HURST'S THE HEART

TWELFTH EDITION

EDITORS

Valentin Fuster, MD, PhD, FACC, FAHA

Richard Gorlin, MD / Heart Research Foundation
Professor of Cardiology
Director, Mount Sinai Heart
Director, The Zena and Michael A. Wiener Cardiovascular Institute
and Marie-Josée and Henry R. Kravis Center for
Cardiovascular Health
The Mount Sinai Medical Center
New York, New York

Richard A. Walsh, MD, FACC, FAHA

John H. Hord Professor
Chair, Department of Medicine
Case Western Reserve University
Physician-in-Chief
University Hospitals of Cleveland
Cleveland, Ohio

Robert A. O'Rourke, MD, MACC, MACP, FAHA

Distinguished Professor of Medicine, Emeritus
University of Texas Health Science Center at San Antonio
San Antonio, Texas

Philip Poole-Wilson, MD, FRCP, FESC, FACC, FMedSci

Professor of Cardiology
British Heart Foundation
Simon Marks Chair of Cardiology
Head of Cardiac Medicine
National Heart and Lung Institute
Faculty of Medicine
Imperial College, London, United Kingdom
Honorary Consultant, Royal Brompton and Harefield NHS Trust
London, United Kingdom

ASSOCIATE EDITORS

Spencer B. King III, MD, MACC, FAHA

Professor of Medicine, Emeritus
Emory University School of Medicine
Director of Interventional Cardiology
Fuqua Chair of Interventional Cardiology
Fuqua Heart Center
Piedmont Hospital
Atlanta, Georgia

Ira S. Nash, MD, FACC, FAHA

Vice Chairman for Veterans Affairs
Associate Professor of Medicine
Samuel Bronfman Department of Medicine
Mount Sinai School of Medicine
Chief of Internal Medicine
James J. Peters VA Medical Center
New York, New York

Robert Roberts, MD, FRCP(C), FACC, FAHA

President and CEO
University of Ottawa Heart Institute
Director, The Ruddy Canadian Cardiovascular Genetics Centre
Ottawa, Ontario, Canada

Eric N. Prystowsky, MD, FACC, FAHA

Consulting Professor of Medicine
Duke University Medical Center
Director, Clinical Electrophysiology Laboratory
St. Vincent Hospital
Indianapolis, Indiana

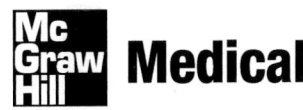

New York Chicago San Francisco Lisbon London Madrid Mexico City
Milan New Delhi San Juan Seoul Singapore Sydney Toronto

Hurst's THE HEART, Twelfth Edition

1 2 3 4 5 6 7 8 9 0   CTP CTP   0 9 8 7

Single Edition Set	ISBN 978-0-07-147886-1; MHID 0-07-147886-8
Single Edition Book	ISBN 978-0-07-154942-4; MHID 0-07-154942-0
Two Volume Set	ISBN 978-0-07-149928-6; MHID 0-07-149928-8
Volume 1	ISBN 978-0-07-149929-3; MHID 0-07-149929-6
Volume 2	ISBN 978-0-07-149930-9; MHID 0-07-149930-X
Card	ISBN 978-0-07-154941-7; MHID 0-07-154941-2

This book was set in Adobe Garamond by Silverchair Science + Communications, Inc.
The editors were Ruth Weinberg and Christie Naglieri.
The production supervisor was Catherine Saggese.
Project management was provided by Niels Buessem, Andover Publishing Services.
The indexer was Alexandra Nickerson Indexing Services.
The cover designer was John Vairo.
Cover image: "Human Heart" by Brian Evans / Photo Researchers, Inc.
China Translation and Printing Services was printer and binder.

This book is printed on acid-free paper.

Library of Congress Cataloging-in-Publication Data

Hurst's the heart / editors, Valentin Fuster ... [et al.] ; associate
editors, Spencer B. King III ... [et al.]. -- 12th ed.
    p. ; cm.
  Includes bibliographical references and index.
  ISBN 978-0-07-149928-6 (2 vol. set : alk. paper) -- ISBN
978-0-07-149929-3 (v. 1 : alk. paper) -- ISBN 978-0-07-149930-9 (v. 2 :
alk. paper) -- ISBN 978-0-07-147886-1 (single vol. : alk. paper) 1.
Cardiovascular system--Diseases. 2. Heart--Diseases. I. Fuster,
Valentin. II. Title: Heart.
  [DNLM: 1. Cardiovascular Diseases. WG 120 H966 2007]
RC667.H88 2007
616.1--dc22
                                    2007020840

CONTENTS

PART 16: DISEASES OF THE GREAT VESSELS AND PERIPHERAL VESSELS

PART 17: SOCIAL ISSUES AND CARDIOVASCULAR DISEASE

CONTRIBUTORS

Jamil A. Aboulhosn, MD
Assistant Clinical Professor of Medicine
David Geffen School of Medicine
Ahmanson/UCLA Adult Congenital Heart Disease Center
Los Angeles, California
Chapter 83

William T. Abraham, MD
Professor of Internal Medicine
The Ohio State University
Director, Divison of Cardiovascular Medicine
Columbus, Ohio
Chapter 26

Masood Akhtar, MD
Clinical Professor of Medicine
University of Wisconsin School of Medicine and Public Health
Milwaukee, Wisconsin
Chapter 42

R. Wayne Alexander, MD, PhD
Chair, Department of Medicine
R. Bruce Logue Professor of Medicine
Emory University Hospital
Atlanta, Georgia
Chapter 7

Charles Antzelevitch, PhD, FACC, FAHA
Professor of Pharmacology
SUNY Health Science Center at Syracuse
Executive Director/Director of Research, Gordon K. Moe Scholar
Masonic Medical Research Laboratory
Utica, New York
Chapter 35

Juan Jose Badimon, PhD, FACC, FAHA
Professor of Medicine
Director
Cardiovascular Biology Research Laboratory
Mount Sinai School of Medicine
New York, New York
Chapter 53

Lina Badimon, PhD, FESC, FAHA
Professor
Director, Cardiovascular Research Center
Hospital de la Santa Creu I Sant Pau
Barcelona, Spain
Chapter 53

Tanvir K. Bajwa, MD, FACC, FSCAI
Director, Cardiac Catheterization Laboratory
Program Director, Interventional Cardiology Fellowship
Clinical Professor of Internal Medicine
Cardiovascular Disease Section
University of Wisconsin Medical School
Milwaukee Clinical Campus
Aurora Sinai Medical Center
Milwaukee Heart Institute
Milwaukee, Wisconsin
Chapter 110

Anton E. Becker, MD, PhD
Professor
Department of Pathology
University of Amsterdam
Amsterdam, The Netherlands
Chapter 34

Emelia J. Benjamin, MD, ScM
Professor of Medicine
Framingham Heart Study
Boston Medical Center
Boston Massachusetts
Chapter 2

Suzanne Benson, Bsc (Hons)
Clinical Nutritionist/Dietician
Department of Nutrition and Dietetics
Adelaide and Meath Hospital
Dublin, Ireland
Chapter 67

Daniel S. Berman, MD
Professor of Medicine
University of California, Los Angeles
Director, Cardiac Imaging
Cedars-Sinai Medical Center
Los Angeles, California
Chapter 19

Gerald J. Berry, MD
Professor of Pathology
Stanford University
Director of Cardiac Pathology
Stanford University Hospital
Stanford, California
Chapter 27

Daniel G. Blanchard, MD
Professor of Medicine
University of California at San Diego School of Medicine
Chief of Clinical Cardiology, UCSD Thornton Hospital
University of California at San Diego Medical Center
San Diego, California
Chapter 16

Wendy M. Book, MD
Assistant Professor of Medicine
Emory University
Director, Emory Adult Congenital Cardiac Program
Emory Clinic—Emory Hospital
Atlanta, Georgia
Chapter 93

Prof. Dr. med Martin Borggrefe, PhD
Direktor, I. Med. Klinik
Universitätsklinikum Mannheim
Mannheim, Germany
Chapter 46

Kenneth L. Brigham, MD
Professor of Medicine
Emory University
Atlanta, Georgia
Chapter 73

Michael R. Bristow, MD, PhD
S. Gilbert Blount Professor of Medicine
Co-Director of University of Colorado Cardiovascular Institute
University of Colorado Health Sciences Center
Denver, Colorado
Chapter 29

Craig S. Broberg, MD, FACC
Assistant Professor
Department of Cardiology and Heart Disease
Oregon Health & Sciences University
Portland, Oregon
Chapter 96

Bruce R. Brodie, MD
Clinical Professor of Medicine
University of North Carolina
Interventional Cardiologist
LeBauer HeartCare
LeBauer Cardiovascular Research Foundation
Moses Cone Heart & Vascular Center
Chapel Hill, North Carolina
Chapter 63

Robert D. Brook, MD
Assistant Professor of Medicine
Division of Cardiovascular Medicine
University of Michigan
Ann Arbor, Michigan
Chapter 104

Ramon Brugada, MD, FACC
Associate Professor of Medicine
University of Montreal
Director, Clinical Cardiovascular Genetics Center
Montreal Heart Institute
Montreal, Quebec, Canada
Chapter 81

Matthew J. Budoff, MD, FACC, FAHA
Associate Professor of Medicine
University of California, Los Angeles School of Medicine
Program Director
Division of Cardiology
Los Angeles Biomedical Research Institute
Torrance, California
Chapter 20

Allen P. Burke, MD
Professor of Pathology
Georgetown University School of Medicine
Deputy Director
CV Path, International Registry of Pathology
Gaithersburg, Maryland
Chapter 57

Hugh Calkins, MD, FACC, FAHA
Professor of Medicine
Professor of Pediatrics
Director of the Arrhythmia Service
    and Clinical Electrophysiology Laboratory
Director of the ARVD Program
Johns Hopkins University School of Medicine
Baltimore, Maryland
Chapter 38

Louis R. Caplan, MD
Professor of Neurology
Harvard Medical School
Senior Neurologist
Beth Israel Deaconess Medical Center
Boston, Massachusetts
Chapter 106

Jonathan R. Carapetis, MBBS, Bmed, Cs, FRACP,
    FAFPMM, PhD
Professor
The University of Melbourne
Counsultant in Pediatric Infectious Diseases
Royal Children's Hospital Melbourne
School of Health Research
Charles Darwin University
Casuarina, Darwin, Australia
Chapter 74

Mark D. Carlson, MD, MA
Chief Medical Officer
Cardiac Rhythm Management Division
St. Jude Medical
Sylmar, California
Chapter 48

Agustin Castellanos, MD, FACC, FAHA
Professor of Medicine
University of Miami Miller School of Medicine
Director, Clinical Electrophysiology
University of Miami/Jackson Memorial Medical Center
Miami, Florida
Chapter 13

Pamela Charney, MD, FACP
Clinical Professor of Medicine
Clinical Associate Professor of Obstetrics & Gynecology and
    Women's Health
Albert Einstein College of Medicine
Program Director, Internal Medicine Residency
Norwalk Hospital
Norwalk, Connecticut
Chapter 102

Jonathan M. Chen, MD
Assistant Professor of Cardiothoracic Surgery
Weill Medical College of Cornell University
Director, Pediatric Cardiac Surgery
Cornell Campus, New York
New York Presbyterian Hospital
New York, New York
Chapter 27

Massimo Chiariello, MD
Professor of Cardiology
Department of Clinical Medicine and Cardiovascular Sciences
Chief of Cardiology
Federico II University
Naples, Italy
Chapter 61

John S. Child, MD, FACC
Streisand Professor of Medicine & Cardiology
David Geffen School of Medicine at UCLA
Director, Ahmanson/UCLA Adult Congenital Heart Disease Center
UCLA Medical Center
Los Angeles, California
Chapter 83

Michael B. Clark, MD
Chief Medical Director
Swiss Re Life and Health
Armonk, New York
Chapter 112

Stephen D. Clements Jr., MD
Director, Outpatient Catheterization Laboratory
Department of Cardiology
Emory University School of Medicine
Atlanta, Georgia
Chapter 66

Lynn Clemow, PhD
Assistant Clinical Professor
Department of Medicine
Columbia University College of Physicians and Surgeons
New York, New York
Chapter 113

Jean-Christophe Cornilly, MD
Associate Professor
Imaging Science Laboratories
Mount Sinai School of Medicine
New York, New York
Chapter 22

Rebecca Costello, MD
Deputy Director
Office of Dietary Supplements
National Institutes of Health
Bethesda, Maryland
Chapter 114

Martin R. Cowie, MD, MSc, FRCP
Professor of Cardiology
National Heart & Lung Institute
Imperial College
Honorary Consultant Cardiologist
Royal Brompton Hospital
London, United Kingdom
Chapter 25

Monica Kelly Cowles, MD, MS
Psychiatric Research Fellow
Department of Psychiatry and Behavioral Sciences
Emory University Hospital
Atlanta, Georgia
Chapter 95

Harry Crijns, MD, PhD
Professor and Chairman
Department of Cardiology
University Hospital Maastricht
The Netherlands
Chapter 43

Peter F. Currie, MD, FRCPE
Consultant Cardiologist
Perth Royal Infirmary
Perth, Scotland, United Kingdom
Chapter 92

Ralph B. D'Agostino, Sr., PhD, FAHA
Professor of Mathematical Statistics and Public Health
Boston University
Boston, Massachusetts
Chapter 2

Owais Dar, MBChB, MRCP
Clinical Research Fellow Cardiology
Imperial College London
National Heart and Lung Institute
London, United Kingdom
Chapter 25

Karina W. Davidson, PhD
Associate Professor of Medicine & Psychiatry
Department of Medicine
Columbia College of Physicians and Surgeons
Zena and Michael Wiener Cardiovascular Institute
Mount Sinai School of Medicine
New York, New York
Chapter 113

James A. de Lemos, MD
J. Fred Schoellkopf Chair in Cardiology Research
University of Texas Southwestern Medical Center
Director, Coronary Care Unit
Parkland Memorial Hospital
Dallas, Texas
Chapter 59

Arjun Deb, MD
Fellow, Division of Cardiovascular Diseases
Duke University Medical Center
Durham, North Carolina
Chapter 10

Santo Dellegrottaglie, MD, PhD
Post-Doctoral Clinical Fellow
Institute of Cardiology
Federico II University of Naples
Naples, Italy
Instructor of Medicine (Adjunct)
Cardiovascular CT/MRI Clinical Program
The Zena and Michael A. Wiener Cardiovascular Institute
The Marie-Josée and Henry R. Kravis Center for
    Cardiovascular Health
The Mount Sinai Medical Center
New York, New York
Chapter 61

Louis J. Dell'Italia, MD
Professor of Medicine
Center for Heart Failure Research
University of Alabama at Birmingham
School of Medicine
Birmingham VA Medical Center
Birmingham, Alabama
Chapter 76

Anthony N. DeMaria, MD, MACC, FAHA
Professor of Medicine
Director, The Sulpizie Family Cardiovascular Center
University of California at San Diego
San Diego, California
Chapter 16

Christophe Depre, MD, PhD
Associate Professor
Department of Cell Biology and Molecular Medicine
University of Medicine and Dentistry of New Jersey
New Jersey Medical School
Newark, New Jersey
Chapter 54

Roberto De Vogli, PhD, MPH
Lecturer
International Institute for Society and Health
Department of Epidemiology and Public Health
University College London
London, England
Chapter 115

Thomas F. Dodson, MD
Professor of Surgery
Emory University School of Medicine
Associate Chairman
Department of Surgery
Division of Vascular Surgery
Atlanta, Georgia
Chapter 109

John S. Douglas, Jr, MD, FACC
Professor of Medicine (Cardiology)
Director, Interventional Cardiology
Director, Cardiac Catheterization Laboratory
Emory University School of Medicine
Emory University Hospital
Atlanta, Georgia
Chapters 62, 64

Prof. Dr. med. Helmut Drexler, MD
Professor of Medicine
Department of Cardiology and Angiology
Medical School Hannover
Hannover, Germany
Chapter 10

Victor Dzau, MD
James B. Duke Professor of Medicine
Duke University Medical Center
Durham, North Carolina
Chapter 10

Kim A. Eagle, MD
Albion Walter Hewlett Professor of Internal Medicine
University of Michigan
Clinical Director of the Cardiovascular Center
University of Michigan Health System
Ann Arbor, Michigan
Chapter 86

William D. Edwards, MD
Professor of Pathology
Mayo College of Medicine
Staff Consultant, Anatomic Pathology
Mayo Clinic
Rochester, Minnesota
Chapter 3

John A. Elefteriades, MD
Professor of Surgery
Department of Cardiothoracic Surgery
Yale University School of Medicine
Chief, Cardiothoracic Surgery
Yale University School of Medicine
New Haven, Connecticut
Chapter 105

Kenneth A. Ellenbogen, MD
Kontos Professor of Cardiology
VCU School of Medicine
Vice-Chairman of Cardiology
Medical College of Virginia
Richmond, Virginia
Chapter 40

Gregory Engel, MD
Division of Cardiovascular Medicine
Stanford University School of Medicine
Staff Cardiologist
Veterans Affairs Palo Alto Health Care System
Palo Alto, California
Chapter 14

N.A. Mark Estes III, MD
Professor of Medicine
Director
Tufts New England Medical Center
Boston, Massachusetts
Chapter 100

Michael S. Ewer, MD, JD, MPH, LLM
Professor of Medicine
The University of Texas M.D. Anderson Cancer Center
Houston, Texas
Chapter 89

Gordon A. Ewy, MD, FACC, FAHA
Professor of Medicine (Cardiology)
University of Arizona College of Medicine
Chief, Section of Cardiology
Director, Sarver Heart Center
Arizona Health Sciences Center
Tucson, Arizona
Chapter 50

Erling Falk, MD, PhD
Professor
University of Aarhus
Department of Cardiology
Aarhus University Hospital
Aarhus, Denmark
Chapter 52

Noeleen Fallon, BSc
Clinical Nurse Manager
Department of Cardiac Rehabilitation
Adelaide and Meath Hospital
Dublin, Ireland
Chapter 67

Michael E. Farkouh, MD, MSc
Clinical Coordinating Center
Mount Sinai School of Medicine
New York, New York
Chapter 90

Michael D. Faulx, MD
Assistant Professor of Medicine
Cleveland Clinic Lerner College of Medicine
Staff
Case Western Reserve University
The Cleveland Clinic
Cleveland, Ohio
Chapter 94

Zahi A. Fayad, PhD
Associate Professor of Radiology and Medicine
Director, Imaging Science Laboratories
Mount Sinai School of Medicine
New York, New York
Chapter 22

Peter F. Fedullo, MD
Professor of Medicine
Director, Medical Intensive Care Unit
Division of Pulmonary and Critical Care Medicine
University of California at San Diego Medical Center
San Diego, California
Chapter 72

Gerald F. Fletcher, MD
Professor of Medicine, Cardiovascular
Mayo Clinic College of Medicine
Preventive Cardiologist
Mayo Clinic Jacksonville
Jacksonville, Florida
Chapter 99

Thomas R. Flipse, MD
Assistant Professor of Medicine
Mayo Clinic College of Medicine
Jacksonville, Florida
Chapter 99

Richard I. Fogel, MD
Clinical Electrophysiologist
The Heart Center of Indiana
Indianapolis, Indiana
Chapter 36

Gary S. Francis, MD
Professor of Medicine
Cleveland Clinic Lerner College of Medicine
Case Western Reserve University
Staff, Department of Cardiovascular Medicine
The Cleveland Clinic
Cleveland, Ohio
Chapters 24, 94

William T. Friedewald, MD
Clinical Professor
Columbia University
New York, New York
Chapter 112

Victor F. Froelicher, MD
Professor of Medicine
Division of Cardiovascular Medicine
Stanford University
Director of ECG/Exercise Laboratory
Palo Alto Veterans Affairs Medical Center
Palo Alto, California
Chapter 14

David R. Fulton, MD
Associate Professor of Pediatrics
Harvard Medical School
Chief, Cardiology Outpatient Services
Children's Hospital Boston
Boston, Massachusetts
Chapter 82

Valentin Fuster, MD, PhD, FACC, FAHA
Richard Gorlin, MD / Heart Research Foundation
    Professor of Cardiology
Director, Mount Sinai Heart
Director, The Zena and Michael A. Wiener Cardiovascular
    Institute and Marie-Josée and Henry R. Kravis Center for
    Cardiovascular Health
The Mount Sinai Medical Center
New York, New York
Chapters 22, 52, 53, 56, 90

Guido Germano, PhD
Professor of Medicine
UCLA School of Medicine
Director, Artificial Intelligence in Medicine Program
Cedars-Sinai Medical Center
Los Angeles, California
Chapter 19

Bernard J. Gersh, MBChB, DPhil, FRCP, PhD (Hon Causa)
Professor of Medicine
Division of Cardiovascular Diseases
Mayo Clinic
Rochester, Minnesota
Chapters 60, 61

Antony H. Gershlick, BSc, MBBS
Consultant Cardiologist
Hon Senior Lecturer
Department of Cardiology
University Hospitals of Leicester
Leicester, United Kingdom
Chapter 61

Gary Gerstenblith, MD
Professor of Medicine
Department of Medicine
The Johns Hopkins University School of Medicine
Johns Hopkins Hospital
Baltimore, Maryland
Chapter 101

Edward M. Gilbert, MD
Professor
Department of Cardiology
University of Utah Health Sciences Center
Salt Lake City, Utah
Chapter 29

Robert C. Gilkeson, MD
Section Chief, Cardiothoracic Imaging
Department of Radiology
University Hospitals of Cleveland
Cleveland, Ohio
Chapter 15

John Gormley, BSc (Hons), DPhil
Lecturer
Department of Physiotherapy
School of Medicine
Trinity College of Dublin
Dublin, Ireland
Chapter 67

Ian Graham, FRCPI, FESC
Consultant Cardiologist
Adelaide & Meath Hospital
Professor of Cardiovascular Medicine
Trinity College
Professor of Preventive Cardiology
Royal College of Surgeons in Ireland
Tallaght, Dublin
Ireland
Chapter 67

Joey P. Granger, Ph.D
Billy S. Guyton Distinguished Professor
Professor of Physiology and Medicine
Department of Physiology & Biophysics
Department of Medicine
Interim Dean
School of Graduate Studies in the Health Sciences
Center for Excellence in Cardiovascular-Renal Research
University of Mississippi Medical Center
Jackson, Mississippi
Chapter 69

Kathy K. Griendling, PhD
Professor of Medicine
Vice Chair for Faculty Development
Emory University
Division of Cardiology, Emory University
Atlanta, Georgia
Chapter 7

Garrett J. Gross, PhD
Professor
Department of Pharmacology and Toxicology
Medical College of Wisconsin
Milwaukee, Wisconsin
Chapter 54

Blair P. Grubb, MD
Professor of Medicine and Pediatrics
The Medical University of Ohio
Director, Cardiac Electrophysiology Service
University Medical Center
Toledo, Ohio
Chapter 48

Scott M. Grundy, MD, PhD
Director, Center for Human Nutrition
Professor of Internal Medicine
Departments of Clinical Nutrition and
    Internal Medicine
University of Texas Southwestern Medical Center at Dallas
Dallas, Texas
Chapters 51, 91

Gary L. Grunkemeier, PhD
Director
Medical Data Research Center
Portland, Oregon
Chapter 79

Sanjaya Gupta, MD
Chief Resident
Department of Medicine
Case Western Reserve University
University Hospitals of Cleveland
Cleveland, Ohio
Chapter 31

Anjan Gupta, MD, FACC, FSCAI
Associate Director, Cardiology Fellowship Program
University of Wisconsin Medical School Milwaukee
Milwaukee, Wisconsin
Chapter 110

Rory Hachamovitch, MD, MSc, FACC
Voluntary Faculty
Los Angeles County
USC Medical Center
Los Angeles, California
Chapter 19

Saptarsi M. Haldar, MD
Assistant Professor of Medicine
Case Cardiovascular Research Institute
Case University Medical School and
    University Hospitals of Cleveland
Cleveland, Ohio
Chapter 85

Michael E. Hall, MD
Internal Medicine Resident
Department of Physiology & Biophysics
Department of Medicine
Center for Excellence in Cardiovascular-Renal Research
University of Mississippi Medical Center
Jackson, Mississippi
Chapter 69

John E. Hall, PhD
Arthur C. Guyton Professor and Chair
Department of Physiology and Biophysiology
Associate Vice Chancellor for Research
University of Mississippi Medical Center
Jackson, Mississippi
Chapter 69

Jonathan L. Halperin, MD
Robert and Harriet Heilbrunn Professor of Medicine (Cardiology)
Mount Sinai School of Medicine
Director, Clinical Cardiology Services
The Zena and Michael A. Wiener Cardiovascular Institute
The Marie-Josée and Henry R. Kravis Center for Cardiovascular
    Health
The Mount Sinai Medical Center
New York, New York
Chapter 105

David G. Harrison, MD
Director, Division of Cardiology
Bernard Marcus Professor of Medicine
Emory University
Atlanta, Georgia
Chapter 7

Ayesha Hasan, MD
Assistant Clinical Professor of Cardiovascular Medicine
Director, Heart Failure Devices Program
Division of Cardiovascular Medicine
The Ohio State University
Columbus, Ohio
Chapter 26

Sean W. Hayes, MD
Assistant Director, Nuclear Cardiology
Cedars-Sinai Medical Center
Los Angeles, California
Chapter 19

Siew Yen Ho, PhD, FRCPath, FESC
Reader in Cardiac Morphology
National Heart & Lung Institute, Imperial College
Honorary Consultant
Royal Brompton Hospital
London, England
Chapter 34

Brian D. Hoit, MD
Professor of Medicine and Phsyiology and Biophysics
Case Western Reserve University
Director, Echocardiography Laboratory
University Hospitals of Cleveland
Cleveland, Ohio
Chapters 4, 31, 84

Borja Ibanez, MD
Research Fellow
Cardiovascular Biology Research Laboratory
Mount Sinai School of Medicine
New York, New York
Chapter 53

Shirley Ingram, RGN, MSc, NFESC
Cardiology Nurse Specialist
Department of Cardiac Rehabilitation
Adelaide and Meath Hospital
Dublin, Ireland
Chapter 67

Alberto Interian Jr., MD
Professor of Medicine
Director, Electrophysiology
Miller School of Medicine
Jackson Memorial Hospital
Director, Arrhythmia Syncope Center
Mercy Hospital
Miami, Florida
Chapter 13

Daniel W. Jones, MD
Vice Chancellor for Health Affairs
Dean, School of Medicine
Langford Professor of Medicine
Professor, Department of Physiology & Biophysics
Department of Medicine
Center for Excellence in Cardiovascular-Renal Research
University of Mississippi Medical Center
Jackson, Mississippi
Chapter 69

Mark E. Josephson, MD, FACC
Chief, Cardiovascular Division
Beth Israel Deaconess Medical Center
Professor of Medicine
Harvard Medical School
Director, Harvard-Thorndike Electrophysiology Institute and
    Arrhythmia Service
Boston, Massachusetts
Chapter 49

Ronald J. Kanter, MD
Associate Professor of Pediatrics
Duke University School of Medicine
Director of Pediatric Electrophysiology
Durham, North Carolina
Chapter 47

Samir R. Kapadia, MD
Associate Professor, Department of Medicine
Cleveland Clinic Lerner College of Medicine of Case Western
    Reserve University
Staff Physician
The Cleveland Clinic
Cleveland, Ohio
Chapter 107

Joel A. Kaplan, MD
Dean Emeritus, School of Medicine
Former Chancellor, Health Sciences Center
Professor of Clinical Anesthesiology
University of Louisville School of Medicine
Louisville, Kentucky
Professor of Clinical Anesthesiology
University of California San Diego School of Medicine
San Diego, California
Chapter 87

Neeru Kaushik, MD
Senior Fellow in Pediatric Cardiology
Division of Pediatric Cardiology
Department of Pediatrics
University of Pittsburgh School of Medicine
Children's Hospital of Pittsburgh
Pittsburgh, Pennsylvania
Chapter 8

Bradley B. Keller, MD
Professor of Pediatrics, Division of Pediatric Cardiology
Department of Pediatrics
University of Pittsburgh School of Medicine
Director, Pediatric Biomedical Innovative Technology
Children's Hospital of Pittsburgh
Pittsburgh, Pennsylvania
Chapter 8

Richard E. Kerber, MD
Professor of Medicine
University of Iowa College of Medicine
Staff Physician
University of Iowa Hospitals and Clinics
Iowa City, Iowa
Chapter 45

Morton J. Kern, MD
Professor of Medicine
Associate Chief Cardiology
University of California, Irvine
Irvine, California
Chapter 17

Han W. Kim, MD
Associate in Medicine
Attending Physician
Duke Cardiovascular Magnetic Resonance Center
Duke University Medical Center
Durham, North Carolina
Chapter 21

Michael C. Kim, MD
Assistant Professor of Medicine
Mount Sinai School of Medicine
Director, Coronary Care Unit
The Mount Sinai Medical Center
New York, New York
Chapter 56

Raymond J. Kim, MD, FACC
Associate Professor of Medicine and Radiology
Co-Director, Duke Cardiovascular Magnetic Resonance Center
Duke University Medical Center
Durham, North Carolina
Chapter 21

Spencer B. King III, MD, MACC, FAHA
Professor of Medicine, Emeritus
Emory University School of Medicine
Director of Interventional Cardiology
Fuqua Chair of Interventional Cardiology
Fuqua Heart Center
Piedmont Hospital
Atlanta, Georgia
Chapters 17, 62

Annapoorna S. Kini, MD, MRCP, FACC
Associate Professor
Mount Sinai School of Medicine
Associate Director, Cardiac Catheterization Laboratory
Mount Sinai Hospital
New York, New York
Chapter 56

Timothy Knilans, MD
Associate Professor of Pediatrics
University of Cincinnati College of Medicine
Director, Clinical Cardiac Electrophysiology and Pacing
Cincinnati Children's Hospital Medical Center
Cincinnati, Ohio
Chapter 47

Peter R. Kowey, MD
Professor of Medicine and Clinical Cardiology
Jefferson Medical College
Philadelphia, Pennsylvania
Main Line Health System
Wynnewood, Pennsylvania
Chapter 43

Mitchell W. Krucoff, MD, FACC, FCCP
Professor Medicine/Cardiology
Duke University Medical Center
Director, Cardiovascular Devices Unit
Director, ECG Core Laboratory
Duke Clinical Research Institute
Chapel Hill, North Carolina
Chapter 114

Harlan M. Krumholz, MD, SM
Harold H. Hines, Jr. Professor of Medicine
Yale University School of Medicine
Director, Center for Outcomes Research and Evaluation
Yale New Haven Hospital
New Haven, Connecticut
Chapter 111

Edward G. Lakatta, MD
Professor
The Johns Hopkins University
Director
Laboratory of Cardiovascular Science
Gerontology Research Center
National Institute on Aging Intramural Research Program
National Institutes of Health
Baltimore, Maryland
Chapter 101

E. Clinton Lawrence, MD
Augustus J. McKeloey Professor of Medicine
Emory University School of Medicine
Medical Director of Lung Transplantation
Emory University Hospital
Atlanta, Georgia
Chapter 73

Megan C. Leary, MD
Instructor in Neurology
Harvard Medical School
Co-Director, Inpatient Stroke Service
Beth Israel Deaconess Medical Center
Boston, Massachusetts
Chapter 106

Daniel J. Lenihan, MD
Associate Professor of Medicine
The University of Texas M.D. Anderson Cancer Center
Director, Clinical Research
The University of Texas M.D. Anderson Cancer Center
Department of Cardiology
Houston, Texas
Chapter 89

Tora Leong, MBChB, MRCPI
Senior Research Fellow
Specialist Registrar in Cardiology
Adelaide and Meath Hospital and Trinity College
Dublin, Ireland
Chapter 67

William Lewis, MD
Professor
Department of Pathology
Emory University School of Medicine
Director, Division of Cardiovascular Pathology
Emory Health Care
Atlanta, Georgia
Chapter 92

Mark S. Link, MD
Associate Professor of Medicine
Tufts University School of Medicine
Tufts-New England Medical Center
Boston, Massachusetts
Chapter 100

Brian D. Lowes, MD
Associate Professor of Medicine/Cardiology
University of Colorado
University of Colorado Health Sciences Center
Denver, Colorado
Chapter 29

Bruce W. Lytle, MD
Professor of Surgery
Chairman, Thoracic & Cardiovascular Surgery
The Cleveland Clinic
Cleveland, Ohio
Chapter 65

Vincent Maher, MD, FRCPI
Consultant Cardiologist
Department of Cardiology
Adelaide and Meath Hospital
Tallaght, Ireland
Chapter 67

Giuseppe Maiolino, MD
Research Fellow
Cebzini Medical Center
Chapter 20

Joseph F. Malouf, MD
Professor of Medicine
Mayo Clinic College of Medicine
Consultant, Cardiovascular Diseases
Mayo Clinic
Rochester, Minnesota
Chapter 3

Donna M. Mancini, MD
Professor of Medicine
Columbia University
New York, New York
Chapter 32

Ali J. Marian, MD
Professor of Cardiovascular Genetics and Medicine
Center for Cardiovascular Genetic Research
The Brown Foundation Institute of Molecular Medicine
The University of Texas Health Science Center
Texas Heart Institute at St. Luke's Episcopal Hospital
Houston, Texas
Chapter 81

Daniel Mark, MD, MPH
Professor of Medicine
Duke University Medical Center
Durham, North Carolina
Chapter 114

Roger R. Markwald, PhD
Distinguished University Professor and Chairman
Department of Cell Biology and Anatomy
Director, Cardiovascular Developmental Biology Center
Adjunct Professor of Pediatrics
Department of Pediatrics
Medical University of South Carolina
Charleston, South Carolina
Chapter 8

Sir Michael G. Marmot, MD, PhD, FRCP
Director, International Institute for Society and Health
Head, Department of Epidemiology and Public Health
Professor
University College London
London, England
Chapter 115

Barry J. Maron, MD
Director, Hypertrophic Cardiomyopathy Center
Minneapolis Heart Institute Foundation
Minneapolis, Minnesota
Chapters 28, 100

David J. Maron, MD
Associate Professor of Medicine
Vanderbilt University Medical Center
Division of Cardiovascular Medicine
Nashville, Tennessee
Chapter 51

S. Carolina Masri, MD
Fellow in Cardiovascular Disease
University of Minnesota
Minneapolis, Minnesota
Chapter 103

Tahsin Masud, MD
Associate Professor of Medicine
Renal Division
Department of Medicine
Emory University School of Medicine
Chief of Nephrology
Emory Crawford Lung Hospital
Atlanta, Georgia
Chapter 98

Bongani M. Mayosi, DPhil, FRCP, FACC
Professor of Medicine and Head of Department
Physician-in-Chief
Department of Medicine
Groote Schuur Hospital, Observatory
Cape Town, South Africa
Chapter 74

John H. McAnulty, MD, FACC, FAHA
Professor Emeritus of Medicine
Division of Cardiology
Oregon Health and Sciences University
Good Samaritan Hospital
Portland, Oregon
Chapter 80, 96

William M. McClellan, MD, MPH
Professor of Medicine
Renal Division, Department of Medicine
Emory University School of Medicine
Atlanta, Georgia
Chapter 98

William M. McDonald, MD
Professor
Department of Psychiatry and Behavioral Sciences
Emory University School of Medicine
Atlanta, Georgia
Chapter 95

Elizabeth McNally, MD, PhD
Director, Institute for Cardiovascular Research
Director, Cardiovascular Genetics Laboratory
Professor of Medicine and Human Genetics
The University of Chicago Hospitals
Center for Advanced Medicine
Chicago, Illinois
Chapter 9

Luisa Mestroni, MD
Professor of Medicine/Cardiology
University of Colorado Health Sciences Center
Aurora, Colorado
Chapter 29

James Metcalfe, MD
Professor Emeritus of Medicine
Oregon Health Sciences University
School of Medicine
Portland, Oregon
Chapter 96

Alexander Mittnacht, MD
Assistant Professor
Mount Sinai School of Medicine
Assistant Clinical Attending
Mount Sinai Hospital
New York, New York
Chapter 87

Douglas C. Morris, MD, FACC, FAHA
J. Willis Hurst Professor of Medicine
Emory University School of Medicine
Director, Emory Hurst Center
Emory Clinic
Atlanta, Georgia
Chapter 66

Debabrata Mukherjee, MD
Gill Foundation Professor of Interventional Cardiology
Director of Peripheral Intervention Program
Associate Director for Cardiac Catheterization Laboratories
Division of Cardiovascular Medicine
University of Kentucky
Lexington, Kentucky
Chapter 86

Dominique L. Musselman, MD, MS
Associate Professor
Department of Psychiatry and Behavioral Sciences
Emory University School of Medicine
Atlanta, Georgia
Chapter 95

Robert J. Myerburg, MD
Professor of Medicine and Physiology
American Heart Association Chair in Cardiovascular Research
Division of Cardiology
University of Miami Miller School of Medicine
Miami, Florida
Chapter 13

Deepak G. Nair, MD, MS, MHA, RVT
Vascular Fellow
Department of Surgery
Emory University
Atlanta, Georgia
Chapter 109

Samer S. Najjar, MD
Head, Human Cardiovascular Studies Unit
Laboratory of Cardiovascular Science
Gerontology Research Center
National Institute on Aging Intramural Research Program
National Institutes of Health
Baltimore, Maryland
Chapter 101

Carlo Napolitano, MD, PhD
Senior Scientist and Research Coordinator
Department of Molecular Cardiology
Fondazione Salvatore Maugeri
Pavia, Italy
Chapter 33

Ira S. Nash, MD, FACC, FAHA
Vice Chairman for Veterans Affairs
Associate Professor of Medicine
Samuel Bronfman Department of Medicine
Mount Sinai School of Medicine
Chief of Internal Medicine
James J Peters VA Medical Center
New York, New York
Chapter 11

Charles B. Nemeroff, MD, PhD
Reunette W. Harris Professor and Chairman
Department of Psychiatry and Behavioral Sciences
Emory University School of Medicine
Atlanta, Georgia
Chapter 95

Stephen J. Nicholls, MBBS, PhD
Research Associate
The Cleveland Clinic
Associate Director
Intravascular Ultrasound Core Laboratory
The Cleveland Clinic
Cleveland, Ohio
Chapter 18

Rick A. Nishimura, MD, FACC
Judd and Mary Morris Leighton Professor of Cardiovascular Diseases
Professor of Medicine
Mayo Clinic College of Medicine
Consultant, Division of Cardiovascular Diseases
Rochester, Minnesota
Chapter 30

Steven E. Nissen, MD
Interim Chairman
Department of Cardiovascular Medicine of Cleveland Clinic
Cleveland Clinic Foundation
Cleveland, Ohio
Chapter 18

Veronica O'Doherty, MSc, MPhil, BA, RGN
Psychologist
Trinity College Dublin
University College Dublin
Acting Principal Psychologist
Adelaide, Meath and National Children's Hospital
Dublin, Ireland
Chapter 67

Patrick T. O'Gara, MD, FACC, FAHA
Associate Professor of Medicine
Harvard Medical School
Director, Clinical Cardiology
Cardiovascular Division
Brigham and Women's Hospital
Boston, Massachusetts
Chapters 64, 85

Gbenga Ogedegbe, MD, MPH, MS, FAHA
Assistant Professor of Medicine
Columbia University College of Physicians and Surgeons
Assistant Attending Physician
Columbia Presbyterian Medical Center
New York, New York
Chapter 68

Keith R. Oken, MD
Assistant Professor of Medicine
Mayo Clinic College of Medicine
Consultant, Cardiovascular Diseases
Director, Cardiopulmonary Rehabilitation
Jacksonville, Florida
Chapter 99

Jeffrey W. Olin, DO
Professor of Medicine
Mount Sinai School of Medicine
Director, Vascular Medicine
The Mount Sinai Medical Center
New York, New York
Chapter 105

Steve R. Ommen, MD
Associate Professor of Medicine
Mayo Clinic College of Medicine
Consultant, Divison of Cardiovascular Diseases
Department of Internal Medicine
Mayo Clinic
Rochester, Minnesota
Chapter 30

William W. O'Neill, MD, FACC
Director of Cardiology
William Beaumont Hospital
Division of Cardiology
Royal Oak, Michigan
Chapter 63

Robert A. O'Rourke, MD, MACC, MACP, FAHA
Distinguished Professor of Medicine, Emeritus
University of Texas Health Science Center at San Antonio
San Antonio, Texas
Chapters 12, 15, 59, 60, 64, 76, 88

Benzy J. Padanilam, MD, FACC
Faculty, Electrophysiology Fellowship Program
Attending Electrophysiologist
The Care Group
St. Vincent Hospital
Indianapolis, Indiana
Chapter 41

Richard L. Page, MD
Robert A. Bruce Endowed Chair in Cardiovascular Research
Head, Division of Cardiology
University of Washington Medical Center
Seattle, Washington
Chapter 39

Thomas A. Pearson, MD, MPH, PhD
Albert A. Kaisar Professor and Chair
Department of Community & Preventive Medicine
University of Rochester School of Medicine & Dentistry
University of Rochester Medical Center
Rochester, New York
Chapter 51

John Pepper, Mchir, FRCS
Professor
Imperial College, School of Medicine
Consultant Cardiac Surgeon
Royal Brompton Hospital
London, United Kingdom
Chapter 66

Michael X. Pham, MD, MPH
Instructor of Medicine
Stanford University School of Medicine
Medical Director of Heart Failure and Transplantation
VA Palo Alto Health Care System
Stanford, California
Chapter 27

Thomas G. Pickering, MD, DPhil
Assistant Professor of Medicine
Center for Behavioral Cardiovascular Health
Columbia Presbyterian Medical Center
New York, New York
Chapters 68, 113

Ileana L. Piña, MD
Professor of Medicine
Case Western Reserve University
Director, Heart Failure & Cardiac Transplantation
University Hospitals of Cleveland
Cleveland, Ohio
Chapter 94

Sean P. Pinney, MD
Assistant Professor of Medicine
Mount Sinai School of Medicine
Director, Advanced Heart Failure & Cardiac Transplant Program
New York, New York
Chapter 32

David J. Pinsky, MD
J. Griswold Ruth MD and Margery Hopkins Ruth Professor of
    Internal Medicine
University of Michigan
Ann Arbor, Michigan
Chapter 58

Duane S. Pinto, MD
Assistant Professor of Medicine
Harvard Medical School
Director, Cardiology Fellowship
Beth Israel Deaconess Medical Center
Boston, Massachusetts
Chapter 49

Philip Poole-Wilson, MD, FRCP, FESC, FACC, FMedSci
Professor of Cardiology
British Heart Foundation
Simon Marks Chair of Cardiology
Head of Cardiac Medicine
National Heart and Lung Institute
Faculty of Medicine
Imperial College, London, United Kingdom
Honorary Consultant, Royal Brompton and Harefield NHS Trust
London, United Kingdom
Chapter 24, 26

Michael Poon, MD
Associate Clinical Professor
Department of Cardiology
Mount Sinai School of Medicine
New York, New York
Chapter 20

Silvia G. Priori, MD, PhD
Associate Professor of Cardiology
Department of Cardiology, University of Pavia-Italy
Head of Molecular Cardiology
Fondazione Salvatore Maugeri
Pavia, Italy
Chapter 33

Eric N. Prystowsky, MD, FACC, FAHA
Consulting Professor of Medicine
Duke University Medical Center
Director, Clinical Electrophysiology Laboratory
St. Vincent Hospital
Indianapolis, Indiana
Chapters 36, 37, 41

Shahbudin H. Rahimtoola, MB, FRCP, MACP,
   MACC, DSc (Hon)
Distinguished Professor
University of Southern California
George C. Griffith Professor of Cardiology
Professor of Medicine
Keck School of Medicine at University of Southern Califonria
Chief Physician
Los Angeles County University of Southern California
   Medical Center
Los Angeles, California
Chapters 75, 77, 79, 80

Mahboob Rahman, MD, MS
Associate Professor of Medicine
Case Western Reserve University
Division of Nephrology and Hypertension
University Hospitals of Cleveland
Louis Stokes Cleveland VA Medical Center
Cleveland, Ohio
Chapter 70

Vivek Rajagopal, MD
Clinical Cardiologist
Piedmont Hospital
Atlanta, Georgia
Chapter 107

Sanjay Rajagopalan, MD
Associate Professor of Medicine
Director, MR & CT Program
Mount Sinai School of Medicine
New York, New York
School of Public Health
Department of Internal Medicine
Ohio State University
Columbus, Ohio
Chapter 104

Arash Rashidi, MD
Nephrology and Clinical Hypertension Fellow
Division of Nephrology and Hypertension
University Hospitals Case Medical Center and Metro Health
   Medical Center
Case Western Reserve University
Cleveland, Ohio
Chapter 70

Elliot J. Rayfield, MD
Clinical Professor of Medicine
Mount Sinai School of Medicine
Attending Physician
Mount Sinai Hospital
New York, New York
Chapter 90

Wolfgang G. Rehwald, PhD
Senior Scientist
Siemens Medical Solutions
Duke Cardiovascular Magnetic Resonance Center
Duke University Health Systems
Durham, North Carolina
Chapter 21

David L. Reich, MD
Horace W. Goldsmith Professor and Chair
Department of Anesthesiology
Mount Sinai School of Medicine
New York, New York
Chapter 87

Matthew R. Reynolds, MD, MSc
Instructor in Medicine
Harvard Medical School
Associate Director of Electrophysiology
Boston VA Healthcare System
Beth Israel Deaconess Medical Center
Boston, Massachusetts
Chapter 49

Robert T. Rho, MD
Assistant Professor of Medicine
Division of Cardiology
University of Washington School of Medicine
Seattle, Washington
Chapter 39

Paul M. Ridker, MD, MPH
Eugene Braunwald Professor of Medicine
Harvard Medical School
Director, Center for Cardiovascular Disease Prevention
Divisions of Cardiovascular Disease and Preventive Medicine
Brigham and Women's Hospital
Boston, Massachusetts
Chapter 51

Nina Rieckmann, PhD
Assistant Professor
Department of Psychiatry
Mount Sinai School of Medicine
New York, New York
Chapter 113

Robert Roberts, MD, FRCP(C), FACC, FAHA
President and CEO
University of Ottawa Heart Institute
Director, The Ruddy Canadian Cardiovascular Genetics Centre
Ottawa, Ontario, Canada
Chapters 5, 9, 81

William C. Roberts, MD, DSc, MACC
Executive Director
Baylor University Medical Center
Editor in Chief
The American Journal of Cardiology
Editor in Chief
Baylor University Medical Center Proceedings
Dallas, Texas
Chapter 88

Jose F. Roldan, MD, FACR
Assistant Professor of Medicine
University of Texas Health Science Center at San Antonio
South Texas Health Care System
Rheumatologist
Director, UTHSCA Lupus and Vasculatic Clinic
San Antonio, Texas
Chapter 88

Thom W. Rooke, MD
Professor of Medicine
Mayo Clinical College of Medicine
John and Posy Krehbiel Professor of Vascular Medicine
Gonda Vascular Center
Division of Cardiovascular Diseases
Mayo Clinic
Rochester, Minnesota
Chapter 108

Eric A. Rose, MD
Chairman, Department of Surgery
Columbia University
New York Presbyterian Hospital
Columbia University Medical Center
New York, New York
Chapter 27

Lewis J. Rubin, MD
Professor of Medicine
University of California at San Diego School of Medicine
University of California at San Diego Medical Center
San Diego, California
Chapter 71

Cyril Ruwende, MBChB, MSc, DPhil, FACC
Assistant Professor
University of Michigan
General and Interventional Cardiologist
Michigan Heart PC
Ann Arbor, Michigan
Chapter 58

Joseph F. Sabik, 3rd, MD
Department of Thoracic and Cardiovascular Surgery
The Cleveland Clinic
Cleveland, Ohio
Chapter 65

Robert E. Safford, MD, PhD
Barbara Woodward Lips Professor of Medicine
Mayo Clinic College of Medicine
Consultant in Cardiovascular Diseases
Mayo Clinic, Jacksonville
Jacksonville, Florida
Chapter 99

Allen Mark Samarel, MD
William B. Knapp Professor of Medicine and Physiology
Loyola University Chicago Stritch School of Medicine
Director of Research, The Cardiovascular Institute
Loyola University Medical Center
Maywood, Illinois
Chapter 6

Heinrich R. Schelbert, MD
The George V. Taplin Professor
Department of Molecular and Medical Pharmacology
David Geffen School of Medicine
University of California, Los Angeles
Los Angeles, California
Chapter 23

John S. Schroeder, MD
Professor of Medicine
Stanford University School of Medicine
Stanford, California
Chapter 27

Steven P. Schulman, MD
Professor of Medicine
Department of Medicine
The Johns Hopkins University School of Medicine
Director, Coronary Care Unit
Johns Hopkins University
Baltimore, Maryland
Chapter 101

James B. Seward, MD, FACC
Mayo Clinic
Rochester, Minnesota
Chapter 3

Pravin M. Shah, MD, MACC
Medical Director and Chair
Hoag Heart Valve Center
Hoag Heart Institute
Newport Beach, California
Chapter 78

Prediman K. Shah, MD, FACC
Professor of Medicine
David Geffen School of Medicine at UCLA
Los Angeles, California
Shapell and Webb Chair and Director
Cardiology and Atherosclerosis Research Center
Cedars-Sinai Medical Center
Los Angeles, California
Chapter 52

James A. Shaver, MD
Professor of Medicine
University of Pittsburgh Medical Center
Cardiovascular Institute
Director of C-V Fellowhip Program
UPMC Presbyterian-Shadyside
Pittsburgh, Pennsylvania
Chapter 12

Leslee J. Shaw, PhD
Acting Professor
Division of Cardiology
Department of Medicine
Cedars-Sinai Research Institute
Cedars-Sinai Medical Center
Los Angeles, California
Chapters 19, 64

Daichi Shimbo, MD
Assistant Professor of Medicine
Department of Medicine
Columbia University College of Physicians and Surgeons
New York, New York
Chapter 113

Mark E. Silverman, MD, MACP, FRCP, FACC
Emeritus Professor of Medicine
Emory University
Chief of Cardiology
Fuqua Heart Center of Atlanta
Piedmont Hospital
Atlanta, Georgia
Chapters 1, 12

Andrew L. Smith, MD
Associate Professor of Medicine
Emory University
Director, Emory Center for Heart Failure Therapy and
    Transplantation
Emory Clinic—Emory Hospital
Atlanta, Georgia
Chapter 93

Sidney C. Smith, Jr., MD, FACC, FAHA, FESC
Professor of Medicine
Director, Center for Cardiovascular Science and Medicine
Division of Cardiology
Department of Internal Medicine
University of North Carolina at Chapel Hill
Chapel Hill, North Carolina
Chapter 91

Joaquin Solis, MD
Physician
Department of Cardiology
University of Wisconsin Medical School Milwaukee Clinical Campus
Milwaukee, Wisconsin
Chapter 110

Edmund H. Sonnenblick, MD, FACC
The Edmond J. Safra Professor of Medicine
Department of Medicine
The Albert Einstein College of Medicine
Attending Cardiologist and Chief Emeritus
Division of Cardiology
Weiler Hospital for the Montefiore Medical Center
Bronx, New York
Chapter 24

Albert Starr, MD
Director of Academic Affairs
Providence Health System of Oregon
Director, Heart Institute
Providence St. Vincent Hospital
Portland, Oregon
Chapter 79

William G. Stevenson, MD
Professor of Medicine
Harvard Medical School
Director, Clinical Cardiac Electrophysiology Program
Brigham and Women's Hospital
Boston, Massachusetts
Chapter 44

Lisa M. Sullivan, PhD
Associate Professor of Biostatistics
Boston University
Boston, Massachusetts
Chapter 2

Qinghua Sun, MD, PhD
Assistant Professor
School of Public Health
Department of Internal Medicine
Ohio State University
Columbus, Ohio
Chapter 104

Panagiotis N. Symbas, MD
Professor of Cardiothoracic Surgery
Emory University School of Medicine
Professor of Cardiothoracic Surgery
Emory University Affiliated Hospitals
Atlanta, Georgia
Chapter 97

A. Jamil Tajik, MD
Chair, Cardiovascular Diseases
Mayo Clinic College of Medicine
Rochester, Minnesota
Chapters 3, 30

W. H. Wilson Tang, MD, FACC
Assistant Professor in Medicine
Cleveland Clinic Lerner College of Medicine of Case Western
    Reserve University
Staff Physician
Department of Cardiovascular Medicine
The Cleveland Clinic
Cleveland, Ohio
Chapter 24

Anne L. Taylor, MD
Professor of Medicine/Cardiology
Associate Dean for Faculty Affairs
Co-Director, Deborah E. Powell National Center of Excellence in
    Women's Health
Division of Cardiology
University of Minnesota
Minneapolis, Minnesota
Chapter 103

Usha B. Tedrow, MD, MS
Director, Women and Arrhythmias Program
Brigham and Women's Hospital
Instructor in Medicine
Harvard Medical School
Boston, Massachusetts
Chapter 44

Gaetano Thiene, MD, FRCP, Hon.
Full Professor, Pathology
Cardiovascular Pathology
Institute of Anatomic Pathology
University of Padua
Civil Hospital
Padua, Italy
Chapter 28

E. Murat Tuzcu, MD
Professor of Medicine
The Cleveland Clinic Lerner College of Medicine
Staff, Interventional Cardiologist and Vice Chairman
Department of Cardiovascular Medicine
Division of Medicine
The Cleveland Clinic Foundation
Cleveland, Ohio
Chapter 18

Ramachandran S. Vasan, MD, DM, FACC
Associate Editor, *Circulation*
Professor of Medicine
Co-Director of Echocardiography Vascular Laboratory
Boston University School of Medicine
Framingham Heart Study
Framingham, Massachusetts
Chapter 2

Stephen F. Vatner, MD
University Professor and Chair
Department of Cell Biology and Molecular Medicine
Director, Cardiovascular Research Institute
University of Medicine and Dentistry of New Jersey
New Jersey Medical School
Newark, New Jersey
Chapter 54

Pugazhendhi Vijayaraman, MD
Director, Cardiac Electrophysiology
Geisinger Wyoming Valley Medical Center
Wilkes-Barre, Pennsylvania
Chapter 40

Renu Virmani, MD
Medical Director
CVPath
International Registry of Pathology
Gaithersburg, Maryland
Chapter 57

Scott Visovatti, MD
Chief Medical Resident
University of Michigan
Ann Arbor, Michigan
Chapter 58

John H. K. Vogel, MD
Chairman
Cardiology
Santa Barbara Cottage Hospital
Santa Barbara, California
Chapter 114

Albert L. Waldo, MD
The Waler H. Pritchard Professor of Cardiology
Professor of Medicine
Case Western Reserve University
Divison of Cardiology
Cleveland, Ohio
Chapter 37

Bruce F. Waller, MD
Cardiologist
The Care Group, LLC
Indianapolis, Indiana
Chapter 55

Richard A. Walsh, MD, FACC, FAHA
John H. Hord Professor
Chair, Department of Medicine
Case Western Reserve University
Physician-in-Chief
University Hospitals of Cleveland
Cleveland, Ohio
Chapters 4, 6

William S. Weintraub, MD
Professor Emeritus
Emory University
Professor of Medicine
Jefferson University
Philadelphia, Pennsylvania
Professor of Health Sciences (Adjunct)
University of Delaware
Chief, Section of Cardiology
Christiana Care Health System
Newark, Delaware
Chapter 111

Paul W. Wennberg, MD
Assistant Professor of Medicine
Gonda Vascular Center
Mayo Graduate School of Medicine
Consultant, Cardiovascular Diseases
Division of Cardiovascular Diseases
Mayo Clinic
Rochester, Minnesota
Chapter 108

Arno (Andy) Wessels, PhD
Associate Professor
Department of Anatomy and Cell Biology
Cardiovascular Develpmental Biology Center
Department of Pediatrics
Division of Pediatric Cardiology
Medical University of South Carolina
Charleston, South Carolina
Chapter 8

James A. White, MD
Co-Director of Cardiovascular MRI
Division of Cardiology
London Health Sciences Centre
London, Ontario, Canada
Chapter 21

Priv. Doz. Dr. Christian Wolpert, MD
Associate Professor
University Hospital Mannheim
Faculty of Medicine of the Ruprecht-Karls-University of
    Mannheim
Mannheim, Germany
Chapter 46

Charles F. Wooley, MD
Professor of Medicine Emeritus
Division of Cardiology
Department of Internal Medicine
The Ohio State University
Heart Lung Research Institute
Columbus, Ohio
Chapter 1

Jackson T. Wright Jr., MD, PhD
Professor of Medicine
Director, Clinical Hypertension Program
Division of Nephrology and Hypertension
Program Director, General Clinical Research
Case Western Reserve University
University Hospitals of Cleveland
Cleveland, Ohio
Chapter 70

YingXing Wu, MD
Postdoctoral Fellow
Medical Data Research Center
Providence Health and Services
Portland, Oregon
Chapter 79

Jay S. Yadav, MD
Chairman, Center for Medical Innoculation
Director, Vascular Intervention
The Cleveland Clinic
Cleveland, Ohio
Chapter 107

Gan-Xin Yan, MD, PhD
Associate Professor of Medicine
Jefferson Medical College of Thomas Jefferson University
Attending Cardiologist, Director of Basic Research
Main Line Health Heart Center
Wynnewood, Pennsylvania
Chapter 43

Eric H. Yang, MD
Assistant Professor of Medicine
Director of the Coronary Care Unit
University of North Carolina at Chapel Hill
Chapel Hill, North Carolina
Chapter 60

Edward T.H. Yeh, MD
Professor and Chairman
Department of Cardiology
The University of Texas M.D. Anderson Cancer Center
Cardiology Department
Houston, Texas
Chapter 89

ACKNOWLEDGMENTS

The editors and authors would like to acknowledge and thank the following individuals for their contributions to the 11th edition of *Hurst's The Heart*. Although their work forms part of the chapters of the 12th edition, they are not authoring the current chapters. (Chapter numbers refer to the 12th edition.)

Suhail Allaqaband, MD, Chapter 110; Jeffrey L. Anderson, MD, Chapter 85; James M. Bailey, MD, Chapter 66; Steven R. Bailey, MD, Chapter 76; George L. Bakris, MD, FACP, Chapter 70; Alan L. Bisno, MD, Chapter 74; Henry R. Black, MD, Chapter 69; Rob A. Bleasdale, MD, Chapter 46; Teresa Bohlmeyer, MD, Chapter 29; Harisios Boudoulas, MD, Chapter 48; Simon Chakko, MD, Chapter 74; Nisha Chandra-Strobos, MD, Chapter 50; Melvin D. Cheitlin, MD, Chapter 92; James T. T. Chen, MD, Chapter 15; Domenico Cianflone, MD, FESC, Chapter 54; Stefano Coli, MD, Chapter 54; Denton A. Cooley, MD, Chapter 89; John E. Deanfield, MB, FACC, Chapter 83; Howard V. Dinh, MD, Chapter 21; William J. Elliott, MD, PhD, Chapter 68; Maksin A. Fedaru, MD, Chapter 58; Robert H. Franch, MD, Chapter 17; O. Howard Frazier, MD, Chapter 89; Michael D. Freed, MD, Chapter 82; William H. Frishman, MD, MACP, Chapters 26 and 94; William Gerin, MD, Chapter 113; Patricia A. Gum, MD, Chapter 107; Robert J. Hall, MD, Chapter 89; Julia H. Indik, MD, Chapter 43; Marinka Kartalija, MD, Chapter 85; G. Neal Kay, MD, Chapter 37; Nils Kucher, MD, Chapter 72; Gaetano Antonio Lanza, MD, FESC, Chapter 54; Thierry H. LeJemtel, MD, Chapter 26; Martin M. LeWinter, MD, Chapter 4; Richard P. Lewis, MD, Chapter 48; Richard Liebowitz, MD, Chapter 114; Richard P. Lifton, MD, Chapter 9; John J. Mahmarian, MD, Chapter 20; Attilio Maseri, MD, FACC, FESC, Chapter 54; Jay W. Mason, MD, Chapter 28; Hugh A. McAllister Jr., MD, Chapter 89; Donogh F. McKeogh, MD, Chapter 80; Darryl Miller, MD, Chapter 31; William E. Mitch, MD, Chapter 98; Susan D. Moffatt, MD, Chapter 27; Joseph B. Muhlestein, MD, Chapter 85; Elizabeth G. Nabel, MD, Chapter 10; Yoshifumi Naka, MD, Chapter 58; Steven D. Nelson, MD, Chapter 48; Konstantin Nikolaou, MD, Chapter 22; R. Joe Noble, MD, FACC, Chapter 41; Peter A. O'Callaghan, MD, Chapter 46; Lionel Opie, MD, DPhil, FRCP, Chapter 94; George Osol, PhD, Chapter 4; Eugen C. Palma, MD, Chapter 44; Vance J. Plumb, MD, Chapter 37; Craig M. Pratt, MD, Chapter 60; John O. Prior, MD, Chapter 23; Robert C. Robbins, MD, Chapter 27; Bruce Rudisch, MD, Chapter 95; Jeremy N. Ruskin, MD, Chapter 46; Thomas J. Ryan, MD, Chapter 60; Merle A. Sande, MD, Chapter 85; Stephen F. Schaal, MD, Chapter 48; Melvin M. Scheinman, MD, Chapter 44; Domenic A. Sica, MD, Chapter 94; Robert B. Smith III, MD, Chapter 109; H. Robert Superko, MD, FACC, FAHA, FACSM, Chapter 91; Victor F. Tapson, MD, Chapter 72; Thomas T. Terramani, MD, Chapter 109; Kent Ueland, MD, Chapter 96; Albert Waldo, MD, Chapter 35; Carole A. Warnes, MD, MRCP, FACC, Chapter 83; Myron L. Weisfeldt, MD, Chapter 50; Nanette K. Wenger, MD, Chapter 67; Andrew L. Wit, PhD, Chapter 35; Raymond L. Woosley, MD, PhD, Chapter 43.

PREFACE

It is 41 years since *The Heart* was published as the first multidisciplinary and comprehensive textbook on cardiovascular disease. This 12th edition of *Hurst's The Heart* with 115 chapters written by preeminent and dedicated experts in each of the specialized areas has innovative features that separate it from prior editions.

1) The 12th edition includes authorship by many physicians from Europe, enabling multiple experts from several institutions and different countries to collaborate, thus providing a worldwide perspective on treatment of diseases such as hypertrophic obstructive cardiomyopathy, dilated cardiomyopathies, systemic hypertension, acute rheumatic fever, and neoplastic heart disease.

2) The previous chapter on hypertension has been divided into three more detailed chapters concerning epidemiology, pathophysiology, and diagnosis and treatment.

3) Chapters concerned with the human genome, cardiovascular practice guidelines, and evolving imaging technology for assessing coronary and non-coronary atherosclerotic disease and plaque characterization have been extensively revised. The most recent advances in pathophysiology and treatment for pulmonary hypertension and for the management of heart failure have been incorporated, and major advances including controversies in interventional cardiology are detailed.

4) Additional revised chapters focus on the diseases of the aorta, cardiovascular drug interactions, and surgical and non-surgical approaches to carotid arterial disease and peripheral vascular disease. In the chapter on treatment of cardiac arrhythmias, cardiovascular drug interactions have been updated to include the antiplatelet drugs, the statins, angiotensin 2 receptor blockers, and the new antianginal drug ranolazine. Chapter 105, Diseases of the Aorta, has been expanded and updated to include the medical treatment of acute aortic syndromes, and the chapter on cardiocerebral and cardiopulmonary resuscitation details the AHA modified approach to CPR.

5) The ACC/AHA Clinical Practice Guidelines and other alternative guidelines (such as those of the European Society of Cardiology) are more clearly elucidated in this edition than previously and are related to a specific chapter (Chapter 11) introducing this topic and defining several different classification systems.

6) The 12th edition of *Hurst's The Heart* includes appropriate classic and recent references, many updated just prior to publication with some still in press at the time of publication.

The editors and associate editors are grateful to the excellent group of authors who participated in the 12th edition of *Hurst's The Heart* for their extraordinary and timely contribution. The quick turnaround time for a textbook of this size and complexity is a tribute to the hard work and dedication of our authors.

We wish to thank J. Willis Hurst, the editor of the first seven editions, for his continuing enthusiastic support.

Finally, we wish to thank our families for their support and the many sacrifices they made to make this volume possible. We especially thank our wives for their strength, love, and support: Maria Fuster, Suzann O'Rourke, Donna Walsh, Mary Elizabeth Poole-Wilson, Gail King, Donna Roberts, Bethany Nash, and Bonnie Prystowsky.

THE EDITORS

Valentin Fuster, MD, PhD
Robert A. O'Rourke, MD
Richard A. Walsh, MD
Phillip Poole-Wilson, MD, PhD

Associate Editors

Spencer B. King III, MD
Robert Roberts, MD
Ira S. Nash, MD
Eric N. Prystowsky, MD

PART 1 Cardiovascular Disease: Past, Present, and Future

CHAPTER (1)

A History of the Heart

Mark E. Silverman / Charles F. Wooley

The heart … is the beginning of life; the sun of the microcosm … for it is the heart by whose virtue and pulse the blood is moved, perfected, made apt to nourish, and is preserved from corruption and coagulation; it is the household divinity which, discharging its function, nourishes, cherishes, quickens the whole body, and is indeed the foundation of life, the source of all action.—William Harvey, 1628[1]

The history of the heart is a remarkable story, with origins in antiquity, centered initially on clinical observations and palpation of the pulse. Thought at one time to be the center of the soul and impervious to disease, the heart was long a source of mystery and wonder. How best to describe this history? Most historians would agree that William Harvey's discovery of the circulation of blood in the early 17th century is a good place to start. Following Harvey, in a general sense, cardiology has followed the pathway of descriptive anatomy and pathology in the 17th and 18th centuries, auscultation and its correlations in the 19th century, an understanding of cardiac disease and its pathophysiology in the last half of the 19th and first half of the 20th century, and major advances in the diagnosis and treatment of heart disease from there into the 21st century.[2–5] The introduction of the first instruments of precision—blood pressure measurement, the chest x-ray, and the electrocardiogram, in the 1890s and early 20th century, transformed the entire field of

medicine and eventually led to the specialty of cardiology. Since the 1950s, following the advent of clinical catheterization and surgery, the field of cardiology has splintered into multiple, highly specialized disciplines and has become more laboratory-focused and less bedside-oriented. Increasingly, genomics and molecular biology, and their diagnostic and therapeutic offshoots, have come to the forefront. Many of the initial discoveries are recalled as eponyms attached to diseases or physical signs. As the number of investigators and institutions has grown exponentially and internationally, it is increasingly difficult to assign priority to contributions for which many are ultimately responsible. Taking all of these considerations into account, we have chosen to provide a condensed narrative by subject, selectively highlighting important events and key figures in the grand story of cardiology written by our illustrious predecessors.[1–11]

WILLIAM HARVEY AND THE CIRCULATION OF THE BLOOD

Early civilizations considered the heart to be a source of heat and believed that the blood vessels carried *pneuma*, the life-sustaining spirit of the vital organs. This concept was most fully elaborated by Claudius Galen (A.D. 130–200), whose erroneous teachings were entrenched for 1300 years, until Andreas Vesalius corrected

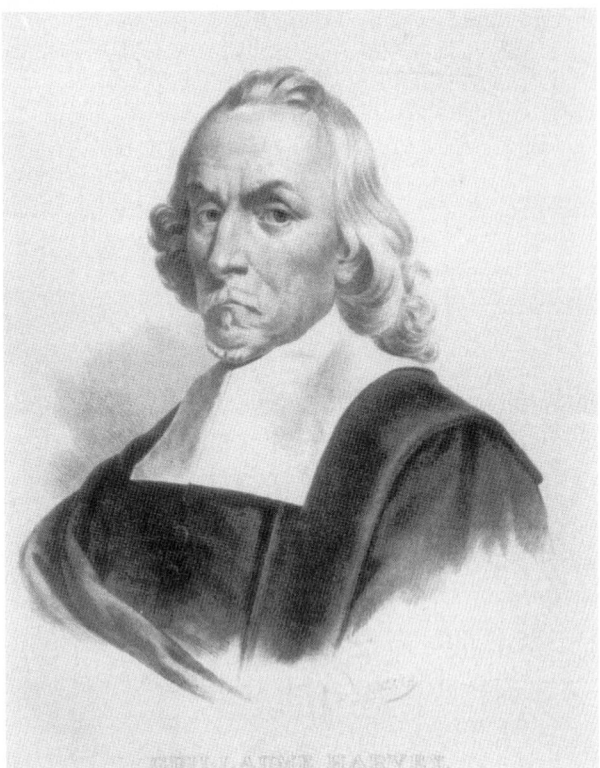

FIGURE 1-1. William Harvey. *Source: Courtesy of the National Library of Medicine.*

his anatomy (1543), and William Harvey proposed that blood circulates because of the force of the heart (1616).[2,3]

The discovery of the circulation of blood by Harvey (Fig. 1–1) in London is often considered to mark the beginning of cardiology as well as the introduction of experimental observation. Starting in 1603, Harvey dissected the anatomy and observed the motion of the cardiac chambers and flow of blood in more than 80 species of animals. His experimental questions "to seek unbiased truth" can be summarized as follows:

1. What is the relationship of the motion of the auricle to the ventricle?
2. Which is the systolic and which is the diastolic motion of the heart?
3. Do the arteries distend because of the propulsive force of the heart?
4. What purpose is served by the orientation of the cardiac and venous valves?
5. How does blood travel from the right ventricle to the left side of the heart?
6. Which direction does the blood flow in the veins and the arteries?
7. How much blood is present and how long does its passage take?

After many experiments and without the knowledge of the capillary circulation of the lungs, which was not known until 1661, Harvey stated: "It must of necessity be concluded that the blood is driven into a round by a circular motion and that it moves perpetually; and hence does arise the action or function of the heart, which by pulsation it performs." This was published in 1628 as *Exercitatio Anatomica de Motu Cordis et Sanguinis in Animalibus.*[1] His revolutionary concept eventually became accepted in Harvey's

lifetime and remains the foundation for our understanding of the purpose of the heart.

THE CARDIAC EXAMINATION

【 】 THE ARTERIAL PULSE

Until the seventeenth century, the clinical examination consisted of palpating the pulse and inspecting the urine to reveal disease and predict prognosis. In Chinese acupuncture, the pulse was timed according to the physician's respiration while digital pressure was applied to elicit information. Galen wrote 18 books on the arterial pulse in the 2nd century, providing elaborate descriptions that influenced clinical practice well into the 18th century.[2,3] The 1-minute pulse watch, invented by Floyer in 1707, offered the first opportunity to measure the heart rate accurately; however, this did not become a routine part of medical practice until the mid 19th century.[3] Since the 19th-century observations of Dominic Corrigan, the carotid arterial pulse has been linked to aortic valve disease and is essential for timing systole at the bedside. In 1847, Carl Ludwig in Leipzig invented the kymograph, a pulse writer that would elevate physiology to a new level and be used to inscribe arterial and venous pulses. Pulsus alternans was described by Ludwig Traube in 1872, and Adolf Kussmaul called attention to the paradoxical pulse in 1873, noting that the arterial pulse could transiently disappear on inspiration even though the heart sounds were still audible. Before electrocardiography, arterial pulse recordings were applied to diagnose arrhythmias, as shown so well by James Mackenzie in his *The Study of the Pulse* (1902).[12]

【 】 PERCUSSION

In 1761, Leopold Auenbrugger, a Viennese physician, published a book proposing "percussion of the human thorax, whereby, according to the character of the particular sounds thence elicited, an opinion is formed of the internal state of that cavity."[2] He had observed his father, an innkeeper, use this technique to check the wine levels in his casks. Although his discovery was initially ignored, percussion was reintroduced by Jean-Nicolas Corvisart in early 19th-century France, and became an essential addition to the chest examination until it was mostly supplanted by the chest x-ray.

【 】 THE JUGULAR VENOUS PULSE

Jugular venous wave recording was initiated in mid-19th century France by Pierre-Carl Potain. In the 1870s, Mackenzie sought to interpret arrhythmias by understanding arterial and venous pulse waves. Using a kymograph, then an ink-writing polygraph, Mackenzie applied his intuitive skills to the interpretation of jugular waves, which he labeled "a, c, and v."[13] Thomas Lewis, a disciple of Mackenzie, described the technique of bedside assessment of jugular venous pressure relative to the sternal angle in 1930.

❲❳ AUSCULTATION

Auscultation of the chest was first practiced by Hippocrates (460–370 B.C.), who applied his ear directly to the chest. The invention of the wooden monaural stethoscope (Greek: *stethos,* chest; *skopein,* to view or to see) by René Laennec in Paris (1816) introduced a powerful, although initially difficult technique to listen to cardiovascular sound.[14,15] This method spread to Europe and Great Britain—where it was promoted by Skoda, Stokes, Hope, Williams, and others—and to America, where Austin Flint became its champion. By the mid-19th century, the stethoscope was established as an indispensable tool for the examination of the heart and lungs. Diagnoses based on percussion and auscultation were subjected to the critical analysis of the autopsy by Corvisart, Laennec, Rokitansky, and Skoda, and murmurs were duly assigned to their underlying pathology. Symptoms not supported by auscultatory or autopsy findings were often thought to be functional or unreliable. The stethoscope evolved from a monaural to a binaural device in 1855, and separate heads were developed by Bowles (1894) and Sprague (1926). Grading of systolic murmurs was introduced by Samuel Levine in 1933. The acoustic principles of cardiovascular sound became better understood through the work of Rappaport and Sprague (1940s); and correlations were made with phonocardiography and cardiac catheterization by Paul Wood, Aubrey Leatham, Samuel Levine, and many others between 1950 and 1975. In 1961, physiologist Robert Rushmer proposed the acceleration-deceleration theory that is our current concept of the generation of normal and abnormal heart sounds. Auscultation continues to be valuable, although less relied on today, when bedside skills are decreasingly prized, teachers are scarce, and valvular disease is much less common.

TECHNOLOGY AND THE HEART
❲❳ THE ELECTROCARDIOGRAM

In 1856, von Kölliker and Müller demonstrated that the heart also produced electricity. Augustus Waller, with a capillary electrometer device (1887), detected cardiac electricity from the limbs, a crude recording that he called an "electrogram." Willem Einthoven, a physiologist in Utrecht, devised a more sensitive string galvanometer (1902), for which he received the Nobel Prize, and the modern electrocardiogram was born. Initially weighing 600 lb and requiring five people to operate, the 3-lead electrocardiograph would eventually become portable, 12 leads, and routine (Table 1–1).[16]

Nineteenth century researchers debated whether the heartbeat was stimulated by the heart muscle or was caused by external nervous or local ganglionic control—the myogenic versus the neurogenic theory. The answer was finally provided by discovering the electrical system of the heart: the Purkinje fibers (1839), bundle of His (1893), bundle branches (1904), atrioventricular (AV) node (1906) and sinus node (1907).[17] With the electrocardiogram, the activation and sequence of stimulation of the human heart could now be measured, and the anatomic basis for the conduction system confirmed. Thomas Lewis in London was the first to realize its great potential, beginning in 1909, and his books on disorders of the heartbeat became bibles for aspiring electrocardiographers.[2,10] Disorders of the heartbeat and abnormalities in the activation of the human heart, heretofore unknown or inferred from pulse tracings or experimental observations, became new clinical currency; palpitations became premature atrial or ventricular beats, and tachycardias and atrioventricular block could be understood. When electrocardiography was added to the chest x-ray and cardiac fluoroscopy in the early 20th century, clinical cardiology became a field of its own, inextricably linked to technology. Those who interpreted the complicated tracings, known as cardiologists, became practitioners of this new specialty.[11] By the 1930s, the electrocardiogram had become 12 leads and a necessary confirmation for myocardial ischemia or infarction. When electrocardiography was combined with the Master "2-step" exercise test (1940s), bicycle and treadmill stress testing (1960s), and nuclear and echocardiography imaging (1970s), a superior diagnostic approach to patients with chest pain became available. Continuous bedside monitoring (Paul Zoll, 1956) and the ambulatory detection of arrhythmias (Holter, 1961) became commonplace in the 1960s; and implanted loop recording appeared in 1999.

Pacing the heart in cardiac standstill was first carried out by John MacWilliam in Aberdeen in 1887. Experiments with external pacemakers in the 1920s to 1930s by Mark Lidwill in Australia and Albert Hyman in the United States showed their feasibility. A temporary pacemaker was inserted in 1952 by Zoll, and an internal pacemaker was inserted in a human by William Chardack in 1960.[18] Although initially plagued by faulty operation, lead breakage, infection, and early battery failure, pacemakers eventually became a marvel of reliability, complexity, and durability. Progressive advances include transvenous leads (1965), lithium iodine batteries (1972), multiprogammability (1972), dual chamber pacing (1980), rate adaptive modes, and antitachycardia programs. Biventricular pacing (1998) for heart failure has been an impressive gain in an evolving field that has prevented Stokes-Adams attacks and saved many lives.

Electrophysiologic testing in humans began as an offshoot of basic catheterization laboratory investigations in the early pacemaker era. Intracardiac potentials were first measured in 1945. Catheter techniques were used to localize the His bundle (Scherlag and Damato, 1967) and to identify accessory pathways (Jackman, 1983). Programmed electrical stimulation of the heart was introduced to localize, provoke, and terminate arrhythmias (Durrer, Wellens, and Coumel, 1967). Mapping techniques, applied to the surface of the heart for the localization and resection of accessory pathways (1968) and the surgical ablation of ventricular arrhythmias (1974) and atrial fibrillation (1991) became an essential method of investigation. As catheter methods of ablation improved, first coupled with intracardiac high-energy shock of the atrioventricular node (1982) and then with radiofrequency current (1987), ablation moved from the surgery suite into the laboratory setting, populated by a new subspecialty group—the electrophysiologists. Catheter ablation of AV nodal reentry was the next great success story. Atrial flutter and fibrillation and ventricular tachycardia are the newest targets. Strides have been made in preventing cardiac arrest with implanted and automatic external defibrillators. Through an understanding of

TABLE 1-1

Advances in Cardiac Diagnosis and Technology

ANCIENT TIMES

General inspection
Palpation of the pulse (Egypt, China, India)

EIGHTEENTH CENTURY

Physician's 1 minute pulse watch (1707)
Percussion of the chest (1761)

NINETEENTH CENTURY

Stethoscopic auscultation of the heart (1816)
Pleximeter (1826)
Kymographic recording of pulses (1847)
Sphygmograph for blood pressure measurement (1855, 1863)
Polygraphic recording of pulses (1883)
Chest x-ray (1895)
Fluoroscopy (1896)

TWENTIETH CENTURY 1900–1929

Electrocardiogram (1902)
Auscultation of blood pressure (1905)
Phonocardiogram (1907)
Leukocytosis in myocardial infarction (1916)
Electrocardiography for myocardial infarction (1920)
Vectorcardiography (1920)
Portable electrocardiogram (1928)
First cardiac catheterization (1929)

1930–1959

Bedside measurement of venous pressure (1930)
Cardiac output measurement (1870, 1930)
Circulation time (1931)
Precordial electrocardiography (1932)
Unipolar ECG leads (1932)
Angiography (1931, 1937)
Sedimentation rate for myocardial infarction (1933)
Development of cardiac catheterization (1941)
Augmented unipolar leads (1942)
Master "2-step" exercise test (1942)
Scintillation scanner (1949, 1952)
Left heart catheterization (1950)
Image intensification (1953)
M-mode echocardiography (1954)
Serum glutamic oxaloacetic transaminase (1954)
Treadmill exercise testing (1956)
Cardiac monitoring (1956)
Selective coronary arteriography (1958)

1960–1979

Computerized electrocardiography (1961)
Ambulatory monitoring (1961)
Creatine phosphokinase (1965)
His bundle recording (1967)
Transfemoral catheterization (1967)
Contrast echocardiography (1968)
Swan-Ganz flotation catheter (1970)
Digoxin level (1971)

Computerized tomographic scanning (1971)
Electrophysiologic testing (1972)
Nuclear stress cardiology (1973)
Two-dimensional echocardiography (1974)
Doppler echocardiography (1975)
Positive emission tomography (1979)
Stress echocardiography (1979)
Ultrafast computed tomography (1979, 1990)

1980–PRESENT

Signal-averaged electrocardiography (1981)
Doppler color-flow echocardiography (1982)
Magnetic resonance imaging of the heart (1984)
ST-segment monitoring (1984)
Transesophageal echocardiography (1985)
Dobutamine stress echocardiography (1986)
Heart rate variability (1973, 1987)
Electron beam tomography for coronary calcium (1990)
Troponin T (1991)
Troponin I (1992)
B-type natriuretic peptide (1994)
Single-photon emission computed tomography (1990s)
Intracoronary ultrasound (1996)
Implanted loop recorder (1999)
Three-dimensional echocardiography (2003)
64-slice CT scanning (2005)

---

the mechanisms of arrhythmias and the identification of genes encoding cardiac ion channels—especially the long-QT and Brugada syndromes—electrocardiography has been elevated to a new level of importance.[19–21]

THE CARDIAC CATHETER

If the electrocardiograph was a touchstone for the identification of the cardiologist at the dawn of the 20th century, it was the cardiac catheter that completed the modern definition of cardiology. Many of the fundamentals of modern cardiovascular instrumentation and physiology originated in mid-19th-century France. Claude Bernard in 1844 was the first to insert a catheter into the heart of animals to measure temperature and pressure.[2] In the

1860s, Etienne Jules Marey combined the kymographic instrumentation created by Ludwig in Leipzig in 1847 with an air-filled manometer for the graphic registration of biological phenomena.[6] Marey's pulse writer—the sphygmograph—was used for recording the external pulsation of the heart and arteries and was a prototype for noninvasive devices in cardiology. In the early 1860s, Auguste Chauveau, a veterinary physiologist, and Marey collaborated to develop a system of devices called *sounds*, forerunners of the modern cardiac catheter, which they used to catheterize the right heart and left ventricle of the horse.[6] They recorded true values of intracardiac pressure with superb tracings and correlated the intracardiac events with precision to show the relation of atrial and ventricular systole to the apex impulse. In 1870, Adolph Fick provided his oximetric formula to measure cardiac output.

Cardiac catheterization in humans was an inconceivable risk until Werner Forssmann, a 29-year-old surgical resident in Germany, performed a self-catheterization in 1929.[22,23] Forssmann was interested in discovering a method of injecting adrenaline to treat cardiac arrest. He passed a ureteral catheter into his antecubital vein, confirming its right atrial position on an x-ray. The next year he attempted to image his heart using an iodide injection. However, he was reprimanded and did not experiment further. Catheterization began in earnest in the early 1940s in New York and London. André Cournand and Dickinson Richards at Bellevue, interested in respiratory physiology, developed and demonstrated the safety of complete right heart catheterization, for which they shared the Nobel Prize with Forssmann in 1956.[6,9]

The cardiac catheter was viewed initially as an instrument to measure pressure and cardiac output, sample blood contents, or deliver contrast agents for cardiovascular angiography. Brannon and Warren in Atlanta were the first to apply the catheter to diagnose heart disease—an atrial septal defect—in 1945. It was the impetus of cardiac surgery requiring an accurate diagnosis, initially for congenital heart and rheumatic mitral disease, that brought cardiac catheterization out of the physiology laboratory and to the forefront of clinical cardiology in the 1950s. Improved catheters and pressure manometers, automatic film changers, and the introduction of retrograde left heart catheterization by Henry Zimmerman (1950) and a percutaneous approach by Sven Seldinger (1953) advanced the technique, accompanying heart surgery into the era of valve replacement in the 1960s. Mason Sones's accidental injection of contrast directly into a right coronary artery (1958) was a serendipitous leap forward. The Judkin transfemoral approach (1967) simplified selective coronary catheterization. Visualization of the coronary circulation ultimately led to the introduction of coronary bypass surgery by René Favoloro (1967) and angioplasty by Andreas Grüntzig (1977).[23,24] Since then, the versatile cardiac catheter has continued to evolve, carrying delivery systems or instruments ranging from ultrasound, balloons, and stents to defibrillators (see Table 1–1; Table 1–2).

【 】 IMAGING OF THE HEART

Radiography

Modern imaging technology began with Konrad Roentgen's discovery of x-rays in 1895, for which he was awarded the Nobel Prize in Physics in 1901 "in recognition of the extraordinary services he has rendered by the discovery of the remarkable rays subsequently named after him."[25,26] Within a year, fluorescent screens were available to view cardiac pulsations. Contrast agents incorporating sodium iodide were necessary to visualize the organ cavities. Moniz in Lisbon (1931) and Castellanos in Cuba (1937) were the first to image the interior of the heart with intravenous angiograms.[2] In the mid-20th century, electronic x-ray technology with the image intensifier allowed enhanced viewing of dynamic events in real time (see Table 1–1). Angiography became the essence of cardiovascular imaging for several decades after the mid-20th century, vital to the diagnosis and management of coronary disease during the 1960s, and it continues to play a central role.

Nuclear Cardiology

Nuclear cardiology began with Herrman Blumgart, who injected radon to measure the circulation time in 1927; followed by G. Liljestrand, who determined normal blood volume in 1939; and Myron Prinzmetal, who monitored the transit of radiolabeled albumin through the heart in 1948.[6,27] Following World War II, radioactive isotopes and scintillation cameras became available for imaging purposes. The gamma camera of Hal Anger, a key development introduced in 1952, provided a high-resolution scanning capability that could visualize the cardiac chambers and assess function and shunting without moving the patient. Electrocardiographic gating, starting in the early 1970s, greatly improved the analysis of wall motion and ejection fraction, as did single-photon emission computed tomography (SPECT) in the 1990s. Nuclear stress testing for ischemia was introduced by Zaret and Strauss in 1973 using potassium 43 as the tracer. Redistribution studies, taking advantage of the properties of thallium 201 and technetium 99m, have improved the performance of the test, and pharmacologic stress testing with dipyridamole and adenosine has expanded their use.[6,27] Recent advances include combining positron emission tomography (PET) or SPECT scanning with CT to integrate anatomic with physiologic information and thereby pin-point high- and low-risk patients. Molecular imaging of vascular plaques and angiogenesis is on the horizon.

Echocardiography

Ultrasound imaging dates back to the production of sound waves from piezoelectric crystals in 1880, and the military use of sonar for the detection of reflected sound waves during World War II.[6] Cardiac ultrasound was introduced in Sweden by Inge Edler and Helmuth Hertz, who detected the anterior mitral leaflet with postmortem correlation—an ice pick through the chest into the mitral leaflet (1954). Starting in the mid 1960s with the detection of pericardial effusion and left ventricular size, M-mode echocardiography became a powerful clinical technique developed by Harvey Feigenbaum who taught the first generation of echocardiographers. Contrast echocardiography (1969), two-dimensional echocardiography (1974), pulsed Doppler hemodynamics (1975), stress echocardiography (1979), Doppler color-flow (1982), and transesophageal imaging (1985) have added to its enormous success. Intraoperative transesophageal monitoring and the intrauterine diagnosis of congenital heart disease have become possible. New additions include measurement of diastolic function and tissue strain rate and three-dimensional capabilities. Digital recording has significantly transformed the acquisition, storage, and interpretation of studies. Echocardiography has safely and brilliantly illuminated the heart and its function.[25,26,28]

Tomography and Magnetic Resonance Imaging

The three decades following the introduction of the gamma camera and ultrasound brought unbelievable expansion to the medical imaging field, including CT (1963–1971), SPECT (1963–1981), PET (1975–1987), and MRI (1972–1981), each delivering its own exciting ability to look at the heart in a differ-

TABLE 1–2

Advances in Medical Therapy: 1900–Present

AVAILABLE IN 1900 (ALPHABETICALLY)		
Alcohol	Warfarin (1954)	Intracoronary thrombolysis (streptokinase) (1979)
Amyl nitrite (1867)	Alpha methyl dopa (1955)	Intravenous nitroglycerine
Atropine (1833, 1867)	Closed chest defibrillation (1956)	
Caffeine (1879)	Chlorothiazide (1957)	**1980–1989**
Chloroform (1831)	Streptokinase for MI (1958)	
Diet	Guanethidine (1959)	Dual chamber pacing (1980)
Digitalis (1785)		Phosphodiesterase inhibitors (1980)
Ether (1842)	**1960–1969**	Propafenone (1980)
Exercise		Automatic implanted defibrillator (1980)
Leeches	Closed chest cardiac massage (1960)	ACE inhibitors (1981)
Morphine (1821)	Cardioversion of ventricular tachycardia (1960)	Transmyocardial laser (1981)
Nitroglycerine (1879)	Implantable pacemaker (1960)	Flecainide (1982)
Quinine (1745)	Amiodarone (1961)	Antitachycardia pacemaker (1982)
Salicylic acid (1876)	Coronary care units (1961)	AV nodal ablation (1982)
Southey trocars	AV synchronous pacemaker (1962)	Catheter ablation of Wolff-Parkinson-White (1984)
Spa therapy	Beta blockers (1962)	Coronary stents (1986)
Squill (17th century)	Synchronized cardioversion (1962)	Low-molecular weight heparin (1986)
Theobromine (1879)	Intra-aortic balloon pump (1962)	Lovastatin (1986)
Venesection	Disopyramide (1963)	Intravenous thrombolysis (tPA) (1987)
Veratrum viride (1859)	Lidocaine (1963)	Aspirin for acute coronary disease (1988)
	Furosemide (1964)	Aspirin for primary prevention (1989)
1900–1949	Balloon atrial septostomy (Rashkind procedure, 1966)	Ticlopidine (1989)
	Programmed electrophysiologic stimulation (1967)	
Adrenaline (1900)	Mobile ICU (1967)	**1990–PRESENT**
Oxygen (1908)	Bretylium tosylate (1968)	
Quinidine (1914)	Outpatient cardiac rehabilitation (1968)	Hirudin (lepirudin) (1991)
Mercurial diuretics (1920)		Endovascular graft for aneurysm and dissection (1991)
Heparin (1935)	**1970–1979**	Angiotensin II receptor blocking agents (1992)
Magnesium (1935)		Directional atherectomy (1993)
Penicillin (1940)	Calcium channel blocking agents (1970)	Glycoprotein IIb–IIIa inhibitors (1993)
Dicoumarol (1941)	Vasodilator therapy (1971)	Carvedilol (1995)
Rice diet (Kempner, 1944)	Stenting of patent ductus arteriosus (1971)	Nesiritide (1996)
Cation exchange resins (1946)	Dopamine (1972)	Biphasic cardioversion–defibrillation (1996)
Open chest defibrillation (1947)	Lithium battery pacemakers (1972)	Carotid artery stenting (1997)
Reserpine (1949)	Intravenous verapamil (1972)	Clopidogrel (1998)
	Nitroprusside (1974)	Biventricular pacing (1998)
1950–1959	Beta blockers for heart failure (1975)	Dofetilide (1999)
	Dobutamine (1975)	Brachytherapy (2000)
Hexamethonium (1950)	Catheter closure of atrial septal defect (1976)	Drug eluding stents (2001)
Hydralazine (1951)	Coronary angioplasty (1977)	
Procainamide (1951)		
Ambulation post-MI (1952)		
Carbonic anhydrase inhibitors (1952)		
External cardiac pacing (1952)		

ACE, angiotensin-converting enzymes; ICU, intensive care unit; MI, myocardial infarction; tPA, tissue plasminogen activator.

ent way (see Table 1–1). Each of these imaging techniques has initiated new clinical disciplines in cardiology and radiology that continue to the present. Electron-beam computed tomography (EBCT), introduced in 1990, has become a popular way to detect early coronary disease. The new 64-slice CT angiogram (2005) provides detailed coronary anatomy and wall motion, calcium scoring, and plaque characterization—a one-stop shop—and is competing with coronary angiography and nuclear imaging for initial imaging. Cardiac magnetic resonance imaging, with its comprehensive portrayal of left and right heart structure and function, and its potential for imaging the coronary arteries and unstable plaques, has only recently joined its imaging companions. As with cardiac catheterization and angiography, industrial developments and the computer have provided the bases for each technological advance.

CORONARY ARTERY DISEASE

【 】 DIAGNOSIS OF CORONARY ARTERY DISEASE AND ITS ETIOLOGY

On July 21, 1768, William Heberden presented "Some Account of a Disorder of the Breast" to the Royal College of Physicians, London: "But there is a disorder of the breast marked with strong and peculiar symptoms, considerable for the kind of danger belonging to it, and not extremely rare. The seat of it, and sense of strangling and anxiety with which it is attended, may make it not improperly be called angina pectoris."[2,29] Heberden appropriated the term *angina* from the Latin word for strangling. His classic account marks the beginning of our appreciation of coronary artery disease. Edward Jenner and Caleb Parry were the first to suspect a coronary etiology, which Parry published in 1799. Allan Burns, in Scotland, likened the pain of angina pectoris to the discomfort brought about by walking with a tight ligature placed on a limb (1809), a prescient concept that remains current. Nevertheless, a coronary cause of angina pectoris was not readily accepted until the late 19th century.[23] The term *arteriosclerosis* was coined by Johann Lobstein (1833). Key pathologic observations were made by Rudolf Virchow, who established the importance of thrombosis of arteries as a cause of disease (1846); Richard Quain, who associated the fatty degeneration of cardiac muscle with coronary obstruction (1850); Karl Weigert, who described the pathology of myocardial infarction and remarked on the importance of collateral vessels (1880); and Karl Huber, who suggested that atheroma could cut off the blood supply and lead to myocardial fibrosis (1882).[29] Adam Hammer was the first to report the premortem diagnosis of myocardial infarction (1878).

By the late 19th century, angina pectoris was linked with coronary artery disease, although there was confusion between angina pectoris and myocardial infarction. Coronary disease was thought to be uncommon at that time. Julius Cohnheim taught that coronary arteries were end arteries, noting that experimental ligation of a coronary artery resulted in ventricular fibrillation (1881). In 1901, Osler called the anterior branch the "artery of sudden death," later stating that "the tragedies of life are largely arterial." The concept that coronary thrombosis was always fatal was finally dispelled by James Herrick (1912).[30,31] He concluded "there is no inherent reason why the stoppage of a large branch of a coronary artery, or even of a main trunk, must of necessity cause sudden death." Herrick was the first to grasp the variable course of myocardial infarction. The three-lead electrocardiogram was used by Herrick and Smith to diagnose experimental infarction (1918) and in humans by Pardee (1920).[16] Precordial leads, introduced by Frank Wilson in the 1930s, furthered the diagnosis. Between 1928 and 1950, large series of patients—analyzed by John Parkinson and Evan Bedford in London, Levine and Paul Dudley

White in Boston, Charles Friedberg in New York, and others—provided a broad understanding of the clinical, electrocardiographic, and laboratory findings of myocardial infarction and its prognosis and autopsy correlations.[10] By the 1930s, myocardial infarction was a familiar diagnosis felt to be increasing in frequency. The clinical-pathologic correlations of atherosclerosis and thrombosis with infarction were greatly strengthened by the 1940 postmortem coronary injection studies of Blumgart, Schlesinger, and Davis. Autoradiographic postmortem studies by Fulton in Glasgow (1976) and DeWood's coronary arteriographic studies (1980) finally proved that a thrombus was the primary event. The "vulnerable plaque" hypothesis (1966) has gained widespread support as the cause of acute coronary disease and sudden death. Inflammation, ignited by risk factors underlies "atherothrombosis," and plaque disruption is now realized to be multifocal.[32]

【 】 TREATMENT OF ANGINA PECTORIS

Treatment of angina pectoris began with amyl nitrite used by Lauder Brunton (1867) and nitroglycerine by William Murrell (1879). Before 1970, xanthine derivatives, sedatives, opiates, diet, prolonged rest, alcohol, long-acting nitrites, paravertebral alcohol injections, dorsal sympathectomy, induction of myxedema, instillation of talc or bone dust into the pericardium, denervation of the heart, radiation to the anterior chest, and carotid sinus pacing enjoyed temporary support. β-Adrenergic blockade, beginning in the early 1970s, greatly improved the management of angina; trials in the 1980s showed that myocardial infarction can be prevented by the regular use of β blockade. Calcium channel blockers and nitroglycerine administered by paste and intravenously were introduced in the late 1970s (see Table 1–2). Percutaneous angioplasty for alleviating angina was the brilliant concept of Grüntzig in Zürich (1977). He was influenced by Charles Dotter's 1964 demonstration that peripheral atherosclerosis was malleable. This has been succeeded by bare metal stenting of coronary arteries (1986), primary angioplasty for acute infarction (1988), brachytherapy (2000), and various drug-eluting stents (2001).[24,33] Restenosis, the Achilles heel of "plain old balloon angioplasty," has fallen from 30 to 40 percent to 5 to 10 percent, however in-stent thrombosis, a new worry, drives further development.

【 】 TREATMENT OF ACUTE CORONARY SYNDROMES

Strict bedrest for 6 to 8 weeks was rigidly advised for heart attacks until 1952 when Levine and Lown suggested an "armchair" approach was better. Anticoagulation, strongly recommended by Wood and others for myocardial infarction in the 1950s, became controversial in the 1960s. Before the defibrillator and coronary care units, the mortality of infarction was 30 percent. With the development of the defibrillator by William Kouwenhoven, Claude Beck and Paul Zoll were able to prove that rescue of cardiac arrest victims was possible. Beck dramatically stated that "The death factor in coronary artery disease is often small and reversible…The heart wants to beat and often it needs only a second chance." His concept that "the heart is too good to die," instilled optimism into the care of coronary patients. Zoll reported closed chest defibrillation in 1956 and cardioversion of ventricular tachycardia in 1960. The monitoring of patients in close proximity to skilled nursing personnel who could perform cardiopulmonary resuscitation was a logical next step suggested by Desmond Julian in 1961. Since then, coronary care has gone through recognizable phases: first, cardiac resuscitation and the essential role of the nurse; second, prevention of arrhythmias; third, hemodynamic catheter monitoring and treatment of pump failure; fourth, reduction of infarct size—first with β blockers and glucose-insulin-potassium and then thrombolytic therapy (1987); and fifth, primary angioplasty (1987). Clinical and electrocardiographic distinctions have been drawn between unstable angina, an acute coronary event, non-transmural/non–Q wave/non-ST elevation infarction, and transmural/ST elevation infarction.

Thrombolytic therapy for acute myocardial infarction, using small doses of intravenous streptokinase, was first tried in 1958 by Fletcher and Sherry and given as an intracoronary infusion by Boucek and Murphy in 1960 and Chazov in 1976.[34] The rationale for thrombolysis derives from the 1977 report by Reimer stating that necrosis from infarction progresses over a period of 3 to 6 hours, and early reperfusion can salvage threatened myocardium. Its current use, emphasizing that "time is muscle," began with intracoronary infusion of streptokinase in 1979 by Rentrop and was followed by intravenous streptokinase (1983) and intravenous tissue plasminogen activator (t-PA) in 1987. The mortality of ST elevation infarction has fallen to as low as 3 to 5 percent, and the period of hospitalization progressively reduced.

An important concept that ischemic myocardium is stunned or hibernating and could benefit by reperfusion and angiotensin-converting enzyme (ACE) inhibitors in the remodeling of myocardium was proven in the early 1990s. Aspirin has been an important adjunct for acute infarction since 1988 and strongly recommended for primary prevention since 1989. Potent platelet inhibition for acute coronary syndromes became available with glycoprotein IIb/IIIa inhibitors (1993) and clopidogrel (1998).[35]

【 】 PREVENTION OF CORONARY ARTERY DISEASE AND SUDDEN DEATH

Cardiovascular epidemiologic studies, advocated by Paul Dudley White, began in earnest with the National Institutes of Health (NIH)-sponsored Framingham study (1948) and the work of Ancel Keys in Minnesota. These landmark studies have emphasized prevention of coronary disease through recognition and treatment of risk factors. The metabolic syndrome, first described in 1983 and now an epidemic driven by visceral obesity, has risen to the forefront of concern. The vascular protective and relaxing role of the endothelium, through its generation of nitric oxide, and the dangers of endothelial dysfunction were key basic science discoveries (1970s) for which the Nobel Prize was awarded in 1998.[36] Regarded as a miracle, the hydroxymethylglutaryl coenzyme A (HMG-CoA) reductase inhibitors, isolated by Akira Endo in Japan (1976) and available since 1986, have dramatically decreased heart attacks and strokes. Low-density lipoprotein levels have been the target, but attention has also turned to elevating high-density lipoprotein levels to stabilize or reverse atheroma.

The internally implanted automatic defibrillator, conceived by Michel Mirowsky, was first used in 1980. Although highly contro-

versial, it is now in widespread use with growing indications that it will prevent sudden cardiac death.

VALVULAR HEART DISEASE

Valvular pathology was described in the 17th and 18th centuries; however, Laennec was the first to hear heart murmurs, calling them "blowing, sawing, filing, and rasping."[14] Originally, he attributed the noise to valvular disease, but he later decided that they were caused by spasm or contraction of a cardiac chamber. James Hope in England was the first to classify valvular murmurs in *A Treatise on the Diseases of the Heart and Great Vessels* (1832).[37] Hope found valvular disease much more likely to occur on the left side of the heart and showed how to separate murmurs of all four valves. He interpreted physical findings in early physiologic terms and provided detailed pathologic correlations.[38] Constriction of the mitral valve was recorded by John Mayow (1668) and Raymond Vieussens (1715); the latter also recognized that it could cause pulmonary congestion.[39] The presystolic murmur of mitral stenosis was heard by Bertin (1824), timed as both early diastolic and presystolic by Williams (1835), and placed on firmer grounds by Fauvel (1843) and Gairdner (1861). Aortic stenosis was first described pathologically by Rivière (1663), and Laennec pointed out that the aortic valve was subject to ossification (1819).[40] Corvisart showed an astute grasp of the natural history of aortic stenosis (1809) commenting:

> When it is considered how narrow the opening is, which these constrictions leave, it is difficult to conceive how such an organic derangement can continue for years. It is evident, if such an obstacle to the circulation were suddenly introduced into a healthy subject, death would immediately follow; but as these obstacles are slowly formed, the circulation is gradually impeded, and nature seems in some measure to be habituated to such a perversion of her laws.

Early descriptions of aortic regurgitation were by William Cowper (1706) and Raymond Vieussens (1715).[41] Giovanni Morgagni recognized the hemodynamic consequences of aortic regurgitation (1761). In 1832, Corrigan provided his classic description of the arterial pulse and murmur of aortic regurgitation. Flint added the presystolic murmur sometimes heard with severe aortic regurgitation (1862).[15] The etiology of valvular disease in the 19th and first half of the 20th century revolved about the role of rheumatic fever. David Pitcairn was the first to suggest rheumatism of the heart (1788), and William Charles Wells described acute rheumatic fever with cardiac involvement in 1812.[10,42] The most important clinician was Jean Baptiste-Bouillaud, who established that acute articular rheumatism was associated with inflammation leading to valvular deformities (1836).[8] Acceptance of the association between *rheumatism*—rheumatic fever—and subsequent valvular heart disease was gradually accepted. By the late 1800s, treatment of rheumatic episodes with salicylic acid had been introduced. Over time, the link between the throat, heart, and rheumatic fever was clarified; the role of the *Streptococcus* was identified; and attention paid to environmental factors—poverty, overcrowding, and malnutrition. Diagnostic criteria for acute rheumatic fever were established by T. Duckett Jones in 1944 with revisions through

1992. Antibiotic therapy has contributed to the great decrease in rheumatic fever in the Western world. The story of valvular heart disease in the second half of the 20th century overlaps with developments in cardiac catheterization, imaging technology, and cardiac surgery. Beginning with cardiac catheterization in the 1950s and supplemented by echocardiographic imaging in the 1970s, the severity of valvular disease could be more easily analyzed and its progression followed. Until the last 40 years, valvular murmurs continued to be ascribed to rheumatic heart disease, to the detriment of recognizing valvular heart disease of other etiologies. Our understanding of the etiology of valvular heart disease changed dramatically with the recognition of many nonrheumatic causes of valvular disease, especially the "floppy mitral valve" with prolapse by Reid and Barlow in the early 1960s.[43] Since 1997, inflammation of the aortic valve, attributed to atherosclerotic risk factors, has been shown to play a central role in the development of adult aortic stenosis.

CARDIOMYOPATHY

At mid-20th century, Henry A. Christian published *Non-Valvular Heart Disease*. He considered this to be the most frequent form of heart disease among those individuals past middle age. At that time, acute or chronic myocarditis was thought to be the major cause; however, he considered the role of hypertension, ventricular hypertrophy and dilatation, heart failure without enlargement, and familial occurrence. Subsequent writers gradually shifted the emphasis from myocarditis to primary (idiopathic) myocardial disease.

The term *cardiomyopathy*, referring to the noncoronary cardiomyopathies, was introduced by Wallace Brigden in 1957. During this period, a dynamic form of subaortic stenosis was discovered and its hemodynamics investigated, and John Goodwin in London presented a new classification based on hypertrophy, dilatation, or restriction (1961).[44] However, the admixture of anatomic and functional groups stultified original thought, and definitions lagged behind progress. Myocardial biopsy, new imaging modalities, and biochemical and genetic studies have reshaped the understanding of cardiomyopathy along with more precise definition of the etiology of myocarditis. In 2006, the American Heart Association (AHA) published a scientific statement incorporating the rapidly evolving advances in molecular genetics in cardiology, thus providing a new perspective and classification to aid in understanding this diverse group of diseases.[45]

CONGENITAL HEART DISEASE

Early textbooks in cardiology by Jean-Baptiste Senac (1749) and Allan Burns (1809) included comments on cardiac malformations. Cyanotic heart disease is mentioned; however, its mechanism was debated because some patients with septal defects had cyanosis while others did not. An early, comprehensive book devoted to cyanotic and acyanotic congenital heart disease, *On Malformations of the Human Heart*, was published in 1858 and 1866 by Thomas Bevill Peacock, a London physician with a special interest in pathology.[2] In his book, Peacock reviews the previous literature and provides detailed case studies, beautiful engravings of the pathology, personal insights, and an anatomic classification of more than 100 patients.

Following Peacock's book, advances in congenital heart disease were limited primarily to pathologic descriptions and summaries until the seminal work of the pathologist Maude Abbott. Beginning in 1908, Abbott catalogued the pathology collection at the Montreal General Hospital, compiling 1000 cases that were fully analyzed in her 1936 classic *Atlas of Congenital Heart Disease*.[6,46] Her meticulous work provided a new classification correlating the history, examination, and postmortem with illustrations; it became the foundation for the study of congenital heart disease. Maternal rubella studies (1940) brought attention to viral influences on cardiac development.

The pivotal breakthrough came from Helen Taussig and Alfred Blalock at Johns Hopkins Hospital with their "blue baby operation." Taussig had observed that patients with cyanotic heart disease worsened when their ductus arteriosus closed. She suggested creating an artificial ductus to improve oxygenation.[47] Blalock, ably assisted by Vivian Thomas, created a shunt from the subclavian to the pulmonary artery, which Blalock performed successfully in November 1944. This innovative operation, in which a blue baby was dramatically changed to a pink one—the Blalock-Taussig shunt—was highly publicized, and other shunt operations soon followed (Table 1–3). Taussig's *Congenital Malformations of the Heart,* a 1947 compendium with schematics explaining the pathophysiology of the defect, became the bible of congenital heart disease. Studies in the 1950s correlated the clinical with the cardiac catheterization findings and led to a firmer physiologic basis for selecting patients who might benefit from the upcoming advances in congenital heart surgery. Natural history studies helped to clarify their prognosis.

In 1966, Rashkind introduced the balloon septostomy—the Rashkind procedure—a novel catheter therapeutic technique that launched the entire field of interventional cardiology and bought time for severely cyanotic infants with transposition of the great arteries.[6] In the 1980s, catheters were adapted to dilate stenotic aortic and pulmonic valves and aortic coarctation. Transcatheter closure of patent ductus arteriosus (1971), atrial septal defects (1976), and ventricular septal defects (1987) have become routine. Indomethacin therapy to enable closure of a patent ductus in the premature infant (1976) and prostaglandin infusion to maintain ductal patency (1981) profoundly changed the medical management of fragile newborns. Stents now keep the ductus open as well as alleviate right ventricular obstruction in tetralogy of Fallot.

Until the 1970s, confirmation of a complex clinical diagnosis, mandatory for critical surgical decisions, required cardiac catheterization and angiography. In the late 1970s and 1980s, two-dimensional and color-flow Doppler echocardiography and later MRI became available to provide a quick diagnosis. With aggressive medical and catheter management, the approach to neonates, including intrauterine intervention, has radically changed. Improvements in operative techniques allowed innovative surgeons to operate earlier on smaller and sicker hearts while offering palliation or complete repair for congenital defects. Prostacyclin treatment for Eisenmenger syndrome has shown early promise. Adult congenital heart clinics have been an offshoot of the increased sur-

TABLE 1–3

Advances in Cardiovascular Surgery

NINETEENTH CENTURY

Drainage of pericardial effusion (1810)
Introduction of ether anesthesia (1842)
Removal of foreign body from heart (1873)
Surgical closure of stab wound of heart (1896)

TWENTIETH CENTURY 1900–1925

End-to-end arterial anastomosis (1902)
Animal heart transplantation (1905)
Arterial patch graft (1910)
Coronary artery bypass in animal (1910)
Insufflation endotracheal anesthesia (1910)
Attempted external dilatation of aortic stenosis (1912)
Pericardial resection for constriction (1913)
Sympathectomy (1917)
Mitral stenosis valvulotomy (1923)
Pulmonary embolectomy (1924)
Lumbar sympathectomy (1925)
Mitral stenosis dilatation by finger (1925)

1926–1950

Thyroidectomy for angina pectoris (1933)
Cardio-omentopexy (1930s)
Ligation of patent ductus arteriosus (1938)
Coarctation repair (1944)
Subclavian artery to pulmonary artery anastomosis for tetralogy of Fallot (Blalock-Taussig shunt, 1944)
Cardiac missile removal (WW II)
Side-to-side anastomosis of aorta to pulmonary artery for tetralogy of Fallot (Potts procedure, 1946)
Valvotomy for pulmonic stenosis (Brock procedure, 1947)
Closed mitral commissurotomy (1948)
Resection of infundibulum of right ventricle (1948)
Atrial septostomy (Blalock-Hanlon procedure, 1950)
Internal mammary tunnel implant into myocardium (Vineberg, 1950)
Hypothermia (1950)

1951–1975

First prosthetic ball valve—into aorta for aortic regurgitation (1952)
Closure atrial septal defects (1950s)
Resection abdominal aortic aneurysm (1952)
Pulmonary artery banding (1953)
Extracorporeal circulation (1953)
Cross-circulation of oxygenated blood (1954)
Closure ventricular septal defect (1954)
Carotid endarterectomy (1954)
Aortic dissection repair (1954)
Tetralogy of Fallot repair (1954)

Potassium cardioplegia (1955)
Aortic valvotomy (1956, 1958)
Transection of ventricular septum for idiopathic hypertrophic subaortic stenosis (1957)
Resection ventricular aneurysm (1958)
Superior vena cava to pulmonary artery shunt (Glenn procedure, 1959)
Transposition of great vessels repair (Senning procedure, 1959)
Mitral ball and cage valve replacement (1960)
Aortic ball and cage valve (1960)
Excision of ventricular aneurysm (1961)
Intraaortic balloon pump (1962)
Homograft valve (1962)
Aortopulmonary window (Waterston procedure, 1963)
Left ventricular assist (1963)
Catheter embolectomy (Fogarty procedure, 1963)
Transposition of aorta with intra-atrial baffle (Mustard procedure, 1963)
Double outlet right ventricle repair (1964)
Internal mammary artery to coronary artery bypass (1964)
Pulmonary autograft for aortic valve disease (Ross procedure, 1966)
Cardiac transplantation (1967)
Saphenous vein to coronary artery bypass (1968)
Wolff-Parkinson-White surgery (1968)
Truncus arteriosus repair (1968)
Extracardiac conduit (Rastelli procedure, 1969)
Tilting disc valve (1969)
Heart and lung transplant (1969)
Connection of right atrial appendage to pulmonary artery for tricuspid atresia (Fontan procedure, 1970)
Bioprosthetic valve (1970)
Annuloplasty ring (1971)
Bovine pericardial valve (1971)
Mitral valve repair (1971)
Porcine valve (1975)

1976–PRESENT

Arterial switch procedure for transposition of great vessels (1976)
Tilting disc valve (1977)
Bi-leaflet hinged valve (1977)
Pericardial valve (1980)
Artificial heart (1982)
Heart transplants in infants with hypoplastic left heart (1984)
Cardiomyoplasty (1985)
Modified Fontan procedure for single ventricle (late 1980s)
Minimally invasive bypass surgery (1997)
Robotic surgery (1998)

vival. Our understanding of the etiology of congenital heart disease has been greatly furthered by genetic, biochemical, and environmental studies.

AORTIC DISEASE

Aristotle (384–322 B.C.) named the great arterial vessel the *aorta*. Vesalius (1514–1564) is credited with the first description of an aneurysm of the abdominal and thoracic aorta (1555). Aneurysm (from the Greek word *dilatation*) of the aorta caught the attention of many early anatomists, especially Giovanni Maria Lancisi (1654–1720), whose 1728 book, *De Moto Cordis et Aneurysmatibus,* provided a definition and classification, separated true from false aneurysms, discussed possible etiologies, and included case studies. Trauma and syphilis were particularly singled out as causes of aneurysms by Lancisi and his followers. Coarctation of the aorta (from the Latin *coarctatus,* meaning pressed together, contracted) was best described by M. Paris (1791): "The part of the aorta which is beyond the arch, between the ligamentum arteriosum and the first inferior intercostals, was so greatly narrowed that it had at most the thickness of a goosequill. Hence in taking apart its walls, which had not decreased in this place, there remained only a very small lumen." Aortic dissection was not distinguished as a separate entity until *The Seats and Causes of Diseases,* published by Morgagni in 1761. He reported a fat 50-year-old woman who cried, "Oh!" and then died instantly. At autopsy, he "observed the blood had, by degrees, made itself a way through one of the intervals of this kind, and had come out under the external coat of the artery…as a large kind of ecchymosis…had burst through this external coat in one place, and had poured itself out within the pericardium." Laennec provided the term *l'anévrysme disséquant* (dissecting aneurysm) in 1826. Over the next century, the separation of a true aneurysm from a dissecting aneurysm; the pathogenesis from an initial transverse tear to a distal entry; the association of coarctation with a bicuspid aortic valve and hypertension; the significance of cystic medial necrosis; and the natural history of a large series of patients with dissection were recognized. Antemortem recognition of aortic dissection dates from 1855 but was rarely made until angiography became available in the 1950s. Recent history has been closely bound to the recognition of heritable disorders of connective tissue and the vulnerability of the vascular system to risk factors and inherited disorders. Cardiovascular imaging has clarified the overlap of intramural hematoma, aortic dissection, and penetrating atherosclerotic ulcers.

BLOOD PRESSURE MEASUREMENT AND HYPERTENSION

Stephen Hales, an English country parson, reported in his *Statical Essays* (1733) that the arterial blood pressure of the cannulated artery of a recumbent horse rose more than 8 feet above the heart—the first true measurement of arterial pressure and the beginning of sphygmometry.[2,3,48] His pioneering efforts stood alone until 1828 when Jean Poiseuille introduced a mercury manometer device to measure blood pressure.[49,50] Over the next 60 years, various sphygmomanometric methods were developed—notably by Lud-

wig (1847), Vierordt (1855), and Marey (1863)—to refine the measurement of the arterial pressure. An inflatable arm cuff coupled to the sphygmograph, a device small enough to allow measurement outside the laboratory, was invented by Riva-Rocci (1896), who also noted the "white-coat effect" on blood pressure.[51] Nicolai Korotkoff, a Russian military surgeon, first auscultated brachial arterial sounds (1905), and his discovery marks the advent of modern blood pressure recording. This auscultatory approach eventually ensured its widespread use by the 1920s. In 1939, blood pressure recordings were standardized by committees of the AHA and the Cardiac Society of Great Britain and Ireland.

Richard Bright was the first to associate kidney disease with hypertrophy of the heart, dropsy, and hardening of the arteries (1827).[50] In the 1870s, the studies of Frederick Mahomed in London established that elevated blood pressure could occur in the absence of nephritis and produce secondary kidney and arteriolar disease.[51] Secondary causes of hypertension were discovered. Robert Tigerstedt in Stockholm discovered a pressor substance in the renal cortex, which he named renin in 1898; however, Goldblatt's experiments, showing that renal artery stenosis induced ischemia and hypertension (1934), eventually led to the understanding of the renin, angiotensin, and aldosterone interaction by Pickering, Page, Braun-Menendez, Laragh, and others.[52] Beginning in the late 19th century, vasomotor, neurohormonal, and baroreceptor reflexes as well as genetic determinants of blood pressure became known. The crucial role of sodium was further delineated by Guyton in the 1960s. Pickering and Platt debated whether or not there was a precise demarcation between normal and abnormal blood pressure in the late 1950s. In 1972, Pickering stated: "There is no dividing line. The relationship between arterial pressure and mortality is quantitative: the higher the pressure, the worse the prognosis."[42] Subsequent studies have supported this and lowered the level where treatment should begin.

In 1913, Janeway showed that patients with hypertensive heart disease and symptoms lived an average of 4 to 5 years. However, the asymptomatic state of most patients with hypertension, the lack of effective treatment, and a prevalent view that lowering the blood pressure would be deleterious to the kidney and brain lulled most physicians into accepting the condition as just caused by aging. In the 1970s, the Framingham studies showed hypertension to be a major contributing cause to stroke, heart attack, and heart and kidney failure. Hypertension was labeled "the silent killer." Other studies followed indicating that treatment of even mild hypertension could reduce stroke and heart failure, although not necessarily heart attacks. National High Blood Pressure Education Programs, beginning in 1972, urged physicians to treat blood pressure elevation, and outposts to measure blood pressure became common. The initial emphasis was on the treatment of diastolic hypertension. More recently, systolic hypertension and wide pulse pressure in seniors has been found to be serious, warranting aggressive treatment.

TREATMENT OF HYPERTENSION

President Franklin Roosevelt's death in 1945 from severe hypertension and stroke called international attention to the consequences of hypertension and its inadequate treatment—he had been managed with diet, digitalis, and phenobarbital. Effective oral treatment became possible in 1949, first with reserpine then hydrochlorothiazide.[53] Lumbar sympathectomy and adrenalectomy (1925), the last resort, was abandoned. Subsequently, β-adrenergic blockers, calcium channel blockers, ACE inhibitors, angiotensin receptor blocking agents, and direct renin inhibitors have brought antihypertensive relief to many. (see Table 1–2). Severe salt restriction, as practiced earlier with the Kempner rice diet, has taken a lesser role, whereas the Dietary Approaches to Stop Hypertension (DASH) diet, exercise, and alcohol restriction are encouraged. Sleep apnea, an overlooked cause of hypertension, has been a new therapeutic direction. Since 1973, recommendations published by the Joint National Committee on Detection, Evaluation, and Treatment of High Blood Pressure (JNC) have been very helpful, although the newest category of *prehypertension* is controversial. Nevertheless, the majority of patients are imperfectly controlled, and many remain undetected.

HEART FAILURE

Medieval physicians commented on suffocative catarrh, dyspnea, asthma, orthopnea, and dropsy and failed to recognize a connection with the heart.[54] This was primarily because of the entrenched teachings of Galen that the purpose of the heart was to generate heat and distribute vital spirit. Marcello Malpighi believed that dyspnea could be caused by retarded circulation in the pulmonary vessels (1660s). Vieussens (1706) and Lancisi (1707) were the first to fault the heart as the direct cause of failure, a concept more fully elaborated by Albertini (1726).[6,54]

Initially, clinical observation was based on case reports describing signs and symptoms. In this setting, clinicians understood that valve obstruction, the most common cardiac problem at that time, caused dyspnea and fluid accumulation. The autopsy findings of hypertrophy and dilatation of the heart were a particular puzzle for 18th-century physicians. Morgagni was the first to comprehend that overload from valvular disease could elicit a compensatory hypertrophic response and dilatation, leading to failure (1761). At the beginning of the 19th century, Corvisart's distinction between the causes of hypertrophy and dilatation led to an appreciation of the beneficial effects of hypertrophy and the harmful effects of dilatation. The primary role of the myocardium versus valvular disease in the production of symptoms and a basis for prognosis followed, was lost, and was then rediscovered. Richard Bright's 1836 discovery of the relationship of cardiac hypertrophy and dropsy to shrunken kidneys introduced the kidneys as a cause of heart failure long before hypertension was known.[48] Toward the end of the 19th century, the beneficial role of hypertrophy was questioned by Schroetter (1876), Osler (1892), and others, who saw that it was harmful in its later stages. Mackenzie, in his influential 1908 textbook *Diseases of the Heart,* stressed the functional role of the heart muscle and its reserve force, downplaying valvular disease as "an embarrassment to the heart muscle." He felt that it was exhaustion of the heart muscle that led to symptoms and signs of heart failure.[10] His insistence that "a heart is what a heart can do" was the beginning of a functional classification that redirected thinking toward physiology and away from just the presence of murmurs and arrhythmias. The definition of normal circulatory physiology was the precursor for an understanding of abnormal circulatory phenomena. In the late 19th and early 20th centuries, the hemodynamic physiologists Otto Frank, Ernest Starling, and Carl Wiggers established the basic principles of cardiac function, pressure, and flow abnormalities in the failing heart.[6] In the mid-20th century, studies by Sarnoff, Braunwald, and others heightened our understanding of the performance of normal and abnormal heart muscle. The widespread application of cardiac catheterization, selective angiography, and imaging studies has resulted in more precise diagnostic criteria and hemodynamic information for differentiating ischemic heart disease, hypertensive heart disease, and dilated and hypertrophic forms of cardiomyopathies. *Congestive heart failure* was a term first used in the 1920s; however, a definition for heart failure based on its pathogenesis has been controversial.[10] The primary debate initially centered over whether the elevated venous pressure was a primary or secondary event. Two opposing camps evolved: the first holding that *backward failure,* or an upstream obstruction (aortic stenosis, for example) was the central factor, and the second championing *forward failure,* that is, when myocardial dysfunction with low cardiac output was the problem. Over time, the rigid concepts embodied in *backward* and *forward failure, right-sided,* and *left-sided failure,* have given way to definitions based on the cardiac output as the discriminator: *low-output* and *high-output failure.* More recently *systolic heart failure* and *diastolic heart failure* have climbed to the top of the clinical lexicon. The discovery of B-type natriuretic peptide (BNP) has revealed that the heart is also an endocrine organ. Cell biochemistry and biophysics have contributed to our understanding of the abnormalities in cardiac contraction, relaxation, and energetics, whereas molecular biology has helped to define the pathways responsible for alterations in growth.

[ ] TREATMENT OF HEART FAILURE

In the late 19th and early 20th centuries, heart failure was treated with venesection, digitalis, saline purges, a low-salt diet, mercurial cathartics, incision and drainage of edema (Southey tubes) or ascites, bromides, theophylline or urea for diuresis, and carbonic acid baths at a spa. By the 1930s, cathartics had been replaced by intramuscular mercurial injections to remove fluid. Thyroidectomy was advised in advanced cases. The introduction of potent oral diuretics, beginning with chlorothiazide (1957) and then furosemide (1964), brought miraculous relief to volume-overloaded cardiac patients, ending the common practice of twice-weekly *merc shots.* The concept of afterload reduction with vasodilators by Cohn (1971) soon led to nitroprusside (1974), ACE inhibitors (1981), and angiotensin receptor blockers (1992), which have greatly improved the quality of life and prognosis for heart failure patients (see Table 1–2). β-Adrenergic blockers, initially thought to be absolutely contraindicated, were shown to be otherwise in 1975 by Wagstein and are now a first-rank drug, along with carvedilol (1995). While digitalis is still used, its effect on mortality has been doubted; newer oral inotropic agents have consistently been found to worsen the prognosis. Biventricular pacing, introduced in 2000, has shown early promise in selected patients. Cardiac transplantation has been a last resort for selected patients since the late 1960s. Cell transplant therapy for cardiac repair, using skeletal myoblasts and bone marrow stem cells, is a promising, still unproven approach to regenerate myocardium (2002).[55]

CARDIAC SURGERY

The Nobel Prize in Physiology or Medicine in 1912 was given to Alexis Carrel, a French experimental surgeon working at the Rockefeller Institute, "in recognition of his work on vascular suture and the transplantation of blood vessels and organs." His many contributions to the basic science of surgery provided the essential foundation and encouragement for the clinical surgeons who would eventually follow his bold path[6] (see Table 1–3). A few attempts were made to suture cardiac wounds in the late 19th century and to remove pericardial adhesions and effusion or improve valvular disease in the first quarter of the 20th century; however, the surgeon was thwarted by the problems of correct diagnosis, cerebral oxygenation, pneumothorax, anesthesia, bleeding, infection, arrhythmias, blood pressure control, metabolic management, and so on.[56] Surgery was a "get in, get out, and pray for the best" proposition. Comroe pointed out that 25 separate bodies of knowledge had to evolve to permit successful open-heart surgery.[57] Extracardiac surgery—ligation of a patent ductus by Gross (1938), repair of coarctation of the aorta by Craaford (1944), the Blalock-Taussig shunt (1944), and removal of intracardiac missile fragments by Harken during World War II—led the way.[56] Simple and quick intracardiac surgery, such as repair of an atrial septal defect, was successfully accomplished using hypothermia in the 1950s by John Lewis and others, although the risk of ventricular fibrillation and air embolism presented a hazard. John Gibbons's development of extracorporeal circulation became the essential platform for safe intracardiac surgery.[58] In 1953, his pump-oxygenator provided 45 minutes to repair an atrial septal defect, and the surgeon finally had time to operate safely and explore new horizons.[59] In the early 1950s, mitral stenosis was the major hurdle, and mitral valvotomy was performed by Bailey, Harken, and Lillehei with increasing success.[6,42] Surgery for congenital heart defects was next, including tetralogy of Fallot (Lillehei, 1954). More complicated surgery, including mechanical prosthetic valve replacement (Starr and Harken, 1960), homograft valve (Donald Ross, 1962), cardiac transplantation (Barnard and Norman Shumway, 1967), bioprosthetic valve replacement (1970), mitral valve repair (Alain Carpentier, 1971), and repair of complex congenital heart disease followed as diagnostic and surgical techniques, artificial valves, and intensive postoperative care improved.[56,57]

In 1910, the ingenious Alexis Carrel attempted the first experimental coronary bypass, fashioning an anastomosis between the descending aorta and the left coronary artery. Efforts to improve the coronary circulation using pericardial irritants (Beck, 1934), omental or pectoral grafts (O'Shaunessy, Beck, 1930s), internal mammary implants tunneled directly into the heart muscle (Vineberg, 1950), and coronary endarterectomy (Bailey, Longmire, 1956) were touted but provided inconsistent benefit. Vaselii Kolesov, in Russia, pioneered internal mammary to coronary artery bypass grafts beginning in 1964; however, René Favaloro, at the Cleveland Clinic, is usually credited for ushering in the era of coronary bypass surgery (1968).[59,60] Aortic surgery, initially dealing with late stage complications, advanced from the ligation of aortic aneurysms to wrapping the aorta with various materials and finally resection. Attempted surgical repair of aortic dissection dates from 1935, but operative success was not achieved until 1954 when DeBakey, Cooley, and Creech reestablished aortic continuity. Vascular reconstruction and endarterectomy, insertion of prosthetic grafts, percutaneous insertion of endovascular grafts for aneurysms and dissection (1991), and stenting of carotid artery stenosis (1997) have transformed the management of vascular disease.

Mortality rates from all cardiac surgery have progressively fallen to low levels, and the surgical benefit has been extended to sicker and older people. Cardiac transplantation has become almost routine, but attempts to manufacture an artificial heart have been disappointing. Off-pump and robotic-assisted surgery has become feasible but of unproven difference. Although cardiovascular surgery has been one of the miracles of the 20th century, catheter techniques are threatening its 21st century growth.

REFERENCES

1. Harvey W. *Anatomical Studies on the Motion of the Heart and Blood.* Leake CD, transl. Springfield, IL: Charles C Thomas; 1970.
2. Acierno LJ. *The History of Cardiology.* London: Parthenon; 1994.
3. Willius FA, Dry TJ. *A History of the Heart and the Circulation.* Philadelphia: Saunders; 1948.
4. Rolleston HD. *Cardiovascular Diseases since Harvey's Discovery: The Harveian Oration of 1928.* London: Cambridge University Press; 1928.
5. Silverman ME. A view from the millennium: the practice of cardiology circa 1950 and thereafter. *J Am Coll Cardiol.* 1999;33:1141–1151.
6. Bing RJ. *Cardiology: The Evolution of the Science and the Art.* Basel: Harwood; 1992.
7. Herrick JB. *A Short History of Cardiology.* Springfield, IL: Charles C Thomas; 1942.
8. Lee HSJ. *Dates in Cardiology.* New York: Parthenon; 2000.
9. Fishman AP, Dickinson WR. *Circulation of the Blood: Men and Ideas.* Bethesda, MD: American Physiological Society; 1982.
10. Fleming P. *A Short History of Cardiology.* Amsterdam: Rodopi; 1997.
11. Fye B. *American Cardiology: The History of a Specialty and Its College.* Baltimore: The Johns Hopkins University Press; 1996.
12. Mackenzie J. *The Study of the Pulse.* Edinburgh: Pentland; 1902.
13. Mackenzie J. The venous and liver pulses, and the arrhythmic contraction of the cardiac cavities. *J Pathol Bacteriol.* 1894;2:84–154.
14. Duffin JM. The cardiology of RTH Laënnec. *Med Hist.* 1989;33:42–71.
15. Hanna IR, Silverman ME. A history of cardiac auscultation and some of its contributors. *Am J Cardiol.* 2002;90:259–267.
16. Burch GE, DePasquale NP. *A History of Electrocardiography.* Chicago: Year Book; 1964.
17. Silverman ME, Grove D, Upshaw CB Jr. Why does the heart beat? The discovery of the electrical system of the heart. *Circulation.* 2006;113:2775–2781.
18. Jeffrey K, Parsonnet V. Cardiac pacing, 1960–1985. *Circulation.* 1998;97:1978–1991.
19. Wellens HJJ. The electrocardiogram 80 years after Einthoven. *J Am Coll Cardiol.* 1986;7:484–491.
20. Scherlag BJ, Tamás F, Patterson E, Jackman WM, Lazara, R. Development of cardiac electrophysiology in the twentieth century. *Cardiol Hung.* 1994;23:15–21.
21. Shah M, Akar FG, Tomaselli GF. Molecular basis of arrhythmias. *Circulation.* 2005;112:2517–2529.
22. Forssmann-Falck R. Werner Forssmann: a pioneer of cardiology. *Am J Cardiol.* 1997;79:651–660.
23. Mueller RL, Sanborn TA. The history of interventional cardiology: cardiac catheterization, angioplasty, and related interventions. *Am Heart J.* 1995;129:146–172.
24. King SB. The development of interventional cardiology. *J Am Coll Cardiol.* 1998;31(suppl B):64B–88B.
25. Muir AL. Cardiac imaging 50 years on. *Br Heart J.* 1987;58:1–5.
26. Roelandt JRTC. Seeing the heart, the success story of cardiac imaging. *Eur Heart J.* 2000;21:1281–1288.
27. Zaret BL. A brief historical perspective on nuclear cardiology. In: Iskandrian AE, Verani MS, eds. *Nuclear Cardiac Imaging.* 3rd ed. London: Oxford University Press; 2003:1–6.

28. Feigenbaum H. Evolution of echocardiography. *Circulation.* 1996;93:1321–1327.

29. Leibowitz JO. *The History of Coronary Heart Disease.* Berkeley, CA: University of California Press; 1970.

30. Fye B. The delayed diagnosis of myocardial infarction: it took half a century! *Circulation.* 1985;72:262–271.

31. Herrick JB. Clinical features of sudden obstruction of the coronary arteries. *JAMA.* 1912;59:2015–2020.

32. Moreno PR, Fuster V. The year in atherothrombosis. *J Am Coll Cardiol.* 2004;44:2099–2110.

33. Surruys PW. A journey in the interventional field. *J Am Coll Cardiol.* 2006;47:1741–1753.

34. Sherry S. The origin of thrombolytic therapy. *J Am Coll Cardiol.* 1989;14:1085–1092.

35. Théroux P, Willerson JT, Armstrong PW. Progress in the treatment of acute coronary syndromes: a 50-year perspective (1950–2000). *Circulation.* 2000;102:IV-2–13.

36. Förstermann U, Mönzel T. Endothelial nitric oxide synthase in vascular disease. *Circulation.* 2006;113:1708–1714.

37. Flaxman N. The hope of cardiology: James Hope (1801–1841). *Bull Hist Med.* 1938;6:1–21.

38. VanderVeer JB. Mitral insufficiency: historical and clinical aspects. *Am J Cardiol.* 1958;2:5–10.

39. Rolleston H. The history of mitral stenosis. *Br Heart J.* 1941;3:1–12.

40. Vaslef SN, Roberts WC. Early descriptions of aortic valve stenosis. *Am Heart J.* 1993;125:1465–1474.

41. Vaslef SN, Roberts WC. Early descriptions of aortic regurgitation. *Am Heart J.* 1993;125:1475–1483.

42. Silverman ME, Fleming PR, Hollman A, et al. *British Cardiology in the 20th Century.* London: Springer, 2000.

43. Boudoulas H, Vavuranakis M, Wooley CF. Valvular heart disease: the influence of changing etiology on nosology. *J Heart Valve Dis.* 1994;3:516–526.

44. Goodwin JF, Gordon H, Hollman A, et al. Clinical aspects of cardiomyopathy. *Brit Med J.* 1961;1:69–79.

45. Maron BJ, Towbin JA, Thiene G, et al. Contemporary definitions and classification of the cardiomyopathies. *Circulation.* 2006;113:1807–1816.

46. Abbott ME. *Atlas of Congenital Heart Disease.* New York: American Heart Association; 1936.

47. Engle MA. Growth and development of state of the art care for people with congenital heart disease. *J Am Coll Cardiol.* 1989;13:1453–1457.

48. Naqvi NH, Blaufox MD. *Blood Pressure Measurement: An Illustrated History.* New York: Parthenon; 1998.

49. Dustan HP. History of clinical hypertension: From 1827 to 1970. In: Oparil S, Weber MA, eds. *Hypertension: A Companion to Brenner and Rector's The Kidney.* Philadelphia: Saunders; 2000:1–4.

50. Ruskin A. *Classics in Arterial Hypertension.* Springfield, IL: Charles C Thomas; 1956.

51. Posten-Vinay N. *A Century of Arterial Hypertension: 1896–1996.* Chichester: Wiley; 1996.

52. Pickering G. Systemic arterial hypertension. In: Fishman AP, Richards DW, eds. *Circulation of the Blood: Men and Ideas.* Bethesda, MD: American Physiological Society; 1982:487–541.

53. Piepho RW, Beal J. An overview of antihypertensive therapy in the 20th century. *J Clin Pharmacol.* 2000;40:967–977.

54. Jarcho S. *The Concept of Heart Failure from Avicenna to Albertini.* Cambridge, MA: Harvard University Press; 1980.

55. Anvers P, Leri A, Kajstura J. Cardiac regeneration. *J Amer Coll Cardiol.* 2006;47:1769–1776.

56. Shumacker HB Jr. *The Evolution of Cardiac Surgery.* Bloomington, IN: Indiana University Press; 1992.

57. Comroe JH. The heart and lungs. In: Comroe JH, ed. *Advances in American Medicine.* New York: Josiah Macey; 1976.

58. Gibbon JH Jr. The development of the heart-lung apparatus. *Am J Surg.* 1978;135:608–619.

59. Brewer LA. Open heart surgery and myocardial revascularization. *Am J Surg.* 1981;141:618–631.

60. Favaloro RG. Landmarks in the development of coronary artery bypass surgery. *Circulation.* 1998;98:466–478.

CHAPTER 2

The Burden of Increasing Worldwide Cardiovascular Disease*

Ramachandran S. Vasan / Emelia J. Benjamin / Lisa M. Sullivan / Ralph B. D'Agostino

* This work was supported in part through NHLBI Contract NO1-HC-25195, NHLBI grant 2K24HL04334 (RS Vasan).

It is widely acknowledged that heart disease and stroke are the leading causes of death and disability in the United States and other developed countries.[1] What is less appreciated is that this holds true for the developing countries as well.[1] We are in the midst of a true global cardiovascular disease (CVD) epidemic.[2] CVD is responsible for approximately 30 percent of all deaths worldwide each year.[3] Of note, nearly 80 percent of these deaths occur in low and middle income countries, and half occur in women. Indeed, CVD is the leading cause of mortality in every region of the world with the sole exception of sub-Saharan Africa where infectious diseases are still the leading cause. Chapter 2 describes the current global burden of CVD and its risk factors, emphasizing the evolution of the CVD epidemic in developing countries and its contributory factors. Furthermore, the projected trends in the global burden of CVD over the next two decades are elucidated, and ongoing efforts by the world community (including the World Health Organization [WHO]) to combat and contain the current epidemic are outlined. The broad term, *CVD,* includes coronary heart disease (CHD; myocardial infarction [MI], angina, coronary insufficiency, and coronary death), cerebrovascular disease (stroke and transient ischemic attacks), peripheral vascular disease, congestive heart failure (CHF), hypertension, and valvular and congenital heart disease.

THE WORLD IN TRANSITION: IMPLICATIONS FOR CARDIOVASCULAR DISEASE

【 】 DEMOGRAPHIC TRANSITION

The last two centuries have witnessed major changes in the demographic characteristics of the human population.[4] This transformation (termed *demographic transition*) involved a progressive change from very high birth and infant mortality rates to low ones. This change was accompanied by a shift from low population growth rates through an intermediate phase of high growth rates, with a consequent major increase in total population. This then was followed by a reversal to low or zero growth rates. The demographic transition results in a conversion of the age distribution of the population from one with a preponderance of young to one with nearly equal representation of all age groups.

The demographic transition has been driven by the most dramatic improvements ever in the history of human health. Improvements in sanitation, nutrition, and infectious disease control and advances in perinatal care have resulted in lower infant and child mortality rates and an enhancement of overall life expectancy. The improvement in life expectancy began in Europe in the late 19th century and by the second half of the 20th century had spread to the rest of the world. Life expectancy at birth has increased from a global average of 46 years in 1950 to 66 years in 1998.[5]

【 】 ECONOMIC, SOCIAL, AND NUTRITIONAL TRANSITION

The developing countries underwent rapid industrialization, urbanization, economic development, and market globalization over the last four decades.[1] As a consequence, standards of living improved but with a detrimental shift toward inappropriate dietary patterns and a reduction in physical activities. The nutritional status of populations has been adversely influenced by the aforementioned changes, a phenomenon referred to as *nutritional transition.*[6]

Globalization has resulted in the expansion of the food economies from local to broad-based ones in which there is easy access to large amounts of unhealthy food products. The shift in dietary patterns comprises a change in all three major food constituents (namely, fats, proteins, and carbohydrates).[7] Local diets that are traditionally rich in fiber and have a low fat content are being replaced by cheap energy-dense micronutrient-poor foods with a high content of saturated fats. Vegetarian diets characterized by high intake of plant proteins have been substituted with nonvegetarian diets rich in animal proteins. Complex carbohydrates in diets have been supplanted by refined carbohydrates and sugars that have a high glycemic index.[7] The overall increased caloric consumption occurs in a milieu of reduced energy expenditure caused by sedentary lifestyles, with the advent of motorized transport, and increased use of labor-saving home and office appliances. Additionally, leisure time physical activities have given way to physically undemanding pastimes including watching television.

These changes in dietary and lifestyle patterns foreshadow in both developing and newly developed countries an increasing burden of diet-related diseases—including obesity, dyslipidemia, diabetes mellitus, hypertension, and eventually CVD—and various forms of cancer. In essence, although referred to under the umbrella of noncommunicable disease, CVD is to some extent a *communicated* disease, spread by the forces of globalization.

【 】 EPIDEMIOLOGIC TRANSITION

The previously mentioned demographic, economic, and nutritional changes lead inexorably to major changes in the patterns of human diseases, a phenomenon referred to as *epidemiologic transition.*[4] Epidemiologic transition is characterized by a progressive shift from a predominance of nutritional deficiencies and infectious diseases to those categorized as degenerative (i.e., chronic diseases such as CVD, cancer, and diabetes).[4]

CHALLENGES OF THE CARDIOVASCULAR DISEASE EPIDEMIC IN DEVELOPING COUNTRIES: DIFFERENCES FROM DEVELOPED COUNTRIES

Although the determinants of the health transition in developing countries are similar to those in the developed countries, it is important to emphasize that the dynamics of health transition are different in the former.[1,8,9]

1. In developing countries the epidemic of CVD is occurring over a compressed time frame (in part related to the rapidity of globalization), whereas in developed countries it took decades for the CVD epidemic to establish itself. Such a compression of the time course of the epidemic requires a greater intensity of public health response.

2. Unfortunately, the transition that is fueling the CVD epidemic in developing countries occurs in settings of poverty and international debt: factors that restrict resources available for public health action. An accentuating factor is the easy access to low-

cost cigarettes in developing countries early in the transition phase. Tobacco is a cash crop, and the tobacco industry is a potential employer: factors that pose a major challenge to the governmental implementation of tobacco control.

3. Individual responses to the CVD epidemic in developing countries are restricted by low levels of education and limited personal resources to purchase drugs required for lowering elevated levels of CVD risk factors. An additional aggravating factor is that CVD afflicts individuals at an earlier age in developing countries, resulting in loss of economic productivity, often of the sole wage-earning member of the family.

4. Very often these countries face a dual burden of communicable and noncommunicable diseases, resulting in a competition for limited public health resources.

5. The global response to the ongoing epidemic is challenged by a paucity of epidemiologic data and the necessary infrastructure to define, characterize, and track the CVD epidemic in most developing countries.

6. The societal response to the CVD epidemic lags behind because of a lack of awareness and the popular belief that CVD is largely a disease of developed countries.

7. It is important to note that for several countries in Asia and Africa, increases in blood pressure and tobacco use preceded the impact of nutrition transition by decades. This has resulted in a differing CVD profile with higher levels of stroke but relatively low levels of CHD. These differing CVD patterns underscore an opportunity to implement strong CHD preventive programs focusing on nutrition and physical activity and aggressive control of blood pressure and tobacco use.

MEASURING THE BURDEN OF DISEASE: THE GLOBAL BURDEN OF DISEASE PROJECT AND THE CONCEPT OF DISABILITY-ADJUSTED LIFE-YEAR

In 1993, the Harvard School of Public Health in collaboration with the World Bank and WHO commenced the Global Burden of Disease (GBD) Project.[10] The GBD project has generated the most comprehensive set of estimates of morbidity and mortality caused by various disease conditions according to age, sex, and region. The investigators subdivided the world into 14 regions based on levels of child (<5 years of age) and adult (15 to 59 years of age) mortality for WHO member states (Fig. 2–1).[11]

The GBD project also introduced a new metric, disability-adjusted life-year (DALY), to quantify the burden of disease.[12] The DALY is a health gap measure that summates the potential years of life lost because of premature death and the years of *healthy* life lost in states of less than full health, broadly termed *disability*. A *premature* death is de-

fined as a death that occurs before the age to which the person could have expected to survive if he or she was a member of a standardized model population with a life expectancy at birth equal to that of the world's longest-surviving population, Japan. Thus, one DALY can be thought of as 1 lost year of healthy life. The burden of disease is the gap between the current health status of a population and an ideal situation where everyone lives into old age free of disease and disability.

WHO undertook an assessment of the GBD for the year 2000 (GBD 2000) with the specific objectives to quantify the burden of premature mortality and disability by age, sex, and WHO subregion for 135 major causes or groups of causes to analyze the contribution of selected risk factors to this burden and to develop various projection scenarios of the burden of disease over the next 30 years.[13] Detailed tables for DALYs by subregion, cause, sex, and age group are available at the WHO Web site at www.who.int/healthinfo/bodestimates/en/.

CARDIOVASCULAR DISEASES
【 】 GLOBAL BURDEN

CVD is the leading cause of mortality worldwide; responsible for one-third of all deaths.[14] According to WHO estimates, 17.5 million people died of CVD in 2005.[14] Developing countries contributed to 80 percent of CVD deaths. There is considerable variation in CVD mortality rates across WHO regions (Table 2–1) and

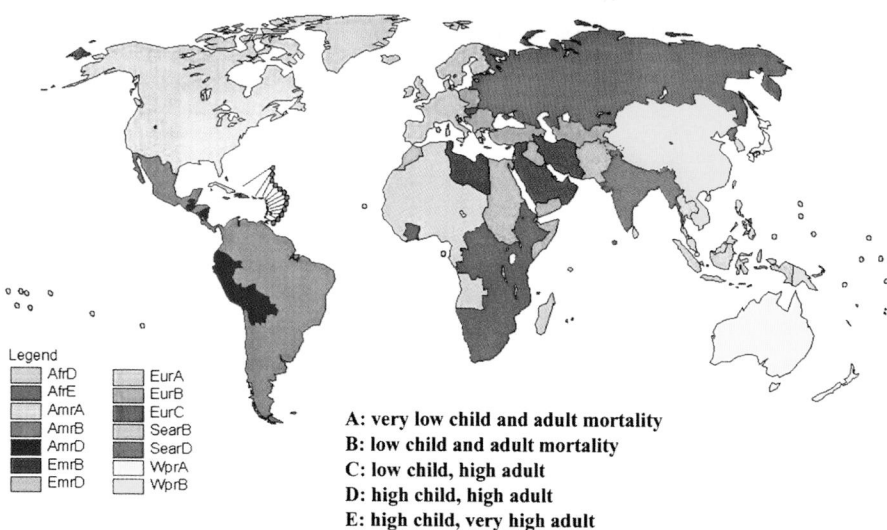

Legend

AfrD	EurA
AfrE	EurB
AmrA	EurC
AmrB	SearB
AmrD	SearD
EmrB	WprA
EmrD	WprB

A: very low child and adult mortality
B: low child and adult mortality
C: low child, high adult
D: high child, high adult
E: high child, very high adult

FIGURE 2–1. World Health Organization (WHO) subregions for global burden of disease. For geographic disaggregation of the global burden of disease, the 6 WHO regions of the world have been further divided into 14 subregions, based on levels of child (younger than 5 years of age) and adult (15 to 59 years of age) mortality for WHO member states. The classification of WHO member states into the mortality strata were carried out using population estimates for 1999 (United Nations population division, 1998) and estimates of 5q0 (mortality in children under 5 years) and 45q15 (adult mortality, risk of death between ages 15 years and 60 years) based on WHO analyses of mortality rates for 1999. Five mortality strata were defined in terms of quintiles of the distribution of 5q0 and 45q15 (both sexes combined). Adult mortality 45q15 was regressed on 5q0, and the regression line used to divide countries with high child mortality into high adult mortality (stratum D) and very high adult mortality (stratum E). Stratum E includes the countries in sub-Saharan Africa where HIV/AIDS has had a very substantial impact. *Source: Adapted from Mathers CD, Stein C, Fat DM, et al. Global burden of disease 2000: version 2 methods and results. Global program on evidence for health policy discussion. World Health Organization; October 2002. Paper No. 50.*

TABLE 2–1

Global Burden of Cardiovascular Disease by World Health Organization Region (2002 data)

CVD	AFR	AMR	EUR	SEAR	WPR	EMR	WORLD
Mortality (thousands)							
CHD	332	921	2373	2039	993	537	7208
Cerebrovascular	360	452	1447	1059	1958	226	5509
HTN heart disease	60	135	180	153	284	97	911
Rheumatic	19	10	30	133	109	24	327
Inflammatory	42	67	101	76	80	37	404
Other CVD	224	342	794	451	400	158	2374
All CVDs	1036	1928	4926	3911	3825	1079	16733
Total burden, DALYs (millions)							
CHD	3.03	6.22	15.75	20.73	7.50	5.32	58.64
Cerebrovascular	3.67	4.48	10.79	10.40	17.28	2.53	49.20
HTN heart disease	0.59	1.03	1.22	1.66	2.24	0.89	7.65
Rheumatic	0.51	0.16	0.38	2.62	1.61	0.58	5.86
Inflammatory	0.87	0.85	1.31	1.51	0.75	0.56	5.85
Other CVD	2.26	2.45	4.96	6.07	3.03	2.18	20.98
All CVDs	10.91	15.17	34.42	42.99	32.41	12.06	148.19

AFR, Africa; AMR, America; CHD, chronic heart disease; CVD, cardiovascular disease; DALYS, disability-adjusted life-years; EMR, Eastern Mediterranean Region; EUR, Europe; HTN, hypertension; SEAR, South East Asia Region; WPR, Western Pacific Region.
Rheumatic heart disease includes: Symptomatic cases of congestive heart failure caused by rheumatic heart disease.
Hypertensive heart disease includes: Symptomatic cases of congestive heart failure caused by hypertensive heart disease.
Ischemic heart disease includes: Acute myocardial infarction—definite and possible episodes of acute myocardial infarction according to MONICA study criteria; Angina pectoris—cases of clinically diagnosed angina pectoris or definite angina pectoris according to Rose questionnaire.
Congestive heart failure includes: Mild and greater (Killip scale k2–k4).
Cerebrovascular disease includes: First-ever stroke cases—first-ever stroke according to WHO definition (includes subarachnoid hemorrhage but excludes transient ischemic attacks, subdural hematoma, and hemorrhage or infarction caused by infection or tumor); Long-term stroke survivors: Persons who survive more than 28 days after first-ever stroke.
Inflammatory heart diseases includes: Myocarditis, symptomatic cases of congestive heart failure caused by myocarditis; Pericarditis, symptomatic cases of congestive heart failure caused by pericarditis; Endocarditis, symptomatic cases of congestive heart failure due to endocarditis.
SOURCE: Available at: www3.who.int/whosis/menu.cfm?path=whosis,burden,burden_estimates,burden_estimates_2002N,burden_estimates_2002N_2002Rev,burden_estimates_2002N_2002Rev_Region&language=English. Accessed on August 15, 2006.
For detailed definition refer to: Mathers CD, Stein C, Fat DM, Rao C, Inoue M, Tomijima N, et al. Global Burden of Disease 2000: Version 2 methods and results. Global Programme on Evidence for Health Policy Discussion Paper No. 50. Geneva: World Health Organization; October 2002.

across countries (Fig. 2–2).[15] Potential reasons for such variation include differing stages of epidemiologic transition in various countries, varying environmental effects caused by dissimilar burden of CVD risk factors, inherent genetic differences, and distinct early childhood programming influences.[8,16]

In terms of combined morbidity and mortality, CVD accounted for 148 million DALYs lost worldwide in 2002, or about 10 percent of all DALYs lost (Fig. 2–3). Eighty-six percent of the DALYs lost because of CVD were in the developing world.

[ ] GLOBAL TRENDS IN MORTALITY

The WHO projections indicate that a pattern of premature CVD mortality is likely to persist and can accentuate further in developing countries. In 2006, CVD is more prevalent in China and India than in all developed countries combined.[15] By 2010, CVD is projected to be the leading cause of death in developing countries. By 2020, WHO estimates there will be nearly 20 million CVD deaths worldwide every year, and the number will increase to 24 million by 2030.[17] Developing countries will account for 70 percent of deaths caused by coronary heart disease and 75 percent of deaths caused by stroke (Table 2–2).[15]

[ ] BURDEN IN THE UNITED STATES

Since 1900, CVD has been the leading cause of death in the United States every year (except for 1918).[18] In 2003, CVD accounted for 37 percent of all deaths. In fact, CVD claims more lives each year than the next four leading causes of death combined. According to the American Heart Association (AHA) estimates, approximately 2600 Americans die of CVD each day, an average of 1 death every 35 seconds.[18] The overall death rate per 100,000 from CVD in the United States was 308.8 in 2003. CVD death rates are higher for men (364.2) than they are for women (262.5), and for blacks as compared to whites; in 2003, CVD death rates were 359.1 for white males versus 479.6 for black males, whereas among women, rates ranged from 256.2 for white females to 354.8 for black females. In the United States, there are marked regional disparities, with the Southeast experiencing the highest CVD mortality rates. The pathogenesis of ethnic and regional disparities in CVD morbidity and mortality are multifactorial and will be discussed later in this chapter.

It is estimated that 71.3 million Americans (34 percent) have one or more type of CVD.[18] Prevalence of CVD varies from about 29 percent in Mexican-Americans, 32 (women) to 34 percent

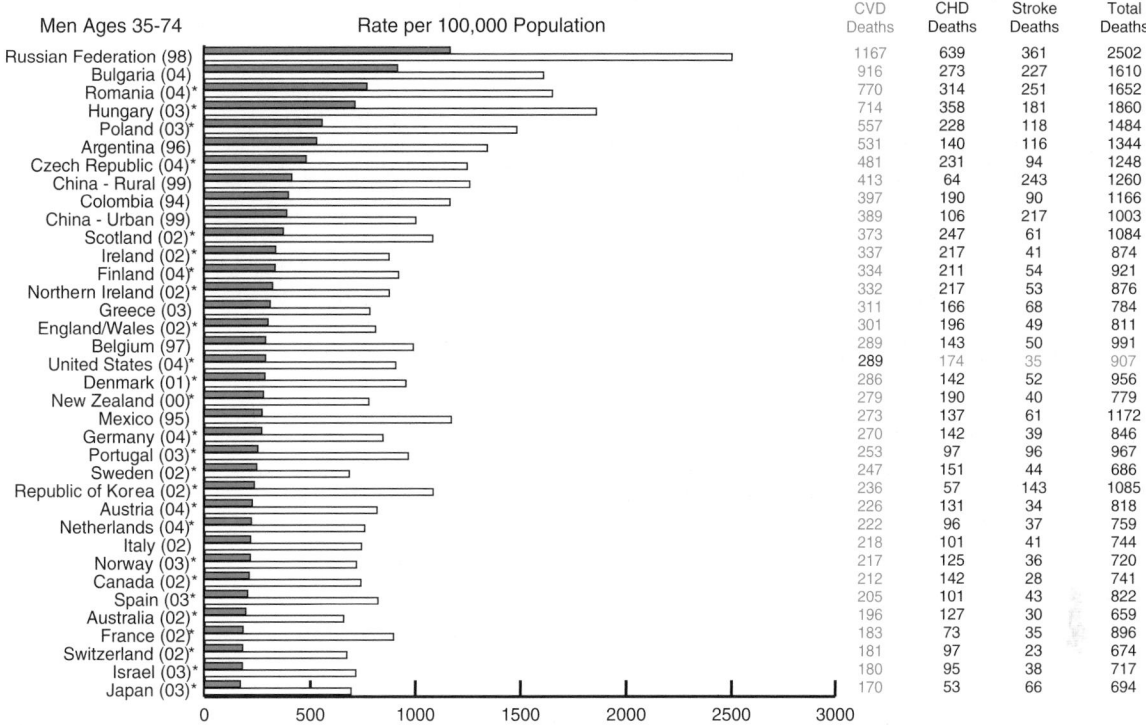

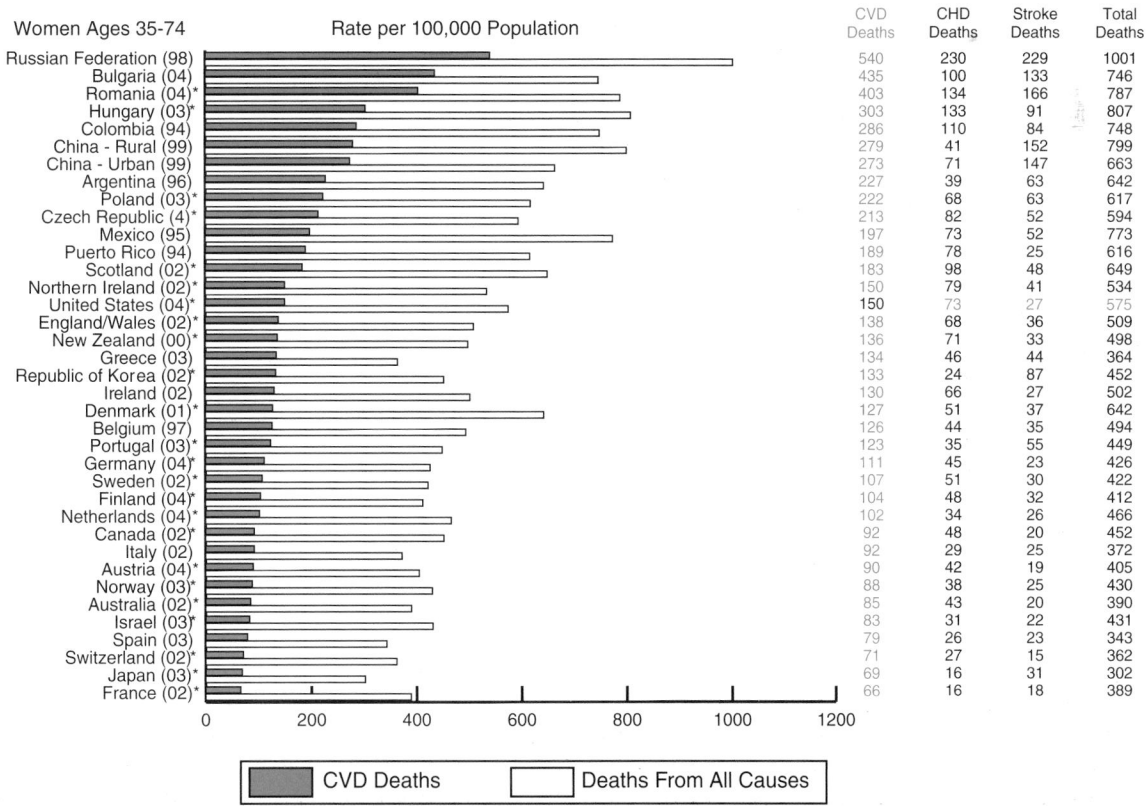

FIGURE 2–2. Death rates for total cardiovascular disease, coronary heart disease, stroke, and total deaths in selected countries (most recent year available). Revised 2006. Rates adjusted to the European Standard population. *Source: The World Health Organization website, who.int/whosis.*

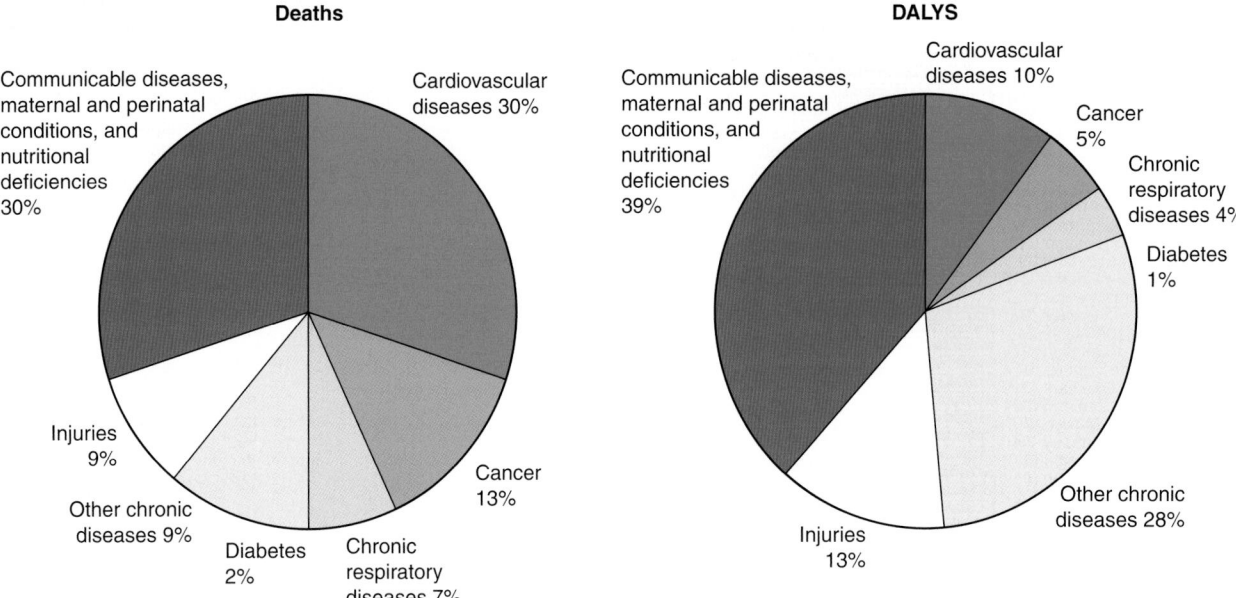

FIGURE 2–3. Disability-Adjusted life-years (DALYs) attributable to cardiovascular disease in developing countries. *Source: From World Health Organization. World Health Report 1999. Making a difference. Geneva: WHO; 1999. Available at www.who.int/whr/en, used with permission.*

(men) in non-Hispanic blacks, and 32 (women) to 34 (men) percent in non-Hispanic whites.[18] CVD is an expensive illness. The estimated direct and indirect costs associated with CVD are approximately $403 billion for 2006.[18]

Incidence in the United States

Data from the Framingham Heart Study, a predominantly white cohort followed from 1948 (original cohort) and 1971 (offspring cohort), provide estimates of CVD-event rates. The average annual rates of first major CVD events increase with age, rising from 7 per 1000 men at ages 35 to 44 years to 68 per 1000 at ages 85 to 94 years (Table 2–3). For women, CVD rates comparable to men are achieved 10 years later in life, with the gender difference in rates narrowing with advancing age. CHD is the predominant cardiovascular event, comprising more than one-half of all CVD events in men and in women younger than 75 years of age (Table 2–4). The proportions of cardiovascular events caused by CHD decline with age because of the increasing proportions of stroke and CHF.

Lifetime Risk in the United States

The long-term risk of developing CVD in an individual is best described by the *lifetime risk* statistic (i.e., the probability that an individual will develop CVD over the course of his or her lifetime). Lifetime-risk estimates are computed as cumulative incidence of the disease, usually for conveying to the general public the risk of experiencing a disease event from 40 to

90 years of age. The lifetime risk of developing CVD at 50 years of age is estimated to be 1 in 2 for men and 2 in 5 for women.[19]

【 】 MORTALITY TRENDS IN THE UNITED STATES

CVD mortality has declined in the United States progressively since about 1940, with sustained long-term declines since the

TABLE 2–2

Global Burden of Cardiovascular Disease: Projected Future Burden

GLOBAL BURDEN	2010	2020	2030
CVD MORTALITY			
Annual, million	18.1	20.5	24.2
All deaths (%)	30.8	31.5	32.5
CHD DEATH, % OF ALL			
Men	13.1	14.3	14.9
Women	13.6	13.0	13.1
Stroke death, % of all			
Men	9.21	9.8	10.4
Women	11.5	11.5	11.8
CVD DALYs			
Annual, million	153	169	187
% of all DALYs	10.4	11.0	11.6
Global rank	3rd: CHD	3rd: CHD	3rd: CHD
	5th: Stroke	4th: Stroke	4th: Stroke
Rank in developing countries	4th: CHD	3rd: CHD	3rd: CHD
	8th: Stroke	6th: Stroke	5th: Stroke

CHD, chronic heart disease; CVD, cardiovascular disease; DALYS, disability-adjusted life-years.
Source: Available at: www.who.int/cardiovascular_diseases/en/cvd_atlas_25_future.pdf. Accessed 2004. Mackay J, Mensah G, eds. The Atlas of Heart Disease and Stroke.

TABLE 2-3

Incidence of Major Cardiovascular Events: Framingham Study, 44-Year Follow-Up of Cohort and 20-Year Follow-Up of Offspring Cohort[a]

AGE, YRS	CARDIOVASCULAR DISEASE, (ALL TYPES)		CORONARY HEART DISEASE		STROKE & TRANSIENT ISCHEMIC ATTACK		CONGESTIVE HEART FAILURE	
	MEN	WOMEN	MEN	WOMEN	MEN	WOMEN	MEN	WOMEN
35–44	7	3	4	1	b	b	b	b
45–54	15	7	10	4	2	1	2	1
55–64	26	15	21	10	4	3	4	2
65–74	39	24	24	14	11	8	9	6
75–84	59	40	33	18	20	15	18	12
85–94	68	63	35	28	12	25	39	31
35–64[c]	17	9	12	5	2	2	2	1
65–94[c]	44	30	27	16	13	11	12	9

[a]Average annual incidence per 100 persons free of specified disease.
[b]Results are omitted when fewer than five individuals experience an event.
[c]Age-adjusted rates.
SOURCE: The Framingham Study.

mid-1960s (see Fig. 2–4).[20,21] CVD mortality decreased by just less than 1 percent per year in the 1950s and 1960s. The decline became steeper in the 1970s, with the rate falling 3 percent per year since then. In the last decade (1993 to 2003), CVD death rates fell 22.1 percent, and actual CVD deaths declined by 4.6 percent.[18] Of note, whereas the initial rapid decrements in CVD mortality rates were consistent across racial groups, since the mid-1980s, a divergence in CVD trends have been noted, with black males experiencing a slower decline as compared to white males.[21]

CORONARY HEART DISEASE
[ ] RISK FACTORS

Numerous epidemiologic investigations have characterized the risk factors for CHD. Age, male sex, elevated low-density lipoprotein (LDL) cholesterol levels, low high-density lipoprotein (HDL) cholesterol levels, diabetes mellitus, and smoking are key risk factors for CHD.[22–29] Risk scores have been developed that can aid the determination of CHD risk.[28,30] The Framingham risk score[28] is one of the most popular ones but requires recalibrating when used to estimate absolute CHD risk in other populations. There is increasing awareness that obesity is a key risk factor that antedates and promotes several CHD risk factors. Obesity does not appear in many risk prediction tools because the risks are partly mediated through other risk factors. Recent data from the Framingham Heart Study indicate that 90 percent of CHD events occur in individuals with elevated levels of an established risk factor.[31]

[ ] GLOBAL BURDEN

In 2002, CHD caused 7.2 million deaths worldwide and accounted for the loss of 59 million DALYs (see Table 2–1). Each year there are

TABLE 2-4

Percentage of First Cardiovascular Events by Type of Event: Framingham Study, 44-Year Follow-Up of Cohort and 20-Year Follow-Up of Offspring Cohort

AGE, YRS	CARDIOVASCULAR DISEASE (N)		CORONARY HEART DISEASE (%)		STROKE & TRANSIENT ISCHEMIC ATTACK (%)		CONGESTIVE HEART FAILURE (%)	
	MEN	WOMEN	MEN	WOMEN	MEN	WOMEN	MEN	WOMEN
35–54	352	200	76.1	60.9	9.6	13.8	5.0	10.6
55–64	437	329	69.9	62.2	11.1	14.6	5.2	8.7
65–74	358	364	57.9	53.6	20.8	24.5	7.2	8.4
75–94	199	312	51.0	39.3	26.0	35.0	13.5	16.8

SOURCE: The Framingham Study.

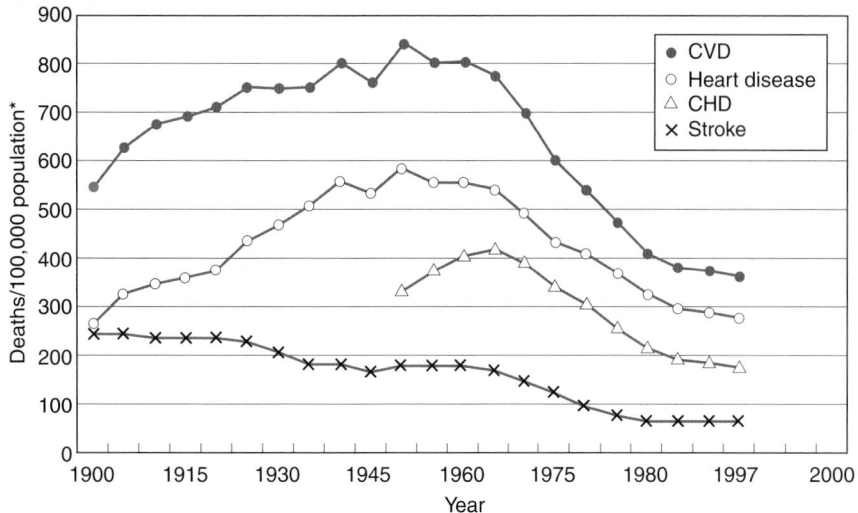

FIGURE 2–4. Decline in cardiovascular disease mortality in the United States. *Source: From CDC, Achievements in Public Health, 1900–1999: decline in deaths from heart disease and stroke—United States, 1900–1999. MMWR Morb Mortal Wkly Rep. 1999;48:649, used with permission.*

about 5.8 million new CHD cases, and about 40 million individuals with prevalent CHD are alive today (Table 2–5).

GLOBAL HETEROGENEITY IN CORONARY EVENT RATES

Data collected from 35 populations that were part of the Monitoring Trends and Determinants in Cardiovascular Disease (MONICA) Project during the mid-1980s until the mid-1990s reveal substantial heterogeneity in coronary event rates (MI and coronary deaths) across countries.[32] Thus, the coronary event rate (per 100,000) in men varied 10-fold, being highest in Finland (835 in North Karelia) and lowest in China (81 in Beijing). Likewise, an eightfold variation in coronary event rates was observed among women; the highest event rate was in the United Kingdom (265 in Glasgow), while the lowest rates (35) were noted both in Spain and China. Potential reasons for such geographic variation have been noted in an earlier section.

GLOBAL TRENDS IN MORTALITY

The MONICA Project tracked coronary event rates, risk factors, and coronary care in predefined populations in 31 countries over a 10-year period from the mid-1980s to the mid-1990s.[33] On average, coronary event rates decreased from 23 (women) to 25 (men) percent, while CHD mortality rates reduced by 34 (women) to 42 (men) percent during the observation period.[34,35] The greatest decline in coronary event rates in men occurred in north European populations—namely, Finland, which had the highest levels at the beginning of the observation period, and northern Sweden. Populations experiencing notable increases in coronary event rates were predominantly from central and Eastern Europe and Asia, although the general pattern of increases and decreases appeared to be less consistent in women.

In regions where coronary mortality rates were falling, it is estimated that improvements in survival contributed one-third, and

TABLE 2–5

Global Incidence and Prevalence of Cardiovascular Disease

CVD	AFR	AMR	EUR	SEAR	WPR	EMR	WORLD
Annual Incidence in 2000 (thousands)							
CHD[a]	292	877	1932	1665	647	431	5844
Cerebrovascular[b]	858	1438	3901	2964	5468	622	15251
Point Prevalence in 2000 (thousands)							
CHD[c]	2739	5969	9945	12001	6985	2925	40,064
Cerebrovascular[d]	1637	5299	11669	5752	13706	1391	39,455

AFR, Africa; AMR, America; CHD, chronic heart disease; CVD, cardiovascular disease; EMR, Eastern Mediterranean Region; EUR, Europe; HTN, hypertension; SEAR, South East Asia Region; WPR, Western Pacific Region.
[a]Acute MI.
[b]First ever stroke
[c]Includes angina
[d]First-ever stroke survivors

Source: Available at: www3.who.int/whosis/menu.cfm?path=whosis,burden,burden_estimates,burden_estimates_2002N,burden_estimates_2002N_2002Rev,burden_estimates_2002N_2002Rev_Region&language=English. Accessed on August 15, 2006.

change in heart attack rates accounted for two-thirds, on average, of the total change in survival rates.[34,35] These data underscore the importance of both the prevention of heart disease and improved care of acute events in determining CHD mortality rates at the population level.

The decline in CHD mortality in developed countries is in sharp contrast to future projections for the developing countries. Between 1990 and 2020, CHD mortality is expected to increase by 120 percent in women and by 137 percent in men in developing countries. It is estimated that the annual number of deaths caused by CHD in developing countries will rise to 11.1 million in 2020. CHD mortality will triple in Latin America, the Middle East and sub-Saharan Africa over the next two decades. By contrast, in developed countries CHD mortality is projected to increase by about 30 to 60 percent, largely because of the aging of the population.[36]

【 】 BURDEN IN THE UNITED STATES

In the United States, an estimated 13 million people have CHD, about one-half of whom have acute MI and one-half have angina pectoris (Table 2–6).[18] For men, prevalence of MI is 1 percent at ages 35 to 44 years, and 16 percent at age 75 years and older. Corresponding figures for women are less than 1 percent and 13 percent, respectively. The estimated direct and indirect costs associated with CHD are about $142.5 billion for the year 2006.[18]

Incidence in the United States:

In the United States, CHD causes about 700,000 new and 500,000 recurrent MIs per year.[18] According to the AHA, the annual rates per 1000 population of new and recurrent heart attacks in nonblack men are 19.2 for ages 65 to 74, 28.3 for ages 75 to 84, and 50.6 for age 85 and older; corresponding rates in black men are 21.6, 27.9, and 57.1. For nonblack women in the same age groups the heart attack rates are 6.8, 14.2, and 33.2, respectively, whereas for black women the rates are 8.6, 17.6, and 24.8, respectively.[18] For American Indians between 65 and 74 years of age, the annual incidence of heart attacks varies from 4.9 (women) to 7.6 (men).

The incidence of CHD events in women lags behind that in men by approximately 5 years; the average age of a first heart attack is 65.8 years in men and 70.4 years in women.[18] The first coronary presentation for women is more likely to be angina, whereas in men it is more likely to be an MI. In premenopausal women, annual CHD event rates are less than 1 percent, but there is a two- to threefold increase after menopause.

Unrecognized MIs are common, numbering at least one in three infarctions in the Framingham Study.[37] Half the unrecognized MIs are silent, and the rest are atypical so that neither the patient nor the physician entertains the possibility. More than one-half of these people eventually develop some overt clinical manifestations of CHD and hence come under medical care. Angina is less frequent in individuals with unrecognized MI than it is in those with recognized symptomatic MI, either before or after the infarction occurs. Despite the apparent mild nature of unrecognized MI, the risk of subsequent mortality is nearly the same as in patients with recognized infarction.[37] Men with diabetes and persons with hypertension of both sexes are particularly susceptible to silent or unrecognized MIs.[37]

Lifetime Risk of Coronary Disease in the United States

The lifetime risk of developing CHD after 40 years of age is 49 percent in men and 32 percent in women. Even at 70 years of age, the risk is 35 percent for men and 24 percent for women.[38]

Prognosis

In patients who survive the acute stage of an MI, the morbidity and mortality ranges from 1.5 to 15 times that of the general population, depending on the person's sex and clinical outcome, with an estimated average number of life years lost of 14 years. The rates of reinfarction, sudden death, angina pectoris, cardiac failure, and stroke are all substantial. The relative and absolute risks of these events are as great in women as in men after MI. In the initial year after a recognized MI, 25 percent of men and 38 percent of women die. Within 6 years, 18 percent of men and 35 percent of women have a recurrent infarction, and 27 percent of men and 14 percent of women develop angina. Approximately 22 percent of men and 46 percent of women are disabled with CHF; 8 percent of men and 11 percent of women will have a stroke. Sudden death will be experienced by 7 percent of men and 6 percent of women, a rate that is 4- to 6-fold higher than the general population.[18]

Mortality in the United States

CHD is the single leading cause of death in adults in the United States, accounting for 1 in 5 deaths.[18] Approximately every 26 seconds an American will sustain a coronary event, and approximately every minute someone will die from one. Approximately 40 percent of persons who suffer a coronary attack die. There are about 479,000 coronary deaths every year (see Table 2–6).[18]

Age, gender, ethnicity, and geographic origin are key correlates of CHD mortality. CHD mortality increases with age, and CHD is also a prominent cause of death in adults at the peak of their productive lives. CHD is the leading cause of death in both men and women and in every racial or ethnic group (except Asian American females). Overall, the CHD death rate is almost three times higher in men than it is in women at 25 to 34 years of age, but this ratio declines to 1.6 by 75 to 84 years of age. In 2003 the overall CHD death rate was 162.6 per 100,000 in the population. CHD death rates are higher in blacks (241.1 for black males and 160.3 for black females) compared to whites (209.2 for white males and 125.1 for white females).[18] The CHD death rate is more than 50 percent higher in blacks than it is in whites at 25 to 34 years of age, but this difference disappears by 75 years of age. CHD mortality is not as high among the Asian, American Indian, and Hispanic populations (rates per 100,000 of 98.6, 114, and 138, respectively) as it is among blacks and whites.

There has been a progressive decline in the age-adjusted CHD death rate in the United States over the last five decades. Framingham data indicate an overall 59 percent decline in CHD death rates between 1950 and 1999.[39] In the last decade (1993 to 2003), CHD death rates fell 30.2 percent, and actual CHD deaths declined by 14.7 percent.[18]

Sudden Coronary Death   In a substantial number of CHD deaths, the progression from unapparent clinical disease to death

TABLE 2–6

BURDEN OF CARDIOVASCULAR DISEASE IN THE UNITED STATES (2003)

	CHD			MI			STROKE			CHF			CVD	
	Prevalence	Incidence	Mortality	Prevalence	Incidence	Mortality	Prevalence	Incidence	Mortality	Prevalence	Incidence	Mortality	Prevalence	Mortality
Total	13,200,000	1,200,000	479,305	7,200,000	865,000	170,961	5,500,000	700,000	157,804	5,000,000	550,000	57,218	71,300,000	910,600
Men (M)	7,200,000	715,000	245,419	4,200,000	520,000	89,670	2,400,000	327,000	61,561	2,400,000	—	22,313	33,100,000	426,800
Women (F)	6,000,000	485,000	233,886	3,000,000	345,000	81,291	3,100,000	373,000	96,243	2,600,000	—	34,905	38,200,000	483,800
White M	8.9%	650,000	216,220	5.1%	—	79,387	2.3%	277,000	51,849	2.5%	—	18,894	34.3%	368,200
White F	5.4%	425,000	204,971	2.4%	—	71,054	2.6%	312,000	83,187	1.9%	—	33,381	32.4%	419,200
Black M	7.4%	65,000	23,957	4.5%	—	8,376	4.0%	50,000	7,791	3.1%	—	2,138	41.1%	49,000
Black F	7.5%	60,000	24,897	2.7%	—	8,908	3.9%	61,000	10,834	3.5%	—	3,159	44.7%	55,800
Mexican-American M	5.6%	—	—	3.4%	—	—	2.6%	—	—	2.7%	—	—	29.2%	—
Mexican American F	4.3%	—	—	1.6%	—	—	1.8%	—	—	1.6%	—	—	29.3%	—
Hispanic/Latino	4.5%	—	—	—	—	—	2.2%	—	—	—	—	—	—	—
Asian	3.8%	—	—	—	—	—	1.8%	—	—	—	—	—	—	—
American Indian	8.2%	—	—	—	—	—	3.1%	—	—	—	—	—	—	—

CHD, Coronary heart disease; CHF, chronic heart failure; CVD, cardiovascular disease; MI, myocardial infarction.

CVD is defined very broadly and includes hypertension, CHD, stroke, CHF and miscellaneous cardiovascular diseases.

Total population data include children, and prevalence estimates are age-adjusted to Americans age 20 years and older. Incidence data refer to annual events (new and recurrent).

SOURCE: Thom T, Haase N, Rosamond W, Howard VJ, Rumsfeld J, Manolio T, et al and Members of the Statistics Committee and Stroke Statistics Subcommittee et al. Heart disease and stroke statistics—2006 update: a report from the American Heart Association Statistics Committee and Stroke Statistics Subcommittee. Circulation, 2006;113:e85–151 and American Heart Association. Heart Disease and Stroke Statistics—2006 Update. Dallas, Texas: American Heart Association; 2006.
Available at: http://circ.ahajournals.org/cgi/content/short/113/6/e85. Accessed August 15, 2006.

is swift. Sudden, unexpected, out-of-hospital coronary death that occurs too rapidly to allow arrival alive at the hospital accounts for one-half of all coronary fatalities. Age, gender, and time since MI are important determinants of sudden death. The proportion of coronary deaths that are sudden is lower in women than it is in men, and lower in elderly men than it is in the young. Sudden cardiac death rates have declined by about 49 percent over a 50-year observation period (1950 to 1999) in the Framingham Study.[39]

STROKE

【 】 RISK FACTORS

Age, elevated blood pressure, smoking, diabetes mellitus, electrocardiographic left ventricular hypertrophy, and atrial fibrillation are the major risk factors for stroke.[23,40] A stroke risk score has been developed to estimate the risk of stroke.[41]

【 】 GLOBAL BURDEN

It is estimated that 15 million people suffer a stroke each year, and 5 million incur a permanent disability as a result. There are 5.5 million stroke deaths worldwide each year.[17] Strokes accounted for the loss of 49.2 million DALYs worldwide in 2002 (see Table 2–1). Every year there are approximately 15.3 million new strokes and 39 million prevalent cases worldwide (see Table 2–5).

【 】 GLOBAL TRENDS IN MORTALITY

Stroke mortality has declined in the developed world over the last two decades. Data from the MONICA Study demonstrate a modest contribution of reduction in risk factors such as hypertension to the decline in stroke mortality in women, but not in men.[42]

Global mortality because of cerebrovascular disease in the next two decades will parallel the CHD trends noted in an earlier section, with a 124 percent increase in women and a 107 percent increase in men in the developing countries, compared to increments of 56 percent in women and 28 percent in men in developed countries.[36]

【 】 BURDEN IN THE UNITED STATES

About 2.6 percent of the U.S. adult population, 5.5 million people, has prevalent cerebrovascular disease (stroke or transient ischemic attack; see Table 2–6). More than 1 million of these individuals are limited in their usual activity. Another 13 million people have silent strokes on MRI scans of the brain. Prevalence rises from 2 percent in men at 45 to 54 years of age to 12.5 percent for men aged 75 years and older, and from 1 to 10.7 percent in the corresponding age groups in women. There is geographic and racial heterogeneity in the burden because of stroke. There is a higher prevalence of stroke in 10 southeastern states relative to the 13 nonsoutheastern states and the District of Columbia, and prevalence is higher in blacks compared to whites. The estimated direct and indirect costs associated with stroke are about $57.9 billion for 2006.[18]

Incidence in the United States

Every year there are approximately 700,000 strokes, of which 500,000 are first events.[18] In the Framingham Study, the chance of having a stroke younger than 70 years of age was 5 percent for both sexes. Overall in the United States, the age-adjusted stroke incidence rates (per 100,000) for first-ever strokes are 167 for white males, 138 for white females, 323 for black males, and 260 for black females.[18] Thus, blacks have almost twice the risk of first-ever stroke as compared with whites. Although men have 1.25-times the stroke incidence rate compared to women overall, there are about 46,000 more women than men with prevalent stroke. This is because the average life expectancy for women is greater than for men, and the stroke rates are highest in the oldest age groups.[18]

Type of Stroke

Of the incident stroke events in the United States, 88 percent are ischemic strokes, whereas 12 percent are hemorrhagic (9 percent are intracerebral hemorrhages, and 3 percent are subarachnoid hemorrhage).[18] Among the 54 percent classified as definite thrombotic brain infarctions, 38 percent were classified as lacunar, with more than twice as many found in blacks as were found in whites.

Lifetime Risk of Stroke in the United States

The lifetime risk of developing stroke older than 55 years of age is 1 in 6 for men and 1 in 5 for women, exceeding the lifetime risk of developing Alzheimer' disease.[43]

Disability following Stroke

The time course of functional recovery is strongly related to initial stroke severity. Of survivors of an initial event, 50 to 70 percent return to functional independence, but 15 to 30 percent become permanently dependent. Institutional care is required by 20 percent at 3 months after onset. Stroke attacks have become less severe in recent years.

Mortality in the United States

Cerebrovascular disease is the third leading cause of death in the United States and is responsible for 157,800 deaths each year (see Table 2–6).[18] On average, every 3.1 minutes someone in the United States dies of a stroke. Stroke accounts for 7 percent of all deaths, and 44,000 of them occur in individuals younger than 75 years of age. The proportion of strokes that result in death within 1 year is about 22 percent in men and 25 percent in women; less if the stroke occurs before 65 years of age. For men or women younger than age 65, however, only 50 percent survive past 8 years.

Approximately 8 to 12 percent of ischemic stroke patients die within 30 days compared to 37 percent of patients with hemorrhagic strokes. Age, ethnicity, and geographic region are other key determinants of stroke mortality. Overall, stroke mortality is higher in the elderly and in blacks. The 2003 overall death rate for stroke was 54.3 per 100,000. Death rates, expressed as per 100,000, were 51.9 for white males and 78.8 for black males, and 50.5 for white females and 69.1 for black females. Younger than 65 years of age, the mortality rate is 3 times greater in blacks than it is in whites, largely as a result of the higher prevalence and increased severity of hypertension in the former. Stroke death rates are lower in other ethnicities (38.6 [women] to 44.3 [men] for Hispanics; 37 [men] to 38 [women] for American Indians/Alaska Natives, and 45.4 [women] to 50.8 [men] for Asian/Pacific Islanders in 2002).[18] Stroke death rates are higher in regions in southeastern United States, referred to as the stroke belt.

Mortality Trends in the United States

In the United States, the age-adjusted death rate for stroke has also declined by more than 50 percent over the last four decades, although the decline appears to have slowed in the 1990s; the rate of decline was 4 to 6 percent per year in the 1970s and early 1980s.[21] In the last decade (1993 to 2003), the stroke death rate fell 18.5 percent, but the actual number of stroke deaths declined only 0.7 percent.[18] The overall decline in stroke mortality is remarkable because the population of older persons increased substantially during that time.

CONGESTIVE HEART FAILURE

【 】 RISK FACTORS

Advancing age, MI, hypertension, diabetes mellitus, valvular heart disease, and obesity are key risk factors for CHF.[44] High blood pressure antedates more than 75 percent of heart failure.[45] A clinical risk score has been formulated to estimate the risk of developing CHF based on several of these risk factors.[46]

【 】 GLOBAL BURDEN

CHF is clearly a major clinical and public health problem. The exact magnitude of the problem is difficult to assess because we lack broadly based population estimates of its prevalence, incidence, and mortality rates. It is estimated that there are nearly 23 million people with heart failure worldwide.[47]

【 】 GLOBAL TRENDS IN MORTALITY

It is estimated that the burden of CHF will increase over the next two decades in developed countries.[48] Despite a stable incidence rate, increasing prevalence can result because of a reduction in CHF mortality.[49]

【 】 BURDEN IN THE UNITED STATES

The AHA estimates that there are 5 million people in the United States who have CHF as of 2003, and that 550,000 new cases are reported each year (see Table 2–5).[18] CHF is reported to be the leading diagnosis for hospitalization of persons older than 65 years of age. The estimated health care costs (direct and indirect) for heart failure for 2006 are $29.6 billion.

National estimates for the United States suggest that CHF afflicts 1.5 to 2 percent of the total population and as much as 6 to 10 percent of the elderly. It is estimated that as many as 20 million additional persons have an asymptomatic impairment of cardiac function likely to become symptomatic over the course of 1 to 5 years. Prevalence estimates from the Framingham Study include both systolic and diastolic dysfunctional varieties but is confined mainly to those who are symptomatic. The population-based estimate from the Framingham Study indicates an increase in prevalence in men from 8 per 1000 at age 50 to 59 years to 66 per 1000 at age 80 to 89 years. In women the prevalence at these ages increases from 8 per 1000 to 79 per 1000. The prevalence of heart failure in blacks is reported to be higher than it is in whites. The age-adjusted prevalence of heart failure in non-Hispanic whites is 2.5 percent in men and 1.9 percent in women. In non-Hispanic blacks, the age-adjusted prevalence is 3.1 percent in men and 3.5 percent in women. Blacks with CHF have a different spectrum of underlying cardiovascular disorders and risk factors; they have a higher prevalence of hypertension and electrocardiographic left ventricular hypertrophy but a lower prevalence of CHD and valvular disease.[50] In Mexican Americans, the age-adjusted prevalence ranges from 1.6 (women) to 2.7 percent (men).[18]

Prevalence of Diastolic versus Systolic Heart Failure in the United States

At present, epidemiologic population-based assessment of the prevalence of diastolic CHF uses the occurrence of clinically overt heart failure in persons with normal left ventricular systolic function for case ascertainment. Approximately 30 to 50 percent of patients with CHF are reported to have a normal or nearly normal left ventricular ejection fraction.[51–53] In the Framingham Study, women predominated in the diastolic CHF subgroup, with 65 percent of the heart failure occurring in association with a normal left ventricular ejection fraction. In men, 75 percent of the heart failure cases occurred in those with left ventricular systolic dysfunction.[54] The high prevalence and female preponderance in diastolic CHF have been corroborated by numerous other community-based investigations.[51–53] Recent data suggest a trend for increasing prevalence of diastolic CHF in the community.[52]

Incidence in the United States

The Framingham Study reported that the incidence of CHF increased steeply with age, approximately doubling with each decade.[44] Between the ages of 35 to 64 and 65 to 94 years, the annual incidence rate in men increased from 3 per 1000 to 12 per 1000. In women, the corresponding rates were 2 and 9 per 1000. The higher rate in men at all ages is chiefly attributable to the greater vulnerability of men to CHD. Similar figures for the incidence of CHF have been reported by other cohort studies and investigations examining new cases in other geographic regions worldwide.

Lifetime Risk in the United States

The Framingham Study reported that the lifetime risk of CHF is 21 percent in men and 20 percent in women.[55] Furthermore, the lifetime risk of CHF, even in the absence of a myocardial infarction, is 11 percent in men and 15 percent in women.[55]

Mortality of Heart Failure in the United States

The annual death rate for CHF was 19.7 per 100,000 population in the year 2003; rates are higher in blacks (20.4 for women and 23.4 for men) compared to whites (18.4 for women, 20.5 for men). In population-based studies the survival rates of CHF patients are appalling. The overall population rate of expected life-years lost because of CHF is 6.7 years per 1000 in men, and 5.1 years per 1000 in women. Geographically, there is about a 10-fold range of reported mortality from CHF, the highest rates reported from the southern stroke belt. The age-adjusted death rates are 25 percent higher in men than they are in women, and 40 percent higher in blacks than they are in whites. The lower mortality in women can be related to a greater likelihood of a false-positive diagnosis of CHF, a lower probability of coronary disease as the basis of heart failure, a higher prevalence of intact left ventricular systolic function, and possibly a greater capacity of women to withstand cardiac pump failure.

In the Framingham Study a number of other conditions were associated with a poor survival experience in individuals with CHF. Advancing age was associated with increased mortality—27 percent per decade in men and 61 percent in women. Valvular heart disease increased the hazard by 68 percent in men, whereas in women diabetes mellitus imposed a 70 percent higher mortality rate. Additional prognostic factors associated with an adverse outcome include the presence of atrial fibrillation, renal dysfunction, underlying diabetes mellitus, a low body mass index, and a low systolic blood pressure. Diastolic CHF had an annual mortality rate of 8.7 percent compared to 18.9 percent for systolic CHF. Compared to age- and sex-matched controls, diastolic and systolic CHF were associated with hazard ratios for mortality of 4.1 and 4.3, respectively.[54] More recent studies have demonstrated more modest differences[52] or no differences[51] in the survival experience of patients with diastolic versus systolic CHF.

Blacks with CHF have a worse prognosis relative to whites even after adjusting for multiple factors including socioeconomic status. Blacks with CHF also suffer more hospital readmissions compared to whites with this condition.[50]

ATRIAL FIBRILLATION

[ ] RISK FACTORS

The risk factors for atrial fibrillation include standard CVD risk factors such as advancing age, male sex, increasing body mass index, hypertension, diabetes, heart failure, MI, valvular heart disease, and increasing left atrial size.[56,57] Miscellaneous factors associated with incident atrial fibrillation including alcohol consumption, hyperthyroidism, and reduced lung function are associated with an increased risk of atrial fibrillation.[58,59] Recent studies reported that elevated biomarkers such as C-reactive protein (CRP) and B-type natriuretic peptide concentrations also predict an increased risk of incident atrial fibrillation,[60,61] although whether these biomarkers are causally related to atrial fibrillation remains to be determined. Additionally, there is increasing evidence that there is a genetic predisposition to atrial fibrillation.[62–64]

In contrast to industrialized countries, in developing countries valvular heart disease appears to be the most common predisposing condition.[62,63,65] However, with the globalization of cardiovascular disease risk factors, hypertension and CHD are increasing in importance in developing countries.

[ ] GLOBAL BURDEN

The global burden of atrial fibrillation is unknown because most atrial fibrillation research has been conducted in North America and Western Europe.[66] Even within these geographic constraints, the reported studies have been from predominantly white cohorts.

[ ] BURDEN IN THE UNITED STATES

Atrial fibrillation is the most common persistent arrhythmia with an estimated prevalence in the United States of 2.2 million.[18] The prevalence increases significantly with advancing age, ranging from 0.1 percent in adults younger than 55 years of age to 17.8 percent in those aged 85 years or older.[67,68] The age-specific prevalence is higher in men than women, but women constitute about half of atrial fibrillation cases because women in general enjoy a longer life span.[68] Several studies suggest that individuals of African descent can have a lower prevalence[68] and incidence than whites[69] for reasons that are incompletely understood. The reported prevalence varies by the chronicity of atrial fibrillation studied; one study reported that paroxysmal, chronic, and recent onset atrial fibrillation were 22.1 percent, 51.4 percent, and 26.4 percent of atrial fibrillation cases, respectively.[70]

The prevalence of atrial fibrillation is increasing in North America, Europe, and Japan. It is projected that more than 12 million Americans will have the condition by 2050.[71] This is partly related to the aging of the population, but speculation also has centered on improved survival with established cardiovascular diseases such as CHF and MI.

Incidence in the United States

The incidence of atrial fibrillation doubles for each successive decade of life and ranges from 3.1 and 38.0 per 1000 person years for men 55 to 64 years and 85 to 94 years; corresponding rates for women were 1.9 and 31.4 per 1000 person years.[72] Similar incidence rates are reported from the Cardiovascular Health Study.[69] In parallel with the increasing prevalence, a recent study suggests a rising incidence of atrial fibrillation in the community.[71]

Lifetime Risk in the United States

The lifetime risk of atrial fibrillation is substantial; at age 40 the lifetime risk is approximately 26 percent for men and 23 percent for women and by 80 years of age declines only to 23 percent and 21 percent, respectively.[73] The Rotterdam Study reported similar lifetime risk of atrial fibrillation in those 55 to 59 years (24 percent in men, 22 percent in women), but at 80 years of age the reported lifetime risk was lower (16 percent in men, 15 percent in women).[67]

Relations to Stroke and Congestive Heart Failure

Atrial fibrillation has been demonstrated to be an independent risk factor for stroke[74] in virtually all settings and countries studied, with an annual stroke rate averaging approximately 5 percent in untreated patients. In Japan the adjusted risk ratio for stroke was 4.3 in women and 6.9 in men.[75] Canadian male air force recruits with atrial fibrillation have an age-adjusted doubling of stroke risk in follow-up.[76] Data from the Framingham Heart Study suggest that whereas the relative risk of atrial fibrillation for stroke does not change substantively with advancing age (rate ratio [RR] ranging from 3 to 5), the percentage of strokes attributable to atrial fibrillation increases markedly from 1.5 percent in subjects in their 50s to 24 percent in subjects 80 to 89 years of age, reflecting the higher prevalence of atrial fibrillation with advancing age.[74]

The relations between atrial fibrillation and heart failure are complex because they share common risk factors and can each predispose to the other's development. Atrial fibrillation doubles to triples the risk of developing congestive heart failure adjusting for the coexistent risk factors.[77] In addition, in individuals with either atrial fibrillation or congestive heart failure, development of the other condition increases mortality.[78] Risk prediction models for stroke[79] and stroke and death[79] have been developed to help clinicians assess the prognosis of patients with atrial fibrillation.

Given the relation to heart failure and stroke it is not surprising that atrial fibrillation is a costly illness. In a study from the United Kingdom it was noted to increase from 1995 to 2000, rising from about 244 to 459 million pounds, or about 0.62 percent to 0.97 percent of the total National Health Service spent on atrial fibrillation.[80]

Mortality in the United States

Atrial fibrillation is associated with a 1.3- to 2-fold increased risk of death, even accounting for the frequently coexistent risk factors.[77,81] Data from the Framingham and the Copenhagen Heart Studies suggest that atrial fibrillation can be particularly deleterious in women and can reduce the survival advantage typically enjoyed by women.[81,82] Whereas atrial flutter was previously considered a more benign condition, recent literature suggests that the prognosis of atrial flutter is similar to atrial fibrillation.[83] Temporal trends in the mortality of atrial fibrillation is controversial, with one study analyzing death certificates noting that age-standardized death rates increased in the United States.[84] Danish and Scottish hospitalization studies suggests that the mortality has significantly declined in the 1980s and 1990s.[85,86] In contrast, in a Medicare study from the United States, since the 1980s there has been an increase in the frequency of atrial fibrillation being listed as a cause of death on death certificates.[87] It remains to be determined whether the contrasting mortality trends are secondary to variation in patient characteristics, coding variation, treatment factors, or a combination.

HYPERTENSION
[ ] DEFINITION

Numerous epidemiologic investigations have demonstrated that blood pressure is related to vascular mortality in continuous fashion.[23,88] Given the continuous relations of blood pressure to vascular risk, any definition of hypertension is somewhat arbitrary, and largely based on thresholds for which there is evidence that the benefits of lowering blood pressure outweigh potential risks of treatment. It is not surprising, therefore, that the definition of *high* blood pressure (hypertension) has been lowered in successive blood pressure guidelines over the past 35 years. Guidelines of the seventh Joint National Committee on prevention, detection, evaluation, and treatment of high blood pressure in the United States

(JNC VII) and the WHO-International Society for Hypertension define hypertension as a systolic blood pressure of 140 mmHg or greater, or a diastolic blood pressure of 90 mmHg or greater, or the use of antihypertensive medication.[89,90] The JNC VII also has categorized blood pressure readings in the range of a systolic pressure of 120 to 139 mmHg or a diastolic pressure of 80 to 89 mmHg as *prehypertension*.[90] An important reason for this change is to simplify the classification system of blood pressure and to emphasize the continuous risk of relations of blood pressure to vascular disease.

[ ] RISK FACTORS

Advancing age, sedentary lifestyle, excess weight, increased dietary salt consumption, and reduced intake of potassium and increased alcohol consumption have been identified as risk factors for developing high blood pressure.[90] Family history of hypertension and African American ancestry have also been observed to elevate the risk of developing high blood pressure. Prehypertension is associated with increased risk of progression to hypertension, relative to those with optimal levels of blood pressure.[91]

[ ] GLOBAL BURDEN

Hypertension is the most common CVD disorder, affecting approximately 20 percent of the adult population.[92] It is considered both as a disease condition and as one of the major risk factors for heart disease, stroke, and kidney disease. Worldwide an estimated 600 million people have high blood pressure.[15] About 15 to 37 percent of the adult population worldwide is afflicted with hypertension. In those older than 60 years of age, as many as one-half are hypertensive in some populations.[15] In general, hypertension prevalence is higher in urban settings as compared with rural settings. It is estimated that the global prevalence of high blood pressure will increase to 1.56 billion by 2025.[93]

Global Awareness, Treatment, and Control of Hypertension

The detection and control of hypertension remains a challenge even in developed countries.[94,95] The detection rates in most developed countries vary from 32 to 64 percent,[94,95] whereas in many developing countries the reported detection rates are substantially lower.[92] The control rates in those already being treated for hypertension varies from 13 to 29 percent.[92,94] However, in African countries, control rates were reported to be as low as 2 percent.[92] Data from the MONICA Study demonstrate small decreases in mean systolic blood pressures in most countries evaluated and in both sexes during the time period 1979 to 1996.[33]

[ ] BURDEN IN THE UNITED STATES

In the United States, 32 percent of the adult population, representing 65 million persons, have hypertension (Table 2–7).[18] The age-adjusted prevalence varies with ethnicity, ranging from 28 percent in Mexican American populations, 31 percent in non-Hispanic white populations, to 42 to 45 percent in non-Hispanic black populations. A distinct geographic variation has also been

TABLE 2-7

Burden of Cardiovascular Disease Risk Factors in the United States (2003)

RISK FACTOR	SMOKING	PHYSICAL INACTIVITY	EXCESS WEIGHT		HYPERTEN-SION	DYSLIPIDEMIA				GLUCOSE INTOLERANCE		
			Overweight	Obesity		TC >200	TC >240	LDL >130	HDL <40	Diagnosed Diabetes	Undiagnosed Diabetes	Prediabetes
Total	44,300,000	23.7%	136,500,000	64,000,000	65,000,000	99,900,000	34,500,000	76,100,000	46,000,000	14,100,000	6,000,000	14,700,000
Men (M)	24,100,000	21.4%	69,600,000	27,900,000	29,400,000	48,400,000	16,400,000	39,100,000	33,200,000	7,000,000	—	—
Women (F)	20,200,000	25.9%	66,900,000	36,100,000	35,600,000	51,500,000	18,100,000	37,000,000	12,800,000	7,100,000	—	—
White M	24.1%	18.4%	69.4%	28.2%	30.6%	48.9%	16.5%	43.8%	34.5%	6.2%	3.0%	8.6%
White F	20.4%	21.6%	57.2%	30.7%	31.0%	52.1%	18.4%	36.9%	12.4%	4.7%	2.7%	4.6%
Black M	23.9%	27.0%	62.9%	27.9%	41.8%	41.6%	12.2%	36.0%	22.7%	10.3%	1.3%	8.3%
Black F	17.2%	33.9%	77.2%	49.0%	45.4%	46.8%	17.4%	34.5%	11.3%	12.6%	6.1%	5.9%
Mexican-American M	18.9%	32.5%	73.1%	27.3%	27.8%	51.9%	16.7%	43.7%	34.4%	10.4%	3.5%	8.7%
Mexican-American F	10.9%	39.6%	71.7%	38.4%	28.7%	44.8%	13.6%	31.3%	15.4%	11.3%	1.8%	7.2%
Hispanic/Latino	—	—	38.9%	24.7%	19.0%	—	25.6%	—	—	8.6%	—	—
Asian	4.8% (women)–17.8% (men)	20.4% (men)–24.0% (women)	25.1%	6%	16.1%	—	27.3%	—	—	6.5%	—	—
American Indian	33.4% (women)–37.3% (men)	—	33.5%	32.9%	23.9%	—	26.0–28.6%	—	—	12.2%	—	—

HDL, high-density lipoprotein; LDL, low density lipoprotein.
Other than for smoking and excess weight (that are crude), all prevalence data are age-adjusted to Americans age 20 and older.

SOURCE: Thom T, Haase N, Rosamond W, Howard VJ, Rumsfeld J, Manolio T, Zheng ZJ, Flegal K, O'Donnell C, Kittner S, Lloyd-Jones D, Goff DC, Jr., Hong Y, Members of the Statistics Committee and Stroke Statistics Subcommittee, Adams R, Friday G, Furie K, Gorelick P, Kissela B, Marler J, Meigs J, Roger V, Sidney S, Sorlie P, Steinberger J, Wasserthiel-Smoller S, Wilson M, Wolf P. Heart Disease and Stroke Statistics–2006 Update: A Report From the American Heart Association Statistics Committee and American Heart Association. Heart Disease and Stroke Statistics — 2006 Update. Dallas, Texas: American Heart Association; 2006. Available at http://circ.ahajournals.org/cgi/content/short/113/6/e85. Accessed August 15, 2006.

noted, prevalence being greater in the southeastern United States. An additional 28 percent of Americans (59 million) have prehypertension.[18] The health care costs associated with high blood pressure are estimated at $63.5 billion in 2006.[18]

The prevalence of hypertension in blacks in the United States is among the highest in the world. Compared with whites, blacks develop hypertension earlier in life, and their average blood pressures are much higher. Within the African American community, rates of hypertension vary substantially; those with the highest rates are more likely to be middle age or older, less educated, overweight or obese, physically inactive, and diabetic.

Lifetime Risk in the United States

The lifetime risk of hypertension reflects the probability that a person will develop high blood pressure during his or her lifetime and has been shown to be as high as 90 percent in middle-aged and elderly Framingham Study participants.[96]

Awareness, Treatment, and Control of Hypertension in the United States

An estimated 40 million, or 31 percent of Americans with hypertension, have inadequately controlled hypertension.[94] Approximately two-thirds of patients with hypertension were aware of their diagnosis, and approximately one-half were taking prescribed medication. Approximately one-half of those taking medication have their blood pressure controlled at or below the 140/90 mmHg threshold.

Treatment rates and control vary by ethnicity, but the pattern that consistently emerges across ethnicities is one of lost opportunities for prevention. Blood pressure control was achieved in only 17.7 percent of Mexican Americans with hypertension, compared to 28.1 percent of blacks and 33.4 percent of non-Hispanic whites.[18] Among blacks, those with uncontrolled high blood pressure who are not taking antihypertensive medication tend to be male, young, and have infrequent contact with a physician.[18] Awareness, treatment, and control of hypertension have improved substantially since the 1976 to 1991 National Health and Nutrition Examination Survey (NHANES) but continue to be suboptimal, especially in Mexican Americans.

[ ] RISKS ASSOCIATED WITH HYPERTENSION

Worldwide, high blood pressure is estimated to cause 7.1 million deaths (see Table 2–1), about 13 percent of the global fatality total.[3] Across WHO regions, research indicates that about 62 percent of strokes and 49 percent of heart attacks are caused by blood pressure levels exceeding optimal levels.[3] Every year 64.3 million DALYs (4.4 percent of total) are lost due to high blood pressure. About two-thirds of these DALYs lost are in developing countries, and about two-thirds in middle age (45 to 69 years of age). Thus, about 5 million of these hypertension-related deaths are premature.

It is important to emphasize that although 10 to 30 percent of adults worldwide suffer from high blood pressure as currently defined, an additional 50 to 60 percent would improve their prognosis if they had levels in the healthy range.[3] Even small reductions in blood pressure for this "silent majority" would reduce their heart attack and stroke risk.[3] A meta-analysis of 61 prospective observational studies evaluated individual records from 958,074 partici-

pants (Prospective Studies Collaboration).[88] Based on 56,000 vascular deaths over a follow-up period of 12.7 million person-years, the report concluded that "usual" blood pressure is related to vascular mortality without evidence of a threshold down to 115/75 mmHg.[88] Across the entire blood pressure distribution, middle-aged persons (40 to 69 years of age) with a 20-mm higher systolic blood pressure (or a 10-mm higher diastolic blood pressure) experienced a twofold greater risk of death because of stroke or coronary disease. These data, the largest of their kind, strongly support the notion that a usual blood pressure of 115/75 mmHg would be "optimal" from a vascular risk standpoint.[88]

Risks in the United States

In the United States, there is both ethnic and geographic variation in morbidity because of high blood pressure. Compared with hypertensive whites, blacks with high blood pressure have a 1.3 times greater rate of nonfatal stroke, a 1.8 times greater rate of fatal stroke, a 1.5 times greater rate of heart disease death, and a 4.2 times greater rate of end-stage kidney disease.[18] Death rates from stroke are higher in hypertensive individuals within the stroke belt than they are among those in other regions.[18]

RHEUMATIC VALVULAR HEART DISEASE

[ ] GLOBAL BURDEN

Acute rheumatic fever and subsequent rheumatic heart disease remain important cardiovascular problems in the tropical and subtropical developing countries of the Middle East, South America, Africa, and Asia, and there have been outbreaks in the United States in recent years. The incidence, however, remains higher in subgroups such as Polynesians, Australian aborigines, Maoris in New Zealand, and within the United States among blacks, Puerto Ricans, Mexican Americans, and Native Americans. Overall, incidence rates vary widely from less than 1 per 100,000 in developed countries to as high as 150 per 100,000 in China.[15] Rheumatic fever is rare before 3 years of age, occurring most frequently between 5 and 15 years of age, when streptococcal infections are most frequent. During epidemics of streptococcal pharyngitis, the rheumatic fever attack rate can be 3 percent, whereas in endemic situations it is usually only 0.3 percent.

In developing countries, rheumatic fever is the most frequent cause of heart disease in the pediatric age group, accounting for 25 to 40 percent of all CVD and 33 to 50 percent of all hospital admissions. The prevalence is high in the African continent, where it can reach 15:1000 school children. It is estimated that 12 million patients with rheumatic heart disease require further treatments to prevent disability and death because of rheumatic heart disease; of these, two-thirds are children of school age.[15] More than 2 million require repeated hospital admissions and 300,000 die because of the illness every year. Another 1 million will need heart surgery in the next 5 to 20 years.[15]

[ ] BURDEN IN THE UNITED STATES

In the United States, rheumatic fever accounted for approximately 3554 deaths in the year 2003; 68 percent were females.[18] From 1993 to 2003, the death rate because of rheumatic fever or rheumatic heart disease fell by 36.8 percent.[18]

GLOBAL BURDEN OF CARDIOVASCULAR DISEASE RISK FACTORS

AGING

The world population was 2.8 billion in 1955 and is 5.8 billion currently. It is estimated that the global population will increase by nearly 80 million people per year to reach 8 billion by 2025.[97] Life expectancy will increase from the current 68 years to approximately 73 years in 2025, representing a 50 percent improvement in life expectancy from that in 1950 (48 years). This will translate into a marked increase in the number of people older than 65 years of age, from 390 million at present to 800 million by 2025.[98] The elderly segment will constitute more than 10 percent of the total human population, and more than two-thirds of them will reside in developing countries.[97] The aging of the world population will have major implications for CVD morbidity and mortality. By 2025, more than 60 percent of all deaths will be among those older than 65 years of ages, and more than 40 percent among those older than 75 years of age.

SMOKING
Global Burden

It is estimated that there are approximately 1.3 billion smokers (250 million women) in the world today, and these individuals consume an average of 14 cigarettes each per day.[15] Of these, 300 million live in developed countries, whereas more than 900 million reside in developing countries. Overall, 47 percent of men and 12 percent of women in the world are current smokers. In developing countries, it is estimated that 48 percent of men and 7 percent of women smoke, whereas in developed countries, 42 percent of men and 24 percent of women are smokers. East-Asian countries account for a disproportionately high percentage (38 percent) of world smokers.[99] More than 60 percent of men in China are present smokers,[100] as are more than 40 percent of men in India.[101]

Global Trends in Tobacco Consumption

Tobacco consumption fell between 1981 and 1991 in most developed countries. In developed countries the decrease in smoking prevalence has been lowest among the least educated.

By contrast, consumption is increasing in developing countries by about 3.4 percent per annum, having risen dramatically in some countries in recent years. Data from the MONICA Study suggest that whereas smoking rates are declining in most of the male populations, rates in women are increasing.[33,102] Smoking is increasing at an alarming rate among young women, especially in Eastern Europe.[33,102] It is estimated that the number of individuals who smoke will increase to 1.7 billion throughout the world by 2025.

Burden in the United States

For Americans 18 years of age and older, the current prevalence of cigarette smoking is 23.4 percent of men and 18.5 percent of women (see Table 2–7).[18] Native Americans have the highest smoking rates, whereas Asian Americans and Hispanic Americans have lower rates relative to whites. There are striking disparities by educational level, with individuals who have a 9th- to 11th-grade education having three times the prevalence of smoking (34.0 percent) as individuals with a college education (8 percent). Similarly, there is also marked geographic variation in smoking rates, with the highest rate in Kentucky (30.9 percent) and the lowest rate in Utah (13.3 percent). Adolescent smoking is a known precursor of adult smoking habits, and it is estimated that approximately 20 percent of 12th graders in the United States currently smoke.

Approximately 1.4 million individuals begin smoking in the United States every year. About 4000 people initiate smoking every day, and half of these individuals are younger than 18 years of age.[18] Smoking poses substantial economic burden, with an estimated annual health care cost of $167 billion.

Trends in Tobacco Consumption in the United States

In the United States, the prevalence of smoking rose steadily from the 1930s and reached a peak in 1964 when more than 40 percent of all adult Americans (60 percent of men) smoked. Since then smoking prevalence has declined markedly, decreasing to approximately 23 percent by 1997.[103]

Health Risks and Future Trends

Smokers of all ages have a two- to threefold elevated risk of dying prematurely compared to nonsmokers.[104,105] Between the ages of 35 to 69 years, smokers lose approximately 20 years of life expectancy relative to nonsmokers. At older than 70 years of age, smokers lose approximately 8 years of life relative to nonsmokers. Smoking is an important CVD risk factor in both men and women, being particularly harmful in the latter after menopause and in those who use oral contraceptives. Smoking increases the risk of stroke and CHD by 100 percent, that for peripheral arterial disease by 300 percent, and the risk of developing an aortic aneurysm by 400 percent.[17] Prospective studies show that cigarette smoking causes approximately 30 percent of CVD deaths worldwide.[104,105] This is especially evident in populations with the clustering of CVD risk factors (i.e., those with diets that are high in saturated fat with subsequent high blood cholesterol and high blood pressure).

Smoking is responsible for 90 percent of all lung cancers and for 75 percent of chronic obstructive pulmonary disease.[105] WHO estimates that tobacco was responsible for 10 percent of the total global mortality and caused about 4.9 million deaths worldwide in 2000. More than 59 million DALYs (4.1 percent of total) were lost because of smoking in 2000. In the United States, from 1995 to 1999, an average of 442,400 individuals died each year from smoking-related illnesses. One-third of these were CVD related.

Based on current smoking patterns and trends, smoking is expected to kill 10 million people annually worldwide by 2020[15]—this is more than the total of deaths from malaria, maternal and major childhood conditions, and tuberculosis combined. Of specific concern is that more than 70 percent of these deaths will be occurring in developing countries. By 2020, smoking will cause about one in three of all adult deaths. Half of these deaths will occur in middle-age and at younger than 70 years of age.[15]

Health risks diminish with smoking cessation. According to WHO, 1 year after quitting, the risk of CHD decreases by 50 percent, and within 15 years, the relative risk of dying from CHD for an exsmoker approaches that of a long-time (lifetime) nonsmoker.[15]

Risks Associated with Environmental Tobacco Exposure

The risk of death from CHD increases by up to 30 percent among those exposed to environmental tobacco smoke at home or work.[106] It is estimated that about 35,000 nonsmokers die from CHD each year as a result of exposure to environmental tobacco smoke.[3]

Tobacco Free Initiative

WHO established the Tobacco Free Initiative in July 1998 to coordinate an improved global strategic response.[107] The goals of the Tobacco Free Initiative are to (1) galvanize global support for evidence-based tobacco-control policies and actions; (2) to build new partnerships for action and strengthen existing ones; (3) to raise awareness of the need to address tobacco issues at all levels of society; and (4) to accelerate the implementation of national, regional, and global strategies.[107] Specific strategies for tobacco control include a ban on advertising and expansion of public health information; use of taxes and regulations to reduce consumption; promotion of cessation of tobacco use, and the building of antitobacco coalitions.[107]

【 】 PHYSICAL INACTIVITY
Significance

It is widely accepted that daily moderate-intensity physical activity helps lower blood pressure, reduce body fat, and improve glucose metabolism.[108] Indeed, physical activity is essential to maintain overall good health and is important in maintaining a healthy weight. Physical activity also reduces the risk of diabetes mellitus, hypertension, CVD, and all-cause mortality.[108]

Global Burden and Trends

WHO estimates that 60 percent of the world population is insufficiently physically active, a situation that is particularly striking among women and that undoubtedly has contributed to the increased prevalence of obesity and diabetes.[108] Physical inactivity is widespread in developed countries and is increasing in urban areas of developing countries, especially in poorer communities. This trend for physical inactivity is influenced by cultural patterns, local traditions, and the lack of civic organizations to promote the benefits of exercise. In developing countries that previously relied on walking or bicycling for transportation, there has been a progressive increase in the use of automobiles and motorized public transportation.

Burden in the United States and Trends

According to national data in the United States, 23.7 percent of Americans 18 years of age or older indulge in no leisure-time physical activity, whereas only 30 percent performed light to moderate physical activity at least 5 times per week as per current AHA guidelines.[18] Physical inactivity is more common in women, elderly, blacks, and Hispanics (see Table 2–7), the less affluent and those without a high school diploma.[18] Physical inactivity among adolescents is a harbinger of continued inactivity during adulthood. It is estimated that 61.5 percent of children 9 to 13 years of age do not participate in any organized physical activity outside of school, and 22.6 percent do not engage in any free-time physical activity.[18]

Risks

Physical inactivity caused about 1.9 million deaths globally in 2000.[3] It is estimated that about 20 percent of cases of CHD, 15 percent of diabetes and some cancers, and 10 percent of strokes are attributable to physical inactivity.[3] The relative risk of CHD associated with physical inactivity ranges from 1.5 to 2.4, relative to people who do follow current minimum physical activity recommendations. This increase in risk associated with physical inactivity is comparable to that observed for high blood cholesterol, high blood pressure, or cigarette smoking.

World Health Organization Physical Activity Initiative

WHO has begun formulating a Global Strategy on Diet, Physical Activity and Health, under a May 2002 mandate from the World Health Assembly.[108]

【 】 OBESITY
Definition

Overweight and obesity are currently defined by body mass index (BMI; calculated as weight in kilograms per height in meters).[2] A BMI of 25.0 to 29.9 defines overweight, and a BMI ≥30.0 defines obesity.[109]

Global Burden

Obesity is a disease condition that is highly prevalent in both developing and developed countries (Fig. 2–5). According to WHO data, an estimated 1 billion people across the world are now overweight or obese.[3] Between 50 and 75 percent of the adults studied in the MONICA study were overweight or obese, and low levels of education were associated with increased body mass index.[102] In the European Union, an estimated 200 million of the 350 million adults are overweight or obese.[15] The WHO estimates that about 18 million children younger than 5 years of age are overweight, and these children are at increased risk of developing adult obesity and related problems of dyslipidemia and hypertension in their teen years.[110]

Global Trends in Prevalence

Obesity rates have risen threefold or more in some parts of the Middle East, North America, Eastern Europe, the Pacific Islands, Australia, and China since 1980.[3] BMI is increased in approxi-

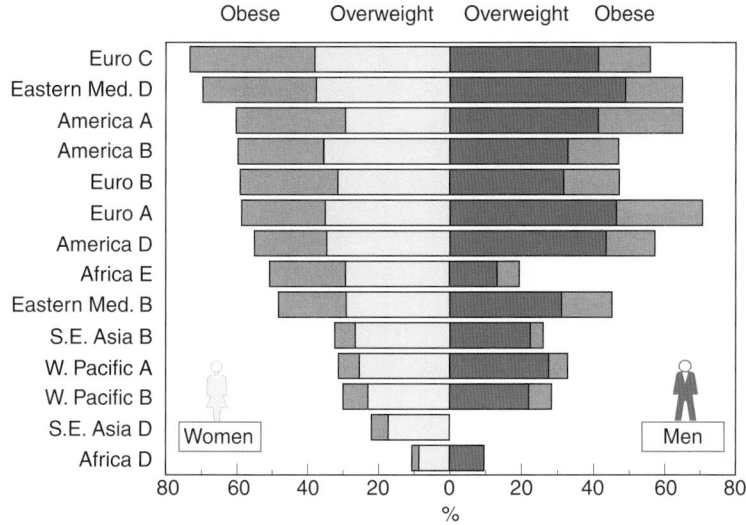

FIGURE 2–5. Global burden of obesity. The Y axis displays WHO subregions as identified in Figure 2–1. *Source: From James PT, Leach R, Kalamara E, Shayeghi M. The worldwide obesity epidemic. Obes Res. 2001;9(90004):228S, used with permission.*

mately half of the female populations and in two-thirds of the male population.[33]

It is estimated that the number of overweight people in the world will increase to 1.5 billion by 2015 if current trends continue unabated.[15]

Burden in the United States

In the United States, 35 percent of United States adults were considered overweight (BMI 25.0 to 29.9 kg/m²), and another 30 percent were considered obese (BMI ≥30.0 kg/m²) in 2003 (see Table 2–7). Hispanic men and Hispanic and black women were more likely to be overweight or obese than were their white counterparts.[18] Among non-Hispanic black women, approximately one-half of females older than 40 years of age were obese, and 77 percent were overweight.[18] A socioeconomic gradient is evident, with excess weight being more common in those in a low social class and with the least education. The estimated annual health care cost of overweight and obesity is $117 billion.

Trends in Prevalence in the United States

The age-adjusted prevalence of overweight increased from 56 percent in NHANES III (1988 to 1994) to 65 percent in 1999 to 2002.[18] The prevalence of obesity (BMI ≥30.0) also increased during this period from 23 percent to 30 percent. Prevalence of extreme degrees of obesity (BMI ≥40.0) increased from 3 to 5 percent. Increases in obesity occurred for both men and women in all age groups and for all ethnicities.

Based on data from the 1999 to 2002 NHANES, the prevalence of overweight in children 6 to 11 years of age increased from 4.2 to 15.8 percent from 1963 to 1965 and in adolescents 12 to 19 years of age from 4.6 to 16.1 percent. Preschool children (2 to 5 years of age) who are overweight increased from 7 percent in 1994 to 10 percent in 2002.[18]

Lifetime Risk of Developing Overweight or Obesity

Recent data from the Framingham Heart Study indicate that at 50 years of age the lifetime risk is 1 in 2 for developing "overweight or more," 1 in 4 for obesity, and 1 in 10 for stage II obesity (BMI ≥30).[111]

Health Risks

Obesity accounts for 60 percent of cases of diabetes mellitus, and 40 percent of cases of hypertension.[29] Conversely, weight loss significantly improves CVD risk factors including lipid profile, blood pressure, blood glucose, and inflammatory markers.[112–114] In addition, obesity accounts for 20 percent of CHD and stroke in the community. Approximately 500,000 people in North America and Western Europe die from obesity-related disease every year.[3] It accounted for the loss of 33 million DALYs (2.3 percent of total) in 2000. Overall, an estimated 3 million deaths are attributed to obesity every year, a figure that will rise to 5 million by 2020.[3]

【 】 DYSLIPIDEMIA
Global Burden and Trends

It is estimated that more than 80 percent of the world population has suboptimal levels of serum cholesterol (i.e., in excess of 150 mg/dL). Excessive levels of serum cholesterol are estimated to cause 18 percent of global cerebrovascular disease (mostly nonfatal events) and 56 percent of global CHD.[3] Overall this amounts to approximately 4.4 million deaths (7.9 percent of total; Fig. 2–6) and 40.4 million DALYs (2.8 percent of total). Data from the MONICA Study demonstrate small decreases in mean cholesterol levels of the populations studied between 1979 and 1996.[33]

Burden and Trends in the United States

In the United States, the age-adjusted mean cholesterol is 5.27 mmol/L (203 mg/dL).[18] An estimated 34.5 million Americans have serum cholesterol levels of 240 mg/dL or higher, an estimated 17 percent of the adult population (see Table 2–7). An estimated 99.9 million, or one-half of the adult population, have serum cholesterol levels in excess of 200 mg/dL. Of note, approximately 10 percent of adolescents (ages 12 to 19 years) have total serum cholesterol levels exceeding 200 mg/dL.[18] The prevalence of elevated serum cholesterol level is similar in men and women and comparable across ethnicities. However, beginning at 50 years of age a higher proportion of women than men have total blood cholesterol of 200 mg/dL or higher. The mean level of LDL cholesterol for American adults age 20 years and older is 123 mg/dL. About 43 percent of men and 35.8 percent of adults have LDL cholesterol levels in excess of 130 mg/dL. Values of HDL cholesterol of less than 40 mg/dL are considered low. About 33.6 percent of men and 12.6 percent of women have values below this threshold. The prevalence of a low HDL cholesterol value is slightly lower in black women relative to white and Hispanic females.

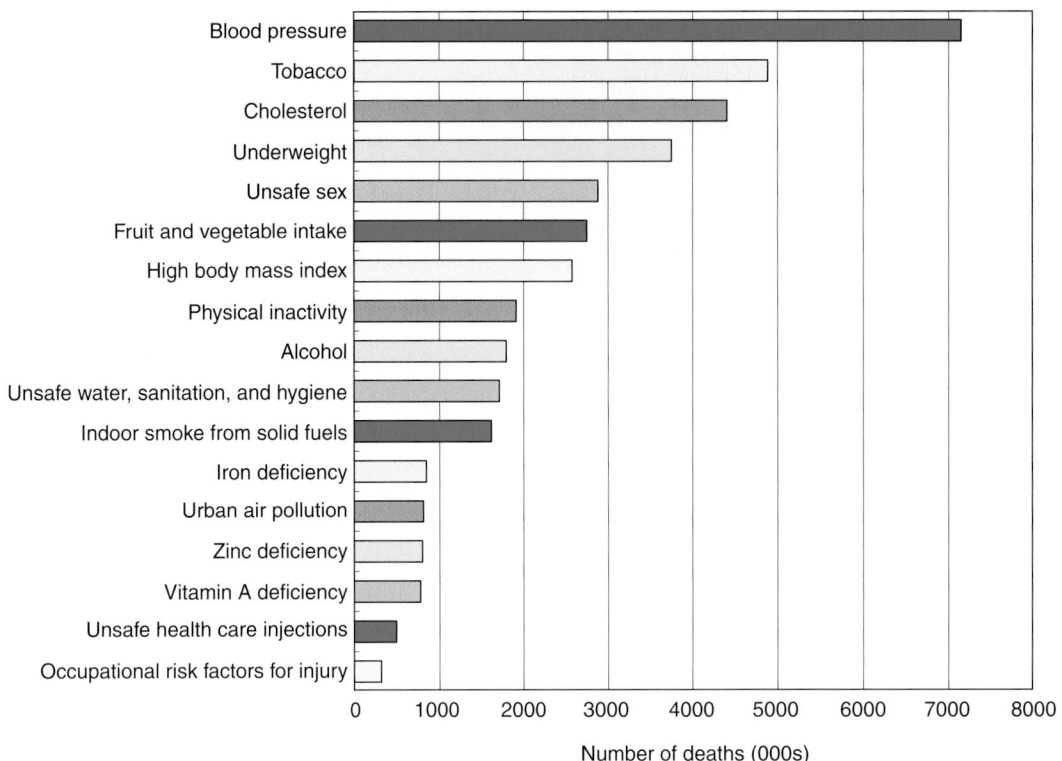

FIGURE 2–6. Contribution of select risk factors to global mortality.

Trends in the United States

Serial NHANES surveys I to III have demonstrated a sequential decrease in the percentage of individuals with elevated serum cholesterol levels. This observation is consistent across all ethnicities, both sexes, and in all educational strata. These data suggest a change in population determinants of serum cholesterol levels in the United States, such as the dietary content of saturated fats, despite the increase in the prevalence of overweight noted across the surveys. After NHANES III, decline in serum cholesterol levels has been limited. Between NHANES III and NHANES 1999 to 2002, the age-adjusted mean total cholesterol concentration decreased marginally from 5.31 mmol/L (206 mg/dL) in NHANES III to 5.27 mmol/L (203 mg/dL) in NHANES 1999 to 2000.[18]

Awareness, Treatment, and Control in the United States

In the United States awareness, treatment, and control levels for hypercholesterolemia mirror the suboptimal patterns observed with hypertension. In the NHANES investigation between 1999 and 2002, among participants who had a total cholesterol concentration ≥5.2 mmol/L (200 mg/dL) or who reported using cholesterol-lowering medications, only 63.3 percent reported awareness that they had hypercholesterolemia. Women, blacks, and Mexican-Americans were less likely to be aware of hypercholesterolemia.[18]

[ ] DIABETES MELLITUS
Global Burden

An estimated 170 million people are affected by diabetes—the majority by type II diabetes.[115] Two-thirds of these individuals live in the de-

veloping world. The top 10 countries, in terms of absolute numbers of individuals with the condition, are India, China, United States, Indonesia, Japan, Pakistan, Russia, Brazil, Italy, and Bangladesh.

Global Trends

The prevalence of diabetes worldwide is increasing at an alarming rate. The prevalence of diabetes in adults globally was estimated to be 4.0 percent in 1995 and was projected to rise to 5.4 percent by the year 2025. The number of adults with diabetes in the world was 30 million in 1985 and is projected to double from 135 million in 1995 to 360 million in 2030.[116] The proportional rise projected by 2030 is much larger in developing countries where a 170 percent increase (from 84 million to 298 million) is estimated, compared to a 42 percent increase in developed countries (from 51 million to 72 million). The highest increase is projected to occur in India and China. Indeed, the prevalence of diabetes in these two countries combined will increase from 45 million in 1995 to an estimated 121 million in 2030.[116] The vast majority of people with diabetes in developing countries are likely to be between the ages of 45 and 64 years, while those in developed countries will be age 65 years or older. The main reasons for the rising epidemic of diabetes are population aging, unhealthy diets, increasing epidemics of obesity, and sedentary lifestyles.

Burden in the United States

In the United States, it is estimated that about 20.1 million people have diabetes, but only about 14.1 million have been diagnosed.[18] Approximately 1.5 million new cases of diabetes are diagnosed annually. The risk of diabetes for Hispanics and non-Hispanic blacks is about 1.5-fold to twice that for non-Hispanic whites. The median percentages with physician-diagnosed diabetes varies from 4.7 (women) to 6.2 (men) percent in whites, from 10.3 (men) to 12.6 (women) percent in non-Hispanic blacks, to 10.4 (men) to 11.3 (women) percent in Hispanics (see Table 2–7). Approximately 40 percent of U.S. adults ages 40 to 74 years (41 million people) are estimated to have pre-diabetes.[18]

Lifetime Risk in the United States

The estimated lifetime risk of developing diabetes in the United States is 32.8 percent for males and 38.5 percent for females overall, the risk being higher for Hispanic persons (45.4 percent for males and 52.5 percent for females).[117]

Trends in the United States

In the United States, the number of persons diagnosed with diabetes has increased several-fold, from 1.6 million in 1958 to 20 million in 2003. The increase has been particularly striking in the last decade; the prevalence of diabetes rose from 4.8 percent in 1994 to 7.3 percent in 2002, an increase of 54 percent. Of note, this increase preceded the introduction of the new diagnostic criteria that use a lower fasting blood sugar threshold. Increases in the prevalence of diabetes have been observed in both sexes, all ages, all ethnic groups, all education levels, and in nearly all states. Type II diabetes is increasing in frequency in young people, including children and adolescents. Similar numbers of people have impaired glucose tolerance. Data from the Framingham Study demonstrate a doubling of incidence in adults over a 30-year period starting from the 1970s.[118]

Health Risks

The number of deaths attributed to diabetes was previously estimated at just over 800,000 worldwide. However, it has long been known that the number of deaths related to diabetes is considerably underestimated. A more plausible figure is likely to be approximately 4 million deaths per year related to the presence of the disorder. This is about 9 percent of the global total mortality. Most deaths caused by diabetes are premature. Approximately 75 percent of the mortality among diabetic men and 57 percent among diabetic women are attributable to CVD. Among people with diabetes, CVD is 2 to 4 times more common; the risk of stroke is 2 to 4 times higher; and more than 60 percent have high blood pressure.[119]

【 】 METABOLIC SYNDROME
Definitions

The metabolic syndrome has been defined as the presence of three or more of the following abnormalities:[120] waist circumference ≥102 cm (40 in) in men and ≥88 cm (36 in) in women; serum triglyceride level ≥150 mg/dL (1.7 mmol/L) or treatment for elevated triglycerides; HDL cholesterol level <40 mg/dL (1.03 mmol/L) in men and <50 mg/dL (1.3 mmol/L) in women or treatment for low HDL; blood pressure ≥130/85 mmHg or treatment for elevated blood pressure; or serum glucose level ≥100 mg/dL (5.6 mmol/L) or treatment for elevated blood sugar. WHO defines the *metabolic syndrome* as the presence of diabetes, impaired glucose tolerance, impaired fasting glucose, or insulin resistance plus two or more of the following abnormalities:[121]

1. High blood pressure defined as a value ≥140/90 mmHg
2. Hyperlipidemia identified by a triglyceride concentration ≥150 mg/dL (1.695 mmol/L) and/or HDL cholesterol <35 mg/dL (0.9 mmol/L) in men and <39 mg/dL (1.0 mmol/L) in women
3. Central obesity characterized by a waist-to-hip ratio of >0.90 in men or >0.85 in women and/or BMI >30 kg/m²
4. Microalbuminuria denoted by a urinary albumin excretion rate ≥20 µg/min or an albumin-to-creatinine ratio ≥30 mg/g

More recently, the International Diabetes Federation has defined the metabolic syndrome as:[122] presence of central obesity (defined as waist circumference ≥94 cm for European men and ≥80 cm for European women, with ethnicity specific values for other groups) plus any two:

1. *Raised triglycerides,* ≥150 mg/dL (1·7 mmol/L) or specific treatment for this lipid abnormality
2. *Reduced HDL cholesterol,* <40 mg/dL (1·03 mmol/L) in men, <50 mg/dL (1·29 mmol/L) in women, or specific treatment for this lipid abnormality
3. *Raised blood pressure,* systolic ≥130 mmHg or diastolic ≥85 mmHg, or treatment of previously diagnosed hypertension
4. *Raised fasting plasma glucose,* ≥100 mg/dL (5·6 mmol/L)

Global Burden

The prevalence of the metabolic syndrome varies from 10 to 25 percent based on the criteria used, the population investigated, and the age of the sample. Prevalence increases with age and is much higher in individuals with diabetes mellitus.

Burden in the United States

There are 47 million Americans with the metabolic syndrome, with an overall age-adjusted prevalence of 24 percent.[123] Older age, postmenopausal status, higher BMI, high carbohydrate consumption, physical inactivity, and Mexican American ethnicity are key correlates of the metabolic syndrome. Prevalence increases with age exceeding 40 percent in individuals older than 65 years of age. Among different ethnicities, Mexican Americans have the highest age-adjusted prevalence of the metabolic syndrome (31.9 percent). The age-adjusted prevalence is similar for men (24.0 percent) and women (23.4 percent). However, among African Americans, women have about a 57 percent higher prevalence than do men, and among Mexican Americans, women have about a 26 percent higher prevalence than do men.[123]

Risks

The presence of the metabolic syndrome is an ominous indicator of future CVD risk.[120] In a prospective study of Finnish men, the metabolic syndrome was associated with a threefold increased risk of CHD/CVD and twofold elevated mortality relative to individuals without the syndrome.[124]

【 】 INFLAMMATION

Inflammation is a fundamental component of atherosclerosis.[125] Plasma levels of several inflammatory markers have been used as a surrogate for vascular inflammation, including that in the atherosclerotic plaque. CRP has emerged as a premier inflammatory marker. There is a paucity of data in the published literature regarding the distribution of CRP levels in developing countries.

Distribution and Determinants in the United States

The distribution of CRP (using high-sensitivity C-reactive protein [hs-CRP] assays) has been investigated in men in the NHANES 1999 to 2000 survey.[126] The median CRP concentrations were 1.6 mg/L for all men, 1.6 mg/L for white men, 1.7 mg/L for African American men, 1.5 mg/L for Mexican American men, and 1.8 mg/L for other men. Age, BMI, and smoking are other positive correlates of CRP.[126] Ethnic and racial variation in CRP levels also has been observed in Canadian samples and is not fully explained by cardiovascular risk factors.[127]

Cardiovascular Disease Risks

Plasma levels of CRP are elevated in CHD patients.[125] Plasma CRP predicts a wide variety of CVD endpoints including CHD, peripheral vascular disease, and stroke. There is an increased risk of CHD, even at levels below those indicating acute inflammation in clinical practice.[128]

Assays for hs-CRP to assess cardiovascular risk are not yet used in routine clinical practice. On the basis of the available evidence, a Centers for Disease Control and AHA workshop recommended against screening of the entire adult population for hs-CRP as a public health measure.[129] The group recommended that hs-CRP measurement appears to have its best utility when performed to detect enhanced absolute risk in persons in whom multiple risk-factor scoring indicates an intermediate 10-year CHD risk (10 to 20 percent).[130] However, the benefits of this strategy or any treatment based on this strategy remain uncertain.[130]

[ ] HOMOCYSTEINE
Distribution and Determinants

Plasma homocysteine levels show a strong inverse correlation both with dietary intake and with plasma levels of the vitamins folate, B_6, and B_{12}, all of which are essential cofactors in homocysteine metabolism.[131] A common polymorphism in the gene for methylene-tetrahydrofolate reductase appears to influence the sensitivity of homocysteine levels to folic acid deficiency.

In the NHANES III examination, plasma homocysteine levels varied according to age, sex, and ethnicity. The mean plasma homocysteine level was 21.5 percent higher in men than it was in women, 11.8 percent higher in non-Hispanic whites than it was in Mexican Americans, and 42 percent higher in persons 70 years or older as compared to individuals younger than the age of 30 years. Others have suggested that Asians may have higher plasma homocysteine levels compared to other ethnicities.[132]

Cardiovascular Disease Risks

Rare homozygous defects of the key enzyme cystathionine-β-synthase cause homocystinuria, which is associated with an up to 10-fold elevation of plasma homocysteine levels pend with premature atherosclerosis, recurrent thromboses of coronary, cerebral, or peripheral arteries and venous thrombosis. A meta-analysis calcu-

lated that each $5 \geq$ mol/L increase in the plasma homocysteine level increases the risk for CHD by approximately 15 to 25 percent.[133] Recently, the results of two large, randomized, double-blind secondary prevention trials, comparing treatment with vitamin B_{12} and/or folic acid for lowering plasma homocysteine with administration of a placebo were reported, HOPE2[134] and NORVIT.[135] These trials cast doubt on the causal link between homocysteine and CVD because, in both, treatment lowered homocysteine levels, but there was no reduction in morbidity or mortality. At present, there is insufficient evidence to recommend measuring homocysteine levels in the general population.[136] Homocysteine levels should be measured in patients with a history of premature coronary artery disease and/or stroke who do not have classic risk factors. It should also be determined in individuals with a history of venous thromboembolism.[136]

GLOBAL BURDEN OF CARDIOVASCULAR DISEASE: GLOBAL RESPONSES TO THE EPIDEMIC

[ ] FUTURE CHALLENGES AND OPPORTUNITIES

Organized efforts at CVD prevention began in high-income countries when the epidemic had peaked, and they have helped accelerate a secular downswing in CVD. The efforts in low- and middle-income countries are starting when the epidemic is still on its upswing. Strategies to control CVD internationally must be based on recognition of global similarities and differences. Principles of prevention must be based on the evidence gathered in high-income countries, but the interventions must be context-specific and resource sensitive.

General Principles of Primary and Secondary Prevention

1. Classic risk factors (i.e., smoking, dyslipidemia, elevated blood pressure, and hyperglycemia/diabetes mellitus) account for more than 75 percent of CVD. For each of these variables, CVD risk operates across a continuum (Table 2–8, Fig. 2–7).[23,24] Indeed, CVD is rare when none of these risk factors are present.[25]

2. CVD risk factors are pathogenetically interrelated and frequently cluster in individuals. For instance, physical inactivity predisposes to the development of obesity, which further exacerbates tendencies toward sedentary lifestyle, and contributes to the development of a host of other risk factors.

3. Many more events arise from the *moderate* middle of the distribution than from the *high-risk* tail. CVD risk is increased when risk factors coexist.[22]

4. *Comprehensive* or *absolute* CVD risk is the best guide for individual interventions, whereas *population-attributable risk* should guide mass interventions, maximizing benefits by bringing about modest distributional shifts. Risk scores have been formulated to assess the absolute risk of developing CVD events.[22,28] It is important to note that although qualitatively the same set of risk factors determine CVD risks in different populations, there are quantitative differences in the relative importance of select risk factors, the relative risks associated with them, and the absolute risks.[27,137] Risk scores, therefore,

TABLE 2–8

Global Burden of Suboptimal Blood Pressure and Serum Cholesterol

	AFR	AMR	EUR	SEAR	WPR	EMR	WORLD
BLOOD PRESSURE							
Mean SBP, mm Hg	129–133	127–128	135–138	125–128	124–133	131–133	128
% SBP >115	>70	>70	>80	>60	>60	>70	>70
% CV burden caused by suboptimal BP HLY	50–58	44–53	51–66	44–55	53–56	55–58	50
CHOLESTEROL							
Mean, mmol/L	4.8	5.1–5.3	5.1–6.0	4.7–5.1	4.6–5.2	5.0	5.0
% >3.8 mmol/L (150 mg/dL)	>80	>80	>80	>80	>70	>80	>80
% CV burden caused by suboptimal cholesterol	24	26–39	32–48	24–40	19–28	37–38	31

AFR, Africa; AMR, America; BP, blood pressure; CV, cardiovascular; EMR, Eastern Mediterranean Region; EUR, Europe; HTN, hypertension; SEAR, South East Asia Region; SBP, systolic blood pressure; WPR, Western Pacific Region.
1mmol/L = 38.7 mg/dL

Source: World Health Organization. The World Health Report 2002: Reducing Risks, Promoting Healthy Life. Geneva: WHO; 2002.

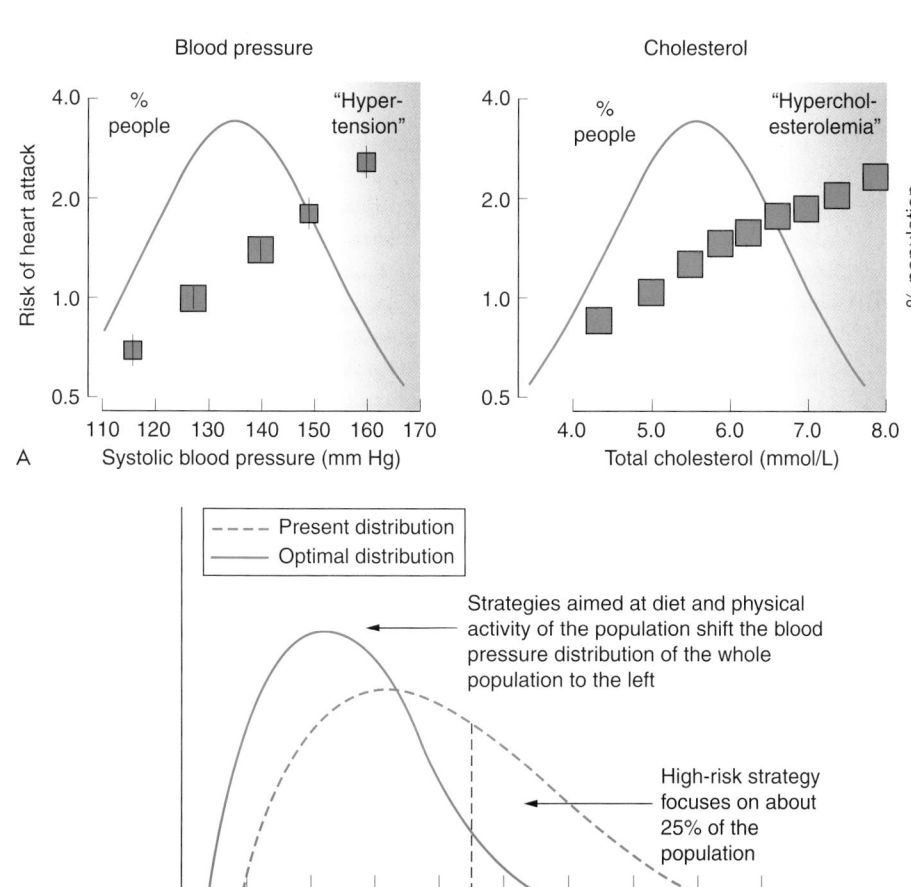

FIGURE 2–7. A. Risk factors and coronary heart disease risk. **B.** Complementary approaches to risk reduction.

have to be recalibrated based on CVD rates of the indigenous population.

5. CVD risk factors evolve in childhood and adolescence so that a synergistically complementary blend of cost-effective *population-wide* and high-risk interventions must extend to the pediatric age group too.

6. Epidemiologic principles dictate that compared with intensive individual treatment of high-risk patients, small improvements in the overall distribution of risk in a population will yield larger gains in disease reduction, when the underlying conditions that confer risk are widespread in the population (see Fig. 2–7). Hence, at a population level primary prevention must be combined in children, and adults free of disease must be combined with secondary prevention in older adults.

Importance of Primordial Prevention

An emerging concept in CVD prevention is a focus on primordial prevention, which proposes strategies to prevent the emergence of risk factors.[138] Primary and secondary prevention strategies intervene at the stage when atherosclerosis is established.[138] Attention to the prevention of the emergence of risk factors is critical, because secular trend data suggest both optimistic and pessimistic developments. For instance in the Minnesota Heart Study from 1980 through 1982 to 1995 through 1997 there were improvements in prevalence of hypertension, cigarette smoking, and dietary fat consumption. However, mirroring national data there was a plateau in lipid levels and less favorable trends in adiposity and physical activity.[139]

It must be emphasized that primordial prevention is not a theoretical objective. Work from several cohort studies suggest that maintenance of optimal risk factor status results in significantly decreased relative risk (rate ratio [RR] 0.15 to 0.60) of CVD mortality and an average gain in life expectancy of 5.8 to 9.5 years.[25] Unfortunately, only 5 to 10 percent of individuals screened were in the low-risk subgroup defined as having a serum cholesterol level <200 mg/dL (5.17 mmol/L), blood pressure ≥120/80, no diabetes or MI, or did not smoke cigarettes.[25] Furthermore, research increasingly demonstrates that the emergence of risk factors can be prevented. For instance, the Diabetes Prevention Program randomized individuals at risk for diabetes to a lifestyle (7 percent weight loss and 150 minutes physical activity per week), metformin, or placebo.[112] The incidence of diabetes was reduced 58 percent by lifestyle intervention and 31 percent by medication—to prevent 1 case of diabetes over 3 years only 7 persons would have to participate in the lifestyle-intervention program.[112] Similar approaches are advocated and efficacious for the prevention of hypertension.

Global Efforts for Cardiovascular Disease Prevention

WHO and several international organizations have commenced a series of measures and investigations to stem the rising burden of global CVD. Several of these efforts are summarized in Table 2–9.[2,140–145]

The World Health Report (WHR) 2002 identifies 5 important risk factors for noncommunicable disease in the top 10 leading risks to health (see Fig. 2–6).[3] These are raised blood pressure, raised cholesterol level, tobacco use, alcohol consumption, and overweight. The disease burden caused by these leading risk factors is global. In every region of the world, including the poorest, raised blood pressure, cholesterol, and tobacco use are causing serious disease and untimely deaths.[3]

The WHR 2002 underscores the fact that blood pressure alone causes approximately 50 percent of CVD worldwide (see Table 2–7).[3] Cholesterol causes approximately one-third of CVD (see Table 2–7). Inactive lifestyles, tobacco use, and low fruit and vegetable intake account for 20 percent each. Overall, approximately 75 percent of CVD can be attributed to the established risks assessed in the report, far higher than the one-third to one-half commonly thought.[3] The CVD burden is equally shared among men and women. A fundamental message of the WHR 2002 is that more than 50 percent of deaths and disability from CVD can be avoided by a combination of simple, cost-effective, national efforts and individual actions to reduce the major risk factors, such as high blood pressure, high cholesterol, obesity, and smoking.[3]

Because the causes of CVD are multifactorial, it follows that the response needs to be multifaceted and multi-institutional.[3] The evidence is overwhelming that prevention is possible when sustained actions are directed both at individuals and families, as well as the broader social, economic, and cultural determinants of CVD. The WHR 2002 also urges countries to adopt policies and programs to promote population-wide interventions such as reducing salt in processed foods, cutting dietary fat, encouraging exercise and higher consumption of fruits and vegetables, and limiting smoking. However, primary prevention must be complemented by secondary prevention.[3] Demographic and epidemiologic changes have steeply increased the need for long-term care of people of all ages suffering from CVD. Fortunately, large randomized clinical trials have established the efficacy of antiplatelet agents, β blockers, angiotensin-converting enzyme inhibitors, diuretics, and statins in the primary and secondary prevention of CVD.[113] Cost-effective pharmacologic treatments for risk factors such as high blood pressure, diabetes, and raised cholesterol levels have lifesaving impacts and should be routinely implemented at the primary health care level. The WHR 2002 shows that countries in all epidemiologic settings will achieve major additional reductions in the disease burden by treating people identified to be at risk. Dietary, physical activity, and smoking cessation programs should also be integral to the management of these diseases. Ensuring good health demands a *life-course* approach to eating and physical activity that begins with prepregnancy, includes breast-feeding, and extends to old age.[3] WHO has also formulated the CVD-Risk Management Package, which is designed to select and target high-risk patients in different countries with varying availability of resources.[140]

CARDIOVASCULAR DISEASE PREVENTION IN THE UNITED STATES: CHALLENGE OF ETHNIC DISPARITIES

Numerous studies have unequivocally documented the existence of profound ethnic disparities in CVD care and outcome in the United States. Ethnic minorities, particularly African Americans, experience excess CVD morbidity and mortality and receive less diagnostic and therapeutic interventions than do their white counterparts.[21] For instance, since the 1980s CHD mortality has declined more slowly in black men and women than it did in their white counterparts. Disparities in cardiac testing and treatment have also been documented (see the review in the Kaiser Family Foundation and American College of Cardiology Report).[146] From 1984 to 2001, 84 percent of the 81 studies reviewed observed ethnic disparities in care for at least one minority group.[146] African Americans have been the most intensively investigated minority group; the vast majority of studies find that African Americans are less likely to undergo diagnostic catheterization (odds ratios 0.23 to 0.85), percutaneous transluminal coronary angioplasty (odds ratios 0.20 to 0.87), coronary artery bypass graft (odds ratios 0.26 to 0.68), and thrombolytic therapy (odds ratios 0.51 to 0.76). The report concludes that these disparities persist after controlling for clinical and socioeconomic factors.[146]

CONCLUSION

CVD has no geographic, gender, or socioeconomic boundaries. The global burden of disease as a result of CVD is rising, principally because of a sharp rise in the developing countries that are

◖ **TABLE 2–9**

Global Efforts to Prevent Cardiovascular Disease

KEY REPORTS/ PROGRAMS	ESSENTIAL FEATURES
The IOM Report, 1998[145]	• U.S. National Academy of Sciences recommendations on the control of international CVD • Research to fully determine the magnitude of CVD in developing countries, the development of targeted primary prevention strategies, reduction in tobacco use, control of hypertension, access to low-cost drugs, and the development of affordable clinical care algorithms • Build capacity to conduct research and development activities • Develop institutional frameworks that facilitate CVD prevention and control
World Heart Forum	• International coalition to confront global cardiovascular issues (AHA is founding member) • Conduct research to better understand the epidemiology of CVD in various regions of the world and to more accurately track its toll in terms of death, disability, and healthcare costs • Develop prevention guidelines to identify common principles for lowering CVD risk, while at the same time provide flexibility to address regional differences (e.g., it is expected that, in some countries or regions of the world, tobacco use and hypertension may take precedence, whereas cholesterol reduction or weight control are of primary importance in others) • Develop programs to assist medical schools in establishing core curricula, which focus on the prevention of CVD • Institute advocacy initiatives that address regional issues of tobacco, exercise, nutrition, and access to care
CVD Research Initiative[142]	• Joint program of WHO and the Global Forum for Health Research • Initiative has developed six multicenter collaborative research projects on capacity assessment, surveillance, community-based interventions, clinical management, and global information networks
WHO Programs for Disease Surveillance (STEPS)	• Based on the concept that CVD surveillance systems need to be simple, focusing on a minimum number of risk factors that predict disease—before placing too much emphasis on costly disease registries that are difficult to sustain long-term • Step 1 gathers information on risk factors by questionnaires. This includes information on sociodemographic features, tobacco use, alcohol consumption, physical inactivity, and fruit/vegetable intake. • Step 2 includes objective data by simple physical measurements needed to examine risk factors that are physiologic attributes of the human body. These are height, weight, and waist circumference (for obesity) and blood pressure. • Step 3 carries the objective measurements of physiologic attributes one step further with the inclusion of blood samples for measuring lipid and glucose levels. • STEPS is now being planned or implemented in 33 countries.
WHO Programs for CHOosing Interventions that are Cost-Effective (CHOICE)	• First-ever system of identifying and reporting cost-effective health interventions consistently across settings • These interventions can be implemented on an a la carte basis, depending on each country's individual circumstances • CHOICE options are contained in a new statistical database that is also a part of the World Health Report 2002.
INTER-HEART[142]	• Global case-control study that seeks to understand the importance of both traditional and emerging risk factors for acute myocardial infarction. • Findings will be relevant for developing health policies that can be applied to different countries and ethnic groups.
CARMEN[141]	• The Pan American Health Organization (PAHO) is promoting CARMEN (Spanish acronym for: actions for the multifactorial reduction of noncommunicable diseases) as a general framework for the prevention and control of noncommunicable diseases, particularly CVD, in the Americas by coordinating health promotion and disease prevention activities in communities and community health services. • This model includes the identification of risk factors, regional surveillance using a common methodology, early detection of cases, delivery of comprehensive and long-term care, and more active participation of all members of the health team and the community. • Management of hypertension and diabetes are particularly important in the model.

(continued)

TABLE 2–9

Global Efforts to Prevent Cardiovascular Disease *(continued)*

KEY REPORTS/ PROGRAMS	ESSENTIAL FEATURES
CINDI[141]	• In Europe, the Countrywide Integrated Noncommunicable Diseases Intervention (CINDI) program aims to reduce modifiable risk factors, such as smoking and high blood pressure, by integrating health promotion and disease prevention; at present, 27 countries participate. • Two other programs also aim to improve the quality of life of people with CVD: (1.) The Helsingborg Declaration on stroke management. (2.) The second program is a pilot project aimed at improving the education skills of general practitioners by showing them how to educate coronary heart disease patients about improving the quality of their lives, and how rehabilitation and secondary prevention can be improved.
Prevention of Recurrences of Myocardial Infarction and Stroke Study (PREMISE)	• The PREMISE is a joint WHO-Welcome trust program aimed at using community and health services-based interventions to prevent recurrences of CVD.
SHARE[144]	• Investigators at the McMaster University have just completed SHARE (Study of Health Assessment and Risk in Ethnic groups), in which atherosclerosis, clinical CVD, and traditional and emerging risk factors were measured in 997 randomly chosen individuals of 3 ethnic groups (South Asian, Chinese, and European Canadian). • Preliminary data indicate marked differences in lipid profile, glucose abnormalities, coagulation parameters, and homocysteine levels between the three groups. Although within each ethnic group the degree of carotid atherosclerosis predicted clinical CVD, the relationship varied (steepest among South Asians, least steep among Chinese, intermediate among European Canadians).

AHA, American Heart Association; CVD, cardiovascular disease; WHO, World Health Organization.
Source: Adapted in part from World Health Organization. The World Health Report 2002: Reducing Risks, Promoting Healthy Life. Geneva: WHO; 2002. Available at www.who.int/cardiovascular_diseases/region/en/.

experiencing rapid health transition. Contributory causes include the aging of the world population, lifestyle changes caused by urbanization, progressive industrialization, and burgeoning globalization, probable effects of fetal undernutrition on adult susceptibility to vascular disease, and possible gene–environment interactions influencing ethnic disparities. Altered diets and diminished physical activity are critical factors contributing to the acceleration of CVD epidemics, along with tobacco use. The prevalence of risk factors for CVD, however, varies across developing regions with consequent variations in the burden of CVD. The CVD epidemic in developing countries differs from that observed in developed countries in the last century by virtue of its rapidity, occurrence in a milieu of limited health care infrastructure, widespread poverty, and low levels of societal education. A global public health response must integrate policies and programs that effectively impact the multiple determinants of these diseases in a resource-sensitive and context-specific manner and provide protection over the life span through primordial, primary, and secondary prevention.

REFERENCES

1. Chockalingam A, Balaguer-Vinto I, eds. *Impending Global Pandemic of Cardiovascular Diseases: Challenges and Opportunities for the Prevention and Control of Cardiovascular Diseases in Developing Countries and Economies in Transition.* World Heart Federation. Barcelona: Prous Science; 1999.
2. Bonow RO, Smaha LA, Smith SC Jr, Mensah GA, Lenfant C. World Heart Day 2002: the International Burden of Cardiovascular Disease: responding to the Emerging Global Epidemic. *Circulation.* 2002;106:1602–1605.
3. World Health Organization. *The World Health Report 2002: Reducing Risks, Promoting Healthy Life.* Geneva: WHO; 2002.
4. Omran AR. The epidemiologic transition: a key of the epidemiology of population change. *Millbank Memorial Fund Q.* 1971;49 509–538.
5. Sen K, Bonita R. Global health status: two steps forward, one step back. *Lancet.* 2000;356 577–582.
6. Popkin BM, Popkin BM, Lu B, Zhai F. Understanding the nutrition transition: measuring rapid dietary changes in transitional countries. *Public Health Nutr.* 2002;5:947–953.
7. Chopra M, Galbraith S, Darnton-Hill I. A global response to a global problem: the epidemic of overnutrition. *Bull World Health Organ.* 2002;80:952–958.
8. Reddy KS, Yusuf S. Emerging epidemic of cardiovascular disease in developing countries. *Circulation.* 1998;97:596–601.
9. Reddy KS. Cardiovascular diseases in the developing countries: dimensions, determinants, dynamics and directions for public health action. *Public Health Nutr.* 2002;5:231–237.
10. Murray CJ, Lopez AD. *The Global Burden of Disease: A Comprehensive Assessment of Mortality and Disability From Disease, Injuries and Risk Factors in 1990 and Projected to 2020.* Cambridge, MA: Harvard School of Public Health; 1996.
11. World Health Organization. *The World Health Report 2000: Health Systems: Improving Performance.* Geneva: WHO; 2000.
12. Murray CJ, Lopez AD. *Global Health Statistics.* Cambridge: Harvard University Press; 1996.
13. Murray CJ, Lopez AD, Mathers CD, Stein C. The global burden of disease 2000 project: aims, methods and data sources. Geneva: WHO; 2001. GPE Discussion Paper No. 36.
14. World Health Organization. World Health Statistics 2006:1–80. Available at: http://www.who.int/whosis/whostat2006.pdf. Accessed August 15, 2006.

15. American Heart Association. International Cardiovascular Disease Statistics, 2006. Available at: http://www.americanheart.org/downloadable/heart/1140811583642InternationalCVD.pdf. Accessed August 15, 2006.

16. Barker DJP. Fetal origins of coronary heart disease. *BMJ*. 1995;311:171.

17. Mackay J, Mensah GA, eds. *The Atlas of Heart Disease and Stroke*. Available at: http://www.who.int/cardiovascular_diseases/resources/atlas/en/index.html. Accessed August 15, 2006.

18. Thom T, Haase N, Rosamond W, Howard VJ, Rumsfeld J, Manolio T, et al, and members of the Statistics Committee and Stroke Statistics Subcommittee et al. Heart disease and stroke statistics—2006 update: a report from the American Heart Association Statistics Committee and Stroke Statistics Subcommittee. *Circulation*. 2006;113:e85–151.

19. Lloyd-Jones DM, Leip EP, Larson MG, D'Agostino RB, Beiser A, Wilson PWF, et al. Prediction of lifetime risk for cardiovascular disease by risk factor burden at 50 years of age. *Circulation*. 2006;113:791–798.

20. CDC. Decline in Deaths from Heart Disease and Stroke—United States, 1900–1999. *JAMA*. 1999;282:724.

21. Cooper R, Cutler J, Desvigne-Nickens P, Fortmann SP, Friedman L, Havlik R, et al. Trends and disparities in coronary heart disease, stroke, and other cardiovascular diseases in the United States: findings of the National Conference on Cardiovascular Disease Prevention. *Circulation*. 2000;102:3137.

22. Grundy SM, D'Agostino S, Mosca L, Burke GL, Wilson PWF, Rader DJ, et al. Cardiovascular risk assessment based on U.S. cohort studies: findings from a national heart, lung, and blood institute workshop. *Circulation*. 2001;104:491.

23. MacMahon S, Peto R, Cutler J, Collins R, Sorlie P, Neaton J, et al. Blood pressure, stroke, and coronary heart disease. Part 1, Prolonged differences in blood pressure: prospective observational studies corrected for the regression dilution bias. *Lancet*. 1990;335:765–774.

24. Magnus P, Beaglehole R. The real contribution of the major risk factors to the coronary epidemics: time to end the "only-50%" myth. *Arch Intern Med*. 2001;161:2657.

25. Stamler J, Stamler R, Neaton JD, Wentworth D, Daviglus ML, Garside D, et al. Low risk-factor profile and long-term cardiovascular and noncardiovascular mortality and life expectancy: findings for 5 large cohorts of young adult and middle-aged men and women. *JAMA*. 1999;282:2012.

26. Tunstall-Pedoe H, Woodward M, Tavendale R, Brook RA, McCluskey MK. Comparison of the prediction by 27 different factors of coronary heart disease and death in men and women of the Scottish heart health study: cohort study. *BMJ*. 1997;315:722–729.

27. van den Hoogen PC, Feskens EJ, Nagelkerke NJ, Menotti A, Nissinen A, Kromhout D. The relation between blood pressure and mortality due to coronary heart disease among men in different parts of the world. Seven Countries Study Research Group. *N Engl J Med*. 2000;342:1–8.

28. Wilson PW, D'Agostino RB, Levy D, Belanger AM, Silbershatz H, Kannel WB. Prediction of coronary heart disease using risk factor categories. *Circulation*. 1998;97:1837–1847.

29. Wilson PW, D'Agostino RB, Sullivan L, Parise H, Kannel WB. Overweight and obesity as determinants of cardiovascular risk: the Framingham experience. *Arch Intern Med*. 2002;162:1867–1872.

30. Durrington PN, Prais H. Methods for the prediction of coronary heart disease risk. *Heart*. 2001;85:489–490.

31. Vasan RS, Sullivan LM, Wilson PWF, Sempos CT, Sundstrom J, Kannel WB, et al. Relative importance of borderline and elevated levels of coronary heart disease risk factors. *Ann Intern Med*. 2005;142:393–402.

32. World Health Organization MONICA Project Principal Investigators. Monitoring trends and determinants in cardiovascular disease: a major international collaboration. *J Clin Epidemiol*. 41 105–114. 1988.

33. Evans A, Tolonen H, Hense HW, Ferrario M, Sans S, Kuulasmaa K. Trends in coronary risk factors in the WHO MONICA Project. *Int J Epidemiol*. 2001;30:35S.

34. Kuulasmaa K, Tunstall-Pedoe H, Dobson A, Fortmann S, Sans S, Tolonen H, et al, for the WHO MONICA Project. Estimation of contribution of changes in classic risk factors to trends in coronary-event rates across the WHO MONICA project populations. *Lancet*. 2000;355:675–687.

35. Tunstall-Pedoe H, Vanuzzo D, Hobbs M, Mahonen M, Cepaitis Z, Kuulasmaa K, et al, for the WHO MONICA Project. Estimation of contribution of changes in coronary care to improving survival, event rates, and coronary heart disease mortality across the WHO MONICA Project populations. *Lancet*. 2000;355:688–700.

36. Yusuf S, Reddy S, Ounpuu S, Anand S. Global burden of cardiovascular diseases: Part I. General Considerations, the Epidemiologic Transition, Risk Factors, and Impact of Urbanization. *Circulation*. 2001;104:2746–2753.

37. Sheifer SE, Manolio TA, Gersh BJ. Unrecognized myocardial infarction. *Ann Intern Med*. 2001;135:801–811.

38. Lloyd-Jones DM, Larson MG, Beiser A, Levy D. Lifetime risk of developing coronary heart disease. *Lancet*. 1999;353:89–92.

39. Fox CS, Evans JC, Larson MG, Kannel WB, Levy D. Temporal trends in coronary heart disease mortality and sudden cardiac death from 1950 to 1999: the Framingham Heart Study. *Circulation*. 2004;110:522–527.

40. Goldstein LB, Adams R, Becker K, Furberg CD, Gorelick PB, Hademenos G, et al. Primary prevention of ischemic stroke: a statement for healthcare professionals from the Stroke Council of the American Heart Association. *Stroke*. 2001;32:280.

41. D'Agostino RB, Wolf PA, Belanger AJ, Kannel WB. Stroke risk profile: adjustment for antihypertensive medication. The Framingham Study. *Stroke*. 1994;25:40–43.

42. Tolonen H, Mahonen M, Asplund K, Rastenyte D, Kuulasmaa K, Vanuzzo D, et al. Do trends in population levels of blood pressure and other cardiovascular risk factors explain trends in stroke event rates? Comparisons of 15 populations in 9 countries within the WHO MONICA Stroke Project. *Stroke*. 2002;33:2367.

43. Seshadri S, Beiser A, Kelly-Hayes M, Kase CS, Au R, Kannel WB, et al. The lifetime risk of stroke: estimates from the Framingham Study. *Stroke*. 2006;37:345–350.

44. Kenchaiah S, Narula J, Vasan RS. Risk factors for heart failure. *Med Clin North Am*. 2004;88:1145–1172.

45. Levy D, Larson MG, Vasan RS, Kannel WB, Ho KK. The progression from hypertension to congestive heart failure. *JAMA*. 1996;275:1557–1562.

46. Kannel WB, D'Agostino RB, Silbershatz H, Belanger AJ, Wilson PW, Levy D. Profile for estimating risk of heart failure. *Arch Intern Med* 1999;159:1197–1204.

47. McMurray JJ, Petrie MC, Murdoch DR, Davie AP. Clinical epidemiology of heart failure: public and private health burden. *Eur Heart J*. 1998;19(suppl P):9–16.

48. Bonneux L, Barendregt JJ, Meeter K, Bonsel GJ, Van Der Maas PJ. Estimating clinical morbidity due to ischemic heart disease and congestive heart failure: the future rise of heart failure. *Am J Public Health*. 1994;84:20–28.

49. Levy D, Kenchaiah S, Larson MG, Benjamin EJ, Kupka MJ, Ho KKL, et al. Long-Term trends in the incidence of and survival with heart failure. *N Engl J Med*. 2002;347:1397.

50. Yancy CW. Heart failure in African Americans. *Am J Cardiol*. 2005;96:3–12.

51. Bhatia RS, Tu JV, Lee DS, Austin PC, Fang J, Haouzi A, et al. Outcome of heart failure with preserved ejection fraction in a population-based study. *N Engl J Med*. 2006;355:260–269.

52. Owan TE, Hodge DO, Herges RM, Jacobsen SJ, Roger VL, Redfield MM. Trends in prevalence and outcome of heart failure with preserved ejection fraction. *N Engl J Med*. 2006;355:251–259.

53. Vasan RS, Benjamin EJ, Levy D. Prevalence, clinical features and prognosis of diastolic heart failure: an epidemiologic perspective. *J Am Coll Cardiol*. 1995;26:1565–1574.

54. Vasan RS, Larson MG, Benjamin EJ, Evans JC, Reiss CK, Levy D. Congestive heart failure in subjects with normal versus reduced left ventricular ejection fraction: prevalence and mortality in a population-based cohort. *J Am Coll Cardiol*. 1999;33:1948–1955.

55. Lloyd-Jones DM, Larson MG, Leip EP, Beiser A, D'Agostino RB, Kannel WB, et al. Lifetime risk for developing congestive heart failure: the Framingham Heart Study. *Circulation*. 2002;106:3068–3072.

56. Stewart S, Hart CL, Hole DJ, McMurray JJV. Population prevalence, incidence, and predictors of atrial fibrillation in the Renfrew/Paisley Study. *Heart*. 2001;86:516–521.

57. Wang TJ, Parise H, Levy D, D'Agostino RB Sr, Wolf PA, Vasan RS, et al. Obesity and the risk of new-onset atrial fibrillation. *JAMA*. 2004;292:2471–2477.

58. Mukamal KJ, Tolstrup JS, Friberg J, Jensen G, Gronbaek M. Alcohol consumption and risk of atrial fibrillation in men and women: the Copenhagen City Heart Study. *Circulation*. 2005;112:1736–1742.

59. Cappola AR, Fried LP, Arnold AM, Danese MD, Kuller LH, Burke GL, et al. Thyroid status, cardiovascular risk, and mortality in older adults. *JAMA*. 2006;295:1033–1041.

60. Aviles RJ, Martin DO, Apperson-Hansen C, Houghtaling PL, Rautaharju P, Kronmal RA, Tracy RP, et al. Inflammation as a risk factor for atrial fibrillation. *Circulation*. 2003;108:3006–3010.

61. Wang TJ, Larson MG, Levy D, Benjamin EJ, Leip EP, Omland T, et al. Plasma natriuretic peptide levels and the risk of cardiovascular events and death. *N Engl J Med*. 2004;350:655–663.

62. Arnar DO, Thorvaldsson S, Manolio TA, Thorgeirsson G, Kristjansson K, Hakonarson H, et al. Familial aggregation of atrial fibrillation in Iceland. *Eur Heart J.* 2006;27:708–712.
63. Gollob MH, Jones DL, Krahn AD, Danis L, Gong XQ, Shao Q, et al. Somatic mutations in the connexin 40 gene (GJA5) in atrial fibrillation. *N Engl J Med.* 2006;354:2677–2688.
64. Olson TM, Michels VV, Ballew JD, Reyna SP, Karst ML, Herron KJ, et al. Sodium channel mutations and susceptibility to heart failure and atrial fibrillation. *JAMA.* 2005;293:447–454.
65. Shatoor AS, Ahmed ME, Said MA, Shabbir K, Cheema A, Kardash MO. Patterns of atrial fibrillation at a regional hospital in Saudi Arabia. *Ethn Dis.* 1998;8:360–366.
66. Ryder KM, Benjamin EJ. Epidemiology and significance of atrial fibrillation. *Am J Cardiol.* 1999;84:131R-138R.
67. Heeringa J, van der Kuip DAM, Hofman A, Kors JA, van Herpen G, Stricker BHC, et al. Prevalence, incidence and lifetime risk of atrial fibrillation: the Rotterdam study. *Eur Heart J.* 2006;27:949–953.
68. Go AS, Hylek EM, Phillips KA, Chang Y, Henault LE, Selby JV, et al. Prevalence of diagnosed atrial fibrillation in adults: national implications for rhythm management and stroke prevention: the Anticoagulation and Risk Factors in Atrial Fibrillation (ATRIA) Study. *JAMA.* 2001;285:2370–2375.
69. Psaty BM, Manolio TA, Kuller LH, Kronmal RA, Cushman M, Fried LP, et al. Incidence of and risk factors for atrial fibrillation in older adults. *Circulation.* 1997;96:2455.
70. Levy S, Maarek M, Coumel P, Guize L, Lekieffre J, Medvedowsky JL, et al. Characterization of different subsets of atrial fibrillation in general practice in France: the ALFA Study. *Circulation.* 1999;99:3028.
71. Miyasaka Y, Barnes ME, Gersh BJ, Cha SS, Bailey KR, Abhayaratna WP, et al. Secular trends in incidence of atrial fibrillation in Olmsted County, Minnesota, 1980 to 2000, and implications on the projections for future prevalence. *Circulation.* 2006;114:119–125.
72. Benjamin EJ, Levy D, Vaziri SM, D'Agostino RB, Belanger AJ, Wolf PA. Independent risk factors for atrial fibrillation in a population-based cohort. The Framingham Heart Study. *JAMA.* 1994;271:840–844.
73. Lloyd-Jones DM, Wang TJ, Leip EP, Larson MG, Levy D, Vasan RS, et al. Lifetime risk for development of atrial fibrillation: the Framingham Heart Study. *Circulation.* 2004;110:1042–1046.
74. Wolf PA, Abbott RD, Kannel WB. Atrial fibrillation as an independent risk factor for stroke: the Framingham Study. *Stroke.* 1991;22:983–988.
75. Nakayama T, Date C, Yokoyama T, Yoshiike N, Yamaguchi M, Tanaka H. A 15.5-year follow-up study of stroke in a Japanese provincial city: the Shibata Study. *Stroke.* 1997;28:45.
76. Krahn AD, Manfreda J, Tate RB, Mathewson FAL, Cuddy TE. The natural history of atrial fibrillation: incidence, risk factors, and prognosis in the Manitoba Follow-Up Study. *Am J Med.* 1995;98:476–484.
77. Stewart S, Hart CL, Hole DJ, McMurray JJV. A population-based study of the long-term risks associated with atrial fibrillation: 20-year follow-up of the Renfrew/Paisley study. *Am J Med.* 2002;113:359–364.
78. Wang TJ, Larson MG, Levy D, et al. The temporal relations of atrial fibrillation and congestive heart failure and their joint influence on mortality: the Framingham Heart Study. *Circulation.* 2003;107:2920–2925.
79. Wang TJ, Massaro JM, Levy D, et al. A risk score for predicting stroke or death in individuals with new-onset atrial fibrillation in the community: the Framingham Heart Study. *JAMA* 2003;290:1049–1056.
80. Stewart S, Murphy N, Walker A, McGuire A, McMurray JJV. Cost of an emerging epidemic: an economic analysis of atrial fibrillation in the UK. *Heart.* 2004;90:286–292.
81. Benjamin EJ, Wolf PA, D'Agostino RB, Silbershatz H, Kannel WB, Levy D. Impact of atrial fibrillation on the risk of death: the Framingham Heart Study. *Circulation.* 1998;98:946.
82. Friberg J, Scharling H, Gadsboll N, Truelsen T, Jensen GB. Comparison of the impact of atrial fibrillation on the risk of stroke and cardiovascular death in women versus men (The Copenhagen City Heart Study). *Am J Cardiol.* 2004;94:889–894.
83. Lelorier P, Humphries KH, Krahn A, Connolly SJ, Talajic M, Green M, et al. Prognostic differences between atrial fibrillation and atrial flutter. *Am J Cardiol.* 2004;93:647–649.
84. Wattigney WA, Mensah GA, Croft JB. Increased atrial fibrillation mortality: United States, 1980–1998. *Am J Epidemiol.* 2002;155:819.
85. Frost L, Vestergaard P, Mosekilde L, Mortensen LS. Trends in incidence and mortality in the hospital diagnosis of atrial fibrillation or flutter in Denmark, 1980–1999. *Int J Cardiol.* 2005;103:78–84.
86. Stewart S, MacIntyre K, Chalmers JWT, Boyd J, Finlayson A, Redpath A, et al. Trends in case-fatality in 22,968 patients admitted for the first time with atrial fibrillation in Scotland, 1986–1995. *Int J Cardiol.* 2002;82:229–236.
87. CDC. Atrial fibrillation as a contributing cause of death and Medicare hospitalization—United States, 1999. *MMWR Morb Mortal Wkly Rep.* 2003;52:128, 130–128, 131.
88. Prospective Studies Collaboration. Age-specific relevance of usual blood pressure to vascular mortality: a meta-analysis of individual data for one million adults in 61 prospective studies. *Lancet.* 2002;360:1903–1913.
89. 1999 World Health Organization-International Society of Hypertension Guidelines for the Management of Hypertension. Guidelines Subcommittee. *J Hypertens.* 1999;17:151–183.
90. Chobanian AV, Bakris GL, Black HR, Cushman WC, Green LA, Izzo JL Jr, et al. The seventh report of the Joint National Committee on Prevention, Detection, Evaluation, and Treatment of High Blood Pressure: the JNC 7 Report. *JAMA.* 2003;289.
91. Vasan RS, Larson MG, Leip EP, Kannel WB, Levy D. Assessment of frequency of progression to hypertension in non-hypertensive participants in the Framingham Heart Study: a cohort study. *Lancet.* 2001;358:1682–1686.
92. Fuentes R, Ilmaniemi N, Laurikainen E, Tuomilehto J, Nissinen A. Hypertension in developing economies: a review of population-based studies carried out from 1980 to 1998. *J Hypertens.* 2000;18:521–529.
93. Kearney PM, Whelton M, Reynolds K, Muntner P, Whelton PK, He J. Global burden of hypertension: analysis of worldwide data. *Lancet.* 2005;365:217–223.
94. Wang TJ, Vasan RS. Epidemiology of uncontrolled hypertension in the United States. *Circulation.* 2005;112:1651–1662.
95. Wolf-Maier K, Cooper RS, Banegas JR, Giampaoli S, Hense HW, Joffres M, et al. Hypertension prevalence and blood pressure levels in 6 European countries, Canada, and the United States. *JAMA.* 2003;289:2363.
96. Vasan RS, Beiser A, Seshadri S, Larson MG, Kannel WB, D'Agostino RB, et al. Residual lifetime risk for developing hypertension in middle-aged women and men: the Framingham Heart Study. *JAMA.* 2002;287:1003–1010.
97. World Health Organization. *World Health Report 1999. Making a difference.* Geneva: WHO; 1999.
98. CDC. Trends in aging—United States and worldwide. *MMWR Morb Mortal Wkly Rep.* 2003;52:101–4, 106.
99. Jha P, Ranson MK, Nguyen SN, Yach D. Estimates of global and regional smoking prevalence in 1995, by age and sex. *Am J Public Health.* 2002;92:1002.
100. Yang G, Fan L, Tan J, Qi G, Zhang Y, Samet JM, et al. Smoking in China: findings of the 1996 National Prevalence Survey. *JAMA.* 1999;282:1247.
101. Shimkhada R, Peabody JW. Tobacco control in India. *Bull World Health Organ* 2003;81:48–52.
102. Molarius A, Seidell JC, Sans S, Tuomilehto J, Kuulasmaa K. Educational level, relative body weight, and changes in their association over 10 years: an international perspective from the WHO MONICA Project. *Am J Public Health.* 2000;90:1260.
103. CDC. Prevalence of current cigarette smoking among adults and changes in prevalence of current and some day smoking—United States, 1996—2001. *MMWR Morb Mortal Wkly Rep.* 2003;52:303.
104. Niu SR, Yang GH, Chen ZM, Wang JL, Wang GH, He XZ, et al. Emerging tobacco hazards in China: 2. Early mortality results from a prospective study. *BMJ.* 1998;317:1423.
105. Peto R, Lopez AD, Boreham J, Thun M, Heath C Jr, Doll R. Mortality from smoking worldwide. *Br Med Bull.* 1996;52:12.
106. He J, Vupputuri S, Allen K, Prerost MR, Hughes J, Whelton PK. Passive smoking and the risk of coronary heart disease—a meta-analysis of epidemiologic studies. *N Engl J Med.* 1999;340:920.
107. World Health Organization. Tobacco free initiative, 2006. Available at: http://www.who.int/tobacco/en/index.html. Accessed August 15, 2006.
108. World Health Organization. WHO global strategy on diet, physical activity and health, 2006. Available at: http://www.who.int/hpr/gs.strategy.document.shtml. Accessed August 15, 2006.
109. National Institutes of Health. Clinical guidelines on the identification, evaluation, and treatment of overweight and obesity in adults. NIH Publication No. 98–4083; 1998.
110. Ebbeling CB, Pawlak DB, Ludwig DS. Childhood obesity: public-health crisis, common sense cure. *Lancet.* 2002;360:473–482.
111. Vasan RS, Pencina MJ, Cobain M, Freiberg MS, D'Agostino RB. Estimated risks for developing obesity in the Framingham Heart Study. *Ann Intern Med.* 2005;143:473–480.

112. Diabetes Prevention Program Research Group. Reduction in the incidence of type 2 diabetes with lifestyle intervention or metformin. *N Engl J Med.* 2002;346:393.

113. Ebrahim S, Smith GD. Systematic review of randomised controlled trials of multiple risk factor interventions for preventing coronary heart disease. *BMJ.* 1997;314:1666.

114. Esposito K, Pontillo A, Di Palo C, Giugliano G, Masella M, Marfella R, et al. Effect of weight loss and lifestyle changes on vascular inflammatory markers in obese women: a randomized trial. *JAMA.* 2003;289:1799.

115. Roglic G, Unwin N, Bennett PH, Mathers C, Tuomilehto J, Nag S, et al. The burden of mortality attributable to diabetes: realistic estimates for the year 2000. *Diabetes Care.* 2005;28:2130–2135.

116. Wild S, Roglic G, Green A, Sicree R, King H. Global prevalence of diabetes: estimates for the year 2000 and projections for 2030. *Diabetes Care.* 2004;27:1047–1053.

117. Narayan KMV, Boyle JP, Thompson TJ, Sorensen SW, Williamson DF. Lifetime risk for diabetes mellitus in the United States. *JAMA.* 2003;290:1884–1890.

118. Fox CS, Pencina MJ, Meigs JB, Vasan RS, Levitzky YS, D'Agostino RB Sr. Trends in the incidence of type 2 diabetes mellitus from the 1970s to the 1990s: the Framingham Heart Study. *Circulation.* 2006;113:2914–2918.

119. Asia Pacific Cohort Studies Collaboration. The effects of diabetes on the risks of major cardiovascular diseases and death in the Asia-Pacific region. *Diabetes Care.* 2003;26:360–366.

120. Grundy SM, Cleeman JI, Daniels SR, Donato KA, Eckel RH, Franklin BA, et al. Diagnosis and management of the metabolic syndrome: an American Heart Association/National Heart, Lung, and Blood Institute Scientific Statement. *Circulation.* 2005;112:2735–2752.

121. Alberti KG, Zimmet PZ. Definition, diagnosis and classification of diabetes mellitus and its complications. Part 1: diagnosis and classification of diabetes mellitus provisional report of a WHO consultation. *Diabet Med.* 1998;15:539–553.

122. International Diabetes Federation. The IDF consensus worldwide definition of the metabolic syndrome, 2006. Available at: http://www.idf.org/webdata/docs/Metac_syndrome_def.pdf. Accessed August 15, 2006.

123. Ford ES, Giles WH, Dietz WH. Prevalence of the metabolic syndrome among U.S. adults: findings from the Third National Health and Nutrition Examination Survey. *JAMA.* 2002;287:356.

124. Lakka HM, Laaksonen DE, Lakka TA, Niskanen LK, Kumpusalo E, Tuomilehto J, et al. The metabolic syndrome and total and cardiovascular disease mortality in middle-aged men. *JAMA.* 2002;288:2709.

125. Libby P, Ridker PM, Maseri A. Inflammation and atherosclerosis. *Circulation.* 2002;105:1135.

126. Ford ES, Giles WH, Myers GL, Mannino DM. Population distribution of high-sensitivity C-reactive protein among U.S. men: findings from National Health and Nutrition Examination Survey 1999–2000. *Clin Chem.* 2003;49:686.

127. Anand SS, Razak F, Yi Q, Davis B, Jacobs R, Vuksan V, et al. C-Reactive protein as a screening test for cardiovascular risk in a multiethnic population. *Arterioscler Thromb Vasc Biol.* 2004;24:1509–1515.

128. Ridker PM, Rifai N, Rose L, Buring JE, Cook NR. Comparison of C-reactive protein and low-density lipoprotein cholesterol levels in the prediction of first cardiovascular events. *N Engl J Med.* 2002;347:1557.

129. Fortmann SP, Ford E, Criqui MH, Folsom AR, Harris TB, Hong Y, et al. CDC/AHA workshop on markers of inflammation and cardiovascular disease: application to clinical and public health practice: report from the Population Science Discussion Group. *Circulation.* 2004;110:e554-e559.

130. Smith SC Jr, Anderson JL, Cannon RO, III, Fadl YY, Koenig W, Libby P, et al. CDC/AHA workshop on markers of inflammation and cardiovascular disease: application to clinical and public health practice: report from the Clinical Practice Discussion Group. *Circulation.* 2004;110:e550-e553.

131. Ganji V, Kafai MR. Demographic, health, lifestyle, and blood vitamin determinants of serum total homocysteine concentrations in the third National Health and Nutrition Examination Survey, 1988–1994. *Am J Clin Nutr.* 2003;77:826.

132. Chandalia M, Abate N, Cabo-Chan AV Jr, Devaraj S, Jialal I, Grundy SM. Hyperhomocysteinemia in Asian Indians living in the United States. *J Clin Endocrinol Metab.* 2003;88:1089.

133. Homocysteine Studies Collaboration. Homocysteine and risk of ischemic heart disease and stroke: a meta-analysis. *JAMA.* 2002;288:2015.

134. The Heart Outcomes Prevention Evaluation (HOPE). Homocysteine lowering with folic acid and B vitamins in vascular disease. *N Engl J Med.* 2006;354:1567–1577.

135. Bonaa KH, Njolstad I, Ueland PM, et al, for the NORVIT Trial Investigators. Homocysteine lowering and cardiovascular events after acute myocardial infarction. *N Engl J Med.* 2006;354:1578–1588.

136. Malinow MR, Bostom AG, Krauss RM. Homocyst(e)ine, diet, and cardiovascular diseases: a statement for healthcare professionals from the Nutrition Committee, American Heart Association. *Circulation.* 1999;99:178–182.

137. Stroke and Coronary Heart Disease Collaborative Research Group E. Blood pressure, cholesterol, and stroke in eastern Asia. *Lancet.* 1998;352:1801–1807.

138. Benjamin EJ, Smith J, Cooper RS, Hill MN, Luepker RV. Task Force #1—magnitude of the prevention problem: opportunities and challenges. *J Am Coll Cardiol.* 2002;40:588–603.

139. Arnett DK, McGovern PG, Jacobs DR Jr, Shahar E, Duval S, Blackburn H, et al. Fifteen-Year trends in cardiovascular risk factors (1980–1982 through 1995–1997): the Minnesota Heart Survey. *Am J Epidemiol.* 2002;156:929.

140. World Health Organization. Integrated management of cardiovascular risk: report of a WHO meeting, Geneva, July 9–12, 2002. Geneva: WHO; 2003.

141. World Health Organization. Regional activities to the global CVD strategy, 2006. Available at: http://www.who.int/cardiovascular_diseases/region/en/. Accessed August 15, 2006.

142. World Health Organization. Research and global partnership initiatives, 2006. Available at: http://www.who.int/cardiovascular_diseases/research/en/. Accessed August 15, 2006.

143. World Health Organization. Multisector partnerships, 2006. Available at: http://www.who.int/cardiovascular_diseases/multisector_partnerships/en/. Accessed August 15, 2006.

144. Anand SS, Yusuf S, Vuksan V, Devanesen S, Teo KK, Montague PA, et al. Differences in risk factors, atherosclerosis, and cardiovascular disease between ethnic groups in Canada: the Study of Health Assessment and Risk in Ethnic groups (SHARE). *Lancet.* 2000;356:279–284.

145. Howson CP, Reddy KS, Ryan TJ, Bale JR. *Control of cardiovascular diseases in developing countries. Research, development and institutional strengthening.* Washington DC: Institute of Medicine, National Academy Press; 1998.

146. Henry J. Kaiser Family Foundation and the American College of Cardiology. Racial/Ethnic differences in cardiac care, 2002. Available at: http://www.kff.org/minorityhealth/6042-index.cfm. Accessed August 15, 2006.

WEB SOURCES

American Heart Association
www.americanheart.org
Heart Disease and Stroke Statistics—2006 Update. Dallas, Texas: American Heart Association; 2006. http://circ.ahajournals.org/cgi/content/short/113/6/e85
International cardiovascular disease statistics: www.americanheart.org/downloadable/heart/1140811583642InternationalCVD.pdf

British Heart Foundation–Coronary Heart Disease Statistics 2006
www.bhf.org.uk/professionals/index.asp?secondlevel=519
This site includes European CVD statistics.

(Canadian) Centre for Chronic Disease Prevention and Control Cardiovascular Disease
www.phac-aspc.gc.ca/ccdpc-cpcmc/cvd-mcv/facts_e.html

Centers for Disease Control
www.cdc.gov/nchs/

European Society of Cardiology
www.escardio.org/

Eurostat
http://europa.eu.int/en/comm/eurostat/eurostat.html

G8 Promoting Heart Health
www.med.mun.ca/g8hearthealth/pages/enter.htm

Global Cardiovascular Infobase
http://cvdinfobase.ca/

Global Health.gov–World Health Statistics
www.globalhealth.gov/worldhealthstatistics.shtml

Heart and Stroke Foundation of Canada
www.heartandstroke.ca
This site includes Canadian CVD statistics.

International Task Force for Prevention of Coronary Disease
www.chd-taskforce.de/

LAC Health Accounts
www.lachealthaccounts.org/en/webguide.php

Morbidity and Mortality Weekly Report (MMWR) **International Bulletins**
www.cdc.gov/mmwr/international/world.html

PAHO Pan American Health Organization
www.paho.org/Project.asp?SEL=HD&LNG=ENG&CD=HTREN

ProCOR Conference on Cardiovascular Health
http://procor.org/

UNICEF—Statistical Data
www.unicef.org/statis/
World Health Organization Web Site
www.who.int/cardiovascular_diseases/en/
World Health Organization Burden of Disease Web Site
www3.who.int/whosis/menu.cfm?path=evidence,bod&language=english
Detailed tables for DALYs subregion, cause, sex, and age group are available at this
    Web site.
World Health Organization (WHO) Publications–Cardiovascular Diseases
www.who.int/cardiovascular_diseases/resources/publications/en/
This page includes links to WHO MONICA Project information.
World Health Organization Statistical Information System (WHOSIS)
www.who.int/whosis/en
World Health Report, 2002
www.who.int/whr/2002/en/index.html

World Federation of Public Health Associations
www.apha.org/wfpha/about_wfpha.htm
World Health Reports
www.who.int/whr/en/
World Heart Federation–White Book
www.worldheart.org/publications-whitebook.php
This site gives information on how to order the *White Book on Cardiovascular
    Diseases*.
World Heart Day (from World Heart Federation, WHO, UNESCO)
www.worldheartday.com/index.asp
United Nations Population Fund (UNFPA)
www.unfpa.org
**United Nations, Department of Economic and Social Affairs—Statistical
    Division**
http://unstats.un.org/unsd/methods/inter-natlinks/sd_intstat.htm

PART 2 Foundations of Cardiovascular Medicine

CHAPTER 3

Functional Anatomy of the Heart

Joseph F. Malouf / William D. Edwards / A. Jamil Tajik / James B. Seward

BACKGROUND

The study of the heart and great vessels has expanded since the days of Andreas Vesalius, the great 16th-century anatomist who recognized the impact of anatomy on the practice of medicine.[1] During the European Renaissance, the tomographic approach to the study of cardiac anatomy became popular because of its artistically based correlations. This is vividly depicted in the drawings of Leonardo da Vinci[2] (Fig. 3–1), the first comparative anatomist since Aristotle (see Chap. 1). During the ensuing nearly four hundred years, however, interest in cardiac anatomy was very sporadic and limited to a few zealous and pioneering physicians, anatomists, and artists. The 19th century ushered in the era of anatomic dissection for the study of physiologic and pathophysiologic processes. Virchow in 1885 described the *inflow-outflow method of cardiac dissection*, which followed the direction of blood flow.[3] It was quick and simple and became the dissection method of choice. The works of Virchow and Osler paved the way to understanding the pathophysiologic basis of such diseases as pulmonary embolism, endocarditis, and heart failure.[4] Renewed interest in the study of cardiac anatomy and pathology was facilitated by the rise in autopsy rates in Europe and North America during the first half of the 20th century.[5] Herrick described the clinical features of coronary thrombosis.[5] Later, Blumgart, Schlesinger, and Zoll ad-

vanced our understanding of coronary artery disease through elegant clinicopathologic correlations.[5]

These achievements notwithstanding, however, they were limited to postmortem examinations. The advent of cardiac surgery in the 1950s, followed by coronary angiography, was a major impetus for promoting the study of in vivo clinicopathologic anatomic correlations. Although cardiac surgeons were quick to appreciate the importance of having a detailed understanding of cardiac anatomy, clinical cardiologists were more interested in pathophysiology. However, with the introduction of noninvasive imaging techniques (echocardiography, CT, MRI, and single-photon-emission computed tomography [SPECT]) over the past two decades, the perception of cardiac anatomy and pathophysiology radically changed for all of medicine in general and cardiology in particular.

With increasing use of tomographic techniques in the diagnosis and management of cardiovascular diseases, there has been a corresponding decrease in the use of autopsy for anatomic correlations. The reasons for this decrease are complex and controversial and include an increased confidence in technology, lack of reimbursement for the cost of autopsy, and rescinding the mandate for autopsies for hospital accreditation.[4] Nonetheless, autopsy still uncovers unexpected processes in approximately 15 percent of cases and is an invaluable tool for quality assurance programs.

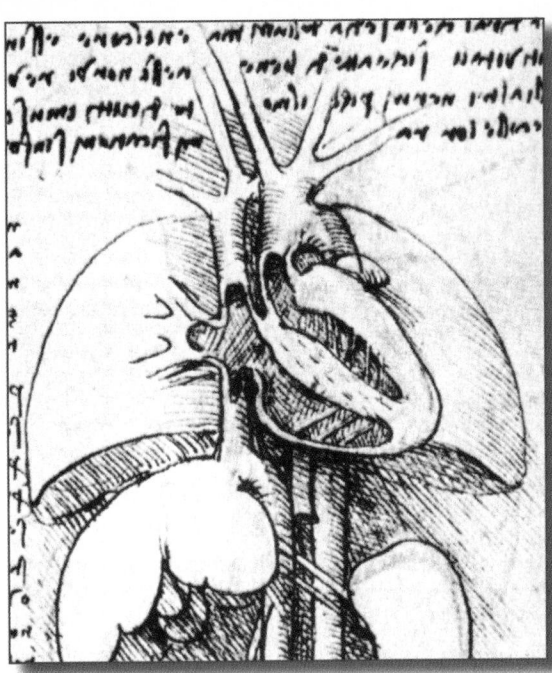

FIGURE 3–1. Four-chamber tomographic section of the heart as illustrated by Leonardo da Vinci. Note the thin-walled right ventricle and thick-walled left ventricle and detailed anatomic connections. *Source: O'Malley, Saunders.*[2] *Used with permission.*

Today, at the beginning of the 21st century, there is a resurgence in the clinicopathologic correlative approach to cardiovascular morphology. In particular, the tomographic presentation of cardiac structure, which had remained dormant for more than a century, has become relevant because the diagnostic techniques used today are tomographic in nature.[6] The specialties associated with cardiovascular diseases have been quick to embrace these newer anatomic presentations. Echocardiography was brought into the operating room, and with the advent of transesophageal echocardiography, the cardiologist became an indispensable member of the surgical team (see Chap. 16).[7,8] Because of increasingly more sophisticated cardiac surgical techniques coupled with closer interaction between the cardiac surgeon and the noninvasive cardiologist, there has been a growing demand for precise diagnostic tools with greater spatial and temporal resolution to guide the planning of surgical procedures and, therefore, to ensure their success.[7,8,9,10]

The interest in cardiac anatomy among cardiologists is by no means limited to those instances involved in imaging the heart. Over the past few years, there has been an explosion of interest in anatomically guided electrophysiologic mapping and ablation techniques, which are increasingly guided by intracardiac ultrasound (see Chap. 44).[11–15] It has thus become feasible to accurately pinpoint the anatomic location of the source of many arrhythmias[11–15] (Figs. 3–2 and 3–3). By providing the electrophysiologist with a real-time visual *road map*, the *search and destroy* mission during an ablation procedure will be made much easier and results, as well as complications, will be recognized immediately.[11–15] By providing a new window to the heart, real-time anatomic-electrophysiologic correlations can also help to enhance our understanding of the mechanisms of propagation of various arrhythmias.

In this technologically driven era, a new appreciation of cardiac anatomy has emerged as the cornerstone for clinical cardiology.

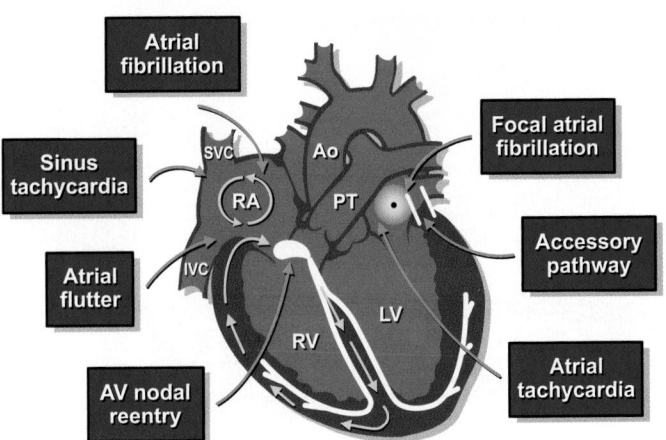

FIGURE 3–2. Anatomic considerations in the treatment of supraventricular arrhythmias. AV, atrioventricular; Ao, ascending aorta; IVC, inferior vena cava; LV, left ventricle; PT, pulmonary trunk; RA, right atrium; RV, right ventricle; SVC, superior vena cava. *Source: Courtesy of Dr. Douglas L Packer, Mayo Clinic, Rochester, MN.*

The purpose of this chapter is to describe the anatomy of the heart by principally using the tomographic format prevalent in current CT, MRI, and echocardiography, with special emphasis and focus on clinically relevant anatomic details. We will make only passing note of the next generation of imaging techniques (i.e., molecular, parametric, quantum, etc.). The intent is to emphasize the important anatomic features of various cardiovascular disease processes relative to diagnosis and management.[16,17]

【 】 ORIENTATION OF THE HEART WITHIN THE THORAX

The body can be viewed in three standard anatomic planes: (1) frontal (coronal), (2) horizontal (transverse), and (3) sagittal, which are orthogonal to one another.[6,7] However, the three primary planes of the heart (short axis [transverse], four-chamber [frontal], and long-axis [sagittal]) do not correspond to the standard anatomic planes of the body[6,7] (Fig. 3–4). *Incorrect photographic or artistic orientation of surgical or autopsy specimens of the heart, presented out of context, can*

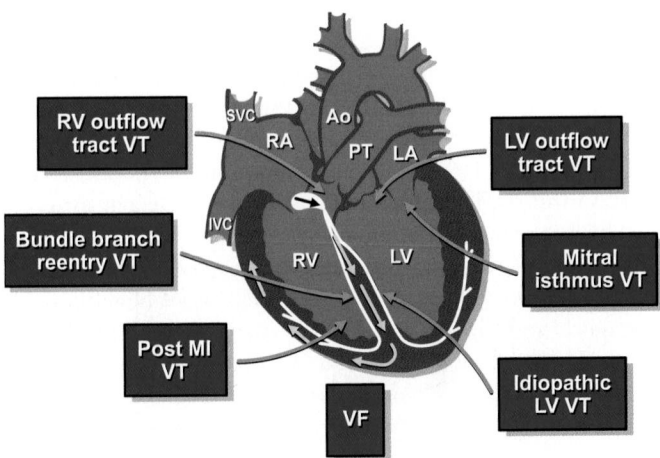

FIGURE 3–3. Anatomic considerations in the treatment of ventricular arrhythmias. LV, left ventricle; LA, left atrium; MI, myocardial infarction; VT, ventricular tachycardia; VF, ventricular fibrillation; other abbreviations as in Fig 3–2. *Source: Courtesy of Dr. Douglas L Packer, Mayo Clinic, Rochester, MN.*

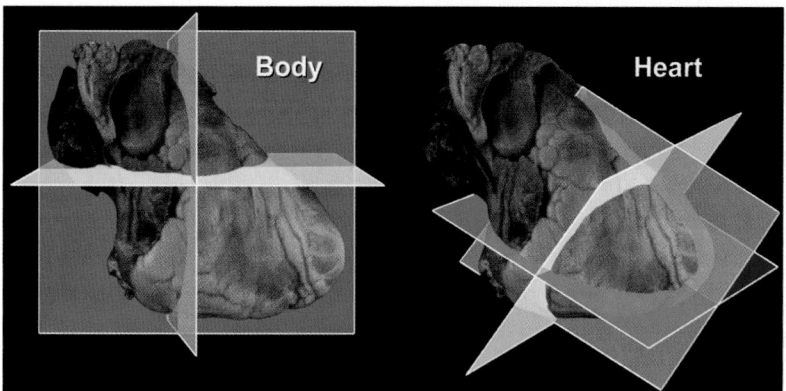

FIGURE 3–4. The three primary planes of the body (*left*) and heart (*right*). Note that the planes of the body are aligned with vertical midline structures, such as the esophagus. In contrast, the major axis of the heart is oriented obliquely. Thus the heart's long and short axes do not lie in the same plane as the body's long and short axes. The body planes cut the heart obliquely and not in its primary planes. Conversely, the heart's primary planes cut the body obliquely.

result in the display of two-dimensional (2D) images in nonanatomic positions and actually contribute to misconceptions regarding the position of the heart within the thorax[6] (Fig. 3–5).

Thus, first, in describing the orientation of a specific organ such as the heart, one must take into account both the position of the heart and the position of adjacent structures such as the thoracic aorta and esophagus. In interpreting 2D images, clinicians must avoid making correlations that yield impossible anatomy[6] (Fig. 3–6). Accurate anatomic diagnoses require close interdisciplinary interactions between cardiovascular pathologists, clinicians, radiologists, anesthesiologists, and surgeons and emphasize a critical need for teamwork and a "common language" in describing cardiac anatomy and pathology.

【 】 METHODS USED TO STUDY CARDIAC ANATOMY

The two conventional approaches to the study of cardiac anatomy that have stood the test of time are (1) the inflow-outflow method (Fig. 3–7) and (2) the tomographic ventricular slice method[3,6] (Fig. 3–8). Although the inflow-outflow method readily demonstrates disease processes in a given cardiac chamber or valve, it does not allow simultaneous visualization of the effects of that process on contiguous structures.[6] Furthermore, the inflow-outflow method does not correspond well to clinical tomographic imaging modalities except possibly cavitary angiography.[6] With the ventricular slice technique (see Fig. 3–8), the ventricles are *bread sliced* perpendicular to the plane of the ventricular septum. This technique is ideal for the evaluation of ischemic heart disease but may have to be carried basally, well beyond the papillary muscle tips.[6]

TOMOGRAPHIC METHOD

Renaissance anatomists such as da Vinci used the *tomographic approach* principally because of its *artistic correlations*.[2] Modern anatomists and pathologists have resorted to this method because it correlates with conventional diagnostic tomographic-anatomic techniques. With this method, cardiac dissection involves bisecting the heart into two pieces using a single plane of section.[6] Anatomy contained within the depth of each section fosters a perception of three-dimensional (3D) anatomy. Commonly used planes bisect the heart perpendicular to the base-apex axis (short-axis *transverse* views) (Fig. 3–9) or parallel to it (long-axis and

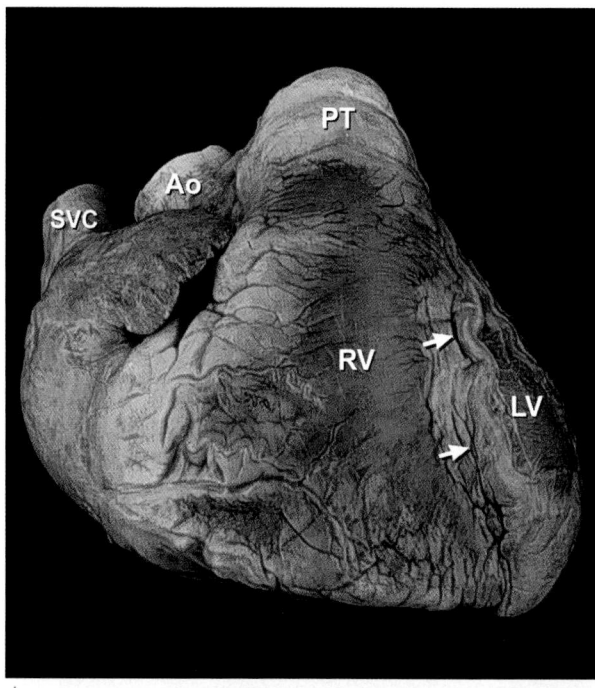

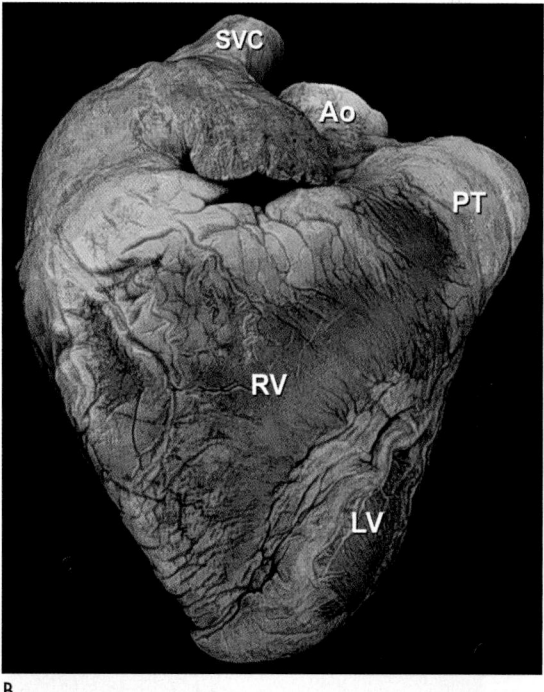

FIGURE 3–5. A. Anterior view of the heart in its usual anatomic position with its apex directed from right to left. Arrows point to the anterior interventricular groove. **B.** Nonanatomic positioning of the normal heart with its apex directed downward, thereby resembling a "valentine." The position of the cardiac apex is normally leftward (levocardia) but can anomalously be rightward (dextrocardia) or midline and inferiorly (mesocardia). Ao, ascending aorta; LV, left ventricle; PT, pulmonary trunk; RV, right ventricle; SVC, superior vena cava.

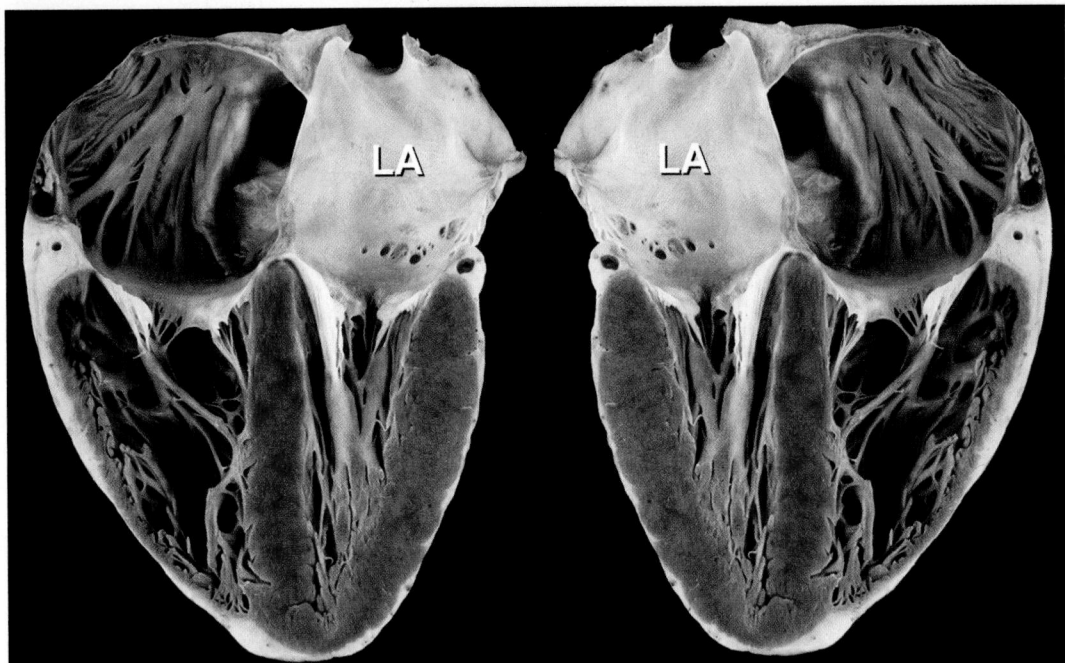

FIGURE 3–6. Apex-down four-chamber view of the heart (*left*) and mirror-image photograph (*right*). Mirror-image depiction (commonly used in publications) to depict normal four-chamber, apex-up echocardiographic anatomic images does not correspond to normal anatomic reality. Obviously, 3D anatomic correctness is essential for accurate clinico-pathologic correlations. LA, left atrium.

four-chamber *frontal* views)[6] (Fig. 3–10). Planes that bisect the heart parallel to the conventional body planes (frontal *coronal*, transverse *short-axis*, and sagittal *long-axis* views) (Fig. 3–11) replicate *body tomography*.[6,18]

The *short-axis tomographic planes*[6,7] of the heart (Fig. 3–12) are similar to the ventricular slice method but differ in two important respects. The *bread slicing* of the heart is continued to the base of the heart and great vessels, and the slices are oriented as though the heart were being viewed from the apex toward the base rather

than in the opposite direction, as has been the case with the ventricular slice technique. Photographs should correspond with diagnostic tomographic scans.

The *long-axis* and *four-chamber planes* are orthogonal to the short-axis planes. The four-chamber planes of cardiac dissection (Fig. 3–13) involve sectioning the heart along both lateral walls, from apex to base, such that both ventricles and both atria are included in the plane of section.[6,7] The long-axis two-chamber method (Fig. 3–14) involves bisecting the heart from the left ven-

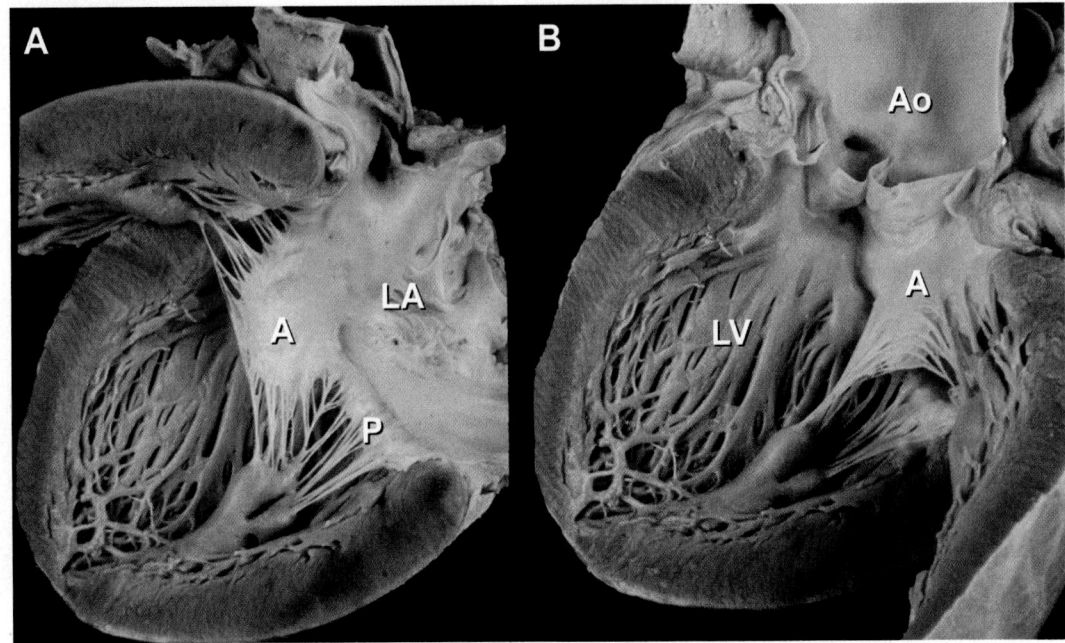

FIGURE 3–7. Inflow-outflow method of cardiac dissection. **A.** Left ventricular inflow view. **B.** Left ventricular outflow view. A, anterior mitral leaflet; Ao, ascending aorta; LA, left atrium; LV, left ventricle; P, posterior mitral leaflet.

tricular apex through the mitral orifice and into the left atrium.[6,7] The long-axis plane can cut through both the left ventricular inflow tract (including the left atrium and mitral valve) and the left ventricular outflow tract (including the ventricular septum, anterior mitral leaflet, and ascending aorta) (Fig. 3–15A). This plane also cuts obliquely through the right ventricular outflow tract.[6,7]

These three anatomic tomographic planes of the heart have been particularly useful in echocardiography and more recently CT and MRI (Fig. 3–15B). Serial sections within each plane produce a collage of anatomic slices (Fig. 3–16) that can be used for 3D and higher-dimensional reconstructions, which is beyond the scope of this chapter. The tomographic planes of section can be tailored to the different imaging modalities. *Thus echocardiography and SPECT generally employ the primary planes of the heart. In contrast, CT and MRI use the primary planes of the body. The parasagittal or oblique planes of the body serve radionuclide angiography and left ventriculography.*[6] When the tomographic examination is not configured to the primary planes of the heart but rather to the planes of the body, the terms *short, long,* and *frontal* can be misleading (Figs. 3–17 and 3–18).

Pathologic lesions in both congenital and acquired heart diseases often involve contiguous chambers, valves, or vessels. The tomographic method is the optimal technique for demonstrating intracardiac relationships and is ideal for any disease that involves several cardiac chambers. The proliferation of noninvasive tomographic imaging techniques makes this method particularly ideal for clinicopathologic correlations. Limitations of tomographic dissection can be overcome by photography, computer imagery, and interestingly, the use of glue. After each tomographic section has been produced and photographed, the bisected specimens can be glued back together using any cyanoacrylate glue, such as Krazy

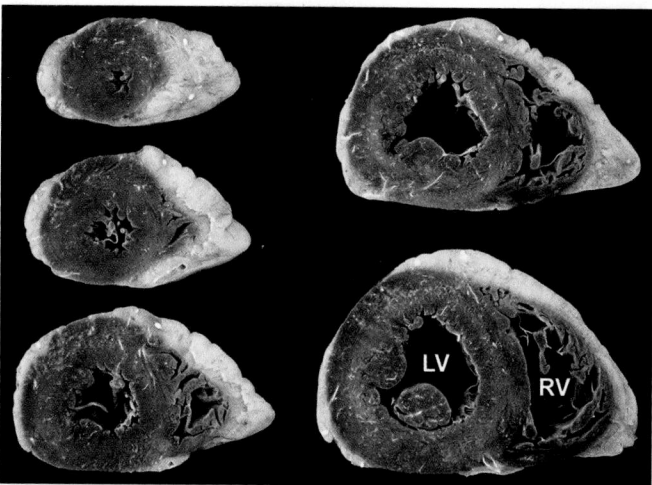

FIGURE 3–8. Ventricular slice method of cardiac dissection. Display of five slices (LV, left ventricle; RV, right ventricle) viewed as though looking from the base of the heart toward the apex.

Glue or Superglue, and resectioned along a different tomographic plane.[6] A step-by-step photographic documentation is necessary, because once the specimen has been glued and recut, the preceding tomographic plane of section will be available only in the photograph and not in the actual specimen.

CORRELATIVE ANATOMY

This section provides an illustrated review of applied cardiac anatomy. The clinical significance of the anatomy described is highlighted in italics.

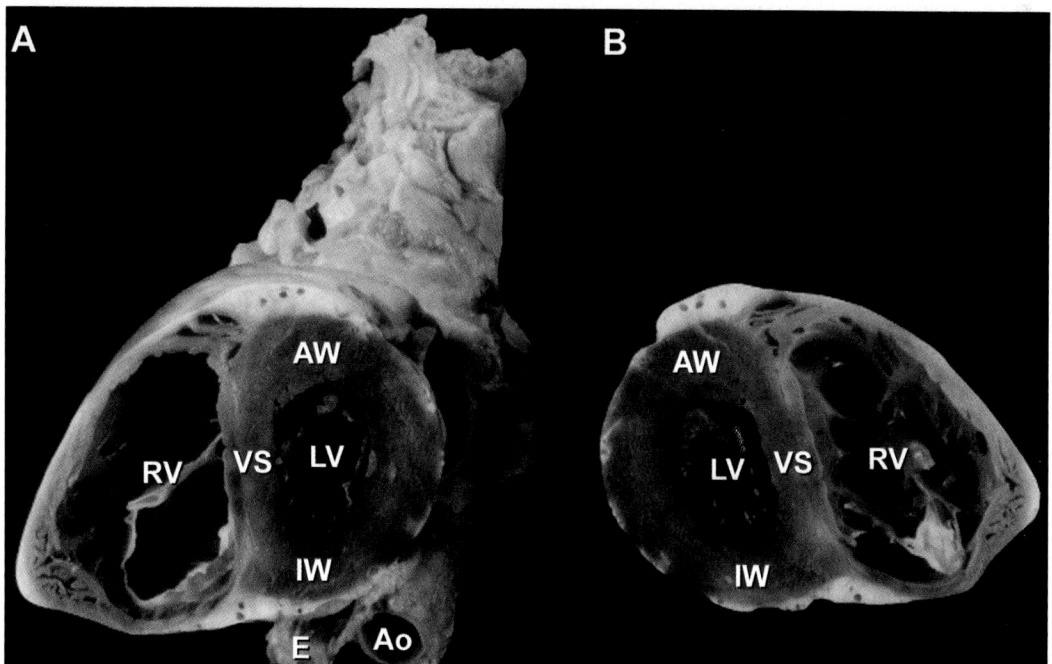

FIGURE 3–9. Bisected cardiac specimen, viewed in the short axis. **A.** The specimen is viewed from the apex toward the base. The esophagus (E) is posterior and adjacent to both the thoracic aorta (Ao) and the inferior wall of the left ventricle (LV). The right ventricular (RV) cavity is to the left. **B.** The other half of the bisected specimen is viewed as though looking from the base toward the apex (comparable with Fig. 3–8). AW, anterior wall; IW, inferior wall; VS, ventricular septum.

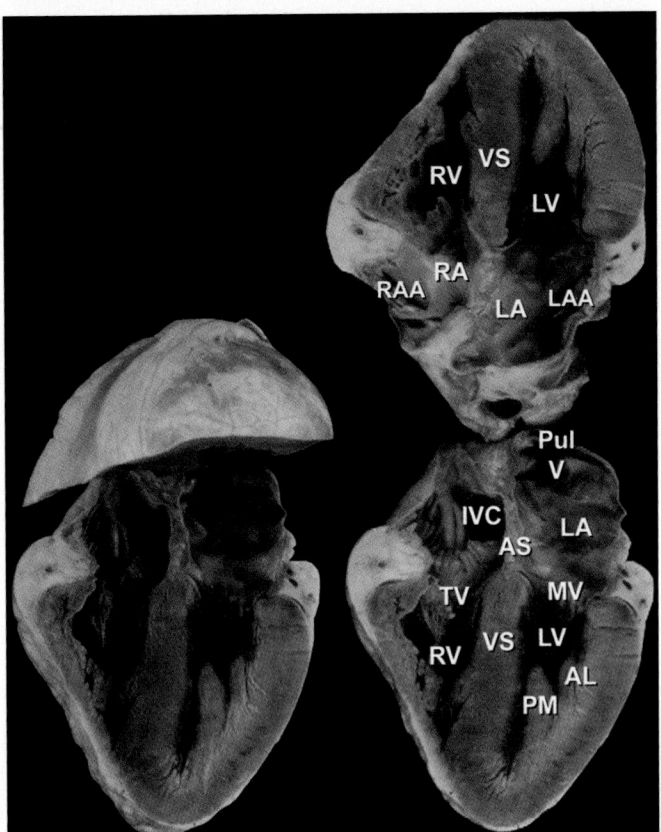

FIGURE 3–10. Bisected cardiac specimen in the four-chamber view parallel to the base-apex axis of the heart. The bisected specimen (*left*) has been partially opened to show the relative relationship of the bisected halves. The two components of the bisected specimen (*right*) are opened completely. Note the positions of the pulmonary veins posteriorly and the positions of the atrial appendages at the atrioventricular groove. AL, anterolateral papillary muscle; AS, atrial septum; IVC, inferior vena cava; LA, left atrium; LAA, left atrial appendage; LV, left ventricle; MV, mitral valve; PM, posteromedial papillary muscle; PulV, pulmonary vein; RA, right atrium; RAA, right atrial appendage; RV, right ventricle; TV, tricuspid valve; VS, ventricular septum.

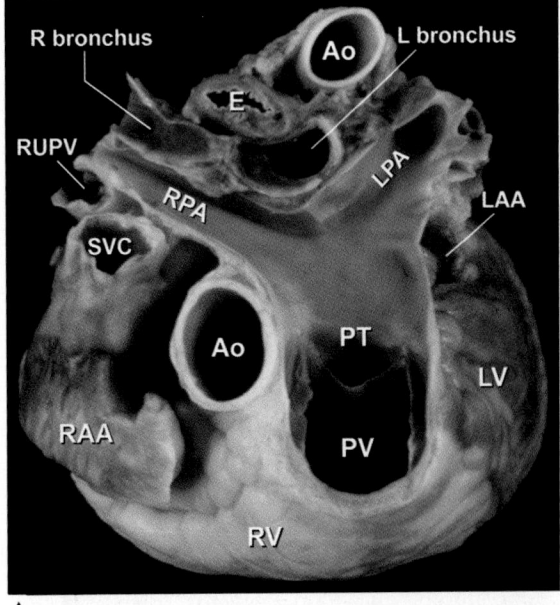

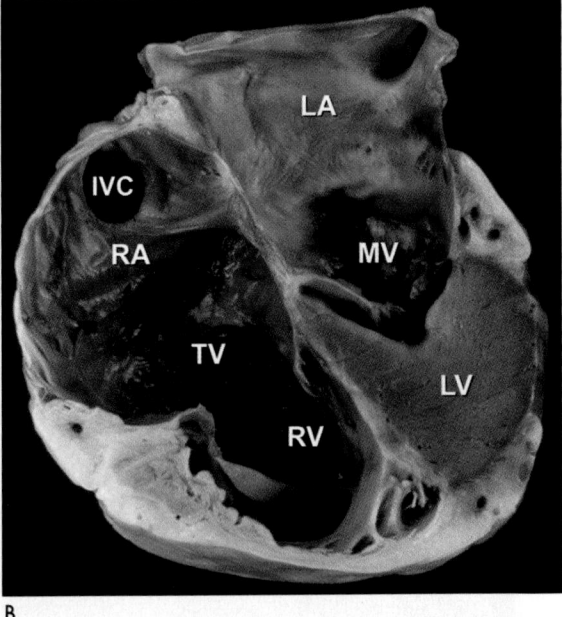

FIGURE 3–11. Tomographic cardiac dissection along the body primary planes. **A,B.** Transverse sections (looking from head toward feet) at the level of the great vessels (**A**) or the cardiac chambers (**B**). The aortic arch travels over the left bronchus and the right pulmonary artery. **C,D.** Frontal sections (looking from anterior to posterior) through both ventricles (**C**) or left ventricle and right atrium (**D**). **E,F.** Parasagittal sections looking from right (**E**) to left (**F**). Ao, ascending aorta; CS, coronary sinus; E, esophagus; IA, innominate artery; IVC, inferior vena cava; LA, left atrium; LAA, left atrial appendage; LB, left bronchus; LCX, left circumflex coronary artery; LIV, left innominate vein; LLPV, left lower pulmonary vein; LPA, left pulmonary artery; LUPV, left upper pulmonary vein; LSA, left subclavian artery; LV, left ventricle; MS, membranous ventricular septum; MV, mitral valve; PS, pericardial sac; PT, pulmonary trunk; PV, pulmonary valve; RA, right atrium; RAA, right atrial appendage; RPA, right pulmonary artery; RUPV, right upper pulmonary vein; RV, right ventricle; RVO, right ventricular outflow; SVC, superior vena cava; TV, tricuspid valve.

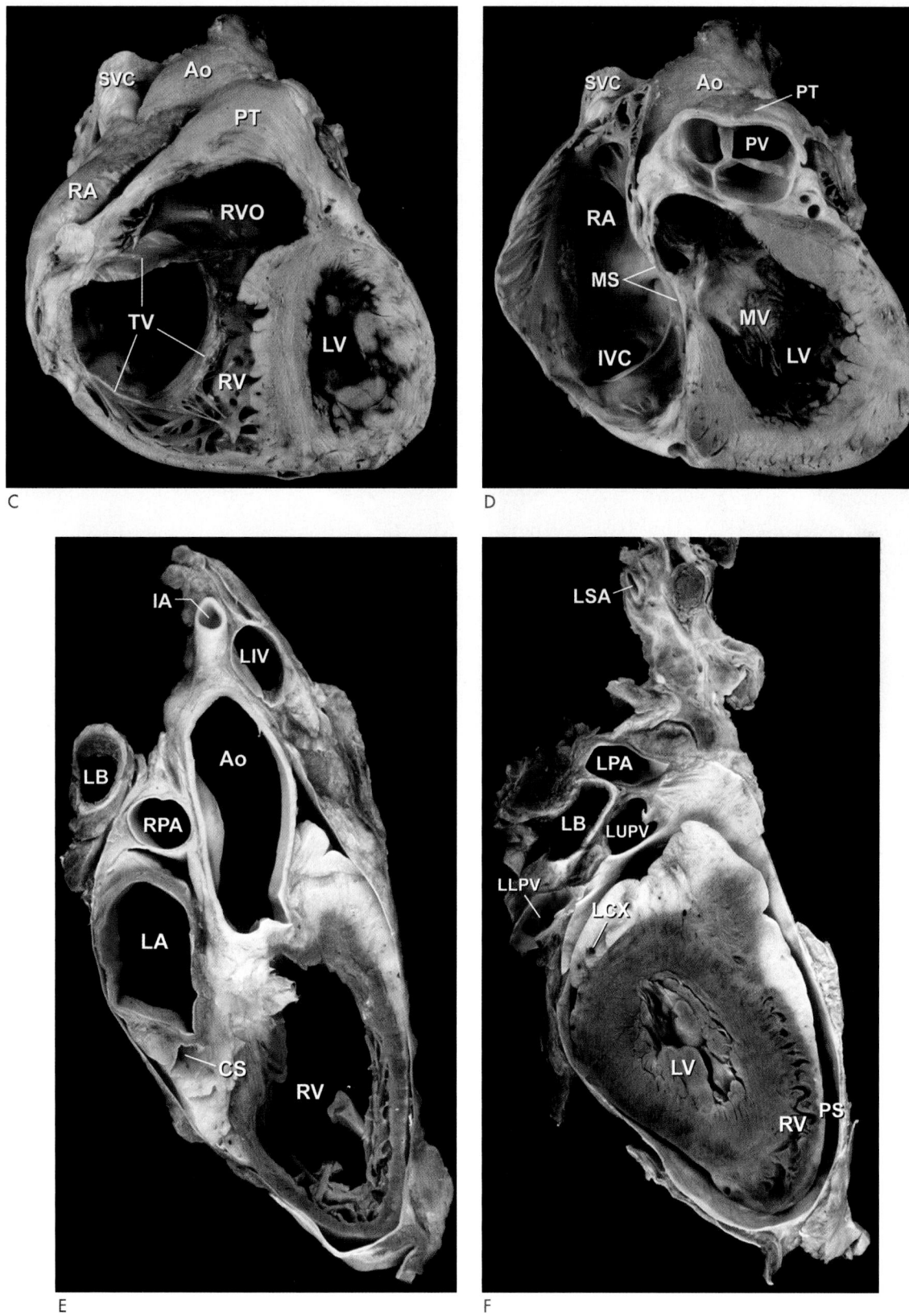

FIGURE 3-11. (continued)

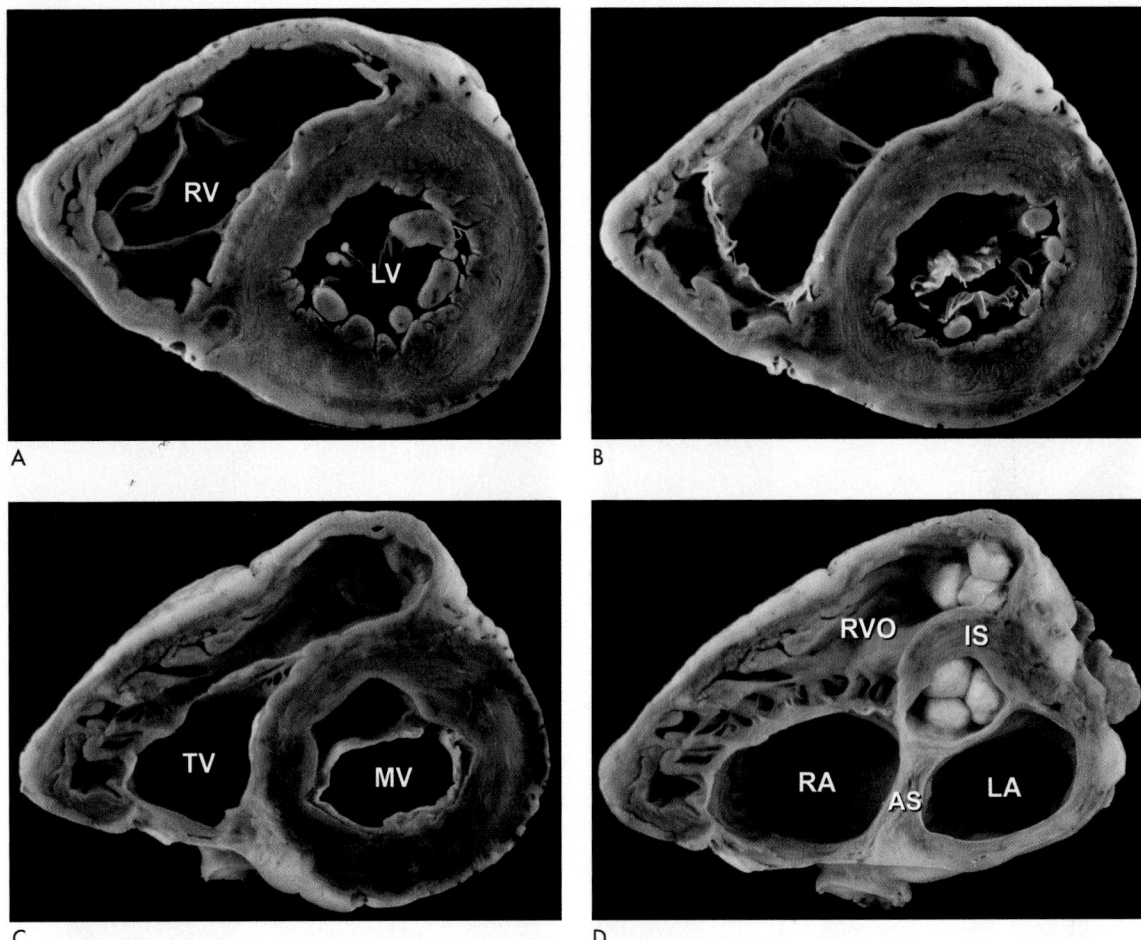

FIGURE 3-12. A-D. Tomographic cardiac dissections along the heart's primary short-axis plane. This method of tomographic dissection shows the crescentic right ventricle (RV) and circular left ventricle (LV). The atrioventricular valves are sectioned at the level of their papillary muscles (*in A*), chordae tendineae (*in B*), atrioventricular valve leaflets (*in C*), and their annuli and the semilunar valves (*in D*). The infundibulum septum (IS) separates the pulmonary and aortic valves. The atrial septum (AS) separates the tricuspid and mitral valves and abuts the posterior (noncoronary) cusp of the aortic valve. LA, left atrium; MV, mitral valve; RA, right atrium; RVO, right ventricular outflow; TV, tricuspid valve.

【 】 PERICARDIUM

The fibrous (parietal) pericardium is a resilient sac that envelops the heart and attaches onto the great vessels.[19] Almost the entire ascending aorta and main pulmonary artery and portions of both venae cavae and all four pulmonary veins are intrapericardial (Fig. 3–19). *These are important anatomic landmarks to remember in evaluating diseases of the pericardium. Given the intrapericardial location of the ascending aorta, diseases such as localized aortic wall hematoma, aortic dissection, or aortic rupture can produce a rapidly fatal hemopericardium. Because the sac is collagenous, with little elastic tissue, it cannot stretch acutely. In patients with total anomalous pulmonary venous connection, the confluence of pulmonary veins is intrapericardial. In contrast, the right and left pulmonary arteries and ductal artery (ductus arteriosus) are extrapericardial structures.*[20]

The serous pericardium forms the delicate inner lining of the fibrous pericardium as well as the outer lining of the heart and great vessels (visceral pericardium). Over the heart, it is referred to as the *epicardium*, and it contains the epicardial coronary arteries and veins, autonomic nerves, lymphatics, and a variable amount of adipose tissue. The junctions between the visceral and parietal pericardium lie along the great vessels and form the pericardial reflections. The reflections along the pulmonary veins and vena cavae are continuous and form a posterior midline cul-de-sac known as the *oblique sinus*. Behind the great arteries, the *transverse sinus* forms a tunnel-like passageway (Fig. 3–20). *After open-heart surgery, localized accumulation of blood within the oblique sinus can produce isolated left atrial tamponade.*[20] *Similarly, a hematoma adjacent to the low-pressure right atrium can cause isolated right atrial tamponade* (see Chap. 84). With increasing age and with obesity, fat can accumulate within the parietal pericardium and epicardium (see Fig. 3–32).[20] *In imaging the heart, it is important not to misinterpret epicardial fat as an abnormal structure or a tumor.*

【 】 CARDIAC SKELETON

The four cardiac valves are anchored to their annuli, or valve rings. These fibrous rings, at the base of the heart, join to form the fibrous skeleton of the heart[20] (Fig. 3–21). The centrally located aortic valve forms the cornerstone of the cardiac skeleton, and its fibrous extensions abut each of the other three valves. The cardiac skeleton contains not only the four valve annuli but also the membranous septum and the aortic intervalvular, right, and left fibrous trigones. The fibrous trigones form the anatomic substrate for direct mitral-aortic continuity[20] (see Fig. 3–21; Fig. 3–22). The intervalvular fibrosa also

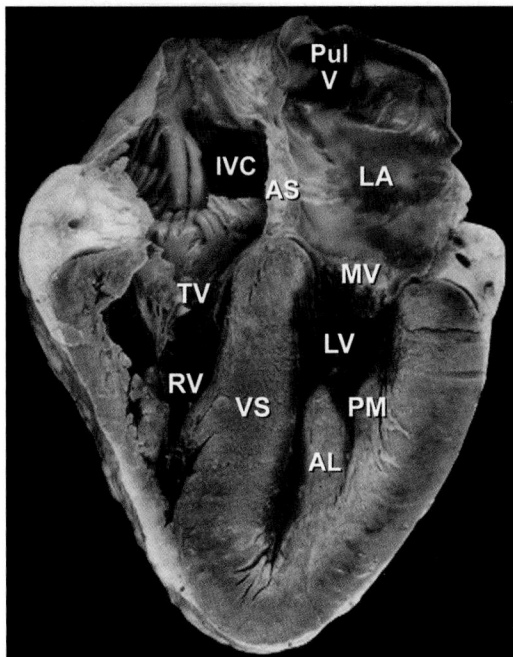

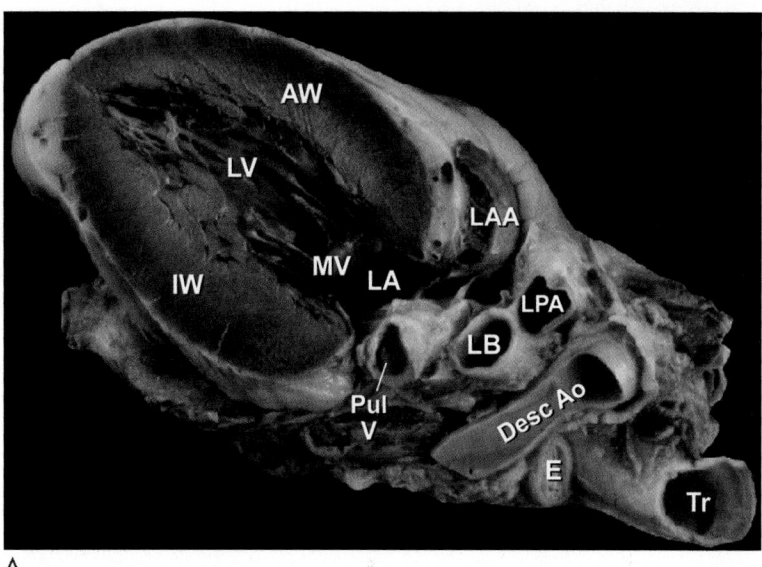

FIGURE 3–13. Tomographic cardiac dissection along the heart's primary four-chamber plane. The heart is viewed as though one were looking from the anterosuperior surface toward the posteroinferior surface. In the floor of the right atrium is the orifice of the inferior vena cava (IVC). The pulmonary veins (PulV) enter the posterior aspect of the left atrium. AL, anterolateral mitral papillary muscle; AS, atrial septum; LA, left atrium; LV, left ventricle; MV, mitral valve; PM, posteromedial mitral papillary muscle; RV, right ventricle; TV, tricuspid valve; VS, ventricular septum.

forms part of the floor of the transverse sinus (see Fig. 3–22). *In patients with infective endocarditis of the mitral or aortic valves, infection can burrow through the intervalvular fibrosa and produce characteristic fistulas between the left ventricle and the adjacent left atrium, ascending aorta, or transverse sinus* (see Chap. 85).[21] The right fibrous trigone (see Fig. 3–21), also known as the *central fibrous body*, welds together the aortic, mitral, and tricuspid valves and forms the largest and strongest component of the cardiac skeleton. It is through the right fibrous trigone that the atrioventricular (His) bundle passes. Otherwise, the fibrous cardiac skeleton serves to electrically isolate the atria from the ventricles. *Diseases or surgical alterations of one valve can affect the shape or angulation of adjacent valves (e.g., aortic valve replacement causing severe mitral regurgitation) and can affect the nearby coronary arteries or conduction tissue.*[21]

【 】 TRICUSPID VALVE

The tricuspid valve is comprised of five components (i.e., annulus, leaflets, commissures, chordae tendineae, and papillary muscles). The anterior tricuspid leaflet is the largest and most mobile and forms an intracavitary curtain that partially separates the inflow and outflow tracts of the right ventricle (Fig. 3–23). The posterior leaflet is usually the smallest. The septal leaflet is the least mobile because of its many direct chordal attachments to the ventricular septum. A distensible fibroadipose annulus is unique to the tricus-

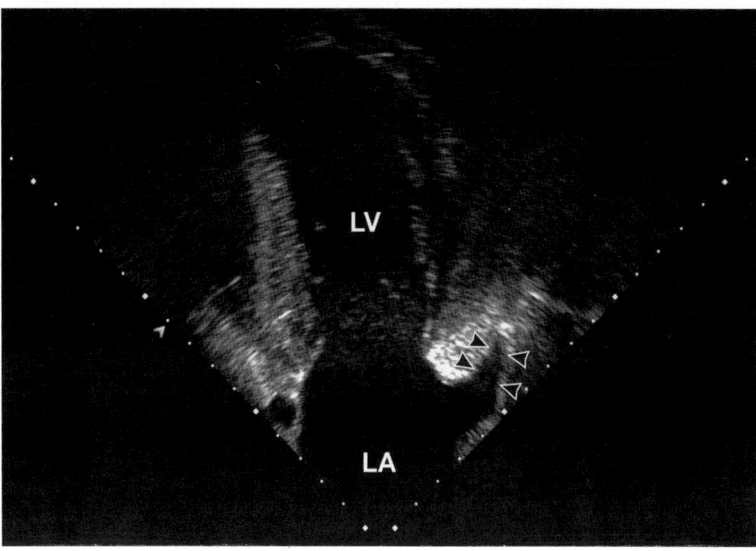

FIGURE 3–14. Tomographic cardiac dissection along the heart's primary long-axis plane. **A.** Tomographic section showing the left ventricle and left atrium. The mitral valve is also well demonstrated. The left atrial appendage is located anteriorly. The specimen is viewed as though one were looking from the tip of the left scapula toward the right nipple. **B.** Two-chamber transesophageal echocardiography (TEE) analogous to the two-chamber transthoracic echocardiography (TTE). *Arrow heads* point to the left atrial appendage. AW, anterior wall; Desc Ao, descending thoracic aorta; E, esophagus; IW, inferior wall; LA, left atrium; LAA, left atrial appendage; LB, left bronchus; LPA, left pulmonary artery; LV, left ventricle; MV, mitral valve; PulV, pulmonary vein; Tr, trachea.

pid valve.[21] Consequently, dilatation of the right ventricle commonly produces circumferential tricuspid annular dilatation that results in variable degrees of tricuspid valve regurgitation (see Chap. 78).[20]

【 】 MITRAL VALVE

The mitral apparatus is composed of the same five components as the tricuspid valve. Competent mitral valve function is a complex process that requires the proper interaction of all components, as well as adequate left atrial and left ventricular function. *Abnormal-*

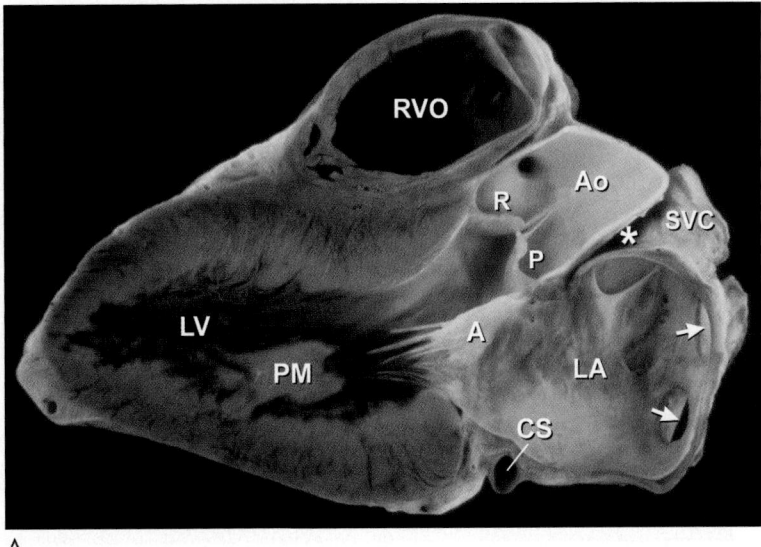

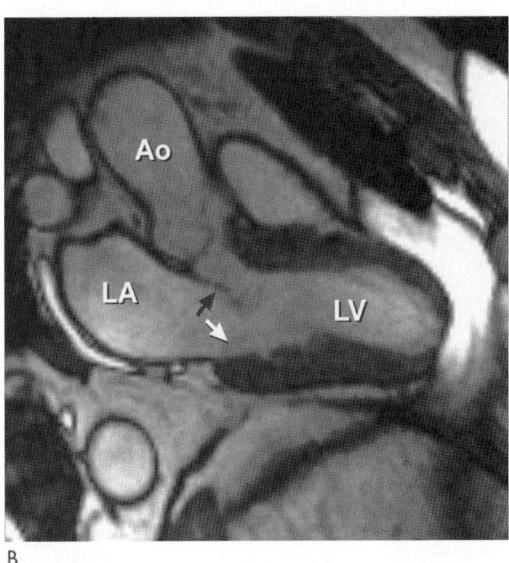

FIGURE 3–15. A. Left ventricular long-axis method of tomographic cardiac dissection (looking from left flank toward the midsternum). Continuity between mitral and aortic valves is clearly seen. The oblique sinus (*) abuts the wall of the left atrium; *arrows* point to the right upper and lower pulmonary veins. **B.** Comparable MRI long-axis view. *Black arrow* points to the anterior mitral leaflet and *white arrow* points to posterior mitral leaflet. A, anterior mitral leaflet; Ao, ascending aorta; CS, coronary sinus; LA, left atrium; LV, left ventricle; P, posterior aortic cusp; PM, posteromedial mitral papillary muscle; R, right aortic cusp; RVO, right ventricular outflow; SVC, superior vena cava.

ities of the mitral valve apparatus can involve any of these components or combinations thereof. The pattern of pathologic involvement often determines the feasibility of mitral valve repair (surgical or percutaneous) (see Chaps. 76 and 77).[22] The mitral valve annulus forms a complete fibrous ring that is firmly anchored along the circumference of the anterior leaflet by the tough fibrous skeleton of the heart[21] (see Fig. 3–21). Therefore, dilatation of the mitral valve annulus primarily affects the posterior leaflet. All current operative mitral valve repair techniques are based on this principle of asymmetric annular dilatation. Mitral valve annuloplasty reduces the mitral valve inlet area by reducing the circumference of the posterior leaflet.[21] This is the rationale for using a partial posterior annuloplasty ring.

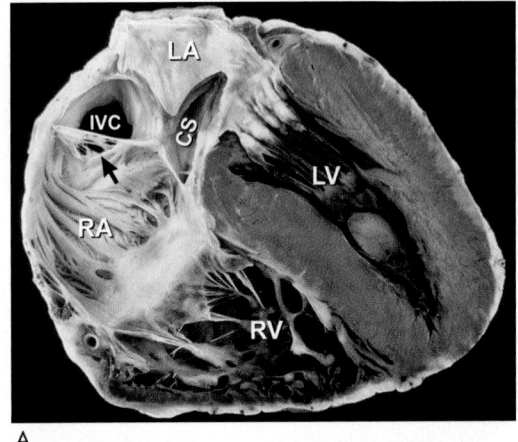

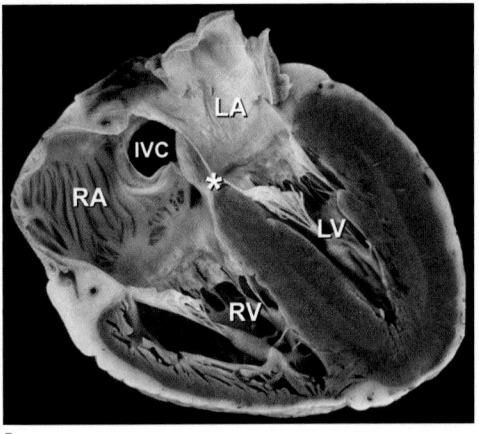

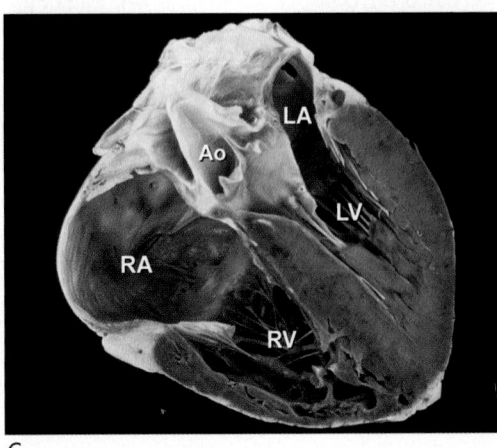

FIGURE 3–16. Collage of four-chamber tomographic sections cutting from inferior wall to anterosuperior wall showing **A.** coronary sinus, **B.** internal cardiac crux (*), and **C.** aortic valve. Ao, ascending aorta; CS, coronary sinus; IVC, inferior vena cava; LA, left atrium; LV, left ventricle; RA, right atrium; RV, right ventricle; *arrow* in **A** points to a fenestrated eustachian valve.

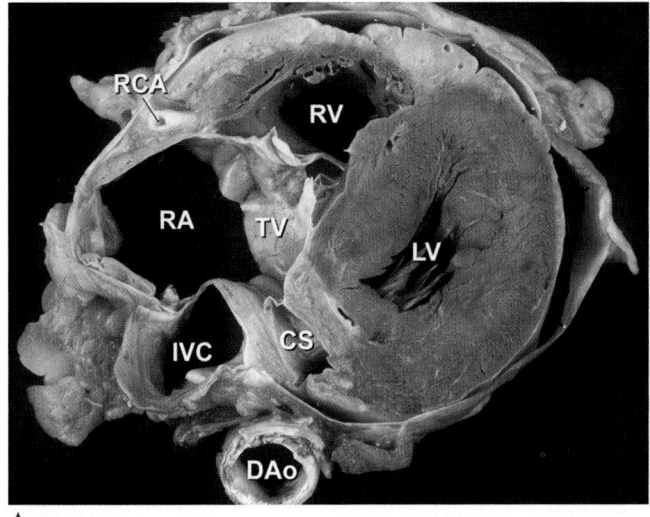

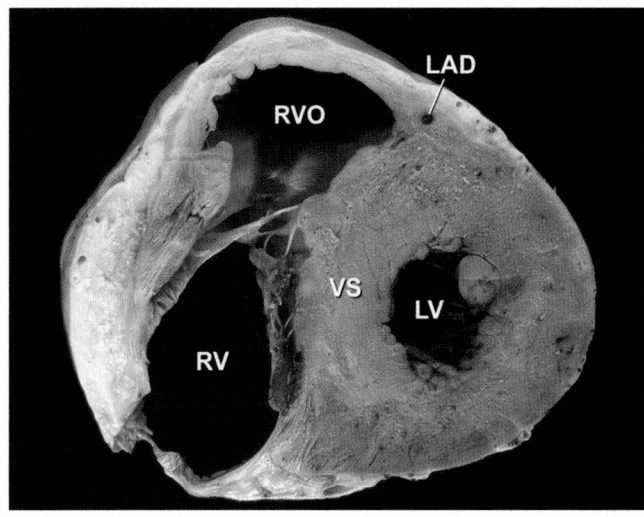

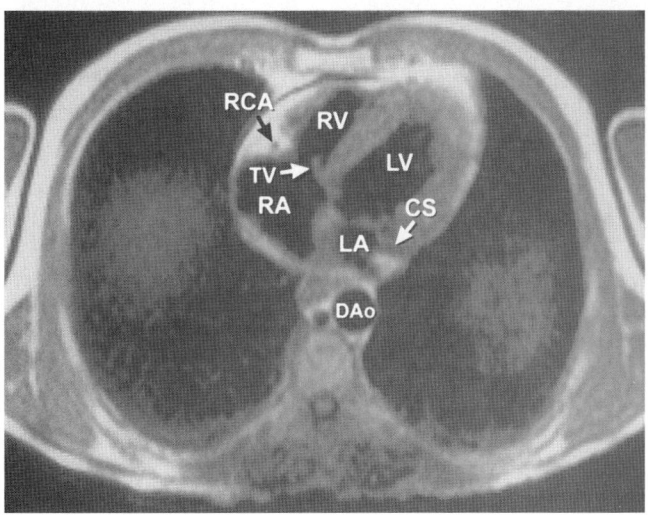

FIGURE 3–17. Tomographic sections of the heart in the transverse (**A**) and frontal (**B**) planes of the body. A tomographic section in the transverse plane of the body (**A**) results in an on-off axis four-chamber view of the heart. A tomographic section along the frontal plane of the body (**B**) results in an oblique short-axis view of the heart. **C.** MRI image corresponding to (**A**). CS, coronary sinus; DAo, descending thoracic aorta; IVC, inferior vena cava; LA, left atrium; LAD, left anterior descending coronary artery; LV, left ventricle; RA, right atrium; RCA, right coronary artery; RV, right ventricle; RVO, right ventricular outflow; TV, tricuspid valve; VS, ventricular septum.

Unlike the other cardiac valves, the mitral valve has only two leaflets. The anterior leaflet is large and semicircular, and it partially separates the ventricular inflow and outflow tracts (see Fig. 3–23). However, unlike its right-sided counterpart, it also forms part of the outflow tract. *In patients with hypertrophic obstructive cardiomyopathy, the anterior mitral leaflet can be pulled toward the basal anterior septum by a Venturi effect, resulting in midsystolic outflow obstruction and mitral regurgitation.*[20] The posterior mitral leaflet is rectangular and is usually divided into three scallops. The middle scallop is the largest of the three in more than 90 percent of normal hearts. Occasionally, however, either the anterolateral or the posteromedial scallop is larger, and rarely there are accessory scallops[19–21] (Fig. 3–24). *Posterior mitral leaflet prolapse usually involves the middle scallop and can be associated with chordal rupture.* Both mitral leaflets are normally similar in area. The anterior leaflet is twice the height of the posterior leaflet but has half its annular length.[21] With advanced age, the mitral leaflets thicken somewhat, particularly along their closing edges.[19]

The commissures are cleft-like splits in the leaflet tissue that represent the sites of separation of the leaflets (Figs. 3–25 and 3–26A). Beneath the two mitral commissures lie the anterolateral and posteromedial papillary muscles, which arise from the left ventricular free wall (see Figs. 3–18B and 3–25). Commissural chords arise from each papillary muscle and extend in a fan-like array to insert into the

free edge of both leaflets adjacent to the commissures (major commissures)[21] (see Figs. 3–24 and 3–26A) or into two adjacent scallops of the posterior leaflet (minor commissures) (see Figs. 3–24, and 3–25). *In contrast to congenital clefts, a true commissure is always associated with an underlying papillary muscle and an intervening array of chordae tendineae.*[21] The attachments of commissural chords precisely demarcate the commissure. *Because the commissural chords are seldom elongated, they serve as accurate reference points for determining the proper closing plane for the leaflets during surgical repair.*

The anterolateral papillary muscle is commonly single and usually has a dual blood supply from the left coronary circulation.[20] In contrast, the posteromedial papillary muscle usually has multiple heads and is most commonly supplied only by the right coronary artery.[20] Small left atrial branches supply the most basal aspects of the mitral leaflets.[21]

Papillary muscle contraction pulls the two leaflets toward one another and thereby promotes valve closure. The line of closure for either mitral leaflet is not its free edge but an ill-defined junction between a thin, clear zone and a thicker, rough zone[21] (see Fig. 3–26). The major chordae supporting a leaflet insert into its free edge and rough zone. The chordae tendineae anchor and support the leaflets and, by doing so, prevent leaflet prolapse during ventricular systole. Two particularly prominent rough zone chords, referred to as

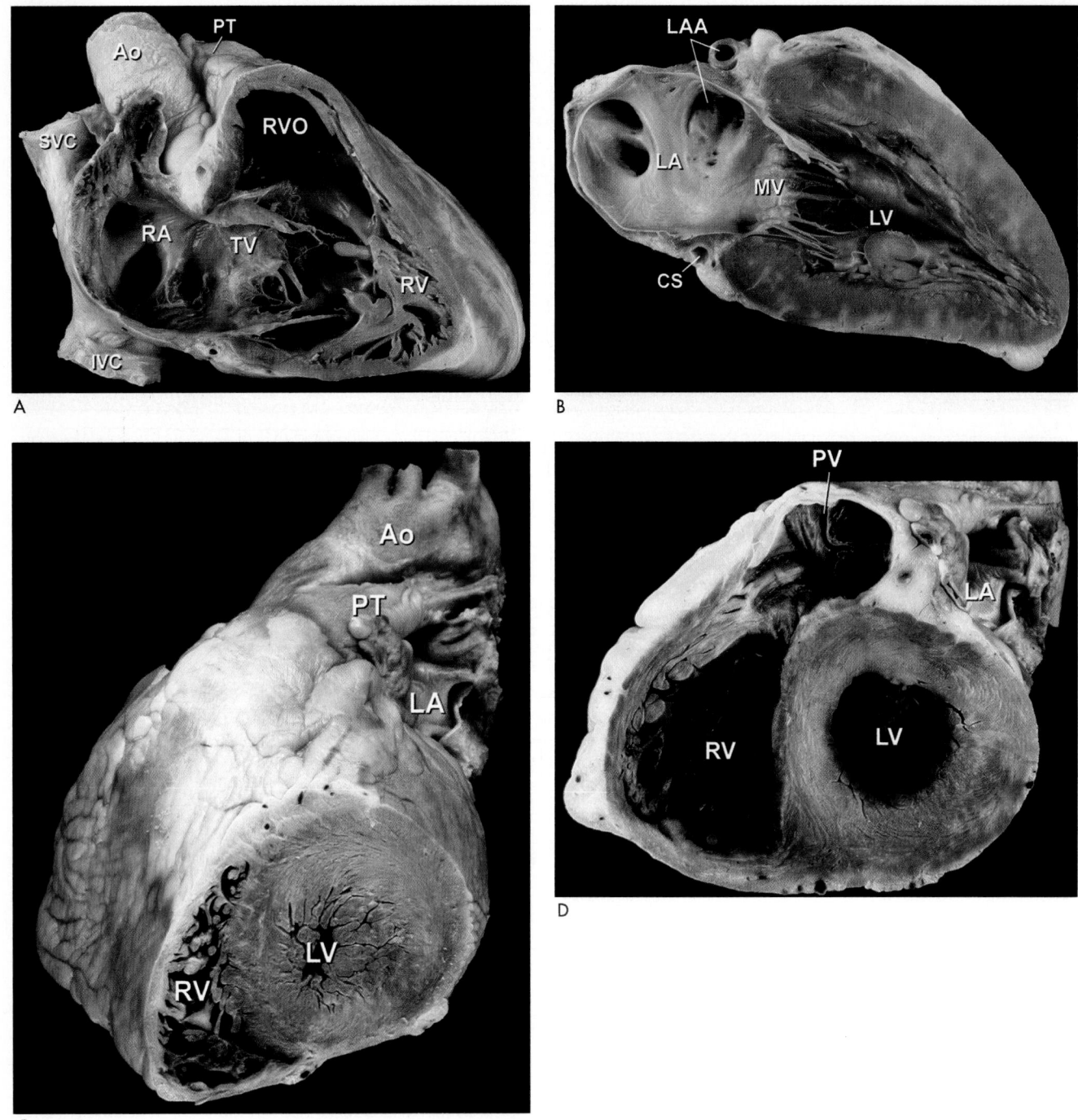

FIGURE 3–18. Oblique methods of tomographic cardiac dissection. **A,B.** Right anterior oblique sections, viewed from the right, are taken parallel to the ventricular and atrial septa, can include the right side of the heart (**A**) or the left side of the heart (**B**), and are similar to the two-chamber tomographic sections. **C,D.** Left anterior oblique sections, viewed from the apex toward the base, can be taken at various levels and are similar to the short-axis tomographic sections. Ao, aorta; CS, coronary sinus; IVC, inferior vena cava; LA, left atrium; LAA, left atrial appendage; LV, left ventricle; MV, mitral valve; PT, pulmonary trunk; PV, pulmonary valve; RA, right atrium; RV, right ventricle; RVO, right ventricular outflow; SVC, superior vena cava; TV, tricuspid valve.

strut chordae, insert along each half of the ventricular surface of the anterior mitral leaflet and provide additional leaflet support.[21] They can contain cardiac muscle and tend to calcify with age. Unlike the tricuspid valve, *the normal mitral leaflets have no chordal insertions into the ventricular septum.*[20]

The functional orifice of the mitral valve is defined by its narrowest diastolic cross-sectional area. This can be at the annulus when there is extensive annular calcification or close to the papillary muscle tips in patients with rheumatic mitral stenosis.

Mitral valve prolapse is characterized by thickened and redundant leaflets, annular dilatation (with or without calcium), and thickened and elongated chordae tendineae (with or without rupture). Prolapse of the posterior leaflet occurs more frequently than that of the anterior leaflet. Rheumatic involvement of the mitral valve causes chordal shortening and thickening without annular dilatation. Rheumatic mitral stenosis is produced by chordal and commissural fusion, often with calcification, whereas rheumatic mitral insufficiency results from scar retraction of leaflets and chords.[19] *Chronic postinfarction mitral regurgitation is asso-*

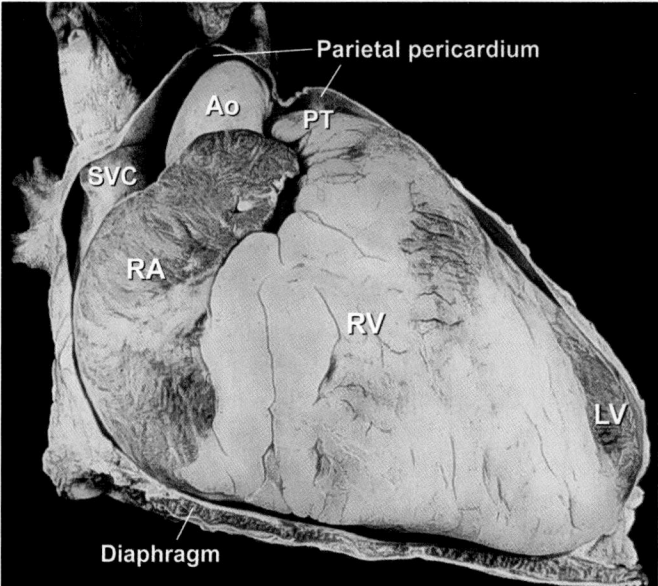

FIGURE 3–19. Anterior view of the heart. The anterior portion of the parietal pericardium has been removed, exposing the intrapericardial portions of the superior vena cava (SVC), ascending aorta (Ao), and pulmonary trunk (PT). LV, left ventricle; RA, right atrium; RV, right ventricle.

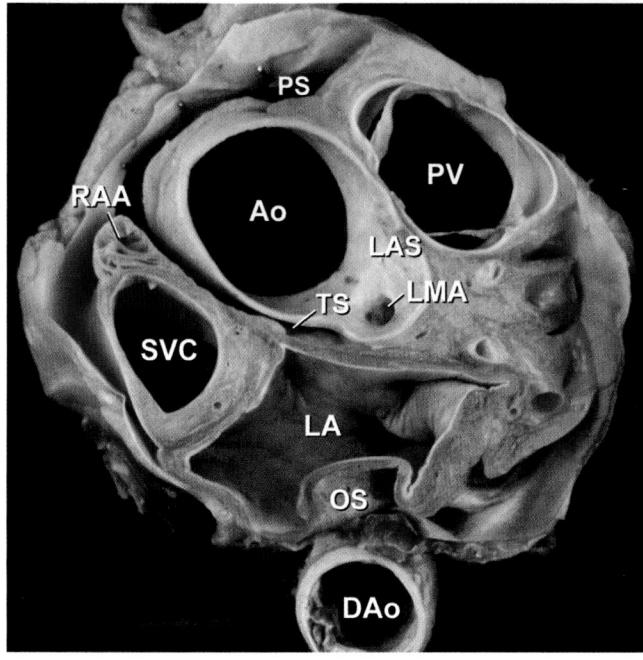

FIGURE 3–20. Tomographic section in the short-axis plane of the body, looking from apex toward the base, showing the oblique (OS) and transverse (TS) pericardial sinus. Ao, ascending aorta; DAo, descending thoracic aorta; LA, left atrium; LAS, left aortic sinus; LMA, left main coronary artery; PS, pericardial sac; PV, pulmonary valve; RAA, right atrial appendage; SVC, superior vena cava.

ciated with left ventricular dilatation and scarring of a papillary muscle and its subjacent ventricular free wall. Leaflet tethering and annular dilatation cause malcoaptation of the contact surfaces of the mitral leaflets. Acute postinfarction mitral regurgitation can be associated with partial or complete rupture of a papillary muscle, usually the posteromedial one.

Anatomically important structures during mitral valve surgery include the left circumflex coronary artery, which courses within the

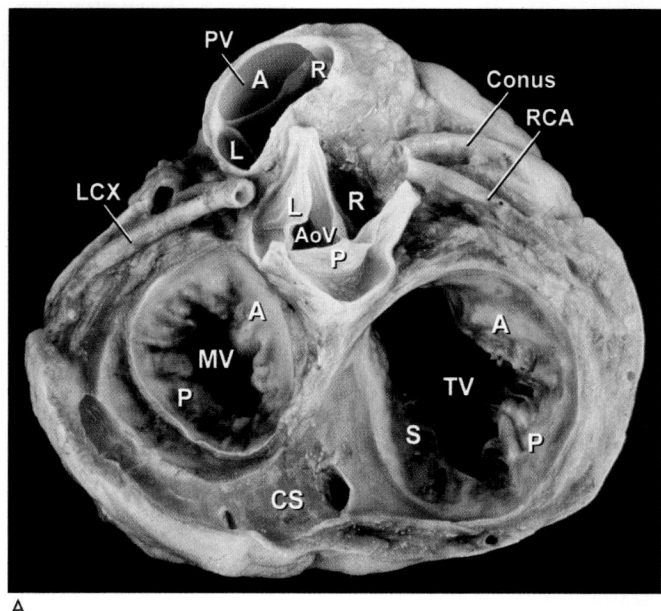

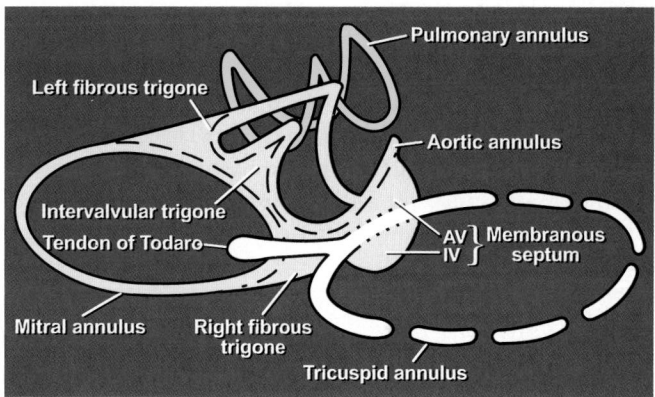

FIGURE 3–21. Base of heart. **A.** Section through the base of the heart, looking from base toward apex, with the atria and great arteries removed, shows all four cardiac valves. **B.** A comparable schematic diagram of the fibrous cardiac skeleton. The centrally located aortic valve forms the cornerstone of the cardiac skeleton. Its fibrous extensions anchor and support the other three valves. A, anterior; AoV, aortic valve; AV, atrioventricular; CS, coronary sinus; IV, interventricular; L, left; LCX, left circumflex coronary artery; MV, mitral valve; P, posterior; PV, pulmonary valve; R, right; RCA, right coronary artery; S, septal; TV, tricuspid valve.

left atrioventricular groove near the anterolateral commissure, and the coronary sinus, which courses within the left atrioventricular groove adjacent to the annulus of the posterior mitral leaflet[21] *(see Fig. 3–21A).*

AORTIC VALVE

The aortic valve, like the pulmonary valve, is composed of three components (i.e., annulus, cusps, and commissures). In contrast to the mitral and tricuspid valves, the two semilunar valves have no tensor apparatus (i.e., chordae tendineae or papillary muscles). The commissures form tall, peaked spaces between the attachments of adjacent cusps (Figs. 3–27 and 3–28) and attain the level of the aortic sinotubular junction, the ridge that separates the sinus and tubular portions of the ascending aorta (originally de-

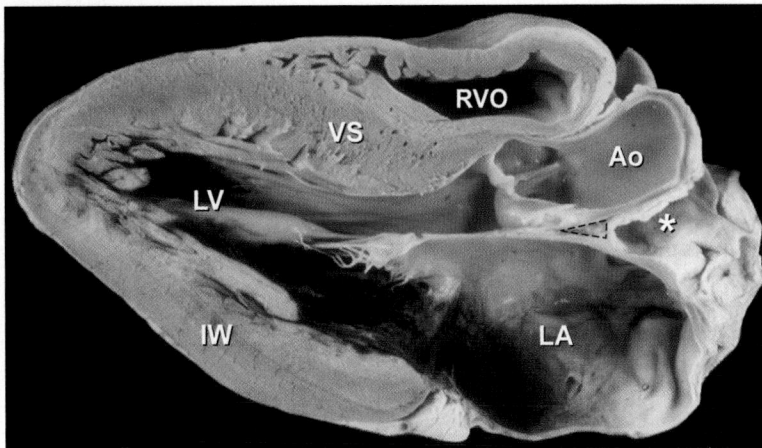

FIGURE 3–22. Long-axis section of the left ventricle. The intervalvular fibrosa (*dashed triangle*) lies between the anterior mitral leaflet and the posterior cusp of the aortic valve and abuts the floor of the transverse pericardial sinus (*). Ao, ascending aorta; IW, inferior wall; LA, left atrium; LV, left ventricle; RVO, right ventricular outflow; VS, ventricular septum.

scribed by da Vinci as the "supraortic ridge")[19] (see Fig. 3–28). The functional aortic valve orifice can be at the sinotubular junction or proximal to it.[21]

The three half moon–shaped (semilunar) aortic cusps form pocket-like tissue flaps that are avascular. In only approximately 10 percent of hearts are they truly equal in size. In two-thirds of hearts, either the right or posterior cusp is larger than the other two.[21] Just below the free edge of each cusp is a ridge-

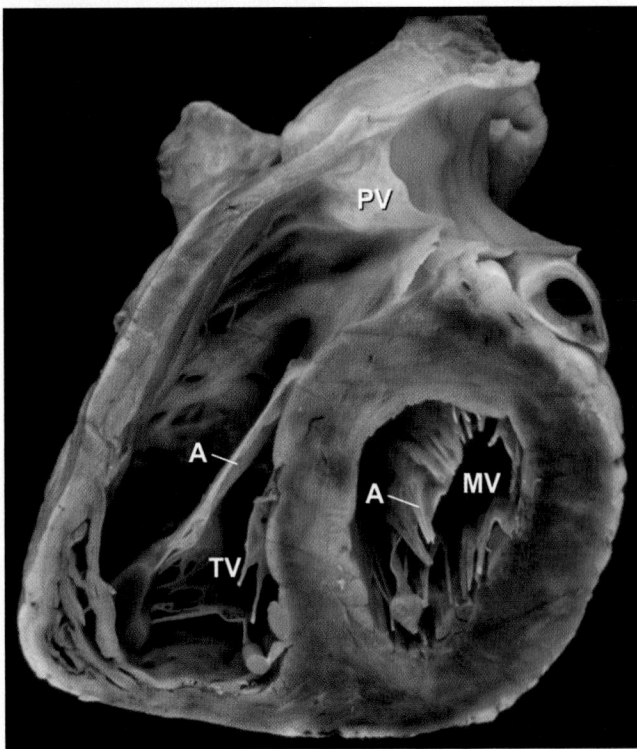

FIGURE 3–23. This oblique short-axis view of the heart shows the triangular-shaped tricuspid orifice (TV) and the elliptical mitral orifice (MV) at midleaflet level. The anterior tricuspid and anterior mitral leaflets (A) separate the inflow and outflow tracts of the right and left ventricles, respectively, and are parallel to one another. PV, pulmonary valve.

like closing edge (see Fig. 3–28). At the center of each cusp the closing edge meets the free edge and forms a small fibrous mound, the *nodule of Arantius*[19] (see Fig. 3–28). Between the free and closing edges, to each side of the nodule are two crescent-shaped areas known as the *lunulae*, which represent the sites of cusp apposition during valve closure.[19] Lunular fenestrations, near the commissures are common and increase in size and incidence with age[19] (Fig. 3–29). However, owing to their position distal to the closing edge, they rarely produce valvular incompetence.[21] When viewed from above, the linear distance along the closing edge of a cusp is much greater than the straight-line distance between its two commissures[19] (see Fig. 3–27). This extra length of cusp tissue is necessary for nonstenotic opening and nonregurgitant closure of the valve.[19] Normally, the diameter of the aortic annulus at the hinge points of the aortic valve is about equal to the diameter of the ascending aorta at the sinotubular junction.[8]

These are important anatomic details in patients undergoing aortic valve repair. In hearts from adults with bicuspid valves and other congenital aortic valve disease, the annular diameter is usually enlarged. In contrast, patients with normal aortic cusps and central aortic regurgitation show enlargement at the level of the sinotubular junction.[7] A prebypass intraoperative transesophageal long-axis view of the left ventricular outflow tract is used to measure the aortic valve annular diameter prior to replacement by a homograft. In doing so, precious bypass time is saved while the homograft is being prepared.[8] Disease processes that produce commissural fusion such as rheumatic valvulitis or which decrease cusp mobility such as fibrosis or calcification can lead to aortic stenosis.[19] In contrast, those disorders that decrease cusp size, such as rheumatic valvulitis, or that cause aortic root dilatation can lead to aortic regurgitation.[19] Combinations of these processes can produce combined stenosis and regurgitation.

The commissure between the right and posterior aortic cusps overlies the membranous septum (Fig. 3–30) and contacts the commissure between the anterior and septal leaflets of the tri-

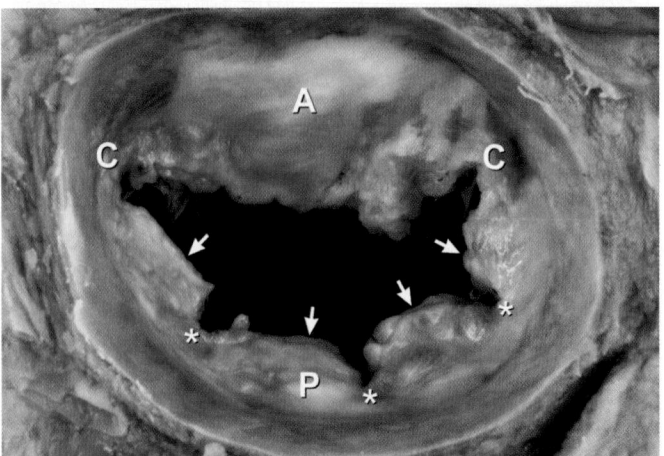

FIGURE 3–24. Mitral valve, viewed from left atrial aspect. Minor commissures (*) divide the posterior leaflet into four scallops (*arrows*). A, anterior; C, major commissures; P, posterior.

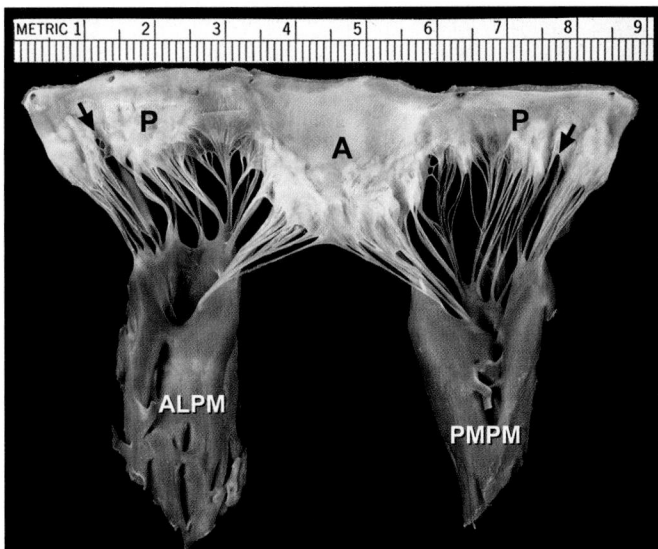

FIGURE 3–25. Gross anatomy of the mitral valve and papillary muscles–chordal apparatus, as demonstrated in an excised and unfolded valve. Each commissure overlies a papillary muscle. *Arrows* point to minor commissures. A, anterior leaflet; ALPM, anterolateral papillary muscle; P, posterior leaflet; PMPM, posteromedial papillary muscle.

cuspid valve (see Fig. 3–41). The commissure between the right and left aortic cusps contacts its corresponding pulmonary commissure and overlies the infundibular septum (see Fig. 3–12D). The intervalvular fibrosa, at the commissure between the left and posterior aortic cusps, fuses the aortic valve to the anterior mitral leaflet.[19,21]

During aortic valve replacement, the anterior mitral leaflet, left bundle branch, or coronary ostia can be injured inadvertently.[21] Annular abscesses caused by infective endocarditis involving the aortic valve can burrow into adjacent structures and thereby produce endocarditis of the other valves; conduction disturbances with septal involvement; aorto-atrial, aorto-pulmonary artery, or aorto-ventricular fistulas; pericarditis; or fatal hemopericardium.[19]

【 】 PULMONARY VALVE

The pulmonary valve is virtually identical in design to the aortic valve.[21] The pulmonary artery sinuses are partially embedded within the muscle bundles of the right ventricular infundibulum, particularly adjacent to the right and left sinuses.[20,23] *In pulmonary valve atresia with an intact ventricular septum, hypertrophy of the muscle bundles and the narrow right ventricular outflow tract accentuate this relationship.[23]* Also, unlike the aortic valve, which is continuous with the mitral valve, the pulmonary and tricuspid valves are separated by infundibular muscle.[21]

【 】 AGE-RELATED VALVE CHANGES

Several age-related changes in the cardiac valves can have clinical significance.[24] In normal hearts, the thickness of the aortic and mitral leaflets increases progressively with each decade, particularly along their closure margins.[24] Probably the most common clinical manifestation of these changes is aortic valve sclerosis, characterized by valve thickening without hemodynamic dysfunction.[24] However, age-

related degenerative calcification of an otherwise anatomically normal-appearing aortic valve can result in progressive aortic stenosis.[24]

Age-related thickening along the nodule of Arantius and closing edges can be associated with the formation of whisker-like projections called *Lambl excrescences*. These fine fibrous-like strands also can develop on the mitral valve.[21] *Lambl excrescences can be detected by echocardiography and have been associated with cardioembolic stroke.[25] Larger clusters, having the appearance of a sea anemone, are considered to be either neoplastic or reactive and are known as* papillary fibroelastomas.[26]

The circumferences of all four cardiac valves increase with age in normal hearts. This is particularly evident in the semilunar valves.[24] Age-related annular dilatation of the aortic valve can result in aortic regurgitation.[24] Mitral annular calcification is rare in women younger than 70 years of age but is present in 40 percent of women older than 90 years of age.[24] Mitral annular calcification almost invariably involves only the posterior leaflet and forms a C-shaped ring of annular and subannular calcium.[21] *Mitral annular*

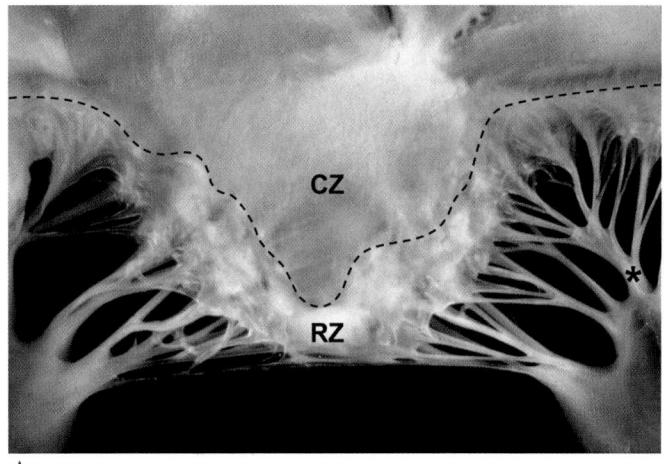

A

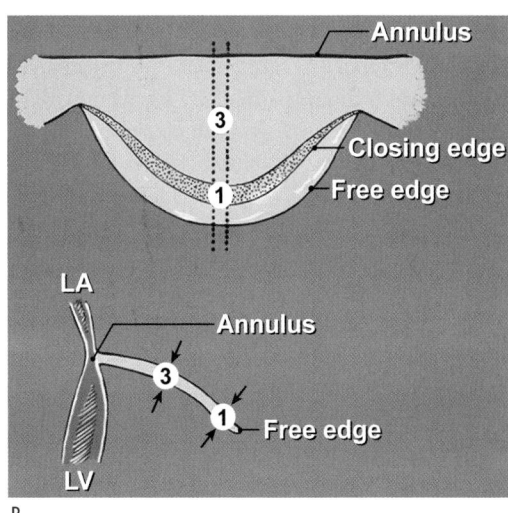

B

FIGURE 3–26. Components of the mitral valve. **A.** Each leaflet has a large clear zone (CZ) and a smaller rough zone (RZ) between its free edge and closing edge (*dotted line*). A fanlike commissural chordae tendinea (*) connects the tip of the papillary muscle to the commissure. **B.** Schematic diagram of an open anterior mitral leaflet comparable to **A.** Section obtained along the *dotted lines* shows the relationship of the mitral annulus and free edge to the closing edge.

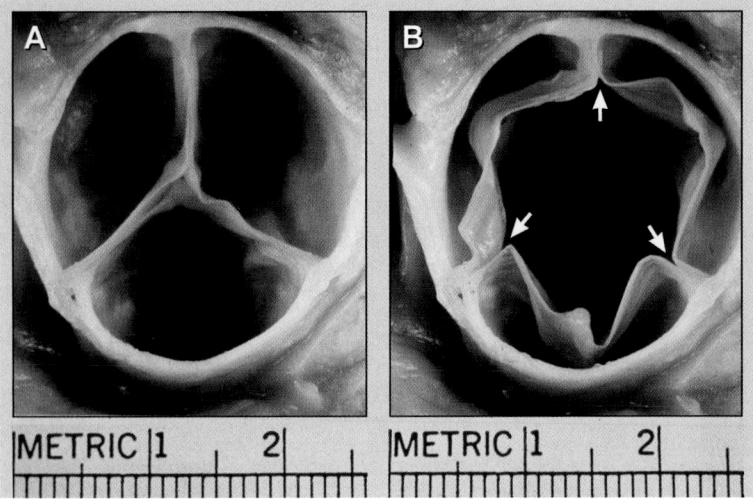

FIGURE 3-27. Each cusp of a semilunar valve is pocket-shaped. The aortic valve is viewed from above in simulated closed (**A**) and open (**B**) positions, showing the three commissures (*arrows*). Note that the length of the closing edge exceeds the straight-line distance between the commissures.

calcification can impede subannular ventricular contraction, thereby resulting in mitral regurgitation. Because of the proximity of the posteromedial commissure to the atrioventricular (His) bundle, mitral annular calcification can be associated with atrioventricular block.[24] *With the increasing size of the aging population, degenerative calcific aortic disease is increasing in frequency.*[24]

[ ] CARDIAC GROOVES, CRUX, AND MARGINS

The atrioventricular groove encircles the heart and defines its base. It separates the atria from the ventricles (Fig. 3–31). The two ventricles are separated by the anterior and posterior (inferior) interventricular grooves, which define the plane of the ventricular septum (see Figs. 3–5A and 3–31).

With age, fat tends to accumulate in increasing amounts in the epicardium, particularly in the atrioventricular grooves.[24,27] *Increased epicardial fat deposits can be associated with increased risk of cardiac rupture after acute transmural myocardial infarction.*[27] Excess fat in the atrial septum is called *lipomatous hypertrophy* (see Fig. 3–46) and can result in a thickness that exceeds that of the ventricular septum. Fat in the right ventricular free wall can be detectable on CT. (Fig. 3–32); its excess accumulation can be associated with increasing age, obesity, or arrhythmogenic right ventricular cardiomyopathy.[28]

Along the surface of the heart, the right and circumflex coronary arteries travel in the right and left atrioventricular grooves, respectively, and the left anterior and posterior descending coronary arteries course along the anterior and posterior (or inferior) interventricular grooves, respectively (see Figs. 3–5A and 3–31). The *external cardiac crux* is the cross-shaped intersection between the atrioventricular, posterior interventricular, and interatrial grooves (see Fig. 3–31). Its internal counterpart (*internal crux*) is the posterior intersection between the mitral and

tricuspid annuli and the atrial and ventricular septa (see Figs. 3–16B and 3–35).

The junction between the anterior and inferior free walls of the right ventricle forms a sharp angle known as the *acute margin*. The rounded lateral wall of the left ventricle forms the *obtuse margin*.[19]

[ ] RIGHT VENTRICLE

The right ventricle is a right-anterior structure. It is comprised of an inlet and trabecular and outflow segments[19] (Fig. 3–33). The inlet component extends from the tricuspid annulus to the insertions of the papillary muscles. An apical trabecular zone extends inferiorly beyond the attachments of the papillary muscles toward the ventricular apex and about halfway along the anterior wall.[19] *This muscular meshwork is the usual site of insertion of transvenous ventricular pacemaker electrodes and the preferred site for positioning of the tip of an intracardiac cardioverter-defibrillator (ICD) lead. During right ventricular endomyocardial biopsy, tissue generally is obtained from the septum, frequently under echocardiographic guidance. Disruption of a portion of the tricuspid support apparatus is a potential complication of right-sided heart instrumentation (e.g., right ventricular endomyocardial biopsy).*[21] The outflow portion, also known as the conus (meaning *cone*) or *infundibulum* (meaning *funnel*), is a smooth-walled muscular subpulmonary channel[19,21] (see Fig. 3–33).

A prominent arch-shaped muscular ridge known as the *crista supraventricularis* separates the tricuspid and pulmonary valves. It is made up of three components (i.e., parietal band, infundibular septum, and septal band) that can appear as distinct structures or can merge together[19,21] (see Fig. 3–33). The parietal band is a free-wall structure, whereas the adjacent infundibular septum is intracardiac and separates the two ventricular outflow tracts beneath

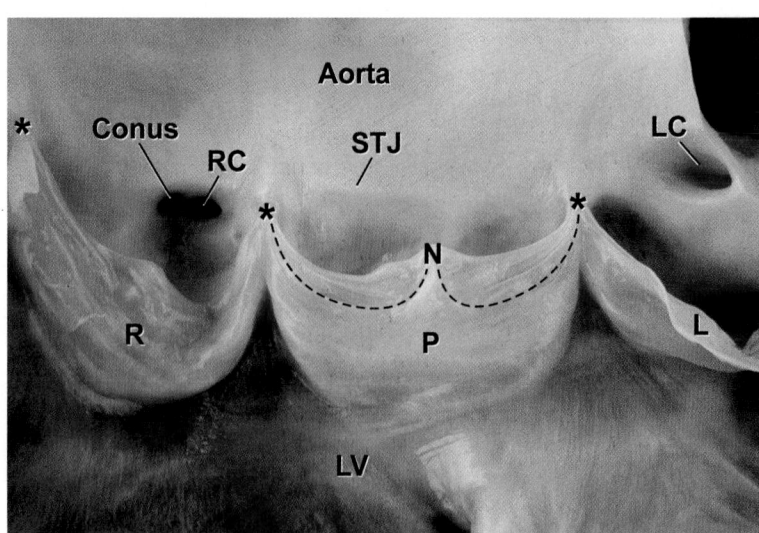

FIGURE 3-28. An opened aortic valve shows the right (R), left (L), and posterior (P) cusps. The *dashed line* marks the closing edge. Between the free and closing edges of each cusp are two lunular areas, representing the surfaces of apposition between adjacent cusps during valve closure. The commissures (*) attain the level of the aortic sinotubular junction (STJ). Conus, conus coronary ostium; LC, left coronary ostium; LV, left ventricle; N, nodule of Arantius; RC, right coronary ostium.

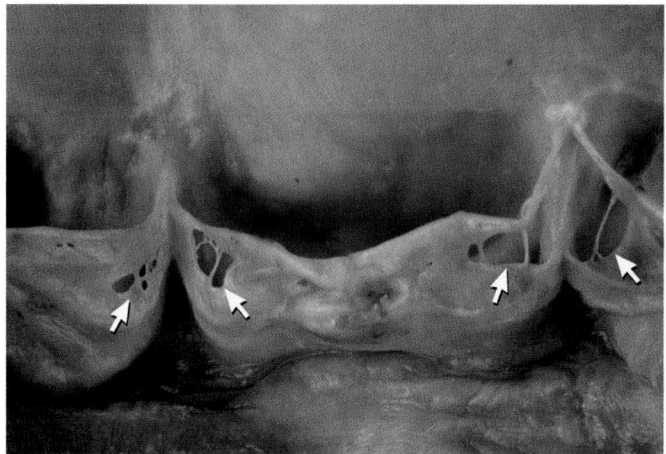

FIGURE 3–29. Aortic cusp fenestrations (*arrows*) occurring in the lunular regions near the commissures. This is a common age-related degenerative finding and normally accounts for little or no aortic valve regurgitation.

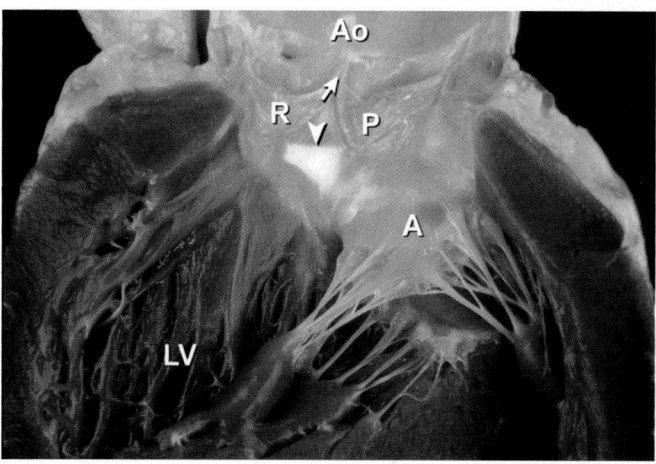

FIGURE 3–30. The commissure between the right and posterior aortic cusps (*arrow*) overlies the transilluminated membranous septum (*arrowhead*). A, anterior mitral leaflet; Ao, ascending aorta; LV, left ventricle; P, posterior aortic cusp; R, right aortic cusp.

the right and left cusps of both semilunar valves[19,21] (see Fig. 3–12D; Fig. 3–34). The septal band forms a Y-shaped muscle, the two upper limbs of which cradle the infundibular septum. From this branching point of the septal band emanates the medial tricuspid papillary muscle[19,21] (see Fig. 3–33). The moderator band forms an intracavitary muscle that connects the septal band with the anterior tricuspid papillary muscle (see Fig. 3–33A).

【 】 LEFT VENTRICLE

The left ventricle, like the right ventricle, is made of an inlet portion comprised of the mitral valve apparatus, a subaortic outflow portion, and a finely trabeculated apical zone.[21] The left ventricular free wall is normally thickest toward the base and thinnest toward the apex, where it averages only 1 to 2 mm in thickness, even in hypertrophied hearts.[21] Structurally, the left and right ventricles differ considerably.[19,21] Normally, the left ventricular free-wall and septal thicknesses are three times the thickness of the right ventricular free wall. The mitral and aortic valves share fibrous continuity, whereas the parietal band separates the tricuspid and pulmonary valves.

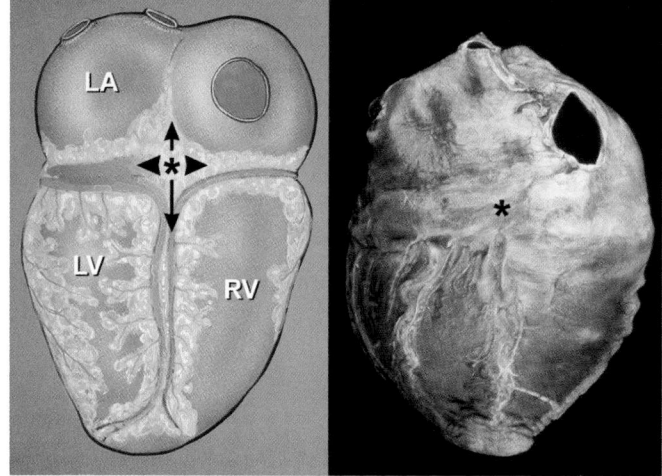

FIGURE 3–31. External cardiac crux. View of the diaphragmatic aspect of the heart shows the intersection of the atrioventricular (*arrowheads*), posterior interventricular (*long arrow*), and interatrial (*small arrow*) grooves at the external cardiac crux (*). (*Left*) Diagram. (*Right*) Cardiac specimen. LA, left atrium; LV, left ventricle; RV, right ventricle.

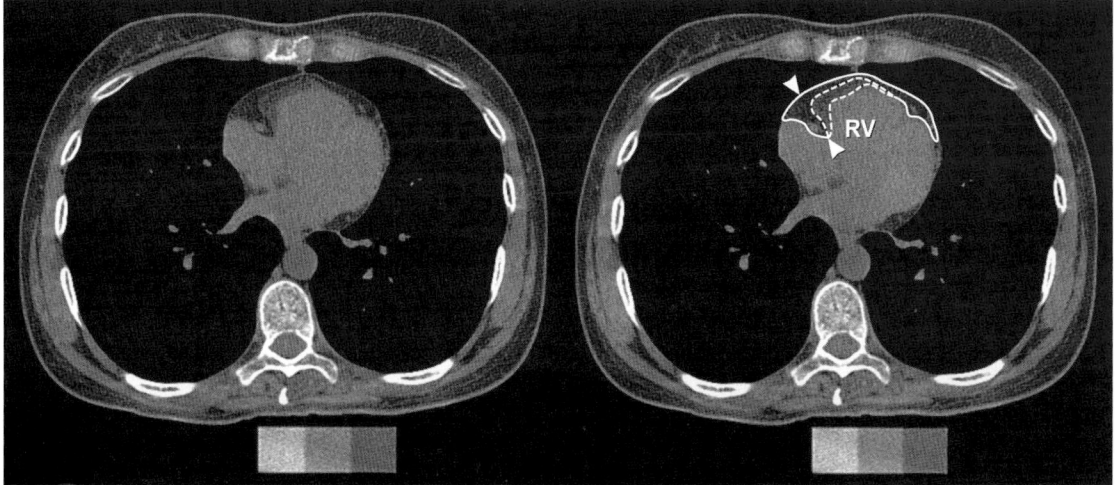

FIGURE 3–32. Noncontrast CT four-chamber view of the heart. Fat is seen within the epicardium (*solid lines*), and right ventricular free wall (*dashed lines*). *Arrowheads* point to fat in the atrioventricular groove. RV, right ventricle.

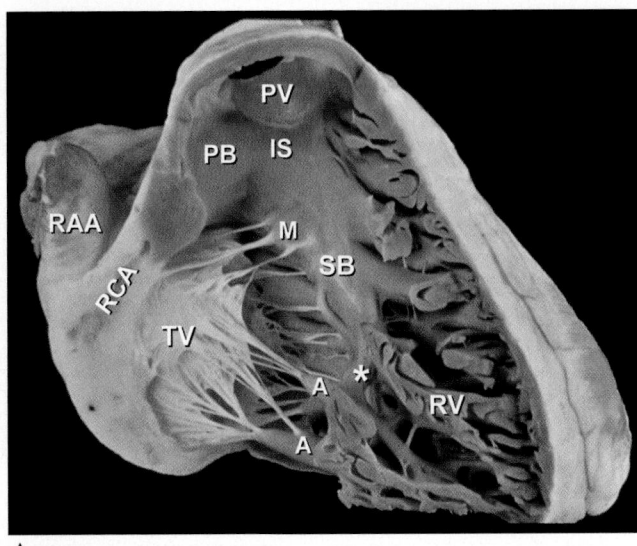

A

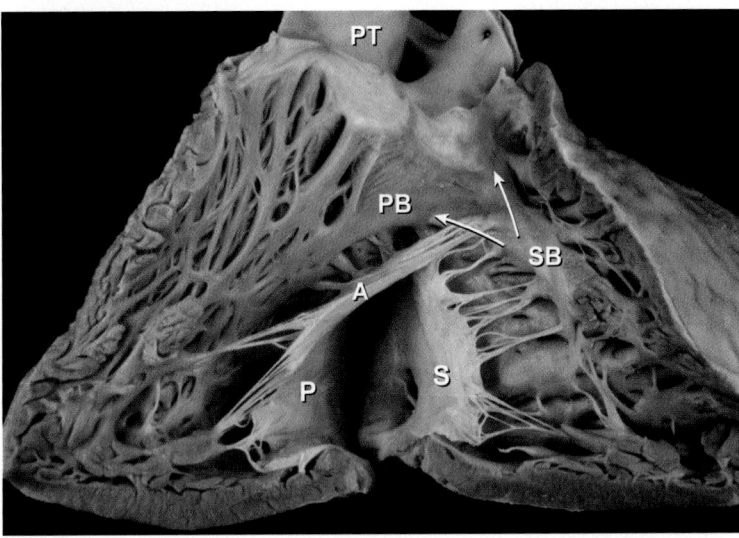

B

FIGURE 3-33. Right ventricle. **A.** The right ventricular free wall has been removed to show the arch-like crista supraventricularis (CSV), which consists of the parietal band (PB), infundibular septum (IS), and septal band (SB). The moderator band (*) joins the septal band to the anterior tricuspid papillary muscle (A). The anteroapical portion of the chamber is heavily trabeculated. M, medial tricuspid papillary muscle; PV, pulmonary valve; RAA, right atrial appendage; RCA, right coronary artery; TV, tricuspid valve. **B.** The right ventricle has been opened by the inflow-outflow method to show the parietal band (PB) separating the tricuspid and pulmonary valves, as well as the two upper limbs (arrows) of the septal band (SB). A, anterior leaflet of the tricuspid valve; P, posterior leaflet of the tricuspid valve; PT, pulmonary trunk; S, septal leaflet of the tricuspid valve; other abbreviations as in **A.**

Whereas the mitral valve has an elliptical orifice and no septal attachments, the tricuspid valve has a triangular orifice and numerous direct septal attachments (see Fig. 3–23). The right ventricular apex is much more trabeculated than its counterpart on the left (see Figs. 3–9B and 18C). *The distinctive differences in apical trabeculations persist even in markedly hypertrophied or dilated hearts.*[21]

The annular attachment of the septal leaflet of the tricuspid valve inserts more apically than that of the anterior mitral leaflet, allowing distinction between the right and left ventricles by four-chamber imaging (Fig. 3–35). *Exceptions include partial atrioventricular septal defects and double-inlet ventricles in which*

the two valve annuli are at the same level. Ebstein anomaly is characterized by exaggeration of apical displacement of the septal and posterior tricuspid leaflets resulting in an atrialized portion of the right ventricular chamber.[20,21] Morphologic differentiation of the right and left ventricles is particularly important in congenital heart disease. The morphologic tricuspid valve virtually always connects to a morphologic right ventricle, whereas the morphologic mitral valve connects to a morphologic left ventricle.[19,20] Because of the rightward bulging of the ventricular septum, the left ventricular chamber appears circular in cross section, whereas the right ventricular chamber has a crescentic appearance (see Fig. 3–23). Tomographic segmental left ventricular anatomy is reviewed in the following section on the coronary arteries.

Left ventricular false tendons, also referred to as *pseudotendons* or *bands*,[29] are discrete, thin, cordlike fibromuscular structures that connect two walls, the two papillary muscles, or a papillary muscle to a wall, usually the ventricular septum (Fig. 3–36). However, false tendons, as the name implies, are not attached to the mitral leaflets. *Chordal attachments between the mitral leaflets and the ventricular septum are abnormal and are usually associated with atrioventricular septal defects or straddling atrioventricular valves.*[20] False tendons are common anatomic variants of the normal left ventricle, occurring in 50 percent of hearts, and can become calcified with age (Fig. 3–37). They are more frequently observed in men, but their incidence does not appear to be age-related.[29] *It has been suggested that they can be the cause of innocent systolic musical murmurs.*[29] *Although they are readily detectable by echocardiography, they can be misinterpreted by the inexperienced sonographer as pathologic structures such as ruptured chords, mural thrombi, or vegetations.*[21,29]

Prominent left ventricular trabeculations[30] are another common anatomic normal variant that can be an even greater source of misinterpretation by 2D echocardiography in patients with suspected mural thrombus. They are defined as discrete, thick muscle bundles that generally connect the free wall to the septum (Fig. 3–38). Less common attachments include papillary muscle to the septum, septum to septum, or free wall to free wall. *In noncompaction of the left ventricular myocardium,*[31,32] *also known as* spongy myocardium, *there is persistence of multiple prominent ventricular trabeculations and deep intertrabecular recesses caused by arrest in the normal in utero process of myocardial compaction. The associated clinical manifestations and age at onset of symptoms (i.e., typically a dilated cardiomyopathy) are highly variable.*

【 】 VENTRICULAR SEPTUM

The ventricular septum is a complex intracardiac partition and is comprised of four parts: (1) inlet, (2) trabecular, (3) membranous, and (4) infundibular. The plane of the infundibular portion (see Figs. 3–12D and 3–34) is different from that of the three other portions. *This anatomic relationship is important in many forms of congenital heart disease in which the infundibular septum is dissociated from the remainder of the ventricular septum (e.g., malalignment forms of ventricular septal defects in tetralogy of Fallot and in double-outlet right ventricle).*[19–21]

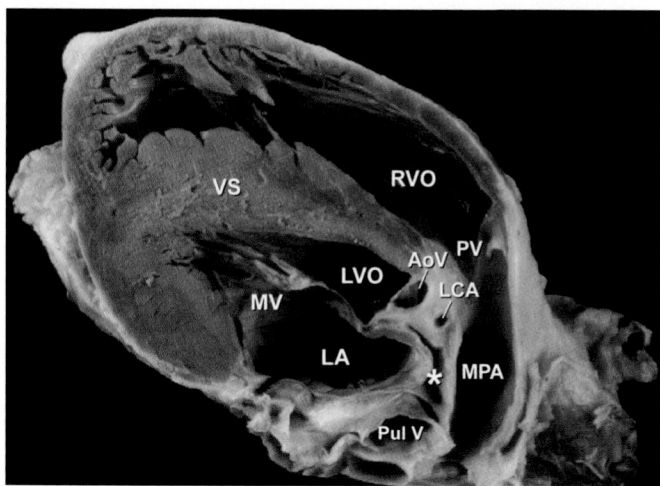

FIGURE 3-34. Long-axis view of the right ventricular outflow (RVO) tract showing the pulmonary valve (PV) and main pulmonary artery (MPA). AoV, aortic valve; LA, left atrium; LCA, left coronary artery; LVO, left ventricular outflow; MV, mitral valve; PulV, pulmonary vein; VS, ventricular septum; *, transverse pericardial sinus.

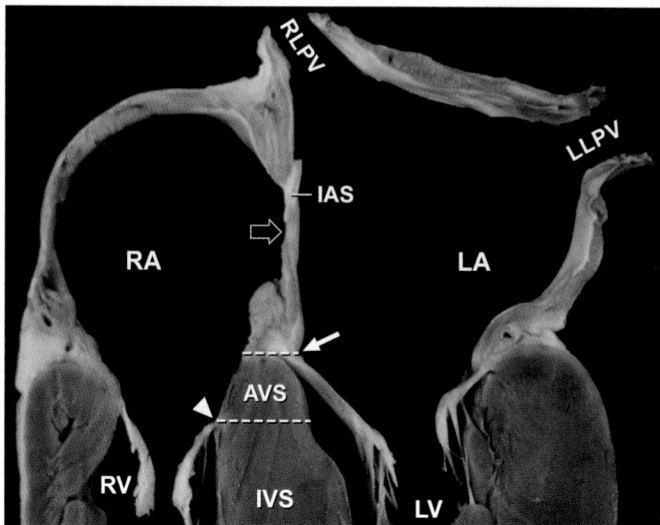

FIGURE 3-35. Internal cardiac crux. Four-chamber slice of the heart shows the characteristic normal apical displacement of the tricuspid valve septal leaflet insertion (*arrowhead*) when compared with septal insertion of the mitral valve (*solid arrow*). This tomographic section also shows the interatrial septum (IAS), atrioventricular septum (AVS), and interventricular septum (IVS). Open arrow points to fossa ovalis. LA, left atrium; LLPV, left lower pulmonary vein; LV, left ventricle; RA, right atrium; RLPV, right lower pulmonary vein; RV, right ventricle.

The ventricular septum also can be divided into muscular and membranous portions[19-21] (Figs. 3-39 and 3-40). The membranous septum lies beneath the right and posterior (non-coronary) aortic cusps (see Fig. 3-30) and contacts the mitral and tricuspid annuli (Fig. 3-41). The membranous septum in conjunction with the right fibrous trigone with which it is continuous fuses the commissure between the right and posterior aortic cusps to the commissure between the anterior and septal tricuspid leaflets (see Fig. 3-21B). *The majority of clinically significant ventricular septal defects involve the membranous septum.*[21] Owing to normal angulation between the infundibular septum and remaining ventricular septum, the septal surface follows the course of an inverted S (moving from apex to aortic

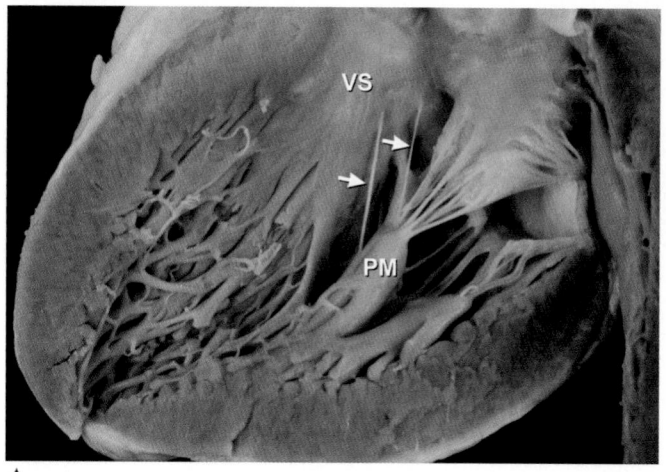

A

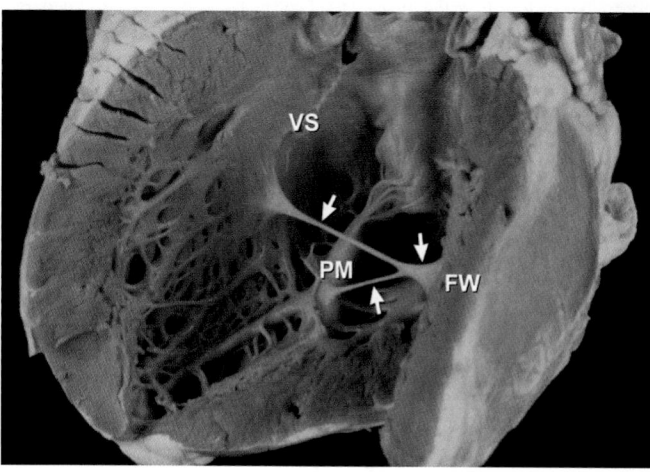

B

FIGURE 3-36. Various locations of left ventricular false tendons. **A.** Two false tendons (*arrows*) from posteromedial mitral papillary muscle (PM) to ventricular septum (VS), representing the most common location. **B.** Complex branching false tendon (*arrows*) with origin from the left ventricular free wall (FW) and insertions into the ventricular septum (VS) and base of posteromedial mitral papillary muscle (PM).

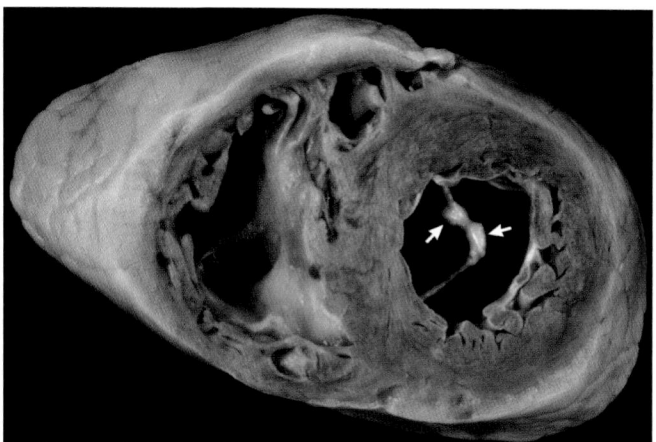

FIGURE 3-37. Calcified left ventricular false tendon (*arrows*) seen in short-axis view.

valve). The basal half of the ventricular septum is smooth-walled, whereas the apical half is characterized by numerous small and irregularly arranged trabeculations.[19-21]

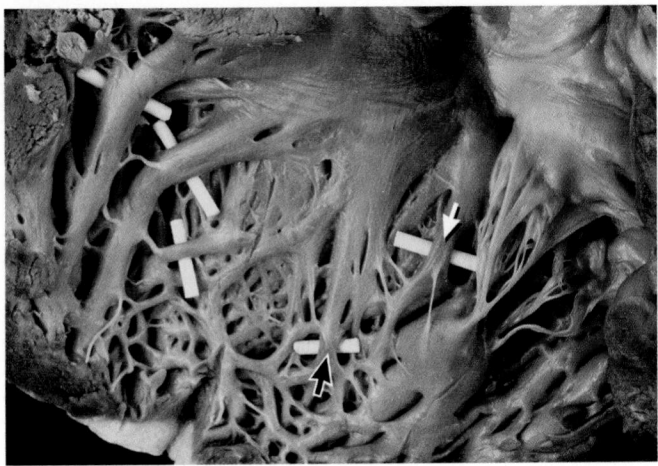

FIGURE 3–38. Prominent left ventricular trabeculations. Multiple large muscle bundles extend from the anterior free wall to the septum (*probes*). A single muscle bundle extends from the posteromedial mitral papillary muscle to the posterior septum (*probe with white arrow*), and one bundle extends from one portion of the posterior septum to another (*probe with black arrow*). Such trabeculations are more prominent in noncompaction cardiomyopathy.

Clinically relevant age-related anatomic changes include a disproportionate increase in ventricular septal thickness regardless of gender and in the absence of a history of hypertension.[24] This is associated with an appreciable increase in the ratio of ventricular septal to left ventricular free-wall thickness often exceeding 1.3 in patients older than 60 years of age[24] (Fig. 3–42). This can be caused in part by the accentuation of the sigmoid shape of the basal septum[19,24] (Fig. 3–43). *Age-related ventricular septal angulation can have clinical importance because it can mimic certain features of hypertrophic cardiomyopathy,[19,24] particularly if complicated by the indiscriminate use of volume-depleting diuretics or afterload-reducing agents.*

【 】 ATRIAL SEPTUM

When viewed from its right aspect, the atrial septum is composed of interatrial and atrioventricular regions[20,21] (see Fig. 3–35). The interatrial portion is characterized by the fossa ovalis, which is the anatomic hallmark of a morphologic right atrium (Fig. 3–44A). Its outer muscular rim is a horseshoe-shaped limbus, and its central depression is the valve of the fossa ovalis[20,21] (see Fig. 3–44A). The potential interatrial passageway between the limbus and the valve (which is patent throughout fetal life) is the foramen ovale (Figs. 3–44B and 3–45). When viewed from the left atrium, the atrial septum is entirely interatrial because the atrioventricular component lies below the mitral annulus between the left ventricle and right atrium. Likewise, the limbus of the fossa ovalis is completely covered by its opaque valve and is not directly visible from the left atrium.[19]

The foramen ovale is anatomically closed in approximately two-thirds of adults, but in the remaining one-third it remains patent and, therefore, a potential source for shunts and paradoxical embolism. Stretching of the atrial septum, when the atria are markedly dilated, can transform a patent foramen ovale into an acquired atrial septal defect. The posterior aortic sinus abuts against the interatrial septum (see Fig. 3–12D). During transseptal procedures, care must be taken to stay within the confines of the valve of the fossa ovalis to avoid per-

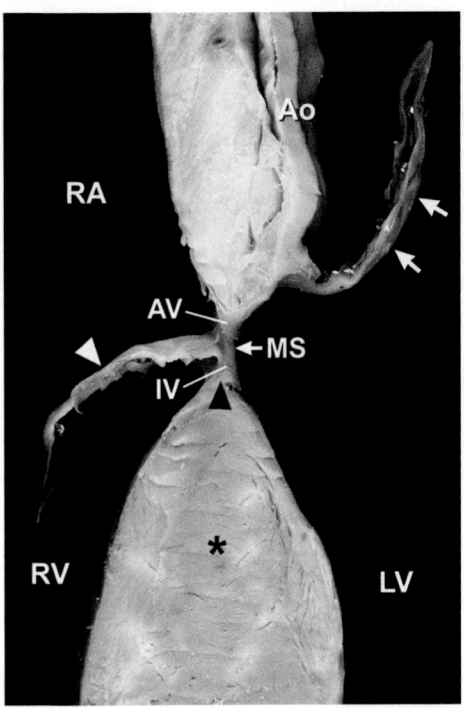

FIGURE 3–39. Four-chamber tomographic slice through the aortic root (Ao) and aortic valve (*arrows*) showing the small membranous (MS) and large muscular (*) portion of the ventricular septum. The membranous septum is divided into atrioventricular (AV) and interventricular (IV) components by the septal tricuspid leaflet (*white arrowhead*). *Black arrowhead* points to the expected location of the AV (His) bundle. LV, left ventricle; RA, right atrium; RV, right ventricle.

foration of an aortic sinus.[20] Echocardiography can help guide transseptal puncture during balloon mitral valvuloplasty or closure of an atrial septal defect with an occluder device.[15] Fenestrations of the valve of the fossa ovalis are the most common cause of congenital atrial septal defects. Redundant valve tissue can form an aneurysm of the valve of the fossa ovalis.

The atrioventricular (AV) portion of the atrial septum is made of major muscular and minor membranous components and sepa-

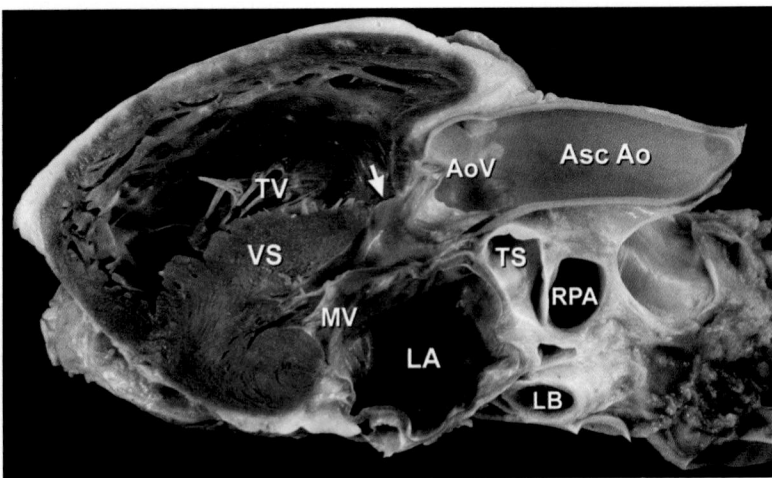

FIGURE 3–40. Tomographic section of the heart along a long-axis plane of the body. The aortic root lies in this plane. The left ventricle and aortic valve are cut obliquely. The membranous ventricular septum (*arrow*) lies beneath the right and posterior aortic cusps. AoV, aortic valve; Asc Ao, ascending aorta; LA, left atrium; LB, left bronchus; MV, mitral valve; RPA, right pulmonary artery; TS, transverse sinus; TV, tricuspid valve; VS, muscular ventricular septum.

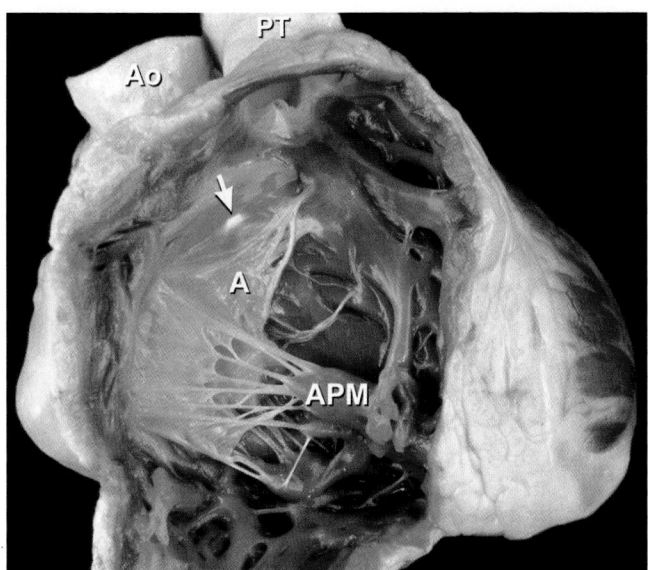

FIGURE 3–41. A view of the right ventricle. Transilluminated membranous ventricular septum (*arrow*) in contact with the commissure between the anterior and septal leaflets of the tricuspid valve. A, anterior tricuspid leaflet; Ao, ascending aorta; APM, anterior tricuspid papillary muscle; PT, pulmonary trunk.

rates the right atrium from the left ventricle[20,21] (see Figs. 3–35 and 3–39). *This explains why there is a potential for left-ventricular-to-right-atrial shunts.*[20,21] *The AV septum corresponds roughly to the triangle of Koch (see Fig. 3–71), an important anatomic surgical landmark because it contains the AV node and proximal portion of the AV (His) bundle. Thus, during tricuspid annuloplasty procedures and patch closures of membranous ventricular septal defects, care must be taken to avoid injury to the conduction system.*[20,21] The muscular component of the AV septum is interposed between the membranous septum anteriorly and the internal cardiac crux posteriorly.

When defects occur in the muscular AV septum, the mitral annulus usually drops to the same level as the tricuspid annulus, so the defect becomes primarily interatrial (primum atrial septal defect), and the AV conduction tissues are displaced inferiorly. Lipomatous hypertrophy of the atrial septum is characterized by excessive accumulation of adipose tissue within the limbus of the fossa ovalis but always sparing the valve of the fossa[7,19–21] (Fig. 3–46). Lipomatous hypertrophy of the atrial septum occurs commonly but not exclusively in older and obese persons.[19–21] *Although readily detected by echocardiography, it can be misinterpreted as a thrombus or tumor.*[7]

RIGHT ATRIUM

A prominent internal muscle ridge, the crista terminalis (Fig. 3–47), separates the right atrial free wall into a smooth-walled posterior region that receives the venae cavae and coronary sinus and a muscular anterior region that is lined

by parallel pectinate muscles and from which the right atrial appendage emanates.[19–21] *Pectinatus* is Latin for "comb," and the pectinate muscles and crista terminalis resemble the teeth and backbone of a comb, respectively.[21] The right atrial appendage abuts the right aortic sinus and overlies the proximal right coronary artery (see Fig. 3–53). *The right atrial free wall is paper-thin between pectinate muscles and therefore can be perforated easily by stiff catheters.*[19–21] *The atrial lead of a dual-chamber pacemaker is normally positioned within the trabeculations of the right atrial appendage.*

Inferior vena caval blood flow is directed by the eustachian valve toward the foramen ovale, and superior vena caval blood is directed toward the tricuspid valve[19] (Fig. 3–48). *Thus transseptal cardiac catheterization is more easily accomplished via the inferior vena cava, whereas instrumentation of the right ventricular apex (e.g., placement of an ICD or ventricular pacemaker lead) is more easily accomplished via the superior vena cava.*[19]

LEFT ATRIUM

The pulmonary vein orifices lie on the posterolateral (left pulmonary veins) and posteromedial (right pulmonary veins) aspects of the left atrial cavity. The left and right upper pulmonary veins are directed anterosuperiorly, whereas the lower veins enter the left atrium nearly perpendicular to the posterior atrial wall[19–21] (see Fig. 3–15A; Fig. 3–49). *Left atrial muscle extends some distance within the pulmonary veins. The resultant cuff of muscle acts as a sphincter during atrial systole and can be the source of focal atrial fibrillation that is amenable to catheter ablation*[11–15] (see Fig. 3–2).

The atrial appendage arises anterolaterally and lies in the left atrioventricular groove atop the proximal portion of the left circumflex coronary artery and, in some individuals, the left main

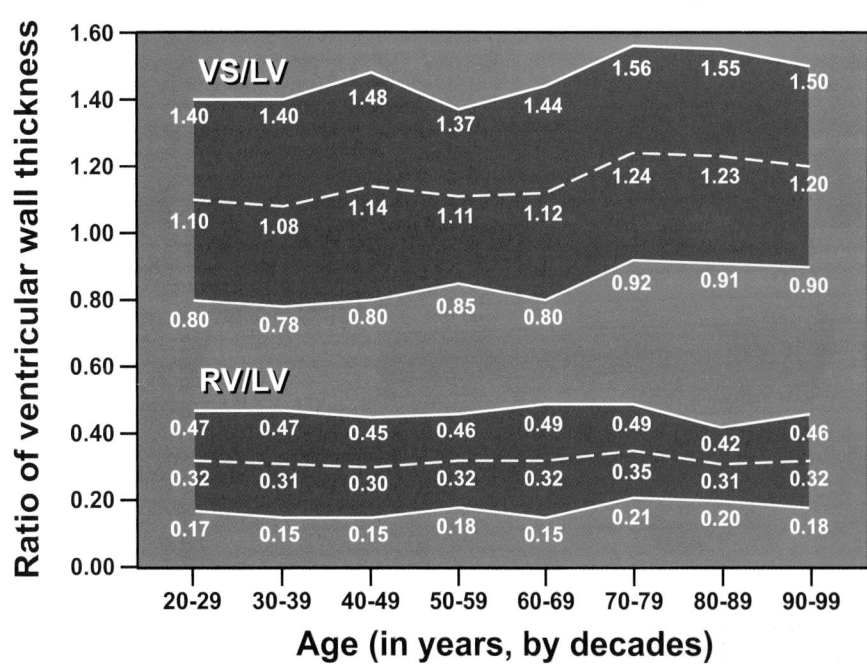

FIGURE 3–42. Ratios of ventricular wall thicknesses (means ± 2 standard deviations) versus age. RV/LV, ratio of right-to-left ventricular wall thickness; VS/LV, ratio of ventricular septal to left ventricular free wall thickness. *Source: Kitzman DW, et al. Mayo Clin Proc. 1988;63:137–146. Reproduced with permission of Mayo Foundation.*

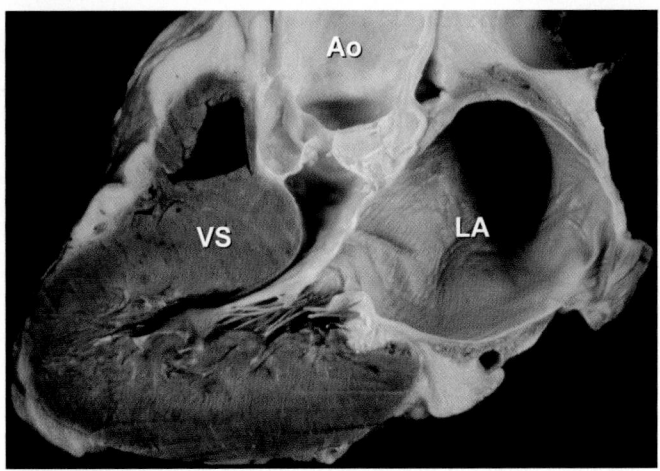

FIGURE 3–43. Age-related changes in the left-sided cardiac structures. Normal heart from an 84-year-old man demonstrates shortening of the base-to-apex (long-axis) dimension, decreased internal left ventricular dimension, aortic root dilatation, left atrial enlargement, and sigmoid-shaped septum. (Compare with Fig. 3–15 from an 18-year-old man.) Ao, ascending aorta; LA, left atrium; VS, ventricular septum.

coronary artery[20] (see Figs. 3–21A and 3–49). The left atrial appendage is smaller, more tortuous, and less pyramidal than its right atrial counterpart.[19–21] At least 80 percent are multilobed (up to four lobes, but the most frequent finding is two lobes)[33] (Fig. 3–50). There are also age- and sex-related differences in the dimensions of the appendage.[24] *With increasing use of transesophageal echocardiography to search for a cardiac source of embolism and to guide cardioversion and percutaneous balloon valvuloplasty procedures, a thorough appreciation of the variations in normal left atrial appendage morphology has become important because a thrombus can be missed if all lobes in the appendage are not visualized.* In contrast to the right atrial free wall, the left has no crista terminalis and no pectinate muscles outside its appendage.[19–21]

The coronary sinus travels along the posterior wall of the left atrium within the left atrioventricular groove (see Fig. 3–21A). *In patients with persistent left superior vena cava, which most commonly drains into a dilated coronary sinus, the left-sided cava courses between the left atrial appendage and the left upper pulmonary vein.*[21]

The venous structure can be misinterpreted as the descending thoracic aorta, a mass, or a pathologic cavity.

The esophagus and descending thoracic aorta are in contact with the posterior left atrial wall (see Figs. 3–20 and 3–49). *Accordingly, esophageal carcinomas can compress, infiltrate, or perforate the left atrium, and descending thoracic aortic aneurysms can compress this chamber.*[19] *A large hiatal hernia also can abut against the left atrium and resemble a mass.*

The marked increase in the incidence of atrial fibrillation from the fourth to the ninth decades of life can be caused by dilatation of the left atrium consequent to left ventricular diastolic dysfunction or mitral valve disease.[34]

CORONARY ARTERIES AND VEINS

A detailed description of the spectrum of coronary artery anatomy including the many variations in the number and size of branches and course of the different arteries is beyond the scope of this chapter. The interested reader is referred to the elegant anatomic work by Wallace McAlpine published in 1975.[35] The focus of the following discussion, therefore, is to introduce the reader to the clinically relevant anatomy of the coronary circulation, with special emphasis on tomographic analysis of regional blood flow.

From the right and left aortic sinuses arise the right and left coronary arteries, respectively, and their ostia, which normally originate about two-thirds the distance from the aortic annulus to the sinotubular junction and about midway between the aortic commissures[19–21] (see Fig. 3–28; Fig. 3–51). Whereas the right coronary artery arises nearly perpendicularly from the aorta, the left arises at an acute angle[19] (Fig. 3–52). Rarely, the anterior descending and circumflex arteries arise separately from a double-barrel left coronary ostium.[19–21] *Ostial stenosis most commonly results from atherosclerosis and degenerative calcification of the aortic sinotubular junction, which often overlies the right aortic sinus.*[21] *Less often it is caused by aortic dissection or by aortitis associated with syphilis or ankylosing spondylitis. Stenosis of the right coronary ostium is much more frequent than that of the left. Iatrogenic ostial injury can complicate coronary angiography, intraoperative coronary perfusion, or aortic valve replacement.*[19–21] *Atherosclerosis or thrombosis of*

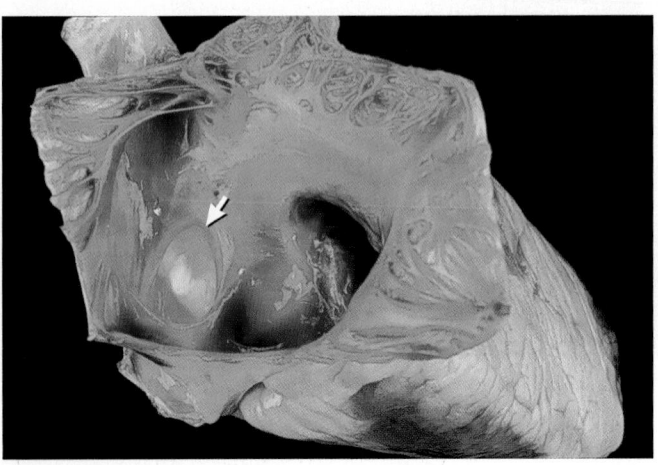

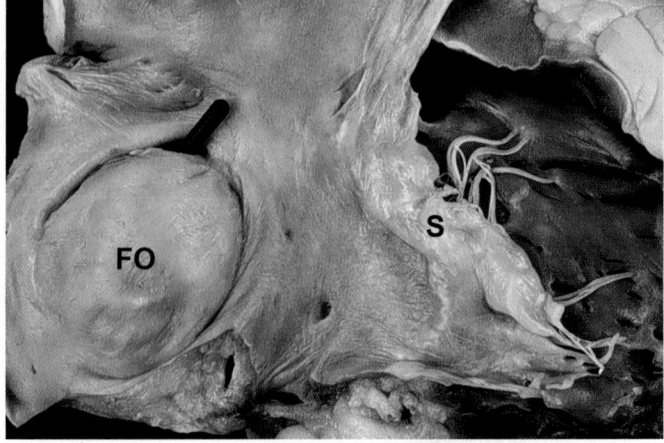

FIGURE 3–44. A. Fossa ovalis. Opened right atrium shows the thick muscular limbus of the atrial septum (*arrow*), in contrast to the thin valve of the fossa ovalis (*transilluminated*). **B.** Patent foramen ovale (*black probe*) as seen from the right atrium. There is also an aneurysm of the valve of the fossa ovalis (FO). S, septal leaflet of the tricuspid valve.

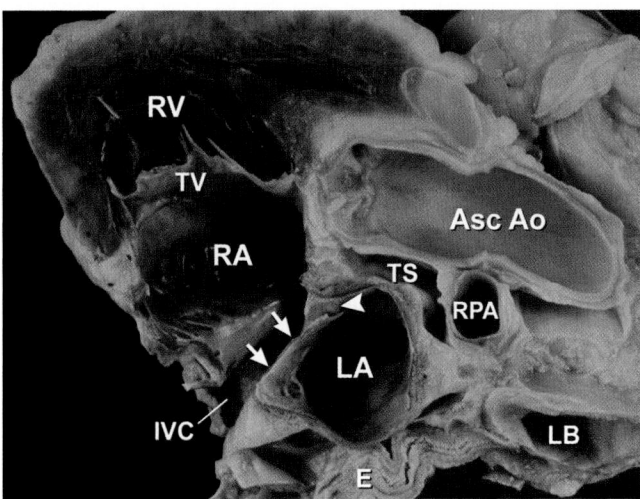

FIGURE 3–45. Tomographic section of the heart along a long axis of the body. The valve of the fossa ovalis (*arrows*) and a patent foramen ovale (*arrowhead*) are seen in this view. Asc Ao, ascending aorta; E, esophagus; IVC, inferior vena cava; LA, left atrium; LB, left bronchus; RA, right atrium; RPA, right pulmonary artery; RV, right ventricle; TS, transverse sinus; TV, tricuspid valve.

the most proximal portion of either coronary artery can mimic true ostial stenosis.

The right coronary artery is embedded in adipose tissue throughout its course within the right atrioventricular groove. *Tricuspid annuloplasty or replacement can be complicated by injury to the right coronary artery.*[21] In 50 to 60 percent of persons, its first branch is the conus artery (Fig. 3–53), which supplies the right ventricular outflow tract and forms an important collateral anastomosis (circle of Vieussens), just below the pulmonary valve, with an analogous branch from the left anterior descending coronary artery (LAD).[19–21] In approximately one-third of patients, the conus artery arises independently from the aorta[21] (see Fig. 3–28).

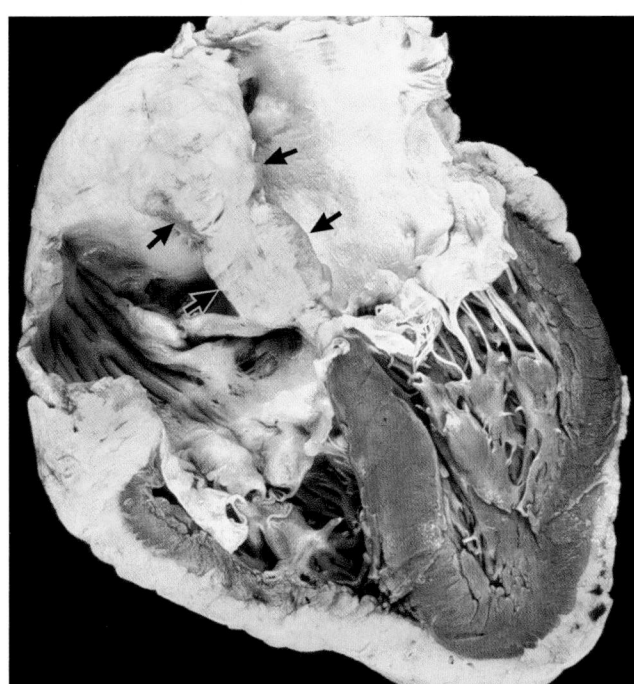

FIGURE 3–46. Four-chamber slice through the heart showing lipomatous hypertrophy of the atrial septum (*arrows*).

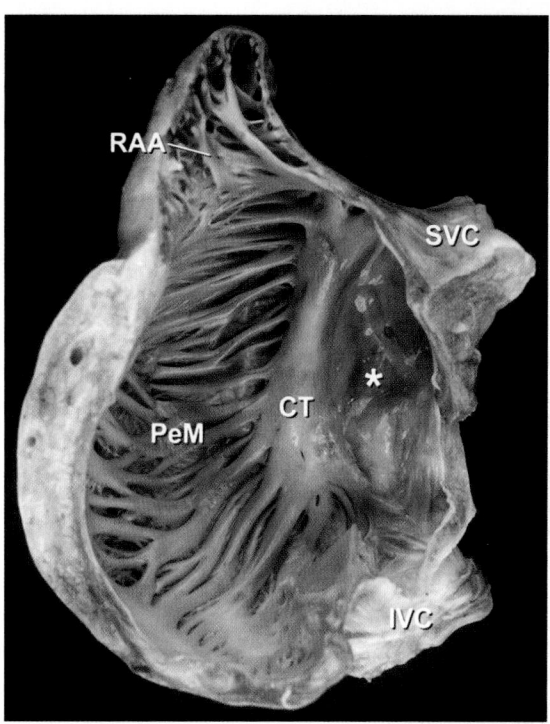

FIGURE 3–47. Right atrial free wall showing separation of the posterior smooth-walled (*) portion from the anterior muscular portion with its pectinate muscles (PeM) and right atrial appendage (RAA) by the crista terminalis (CT). IVC, inferior vena cava; SVC, superior vena cava.

The infundibular septum is supplied by the descending septal artery, which usually originates from the proximal right or conus coronary artery.[19–21] Among the numerous marginal branches of the right coronary artery that supply the remainder of the right ventricular free wall, the largest branch travels along the acute margin from base to apex[19–21] (see Fig. 3–51). In at least 70 percent of human hearts, the posterior descending artery arises from the distal right coronary artery (see Fig. 3–51). The posterior descending and distal posterolateral branches of a dominant right coronary artery supply the basal and middle inferior wall, basal

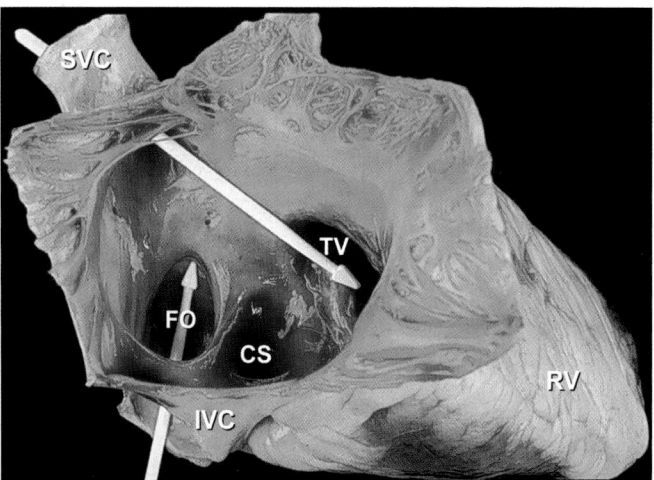

FIGURE 3–48. Opened right atrium. Two arrow-shaped probes show that superior vena caval flow is directed toward the tricuspid orifice and inferior vena caval flow is directed toward the fossa ovalis (FO). CS, coronary sinus; IVC, inferior vena cava; RV, right ventricle; SVC, superior vena cava; TV, tricuspid valve.

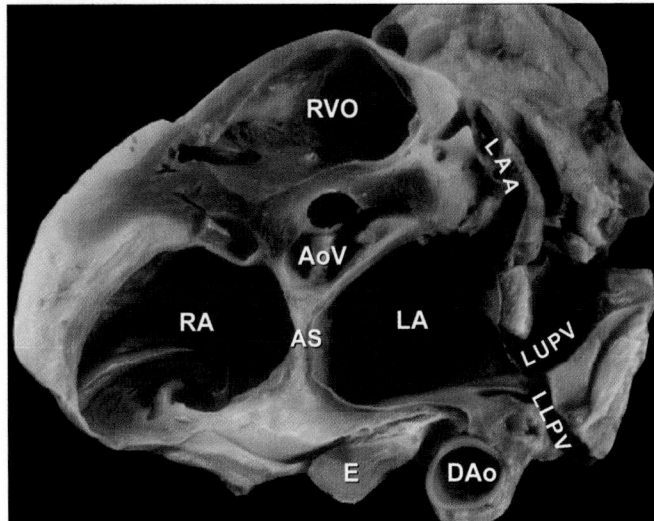

FIGURE 3–49. Oblique, short-axis cut at the base of the heart. The esophagus (E) is posterior and adjacent to the left atrium (LA) and adjacent to the descending thoracic aorta (DAo). The left upper pulmonary (LUPV) and left lower pulmonary vein (LLPV) are clearly seen. The right ventricular outflow tract (RVO) is anterior. AS, atrial septum; AoV, aortic valve; LA, left atrium; LAA, left atrial appendage; RA, right atrium.

(inlet) inferior septum, right bundle branch, AV node, AV (His) bundle, posterior portion of the left bundle branch, and posteromedial mitral papillary muscle.[21]

The left main coronary artery travels for a very short distance along the epicardium between the pulmonary trunk and left atrium (see Figs. 3–51 and 3–53). It then divides into anterior descending and circumflex arteries (see Figs. 3–51 and 3–53). An intermediate artery also may arise at this division, thus forming a trifurcation rather than a bifurcation, and follows the course of a circumflex marginal branch[19–21] (see Fig. 3–53).

The LAD courses within the epicardial fat of the anterior interventricular groove, wraps around the cardiac apex, and travels a variable distance along the inferior interventricular groove toward the cardiac base. Its septal perforating branches supply the anterior septum and apical septum. The first septal perforating branch supplies the AV (His) bundle and proximal left bundle branch[21] (Fig. 3–54). *In patients with symptomatic hypertrophic obstructive cardiomyopathy, nonsurgical septal reduction by percutaneous transluminal occlusion of septal branches of the LAD is a new therapeutic approach aimed at reducing the outflow gradient.[36] The long-term effects of this procedure are currently unknown.* The epicardial diagonal branches of the LAD supply the anterior left ventricular free wall, part of the anterolateral mitral papillary muscle, and the medial one-third of the anterior right ventricular free wall.[19–21] Although short segments of the LAD can travel within the myocardium (covered by a so-called myocardial bridge) (Fig. 3–55), the resulting systolic luminal narrowing is probably benign in the vast majority of people.[21] *However, whereas the prevalence of myocardial bridging is only 0.5 to 1.6 percent in the general population, it is reported to be 28 percent in children and 30 to 50 percent in adults with hypertrophic cardiomyopathy.[37] More important, myocardial bridging appears to be associated with a poor prognosis (higher incidence of myocardial ischemia and sudden death) in patients with hypertrophic cardiomyopathy regardless of age.[37]*

The left circumflex coronary artery courses within the adipose tissue of the left atrioventricular groove (see Fig. 3–21A) and commonly terminates just beyond its large obtuse marginal branch (see Fig. 3–51). It supplies the lateral left ventricular free wall and a portion of the anterolateral mitral papillary muscle.[19–21]

Along the inferior surface of the heart, the length of the right coronary artery varies inversely with that of the circumflex artery. The artery that crosses the cardiac crux and gives rise to the posterior descending branch represents the dominant coronary artery. Dominance is right in 70 percent of human hearts, left in 10 percent, and shared in 20 percent.[19–21] *In patients with a congenitally bicuspid aortic valve, the incidence of left coronary dominance is 25 to 30 percent.[21]* Recent advances in CT technology allow for 3D reconstruction of the epicardial coronary arteries and veins (see Fig. 3–56).

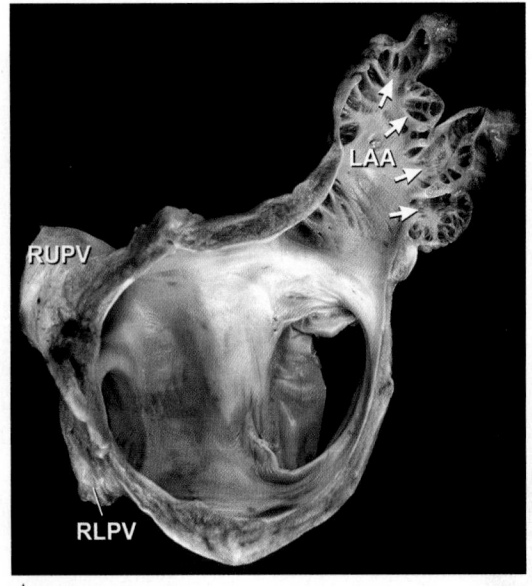 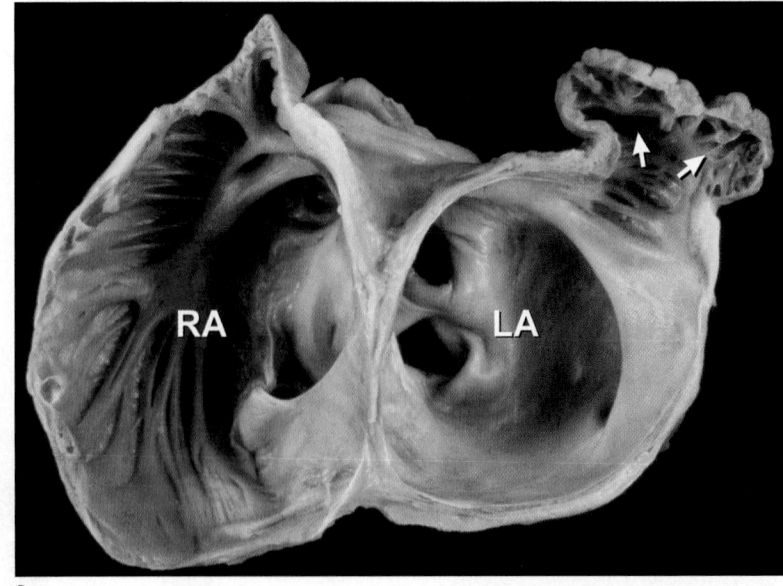

FIGURE 3–50. Left atrial appendages (LAA). **A.** Left atrial free wall showing appendage with four lobes (*arrows*). **B.** Biatrial specimen demonstrating left atrial appendage with two lobes (*arrows*). LA, left atrium; RA, right atrium; RLPV, right lower pulmonary vein; RUPV, right upper pulmonary vein.

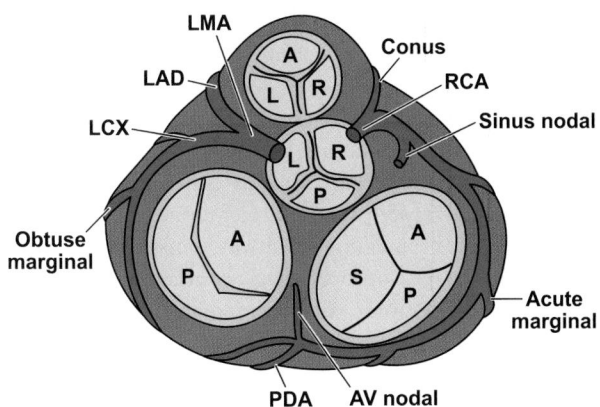

FIGURE 3–51. Schematic diagram of coronary artery distribution viewed at the base of the heart. In this right-dominant system, the right coronary artery (RCA) gives rise to the posterior descending artery (PDA), and the left main coronary artery (LMA) gives rise to the left anterior descending (LAD) and left circumflex (LCX) branches. A, anterior; AV, atrioventricular; L, left; P, posterior; R, right; S, septal.

The coronary venous circulation is comprised of coronary sinus, cardiac veins, and thebesian venous systems[19–21] (Fig. 3–57). The great cardiac vein travels in the anterior interventricular groove beside the left anterior descending coronary artery and in the left atrioventricular groove beside the left circumflex artery.[19–21] The great cardiac vein and other cardiac veins, such as the left posterior and middle cardiac veins, drain into the coronary sinus, which courses along the posteroinferior aspect of the left atrioventricular groove and empties into the right atrium[19–21] (see Fig. 3–21A). The ostium of the coronary sinus is guarded by a crescent-shaped valvular remnant, the thebesian valve. Rarely, the coronary sinus drains directly into the left atrium.[21]

During cardiac operations, cardioplegic solution can be administered retrogradely into the coronary sinus. In patients with the Wolff-Parkinson-White preexcitation syndrome and left-sided bypass tracts, the ablation catheter during electrophysiologic studies can be positioned within the coronary sinus and great cardiac vein adjacent to the mitral valve ring to localize the aberrant conduction pathway.[21] Coronary venous anatomy is extremely variable, however. This can have important practice implications. The coronary veins, via the coronary sinus, provide access to percutaneous epicardial mapping and

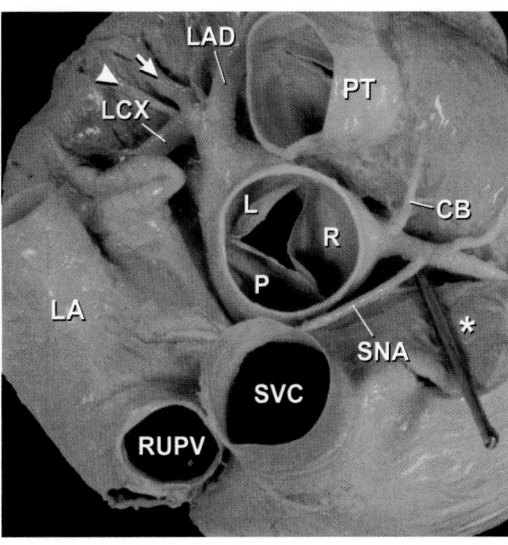

FIGURE 3–53. The right coronary artery gives rise to the conus branch (CB). A rod retracts the right atrial appendage (*) to disclose the sinus node artery (SNA). *Arrow* points to an intermediate left coronary artery; *arrowhead* points to a circumflex marginal branch. L, left aortic cusp; LA, left atrium; LAD, left anterior descending coronary artery; LCX, left circumflex coronary artery; P, posterior aortic cusp; PT, pulmonary trunk; R, right aortic cusp; RUPV, right upper pulmonary vein; SVC, superior vena cava. *Source: McAlpine.[35] Used with permission.*

pacing of the ventricles and ablation of subepicardial arrhythmogenic foci[38] (Fig. 3–58). For biventricular pacing, optimal left ventricular pacing lead position is within the posterolateral branch of the coronary sinus, followed by the lateral branch. Some patients with ischemic cardiomyopathy can be poor candidates for conventional revascularization procedures (e.g., coronary artery bypass graft surgery or angioplasty) because their epicardial coronary arteries are diffusely diseased. Because in virtually all people the coronary veins run parallel to the entire course of coronary arteries, alternative percutaneous revascularization methods that use the coronary veins as a bypass conduit for coronary arterial flow are being explored.[39–41] Myocardial revascularization is achieved by either connecting the coronary artery proximal and distal to a stenosis to its companion coronary vein (similar to a conventional bypass graft) or by retroperfusion through the venous mi-

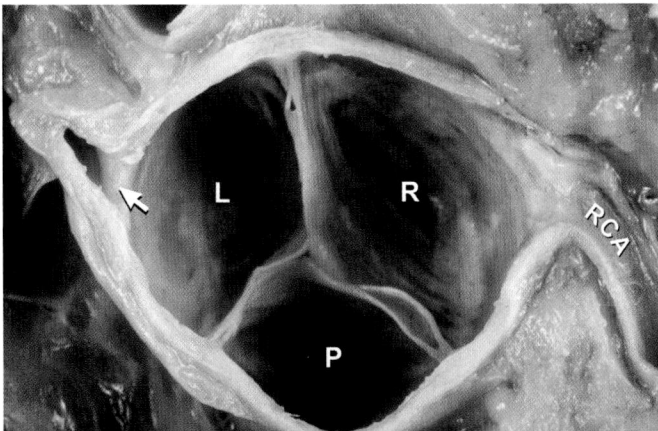

FIGURE 3–52. Differences in angulation at the origins of the right (RCA) and left main (*arrow*) coronary arteries. L, left aortic cusp; P, posterior aortic cusp; R, right aortic cusp.

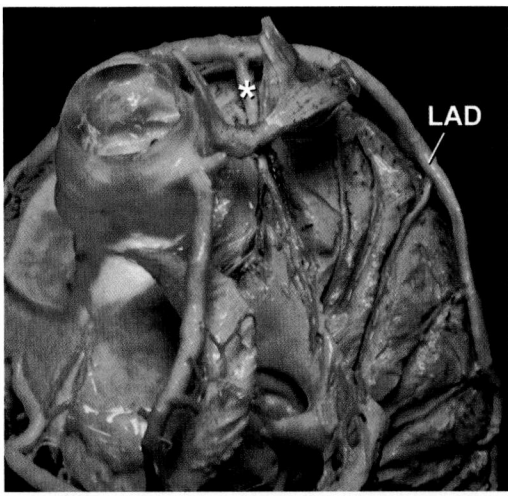

FIGURE 3–54. Septal branches of the left anterior descending coronary artery (LAD); * points to the first septal perforator. *Source: McAlpine.[35] Used with permission.*

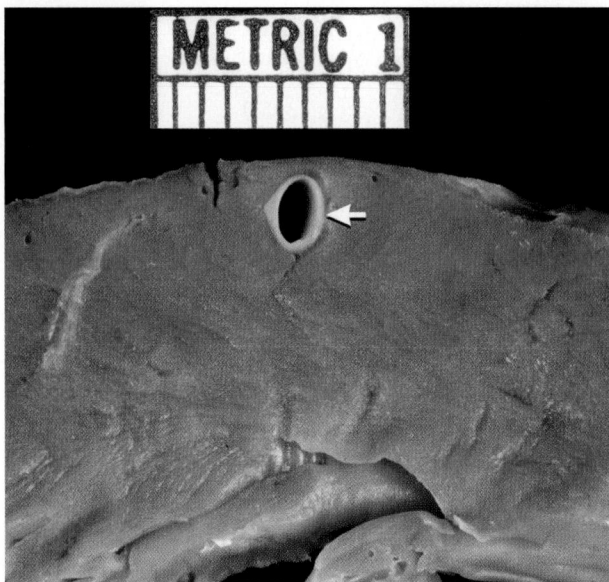

FIGURE 3–55. Intramyocardial course of the left anterior descending coronary artery (*arrow*).

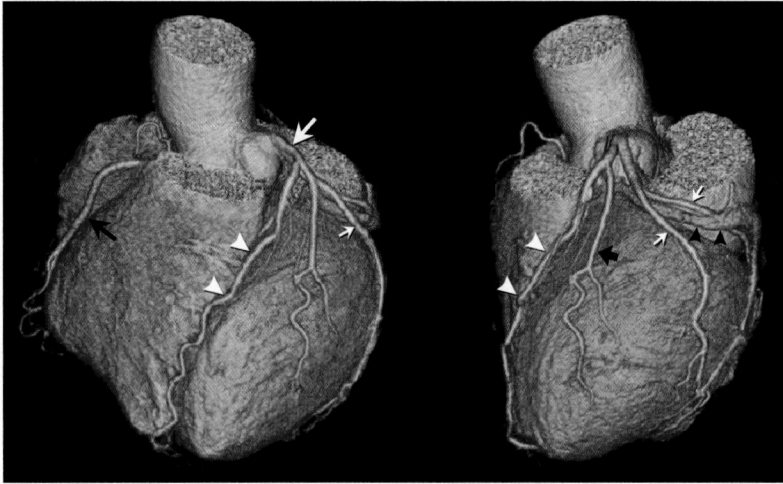

FIGURE 3–56. Three-dimensional reformatted images of CT coronary angiograms showing the right coronary artery (*long black arrow*), left main (*large white arrow*), left anterior descending coronary artery (*white arrowheads*) and a diagonal branch (*short black arrow*), and left circumflex coronary artery (*small white arrows*). A segment of the coronary venous circulation is also seen (*black arrowheads*).

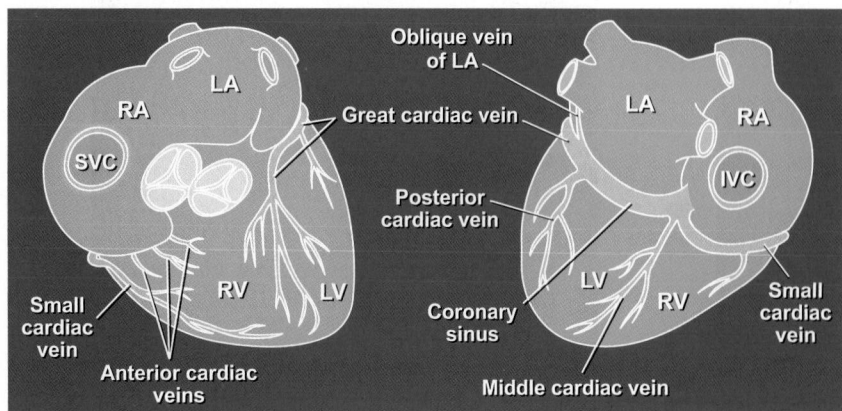

FIGURE 3–57. Schematic diagram of the coronary venous circulation. IVC, inferior vena cava; LA, left atrium; LV, left ventricle; RA, right atrium; RV, right ventricle; SVC, superior vena cava.

crovasculature if the artery and vein are only connected proximal to the stenosis. Coronary veins, unlike saphenous veins, are not removed, thus preserving their adventitia and blood supply.[39–41]

Coronary artery disease is associated with regional abnormalities in ventricular structure and function. Because analysis of segmental myocardial perfusion or contractility is the cornerstone of tomographic imaging techniques (stress echocardiography, SPECT imaging, positron emission tomography [PET], and MRI), for clinicopathologic correlations (Fig. 3–59), a combination tomographic and segmental approach to coronary artery anatomy is recommended.[21,42,43] Ventricular mass is made of the left and right ventricular free walls and the partitioning ventricular septum. Three levels (i.e., basal, midventricular, and apical) are used to divide the base-apex length of the left ventricle into thirds (Fig. 3–60). The basal third includes that portion between the mitral annulus and the tips of the papillary muscles. The midventricular third is from the papillary muscle to the most apical insertion point of these muscles into the left ventricular free wall. The apical third includes the remainder of the ventricle, from the insertion of the papillary muscles to the left ventricular apex. A similar approach can be applied to the right ventricle.[19–21,42] The ventricular septum can be divided into anteroseptal, septal, and inferoseptal segments, and the left ventricular free wall is divided into anterior, lateral, and inferior segments at the basal and midventricular levels (see Fig. 3–60). The left ventricular apical level consists of four segments (i.e., septum, inferior, lateral, and anterior) (see Fig. 3–60).

This regional approach is not arbitrary and has been verified by studies of normal, dilated, and hypertrophied hearts. According to this system, there are 16 left ventricular segments that can be evaluated for regional abnormalities. This regional approach can also be used to assess transmural infarct size, because the percentage of left ventricular mass contributed by any particular region is not altered in any significant manner by symmetric hypertrophy or dilatation.[21]

⟦ ⟧ REGIONAL CORONARY ARTERY SUPPLY

The ventricular regions described tend to correlate well with common patterns of coronary arterial distribution[19–21] (Figs. 3–61 and 3–62). Any specific epicardial coronary artery generally will supply a certain cluster of regions. For example, in a typical right-dominant system, the LAD would supply the midventricular and basal segments of the anterior and anterolateral walls and anterior septum and all apical segments. The left circumflex artery would supply the midventricular and basal inferolateral segments, and the right coronary artery would supply the midventricular and basal inferior wall and inferior septum (see Fig. 3–62). However,

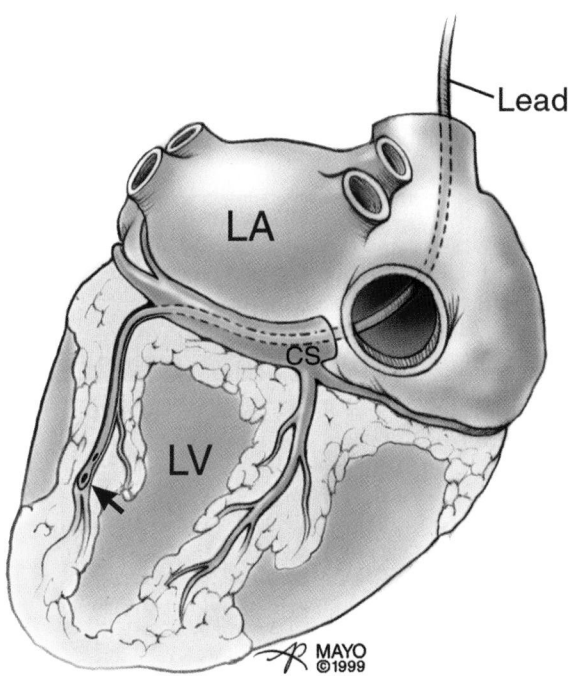

FIGURE 3–58. Schematic diagram shows placement of the tip of a pacing/mapping catheter within a coronary vein (*arrow*) via the coronary sinus (CS). LA, left atrium; LV, left ventricle.

because the patterns of coronary distribution are so highly variable, these correlations between coronary blood flow and regional anatomy are not precise. For example, a hyperdominant right coronary artery can supply the apex, and a large, obtuse marginal branch of the circumflex artery can supply the anterolateral or inferior wall. Also, any given myocardial region can, in some people, receive its blood supply from the branches of two independent major epicardial arteries.[19–21] In old age, the coronary arteries become dilated and tortuous (Fig. 3–63). *Ultrafast electron beam CT is very useful for the detection of calcified plaques within the coronary arteries.*

[ ] CORONARY COLLATERALS AND MICROCIRCULATION

Collateral channels provide communication between the major coronary arteries and their branches.[21] If stenosis of an epicardial coronary artery produces a pressure gradient across such a vessel, the collateral channel can dilate with time and provide a bypass avenue for blood flow beyond the obstruction. Such functional collaterals can develop between the terminal extensions of two coronary arteries, between the side branches of two arteries, between branches of the same artery, or within the same branch (via the vasa vasorum). These are most common in the ventricular septum (between septal perforators of the anterior and posterior descending arteries), in the ventricular apex (between anterior descending septal perforators), in the anterior right ventricular free wall (between anterior descending and right or conus arteries), in the anterolateral left ventricular free wall (between anterior descending diagonals and circumflex marginals), at the cardiac crux, and along the atrial surfaces (between the right and left circumflex arteries).[21]

The intramural coronary vessels form the microcirculation. There are age-related variations in the pattern of distribution of the coronary microcirculation.[44] *Angina-like chest pain in some patients with angiographically normal epicardial coronary arteries (i.e., syndrome X, or microvascular angina) can be secondary to abnormal vasodilator reserve or vasoconstriction of the coronary microcirculation.*[45] *Abnormal flow reserve of the coronary microcirculation is seen in both dilated and hypertrophied hearts. In the latter, structural changes in the coronary arterioles can be found on histologic examination of the myocardium.*[46–48] *In patients with symptomatic hypertrophic cardiomyopathy without angiographic evidence of epicardial coronary artery disease, myocardial tissue obtained during surgical myectomy can show smaller than normal coronary arteriolar lumina.*[48] *Postmortem analysis of hearts with hypertrophic cardiomyopathy also has revealed coronary arterioles with abnormally thick walls.*[48] *With contrast echocardiography, it can be possible to noninvasively visualize intramyocardial arterioles and study coronary flow reserve.*[49] *Demonstration of an intact microvascular circulation in akinetic myocardium following acute myocardial infarction, using PET or SPECT imaging or contrast echocardiography, is evidence of viability of the affected segment.*[49] *The creation of intramyocardial channels with CO_2 laser transmyocardial revascularization has been associated with augmentation of collateral flow to ischemic myocardium through angiogenesis.*[50]

[ ] CARDIAC LYMPHATICS

The myocardial lymphatics drain toward the epicardial surface, where they merge to form the right and left lymphatic channels, which travel in retrograde fashion with their respective coronary arteries. These two lymphatic channels travel along the ascending aorta and merge before draining into a pretracheal lymph node beneath the aortic arch. This single lymphatic channel then travels through a cardiac lymph node, between the superior vena cava and innominate artery, and finally empties into the right lymphatic duct. Metastatic tumor obstruction of epicardial lymphatics can produce a pericardial effusion.[19–21]

[ ] GREAT VESSELS

The subclavian and internal jugular veins merge bilaterally to form the right and left innominate veins (Fig. 3–64). Valves in the subclavian and internal jugular veins, near their junctions with the innominate veins, are important anatomic structures that help maintain unidirectional antegrade blood flow not only in the normal state but also in the setting of elevated right-sided heart filling pressures.[51] Subclavian and internal jugular venous valves are absent in 2 and 6 percent of people, respectively, and venous valves can be damaged by catheter-induced trauma or by age.[51] *Absent or malfunctioning valves can interfere with the success of closed-chest cardiopulmonary resuscitation and contribute to the development of brain edema during such a procedure.*[51]

The left innominate vein is two to three times the length of its right-sided counterpart. It travels anteriorly to the aortic arch along the right anterolateral border of the ascending aorta, where it joins the shorter right innominate vein to form the superior vena cava[19–21] (see Fig. 3–64). *Transesophageal echocardiographic imaging of the upper ascending aorta can show a double lumen (i.e., aorta and adjacent innominate vein) that can be misinterpreted as aortic dissection by an inexperienced echocardiographer.*[7]

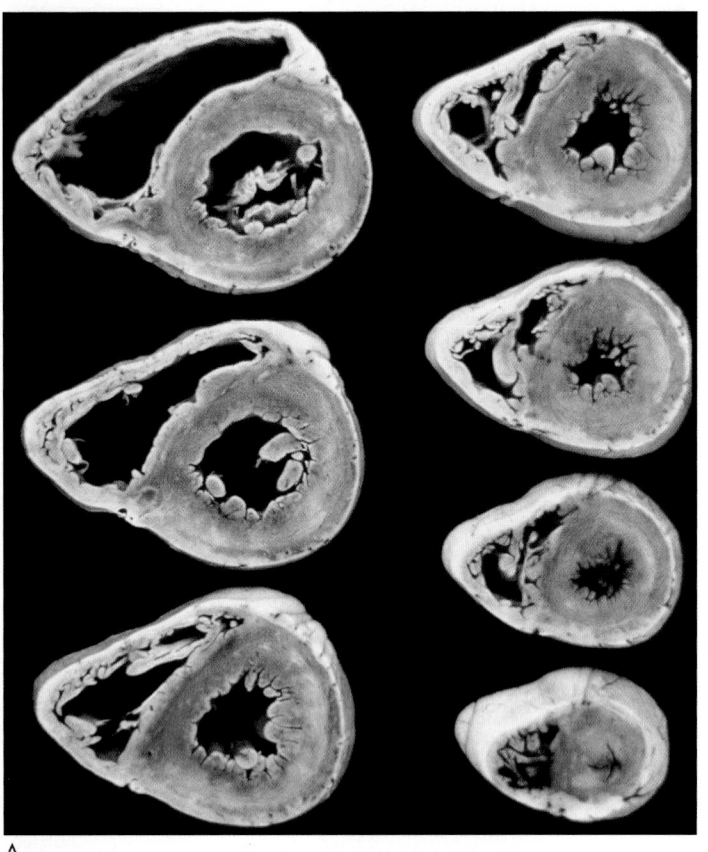

A

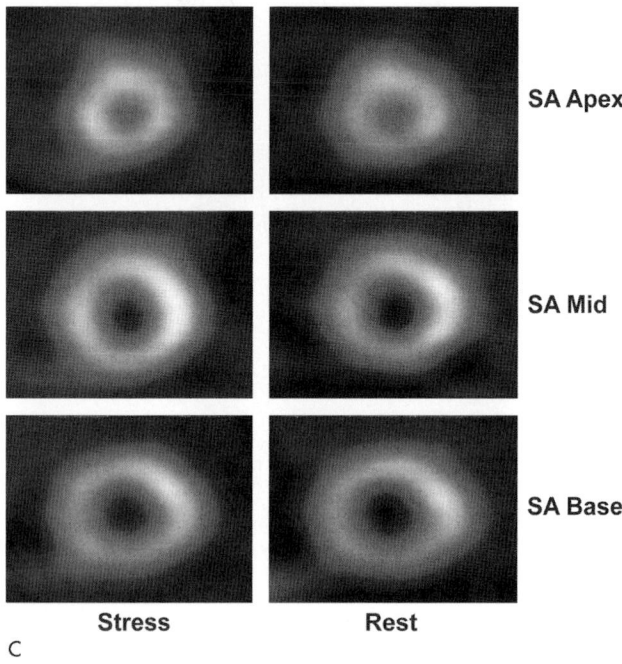

SA Apex

SA Mid

SA Base

Stress   Rest

C

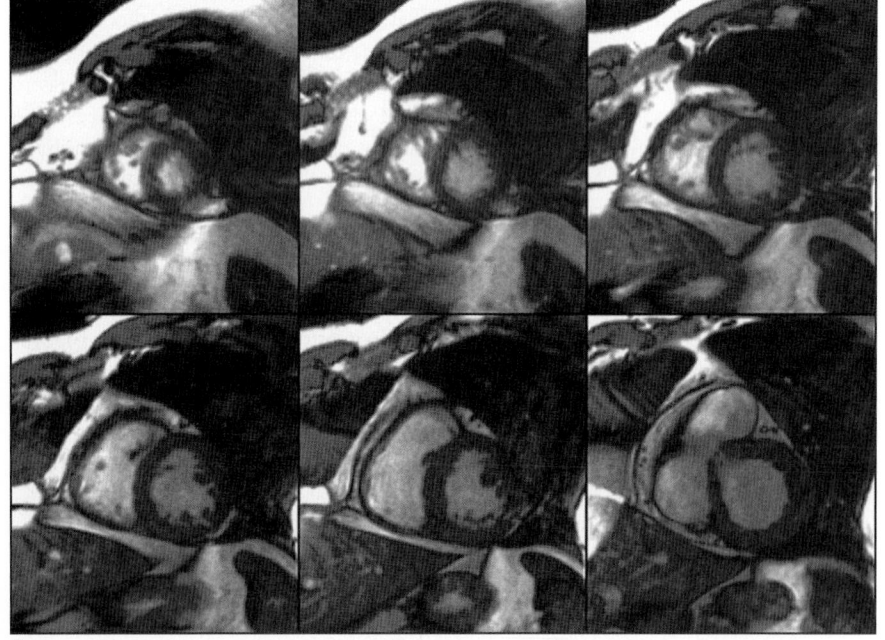

B

FIGURE 3–59. Short-axis views. **A.** Collage of anatomic sections obtained by "bread slicing" the heart in its short-axis plane viewed from the apex toward the base of the heart. **B.** Comparable MRI images. **C.** Comparable sestamibi SPECT images of the left ventricle showing normal myocardial perfusion at rest and with exercise. SA, short axis.

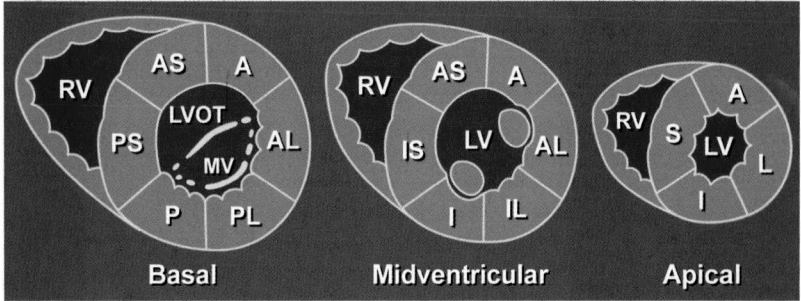

Basal   Midventricular   Apical

FIGURE 3–60. Schematic diagram of the three levels of short-axis tomographic views used in echocardiography for 16-segment wall motion analysis. A, anterior; AL, anterolateral; AS, anterior ventricular septum; I, inferior; IL, inferolateral; IS, inferior ventricular septum; L, lateral; LV, left ventricle; LVOT, left ventricular outflow tract; P, posterior; PL, posterolateral; PS, posterior ventricular septum; RV, right ventricle; S, septum. The most basal segment of the inferior wall is the anatomically true posterior segment. At this level, the adjacent ventricular septum is commonly referred to as either the *basal posterior septum* or the *basal inferior septum* and the adjacent lateral wall as either the *basal posterolateral wall* or the *basal inferolateral wall*.

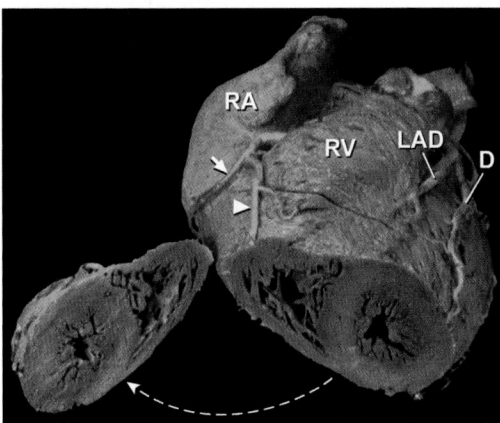

FIGURE 3–61. Regional coronary flow, with a short-axis slice of the heart. A large diagonal branch (D) of the left anterior descending coronary artery (LAD) supplies the lateral wall, and an acute marginal branch (*arrowhead*) of the right coronary artery (*arrow*) supplies the anterior right ventricular free wall. The distal segment of the LAD is intramural. RA, right atrium; RV, right ventricle. *Source: McAlpine.[35] Used with permission.*

The superior vena cava lies anterior to the right pulmonary artery (Fig. 3–65) and receives the azygos vein posteriorly before draining into the superior aspect of the right atrium, just posterior to the atrial appendage[19–21] (see Figs. 3–47, 3–48, and 3–65). *The vein of Marshall forms the terminal connection between a persistent left superior vena cava and the coronary sinus. Its vestigial remnant in normal adults is the ligament of Marshall (Fig. 3–66). Both vein and ligament are a potential source of arrhythmias.* The ostium of the inferior vena cava is guarded by a crescent-shaped, often fenestrated flap of tissue, the eustachian valve[19–21] (see Fig. 3–16A), which is readily seen by echocardiography. Although generally small, the eustachian valve can become so large that it can produce a double-chambered right atrium.[20] Also, when either the eustachian or thebesian valve is large and fenestrated, it is referred to as a *Chiari*

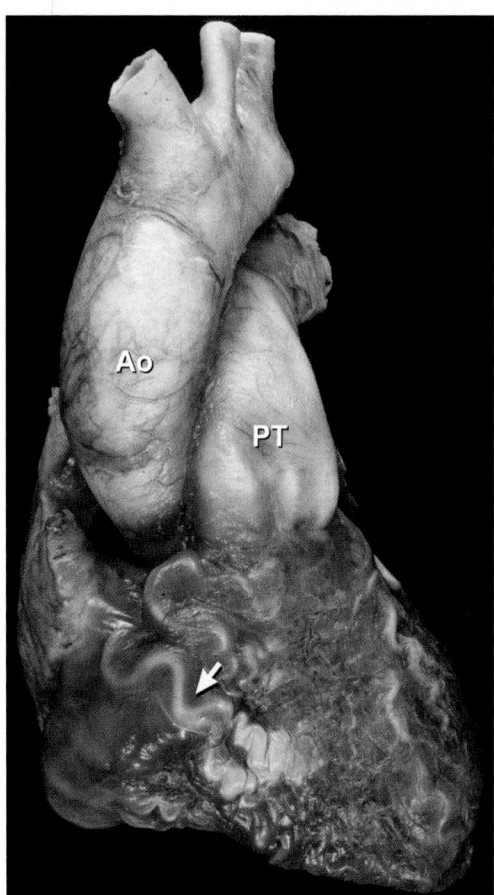

FIGURE 3–63. Tortuous coronary arteries (*arrow*) typically seen in the elderly with nondilated hearts. Ao, ascending aorta; PT, pulmonary trunk.

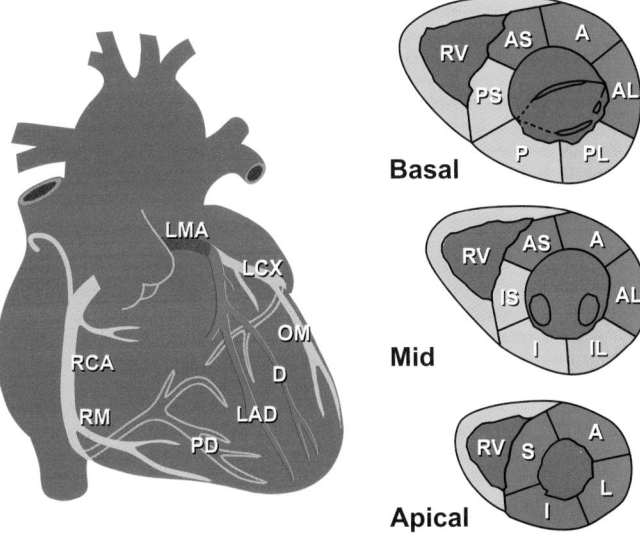

FIGURE 3–62. Coronary distribution using a 16-segment model. D, diagonal branch of the left anterior descending coronary artery; LAD, left anterior descending coronary artery; LCX, left circumflex coronary artery; LMA, left main coronary artery; OM, obtuse marginal branch of the circumflex coronary artery; PD, posterior descending coronary artery; RCA, right coronary artery; RM, right marginal branch; other abbreviations as in Fig. 3–58.

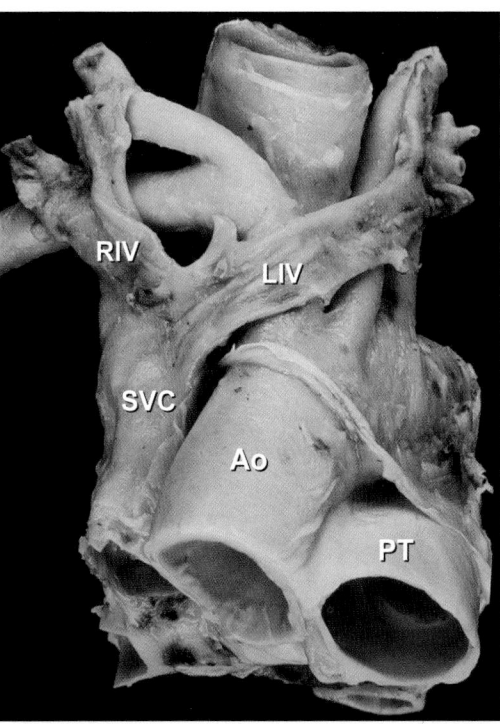

FIGURE 3–64. The longer left (LIV) and shorter right (RIV) innominate veins normally join to form the right superior vena cava (SVC). Ao, ascending aorta; PT, pulmonary trunk.

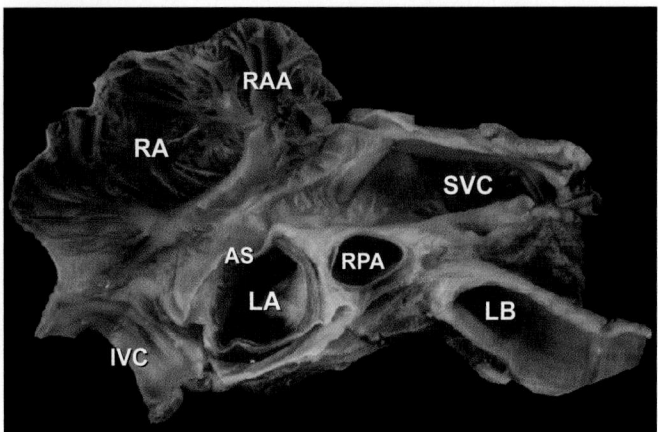

FIGURE 3–65. Long-axis view of the superior vena cava (SVC) and inferior vena cava (IVC). The specimen is viewed from the left looking toward the free wall of the right atrium. The right atrium (RA) and its appendage (RAA) are anterior. This is a commonly used tomographic plane in transesophageal echocardiography (TEE). AS, atrial septum; LA, left atrium; LB, left bronchus; RPA, right pulmonary artery.

net.[19–21] *By echocardiography, a Chiari net can be misinterpreted as a mass.* The thoracic aorta arises at the level of the aortic valve and is divided into three segments: ascending aorta, aortic arch, and descending thoracic aorta (Fig. 3–67). The ascending aorta consists of sinus and tubular portions, which are demarcated by the sinotubular junction (see Fig. 3–28; Fig. 3–68). *This is the site at which supravalvular aortic stenosis is often most severe.*[19–21] *The entire thoracic aorta can be readily imaged by CT and MRI* (Fig. 3–69).

Behind the aortic valve cusps are three outpouchings, or sinuses (of Valsalva). The right aortic sinus abuts against the ventricular septum and right ventricular parietal band and is covered in part by the right atrial appendage (see Figs. 3–30 and 3–53). In contrast, the left aortic sinus rests against the anterior left ventricular free wall and a portion of the anterior mitral leaflet, abuts the left atrial free wall, and is covered in part by the pulmonary trunk and left atrial appendage (see Figs. 3–20 and 3–21A). The posterior (noncoronary) aortic sinus overlies the ventricular septum and a part of the anterior mitral leaflet, forms part of the transverse sinus, abuts the atrial septum, and indents both atrial free walls[19–21] (see Figs. 3–12D and 3–22). *Rupture of the right and posterior aortic sinuses of Valsalva can result in a communication with the right ventricular outflow tract or right atrium, whereas rupture of the left aortic sinus of Valsalva leads to a communication with the left atrium or left ventricular outflow tract. Annuloaortic ectasia is associated with hypertension, aortic medial degeneration, and advanced age and can produce aortic regurgitation, ascending aortic aneurysm, or aortic dissection.*[19–21]

The aortic arch gives rise to the innominate, left com-

mon carotid, and left subclavian arteries in that order (see Fig. 3–67). In approximately 10 percent of people, the innominate and left common carotid arteries share a common ostium, and in 5 percent of people, the left vertebral artery arises directly from the aortic arch, between the left common carotid and left subclavian arteries.[21] The ligamentum arteriosum (ductal artery ligament) represents the vestigial remnant of the fetal ductal artery, which, when patent, connects the proximal left pulmonary artery to the undersurface of the aortic arch.[21] *Most coarctations occur just distal to the left subclavian artery. When thoracic aortic dissection does not involve the ascending aorta (DeBakey type III and Stanford type B), the intimal tear is commonly near the ligamentum arteriosum or the ostium of the left subclavian artery.*[21] *Nonpenetrating deceleration chest trauma, as can occur in motor vehicle accidents, commonly involves the aorta in the region between the aortic arch and descending thoracic aorta and can be associated with aortic transection or pseudoaneurysm formation.*[21]

The descending thoracic aorta lies adjacent to the left atrium, esophagus, and vertebral column. The pulmonary trunk (or main pulmonary artery) emanates from the right ventricle and travels to the left of the ascending aorta. As it bifurcates, the left pulmonary artery courses over the left bronchus, whereas the right pulmonary artery travels beneath the aortic arch and behind the superior vena cava (see Figs. 3–11A and 3–65). Thus the *left* bronchus and the *right* pulmonary artery normally travel beneath the aortic arch.

CARDIAC CONDUCTION SYSTEM

The cardiac conduction system consists of the sinus node, internodal tracts, AV node, AV (His) bundle, and right and left bundle branches[19–21] (Fig. 3–70). The sinus node is located subepicardially in the terminal groove, close to the junction between the superior vena cava and right atrium. The sinus node artery arises from the right coronary artery in 55 percent of people. Its course can place it in contact with the base of the right atrial appendage and the superior vena cava–right atrial junction (see Fig. 3–53). When the sinus node artery arises from the left circumflex artery (45 percent), it can course close to the left atrial appendage. *During such surgical operations as the Mustard and*

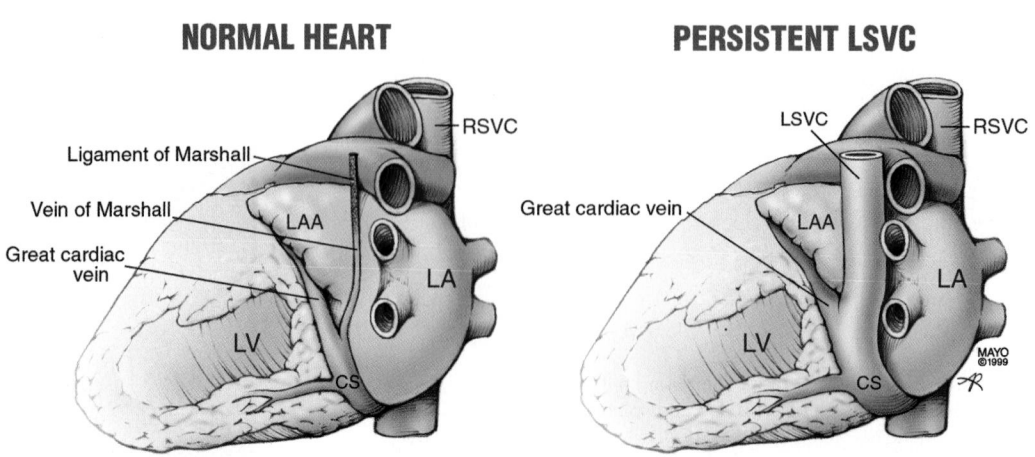

FIGURE 3–66. Schematic diagrams showing the ligament/vein of Marshall in normal hearts (*left*) and persistent left superior vena cava (LSVC) (*right*). CS, coronary sinus; LA, left atrium; LAA, left atrial appendage; LV, left ventricle; RA, right atrium; RSVC, right superior vena cava.

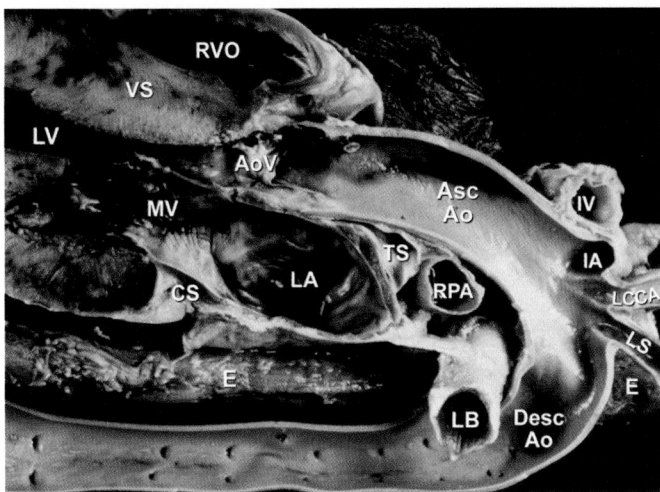

FIGURE 3-67. Thoracic aorta. The entire thoracic aorta has been cut in a tomographic manner. The aortic arch travels over the left bronchus and the right pulmonary artery. Asc Ao, ascending aorta; AoV, aortic valve; CS, coronary sinus; Desc Ao, descending thoracic aorta; E, esophagus; IA, innominate artery; IV, innominate vein; LA, left atrium; LB, left bronchus; LCCA, left common carotid artery; LS, left subclavian artery; LV, left ventricle; MV, mitral valve; RPA, right pulmonary artery; RVO, right ventricular outflow; TS, transverse sinus; VS, ventricular septum.

Fontan procedures, the sinus node and its artery are susceptible to injury.[20,21] By light microscopy, there are no morphologically distinct conduction pathways between the sinus and AV nodes.[21] However, electrophysiologic studies support the concept of functional preferential pathways that travel along the crista terminalis and atrial septum including the limbus but not the valve of the fossa ovalis.[21] *Internodal conduction disturbances therefore are not expected as a result of transseptal procedures. With the Mustard operation for complete transposition of the great arteries, there can be severe disturbance of internodal conduction because the entire septum is resected, and the surgical atriotomy can disrupt the crista terminalis.*[21] *Lipomatous hypertrophy of the atrial septum can interfere with internodal conduction and induce a variety of atrial arrhythmias. Ventricular preexcitation is most commonly associated with aberrant bypass tracts that span the annulus of the tricuspid or mitral valve (see Fig. 3–2).*

The AV node, in contrast to the sinus node, is a sub*endo*cardial structure that is located within the triangle of Koch[19–21] (Fig. 3–71). The triangle of Koch is bordered by the coronary sinus ostium posteroinferiorly and the septal tricuspid annulus anteriorly. *Because of its right atrial location near the tricuspid annulus, the AV node is susceptible to injury during tricuspid annuloplasty and during plication procedures for Ebstein's anomaly.*[19–21]

The AV (His) bundle arises from the distal portion of the AV node and travels along the ventricular septum adjacent to the membranous septum[19–21] *(see Fig. 3–71). The AV conduction tissue is generally remote from the defect in the outlet, inlet, and muscular forms of ventricular septal defect but travels along the inferior margin of a membranous ventricular septal defect.* The AV bundle travels through the central fibrous body (right fibrous trigone) and therefore is closely related to the annuli of the aortic, mitral, and tricuspid valves. *Thus, during operative procedures involving these valves or a membranous ventricular septal defect, care must be taken to avoid injury to the His bundle. Whereas in normal hearts the AV bundle*

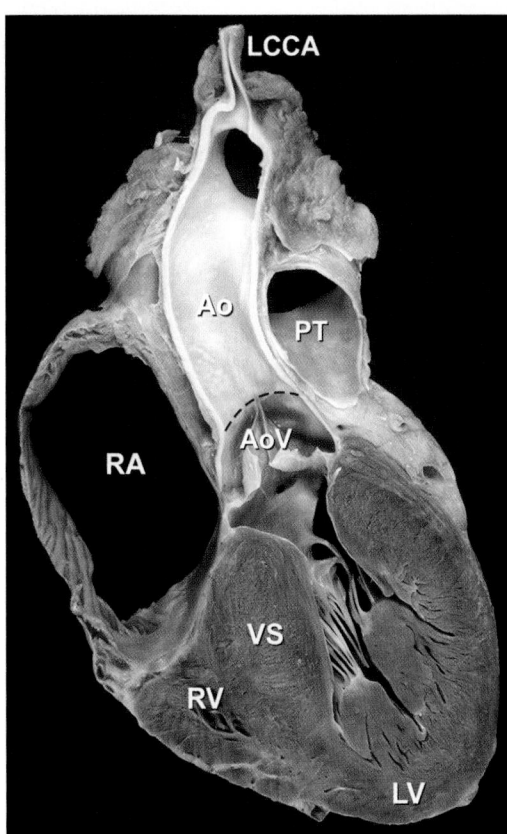

FIGURE 3-68. Tomographic section of the heart in the frontal plane of the body showing the aortic sinotubular junction (*dashed line*). Ao, ascending aorta; AoV, aortic valve; LCCA, left common carotid artery; LV, left ventricle; PT, pulmonary trunk; RA, right atrium; RV, right ventricle; LV, left ventricle; VS, ventricular septum.

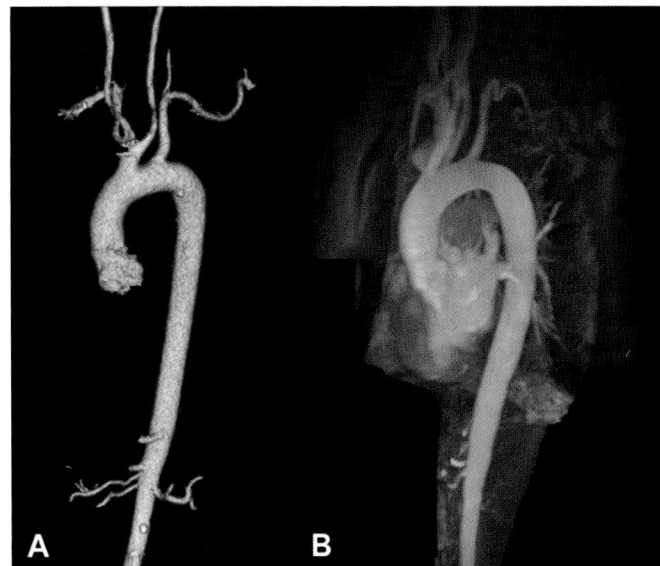

FIGURE 3-69. Real-time 3D reconstructions of a normal thoracic aorta by **(A)** CT and **(B)** MRI.

courses along the posteroinferior rim of the membranous septum, it courses along the anterosuperior rim of the membranous septum in hearts with AV discordance. The AV bundle receives a dual blood supply from the AV nodal artery and the first septal perforator of the left anterior descending coronary artery.[21]

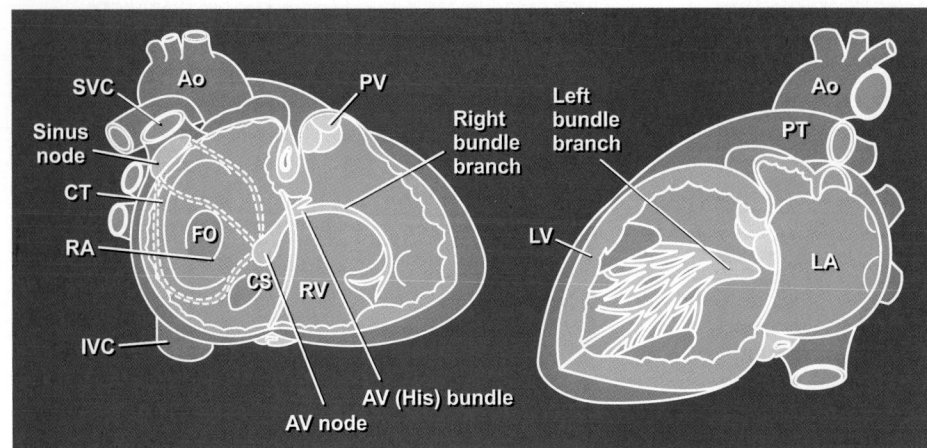

FIGURE 3–70. Schematic diagram of the cardiac conduction system. The right side of the heart (*left*) showing the sinus node, atrioventricular (AV) node, AV (His) bundle, and right bundle branch. The left side of the heart (*right*) showing incomplete anatomic separation of the left bundle into anterior and posterior fascicles. Ao, ascending aorta; AV, atrioventricular; CS, coronary sinus; CT, crista terminalis; FO, fossa ovalis; IVC, inferior vena cava; LA, left atrium; LV, left ventricle; PT, pulmonary trunk; PV, pulmonary valve; RA, right atrium; RV, right ventricle; SVC, superior vena cava.

The right bundle branch emanates from the distal portion of the AV bundle and forms a cord-like structure that travels along the septal and moderator bands toward the anterior tricuspid papillary muscle (see Fig. 3–70). In contrast, the left bundle branch represents a broad fenestrated sheet of subendocardial conduction fibers that spread along the septal surface of the left ventricle[19–21] (see Fig. 3–70). The right and left bundle branches receive dual blood supply from the septal perforators of the left anterior descending coronary artery and posterior descending coronary arteries.[21] Left ventricular pseudo-tendons can contain conduction tissue from the left bundle branch.[21] *The left bundle branch can be disrupted following surgical myectomy, whereas the right bundle branch can be damaged during percutaneous alcohol septal ablation.[52] Following right ventriculotomy for reconstruction of the right ventricular outflow tract, the electrocardiogram shows a pattern of right bundle-branch block even though the right bundle is not disrupted.[20]*

NEW DEVELOPMENTS AND FUTURE CHALLENGES

The future holds promise for an integrated multidimensional approach to the study of cardiac anatomy that incorporates static 3D data, the elements of time (the fourth dimension) and motion, and physiologic (pressure and perfusion) and metabolic parameters.[53–55] Until recently, the geometric fusion of anatomy and function was not possible without physically invading the body. With the currently available imaging techniques, multidimensional anatomy and physiology are mentally reassembled from the sequential tomographic images using echocardiography, MRI or CT, or multiple scintigraphy, as with SPECT imaging.[53] With the advances made in medical technology propelled by the rapid developments in computer technology, digital imaging, and data-storage techniques, it has become possible to electronically perform virtual dissection and reconstruction of the heart and cardiovascular system.[53–55] Furthermore, multidimensional imaging allows contin-

ued study of any human organ of interest because of the ability to permanently store anatomic images and the contained physiologic features for retrieval, comparison for change, and ultimately, replication in a more familiar 3- and 4-dimensional presentation.[53–55]

The potential realization of virtual anatomy notwithstanding, standardization of the various tomographic approaches to image acquisition in a manner that conforms to familiar anatomic presentation remains a major challenge that has to be overcome if multidimensional cardiac imaging is to become a clinical reality. There is current progress in this direction. Real-time 3D reconstruction of the heart using identical CT and 2D tomographic sectioning of the heart is now possible. Virtual human vivisection might soon become reality. The goal is virtual surgery (dry runs prior to the actual operation) and dissection of the heart into its various components, be it anatomic, functional, or metabolic, either separately or in various combinations. Because of advances in multimedia technology, the centuries-old great divide between physiologists and anatomists is about to become relegated to the history books.

ANATOMY NOT ADDRESSED AND QUANTUM COMPUTING

Fine-detailed anatomy such as that of the conduction system and microvasculature is not readily available to the usual anatomic dissection by computer-based imaging. Additionally, tissue histology or molecular biological assessment is not obtained routinely by imaging. At the other end of the spectrum, 3D gross anatomic dissection of contiguous structures is also normally not available

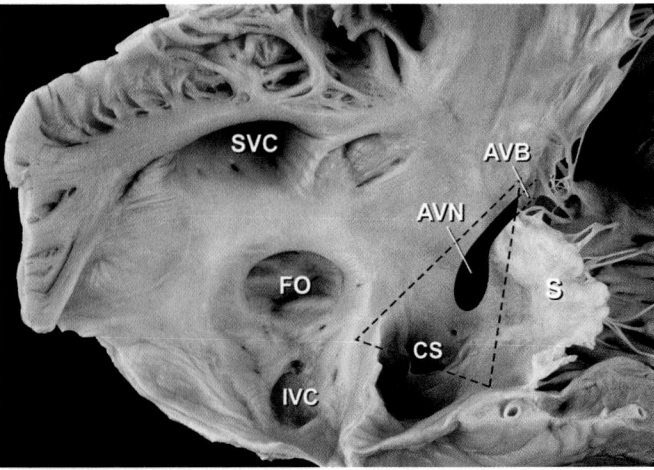

FIGURE 3–71. The atrioventricular node (AVN) lies within the triangle of Koch (*dashed triangle*), and the AV (His) bundle (AVB) travels through the tricuspid annulus to rest along the summit of the ventricular septum. CS, coronary sinus; FO, fossa ovalis; IVC, inferior vena cava; S, septal leaflet of the tricuspid valve; SVC, superior vena cava.

(e.g., How does metastatic cancer throughout the system relate to a primary tumor in the gut?).

These and other macroscopic and microscopic dissections await the future of increasingly sophisticated computer technology and information management. Both pathologic and living tissues someday will be dissected and analyzed not by destructive cutting but by higher-dimensional imagery. Today's computers have introduced the information era. Information has become a commodity expanding our ability to access useful data. Within the next two decades, however, we will have evolved to the *Quantum Era,* where all that has been discussed in this chapter plus gross and microscopic anatomy will be possible within an electronic environment. Reality will be expressed as base parts or characteristics (quanta, molecules, pixels, etc.) and reformatted in 3- or 4-dimensional geometry relative to the desired information. Gross anatomy, physiology, tissue characteristics, and even histopathology will be dissected and presented as a quantifiable geometric image. The concept of a *living autopsy* will be a reality.

REFERENCES

1. Callahan JA, Key JD. Foundations of cardiology. In: Giuliani ER, Fuster V, Gersh BJ, et al, eds. *Cardiology Fundamentals and Practice.* Vol 1. 2nd ed. St Louis, MI: Mosby-Year Book; 1991:3–25.

2. O'Malley CD, Saunders JB. *Leonardo da Vinci on the Human Body.* New York: Greenwich House; 1982:223.

3. Ackermann DM, Edwards WD. Anatomic basis for tomographic analysis of the pediatric heart at autopsy. *Perspect Pediatr Pathol.* 1988;12:44–68.

4. Landefeld CS, Goldman L. The autopsy in clinical medicine. *Mayo Clinic Proc.* 1989;64:1185–1189.

5. Hurst JW, King SB, Friesinger GC, et al. Atherosclerotic coronary heart disease: angina pectoris, myocardial infarction, and other manifestations of myocardial ischemia. In: *Hurst's the Heart.* 6th ed. New York: McGraw-Hill; 1986:882–1008.

6. Edwards WD. Anatomic basis for tomographic analysis of the heart at autopsy. *Cardiol Clin.* 1984;2:485–506.

7. Seward J. Transesophageal echocardiographic anatomy. In: Freeman W, Seward J, Khandheria B, Tajik AJ, eds. *Transesophageal Echocardiography.* Boston: Little, Brown; 1994:55–101.

8. Stewart W. Intraoperative echocardiography. In: Topol EJ, ed. *Textbook of Cardiovascular Medicine.* Philadelphia: Lippincott-Raven; 1998:1497–1525.

9. Katsnelson Y, Raman J, Katsnelson F, et al. Current state of intraoperative echocardiography. *Echocardiography.* 2003;20(8):771–780.

10. Szili-Torok T, Krenning BJ, Voormolen MM, Reclandt JR. Dynamic three-dimensional echocardiography combined with semiautomated border detection offers advantages for assessment of resynchronization therapy. *Cardiovasc Ultrasound.* 2003;1(1):14.

11. Packer DL, Johnson SB. Intracardiac ultrasound guidance of linear lesion creation for ablation of atrial fibrillation. *J Am Coll Cardiol.* 1998;31:333A.

12. Chu E, Fitzpatrick AP, Chin MC, et al. Radio-frequency catheter ablation guided by intracardiac echocardiography. *Circulation.* 1994;89:1301–1305.

13. DeLurgio DB, Frohwein SC, Walter PF, et al. Anatomy of atrioventricular nodal reentry investigated by intracardiac echocardiography. *Am J Cardiol.* 1997;80:231–234.

14. Bruce CJ, Packer DL, Seward J. Transvascular imaging: feasibility study using a vector phased array ultrasound catheter. *Echocardiography.* 1999;16:425–430.

15. Fu M, Hung JS, Lo PH, et al. Intracardiac echocardiography via the transvenous approach with use of 8F 10-MHz ultrasound catheters. *Mayo Clin Proc.* 1999;74:775–783.

16. Corsi C, Lamberti C, Sarti A, et al. Real-time 3D echocardiographic data analysis for left ventricular volume estimation. *Comput Cardiol.* 2000;27:107–110.

17. Abidov A, Bax JJ, Hayes SW, Hachamovitch R, et al. Transient ischemic dilation ratio of the left ventricle is a significant predictor of future cardiac events in patients with otherwise normal myocardial perfusion SPECT. *J Am Coll Cardiol.* 2003;42(10):1818–1825.

18. Nazarian GK, Julsrud PR, Ehman RL, et al. Correlation between magnetic resonance imaging of the heart and cardiac anatomy. *Mayo Clinic Proc.* 1987;62:573–583.

19. Edwards WD. *Anatomy of the Cardiovascular System: Clinical Medicine.* Vol 6. Philadelphia: Harper & Row; 1984:1–24.

20. Edwards WD. Cardiac anatomy and examination of cardiac specimens. In: Emmanouilides G, Reimenschneider T, Allen H, Gutgesell H, eds. *Moss & Adams' Heart Disease in Infants, Children, and Adolescents.* 5th ed. Baltimore: Williams & Wilkins; 1995:70–105.

21. Edwards WD. Applied anatomy of the heart. In: Giuliani ER, Fuster V, Gersh BJ, et al, eds. *Cardiology Fundamentals and Practice.* Vol 1. 2nd ed. St Louis: Mosby-Year Book; 1991:47–112.

22. McAfee MK, Schaff HV. Valve repair for mitral insufficiency. *Cardiology.* 1990;20:35–43.

23. Arom KV, Edwards JE. Relationship between right ventricular muscle bundles and pulmonary valve: significance in pulmonary atresia with intact ventricular septum. *Circulation.* 1976;54:79–83.

24. Kitzman D, Edwards WD. Minireview: age-related changes in the anatomy of the normal human heart. *J Gerontol Med Sci.* 1990;45:M33–M39.

25. Freedberg RS, Goodkin GM, Perez JL. Valve strands are strongly associated with systemic embolization: a transesophageal echocardiographic study. *J Am Coll Cardiol.* 1995;26:1709–1712.

26. Burke A, Virmani R. *Atlas of Tumor Pathology: Tumors of the Heart and Great Vessels in Papillary Fibroelastoma.* Washington, DC: Armed Forces Institute of Pathology; 1996:47–54.

27. Roberts WC, Roberts JD. The floating heart too fat to sink: analysis of 55 necropsy patients. *Am J Cardiol.* 1983;52:1286–1289.

28. Cristina B, Gaetano T, Domenico C, et al. Arrhythmogenic right ventricular cardiomyopathy: dysplasia, dystrophy, or myocarditis. *Circulation.* 1996;94:983–991.

29. Luetmer PH, Edwards WD, Seward JB, et al. Incidence and distribution of left ventricular false tendons: an autopsy study of 483 normal human hearts. *J Am Coll Cardiol.* 1986;8:179–183.

30. Boyd MT, Seward JB, Tajik AJ, et al. Frequency and location of prominent left ventricular trabeculations at autopsy in 474 normal human hearts: implications for evaluation of mural thrombi by two-dimensional echocardiography. *J Am Coll Cardiol.* 1987;9:323–326.

31. Ritter M, Oechslin E, Sutsch G. Isolated noncompaction of the myocardium in adults. *Mayo Clin Proc.* 1997;72:26–31.

32. Agmon Y, Connolly H, Olson L, et al. Noncompaction of the ventricular myocardium. *J Am Soc Echocardiogr.* 1999;20:859–863.

33. Veinot JP, Harrity PJ, Gentile F, et al. Anatomy of the normal left atrial appendage: a quantitative study of age-related changes in 500 autopsy hearts: implications for echocardiographic examination. *Circulation.* 1997;96:3112–3115.

34. Tsang TSM, Gersh BJ, Appleton CP, et al. Left ventricular diastolic dysfunction as a predictor of the first diagnosed non valvular atrial fibrillation in 840 elderly men and women. *J Am Coll Cardiol.* 2002;40:1636–1644.

35. McAlpine W. *Heart and Coronary Arteries: An Anatomic Atlas for Radiologic Diagnosis and Surgical Treatment.* New York: Springer-Verlag; 1975.

36. Naqueh SF, Lakkis NM, He ZX, et al. Role of myocardial contrast echocardiography during nonsurgical septal reduction therapy for hypertrophic obstructive cardiomyopathy. *J Am Coll Cardiol.* 1988;32:225–229.

37. Yetman AT, McCrindle BW, MacDonald C, et al. Myocardial bridging in children with hypertrophic cardiomyopathy: a risk factor for sudden death. *N Engl J Med.* 1998;339:1201–1209.

38. Gras D, Mabo P, Tang T, et al. Multisite pacing as a supplemental treatment of congestive heart failure: preliminary results of the Medtronic Inc in Sync Study. *Pacing Clin Electrophysiol.* 1998;21:2249–2255.

39. Kar S, Nordlander R. Coronary veins: an alternate route to ischemic myocardium. *Heart Lung.* 1992;21:148–157.

40. Kar S, Drury JK, Hajduczki I, et al. Synchronized coronary venous retroperfusion for support and salvage of ischemic myocardium during elective and failed angioplasty. *J Am Coll Cardiol.* 1991;18:271–282.

41. Lazar HL, Haan CK, Yang X, et al. Reduction of infarction size with coronary venous retroperfusion. *Circulation.* 1992;86:11351–11352.

42. Schiller NB, Shah PM, Crawford M, et al. Recommendations for quantitation of the left ventricle by two-dimensional echocardiography: American Society of Echocardiography Committee on Standards, Subcommittee on Quantitation of Two-Dimensional Echocardiograms. *J Am Soc Echocardiogr.* 1989;2:358–367.

43. Nagel E, Lehmkuhl H, Bocksch W, et al. Noninvasive diagnosis of ischemia-induced wall motion abnormalities with the use of high-dose dobutamine stress MRI comparison with dobutamine stress echocardiography. *Circulation.* 1999;99:763–770.

44. Ichikawa H, Matsubara O. Studies on the microvasculature of human myocardium. *Bull Tokyo Med Dent Univ.* 1977;24:53–65.

45. Cannon RO, Leon MB, Watson RM, et al. Chest pain and "normal" coronary arteries: the role of small coronary arteries. *Am J Cardiol.* 1985;55:50B–60B.

46. Parodi O, Sambuceti G. The role of coronary microvascular dysfunction in the genesis of cardiovascular diseases. *Q J Nucl Med.* 1996;40:9–16.

47. Schwartzkopff B, Motz W, Frenzel H, et al. Structural and functional alterations of the intramyocardial coronary arterioles in patients with arterial hypertension. *Circulation.* 1993;88:993–1002.

48. Krams R, Kofflard MJM, Duncker DJ, et al. Decreased coronary flow reserve in hypertrophic cardiomyopathy is related to remodeling of the coronary microcirculation. *Circulation.* 1998;97:23–233.

49. Oh JK, Seward JB, Tajik AJ. Contrast echocardiography. In: Weinberg RW, Simmons LA, Madrigal R, eds. *The Echo Manual.* 2nd ed. Philadelphia: Lippincott-Raven; 1999:245–249.

50. Kantor B, McKenna CJ, Caccitolo JA, et al. Transmyocardial and percutaneous myocardial revascularization: current and future roles in the treatment of coronary artery disease. *Mayo Clin Proc.* 1999;74:585–592.

51. Harmon J Jr, Edwards WD. Venous valves in subclavian and internal jugular veins. *Am J Cardiovasc Pathol.* 1987;1:51–54.

52. Talreja DR, Nishimura RA, Edwards WD, et al. Alcohol septal ablation versus surgical septal myectomy: comparsion of effects on atrioventricular conduction tissue. *J Am Coll Cardiol.* 2004;44:2329–2332.

53. Maclellan-Tobert SG, Buithieu J, Belohlavek M, et al. Three-dimensional imaging used for virtual dissection, image banking and physical replications of anatomy and physiology. *Echocardiography.* 1998;15:89–98.

54. Bruining N, Roelandt J, Grunst G, et al. Three-dimensional echocardiography: the gateway to virtual reality. *Echocardiography.* 1999;16:417–423.

55. Seward JB, Belohlavek M, Kinter T, et al. Evolving era of multidimensional medical imaging. *Mayo Clin Proc.* 1999;74:399–414.

CHAPTER 4

Normal Physiology of the Cardiovascular System

Brian D. Hoit / Richard A. Walsh

The principal function of the cardiovascular (CV) system is to deliver oxygen and nutrients to metabolizing tissues and remove carbon dioxide and wastes from metabolizing tissues. This is accomplished by means of two specialized circulations in series: a low-resistance pulmonary and a high-resistance systemic circulation driven by specialized muscle pumps, the right and left heart (each in turn comprised of a thin-walled atrium and thicker-walled ventricle), respectively. Although CV physiology can be understood at a number of hierarchical levels, it is the complex interplay among the intrinsic properties of the cardiomyocytes and isolated muscle, chamber mechanics, and their modulation by variable cardiac-loading conditions, neurohormonal, and renal compensatory mechanisms that determines the integrated performance of the CV system. Accordingly, CV physiology will be examined at cellular, isolated muscle, and organ (isolated heart and integrated systems) levels.

CELLULAR BASIS OF CONTRACTION

【 】 EXCITATION: THE ACTION POTENTIAL

The rhythmic beating of the heart distinguishes it from all other organs. The normal heartbeat is initiated by a complex flow of electrical signals called *action potentials*. The action potential in turn results from highly coordinated, sequential changes in ion conductances through gated sarcolemmal membrane channels[1] (Fig. 4–1).

Increases in transmembrane potential from a resting value of negative 80 to 90 mV to approximately positive 30 mV (depolarization) represents phase 0 (the rapid upstroke) of the action potential and results primarily from a sudden increase in sodium (Na^+) permeability; this permits a large inward current of Na^+ ions to flow down an electrochemical gradient by means of voltage- and time-dependent fast Na^+ channels. The upstroke is caused by a regenerative process, that is, depolarization leads to Na^+ influx, which leads to further depolarization. The rapid opening of the activation gates for the fast Na^+ channel is immediately followed by a slower closing of inactivation gates, which interrupt the influx of Na^+ into the cell. The membrane must be fully repolarized for inactivation gates to reopen and conduct another action potential, a process called *recovery*. Phase I (the notch) is the initial rapid repolarization phase of the action potential, which is carried by potassium (K^+) and to a lesser extent, chloride (Cl^-) ion conductance. Phase II of the action potential is unique to cardiac muscle; this plateau phase results from a balance of inward calcium (Ca^{2+}) and

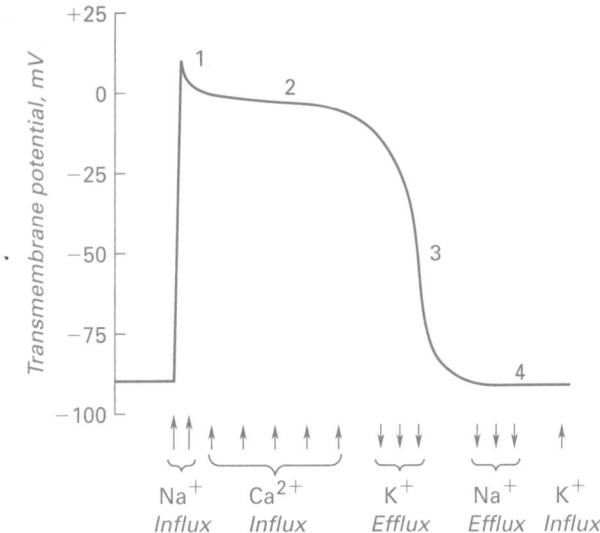

FIGURE 4–1. Phases of the action potential and major associated currents in ventricular myocytes. The initial phase 0 spike is not labeled. See Excitation discussion in text. In specialized conduction system tissue, there is spontaneous depolarization during phase IV. Ca²⁺, calcium; K⁺, potassium; Na⁺, sodium. *Source: Reproduced with permission from LeWinter MM, Osol G. Normal physiology of the cardiovascular system. In: Fuster V, Alexander RW, O'Rourke RA, Roberts R, King SB III, Nash IS, Prystowksy EN. Hurst's The Heart. 11th ed. New York: McGraw-Hill; 2004:87–112.*

outward K⁺ currents. The slow inward (L-type) Ca²⁺ channel is activated at threshold potentials above –50 mV, is maximal at approximately 0 to 10 mV, peaks rapidly, and inactivates slowly. Phase III is the final rapid repolarization that restores resting potential and is caused by inactivation of the Ca²⁺ current and an increase in the outward K⁺ current. Several ionic K⁺ pumps contribute to the plateau and repolarization: (1) the inwardly rectifying K⁺ current (I_{K1}), a K⁺ conductance that generates the resting potential, turns off during phase 0, and is inactive until repolarization begins—it also generates a small outward current late in repolarization; (2) the transient outward K⁺ current (I_{TO}), responsible for the initial phase I repolarization; and (3) the delayed outward K⁺ current (I_K), the primary current responsible for initiating final repolarization turns on slowly at the final phase of the action potential. After repolarization the Na⁺K⁺ adenosine triphosphatase (ATPase) pump extrudes accumulated intracellular Na⁺ and pumps extracellular K⁺ into the cell. Ionic balance across the sarcolemmal membrane is also maintained by the action of a sodium-calcium exchanger.[2]

All myocardial cells are excitable, that is, when adequately stimulated they can generate an action potential. However, only specialized cells are capable of reaching threshold potential and firing without such an outside stimulus (automaticity). Phase IV of the action potential represents the slow, spontaneous diastolic depolarization responsible for the property of automaticity. Normally, action potentials reach threshold potential and depolarize spontaneously and rhythmically only in the primary pacemaker of the heart, the sinoatrial (SA) node. However, cells in other areas (atrial cells near the ostium of the coronary sinus, the distal atrioventricular [AV] node, and the His-Purkinje fibers) are capable of automaticity when not suppressed by the faster firing of the SA node. The slope and maximal diastolic potential of the pacemaker potential and the threshold potential determine the rate of impulse formation; the former is

modulated by the autonomic nervous system (sympathetic stimulation increasing the slope of the pacemaker potential and accelerating the rate of firing, and parasympathetic stimulation producing the opposite effects). Several ionic currents, specific for the site of impulse genesis, can be involved in the pacemaker current. In the SA node, an inward Ca²⁺ current and an outward delayed K⁺ current that is activated during the plateau and deactivated during phase IV contribute to depolarization. The funny current (pacemaker current; I_F), which slowly activates on hyperpolarization, is a critical determinant of the slope of diastolic depolarization; it is therefore a key regulator of pacemaker activity.[3]

Effective cell-to-cell communication is essential for rapid, uniform conduction of action potentials and a resultant effective, synchronized myocardial contraction. The organized distribution of local currents that comprise the depolarization wave flow from cell to cell by means of gap junctions. These clusters of transmembrane channels connect the plasma membranes of adjacent myocytes and form low-resistance pathways.[4] Channels are comprised of two connexons; each connexon is a hexamer of connexins, members of a multigene family of conserved proteins.

【 】 EXCITATION-CONTRACTION COUPLING

The cascade of biological processes that begins with the cardiac action potential and ends with myocyte contraction and relaxation defines cardiac excitation-contraction (E-C) coupling (Fig. 4–2). E-C is intimately related to calcium homeostasis, myofilament calcium sensitivity, and functions of cytoskeletal and sarcomeric proteins, and forms the biophysical underpinnings of the inotropic state of the heart.[5] Because E-C coupling is by first principles a manifestation of myocyte calcium handling, an understanding of the calcium transient and calcium homeostasis is essential.

The calcium transient is initiated in response to sarcolemmal depolarization by extracellular calcium (Ca²⁺) influx through voltage dependent L-type Ca²⁺ channels, which instigates the release of stored Ca²⁺ from the cardiomyocyte endoplasmic reticulum, sarcoplasmic reticulum (SR), via spatially proximate Ca²⁺ release channels (ryanodine receptor [RyR2]). This latter step, fittingly termed *calcium-induced calcium release* (CICR), amplifies the amount of calcium available for myofilament binding and force generating actin-myosin crossbridges. Relaxation results from closure of the release channels, resequestration of Ca2+ by the SR Ca2+-ATPase (SERCA2), and crossbridge dissolution. To maintain steady-state calcium homeostasis, the amount of Ca²⁺ entering the cell with each contraction must be removed before the subsequent contraction. To this end, the Na⁺-Ca²⁺ exchanger (NCX) acting in the *forward* mode competes with SERCA2 for Ca²⁺ and pumps [Ca²⁺]$_i$ into the extracellular space.

The magnitude of the [Ca²⁺]$_i$ transient modulates the force developed by myofilaments, and factors that modify calcium cycling and/or Ca²⁺ sensitivity of myofilaments can alter significantly the force and extent of myocyte contraction. The determinants of the cardiac myocyte [Ca²⁺]$_i$ transient are summarized in Table 4–1. Factors responsible for the [Ca²⁺]$_i$ transient amplitude include: (1) the calcium current (I_{Ca}), primarily caused by Ca²⁺ influx through the L-type Ca²⁺ channel, but in small part caused by *reverse mode* NCX; (2) SR [Ca²⁺]$_i$ content, which determines the amount of releasable calcium; (3) the efficiency of E-C coupling, or the *gain* (i.e., the

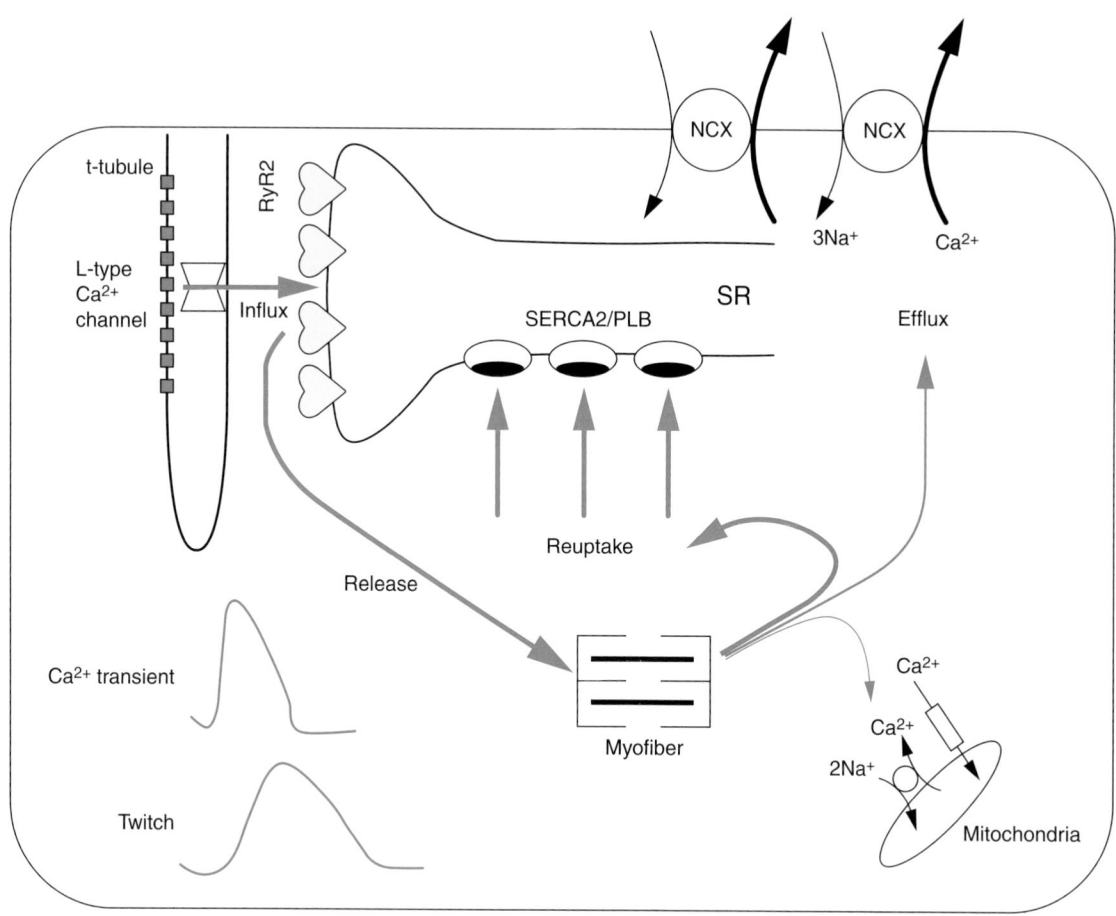

FIGURE 4–2. Cartoon of a healthy myocyte containing key components of E-C coupling. Influx of calcium is predominantly through the L-type calcium channel. The *arrow* through the channel denotes the amount of activator calcium and is an index of the E-C coupling gain. The relative magnitudes of calcium release, reuptake, and efflux are denoted by the *arrow* widths. The resultant calcium transient and muscle twitch are shown in the lower left of the cell. Ca+, calcium; Na+, sodium; RyR2, ryanodine receptor; SERCA2, sarcoplasmic-endoplasmic reticulum calcium ATPase. *Source: Reproduced with permission from Hoit.*[5]

<table>
<tr><td>

TABLE 4–1

Determinants of the Calcium ($[Ca^{2+}]_i$) Current

$[Ca^{2+}]_i$ transient magnitude
   Calcium current (I_{Ca})
      L-type channels
      NCX
      Others (T-type channel, tetrodotoxin-sensitive)
   SR $[Ca^{2+}]_i$ content
   Efficiency of E-C coupling
   Intracellular Ca^{2+} buffers

$[Ca^{2+}]_i$ transient decline
   SERCA2/phospholamban
   NCX
   Sarcolemmal Ca^{2+}-ATPase
   Mitochondria
   Intracellular buffers

ATPase, adenosinetriphosphatase; E-C, excitation-contraction; NCX, sodium-calcium exchanger; SERCA2, SR Ca^{2+}-adenosinetriphosphatase; SR, sarcoplasmic reticulum.
Source: Reproduced with permission from Hoit.[5]

</td></tr>
</table>

amount of calcium released by the SR for the calcium current, $\Delta[Ca^{2+}]_i / I_{Ca}$); and (4) intracellular Ca^{2+} buffers. The decline of the $[Ca^{2+}]_i$ transient is caused by the following: (1) Ca^{2+} reuptake into SR by SERCA2 (a process modulated by a phosphorylatable regulatory protein termed *phospholamban*); (2) Ca^{2+} extrusion from the cell by the NCX; (3) Ca^{2+} extrusion from the cell by the sarcolemmal Ca^{2+}-ATPase; (4) Ca^{2+} accumulation by mitochondria; and (5) Ca^{2+} binding to intracellular buffers (including fluorescent indicators that are used in experimental systems to measure the transient).[6]

Calcium sparks (localized $[Ca^{2+}]_i$ transients) are the elementary SR Ca^{2+} release events that trigger E-C coupling in heart muscle.[7] The basis for the generally accepted *local control* theory of E-C coupling is that Ca^{2+} sparks are triggered by a local $[Ca^{2+}]_i$ established in the region of the RyR2s by the opening of a single L-type Ca^{2+} channel. The amplitude of Ca^{2+} sparks is determined by SR Ca^{2+} load and gating properties of the RyR2. Although the exact nature and origin of Ca^{2+} sparks are not completely understood, the prevailing view is that the global $[Ca^{2+}]_i$ transient is produced by the temporal and spatial summation of a large number of Ca^{2+} sparks.[8] The mechanisms responsible for terminating sparks are not clear, but proteins accessory to the RyR2 (e.g., sorcin [FKB12]) have been suggested as playing a key role.[9]

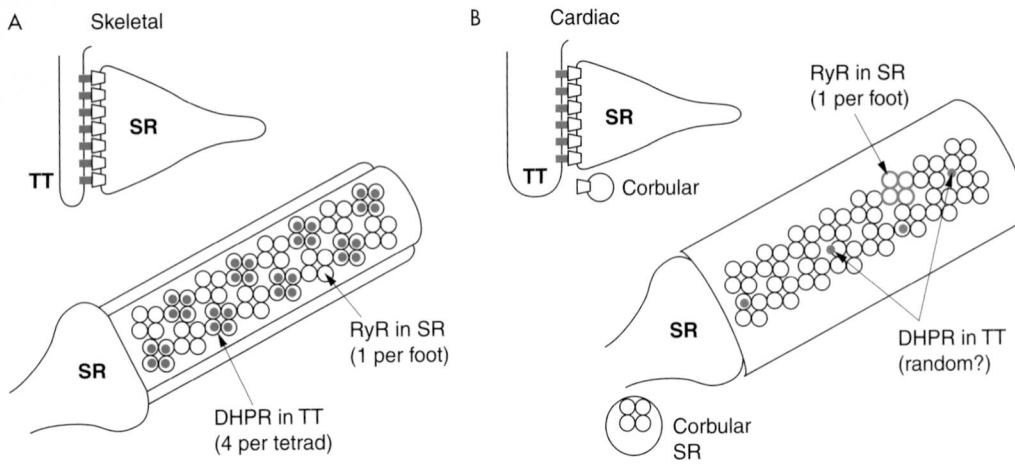

FIGURE 4–3. Cartoon comparing the organizational differences between skeletal and cardiac T-tubule junctions. The upper diagrams are side views of the junction (trapezoids are ryanodine receptors [RyRs] and filled ovals are the dihydropyridine receptors [DHPRs]). Lower panels are views from inside the T-tubule at the junction. Note that DHPRs are sparse and less aligned in heart. RyR, ryanodine receptor; SR, sarcoplasmic reticulum; TT, T-tubules. *Source: Reproduced with permission from Bers.[12]*

Components of Excitation-Contraction Coupling

Sarcolemma The sarcolemma is the site where calcium enters and leaves the cell through a distribution of ion channels, transporters, and pumps. The T-tubules are invaginations of the sarcolemma and glycocalyx, and are both longitudinal and oblique in their orientation; this system forms a permeability barrier between the cytosol and the extracellular space.[10] The membranous surface areas are tissue (atrial cells have poorly developed T-tubules) and species specific. The structural specialization of the sarcolemma include: (1) SR coupling in the form of dyads by means of the T-tubule; (2) caveolae, which are invaginations of the sarcolemma that increase surface area and form a scaffold for signaling molecules such as nitric oxide (NO) synthase and protein kinase C (PKC); and (3) the intercalated disc, which takes the form of either a gap junction, intermediate junction, or desmosome.

Sarcoplasmic Reticulum The sarcoplasmic reticulum is an intracellular membrane-bounded compartment comprised of terminal, longitudinal, and corbular components (Fig. 4–3). The free walls of the terminal cisternae are apposed to the walls of the T-tubules and form the dyadic cleft; the RyR2 receptors are located in the walls of the terminal cisternae (*feet*) and face the dyadic cleft. Longitudinal SR is fairly homogenous and contains primarily the SR Ca^{2+}-ATPase proteins, SERCA2, and the associated phosphoprotein, phospholamban. In its dephosphorylated state, phospholamban is an endogenous inhibitor of SERCA2. Phosphorylation by PKA (at amino acid serine 16) and calcium-calmodulin kinase II (CaMKII) (at threonine 17) lowers the Michaelis constant (K_m) of sarcoplasmic-endoplasmic reticulum calcium ATPase (SERCA) and results in enhanced calcium uptake.[11] SR calcium is transported from the tubular lumen of the SR to the terminal cisternae where it is stored mostly bound to calsequestrin, a low-affinity, high-capacity, calcium-binding protein. Calsequestrin forms a complex with the proteins junctin, triadin, and RyR2. Junctional SR does not come into contact with the sarcolemma; corbular SR is a form of junctional SR that contains calsequestrin and RyR2s but is not coupled to the well-recognized calcium cycling events.[12]

Myofilaments Myofilaments comprise the contractile machinery of the cell and occupy 45 to 60 percent of the ventricular myocyte volume (Fig. 4–4). The fundamental unit of the myofilament is the sarcomere, bounded by Z lines on each end, from which the thin actin filaments extend toward the center. At the center of the thick myosin filament is the M line, where the thick filaments are interconnected by M protein and myoesin. Titin runs from the M line to the Z line in association with myosin and myosin-binding protein C; this large structural sarcomeric protein acts as a scaffold for myosin deposition, stabilizes the thick filament, functions as a molecular spring, and plays a critical role in determining the pas-

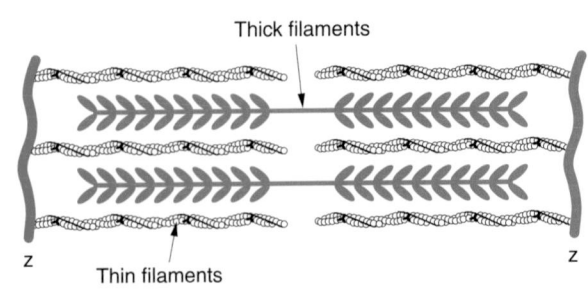

FIGURE 4–4. Electron micrograph and cartoon of a sarcomere. The darkly staining regions that flank the sarcomere are the Z lines. Myosin-containing thick filaments are in the center of the sarcomere and interact with actin-containing thin filaments by way of myosin heads that protrude from the thick filaments. Thin-filament regulatory proteins, the troponin and tropomyosin, provide calcium regulation of the actin-myosin interface. Thin filaments are anchored to the Z line, which is enriched in proteins such as α-actinin and Cap Z. (*Right*) Membrane complexes that concentrate over Z lines. The dystrophin-glycoprotein complex. *Source: Reproduced with permission from McNally E. The cytoskeleton. In: Walsh RA, ed. Molecular Mechanisms of Cardiac Hypertrophy and Failure. London: Taylor and Francis; 2005:309–321.*

sive stiffness of the heart.[13] The Z lines are the sites of anchor for cytoskeletal intermediate filaments and actin filaments at the intercalated disks and at focal adhesions. The two major structural complexes involved in the connections between sarcomeric proteins and the extracellular matrix include the membrane-spanning integrin complex and the dystrophin complex, which links actin to laminin and collagen.

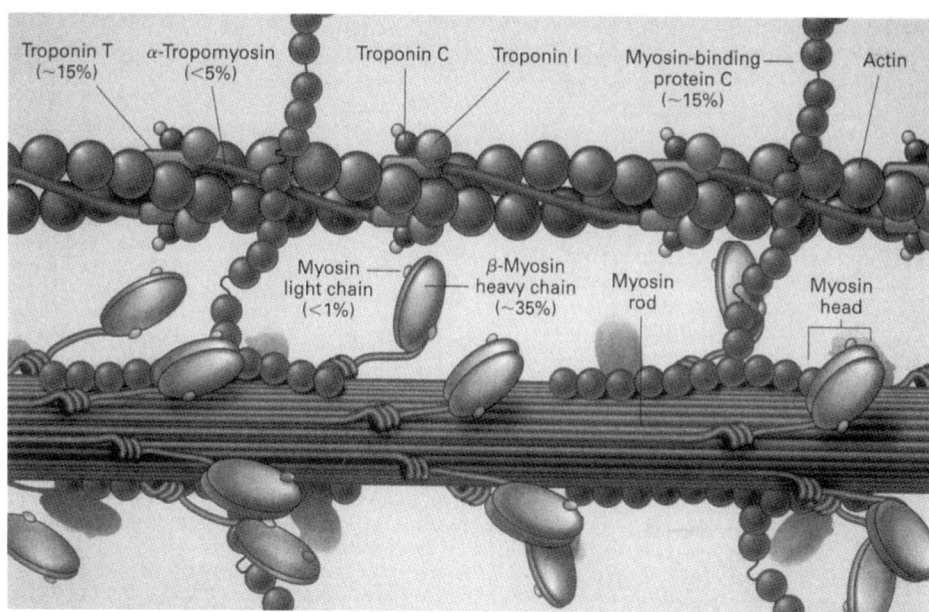

FIGURE 4–5. Cartoon of sarcomeric protein. Titin, which runs from the M line to the Z line in association with myosin and myosin-binding protein C, is not shown. *Source: Reproduced with permission from LeWinter MM, Osol G. Normal physiology of the cardiovascular system. In: Fuster V, Alexander RW, O'Rourke RA, Roberts R, King SB III, Nash IS, Prystowksy EN. Hurst's The Heart. 11th ed. New York: McGraw-Hill; 2004:87–112.*

Myosin   The myosin molecule consists of two heavy chains with a globular head, a long α-helical tail, and four myosin light chains (Fig. 4–5). The myosin head forms crossbridges with the thin actin filament through an actin-binding domain. Transduction of chemical to mechanical energy and work is the function of myosin ATPase, located in the myosin heads. Myosin heavy chain (MHC) exists as two isoforms, α (fast ATPase and crossbridge formation) and β (slow ATPase and crossbridge formation). In higher mammals, including humans, the β-myosin isoform predominates whereas in small mammals, such as mice and rats, the α form is dominant. The most accepted model of energy transduction is the sliding filament theory based on the formation and dissociation of crossbridges between the myosin head and the thin filament that transition through different energetic states.[14] Two myosin light chains (the alkali or essential light chain, MLC1 and the phosphorylatable or regulatory light chain, MLC2), are associated with each myosin head and confer stability to the thick filament. Phosphorylation of the myofilament regulatory protein troponin modulates the activity of myosin ATPase. Although phosphorylation of MLC2 by myosin light-chain kinase is critical for smooth muscle cell contraction (see the following section), its physiological significance in cardiac muscle (increased calcium sensitivity and rate of force development) is controversial.

Thin Filaments   The backbone of thin filament is helical double-stranded actin. Tropomyosin is a long flexible double-stranded (largely α-helix) protein that lies in the groove between the actin strands and inhibits the interaction between actin and myosin (see Fig. 4–5). The troponin complex is comprised of a calcium-binding subunit, troponin C (TnC), an inhibitory subunit that binds to actin, troponin I (TnI), and a tropomyosin-binding subunit, troponin T (TnT), which is attached to tropomyosin. In the resting state, when $[Ca^{2+}]_i$ is low, calcium-binding sites of TnC are unoccupied and TnI preferentially binds to actin; this favors a configuration in which the troponin-tropomyosin complex sterically hinders myosin-actin interaction. In this configuration, crossbridges are in both detached and weakly attached non–force-producing states. When $[Ca^{2+}]_i$ rises, calcium binds to the calcium-specific sites on TnC and strengthens the interaction of TnC and TnI; TnI then dissociates from actin, and a conformational change removes the steric hindrance to myosin-actin interaction. Strong binding of actin to myosin begins when the actin-myosin inhibition is relieved. Binding Ca^{2+}

to troponin causes the process of crossbridge formation to spread down the actin filament, and by means of ATP hydrolysis, transitions are made from detached/weakly bound states to force producing states. Release of conformational energy leads to rotation of the myosin head that propels the thin filament along the thick filament. Usually the systolic $[Ca^{2+}]_i$ only submaximally activates muscle; the steep relation between $[Ca^{2+}]$ and tension is thought to result from both nearest neighbor interaction and strong actin-myosin binding, which allows for contractile reserve with modest changes in $[Ca^{2+}]_i$.[15] Although this is the most accepted model, other potential explanations exist; all models incorporate the concept that myofilaments are dynamically involved in their state of activation and not simply subject to passive changes in $[Ca^{2+}]_i$.[16] A simplified mechanical model of crossbridge formation is presented in Fig. 4–6.

Mitochondria   Mitochondria comprise approximately 35 percent of ventricular myocyte volume and according to their cellular location are designated as either subsarcolemmal or interfibrillar. Mitochondria are the site of oxidative phosphorylation and ATP generation. Although they have the capacity to buffer large amounts of Ca^{2+} and are a potential source of activator calcium, their contribution to E-C coupling is probably minimal in view of the short-time constants involved. Variation in mitochondrial Ca^{2+} during a twitch is imperceptible and thus plays a very minor role in beat to beat changes in calcium homeostasis. Although mitochondrial Ca^{2+} plays a small role in E-C coupling, slower increases in mitochondrial Ca^{2+} content are important with respect to mitochondrial function and energetics; for example, the matrix enzymes pyruvate dehydrogenase, nicotinamide adenine dinucleotide (NAD)-dependent isocitrate dehydrogenase, and α-ketoglutarate dehydrogenase are activated by low $[Ca^{2+}]$.[17] In addition, the ability to accumulate large amounts of Ca^{2+} under pathological conditions (e.g., ischemia) can help protect against myocyte Ca^{2+} overload; however, Ca^{2+} accumulation by mitochondria ultimately slows ATP production.

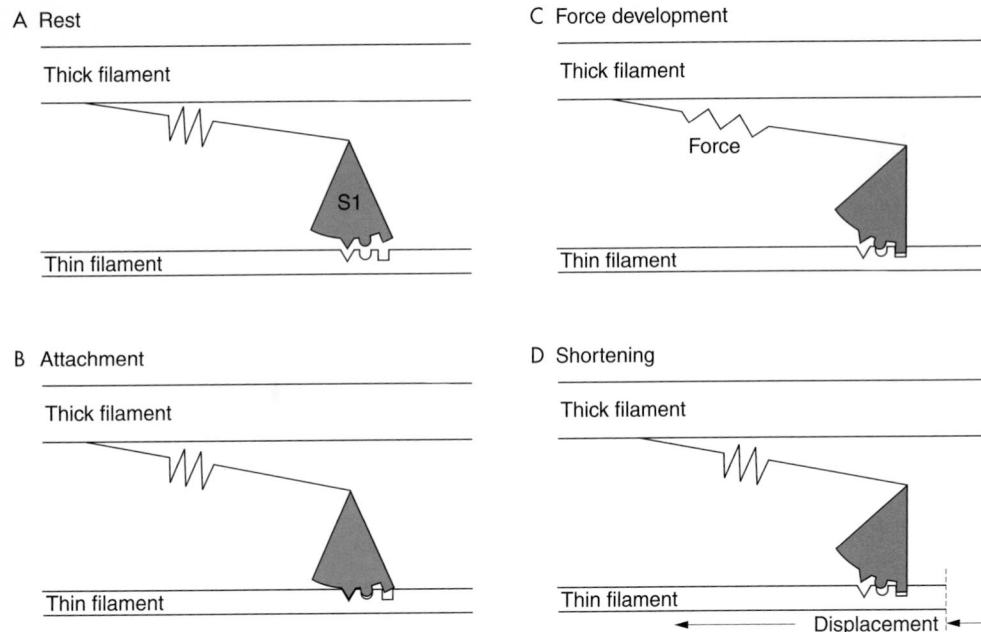

A Rest

Thick filament

S1

Thin filament

B Attachment

Thick filament

Thin filament

C Force development

Thick filament

Force

Thin filament

D Shortening

Thick filament

Thin filament

Displacement

FIGURE 4–6. A mechanical model of the crossbridge cycle. **A.** Detached crossbridge. **B.** Crossbridge prior to developing force. **C.** Attached crossbridge developing force stored in the elastic component. **D.** Crossbridge rotated and translated so the filaments slide relative to one another. Each step in the cycle can be related to energetically different chemical states. *Source: Reproduced with permission from Bers.*[12]

█ ROLE OF NITRIC OXIDE

Nitric oxide (NO) is produced by the myocardium and regulates cardiac function through both vascular-dependent and -independent effects.[18] NO has a modest positive inotropic effect on basal contractility in isolated myocytes and the isolated perfused heart, but a negative inotropic effect in vivo,[19] possibly because of nitrosylation ion channels responsible for E-C coupling (e.g., L-type channel, RyR2). The negative inotropic effects on β-adrenergic stimulated contractility are greater and less controversial, and can comprise a critical component of negative feedback over contractile reserve. NO's positive effects on relaxation or lusitropy (and in part, for negative inotropic effects) are likely to be caused by cyclic 3′,5′-guanosine monophosphate (cGMP)-mediated reduction in myofilament Ca^{2+} sensitivity.[20] Finally, mitochondrial NO reduces maximal venous oxygen (MVO_2) consumption and increases mechanical efficiency (stroke work/MVO_2), suggesting that NO regulates energy production as well influencing consumption.

The effects of NO on E-C coupling are confusing and controversial because of the presence of three nitrous oxide synthase (NOS) isoforms that are spatially localized to highly controlled microdomains and linked to disparate signaling pathways and effectors. For example, nitrous oxide synthase type III (NOS3) is compartmentalized to the sarcolemmal and T-tubule caveolae, associated with the L-type channel, inactivated by the scaffolding protein caveolin-3, and activated by Ca^{2+}/calmodulin and Akt phosphorylation. NOS3 produces its negative inotropic and positive lusitropic effects by means of cGMP activation.

In contrast, nitrous oxide synthase type I (NOS1), which is also activated by Ca^{2+}/calmodulin and can be inactivated by caveolin-3, is localized to cardiac SR and is involved with calcium homeostasis. NOS1 increases the open probability of the cardiac RyR2 and modulates β-adrenergic mechanics, calcium transients, and the force-frequency relationship, although the mechanisms remain controversial. Nevertheless, accumulating data suggest that NO plays an important role in E-C coupling vis-à-vis modulation of Ca^{2+} channel activity, myofilament Ca^{2+} sensitivity, and mitochondrial respiration.[19]

█ NON–STEADY-STATE EXCITATION-CONTRACTION COUPLING

Heart-rate dependence of cardiac contractility reflects basic cycling kinetics of calcium and is critically dependent on SR function. Processes related to force-interval behavior (e.g., mechanical restitution, force-frequency, postextrasystolic potentiation) are important insofar as they represent fundamental physiological control mechanisms, they are utilized as indices of myocardial function, and they play a role in the response to exercise and the development and maintenance of heart failure. Non–steady-state aspects of E-C coupling provide the basis for these phenomena.

Mechanical restitution is the relative refractory period that immediately follows a contraction and is usually explained by the recovery of the RyR2 receptors (because I_{Ca} and SR Ca^{2+} content recover rapidly).[21] Mechanical restitution is the basis for postextrasystolic potentiation (PESP), the strong contraction following a weaker extrasystole, because lower $[Ca^{2+}]$ on the extrasystole results in increased I_{Ca} (less Ca^{2+}-induced inactivation of the L-channel), less Ca^{2+} efflux from NCX, and increased SR Ca^{2+} loading on the postextrasystolic beat.[22] The result is a greater amount of released Ca^{2+} and therefore a stronger contraction. In the intact heart, the effect of changing preload (and the impact on Frank-Starling and calcium sensitivity) is an important additional mechanism. Postextrasystolic potentiation contributes to the beat-to-beat variability of the pulse in atrial fibrillation. Mechanical alternans, the alternating contraction amplitude at a constant heart rate that is seen in heart failure, is explained by a similar interplay of RyR2 refractoriness (which is increased in heart failure), I_{Ca} inactivation, NCX competition, and SR Ca^{2+} load.[12]

The relation between pacing rate and force (force-frequency relationship) can be understood similarly by these non–steady-state phenomena. Increased pacing rate overcomes the encroachment on mechanical restitution and produces an increase in force because of rate-dependent increases in I_{Ca}, I_{Na} (which results in less Ca^{2+} efflux by the NCX), diastolic $[Ca^{2+}]_i$ (less time for efflux and greater influx/sec), releasable SR Ca^{2+} content, and fractional SR Ca^{2+} release.[23] A phenomenon similar to the force-frequency relationship is observed when the effects of heart rate on the time constant of isovolumic relaxation are examined. Thus, similar to the effect on contraction, relaxation is augmented at higher rates of stimulation.

EXCITATION-TRANSCRIPTION COUPLING

An emerging concept is that the molecular machinery of E-C coupling is involved in the long-term regulation of gene expression by a process known as *excitation-transcription* (E-T) coupling. Despite periodic oscillations of $[Ca^{2+}]$ from 100 nM to 1 µM during E-C coupling, transcription regulatory proteins (e.g., NFB, JNK, NFAT) are calcium-activated. The amplitude and duration of the calcium signal, the presence of microdomains and anchoring proteins, and linkages through calmodulin, kinases, and phosphatases are important mechanisms for discriminating important regulatory cues and resolving this apparent paradox.[24]

CaMKII regulates proteins involved in calcium transport, ion channels, and cell contraction, metabolism, and proliferation by phosphorylation. Phosphorylation substrates for CaMKII that are involved in modulating contraction-relaxation include PLB, SERCA2a, L-type Ca^{2+} channels, and the RyR2.[25] CaMKII phosphorylates the transcription factor cyclic adenosine monophosphate (cAMP) response element-binding (CREB), which promotes transcription of c-fos.[26] In addition, CaMKII has autoregulatory properties that are dependent on the frequency of Ca^{2+} spikes, a process thought to have a role in neuronal memory. Little is known about in-vivo CaMKII activation, but biochemical data suggest that that CaMK might be *primed* to respond to Ca^{2+} spikes. Thus calcium-dependent regulation by calmodulin (CaM) and CaMKII has both acute responses affecting E-C coupling and chronic responses that influence the expression levels of proteins involved in E-C coupling.[5] In vascular smooth muscle cells, the L-type channel (via the RhoA/ROK pathway) and the calcineurin/NFAT pathway are involved in the regulation of cell differentiation.[27]

VASCULAR EXCITATION-CONTRACTION COUPLING

Arterial smooth muscle cells exist in the partially constricted state. The principal determinant of vascular tone is membrane potential, which is achieved through activation of voltage-gated calcium channels. There is a steep relation between $[Ca^{2+}]$ and vascular tone, and therefore membrane potential must be highly regulated to maintain appropriate vascular resistance. The resting potential of smooth muscle cells ranges from –40 to –70 mV, lower than cardiac muscle because of greater Na^{+} permeability. Thus the rising phase of the action potential is produced by inward calcium current through the slow L-type Ca^{2+} channels. Contraction results directly from depolarization-induced Ca^{2+} influx and indirectly by means of CICR-activation of the contractile apparatus. Relaxation results from lowering cellular Ca^{2+} via Ca^{2+}ATPase pumps and hyperpolarization of the cell by activation of K^{+} channels.[28]

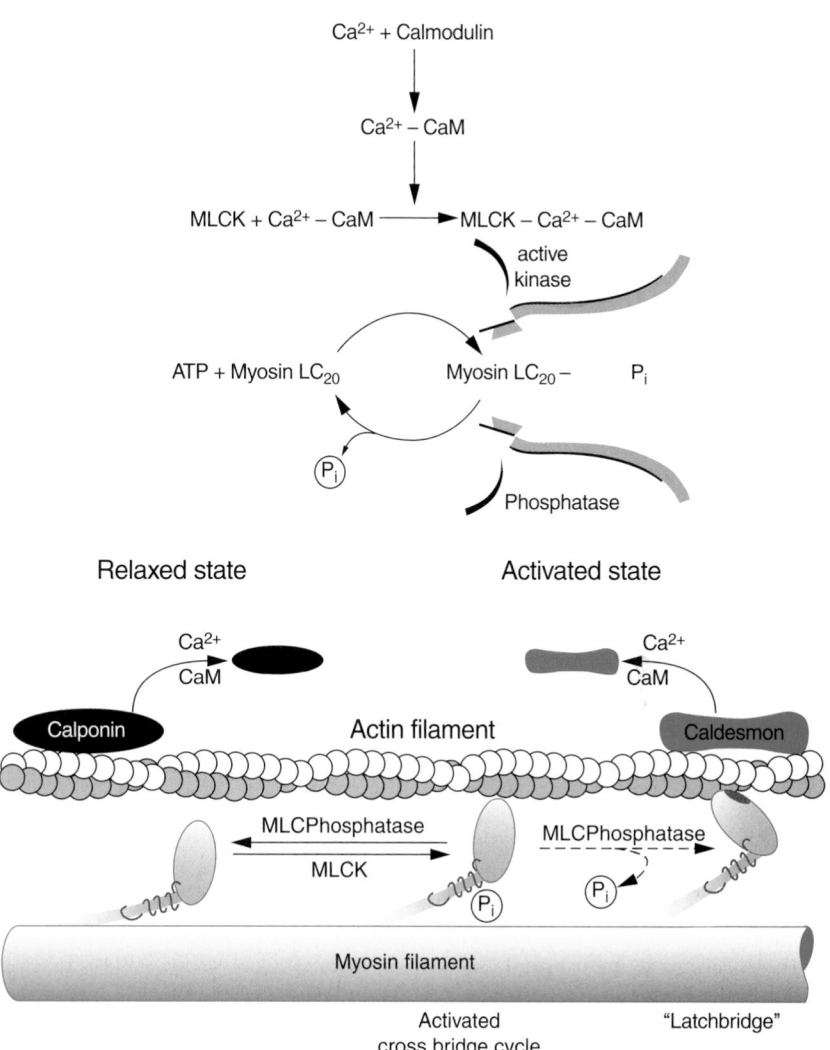

FIGURE 4–7. The molecular basis of regulation of smooth muscle contraction. Stimulation of muscarinic receptors increases the $[Ca]_i$ because of entry of external calcium (Ca^{2+}) and release of Ca^{2+} from internal stores. Ca^{2+} binds to calmodulin (CaM) and the Ca^{2+}-CaM complex subsequently binds to and activates myosin light-chain kinase (MLCK). Phosphorylation of myosin by MLCK stimulates actin-activated myosin-ATP hydrolysis, which produces contraction. Relaxation begins with the cessation of agonist stimulation, resulting in decreased $[Ca]_i$, dissociation of Ca^{2+} from CaM, inactivation of MLCK because of dissociation of CaM, dephosphorylation of myosin by phosphoprotein phosphatases, and relaxation. ATP, adenosine triphosphate. *Source: Reproduced with permission from Paul R, Heiny JA, Ferguson DG, Solaro RJ. Diversity of muscle. In: Sperelakis N, Banks RO, eds. Essentials of Basic Science: Physiology. 2nd ed. Boston: Little, Brown and Company; 1996:217–225.*

A distinctive feature in smooth muscle is that Ca^{2+} acts as a second messenger to activate myosin light-chain kinase (MLCK), which phosphorylates the myosin light chains and produces force. Ca^{2+} binds to calmodulin, and this complex activates MLCK. Phosphorylation of the 20 kD light chain stimulates actin-activated myosin ATP hydrolysis and contraction. Relaxation occurs when there is dissociation of Ca^{2+} from calmodulin, inactivation of MLCK, and dephosphorylation of myosin by myosin light-chain phosphatase (Fig. 4–7).

Unlike myocardial cells, both cAMP and cGMP inhibit the activity of the slow Ca^{2+} channels. Thus both NO (which increases cGMP) and β-adrenergic agonists (which increase cAMP) are vasodilators. Stimulation of delayed rectifier channels and sarcolemmal Ca^{2+} pumps produce vasodilation. Angiotensin II and α-agonists cause vasoconstriction by phospholipase C (PLC)-mediated production of inositol trisphosphate (IP_3; which releases Ca^{2+}) and diacylglycerol (DAG), which stimulates protein kinase C-phosphorylation of the Ca^{2+} channel and inhibition of the delayed rectifier channel.[28]

PROPERTIES OF MYOCARDIAL CONTRACTION

【 】 FUNDAMENTALS OF MYOCARDIAL CONTRACTILITY

Fundamental to cardiac muscle function are the relations between force and muscle length, velocity of shortening, calcium, and heart rate. The maximal force developed at any sarcomere length is determined by the degree of overlap of thick and thin filaments, and therefore, the number of available crossbridges. Force increases linearly until a sarcomere length with maximal overlap (~2.2 μm) is achieved (Fig. 4–8), beyond which force and overlap gradually declines to zero (i.e., the *descending limb*). The descending limb of the length-tension relationship is prevented by the strong parallel elastic component in cardiac muscle. The ascending limb of the length-tension relationship (equivalent to the Frank-Starling relationship that relates preload to cardiac performance) is also caused by a length-dependent increase in myofilament calcium sensitivity (Fig. 4–9A). This has been explained by enhanced calcium binding to TnC, narrower interfilament gaps at long sarcomere length, and increased SR calcium release and uptake at longer sarcomere lengths.[29]

The relation between force and velocity of contraction is hyperbolic (Fig. 4–9B); at maximum force (isometric force), shortening cannot occur, and at zero force (i.e., *unloaded* muscle), velocity is at a maximum, V_{max}, reflecting the maximum turnover rate of myosin ATPase. Therefore, alterations in the myosin isoform (i.e., α, fast; β, slow) such as those seen in response to pressure overload, have an effect on V_{max}.[29]

Another fundamental property of cardiac muscle is the force p-Ca^{2+} relation.[29] Shorter sarcomere lengths decrease Ca^{2+} sensitivity, and caffeine and various inotropic drugs (e.g., levosimendan), are potent calcium sensitizers. β-Adrenergic stimulation results in a cAMP-dependent phosphorylation of cardiac TnI and a resultant decrease in myofilament calcium sensitivity; thus for a positive β-adrenergic receptor (βAR)–inotropic effect, the amplitude of the calcium transient must more than compensate for reduced βAR-mediated myofilament sensitivity.[12]

The final property relates heart rate to contraction and relaxation.[29] Increasing the heart increases contractility; this is related to the Ca^{2+} capacity and load of the sarcoplasmic reticulum (SR). A related phenomenon, frequency-dependent acceleration of relaxation (FDAR) results from CaMKII phosphorylation of phospholamban (or by some other mechanism that increases SR Ca^{2+} transport).[30] CaMKII might be activated by the increased $[Ca^{2+}]_i$ that occurs with increased stimulation rates; however, the precise mechanisms are unresolved. The physiological implications for faster relaxation at increased heart rates, when the diastolic filling periods are shortened, are discussed in the following section.

【 】 ISOLATED MUSCLE: MECHANICS OF CONSTITUENT MUSCLE FIBERS

When a strip of heart muscle is attached at both ends so that the length is fixed and then electrically stimulated, the muscle develops force with-

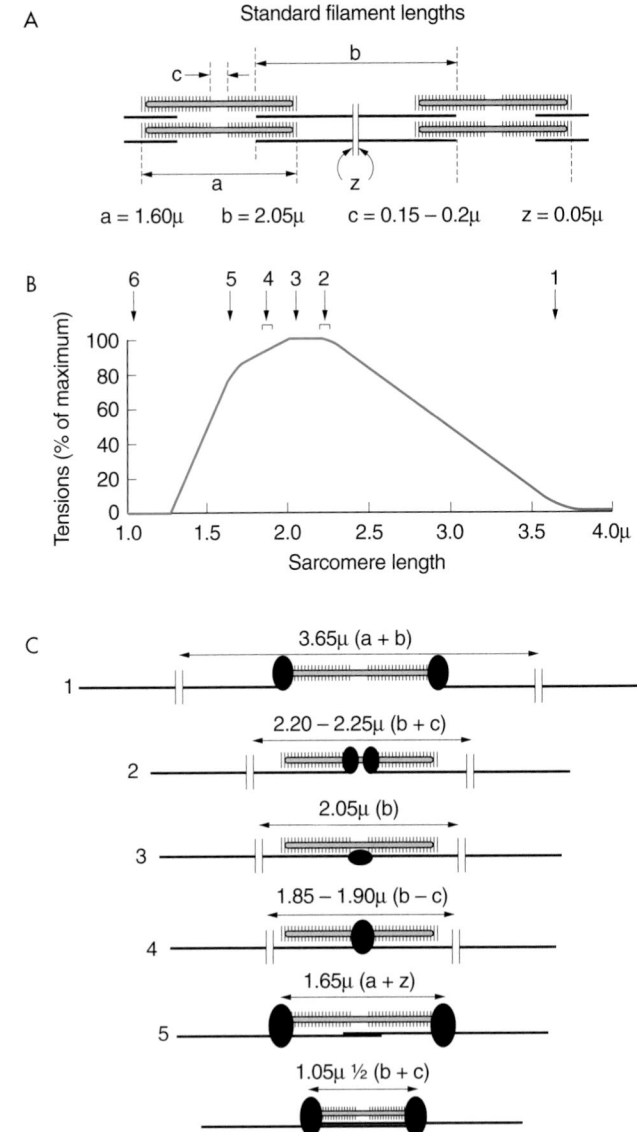

FIGURE 4–8. Structural basis for the active isometric force-length relationship. *Source: Reproduced with permission from Paul R, Heiny JA. Muscle: overview of structure and function at the cellular level. In: Sperelakis N, Banks RO, eds. Essentials of Basic Science: Physiology. 2nd ed. Boston: Little, Brown and Company; 1996:217–225.*

out shortening (Fig. 4–10A). A fundamental property of striated muscle is that the strength of this isometric twitch is dependent on the initial resting muscle length, or preload (Fig. 4–10B). As cardiac muscle is stretched passively, the resting tension rapidly rises and prevents overstretching of the sarcomeres. If additional load is applied before contraction (i.e., the preload), stimulation causes contraction with an increased peak tension and rate of tension development (dT/dt). Thus, total tension includes both active and passive tension. The length-tension relationship, which forms the basis for the Frank-Starling relationship, is depicted in Fig. 4–10C. Inotropic state is defined operationally as a change in the rate or extent of force development that occurs independently of the loading conditions.[29] The biophysical basis of the inotropic state includes the subcellular processes that regulate myocyte cytosolic calcium and actin-myosin crossbridge cycling. In isolated cardiac muscle, changes in the inotropic state are measured by changes in the peak isometric tension and dT/dt at a fixed preload.

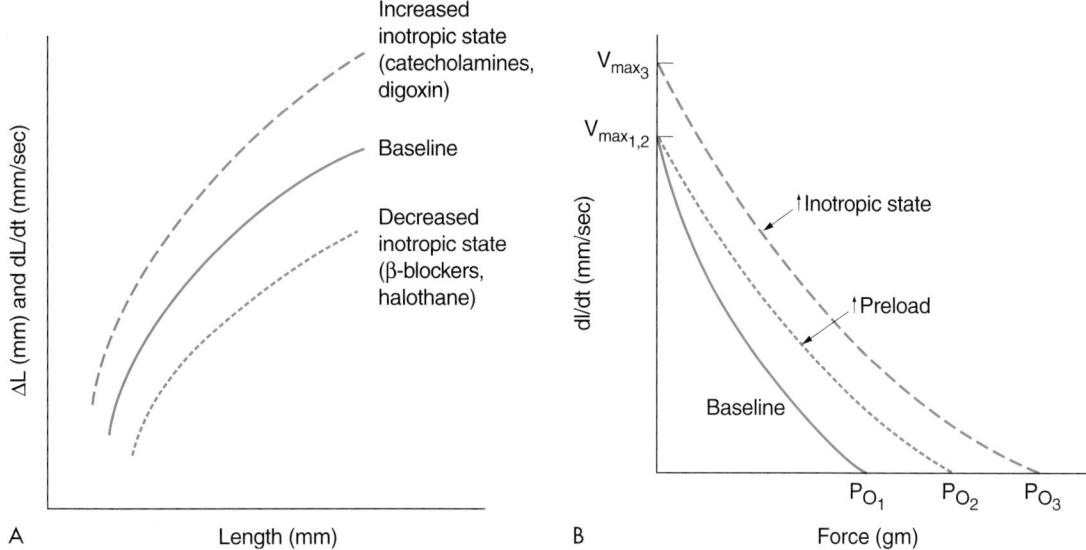

FIGURE 4–9. A. Length-shortening and length-velocity relationships from isotonic contractions at a constant afterload. As muscle length (preload) increases, shortening (ΔL) and velocity of shortening (dL/dt) increase. An increased inotropic state shifts the curve upward and to the left; conversely, a decreased inotropic state shifts the curve downward and to the right. **B.** Force-velocity relationship from variably afterloaded contractions. Increased preload causes an increase in the maximum isometric tension (P_{01} to P_{02}) without a change in the extrapolated velocity of an unloaded contraction (V_{max}). An increase in the inotropic state increases P_0 and V_{max} (dL/dt = velocity of contraction). *Source: Reproduced with permission from Hoit and Walsh.*[29]

If isolated cardiac muscle is allowed to shorten, the contraction is termed *isotonic* (Fig. 4–10D). Initial muscle length is determined by applying a preload; an additional load known as the *afterload*, affects muscle behavior after stimulation. Muscle shortening occurs when tension development equals the total load (preload plus afterload). During shortening, tension remains constant. With dissipation of the active state, the muscle returns to its initial preloaded length, and tension finally declines. If preload is altered while the afterload is kept constant, length-shortening and length-velocity curves (analogous to the length-tension curve seen in isometric muscle).[29]

The force-velocity curve describes an inverse hyperbolic curve relating afterload and the initial velocity of shortening and can be obtained from a series of variably afterloaded contractions (see Fig. 4–9B). When the afterload is so great that the muscle cannot shorten, the contraction becomes isometric (P_0). The velocity of an unloaded contraction (V_{max}) is determined by the physicochemical properties unique to cardiac muscle and is therefore considered a measure of the inotropic state. However, because load always exists, V_{max} must be extrapolated from the force-velocity curve. Although changes in preload shift P_0 without changing V_{max}, a positive inotropic agent increases V_{max} and P_0 by means of a parallel upward shift of the force-velocity curve; a negative inotropic agent causes the opposite effect. Similar operational definitions of the inotropic state can be applied to the preloaded isotonic contraction, in that a positive inotropic agent produces an upward shift of the length-shortening and length-velocity curves.[29]

An important property of cardiac muscle is that the isometric passive length-tension curve establishes the limits of tension for an isotonic contraction. In other words, the tension at the end of an isotonic contraction is the same as the tension developed from an isometric contraction at the same resting muscle length.[29]

Besides load and the contractile state, cardiac muscle performance is influenced by the frequency of stimulation. An increase in stimulation frequency causes an increase in tension in isolated cardiac muscle, known as the *Bowditch phenomenon*.[31] This is the force-frequency relation previously described.

CARDIOVASCULAR PHYSIOLOGY AT THE ORGAN LEVEL

For all the advantages of studying isolated myocytes and muscle fibers, an integrated and more realistic analysis of CV function regards the left ventricle as a muscle pump coupled to the systemic and venous circulations. In contrast to isolated cardiac muscle, contraction of the intact left ventricle is auxotonic, in that force rises and falls during ejection of viscous blood into a viscoelastic arterial system. Moreover, attempts to extrapolate results from isolated muscle to the intact left ventricle are hampered by the complexity of chamber geometry and myocardial fiber orientation, which make it difficult to estimate initial fiber length (preload) and the force opposing left ventricular ejection (afterload). Finally, unlike isolated cardiac muscle, ventricular performance is modulated by neurohumoral influences, right and left ventricular interaction, restraining effects of the pericardium, and atrial function. At the organ level, the preceding events are initiated by the electrical activation of the heart and structured by the sequence of events in a heartbeat, the cardiac cycle.

【 】 THE ELECTROCARDIOGRAM

The ECG (Fig. 4–11A) records the pattern of electrical activation of the heart on the body surface. Electrical currents generated by differences in potential between depolarized and polarized regions of the heart are conducted through the body, detected by electrodes, ampli-

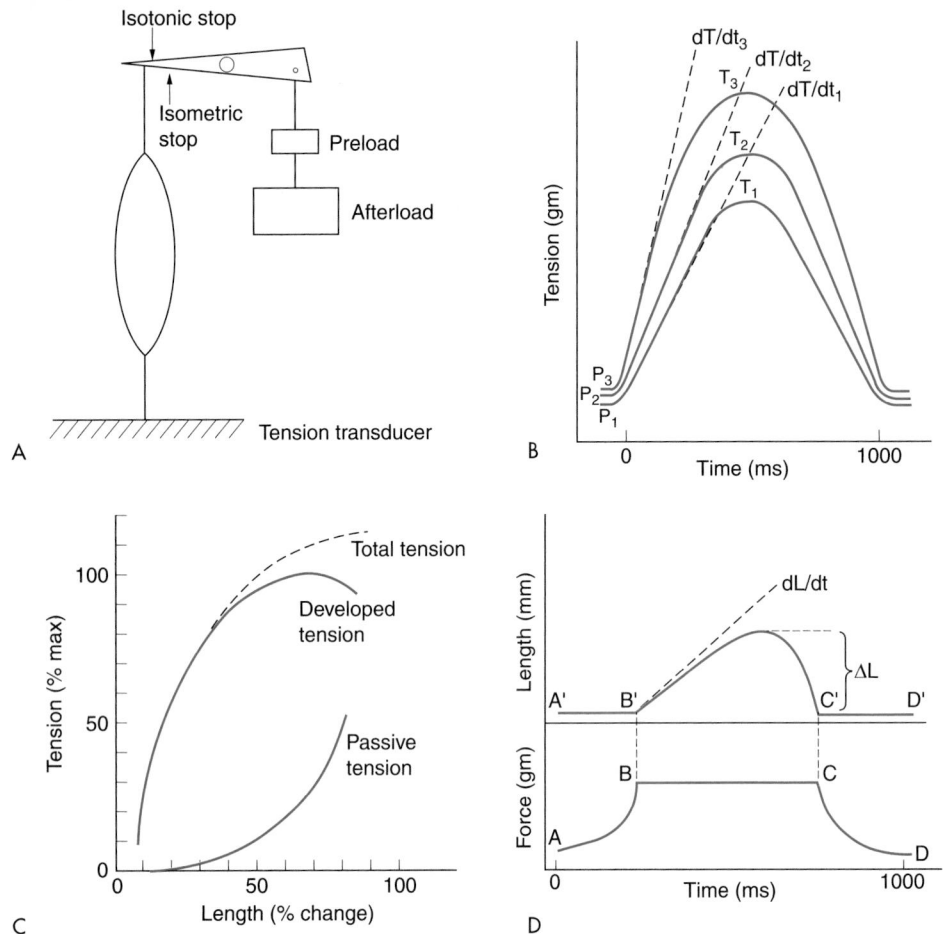

FIGURE 4–10. Contractions in isolated muscle. **A.** Isolated muscle preparation. Muscle is attached to a level arm at one end and fixed to a tension transducer at the other. The muscle is stretched by applying a weight (preload) at one end of the lever arm. A stop prevents muscle shortening. **B.** Tension-time curves of isometric twitches at three levels of preload. With increased preload, peak tension (T) and the maximum rate of tension development (dT/dt) are increased. The time to peak tension is unchanged. **C.** Length-total tension relationship and its components, passive and active tension. As muscle is stretched, the absolute passive and total tension increase. **D.** Superimposed tension-time and length-time recordings from afterloaded isotonic contractions. After preload is applied, a stop is placed to prevent further stretching. Afterload is added, and the muscle is stimulated. Muscle shortens when generated tension equals total load (preload and afterload). Measures of shortening in the isotonic contraction include total shortening (DL) and the initial velocity of contraction (dL/dt). *Source: Reproduced with permission from Hoit and Walsh.[29]*

dle branches). The impulse travels slowly (0.02–0.05 ms) through the AV node. In contrast, conduction velocity through the Purkinje system is very fast (2.0–4.0 ms). The P-R interval includes atrial depolarization, AV nodal conduction, and His-Purkinje activity. Activation of ventricular myocardium (conduction velocity 1.0–2.0 ms) occurs after most of the conduction system is depolarized and is represented by the QRS complex. Ventricular repolarization occurs during the T wave.[32]

The ECG is essentially a voltmeter that measures and records potential differences between pairs of electrodes or leads. Three bipolar leads (I, II, II) and six unipolar leads (aVR, aVL, aVF, V1–6) record the distribution of the potentials on the frontal and horizontal planes of the heart (Fig. 4–11B). Depolarization and repolarization of the heart results in differences in electrical potential, and the ECG measures these changes in potential over time. The external surface of a depolarized membrane becomes electrically negative relative to quiescent, polarized areas. The direction of the propagated impulse travels from the depolarized to polarized areas. By convention, the direction of the propagation wave toward the positive pole of a bipolar lead system or exploring electrode produces an upright defection and conversely, if the propagation wave is toward the negative pole or away from an exploring electrode, a negative deflection is produced. Depolarization progresses from cell to cell in an orderly fashion from endocardium to epicardium from the apex to base of the

fied and recorded on calibrated moving paper. The ECG provides important clinical information regarding the electrical orientation of the heart in three-dimensional space, the relative size of the cardiac chambers, the presence of conduction system defects, and provides evidence for a variety of underlying pathologic conditions, such as ischemia, infarction, cardiomyopathy, and hypertrophy.[32]

The SA node is the primary pacemaker of the heart and is located at the junction of the superior vena cava and the right atrium. The action of the sinus node is electrically silent, although a measurable conduction time between sinus node discharge and atrial depolarization (denoted by a P wave) can be measured on intracardiac electrograms. Action potentials travel rapidly (1.0–1.5 ms) through the atrial myocardium and generate an atrial contraction. Preferential conduction in specialized bundles of muscle fibers (*the internodal tracts of Bachmann, Wenckebach, and Thorel*) nearly simultaneously activate the atrial musculature and ensure that the action potential reaches the atrioventricular node in a timely fashion. Excitation of the ventricles spreads by means of the AV node, and the His-Purkinje system (bundle of His, and bun-

heart. In contrast, repolarization does not occur as a propagated wave; nevertheless, it is represented by a single vector that integrates multiple areas of potential difference. Local circuit-currents precede the depolarization wavefront, depolarize the adjacent membrane, and bring the membrane to threshold potential; with depolarization, the local circuit-currents flow through low-resistance gap junctions (the major component of which is connexin), and depolarize a neighboring cell. Thus, the myocardium functions as a functional syncytium.[1,32] The ECG is discussed in detail in Chapter 13.

【 】 THE CARDIAC CYCLE

The cardiac cycle describes pressure, volume, and flow phenomena in the ventricles as a function of time. This cycle is similar for both the left and right ventricles, although there are differences in timing stemming from differences in the depolarization sequence and the levels of pressure in the pulmonary and systemic circulations.

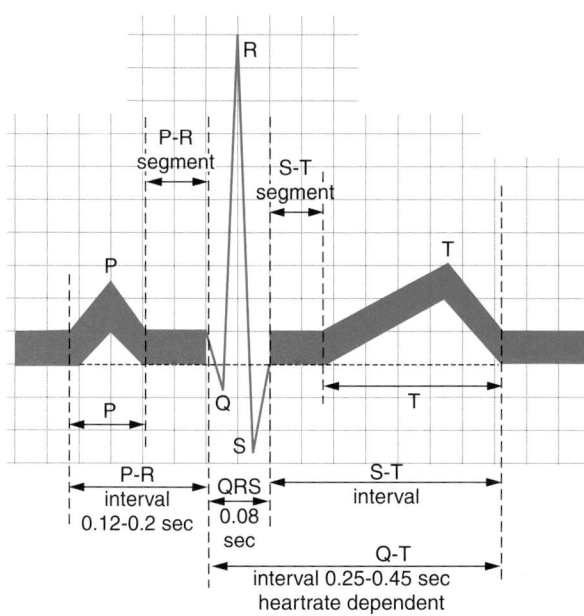

FIGURE 4–11. Nomenclature of the deflections, intervals, and segments of the normal electrocardiogram. *Source: Reproduced with permission from Grupp et al.[32]*

For simplicity the cardiac cycle for the left heart during one beat will be described (Fig. 4–12).

The QRS complex on the surface ECG represents ventricular depolarization. Contraction (*systole*) begins after a ~50 ms delay and results in closure of the mitral valve. The left ventricle contracts isovolumetrically until the ventricular pressure exceeds the systemic pressure; at this time, the aortic valve opens, and ventricular ejection occurs. Bulging of the mitral valve into the left atrium during isovolumic contraction causes a slight increase in left atrial pressure (*c* wave). Shortly after ejection begins, the active state declines, and ventricular pressure begins to decrease. Left atrial pressure rises during ventricular systole (*v* wave) as blood returns to the left atrium by means of the pulmonary veins. The aortic valve closes when left ventricular pressure falls below aortic pressure; momentum briefly maintains forward flow despite greater aortic than left ventricular pressure. Ventricular pressure then declines exponentially during isovolumic relaxation, when both the aortic and mitral valves are closed. This begins the ventricular diastole (see the following). When ventricular pressure declines below left atrial pressure, the mitral valve opens, and ventricular filling begins. Initially, ventricular filling is very rapid because of the relatively large pressure gradient between the atrium and ventricle. Ventricular pressure continues to decrease after mitral valve opening because of continued ventricular relaxation; its subsequent increase (and the decrease in atrial pressure) slows ventricular filling. Especially at low end-systolic volumes, ventricular early rapid filling can be facilitated by ventricular suction produced by elastic recoil. Ventricular filling slows during diastasis, when atrial and ventricular pressures and volumes increase very gradually. Atrial depolarization is followed by atrial contraction, increased atrial pressure (*a* wave), and a second, late rapid-filling phase. A subsequent ventricular depolarization completes the cycle.

Valve closure and rapid-filling phases are audible with a stethoscope placed on the chest and can be recorded phonocardiograph-

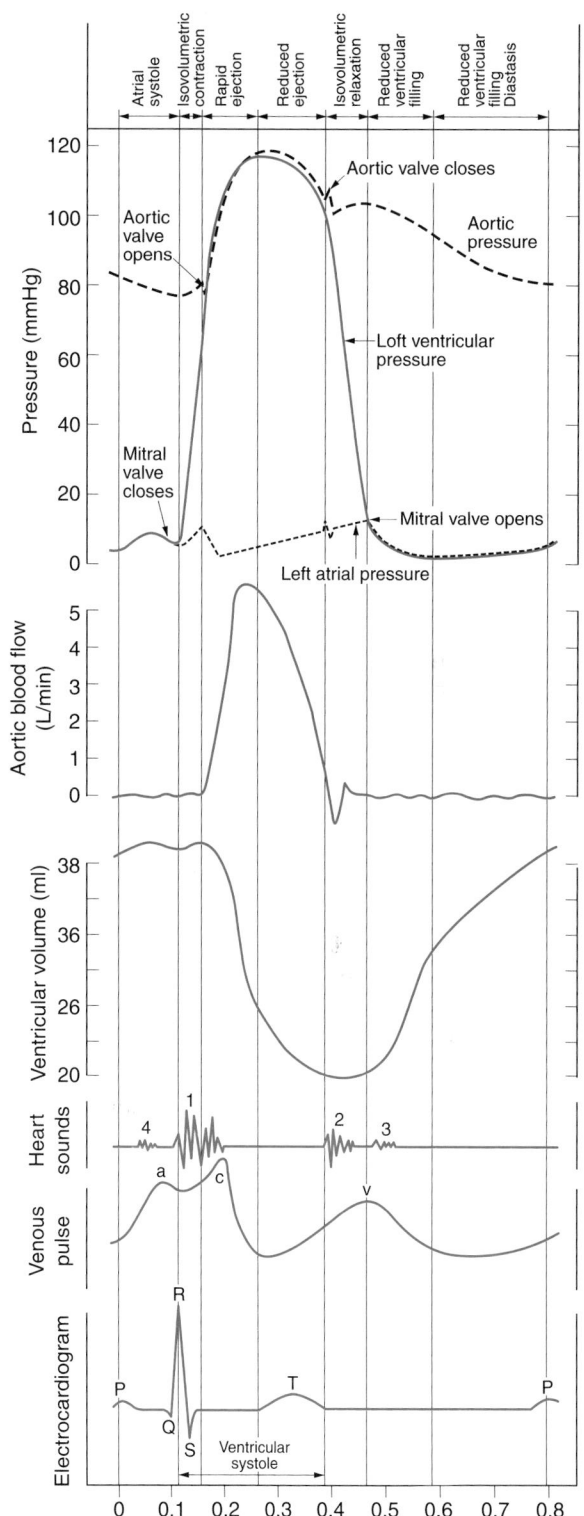

FIGURE 4–12. Pressure, flow, volume, electrocardiographic and phonocardiographic events constituting the cardiac cycle. *Source: Reproduced with permission from Hoit and Walsh.[29]*

ically after electronic amplification. The first heart sound, resulting from cardiohemic vibrations with closure of the atrioventricular (mitral, tricuspid) valves, heralds ventricular systole. The second heart sound, shorter and composed of higher frequencies than the first, is associated with closure of the semilunar valves (aortic and pulmonic) at the end of ventricular ejection. Third and fourth

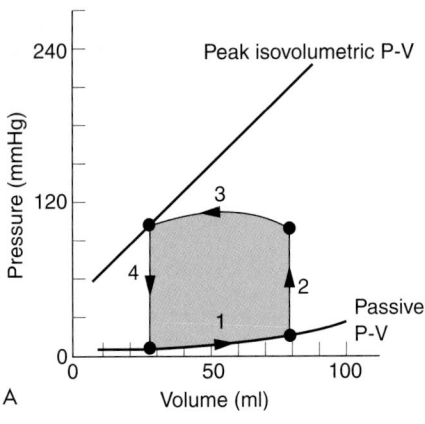
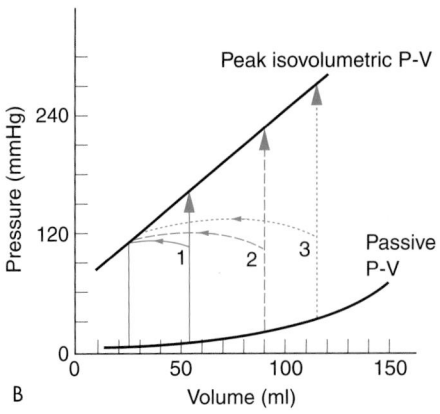

A

B

FIGURE 4–13. A. Left ventricular pressure-volume (P-V) loop, the segments of which correspond to events of the cardiac cycle: diastolic ventricular filling along the passive P-V curve (phase I), isovolumetric contraction (phase II) ventricular ejection (phase III), and isovolumetric relaxation (phase IV). **B.** The ventricle ejects to an end-systolic volume determined by the peak isovolumetric P-V line; an isovolumetric contraction (*large arrowheads*) from varying end-diastolic volumes (preload). *Source: Reproduced with permission from Hoit and Walsh.*[29]

heart sounds are low-frequency vibrations caused by early, rapid filling and late diastolic atrial contractile filling respectively. These sounds can be heard in normal children but in adults usually indicate disease.

An alternative time-independent representation of the cardiac cycle is obtained by plotting instantaneous ventricular pressure and volume (Fig. 4–13). During ventricular filling, pressure and volume increase nonlinearly (phase I). The instantaneous slope of the pressure-volume (P-V) curve during filling (dP/dV) is diastolic stiffness, and its inverse (dV/dP) is compliance. Thus, as chamber volume increases, the ventricle becomes stiffer. In a normal ventricle, *operative* compliance is high, because the ventricle operates on the flat portion of its diastolic P-V curve. During isovolumic contraction (phase II) pressure increases, and volume remains constant. During ejection (phase III) pressure rises and falls until the minimum ventricular size is attained. The maximum ratio of pressure to volume (maximal active chamber stiffness or elastance) usually occurs at the end of ejection. Isovolumic relaxation follows (phase IV), and when left ventricular pressure falls below left atrial pressure, ventricular filling begins. Thus, end diastole is at the lower right hand corner of the loop, and end systole is at the upper left corner of the loop. Left ventricular P-V diagrams can illustrate the effects of changing preload, afterload, and inotropic state in the intact ventricle (see the following).

A P-V loop (PVA) can also be described for atrial events.[33] During ventricular ejection, descent of the ventricular base lowers atrial pressure and thus assists in atrial filling. Filling of the atria from the veins results in a *v* wave on the atrial and venous pressure tracing. When the mitral and tricuspid valves open, blood stored in the atria empties into the ventricles. Atrial contraction,

denoted by an *a* wave on the atrial pressure tracing actively assists ventricular filling. The resultant atrial P-V diagram has a figure of eight configuration with a clockwise V loop representing passive filling and emptying of the atria and a counterclockwise A loop, representing active atrial contraction. Thus the atria function as reservoirs, conduits, and booster pumps.[33]

【 】 PRESSURE-VOLUME RELATIONS IN THE ISOLATED HEART

Isolated, perfused, isovolumically contracting hearts are useful preparations to study preload dependency of ventricular performance (the Frank-Starling relation) and fully relaxed, end-diastolic P-V relations without the confounding, uncontrolled changes in either neurohumoral activation or coronary perfusion. These preparations are especially well-suited for quantifying end-systolic elastance (stiffness), a relatively load-independent index of ventricular function. The time varying elastance model of ventricular contraction is based on the experimental observations in which ventricular volume and loading are altered under conditions of unvarying contractility (Fig. 4–14).[34] At any time, *t*, following the onset of contraction, the relation between pressure (*P*) and volume (*V*) is linear according to the relation: $P(t) = E(t) - [V(t) - V_0]$, where E is the time-varying elastance, and V_0 is the volume at zero pressure or dead volume; this relation becomes progressively steeper until it reaches a maximum at endsystole (ES). Thus, the ventricle behaves like a spring with a stiffness (elastance) that increases during contraction and decreases during relaxation. The slope of the end-systolic P-V relationship, endsystolic elastance, (E_{es}), changes directly as a function of acute

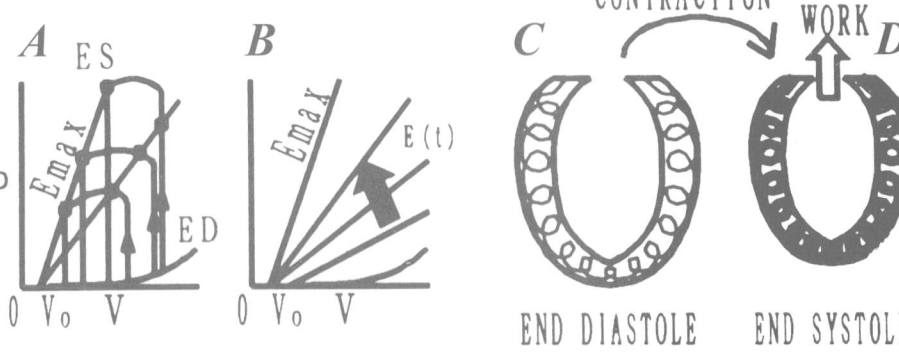

FIGURE 4–14. The time varying elastance concept. **A.** A series of variably loaded PVAs. The relation between pressure and volume at any time, *t*, during variably loaded contractions under constant contractility conditions is linear and reaches a maximum value at end-systole. *Filled circles connected by straight lines* occur at the same time, *t*, during contraction. E_{max} is the line connecting the points at end-systole (ES). **B.** Elastance, $E(t)$, increases at each time, *t*, during contraction until it reaches maximal values at ES. Increasing contractility increases the slope at any time, *t*, including ES (E_{max}). **C,D.** The concept that the ventricle behaves as an elastic *spring* with a stiffness (elastance) that increases during systole and decreases during diastole (EES or E_{max}). V, volume; P, pressure; V_0, dead volume; S, systole; D, diastole. *Source: Reproduced with permission from LeWinter MM, Osol G. Normal physiology of the cardiovascular system. In: Fuster V, Alexander RW, O'Rourke RA, Roberts R, King SB III, Nash IS, Prystowksy EN. Hurst's The Heart. 11th ed. New York: McGraw-Hill; 2004:87–112.*

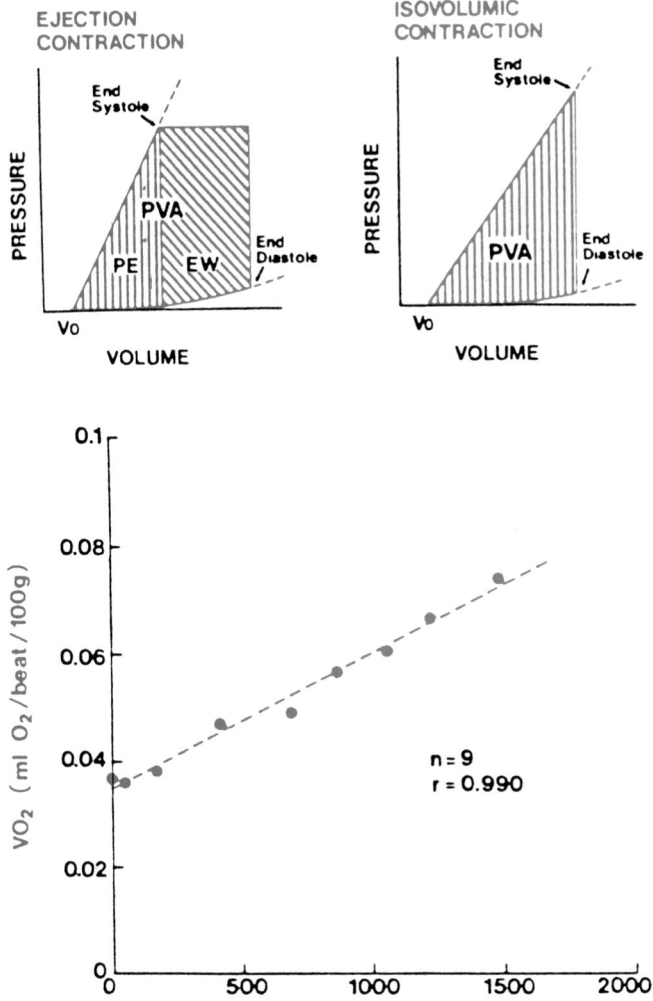

FIGURE 4–15. (*Top*) Schematic of VO2–PVA concept. In ejecting contractions, PVA = EW + PE; in isovolumic contraction, PVA = PE only. (*Bottom*) Correlation of PVA with VO_2. P-V, pressure-volume; VO_2, oxygen consumption. P-V, pressure-volume; VO_2, oxygen consumption. *Source: Reproduced with permission from LeWinter MM, Osol G. Normal physiology of the cardiovascular system. In: Fuster V, Alexander RW, O'Rourke RA, Roberts R, King SB III, Nash IS, Prystowksy EN. Hurst's The Heart. 11th ed. New York: McGraw-Hill; 2004:87–112.*

changes in contractility without a change in dead volume (V_0). Appropriate changes in Ees are also observed with increases in beating frequency (e.g., force-frequency relations).

The elastance concept has been extended to the study of ventricular mechanoenergetics by proposing that the area (PVA) bounded by the left ventricle (LV) P-V loop is a measure of the total mechanical energy of LV contraction.[35] The PVA concept is shown schematically in Fig. 4–15. The total mechanical energy of contraction can be considered to consist of two components: (1) external work, the area enclosed within the P-V loop; and (2) potential energy stored in the ventricular *spring* at ES, that is, the area between the end-systolic pressure relation on the left, and the end-diastolic P-V relation on the right.

The myocardial oxygen consumption (MVO_2)–PVA relation is obtained by measuring P-V area loops and LV MVO_2 at several steady-states. There is a highly linear correlation ($r > .98$) between

LV VO_2/beat and PVA/beat over a wide range of experimental conditions (Fig. 4–15, bottom) indicating the accuracy of the PVA as a measure of total mechanical energy.[35] The VO_2 intercept of the VO_2–PVA relationship is the unloaded VO_2 (PVA–independent VO_2), which in an isovolumically contracting heart, corresponds to a point at which LV peak pressure is 0 mmHg (Fig. 4–16). At this point, except for a low level of crossbridge cycling caused by shape changes, there is neither mechanical energy produced nor energy expended for crossbridge cycling.[36] The VO_2 under unloaded conditions reflects energy used for excitation-contraction coupling and basal metabolism; the latter can be eliminated experimentally by arresting the heart. In this manner, changes in excitation-contraction coupling energy consumption have been detected as shifts in the unloaded VO_2.[37] Oxygen consumption used by the contractile apparatus for crossbridge cycling is PVA–dependent VO_2, which increases linearly and directly with PVA. Because PVA–dependent VO_2 is the energy input, and the PVA is the total energy output of the contractile machinery, the inverse slope of the VO_2–PVA relationship is a dimensionless measure of the thermodynamic efficiency of the contractile machinery.[37,38] Unlike efficiency expressed as the external work/total VO_2 efficiency expressed by the VO_2–PVA relationship is relatively insensitive to load. The VO_2–PVA relationship is sensitive to metabolic changes and impacts the efficiency of ATP production.[39]

【 】 DETERMINANTS OF LEFT VENTRICULAR FUNCTION

Measures of Ventricular Performance

Measures of overall ventricular performance typically include cardiac output (the quantity of blood delivered to the circulation, calculated as the stroke volume and heart rate), stroke volume (quantity of blood ejected/beat, which equals the ventricular end-diastolic vol-

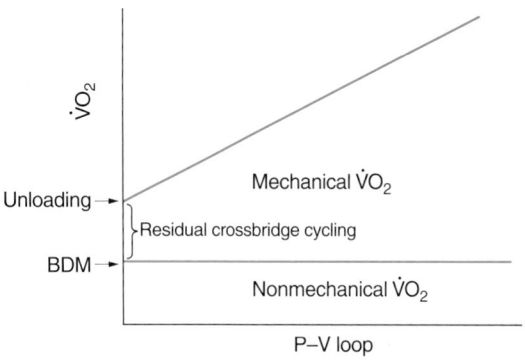

FIGURE 4–16. Schematic of the relation between VO_2/beat and the P-V area (PVA). The diagonal VO_2–PVA line is obtained by mechanical unloading of the ventricle; the y intercept is the unloaded VO_2. Mechanically unloaded VO_2 is subdivided into VO_2 for residual crossbridge cycling and that for nonmechanical VO_2 (BDM, which inhibits crossbridge cycling). The latter consists of VO_2 for E-C coupling and basal metabolism. E-C, excitation-contraction; P-V, pressure-volume; VO_2, oxygen consumption. *Source: Reproduced with permission from LeWinter MM, Higashiyama A, Yaku H, Watkins MW. Influence of preload on non-mechanical VO_2 assessed with 2.3-butanedione monoxime. In: LeWinter MM, Suga H, Watkins MW, eds. Cardiac Energetics: From Emax to Pressure-Volume Area. Norwell MA: Kluwer Academic Publishers; 1995:133–127.*

ume minus the end-systolic volume), and stroke work (the product of pressure and stroke volume, which equals the area bounded by the ventricular PVA and which can be approximated in the clinical setting as ([mean LV systolic-diastolic pressure] × stroke volume × 0.0136). Cardiac output responds to changes in the oxygen requirements of tissues, for example, as occurs with exercise. The extraction of nutrients by tissue can be expressed as the arteriovenous difference across the tissue. According to the Fick principle, the consumption of a particular nutrient (e.g., oxygen) by a tissue equals the rate of delivery of that nutrient, that is, the cardiac output times the arteriovenous difference of that nutrient. Changes in cardiac output necessary to meet the metabolic needs of the tissues can be produced by changes in the stroke volume or heart rate or both. Changes in stroke volume are mediated by altered loading conditions, inotropic state, and heart rate. Thus, those factors that influence the strength of contraction in isolated muscle are the same factors that determine cardiac output. The stroke volume (end-diastolic volume minus end-systolic volume) expressed as a function of the end-diastolic volume is the ejection fraction (EF). Thus, EF = (end-diastolic volume − end-systolic volume)/end-diastolic volume.

Preload The influence of preload on measures of ventricular performance defines the left ventricular function curve, known as the *Frank-Starling curve.* Increasing left ventricular end-diastolic volume increases stroke volume in ejecting beats and increases peak left ventricular pressure in isovolumic beats. The modulation of ventricular performance by changes in preload, termed *heterometric regulation,* operates on a beat-by-beat basis and is responsible for matching outputs of the right and left ventricles, as with changes in posture and breathing. The Frank-Starling curve also represents an important compensatory mechanism that maintains left ventricular stroke volume (vis-à-vis increasing left ventricular end-diastolic volume) when left ventricular shortening is impaired, owing either to myocardial contractile dysfunction or to excessive afterload. The atria also exhibit a Frank-Starling curve that becomes clinically important during exercise and when there is resistance to early diastolic left ventricular filling.

Because a representative fiber length (i.e., preload) is difficult to determine in the left ventricle, changes in the myocardial fiber length are estimated from changes in either the left ventricular end-diastolic volume or left ventricular end-diastolic pressure. In the clinical setting, end-diastolic pressure or pulmonary capillary wedge pressure are used frequently as measures of preload. However, the passive P-V relationship, analogous to the passive length-tension curve in isolated muscle, is not linear, but exponential. Thus the ratio of change in left ventricular pressure to volume is greater at higher than at lower left ventricular volumes. Not surprisingly, under certain circumstances, ventricular pressure can inaccurately reflect the ventricular volume. Moreover, changes in ventricular volume can erroneously be inferred from changes in cardiac pressures, which can result only from alterations in ventricular compliance.[40] For example, chronic volume overload can shift the ventricular diastolic pressure-relation rightward so that volume is increased at a normal end-diastolic pressure, whereas chronic pressure overload can shift the diastolic P-V relation leftward and for the same end-diastolic pressure, result in a smaller ventricular volume. Compliance of the left ventricle is affected by pericardial

pressure, right ventricular pressure and volume, and coronary artery perfusion (*turgor*) in addition to changes in the intrinsic elastic properties of the left ventricle.

Afterload Afterload in the intact heart can be considered as the tension in the left ventricular wall that resists ventricular ejection (wall stress during systole) or as the arterial input impedance (the ratio of instantaneous change in pressure to instantaneous change in flow). Although forces within the ventricular wall are difficult to measure, initial estimates of systolic wall stress can be derived from application of the Laplace relationship in which wall tension = $(P \cdot r)/2h$, where P refers to pressure, r to ventricular radius, and h to wall thickness. More complex derivations based on various geometric assumptions are used to calculate end-systolic wall stress. Input impedance is a complex function of arterial pressures, elasticity, vessel dimension, and blood viscosity, which requires measurement of instantaneous aortic pressure and flow, and is therefore impractical to measure in the clinical setting. Owing to its simplicity, aortic pressure is often used as a surrogate for afterload. An increase in afterload causes a decrease in stroke volume and the velocity of left-ventricular shortening. The resulting stress-shortening and stress-velocity curves are analogous to those obtained from variably afterloaded isotonic contractions in isolated muscle.

Inotropic State The ideal method of measuring the inotropic state in the intact left ventricle should incorporate the variables of force, length, velocity, and time, be independent of external loading conditions, and relate to physicochemical processes at the sarcomeric level. Because of these constraints, changes in inotropic state are usually defined operationally by shifts of the various ventricular function curves, which by definition, are independent of loading conditions. For example, a drug with positive inotropic activity (e.g., dobutamine) shifts the Frank-Starling curve (analogous to the length-shortening curve in papillary muscle preparations) upward and to the left, and changes in the stress-shortening relationship (analogous to the force-velocity curve) upward and to the right.

The rate of pressure development in the left ventricle during isovolumic systole (dP/dt) is used frequently as an index of the inotropic state. Although LV + dP/dt_{max} provides a measure of the rate of tension development and of myocardial contractility, this index is preload dependent, caused in part by length-dependent changes in myofilament Ca^{2+} sensitivity.[41] However, $+dP/dt_{max}$ is largely independent of afterload, provided that the maximum rate of increase occurs before aortic valve opening. Although changes in the maximal rate of increase of ventricular pressure are highly sensitive to acute changes in contractility and are useful to assess directional changes in inotropic state, absolute dP/dt_{max} is not as useful for assessment of basal contractility as are the ejection phase indices, such as LV ejection fraction (stroke volume/end-diastolic volume × 100).[42] Moreover, dP/dt_{max} cannot be corrected for changes in muscle mass produced by left ventricular hypertrophy, in which case it is best to compare peak stress (dP/dt), which incorporates pressure, volume, mass, and geometry. Because of the direct influence of preload on dP/dt—dP/dt at a common developed pressure (LV systolic minus diastolic pressure) and the slope of the dP/dt end-diastolic volume curve (preload recruitable stroke work, see the following) have been proposed as preload independent indices of the inotropic state.[43]

End-systolic P-V points from ejecting beats obtained from variably preloaded or afterloaded contraction fall reasonably close to the isovolumetric P-V line for a given inotropic state (vide supra). Thus, changes in the inotropic state, independent of the loading conditions can be identified by changes in the slope of the end-systolic P-V relationship (Ees). By acutely altering loading conditions (e.g., transient vena caval occlusions or phenylephrine boluses), a family of PVAs are obtained (single beat methods designed for clinical use have been proposed).[44] End-systole can be defined as end ejection or as the time of maximal elastance (the maximal P-V ratio) during systole. In the normal heart, these two points are closely related in time. In practice, the end-systolic P-V relationship (ESPVR) is constructed by connecting the end-systolic points of each loop; the relation is a relatively linear and defines the properties of the chamber when maximally activated.[45]

However, Ees does have a modest degree of load dependence, likely caused by the load dependence of activation. Moreover, the *linear* ESPVR is really curvilinear, particularly at the extremes of the contractile state.[45] The effects of nonlinearity are particularly important when the P-V relation is acquired over a narrow range of pressures and volume. A single slope in the latter instance will not uniquely characterize the ESPVR and therefore the contractile state. In addition, the extrapolated V_0 is unlikely to represent dead volume. Finally, V_0 is not entirely independent of inotropic state. Thus, more than Ees is needed to compare two contractile states; interpretation must take into account V_0, and analysis of covariance or a multiple linear regression analysis with dummy variables is desirable.[45]

Other considerations for the use of P-V relations to characterize contractility are: (1) specialized and invasive instruments are necessary for its measurement; (2) methods used to alter load should be free of inotropic effects; (3) because changes in autonomic tone and heart rate can complicate analysis, loading changes should be as rapid as possible; (4) arrhythmias can occur and complicate the analysis; (5) changes in coronary perfusion pressure that can alter the P-V relation occur with changes in load; (6) changes in mass and geometry of the ventricle make changes in the ESPVR ambiguous. In addition to Ees, preload recruitable stroke work (slope of the end-diastolic volume-stroke work relation) and the slope of the end-diastolic volume–dP/dt_{max} relation are derived as indices of contractility from P-V analysis. Each of these approaches are linear and afterload independent. Preload recruitable stroke work is independent of heart size and the slope of the end-diastolic volume–dP/dt_{max} is more sensitive to inotropic state than is Ees.[45]

Heart Rate Heart rate is normally determined by the interplay between the intrinsic automaticity of the sinoatrial node and the activity of the autonomic nervous system. Increasing heart rate causes a small but measurable increase in the inotropic state through the force-frequency relationship. In addition, heart rate is a major determinant of cardiac output. However in a normal heart, pacing between heart rates of 60 and 160 beats per minute has little effect on cardiac output because the diminished diastolic filling time offsets the modest increase in inotropic state.

[ ] DIASTOLE AND DIASTOLIC FUNCTION

Diastole is the summation of processes by which the heart loses its ability to generate force and shorten and returns to its precontrac-

tile state. Diastolic properties of the ventricle are complex and multifactorially determined and are related to the speed and synchrony of myocardial relaxation and inactivation, loading conditions, viscoelasticity, heart rate, atrial function, and ventricular interaction. Diastole occurs in a series of energy-consuming steps beginning with release of calcium from troponin C, detachment of actin-myosin crossbridges, SERCA2a-induced calcium sequestration into the SR, NCX-induced extrusion of calcium from the cytoplasm, and return of the sarcomere to its resting length. Adequate ATP must be present for these processes to occur at a sufficient rate and extent.

The P-V relation during early diastole reflects the lusitropic (relaxation) state of the heart, analogous to the inotropic (contraction) state measured during systole. The rate of left ventricular relaxation can be estimated from the maximal rate of pressure decay ($-dP/dt_{max}$) and indices (e.g., relaxation half-time [$RT_{1/2}$]) that are related to the time necessary for ventricular relaxation, but these measurements are highly dependent on the prevailing load of the intact circulation. In contrast, τ, the time constant of left ventricular relaxation during isovolumic relaxation provides a more accurate, less load-dependent measure of relaxation;[46] τ is shortened by β-adrenergic stimulation (cyclase-dependent phosphorylation of phospholamban and troponin I) and prolonged with β-adrenergic antagonists.[47] Although several mathematical models of the exponential decay of left ventricular pressure exist, a simple monoexponential model that declines to zero is frequently employed: $P(t) = P_o e - t/\tau$ where $P(t)$ is the left ventricular pressure at any time, t; τ is the relaxation constant; P_o is the left ventricular pressure at the onset of relaxation; and e is the base of the natural logarithm.[48,49] The natural logarithmic transformation of both sides of the equation yields: $lnP = -1/T + ln\ P_o$. Thus, τ is derived by obtaining the negative of the reciprocal of the slope of $ln\ P(t)$ versus time, t, from aortic valve closure to mitral valve opening (isovolumic relaxation). High-fidelity catheter tip micromanometers are necessary for accurate measurement of $-dP/dt_{max}$ and τ.

In addition to relaxation, the passive viscoelasticity of the ventricle, dependent both on intracellular and extracellular structures, is a major determinant of diastolic function. During contraction, cytoskeletal proteins such as titin and microtubules are deformed by actin-myosin crossbridge cycling and sarcomere contraction, which act like viscoelastic springs during diastole.[50] This reclaimed potential energy constitutes a recoiling force that helps restore the myocardium to its resting configuration. In addition, extracellular matrix proteins such as collagen contribute to the establishment of resting force and length.[51]

Chamber stiffness is quantified from the relation between diastolic LV pressure and volume. LV-diastolic pressure can be changed either by a volume-dependent change in operating stiffness (equal to the slope of a tangent drawn to the P-V curve at any point) or by a volume-independent change in the overall chamber stiffness, because of a change in properties either intrinsic (e.g., hypertrophy) or extrinsic (e.g., pericardial) to the ventricle (Fig. 4–17, Table 4–2).[51,52] Operating stiffness changes throughout filling, such that stiffness (dP/dV) is less at smaller volumes and greater at larger volumes. Because the diastolic P-V relation is generally exponential, the relation between dP/dV and pressure is linear. The slope of this relation is called the *modulus of chamber stiffness* (k_c) and has been used to quantitate chamber stiffness. Thus, when chamber stiffness is increased, the P-V curve

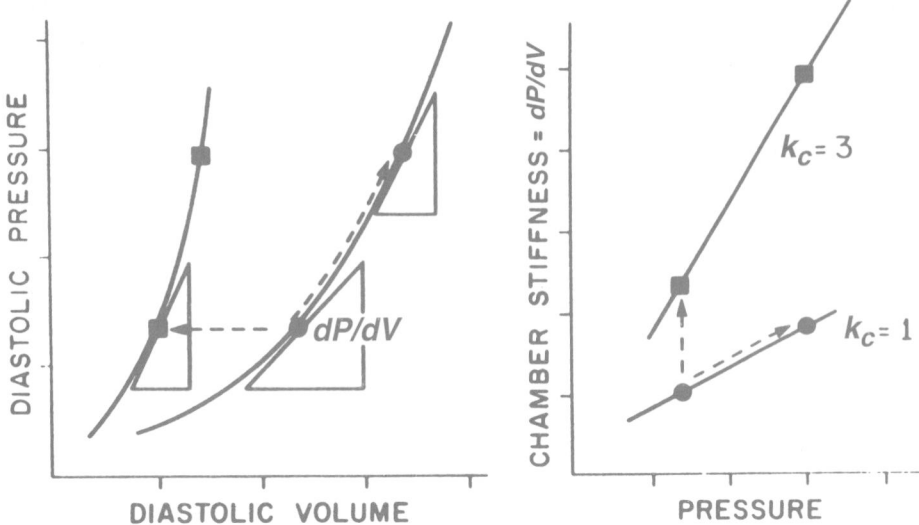

FIGURE 4–17. (*Left*) EDPVR in two ventricles with differing passive diastolic properties. Chamber stiffness is *dP/dV* at any point on the EDPVR. The stiffer chamber on the left has a steeper overall slope. (*Right*) Same data plotted as pressure versus chamber stiffness. Because of the exponential nature of ED-PVR, the relation between chamber stiffness and pressure is a straight line whose slope is the chamber stiffness constant (k_c) that characterizes the overall slope of the EDPVR. A similar relationship holds for stress and strain. EDPVR, end-diastolic pressure-volume relation. *Source: Reproduced with permission from LeWinter MM, Osol G. Normal physiology of the cardiovascular system. In: Fuster V, Alexander RW, O'Rourke RA, Roberts R, King SB III, Nash IS, Prystowksy EN. Hurst's The Heart. 11th ed. New York: McGraw-Hill; 2004:87–112.*

shifts to the left, the slope of the *dP/dt* versus pressure relation becomes steeper, and k_c is increased.[51,52]

Diastolic chamber stiffness, like the systolic chamber stiffness index, Ees, is dependent on both material (myocardial) stiffness and ventricular chamber characteristics (e.g., volume, mass). Myocardial stiffness is quantified from the relation between diastolic LV wall stress (ε) and strain (σ). Strain is the deformation of the muscle produced by an applied force and is expressed as the percent change in length from the unstressed length. At any given strain throughout diastole, myocardial stiffness is equal to the slope ($d\sigma/d\varepsilon$) of a tangent drawn to the stress-strain curve at that strain. Because the stress-strain relation is generally exponential, the relation between ($d\sigma/d\varepsilon$) and stress is linear. The slope of this relation is the modulus of myocardial stiffness (K_m) and has been used to quantitate myocardial stiffness. Thus, when myocardial stiffness is increased, the stress-strain relation shifts to the left, the slope of the ($d\sigma/d\varepsilon$) versus stress relationship becomes steeper and K_m increases.[51,52]

The end-diastolic P-V relation (EDPVR) is constructed by connecting the end-diastolic points (lower right hand) of a series of PVAs; the relation is nonlinear and defines the passive properties of the chamber when it is fully relaxed. The nonlinearity of the EDPVR results from the different types of structural proteins being stretched over the range of pressures and volumes. Thus, at the low end of the relation, where operative stiffness is low, stiffness is caused by compliant elastin and sarcomeric titin. As volume increases and operative stiffness increases, the slack length of collagen and titin are exceeded, and stretch is resisted. At the other extreme (subphysiologic volumes), negative pressures are required to reduce volume (diastolic suction); however negative pressures are rarely recorded in vivo, and less stringent criteria to establish the presence of diastolic suction are required.[45] It is important to recall that changes in intrathoracic pressure, pericardial constraint, and ventricular interaction all influence

the EDPVR. Analytic limitations similar to the ESPVR are present for the EDPVR; that is, comparisons of EDPVR should account for covariance of the parameters.[45]

A variety of curve fits for EDPVR using nonlinear regression analysis have been proposed, but single value indices of stiffness, such as the stiffness constant, have met with limited success.[35] Chamber stiffness (k_c) and myocardial stiffness (K_m) provide load and chamber size-independent parameters of passive chamber and myocardial properties, respectively; however, when comparing hearts of different sizes, a simple approach is to measure the volume at a specified pressure.[45]

【 】 VENTRICULO-ARTERIAL COUPLING

In isolated muscle, loading conditions represent the force applied to muscle before and after (preload and afterload, respectively) the onset of contraction. In the intact ventricle, preload and afterload are also determined by the characteristics of the arterial and venous circulations (pulmonary and systemic circulations for the right and left ventricles, respectively). Thus, loading conditions are not only important direct determinants of ventricular performance, but they also function indirectly by coupling the ventricle to the vascular system.

Ventricular contraction transfers blood from the venous to the arterial side of the circulation, and arterial and venous capacitances (the change in volume per change in pressure, *dV/dP*) determine the respective pressures that result from the shift in blood volume. These pressures determine the driving force across the pe-

▌ TABLE 4–2

Factors Influencing Left Ventricular Chamber Stiffness

Physical Properties of the Left Ventricle
Left ventricular chamber volume and mass
Composition of the left ventricular wall
Viscosity, stress relaxation, and creep

Intrinsic Factors
Myocardial relaxation
Coronary turgor

Extrinsic Factors
Pericardial restraint
RV interaction
Atrial contraction
Pleural and mediastinal pressure

RV, right ventricular.
Source: Reproduced with permission from Gaasch WH. Basic and clinical aspects. In: Levine HJ, Gaasch WH, eds. The Ventricle. Boston: Martinus Nijhoff Publishing; 1985.

ripheral resistance (where resistance equals pressure gradient for flow divided by the cardiac output) and are primarily responsible for venous return to the heart.

The venous return curve describes the inverse relationship between venous pressure and cardiac output (Fig. 4–18A,B). In contrast to convention, the venous return curve plots the independent variable (cardiac output) on the vertical axis and the dependent variable (venous pressure) on the horizontal axis. The X intercept is the mean circulatory pressure, that is, that pressure in the vascular system in the absence of cardiac pumping. The mean circulatory pressure is a function of the capacitance of the vascular system and the total blood volume. The plateau of the venous return curve and the Y intercept represents the maximal obtainable cardiac output as venous pressure is reduced. In the normal heart, cardiac output is limited by venous return, and the operating venous pressure is near the plateau of the venous return curve.[53]

Coupling of the venous system of the heart is graphically represented in Fig. 4–18C. In this analysis developed by Guyton and coworkers, the intersection of the ventricular function (Frank-Starling) curve and the venous return curve represent the steady-state operating values of cardiac output and venous pressure. At this equilibrium point, the ability of the venous system to provide venous return at a given pressure is matched with the ability of the ventricle to pump that venous return when distended to the same pressure.[53]

Increased blood volume and venoconstriction shift the venous function curve upward and to the right, increasing the mean circulatory pressure and the maximal cardiac output (Fig. 4–18D). The venous system contains the major fraction of blood in the vascular system because of the greater capacitance of veins than of arteries. As a result, venoconstriction shifts significant quantities of blood from the peripheral to central circulation. Because arteries contain only a small percentage of the total blood volume, their contractile state does not affect the mean circulatory pressure. Moreover, because venous pressure varies inversely with systemic vascular resistance, arteriolar constriction (increased afterload) shifts the curve downward and to the left without changing the mean circulatory pressure. Conversely, arteriolar dilation shifts the curve upward and to the right.

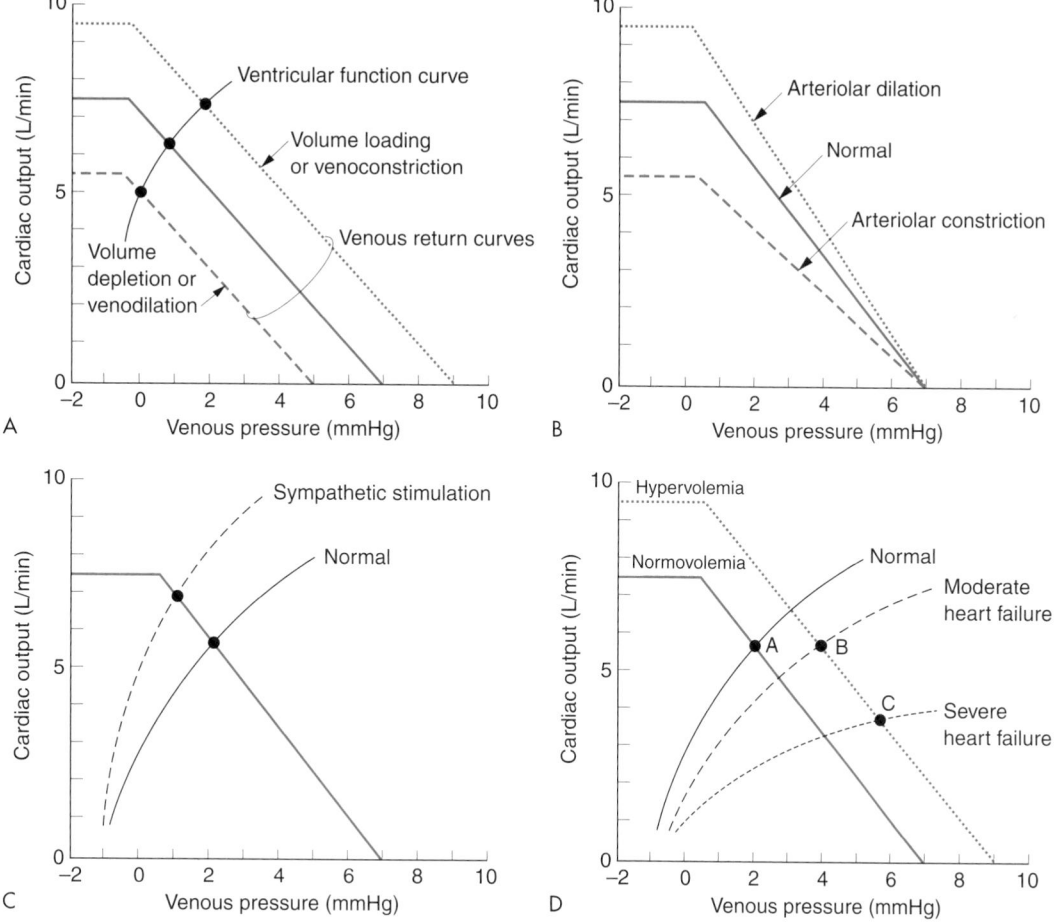

FIGURE 4–18. Venous pressure-cardiac output curves. The equilibrium point is defined by the intersection of the ventricular function curve with the venous return curve. **A.** Volume loading and venoconstriction shift the venous return curves to the right, resulting in an equilibrium point with a higher cardiac output and higher mean circulatory pressure. Volume depletion and venodilation shift the curve to the left, resulting in an equilibrium point with a lower cardiac output and a smaller mean circulatory pressure. **B.** The effects of arteriolar constriction and dilation on the venous return curves are more complex. At **B** (moderate heart failure), cardiac output is preserved at the expense of venous pressure. **C.** Sympathetic nerve stimulation causes a leftward shift of the ventricular function curve resulting in an equilibrium point with a lower venous pressure and higher cardiac output. At **C** (severe heart failure), cardiac output is decreased and venous pressure further increased. **D.** Chronic heart failure causes rightward shifts of both the ventricular function and venous return curves. *Source: Reproduced with permission from Hoit and Walsh.[29]*

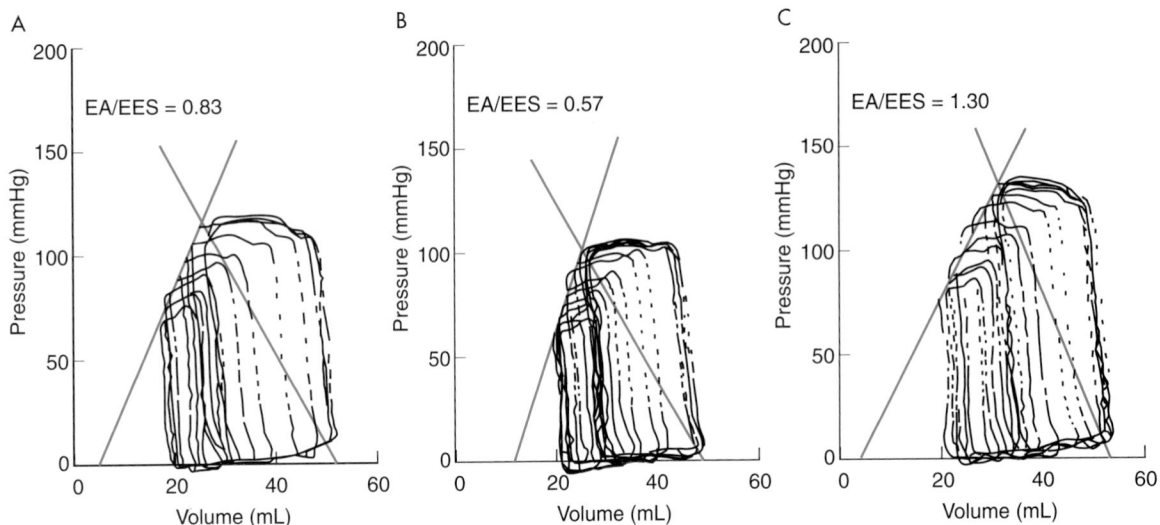

FIGURE 4–19. Ventriculo-arterial coupling using the arterial elastance-LV end-systolic relation (EA/EES). **A.** Baseline. **B.** Nitroprusside increases EES with little change in EA, resulting in a decrease in EA/EES. **C.** Angiotensin II increases EA without a change in EES, resulting in an increase in EA/EES. EA, arterial elastance; Ees, end-systolic elastance; LV, left ventricular. *Source: Reproduced with permission from Asanoi et al.*[56]

An increased inotropic state shifts the ventricular function curve to the left without significantly altering the venous return curve. Conversely, in chronic heart failure, there is a rightward shift of the ventricular function curve and because of renal salt and water retention, a parallel rightward shift of the vascular function curve. In this way, cardiac output is initially maintained at the expense of increased venous pressure and congestion. If the compensatory mechanisms fail, venous pressure increases further, and cardiac output falls.[53]

Ventriculo-arterial coupling can also be expressed in the P-V framework (Fig. 4–19). Arterial properties are represented by effective arterial elastance (EA), which incorporates the mean resistance and pulsatile features of the arterial load.[54] EA is estimated by PES/SV, where PES is the end-systolic pressure, and SV is the stroke volume. The EA/Ees ratio has been used as an index of ventriculo-arterial coupling, and has been shown to be a critical determinant of pump performance and efficiency.[55] With increases in EA, stroke work initially increases, reaches a plateau, and then decreases. Maximum stroke work occurs when arterial and ventricular properties are equal, that is, when $EA = Ees$.[56] Similar changes with increases in EA occurs with ventricular efficiency, defined as external stroke work/MVO_2/beat and is maximum when $EA = Ees/2$. Therefore, in this conceptual framework, energetically optimal ventriculo-arterial coupling exists when the EA/Ees ratio ranges from 0.5 to 1.0.[56]

HEMODYNAMICS
【 】 CARDIAC OUTPUT/BLOOD FLOW

Cardiac output is determined by a relation analogous to Ohms law governing current, voltage, and resistance; that is, cardiac output (Q) increases with an increase in the pressure gradient ($P_1 - P_2$) generated by the heart or a decrease in the resistance (R) according to the relationship $Q = (P_1 - P_2)/R$. The normal cardiac output at rest is ~5 to 6 liters/minute and can increase approximately fivefold during strenuous exercise.[57] The relative distribution of the cardiac output changes dramatically with exercise, such that blood flow to the skin and skel-etal muscle increases to constitute as much as 85 percent of the cardiac output; blood flow to the heart increases nearly fivefold; the brain receives the same amount as it does at rest, the renal and splanchnic circulations receive about half of their basal flow. Physical factors, metabolic products, and peptides that operate through autocrine (regulation of cell function by the producing cell), paracrine (regulation of neighboring cells by the producing cell), or endocrine (regulation of distant cells by the producing cell) mechanisms and neural regulation control the relative distribution of regional blood flow.[57]

Blood flow refers to the bulk flow of fluid in the circulation. Blood flow velocity refers to the speed with which blood moves along the circulation in any particular segment and is related directly to blood flow and inversely to cross-sectional area. Thus blood flow velocity is greatest in the aorta and least in the capillary beds (Fig. 4–20). In the normal circulation, blood flows predominantly in a streamline or laminar pattern. Friction between the blood vessel wall and adjacent blood flow causes blood flow velocity to approach zero next to the wall; centerline velocities are the highest. Shear stresses between adjacent concentric layers of blood cause blood to flow in a laminar pattern resembling a parabola in much of the circulation. The laminar pattern of blood flow is interrupted and converted to a turbulent flow pattern in the ventricles, at bifurcations in the circulation, and when there is an abrupt change in vessel diameter (e.g., from atherosclerosis), which causes blood flow to increase above a critical, dimensionless value (related to cross-sectional area, mean velocity of flow, and kinematic viscosity of the fluid) called the *Reynolds number.*

【 】 PRESSURE

As blood courses through the large arteries, systolic pressure increases slightly, and diastolic pressure decreases. Because the decrease in diastolic pressure is greater than the increase in systolic pressure, the pulse pressure (systolic-diastolic) increases gradually, and mean arterial blood pressure (1/3 systolic pressure + 2/3 dia-

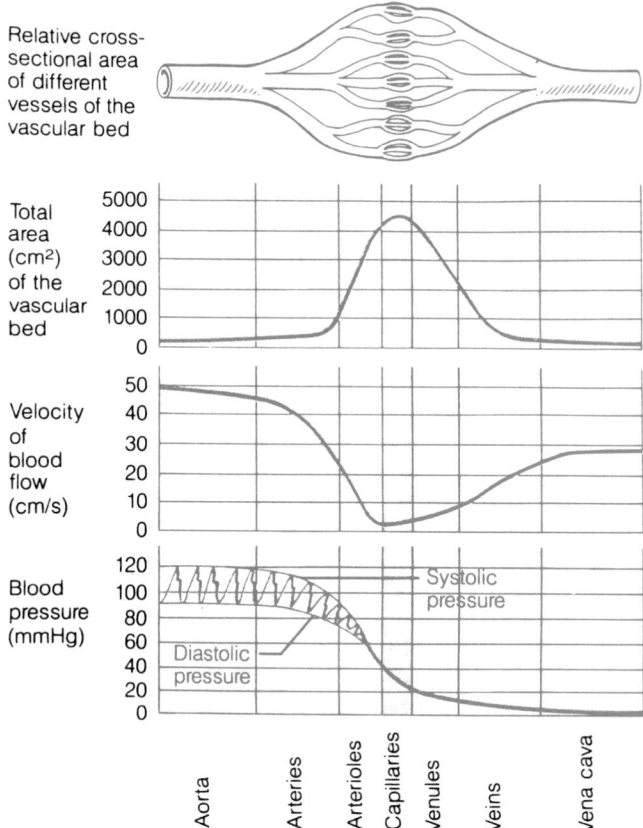

Relative cross-sectional area of different vessels of the vascular bed

FIGURE 4–20. Relations between total cross-sectional area of the vascular bed, velocity of blood flow and blood pressure in various vessels in the systemic circulation. *Source: Reproduced with permission from LeWinter MM, Osol G. Normal physiology of the cardiovascular system. In: Fuster V, Alexander RW, O'Rourke RA, Roberts R, King SB III, Nash IS, Prystowksy EN. Hurst's The Heart. 11th ed. New York: McGraw-Hill; 2004:87–112.*

stolic pressure) decreases in the systemic arteries as the distance from the heart increases. The arterioles provide the greatest resistance to blood flow in the circulation. Consequently, absolute blood pressure decreases by the greatest amount in the arterioles; in addition, the oscillations of blood pressure are abolished in the arteriolar portion of the systemic circulation. Blood enters the capillaries of the systemic circulation with pressures of ~35 mmHg. As blood flows though the capillaries, the blood pressure decreases to ~20 mmHg, and in the venules it decreases to ~5 mmHg. Blood pressure decreases further in the large veins and vena cava, so blood returns to the right atrium with an absolute pressure nearly equal to the atmospheric pressure. The right ventricle generates lower pressures than the left (0 to 30 mmHg vs. 3 to 120 mmHg). Like the systemic circulation, the arterioles exert the greatest resistance to blood flow; however, pulmonary arterioles do not completely dampen the pressure pulses.[57]

Transformation of the ventricular pressure pulse, with its intermittent flow and large pressure changes, into the peripheral pulse, with its continuous flow and smaller pressure changes is caused by the initial transfer of kinetic to potential energy in the aorta in systole and subsequent reclamation of this stored energy in diastole. The arterial pulse is altered by several factors, including heart rate (increased diastolic pressure with increased heart rate), stroke volume (systolic and pulse pressure increase with increased stroke volume), aortic valve function (increased pulse pressure and decreased

diastolic pressure with aortic insufficiency, decreased pulse pressure and a slow rate of increase of pressure with aortic stenosis), arterial compliance (increased pulse pressure and peaked waveform with decreased compliance), and transmission of the pressure wave through the arterial circulation. The latter results from waves reflected at branch points, changes in arterial compliance, and differential transmission between the high-frequency and low-frequency components of the arterial pressure waveform.[57]

RESISTANCE

Total peripheral vascular resistance is the sum of all regional resistances in the systemic circulation that must be overcome by the ejecting left ventricle. This is calculated as (mean aortic–mean right atrial pressure/cardiac output) for the systemic circulation, and as (pulmonary arterial pressure–pulmonary venous pressure)/cardiac output) for the pulmonary circulation. However, the circulation is composed of a number of circuits (e.g., coronary, skeletal, and splanchnic) arranged in series as well as in parallel. Each circuit provides resistance to blood flow, and the type of circuit determines its contribution to total peripheral resistance. For a circuit that has resistances arranged in series, the total resistance is equal to the sum of component resistances. For resistances connected in parallel, the reciprocal of the total resistance is equal to the sum of the reciprocals of the component resistances. Resistances connected in parallel are more efficient than resistances connected in series because the heart does not have to generate a large driving pressure to perfuse multiple beds. In addition, because arterial pressure is maintained within narrow limits, a marked change in the resistance of one circuit changes only slightly blood flow to other circuits. Thus, when one circuit is eliminated, total resistance and arterial blood pressure increase immediately; the increase is sensed by baroreceptors that mediate changes that cause pressure to return to its original value, maintaining blood flow to other areas of the circulation relatively constant (Fig. 4–21). Although less efficient, series resistance

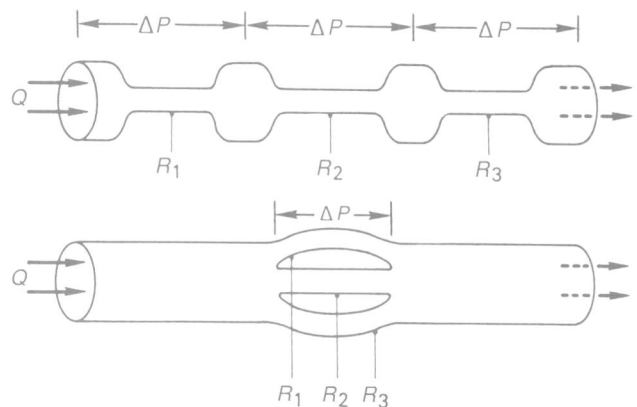

FIGURE 4–21. Illustration of the principle of resistance elements arranged in series versus parallel. (*Top*) If the driving pressure (ΔP) across each series resistance is 3 mmHg, and flow (Q) is 1 mL/min, each resistance (R) would be 3 mmHg/mL (ΔP/Q) and total resistance (R_t) would be 9 mmHg/mL. (*Bottom*) In parallel resistances, if driving pressure is 3 mmHg and flow is 1 mL/min, total resistance is $1/R_1 + 1/R_2 + 1/R_3$, or 1 mL/min. When three resistances are in parallel, total resistance is only one-ninth that with resistances in series. Thus it would take a ΔP of only 1 mmHg to produce a 1 mL/min flow. *Source: Reproduced with permission from LeWinter MM, Osol G. Normal physiology of the cardiovascular system. In: Fuster V, Alexander RW, O'Rourke RA, Roberts R, King SB III, Nash IS, Prystowksy EN. Hurst's The Heart. 11th ed. New York: McGraw-Hill; 2004:87–112.*

units are sometimes necessary, for example, the portal venous connection between the gastrointestinal tract and liver.[57]

Several factors influence resistance (R) to blood flow. The most important factor is the vessel radius (r), such that $R\alpha 1/r$;[4] thus, when the radius is halved, resistance increases by a factor of 16. Another factor is viscosity; the energy required to overcome frictional forces necessary for fluid movement is directly related to viscosity. For a homogeneous fluid such as water or plasma at a given temperature, viscosity is constant (i.e., it is a Newtonian fluid). At 98.6°F (37°C) the viscosity of plasma is approximately 1.7 times that of water. However, for a suspension solution such as blood, viscosity is not constant, that is, it is non-Newtonian. In large blood vessels, laminar blood flow and the alignment of red blood cells parallel to the axis of motion greatly reduce viscosity. However, when blood flow falls below a critical level, the cells fall out of alignment and tumble end over end, which increases apparent viscosity. In addition, temperature, red blood cell mass, and protein concentration affect viscosity The relationship between viscosity, length, and vessel radius is quantified by Poiseuille's law: $R = 8nL/\pi r^4$. By substituting $R = (P_1 - P_2)/Q$ and rearranging: $Q = (P_1 - P_2)\pi r^4/8nL$. Although this relationship was originally developed to describe the flow of a homogeneous fluid through a rigid tube, it approximates the steady-state flow of the circulation.[57]

THE MICROCIRCULATION

The microcirculation is comprised of arterioles, capillaries, and venules. Arterioles range from 10 to 150 μm in diameter and regulate the distribution of blood flow to capillaries (0.5–1 μm); small arterioles (metarterioles) can bypass the capillary beds, shunting flow directly into the small venules (10–40 μm).[58] The independent vasoactivity of different sized arterioles produces blood flow patterns that vary in speed and direction. Although flow in the arterioles is usually rapid, continuous, and unidirectional, capillary flow is highly variable. Capillaries have a single layer of endothelial cells through which oxygen and nutrients diffuse to adjacent tissues. Venules have an endothelial cell layer surrounded by an adventitia and contractile pericytes and are involved in transvascular exchange of fluid and macromolecules across the vascular wall. The larger venules and veins collect and store blood for return to the heart. The cellular and molecular mechanisms that control blood flow in the microcirculation are only beginning to be understood.[59]

Important determinants of capillary exchange through the endothelial cell membrane (*diffusion*) include: (1) the capillary density, which is directly related to the metabolic activity of tissue; (2) lipid solubility of the material to be exchanged; (3) the free diffusion coefficient (small molecules and molecules with very little net electric charge have very high free diffusion coefficients); and (4) the relative concentrations of the material in the blood and the tissue interstitium. Thus the rate of diffusion for a substance Q moving from the vessel to the interstitial space, dQ/dt is proportional to the capillary wall area ($2\pi rl$), the difference in concentration of the substance (ΔC), which represents the driving force for the movement across the vessel wall, and the permeability (P) which is a function of lipid solubility and the free diffusion coefficient: $dQ/dt = (2\pi rl)(P)(\Delta C)$. Permeability for

substances varies by capillary bed (e.g., capillaries in the brain restrict the diffusion of almost all solutes whereas liver capillaries have a very high permeability to large solutes such as albumin). Endothelial transport across restrictive beds is accomplished by other processes such as pinocytosis and vesicular transport. Pores occupy less than 1 percent of the total capillary surface area; there are more present on the venular than arteriolar end of the capillary system, and therefore lipid-insoluble materials (e.g., glucose, small ions) exchange slowly. Thus, lipid-soluble materials are considered *flow limited* whereas lipid-insoluble materials (except water) are considered to be relatively *limited by diffusion*.[58]

The transvascular exchange of water occurs primarily through the bulk flow of water through the pores in the capillary walls (Q_{H2O}); the amount of bulk flow is a function of the difference in hydrostatic pressure in the vessel (*CHP*, variable, depending on tissue bed) and interstitium (*THP*, small but variable), the capillary filtration coefficient (*CFC*), the plasma colloid osmotic pressure (*COP*, caused by protein in blood plasma, ~20 mmHg), and the tissue colloid osmotic pressure (*TOP*, caused by proteins in the interstitial space, ~4.5 mmHg). Thus the net force out of the vessel (*filtration*) is a hydrostatic force and the net force into the vessel (*reabsorption*) is a colloid osmotic force. The effect of these forces on transvascular water flow is described in the Starling equation: $Q_{H2O} = CFC[(CHP - THP) - \sigma(COP - TOP)]$. Where σ is the reflection coefficient for the movement of proteins across the capillary wall (the inverse of the permeability of the vessel wall to protein). The capillary filtration coefficient is the product of capillary surface area and permeability and is related to number and size of the pores through which water can pass through the vessel. Because the balance of forces is different across the length of a capillary bed, filtration occurs near the arterial end and reabsorption near the venule end of the capillary.[58]

Of these forces, capillary hydrostatic pressure (CHP) is the principal mechanism responsible for transcapillary exchange of water. CHP increases whenever arterial pressure increases, venous pressure increases, venule resistance to flow increase, or arteriole resistance to flow decreases. Mathematically, CHP = $(R_V/R_A)P_A + P_V$, where R_V/R_A is the ratio of venule to arteriolar resistance, P_A is approximately mean arterial pressure and P_V is approximately central venous pressure. Capillary pressure is far more sensitive to changes in venous pressure than changes in arterial pressure. The ratio of venule to arteriole resistance (R_V/R_A) is ~0.1; thus, arterial pressure must increase 10 mmHg to cause a 1 mmHg increase in capillary hydrostatic pressure, whereas a 1 mmHg increase in venous pressure will cause a similar increase in capillary hydrostatic pressure. Greater filtration than reabsorption produces tissue lymph flow; the total volume of lymph fluid (important in returning plasma proteins that leaked from the microcirculation and transport of chylomicrons) is ~3 to 4 liters per day.[58]

SPECIAL CIRCULATIONS
[ ] CORONARY CIRCULATION

Two major coronary arteries arise from the aortic sinuses, subdivide on the epicardial surface of the heart and give off small penetrating branches and an extensive network of intramural arteries, arterioles and capillaries. Commensurate with the high oxygen requirements of the myocardium, capillary density is very high, (accounting for ~15 percent of the total cardiac mass), which facilitate the diffusion of nutrients and wastes to and from the cardiomyocytes. Myocardial capillaries feed into a network of intramural venules that drain into large epicardial collecting veins. The majority of the left ventricular venous blood drains into the coronary sinus, which runs along the atrioventricular groove and empties into the right atrium. Other drainage is by means of thebesian veins, which drain directly into the right heart, and anterior cardiac veins that empty into the right atrium. Small intramural collateral vessels connect the coronaries and can enlarge after coronary obstruction, providing near-normal flow at rest to the distal segment of the diseased artery. However, the capacity to augment myocardial blood flow during exercise or stress, that is, the coronary reserve, is usually limited in collateral vessels.[60]

Myocardial Metabolism

Cardiac muscle metabolism requires sustained oxidative phosphorylation to synthesize the ATP that powers the continuous cycles of excitation-contraction coupling and relaxation. A smaller amount of energy (~15–20 percent) is needed for electrical excitation and basal housekeeping activities of the cardiomyocyte. Accordingly, myocardial oxygen requirements are high (~8 mL/min/100 g myocardium). During stress or exercise, oxygen requirements increase abruptly. However, unlike skeletal muscle, extraction of oxygen in cardiac muscle is near maximal at rest and therefore to augment oxygen supply, coronary blood flow must increase.

Compared with other tissues, the myocardium contains a low concentration of high-energy phosphates, given the constant requirement for energy. ATP levels are buffered in the heart by the much larger concentration of phosphocreatine (PCr), which regenerates ATP, by the creatine kinase-catalyzed reaction: adenosine diphosphate (ADP) + PCr = ATP + creatine (Cr). Regeneration of ATP from phosphocreatine can protect the heart from ATP depletion during a mild or brief increase in energy demand, but the heart is fundamentally dependent on continuous resynthesis of mitochondrial ATP.

A variety of substrates are used for myocardial ATP synthesis. Under normal resting conditions, the heart generates 60 to 70 percent of its ATP from β oxidation of free fatty acids and 30 percent from metabolism of carbohydrates. Amino acids and ketones are also used as substrates, but to much lesser extent. During exercise, the large amount of lactate produced by skeletal muscle becomes a major substrate, entering the Krebs cycle after conversion to pyruvate. Oxidation of free fatty acids is inhibited, and carbohydrates become the predominant substrate for energy metabolism.[61]

Control of Coronary Blood Flow

Resting coronary blood flow is normally between 60 and 90 mL/min/100 g of myocardium and can rapidly increase four- to fivefold during exercise or other conditions requiring augmented flow. The coronary flow rate is determined by the coronary artery perfusion pressure and by the resistance to flow exerted by forces generated within and outside the coronary vascular bed; the complexity of these forces is highlighted by the unexpected finding that the coronary diastolic pressure at the time of zero flow (e.g., after a long diastole) is greater than coronary sinus pressure.[62] Control of coronary blood flow is metabolic, mechanical, autonomic, and endothelial. However, the exact local feedback control mechanisms that match coronary blood flow to myocardial oxygen consumption are poorly understood.[63]

Metabolic Control: Autoregulation

A sudden change in aortic pressure is met by a rapid adjustment of coronary vascular resistance so that blood flow remains constant. This autoregulatory phenomenon protects the myocardium from inadequate blood flow owing to a decline in coronary perfusion pressure. Autoregulation at high aortic pressures may attenuate endothelial wall stress and protect the vasculature from damage resulting from elevated coronary distending pressures. The normal coronary vascular bed usually autoregulates over a range of systemic arterial pressures ranging from 60 to 140 mmHg. Above or below these limits, autoregulation fails, and coronary flow increases or decreases in a linear fashion, with corresponding increases or decreases in aortic pressure, respectively. Autoregulation also occurs in localized areas of the coronary vasculature when a partial obstruction of an artery causes a decrease in the coronary perfusion pressure. The vessel distal to the obstruction will dilate, thus normalizing flow by decreasing coronary vascular resistance.

Autoregulatory reserve refers to the maximal degree of vasodilation in the coronary vascular bed and determines the range of decreased perfusion pressures over which myocardial flow can be maintained. Autoregulatory reserve depends on the level of chronic vasodilation in the coronary vasculature as a whole or in any specific region of the heart. If a region of the vascular bed is already vasodilated in an effort to compensate for a localized decrease in coronary perfusion pressure, the capacity to autoregulate during additional reductions in aortic diastolic pressure will be impaired. Thus, the affected area of myocardium becomes vulnerable to transient decreases in aortic pressure. This impairment in autoregulation is the basis for perfusion scans used to diagnose myocardial ischemia.

Autoregulation is mediated by both myogenic (a change in tone in response to changes in pressure and flow) and metabolic (related to washout of vasoactive metabolites) means. The most compelling evidence suggests that adenosine, a breakdown product of ATP, is a major mediator of autoregulation. Adenosine is a potent vasodilator that is generated continually in myocardial cells from adenosine monophosphate by the action of 5′ nucleotidase located at the inner surface of the cell membrane. Adenosine diffuses freely across the cell membrane, and any decrease in perfusion pressure, by causing an initial decrease in coronary artery flow, leads to a diminished rate of adenosine washout and an increase in local tissue concentration. This in turn, results in increased vasodilation and a subsequent increase in the coronary flow rate. Tissue pO_2 and the level of other metabolic products in tissue (e.g., carbon dioxide), by changing slightly as perfusion pressure rises and falls, can also directly affect coronary artery tone.[64] In addition, local release of potassium (K^+) and adenosine-induced activation of ATP-sensitive K^+ channels can also mediate autoregulation in the coronary circulation.[65]

Mechanical Control

The pattern of blood flow to the left ventricle, which receives the greatest proportion of coronary flow, is unique in that arterial flow is markedly decreased during systole owing to the intramyocardial pressure generated by contracting myocardial fibers. Thus, most of the coronary flow to the left ventricle occurs during diastole, and coronary perfusion pressure is largely determined by aortic diastolic pressure. Blood flow to the right ventricular myocardium is also phasic, but because the systolic pressure transmitted to the right ventricular myocardium is much lower, the difference between systolic and diastolic flow is less marked.

Several factors affecting blood flow are markedly different in the inner, subendocardial, and outer, subepicardial, layers of myocardium. Systolic compression is greater in the subendocardial layers (mechanical interference with flow in late diastole owing to chamber distension can also occur). In the subepicardium, flow is slightly higher in systole than diastole. In the midwall, flow is approximately equal in systole and diastole. Vascular density is increased in the subendocardium so that net flow is augmented, despite the almost complete absence of blood flow in the subendocardium during systole. In addition, the intrinsic coronary vascular resistance in subendocardial arteries is lower, so that the ratio of subendocardial to subepicardial flow is ~1.1:1. Although this suits the increased oxygen requirements because of increased wall stress and shortening, the lower resting coronary resistance limits the coronary reserve of the subendocardial vessels and makes it more vulnerable to injury if coronary perfusion pressure drops or coronary flow is impeded.[65] Thus subendocardial injury is not uncommon when myocardial oxygen requirements increase, such as with severe hypertension.

Autonomic Control

The autonomic nervous system influences the smooth muscle tone of the coronary arteries, and this modulates coronary flow to some extent, although under normal conditions, its role is overshadowed by metabolic and mechanical influences.[66] The larger epicardial coronary arteries have both α-adrenergic receptors, which mediate vasoconstriction, and β-adrenergic receptors, which mediate vasodilation. Parasympathetic muscarinic coronary vasodilation has also been demonstrated, but its role in regulation of coronary flow is unclear.[65]

Release of norepinephrine during sympathetic stimulation can cause coronary artery vasoconstriction, but this response is normally overridden by metabolic factors because sympathetic stimulation also increases heart rate and contractility, thereby augmenting myocardial oxygen consumption, ATP turnover, and vasodilation by metabolic mechanisms. Although there is a small degree of resting coronary vasoconstrictor tone, the significance of sympathetic innervation of the normal coronary arteries is unclear. Abnormal increases in vasoconstrictor tone have been suggested as a mechanism underlying ischemic heart disease.[66]

Stimulation of β_2-adrenergic receptors in the smaller coronary arteries by endogenous circulating catecholamines or by pharmacologic β-agonists results in coronary vasodilation. The extent to which coronary β-receptors contribution to coronary blood flow regulation is difficult to assess, since β stimulation of the myocardium increases oxygen consumption, leading to metabolically-

mediated vasodilation. However, during exercise, sympathetic β-adrenergic–mediated feedforward arteriolar vasodilation contributes approximately one-quarter of the increase in coronary blood flow, and α-adrenergic–mediated vasoconstriction in medium and large coronary arteries helps maintain blood flow to the vulnerable subendocardium.[63]

Endothelial Control

Endothelium-derived relaxing factor (EDRF) is a potent vasodilator that is elaborated by vascular endothelial cells in response to a number of stress signals, such as hypoxia, and ADP accumulation. EDRF release is also stimulated by distending forces in the vascular wall, which can amplify the coronary flow in response to conditions such as exercise when it can be appropriate for both coronary perfusion pressure and flow to increase. This is in contrast to autoregulation, which keeps flow constant during inappropriate changes in coronary perfusion pressure.

NO is the principal EDRF. Reactive hyperemia, myogenic vasodilation, and the vasodilator effects of acetylcholine and bradykinin are mediated by NO. NO-independent vasodilation increases shear stress, which stimulates endothelial NO synthase, generates NO, and prolongs vasodilation.[67]

【 】 CEREBRAL CIRCULATION

The brain cannot survive on anaerobic metabolism and therefore powerful mechanisms exist to maintain the cerebral blood flow constant. Cerebral blood flow is also controlled by autoregulation of blood flow in the face of perfusion pressures ranging from approximately 60 to 150 mmHg. When arterial blood pressure decreases below 60 mmHg, and cerebral blood flow falls, brain tissue begins to become ischemic; this elicits a powerful stimulation of the peripheral sympathetic nervous system resulting in generalized vasoconstriction and an increase in arterial blood pressure. This response is effective down to blood pressures of 15 to 20 mmHg and is so powerful that blood flow to other areas can drop to zero in an effort to preserve cerebral blood flow. Myocardial blood flow increases, as the intense sympathetic stimulation increases myocardial work (heart rate and contractility).

There is also a positive curvilinear relationship between cerebral blood flow and arterial CO_2 tension, mediated in part through changes in extracellular pH; small increases in arterial blood CO_2 tension above normal values produce large increases in cerebral blood flow. Decreases in CO_2 decrease blood flow. There is also an inverse relation between arterial O_2 content and cerebral blood flow that helps maintain cerebral O_2 delivery constant.

Although cerebral blood vessels are innervated, neural mechanisms modify cerebral blood flow only weakly and are overpowered by other factors that regulate cerebral blood flow.[57]

【 】 SKELETAL-MUSCLE CIRCULATION

Blood flow to resting skeletal muscle is relatively low, normally only 3 to 4 mL/min/100 g of muscle. Whereas only 10 percent of the capillary beds are perfused, this is sufficient to meet the basal metabolic needs of resting muscle. Blood vessels in skeletal muscle are innervated and constrict in response to α-adrenergic stimulation and dilate in response to β-adrenergic or cholinergic stimulation. Adrenergic and cholinergic vasodilation is largely mediated by endothelial NO.[68] When skeletal muscle is inactive and blood flow is needed in other vascular beds, neural mechanisms constrict muscle vessels to divert blood to the needed areas. When skeletal muscle is active, however, neural influences on blood flow are overridden by powerful local metabolic and vascular control mechanism. The primary regulators of skeletal muscle blood flow during exercise are metabolic factors. A decrease in oxygen tension and increases in concentration of carbon dioxide, lactic acid, hydrogen ions, and potassium ions directly increase muscle blood flow. As the increase in blood flow washes out these substances, tissue concentrations return to normal. Strenuous exercise can increase blood flow to muscle by as much as 25-fold, to a maximum of ~80 mL/min/100 g, and opens previously unperfused capillary beds. With aerobic exercise, blood flow is maintained at a steady level, albeit one higher than normal, commensurate with the increase in metabolic rate. Skeletal muscle can depend on anaerobic metabolism for short periods of time by generating an oxygen debt; at the end of exercise muscle blood flow remains elevated until the concentration of all effector substances return to normal.[57]

INTEGRATED PHYSIOLOGY

Integrated control of the circulation results from mechanisms both intrinsic (e.g., myogenic tone, endothelial function) and extrinsic (e.g., autonomic nervous system) to the vascular wall.

The cardiac output is delivered to the peripheral tissues by the aorta and large conductance arteries. These vessels have relatively little smooth muscle in their walls and are not significantly impacted by the preceding vascular control mechanisms. Importantly, however, they contain mechanoreceptors (the aortic arch and carotid sinus baroreceptors) that initiate circulatory reflexes important in controlling systemic arterial pressure. The elastic tissue of the aortic and its branches converts pulsatile cardiac flow into a continuous, steady-state flow optimal for perfusion of the smaller arteries and arterioles. These smaller vessels are surrounded by layers of smooth muscle cells in direct contact with endothelium on the luminal side and are richly innervated on the adventitial side. Regulatory input from both the endothelium and neural connections together determines the tension in the vascular smooth muscle and the cross-sectional area of the vessel. The effective cross-sectional area in the muscular arteries, arterioles, and venules is the principal determinant of steady-state peripheral resistance.

In contrast to arteries veins are highly distensible, and together with the venules and venous sinuses contain approximately 60 percent of the blood volume. By regulating the functional cross-sectional area of the venous compartment, blood can be translocated from the venous to the arterial side of the circulation. Thus, an increase in the venomotor tone decreases venous capacitance and redistributes blood volume thereby increasing cardiac output; a decrease in venomotor tone has the opposite effect. Local external pressures (intra-abdominal, intrathoracic) influence the large veins as they return blood to the right heart. Because venous pressures are relatively low and capacitance is large, these external forces can facilitate or inhibit venous return.

AUTONOMIC NERVOUS SYSTEM

The autonomic nervous system affects vasomotor tone and cardiac function through its sympathetic and parasympathetic divisions. It also influences systemic volume and peripheral resistance by modulating the release of certain peptide hormones (e.g., angiotensin II). Neural control involves assimilation of inputs from the cerebral cortex and specialized sensors, (i.e., the mechanoreceptors, chemoreceptors, osmoreceptors, and thermoreceptors), integration into several specialized regions of the brain (hypothalamus, pons, medulla), and transmission of efferent nerve activity to the periphery over the sympathetic and parasympathetic pathways. The dynamic balance between these two systems determines the net, integrated response.[69]

The overall organization of the vasomotor area is complex, but there appear to be three functionally overlapping anatomic zones that interact extensively. These include: (1) a vasoconstrictor area in the upper anterolateral medulla, (2) a vasodilator area in the lower anterolateral medulla, and (3) a sensory area that integrates the vasoconstrictor and vasodilator areas located bilaterally in the nucleus tractus solitarii of the posterolateral medulla and lower pons. Regions modifying heart rate are located in the thalamus, posterior and posterolateral regions of the hypothalamus, and dorsal region of the medulla.[69]

Stimulation and withdrawal of sympathetic nervous activity are the most powerful factors controlling the peripheral circulation. In addition to CV reflex regulation, mechanisms involving central interactions between angiotensin II and NO contribute to sympathetic excitation.[70] Fibers travel either in specific sympathetic nerves, which innervate the viscera and heart, or join the paravertebral sympathetic chain and synapse in secondary ganglia that give rise to the spinal nerves that innervate peripheral vessels. The vascular nerves terminate on small arteries, arterioles, venules, and veins, and modulate resistance and vascular volume. Cardiac nerves, many of which descend from the stellate ganglia, innervate the atria and ventricles.

Reflex sympathetic stimulation causes vasoconstriction by releasing norepinephrine from sympathetic nerve endings. Sympathetic nerve stimulation to a limb increases local vascular resistance and decreases blood flow and capillary pressure; as a result, local interstitial fluid is absorbed, and blood volume is displaced from the limb. In a metabolically active organ, local influences are likely to override the autonomic ones. Although most reflex sympathetic stimulation produces vascular constriction, a subset of fibers originating in the cerebral motor cortex releases acetylcholine rather than norepinephrine. These neurons innervate the vasculature of skeletal muscle and bring about an anticipatory increase in local blood flow prior to exercise.[69] Sympathetic stimulation of these fibers also releases epinephrine from the adrenal medullae. Unlike norepinephrine, epinephrine stimulates both α and β receptors. The effect of epinephrine is biphasic; at low concentrations, epinephrine produces vasodilation and cardiac stimulation; at higher concentrations, vasoconstriction predominates.

Reflex sympathetic stimulation is important as it increases cardiac output necessary during exercise or other forms of stress. These cardiac stimulating effects of the sympathetic nervous system increase the metabolic requirements of heart muscle. Sympathetically mediated actions are largely responsible for maintaining systemic arterial pressure and vital organ perfusion during hypovolemic states and cardiac dysfunction. The inhibition of sympathetic outflow allows vessels to dilate and responds to local humoral and myogenic stimuli.

The parasympathetic nervous system consists of a cranial division, which supplies the blood vessels of the head and viscera, and a sacral division, which innervates the vessels of the genitalia, bladder, and large intestine. Because these fibers supply only a small percentage of the resistance vessels, the parasympathetic division of the autonomic nervous system plays a minor role in arterial pressure regulation. It does, however, play an important role in modulating the heart rate. Fibers traveling in the vagus nerve innervate the sinoatrial and atrioventricular nodes and atrial myocardium. Changes in heart rate arise from slower intrinsic rates of depolarization and changes in membrane depolarization secondary to acetylcholine stimulation. When the vagus nerve is stimulated, heart rate and the force of atrial contraction both decline. These effects, coupled with the development of AV block can lower cardiac output by as much as 40 to 50 percent.[69] Effects of vagal stimulation are evident following external massage of the carotid sinus, which stimulates the glossopharyngeal afferent limb of the baroreceptors reflex and modifies efferent parasympathetic outflow.

BARORECEPTOR CONTROL

The baroreceptor system consists of the carotid sinus and aortic arch mechanoreceptors, central vasomotor integrating areas and autonomic efferents. The baroreflex system operates as an open loop with negative feedback and cushions changes in arterial pressure, such as those produced by changes in posture. Under resting conditions, the system is static; however, it can be modified by periodic or transient perturbations, such as respiration or exercise and therefore is also dynamic. The neural outflow from the vasomotor centers modulates the smooth muscle tone of resistance vessels, the force of myocardial contraction, and the heart rate and thereby buffers changes in systemic arterial pressure. Activation of the baroreceptors by an arterial blood pressure-induced stretch produces an increase in afferent impulses traveling through the vagus and glossopharyngeal nerves. In the central vasomotor centers of the pons and medulla, sympathetic efferent nerve activity to the heart, resistance vessels, and veins is inhibited; parasympathetic outflow to the heart increases. The result is cardiac slowing and a decrease in blood pressure.

The carotid sinus baroreceptor is located at the bifurcation of the common carotid artery. The receptors are located in the adventitia of the sinus wall and are innervated by a branch of the glossopharyngeal nerve, which carries afferent activity to the nucleus tractus solitarii in the medulla. Strain energy density (i.e., the force required to bring about an incremental stretch) in the wall of the sinus is linearly related to pressure over a wide range of values from 50 to 250 mmHg.[69] Over this range, the relation between deformations produced by an increase in pressure and afferent nerve activity is directly linear. The rate of afferent nerve discharge is largely influenced by the mean arterial pressure, and to a lesser extent, by pulse pressure. Thus for a given mean pressure, a narrower pulse pressure decreases afferent activity. Factors that modify the distensibility of the carotid sinus (e.g., hypertension, atherosclero-

sis) also change the relationship between intraluminal pressure and stretch. The ability of baroreceptors to cushion chronic increases in mean arterial pressure is limited by *resetting*, a rightward shift in the relation between baroreceptor firing and mean arterial pressure.[71] Baroreflex resetting (in this case closer to threshold) also occurs during exercise, which increases the ability of the reflex to buffer hypertensive stimuli.[72] Carotid baroreceptor denervation causes an increase in blood pressure variability, but not sustained hypertension.[73]

The aortic arch baroreflex system is similar to that of the carotid sinus. Nerve endings concentrated at the junction between the adventitia and media of the aortic arch serve as stretch receptors with their afferent impulses traveling in the vagus nerve. The threshold of pressure stimulation for aortic receptors is approximately 90 mmHg, compared with 60 mmHg for the carotid receptors.[69] Therefore, the carotid sinus is important in modulating blood pressure and heart rate at lower pressures, a feature that may be important for maintaining cerebral perfusion in an upright posture.

CHEMORECEPTOR CONTROL

Arterial chemoreceptors are located in the carotid arteries and aortic arch in the same regions as baroreceptors. These receptors are composed of excitable cells that release neurotransmitters and activate afferent nerves (type I receptors) and inexcitable cells that function as a sensor for hypoxia and acidosis (type II receptors). The carotid bodies are innervated by a branch of the glossopharyngeal nerve, and the aortic bodies are supplied by a branch of the vagus. Nerve activity is stimulated by decreases in pH or pO_2 or by an increase in the CO_2 tension and temperature. For any give arterial pO_2, the number of discharges increases at higher pCO_2; conversely, for any given pCO_2, the number of impulses increases with lower pO_2. The carotid and aortic body chemoreflexes are responsible for reflex systemic arterial hypertension, which is mediated by sympathetic outflow from the vasomotor areas. Increases in heart rate, contractility and cardiac output are most likely caused by the combined effects of central nervous system (CNS) hypoxia and increased ventilation, as chemoreceptor denervation does not abolish the cardiac responses, but lung denervation largely prevents or reverses them.[69] Moreover, carotid chemoreceptor denervation eliminates the ventilatory responses to hypoxia and hypercapnea.[73]

MECHANORECEPTOR CONTROL

Mechanoreceptors in the heart possess both vagal and sympathetic afferents. Sensors on the atria and ventricles receive vagal afferents; sensors on the pulmonary veins and coronary vessels receive sympathetic afferents. However, the cardiac mechanoreceptors are much less involved than are the baroreceptors in the short-term regulation of arterial pressure.

Atrial A and B receptors are located at the venoatrial junctions and have distinct functions. Type A receptors react primarily to heart rate but adapt to long-term changes in atrial volume. Type B receptors increase their discharge during atrial distension. C fibers arise from receptors scattered through the atria; these discharge with a low frequency and respond with increased discharge to increase in atrial pressure. The A and B receptors are thought to mediate the increase in heart rate associated with atrial distension (such as can occur with intravenous infusions) known as the *Bainbridge reflex*.[74] In contrast, activation of atrial C fibers generally produces a vasodepressor effect (bradycardia and peripheral vasodilation).

Ventricular mechanoreceptor afferent discharge decreases periodically with inspiration. Ventricular C fibers are located primarily in the epicardium and discharge more rapidly in response to increase in both systolic and diastolic pressure. They exhibit a sharp threshold, discharging only at high systolic pressures, but progressively increase as diastolic pressures increase from 5 to 20 mmHg. Ventricular distension can produce a powerful depressor reflex called the *Bezold-Jarisch reflex*; vagal afferents of this cardiopulmonary reflex are also activated by chemical stimulation (e.g., prostanoids, cytokines, serotonin, and classically, Veratrum alkaloids).[75] The central connections for this reflex are in the nucleus tractus solitarii, which has both sympathetic and parasympathetic synapses. Cardiac C-fiber activation also induces gastric relaxation by means of vagal noncholinergic fibers, which is part of a more generalized activation of the vomiting reflex.

The sympathetic afferents are less well understood than the vagal afferents. Atria and ventricular receptors can affect the release of vasopressin and the renal release of renin by modifying efferent sympathetic outflow. Atrial fibers increase activity with increases in atrial pressure and volume and respond to phasic changes in atrial volume. Ventricular fibers increase their discharge rate when ventricular end-diastolic pressure (via unmyelinated fibers) or systolic pressure (via myelinated fibers) is elevated. Afferents on the coronary vessels discharge more rapidly as blood flow or intracoronary pressures decrease and may be important during myocardial ischemia.

LOCAL INFLUENCES AND CIRCULATORY CONTROL

Vascular tone is greatest in the small muscular arteries. The level of tone represents the integration of excitatory and inhibitory pathways of metabolic, endothelial, and neurotransmitter origin. However, vascular smooth muscle constricts in response to pressure or stretch in the absence of the endothelium. The mediator of this myogenic response is uncertain, but may be integrins, stretch-activated cation channels, and cytoskeletal proteins. Signaling pathways involved in the myogenic response include phospholipase C/PKC and calmodulin-mediated myosin light chain phosphorylation. In addition, calcium sensitivity of the contractile proteins is produced by inhibition of myosin light chain phosphatase, which dephosphorylates and inactivates myosin.

Flexible and precise circulatory control is possible because vascular smooth muscle can change its tension in response to both centrally transmitted signals and local factors. Vasodilators include atrial natriuretic peptide (ANP), kinins, nitric oxide, and prostacyclins; vasoconstrictors include thromboxane A_2, prostaglandin H_2, superoxide anion, endothelins, arginine vasopressin, and angiotensin II. The endothelium is an important modulator of tone as it releases many of these vasoactive substances.[76–78] Vasoactive molecules are released in response to both physical and chemical stimulation. For example, flow-induced shear produces vasodilation and normalization of elevated shear stress.

An important endothelium-derived relaxing factor is the simple gas, NO, which is synthesized from L-arginine by NOS. There are three isoforms of NO synthase that vary in their calcium dependence and type of regulation: neuronal NOS (nNOS), inducible NOS (iNOS), and endothelial NOS (eNOS). As mentioned earlier, these isoforms are spatially localized to highly controlled microdomains and are linked to disparate signaling pathways and effectors. In the vasculature, NO exerts paracrine control by means of vasodilation by the action of cGMP. The endothelium is also the source of substances that initiate smooth muscle contraction.

Angiotensin II is a powerful vasoconstrictor peptide that has endocrine functions crucial to salt and water homeostasis but is also locally produced and plays critical autocrine and paracrine roles in organ perfusion and growth.

The endothelins are a group of peptides cleaved from larger inactive precursors that constrict arterial and venous smooth muscle. Endothelins (and angiotensin II and α_1-adrenergic agonists) function by activating phospholipase, which produces IP_3 and DAG; IP_3 releases Ca^{2+} into the cytoplasm from endoplasmic reticulum stores and DAG activates protein kinase C. Arterial constriction increases peripheral resistance, and venoconstriction decreases capacitance and increases cardiac preload; the former usually predominates.

ANP is a direct-acting vasodilator that is released in response to atrial stretch, β-adrenergic stimulation and increased heart rate. ANP stimulates the second messenger, membrane-bound cGMP to produce arterial and venous dilation. The resultant hemodynamic effects include a dose-dependent decrease in arterial pressure and cardiac output. ANP also blocks the effects of angiotensin II on aldosterone release and lowers angiotensin II level. Although ANP is elevated in heart failure, its effects are offset by the action of potent vasoconstrictors and sodium retention.

Kinins are polypeptide vasodilators that are synthesized and circulate as large, inactive molecules and are locally bioconverted to active moieties. Bradykinin is formed from kallikrein and performs vital roles in inflammation and local circulatory control.

Arginine vasopressin (AVP) is synthesized in neurons of the hypothalamic nuclei and is released from nerve endings of the neurohypophysis. AVP is also a neurotransmitter found in central regions involved in circulatory control. AVP is important in maintaining arterial pressure in the presence of reduced blood volume and regulates osmolality. AVP modulates volume by inhibiting systemic ANP when arterial and atrial receptors are activated.

Substance P is a neurotransmitter peptide that is widely distributed in the brain and peripheral nervous system. Its CV regulatory potential is suggested by its relatively high concentration in the vasomotor area where it may interact with the opioid peptide system. In addition, it is present in the nerves that supply virtually every vascular bed, where its release triggers vasodilation through a specific receptor.

Opioids such as the enkephalins and endorphins are also widely distributed in the brain and spinal cord. Although infusion of these neurotransmitters produces transient vasodilation, they are thought to cooperate with and modulate the response of other neurotransmitters operating in the same synaptic cleft. They appear to be most involved in the behavioral responses to pain and exercise.

Vasoactive intestinal polypeptide is found in the brain, gut, salivary glands, uterus, and skeletal muscle. It is a potent vasodilator and also increases heart rate above that obtained with sympathetic stimulation alone.

REFERENCES

1. Josephson IR. Initiation and propagation of the cardiac action potential. In: Sperelakis N, Banks RO, eds. *Essentials of Physiology.* 2nd ed. Boston: Little, Brown, and Company, 1996;247–257.
2. Carmeliet E. Action potential duration, rate of stimulation, and intracellular sodium. *J Cardiovasc Electrophysiol.* 2006;2001;17(suppl 1):S2–S7.
3. DiFrancesco D. Cardiac pacemaker I(f) current and its inhibition by heart rate-reducing agents. *Curr Med Res Opin.* 2005;21:1115–1122.
4. Bernstein SA, Morley GE. Gap junctions and propagation of the cardiac action potential. *Adv Cardiol.* 2006;42:71–85.
5. Hoit BD. Normal and abnormal excitation-contraction coupling. In: Walsh RA, ed. *Molecular Mechanisms of Cardiac Hypertrophy and Failure.* London: Taylor and Francis; 2005:179–97.
6. Su SF, Barry WH. Isolated myocyte mechanics and calcium transients. In: Hoit BD, Walsh RA, eds. *Cardiovascular Physiology in the Genetically Engineered Mouse.* 2nd ed. Norwell, MA: Kluwer Academic Publishers; 2002:71–89.
7. Wier WG, Balke CW. Ca(2+) release mechanisms, Ca(2+) sparks, and local control of excitation-contraction coupling in normal heart muscle. *Circ Res.* 1999;85:770–776.
8. Cannell MB, Cheng H, Lederer WJ. The control of calcium release in heart muscle. *Science.* 1995;268:1045–1049.
9. Valdivia HH. Modulation of intracellular Ca2+ levels in the heart by sorcin and FKBP12, two accessory proteins of ryanodine receptors. *Trends Pharmacol Sci.* 1998;19:479–482.
10. Brette F, Orchard C. T-tubule function in mammalian cardiac myocytes. *Circ Res.* 2003;92:1182–1192.
11. Kranias EG. Regulation of Ca2+ transport by cyclic 3',5'-AMP-dependent and calcium-calmodulin-dependent phosphorylation of cardiac sarcoplasmic reticulum. *Biochim Biophys Acta.* 1985;844:193–199.
12. Bers DM. *Excitation-Contraction Coupling and Cardiac Contractile Force.* 2nd ed. Norwell, MA: Kluwer Academic Publishers.
13. Brady AJ. Length dependence of passive stiffness in single cardiac myocytes. *Am J Physiol.* 1991;260:H1062–H1071.
14. Brenner B. Mechanical and structural approaches to correlation of cross-bridge action in muscle with actomyosin ATPase in solution. *Annu Rev Physiol.* 1987;49:655–672.
15. Solaro RJ, Rarick HM. Troponin and tropomyosin: proteins that switch on and tune in the activity of cardiac myofilaments. *Circ Res.* 1998;83:471–480.
16. Swartz DR, Moss RL. Influence of a strong-binding myosin analogue on calcium-sensitive mechanical properties of skinned skeletal muscle fibers. *J Biol Chem.* 1992;267:20497–20506.
17. Hansford RG. Relation between mitochondrial calcium transport and control of energy metabolism. *Rev Physiol Biochem Pharmacol.* 1985;102:1–72.
18. Massion PB, Feron O, Dessy C, Balligand JL. Nitric oxide and cardiac function: ten years after, and continuing. *Circ Res.* 2003;93:388–398.
19. Hare JM. Nitric oxide and excitation-contraction coupling. *J Mol Cell Cardiol.* 2003;35:719–729.
20. Layland J, Li JM, Shah AM. Role of cyclic GMP-dependent protein kinase in the contractile response to exogenous nitric oxide in rat cardiac myocytes. *J Physiol.* 2002;540:457–467.
21. Hoit BD, Kadambi VJ, Tramuta DA, et al. Influence of sarcoplasmic reticulum calcium loading on mechanical and relaxation restitution. *Am J Physiol Heart Circ Physiol.* 2000;278:H958–H963.
22. Hoit BD, Tramuta DA, Kadambi VJ, et al. Influence of transgenic overexpression of phospholamban on postextrasystolic potentiation. *J Mol Cell Cardiol.* 1999;31:2007–2015.
23. Schmidt A, Kadambi V, Ball N, et al. Cardiac specific overexpression of calsequestrin results in left ventricular hypertrophy, depressed force frequency relation and pulsus alternans in vivo. *J Mol Cell Cardiol.* 2000;37:1735–1744.
24. Anderson ME. Connections count: excitation-contraction meets excitation-transcription coupling. *Circ Res.* 2000;86:717–719.
25. Maier LS, Bers DM. Calcium, calmodulin, and calcium-calmodulin kinase II. heartbeat to heartbeat and beyond. *J Mol Cell Cardiol.* 2002;34:919–939.
26. Hook SS, Means AR. Ca(2+)/CaM-dependent kinases: from activation to function. *Annu Rev Pharmacol Toxicol.* 2001;41:471–505.
27. Wamhoff BR, Bowles DK, Owens GK. E Excitation-transcription coupling in arterial smooth muscle. *Circ Res.* 2006;98:868–878.
28. Sperelakis N. Regulation of intracellular Ca²⁺ in cardiac muscle and smooth muscle. In: Sperelakis N, Banks RO, eds. *Essentials of Physiology.* 2nd ed. Boston: Little, Brown, and Company; 1996:227–238.
29. Hoit BD, Walsh RA. Determinants of left ventricular performance and cardiac output. In: Sperelakis N, Banks RO, eds. *Essentials of Physiology.* 2nd ed. Boston: Little, Brown, and Company; 1996:269–278.
30. DeSantiago J, Maier LS, Bers DM. Frequency-dependent acceleration of relaxation in the heart depends on CaMKII, but not phospholamban. *J Mol Cell Cardiol.* 2002;34:975–984.
31. Lohn M, Szymanski G, Markwardt F. Deformation of the Bowditch staircase in Ca(2+)-overloaded mammalian cardiac tissue—a calcium phenomenon? *Mol Cell Biochem.* 1996;160–161:13–25.
32. Grupp G, Grupp IL, Farr WC. Physiologic basis of the electrocardiogram. In: Sperelakis N, Banks RO, eds. *Essentials of Physiology.* 2nd ed. Boston: Little, Brown, and Company, 1996;259–267.
33. Hoit BD, Shao Y, Gabel M, Walsh RA. In-vivo assessment of left atrial contractile performance in normal and pathological conditions using a time-varying elastance model. *Circulation.* 1994;89:1829–1838.
34. Sagawa K. The ES pressure-volume relation of the ventricle: definition, modifications and clinical use. *Circulation.* 1981;63:1223–1227.
35. Suga H. Ventricular energetics. *Physiol Rev.* 1990;70:247–277.
36. LeWinter MM. The isolated isovolumic (Langendorff) heart preparation. In: Hoit BD, Walsh RA, eds. *Cardiovascular Physiology in the Genetically Engineered Mouse.* 2nd ed. Norwell, MA: Kluwer Academic Publishers; 2002:113–127.
37. Suga H. Total mechanical energy of a ventricle model and cardiac oxygen Consumption. *Am J Physiol.* 1979;236:H498–H505.
38. Kass D, Maughan DL. From "Emax" to pressure-volume relations: a broader view. *Circulation.* 1988;77:1203–1212.
39. Goto Y, Slinker BK, LeWinter MM. Decreased contractile efficiency and increased nonmechanical energy cost in hyperthyroid rabbit heart. *Circ Res.* 1990;66:999–1011.
40. Raper R, Sibbald WJ. Misled by the wedge? The Swan-Ganz catheter and left ventricular preload. *Chest.* 1986;89:427–434.
41. Hibberd M, Jewell B. Calcium- and length-dependent force production in rat ventricular muscle. *J Physiol.* 1982;329:527–540.
42. Quinones M, Gaasch W, Alexander J. Influence of acute changes in preload, afterload, contractile state and heart rate on ejection and isovolumic indices of myocardial contractility in man. *Circulation.* 1976;53:293–302.
43. Little W. The left ventricular *dP/dt*ₘₐₓ end-diastolic volume relation in closed chest dogs. *Circ Res.* 1985;56:808–815.
44. Freeman G, Colston J. Evaluation of left ventricular mechanical restitution in closed-chest dogs based on single-beat elastance. *Circ Res.* 1990;67:1437–1445.
45. Burkhoff D, Mirsky I, Suga H. Assessment of systolic and diastolic ventricular properties via pressure-volume analysis: a guide for clinical, translational, and basic researchers. *Am J Physiol Heart Circ Physiol.* 2005;289:501–512.
46. Lenihan DJ, Gerson MC, Dorn GW 2nd, et al. Effects of changes in atrioventricular gradient and contractility on left ventricular filling in human diastolic cardiac dysfunction. *Am Heart J.* 1996;132:1179–1188.
47. Li L, Desantiago J, Chu G, et al. Phosphorylation of phospholamban and troponin I in beta-adrenergic-induced acceleration of cardiac relaxation. *Am J Physiol Heart Circ Physiol.* 2000;278:H769–H779.
48. Weiss JL, Fredericksen JW, Weisfeldt ML. Hemodynamic determinants of the time course of fall in canine left ventricular pressure. *J Clin Invest.* 1976;58:83–95.
49. Mirsky I, Pasipoularides A. Clinical assessment of diastolic function. *Prog Cardiovasc Dis.* 1990;32:291–318.
50. Bell SP, Nyland L, Tischler MD, et al. Alterations in the determinants of diastolic suction during pacing tachycardia. *Circ Res.* 2000;87(3):235–240.
51. Kato S, Spinale FG, Tanaka R, et al. Inhibition of collagen cross-linking: effects on extracellular matrix structure and left ventricular diastolic function. *Am J Physiol.* 1995;269:J863–H868.
52. Zile MR, Tomita M, Ishihara K, et al. Changes in diastolic function during the development and correction of chronic LV volume overload produced by mitral regurgitation. *Circulation.* 1993;87:1378–1388.
53. Guyton AC, Jones CE, Coleman TG. *Circulatory Physiology: Cardiac Output and Its Regulation.* Philadelphia, PA: WB Saunders; 1973:146–233.
54. Sunagawa K, Maughan WL, Burkhoff D, et al. Left ventricular interaction with arterial load studied in isolated canine ventricle. *Am J Physiol.* 1983;245:H773–H780.

55. Burkhoff D, Sagawa K. Ventricular efficiency predicted by an analytical model. *Am J Physiol.* 1986;250;R1021–127.

56. Asanoi H, Kameyama T, Ishizaka S. Ventriculo-arterial load matching of failing hearts. In: LeWinter MM, Suga H, Watkins MW, eds. *Cardiac Energetics: From Emax to Pressure-Volume Area.* Norwell MA: Kluwer Academic Publishers; 1995;157–169.

57. Iwamoto HS, Walsh RA. Hemodynamics and regional circulation. In: Sperelakis N, Banks RO, eds. *Essentials of Physiology.* 2nd ed. Boston: Little, Brown, and Company: 1996:289–301.

58. Harris PD, Anderson GL. Microcirculation and lymphatic circulation. In: Sperelakis N, Banks RO, eds. *Essentials of Physiology.* 2nd ed. Boston: Little, Brown, and Company; 1996:303–308.

59. Segal SS, Regulation of blood flow in the microcirculation. *Microcirculation.* 2005;12:33–45.

60. Wexler LF, Walsh RA. Coronary circulation, myocardial oxygen consumption, and energetics. In: Sperelakis N, Banks RO, eds. *Essentials of Physiology.* 2nd ed. Boston: Little, Brown, and Company; 1996:279–288.

61. Stanley WC, Recchia FA, Lopaschuk GD. Myocardial substrate metabolism in the normal and failing heart. *Physiol Rev.* 2005;85:1093–1129.

62. Feigl EO. Coronary physiology. *Physiol Rev.* 1983;63:1–205.

63. Tune JD, Gorman MW, Feigl EO. Matching coronary blood flow to myocardial oxygen consumption. *J Appl Physiol.* 2004;97:404–415.

64. Berne RM. The role of adenosine in the regulation of coronary blood flow. *Circ Res.* 1980;47:807–813.

65. Olsson RA, Bunger R. Metabolic control of coronary blood flow. Prog *Cardiovasc Dis.* 1987;29:369–387.

66. Young MA, Vatner SF. Regulation of large coronary arteries. *Circ Res.* 1986;59:579–596.

67. Gattullo D, Pagliaro P Marsh NA, et al. New insights into nitric oxide and coronary circulation. *Life Sci.* 1999;65:2167–2174.

68. Joyner MJ, Dietz NM. Sympathetic vasodilation in human muscle. *Acta Physiol Scand.* 2003;177:329–336.

69. Blaustein AS, Walsh. Regulation of the cardiovascular system. In: Sperelakis N, Banks RO , eds. *Essentials of Physiology.* 2nd ed. Boston: Little, Brown, and Company; 1996:309–321.

70. Zucker IH, Liu JL. Angiotensin II-nitric oxide interactions in the control of sympathetic outflow in heart failure. *Heart Fail Rev.* 2000;5:27–43.

71. Thrasher TN. Baroreceptors, baroreceptor unloading, and the long-term control of blood pressure. *Am J Physiol Regul Integr Comp Physiol.* 2005;288:R819–R827.

72. Raven PB, Fadel PJ, Ogoh S. Arterial Baroreflex resetting during exercise: a current perspective. *Exp Physiol.* 2006;91:37–49.

73. Timmers HJ, Wieling W, Karemaker JM, Lenders JW. Denervation of carotid baro- and chemoreceptors in humans. *J Physiol.* 2003;553:3–11.

74. Hakumaki MO. Seventy years of the Bainbridge reflex. *Acta Physiol Scand.* 1987;130:177–185.

75. Verberne AJ, Saita M, Sartor DM. Chemical stimulation of vagal afferent neurons and sympathetic vasomotor tone. *Brain Res Brain Res Rev.* 2003;41:288–305.

76. Harrison DG, Cai H. Endothelial control of vasomotion and nitric oxide production. *Cardiol Clin.* 2003;21:289–302.

77. Kusserow H, Unger T. Vasoactive peptides, their receptors and drug development. *Basic Clin Pharmacol Toxicol.* 2004;94:5–12.

78. Moreeau ME, Garbacki N, Molinaro G, et al. The kallikrein-kinin system: current and future pharmacological targets. *J Pharmacol Sci.* 2005;99:6–38.

CHAPTER (5)

Principles of Molecular Cardiology

Robert Roberts

THE EVOLUTION OF MODERN MOLECULAR BIOLOGY

In 1953, Watson and Crick[1] proposed the double-helix model for DNA structure based on the results of x-ray diffraction studies by Franklin and Wilkins. The implications of DNA being a double helix, in which each strand is a mirror image of the other, were evident—namely, that one strand could serve as a template for the synthesis of a daughter strand, thus providing the means whereby genetic information could be perpetuated from parent to offspring. Marmor and Lane showed that the double helix of DNA, when subjected to high temperatures, could be separated into its separate strands (denatured), and subsequently decreasing the temperature resulted in the reannealing, or hybridizing, of the strands to their previous double-stranded nature.[2,3] This specific hybridization, or *base pairing* of complementary nucleotide strands, provides both the rationale and the practical basis for much of recombinant-DNA technology. This was followed by several discoveries including unraveling the code whereby the nucleic acids code for proteins[4,5] and the identification of the enzyme, DNA ligase, which joins DNA fragments together.[6] All of this information was known in the 1960s, as was the role of messenger RNA and cytoplasmic ribosomal RNA for protein synthesis. Re-

combinant technology was not yet born and, in fact, for the next few years did not appear promising.

Many important discoveries, including those from the 1950s, played a role in recombinant technology, but four that brought it to fruition and made possible modern molecular biology occurred between the years of 1970 and 1977. A major obstacle to the manipulation of DNA was its large size with no means to cut it into smaller pieces of known specific size. This obstacle was overcome by the discovery of restriction endonucleases that made it possible to cut DNA into smaller pieces in a predictable fashion.[7] These endonucleases, more commonly referred to as *restriction enzymes,* recognize specific sequences of DNA consisting of anywhere from four to eight nucleotides and specifically cut the DNA molecules at their recognition sites, making it possible to use and manipulate DNA fragments in a variety of procedures and reactions. In 1970, the enzyme, reverse transcriptase (RT), was discovered by Baltimore[8] and Temin and Mizutani[9] simultaneously, making it possible to translate messenger RNA (mRNA) into its complementary DNA (cDNA). It was quickly realized that the cDNA had all the properties of the original gene and could be used to clone the gene following insertion of the cDNA into an appropriate host. This immediately led to the first cloning of a gene.[10] In 1975, Sanger and Coulson[11] and Maxam and Gilbert[12] developed techniques for the rapid sequencing of DNA. Shortly after the first molecule was cloned,[10] recombinant DNA techniques were born, as was modern molecular biology. In addition to these four developments, polymerase chain reaction (PCR), a more recently developed technique to rapidly amplify small amounts of DNA or RNA several million-fold, is also having a revolutionary effect on medicine and other fields.

THE DOGMA OF HOW GENES DIRECT THE SYNTHESIS OF PROTEINS

【 】 THE COMPOSITION AND UNIQUE FEATURES OF DNA

DNA consists of four building blocks referred to as *nucleotides* or merely as *bases*. A nucleotide consists of a nitrogenous base, a 5-carbon sugar (deoxyribose), and a phosphate group.[13] There are two purine bases (adenine and guanine) and two pyrimidine bases (cytosine and thymine) (Fig. 5–1). The triphosphate molecule is bonded to the 5′ carbon of the sugar, and the base is bonded to the 1′ carbon of the sugar. Each DNA molecule consists of millions of nucleotides joined together in a linear fashion through the phosphate group, which forms a bond with the hydroxyl group of the 3′ carbon of the next sugar. The phosphate groups form the backbone of the molecule, but because they are water-soluble, they face outward. Attached to the inner side of the sugar is the hydrophobic base, which faces inward to shield it from the aqueous environment. The molecule forms a right-sided spiral coil with a turn every 10 nucleotides (3.4 nanometer [nm]), referred to as a *right-sided-helix*, and pairs with its complementary strand to form the so-called double helix (Fig. 5–2). The center of the molecule consists of the bases that face inward and are opposite to each other.

This arrangement provides for the hydrogen bonding between the bases that keeps the two strands together. The hydrogen bonds are perpendicular to the helical axis. The directionality of the strands is referred to as 5′ *to* 3′ *or* 3′ *to* 5′, which is based on the position of the carbons in the sugar. The end of the molecule with a phosphate or hydroxyl group on the 5′ carbon is termed the 5′ *end*, whereas the end with a free terminal 3′ carbon is referred to as the 3′ *end*. It is important to distinguish the two ends because the enzyme, DNA polymerase, always initiates replication of DNA from the 5′ end and proceeds to the 3′ end. There seems to be no constraints on which bases can be adjacent to each other; however, the hydrogen binding between the bases of the two chains is highly specific, because adenine (A) always pairs with thymine (T), and guanine (G) always pairs with cytosine (C). The sugars and the phosphate groups are always the same, whereas the sequence of the bases varies and determines the nature of the hereditary information to be passed onto the progeny. The specificity of this "base pairing" is the basis of the ability of DNA to replicate itself and pass on the genotype characteristics and also forms the basis for

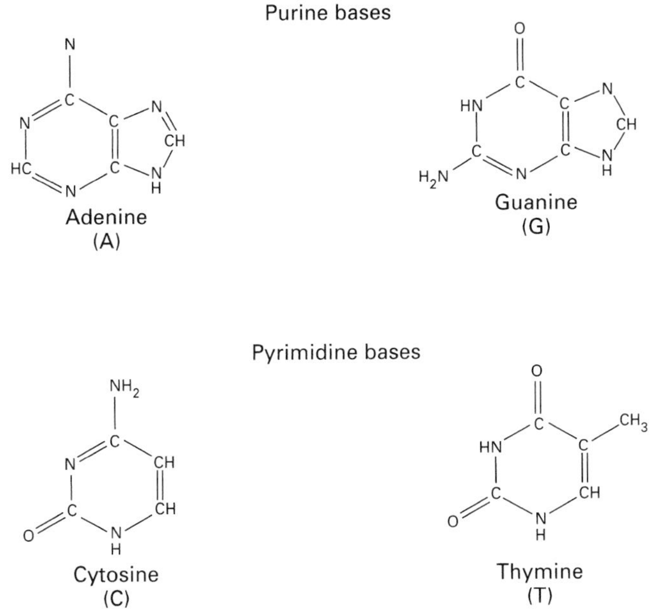

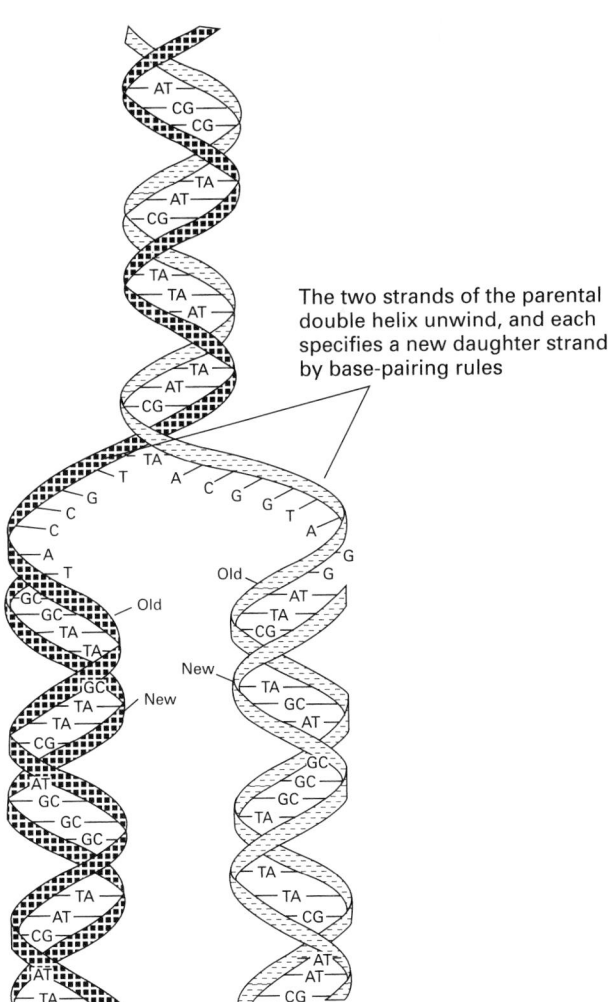

The two strands of the parental double helix unwind, and each specifies a new daughter strand by base-pairing rules

Purine bases

Adenine
(A)

Guanine
(G)

Pyrimidine bases

Cytosine
(C)

Thymine
(T)

FIGURE 5–1. The common purine and pyrimidine bases found in DNA. Uracil is substituted for thymine in RNA. *Source: Mares A Jr, Towbin J, Bies RG, Roberts R. Molecular biology for the cardiologist. Curr Probl Cardiol. 1992;17:9–72. Reproduced with permission from the publisher and authors.*

FIGURE 5–2. DNA replication conserves the nucleotide sequence. DNA is a double-stranded helical molecule bound together by the nucleotide bases contained on each individual strand. During cell division, two identical copies of the original parental strand are made by unwinding the DNA and then synthesizing a complementary second strand to make two identical new daughter strands.

the specificity of essentially all the procedures used in recombinant DNA technology. During the process of DNA replication, the strands separate, and new strands form complementary to the original strands, resulting in two additional identical molecules.

【 】 TRANSCRIPTION OF DNA INTO SINGLE-STRANDED RNA

The central dogma of molecular biology is that DNA produces RNA, which in turn produces a polypeptide, the latter being the molecule that makes up proteins. Proteins provide the cell structure and are solely responsible for all of the functions of the cell (Fig. 5–3). The genetic information inherited by each individual is encoded by the sequence of the bases of the DNA (the genotype), which is translated into proteins and provides the observable characteristics of the individual (the phenotype). This overall process from DNA to protein, however, must first go through the intermediary step of RNA. The process whereby mRNA is synthesized using DNA as the template is referred to as *transcription* (Fig. 5–4). Transcription and the processing of mRNA occur in the nucleus of the cell, separated by the nuclear membrane from the cytoplasm. The process of transcription is initiated by attachment of the enzyme, RNA polymerase II, to specific recognition sites where the DNA is double-stranded, but on activation by the enzyme, the strands selectively unwind and separate. The binding site of RNA polymerase II is always located on the 5′ end of the gene, and the enzyme remains attached to a single strand of DNA as it travels in the 3′ direction. The DNA immediately in front of it separates into two strands with just one strand of DNA (antisense) acting as a template for the synthesis of mRNA. Thus, in contrast to DNA, mRNA is a single-stranded polynucleotide. Messenger RNA also differs from DNA in that deoxyribose, the sugar found in DNA, is replaced by ribose. Moreover, uracil (U) replaces thymine (T), and like thymine, uracil pairs exclusively with adenine (A).

The mRNA, as transcribed from the DNA, is referred to as the *primary transcript*, or sometimes as *immature mRNA*, and is a complementary copy of the DNA (Fig. 5–5). Because protein synthesis occurs in the cytoplasm, the mRNA must exit the nucleus, but prior to transport, it undergoes extensive posttranscriptional processing primarily through three main events: (1) addition of a methylated guanosine (4-methylguanosine residue) to the 5′ end, referred to as a *cap*, which is important for the initiation of translation; (2) addition of a long tail of repeated adenine nucleotides, called the *poly(A) tail*, to the 3′ region of the mRNA, which is essential for stability of the message in the cytoplasm; and (3) the primary transcript, which contains introns and exons, undergoes a

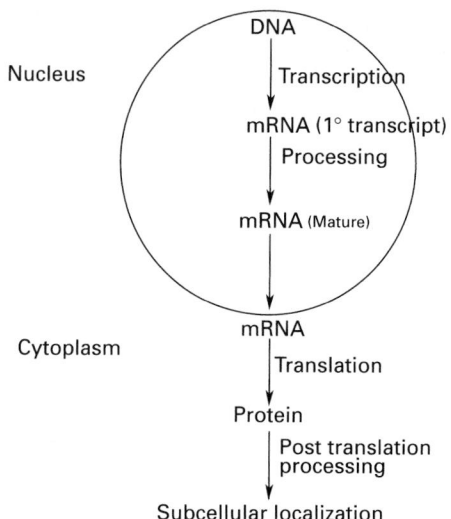

FIGURE 5–4. Schematic localization of the processes of transcription and translation.

specific splicing process whereby the introns are removed and the exons are properly re-spliced together prior to exit from the nucleus as mature mRNA. The process of splicing is, in part, performed by molecules referred to as *small nuclear ribonucleoproteins* (snRNPs), which consist of RNA molecules tightly associated with a group of approximately 10 different proteins. Exons survive the mRNA processing and exit the nucleus (hence the name) as part of the mature mRNA. The mature mRNA consists of three distinct regions. The exons of the 5′ end are not translated into protein but signal the beginning of mRNA translation and contain sequences that direct the mRNA to the ribosome in the cytoplasm for protein synthesis. The exons in the second region, referred to as the *coding region,* contain the information that determines the amino-acid sequence of the protein. The exons of the 3′ end do not code for protein but contain signals that terminate translation and direct the addition of the poly(A) tail. Introns are portions of the gene included in the primary mRNA transcript but spliced out of the mature mRNA. The process of splicing out introns and rejoining exons is an important means of introducing genetic diversity, because one mRNA can provide several different mRNAs that code for different polypeptides. The primary transcript undergoes extensive shortening such that the mature mRNA often represents only 10 percent of the primary transcript. The mature mRNA exits to the cytoplasm and attaches to a ribosome to initiate protein synthesis.

【 】 TRANSLATION OF RNA INTO PROTEIN

The final process, referred to as *translation,* is the most complex of the various processes that occur in the flow from genomic DNA (gene) to mature protein. The alphabet of DNA or its single-stranded complementary mRNA is that of the four nucleotides (bases), whereas that of protein is amino acids. Thus, the term translation, because the nucleic acids of DNA must be translated into the amino acids of protein. The genetic code is written in triplets of bases, with each amino acid being encoded by three base pairs referred to as a *codon.* The mRNA codons dictate which amino acids are to be selected, and the sequence of the codons in the RNA dictates the sequence of the amino acids in the protein.

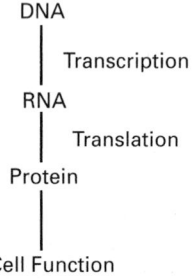

FIGURE 5–3. Central dogma of molecular biology.

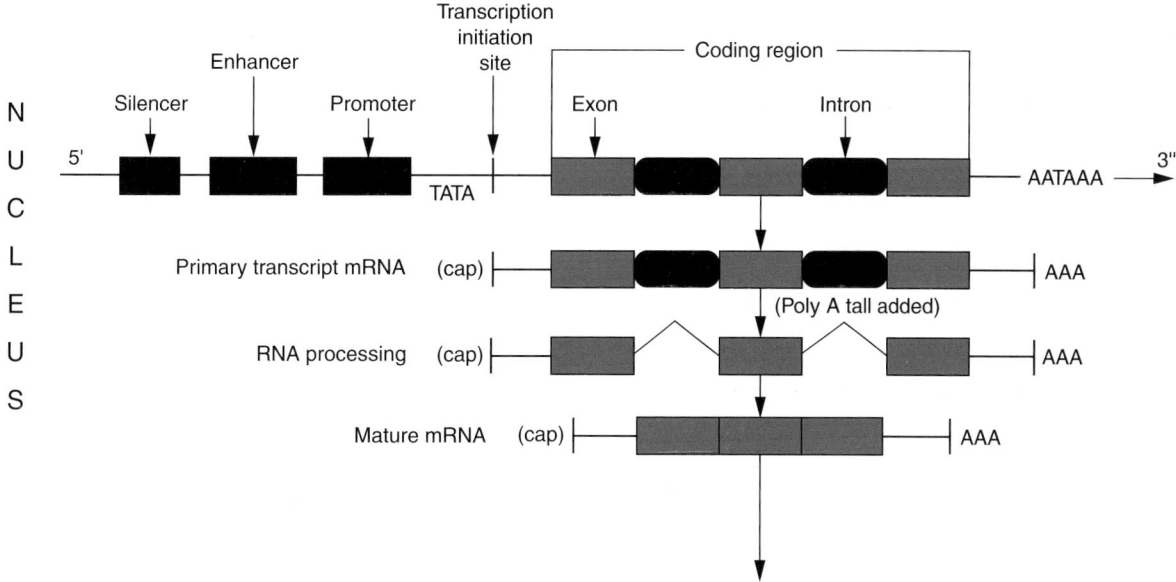

FIGURE 5–5. Transcription. Transcription occurs in the nucleus, producing mRNA that is processed into mature mRNA and transported to the cytoplasm. In the cytoplasm, translation occurs, with the mRNA coding for specific amino acids that are linked together to form a polypeptide and ultimately to form a mature protein. *Source: Mares A Jr, Towbin J, Bies RG, Roberts R. Molecular biology for the cardiologist. Curr Probl Cardiol. 1992;17:9–72. Reproduced with permission from the publisher and authors.*

There is a linear one to one relationship. There are four different nucleotides to form the triplets; thus the number of combinations (4^3) is 64, but there are only 20 amino acids. There is considerable redundancy, referred to as *degeneracy*, and this results in most of the amino acids having more than one codon. In addition to codons for each amino acid, there is also the codon AUG, which is the start codon that initiates protein synthesis and also codes for methionine. To stop translation, there are three codons, UAA, UAG, and UGA, that signal the end of a particular polypeptide. Translation into protein requires two other RNA species, ribosomal RNA (rRNA) and transfer RNA (tRNA). The mRNA, after exiting the nucleus, recognizes the ribosome, which is the site of protein synthesis. The ribosome moves along an mRNA molecule, translating each of its codons in a 5′ to 3′ direction to assemble the polypeptide from its amino (N-terminal) to its carboxy (C-terminal) ends. More than 80 percent of RNA are rRNAs, 15 percent tRNAs, and less than 5 percent mRNAs.

The mRNA does not interact directly with amino acids but rather through adaptor molecules referred to as *transfer RNA* (tRNA) to which amino acids are covalently joined by a highly specific enzyme (aminoacyl tRNA synthetase) using adenosine triphosphate (ATP). There is at least one tRNA species corresponding to each of the 20 naturally occurring amino acids. The aminoacyl tRNA synthetase performs a special function of activating the amino acids and ensuring that each amino acid is joined specifically to its complimentary codon exposed at one end of the folded tRNA molecule referred to as the *anticodon*. The amino acid receptor site is exposed at the other end. Amino acids thus are specified at two recognition steps: one in which a specific enzyme joins the amino acid to a specific tRNA and the other in which the tRNA serving as an adaptor molecule joins the amino acid to the ribosomal-mRNA complex through a codon-anticodon specific-base-pairing interaction between the mRNA and the tRNA. Once the process of protein synthesis is initiated, the ribosome moves along the mRNA joining the amino acids by means of peptide bonds in the sequence specified by the mRNA to form the mature polypeptide. The process of protein synthesis from this complex of mRNA and ribosome involves more than 100 enzymes. The steps involved consist of initiation, elongation, and termination of the polypeptide, with each process having its own enzymes.[14]

Once a polypeptide is synthesized, many modifications occur referred to as *posttranslational modifications* (Fig. 5–6). It is estimated that more than 200 modifications occur including: glycosylation; phosphorylation or dephosphorylation of serine, threonine or tyrosine; carboxylation; formation of thiol groups; prenylation; palmitoylation or oxidation. The polypeptide may also bind to other polypeptides and with the help of chaperone proteins undergo various conformational changes. Leader sequences direct the protein to its destination of either the intracellular membranes, the plasma membrane, or organelle (e.g., mitochondria). Finally, the protein is destroyed, usually through ubiquitization.[15]

[ ] THE STRUCTURE OF A GENE

The concept that one gene leads to one protein remains basic to the central dogma of molecular biology but does, in some cases, need modification. In the classic sense, a gene consists of a discrete unit of DNA that encodes for a specific polypeptide. Two observations must be noted: First, transcription produces two end points—ribonucleic acid (RNA) and protein. The products, rRNA, tRNA, and small nuclear RNA (snRNA), do not get translated into protein but rather perform functions during posttranscription and translation that are pivotal to expression of the mRNA. The polymerases necessary for transcription of these genes are of three types—polymerase I for rRNA, polymerase II for mRNA, and polymerase III for tRNA and some other snRNAs. Second, in part because of snRNA and certain proteins, alternative splicing of the exons in the primary mRNA can lead to different

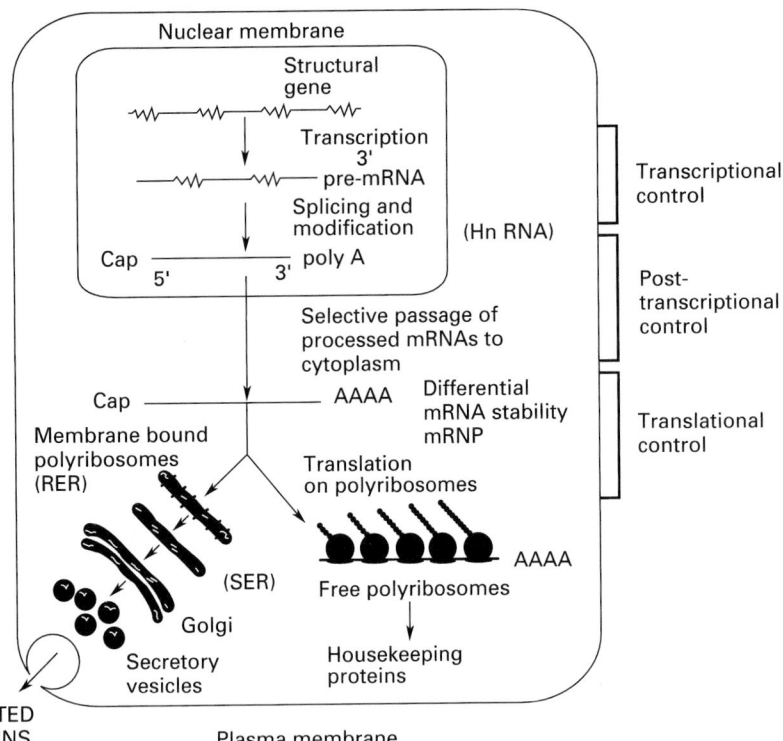

FIGURE 5–6. A summary of the multiple steps involved in gene expression from the genomic DNA to the protein showing how the protein destined for secretion follows a systematic path different from proteins destined to remain in the cytoplasm. RER, rough endoplasmic reticulum; SER, smooth endoplasmic reticulum. *Source: Mares A Jr, Towbin J, Bies RG, Roberts R. Molecular biology for the cardiologist. Curr Probl Cardiol. 1992;17:9–72. Reproduced with permission from the publisher and authors.*

as the *coding region,* that codes for the amino acids and their sequence in the protein; and the 3′ untranslated end, which also has regulatory sequences and coding signals for stability of the mature mRNA. The first nucleotide to be transcribed is given the +1 number, and everything 5′ to it is referred to as *upstream* or *proximal* and is numbered with the first base pair as −1, and so on. The initiation site for transcription is always upstream from the 5′ untranslated region. The 5′ regulatory untranslated region has variable sequences, but there are several consistent sequences present in the same position in most human genes. Polymerase II has no intrinsic affinity for DNA and can only bind after several transcription factors have bound. The site of transcription and its direction in most human genes are determined by a consensus sequence of TATAA referred to as the *TATA box* found at base pairs −25 to −30 upstream from the start site. A large complex of transcription factors (more than 25 proteins) binds to the TATA box in preparation for RNA polymerase II binding and transcription. Collectively, these transcription factors are referred to as *transcription factors for polymerase II* (TFII), with letters designating the different factors. TFIID binds first, then TFIIB, followed by RNA polymerase II, followed by several TFII factors such as E, F, G, H, and J, and so on. In addition, in many human genes, located at approximately base pair 200 upstream is the GGGCG box to which stimulatory protein 1 (SP1) binds, and this is felt to be a regulator of housekeeping genes (Fig. 5–7).

mature mRNAs with each coding for a slightly different polypeptide, which forms isoforms of the same protein.

The anatomy of a protein-coding gene is composed of introns and exons. The average exon is approximately 300 base pairs long, whereas introns are much larger and are spliced out of the mature mRNA and, thus, do not code for protein. A typical gene has three regions: the 5′ untranslated region that contains the *cis*-acting sequences that regulate transcription; the central portion, referred to

❲ ❳ REGULATION OF GENE EXPRESSION

Gene expression refers to the expressed form of the gene, which is the protein, and to all the processes required to go from DNA to

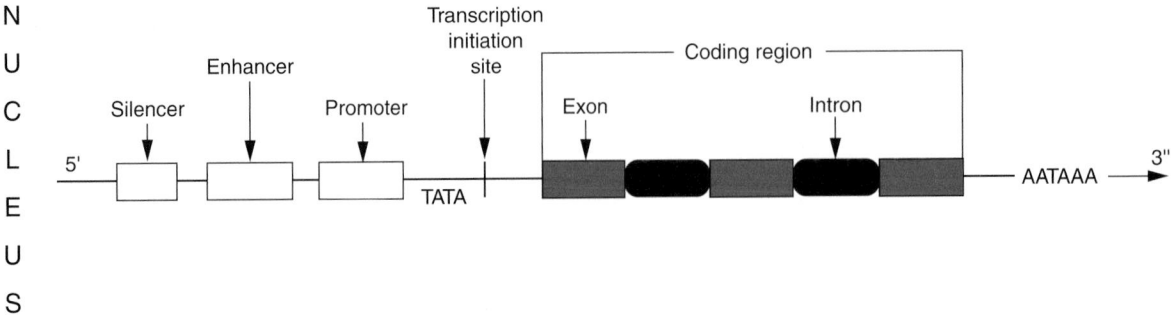

FIGURE 5–7. Structure of a gene. These small functional units within the nucleus contain the coding information for the synthesis of a polypeptide and on their 5′ ends have regulatory sequences that include silencers, enhancers, and promoters. The coding region consisting of exons (code for protein) as well as intervening noncoding sequences (introns) is followed by a 3′ noncoding region that is translated into the mRNA. The 3′ end appears important for exit of the mRNA from the nucleus and its stability in the cytoplasm but does not code for protein. The TATA is the initiation site for polymerase and is present in most eukaryotes at approximately 10 to 30 bp 5′ from the start codon (TAC) of the coding region. The AATAA will become the recognition site on the mRNA to which attaches an enzyme that cleaves the 3′ region and replaces the distal portion with a poly(A) tail. *Source: Mares A Jr, Towbin J, Bies RG, Roberts R. Molecular biology for the cardiologist. Curr Probl Cardiol. 1992;17:9–72. Reproduced with permission from the publisher and authors.*

protein, from the initial unfolding of the nuclear chromatin in preparation for transcription to the mature protein emerging following completion of posttranslational changes. Regulation of gene expression occurs at all levels in response to signals both from within and outside of the cell. The cell maintains its integrity and responds to external stimuli through signals that activate receptors (generally in the cell membrane). These in turn use signaling proteins to transfer their message to the cytoplasm or nucleus, which in some way modifies gene expression. Delineation of the receptor, the signaling proteins, and where and how gene expression is altered are of prime importance in cardiovascular medicine.

The most fundamental level of gene expression regulation involves cell differentiation. The body contains at least 200 different types of cells that have been programmed by their genes to perform highly specialized functions. All cells have the same DNA and the same genes, but only those genes that are expressed determine the cell's phenotype. Cardiac myocytes, for example, are characterized by a set of proteins that specialize in contractile activity, whereas hepatocytes specialize in the synthesis and catabolism of proteins. Selective gene expression is the basis of cell differentiation. Cell growth and replication occur in what is termed the *undifferentiated cell* often referred to as a stem cell but, through complex mechanisms, give rise to cells that cease to replicate and are programmed to take on specialized functions (cell differentiation). In the process of cell differentiation, genes, particularly those concerned with cell proliferation and undifferentiated functions, are downregulated, whereas those genes coding for the proteins that perform the specialized functions are upregulated. Once cells are differentiated, protein synthesis, however, remains a dynamic process to maintain cell integrity. Most of gene regulation is concerned with the maintenance of cellular integrity, and the genes responsible for this basal function are referred to as *housekeeping genes*. Housekeeping genes are constitutively regulated, as opposed to genes responsible for cell differentiation and growth, which are developmentally regulated. It is estimated that organs use approximately 10,000 genes (constitutive) to maintain their integrity, with one exception, the brain, which is estimated to use approximately 20,000 genes. Gene regulation can be classified under the following headings: pretranscription, transcription, posttranscription, translation, and posttranslation[16] (Table 5–1).

Pretranscriptional Control

Pretranscriptional regulation[17] refers to the decompaction of the DNA and exposure of the region about to undergo transcription. The total DNA of a single cell would measure about 1 meter in length, yet in the nucleus it is markedly compacted and is folded around specific proteins, the dominant class being histones. The chromatin takes on a specific repeating structure called the *nucleosome*. The nucleosome is identical from gene to gene and highly conserved, being virtually identical from yeast to humans. This structure consists of core histones (two each of H2A, H2B, H3, and H4), around which are wrapped 146 base pair (bp) in the superhelical turn.[18] Recently, it became evident that nucleosomes play a major role in the regulation of gene expression and can transmit epigenetic information from one cell generation to the next.

TABLE 5–1

Factors Regulating Gene Expression

Pretranscription
Transcription
Posttranscription
Translation
Posttranslation

The information storage function and gene regulation reside primarily in the amino terminal tails of the four core histones. The positive charge of the lysine residues of the histone proteins bind tightly to the negatively charged DNA to prevent exposure for transcription. Modification of histone binding to DNA is a major regulatory mechanism of gene expression.[19] A group of enzymes facilitates histone acetylation (HAC) of histone-lysine tails exposed on the nucleosome surface, which decreases binding of the histone to the DNA (decompaction) and exposes the region for transcription. Similarly, another set of enzymes induces histone deacetylation (HDAC), removing the acetyl groups from the lysine to prevent transcription. Other modifications involved with binding between the histone proteins and DNA play a similar regulatory role in gene transcription including lysine and arginine methylation, serine phosphorylation, and attachment of the small peptide ubiquitin.[20,21] This pretranscriptional level of gene regulation is now an area of major research. Therapeutic targets are being sought to manipulate cell growth such as cardiac hypertrophy.[22,23,24]

Transcriptional Control

Transcriptional control is a major rate-limiting step to gene expression. The 5' upstream region immediately adjacent to the transcription initiation site is referred to as the *promoter region*. This region contains sequences that are specific binding sites for proteins referred to as *transacting factors* or *transcriptional factors*. The protein-binding sites are often referred to as *cis-acting sequences* because they are on the same DNA molecule on which they act. The transcription factors (also referred to as *DNA-binding proteins*) are referred to as *transacting factors* (acting at a distance) because they are encoded by genes that can even be on another chromosome.

The promoter sequences and their corresponding DNA-binding proteins can act ubiquitously or can be tissue-specific. Promoters often increase transcription of a class of genes rather than a single gene. Another type of DNA sequence that increases transcription is referred to as an *enhancer* (see Fig. 5–7). Enhancers, like promoters, consist of several small motifs of 4 to 10 base pairs and, when bound by their corresponding DNA-binding proteins (transcription factors), have a positive influence on gene transcription. Another regulatory DNA sequence that is similar to enhancers in size and location but exerts a negative influence on transcription is referred to as a *silencer* or *repressor*.

Most of the DNA-binding proteins (transcription factors) have one of four protein structures; the zinc-finger, leucine-zipper, helix-loop-helix, or helix-turn-helix. The zinc-finger type of transcription factor directs developmental genes (*GATA factors*). The receptors for circulating hormones, including the glucocorticoids, progesterones, androgens, mineralocorticoids, estrogen, thyroxine, vitamin D_3, and retinoic acid lipophilic and penetrate the cell membrane and activate an intracellular receptor or nuclear receptor, which, in turn, activates gene expression through the zinc-finger transcription proteins. Transcription factors such as the *myo-D* family of genes that induce differentiation of skeletal muscle contain a helix-loop-helix motif.

Translational Control

Translational control is a major level at which gene expression is regulated. The mature mRNA that exits the nucleus and migrates to the ribosome in the cytoplasm to serve as the template for protein synthesis is significantly altered from the original transcribed mRNA. The protein-coding region undergoes significant modification with removal of the introns and subsequent splicing together of the exons to provide the mature mRNA. In the majority of instances, each exon present in the gene is incorporated into a mature mRNA by means of ligation of consecutive pairs of exons and removal of all introns. In other instances, however, nonconsecutive exons are joined in the processing of some gene transcripts, and this alternative pattern of primary mRNA splicing can exclude individual exons from mature mRNA in some transcripts and include them in others. This process of alternative splicing creates mRNAs that generate a variety of proteins from a single gene. Differential splicing is particularly prevalent in genes of muscles and has been shown to occur in several sarcomeric proteins including myosin heavy chains, tropomyosin, and troponin T.

The precise mechanism whereby an mRNA is induced to remain stable and encode several thousand polypeptides as opposed to being extremely unstable and encoding only a few molecules is not well understood. Nevertheless, it is likely to be an important step in regulating the response to cytoplasmic signals that require rapid synthesis of a particular polypeptide. The synthesis of a polypeptide initiated by means of transcription is estimated to take several minutes, whereas synthesis of a protein initiated through translation requires only seconds. Regulation of gene expression at the protein synthesis level is more fully discussed in Chapter 6.

Posttranslational Control by Small Inhibitory RNA

Posttranslational control by small inhibitory RNA is a new mechanism for regulation of gene expression. It has recently become evident that a new mechanism for control of gene expression occurs posttranslational by a new group of molecules: the small inhibitory RNA's. These consist of 19 to 25 bases in length and interact with specific mRNA to inhibit their activity. This RNA is produced in a variety of cell types from yeast to humans.[25,26,27] These small RNA are currently being used to inhibit genes in cell and animal models to determine the function of genes. These RNA have also been shown to inhibit gene expression at the chromatin level and appear to be a major means of controlling gene expression. Their use as a therapeutic weapon is likely to become successful.

MOLECULAR BIOLOGY AND RECOMBINANT DNA TECHNOLOGY

THE BASIS FOR RECOMBINANT DNA TECHNOLOGY

Modern molecular biology, initiated in the 1970s,[12] was in part caused by four pivotal discoveries or inventions: (1) restriction enzymes, (2) reverse transcription, (3) cloning, and (4) DNA sequencing. The discovery of the restriction endonucleases provided the genetic scalpel to cut DNA into smaller pieces of predictable size that could be used in a variety of procedures. The unique feature of these enzymes is that each recognizes a specific sequence of DNA of 4 to 8 base pairs and cleaves the molecule at that particular site. Thus, one knows precisely where the enzyme cuts, and using a number of different enzymes, one can identify the site and number of recognition sites for each enzyme in a fragment of DNA of interest and develop what is referred to as a *restriction map*. These enzymes also made it possible to cut DNA from different sources in a predictable manner in preparation for ligating them together into a recombinant molecule. Restriction endonucleases are obtained from bacteria, and enzymes have been purified that recognize more than 100 different cleavage sites.

The discovery of the enzyme, RT, revolutionized molecular biology (Fig. 5–8). Messenger RNA, as discussed previously, codes for a specific polypeptide and is derived from a discrete, specific unit of DNA referred to as a *gene*. RT reverses this process so that a cDNA is generated from an mRNA (coding part of the gene) and can be used as a gene to express the protein. The cDNA is reinserted into the genome of a vector (virus or plasmid) and subsequently replicated in an appropriate host, such as a bacterium, which made possible the first cloning of a gene. Radioactive labeling of a cDNA provides an extraordinarily powerful tool to isolate and identify DNA fragments of interest including genes. The labeled cDNA, referred to as a *probe*, or *indicator molecule*, is a routine, essential tool used to identify and isolate DNA or RNA fragments of interest. Development of rapid-sequencing techniques made it possible to rapidly sequence fragments of DNA containing thousands of base pairs from which the protein sequence could be derived.

Three features essential to all techniques of recombinant DNA technology need to be highlighted: The first is the ability of DNA

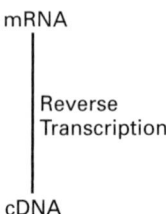

FIGURE 5–8. Generation of a complementary DNA (cDNA). Taking advantage of the enzyme reverse transcriptase, mRNA is converted to DNA, referred to as *complementary* DNA (cDNA). The DNA is single-stranded and complementary to the sequence of RNA, except thymine now replaces uracil. Using DNA polymerase, one can then make the single-stranded DNA into double-stranded cDNA. The cDNA can be used as a probe to identify specific sequences or genes of the genomic DNA, or it can be inserted into vectors to be cloned or expressed in a variety of hosts.

to denature and anneal, or hybridize. The double-stranded DNA, held together by hydrogen bonding of the corresponding complementary bases, will, on exposure to high temperatures (200°F [95°C]), separate into two strands, but under appropriate conditions (131°F [55°C]), the complementary strands will again anneal precisely as originally and return to their normal double-stranded state. The process of separating into separate strands is referred to as *denaturation,* and the recombining process is known as *annealment* or *hybridization,* with the latter term preferred if the two DNA fragments are from different sources. Second, the strands come together identically to the parent molecule because of complementary base pairing, whereby A must bind to T and C to G. Third, the phosphorus present in DNA provides DNA with a net negative charge. This property is exploited in many techniques (e.g., electrophoresis) to separate and detect DNA molecules of different sizes. To understand the power of recombinant technology as it applies to cardiology, it is necessary to have knowledge of the terminology and methods. The starting material is usually DNA but could be RNA isolated from either a blood or tissue sample. DNA could be obtained from any source because DNA within the human body is the same regardless of the cell or organ from which it is obtained. Messenger RNA represents the expressed form of the DNA gene, and although it is identical throughout the body for a particular gene, certain mRNAs may or may not be expressed, depending on the organ source. Because DNA and RNA are negatively charged (phosphorus ion), this property is commonly used to separate DNA and RNA molecules of different size by electrophoresis. Fragments of increasing size move slower through the pores of gels as they migrate toward the positive electrode during electrophoresis. One can alter the resolution of this technique by changing the size of the pores in the gel. Thus, electrophoresis is the predominant method to separate RNA or DNA fragments. One can use a short sequence complementary to the DNA of interest as a probe tagged with an identification marker such as radioactivity or fluorescence. The probe can be synthesized chemically, referred to as an *oligonucleotide,* or be a natural DNA or RNA fragment. The labeled sequence, referred to as a *probe,* will be used as bait to identify the RNA or DNA of interest. If the probe of interest is DNA, it is first denatured to single strands. On reannealing or hybridizing, the labeled probe will bind to complementary sequences of DNA or RNA of interest present in the sample. On electrophoresis, only the band with the attached marker (radioactivity or fluorescence) will be visualized. The band will contain specifically only the DNA or RNA of interest because the probe will only bind to the specific and precise sequence that is complementary to the sequence of the probe.

To obtain multiple copies of a gene, or any DNA sequence, one can insert the fragment of interest into various vectors, which can be replicated in a host cell such as a bacteria to provide on average a million copies identical to the initial sequence. This process is referred to as cloning. Initially, it was thought one could only clone DNA based on the misconception that one could not go from RNA to DNA. The discovery of the enzyme, RT, made it possible to convert mRNA, which reflects a specific gene, into DNA referred to as *complementary DNA* (cDNA). This made it possible to isolate mRNA, which represents a specific gene; convert it to cDNA by RT; and clone it in cell culture or living organisms. This discovery has revolutionized biology and medicine and is routinely

used to generate animal models of disease such as transgenic animals or to harvest specific drugs for the treatment of disease such as insulin, tissue plasminogen activator (tPA), or vascular endothelial growth factor (VEGF). It is hoped that within the next 10 years cDNAs for all human genes will be available, which will further revolutionize the diagnosis, treatment, and prevention of human disease. Another technique routinely used to obtain multiple copies of a DNA or RNA sequence is referred to as PCR. This is a technique whereby two primers of 15 to 20 bp are selected complementary to the sequence that is upstream and downstream to the sequence. The sequences between the two primers under appropriate conditions with a polymerase enzyme can be amplified to a million copies in 3 hours and a billion copies in 24 hours. If one needs to amplify copies of mRNA, the mRNA is converted to cDNA followed by amplification with PCR. This technique is much simpler, cheaper, and faster than cloning. Both techniques are necessary, because the size of the fragment amplified by PCR is limited (1000 to 20,000 bp). To provide multiple copies of larger fragments, cloning is necessary. Another useful and routinely used tool is a gene library. A library can consist of DNA sequences that would be the same for all organs, or it can contain cDNAs specific for a particular organ. These libraries consist of genes stored in a host such as bacteria and are now commercially available. The library can consist of all the genes expressed in a particular organ or subspecialized region of the organ. An example is a cDNA library that contains supposedly all of the genes expressed in the heart and a library containing only those genes expressed in the cardiac Purkinje system. The techniques routinely used in molecular biology include electrophoresis, Southern and Northern blot analysis, DNA cloning, PCR, electrophoretic mobility shift assay, and the development of gene libraries.

【 】 ISOLATION OF DNA

Because the DNA of all human tissues is the same, practically any tissue can be used to obtain a DNA sample. It requires only a microgram for most procedures. In humans, lymphocytes are commonly used because they are very accessible, and the DNA can be extracted easily. Lymphocytes are also used because they can be transformed by Epstein-Barr virus into an immortal cell line that can provide a continuous, renewable source of DNA. The cells can be grown in culture, frozen for years (from which samples can be obtained), thawed, and regrown, providing a renewable source of DNA for several decades. A sample of 10 to 15 mL of whole blood typically would yield approximately 50 to 100 μg of genomic DNA. If one's interest is restricted to the DNA sequences that are expressed, one would isolate mRNA and, using it as a template, employ RT to derive its cDNA. cDNA molecules represent the expressed form of a gene and thus can be used as probes to select the specific genomic DNA segments from which the mRNA was transcribed. Myocardial biopsies obtained under appropriate conditions provide adequate tissue for most DNA or RNA analyses.

【 】 SEPARATION OF DNA MOLECULES BY ELECTROPHORESIS

One of the important physical properties of the DNA molecule is that each individual nucleotide possesses a net negative charge resulting from the phosphate group. Thus, fragments of different sizes exposed to an electric field tend to migrate toward the positive electrode at differential rates depending on their size, with small fragments migrating faster than larger ones. This process of separation based on electric charge is called *electrophoresis*. The DNA sample, after being digested into fragments of different size by a restriction endonuclease, is added to a gel matrix such as agarose or acrylamide. After separation by electrophoresis, the pattern of the DNA can be visualized under an ultraviolet lamp with a fluorescent dye such as ethidium bromide (Fig. 5–9). Agarose gel electrophoresis will separate fragments from 1000 to 60,000 bp (60 kilobase [kb]) in size, and polyacrylamide gels effectively separate fragments smaller than 1000 bp (1 kb). The recent development of pulsed-field gel electrophoresis (PFGE) made possible the separation of DNA fragments even up to 2000 kb in size. In this technique, the electric field is alternated in different directions, forcing the molecules of DNA to reorient between each pulse of electric current. Thus this technique is particularly suitable for isolating and characterizing large segments of DNA to identify a known gene.

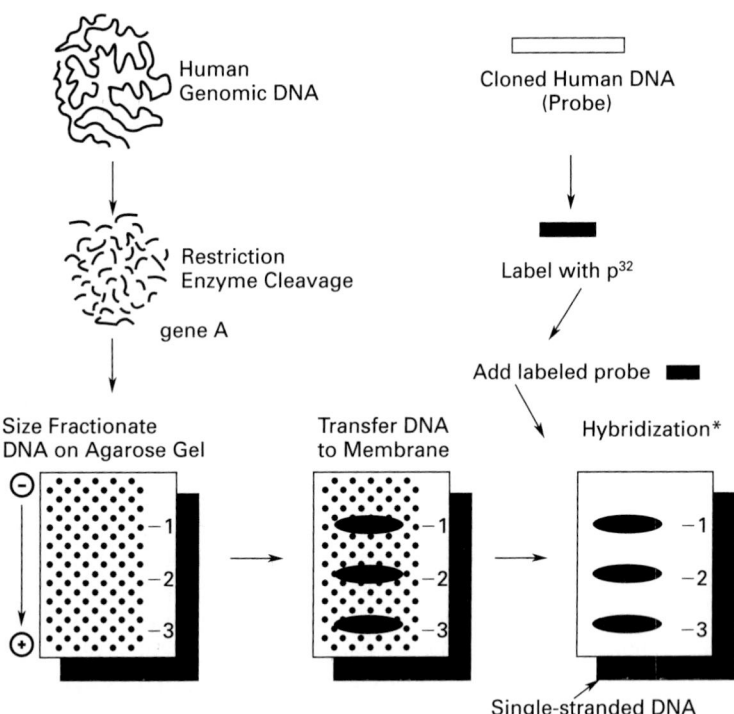

FIGURE 5–9. Southern blotting technique. The DNA is cleaved with an appropriately selected restriction endonuclease. The digested fragments are separated by electrophoresis on agarose gel, and the fragments of gene A are located at positions 1, 2, and 3 but cannot be seen against the background of many other randomly occurring DNA fragments. The DNA is denatured and transferred to a membrane in an identical pattern to what it was on the agarose gel. It is difficult to manipulate anything on a soft gel or to remove it. Once transferred to the membrane (filter), a solid support system, the DNA is much easier to handle. A DNA probe (cDNA) that has been labeled with 32P is hybridized to its cDNA and visualized after exposure of the nylon membrane to an autoradiograph. The transfer of the DNA from the gel to the membrane developed by Southern was a major innovation illustrated in Fig. 5–10. *Source: Mares A Jr, Towbin J, Bies RG, Roberts R. Molecular biology for the cardiologist. Curr Probl Cardiol. 1992;17:9–72. Reproduced with permission from the publisher and authors.*

As noted previously, prior to electrophoresis, the DNA must be digested with one of the restriction endonucleases. The size of the fragments resulting from digestion will depend on the type of restriction endonuclease used—that is, whether they recognize sequences of 4, 5, 6, or 8 bp. Enzymes recognizing a 4-bp sequence will cut the DNA into much smaller fragments than one that recognizes an 8-bp sequence.

[ ] DEVELOPMENT OF A DNA PROBE

A nucleic acid probe is a fragment of nucleic acid to which has been attached a label such as a radioisotope or a fluorescent compound, making it possible to easily detect and recognize the desired fragment among other native DNA molecules. The fragment labeled is usually cDNA or a synthetic oligonucleotide, although it could be RNA. It is now possible to synthesize DNA fragments of up to 30 to 40 bp, referred to as *oligonucleotides* that, with an attached label, can be used as probes to identify cDNA in the human genome or mRNA. This takes advantage of the fact that at high temperatures, the double-stranded DNA probe and the native DNA will break into separate strands. On recombining at random, the labeled DNA probe can bind with either its original complementary strand or the native DNA that is complementary to the probe and thus provide a means of isolating a fragment of native genomic DNA. A probe is necessary in most recombinant DNA procedures to detect the molecule of interest following electrophoresis.

[ ] SOUTHERN, NORTHERN, AND WESTERN BLOT ANALYSIS

A procedure to separate and detect specific DNA fragments, referred to as *Southern blotting*, is named after E. M. Southern, who developed it in 1975.[28] Genomic DNA is isolated and digested into small fragments with restriction enzymes, and the fragments are separated by gel electrophoresis, as described previously. Following separation, DNA fragments are denatured chemically into single-strand fragments. It is very difficult to handle gels and even more difficult and also impractical to store them. Southern developed a technique whereby these separated single-stranded fragments in the gel could be transferred by capillary action to a solid support medium (nylon or nitrocellulose membrane) and fixed permanently by heating. The pattern on the membrane reflects identically the pattern induced by electrophoresis on the gel. The process used to produce a Southern blot is illustrated schematically in Fig. 5–9. The nylon membrane and its attached single-strand DNA fragments are then incubated with a radioactively labeled complementary probe. The hybridized, radioactive double-strand product, on exposure to x-ray film (autoradiography), will exhibit the pattern of the radiolabeled DNA fragments (Fig. 5–10).

In summary, the electrophoretic separation of DNA followed by its transfer to a nylon membrane for subsequent identification by radioactive hybridization is referred to as *Southern blotting*, and the autoradiogram as a *Southern blot*. The same approach to detect mRNA is referred to as *North-*

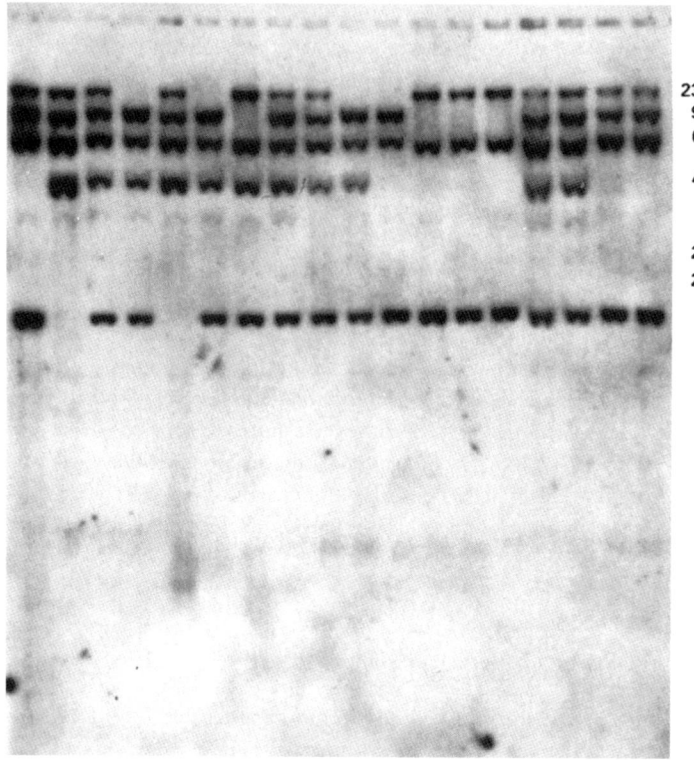

Length of Fragments, kb

23.1
9.4
6.6

4.4

2.3
2.0

FIGURE 5–10. A typical Southern blot with distinct bands. Each vertical lane consists of DNA from a separate individual. All the individual DNAs were digested with the same restriction endonuclease. Following separation on electrophoresis and transfer to a nylon membrane, hybridization was performed with the selected radioactive probe, and thus only those fragments complementary to the probe are visualized. This is an analysis of a family with hypertrophic cardiomyopathy, and the different patterns reflect restriction fragment length polymorphisms (RFLPs) characteristic of the marker locus, which is linked to the disease locus. *Source: Mares A Jr, Towbin J, Bies RG, Roberts R. Molecular biology for the cardiologist. Curr Probl Cardiol. 1992;17:9–72. Reproduced with permission from the publisher and authors.*

ern blotting. This procedure also can be used for detection of proteins, in which case it is referred to as *Western blotting* (Table 5–2). The only significant difference in detecting protein versus nucleic acid by this procedure is the probe, which is an antibody rather than an oligonucleotide or cDNA. However, as in Southern and Northern blotting, the probe can be labeled with a radioactive isotope, a fluorescent tag, or some visual colorimetric substance.

CLONING A GENE

DNA cloning is a technique used to produce large quantities of a specific DNA fragment of interest. It generally is quite feasible to produce a million copies of a DNA fragment by routine cloning

TABLE 5–2

Separation and Identification of Molecular Species

PROCEDURES	MOLECULE	LABELED PROBE
Southern blotting	DNA	DNA or cDNA
Northern blotting	RNA	DNA or cDNA
Western blotting	Protein	Antibody

techniques. The DNA fragment of interest to be cloned, referred to as the *insert,* is incorporated into the DNA of a vector, and the vector is replicated in an appropriate host cell. The host provides replication of the DNA of both the vector and the insert. The prerequisites for cloning are (1) isolation of the DNA fragment (insert) of interest for cloning, (2) a vector for transferring the DNA fragment, (3) a restriction endonuclease to cut the DNA of the vector so the DNA ends will be compatible for ligating the insert (as illustrated in Fig. 5–11), (4) a DNA ligase to ligate the insert into the vector, (5) a means to introduce the vector into the host cell, and (6) a means to differentiate the host cells that have incorporated the vector from those which have not. Standard vectors used in cloning have circular DNA and fall into three classes: (1) plasmids harvested from bacterial cells (a *plasmid* is an extrachromosomal segment of DNA present in bacteria that is self-replicating and has been constructed to contain genes that express resistance to ampicillin or other antibiotics); (2) bacteriophages (commonly referred to merely as *phages,* which are viruses that invade and multiply in bacterial cells); and (3) an artificially developed vector (referred to as a *cosmid*). The usual host cell is bacteria, which has circular DNA as opposed to the linear DNA of the human genome. The circular DNA of the vector is cut by an appropriate restriction enzyme. The linear DNA is then incubated with the insert in the presence of a ligating enzyme, which induces the incorporation of the insert through attachment to each end of the vector's DNA to form a circle. The circularized recombinant product (hence the name *recombinant*) is inserted into a host such as a bacterium or a mammalian cell for amplification (Fig. 5–12). To increase uptake of the vector into the host, the pore sizes of the bacteria are increased, usually with heat shock treatment for about 45 seconds. To identify whether or not the particular DNA of interest has been replicated in the host, a so-called selection gene, such as one responsible for ampicillin resistance, is incorporated into the vector. The bacteria are grown in media containing ampicillin so only those bacteria with the resistance gene will survive. Because the resistance gene is attached to the DNA fragment being cloned, colonies (bacteria) or plaques (phage) that survive must contain the gene of interest. Some of the colonies or plaques can, however, contain the insert in the wrong direction or have circularized on itself without the insert, and thus, it is necessary to check and sometimes sequence the DNA to be certain the insert is in the appropriate direction. One can then transfer the colonies that contain the insert onto a petri dish and grow them for 24 hours at 98.6°F (37°C). The colonies can be stored at 39.2°F (4°C). Replating for regrowth every few months will maintain a source of clones essentially indefinitely.

The size of the insert is a limitation in cloning. Plasmids as vectors can only accommodate inserts up to approximately 15,000 bp, phages up to 25,000 bp, and cosmids up to 45,000 bp. Recently, a new vector has been developed, namely, bacterial artificial chromosomes (BACs), that accommodates DNA fragments of up to 200,000 bp. The yeast artificial chromosome (YAC), developed several years ago, accommodates DNA inserts of up to 2 million bp but is extremely difficult to work with on a routine basis. In con-

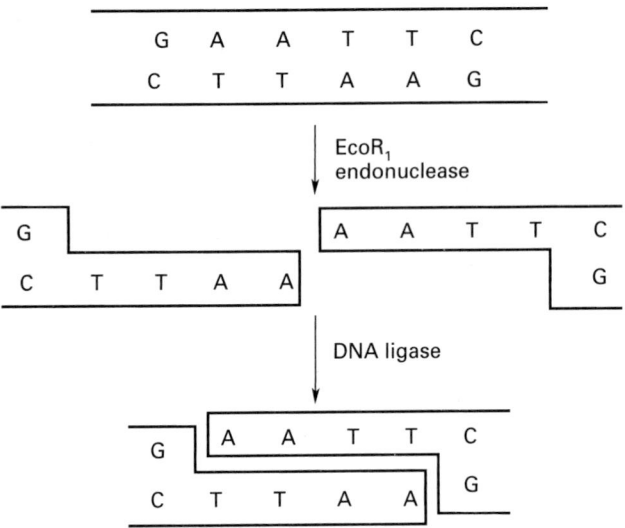

FIGURE 5–11. Restriction endonucleases recognize specific sequences and cut in a specific manner. The sequences recognized can be anywhere from 3 to 8 base pairs long and can cut to give a blunt end or a staggered end (EcoR1). Enzymes that provide staggered ends (cohesive or sticky ends) have unpaired bases that are easy to ligate together because they are complementary to each other, as shown in this illustration. This feature is exploited in cloning or in the formation of any recombinant DNA molecule. For cloning purposes, the fragment of DNA to be inserted is digested with the same restriction enzyme as is used to digest the DNA of the vector into which it will be inserted. Thus the sticky ends of the DNA insert and the vector will be complementary and easy to ligate together in the presence of the enzyme DNA ligase, as illustrated in Fig. 5–12.

trast, the BACs are as convenient as plasmids or phages. This has markedly accelerated the cloning of large fragments of DNA. Cloning, as discussed, is performed to obtain multiple copies of DNA, and unless specifically designed, the DNA is neither transcribed into mRNA nor translated into protein. If one desires to express a particular DNA fragment or gene, one must use what is referred to as an *expression vector*. It is imperative to provide a promoter element that is appropriate for the host, and the gene must contain the appropriate 5′ untranslated region for binding to the ribosome as well as the appropriate 3′ region for stability of the message. An example would be the expression of rt-PA in mammalian cells, whereby the protein is expressed and secreted to be harvested and processed commercially for use as a thrombolytic agent.

[ ] DEVELOPMENT OF GENE LIBRARIES

Gene libraries can be either genomic or cDNA libraries. A *genomic library* is one made from genomic DNA. A library is a collection of DNA fragments that have been cloned in an appropriate vector and grown in a particular host, usually bacteria. A major difference between a genomic and a cDNA library is that a genomic library contains DNA fragments composed of introns and exons, whereas a cDNA library is made from mRNA that represents genes expressed in a particular organ and does not have introns. The cDNA library contains genes specifically expressed in a particular tissue only. In contrast, a genomic library, whether derived from the heart or another tissue, will have the same genes. To make a human genomic library, one must first isolate the whole genome of a cell, cut it into fragments with a restriction enzyme, and insert the fragments into a

vector to be replicated in an appropriate host, usually bacteria. To increase the odds that enough fragments are cloned to represent the whole genome, certain calculations are necessary. It is assumed that the recognition site for a particular restriction enzyme occurs at random. For the restriction enzyme, EcoR1, with a 6-bp recognition site, the average size of each fragment will be $4^6 = 4096$ bp. In contrast, if the recognition site involves 4 bp, each fragment would be $4^4 = 256$ bp long. If the 6-bp cutter were used for the human genome, the result would be the 3 billion bp of the human genome divided by 4096 to produce roughly 750,000 fragments requiring 750,000 colonies or clones. However, the recognition sites are not evenly or randomly distributed. Thus, some fragments are larger and others are smaller, so to be certain, at least 1 million colonies would be required. Other factors also must be considered, such as the choice of vector with respect to insert size. The library is a permanent, renewable source of DNA. cDNA libraries from all human tissues are now commercially available including the heart and specific structures of the heart such as the Purkinje system.

[ ] MICROARRAYS—ORGAN PROFILING FOR GENE EXPRESSION

Microarrays are so called *gene chips* prepared in which DNA sequences derived from different messenger RNAs are laid out in a regular array at a density of more than 10,000 different DNA sequences per square centimeter.[29] This can be achieved by spotting cDNA clones on a glass slide or by synthesizing short oligonucleotides derived from each mRNA in situ. To determine the expression profile of a particular organ radio labeled, total mRNA can be prepared from the organ and then exposed to these chips for hybridization. mRNAs that are expressed in the organ will hybridize to their equivalent complimentary oligonucleotide or cDNA and can be detected and quantified by the intensity of the radioactivity. Each cDNA or oligonucleotide is specifically identified, and the sequence known. The display of the microarray is converted to color such that the intensity of each color reflects the abundance of expression. Thus, is it possible from the different colors and intensity to determine the particular genes expressed and their abundance. Determination of microarrays gene expression profiles before and after exposure of tissue to different stimuli can be used to assess the influence of particular stimuli on gene expression in that organ. Microarrays of most human organs are now available and are being exploited for human disease as well as for determining specific therapies for such diseases such as cancer.

In addition to the many uses and insights to be obtained from organ profiling of gene expression, there are also major diagnostic and therapeutic needs emerging. There are multiple ongoing studies showing that certain expression patterns found in the blood can be used to diagnose various forms of cancer and possibly heart disease. Several studies have shown such profiles can be used to diagnose cancer of the prostate or cancer of the breast, and recently are also being pursued to diagnose early coronary artery disease.[30,31] The evolution of molecular techniques will soon make possible the identification of the full human gene profile and from this can be determined the precise organ gene expression profile. These profiles will undoubtedly reflect both normal and physiological states and are likely to facilitate early diagnosis and the selection of specific therapies within the framework of personalized medicine.

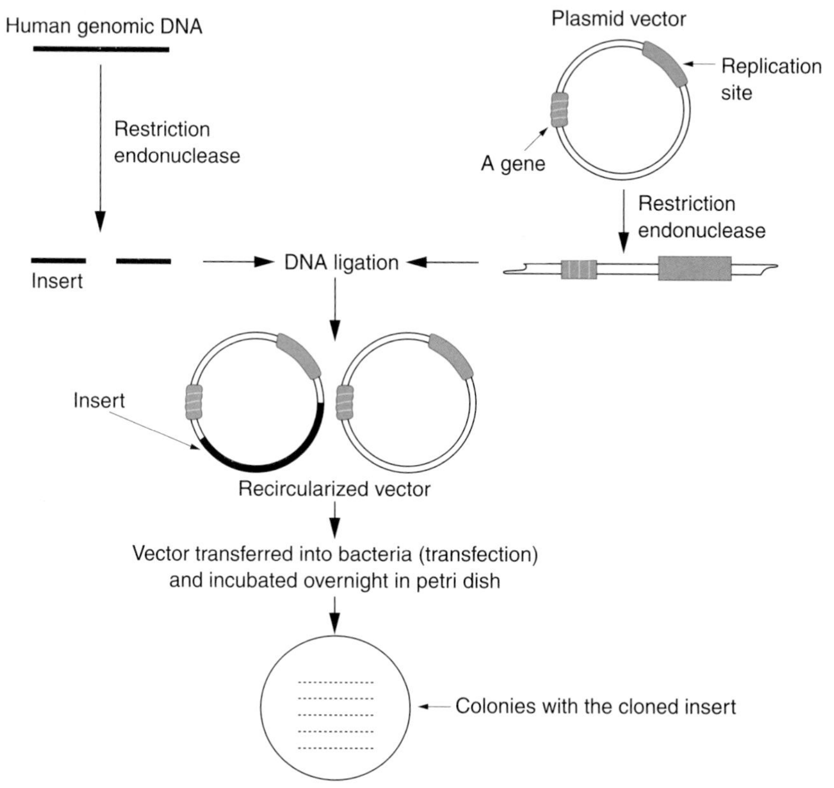

FIGURE 5–12. DNA cloning. The basic objective of cloning is to provide multiple copies of a DNA fragment of interest. The fundamental principles for cloning of a specific DNA fragment are as follows: (1) The human DNA fragment of interest is isolated from human DNA (*shown on the left*) by using a restriction endonuclease enzyme. The fragment obtained to be cloned is referred to as the *DNA insert* (*bottom*). (2) A DNA vector is selected (*shown on the right*), usually a plasmid, that has circular DNA and contains the necessary replication site (as indicated) and a drug resistance gene (A gene, *top*). The vector's DNA is digested with a restriction endonuclease so that the circular DNA of the plasmid is linearized (*as shown on the right*). (3) DNA ligase is selected to join both ends of the insert to both ends of the linearized vector DNA such that it is again recircularized. The vector DNA containing the insert along with the antibiotic resistance gene is transferred into a host cell, which is usually bacteria. The bacteria are now plated on a petri dish and incubated (usually overnight) to grow colonies. The culture medium in the petri dish contains an antibiotic to which the bacteria containing the plasmid vector will be resistant. Thus, the only bacteria to form colonies will be those resistant to the antibiotic. Because the insert and the antibiotic resistance gene are together in the vector's DNA, the only bacteria to form colonies will be those that contain the insert. As the bacteria host proliferates, so will the insert of interest proliferate (cloned), usually to approximately 1 million copies after 24 hours.

【 】 POLYMERASE CHAIN REACTION—DNA PROLIFERATION WITHOUT CLONING

PCR has revolutionized the application of the techniques of molecular biology. This technique was not developed until 1985,[32,33] but its impact has been felt throughout medicine and biotechnology. This procedure, conveniently and without the tedium of cloning, can provide 1 million copies of a DNA fragment in 3 to 4 hours and 1 billion copies within 24 hours. PCR simply and ingeniously takes advantage of the natural DNA replication process. One must know the sequence of the two ends of the DNA fragment that is to be amplified, but short sequences of 15 to 30 bp are adequate, and fragments in between these sequences as large as 20 kb can be amplified. The sequence is used to make two oligonucleotides, referred to as *primers,* with one for each end of the DNA fragment. The sequence of one primer is complementary to the sense direction, and the sequence of the other is made complementary to the antisense direction. The primers are used to prime the synthesis of cDNA strands and are designed such that the DNA between the primers is the fragment of interest to be amplified. If mRNA is to be amplified, it is first converted to a cDNA using the enzyme RT. The primers (oligonucleotides) and the necessary bases are added in excess, together with the enzyme, Taq DNA polymerase (which catalyzes DNA synthesis) and a sample containing the DNA to be amplified. There are three steps to each cycle. Initially, one must denature the DNA (separate the primers and the native DNA) into separate strands, which is done by increasing the temperature to 203°F (95°C). The temperature is then decreased to 122°F (50°C) so that the primers and native DNA will reanneal to their complementary base sequences. The native DNA strands will bind not only to each other but also to the primers. The temperature is now increased to 149°F (65°C) for synthesis of the new DNA fragments. Synthesis in the presence of Taq1 polymerase is initiated at the 5′ end, and further nucleotides are added in the 5′ to 3′ direction to provide the desired double-stranded DNA fragment. Taq1 DNA polymerase, isolated from *Thermus aquaticus,* is thermostable, which is of tremendous advantage in performing the PCR reaction. Because the high temperatures of up to 203°F (95°C) do not destroy this polymerase, it negates the need to add DNA polymerase between each cycle. Furthermore, because Taq polymerase has an optimal activity at approximately 158°F (70°C), one can significantly accelerate DNA synthesis. The cycle is then repeated, and after approximately 30 cycles over 3 hours, one should have approximately 1 million copies. There are many clinical applications for PCR. To make a diagnosis of viral myocarditis, for example, one can use PCR to amplify from a myocardial biopsy any specific viral RNA or DNA for which primers can be made. The sensitivity of most conventional techniques is inadequate to detect molecules unless present in 50,000 to 100,000 copies per cell. In contrast, only one copy of RNA or DNA is needed for detection by PCR, and in 3 to 4 hours, up to 1 million copies can be generated, which is adequate abundance for detection by most conventional techniques. PCR offers exquisite diagnostic sensitivity and specificity for determining the etiology of cardiac disorders such as myocarditis, and in patients undergoing cardiac transplantation, it is used for detecting infection or immunologic rejection. Another application of PCR is to detect and amplify mutations associated with hereditary disorders. One also can sequence DNA directly from PCR without the need for cloning.

REFERENCES

1. Watson JD, Crick FHC. Molecular structure of nucleic acids: a structure for deoxyribose nucleic acid. *Nature.* 1953;171:737–738.
2. Schekman R, Weiner A, Kornberg A. Multienzyme systems of DNA replication. *Science.* 1956;186:987–993.
3. Marmor J, Lane L. Strand separation and specific recombination of deoxyribonucleic acids: biological studies. *Proc Natl Acad Sci U S A.* 1960;46:453–461.
4. Leder P, Nirenberg M. RNA code words and protein synthesis: II. Nucleotide sequence of a valine RNA code word. *Proc Natl Acad Sci U S A.* 1964;52:420–427.
5. Nishimura S, Jones DS, Khorana HG. The in vitro synthesis of a copolypeptide containing two amino acids in alternative sequence dependent upon a DNA-like polymer containing two nucleotides in alternating sequence. *J Mol Biol.* 1981;146:1–21.
6. Olivera BM, Hall ZW, Lehman IR. Enzymatic joining of polynucleotides: V. A DNA adenylate intermediate in the polynucleotide joining reaction. *Proc Natl Acad Sci U S A.* 1968;61:237–244.
7. Smith HO, Wilcox KW. A restriction enzyme from *Hemophilus influenzae:* I. Purification and general properties. *J Mol Biol.* 1970;51:379–391.
8. Baltimore D. Viral RNA-dependent DNA polymerase. *Nature.* 1970;226:1209–1211.
9. Temin HM, Mizutani S. RNA-dependent DNA polymerase in virions of Rous sarcoma virus. *Nature.* 1970;226:1211–1213.
10. Cohen S, Chang A, Boyer H, Helling R. Construction of biological functional bacterial plasmids in vitro. *Proc Natl Acad Sci U S A.* 1973;70:3240–3244.
11. Sanger F, Coulson AR. A rapid method for determining sequences in DNA by primed synthesis and DNA polymerase. *J Mol Biol.* 1975;94:444–448.
12. Maxam AM, Gilbert W. A new method of sequencing DNA. *Proc Natl Acad Sci U S A.* 1977;74:560–564.
13. Metzler DE. The nucleic acids. In: Metzler DE, ed. *Biochemistry: The Chemical Reaction of Living Cells.* 2nd ed. Burlington, MA: Harcourt/Academic Press; 2001:198–279.
14. Lodish H, Berk A, Zipursky SL, et al. Nucleic acids, the genetic code, and the synthesis of macromolecules. In: *Molecular Cell Biology.* 4th ed. Houndsmills, Basingstoke, England: Freeman; 2000:100–137.
15. Lodish H, Berk A, Zipursky SL, et al. Regulation of the eukaryotic cell cycle. In: *Molecular Cell Biology.* 4th ed. Houndsmills, Basingstoke, England: Freeman; 2000:500–505.
16. Roberts R. Modern molecular biology: historical perspective and future potential. In: Roberts R, ed. *Molecular Basis of Cardiology.* Hamden, CT: Blackwell Scientific; 1992:1–15.
17. Carrozza MJ, Utley RT, Workman JL, Coate J. The diverse functions of histone acetyltransferase complexes. *Trends Genet.* 2003;19;321–329.
18. Henikoff S, Furuyama T, Ahmad K. Histone variants, nucleosome assembly and epigenetic inheritance. *Trends Genet.* 2004;20;320–326.
19. Khorasanizadeh S. The nucleosome: from genomic organization to genomic regulation. *Cell.* 2004;116:259–272.
20. Spotswood HT, Turner BM. An increasingly complex code. *J Clin Invest.* 2002;110(5):577–582.
21. Sun ZW, Allis CD. Ubiquitination of histone H2B regulates H3 methylation and gene silencing in yeast. *Nature.* 2002;418(6893):104–108.
22. Zhang CL, McKinsey TA, Chang S, Antos CL, Hill JA, Olson EN. Class II histone deacetylases act as signal-responsive repressors of cardiac hypertrophy. *Cell.* 2002;110(4):479–488.
23. Kee HJ, Sohn IS, Nam KI, et al. Inhibition of histone deacetylation blocks cardiac hypertrophy induced by angiotensin II infusion and aortic banding. *Circulation.* 2006;113:51–59.
24. Marian AJ, Roberts R. The molecular genetic basis for hypertrophic cardiomyopathy. *J Mol Cell Cardiol.* 2001;33(4):655–670.
25. Bartel DP. MicroRNAs: genomics, biogenesis, mechanism and function. *Cell.* 2004;116:281–297.
26. Novina CD, Sharp PA. The RNAi Revolution. *Nature.* 2004;430:161–164.
27. Mellow C-C, Conte D. Revealing the world of RNA interference. *Nature.* 2004;431:338–342.
28. Southern EM. Detection of specific sequences among DNA fragments separated by gel electrophoresis. *J Mol Biol.* 1975;98:503–517.
29. Young RA. Biomedical discovery with DNA arrays. *Cell.* 2000;102:9–15.
30. Liew C-C, Dzau VJ. Molecular genetics and genomics of heart failure. *Nat Genet.* 2004;5(11):811–825.
31. Ma J, Liew C-C. Gene profiling identifies secreted protein transcripts from peripheral blood cells in coronary artery disease. *J Mol Cell Cardiol.* 2003;35(8):993–998.
32. Saiki RK, Scharf S, Faloona F, et al. Enzymatic amplification of beta-globin genomic sequences and restriction site analysis for diagnosis of sickle cell anemia. *Science.* 1985;230:1350–1354.
33. Saiki RK, Gelfand DH, Stoffel S, et al. Primer-directed enzymatic amplification of DNA with a thermostable DNA polymerase. *Science.* 1988;239:487–491.

CHAPTER (6)

Molecular and Cellular Biology of the Normal, Hypertrophied, and Failing Heart

Allen M. Samarel / Richard A. Walsh

INTRODUCTION

Growth of the heart is a dynamic process that occurs during embryogenesis, postnatal development, maturity, and senescence, as well as in response to changing environmental and pathologic conditions. Cardiac growth occurs at the cellular level because of the interplay between *hyperplasia* (increase in cell number) and *hypertrophy* (increase in cell size) or a combination of both processes. The relative importance of each of these two mechanisms depends on the cell type, developmental stage, and nature of the growth stimulus. These two forms of cellular growth are variably modulated by *apoptosis,* or programmed cell death. Apoptosis is of importance in the determination of heart shape and chamber formation during cardiogenesis and may contribute to altered cardiac chamber geometry and mass in response to pathologic stimuli. Physiologic growth of the heart is generally mediated by developmental programs, mechanical load, and locally derived and circulating growth factors, whereas pathologic cardiovascular growth is generally mediated by similar factors as well as superimposed myocardial injury. These processes stimulate a repertoire of biochemical signals that alter the cardiovascular phenotype. The application of molecular and cell biological approaches to this problem is rapidly defining the precise factors responsible for normal and pathologic growth of the heart and the mechanisms responsible for altered cardiac function.

CARDIAC GROWTH AND PHYSIOLOGIC HYPERTROPHY

Cardiac hypertrophy is a process wherein there is an increase in chamber mass produced largely by an increase in the size of fully differentiated cardiomyocytes. Although cardiomyocytes make up only one-third of the total cell number, they are responsible in aggregate for more than 70 percent of cardiac volume. Cardiac hypertrophy may be functionally categorized as either physiologic or pathologic (Fig. 6–1).

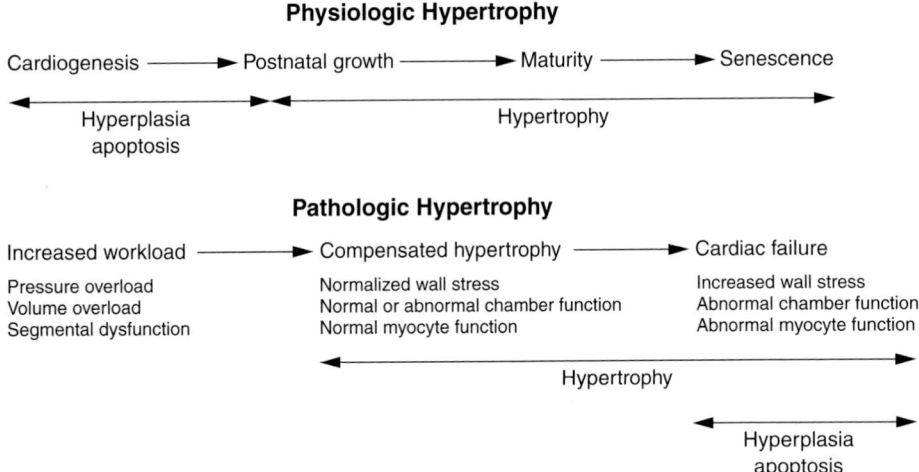

FIGURE 6-1. Relative roles of cardiomyocyte hypertrophy, hyperplasia, and apoptosis in physiologic and pathologic cardiac hypertrophy, along with the functional differences between compensated hypertrophy and heart failure.

【 】 GROWTH OF THE HEART DURING NORMAL DEVELOPMENT

Cardiac growth during normal development (also referred to as *cardiac eutrophy*) includes cardiogenesis during embryonic and fetal development, postnatal cardiac growth, and the modest additional increase in heart size that evolves during senescence (see Fig. 6–1). The earliest stage of cardiac growth in utero depends on a genetically determined developmental program, because it can occur in the absence of contractile activity. Subsequently, mechanical forces become increasingly important in the development of the normal cardiac phenotype. Throughout the embryonic period and for a few weeks after birth, cardiac growth occurs as a consequence of both hyperplasia and hypertrophy of cardiomyocytes, with the final round of karyokinesis (nuclear division), but not cytokinesis (cell division), producing a mixture of mononucleate and binucleate cells. Growth of the left ventricle exceeds that of the right ventricle during the early postnatal period as the mammalian heart transits from the fetal- to adult-type circulation. Thereafter, the heart undergoes a sixfold increase in mass. The normal heart-to-body weight ratio then remains relatively constant throughout adolescence and adulthood and is species-specific. The largest hearts relative to body size occur in animals with survival requirements that depend on sustained exercise rather than on burst activity.

Adult cardiomyocytes have long been viewed as terminally differentiated—that is, as incapable of reentering the cell cycle—and there is little evidence that they are capable of cell division under normal conditions after the early postnatal period. However, there is some evidence to suggest that a small subpopulation of adult cardiomyocytes re-enter the cell cycle and proliferate, especially at the border zone following recent myocardial infarction.[1] The origin of the replicating cardiomyocytes is presently unclear. They may be derived from a resident pool of cardiac stem cells or, alternatively, from bone marrow–derived, circulating stem cells that home to the heart following tissue injury. The capacity to reactivate hyperplasia in the terminally differentiated cardiomyocyte is an area of intense research interest, with potentially important therapeutic implications in the hypertrophied and failing heart.[2]

【 】 PHYSIOLOGIC HYPERTROPHY OF EXERCISE

Cardiac hypertrophy of the adult heart also occurs in response to athletic conditioning. In humans and experimental animals, intense, prolonged exercise training can produce an increase in cardiac mass. Isotonic exercise, such as running, produces *eccentric hypertrophy*, characterized by a normal ratio of wall thickness-to-dimension; whereas isometric exercise, such as weight lifting, stimulates *concentric hypertrophy*, associated with an increased wall thickness-to-dimension ratio. Senescent animals and aged humans free of organic heart disease also develop mild concentric left ventricular hypertrophy as a consequence of an age-related decrease in the distensibility of the peripheral vasculature. The molecular, biochemical, and physiologic changes associated with physiologic hypertrophy differ both qualitatively and quantitatively from those that occur during pathologic hypertrophy. Physiologic studies in animal models and humans have demonstrated no substantial alterations in isolated muscle or intact heart function. There is also little evidence of alterations in the molecular determinants of excitation–contraction coupling. Most importantly, epidemiologic data fail to demonstrate adverse risk associated with the modest hypertrophy that occurs as a consequence of athletic conditioning. It is, therefore, important clinically to distinguish physiologic hypertrophy of exercise from hypertrophic cardiomyopathy in athletes.

【 】 PATHOLOGIC HYPERTROPHY

In most clinically relevant situations, pathologic hypertrophy serves as an important adaptive response to regional or global increases in systolic and/or diastolic wall stress (see Fig. 6–1). Initially, the increase in cardiac mass serves to normalize wall stress and permit normal cardiovascular function at rest and during exercise. Nevertheless, during the *compensated* phase of pathologic hypertrophy, distinct alterations in myocardial gene expression occur; and these changes may serve to maintain function in the context of increased wall stress.[3] In rodents and other small mammals, ventricular myocytes undergoing pathologic hypertrophy express a subset of genes that are normally expressed predominantly during fetal life. These include β-myosin heavy chain (β-MHC), α-skeletal actin, and atrial natriuretic peptide.[4] Pathologic hypertrophy may be caused by pressure overload, as in systemic or pulmonary arterial hypertension, left ventricular outflow obstruction, or aortic coarctation. Pressure overload produces a disproportionate increase in systolic wall stress and results in concentric ventricular hypertrophy. At the cellular level, cardiomyocyte cross-sectional area is increased, predominantly because of the parallel addition of new sarcomeres. Similarly, volume overload, as occurs in mitral or aortic regurgitation or as a result of an arteriovenous fistula, also produces pathologic hypertrophy. These latter conditions induce an increase in either diastolic wall stress (mitral regurgitation) or both systolic and diastolic wall stress (aortic regurgitation and arteriovenous fistulas) and result in eccentric left ventricular hypertrophy. Eccentric hypertrophy results in an overall increase in myocyte length without a substantial increase in myocyte cross-sectional area and is caused by the addition of new sarcomeres in series. Regional hypertrophy that occurs in viable myocardium adjacent to and remote from an area of infarction also has the characteristics of eccentric hypertrophy. The cellular mechanisms responsible for the distinctive changes in cardiomyocyte shape that result from pressure versus volume overload remain unknown but is the subject of considerable interest to cell biologists. Regardless of the nature of the hemodynamic overload, however, if the stimulus for pathologic hypertrophy is sufficiently intense or prolonged, *decompensated hypertrophy* and heart failure ensue.

There are exceptions to the principle that pathologic hypertrophy primarily occurs as a consequence of excessive increases in external cardiac work. For example, familial hypertrophic cardiomyopathy is most often produced by a point mutation in one of several different sarcomeric proteins, in particular β-MHC. These mutations result in massive asymmetric or concentric hypertrophy in the absence of augmented peripheral hemodynamic requirements. In some forms of the disease, the contractile protein gene mutations are *gain of function,* resulting in a hypercontractile state with an increased Ca^{2+} sensitivity of the contractile apparatus and increased force generation at submaximal Ca^{2+} concentrations.[5] Thus, the hypertrophic response appears related to an increase in *internal* rather than external cardiac work. In contrast, genetically engineered mice with cardiac-specific postnatal overexpression of the β2-adrenergic receptor[6] or targeted ablation of the phospholamban gene[7] have enhanced cardiac function throughout life but no significant increase in cardiac mass, thus dissociating increased internal cardiac work from the hypertrophic response. Furthermore, certain genetically engineered mice with a reduced capacity to undergo hypertrophy in response to pressure overload maintain preserved cardiac function without normalization of wall stress.[8] Finally, tachycardia-induced heart failure in animal models and humans is associated with increased external cardiac work, decreased cardiac function, and no alteration in cardiac mass.[9] These and other disparate observations suggest a critical reexamination of the primary role of mechanical load in the etiology of certain forms of pathologic hypertrophy.

MECHANISMS FOR THE DEVELOPMENT OF CARDIAC HYPERTROPHY

Cardiovascular investigators have witnessed an explosion in new knowledge concerning the cellular and molecular mechanisms responsible for cardiac growth and remodeling. Much of the recently acquired information has relied on reproducible techniques to isolate and culture neonatal and adult cardiac myocytes in vitro and to manipulate cardiac gene expression in vivo using transgenic and knockout strategies.[10] These results have identified intracellular signaling pathways responsible for hypertrophic growth during both physiologic and pathologic hypertrophy, as outlined below.

[ ] MECHANOTRANSDUCTION

Based primarily on studies of isolated cells maintained in primary culture, it is clear that cardiomyocytes can undergo hypertrophic growth in response to mechanical loading in the absence of other exogenous stimuli. The process by which stimuli in the physical domain activate intracellular growth-signaling pathways is known as *mechanotransduction*. For example, cyclic or static stretch of pure populations of neonatal or adult myocytes attached to a flexible substratum stimulates protein synthesis, induces the assembly of newly synthesized contractile proteins into sarcomeres, and results in cellular hypertrophy.[11] Cardiomyocyte mechanotransduction appears critically important during physiologic growth of the heart, as well as during many forms of pathologic hypertrophy.

Cardiomyocytes rely on several intracellular components to sense mechanical load and convert mechanical stimuli into biochemical events that affect cellular structure and function. These sensors include protein components within the myofilaments and Z-discs, stretch-activated ion channels, and other membrane-associated proteins involved in cell-cell junction formation. However, much of the recent evidence points to components of the extracellular matrix (ECM)–integrin-cytoskeletal complex as critically important to the process of mechanotransduction during cardiomyocyte hypertrophy.[12] Cardiomyocytes attach to ECM proteins via cell surface receptors known as *integrins* (Fig. 6–2). Integrins are heterodimeric integral membrane proteins consisting of single α and β chains. At least 18 α and 8 β subunits have been identified, with more than 24 paired integrin receptors expressed.[13] Additional complexity arises from the existence of multiple isoforms of individual α and β chains generated by alternative splicing of α and β integrin mRNAs. Cardiomyocytes express $α_1$, $α_3$, $α_5$, $α_6$, $α_7$, $α_9$, and $α_{10}$, whereas the predominant β subunit expressed is the ubiquitous $β_{1A}$ subunit, and

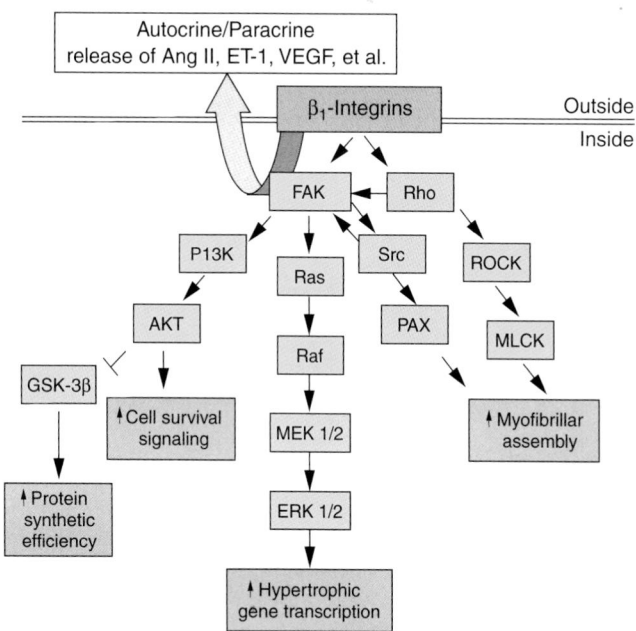

FIGURE 6–2. Schematic diagram of some of the signaling pathways known to be activated in cardiomyocytes following integrin engagement and clustering. Integrins may directly stimulate downstream effectors involved in hypertrophic gene expression, cell survival, enhanced protein synthesis, and myofibrillar assembly via the activation of focal adhesion kinase and Rho-dependent signaling pathways. Alternatively, integrins transduce signals by sensing mechanical stimuli, which leads to the autocrine/paracrine release of growth factors into the extracellular space and activation of their cognate receptors.

the striated muscle-specific β_{1D} isoform. The relative expression of the various α chains varies throughout development, and in response to hemodynamic overload, suggesting an important regulatory role of integrins in cardiomyocyte mechanotransduction.[13]

Cardiomyocyte integrins are not randomly distributed on the cell surface but are found within the sarcolemmal membrane directly adjacent to costameres. Costameres are band-like structures that link the Z-discs to the sarcolemmal membrane and are therefore considered important sites for bidirectional communication of mechanical forces.[14] The physical interaction between integrin cytoplasmic domains and adaptor proteins within the cytoskeleton generate a submembrane adhesion plaque that appears critical for transmitting mechanical force between the ECM and the actin cytoskeleton. In addition to their structural role, costameres are also sites for the localization of signaling molecules that are important in cardiomyocyte survival and growth, including protein tyrosine kinases such as FAK, PYK2, Src, and Csk as well as serine-threonine protein kinases such as ILK, PKCε, and PAK. Adapter proteins, such as Crk, DOCK180, and Cas, and the small GTPase Rho can link focal adhesion proteins to other downstream signaling cascades that may be important in both mechanotransduction and growth factor signaling (see Fig. 6–2). In general, there appears to be substantial crosstalk between integrin and growth factor receptors in many cell types, suggesting that integrin- and growth factor–mediated cellular responses are locally coordinated within focal adhesions.[15]

The ECM-integrin-cytoskeletal complex can directly activate cytosolic signal transduction pathways that initiate gene transcription and translation of increased quantities of cardiomyocyte contractile proteins. Alternatively, activation of the mechanosensory complex can lead to enhanced production and secretion of peptide growth factors and cytokines into the surrounding extracellular space, thereby initiating growth by means of an autocrine or paracrine mechanism (see Fig. 6–2). Indeed, autocrine/paracrine production and release of angiotensin II, endothelin 1, vascular endothelial growth factor (VEGF), and other growth factors may be responsible for a considerable proportion of the growth response of cultured cardiomyocytes to mechanical stretch in vitro and the intact heart to pressure overload in vivo.[16]

Important downstream signal transduction pathways that are directly or indirectly activated by mechanical deformation include the focal adhesion kinase family of nonreceptor protein tyrosine kinases, protein kinase C (PKC) isoenzymes, and the mitogen-activated protein kinases. In particular, cultured neonatal cardiomyocytes stretch causes Gαq-protein–coupled receptor activation through autocrine/paracrine release of growth factors into the culture medium (Fig. 6–3). Stretch-induced guanosine triphosphate (GTP) loading of Gαq in turn activates membrane-bound phospholipase C-β (PLC-β), which in turn hydrolyzes phosphatidylinositol 4,5-bisphosphate (PIP$_2$) to inositol triphosphate (IP$_3$) and diacylglycerol (DAG). Membrane-bound diacylglycerol then directly activates to varying degrees the phorbol-ester sensitive isoenzymes PKCα, PKCβ, PKCδ, and PKCε. Phosphorylation of downstream cytosolic and nuclear proteins and transcription factors by PKC isoenzymes is critical for growth in a number of cell types, whereas IP$_3$ is an important modulator of cytosolic calcium homeostasis by the interaction with its receptor within the sarco-

plasmic reticulum. Angiotensin II receptor coupling appears to play a critical role in the activation of PLC by mechanical load; however, endothelin-1 and α$_1$-adrenergic receptor stimulation can also activate these pathways, with resultant hypertrophy in neonatal cardiomyocytes and in transgenic mice.[17]

Current information suggests that mechanotransduction and the interrelated autocrine/paracrine effects of locally produced growth factors mediate features of both physiologic and pathologic hypertrophy. The resultant activation of multiple signal transduction pathways, which have demonstrable crosstalk and considerable redundancy, provides a powerful mechanism by which the heart can respond to changing chronic hemodynamic requirements (see Fig. 6–3). A point of downstream convergence of multiple signal transduction pathways in cardiomyocytes is the phosphorylation and activation of the mitogen-activated protein kinases (MAPKs).[18] Mammalian MAPKs are a family of serine-threonine protein kinases that are generally subdivided into 3 classes: extracellular regulated kinases (ERKs), c-Jun N-terminal kinases (JNKs), and p38^{MAPKs}. Although all three MAPK subfamilies have been implicated in hypertrophic signaling, the JNKs and p38^{MAPK} appear to serve a more specialized role in signaling stress and tissue injury.[19] The ERK cascade, however, is activated by signal transduction pathways coupled to both phosphatidylinositol hydrolysis/PKC activation and receptor protein tyrosine kinases. Of particular importance to cardiac hypertrophy is the observation that important transcription factors involved in hypertrophic gene transcription (c-Jun, c-myc, c-fos, Elk-1, SRF, GATA4, and others) are known phosphorylation targets of activated MAPKs, and MAPKs translocate into the nucleus in response to stretch and growth factor stimulation. Information from noncardiomyocyte cell systems, cultured neonatal and adult myocytes, and genetically engineered mice has demonstrated considerable complexity, redundancy, and crosstalk among these and other intracellular signaling pathways in the development of the cardiac hypertrophy phenotype in response to stretch and other stimuli.[20] In particular, ischemia, hypoxia, oxidative stress, neurohormones, and cytokines can all activate downstream signaling and resultant nuclear transcriptional events, including cardiomyocyte hypertrophy and fibroblast hyperplasia.

【 】 INSULINLIKE GROWTH FACTOR-1 AND PHYSIOLOGIC HYPERTROPHY

In addition to mechanical factors, there is now substantial evidence based on studies performed in isolated cardiomyocytes and transgenic mice that the peptide growth factor insulinlike growth factor-1 (IGF-1) plays an important role in physiologic hypertrophy of the heart during normal development and in response to exercise training.[21] It is produced in the liver and other organs in response to circulating growth hormone; IGF-1 receptors are receptor tyrosine kinases present on the sarcolemmal membrane of cardiomyocytes, where they transduce growth signals to the nucleus and protein synthetic machinery with the activation of a PI3-K/PDK1/Akt-dependent signal transduction pathway (see Fig. 6–3). Cardiac expression of a kinase-deficient form of the catalytic subunit of PI3-K in transgenic mice impaired normal cardiac growth and prevented physiologic hypertrophy caused by swimming but not pathologic hypertrophy in response to pressure overload.[21] Similarly, cardiac-specific overexpression of IGF-1 re-

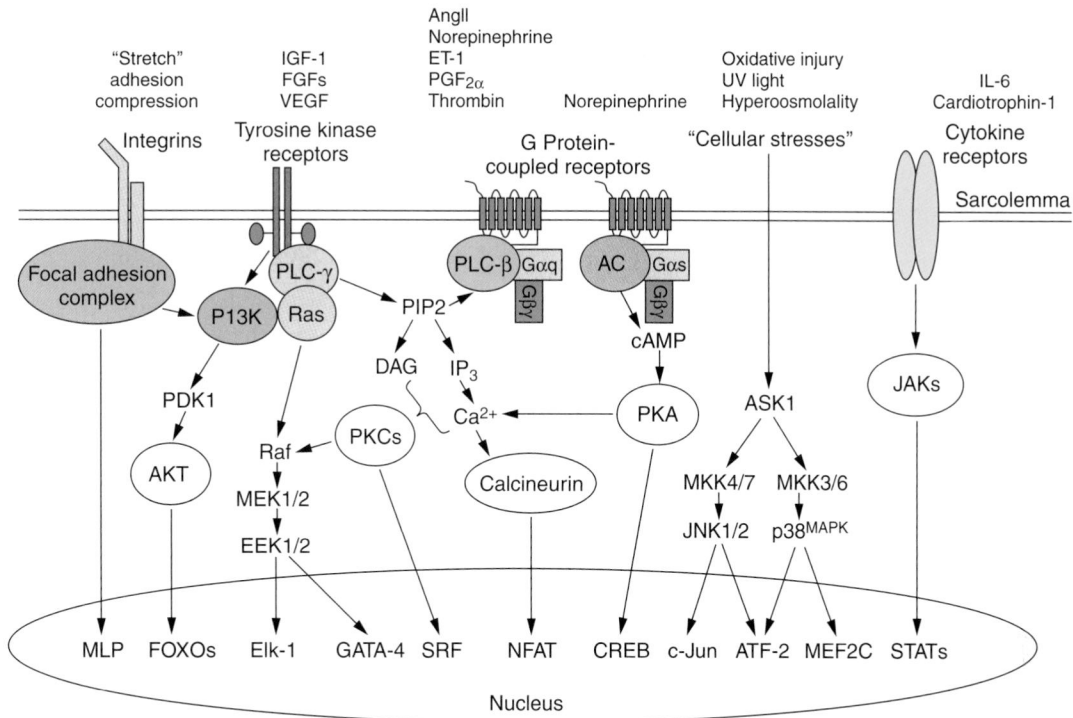

FIGURE 6–3. A schematic outlining some of the overlapping signal transduction pathways that activate transcriptional regulation and induce hypertrophic genes. Integrin receptors share many downstream signaling components common to receptor tyrosine kinases and G protein–coupled receptors. In addition, one component of the focal adhesion complex, the muscle LIM protein, may translocate to the nucleus following integrin engagement and clustering and serve as a coactivator of gene transcription. Insulin-like growth factor-1 (IGF-1), fibroblast growth factors (FGFs), vascular endothelial growth factors (VEGFs), and other peptide growth factors interact with their cognate membrane receptor tyrosine kinases, which then activate phospholipase C-γ (PLC-γ) and Ras. Ras in turn activates Raf, MAPK/ERK-activating kinases (MEK1/2), and the extracellular signal-regulated kinases (ERKs). Other pathways mediated by Ras activation include the phosphoinositol-3-kinases (PI3K), phosphoinositol-dependent protein kinase (PDK1), and protein kinase B (also known as *AKT*) pathway important in cell survival signaling and the regulation of protein synthesis. The G protein–coupled receptor agonists norepinephrine, endothelin-1, prostaglandin $F_{2}\alpha$ (PG-$F_{2}\alpha$), and thrombin can all bind to their receptors and activate PLC-β via the dissociated α subunit of a GTP-binding protein of the Gq class (Gαq). PLC-β, like PLC-γ, catalyzes the hydrolysis of phosphatidylinositol bisphosphate (PIP$_2$) into diacylglycerol (DAG) and inositol triphosphate (IP$_3$). DAG is required for the activation of the Ca^{2+}-dependent (α and β) and Ca^{2+}-independent (δ and ε) isoenzymes of protein kinase C (PKC), whereas IP$_3$ induces the release of Ca^{2+} from intracellular stores. PKCs activated by DAG ± Ca^{2+} initiate cascades of phosphorylation. One of the downstream targets of PKC signaling is the Ras/Raf/MEK/ERK cascade. In contrast, activation of β-adrenergic receptors leads to increased cyclic adenosine monophosphate production and signaling via adenylyl cyclases (ACs) and protein kinase A (PKA). Intracellular targets of PKA include L-type Ca^{2+} channels, phospholamban, and the ryanodine receptor, all leading to dramatic increases in $[Ca^{2+}]_i$. Ca^{2+} itself initiates signaling via several important Ca^{2+}-dependent signaling kinases, as well as via the Ca^{2+}-calmodulin dependent phosphatase, calcineurin. Activated calcineurin dephosphorylates nuclear factor of activated T lymphocytes (NFAT), which translocates into the nucleus to interact with multiple transcription factors. Cellular stresses can activate other members of the MAPK family, including *c-Jun* N-terminal kinases (JNKs) and p38^{MAPK}, perhaps via activation of apoptosis signaling kinase-1 (ASK1) and the MAPK kinases, but small G proteins of the Rho family (i.e., Rac and Rho) are also likely to be involved. Signaling through interleukin-1 (IL-1) and cardiotrophin-1 (CT-1) receptors involves gp 130, which acts as a signal transducing receptor component. The binding of ligands to their cognate receptors results in receptor dimerization, autophosphorylation, and activation of the associated Janus kinase (JAK). In turn, JAK activates members of the STAT (signal transducer and activator of transcription) family. Many of the aforementioned signaling components then translocate into the nucleus and phosphorylate transcription factors necessary for hypertrophic gene transcription, cell survival, and apoptosis.

ceptors in transgenic mice produced *physiologic* cardiac growth indistinguishable from that produced by exercise training.[22]

[ ] THYROID HORMONES

Administration of excess thyroid hormone to experimental animals produces increased heart weight, which is associated with transcriptionally mediated alterations in the MHCs, calcium-cycling proteins, and other functional constituents of the cardiomyocyte.[23] Thyroid hormone–induced hypertrophy is predominantly an indirect effect of the T_3-mediated increased oxygen consumption and resultant augmentation of cardiac work. For example, heterotopic transplantation of a nonworking rat heart into the abdominal aorta of the hyperthyroid animal is unassociated with hypertrophy, de-

spite the presence of the transcriptionally mediated effects of the hormone in the transplanted organ and hypertrophy and typical transcriptional events in the native working heart.[24] Features of thyroid-induced cardiac hypertrophy are most consistent with physiologic, rather than pathologic hypertrophy, with increased organ growth in the absence of fibrosis, and enhanced, rather than depressed cardiac function.[25]

[ ] OTHER HORMONES AND CYTOKINES

Circulating Gαq-coupled receptor agonists—which include angiotensin II, endothelin-1, prostaglandin F2α, and thrombin—can induce hypertrophy of neonatal cardiomyocytes in culture in the absence of altered mechanical forces and in vivo in genetically engineered mice when their receptors are overexpressed (see Fig. 6–3). Activation of Gαq-coupled receptors or overexpression of Gαq itself in transgenic mice produces many of the features of pathologic hypertrophy. Indeed, Gαq activation has been shown to be essential for the development of pathologic hypertrophy in response to pressure overload.[26]

Cytokines were initially characterized by their pleiotropic effects on the cellular components of the immune system. They have recently been implicated in normal and pathologic cardiac growth by a variety of in vitro and in vivo animal studies and by clinical investigation. Cytokines of the interleukin-6 and cardiotrophin family activate the cardiomyocyte gp 130 transmembrane receptor and rapidly stimulate cytoplasmic Janus kinases (JAKs); these, in turn phosphorylate other cytoplasmic proteins called *signal transducers and activators of transcription* (STATs) (see Fig. 6–3). Various components of gp 130 and JAK-STAT pathways have induced hypertrophy in vitro and in vivo when overexpressed in transgenic mice.[27] By contrast, interleukin-1 and tumor necrosis factor alpha (TNF-α) use a distinct pathway that involves activation of a phosphatidylcholine-specific phospholipase C with generation of diacylglycerol. Despite the fact that these cytokines are elevated in the plasma of patients with congestive heart failure, a clinical trial with a TNF-α inhibitor was halted because of a lack of therapeutic benefit and adverse events.[28]

There is increasing evidence that stimulation of cell-surface tyrosine-kinase receptors can elicit a hyperplastic or hypertrophic response in neonatal cardiomyocytes. Members of the fibroblast growth factor (FGF) family of peptide growth factors, which act as ligands for tyrosine-kinase receptors, can induce myocyte growth (see Fig. 6–3). In contrast, members of the transforming growth factor β (TGF-β) family of growth factors do not induce a growth response under these conditions but appear important to the regulation of ECM production by cardiac fibroblasts during pathologic hypertrophy and remodeling.[29]

In addition to FGFs and TGF-β, VEGF is expressed in the myocardium in response to pressure overload and tissue hypoxia. These and other peptide growth factors (neural growth factor [NGF], epidermal growth factor [EGF], platelet-derived growth factor [PDGF], and insulin) bind to receptor tyrosine kinases (RTKs), and undergo ligand-mediated homodimerization with resultant autophosphorylation of tyrosine residues on the cytoplasmic domain. These tyrosine complexes recruit signaling molecules such as the monomeric GTP-binding protein Ras to the membrane, where transient complexes stimulate downstream signaling to the nucleus via the ERK and PI3-K/Akt signaling cascades, thus stimulating growth.

NOREPINEPHRINE AND THE SYMPATHETIC NERVOUS SYSTEM

All three major adrenergic receptors for norepinephrine (α_1-, β_1-and β_2-adrenergic receptors) are expressed by cardiomyocytes, and all have been implicated in the induction of hypertrophic growth but by distinctly differing intracellular mechanisms.[30] In general, α_1-adrenergic receptors (ARs) activate signaling via Gαq/G_{11}-dependent pathways, whereas the β_1-AR adrenergic receptor couples to Gαs. The β_2-AR, in contrast, couples to both Gαs and G_i. Activation of small GTPases of the Rho family also occurs in re-

sponse to norepinephrine stimulation. Chronic infusion of norepinephrine in experimental animals produces pathologic hypertrophy, which can be prevented by concomitant administration of both β- and α_1-adrenergic blocking agents, suggesting a role for both types of receptors in the hypertrophic growth response to sympathetic stimulation of the heart.

CALCIUM SIGNALING

In addition to directly stimulating kinase-dependent signaling cascades, many peptide growth factors and neurohormones implicated in hypertrophic signaling also affect intracellular Ca^{2+} ($[Ca^{2+}]_i$), and increases in $[Ca^{2+}]_i$ have long been associated with hypertrophic cardiomyocyte growth in vitro. Global or subcompartmental increases in $[Ca^{2+}]_i$ can increase the force of contraction, thereby stimulating mechanotransduction, and also activate Ca^{2+}-dependent signaling molecules critical to cardiomyocyte hypertrophy. Indeed, a number of Ca^{2+}-dependent signaling molecules, including the Ca^{2+}-dependent isoenzymes of PKC (i.e., PKCα and PKCβ), calcium-calmodulin–dependent protein kinases (CaM-kinases), and the calcium-activated focal adhesion kinase PYK2, have been implicated in signaling specific aspects of cardiomyocyte hypertrophy. In addition, the Ca^{2+}-dependent phosphatase calcineurin has been shown in several experimental models of cardiac hypertrophy to be critically important to transcriptional regulation of the growth response. Calcineurin dephosphorylates nuclear factor for activation of transcription (NFAT), which translocates to the nucleus where it activates numerous transcription factors involved in hypertrophic gene expression including GATA-4. In vitro and in vivo studies using genetically engineered mice have demonstrated that augmented levels of activity of calcineurin, NFAT, or both can initiate a hypertrophic response.[31]

MOLECULAR TARGETS OF HYPERTROPHIC SIGNAL TRANSDUCTION

Signaling pathways that transduce hypertrophic growth signals converge on specific components of the intracellular machinery responsible for protein transcription and translation and also stimulate the assembly of newly synthesized contractile proteins into functional sarcomeres. Transcriptional control of gene expression is mediated by the activation of a variety of DNA-binding proteins that bind to specific sequences within the promoter regions of cardiac growth and remodeling genes and either activate or repress the transcription of their specific mRNAs.[32] Transcription factors work in concert with histone acetyltransferases (HATs) and histone deacetylases (HDACs) to control the acetylation state of nucleosomal histones, thereby affecting the state of chromatin condensation and relaxation.[33] Histone deacetylation by Class II HDACs is one way in which cytoplasmic signaling cascades serve to connect extracellular growth stimuli to nuclear events leading to the transcriptional regulation of an entire program of hypertrophy-related genes. HDACs function to suppress transcription, and nuclear export of HDACs is regulated by reversible phosphorylation. CaM-kinase–, PKC-, and Rho-dependent signaling pathways stimulate Class II HDAC phosphorylation, which in turn leads to their translocation out of the nucleus, thus allowing for association of MEF2 and other transcription factors with relaxed regions of chromatin. Inhibition of HDAC phosphorylation may be a useful way to repress specific aspects of the hypertrophic gene program that is associated with pathologic hypertrophy.

In addition to modulating gene transcription, hypertrophic growth signals regulate both the efficiency and capacity of contractile protein synthesis. Cardiomyocyte hypertrophy ultimately develops as the result of an imbalance between the rate of protein synthesis and the rate of protein degradation. Under normal circumstances, these two processes are matched and result in nitrogen balance. Because the average half-life of cardiac proteins is 5 to 7 days, the composition of the adult heart is regenerated approximately every 3 weeks. The more rapid rate of cardiac growth in response to increased hemodynamic load is invariably associated with a substantial increase in the rate of new protein synthesis and results from an augmentation in either the efficiency or capacity of protein synthesis or a combination of the two.[34] Protein synthetic efficiency is in part regulated by the phosphorylation state of components of the protein translational initiation complex; for example, phosphorylation of eIF4F follows activation of the ERK cascade.[35] Experiments in a variety of systems also indicate that a critical determinant for cardiac hypertrophy is an increased capacity for protein synthesis, which is mediated by augmented ribosomal biosynthesis and increased ribosomal content. Signaling pathways downstream of both the ERK and PI3-K cascades are likely involved.[36]

Relatively little is known about the molecular mechanisms whereby activation of cytoplasmic signaling pathways stimulates the assembly of newly synthesized contractile proteins into functional sarcomeres. Nevertheless, sarcomeric protein assembly may be the rate-limiting step in contractile protein turnover. Rates of contractile protein synthesis often exceed the rate at which contractile proteins are assembled, leading to enhanced degradation of the unassembled subunits by the proteasome and other components of the cell proteolytic machinery.[37] In cultured cardiomyocytes, sarcomerogenesis induced by Gαq-coupled agonists begins at the sarcolemmal membrane by the formation of premyofibrils, which may involve Rho and Ca^{2+}-dependent activation of myosin light chain kinase.[38] Sarcomere addition during length remodeling in response to mechanical stretch may also involve signaling via PKCε and FAK.[39]

PROTEIN CONTENT AND ISOFORM DIVERSITY

In addition to increased total protein content, cardiac hypertrophy is characterized by alterations in the relative abundance and isoform composition of the cardiomyocyte contractile, regulatory, and calcium-cycling proteins and other subcellular constituents. These processes provide an additional degree of plasticity for the heart to adapt to changing functional requirements.

[ ] CONTRACTILE PROTEIN ISOFORMS

It is clear that there is considerable species specificity in the capacity for isoform switching. In small mammals with rapid heart rates, such as mice and rats, imposition of a pressure overload produces a transcriptionally mediated shift from the αMHC to the βMHC and from cardiac to skeletal α-actin. αMHC has a three- to sevenfold greater ATPase activity than βMHC. The greater abundance

of βMHC in response to pressure overload in small animals increases the efficiency of force development by producing the same absolute muscle tension at a slower rate. Despite identical cardiac muscle mechanics in response to hypertrophy, large animals with slower heart rates, including humans, possess βMHC almost exclusively throughout embryogenesis and postnatal development. Nevertheless, the small amount of residual αMHC that is expressed in human myocardium is lost during human heart failure, which may contribute to contractile dysfunction.[40] It is also possible that, in higher mammalian species, altered myofibrillar ATPase in response to pressure- or volume-overload hypertrophy may be mediated in part by isoform shifts in other myofibrillar proteins. For example, cardiac isoforms exist for essential and regulatory light chains, troponin (I, C, and T), tropomyosin, and the sarcolemmal Na^+, K^+-ATPase. Isoform switching of each of the components of the cardiomyocyte has been reported in hypertrophy and failure, but the functional significance of this has been unclear.

[ ] EXTRACELLULAR MATRIX AND THE CYTOSKELETON

Although cardiomyocytes make up the bulk of cardiac mass by volume, they are tethered in an extensive extracellular network of collagen and other structural proteins, including fibronectins and proteoglycans. The extracellular scaffolding is a critical determinant of cardiac shape during normal and pathologic cardiac growth.[41] Collagen is synthesized principally by fibroblasts but also by vascular smooth muscle cells in response to a variety of pathologic stimuli, including increased oxidative and mechanical stress, ischemia, and inflammation. Most molecules and signal transduction pathways operant in cardiomyocyte growth play a role in hyperplasia of fibroblasts and in the elaboration of collagen. The resultant fibrosis produces altered myocardial stiffness and arrhythmogenesis in ischemic heart disease, cardiac hypertrophy, and congestive heart failure. Collagen synthesis is continuously and variably offset by extracellular matrix resorption mediated by matrix metalloproteinases. The activity of these enzymes is increased in dilated cardiomyopathy. Conversely, the activity of a class of enzymes known as *tissue inhibitors of matrix metalloproteinases* is reduced in this setting. The resultant excessive collagenolysis may induce myofibrillar slippage and contribute to the dilated thin-walled chamber geometry that characterizes acute and chronic heart failure.

Pressure overload (but not volume overload) hypertrophy has also been associated with changes in the levels of the cytoskeletal proteins titin, desmin, and tubulin. Depolymerization of tubulin with colchicine reversed abnormalities in cardiac function in feline right ventricular hypertrophy but not in guinea pig left ventricular hypertrophy.[42,43]

[ ] EXCITATION-CONTRACTION COUPLING AND CALCIUM HOMEOSTASIS

Cardiomyocyte excitation-contraction coupling is accomplished by a complex interplay between voltage-gated ion channels and transporters on the sarcolemmal membrane and specific membrane transporters and pumps within the sarcoplasmic reticulum (SR).[44] Based on studies of a variety of experimental model systems as well as work with human myocardium, it is now clear that defective Ca^{2+} regulation is a common feature of pathologic hypertrophy and its progression to heart failure as well as that these defects involve multiple molecules and processes. These include alterations in the expression levels of voltage-gated, L-type Ca^{2+} channels, SR calcium release channels, the Na^{+}-Ca^{2+} exchanger, the SR Ca^{2+} ATPase (SERCA2), and the regulatory protein phospholamban.[45] The molecular mechanisms responsible for SERCA2 downregulation during cardiac hypertrophy have been most extensively studied. SERCA2 gene expression is tightly regulated by both transcriptional and post-transcriptional mechanisms. SERCA2 downregulation and reduced SR Ca^{2+} pumps have been shown to cause prolongation of the $[Ca^{2+}]_i$ transient and reduced SR Ca^{2+} content, which are characteristic of the hypertrophied and failing cardiomyocyte.

CARDIAC FUNCTION IN PATHOLOGIC HYPERTROPHY

The phenotypic consequences of the increased cardiac mass and altered protein abundance and composition of the pathologically hypertrophied heart are considerable. They depend on the model used; animal species; and nature, intensity, and duration of the hypertrophic stimulus. Taken together, available clinical and animal studies suggest that functional alterations evolve along a continuum from normal chamber and myocyte function to abnormal chamber and normal myocyte function to abnormalities of both chamber and myocyte function.

[ ] ELECTRICAL PROPERTIES AND EXCITATION-CONTRACTION COUPLING

Patients with pathologic cardiac hypertrophy are at significantly increased risk of developing malignant arrhythmias, and this propensity accounts for a substantial proportion of the mortality related to both congenital and acquired hypertrophic heart diseases.[46] The proarrhythmic potential of the hypertrophied heart is most closely related to prolongation of the action potential, which predisposes to early and late afterdepolarizations.[47] Studies using the single-cell voltage-clamp technique help elucidate the ionic mechanisms responsible for this phenomenon. In mild hypertrophy, increases in calcium and calcium-activated inward currents (including the Na^{+}-Ca^{2+} exchanger) appear to be important. In severe hypertrophy, prolongation of the action potential is also determined importantly by a reduction in the outward potassium currents I_{K1} and I_{to}. The mechanisms for arrhythmogenesis are multifactorial and operant at the tissue and cardiomyocyte levels. Increased dispersion of refractoriness and slowed conduction result from myocyte loss and fibrosis, as well as a reduction in gap junction surface area per unit of cell volume.[48] Reduced coronary artery flow reserve and accelerated atherosclerosis of epicardial coronary vessels also predispose toward ischemia-induced arrhythmias. In concert, these mechanisms contribute to the finding of cardiac hypertrophy as a powerful, independent predictor of cardiovascular morbidity and mortality.[49]

Action potential prolongation is associated with changes in the amplitude and length of the $[Ca^{2+}]_i$ transient, which secondarily affects the velocity of contraction and relaxation. In cardiomyocytes with mild-to-moderate hypertrophy the peak systolic Ca^{2+} is normal in the basal state but becomes depressed when conditions that increase Ca^{2+} loading are imposed.[45]

[ ] MECHANICAL PROPERTIES

Mechanical function of the hypertrophied heart has been studied at the isolated myocyte, muscle, and chamber levels as well as in the intact circulation. These studies have revealed variable alterations in the rate and extent of contraction and relaxation, the amount of force development, and resting muscle and chamber properties. In the intact circulation, altered systolic and diastolic function is a composite result of subcellular changes in the cardiomyocyte, changes in the extracellular matrix, altered chamber geometry and mass, altered ventricular-vascular coupling, and the modulatory effects of neural and hormonal influences.

The earliest changes in mechanical performance observed in isometrically contracting papillary muscles extracted from hypertrophied hearts consist of a prolongation of time to peak tension and relaxation, despite normal peak twitch tension normalized for cross-sectional areas of the muscle. Afterloaded isotonically shortening papillary muscle preparations from hypertrophied hearts of a variety of animal species typically reveal a decrease in the force–velocity relationship and a depression of $\dot{V}_{max}$ (the extrapolated maximal unloaded shortening velocity). $\dot{V}_{max}$ has been directly related to the calcium-activated myosin ATPase activity. Both myosin and myofibrillar ATPase activity are typically depressed in hypertrophied myocardium. In small rodents, this is caused by the transcriptionally mediated switch from αMHC to βMHC. In higher mammals including humans, the decreased myofibrillar ATPase activity of the hypertrophied heart may be caused by loss of αMHC expression, or isoform switches involving other components of the contractile apparatus. The dissociation between depressed rate-dependent indices of contraction and relaxation and normal maximal force development and extent of shortening in early pathologic hypertrophy has also been demonstrated in isolated cardiomyocytes and in the intact circulation of the nonhuman primate.[50,51] *These results suggest that the rate of crossbridge cycling is reduced but that the effective number of active crossbridges per unit of myocardium is preserved in compensated cardiac hypertrophy.* In decompensated hypertrophy, reduced absolute levels of force development and diminished contractility ultimately ensue.

In addition to alteration in excitation-contraction coupling and relaxation, the increased cardiac mass and changes in geometry significantly affect passive muscle and chamber properties of the hypertrophied heart. Concentric hypertrophy is characterized by an increased resting muscle and chamber stiffness, which results in an increase in pulmonary venous pressure for any given left ventricular volume. The resultant pulmonary congestion at rest or with exercise is an important determinant of symptoms in patients with hypertensive left ventricular hypertrophy or familial hypertrophic cardiomyopathy and normal or elevated ejection fraction. Pure volume overload hypertrophy, as occurs with mitral regurgitation, is typically associated with no change or a decrease in passive muscle or chamber stiffness. As a result, patients with chronic volume overload may remain asymptomatic for long periods despite appreciable increase in regurgitant fraction.

【 】 CORONARY CIRCULATION

Clinicians have long recognized that myocardial blood flow may be abnormal in the hypertrophied heart, because such patients may have exertional angina, resting or exercise-induced electrocardiographic or perfusion abnormalities, or pathologic evidence of subendocardial fibrosis, despite the presence of angiographically normal epicardial coronary arteries. Morphologic studies of hypertrophied hearts from experimental animals and patients with pressure-overload hypertrophy demonstrate that the ratio of capillaries to myocytes remains unchanged.[52] Because the myocyte cross-sectional area is increased, there is a resultant increase in nutrient diffusion distance in the hypertrophied heart. This anatomic change results in a reduced vasodilatory reserve in response to various stimuli in experimental and clinical studies. Myocardial blood flow and oxygen consumption per unit of myocardium are normal in compensated pressure overload–left ventricular hypertrophy, where wall stress is normalized by increased wall thickness. The impairment in vasodilatory reserve produces evidence of ischemia during increased myocardial oxygen demand. In right ventricular pressure–overload hypertrophy, differences in perfusion between the ventricles result in increased right ventricular blood flow per unit of myocardial mass at rest and no increase in minimum coronary resistance of hypertrophied right ventricular myocardium.[53]

Few data are available regarding changes in the coronary circulation in experimental or clinical volume-overload hypertrophy. Most studies have reported normal resting flow values per unit of myocardial mass. In contrast to pressure overload, volume-overload hypertrophy has been associated with normal or mildly increased minimum coronary resistance and normal or mildly decreased coronary reserve. The coronary circulatory abnormalities associated with cardiac hypertrophy appear to be reversible with removal of the hypertrophic stimulus and resultant decreased chamber mass.[54]

MECHANISMS FOR THE TRANSITION FROM COMPENSATED HYPERTROPHY TO HEART FAILURE

In contrast to hypertrophied skeletal muscle, chronically increased work eventually results in depressed contractility and relaxation of the hypertrophied heart. Compensated hypertrophy, which is characterized by abnormal chamber function but preserved muscle and myocyte function, evolves into a decompensated phase characterized by abnormal chamber, muscle, and myocyte function (see Fig. 6–1). Attempts to elucidate the underlying mechanisms for this transition have involved multidisciplinary studies of clinical end-stage heart failure, longitudinal studies in experimental animals, and characterization of cardiovascular function in genetically engineered mice where attempts are made to mimic human disease.

Current information suggests that decompensated hypertrophy may result from many mechanisms that are both intrinsic and extrinsic to the cardiomyocyte. These include necrosis; apoptosis; altered growth secondary to altered signal transduction pathways; progressive alterations in cardiomyocyte contractile, regulatory, calcium-cycling, and structural proteins; alterations in the extracellular matrix; and remodeling (Fig. 6–4). Because of the complex

combinatorial alterations that occur in human heart failure and conventional animal models of hypertrophy, studies in genetically engineered mice in which a protein of interest is either overexpressed or ablated using homologous recombination have helped determine the relative importance of various candidate genes. For example, mice bearing a mutation in the βMHC that occurs in familial hypertrophic cardiomyopathy have many features of the human disease.[55] Overexpression of the α subunit of the G protein that couples to the β-adrenergic receptor has produced dilated, fibrotic hearts with altered cardiovascular function.[56] Overexpression or ablation of genes involved in cardiomyocyte calcium-cycling proteins is associated with altered heart function and abnormal calcium kinetics.[57] It is of interest that, with few exceptions, the resultant cardiac phenotype has failed to reproduce completely human decompensated hypertrophy and failure. This observation further supports the multifactorial nature of the condition and the importance of genetic background on the phenotype observed after loss-of-function or gain-of-function genetic engineering.

A common, prominent feature of many experimental and clinical studies of decompensated hypertrophy and failure is a derangement of cardiomyocyte calcium homeostasis. Studies of human cardiomyocytes isolated from the hearts of normal individuals reveals an increase in the size of the $[Ca^{2+}]_i$ transient and the force of contraction with increasing pacing frequency (i.e., a positive force-frequency relationship). However, in patients with end-stage heart failure, there is either no change in the amplitude of the $[Ca^{2+}]_i$ transient or a reduction in $[Ca^{2+}]_i$ transient amplitude and contractile force with increasing pacing frequency, thereby leading to a negative force-frequency relationship. Diastolic calcium levels are also elevated in failing versus nonfailing cardiomyocytes.[45] These changes were initially attributed to alterations in the expression levels of one or more calcium handling proteins.[51] For example, longitudinal studies of pathologic hypertrophy in experimental animals have revealed depression of steady-state mRNA levels and sarcoplasmic reticulum ATPase and phospholamban proteins in decompensated, but not compensated, pressure-overload hypertrophy.[51] These changes were associated with distinctive contractile depression of isovolumically contracting heart function, increases in the EC_{50}, and decreases in the $\dot{V}_{max}$ for sarcoplasmic reticular membrane uptake of calcium. However, current evidence suggests that defects in calcium homeostasis during the transition from compensated to decompensated hypertrophy may arise from even more subtle changes in Ca^{2+} transporter function. There is evidence that abnormal spatial organization of the L-type Ca^{2+} channel and SR Ca^{2+} release channel may contribute to the abnormal calcium cycling observed in the pressure-overloaded, failing heart.[58] Indeed, a decreased efficacy of excitation-contraction (EC) coupling can be detected quite early in the progression of pathologic hypertrophy, well before expression levels of calcium transporters and overt heart failure are manifest.[59] Functional changes caused by protein phosphorylation or other post-translational modifications, rather than protein abundance alone, may underlie specific defects in calcium handling, especially with respect to SR calcium loading, and Ca^{2+} release by the ryanodine receptor.[60]

In addition to altered calcium homeostasis, there is increasing evidence that abnormal signal transduction plays a critical role in the transition to decompensated cardiac hypertrophy and failure. Increased sympathetic nerve traffic as well as circulating and lo-

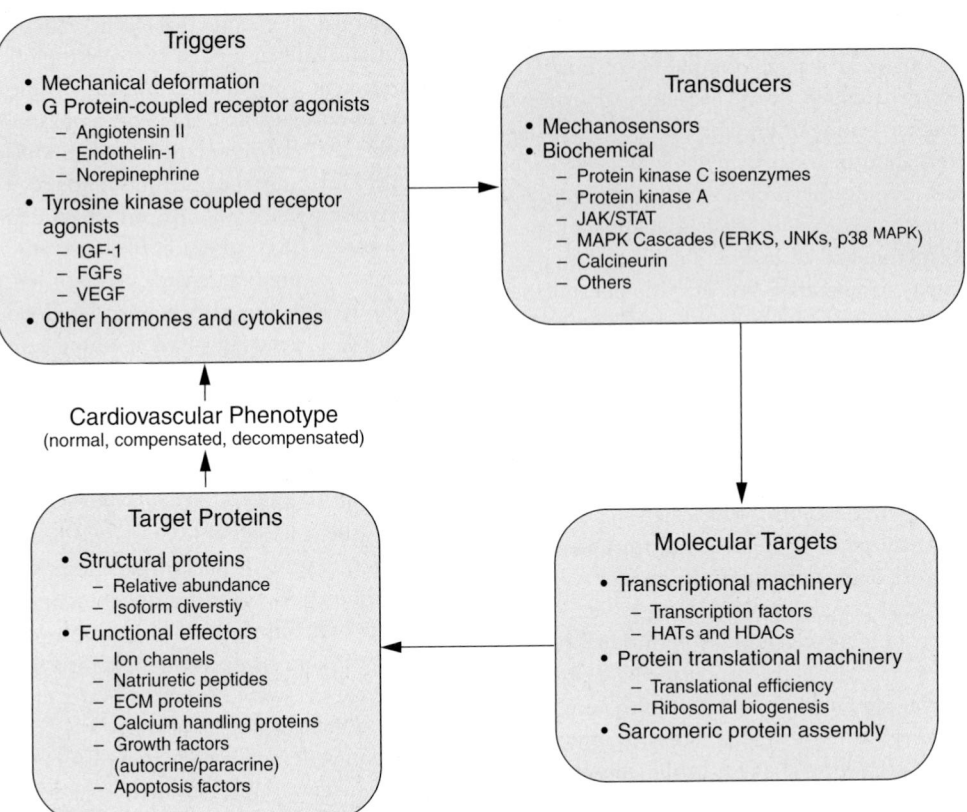

FIGURE 6–4. Schematic diagram of the mechanisms responsible for the development of the anatomic and functional cardiac phenotypes in physiologic and pathologic hypertrophy. Abnormalities at one or multiple levels in this putative closed-loop system may be responsible for the transition between compensated and decompensated hypertrophy.

cally derived peptide growth factors are likely to contribute. Indeed, overstimulation of their receptors may account for the beneficial effects of β blockers, angiotensin-converting enzyme inhibitors, and angiotensin II receptor blockers in preventing heart failure progression. In vitro studies with neonatal myocytes have demonstrated that norepinephrine, endothelin 1, and angiotensin II cause cardiomyocyte hypertrophy and produce gene expression changes that mimic the hypertrophic gene program elicited by pressure or volume overload.[21] These agonists all have cognate receptors that signal via the α subunit of the Gq protein. Furthermore, cardiac-specific overexpression of Gαq produced cardiac hypertrophy, apoptosis, and contractile depression in transgenic mice.[61] By contrast, overexpression of a protein inhibitor of Gαq in a similar manner prevented cardiac hypertrophy caused by pressure overload.[26] Transgenic overexpression of receptors that couple through Gαq, such as the α_1-AR, ET_A, and the AT_{1A} receptors, produce a similar phenotype. Important downstream effectors of Gαq include the Ca^{2+}-dependent and Ca^{2+}-independent isoenzymes of PKC, as well as other signaling kinases implicated in mechanotransduction and growth factor signaling. Augmented PKC activity and elevated levels of the calcium-sensitive PKCα and PKCβ isoforms were found in human end-stage cardiomyopathic heart failure.[62] Cardiac-specific postnatal overexpression of PKCβ produced cardiac hypertrophy and failure, whereas pretreatment of mice overexpressing PKCβ with a highly specific inhibitor prevented or reversed this hypertrophy–heart failure phenotype.[63] Similarly, cardiac-specific overexpression of PKCα produced animals with depressed contractile function,

which was mediated by changes in SR Ca^{2+} function as well as the Ca^{2+} sensitivity of the contractile apparatus. Part of the contractile depression observed with excess PKCβ activity was also caused by phosphorylation of troponin I and resultant reduced myofilament calcium sensitivity.[64]

In addition to overstimulation of Gαq-coupling receptors, chronic overactivation of β-adrenergic receptors (β-ARs) has long been considered a feature of heart failure progression. β-AR stimulation leads to activation of protein kinase A (PKA), and increased phosphorylation of L-type Ca^{2+} channels, phospholamban, and troponin I, which have opposing effects on contractility. More importantly, recent studies have indicated that β-AR stimulation also induces the phosphorylation of the ryanodine receptor, increasing the leak of calcium from intracellular stores, and thereby increasing the susceptibility to triggered arrhythmias and reducing $[Ca^{2+}]_i$ available for excitation-contraction coupling.[60] Thus, the progressive deterioration in contractile function observed during the transition from compensated to decompensated hypertrophy is likely related to increased neurohormonal stimulation via both PKC- and PKA-dependent signal transduction pathways.

A variety of studies with end-stage human cardiomyopathic heart tissue, conventional animal models, and genetically engineered mice suggest that apoptosis contributes to the transition from compensated hypertrophy to heart failure.[65] Genes involved in apoptosis signaling are upregulated during pathologic but not physiologic hypertrophy,[66] and there are also distinct differences in pro- versus antiapoptotic genes that may predict the transition from compensated to decompensated hypertrophy and heart failure.[67] The key issue that remains unclear is the quantitative importance of the phenomenon.[68] This problem is further complicated by the fact that a number of signaling molecules (e.g., Gαq and TNF-α) produce both hypertrophy and apoptosis, and the fact that apoptosis may represent only one form of myocyte cell death that occurs during the transition to heart failure.[69,70] It is expected that continued application of molecular, genetic, and cellular approaches to elucidate mechanisms responsible for myocardial hypertrophy, cardiac failure, arrhythmogenesis, and ischemic dysfunction will permit improved diagnostic and therapeutic approaches to congenital and acquired heart diseases.[71]

REFERENCES

1. Anversa P, Nadal-Ginard B. Myocyte renewal and ventricular remodelling. *Nature* 2002;415:240.

2. Murry CE, Reinecke H, Pabon LM. Regeneration gaps: observations on stem cells and cardiac repair. *J Am Coll Cardiol* 2006;47:1777.

3. Krenz M, Robbins J. Impact of β-myosin heavy chain expression on cardiac function during stress. *J Am Coll Cardiol* 2004;244:2390.

4. Chien KR, Knowlton KU, Zhu H, et al. Regulation of cardiac gene expression during myocardial growth and hypertrophy: molecular studies of an adaptive physiologic response. *FASEB J* 1991;5:3037.

5. Lowey S. Functional consequences of mutations in the myosin heavy chain at sites implicated in familial hypertrophic cardiomyopathy. *Trends Cardiovasc Med* 2002;12:348.

6. Milano CA, Allen LF, Rockman HA, et al. Enhanced myocardial function in transgenic mice overexpressing the β2-adrenergic receptor. *Science* 1994;264:582.

7. Hoit BD, Khoury SF, Kranias EG, et al. In vivo echocardiographic detection of enhanced left ventricular function in gene-targeted mice with phospholamban deficiency. *Circ Res* 1995;77:632.

8. Esposito G, Rapacciuolo A, Naga Prasad SV, et al. Genetic alterations that inhibit in vivo pressure-overload hypertrophy prevent cardiac dysfunction despite increased wall stress. *Circulation* 2002;105:85.

9. Spinale FG, Bishop SP. Myocardial remodeling with the development of tachycardia-induced heart failure. In: Spinale, FG ed. *Pathophysiology of Tachycardia-Induced Heart Failure.* Armonk, NY: Futura, 1996:61.

10. Sadoshima J, Izumo S. The cellular and molecular response of cardiac myocytes to mechanical stress. *Annu Rev Physiol* 1997;59:551.

11. Samarel AM. Costameres, focal adhesions, and cardiomyocyte mechanotransduction. *Am J Physiol Heart Circ Physiol* 2005;289:H2291.

12. Ross RS, Borg TK. Integrins and the myocardium. *Circ Res* 2001;88:1112.

13. Sussman MA, McCulloch A, Borg TK. Dance band on the Titanic: biomechanical signaling in cardiac hypertrophy. *Circ Res* 2002;91:888.

14. Eliceiri BP. Integrin and growth factor receptor crosstalk. *Circ Res* 2001;89:1104.

15. Yamazaki T, Komuro I, Shiojima I, et al. The molecular mechanism of cardiac hypertrophy and failure. *Ann N Y Acad Sci* 1999;874:38.

16. Molkentin JD, Dorn IG II. Cytoplasmic signaling pathways that regulate cardiac hypertrophy. *Annu Rev Physiol* 2001;63:391.

17. Molkentin JD. Calcineurin-NFAT signaling regulates the cardiac hypertrophic response in coordination with the MAPKs. *Cardiovasc Res* 2004;63:467.

18. Baines CP, Molkentin JD. STRESS signaling pathways that modulate cardiac myocyte apoptosis. *J Mol Cell Cardiol* 2005;38:47.

19. Hunter JJ, Chien KR. Signaling pathways for cardiac hypertrophy and failure. *N Engl J Med* 1999;341:1276.

20. Dorn GW II, Force T. Protein kinase cascades in the regulation of cardiac hypertrophy. *J Clin Invest* 2005;115:527.

21. McMullen JR, Shioi T, Zhang L, et al. Phosphoinositide 3-kinase (p110α) plays a critical role for the induction of physiological, but not pathological, cardiac hypertrophy. *Proc Natl Acad Sci U S A* 2003;100:12355.

22. McMullen JR, Shioi T, Huang WY, et al. The insulin-like growth factor 1 receptor induces physiological heart growth via the phosphoinositide 3-kinase (p110α) pathway. *J Biol Chem* 2004;279:4782.

23. Klein I, Ojamaa K. Thyroid hormone and the cardiovascular system. *N Engl J Med* 2001;344:501.

24. Ojamaa K, Samarel AM, Kupfer JM, et al. Thyroid hormone effects on cardiac gene expression independent of cardiac growth and protein synthesis. *Am J Physiol* 1992;263:E534.

25. Kahaly GJ, Dillmann WH. Thyroid hormone action in the heart. *Endocr Rev* 2005;226:704.

26. Akhter SA, Luttrell LM, Rockman HA, et al. Targeting the receptor-Gq interface to inhibit in vivo pressure overload myocardial hypertrophy. *Science* 1998;280:574.

27. Wollert KC, Chien KR. Cardiotrophin-1 and the role of gp130-dependent signaling pathways in cardiac growth and development. *J Mol Med* 1998;75:492.

28. Mann DL, McMurray JJ, Packer M, et al. Targeted anticytokine therapy in patients with chronic heart failure: results of the Randomized Etanercept Worldwide Evaluation (RENEWAL). *Circulation* 2004;109:1594.

29. Topper JN. TGF-β in the cardiovascular system: molecular mechanisms of a context-specific growth factor. *Trends Cardiovasc Med* 2000;10:132.

30. Barki-Harrington L, Perrino C, Rockman HA. Network integration of the adrenergic system in cardiac hypertrophy. *Cardiovasc Res* 2004;63:391.

31. Wilkins BJ, Molkentin JD. Calcium-calcineurin signaling in the regulation of cardiac hypertrophy. *Biochem Biophys Res Commun* 2004;322:1178.

32. McKinsey TA, Olson EN. Toward transcriptional therapies for the failing heart: chemical screens to modulate genes. *J Clin Invest* 2005;115:538.

33. Backs J, Olson EN. Control of cardiac growth by histone acetylation/deacetylation. *Circ Res* 2006;98:15–24.

34. Nagatomo Y, Carabello BA, Hamawaki M, et al. Translational mechanisms accelerate the rate of protein synthesis during canine pressure-overload hypertrophy. *Am J Physiol* 1999;277:H2176.

35. Tuxworth WJ Jr, Saghir AN, Spruill LS, et al. Regulation of protein synthesis by eIF4E phosphorylation in adult cardiocytes: the consequence of secondary structure in the 5'-untranslated region of mRNA. *Biochem J* 2002;378:73.

36. Iijima Y, Laser M, Shiraishi H, et al. c-Raf/MEK/ERK pathway controls protein kinase C-mediated p70S6K activation in adult cardiac muscle cells. *J Biol Chem* 2002;277:23065.

37. Eble DM, Spragia ML, Ferguson AG, et al. Sarcomeric myosin heavy chain is degraded by the proteasome. *Cell Tissue Res* 1999;296:541.

38. Aoki H, Sadoshima J, Izumo S. Myosin light chain kinase mediates sarcomere organization during cardiac hypertrophy in vitro. *Nat Med* 2000;6:183.

39. Mansour H, de Tombe PP, Samarel AM, et al. Restoration of resting sarcomere length after uniaxial static strain is regulated by protein kinase Cε and focal adhesion kinase. *Circ Res* 2004;94:642.

40. Miyata S, Minobe W, Bristow MR, Leinwand LA. Myosin heavy chain isoform expression in the failing and nonfailing human heart. *Circ Res* 2000;86:386.

41. Camelliti P, Borg TK, Kohl P. Structural and functional characterisation of cardiac fibroblasts. *Cardiovasc Res* 2005;65:40.

42. Collins JF, Pawloski-Dahm C, Davis MG, et al. The role of the cytoskeleton in left ventricular pressure overload hypertrophy and failure. *J Mol Cell Cardiol* 1996;28:1435.

43. Tsutsui H, Ishihara K, Cooper GT. Cytoskeletal role in the contractile dysfunction of hypertrophied myocardium. *Science* 1993;260:682.

44. Bers DM. Cardiac excitation-contraction coupling. *Nature* 2002;415:198.

45. Houser SR, Piacentino V III, Weisser J. Abnormalities of calcium cycling in the hypertrophied and failing heart. *J Mol Cell Cardiol* 2002;32:1595.

46. Wolk R. Arrhythmogenic mechanisms in left ventricular hypertrophy. *Europace* 2000;2:216.

47. Hill JA. Electrical remodeling in cardiac hypertrophy. *Trends Cardiovasc Med* 2003;13:316.

48. Peters NS, Green CR, Poole-Wilson PA, et al. Reduced content of connexin43 gap junctions in ventricular myocardium from hypertrophied and ischemic human hearts. *Circulation* 1993;88:864.

49. Levy D, Garrison RJ, Savage DD, et al. Prognostic implications of echocardiographically determined left ventricular mass in the Framingham Heart Study. *N Engl J Med* 1990;322:156.

50. Dorn GW II, Robbins J, Ball N, et al. Myosin heavy chain regulation and myocyte contractile depression after LV hypertrophy in aortic-banded mice. *Am J Physiol* 1994;267:H400.

51. Kiss E, Ball NA, Kranias EG, et al. Differential changes in cardiac phospholamban and sarcoplasmic reticular Ca²⁺-ATPase protein levels. Effects on Ca²⁺ transport and mechanics in compensated pressure-overload hypertrophy and congestive heart failure. *Circ Res* 1995;77:759.

52. Bache RJ. Effects of hypertrophy on the coronary circulation. *Prog Cardiovasc Dis* 1988;30:403.

53. Murray PA, Vatner SF. Reduction of maximal coronary vasodilator capacity in conscious dogs with severe right ventricular hypertrophy. *Circ Res* 1981;48:25.

54. Isoyama S, Ito N, Kuroha M, et al. Complete reversibility of physiological coronary vascular abnormalities in hypertrophied hearts produced by pressure overload in the rat. *J Clin Invest* 1989;84:288.

55. Geisterfer-Lowrance AA, Christe M, Conner DA, et al. A mouse model of familial hypertrophic cardiomyopathy. *Science* 1996;272:731.

56. Iwase M, Bishop SP, Uechi M, et al. Adverse effects of chronic endogenous sympathetic drive induced by cardiac Gsα overexpression. *Circ Res* 1996;78:517.

57. Schultz Jel J, Glascock BJ, Witt SA, et al. Accelerated onset of heart failure in mice during pressure overload with chronically decreased SERCA2 calcium pump activity. *Am J Physiol Heart Circ Physiol* 2004;286:H1146.

58. Gomez AM, Valdivia HH, Cheng H, et al. Defective excitation-contraction coupling in experimental cardiac hypertrophy and heart failure. *Science* 1997;276:800.

59. McCall E, Ginsburg KS, Bassani RA, et al. Ca flux, contractility, and excitation-contraction coupling in hypertrophic rat ventricular myocytes. *Am J Physiol* 1998;274:H1348.

60. Wehrens XH, Lehnart SE, Reiken S, et al. Ryanodine receptor/calcium release channel PKA phosphorylation: a critical mediator of heart failure progression. *Proc Natl Acad Sci U S A* 2006;103:511.

61. D'Angelo DD, Sakata Y, Lorenz JN, et al. Transgenic Gαq overexpression induces cardiac contractile failure in mice. *Proc Natl Acad Sci U S A* 1997;94:8121.

62. Bowling N, Walsh RA, Song G, et al. Increased protein kinase C activity and expression of Ca^{2+}-sensitive isoforms in the failing human heart. *Circulation* 1999;99:384.

63. Wakasaki H, Koya D, Schoen FJ, et al. Targeted overexpression of protein kinase C β$_2$ isoform in myocardium causes cardiomyopathy. *Proc Natl Acad Sci U S A* 1997;94:9320.

64. Takeishi Y, Chu G, Kirkpatrick DM, et al. In vivo phosphorylation of cardiac troponin I by protein kinase C-β$_2$ decreases cardiomyocyte calcium responsiveness and contractility in transgenic mouse hearts. *J Clin Invest* 1998;102:72.

65. Kang PM, Izumo S. Apoptosis and heart failure: a critical review of the literature. *Circ Res.* 2000;86:1107.

66. Kong SW, Bodyak N, Yue P, et al. Genetic expression profiles during physiological and pathological cardiac hypertrophy and heart failure in rats. *Physiol Genomics* 2005;21:34.

67. Buermans HP, Redout EM, Schiel AE, et al. Microarray analysis reveals pivotal divergent mRNA expression profiles early in the development of either compensated ventricular hypertrophy or heart failure. *Physiol Genomics* 2005;21:314.

68. Rodriguez M, Schaper J. Apoptosis: measurement and technical issues. *J Mol Cell Cardiol* 2005;38:15.

69. Hein S, Arnon E, Kostin S, et al. Progression from compensated hypertrophy to failure in the pressure-overloaded human heart: structural deterioration and compensatory mechanisms. *Circulation* 2003;107:984.

70. Kostin S, Pool L, Elsasser A, et al. Myocytes die by multiple mechanisms in failing human hearts. *Circ Res* 2003;92:715.

71. Takeishi Y, Walsh RA. Cardiac hypertrophy and failure: lessons learned from genetically engineered mice. *Acta Physiol Scand* 2001;173:103.

CHAPTER 7

Biology of the Vessel Wall

Kathy K. Griendling / David G. Harrison / R. Wayne Alexander

It has become apparent that a diverse number of pathologic processes all contribute to common vascular diseases such as atherosclerosis and hypertension. During the past several years, these pathologic events have been defined with increasing clarity at a cellular and molecular level, and strategies are emerging to treat these primary processes rather than simply treating the secondary manifestations of vascular disease. For this reason, understanding normal functions of vascular cells and how they are altered by various vascular insults has become essential for both basic investigators and clinicians caring for patients with peripheral vascular disease, coronary artery disease, and hypertension. This chapter is designed to introduce important concepts in vascular biology and to emphasize how fundamental aspects of vascular control are altered by common disease conditions.

THE ENDOTHELIAL CELL

Normal endothelial cell function is crucial to homeostasis in the vascular system. During the past 20 years, it has become apparent that diseases such as atherosclerosis are ultimately manifestations of endothelial dysfunction. Normally, the endothelium has three major roles: (1) it is a metabolically active secretory tissue; (2) it serves as an anticoagulant, antithrombotic surface; and (3) it pro-

vides a barrier to the indiscriminate passage of blood constituents into the arterial wall. The implications of these physiologic properties for vascular biology will be considered separately.

ENDOTHELIAL CELL METABOLISM AND SECRETION OF VASOACTIVE FACTORS

As discussed in more detail below, endothelial cells secrete vasoactive substances that play a major role in the control of vascular tone. These molecules include vasodilators such as prostacyclin, nitric oxide (NO), and endothelial-derived hyperpolarizing factors (EDHFs) such as hydrogen peroxide and eicosanoids.[1–3] In addition, the endothelium produces vasoconstrictor substances, including endothelin[4] and vasoconstrictor prostanoids.[5]

Endothelial cells also manufacture and secrete substances such as factor VIII antigen, von Willebrand factor, tissue factor, thrombomodulin, and tissue plasminogen activator, which are all involved in coagulation/fibrinolytic pathways. Structural components of the extracellular matrix synthesized by these cells include collagen, elastin, glycosaminoglycans, and fibronectin.[6,7] The composition of the extracellular matrix is dynamically modulated by matrix metalloproteinases, enzymes that degrade matrix protein and participate in its remodeling. These enzymes are secreted by both endothelial and smooth muscle cells (SMCs).[8,9] In addition, endothelial cells synthesize and secrete heparans and growth factors that regulate SMC proliferation.[10–13] Finally, endothelial cells can clear and metabolically alter bloodborne and locally produced substances, including plasma lipids and lipoproteins,[14] adenine nucleotides and nucleosides,[15] serotonin, catecholamines, bradykinin, and angiotensin I.[16]

Endothelial cells are involved in the metabolism of plasma lipids in several ways. Lipoprotein lipase, an enzyme that hydrolyzes triglycerides into constituent fatty acids, is bound to the endothelial cell surface by heparan sulfates.[17] The interaction of this enzyme with chylomicrons or very low density lipoprotein particles results in the release of free fatty acids, which can then cross the subendothelial space to the underlying smooth muscle or inflammatory cells in atherosclerosis. In addition, endothelial cells possess receptors for low-density lipoprotein (LDL),[18] which regulate the transport and modification of LDL. Normally, LDL receptors are downregulated because receptor processing is inhibited in the nonproliferating monolayer.[18] There are, however, two other pathways for uptake of LDL. First, LDL can be transported across the endothelium by an active process that is likely independent of plasmalemmal vesicles but may use paracellular gaps or fixed transendothelial channels.[19]

Second, modified, or oxidized, LDL can be taken up by *scavenger* LDL receptors,[20] which include SRA, SR-BI, CD36 and the lectin-like oxidized LDL receptor-1.[21,22] Endothelial cells also have the capacity to modify LDL,[23] thus enhancing its uptake and ultimately leading to an increase in cholesterol esters in the vessel wall.

【 】 THE ENDOTHELIAL CELL AND THROMBOSIS

Quiescent endothelial cells normally present an antithrombotic surface that inhibits platelet adhesion and coagulation. (For a more detailed discussion of thrombosis, see Chap. 53.) Endothelial cells are, however, capable of synthesizing and secreting prothrombotic factors, especially when stimulated with cytokines or other inflammatory agents. The endothelium thus represents a functional antithrombotic-thrombolytic or thrombotic balance. Potent anticoagulants elaborated by the endothelium include prostacyclin and nitric oxide, which inhibit platelet aggregation;[24] antithrombin III,[25] heparin-like molecules,[26] and thrombomodulin, which activates endothelial protein C;[27] and tissue plasminogen activator (tPA). Procoagulant factors that can be produced by the endothelium include tissue factor,[28] factor VIII, factor V_a and PAI-1 (Fig. 7–1). Conditions of injury or inflammation enhance the prothrombotic state of the endothelium by stimulating production of tissue factor and plasminogen activator inhibitor 1 (PAI-1). Of particular importance is tissue factor, which initiates the extrinsic coagulation pathway. The transcription and release of tissue factor is regulated by a myriad of proinflammatory, proatherogenic stimuli and large amounts of tissue factor are associated with complex atherosclerotic lesions.[29] There has also been substantial interest in the role of PAI-1 in vascular disease. PAI-1 levels are substantially elevated in humans with atherosclerosis and even higher in the setting of acute coronary syndromes. Moreover, the metabolic syndrome, consisting of dyslipidemia, obesity and insulin resistance, is associated with higher levels of PAI-1.[30] Angiotensin II and thrombin likewise stimulate endothelial PAI-1 production, promoting thrombosis.[31] Thus, under inflammatory conditions, endothelial cells can amplify the prothrombotic response. Not all factors controlling the expression of pro- and antithrombotic/fibrinolytic molecules are known, but it is clear that the endothelium functions as a major regulator of hemostasis.

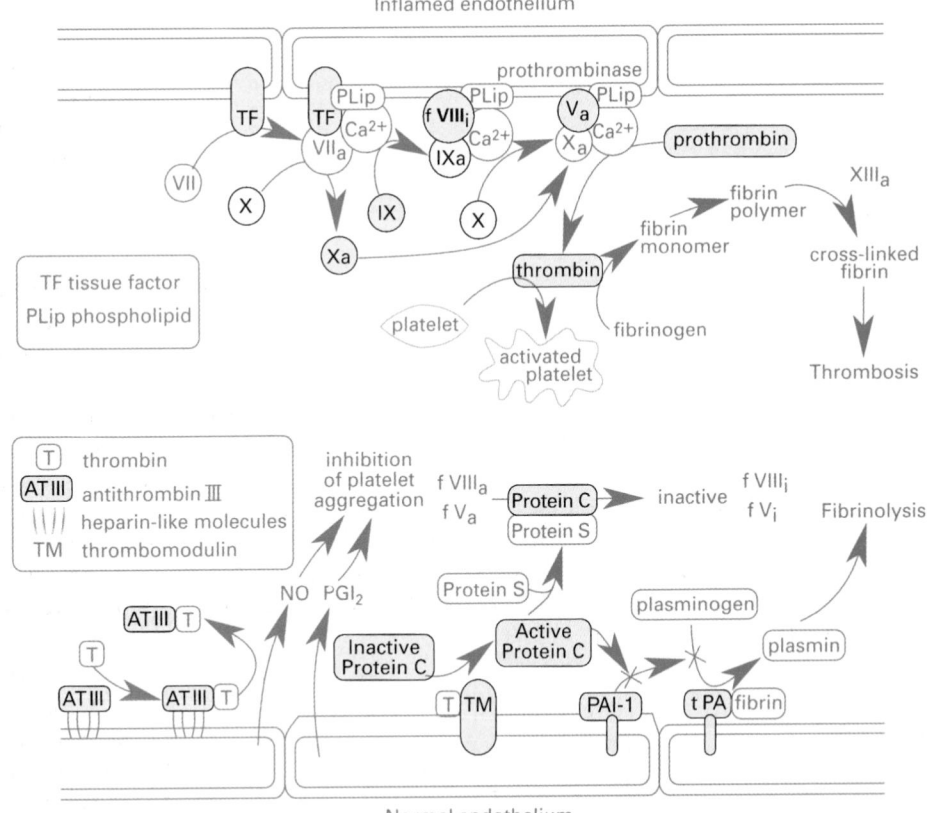

FIGURE 7–1. Pathways of thrombosis and thrombolysis. Under normal conditions, the endothelium is antithrombotic. Antithrombin III (AT III) binds thrombin and serves to clear thrombin from the circulation. Prostacyclin (prostaglandin I_2 [PGI_2]) inhibits platelet aggregation, and thrombomodulin (TM) activates protein C, which inhibits plasminogen activator inhibitor 1 (PAI-1) and interacts with protein S to inactivate activated factors V and VIII, thus limiting thrombosis. Because PAI-1 inhibits the tissue plasminogen activator (tPA)–catalyzed conversion of plasminogen to plasmin, PAI-1 inhibition leads to accumulation of plasmin and fibrinolysis. With stimulation with inflammatory cytokines, there is increased expression of tissue factor on the endothelial cell surface. Tissue factor participates in the activation of factor X, which, in turn, promotes assembly of the prothrombinase complex, producing thrombin. Under these conditions, endothelial cells thus amplify the thrombotic response. *Source: Courtesy of Bernard Lassègue, Ph.D.*

【 】 ENDOTHELIAL CELL PERMEABILITY

An essential role of the endothelium is regulation of permeability to macromolecules. The consequences of fluid and macromolecular transport vary depending on vessel size. In large vessels, these processes contribute to vessel nutrition and act as a selective barrier. In the microcirculation, endothelial permeability regulates delivery of nutrients to target organs and exchange of metabolic by-products.

The major two mechanisms regulating endothelial barrier function involve modulation of intercellular contacts and transendothelial vesicular transport in caveolae. Two types of junctions regulate endothelial cell contact: adherens and tight junctions. Adherens junctions contain the protein VE-cadherin, which is essential for maintenance of interendothelial cell contacts. VE-cadherin associates with catenins, plakoglobulin and the actin cytoskeleton to support cell adhesion. The catenins in turn bind to the actin cytoskeleton and modulate actin dynamics.[32] Tight junctions are composed of occludins, claudins, and junctional adhesion molecule-1. Regulation of these interendothelial cell contacts is dynamic and important in modulation of new vessel growth, the extravasation of leukocytes and macromolecule leakage. The nature of these intercellular contacts varies substantially depending on the vessel size and location. For example, tight junctions are well developed in the blood–brain barrier, but are less structurally defined in postcapillary venules, where fluid and solute transport is active. Capillaries and postcapillary venules respond to vasoactive agents, including vascular endothelial cell growth factor (VEGF), histamine, and prostaglandins, with increased flux through these sites.[33] The tight junctions found in arteries tend to be more occlusive but may also be influenced by various agonists. Dynamic regulation of these pathways enables the endothelium to serve as a selective barrier, modulating access of highly mitogenic, thrombotic, or vasoactive substances to the underlying vascular smooth muscle.

Transendothelial vesicular transport is mainly used by the cell to transfer water-soluble macromolecules from the luminal surface to the abluminal surface. It has recently been shown that caveolae, vesicles containing the structural protein caveolin that are pinched off from the plasma membrane, are involved in transendothelial transport of macromolecules.[34,35] Caveolae are also sites where a variety of kinases, docking proteins, G-proteins, and receptors reside,[36] and therefore play an extremely important role in endothelial cell signal transduction.

Another major mechanism modulating endothelial barrier formation is endothelial cell contraction, analogous to smooth muscle contraction. This occurs in response to a variety of agonists, including thrombin, histamine, and ionomycin, and results in cell shape change that opens gap junctions between cells. It is likely that this contractile response is a major mechanism for edema formation in response to histamine and bradykinin, and is also

involved in solute transport. This phenomenon is mediated by a series of intracellular signaling events, including activation of protein kinase C, myosin light chain phosphorylation, activation of tyrosine kinases, and stimulation of the small G-protein Rho.[37–39]

Thus, the endothelium has both passive and active roles in the control of vascular permeability by acting as a physical permeability barrier and by modulating the expression of cell surface and secreted agonists and molecules that are capable of altering permeability.

ENDOTHELIAL CONTROL OF VASCULAR TONE

The endothelium serves a dual function in the control of vascular tone (Fig. 7–2). It secretes relaxing factors such as nitric oxide, prostacyclin, and the endothelium-derived hyperpolarizing factor, as well as constricting factors such as endothelin. Vessel tone thus depends on the balance between these factors, as well as on the ability of the SMC to respond to them. The most important regulatory molecules are discussed separately.

Nitric Oxide

An endothelium-derived relaxing factor (EDRF) was first described by Furchgott and Zawadzki,[2] who observed that aortic rings dilated in response to acetylcholine only when the rings maintained an intact endothelium. The EDRF was subsequently found to be nitric oxide (NO).[40]

NO is produced by the action of the enzyme nitric oxide synthase (NOS), which oxidizes the guanidino nitrogens of L-argi-

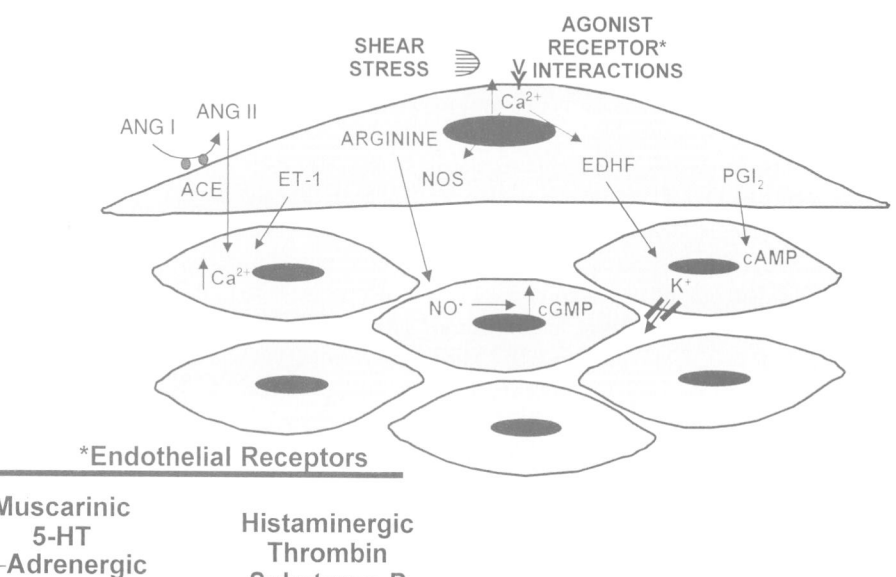

FIGURE 7–2. Endothelial control of vascular tone. Endothelial cells synthesize and secrete both vasodilator substances (NO, EDHF, and PGI$_2$) and vasoconstrictor compounds (Ang II and ET-1). Secretion of these factors occurs in response to receptor stimulation and hemodynamic forces such as shear stress. Vessel tone depends on the balance between these factors, as well as on the ability of the smooth muscle cells to respond to them. NO, nitric oxide; NOS, nitric oxide synthase; EDHF, endothelial-derived hyperpolarizing factor; PGI$_2$, prostaglandin I$_2$; ACE, angiotensin-converting enzyme; ANG, angiotensin; ET-1, endothelin-1; cGMP, cyclic guanosine monophosphate; cAMP, cyclic adenosine monophosphate; 5-HT, 5-hydroxytryptamine.

nine to form citrulline and NO. This enzyme has been cloned from brain (nNOS, for neuronal NOS, type I),[41] macrophages (iNOS, for inducible NOS, type II),[42] and endothelial cells (eNOS, for endothelial NOS type III).[43] The three isoforms of NOS share important consensus sequences for nicotinamide adenine dinucleotide phosphate (NADPH), flavin adenine dinucleotide, and flavin mononucleotide cofactor-binding sites, as well as a Ca^{2+}-calmodulin binding site. An important cofactor for the NO synthases is tetrahydrobiopterin, which participates in electron transfer from the heme group of the enzyme to L-arginine. Interestingly, when tetrahydrobiopterin or L-arginine is absent, electron transfer is shunted to molecular oxygen, resulting in formation of the superoxide anion.[44] This phenomenon has been termed *uncoupling* of NOS, and there are substantial data that this may occur in a variety of disease states.[45]

Many factors have been shown to regulate the release of NO.[46] These include hormones such as acetylcholine, norepinephrine, bradykinin, thrombin, adenosine triphosphate (ATP), and vasopressin; the platelet-derived factors, serotonin and histamine; fatty acids; ionophores; and shear stress. NO easily crosses the SMC membrane and binds to the heme moiety of the soluble guanylate cyclase, thereby enhancing the formation of cyclic guanosine monophosphate (GMP). Cyclic GMP, in turn, reduces intracellular Ca^{2+} concentrations leading to dephosphorylation of the myosin light chain and relaxation.[47] It should be noted that the drug nitroglycerin exerts its vasodilator effects by being converted to NO, thus substituting for a natural product.

Although increases in intracellular calcium in response to the aforementioned agents clearly activate eNOS via binding of Ca and calmodulin, phosphorylation of the enzyme is important in regulating its activity. For example, shear stress acutely stimulates the release of NO from the endothelium, and this depends only on calcium during the first few seconds of the response.[48] The continued activation of eNOS in response to several minutes or hours of shear is maintained by serine phosphorylation.[49]

The expression of eNOS is highly regulated. Increases in shear stress enhance eNOS expression, whereas low levels of shear decrease it.[50] Exercise training dramatically increases eNOS expression in endothelial cells, likely because of the increased shear stress caused by the high cardiac output that accompanies sustained exercise.[51] In contrast, oxidized LDL, hypoxia, and inflammatory cytokines such as TNFα decrease eNOS expression.[43,52,53] The hydroxymethylglutaryl coenzyme A (HMG-CoA) reductase inhibitors increase eNOS levels by stabilizing the eNOS mRNA. This is thought to be an important component of the so-called *pleiotropic effects* of the statins that may contribute to their therapeutic effects.

Endothelium-Derived Hyperpolarizing Factors

Shortly after the identification of NO, it was suspected that the endothelium could release more than one relaxing factor, depending on the vessel size, stimulus, and species studied. Initial studies showed that some vasodilators produce hyperpolarization of the vascular smooth muscle membrane in an endothelium-dependent manner. It is now clear that this is caused by the release of hyperpolarizing factors from the endothelium that are different from NO.[54] Increasing evidence suggests that there are at least two EDHFs. One is 14,15-epoxyeicosatrienoic acid (14,15-EET), a cytochrome P450 metabolite of arachidonic acid.[55] This epoxide and its metabolite 14,15-dihydroxyeicosatrienoic acid are released from the endothelium, diffuse to the adjacent vascular smooth muscle and open calcium-activated potassium channels. This results in efflux of potassium ions, hyperpolarization, and subsequent closing of voltage-dependent calcium channels, leading to vasodilatation.[56] The second EDHF is likely hydrogen peroxide, which is also made by endothelial cells and acts in the same fashion as the EETs.[57,58] Recent studies have shown that hydrogen peroxide is particularly important in human coronary arterioles.[59] In general, as one progresses from large conduit vessels to smaller arterioles, the role of NO seems to decrease and the EDHF component of vasodilatation increases.[60] Moreover, there is an interplay between regulation of NO levels and EDHF production. NO can bind to the heme group of the cytochrome p450s and inhibit these enzymes and their production of 12,15-EET. If NO production is diminished, this seems to *unleash* cytochrome p450 EET production, which can then take over the role of NO in mediating vasodilatation. In the setting of excessive superoxide production, NO is oxidatively degraded, leading to loss of NO bioactivity. A substantial portion of the increased superoxide is dismutated to hydrogen peroxide, which can then also serve as an EDHF. Through these mechanisms, the loss of NO can lead to a compensatory increase in EDHF and maintenance of small vessel vasodilatation.

Prostacyclin

Prostacyclin, or prostaglandin I_2 (PGI_2), a prostanoid derived from the action of cyclooxygenase (COX)-1 and -2 on arachidonic acid, is released by the endothelium and relaxes vascular smooth muscle by increasing its intracellular content of cyclic adenosine monophosphate.[61] Prostacyclin is also platelet suppressant and antithrombotic, and reduces the release of growth factors from endothelial cells and macrophages.[24] Inhibition of these beneficial effects likely underlies the untoward clinical outcomes observed in patients treated with COX-2 inhibitors.[62] Among the agonists that stimulate prostacyclin synthesis are bradykinin (one of the most potent), substance P, platelet-derived growth factor, epidermal growth factor, and adenine nucleotides.[24] Prostacyclin has been shown to compensate for the loss of NO in the eNOS knockout mouse.[63] Analogues of prostacyclin such as iloprost have proven useful in the treatment of pulmonary hypertension.[64]

Arachidonic Acid-Derived Vasoconstrictors

Although the endothelium predominantly produces prostacyclin, under pathologic conditions, it can begin to generate other prostaglandins with vasoconstrictor activity.[65] These include prostaglandin H_2 (PGH_2), a direct product of COX-1 and -2, and thromboxane, made by the action of thromboxane synthase on PGH_2.[66] In hypertensive models, various hormones such as acetylcholine and endothelin-1 can stimulate the release of an endothelium-derived constricting factor (EDCF) that acts on the thromboxane receptor. Interestingly, the EDCF is not thromboxane but the endoperoxide PGH_2, and in some models prostacyclin, which paradoxically causes constriction because of a loss of the PGI_2 receptor.[67]

Another important vasoconstrictor derived from cytochrome P450 metabolism of arachidonic acid is 20-hydroxyeicosatetraenoic acid (20-HETE).[68] This compound depolarizes vascular SMCs by inhibiting calcium-activated potassium channels and thereby promotes vasoconstriction. The synthesis of 20-HETE is stimulated by angiotensin

II, endothelin, and catecholamines and is inhibited by nitric oxide.[68] Not surprisingly, 20-HETE production is elevated in a number of common diseases such as hypertension, kidney disease, and diabetes.

Angiotensin-Converting Enzymes

Endothelial cells, particularly those in the pulmonary vasculature, synthesize and express angiotensin-converting enzyme (ACE) on their surface.[69] ACE converts angiotensin I to the potent vasoconstrictor angiotensin II and degrades and inactivates bradykinin. Recent work has suggested that upon binding of ACE inhibitors, ACE can directly signal via its short cytoplasmic tail, leading to changes in gene expression.[70] The overall importance of this phenomenon in the cardiovascular system is unclear. Of note, vascular and cardiac cells contain almost all components of the renin/angiotensin system,[71] and thus local production of angiotensin II can contribute importantly to vascular function. This local production of angiotensin II can explain why ACE inhibitors and angiotensin receptor antagonists are often effective even when the circulating levels of renin or angiotensin II are not elevated.

Recently, a new carboxypeptidase, ACE-II has been identified.[72] This enzyme cleaves one amino acid from either angiotensin I or angiotensin II. The overall effect of ACE-II action is a reduction in angiotensin II and an increase in the metabolite angiotensin 1–7, which has vasodilator properties. Thus, the balance between ACE and ACE-II is an important factor controlling angiotensin II levels and ultimately vasomotor tone.[73]

Endothelins

The endothelins are a family of closely related peptides made and secreted by many cells including endothelial cells. There are 3 endothelins (ET-1, -2, and -3), all of which are 18 amino acid peptides. The endothelins are initially synthesized as preproendothelin, which undergoes preprocessing to big endothelin. Big endothelin is released and converted to active endothelin by the endothelin-converting enzyme. The synthesis of preproendothelin is stimulated by diverse stimuli including angiotensin II, oxidized LDL, hypoxia, low shear stress, and inflammatory cytokines.[74] The vascular effects of endothelin are mediated by endothelin receptors, of which three subtypes have been identified: A, B, and C. The receptors have differing specificity for the individual endothelin peptides, and activate different signaling pathways. In the vessel, the ET-A receptor is predominantly found on vascular smooth muscle, whereas the ET-B receptor resides on endothelial cells. Activation of the former stimulates potent vasoconstriction, whereas activation of the latter stimulates release of NO and thus favors vasodilation.[75]

The slow, intense, and sustained contraction caused by ET-1 appears to be the result of activation of the phosphoinositide/protein kinase C signaling pathway, as well as of opening voltage-dependent L-type calcium channels.[76] Importantly, even low, subthreshold concentrations of ET-1 enhance vasoconstriction to a variety of other vasoconstrictor agents, including serotonin, angiotensin II, and α-adrenergic agonists, seemingly via activation of protein kinase C.

ET-1 is also a potent growth factor for VSMCs,[77] and a chemoattractant for monocytes.[78] Angiotensin II has been shown to stimulate the production of ET-1 by VSMCs in culture,[79] and, in vivo, some of the hypertensive effect of angiotensin II is mediated by endothelin.[80] Thus, ET-1 and angiotensin II act in concert in conditions such as hypertension, diabetes, and heart failure.[81,82]

Currently, the mixed ET-A and ET-B receptor antagonist bosentan is clinically used for pulmonary hypertension.[74]

【 】 ENDOTHELIAL RESPONSES TO HEMODYNAMIC INFLUENCES

Many previously described endothelial functions are modulated by the physical forces of stretch, strain, and shear stress imposed by the hemodynamics of the circulation. Both stretch of the vessel wall (as observed in hypertension) and shear stress have been shown independently to affect endothelial cell morphology and/or function. Studies in cultured cells have shown that stretching endothelial cells leads to changes in cell shape,[83] intracellular signal generation with an increase in calcium and superoxide levels,[84] and proliferation.[85] Shear stress has numerous effects on endothelial cells. Initially, it was found that exposure of endothelial cell monolayers to elevated shear stresses in vitro caused them to align in the direction of flow. This reorientation was accompanied by changes in the cytoskeleton of the cells, including reorganization and alignment of the actin filaments and microtubules (Fig. 7–3). Similar mechanisms presumably also account for the orientation of endothelial cells parallel to the longitudinal axis in areas of laminar flow in the arterial system. The function of the endothelium is also altered by shear stress. Some of the cellular responses to shear stress include activation of K+ currents; increased secretion of vasoactive and growth factors, including NO, endothelin, prostacyclin, and basic fibroblast growth factor (bFGF); enhanced tissue factor expression; elevation of LDL uptake; and increased tPA secretion.[86]

The importance of these observations lies in the variation in hemodynamic forces throughout the circulation. Areas of the vasculature exposed to low shear stress (branch points and curvatures) exhibit a predilection to the formation of atherosclerotic lesions.[87] True oscillations of flow have also been shown to occur in the carotid bulb, the proximal coronary arteries, and in the distal aorta.[88] Studies in cultured endothelial cells have shown that oscillatory shear stress increases endothelial cell production of reactive oxygen species,[89] enhances adhesion molecule expression, and stimulates monocyte adhesion.[90] Recent work has shown that the bone morphogenic protein 4 is a key signaling molecule in the pathways leading to these events.[91,92]

The mechanisms by which the endothelial cell can sense and transduce mechanical signals have been extensively studied. Two recent hypotheses have emerged suggesting that mechanical forces are transduced by extracellular glycosaminoglycans or by the selectin, platelet endothelial cell adhesion molecule-1 (PECAM-1). Enzymatic disruption of the glycocalyx has been shown to decrease endothelial cell NO production in response to shear and to alter cell motility.[93,94] Coexpression of PECAM-1 with VE-cadherin confers shear responsiveness in heterologous cells that normally are not affected by shear stress.[95] These mechanosensors in turn activate integrins that modify the cytoskeleton and coordinate downstream signaling. As an example, integrin activation leads to stimulation of kinases and phosphatases in focal adhesion complexes.[96] Changes in the actin cytoskeleton may affect RNA stability and translation.[97] In addition, flow sensitive ion channels[98] and G-proteins participate in mechanotransduction.[99] Furthermore, caveolae, which are flask-shaped membrane vesicular structures, are rich in signaling molecules such as G proteins, and are involved in signal generation in response to shear stress.[100]

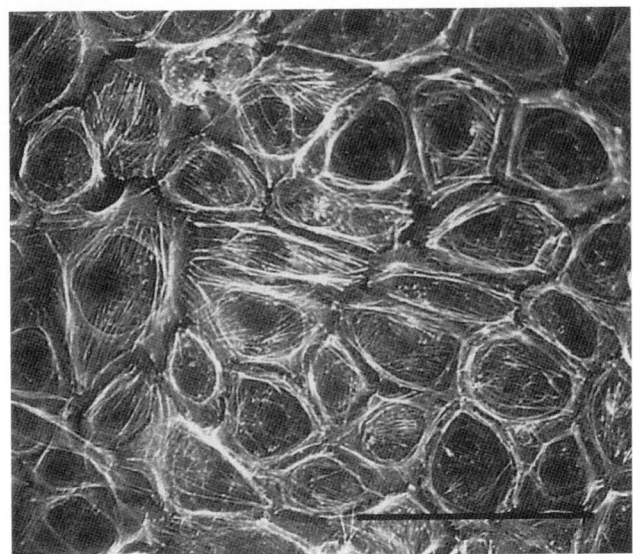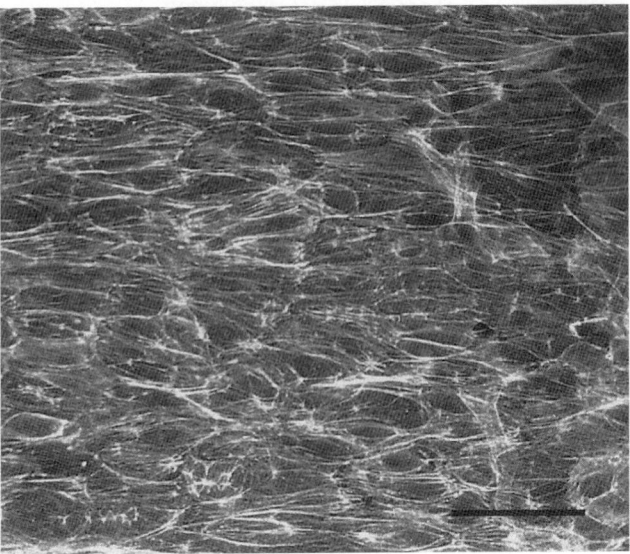

FIGURE 7–3. Effect of shear stress on endothelial cells. In bovine aortic endothelial cells grown in static conditions, F-actin filaments assume a random orientation as visualized by rhodamine-labeled phalloidin staining (*left*). On exposure to shear stress (30 dynes/cm², 24 h), these filaments align (*right*). Bars, 100 μm. *Source: Courtesy of Lula Hilenski, Ph.D.*

PHYSIOLOGY OF THE VASCULAR SMOOTH MUSCLE CELL

The SMC normally responds to hormonal stimulation with contraction or relaxation. In certain disease states, however, growth and/or hypertrophy and migration to the intima are predominant responses. Some of the biochemical signals generated by these vasoactive agonists are similar for both types of responses, with the final physiologic response dictated by the phenotype and environment of the cell, and the exact biochemical pathways activated.

【 】 MECHANISMS OF VASCULAR SMOOTH MUSCLE CELL CONTRACTION

Some of the earliest signals generated within the cell following stimulation with calcium-mobilizing vasoactive agonists involve hydrolysis of a specific class of membrane lipids, the phosphoinositides, by phospholipase C.[101] This event leads to production of inositol triphosphate (IP_3) and diacylglycerol (Fig. 7–4). IP_3 binds to IP_3 receptors (IP_3Rs) on intracellular organelles with releasable calcium stores. When IP_3 binds to these receptors, they form channels allowing calcium transit from these organelles into the cytoplasm.[102] IP_3R activity is modulated not only by IP_3 binding but also by phosphorylation and binding of nucleotides like ATP and NADH.[103] The consequent increase in cytosolic Ca^{2+} activates a cascade of enzymes leading to contraction or growth (see below). Diacylglycerol is a potent activator of protein kinase C, a Ca^{2+}- and phospholipid-dependent enzyme that phosphorylates numerous cellular proteins and thereby enhances contraction at any given level of intracellular calcium.[104] Diacylglycerol can be further metabolized to phosphatidic acid or to glycerol, fatty acids, and ultimately eicosanoids and leukotrienes that may themselves modulate tone.

Contractions induced by various vasoactive hormones differ not only in magnitude and time course, but also differ between vessels. In general, there is an initial, rapid component of force generation and a more sustained phase of contraction. Some agonists, such as angiotensin II, induce only a transient constriction of many vessels, whereas others including norepinephrine, endothelin, and vasopressin cause sustained contractions. The initial phase of force development is dependent on formation of actin-myosin cross-bridges in response to acute elevations of intracellular calcium, whereas the sustained phase of contraction persists even after calcium levels return toward baseline.

A sliding-filament mechanism similar to that found in skeletal muscle is thought to regulate phasic contraction of smooth muscle. Tension development is regulated by myosin light-chain kinase (MLCK)–mediated phosphorylation of myosin light chain (Fig. 7–5). When Ca^{2+} increases within the cell in response to hormonal stimulation, it binds to calmodulin, which, in turn associates with MLCK, converting it from an inactive to an active form. MLCK then phosphorylates the MLC, enabling actin to activate myosin Mg^{2+}-ATPase and crossbridge formation. When the intracellular Ca^{2+} concentration drops to less than approximately 100 nM, Ca^{2+} dissociates from calmodulin, calmodulin detaches from MLCK, and MLCK becomes inactive. MLC phosphatase activity then predominates, myosin is dephosphorylated, and crossbridge cycling ceases. During sustained contraction, however, the intracellular Ca^{2+} concentration is low, and energy consumption is reduced, suggesting the development of a latch-bridge, or of a low cycling state.[105] Alternatively, the Ca^{2+} sensitivity of the contractile apparatus may be increased, a response posited to be regulated by protein kinase C.[106] Recent evidence indicates that this latch state is also modulated the actin binding proteins caldesmon and calponin.[107] Caldesmon tonically inhibits contraction. Agonists such as phenylephrine stimulate extracellular regulated kinase (ERK) 1/2–mediated phosphorylation of caldesmon and enhance binding of calcium/calmodulin, removing its inhibitory effect and increasing tension.[108] Calponin has been suggested to directly inhibit the ATPase activity of myosin and to act as a signaling molecule that facilitates agonist-stimulated activation of protein kinase C.[109,110]

Recently, it has become apparent that the small molecular weight guanosine triphosphatase (GTPase) Rho, initially described as a modulator of the actin cytoskeleton, plays an important role in vascular smooth muscle contraction. In its active GTP-bound form, Rho activates Rho kinase, which inhibits myosin phosphatase type

1.[111] This inhibition in turn sustains MLC phosphorylation and sensitizes the contractile apparatus to calcium.[112] Rho kinase has become a target of therapeutic interventions. Its activity seems to be increased in hypertension,[113] and inhibitors of Rho kinase such as fasudil have been shown to lower vascular resistance in hypertension.[114]

【 】 FACTORS MODULATING VASCULAR SMOOTH MUSCLE GROWTH AND HYPERTROPHY

Normally, vascular SMCs are relatively refractory to growth stimuli and exist in a quiescent, differentiated state. The healthy endothelium is critically important in maintaining this phenotype. Products of the endothelium such as nitric oxide,[115] prostacyclin,[115] heparan sulfates[116] and transforming growth factor (TGF-β)[117] directly inhibit vascular smooth muscle growth. The endothelium is also an effective barrier limiting access of bloodborne growth factors to vascular smooth muscle. For example, the antithrombotic properties of the endothelium prevent access of promitogenic factors such as platelet-derived growth factor (PDGF) and thrombin to the underlying smooth muscle. Endothelial disruption allows initiation of a mitogenic smooth muscle response and regrowth of normal endothelium inhibits further proliferation.[118] In addition to these effects of the normal endothelium, the healthy vascular matrix minimizes vascular smooth muscle proliferation.

Under pathophysiologic conditions, the vascular milieu begins to favor vascular smooth muscle growth. One important phenomenon is degradation of the extracellular matrix to allow SMC migration, proliferation, and hypertrophy.[119] This is largely caused by matrix metalloproteinases released by activated cells intrinsic to the vessel or as invading inflammatory cells. A second pathologic alteration is the secretion of promitogenic agents by cells intrinsic to the vessel and invading inflammatory cells. The best studied of these factors is PDGF, so named because it was originally isolated from platelets. PDGF is composed of two distinct peptide chains (designated A and B chains), and can be secreted as an AB heterodimer, or as an AA or BB homodimer. Release of PDGF from the endothelium is regulated by growth factors including TGF-β, fibroblast growth factor (FGF), and tumor necrosis factor (TNF); circulating factors; and locally produced factors such as thrombin.[120] Another growth factor is insulin-like growth factor 1 (IGF-1),[13]

which is a progression factor that facilitates movement of cells through the cell cycle and enhances the mitogenic effect of PDGF on smooth muscle.[121] IGF-1 production by endothelium is regulated by PDGF and plays a major role in vascular hypertrophy and hyperplasia.[122] Other factors that affect smooth muscle proliferation include interleukin-1 (IL-1), FGF, and endothelin. IL-1 is an inflammatory cytokine that has numerous vascular effects in addition to mitogenesis, including the stimulation of procoagulant activity,[123] induction of leukocyte adhesiveness (see below), and inhibition of contraction.[124] Basic FGF acts as a potent smooth muscle mitogen, particularly after denuding injury.[125] It is stored in the subendothelial matrix and may be released by heparin and proteinases,[126] suggesting that the matrix may serve as a store for rapidly mobilizing this growth factor. FGF released from VSMCs may be particularly important in the growth response induced by injury to the arterial wall. Finally, endothelin-1, through its action on the ET-A receptor, induces SMC growth by stimulating increases in intracellular calcium, activating protein kinase C and in-

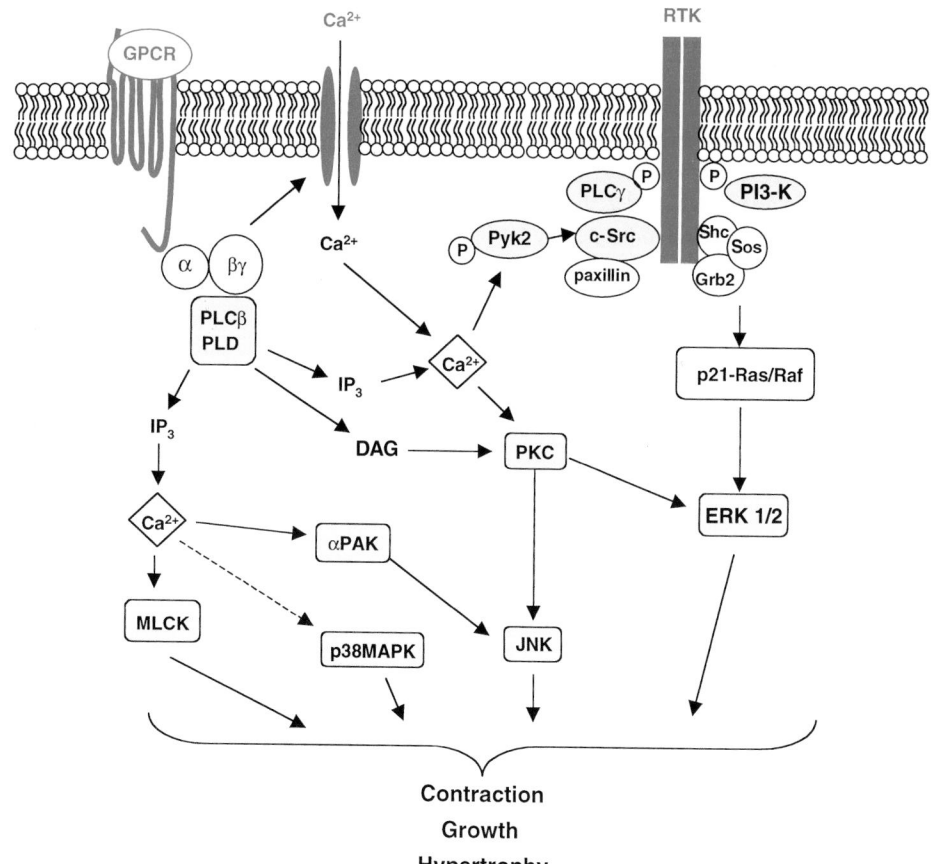

FIGURE 7-4. Signaling pathways in vascular smooth muscle. Vasoconstrictor agonists interact with specific G protein-coupled receptors (GPCRs) on vascular smooth muscle. These receptors are linked to a heterotrimeric G protein (αβγ), which then couples to one or more phospholipase Cs (PLCs) or phospholipase D (PLD). PLC cleaves the inositol phospholipids to yield diacylglycerol (DAG) and inositol phosphates, in particular, inositol trisphosphate (IP₃). IP₃ releases calcium from intracellular stores, and, along with DAG, activates the Ca²⁺ and phospholipid-dependent enzyme protein kinase C (PKC). Ca²⁺ activates numerous other kinases, including p21-activated kinase (α-PAK), Pyk2, and myosin light chain kinase (MLCK). PLD cleaves phosphatidycholine to release phosphatidic acid, which is converted to DAG. PKC is involved in activation of the mitogen-activated protein (MAPK) cascade, including extracellular signal-regulated kinases (ERK 1/2) and Jun kinase (JNK). Growth factors activate receptor tyrosine kinases (RTKs), Src, PLC-γ, and phosphatidylinositol 3-kinase (PI3-K). RTKs also phosphorylate and form a signaling complex with paxillin and adapter proteins such as Shc, which binds Grb-2 and Sos and ultimately mediates the conversion of Ras to its active form, Ras phosphorylates Raf1, which in turn leads to activation of the MAP kinase cascade.

creasing intracellular production of reactive oxygen species. Diverse stimuli such as elevated insulin,[127] oscillatory shear stress and pressure,[128] and angiotensin II[129] potently induce endothelial production of ET-1.

MECHANISMS OF VASCULAR SMOOTH MUSCLE GROWTH

Vascular SMC growth occurs via two processes: hypertrophy and hyperplasia. In general, hypertrophy occurs in response to long-term stimulation with vasoconstrictor-type agents, whereas hyperplasia occurs in response to the classic growth factors. Hypertrophy is characterized by an increase in SMC mass caused by increased protein synthesis and has been shown to occur in response to angiotensin II[130] and thrombin[131] as well as in large vessels during hypertension. Hyperplasia is characterized by cell replication and is stimulated by growth factors such as PDGF and FGF following vascular injury.[125,132,133] The biochemical processes leading to hypertrophy and hyperplasia have been extensively investigated.

Classic growth factors, such as PDGF, activate many of the same signaling pathways as do vasoconstrictors: phosphoinositide hydrolysis, Ca^{2+} mobilization and influx, and protein kinase C activation. Receptors for these growth factors are intrinsic tyrosine kinases, leading to the tyrosine phosphorylation of numerous proteins that are essential for growth. Tyrosine phosphatases can counteract the mitogenic effects of growth factors by inhibiting tyrosine phosphorylation of specific substrates.[134]

When growth factor receptors are activated, they recruit a complex of proteins that subsequently activate multiple signaling cascades leading to the final cellular response.[135] Initially, growth factor receptors dimerize and phosphorylate themselves on tyrosine residues. Some proteins, such as phospholipase C-γ, the tyrosine kinase c-Src, and phosphatidylinositol 3-kinase, bind directly to receptor tyrosine kinases, whereas others, including the tyrosine kinase Pyk-2 and the cytoskeletal protein paxillin, associate with the receptor via linker proteins such as Grb and Shc. Shc and Grb2 link these receptors to Ras, a ubiquitous GTPase that initiates a serine/threonine kinase cascade that includes mitogen-activated protein kinase (MAPK) and ultimately leads to growth. Recent evidence suggests that many of these proteins are also activated by seven transmembrane-spanning G-protein-coupled receptors,[136,137] an observation that may partially explain the growth-promoting properties of vasoconstrictor hormones like angiotensin II, thrombin, and ET-1.

Reactive oxygen species play a crucial role in modulation these growth-related signaling pathways. Growth-promoting agonists

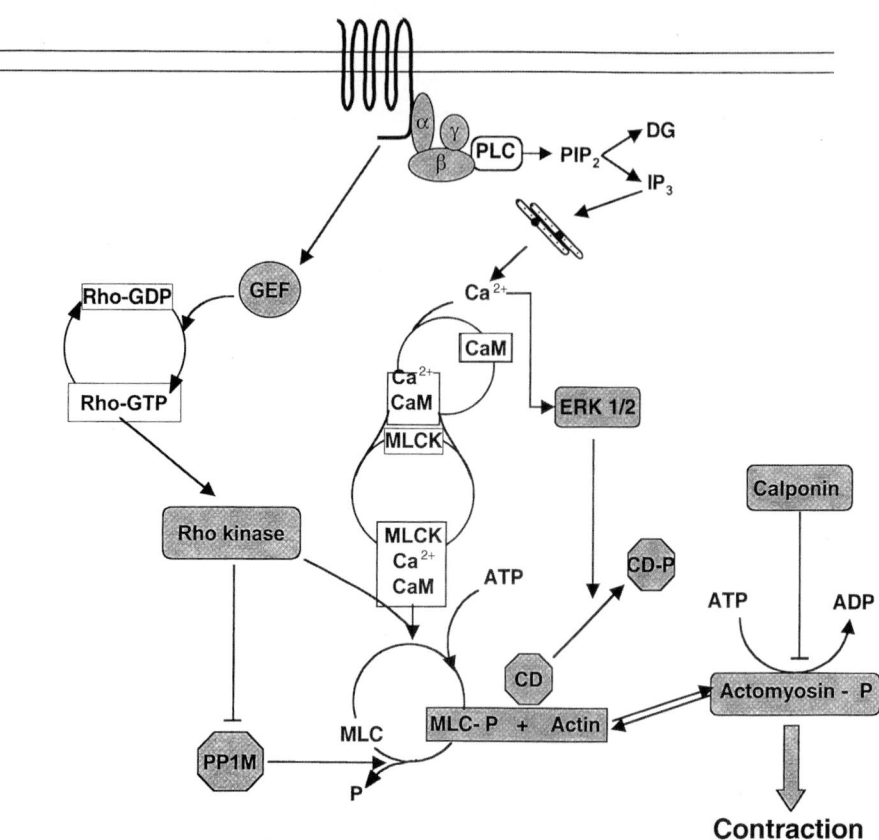

FIGURE 7–5. Contraction cascade. Activation of smooth muscle by a vasoconstrictor hormone leads to a cascade of biochemical signals, ultimately resulting in phosphorylation of actomyosin, crossbridge formation, and force generation. The release of Ca^{2+} from intracellular stores is one of the major initiating events, because Ca^{2+} combines with calmodulin (CaM) to activate myosin light chain kinase (MLCK). This enzyme phosphorylates the myosin light chain (MLC), which is then able to interact with actin. In addition, activation of a guanine nucleotide exchange factor (GEF) for the small molecular weight G protein Rho leads to stimulation of Rho and Rho kinase, which inhibits myosin phosphatase (PP1M), thus enhancing myosin light chain phosphorylation (MLCP). Caldesmon (CD), which normally inhibits actin-myosin interaction, becomes phosphorylated by extracellular signal regulated kinase (ERK 1/2) and is released from this complex. Calponin acts by inhibiting myosin ATPase activity. αβγ, heterotrimeric G protein; PLC, phospholipase C; DAG, diacylglycerol; PIP_2, phosphatidylinositol 4,5-bisphosphate; IP_3, inositol triphosphate; Ca^{2+}, calcium; ATP, adenosine triphosphate; P, phosphate. *Source: Courtesy of Bernard Lassègue, Ph.D.*

stimulate the NADPH oxidases to produce superoxide and hydrogen peroxide, which may serve as progenitors to numerous other reactive oxygen species.[138,139] Of these, hydrogen peroxide seems to be particularly important in the growth process. Production of small concentrations of endogenous hydrogen peroxide activates specific mitogenic signaling pathways such as p38 mitogen-activated protein kinase (MAPK) and Akt/protein kinase B and promotes entry into the cell cycle.[140–142] Hydrogen peroxide inactivates protein tyrosine phosphatases by oxidizing critical cysteine residues, leading to sustained protein phosphorylation of target molecules. Important scavengers of hydrogen peroxide are the peroxiredoxins, which are localized in specific regions of the cell. One of these, peroxiredoxin II, has a unique role in modulating cell growth because it binds to the PDGF receptor and inhibits its downstream signaling.[143]

THE EXTRACELLULAR MATRIX

The extracellular matrix is a major component of the vessel wall. It is the medium through which nutrients are transported, a re-

TABLE 7–1

Components of the Extracellular Matrix

MATRIX COMPONENT	FUNCTION
Proteoglycans	• Resistance to deformation • Arterial permeability, filtration, ion exchange • Transport and deposition of plasma elements • Regulation of cellular metabolism
Collagens (types I and III)	• Mechanical strength
Collagens (types IV, V, and VI)	• Attachment of vascular cells to the matrix • Components of the basal lamina • Linking collagens to noncollagenous structures
Elastin	• Regulation of vascular elasticity
Fibronectin	• Cell–cell adhesion • Cell–substrate adhesion • Cell motility • Specific binding of collagen, heparin
Laminin	• Attachment of endothelial cells to type IV collagen

pository for products secreted by the cells of the vascular wall, the site of accumulation of cell debris, and a substrate for migration and proliferation of endothelial cells, monocytes, and vascular SMCs. The matrix consists of several proteins that have distinct functions in maintaining the integrity of the wall (Table 7–1).

Extracellular matrix degradation and reformation is an extremely important biological process with profound clinical implications. It is impossible for vascular cells to hypertrophy, proliferate, or migrate without initial degradation of the matrix. One of the earliest events in angiogenesis is the degradation of the extracellular matrix to enable tube (capillary) formation. Vascular cells, including endothelial cells, VSMCs, resident macrophages and fibroblasts, may secrete matrix metalloproteinases (MMPs), enzymes that selectively digest the individual components of the matrix. In addition, these cells elaborate tissue inhibitors of metalloproteinases (TIMPs).[8]

There are two classes of MMPs: Those that are secreted and those that are membrane spanning with their active site outside the cell. The secreted MMPs belong to three main groups: the type IV collagenases (also called *gelatinases*), stromelysins, and interstitial collagenase. The characteristics of these proteins are described in Table 7–2. MMPs are produced as inactive zymogens that can be activated by plasmin.[9] The activity

TABLE 7–2

Matrix Metalloproteinases and Inhibitors

CLASS	NOMENCLATURE	MOLECULAR WEIGHT (KDA)[a]	VASCULAR CELL TYPE	EXPRESSION
Interstitial collagenase	MMP-1	~45	VSMC, EC, microvascular EC	Inducible by PDGF, PMA, IL-1, VEGF
Type IV collagenase	MMP-9 gelatinase B type V gelatinase	92	VSMC EC	Inducible by IL-1α, PMA Inhibited by retinoic acid
	MMP-2 gelatinase A type IV gelatinase	72	VSMC wounded EC microvascular EC	Constitutive ↑ by TNF-α, IL-1α (VSMC) ↓ by retinoic acid (EC)
Stromelysin	MMP-3	50	VSMC EC microvascular EC	Inducible by IL-1 (VSMC); TNF-α, PMA (EC)
Matrilysin	MMP-7	—	VSMC, macrophage	Hypercholesterolemia
Membrane-type metalloproteinase	MT-MMP	—	VSMC, macrophage, EC	?
TIMP-1	Inhibits MMPs	30	VSMC EC microvascular EC	Constitutive
TIMP-2	Inhibits MMP-2	~20	VSMC EC microvascular EC	Constitutive ↑ by retinoic acid (EC)

EC, endothelial cell; IL, interleukin; MMP, matrix metalloproteinase; MT-MMP, membrane type MMP; PDGF, platelet-derived growth factor; PMA, phorbol 12,13-myrisate acetate; TIMP, tissue inhibitor of metalloproteinase; TNF, tumor necrosis factor; VEGF, vascular endothelial growth factor; VSMC, vascular smooth muscle cell.
[a]The molecular weight of MMP-1 and MMP-3 depends on the species.

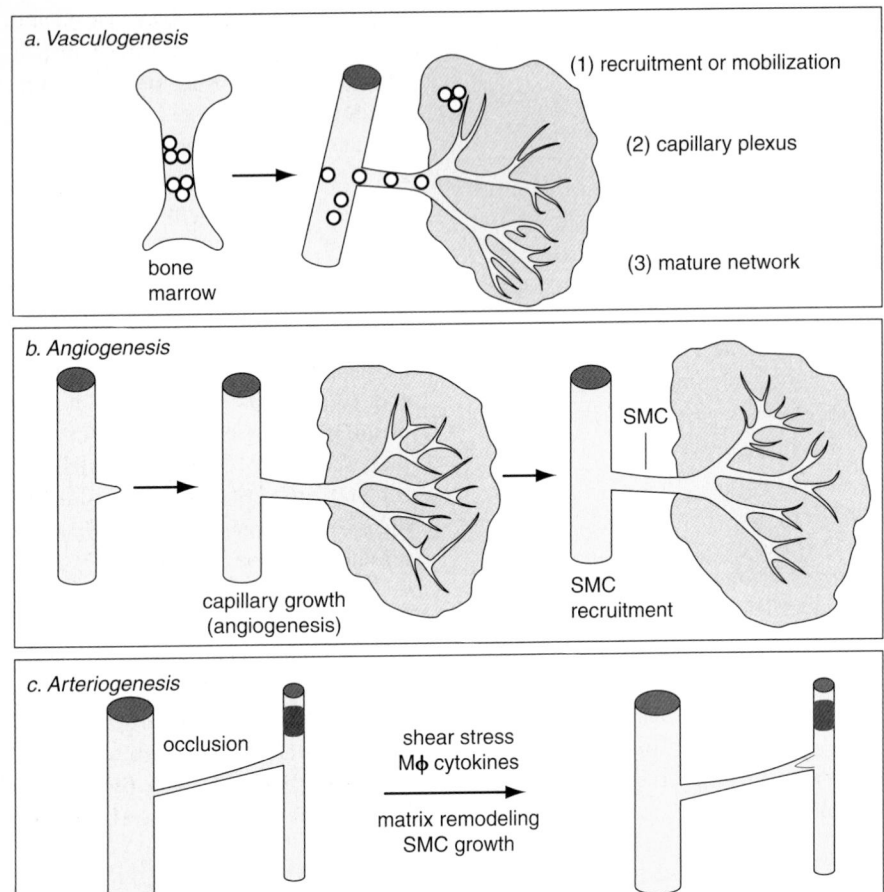

a. Vasculogenesis

bone marrow

(1) recruitment or mobilization

(2) capillary plexus

(3) mature network

b. Angiogenesis

capillary growth (angiogenesis)

SMC recruitment

SMC

c. Arteriogenesis

occlusion

shear stress Mφ cytokines

matrix remodeling SMC growth

FIGURE 7–6. Pathologic vascular growth in the adult may occur via vasculogenesis (endothelial progenitor cell [EPC] mobilization), angiogenesis (sprouting) or arteriogenesis (collateral growth). Mφ, macrophages; SMCs, smooth muscle cells. *Source: Reprinted with permission from Luttun, Carmeliet, and Carmeliet.*[152]

teases capable of degrading all the major matrix components. In contrast, although TIMP-1 and TIMP-2 are constitutively expressed by vascular smooth muscle, their expression is unaffected by cytokines.[9] The net effect of cytokines on the vascular wall may be to tip the balance between the production of MMPs and TIMPs in favor of extracellular matrix degradation and remodeling.

Of particular importance, several reactive oxygen species have been shown to stimulate both activation and expression of MMPs, in particular MMP-9.[146,147] This is likely to be important in diseases like atherosclerosis and hypertension, where vascular oxidant stress is increased. Activated macrophages accumulate at shoulder regions of the atherosclerotic plaque and secrete both MMPs and reactive oxygen species,[147,148] contributing to plaque rupture in this region.

There has been a great deal of interest recently in the pivotal role of MMPs and TIMPs in atherosclerotic plaques and aneurysms.[149] In the atherosclerotic lesion, MMPs are highly expressed at the shoulder region and predispose to plaque rupture.[148] Abdominal aortic aneurysms which are atherosclerotic in origin, exhibit unbridled MMP activity.[150] In both conditions, oxidative stress, inflammation, and altered hemodynamics likely contribute to MMP expression and activation. It has recently been demonstrated that MMPs are also active in aneurysms of Marfan syndrome patients.[151]

of MMPs is also regulated by cytokines at transcriptional and posttranslational levels, as well as by the relative levels of TIMPs. MMP-2 is usually found complexed with its specific inhibitor, TIMP-2. The membrane spanning MMPs are known as *a disintegrin and metalloproteinase* (ADAM). These multifunctional proteins mediate cell adhesion, and degrade matrix components to release important paracrine factors such as heparin-binding epidermal growth factor (EGF), tumor necrosis factor-α (TNF-α), Fas ligand, Notch, and monocyte-colony stimulating factor.[144]

In venous or microvascular endothelial cells, MMP-1 (interstitial collagenase), MMP-2 (72-kDa gelatinase), and TIMPs-1 and -2 are constitutively expressed. Although MMP-3 is only weakly expressed, it can be induced synergistically by incubation of the cells with TNF-α and with phorbol ester tumor promoters.[8] This treatment also induces MMP-9 expression. Because MMP-2 and TIMP-2 are unaffected by TNF-α, cytokine activation of endothelial cells can change the complement of metalloproteinases produced. In VSMCs, MMP-2 is constitutively expressed, whereas MMP-1, MMP-9 (92-kDa gelatinase), and MMP-3 (stromelysin) are induced by cytokines such as interleukin-1 and TNF-α.[9] Cytokines can also activate MMP-2 zymogen.[145] Thus, cytokine stimulation increases the range of active metalloproteinases secreted by SMCs to encompass pro-

ANGIOGENESIS

Although pathologic vascular remodeling in conditions like atherosclerosis and hypertension has been widely appreciated, it was previously thought that new vessel formation, such as the growth of collaterals caused by ischemia, arose from cells in existing vascular structures (angiogenesis and arteriogenesis). This general perception has changed radically in recent years (Fig. 7–6). It is now recognized that endothelial and vascular smooth muscle progenitor cells, likely derived from the bone marrow, contribute to new blood vessel development in adults and to continuous renewal of the existing vasculature.[152]

▌▐ GENERAL ASPECTS OF VASCULAR DEVELOPMENT

The angioblast/hemangioblast is an early endothelial cell progenitor and is also the progenitor cell for hematopoietic cells and skeletal muscle. Many of the genes involved in vasculogenesis have been defined using mouse gene knockout models.[153] Of the large number of genes involved, a smaller number are particularly interesting because their loss has a major impact on vasculogenesis. The VEGF family is among the most important, and VEGF is required for initial endothelial cell differentiation and proliferation.[154,155]

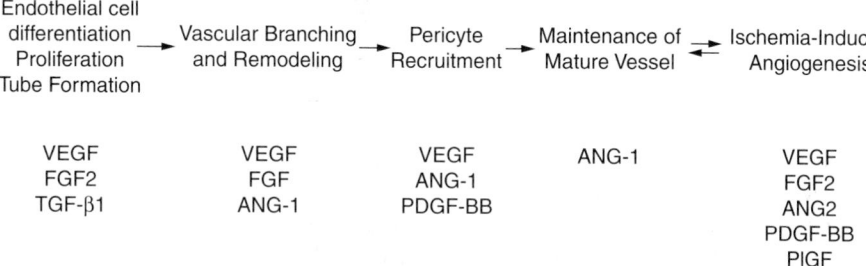

FIGURE 7–7. A simplified scheme of vasculogenesis and angiogenesis. Examples of angiogenic factors that are critical at each step are shown. VEGF, vascular endothelial growth factor; FGF, fibroblast growth factor; TGF-β1, transforming growth factor-β1; ANG-1, angiopoietin; PDGF-BB, platelet-derived growth factor-BB (B= B chain); PGF, placenta-derived growth factor. *Source: Reproduced with permission from Semenza.*[153]

VEGF binds to its cognate tyrosine kinase receptor VEGF receptor-2 (VEGFR-2), which is also known as *flk1* or *kdr*.[156] Other homologs of VEGF include VEGF-B and placental growth factor (PGF) and all three growth factors bind to VEGFR-1 or flt-1. The PGF- flt-1 interaction contributes to pathologic angiogenesis in the adult, as discussed subsequently. The angiopoietins (1 and 2) are also involved in development and maintenance of mature blood vessels in part because they recruit pericytes, which are essential to vessel maturation. An additional family of molecules, the ephrins, mediate cell-to-cell recognition.[154,155] Other growth factors that play a role in vascular development include PDGF-BB, bFGF, acidic FGF, and TGF-β1. The process of embryonic vascu-

logenesis, angiogenesis, and arteriogenesis is depicted sequentially with the involved growth factors in Figure 7–7 and graphically in Figure 7–8.

【 】 ANGIOGENESIS AND ARTERIOGENESIS IN THE ADULT

Growth Factors

In animal models of ischemic heart disease VEGF expression is stimulated after coronary artery occlusion and is associated with formation of collateral vessels.[157,158] VEGF expression is regulated, at least in part, by hypoxia-inducible factor-1 (HIF-1), which is a transcription factor that acts as a molecular switch for angiogenesis.[159] HIF-1 expression is upregulated by hypoxia and ischemia. The response of this system varies, as reflected in clinical experience in which different patients have variable degrees of collateralization with apparently similar degrees of coronary artery obstruction. This heterogeneity of individual responses partially depends on age as determined in animal experiments.[160–162] In addition to age-related factors, individual genetic or environmental factors likely determine the responsiveness of the systems controlling collateralization in humans.[153,163]

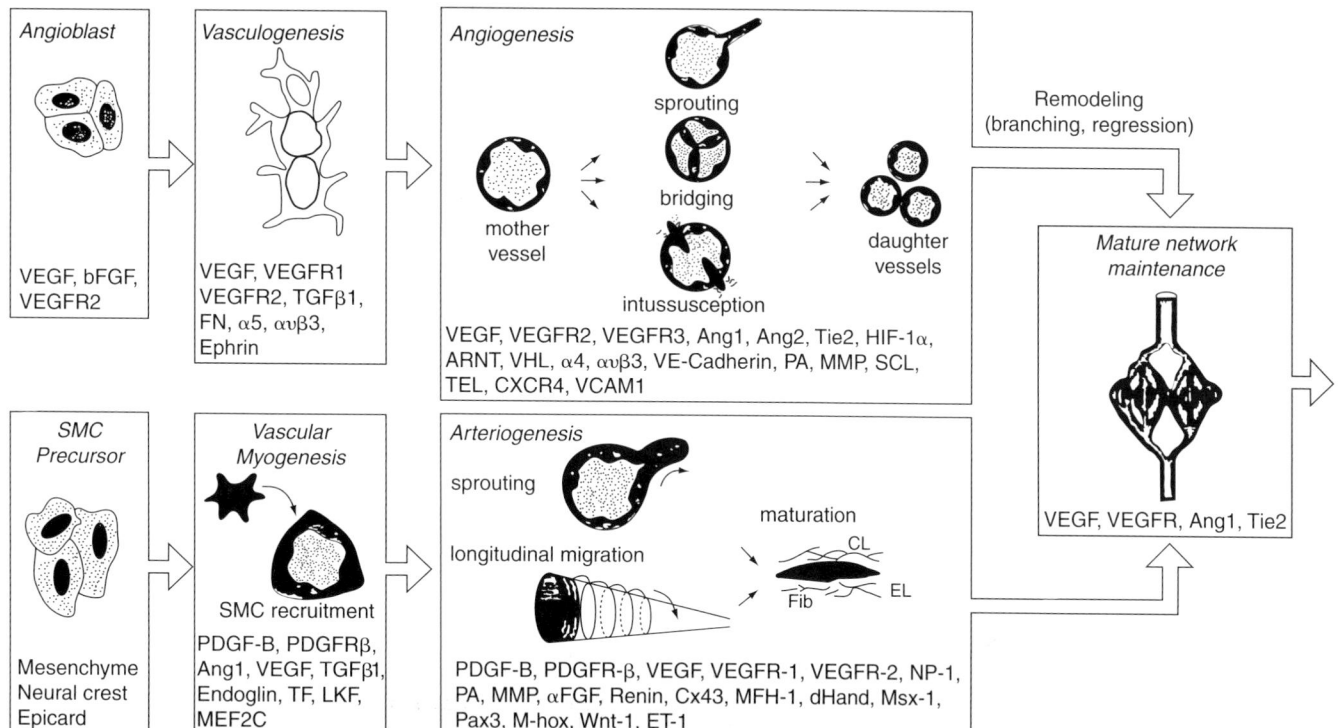

FIGURE 7–8. Endothelial precursors (angioblasts) in the embryo assemble in a primitive network (vasculogenesis), that expands and remodels (angiogenesis). Smooth muscle cells cover endothelial cells during vascular myogenesis, and stabilize vessels during arteriogenesis. CL, collagen; EL, elastin, Fib, fibrillin. *Source: Reproduced with permission from Carmeliet P.*[155]

Bone Marrow–Derived Progenitor Cells

As noted, neovascularization in the adult previously was thought to result exclusively from angiogenesis.[152] Several recent studies, however, have described endothelial progenitor cells (EPCs) postnatally circulating in the peripheral blood that incorporate into the neovasculature associated with tumors, ischemic myocardium and hindlimbs, cutaneous wounds, and injured corneas.[164–167] There is an emerging large body of literature regarding the biology of EPCs, including their proliferation in the bone marrow, mobilization from the marrow, homing to sites of injury, and differentiation. Proliferation of EPCs seems to be stimulated by factors that activate phosphatidylinositol 3-kinase (PI3-K) and Akt, and inhibited by activation of p38 mitogen-activated protein kinase (MAPK).[168] Numerous agents, including erythropoietin, nitric oxide, VEGF, PGF, macrophage colony-stimulating factor, angiopoietin-1, and granulocyte-macrophage colony-stimulating factor, promote mobilization of EPCs from the marrow.[169] Homing EPCs to ischemic regions is thought to be initiated by hypoxic stimulation of the chemokine stromal cell-derived factor-1.[170] Risk factors for coronary artery diseases are associated with lower numbers of circulating EPCs and the HMG-CoA reductase inhibitors have been shown to increase their number.[171,172] In keeping with the aforementioned role of p38 MAPK in inhibiting EPC proliferation, patients with coronary artery disease have increased p38 phosphorylation, which corresponds to activity, in their EPCs and inhibition of p38 leads to increased EPC proliferation.[173]

There has been enormous interest in therapeutic approaches to enhance collateral growth. Initial studies involved injection of either growth factors or growth factor genes into ischemic tissues. Although early studies lacking appropriate controls seemed promising, a well-designed trial of VEGF injection for stimulation of coronary collaterals showed virtually no more effect than placebo control.[174] Studies using strategies to mobilize progenitor cells from the bone marrow have proven ineffective in treatment of either limb or myocardial ischemia.[175,176] More recent studies have used injection of cells from the bone marrow or from peripheral blood and have yielded promising results, but these studies have lacked appropriate controls.[177–181]

VASCULAR INFLAMMATION

Endothelial cells actively participate in the development of inflammatory reactions. The recruitment of leukocytes to sites of inflammation is initiated by endothelial secretion of chemotactic molecules and enhanced expression of adhesion molecules that interact with surface proteins on leukocytes.[182] Cytokines and arachidonic acid metabolites of the leukotriene pathway derived from cells of the vessel wall, the infiltrating macrophages, and T-lymphocytes stimulate endothelial secretion in many of these molecules.[182] An important class of molecules that mediate the vascular inflammatory response is the chemokines, of which more than 50 have been identified.[183] Two classes of the chemokines exist, known as the CXC and CC, based on differences in the position of the first two cysteines in their amino acid sequence. These interact with at least 20 G-protein receptors, classified as CXCR and CCR, according to their corresponding ligand.

It has been suggested that the sequential accumulation of different leukocyte classes at sites of inflammation can be explained by the differential induction of these endothelial cell adhesion molecules.[184] An early step in the inflammatory response is capture of leukocytes from the flowing blood, mediated by the L- and P- selectins.[185,186] A second step is leukocyte rolling, which is mediated by interaction with E- and P- selectins.[185,186] Ultimate adhesion of leukocytes depends interactions with β_2-integrins PECAM and ICAM-1.[185,186] At the site of atherosclerotic lesions, recruitment of leukocytes is markedly enhanced by the surface expression of VCAM-1 and interactions between the monocyte chemotactic protein (MCP-1) and its monocyte receptor CCR2.[187,188] IL-8 and its receptor CXCR2 as well as fractalkine and its receptor CX_3CL1 also contribute to this response.[189,190] The list of proinflammatory molecules contributing to these endothelial/leukocyte interactions continues to grow, and it is likely that the complete inflammatory response depends on the concerted action of many such molecular mediators. This is supported by the observations that genetic knockout of the IL-8 receptor, MCP-1, or CX3CR1 each leads to a >50 percent reduction in lesion formation in atherosclerotic mice.[189,190] Knockout of CX3CR1 also protects against vascular proliferation in response to injury.[191]

ENDOTHELIAL DYSFUNCTION AND VASCULAR SMOOTH MUSCLE ABNORMALITIES

In general, the normal endothelium promotes vasodilatation and inhibits contraction, thrombosis, white cell adhesion, and vascular smooth muscle growth (see Fig. 7–2; Fig. 7–9). A common feature of many different vascular diseases is that these functions of the endothelium are either lost or disrupted, a phenomenon often referred to as *endothelial dysfunction*. Implicit in this term is the recognition that the fundamental or normal functions of the endothelium are not fixed but are mutable. Thus, the endothelium in a given area may lose its vasodilator predominance; become prothrombotic or less thrombolytic; begin to support leukocyte adherence, which may be a

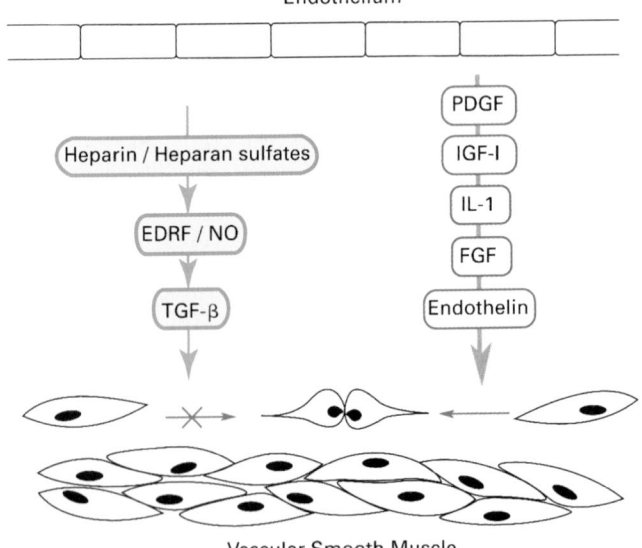

FIGURE 7–9. Endothelial control of vascular growth. As with vasoactive substances, endothelial cells make and secrete both growth-promoting (*white boxes*) and growth-inhibitory (*colored boxes*) compounds. Under normal conditions, the net effect of the endothelium is growth inhibitory. EDRF, endothelial-derived relaxing factor; NO, nitric oxide; TGF-β, transforming growth factor-β; PDGF, platelet-derived growth factor; IGF-I, insulinlike growth factor-I; IL-1, interleukin-1; FGF, fibroblast growth factor. *Source: Courtesy of Bernard Lassègue, Ph.D.*

normal response in the inflammatory process; or stimulate rather than inhibit smooth muscle migration and proliferation.

ROLE OF REACTIVE OXYGEN SPECIES

In the past several years, it has become clear that vascular cells, including endothelial, vascular smooth muscle, and adventitial cells, can produce reactive oxygen species (ROS).[192] These include the superoxide anion, hydrogen peroxide, NO, and peroxynitrite. In numerous pathophysiologic conditions, the production of ROS in the vascular wall is increased. Many normal functions of the endothelium are altered by this increase in ROS, which contributes to the development of vascular disease.

Recent studies suggest that NADPH oxidases are major sources of ROS in endothelial and vascular SMCs.[192] These are multisubunit enzymes that have partial similarity to the neutrophil respiratory burst oxidase. The catalytic subunits of these enzymes are the Nox proteins, which harbor the NADPH binding site and transfer electrons through FAD to heme groups and subsequently to molecular oxygen.[193–195] Vascular cells express Nox1, Nox2, Nox4, and Nox5.[195,196] The adventitia also contains fibroblasts and macrophages that express multiple oxidases.[197] Nox1 and Nox2 clearly require cytosolic subunits for activation, whereas regulation of Nox4 is less well understood. Importantly, the NADPH oxidases are activated by several pathophysiologic stimuli, including angiotensin II, mechanical stretch, cytokines, and thrombin.[84,139,198,199] Recent studies have shown that the small molecular weight G-protein Rac1 is a central regulator of oxidase activity.[200] Rac1 geranylation can be inhibited by the HMG-CoA reductase inhibitors,[201] suggesting one mechanism whereby these agents can have vasculoprotective effects.

A second source of ROS is eNOS. As discussed previously, in the absence of tetrahydrobiopterin or L-arginine, this enzyme becomes *uncoupled* so that it produces hydrogen peroxide and superoxide, rather than NO.[44,202] In hypercholesterolemia,[203] hypertension,[45] insulin resistance,[204] and diabetes,[205] there is evidence that tetrahydrobiopterin is oxidized, leading to eNOS uncoupling.

Another source of radicals in the vasculature is the lipoxygenases, and in particular 12,15-lipoxygenase.[206] These enzymes do not form superoxide but react directly with unsaturated fatty acids (e.g., linoleic or arachidonic acid) to form a lipid radical (L·), which in turn can react with molecular O_2 to produce alkoxy radicals (LO·) and lipid peroxy radicals (LOO·). These lipid radicals are biologically active, and can stimulate gene expression, consume NO, oxidize NADH, and serve as a source of other radicals.[207]

ROS in vascular cells are also produced by xanthine oxidase, cytochrome P450, cyclooxygenase, and mitochondrial electron transport. In particular there is evidence in humans that xanthine oxidase can produce ROS and affect endothelial function in the setting of atherosclerosis and heart failure,[208–210] possibly caused by stimulation of XO expression by inflammatory cytokines. In addition, in many tissues, the mitochondrial electron transport chain represents a predominant source of ROS. Under normal circumstances, between 1 and 4 percent of the oxygen reacting with the respiratory chain is incompletely reduced to O_2. Hyperglycemia has been shown to increase electron shuttling to oxygen in the mitochondrial pathway, increasing superoxide formation. This has profound effects on other metabolic events in the cell.[211] There is substantial interest in how various sources of ROS are affected by different pathologic states.

In the next several paragraphs, we consider how endothelial dysfunction and vascular smooth muscle abnormalities contribute to several vascular diseases. A recurring theme in these conditions is that ROS play a central role. For example, superoxide rapidly reacts with NO, forming the strong oxidant peroxynitrite. The latter can oxidize lipids, damage lipid membranes, deplete cellular thiols, and alter function of several enzymes.[212] This inactivation of NO alters vasomotion and can predispose one to or even cause hypertension.[213] Other ROS such as the hydroxyl radical and lipid radicals can also react with NO. Furthermore, both VSMC hypertrophy and migration are regulated by hydrogen peroxide.[214] ROS also contribute to vascular inflammation by stimulating expression of adhesion molecules in endothelial cells.[215] These issues are discussed in the context of several vascular diseases.

ATHEROSCLEROSIS

Atherosclerosis is the prototypical disease characterized by endothelial dysfunction, which explains many of its cardinal features. Abnormalities of the endothelium induced by hyperlipidemia, hypertension, smoking, and unknown hereditary factors initiate mononuclear and lymphocytic infiltration, vascular smooth muscle hypercontractility, and LDL modification, as well as SMC growth and migration. The pathogenesis of atherosclerosis viewed as a disease of endothelial dysfunction is depicted in Fig. 7–10. (For a more detailed discussion, see Chap. 52.)

Clinically, endothelial dysfunction in atherosclerosis has primarily been defined by impairment of endothelial-dependent relaxation.[216,217] Coronary endothelial-dependent vasodilator function is impaired in patients with risk factors such as hypercholesterolemia, prior to angiographically demonstrable coronary disease.[218] As previously discussed, increased inactivation of NO by the superoxide anion is likely one cause of this abnormality. The increase in O_2 leads to increased hydrogen peroxide formation, which can serve as a direct vasodilator via hyperpolarization to counter the effects of NO depletion.[58] Of note, LDL and cytokines have been shown to downregulate eNOS by destabilizing the eNOS mRNA.[219] This is prevented by statins via inhibition of Rho GTPase and downstream modification of the actin cytoskeleton. This effect likely represents an additional mechanism of action of the HMG-CoA reductase inhibitors.[220]

A second manifestation of a dysfunctional endothelium that is apparent very early after initiation of cholesterol feeding in animals is the recruitment of monocytes and macrophages into the vessel wall.[221] LDL particles normally cycle in and out of the subintimal space; however, in the setting of numerous risk factors, this environment becomes more oxidized, leading to LDL modification. Modified LDL activates Toll-like receptors (TLRs), in particular TLR4, which in turn induce proinflammatory gene expression, and lead to macrophage infiltration.[222] This recruitment is likely the result of induction of VCAM-1 expression[223] as well as secretion of MCP-1.[224] Activated macrophages and vascular cells then secrete inflammatory cytokines that amplify adhesion molecule expression.[225] The role of these various signaling and inflammatory molecules in atherosclerosis has been demonstrated elegantly using genetically modified mice. Inhibition of MCP-1 or its receptor attenuates the development of early atherosclerotic lesions in experimental animals.[187,226] Mice harboring a mutation of

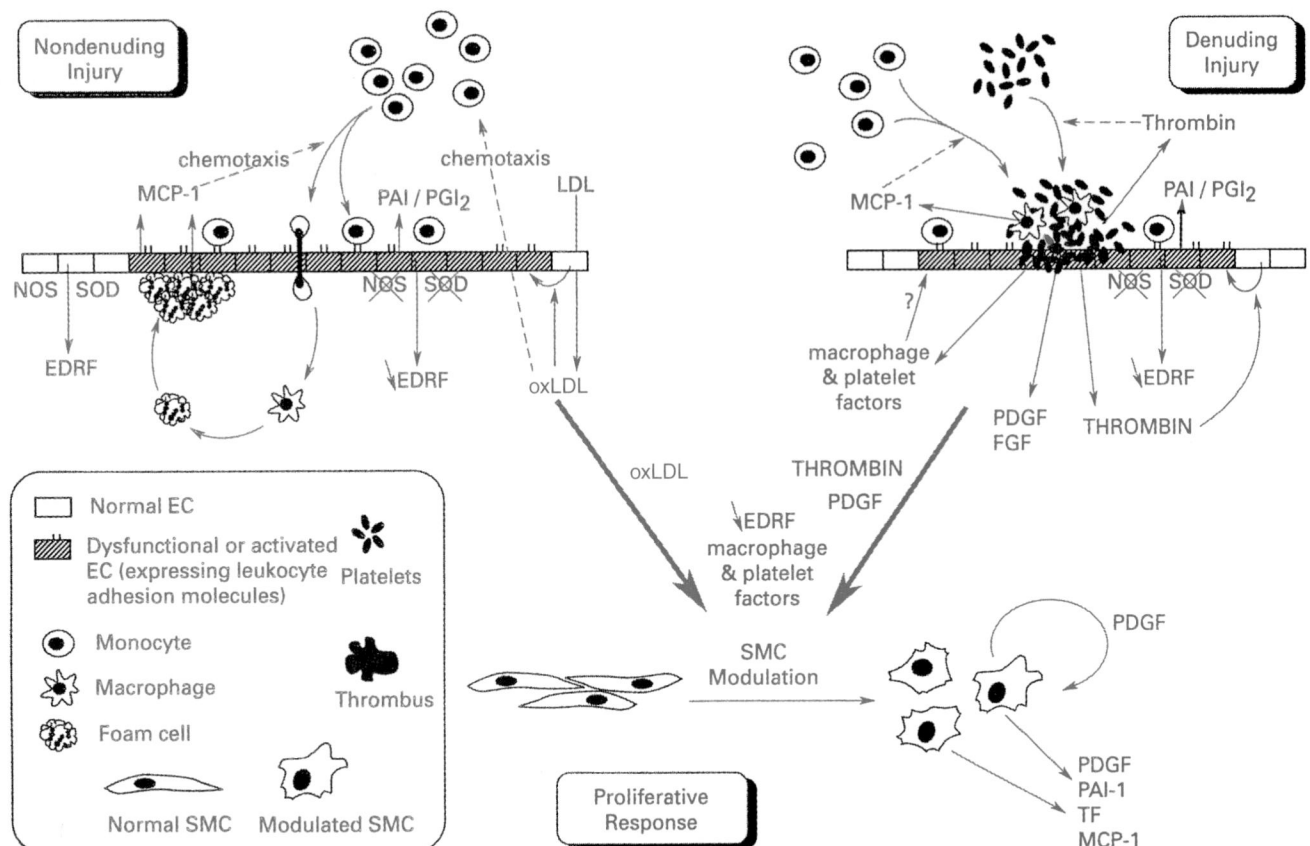

FIGURE 7–10. Theoretical initiating events in vascular lesion formation. **Nondenuding injury:** Low-density lipoprotein (LDL) enters the subendothelial space where it is converted to oxidized LDL (oxLDL), which induces monocyte chemoattraction and endothelial dysfunction. Dysfunctional endothelial cells (ECs) express cell adhesion molecules (intercellular adhesion molecule [ICAM], endothelial-leukocyte adhesion molecule [ELAM], and vascular cell adhesion molecule [VCAM]), leading to increased monocyte adhesion and movement into the vessel wall. Monocytes in the vessel wall differentiate into macrophages, take up lipids, and remain locally as foam cells, subsequently evolving into fatty streaks. The foam cells in the fatty streak and the overlying endothelium express monocyte chemotactic protein 1 (MCP-1), resulting in further enhanced monocyte chemoattraction and adhesion. Dysfunctional ECs may synthesize less nitric oxide synthase (NOS) or superoxide dismutase (SOD, an enzyme that metabolizes oxygen radicals that have been shown to inactivate NO). This decreases endothelial-derived relaxing factor (EDRF) release/activity. The loss of EDRF together with the direct effects of oxLDL, or growth factors secreted by the foam cells or endothelium, act on the quiescent contractile smooth muscle cells (SMCs) in the vessel wall, giving rise to the proliferative phenotype, with division and migration into the intima. **Denuding injury:** Loss of endothelium leads to platelet deposition, tissue factor-mediated activation of extrinsic coagulation to generate thrombin, cleavage of fibrinogen to fibrin, and the formation of thrombus. Thrombin gives rise to endothelial expression of adhesion molecules and consequent monocyte attachment, together with secretion of platelet granular constituents. Monocytes enter the thrombus and differentiate into phagocytic macrophages expressing tissue factor and MCP-1. This leads to further monocyte chemoattraction into the vessel wall. SMC proliferation is produced by (1) thrombin generation at the site of denuding injury, (2) platelet-derived growth factor (PDGF) or other growth factors released from platelets in the thrombus, (3) factors secreted by the macrophages ingesting the thrombus, and (4) the loss of EDRF activity caused by endothelial dysfunction. **Proliferative response:** Modulated SMCs proliferate and synthesize factors that promote plaque development. SMCs synthesize (1) PDGF and other growth factors that cause self-perpetuating autocrine or paracrine stimulation of SMC proliferation, (2) tissue factor (TF) and plasminogen activator inhibitor 1 (PAI-1) that act locally to produce thrombin or inhibit fibrinolysis of the fibrin network used to facilitate cell migration, and (3) MCP-1, which increases monocyte chemoattraction into the lesion, thereby leading to lesion development. *We thank Drs. Laurence Harker, Josiah Wilcox, and Bernard Lassègue for their creative and intellectual development of this figure.*

TLR4 are resistant to diet-induced atherosclerosis and vascular injury.[222] Deletion of the fractalkine receptor (CX3CR1) reduces macrophage recruitment into the vessel wall and diminishes lesion formation in Apo E–deficient mice.[190] Moreover, a common polymorphism of the fractalkine receptor has been shown to have reduced adhesive and chemoattractant properties and is associated with a lower incidence of human atherosclerosis and acute coronary syndromes.[227]

The intimal proliferation observed in atherosclerotic lesion formation results from migration and hyperplasia of vascular SMCs and myofibroblasts[228] and accumulation of extracellular matrix.[229] Proliferation has been attributed to growth factors such as PDGF, FGF,

and IGF-1. Because these growth factors can be produced by the endothelium in vitro, it is likely that the dysfunctional endothelium in atherosclerosis also produces growth factors while shifting from a growth-inhibitory to a growth-promoting mode. Furthermore, there is evidence that products of oxidative metabolism may increase matrix metalloproteinase activation[146] and expression,[147] thus contributing to intimal lesion formation on multiple levels.

HYPERTENSION

Hypertension is characterized by dysfunction of both endothelium and vascular smooth muscle. In chronic hypertension, endothelium-dependent relaxations are impaired, and endothelium-dependent constrictor activity is increased.[230–234] Vascular smooth muscle of hypertensive animals has enhanced calcium sensitivity, exacerbating the response to vasoconstrictor agonists.[235] Hypertension also causes an increase in vessel wall mass. In the aortas of spontaneously hypertensive and Goldblatt hypertensive rats, this increase can be attributed to an increase in the size of the existing SMCs.[236,237] Hypertrophy is accompanied by an increase in ploidy; that is, an increased DNA content per cell.[236,237] In contrast, resistance vessels from these same animals appear to increase their mass by hyperplasia of the SMCs.[238] Vascular remodeling appears to have two stages: (1) an initial, reversible intense vasoconstriction mediated by neural or endogenous signals, followed by (2) a remodeling of the vessel wall characterized by increased smooth muscle mass and narrowing of the vessel lumen. Thus, the increase in vascular tone and remodeling of the vessel can lead to an increase in systemic vascular resistance, augmenting the hypertensive syndrome.

【 】 RESTENOSIS

Restenosis is the development of a neointima that occurs following mechanical vascular injury, such as the response to angioplasty/stent insertion or graft placement. The response of the arterial wall to the injury induced by angioplasty (removing the endothelium and stretching the vessel wall) involves several distinct events. Removing the endothelium not only alters the paracrine hormonal environment in which VSMCs exist, but it also exposes a thrombogenic surface to which platelets and other circulating factors can adhere, resulting in the formation of a thrombus. In addition, injury to the underlying smooth muscle may release factors such as FGF, which have mitogenic effects on the remaining SMCs. Finally, infiltration and subsequent activation of macrophages into the denuded vessel wall bring an additional set of hormonal influences to bear on the vascular smooth muscle. The pathophysiologic consequences of these complex events include migration and proliferation of SMCs into the intimal area, resulting in the formation of a neointima over a period of weeks to months.

Balloon injury has been extensively studied in several animal models, including pigs, rabbits, rats, and baboons. During the initial response to injury, growth-related genes in the SMCs are induced, including c-fos, PDGF-A, PDGF-β receptor and MCP-1.[239,240] It also appears that deep injury to SMCs results in an outpouring of FGF, a potent smooth muscle mitogen.[241] This initial response appears to be directly related to the removal of the endothelium.[118] During a second migratory phase, a large increase of thymidine incorporation in the vessel wall occurs, accompanied by further increases in the mRNA encoding IGF-I[242] and the PDGF-β receptor.[239] This phase of the response can be modulated by platelet factors and inhibited by the endothelium.[118] A final proliferative phase is characterized by marked intimal thickening, caused by increased SMC mass and deposition of extracellular matrix. This proliferative phase seems ultimately inhibited by regrowth of normal-functioning endothelium, which is at least in part mediated by the recruitment of circulating endothelial progenitor cells.[243]

Thus, during the process of restenosis after angioplasty and stent placement, both the loss of endothelium and the transformation of SMCs appear to contribute to neointimal formation. At least two lines of evidence implicate the endothelium as having a crucial role in the response of the vessel wall to injury. First, removal of the endothelium allows initiation of the mitogenic response and, second, regrowth of normal endothelium inhibits further proliferation. Furthermore, gentle denudation with a nylon loop, accompanied by rapid regeneration of endothelium, results in significantly less neointimal proliferation.[244] In addition, proliferating SMCs have characteristics distinct from the differentiated SMCs in the medial layer. Their cytoskeleton is similar to that found in cultured cells. It seems likely, therefore, that two of the most important causes of restenosis are the loss of endothelium-derived growth-inhibitory factors and the transformation of SMCs into a phenotype able to respond to platelet- and endothelial-derived factors with proliferation.

Restenosis following balloon angioplasty and stent placement has been reduced from 30 to 50 percent of cases to about 10 percent by the use of stents that elute either sirolimus (rapamycin), which blocks cell cycle progression, or paclitaxel, which inhibits mitosis.[245] The use of drug-eluting stents is complicated by the fact that they reduce endothelial regrowth and thus enhance the tendency for thrombosis for several months following their placement. Newer stents are in development that enhance recruitment of endothelial progenitor cells in an effort to remedy this problem.[246]

【 】 VASCULAR COMPLICATIONS OF DIABETES

Diabetes and its myriad metabolic abnormalities affect both the endothelium and vascular smooth muscle in conduit and resistance vessels. In the endothelium, diabetes increases the production of ROS and reduces the bioavailable NO.[205,247] This results in impaired endothelium-dependent vasodilatation, particularly in type II diabetes.[248] Both insulin resistance and type II diabetes increase clotting factor formation, enhance platelet aggregation, and decrease endothelial production of PAI-1, predisposing to thrombosis.[249] Vascular expression of proinflammatory genes is also increased by diabetes. Many of these events are mediated by advanced glycation end-products acting on endothelium, macrophages, and SMCs.[250] In the larger conduit vessels, these events promote atherosclerosis, whereas in the resistance arteries, an arteriopathy develops. This is characterized by wall thickening, luminal narrowing, inflammation, and remodeling; and leads to retinopathy, nephropathy and ischemia of peripheral tissues.[251]

FUTURE DIRECTIONS

Defining the molecular and cellular basis for dysfunction of the arterial wall in vascular diseases provides information critical to developing clinical strategies for patient management, as well as new therapeutic targets. It is now clear that both endothelial and smooth muscle function are compromised by a variety of risk factors for vascular disease. Further research is required to determine at a more basic level the molecular events that link these risk factors to these diseases. The human genome has been fully sequenced; and with the use of bioinformatics, it will be possible to identify genetic profiles that predispose people to the development of vascular pathologies. Clinical trials in the future will be targeted to these populations in new and powerful ways, and basic research will address the roles of these newly identified genes in vascular physiology and pathophysiology. In addition, the advent of stem cell technology opens new avenues for therapeutic treatment. Once researchers understand the mechanisms controlling stem cell targeting and differentiation, genetic and pharmacologic manipulation of these cells may be the treatment of the future.

REFERENCES

1. Moncada S, Vane JR. Arachidonic acid metabolites and the interaction between platelets and blood vessel walls. *N Engl J Med* 1979;300:1142–1147.

2. Furchgott RF, Zawadski JV. The obligatory role of endothelial cells in the relaxation of arterial smooth muscle by acetylcholine. *Nature* 1980;228:373–376.

3. Taylor SG, Weston AH. Endothelium-derived hyperpolarizing factor: a new endogenous inhibitor from the vascular endothelium. *Trends Pharmacol Sci* 1988;9:272–274.

4. Yanagisawa Y, Kurihara H, Kimura S, et al. A novel potent vasoconstrictor peptide produced by vascular endothelial cells. *Nature* 1988;332:411–415.

5. Lin L, Balazy M, Pagano PJ, Nasjletti A. Expression of prostaglandin H2-mediated mechanism of vascular contraction in hypertensive rats: relation to lipoxygenase and prostacyclin synthase activities. *Circ Res* 1994;74(2):197–205.

6. Stenmark KR, Orton EC, Reeves JT, et al. Vascular remodeling in neonatal pulmonary hypertension. *Chest* 1988;93(suppl 3):127S–133S.

7. Sato T, Arai K, Ishiharajima S, Asano G. Role of glycosaminoglycan and fibronectin in endothelial cell growth. *Exp Mol Pathol* 1987;47:202–210.

8. Hanemaaijer R, Koolwijk P, le Clercq L, de Vree WJ, van Hinsbergh VW. Regulation of matrix metalloproteinase expression in human vein and microvascular endothelial cells: effects of tumor necrosis factor alpha, interleukin 1 and phorbol ester. *Biochem J* 1993;296:803–809.

9. Galis ZS, Muszynski M, Sukhova GK, et al. Cytokine-stimulated human vascular smooth muscle cells synthesize a complement of enzymes required for extracellular matrix digestion. *Circ Res* 1994;75:181–189.

10. Castellot JJ Jr, Addonizio ML, Rosenberg R, Karnovsky MJ. Cultured endothelial cells produce a heparin-like inhibitor of smooth muscle cell growth. *J Cell Biol* 1981;90:372–379.

11. Zerwes HG, Risau W. Polarized secretion of a platelet-derived growth factor-like chemotactic factor by endothelial cells in vitro. *J Cell Biol* 1987;105:2037–2041.

12. Hannan RL, Kourembanas S, Flanders KC, et al. Endothelial cells synthesize basic fibroblast growth factor and transforming growth factor beta. *Growth Factors* 1988;1:7–17.

13. Delafontaine P, Bernstein KE, Alexander RW. Insulin-like growth factor I gene expression in vascular cells. *Hypertension* 1991;17:693–699.

14. Wang-Iverson P, DeRosa PM, Brown WV. Plasma lipoprotein interaction with endothelial cells. In: Ryan U, ed. *Endothelial Cells.* Boca Raton: CRC Press, 1988:179–187.

15. Gordon EL, Pearson JD, Slakey LL. The hydrolysis of extracellular adenine nucleotides by cultured endothelial cells from pig aorta. *J Biol Chem* 1986;33:15496–15504.

16. Cary DA, Mendelsohn FA. Effect of forskolin, isoproterenol and IBMX on angiotensin converting enzyme and cyclic AMP production by cultured bovine endothelial cells. *Mol Cell Endocrin* 1987;53:103–109.

17. Shimada K, Gill PJ, Silbert JE, Douglas WHJ, Fanburg BL. Involvement of cell surface heparan sulfate in the binding of LPL to cultured bovine endothelial cells. *J Clin Invest* 1981;68:995–1002.

18. Vlodavsky I, Fielding PE, Johnson LK, Gospodarowicz D. Inhibition of low density lipoprotein uptake in confluent endothelial cell monolayers correlates with a restricted surface receptor redistribution. *J Cell Physiol* 1979;100:481–495.

19. Rippe B, Rosengren BI, Carlsson O, Venturoli D. Transendothelial transport: the vesicle controversy. *J Vasc Res* September–October 2002;39(5):375–390.

20. Baker DP, van Lenten BJ, Fogelman AM, Edwards PA, Kean C, Berliner JA. LDL, scavenger and beta-VLDL receptors on aortic endothelial cells. *Arteriosclerosis* 1984;4:357–364.

21. Krieger M, Stern DM. Series introduction: multiligand receptors and human disease. *J Clin Invest* September 2001;108(5):645–647.

22. Hayashida K, Kume N, Minami M, Kita T. Lectin-like oxidized LDL receptor-1 (LOX-1) supports adhesion of mononuclear leukocytes and a monocyte-like cell line THP-1 cells under static and flow conditions. *FEBS Lett* January 2002;511(1–3):133–138.

23. Morel DW, DiCorleto PE, Chisolm GM. Endothelial and smooth muscle cells alter low density lipoprotein in vitro by free radical oxidation. *Arteriosclerosis* 1984;4:357–364.

24. Gryglewski RJ, Botting RM, Vane JR. Mediators produced by the endothelial cell. *Hypertension* 1988;12:530–548.

25. van Iwaarden F, Acton DS, Sixma JJ, Meijers JCM, de Groot PG, Bouma BN. Internalization of antithrombin III by cultured human endothelial cells and its subcellular localization. *J Lab Clin Med* 1989;113:717–726.

26. Rosenberg RD, Rosenberg JS. Natural anticoagulant mechanisms. *J Clin Invest* 1984;74:1–6.

27. Esmon CT, Owen WG. Identification of an endothelial cofactor for thrombin-catalyzed activation of protein C. *Proc Natl Acad Sci U S A* 1981;78:2249–2252.

28. Schorer AE, Moldow CF. Production of tissue factor. In: Ryan US, ed. *Endothelial Cells.* Vol I. Boca Raton: CRC Press; 1988:85–105.

29. Steffel J, Luscher TF, Tanner FC. Tissue factor in cardiovascular diseases: molecular mechanisms and clinical implications. *Circulation* February 2006;113(5):722–731.

30. Vaughan DE. PAI-1 and atherothrombosis. *J Thromb Haemost* August 2005;3(8):1879–1883.

31. Vaughan DE. Fibrinolytic balance, the renin-angiotensin system and atherosclerotic disease. *Eur Heart J* 1998;19(suppl):G9–G12.

32. Gates J, Peifer M. Can 1000 reviews be wrong? Actin, alpha-Catenin, and adherens junctions. *Cell* December 2005;123(5):769–772.

33. Svensjo E, Grega GJ. Evidence for endothelial cell-mediated regulation of macromolecular permeability by post-capillary venules. *Fed Proc* 1986;45:89–95.

34. Schnitzer JE. Caveolae: from basic trafficking mechanisms to targeting transcytosis for tissue-specific drug and gene delivery in vivo. *Adv Drug Deliv Rev* July 2001;49(3):265–280.

35. Gumbleton M, Abulrob AG, Campbell L. Caveolae: an alternative membrane transport compartment. *Pharm Res* September 2000;17(9):1035–1048.

36. Simons K, Toomre D. Lipid rafts and signal transduction. *Nat Rev Mol Cell Biol* October 2000;1(1):31–39.

37. Garcia JG, Davis HW, Patterson CE. Regulation of endothelial cell gap formation and barrier dysfunction: role of myosin light chain phosphorylation. *J Cell Physiol* 1995;163(3):510–522.

38. Garcia JG, Schaphorst KL, Shi S, et al. Mechanisms of ionomycin-induced endothelial cell barrier dysfunction. *Am J Physiol* 1997;273(1 pt 1):L172–L184.

39. Garcia JG, Verin AD, Schaphorst K, et al. Regulation of endothelial cell myosin light chain kinase by rho, cortactin, and p60. *Am J Physiol* 1999;276:L989–L998.

40. Palmer RMJ, Ferrige AG, Moncada S. Nitric oxide release accounts for the biological activity of endothelium-derived relaxing factor. *Nature* 1987;327:524–526.

41. Bredt DS, Hwang PM, Glatt CE, Lowenstein C, Reed RR, Snyder SH. Cloned and expressed nitric oxide synthase structurally resembles cytochrome P-450 reductase. *Nature* 1991;351:714–718.

42. Lyons CR, Orloff GJ, Cunningham JM. Molecular cloning and functional expression of an inducible nitric oxide synthase from a murine macrophage cell line. *J Biol Chem* 1992;267:6370–6374.

43. Nishida K, Harrison DG, Navas JP, et al. Molecular cloning and characterization of the constitutive bovine aortic endothelial nitric oxide synthase. *J Clin Invest* 1992;90:2092–2096.

44. Vasquez-Vivar J, Kalyanaraman B, Martasek P, et al. Superoxide generation by endothelial nitric oxide synthase: the influence of cofactors. *Proc Natl Acad Sci U S A* 1998;95(16):9220–9225.

45. Landmesser U, Dikalov S, Price SR, et al. Oxidation of tetrahydrobiopterin leads to uncoupling of endothelial cell nitric oxide synthase in hypertension. *J Clin Invest* April 2003;111(8):1201–1209.

46. Furchgott RF, Vanhoutte PM. Endothelium-derived relaxing and contracting factors. *FASEB J* 1989;3:2007–2018.

47. Rapoport RM, Draznin MB, Murad F. Endothelium-dependent relaxation in rat aorta may be mediated through cyclic GMP-dependent protein phosphorylation. *Nature* 1983;306:174–176.

48. Kuchan MJ, Frangos JA. Role of calcium and calmodulin in flow-induced nitric oxide production in endothelial cells. *Am J Physiol* 1994;266(3 pt 1):C628–C636.

49. Gallis B, Corthals GL, Goodlett DR, et al. Identification of flow-dependent endothelial nitric-oxide synthase phosphorylation sites by mass spectrometry and regulation of phosphorylation and nitric oxide production by the phosphatidylinositol 3-kinase inhibitor LY294002. *J Biol Chem* 1999;274(42):30101–30108.

50. Uematsu M, Ohara Y, Navas JP, et al. Regulation of endothelial cell nitric oxide synthase mRNA expression by shear stress. *Am J Physiol* 1995;269(6 pt 1):C1371–C1378.

51. Sessa WC, Pritchard K, Seyedi N, Wang J, Hintze TH. Chronic exercise in dogs increases coronary vascular nitric oxide production and endothelial cell nitric oxide synthase gene expression. *Circ Res* 1994;74(2):349–353.

52. Liao JK, Shin WS, Lee WY, Clark SL. Oxidized low-density lipoprotein decreases the expression of endothelial nitric oxide synthase. *J Biol Chem* 1995;270(1):319–324.

53. Liao JK, Zulueta JJ, Yu FS, Peng HB, Cote CG, Hassoun PM. Regulation of bovine endothelial constitutive nitric oxide synthase by oxygen. *J Clin Invest* 1995;96(6):2661–2666.

54. Feletou M, Vanhoutte PM. The alternative: EDHF. *J Mol Cell Cardiol* 1999;31(1):15–22.

55. Gauthier KM, Edwards EM, Falck JR, Reddy DS, Campbell WB. 14,15-epoxyeicosatrienoic acid represents a transferable endothelium-dependent relaxing factor in bovine coronary arteries. *Hypertension* April 2005;45(4):666–671.

56. Larsen BT, Miura H, Hatoum OA, et al. Epoxyeicosatrienoic and dihydroxyeicosatrienoic acids dilate human coronary arterioles via BK(Ca) channels: implications for soluble epoxide hydrolase inhibition. *Am J Physiol Heart Circ Physiol* February 2006;290(2):H491–H499.

57. Matoba T, Shimokawa H, Nakashima M, et al. Hydrogen peroxide is an endothelium-derived hyperpolarizing factor in mice. *J Clin Invest* December 2000;106(12):1521–1530.

58. Shimokawa H, Morikawa K. Hydrogen peroxide is an endothelium-derived hyperpolarizing factor in animals and humans. *J Mol Cell Cardiol* November 2005;39(5):725–732.

59. Miura H, Bosnjak JJ, Ning G, Saito T, Miura M, Gutterman DD. Role for hydrogen peroxide in flow-induced dilation of human coronary arterioles. *Circ Res* February 2003;92(2):e31–e40.

60. Shimokawa H, Yasutake H, Fujii K, et al. The importance of the hyperpolarizing mechanism increases as the vessel size decreases in endothelium-dependent relaxations in rat mesenteric circulation. *J Cardiovasc Pharmacol* November 1996;28(5):703–711.

61. Ito T, Ogawa K, Enomoto I, Hashimoto H, Kai I, Satake T. Comparison of the effects of PGI$_2$ and PGE1 on coronary and systemic hemodynamics and coronary arterial cyclic nucleotide level in dogs. *Adv Prostaglandin Thromboxane Leukot Res* 1980;7:641–646.

62. Grosser T, Fries S, FitzGerald GA. Biological basis for the cardiovascular consequences of COX-2 inhibition: therapeutic challenges and opportunities. *J Clin Invest* January 2006;116(1):4–15.

63. Sun D, Huang A, Smith CJ, et al. Enhanced release of prostaglandins contributes to flow-induced arteriolar dilation in eNOS knockout mice. *Circ Res* August 1999;85(3):288–293.

64. Galie N, Manes A, Branzi A. Emerging medical therapies for pulmonary arterial hypertension. *Prog Cardiovasc Dis* November–December 2002;45(3):213–224.

65. Nasjletti A. Arthur C. Corcoran Memorial Lecture. The role of eicosanoids in angiotensin-dependent hypertension. *Hypertension* January 1998;31(1 pt 2):194–200.

66. Simmons DL, Botting RM, Hla T. Cyclooxygenase isozymes: the biology of prostaglandin synthesis and inhibition. *Pharmacol Rev* September 2004;56(3):387–437.

67. Feletou M, Vanhoutte PM. Endothelial dysfunction: a multifaceted disorder. *Am J Physiol Heart Circ Physiol* 2006;291:H985–H1002.

68. Miyata N, Roman RJ. Role of 20-hydroxyeicosatetraenoic acid (20-HETE) in vascular system. *J Smooth Muscle Res* August 2005;41(4):175–193.

69. Gumkowski F, Kaminska F, Kaminiski M, Morrissey LW, Auerbach R. Heterogeneity of mouse vascular endothelium: in vitro studies of lymphatic, large blood vessel and microvascular endothelial cells. *Blood Vessels* 1987;24:11–23.

70. Fleming I. Signaling by the angiotensin-converting enzyme. *Circ Res* April 2006;98(7):887–896.

71. Jan Danser AH. Local renin-angiotensin systems: the unanswered questions. *Int J Biochem Cell Biol* June 2003;35(6):759–768.

72. Crackower MA, Sarao R, Oudit GY, et al. Angiotensin-converting enzyme 2 is an essential regulator of heart function. *Nature* June 2002;417(6891):822–828.

73. Danilczyk U, Penninger JM. Angiotensin-converting enzyme II in the heart and the kidney. *Circ Res* March 2006;98(4):463–471.

74. Attina T, Camidge R, Newby DE, Webb DJ. Endothelin antagonism in pulmonary hypertension, heart failure, and beyond. *Heart* June 2005;91(6):825–831.

75. Luscher TF, Wenzel RR. Endothelin and endothelin antagonists: pharmacology and clinical implications. *Agents Actions Suppl* 1995;45:237–253.

76. Simonson MS, Dunn MJ. Cellular signaling by peptides of the endothelin gene family. *FASEB J* 1990;4:2989–3000.

77. Hafizi S, Allen SP, Goodwin AT, Chester AH, Yacoub MH. Endothelin-1 stimulates proliferation of human coronary smooth muscle cells via the ET(A) receptor and is co-mitogenic with growth factors. *Atherosclerosis* 1999;146(2):351–359.

78. Achmad TH, Rao GS. Chemotaxis of human blood monocytes toward endothelin-1 and the influence of calcium channel blockers. *Biochem Biophys Res Commun* 1992;189:994–1000.

79. Sung CP, Arleth AJ, Storer BL, Ohlstein EH. Angiotensin type 1 receptors mediate smooth muscle proliferation and endothelin biosynthesis in rat vascular smooth muscle. *J Pharmacol Exp Ther* 1994;271(1):429–437.

80. Rajagopalan S, Bech-Laursen J, Borthayre A, et al. A role for endothelin-1 in angiotensin II mediated hypertension. *Hypertension* 1997;30:29–34.

81. Luft FC. Proinflammatory effects of angiotensin II and endothelin: targets for progression of cardiovascular and renal diseases. *Curr Opin Nephrol Hypertens* January 2002;11(1):59–66.

82. Kobayashi T, Matsumoto T, Kamata K. The PI3-K/Akt pathway: roles related to alterations in vasomotor responses in diabetic models. *J Smooth Muscle Res* December 2005;41(6):283–302.

83. Dartsch PC, Betz E. Response of cultured endothelial cells to mechanical stimulation. *Basic Res Cardiol* May-June 1989;84(3):268–281.

84. Howard AB, Alexander RW, Nerem RM, Griendling KK, Taylor WR. Cyclic strain induces an oxidative stress in endothelial cells. *Am J Physiol* 1997;272:C421–C427.

85. Nerem RM, Girard PR. Hemodynamic influences on vascular endothelial biology. *Toxicol Path* 1990;18:572–582.

86. Gimbrone MA Jr, Topper JN, Nagel T, Anderson KR, Garcia-Cardena G. Endothelial dysfunction, hemodynamic forces, and atherogenesis. *Ann N Y Acad Sci* 2000;902:230–239; discussion 239–240.

87. Asakura T, Karino T. Flow patterns and spatial distribution of atherosclerotic lesions in human coronary arteries. *Circ Res* 1990;66:1045–1066.

88. Ku D, Giddens D, Zarins C, Glagov S. Pulsatile flow and atherosclerosis in the human carotid bifurcation: positive correlation between plaque location and low and oscillating shear stress. *Arteriosclerosis* 1985;5:293–302.

89. De Keulenaer GW, Chappell DC, Ishizaka N, Nerem RM, Alexander RW, Griendling KK. Oscillatory and steady laminar shear stress differentially affect human endothelial redox state. *Circ Res* 1998;82:1094–1101.

90. Chappell DC, Varner SE, Nerem RM, Medford RM, Alexander RW. Oscillatory shear stimulates adhesion molecule expression in cultured human endothelium. *Circ Res* 1998;82:532–539.

91. Sorescu GP, Song H, Tressel SL, et al. Bone morphogenic protein 4 produced in endothelial cells by oscillatory shear stress induces monocyte adhesion by stimulating reactive oxygen species production from a nox1-based NADPH oxidase. *Circ Res* October 2004;95(8):773–779.

92. Sorescu GP, Sykes M, Weiss D, et al. Bone morphogenic protein 4 produced in endothelial cells by oscillatory shear stress stimulates an inflammatory response. *J Biol Chem* August 2003;278(33):31128–31135.

93. Mochizuki S, Vink H, Hiramatsu O, et al. Role of hyaluronic acid glycosaminoglycans in shear-induced endothelium-derived nitric oxide release. *Am J Physiol Heart Circ Physiol* August 2003;285(2):H722–H726.

94. Moon JJ, Matsumoto M, Patel S, Lee L, Guan JL, Li S. Role of cell surface heparan sulfate proteoglycans in endothelial cell migration and mechanotransduction. *J Cell Physiol* April 2005;203(1):166–176.

95. Tzima E, Irani-Tehrani M, Kiosses WB, et al. A mechanosensory complex that mediates the endothelial cell response to fluid shear stress. *Nature* September 2005;437(7057):426–431.

96. Giancotti FG, Ruoslahti E. Integrin signaling. *Science* 1999;285(5430):1028–1032.

97. Takemoto M, Sun J, Hiroki J, Shimokawa H, Liao JK. Rho-kinase mediates hypoxia-induced downregulation of endothelial nitric oxide synthase. *Circulation* July 2002;106(1):57–62.

98. Clapham DE, Neer EJ. New roles for G-protein bg-dimers in transmembrane signaling. *Nature* 1993;365:403–406.

99. Traub O, Berk BC. Laminar shear stress: mechanisms by which endothelial cells transduce an atheroprotective force. *Arterioscler Thromb Vasc Biol* 1998;18(5):677–685.

100. Rizzo V, McIntosh DP, Oh P, Schnitzer JE. In situ flow activates endothelial nitric oxide synthase in luminal caveolae of endothelium with rapid caveolin dissociation and calmodulin association. *J Biol Chem* 1998;273(52):34724–34729.

101. Berridge MJ, Irvine RF. Inositol trisphosphate, a novel second messenger in cellular signal transduction. *Nature* 1984;312:315–321.

102. Yamamoto H, van Breeman C. Inositol 1,4,5-trisphosphate releases calcium from skinned cultured smooth muscle cells. *Biochem Biophys Res Commun* 1985;130:270–274.

103. Patterson RL, Boehning D, Snyder SH. Inositol 1,4,5-trisphosphate receptors as signal integrators. *Annu Rev Biochem* 2004;73:437–465.

104. Nishizuka Y. The role of protein kinase C in cell surface signal transduction and tumour promotion. *Nature* 1984;308:693–698.

105. Dillon PF, Aksoy MO, Driska SP, Murphy RA. Myosin phosphorylation and the cross-bridge cycle in arterial smooth muscle. *Science* 1981;211:495–497.

106. Morgan KG. Role of calcium ion in maintenance of vascular smooth muscle tone. *Am J Cardiol* 1987;59:24A–28A.

107. Morgan KG, Gangopadhyay SS. Invited review: cross-bridge regulation by thin filament-associated proteins. *J Appl Physiol* August 2001;91(2):953–962.

108. Dessy C, Kim I, Sougnez CL, Laporte R, Morgan KG. A role for MAP kinase in differentiated smooth muscle contraction evoked by alpha-adrenoceptor stimulation. *Am J Physiol* October 1998;275(4 pt 1):C1081–1086.

109. Je HD, Gangopadhyay SS, Ashworth TD, Morgan KG. Calponin is required for agonist-induced signal transduction: evidence from an antisense approach in ferret smooth muscle. *J Physiol* December 2001;537(pt 2):567–577.

110. Winder SJ, Allen BG, Clement-Chomienne O, Walsh MP. Regulation of smooth muscle actin-myosin interaction and force by calponin. *Acta Physiol Scand* December 1998;164(4):415–426.

111. Sward K, Mita M, Wilson DP, Deng JT, Susnjar M, Walsh MP. The role of RhoA and Rho-associated kinase in vascular smooth muscle contraction. *Curr Hypertens Rep* February 2003;5(1):66–72.

112. van Nieuw Amerongen GP, van Hinsbergh VW. Cytoskeletal effects of rho-like small guanine nucleotide-binding proteins in the vascular system. *Arterioscler Thromb Vasc Biol* March 2001;21(3):300–311.

113. Kitazono T, Ago T, Kamouchi M, et al. Increased activity of calcium channels and Rho-associated kinase in the basilar artery during chronic hypertension in vivo. *J Hypertens* May 2002;20(5):879–884.

114. Masumoto A, Hirooka Y, Shimokawa H, Hironaga K, Setoguchi S, Takeshita A. Possible involvement of Rho-kinase in the pathogenesis of hypertension in humans. *Hypertension* December 2001;38(6):1307–1310.

115. Newby AC, Southgate KM, Assender JW. Inhibition of vascular smooth muscle cell proliferation by endothelium-dependent vasodilators. *Herz* October 1992;17(5):291–299.

116. Ettenson DS, Koo EW, Januzzi JL, Edelman ER. Endothelial heparan sulfate is necessary but not sufficient for control of vascular smooth muscle cell growth. *J Cell Physiol* July 2000;184(1):93–100.

117. Ueba H, Kawakami M, Yaginuma T. Shear stress as an inhibitor of vascular smooth muscle cell proliferation. Role of transforming growth factor-beta 1 and tissue-type plasminogen activator. *Arterioscler Thromb Vasc Biol* August 1997;17(8):1512–1516.

118. Clowes AW, Clowes MM, Fingerle J, Reidy MA. Regulation of smooth muscle cell growth in injured artery. *J Cardiovasc Pharmacol* 1989;14(suppl 6):S12-S15.

119. Kuzkaya N, Weissmann N, Harrison DG, Dikalov S. Interactions of peroxynitrite, tetrahydrobiopterin, ascorbic acid, and thiols: implications for uncoupling endothelial nitric-oxide synthase. *J Biol Chem* June 2003;278(25):22546–22554.

120. Kavanaugh WM, Harsh GR IV, Starksen NF, Rocco CM, Williams LT. Transcriptional regulation of the A and B chain genes of PDGF in microvascular endothelial cells. *J Biol Chem* 1988;263:8470–8472.

121. Clemmons DR. Exposure to platelet-derived growth factors modulate the porcine aortic smooth muscle cell response to somatomedin-C. *Endocrinology* 1985;117:77–83.

122. Delafontaine P. Insulin-like growth factor I and its binding proteins in the cardiovascular system. *Cardiovasc Res* 1995;30:825–834.

123. Bevilaqua MP, Gimbrone MA Jr. Modulation of endothelial cell procoagulant and fibrinolytic activities by inflammatory mediators. In: Ryan US, ed. *Endothelial Cells.* Vol I. Boca Raton: CRC Press; 1988:107–118.

124. Beasley D, Cohen RA, Levinsky NG. Interleukin 1 inhibits contraction of vascular smooth muscle. *J Clin Invest* 1989;83:331–335.

125. Lindner V, Lappi DA, Baird A, Majack RA, Reidy MA. Role of basic fibroblast growth factor in vascular lesion formation. *Circ Res* 1991;68:106–113.

126. Bashkin P, Doctrow S, Klagsbrun M, Svahn CM, Folkman J, Vlodavsky I. Basic fibroblast growth factor binds to subendothelial extracellular matrix and is released by heparinase and heparin-like molecules. *Biochemistry* 1989;28:1737–1743.

127. Nagai M, Kamide K, Rakugi H, et al. Role of endothelin-1 induced by insulin in the regulation of vascular cell growth. *Am J Hypertens* March 2003;16(3):223–228.

128. Ziegler T, Bouzourene K, Harrison VJ, Brunner HR, Hayoz D. Influence of oscillatory and unidirectional flow environments on the expression of endothelin and nitric oxide synthase in cultured endothelial cells. *Arterioscler Thromb Vasc Biol* May 1998;18(5):686–692.

129. Seeger H, Lippert C, Wallwiener D, Mueck AO. Valsartan and candesartan can inhibit deteriorating effects of angiotensin II on coronary endothelial function. *J Renin Angiotensin Aldosterone Sys* June 2001;2(2):141–143.

130. Geisterfer A, Peach MJ, Owens GK. Angiotensin II induces hypertrophy, not hyperplasia of cultured rat aortic smooth muscle cells. *Circ Res* 1988;62:749–756.

131. Berk BC, Taubman MB, Griendling KK, Cragoe EJ Jr, Fenton JW, II, Brock TA. Thrombin-stimulated events in cultured vascular smooth muscle cells. *Biochem J* 1991;274:799–805.

132. Golden MA, Au YPT, Kirkman TR, Wilcox JN, Raines EW, Ross R, Clowes AW. Platelet-derived growth factor activity and mRNA expression in healing vascular grafts in baboons. *J Clin Invest* 1991;87:406–414.

133. Myers PR, Minor RL, Guerra R Jr, Bates JN, Harrison DG. The vasorelaxant properties of the endothelium derived relaxing factor more closely resemble S-nitrosocysteine than nitric oxide. *Nature* 1990;345:161–163.

134. Liebow C, Reilly C, Serrano M, Schally AV. Somatostatin analogues inhibit growth of pancreatic cancer by stimulating tyrosine phosphatase. *Proc Natl Acad Sci U S A* 1989;86:2003–2007.

135. Ullrich A, Schlessinger J. Signal transduction by receptors with tyrosine kinase activity. *Cell* 1990;81:203–212.

136. Luttrell LM, Daaka Y, Lefkowitz RJ. Regulation of tyrosine kinase cascades by G-protein-coupled receptors. *Curr Opin Cell Biol* 1999;11(2):177–183.

137. Kalmes A, Daum G, Clowes AW. EGFR transactivation in the regulation of SMC function. *Ann N Y Acad Sci* December 2001;947:42–54; discussion 54–45.

138. Sundaresan M, Zu-Xi Y, Ferrans VJ, Irani K, Finkel T. Requirement for generation of H_2O_2 for platelet-derived growth factor signal transduction. *Science* 1995;270:296–299.

139. Griendling KK, Minieri CA, Ollerenshaw JD, Alexander RW. Angiotensin II stimulates NADH and NADPH oxidase activity in cultured vascular smooth muscle cells. *Circ Res* 1994;74:1141–1148.

140. Ushio-Fukai M, Alexander RW, Akers M, Griendling KK. p38MAP kinase is a critical component of the redox-sensitive signaling pathways by angiotensin II: role in vascular smooth muscle cell hypertrophy. *J Biol Chem* 1998;273:15022–15029.

141. Ushio-Fukai M, Alexander RW, Akers M, et al. Reactive oxygen species mediate the activation of Akt/Protein kinase B by angiotensin II in vascular smooth muscle cells. *J Biol Chem* 1999;274:22699–22704.

142. Deshpande NN, Sorescu D, Seshiah P, et al. Mechanism of hydrogen peroxide-induced cell cycle arrest in vascular smooth muscle. *Antioxid Redox Signal* October 2002;4(5):845–854.

143. Choi MH, Lee IK, Kim GW, et al. Regulation of PDGF signalling and vascular remodelling by peroxiredoxin II. *Nature* May 2005;435(7040):347–353.

144. White JM. ADAMs: modulators of cell-cell and cell-matrix interactions. *Curr Opin Cell Biol* October 2003;15(5):598–606.

145. Sato H, Takino T, Okada Y, et al. A matrix metalloproteinase expressed on the surface of invasive tumor cells. *Nature* 1994;370:61–65.

146. Rajagopalan S, Meng XP, Ramasamy S, Harrison DG, Galis ZS. Reactive oxygen species produced by macrophage-derived foam cells regulate the activity of vascular matrix metalloproteinases in vitro. *J Clin Invest* 1996;98:2572–2579.

147. Galis ZS, Asanuma K, Godin D, Meng X. *N*-acetyl-cysteine decreases the matrix-degrading capacity of macrophage-derived foam cells: new target for antioxidant therapy? *Circulation* 1998;97(24):2445–2453.

148. Galis ZS, Sukhova GK, Lark MW, Libby P. Increased expression of matrix metalloproteinases and matrix degrading activity in vulnerable regions of human atherosclerotic plaques. *J Clin Invest* 1994;94:2493–2503.

149. Galis ZS, Khatri JJ. Matrix metalloproteinases in vascular remodeling and atherogenesis: the good, the bad, and the ugly. *Circ Res* 2002;90(3):251–262.

150. Wilson WR, Anderton M, Schwalbe EC, Jones JL, Furness PN, Bell PR, Thompson MM. Matrix metalloproteinase-8 and -9 are increased at the site of abdominal aortic aneurysm rupture. *Circulation* January 2006;113(3):438–445.

151. Ikonomidis JS, Jones JA, Barbour JR, et al. Expression of matrix metalloproteinases and endogenous inhibitors within ascending aortic aneurysms of patients with Marfan syndrome. *Circulation* July 2006;114(1 suppl):I365–I370.

152. Luttun A, Carmeliet G, Carmeliet P. Vascular progenitors: from biology to treatment. *Trends Cardiovasc Med* 2002;12:88–96.

153. Semenza GL. Angiogenesis in ischemic and neoplastic disorders. *Annu Rev Med* 2003;54:17–28.

154. Gale N, Yancopoulos G. Growth factors acting via endothelial cell-specific receptor tyrosine kinases: VEGFs, angiopoietins, and ephrins in vascular development. *Genes Dev* 1999;13:1055–1066.

155. Yancopoulos G, Davis S, Gale N, et al. Vascular-specific growth factors and blood vessel formation. *Nature* 2000;407:242–248.

155a. Carmeliet P. Mechanisms of angiogenesis and arteriogenesis. *Nature Med* 2002;6:389–395.

156. Luttun A, Tjwa M, Moons L, et al. Revascularization of ischemic tissues by PIGF treatment, and inhibition of tumor angiogenesis, arthritis and atherosclerosis by anti-Flt1. *Nature Medicine* 2002;8(8):831–840.

157. White F, Carroll S, Magnet A, et al. Coronary collateral development in swine after coronary artery occlusion. *Circ Res* 1992;71:1490–1500.

158. Banai S, Shweiki D, Pinson A, et al. Upregulation of vascular endothelial growth factor expression induced by myocardial ischemia: implications for coronary angiogenesis. *Cardiovasc Res* 1994;28:1176–1179.

159. Semenza GL. Surviving ischemia: adaptive responses mediated by hypoxia-inducible factor 1. *J Clin Invest* 2000;106:809–812.

160. Frenkel-Denkberg G, Gershon D, Levy A. The function of hypoxia-inducible factor 1 (HIF-1) is impaired in senescent mice. *FEBS Lett* 1999;462:341–344.

161. Rivard A, Fabre J, Silver M, et al. Age-dependent impairment of angiogenesis. *Circulation* 1999;99:111–120.

162. Rivard A, Berthou-Soulie L, Principe N, et al. Age-dependent defect in vascular endothelial growth factor expression is associated with reduced hypoxia-inducible factor 1 activity. *J Biol Chem* 2000;275:29643–29647.

163. Schultz A, Lavie L, Hochberg I, et al. Interindividual heterogeneity in the hypoxic regulation of VEGF: significance for the development of the coronary artery collateral circulation. *Circulation* 1999;100:547–552.

164. Asahara T, Masuda H, Takahashi T, et al. Bone marrow origin of endothelial progenitor cells responsible for postnatal vasculogenesis in physiological and pathological neovascularization. *Circ Res* 1999;85:221–228.

165. Takahashi T, Kalka C, Masuda H, et al. Ischemia- and cytokine-induced mobilization of bone marrow-derived endothelial progenitor cells for neovascularization. *Nature Medicine* 1999;5:434–438.

166. Kalka C, Masuda H, Takahashi T, et al. Transplantation of ex vivo expanded endothelial progenitor cells for therapeutic neovascularization. *Proc Natl Acad Sci U S A* 2000;97:3422–3427.

167. Schatteman G, Hanlon H, Jiao C, et al. Blood-derived angioblasts accelerate blood-flow restoration in diabetic mice. *J Clin Invest* 2000;106:571–578.

168. Urbich C, Dimmeler S. Endothelial progenitor cells: characterization and role in vascular biology. *Circ Res* August 2004;95(4):343–353.

169. Aicher A, Zeiher AM, Dimmeler S. Mobilizing endothelial progenitor cells. *Hypertension* March 2005;45(3):321–325.

170. Ceradini DJ, Gurtner GC. Homing to hypoxia: HIF-1 as a mediator of progenitor cell recruitment to injured tissue. *Trends Cardiovasc Med* February 2005;15(2):57–63.

171. Dimmeler S, Aicher A, Vasa M, et al. HMG-CoA reductase inhibitors (statins) increase endothelial progenitor cells via the PI 3-kinase/Akt pathway. *J Clin Invest* August 2001;108(3):391–397.

172. Vasa M, Fichtlscherer S, Adler K, et al. Increase in circulating endothelial progenitor cells by statin therapy in patients with stable coronary artery disease. *Circulation* June 2001;103(24):2885–2890.

173. Seeger FH, Haendeler J, Walter DH, et al. p38 mitogen-activated protein kinase downregulates endothelial progenitor cells. *Circulation* March 2005;111(9):1184–1191.

174. Henry TD, Annex BH, McKendall GR, et al. The VIVA trial: vascular endothelial growth factor in Ischemia for Vascular Angiogenesis. *Circulation* March 2003;107(10):1359–1365.

175. Bonfrer JM, Korse CM. Monitoring malignant melanoma with the S-100B tumour marker. *Recent Results Cancer Res* 2001;158:149–157.

176. Zohlnhofer D, Ott I, Mehilli J, et al. Stem cell mobilization by granulocyte colony-stimulating factor in patients with acute myocardial infarction: a randomized controlled trial. *JAMA* March 2006;295(9):1003–1010.

177. Beeres SL, Bax JJ, Kaandorp TA, et al. Usefulness of intramyocardial injection of autologous bone marrow-derived mononuclear cells in patients with severe angina pectoris and stress-induced myocardial ischemia. *Am J Cardiol* May 2006;97(9):1326–1331.

178. Schachinger V, Assmus B, Britten MB, et al. Transplantation of progenitor cells and regeneration enhancement in acute myocardial infarction: final one-year results of the TOPCARE-AMI Trial. *J Am Coll Cardiol* October 2004;44(8):1690–1699.

179. Schachinger V, Assmus B, Honold J, et al. Normalization of coronary blood flow in the infarct-related artery after intracoronary progenitor cell therapy: intracoronary Doppler substudy of the TOPCARE-AMI trial. *Clin Res Cardiol* January 2006;95(1):13–22.

180. Templin C, Kotlarz D, Marquart F, et al. Transcoronary delivery of bone marrow cells to the infarcted murine myocardium: feasibility, cellular kinetics, and improvement in cardiac function. *Basic Res Cardiol* July 2006;101(4):301–310.

181. Tendera M, Wojakowski W. Clinical trials using autologous bone marrow and peripheral blood-derived progenitor cells in patients with acute myocardial infarction. *Folia Histochem Cytobiol* 2005;43(4):233–235.

182. Rosenfeld ME. Leukocyte recruitment into developing atherosclerotic lesions: the complex interaction between multiple molecules keeps getting more complex. *Arterioscler Thromb Vasc Biol* March 2002;22(3):361–363.

183. Baggiolini M. Chemokines in pathology and medicine. *J Intern Med* August 2001;250(2):91–104.

184. Pober JS, Cotran RS. The role of endothelial cells in inflammation. *Transplantation* 1990;50:537–544.

185. Tailor A, Granger DN. Role of adhesion molecules in vascular regulation and damage. *Curr Hypertens Rep* February 2000;2(1):78–83.

186. Steeber DA, Tedder TF. Adhesion molecule cascades direct lymphocyte recirculation and leukocyte migration during inflammation. *Immunol Res* 2000;22(2–3):299–317.

187. Egashira K. Molecular mechanisms mediating inflammation in vascular disease: special reference to monocyte chemoattractant protein-1. *Hypertension* March 2003;41(3 pt 2):834–841.

188. Nakashima Y, Raines EW, Plump AS, Breslow JL, Ross R. Upregulation of VCAM-1 and ICAM-1 at atherosclerosis-prone sites on the endothelium in the ApoE-deficient mouse. *Arterioscler Thromb Vasc Biol* May 1998;18(5):842–851.

189. Boisvert WA, Santiago R, Curtiss LK, Terkeltaub RA. A leukocyte homologue of the IL-8 receptor CXCR-2 mediates the accumulation of macrophages in atherosclerotic lesions of LDL receptor-deficient mice. *J Clin Invest* January 1998;101(2):353–363.

190. Lesnik P, Haskell CA, Charo IF. Decreased atherosclerosis in CX3CR1-/- mice reveals a role for fractalkine in atherogenesis. *J Clin Invest* February 2003;111(3):333–340.

191. Liu P, Patil S, Rojas M, Fong AM, Smyth SS, Patel DD. CX3CR1 deficiency confers protection from intimal hyperplasia after arterial injury. *Arterioscler Thromb Vasc Biol* June 2006.

192. Griendling KK, Sorescu D, Ushio-Fukai M. NAD(P)H oxidase: role in cardiovascular biology and disease. *Circ Res* 2000;86(5):494–501.

193. Suh Y, Arnold RS, Lassègue B, et al. Cell transformation by the superoxide-generating oxidase mox1. *Nature* 1999;401:79–82.

194. Lassègue B, Sorescu D, Szöcs K, et al. Novel gp91phox homologues in vascular smooth muscle cells: nox1 mediates angiotensin II-induced superoxide formation and redox-sensitive signaling pathways. *Circ Res* 2001;88:888–894.

195. Sorescu D, Weiss D, Lassègue B, et al. Superoxide production and expression of nox family proteins in human atherosclerosis. *Circulation* 2002;105(12):1429–1435.

196. Banfi B, Molnar G, Maturana A, et al. A Ca(2+)-activated NADPH oxidase in testis, spleen, and lymph nodes. *J Biol Chem.* October 2001;276(40):37594–37601.

197. Pagano PJ, Clark JK, Cifuentes-Pagano ME, Clark SM, Callis GM, Quinn MT. Localization of a constitutively active, phagocyte-like NADPH oxidase in rabbit aortic adventitia: enhancement by angiotensin II. *Proc Natl Acad Sci U S A* 1997;94:14438–14488.

198. De Keulenaer GW, Alexander RW, Ushio-Fukai M, Ishizaka N, Griendling KK. Tumor necrosis factor-a activates a p22phox-based NADH oxidase in vascular smooth muscle cells. *Biochem J* 1998;329:653–657.

199. Patterson C, Ruef J, Madamanchi NR, et al. Stimulation of a vascular smooth muscle cell NAD(P)H oxidase by thrombin. Evidence that p47(phox) may participate in forming this oxidase in vitro and in vivo. *J Biol Chem* 1999;274(28):19814–19822.

200. Seshiah PN, Weber DS, Rocic P, Valppu L, Taniyama Y, Griendling KK. Angiotensin II stimulation of NAD(P)H oxidase activity: upstream mediators. *Circ Res* September 2002;91(5):406–413.

201. Laufs U, Kilter H, Konkol C, Wassmann S, Bohm M, Nickenig G. Impact of HMG CoA reductase inhibition on small GTPases in the heart. *Cardiovasc Res* March 2002;53(4):911–920.

202. Xia Y, Tsai AL, Berka V, Zweier JL. Superoxide generation from endothelial nitric-oxide synthase. A Ca2+/calmodulin-dependent and tetrahydrobiopterin regulatory process. *J Biol Chem* 1998;273(40):25804–25808.

203. Verhaar MC, Wever RM, Kastelein JJ, van Dam T, Koomans HA, Rabelink TJ. 5-methyltetrahydrofolate, the active form of folic acid, restores endothelial function in familial hypercholesterolemia. *Circulation* 1998;97(3):237–241.

204. Shinozaki K, Nishio Y, Okamura T, et al. Oral administration of tetrahydrobiopterin prevents endothelial dysfunction and vascular oxidative stress in the aortas of insulin-resistant rats. *Circ Res* 2000;87(7):566–573.

205. Hink U, Li H, Mollnau H, et al. Mechanisms underlying endothelial dysfunction in diabetes mellitus. *Circ Res* 2001;88(2):E14–22.

206. Cyrus T, Pratico D, Zhao L, et al. Absence of 12/15-lipoxygenase expression decreases lipid peroxidation and atherogenesis in apolipoprotein e-deficient mice. *Circulation* May 2001;103(18):2277–2282.

207. Harrison DG, Galis Z, Parthasarathy S, Griendling KK. Oxidative stress and hypertension. In: Izzo JL, Black HR, eds. *Hypertension Primer*. Baltimore: Lippincott, Williams & Wilkins; 1999:163–166.

208. Farquharson CA, Butler R, Hill A, Belch JJ, Struthers AD. Allopurinol improves endothelial dysfunction in chronic heart failure. *Circulation* July 2002;106(2):221–226.

209. Guthikonda S, Sinkey C, Barenz T, Haynes WG. Xanthine oxidase inhibition reverses endothelial dysfunction in heavy smokers. *Circulation* January 2003;107(3):416–421.

210. Spiekermann S, Landmesser U, Dikalov S, et al. Electron spin resonance characterization of vascular xanthine and NAD(P)H oxidase activity in patients with coronary artery disease: relation to endothelium-dependent vasodilation. *Circulation* March 2003;107(10):1383–1389.

211. Brownlee M. The pathobiology of diabetic complications: a unifying mechanism. *Diabetes.* June 2005;54(6):1615–1625.

212. Beckman JS, Koppenol WH. Nitric oxide, superoxide, and peroxynitrite: the good, the bad, and ugly. *Am J Physiol* 1996;271(5 pt 1):C1424–1437.

213. Bech-Laursen J, Rajagopalan S, Galis Z, Tarpey M, Freeman BA, Harrison DG. Role of superoxide in angiotensin II-induced but not catecholamine-induced hypertension. *Circulation* 1997;95:588–593.

214. Clempus RE, Griendling KK. Reactive oxygen species signaling in vascular smooth muscle cells. *Cardiovasc Res.* July 2006;71(2):216–225.

215. Marui N, Offerman M, Swerlick R, et al. Vascular cell-adhesion molecule-1 (VCAM-1) gene-transcription and expression are regulated through an anti-oxidant sensitive mechanism in human vascular endothelial cells. *J Clin Invest* 1993;92:1866–1874.

216. Ludmer PL, Selwyn AP, Shook TL, et al. Paradoxical vasoconstriction induced by acetylcholine in atherosclerotic coronary arteries. *N Engl J Med* October 1986;315(17):1046–1051.

217. Freiman PC, Mitchell GG, Heistad DD, Armstrong ML, Harrison DG. Atherosclerosis impairs endothelium-dependent vascular relaxation to acetylcholine and thrombin in primates. *Circ Res* 1986;58:783–789.

218. McLenachan JM, Williams JK, Fish RD, Ganz P, Selwyn AP. Loss of flow-mediated endothelium-dependent dilation occurs early in the development of atherosclerosis. *Circulation* 1991;84:1273–1278.

219. Searles CD. Transcriptional and Posttranscriptional Regulation of Endothelial Nitric Oxide Synthase Expression. *Am J Physiol Cell Physiol* 2006;291(5):C803–816.

220. Laufs U, Liao JK. Post-transcriptional regulation of endothelial nitric oxide synthase mRNA stability by Rho GTPase. *J Biol Chem* 1998;273(37):24266–24271.

221. Hansson GK, Seifert PS, Olsson G, Bondjers G. Immunohistochemical detection of macrophages and T lymphocytes in atherosclerotic lesions of cholesterol-fed rabbits. *Arteriosclerosis Thrombosis* 1991;1:745–750.

222. Miller YI, Chang MK, Binder CJ, Shaw PX, Witztum JL. Oxidized low density lipoprotein and innate immune receptors. *Curr Opin Lipidol* October 2003;14(5):437–445.

223. Cybulsky MI, Gimbrone MAJ. Endothelial expression of a mononuclear leukocyte adhesion molecule during atherogenesis. *Science* 1991;251:788–791.

224. Wang JM, Sica A, Peri G, et al. Expression of monocyte chemotactic protein and interleukin-8 by cytokine-activated human vascular smooth muscle cells. *Arteriosclerosis Thrombosis* 1991;11:1166–1174.

225. Meager A. Cytokine regulation of cellular adhesion molecule expression in inflammation. *Cytokine Growth Factor Rev* 1999;10(1):27–39.

226. Eto Y, Shimokawa H, Tanaka E, et al. Long-term treatment with propagermanium suppresses atherosclerosis in WHHL rabbits. *J Cardiovasc Pharmacol* February 2003;41(2):171–177.

227. McDermott DH, Fong AM, Yang Q, et al. Chemokine receptor mutant CX3CR1-M280 has impaired adhesive function and correlates with protection from cardiovascular disease in humans. *J Clin Invest* April 2003;111(8):1241–1250.

228. Ross R. The pathogenesis of atherosclerosis: an update. *N Engl J Med* 1986;314:488–500.

229. Stary HC. Changes in components and structure of atherosclerotic lesions developing from childhood to middle age in coronary arteries. *Basic Res Cardiol* 1994;89(suppl 1):17–32.

230. Alexander RW. Hypertension and the pathogenesis of atherosclerosis. Oxidative stress and the mediation of arterial inflammatory response: a new perspective. *Hypertension* 1995;25:155–161.

231. Li J, Zhao SP, Li XP, Zhuo QC, Gao M, Lu SK. Non-invasive detection of endothelial dysfunction in patients with essential hypertension. *Int J Cardiol* 1997;61(2):165–169.

232. Panza JA, Quyyumi AA, Brush JE Jr, Epstein SE. Abnormal endothelium-dependent vascular relaxation in patients with essential hypertension. *N Engl J Med* 1990;323(1):22–27.

233. Panza JA, Quyyumi AA, Callahan TS, Epstein SE. Effect of antihypertensive treatment on endothelium-dependent vascular relaxation in patients with essential hypertension. *J Am Coll Cardiol* 1993;21(5):1145–1151.

234. Luscher TF, Vanhoutte PM. Endothelium-dependent contractions to acetylcholine in the aorta of the spontaneously hypertensive rat. *Hypertension* 1986;8:344–348.

235. Kwan CY. Dysfunction of calcium handling by smooth muscle in hypertension. *Can J Physiol Pharmacol* April 1985;63(4):366–374.

236. Owens GK, Schwartz SM. Alterations in vascular smooth muscle mass in the spontaneously hypertensive rat. Role in cellular hypertrophy, hyperploidy and hyperplasia. *Circ Res* 1982;51:280–289.

237. Owens GK, Schwartz SM. Vascular smooth muscle cell hypertrophy and hyperploidy in the Goldblatt hypertensive rat. *Circ Res* 1983;53:491–501.

238. Halpern W, Warshaw DM, Mulvany MJ. Mechanical and morphological properties of arterial resistance vessels in young and old spontaneously hypertensive rats. *Circ Res* 1979;45:250–259.

239. Majesky MW, Reidy MA, Bowen-Pope DF, Hart CE, Wilcox JN, Schwartz SM. PDGF ligand and receptor gene expression during repair of arterial injury. *J Cell Biol* 1990;111:2149–2158.

240. Taubman MB, Rollins BJ, Poon M, et al. JE mRNA accumulates rapidly in aortic injury and in platelet-derived growth factor-stimulated vascular smooth muscle cells. *Circ Res* 1992;70:314–325.

241. Lindner V, Reidy MA. Proliferation of smooth muscle cells after vascular injury is inhibited by an antibody against basic fibroblast growth factor. *Proc Natl Acad Sci U S A* 1991;88:3739–3743.

242. Cercek B, Fishbein MC, Forrester JS, Helfant RH, Fagin JA. Induction of insulin-like growth factor I messenger RNA in rat aorta after balloon denudation. *Circ Res* 1990;66:1755–1760.

243. George J, Herz I, Goldstein E, et al. Number and adhesive properties of circulating endothelial progenitor cells in patients with in-stent restenosis. *Arterioscler Thromb Vasc Biol* December 2003;23(12):e57–60.

244. Fingerle J, Au YP, Clowes AW, Reidy MA. Intimal lesion formation in rat carotid arteries after endothelial denudation in absence of medial injury. *Atherosclerosis* 1990;10:1082–1087.

245. Wessely R, Schomig A, Kastrati A. Sirolimus and Paclitaxel on polymer-based drug-eluting stents: similar but different. *J Am Coll Cardiol* February 2006;47(4):708–714.

246. Blindt R, Vogt F, Astafieva I, et al. A novel drug-eluting stent coated with an integrin-binding cyclic Arg-Gly-Asp peptide inhibits neointimal hyperplasia by recruiting endothelial progenitor cells. *J Am Coll Cardiol* May 2006;47(9):1786–1795.

247. Whiteside CI. Cellular mechanisms and treatment of diabetes vascular complications converge on reactive oxygen species. *Curr Hypertens Rep* April 2005;7(2):148–154.

248. Bagi Z, Koller A, Kaley G. Superoxide-NO interaction decreases flow- and agonist-induced dilations of coronary arterioles in Type 2 diabetes mellitus. *Am J Physiol Heart Circ Physiol* October 2003;285(4):H1404–1410.

249. Dunn EJ, Grant PJ. Type 2 diabetes: an atherothrombotic syndrome. *Curr Mol Med* May 2005;5(3):323–332.

250. Basta G, Schmidt AM, De Caterina R. Advanced glycation end products and vascular inflammation: implications for accelerated atherosclerosis in diabetes. *Cardiovasc Res* September 2004;63(4):582–592.

251. Singleton JR, Smith AG, Russell JW, Feldman EL. Microvascular complications of impaired glucose tolerance. *Diabetes.* December 2003;52(12):2867–2873.

CHAPTER 8

Molecular Development of the Heart

Neeru Kaushik / Andy Wessels / Roger R. Markwald / Bradley B. Keller

The wide spectrum of congenital cardiovascular anomalies found from the prenatal period into adulthood has challenged clinicians and scientists for centuries.[1–6] The goal of this chapter is to present a condensed overview of our current understanding of the normal development of the vertebrate heart and vasculature and to illustrate how this knowledge allows us to begin to define the pathogenesis of congenital cardiovascular malformations. Although most of the mechanisms that lead to the fully septated, four-chambered vertebrate heart are interdependent (e.g., various transcription factors involved in the molecular regulation of right–left pattern formation, or the role of neural crest cells in aortopulmonary septation), many such events are discussed in separate sections for clarity. This chapter focuses on human development; however, numerous lower vertebrate and invertebrate animal models are now under investigation to accelerate our identification of the genetic and epigenetic regulation of normal and aberrant cardiovascular morphogenesis.[7–11]

MOLECULAR DEVELOPMENT OF THE HEART

【 】 EMBRYO PATTERNING AND LATERALITY

Cardiac morphogenesis begins at the earliest stage of development with determination of the three axes of the embryo: anteroposterior, dorsoventral, and left-right. Specific genes have been identified that alter axis determination in a range of species including the mouse, frog, and chicken.[12] Following determination of the embryo axes, subpopulations of cells (somites) are programmed in a segmental body plan controlled at the molecular level by a segmentation clock and gradients of signaling molecules.[13–16] In mammals, maternal gene products control the cell through the first two cell cycles; then control switches to the embryonic genome.

The process of mesoderm formation is integral to the organization of the primary axis of the embryo and the differentiation of right and left sides. At the blastodisk stage of development, there are two primitive germ layers: endoderm and ectoderm; the endoderm layer then splits into splanchnic and visceral layers, with interposed mesodermal cells (Fig. 7–1). Mesoderm is formed as ectodermal cells migrate through the primitive streak coursing adjacent to Hensen node and lateral plate *precardiac* mesodermal cells migrate to form the heart and great vessels. Hensen node contains retinoic acid and serves as an embryonic organizer that confers information required to direct the ultimate fate of these mesodermal cells.[17] At this critical phase in cell determination, exogenous retinoic acid is extremely teratogenic, with the greatest effect at the arterial pole and the least effect at the venous pole.[18]

Correct laterality is a fundamental aspect of normal embryonic development and errors in laterality occur approximately 1 in 8000 births. Normal cardiac laterality (situs) has the lowest risk of congenital cardiovascular malformations.[19] The first grossly asymmetric feature to develop is the heart tube, which undergoes rightward looping (Fig. 8–1). However, the asymmetric expression of molecular markers occurs much earlier in development. This pattern of left-right asymmetry occurs in all vertebrate internal organs because of signaling cascades present prior to gastrulation. The current paradigm for explaining asymmetry begins with the function of surface cilia on primitive, dorsal forerunner cells in the region of the neural tube prior to gastrulation.[20] Ciliary function at this sites drives unilateral extraembryonic *nodal flow* of fluid containing secreted morphogens.[21] A key insight into this process came from investigating mutant mouse embryos that lack the kinesin motor protein, KIF3, have immotile epithelial nodal cilia, randomized localization of the laterality gene *lefty2*, and randomized left-right determination.[22] These epithelial monocilia can be subdivided into a subclass that contain or lack the motor protein left-right dynein, lrd, which is targeted by the mutant *iv* gene in mice that display situs inversus.[23,24] The mouse *inv* mutant shows consistent reversal of left-right patterning, which may be dependent in part on calcium-calmodulin signaling.[25,26] One of the earliest *morphogens* regulating left-to-right (L-R) patterning is the asymmetric phosphorylation of syndecan-2 by protein kinase C gamma.[27] Recent evidence suggests that the leftward movement of membrane-sheathed particles, called *nodal vesicular parcels* (NVPs), may result in the activation of the noncanonical hedgehog signaling pathway, an asymmetric elevation in intracellular Ca²⁺ and changes in gene expression.[28] The critical timing of this patterning process has been shown to produce phenotypic variation from L-R reversal

to randomized L-R patterning within a 1-hour window. The development of L-R asymmetry requires transcription factors that unilaterally suppress gene expression (for example *Shh* induction of *Nodal* on the left side, which then induces the bicoid-type transcription factor *Pitx2c*). Targeted disruption of *Pitx2c* in mice results in a complex phe-

Stage 7/8

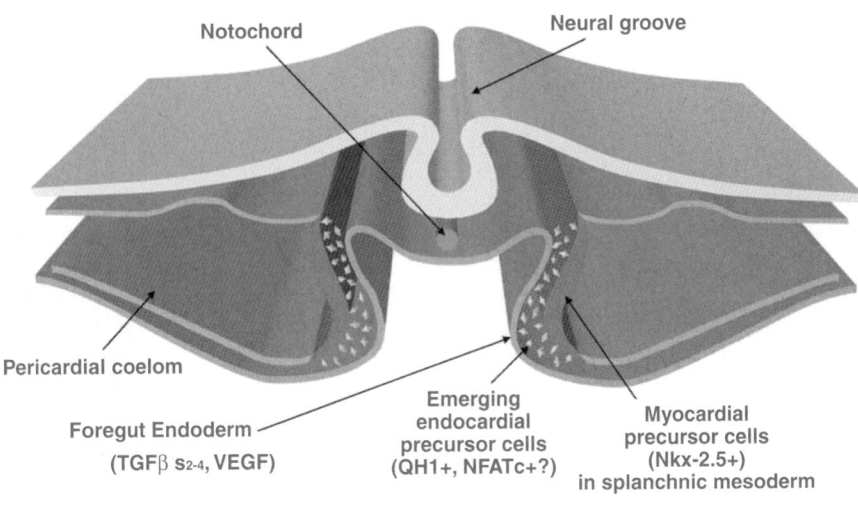

Stage 9/10

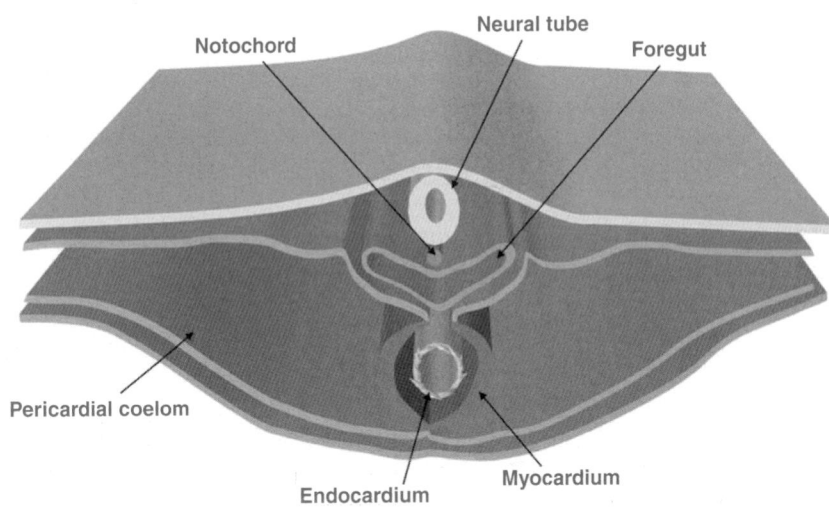

FIGURE 8–1. This figure illustrates the postgastrulation morphogenetic events involved in the formation of the tubular heart. The upper panel represents a quail embryo at stage 7/8 H/H, demonstrating the emergence of endocardial precursor mesenchymal cells, characterized by the expression of the antigen QH1 and the transcription factor NFATc, from the splanchnic mesoderm. This mesoderm is also the source for the future myocardium, which, for instance, expresses the transcription factor Nkx-2.5. It is proposed that the formation of both endocardium and myocardium are induced by growth factors, such as transforming growth factor β (TGFβ) isoforms and vascular endothelial growth factor (VEGF) in the adjacent endoderm. The lower panel shows that, subsequent to the migration and assembly of endocardial precursor mesenchymal cells during stages 7 to 8 H/H, the cellular plexus coalesces to form the definitive endocardial tube enveloped by the myocardial tube. Note that the endocardium is still in close proximity to the ventral side of the foregut. *Source: Courtesy of Dr. Yukiko Sugi, Cardiovascular Developmental Biology Center, Medical University of South Carolina.*

notype including body plan laterality defects associated with complex cardiac anomalies associated with right atrial isomerism and complex intracardiac defects.[29] It is important to note that *Pitx2c* is also expressed later in development in the secondary heart-forming field responsible for expanding and remodeling the outflow tract; therefore the *cardiac* phenotype in this mouse mutant is related to more than disrupted laterality.[30] Misexpression of the normally left-sided signals *Nodal, Lefty2,* and *Shh* on the right side, or ectopic application of retinoic acid, results in upregulation of *Nkx-3.2* contralateral to its normal expression on the left,[31] whereas *FGF8* inhibits *Nkx-3.2* expression.[32]

【 】 MOLECULAR FACTORS INVOLVED IN CARDIOGENESIS

Defining the molecular basis underlying the establishment and maintenance of cardiac muscle differentiation has presented a fundamental challenge in developmental biology and molecular genetics (Fig. 8–2). Despite the shared expression of numerous contractile protein genes by both cardiac and skeletal striated muscles, the molecular mechanisms for cell determination, differentiation, and tissue patterning between these two *organs* are quite distinct. For example, a basic helix-loop-helix transcription factor, MyoD,[33] is sufficient to convert a variety of mesodermal and non-

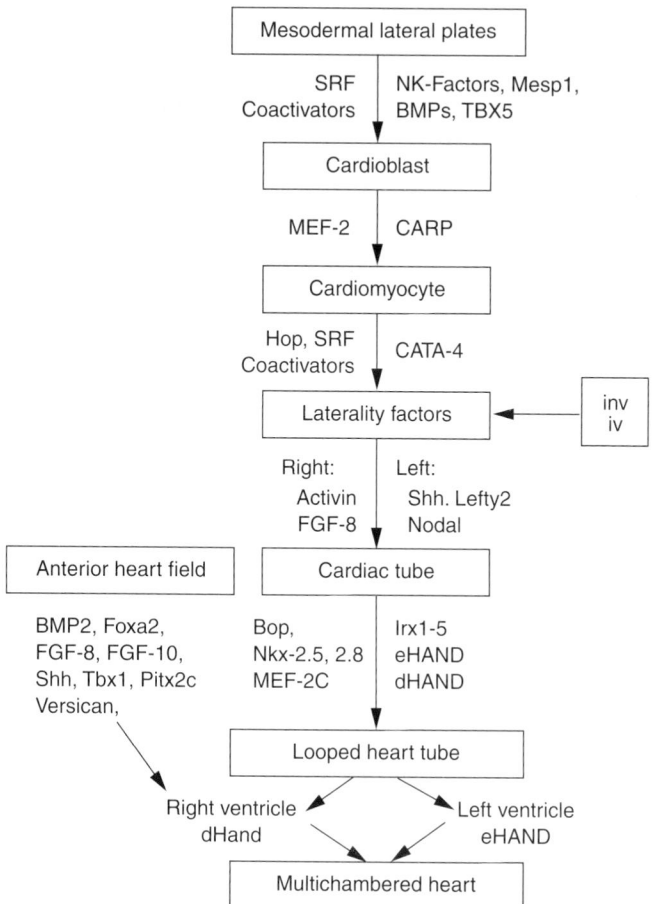

FIGURE 8–2. Schematic cascade of some of the major genes and transcription factors proven to regulate cardiomyocyte determination, differentiation, and final phenotype. This outline is intended to display the concept of temporal and spatial regulation of a complex developmental process rather than to be comprehensive, as there are now more than 200 genes and proteins identified to affect cardiovascular morphogenesis.

mesodermal cell types to stable skeletal myoblasts with active muscle specific gene expression.

Tinman and Other Related *Nk-2* Genes

The identification of molecular mechanisms involved specifically in heart development has depended on the investigation of simpler biological models, including the fruit fly, *Drosophila melanogaster;* the zebrafish, *Danio rerio;* and the frog, *Xenopus laevis.*[34,35] Homeotic genes are genes that determine a change in structure and have in common a 60–amino acid coding region. Genes with this sequence, referred to as homeobox (HOX) genes, are generally upregulated during early differentiation in a time-dependent sequence. HOX genes have been studied extensively in *Drosophila,* where they are involved in the commitment of cells to specific developmental pathways and play an important role in pattern formation.[36,37] Murine homologs of *tinman,* called NK HOX genes, have been identified to have similar functions during early cardiac development in vertebrates.[38] The murine NK-2 HOX gene *Nkx-2.5/Csx* is expressed in early cardiac progenitor cells prior to cardiogenic differentiation and continues through adulthood.[35] Homeotic genes are DNA-binding proteins (transcription factors) capable of activating transcription. For example, *Nkx-2.5* has been shown to bind to novel NKE sites, certain serum response elements of the cardiac α-actin promoter, and the NKE sites in the cardiac atrial natriuretic factor promoter.[39] Mutations in the *Drosophila* homeotic gene, *tinman,* result in loss of heart formation.[40] In addition, *tinman* is known to regulate *NK-3/bagpipe* expression in the visceral mesoderm.[38]

The *Nkx-2.5* factors identified in vertebrates including zebrafish, *Xenopus,* chickens, mice, and humans are highly related in sequence and expression pattern.[39,41] An attractive hypothesis is that these homeodomain factors function in phylogenetically conserved myogenic pathways occurring in muscle types that do not use the MyoD family. Whether the vertebrate *Nkx-2.5* or other *Nkx-2*–related genes expressed in the early heart play a role in heart specification or whether they are downstream regulators of cardiac gene expression remains to be determined. For example, in mice homologous recombination knockouts of the endogenous *Nkx-2.5* gene do not inhibit formation of the cardiac tube but result in cardiac dysmorphogenesis at the looping stages of development and embryonic lethality.[40] Overexpression of *Nkx-2.5* in zebrafish embryo results in an enlarged heart as well as conduction defects.[42] As mentioned in the following text, patients with secundum atrial septal defect have now been identified to have specific mutations in the human homolog to the *Nkx-2.5* gene.[43]

Cardiac-Restricted Ankyrin Repeat Protein Genes

The expression of CARP (cardiac-restricted ankyrin repeat protein) genes, is at least partially regulated by *Nkx-2.5.*[44] *CARP* genes are coregulators of the cardiac gene expression program, which are normally developmentally downregulated but are dramatically reinduced during cardiac hypertrophy. A distinct 5' cis regulatory element binds *Nkx2.5* and *GATA-4* and directs heart segment–specific expression, such as atrial versus ventricular and left versus right. In addition, a 213 base pair sequence element of the gene confers conotruncal segment-specific expression.[44]

SRF and MEF2, MADS Box Factors

Serum response factor (SRF) is an ancient DNA-binding protein, containing a highly conserved DNA-binding/dimerization domain termed the *MADS box.* SRF is a ubiquitous and constitutively trophic factor highly expressed in heart[45] and SRF-related proteins bind to the regulatory regions of both nonmuscle- and muscle-specific genes.[46] SRF-related proteins are capable of binding MEF2 sites which can be found in the regulatory regions of both nonmuscle- and muscle-specific genes.[47,48] Like SRF, MEF2 factors contain a MADS box and an adjacent MEF2 box. Expression and mutagenesis studies in *Drosophila* have shown that MEF2 proteins are necessary for myogenic differentiation during development[49,50] and are activated by *tinman.*[51] In the mouse embryo, *MEF2* genes (of which four have been identified in vertebrate species) are highly expressed in the early heart and skeletal muscle progenitor cells prior to the induction of cardiac and skeletal muscle structural genes, implicating MEF2 as a key regulator of cardiac and skeletal muscle differentiation programs. It has been shown that Nkx-2.5 transactivates the cardiac α-*actin* gene by binding to SRF but only after SRF has bound to DNA.[52]

GATA Family and FOG Cofactors

The GATA proteins are vital regulators for the cardiac secretory proteins ANF and BNP which themselves are essential for cardiac growth and differentiation. GATA-1/2/3 are linked to hematopoiesis and GATA-4/5/6 are involved with cardiac, gut, and blood vessel formation. Each of the six GATA proteins contains a highly specific DNA-binding domain, consisting of two C4 zinc fingers that may interchangeably bind to a unique DNA sequence. GATA-4 and -6 are expressed in developmentally and lineage-specific patterns within cardiac mesoderm and gut epithelium,[53,54] whereas GATA-5 expression is restricted to the epicardium. Experiments have shown that GATA-4 regulates expression of cardiac-specific genes, such as cardiac *troponin C*[55] and α *MHC.*[56] Several studies have demonstrated that the GATA-4 transcription factor plays an important role in regulating cardiac-specified genes and appears to be downstream to the *Nkx-2.5* gene.[57,58] Mice lacking *GATA-4* gene display a severe defect in cardiac tube formation. Transcriptional repressors have also been found to regulate cardiac development; and FOG-2, a zinc-finger repressor protein, functions to suppress GATA-4–mediated activation of cardiac-restricted genes.[59]

Bone Morphogenic Proteins

Another category of signaling molecule responsible for cardiogenic commitment is the class of bone morphogenic proteins (BMPs), which are members of the transforming growth factor β family of signaling molecules. BMP-2 and BMP-4 can induce the cardiac regulatory factors Nkx-2.5 and GATA-4 when ectopically applied to regions of chick embryos that are not usually specified to become heart tissue.[60] In mice lacking the *BMP-4* gene there was little or no mesoderm differentiation. Some mice deficient for *BMP-2* gene that lacked *Nkx-2.5* expression also failed to develop beyond the early stages of looping.[61] Thus, BMPs appear to have an early influence on cardiac lineage commitment and cardiogenesis.[62,63]

dHAND, eHAND, and Ventricular Chamber Formation

Basic helix-loop-helix (bHLH) factors that are present in the developing mammalian heart include dHAND and eHAND; these proteins share sequence homology in their bHLH regions and have temporally and spatially specific expression patterns.[64] In the mouse, HAND expression coincides with that of other cardiac transcription factors under the regulation of a cardiac-specific SET domain protein, BOP, that interacts with histone deacetylases. Expression of dHAND and eHAND precedes separation of the two ventricles and is required for early chamber specification. dHAND expression in the myocardium is maintained throughout the straight heart tube but is restricted to the conotruncus and future right ventricle (RV) as the heart tube forms a loop. eHAND expressed in the myocardium becomes rapidly restricted to the left ventricle (LV).[65] Deletion of dHAND by gene targeting showed that dHAND expression is necessary for RV formation[66]; and although GATA-4 expression is reduced following the elimination of dHAND, the expression of cardiac-specified genes, α*MHC, MLC2A, MLC2V, ANF,* and *Nkx-2.5,* are unaffected.[67] Double mutants lacking dHAND and *Nkx-2.5* lack ventricular chamber development, fail to express the ventricular specific transcription factor Irx4, and are embryo lethal.[68]

The expansion of unique RV and LV myocardium is under the tight regulation of molecular pathways. For example, expression of the T-box gene, *Tbx5,* is responsible for the specific identity of LV myocardium through interactions with both eHAND and eHAND-sensitive elements and is negatively regulated by the related *Tbx20* gene that is normally expressed in the developing RV myocardium. Of note, not all mouse embryos lacking *Tbx5* have a secundum atrial septal defect similar to humans with Holt-Oram Syndrome, but all affected embryos have impaired ventricular function.[69–73] The differential effects of changes in *Tbx* expression in the embryo reflects differences between the concept of heterochrony (similar genes expressed under differential temporal schemes) versus heterotopy (similar genes with differential effects based on spatial context). Mice that lack a single copy of *Tbx-5* have the atrial septal defect and conduction abnormality found in patients with Holt-Oram syndrome and the zebrafish mutant, *heartstrings,* has a similar defect.[74] Of note, *Tbx-5* directly regulates forelimb development via direct activation of the *Fgf-10* gene.[75,76]

An attractive hypothesis from the analysis of these transcriptional cascades is that homeodomain factors function in phylogenetically conserved pathways in muscle cell types that do not use the MyoD family. However, whether these factors play the primary role in heart specification and serve as regulators of other downstream cardiac genes remains to be determined.

【 】 CONTRIBUTIONS OF THE ANTERIOR (SECONDARY) HEART FIELD

Although it is clear that the ventricular myocardium expands by a process of clonal expansion, the recruitment of mesenchymal cells into a cardiomyocyte lineage from the anterior (or secondary) heart field is now understood to also be required for normal formation of the right ventricular outflow tract and great vessels (Fig. 8–3).[77–81] The regulation of myocyte specification and differentiation in the anterior heart forming region likely involves cell adhesion molecules, including N-cadherin, extracellular proteases, and morphogenetic signals from the transforming growth factor β (TGFβ) and fibroblast growth factor (FGF) families of growth and differentiation factors.[82,83] Recent data suggest major roles for the T-box transcription factor, *Tbx-1,* and both *FGF8* and *FGF10* in regulating the fate of these cells in contributing to the aortic arches and expanding right ventricular outflow tract.[84–89] The transcription factor *Tbx-1* is expressed in the pharyngeal arch under the regulation of *Shh* and the forkhead transcription factor, *Foxa2*, and *Tbx-1*–expressing cells are recruited from the anterior heart-forming region to expand the developing outflow tract.[90] Remodeling the outflow tract involves programmed cell death likely regulated by mechanical load and by tissue oxygen content.[91,92]

THE NEURAL CREST AND CARDIAC DEVELOPMENT

The neural crest functions as the origin for migrating pluripotent cell populations with broad developmental fates. The "*cardiac*" neural crest is an important migratory cell population contributing to cardiovascular (CV) morphogenesis.[93,94] The cardiac neural crest arises from the dorsal margin of the neural tube prior to fusion and migrates ventrally to form the autonomic ganglia, melanocytes, and Schwann cells. The crest cells move in waves through the branchial arches during the first 4 weeks of human development. The eventual fate of the neural crest cells is likely determined long before the initial phenotypic expression of a heart tube by activation of cellular gradients of HOX genes and other morphoregulating factors.[95] The cranial neural crest region defines a developmental field that includes the heart, hind brain, face, and branchial arch derivatives.

Experimental disruption of cranial neural crest produces a spectrum of cardiac abnormalities. In a series of elegant ablation and chick/quail chimera studies, Kirby and colleagues defined the region of cardiac neural crest that is integral to the septation of the conotruncal region of the heart and branchial arch derivatives including facial abnormalities, thymus, parathyroid, and autonomic derivatives.[94] These neural crest cells migrate to specific sites from the neural crest through the pharyngeal arches to the developing heart and carry information critical both to normal CV morphogenesis and function.[94]

Several genes are recognized as key factors required for the proper migration and differentiation of the cardiac neural crest. Transgenic mouse mutants lacking the endothelin (ET) peptide, ET-1, or endothelin receptors ET-A and ET-B express abnormal cardiac neural crest phenotypes including abnormal pharyngeal arches and outflow tract septation similar to the avian neural crest ablation model.[96] The *splotch* mutant mouse contains a mutated *Pax 3* gene, and homozygote splotch mutants have a complete neural crest ablation phenotype, including persistent truncus arteriosus and aortic arch anomalies[97] similar to the CV phenotype of neural crest ablation in the chick embryo. *HOX* gene abnormalities are also associated with defects in the derivatives of cranial neural crest.[98] A transgenic murine model of *Hox 1.1* overexpression has neural crest ectomesenchymal tissue abnormalities including cleft palate, nonfused pinnae, and open eyes. *Hox 1.5*–deficient mice have features of DiGeorge syndrome.[98] In humans, DiGeorge syndrome, velo-cardio-facial syndrome, and conotruncal anomaly face syndrome are associated with chromosomal deletions in the 22q11 region on long arm of chromosome 22.[99] Recent studies have indicated a number of candidate factors involved in the pathogenesis of these syndromes, including *Tbx-1*.[100] Interestingly, *Tbx-1* is expressed in the pharyngeal endoderm but not in migrating neural crest cells, so this gene regulates morphogenesis via secreted paracrine signals, including FGF-8 and FGF-10, to determine neural crest cell fate.[101] Another secreted factor, semaphorin 3C, and

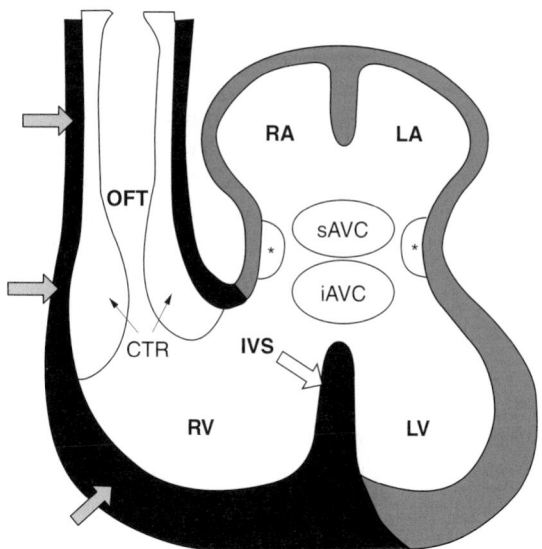

FIGURE 8–3. Schematic representation of the contribution of the anterior/secondary heart fields to the developing heart. This illustration shows that the myocardial structures of LA, RA, and LV are derived from cells in the lateral plate mesoderm identified as the primary heart fields (*grey*). In contrast, the endothelial and myocardial tissues (*black*) of the outflow tract, RV, and portions of the interventricular septum (*black*) develop as derivatives of cells from the anterior/secondary heart fields. Asterisks, lateral atrioventricular cushions; CTR, conotruncal ridge; IVS, interventricular septum; iAVC, inferior atrioventricular cushion; LA, left atrium; LV, left ventricle; OFT, outflow tract; RA, right atrium; RV, right ventricle; sAVC, superior atrioventricular cushions. *Source: Adapted from Verzi MP, McCulley DJ, De Val S, Dodou E, Black BL.[81]*

the associated coreceptor, Plexin A2, are also required for normal migration of pharyngeal and cardiac neural crest cells.[102,103] In addition to genetic mechanisms, exogenous dosing of retinoic acid acts as a potent teratogen in humans and produces a syndrome involving all the derivatives of the cranial neural crest.[104,105]

MYOCYTE DIFFERENTIATION

In the human embryo, the heart begins to contract on approximately postconception day 17, as the electromechanical machinery of contraction and relaxation become functional. These functional units include the sarcomere, containing the contractile elements; the mitochondria, containing the enzymes for energy production and modulation; and the sarcolemma, including the cell envelope with specialized components of the t-tubular system linked to the sarcoplasmic reticulum. In the mature myocardium, sarcomeres are organized parallel to the lines of peak systolic stress. In the embryonic myocyte, myofibrils initially appear disarrayed and become aligned in response to mechanical load as development proceeds.[106] Confocal microscopic studies of the early looping heart reveal a circumferential pattern of premyofibril distribution with randomized surface focal adhesions.[107,108] Despite this disordered appearance, the contraction pattern of the early embryonic heart is isotropic for only a brief period and then the contraction and relaxation patterns of the embryonic heart become anisotropic.[109,110]

The temporal and spatial expression of contractile proteins in the developing heart is similar across a range of species. At the precardiac tube stage, smooth muscle α-*actin* is the only isoform present. The onset of cardiac contractions is associated with a progressive increase in the expression of the cardiac form of sarcomeric actin. Smooth muscle α-*actin* may act as a scaffolding during assembly of the sarcomere.[111–115] Much additional work is required to define the regulation of myofibrillogenesis during cardiac morphogenesis.

Mitochondria multiply concurrently with the myofibrils in the differentiating myocyte. In the mature heart, mitochondrial enzymes are the major source of high-energy phosphate necessary for contraction and likely begin this function during embryonic development. In the chick, mitochondria account for approximately 10 percent of myocyte volume.[116] In the rat embryo, the total volume increases from 22 to 34 percent between days 6 and 10, and the mitochondria also change morphologically with development, becoming larger with more cristae and denser matrix.[116] The myocyte mitochondrial volume fraction correlates directly with heart rate and oxygen consumption among animals.[117]

Maturation of the sarcoplasmic reticulum and apparatus for excitation-contraction coupling occurs coincident with the structural morphogenesis of the embryonic heart.[118] During maturation of the heart, the resting potential increases (becomes more negative) in both birds and mammals[119] and Ca^{2+} influx through Ca^{2+} channels may play a relatively important role in transsarcolemmal Ca^{2+} influx in the immature heart.[120,121] However, peak Ca^{2+} current density is actually decreased compared to that measured in mature cells.[122–124] Although Ca^{2+} influx by way of the Na^+–Ca^{2+} exchanger is less important for excitation-contraction coupling in mature myocardium, Na^+–Ca^{2+} exchange plays an important role in the developing myocyte.[125] In contrast to the mature myocardium, T-type Ca^{2+} channels also play an important role in regulating both heart rate and myocardial contractility in the embryonic myocardium.[126] The molecular regulation of ion channels has been identified in the pathogenesis of adult dysrhythmias, and this process is likely to be as critical in the regulation of ion channels and embryo fate during cardiac morphogenesis.

Relaxation, an active process by which the myocardium returns to a passive, steady state after contraction, depends on the rapid removal of Ca^{2+} from troponin C, mediated primarily by active transport of Ca^{2+} back into the sarcoplasmic reticulum (SR). The SR Ca^{2+}-adenosine triphosphatase usually couples hydrolysis of adenosine triphosphate to active Ca^{2+} transport. The rate of SR Ca^{2+} uptake correlates well with the observed rate of myocardial relaxation. Regulation of SR Ca^{2+} pump activity is mediated by the intrinsic SR protein, phospholamban. Ca^{2+} is also removed from the myofilaments by extrusion across the cell membrane. In the steady state, the amount of Ca^{2+} removed from the myocyte equals the amount entering through the Ca^{2+} channels.[127] Ca^{2+} removal from myofibers and myocardial relaxation is emerging as a critical determinant of the function of the early embryonic heart based on new evidence of the role of diastolic relaxation and suction on early heart function.[128]

SEGMENTAL BASIS OF HEART TUBE FORMATION

Formation of the cardiac tube is a complex morphogenetic sequence. Initially, primitive, bilateral heart tubes form from lateral plate mesoderm and each contains an inner layer of endocardium, a middle layer of cardiac jelly, and an outer layer of myocardium. The primitive heart tubes then fuse in the ventral midline to form the linear or *straight* heart tube.[4,5,129] It is important to note the primitive linear heart tube does not contain all of the cardiac segments present in the mature

heart. During morphogenesis, the proximate portion of the aortic sac is incorporated into the outflow tract of the RV (along with migrating neural crest cells) and the proximate sinus venosus is incorporated into developing atria. Expansion of the RV and outflow tract require the incorporation of cells from the anterior heart field. Thus, each *segment* of the mature heart arises at a unique time during embryogenesis.[130] One critical aspect of this segmental assembly and maturation of the heart is that there are temporal and spatial *windows* that are developmentally regulated, partially explaining why morphogens such as retinoic acid can also function as potent teratogens to produce a embryowide spectrum of defects depending on the time in gestation of exposure. Another aspect of this segmental paradigm for molecular cardiogenesis is that cardiac morphogenesis depends on complex molecular, cellular, and biomechanical interactions between the respective segments.[130]

CARDIAC JELLY AND EXTRACELLULAR MATRIX

Prior to looping, the acellular space between the myocardium and endocardium in the heart is filled with a deformable extracellular matrix, the *cardiac jelly*, secreted by the myocardium.[131] At the pretubular heart stages, the extracellular matrix contains collagen types I and IV, fibronectin, and laminin. Radioactive labeling demonstrates that proteins produced in the myocardium flow toward the endocardium and are incorporated into the basal lamina.[132] The cardiac jelly has a variety of functions related to hemodynamic performance, cardiac looping, and cell migration in cardiac septation and formation of the endocardial cushion valves at the atrioventricular (AV) junction and outflow tract of the heart.

More than 100 genes have been identified in the formation of endocardial cushions, and these genes function to either stimulate or repress competitive molecular pathways.[133] The protein composition of the cardiac jelly regulates endothelial differentiation via the TGFβ family of peptide growth factors.[134] Some extracellular matrix proteins stimulate transdifferentiation of the endocardium in these regions by prompting endothelial cells to transform into mesenchymal cells and then migrate into the cushion matrix. Blockade of the TGFβ type I (activin receptor–like kinase), type II, and type III receptors can block this cell transformation.[135–137] *Smad6* negatively regulates AV cushion transformation and myocyte proliferation.[138] Conversely, laminin and type IV collagen are likely stabilizing signals or markers, because these compounds are absent in the cushion regions but their presence in adjacent regions stimulates endocardial cells to maintain epithelial integrity. Periostin, the osteoblast-specific factor 2, functions to promote the differentiation of cells along a fibroblastic cell lineage toward the formation of the primary fibrous rings in the developing heart under the negative regulation of BMP-2,[139] BMP-2 and NFATc/VEGF stimulate cardiac progenitor cells to form heart-valve inducing fields.[140,141] The extracellular matrix also presents a complex three-dimensional, antigenic, structural environment that directly influences cell migration, differentiation, and response to cyclic mechanical loads. The temporal and spatial secretion and remodeling of the extracellular matrix influences the fate of numerous cell populations with dramatic effects on CV phenotype and function.[142–144]

ENDOCARDIAL MATURATION

The endothelial cells that make up the lining of the embryonic heart are initially arranged as a single sheet. This squamous-like

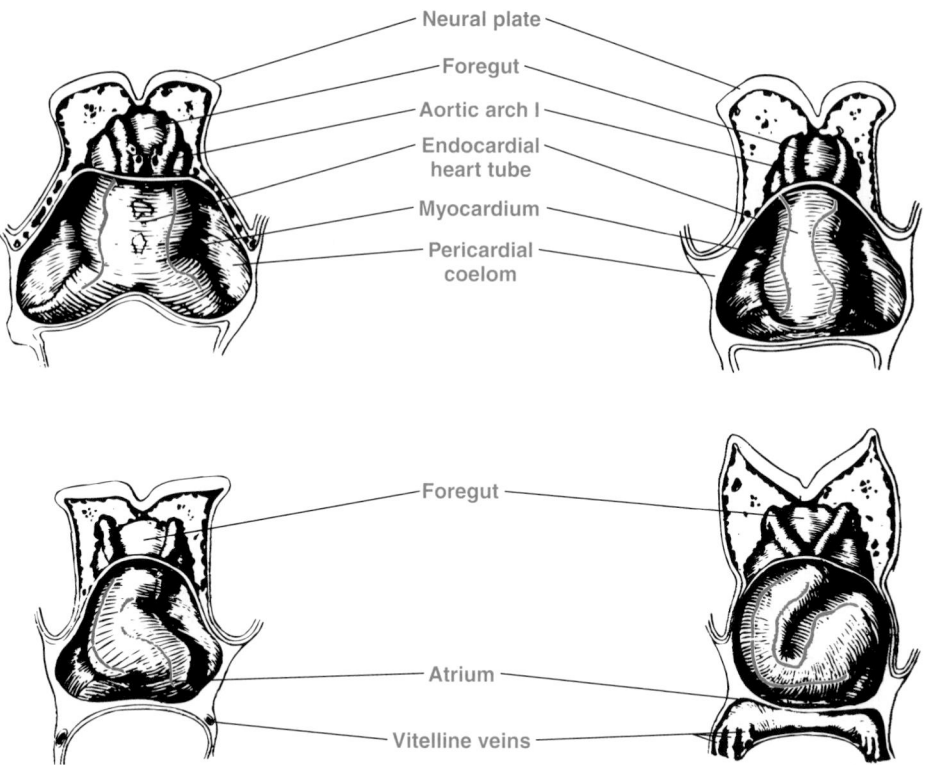

FIGURE 8–4. Schematic ventral dissections of human embryos of different ages, showing formation of the heart loop. *Source: Adapted from Davis CL. Development of the human heart from its first appearance to the state found in embryos of 20 paired somites. Contrib Embryol 1927;19:245. Reproduced with permission from the Carnegie Institution of Washington, DC.*

sheet has the morphologic features of an active tissue, including microvilli, ruffles, and intercellular openings.[145] The endocardium participates in the formation of endocardial cushions at the AV junction and in the outflow tract.[146] Transdifferentiation of the endocardium occurs in the endocardial cushions, where cells round up, produce pseudopodia, and migrate into the cardiac jelly.[147] These cells eventually make up a portion of the fibrous skeleton of the cardiac valves. Inductive chemical signals from the myocardium contribute to the endocardial transdifferentiation and regulate the migration of the mesenchymal cells.[148] In addition, hemodynamic alterations can influence the orientation of endocardial cells on the endocardial cushions[149,150] and the loci of dead and dying cells in the chick and zebrafish embryos.[151] Endocardial cells are also involved in patterning and remodeling of the developing outflow tract under the regulation of nuclear transcription factor NFATc1.[152] Finally, expansion of the endocardium is critical to the process of ventricular trabeculation, as discussed in the following text.

[ ] LOOPING

Following the formation of the straight heart tube, the human embryo is approximately 2 mm long and 23 days old. At the cephalic (or cranial) end of the myocardial heart tube, the nonmyocardial aortic sac can be recognized. The aortic sac is connected to the first pair of aortic arches and, later, also to the second, third, fourth, and sixth arches (the fifth pair of aortic arches does not normally develop in mammals). The caudal end of the myocardial tube receives the paired confluence of veins that lie extrapericardially and embedded in mesenchyme. In the early tubular stage, the heart hangs suspended from the ventral foregut by a dorsal mesocardium. During heart tube looping, the midportion of the dorsal mesocardium disintegrates, leaving the heart connected at the anterior pole at the level of the aortic sac and at the posteriorly located venous pole (atria and sinus venosus). At least three distinct biomechanical mechanisms may act in combination to generate the characteristic rightward bend in the cardiac tube: locally constrained growth, active cell deformation, and the release of the prestressed dorsal mesocardium.[153]

As the tubular heart continues to grow, it bends to the right and anteriorly (Fig. 8–4). This results in a compound sigmoid structure with a D loop (dextro- or rightward) configuration. At this stage it is easy to distinguish the sinus venosus, common atrium, atrioventricular canal, future LV and RV, and outflow segment. Internally, the developing muscular interventricular septum is recognizable, its crest characteristically expressing the molecular marker *GLN2/HNK-1*.[154–156] It is important to note that, at this stage, all the future segments of the heart are still basically connected in series and that the common atrium connects via the atrioventricular canal exclusively to the LV, whereas the outflow tract is exclusively committed to the RV (Fig. 8–5). If cardiac morphogenesis fails to

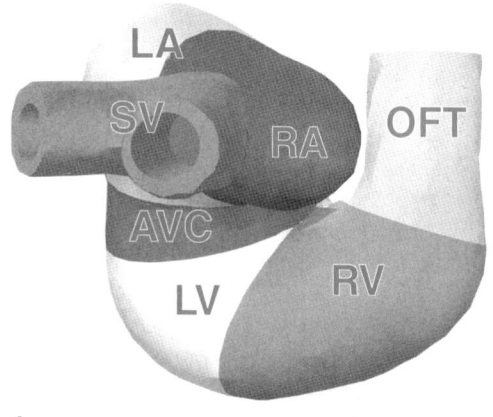
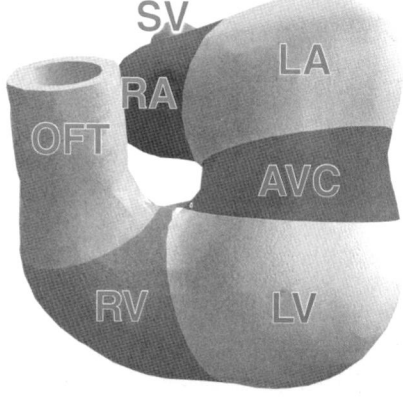

A   **B**

FIGURE 8–5. Schematic representation of the tubular heart during looping. **A.** Posterior view of the heart. **B.** Anterior view of the heart. Note that at this stage (approximately 4 weeks of development in the human), all the segments are more or less arranged in series. From inflow to outflow: SV, sinus venosus; RA, right atrium; LA, left atrium; AVC, atrioventricular canal; LV, left ventricle; RV, right ventricle; OFT, outflow tract.

progress beyond this state, the cardiac anatomy will include a double-inlet LV and a double-outlet right ventricle (DORV), as discussed further on in this chapter.

The transition from a tubular heart, in which the future segments are arranged in series (atrium to LV to RV to outflow tract), into a four-chambered heart, in which the definitive chambers are arranged in parallel separated by septa and valves, raises two important questions. The first is how the right atrium becomes connected to the RV and the second is how the LV gains access to the aortic portion of the outflow tract. The remodeling of the so-called *inner curvature* of the looping heart tube plays an important role in this process and involves a rightward expansion of the AV canal and a concomitant leftward shift of the aorta.[155] Immunohistochemical studies have demonstrated that this remodeling is intimately related to the development of the so-called *primary ring* (Fig. 8–6).[155] In the postnatal human heart, derivatives of the primary ring are found in the AV conduction system, in the right AV junction (the right AV ring), and behind the aorta (the retroaortic root branch) (Fig. 8–7).[156]

Structural Anomalies

Ventricular Inversion with Transposition of the Great Arteries
If the primitive heart tube loops to the left and anterior (L loop) rather than to the right and anterior, most of the structures adjacent to and including ventricular segments of the heart tube (the AV valves, ventricles, and arterial roots) will develop in an inverted position. Subsequently, the right atrium is connected via a morphologic mitral valve to a morphologic LV and the left atrium is connected via a morphologic tricuspid valve to a morphologic RV. Within the aortic sac, the aorticopulmonary septum develops in a normal fashion. However, as partitioning of the inverted conotruncus (outflow tract) takes place in mirror image, the end result is L-transposition of the great arteries, with the aorta arising anteriorly from a left-sided, morphologically right (systemic) ventricle and the pulmonary trunk (PT) arising posteriorly from a right-sided, morphologically left (venous) ventricle. Because systemic and pulmonary venous return are still routed to the pulmonary and systemic arterial circulations, respectively, this anomaly is commonly referred to as *corrected* transposition.

Double-Outlet Right Ventricle
This anomaly is caused by a failure in the leftward repositioning of the aortic portion of the out-

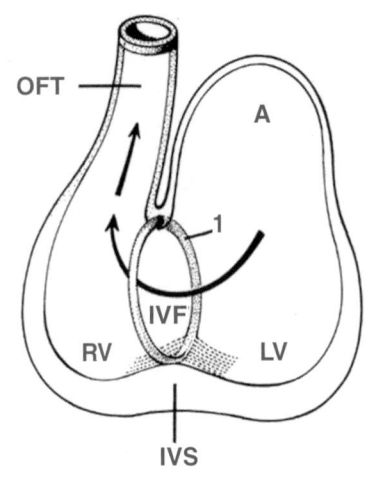
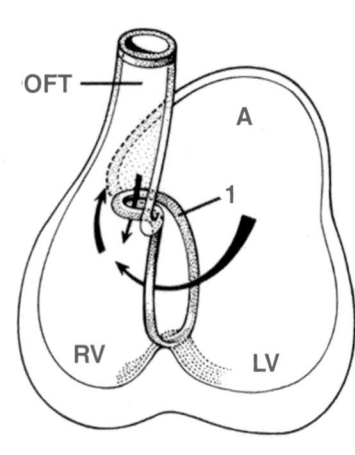
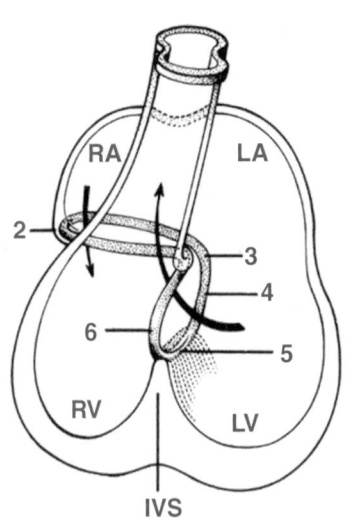
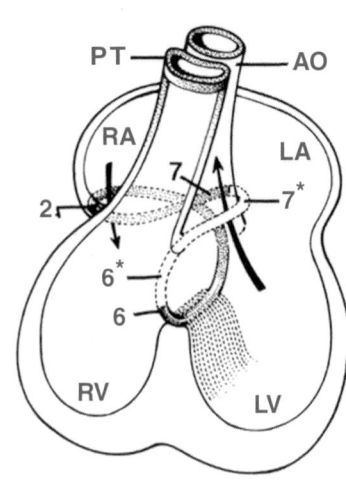

FIGURE 8–6. Schematic representation of the location of the *primary ring* (characterized by the expression of the antigen G1N2) in different stages of human development. The drawings illustrate the development of the conduction system as a derivative of the primary ring but also show that the changes in the topography of the ring tissue is reflecting the rightward expansion of the atrioventricular canal and the leftward shift (*wedging*) of the developing aorta. 1, primary ring; 2, right atrioventricular ring; 3, atrioventricular nodal area; 4, penetrating His bundle; 6, septal branch; 7, retroaortic branch. Those areas marked with an asterisk have lost their expression. The Carnegie stages of development presented in drawings **A** to **D** are as follows: **A**, stage 14; **B**, stage 15; **C**, stage 17; **D**, stages 18–19. *Source: Adapted from Icardo JM, Fernandez-Teran A.[158]*

flow tract, resulting in persistence of the more *primitive* embryonic morphology in which the entire outflow tract originates from the RV. One morphologic hallmark of the failure of completion of the leftward shift of the aorta is the presence of myocardial tissue between the left AV valve and the aorta (mitral-aortic separation). This anomaly is found following a wide range of hemodynamic, metabolic, and genetic insults to the embryo, suggesting that the phenotype of DORV may be a final common expression of a range of primary abnormalities that result in persistence of the embryonic configuration.[157]

【 】 MYOCARDIAL TRABECULATION

The processes of primary myocardial trabeculation, expansion of secondary and tertiary myocardial trabeculae, and myocardial

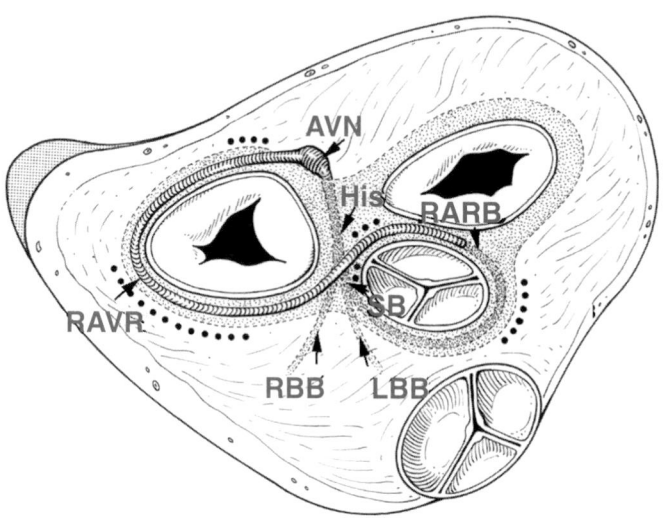

FIGURE 8–7. Schematic representation of the localization of remnants of the primary ring in the neonatal human heart. The ring is projected on a superior view of the aortic mitral fibrous unit of the heart. The *black dots* indicate the areas in which remnants of the ring are detected in a series of neonatal hearts as described in Wessels A, Anderson RH, Markwald R, et al.[171] AVN, atrioventricular node; His, bundle of His; LBB, left bundle branch; RARB, retroaortic root branch; RAVR, right atrioventricular ring; RBB, right bundle branch; SB, septal branch.

compaction are critical to the structural maturation of the ventricular chambers. This process results in the transformation of the smooth walled endocardial lining into complex three-dimensional structure of the right and left ventricular myocardium. Rapid cell division and interposition of endothelial cells along the right and left ventrolateral borders of the endocardial tube is associated with a rapid resorption of cardiac jelly resulting in myocardial ridges and trabeculae lined with single layers of endocardial cells.[158] The initial number and orientation of the myocardial ridges differs between species.[159] In general, myocardial trabeculation begins at the ventricular outer curvature (future apex) and then extends proximally and distally. The intersection between the outer, compact myocardium and the base of the trabeculae is likely a site of peak wall stress; and myocyte division is most active at this site.[160] Retroviral marker studies have also shown that ventricular myocardial growth is associated with a transmural distribution of clonally related myocardial cells extending from the epi- to endocardium.[161,162] Of note, these cells reside in muscle bundles that are oriented at an angle to the longitudinal axis of the heart, consistent with the adult myocardial architecture, which results in efficient twist and contraction.[106] However, the mechanisms that regulate clonal myocardial expansion and compaction remain undefined.

The filling capacity of the heart is increased by the added intertrabecular spaces (Fig. 8–8). The trabeculating embryonic heart can now be divided into primitive right and LVs, because there are distinct morphologic differences between the trabecular architecture of the developing ventricular chambers. The developing LV is trabeculated along most of its greater curvature, whereas the developing RV has a significant portion of the greater curvature that is smooth walled.[163,164] At this stage of development, the human embryo is approximately 3 mm long and has an ovulation age of approximately 25 days.[165] The common outflow tract of the developing heart can be classified as having a proximal (conus) segment

and a distal (truncus) segment. The conus eventually septates into the outflow portions of each ventricle as the fused conal cushions become *myocardialized* to form the muscular portion of the outlet septum. The truncus contributes to the formation of the semilunar valves and to the development of the aortic and pulmonary roots. Migrating neural crest cells contribute to the aortic sac and septation of the distal truncus.

Structural Anomalies

Noncompaction of the Ventricular Myocardium Noncompaction of the ventricular myocardium is a rare familial congenital cardiomyopathy resulting from incomplete compaction of the trabecular embryonic myocardium.[166,167] The characteristic echocardiographic findings consist of multiple prominent myocardial trabeculations and deep intertrabecular recesses communicating with the left ventricular cavity. The disease uniformly affects the LV, with or without concomitant right ventricular involvement, and results in systolic and diastolic ventricular dysfunction and clinical heart failure. Recent studies have noted an increased incidence of ventricular pre-excitation.[168] Recently, a case of ventricular noncompaction was identified in a patient who also had a haplotype deletion on the long arm of chromosome 5.[169] The affected region included the locus for *Nkx-2.5*, the cardiac-specific HOX gene, suggesting an association between ventricular myocardial noncompaction and haploinsufficiency of *Nkx-2.5*.

MECHANISMS OF CARDIAC SEPTATION

In the following discussion on cardiac septation the diaphragm (septum transversum) is assumed to maintain an approximately horizontal position, as in the mature heart. The terms *anterior, posterior, superior,* and *inferior* are employed accordingly. Although the formation of the various cardiac septa occurs almost simultaneously, for clarity it is necessary to consider their development separately. Cardiac septation involves the formation of several septal (myocardial and mesenchymal/fibrous) and valvar structures. All the original tissues of the tubular heart (myocardium, endocardium, endocardial cushion tissues) as well as the *extracardiac* cell populations, which arrive in the heart at relatively late stages of development (neural crest, epicardium, ventral neural tube cells), appear to play a role during valvuloseptal morphogenesis.[170–172]

[ ] THE SINUS VENOSUS

In the 3-mm human embryo, the sinus venosus consists of a central transverse portion and of the right and left sinus horns (Fig. 8–9). The sinus venosus receives three pairs of veins: the omphalomesenteric (vitelline) veins, the umbilical (allantoic) veins, and the common cardinal veins. The proximal portions of the umbilical veins soon disappear. As a result of the increased blood flow associated with the right and left systemic veins, the right sinus horn and proximal cardinal and vitelline veins attain a vertical position, increase in size, and form the smooth-walled, intercaval part of the atrium. The transverse portion and the proximal left sinus horn become the coronary sinus. Infolding of the sinoatrial junctional tissue at the right border of the sinoatrial foramen results in the formation of the right venous valve.[171] The left valve develops as a

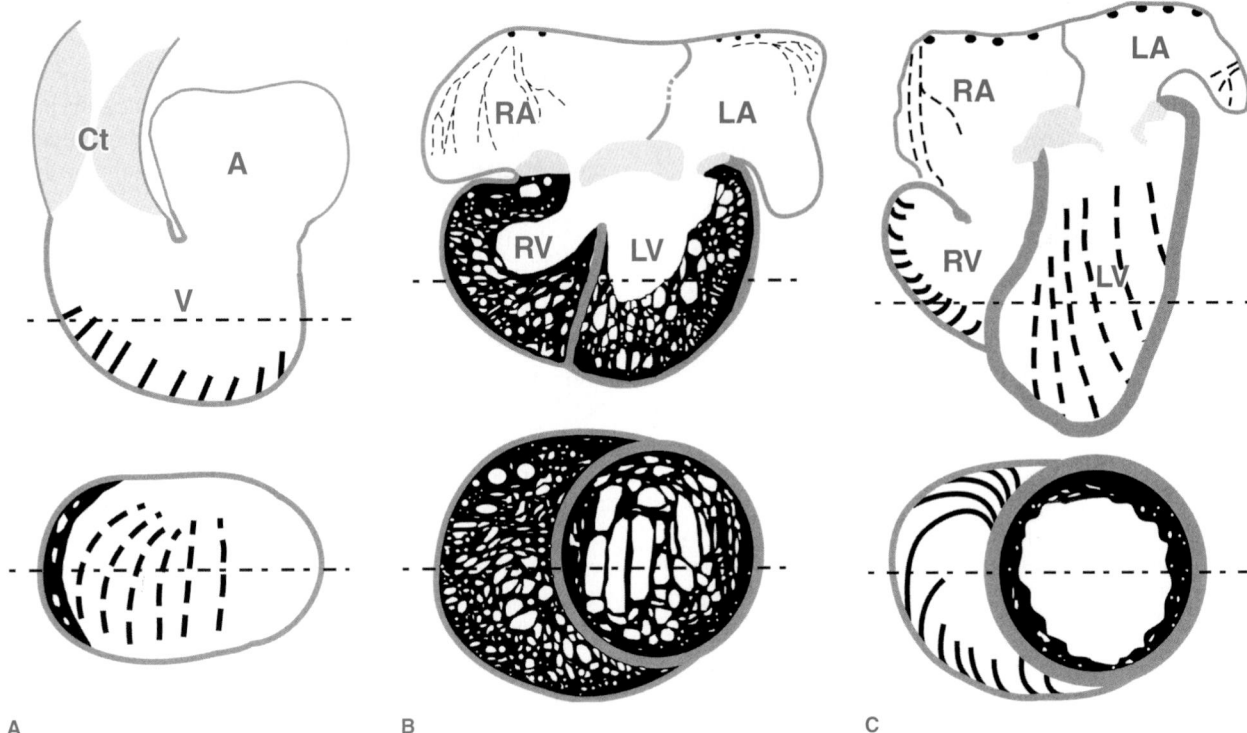

FIGURE 8–8. Schematic representation of myocardial trabecular development in the chick embryo. The top row of diagrams represents frontal (four-chamber) long-axis views; the bottom row of diagrams represents transverse (two-chamber) short-axis views. **A.** At the onset of ventricular trabeculation (approximately Hamburger-Hamilton stage 17), the trabeculation process is limited to the apex of the primitive ventricle (*V*), whereas the inner curvature of the cardiac loop, the primitive atrium (*A*), and the conotruncus (*Ct*) remain smooth. **B.** Pattern of secondary trabeculae (approximately Hamburger-Hamilton stage 29). A complex three-dimensional network of fine trabeculae fills most of the ventricular cavities. **C.** Mature tertiary trabecular pattern (Hamburger-Hamilton stage 45). In both ventricles, the trabeculae are arranged in a counterclockwise apicobasal spiral (viewed from base to apex). Differences between the right and LV relate primarily to geometric differences (cone/crescent versus cylinder/prolate ellipsoid). The trabeculae and pectinate muscles in the atria are shown in black, the rest of the myocardium in dark gray, and mesenchymal structures in light gray. LA, left atrium; LV, left ventricle; RA, right atrium; RV, right ventricle. Source: Adapted from Sedmera D, Pexieder T, Hu N, et al.[179]

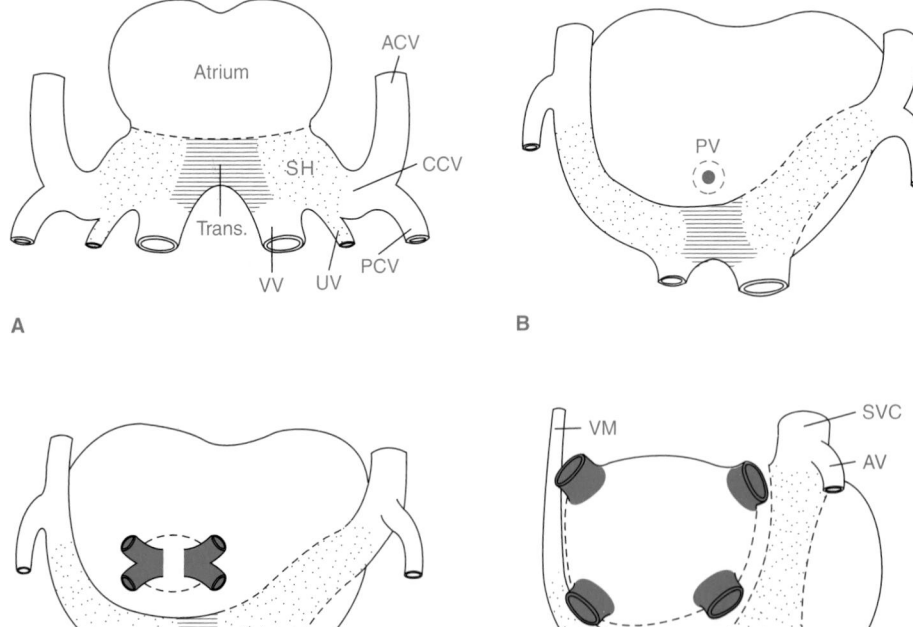

FIGURE 8–9. Posterior view of the atria and sinus venosus in embryos. **A.** 3-mm CR length; **B.** 5-mm CR length; **C.** 12-mm CR length; **D.** Newborn, diagrammatic view. A(C)CV, anterior (common) cardinal vein; AV, azygos vein; CS, coronary sinus; IVC, inferior vena cava; PCV, posterior cardinal vein; PV, pulmonary vein; SH, sinus horn; Trans., transverso portion; UV, umbilical vein; VM, vein of Marshall; VV, vitelline vein. *Source: Van Mierop LHS, Wiglesworth FW. Isomerism of the cardiac atria in the asplenia syndrome. Lab Invest 1962;11:1303. © U.S. and Canadian Academy of Pathology.*

result of active growth, similar to that of the primary atrial septum (i.e., the left valve does not develop as a fold) (Fig. 8–10). Thus, the vertical sinoatrial orifice is flanked on each side by a valve-like structure in the 4- to 6-mm human embryo. Superiorly, the venous valves join to form the septum spurium. The venous valves, particularly the right venous valve, are relatively large in the 16-mm embryo. The superior aspect of the right venous valve eventually develops into the crista terminalis, or terminal crest. The left sinus valve fuses partly with the atrial septum. Inferiorly, the left venous valve intersects with the inferior part of the right venous valve. As a result, the right venous valve becomes divided into the relatively large inferior vena caval (or eustachian) valve and a smaller coronary sinus (or thebesian) valve.

Structural Anomalies

Cor Triatriatum On the right side of the heart, complete persistence of the right venous valve of the embryonic heart produces a septum in the right atrium separating the intercaval part of the right atrium from the atrial body. The remaining opening may be quite small and restrictive. On the left side of the heart, if incorporation of the common pulmonary vein into the left atrium is incomplete, the result is a septum-like structure that might derive from the left pulmonary ridge and divides the left atrium into two components: one receiving the pulmonary veins and the other giving access to the mitral valve and left atrial appendage.

Persistent Left Superior Vena Cava Persistence of the left common cardinal vein and left sinus horn results in a left superior vena cava draining into the coronary sinus.

【 】 ATRIAL SEPTATION

Septation of the embryonic common atrium involves two distinct mechanisms.[172] The primary atrial septum (septum primum) forms by active growth of a myocardial septum. Initially the primordium of this septum can be seen as a ridge in the medial roof of the common atrium. The leading edge of the ridge is covered with a mesenchymal cap termed the *spina vestibuli,* which is contiguous superiorly with the superior AV cushion and inferiorly with the inferior AV cushion. As the primary septum descends from the roof of the atrium toward the atrioventricular canal, thereby decreasing the size of the primary interatrial foramen, the mesenchymal leading edge continues to fuse with the AV cushions, which themselves are also in the process of fusing. These events result in closure of the primary interatrial foramen (or ostium primum) and the formation of the central fibrous body (Fig. 8–11). Concomitantly, perforations appear in the superior aspect of the primary atrial septum. The perforations coalesce, resulting in the secondary atrial foramen (or ostium secundum). Next, the secondary atrial septum develops as an infolding of the atrial roof located between the primary septum and the left venous valve. The foramen ovale is the opening bordered by the free edge of the septum secundum. After fusion of the septum primum with the septum secundum, the foramen ovale becomes the fossa ovalis. Multiple genetic factors, including *Tbx-5, Nkx-2.5, Evc,* and *Prk-AR1,* have been identified in patients with abnormal atrial morphogenesis and septation.

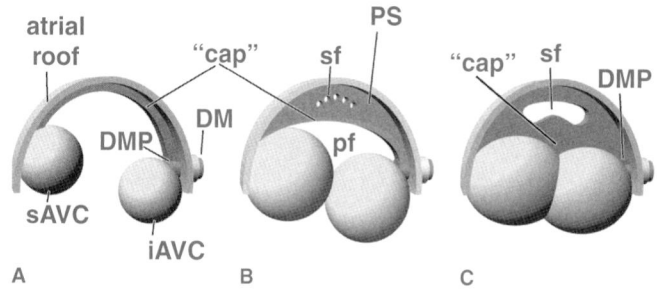

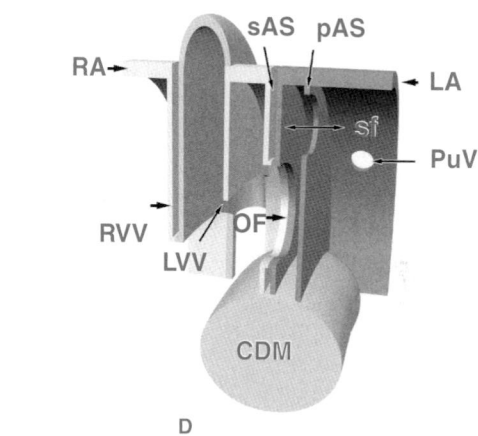

FIGURE 8–10. A model for the development of the atrial septal complex in the human heart. **A.** A heart at approximately 4-1/2 weeks of development. The atrioventricular cushions can be distinguished but have not yet fused. The leading edge of the primary septum is covered by a mesenchymal cap, which is in continuity with the dorsal mesenchymal protrusion of the dorsal mesocardium. **B.** A heart at approximately 6 weeks of development. The leading edge of the primary atrial septum, covered with a mesenchymal cap, is now approaching the atrioventricular cushions, which themselves are in the process of fusing. Within the myocardial portion of the primary septum, multiple fenestrations represent the developing secondary foramen. **C.** Completion of fusion of the mesenchymal tissues at 6 to 7 weeks of development results in the closure of the primary interatrial foramen. At this time a prominent secondary foramen can be found within the superior portion of the primary septum. **D.** Schematic diagram showing the formation of the atrial septum and venous valves. Formation of the secondary atrial septum results from infolding of the atrial roof. This occurs at the margin between myocardium with left and right atrial expression domain. The myocardium of the primary atrial septum is part of the left atrial expression domain; the orifice of the pulmonary vein is also surrounded by myocardium with a left atrial molecular phenotype. This panel also illustrates that, based on the gene expression patterns, the left venous valve develops as a myocardial structure with a right atrial molecular phenotype, whereas the right venous valve (like the secondary atrial septum) develops by infolding, in this case of the junctional tissue between the right atrium and the sinus venosus. iAVC, inferior atrioventricular cushion; sAVC, superior atrioventricular cushion; DM, dorsal mesocardium; DMP, dorsal mesenchymal protrusion; pf, primary foramen; PS, primary atrial septum; sf, secondary foramen; LA, left atrium; RA, right atrium; OF, oval fossa; pAS, primary atrial septum; sAS, secondary atrial septum; PuV, pulmonary vein; LVV, left venous valve; RVV, right venous valve. Source: Adapted from Wessels A, Anderson RH, Markwald RR, et al.[171]

Structural Anomalies

Atrial Septal Defect at the Fossa Ovalis This defect, often referred to as a secundum-type atrial septal defect, is caused by malformation of the primary atrial septum, resulting in an oversized ostium secundum. Frequently, the atrial defect is further enlarged

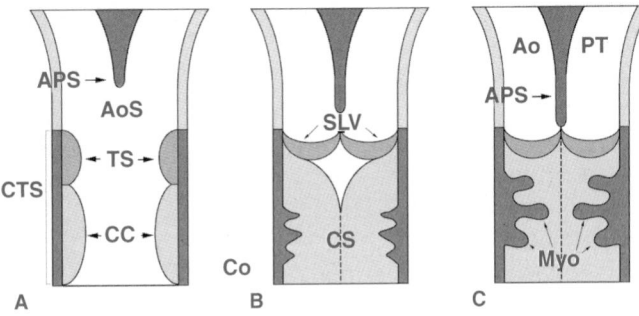

FIGURE 8–11. Schematic diagram of some of the developmental events involved in the septation of the outflow tract. **A.** The stage at which the endocardial cushion tissues in the outflow tract (conal cushions and truncal swellings) and the aortopulmonary septum have not yet fused. **B.** The truncal swellings contribute to the formation of the semilunar valves of Ao and PT, whereas the fusing conal cushions form the mesenchymal outlet septum. At this stage the conal myocardium starts to myocardialize the outlet septum. **C.** One of the final stages. The aortopulmonary septum has now completely separated the Ao and PT above the level of the semilunar valves while below the valves the outlet septum divides the outlet segment of the heart in a subaortic and subpulmonary outlet. Ao, aorta; AoS, aortic sac; APS, aorticopulmonary septum; CC, conal cushions; CS, conal septum; CTS, conotruncal segment; Myo, myocardialization; PT, pulmonary trunk; SLV, semilunar valve; TS, truncal swelling.

by a hypoplastic septum secundum. Total absence of both septum primum and septum secundum (common atrium) is rare and almost always associated with a form of persistent AV canal.

Sinus Venosus Defect Deficiency of the wall of the common pulmonary vein results in communication between the pulmonary veins, left atrium, and right atrium. This defect can be located superior and posterior (superior sinus venosus defect) and is commonly associated with preferential drainage of the right upper lobe pulmonary vein into the right atrium. Less frequently, the defect is inferior and posterior (inferior sinus venosus defect) and is associated with drainage of the right lower lobe pulmonary vein to the right atrium.

Anomalous Pulmonary Venous Connection The total form of anomalous pulmonary venous connection presumably is due either to lack of development or to a premature involution of the common pulmonary vein.[173] A number of aberrant types of pulmonary venous to systemic venous connections occur, depending on which of the early embryonic channels connecting the pulmonary venous bed to the systemic venous circulation persists. In addition to the abnormal anatomic connection between the pulmonary veins and the heart, there is usually an intrinsic dysregulation of pulmonary venous growth and remodeling, which results in inadequate pulmonary venous growth despite *successful* surgical management. The mortality associated with anomalous pulmonary venous connections remains high because of recurrent pulmonary vein stenosis and secondary pulmonary hypertension.

【 】 THE ATRIOVENTRICULAR CANAL

Division of the AV canal into left- and right-sided orifices occurs as a result of fusion of the superior and inferior AV cushions, which are first evident in the 6-mm crown rump-length human embryo. At this stage, the common AV canal is located exclusively over the LV. The superior aspect of the developing interventricular septum is continu-

ous with the right aspect of the AV junctional myocardium. The communication between the developing right atrium and RV is established by the rightward expansion of the AV canal. This expansion, combined with tissue remodeling, brings the right margin of the original AV junction, still in continuity with the posterior part of the interventricular septum toward the posteromedial aspect of the AV junction, where it will form the AV node.[155,174]

Myocardialization

The term *myocardialization* refers to the process of active ingrowth of existing myocardium into mesenchymalized tissues of the heart. In the human heart, it primarily takes place in the conal septum, where it transforms the mesenchymal outlet septum, formed as a result of fusion of the conal ridges of the outflow tract, into the muscular outlet septum (Fig. 8–12).[175] It is believed that myocardialization is the driving force for the incorporation of the aortic portion of the outflow tract into the LV and for the rightward expansion of the AV junction. Absence or inhibition of myocardialization is associated with structural congenital heart disease in a number of experimental animal models.[176] Most of these malformations involve malalignment of the outlet septum with the muscular interventricular septum, resulting in ventricular septal defects with varying of great vessel size disparity.[130]

Within the AV canal the growing endocardial cushions project into the lumen. Smaller cushions appear on the lateral borders of the AV canal. In the 10-mm CR-length embryo, the major cushions reach each other and fuse, resulting in a complete division of the canal into right and left AV orifices. At the same time, the cushions also bend, and after fusion they form an arch that is concavely directed anteriorly and toward the LV[176] and its convexity directed anteriorly and toward the atria. The mesenchymal cap on the free margin of the atrial septum primum fuses with the convex atrial side of the fused endocardial cushions. The left limb of the fused AV cushion eventually becomes incorporated into the anterior cusp (aortic leaflet) of the mitral valve. The right half of the fused endocardial cushions comes to lay within the ventricles in a sagittal orientation somewhat to the right of the muscular inter-

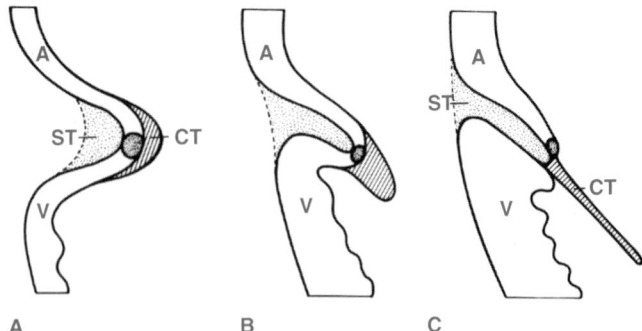

FIGURE 8–12. Schematic diagrams of formation of atrioventricular junction in the human heart. **A.** The atrioventricular junction at 4 to 5 weeks of development. Myocardial continuity between atrium and ventricle occurs through the myocardium of the atrioventricular canal. The atrioventricular junction is sandwiched between the tissues of the atrioventricular sulcus at the epicardial side and the atrioventricular cushion at the endocardial side. **B.** With progressive remodeling of the atrioventricular junction, the sulcus tissues expand toward the midline of the atrioventricular canal as the cushion tissue remodels. **C.** On completion of this process, continuity is lost between atrial and ventricular myocardium. A, atrium; CT, cushion tissue; ST, sulcus tissue; V, ventricle.

ventricular septum. Thus, the communication remaining between right and LVs, the secondary interventricular foramen, is bordered by the muscular ventricular septum inferiorly and anteriorly, the right extremity of the fused endocardial cushions posteriorly, and the conal septum superiorly.

Structural Anomalies

Partial and Complete AV Canal Defect
The several forms of persistent AV canal are caused by various degrees of failure of fusion of the superior and inferior AV canal cushions. The muscular septum primum and venous valves develop normally, and the size and histology of the nonfused endocardial cushions are normal.[177] However, the mass of extracardiac mesenchyme (vestibular spine) located in the dorsal mesocardium is reduced and, as a result, does not protrude ventrally toward the right wall of the common pulmonary vein. Total lack of fusion results in a single AV ostium (i.e., the complete form of the anomaly). Because the arch or bay, normally formed after the fusion of the endocardial cushions, fails to develop, the lower mesenchymal border of the atrial septum cannot fuse with the endocardial cushions. The result is a low-lying, large interatrial communication, with the AV part of the cardiac septum absent. The upper part of the ventricular septum remains deficient to a greater or lesser degree, and there is an interventricular communication. In the partial forms, the major endocardial cushions fuse only centrally. The result is an interatrial communication or so-called *ostium primum–type atrial septal defect*. The upper part of the muscular ventricular septum remains deficient, but this area of the ventricular septum is closed by fibrous tissue. Because the left side of the endocardial cushions does not fuse, the anterior or aortic cusp of the mitral valve is cleft. AV septal defects are frequently associated with trisomy 21 in humans and trisomy 16 in mice.[178] Genetic markers in patients without trisomy 21 are also under investigation.

Ventricular Septal Defect
Some forms of perimembranous ventricular septal defect may be caused by failure of fusion of the right extremity of the fused endocardial cushions, upper border of the muscular ventricular septum, and conal septum. Because the endocardial cushions fuse normally, there is no cleft in the anterior mitral valve cusp, nor is there an interatrial communication.

Single Ventricle, Left Ventricular Type with Rudimentary Outflow Chamber, or Double-Inlet Left Ventricle
If the AV canal becomes divided into two separate ostia (by the fusing AV cushions) but fails to expand to the right, thus retaining its far leftward position, both ostia connect only to the primitive LV. As a result, a communication between right atrium and RV does not develop. The communication between the large ventricular chamber (i.e., LV) and the rudimentary outflow chamber (i.e., RV) represents the persistence of the primary interventricular foramen.

【 】 THE VENTRICLES

As mentioned previously, the AV canal communicates exclusively with the primitive (or embryonic) LV in the 5-mm CR-length human embryo and blood from the LV reaches the primitive (or embryonic) RV only by way of the primary interventricular foramen. In the developing human heart, the myocardium surrounding the interventricular foramen is characterized by expression of the GFIN2/HNK antigen and is called the *primary interventricular ring*.[158]

The ventricles enlarge by centrifugal growth or *ballooning* of the myocardium along the greater curvature of the heart. The trabecular myocardium progresses from primary to secondary to tertiary trabeculations, whereas the compact outer myocardial layer remains relatively thin.[179,180] Coalescence of the secondary trabeculations into larger tertiary trabeculations occurs following septation, coincident with formation of the AV valve leaflets. The trabeculae positioned at the border between the developing LV and RV coalesce to form the major portion of the muscular ventricular septum. On the right side, a large trabecula, the trabecula septomarginalis, appears early (in embryos of approximately 9 mm in CR length) and runs from the anteroinferior border of the primary interventricular foramen toward the apex.

Structural Anomalies

Muscular Ventricular Septal Defect
Failure of compaction and fusion of the trabecular portion of the ventricular septum results in the most common congenital cardiovascular anomaly, the isolated muscular ventricular septal defect.

【 】 THE TRUNCUS ARTERIOSUS

The embryonic *outflow tract* consists of the conus, truncus, and aortic sac and functions as the conduit between the primitive RV and the aortic arches. Septation of the conotruncal area of the outflow tract begins in embryos of approximately 6 mm in CR length with the appearance of two opposing truncal cushions. One is located along the dextrosuperior truncal endocardium (dextrosuperior truncal cushion) and the other on the sinistroinferior wall (sinistroinferior truncal cushion). Coincident with the expansion of the conotruncus, the cushions rapidly enlarge and fuse to form the truncal septum, thus dividing the truncus into aortic and pulmonary channels. Proximally, the truncal cushions merge with the superior aspects of the conal cushions, which are the comparable mesenchymal masses within the conus. Distally, the undivided portion of the truncus and the aortic sac enlarge to form the truncoaortic sac. Simultaneously, the origin and course of the sixth arches shift leftward, aligning with right ventricular outflow and the origin and course of the fourth aortic arches shift rightward, aligning with left ventricular outflow. At the same time, a population of cells located between the fourth and sixth aortic arches and derived from the cardiac neural crest contributes to the formation of a vertical septum, the aortopulmonary septum, in the aortic sac.[181] The aortopulmonary septum fuses with the truncal septum to complete septation of the posterior aorta and the anterior PT. The role of altered cell number, migration, and differentiation of cells from the anterior heart-forming region on conotruncal septation remains an area of intense investigation.

Structural Anomalies

Persistent Truncus Arteriosus
If the truncal cushions remain hypoplastic and fail to fuse, partitioning of the truncus arteriosus does not take place. If, in addition to the hypoplastic truncal cushions, both intercalated valve cushions persist, the result is a quadricuspid truncal valve. Usually, fusion occurs between adjacent valve anlagen, resulting in an apparently tricuspid truncal valve with one larger cusp containing a fused raphe. In most cases, a truncated aortopulmonary septum develops, and a short common PT arises from the persistent trunk. The ductus arteriosus is almost always absent except when as-

sociated with interruption of the aortic arch. In experimental models, persistent truncus arteriosus can be produced following selected ablation of neural crest tissue, as mentioned previously.[94]

Aortopulmonary Septal Defect This anomaly may be caused by malalignment and/or failure of fusion between the distal truncal septum and the aortopulmonary septum. Both arterial valves are present, but there is a communication of varying size (aortopulmonary window) between the ascending aorta and the PT.

【 】 THE CONUS

The conal cushions make their appearance slightly before the truncal cushions. On the right side, the dorsal conal cushion becomes continuous with the superior truncal cushion; on the left side, the ventral conal cushion becomes continuous with the inferior truncal cushion. Fusion of the conal cushion begins proximally and then progresses rapidly, completing the partition of the conal septum by the 14- to 15-mm CR-length stage in the human embryo. Conal septation reduces and then closes the small secondary interventricular foramen, which was bordered by the conal septum, the top of the muscular ventricular septum, and the right extremities of the fused endocardial cushions. The mesenchymal conal septum and infundibulum eventually become *myocardialized,* resulting in the muscular outlet septum.[175]

Structural Anomalies

Ventricular Septal Defect, Eisenmenger Type A large basilar septal defect, dextroposition of the aortic valve, and a hypoplastic or absent infundibular septum is likely caused by hypoplasia or absence of the conal cushions. If mitral-aortic separation occurs, this ventricular septal defect can be included under the heading of double-outlet LV.

Ventricular Septal Defect, Supracristal Type The supracristal type of ventricular septal defect is likely caused by either simple failure of conal septal fusion or to septal malalignment, which prevents fusion.

Tetralogy of Fallot The primary anomaly in tetralogy of Fallot is likely an anterior displacement to a varying degree of the conal septum, which leads to unequal partitioning of the conus and reduction of the right ventricular infundibulum. A large basilar ventricular septal defect and dextroposition of the aortic valve result from failure of the displaced conal septum to participate in closure of the interventricular foramen. Pulmonary vascular hypoplasia is likely a secondary result of diminished forward blood flow. As mentioned earlier, tetralogy of Fallot is frequently associated with 22q11 deletion, particularly in the setting of severe pulmonary atresia or in the presence of extracardiac anomalies.

DEVELOPMENT OF THE HEART VALVES
【 】 THE ATRIOVENTRICULAR VALVES

Initially, the tubular embryonic heart functions as a peristaltoid pump, relying on endocardial cushions to function as valves and regional variations in conduction velocity to facilitate forward flow. Initially the embryonic heart contains only two AV cushions (AVCs), the inferior (iAVC) and the superior (sAVC) cushions; and fusion of these two cushions result in the formation of two AV orifices. At later stages the so-called *lateral AV cushions* appear. Over time, the cushion-derived tis-

sues develop into the thin mature AV valve cusps.[182] The sAVC contributes to the aortic leaflet of the mitral valve, and the iAVC contributes to the septal and posteroinferior leaflet of the tricuspid valve. The right lateral AVC contributes to the formation of the anterosuperior (mural) leaflet of the tricuspid valves, and the left lateral AVC is involved in the formation of the parietal (mural) leaflet of the mitral valve. Although the cushion-derived tissues form the main component of the leaflets (see Fig. 8–11), it is important to note that an essential step in the morphogenesis of the valves is the delamination of the developing leaflets from the underlying ventricular myocardium.[183–186]

Structural Anomalies

Tricuspid Valve Atresia, Mitral Valve Atresia Tricuspid and mitral valve atresias are anomalies that may be caused by incomplete expansion of the common AV canal toward the right during remodeling of the inner curvature of the heart or caused by abnormal formation and/or premature fusion of endocardial cushion tissue that borders the AV canal.

Ebstein Anomaly of the Tricuspid Valve Ebstein anomaly of the tricuspid valve is likely caused by an abnormality in the process of myocardial delamination required for AV valve and chordal formation.

【 】 THE ARTERIAL VALVES

The primordia of the semilunar valves become visible as small tubercles on the distal extensions of each truncal cushion after truncal partitioning in the 9-mm embryo. One of each pair is assigned to pulmonary and aortic channels, respectively. On the walls of both aortic and pulmonary channels, opposite the fused truncus cushions, a third small cushion appears.[187–189] These two intercalated valve cushions form the third member of each arterial valve primordium. Both the aortic and pulmonary roots, consisting of the sinuses of Valsalva and the semilunar valves, are likely derived from the truncus arteriosus and the truncal and intercalated valve cushions.

Structural Anomalies

Bicuspid Arterial Valves A bicuspid aortic or pulmonary valve is caused by a failure of development of an intercalated valve cushion, resulting in a valve with two equal-sized cusps, neither containing a raphe, or fusion of adjacent valve anlagen, in which case the cusps are generally unequal in size with the larger containing a raphe of varying length.

Arterial Valve Stenosis or Atresia Fusion of two or all three of the arterial valve anlagen likely results in stenosis or atresia of the valve. Pulmonary valve stenosis is associated with several autosomal dominant genetic syndromes including Noonan syndrome, caused by an altered nonreceptor-type tyrosine phosphatase, PTPN11, mapped to 12q24.1,[190] and Costello syndrome.

AORTIC ARCH DEVELOPMENT

Aortic arch development involves the sequential development and then involution of six arch pairs, which arise from paired dorsal aortae that fuse distally (Fig. 8–13A, B). Of note, in mammals, the fifth aortic arch is rudimentary. By the 10-mm embryonic stage, the first two aortic arches have regressed; and the third, fourth, and sixth are present;

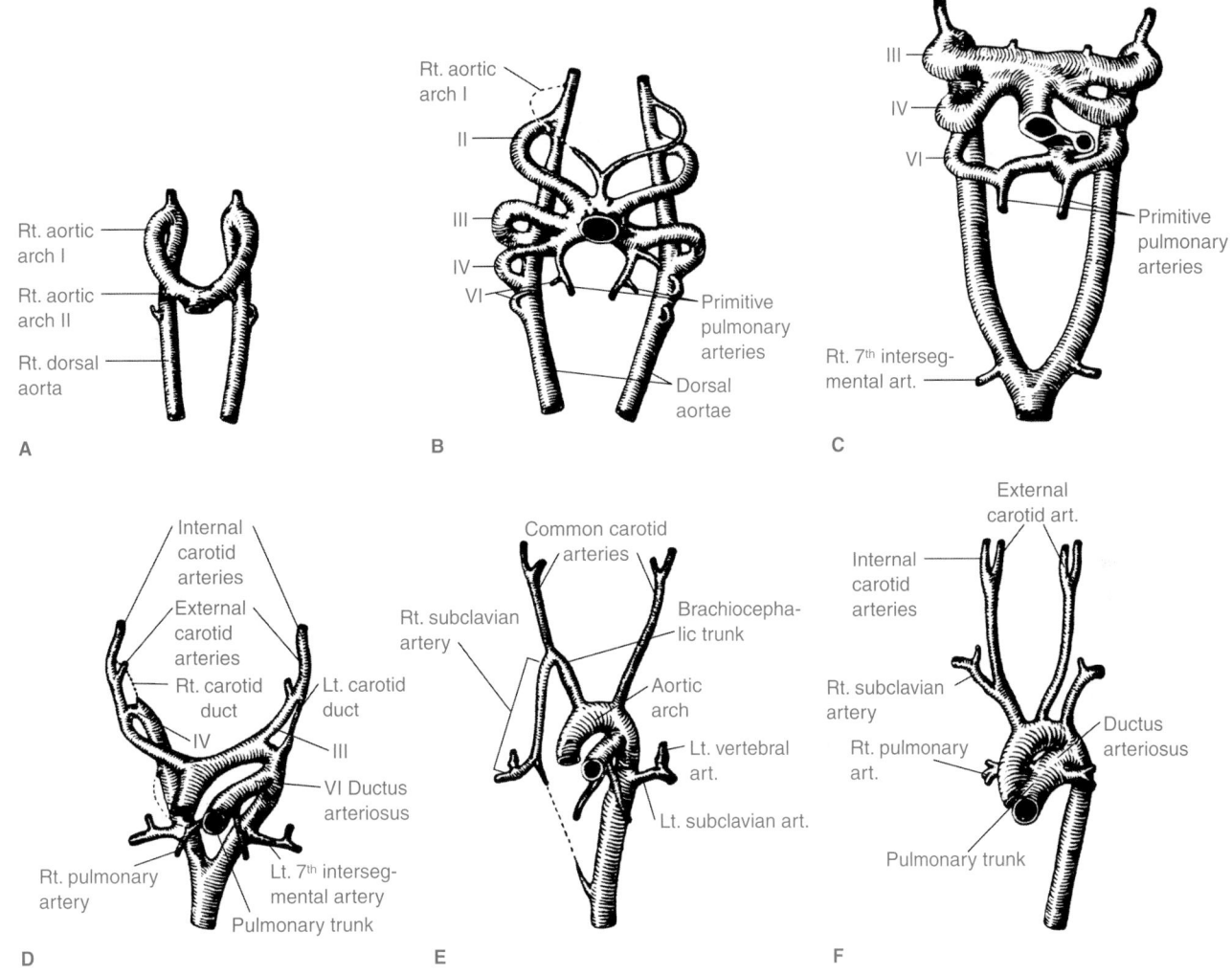

FIGURE 8–13. Development of the aortic arch system. Sizes of embryos: **A.** 3 mm, **B.** 4 mm, **C.** 10 mm, **D.** 14 mm, **E.** 17 mm, and **F.** neonate. LT, left; RT, right. Source: Adapted from Congdon ED. Transformation of the aortic arch system during development of the embryo. Carnegie Contrib Embryol 1922;14:47.

and the truncoaortic sac has been divided by the formation of the aortopulmonary septum, so that the sixth arches are now continuous with the PT (Fig. 8–13C). In the 14-mm embryo, the dorsal aortas, between the third and fourth arches, have disappeared and the third arches begin to elongate (Fig. 8–13D). The right sixth arch has disappeared, but the left sixth arch persists as the ductus arteriosus. Finally, by the 17-mm embryo stage, the right dorsal aorta has become atrophic between its junction with the left dorsal aorta; the origin of the right seventh intersegmental artery has now become attenuated and later disappears (Fig. 8–13E). The remaining components of the right dorsal aorta and right fourth aortic arch form the proximal subclavian artery. After birth, the distal part of the left sixth aortic arch, the ductus arteriosus, normally also involutes to form the ligamentum arteriosum. Thus, most aortic arch anomalies are secondary to abnormal retention or disappearance of various embryonic vascular segments.

【 】 STRUCTURAL ANOMALIES

Patent Ductus Arteriosus

Persistence of the ductus arteriosus postnatally often occurs in premature infants caused by delayed ductal involution. Ductal closure involves the prostaglandin cascade[191] as well as mitochondrial

oxygen sensing and altered voltage-gated K+ channels.[192] However, persistence of a large ductus arteriosus also occurs in isolation and in association with a variety of congenital cardiovascular malformations. Patent ductus also occurs as a component of Char syndrome, an autosomal dominant syndrome that also includes facial dysmorphism and hand abnormalities. Mutations in the neuroectoderm transcription factor TFAP2B gene on chromosome 6p12-p21 have been identified in Char syndrome.[193] TFAP2B protein is expressed in the neural fold; lateral head mesenchyme; and developing third, fourth, and sixth aortic arches. However, the direct pathogenesis of ductal patency has not yet been defined.[193]

Coarctation of the Aorta

Coarctation of the aorta is defined as a luminal narrowing of the aortic arch, usually posterior and adjacent to the insertion of the ductus arteriosus.[194] Coarctation of the aorta is often associated with abnormal aortic valve morphologies, abnormal dimensions of the transverse aortic arch (isthmus), and abnormal antegrade left ventricular output in utero. The functional consequence of reduced antegrade left ventricular output in utero is a bifurcation of flow from the fetal ductus arteriosus, resulting in retrograde flow from the ductus toward the ascending aorta and abnormal shear stress to the juxtaductal aortic wall.[194]

Double Aortic Arch

Double aortic arch is the result of persistence and continued patency of the segment of the right dorsal aorta between the origin of the right seventh intersegmental artery and its junction with the left dorsal aorta.

Right Aortic Arch

In the right aortic arch anomaly, the right rather than the left dorsal aorta is maintained in its entirety. The branching pattern of the aortic arch, therefore, will be the mirror image of normal with the brachiocephalic (innominate) artery arising as the first vessel on the left rather than the right side.

Anomalous Subclavian Artery

The origin of the right subclavian artery is the right fourth aortic arch. When this neural crest patterned segment is absent, the right subclavian artery can arise from the aortic arch distal to the left subclavian artery if the right dorsal aorta between the origin of the right seventh intersegmental artery and the junction with the left dorsal aorta is maintained to form the proximal portion of the right subclavian artery.[195]

Interrupted Aortic Arch

Interrupted aortic arch type B (IAA Type B) results from the disappearance of the left fourth aortic arch which has been shown in the mouse embryo to represent a unique population of neural crest cells.[195] The ascending aorta terminates as the brachiocephalic and left common carotid arteries and is isolated from the descending aorta, which is perfused by the PT by way of a patent ductus arteriosus. In the setting of interrupted aortic arch, an anomalous right subclavian artery is frequently present due to comparable unique neural crest patterning of this vessel.[195]

Absent Left Pulmonary Artery

The left pulmonary artery can be absent when it arises from a left-sided ductus arteriosus (or ligamentum arteriosum). This anomaly is the result of disappearance of the proximal left sixth arch.

CORONARY ARTERY DEVELOPMENT

[ ] ENDOTHELIAL CELL ORIGIN

Coronary vascular endothelial maturation closely parallels the development of the embryonic epicardium.[196–198] A series of cell-fate studies has revealed that the coronary endothelial cells as well as coronary smooth muscle cells derive from the proepicardial organ, a cluster of coelomic mesothelial cells attached to the ventral wall of the sinus venosus. As cells from the proepicardium spread out and cover the surface of the heart, a subpopulation of epicardially derived cells transdifferentiate and migrate into the myocardial cell layers,[197–204] where they contribute to the formation of the coronary network. Studies have shown that these future coronary epithelial cells express *Tbx-5* and retroviral studies show that overexpression of *Tbx-5* in these cells suppresses cell migration and coronary formation. Initially, multiple connections between the coronary vascular plexus and the aortic root are present; however, only two connections persist. It is interesting to note that the heart begins to pump blood before perfusion by the coronary vasculature occurs, indicating that, in these early stages, local diffusion of nutrients is sufficient for the early trabecular myocardium.

[ ] VASCULAR SMOOTH MUSCLE CELL ORIGIN

Antibodies to smooth muscle α-actin document that the maturation of coronary smooth muscle precedes the maturation of the outflow vessels.[199] Several studies have demonstrated that coronary smooth muscle is derived from the epicardially derived cells. Interestingly, the orderly development of the coronary arterial branching pattern and elastic lamina is dependent on the presence of the neural crest (NC), demonstrating that the perturbation in the development of one subpopulation of *extracardiac* cells (NC-derived cells) can lead to the abnormal development of another (epicardially derived cells).[204] Following experimental NC ablation in the chick embryo, persistent truncus arteriosus associated with a single origin of the coronary arterial tree occurs.[205] The distribution and symmetry of the coronary vascular is distinctly abnormal following injury to the NC. In addition, the elastic lamina and collagen organization of the great vessels is markedly abnormal following NC ablation, as has been noted in some congenital cardiovascular anomalies.[205]

[ ] VASCULOGENESIS AND ADAPTATION

It is important to note that the maturation of the coronary vasculature, as with the systemic vasculature, represents both angiogenesis (sprouting of existing vessels) and vasculogenesis (fusion of precursor cells).[206] Following increased ventricular pressure loading in the chick embryo, myocardial vasculogenesis increases to match increased ventricular mass. This finding is consistent with the investigation of children with pressure-overload left ventricular hypertrophy, where capillary density remains unchanged.[207] It is also important to note that the developing systemic vasculature is sensitive to changes in downstream mechanical load and can remodel arterial wall architecture and material properties to normalize wall stress during morphogenesis.[208]

Structural Anomalies

Abnormal Origin and Course of Coronary Arteries
Occasionally, the left coronary artery is found to arise from the pulmonary artery and rarely from other aortic arch vessels. The developing coronary vessels perforate the aortic annulus in association with specific immunohistochemical markers, so abnormal connections between the coronary arteries and the great vessels occur when this patterning event is altered. Numerous variations in the architecture and course of the coronary arteries occur in association with structural cardiovascular malformations. For example, an anomalous origin of the left anterior descending coronary artery from the right coronary artery occurs in association with tetralogy of Fallot. The mechanisms for these associations have not yet been defined.

Coronary Arterial Fistulas
Coronary arterial fistulas occasionally occur in isolation and in association with pulmonary valve atresia with intact ventricular septum and the etiology of these abnormal vascular connections between the cardiac chambers and coronary arterial tree is not yet known.[209]

CONDUCTION SYSTEM DEVELOPMENT

The development of the conduction system has fascinated cardiovascular embryologists from the moment it became clear that

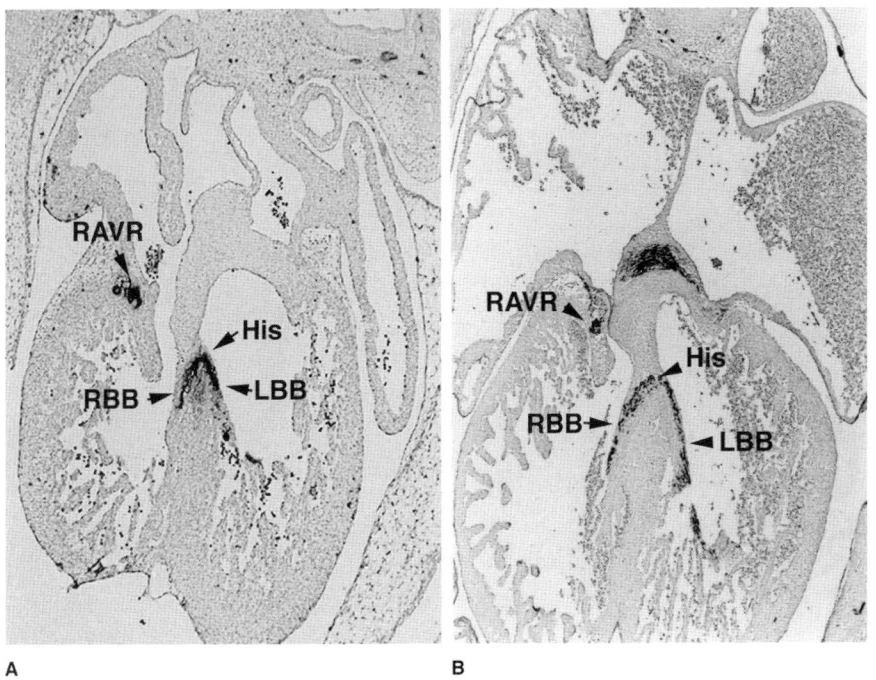

FIGURE 8–14. Expression of neuromuscular markers in the developing vertebrate heart. **A.** A transverse section of a human heart at 6 weeks of development immunohistochemically stained for the presence of a carbohydrate moiety recognized by the monoclonal antibody G1N2 (see also Wessels A, Markman MW, Vermeulen JL, et al[156]). **B.** Section of a rabbit embryo at 15 days of development that was immunohistochemically stained for the presence of neurofilaments. His, bundle of His; LBB, left bundle branch; RAVR, right atrioventricular ring bundle; RBB, right bundle branch. *Source: Adapted with permission from Wessels et al. (unpublished).*

a subpopulation of specialized myocytes is responsible for the regulation of the cardiac impulse in the heart.[210] The cardiac conduction system is composed of central and peripheral components and, during the last decade, several studies have revealed new aspects regarding the development of the conduction system. Immunohistochemical studies have shown that the developing conduction system in human and other vertebrates is characterized by the expression of a unique set of antigens and genes, some of which are also expressed in the nervous system, sometimes referred to as *neuromuscular markers* (Fig. 8–14).[210–214] Methods of retroviral cell targeting and tracing have defined subpopulations of cardiomyocytes that differentiate into Purkinje cells within the trabecular myocardium[161,162] under the regulation of endothelin secreted by adjacent coronary vascular cells.[208,209,215] These developing Purkinje cells express unique molecular markers, and their fate is dynamically influenced by the local environment.[216,217]

Altered patterns of atrial and ventricular depolarization have been recognized in association with structural heart defects, such as the pattern of depolarization noted with endocardial cushion defects, Ebstein anomaly and conduction abnormalities associated with atrial septal defects are observed in patients with mutations in the *Nkx-2.5* and *TBX5* (Holt-Oram syndrome) genes.[42]

CARDIOVASCULAR INNERVATION

Despite numerous descriptive studies regarding the location of cardiac ganglia, our understanding of the cues required for

the patterning of myocardial innervation remains incomplete. NC cell migration is critical for this process, because NC cells serve as precursors for the cardiac nerves and ganglia.[94] Cardiac ganglia and nerves are present in the human embryo at 7 weeks of gestation.[218] The density of cardiac innervation exhibits a gradient of decreasing density from the atrium to the ventricle. Functional adrenergic receptors are present on the embryonic heart prior to histologic evidence of autonomic nerves.[219] The differential appearance and distribution of peptide-containing nerves indicates that there is a maturational order to the autonomic and sensory components of the developing human heart.[220]

FUNCTIONAL MATURATION OF THE EMBRYONIC HEART

Cardiovascular morphogenesis is directly influenced by the dynamic mechanical environment of the pulsatile embryonic heart. Relevant to the morphogenesis, adaptation, and remodeling of developing normal and abnormal hearts and vessels, all critical cellular subpopulations are likely to be associated with regionally specific gene and protein expression patterns that correlate with both structure and function. Unfortunately, an overview of functional maturation, while critical, is beyond the scope of this chapter. The reader is therefore referred to several recent reviews of embryonic functional maturation in vertebrate and invertebrate species.[221,222]

MOLECULAR MECHANISMS OF CONGENITAL HEART DISEASE

The list of congenital and acquired cardiovascular diseases identified to have specific molecular mechanisms continues to expand rapidly, and at the time of publication any list of these molecular factors becomes incomplete (Table 8–1). The challenge now is to correlate specific changes in genotype with the dynamic process of CV morphogenesis and subsequent phenotype. Many molecular mechanisms involved in CV development are spatially and temporally restricted, so that a conserved set of transcription factors can have dramatically disparate effects during morphogenesis. The developing CV system also adapts to altered morphogenetic events via evolutionarily conserved mechanisms to preserve CV function, which result in structural and functional remodeling. Finally, epigenetic maternal factors likely play a critical role in influencing embryonic and fetal development. Thus, the identification of molecular mechanisms of congenital heart disease constitutes an important advance in our understanding of this complex, dynamic, and critical developmental process.

TABLE 8–1

Partial Listing of Chromosomes, Deletions, Genes and Transcription Factors Associated with Human Congenital Heart Disease

	CHROMOSOMES, LINKAGE REGIONS OR DELETIONS, GENES
Situs	
Heterotaxy, Kartagener	DNAH11 (7p21), ZIC3, LEFTYA, CRYPTIC, ACVR2B, CITED2, NKX2.5, CRELDA, DFC1, 15q24-25
Atrial septum	
Isolated atrial septal defect	GATA4 (8p22-23), CSX (5q34)
Ellis-van Creveld	EVC, EVC2 (4p16)
Holt-Oram	TBX5 (12q24.1)
Atrioventricular canal	
Atrioventricular canal defect	Trisomy 21 (DSCR1), Trisomy 18, Trisomy 13, (del8p), 3p25-pter
Smith-Lemli-Opitz	DHCR7 (11q12-13)
Pulmonary valve	
Noonan syndrome	PTPN11 (12q24.1)
Pulmonary stenosis	MTHFR
Pulmonary vasculature	
Primary pulmonary hypertension	BMPR2, ALK1 (hereditary hemorrhagic telangiectasia)
Hypoplastic left heart syndrome	
Jacobsen syndrome	11q23 (terminal deletions), OBCAM
Tetralogy of Fallot	GATA4
DiGeorge syndrome	22q11
Velo-cardio-facial syndrome	22q11
Alagille syndrome	JAGGED1 (20p12)
8p deletion syndrome	
Aortic valve	NOTCH1
Turner syndrome	45 (X,O)
Aortic vasculature	
Williams syndrome	elastin (7q11.23)
Marfan syndrome	fibrillin-1 (15q21)
Loeys-Dietz syndrome	TGFBR1 and TGFBR2
Interrupted aortic arch	FOXC1, FOXC2, FREAC10, NKX2.5, 1q21.1 deletion (Cx40)
Patent ductus arteriosus	12q24
Char syndrome	TFAB2B
Ventricular septal defect	trisomy 18
CHARGE syndrome	CHD7
Cardiomyopathy/tumors	
Hypertrophic/dilated	beta-myosin heavy-chain (14q11), dystrophin, G4.5, titin (2q31), actin, desmin, lamin A/C, Delta-sarcoglycan, troponin, tropomyosin
Arrhythmogenic	plakoglobin, 14q23, 10p12, 1q42
Mitochondrial	numerous mtDNA deletions
Metabolic	VLCAD (17p11.2), LCAD
Histiocytoid	(Xp22)
Barth syndrome	G4.5 (Xq28)
Tuberous sclerosis	TSC1 (9q34), TSC2 (16p13)
Ventricular noncompaction	CSX (del5q35.1-3)
Carney complex (atrial myxoma)	(2p16)
Conduction system	
Wolf-Parkinson-White syndrome	PRKAG2
Kearns-Sayre syndrome	mtDNA (deletions)
Friedreich's Ataxia	frataxin (9q13)
LQTS	HERG, SCN5A, numerous others

LQTS, long QT syndrome.

REFERENCES

1. Von Haller A. *Sur la formation du coeur dans le poulet.* Lausanne, Switzerland, 1758.

2. Neill CA, Clark EB. Tetralogy of Fallot: The first 300 years. *Tex Heart Inst J* 1994;21:272–279.

3. Anderson RH. Simplifying the understanding of congenital malformations of the heart. *Int J Cardiol* 1991;32:131–142.

4. Van Mierop LHS. Morphological development of the heart. In: Berne RM, ed. *Handbook of Physiology.* Sec 2. Vol 1. Bethesda, MD: American Physiological Society, 1979:1–28.

5. Clark EB, Van Mierop LHS. Cardiac development. In: Adams FH, Emmanoulides GC, Riemenschneider TA, eds. *Heart Disease in Infants, Children, and Adolescents.* 4th ed. Baltimore: Williams & Wilkins, 1989:1–22.

6. Wenick ACG. Embryology of the heart. In: Anderson RH, Macartney FJ, Shinebourne EA, Tynan M, eds. *Pediatric Cardiology.* Vol 1. New York: Churchill Livingstone, 1987:83–107.

7. Ferrens VJ, Rosenquist GC, Weinstein C. *Cardiac Morphogenesis.* New York: Elsevier 1985:282.

8. Nora JJ, Takao A. *Congenital Heart Disease: Causes and Processes.* Mount Kisco, NY: Futura, 1984:654.

9. Clark EB, Takao A. *Developmental Cardiology: Morphogenesis and Function.* Mount Kisco, NY: Futura 1990:732.

10. Bockman DE, Kirby ML. *Embryonic Origins of Defective Heart Development.* New York: Academy of Sciences, 1990:464.

11. Clark EB, Markwald RR, Takao A. *Developmental Mechanisms of Heart Disease.* Mount Kisco, NY: Futura, 1995:679.

12. Ramsdell AF. Left-right asymmetry and congenital cardiac defects: getting to the heart of the matter in vertebrate left-right axis determination. *Dev Biol* December 2005;288(1):1–20.

13. Dubrelle J, Pourquie O. Coupling segmentation to axis formation. *Development* December 2004;131(23):5783–5793.

14. Aulehla A, Herrmann BG. Segmentation in vertebrates: clock and gradient finally joined. *Genes Dev* September 2004;18(17):2060–2067.

15. Lo PC, Skeath JB, Gajewski K, et al. Homeotic genes autonomously specify the anteroposterior subdivision of the Drosophila dorsal vessel into aorta and heart. *Dev Biol* November 2002;251(2):307–319.

16. Habets PE, Moorman AF, Christoffels VM. Regulatory modules in the developing heart. *Cardiovasc Res* May 2003;58(2):246–263.

17. Zile MH. Vitamin A requirement for early cardiovascular morphogenesis specification in the vertebrate embryo: insights from the avian embryo. *Exp Biol Med (Maywood)* 2004;229(7):598–606.

18. Chen Y, Solursh M. Comparison of Hensen's node and retinoic acid in secondary axis induction in the early chick embryo. *Dev Dyn* 1992;195:142–151.

19. Bisgrove BW, Morelli SH, Yost HJ. Genetics of human laterality disorders: insights from vertebrate model systems. *Annu Rev Genomics Hum Genet* 2003;4:1–32.

20. Levin M. The embryonic origins of left-right asymmetry. *Crit Rev Oral Biol Med* 2004;15(4):197–206.

21. Brueckner M. Cilia propel the embryo in the right direction. *Am J Med Genet* 2001;101(4):339–344.

22. Miki H, Setou M, Kaneshiro K, et al. All kinesin superfamily protein, *KIF,* genes in mouse and human. *Proc Natl Acad Sci U S A* 2001;98:7004–7011.

23. Supp DM, Brueckner M, Kuehn MR, et al. Targeted deletion of the ATP binding domain of left-right dynein confirms its role in specifying development of left-right asymmetries. *Development* 1999;126:5495–5504.

24. McGrath J, Somio S, Makova S, et al. Two populations of node monocilia initiate left-right asymmetry in the mouse. *Cell* 2003;114:61–73.

25. Essner JJ, Vogan KJ, Wagner MK, et al. Conserved function for embryonic nodal cilia. *Nature* 2002;418:37–38.

26. Yasuhiko Y, Imai F, Ookubo K, et al. Calmodulin binds to inv protein: implication for the regulation of *inv* function. *Dev Growth Differ* 2001;43:671–681.

27. Kramer KL, Yost HJ. Ectodermal Syndecan-2, regulates left-right axis formation in migrating mesoderm as a cell nonautonomous Vg1, co-receptor. *Dev Cell* 2002;2:115–124.

28. Hirokawa N, Tanaka Y, Okada Y, Takeda S. Nodal flow and the generation of left-right asymmetry [review]. *Cell* 2006;125(1):33–45.

29. Franco D, Campione M. The role of Pitx2, during cardiac development. Linking left-right signaling and congenital heart diseases. *Trends Cardiovasc Med* 2003;13(4):157–163.

30. Kelly RG, Brown NA, Buckingham NE. The arterial pole of the mouse heart forms from Fgf10-expressing cells in pharyngeal mesoderm. *Dev Cell* 2001;1:435–440.

31. Schlange T, Schnipkoweit I, Andree B, et al. Chick CFC controls Lefty1, expression in the embryonic midline and nodal expression in the lateral plate. *Dev Biol* 2001;234(2):376–389.

32. Fischer A, Viebahn C, Blum M. FGF8, acts as a right determinant during establishment of the left-right axis in the rabbit. *Curr Biol* 2002;12(21):1807–1816.

33. Davis RL, Weintraub H, Lassar AB. Expression of a single transfected cDNA converts fibroblasts to myoblasts. *Cell* 1987;51:987–1000.

34. Tanaka M, Chen Z, Bartunkova S, Yamasaki N, Izumo S. The cardiac homeobox gene Csx/Nkx2.5, lies genetically upstream of multiple genes essential for heart development. *Development* March 1999;126(6):1269–1280.

35. Akazawa H, Komuro I. Cardiac transcription factor Csx/Nkx2.5: its role in cardiac development and diseases. *Pharmacol Ther* August 2005;107(2):252–268.

36. Stanfel MN, Moses KA, Schwartz RJ, Zimmer WE. Regulation of organ development by the NKX-homeodomain factors: an NKX code. *Cell Mol Biol (Noisy-le-grand)* October 2005;51(suppl):OL785–OL799.

37. Chen CY, Schwartz RJ. Identification of novel DNA binding targets and regulatory domains of a murine tinman homeodomain factor, Nkx-2.5. *J Biol Chem* 1995;270:15628–15633.

38. Lee HH, Frasch M. Nuclear integration of positive Dpp signals, antagonistic Wg inputs and mesodermal competence factors during Drosophila visceral mesoderm induction. *Development* March 2005;132(6):1429–1442.

39. Nemer G, Nemer M. Regulation of heart development and function through combinatorial interactions of transcription factors. *Ann Med* December 2001;33(9):604–610.

40. Prall OW, Elliott DA, Harvey RP. Developmental paradigms in heart disease: insights from tinman. *Ann Med* 2002;34(3):148–156.

41. Evans SM. Vertebrate tinman homologues and cardiac differentiation *Semin Cell Dev Biol* February 1999;10(1):73–83.

42. Jay PY, Harris BS, Buerger A, et al. Function follows form: cardiac conduction system defects in Nkx2–5, mutation. *Anat Rec A Discov Mol Cell Evol Biol* October 2004;280(2):966–972.

43. Schott JJ, Benson DW, Basson CT, et al. Congenital heart disease caused by mutations in the transcription factor *NKX2–5. Science* 1998;281:108–111.

44. Kuo H, Chen J, Ruiz-Lozano P, et al. Control of segmental expression of the cardiac-restricted ankyrin repeat protein gene by distinct regulatory pathways in murine cardiogenesis. *Development* 1999;126:4223–4234.

45. Niu, Z, Yu W, Zhange SX, et al. Conditional mutagenesis of the murine SRF gene blocks cardiogenesis and the transcription of downstream gene targets. *J Biol Chem* September 2005;280(37):32531–32538.

46. Dalton S, Treisman R. Characterization of SAP-1, a protein recruited by serum response factor to the *c-fos* serum response element. *Cell* 1992;68:597–612.

47. Pollock R, Treisman R. Human SRF-related proteins: DNA-binding properties and potential regulatory targets. *Genes Dev* 1991;5:2327–2341.

48. Gossett LA, Kelvin DJ, Sternberg EA, et al. A new myocyte-specific enhancer-binding factor that recognizes a conserved element associated with multiple muscle-specific genes. *Mol Cell Biol* 1989;9:5022–5033.

49. Bour BA, O'Brien MA, Lockwood ML, et al. Drosophila MEF2, a transcription factor is essential for myogenesis. *Genes Dev* 1995;9:730–741.

50. Lilly B, Zhao B, Ranganayakulu G, et al. Requirement of MADS domain transcription factor D-MEF2, for muscle formation in *Drosophila. Science* 1995;267:688–693.

51. Gajewski K, Kim Y, Lee YM, et al. D-mef2, is a target for tinman activation during Drosophila heart development. *EMBO J* 1997;16:515–522.

52. Chen CY, Schwartz RJ. Recruitment of the *tinman* homolog Nkx-2.5, by serum response factor activates cardiac α-actin gene transcription. *Mol Cell Biol* 1996;16:6372–6384.

53. Temsah R, Nemer M. GATA factors and transcriptional regulation of cardiac natriuretic peptide genes. *Regul Pept* 2005;128(3):177–185.

54. Peterkin T, Gibson A, Loose M, et al. The roles of GATA-4, -5, and -6, in vertebrate heart development. *Semin Cell Dev Biol* 2005;16(1):83–94.

55. Ip HS, Wilson DB, Heikinheimo M, et al. The GATA-4, transcription factor transactivates the cardiac muscle specific troponin C promoter-enhancer in nonmuscle cells. *Mol Cell Biol* 1994;14:7515–7526.

56. Mokentin JD, Lin Q, Duncan S, et al. Requirement of the transcription factor GATA4, for heart tube formation and ventral morphogenesis. *Genes Dev* 1997;11:1061–1072.

57. Sorrentino RP, Gajewski KM, Schulz RA. GATA factors in Drosophila heart and blood cell development. *Semin Cell Dev Biol* 2005;16(1):107–116.

58. Sachinidis A, Fleischmann BK, Kolossov E, et al. Cardiac specific differentiation of mouse embryonic stem cells. *Cardiovasc Res* 2003;58(2):278–291.

59. Crispino JD, Lodish MB, Thurberg BL, et al. Proper coronary vascular development and heart morphogenesis depend on interaction of GATA-4, with FOG cofactors. *Genes Dev* 2001;15(7):839–844.

60. Schwartz RJ, Olson EN. Building the heart piece by piece: modularity of cis-elements regulating *Nkx2.5,* transcription. *Development* 1999;126:4187–4192.

61. Ying Y, Zhao GQ. Cooperation of endoderm-derived BMP2, and extraembryonic ectoderm-derived BMP4, in primordial germ cell generation in the mouse. *Dev Biol* 2001;232(2):484–492.

62. Czyz J, Wobus A. Embryonic stem cell differentiation: the role of extracellular factors. *Differentiation* 2001;68(4–5):167–174.

63. Fossett N, Schulz RA. Conserved cardiogenic functions of the multitype zinc-finger proteins: U-shaped and FOG-2. *Trends Cardiovasc Med* 2001;15(7):839–844.

64. Srivastava, D. Genetic assembly of the heart: implications for congenital heart disease. *Annu Rev Physiol* 2001;63:451–469.

65. Yamagishi H, Yamagishi C, Nakagawa O, Harvey RP, Olson EN, Srivastava D. The combinatorial activities of Nkx2.5, and dHAND are essential for cardiac ventricle formation. *Dev Biol* November 2001;239(2):190–203.

66. McFadden DG, Barbosa AC, Richardson JA, Schneider MD, Srivastava D, Olson EN. The Hand1, and Hand2, transcription factors regulate expansion of the embryonic cardiac ventricles in a gene dosage-dependent manner. *Development* January 2005;132(1):189–201.

67. Thattaliyath BD, Firulli BA, Firulli AB. The basic-helix-loop-helix transcription factor HAND2, directly regulates transcription of the atrial naturetic peptide gene. *J Mol Cell Cardiol* October 2002;34(10):1335–1344.

68. Christoffels VM, Keijser AG, Houweling AC, et al. Patterning the embryonic heart: identification of five mouse Iroquois homeobox genes in the developing heart. *Dev Biol* 2000;224:263–274.

69. Basson CT, Bachinsky DR, Lin RC, et al. Mutations in human TBX5, [corrected] cause limb and cardiac malformation in Holt-Oram syndrome. *Nat Genet* 1997;15:30–35.

70. Bruneau BG, Nemer G, Schmitt JP, et al. A murine model of Holt-Oram syndrome defines roles of the T-box transcription factor Tbx5, in cardiogenesis and disease. *Cell* September 2001;106(6):709–721.

71. Mori AD, Bruneau BG. TBX5, mutations and congenital heart disease: Holt-Oram syndrome revealed. *Curr Opin Cardiol* 2004;19(3):211–215.

72. Zhou YQ, Zhu Y, Bishop J, et al. Abnormal cardiac inflow patterns during postnatal development in a mouse model of Holt-Oram syndrome. *Am J Physiol Heart Circ Physiol* September 2005;289(3):H992-H1001.

73. Keller BB. Developmental structure-function insights from Tbx5(del/+) mouse model of Holt-Oram syndrome. *Am J Physiol Heart Circ Physiol* 2005;289(3):H975–H976.

74. Garrity DM, Childs S, Fishman MC. The heartstrings mutation in zebrafish causes heart/fin Tbx5, deficiency syndrome. *Development* October 2002;129(19):4635–4645.

75. Stennard FA, Harvey RP. T-box transcription factors and their roles in regulatory hierarchies in the developing heart. *Development* 2005;132(22):4897–4910.

76. Koshiba-Takeuchi K, Takeuchi JK, Arruda EP, et al. Cooperative and antagonistic interactions between Sall4, and Tbx5, pattern the mouse limb and heart. *Nat Genet* February 2006;38(2):175–183.

77. Kelly RG, Brown NA, Buckingham ME. The arterial pole of the mouse heart forms from Fgf10-expressing cells in pharyngeal mesoderm. *Dev Cell* September 2001;1(3):435–440.

78. Eisenberg LM, Markwald RR. Cellular recruitment and the development of the myocardium. *Dev Biol* 2004;274:225–232.

79. Kelly RG. Molecular inroads into the anterior heart field. *Trends Cardiovasc Med* February 2005;15(2):51–56.

80. Eisenberg LM, Moreno R, Markwald RR. Multiple stem cell populations contribute to the formation of the myocardium. *Ann N Y Acad Sci* 2005;1047:38–49.

81. Verzi MP, McCulley DJ, De Val S, Dodou E, Black BL. The right ventricle, outflow tract, and ventricular septum comprise a restricted expression domain within the secondary/anterior heart field. *Dev Biol* 2005;287(1):134–145.

82. Linask KK, Manisastry S, Han M. Cross talk between cell-cell and cell-matrix adhesion signaling pathways during heart organogenesis: implications for cardiac birth defects. *Microsc Microanal* 2005;151:213–224.

83. Bagatto B, Franci J, Liu B, et al. Cadherin2, (N-cadherin) plays an essential role in zebrafish cardiovascular development. *BMC Dev Biol* 2006;6:23.

84. Plageman TF Jr, Yutzey KE. T-box genes and heart development: putting the "T" in heart. *Dev Dyn* 2005;232(1):11–20.

85. Ryan K, Chin AJ. T-box genes and cardiac development. *Birth Defects Res C Embryo Today* 2003;69(1):25–37.

86. Vitelli F, Morishima M, Taddei I, et al. *Tbx1,* mutation causes multiple cardiovascular defects and disrupts neural crest and cranial nerve migratory pathways. *Hum Mol Genet* 2002;11(8):915–922.

87. Szeto DP, Griffin KJ, Kimelman D. *HrT* is required for cardiovascular development in zebrafish. *Development* 2002;129:5093–5101.

88. Park EJ, Ogden LA, Talbot A, et al. Required, tissue-specific roles for Fgf8, in outflow tract formation and remodeling. *Development* June 2006;133(12):2419–2433.

89. Ilagan R, Abu-Issa R, Brown D, et al. Fgf8, is required for anterior heart field development. *Development* June 2006;133(12):2435–2445.

90. Yamagishi H, Maeda J, Hu T, et al. *Tbx1,* is regulated by tissue-specific forkhead proteins through a common Sonic hedgehog-responsive enhancer. *Genes Dev* 2003;17:269–281.

91. Sugishita Y, Watanabe M, Fisher SA. Role of myocardial hypoxia in the remodeling of the embryonic avian cardiac outflow tract. *Dev Biol* March 2004;267(2):294–308.

92. Sugishita Y, Watanabe M, Fisher SA. The development of the embryonic outflow tract provides novel insights into cardiac differentiation and remodeling. *Trends Cardiovasc Med* August 2004;14(6):235–241.

93. Kirby ML. Molecular embryogenesis of the heart. *Pediatr Dev Pathol* 2002;5(6):516–543.

94. Hutson MR, Kirby ML. Neural crest and cardiovascular development: a 20-year perspective. *Birth Defects Res C Embryo Today* 2003;69(1):2–13.

95. Stoller JZ, Epstein JA. Cardiac neural crest. *Semin Cell Dev Biol* 2005;16(6):704–715.

96. Clouthier DE, Hosoda K, Richardson JA, et al. Cranial and cardiac neural crest defects in endothelin-A receptor-deficient mice. *Development* 1998;125(5):813–824.

97. Chan WY, Cheung CS, Yung KM, et al. Cardiac neural crest of the mouse embryo: axial level of origin, migratory pathway and cell autonomy of the splotch (Sp2H) mutant effect. *Development* 2004;131(14):3367–3379.

98. Chisaka O, Capecchi MR. Regionally restricted developmental defects resulting from targeted disruption of the mouse homeobox gene Hox-1.5. *Nature* 1991;350:473–474.

99. McDermid HE, Morrow BE. Genomic disorders on 22q11. *Am J Hum Genet* 2002;70(5):1077–1088.

100. Liao J, Kochilas L, Nowotschin S, et al. Full spectrum of malformations in velo-cardio-facial syndrome/DiGeorge syndrome mouse models by altering Tbx1, dosage. *Hum Mol Genet* August 2004;13(15):1577–1585.

101. Vitelli F, Zhang A, Huynk T, et al. Fgf8, expression in the Tbx1, domain causes skeletal abnormalities and modifies the aortic arch but not the outflow tract phenotype of Tbx1, mutants. *Dev Biol* 2006;295(2):559–570.

102. Feiner L, Webber AL, Brown CB, et al. Targeted disruption of semaphorin 3C leads to persistent truncus arteriosus and aortic arch interruption. *Development* 2001;128:3061–3070.

103. Brown CB, Feiner L, Lu MM, et al. Plexin A2, and semaphorin signaling during cardiac neural crest development. *Development* 2001;128:3071–3080.

104. Lammer EJ, Chen DT, Hoar R, et. al. Retinoic acid embryopathy *N Engl J Med* 1985;313:837–841.

105. Otto DM, Henderson CJ, Carrie D, et al. Identification of novel roles of the cytochrome p450, system in early embryogenesis: effects on vasculogenesis and retinoic Acid homeostasis. *Mol Cell Biol* 2003;23(17):6103–6116.

106. Tobita K, Garrison JB, Liu LJ, et al. Three-dimensional myofiber architecture of the embryonic left ventricle during normal development and altered mechanical loads. *Anat Rec A Discov Mol Cell Evol Biol* 2005;283(1):193–201.

107. Shiraishi I, Takamatsu T, Minamikawa T, et al. 3-D observation of actin filaments during cardiac myofibrinogenesis in chick embryo using a confocal laser scanning microscope. *Anat Embryol* 1992;185:401–408.

108. Price RL, Chintanawonges C, Shiraishi I, et al. Local and regional variations in myofibrillar patterns in looping rat hearts. *Anat Rec* 1996;245:83–93.

109. Taber LA, Keller BB, Clark EB. Cardiac mechanics in the stage 16, chick embryo. *J Biomech Eng* 1992;114:427–434.

110. Tobita K, Keller BB. Right and left ventricular wall deformation patterns in normal and left heart hypoplasia chick embryos. *Am J Physiol* 2000;279:H959–H969.

111. Zhao Z, Rivkees SA. Rho-associated kinases play an essential role in cardiac morphogenesis and cardiomyocyte proliferation. *Dev Dyn* 2003;226(1):24–32.

112. Ruzicka DL, Schwartz RJ. Sequential activation of alpha actin genes during avian cardiogenesis: vascular smooth muscle alpha actin gene transcripts mark the onset of cardiomyocyte differentiation. *J Cell Biol* 1988;107:2575–2586.

113. Sugi Y, Lough J. Onset of expression and regional deposition of alpha-smooth and sarcomeric actin during avian heart development. *Developmental Dynamics* 1992;193:116–124.

114. Warkman AS, Zheng L, Qadir MA, et al. Organization and developmental expression of an amphibian vascular smooth muscle alpha-actin gene. *Dev Dyn* 2005;233(4):1546–1553.

115. Matsui H, Ikeda K, Nakatani K, et al. Induction of initial cardiomyocyte alpha-actin-smooth muscle alpha-actin in cultured avian pregastrula epiblast: a role for nodal and BMP antagonist. *Dev Dyn* August 2005;2333(4):1546–1553.

116. Sordahl LA, Crow CA, Draft GH, et al. Some ultrastructural and biochemical aspects of heart mitochondria associated with development. *J Mol Cell Cardiol* 1972;4:1–10.

117. Barth E, Stammler G, Speiser B, et al. Ultrastructural quantitation of mitochondria and myofilaments in cardiac muscle from 10, different animal species including man. *J Mol Cell Cardiol* 1992;24:669–681.

118. Mahony, L. Calcium homeostasis and control of contractility in the developing heart. *Semin Perinatol* 1996;20(6):510–519.

119. Artman M, Henry G, Coetzee WA. Cellular basis for age-related differences in cardiac excitation-contraction coupling. *Prog Pediatr Cardiol* 2000;11:185–194.

120. Conway SJ, Godt RE, Hatcher CJ, et al. Neural crest is involved in development of abnormal myocardial function. *J Mol Cell Cardiol* 1997;29:2675–2685.

121. Takehima H. Intracellular Ca^{2+} store in embryonic cardiac myocytes. *Front Biosci* 2002;7:1642–1652.

122. Osaka T, Joyner RW. Developmental changes in calcium currents of rabbit ventricular cells. *Circ Res* 1991;68:788–796.

123. Wetzel GT, Chen F, Klitzner TS. Ca^{2+} channel kinetics in acute isolated fetal, neonatal and adult rabbit cardiac myocytes. *Circ Res* 1993;72:1065–1074.

124. Wetzel GT, Klitzner TS. Developmental cardiac electrophysiology recent advances in cellular physiology. *Cardiovasc Res* 1996;31(spec E):52–60.

125. Levi AJ, Spitzer KW, Kohmoto O. Depolarization-induced Ca entry via Na-Ca exchange triggers SR release in guinea pig cardiac myocytes. *Am J Physiol* 1994;266(4, pt 2):H1422–H1433.

126. Cribbs LL, Martin BL, Schroder EA, Keller BB, Delisle BP, Satin J. Identification of the t-type calcium channel (Ca(v)3.1d) in developing mouse heart. *Circ Res* March 2001;88(4):403–407.

127. Bridge JHB, Smolley JR, Spitzer KW. The relationship between charge movements associated I_{Ca} and I_{Na-Ca} in cardiac myocytes. *Science* 1990;248:376–378.

128. Forouhar AS, Liebling M, Hickerson A, et al. The embryonic vertebrate heart tube is a dynamic suction pump. *Science* May 2006;312(5774):751–753.

129. Van Mierop LHS. Embryology of the heart. In: Netter FH, ed. *The CIBA Collection of Medical Illustrations*. Vol 5. Pt 1. Summit, NJ. CIBA Pharmaceutical; 1969:112–130.

130. Markwald RR, Trusk T, Gittenberger-de Groot AC, et al. Cardiac morphogenesis: formation and septation of the primary heart tube. In: Kavlock R, Datson G, eds. *Handbook of Experimental Pharmacology*. Berlin: Springer-Verlag; 1998:11–40.

131. Kalman F, Viragh S, Modis L. Cell surface glycoconjugates and the extracellular matrix of the developing mouse embryo epicardium. *Anat Embryol (Berl)* 1995;191(5):451–464.

132. Markwald RR, Mjaatvedt CH, Krug EL. Induction of endocardial cushion tissue formation by adheron-like molecular complexes derived from the myocardial basement membrane. In: Clark EB, Takao A, eds. *Developmental Cardiology: Morphogenesis and Function*. Mt. Kisco, NY: Futura, 1990:191–204.

133. Person AD, Klewer SE, Runyan RB. Cell biology of cardiac cushion development. *Int Rev Cytol* 2005;243:287–335.

134. Nakajima Y, Yamagishi T, Hokari S, et al. Mechanisms involved in valvuloseptal endocardial cushion formation in early cardiogenesis: roles of transforming growth factor (TGF)-beta and bone morphogenetic protein (BMP). *Anat Rec* 2000;258(2):119–127.

135. Walker GA, Masters KS, Shah DN, et al. Valvular myofibroblast activation by transforming growth factor-beta: implications for pathological extracellular matrix remodeling in heart valve disease. *Circ Res* 2004;95(3):253–260.

136. Cushing MC, Liao JT, Anseth KS. Activation of valvular interstitial cells is mediated by transforming growth factor-beta1, interactions with matrix molecules. *Matrix Biol* 2005;24(6):428–437.

137. Sales VL, Engelmayr GC Jr, Mettler BA, et al. Transforming growth factor-beta1, modulates extracellular matrix production, proliferation, and apoptosis of endothelial progenitor cells in tissue-engineering scaffolds. *Circulation* 2006;114(suppl 1):I193–I199.

138. Runyan RB, Potts JD, Sharma RV, et al. Signal transduction of a tissue interaction during embryonic heart development. *Cell Regul* 1990;1:301–313.

139. Kruzynska-Frejtag A, Machnicki M, Rogers R, et al. Periostin (an osteoblast-specific factor) is expressed within the embryonic mouse heart during valve formation. *Mech Dev* 2001;103:183–188.

140. Izumi M, Fujio Y, Kunisada K, et al. Bone morphogenetic protein-2, inhibits serum deprivation-induced apoptosis of neonatal cardiac myocytes through activation of Smad1, pathway. *J Biol Chem* 2001;276:31133–31141.

141. Rivera-Feliciano J, Tabin CJ. Bmp2, instructs cardiac progenitors to form the heart-valve-inducing field. *Dev Biol* July 2006;295(2):580–588.

142. Atance J, Yost MJ, Carver W. Influence of the extracellular matrix on the regulation of cardiac fibroblast behavior by mechanical stretch. *J Cell Physiol* 2004;200(3):377–386.

143. Simpson DG, Majeski M, Borg TK, et al. Regulation of cardiac myocyte protein turnover and myofibrillar structure in vitro by specific directions of stretch. *Circ Res* 1999;85:59–69.

144. Ross RS, Borg TK. Integrins and the myocardium. *Circ Res* 2001;88:1112–1119.

145. Pexieder T. Prenatal development of the endocardium: A review. *Scan Electron Microsc* 1981;2:223–253.

146. Noden DM. Origins and patterning of avian outflow tract endocardium. *Development* 1991;111:867–876.

147. Markwald RR, Mjaatvedt CH, Krug EL, et al. Inductive interaction in heart development: role of cardiac adherons in cushion tissue formation. In: Bockman DE, Kirby ML, eds. *Embryonic Origins of Defective Heart Development*. Ann NY Acad Sc, 1990;588:13–25.

148. Icardo JM. Changes in endocardial cell morphology during development of the endocardial cushions. *Anat Embryol (Berl)* 1989;179(5):443–448.

149. Hove JR, Koster RW, Forouhar AS, et al. Intracardiac fluid forces are an essential epigenetic factor for embryonic cardiogenesis. *Nature* 2003;421:172–177.

150. Groenendijk BC, Hierck BP, Gittenberger-De Groot AC, Poelmann RE. Development-related changes in the expression of shear stress responsive genes KLF-2, ET-1, and NOS-3, in the developing cardiovascular system of chicken embryos. *Dev Dyn* May 2004;230(1):57–68.

151. Poelmann RE, Molin D, Wisse LJ, et al. Apoptosis in cardiac development. *Cell Tissue Res* 2000;301(1):43–52.

152. Zhou B, Cron RQ, Wu B, et al. Regulation of the murine *NFATc1*, gene by NFATc2. *J Biol Chem* 2002;277:10704–10711.

153. Gittenberger-de Groot AC, Bartelings MM, Deruiter MC, et al. Basics of cardiac development for the understanding of congenital heart malformations. *Pediatr Res* 2005;57(2):169–176.

154. Kim JS, Viragh S, Moorman AF, et al. Development of the myocardium of the atrioventricular canal and the vestibular spine in the human heart. *Circ Res* 2001;88(4):395–402.

155. Lamers WH, Moorman AF. Cardiac septation: a late contribution of the embryonic primary myocardium to heart morphogenesis. *Circ Res* 2002;91(2):93–103.

156. Wessels A, Markman MW, Vermeulen JL, et al. The development of the atrioventricular junction in the human heart. *Circ Res* 1996;78(1):110–117.

157. Gittenberger-de Groot A. Principles of abnormal cardiac development. In: Burggren WW, Keller BB, eds. *Development of Cardiovascular Systems: Molecules to Organisms*. New York: Cambridge University Press 1996:259–267.

158. Icardo JM, Fernandez-Teran A. Morphologic study of ventricular trabeculation in the embryonic chick heart. *Acta Anat* 1987;130:264–274.

159. Pexieder T, Christen Y, Vuillemin M, et al. Comparative morphometric analysis of cardiac organogenesis in chick, mouse, and dog embryos. In: Nora JJ, Takao A. *Congenital Heart Disease: Causes and Processes*. Mt. Kisco, NY: Futura Publishing 1984:423–438.

160. Taber LA. Biomechanics of cardiovascular development. *Annu Rev Biomed Eng* 2001;3:1–25.

161. Mikawa T, Borisov A, Brown AM, et al. Clonal analysis of cardiac morphogenesis in the chicken embryo using a replication-defective retrovirus: I. Formation of the ventricular myocardium. *Dev Dyn* 1992;193:11–23.

162. Mikawa T, Cohen-Gould L, Fischman DA. Clonal analysis of cardiac morphogenesis in the chicken embryo using a replication-defective retrovirus. III. Polyclonal origin of adjacent ventricular myocytes. *Dev Dyn* 1992;195:133–141.

163. Christoffels VM, Burch JB, Moorman AF. Architectural plan for the heart: early patterning and delineation of the chambers and the nodes. *Trends Cardiovasc Med* 2004;14(8):301–307.

164. Anderson RH, Webb S, Brown NA, et al. Development of the heart: (3) formation of the ventricular outflow tracts, arterial valves, and intrapericardial arterial trunks. *Heart* 2003;89(9):1110–1118.

165. Streeter GL. Developmental horizons in human embryos: description of age groups XI 13–20, somites, and age group XII 21–29, somites. *Contrib Embryol* 1942;30:211–246.

166. Agmon Y, Connolly HM, Olson LJ, et al. Noncompaction of the ventricular myocardium. *J Am Soc Echo* 1999;12:859–863.

167. Ichida F, Hamamichi Y, Miyawaki T, et al. Clinical features of isolated noncompaction of the ventricular myocardium: long-term clinical course, hemodynamic properties, and genetic background. *J Am Coll Cardiol* 1999;34:233–240.

168. Weiford BC, Subbarao VD, Mulhern KM. Noncompaction of the ventricular myocardium. *Circulation* June 2004;109(24):2965–2971.

169. Pauli RM, Scheib-Wixted S, Cripe L, et al. Ventricular noncompaction and distal chromosome 5q deletion. *Am J Med Genet* 1999;85:419–423.

170. Hatcher CJ, Kim MS, Basson CT. Atrial form and function: lessons from human molecular genetics. *Trends Cardiovasc Med* 2000;10:93–101.

171. Wessels A, Anderson RH, Markwald RR, et al. Atrial development in the human heart: An immunohistochemical study with emphasis on the role of mesenchymal tissues. *Anat Rec* 2000;259:288–300.

172. Wessels A, Sedmera D. Developmental anatomy of the heart: a tale of mice and man. *Physiol Genomics* 2003;15(3):165–176.

173. Anderson RH, Brown NA, Moorman AF. Development and structures of the venous pole of the heart. *Dev Dyn* 2006;235(1):2–9.

174. Nakajima Y, Yamagishi T, Hokari S, et al. Mechanisms involved in valvuloseptal endocardial cushion formation in early cardiogenesis: roles of transforming growth factor (TGF)-beta and bone morphogenetic protein (BMP). *Anat Rec* 2000;258(2):119–127.

175. Van den Hoff MJB, Bennington RW, Moorman AFM, et al. Myocardialization in the developing heart. *Dev Biol* 1999;212:477–490.

176. Van den Hoff MJ, Moorman AF. Wnt, a driver of myocardialization? *Circ Res* 2005;96(3):274–276.

177. Blom NA, Ottenkamp J, Wenink AG, et al. Deficiency of the vestibular spine in atrioventricular septal defects in human fetuses with down syndrome. *Am J Cardiol* 2003;91:180–184.

178. Maslen CL. Molecular genetics of atrioventricular septal defects. *Curr Opin Cardiol* 2004;19(3):205–210.

179. Sedmera D, Pexieder T, Hu N, et al. Developmental changes in the myocardial architecture of the chick. *Anat Rec* 1997;248:421–432.

180. Toyofuku T, Zhang H, Kumanogoh A, et al. Guidance of myocardial patterning in cardiac development by Sma6D reverse signaling. *Nat Cell Biol* 2004;6(12):1204–1211.

181. Webb S, Qayyum SR, Anderson RH, Lamers WH, Richardson MK. Septation and separation within the outflow tract of the developing heart. *J Anat* April 2003;202(4):327–342.

182. Wessels A, Markman MWM, Vermeulen JLM, et al. The development of the atrioventricular junction in the human heart; an immunohistochemical study. *Circ Res* 1996;78:110–117.

183. Oosthoek PW, Wenink ACG, Vrolijk BCM, et al. Development of the atrioventricular valve tension apparatus in the human heart. *Anat Emb* 1998;198:317–329.

184. Bergwerff M, Verberne ME, DeRuiter MC, et al. Neural crest cell contribution to the developing circulatory system: implications for vascular morphology? *Circ Res* 1998;82:221–231.

185. Person AD, Kiewer SE, Runyan RB. Cell biology of cardiac cushion development. *Int Rev Cytol* 2005;243:287–335.

186. Schroeder JA, Jackson LF, Lee DE, et al. Form and function of developing heart valves: coordination by extracellular matrix and growth factor signaling. *J Mol Med* 2003;81(7):392–403.

187. Webb S, Qayyum SR, Anderson RH, et al. Septation and separation within the outflow tract of the developing heart. *J Anat* 2003;202(4):327–342.

188. Qayyum SR, Webb S, Anderson RH, et al. Septation and valvar formation in the outflow tract of the embryonic chick heart. *Anat Rec* 2001;264(3):273–283.

189. Hutson MR, Zhang P, Stadt HA, et al. Cardiac arterial pole alignment is sensitive to FGF8, signaling in the pharynx. *Dev Biol* 2006;295(2):486–497.

190. Tartaglia M, Mehler EL, Goldberg R, et al. Mutations in PTPN11, encoding the protein tyrosine phosphatase SHP-2, cause Noonan syndrome. *Nat Genet* 2001;29:465–468.

191. Leonhardt A, Glaser A, Wegmann M, et al. Expression of prostanoid receptors in human ductus arteriosus. *Br J Pharmacol* 2003;138:655–659.

192. Michelakis ED, Rebeyka I, Wu X, et al. O2, sensing in the human ductus arteriosus: regulation of voltage-gated K+ channels in smooth muscle cells by a mitochondrial redox sensor. *Circ Res* 2002;91:478–486.

193. Zhao F, Weismann CG, Satoda M, et al. Novel TFAP2B mutations that cause Char syndrome provide a genotype-phenotype correlation. *Am J Hum Genet* 2001;69:695–703.

194. Elzenga NJ, Gittenberger-de Groot AC, Oppenheimer-Dekker A. Coarctation and other obstructive aortic arch anomalies: their relationship to the ductus arteriosus. *Int J Cardiol* 1986;13:289–308.

195. Bergwerff M, DeRuiter MC, Hall S, Poelmann RE, Gittenberger-de Groot AC. Unique vascular morphology of the fourth aortic arches: possible implications for pathogenesis of type-B aortic arch interruption and anomalous right subclavian artery. *Cardiovasc Res* October 1999;44(1):185–196.

196. Gittenberger-de Groot AC. Mannheimer Lecture. The quintessence of the making of the heart. *Cardiol Young* 2003;13(2):175–183.

197. Poelmann RE, Gittenberger-de Groot AC, Metlink MMT, et al. Development of the cardiac coronary vascular endothelium, studied with antiendothelial antibodies, in chicken-quail chimeras. *Circ Res* 1993;73:559–568.

198. Poelmann RE, Lie-Venema H, Gittenberger-de Groot AC. The role of the epicardium and neural crest as extracardiac contributors to coronary vascular development. *Tex Heart Inst J* 2002;29(4):255–261.

199. Mu H, Ohashi R, Lin P, et al. Cellular and molecular mechanisms of coronary vessel development. *Vasc Med* 2005;10(1):37–44.

200. Bernanke DH, Velkey JM. Development of the coronary blood supply: changing concepts and current ideas. *Anat Rec* 2002;269(4):198–208.

201. Velkey JM, Bernanke DH. Apoptosis during coronary artery orifice development in the chick embryo. *Anat Rec* 2001;262(3):310–317.

202. Hatcher CJ, Diman NY, Kim MS, et al. A role for Tbx5, in proepicardial cell migration during cardiogenesis. *Physiol Genomics* 2004;18(2):129–140.

203. Munoz-Chapuli R, Gonzalez-Iriarte M, Carmona R, et al. Cellular precursors of the coronary arteries. *Tex Heart Inst J* 2002;29(4):243–349.

204. Guadix JA, Carmona R, Munoz-Chapuli R, et al. In vivo and in vitro analysis of the vasculogenic potential of avian proepicardial and epicardial cells. *Dev Dyn* 2006;235(4):1014–1026.

205. Thieszen SL, Rosenquist TH. Expression of collagens and decorin during aortic arch artery development: implications for matrix pattern formation. *Matrix Biol* 1995;14(7):573–582.

206. Risau W. Vasculogenesis, angiogenesis and endothelial cell differentiation during embryonic development. In: Feinberg RN, Sherer GK, Auerbach R, eds. *The Development of the Vascular System. Issues Biomed.* Vol. 14. Basel, Switzerland: Karger, 1991:58–66.

207. Rakusan K, Flanagan MF, Geva T, et al. Morphometry of human coronary capillaries during normal growth and the effect of age in left ventricular pressure-overload hypertrophy. *Circulation* 1992;86:38–46.

208. Lucitti JL, Tobita K, Keller BB. Arterial hemodynamics and mechanical properties after circulatory intervention in the chick embryo. *J Exp Biol* May 2005;208(pt 10):1877–1885.

209. Lie-Venema H, Gittenberger-de Groot AC, Van Empel LJ, et al. Ets-1, and ETS-2, transcription factors are essential for normal coronary and myocardial development in chicken embryos. *Circ Res* 2003;92:749–756.

210. Franco D, Icardo JM. Molecular characterization of the ventricular conduction system in the developing mouse heart: topographical correlation in normal and congenitally malformed hearts. *Cardiovasc Res* 2001;49(2):417–429.

211. Poelmann RE, Jongbloed MR, Molin DG, et al. The neural crest is contiguous with the cardiac conduction system in the mouse embryo: a role in induction? *Anat Embryol (Berl)* 2004;208(5):389–393.

212. Harris BS, Jay PY, Rackley MS, et al. Transcriptional regulation of cardiac conduction system development: 2004, FASEB cardiac conduction system minimeeting, Washington DC. *Anat Rec A Discov Mol Cell Evol Biol* 2004;280(2):1036–1045.

213. Pennisi DJ, Rentschler S, Gourdie RG. Induction and patterning of the cardiac conduction system. *Int J Dev Biol* 2002;46(6):765–775.

214. Gourdie RG, Harris BS, Bond J, et al. Development of the cardiac pacemaking and conduction system. *Birth Defects Res C Embryo Today* 2003;69(1):46–57.

215. Pennisi DJ, Rentschler S, Gourdie RG, Fishman GI, Mikawa T. Induction and patterning of the cardiac conduction system. *Int J Dev Biol* September 2002;46(6):765–775.

216. Reckova M, Rosengarten C, deAlmeida A, et al. Hemodynamics is a key epigenetic factor in development of the cardiac conduction system. *Circ Res* July 2003;93(1):77–85.

217. Hall CE, Hurtado R, Hewett KW, et al. Hemodynamic-dependent patterning of endothelin converting enzyme 1, expression and differentiation of impulse-conducting Purkinje fibers in the embryonic heart. *Development* February 2004;131(3):581–592.

218. Baptista CA, Kirby ML. The cardiac ganglia: cellular and molecular aspects. *Kaohsiung J Med Sci* 1997;13(1):42–54.

219. Chen F, Klitzner TS, Weiss JN. Autonomic regulation of calcium cycling in developing embryonic mouse hearts. *Cell Calcium* May 2006;39(5):375–385.

220. Hyer J, Johansen M, Prasad A, et al. Induction of Purkinje fiber differentiation by coronary vascularization. *Proc Natl Acad Sci U S A* 1999;96:13214–13218.

221. Keller BB. Function and biomechanics of developing cardiovascular systems. In: Tomanek R, ed. *Formation of the Heart & Its Regulation.* New York: Springer-Verlag, 2001:251–271.

222. Keller BB. Functional maturation and coupling of the embryonic cardiovascular system. In: Clark EB, Markwald RR, Takao A, eds. *Developmental Mechanisms of Heart Disease.* Mount Kisco, NY: Futura Publishing, 1995:367–386.

CHAPTER (9)

Genetic Basis for Cardiovascular Disease

Robert Roberts / Elizabeth McNally

THE HUMAN GENOME

The term *genome* refers to all chromosomal DNA including the genes responsible for an organism. The proteome refers to all of the proteins responsible for an organism. Genes exert their influence through the proteins they produce. Each gene produces a unique protein, referred to as a *polypeptide.* Some proteins are made of two or more polypeptides and a significant proportion of genes use alternative splicing to produce more than one form of the same polypeptide. In addition to genes that encode proteins, there are genes that transcribe RNA without encoding protein. The human genome within each cell consists of approximately 3 billion bases in the form of 23 pairs of chromosomes of which 22 pairs are homologous (one from the father and one from the mother) referred to as *autosomes,* and the remaining pair contain the sex chromosomes that consists of X and Y in the male and two X chromosomes in the female. Each chromosome is a long molecule made of DNA. DNA is comprised of only four bases: adenine (A), guanine (G), cytosine (C), and thymidine (T) (see Chap. 5). A chromosome consists of monotonous repeats of these four bases. Nevertheless, the sequence of these four bases determines all inherited characteristics. The average length of a chromosome is approximately 135,000,000 base pairs (bp). The longest chromosome, chromosome 1, has more than 250,000,000 bp. The smallest, chromosome 21, has only 50,000,000 bp. The 23 chromosomes together contain a total of 3 billion bp (Table 9–1). The chromosomes contain the genes, which are discrete units with a start and a stop point and vary in size from 10,000 to 2,000,000 bp. The estimated average size of a gene is approximately 20,000 bp. The genes are nonrandomly distributed along chromosome into gene-rich and gene-poor regions. The ends of chromosome are referred to as *telomeres.* The centromeres are those regions of chromosome that attach to the mitotic apparatus during cell divi-

TABLE 9–1

The Human Genome

Base pairs	3 billion
Genes estimated	30,000
Percent of DNA coding for genes	<2%

sion. Both telomeres and centromeres are comparatively gene-poor regions. Embedded in the DNA sequence of each chromosome are genes that encode for proteins (2 percent of the DNA)[1] and others that encode for all RNAs. Interspersed between the sequences coding for proteins and RNAs are sequences that regulate when and how much of a gene is transcribed into protein or RNA referred to as *regulatory DNA elements*. The proteins that bind to these elements are referred to as *transcription factors* and have specific DNA binding sites that attach to the sequence of the regulatory DNA element that controls transcription. In between these sequences is extensive DNA of unknown function, which may simply serve as support structure. It is postulated that more than half [1] of genomic DNA is transcribed into RNA transcripts with the end product being primarily RNA and the remainder proteins. Approximately 10 percent of DNA sequence is transcribed into messenger RNA, of which only 2 percent exits the nucleus to serve as templates for proteins. Another much larger proportion of DNA is used to transcript RNAs.[1] A new class of RNA[2] of 15 to 22 bases in length referred to as small interference RNA or microRNAs was recently described with several functions including the regulation of gene expression. Although knowledge is continuing to unfold on the function of these molecules, they are clearly more in abundance than expected.[3] It is estimated that 46 percent of the human genome is composed of DNA from mobile DNA elements transposed into the human genome over the past 150 to 200 million years with no known function.[4] It is estimated that the human genome contains 25,000 genes with each encoding for a single polypeptide; but through alternative splicing of the exons, each gene may produce several slightly modified forms of that polypeptide. Thus, it is likely that despite the 25,000 genes, we may have more than 100,000 proteins. The DNA is bound to a series of support proteins belonging to the histone family,[4] which maintains the structure of the chromosome and participate in gene silencing. In addition to their support role, histones play a major function in the epigenetic regulation[5] of gene expression (see Chap. 5).

CHROMOSOMAL LOCI, GENES, AND ALLELES

The precise position of each gene on the chromosome is identical from person to person and is referred to as the *chromosomal locus*. Chromosome loci are designated by giving the chromosome number (1–23, X, or Y) and whether it is on the long (q) or short arm (p) and the subband region. Subregions reflect the banding patterns of chromosomes based on Giemsa staining patterns. An example is the chromosomal locus for the gene that encodes for angiotensin-converting enzyme (ACE) is designated 17q23. Each pair of autosomal homologous chromosomes carry the same set of genes with one inherited from each parent. De-

spite their homology and the identical overall function of the genes, some genes have a slightly different DNA sequence from that of their corresponding genes on the other chromosome of the homologous pair, which may slightly or markedly alter the gene's function. For example, the gene encoding for ACE located at 17q23 is present at this locus on each homologous chromosome from both parents. However, the ACE gene is known to exist in the general population in three forms of alleles designated D, DI, and II. The particular allele accompanying the 17q23 locus depends on which alleles are inherited from the parents. If one inherits the D allele from the mother and the D allele from the father, they would be homozygous for the D allele; but if a parent had the D and the other the I allele, they would be heterozygous. Although both genes or alleles encode for ACE and convert angiotensinogen to angiotensin II, there is increased plasma enzyme activity associated with the D form, and studies suggest homozygosity for the D gene (DD), predisposes to cardiac hypertrophy.[6,7] Many genes exhibit multiple alleles.

THE HUMAN GENOME SEQUENCE: THE BLUEPRINT FOR HUMAN LIFE AND ITS DIVERSITY

The Human Genome Project's goals were to map and sequence the entire DNA of the human genome. The first large international effort in the history of biological research,[8] the Human Genome Project was initiated on October 1, 1990, to be completed in the year 2005.[9] However, a rough draft of 90 percent of the DNA sequences was available to the public in 2000[8] and the complete sequence in 2003.[10] The sequence of each gene was entered into a publicly accessible database and is freely available. In the United States GenBank (accessible at www.ncvi.nlm.nih.gov), run by the National Center for Biotechnology Information, serves as the public repository of sequence information.

The Human Genome Project contains the blueprint for the development of a single fertilized egg into a complex organism of more than 10^{13} cells. There were other goals completed along the way that markedly accelerated the pace of biological or medical research. One goal was the development of a genetic map. This meant developing markers (a unique DNA sequence) along each chromosome that would have a readily identifiable chromosomal position to provide highly informative signposts for the identification of nearby genes. This goal was completed with thousands of markers spaced less than 1 million bp apart spanning the entire human genome.[11] Thus, the complete set of genetic markers available for each chromosome provides a complete genetic map of the human genome. The genetic map was the necessary tool for widespread application of genetic linkage analysis, a technique that has led to mapping numerous loci and genes responsible for single-gene disorders including several diseases of the cardiovascular system (see Chapter 81). It is estimated there are approximately 6000 rare inherited single-gene disorders, of which more than 2000 genes have been identified.[12,13] The catalog of single-gene disorders is found in the Online Mendelian Inheritance in Man (OMIM) at www.ncbi.nlm.nih.gov/entrez/query.fcgi?db=OMIM/. OMIM documents all single-gene disorders, including disease gene information along with correlates of mutations and phenotypes.

TABLE 9–2

Genetic Base for Disease

Chromosomal abnormalities
Single-gene disorders
Polygenic disorders

A genetic map of the human genome designates the locus of a gene as previously indicated by the example of the ACE gene located at 17q23. This simply indicates the gene is on chromosome 17. If one were to compare this to a postal address, the chromosome number is the country, the q or p arm is the city, and the subband number lacks precise molecular specificity but does refine the genetic region. The resolution is such that the gene will be within a few million base pairs along with many other genes. With the physical map, it is now possible to precisely locate the gene by its sequence in the human genome. This is equivalent to the street address. Concomitant with the sequencing of the human genome was the integration of the chromosomal signpost sequences spanning the genome that are expressed as mRNA. These tags identified throughout the genome are referred to as *expressed sequenced tags* (ESTs).[10] ESTs consist of sequences of 200 to 300 bp, which are unique and represent a specific gene. To be unique ESTs were preferentially defined from the 3′ untranslated regions of genes that tend to have less homology to related family members. Not all ESTs are derived from 3′ untranslated regions, but these regions are more highly represented in the EST databases. ESTs were integrated into the human genome sequence and have been invaluable in assisting in the pursuit of human genes. The sequence of each EST in GenBank has been cloned and stored in bacteria referred to as a library of human ESTs. Most ESTs have been mapped to their chromosomal locations and can be used as markers to find genes responsible for disease. The development of the genetic map (chromosomal markers), followed by the physical map, has tremendously accelerated the efforts of investigators to identify genes responsible for disease.

CLASSIFICATION OF GENETIC DISORDERS

A number of mutagenic factors induce mutations, including radiation, chemicals, and most importantly errors by the DNA synthetic and editing enzymes. Large-scale mutations, or genomic rearrangements, can involve a visible alteration at the level of the chromosome (chromosomal abnormalities detected by cytogenetic staining patterns) and may result in deletions, additions, or translocations of a chromosomal regions. Because of the scale of these chromosomal rearrangements, genes are eliminated or altered. In contrast, small-scale mutations are usually restricted to minor alterations in the DNA sequence that vary from single or multiple nucleotides being substituted, deleted, or inserted. Thus, hereditary and congenital diseases are conventionally classified into three broad categories: *chromosomal abnormalities, single-gene or monogenic disorders,* and *polygenic disorders or complex traits* (Table 9–2). The latter is caused by interactions between defects in multiple genes and nongenetic factors. Chromosomal abnormalities are usually detected early in life and are associated with many pediatric or congenital disorders as opposed to being discovered in adulthood. These disorders are discussed in Chap. 81.

MUTATIONS: A STABLE CHANGE IN THE DNA SEQUENCE

SOMATIC VERSUS GERMLINE MUTATIONS

In general, the sequence of the nucleotides or bases that comprise DNA has remained stable over hundreds of thousands of years. Nonetheless, occasionally, a change in the base sequence occurs, which is referred to as a mutation. The natural rate is approximately 1 per million per gamete. This is approximately 1 mutation per 250 years. Mutations are stable alterations in the sequence of the DNA, which occur because of one or more nucleotides undergoing substitution, insertion, deletion, or a structural alteration. If the mutation occurs in the germ line, it becomes heritable and can be transmitted to the offspring. Inheritance of a mutation is referred to as *familial,* whereas when it occurs de novo it is referred to as *sporadic.* If the mutation occurs in somatic cells, although it will not be transmitted to offspring, it may be a major cause of disease for that individual. Most of cancer is caused by somatic mutations induced by carcinogens or more commonly caused by errors in the normal repair of DNA. Somatic mutations as a cause for cardiovascular disease are only recently appreciated. This was recently highlighted by the identification of several mutations in the connexin 40 gene responsible for atrial fibrillation, which was shown to be present only in cardiac tissue.[14] It remains to be determined how common somatic mutations are as a cause of cardiovascular disease.

CLASSIFICATION OF RARE MUTATIONS CAUSING SINGLE-GENE DISORDERS

Mutations that cause single-gene disorders (see Chapter 81) are rare. They occur at a frequency of significant less than 1 percent, generally in the range of 0.001 to 0.005 percent. Familial hypertrophic cardiomyopathy, an example of an inherited cardiac disease, has a frequency of 0.005, translating into 1 per 500 of the population. For an inherited disease this is common; in fact it is the most common inherited cardiac disease. Most mutations involving single-gene disorders in adults are caused by minor alterations in the DNA sequence. A mutation could involve a minute change in the DNA sequence, such as alteration of one purine or pyrimidine base in the DNA sequence. Mutations involving only a single nucleotide are known as *point mutations* and are responsible for 70 percent or more of all adult single-gene disorders (Table 9–3). A point mutation may be a substitution of one nucleotide for an-

TABLE 9–3

Classifications of Mutations

Large mutations	Involving the addition or deletion of several nucleotides
Point mutations	Substitutions
	Missense
	Nonsense
	Synonymous
Frame-shift mutations	Insertion
	Deletion

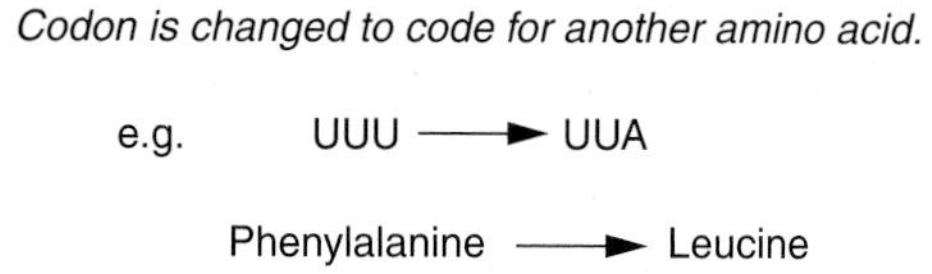

Codon is changed to code for another amino acid.

e.g.   UUU ——→ UUA

Phenylalanine ——→ Leucine

FIGURE 9–1. The codon UUU encodes for phenylalanine; and with the mutation, which changes a single base, the codon changes to UUA, a codon for leucine. This represents a point substitution mutation, which alters a single amino acid and is referred to as *missense*. The remainder of the protein will be normal, and whether this change in one amino acid alters its function depends on whether it falls into a conserved functional domain.

other, changing the amino acid sequence (*missense mutation*) (Fig. 9–1); or it may change the codon from encoding an amino acid to that of a stop codon (Fig. 9–2), which will truncate the protein (*truncated or nonsense mutation*); or it may eliminate a stop codon so the protein is elongated (*elongated mutant*); or it may change the codon without changing amino acid sequence (*synonymous mutation*). All genes during transcription and translation are read from 5′ to 3′ orientation with each triplet of bases (*codon*) coding for a specific amino acid. If a nucleotide is deleted (*deletion*) or an additional one is inserted (*insertion*), it shifts the reading frame; and the resulting protein is entirely different (*frame-shift mutation*) and is usually nonfunctional (Fig. 9–3). If a purine nucleotide is substituted for a pyrimidine or the reverse, the mutation is referred to as a *transversion*, whereas if purine or pyrimidine substitutes for another purine or pyrimidine, respectively, it is called a *transition*.

SYNONYMOUS MUTATIONS

Mutations are divided into those that are synonymous and non-synonymous. Synonymous mutations are usually single nucleotide changes that do not induce a change in the amino acid structure of the protein for which it encodes. Synonymous mutations can fall within a coding region or into the third base position of a codon. Because a number of amino acids are encoded by multiple codons that differ often only in the third base DNA position, this wobble in the sequence is not under evolutionary selective pressure. For example, the amino acid glycine is encoded by four different codons GGG, GGA, GGU, or GGC. A substitution of any nucleotide in the third position will still encode a glycine residue and not alter the predicted protein structure. Nonsynonymous mutations induce changes that affect nucleotides of the first or second codon and produce an alternative amino acid. Glycine has the least of side chains, consisting of a single hydrogen, allowing con-

Base substitution changes the codon
from an amino acid to a stop codon.

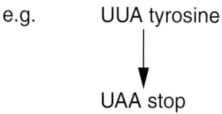

e.g.   UUA tyrosine

UAA stop

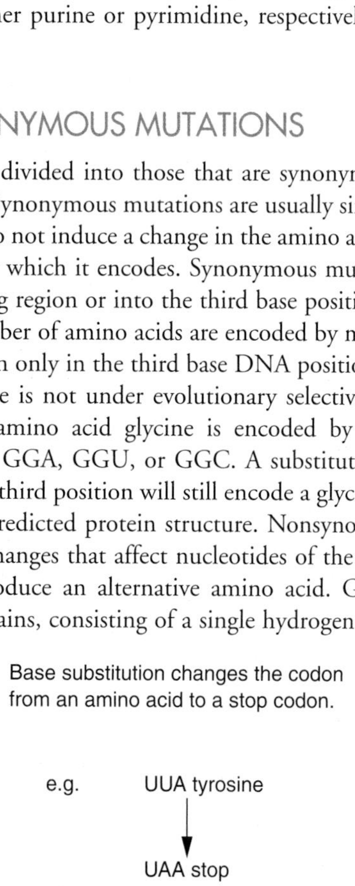

FIGURE 9–2. The codon UUA encodes for the amino acid tyrosine and with the single-base mutation changes the codon to UAA, which happens to be the codon for the stop signal. This represents a point substitution mutation, which alters a single amino acid and is referred to as *nonsense*. Translation of the protein stops with this codon and usually produces a truncated protein with no function. Thus, it is referred to as *nonsense mutation*.

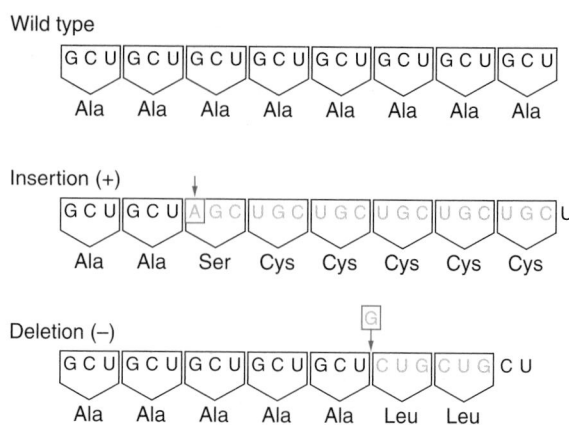

FIGURE 9–3. Shown here is the marked defect of inserting or subtracting a single base, in contrast to the previous examples of substitution in Figures 9–1 and 9–2. The code is always read from left to right with each codon of three bases representing an amino acid. Inserting or deleting a single base changes all subsequent amino acids in that protein, which frequently makes it either nonfunction or dysfunctional. Although the mutation is a single base, because it changes the reading frame, it is referred to as a *frame shift mutation*, which frequently has devastating effects on the function of the protein.

siderable rotation of the peptide backbone into which it is incorporated. Therefore, any substitution that inserts a side chain often reduces protein flexibility and potentially has a deleterious effect on protein function. Synonymous mutations can be associated with disease phenotypes, but the mechanism may or may not involve changing protein function. Mutations that fall within promoter or regulatory regions of genes may decrease or increase gene transcription. These types of substitutions are likely to have a smaller effect, which may still be meaningful to the phenotype of the organism. Synonymous mutations that occur near intron exon borders can affect mRNA splicing and may have a significant effect on protein function. For example, the most common variant associated with Hutchinson-Guilford progeria, a premature aging syndrome, is a synonymous mutation that affects mRNA splicing and ultimately protein processing.[15]

MUTATIONS AND THEIR FUNCTIONAL SIGNIFICANCE

Alterations in Conserved Sequences

Nonsynonymous point mutations that encode conservative amino acid substitutions and do not change the general classification of the amino acid are less likely to affect protein function. Amino acid substitutions that introduce a new charge, insert a proline (reduces protein flexibility), or substitute a hydrophilic amino acid into a hydrophobic domain are more likely to disrupt protein function. Mutations that result from deletion or addition of several nucleotides may have a greater effect on the protein function. Small deletions that remove 3 bp of sequence do not disrupt the reading frame of the protein and instead simply delete a single amino acid. Given the mechanisms for DNA repair, this type of mutation is less common. When DNA repair mechanisms fail leading to mutations, most often single base pairs are affected by substitution. The sequences immediately upstream from a transcribed region are referred to as *promoter sequences*. Frequently, single base pair changes in promoter regions will have only a modest effect on the overall expression of the gene product, but nonetheless these changes can affect the phenotype. The promoter sequences direct the transcription of the entire DNA sequence into RNA until termination sequences direct the cessation of transcription. The RNA is then processed to mature mRNA by removing the intronic regions that do not encode protein. The sequences that direct the removal of introns (consensus splicing sequences) are conserved and include sequences within both the intron and the exon but very near the border between the intron and exon. Mutations that affect the consensus splicing sequences can produce a devastating effect on the resulting protein since missplicing frequently produce a change of reading frame and often a truncation of the resulting protein. The outcome of mutations can be difficult to predict based on sequence alone. Mutations that produce a premature stop codon may lead to aberrant function. However, further complicating prediction is nonsense-mediated decay (NMD) where certain mutations destabilize the encoding mRNA to the extent that the mutant RNA is specifically degraded by NMD.[16] Stop codons offer a unique approach to gene therapy because certain compounds promote readthrough of mutant stop codons and restore protein expression.[17]

Mutations that disrupt mRNA splicing can result in the internal loss of protein. Such mutations are common in the dystrophin gene where the large dystrophin gene contains a repeating protein structure within its midportion. Mutations that cause an internal deletion result in an internal truncated protein that may maintain the reading frame. This feature of the dystrophin gene is currently exploited for potential therapy. Oligonucleotides that deliberately produce missplicing, mutant exons can be removed leading to proteins with normal function.[18]

Phenotype Is Induced by Loss or Gain of Function of Mutant Protein

The phenotype induced by a mutation can in general be classified as loss or gain of function, which refers only to the mutant protein. This is a point of emphasis because other proteins downstream from the mutant protein may exhibit a loss or gain of function irrespective of how the mutation affects the mutant protein. The phenotype may reflect the loss or gain of function of these secondary normal proteins rather than that of the mutant protein. The gain of function is usually abnormal and has a negative effect on the overall function of the individual. It is important to recognize that protein function is usually normal and so is the phenotype when only one allele is missing because every one has two alleles of each gene. Thus, in recessive disorders the phenotype is normal unless both alleles are abnormal. Loss of function mutations most commonly occur in recessive disorders where there is a complete absence of protein production and therefore, protein function. Occasionally, however, loss of function can occur when only one allele is missing or defective, which is referred to as *haploinsufficiency.*

Dominant negative function refers to a mutant protein that has a gain of function that interferes with other protein activity. Dominant negative function is most commonly seen in proteins that interact or bind to other proteins in macromolecular structures. Dominant negative function can also result from point mutations if the single point mutation creates a protein capable of interfering

with the function of other proteins. A dominant negative function can occur when grossly abnormal remnants of proteins are produced. This is typified by the phenotype of autosomal dominant disorders where only one allele is affected, yet it induces an abnormal phenotype. Although the mechanism is not completely understood, the predominant hypothesis is that of a poison peptide. The abnormal protein interacts to inhibit the normal protein from the normal allele or disrupts downstream proteins of the pathway induced by the normal protein. Examples of genes affected by dominant negative mutations are the β-myosin heavy chain gene (MYH7) and lamin A/C (LMNA). Both proteins assemble into larger structures, so the combination of mutant and normal protein is dysfunctional. The difference between loss of function and dominant negative function has great therapeutic implications. Gene therapy offers great promise to those disorders where replacement of the normal protein can restore normal function and reverse the abnormal phenotype. In contrast, such replacement would not be expected to be effective against dominant negative-induced phenotypes.

Repeat expansions are a unique mechanism of genetic disease. Short repeated sequences of 2, 3, or 4 bp occur throughout the human genome and are referred to as short tandem repeats or microsatellites. These repeated sequences can expand considerably during DNA replication, and this expansion can produce a profound effect if these sequences are expressed as mRNA. In myotonic dystrophy, an expansion from the normal 30 to 50 copies of a specific triplet repeat on chromosome 19 to more than 100 copies is sufficient to produce the syndrome of heart and muscle weakness. Initially, it was believed that this chromosome 19 expansion produced disease by disrupting the genes in which it resides. More recently, it has become clear that the mRNA copy of the expanded repeat is toxic to cells leading to sequestration of splicing factors and aberrant mRNA splicing of unrelated genes.

Functional assessment of DNA variation can also be achieved by comparing conservation of the DNA sequence variant, for example, assuming a nonsynonymous mutation has been identified to be associated with disease. It is helpful to determine whether the nonsynonymous mutation alters an amino acid that is highly conserved in other species. The availability of genomic information from multiple species in the public databases greatly facilitates identifying amino acid conservation. The increase in genomic information for noncoding regions from multiple species now makes it possible to determine conservation for noncoding regions as well. For nonsynonymous mutations, protein domain information and structural information may be available and can be used to predict whether the amino acid substitution will affect protein function. Marfan syndrome is a mendelian disorder that arises from mutations in fibrillin-1, a protein that forms the extracellular matrix around vessels and valves.[19] Fibrillin-1 is a large gene with a series of conserved cysteine residues. Many *private* mutations have been identified in Marfan families indicating that the mutation is specific and unique to a particular family. It can be difficult to assess whether the DNA variation is of known or unknown significance. Those sequence variants that disrupt the conserved cysteine residues likely affect protein processing and fibrillin-1 deposition and function. Most recently, a second gene, the transforming growth factor (TGF) receptor 2, has also been implicated in Marfan-like syndromes including familial aortic aneurysms.[20]

TABLE 9–4

Single Nucleotide Polymorphisms

Human genome	3,000,000
General population	17,000,000
Present in protein coding regions	20,000–40,000
Present in conserved non-protein coding regions	20,000–40,000

TGF is a heterogeneous group of proteins that regulate growth and differentiation. TGF proteins reside in the extracellular matrix scaffolding and signal through cell surface receptors.

COMMON MUTATIONS AND COMMON DISEASE

Although 99.9 percent of the DNA sequence is identical among humans, the 0.1 percent difference in DNA sequence of 3 million bases is responsible for all individual differences such as height and weight as well as the lack of or presence of susceptibility to disease. Those common mutations which occur in *normals* occur at a frequency of ≥ 1 percent. Common mutations are primarily caused by substitutions of a single nucleotide and are thus referred to as *single nucleotide polymorphisms* (SNPs). It is estimated there is 1 SNP per 1000 bp,[21,6] which amounts to approximately 3 million per human genome (Table 9–4). These SNPs are fairly evenly distributed throughout the genome with perhaps only approximately 30,000 to 40,000 occurring in protein coding regions but at least another 30,000 occurring in conserved noncoding regions that potentially regulate gene expression. In addition, because of their frequency and widespread distribution, they are excellent markers for genome-wide scans to identify SNPs or genes that predispose to common multigene disorders or traits.

EPIGENETICS

Epigenetics refers to genetic regulation in which an alteration in gene function occurs without a change in the DNA sequence. There are two main mechanisms. The first are those induced by methylation of the DNA nucleotide cytosine in CpG islands and the methylation of terminal lysines of histone proteins that form the core structure of the nucleosome. The second epigenetic mechanism is the addition of chemical groups such as acetyl, phosphate, or ubiquitination to terminal lysine groups of histones. The methylation of CpG islands, and possibly of lysines, is considered permanent in the sense it can be passed onto the next generation, whereas the modification of lysine groups such as acetylation are transient and part of the reversible mechanism to regulate gene transcription. Methylation of genes is referred to as *silencing* because it inhibits the expression of the gene. It is an important mechanism in cancer, whereby several genes can be silenced, leading to unwanted and uncontrolled cell growth. It is considered a major mechanism in the induction of cancer.[22] The role of methylation in cellular and organ differentiation whereby certain genes are permanently prohibited from being expressed remains controversial.[23]

The role of adding chemical groups to lysines of the histone proteins is now recognized as a major mechanism regulating gene expression, including the induction of cardiac hypertrophy.[24] To understand how modification to lysine affects gene transcription, it is necessary to briefly discuss the chromatin structure of DNA. Compaction of DNA into condensed chromatin fibers is required to fit more than a meter of DNA within the volume provided in the nucleus of the cell. The DNA is wrapped around a group of proteins referred to as *histones*. The basic building block of chromatin (DNA and proteins) is the nucleosome which contains 147 bp of DNA wrapped in a left handed superhelix 1.7 times around a core histone octamer.[25] These are joined together with linker DNA. The core histone proteins have either amino or carboxy terminal tails domains that contain sites for posttranslational modifications such as acetylation, methylation, phosphorylation, and ubiquitination. In general, blocking these charged lysine groups releases DNA to bind to promoters that activate gene transcription.

Acetylation of histones promotes gene expression by favoring a less tightly wound state of DNA and allows access of transcription factors to the DNA. Histone deacetylases (HDACs) reduce histone acetylation and broadly decrease gene expression. HDACs are regulated by movement to and from the nucleus. The role of HDACs in regulating cardiac hypertrophic states has been described where suppression of HDACs can block cardiac hypertrophy.[25,26] These mechanisms are critical to understand because HDAC inhibitors are currently being evaluated for their clinical utility. In addition to histone modification by deacetylases, the role of poly(ADP-ribose)polymerases (PARPs) are also being examined for their general role in chromatin structure and the regulation of gene expression. PARPs mediate the transfer of ADP-ribose units from NAD^+ to acceptor proteins that include histones.

The two best understood epigenetic mechanisms are those of imprinting and X inactivation. Imprinting is the process whereby parent of origin effects occur to silence either the maternal or paternal copy of the inherited gene. Imprinting can occur during development where only a single allele is expressed during a strict developmental stage. In more mature tissues, both alleles can then become equally expressed. One of the genes mutated in the long QT syndrome, kvlqt2 also known as KCNQ1, is imprinted during development but not in the mature organism.[27] Therefore, the inheritance of the mutated allele is differentially expressed depending on whether it is the maternal or paternal copy. In general, contiguous regions of chromosomes are subjected to imprinting.

A second common epigenetic mechanism occurs in the form of X inactivation. All females inherit two X chromosomes, but only one remains active. The second X is inactivated taking the structure of the Barr body. In humans with X-linked disorders, X inactivation that preferentially inactivates the nonmutated or normal X chromosome can render female carriers of X-linked disease symptomatic. Duchenne muscular dystrophy is the most common X-linked recessive disorder that leads to progressive muscle weakness and cardiomyopathy in boys. Mothers of Duchenne boys are at risk of developing cardiomyopathy because X-inactivation in cardiomyocytes may inactivate the X containing the normal dystrophin gene leaving more cardiomyocytes that express the nonfunctional dystrophin gene.[28]

GENETIC TRANSMISSION: LINKAGE EQUILIBRIUM OR DISEQUILIBRIUM

Each gene or allele along with its genetic variants is an independent unit with the tendency to be randomly assorted during transmission to offspring. The expected random assortment is referred to as *genetic linkage equilibrium.* The process whereby the gene pool is diversified, and no two offspring are identical (except identical twins) is caused by chromosomal crossover referred to in genetic parlance as *recombination.* During each division of the egg or sperm, the chromosomes in the sperm and the egg align and form bridges, or chiasma, between homologous pairs followed by a piece of one chromosome substituting for the homologous region of the other chromosome and resulting in a crossover of genes from one chromosome to the other. Because there is no addition or loss of chromosomal material, it is referred to as recombination. In each preceding as in subsequent generation, the chromosomes break and recombine averaging approximately two bridges per pair of homologous chromosomes per division of mitosis.

When a particular combination of genes or genetic variants are linked along a chromosomal segment, this is referred to as a *haplotype.* It is well recognized that haplotypes may be transmitted intact to offspring because the DNA containing the haplotype transmits as a block or unit. When two or more genes or genetic variants (e.g., SNPs) are transmitted together more frequently than by chance it is referred to as genetic linkage disequilibrium (LD). This occurs when two or more genes are on the same chromosome in close physical proximity. The close physical distance makes it less likely for a chromosomal break to occur between the two genes. Therefore, the closer two genes or genetic variants are, the less likely they are to be separated by recombination events. On an evolutionary timescale, at the first outset, a genetic mutation will exist adjacent to all the unique sequences surrounding it. However, in subsequent generations, the mutation tends to separate from its neighboring unique sequences because of the shuffling caused by chromosomal recombination or crossover. The rate at which a particular unique sequence is separated from its neighbors is referred to as the *recombination rate* and depends on the initial chromosomal distance between sequences and the number of subsequent crossovers. Thus, when a mutation is first formed, it is coinherited with neighboring genes and SNPs that may be several million base pairs apart, meaning these sequences are in LD. In subsequent generations, only neighbors that are within 20,000 to 30,000 bp may be coinherited with the mutation. Most of the sequence variation in the human genome that occurs frequently (0.05 frequency) is felt to be older than 200,000 years old.[29] Because of repeated recombination, SNPs may exhibit disequilibrium but only over short distances. Thus, the haplotypes or blocks of DNA that are inherited containing SNPs may be short and could vary markedly.

THE INTERNATIONAL HAPMAP PROJECT (SINGLE NUCLEOTIDE POLYMORPHISMS AND HAPLOTYPES)

Following the completion of the sequencing of the human genome, several sequencing projects were pursued including the genome of the mouse,[30] rat,[31] and chimpanzee.[32] These genomes have provided a rich resource from which to define the function of genes[33] and is now part of a highly specialized science referred to as *bioinformatics*[34] (discussed in the Bioinformatics section). Another notable project that is particularly germane to finding genes that affect health and disease is the International HapMap Consortium.[35] Funded and performed by five countries, this study was initiated in 2002 and Phase I was completed in 2005 and Phase II in 2006. It is recognized from the sequencing of the human genome and subsequent studies that the DNA sequence is 99.9 percent identical. The 0.1 percent of the sequence, which amounts to approximately 3 million bases, accounts for the individual characteristics of each person including the presence or lack of susceptibility to disease. Most of the 3 million bases are caused by mutations that induced single nucleotide polymorphisms substitution that occur with a frequency of ≥ 1 percent and are referred to as *single nucleotide polymorphisms* (SNPs). Although it is known that a SNP exists on average every 1000 bp, it would be prohibitive in terms of time and cost to genotype 3 million SNPs to identify those contributing to disease. However, SNPs may be inherited in blocks (haplotypes), which make it unnecessary to genotype every SNP. Genotyping one or two SNPs that are in LD with several adjacent SNPs would identify the latter as well. A major aim of the HapMap project was to determine if SNPs are inherited in blocks of haplotypes and how large these haplotypes are. This has major implications for the pursuit of the genetic variants contributing to common diseases such as coronary artery disease (CAD).

The investigators of the HapMap Project[36] for their genome-wide scans selected 1,007,329 SNPs spanning the genome. The SNPs were selected with a minor allele frequency (MAF) of ≥ 0.05 and for convenience was referred to as *common SNP.* They selected five ethnic groups for a total of 269 individuals as shown in Table 9–5. Of the 1,007,329 SNPs, 11,500 were encoding regions that specifically code for different amino acids. In addition, for comparison, 10 representative regions of the human genome of 500 kb each (totaling 5000 kb) were selected from the ENCODE (Encyclopedia of DNA Elements) Project[37] and sequenced in 48 individuals. All SNPs known and unknown, common and uncommon, were sequenced and subsequently genotyped in the complete set of 269 DNA samples.

The results were very insightful and are likely to remain a landmark for decades to come. They showed the extent of LD for SNPs was greater at the centromere and less at the telomere and overall correlated with the length of the chromosome. There were several hotspots where recombination occurs. It was estimated that 80 percent of recombination occurs in 15 percent of the sequence.

TABLE 9–5

Population Analyzed by the International HapMap Project

ETHNIC GROUP	SAMPLE SIZE
Yoruba, Nigeria	90
Utah, United States	90
Beijing, China	49
Tokyo, Japan	44

Hotspots typically span approximately 2 kb and are rich in the sequence motif of CCTCCCT as well as the THE1A/B retrotransposon-like element. Most of the human genome is contained in blocks. It is estimated that over half of the human genome is in blocks of 22k in Africans and 44k in Americans, Europeans, or Asians. In the haplotype map of the International Consortium, it was observed that the average length of the DNA block in a European/American population was 16.3 kb, in the African population 7.3 kb, and in the Chinese population, 13.2 kb as determined by one method; and by the four-gamete method, it was 5.9 kb, 4.8 kb, and 5.9 kb, respectively in these populations. Again, it was confirmed that the average number of commonly occurring SNPs (MAF ≥ 0.0.5) in these blocks was 4 to 5. Nevertheless, there is marked variation in the size of the blocks from 1 kb to 97 kb. Within each block, it requires on average 3 to 5 common haplotypes to capture 90 percent of the sequence. Almost all common SNPs showed a good correlation with one or more rare SNPs. If one selected sets of SNPs, it would be possible to detect more than 90 percent of genetic variation by spanning the human genome with 250,000 SNPs rather than the 1,007,329 SNPs. Secondly, using evenly spaced common SNPs across the genome requires 486,000 in the American population to detect the same genetic variants detected by the 1,007,329 SNPs.

BIOINFORMATICS

Bioinformatics is the application of computer science and modeling to biological databases. Large-scale databases of biological materials, namely genetic sequence and expression data, have been developed in the last decade. These databases include the repository of the human genome sequence (GenBank), a growing database of human sequence variation (SNP, www.ncbi.nlm.nih.gov/geo/), a collection of data regarding gene expression profiles (Gene Expression Omnibus, www.ncbi.nlm.nih.gov/geo/), and protein databases (SwissProt, www.ebi.ac.uk/swissprot/). GenBank is the annotated collection of all publicly available nucleotide sequences and their protein translations. These sequences derive from direct submissions from individual laboratories and high throughput sequencing centers from around the world. DNA sequence is directly submitted to GenBank, where it is assigned an accession number and check for quality. Annotation of genomic sequence includes identifying sequences that are transcribed into RNA or expressed, predicting sequences likely to encode genes based on algorithms that predict exon sequences and open reading frames.[38] For established gene sequences, new information is routinely added to demarcate likely or known function of the gene product; and, importantly, information is routinely updated indicating sequence variation, both functional and of unknown function. The source of information used to annotate DNA sequence can be from direct submission to GenBank or more likely from published information that is found in the bibliographic database PubMed.

DNA sequence variation explains our unique qualities, including the tendency to develop certain disease phenotypes. Cardiovascular diseases of all types is highly influenced by inheritance. Although environmental influences remain substantial for the manifestation of many types of cardiovascular disease, the genetic influence for the most common cardiovascular traits is greater than or equal to that observed for many types of cancer; pulmo-

nary diseases; and psychiatric disease including autism, depression, and schizophrenia. DNA sequence variation among humans is determined through *resequencing* multiple unrelated individuals. Most commonly, specific genetic regions implicated in a disease phenotype are subjected to sequencing to determine the degree of sequence variation from individual to individual, and to correlate sequence variation with phenotype or disease traits. This approach of DNA sequencing most commonly uncovers SNPs where single base pairs are substituted. SNPs that change the coding region of a gene and therefore the protein product are referred to as *nonsynonymous SNPs*. SNPs that do not change the predicted protein sequence are synonymous SNPs. There is also a growing interest in SNPs that are present in noncoding regions but highly conserved sequence such as regions containing gene promoter elements. The catalog of SNPs is also a publicly accessible database into which individuals can deposit SNP information.

A third growing database serves to organize data on gene expression in disease states. It is now possible to probe the expression state of all mRNAs within a given tissue or cell type. This has been made possible by the availability of multiple formats that enable gene expression profiling. Most commonly, chip-based formats are used to profile gene expression. In these chip-based or array formats, fragments of complementary DNA or EST sequences have been predictably and reproducible permanently arrayed onto microchips. RNA is purified from the disease tissue or cell type of interest and a control tissue. For example, gene profiles have been determined from RNA isolated from cardiomyopathic hearts and from vessels with coronary artery stenosis. Once the RNA is isolated from the desired source, it is then copied, fluorescently labelled, and hybridized to the array format containing thousands of genes. Because fluorescence signals are sensitive and quantitative, the differences between hybridization profiles can be compared to determine which genes are upregulated or downregulated. The marked sensitivity of this approach necessitates technical and biological replicates of the studies for validation. As chip hybridization techniques have become more standard, the need for multiple technical replicates has been reduced. However, when dealing with human samples that have inherent biological variability, multiple human samples must often be considered to determine those changes in gene expression that occur commonly in a disease state.

Chip or array-based gene profiles enable the simultaneously sampling of 25,000 genes. Therefore, the analysis of this large quantity of data has lead to a subspecialty of bioinformatics. Grouping genes with expression changed into subsets based on function, or gene ontology analysis, has been most commonly used to analyze changes in gene expression. The GEO, or gene expression omnibus, database is a searchable database where individual genes and disease states can be queried.

PROTEOMICS

Because most genetic mutations lead to changes in protein expression or function, the ability to study, on a larger scale, changes in protein profiles is increasingly being developed and used. Several technical issues must be considered when determining protein profiles. It is important to consider the techniques used to isolate the proteins in question and the degree to which a subset of proteins has been purified prior to determining their content and identification. A second consideration is the methodology used to identify proteins. Mass spectrometry is used to identify proteins, which can fundamentally identify molecules, including proteins, based on determining mass and charge. Energy is applied to a protein, or complex of proteins, to ionize and partially degrade the protein into manageably sized components suitable for subsequent mass and charge analysis. To determine the complex of proteins expressed in disease states requires detailed attention to the methodologies used to isolate the proteins. Proteomics is increasingly focusing approaches to understanding posttranslational modifications such as phosphorylation, glycosylation, and acetylation because an improved understanding of these modifications will better determine how protein function can be modified.

The availability of genomic data from multiple organisms, including humans, has dramatically increased the database of predicted protein information. Algorithms for identifying predicted domain structures, many of which are coupled to crystallographic protein structures, have improved the ability to predict protein function. Within proteins, protein domains are units of molecular evolution and most are units of protein function. Often, domains are defined because they are independently folding units that can be isolated and whose structures can be solved. The Conserved Domain Database is linked to Entrez databases including Proteins, Taxonomy, and PubMed and integrates data from these sources to understand and identify better domains of proteins and their hierarchy. In the coming years, increasing data on protein complexity generated by alternative splicing and posttranslational modification will be incorporated into these databases.

RARE SINGLE-GENE DISORDERS VERSUS COMMON POLYGENIC DISORDERS

Single-gene disorders are rare, and by definition the mutation is both necessary and sufficient to cause the disease. In contrast, common disorders such as atherosclerosis or hypertension are not dominated by a single gene and neither is any one gene necessary nor sufficient to induce the disease. It is believed a variety of genes impart predisposition to these diseases which interact with the environment to induce the disease. Single-gene disorders follow mendelian inheritance through which mathematical formulations referred to as *genetic linkage* lend themselves to means of mapping the chromosomal location of the genes via the use of pedigrees. With the development of complete genetic maps of the human genome, a new approach to identifying genes contributing to mendelian diseases, called *positional cloning*, became available[39] (see Chap. 81). Positional cloning proceeds in several stages: (1) collect families, segregating traits of interest; (2) determine the chromosomal location of disease genes by comparing the inheritance of chromosome segments to the inheritance of disease in families; (3) refine the interval containing the disease gene and identification of genes in the disease interval; and (4) screen genes in the interval for mutations that alter the structure or expression of the encoded protein. In the mendelian paradigm, independent mutations that alter the encoded protein and segregate specifically with the disease in families constitute proof that the disease gene has been identified. It is estimated there are 6000 of these rare single-gene disorders; and in the last decade, this approach has resulted in identification of

more than 2000 human disease genes, of which more than 200 are associated with cardiac diseases. Although these mendelian disorders are rare, in many cases they have provided fundamental new insight into disease biology that has proved relevant to the understanding of more common forms of disease.

Nonetheless, the truly common diseases of mankind, such as CAD, stroke, diabetes, and hypertension are multifactorial in nature. For these diseases, the positional cloning paradigm has limited power, because even single families with affected individuals may have different combinations of inherited and acquired risk factors; moreover, the number of factors and the magnitude of the impact of any single-gene locus can be minimal. Evidence that these diseases have an inherited component comes from a variety of studies as discussed in the following text.

EVIDENCE OF A GENETIC BASIS FOR CORONARY ARTERY DISEASE

All diseases represent an interaction between the individual's genes and that of the environment. This is more complex in polygenic disorders such as CAD, hypertension, or diabetes. This section provides a brief summary of the evidence for the inheritance of CAD and how high throughput genotyping with application of genome-wide mapping using SNPs is likely to unravel the genes predisposing to such common diseases. The evidence for heritability is from several sources as outlined in the following text (Table 9–6).

FAMILIAL AGGREGATION STUDIES

Studies investigating case control families have shown on average a two- to threefold increase in risk for CAD in first-degree relatives.[40–44] A family history of CAD in a first-degree relative younger than age 60 years is an independent risk factor for early myocardial infarction (MI) even after controlling for traditional risk factors.[45,46] Several prospective studies have shown up to a twofold increase in CAD risk associated with a family history of CAD after adjusting for traditional risk factors.[47–53] There is also a clustering of susceptibility to CAD in families with risk factors associated with abnormalities such as lipid metabolism, hypertension, diabetes, and obesity indicating a genetic basis for these conditions and risk factors.[54–60] The extent of coronary occlusion in patients with CAD also relates to a parental history of MI.[61] In families with CAD onset before age 46 years, heritability was estimated to be .92 to 100 percent whereas within families of older cases, the heritability range from 15 to 30 percent.[44] Premature

---

TABLE 9–6

Evidence of Genetic Basis for Coronary Artery Disease

Familial aggregation studies
The predictability of the family history
Genetic association studies
Atherosclerosis inherited as mendelian disorders
Genetic factors predominant in premature coronary artery disease

CAD in the young is transmitted as an even greater genetic load to their offspring.[62] The Danish twin registry, of 8000 twin pairs, shows a higher incidence of CAD and deaths in monozygotic twins compared with dizygotic twins, 44 versus 14 percent.[63]

THE PREDICTABILITY OF THE FAMILY HISTORY

The importance of inheritance is illustrated by recent studies showing the importance of a family history of CAD. It has been shown that 14 percent of the Utah population has a family history of CAD, which accounts for 72 percent of early CAD cases (younger than age 50 years) and 48 percent of all CAD events at any age in the state of Utah. Similarly, 11 percent of the Utah population has a family history of stroke which accounts for 86 percent of all early strokes.[64] In the Framingham Study, a family history of CAD, cerebral vascular accidents or peripheral arterial disease was associated with 2.4-fold increased risk of CAD in men and 2.2 in women. In the Interheart Study, a family history of CAD had a 1.55-fold increased risk and after corrected for other risk factors 1.45.[65] In the Procam Study, a family history of MI was an independent risk factor of CAD.[66] Family history of CAD in a first-degree relative younger than age 60 years is an independent risk factor for MI.

GENETIC ASSOCIATION STUDIES

Essentially, all association studies remain suspect because of the small sample size and lack of functional evidence.[29] The candidate genes selected for these studies are generally associated with pathways known to involve atherosclerosis and numerous studies have used genes implicated in known risk factors such as hypertension,[67,68] obesity,[69–75] and diabetes.[76–81] In one family-based study, it was shown that heritability of thrombosis and related phenotypes accounted for more than 60 percent of the variation in susceptibility.[82]

ATHEROSCLEROSIS INHERITED AS MENDELIAN DISORDERS

Linkage analysis in families with premature CAD have found evidence for linkage to a region on chromosomes 2q21, Xq23,[83] 1p34,[84] 16p13, 14qter,[85] and 15q26.[86] The gene at 15q26 has been identified as *MEF-2A,* which has a small deletion.[86] Recently, the DeCode Study has identified another gene *LTA4H* as encoding leukotriene A4 hydroxylase.[87] Several other chromosomal loci have been identified that associate with known risk factors for CAD such as hyperlipidemia, hypertension, homocysteine defects, and diabetes.

GENETIC FACTORS PREDOMINATE IN EARLY PREMATURE CAD

Approximately 10 percent of patients with CAD develop a diagnosable phenotype before the age of 50 years.[88,89] One study of 207 cases of MI occurring before the age of 55 were matched to controls.[90] A family history of MI occurring in a first-degree relative before the age of 55 years increased the risk of MI by 7.1-fold. This study estimated that heritability for early onset of CAD at 0.63, after exclusion of apparent lipid abnormalities the heritability estimate was 0.56 suggesting that more than half of CAD diagnosed before the age of 55 is genetic.

A NEW ERA FOR UNRAVELLING COMMON POLYGENIC DISORDERS

GENOME-WIDE SCANNING WITH SNPS

DNA markers at a density of 1 per 10 million bases have been quite successful in mapping the chromosomal location of genes responsible for the rare single-gene disorders. In contrast, mapping genes for common disorders such as CAD or hypertension would require hundreds of thousands of markers, generally 1 marker per 6,000 bp.[91] This is because each gene may contribute only 5 to 10 percent of the phenotype. Scanning a genome with 500,000 or more markers was not feasible until recently. A new era has emerged with the discovery of the SNP. These polymorphisms occur throughout the genome at a frequency of 1 SNP per 1000 bp.[36] It is recognized that of the 3 million SNPs, perhaps only 20,000 to 40,000 are located in protein or RNA coding regions. Another 20,000 to 40,000 are in conserved noncoding regions that could alter the DNA-binding elements for promoters and thus alter gene transcription and protein function. A new marker set consisting of more than 500,000 SNPs has been developed for genome-wide studies in large populations. This marker set is selected to detect or be in disequilibrium with most of the common SNPs that occur in the human genome. Common SNPs are defined as those occurring at a frequency of ≥ 5 percent.[92–94] Furthermore, common SNPs are thought to be the major genetic variants accounting for human variation and predisposition to disease.[92]

Because the phenotype of these diseases is not inherited as a mendelian disorder, pedigrees cannot map the chromosomal location of the genes. The techniques currently available to map the chromosomal location of these genes using 500,000 markers require high throughput phenotyping and genotyping of a sample size of several thousand individuals. Furthermore, it is recognized that such analysis must be replicated in at least one independent population to avoid false positives. This density of markers (every 6000 bp) using the association approach involves phenotyping unrelated individuals to compare affecteds with controls. An analysis is performed to detect associations between the phenotype and DNA markers (SNPs). Using 500,000 markers, one can expect 2500 associations by chance alone with a p value of 0.05 or 500 with a p value at 0.01 or 50 at 0.001. To avoid false positives, it is preferable to have a larger second population, so one can select a more stringent p value. It is reasonable to design the study to detect genes that impart an increased risk of ≥ 1.3.[95] However, the sample size required is large (Table 9–7). It requires 14,000 to detect a

TABLE 9–7

Sample Size Required to Detect Genes for Coronary Artery Disease Using the 550,000 Single Nucleotide Polymorphisms Set

Minor allele frequency	≥ 5%
Increased risk (odds ratio)	≥ 1.3
Size effect difference controls vs. cases	≥ 0.2
Sample size	
Controls	5,000
Cases	9,000

difference between controls and affecteds of ≥ 0.2 and alleles with a minor allele frequency ≥ 5 percent. Ideally, the analysis should be performed in at least two separate populations. The initial population of 2000 (1000 affecteds and 1000 controls) is genotyped with the 500,000 marker set. This population is then analyzed for markers that show a significant association with the phenotype. Markers showing an association ($p = 0.01$) in the initial population are genotyped in a second independent population of 12,000 (8000 affected and 4000 controls or evenly divided). A more stringent p valve such as .001 is recommended to analyze the second population. This provides 90 percent power to detect genetic variants that impart a risk of 1.3 or greater. It may be helpful and necessary to genotype additional SNPs in the second population in the region of SNPs showing an association in the previous population to detect the actual causative gene. This method is referred to as the *indirect case control association approach*. This is an unbiased approach without any prior assumptions to identify genetic variants that contribute as little as 5 percent to the overall phenotype. These studies are now possible and it is expected that several such studies will soon be pursued to unravel the genetic variants of many common polygenic disorders such as CAD, hypertension, obesity, and diabetes. One such study underway is the Ottawa Heart Genomic Study[95] in Canada to identify genes responsible for CAD. It is expected that most of the SNPs relating to CAD will be identified and properly characterized within the next 10 years. This will generate the requisite information to provide personalized medicine in the next era.

Identification of genes for CAD has been pursued using the candidate gene approach. Using this method sequences a known gene (suspected candidate) in individuals with the disease and compares it to the sequence in controls. This is referred to as the *direct association approach*. Although many polymorphisms have been identified, because of the sample size and the lack of replication in an independent population, none have been confirmed to be reliable for clinical application.[93,94] Attempts to perform genome-wide scans have been inadequate because of the use of 50,000 to 100,000 markers, as opposed to the hundreds of thousands of markers required, and an inadequate sample size. The populations genotyped have generally been several hundred as opposed to the several thousand required.[93] The genome-wide approach has until recently been limited because of lack of high throughput genotyping and the inadequate number of markers.

[ ] OTHER APPROACHES: SIB-PAIR ANALYSIS AND TRANSMISSION DISEQUILIBRIUM TEST

The principle behind the sib-pair technique of genome-wide search is based on the likelihood of sharing a susceptibility allele between the two relatives with the phenotype. For example, two sibs with the disease are expected to share the susceptibility allele more often than by chance alone. Sib-pair analysis is often performed in more than 300 sib-pairs. Several variations of this approach, such as transmission disequilibrium test (TDT), have been developed and applied to complex traits. These techniques use the principle of LD to map the location of the susceptibility gene. LD indicates that two DNA markers that are located in close proximity in the genome are more likely to cosegregate than by chance alone. Techniques based on LD are independent from incomplete penetrance, false positive phenotype, genetic heterogeneity, and the high frequency of the disease-related allele. According to the principle of LD, for example, in sib-pairs linkage analysis it is expected that the affected sibs will share the disease-related allele more often

than expected by chance alone. Sib-pair linkage analysis is best suited for mapping genes that denote a high genotype-related risk (approximately >4). It is not considered a powerful technique to map the susceptibility genes that confer modest risk for a complex trait, such as CAD. The TDT approach is considered more powerful in mapping the susceptibility genes that confer a modest genotype-related risk. TDT examines transmission of a particular allele from heterozygous parents to their offspring. An affected offspring is more likely to inherit the disease-related phenotype from a heterozygous parent than by chance alone (50 percent per random inheritance) or as compared to the unaffected offspring. Several other variations of these allele-sharing approaches are available and used to map susceptibility genes for complex traits. The genome-wide scan approach with the 500,000 marker set to identify associations with the phenotype will likely be the most productive method for the immediate future in identifying genes responsible for common complex cardiovascular diseases.

REFERENCES

1. Hattori M, Fujiyama A, et al. The DNA sequence of the human chromosome 21. *Nature* 2000;405:311–319.
2. Bartel DP. MicroRNAs: genomics, biogenesis, mechanism and function. *Cell* 2004;116:281–297.
3. Kai-How Farh K, et al. The widespread impact of mammalian microRNAs on mRNA repression and evolution. *Science* 2005;310:1817–1820.
4. Henikoff S, Furuyama T, Ahmad K. Histone variants, nucleosome assembly and epigenetic inheritance. *Trends Genet* 2004;20:320–326.
5. Khorasanizadeh S. The Nucleosome: from genomic organization to genomic regulation. *Cell* 2004;116:259–272.
6. Marian AJ. Genetic risk factors for myocardial infarction. *Curr Open Cardiol* 1998;13:171–178.
7. Schunkert H, Dzau VJ, Tank SS, Hirsch AT, Apstein C, Lorrell BH. Increased rat cardiac angiotensin converting enzyme activity and mRNA levels in pressure overload left ventricular hypertrophy: Effects on coronary resistance, contractility and relaxation. *J Clin Invest* 1990;86:1913–1920.
8. Collins FS. Shattuck lecture: medical and societal consequences of the human genome project. *N Engl J Med* 1999;341(1):28–37.
9. Department of Health & Human Services, Department of Energy. Understanding our genetic inheritance: the U.S. Human Genome Project, 1990.
10. Katsanis N, Worley KC, Lupski JR. An evaluation of the draft human genome sequence. *Nat Genet* September 2001;29(1):88–91.
11. Murray JC, Buetow KH, Weber JL, et al. A comprehensive human linkage map with centimorgan density: Cooperative Human Linkage Center (CHLC). *Science* September 1994;265(5181):2049–2054.
12. Fraser C, Norris S, Weinstock G, et al. Complete genome sequence of treponema pallidum, the syphilis spirochete. *Science* 1999;281:375–388.
13. Hodgkin J, Horowitz RS, Jasny BR, Kimble J. *C. Elegans*: sequence to biology. *Science* December 1998;282:2011.
14. Gollob MH, Jones DL, Krahn AD, et al. Somatic mutations in the connexin 40 gene (GJA5) in atrial fibrillation. *N Engl J Med* June 2006;354(25):2677–2688.
15. Eriksson M, Brown WT, Gordon LB, et al. Recurrent de novo point mutations in lamin: a cause Hutchinson-Gilford progeria syndrome. *Nature* 2003;423(6937):293–298.
16. Baldini A. DiGeorge syndrome: an update. *Curr Opin Cardiol* 2004;19(3):201–204.
17. Ainsworth C. Nonsense mutations: running the red light. *Nature* 2005;438:726–728.
18. Alter J, Rabinowitz A, Yin H, et al. Systemic delivery of morpholino oligonucleotide restores dystrophin expression bodywide and improves dystrophic pathology. *Nat Med* 2006;12:175–177.
19. Ramirez F, Dietz HC. Therapy insight: aortic aneurysm and dissection in Marfan's syndrome. *Nat Clin Pract Cardiovasc Med* 2004;1(1):31–36.
20. Boileau C, et al. Molecular genetics of Marfan syndrome. *Curr Opin Cardiol* 2006;20(3):194–200.
21. Halushka MK, Fan J-B, Bentley K, et al. Patterns of single-nucleotide polymorphisms in candidate genes for blood-pressure homeostasis. *Nat Genet* 1999;22:239–247.

22. Frigola J, Song J, Stirzaker C, Hinshelwood RA, Peinado MA, Clark SJ. Epigenetic remodeling in colorectal cancer results in coordinate gene suppression across an entire chromosome band. *Nat Genet* May 2006;38(5):540–549.

23. van Steensel B, Henikoff S. Epigenomic profiling using microarrays. *Biotechniques* 2006;35(2):346–357.

24. Tardiff J. Sarcomeric proteins and familial hypertrophic cardiomyopathy: linking mutations in structural proteins to complex cardiovascular phenotypes. *Heart Fail Rev* September 2005;10(3):237–248.

25. Backs J, Olson EN. Control of cardiac growth by histone acetylation/deacetylation. *Circ Res* January 2006;98(1):15–24.

26. Kong Y, Tannous P, Lu G, et al. Suppression of class I and II histone deacetylases blunts pressure-overload cardiac hypertrophy. *Circulation* June 2006;113(22):2579–2588.

27. Backs J, Olson EN. Control of cardiac growth by histone acetylation/deacetylation. *Circ Res* 2006;98(1):15–24.

28. Bushby K, Goodship J, Nicholson LV, Johnson MA, Haggerty I, Gardner-Medwin D. Variability in clinical, genetic and protein abnormalities in manifesting carriers of Duchenne and Becker muscular dystrophy. *Neuromuscul Disord* 1993;3(1):57–64.

29. Kruglyak L. Prospects for whole-genome linkage disequilibrium mapping of common disease genes. *Nat Genet* 1999;22:139–44.

30. Bradley A. Commentary: mining the mouse genome. *Nature* 2002;420:512–514.

31. Okazaki Y, Furuno M, Kasukawa T, et al. Analysis of the mouse transcriptome based on functional annotation of 60,770 full-length cDNAs. *Nature* 2002;420:563–573.

32. Boguski MS. The mouse that roared. *Nature* 2002;420:515–516.

33. Pennacchio LA, Rubin EM. Comparative genomic tools and databases: providing insights into the human genome. *J Clin Invest* 2003;111(8):1099–1106.

34. Roberts R. Genomics and its application to cardiovascular disease. In: Runge MS, Patterson C, eds. *Principles for Molecular Cardiology.* Totowa, NJ: Humana Press, 2005:45–55.

35. The International HapMap Consortium. The International HapMap Project. *Science* 2003;426:789–796.

36. The International HapMap Consortium. A haplotype map of the human genome. *Nature* October 2005;437(7063):1299–1320.

37. ENCODE Project Consortium. The ENCODE (Encyclopedia of DNA Elements) Project. *Science* 2004;306:636–640.

38. Brent MR. Genome annotation past, present, and future: How to define an ORF at each locus. *Genome Res* December 2005;15(12):1777–1786.

39. Botstein D, White RL, Skolnick M, Davis RW. Construction of a genetic linkage map in man using restriction fragment length polymorphisms. *Am J Hum Genet* 1980;32:314–331.

40. Gertler M, White PD. *Coronary Heart Disease in Young Adults: A Multidisciplinary Study.* Cambridge, Mass.: Harvard University Press, 1954.

41. Thomas CB, Cohen BH. The familial occurrence of hypertension and coronary artery disease, with observations concerning obesity and diabetes. *Ann Intern Med* 1955;42:90–127.

42. Rose GC. Familial patterns in ischaemic heart disease. *Br J Prev Soc Med* 1964;(18):75–80.

43. Slack J, Evans KA. The increased risk of death from ischaemic heart disease in first-degree relatives of 121 men and 96 women with ischaemic heart disease. *J Med Genet* 2004;3:239–257.

44. Rissanen A. Familial occurrence of coronary heart disease: effect of age at diagnosis. *Am J Cardiol* 1979;44:60–66.

45. Hamsten A, de Faire U. Risk Factors for coronary artery disease in families of young men with myocardial infarction. *Am J Cardiol* 1987;59:14–19.

46. ten Kate LP, Boman H, Daiger SP, et al. Familial aggregation of coronary heart disease and its relation to known genetic risk factors. *Am J Cardiol* 1982;50:945–953.

47. Sholtz RI, Rosenman RH, Brand RJ. The relationship of reported parental history to the incidence of coronary heart disease in the Western Collaborative Group Study. *Am J Epidemiol* 1975;102:350–356.

48. Colditz GA, Rimm EB, Giovannucci E, et al. A prospective study of parental history of myocardial infarction and coronary artery disease in men. *Am J Cardiol* 1991;67:933–938.

49. Barrett-Connor E, Khaw K. Family history of heart attack as an independent predictor of death due to cardiovascular disease. *Circulation* 1984;69(6):1065–1069.

50. Colditz GA, Stampfer MJ, Willett WC, et al. A prospective study of parental history of myocardial infarction and coronary heart disease in women. *Am J Epidemiol* 1986;123:48–58.

51. Schildkraut JM, Myers RM, Cupples LA, et al. Coronary risk associated with age and sex of parental heart disease in the Framingham Study. *Am J Cardiol* 1989;64:555–559.

52. Phillips AN, Sharper AG, Pocock SJ, et al. Parental death from heart disease and the risk of heart attack. *Eur Heart J* 1988;9:243–251.

53. Hopkins PN, Williams RR, Kuida H, et al. Family history as an independent risk factor for incident coronary artery disease in a high-risk cohort in Utah. *Am J Cardiol* 1988;62:703–707.

54. Adlersberg D, Parets AD, Boas EP. Genetics of atherosclerosis: studies of families with xanthoma and unselected patients with coronary artery disease under the age of fifty years. *JAMA* 1949;141–246.

55. Blumenthal S, Jesse MJ, Hennekens CH, et al. Risk factors for coronary artery disease in children of affected families. *J Pediatr* 1975;87:1187–1192.

56. Rissanen A, Nikkila EA. Identification of the high-risk groups in familial coronary heart disease. *Br Heart J* 1977;(39):875.

57. Hamby RI. Hereditary aspects of coronary artery disease. *Am Heart J* 1981;101:639–649.

58. Berg KA, Dahlen G, Borresen AL. Lp(a) phenotypes, other lipoprotein parameters and a family history of coronary heart disease in middle-aged males. *Clin Genet* 2004;16:347–352.

59. Becker DM, Becker L, Pearson TA, et al. Risk factors in siblings of people with premature coronary heart disease. *J Am Coll Cardiol* 2004;12(1273):1280.

60. Rosengren A, Wilhelmsen L, Eriksson E, et al. Lipoprotein (a) and coronary heart disease: a prospective case-control study in a general population sample of middle aged men. *Br Med J* 2004;301:1248–1251.

61. Anderson AJ, Loeffler RF, Barboriak JJ, et al. Occlusive coronary artery disease and parental history of myocardial infarction. *Prev Med* 1979;8:419–428.

62. Falconer DS. The inheritance of liability to certain diseases estimated from the incidence among relatives. *Ann Hum Genet* 1965;29:51–71.

63. Allen G, Harvald B, Shields JP. Measures of twin concordance. *Acta Genet Stat Med* 1967;1775–1781.

64. Hunt SC, Gwinn M, Adams TD. Family history assessment: strategies for prevention of cardiovascular disease. *Am J Prev Med* February 2003;24(2):136–142.

65. Yusuf S, Hawken S, Ounpuu S, et al. INTERHEART Study Investigators. *Lancet* 2004;364:937–952.

66. Cooper JA, Miller GJ, Humphries SE. A comparison of the PROCAM and Framingham point-scoring systems for estimation of individual risk of coronary heart disease in the Second Northwick Park Heart Study. *Atherosclerosis* July 2005;181(1):93–100.

67. Krushkal J, Xiong M, Ferrell RE, et al. Linkage and association of adrenergic and dopamine receptor genes in the distal portion of the long arm of chromosome 5 with systolic blood pressure variation. *Hum Mol Genet* 2005;7:1379–1383.

68. Frossard P, Lestringant GG, Malloy MJ, et al. Human renin gene BglI dimorphism associated with hypertension in two independent populations. *Clin Genet* 1999;56:428–433.

69. Heinonen P, Koulu M, Pesonen U, et al. Identification of a three-amino acid deletion in the alpha2B-adrenergic receptor that is associated with reduced basal metabolic rate in obese subjects. *J Clin Endocrinol Metab* 1999;84:2429–2433.

70. Large V, Hellstrom L, Reynisdottir S, et al. Human beta-2 adrenoceptor gene polymorphisms are highly frequent in obesity and associate with altered adipocyte beta-2 adrenoceptor function. *J Clin Inv* 1997;100:3005–3013.

71. Nagase T, Aoki A, Yamamoto M, et al. Lack of association between the Trp64 Arg mutation in the beta 3-adrenergic receptor gene and obesity in Japanese men: a longitudinal analysis. *J Clin Endocrinol Metab* 1997;82:1284–1287.

72. Mitchell BD, Blangero J, Comuzzie AG, et al. A paired sibling analysis of the beta-3 adrenergic receptor and obesity in Mexican Americans. *J Clin Inv* 1998;101:584–587.

73. Sina M, Hinney A, Ziegler A, et al. Phenotypes in three pedigrees with autosomal dominant obesity caused by haploinsufficiency mutations in the melanocortin-4 receptor gene. *Am J Hum Genet* 2005;65:1501–1507.

74. Ristow M, Muller-Wieland D, Pfeiffer A, et al. Obesity associated with a mutation in a genetic regulator of adipocyte differentiation. *N Engl J Med* 1998;339:953–959.

75. Walder K, Norman RA, Hanson RL, et al. Association between uncoupling protein polymorphisms (UCP2-UCP3) and energy metabolism/obesity in Pima Indians. *Hum Mol Genet* 1998;7:1431–1435.

76. Horikawa Y, Oda N, Cox NJ, et al. Genetic variation in the gene encoding calpain-10 is associated with type 2 diabetes mellitus. *Nat Genet* 2000;26:163–175.

77. Stone LM, Kahn SE, Fujimoto WY, et al. A variation at position -30 of the beta-cell glucokinase gene promoter is associated with reduced beta-cell function in middle-aged Japanese-American men. *Diabetes* 2005;45:422–428.

78. Vinik A, Bell G. Mutant insulin syndromes. *Horm Metab Res* 1988;20:1–10.

79. Hart LM, Stolk RP, Dekker JM, et al. Prevalence of variants in candidate genes for type 2 diabetes mellitus in The Netherlands: the Rotterdam study and the Hoorn study. *J Clin Endocrinol Metab* 1999;84:1002–1006.

80. Reis A, Ye W-Z, Dubois-Laforgue D, et al. Association of a variant in exon 31 of the sulfonylurea receptor 1 (SUR1) gene with type 2 diabetes mellitus in French Caucasians. *Hum Genet* 2000;107:138–144.

81. Altshuler D, Hirschhorn JN, Klannemark M, et al. The common PPAR-gamma Pro12Ala polymorphism is associated with decreased risk of type 2 diabetes. *Nat Genet* 2000;26:76–80.

82. Souto JC, Almasy L, Borrell M, et al. Genetic susceptibility to thrombosis and its relationship to physiological risk factors: the GAIT study—Genetic analysis of idiopathic thrombophilia. *Am J Hum Genet* 2005;67:1452–1459.

83. Pajukanta P, Lilja HE, Sinsheimer JS, Cantor RM, Lusis AJ, et al. Familial combined hyperlipidemia is associated with upstream transcription factor 1 (USF1). *Am J Hum Genet* 2005;67:1481–1493.

84. Wang Q, Rao S, Shen G-Q, Li L, Moliterno DJ. Premature myocardial infarction novel susceptibility locus on chromosome 1P34–36 identified by genomewide linkage analysis. *Am J Hum Genet* 2004;74:262–271.

85. Broeckel U, Hengstenberg C, Mayer B, et al. A comprehensive linkage analysis for myocardial infarction and its related risk factors. *Nat Genet* 2002;30:210–214.

86. Wang L, Fan C, Topol SE. Mutation of MEF2A in an inherited disorder with features of coronary artery disease. *Science* 2003;302:1578–1581.

87. Helgadottir A, Manolescu A, Helgason A, et al. A variant of the gene encoding leukotriene A4 hydrolase confers ethnicity-specific risk of myocardial infarction. *Nat Genet* 2006;38(1):68–74.

88. American Heart Association. *Heart and Stroke Statistical Update: 2000.* Dallas: American Heart Association, 2000.

89. Lloyd-Jones DM, Larson MR, Beiser A, et al. Lifetime risk of developing coronary heart disease. *Lancet* 1999;353:89–92.

90. Nora JJ, Lortshcher RH, Spangler RD, et al. Genetic—epidemiologic study of early-onset ischemic heart disease. *Circulation* 1980;61(3):503–508.

91. Dressel R, Walter L, Gunther E. Genomic and functional aspects of the rat MHC, the RT1 complex. *Immunol Rev* December 2001;184:82–95.

92. Hinds DA, Stuve LL, Nilsen GB, Halperin E, Eskin E, Ballinger DG, et al. Whole-Genome Patterns of Common DNA Variation in Three Human Populations. *Science* 2005;307:1072–9.

93. Hirshhorn JN, Daly MJ. Genome-wide association studies for common diseases and complex traits. *Nature* 2005;6:95–108.

94. Wang WY, Barratt B, Clayton DG, Todd JA. Genome-wide association studies: theoretical and practical concerns. *Nature* 2005;6:109–118.

95. Roberts R., Stewart AFR. Personalized medicine, a prerequisite for the prevention of coronary artery disease and its sequelae. *Am Heart Hosp J* 2006;5:167–175.

CHAPTER (10)

Tissue Regeneration of the Cardiovascular System and Stem Cells

Arjun Deb / Helmut Drexler / Victor Dzau

Despite great advances in the therapy of cardiovascular diseases within the last several decades, ischemic heart disease and congestive heart failure continue to lead the causes of mortality and morbidity in the Western hemisphere.[1] Myocyte loss as well as structural and functional abnormalities of the myocyte are observed in the syndrome of congestive heart failure, regardless of its etiology.[2] Although much molecular cardiology over the last two decades was devoted to understanding myocyte abnormalities in heart failure, only recently has regenerative heart therapy emerged as an exciting therapeutic modality.[3] Unlike hearts of lower animals such as newts or zebrafish,[4] which regenerate completely following injury, the human heart has been traditionally considered a terminally differentiated organ incapable of regeneration.[5] This traditional line of thinking has been challenged recently by observations in animals and humans of the existence of cardiac[6,7] and extracardiac progenitor cells capable of forming cardiomyocytes, and endothelial as well as smooth muscle cells.[8–14] Such observations have engendered clinical trials of stem cell therapy aimed at regenerating the heart following acute myocardial infarction (MI) and in chronic left ventricular (LV) failure.[15]

This chapter provides a brief overview of the emerging field of cardiac regenerative therapy. We first discuss the scientific basis for cardiac regenerative therapy; examine the types of stem cells used, mechanisms of action, and mode of delivery; address safety concerns; review clinical trials of cardiac cell therapy; and finally summarize the questions that confront the future of this rapidly developing field.

SCIENTIFIC BASIS OF CARDIAC REGENERATIVE THERAPY

The concept of the heart as a terminally differentiated organ incapable of replacing myocytes has been an accepted paradigm over the last 50 years.[3] However, several lines of evidence from animal and human studies have emerged over the last few years to challenge this existing paradigm. A number of experimental studies in animals supported the possibility of stem cell-based cardiac regeneration. Orlic and coworkers demonstrated that bone marrow cells injected into the infarcted mouse heart regenerated infarcted myocardium and led to improvement in cardiac function.[8] More recently, Beltrami and colleagues identified a resident cardiac progenitor cell capable of differentiating into cardiomyocyte, endothelial, and smooth muscle lineages.[6] Injection of these cells into the injured heart leads to regeneration of functioning myocardium and improvement in cardiac function. Studies in human subjects support the aforementioned experimental observations. The presence of Y chromosome–positive cardiomyocytes in female hearts transplanted into male recipients directly point to the presence of putative progenitors capable of de novo cardiomyocyte formation (Fig. 10–1A and B).[11,14] Furthermore, the presence of chimeric cardiomyocytes, albeit at low numbers, in hearts of patients who underwent gender-mismatched bone marrow transplantation strongly suggested the existence of bone marrow progenitors capable of contributing to cardiomyocyte formation in the adult human heart (Fig. 10–1C).[10] Taken together, a large body

of experimental evidence suggests the existence of progenitors capable of cardiomyocyte formation in postnatal life. Although these observations challenge the concept of the heart as a postmitotic organ, cardiac regeneration with complete restoration of cardiac function following injury does not occur in higher mammals, including man. Several strategies have evolved to assist the postnatal heart in regenerating its damaged cells following injury.[2] These have included strategies to force existing cardiomyocytes to override cell cycle checkpoints and re-enter cell cycle,[16] stimulate angiogenesis by delivery of angiogenic cytokines or cells capable of forming new blood vessels,[17,18] and deliver exogenous progenitor cells that help in cardiac repair[19] or are capable of forming cardiac muscle itself.[6] Regenerative therapy of the heart has so far primarily involved the latter two strategies, namely the use of cytokines or progenitor cells for cardiac repair.

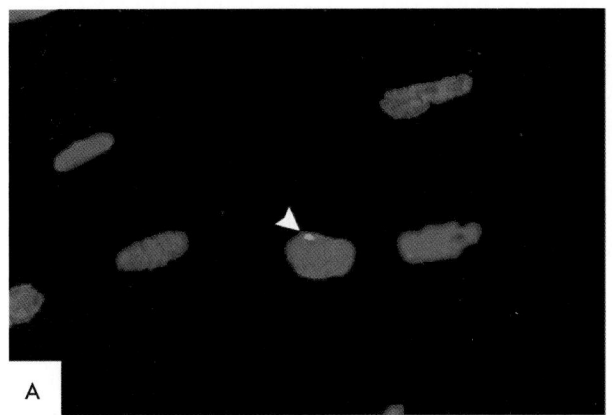

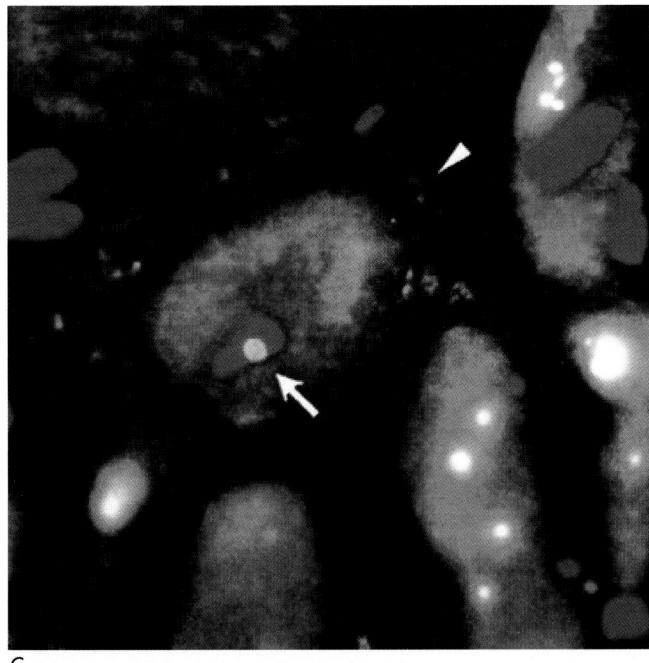

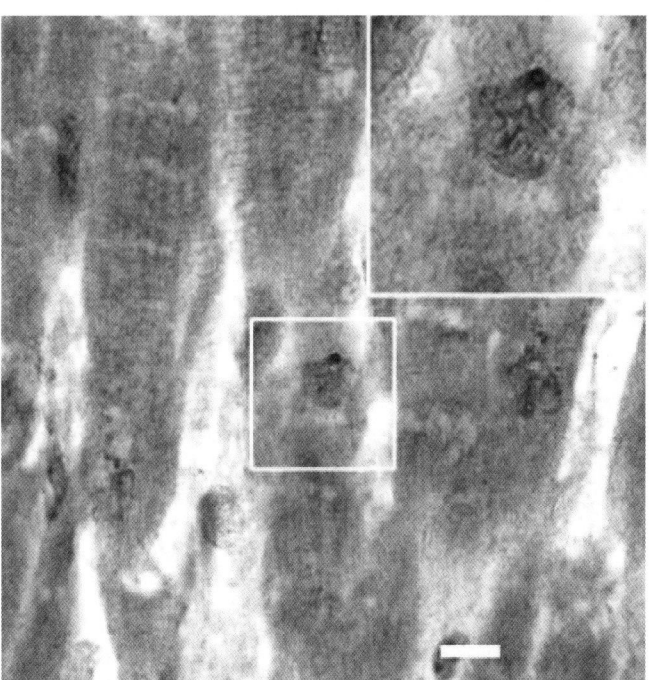

FIGURE 10–1. Cardiomyocyte chimerism in humans. Y chromosome–positive cardiomyocyte (*arrowhead*, **A**) (*red dot*, **B**) in a male patient who underwent gender-mismatched cardiac transplantation (**A,B**). Y chromosome–positive cardiomyocyte (*arrow*, **C**) present in a female patient who underwent gender-mismatched bone marrow transplantation (**C**). *Source: From Quaini F, Urbanek K, Beltrami AP, et al[14]; Laflamme MA, Myerson D, Saffitz JE, Murry CE[11]; Deb A, Wang S, Skelding KA, et al.[10]*

TYPES OF CELLS USED FOR CARDIAC REGENERATION AND REPAIR

【 】 EMBRYONIC STEM CELLS

Embryonic stem (ES) cells are derived from the inner cell mass of the blastocyst, can be propagated indefinitely in an undifferentiated state, and are pluripotent capable of differentiating into tissues belonging to the three germ layers.[20] In culture, they spontaneously form cystic structures known as *embryoid bodies* that contain foci of beating cardiomyocytes. However, owing to their pluripotent nature, when injected into the heart, ES cells differentiate into undesirable tissue lineages and give rise to teratomas. Thus, much research in the use of ES cells for cardiac regeneration has focused on strategies to direct differentiation into a particular cell type as well as enhance the yield of isolation of ES cell–derived cardiomyocyte. Various chemicals and molecules have been used to enhance cardiomyogenic differentiation of ES cells including retinoic acid,[21] ascorbic acid,[22] transforming growth factor,[23] bone morphogenetic proteins[24] or their antagonist noggin,[25] and members of the Wnt[26] family of proteins. Although cardiomyogenic differentiation was substantially increased with the use of such a variety of chemicals and proteins, a universal recipe for efficient and large-scale regeneration of cardiomyocytes from ES cells is still elusive.[5] Klug and coworkers were the first to pioneer a genetic selection strategy to enhance isolation of cardiomyocytes from ES cells. Using a selection marker driven by a cardiac promoter, Klug and coworkers reported a highly purified population of ES cell–derived cardiomyocytes.[27] Furthermore, injection of cardiomyocytes derived by the aforementioned strategy stably engrafted into hearts of immunocompromised animals. Since this observation, other groups have also reported successfully improved cardiac function by stable engraftment of ES cells that seemed to integrate functionally into the recipient myocardium[28–30] and not generate teratomas.[31] More recently, human ES cell–derived cardiomyocytes have been shown to successfully engraft and electromechanically integrate when injected into uninjured hearts of immunosuppressed animals.[32–34] In these studies the injected cells behaved as a biological pacemaker and electrically excited the rest of the ventricle. Although these early studies generate enthusiasm and provide important proof of concept data for generation of biological pacemakers, the field is still in its infancy and plagued with problems of large scale generation of ES cell-derived cardiomyocytes, immunologic rejection, differentiation into undesirable lineages, and finally ethical concerns. Nevertheless, these pluripotent cells still remain an attractive and powerful tool for cardiac regenerative therapy (Table 10–1).

【 】 SKELETAL MYOBLASTS

Skeletal myoblasts were the first cells to be tried for cell based cardiac therapy. Skeletal myoblasts are already committed towards a myogenic fate and do not form tumors as with embryonic stem cells.[35–37] Moreover, they can be easily handled and expanded in vitro (millions of myoblasts can be grown from a single muscle biopsy within a relatively short time).[15] Myoblasts following injection into the infarcted heart have been shown to exhibit long-term engraftment. However, skeletal myoblasts do not adopt a cardio-

TABLE 10–1

Types of Stem Cells and Their Current Applications for Cardiac Cell Therapy

TYPE	ANIMAL/CLINICAL TRIALS
Embryonic stem cell	Animal study only
Skeletal myoblasts	Clinical study
Whole bone marrow cell	Clinical study
Bone marrow mononuclear cell	Clinical study
Mesenchymal stem cell	Clinical study
CD34+ stem cells	Clinical study
CD133+ stem cell	Clinical study
Peripheral blood derived progenitor	Clinical study
Endothelial progenitor cell	Clinical study
Resident cardiac progenitor	Animal study only
Bone marrow–derived MAPC	Animal study only

MAPC, multipotent adult progenitor cell.

myogenic differentiation program but adopt a skeletal muscle fate following injection into the heart.[38] Moreover, they lack gap junctions, have not been shown to integrate electromechanically with the surrounding myocardium, and current data suggests that they do not beat in synchrony and are isolated from the rest of the myocardium.[39,40] Nevertheless, studies with injection of skeletal myoblasts into the infarcted heart demonstrate an improvement in cardiac function. Although the precise mechanisms of benefit are unclear, it is thought that myoblasts ameliorate the adverse consequences of postinfarction ventricular remodeling.[41] This is supported by observations showing decreased ventricular chamber size following myoblast injection.[41] Clinical trials of myoblast therapy are already underway and have shown improvements in ejection fraction that persist 10 months following injection.[42] However, most trials of skeletal myoblast therapy have not been randomized or placebo controlled, and a definitive conclusion approximately the efficacy of myoblast therapy is still unclear. Ventricular tachycardia early on following skeletal myoblast implantation has been an additional concern of skeletal myoblast therapy.[43] Although the heart after MI is prone to ventricular arrhythmias and the cause-and-effect relationship of injected myoblasts and arrhythmias is not definitive, current trials of myoblast therapy are using implantable defibrillators as a safety net.

【 】 BONE MARROW CELLS

Ferrari and colleagues[44] first reported the generation of skeletal muscle from bone marrow cells in mice. Since this initial observation, several groups of investigators have studied the ability of bone marrow cells to regenerate cardiomyocytes. It is important to appreciate that the bone marrow contains a varied assortment of progenitor cells including hematopoietic stem cells; mesenchymal stem cells; multipotent adult progenitor cells (considered a subset of mesenchymal stem cells); and side population cells, which are characterized by their ability to rapidly efflux Hoechst dye. Multiple reports suggested that bone marrow progenitor cells could transdifferentiate, cross lineage boundaries, and differentiate into tissues belonging to all three germ line lineages. For instance, several reports suggested the ability of bone marrow cells to generate neurons, endothelium, skeletal muscle, and even cardiomyocytes.[45–47] This newly discovered plasticity of bone marrow progenitor cells generated immense excitement in the clinical and scientific cardiovascular community for purposes of regenerative therapy. Bittner and coworkers[48] published one of the first reports demonstrating the presence of Y chromosome–positive cardiomyocytes in female dystrophin mutant mice transplanted with bone marrow from wild-type male mice. Subsequently, Jackson and colleagues demonstrated that bone marrow–derived side population cells, a fraction enriched in hematopoietic stem cells, contributed to cardiomyocyte formation in the infarcted mouse heart, albeit at a very low degree.[9] Interestingly, the degree of endothelial chimerism was 100-fold higher than that of cardiomyocyte formation. Analysis in patients undergoing gender mismatched bone marrow and cardiac transplantation also demonstrated endothelial and myocardial chimerism.[10,11,14,49] These preliminary studies in animal models and human subjects set the stage for injecting bone marrow cells into the post-infarct heart to determine the ability of these cells to regenerate the injured heart. Orlic and colleagues in a pioneering study, reported that an enriched population of bone marrow hematopoietic progenitors (linc-kit+) following injection into the infarcted heart regenerated 68 percent of the myocardium.[50] This robust regeneration of myocardium improved echocardiographic and hemodynamic indices of LV function. More recently, another group has reported cardiomyocyte regeneration using a non hematopoietic bone marrow population of cells.[51] However, other groups of investigators have failed to reproduce these promising results.[52,53] Whether bone marrow cells can regenerate cardiomyocytes in the infarcted heart is currently unsettled. Nevertheless, irrespective of the mechanism, bone marrow progenitor cells evidently improve cardiac performance following myocardial injury. These promising experiments have led to the design of clinical trials of bone marrow cell therapy in patients of MI.

MESENCHYMAL STEM CELLS

Mesenchymal stem cells (MSCs) reside in the stromal component of the bone marrow and are also known as *stromal cells*. They lack typical hematopoietic cell surface markers such as CD34 and CD45; and they can be coaxed to differentiate into a number of tissues including bone, cartilage, adipose, and skeletal muscle.[54] Several reports suggested that these cells could be induced to differentiate into beating cardiomyocytes in vitro and kindled interest in using these cells for cardiac regenerative therapy.[55] MSCs possess several unique properties that confer on them several advantages as cell therapy agents. They do not elicit a robust host immune response, a property that might allow them to survive in an allogeneic transplantation setting.[56] Moreover, systemically injected MSCs possess a natural ability to home to the injured heart, whereas in the absence of injury they home to the bone marrow.[57] A number of studies suggest the salutary effects of injecting MSCs into the postinfarct heart. Direct injection of MSCs into the infarcted rat and pig hearts improved ventricular function.[58,59] Injection of genetically labeled MSCs into infarcted mouse hearts demonstrated a small percentage of MSC derived cardiomyocytes but improved cardiac performance.[60] MSCs do not appear to integrate electromechanically with the recipient myocardium but do exert

beneficial effects on postinfarct ventricular remodeling. Mangi and coworkers also demonstrated dramatic reduction of infarct size when MSCs overexpressing the prosurvival gene Akt are injected into rodent hearts at the time of MI.[19] Interestingly, MSCs appear to exert their cytoprotective effects through paracrine mechanisms because injection of MSC–conditioned medium into infarcted rodent hearts yields similar degrees of myocardial protection.[61] Currently, it seems that MSCs likely exert their beneficial effects through panoply of mechanisms pertaining to myocardial protection, ventricular remodeling, angiogenesis, and possibly myocyte regeneration. Several other groups of investigators have isolated other rare progenitors from the stromal component of the bone marrow that have differentiated both in vivo and in vitro to cardiomyocytes.[51] The immunotolerant properties of mesenchymal stem cells, ease of handling, and ability to home to injured myocardium following systemic delivery have made them attractive tools for cardiac regenerative therapy.

RESIDENT CARDIAC PROGENITOR CELL

The concept of the heart as a static organ incapable of turnover or regeneration was challenged by several groups of investigators, who described a cardiac progenitor cell capable of multilineage differentiation. Beltrami[6] and coworkers were the first to describe the existence of a resident cardiac progenitor cell (CPC) capable of differentiating into myocytes as well as endothelial and smooth muscle cells. The c-kit+ CPC isolated by Beltrami and colleagues from the adult rat heart and was demonstrated to be self-renewing, clonogenic, and multipotent. In the presence of specialized differentiating medium, c-kit+ cells differentiated into cardiomyocyte like cells bearing myocyte-specific structural proteins. Furthermore, injection of clonogenic c-kit+ cells into the infarcted rodent heart resulted in multilineage differentiation of these cells into myocytes, endothelial, smooth muscle cells, and improved ventricular performance. Intracoronary injection of c-kit+ cells following ischemia-reperfusion injury also resulted in improved myocardial performance, diminished scar formation and new myocyte regeneration independent of cell fusion. C-kit+ cells have also been isolated from human myocardial biopsy specimens as well and demonstrated to differentiate into functional cardiomyocytes after injection into immunocompromised mice.[62] Since then, other investigators have reported the existence of CPCs identified by other stem cell markers such as Sca-1, Isl-1, and ABC transport protein. Oh and coworkers demonstrated that a Sca-1 population of cells isolated from the adult mouse heart when treated with azacytidine expressed cardiac-specific genes, and following injection into the infarcted mouse heart they improved cardiac function by de novo cardiomyocyte formation as well as fusion with existing cardiomyocytes in roughly equal proportions.[7] Laugwitz and colleagues demonstrated that cells possessing the LIM homeodomain transcription factor Isl-1, isolated from neonatal mouse hearts, could rapidly differentiate into beating cardiomyocytes persistently expressing mature cardiac specific proteins and generating action potentials.[63] However, Isl-1 cells are rare in the adult heart and the functional significance and the role of these cells in cardiac homeostasis are not entirely clear. Currently, it is unclear whether there are biological differences in CPCs bearing different stem cell markers. Nevertheless, most populations of resident cardiac progenitor cells have improved cardiac function following injection into the postinfarct heart. Importantly, the multilineage differentiation capacity of these cells into endothelial and smooth muscle cells represent an important advantage as regenerating myocytes need blood vessels for survival and effective functioning.

ENDOTHELIAL PROGENITOR CELLS

Asahara and coworkers first described the existence of circulating endothelial progenitor cells in humans.[64] They isolated CD34+ cells from human peripheral blood and demonstrated that under specific conditions the proliferating cells displayed endothelial cell–like properties in vitro and incorporated into neovasculature when injected into ischemic hind limbs of mice and rabbits. Since the last decade, the field of endothelial progenitor biology has rapidly expanded. Several groups of investigators have consistently demonstrated that these cells help in formation of de novo blood vessels and lead to improvement in blood flow of ischemic regions. Like hematopoietic stem cells, they can be mobilized into the peripheral circulation with the use of cytokines and have been shown to home to ischemic regions in party mediated by stromal cell-derived factor and CXCR4 signaling.[65] The number as well as function of endothelial progenitors is impaired in conditions such as diabetes and coronary artery disease.[66] Endothelial progenitors have now been used in several clinical trials of MI and hind limb ischemia. Although very few trials have been randomized and placebo controlled, the cells appear to be safe and therapeutic outcomes are promising. Myocardial blood flow, wall motion abnormalities, ejection fraction, and even chamber dimensions seemed to improve following administration of endothelial progenitors derived from autologous bone marrow or peripheral blood.[67] In some reports an increase in exercise time and decreased number of anginal episodes was noted following cell therapy. Interestingly, these cells also appear to secrete angiogenic cytokines like vascular endothelial growth factor, hepatocyte growth factor, and granulocyte colony-stimulating factor (G-CSF).[68] It is unclear whether endothelial progenitors exert their effects by direct incorporation into new vessels or through paracrine signaling. It is likely that the pleiotropic salutary effects of endothelial progenitors are secondary to a combination of paracrine signaling and direct incorporation into de novo blood vessels.

MECHANISMS OF ACTION OF STEM CELLS IN CARDIAC REGENERATION AND REPAIR

Although multiple experimental animal models and several clinical trials of cell based cardiac therapy have shown promising results, the mechanisms of such cell mediated benefit are rather unclear. As illustrated in Fig. 10–2, stem cells could act via several potential mechanisms, which then could dictate specific functional benefits. It is also likely that a type of stem cell could exert more than one mechanism of action. Undoubtedly, interplay between the diseased condition, microenvironment and type of stem cell ultimately determines functional benefits. The following section discusses some potential mechanisms mediating beneficial effects of stem cell therapy on the heart.

DIFFERENTIATION

Stem cells depending on their lineage commitment possess the ability to differentiate into cells of various tissues. Embryonic cells are pluripotent, can generate tissues belonging to all three germ layers, and can differentiate and electromechanically integrate with existing cardiomyocytes in animals. Adult stem cells are thought to be more committed and possess a limited ability to differentiate along a specific lineage. In contrast to embryonic stem cells, differentiation of adult bone marrow stem cells into functional cardiomyocytes has been more difficult to demonstrate and fraught with controversy.[69] However, several groups of investigators have demonstrated that resident cardiac progenitors are capable of adopting a cardiomyogenic fate both in vitro and in vivo.[62] Bone marrow and peripheral blood-derived endothelial progenitor cells have also been shown to differentiate into functioning endothelium, incorporate into new blood vessels, and lead to improvement in blood flow. The signaling mechanisms determining differentiation of adult stem cells into cardiomyocytes or endothelial cells are a subject of intense research.

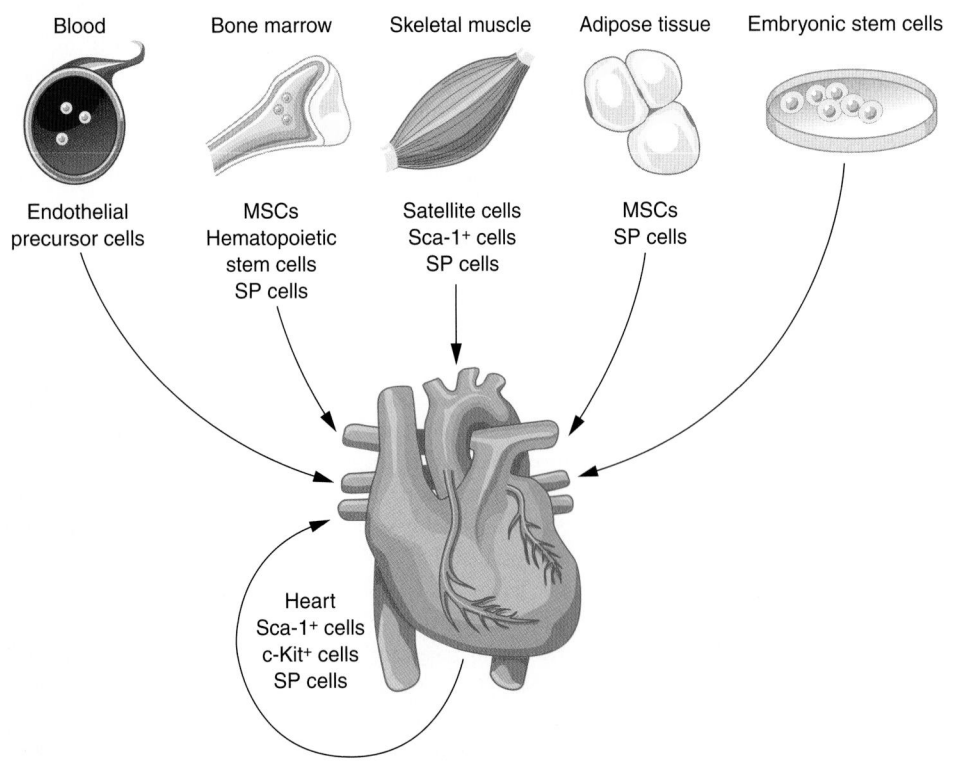

Blood — Endothelial precursor cells

Bone marrow — MSCs Hematopoietic stem cells SP cells

Skeletal muscle — Satellite cells Sca-1+ cells SP cells

Adipose tissue — MSCs SP cells

Embryonic stem cells

Heart Sca-1+ cells c-Kit+ cells SP cells

FIGURE 10–2. Sources of cells for cardiac stem cell therapy. MSC, mesenchymal stem cell; SP, side population. *Source: Adapted from Dimmeler S, Zeiher AM, Schneider MD.[2]*

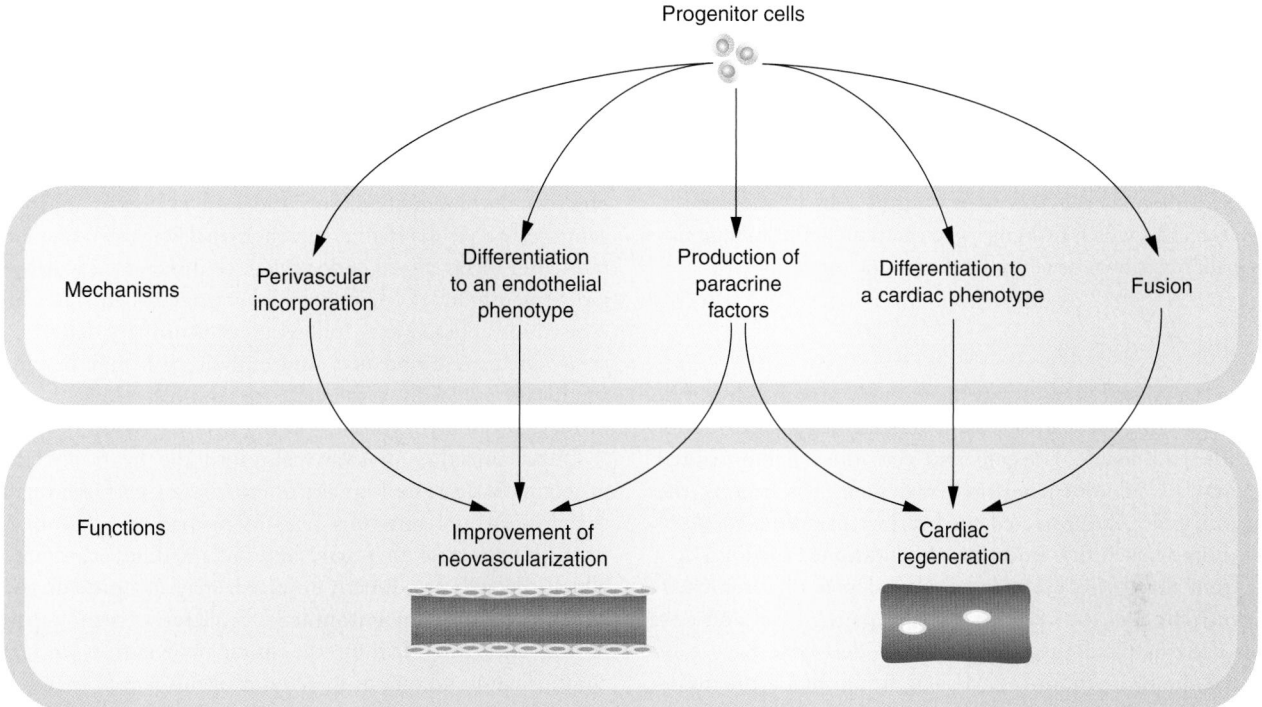

FIGURE 10–3. Mechanisms of action. Progenitor cells may improve functional recovery of infarcted or failing myocardium by various potential mechanisms, including direct or indirect improvement of neovascularization. Paracrine factors released by progenitor cells may inhibit cardiac apoptosis, affect remodeling, or enhance endogenous repair (e.g., by tissue-resident progenitor cells). Differentiation into cardiomyocytes may contribute to cardiac regeneration. The extent to which these different mechanisms are active may critically depend on the cell type and setting, such as acute or chronic injury. *Source: From Dimmeler S, Zeiher AM, Schneider MD.[2]*

Resident cardiac progenitors possess hepatocyte growth factor and insulin growth factor receptors and the corresponding ligands have been shown to play important roles in cardiac progenitor cell migration, proliferation and survival.[70] High mobility group box 1 protein, a chromatin protein released by inflammatory and necrotic cells has been shown to regenerate myocytes after MI by inducing resident cardiac progenitor cells to proliferate and differentiate[71] (Fig. 10–3). Enzymes controlling chromatin remodeling such as histone deacetylases have been shown to regulate commitment of endothelial progenitors to mature endothelial cells.[72] Undoubtedly, discovery of signaling pathways regulating differentiation of a stem cell along a particular tissue lineage will hold great therapeutic promise for enhancing regeneration of target tissue.

▌ ▐ TRANSDIFFERENTIATION

Transdifferentiation is a term used to define a committed stem cell crossing lineage boundaries and differentiating into cells belonging to another lineage. For instance, a hematopoietic stem cell giving rise to daughter blood cells would be an example of differentiation, whereas giving rise to cardiomyocytes would be an example of transdifferentiation.[5] Transdifferentiation in vivo is still a matter of great debate. Orlic and colleagues demonstrated that a Linc-Kit+ fraction of bone marrow cells generated 68 percent of the myocardium following MI in mice.[50] These findings have been challenged by other investigators, who report that Linc-Kit+ cells adopt a hematopoietic fate following injection into the infarcted heart and do not differentiate into cardiomyocytes. Rigorous criteria have been postulated to demonstrate unequivocally the phe-

nomenon of transdifferentiation, including definitive identification of transdifferentiated cells with expression of donor- and tissue-specific markers, anatomic and functional integration into target tissue, using a clonal population of cells and excluding cell fusion.[73] Nevertheless, bone marrow–derived progenitor cells can be reprogrammed to express cardiac specific genes in vitro, and endothelial progenitor cells can differentiate in vitro into a cardiomyogenic phenotype when cocultured with cardiomyocytes.[2] It is currently unclear the extent to which such observed plasticity of stem cells plays a role in cardiac regeneration in vivo.

▌ ▐ FUSION

Fusion refers to the phenomenon where stem cells fuse with somatic cells; the resultant hybrid cells usually assume the more undifferentiated phenotype but possess some characteristics of both cell types. Terada and colleagues demonstrated that bone marrow cells, when grown in culture with embryonic stem cells, could fuse with embryonic stem cells and adopt the recipient phenotype.[74] Bone marrow–derived cells have been shown to correct a mouse model of tyrosinemia by regenerating hepatocytes through cell fusion. Mice deficient in the enzyme fumarylacetoacetate hydrolase had correction of the tyrosinemic phenotype on transplantation with bone marrow from wild-type mice. It was subsequently shown that donor bone marrow cells regenerated functionally normal hepatocytes following cell fusion with existing hepatocytes.[75] Similarly, Alvarez-Dolado and coworkers demonstrated that bone marrow cells fuse with cardiomyocytes with the fused hybrid cells being virtually indistinguishable from unfused cardiomyocytes, even at the electron microscopy level.[76] The frequency of fusion noted in this study was comparable to the frequency of chimeric cardiomyocytes noted in animal and human transplantation studies raising the possibility that fusion could be a principal mechanism for the formation of bone marrow–derived cardiomyocytes.[5] Nygren and colleagues also demonstrated that circulating cells fused with cardiomyocytes at the infarct border zone.[77] However, fusion of cardiomyocytes and bone marrow cells is uncommon, and the extent to which fusion in vivo can reprogram somatic nuclei to yield functional benefit is currently unclear.

【 】 PARACRINE

Over the last several years, it has increasingly become clear that through paracrine mechanisms stem cells can regulate tissue regeneration and repair. Gnecchi and coworkers demonstrated that genetically modified mesenchymal stem cells bearing the prosurvival gene Akt protected the heart by paracrine effects.[61] The authors showed that injection of conditioned medium collected from these cells exerted the same degree of cytoprotection as injection of the cells. In a recent paper, Fazel and colleagues demonstrated that bone marrow–derived c-Kit+ cells populated the heart following MI and established a proangiogenic milieu by increasing vascular endothelial growth factor and reversing the cardiac ratio of angiopoietin-1 and -2.[78] Changes in local cytokines brought approximately by these cells were critical for endothelial mitogenesis and proper wound repair. Mice harboring a mutant c-Kit receptor did not mobilize bone marrow cells to the heart, had poor myofibroblast rich tissue, and underwent rapid cardiac dilatation and death. Apart from angiogenesis and wound healing, stem cells could exert a host of other paracrine effects on myocardial protection, cardiac contractility, myogenic differentiation of resident cardiac progenitors, and scar formation. Urbich and coworkers have demonstrated that soluble factors secreted by endothelial progenitor cells mediate migration of both endothelial and resident cardiac progenitor cells.[79] It is currently unclear whether a single factor or a combination of specific factors can recapitulate the beneficial effects of cell injection in MI. Discovery of such key stem cell paracrine factors would have several advantages over cell therapy including lack of immunologic response following injection, easier dose titration, and ready availability.

ROUTES OF ADMINISTRATION

Clinical trials of stem cell therapy so far have administered cells via the intracoronary route, or by direct injection into the myocardium using a percutaneous catheter-based or surgical epicardial approach. Trials using the intracoronary approach have administered the cells in the culprit artery from 5 to 14 days following MI.[80] Direct intracoronary injection following revascularization has the obvious advantage of the cells reaching previously underperfused regions of the myocardium. Potentially, the perfused myocardium also creates a more suitable environment for engraftment of the progenitor cells. A favorable environment for successful engraftment will likely enhance the reparative actions of these cells.[2] Conversely, less perfused regions

of the myocardium receive fewer cells; thus this route may be inefficient for successful targeting of underperfused myocardium, an important consideration for patients with extensive microvascular disease. The type of stem cell administered is another important consideration for selecting the best route of administration. Skeletal myoblasts are larger cells and may even obstruct the microcirculation and lead to greater injury. A recent study that compared mesenchymal stem cell engraftment rates after intravenous, endocardial, or intracoronary delivery in a porcine model of MI noted higher engraftment rates but decreased distal blood flow following intracoronary delivery.[81] Decrease in distal blood flow and embolic risk may be clinically significant especially if the cells are administered at the time of primary revascularization following MI.

Direct injection of stem cells into the heart obviates the problems of decreased uptake of cells in less perfused regions of the myocardium but runs risks of cardiac perforation. Moreover, the necrotic, hypoxic, and inflamed myocardium, into which the cells are directly injected, may not provide the cells with the best microenvironment for effective tissue repair. Potential cues provided by the microenvironment influencing commitment and fate of injected progenitor cells may be aberrant in inflamed and necrotic tissue. In fact, clinical trials of cardiac cell therapy suggest that injection of stem cells at least 4 days following myocardial injury leads to improvement in ejection fraction compared to earlier injection.[2] Electromechanical mapping of viable but *stunned* myocardium has been suggested as a promising tool to determine preferred sites for direct intramyocardial injection of stem cells. Finally, focal injection of stem cells may not be the optimal route in diseases that affect the myocardium more globally such as nonischemic dilated cardiomyopathy. Systemic mobilization of bone marrow stem cells with the use of G-CSF has been tested in several small trials of acute MI.[80] However, the safety of this approach has been questioned with the observed increase in incidence of restenosis.[82] It is likely that the undermining cause of ventricular dysfunction, clinical condition, and type of cell to be administered will eventually determine the optimal mode of delivery of stem cells to the heart.

SAFETY CONCERNS

With increasing numbers of clinical trials and types of stem cells being used, safety is a major concern.[10] Trials of cardiac stem cell therapy for the heart have been safe so far, but the long-term safety of stem cell therapy is far from proven. The following section discusses concerns that have risen from both animal and human studies.

Injection of skeletal myoblasts has been associated with increased incidence of ventricular arrhythmias in a number of human studies.[43] The precise reason for this adverse effect is not understood but is thought to arise from lack of electromechanical coupling between myoblasts and host cardiomyocytes.[39,40] Other factors that could potentially enhance arrhythmogenesis in this setting include injury from cell delivery itself, nerve sprouting, and the inherent arrhythmogenic substrate of the failing heart.[15,83] Technical factors such as growth medium for myoblasts during culture could be important, too, because culture of myoblasts in bovine serum-free medium prevented the occurrence of arrhythmias.[84] Ventricular arrhythmias have also been reported with other types of cells including bone marrow mononuclear cells[80] and CD133+ cells.[85] Dangerous occurrences of potentially lethal arrhythmias with cell therapy have necessitated the use of implantable cardioverter-defibrillators particularly in human skeletal myoblast injection trials.

Endothelial progenitor cells could contribute to de novo vasculogenesis in the postinfarcted heart but have also been shown to worsen angiogenesis-induced plaque growth in animal models of atherosclerosis.[86] Conceivably, harmful angiogenesis could increase plaque burden as well as instability and lead to plaque rupture in patients with coronary artery disease. Such lessons learned from animal models of stem cell therapy may warrant long-term monitoring of plaque growth, especially in patients with coronary artery disease. In this respect, a high proportion of de novo lesions have been found in non-revascularized vessels following stem cell transplantation in humans.[87] Close angiographic followup determines the long-term significance of these observations on plaque growth.

Stem cells administered systemically seed to multiple organs including the heart, liver, spleen, and brain.[88,89] Animal studies show a low percentage of stem cell homing to the heart, which has also been confirmed in human subjects.[90] Seeding of cells to other organs may have unforeseen consequences. For instance, endothelial progenitor cells are known to participate in tumor angiogenesis and a CD133-positive tumor stem cell has been isolated from medulloblastoma tumor.[91] Tumor-enhancing properties of stem cells are concerning, especially when they are used in patients with known malignancy. Close follow up in a wide variety of patients over an extended duration of time determines the risks associated with multiorgan seeding of administered stem cells.

Intracoronary administration of mesenchymal stem cells in dogs has been associated with microinfarctions.[92] Decreases in distal coronary flow were noted in porcine hearts that received intracoronary mesenchymal stem cells. Studies in human subjects have not corroborated the decreases in microvascular flow seen in animal models. Apart from concerns about microvascular perfusion, restenosis has emerged as another potential problem. Cytokines such as G-CSF have been used in clinical trials on the premise that mobilization of bone marrow stem cells to the peripheral blood could help in cardiac repair or regeneration. However unexpectedly high rates of in-stent restenosis have been observed in several clinical trials using G-CSF.[82] It is difficult to determine causality based on the design of the studies, but elevation of white cell counts could have potentially contributed to plaque growth.[2]

Aberrant differentiation of injected stem cells into undesirable lineages is a concern observed in animal studies. Use of more undifferentiated pluripotent embryonic cells has been associated with teratoma formation in animal models. Intracardiac injection of unselected whole bone marrow mononuclear cells in one study led to significant intramyocardial calcification.[93] Potentially, bone marrow cell–derived myocardial calcification in human subjects could lead to conduction disturbances, arrhythmias, or adversely affect contractile function.

Although clinical trials of stem cell therapy have looked promising, the lack of understanding of precise mechanisms of benefit is another cause of concern. Failure to properly understand mechanisms of stem cell action may impede fine tuning of therapy and yield deleterious and unexpected results that could significantly set back the field as was the case with gene therapy.[94]

CLINICAL TRIALS OF CELL-BASED CARDIAC THERAPY

Clinical trials of cell-based cardiac therapy have been broadly carried out on 2 different sets of patients, one with acute MI and another with chronic LV dysfunction secondary to chronic coronary artery disease. Tables 10–2 and 10–3 summarize the salient features of the clinical trials to date.[80] Interpretation of trials has been difficult because most of them have been uncontrolled and not randomized. Moreover, differences in trial design pertaining to the type of cell used, the underlying clinical status, mode, timing of delivery of cells and methods of measuring outcome have contributed to the lack of a clear consensus about the efficacy of cardiac cell therapy. Strauer[95] and colleagues first reported the delivery of bone marrow mononuclear cells via the intra coronary route in 10 patients within 5 to 9 days of MI and observed an improvement in regional wall motion and perfusion compared to controls who refused cell infusion therapy. Assmus and coworkers[67] injected unfractionated bone marrow mononuclear cells or peripheral blood-derived progenitors into the culprit vessel 4 days after MI and observed a significant improvement (over 4 months of follow up) in ejection fraction in both the cell-injected groups compared to controls. Improvements were also noted in myocardial perfusion, coronary flow reserve, and glucose uptake. More recently, this group has reported that the improvement of LV function and absence of hypertrophy was evident even a year out, suggesting a sustained benefit on ventricular remodeling.[96] The BOOST[97] trial was the first randomized trial of bone marrow cell therapy for the heart and included 60 patients; half of the patients received intracoronary infusion of unfractionated mononuclear cells within approximately 6 days of MI. The control group comprising 30 patients did not receive sham marrow aspiration or cell infusion. After 6 months of follow up, cardiac MRI demonstrated a significant increase in ejection fraction compared to controls. In another randomized study, Chen and colleagues delivered mesenchymal stem cells via the intracoronary route on an average of 18 days following MI.[98] The control group comprised 35 patients who underwent bone marrow aspiration but received only saline infusion. The investigators reported a significant improvement in ejection fraction in cell-treated group associated with improved wall motion, increased fluorodeoxyglucose uptake, and improved end systolic and diastolic volumes. However, in a randomized, double blind, placebo-controlled trial, Janssens and coworkers did not note any significant improvement in ejection fraction at 4 months when patients were injected with autologous bone marrow cells within 24 hours of successful reperfusion.[99]

Trials of cardiac cell therapy have also been performed in patients with chronic LV dysfunction secondary to coronary artery

TABLE 10–2

Clinical Trials of Stem Cell Therapy in Acute Myocardial Infarction

STUDY	N	TREATMENT (AND ROUTE)	DOSE[a]	TIMING	IMPROVED	NO CHANGE	COMPLICATIONS
Strauer et al[95]	10 treated 10 controls	MNC (IC)	$2.8 \pm 2.2 \times 10^7$	5–9 d	Regional wall motion; infarct size; perfusion LVEDV	EF	Not observed
Assmus et al[67]	29 MNC 30 CPC 11 controls	MNC (IC) CPC (IC)	$2.1 \pm 0.8 \times 10^8$ $1.6 \pm 1.2 \times 10^7$	5 ± 2 d	Regional wall motion; EF; infarct size; coronary flow	LVEDV	2 patients presented with reinfarction
Fernández-Aviles et al[87]	20 treated 13 controls	MNC (IC)	$7.8 \pm 4.1 \times 10^7$	14 ± 6 d	Regional wall motion; EF	LVEDV	1 patient presented with TIA
Kuethe et al[103]	5 treated	MNC (IC)	$3.9 \pm 2.3 \times 10^7$	6 d	NA	Regional wall motion; EF	Not observed
Obradovic et al[98] Wollert[97]	4 treated 30 treated 30 controls	MNC (IC) NC (IC)	NA $2.5 \pm 0.9 \times 10^9$	3–5 d 6 ± 1 d	EF; perfusion Regional wall motion; EF	NA LVEDV; EF	Not observed Not observed
Chen et al[104]	34 treated 35 controls	MSC (IC)	$4.8 \pm 6.0 \times 10^{10}$	18 d	Regional wall motion; EF; infarct size; LVEDV	NA	Not observed
Katritis et al[105]	11 treated 11 controls	MSC + EPC (IC)	$1\text{–}2 \times 10^6$	8–1,560 d	Regional wall motion; viability in infarct area	LVEDV; EF	Not observed
Bartunek et al[85]	19 treated 16 controls	CD133+ (IC)	$12.6 \pm 2.2 \times 10^6$	12 ± 1 d	Regional wall motion; EF; perfusion	LVEDV	Atherosclerosis progression;[b] VT in 2 patients
Kang et al[82]	7 G-CSF +CPC 3 G-CSF 1 control	CPC (IC) G-CSF (SC)	$1.5 \pm 0.5 \times 10^9$ 10 µg/kg body wt daily for 4 d	3–270 d	EF; perfusion in the group with cell infusion	NA	7 patients presented in-stent restenosis

CPC, circulating blood-derived progenitor cell; EF, ejection fraction; EPC, bone marrow–derived endothelial progenitor cell; G-CSF, granulocyte colony-stimulating factor; IC, intracoronary; LVEF, left ventricular ejection fraction; LVEDV, left ventricular end-diastolic volume; MI, myocardial infarction; MNC, bone-marrow-derived mononuclear cell; MSC, bone marrow–derived mesenchymal stem cells; NA, not applicable; NC, bone mar-row–derived nucleated cells; PCI, percutaneous coronary intervention; SC, subcutaneous; TIA, transitory ischemic attack; VT, ventricular tachycardia; wt, weight.

[a]Number of cells, or amount of substance given.

[b]Two patients developed in-stent reocclusion, seven developed in-stent restenosis, and two developed significant de novo lesions of the infarct-related artery.

SOURCE: *Adapted from Sanchez PL, San Roman JA, Villa A, Fernandez ME, Fernandez-Aviles F.[80]*

● TABLE 10-3

Clinical Trials of Stem Cell Therapy in Chronic Myocardial Ischemia

STUDY	N	EF (%)	CELL TYPE (AND ROUTE)	DOSE (NUMBER OF CELLS)	IMPROVED	NO CHANGE	COMPLICATIONS
Hamano et al[106]	5 treated	NA	MNC (transepicardial, during CABG)	$0.3-2.2 \times 10^9$	Perfusion	NA	Not observed
Tse et al[100]	8 treated	58 ± 11	MNC (transendocardial, guided by EMM)	$11.7 \pm 6.7 \times 10^6$	Symptoms; perfusion; regional wall motion	EF	Not observed
Fuchs et al[101]	10 treated	47 ± 10	NC (transendocardial, guided by EMM)	$7.8 \pm 6.6 \times 10^9$	Symptoms; perfusion	EF; treadmill exercise	Not observed
Perin et al[102]	14 treated 7 controls	30 ± 6	MNC (transendocardial, guided by EMM)	$3.0 \pm 0.4 \times 10^7$	Symptoms; perfusion; EF; regional wall motion; LVEDV	NA	1 sudden cardiac death

CABG, coronary artery bypass grafting; EF, ejection fraction; EMM, electromechanical mapping; LVEDV, left ventricular end-diastolic volume; IC, intracoronary; MI, myocardial infarction; MNC, bone-marrow-derived mononuclear cells; NA, not applicable; NC, bone-marrow-derived nucleated cells.

Source: Adapted from Sanchez PL, San Roman JA, Villa A, Fernandez ME, Fernandez-Aviles F.[80]

disease. Initial efforts mainly consisted of injection of skeletal myoblasts during coronary artery bypass surgery. Although an improvement in ejection fraction was noted in most of these studies, there was an increased incidence of ventricular arrhythmias. Current trials of skeletal myoblast injection require concomitant placement of an implantable defibrillator. Bone marrow cell therapy has been also tried in patients with chronic ischemic ventricular dysfunction. In these trials subjects underwent electromechanical mapping to determine optimal sites for injection of cells into the LV myocardium.[100–102] An improvement in symptoms, exercise score, as well as perfusion abnormalities was noted. Although these initial pilot studies have been greeted with great enthusiasm by the clinical community, they are still preliminary to draw definite conclusions about the effectiveness of cardiac cell therapy for chronic ischemic cardiomyopathy. Multiple randomized trials of myoblast and bone marrow cell injection are currently underway to determine clearly the efficacy of cardiac cell therapy for chronic ischemic cardiomyopathy.

Cardiac cell therapy trials have differed from each other in a number of variables including the clinical scenario of patients included in the trial, type of stem cell injected, mode of delivery, and predefined end points. Nevertheless, there are several messages to take from these early trials of cardiac cell therapy. First, bone marrow cell therapy appears to be safe and feasible in acute MI as well as chronic ischemic conditions, whereas the same cannot be concluded about myoblast injection. Trials administering mesenchymal stem cells are still early for reaching definitive con-

clusions about safety. Second, bone marrow cell therapy both for acute MI and chronic ischemic dysfunction has yielded promising results. Most studies demonstrate an improvement in ejection fraction and improved perfusion in the infarcted region. However, the effect appears not to be dose dependent with no clear association between dose of cells injected and degree of observed benefit. Third, the best cell population to be injected is still unclear in spite of the many trials. Clearly, this depends on the underlying disease and the mechanistic underpinnings of LV dysfunction. Finally, multiple, randomized, large, double-blinded, placebo-controlled trials with clearly measurable predefined therapeutic end points are necessary to prove unequivocal clinical benefit including improved survival.

UNANSWERED QUESTIONS AND THE FUTURE OF CARDIAC STEM CELL THERAPY

Cardiovascular stem cell therapy has become one of the most fascinating and intriguing fields of study in cardiovascular biology. Given the promising scientific findings, early results of clinical trials, and unmet clinical needs, cardiac cell therapy is rapidly translated from the bench to the bedside.[69] As with any new scientific field, there are more questions than answers. Beyond safety and feasibility, which the early trials demonstrate, rudimentary but critical questions about patient selection, cell selection, timing of therapy, and efficacy of repeated therapies still remain unanswered.

TABLE 10–4

Critical Determinants of Successful Cardiac Stem Cell Therapy

BENCH	BEDSIDE
EMERGING EVIDENCE	
Animal models suggest bone marrow cells improve myocardial function	Improved cardiac function in acute and chronic myocardial dysfunction following therapy with bone marrow and circulating progenitor cells
CONTROVERSIES	
Mechanisms of improvement	Nature of studies
Transdifferentiation	Uncontrolled
Angiogenesis	Unblinded
Paracrine factors or cell survival factors	Small numbers
Cell fusion	Mechanisms unclear
Endogenous progenitor recruitment	
FUTURE DIRECTIONS	
Animal models to address mechanisms	Large, placebo-controlled, double-blinded trials
Genetically marked donor or recipient cells	Development of mobilization factors, involve pharmaceutical industry
Experiments to address cell mobilization, recruitment, and survival	Standard isolation and delivery protocols for widespread clinical use
Comparative cell studies for efficacy	Strict safety criteria with monitoring for arrhythmias, aberrant angiogenesis, plaque growth, thrombosis, restenosis, oncogenic transformation, distant organ-seeding events
Identification of specific cell mobilization and recruitment factors for pharmacologic therapy	

Source: Adapted from Caplice NM, Deb A.[93]

Whether cardiac cell therapy will be effective in nonischemic causes of ventricular dysfunction is another important yet unaddressed question. Inability to comprehend basic mechanisms of benefit has been another stumbling block. Undoubtedly, in the near future these are the important questions for the clinical and scientific community to address for translating the promise of stem cells into effective therapy (Table 10–4).[93]

REFERENCES

1. Srivastava D, Ivey KN. Potential of stem-cell-based therapies for heart disease. *Nature* 2006;441(7097):1097–1099.
2. Dimmeler S, Zeiher AM, Schneider MD. Unchain my heart: the scientific foundations of cardiac repair. *J Clin Invest* 2005;115(3):572–583.
3. Leri A, Kajstura J, Anversa P. Cardiac stem cells and mechanisms of myocardial regeneration. *Physiol Rev* 2005;85(4):1373–1416.
4. Poss KD, Wilson LG, Keating MT. Heart regeneration in zebrafish. *Science* 2002;298(5601):2188–2190.
5. Laflamme MA, Murry CE. Regenerating the heart. *Nat Biotech* 2005;23(7):845–856.
6. Beltrami AP, Barlucchi L, Torella D, et al. Adult cardiac stem cells are multipotent and support myocardial regeneration. *Cell* 2003;114(6):763–776.
7. Oh H, Bradfute SB, Gallardo TD, et al. Cardiac progenitor cells from adult myocardium: homing, differentiation, and fusion after infarction. *Proc Natl Acad Sci U S A* 2003;100(21):12313–12318.
8. Orlic D, Kajstura J, Chimenti S, et al. Bone marrow cells regenerate infarcted myocardium. *Nature* 2001;410(6829):701–705.
9. Jackson KA, Majka SM, Wang H, et al. Regeneration of ischemic cardiac muscle and vascular endothelium by adult stem cells. *J Clin Invest* 2001;107(11):1395–1402.
10. Deb A, Wang S, Skelding KA, et al. Bone marrow-derived cardiomyocytes are present in adult human heart: A study of gender-mismatched bone marrow transplantation patients. *Circulation* 2003;107(9):1247–1249.
11. Laflamme MA, Myerson D, Saffitz JE, Murry CE. Evidence for cardiomyocyte repopulation by extracardiac progenitors in transplanted human hearts. *Circ Res* 2002;90(6):634–640.
12. Minami E, Laflamme MA, Saffitz JE, Murry CE. Extracardiac progenitor cells repopulate most major cell types in the transplanted human heart. *Circulation* 2005;112(19):2951–2958.
13. Muller P, Pfeiffer P, Koglin J, et al. Cardiomyocytes of noncardiac origin in myocardial biopsies of human transplanted hearts. *Circulation* 2002;106(1):31–35.
14. Quaini F, Urbanek K, Beltrami AP, et al. Chimerism of the transplanted heart. *N Engl J Med* 2002;346(1):5–15.
15. Murry CE, Field LJ, Menasche P. Cell-based cardiac repair: reflections at the 10-year point. *Circulation* 2005;112(20):3174–3183.
16. Pasumarthi KB, Nakajima H, Nakajima HO, Soonpaa MH, Field LJ. Targeted expression of cyclin D2 results in cardiomyocyte DNA synthesis and infarct regression in transgenic mice. *Circ Res* 2005;96(1):110–118.
17. Losordo DW, Dimmeler S. Therapeutic angiogenesis and vasculogenesis for ischemic disease: part II—cell-based therapies. *Circulation* 2004;109(22):2692–2697.
18. Losordo DW, Dimmeler S. Therapeutic angiogenesis and vasculogenesis for ischemic disease: part I—angiogenic cytokines. *Circulation* 2004;109(21):2487–2491.
19. Mangi AA, Noiseux N, Kong D, et al. Mesenchymal stem cells modified with Akt prevent remodeling and restore performance of infarcted hearts. *Nat Med* 2003;9(9):1195–1201.
20. Amit M, Carpenter MK, Inokuma MS, et al. Clonally derived human embryonic stem cell lines maintain pluripotency and proliferative potential for prolonged periods of culture. *Dev Biol* 2000;227(2):271–278.
21. Zandstra PW, Bauwens C, Yin T, et al. Scalable production of embryonic stem cell-derived cardiomyocytes. *Tissue Eng* 2003;9(4):767–778.
22. Wobus AM, Kaomei G, Shan J, et al. Retinoic acid accelerates embryonic stem cell-derived cardiac differentiation and enhances development of ventricular cardiomyocytes. *J Mol Cell Cardiol* 1997;29(6):1525–1539.
23. Behfar A, Zingman LV, Hodgson DM, et al. Stem cell differentiation requires a paracrine pathway in the heart. *FASEB J* 2002;16(12):1558–1566.
24. Rudy-Reil D, Lough J. Avian precardiac endoderm/mesoderm induces cardiac myocyte differentiation in murine embryonic stem cells. *Circ Res* 2004;94(12):e107–e116.

25. Yuasa S, Itabashi Y, Koshimizu U, et al. Transient inhibition of BMP signaling by noggin induces cardiomyocyte differentiation of mouse embryonic stem cells. *Nat Biotechnol* 2005;23(5):607–611.
26. Terami H, Hidaka K, Katsumata T, Iio A, Morisaki T. Wnt11 facilitates embryonic stem cell differentiation to Nkx2.5-positive cardiomyocytes. *Biochem Biophys Res Commun* 2004;325(3):968–975.
27. Klug MG, Soonpaa MH, Koh GY, Field LJ. Genetically selected cardiomyocytes from differentiating embryonic stem cells form stable intracardiac grafts. *J Clin Invest* 1996;98(1):216–224.
28. Etzion S. Influence of embryonic cardiomyocyte transplantation on the progression of heart failure in a rat model of extensive myocardial infarction. *J Mol Cell Cardiol* 2001;33:1321–1330.
29. Min JY. Transplantation of embryonic stem cells improves cardiac function in postinfarcted rats. *J Appl Physiol* 2002;92:288–296.
30. Min JY. Long-term improvement of cardiac function in rats after infarction by transplantation of embryonic stem cells. *J Thorac Cardiovasc Surg* 2003;125:361–369.
31. Hodgson DM, Behfar A, Zingman LV, et al. Stable benefit of embryonic stem cell therapy in myocardial infarction. *Am J Physiol Heart Circ Physiol* 2004;287(2):H471–H479.
32. Kehat I. Human embryonic stem cells can differentiate into myocytes with structural and functional properties of cardiomyocytes. *J Clin Invest* 2001;108:407–414.
33. Kehat I. Electromechanical integration of cardiomyocytes derived from human embryonic stem cells. *Nat Biotechnol* 2004;22:1282–1289.
34. Xue T. Functional integration of electrically active cardiac derivatives from genetically engineered human embryonic stem cells with quiescent recipient ventricular cardiomyocytes: insights into the development of cell-based pacemakers. *Circulation* 2005;111:11–20.
35. Marelli D, Desrosiers C, el-Alfy M, Kao RL, Chiu RC. Cell transplantation for myocardial repair: an experimental approach. *Cell Transplant* 1992;1:383–390.
36. Chiu RC, Zibaitis A, Kao RL. Cellular cardiomyoplasty: Myocardial regeneration with satellite cell implantation. *Ann Thorac Surg* 1995;60:12–18.
37. Taylor DA. Regenerating functional myocardium: improved performance after skeletal myoblast transplantation. *Nat Med* 1998;4:929–933.
38. Reinecke H, Poppa V, Murry CE. Skeletal muscle stem cells do not transdifferentiate into cardiomyocytes after cardiac grafting. *J Mol Cell Cardiol* 2002;34:241–249.
39. Rubart M, Soonpaa MH, Nakajima H, Field LJ. Spontaneous and evoked intracellular calcium transients in donor-derived myocytes following intracardiac myoblast transplantation. *J Clin Invest* 2004;114:775–783.
40. Leobon B. Myoblasts transplanted into rat infarcted myocardium are functionally isolated from their host. *Proc Natl Acad Sci U S A* 2003;100:7808–7811.
41. Jain M. Cell therapy attenuates deleterious ventricular remodeling and improves cardiac performance after myocardial infarction. *Circulation* 2001;103:1920–1927.
42. Murry CE, Field LJ, Menasche P. Cell-based cardiac repair: reflections at the 10-year point. *Circulation* 2005;112(20):3174–3183.
43. Menasche P. Autologous skeletal myoblast transplantation for severe postinfarction left ventricular dysfunction. *J Am Coll Cardiol* 2003;41:1078–1083.
44. Ferrari G. Muscle regeneration by bone marrow-derived myogenic progenitors. *Science* 1998;281:973–1530.
45. Jackson KA. Regeneration of ischemic cardiac muscle and vascular endothelium by adult stem cells. *J Clin Invest* 2001;107:1395–1402.
46. Brazelton TR, Rossi FM, Keshet GI, Blau HM. From marrow to brain: expression of neuronal phenotypes in adult mice. *Science* 2000;290(5497):1775–1779.
47. Majka SM, Jackson KA, Kienstra KA, et al. Distinct progenitor populations in skeletal muscle are bone marrow derived and exhibit different cell fates during vascular regeneration. *J Clin Invest* 2003;111(1):71–79.
48. Bittner RE, Schofer C, Weipoltshammer K, et al. Recruitment of bone-marrow-derived cells by skeletal and cardiac muscle in adult dystrophic Mdx mice. *Anat Embryol (Berl)* 1999;199:391–396.
49. Quaini F. Chimerism of the transplanted heart. *N Engl J Med* 2002;346:5–15.
50. Orlic D, Kajstura J, Chimenti S, Bodine DM, Leri A, Anversa P. Bone marrow cells regenerate infarcted myocardium. *Nature* 2001;410:701–705.
51. Yoon YS, Wecker A, Heyd L, et al. Clonally expanded novel multipotent stem cells from human bone marrow regenerate myocardium after myocardial infarction. *J Clin Invest* 2005;115(2):326–338.
52. Balsam LB. Haematopoietic stem cells adopt mature haematopoietic fates in ischaemic myocardium. *Nature* 2004;428:668–673.
53. Murry CE. Haematopoietic stem cells do not transdifferentiate into cardiac myocytes in myocardial infarcts. *Nature* 2004;428:664–668.

54. Pittenger MF, Martin BJ. Mesenchymal stem cells and their potential as cardiac therapeutics. *Circ Res* 2004;95(1):9–20.

55. Makino S. Cardiomyocytes can be generated from marrow stromal cells in vitro. *J Clin Invest* 1999;103:697–705.

56. El-Badri NS, Maheshwari A, Sanberg PR. Mesenchymal stem cells in autoimmune disease. *Stem Cells Dev* 2004;13:463–472.

57. Bittira B, Shum-Tim D, Al-Khaldi A, Chiu RC. Mobilization and homing of bone marrow stromal cells in myocardial infarction. *Eur J Cardiothorac Surg* 2003;24:393–398.

58. Shake JG. Mesenchymal stem cell implantation in a swine myocardial infarct model: engraftment and functional effects. *Ann Thorac Surg* 2002;73:1919–1925.

59. Ma J. Time course of myocardial stromal cell-derived factor 1 expression and beneficial effects of intravenously administered bone marrow stem cells in rats with experimental myocardial infarction. *Basic Res Cardiol* 2005;100:217–223.

60. Toma C, Pittenger MF, Cahill KS, Byrne BJ, Kessler PD. Human mesenchymal stem cells differentiate to a cardiomyocyte phenotype in the adult murine heart. *Circulation* 2002;105:93–98.

61. Gnecchi M, He H, Liang OD, et al. Paracrine action accounts for marked protection of ischemic heart by Akt-modified mesenchymal stem cells. *Nat Med* 2005;11(4):367–368.

62. Dawn B, Stein AB, Urbanek K, et al. Cardiac stem cells delivered intravascularly traverse the vessel barrier, regenerate infarcted myocardium, and improve cardiac function. *Proc Natl Acad Sci, USA* 2005;102(10):3766–3771.

63. Laugwitz KL, Moretti A, Lam J, et al. Postnatal isl1+ cardioblasts enter fully differentiated cardiomyocyte lineages. *Nature* 2005;433(7026):647–653.

64. Asahara T, Murohara T, Sullivan A, et al. Isolation of putative progenitor endothelial cells for angiogenesis. *Science* 1997;275(5302):964–967.

65. Ceradini DJ. Progenitor cell trafficking is regulated by hypoxic gradients through HIF-1 induction of SDF-1. *Nat Med* 2004;10:858–864.

66. Hill JM, Zalos G, Halcox JP, et al. Circulating endothelial progenitor cells, vascular function, and cardiovascular risk. *N Engl J Med* 2003;348(7):593–600.

67. Assmus B, Schachinger V, Teupe C, et al. Transplantation of Progenitor Cells and Regeneration Enhancement in Acute Myocardial Infarction (TOPCARE-AMI). *Circulation* 2002;106(24):3009–3017.

68. Kinnaird T. Marrow-derived stromal cells express genes encoding a broad spectrum of arteriogenic cytokines and promote in vitro and in vivo arteriogenesis through paracrine mechanisms. *Circ Res* 2004;94:678–685.

69. Chien KR. Stem cells: lost in translation. *Nature* 2004;428(6983):607–608.

70. Urbanek K, Rota M, Cascapera S, et al. Cardiac stem cells possess growth factor-receptor systems that after activation regenerate the infarcted myocardium, improving ventricular function and long-term survival. *Circ Res* 2005;97(7):663–673.

71. Limana F, Germani A, Zacheo A, et al. Exogenous high-mobility group box 1 protein induces myocardial regeneration after infarction via enhanced cardiac C-Kit+ cell proliferation and differentiation. *Circ Res* 2005;97(8):e73–e83.

72. Rossig L, Urbich C, Bruhl T, et al. Histone deacetylase activity is essential for the expression of HoxA9 and for endothelial commitment of progenitor cells. *J Exp Med* 2005;201(11):1825–1835.

73. Wagers AJ, Weissman IL. Plasticity of adult stem cells. *Cell* 2004;116(5):639–648.

74. Terada N, Hamazaki T, Oka M, et al. Bone marrow cells adopt the phenotype of other cells by spontaneous cell fusion. *Nature* 2002;416(6880):542–545.

75. Vassilopoulos G, Wang P-R, Russell DW. Transplanted bone marrow regenerates liver by cell fusion. *Nature* 2003;422(6934):901–904.

76. Alvarez-Dolado M, Pardal R, Garcia-Verdugo JM, et al. Fusion of bone-marrow-derived cells with Purkinje neurons, cardiomyocytes and hepatocytes. *Nature* 2003;425:968–973.

77. Nygren JM, Jovinge S, Breitbach M, et al. Bone marrow-derived hematopoietic cells generate cardiomyocytes at a low frequency through cell fusion, but not transdifferentiation. *Nat Med* 2004;10:494–501.

78. Fazel S, Cimini M, Chen L, et al. Cardioprotective c-kit+ cells are from the bone marrow and regulate the myocardial balance of angiogenic cytokines. *J Clin Invest* 2006;116(7):1865–1877.

79. Urbich C, Aicher A, Heeschen C, et al. Soluble factors released by endothelial progenitor cells promote migration of endothelial cells and cardiac resident progenitor cells. *J Mol Cell Cardiol* 2005;39(5):733–742.

80. Sanchez PL, San Roman JA, Villa A, Fernandez ME, Fernandez-Aviles F. Contemplating the bright future of stem cell therapy for cardiovascular disease. *Nat Clin Pract Cardiovasc Med* 2006;3(suppl 1):S138–S151.

81. Freyman T, Polin G, Osman H, et al. A quantitative, randomized study evaluating three methods of mesenchymal stem cell delivery following myocardial infarction. *Eur Heart J* 2006;27(9):1114–1122.

82. Kang HJ, Kim HS, Zhang SY, et al. Effects of intracoronary infusion of peripheral blood stem-cells mobilised with granulocyte-colony stimulating

factor on left ventricular systolic function and restenosis after coronary stenting in myocardial infarction: the MAGIC cell randomised clinical trial. *Lancet* 2004;363(9411):751–756.

83. Makkar RR, Lill M, Chen PS. Stem cell therapy for myocardial repair: is it arrhythmogenic? *J Am Coll Cardiol* 2003;42(12):2070–2072.

84. Chachques JC, Herreros J, Trainini J, et al. Autologous human serum for cell culture avoids the implantation of cardioverter-defibrillators in cellular cardiomyoplasty. *Int J Cardiol* 2004;95(suppl 1):S29-S33.

85. Bartunek J, Vanderheyden M, Vandekerckhove B, et al. Intracoronary injection of CD133-positive enriched bone marrow progenitor cells promotes cardiac recovery after recent myocardial infarction: feasibility and safety. *Circulation* 2005;112(suppl 9):I178–I183.

86. George J, Afek A, Abashidze A, et al. Transfer of endothelial progenitor and bone marrow cells influences atherosclerotic plaque size and composition in apolipoprotein E knockout mice. *Arterioscler Thromb Vasc Biol* 2005;25(12):2636–2641.

87. Fernandez-Aviles F, San Roman JA, Garcia-Frade J, et al. Experimental and clinical regenerative capability of human bone marrow cells after myocardial infarction. *Circ Res* 2004;95(7):742–748.

88. Aicher A, Brenner W, Zuhayra M, et al. Assessment of the tissue distribution of transplanted human endothelial progenitor cells by radioactive labeling. *Circulation* 2003;107(16):2134–2139.

89. Barbash IM, Chouraqui P, Baron J, et al. Systemic delivery of bone marrow-derived mesenchymal stem cells to the infarcted myocardium: feasibility, cell migration, and body distribution. *Circulation* 2003;108(7):863–868.

90. Hofmann M, Wollert KC, Meyer GP, et al. Monitoring of bone marrow cell homing into the infarcted human myocardium. *Circulation* 2005;111(17):2198–2202.

91. Singh SK, Clarke ID, Terasaki M, et al. Identification of a cancer stem cell in human brain tumors. *Cancer Res* 2003;63(18):5821–5828.

92. Vulliet PR, Greeley M, Halloran SM, MacDonald KA, Kittleson MD. Intracoronary arterial injection of mesenchymal stromal cells and microinfarction in dogs. *Lancet* 2004;363(9411):783–784.

93. Caplice NM, Deb A. Myocardial-cell replacement: the science, the clinic and the future. *Nat Clin Pract Cardiovasc Med* 2004;1(2):90–95.

94. Couzin J, Kaiser J. Gene Therapy. As Gelsinger case ends, gene therapy suffers another blow. *Science* 2005;307(5712):1028.

95. Strauer BE, Brehm M, Zeus T, et al. Repair of infarcted myocardium by autologous intracoronary mononuclear bone marrow cell transplantation in humans. *Circulation* 2002;106(15):1913–1918.

96. Schachinger V, Assmus B, Britten MB, et al. Transplantation of progenitor cells and regeneration enhancement in acute myocardial infarction: final one-year results of the TOPCARE-AMI Trial. *J Am Coll Cardiol* 2004;44(8):1690–1699.

97. Wollert KC. Intracoronary autologous bone-marrow cell transfer after myocardial infarction: the BOOST randomised controlled clinical trial. *Lancet* 2004;364:141–148.

98. Obradovic S, Rusovic S, Balint B, et al. Autologous bone marrow-derived progenitor cell transplantation for myocardial regeneration after acute infarction. *Vojnosanit Pregl* 2004;61(5):519–529.

99. Janssens S, Dubois C, Bogaert J, et al. Autologous bone marrow-derived stem-cell transfer in patients with ST-segment elevation myocardial infarction: double-blind, randomised controlled trial. *Lancet* 367(9505):113–121.

100. Tse HF, Kwong YL, Chan JK, et al. Angiogenesis in ischaemic myocardium by intramyocardial autologous bone marrow mononuclear cell implantation. *Lancet* 2003;361(9351):47–49.

101. Fuchs S, Satler LF, Kornowski R, et al. Catheter-based autologous bone marrow myocardial injection in no-option patients with advanced coronary artery disease: a feasibility study. *J Am Coll Cardiol* 2003;41(10):1721–1724.

102. Perin EC, Dohmann HF, Borojevic R, et al. Improved exercise capacity and ischemia 6 and 12 months after transendocardial injection of autologous bone marrow mononuclear cells for ischemic cardiomyopathy. *Circulation* 2004;110(11 suppl 1):II213–II218.

103. Kuethe F, Richartz BM, Sayer HG, et al. Lack of regeneration of myocardium by autologous intracoronary mononuclear bone marrow cell transplantation in humans with large anterior myocardial infarctions. *Int J Cardiol* 2004;97(1):123–127.

104. Chen SL, Fang WW, Ye F, et al. Effect on left ventricular function of intracoronary transplantation of autologous bone marrow mesenchymal stem cell in patients with acute myocardial infarction. *Am J Cardiol* 2004;94(1):92–95.

105. Katritsis DG, Sotiropoulou PA, Karvouni E, et al. Transcoronary transplantation of autologous mesenchymal stem cells and endothelial progenitors into infarcted human myocardium. *Catheter Cardiovasc Interv* 2005;65(3):321–329.

106. Hamano K, Nishida M, Hirata K, et al. Local implantation of autologous bone marrow cells for therapeutic angiogenesis in patients with ischemic heart disease: clinical trial and preliminary results. *Jpn Circ J* 2001;65(9):845–847.

PART 3 Evaluation of the Patient

CHAPTER (11)

Clinical Practice Guidelines in Cardiovascular Disease

Ira S. Nash

The delivery of medical care in the United States is an enormous enterprise accounting for approximately 15 percent of the entire economic activity of the nation. The annual cost is one trillion dollars.[1] The rapid growth of medical expenditures and the recognition that there are significant deficiencies in the quality of care delivered in the United States and elsewhere have fueled the so-called *quality movement.*[2]

The development of clinical practice guidelines has paralleled the growth and importance of the focus on medical quality. A discussion of the context in which practice guidelines have achieved their current prominence is followed by a presentation of their development, implementation, and maintenance. Finally, their quality and impact on medical practice are assessed.

QUALITY OF CARE
【 】 PRACTICE VARIATION

One of the most striking aspects of the delivery of medical care in the United States and internationally is its enormous inhomogeneity.[3,4] Many well-documented examples of substantial variability in clinical practice exist among diagnostic tests and treatments for cardiovascular illnesses. The data on racial and ethnic disparities in cardiovascular care were authoritatively reviewed by a collaborative effort of the Henry J. Kaiser Family Foundation, the Robert Wood Johnson Foundation, and several prominent medical organizations.[5] They found significant evidence of less intensive cardiac testing and coronary revascularization among minority patients. Others have reported that risk-adjusted mortality rates for acute myocardial infarction are higher at hospitals with disproportionately large African American patient populations.[6] There are striking geographic differences in the use of effective medications[7] and invasive procedures for patients with acute myocardial infarction.[8] Women often are treated less intensively than men.[9]

As the cost, complexity, and potential benefit of medical care have grown, so too has the importance of addressing this variation. Which of the different approaches to care is *correct*? Which leads to the greatest benefit for patients? Could similar benefits be achieved at a lower cost? How could one tell? Addressing these and related questions is the essence of evaluating the quality of medical care. Evaluating the quality of care is a necessary prerequisite for improving it.

【 】 DEFINING QUALITY

Many different definitions of quality have been proposed. The Institute of Medicine put forth a definition of the quality of medical care that has been widely adopted: "the degree to which health services for individuals and populations increase the likelihood of desired health outcomes and are consistent with current professional knowledge."[10] Good medical practice is necessarily based on sound medical knowledge, and if done right, it benefits patients. Note that even under the best of circumstances, quality medical care improves the *likelihood* of good outcomes, but it cannot guarantee them. A patient with cardiogenic shock on the basis of an extensive myocardial infarction is at high risk of dying even with the best medical care. Likewise, many patients will recover without incident after an infarction even if they do not receive effective therapies such as thrombolysis or postinfarction β-blockade. It is therefore inappropriate to examine only patient outcomes to judge the quality of care they received.

MEASURING QUALITY: STRUCTURE, PROCESS, AND OUTCOME

A more complete assessment of the quality of care depends on considering three fundamental components of medical practice, which, taken together, provide a more complete picture: the structure, process, and outcome of care.[11] The *structure* of care is a characterization of the environment in which care is delivered. The *process* of care encompasses the myriad steps in the actual delivery of services; and the *outcome* of care is some result of interest to patients or providers. Consider, as an example, the assessment of the quality of care provided by a cardiac catheterization laboratory.

The structure of care provided by the lab includes the physical attributes of the facility, and the sophistication of the patient hemodynamic monitor. Perhaps less obviously, it also encompasses the staffing levels of the laboratory, the level of training of the personnel (e.g., advanced cardiac life support certification, or cross-training of nursing and technical staff), and the maintenance of the equipment (e.g., the frequency of radiation safety inspections). The structure of the laboratory also extends beyond its own physical boundaries. Is the laboratory a freestanding facility? Is it in a community hospital, where it can be used for general vascular radiology as well as coronary angiography? Is there a cardiac surgical program at the same institution?

The process of care addresses what providers do and how they do it. For the catheterization laboratory, this runs the gamut from how patients are scheduled for their procedure (indeed, how they are identified as candidates for a procedure) through the steps taken to prepare them for the catheterization (including patient education and the solicitation of informed consent) and all the details of the procedure and postprocedural care. Clearly, this includes an enormous number of potential points of quality assessment. How are patients prepared for the catheterization? Do cardiology trainees perform part (or all) of the procedure under supervision? How are patients monitored after their procedure? Are there dedicated personnel who remove the arterial introducing sheaths? How much heparin is used? How long are patients required to stay in bed? The list goes on.

Finally, an assessment of the quality of the laboratory can rightfully include an examination of the outcomes of the patients who were treated. This can include traditional outcomes such as complications and mortality, but it can also be construed more broadly to include *patient-centered outcomes,* such as patient satisfaction, functional capacity, or emotional well being.

QUALITY ASSESSMENT AND IMPROVEMENT

With the dimensions of quality more broadly drawn, the assessment and improvement of care can be specified more precisely with reference to the definition of quality offered by the Institute of Medicine. This assessment can then, in turn, form the basis for quality improvement or for comparisons among providers. Some component of the structure, process, or outcome of a particular aspect of medical care must be selected, defined, and measured. In

order for the quality assessment to be meaningful, certain criteria must be met.

First, the focus of the assessment must be something under the control of the providers of care. Particular health outcomes of interest to patients and providers can remain outside the ability of medical care to influence them. Measuring such outcomes would be a waste of time. For example, the frequency with which patients with hypertrophic cardiomyopathy experience potentially life-threatening arrhythmias is of great interest to affected patients and their physicians. Yet tracking such events says little about the quality of medical care they received because there are no therapies currently available that can reliably influence the outcome. A measurable *outcome* of care must therefore be linked with a controllable structure or process of care. The mortality associated with coronary artery bypass grafting (CABG) surgery is arguably the most intensively tracked outcome in all of medicine and has drawn the attention of a large number of investigators[12–15] as well as government agencies.[16,17] Mortality following CABG depends in part on how well patients are treated. Tracking outcomes can therefore stimulate examination of the way care is delivered and possible changes in this, which can then result in improved outcomes.

A measurable *process* of care can also be the focus of quality assessment and improvement activities as long as it is closely linked to an important health outcome. The Cooperative Cardiovascular Project (CCP), sponsored by the Health Care Finance Administration (HCFA, now the Centers for Medicare and Medicaid Services [CMS]), was an excellent example of a large-scale quality assessment and improvement project predicated on this principle.[18] Using a large body of randomized controlled clinical trials of therapies for patients with acute myocardial infarction, investigators developed a series of quality indicators. These were measures of specific processes of care, that is, they identified which patients received which therapy. Based on the evidence from clinical trials, the investigators also specified which patients *should* get which therapy. They determined in this way the percentage of candidates for a given therapy who actually received it. The clinical trials established, for example, the connection between early aspirin administration and improved survival,[19] measuring the extent to which patients actually did receive aspirin served as a measure of the quality of the care delivered.

The current efforts by CMS,[20] The Joint Commission on Accreditation of Healthcare Organizations (JCAHO),[21] the American Heart Association (AHA),[22] and the American College of Cardiology (ACC)[23] to promote the use of effective treatments, are also based on improving processes of care. In clinical circumstances where process and outcome are well linked by clinical evidence, measuring some specific step in the delivery of care instead of the final outcome offers several important advantages. First, it provides an important efficiency. Because every patient treated for a particular condition, such as myocardial infarction, is exposed to a system of care but only a small percentage of patients (regardless of the care they receive) is likely to experience a particular outcome such as death, many more patients must be studied if the quality of care they receive is to be judged solely on the outcomes they experience.

Mant and Hicks[24] estimated the relative numbers of patients required to detect differences in the quality of care provided to patients with acute myocardial infarction based on process versus outcome measures. After applying estimates of the efficacy of a variety of medical therapies for myocardial infarction derived from randomized trials, they constructed a model for calculating the sample size needed to detect a given difference in mortality between two hospitals treating populations with the same risk of dying. For example, detecting a reduction in mortality from 30 percent (the assumed baseline mortality in the absence of any effective therapies) to 25 percent (achievable with the adoption of only 31 percent of all available effective interventions) with a power of 80 percent and a significance level of 5 percent would require the examination of records from nearly 1300 patients with myocardial infarction. To detect the difference in frequency of use of effective therapeutic interventions that could lead to a reduction in mortality of the same magnitude (the process instead of the outcome of care), they derived a minimum sample size of only 27 patients. Clearly, tremendous economy of effort could be achieved by focusing on process instead of outcome.

In addition, if only the outcomes of care are tracked, then any efforts directed at improving outcomes must still ultimately identify and improve those aspects of the delivery of care that influence it. For example, if hospitals tracked only infarction mortality without measuring the extent to which their patients receive aspirin, then the discovery of high mortality rates would necessarily lead to an investigation of care, including such critical steps as the use of aspirin. Another criterion that any useful quality measure must fulfill rests on the fact that resources devoted to assessing one aspect of care are necessarily unavailable for a similar examination of some other aspect of care. Maximizing the impact of quality assessment and improvement activities therefore requires prioritization in favor of high-cost, prevalent conditions.

Finally, a range of practical issues must be considered in choosing a useful measure of the structure, process, or outcome of care. The collection of necessary data must be feasible within the constraints of time and resources. Quality measures must also be reliable (measurable in a consistent way over time), valid (a true measure of what one hopes to measure), and sensitive to change over time and differences among systems of care.

Ultimately, improving the quality of care depends on creating the setting, conditions, and particular processes of care, which, if adhered to, will maximize the likelihood of good patient outcomes. The summary of these settings, conditions, and processes are practice guidelines.

CLINICAL PRACTICE GUIDELINES

[ ] DEFINITION

In 1989, the Agency for Health Care Policy and Research (AHCPR, since renamed the Agency for Healthcare Research and Quality [AHRQ]) was created with the charge to "enhance the quality, appropriateness, and effectiveness of health care services, through the establishment of a broad base of scientific research and through the promotion of improvements in clinical practice and in the organization, financing and delivery of health care services." Specifically included in the legislation was the charge that the agency put forth "clinically relevant" practice guidelines. The Institute of Medicine convened an advisory committee at the time to assist the newly formed agency in fulfilling its mandate. The

committee's report defined practice guidelines as "systematically developed statements to assist practitioner and patient decisions about appropriate health care for specific clinical circumstances."[25] The intended utility of practice guidelines was expressed in a follow-up report by the Institute of Medicine in 1992: "*Scientific evidence and clinical judgment can be systematically combined to produce clinically valid, operational recommendations for appropriate care that can and will be used to persuade clinicians, patients, and others to change their practices in ways that lead to better health outcomes and lower health care costs.*"[26] Although the report acknowledged the existence of substantial barriers to the realization of this ideal, it remains a concise statement of the definition and promise of practice guidelines.

[ ] OTHER AIDS TO CLINICAL PRACTICE

As the perceived need to improve the quality of care has grown, so too has the range of tools available to practitioners. *Medical review criteria* are "systematically developed statements that can be used to assess the appropriateness of specific health care decisions, services, and outcomes." These are also referred to as *performance measures, quality measures,* or *performance indicators* and are generally derived from clinical practice guidelines and allow for their application in assessing and improving care. They can be "restatements of specific guideline recommendations into forms suitable for … review of clinical practice." For example, the ACC/AHA guidelines for acute myocardial infarction (AMI) recommend the use of angiotensin-converting enzyme (ACE) inhibitors for AMI patients with a reduced ejection fraction or clinical heart failure.[27] One of the performance indicators developed by CMS and JCAHO for the assessment of the quality of care and publicly reported for U.S. hospitals, is the percentage of myocardial infarction patients with left ventricular systolic dysfunction and without contraindications to ACE inhibition who actually receive the medication during their hospitalization.[28]

Another quality improvement tool closely related to practice guidelines is a *critical pathway*. A critical pathway can also be referred to as a *critical path*, a *clinical pathway*, a *clinical plan*, a *care map*, or a *care plan*. These are usually locally developed, highly detailed accounts of how the process of care should unfold for a focused episode of care. They typically deal with the direction and coordination of inpatient services for a particular diagnosis or procedure. For instance, a CABG critical pathway can specify what each of several different providers of care should do during each day of a patient's stay. This would include items such as nursing instruction in the use of incentive spirometry on postoperative day 1, the removal of chest tubes by the surgeon on day 3, climbing stairs with the physical therapist on day 5, and so on. Developing an explicit statement of this sort forces groups of providers to examine their practices and achieve local consensus about how care should be delivered. The final products serve as real-time references to those caring for patients.

[ ] GUIDELINE DEVELOPMENT

The utility of a practice guideline depends critically on the process by which it was created. Task Force 1 of the 28th Bethesda Conference of the ACC detailed eight phases of successful clinical

TABLE 11–1

Phases of Guideline Development and Associated Tasks Identified by the 28th Bethesda Conference

PHASE 1. ADMINISTRATIVE OVERSIGHT

Task 1. Identify specific goals
Task 2. Prioritize possible guideline topics
Task 3. Review the literature to define task, costs, and time line

PHASE 2. SELECT EXPERT PANEL

Task 1. Members must bring expertise, diversity, enthusiasm, and commitment
Task 2. Convene panel electronically (videoconference, e-mail) to begin plans
Task 3. Confirm outline, map patient-care algorithm

PHASE 3. LITERATURE SEARCH AND EVIDENCE REVIEW

Task 1. Computerized literature search
Task 2. Match literature to guideline outline, rate evidence
Task 3. Create evidence tables for each topic
Task 4. Base wording of recommendations on strength of relevant evidence

PHASE 4. CONSENSUS PROCESS

Task 1. Converge on recommendations by an explicit process

PHASE 5. COMPUTERIZE GUIDELINE DOCUMENTS IN FORMAT FOR CLINICAL USE

Task 1. Link recommendations with related evidence
Task 2. Create preformatted documents to capture data and facilitate care
Task 3. Create database to store information regarding guideline compliance

PHASE 6. TEST AND REVISE GUIDELINE

Task 1. Expert panel tests computerized guideline in actual patient care
Task 2. Final revision of guidelines based on testing

PHASE 7. DISSEMINATE GUIDELINE

Task 1. Publish printed version, disseminate computerized version
Task 2. Encourage local customization

PHASE 8. REVISE AND REFINE GUIDELINE

Task 1. Maintain ongoing literature review
Task 2. Refine management strategies based on patient outcomes associated with guideline use

SOURCE: From Jones, Ritchie, Fleming, et al.[29] Used with permission.

practice guideline development.[29] Within each of these phases, they outlined specific tasks to be accomplished (Table 11–1). Others have proposed comparable work plans. The AHA and the ACC have collaborated, often in association with international or subspecialty societies, to produce a series of well-respected clinical practice guidelines for cardiovascular care. They have produced a manual for guideline developers that is consistent with these recommendations.[30] International efforts to facilitate guideline development also recommend an explicit work plan that includes defining the precise scope of the endeavor, systematically gathering and evaluating evidence from the medical literature, and synthesizing clear recommendations.[31]

Level of Evidence

Perhaps no other step in guideline development is as critical as systematically evaluating the strength of the evidence on which recommendations are based. Some research findings (or other pieces of evidence) reported in the medical literature are more reliable than others. Some reported findings are likely to be a true effect, although others can be only an artifact of a study design flaw or a statistical quirk. There is a generally accepted hierarchy of study design, based on the premise that the systematic minimization of potential bias improves the reliability of research results. The most reliable research results come from randomized controlled trials (RCTs). In descending order of reliability (ascending vulnerability to bias), the remaining sources of data are observational studies, case reports, and expert opinion.[32] Within these broad categories, some RCTs can be less reliable than others if the studied population is small, or if they have methodological flaws such as ineffective blinding, ambiguous endpoint assignment or large drop-out rates.[33] Conversely, observational studies can provide relatively more reliable estimates of treatment or intervention effects if the magnitude of the effect is large, if plausible confounding would only diminish rather than exaggerate the observed effect, or if a dose-response is demonstrated.[33]

The international GRADE (grades of recommendations, assessment, development, and evaluation) Working Group also recommended that evidence should be weighed on the basis of consistency and directness.[34] Consistency refers to finding a similar direction and magnitude of treatment effects across different studies. Note that there are no clear quantitative criteria for concluding that the available evidence is or is not consistent; this is largely a matter of informed judgment. Directness refers to the extent to which the studied population, treatments, and outcomes are similar to those to which the guideline applies. For example, evidence of a greater treatment effect of medication A over placebo compared with the treatment effect of medication B over placebo is only indirect evidence of the superior efficacy of medication A compared with medication B. It is not as reliable as evidence derived from an RCT directly comparing medication A with medication B.

Finally, any scheme used to grade evidence to form the basis of clinical practice guidelines should also consider the ease with which it can be applied consistently by guideline developers and the ultimate transparency and utility of the scheme to the guideline's users.[35] The evidence grading schemes used in this book are adopted from the ACC and AHA. The 2006 Methodology Manual for ACC/AHA Guideline Writing Committees stipulates that evidence should be characterized as "level" A, B, or C. Level A is defined as "data derived from multiple RCTs or meta-analyses"; Level B as "data derived from a single randomized trial, or nonrandomized studies"; Level C as "consensus opinion of experts, case studies, or standard of care."[30]

Classification of Recommendations

The formulation of treatment recommendations rests on making an informed judgment about whether the benefits of a particular intervention outweigh the associated risks, burden, and cost.[35] When this balance is substantially tipped in one direction or the other, and the evidence to support that conclusion is clear, then a strong recommendation about the intervention can be made. When the balance is less clear, then a less definitive recommendation is appropriate. This latter situation can arise in a number of circumstances. Sometimes, there is considerable uncertainty about the potential risks and benefits of an intervention. In other cases, the risks and benefits, although well defined, are more closely balanced, such that reasonable, equally well-informed individuals, can choose different courses of action.

The apparent favorable comparison of benefits over risks also depends critically on how individuals value particular outcomes. As a result, recommendations inevitably involve making judgments about values held by others, which is a subjective, and often challenging exercise. For example, there is no fully objective or quantitative way to balance the benefit of stroke avoidance in atrial fibrillation with warfarin anticoagulation against the risk of hemorrhage and the nuisance of anticoagulation monitoring.

Unfortunately, well-designed clinical trials usually involve highly specified patient populations, defined by extensive inclusion and exclusion criteria, although practice guidelines, by their nature, are intended to be broadly applicable. There is no simple formula to reconcile the nature of the evidence and the need for recommendations.

As with grading of evidence, a variety of different schemes have been recommended for expressing the relative strength of a particular recommendation. The GRADE group suggested that recommendations be categorized into those that clearly have "net benefit," those that involve important and apparent "trade-offs" between benefits and risks, those that involve "uncertain trade-offs" and those that are clearly of "no net benefit."[34] More recently, a task force of the American College of Chest Physicians suggested that recommendations be divided simply into those that are "strong" or "weak" based on the balance among benefits, risks, and burdens and the degree of confidence in estimating these parameters.[35] The classification of recommendations of the ACC and AHA is used throughout this book and is summarized in Table 11–2.

There is no consistent correlation between level of evidence and class of recommendation. If several large RCTs provide conflicting conclusions, then the quality of the available evidence can be high but the recommendation necessarily weak. However, if there is such universal agreement that a particular element of care is so essential that no RCT is ever likely to be done (e.g., the necessity of examining a patient),[29] then a strong recommendation can be appropriate in the absence of rigorous evidence (Figure 11–1).

[ ] GUIDELINE IMPLEMENTATION

Clinical practice guidelines are tools for improving patient care. Much of that potential can be realized only by changing physician behavior because physicians are responsible for directing care. Even a well-crafted guideline, then, will not benefit patients unless and until it actually changes how doctors act under particular circumstances.

TABLE 11–2

American College of Cardiology/American Heart Association Classification of Guideline Recommendations

Class I: Conditions for which there is evidence and/or general agreement that a given procedure or treatment is useful and effective

Class II: Conditions for which there is conflicting evidence and/or a divergence of opinion about the usefulness/efficacy of a procedure or treatment

Class IIa: Weight of evidence/opinion is in favor or usefulness/efficacy

Class IIb: Usefulness or efficacy is less well established by evidence/opinion

Class III: Conditions for which there is evidence and/or general agreement that the procedure/treatment is not useful/effective and in some cases can be harmful

The prevalence of substantial deficiencies in the quality of care[36] despite the ubiquity of clinical practice guidelines suggests strongly that their successful implementation must go beyond making the guidelines themselves accessible through publication in the medical literature or by electronic means.[37] Cabana and colleagues presented a useful taxonomy for the barriers to guideline adoption and implementation.[38] They grouped barriers into those related to physician knowledge (lack of awareness or lack of familiarity), attitudes (lack of agreement, lack of self-efficacy, lack of outcome expectancy, or the inertia of previous practice), and behavior (external barriers).

Lack of physician awareness of or familiarity with specific guidelines has been well documented. Although the large number of practice guidelines makes this virtually inevitable, physicians are often unfamiliar with even the principal recommendations of well-publicized and broadly applicable guidelines.[39]

A negative attitude among clinicians about the value of guidelines is also a significant barrier to their implementation.[40] This, in turn, can be a result of a general mistrust of cookbook approaches to clinical practice, a rejection of national standards of practice, concerns regarding malpractice liability, and the paucity of data that adherence to guidelines actually improves care. Many clinicians also believe that guidelines are fundamentally incapable of capturing the nuances and complexity of clinical medicine. Certainly, deficiencies in the guidelines themselves, including conflicting recommendations among different guidelines addressing the same conditions[41] or lack of clarity of recommendations, contribute to physician skepticism. Physicians are most likely to adopt concrete, precise, and uncontroversial recommendations. Perhaps the greatest external barrier to guideline implementation is the complexity of the healthcare delivery system itself. Medical care is provided in a broad range of settings, from private physicians' offices to large academic medical centers and by a host of practitioners with different levels of interest and expertise in particular clinical conditions. Given the financial pressure present in many medical delivery systems, guideline implementation can well be seen as another burden or expense rather than as an aid to clinical practice. Even if guideline adoption is seen as desirable, limitations

"SIZE of TREATMENT EFFECT"

	Class I Benefit >>> Risk	Class IIa Benefit >> Risk Additional studies with focused objectives needed	Class IIb Benefit ≥ Risk Additional studies with broad objectives needed; Additional registry data would be helpful	Class III Benefit ≥ Risk No additional studies needed
	Procedure/Treatment SHOULD be performed/administered	IT IS REASONABLE to perform procedure/administer treatment	Procedure/Treatment MAY BE CONSIDERED	Procedure/Treatment should NOT be performed/administered SINCE IT IS NOT HELPFUL AND MAY BE HARMFUL
Level A *Multiple (3-5) population risk strata evaluated** *General consistency of direction and magnitude of effect**	• Recommendation that procedure or treatment is useful/effective • Sufficient evidence from multiple randomized trials or meta-analyses	• Recommendation in favor of treatment or procedure being useful/effective • Some conflicting evidence from multiple randomized trials or meta-analyses	• Recommendation's usefulness/efficacy less well established • Greater conflicting evidence from multiple randomized trials or meta-analyses	• Recommendation that procedure or treatment not useful/effective and may be harmful • Sufficient evidence from multiple randomized trials or meta-analyses
Level B *Limited (2-3) population risk strata evaluated**	• Recommendation that procedure or treatment is useful/effective • Limited evidence from single randomized trial or non-randomized studies	• Recommendation in favor of treatment or procedure being useful/effective • Some conflicting evidence from single randomized trial or non-randomized studies	• Recommendation's usefulness/efficacy less well established • Greater conflicting evidence from single randomized trial or non-randomized studies	• Recommendation that procedure or treatment not useful/effective and may be harmful • Limited evidence from single randomized trial or non-randomized studies
Level C *Very limited (1-2) population risk strata evaluated**	• Recommendation that procedure or treatment is useful/effective • Only expert opinion, case studies, or standard-of-care	• Recommendation in favor of treatment or procedure being useful/effective • Only diverging expert opinion, case studies, or standard-of-care	• Recommendation's usefulness/efficacy less well established • Only diverging expert opinion, case studies, or standard-of-care	• Recommendation that procedure or treatment not useful/effective and may be harmful • Only expert opinion, case studies, or standard-of-care
Suggested phrases for writing recommendations	should is recommended is indicated is useful/effective/beneficial	is reasonable can be useful/effective/beneficial is probably recommended or indicated	may/might be considered may/might be reasonable usefulness/effectiveness is unknown/unclear/uncertain or not well established	is not recommended is not indicated should not is not useful/effective/beneficial may be harmful

"Estimate of Certainty (Precision) of Treatment Effect"

FIGURE 11-1. Grid demonstrating the possible combinations of level of evidence and class of recommendation. *Source: From the American College of Cardiology (ACC)/American Heart Association (AHA) Methodology Manual for ACC/AHA Guideline Writing Committees. Available at: http://www.acc.org/clinical/manual/manual_index.htm.*

of physician time and practice resources can hinder efforts to move forward. The inadequacy of many clinical information systems, which under ideal circumstances could identify patients who meet guideline criteria and remind providers of current recommendations, is another important institutional barrier to successful guideline implementation.

Just as the barriers to guideline implementation are diverse, there is no single proven strategy for successful guideline adoption. For guideline developers, close attention to the principles of rigorous data synthesis and the straightforward presentation of well-documented recommendations is essential. Explicit discussion of potential conflicts with other guidelines and the reasons for different recommendations should be included. Guideline writers should include clear statements regarding the limitations of their own guidelines with respect to the patients or conditions to which they apply and consider the practicality of their recommendations.

Those who are charged with implementing practice guidelines must be prepared to address the preceding barriers.[42] Clear demonstration of the value of guideline adoption, through the feedback of local data demonstrating improvements in patient outcomes, is often part of a successful strategy.[42] Simultaneous development of the infrastructure to support clinical practice guidelines, including modifying the incentives of clinicians and investing in clinical information systems, is also helpful. Recognizing that creating high-quality practice guidelines does not, in it-

self, improve care, the AHA and the ACC have embarked on their own programs to enhance guideline implementation.[43]

The AHA program, called "Get with the Guidelines," is intended to promote the use of a small number of key treatments for patients hospitalized with coronary heart disease, acute coronary syndromes, heart failure, and atrial fibrillation. These treatments include, for example, the timely use of aspirin, the assessment and treatment of blood lipid disorders, and the discharge prescription of an ACE inhibitor in patients with left ventricular systolic dysfunction. Hospitals must register as program participants. They then gain access to a Web-based data collection instrument for monitoring guideline adherence, which also allows for comparisons of local performance against regional and national data. The "Get with the Guidelines" program also provides a "tool kit" of educational material (including presentation slides), guideline implementation aids (such as standardized admission order sets), and extensive program support. More information is available on the AHA Web site.[44]

The AHA has also issued a Scientific Statement regarding the implementation of its published guidelines on the treatment of unstable angina and non–ST-elevation myocardial infarction. This practical approach—a guideline on the implementation of guidelines—recognizes and addresses the critical barriers to successful implementation.[45]

The ACC-sponsored Guidelines Applied in Practice (GAP) program is a rapid-cycle quality improvement initiative that is also intended to boost adherence with major elements of the ACC/AHA guidelines.[46] The GAP program has separate modules for AMI and congestive heart failure. The myocardial infarction tool kit consists of (1) AMI standard admission orders, (2) a clinical pathway, (3) a pocket guide to care, (4) a patient information form, (5) a patient discharge checklist, (6) chart stickers to alert providers, and (7) hospital performance charts. A pilot implementation of the program in 10 acute care hospitals in Michigan yielded statistically and clinically significant improvements in the use of aspirin and β-blockers and favorable trends in the use of other efficacious therapies.[47]

【 】 GUIDELINE MAINTENANCE

If a particular practice guideline is to remain a useful tool for improving the quality of care, it must maintain its scientific currency and its relevance to clinical practice. Several different circumstances could necessitate a guideline update:

- Changes in the risk and benefit of current interventions
- Changes in which outcomes are considered important (e.g., quality-of-life measures)
- Changes in the quality of current practice
- Changes in the value placed on outcomes (e.g., economic endpoints)
- Changes in available resources

Establishing the appropriate threshold for any of these criteria is not simple; recognizing when that threshold is achieved is harder still. Some organizations therefore rely on an arbitrary time-based cycle of guideline revision. For example, the National Guideline Clearinghouse,[48] a Web site maintained by the AHRQ, deletes guidelines that are more than 5 years old. Such a policy may not be ideal. Rather, a systematic reassessment of existing guidelines by recognized experts, supplemented by limited searches of the medical literature and operating with prospectively defined criteria for obsolescence, may be the only practical way to assure timely updates.

Electronic publication and partial, rather than complete, revisions have been used effectively by the AHA and ACC to reduce the revision cycle time for their guidelines that need updating.

【 】 GUIDELINE QUALITY

Several observers have suggested lists of attributes that good practice guidelines should have. The Institute of Medicine report lists eight important qualities[25] (Table 11–3). *Validity* implies that the guidelines, if adopted, will actually lead to the anticipated improvements in health outcomes and/or cost of care. *Reliability* or *reproducibility* is achieved if another group of guideline developers would create equivalent guidelines, if they relied on the same evidence, and if the guidelines are "interpreted and applied consistently by practitioners." Good guidelines should also have clear *clinical applicability,* so that they pertain to a broad, well-defined, and explicitly stated population. Guidelines must also allow for some *flexibility* of medical practice and acknowledge the appropriate role of clinical judgment and possible exceptions to broad dictates. *Clarity* of recommendations is another important attribute and should be promoted through the use of precise definitions of terms, unambiguous recommendations, and a variety of presentation

---

TABLE 11–3

Desirable Attributes of Clinical Practice Guidelines Identified by the Institute of Medicine

Validity
Reliability
Clinical applicability
Flexibility
Clarity
Multidisciplinary development
Scheduled review
Documentation

SOURCE: Field and Lohr.[25] Used with permission.

---

techniques. Ideally, guidelines should be developed through *a multidisciplinary process,* which elicits the input of a broad range of stakeholders in the field. The Institute of Medicine report also suggests a provision for *scheduled revision* or an "expiration date," although, as previously discussed, this can be of limited utility. Finally, the Institute report suggests that good guidelines should be *well documented,* so that users will know the "procedures followed in developing guidelines, the participants involved, the evidence used, the assumptions and rationales accepted, and the analytic methods employed."

The Evidence-Based Medicine Working Group put forth its own criteria for judging the quality of practice guidelines. They posed a series of questions, the affirmative answers to which indicate a good guideline[49]:

- Were all important options and outcomes clearly specified?
- Was an explicit and sensible process used to identify, select, and combine evidence?
- Was an explicit and sensible process used to consider the relative value of different outcomes?
- Is the guideline likely to account for important recent developments?
- Has the guideline been subject to peer review and testing?
- Are practical, clinically important recommendations made?
- How strong are the recommendations?

They conclude: "A good guideline, based on solid scientific evidence and an explicit process for judging the value of alternative practices, allows you to review, at one sitting, links between multiple options and outcomes."[50]

There is now a huge number of practice guidelines put forth by a large number of organizations dealing with a broad array of clinical issues. The National Guideline Clearinghouse lists thousands of practice guidelines on its Web site. With so many guidelines in the published literature, a number of investigators have attempted to assess how well they fulfill the criteria discussed earlier.

Although the Institute of Medicine tried unsuccessfully to create a uniform guideline assessment tool, several different investigators have created and applied their own assessment instruments.

Shaneyfelt and colleagues explicitly judged a total of 279 clinical practice guidelines published between 1985 and 1997.[51] They first devised an evaluation tool that consisted of 25 specific standards that guidelines should ideally fulfill. These criteria were separated into standards of development and format, standards of evidence identification and summary, and standards on the formulation of recommendations. No attempt was made to prioritize the standards, and the authors acknowledge that it is extremely unlikely that any guideline would fulfill all of them. Nevertheless, they reported that the guidelines met a mean of only 43.1 percent of the quality standards and concluded that most guidelines "do not adhere well to established methodological standards," especially in regard to how the underlying medical evidence is gathered and critically combined. Cook and Giacomini, in an accompanying editorial, commented that the findings revealed "the diversity of guideline methodologies … and [are a] call for greater transparency of guideline reporting and more rigorous peer review."[52]

A generic guideline assessment tool was also developed and evaluated by Cluzeau and colleagues.[53] They evaluated guidelines in three "dimensions"—rigor of development, context and content, and application—by means of a series of yes/no questions and applied their tool to a set of 60 different practice guidelines for coronary heart disease, asthma, breast cancer, and depression. They reported that the tool was easy to apply and reliable in practice and that most guidelines did not achieve the majority of criteria in each dimension.

Graham and coworkers evaluated the usefulness of 15 different guideline "appraisal instruments" published by other investigators, including Shaneyfelt and Cluzeau.[54] They concluded that there was insufficient evidence to support the exclusive use of a single instrument. Grilli and colleagues presented a much simpler assessment tool, which addresses three central issues related to guideline quality: a description of the type of professionals who developed the guideline, a description of the sources of information used, and whether an explicit method of grading the evidence was described.[55] They concluded that Shaneyfelt overstated the general problem of poor guideline quality; they instead identified only those guidelines developed by specialty societies as being of particularly poor quality. They proposed uniform reporting of methodology by guideline developers.

More recently, an international effort, the AGREE (Appraisal of Guidelines, Research and Evaluation) project, has led to the development and validation of a new tool to evaluate guideline quality.[56] The evaluation instrument allows reviewers to use standard criteria to judge guidelines in six "domains": scope and purpose, stakeholder involvement, rigor of development, clarity and presentation, applicability, and editorial independence. Each domain is scored independently on the basis of answers to explicit questions. This tool is rapidly becoming the new international standard for the assessment of guideline quality, and is now available through the AGREE Web site in 14 languages.[57] Despite its rapid and widespread adoption, investigators have pointed out that the AGREE instrument, like others before it, assesses only the methodology used to develop a guideline and not the quality of its actual content.[58] Others caution that there is an imperfect correlation between the methodological rigor assessed by the AGREE tool and the validity of specific guideline recommendations.[59]

[ ] GUIDELINE EFFECTIVENESS

With legitimate questions raised over the quality of guidelines and the challenges associated with their development, implementation, and maintenance, what is the evidence that the cardiovascular clinical practice guidelines have actually improved the quality of care? The question, although vital to the allocation of resources for quality improvement activities, is difficult to answer. Because the impact of practice guidelines depends on both the quality of the guideline itself

and its successful implementation (its local application to a system of care delivery), there is no simple way to allocate observed success or failure between these two. In other words, a failure to demonstrate improvements in cardiovascular care through the use of guidelines can represent deficiencies in the applicability or practicality of practice guidelines, the operational failure of implementing them locally, or some combination of both. In addition, it is challenging to perform randomized trials of guideline use. Fortunately, there are data to suggest that guidelines can improve care.

Grimshaw and Russell compiled the most rigorous assessment of the success of practice guidelines, in a variety of medical conditions, in improving the quality of care.[60] They reviewed 59 published reports evaluating the impact of practice guidelines and found that in nearly all cases the implementation of a practice guideline had improved the measured process of care. Of the 11 studies they reviewed that reported a clinical outcome in addition to the process of care, 9 reported significant improvement. One can question the generalizability of these conclusions because it is likely that there is a significant publication bias in favor of studies demonstrating an improvement in care over *negative* studies of the same question. Nevertheless, regardless of the frequency with which practice guidelines actually *do* improve care, there is clear and compelling evidence that they *can* improve care.

Sarasin and colleagues reported significant improvements in the use of β-blockers in postinfarction patients following the implementation of a practice guideline on the subject at their institution.[61] In their time series, the use of discharge β-blockers nearly doubled, despite no significant change in the profile of infarction patients. A Canadian group looked at the improvement in several process measures of care for patients with AMI cared for at the University of Alberta Hospitals between 1987 and 1993. They found continuous and significant improvement in the use of therapies of proven efficacy, with a corresponding fall in the use of unproven interventions. Although the observations were made in an uncontrolled setting, the investigators attributed the results to "repeated measurement and reporting of key health care performance indicators, and initiation of explicit … AMI practice guidelines." On a much larger scale, the Cooperative Cardiovascular Project demonstrated that the feedback on compliance with guidelines for critical process of care measures for patients with myocardial infarction was associated with a significant improvement in the quality of care that AMI patients received.[62]

The success of the guideline implementation programs sponsored by the AHA and ACC, detailed earlier in this chapter, also support the usefulness of practice guidelines in improving the quality of cardiovascular care. Greater success in implementing practice guidelines depends in part on the refinement of the guidelines themselves, the more extensive use of clinical information systems to present critical data and guideline recommendations to clinicians at the point of care, and greater sensitivity to the systematic barriers to their adoption.

[ ] FINDING PRACTICE GUIDELINES

Clinical practice guidelines in cardiovascular medicine have been developed by many different organizations on a wide array of topics. New guidelines are constantly being produced to cover new subjects and to incorporate new data about previously addressed conditions. Just keeping track of the guidelines themselves has become challenging for clinicians and policy-makers. Fortunately, there are several ways to find relevant guidelines.

Most clinical practice guidelines are published in peer-reviewed medical journals. Often, the journals are the official publication of the same parent organization that produced the guideline. So, for example, the guidelines compiled by the American College of Physicians/ American Society of Internal Medicine are published in the *Annals of Internal Medicine;* those of the American College of Chest Physicians appear in *Chest,* and the guidelines of the joint efforts of the ACC/ AHA are published in both the *Journal of the American College of Cardiology* and *Circulation.* Guidelines by lesser-known groups are also generally published in mainstream journals. Even government agencies, which have their own publishing capabilities, often seek to have part or all of their guidelines published in journals as well. As a consequence, a computer search of the MEDLINE database of peer-reviewed journals can produce a list of many of the sought guidelines. This process is far from perfect, however, in part because of the wide variety of key terms used to index published guidelines.

Each of these organizations also maintains its own Web site where practice guidelines are available. As the pace of medical developments accelerates, guideline updates have become more frequent, and some organizations have adopted a policy of publishing their updated guidelines exclusively in electronic form. The ACC/AHA guidelines and their associated updates are all available at their respective Web sites: www.acc.org and www.americanheart.org.

The electronic compendium of guidelines maintained by the National Guideline Clearinghouse is very useful.[48] This searchable Web site allows the user to specify the subject and/or sponsor of guidelines. The interface is user-friendly, and the list generated by the search contains links to the specified guideline. So, for example, if one specifies *cardiovascular disease,* more than 850 listed guidelines are presented, along with suggested search terms (*heart disease, vascular disease,* etc.) and the number of guidelines fitting those search criteria. The links allow a user to go directly from the list to a brief summary of the guideline prepared by the National Guideline Clearinghouse as well as to the full text of a particular guideline, often at the Web site of the sponsoring organization.

CONCLUSION

Assessing and improving the quality of care is a vital component of responsible medical practice. It has taken on increased prominence in recent years because of the widespread evidence of unexplained practice variation, the underuse of effective therapies, and the increasing pressure for accountability at all levels of healthcare delivery. Clinical practice guidelines have emerged as an important tool to improve the quality of medical care, and cardiovascular medicine has become a particularly fertile ground for their development. A large number of high-quality clinical practice guidelines are now available that address critical issues in cardiovascular medicine. When they are based on dependable, rigorous evidence, written in clear language, and implemented with sensitivity to the myriad local issues that can thwart their success, clinical practice guidelines can help improve patient care.

REFERENCES

1. United States Census Bureau. The 2006 statistical abstract. The national data book. Available at: http://www.census.gov/compendia/statab/.
2. Wachter RM. Expected and unanticipated consequences of the quality and information technology revolutions. *JAMA.* 2006;295:2780–2783.
3. Chassin MR, Kosecoff J, Park RE, et al. Variations in the use of medical and surgical services by the Medicare population. *N Engl J Med.* 1986;314:285–290.
4. Dartmouth Atlas Working Group. The Dartmouth atlas of healthcare. Available at: http://www.dartmouthatlas.org/index.shtm.
5. Lillie-Blanton M, Rushing OE, Ruiz S, et al. Racial/ethnic differences in cardiac care: the weight of the evidence. 2002 report. Available at: http://www.kff.org/whythedifference.
6. Skinner J, Chandra A, Staiger D, Lee J, McClellan M. Mortality after acute myocardial infarction in hospitals that disproportionately treat black patients. *Circulation.* 2005;112:2634–2641.
7. O'Connor GT, Quinton HB, Traven ND, et al. Geographic variation in the treatment of acute myocardial infarction. The Cooperative Cardiovascular Project. *JAMA.* 1999;281:627–633.
8. Stukel TA, Lucas FL, Wennberg DE. Long-term outcomes of regional variations in intensity of invasive vs medical management of Medicare patients with acute myocardial infarction. *JAMA.* 2005;293:1329–1337.
9. Roger VL, Farkouh ME, Weston SA, et al. Sex differences in evaluation and outcome of unstable angina. *JAMA.* 2000;283:646–652.
10. Institute of Medicine. *Medicare: A Strategy for Quality Assurance.* Washington, DC: National Academy Press; 1990.
11. Donabedian A. *Explorations in Quality Assessment and Monitoring.* Vol 1: *The Definition of Quality and Approaches to Its Assessment.* Ann Arbor, MI: Health Administration Press; 1980.
12. Hannan EL, Wu C, Bennett EV, Carlson RE, Culliford AT, Gold JP, et al. Risk stratification of in-hospital mortality for coronary artery bypass graft surgery. *J Am Coll Cardiol.* 2006;47(3):661–668.
13. Guru V, Fremes SE Austin PC, Blackstone EH, Tu JV. Gender differences in outcomes after hospital discharge from coronary artery bypass grafting. *Circulation.* 2006;113:507–516.
14. Nilsson J, Algotsson L, Hoglund P, Luhrs C, Brandt J. Comparison of 19 pre-operative risk stratification models in open-heart surgery. *Eur Heart J.* 2006;27:867–874.
15. Zaroff JG, diTommaso DG, Barron HV. A risk model derived from the National Registry of Myocardial Infarction 2 database for predicting mortality after coronary artery bypass grafting during acute myocardial infarction. *Am J Cardiol.* 2002;90(1):35–38.
16. New York State Department of Health. *Adult Cardiac Surgery in New York State, 2001–2003.* Albany, NY: New York State Department of Health; 2005. Also available at: http://www.health.state.ny.us/nysdoh/heart/heart_disease.htm.
17. Pennsylvania Health Care Cost Containment Council. *Pennsylvania's Guide to Coronary Artery Bypass Graft Surgery 2004.* Harrisburg, PA: Pennsylvania Health Care Cost Containment Council; 2006. Also available at: http://www.phc4.org/reports/cabg/04/default.htm.
18. Ellerbeck EF, Jencks SF, Radford MJ, et al. Quality of care for Medicare patients with acute myocardial infarction. *JAMA.* 1995;273:1509–1514.
19. ISIS-2 (Second International Study of Infarct Survival) Collaborative Group. Randomised trial of intravenous streptokinase, oral aspirin, both, or neither among 17,187 cases of suspected acute myocardial infarction: ISIS-2. *Lancet.* 1988;2:349–360.
20. U.S. Department of Health and Human Services. Centers for Medicare and Medicaid services: quality of care center. Available at: http://www.cms.hhs.gov/center/quality.asp.
21. Joint Commission on Accreditation of Healthcare Organizations (JCAHO). Home page. Available at: http://www.jointcommission.org/.
22. American Heart Association. Get with the guidelines. Available at: http://www.americanheart.org/presenter.jhtml?identifier=1165.
23. American College of Cardiology. Guidelines applied in practice. Available at: http://www.acc.org/qualityandscience/gap/gap.htm.
24. Mant J, Hicks N. Detecting differences in quality of care: the sensitivity of measures of process and outcome in treating acute myocardial infarction. *BMJ.* 1995;311:793–796.
25. Field MJ, Lohr KN, eds. *Clinical Practice Guidelines: Directions for a New Program.* Washington, DC: National Academy Press; 1990.
26. Field MJ, Lohr KN, eds. *Guidelines for Clinical Practice: From Development to Use.* Washington, DC: National Academy Press; 1992:4.
27. Antman EM, Anbe DT, Armstrong PW, Bates ER, Green LA, Hand M, et al. ACC/AHA guidelines for the management of patients with ST-elevation myocardial infarction: executive summary: a report of the ACC/AHA Task Force on Practice Guidelines (Committee to Revise the 1999 Guidelines on the Management of Patients with Acute Myocardial Infarction). *J Am Coll Cardiol.* 2004;44:671–719.
28. U.S. Department of Health and Human Services. Hospital quality initiatives overview. Available at: http://www.cms.hhs.gov/HospitalQualityInits/.

29. Jones RH, Ritchie JL, Fleming BB, et al. Task Force 1: clinical practice guideline development, dissemination and computerization. *J Am Coll Cardiol.* 1997;29:1133–1141.

30. *Methodology Manual for ACC/AHA Guidelines Writing Committees.* Available at: http://www.acc.org/clinical/manual/manual_index.htm.

31. Scottish Intercollegiate Guidelines Network (SIGN). Home page. Available at: http://www.sign.ac.uk/.

32. Guyatt G, Sinclair J, Cook D, Jaeschke R, Schunemann H, Pauker S. Grading recommendations—a qualitative approach. In: Guyatt G, Rennie D, ed. *Users' Guide to the Medical Literature: A Manual for Evidence-Based Practice.* Chicago: AMA Press; 2002.

33. Guyatt G, Vist G, Falck-Ytter Y, Kunz R, Magrini N, Schunemann H. An emerging consensus on grading recommendations? *Evid Based Med.* 2006;11:2–4.

34. GRADE Working Group. Grading quality of evidence and strength of recommendations. *BMJ.* 2004;328:1490–1497.

35. Guyatt G, Gutterman D, Baumann MH, Addrizzo-Harris D, Hylek EM, Phillips B, et al. Grading strength of recommendations and quality of evidence in clinical guidelines: report from an American College of Chest Physicians Task Force. *Chest.* 2006;129:174–181.

36. McGlynn EA, Asch SM, Adams J, Keesey J, Hicks J, DeCristofaro A, et al. The quality of health care delivered to adults in the United States. *N Engl J Med.* 2003;348:2635–2645.

37. Williams JG, Cheung WY, Price DE, Tansey R, Russell IT, Duane PD, et al. Clinical guidelines online: do they improve compliance? *Postgrad Med J.* 2004;80:415–419.

38. Cabana MD, Rand CS, Powe NR, et al. Why don't physicians follow clinical practice guidelines? A framework for improvement. *JAMA.* 1999;282:1458–1465.

39. Mosca L, Linfante AH, Benjamin EJ, Berra K, Hayes SN, Walsh BW, et al. National study of physician awareness and adherence to cardiovascular disease prevention guidelines. *Circulation.* 2005;111:499–510.

40. Powell-Cope GM, Luther S, Neugaard B, Vara J, Nelson A. Provider-perceived barriers and facilitators for ischaemic heart disease (IHD) guideline adherence. *J Eval Clin Pract.* 2004;10:227–239.

41. Thomson R, McElroy H, Sudlow M. Guidelines on anticoagulant treatment in atrial fibrillation in Great Britain: variation in content and implications for treatment. *BMJ.* 1998;316:509–513.

42. Jamtvedt G, Young JM, Kristoffersen DT, O'Brien MA, Oxman AD. Audit and feedback: effects on professional practice and healthcare outcomes. *Cochrane Database Syst Rev.* 2007:Issue 2.

43. Eagle KA, Garson AJ, Beller GA, Sennett C. Closing the gap between science and practice: the need for professional leadership. *Health Aff.* 2003;22:196–201.

44. American Heart Association. Available at: http://www.americanheart.org/presenter.jhtml?identifier=1165.

45. Gibler WB, Cannon CP, Blomkalns AL, Char DM, Drew BJ, Hollander JE, et al. Practical implementation of the guidelines for unstable angina/non–ST-segment elevation myocardial infarction in the emergency department: a scientific statement from the American Heart Association Council on Clinical Cardiology (Subcommittee on Acute Cardiac Care), Council on Cardiovascular Nursing, and Quality of Care and Outcomes Research Interdisciplinary Working Group in collaboration with the Society of Chest Pain Centers. *Circulation.* 2005;111:2699–2710.

46. Eagle KA, Koelling TM, Montoye CK. Primer: implementation of guideline-based programs for coronary care. *Nat Clin Pract Cardiovasc Med.* 2006;3:163–171.

47. Mehta RH, Montoye CK, Gallogly M, et al. Improving quality of care for acute myocardial infarction. The Guidelines Applied in Practice (GAP) Initiative. *JAMA.* 2002;287:1269–1276.

48. *JAMA.* 1998;279(17):1351–1357.

49. Hayward RSA, Wilson MC, Tunis SR, et al. User's guide to the medical literature: VIII. How to use clinical practice guidelines. A. Are the recommendations valid? *JAMA.* 1995;274:570–574.

50. Wilson MC, Hayward RS, Tunis SR, et al. User's guide to the medical literature: VIII. How to use clinical practice guidelines. B. What are the recommendations and will they help you in caring for your patients? *JAMA.* 1995;274:1630–1632.

51. Shaneyfelt TM, Mayo-Smith MF, Rothwangle J. Are guidelines following guidelines? The methodological quality of clinical practice guidelines in the peer-reviewed medical literature. *JAMA.* 1999;281:1900–1905.

52. Cook D, Giacomini M. The trials and tribulations of clinical practice guidelines. *JAMA.* 1999;281:1950–1951.

53. Cluzeau FA, Littlejohns P, Grimshaw JM, et al. Development and application of a generic methodology to assess the quality of clinical practice guidelines. *Int J Qual Health Care.* 1999;11:21–28.

54. Graham ID, Clader LA, Hebert PC, et al. A comparison of clinical practice guideline appraisal instruments. *Int J Technol Assess Health Care.* 2000;16(4):1024–1038.

55. Grilli R, Magrini N, Penna A, et al. Practice guidelines developed by specialty societies: the need for a critical appraisal. *Lancet.* 2000;355:103–106.

56. The AGREE Collaboration. Development and validation of an international appraisal instrument for assessing the quality of clinical practice guidelines: the AGREE project. *Qual Saf Health Care.* 2003;12:18–23.

57. Agree Collaboration. Appraisal of guidelines research and evaluation. Available at: http://www.agreecollaboration.org.

58. Vlayen J, Aertgeerts B, Hannes K, Sermeus W, Ramaekers D. A systematic review of appraisal tools for clinical practice guidelines: multiple similarities and one common deficit. *Int J Qual Health Care.* 2005;17:235–242.

59. Watine J, Friedberg B, Nagy E, Onody R, Oosterhuis W, Bunting PS, et al. Conflict between guideline methodologic quality and recommendation validity: a potential problem for practitioners. *Clin Chem.* 2006;52:65–72.

60. Grimshaw JM, Russell IT. Effect of clinical guidelines on medical practice: a systematic review of rigorous evaluations. *Lancet.* 1993;342:1317–1322.

61. Sarasin FP, Maschiangelo ML, Schaller MD, et al. Successful implementation of guidelines for encouraging the use of beta blockers in patients after acute myocardial infarction. *Am J Med.* 1999;106:499–505.

62. Marciniak TA, Ellerbeck EF, Radford MJ, et al. Improving the quality of care for Medicare patients with acute myocardial infarction: results from the Cooperative Cardiovascular Project. *JAMA.* 1998;279:1351–1357.

CHAPTER 12

The History, Physical Examination, and Cardiac Auscultation

Robert A. O'Rourke / James A. Shaver / Mark E. Silverman

In the evaluation of patients with definite or suspected heart disease, important information (when sought) can be acquired from the history, physical examination, chest roentgenogram, electrocardiogram, and other routine laboratory tests.[1-4] These data, when integrated properly, facilitate an accurate diagnosis and appropriate decisions regarding therapy in many patients at a relatively low cost. When more information is necessary, additional, more expensive noninvasive cardiac tests such as echocardiography or radionuclide studies are often indicated. In some patients, the general assessment indicates the need for cardiac catheterization and contrast angiography with or without additional noninvasive cardiac testing. For example, the proper approach to certain, but not all, patients with symptomatic coronary artery disease can include both coronary arteriography and cardiac catheterization (anatomy and hemodynamics) as well as myocardial perfusion imaging with thallium or technetium sestamibi (extent of inducible ischemia).

Not all patients need every test; the skillful use of low-technology approaches, including the history and general examination (even when performed in the 21st century), can preclude the need for additional testing or can indicate which of a variety of available sophisticated tests should be selected for a particular patient. Chapter 12 is divided into three sections. The first concerns the proper application of the history and its use to delineate the differential diagnosis in patients who present with certain common cardiovascular symptoms. The second details the essential components of the *physical examination* and their usefulness in establishing a likely diagnosis when specific abnormal findings are detected. Finally, the third section focuses on cardiac auscultation.

THE HISTORY

[ ] COMPONENTS OF ACCURATE HISTORY TAKING

A carefully obtained history is the cornerstone for evaluating a patient with known or suspected cardiac disease.[4,5] A deliberate, compassionate interview forms the basis for a patient-physician relationship that can continue indefinitely. Unfortunately, the interview can result in adversarial roles for physician and patient if the interviewer appears hurried, shows impatience, fails to establish eye contact, seems to treat dreaded diseases casually, or appears to be unsympathetic.[5] When the medical interview is unsatisfactory because of poor communication and lack of rapport, inaccurate information and often unnecessary testing will be obtained.[5] Also, important facts not revealed during a meticulous initial history are usually not detected later, because both the patient and physician become focused on high-technology studies and more aggressive therapeutic interventions.[4]

The patient's chief complaint, which requires further elaboration and investigation, may not identify his or her most serious problem. Therefore symptoms other than the patient's chief complaint must be defined.[5] The interviewer should note all existing symptoms and establish a present illness for each of these.[5]

A medical questionnaire given to the patient well in advance of the interview is useful and can record important data more accurately because of the time thus made available to reflect and check details.[5]

A proper interpretation of the past history is important; the physician should not accept a past event as a fact when the evidence is not well established. Information obtained from family members about the patient's symptoms and his or her response to the illness is extremely important.[5]

Serious heart disease can occur in patients with mild or no symptoms. The physician must determine whether or not the history obtained is sufficient to support a decision-making process about the patient.[2] Although many patients with severe heart disease have no symptoms, others have many symptoms associated with minor or no disease.

Some patients deny symptoms because they cannot accept the reality of the situation, whereas others purposely withhold information so as not to jeopardize their jobs.[2] Some patients overstate their symptoms for personal gain. Elderly patients, sedentary patients, and those with other illnesses can have no symptoms because they are not physically active enough to induce them.[5]

[ ] PAST AND FAMILY HISTORY

The past history can provide important clues to the presence of cardiovascular disease. A definite history of rheumatic fever can be useful in defining the cause of a heart murmur (see Chap. 74), whereas a negative history does not exclude it.[5] A history of hypertension in a family member increases the likelihood that the patient has essential hypertension.[5] Previous trauma can be the cause of constrictive pericarditis, a thoracic aortic aneurysm, an arteriovenous fistula, and other types of cardiac lesions. A detailed history of the use of medications, addicting drugs, and alcohol, each of which can cause heart disease, is essential. A past history of pulmonary embolism, thrombophlebitis, or systemic embolism should be ascertained.

A history of dental work, some other diagnostic or therapeutic procedure, or recent infection suggests infective endocarditis in a patient with valvular heart disease. Patients often give a history of a *heart attack* that, in fact, can have been an episode of unstable angina, heart failure, or arrhythmia. The heart attack history often becomes *myocardial infarction* in the patient's medical record unless more information is obtained, or documentation of the event is reviewed.[4]

Many patients are referred who have had several catheterizations, percutaneous coronary interventions, and one or more coronary bypass operations in addition to multiple noninvasive tests. A thorough and often time-consuming review of records from other institutions, operative notes, cineangiographic films, and noninvasive studies will often provide an accurate assessment of the patient's current status without the *unnecessary repetition* of expensive and potentially risky procedures.[3]

Past and present therapeutic regimens must be reviewed carefully. Various treatment programs have often been inappropriate or suboptimal. Drugs used for the treatment of cardiovascular diseases have potential side effects that can produce both cardiovascular and noncardiovascular symptoms (see Chap. 94).

Multiple risk factors for developing coronary heart disease (CHD) have been identified, including age, male sex, hypertension, hypercholesterolemia, a low level of high-density lipoprotein (HDL) cholesterol, cigarette smoking, diabetes, and a family history of premature atherosclerosis (See Chap. 53).

Information from previous health evaluations should be sought. Patients have often been examined for military service, athletics, or insurance, and they might have been told of a heart murmur or hypertension on those occasions,[5] or they were rejected for medical insurance or military service. Many patients have never had a careful examination of the cardiovascular system.

The increasing hemodynamic burden of pregnancy can cause an otherwise marginally compensated cardiac patient to become symptomatic (See Chap. 96). Specific inquiry should be made about heart failure, edema, dyspnea, or prescribed prolonged periods of bedrest during pregnancy.[4] Many normal women have had a murmur detected during pregnancy. A history of illicit parenteral drug use should raise the suspicion of infective endocarditis, especially in a febrile patient (See Chap. 85). Cocaine can cause coronary artery vasospasm and also raise myocardial oxygen demand by increasing heart rate and blood pressure (BP). Angina, myocardial infarction, and sudden cardiac death after cocaine use have been well documented (See Chap. 94).

A history of moderate to excessive alcohol consumption, an enlarged heart on a prior chest roentgenogram, periods of rapid weight gain or loss, and other illnesses can provide important information.[1]

A family history of congenital heart disease indicates a higher risk of a congenital heart lesion (See Chap. 62). The patient's mother can give a history of rubella during the first few months of pregnancy; this increases the likelihood that the patient has patent ductus arteriosus, pulmonic valve stenosis, coarctation of the pulmonary arteries, or atrial septal defect.

Although many of the common cardiovascular diseases are sporadic, there are a rapidly increasing number of disease entities in which genetic transmission has been documented. These are detailed elsewhere (see Chaps. 9, 10, 81, and 82).

❚ ❩ SYMPTOMS CAUSED BY CARDIOVASCULAR DISEASE

Chest Pain

Chest pain or chest discomfort is the foremost manifestation of myocardial ischemia and results from a disparity between myocardial oxygen demand and coronary blood flow in patients with coronary artery disease (CAD).[5] The most common causes of myocardial ischemia are coronary atherosclerosis, coronary vasoconstriction, and coronary artery thrombosis, the latter occurring particularly in patients with acute coronary syndromes such as acute myocardial infarction and unstable angina (see Chaps. 52 and 53). An increase in myocardial oxygen consumption ($M\dot{V}O_2$) or demand ischemia, a decrease in or inadequate blood flow (supply ischemia), or their combination can be responsible for anginal chest pain (See Chap. 58).

The mechanism responsible for cardiac pain is not clearly understood. Nonmedullated small sympathetic nerve fibers that parallel the coronary arteries are thought to provide the afferent sensory pathway for angina; these enter the spinal cord in the C8 to T4 segments.[7] Impulses are transmitted to corresponding spinal ganglia and then through the spinal cord to the thalamus and cerebral cortex. Angina pectoris, like other pain of visceral origin, is often poorly localized and is commonly referred to the corresponding segmental dermatomes.

The differential diagnosis of chest pain is extensive.[5] In addition to angina pectoris and myocardial infarction, other cardiovascular diseases, gastrointestinal diseases, psychogenic diseases, neuromuscular diseases, and diseases of the pulmonary system must be considered (Table 12–1). An accurate interpretation of the etiology and significance of chest discomfort is critically dependent on a carefully taken history. Important, clinically relevant information can be missed if the *overenthusiastic use of noninvasive or invasive diagnostic methods* replaces rather than augments direct physician-patient communication (See Chap. 64).

The original subjective description of angina pectoris by William Heberden[6] in the late 18th century has not been surpassed. It is quoted in Chap. 64.

Angina pectoris is defined as chest pain or discomfort of cardiac origin that usually results from a temporary imbalance between myocardial oxygen supply and demand.[7] It can occur only with

---

❩ TABLE 12–1

Differential Diagnosis of Chest Pain

1. Angina pectoris/myocardial infarction
2. Other cardiovascular causes
   a. Likely ischemic in origin
      (1) Aortic stenosis
      (2) Hypertrophic cardiomyopathy
      (3) Severe systemic hypertension
      (4) Severe right ventricular hypertension
      (5) Aortic regurgitation
      (6) Severe anemia/hypoxia
   b. Nonischemic in origin
      (1) Aortic dissection
      (2) Pericarditis
      (3) Mitral valve prolapse
3. Gastrointestinal
   a. Esophageal spasm
   b. Esophageal reflux
   c. Esophageal rupture
   d. Peptic ulcer disease
4. Psychogenic
   a. Anxiety
   b. Depression
   c. Cardiac psychosis
   d. Self-gain
5. Neuromusculoskeletal
   a. Thoracic outlet syndrome
   b. Degenerative joint disease of cervical/thoracic spine
   c. Costochondritis (Tietze syndrome)
   d. Herpes zoster
   e. Chest wall pain and tenderness
6. Pulmonary
   a. Pulmonary embolus with or without pulmonary infarction
   b. Pneumothorax
   c. Pneumonia with pleural involvement
7. Pleurisy

exertion or spontaneously at rest; various subtypes are defined in Chap. 64. The quality of the chest discomfort is usually described as "tightness," "pressure," "burning," "heaviness," "aching," "strangling," or "compression." Usually the patient is able to describe a deep rather than a superficial origin of the pain. Because the qualitative description of the pain is greatly influenced by the patient's intelligence, education, and social/cultural background, a delineation of the other characteristics of the chest discomfort is often extremely important in evaluating the symptoms appropriately. The most important of these characteristics are the *precipitating factors* for the onset of pain, its mode of onset and duration, *its pattern of disappearance,* and its *location*. Classically, the discomfort is induced by exercise, emotion, eating, or cold weather.

A recognizable pattern of reproducibility of chest pain by certain activities is an important characteristic of angina. Often, patients develop pain with exertion after meals, and there is a greater tendency for arm work (a greater degree of isometric exercise) to produce distress.[8–10] Occasionally, angina will dissipate despite continued exercise (the *walk-through* phenomenon) or will not occur when a second exercise effort is undertaken that previously produced chest discomfort (*warmup* phenomenon). Both circumstances can be attributed to the opening of functioning coronary arterial collaterals during the initial myocardial ischemia. This is consistent with ischemic preconditioning as described elsewhere (See Chap. 64).[11]

Angina commonly occurs after the patient has eaten a heavy meal or when he or she is excited, angry, or tense. Cold showers increase BP and heart rate, whereas hot showers cause an augmented cardiac output in response to vasodilation. Either can precipitate angina after exercise. The chest pain during any activity is often made worse by the use of tobacco. All the hemodynamic changes caused by the use of nicotine increase myocardial oxygen demand.

Angina pectoris characteristically has a crescendo pattern at onset and "builds up." Pains, often described as "shooting" or "stabbing," that reach their maximum intensity virtually instantaneously are often not angina but are of musculoskeletal or neural origin. Angina is usually relieved within 5 to 20 minutes by rest, with or without the use of vasodilator drugs such as nitroglycerin (TNG), although sublingual TNG or TNG spray characteristically hastens relief. Failure to obtain relief with rest or TNG suggests another cause of pain or actual impending myocardial infarction. The reproducible relief of chest pain in an appropriate time frame (usually within 10 min) is strong evidence favoring ischemia. A trial of TNG can be a useful diagnostic strategy. Patients with angina pectoris are usually classified functionally from class I to class IV (Table 12–2), depending on the amount of activity necessary to induce chest pain.[12]

Localizing the *site* of chest discomfort provides additional information as to its cause. Anginal pain is ordinarily retrosternal or felt slightly to the left of the midline, beside or partly under the sternum. It is rarely isolated to the cardiac apex in the inframammary region. The chest pain of myocardial ischemia tends to radiate bilaterally across the chest into the arms (left more than right) and into the neck and lower jaw. Occasionally, radiation to the back or occiput is noted. In the arms, the pain passes down the ulnar and volar surface to the wrist and then only into the ulnar fingers, rarely into the thumb or down the outer (extensor) surface of the arm, which has a different dermatome pattern. Pain can occasion-

TABLE 12–2

Canadian Cardiovascular Society Functional Classification of Angina Pectoris

I. Ordinary physical activity, such as walking and climbing stairs, does not cause angina. Angina results from strenuous or rapid or prolonged exertion at work or recreation.

II. Slight limitation of ordinary activity. Walking or climbing stairs rapidly, walking uphill, walking or stair climbing after meals, in cold, in wind, or when under emotional stress, or only during the few hours after awakening. Walking more than two blocks on the level and climbing more than one flight of ordinary stairs at a normal pace and under normal conditions.

III. Marked limitations of ordinary physical activity. Walking one to two blocks on the level and climbing more than one flight under normal conditions.

IV. Inability to carry on any physical activity without discomfort—anginal syndrome can be present at rest.

SOURCE: *Modified from Campeau L. Letter to the editor. Circulation. 1976; 54:522. Reproduced with permission from the American Heart Association, Inc., and the author.*

ally be felt only in the arm or can start in the arm and radiate to the chest. Noting the patient's gestures in characterizing and localizing the site of pain can be useful. One or two clenched fists held by the patient over the sternal area (Levine sign) is much more indicative of ischemic pain than is a finger pointed to a small, circumscribed area in the left inframammary region. The latter is likely an indicator of psychogenic pain.

The *duration* of chest pain can also be a useful differentiating feature. Angina pectoris rarely lasts less than 1 minute or more than 20 minutes in the absence of myocardial infarction or persistent arrhythmias. Most patients with angina report *prompt relief* in fewer than 5 minutes after cessation of activity or with the use of sublingual or spray TNG.[13] Carotid sinus massage should be performed only in the absence of extracranial occlusive cerebrovascular disease as indicated by carotid bruits or decreased carotid arterial pulsations and with careful auscultatory monitoring of the heart rate. The Valsalva maneuver can also relieve anginal pain by decreasing myocardial wall stress because of the reduced venous return and left ventricular (LV) volume accompanying the increase in intrathoracic pressure. *Associated symptoms*—such as nausea, vomiting, faintness, fatigue, or diaphoresis—often accompany severe episodes of myocardial ischemia.[12] Severe myocardial ischemia often produces marked dyspnea caused by a large increase in LV diastolic filling pressure, sometimes producing an *angina equivalent* in the absence of chest discomfort.

Linked angina is a term applied to definite episodes of angina in patients with established CAD caused by gastrointestinal factors not related to an increase in cardiac work. Episodes are typically induced by stooping or occur after eating; they can be mimicked by esophageal acid stimulation, which can reduce coronary blood flow.[13–15]

No consideration of myocardial ischemia as a likely cause of chest discomfort is complete without carefully considering the chest pain in the context of *known risk factors* for CAD (See Chap. 51).

Angina pectoris should be considered a symptom and not a specific disease. Coronary arteriographic studies have demonstrated that more than 90 percent of patients with chest pain precipitated by exercise and relieved by rest have angiographic evidence of significant CAD. However, other diseases can be associated with classic angina pectoris.

Several reports have described certain patients with typical exertional chest discomfort and arteriographically normal coronary arteries. These patients are more likely to be females, have fewer coronary risk factors, and have variable responses to various antianginal agents, including TNG. Although the underlying cause of this condition remains unsettled, the life expectancy of these patients appears no different from that of an age- and sex-matched population without chest discomfort[16] (See Chap. 74).

There is some evidence that abnormal function of small coronary arteries can cause limited coronary blood flow (CBF) responses to stress or pharmacologic vasodilators in a subset of patients with anginal chest pain despite angiographically normal coronary arteries (*microvascular angina*).[16–18] In the past, investigators arguing for or against the existence of this syndrome have often used the term *syndrome X* to describe their patient cohort. Syndrome X appears to include a heterogeneous group of patients with a wide spectrum of chest pain and a variety of hypersensitive vascular and smooth muscle constrictor responses. Multiple research studies continue in an effort to explain syndrome X. The term *syndrome X* is a poor substitute for chest pain in patients with normal large vessel coronary arteriography. It is likely to represent a polyglot of disorders. It must be distinguished from the *metabolic syndrome (X)* of insulin resistance (glucose intolerance), hypertension, hyperlipidemia, and upper body obesity. The latter is often associated with severe vascular disease and frequently abnormal coronary arteriography. Some patients with classic angina but *near normal* contrast laminography, angiography fail to demonstrate areas of plaque formation because of coronary artery remodeling. Intracoronary ultrasound often demonstrates plaque of various size, volume, and location when CHD is present.[5]

Some patients with CAD experience angina at rest as a complication or an isolated clinical manifestation of ischemic heart disease. Myocardial ischemic pain at rest more likely results from an acute reduction in CBF than from an increase in $M\dot{V}O_2$. Possible causative factors include isolated coronary artery spasm or embolism, coronary artery spasm superimposed on coronary atherosclerosis (a common occurrence),[4] and coronary thrombosis with spontaneous thrombolysis. In patients with progressive coronary atherosclerosis; however, ischemic rest pain also can result from intermittent arrhythmias that increase $M\dot{V}O_2$ or decrease CBF or from labile hypertension, with its increased systolic wall stress. Chest pain at rest can occur only as nocturnal angina. In addition, nocturnal angina (also known as *angina decubitus*) can be produced by the increase in LV wall stress and $M\dot{V}O_2$ as a result of the redistribution of the intravascular blood volume in the recumbent position.

The relative hypercapnia and acidosis that occur during sleep can also contribute to nocturnal angina. The diagnosis of *sleep apnea* is often overlooked in patients with angina, heart failure, and arrhythmia. Nocturnal angina has been accompanied by concomitant rapid-eye-movement sleep patterns on the electroencephalogram, which can be associated with augmented sympathetic dis-

charge increasing $M\dot{V}O_2$ and/or causing coronary constriction[11–14] (see Chap. 64).

The quality of pain with rest angina is usually similar to that of exertional angina, but the discomfort can be more severe and its duration longer. In addition, angina at rest is commonly associated with nausea, vomiting, and diaphoresis. The onset of shortness of breath during or after the beginning of chest discomfort suggests that the pain is caused by extensive myocardial ischemia and results from an acute elevation of LV filling pressure secondary to the development of a large, transiently ischemic myocardial segment. Such patients commonly have multivessel occlusive CAD on arteriography.

Chest pain or discomfort resulting from *myocardial infarction* (MI) is qualitatively similar to angina at rest. Differentiating the pain resulting from ischemia and that caused by MI is often impossible based on the history alone.[11–13] Pain associated with acute coronary syndrome (ACS) is usually more severe and longer-lasting than anginal pain and is often associated with nausea, vomiting, and diaphoresis (see Chap. 49). In addition, MI or other ACS is frequently accompanied by symptoms of sustained LV dysfunction (dyspnea, orthopnea) and evidence of autonomic nervous system hyperactivity (tachycardia, diaphoresis, bradycardia).[11–13] Painless or atypical presentations of MI, however, occur in up to 40 percent of patients, particularly in diabetic patients and the elderly. Thus, determination of serial serum enzymes, isoenzymes, and other serum biomarkers (e.g., troponin I or T), providing evidence of myocardial necrosis, and serial electrocardiograms (ECGs), indicating myocardial injury, are necessary to establish the diagnosis (see Chaps. 59 and 60).

There are two groups of *cardiovascular diseases causing chest pain that is not caused by coronary atherosclerosis* (see Table 12–1). The first group consists of cardiac diseases causing myocardial ischemia–related angina in the absence of CAD. Ischemia is caused by hemodynamic changes associated with an inadequate CBF in relation to a normal or increased myocardial oxygen demand. Among these are *aortic valve stenosis* (see Chap. 75), *hypertrophic cardiomyopathy* (see Chap. 30), and *systemic arterial hypertension* (see Chap. 69), in which LV systolic pressure and LV wall tension are greatly increased, or LV hypertrophy is present.[11–13] Chest pain caused by myocardial ischemia also can occur with severe aortic regurgitation (AR) (see Chap. 75). The large LV volume load and increased LV dimensions augment $M\dot{V}O_2$ and the reduced diastolic perfusion pressure results in a relatively inadequate CBF. Occasionally, very severe anemia or hypoxia can also produce myocardial ischemia as a result of inadequate oxygen blood supply even in the absence of associated CAD. Both also can increase angina in the presence of obstructive CAD.[11–13] In addition, severe right ventricular (RV) systolic hypertension, as often occurs with pulmonic stenosis (PS) or pulmonary hypertension (PH), can cause exertional angina, presumably on the basis of RV subendocardial ischemia.[19]

A second group of cardiac diseases causing chest pain not usually caused by myocardial ischemia includes *pericarditis* (see Chap. 84), aortic dissection (see Chap. 105), and mitral valve prolapse (MVP) (see Chap. 76). Pericarditis is a relatively common cause of chest pain.[20] It is most often sharp and penetrating in quality; patients often obtain relief by sitting up and bending forward (see Chap. 84). The cardinal diagnostic feature of pericardial pain is its frequent worsening by changes in body position, during deep inspiration, and occasionally on swallowing. The chest discomfort can radiate to the shoulders, upper back, and neck because of irritation of the diaphragmatic pleura, which is innervated through the phrenic nerve by fibers originating in sympathetic ganglia C3 to C5. Therefore the chest discomfort associated with pericarditis is caused predominantly by parietal pleural irritation. Occasionally, the pain of acute benign, presumptive viral pericarditis can mimic that observed in acute MI. Importantly, the most common cause of pericarditis in middle-aged or older people is acute MI. The pericarditis usually occurs several days after the myocardial necrosis and must be distinguished from recurrent infarction or ischemia. Pericarditis can also be a cause of chest pain after cardiac surgery and can be a complication of aortic dissection, with leakage into the pericardium.

Aortic dissection (see Chap. 105) can be misdiagnosed on initial presentation as an acute MI; indeed, MI is a recognized complication of aortic dissection. The pain with dissection, however, is usually of sudden onset as compared with that of myocardial ischemia, which builds in intensity with time.[21] Patients frequently characterize the pain as excruciating, as having a tearing quality, and commonly localized to the interscapular area. The discomfort can radiate widely into the neck, back, abdomen, flanks, and legs and can migrate, depending on the location and progression of the aortic dissection and the amount of arterial luminal compression. Neurologic symptoms and signs can occur when dissection involves the cerebral arteries. With the exception of patients with Marfan syndrome (see Chaps. 88 and 105) or idiopathic cystic medial necrosis, most patients with aortic dissection have a history of longstanding systemic arterial hypertension or evidence of it on physical examination, or by ECG (left ventricular hypertrophy [LVH]).

Psychogenic chest discomfort is a common recurrent chest pain that can be difficult to separate from angina pectoris, particularly when it occurs in patients with multiple risk factors for CAD or in otherwise asymptomatic patients with well-documented CAD. The most common psychogenic cause of chest discomfort is anxiety[22] (see Chap. 95). Psychogenic chest pain is often described as sharp or stabbing, localized to the left inframammary area, and usually sharply circumscribed. Descriptors such as "stabbing" or "lightning-like" can be used to describe extremely short (<1 min) episodes of pain. At times, the pain can persist for many hours or several days. Patients often note psychogenic pain at rest. Also, nonvocal communication—such as a flat or worried facial expression, retarded motor activity, and hand wringing—can indicate underlying depression. Observation of the patient during pain that occurs spontaneously or during exercise testing often provides insight into a potential psychogenic etiology. Patients with anxiety often have multiple complaints. Associated symptoms—such as air hunger, circumoral paresthesias, globus hystericus, and multiple somatic complaints—can suggest a neurasthenic personality or hyperventilation syndrome.

Pain originating in the gastrointestinal tract, particularly that of esophageal origin, is commonly confused with ischemic chest pain.[23] *Diffuse esophageal spasm,* a neuromuscular motor disorder of the esophagus characterized by chest pain, is the extracardiac condition most frequently confused with angina pectoris. Esophageal spasm can occur at any age but is more common in 50- to 60-year-old individuals. The pain is usually retrosternal; can be burning, squeezing, or aching in quality; and often radiates to the

back, arms, and jaw. It usually begins during or after a meal and can last minutes or hours. The pain can be relieved by TNG, which also relaxes esophageal smooth muscle. A useful diagnostic feature in esophageal spasm is its frequent association with pain as a result of swallowing, dysphagia, and the regurgitation of gastric contents. The diagnosis of diffuse esophageal spasm is based on the history, the exclusion of cardiac and musculoskeletal causes of chest pain, and the demonstration of abnormal esophageal motility on cine-esophagograms or by esophageal manometry.

Reflux esophagitis results from mucosal irritation produced by failure of the lower esophageal sphincter to prevent regurgitation of highly acidic gastric contents into the distal esophagus.[24–26] The pain is usually epigastric or retrosternal, burning in quality, and frequently precipitated by the recumbent position or by bending over. *Heartburn* and regurgitation often occur after meals or ingestion of coffee or after postural changes. Patients are often awakened by chest discomfort caused by acid reflux occurring in the recumbent position. Dysphagia can result from stricture formation secondary to long-standing esophageal reflux. An upper gastrointestinal x-ray series can demonstrate hiatal hernia, but this does not establish the diagnosis of esophagitis or esophageal reflux. Esophagoscopy and esophageal biopsy can demonstrate mucosal lesions and are useful for assessing the severity of inflammation and for excluding malignancy. Sphincter incompetence can be documented by the use of esophageal manometry. Esophageal acid perfusion testing (Bernstein test) often will provoke the patient's characteristic symptoms, and distal esophageal pH monitoring will detect gastroesophageal reflux.[25]

Acute esophageal rupture, a serious and often rapidly lethal event, causes severe retrosternal pain secondary to the chemical mediastinitis produced by acidic gastric contents.[8–11] Spontaneous rupture usually results from a prolonged bout of vomiting or retching after a heavy meal. The pain varies in location depending on the rupture's site and position. The diagnosis is based on symptoms and signs of mediastinal air following vomiting or esophageal instrumentation.

Although peptic ulcer disease and biliary colic are less commonly confused with chest pain of cardiac origin, myocardial ischemic pain can occasionally be described as burning in character and located near the epigastrium.

Diseases involving the neuromuscular-skeletal systems can cause pain affecting dermatomal patterns similar to those occurring with angina pectoris.[8–11] The thoracic outlet syndromes, in which various neural and vascular structures are compressed, can produce symptoms that are sometimes confused with cardiac chest pain. Although compression of the neurovascular bundle by a cervical rib or the scalenus anterior muscle can cause discomfort radiating to the head and neck, the shoulder region, or the axilla, most patients experience pain in the upper extremity ulnar distribution resulting from somatic nerve compression. The presence of associated paresthesias, of pain unrelated to physical exercise, and the worsening of discomfort with certain body positions are useful differentiating characteristics.

Tietze syndrome, or idiopathic costochondritis, is an occasional cause of anterior chest-wall pain that is aggravated by movement and deep breathing. Reproducing the chest pain syndrome by direct pressure over the involved costochondral junction or the relief of pain after local infiltration with lidocaine is a helpful diagnostic maneuver. Degenerative arthritis of the cervical and thoracic vertebrae can cause band-like pain confined to the chest, neck, or back that often radiates to the arms.[8-10] Radiologic evidence of degenerative changes involving the cervical and thoracic vertebrae is often found in asymptomatic elderly patients. The production or exacerbation of pain by various postures, movement, sneezing, or coughing is more useful in the diagnosis of chest discomfort caused by vertebral disease.[8-10]

The *preeruptive stage of herpes zoster* can be characterized by band-like chest pain over one or more dermatomes. The advanced age of the patient; additional symptoms of malaise, headache, and fever; the presence of hyperesthesia of the involved area on physical examination; and the eventual eruption of typical lesions 4 or 5 days after the onset of symptoms will result in the correct diagnosis. Chest wall pain and tenderness can occur for unknown reasons. The discomfort can be reproduced by pressure over the painful area and by movements of the thorax such as bending, twisting, or turning.

The syndrome of acute massive *pulmonary embolism* with its associated acute PH and low cardiac output occasionally can simulate acute MI because myocardial ischemia can be present in both conditions. The quality of chest pain can be identical to that observed in patients with nonradiating ischemic chest pain or can be pleuritic. The associated signs of severe dyspnea, tachypnea, and intense cyanosis, accompanied by profound anxiety and agitation, however, favor the diagnosis of pulmonary embolism[9-12] (see Chap. 72). Measurements of arterial blood gases, abnormal pulmonary ventilation/perfusion scans, and, if needed, pulmonary arteriography will establish the correct diagnosis.[8-10]

Other pulmonary conditions associated with chest discomfort, such as pneumothorax, are rarely confused with ischemic chest pain because of additional characteristic clinical features. Spontaneous pneumothorax usually occurs in otherwise healthy males in the third and fourth decades. The clinical presentation is usually characterized by the abrupt onset of agonizing unilateral pleuritic chest pain associated with severe shortness of breath. The plain or expiratory chest film provides the definitive diagnosis. Chest pain associated with pneumonias of various etiologies, as well as pulmonary infarctions as a consequence of pulmonary embolus, can result from pleural irritation. The discomfort is sharp, varies acutely with breathing, and is frequently accompanied by a reduced inspiratory effort. Associated signs of pulmonary parenchymal infection or infarction usually indicate the underlying diagnosis.

Extrathoracic Pain

Intermittent claudication of the lower extremities caused by peripheral atherosclerosis (see Chap. 108) can present as discomfort during exercise in the arch of the foot, calf of the leg, thighs, hips, or gluteal region.[8-11] Acute arterial occlusion in the lower extremities caused by systemic embolism can cause the sensation of hypesthesia.[2] The pain of Raynaud disease can be noted in the fingers after exposure to cold, with pallor of the fingers prior to the sensation of pain. Pain and swelling of lower extremities can be caused by thrombophlebitis (see Chap. 108).

Head pain secondary to myocardial ischemia can be felt in the jaw, hard palate, cheek, and sometimes deep in the ear canals. The pain of temporal arteritis, commonly localized to the temporal area, often is associated with abnormal vision and polymyalgia rheumatica. A severe headache can be present in patients with uncontrolled hypertension (see Chap. 69).

Pain in the abdomen, often localized to the midabdomen and lower portion of the back, can be produced by an expanding or rupturing atherosclerotic abdominal aneurysm. Abdominal angina caused by vascular disease of the mesenteric arteries is discussed in Chap. 105. The liver is often painful and tender in severe right-sided heart failure, with worsening of the pain during activity.[2]

Various types of *joint pain* can be associated with heart disease (see Chaps. 74 and 88). Rheumatic fever, rheumatoid arthritis, lupus erythematosus, psoriatic arthritis, ankylosing spondylitis, gonococcal arthritis, Reiter syndrome, and Lyme disease can be associated with valvular, myocardial, or pericardial disease.[2]

Respiratory Symptoms

Dyspnea is defined as difficult or labored respiration or the unpleasant awareness of one's breathing. A clue to the etiology is obtained from the factors that precipitate or relieve it.[1] Chronic dyspnea can be caused by heart failure, pulmonary disease, anxiety, obesity, poor physical fitness, pleural effusions, and asthma.[2] Acute dyspnea can occur with acute pulmonary edema, hyperventilation, pneumothorax, pulmonary embolism, pneumonia, and airway obstruction.[2]

Dyspnea on effort, a frequent symptom, is usually caused by congestive heart failure, chronic pulmonary disease, or physical deconditioning (see Chap. 26). A recent or dramatic increase in the dyspnea is more likely to be caused by the development of heart failure than by lung disease. When heart and lung disease coexist, however, determination of the relative contribution of pulmonary and cardiac dysfunction to dyspnea can be very difficult.

Cheyne-Stokes respiration is a form of periodic breathing characterized by cycles beginning with shallow respirations that increase in rate and depth to significant hyperpnea, followed by decreasing rate and depth of respiration, and then a period of apnea that can last 15 seconds or longer. This form of respiration occurs in advanced congestive heart failure and in some forms of central nervous system disease. Cheyne-Stokes respiration often occurs during sleep without the patient's awareness and is often reported by others.

Orthopnea results from an increase in hydrostatic pressure in the lungs that occurs with assumption of the supine position. It consists of cough and dyspnea in some patients with LV failure or mitral valve (MV) disease and necessitates the use of two or more pillows on lying down. The patient with severe obstructive lung disease, especially acute asthma, also cannot lie flat comfortably.

Paroxysmal nocturnal dyspnea (PND) is the occurrence of dyspnea during sleep, commonly 2 to 3 hours after going to bed, which is relieved by assuming the upright position. Dyspnea usually does not recur after the patient goes back to sleep. Episodes can be mild, or they can be severe with wheezing, coughing, gasping, and apprehension.[1] Some episodes will progress to pulmonary edema. The probable mechanism for this *relatively specific symptom* of left-sided heart failure is the increase in central blood volume in the supine position.

A dry, unproductive cough, occurring with effort or at rest, can be related to the pulmonary congestion associated with heart failure (see Chap. 25). Although dyspnea is usually present, cough can dominate the clinical picture. The cough that accompanies acute pulmonary edema is often associated with frothy, pink-tinged sputum, whereas the sputum associated with chronic bronchitis is usually white and mucoid.[2] Sputum associated with pneumonia is often thick and yellow and because of pulmonary infarction can be bloody, as can the sputum associated with cancer of the lung or bronchiolectasis. Cough also can be caused by angiotensin-converting enzyme inhibitors.

Recurrent coughing caused by heart failure is often thought to be caused by bronchitis, and patients with chronic bronchitis can cough more when heart failure ensues.[2] Patients with a high pulmonary blood flow caused by congenital left-to-right shunts are subject to pulmonary infection. Patients with a high pulmonary venous pressure (e.g., mitral stenosis) are more vulnerable to pulmonary edema when they have viral pneumonitis than are patients with normal pulmonary venous pressure.

Hemoptysis occurs in many cardiac disorders. Posterior epistaxis as a result of systemic hypertension can cause blood-streaked sputum; patients on anticoagulants can have epistaxis that mimics hemoptysis. Bright red pulmonary venous blood from rupture of submucosal pulmonary venules can be expectorated by patients with pulmonary venous hypertension caused by mitral stenosis (MS) or severe left ventricle failure.[2] Darker blood or clots often occur with pulmonary emboli.

Pink, frothy sputum can be produced during acute pulmonary edema. Blood-streaked sputum is a feature of the *winter bronchitis* of mitral stenosis.[2] Massive hemoptysis with exsanguination can follow rupture of an aortic aneurysm or one of the cardiac chambers into the bronchial tree.[2] Rupture of a pulmonary artery by the balloon of an indwelling pulmonary artery catheter can cause abrupt, severe hemoptysis in hospitalized patients.

Wheezing associated with dyspnea can be caused by lung or heart disease. If the symptoms have developed recently in an adult older than 40 years of age, other clues indicating heart disease (cardiac asthma) should be sought.

Edema and Ascites

Edema is a common symptom or finding in patients with right- or left-sided heart failure. Fluid retention in heart failure results from increased venous pressure and abnormal activity of salt-retaining hormones (see Chap. 25). In an average-sized person, 5 to 10 lb (2.3–4.5 kg) of excess fluid is required for edema to become apparent; a history of recent weight gain will often correlate with deterioration in clinical status. The amount of weight loss in response to treatment for heart failure in the past will relate to the severity of the problem. Minor degrees of edema are evident only after a period of dependency of the legs and will decrease after rest. Presacral edema can be most obvious when the patient has been at bedrest. Although edema of cardiac origin can progress to anasarca, cardiac edema rarely involves the face or upper extremities. Persistent edema in the legs from which veins were harvested at the time of bypass surgery is common. Other causes of edema—such as varicosities, obesity, tight girdle, renal insufficiency, or cirrhosis with hypoproteinemia—must be considered.[1] A patient with chronic congestive heart failure can detect edema of the ankles and lower legs during the day and note that it diminishes during the night. It is important to ascertain whether edema of the extremities preceded or followed dyspnea on effort. The calcium antagonists can produce bilateral edema of the lower legs. Edema can occur in one or both legs following the harvesting of veins for conduits in patients undergoing coronary artery bypass grafting (CABG) surgery.

Patients will be aware of ascites because of increased abdominal girth. Previously comfortable trousers or skirts can no longer fit. Bending at the waist is uncomfortable, with ill-defined abdominal fullness. Patients with severe edema caused by congestive heart failure can develop ascites; however, ascites is particularly common in patients with constrictive pericardial disease, sometimes occurring before peripheral edema becomes obvious (see Chap. 84). Ascitic fluid is formed when elevated venous pressure leads to transudation of fluids from the serosal surfaces.

Fatigue and Weakness

Fatigue and *weakness* can be caused by many causes and therefore are not specific symptoms for heart disease. The most common cause of these symptoms is anxiety and depression. Anemia, thyrotoxicosis, and other chronic disease states can be associated with fatigue and weakness.

When a patient with heart disease is volume overloaded, or when there is pulmonary congestion caused by heart disease, the patient is likely to complain of dyspnea. With vigorous diuretic therapy, this complaint can be replaced by symptoms of fatigue and weakness,[2] probably related to inadequate cardiac output (see Chap. 26). As congestive heart failure worsens, fatigue can replace dyspnea as the major symptom. β-Blockers used to treat angina or hypertension and LV dysfunction often cause fatigue and lethargy. When starting β-blockers to treat heart failure "start low and go slow." Hypotension or hypokalemia caused by diuretics can result in fatigue and weakness, as can relative hypovolemia caused by the use of angiotensin-converting enzyme inhibitors.

Severe fatigue related to effort can result from transient global myocardial ischemia in patients with extensive CAD. Dyspnea and hypotension also can occur at the same time as the severe fatigue as *angina equivalents*.[2]

Palpitation

Most normal individuals are intermittently aware of their heart action, particularly at the time of physical and emotional stress. When the heart action is more vigorous than usual or its perception is unpleasant, the term *palpitation* is appropriate.[1] The patient can complain of a "pounding," "stopping," "jumping," or "racing" in the chest. Palpitation is frequently a benign symptom without any serious cardiac disease present; at other times it can indicate a potentially life-threatening condition. Simple premature beats can be perceived as a "floating" or "flopping" sensation in the chest caused by the more forceful beat that occurs after the pause following the premature beat. Sometimes a transient feeling of fullness in the neck (caused by cannon A waves) is perceived with premature beats. Certain patients perceive almost every premature beat, whereas others are totally unaware of frequent or advanced arrhythmias. A report of skips or irregularity during uninterrupted sinus rhythm is not uncommon. Generally, thin, tense individuals are likely to be more aware of their cardiac activity than others. Individuals with and without arrhythmias often are aware of their cardiac activity when they first lie down to sleep, especially if they lie on their left side.[1]

Rapid heart action of a paroxysmal tachycardia usually begins and terminates abruptly and causes a pounding sensation in the chest.[1] Patients often will indicate whether the tachycardia is regular or irregular and can be able to tap out the rate and rhythm of the episode (see Chap. 36). Chest pressure suggesting angina can occur with an episode of tachycardia even in young, healthy patients without CAD. Patients with CAD, however, often develop severe angina with a sustained arrhythmia because of increased $M\dot{V}O_2$. Depending on the rate and mechanism of the arrhythmia, faintness, and syncope can be described during questioning. Nevertheless, sustained ventricular tachycardia can occur in the setting of serious underlying cardiac disease without a significant compromise in hemodynamics (see Chap. 36). Syncope caused by tachyarrhythmias can occur without the patient being aware of palpitations.

Syncope

Cardiac *syncope* (fainting) is defined as the transient loss of consciousness caused by inadequate cerebral blood flow secondary to an abrupt decrease in cardiac output (see Chap. 48). *Near syncope* refers to the clinical situation in which the patient feels dizzy and weak and tends to lose postural tone but does not lose consciousness. In assessing the patient with syncope, one determines if there were precipitating factors, premonitory symptoms, injury with the episode, seizure activity or incontinence, or a postictal state.[1] Injury during an episode suggests a sudden profound loss of body tone and increases the likelihood of more serious causes. Brief, unsustained seizure activity can occur with syncope caused by a cardiac arrhythmia.

The patient can be incontinent during cardiogenic syncope, but an aura, sustained tonic-clonic movements, tongue biting, and confusion or drowsiness after the event are more characteristic of syncope caused by central nervous system disease. In contrast, return of consciousness to the alert state is prompt after reversal of the arrhythmia causing cardiac syncope.[1] The common faint (*vasovagal syncope*) results from bradycardia and hypotension caused by excessive vagal discharge. It is often associated with some precipitating event such as a heavy meal in a warm room and has brief premonitory signs and symptoms such as nausea, yawning, diaphoresis, and sometimes the feeling of decreased hearing or vision.[1] The results of head-up, tilt-table testing indicate a vasovagal mechanism in some patients with syncope who do not have premonitory symptoms (see Chap. 48). Following a fainting episode, the patient can be pale and diaphoretic and have a slow heart rate. A history of similar episodes during the preceding several years is common in patients with vagal syncope.

A hypersensitive carotid sinus can cause syncope. A history of episodes during an activity such as shaving, wearing of a tight collar, or extreme turning of the head can occur but is unusual even when a sensitive carotid sinus is shown to be the cause of syncope. Syncope following urination (micturition syncope) can occur at the time of rapid decompression of a distended bladder, which typically occurs after a period of sleep. Paroxysms of coughing, usually in patients with underlying pulmonary disease, can result in syncope. Very fast or slow arrhythmias can decrease the cardiac output enough to cause alterations in consciousness, ranging from abrupt profound syncope to mild light-headedness. Stokes-

Adams syncope is caused by intermittent complete heart block, sinus arrest, or ventricular tachyarrhythmias (see Chap. 48). It is characterized by abrupt loss of consciousness without warning, a variable period of unconsciousness (seconds to minutes), and then a rapid return of normal mental status without amnesia or a postictal state.

In the presence of severe LV outflow obstruction (aortic stenosis or hypertrophic cardiomyopathy), loss of consciousness with effort can occur. Syncope can be caused either by the heart's inability to increase its output in response to the peripheral vasodilatation that occurs during exercise or by a tachyarrhythmia. Intermittent obstruction of a cardiac valve by an intracavitary tumor or thrombus is a rare cause of syncope that occasionally can be precipitated when the patient changes position (see Chap. 89).

Many normal subjects experience transient light-headedness with rapid changes in position. This is more common in older patients, because the ability of the peripheral vasculature to respond is attenuated with aging (see Chap. 100). Postural hypotension is a well-defined cause of fainting or dizziness that usually occurs when the individual is upright and often just after rising from a supine or sitting position. Possible causes include peripheral neuropathy, autonomic dysfunction, volume depletion, or drug side effects.

Other Cerebral Symptoms

Patients with decreased cardiac output secondary to heart failure can become mentally confused and disoriented. Such symptoms also can be caused by hypoxia, to drugs that are invariably prescribed for such patients, and to renal or hepatic failure.[2] A completed stroke can be caused by a lacunar infarct, cerebral hemorrhage, cerebral arterial thrombosis, or a cerebral embolus (see Chap. 106). A transient cerebral ischemic attack is commonly caused by an embolus. The embolus can originate in an atheromatous ulcer in the carotid artery system or the aortic arch; be related to infective endocarditis, a recent MI, atrial fibrillation, or clots on a prosthetic valve; or originate in the leg veins and pass through a patent foramen ovale to the brain (see Chap. 106).

The patient with cardiogenic shock or with a severe tachyarrhythmia who also has considerable intracranial or extracranial vascular disease can develop such severe cerebral hypoxia that coma occurs. Hypoxic encephalopathy can follow cardiac resuscitation and occasionally occurs after cardiopulmonary bypass for cardiac surgery. A cerebral abscess can occur in patients with congenital heart disease and a right-to-left shunt.[2]

Fever, Chills, and Sweats

Fever with chills is common in patients with infective endocarditis. Symptoms of fever, chills, or sweats in any patient with a heart murmur should lead one to suspect infective endocarditis (see Chap. 85). A history of valvular heart disease is not a prerequisite because previously normal valves become infected. A history of recent dental work, genitourinary surgery, or illicit drug use increases the suspicion of infective endocarditis. Fever can accompany rheumatic fever or pericarditis. An intracardiac tumor (myxoma) can produce systemic symptoms in the absence of infection. Low-grade fever in a patient with heart failure can be a sign of pulmonary emboli.[2] Excessive sweating can occur in patients with severe aortic regurgitation (AR) or acute MI. Diaphoresis is often a sign of congestive heart failure in infants.

Hoarseness

Hoarseness can occur in patients with an aortic aneurysm that involves the left recurrent laryngeal nerve. MS occasionally can produce hoarseness caused by the pressure of a large pulmonary artery on the recurrent laryngeal nerve. Pericardial effusion can be related to myxedema, which can be associated with a coarse, low-pitched voice. Hoarseness and loss of voice can occur following the use of an endotracheal tube during cardiac surgery.

Indigestion, Hiccups, and Dysphagia

Many patients with angina pectoris caused by CAD erroneously attribute their symptoms to *indigestion* or heartburn. Also, patients with heartburn, esophageal reflux, and esophageal spasm can believe they have angina pectoris. *Hiccups* occasionally can occur in patients with MI and during the postoperative period after cardiac surgery. *Dysphagia* can occur in patients with progressive systemic sclerosis, an aortic arch anomaly, or an extremely large left atrium.

Gastrointestinal Symptoms

Anorexia, nausea, and vomiting can occur as a result of digitalis excess. Hepatomegaly associated with tricuspid valve disease or severe right-sided heart failure can cause right-upper-quadrant epigastric pain and fullness as well as anorexia. Abdominal pain caused by visceral ischemia or infarction can occur in a patient who has had a period of very low cardiac output.

Abnormal Skin Color

Although *cyanosis* is a sign rather than a symptom, patients or family members can describe cyanosis during the history. *Cyanosis* is a bluish color of the skin or mucous membranes caused by excess amounts of reduced hemoglobin. Approximately 4 grams of reduced hemoglobin is required for cyanosis to be apparent (see Chap. 82). Severely anemic patients will not exhibit cyanosis. A distribution of cyanosis involving the mucous membranes as well as the periphery (central cyanosis) is caused by the admixture of venous blood at the level of the heart or great vessels. A patient or a family member can detect that the cyanosis is more intense in the feet than in the hands. This differential cyanosis suggests a right-to-left shunt through a patent ductus arteriosus in a patient with Eisenmenger physiology (see Chap. 82). Peripheral cyanosis does not involve the mucous membranes but is the result of slow peripheral flow with accumulation of excess reduced hemoglobin in the setting of circulatory failure, shock, or peripheral vasospasm.

Jaundice can be detected by a patient or by a member of the family. As a rule, hepatic congestion caused by heart failure will not produce jaundice. When jaundice does occur in a patient with heart failure, it is appropriate to consider pulmonary infarction in addition to hepatic congestion or cirrhosis of the liver. Hemolysis of red blood cells can occur in patients with prosthetic valves and can produce jaundice.[2]

A history of flush of face and trunk, sometimes accentuated by alcohol, should lead one to search for the other signs and symptoms of carcinoid heart disease[2] (see Chap. 85). Cardiomyopathies caused by hemochromatosis should be considered in the patient with diabetes whose skin color has changed from normal to bronze.[2] A slate-like color of the skin, hands, and nose can develop in patients who take amiodarone.

Embolization

The entry of a blood clot, vegetation, or tumor fragment from the heart into the systemic circulation results in arterial embolus. Clots can occur in the left atrium behind a stenotic mitral valve, within a ventricular aneurysm, or in the left ventricle of a patient with cardiomyopathy. Although many emboli originate in the heart, arteriosclerotic material in the ascending and descending aorta often embolizes to the periphery.[1] Many emboli are asymptomatic. Symptoms of a stroke occur with emboli to the cerebral vessels. MI can result from an embolus to a coronary artery. Hematuria, flank pain, and hypertension can result from embolization to a renal artery. The abrupt development of a cold, painful extremity follows embolic obstruction of an arm or leg artery.[1] Emboli from the vegetations of acute endocarditis can produce characteristic areas of vascular necrosis in the fingers or toes (see Chap. 85). Severe atherosclerosis in the abdominal aorta and iliac vessels can be responsible for showers of peripheral emboli with multiple small, reddish blue lesions on the lower extremities sometimes causing small areas of gangrene. An embolic event can be the presenting manifestation of previously unrecognized cardiac disease.

Insomnia

The most common causes of insomnia are mental conflict, emotional disturbances, and depression. Heart failure, however, can also cause insomnia. The patient with Cheyne-Stokes respirations (see preceding section on Respiratory Symptoms) can sleep during the apneic phase and wake during the hyperpneic phase of the condition. Occasionally, patients with pulmonary congestion caused by heart failure have insomnia before they develop nocturnal dyspnea. Central and obstructive sleep apnea are discussed elsewhere (see Chaps. 26, 82, and 101).

❏ CLASSIFICATION OF CARDIAC DISABILITY

Several classifications have been proposed and used for the systematic and reproducible grading of disability caused by cardiac disease. Although the complete New York Heart Association method of classifying cardiac diagnoses, originally proposed many years ago, is not widely used now, the portion of the classification that concerns functional capacities[27] in heart failure is still commonly used (Table 12–3). Although the Canadian Cardiovascular Society's grading system for angina (see Table 12–2) is more widely used for patients with chest pain, both classifications continue to be used in the medical literature and in clinical practice, particularly as criteria for the inclusion of heart patients in multicenter clinical trials. Recommendations for the management based on the results of multicenter randomized clinical trials and/or the consensus of expert writing groups and resulting publications of practice guidelines recommendation table (Table 12–4) (See Chapter 11).

TABLE 12–3

The Old New York Heart Association Functional Classification

Class 1 No symptoms with ordinary physical activity.
Class 2 Symptoms with ordinary activity. Slight limitation of activity.
Class 3 Symptoms with less than ordinary activity. Marked limitation of activity.
Class 4 Symptoms with any physical activity or even at rest.

SOURCE: *The Criteria Committee of the New York Heart Association. Diseases of the Heart and Blood Vessels: Nomenclature and Criteria for Diagnosis of the Heart and Great Vessels, 6th ed. New York: New York Heart Association/Little, Brown; 1964. Reproduced with permission from the New York Heart Association, Inc., and the publisher.*

THE PHYSICAL EXAMINATION

Important information concerning the patient with heart disease is often obtained by a careful and deliberate physical examination, which includes a general inspection of the patient, an indirect measurement of the arterial BP in both arms and one or both lower extremities, an examination of central and peripheral arterial pulses, an evaluation of the jugular venous pressure and pulsa-

TABLE 12–4

ACC/AHA Clinical Practice Guidelines

Class I	Conditions for which there is evidence and/or general agreement that a given procedure or treatment is useful and effective.
Class II	Conditions for which there is conflicting evidence and/or a divergence of opinion about the usefulness/efficacy of a procedure or treatment.
	IIa. Weight of evidence/opinion is in favor of usefulness/efficacy.
	IIb. Usefulness/efficacy is less well established by evidence/opinion.
Class III	Conditions for which there is evidence and/or general agreement that the procedure/treatment is not useful/effective, and in some cases can be harmful.
Level of evidence A	Data derived from multiple randomized clinical trials.
Level of evidence B	Data derived from a single randomized trial, or nonrandomized studies.
Level of evidence C	Consensus opinion of experts.

ACC/AHA, American College of Cardiology/American Heart Association.

tions, palpation of the precordium, and cardiac auscultation. Based on the results of this rather inexpensive evaluation, a definite diagnosis often is made; selected noninvasive and invasive testing is ordered only when appropriate.

【 】 GENERAL INSPECTION OF THE PATIENT

Bedside examination begins with a careful general appraisal of the patient. This visual inspection can provide important information leading to the etiology of cardiovascular disease.

Clues to the diagnosis of underlying congenital heart disease can be obtained from careful observation of the thorax and extremities. Bilateral prominence of the anterior chest with bulging of the upper two-thirds of the sternum is commonly present in children with a large ventricular septal defect (VSD). A unilateral bulge at the fourth and fifth intercostal spaces at the lower left sternal border is found in adults with VSD. Scoliosis can be present in cyanotic congenital heart disease. Underdeveloped musculature of the lower extremities compared with the upper extremities occurs with coarctation of the aorta. Clubbing of the digits and cyanosis of the skin or nails suggest congenital heart disease with right-to-left shunting of blood (Fig. 12–1). Differential cyanosis provides information about anatomy.[28] Cyanosis and clubbing of the toes associated with pink fingernails of the right hand and cyanosis and clubbing of the left hand are caused by a patent ductus arteriosus with normally related great vessels and a reversed shunt as a result of pulmonary hypertension, with the patent ductus arteriosus delivering cyanotic blood to the left arm and lower extremities (Figs. 12–2 and 12–3). The same color pattern results from interruption of the aortic arch and a patent ductus arteriosus delivering desaturated blood to the legs. However, if

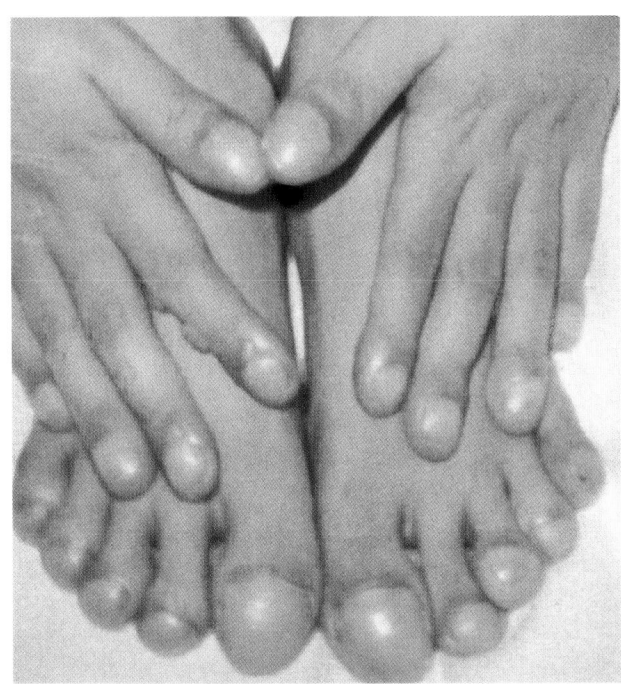

FIGURE 12–1. Symmetric cyanosis. Equal cyanosis and clubbing of hands and feet caused by transposition of the great vessels and a ventricular septal defect without patent ductus arteriosus.

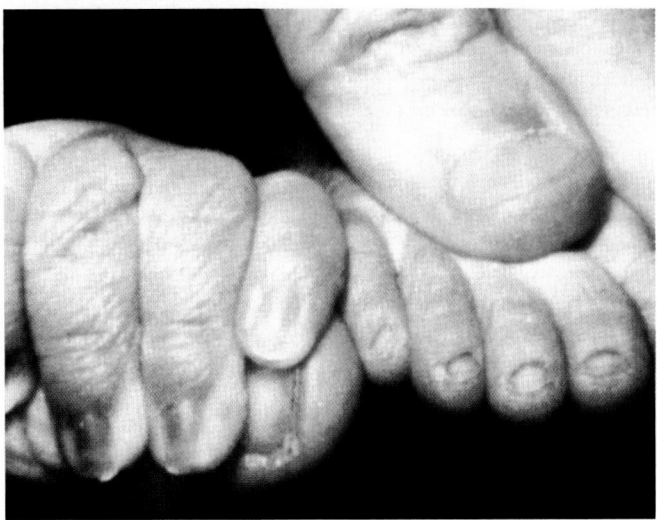

FIGURE 12–2. *Differential cyanosis.* Clubbing of left hand and cyanosis of left hand and all toes as a result of patent ductus arteriosus with pulmonary hypertension and normally related great vessels. *Courtesy of Dr. Joseph K. Perloff, University of California, Los Angeles.*

the right subclavian artery arises proximal to the aortic obstruction, the right hand can be pink and the left hand cyanotic. When an anomalous right subclavian artery originates from the descending aorta, both hands are cyanotic. Cyanosis of the fingers greater than in the toes indicates complete transposition of the great vessels with preductal coarctation or complete interruption of the aortic arch, pulmonary hypertension, and a reverse shunt through a patent ductus arteriosus, in this case delivering oxygenated blood to the lower extremities.

The presence of any congenital somatic abnormality should prompt a search for congenital heart disease.

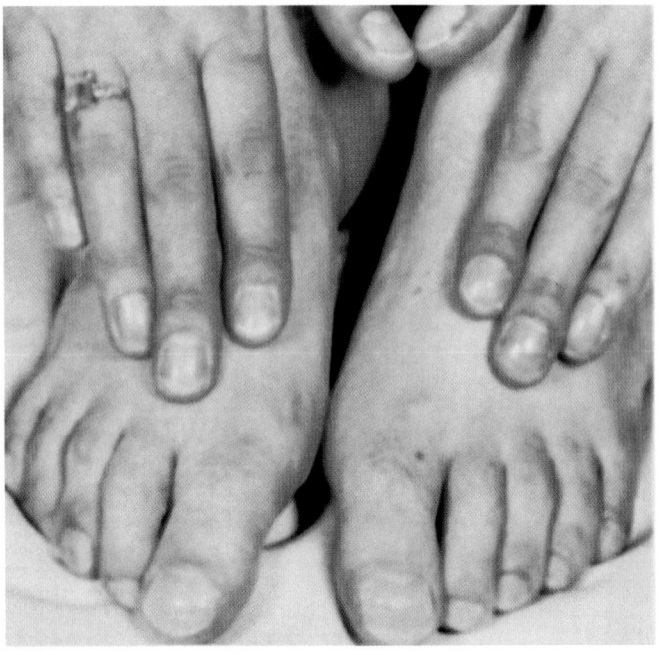

FIGURE 12–3. *Differential cyanosis.* Cyanosis of fingers (*left*) greater than that of toes caused by transposition of the great vessels with patent ductus arteriosus.

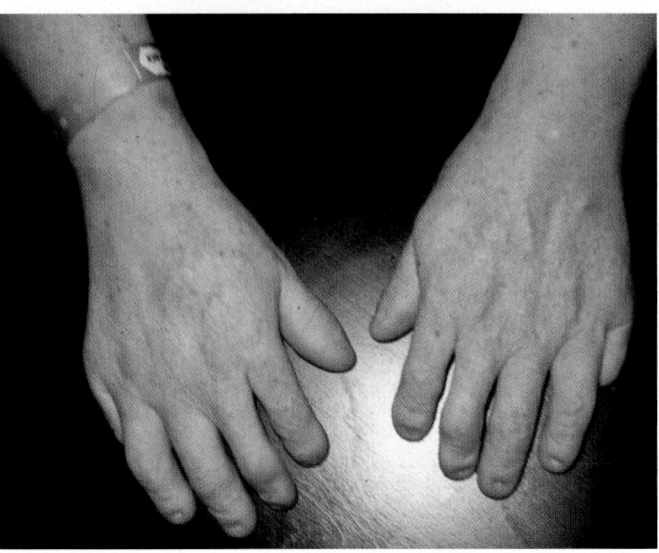

FIGURE 12–4. *Ellis-van Creveld syndrome.* Polydactyly. This patient has a large septal defect.

【 】 SYNDROMES ASSOCIATED WITH CONGENITAL HEART DISEASE

The Ellis-van Creveld syndrome is a heritable form of dwarfism characterized by short extremities, polydactyly, dysplastic teeth and nails, and multiple frenula binding the upper lip to the alveolar ridge (Fig. 12–4). More than one-half of the patients have heart disease, usually a large atrial septal defect or a single atrium.

The thrombocytopenia–absent radius (TAR) syndrome includes bilateral radial aplasia with a persistent thumb and thrombocytopenia and can be associated with an ostium secundum atrial septal defect (ASD) and/or tetralogy of Fallot. The Holt-Oram syndrome, an autosomal dominant condition, combines an ASD or other congenital heart disease with an abnormal thumb[29] (Fig. 12–5). In the Laurence-Moon–Bardet-Biedl syndrome, mental re-

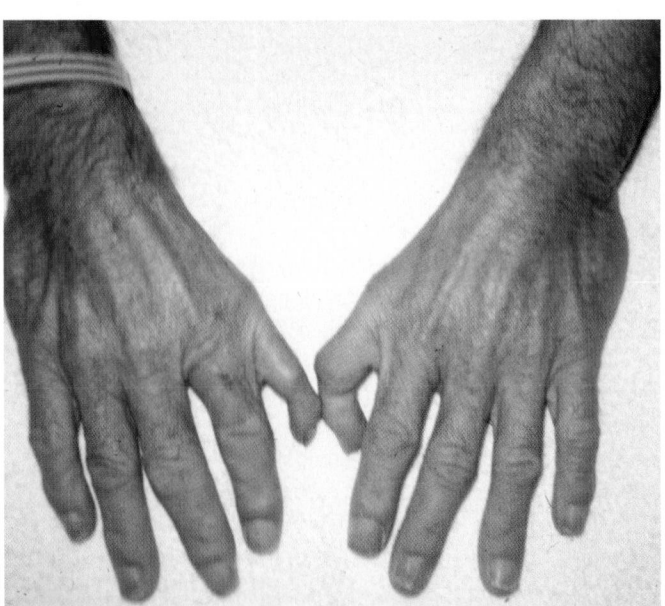

FIGURE 12–5. *Holt-Oram syndrome:* fingerized thumb associated with an atrial septal defect.

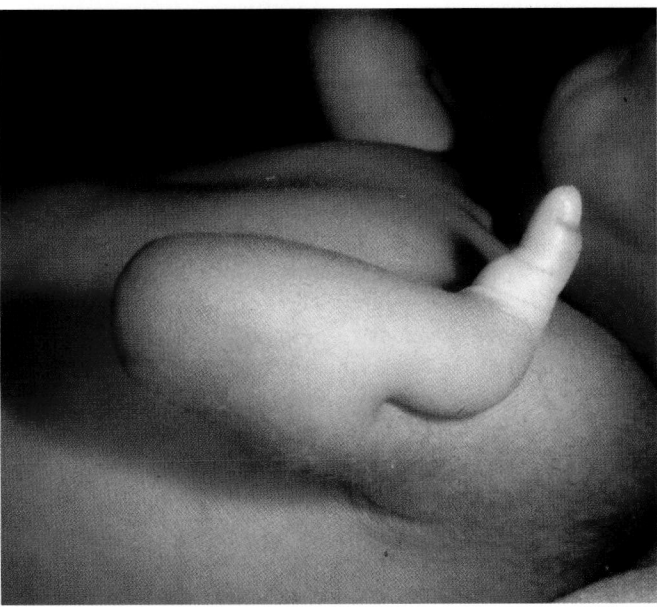

FIGURE 12-6. *Cornelia de Lange syndrome*: low hairline, hirsutism, bushy brows, phocomelia, and a single thumb-like digit. It can be associated with ventricular septal defect.

tardation, polydactyly, obesity, retinitis pigmentosa, and hypogonadism occur with a variety of congenital heart diseases.

The Cornelia de Lange syndrome is characterized by bushy, confluent eyebrows, downward-slanting eyes, a small mandible, low-set ears, hirsutism, long eyelashes, a broad, flat, upturned nose, severe growth and mental retardation, and a peculiar *chicken-wing* extremity with a single thumb like digit (Fig. 12–6). A VSD, patent ductus arteriosus, pulmonic stenosis, anomalous venous return, or ASD can be present.

There is an increased incidence of congenital heart disease in children with a cleft palate or lip. In the Pierre Robin syndrome (Fig. 12–7) the cleft palate is associated with a hypoplastic mandible causing a *shrew like* face. Patients with the Ehlers-Danlos syndrome (Figs. 12–8A,B) have hyperextensible joints and hyperelastic

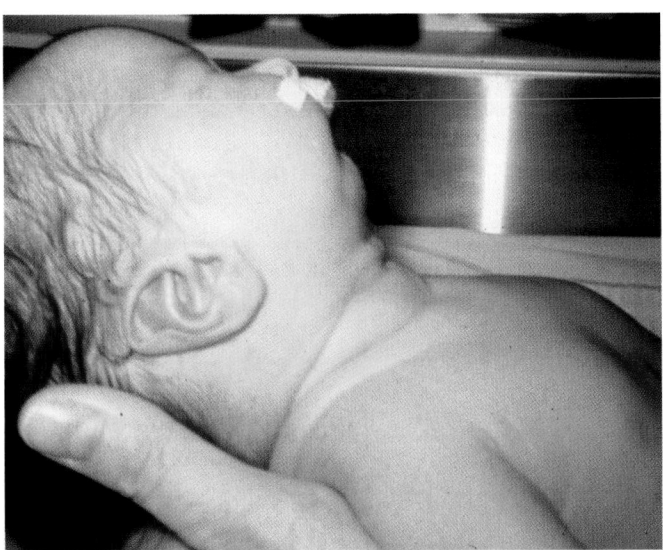

FIGURE 12-7. *Pierre Robin syndrome*: hypoplastic mandible associated with a ventricular septal defect.

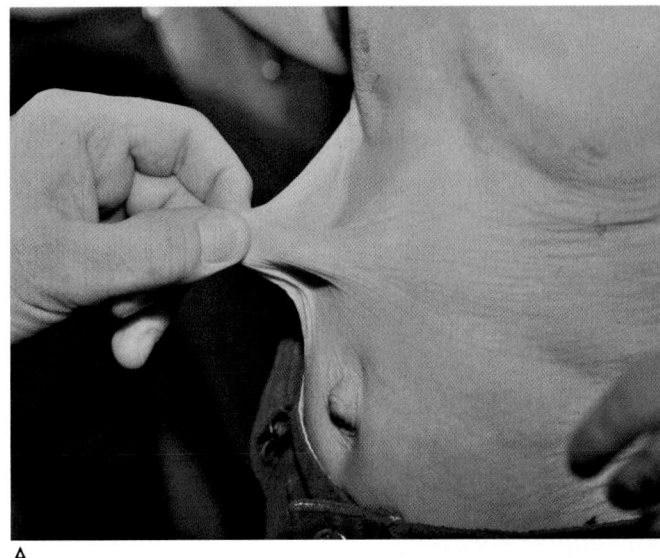

A

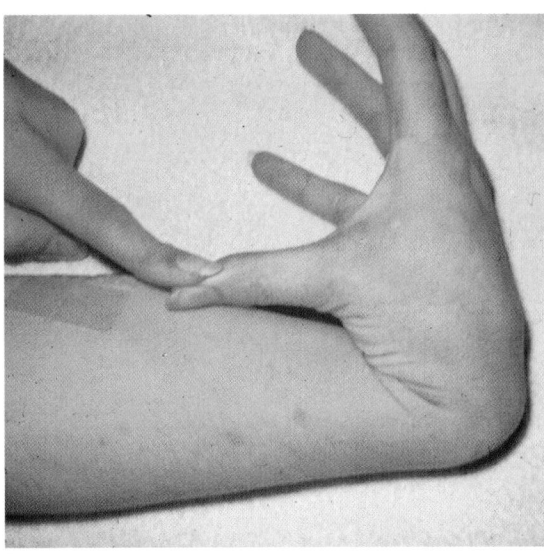

B

FIGURE 12-8. *Ehlers-Danlos syndrome*. **A.** Hyperextensible skin. **B.** Lax joints. Redundant chordae tendineae and arterial rupture can occur.

and friable skin often associated with arterial dilatation and rupture, aortic regurgitation, or MVP. Patients with osteogenesis imperfecta have brittle bones, blue sclera, and short legs and an increased incidence of aortic and mitral regurgitation. Patients with pseudoxanthoma elasticum (see Chap. 88) have degeneration of dermal elastic fibers and retinal angioid streaks and can develop aortic regurgitation and coronary artery disease (CAD) (Fig. 12–9).

Marfan syndrome, an autosomal dominant disorder, is suggested by skeletal features such as increased height, long fingers, lax joints, kyphoscoliosis, pectus excavatum or carinatum, an elongated face, high-arched palate, and flat feet (Fig. 12–10A to C). The legs are disproportionately long, and the arm span can exceed the height. When a patient clenches the fingers around their flexed thumb, the thumb protrudes past the ulnar side of the hand (*thumb sign*). The wrist can be encircled by grasping it with the fifth finger and thumb of the other hand (*wrist sign*) (see Fig. 12–9B). Other findings include bilateral subluxation of the lens, severe myopia, and blue sclera. Patients with Marfan syndrome usually have MVP (see

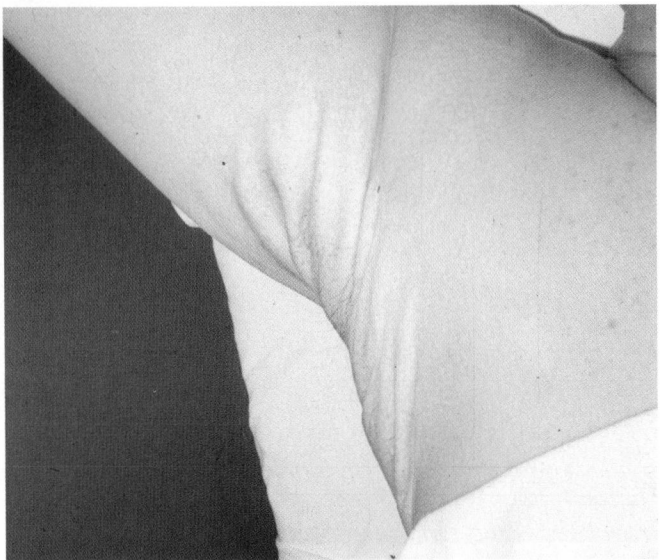

FIGURE 12-9. *Pseudoxanthoma elasticum*: grooved skin in a typical location. Arterial calcification can occur.

Chap. 88), mitral regurgitation, a calcified mitral annulus, and chordal rupture. AR is a consequence of a dilated aortic root, prolapse of the aortic cusps, or aortic dissection (see Chap. 88).

AR has been described in patients with inborn errors of metabolism, including Morquio syndrome (mucopolysaccharidosis IV) and Scheie syndrome (mucopolysaccharidosis V). Patients with Morquio syndrome are identified by their short stature, short neck, barrel chest, broad mouth, short nose, widely spaced teeth, and cloudy cornea. In Scheie syndrome, growth retardation, sternal protrusion, facial abnormalities, and cloudy cornea are present. In Fabry disease, angiokeratomas—purplish pinpoint skin lesions—occur on the lips, underarm, buttocks, scrotum, and penis (Fig. 12–11). Cardiomyopathy, ischemic heart disease, and conduction defects are associated with this sex-linked recessive disorder in which there is a genetic deficiency of the enzyme α-galactosidase A.

Many chromosomal abnormalities cause congenital heart disease. The well-recognized characteristics of Down syndrome (trisomy 21) (Fig. 12–12) include a small head, shallow orbits, epicanthal folds, low-set ears, widely spaced eyes (hypertelorism), Brushfield white spots of the iris, protruding tongue, transverse

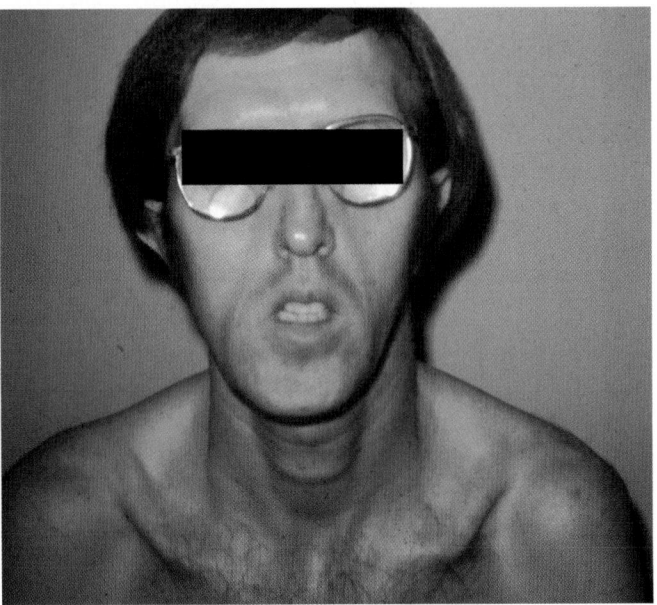

A

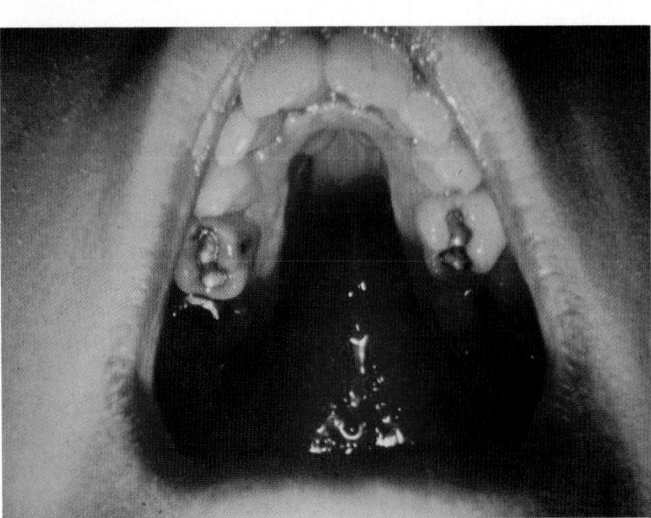

C

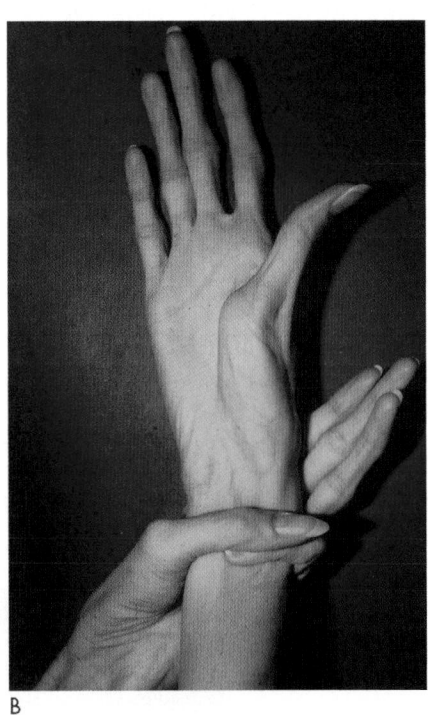

B

FIGURE 12-10. *Marfan syndrome.* **A.** Long, narrow face. **B.** Arachnodactyly and positive wrist sign. **C.** High-arched palate.

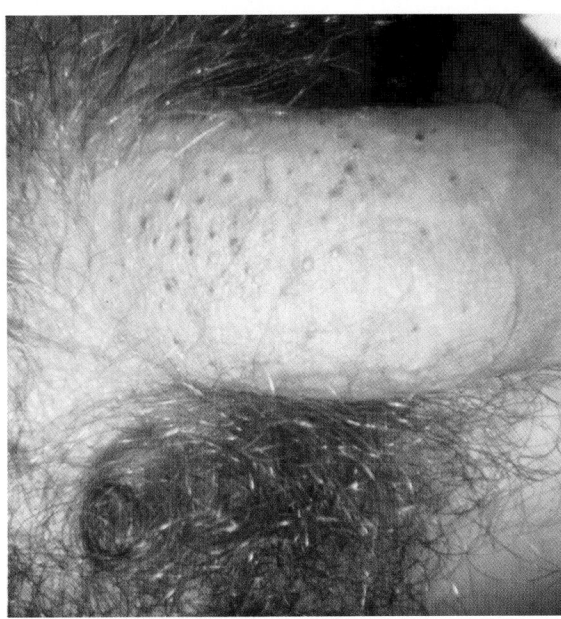

FIGURE 12–11. *Fabry disease*: dark-red angiokeratomas on the penis can be linked with coronary artery disease.

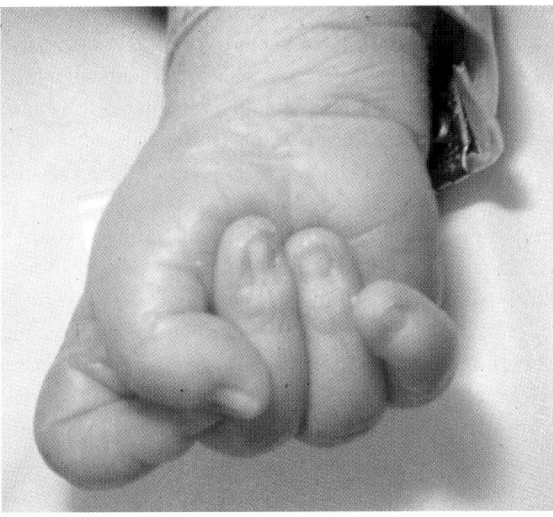

FIGURE 12–13. *Trisomy 18 syndrome*: tightly clenched fist with overlapping index and fifth fingers. A ventricular septal defect is present.

palmar creases, and mental retardation. Congenital heart disease occurs in 40 to 60 percent of patients; a VSD or endocardial cushion defect are the most frequent. Klinefelter syndrome is characterized by gynecomastia, small testicles, a eunuchoid appearance, tall stature, and long extremities septum, proximum and secundum. ASDs have been described.

Congenital heart disease of varied types is common in trisomy 13 and trisomy 18 syndromes. In trisomy 13 syndrome, the child has a cleft palate and lip; the ocular tissue and the nose can be missing.[30] Polydactyly, retroflexible thumbs, transverse creases, hyperconvex narrow nails, and flexion of the fingers and hands are

characteristic of this syndrome. The features of the trisomy 18 syndrome are a small, triangular mouth with receding chin, small mandible, webbed neck, and tightly clenched fists with the index finger overlapping the third finger and the fifth finger over the fourth (Fig. 12–13).

Low hairline, low-set ears, deafness, small jaw, and short, webbed neck are physical findings common to both Turner syndrome and the Klippel-Feil syndrome. Turner syndrome (Fig. 12–14) also includes short stature, broad chest with widely spaced nipples, epicanthal folds, widely spaced eyes, pigmented moles, ptosis, clinodactyly (curved fifth finger), and a shortened fifth finger.[31] Coarctation of the aorta, aortic stenosis, and hypertrophic cardiomyopathy are the cardiovascular considerations. The Klippel-Feil syndrome can cause

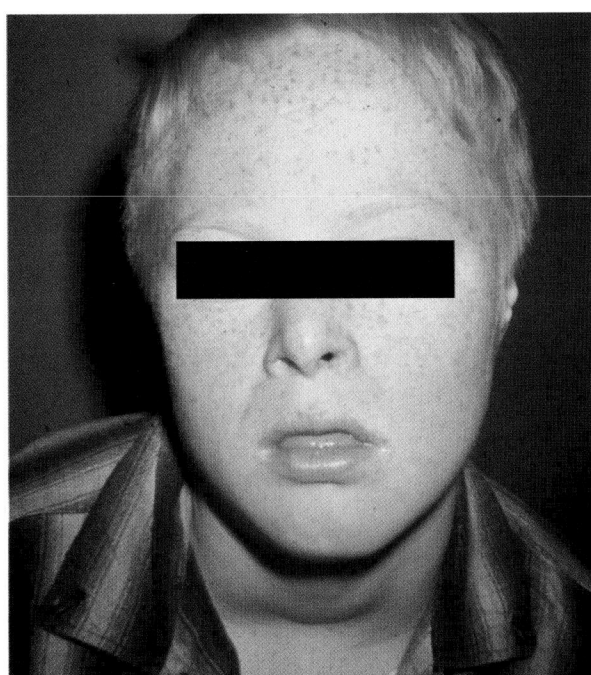

FIGURE 12–12. *Down syndrome*.

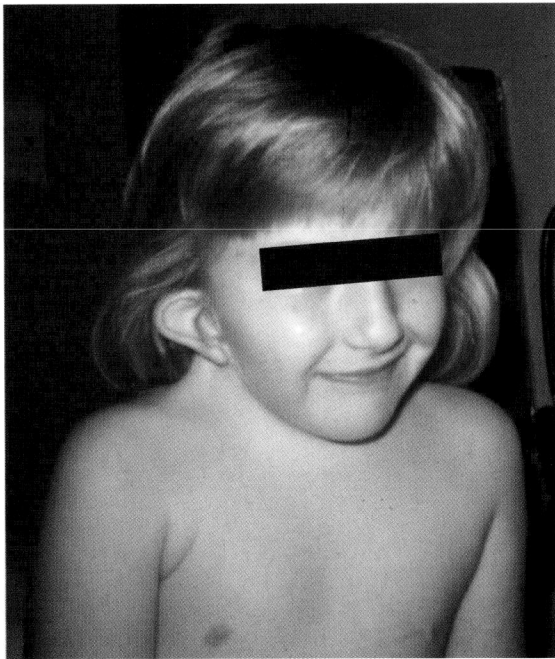

FIGURE 12–14. *Turner syndrome*: epicanthal folds, pigmented moles, hypertelorism, and scars on the neck where webs have been removed. It can be associated with coarctation of the aorta.

facial asymmetry, cleft palate, torticollis, scoliosis, deafness, strabismus, and hydrocephaly. VSD is the most common cardiac disorder.

There are sporadic disorders associated with congenital heart disease. The VATER association includes vertebral defect, anal (imperforation), tracheoesophageal fistula, and radial and renal dysplasia. A ventricular defect occurs in 80 percent of these patients. The asplenia syndrome is associated with a high incidence of complex congenital heart disease. Cardiovascular malformations are found in 15 to 25 percent of newborns with omphalocele.

Teratogenic effects resulting in congenital heart disease can be alcohol-related, the result of rubella during pregnancy, or induced by phenytoin, thalidomide, or lithium. From 30 to 40 percent of children born to alcoholic mothers are affected with the fetal alcohol syndrome. These children have an undeveloped-appearing central face because of maxillary hypoplasia, a small and upturned nose, an indistinct or smooth philtrum, micrognathia, and a thin upper lip and vermilion (Fig. 12–15). ASDs and VSDs are most common. The teratogenic effects of the rubella syndrome include cataracts, deafness, microcephaly, patent ductus arteriosus, pulmonic valvular and/or arterial stenosis, and ASD.

【 】 DISORDERS AFFECTING THE VALVES

The cutaneous manifestations of infective endocarditis (see Chap. 85) include Osler nodes, Janeway lesions, clubbing of the fingers

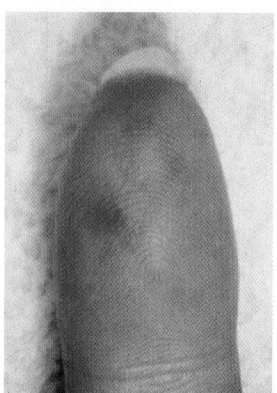

FIGURE 12–16. *Bacterial endocarditis*: Valvular infection associated with a tender, purplish nodule (Osler node) in the finger pad.

(Fig. 12–16), splinter hemorrhages of the nails, and petechiae. Osler nodes are reddish purple, tender nodules typically found in the distal pad of the finger or toe (see Fig. 12–16). Janeway lesions are hemorrhagic, nontender, and involve the palms or soles. Splinter hemorrhages are linear, black, and appear in the distal third of the fingernail.

Pulmonic stenosis can be part of Noonan syndrome, Turner syndrome, Rubinstein-Taybi syndrome, rubella syndrome, the multiple-lentigines syndrome, pulmonary valve dysplasia, or Watson syndrome. In Noonan syndrome, the characteristic findings include ptosis, low-set ears, downward-slanting eyes, webbed neck, hypertelorism, low posterior hairline, short stature, mental retardation, normal chromosomes, and a dysplastic pulmonic valve (Fig. 12–17). Broad toes and thumbs (Fig. 12–18A,B), a slanting forehead, a thin, beaked nose, and large, low-set ears are seen in Rubinstein-Taybi syndrome.

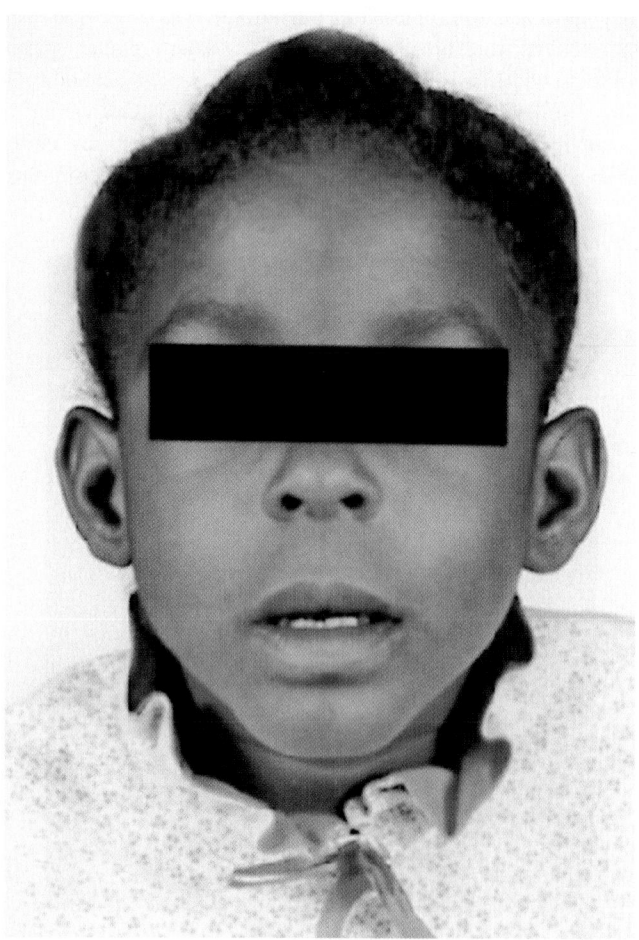

FIGURE 12–15. *Fetal alcohol syndrome*: midface hypoplasia, absent philtrum, and microcephaly associated with a ventricular septal defect.

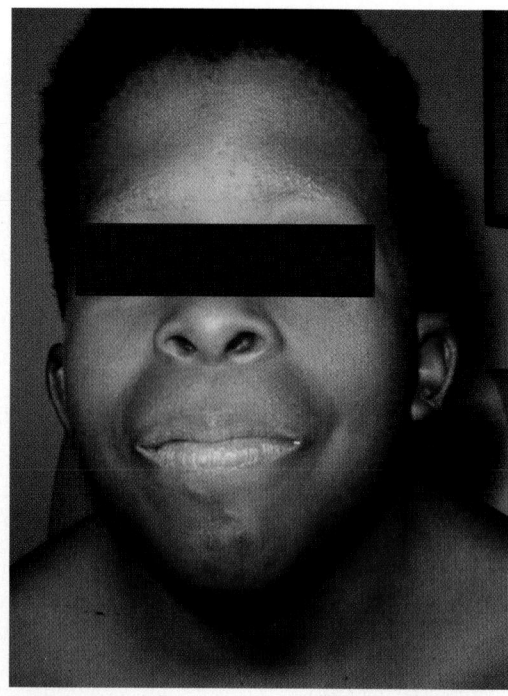

FIGURE 12–17. *Noonan syndrome*: ptosis, hypertelorism, and low-set ears associated with valvular pulmonic stenosis.

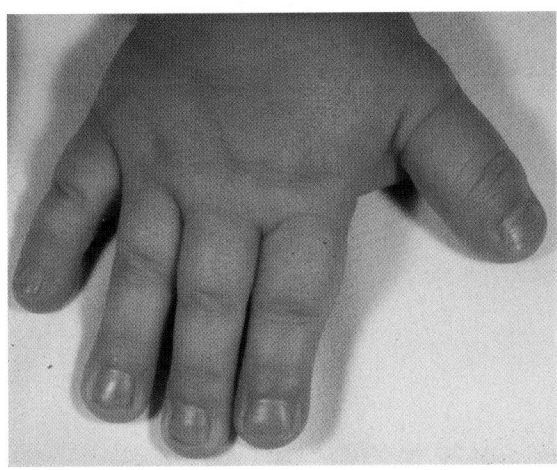
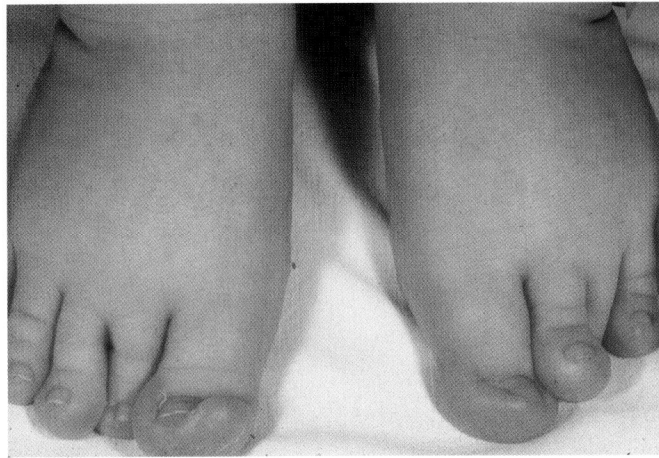

FIGURE 12–18. *Rubinstein-Taybi syndrome can be associated with a variety of congenital heart defects. Source: Silverman ME, Hurst JW. The hand and heart. Am J Cardiol. 1968;22:718. Reproduced with permission from the publisher and authors.*

The multiple lentigines syndrome is identified by the presence of multiple dark brown macules varying in size from pinpoint to 5 cm (Fig. 12–19). They cover the entire body but are most heavily concentrated on the neck and upper thorax.

The carcinoid syndrome (see Chaps. 78 and 89) can present as intense flushing of the face and a chronic cyanotic hue. Telangiectasia can be present. Stenosis and/or regurgitation of the tricuspid and/or pulmonic valves can result when hepatic metastases are present. When a patent ductus arteriosus, lung metastases, or a patent foramen ovale is present, the left-sided heart valves can also be affected.

In scleroderma, there is tightening of the skin of the fingers and then the hands, forearms, upper chest, and face. Subcutaneous tissue and skin creases disappear. Flexion contractures of the fingers can cause a claw like hand deformity (Fig. 12–20). Raynaud phenomenon is an early manifestation. The CREST syndrome (calcinosis cutis, Raynaud phenomenon, esophageal motility disorder, sclerodactyly, and telangiectasia) is a variant of scleroderma (Fig. 12–21). Valvular changes, including thickening of the edges of the mitral, aortic, and tricuspid valves, as well as thickening and shortening of the mitral chordae, are rarely significant.

Joint disease is often associated with cardiac valvular disease and can occur with systemic lupus erythematosus (SLE), rheumatoid arthritis, rheumatic fever, polychondritis, ankylosing spondylitis, alkaptonuria, and Whipple disease (see Chap. 88). In SLE, the joint inflammation is usually symmetric and nondeforming. Typical skin lesions include an erythematous, scaling eruption over the cheeks and bridge of the nose, circumscribed reddish purple plaques, telangiectasia, and patchy hair loss (Fig. 12–22). Verrucous endocarditis can involve any of the four cardiac valves; however, severe valvular dysfunction is unusual.

In patients with rheumatoid arthritis, the wrists, shoulders, knees, ankles, and elbows can become inflamed. Advanced disease results in ulnar deviation of the fingers and flexion of the distal interphalangeal joints with hyperextension of the proximal interpha-

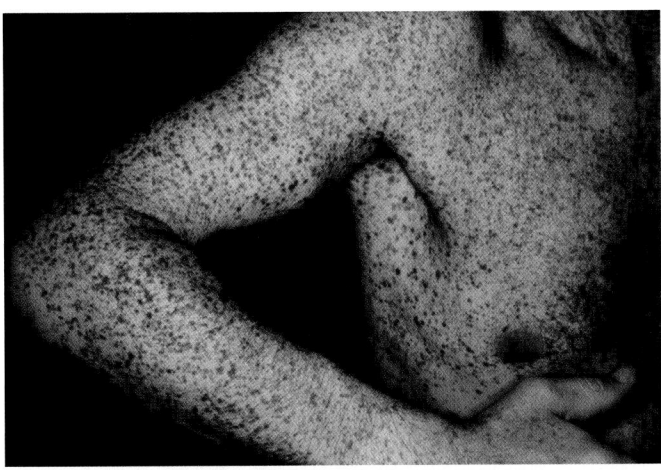

FIGURE 12–19. *Multiple lentigines syndrome:* dark-brown macular lesions of the abdomen associated with hypertrophic obstructive cardiomyopathy. *Source: Silverman ME. Visual clues to diagnosis. Prim Cardiol. 1986; Reproduced with permission from the publisher and author.*

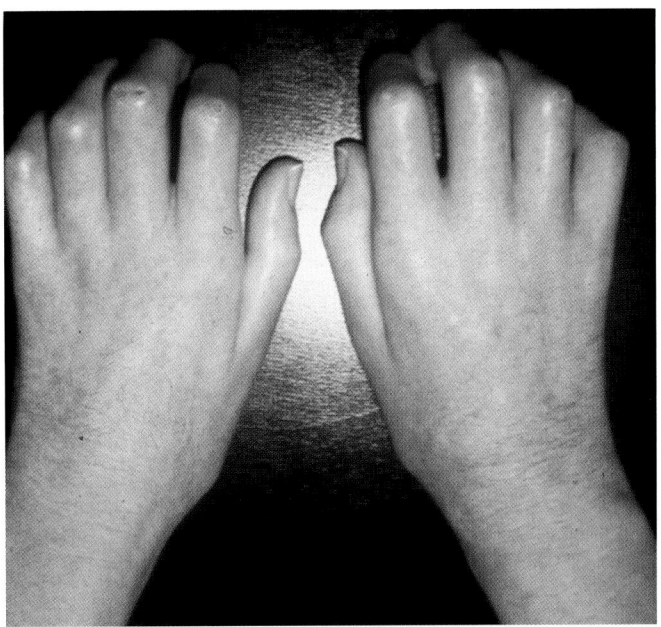

FIGURE 12–20. *Scleroderma:* claw like hand deformity and shiny, tight skin. It can be linked with myocardial fibrosis.

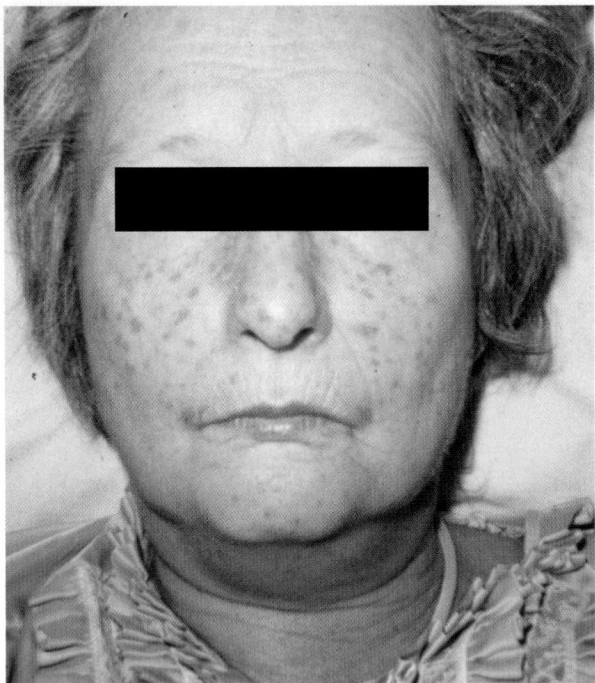

FIGURE 12–21. *CREST syndrome.* Telangiectasia of the face in a patient with Raynaud phenomenon and sclerodactyly.

langeal joints, producing a *swan-neck* deformity and a Z-shaped configuration of the thumb (Fig. 12–23). Granulomatous aortic or mitral valve disease with regurgitation is most common in patients who are seropositive and have subcutaneous nodules or classic rheumatoid deformities. Rheumatic fever should be suspected in patients with erythema marginatum and migratory polyarthritis involving the large joints (see Chap. 74). Marked ulnar deviation, suggesting rheumatoid arthritis, can be caused by repeated attacks

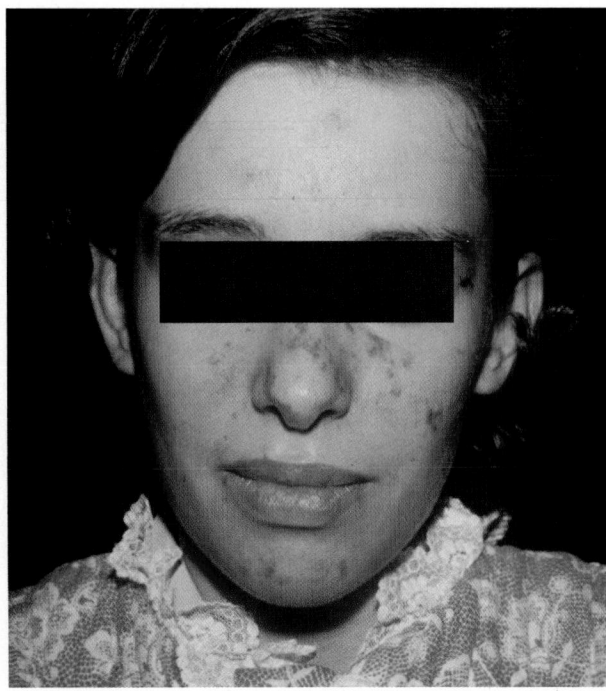

FIGURE 12–22. *Systemic lupus erythematosus:* butterfly rash associated with pericardial, myocardial, and endocardial disease.

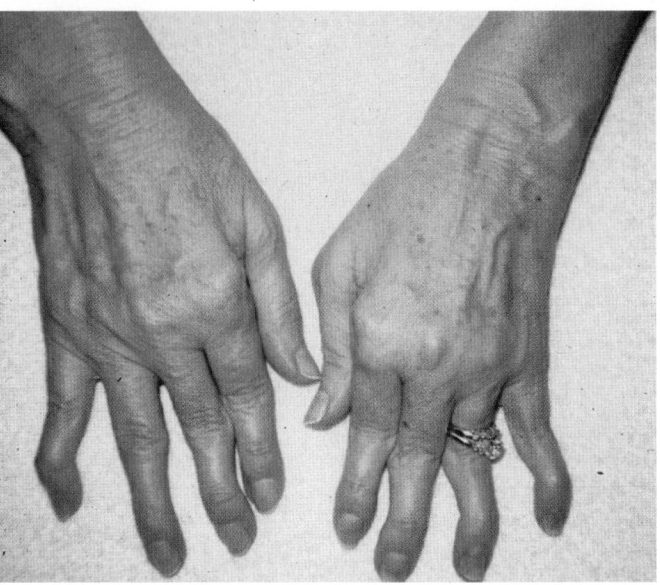

FIGURE 12–23. *Rheumatoid arthritis:* with ulnar deviation of the fingers and flexion of the distal interphalangeal joints with hyperextension of the proximal interphalangeal joints.

of rheumatic fever and is known as Jaccoud arthritis. In contrast to rheumatoid arthritis, the fingers can be moved freely back into a correct alignment.

Polychondritis causes an inflammatory destruction of cartilage, resulting in a saddle-shaped collapse of the nose or a cauliflower ear. Aortic root dilatation and rarely dissection are associated (Fig. 12–24A,B).

Chronic synovitis of the spine occurs in patients with ankylosing spondylitis (see Chap. 88). The patient with advanced disease is bent forward, unable to stand upright, and walks with a stiff and halting gait (Fig. 12–25). Aortic regurgitation, as a result of the thickening and shortening of the aortic cusps from perivascular inflammation and fibrosis, mitral regurgitation, and complete heart block can occur.[32]

Whipple disease is suggested by polyarthritis, abdominal pain, and diarrhea. Aortic and mitral regurgitation and endocarditis are known complications. Aortic or mitral valvular disease can be

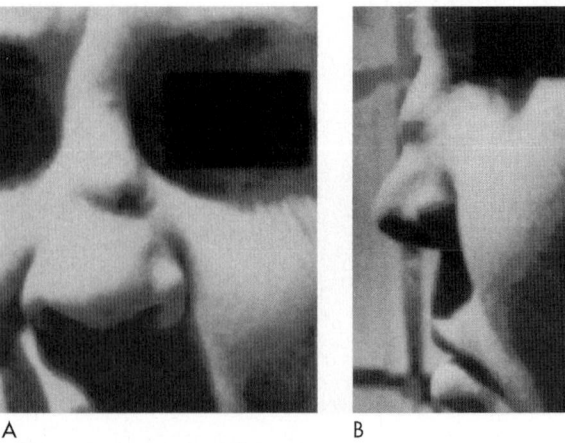

A   B

FIGURE 12–24. *Polychondritis.* **A, B.** Destruction of cartilage of the nose, producing a *saddle nose* deformity in association with aortic regurgitation. *Courtesy of Dr. Warren Sarrell, Anniston, AL.*

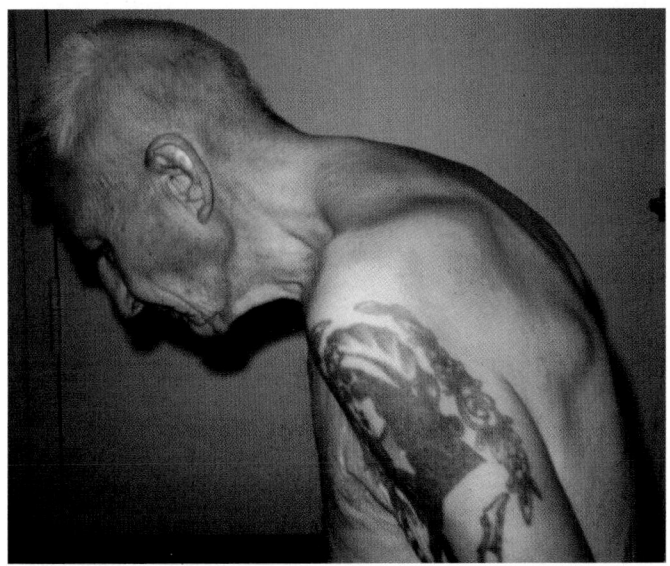

FIGURE 12–25. *Ankylosing spondylitis:* immobile, curved spine with forward jutting of head. It can be seen with AV block or aortic regurgitation. *Source: Silverman ME. Visual clues to diagnosis. Prim Cardiol. 1987. Reproduced with permission from the publisher, author, and patient.*

caused by an accumulation of homogentisic acid in alkaptonuria (Fig. 12–26). Blue-black, stiff ears and joints are important clues to this inherited disorder of tyrosine metabolism.

Patients with the MVP syndrome (see Chap. 76) can have a straight thoracic spine, pectus excavatum, scoliosis, micromastia, and joint laxity (Fig. 12–27). Systolic and rarely diastolic murmurs have been described with chest-wall deformities as a result of a straight-back syndrome and pectus excavatum that can impinge on or displace the heart.

[ ] DISORDERS ASSOCIATED WITH CARDIOMYOPATHY

Hypertrophic cardiomyopathy (see Chap. 30) that can be concentric or asymmetric has been associated with Friedreich ataxia, Turner syndrome, Noonan syndrome, Fabry disease, neurofibromatosis, and the multiple-lentigines syndrome. Friedreich ataxia is a spinocerebellar degenerative disorder that results in a broad-based, lurching gait, impaired vibration, position, and joint sense and incoordination. Kyphoscoliosis and pes cavus (high instep, retraction of the toes at the metatarsophalangeal joints, and hammer toes) are two important physical signs (Fig. 12–28A,B).

Cor pulmonale can be secondary to pulmonary hypertension caused by kyphoscoliosis, restrictive lung disease, scleroderma, upper airway blockade by enlarged tonsils and adenoids, or the sleep apnea syndrome.[33]

Myocarditis (see Chap. 72) occurs with SLE, rheumatic fever, Reiter syndrome, Kawasaki disease, Lyme arthritis,[34] and, occasionally, Whipple disease. In Reiter syndrome, conjunctivitis and hyperkeratotic coalescing lesions encrusted on the soles and palms, known as hyperkeratosis blenorrhagicum, are associated with arthritis and urethritis (Fig. 12–29). Kawasaki disease begins with fever; nonexudative conjunctivitis; dry, fissured lips; cervical adenopathy; and a strawberry tongue. Later, the palms and soles become indurated, purplish red, and then peel. A widespread

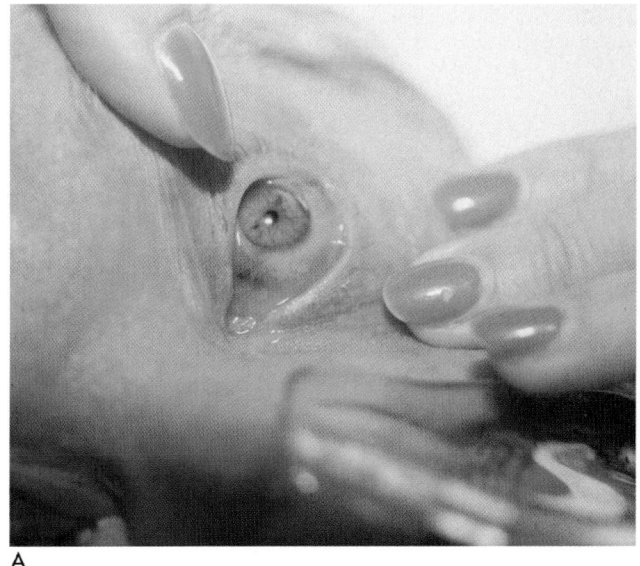

A

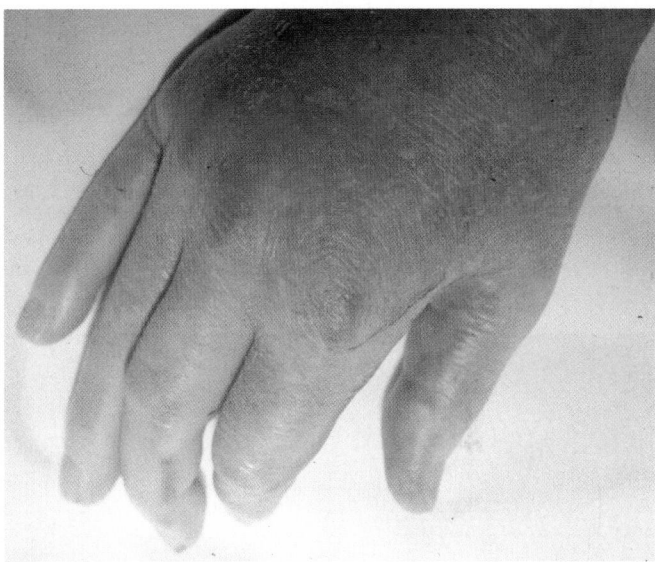

B

FIGURE 12–26. *Alkaptonuria.* **A.** Bluish sclera. **B.** Blue-black joints of hand associated with valvular disease.

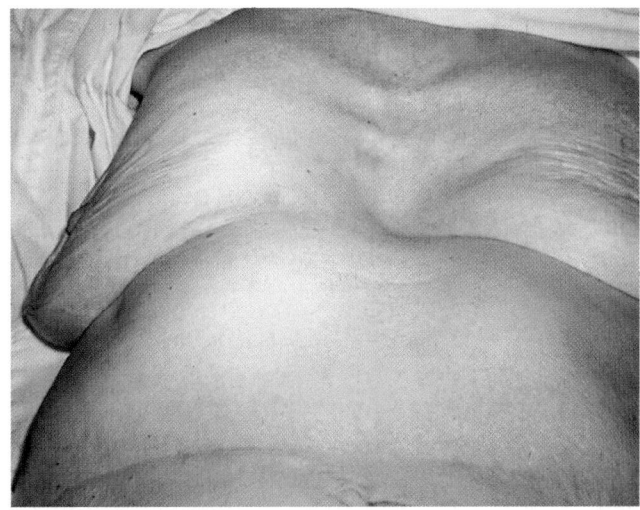

FIGURE 12–27. Marked pectus excavatum.

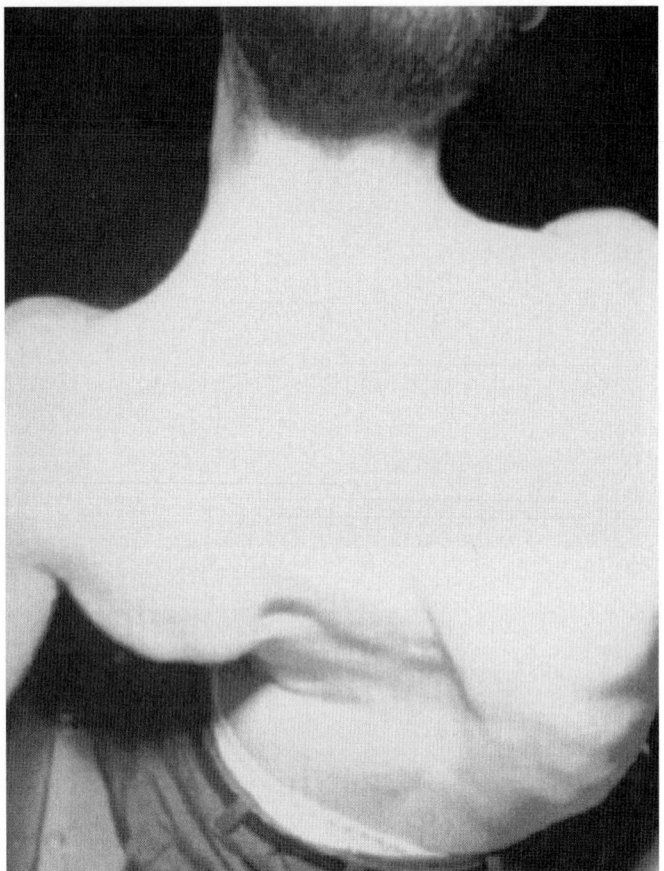

A

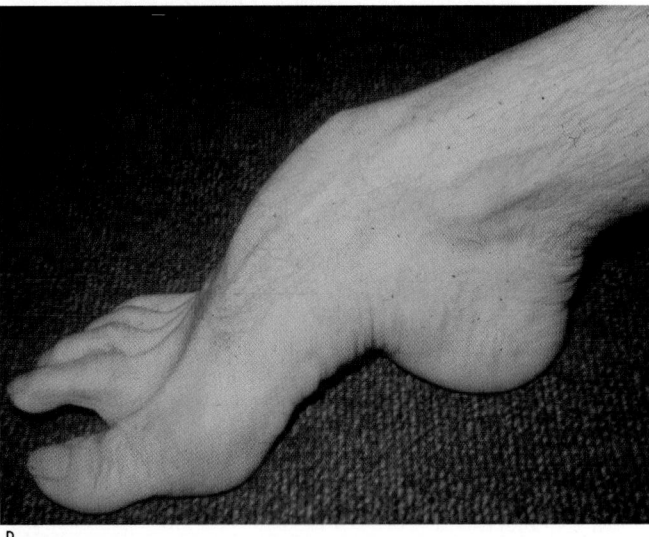

B

FIGURE 12–28. *Friedreich ataxia (photographs from different patients).* **A.** Kyphoscoliosis. **B.** Pes cavus. Myocardial fibrosis and hypertrophy are often present. *Source: Silverman ME. Visual clues to diagnosis. Prim Cardiol. 1987. Reproduced with permission from the publisher and authors.*

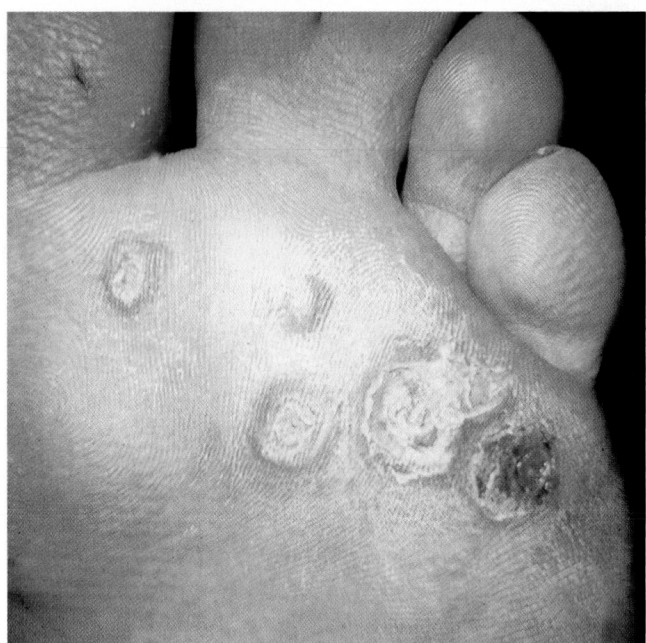

FIGURE 12–29. *Hyperkeratotic lesions* encrusted on the soles of the feet in Reiter syndrome.

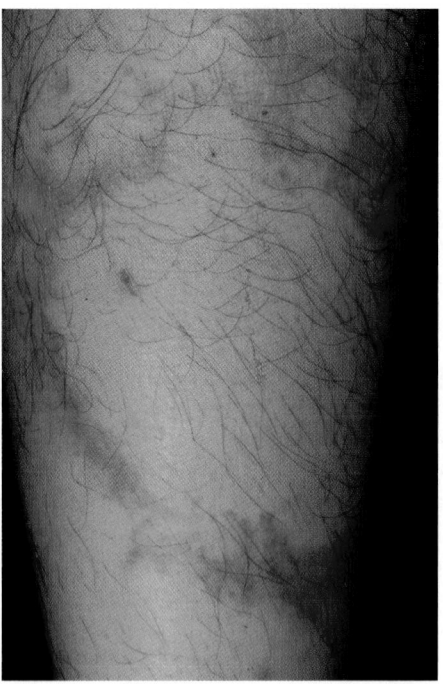

FIGURE 12–30. *Lyme arthritis:* annular expanding rash with a clear central area. It can be associated with pericarditis and atrioventricular (AV) block. *Source: Silverman ME. Visual clues to diagnosis. Prim Cardiol. 1986. Reproduced with permission from the publisher and author.*

erythematous rash can appear and then desquamate. Lyme arthritis, caused by the spirochete *Borrelia burgdorferi,* begins with a red macule or papule and then develops into an expanding erythematous rash with a bright red border known as erythema migrans (Fig. 12–30). The center of the rash can clear, indurate, blister, or become necrotic. Multiple annular lesions can develop.

Diseases that cause myocardial fibrosis include dermatomyositis, Duchenne and Becker muscular dystrophy, myotonic muscular dystrophy, Kearns-Sayre syndrome, Friedreich ataxia, sarcoidosis, and scleroderma (see Chaps. 31 and 32). With dermatomyositis, a heliotropic discoloration is displayed on the upper eyelids (Fig. 12–31A,B), and a scaly, erythematous papular rash—*Gottron papules*—can cover the knuckles, sparing the interphalangeal region. A

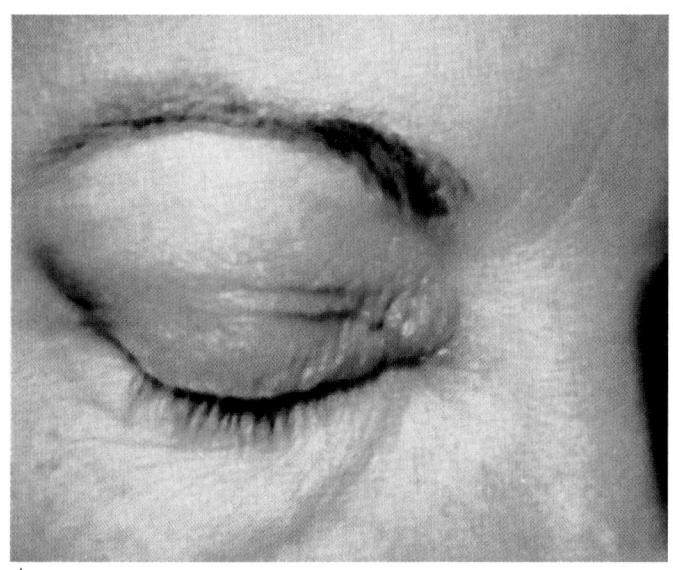

A

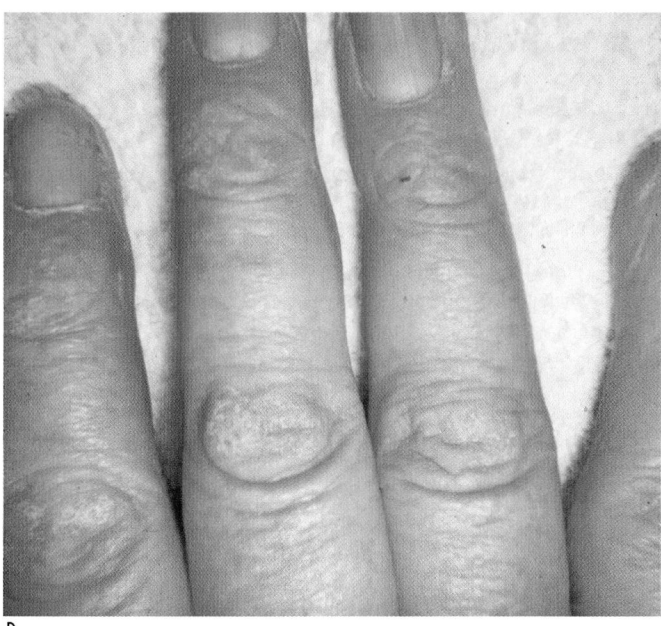

B

FIGURE 12-31. *Dermatomyositis.* **A.** A violaceous hue and edema of the upper eyelid can be associated with myocardial disease. **B.** Scaly, papular rash on knuckles only.

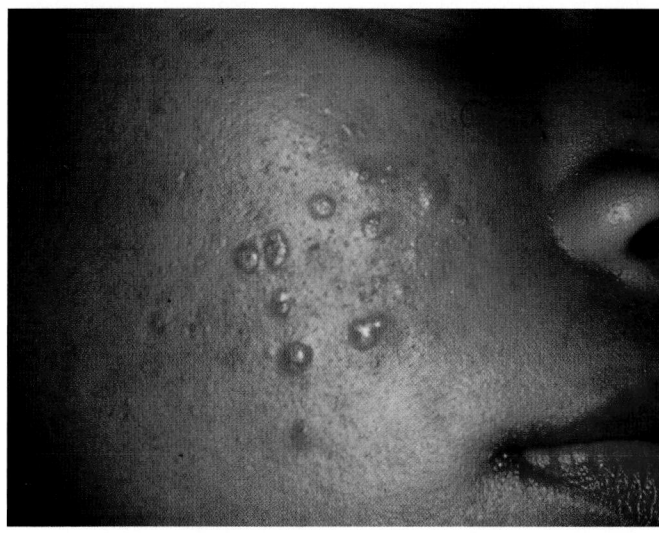

FIGURE 12-32. *Sarcoidosis.* Waxy papules on cheek associated with heart block.

waddling gait and pseudohypertrophic calves are characteristic of Duchenne muscular dystrophy, which can lead to fibrosis of the posterior left ventricle. In myotonic dystrophy, drooping eyelids, cataracts, a receding hairline, and a mask-like expression are present. The Kearns-Sayre syndrome is a form of ocular muscular dystrophy in which external ophthalmoplegia, ptosis, and retinitis pigmentosa occur. Skin manifestations of sarcoidosis are common and include erythema nodosum, lupus pernio (a red or violet plaque formation with a predilection for the nasolabial folds, eyelids, and ears), and waxy translucent papules found on the cheeks, periorbital area, ears, and elsewhere. Uveitis, bilateral parotid and lacrimal gland enlargement, and arthritis are other signs (see Chap. 31).

Infiltrative diseases of the myocardium include Wilson disease, Cori disease, Fabry disease, hemochromatosis, amyloidosis, glycogen storage disease, and sarcoidosis (Fig. 12–32) (see Chap. 31).[35]

Wilson disease is an autosomal recessive disorder in which copper accumulates in tissues, including the myocardium.[36] Arrhythmias, autonomic dysfunction, and cardiomyopathy have been reported. Kayser-Fleischer rings, usually golden-brown in color and circling the edge of the cornea, provide a major clue to the correct diagnosis.

In hemochromatosis, the skin has a bronze or slate-gray coloration; myocardial infiltration with iron deposits can cause a dilated or rarely a restrictive cardiomyopathy associated with arrhythmias and heart failure. Macroglossia with indentations, waxy nodules of the skin and eyelids caused by fibrillar protein deposition, and "pinch purpura" are clues to the diagnosis of amyloidosis[37] (Fig. 12–33) (see Chap. 31).

【 】 DISORDERS ASSOCIATED WITH PERICARDIAL DISEASE

Pericarditis can be a result of Reiter syndrome, Whipple disease, Kawasaki disease, SLE, rheumatoid arthritis,[38] rheumatic fever, sarcoidosis, scleroderma, dermatomyositis, hemochromatosis, Behçet syndrome, Degos disease, uremia, mulibrey nanism, polychondritis, hypothyroidism, or metastatic disease (see Chap. 89). The components of Behçet syndrome include erythema nodosum, superficial phlebitis, oral and genital ulcers, and iritis. Patients with Degos disease (malignant atrophic papulosis) present with painless, oval cutaneous lesions that have a white center and surrounding erythema. In this rapidly fatal disease, occlusive fibrosis of small and medium-sized arteries produces pleuritis and pericarditis. In far-advanced renal disease, urochrome pigmentation of the skin and uremic frost can be cutaneous manifestations. Hypothyroidism, a cause of massive pericardial effusion, thickens the face and causes dry hair, puffy eyelids, and an enlarged tongue. Pericarditis is common in SLE but only rarely the presenting manifestation.

【 】 DISORDERS CAUSING CONDUCTION SYSTEM DISEASE

Acquired causes of atrioventricular (AV) block or bundle-branch block include sarcoidosis, rheumatic fever, gout, Reiter syndrome,[39] dermatomyositis, polychondritis, amyloidosis, Kawasaki

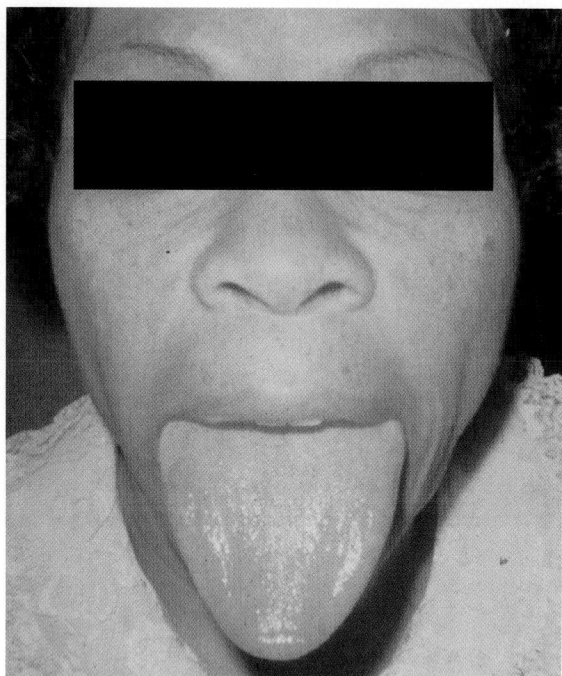

FIGURE 12–33. *Amyloidosis.* Enlarged tongue can be a sign of an infiltrative cardiomyopathy. *Source: Silverman ME. Visual clues to diagnosis. Prim Cardiol. 1987. Reproduced with permission from the publisher, author, and patient.*

disease, ankylosing spondylitis, SLE, and Lyme arthritis. In gout, uric acid crystals can form nodules affecting the conduction system. AV block can be an early cardiac manifestation of ankylosing spondylitis. Maternal lupus is an important cause of congenital complete AV block in the newborn.

Inherited disorders associated with conduction defects include Fabry disease, Friedreich ataxia, Kearns-Sayre syndrome, the multiple-lentigines syndrome, muscular dystrophy, myotonic dystrophy, tuberous sclerosis, and Refsum disease.

There is a high incidence of paroxysmal complete AV block with myotonic dystrophy, and pacing is often necessary.[40]

【 】 DISORDERS AFFECTING THE VASCULAR SYSTEM

Aortic aneurysms and dissection (see Chap. 105) are frequent cardiovascular complications of Marfan and Ehlers-Danlos syndromes. Aneurysms of other vessels and arterial rupture can also occur. A progressive looseness of skin producing pendulous folds and droopy eyelids can be caused by cutis laxa, a generalized destruction of elastic tissue that can cause dilatation of the aorta or rupture of the pulmonary artery and aorta. Coronary aneurysms and occlusion—leading to arrhythmia, infarction, and sudden death—are late sequelae of Kawasaki disease, which can present in a young adult.[41]

Coronary atherosclerosis can be associated with hyperlipidemia, cerebrotendinous xanthomatoses, Werner syndrome, uremia, progeria, acromegaly, and diabetes mellitus. Hyperlipidemia can be suspected when xanthomas or arcus senilis are present. Xanthelasma is a skin condition usually involving lipid-laden plaques on the upper eyelid. When it occurs before age 50, there is a strong association with familial hyperlipidemia

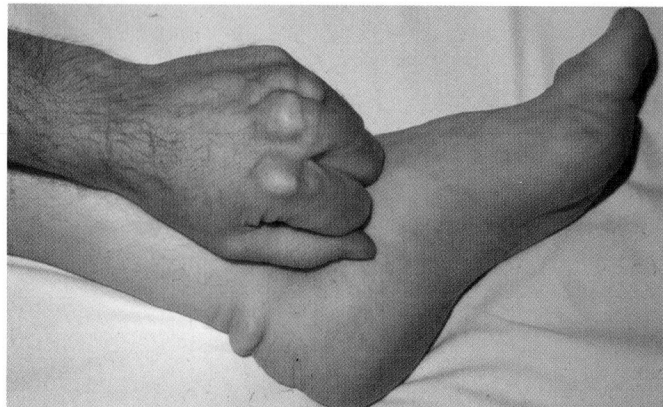

FIGURE 12–34. *Hyperlipidemia:* xanthomata associated with coronary artery disease on the extensor tendons of the hand and on the Achilles tendon.

and premature CAD. Eruptive xanthomata are recognized as 1- to 4-mm papules with yellow centers surrounded by an erythematous halo. They often appear with a sudden outbreak of discrete lesions on the buttocks, back, thighs, and exterior surfaces of the knees and elbows. They indicate a very high level of triglycerides and are associated with hyperlipidemia, diabetes mellitus, pancreatitis, myxedema, and the nephrotic syndrome. Tendon xanthomata are firm, painless nodules that thicken the exterior tendons of the hand, the Achilles tendons, and sometimes the tendons of the knees and elbows in patients with familial type II hyperlipidemia (Fig. 12–34).

In Werner syndrome, the skin is tightly stretched over the underlying bones. There is marked loss of subcutaneous tissue, and ulcerations occur over the legs. Severe coronary atherosclerosis often results in myocardial infarction at an early age. Physical findings in diabetes mellitus can include tight skin and necrobiosis diabeticorum, (Fig. 12–35) an atrophy of the skin of the lower

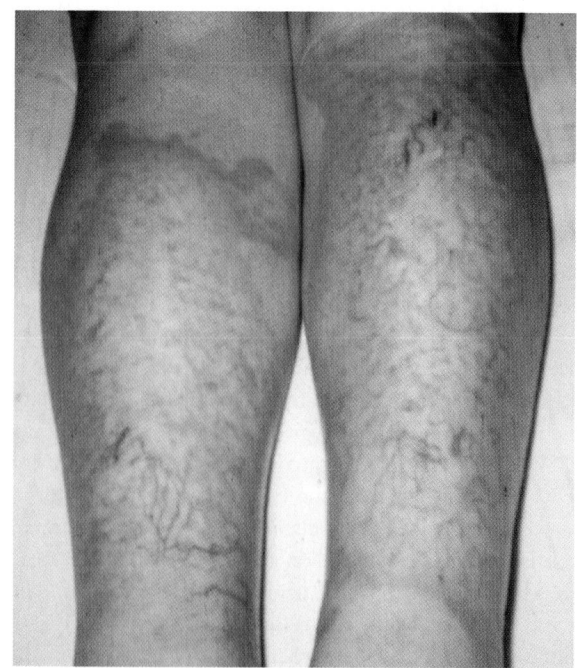

FIGURE 12–35. *Diabetes mellitus:* atrophy of skin (necrobiosis diabeticorum) of legs with coronary disease.

extremities characterized by ovoid plaques with central telangiectasia and a violet, indurated perimeter. Progeria is a rare disorder in which the face is small and prematurely aged, the eyes bulge, and the nose is beaked. Severe atherosclerosis is a common cause of death in early life. A diagonal earlobe crease is curiously associated with coronary atherosclerosis and stroke and present in 60 percent of patients, including virtually all with onset before age 40 (Fig. 12–36). Patients with homocystinuria resemble those with Marfan syndrome because they have long extremities, pectus carinatum, and kyphoscoliosis. Their cardiac disease differs from Marfan, with homocystinuria causing premature coronary disease. Pseudoxanthoma elasticum has been associated with fibrosis of the coronary artery and calcification of peripheral arteries (see Chap. 88). A glycosphingolipid is deposited in the arterial endothelium of patients with Fabry disease and can result in angina pectoris or MI. Patients with Hurler syndrome have mental retardation; a large, boat-shaped head; a broad nose; large lips; small, widely spaced teeth; and a large, protuberant tongue. Glycosaminoglycan deposition in the coronary arteries is present. Myocardial fibrosis caused by repeated spasm of the small coronary vessels has been postulated to be a result of scleroderma.

Vasculitis can be caused by SLE, rheumatoid arthritis, Behçet syndrome, Kawasaki disease, and polyarteritis. Cutaneous infarction, nodules, petechiae, livedo reticularis, gangrenous digits, MI, heart failure, and hypertension can be caused by polyarteritis (see Chap. 88). Cholesterol emboli, caused by extensive aortic atherosclerosis, cause livedo reticularis and embolic/gangrenous changes in the toes simulating polyarteritis.

Arteriovenous shunts can be found in extensive skin disease, hereditary hemorrhagic telangiectasia, and the Klippel-Trenaunay-Weber syndrome. Kaposi sarcoma or exfoliative dermatitis caused by psoriasis can divert the blood supply through shunts in the skin to produce high-output cardiac failure. Telangiectasias of the fingertips (Fig. 12–37), face, palate, lips, and tongue, as well as pulmonary and hepatic arteriovenous fistulas, are components of hereditary hemorrhagic telangiectasia (Osler-Weber-Rendu syndrome).[42] The triad of anomalies that Klippel-Trenaunay-Weber syndrome comprises are vascular nevus, large varices, and bony or soft tissue hypertrophy (Fig. 12–38). Marked enlargement of a limb(s) and facial hemihypertrophy are features of this disorder, in which part or all of the deep venous system is absent and arteriovenous malformation is

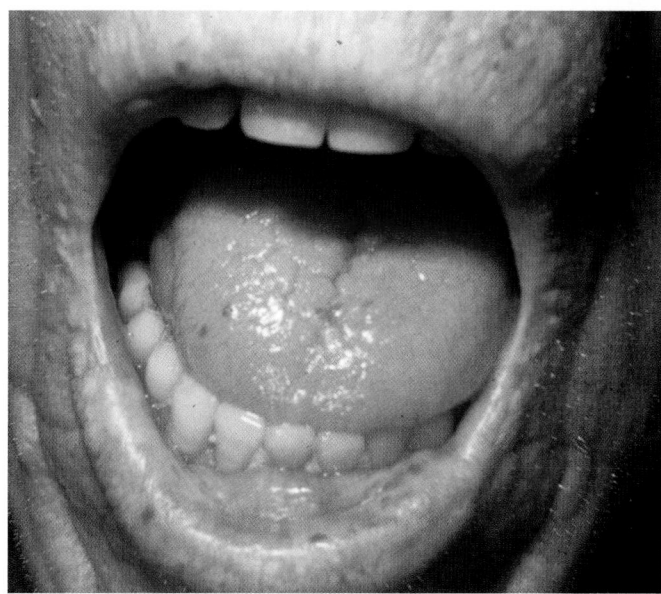

FIGURE 12–37. *Hereditary telangiectasia*: telangiectasia on lips and tongue found with pulmonary AV fistula.

often present. Hemangiomas of the skin also can indicate multinodular hemangiomatosis of the liver, a cause of high-output heart failure in infancy.

Stenosis of large arteries can occur with supravalvular aortic stenosis, rubella syndrome, Turner syndrome, and neurofibromatosis. The face of a child with supravalvular aortic stenosis (Williams syndrome) is diagnostic (Fig. 12–39). The head is small, with an elf like appearance; the cheeks are full and baggy; and the mouth and forehead are large. Curved lips and peg-shaped, widely spaced teeth are typical. Mental retardation is often present. Pulmonic artery branch stenosis is frequently present. Coarctation of the aorta

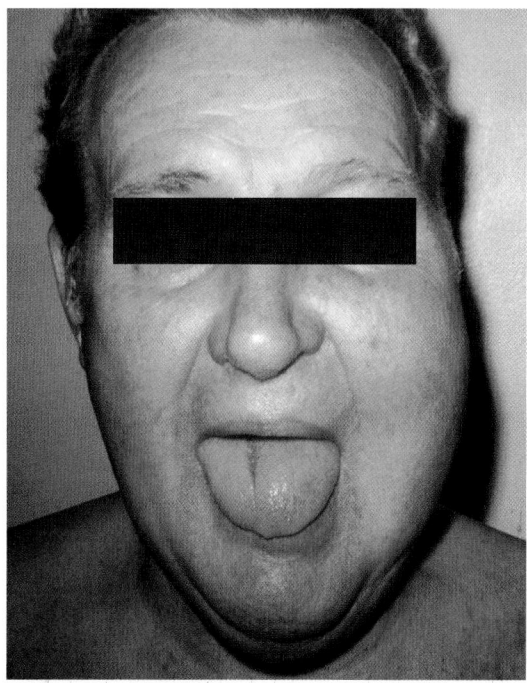

FIGURE 12–38. *Klippel-Trenaunay syndrome*: hypertrophy of left side of face and tongue in a patient with port-wine stains, gigantism of digits, and varicose veins.

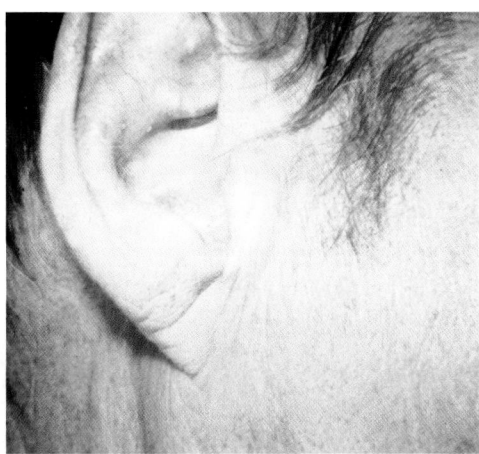

FIGURE 12–36. Horizontal ear creases are often associated with the presence of extensive coronary artery disease (CAD).

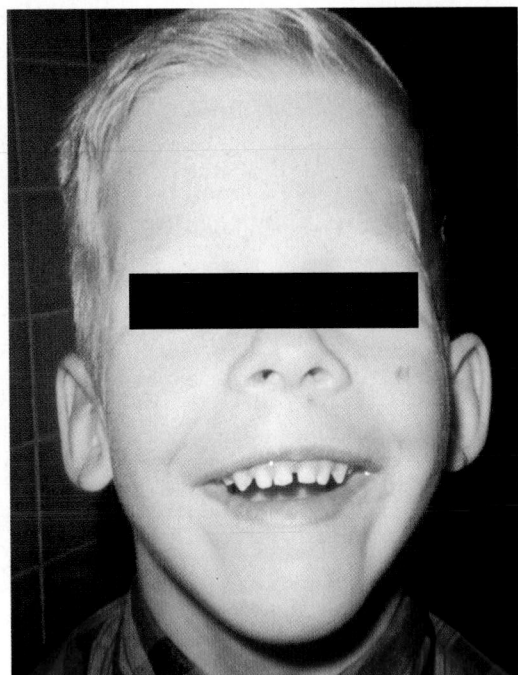

FIGURE 12–39. *Supravalvular aortic stenosis:* turned-up nose, broad cheeks, large mouth with peg-shaped teeth, and large ears.

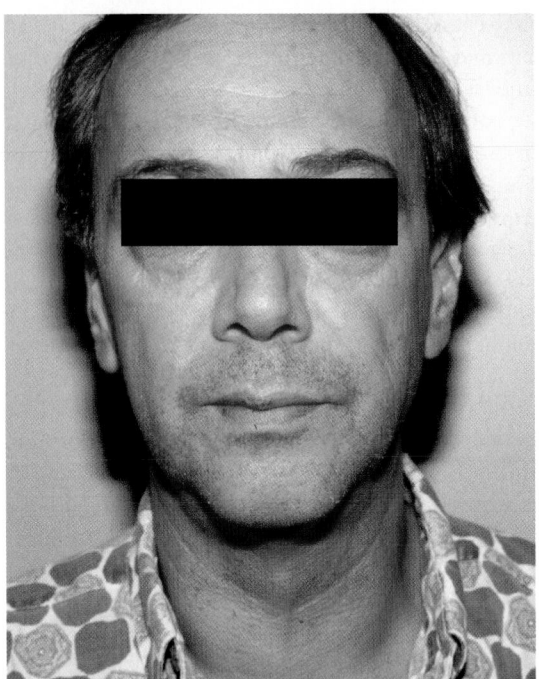

FIGURE 12–40. *Hyperthyroidism:* exophthalmos and atrial fibrillation manifestation of hyperthyroidism.

is a common cardiac lesion in Turner syndrome, and neurofibromatosis has been associated with renal artery stenosis.

【 】 MISCELLANEOUS DISORDERS

Multiple lentigines, cutaneous myxomas, myxoid fibroadenomas of the breast, and various endocrine abnormalities are features of an inherited disorder in which single or multiple cardiac myxomas occur. A susceptibility to atrial fibrillation and atrial flutter has been documented in patients who have fascioscapulohumeral muscular dystrophy.[43] Sinus node dysfunction with atrial paralysis, elbow contractures, and humeroperoneal weakness are manifestations of Emery-Dreifuss muscular dystrophy.[44]

Figure 12–40 indicates exophthalmus in a patient with atrial fibrillation and hyperthyroidism.

Single or multiple rhabdomyomas can develop within the myocardium and cause heart failure, valvular obstruction, or arrhythmias in patients with tuberous sclerosis. The diagnosis is suggested by the presence of yellow-brown angiofibromas (adenoma sebaceum) on the face (Fig. 12–41), subungual fibromas around the fingernail, café-au-lait spots, and subcutaneous nodules.

MEASUREMENT OF ARTERIAL BLOOD PRESSURE

For the noninvasive evaluation of arterial BP, a pneumatic cuff with a mercury or aneroid manometer is the most frequently used technique for assessing the status of the circulation and the interaction between the heart and arterial system. BP measurements above or below normal limits often provide important diagnostic information in patients with a variety of cardiac and noncardiac diseases. Accordingly, the BP is best recorded by the *physician* during his or her *initial physical examination* (see Chap. 70).

【 】 PHYSICAL DETERMINANTS OF THE ARTERIAL PRESSURE

The arterial BP, a measure of lateral force per unit area of vascular wall, is quantitated as millimeters of mercury (mmHg) or dynes per square centimeter (d/cm^2). Factors responsible for the peak systolic BP include the volume and velocity of LV ejection, the peripheral arteriolar resistance, the distensibility of the arterial wall,

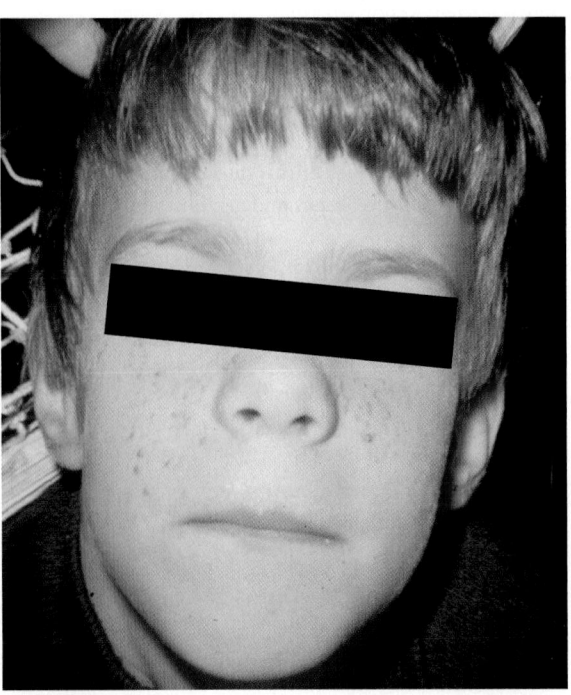

FIGURE 12–41. *Tuberous sclerosis.* Adenoma sebaceum can be associated with rhabdomyomas of the myocardium.

the viscosity of the blood, and the end-diastolic volume in the arterial system.[45] The subsequent diminution in pressure during diastole is determined by blood viscosity, arterial distensibility, peripheral resistance to flow, and length of the cardiac cycle.[46] Important physical factors affecting arterial distensibility include (1) the elastic modulus of the arterial wall, the ratio of stress (force acting to deform the wall) to strain (the proportional deformation produced), and (2) the geometry of the arterial wall, that is, the internal radius (r) and wall thickness (h), which govern wall tension (T) according to the modified Laplace equation $T = Pr/h$, where P is intravascular pressure. A decrease in elasticity or an increase in radius results in diminished distensibility and a greater increase in pressure per unit volume of blood.[47]

The mean arterial pressure is the product of the cardiac output and the total peripheral resistance, the latter often being increased by several mechanisms, including β-adrenergic stimulation, the renin-angiotensin system, or other circulating hormonal or humoral factors.[48]

[ ] METHODS FOR MEASURING THE ARTERIAL PRESSURE*

*(See Chap. 70)

Direct Methods

In 1733, Stephen Hales recorded the arterial pressures in animals by cannulation and use of a blood-filled glass column.[48] Current methods for the direct and continuous measurement of arterial pressure use the electromanometer, a transducer that converts mechanical energy into an electric signal. The artery is cannulated with a saline-filled catheter or needle that mechanically couples the circulation to the arterial manometer. Pressures are recorded using atmospheric pressure as the *zero* reference level, and intravascular pressures are further referenced to the level of the heart by addition or subtraction of a gravitation factor. The gravitation factor is expressed as *pgh*, where *p* is the density of blood (in grams per milliliter), *g* is the acceleration caused by gravity (980 cm/s), and *h* is the transducer height (centimeters) above or below the horizontal plane of the heart.

The strain-gauge manometer often is used for the precise and accurate measurement of the arterial pressure. However, error can originate in the catheter or coupling system when the properties of inertia, friction, and elasticity interact to produce damping of the frequency response. Either overdamping or underdamping can result in signal distortion. Nevertheless, the appropriate combination of an inelastic cardiac catheter and connecting tube filled with bubble-free fluid produces *critical* damping with the system response constant and adequate for the clinical recording of intravascular pressures.[45,46]

Measurement errors also occur when an end-hole catheter is positioned axial to flow in a vessel and can become especially important during high arterial flow, when kinetic energy can exceed 10 percent of the total fluid energy. Also, pressure transients caused by catheter whip can falsely elevate the measured arterial pressure.[45]

Miniature, self-flushing strain-gauge manometers attached directly to an intravascular catheter or needle, reduce the problems related to transducer mounting and flushing. A more effective method for reducing measurement errors, however, is the use of intravascular electromanometers mounted on cardiac catheters or surgically implanted in the vascular wall.

Indirect Methods

The invention of the pneumatic cuff manometer (Riva-Rocci, 1896) and the subsequent discovery and use of the arterial sounds (Korotkoff, 1905) enabled indirect measurement of the arterial pressure. The mercury manometer is the gold standard; the aneroid manometer should be calibrated against the mercury manometer at least every 6 months. Semiautomatic electronic devices, if used, should be validated according to Association for the Advancement of Medical Instrumentation (AAMI) guidelines.[49] The most commonly used noninvasive method is based on the auscultatory detection of low-pitched Korotkoff sounds over a peripheral artery at a point distal to cuff compression of the artery. McCutcheon and Rushmer[50] defined two major components of these sounds: the initial transient (k_{-i}) and the compression murmur (k_c), which coincide with the opening tap and rumble sounds of Rodbard.[51] The initial sound, k_{-i}, occurs when cuff pressure reaches arterial pressure and likely results from abrupt arterial opening and vascular distension. The intensity of this initial sound depends on the slope of the pressure pulse and the level of the distal arterial pressure at the time of arterial opening, the sound being louder with vasodilatation and high-velocity flow and softer with arterial constriction or circulatory collapse. The initial transient is probably caused by oscillation of the arterial walls as the occluded segment is suddenly opened by systolic pressure, and the compression murmur is caused by a turbulent jet of flow distal to the partially compressed segment.

The Korotkoff sounds have been divided into five phases occurring in sequence as the occluding pressure declines (Table 12–5). To avoid error, the observer must be prepared to recognize two normal Korotkoff sound variations associated with BP reading: (1) The *auscultatory gap* is a period of silence occurring during Korotkoff phases I and II. This disappearance of sound is temporary and is usually short, but the gap can occur over a 40 mmHg measurement. (2) An absent Korotkoff phase V occurs when sounds are heard to *0*. When this is the case, phase IV should be recorded along with phase V. In this case, phase IV is the best reference for diastolic pressure.

Proper technique is important for accurate measurement. The inflatable rubber bag within the compression cuff should have a width that is 20 percent greater than the limb diameter and a length adequate to encompass two-thirds the limb. Before auscultation, the cuff is quickly inflated to a pressure 20 mmHg above the systolic, as indicated by obliteration of the radial pulse. The stethoscope is then applied lightly but firmly over the artery, and auscultatory pressure is determined by noting the onset (peak systole) and behavior of the Korotkoff sounds as the cuff is deflated at a rate of approximately 3 mmHg/s. When the sounds disappear, the bag should be rapidly decompressed and 1 or 2 minutes allowed to pass before repeat determinations are made. The BP should be taken with the subject upright as well as supine. Measurement of the BP in both arms is recommended, especially in the elderly. An American Heart Association hypertension primer recommends that the systolic pressure be recorded as the point at

TABLE 12–5

Phases of the Korotkoff Sounds

Phase I

The pressure level at which the first faint, consistent tapping sounds are heard. The sounds gradually increase in intensity as the cuff is deflated. The first of at least two of these sounds is defined as the systolic pressure.

Phase II

The time during cuff deflation when a murmur of swishing sounds are heard.

Phase III

The period during which sounds are crisper and increase in intensity.

Phase IV

The time when a distinct, abrupt, muffling of sound (usually of a soft blowing quality) is heard. This is defined as the diastolic pressure in anyone in whom sounds continue to zero.

Phase V

The pressure level when the last regular blood pressure sound is heard and after which all sound disappears. This is defined as the diastolic pressure unless sounds are heard to zero.

which the first tapping sounds occur for two consecutive beats (phase I) and that the diastolic pressure *in adults* be recorded as the point at which sounds become inaudible. *In children* and in adults with a hyperkinetic circulation, the diastolic pressure should be recorded as the point at which muffling of the sounds occurs (onset of phase IV). The arterial pressures at both the onset of muffling (phase IV) and the disappearance of sound (phase V) should be recorded. The mean BP can be estimated by the addition of one-third the pulse pressure (systolic pressure minus diastolic pressure) to the diastolic pressure.

Patients with atrial fibrillation can have a significant beat-to-beat variation in their arterial pressure. Accordingly, the indirect BP should be measured several times and the average noted.

This indirect method provides several potential sources of error because of improper equipment, inaccurate detection of the Korotkoff sounds, and observer techniques.[52] The standard pneumatic cuff often can be unsatisfactory for pressure measurement in the arms or in the legs of very obese subjects. The arterial pressure can be underestimated if the cuff is deflated too rapidly, or if inadequate inflation does not result in complete arterial occlusion. When the cuff is deflated too slowly or is immediately reinflated for multiple pressure determinations, the resulting venous congestion can elevate the diastolic pressure artificially and falsely decrease the systolic pressure by decreasing the intensity of phase I or phase II sounds to an inaudible level.

Studies correlating direct and indirect BP measurements have, in general, shown a good correlation between indirect and direct measurements of BP in the arm. The indirect method tends to underestimate systolic pressure by several millimeters of mercury, to overestimate diastolic pressure by several millimeters of mercury

when phase IV is used as an endpoint, and to slightly underestimate diastolic pressure in normal individuals when phase V is taken as the endpoint.

Home BP recordings using manual or automatic inflation and deflation of the cuff and detection of Korotkoff sounds by a microphone, stethoscope, or ultrasonic transducer are being used with increasing frequency for the ambulatory assessment of patients with hypertension. Although clinically useful, ambulatory BP devices in general do not meet the standards for automated devices of the AAMI.

More recently, arterial tonometry has been used as a completely noninvasive method for monitoring the arterial pressure. This probe, with a micromanometer in its tip, operates on the principle of a piezo-resistive transducer of cantilever construction.[53,54]

[ ] NORMAL ARTERIAL PRESSURE

Normal pressures have been defined on the basis of values included within two standard deviations of the mean of pressures obtained in a large population of apparently healthy individuals (see Chap. 70). The normal BP range varies with age, sex, and race.[55] In the United States, the pressure increases rapidly during the first few days of life and then increases gradually, with a slightly greater increment in systolic than in diastolic values, throughout life. The pressure tends to be higher in Western industrialized societies than in Asian, African, and technically undeveloped societies.

With increasing age and into senescence, the aorta undergoes progressive dilatation and elongation, with increasing stiffness of its walls.[56] Resulting from this diminished vascular distensibility, there is an increase in systolic arterial pressure with less change in diastolic pressure.

The normal BP limits for adults living in the United States are approximately 100 to 140 mmHg systolic and 60 to 90 mmHg diastolic. In an individual subject, however, baseline pressures above or below these levels do not define a pathologic state.[45] The systolic arterial pressure rises slowly and progressively in most Americans between the ages of 20 and 60 and more rapidly later, increasing by approximately 20 mmHg between the ages of 60 and 80.[57] Diastolic pressure usually rises very little after 45 years of age. Data from the Framingham Study and more recent studies (e.g., MRFIT, SHEP, Syst-Eur) have shown a clear correlation between systolic BP and cardiovascular events, a reduction in events with reduction of systolic BP, or even a negative association between diastolic BP and events.[58]

In mildly to moderately hypertensive persons, the BP *casually* recorded by a physician is significantly higher than the average value of a series of intermittent, indirect determinations or continuous direct recordings made during normal activity. To estimate basal BP, measurements have been obtained during sleep, when the subject first awakens in the morning while still recumbent, or after several hours of reclining.

Factors contributing to variations in an individual's BP during daily activities include (1) body posture; (2) state of muscular, cerebral, or gastrointestinal activity; (3) emotional or painful stimuli; (4) environmental factors such as temperature and noise level; and (5) the use of tobacco, coffee, alcohol, and other drugs with direct or neurally mediated vasomotor properties.[45] Twenty-four–hour pressures, obtained from normal and hypertensive subjects with an automatic recorder, have shown considerable variability with activity and emotional stimuli. The average diurnal pattern of BP consists of an increase throughout the day and early evening and a significant, rapid decline to a low point during the early, deep stage of sleep. This is an important fact to remember in prescribing medications for systemic hypertension (see Chap. 90).

With normal respiration, the peak systolic BP is greater during expiration than during inspiration by as much as 10 mmHg. An augmentation of this difference occurs in patients with pericardial tamponade (pulsus paradoxus; see Chap. 84) and during hyperventilation.

Isotonic exercise in both the supine and upright positions produces a moderate increase in BP (systolic pressure greater than mean pressure, which is greater than diastolic pressure). Sustained isometric muscular contractions produce an abrupt increase in systolic, mean, and diastolic BP that depends on the strength of the contraction.[59]

ABNORMAL ARTERIAL PRESSURE

Increased Pulse Pressure

An increase in arterial pulse pressure is commonly observed during routine BP recordings. This usually is caused by an increase in stroke volume and ejection velocity, often with a decrease in peripheral resistance. Fever, anemia, hot weather, exercise, pregnancy, hyperthyroidism, or arteriovenous fistulas can produce this change. Several cardiac diseases, such as AR, patent ductus arteriosus, and truncus arteriosus, also can result in a widened pulse pressure. An increased pulse pressure caused by a large stroke volume can occur with complete heart block or marked sinus bradycardia.[45]

Atherosclerosis of the large arteries often reduces arterial compliance and results in an elevated systolic pressure with a normal or even decreased stroke volume. The systolic hypertension of the elderly does not necessarily represent a change in arteriolar resistance. Efforts to lower this type of systolic pressure elevation are often appropriate but can result in diminished peripheral perfusion (see Chap. 69). The increased pulse pressure associated with systemic arteriovenous fistulas is less common; a relative tachycardia can be the only clinical clue. Compression of a systemic arteriovenous fistula can produce a prompt slowing of the heart rate (Branham sign).

Reduced Pulse Pressure

A narrow pulse pressure is uncommon in normal subjects but can result from an increased peripheral resistance (increased circulating catecholamines in heart failure), decreased stroke volume (severe as in arteriosclerosis [AS]), and/or markedly decreased intravascular volume (diabetic ketoacidosis).[45]

Unequal Pulse Pressures

The diagnostic importance of BP differences between the right and left arms can occur as a result of supravalvular AS as well as the *choanal effect* in children and the subclavian steal syndrome in adults.[60] Most patients with the former have greater than 20 mmHg higher BP in the right arm. The subclavian steal syn-

drome, often accompanied by symptoms of cerebrovascular insufficiency, usually results in a pronounced lowering or absence of brachial artery pressure in the ipsilateral extremity.[45] There is diminished vertebral blood flow to the brain because flow is diverted to the involved subclavian artery distal to the stenosis.

A progressive increase in systolic pressure normally occurs as the point of measurement is moved peripherally from the central aorta (Fig. 12–42); the increment is similar in the large arteries of the upper arm and the thigh. Direct recordings of femoral and brachial arterial pressures (systolic, diastolic, and mean) in adults and children and indirect measurement of popliteal and brachial artery pressures have demonstrated that mean pressures are equal at these sites. A difference in arm and leg pressures can occur because of coarctation of the aorta or acquired disease, such as aortic dissection, aortic arch syndrome, or the subclavian steal syndrome.[45]

PULSUS ALTERNANS

Pulsus alternans can be detected by palpating a peripheral artery, preferably the femoral artery, when the heart rhythm is normal. The sphygmomanometer can be used to measure accurately the beat-to-beat variation in pressure that characterizes pulsus alternans.

Pulsus alternans occurs in patients with severe heart disease who exhibit impaired LV contraction. It can also occur for several beats following supraventricular tachycardia in normal persons or when the respiratory rate is half the pulse rate.

PULSUS PARADOXUS

A normal person can exhibit a 10 mmHg drop in systolic pressure during normal inspiration. A greater decline can be identified in patients with acute cardiac tamponade, constrictive pericarditis, severe obstructive lung disease, and restrictive cardiomyopathy.

Pulsus paradoxus is best detected by inflating the BP cuff above systolic pressure and then slowly releasing it. As the cuff pressure is

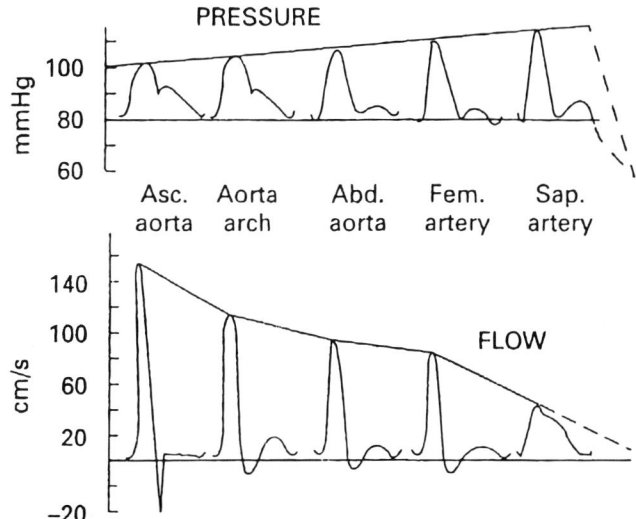

FIGURE 12–42. Micromanometer and catheter tip flow velocity as change in contour of pressure waves (*above*) and flow waves (*below*) between the ascending aorta and the saphenous artery. *Source: Vlachopoulos C, O'Rourke MF. The arterial pulse. Curr Probl Cardiol. 2000;25:296–346. Used with permission from the publisher.*

gradually reduced, the BP sounds become audible during expiration. The difference in pressure between the first audible sound heard on expiration and the pressure level at which the sounds are heard during all phases of respiration gives a measurement of magnitude of pulsus paradoxus. The mechanism of pulsus paradoxus is discussed in Chap. 84.

THE ARTERIAL PULSE

The arterial pulse, like any periodic fluctuation that is caused by the heart, occurs at the same frequency as the heartbeat. Ejection of blood with every cardiac contraction is converted to *flow, pressure,* and *dimension* pulsations in arteries throughout the body. Although the term *pulse* refers to any such pulsation, the arterial pulse perceived by a clinician is the pressure pulse in a large, accessible artery. Palpation of the arterial pulse is a basic and important element of the physical examination.[61]

[ ] PHYSICAL DETERMINANTS OF THE ARTERIAL PULSE

Genesis of the Arterial Pulse

Pressure and blood flow in the ascending aorta result from the interaction between the heart and arterial system. When LV pressure exceeds the aortic pressure, it becomes the driving force for the movement of blood into the ascending aorta.[51,62] This driving force depends on the intrinsic contractility of ventricular muscle, the size and shape of the left ventricle, and the heart rate. It is opposed by several forces that impede the development of flow and are interrelated in a complex manner. Three major determinants of arterial impedance include (1) resistance, (2) inertia, and (3) compliance.

Resistance is related to blood viscosity and the geometry of the vasculature; it opposes flow and is unaffected by changes in heart rate. Inertia, which is related to the mass of the column of blood, opposes the rate of change of arterial blood flow (i.e., acceleration) and depends on the heart rate. Compliance is related to the distensibility of the vascular walls, opposes changes in arterial blood volume, and also depends on the heart rate. The heart rate dependency of inertia and compliance introduces phase shifts between instantaneous pressure and flow in a pulsatile system.[63] Inertia and compliance are important determinants of the character of ventricular ejection, especially in early systole, when flows and pressures are changing rapidly.

The arterial pulse wave begins with aortic valve opening and the onset of LV ejection. Aortic pressure rises rapidly in early systole because the LV stroke volume enters the aorta faster than it flows to distal sites. The rapid-rising portion of the arterial pressure curve is often termed the *anacrotic limb* (from the Greek meaning *upbeat*). In experimental animals and in humans, peak proximal aortic flow velocity occurs slightly earlier than peak pressure.[64] After its peak, aortic pressure declines as LV ejection slows, and peripheral blood flow continues. During isovolumic relaxation, a transient reversal of flow from the central arteries toward the ventricle just prior to aortic valve closure is associated with an incisura on the descending limb of the aortic pressure pulse. The subsequent smaller, secondary positive wave has been attributed to the

elastic recoil of the aorta and aortic valve but is partially caused by reflected waves from more distal arteries. Subsequently, aortic pressure decreases again as further *runoff* in the peripheral circulation occurs in diastole.

The proximal aortic pulse pressure is directly proportional to the ratio of stroke volume to arterial distensibility, but multiple factors influence this complex relationship.[65] Arterial distensibility diminishes as the distending arterial pressure increases. Accordingly, the pulse pressure for a constant stroke volume will be larger if the mean BP is elevated. Also, arterial distensibility varies inversely with the rate of rise of intraluminal pressure. When the systolic ejection rate increases, the stiffer arterial wall results in a greater pulse pressure.

Contour of the Arterial Pulse

Pulsatile changes in arterial diameter are virtually identical to the pressure pulse, with minor differences explained in terms of nonlinear elasticity and viscosity of the arterial wall. In 1939, Hamilton and Dow defined the pressure wave contour in different arteries in terms of wave reflection between the aortic valve and peripheral sites.[66] The pulse waveform recorded at any site of the arterial tree is the sum of a forward waveform and a backward-traveling one that is the *echo* of the incident wave reflected at peripheral sites. *Wave reflection is an important determinant of LV load and CBF.* A reflected wave occurring at systole increases systolic pressure and thereby increases ventricular afterload. In contrast, occurrence of the reflected wave at diastole is highly desirable because augmentation of pressure during diastole aids coronary perfusion.

Conventionally, the pulse is described in the *time domain,* where it is considered as a change in arterial pressure with time. An alternative, quantitative approach is to analyze the pulse in the *frequency domain.* Pulse is conceived as a composite wave that can be resolved into component harmonics like a musical wave. Impedance is the measure of the opposition to flow presented by a system and can be measured when harmonic analysis is used to relate frequency components of pressure and flow pulses.

Usually there is a linear relation between pressure and flow at the same point in an artery and between pressures at different points in the arterial system. From impedance curves, it is possible to identify the factors responsible for the relation between the pulsatile pressure and flow. The peripheral arterial pressure wave recorded is the summation of the incident (initial) and reflected waves. The systemic circulation has been represented by a simple asymmetric T-tube model that emphasizes the importance of wave reflection at two arteriolar reflecting sites in the upper and lower parts of the body.[65] An important patient study indicates major reflection sites at the aortic level of the renal arteries and at a point distal to the terminal abdominal aorta bifurcation.[66]

Peripheral Transmission of the Arterial Pulse

As the normal aortic pulse wave is transmitted peripherally, significant changes in its contour occur caused by (1) distortion and damping of pulse wave components; (2) different rates of transmission of various components; (3) distortion or exaggeration by reflected, resonant, or standing waves; (4) conversion of kinetic energy into hydrostatic or potential energy; (5) differences in distensibility and caliber of the arteries; and (6) changes in the vessel wall caused by age and/or disease.

The arterial pressure pulse enters the proximal aorta and travels distally at a velocity many times faster than that of maximum blood flow. The pressure wave is accompanied by a traveling wave distending the arterial wall, the pulse wave velocity increasing as arterial wall distensibility diminishes.

The pulse wave arrives progressively later at more peripheral sites when timed from the QRS complex on the ECG. Representative time delays from the central aorta are as follows: carotid, 30 milliseconds (ms); brachial, 60 ms; radial, 80 ms; and femoral, 75 ms.

The arterial pulse wave undergoes a progressive change in shape during its transmission distally (see Fig. 12–42). The pulse pressure and systolic amplitude increase, and the ascending limb of the pulse wave becomes steeper. The incisura of the central aorta pulse is gradually replaced by a smoother, somewhat later dicrotic notch that occurs at lower pressure levels. The dicrotic notch and the following positive secondary or dicrotic wave probably result from the summation of the forward pulse wave and reflected waves from the peripheral vessels.

The Ankle-Brachial Index

The ankle-brachial index (ABI) is the ratio of the systolic blood pressure at the ankle divided by the higher of the two arm systolic blood pressures.[67] It reflects the degree of lower-extremity arterial occlusive disease, which is manifest by reduced blood pressure distal to stenotic lesions. Either the posterior tibial or dorsalis pedis artery pressures can be used. It is important to note that each equally reflects the status of the aortoiliac and femoropopliteal segments but different tibial arteries; therefore, the resulting ABIs can differ. An arm systolic pressure of 120 mmHg and an ankle systolic pressure of 60 mmHg yields an ABI of 0.5 (60/120). The ABI is inversely related to disease severity. A resting ABI <0.9 is considered abnormal. Lower values correspond to progressively more severe occlusive peripheral arterial disease (PAD) and disabling claudication. An ABI <0.3 is consistent with critical ischemia, rest pain, and tissue loss. This concept has been in widespread clinical use for several decades.

A reduced ABI is generally equated with atherosclerotic lower-extremity PAD. However, other forms of arterial disease such as giant cell arteritis, dissection, and emboli can cause lower-extremity arterial occlusions or stenoses, thus yielding an abnormal ABI. False negatives can be encountered in diabetics with calcified noncompressible tibial and pedal vessels. Because arm pressure is used as the denominator in calculating ABI, stenotic disease of the brachiocephalic, subclavian, axillary, or brachial arteries can lower arm pressure and give an ABI that does not reflect the lower-extremity arterial occlusive disease. There are patients with increasing ABIs who were thought to have improving lower-extremity circulation but who were in fact experiencing worsening upper-extremity arterial occlusive disease. For screening purposes, ABI is usually measured only at rest. However, a resting ABI >0.9 does not exclude significant PAD. More proximal stenoses, particularly at the aortoiliac level, may not be severe enough to reduce ankle pressure at rest but can cause a precipitous fall in ABI after exercise.

Because atherosclerosis is a systemic process, a patient with PAD and an abnormal ABI has an increased risk of disease in other vascular territories including the coronary and cerebral circulation, putting him or her at risk for major adverse cardiovascular events.

There is a highly significant trend toward increasing relative risk of prior history of manifest cardiovascular disease with decreasing ABIs. In the Cardiovascular Health Study, the 7.4 percent of participants with an ABI <0.8 were more than twice as likely to have a history of prior coronary event, cerebrovascular event, or congestive heart failure than were those with a normal ABI (*p* < .01).

Examination of the Arterial Pulse

All major arterial pulses should be examined bilaterally for both patency and waveform characteristics. The thickness and hardness of the arterial walls often can be assessed by *rolling* the vessel against underlying tissue. A pulse in the foot should not be considered absent unless examined with the foot in a dependent position. Otherwise, the arterial pulses usually are examined with the patient supine and with the trunk of the body slightly elevated.

The examiner uses tactile receptors in the tips of the fingers to sense movement of the arterial wall associated with the pressure pulse as it passes the site of palpation. Measurements in the proximal aorta show cyclic movement in both diameter and length proportional to the pulse pressure. In more peripheral arteries with connective tissue attachments, however, the detectable movement is small and variable, with radial expansion by only approximately 2 percent of the end-diastolic cross-sectional area.

The usual technique for palpating the arterial pulse is to press with the examining fingers until the maximum pulse is sensed. The pulse is felt as changing displacement superimposed on the *baseline* displacement produced by compressing the artery. The examiner should apply varying degrees of pressure while concentrating on the separate phases of the pulse wave. This method, referred to as *trisection,* is useful for assessing the upstroke, systolic peak, and diastolic slope of the arterial pulse.[45,68]

Palpation of the carotid artery is preferred for assessing cardiac performance because the carotid pulse corresponds more closely to the central aortic pressure. In certain cardiac diseases (e.g., AR), however, the abnormalities detected in the carotid pulse are accentuated in the more peripheral pulses. To evaluate the integrity of the peripheral arterial blood supply and to localize any lesions that exist, the arterial pulses in all four extremities should be examined and compared (see Chap. 108).

Inspection of the carotid arterial and jugular venous pulsations should be performed at the same time. The carotid pulse is usually best examined with the sternocleidomastoid muscles relaxed and the head rotated slightly toward the examiner. The carotid pulse can be timed from the first heart sound, which is heard slightly before the pulsation. The carotid pulse should be palpated in the lower half of the patient's neck to avoid carotid sinus compression. Occasionally, it is useful to palpate two arteries simultaneously (e.g., radial and femoral) to detect an apparent pulse wave delay, such as occurs in patients with coarctation of the aorta.

The examination of arterial pulses in the abdomen and upper and lower extremities should be performed carefully in all patients and compared using a scale such as the following: 0 = complete absence of pulsation; 1+ = small or reduced pulsation; 2+ = normal or average pulsation; and 3+ = large or bounding pulsation. Furthermore, auscultation over the major arteries should be performed because an audible bruit can be a clue to partial occlusion or can indicate transmission (e.g., carotid) of a cardiac murmur (see Chap. 108).

Normal Arterial Pulse

The normal carotid pulse has a smooth, rapid upstroke or ascending limb to a smooth, dome-shaped summit (Fig. 12–43A). Then a downstroke occurs that is somewhat less rapid than the upstroke. The dicrotic notch and secondary diastolic wave are usually not felt but can be palpable in some normal individuals, particularly during fever, exercise, or excitement. The dicrotic notch usually occurs approximately 300 ms after the onset of the pulse wave when corrected for heart rate.

In arteries distal to the carotid, the pulse wave arrives later and has a steep initial wave that rises to a high peak pressure, whereas the diastolic and mean pressures are slightly lower. The systolic upstroke time (onset of pulse wave to its peak) tends to be shorter, but the apparent LV ejection time (onset of pulse wave to incisura) is longer in more peripheral arterial pulses. In the brachial artery, the heart rate-corrected systolic upstroke time averages 120 ms (range, 90 to 160 ms), and the systolic ejection time averages approximately 320 ms (range, 280 to 360 ms).

Graphic recordings of the arterial pulses frequently show two positive deflections during systole, the first shoulder being referred to as the *percussion wave* and the second as the *tidal wave*. In the normal proximal aortic pulse, the percussion wave is caused by arrival of the impulse generated by LV ejection, the tidal wave can represent its echo from the upper part of the body, and the dicrotic or diastolic wave is a reflection from the lower part of the body.

With aging (see Chap. 101), there is a relative increase in the second (tidal) systolic wave and the height of the incisura relative to the first systolic wave.[69] The systolic upstroke time is longer, and the amplitude and duration of the diastolic wave tend to be less prominent.

Abnormal Arterial Pulses

In hypertension and arteriosclerosis, the pressure pulse amplitude is increased, the tidal wave is prominent, and the diastolic wave is absent. All features of the pulse can be explained by increased wave velocity.[69] Reflected waves return to the proximal aorta during late systole, augmenting the tidal wave and increasing systolic pressure. With systemic hypotension, the pulse-wave velocity is decreased, and the later tidal and diastolic waves are further displaced from the percussion wave.

Impairment of the pulse of one or both carotid arteries is usually produced by atherosclerosis, but multiple other causes include thrombosis, embolus, arteritis, and diseases of the aortic arch. Kinking of the carotid or brachiocephalic artery is relatively fre-

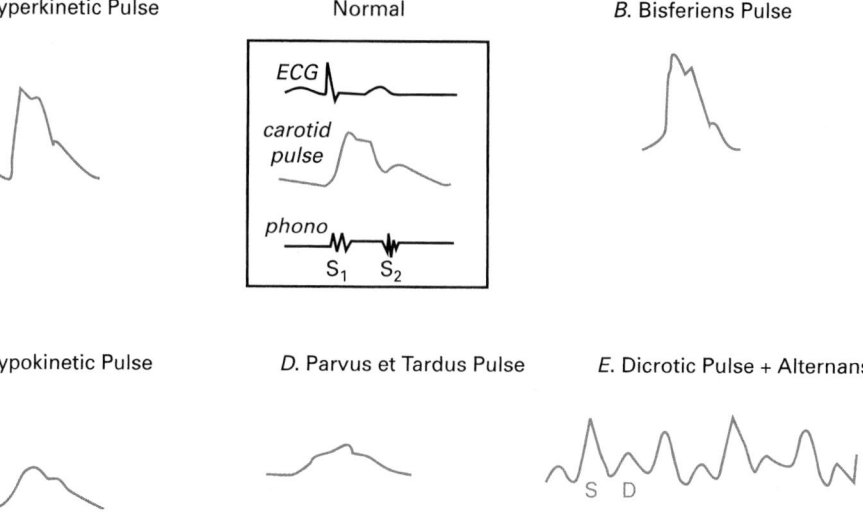

FIGURE 12–43. Schematic representation of the normal carotid arterial pulse, five types of abnormal pulses, and pulsus alternans. D, diastole; ECG, electrocardiogram; phono, phonocardiogram; S, systole; S$_1$, first heart sound; S$_2$, second heart sound.

quent, particularly in hypertensive patients, and can simulate aneurysmal dilatation. Femoral pulses can be diminished in the child or young adult as a result of coarctation of the aorta. In most adults, however, the diminution of the femoral pulsation is caused by atherosclerosis of the abdominal aorta, aortic bifurcation, or ileofemoral arteries (see Chap. 101).

Hyperkinetic Arterial Pulse

Large, bounding arterial pulses usually indicate the rapid ejection of an increased volume of blood from the left ventricle (see Fig. 12–43A). Commonly, the arterial pulse pressure is increased, and the peripheral arterial resistance diminished. The hyperdynamic arterial pulse is sometimes referred to in terms that describe a particular component of the pulse wave. Thus the *water-hammer pulse,* named after a Victorian toy, refers to an extremely rapid, forceful ascending limb of the arterial pulse wave.[70] By contrast, *collapsing pulse* refers to a quick, marked decrease in the arterial pulse wave following its peak. The term *Quincke pulse* refers to visible small pulsations in the nail bed of patients with hyperdynamic arterial pulses from any cause, including AR.

Hyperkinetic arterial pulses occur in normal subjects with a hyperkinetic circulation (e.g., exercise, fever), patients with cardiovascular diseases associated with increased stroke volume, and subjects with marked bradycardia and an extremely large stroke volume (e.g., athletes). A hyperdynamic arterial pulse also occurs in patients with an abnormally rapid runoff of blood from the arterial system (e.g., patent ductus arteriosus, arteriovenous fistulas). Patients on chronic hemodialysis often have hyperdynamic pulses produced by the combination of a surgical arteriovenous fistula, anemia, and hypertension.

In AR, the rapid-rising, bounding arterial pulse results from increases in both stroke volume and the rate of LV ejection. The early systolic flow often produces palpable vibrations manifest as a thrill on the steep ascending limb. Later in systole, the rate of ventricular ejection and the arterial pulse wave decrease sharply, often resulting in systolic collapse.

Bisferiens Arterial Pulse

The bisferiens (from the Latin *twice beating*) pulse has a waveform characterized by two positive waves during systole (Fig. 12–43B). The pulse wave upstroke rises rapidly and forcefully, producing the first systolic peak (percussion wave). A brief decline in pressure is followed by a smaller and somewhat slower-rising positive pulse wave (tidal wave). Abnormalities of LV ejection and reflected waves from peripheral arteries contribute to the prominence of the second systolic wave in the bisferiens pulse. The bisferiens pulse is sometimes more easily palpable in a brachial or radial artery. A bisferiens pulse often occurs in patients with pure AR and in patients with combined AS and severe AR. It also occurs in association with the rapid ejection of an increased stroke volume from the left ventricle (e.g., exercise, fever, patent ductus arteriosus).

The bisferiens pulse often is present in patients with hypertrophic cardiomyopathy, many of whom have a pressure gradient in the LV outflow tract. In this syndrome, the midsystolic negative wave usually coincides with a marked decrease in the rate of LV ejection. The second systolic wave, or tidal wave, most likely is produced by reflected waves from the periphery. The bisferiens pulse can be elicited by maneuvers that decrease the LV size or increase its contractility. The most characteristic aspect of the arterial pulse in hypertrophic cardiomyopathy is its rapid rate of rise. A physical finding nearly specific for hypertrophic cardiomyopathy is a much smaller arterial pressure pulse in the cardiac cycle following a premature ventricular beat (see Chap. 30).

Hypokinetic Arterial Pulse

A small, weak arterial pulse is frequently present in patients with a diminished stroke volume (Fig. 12–43C). Usually, the decreased stroke output is associated with decreased rate and duration of LV ejection, and there is a narrow arterial pulse pressure despite an increased arterial resistance. Common causes include hypovolemia, LV failure, and mitral or aortic valve stenosis.

Parvus et Tardus Pulse

Patients with moderate or severe valvular AS often have an arterial pulse that is small and has a delayed systolic peak. Occasionally, there can be a detectable shoulder on the upstroke of the carotid pulse, referred to as *anacrotic*[71] (Fig. 12–43D). Palpable coarse vibrations often are present as a systolic thrill over the slowly rising carotid pulse. The parvus et tardus pulse is much easier to detect in the carotid arteries than in more distal arteries.

Most middle-aged patients with uncomplicated severe AS have a parvus et tardus pulse, but this pulse also can occur in relatively mild stenosis. Conversely, an apparently normal arterial pulse is not unusual in elderly patients with severe AS who have decreased distensibility of the large arteries. Severe LV failure often results in a small, weak pulse that can be difficult to distinguish from that of AS.

Dicrotic Arterial Pulse

The dicrotic (from the Greek *dikrotos,* "double beating") pulse is a twice-peaked pulse with one peak in systole and the second in diastole, the latter caused by an accentuated and palpable dicrotic wave that follows the second heart sound (Fig. 12–43E).[72] It is usually best felt in the carotids, although it also can be palpated over more peripheral arteries. Major abnormalities include a short systolic ejection phase, a low dicrotic notch, a large diastolic wave, a narrow pulse pressure, a diminished rate of rise of the pulse, and the lack of distinct percussion and tidal waves. The dicrotic pulse is most common in young or middle-aged patients with impaired LV performance. It is usually associated with a low cardiac output, markedly diminished stroke volume, elevated LV end-diastolic pressure, and high systemic arterial resistance. Rarely, the dicrotic wave can be palpated in young, febrile patients in whom none of the other abnormal features of the dicrotic pulse are present.

Pulsus Alternans

In pulsus alternans, beats occur at regular intervals with a regular alternation of the systolic height of the pressure pulses (Fig. 12–43E).[73] Rarely, pulsus alternans is so marked that the weaker pulses are not felt at all. When pulsus alternans is noticed first after a premature beat, the extent of the difference in systolic pressure in alternating beats can decline for several cycles until the pulse amplitude is again constant. The initiation of post-premature ventricular beat pulsus alternans is probably related to the increased duration of LV filling after the premature beat.

Sustained pulsus alternans is seen in severe depression of LV performance with an alteration in aortic flow, systolic LV pressure, aortic systolic pressure, LV upstroke pattern on apex cardiogram (*dP/dt*), and LV end-diastolic pressure. Sustained pulsus alternans likely is caused by alteration of the contractile state of at least part of the myocardium, which can be caused by the failure of electromechanical coupling in some cells during the weaker contraction. A subsequent stronger contraction would then represent contraction of all cells, some of which were potentiated.

Pulsus alternans can be better appreciated when palpating a distal artery, which normally has a slightly wider pulse pressure than the carotid artery. The patient's respiration should be held, because the small changes in arterial pressure caused by normal respiration can obscure the recognition of pulsus alternans. Pulsus alternans can be confirmed by using a sphygmomanometer and is usually associated with a LV third heart sound.

Pulsus Paradoxus

A *paradoxical pulse* is defined as a marked decrease in the pulse amplitude during normal quiet inspiration or a decrease in the systolic arterial pressure by more than 10 mmHg.[74] The normal small decline in systolic BP probably is produced predominantly by relative pooling of blood in the pulmonary vessels during inspiration and also can reflect the delayed transmission through the lungs of the preceding expiratory fall in venous pressure and RV cardiac output.

In patients with cardiac tamponade, fluid accumulation in the pericardium increases intrapericardial pressure, and the heart's filling capacity is reduced. During inspiration, the expected augmentation of venous return to the right side of the heart occurs despite the elevated intrapericardial pressure.[75] The diminished thoracic pressure also causes a pooling of blood in the pulmonary veins and capillaries and diminishes pulmonary venous return to the left atrium. Because the high intrapericardial pressure limits flow to the heart and the total cardiac filling capacity is limited, the increase in right-sided heart volume with inspiration causes an obligatory decrease in left-sided heart filling. This, along with the pooling of blood in the pulmonary bed, produces a decline in LV stroke volume and systolic BP during inspiration.[75]

Pulsus paradoxus is common with cardiac tamponade but infrequent with constrictive pericarditis (see Chap. 84). Different hemodynamic mechanisms contribute to the production of a paradoxical pulse in certain patients with superior vena cava obstruction, asthma, or obstructive airways disease; in some patients with pulmonary embolism or shock; and in some patients after thoracotomy.

The extent of pulsus paradoxus can be quantitated by cuff sphygmomanometry as the pressure difference between the first discernible Korotkoff sound on expiration and the pressure level at which Korotkoff sounds are audible during all phases of respiration.

Effects of Arrhythmias on the Arterial Pulse

Premature Ventricular Depolarizations
A premature ventricular depolarization can be associated with no pulse, a small-amplitude pulse, or a normal arterial pulse, depending on timing and whether or not the LV pressure generated is able to open the aortic valve.[76] The arterial pulse following a premature beat usually is greatly enhanced because of decreased aortic impedance, increased LV filling, and augmented LV contractility. At times, premature ventricular beats are so common as to produce an irregularly irregular pulse. Then the presence of cannon *a* waves in the jugular venous pulse (JVP) should alert one to the correct diagnosis.

Tachyarrhythmias
The ECG is usually needed for the definitive diagnosis of any abnormality of heart rate or rhythm. However, careful observation of the arterial pulse and the JVP frequently leads to the correct diagnosis. Simultaneous cardiac auscultation is also frequently helpful.

Most tachycardias associated with a regular pulse are of supraventricular origin. In sinus tachycardia, the arterial pulse will slow gradually with carotid sinus pressure and then again increase gradually. Paroxysmal atrial tachycardia has an *all or none* response. In patients with atrial flutter, carotid sinus pressure will increase the block at the AV junction, the pulse rate slowing and subsequently returning to its original rate in a "jerky" fashion.

In patients with ventricular tachycardia and AV dissociation, the variation in the atrial ventricular sequence of contraction and resulting variation in pulse amplitude often can be detected by palpation.[77]

An irregularly irregular pulse with a varying pulse pressure is usually the result of atrial fibrillation; however, multifocal atrial tachycardia is also a common cause of this finding in patients with severe chronic obstructive lung disease.

Bradyarrhythmias
An unusually slow heart rate frequently is associated with a decrease in the rate of rise and amplitude of the arterial pressure pulse. Complete heart block often is readily diagnosed by the variability in the arterial pulse ampli-

tude, changing intensity of the first heart sound, and intermittent cannon *a* waves in the JVP. These are all caused by the time-dependent variable contribution of atrial contraction to ventricular filling.

【 】 EFFECTS OF DRUG THERAPY ON THE ARTERIAL PULSE

Pulse wave analysis provides important information about the actions of drugs that, most importantly, may not be apparent with conventional methods. *Nitrates* decrease central systolic pressure substantially although they have no or minimal effect on peripheral systolic pressure (Fig. 12–44). β-*Blocking* agents have variable effect, depending on their intrinsic properties. Nonselective agents tend to increase late systolic pressure augmentation; in contrast, those agents with vasodilating properties have the opposite effect. Both angiotensin-converting enzyme (ACE) inhibitors and calcium channel blockers have significant effects on the arterial pulse by reducing late systolic pressure augmentation. These actions can be explained on the basis of wave reflection. Reduction of wave reflection is an important advantage in the logical treatment of hypertension and heart failure.

THE VENOUS PULSE

An accurate assessment of the venous pulse is an integral part of the physical examination because it provides information concerning both the mean right atrial pressure and the hemodynamic events in the right atrium. Factors influencing the right atrial and central venous pressure (CVP) include the total blood volume, the distribution of blood volume, and the strength of right atrial contraction.

Venous blood returning from the systemic capillaries is nonpulsatile. Changes in volume flow created by skeletal muscles and the respiratory pump are nonsynchronous with the pulsatile activity of the heart. Changes in flow and pressure caused by right

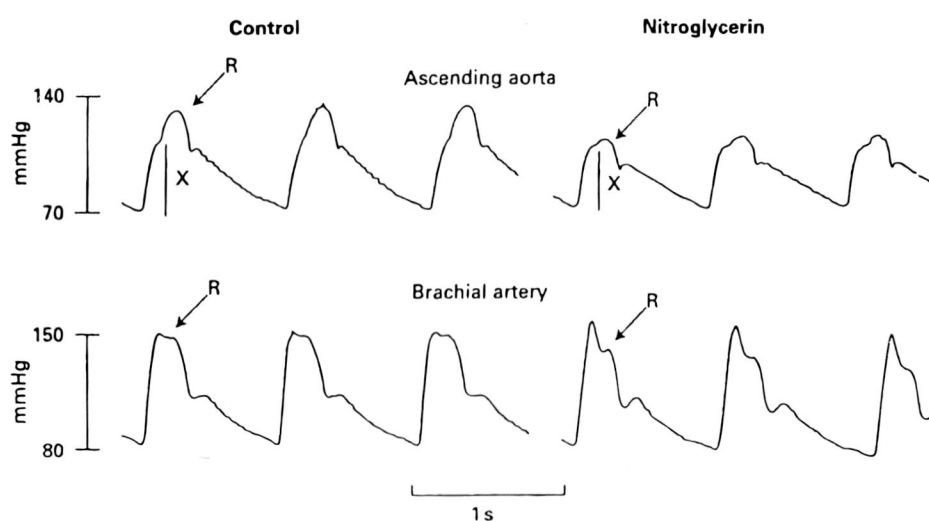

FIGURE 12–44. Pressure waves recorded directly in the ascending aorta (*top*) and brachial artery (*bottom*) under control conditions (*left*) and after 0.3 mg sublingual nitroglycerin (*right*) in a human adult. X, height the pressure would have without reflection (R). *Source: Kelly RP, Gibbs HH, O'Rourke MF, et al. Nitroglycerin has a favorable effect on left ventricular afterload than apparent from measurement of pressure in a peripheral artery. Eur Heart J. 1990;11:138–144, with permission.*

atrial and ventricular filling, however, produce pulsations in the central veins that are transmitted toward the peripheral veins, opposite to the direction of blood flow. With the possible exception of the *c* wave, which is the combined result of carotid arterial impact and an upward movement of the tricuspid valve, the pulsations observed in the neck are produced by right atrial and ventricular activity.[78]

EXAMINATION OF THE JUGULAR VENOUS PULSE

The two main objectives of the bedside examination of the neck veins are estimation of the CVP and inspection of the waveform.[78] Usually, the right internal jugular vein (IJV) is superior for both purposes. In most normal subjects, the maximum pulsation of the IJV is observed when the trunk is inclined by less than 30 degrees. In patients with an elevated CVP, it can be necessary to elevate the trunk further, sometimes to as much as 90 degrees. When the neck muscles are relaxed, shining a beam of light tangentially across the skin overlying the IJV often exposes its pulsations. Simultaneous palpation of the left carotid artery aids the examiner in deciding which pulsations are venous.

MEASUREMENTS OF VENOUS PRESSURE

The difference between venous distension and venous pressure elevation must be considered. Veins can be markedly dilated with minimal increase in pressure or may not be visibly distended despite a very high venous pressure.[77,78] Venous pressure can be estimated by examining the veins on the dorsum of the hand. With the patient sitting or lying at 30 degrees of elevation or greater, the arm is slowly and passively raised from a dependent position. When the CVP is normal, the veins collapse when the dorsum of the hand reaches the level of the sternal angle of Louis. Unfortunately, local venous obstruction or augmented peripheral venous constriction can diminish the accuracy of estimating CVP by this method.

The external or internal jugular veins can also be used to estimate venous pressure.[79] Because of its more direct route to the right atrium, the IJV is superior for the estimation of venous pressure and assessment of the venous waveform. The patient is examined at the optimal degree of trunk elevation for visualization of venous pulsations. The vertical distance from the top of the oscillating venous column to the level of the sternal angle is generally less than 3 centimeters. Greatly elevated venous pressure can be missed by failing to elevate the patient's head adequately. It can be necessary to actually have the patient sit upright. If the *pulsating meniscus* is very high, pulsations may not be apparent in the lower neck. When venous engorgement is marked, the patient's earlobe can pulsate, and even the veins on the top of the head can be distended.

In patients suspected of RV failure but with a normal resting venous pressure, the abdominojugular test is useful.[80] With the patient breathing normally, firm pressure is applied with the palm of the hand to the upper right quadrant of the abdomen for 10 seconds or more. The patient should be instructed to continue to breathe normally during the test. In most subjects, the jugular venous pressure is not altered significantly. In some normal patients there is a transient increase in jugular venous pressure with a rapid return to or near baseline in less than 10 seconds. The dysfunctioning RV, however, is unable to accept the increment in blood volume because of enhanced venous return without a marked increase in its filling pressure, which is transmitted to the neck veins. In patients with RV failure, often caused by left-sided heart failure, the venous pressure either rises rapidly and then partially declines slowly during continued abdominal compression or remains elevated by 4 centimeters of blood or more until the abdominal pressure is released (Fig. 12–45). Ducas and colleagues[81] also studied the abdominojugular test and confirmed its clinical value.

ANALYSIS OF VENOUS WAVEFORMS

Again, the patient's trunk should be inclined to whatever elevation is necessary to reveal the top of the oscillating venous column. Slow, deep inspiration will increase the amplitude of the presystolic *a* wave while decreasing the mean right atrial pressure. This is a useful technique for identifying the site at which the pulsations will be best visualized. Simultaneous palpation of the left carotid artery and cardiac auscultation aid the examiner in relating the venous pulsations to the timing of the cardiac cycle.

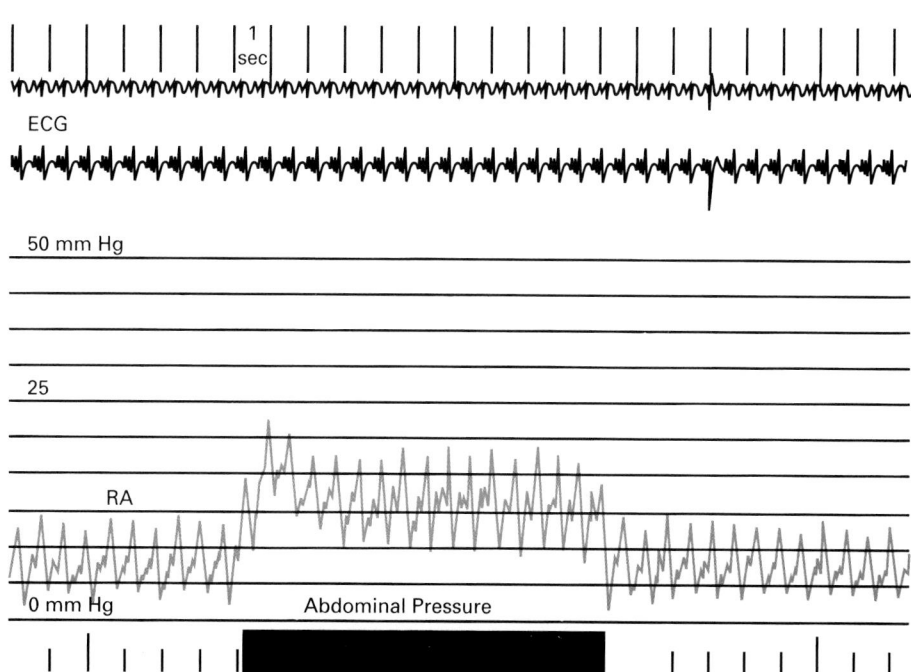

FIGURE 12–45. Elevation in right atrial pressure observed during abdominal pressure in patient with mild congestive heart failure. ECG, electrocardiogram; RA, right atrial. *Source: Ewy GA. The abdominojugular test: technique and hemodynamic correlates. Ann Intern Med. 1989;109:456. Used with permission from the publisher and author.*

[ ] NORMAL VENOUS PULSE

The normal *jugular venous pulse* (JVP) reflects phasic pressure changes in the right atrium and consists of three positive waves and two negatives troughs (Fig. 12–46). It is useful to refer to the events of the cardiac cycle (see Chap. 3). The positive presystolic *a* wave is produced by right atrial (RA) contraction and is the dominant wave in the JVP, particularly during inspiration. During atrial relaxation, the venous pulse descends from the summit of the *a* wave. Depending on the PR interval, this descent can continue until a plateau (*z* point) is reached just prior to RV systole. More often, the descent is interrupted by a second positive venous wave, the *c* wave, that is produced by bulging of the tricuspid valve into the right atrium during RV isovolumic systole and by the impact of the carotid artery adjacent to the jugular vein. Following the summit of the *c* wave, the JVP contour declines, forming the normal negative systolic wave, the *x* wave. The *x* descent is caused by a combination of atrial relaxation, the downward displacement of the tricuspid valve during RV systole, and the ejection of blood from both ventricles (see Chap. 4).

The positive, later systolic *v* wave in the JVP results from the increase in blood volume in the venae cavae and right atrium during ventricular systole when the tricuspid valve is closed. After the peak of the *v* wave is reached, the RA pressure decreases because of the diminished bulging of the tricuspid valve into the right atrium and the decline in RV pressure that follows tricuspid valve opening. In the JVP, the latter occurs at the peak of the *v* wave. Following the summit of the *v* wave, there is a negative descending limb, referred to as the *y* descent or diastolic collapse, which is caused by the tricuspid valve opening and the rapid inflow of blood into the RV. The initial *y* descent corresponds to the RV rapid-filling phase. The trough of the *y* wave occurs in early diastole and is followed by the ascending limb of the *y* wave, which is produced by the continued diastolic inflow of blood into the right side of the heart. The velocity of this ascending pressure curve depends on the rate of venous return and the distensibility of the chambers of the right side of the heart. When diastole is long, the ascending limb of the *y* wave is often followed by a small, brief, positive wave, the *h* wave, which occurs just prior to the next *a* wave. At times, there is a plateau phase rather than a distinct *h* wave. With increasing heart rate, the *y* trough and *y* ascent are followed immediately by the next *a* wave.

Usually, there are three visible major positive waves (*a*, *c*, and *v*) and two negative waves (*x* and *y*) when the pulse rate is below 90 beats per minute, and the PR interval is normal. With faster heart rates, there is often fusion of some of the pulse waves, and an accurate analysis of the waveform is more difficult.

[ ] ABNORMAL VENOUS PULSE

Elevated Venous Pressure

The most common cause of an elevated jugular venous pressure is an increased RV pressure such as occurs in patients with PS, PH, or RV failure secondary to left-sided heart failure or RV infarction. The venous pressure also is elevated when obstruction to RV inflow occurs, as with tricuspid stenosis (TS) or RA myxoma, or when constrictive pericardial disease impedes RV inflow. It also can result from vena cava obstruction and, at times, an increased blood volume. Patients with obstructive pulmonary disease can have an elevated venous pressure only during expiration.

Kussmaul Sign

Normally, during inspiration, there is an increase in the *a* wave of the JVP but a decrease in the mean JVP as a result of the increased filling of the right-sided chambers associated with the decrease in intrathoracic pressure. *Kussmaul sign* denotes an inspiratory increase in the venous pressure, which can occur in patients with severe constrictive pericarditis when the heart is unable to accept the increase in RV volume without a marked increase in the filling pressure. Although Kussmaul sign was first described in patients with constrictive pericarditis, its most common cause is severe right-sided heart failure, regardless of etiology. The presence of Kussmaul sign is also useful in the diagnosis of RV infarction[82] (see Chap. 84).

Abnormalities of the A Wave

The *a* wave in the JVP is absent when there is no effective atrial contraction, such as in atrial fibrillation (Fig. 12–46E). In certain other conditions, the *a* wave may not be apparent. In sinus tachycardia, the *a* wave can fuse with the preceding *v* wave, particularly if the PR interval is prolonged. In some patients with sinus tachycardia, the jugular *a* wave can occur during the *v* or *y* descent and can be small or absent. In the presence of first-degree AV block, a discrete *a* wave with ascending and descending limbs is often completed prior to the first heart sound, and the *ac* interval is prolonged (Fig. 12–46F).

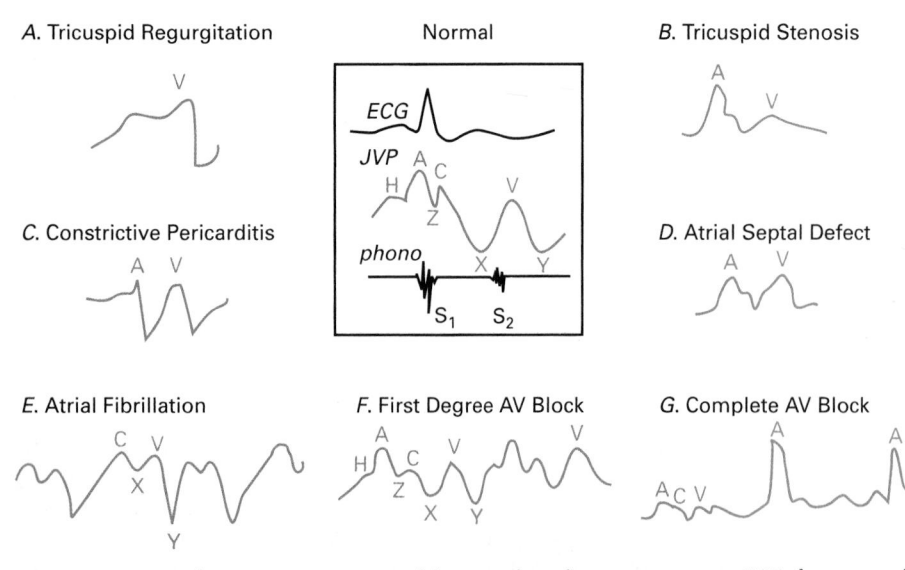

FIGURE 12–46. Schematic representation of the normal jugular venous pressure (JVP), four types of abnormal JVP, and the JVP in three arrhythmias. AV, atrioventricular; ECG, electrocardiogram; S₁, first heart sound; S₂, second heart sound. See chapter section Normal Venous Pulse for definition of H, A, Z, C, X, V, and Y.

Large *a* waves are of considerable diagnostic value (Fig. 12–46B). When giant *a* waves are present with each beat, the right atrium is contracting against an increased resistance. This can result from obstruction at the tricuspid valve (TS or atresia, right atrial myxoma) or conditions associated with increased resistance to RV filling. A giant *a* wave is more likely to occur in patients with PS or PH in whom both the atrial and ventricular septa are intact.

Cannon *a* waves occur when the right atrium contracts while the tricuspid valve is closed during RV systole.[81] Cannon *a* waves can occur either regularly or irregularly and are most common in the presence of arrhythmias (Fig. 12–46G).

Abnormalities of the X Wave

The most important alteration of the normally negative systolic collapse (*x* wave) of the JVP is its obliteration or even replacement by a positive wave, usually caused by tricuspid regurgitation TR. Although atrial relaxation can contribute to the normal *x* descent, the development of atrial fibrillation does not obliterate the *x* wave except in the presence of TR. Accordingly, the occurrence of a positive wave in the JVP during ventricular systole is strong evidence of TR (Fig. 12–46A). Mild TR lessens and shortens the downward *x* wave as the regurgitation of blood into the right atrium produces a positive wave that diminishes the usual systolic fall in venous pressure. In some patients with moderate TR, there is a fairly distinct positive wave during ventricular systole between the *c* and *v* waves. This abnormal systolic waveform is usually referred to as a *v* or *cv* wave, although it has also been referred to as an *r* (regurgitant) or an *s* (systolic) wave. In patients with constrictive pericarditis, the *x* descent wave during systole is often more prominent than the early diastolic *y* wave (Fig. 12–46C and see Chap. 84).

Abnormalities of the V Wave

The positive, late systolic *v* wave results from the increasing RA blood volume during ventricular systole when the tricuspid valve normally is closed. With mild TR, the *v* wave and the obliteration of the *x* descent result in a single, large positive systolic wave (ventricularization) (Figs. 12–46A and 12–47).

Normally in the JVP the *v* wave is lower in amplitude than the *a* wave. In patients with an ASD, however, the *a* and *v* waves are often equal in the right atrium and the JVP (Fig. 12–46D). In patients with constrictive pericarditis and sinus rhythm, the RA *a* and *v* waves also can be equal, but the venous pressure is increased, which is unusual with isolated ASD. In patients with constrictive pericarditis who are in atrial fibrillation, the *cv* wave is prominent and the *y* descent rapid.

Abnormalities of the Y Trough

The *y* descent, or diastolic collapse, is produced mainly by tricuspid valve opening and the rapid inflow of blood into the RV. A rapid, deep *y* descent in early diastole occurs with severe TR (Fig. 12–46A). A venous pulse characterized by a sharp *y* descent, a deep *y* trough, and a rapid ascent to the baseline is seen in patients with constrictive pericarditis or with severe right-sided heart failure. A slow *y* descent in the JVP suggests an obstruction to RV filling and can be the *only* abnormal finding in patients with TS or right atrial myxoma (Fig. 12–46B). In both constrictive pericarditis and severe right-sided

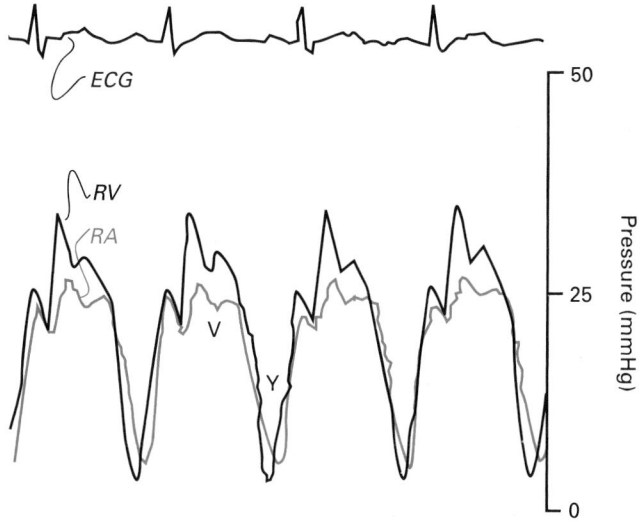

FIGURE 12–47. Right ventricular (RV) and right atrial (RA) pressure curves and simultaneous ECG from a patient with severe tricuspid regurgitation. Note ventricularization of the RA pressure curve.

heart failure, the venous pressure is elevated with a sharp *y* dip in the JVP (see Chap. 84). The presence of a large positive systolic venous wave favors the diagnosis of severe heart failure.

〖 〗 EFFECTS OF ARRHYTHMIAS ON THE VENOUS PULSE

Large *a* waves in the JVP during arrhythmias are present when the *P* wave (atrial contraction) occurs between the onset of the QRS complex and the termination of the T wave (Fig. 12–46G). Such cannon *a* waves can occur regularly in junctional rhythm. More commonly, they occur irregularly when AV dissociation accompanies premature ventricular beats, ventricular tachycardia, or complete heart block. The *a* wave is absent in patients with atrial fibrillation, and flutter *a* waves at a regular rate of 250 to 300 per minute occasionally are observed in patients with atrial flutter and varying degrees of AV block. Patients with multifocal atrial tachycardia often have prominent and somewhat variable *a* waves in the JVP. In these patients, many of whom have PH secondary to lung disease, the *a* waves are often very large.

EXAMINATION OF THE RETINA

Inspection of the smaller vessels of the body is possible in only three areas: the retina, conjunctiva, and nail beds. The ophthalmoscope[83] has made the retina by far the easiest and most rewarding site.[83] Viewing this two-dimensional vascular display is generally much easier if the pupils are dilated. Pulse and BP determinations should precede instillation of rapidly acting mydriatics, because both can increase after absorption of the drops. Best pupillary dilatation is maintained if the optic disk is observed first. Assess for evidence of edema and blurred margins and for cupping with sharp contours. Rule out neovascularization or the pallor of optic atrophy.

Next, scan along the superior temporal arcade and inspect the arteries carefully for embolic plaques at each bifurcation. Observe the arteriovenous crossing for obscuration of the vein and for pro-

TABLE 12-6

Retinal Topography

FINDING	MOST COMMON LOCATION
Arteriovenous crossings	Upper temporal quadrant
Cotton-wool spots	Around optic disk
Hard exudates	Between disk and fovea
Microaneurysms	Temporal to fovea
Emboli	Arterial bifurcations
Diabetic new vessels	Nerve head and arcades

nounced nicking and banking of the vessels. Avoid the macular area until last because the pupil constricts most intensely when this area is illuminated. To discover diabetic microaneurysms early, look just temporal to the fovea. To find cotton-wool infarcts, look circularly around the disk, two disk diameters out (Table 12–6).

Variations in the caliber of a single vessel are more important than determinations of arteriovenous ratios. Changes can take the form of focal narrowing, sometimes called *beading* or *spasm*.

【 】 THICKENING OF THE VASCULAR WALL

Normally, only the blood column is visible when the retinal vessels are viewed. When changes in the walls do occur, they are most visible along the sides of the vessels because the location of the tangential line of sight presents a greater thickness to the viewer. Fatty exudate (hard exudate) can collect along venous walls (never arteries), particularly in diabetic exudative retinopathy.

【 】 ARTERIOSCLEROSIS

In arteriosclerosis, medial smooth muscle (which can hypertrophy in chronic hypertension) becomes hyalinized with the deposition of collagen. As the wall thickens, the vessel takes on a burnished coppery luster; with further thickening, this can transmute to silver.

【 】 ARTERIOVENOUS COMPRESSIONS

Arteriovenous compressions or *nicking* results from the sharing by the artery and vein of a common adventitial sheath at their crossings. Arteriosclerotic thickening impedes venous outflow at these locations, with venous tortuosity, engorgement, and darkening of the flood column distal to the compression.[83]

【 】 ATHEROSCLEROSIS

Retinal atheromata have a predilection for the bifurcation and bends within the first two branches of the central retinal artery, appearing as segments of irregular yellowish sheathing and having the crystalline knobbiness of a salted pretzel stick.[83]

【 】 COTTON-WOOL SPOTS

Cotton-wool spots are generally a sign of serious systemic disease. They can be seen in patients with severe hypertension, blood dys-

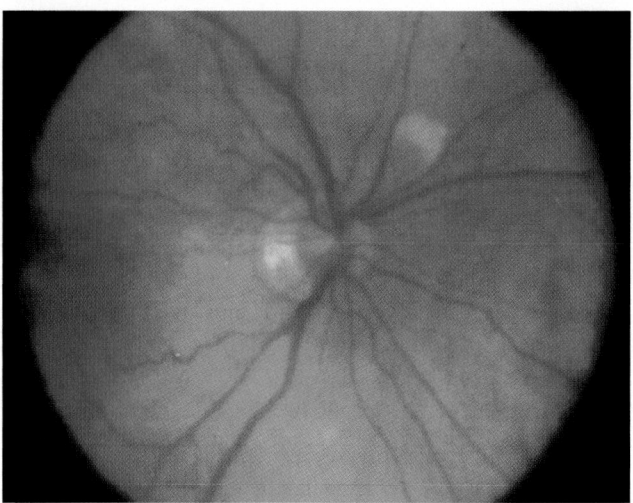

FIGURE 12–48. Retinal cotton-wool spot. Cotton-wool spots are most frequently found close to the optic disk. Although they occur in acute uncontrolled systemic hypertension, the more common cause now, in younger patients, is infection with HIV. This normotensive 37-year-old man had no visual symptoms and no other retinopathy. There is a myopic crescent at the temporal disk edge, which is not abnormal. He died of complications related to AIDS 2 years later.

crasias, collagen diseases, or hemorrhagic shock. Cotton-wool spots also are seen frequently in patients with acquired immunodeficiency syndrome (Fig. 12–48). Cotton-wool *exudates* are not exudates but consist of a cluster of cell-like swollen ends of fragmented axons in an area of edematous retina.[83]

【 】 HARD EXUDATES

Hard exudates are most likely residues of edema. They occur in situations where the vessels become leaky, and as the more watery component of the extravasation is resorbed, the lipid residue forms a hard, yellow, waxy deposit. These deposits can surround the leaking vessel in a circinate ring or can accumulate in the macula, radiating from the fovea in the spokes of a macular *star* (Fig. 12–49).

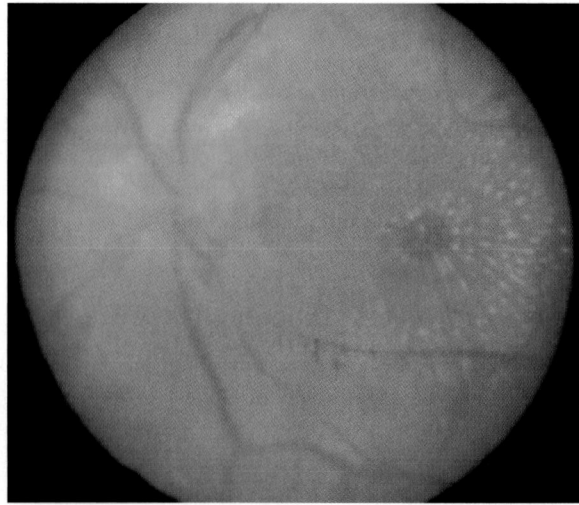

FIGURE 12–49. Disk swelling and hard exudate in a macular "star" pattern. In this hypertensive patient with periarteritis nodosa, vascular leakage has led to the deposition of hard exudates around the fovea. The star pattern of the exudate is caused by radial perifoveal connective tissue. Note also that the optic disk is edematous, with blurred margins, secondary to hypertension.

【 】 MICROANEURYSMS

Microaneurysms occur in many disease states, including retinal venous obstructive disease, sickle cell disease, the dysproteinemias, Behçet disease, sarcoidosis, and other forms of uveitis. They can represent abortive attempts at revascularization of compromised capillary bed in diabetics (Fig. 12–50).

【 】 NEOVASCULARIZATION

In neovascularization the new vessels generally originate from capillaries from the venous side of the circulation and are associated with greater or lesser degrees of fibrosis. In all cases, however, the new vessels are incorporated in an associated fibrous membrane (Fig. 12–51).

【 】 RETINAL HEMORRHAGE

Hemorrhage into the retina indicates further breakdown in the integrity of the vascular wall. When the hemorrhage occurs in the inner retina, as in hypertension, it assumes a feathery flame shape as it is molded and dispersed by the nerve fibers coursing toward the disk (Fig. 12–52). In obstruction of the central retinal vein, the fundus may be splattered with blood.

【 】 VASCULAR OCCLUSION

When the central artery or one of its branches is occluded, the nonperfused retinal area becomes cloudy in a matter of minutes. Occlusions of branches of the central vein produce edema and hemorrhage in the drained area. As collateral drainage, the edema and hemorrhagic retinopathy subside, leaving white-walled veins, neovascularization, and microaneurysms in the affected area.

OPTIC DISK EDEMA

The term *papilledema* is reserved for the form of disk edema that is the result of increased intracranial pressure. It therefore has an eti-

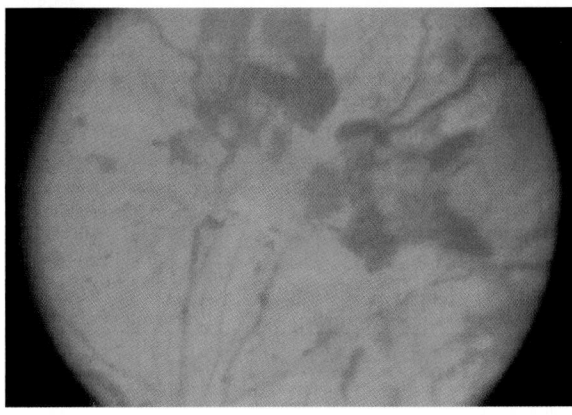

FIGURE 12-51. Proliferative diabetic retinopathy with preretinal hemorrhage. When neovascularization develops, preretinal and vitreous hemorrhages are much more likely to occur. Easily visible neovascularization either in the periphery of the retina, as in this diabetic patient, or at the disk is an indication for immediate panretinal laser photocoagulation.

ologic connotation. *Papillitis* is the term applied to inflammatory disk edema.

【 】 EMBOLISM

The characteristics of retinal emboli of cardiovascular significance are listed in Table 12–7. Of these, platelet emboli are at once the most common and the most evanescent. Hollenhorst cholesterol plaques can be identified at the same bifurcations for months to years after the embolic shower. Platelet emboli, Hollenhorst plaques (Fig. 12–52), and calcium emboli are usually seen along

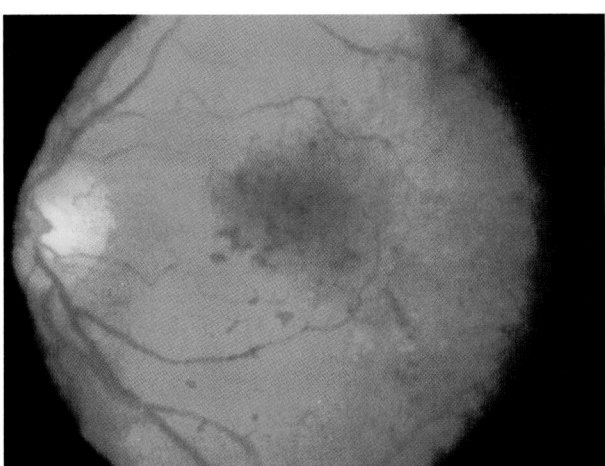

FIGURE 12-50. Background diabetic retinopathy. Retinal microaneurysms, dot-and-blot hemorrhages, and a few fine upper temporal hard exudates are diagnostic of early diabetic retinopathy. The patient had no visual symptoms, but retinopathy of this magnitude can often be seen in patients with insulin-requiring diabetes of 15 or more years' duration.

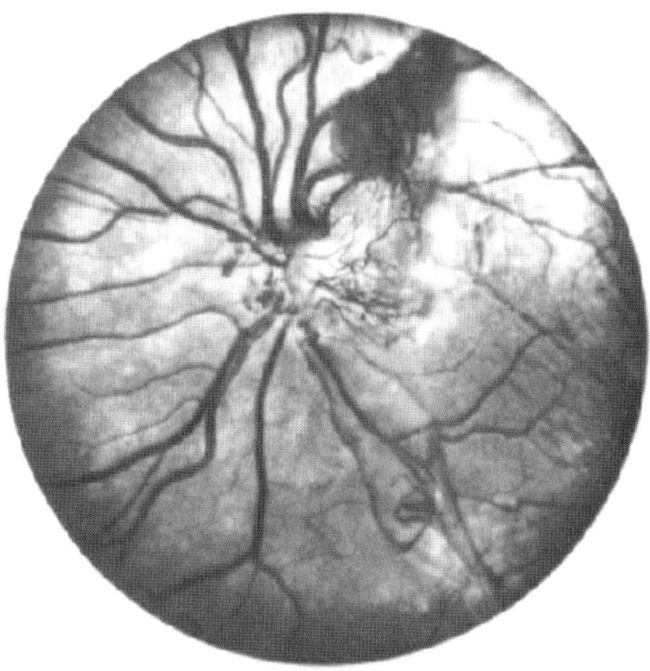

FIGURE 12-52. Proliferative diabetic retinopathy, left eye. There is extensive neovascularization of the disk with an associated small intravitreal hemorrhage that obscures the upper temporal vessels. Along the inferior temporal arcade is another area of neovascularization. These new vessels are incorporated into fibrous membranes, which can tent up the vessels and cause traction detachments of the retina, as at the lower right edge of the photograph.

TABLE 12–7

Emboli of Cardiovascular Significance

TYPE	APPEARANCE	SIGNIFICANCE
Platelet	Dull pink to gray often with associated fibrin	Downstream vegetations, mural thrombi
Hollenhorst plaque	Glistening yellow-orange plaques at bifurcations	Downstream atheroma (containing cholesterol)
Calcium plaque	Glistening white plaques	Calcific aortic stenosis
Roth spot	Hemorrhage with gray-white center	Blood dyscrasia or septic embolus as in subacute bacterial endocarditis
Fat embolus	Fuzzy-bordered gray-white spot without hemorrhage	Severe trauma with long-bone fractures
Myxoma	Disk edema, retinal edema in arterial supply zone	Life-threatening atrial myxoma

the course of a retinal artery. Roth spots (Fig. 12–53) and fat emboli may not appear to be intravascular and may not be associated with a vessel that is ophthalmoscopically visible (see Table 12–7).

【 】 DIABETES MELLITUS

In diabetes mellitus, focal loss of a portion of the capillary bed is followed by microaneurysm formation and vascular dilatation around the borders of the area of capillary dropout (Fig. 12–54).

Vasoconstriction of the arterial tree and thickening of the arterial vessel walls with consequent reduction in lumen diameter are homeostatic responses to hypertension. Arteriosclerotic narrowing of the vessels acts to insulate the capillary bed from the elevated pressure of the arterial supply. These arteriosclerotic changes are visible as narrowing, increases in central light reflexes, and copper and silver *wiring* of the arteries (Fig. 12–55).

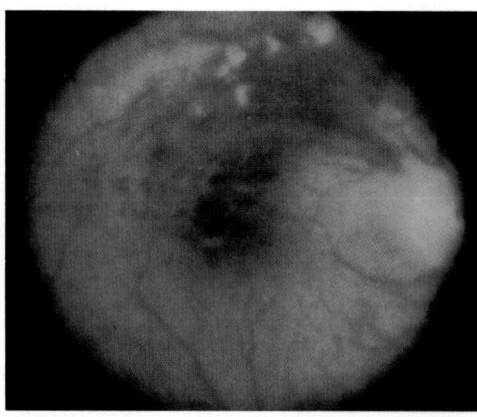

FIGURE 12–53. Branch retinal vein obstruction. Thickening of the retinal arterial wall in diabetes and hypertension can compromise the lumen of the vein, where artery and vein share a common adventitial sheath at an arteriovenous crossing. The resulting obstruction produces hemorrhage retinopathy in the drainage area of the affected vein. Note how the flame-shaped pattern of blood outlines the arcuate pattern of the nerve fibers as they run toward the optic disk.

Hypertensive patients should be classified as to whether or not their retinal circulation is compensated or has decompensated with observable edema, cotton-wool spots, flame hemorrhages, or swelling of the optic disk (Fig. 12–56).[83]

PHYSICAL EXAMINATION OF THE CHEST, ABDOMEN, AND EXTREMITIES

Physical examination of the lungs is an important noninvasive technique requiring only a stethoscope. Wheezing and a pleural friction rub are detected only by the clinical evaluation. The pleural friction rub can be a clue to the diagnosis of pulmonary infarction. Pleural fluid caused by heart failure is usually located in the right pleural space. When pleural fluid is localized predominantly to the left, a cause other than or in addition to heart failure, such as pulmonary infarction, should be considered.

A pneumothorax can develop as a consequence of spontaneous mediastinal emphysema or can be iatrogenic, as a result of procedures.[84] Hyperresonance and diminished breath sounds can be caused by pulmonary emphysema. Signs of pulmonary consolidation can be caused by pneumonia or pulmonary infarction. Wheezing and rales can be caused by bronchial disease. Heart failure can be associated with rales in the lung bases, wheezing, and pleural fluid. Importantly, heart failure frequently is not associated with rales because interstitial pulmonary edema usually does not produce rales.

The diameter of the *abdominal* aorta should be determined in every patient[84] (see Chap. 105). An abdominal aortic aneurysm can be missed if the examiner fails to assess the area above the umbilicus.

Specific abnormalities of the abdomen can be secondary to heart disease. A large, tender liver is common in patients with heart failure or constrictive pericarditis. Systolic hepatic pulsations are frequent in patients with TR. A palpable spleen is a common but late sign in patients with severe heart failure and is also often present in patients with infective endocarditis.

Although hepatic cirrhosis is the most common cause of ascites, the latter can occur with heart failure alone, although it is less common with the use of diuretic therapy. Severe TR, as caused by infective endocarditis in drug addicts, can produce prominent systolic pulsation of the internal jugular veins in the neck; a large, moving, and pulsating liver; and ascites. Constrictive pericarditis should be considered when the ascites is out of proportion to peripheral edema. In many such patients, the heart is normal in size or only slightly enlarged, a pericardial *knock* is heard, and there is a rapid *x* and/or *y* descent in the internal jugular vein pulsation. Restrictive cardiomyopathy can mimic constrictive pericarditis, but the heart is usually moderately large in patients with restrictive cardiomyopathy. When there is an arteriovenous fistula in the abdomen, a continuous murmur can be heard over the abdomen. Fistulas caused by trauma and surgery can occur.

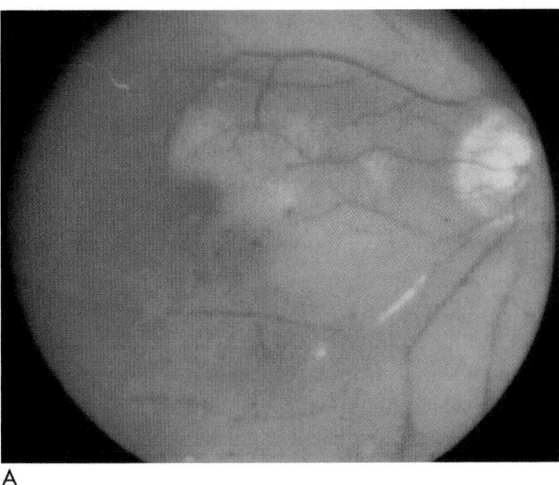

A

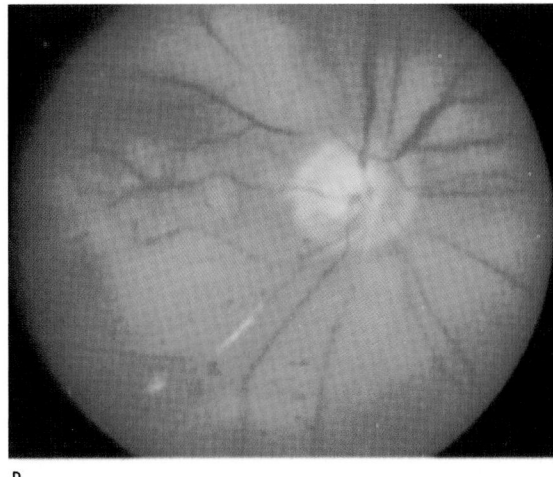

B

FIGURE 12-54. Embolic retinal arterial obstruction (**A**, **B**). Cholesterol crystals can dislodge from the walls of the heart, aortic arch, or carotids. Carried into the retinal circulation as Hollenhorst plaques, they seldom obstruct the arterioles completely. Although amaurosis fugax is more common, the embolic burden can occasionally be so large as to produce retinal infarction. Note in the photograph of the macular area (**A**) that this patient's fovea remains red, although there is a pale, cloudy swelling nasal to it. This has produced a half "cherry-red" spot. With complete central retinal artery occlusion, the red foveal area is completely surrounded by pale swollen retina. Hollenhorst cholesterol plaques can be seen in both the upper and lower temporal retinal arteries. In **A**, the inferior temporal arteriole demonstrates "boxcar" segmentation of the blood column, indicative of very slow flow.

A systolic bruit can be heard over the kidney areas and can signify renal artery stenosis, particularly in patients with systemic hypertension. A systolic bruit often is auscultated over the abdominal aorta, but its presence does not indicate the severity of disease of the aorta.

Examination of the upper and lower extremities can provide important diagnostic information (see Chap. 108). Atherosclerosis of the peripheral arteries can produce intermittent claudication of the buttock, calf, thigh, or foot, with severe disease resulting in tissue damage of the toes. Peripheral atherosclerosis is an important risk factor for ischemic heart disease, and its presence increases the likelihood of coronary atherosclerosis. Thrombophlebitis often causes pain in the calf or thigh or edema, and its presence should raise the consideration of pulmonary emboli as well. Edema is a late sign of heart failure, and its predictive value as a diagnostic sign is poor. It frequently involves the right leg prior to the left. Considerable heart failure and a resulting weight gain can be present without edema being present. Edema of the lower extremities can be secondary to local factors such as varicose veins or thrombophlebitis or the removal of veins at CABG surgery. Under such circumstances, the edema often occurs in only one leg.

Edema can result from restrictive garments, and venous stasis often is secondary to a long trip in a car or airplane. Edema can be caused by salt and water retention in patients with primary renal disease. In the differential diagnosis of edema, local factors should be considered first. If local factors can be excluded, an assessment for evidence of primary renal disease is indicated. Rarely, peripheral edema can be an early sign of lymphatic obstruction produced by metastatic disease in the pelvis or abdomen.

Since the invention of the stethoscope by Laennec in 1826, cardiac auscultation has played a key role in the evaluation of patients with cardiovascular disease and is unlikely to be replaced by small handheld echocardiographic detectors. The analysis of heart

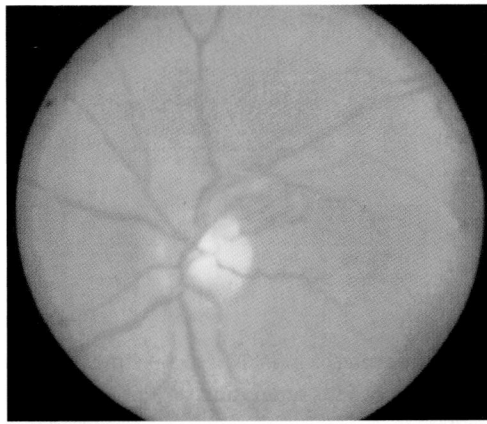

FIGURE 12-55. Neovascularization after branch retinal vein obstruction. New vessels can develop late after obstruction of a branch of the central retinal vein. These most often serve to shunt flow around the obstructed vessel site and are thus not as exuberantly proliferative as those seen in diabetic retinopathy.

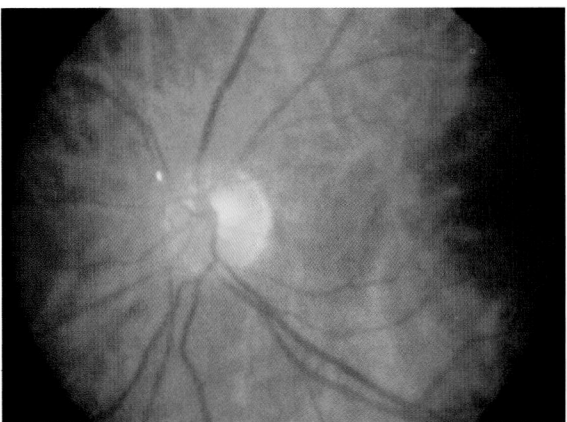

FIGURE 12-56. Calcific retinal embolus associated with aortic valvular disease. Calcific aortic valvular disease and valve replacement surgery can give rise to retinal emboli. Like cholesterol emboli, these calcific flecks lodge at arterial bifurcations but seldom obstruct flow completely. They are white and glitter in the ophthalmoscope beam. Somewhat similar emboli can be seen after the intravenous injection of illicit drugs expanded with talc.

sounds and murmurs by phonocardiography, together with information obtained by cardiac catheterization, angiography, echocardiography, and cardiac surgery, has made cardiac auscultation a *precise discipline* based on firm physiologic principles.[84]

INSPECTION AND PALPATION OF THE PRECORDIUM

Inspection and palpation of the cardiac pulsations of the anterior chest have been practiced by physicians since ancient times and have a solid scientific basis. The results of precordial inspection and palpation have been correlated with noninvasive studies, hemodynamic data, and surgical and autopsy studies[62,85] and remain an important part of the cardiovascular examination.

▌ ▌ PRECORDIAL PULSATIONS CAUSED BY THE HEARTBEAT

Precordial pulsations, reflecting underlying movement of the heart and great vessels, occur principally in the following seven areas of the anterior chest[62,85] (Fig. 12–57):

1. The sternoclavicular area
2. The aortic area
3. The pulmonic area
4. The RV (left parasternal) area
5. The LV (apical) area
6. The epigastric area
7. Ectopic (variable-location) areas

   Although the cardiac apex is usually produced by the left ventricle, it is sometimes produced by an enlarged right ventricle that displaces the left ventricle laterally and posteriorly. Occasionally, the cardiac position is abnormal as a result of dextroposition, dex-

troversion, dextrocardia, or other changes in intrathoracic structures. Although the cardiac apex impulse is commonly referred to as the *point of maximal impulse* (PMI), the two terms are not necessarily synonymous, because the maximal precordial pulsation can be produced by an enlarged or hypertrophied right ventricle, a dilated aorta or pulmonary artery, or an LV wall-motion abnormality. Therefore, precordial pulsations should be described by their location, timing, contour, and duration.

▌ ▌ INSPECTION OF THE PRECORDIUM

The examiner should first inspect the thorax from the foot of the bed with the subject supine, the legs horizontal, and the head and trunk elevated to approximately 30 degrees. The patient may have a barrel-shaped chest with an increased anteroposterior diameter, a straight-back syndrome, pectus excavatum, pectus carinatum, kyphoscoliosis, or ankylosing spondylitis. Each can produce or be associated with cardiac abnormalities. Asymmetry of the thorax caused by convex bulging of the precordium suggests the presence of heart disease since childhood. Exaggerated movements of the cardiac apex often can be detected from this observation point.

   Next, the examiner should move to the patient's right side and observe the patient's chest tangentially rather than from above. A light beam directed across the precordium can enhance subtle findings. Precordial movements frequently can be recognized more easily if the tip of an applicator stick, tongue blade, or light pencil is held against the impulse as a fulcrum. Motion of the underlying chest wall is transmitted to the free end of the instrument and exaggerated, making the movements more obvious.

   In patients with an abnormally prominent apical impulse and in some thin, normal individuals, the apex beat can be seen. The presystolic apical motion associated with the atrial contribution to ventricular filling (a fourth heart sound) sometimes can be visualized, as can the diastolic waveform caused by rapid ventricular filling (a third heart sound). A late systolic bulge either at the apex or in an ectopic area, usually located either medial and superior or lateral to the apical impulse, can be observed in patients with a large dyskinetic ventricular aneurysm. When precordial pulsations are exaggerated, they become visible as well as palpable. In general, outward movements are best discerned by palpation, whereas inward movements usually are seen more easily than felt.[62,85]

▌ ▌ PALPATION OF THE PRECORDIUM

With Tietze syndrome, pain, sometimes with swelling and tenderness, can affect the costochondral, chondrosternal, or xiphosternal joints and can be reproduced by touching. Palpation also can reveal tender superficial veins on the anterior chest (Mondor disease), a rare etiology of chest discomfort. Collateral vessels in the posterior intercostal spaces can be palpable in patients with aortic coarctation.

   Palpation of the precordium is also best performed from the right side, with the patient supine and the upper trunk elevated 30 degrees. Palpation with the right hand usually provides more information. Patients with suspected cardiovascular disease also should be examined in the left lateral decubitus position, rotated 45 to 90 degrees. In this position, the normal LV impulse can be displaced several centimeters leftward and can appear more promi-

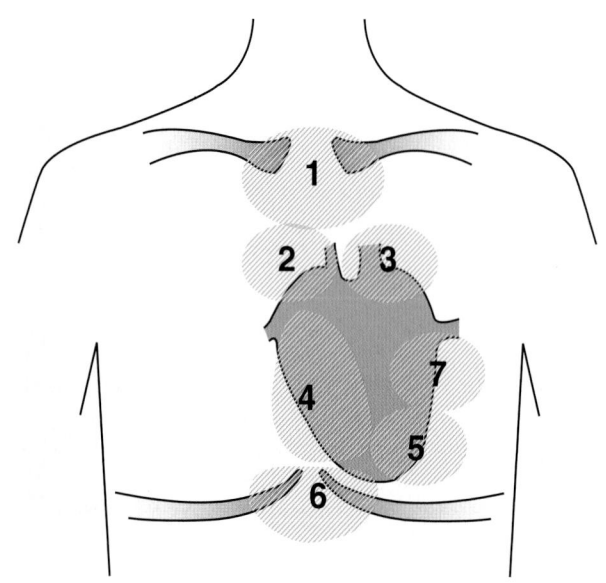

FIGURE 12–57. Seven areas to be examined for abnormal cardiovascular pulsations by inspection and palpation. 1, sternoclavicular; 2, aortic; 3, pulmonic; 4, left parasternal; 5, apical; 6, epigastric; 7, ectopic (abnormal impulse, which may be in variable locations).

nent and sustained. The size of the apex impulse rather than its distance from the midsternal or midclavicular line determines its normality. Often, the apex impulse and other palpable events such as an LV rapid filling wave (third heart sound [S_3]) or presystolic *a* wave (fourth heart sound [S_4]) can be felt only in this position.

The location and size of the cardiac apex impulse should be defined, its contour characterized, and any abnormal precordial pulsations identified. The palm of the hand, ventral surface of the proximal metacarpals, and fingers should all be used for optimal appreciation of specific movements. The fingers appear to be particularly insensitive to movements of relatively large amplitude and very low frequency. Thus, an examiner's hand occasionally can be seen to move up and down with precordial motion, although the same movements are imperceptible by palpation alone. By contrast, higher-frequency events, such as the vibrations associated with abnormally loud aortic or pulmonic components of the second heart sound, are easily palpable, but the amplitude of their movement is not readily visible.

The pads of the fingers are most useful for detecting LV and normal RV motion, whereas the palm and proximal metacarpals are usually best used for palpating larger, low-frequency movements such as the parasternal systolic lift of RV hypertrophy. High-frequency movements such as ejection sounds, valve closure sounds, and mitral opening snaps are detected more easily with the hand held firmly against the chest, whereas low-frequency movements such as ventricular diastolic filling events are best recognized with light pressure with the fingertips.

Thrills are palpable vibrations from murmurs or bruits ordinarily associated with grade 4/6 murmurs or louder. The location of a thrill often helps identify its origin. Thrills are palpated most easily using either the palm of the hand or the proximal metacarpals. Sometimes thrills are felt better during a held end-expiration with moderate pressure applied from the right hand on top of the left hand.

To detect abnormal RV motion, the heel of the hand should be placed over the lower half of the sternum with the patient's breath held at end-expiration. The parasternal lift caused by RV hypertrophy is often better visualized than actually felt. In patients with chronic obstructive pulmonary disease, subxiphoid and epigastric palpation with the patient's breath held at end-inspiration is useful for assessing RV motion.

Proper patient positioning is important. The location of the apex impulse is usually described in terms of its distance from the midsternal or midclavicular line and the intercostal space in which it is located. The apex impulse is often faint or not palpable with the patient supine because of the distance of the ventricular apex from the chest wall. Palpation of the cardiac apex with the patient in the left lateral position, however, permits optimal assessment of the size (diameter) and contour of the systolic outward movement at the apex; diastolic movements are also best appreciated with the patient in this position. Because the apex impulse can shift several centimeters laterally when the patient rotates to the left lateral position, however, the location of the apex impulse can be incorrect in this position. Palpation with simultaneous cardiac auscultation often is useful for identifying the systolic or diastolic timing of precordial pulsations. Simultaneous palpation of the apical impulse and carotid pulse can be helpful in assessing the severity of AS. An appreciable lag time between the onset of the apex impulse and carotid pulse usually indicates severe AS.

[ ] PHYSIOLOGY OF PRECORDIAL MOTION

Although only the apical impulse is palpable normally, a brief RV systolic motion can be felt at the left sternal edge in asthenic individuals. With the onset of isovolumic LV contraction, there is anterior movement of the left ventricle toward the chest walls (see Fig. 12–57). Counterclockwise rotation of the left ventricle along its longitudinal axis occurs as the cardiac apex moves anteriorly and makes contact with the chest wall in early systole.[86] The maximal outward movement occurs coincident with or just after aortic valve opening. After rapid early ejection, the left ventricle moves away from the chest wall, and the apex retracts during later systole and returns to baseline well before the second heart sound.[87] The outward apex movement in early systole normally is palpable, but the later systolic inward movement is only visible (see Fig. 12–57). Palpable movements of the apex in diastole result from LV filling. The early diastolic outward movement caused by rapid ventricular filling (F wave), which corresponds to the normal S_3, is occasionally palpable in normal children and young adults (see Fig. 12–57). Later diastolic filling caused by left atrial contraction (*a* wave) is not normally palpable. Precordial motion is modified by age, chest wall thickness, lung disease, and pleural or pericardial effusion.

Area 1: Sternoclavicular Area Pulsations

The sternoclavicular area (Fig. 12–58) includes the right and left sternoclavicular joints, the manubrium, and the upper sternum. Usually, no pulsation is noted in this area. A slight, brief systolic pulsation of a sternoclavicular joint or the manubrium can be caused by AR. Abnormal pulsations and movements in the sternoclavicular area are commonly produced by enlargement, dilatation, or diseases of the aorta, particularly aortic dissection, atherosclerotic aneurysm, or syphilitic aneurysm. An abnormal pulsation of a sternoclavicular joint in patients with chest pain can be an early clue to diagnosis of aortic dissection. A slight pulsation in the right sternoclavicular area can suggest a right-sided aortic arch in patients with cyanotic heart disease, particularly tetralogy of Fallot.[84] A kinked, tortuous right carotid artery or dilatation and tortuosity of other brachiocephalic vessels can produce visible and palpable pulsations in the suprasternal notch or the supraclavicular areas.

Area 2: Aortic Area Pulsations

Vibrations of the aortic component (aortic second sound [A_2]) of the second heart sound can be palpated when they are accentuated, as in arterial hypertension. With valvular AS, a systolic thrill is present frequently in the second and less commonly in the first and third right intercostal spaces near the sternum (see Fig. 12–58). It often radiates upward toward the right side of the neck and to the suprasternal notch and right supraclavicular area. Less frequently, the thrill is palpable at the second or third left interspaces next to the sternum or at the apex. A systolic thrill in the aortic area and in the right carotid artery also can occur in patients with severe AR without stenosis. Abnormal systolic pulsations in the aortic area can be caused by dilatation of the ascending aorta as a result of aneurysm and/or chronic AR.

Area 3: Pulmonic Area Pulsations

Vibrations associated with a loud pulmonic component of the second heart sound (S_2) (see Fig. 12–58) often are palpable in pa-

Graphic Representation
(palpable features in heavy line)

Type of movement and associated clinical condition	Graphic Representation	Location and accompanying features
NORMAL ADULT APEX IMPULSE	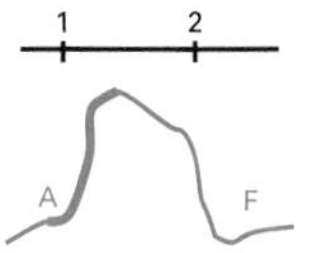	Cardiac apex; moderate systolic thrust; A and F waves usually imperceptible
HYPERKINETIC APEX IMPULSE °°Normal Child °°Hyperdynamic states °°Ventricular septal defect °°Patent ductus arteriosus °°Mitral regurgitation °°Aortic regurgitation	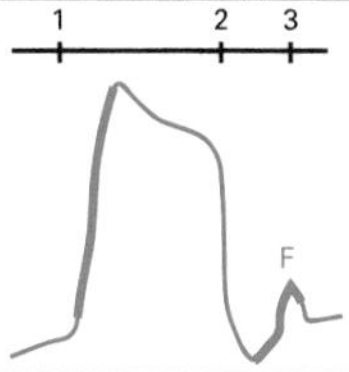	Exaggerated thrust at cardiac apex; F wave may be palpable, coincident with third heart sound
HYPERKINETIC RIGHT VENTRICULAR IMPULSE °°Atrial septal defect °°Pulmonary regurgitation	Same as above	Maximal at left sternal edge in third and fourth intercostal spaces
SUSTAINED APEX IMPULSE °°Left ventricular hypertrophy, °°°°as in: °°Aortic stenosis °°Hypertension °°Insert: a variation that °°°°may occur in hypertrophic °°°°cardiomyopathy	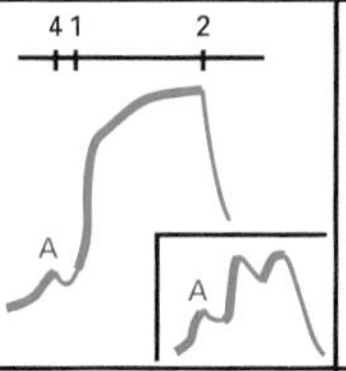	Maximal at cardiac apex; A wave may be visible and palpable coincident with fourth heart sound
SUSTAINED RIGHT VENTRICULAR IMPULSE °°Right ventricular °°°°hypertrophy, as in: °°Pulmonary hypertension °°Pulmonary stenosis	Same impulse as in Sustained above	Maximal at left sternal edge in third and fourth intercostal spaces
ECTOPIC LEFT VENTRICULAR IMPULSE °°Ventricular aneurysm	Same impulse as in Sustained above	Maximal over mid-precordium rather than at apex
LEFT ATRIAL EXPANSION °°Severe mitral regurgitation	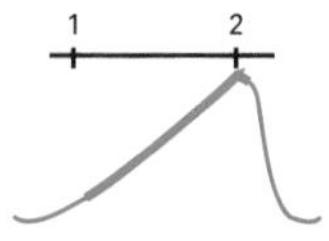	Left sternal edge or entire precordium; hyperkinetic apex impulse due to left ventricular volume overload
PULMONARY ARTERY PULSATION °°Pulmonary hypertension	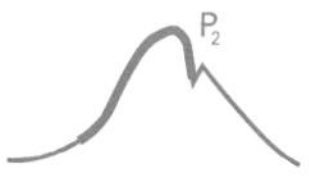	Second left intercostal space; palpable P_2
INWARD MOVEMENT DURING SYSTOLE °°Constrictive pericarditis °°Tricuspid regurgitation; °°°°primary	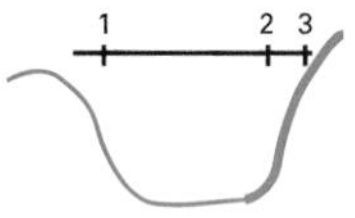	Cardiac apex or entire precordium; reversal of direction during systole as compared with preceding examples
DIASTOLIC MOVEMENTS °°Cardiomyopathy	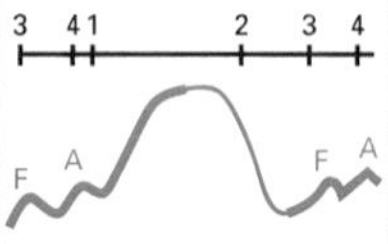	Cardiac apex; systolic movement may be inconspicuous; diastolic movements F and A correspond to 3rd and 4th heart sounds which may merge in tachycardia to form a summation gallop

FIGURE 12–58. Graphic representation of apical movements in health and disease. Heavy line indicates palpable features. A, atrial wave, corresponding to a fourth heart sound (S_4) or atrial gallop; F, filling wave, corresponding to third heart sound (S_3) or ventricular gallop; P_2, pulmonary component of second heart sound. *Source: Willis.[85] Reproduced with permission from the publisher and author.*

tients with PH from any cause. During simultaneous palpation of the carotid pulse, a palpable P_2 or A_2 coincides with the early down-slope of the carotid pulse. A systolic thrill in the second and third left intercostal spaces near the sternum often occurs with pulmonic valve stenosis. The thrill often radiates toward the left side of the neck, in contrast to the thrill with AS, which radiates upward and to the right.

Pulsations of a dilated pulmonary artery can be seen or felt in the second or third left intercostal space near the sternum. In normal infants and children or anxious adults with thin chest walls, a slight, brief, early systolic pulsation can be present in this area. This pulsation is accentuated by conditions that cause an increased cardiac output (e.g., fever, pregnancy). Idiopathic dilatation of the pulmonary artery also can cause a palpable systolic impulse in the same area.[84]

The common causes of an accentuated and sustained systolic pulsation in the pulmonary artery area are PH, increased pulmonary blood flow, and their combination. In general, PH causes a relatively slow, sustained, and forceful pulmonary artery pulsation, whereas a large pulmonary blood flow (e.g., ASD) produces an extremely active, more vigorous, but less sustained pulsation. Valvular pulmonary stenosis with poststenotic dilatation of the pulmonary artery can be associated with a palpable, sustained pulsation in this area, often with a slow rise of the initial phase.

Area 4: Left Parasternal–Right Ventricular or Tricuspid Area Pulsations

A systolic thrill in the third, fourth, or fifth intercostal space in the parasternal area to the left of the sternum (see Fig. 12–58) is characteristic of VSD, although TR also can produce a thrill here.

Normally, the lower left parasternal region retracts very slightly during systole, and RV activity is not palpable. Slight, gentle outward pulsations of the lower sternum and left parasternal area can be recorded in normal children and young adults, in thin adults with a small anteroposterior thoracic diameter, or in patients with pectus excavatum.

Abnormal pulsations of the sternal and left parasternal areas most commonly are caused by RV hypertrophy or dilatation. The pulsation associated with RV hypertension is usually more sustained throughout systole and tends to rise more gradually than the pulsation produced by an RV volume load, which usually is more vigorous but often briefer.[86]

A predominant RV pressure load occurs with PS and PH caused by LV failure, mitral valve disease, a left-to-right shunt, or pulmonary vascular disease. The sustained anterior precordial pulsation associated with isolated valvular PS may not occur with tetralogy of Fallot because the thick RV is not excessively dilated. ASD and VSD are two congenital lesions frequently associated with an RV volume load.

Moderate or severe MR can produce an abnormal late systolic anterior left parasternal pulsation even in the absence of PH. This precordial lift is brisk, and its greatest force coincides with the accentuated v wave in the left atrial pressure wave. It likely is caused by the large volume of blood regurgitated into the expanding left atrium, which is located centrally behind the

RV and anterior to the spine. Although expansion of the left atrium can contribute somewhat to the anterior motion of the heart, it is likely that most of the anterior motion and force is the result of a jet or squid effect.

Conditions associated with a decrease in RV compliance, such as RV hypertrophy caused by PH, can be associated with a palpable *right-sided* S_4 in this area or, occasionally, in the epigastric area. Although a palpable S_3 in this area can reflect a large RV volume load, it usually indicates RV dysfunction or failure. RV S_3 and S_4 vibrations can be augmented during inspiration and can be attenuated or even disappear during expiration.

Area 5: Apical Area Pulsations

As mentioned earlier, the apex impulse (see Fig. 12–58) is not necessarily synonymous with maximum impulse or PMI. The location, size, and character of the apex impulse should be determined.[62] The examiner should focus on one phase of the cardiac cycle at a time and correlate the findings with other cardiovascular events.

The normal apex (apical) impulse usually is located within 10 cm of the sternal midline, at or within the left midclavicular line in the fifth intercostal space, when the patient is supine. It can be located lateral to the midclavicular line when associated with a high diaphragm, pregnancy, marked pectus excavatum, or other conditions that displace a normal heart to the left. The normal apex impulse is *less than 3 cm in diameter* and in most instances is considerably smaller. The early systolic outward movement of the apical area (see Fig. 12–58) begins at approximately the same time as that of the first heart sound (S_1), just before the upstroke of the carotid pulse. Peak outward motion normally occurs with or just after blood is ejected into the aorta; then the apex normally moves inward. The outward movement of the apical impulse is normally not excessively forceful and is felt only during the first third of systole.

The apex impulse can be hyperkinetic or hyperdynamic with increased amplitude in normal individuals who have a thin chest wall, a flat chest, or a depressed sternum. Lying on the left side can cause a normal apical impulse to move laterally and to have increased amplitude and duration[62]; however, it still should not exceed a diameter of >3 cm. A hyperdynamic apex impulse also can be found in anxious children, in patients with high cardiac output states, and in patients with a mild to moderate LV volume load from mitral or AR. The apex impulse is more sustained when mitral or AR is severe or when LV systolic function is decreased.[84] In general, a greatly sustained apex impulse indicates either marked LV hypertrophy or depressed LV systolic function, whereas LV dilatation displaces the apex impulse laterally and inferiorly[88,89] (see Fig. 12–58).

Concentric LV hypertrophy without an increase in LV cavity size can occur in systemic hypertension, valvular AS, and hypertrophic cardiomyopathy. Characteristically, the apex impulse is not displaced but is both abnormally forceful and sustained.[84,90] An S_4 vibration can be palpable or visible or both.

Severe LV dilatation—whether caused by volume load or ventricular failure—can displace the apex impulse laterally and inferiorly and cause a marked increase in size and duration.

Important information about relative amounts of ventricular hypertrophy and dilatation often can be obtained from the apex impulse. Thus, in valvular AS, with marked concentric LV hypertrophy but little or no dilatation, the apex impulse characteristically is

small, forceful, and sustained but not displaced. A presystolic S_4 often is palpable at the apex. By contrast, in severe AR with marked dilatation of the left ventricle plus considerable eccentric hypertrophy, there is a diffuse apex impulse with increased force, duration, and amplitude, and it is displaced laterally and inferiorly.[91]

In some patients with acute MI, a sustained apex impulse can simulate that caused by LV hypertrophy. Those developing mitral regurgitation (MR) secondary to MI (papillary muscle dysfunction) can manifest LV dilatation and hypertrophy by a displaced and sustained, forceful, large apex impulse.[92] A late systolic bulge at the cardiac apex can be caused by a functional LV aneurysm, occasionally resulting in a bifid apex impulse. In other patients, a late systolic bulge can be palpable in an ectopic area between the apex impulse and the left parasternal area.

A bifid apex impulse during systole also can be caused by marked LV dilatation and hypertrophy in patients with both AS and regurgitation or in patients with hypertrophic cardiomyopathy.[93] Infrequently, a faint systolic notch is palpable in the apex impulse of patients with MVP at the moment of a midsystolic click. Systolic retraction of the apical impulse usually indicates either constrictive pericarditis or severe TR with marked RV dilatation (see Fig. 12–58). An apical systolic thrill most commonly is produced by MR and often is diffuse, whereas a diastolic thrill is usually produced by MS and is localized to a small, discrete periapical area.

【 】 DIASTOLIC EVENTS: PALPABLE THIRD AND FOURTH HEART SOUNDS

During early diastole, brief outward chest-wall movement corresponding to an LV filling or S_3 occasionally can be seen or felt, even if it is not audible with a stethoscope (see Fig. 12–58). In children and young adults, the presence of an early diastolic ventricular filling sound (S_3) and movement is usually normal. Conversely, the presence of such a movement or sound in a sedentary adult or a patient with heart disease usually indicates an elevated LV diastolic pressure and volume and likely ventricular decompensation, often with a decreased ejection fraction. Patients with acute MI or transient myocardial ischemia during angina pectoris frequently develop a transient palpable and audible ventricular filling S_3, which reflects the acutely decreased ventricular compliance. A palpable ventricular rapid filling wave (S_3) can be present in patients with LV failure from any cause; however, hemodynamic systolic ventricular failure is often not always present when a ventricular filling wave or sound occurs in the presence of volume loading and dilatation of the left ventricle, as with MR or AR.

The presystolic left atrial contribution to the apical impulse (referred to as the *atrial impulse* or *a* wave) can be detected during late diastole, just prior to S_1 (see Fig. 12–58). Usually, a palpable atrial impulse coincides with an audible S_4 and is associated with an increased LV end-diastolic pressure and decreased compliance. In general, an LV S_4 presystolic impulse is not normally palpable but can be felt at the apex with its associated S_4 in some normal adults if the PR interval is long, and circulation is hyperdynamic. In some patients with ischemic heart disease, a palpable apical S_4 can develop or become more prominent during an episode of angina pectoris or even during exertion without chest pain. A palpable presystolic impulse, S_4, or both occur frequently in patients with acute MI, but these are also often present in other conditions producing a decrease in LV compliance and increased end-diastolic pressure.

A double, or bifid, apical impulse can be present in various circumstances, most commonly in the combination of an outward movement during ventricular systole and a second outward pulsation during diastole. The diastolic impulse can occur either in early diastole (S_3) or in late diastole or presystole (S_4).

A bifid apical impulse with two systolic impulses can be present in patients with hypertrophic obstructive cardiomyopathy, complete left bundle-branch block (LBBB), or MI. If these patients also develop a palpable impulse during either early (S_3) or late (S_4) diastole, a triple or trifid apical impulse can occur. When such patients develop both a palpable S_3 and a palpable S_4, it is occasionally possible to see and feel a quadruple apical impulse.

Area 6: Epigastric Area Pulsations

Some normal and many hyperkinetic individuals have visible or palpable pulsations of the aorta in the epigastric area (see Fig. 12–58). Abnormally large pulsations of the aorta can be caused by an aortic aneurysm or AR. Hepatic movements can be identified in the epigastric area, particularly in patients with TR, tricuspid stenosis, or marked RV dilatation, hypertrophy, and hyperactivity.

In some patients with PH caused by chronic lung disease, the detection of RV hypertrophy by precordial palpation is difficult because the shape of the chest often conceals the enlarged RV. To detect abnormal RV pulsations in patients with emphysema, the palm of the right hand should be placed on the epigastric area and moved cephalad while gently sliding the fingers under the rib cage. Aortic pulsations can be detected by the palmar surface of the fingers, and pulsations caused by RV hypertrophy can be felt in the fingertips.

Area 7: Ectopic Area Pulsations

Occasionally, cardiac pulsations are encountered in areas other than those described previously, that is, between the pulmonary and apical areas (see Fig. 12–58). Ischemic heart disease is the most common cause of an ectopic systolic pulsation, which can occur transiently during an episode of angina pectoris. A similar paradoxical systolic outward movement can be detected after acute MI and can persist; more commonly, it disappears within a few weeks. A persistent paradoxical ectopic pulsation also can be found in patients who develop a ventricular aneurysm after MI. Ectopic pulsations on the anterior chest wall also can be found in patients with cardiomyopathies of varying etiologies. In patients with severe MR and a giant left atrium that extends to the right, an ectopic systolic pulsation of the atrium occasionally can be felt in the right anterior or lateral chest or in the left axilla.

【 】 PERCUSSION VERSUS INSPECTION AND PALPATION OF THE PRECORDIUM

When performed by a skilled examiner, percussion of the heart can provide an estimate of cardiac size and shape. Percussion of the heart only gives information about the location of the borders of cardiac dullness, whereas precordial inspection and palpation provide both information about the location of the outer limits of cardiac pulsations and a determination of the size and character of

the pulsations. Although percussion has been used in the diagnosis of pericardial effusion, it has limited value when the results are objectively correlated with the diagnosis as determined by more sensitive and specific noninvasive and invasive testing.

CARDIAC AUSCULTATION
【 】 THE STETHOSCOPE

The physician must choose a stethoscope that fits the ears comfortably with the right angulation, has only a short segment of flexible tubing, and is equipped with a diaphragm and a bell. Selection of the proper earpieces for comfort and the best transmission of sound is based on individual preference. A snug, comfortable fit depends on the size of the earpieces as well as the angle at which they enter the ear canal. The rubber tubing should be as short as possible; experience indicates that tubing approximately 12 in (30 cm) long is the best compromise. Thick-walled tubing approximately 3 mm in diameter is best suited to transmit sounds and murmurs.

The human ear is most sensitive to auditory vibrations that occur in the frequency range between 1000 and 4000 to 5000 Hz; the sensitivity falls off sharply when the frequency of vibration is below 1000 Hz. This is particularly true of low-frequency sounds, which must be of considerably greater amplitude to reach the threshold of audibility than sounds of higher frequency. Most cardiovascular sounds and murmurs of diagnostic importance are between 30 and 1000 Hz, thereby placing the auscultator at considerable disadvantage.[1] Therefore, a stethoscope requires *both a diaphragm and a bell*, and each must be applied to the chest wall with optimal pressure. The diaphragm, which is fairly rigid, brings out the high frequencies and attenuates the lows. When it is used to accentuate high-pitched sounds, the diaphragm should be pressed very firmly against the skin. This technique will make a high-frequency murmur, such as the faint diastolic blowing murmur of AR, audible along the left sternal border when it would otherwise be missed. The bell tends to accentuate the low-frequency sounds and to filter out the high-pitched tones. Often, low-frequency sounds are more easily appreciated by palpation than by auscultation; in these situations, the stethoscope is placed very lightly on the skin, with just enough pressure to seal the edge at the point of maximal impulse. With very light pressure of the bell, the low-pitched sounds are accentuated; however, with firm pressure of the bell against the skin, the skin itself becomes a relatively tight diaphragm, and the low-frequency sounds are suppressed.

【 】 EXAMINATION OF THE PATIENT

The examination should take place in a quiet room that is well lighted and comfortably heated. The patient should be properly gowned, with adequate exposure to the waist. The examining table should be large enough that the patient can be instructed to lie flat, sit up, or roll to one side with complete ease. Usually, the physician will examine from the right side, and it is equally important that the physician be comfortable.

Prior to auscultation, the clinician should take advantage of the information obtained from the history as well as from the examination of the arterial, venous, and cardiac pulsations. When abnormalities are found, their auscultatory counterparts should be pursued diligently. The presence of pulsus alternans should always demand a careful search for third and fourth heart sounds (S_3, S_4) as well as for the presence of functional mitral or TR, often present in severe cardiac decompensation. A rapid, jerky rise of the carotid pulse can be the clue to the diagnosis of hypertrophic cardiomyopathy, which can be confirmed by manipulating the systolic murmur with maneuvers that change the pre- and afterloading conditions of the heart.

There are four primary areas of cardiac auscultation: (1) the primary and secondary aortic areas in the second right interspace and the third left interspace adjacent to the sternum, respectively, (2) the pulmonary area in the second left interspace, (3) the tricuspid area in the fourth and fifth interspaces adjacent to the left sternal border, and (4) the mitral area at the cardiac apex. This does not imply that auscultatory events arising from each valve are heard only in these respective areas. The murmur of AS in the elderly is often heard best (and at times only) at the apex, whereas the murmur of a flail posterior mitral leaflet can radiate to the base and simulate the murmur of AS. Ejection sounds arising from the stenotic aortic valve are usually most prominent at the apex, whereas the opening snap of MS is heard best midway between the tricuspid and mitral areas. The murmur of TR can be appreciated best at the classic mitral area if the RV occupies the apex. Furthermore, cardiac auscultation should not be restricted to just these four areas. For example, the murmur of AR secondary to abnormalities of the aortic root can be heard best to the right of the sternum, whereas the murmur of TR in the emphysematous patient with PH can be heard best in the epigastrium. The continuous murmur of a patent ductus arteriosus is heard just below the left clavicle, whereas the murmur of large bronchial collaterals can be most prominent in the posterior thorax.

During auscultation, one listens both specifically and selectively for heart sounds and then for murmurs, first during systole and then during diastole. As described by Levine and Harvey,[94] the physician should adopt a *systematic approach* to listening. The patient should be lying on his or her back, and each area should be surveyed with both chest pieces. In each area examined, the physician listens specifically for the S_1. This is followed by selective listening for the S_2, noting the presence of splitting and variation with respirations. Then extra sounds are searched for and carefully listened to, first in systole and then in diastole. With the bell applied lightly to the skin at the apex, the patient is instructed to roll onto the left side, and the clinician selectively *tunes in* to diastole and the low-frequency range. This allows the physician to determine the presence or absence of diastolic filling sounds or diastolic rumbles arising from the AV valves. The examination is continued with the patient in the sitting position. While the patient leans slightly forward during quiet respiration, the clinician can optimally appreciate splitting of S_2. With the patient's breath held in deep expiration, the physician examines the aortic and pulmonic areas with the diaphragm firmly pressed against the chest wall, selectively tuning in to the high-frequency range in an effort to hear the faint blowing diastolic murmur of AR or, if the clinical situation warrants, the presence of a pericardial friction rub.

Auscultation of the heart should be considered a dynamic exercise. In addition to being auscultated in the left lateral decubitus position, the patient should, when possible, also be examined while standing, squatting, and during the Valsalva maneuver and following its release. This type of dynamic examination changes the pre- and afterloading conditions of the heart and can yield diagnostic information because of the typical responses of various heart sounds and murmurs using these maneuvers.

HEART SOUNDS

Heart sounds are of two types: high-frequency transients associated with the abrupt terminal checking of valves that are closing or opening and low-frequency sounds related to early and late diastolic filling events of the ventricles.[95] Sounds related to closing and opening of the AV valves include mitral and tricuspid closing sounds (M_1, T_1), nonejection sounds, and the opening snaps; sounds related to closing and opening of the semilunar valves include aortic and pulmonic closure sounds (A_2, P_2) and early valvular ejection sounds or clicks. Low-frequency sounds include the physiologic heart sound (S_3) and the pathologic S_3 gallop associated with early ventricular filling events and the presystolic atrial S_4 gallop associated with late diastolic events resulting from the atrial contribution to ventricular filling. With tachycardia, these sounds can fuse, producing a summation gallop.

THE FIRST HEART SOUND

The S_1, as recorded by high-resolution phonocardiography, consists of four sequential components. The two *major components normally audible* at the left lower sternal border are the louder M_1 followed by T_1. Splitting of the first heart sound is less evident with the tachycardia following coughing or with sustained handgrip exercise.

Echocardiographic Correlates and Splitting of S_1

The first high-frequency component of S_1 coincides with the complete coaptation of the anterior and posterior leaflets of the mitral valve.[96,97] This sound is caused by the sudden deceleration of blood setting the entire cardiohemic system into vibration when the elastic limits of the closed, tensed valves are met. It is unlikely that complete coaptation of the complex valve leaflets and final tensing are simultaneous; presumably it is the latter event that is associated with vibrations perceived as M_1. When T_1 is more widely separated from M_1, however, identical echocardiographic correlates have been demonstrated in patients with wide splitting of S_1 caused by Ebstein anomaly of the tricuspid valve. Wide splitting of S_1 with normal sequencing (M_1, T_1) is also present in right bundle-branch block of the proximal type as well as in LV pacing, ectopic beats, and idioventricular rhythms originating from the left ventricle as a result of a delayed contraction of the RV. Similarly, pacing from the RV and ectopic beats and idioventricular rhythms originating from the RV will produce reversed splitting of S_1 (T_1, M_1) because of a delay in LV contraction.

Hemodynamic Correlates of S_1

Figure 12–59 illustrates the sound and pressure correlates of M_1. The first high-frequency component of M_1 coincides with the downstroke of the left atrial *c* wave and is delayed from the LV–left

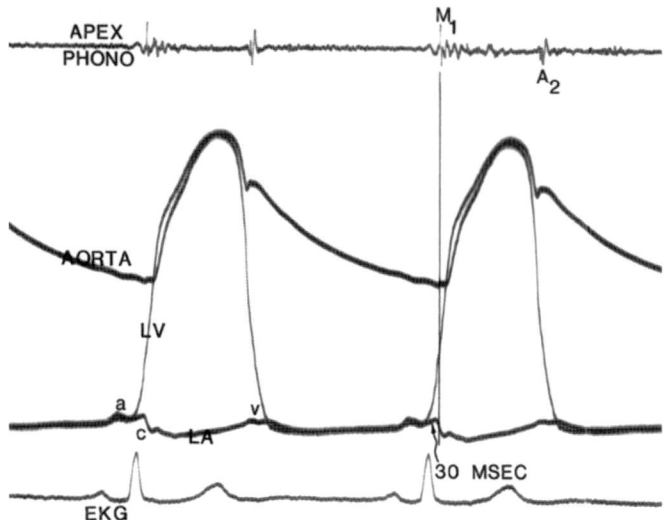

FIGURE 12-59. The apex phonocardiogram is displayed simultaneously with the cardiac cycle, as recorded by high-fidelity catheter-tipped micromanometers in the central aorta, left ventricle (LV), and left atrium (LA). The first high-frequency component of the mitral first sound (M_1) is coincident with the downstroke of the left atrial c wave and is separated from LV–left atrial pressure crossover by an interval of 30 ms. *Source: Shaver JA, Salerni R, Reddy PS. Normal and abnormal heart sounds in cardiac diagnosis: I. Systolic sounds. Curr Probl Cardiol. 1985;10:10–53. Reproduced with permission from the publisher and authors.*

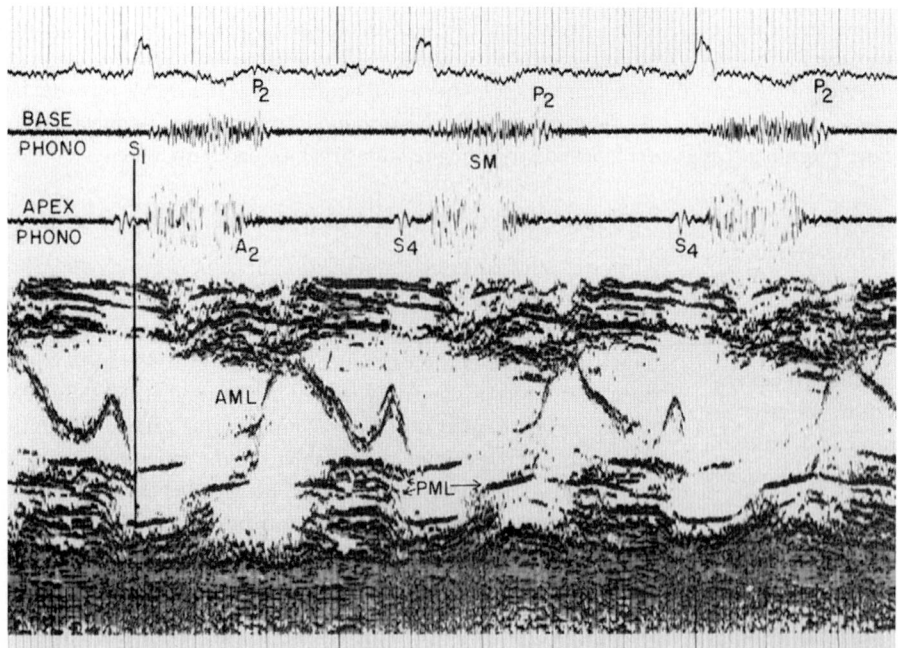

FIGURE 12-60. Base and apex phonocardiograms are recorded simultaneously with the mitral valve echocardiogram in a 62-year-old man who developed acute mitral regurgitation (MR) secondary to rupture of the chordae tendineae of a myxomatous valve. During diastole, multiple echoes arise from the flail posterior mitral leaflet (PML); during early ventricular systole, effective mitral valve closure does not occur, resulting in an inaudible low-frequency vibration on the apex phonocardiogram. During systole, there is separation of the anterior mitral leaflet (AML) and PMLs, resulting in severe MR. The murmur has a crescendo-decrescendo contour simulating the murmur of aortic stenosis (AS) ending prior to the aortic first sound (A_1). Wide physiologic splitting of the first heart sound (S_1) is present. The prominent fourth heart sound (S_4) present on the apex phonocardiogram was associated with an apical presystolic impulse. P_2, pulmonic second heart sound; SM, systolic murmur. *Source: Shaver JA. The physical examination in cardiac diagnosis. Cardiol Consult. 1985;6:3. Reproduced with permission from the publisher and author.*

atrial pressure crossover by 30 ms. Forward flow continues for a short period following LV–left atrial pressure crossover as a result of the inertia of mitral flow, with M_1 occurring 20 to 40 ms later, coincidentally with cessation of mitral flow and closure of the valve. An even greater delay between the occurrence of T_1 and RV–right atrial pressure crossover has been shown. Also, T_1 coincides with the downstroke of the right atrial c wave. These hemodynamic data confirm the prime role played by the AV valves in the genesis of S_1.

Intensity of S_1

The primary factors determining intensity of S_1 are (1) integrity of valve closure, (2) mobility of the valve, (3) velocity of valve closure, (4) status of ventricular contraction, (5) transmission characteristics of the thoracic cavity and chest wall, and (6) physical characteristics of the vibrating structures.

Integrity of Valve Closure
In rare situations, usually in the setting of severe MR, there is inadequate coaptation of the mitral leaflets to a degree that valve closure is not effective. As a result, abrupt halting of the retrograde blood column during early ventricular contraction does not occur, and S_1 can be markedly attenuated or absent. Such can be the case in severe MR caused by a flail mitral leaflet, as shown in Fig. 12–60.

Mobility of the Valve
Severe calcific fixation of the mitral valve with complete immobilization will cause a markedly attenuated M_1. This is seen most commonly in the setting of long-standing severe MS.

Velocity of Valve Closure
The velocity of valve closure is the most important factor affecting the intensity of S_1 and is determined by the timing of mitral valve closure in relation to the LV pressure rise in early systole.[97] The relative timing of left atrial and LV systole can vary this relationship. As the PR interval progressively decreases from 130 to 30 ms, there is a progressive increase in the intensity of M_1 and progressive delay in M_1 relative to the onset of LV contraction. When left atrial and LV systole occur almost simultaneously, at a PR interval of 10 ms, however, S_1 again becomes soft. At short PR intervals (30 to 70 ms), the mitral valve leaflets are maximally separated by atrial contraction at the onset of LV systole. With LV contraction, the mitral valve closes at a high velocity with a large excursion. This results in a loud, late M_1 occurring on a steeper part of the LV pressure curve when the retrograde blood column is suddenly decelerated at the moment the elastic limits of the mitral valve are met (see Chap. 76). At longer PR intervals, there is less separation of the mitral valve leaflets, which have already begun to close with atrial relaxation. When LV systole begins,

there is less excursion of the mitral valve until tensing occurs, and S_1 occurs earlier relative to the onset of LV contraction at a lower LV pressure. Thus, less force is applied to the mitral valve, its closing velocity is decreased, and less energy is generated when a column of retrograde blood is abruptly halted.

The clinical finding of marked variation in the intensity of S_1 in a patient with a slow heart rate often will alert the clinician to the diagnosis of complete AV block with AV dissociation. Other conditions in which there are beat-to-beat variations in the intensity of S_1 include Mobitz type I AV block and ventricular tachycardia with AV dissociation. Variations in the intensity of S_1 also occur with atrial fibrillation with both normal and stenotic AV valves. The loud S_1 occurs at short RR intervals, whereas a softer S_1 occurs at longer RR.

The position of the mitral valve at the onset of ventricular systole can be altered not only by the relative timing of atrial and ventricular systole but also by altering the rate of LV filling during atrial systole. The timing and intensity of both S_1 and S_4 in hypertensive patients can be influenced by variations in venous return. It is suggested that the mitral leaflets have a greater separation when venous return is *decreased* to the noncompliant hypertensive LV because there is more effective atrial volume transport into a relatively underfilled ventricle. This results in a softer S_4 that migrates toward an increased S_1. When venous return is *increased,* the atrial contribution of ventricular filling is now operating on the steeper portion of the LV pressure-volume curve. The S_4 becomes louder and earlier, and S_1 is decreased in amplitude as a result of partial arteriogenic closure of the mitral valve (Fig. 12–61).

Status of Ventricular Contraction

The status of ventricular contractility is also an independent factor determining the amplitude of S_1.[97] In normal subjects, both exercise and catecholamine infusion increase the amplitude of S_1, whereas administration of β-blocking agents decreases it.[97] In both situations, the prime factor in altering the intensity of S_1 is the rate of pressure development in the ventricle. This increased rate of pressure development partially explains why S_1 is increased in patients with anemia, arteriovenous fistulas, pregnancy, anxiety, and fever. Similarly, the loud T_1 in an atrial septal defect (ASD) is caused by high flow through the tricuspid valve, secondary to the left-to-right shunt at the atrial level. A decrease in the intensity of S_1 associated with a decrease in the rate of LV pressure development can be found in myxedema, cardiomyopathy, and acute MI.[97]

Transmission Characteristics of the Thoracic Cavity and Chest Wall

The degree of attenuation of heart sounds generated by the vibrating cardiohemic system is a function of both sound frequency and the distance of the heart from the chest wall. Condi-

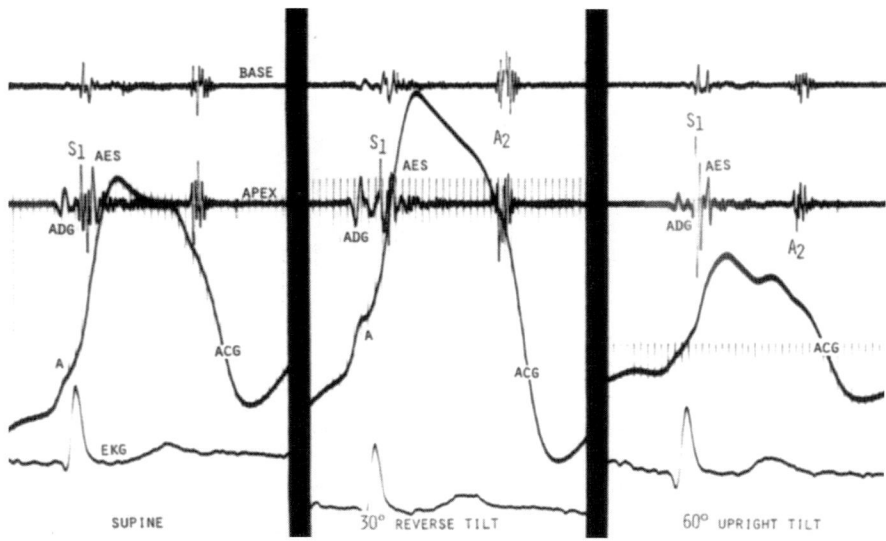

FIGURE 12–61. External phonograms are recorded at the base and apex in a 52-year-old man with significant systemic hypertension, together with an apexcardiogram and ECG. In all three postures, an atrial gallop precedes the first heart sound (S_1), which in turn is followed by a prominent aortic root ejection sound. In the supine position, the atrial diastolic gallop is coincident with the peak of the A wave on the apexcardiogram. During a 30-degree reverse tilt with increased venous return, there is a significant increase in the amplitude of the atrial diastolic gallop as well as an increase in the amplitude of the A wave on the apexcardiogram. In contrast with a 60-degree upright tilt and a decrease in the venous return, there is a marked decrease in the intensity of the atrial diastolic gallop and a loss of the A wave on the apexcardiogram. Note also the migration of the atrial gallop toward S_1 with an increase in the intensity of the latter. With these changes in posture, there is no significant change in the intensity of the aortic ejection sound, which is recorded well at both the apex and the base in all tracings. These simple maneuvers at the bedside can be helpful in distinguishing an atrial gallop from an aortic ejection sound. *Source: Shaver JA, et al. Ejection sounds of left-sided origin. In: Leon DF, Shaver JA, eds. Physiologic Principles of Heart Sounds and Murmurs. New York: American Heart Association, Monograph 46; 1975:31. Reproduced with permission from the American Heart Association, Inc. and the authors.*

tions such as obesity, emphysema, and large pleural or pericardial effusions will decrease the intensity of all auscultatory events, whereas a thin body habitus would tend to increase the intensity.

Physical Characteristics of the Vibrating Structures   Alterations in the physical characteristics of the vibrating structures also can vary the intensity of S_1. Both MI and ischemia induced by pacing have been shown to decrease the intensity of S_1.

S_1 in Pathologic Conditions

Careful attention to the intensity of S_1 is an extremely important aspect of cardiac auscultation, often giving clues to the proper diagnosis and degree of abnormality of the involved structures. In the following conditions, alterations in the intensity of S_1 can play a key role in the correct diagnosis.

S_1 in Mitral Stenosis   A loud, late M_1 is the hallmark of hemodynamically significant mitral stenosis.[98] When M_1 is loud, it is associated with a loud opening snap, and the intensity of both M_1 and the opening snap correlates with valve motility (Fig. 12–62, *left*). When calcific fixation of the stenotic mitral valve occurs, M_1 is soft, and the opening snap is absent. The relationship between sound and pressure and echocardiographic mitral valve motion is shown in Fig. 12–63. The increased left atrial pressure delays the time of pressure crossover between the left atrium and the left ven-

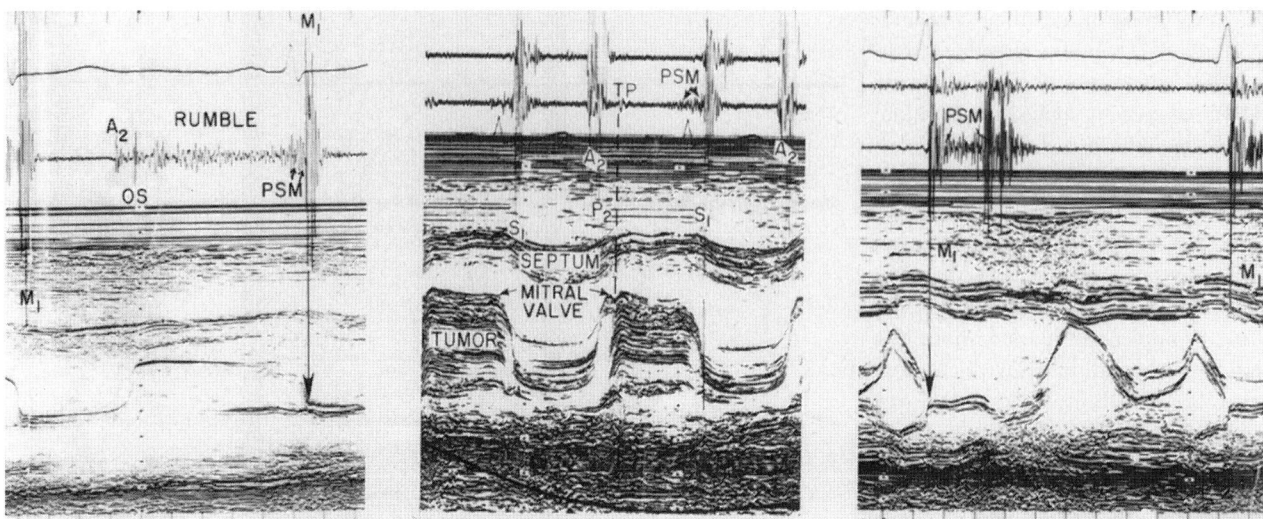

FIGURE 12–62. Simultaneous phonocardiograms are recorded with the mitral valve echocardiograms in three patients: mitral stenosis (MS) (*left*), left atrial myxoma (*center*), and prolapse of the mitral valve (*right*). In each condition, a loud mitral first sound (M_1) is present and coincident with the closing point of the mitral valve echocardiogram. Common to each condition is wide separation of the mitral leaflets at the onset of left ventricular (LV) systole, with high-velocity closure occurring over a large excursion. *In the left panel,* a mobile stenotic valve is demonstrated, and a loud opening snap (OS) is coincident with the E point. In the center panel, an early diastolic tumor plop (TP) is coincident with the maximal excursion of the tumor during its rapid descent into the ventricle. Note the presystolic crescendo murmur (PSM) occurring during the rapid closure of the mitral valve in both MS and left atrial myxoma. In the right panel, a pansystolic murmur (PSM) with late systolic accentuation is secondary to the prolapse of the mitral valve with late systolic hammocking. A_2, aortic second sound; P_2, pulmonic second heart sound; S_1, first heart sound. *Source: Shaver JA. Current uses of phonocardiography in clinical practice. In: Rapaport E, ed. Cardiology Update: Reviews for Physicians. New York: Elsevier; 1981:370. Reproduced in part (center panel) with permission from the publisher and author. Copyright 1981 by Elsevier Science Publishing Co., Inc.*

tricle. As a result, M_1 occurs later and at a much higher than normal LV pressure, at a time when there is a more rapid rate of development of LV pressure. The presystolic gradient between the left atrium and the left ventricle prevents preclosure of the mitral valve leaflets. As a result, the closure of the leaflet begins from a domed position within the LV cavity and takes place over a much greater distance following the onset of LV contraction. Both these factors increase the velocity of mitral valve closure and the momentum of blood directed toward the mitral valve leaflets, resulting in a loud M_1. A similar mechanism is responsible for the booming S_1 with after vibrations in left atrial myxoma (see Fig. 12–62, *center*).

S_1 in Mitral Valve Prolapse Tei and colleagues[99] have reported a loud M_1 heard over the apex in patients with nonrheumatic MR; this is indicative of holosystolic MVP (see Fig. 12–61, *right*). Patients with the more common middle to late systolic prolapse have a normal S_1, whereas a soft or absent S_1 can indicate a flail mitral leaflet (see Fig. 12–60). The increased amplitude of leaflet excursion with prolapse beyond the line of closure explains the loud M_1 associated with holosystolic prolapse. An alternate explanation can be a summation of a normal M_1 and an early nonejection click of valvular prolapse.

S_1 and Left Bundle-Branch Block In LBBB, M_1 is decreased in intensity and is frequently delayed, at times resulting in reversal of sequence of S_1.[100] The reason for the delay and the decreased intensity of M_1 in this condition is multifactorial. The primary factors involved are (1) delay in onset of LV contraction, (2) degree of LV dysfunction, (3) presence of concomitant first-degree heart block, and (4) presence of a noncompliant left ventricle facilitating arteriogenic preclosure of the mitral valve. It is likely that more than one factor is operative in most patients with LBBB, with one or two factors predominating.

S_1 in Acute Aortic Regurgitation One of the important auscultatory findings in acute AR is attenuation or absence of M_1.[101] Severe regurgitation into a left ventricle that has not had time to adapt to the acute volume overload causes a marked increase in the LV end-diastolic pressure, resulting in premature closure of the normal mitral valve in mid-diastole. With the onset of LV systole, minimal mitral valve excursion occurs, causing a marked reduction in the intensity of M_1.

【 】 SYSTOLIC EJECTION SOUNDS

Ejection sounds are early systolic ejection events that can originate from either the left or the right side of the heart. These sounds can be classified as *valvular,* arising from deformed aortic or pulmonic valves, or as *vascular* or *root* events caused by the rapid, forceful ejection of blood into the great vessels. The presence or absence of valvular ejection sounds is of great benefit in defining the level of RV or LV outflow tract obstruction, whereas root ejection sounds indicate abnormalities of the great vessels with or without systemic or PH.

Aortic Valvular Ejection Sounds

Aortic valvular ejection sounds are found in nonstenotic congenital bicuspid valves and in the entire spectrum of mild to severe stenosis of the aortic valve. This sound introduces the typical ejection murmur of AS, is widely transmitted, and is often heard best at the apex. The aortic valvular ejection sound is delayed 20 to 40 ms after the onset of pressure rise in the central aorta and is coincident with the sharp anacrotic notch on the upstroke of the aortic pressure curve. The sound is coincident with the maximal excursion of the domed valve when its elastic limits are met. Deceleration of the oncoming column of blood sets the entire cardiohemic system into vibration,

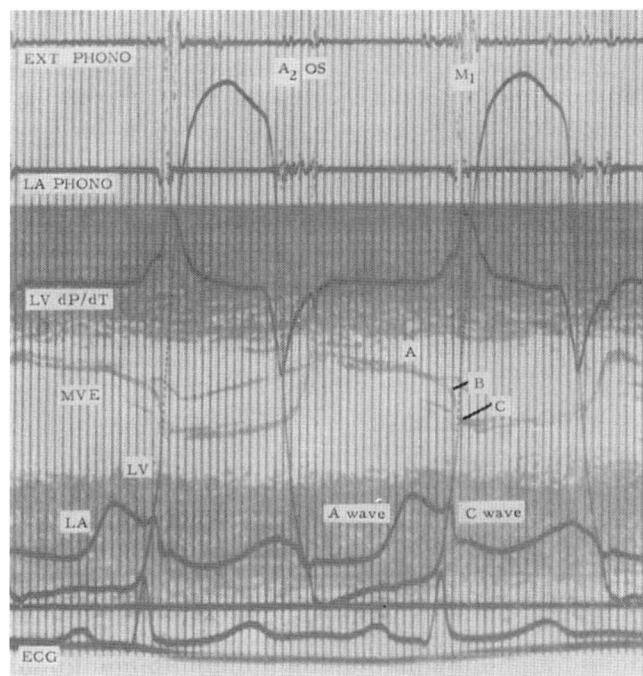

FIGURE 12–63. External sound, equisensitive left ventricular (LV) and left atrial pressures (catheter-tipped micromanometer), LV upstroke pattern on apex cardiogram (*dP/dt*), and left atrial sound are recorded simultaneously with the mitral valve echocardiogram in a patient with hemodynamically significant mitral stenosis. A significant presystolic gradient is present as a result of atrial contraction, and the onset of the rapid closure of the mitral valve (point B) is delayed until the LV pressure exceeds left atrial pressure. This occurs 40 ms after the beginning of the LV pressure rise at a time when LV *dP/dt* is much higher than normal. Following left atrial–LV pressure crossover, there is rapid ventriculogenic closure of the mitral valve (points B and C), resulting in a very loud mitral first sound (M_1) coincident with the C point of the mitral valve echocardiogram. Its separation from the aortic second sound (A_2) is determined by both the level of the left atrial pressure and the rate of LV pressure decline. LA, left arterial; MVE, mitral valve echo; OS, opening snap. *Source: Shaver JA, et al. Normal and abnormal heart sounds in cardiac diagnosis: 1. Systolic sounds. Curr Probl Cardiol. 1985;10:10–53. Reproduced with permission from the publisher and the authors.*

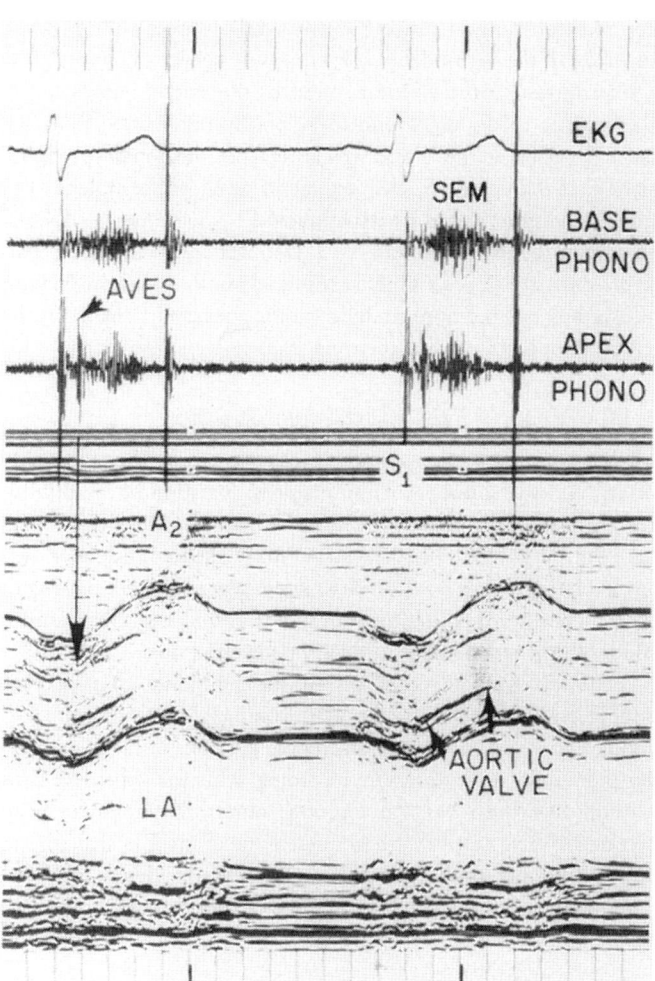

FIGURE 12–64. Base and apex phonocardiograms are recorded simultaneously with the aortic valve echocardiogram in a young man with valvular aortic stenosis. A prominent aortic valvular ejection sound (AVES) is recorded at the apex and is coincident with the maximal excursion of the aortic valve in early systole. It is followed by a crescendo-decrescendo systolic ejection murmur (SEM) that ends well before a loud aortic second sound (A_2). LA, left arterial; S_1, first heart sound.

the lower-frequency components being recorded as the anacrotic notch and the high-frequency components representing the valvular ejection sound. Inherent in this mechanism of sound production is the ability of the deformed valve to move. Sound and motion correlates identical to those demonstrated by cineangiography have been found with phonoechocardiography, clearly showing the onset of the ejection sound to be coincident with the maximal opening of the valve (Fig. 12–64). The intensity of the ejection sound correlates directly with the mobility of the valve, but there is no correlation between intensity and the severity of the obstruction. In mobile, non-stenotic bicuspid valves, the ejection sound is not only loud but also widely separated from S_1 because of the prolonged excursion of the mobile valve. The presence of an aortic valvular ejection sound is a valuable physical finding at the bedside; it not only defines the LV outflow obstruction at the valvular level but also gives insight into the mobility of the valve (see Fig. 12–64).

Pulmonic Valvular Ejection Sounds

Pulmonic valvular ejection sounds have identical sound and pressure correlates as aortic valvular ejection sounds. Echocardiographic correlations also show that the onset of the pulmonary ejection sound occurs at the maximal excursion of the stenotic pulmonic valve. In contrast to the aortic valvular ejection sounds and to most right-sided auscultatory events, the *pulmonic sound or ejection click decreases in intensity or disappears with inspiration* in mild to moderate PS. In very mild valvular PS, respiratory variation can be absent. In very severe valvular obstruction, a vigorous atrial contraction can completely preopen the pulmonic valve in diastole, causing a crisp preejection sound. In this situation, RV pressure at the time of the atrial kick actually can exceed pulmonary artery end-diastolic pressure.

Aortic Vascular Ejection Sounds

Ejection sounds originating from the aortic root are common in systemic arterial hypertension in the setting of a tortuous sclerotic aortic root, a tight, noncompliant arterial tree, and forceful LV ejection. They are coincident with the upstroke of the high-fidelity central aortic pressure and have been interpreted as an exaggeration of the ejection component of the normal S_1. Echocardiographic correlations show that this sound occurs at the moment of complete opening of the aortic valve and always on the pressure upstroke of the high-fidelity aortic pressure curve.

In contrast to the ejection sound of the stenotic aortic valve, these aortic root sounds tend to be poorly transmitted from the aortic area and are not heard well at the apex. It should be emphasized that the benign S_1 ejection sound or M_1-T_1 complex is frequently misinterpreted as a pathologic S_4–S_1 sequence. Factors that favor the presence of an S_4–S_1 complex are an associated palpable presystolic apical impulse, optimal audibility of the S_4 with the stethoscope bell applied lightly at the apex, and a change in the intensity of the S_4 with maneuvers that vary venous return.

Pulmonary Vascular Ejection Sounds

Vascular or root ejection sounds also can arise from the pulmonary artery, and the common denominator is dilatation of the pulmonary artery.[87] This dilatation can be idiopathic or secondary to severe PH. Although it has been stated that this sound is louder during expiration, *there is no consensus on this point*. Unlike splitting of S_1, which is heard best at the mitral or tricuspid area, this sound is louder in the second and third left intercostal spaces.

Echocardiographic correlates of the pulmonic root ejection sound show it to be coincident with complete opening of the pulmonary valve and occurring during the upstroke of the high-fidelity pulmonary artery pressure recording. This has led to the conclusion that these vascular ejection sounds can originate from semilunar valve cusps that have undergone changes in structure in response to increased pressure. In both idiopathic dilatation of the pulmonary artery and ASD, this sound occurs during the upstroke of the pulmonary pressure tracing.[87]

【 】 NONEJECTION SOUNDS

The midsystolic click caused by prolapse of the mitral or tricuspid valve is the most frequent cause of systolic nonejection sounds and is often associated with a systolic regurgitant murmur.[102] Although originally thought to be extracardiac in origin, confirmation of their valvular origin has been shown by angiographic,[91,102] intracardiac phonocardiographic,[88,103] and echocardiographic[89] studies. As originally proposed by Reid, the cause of this sound is caused by tensing of the AV valves during systole. It is produced by vibrations of the entire cardiohemic system when the elastic limits of the prolapsed valve are suddenly reached.

The presence of a nonejection click on physical examination is sufficient to make the diagnosis of MVP. The sound has a sharp, high-frequency clicking quality and, although often confined to the apex, can be transmitted widely on the precordium (see Chap. 76). It can be an isolated finding, occurring most often in middle to late systole, or there can be multiple clicks, presumably as a result of different areas of the large, redundant, scalloped mitral leaflets prolapsing at different times. Numerous echocardiographic studies have shown the presence of the characteristic mid- to late-systolic prolapse as well as holosystolic prolapse in patients with clicks. All these patterns can be seen in the presence of an isolated systolic click, click and late systolic murmur, or a late systolic murmur alone. The click usually occurs at the time of maximal prolapse.

A feature of MVP is the variability of the auscultatory findings from examination to examination and even from beat to beat (Fig. 12–65). The timing of the click or the click and late systolic murmur varies considerably with changes in posture (Fig. 12–66) (see Chap. 76). In the upright posture, the heart becomes smaller be-

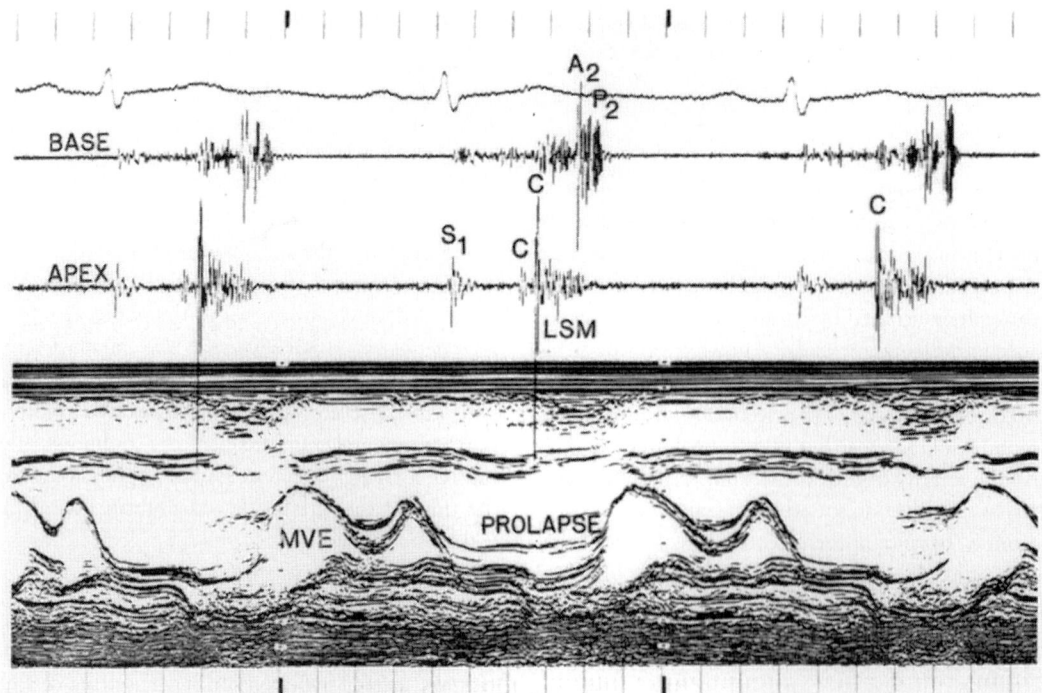

FIGURE 12–65. Simultaneously recorded base and apex phonocardiograms and mitral valve echocardiogram (MVE) demonstrating the frequent association of a late systolic murmur with a prominent late systolic click. Although the murmur is well transmitted to the base, the click transmits poorly. In the first two complexes, an additional softer click precedes the click murmur complex. The last complex shows only a single click, demonstrating the variability of the auscultatory findings even at rest. The large click occurs at maximal prolapse, and the smaller click occurs near the onset of echocardiographic prolapse. A_2, aortic second sound; LSM, late systolic murmur; P_2, pulmonic second heart sound; S_1, first heart sound.

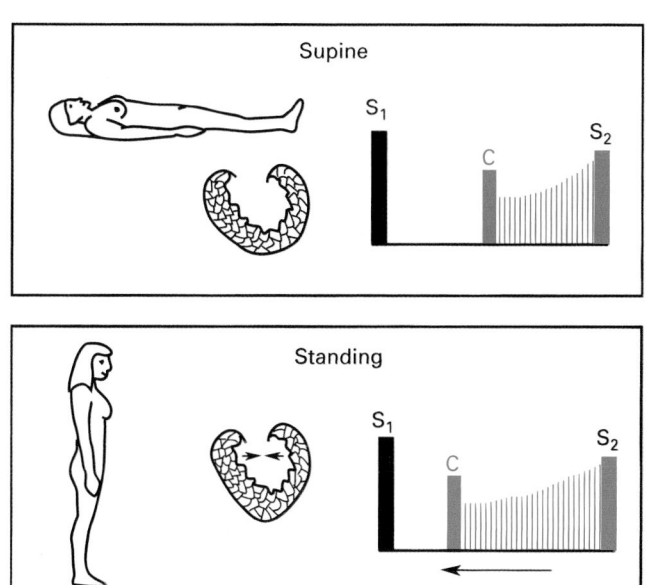

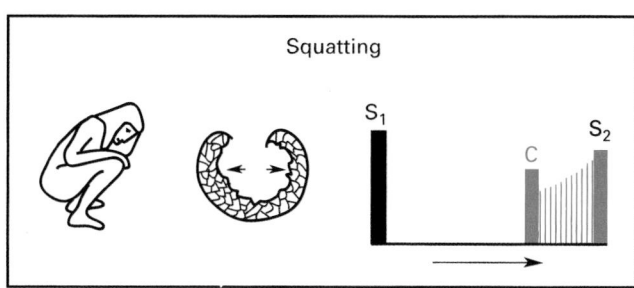

FIGURE 12–66. A midsystolic nonejection sound (C) occurs in mitral valve prolapse and is followed by a late systolic murmur that crescendos to a first heart sound (S₁). With assumption of the upright posture, venous return decreases, the heart becomes smaller, the C moves closer to S₁, and the mitral regurgitant murmur has an earlier onset. With prompt squatting, both venous return and afterload increase, the heart becomes larger, the C moves toward a second heart sound (S₂), and the duration of the murmur shortens.

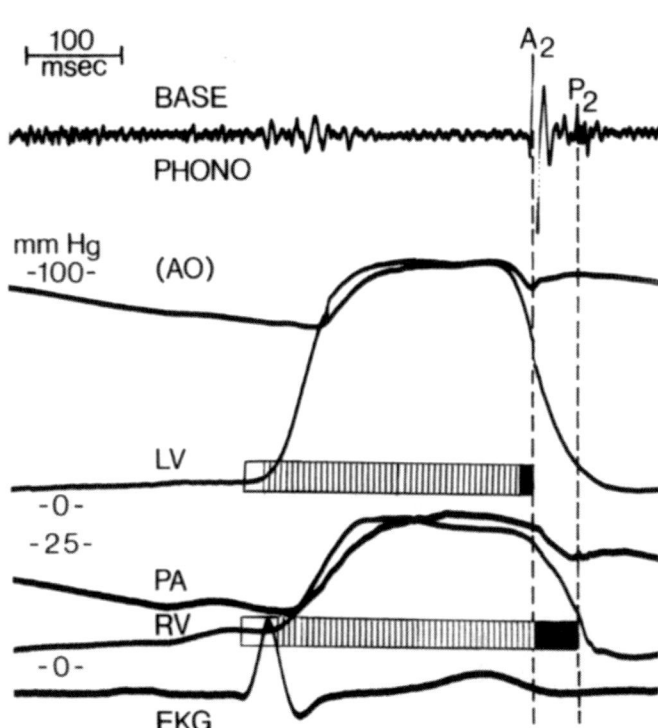

FIGURE 12–67. The cardiac cycle recorded by high-fidelity catheter-tipped micromanometers. The aortic (A₂) and pulmonic (P₂) closure sounds are coincident with the incisurae of their respective arterial traces. Although the left and right ventricular (LV and RV) mechanical systoles are nearly equal in duration, the RV systolic ejection period terminates after LV ejection because of an increased right-sided *hangout* interval. The cardiac cycle has been divided into three phases: (1) (open bar) the electrical mechanical coupling interval (time from the onset of Q wave to the rise of ventricular pressure); (2) (vertical stripe) ventricular mechanical systole (the sum of isovolumic contraction time plus ejection period, minus the hangout interval); and (3) (solid bar) the impedance interval of hangout (the time between the incisura of the arterial trace and the ventricular pressure at the same level as the incisura). *Source: Shaver JA. The second heart sound: newer concepts: I. Normal and wide physiological splitting. Mod Concepts Cardiovasc Dis. 1997;46:7. Reproduced with permission from the American Heart Association and the authors.*

cause of decreased venous return, and the click moves earlier in systole. Angiographic studies have confirmed an earlier and greater degree of prolapse in the upright posture compared with the supine position. Squatting, which causes an immediate increase in venous return and afterload, increases LV volume, resulting in later prolapse and movement of the click toward S₂. At the bedside, these simple maneuvers are helpful in differentiating the nonejection click from early ejection sounds, a split S₂, or an S₃.

In general, maneuvers that decrease LV volume such as sitting, standing, or strain of the Valsalva maneuver cause the click to move closer to S₁. Maneuvers that increase LV volume move the click toward S₂.

Although the most common cause of nonejection clicks is prolapse of the AV valves, systolic sounds have been reported in patients with left-sided pneumothorax, adhesive pericarditis, atrial myxomas, LV aneurysm, aneurysm of the membranous ventricular septum associated with a VSD, and incompetent heterograft valves.

【 】 THE SECOND HEART SOUND

To appreciate the significance of the normal and abnormal S₂, knowledge of its relationship to the hemodynamic events of the cardiac cycle is essential.[104] Figure 12–67 records the two components of S₂ simultaneously with the cardiac cycle by high-fidelity catheter-tipped micromanometers. The A₂ and P₂ are coincident with the incisura of the aorta and pulmonary artery pressure trace, respectively, and terminate the LV and RV ejection periods. RV ejection begins prior to LV ejection, has a longer duration, and terminates after LV ejection, resulting in P₂ normally occurring after A₂. RV and LV systole are nearly equal in duration, and the pulmonary artery incisura is delayed relative to the aortic incisura, primarily a result of a larger interval separating the pulmonary artery incisura from the RV pressure compared with the same left-sided event. This interval has been called the *hangout* interval, a purely descriptive term coined in Shaver laboratory more than 30 years ago. Its duration is felt to be a reflection of the impedance of the vascular bed into which the blood is being received.[105] Normally, it is less than 15 ms in the systemic circulation and only slightly prolongs the LV ejection time. In the low-resistance, high-capacitance pulmonary bed, however, this interval is normally much greater than on the left, varying between 43 and 86 ms, and therefore contributes significantly to the duration of RV ejection.

Echocardiographic Correlations and Mechanisms of Sound Production

Figure 12–68 illustrates the relationship between the aortic and pulmonary valve echocardiogram and A_2 and P_2. The first high-frequency component of both A_2 and P_2 is coincident with completion of closure of the aortic and pulmonic valve leaflets. A_2 and P_2 are produced by the sudden deceleration of retrograde flow of the blood column in the aorta and pulmonary artery when the elastic limits of the tensed leaflets are met. This abrupt deceleration of flow sets the cardiohemic system into vibration and the higher-frequency components result in A_2 and P_2. This pressure gradient across the valves is the result of both the level of the diastolic pressure in the great vessel and the rate of pressure decline in the ventricle and is consistent with the well-known clinical observation of increased intensity of A_2 and P_2 in systemic and PH.

Normal Physiologic Splitting

Normally during expiration, A_2 and P_2 are separated by an interval of less than 30 ms and are heard by the clinician as a single sound.[106] During inspiration, both components become distinctly audible as the splitting interval widens, primarily caused by a delayed P_2, although an earlier A_2 contributes to a lesser degree (Fig. 12–69).

On auscultation, splitting of S_2 is usually best heard at the second or third left intercostal space; the normal P_2 is softer than A_2 and is rarely audible at the apex. When P_2 is heard at the apex, either significant PH is present or the apex is occupied by the RV, a situation seen commonly in normotensive ASD. The absolute value of inspiratory splitting varies with age and depth of respiration. In younger subjects, maximal splitting during inspiration averages 40 to 50 ms; with age, this value decreases such that a single S_2 during both phases of respiration can be normal in subjects older than 40 years of age.

Abnormal Splitting

All conditions in which abnormal splitting of S_2 exists can be identified at the bedside by the presence of audible expiratory splitting (>30 ms) (see Fig. 12–69). This finding must be present when the patient is auscultated in both the supine and upright positions. There are three causes of audible expiratory splitting: (1) wide physiologic splitting primarily caused by delayed P_2, (2) reversed splitting primarily caused by delayed A_2, and (3) narrow physiologic splitting as seen in PH, where A_2 and P_2 are heard as two distinct sounds during expiration at a narrow splitting interval. Tables 12–8 and 12–9 classify the common causes of wide physiologic splitting and reversed splitting of S_2 according to the abnormality of the cardiac cycle responsible for the altered timing of A_2 and P_2. In each table, the cardiac cycle has been divided into three phases (see Fig. 12–67): (1) the electromechanical couple interval, the time from the on-

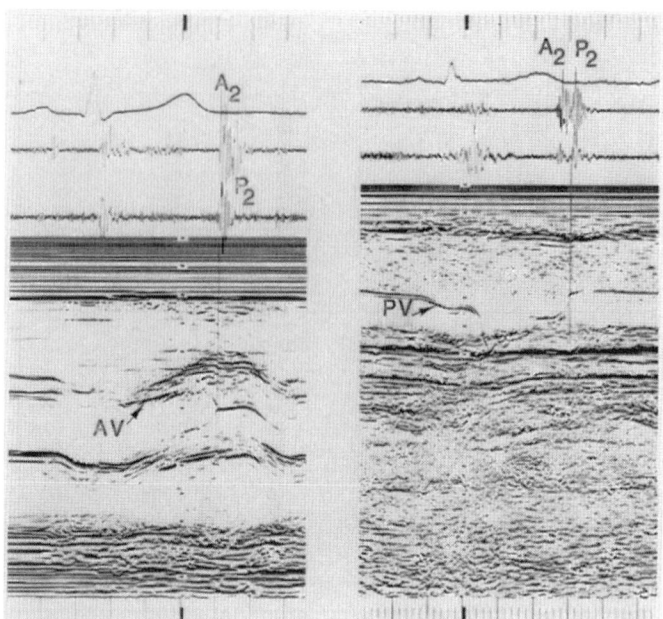

FIGURE 12–68. *Left.* The base and apex phonocardiograms are recorded simultaneously with the aortic valve echocardiogram. The first high-frequency component of A_2 is coincident with the completion of closure of the aortic valve. *Right.* Base and apex phonocardiograms are recorded with the pulmonary valve echocardiogram. The first high-frequency component of pulmonic first heart sound (P_1) is coincident with the completion of closure of the pulmonic valve. A_2, aortic second sound; AV, atrioventricular; P_2, pulmonic second heart sound; PV, pulmonic valve. *Source: Shaver JA, Salerni R, Reddy PS. Normal and abnormal heart sounds in cardiac diagnosis: I. Systolic sounds. Curr Probl Cardiol 1985:10:43. Reproduced with permission from the publisher and the authors.*

set of the Q wave to the rise of ventricular pressure; (2) ventricular mechanical systole, the sum of the isovolumic contraction time plus the ejection period minus the *hangout* interval (abnormalities of this interval exclude those conditions in which prolongation of the hangout interval is primarily responsible for the increased ejection time); and (3) hangout or impedance interval, the time between the incisura of the arterial trace and the ventricular pressure at the same level as the incisura (includes all conditions in which prolongation of this interval is primarily responsible for the increased ejection time).

Wide Physiologic Splitting of S_2 An example of wide physiologic splitting of S_2 caused by delayed electrical activation of the right ventricle secondary to right bundle-branch block is shown in Fig. 12–70. Prolongation of RV mechanical systole secondary to severe PH and PS are also responsible for a delayed P_2. Classic wide, fixed splitting of S_2 is found in patients with ASD. A composite in Fig. 12–71 documents the role played by decreased impedance of the pulmonary vascular bed in the audible expiratory splitting found in ASD, idiopathic dilatation of the pulmonary artery, and mild PS with aneurysmal dilatation of the pulmonary artery. In each case, there is a marked increase in the hangout interval, as measured by high-fidelity pressure tracings. Wide physiologic splitting secondary to a decreased LV ejection time occurs in patients with acute MR.

Reversed Splitting of S_2 Almost all cases of reversed splitting of S_2 are caused by a delay in A_2. As a result, the sequence of closure

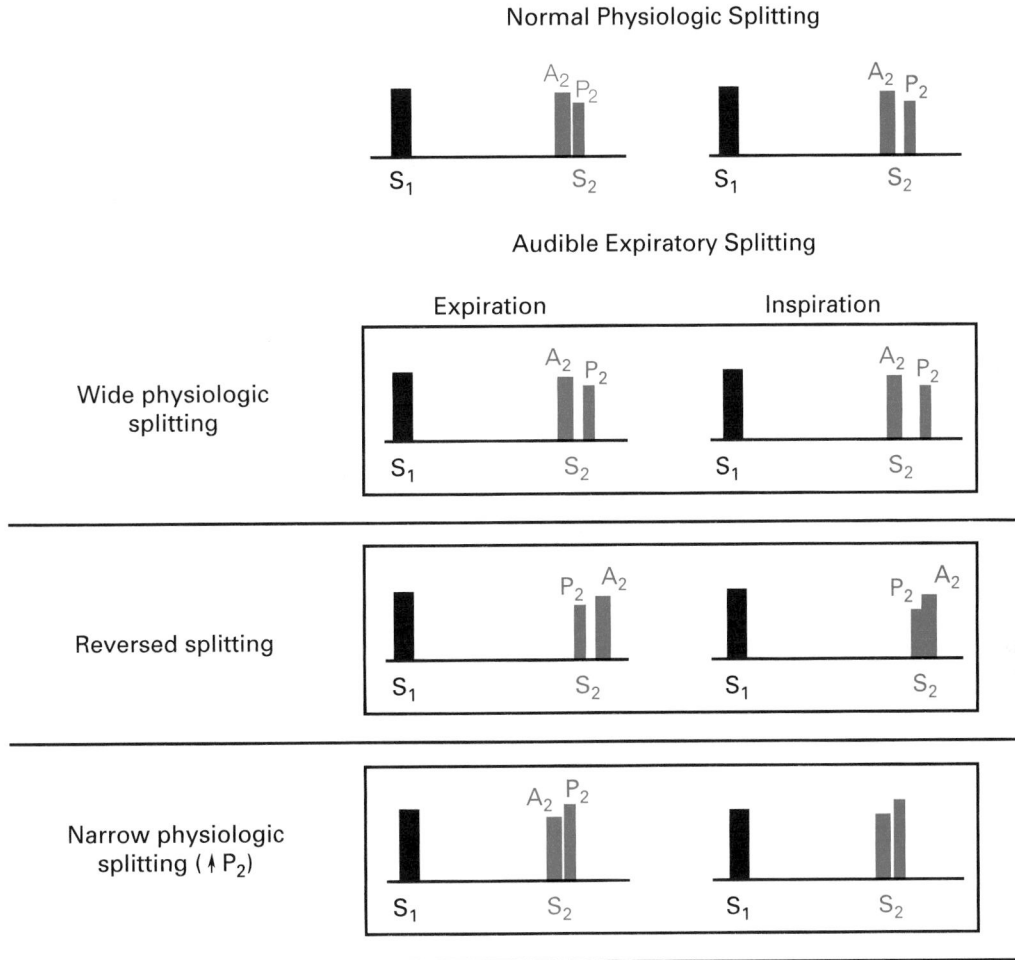

FIGURE 12–69. *Top.* Normal physiologic splitting. During expiration, the aortic second sound (A_2) and the pulmonic second heart sound (P_2) are separated by less than 30 ms and are appreciated as a single sound. During inspiration, the splitting interval widens, and A_2 and P_2 are clearly separated into two distinctly audible sounds. *Bottom.* Audible expiratory splitting. In contrast to normal physiologic splitting, two distinct sounds are easily heard during expiration. Wide physiologic splitting is caused by delay in P_2. Reversed splitting is caused by delay in A_2, resulting in paradoxical movement; that is, with inspiration, P_2 moves toward A_2, and the splitting interval narrows. Narrow physiologic splitting is seen in pulmonary hypertension, and both A_2 and P_2 are heard during expiration at a narrow splitting interval as a result of an increased intensity and high-frequency composition of P_2. S_1, first heart sound; S_2, second heart sound.

sounds is reversed, with P_2 preceding A_2. This abnormality is recognized by paradoxical movement of A_2 and P_2 with respiration.[107] During inspiration, P_2 moves toward A_2, and the splitting interval narrows, whereas during expiration, the two components separate, and audible expiratory splitting is present (see Fig. 12–69). The presence of reversed splitting of S_2 almost always indicates significant underlying cardiovascular disease.

Both RV ectopic and paced beats produce a delay in the onset of LV contraction, resulting in reversed splitting of S_2. The mechanism responsible is a delayed activation of the LV, prolonging the Q to LV pressure rise interval. The most common cause of reversed splitting is complete LBBB, which can be caused either by delayed activation of the LV, as seen in isolated proximal block, or to prolonged mechanical systole (primarily isovolumic contraction time), as seen in proximal or peripheral block invariably associated with significant LV dysfunction.

Reversed splitting of S_2 can occur in a patient with hypertrophic cardiomyopathy and is caused by the large systolic pressure gradient and prolonged LV relaxation. Although both these mechanisms can contribute to the reversed splitting observed in patients with valvular AS, an additional mechanism is an exaggerated hangout interval.[108]

In hypertensive cardiovascular disease, splitting is usually physiologic, with the intensity of A_2 being increased; however, rare instances of reversed splitting do occur. Reversed splitting of S_2 also has been reported in ischemic heart disease and during episodes of angina pectoris. The latter is extremely uncommon and rarely has been documented by phonocardiography. It is most likely caused by a prolonged isovolumic contraction time of the ischemic LV, although during angina it also can be caused by an increase in systemic arterial pressure or transient LBBB.[109]

Decreased impedance in the systemic vascular bed also can contribute to the delayed A_2 seen in poststenotic dilatation of the aorta. It also plays a role in the reversed splitting occasionally seen in both chronic AR and patent ductus arteriosus. Reversed splitting of S_2 also has been reported in some cases of type B Wolff-Parkinson-White syndrome, where early activation of the RV through an accessory pathway has caused P_2 to occur prematurely.

TABLE 12–8

Wide Physiologic Splitting of the Second Heart Sound

Delayed pulmonic closure
  Delayed electrical activation of the right ventricle
    Complete RBBB (proximal type)
    Left ventricular paced beats
    Left ventricular ectopic beats
  Prolonged right ventricular mechanical systole
    Acute massive pulmonary embolus
    Pulmonary hypertension with right heart failure
    Pulmonic stenosis with intact septum (moderate to severe)
  Decreased impedance of the pulmonary vascular bed
  (increased hangout)
    Normotensive atrial septal defect
    Idiopathic dilation of the pulmonary artery
    Pulmonic stenosis (mild)
    Atrial septal defect, postoperative (70%)
    Unexplained AES in normal subjects
Early aortic closure
  Shortened LVET
    Mitral regurgitation
    Ventricular septal defect

AES, audible expiratory splitting; LVET, left ventricular ejection time; RBBB, right bundle-branch block.
SOURCE: Shaver JA, et al. The second heart sound: newer concepts: 1. Normal and wide physiological splitting. Mod Concepts Cardiovasc Dis. 1977;46:9. Reproduced with permission from the American Heart Association, Inc., and the authors.

TABLE 12–9

Reversed Splitting of the Second Heart Sound

Delayed aortic closure
  Delayed electrical activation of the left ventricle
    Complete LBBB (proximal type)
    Right ventricular paced beat
    Right ventricular ectopic beats
  Prolonged left ventricular mechanical systole
    Complete LBBB (peripheral type)
    Left ventricular outflow tract obstruction
    Hypertensive cardiovascular disease
    Arteriosclerotic heart disease
     Chronic ischemic heart disease
     Angina pectoris
  Decreased impedance of the systemic vascular bed
  (increased hangout)
    Poststenotic dilation of the aorta secondary to aortic
     stenosis or regurgitation
    Patent ductus arteriosus
Early pulmonic closure
  Early electrical activation of the right ventricle
    Wolff-Parkinson-White syndrome, type B

LBBB, left bundle-branch block.
SOURCE: Shaver JA, et al. The second heart sound: newer concepts: 2. Paradoxical splitting and narrow physiological splitting. Mod Concepts Cardiovasc Dis. 1977;46:13. Reproduced with permission from the American Heart Association, Inc., and the authors.

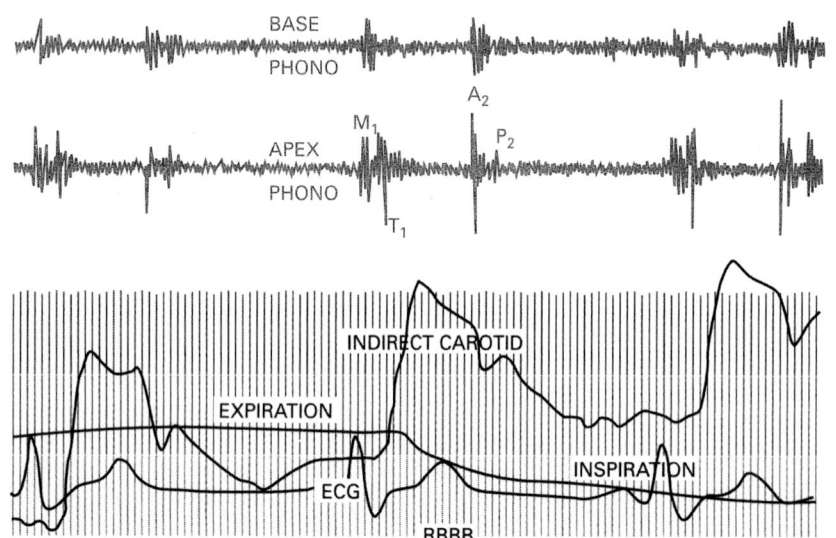
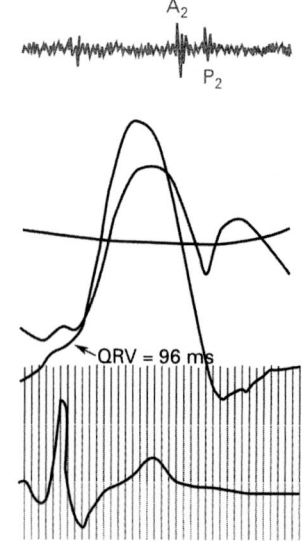

FIGURE 12–70. *Left.* Wide physiologic splitting of the second heart sound (S₂) is seen in a patient with complete right bundle-branch block. Audible expiratory splitting, which widens normally with inspiration, is present. Note also the wide splitting of the first heart sound into its mitral (M₁) and tricuspid (T₁) sound components, as recorded at the apex. *Right.* The base phonocardiogram is recorded simultaneously with high-fidelity catheters in the right ventricle (RV) and pulmonary artery during cardiac catheterization. There is marked prolongation of the Q to the onset of the right ventricular (RV) pressure rise of 96 ms, resulting in wide physiologic splitting of S₂. The delayed pulmonic second heart sound (P₂) is secondary to delayed activation of the right ventricle. RBBB, right bundle-branch block. *Source: Shaver JA. Current uses of phonocardiography in clinical practice. In: Rapaport E, ed. Cardiology Update: Reviews for Physicians. New York: Elsevier; 1981:337. Reproduced originally in part (left panel) with permission from the publisher and author; and from Shaver JA, Salerni R, Reddy PS. Normal and abnormal heart sounds in cardiac diagnosis: I. Systolic sounds. Curr Probl Cardiol. 1985;10:48. Reproduced in total with permission from the publisher and authors.*

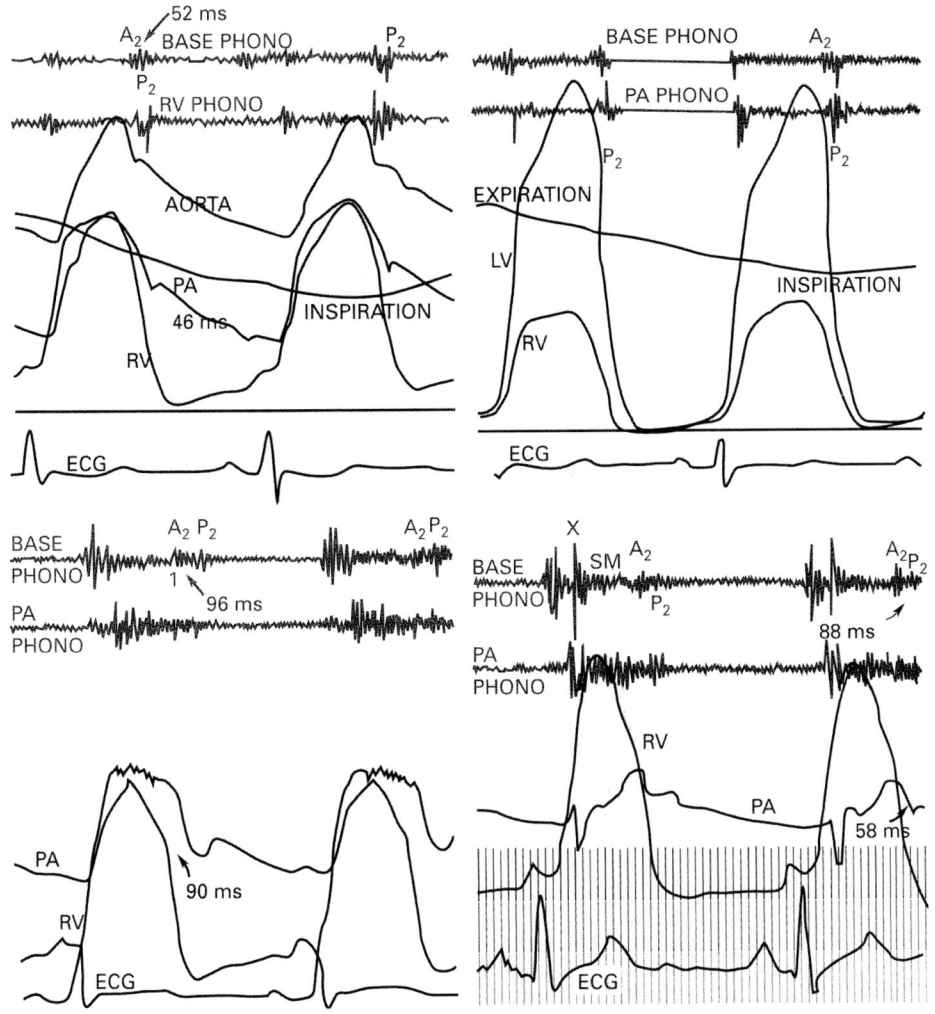

interval) can be encroached on as the PH progressively decreases the capacitance and increases the resistance of the pulmonary vascular bed[110] (Fig. 12–71). Thus a spectrum of the width of splitting can be seen in PH, depending on the degree of selective prolongation of RV systole, always in the setting of a narrow hangout interval. Similar hemodynamic correlates have been found in patients having hyperkinetic PH secondary to large ASDs. Fixed splitting of S_2 occasionally has been documented in severe RV failure secondary to PH.

Single S_2

All conditions listed in Table 12–2 that delay A_2 can produce a single S_2 when the splitting interval becomes less than 30 ms. Also, conditions in which one component of S_2 is either absent or inaudible will produce a single. In Eisenmenger VSD, the duration of RV and LV systole is necessarily equal, and a loud, single S_2 is appreciated because A_2 and P_2 occur simultaneously. The most common cause of an apparently single S_2 is the inability to hear the fainter of the two components of the sound (usually P_2) because of emphysema, obesity, or respiratory noise. Single S_2 often is seen in individuals older than 50 years of age.

[ ] OPENING SNAPS

Opening of the normal AV valve is almost always a silent event. With thickening and deformity of the leaflets, usually rheumatic in origin, however, a sound is generated in early diastole in a manner analogous to ejection sounds arising from deformed semilunar valves. The term *opening snap* was first used by Thayer[111] in 1908 to describe the high-frequency early diastolic sound in MS. Thayer also recognized that the sound

FIGURE 12–71. *Upper left.* Sound and pressure correlates of the second heart sound (S_2) in a 45-year-old woman with a normotensive atrial septal defect (shunt 2:1). Wide, fixed splitting of S_2 is demonstrated; pulmonic second heart sound (P_2) and aortic second sound (A_2) are coincident with their respective incisurae, and the duration of the *hangout* interval is nearly equal to the A_2–P_2 interval. *Upper right.* Simultaneous right ventricular (RV) and left ventricular (LV) pressures clearly show that the duration of RV and LV systole is equal. *Lower left.* Sound and pressure correlates of a patient with idiopathic dilatation of the pulmonary artery. P_2 is coincident with the incisura of the pulmonary artery and separated from the RV pressure tracing by a hangout interval of 90 ms (almost identical to the splitting interval). *Lower right.* Similar sound and pressure correlates in a patient with mild valvular pulmonic stenosis and aneurysmal dilatation of the pulmonary artery. Most of the delay in P_2 is caused by a wide hangout interval of 56 ms. In each patient all pressures are recorded by catheter-tipped micromanometers. PA, pulmonary angiograph; SM, systolic murmur.
Source: Shaver JA, O'Toole JD. Second heart sound: the role of altered greater and lesser circulation. In: Leon DF, Shaver JA, eds. Physiologic Principles of Heart Sounds and Murmurs. Monograph 46. New York: American Heart Association; 1975:63. Reproduced originally in part (top panel) with permission from the publisher and the authors; and from Shaver JA. The second heart sound: hemodynamic determinants. Acta Cardiol. 1985;40:12. Reproduced in total with permission from the publisher and authors.

Narrow Physiologic Splitting Narrow physiologic splitting of S_2 is a common finding in severe PH, as shown in Fig. 12–69. In contrast to the normal situation, where only a single sound is heard during expiration, both A_2 and P_2 are easily heard, even though the splitting interval is less than 30 ms because of the increased intensity and high-frequency composition of P_2. Wide, persistent splitting becomes a useful sign of abnormal RV performance in patients with primary PH. To reconcile these different responses in S_2 when PH develops, it is essential to appreciate that normally the duration of RV and LV systole is nearly equal and that a potential interval (the normally wide right-sided hangout

had been absent in those patients who, on autopsy, had markedly thickened and essentially immobile valves. This mechanism was confirmed by hemodynamic and angiographic studies that showed sudden checking of the early diastolic descent of the funnel-shaped stenotic valve when its elastic limits were met. Phono-echocardiography has shown an even more precise correlation of the opening snap with the maximum opening motion of the anterior mitral leaflet (see Fig. 12–62, *left*).

The opening snap is a crisp, sharp sound that can be heard in the midprecordial location, usually best in the area from the left sternal border to just inside the apex. Often it is heard well at the base of the heart and frequently is not well heard at the maximal intensity of the diastolic murmur. The diastolic rumble generally follows the opening snap by a short interval. There is no variation in the intensity or timing of the mitral opening snap with respiration.

As with ejection sounds of valvular origin, the intensity of the mitral opening snap correlates well with the mobility of the valve. A loud opening snap is found in mobile stenotic valves with good excursions (see Fig. 12–62, *left*), whereas the opening snap is absent with severe calcific fixation of the valve. The intensity of M_1 parallels the intensity of the opening snap.

The opening snap follows A_2 by an interval of 0.03 to 0.15 s. In patients with mild MS, the interval is usually long, whereas in patients with more severe stenosis, the A_2–opening snap interval is shorter. The A_2–opening snap interval in atrial fibrillation can vary with cycle length. With a short preceding RR interval, the left atrium has not had time to empty, the left atrial pressure remains high, and the A_2–opening snap interval is short. With a longer preceding RR interval, the left atrial pressure falls, and the A_2–opening snap interval widens.

The opening snap occurs at the maximal mitral valve opening shortly after LV–left atrial pressure crossovers. Factors that influence the timing of the opening snap relative to A_2 are (1) the rate of LV pressure decline, (2) the level of the LV pressure at the time of A_2, and (3) the level of the left atrial pressure.[112] Increasing severity of MS is usually accompanied by a shortening of the A_2–opening snap interval. Because this interval is multifactorially determined, there is an imperfect correlation between the A_2–opening snap interval and the mitral valve area. Tricuspid valve stenosis also can produce an opening snap. This sound is frequently not detected because the findings of coexisting MS, which is almost invariably present, overshadow those of TS. When present, it generally follows the mitral opening snap. An early diastolic sound can also be caused by a right or left atrial myxoma. Although the clinical findings of a left atrial myxoma can be similar to those of MS, the echocardiographic picture is classic (see Fig. 12–62, *center*). The tumor *plop* occurs at the maximal diastolic descent of the myxoma.

Although an opening snap is rarely heard with normal valves, it can be heard in situations where high flow exists across the AV valves. An early diastolic sound is frequently present in large ASDs coincident with maximal opening of the tricuspid valve. The opening snap must be differentiated from other early diastolic sounds such as the S_3, the pulmonary component of a widely split S_2, and a pericardial knock.

【 】 THE THIRD AND FOURTH HEART SOUNDS

S_3 and S_4 are low-frequency events related to early and late diastolic filling of the ventricles (Fig. 12–72). When they are heard in disease states, they are called *gallop sounds,* and their presence gives valuable information to the clinician regarding the status of ventricular function and compliance.

The Third Heart Sound

Physiologic S_3 The physiologic S_3 is a benign finding commonly heard in children, adolescents, and young adults, but it is rarely present in adults after 40 years of age and, when

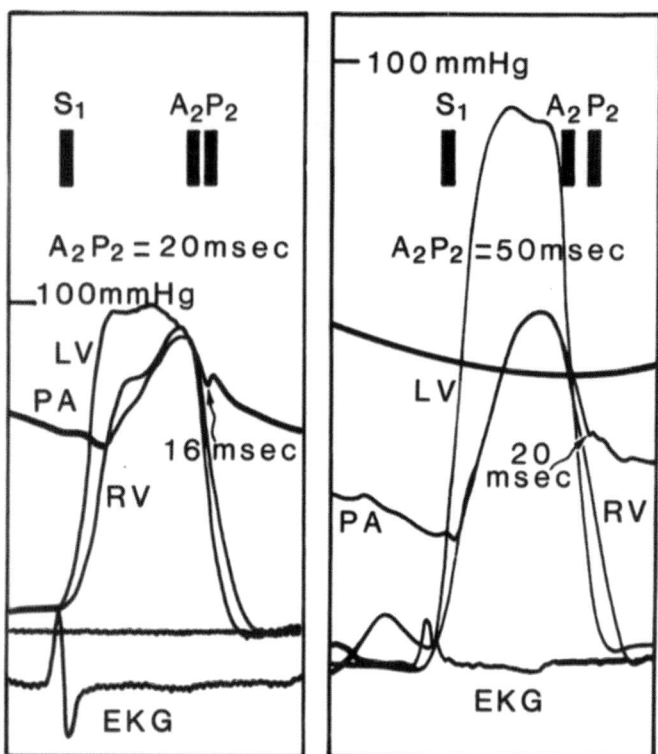

FIGURE 12–72. Sound-pressure correlates recorded by high-fidelity, catheter-tipped micromanometers in two patients with severe pulmonary hypertension. (*Left panel*) Narrow physiologic splitting (less than 30 ms) is present. (*Right panel*) Wide splitting is shown. There is marked reduction in hangout interval in both patients. *In the left panel,* duration of left and right ventricular (LV and RV) systole is nearly equal, and narrow splitting of second heart sound results. In right panel, significant prolongation of RV mechanical systole beyond LV systole delays pulmonic valve closure sound (P_2), resulting in wide splitting of second heart sound. A_2, aortic valve closure sound; PA, pulmonary artery; S_1, first heart sound.

present, is often associated with a thin, asthenic body habitus. This is a low-frequency sound that follows A_2 by 120 to 200 ms and occurs during rapid filling of the ventricle (Fig. 12–73, *top panel*).[113,114] It is best heard at the apex in the left lateral position with the stethoscope's bell pressed lightly against the skin and is differentiated from the pathologic S_3 primarily by the "company it keeps."[115]

Pathologic S_3 Most agree that the pathologic S_3 is an exaggeration of the physiologic S_3, with a common mechanism of production.[116] The exact genesis of the S_3 remains controversial. Three major mechanisms of production have been proposed: the valvular theory, the ventricular theory, and the impact theory. The most popular theory has indicated that these sounds have their origins within the left or right ventricle or their walls.[117] The dynamic interplay between the force of delivery of blood into the ventricle and the ability of the ventricle to accept this flow is an important factor in the genesis of this sound. When there is appropriate interaction between these factors, the S_3 occurs when the ventricle suddenly reaches its elastic limits and abruptly decelerates the onrushing column of blood, thereby setting the entire cardiohemic system into vibration. Thus an S_3 can be produced by excessive rapid filling into a ventricle with normal or increased compliance,

Diastolic Filling Sounds

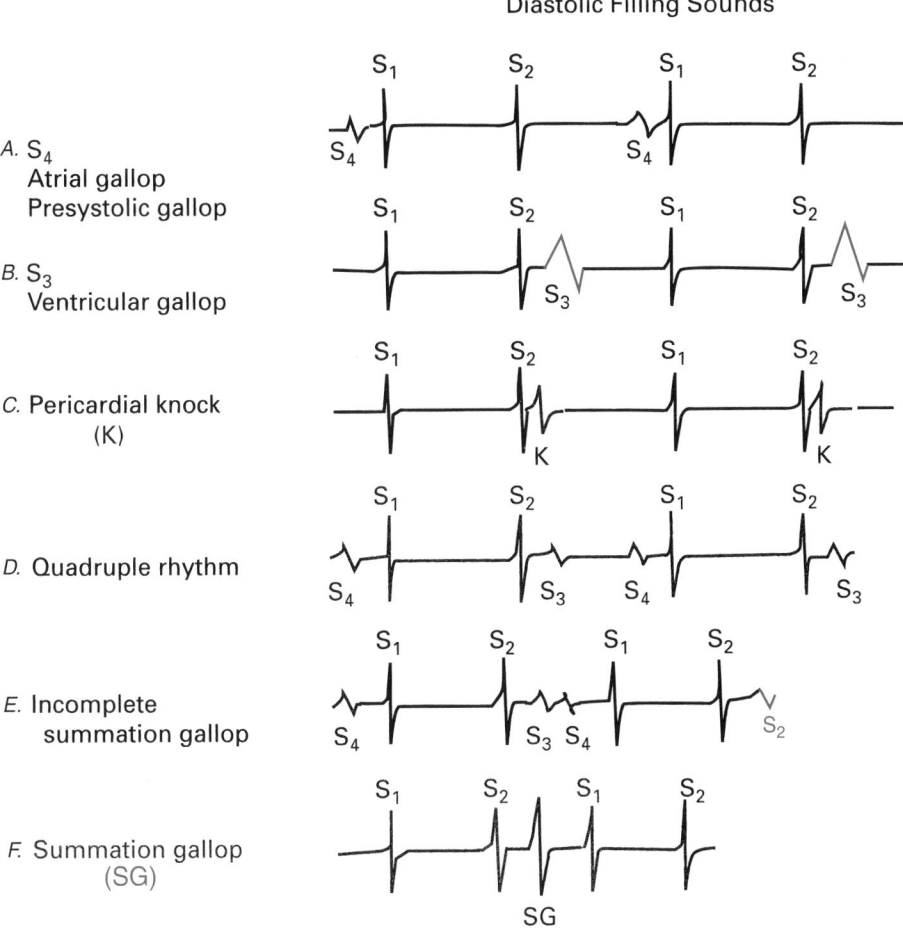

A. S_4
Atrial gallop
Presystolic gallop

B. S_3
Ventricular gallop

C. Pericardial knock
(K)

D. Quadruple rhythm

E. Incomplete
summation gallop

F. Summation gallop
(SG)

FIGURE 12–73. A. The fourth heart sound (S_4) occurs in presystole and is frequently called an atrial, or presystolic gallop. **B.** The third heart sound (S_3) occurs during the rapid phase of ventricular filling. It is a normal finding and is commonly heard in children and young adults, disappearing with increasing age. When it is heard in a patient with cardiac disease, it is called a pathologic S_3, or ventricular gallop, and usually indicates ventricular dysfunction or atrioventricular (AV) valvular incompetence. **C.** In constrictive pericarditis, a sound in early diastole, the pericardial knock (K), is heard earlier and is louder and higher pitched than the usual pathologic S_3. **D.** A quadruple rhythm results if both the fourth heart sound (S_4) and S_3 are present. **E.** At faster heart rates, the S_3 and S_4 occur in rapid succession and can give the illusion of a middiastolic rumble. **F.** When the heart rate is sufficiently fast, the two rapid phases of ventricular filling reinforce each other, and a loud summation gallop (SG) can appear; this sound can be louder than either the S_3 or S_4 alone.

as with high-output states and MR, or by a normal or less than normal rate of filling into a ventricle with decreased compliance, as in patients with hypertrophic cardiomyopathy. Likewise, decreased rates of filling into overfilled ventricles with large end-systolic volumes, as seen in patients with LV systolic dysfunction, will produce this sound.[118]

Although this mechanism is likely responsible for the sound recorded within the ventricular cavity and on its epicardial surface, Reddy and coworkers[119] have reported convincing data that the sound heard with the stethoscope can be caused by the dynamic impact of the heart with the chest wall. This theory explains the S_3 present in hyperdynamic states as well as those with an increased end-systolic volume secondary to LV dysfunction. In the latter, the space between the enlarged heart and the lateral chest wall is diminished, thereby facilitating a more forceful impact in early diastole. This results in an exaggerated rapid filling wave on the apexcardiogram and the

prominent S_3 pathognomonic of congestive failure (see Fig. 12–73, *lower panel*). Table 12–10 tabulates the major factors responsible for the production of the S_3 as recorded within the LV and on the chest wall.

A convenient classification of physiologic and pathologic states with an S_3 is presented in Table 12–11. Both the intensity and timing of the pathologic S_3 associated with LV dysfunction are related to the patient's volume status. With diuresis, the S_3 can decrease in intensity or disappear, and it tends to move away from A_2. A loud, persistent S_3 with cardiomyopathy or acute MI is an ominous sign associated with high mortality, whereas prompt subsidence with therapy suggests a more favorable outlook. LV third heart sounds are heard best at the apex, whereas RV third heart sounds are heard at the lower left sternal edge and can increase in intensity with inspiration.

In chronic AR, even though end-diastolic volume is increased, end-systolic volume may not be increased until LV dysfunction develops. As LV dysfunction develops, the ejection fraction decreases, resulting in an increased end-systolic volume, and a pathologic S_3 appears in these patients.[120] An S_3 is very common in acute AR and is usually followed by the middiastolic component of the Austin Flint rumble.

A pathologic S_3 resulting from excessive early diastolic filling is common in hyperkinetic states and AV valve regurgitation and often initiates a short flow rumble. It is often present in large left-to-right shunts caused by high flow across the mitral valve with VSD or patent ductus arteriosus and with high flow across the tricuspid valve with ASD. The presence of this sound in these conditions does not imply congestive heart failure, and such patients can maintain normal myocardial contractility for years after the S_3 is detected. Pathologic third heart sounds are heard in both restrictive and hypertrophic cardiomyopathy. In constrictive pericarditis, an early prominent sound of a somewhat higher frequency is heard, the *pericardial knock* (see Fig. 12–72). The evidence to date points to the simultaneous occurrence of the pericardial knock and the termination of rapid filling of the ventricles.

The Fourth Heart Sound

Precordial vibrations resulting from atrial contraction are normally neither palpable nor audible. Under pathologic conditions, forceful atrial contraction generates a low-frequency sound (S_4) just

TABLE 12–10

Hemodynamic Determinants of the S₃

Ability of the ventricle to accept flow during the rapid
   phase of diastolic filling
     Rate of relaxation of the ventricle
     End-systolic or residual volume of the ventricle
     Compliance of the relaxed ventricle
     Nonobstructed atrioventricular valve
Atrial pressure head
     Atrial blood volume
     Atrial compliance
Dynamic impact of the heart with the chest wall
     Architecture of the thorax
     Cardiac size
     Cardiac motion within the thorax
     Phase of respiration
     Position of the patient

SOURCE: Shaver JA et al. Early diastolic events associated with the physiologic and pathologic S₃. Am J Cardiol. 1984;14(suppl 5):45. Reproduced with permission from the publisher and authors.

TABLE 12–11

Third Heart Sound (S₃), Ventricular Diastolic Gallop, Protodiastolic Gallop, and Pericardial Knock

Physiologic S₃—children and young adults
   Decreased prevalence with increasing age
Pathologic S₃
   Ventricular dysfunction—poor systolic function,
     increased end-diastolic and end-systolic volume,
     decreased ejection fraction, and high filling pressures
      Idiopathic dilated cardiomyopathy
      Ischemic heart disease
      Valvular heart disease
      Congenital heart disease
      Systemic and pulmonary hypertension
   Excessively rapid early diastolic ventricular filling
     Hyperkinetic states
      Anemia
      Thyrotoxicosis
      Arteriovenous fistula
     Atrioventricular valve incompetence
     Left-to-right shunts
   Restrictive myocardial or pericardial disease
   Constrictive pericarditis (pericardial knock)
   Restrictive cardiomyopathy
   Hypertrophic cardiomyopathy?

---

prior to S_1 (also termed the *atrial diastolic gallop* or the *presystolic gallop*). Atrial contraction must be present for production of an S_4. It is absent in atrial fibrillation and in other rhythms in which atrial contraction does not precede ventricular contraction. The S_4 follows the onset of the P wave of the ECG by approximately 70 ms. Audibility of the S_4 depends not only on its intensity and frequency but also on its separation from S_1. The degree of this separation is determined primarily by the PR interval, but it is also somewhat influenced by the P-S_4 and the Q-S_1 intervals. A loud S_1 also can mask the audibility of a preceding softer S_4. The S_4 is best heard at the apex impulse with the patient turned in the left lateral position. It varies considerably with respiration, usually being heard best during expiration. A left-sided S_4 can radiate to the brachiocephalic and carotid vessel and be best heard in the areas in patients with severe lung disease or who are very obese. A left-sided S_3 can do likewise. A left-sided S_4 and S_3 can also be augmented post-tussively and with sustained handgrip exercise. Both the intensity and timing of the S_4 are closely related to the end-diastolic volume of the ventricle. Maneuvers that increase venous return increase the audibility by increasing the intensity of the sound and by causing it to occur earlier, thereby separating it further from S_1. Decreased venous return does the opposite (see Fig. 12–62). Audible fourth heart sounds are usually accompanied by a palpable presystolic apical impulse in the absence of obesity, emphysema, and so forth, but occasionally, palpable presystolic impulses are not audible. The S_4 generated by a forceful right atrial contraction is usually heard best at the lower left sternal border. Unlike the left-sided S_4, it tends to be accentuated with inspiration. It is also accompanied by prominent *a* waves in the JVP and is occasionally audible over the right jugular vein.[121]

As with the S_3, both the ventricular origin of the S_4 sound as a result of the abrupt deceleration of the atrial contribution to late diastolic filling and the impact theory have been proposed. It is likely that the former is responsible for the sounds recorded within the ventricular cavities or on their epicardial surfaces, whereas the latter mechanism is responsible for the S_4 auscultated at the chest wall.

The presence of an S_4, particularly when associated with a palpable presystolic apical impulse, is an abnormal finding. Although it is considered to be a normal finding in older subjects by some investigators, others feel strongly that a definite S_4 in a middle-aged or older person is unlikely to be a normal event.[121] Conditions such as obesity, emphysema, or barrel-chest deformity can hinder the clinical detection of both an S_4 and an apical presystolic impulse.

The common pathologic conditions in which S_4 is heard are listed in Table 12–13. A forceful atrial contraction into a hypertrophied, noncompliant ventricle almost always produces an early and easily audible and recordable S_4. The severe LV hypertrophy present in systemic hypertension, severe valvular AS, and hypertrophic cardiomyopathy often is responsible for a loud S_4 (Fig. 12–74). In each case, the S_4 is associated with a prominent apical presystolic impulse and is widely separated from S_1.

An audible S_4 with a palpable presystolic impulse is common in patients with ischemic heart disease during an acute episode of angina and in the early phases of transmural MI. Its prevalence is also increased with prior MI; however, audible fourth heart sounds in patients with ischemic heart disease without prior infarction or hypertension are uncommon.[97] In patients with LV aneurysm or idiopathic or ischemic cardiomyopathy, abnormal fourth heart sounds are commonly present and often associated with an S_3, producing a quadruple rhythm. If tachycardia is present, or if the PR interval is prolonged, S_3 and S_4 can fuse, giving rise to a loud summation gallop (see Fig. 12–72).

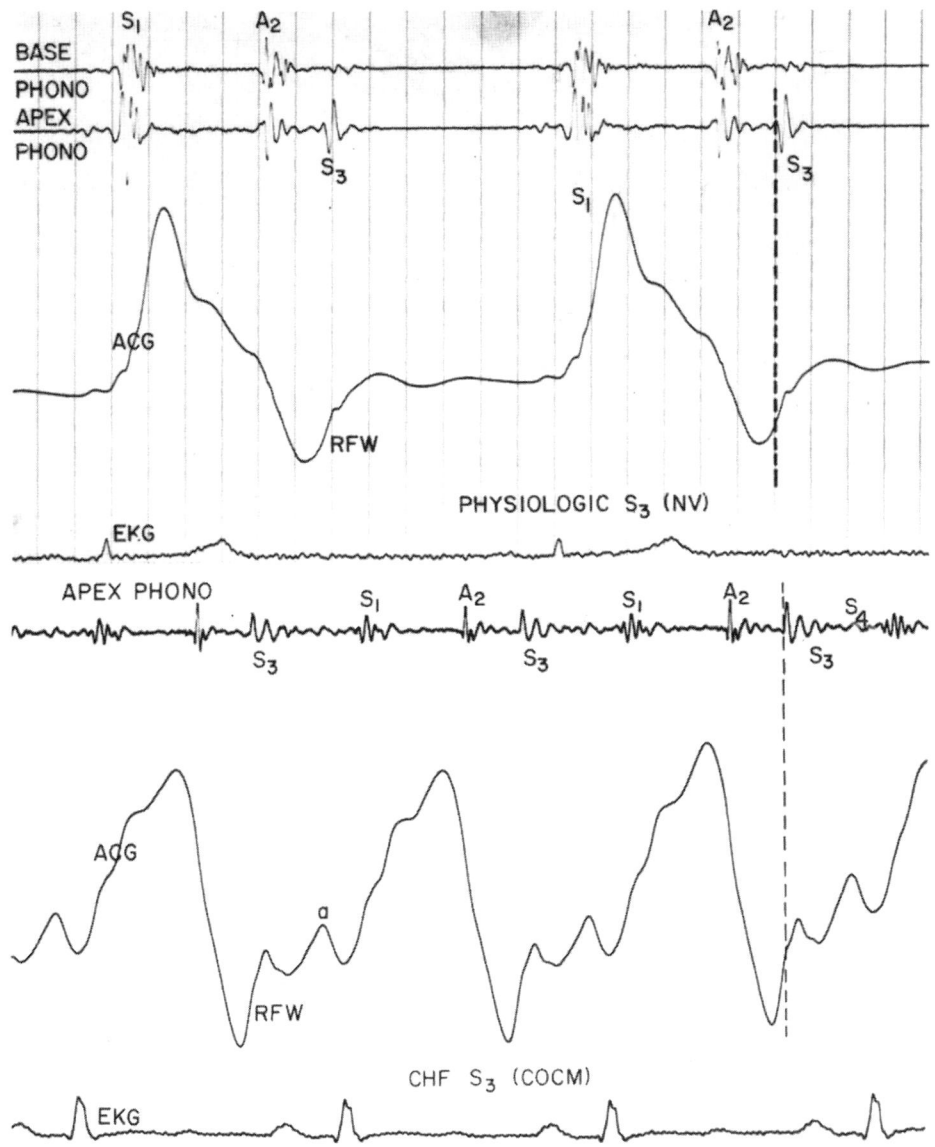

FIGURE 12–74. *Top.* A physiologic third heart sound (S₃) (normal variant) recorded in a 24-year-old woman without evidence of cardiovascular disease. The onset of the S₃ occurs during the rapid filling wave (RFW) of the apexcardiogram (ACG) between the *O* and *F* points. The remainder of the cardiovascular examination was entirely within normal limits. *Bottom.* A very prominent S₃ gallop is recorded in a patient with severe congestive cardiomyopathy (COCM). On physical examination, there was a small-volume carotid pulse and marked engorgement of the neck veins with elevated venous pressure. The ACG shows a very prominent presystolic pulsation (a), and an extremely rapid filling wave is present. The onset of the S₃ occurs during the RFW of the ACG. The first heart sound is soft. A₂, aortic second sound; CHF, chronic heart failure; S₁, first heart sound; S₄, fourth heart sound. *Source: Shaver JA. Early diastolic events associated with the physiologic and pathologic S₃. J Cardiogr. 1984;14(suppl 5):30. Reproduced with permission from the publisher and the authors.*

Quadruple rhythms are common in hyperkinetic states where the S₃ is caused by excessively rapid early diastolic filling and the S₄ results from a forceful atrial contraction into a volume-loaded ventricle. With varying degrees of tachycardia, incomplete summation can occur, simulating a diastolic rumble, or complete fusion can occur, generating a loud summation gallop (see Fig. 12–72). In acute AV valve regurgitation, vigorous atrial contraction into an acutely volume-loaded ventricle can produce an S₄ associated with a presystolic apical impulse (see Fig. 12–61). At times it can be difficult to appreciate because of the masking effect of the loud systolic murmur. This contrasts with most patients with

chronic MR, who do not have an S₄ but frequently have an S₃.

Presystolic and isolated diastolic fourth heart sounds as well as summation gallops can be heard with varying degrees of heart block. First-degree heart block facilitates audibility of the S₄ because it further separates S₄ from S₁. In 2:1 heart block, an isolated S₄ can be heard in diastole, and a presystolic S₄ can be audible because of the increase in diastolic volume. In complete heart block, S₄ can be heard randomly throughout diastole, and when it occurs simultaneously with rapid early ventricular filling, a loud summation gallop can occur.

█ ❙ PROSTHETIC VALVE SOUNDS

The sounds produced by prosthetic valves are varied, depending on the type of valve, its position, and whether or not it is functioning normally (see Chap. 79). Mechanical valves produce opening and closing clicks that are easily audible and in many patients can be heard even without a stethoscope. Ball-in-cage valves such as the Starr-Edwards produce the loudest and most distinctive opening and closing clicks in any position as long as there is normal valve and ventricular function. In the aortic position, a crisp opening click occurs 0.06 to 0.07 seconds after S₁ and is coincident with maximal ball excursion, as demonstrated by echocardiography. The metallic ball of the Starr-Edwards valve also produces multiple early systolic clicks when the freely moving ball bounces against the cage during early systolic ejection. These clicks occur *during* the harsh systolic ejection murmur. Absence or decrease in intensity of these clicks can occur with valve obstruction or LV dysfunction. A decrease in the intensity of the opening and closing clicks, which normally have an intensity ratio of more than 0.5, and the absence of the opening click are also indications of valve malfunction.

In the mitral position, a prominent opening click occurs 0.05 to 0.15 seconds after A₂. Narrowing of this interval indicates an elevation of left atrial pressure, which can be caused by either relative MS or MR. Interference with ball motion also can produce prolongation or significant beat-to-beat variation of this interval. A closing click is also prominent. Just as is seen with the normal S₁, there is variability in the intensity of the closing click, with the changing rate ratio (RR) intervals of atrial fibrillation being louder with short RR intervals and softer with long intervals. A decreased intensity with first-degree AV block also occurs because of partial arteriogenic closure of the valve, thus reducing the ball excursion and therefore the click intensity. Although a decreased intensity of the valve clicks occurs with valve malfunction, the presence of normal ball motion on an echocardiogram suggests that a nonvalvular cause such as severe LV dysfunction is responsible for the decreased intensity.

The auscultatory findings of disk-valve prostheses vary, depending on the type of disk valve. Central occluder valves such as the Beall valve, which was used predominantly in the mitral and tricuspid positions, produce distinct, audible opening and closing sounds. The more commonly used tilting-disk valves do not ordinarily produce audible opening sounds in either the aortic or mitral position. The closing sounds of disk valves are distinct and easily heard in both aortic and mitral positions. LV dysfunction, first-degree AV block, or another arrhythmia that causes the disk to move to a partially closed position prior to the onset of ventricular contraction will result in a softer sound. This finding must be distinguished from malfunction caused by either fibrosis or thrombus disturbing the disk motion. Auscultation of the bileaflet St. Jude valve is similar to that of the tilting-disk valve.

The sounds produced by tissue prosthetic valves are more like normal heart sounds than the sounds from a mechanical valve. In the aortic position, an opening sound is usually not audible. In the mitral position, an opening sound is audible in approximately 50 percent of patients at an interval of 0.07 to 0.11 seconds after A_2.

EXTRACARDIAC SOUNDS

[ ] PACEMAKER SOUNDS

High-frequency sounds of brief duration are occasionally present in patients with transvenous pacemakers located in the RV apex. They are extracardiac in origin, occurring nearly synchronously (within 6 to 10 ms) with the pacemaker spike, and are caused by stimulation of intercostal nerves adjacent to endocardial electrodes.[122] This stimulus results in contraction of the intercostal muscles; frequently, twitching of the muscle can be observed. The presence of these sounds should suggest myocardial perforation by the endocardial lead, although this is not always present. Stimulation of the pectoral muscles, as well as diaphragmatic stimulation, also has been reported to produce these extracardiac sounds.

[ ] PERICARDIAL FRICTION RUB

Inflammation of the pericardial sac with or without fluid can cause a pericardial friction rub. These friction sounds are very high pitched, leathery, and scratchy in nature. They seem close to the ear and are auscultated best with the patient leaning forward or in the knee-chest position, holding his or her breath after forced expiration. The pericardial rub can have three components during the intervals of the cardiac cycle when the heart has the greatest excursions within the pericardial sac—at the time of atrial systole, at the time of ventricular contraction, and during rapid early diastolic filling. The usual friction rub occurs during the first two intervals, although three-component rubs can be heard. Triple-component friction rubs are common in uremic pericarditis, particularly when the underly-

ing cardiac disease is hypertension. In this situation, the heart is hyperkinetic because of both pressure and volume overload as well as because of the anemia associated with renal failure. Pericardial friction rubs are very common in the acute phase of transmural MI, although they often last for only a few hours. There is a common misconception that friction rubs are not heard when there is a large amount of fluid in the pericardial sac; this is not the case, because usually some portions of the visceral and parietal pericardial surfaces are in contact despite the large amount of fluid (see Chap. 84).

Occasionally, certain midsystolic (ejection) murmurs have a scratchy character and can be misinterpreted as friction rubs. This is particularly true of the short, scratchy pulmonic ejection murmur heard in hyperthyroidism (Means-Lerman sign).[123] Such scratchy sounds should not be interpreted as a friction rub unless both systolic and diastolic components are heard.

[ ] MEDIASTINAL CRUNCH: HAMMAN SIGN

When air is present in the mediastinum, a series of scratchy sounds (Hamman sign[124]) can occur, related indirectly to both heartbeat and respiratory excursion. These sounds occur most frequently during ventricular systole and in a random fashion. The diagnosis of mediastinal emphysema can be confirmed by crepitation in the neck secondary to subcutaneous air. These crunching sounds caused by air in the mediastinum are common following cardiac surgery.

HEART MURMURS

A *cardiac murmur* is defined as a relatively prolonged series of auditory vibrations of varying intensity (loudness), frequency (pitch), quality, configuration, and duration.[125] Most authorities now agree that turbulence is the prime factor responsible for most murmurs. Turbulence occurs when blood velocity becomes critically high because of high flow, flow through an irregular or narrow area, or a combination of both. Leatham has attributed the production of murmurs to three main factors: (1) high flow rate through normal or abnormal orifices, (2) forward flow through a constricted or irregular orifice or into a dilated vessel or chamber, and (3) backward or regurgitant flow through an incompetent valve, septal defect, or patent ductus arteriosus. Frequently, a combination of these factors is operative.

Grading the loudness of a murmur from 1 to 6 as described by Freeman and Levine[126] is generally used. A *grade 1 murmur* is so faint that it can be heard only with special effort. A *grade 2 murmur* is faint but can be heard easily. A *grade 3 murmur* is moderately loud, a *grade 4 murmur* is very loud, and a *grade 5 murmur* is extremely loud and can be heard if only the edge of the stethoscope is in contact with the skin but cannot be heard if the stethoscope is removed from the skin. A *grade 6 murmur* is exceptionally loud and can be heard with the stethoscope just removed from contact with the chest. Experience has shown that systolic murmurs of grade 3 or more in intensity are usually hemodynamically significant.[127] Systolic thrills usually are associated with murmurs of grade 4 or louder. The intensity of the murmur varies directly with the velocity of blood flow across the area of murmur production. The velocity, in turn, is directly related to the pressure head that drives the blood across the murmur-producing area. For example, high velocity of flow through a small VSD produces a loud murmur, whereas a large flow at low velocity through an ASD produces no murmur. The *intensity* of a murmur as auscultated at the chest wall is also determined by the transmission characteristics of the tissues intervening between the source of the murmur and the stethoscope. Obesity, emphysema, and the presence of significant pericardial or pleural effusion will decrease the intensity of a murmur, whereas a thin, asthenic body habitus often will accentuate it.

The frequency of a murmur bears a direct relationship to the velocity of blood flow, as does the intensity of the murmur. The low-velocity flow resulting from a small pressure head across a stenotic mitral valve produces a low-pitched rumbling murmur, whereas the large diastolic pressure gradient across a regurgitant aortic valve causes a high-pitched murmur. Occasionally, the frequency composition of the same systolic murmur can vary, depending on the area auscultated. For example, the systolic murmur of AS frequently sounds higher-pitched at the apex than at the base. Some murmurs—such as the "cooing dove" regurgitant murmur of a ruptured or retroverted aortic cusp, the systolic "whoop" or "honk" of MVP, or the high-pitched systolic murmur of a degenerated bioprosthetic valve—have a very distinctive musical quality.

In addition to the intensity and frequency of murmurs, their *timing* should also be described. There is seldom any difficulty distinguishing between systole and diastole, because systole is considerably shorter at normal heart rates. At rapid heart rates, the examiner can usually time the murmur by simultaneous palpation of the lower right carotid artery or can rely on the fact that the S_2 is usually the louder sound at the base. Once S_2 is identified, murmurs can be located properly in the cardiac cycle as systolic or diastolic. The *inching* technique, popularized by Harvey and Levine, consists of slowly moving the stethoscope down from the base to the apex while repeatedly fixing the cardiac cycle in mind, using S_2 as a reference point. With sinus tachycardia, carotid sinus pressure can temporarily slow the rate and make it possible to differentiate systole from diastole. Continuous murmurs are heard throughout the cardiac cycle in systole and diastole and usually have their peak intensity around S_2.

The *location* and *radiation* of a murmur are determined multifactorially by the site of origin, intensity, and direction of blood flow, as well as by the physical characteristics of the chest. The duration and time intensity contour (murmur *envelope*) of a specific murmur are intimately related to the instantaneous pattern of blood flow velocity causing the murmur.

ACCURATE AUSCULTATION VERSUS ECHOCARDIOGRAPHY

The availability of echocardiography does not eliminate the need for properly

performed auscultation of the heart. Although echocardiography provides additional information in many patients and can even provide the correct etiology of various systolic and diastolic murmurs, it is an unnecessary step in many patients with *innocent* murmurs. Echocardiography can even lead to a false diagnosis of *echocardiographic heart disease.*

Often, a mild valvular regurgitant jet, detected by color-flow Doppler techniques, is not associated with an audible murmur despite optimal auscultation. Such regurgitant jets usually do not indicate clinical heart disease. Trivial mitral regurgitation can be detected by Doppler in up to 45 percent of normal individuals; tricuspid regurgitation in up to 70 percent; and pulmonic regurgitation in up to 88 percent. Normal aortic regurgitation is encountered much less frequently, and its incidence increases with advancing age (Fig. 12–75). Newly developed small handheld echocardiographic detectors are highly unlikely to replace the stethoscope.

SYSTOLIC MURMURS

Systolic murmurs can be classified into two basic categories—ejection (midsystolic) murmurs and regurgitant murmurs. This simple classification is attractive because it has a physiologic as well as a descriptive basis (Fig. 12–76).[128] Systolic *ejection* murmurs are caused by forward flow across the LV or RV outflow tract, whereas systolic *regurgitant* murmurs are caused by retrograde flow from a high-pressure cardiac chamber to a low-pressure chamber.

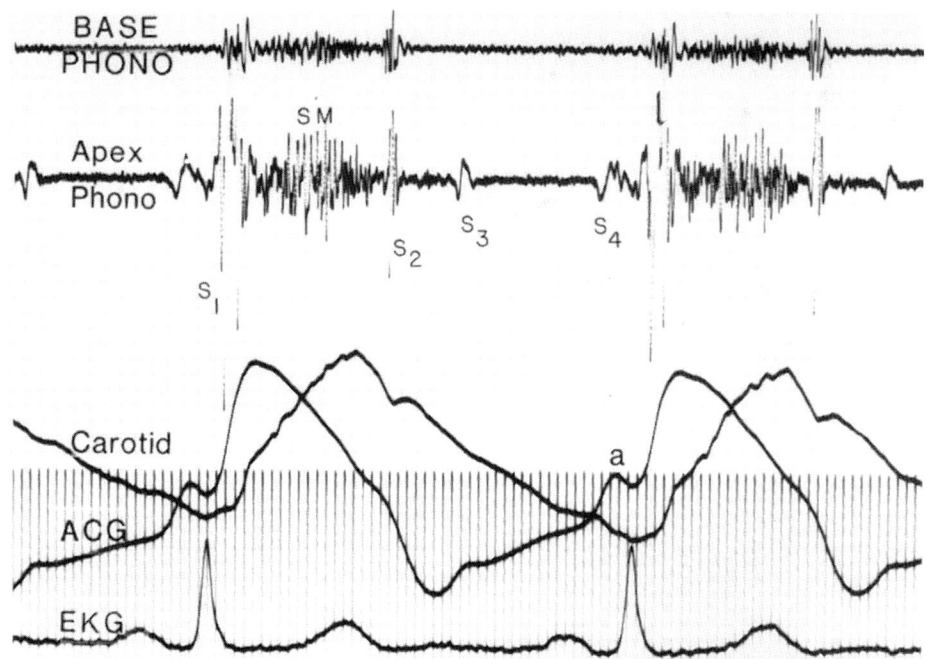

FIGURE 12–75. Atrial diastolic gallop (ADG) and ventricular diastolic gallop (VDG) recorded in an adult with severe calcific aortic stenosis. The ADG is associated with a prominent presystolic apical impulse (a); the VDG occurs during the rapid filling wave of the apexcardiogram (ACG). The carotid pulse has a very slow rate of rise and a markedly prolonged left ventricular (LV) ejection time. The classic diamond-shaped systolic ejection murmur (SM) is present at the base and apex. Note the higher-frequency composition of the SM at the apex but preservation of the crescendo-decrescendo pattern. S_1, first heart sound; S_2, second heart sound; S_3, third heart sound; S_4, fourth heart sound. *Source: Shaver JA. Current uses of phonocardiography in clinical practice. In: Rapaport E, ed. Cardiology Update: Reviews for Physicians. New York: Elsevier; 1981:356. Reproduced with permission from the publisher and author. Copyright 1981 by Elsevier Publishing Co., Inc.*

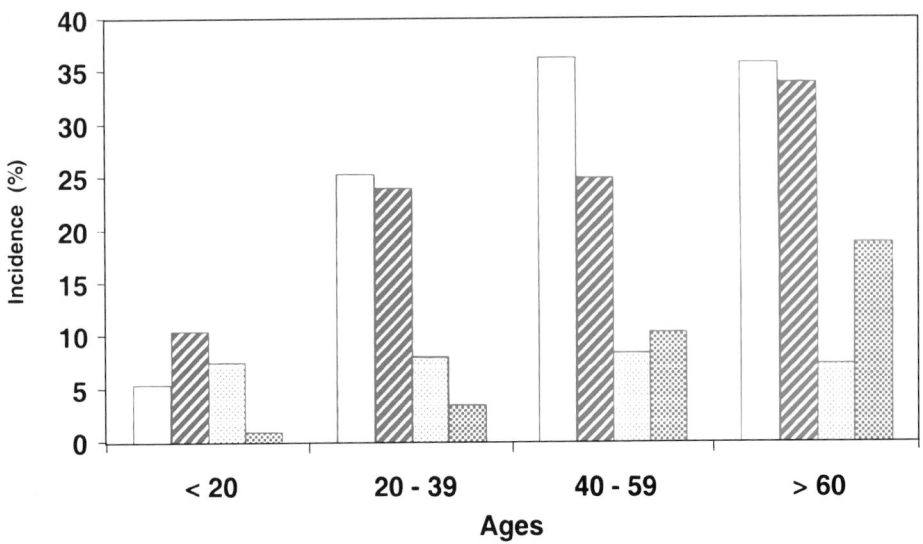

FIGURE 12–76. Percent incidence of mitral, tricuspid, pulmonic, and aortic regurgitation, respectively, by Doppler echocardiography in clinically normal subjects at various ages.

Systolic Ejection (Midsystolic) Murmurs

The systolic *ejection* murmur begins shortly after the pressure in the left or right ventricle exceeds the aortic or pulmonic diastolic pressure sufficiently to open the aortic or pulmonic valve. There is a delay between the S_1, which occurs shortly after AV pressure crossover, and the beginning of the murmur (Fig. 12–77). The murmur then waxes and wanes in a crescendo-decrescendo fashion often described as "diamond-shaped" or "spindle-shaped" in configuration. The murmur ends before the semilunar valve closure on the side from which it originates. The contour of the time-intensity pattern or *envelope* of the murmur corresponds to the contour of the flow velocity, and the murmur is heard when the sound produced during the peak turbulence exceeds the audible threshold. Thus, not only is the overall intensity of the murmur proportional to the rate of ventricular ejection, but also its shape depends on the instantaneous flow velocity during the period of ejection. As can be seen in Fig. 12–77, during normal LV ejection, a disproportionately large volume flow occurs in early systole. If velocity of flow exceeds the murmur threshold, a short midsystolic or ejection murmur results, and its envelope corresponds to the flow velocity pattern. If the stroke volume of the ventricle is increased, this pattern of ejection persists in an exaggerated fashion; the resulting murmur has a tendency to peak early in systole and fade out approximately halfway through the ejection phase. Such murmurs have been referred to as "kite-shaped" and are common in high-output states or conditions such as AR or heart block, where stroke volume is high (Fig. 12–78).

The flow characteristics of normal RV ejection are somewhat different. Early ejection rates are not nearly as high, and the flow curve peaks somewhat later, having a more rounded contour. This flow pattern can well explain some of the long systolic ejection murmurs heard in ASDs and the straight-back syndrome, where only minimal gradients are found across the RV outflow tract. With true valvular obstruction, rapid early ejection is no longer possible; the aortic flow velocity patterns become rounded, resulting in the more symmetric murmur of AS. In such cases, the in-

stantaneous flow pattern is determined by the instantaneous pressure head with the resulting high correlation between the contour of the pressure gradient and the murmur envelope.[129] If LV or RV obstruction is severe, systole is prolonged, and closure sound of the semilunar valve is delayed. The murmur, however, always stops before the closure sound on the side from which it originates, although it can envelop the closure sound of the *opposite side* of the circulation.

The intensity of ejection murmurs closely parallels changes in cardiac output. Any condition that increases forward flow—such as exercise, anxiety, fever, or increased stroke volume associated with the long diastolic filling period after a premature beat—increases the intensity of the murmur. Likewise, conditions that decrease cardiac output—congestive heart failure, β-blockade, or other negative inotropic agents—will decrease the intensity of the ejection murmur. Furthermore, definitive diagnosis of the systolic murmur often can be made during auscultation by careful attention to the response of the murmur to various bedside maneuvers that alter the flow and loading conditions of the heart.[130] These maneuvers include respiration, the strain and release phases of the Valsalva maneuver, standing, squatting, passive leg elevation, isometric hand-grip exercise, and transient arterial occlusion.

〔 〕INNOCENT MURMURS

Innocent murmurs are always systolic ejection in nature and occur without evidence of physiologic or structural abnormalities in the cardiovascular system when peak flow velocity in early systole exceeds the murmur threshold.[127] These murmurs are almost always less than grade 3 in intensity and vary considerably from examination to examination and with body position and level of physical activity. They are not associated with a thrill or with radiation to the carotid arteries or axillae. They can arise from flow across either the normal LV or RV outflow tract and always end well before semilunar valve closure.

Innocent murmurs are found in approximately 30 to 50 percent of all children. In young children, especially children 3 to 8 years of age, the vibratory systolic (Still) murmur is common. It has a very distinctive quality described as "groaning," "croaking," "buzzing," or "twanging." It is heard best along the left sternal border at the third or fourth interspace and disappears by puberty. Regardless of the exact cause, most authorities agree that this murmur originates from flow in the LV outflow tract.

Innocent systolic ejection murmurs also have been attributed to flow in the normal RV outflow tract and have been termed *innocent pulmonic systolic murmurs* because the site of their maximal intensity is auscultated best in the pulmonic area at the second left interspace with radiation along the left sternal border. These are low to medium in pitch, with a blowing quality, and are common

Systolic Murmurs

A. Ejection murmurs: due to forward flow across the right or left ventricular outflow tract

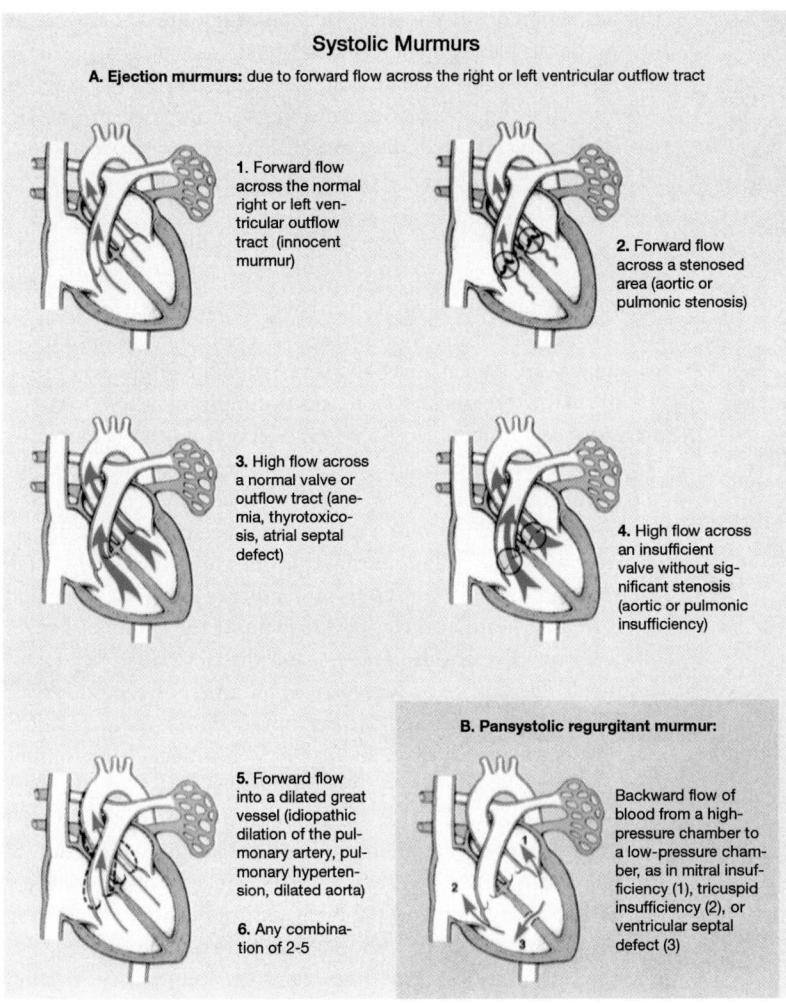

1. Forward flow across the normal right or left ventricular outflow tract (innocent murmur)

2. Forward flow across a stenosed area (aortic or pulmonic stenosis)

3. High flow across a normal valve or outflow tract (anemia, thyrotoxicosis, atrial septal defect)

4. High flow across an insufficient valve without significant stenosis (aortic or pulmonic insufficiency)

5. Forward flow into a dilated great vessel (idiopathic dilation of the pulmonary artery, pulmonary hypertension, dilated aorta)

6. Any combination of 2-5

B. Pansystolic regurgitant murmur:

Backward flow of blood from a high-pressure chamber to a low-pressure chamber, as in mitral insufficiency (1), tricuspid insufficiency (2), or ventricular septal defect (3)

FIGURE 12–77. Classification of systolic murmurs based on physiologic mechanism of production. *Source: Shaver JA. Heart murmurs: innocent or pathologic? (Part 1). Hosp Med. 1982. Reproduced with permission from the publisher and author.*

in children, adolescents, and young adults. Stein and coworkers,[131] who used high-fidelity catheter-tipped micromanometers to record intracardiac sound and pressure in the aorta and pulmonary artery in adults with normal valves, invariably recorded the ejection murmur in the region of the aortic valve. They concluded that these murmurs, despite their pulmonic precordial location, were aortic in origin.

In adults older than 50 years of age, innocent murmurs caused by flow in the LV outflow tract are often heard and can be of a higher frequency, with a musical quality, and frequently loudest at the apex. They can be associated with a tortuous, dilated sclerotic aortic root, often in the setting of systolic hypertension. Mild sclerosis of the aortic valve also can be present.

The preceding descriptive breakdown of innocent murmurs is based primarily on age, precordial location, and distinctive acoustic qualities. Because both innocent and pathologic ejection murmurs have the same mechanism of production, it is "the company the murmur keeps" that affords the differential diagnosis of the pathologic systolic ejection murmur from the innocent murmur[132] (Fig. 12–79).

For a murmur to be considered innocent, the examination of the cardiovascular system must disclose no abnormalities. BP and

contour of the carotid, femoral, and brachial arteries always should be evaluated carefully. There should be no elevation of the JVP, and the contour of the jugular pulse should be normal, without exaggeration of either the *a* or *v* wave. Evidence of cardiac enlargement on physical examination should be absent, and palpation of the apex in the left lateral position should show no evidence of a presystolic impulse, sustained systolic motion, or hyperdynamic circulation. On auscultation, normal physiologic splitting should be present. A physiologic S_3 is often present in association with an innocent murmur in children and young adults but should not be heard after age 30. An S_4 is rarely heard in normal children and adults (younger than 50 years of age) and always should be considered to be abnormal when associated with a palpable presystolic impulse. Systolic ejection sounds of valvular origin as well as midsystolic nonejection sounds should be absent because their presence points to minor abnormalities of the semilunar and AV valves, respectively (see Fig. 12–78). The remainder of the physical examination should show no evidence of a cardiac cause of pulmonary or systemic congestion.

The supraclavicular arterial murmur or bruit is a common finding in normal individuals, particularly children and adolescents. These murmurs are maximal in intensity above the clavicles and tend to be louder on the right, although they are often heard bilaterally. The bruit begins shortly after S_1, is diamond-shaped, and is of brief duration, usually occupying less than half of systole. Although the exact mechanism is unknown, it is related to peak flow velocity near the origin of the normal subclavian, brachiocephalic, or carotid artery. Unlike the cardiac ejection murmur, the supraclavicular murmur is always louder above the clavicles than below them. Complete compression of the subclavian artery can cause the murmur to disappear completely, whereas partial compression occasionally can intensify it. Hyperextension of the shoulders is a simple bedside maneuver that can decrease the intensity of the murmur and cause it to disappear completely. In the adult, the supraclavicular murmur must be distinguished from the murmur of true organic carotid obstruction, this latter murmur being longer, often extending through S_2, and frequently associated with a history suggestive of transient ischemic attacks.

【 】 FUNCTIONAL SYSTOLIC EJECTION MURMURS

Systolic ejection murmurs produced by high-cardiac-output states are functional and flow-related but are excluded from the category of innocent murmurs because of their associated altered physiologic state. These include the cardiac murmurs of thyrotoxicosis, pregnancy, anemia, fever, exercise, and peripheral arteriovenous fistula, which are best interpreted in light of the total presentation of the patient.[133] Although these murmurs are often grade 3 and occasionally grade 4 in intensity, they always end well before S_2 and are only rarely confused with obstruction of the LV or RV outflow tract. The large stroke volume associated with high-degree

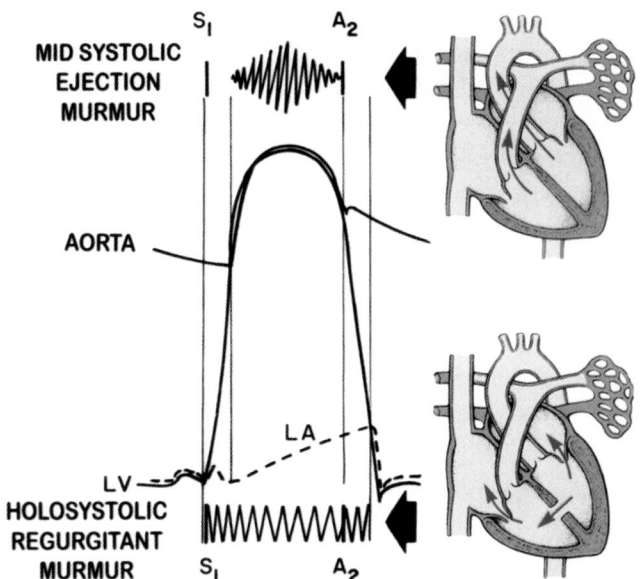

FIGURE 12–78. Midsystolic ejection murmurs are caused by forward flow across the left ventricular (LV) or right ventricular (RV) outflow tract, whereas pansystolic regurgitant murmurs are caused by retrograde flow from a high-pressure cardiac chamber to a low-pressure one. *Left.* Diagrammatic representation of the midsystolic ejection murmur and the pansystolic regurgitant murmur as related to LV, aortic, and left atrial (LA) pressures. The systolic ejection murmur occurs during the period of LV ejection; the onset of the murmur is separated from first heart sound (S_1) by the period of isovolumic contraction and the crescendo-decrescendo murmur terminates before aortic second sound A_2. The pansystolic regurgitant murmur begins with or can replace S_1, and the murmur continues up to and through A_2 as LV pressure exceeds left atrial pressure during the period of isovolumic relaxation. The murmur has a plateau configuration and varies little with respiration. *Right.* Flow diagram. *Source: Left panel reproduced from Reddy PS, Shaver JA, Leonard JJ. Cardiac systolic murmurs: pathophysiology and differential diagnosis. Prog Cardiovasc Dis. 1971;14:19. Entire figure reproduced with permission from Shaver JA. Systolic murmurs. Heart Dis Stroke. 1993;2:10.*

heart block often produces a functional systolic murmur; when found in the setting of complete heart block, beat-to-beat variations in the intensity of the murmur are present as a result of the random contribution of atrial systole to LV filling.

The functional systolic murmur in patients with a hemodynamically significant ASD is caused by the increased flow in the RV outflow tract secondary to the left-to-right shunt at the atrial level. It is easily diagnosed at the bedside "by the company it keeps." The hallmark of this condition is wide, fixed splitting of S_2 (see Fig. 12–70 *top left panel*). When the shunt is large (more than 2.5:1), a hyperdynamic parasternal impulse is usually present, and a diastolic flow rumble is often heard in the tricuspid area. In addition, the tricuspid closure is loud, and prominent *a* and *v* waves are seen in the JVP. An important condition to be differentiated from an ASD is narrowing of the anteroposterior diameter of the bony thorax. Prominent systolic murmurs—often grade 3 or 4— are heard in patients who have the straight-back syndrome and/or pectus excavatum. Audible expiratory splitting is frequently present and, coupled with a prominent pulmonary artery on the chest x-ray (secondary to the narrow anteroposterior [AP] diameter), can lead to additional unnecessary procedures to rule out an ASD. Careful attention at the bedside to the physical examination of the spine, thoracic cage, and sternum should be part of the rou-

tine evaluation of any patient with a murmur. Often, confirmation of the thoracic abnormality with a lateral chest film is all that is necessary for definitive evaluation.

Prominent systolic ejection murmurs are the rule in patients with significant AR secondary to the large forward stroke volume. Although no significant LV outflow pressure gradient is found in these patients, the intensity of such murmurs can be grade 4 or 5, and occasionally they are associated with a thrill. They always end well before aortic closure and are clearly separated from the early regurgitant murmur. Such a murmur is rarely confused with significant valvular obstruction because of the peripheral findings of wide-open AR. When true valvular obstruction is present (mixed AS and AR), the longer systolic ejection murmur is often associated with a prominent thrill. Systolic ejection murmurs caused by large RV stroke volume are also seen in severe organic pulmonic valvular regurgitation.

Ventricular ejection into a dilated great vessel is commonly associated with a systolic ejection murmur. In the elderly, such murmurs are caused by ejection into a dilated, sclerotic aorta and often are best heard at the apex. Frequently, degenerative changes of the aortic valve are also present, and the clinician is faced with a difficult decision as to whether or not true obstruction exists. The presence of significant calcification on fluoroscopic examination favors true obstruction and can be confirmed when a significant gradient is demonstrated by Doppler studies. A systolic ejection murmur caused by RV ejection into a massively dilated pulmonary artery is frequently present in idiopathic dilatation of the pulmonary artery (see Fig. 12–70), which is often confused with an ASD as a result of the wide auditory expiratory splitting present in this condition. Short systolic ejection murmurs, frequently associated with a prominent late pulmonary ejection sound, are also seen in dilated pulmonic arteries secondary to severe PH of any cause. Physical findings of severe PH are always present, including a prominent parasternal impulse and increased intensity of the pulmonic component of S_2, which is well heard at the apex. Prominent *a* waves in the neck and a right-sided S_4 that increases with inspiration are present if the ventricular septum is intact. If the PH is associated with intracardiac shunting, cyanosis frequently is present. A high-pitched, early diastolic murmur of pulmonic regurgitation secondary to severe PH often is present.

【 】 LEFT VENTRICULAR OUTFLOW TRACT MURMURS

Obstruction to LV outflow can be congenital or acquired and can be located at the valvular, supravalvular, or subvalvular level. Stenosis is occasionally present at more than one level. In the clinical evaluation, one should attempt to define the severity and the level of obstruction. A summary of this differential diagnosis can be found in Table 12–12.

The murmur of fixed stenosis of the LV outflow tract, regardless of the site, is crescendo-decrescendo, and its contour closely parallels the instantaneous pressure gradient. As long as cardiac output is maintained, there is an excellent correlation between the intensity and length of the murmur with severity of obstruction. Although there is a tendency toward late peaking of the murmur with increasing severity of the obstruction, this delayed peaking has not

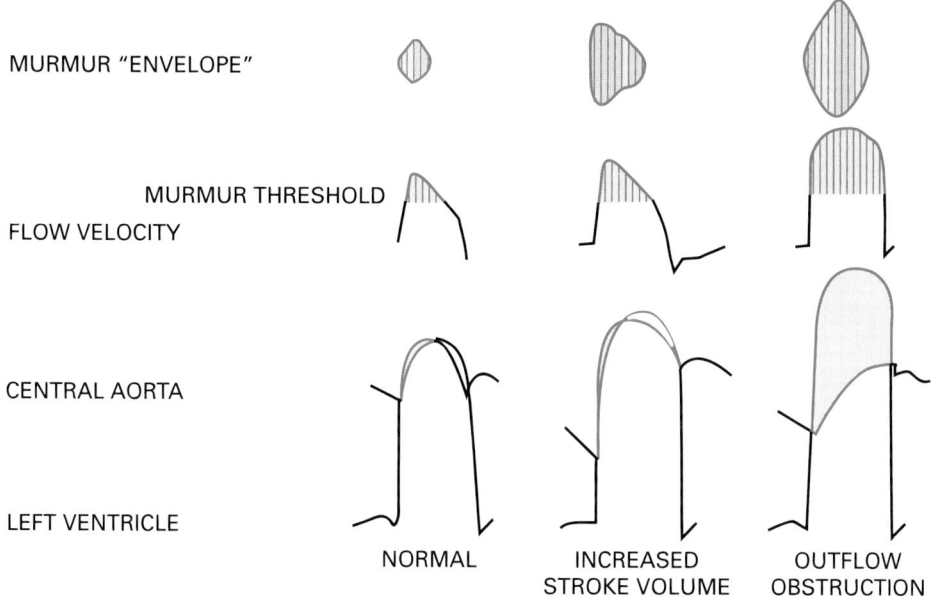

MURMUR "ENVELOPE"

MURMUR THRESHOLD
FLOW VELOCITY

CENTRAL AORTA

LEFT VENTRICLE

NORMAL   INCREASED
STROKE VOLUME   OUTFLOW
OBSTRUCTION

FIGURE 12–79. The simultaneous time-intensity course of the murmur *envelope*, aortic-flow velocity, and left ventricular (LV) and central aortic pressure. During normal LV ejection (*left*), peak flow velocity is early, with two-thirds of the ventricular volume ejected during the first half of systole. The murmur threshold can be exceeded during the early peak flow and the corresponding murmur envelope inscribed. *Center.* Exaggeration of the normal pattern of LV ejection with a high stroke volume, as in high-output states. With critical aortic stenosis (AS) (*right*), rapid early ejection is no longer possible; the flow velocity is increased, and the contour becomes rounded and prolonged, producing the typical diamond-shaped murmur of AS. *Source: Modified from Reddy PS, Curtis EI, Salerni R, et al. Cardiac systolic murmurs: pathophysiology and differential diagnosis. Prog Cardiovasc Dis. 1971;14:4. Reproduced with permission from the publisher and the authors.*

been found to correlate as well with the severity of valvular obstruction in AS as it has in PS. The murmur of significant fixed LV outflow tract obstruction usually is best heard in the second right and second and third left interspaces near the sternum. It radiates widely into the neck and along the great vessels. With radiation to the apex, particularly in the elderly patient, the high-frequency components of the murmur predominate, and the apical murmur has a high pitch and often a musical quality. Observations repeatedly demonstrate that this murmur, regardless of its harmonics, retains a spindle-shaped configuration whenever it is heard or recorded. The murmur of AS varies directly with the length of the preceding diastole; the longer the preceding ventricular filling period, the louder is the systolic murmur (Fig. 12–80). In contrast, the apical murmur of MR is associated with little or no variation in intensity with varying cycle lengths. This observation is useful in patients with atrial fibrillation or frequent premature contractions for identifying whether an apical murmur is caused by radiation of an AS murmur or is an additional murmur of MR. Beat-to-beat variations in the intensity of the murmur of AS have been noted in both pulsus alternans and AV dissociation.

A loud early systolic valvular ejection sound or click is the hallmark of congenital valvular AS, and its presence defines the obstruction at the valvular level (Table 12–13). Its intensity correlates well with the mobility of the valve, and there is little correlation with the severity of the obstruction. It disappears when the valve becomes immobile as a result of calcific fixation and is absent in fixed subaortic stenosis. With progressive increase in the severity of the outflow obstruction, the duration of LV ejection is prolonged, resulting in narrow, single, or reversed splitting of S_2. Reversed

splitting of S_2 in AS in the absence of LBBB is always associated with severe obstruction.

Regardless of the site of obstruction, significant AS always results in LV hypertrophy, with a decreased diastolic compliance. Clinically, this is manifest as a presystolic apical pulsation on palpation and as an S_4 on auscultation (see Fig. 12–73). The relationship between the severity of obstruction and the presence of S_4 gallops is indirect, reflecting hypertrophy and decreased compliance of the LV rather than obstruction per se.

Because of the frequent coexistence of hypertensive or arteriosclerotic heart disease in elderly patients with calcific AS, the presence of an S_4 is nonspecific and correlates poorly with the severity of obstruction. S_3 gallops also can be heard in LV outflow tract obstruction, particularly when decompensation occurs (see Fig. 12–73).

The diagnosis of hemodynamically significant AS in the elderly presents a particularly difficult problem. The murmur is often of low intensity caused by the decreased cardiac output and poor LV function. An ejection sound or click is rarely present, because of calcific fixation of the valve leaflets, and S_2 is of low amplitude. The murmur is often loudest at the apex, has a high-frequency content, and can be difficult to define as ejection in nature because S_1 and A_2 can be poorly heard. In most patients with severe AS, no A_2 is heard, and the systolic murmur obliterates P_2. In the elderly, the rate of rise of the carotid pulse can be nearly normal as a result of the hard, sclerotic vessels even with severe obstruction. As shown in Fig. 12–80, the response of the murmur following a premature ventricular contraction (PVC) can be very helpful in confirming the ejection nature of the murmur. Differentiation from the benign murmur of mild aortic sclerosis can be difficult and often necessitates confirmation of obstruction and its quantitation by echo-Doppler examination.

【 】 RIGHT VENTRICULAR OUTFLOW TRACT OBSTRUCTION

Obstructions to RV outflow are congenital anomalies and can be at the level of the valve, infundibulum, and proximal or distal branches of the pulmonary artery. Isolated infundibular PS with an intact septum is rare and is usually associated with a large VSD (tetralogy of Fallot). When the ventricular septum is intact, there is an excellent correlation between both the intensity and duration of the murmur and the severity of obstruction.[134] Figure 12–81 contrasts the auscultatory findings of progressively more severe valvular PS with an intact ventricular septum with those in tetralogy of Fallot with progressively more severe RV outflow obstruction.[134] As with valvular AS, an early systolic ejection sound defines the level of ob-

TABLE 12–12

Differential Diagnosis of Left Ventricular Outflow Obstruction

| PARAMETER | CONGENITAL AORTIC STENOSIS | | | ACQUIRED AORTIC STENOSIS | HYPERTROPHIC OBSTRUCTIVE CARDIOMYOPATHY |
	VALVULAR	SUBVALVULAR	SUPRAVALVULAR		
Physical appearance	Normal	Normal	Characteristic	Normal	Normal
Arterial pulse	Slow rise, sustained peak	Slow rise, sustained peak	Right brachial and carotid > left	Slow rise, sustained peak	Brisk rise, unsustained double peak
S_4 presystolic impulse	Yes	Yes	Yes	Yes	Yes
Left ventricular systolic impulse	Sustained, single	Sustained, single	Sustained, single	Sustained, single	Sustained, can be double
Aortic ejection sound	Typical ↓ with calcif.	Rare	Rare	Common ↓ with calcif.	Rare exception
Midsystolic ejection murmur; maximal site	First or second right interspace	First or second right interspace	First right interspace and over right carotid	First or second right interspace; apex in elderly	Apex, lower left sternal edge
Second sound splitting	Usually normal or single	Usually normal or single	Usually normal or single	Usually single or reversed	Usually reversed or single
Intensity of aortic closure	Normal or increased or ↓ with calcif.	Normal or decreased	Normal or decreased	Decreased or absent with calcif.	Normal
Murmur of aortic regurgitation	Common	Common	Uncommon	Common	Rare exception

calcif, calcification; S_4, fourth heart sound.
SOURCE: Modified from Reddy PS, et al. Cardiac systolic murmurs: pathophysiology and differential diagnosis. Prog Cardiovasc Dis. 1971;14:6. Reproduced with permission from the publisher and authors.

struction at the valve. In mild to moderate valvular obstruction, the intensity of this sound is markedly attenuated or can disappear with inspiration. In more severe valvular obstruction, this sound can fuse with S_1 or actually can present as a presystolic click when the pressure generated by a forceful right atrial contraction exceeds RV end-diastolic pressure, causing doming of the stenotic valve in late diastole. Although obstruction to RV outflow in tetralogy of Fallot is usually at the infundibular level, valvular stenosis also can be present. In this setting, a pulmonary valvular ejection sound introduces a systolic murmur, and little variation in the intensity of the ejection sound is found with respiration.

The classic late peaking of the systolic ejection murmur of severe PS with an intact ventricular septum is demonstrated in Fig. 12–82. Note that the late vibrations of the murmur completely envelop A_2, whereas P_2 is markedly delayed and decreases in intensity secondary to the low pulmonary artery closing pressure. In moderate to severe valvular PS, an excellent correlation has been found between the A_2-P_2 interval and the RV peak pressure. When the ventricular septum is intact in severe RV outflow obstruction, prominent *a* waves are present in the JVP in association with a right-sided S_4 that can increase with inspiration. Neither of these is present in uncomplicated tetralogy of Fallot. In isolated in-

fundibular obstruction, a pulmonic ejection sound is usually not encountered, and the pulmonic closure (P_2) is usually not audible except in the mildest cases.

In branch stenosis of the pulmonary artery, there is a systolic murmur of varying intensity at the upper left sternal border that is widely transmitted to the right side of the chest, back, and both axillae. The murmur is usually less harsh and of higher pitch than the murmur of valvular PS. With more peripheral branch stenosis, systolic ejection murmurs or even continuous murmurs can be heard over the lung fields. The wide radiation of this murmur is particularly helpful in alerting the clinician to this type of right-sided obstruction.

SYSTOLIC REGURGITANT MURMURS

Systolic regurgitant murmurs are produced by retrograde flow from a chamber of high pressure to a chamber of lower pressure. The classic examples of such murmurs are the holosystolic (pansystolic) murmur of MR, TR, and VSD. Because there is usually a high-pressure differential between the two chambers throughout systole, the murmurs are holosystolic in duration, high-pitched and blowing in quality, and plateau-like in configuration.

TABLE 12–13

Fourth Heart Sound (S₄), Atrial Diastolic Gallop, and Presystolic Gallop

Physiologic—recordable, but rarely audible
Pathologic
  Decreased ventricular compliance
    Ventricular hypertrophy
      Left or right ventricular outflow obstruction
      Systemic or pulmonary hypertension
      Hypertrophic cardiomyopathy
    Ischemic heart disease
      Angina pectoris
      Acute myocardial infarction
      Old myocardial infarction
      Ventricular aneurysm
    Idiopathic dilated cardiomyopathy
  Excessively rapid late diastolic filling secondary to
    Vigorous atrial systole
    Hyperkinetic states
      Anemia
      Thyrotoxicosis
    Arteriovenous fistula
    Acute atrioventricular valve incompetence
  Arrhythmias
    Heart block

Holosystolic Regurgitant Murmurs

The murmur of chronic MR is the prototype of the holosystolic regurgitant murmur, as shown in Fig. 12–74. It begins with or replaces S₁ and continues throughout systole in a plateau-like fashion beyond A₂, finally terminating when the LV pressure drops to the level of the left atrial pressure during isovolumic relaxation.[135] In contrast to the systolic ejection murmur, there is little variation in its intensity with varying cycle lengths.[136] It is heard best at the apex and radiates well into the axilla; only the loudest murmurs are associated with a thrill at the apex. There is little variation in its intensity with respiration, and it is frequently accompanied by a loud diastolic filling sound followed by a short rumble. In this situation, the loud S₃ is not a manifestation of congestive failure but a reflection of hemodynamically significant MR. Likewise, the short rumble does not mean concomitant obstruction at the mitral valve but rather is secondary to extremely rapid early diastolic filling. The intensity of the murmur is directly related to the pressure gradient between the LV and the left atrium.

The diagnosis of hemodynamically significant MR is established by the presence of the holosystolic regurgitant murmur and loud S₃ associated with a short flow rumble. The etiology, however, is determined by the clinical presentation and associated physical findings and is best confirmed by echocardiography.

The classic holosystolic (pansystolic) murmur of TR in the setting of RV pressure overload is best heard at the lower left sternal border. At times it can be heard laterally to the midclavicular line, indicating that the RV occupies the region of the cardiac apex. Furthermore, it generally can be differentiated from MR because its in-

tensity is usually strongly influenced by respiration. During continuous and accentuated respiration, the murmur increases in intensity with inspiration because of the increased venous return and RV filling associated with inspiration. The inspiratory increase in loudness of right-sided auscultatory events is known as *Carvallo sign*.[137] Careful inspection of the JVP while auscultating the murmur will be of further help in defining its tricuspid origin, showing a prominent *v* wave with a rapid *y* descent that augments during inspiration. In severe RV failure, this respiratory variation can be absent, but it can reappear as the state of compensation improves. With severe TR, a short flow rumble introduced by an S₃ can be present, just as with MR, and both will increase with inspiration.

The holosystolic murmur of VSD is heard best just off the sternal border in the fourth, fifth, and sixth intercostal spaces and is usually accompanied by a forceful thrill.[138] The murmur does not radiate to the axilla as with MR and does not have the respiratory variation characteristic of TR. Wide physiologic splitting with an easily heard P₂ is usually present when the left-to-right shunt is hemodynamically significant. When the shunt is large, there is an LV S₃ followed by a short flow rumble. The regurgitant murmur is caused by high-velocity flow from the high-pressure LV to the lower-pressure RV, and its intensity correlates poorly with the degree of left-to-right shunting. When the defect is very large and the RV and LV pressures are equal, however, no murmur can be produced across the defect; instead, the short pulmonary ejection murmur of severe PH is present (Eisenmenger VSD).

Early Systolic Regurgitant Murmurs

Rarely, a regurgitant murmur confined to early systole is seen in the presence of a small VSD. This murmur begins in the usual manner at the onset of ventricular systole and stops suddenly in early or middle systole. The sudden cessation of the murmur is caused by the fact that as ejection continues and ventricular size decreases, the small defect is sealed shut as the ventricular septum thickens during systole and the flow ceases. This murmur is important because it is characteristic of the type of VSD that can disappear with age.

In contrast to the holosystolic murmur of chronic MR, acute severe MR can present as an early systolic spindle-shaped murmur.[139] Common conditions producing acute MR include spontaneous rupture of the chordae tendineae of a myxomatous valve, acute or subacute bacterial endocarditis of the mitral valve, papillary muscle rupture or dysfunction secondary to acute MI, and disruption of the mitral apparatus caused by chest trauma.[140] In each of these conditions, large-volume flow regurgitates into a relatively normal left atrium that has not had the time to make the adaptive changes in compliance seen in chronic long-standing MR. As a result, an extremely high *v* wave is generated in the left atrium.

This high *v* wave abolishes the LV–left atrial gradient during the latter part of systole, resulting in termination of retrograde flow and abbreviation of the systolic murmur. In a patient with acute MR secondary to spontaneous rupture of the chordae tendineae of a myxomatous valve, the murmur ends before A₂. Audible expiratory splitting with an accentuated P₂ is present at the base, and a loud S₄ is recorded at the apex. The presence of the S₄ associated with a prominent presystolic impulse on palpation is an important clue that indicates the acute nature of the MR and is

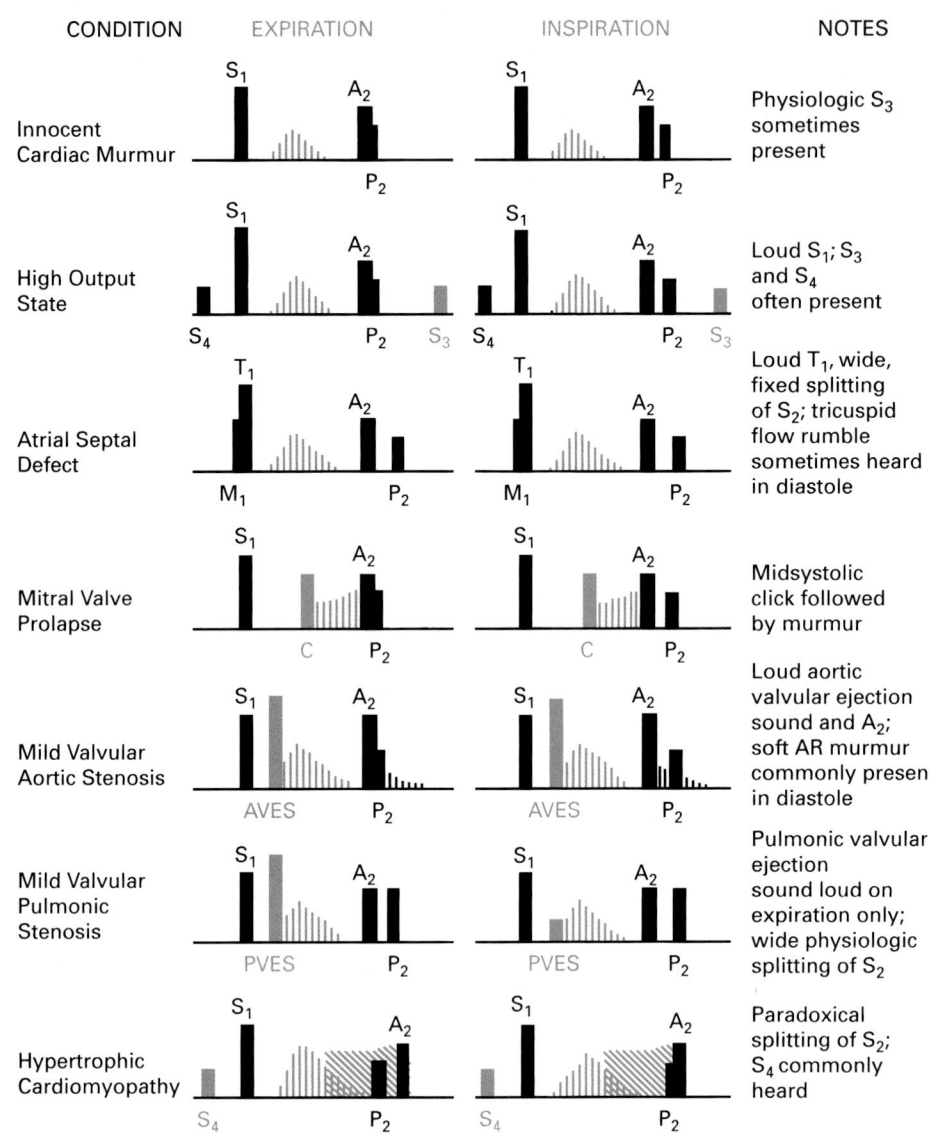

CONDITION   EXPIRATION   INSPIRATION   NOTES

Innocent Cardiac Murmur — Physiologic S_3 sometimes present

High Output State — Loud S_1; S_3 and S_4 often present

Atrial Septal Defect — Loud T_1, wide, fixed splitting of S_2; tricuspid flow rumble sometimes heard in diastole

Mitral Valve Prolapse — Midsystolic click followed by murmur

Mild Valvular Aortic Stenosis — Loud aortic valvular ejection sound and A_2; soft AR murmur commonly present in diastole

Mild Valvular Pulmonic Stenosis — Pulmonic valvular ejection sound loud on expiration only; wide physiologic splitting of S_2

Hypertrophic Cardiomyopathy — Paradoxical splitting of S_2; S_4 commonly heard

FIGURE 12–80. The differential diagnosis of the innocent murmur versus the pathologic systolic murmur is made by the "company the murmur keeps." The innocent murmur must be found in the setting of an otherwise normal cardiovascular examination. A_2, aortic second sound; AR, aortic regurgitation; AVES, aortic valvular ejection sound; C, midsystolic nonejection sound; M_1, mitral first sound; P_2, pulmonic second heart sound; PVES, pulmonic valvular ejection sound; S_1, first heart sound; S_2, second heart sound; S_3, third heart sound; S_4, fourth heart sound; T_1, tricuspid first sound.

with only a small pressure differential between the RV and the right atrium. The small pressure head results in a low-velocity flow, minimal turbulence, and a soft, abbreviated murmur. Occasionally, only minimal early systolic vibrations are heard. In most patients, large *v* waves are readily apparent in the JVP. The murmur retains the characteristic inspiratory augmentation seen in right-sided regurgitant murmurs and is frequently associated with an S_4 that increases in intensity with inspiration. A right-sided S_4 and a prominent diastolic tricuspid flow rumble are the rule when the TR is acute, as with endocarditis of the tricuspid valve. After total excision of the tricuspid valve for infective endocarditis related to intravenous drug abuse, the systolic murmur is often very unimpressive or can be completely absent. Giant *v* waves in the neck are easily visible, however, and palpable venous thrills and a murmur at the base of the neck can be present secondary to rapid retrograde flow in the jugular system. Other causes of organic TR include carcinoid heart disease, RV infarction, chest trauma, and damage of the tricuspid valve during open heart surgery.

Mid- and Late-Systolic Regurgitatant Murmurs

Midsystolic murmurs can occur with MR as a result of papillary muscle dysfunction.[142] The timing of the murmur of papillary muscle dysfunction also can be late systolic, and the murmur can be either intermittent or constant. It occurs with ischemia or infarction of either the posteromedial or anterolateral papillary muscle. Often these murmurs are transient, being provoked by episodes of ischemia.

rarely present in MR of a chronic nature. The systolic murmur of acute MR, which can mimic ejection murmurs, can have classic radiation to the axilla and back, especially if it is caused by prolapse of the anterior leaflet of the mitral valve with flow directed over the posterior leaflet. When the murmur is loud, it can be conducted to the top of the head and to the sacrum along the spinal column. Occasionally, the murmur is conducted to the base of the heart and great vessels, simulating AS. The quick-rising carotid pulse with rapid falloff, as well as the wide physiologic splitting of the S_2, helps differentiation from AS.

The systolic murmur of organic TR is often unimpressive and presents as an early systolic murmur ending well before A_2, even in the presence of severe regurgitation.[141] In this condition, the RV pressure is nearly normal, and massive regurgitation can be present

Varying degrees of MVP are the most frequent cause of a late-systolic murmur, and this entity is one of the most common causes of systolic murmurs seen in clinical practice. The murmur is best heard at the apex and often has a tendency to a late systolic crescendo. It is frequently introduced or accompanied by nonejection clicks. These clicks can be single or multiple, and they can occur independently without an accompanying systolic murmur. As shown in Fig. 12–65, the click occurs near the time of maximal prolapse in midsystole, and the late-systolic murmur continues up to and through A_2 because of prolapse of the posterior leaflet during the remainder of systole.

The timing and intensity of these murmurs vary with physiologic and pharmacologic maneuvers that alter the end-diastolic volume of the heart (see Fig. 12–66). These murmurs are also sensitive to con-

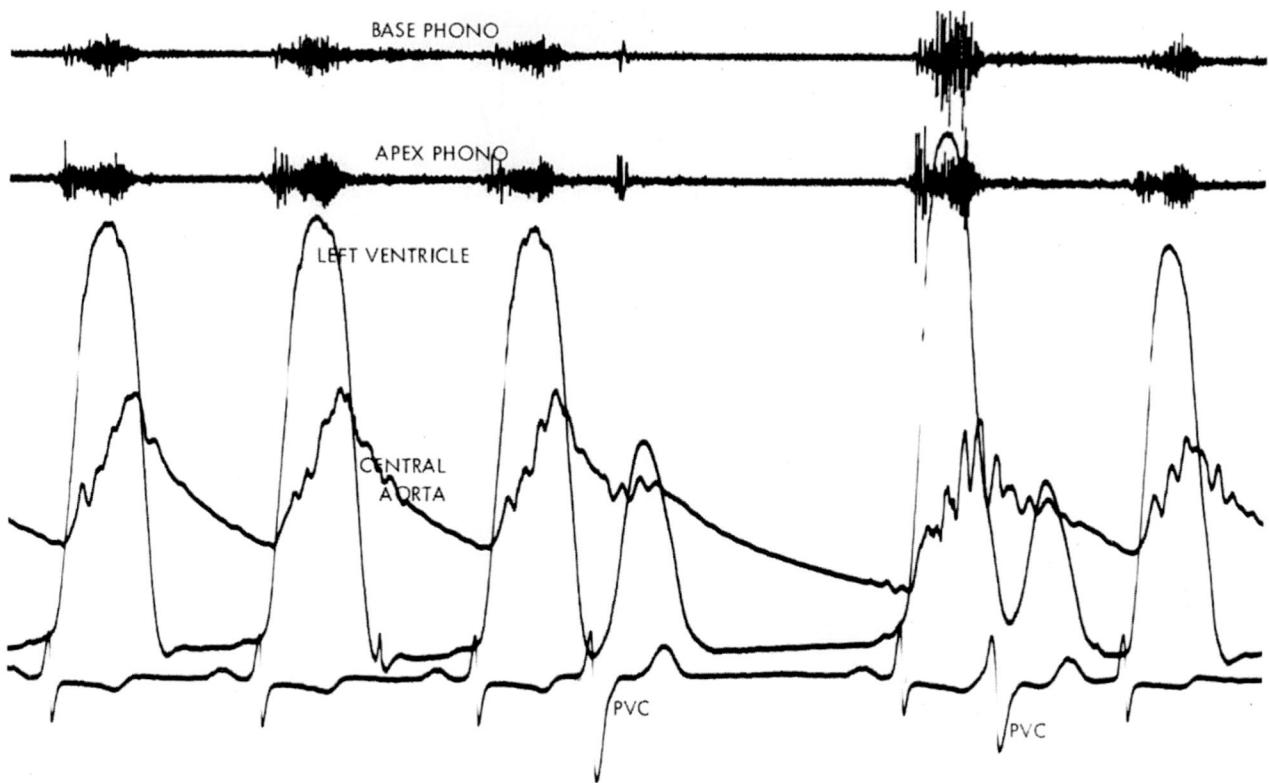

FIGURE 12–81. Effect of the long diastolic filling period following a premature ventricular contraction (PVC) on the intensity of a systolic ejection murmur. There is a marked increase in the intensity of the aortic stenosis: murmur recorded at the base and at the apex. Despite the higher-frequency content of the apical murmur, this response clearly identifies this murmur as ejection in nature. *Source: Paley H. Left ventricular outflow tract obstruction: heart sounds and murmurs. In: Leon DF, Shaver JA, eds. Physiologic Principles of Heart Sounds and Murmurs. Monograph 46. Dallas, TX: American Heart Association; 1975:112. Reproduced with permission from the publisher and the author.*

ditions that alter the peripheral vascular impedance as well as the inotropic state of the heart. These variations in the timing and duration of the murmur can be understood most easily by considering MVP as a condition in which the valve is too big for the ventricle (see Chap. 76). This valvuloventricular disproportion manifests itself at a given geometric size and configuration during LV contraction. These dynamic changes can best be appreciated at the bedside by examining the patient in the supine, left lateral, sitting, and standing positions as well as during prompt squatting. Late-systolic murmurs also can originate from prolapse of the tricuspid valve.

Levine and Harvey described a musical, apical systolic murmur that they called a "whoop" because it simulated the "whoop" of whooping cough. These murmurs are loud, high-pitched, musical, sonorous, and vibratory; are best heard at the apex in late systole; and are frequently intermittent. They are often preceded by clicks and originate in the mitral valve. They are associated with ballooning of the mitral valve or MR (or both), and their unusual quality is secondary to the high-frequency vibrations of the mitral apparatus. The systolic "whoop" or "honk," together with late systolic murmurs, with or without associated clicks, is part of a continuum representing abnormalities of the mitral valve apparatus of varying etiologies. Similar honking noises, with or without clicks, can arise from the tricuspid valve and also have been produced by transvenous pacemaker catheters situated across the valve. These murmurs are best auscultated at the fourth left intercostal space and have the typical inspiratory augmentation of tricuspid murmurs.

Murmur of Hypertrophic "Obstructive" Cardiomyopathy

The classic cardiac findings of hypertrophic cardiomyopathy (HCM) (see Chap. 30) with an LV outflow gradient are demonstrated in Fig. 12–83; the echocardiogram gives insight into the mechanism of production of the systolic murmur. Systolic anterior motion (SAM) of the mitral apparatus impinges on the massively thickened septum, producing high-velocity flow in middle and late systole, resulting in a midsystolic ejection murmur usually with its maximal intensity at the left sternal edge.[143] Varying degrees of MR also can be present during systole because of the distorted mitral apparatus. Frequently, on auscultation, there is difficulty deciding whether the systolic murmur found in HCM is ejection or regurgitant in nature.[144] Usually, the murmur recorded by the precordial phonocardiogram is actually the summation of the murmurs of LV outflow obstruction and MR as transmitted to the chest wall.

In patients with dynamic LV outflow gradients, the intensity of both the systolic ejection murmur and the MR murmur varies directly with the magnitude of the pressure gradient. Thus physiologic maneuvers and pharmacologic interventions that increase the pressure gradient will increase the intensity of the precordial murmur, and vice versa. Decreases in LV preload and afterload or increases in LV contractility are associated with increases in the pressure gradient and the intensity of the murmur, whereas increases

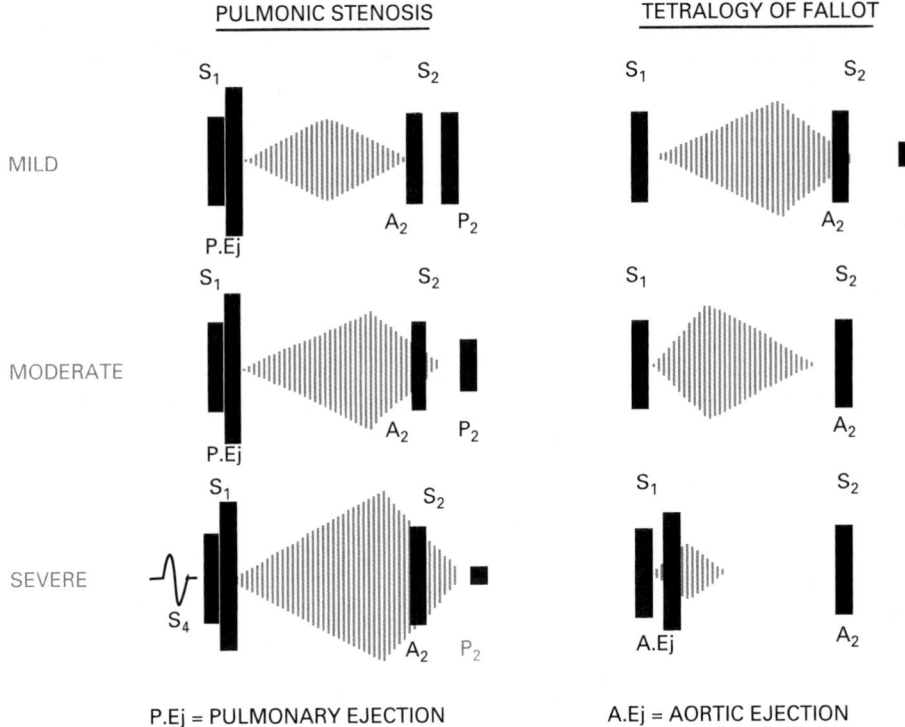

PULMONIC STENOSIS

TETRALOGY OF FALLOT

MILD

MODERATE

SEVERE

P.Ej = PULMONARY EJECTION

A.Ej = AORTIC EJECTION

FIGURE 12–82. In valvular pulmonic stenosis (PS) with intact ventricular septum, right ventricular (RV) systolic ejection becomes progressively longer with increasing obstruction to flow. As a result, the murmur becomes louder and longer, enveloping the aortic closure sound. At the same time, pulmonic closure occurs later; splitting becomes wider but is more difficult to appreciate because the aortic closure sound is lost in the murmur; and the pulmonary closure sound becomes progressively softer caused by the low pulmonary artery pressure. With increasing severity of PS, the pulmonary ejection sound can fuse with the first heart sound (S_1). In severe obstruction with concentric hypertrophy and decreased RV compliance, a fourth heart sound (S_4) appears. In tetralogy of Fallot, with increasing obstruction at the infundibular area, more and more RV blood is shunted across a silent ventricular septal defect with less flow across the obstructed RV outflow tract. With increasing obstruction, the murmur becomes shorter, earlier, and fainter. The pulmonary closure sound is absent in severe tetralogy of Fallot. The dilated aorta receives almost all the cardiac output from both ventricular chambers, and there is an aortic ejection sound. A_2, aortic second sound; AEJ, aortic ejection; P_2, pulmonic second heart sound; PEJ, pulmonary ejection; S_2, second heart sound.

in LV preload and afterload or decreases in LV contractility will decrease the pressure gradient and the intensity of the murmur. For example, the upright posture and the strain phase of the Valsalva maneuver decrease venous return and LV preload, and the murmur increases in intensity. On reclining or with prompt squatting, augmented venous return increases LV preload, and the murmur decreases in intensity.

In the absence of an LV outflow gradient at rest or with provocation, the murmur of HCM is less impressive. Although a short ejection murmur is usually recorded as a result of rapid early LV ejection, it is often softer and extends through less of systole than when a gradient is present. There is also little variation in the intensity with changes in preload, afterload, or contractility.

In HCM with and without a gradient across the LV outflow tract, massive LV hypertrophy is present, and a prominent presystolic impulse associated with an LV S_4 is the rule when normal sinus rhythm is present. An S_3 is also a common finding in patients with HCM, and occasionally there is an early diastolic rumble that can mimic the diastolic murmur of MS. Such rumbles are felt to be caused by the increased impedance to LV filling secondary to the decreased diastolic compliance of the LV.

[ ] DIASTOLIC MURMURS

Diastolic murmurs have two basic mechanisms of production. Diastolic filling murmurs or rumbles are caused by forward flow across an AV valve, whereas diastolic regurgitant murmurs are caused by retrograde flow across an incompetent semilunar valve[145] (Fig. 12–86).

Diastolic Filling Murmurs (Rumbles)

Diastolic rumbles are caused by forward flow across the AV valves and are delayed from their respective semilunar closure sound by the isovolumic relaxation period. Only following this period, when the atrial pressure exceeds the declining ventricular pressure, do the AV valves open and filling begins (Fig. 12–85). Because there are two phases of rapid ventricular filling—early diastole and presystole—these murmurs have a tendency to be most prominent during these two filling periods. Because the velocity of flow is relatively low, these murmurs have a low-frequency content and are rumbling in character.

Diastolic Rumbles Caused by Obstruction of the AV

The murmur of mitral stenosis (MS) is heard best at the apex in the left lateral position, and its duration correlates well with the duration of the mitral diastolic gradient. Its intensity is related to the severity of the obstruction and to the flow across the valve.

As a result, there is poor correlation between the intensity of the murmur and the severity of the obstruction; that is, high flow across a mild obstruction can produce a loud rumble, whereas low flow across a severely stenotic valve can produce a very soft murmur or can be silent. When the stenotic mitral valve is mobile, the murmur is introduced by a prominent opening snap (see Fig. 12–62, *left*). The duration of the interval between A_2 and the opening snap (OS) correlates well with the level of left atrial pressure; the shorter the A_2–OS interval, the higher is the left atrial pressure, and vice versa. The S_1 is also loud when the stenotic valve is mobile and is usually preceded by a crescendo murmur. Although originally attributed to increased flow secondary to left atrial systole, phonoechocardiographic studies have suggested that this short *presystolic* murmur is actually caused by high-velocity antegrade flow through a progressively narrowing mitral orifice during very early (isovolumic) ventricular systole[146] (see Fig. 12–62, *left*). This mechanism also can be responsible for the brief crescendo presystolic murmur observed in patients with MS in atrial fibrillation following a short cycle length.

Although the intensity of the diastolic rumble in MS correlates poorly with the severity of obstruction, there is an excellent correlation of severity with the duration of the murmur. When sinus

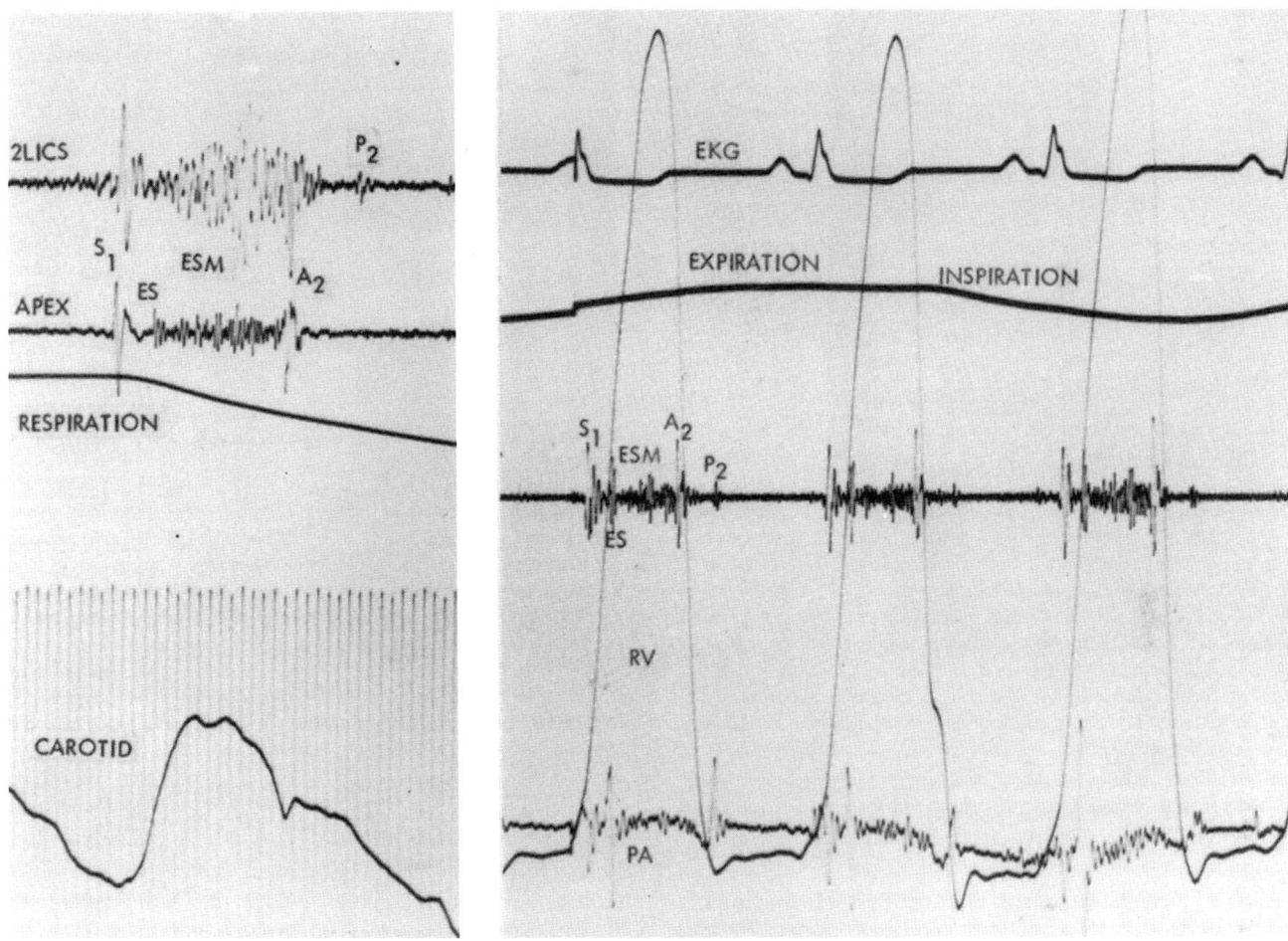

FIGURE 12–83. *Left*. The phonocardiogram of a patient with severe valvular pulmonic stenosis (PS) as recorded at the second left intercostal space (2LICS) and the apex. The long ejection murmur has late systolic peaking and spills through the aortic second sound (A_2). There is a marked delay in the pulmonic second heart sound (P_2), which is very small in amplitude. *Right*. At cardiac catheterization, the markedly delayed P_2 is shown to be secondary to a very large systolic pressure gradient, and its decreased intensity is caused by the low pulmonary artery pressure at the time of valve closure. The late peaking of the ejection murmur correlates with the maximal pressure gradient between the right ventricle and the pulmonary artery. EKG, electrocardiogram; ES, ejection sound; ESM, ejection systolic murmur; RV, right ventricle; S_1, first heart sound. *Source: Curtiss EI. First and second heart sound. In: Horwitz LD, ed. Signs and Symptoms in Cardiology. Philadelphia, PA: Lippincott; 1985:200. Reproduced with permission from the publisher and authors.*

tachycardia or rapid atrial fibrillation is present, a rumble starting with an OS and continuing to S_1 may not be meaningful because of the short diastolic time. Carotid sinus pressure can be very helpful in temporarily slowing the heart rate, thereby allowing the clinician to uncover the potential length of the rumble.

Obstruction of the mitral orifice also can be produced by a left atrial tumor. The diastolic murmur can be very similar to that produced by MS (see Fig. 12–62, *center*). A loud tumor "plop" is present instead of the OS, and the presystolic crescendo murmur occurs as the protruding tumor mass returns rapidly through the mitral orifice into the left atrium during early ventricular systole. A systolic murmur of MR also can be present, and both murmurs can vary from examination to examination and with changes in body position.

The murmur of tricuspid stenosis (TS) is usually heard in the xiphoid area just off the sternal border. Because right atrial systole occurs earlier than left, the diastolic murmur of TS can have a crescendo-decrescendo configuration.[147] Even when the PR interval is normal, the presystolic accentuation of the diastolic rumble can terminate before S_1. Because TS almost always oc-

curs in the presence of MS, this diastolic diamond-shaped murmur, which augments during inspiration, and the presence of large *a* waves in the JVP are clues to this additional diagnosis. When atrial fibrillation is present, the murmur is in mid-diastole and has the typical inspiratory augmentation. A tricuspid OS, which usually follows the mitral OS, also can be present and can initiate the murmur.

Diastolic Rumbles Caused by High Flow Across the Atrioventricular Valves

High-velocity flow across the normal or regurgitant AV valve can result in short middiastolic rumbles often accompanied by an S_3 and should not be confused with murmurs produced by true obstruction of the AV valves (Fig. 12–86). Such rumbles are common in both VSD and patent ductus arteriosus caused by the large flow across the MV secondary to the left-to-right shunt. Likewise, the left-to-right shunt in a large ASD often produces a tricuspid rumble. Similar low-pitched rumbling murmurs also can be present in hyperkinetic states and occasionally are heard in patients with complete heart block and increased diastolic blood flow in each cardiac cycle. Common to all these

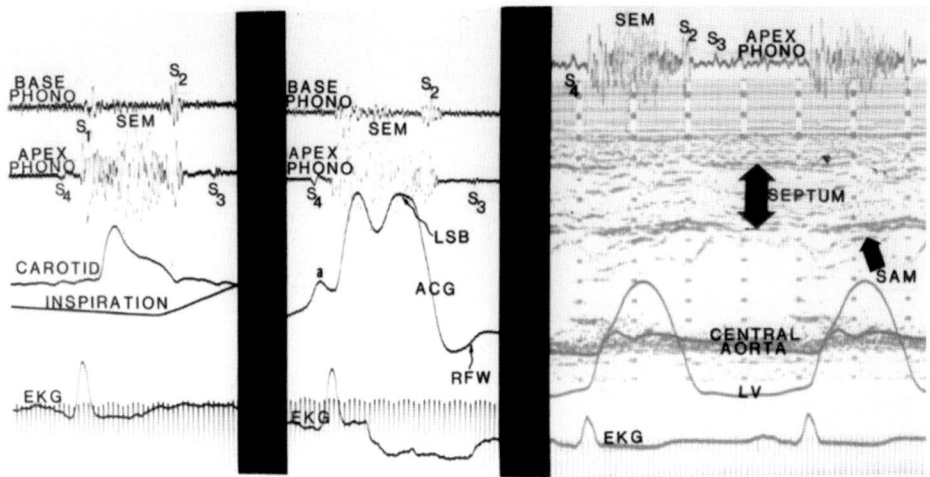

FIGURE 12–84. Simultaneous base and apex phonocardiograms are recorded with the carotid pulse and apexcardiogram in the left and center panels, respectively, in a 54-year-old man with hypertrophic cardiomyopathy. The carotid pulse rises rapidly and has a late systolic plateau and a prolonged ejection period. Prominent fourth heart sound (S_4) and first heart sound (S_1) are demonstrated and are associated with the *a* wave and the rapid filling wave (RFW), respectively, of the apexcardiogram (ACG). Note the late systolic bulge (LSB) on the ACG. The second heart sound (S_2) is single. A loud grade 5 systolic ejection murmur is present and is of greatest intensity at the apex. In the right panel, the apical systolic murmur is recorded together with the M-mode echocardiogram. Simultaneous high-fidelity left ventricular (LV) and central aortic pressures are recorded by catheter-tipped micromanometers. Marked thickening of the interventricular septum and systolic anterior motion of the mitral valve are present on the echocardiogram. A large systolic pressure gradient is demonstrated beginning shortly after the onset of the systolic anterior motion (SAM). *Source: Shaver JA, et al. Phonoechocardiography and intracardiac phonocardiography in hypertrophic cardiomyopathy. Postgrad Med J. 1986;62:538. Reproduced with permission from the publisher and the authors.*

conditions is high-volume flow during the latter phase of the rapid filling period. Phonoechocardiography indicates that these murmurs occur during the rapid closing motion of the mitral valve, suggesting a functional *obstruction* during the period of rapid early

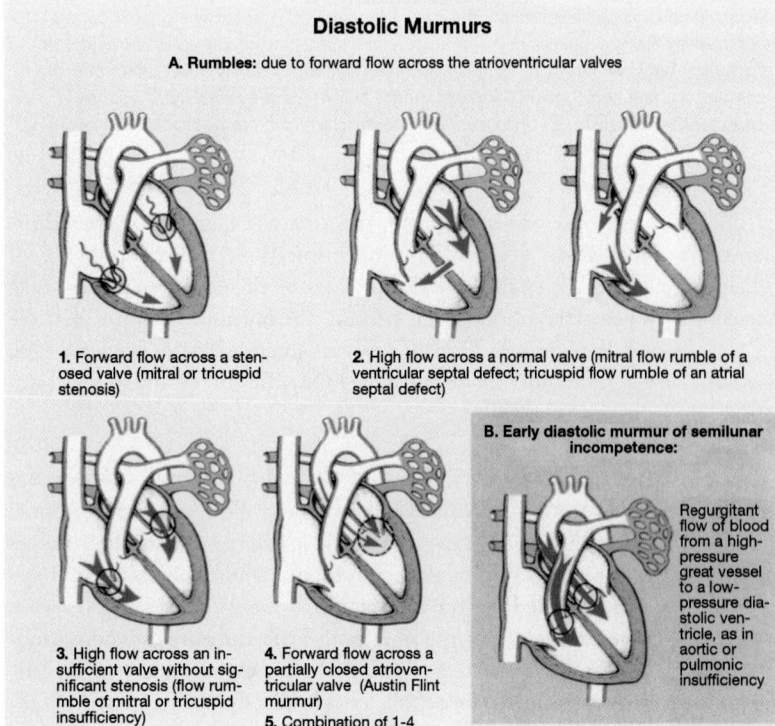

FIGURE 12–85. Classification of diastolic murmurs based on physiologic mechanism of production. *Source: Shaver JA. Heart murmurs: innocent or pathologic? (Part 1) Hosp Med. 1982. Reproduced with permission from the publisher and author.*

diastolic filling. Identical phonoechocardiographic correlates also have been shown with MR and TR, where early diastolic filling is also extremely rapid. With TR, the early rumble will increase with inspiration, typical of right-sided murmurs. During rapid atrial fibrillation, ventriculogenic closure of the normal mitral valve during the rapid filling phase of a short cardiac cycle can cause a *presystolic* murmur by a similar mechanism.

Mitral valvulitis during an episode of acute rheumatic fever can cause a short diastolic rumble, the *Carey Coombs murmur.*[148] This rumble, especially in children or in the presence of fever and anemia, can be introduced by an S_3 rather than by an OS. This combination of an S_3 with a short rumble indicates that there is not enough obstruction to the valve to alter the characteristics of rapid early ventricular filling.

The Austin Flint murmur, as originally described in 1862,[149] consisted of an apical presystolic murmur observed in two patients with considerable AR and no evidence of MS at autopsy. Since its original description, the timing of this murmur has been extended to include a middiastolic component. It is heard best at the apex and has many of the qualities of the murmur of MS. It is introduced by an S_3 rather than by an OS, however, and S_1 is of normal or decreased amplitude. Maneuvers that increase the degree of AR, such as hand grip or transient arterial occlusions will increase the intensity of the rumble. In most cases of severe AR, particularly when acute, the presystolic component of the Austin Flint murmur is lost. In this situation, there is marked elevation of the LV end-diastolic pressure, and the reverse pressure gradient between the LV and the left atrium causes premature closure of the mitral valve.

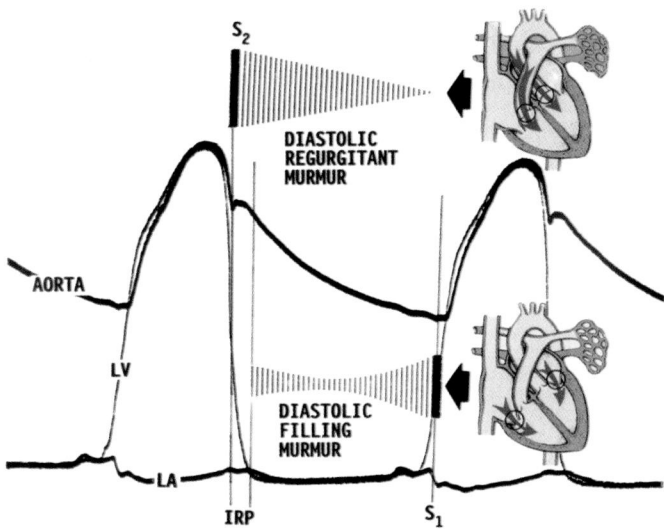

FIGURE 12–86. Diastolic filling murmurs or rumbles are caused by forward flow across the atrioventricular (AV) valves, whereas diastolic regurgitant murmurs are caused by retrograde flow across incompetent semilunar valves. *Left.* Diagrammatic representation of the diastolic filling murmur and the diastolic regurgitant murmur as related to left ventricular (LV), aortic, and left atrial (LA) pressures. The diastolic filling murmur occurs during the diastolic filling period and is separated from the second heart sound (S_2) by the isovolumic relaxation period. The rumbling murmur is most prominent during rapid early ventricular filling and presystole, terminating with the first heart sound (S_1). The diastolic regurgitant murmur begins immediately after S_2 and continues in a decrescendo fashion up to S_1, closely paralleling the aortic LV diastolic pressure gradient. *Right.* Flow diagram. *Source: Shaver JA. Diastolic murmurs. Heart Dis Stroke. 1993;1:98–103. Reproduced with permission from the American Heart Association.*

Elegant phonoechocardiographic studies have shown that the murmur is associated with the rapid closing motion of the mitral valve leaflets during mid-diastole and presystole, presumably caused by antegrade flow across a closing orifice in a manner similar to the flow rumble of AV valvular regurgitation and high-output states.[149] Austin Flint murmurs have been observed in the absence of rapid closing of the mitral valve, however, and Reddy and colleagues[150] have suggested that incomplete valve opening rather than excessively rapid closure rates can be the essential requirement for producing the increased mitral flow velocity. One echo-Doppler study has suggested that patients with an Austin Flint murmur usually have an aortic regurgitant jet aimed directly at the mitral valve, causing deformity and shuddering of the valve. Right-sided Austin Flint murmurs of similar quality occur in association with severe pulmonic regurgitation associated with PH.

Diastolic Regurgitant Murmurs

Holodiastolic Aortic Regurgitant Murmurs The early diastolic murmur of AR is blowing and high-pitched and is often more difficult to record than to hear because of its high-frequency content. Because isovolumic relaxation of the LV is very rapid, a large gradient quickly develops between the aortic and LV diastolic pressures, and the murmur builds up to maximum intensity almost immediately after A_2 (Fig. 12–87). As diastole progresses, the gradient between the two chambers falls slowly, and the murmur envelope closely parallels the pressure drop in a decrescendo fashion

up to S_1. When the AR is valvular in origin, the murmur is usually best heard at the third and fourth left parasternal areas. If the murmur is heard best to the right of the sternum, it should alert the clinician to an aortic root etiology of the regurgitation.[151] It should be pointed out that this finding is helpful only if present, because many patients with AR secondary to dilatation of the aortic root have the usual radiation with peak intensity to the left of the sternum. The murmur can be faint and overlooked if the examiner does not listen with the patient sitting up and leaning forward and does not listen with the diaphragm of the stethoscope pressed firmly against the chest wall. One should listen while the patient holds his or her breath after deep expiration.

The degree of AR is directly proportional to the pressure head driving the flow in a retrograde fashion. Maneuvers that increase or decrease the diastolic aortic LV pressure gradient will increase or decrease the intensity of the regurgitant murmur. Prompt squatting often will bring out a very faint AR blowing murmur at the bedside, and transient arterial occlusion with two BP cuffs will also markedly increase its intensity. It should be remembered that the murmur of mild AR often disappears during the latter stages of pregnancy because of the low peripheral vascular resistance. Pure AR without associated valvular stenosis can present with a prominent systolic ejection murmur as well as an Austin Flint rumble at the apex. The carotid pulse is rapid-rising and has a large volume. The A_2 is often diminished or even absent when the regurgitation is valvular in origin.

The etiology of the AR usually cannot be determined by the quality of the murmur. An exception to this rule is the presence of a "cooing dove" or musical diastolic murmur, which usually denotes a rupture or retroversion of an aortic cusp. Such ruptures occur secondary to trauma, infective endocarditis, and occasionally in the presence of arteriosclerosis of the aortic valve. Retroversion and subsequent rupture of the aortic valve with a musical murmur are also a complication of syphilitic AR.

Abbreviated Aortic Diastolic Regurgitant Murmur The murmur of very mild AR can be abbreviated and can end by mid-diastole. This is particularly true of the functional AR murmur of systemic arterial hypertension. As the volume of blood in the aorta decreases during diastole, the aortic annulus becomes smaller, and coupled with the decreasing aortic LV diastolic gradient, retrograde flow ceases, and the murmur disappears.

The murmur of AR also can be abbreviated if the AR is acute. Acute regurgitation of blood into an LV that has not adapted to a large-volume load results in marked elevation of the LV end-diastolic pressure with equilibration of the aortic and LV diastolic pressures. As a result, retrograde flow ceases, and the murmur disappears in the latter part of diastole. When AR is acute, there can be preclosure of the mitral valve, resulting in a soft or absent S_1 as well as absence of the presystolic component of the Austin Flint murmur. The auscultatory findings of acute versus chronic AR are contrasted in Fig. 12–88. Common causes of acute AR include aortic valve endocarditis, trauma, acute aortic dissection, and dehiscence of an aortic valve prosthesis (see Chap. 79).

Holodiastolic Pulmonic Regurgitant Murmur Pulmonic regurgitation (PR) is found most commonly in the setting of severe PH and dilatation of the pulmonary artery with inadequate coaptation

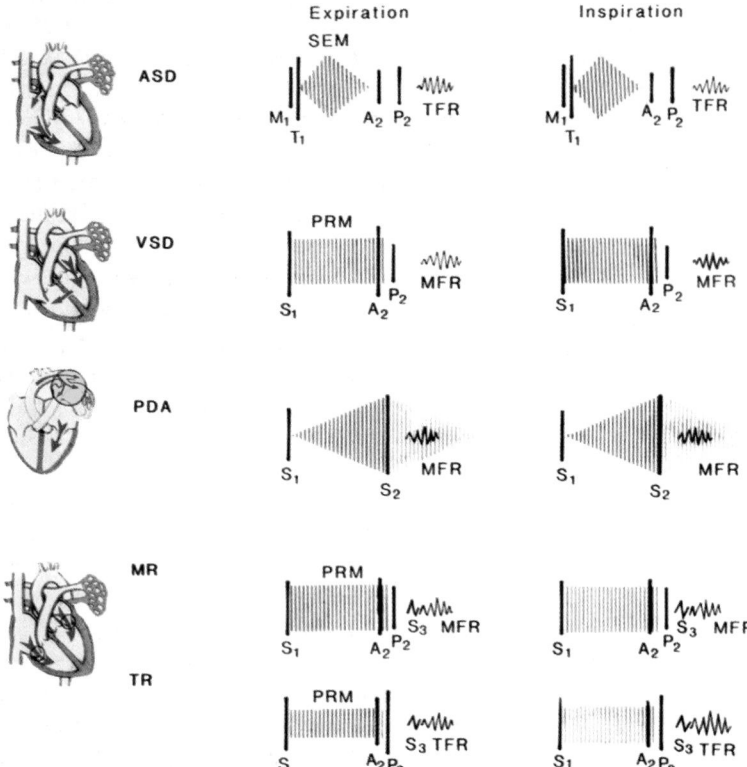

FIGURE 12–87. Diastolic flow rumbles are caused by high flow across the atrioventricular valves in patients having atrial septal defect (ASD), ventricular septal defect (VSD), and patent ductus arteriosus. Shunting through the atrial septal defect results in high flow across the tricuspid valve, producing the tricuspid flow rumble (TFR). In both VSD and patent ductus arteriosus (PDA), left-to-right shunting through the VSD or PDA, causes high flow across the mitral valve, resulting in a mitral flow rumble (MFR). With both mitral regurgitation (MR) and tricuspid regurgitation (TR), the large regurgitation volume causes increased flow during early diastole across the atrioventricular valve, resulting in MFR and TFR, respectively, both being introduced by a prominent third heart sound (S_3). With inspiration, there is a significant increase in the intensity of the pansystolic regurgitant tricuspid murmur (PRM), the S_3, and the TFR. No significant changes in the intensity of the diastolic flow rumbles occur with inspiration in patients have ASD, VSD, PDA or MR. A_2, aortic valve closure sound; M_1, mitral valve closure sound; P_2, pulmonary valve closure sound; SEM, systolic ejection murmur, T_1, tricuspid valve closure sound. *Source: Shaver JA. Diastolic murmurs. Heart Dis Stroke. 1993;1:98–103. Reproduced with permission from the American Heart Association.*

of the leaflets of the pulmonic valve. The functional murmur of PR (Graham Steell murmur[152]) is similar in both frequency and contour to that of AR because the hemodynamics responsible for their production are identical. The differential diagnosis is made by the "company the murmur keeps," and when it is associated with the peripheral signs of hemodynamically significant AR or with the findings of severe PH, there is rarely a problem. However, when rheumatic MS is the primary lesion, the semilunar regurgitant murmur can be secondary either to associated rheumatic AR or to the Graham Steell murmur if the PH is severe. Careful investigation of the semilunar blowing murmur in the setting of MS has shown that it is usually caused by AR, even when significant PH is present.[153] More common causes of the Graham Steell murmur of functional PR are primary PH and Eisenmenger syndrome.

Early diastolic murmurs occasionally are heard in end-stage renal failure, particularly when there is concurrent anemia, hyper-

tension, and fluid overload. Doppler echocardiography demonstrated that these murmurs are usually pulmonic in origin.[154] They are often transient in nature and are related to fluid overload. Such murmurs are diminished by extracellular fluid removal and reflect correctable PH.[154]

Delayed Pulmonic Regurgitant Murmur The murmur of organic (nonpulmonary hypertensive) PR is quite different in quality and duration as compared with either AR or the Graham Steell murmur of PH.[152] The murmur is delayed from P_2 by a short interval, builds up quickly to a crescendo followed by a decrescendo that ends well before S_1. In organic PR, the pulmonary artery pressure can be normal, and the diastolic gradient between the pulmonary artery and RV can be very small, resulting in low-velocity retrograde flow and a *lower-pitched murmur*. The murmur is heard only during the period of maximal gradient in early and middle diastole. This type of murmur can be congenital or acquired, as with pulmonic valve endocarditis, carcinoid syndrome, or surgical procedures on the pulmonic valve. It is often associated with a prominent systolic ejection murmur secondary to the large RV stroke volume.

Continuous Murmurs

A *continuous murmur* is defined as one that begins in systole and extends through S_2 into part or all of diastole. It need not occupy the entire cardiac cycle; therefore, a systolic murmur that extends into diastole without stopping at S_2 is considered to be continuous even if it fades completely before the subsequent S_1. A physiologic classification of continuous murmurs as described by Myers[155] is detailed in Table 12–14.

Continuous Murmurs Caused by Rapid Blood Flow High-velocity blood flow through veins and arteries can cause a continuous murmur. The cervical venous hum is a continuous murmur with diastolic accentuation and is easily heard in most children. It is best heard with the patient sitting and the neck rotated laterally. This murmur also can be heard in healthy adults and is present in nearly all women in the later stages of pregnancy. High cardiac output states such as thyrotoxicosis and anemia are also associated with easily heard cervical venous hums. Peak intensity is in the supraclavicular fossa just lateral to the sternocleidomastoid muscle, and it is usually more prominent on the right side. When the murmur is loud, it can radiate below the clavicles and occasionally can be confused with the continuous murmur of patent ductus arteriosus. This error should never be made, however, because the cervical venous hum can be terminated easily by digital compression of the JVP.

The mammary souffle is a continuous murmur occurring in 10 to 15 percent of pregnant women during the second and third trimesters and in the early postpartum period, particularly in lactating women, and is heard between the second and sixth anterior in-

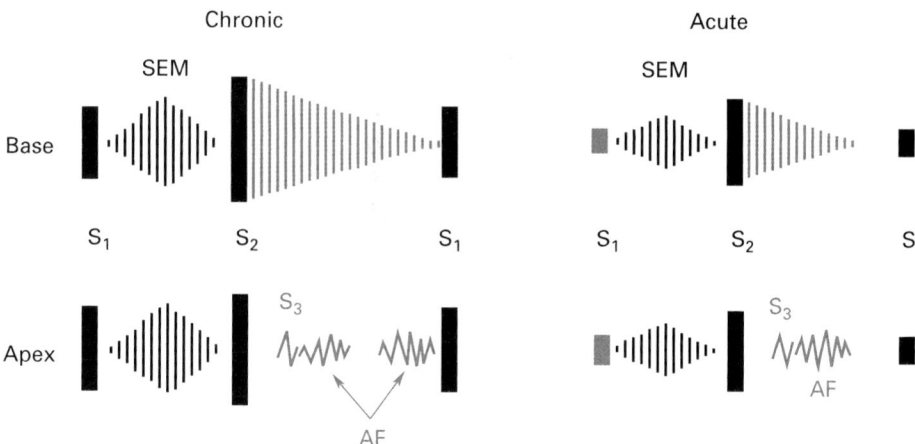

Chronic
SEM
Base
S_1 S_2 S_1

Apex
S_3
AF

Acute
SEM
S_1 S_2 S_1

S_3
AF

FIGURE 12–88. Diagram contrasting the auscultatory findings in chronic and acute aortic regurgitation (AR). In chronic AR, a prominent systolic ejection murmur (SEM), resulting from the large forward stroke volume, is heard at the base and apex and ends well before the second heart sound (S_2). The aortic diastolic regurgitant murmur begins with S_2 and continues in a decrescendo fashion, terminating before the first heart sound (S_1). At the apex, the early diastolic component of the Austin Flint (AF) murmur is introduced by a prominent third heart sound (S_3). A presystolic component of the AF is also heard. In acute AR, there is a significant decrease in the intensity of the SEM compared with chronic AR because of the decreased forward stroke volume. S_1 is markedly decreased in intensity because of preclosure of the mitral valve; at the apex, the presystolic component of the AF murmur is absent. The early diastolic murmur at the base ends well before S_1 because of the equilibration of the left ventricular (LV) and aortic end-diastolic pressure. Significant tachycardia is usually present. *Source: Shaver JA. Diastolic murmurs. Heart Dis Stroke. 1993;1:98–103. Reproduced with permission from the American Heart Association.*

tercostal spaces. This murmur can be obliterated by firm pressure on the stethoscope or by digital pressure applied just lateral to the site of auscultation and therefore should not be confused with the continuous murmur of patent ductus arteriosus or with an arteriovenous fistula. The mammary souffle disappears after termination of lactation. Other causes of continuous murmurs caused by rapid blood flow through arterial or venous channels are outlined in Table 12–14.

Continuous Murmurs Caused by High- to Low-Pressure Shunts A group of congenital cardiovascular anomalies has shunting from the high-pressure systemic (aortic) circulation to the low-pressure pulmonary arterial circulation, resulting in a large gradient between the two systems throughout the cardiac cycle. The murmur of patent ductus arteriosus is the classic example of this type of anomaly. It is heard best in the left infraclavicular area and the second left intercostal space. The peak intensity of the murmur is at the time of S_2, after which it gradually wanes until it terminates before S_1. The length of the murmur is determined by the difference in the vascular resistance between the greater and lesser circulation. As the pulmonary vascular resistance increases, the diastolic pressure in the pulmonary artery approaches and finally reaches systemic levels, diminishing and finally abolishing diastolic flow and the diastolic portion of the murmur. With equilibration of aortic and pulmonary artery pressure, systolic flow across the shunt diminishes and finally disappears, leaving the ductus silent (Eisenmenger patent ductus arteriosus). Surgically produced aortopulmonary connections (Blalock, Waterston, and Potts shunts), as well as the murmur of aortic pulmonary window, have identical qualities, and the effect of PH on their length is analogous. These types of continuous murmurs must be distinguished from to-and-fro murmurs. The latter is a combination of the

systolic ejection murmur and a semilunar diastolic murmur. The classic example of a to-and-fro murmur is the murmur of AS and AR. The continuous murmur builds to a crescendo around S_2, whereas the to-and-fro murmur has two components. The midsystolic ejection component decrescendos and can disappear as it approaches S_2, leaving a silent period before the onset of the regurgitant murmur. Truncus arteriosus is a rare congenital anomaly and probably produces a continuous murmur only if there is coexisting pulmonary artery stenosis. In the presence of severe RV outflow obstruction, bronchial collateral arteries can enlarge their normal precapillary anastomoses with pulmonary arteries, and the resulting aortic pulmonary fistula can produce a continuous murmur. This murmur can be heard in the same location as the patent ductus but radiates widely, especially over the posterior thorax. Large bronchial collateral arteries producing such continuous murmurs are more common with pulmonary atresia but also occur with tetralogy of Fallot. Bronchial artery–pulmonary artery collaterals sufficient to produce continuous murmurs are also found in far-advanced bronchiectasis and sequestration of the lung.

An anomalous left coronary artery arising from the pulmonary artery can cause a continuous murmur when the left-to-right shunt flow is large; it is usually best heard at the left sternal border. In this condition, the origin of the right coronary artery is from the aorta, and the left-to-right shunt is from the high-pressure right coronary arterial bed through large arterial collaterals to the left coronary system, which empties into the low-pressure pulmonary artery.

Sinus of Valsalva aneurysms can cause continuous murmurs when they rupture into the right side of the heart. In almost all cases, rupture occurs from the right and noncoronary sinuses into the right atrium or the RV.[154] The murmur is heard maximally at the lower sternal border or xiphoid over the area corresponding to the fistulous tract. Diastolic accentuation of this murmur is an important sign to differentiate ruptured sinus from patent ductus arteriosus or arteriovenous fistula. Systolic suppression of the murmur is caused by both mechanical narrowing of the fistulous tract during systole as well as the probable Venturi effect created by the rapid ejection of blood past the aortic origin of the fistula.

Coronary artery fistulas usually empty into the right atrium or ventricle and can cause a continuous murmur that is best heard to either the left or the right of the lower sternal area. Because the majority of coronary flow occurs during diastole, the diastolic component of the murmur is louder. When the coronary artery fistula empties into a high-pressure RV, only a diastolic murmur can be heard because the pressure gradient across the shunt is reduced during systole. Left-to-right shunting through an uncomplicated ASD produces no murmur audible on the chest wall because of the minimal pressure gradient and absence of turbulence.

TABLE 12–14

Physiologic Classification of Continuous Murmurs

Continuous murmurs caused by rapid blood flow
- Venous hum
- Mammary souffle
- Hemangioma
- Hyperthyroidism
- Acute alcoholic hepatitis
- Hyperemia of neoplasm (hepatoma, renal cell carcinoma, Paget disease)

Continuous murmurs caused by high- to low-pressure shunts
- Systemic artery to pulmonary artery (patent ductus arteriosus, aortopulmonary window, truncus arteriosus, pulmonary atresia, anomalous left coronary, bronchiectasis, sequestration of the lung)
- Systemic artery to right heart (ruptured sinus of Valsalva, coronary artery fistula)
- Left-to-right atrial shunting (Lutembacher syndrome, mitral atresia plus atrial septal defect)
- Venovenous shunts (anomalous pulmonary veins, portosystemic shunts)
- Arteriovenous fistula (systemic or pulmonic)

Continuous murmurs secondary to localized arterial obstruction
- Coarctation of the aorta
- Branch pulmonary stenosis
- Carotid occlusion
- Celiac mesenteric occlusion
- Renal occlusion
- Femoral occlusion
- Coronary occlusion

SOURCE: Myers JD. The mechanisms and significances of continuous murmurs. In: Leon DF, Shaver JA, eds. Physiologic Principles of Heart Sounds and Murmurs. Monograph 46. New York: American Heart Association; 1975:202. Reproduced with permission from the American Heart Association, Inc., and author.

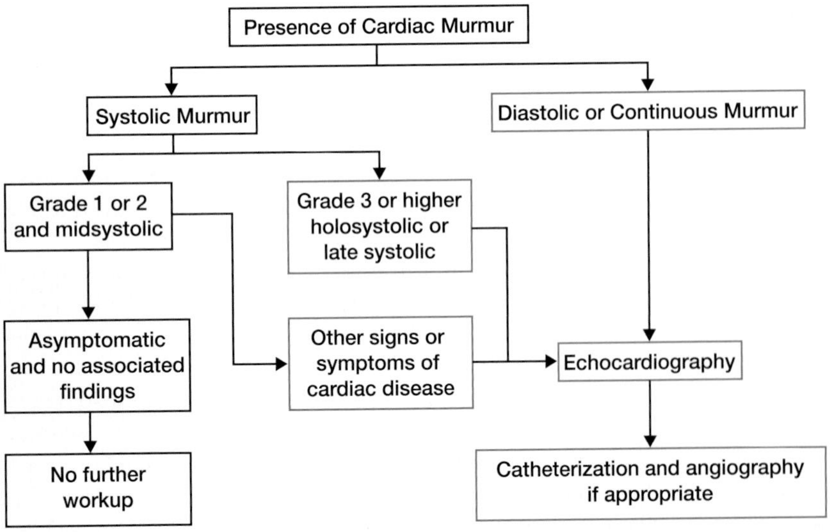

FIGURE 12–89. Algorithm for the evaluation of a cardiac murmur.

When mitral valve obstruction is present, as with Lutembacher syndrome or mitral atresia, however, there can be a high-pressure gradient between the left and right atria across a small defect, and a continuous murmur can be present. This murmur increases in intensity with inspiration and decreases with the Valsalva maneuver. Occasionally, a small ASD is produced following transseptal catheterization or balloon valvuloplasty for MS, and a continuous murmur is produced caused by high-velocity flow resulting from the large pressure gradient from the left to the right atrium.

Total anomalous pulmonary venous drainage into a systemic vein can produce a continuous venous hum usually heard in the pulmonary area or the left infraclavicular area. Frequently, a constriction at the junction of the anomalous venous conduit and the innominate vein or superior vena cava can cause augmentation of the murmur.

Arteriovenous fistulas between peripheral vessels produce a classic continuous murmur with systolic accentuation caused by shunting of a large volume of blood at rapid flow rates from a high-pressure artery into a low-pressure vein. These murmurs are best heard at the site of the fistula. Local compression of the veins can decrease the intensity of the murmur by raising venous pressure and reducing the arteriovenous pressure gradient. Complete obliteration of the fistula will terminate the murmur, and if the shunt is of considerable magnitude, a baroreceptor-mediated reflex bradycardia can occur (Branham sign). Likewise, a reflex tachycardia will occur on release of the obstruction. Pulmonary arteriovenous fistulas usually produce only a systolic murmur because the peripheral vascular resistance of the normal lung is very low, and the normally small diastolic pressure gradient from pulmonary artery to pulmonary vein is not significantly increased by the presence of the fistula.

Continuous Murmur Secondary to Localized Arterial Obstruction

Localized stenosis of systemic or pulmonary arteries can produce a continuous murmur if the obstruction is critical and adequate collateral flow is not available. Most partially obstructed arteries have only systolic murmurs that are delayed relative to cardiac systole, depending on the transit time of pulsatile flow from the heart to the site of obstruction. This lack of diastolic gradient is caused by the collateral arteries around the obstruction that deliver adequate flow such that the diastolic pressure on either side of the localized obstruction is essentially equal. Thus a localized, partial arterial obstruction characteristically produces only a systolic murmur. If adequate collateral flow is not present, there is a continuous murmur with systolic accentuation. In severe coarctation of the aorta, a continuous murmur can also be produced at the site of the coarctation. This latter murmur is best heard over the back midline between the scapulae.

Continuous murmurs also can result from branch pulmonary stenosis or partial obstruction of a major pulmonary artery occluded by a massive pulmonary embolus. Other common locations of continuous murmurs secondary to localized arterial obstructions are listed in Table 12–14. Common to all these murmurs is critical narrowing of the vessel with inadequate collateral flow such that a continuous pressure gradient is produced throughout the cardiac cycle. Murmurs produced by obstruction of major coronary arteries are rarely loud enough to be transmitted to the chest wall. When audible, they produce only diastolic murmurs, even with inadequate collateral circulation.

【 】 APPROACH TO PATIENT WITH A HEART MURMUR

The majority of heart murmurs are midsystolic and soft (grades 1 to 3). When such a murmur occurs in an asymptomatic child or young adult *without* other evidence of heart disease on clinical examination, it is usually benign and echocardiography is not generally required. Conversely, echocardiographic examination is indicated in patients with loud systolic murmurs (grade 3), especially when those are holosystolic or late systolic; in most patients with diastolic or continuous murmurs and in patients with additional unexplained physical findings on cardiac examination (Fig. 12–89).

REFERENCES

1. Vanden Belt RJ. The history. In: Chizner M, ed. *Classic Teachings in Clinical Cardiology: A Tribute to W. Proctor Harvey.* Cedar Grove, NJ: Laennec; 1996:41–54.
2. Hurst JW, Morris DC. The history: symptoms and past events related to cardiovascular disease. In: Schlant RC, Alexander RW, O'Rourke RA, et al., eds. *The Heart.* 8th ed. New York: McGraw-Hill; 1994:205–216.
3. O'Rourke RA. Chest pain. In: Fuster V, Alexander RW, O'Rourke RA, et al., eds. *The Heart.* 10th ed. New York: McGraw-Hill; 2001:195–199.
4. Sampson JJ, Cheitlin M. Pathophysiology and differential diagnosis of cardiac pain. *Prog Cardiovasc Dis.* 1971;13:507–531.
5. O'Rourke RA. Diagnostic approach to the patient with chest pain compatible with definite or suspected angina pectoris. In: Sobel BE, ed. *Medical Management of Heart Disease.* New York: Marcel Dekker; 1996:4–22.
6. Heberden W. Some accounts of a disorder of the breast. *Med Trans.* 1772;2:59.
7. Goswami N, O'Rourke RA. The pathophysiology of chronic stable angina. In: Fuster V, Nabel E, Topol EJ, eds. *Atherothrombosis and Coronary Heart Disease.* 2nd ed. Philadelphia: Lippincott. In press.
8. Murray DR, O'Rourke RA, Walling AD, Walsh RA. History and physical examination in myocardial ischemia and acute myocardial infarction. In: Francis G, Alpert J, eds. *Coronary Care.* 2nd ed. Boston: Little, Brown; 1995:73–95.
9. Dell'Italia LJ. Chest pain. In: Stein JH, ed. *Internal Medicine.* 5th ed. Boston: Little, Brown; 1998:125–129.
10. Christie LG Jr, Conti CR. Systemic approach to evaluation of angina-like chest pain: pathophysiology and clinical testing with emphasis on objective documentation of myocardial ischemia. *Am Heart J.* 1981;102:897–912.
11. Taggart P, Yellon D. Preconditioning and arrhythmias. *Circulation.* 2002;106:2999–3001.
12. Campeau L. Letter to the editor. *Circulation.* 1976;54:522.
13. Levine SA. Carotid sinus massage: a new diagnostic test for angina pectoris. *JAMA.* 1962;182:1332–1356.
14. Douglas PS, Ginsberg GS. The evaluation of chest pain in women. *N Engl J Med.* 1996;334:1311–1315.
15. Chauhan A, Mullins PA, Taylor G, et al. Cardioesophageal reflux: a mechanism for "linked angina" in patients with angiographically proven coronary artery disease. *J Am Coll Cardiol.* 1996;27:1621–1628.
16. Epstein SE, Talbot TL. Dynamic coronary tone in precipitation, exacerbation and relief of angina pectoris. *Am J Cardiol.* 1981;48:797–803.
17. Proudfit WL, Shrey ED, Sones FM Jr. Selective cine coronary arteriography: correlation with clinical findings in 1000 patients. *Circulation.* 1996;33:901–910.
18. Gibbons R, Abrams J, Chatterjee K, et al. ACC/AHA 2002 guideline update for the management of patients with chronic stable angina. Available at: www.acc.org/clinical/guidelines/stable/stable.pdf.
19. Ross RS, Babe BM. Right ventricular hypertension as a cause of angina. *Circulation.* 1960;22:801–802.
20. Spodick DH. Pitfalls in the recognition of pericarditis. In: Hurst JW, ed. *Clinical Essays on the Heart.* Vol V. New York: McGraw-Hill; 1985:95–111.
21. Eagle KA, DeSanctis RW. Dissecting aortic aneurysm. *Curr Probl Cardiol.* 1989;14:227–228.
22. Katon W, Hall ML, Russo J, et al. Chest pain: Relationship of psychiatric illness to coronary arteriographic results. *Am J Med.* 1988;84:1–9.
23. Mellow MH. A gastroenterologist's view of chest pain. *Curr Probl Cardiol.* 1983;9:1–36.
24. Rose S, Achkar E, Easley KA. Follow-up of patients with noncardiac chest pain: value of esophageal testing. *Dig Dis Sci.* 1994;39:2063–2068.
25. Bernstein LM, Grain RC, Pacini R. Differentiation of esophageal pain from angina pectoris: role of esophageal acid perfusion test. *Medicine.* 1962;41:145–162.
26. Atkinson M. Monitoring esophageal pH. *Gut.* 1987;28:509–514.
27. The Criteria Committee of the New York Heart Association. *Diseases of the Heart and Blood Vessels: Nomenclature and Criteria for Diagnosis of the Heart and Great Vessels.* 6th ed. New York: New York Heart Association/Little, Brown, 1964.
28. Aziz K, Sanyal SK, Goldblatt E. Reversed differential cyanosis. *Br Heart J.* 1968;30:288–290.
29. Basson CT, Cowley GS, Solomon SD, et al. The clinical and genetic spectrum of the Holt-Oram syndrome (heart-hand syndrome). *N Engl J Med.* 1994;330:885–891.
30. Musewe NN, Alexander DJ, Teshima I, et al. Echocardiographic evaluation of the spectrum of cardiac anomalies associated with trisomy 13 and trisomy 18. *J Am Coll Cardiol.* 1990;15:673–677.
31. Subramaniam PN. Turner's syndrome and cardiovascular anomalies. *Am J Med Sci.* 1989;297:260–262.
32. Roldan CA, Chavez J, Wiest PW, et al. Aortic root disease and valve disease associated with ankylosing spondylitis. *J Am Coll Cardiol.* 1998;32:1397–1404.
33. Parish JM, Shepard JW. Cardiovascular effects of sleep disorders. *Chest.* 1990;97:1220–1225.
34. Cox J, Krajden M. Cardiovascular manifestations of Lyme disease. *Am Heart J.* 1991;122:1449–1455.
35. Shammas RL, Movahed A. Sarcoidosis of the heart. *Clin Cardiol.* 1993;16:462–472.
36. Kuan P. Cardiac Wilson's disease. *Chest.* 1987;91:579–583.
37. Kyle RA. Amyloidosis. *Circulation.* 1995;91:1269–1271.
38. Hara KS, Ballard DJ, Ilstrup DM, et al. Rheumatoid pericarditis: clinical features and survival. *Medicine.* 1990;69:81–91.
39. Deer T, Rosencrance JG, Chillag SA. Cardiac conduction manifestations of Reiter's syndrome. *South Med J.* 1991;84:799–800.
40. Lazarus A, Varin J, Babuty D, et al. Long-term follow-up of arrhythmias in patients with myotonic dystrophy treated by pacing. A multicenter diagnostic pacemaker study. *J Am Coll Cardiol.* 2002;40:1645–1652.
41. Burns JC, Shike H, Gordon JB, et al. Sequelae of Kawasaki disease in adolescents and young adults. *J Am Coll Cardiol.* 1996;28:253–257.
42. Jacob AG, Driscoll DJ, Shaughnessy WJ, et al. Klippel-Trénaunay syndrome: spectrum and management. *Cano Clin Proc.* 1998;73:28–36.
43. Stevenson WG, Perloff JK, Weiss JN, Anderson TL. Facioscapulohumeral muscular dystrophy: evidence for selective, genetic electrophysiologic cardiac involvement. *J Am Coll Cardiol.* 1990;15:292–299.
44. Buckley AE, Dean J, Mahy IR. Cardiac involvement in Emery Dreifuss muscular dystrophy: a case series. *Heart.* 1999;82:105–108.
45. Nutter DO. Measurements of the systolic blood pressure. In: Hurst JW, ed. *The Heart.* 5th ed. New York: McGraw-Hill, 1982.
46. Asmar R, Benetos A, London G, et al. Aortic distensibility in normotensive, untreated and treated hypertensive patients. *Blood Press.* 1995;4:48–54.
47. Frohlich ED. Hypertension in the elderly. *Curr Probl Cardiol.* 1988;13:313–367.
48. Hales S. *Statistical Essays: Containing Haema-staticks; or, an Account of Some Hydraulick and Hydrostatical Experiments Made on the Blood and Blood-Vessels of Animals.* London: Innys W, Manby R;1733.
49. Grim NC, Grim CE. Blood pressure measurements. In: Izzo JL, Black HE, eds. *AHA Hypertension Primer.* 2nd ed. New York: American Heart Association; 1998:295–298.
50. McCutcheon EP, Rushmer RF. Korotkov sounds: an experimental critique. *Circ Res.* 1967;20:149–161.
51. Rodbard S. The components of the Korotkov sounds. *Am Heart J.* 1967;74:278–282.
52. Neilsen PR, Janniche H. The accuracy of auscultatory measurement of arm blood pressure in very obese subjects. *Acta Med Scand.* 1974;196:403–409.
53. White SB, Berson AS, Robbins C, et al. National standard for measurement of resting and ambulatory blood pressure with automated sphygmomanometers. *Hypertension.* 1993;21:504–509.

54. Nichols WW, O'Rourke MF, eds. *McDonald's Blood Flow in Arteries.* 4th ed. London: Edward Arnold, 1998.

55. Siebenhofer A, Kemp C, Sutton A, Williams B. The reproducibility of central aortic blood pressure measurements in healthy subjects using applanation tonometry and sphygmocardiography. *J Hum Hypertens.* 1999;13:625–629.

56. Frohlich ED, Gifford RW, Hall WD. Hypertensive cardiovascular disease. In: 18th Bethesda Conference Report: Cardiovascular Disease in the Elderly. *J Am Coll Cardiol.* 1987;10(suppl A):57A–59A.

57. O'Rourke MF. *Arterial Function in Health and Disease.* New York: Churchill-Livingstone; 1982.

58. Wei Y, Gersh BJ. Heart disease in the elderly. *Curr Probl Cardiol.* 1987;12:1–65.

59. Richardson DW, Honour AJ, Fenton DW, et al. Variation in arterial pressure throughout the day and night. *Clin Sci.* 1964;26:445–460.

60. Littler WA, Honour AJ, Pugsley DJ, Sleight PL. Continuous recording of direct arterial pressure in unrestricted patients. *Circulation.* 1975;51:1101–1106.

61. Vlachopoulos C, O'Rourke M. Genesis of the normal and abnormal arterial pulse. *Curr Probl Cardiol.* 2000;25:306–367.

62. Schlant RC, Hurst JW. *Examination of the Precordium: Inspection and Palpation.* New York: American Heart Association; 1990:1–28.

63. Crawford MH. Inspection and palpation of venous and arterial pulses: In: *Examination of the Heart.* Part 2. New York: American Heart Association; 1990.

64. O'Rourke MF. The arterial pulse in health and disease. *Am Heart J.* 1971;82:687–702.

65. Murgo JP, Westerhof N, Giolma JP, Altobelli SA. Aortic input impedance in normal man: relationship to pressure wave shapes. *Circulation.* 1980;62:105–116.

66. Hamilton WF, Dow P. An experimental study of the standing waves in the pulse propagated through the aorta. *Am J Physiol.* 1939;125:48.

67. McPhail I. Use of the ankle-brachial index in cardiovascular risk assessment. Available at: www.acessmedicine.com. Accessed September 25, 2003.

68. Schlant RC, Felner MJ. The arterial pulse: clinical manifestations. *Curr Prob Cardiol.* 1977;2:1–50.

69. Safar ME, Frohlich ED. The arterial system in hypertension: a prospective view. *Hypertension.* 1995;26:10–14.

70. Armentano R, Megnien JL, Simon A, et al. Effects of hypertension on viscoelasticity of carotid and femoral arteries in humans. *Hypertension.* 1995;26:48–54.

71. Bude RO, Rubin JM, Platt JF, et al. Pulsus tardus: its cause and potential limitations in detection of aortic stenosis. *Radiology.* 1994;190:779–784.

72. Ewy GA, Rios JC, Marcus FI. The dicrotic arterial pulse. *Circulation.* 1969;39:655–661.

73. Mitchell JH, Sarnoff SJ, Sonnenblock EH. The dynamics of pulsus alternans: alternating end-diastolic fiber length as a causative factor. *J Clin Invest.* 1963;42:55–63.

74. Shabetai R, Fowler NO, Fenton JC, Masangkay M. Pulsus paradoxus. *J Clin Invest.* 1965;44:1882–1898.

75. Shabetai R, Fowler NO, Guntheroth WG. The hemodynamics of cardiac tamponade and constrictive pericarditis. *Am J Cardiol.* 1970;26:480–498.

76. Otsuji Y, Toda H, Kisanuki A, et al. Influence of left ventricular filling profile during preceding control beats on pulse pressure during ventricular premature contractions. *Eur Heart J.* 1994;15:462–467.

77. Garratt CJ, Griffith MJ, Young G, et al. Value of physical signs in the diagnosis of ventricular tachycardia. *Circulation.* 1994;90:3103–3107.

78. Hurst JW, Schlant RC. Examination of the veins and their pulsation. In: Hurst JW, ed. *The Heart* 4th ed. New York: McGraw-Hill; 1978:193–201.

79. Ewy GA, Marcus FI. Bedside estimation of the venous pressure. *Heart Bull.* 1968;17:41.

80. Ewy GA. The abdominojugular test: technique and hemodynamic correlates. *Ann Intern Med.* 1989;108:456–460.

81. Ducas J, Magder S, McGregor M. Validity of the hepatojugular reflux as a clinical test for congestive heart failure. *Am J Cardiol.* 1983;52:1299–1303.

82. Dell'Italia L, Starling MR, O'Rourke RA. Physical examination for exclusion of hemodynamically important right ventricular infarction. *Ann Intern Med.* 1983;99:608–612.

83. Anderson WB. Examination of the retina: In: Alexander AW, Schlant RC, Fuster W, eds. *Hurst's The Heart.* 9th ed. New York: McGraw-Hill; 1998:343–349.

84. Hurst JW, Robinson PH. Physical examination of the chest, abdomen and extremities. In: Hurst JW, et al, eds. *The Heart.* 7th ed. New York: McGraw-Hill; 1990:242–243.

85. Willis PW IV. Inspection and palpation of the precordium. In: Hurst JW, ed. *The Heart.* 7th ed. New York: McGraw-Hill; 1990:163–169.

86. Abrams J. Precordial palpation: let your fingers do the walking. In: Chizner M, ed. *Classic Teachings in Clinical Cardiology: A Tribute to W. Proctor Harvey.* Cedar Grove, NJ. Laennec; 1996:85–103.

87. Martin CE, Shaver JA, O'Toole JD, et al. Ejection sounds of right-sided origin. In: Leon DF, Shaver JA, eds. *Physiologic Principles of Heart Sounds and Murmurs* (Monograph 46). New York: American Heart Association; 1975:35–44.

88. Ronan JA, Perloff JK, Harvey WP. Systolic clicks and the late systolic murmur. *Am Heart J.* 1965;70:319–325.

89. Popp Rl, Brown OR, Silverman JF, et al. Echocardiographic abnormalities in the MVP syndrome. *Circulation.* 1974;49:428433.

90. Abrams J. *Essentials of Cardiac Physical Diagnosis.* Philadelphia: Lea & Febiger, 1987.

91. Barlow JB, Pocock WA, Marchand P, Denny M. The significance of late systolic murmurs. *Am Heart J.* 1963;66:443–452.

92. Ronan JA Jr, Steelman RB, DeLeon AC Jr, et al. The clinical diagnosis of acute severe mitral insufficiency. *Am J Cardiol.* 1971;27:284–290.

93. Abrams J. Precordial palpation. In: Horwitz LD, Graves BM, eds. *Signs and Symptoms in Cardiology.* Philadelphia: Lippincott; 1985:156–177.

94. Levine SA, Harvey SP. *Clinical Auscultation of the Heart.* 2nd ed. Philadelphia, PA: Saunders; 1959.

95. Shaver JA, Salerni R, Reddy PS. Normal and abnormal heart sounds in cardiac diagnosis: I. Systolic sounds. *Curr Probl Cardiol.* 1985;10:1–68.

96. Reddy PS, Salerni R, Shaver JA. Normal and abnormal heart sounds in cardiac diagnosis: II. Diastolic sounds. *Curr Probl Cardiol.* 1985;10:1–55.

97. Laniado S, Yellin EL, Miller H, Frater WM. Temporal relation of the first heart sound to closure of the mitral valve. *Circulation.* 1973;47:1006–1014.

98. Shah PM. Hemodynamic determinants of the first heart sound. In: Leon DF, Shaver JA, eds. *Physiologic Principles of Heart Sounds and Murmurs* (Monograph 46). New York: American Heart Association; 1975:2–7.

99. Tei C, Shah PM, Cherian G, et al. The correlates of an abnormal first heart sound in MVP syndromes. *N Engl J Med.* 1982;307:334–339.

100. Shaver JA, Rahko PS, Grines CL. Effect of left bundle branch block on the events of the cardiac cycle. *Acta Cardiol.* 1988;4:459–467.

101. Mills P, Craige E. Echophonocardiography. *Prog Cardiovasc Dis.* 1978;20:337.

102. Criley JM, Lewis KB, Humphries JO, Ross RS. Prolapse of the mitral valve: clinical and cine-angiocardiographic findings. *Br Heart J.* 1966;28:488–496.

103. Leon DF, Leonard JJ, Kroetz FW, et al. Late systolic murmurs, clicks, and whoops arising from the mitral valve. *Am Heart J.* 1966;72:325–336.

104. Leatham A. The second heart sound, key to auscultation of the heart. *Acta Cardiol.* 1964;19:395–416.

105. Shaver JA, Nadolny RA, O'Toole JD, et al. Sound pressure correlates of the second heart sound: an intracardiac sound study. *Circulation.* 1974;49:316–325.

106. Dell'Italia LJ, Walsh RA. Acute determinants of the hangout interval in the pulmonary circulation. *Am Heart J.* 1988;16:1289–1297.

107. Shaver JA, O'Toole JD. The second heart sound: Newer concepts: 2. Paradoxical splitting and narrow physiological splitting. *Mod Concepts Cardiovasc Dis.* 1977;46:13–16.

108. Gamble WH, Shaver JA, Alvares RF, et al. A critical appraisal of diastolic time intervals as a measure of relaxation in left ventricular hypertrophy. *Circulation.* 1983;68:76–87.

109. Martin CE, Shaver JA, Leonard JJ. Physical signs, apex cardiography, phonocardiography, and systolic time intervals in angina pectoris. *Circulation.* 1972;46:1098–1114.

110. Wood P. Pulmonary hypertension. *Br Med Bull.* 1952;8:348–353.

111. Thayer WS. The early diastolic heart sound. *Trans Assoc Am Phys.* 1908;13:326–357.

112. Oriol A, Palmer WH, Nakhjavan F, McGregor M. Prediction of left atrial pressure from the second sound-OS interval. *Am J Cardiol.* 1965;16:184–188.

113. Sloan AW, Campbell FW, Henderson AS. Incidence of the physiological third heart sound. *Br Med J.* 1952;2:853–855.

114. Harvey WP, Stapleton J. Clinical aspects of gallop rhythm with particular reference to diastolic gallops. *Circulation.* 1958;18:1017–1024.

115. Craige E. Gallop rhythm. *Prog Cardiovasc Dis.* 1967;10:246–260.

116. Shaver JA, Reddy PS, Alvares FR. Early diastolic events associated with the physiologic and pathologic S₃. *J Cardiol.* 1984;14(suppl V):30–46.

117. Shah PM, Jackson D. Third heart sound and summation gallop. In: Leon DF, Shaver JA, eds. *Physiologic Principles of Heart Sounds and Murmurs* (Monograph 46). New York: American Heart Association; 1975:79–84.

118. Reddy PS, Meno F, Curtiss EI, O'Toole JD. The genesis of gallop sounds: investigation by quantitative phono- and apex cardiography. *Circulation.* 1981;63:922–933.

119. Shaver JA, Reddy PS, Alvares RF, Salerni R. Genesis of the physiologic third heart sound. *Am J Noninvas Cardiol.* 1987;1:39–55.

120. Stapleton JF. Third and fourth heart sounds. In: Horwitz LD, Groves BM, eds. *Signs and Symptoms in Cardiology.* Philadelphia, PA: Lippincott; 1985:214–226.

121. Fowler NO, Adolph RJ. Fourth sound gallop or split first sound? *Am J Cardiol.* 1972;30:441–444.

122. Harris A. Pacemaker "heart sound." *Br Heart J.* 1967;29:608–615.

123. Lerman J, Means JH. Cardiovascular symptomatology in exophthalmic goiter. *Am Heart J.*1932;8:55–65.

124. Hamman L. Spontaneous mediastinal emphysema. *Bull Johns Hopkins Hosp.* 1939;64:1–21.

125. Soffer A, Feinstein A, Luisada AA, et al. Glossary of cardiologic terms related to physical diagnosis and history. *Am J Cardiol.* 1967;20:285–286.

126. Freeman AR, Levine SA. Clinical significance of systolic murmurs: study of 1000 consecutive "noncardiac" cases. *Ann Intern Med.* 1933;6:1371–1385.

127. Norton P, O'Rourke RA. Cardiac murmurs. In: Goldman L, Braunwald E, eds. *Cardiology for the Primary Physician.* 2nd ed. Philadelphia, PA: Saunders; 2003:151–168.

128. Mangione S, Nieman LZ. Cardiac auscultatory skills of internal medicine and family practice trainees. A comparison of diagnostic proficiency. *JAMA.* 1997;278(9):717.

129. Murgo JP. Systolic ejection murmurs in the era of modern cardiology. What do we really know? *J Am Coll Cardiol.* 1998;32:1596.

130. Gallavardin L, Ravault P. Le souffle du retrecissement aortique puet changer de timbre et devenir musical dans sa propagation apexienne. *Lyon Med.* 1925;135:523–529.

131. Stein PD, Sabbah HN. Aortic origin of innocent murmurs. *Am J Cardiol.* 1977;39:665–671.

132. Murgo JP, Altobelli SA, Dorethy JF, et al. Normal ventricular ejection dynamics in man during rest and exercise. In: Leon DF, Shaver JA, eds. *Physiologic Principles of Heart Sounds and Murmurs* (Monograph 46). New York: American Heart Association; 1975:92–101.

133. Reddy PS, Shaver JA, Leonard JJ. Cardiac systolic murmurs: Pathophysiology and differential diagnosis. *Prog Cardiovasc Dis* 1971;14:19.

134. deLeon AC Jr. "Straight back" syndrome. In: Leon DF, Shaver JA, eds. *Physiologic Principles of Heart Sounds and Murmurs* (Monograph 46). New York: American Heart Association; 1975:197–208.

135. Shaver JA. Innocent murmurs. *Hosp Med.* 1978;8–35.

136. Vogelpoel L, Schrire V. Ausculatory and phonocardiographic assessment of pulmonary stenosis with intact ventricular septum. *Circulation* 1960;22:55–72

137. Rivero Carvallo JM. Signo para el diagnostico de las insuficiencias tricuspideas. *Arch Inst Cardiol Mex.* 1946;16:531–540.

138. Karliner JS, O'Rourke RA, Kearney DJ, Shabetai R. Hemodynamic explanation of why the murmur of MR is independent of cycle length. *Br Heart J.* 1973;35:397–401.

139. Wooley CF. The spectrum of TR. In: Leon DF, Shaver JA, eds. *Physiologic Principles of Heart Sounds and Murmurs* (Monograph 46). New York: American Heart Association; 1975:139–148.

140. Leatham A, Segal BL. Auscultatory and phonocardiographic findings in ventricular septal defect with left-to-right shunt. *Circulation.* 1962;25:318–327.

141. Ronan JA Jr, Steelman RB, DeLeon AC, et al. The clinical diagnosis of acute severe mitral insufficiency. *Am J Cardiol.* 1971;27:284–290.

142. Braunwald E. MR. *N Engl J Med.* 1969;281:425–433.

143. Amidi M, Irwin JM, Salerni R, et al. Venous systolic thrill and murmur in the neck: a consequence of severe tricuspid insufficiency. *J Am Coll Cardiol* 1986;7:942–945

144. Burch GE, DePasquale NP, Phillips HJ. Clinical manifestations of papillary muscle dysfunction. *Arch Intern Med.* 1963;112:158–163.

145. Murgo JP, Miller JW. Hemodynamic, angiographic and echocardiographic evidence against impeded ejection in hypertrophic cardiomyopathy. In: Goodwin JF, ed. *Heart Muscle Disease.* Lancaster, England: MTP Press; 1985:187–211.

146. Shah PM. Controversies in hypertrophic cardiomyopathy. *Curr Probl Cardiol.* 1986;11:563–613.

147. Shaver JA, Salerni R, Curtiss EI, Follansbee WP. A clinical presentation and noninvasive evaluation of the patient with hypertrophic cardiomyopathy. In: Shaver JA, Brest AN, eds. *Cardiomyopathies: Clinical Presentation, Differential Diagnosis, and Management* (Cardiovascular Clinics). Philadelphia, PA: Davis, 1988:149–192.

148. Coombs CF. *Rheumatic Heart Disease.* New York: William Wood; 1924:190.

149. Flint A. On cardiac murmurs. *Am J Med Sci.* 1862;44:29–54.

150. Reddy PS, Curtiss EI, Salerni R, et al. Sound pressure correlates of the Austin Flint murmur: an intracardiac sound study. *Circulation.* 1976;53:210–217.

151. Harvey WP, Corrado MA, Perloff JK. "Right-sided" murmurs of aortic insufficiency. *Am J Med Sci.* 1963;245:533–543.

152. Runco V, Molnar W, Meckstroth CV, Ryan JM. The Graham Steell murmur versus AR in rheumatic heart disease. *Am J Med.* 1961;31:71–80.

153. Green EW, Agruss NS, Adolph RJ. Right-sided Austin Flint murmur. *Am J Cardiol.* 1973;32:370–374.

154. Perez JE, Smith CA, Meltzer VN. Pulmonic valve insufficiency: a common cause of transient diastolic murmurs in renal failure. *Ann Intern Med.* 1985;103:497–502.

155. Myers JD. The mechanisms and significances of continuous murmurs. In: Leon DF, Shaver JA, eds. *Physiologic Principles of Heart Sounds and Murmurs* (Monograph 46). New York: American Heart Association; 1975:201–208.

CHAPTER 13

The Resting Electrocardiogram

Agustin Castellanos / Alberto Interian Jr. / Robert J. Myerburg

The electrocardiogram (ECG) has evolved during the last century in many different directions.[1-13] Besides classical 12-lead electrocardiography, recent experimental studies have provided new information capable of expanding the clinical usefulness of this method. The ECG has many uses: it can serve as an independent marker of myocardial disease; it can reflect anatomic, hemodynamic, molecular, ionic, and drug-induced abnormalities of the heart; and it can provide information that is essential for the proper diagnosis and therapy of many cardiac problems.[4] *It is the most commonly used laboratory procedure for the diagnosis of heart disease and one of the most commonly employed tests in medicine.*[4,6] *Importantly, it is a required portion of the subspecialty boards in cardiovascular diseases that must be passed by those taking the examination.* It is used by a host of different health care providers. Paradoxically, Hurst has emphasized that many of those who order ECGs cannot interpret the tracings properly and do not even know of their inadequacies in this regard.[3] Worse, a few can transmit information that is incorrect. Many medical schools have remarkable technologically innovative electrophysiologic laboratories and lack good teachers of electrocardiography. Hurst posed the question of "where have the latter gone?" His answer: "They have become invasive interventional electrophysiologists, echocardiographers, nuclear cardiologists," and so on. Certainly computer interpretation has offered some help, but leaves much to be desired.[3] Recognition of the importance of the ECG and of its appropriate use should be given the necessary importance. Finally, in view of the innumerable technical problems encountered in the recording of ECGs today, and paraphrasing Hurst, we can pose the following question "where have the good ECG technicians gone?"

ELECTROCARDIOGRAPHIC LEADS

【 】 BIPOLAR LIMB LEADS

Electrodes placed on the right arm (RA), left arm (LA), and left leg (LL) are used to pick up the potential variations on these extremities to form an equilateral triangle, which sides are bipolar leads I (RA-LA); II (RA-LL); and III (LA-LL). The latter can be said to form a geometric equilateral triangle in which the distances between the cardiac vectors and the extremities is great enough to approach "infinity"[12] so that the electrical activity of the heart can be represented by a single dipole. Consequently, when the electrodes are placed proximally to the roots of the extremities, as for exercise testing and Holter monitoring, the leads lose their relatively *far* distance from the heart, and the Einthoven equilateral theory does not hold.[12,14] This also applies to the precordial leads, something that is not considered in many interpretations of the ECG.[14]

ELECTRICAL AXIS

The *electrical axis* (EA) can be defined as a vector originating in the center of the Einthoven equilateral triangle[8,11-13] that also gives the direction of the activation process as projected only in the (frontal) plane given by the limb leads. The method for determining the mean EA recommended by electrocardiographers of the classic school consists of calculating the net areas enclosed by the QRS complex in leads I, II, and III.[1,2,7,8-13,15] However, the absolute values of the net area cannot be determined *accurately* by inspection. A simpler although less precise method of calculating the quadrant (or parts of a quadrant) in which the EA is located consists of using the maximal QRS deflection in leads I and aVF and, when necessary, lead II.[5]

VENTRICULAR GRADIENT

The relationship between the EA of the QRS complex and the T wave was referred to as the *ventricular gradient*.[12] In the isolated muscle strip, the *sequence* of ventricular depolarization occurs in the same direction as that of repolarization.[10,12] Although the QRS and T deflections have opposite polarity, the algebraic sum of QRS and T *areas* is zero. In the human heart the sequence is different, and the pathways of ventricular depolarization and repolarization are not exactly the same. Thus the algebraic sum of QRS and T *areas* is no longer zero. Therefore, a *gradient* is said to exist.[10,12] The ventricular gradient *must* be calculated by determining the electrical axis of the QRS and T (using *areas*) and then obtaining the resultant by the parallelogram method (Fig. 13–1, left). Its magnitude ranges between 8 and 88 µV/s with its direction being between −16 and +86 degrees in the frontal plane. Its main usefulness is the differentiation between primary and secondary changes in repolarization (see Fig. 13–1). Unfortunately, in practice, calculation of the ventricular gradient is difficult and time-consuming and is rarely used.

UNIPOLAR LEADS

【 】 WILSON CENTRAL TERMINAL

The sum of the potentials from the RA, LA, and LL is equal to zero throughout the cardiac cycle with respect to any point at the body surface.[1,8-12] Lead wires attached to electrodes on each limb are connected together, through 5000-Ω resistors, at a point. When this common point (*Wilson central terminal*) is attached to the negative pole of the ECG machine and an *exploring* electrode is connected to the positive pole, the potential variations recorded will be those of the latter only.[12] A lead taken by this method is

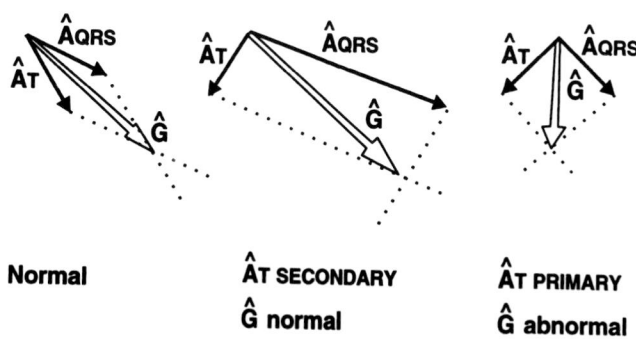

FIGURE 13–1. Ventricular gradient ($\hat{G}$) calculated by areas of QRS complex and T-waves in the frontal plane. Although the T vectors are abnormally located in the middle and right diagrams, secondary T-wave abnormalities do not produce an abnormally directed gradient although primary abnormalities do.

called a *unipolar lead.* Actually, the central terminal is not zero, because the RA, LA, and LL are not equidistant from each other and from the heart, the body tissues vary in resistance, and the heart and extremities do not lie in exactly the same plane in the body. The potential of the central terminal has been said to average approximately 0.3 mV.[13]

[ ] UNIPOLAR EXTREMITY LEADS

Unipolar extremity leads are obtained by disconnecting the input to the central terminal of Wilson from the extremity being explored. This results in a 1.5 increase in their voltage. These *augmented* (a) extremity leads are the ones usually used for clinical electrocardiography and are labeled aVR, aVL, and aVF.[1,2,11-13]

[ ] UNIPOLAR PRECORDIAL LEADS

Unipolar precordial ECGs are obtained by placing the exploring electrode (connected to the positive pole of the ECG machine) on the classic six locations on the anterior and left portions of the chest.[1,2,8-12] The central terminal is used as the indifferent electrode or negative pole. Precordial leads yield positive (upright) deflections when facing positive charges and negative deflections when facing negative charges.[1,2,5,10-12] They can be interpreted by what Wilson called the *solid-angle concept.*[1,8,11,12,14] A solid angle is merely an imaginary cone extending from a site in the chest throughout the heart. The precordial electrode is at its apex, and its base is at the opposite epicardial surface.[12]

Accepting that the amount of muscle activity recorded by the various precordial leads is different implies that the duration of depolarization and repolarization is not the same in each lead, irrespective of that supposedly resulting from the projections of their lead vectors on an idealized horizontal lead axis (see chapter sections, QT Dispersion and Novel Modes of Repolarization Analysis, and Spatial Vectorcardiography).

According to the American College of Cardiology (ACC) criteria V_1 and V_2 are called (anterior) septal, V_3 and V_4 anterior, and V_5 lateral. But in reality V_1 and V_2 can reflect events occurring in the posterior wall of the heart as a result of these leads being, in a sense, its mirror image. V_{4R} (and occasionally also V_1 and even V_2) can reflect right ventricular (RV) events.

OTHER LEAD PLACEMENT METHODS

These are used mainly for initial monitoring of patients with chest pain because it has been said that during emergencies the usual 10-electrode, 12-lead ECG is time consuming, difficult to position properly, and that distal limb placement of electrodes can inevitably create baseline movement.[16]

VENTRICULAR DEPOLARIZATION AND REPOLARIZATION

[ ] THEORETICAL CONSIDERATIONS

It is conventional to first discuss the electrical properties of a hypothetical muscle strip from the free wall of the left ventricle extend-

ing from endocardium to epicardium.[1,2] If activation of this relatively large muscle strip starts in the endocardial side, it initiates the process called *depolarization*[1,2,7-12] that has been described as a moving wave *with the positive charges in front of the negative charges.* A unipolar lead such as V_6 overlying the epicardium of the left ventricle will record a positivity because it consistently faces positive charges throughout the entire depolarization sequence. Conversely, the *sequence* of ventricular repolarization is from epicardium to endocardium. The *negative charges,* however, travel *in front* because repolarization tends to reestablish the resting, polarized state of the previously depolarized cells. Accordingly, V_6 will record a positive deflection (T wave) because it constantly faces positive charges throughout the entire repolarization sequence. The earlier epicardial end of repolarization has been attributed to the shorter duration of repolarization that epicardial cells have in comparison with endocardial cells. This simplistic view is of didactic value only because it fails to take into consideration the role played by the M cells, described by Antzelevitch and colleagues.[15] The latter cells play a determining role in the inscription of the T wave because currents flowing down voltage gradients on either side of the usual (but not necessarily) mid-myocardial cells determine both the height and width of the T wave as well as the degree to which the ascending or descending limbs of the T wave are interrupted.

Yet, some questions remain regarding the role of these cells in determining the sequence of depolarization. For, if the initial repolarization in the free lateral wall proceeds first from epicardium to M-cell layers and thereafter from endocardium to M-cell layers, why are there normally no biphasic (positive–negative) T waves in the left lateral leads? Also, what is the role of the inflection point on the downstroke of the T wave?

VENTRICULAR DEPOLARIZATION: THE QRS COMPLEX

In normal individuals, intervals between sinus beats show different degrees of variations because of respiration, blood pressure regulation, thermoregulation, actions of the renin-angiotensin system, circadian rhythms, premature beats, and so on (Fig. 13–2).[17-20] This has led to the analysis of so-called heart rate variability and heart rate turbulence.[17-20] After emerging from the sinus node, the cardiac impulse propagates throughout the atria in its journey toward the atrioventricular (AV) node. The PR interval (used to estimate AV conduction time) includes conduction through the *true* AV structures (AV node, His bundle, bundle branches, and main divisions of the left bundle branch [LBB]) as well as through those parts of the atria located between sinus and AV nodes.[9] The onset of ventricular depolarization (the beginning of the normal q wave) reflects activation of the left side of the interventricular septum. Hence, the normal initial depolarization is oriented from left to right, therefore explaining the small q wave in lead V_6 and the small r wave in lead V_1. After the cardiac impulse descending through the right bundle branch reaches the right septal surface, the interventricular septum is activated in both directions. Septal activation is thereafter encompassed within or neutralized by free-wall activation.[8,9,11-13] The most distal ramifications of both bundle branches (Purkinje fibers) form networks within the subendocardial regions of both ventricular

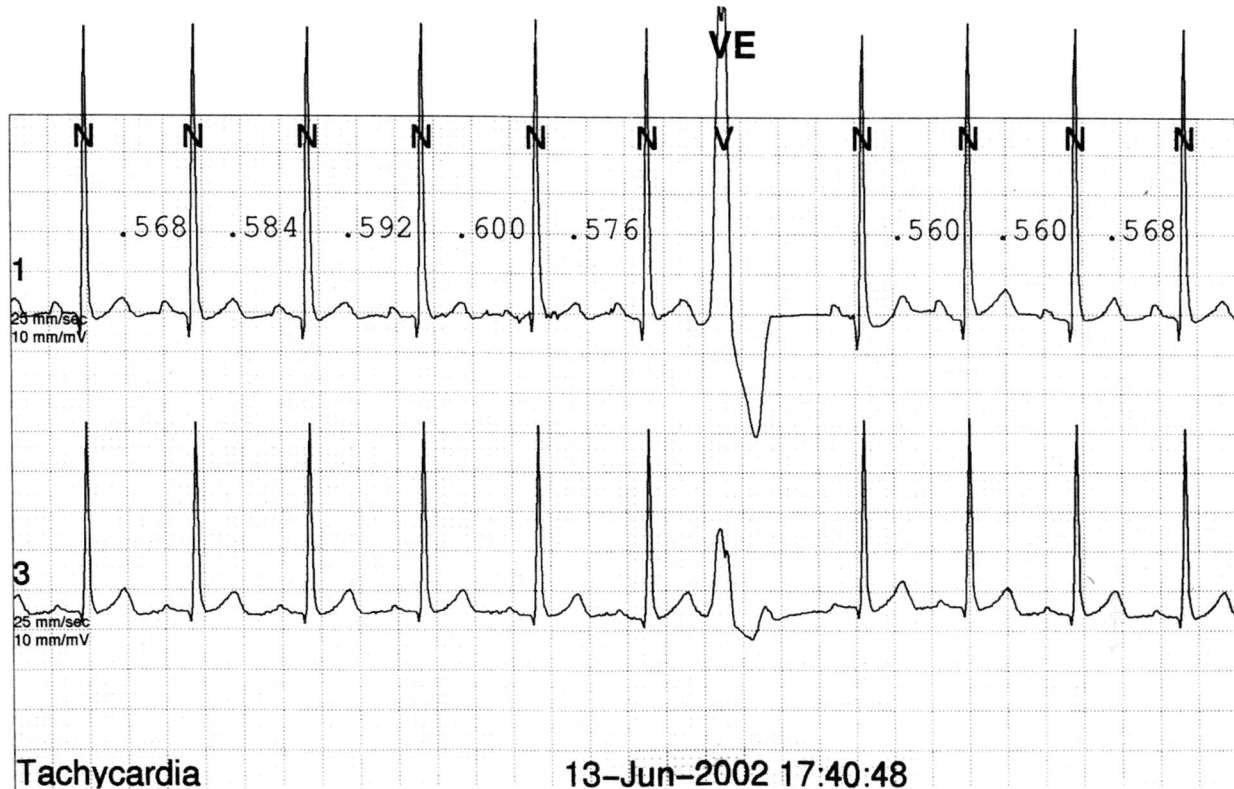

FIGURE 13-2. Rhythm strips showing that the R-R intervals are slightly irregular even during sinus tachycardia (when sinus arrhythmia should not be marked). In addition, ventricular ectopic beats tend to affect (usually accelerate) the first two post-extrasystolic intervals, a phenomenon known as *heart rate turbulence onset.* VE, ventricular ectopic beats.

walls. The greater mass of the left ventricular (LV) free wall explains why LV free-wall events overpower those of the interventricular septum and RV free wall. Ventricular depolarization is represented by the QRS complex.

VENTRICULAR REPOLARIZATION: THE T WAVE

【 】 PRIMARY T-WAVE ABNORMALITIES

Primary T-wave abnormalities can be produced by uniform changes in the shape and (or) the duration of all ventricular potentials without a change in the sequence of repolarization or to nonuniform alterations in the shape and/or duration of the action potentials leading to an altered sequence of repolarization.[1,12,13,21,22] See Fig. 13-1, right, which depicts an abnormally located T vector with an abnormal gradient. This results from molecular, metabolic, or structural changes that induce alterations in repolarization having no dependence whatsoever on the sequence (and duration) of activation.

【 】 SECONDARY T-WAVE ABNORMALITIES

Secondary T-wave abnormalities are generated mainly by abnormalities in ventricular depolarization and occur (for example) in left bundle-branch block (LBBB) and RV pacing in leads with a predominant positive deflection (such as V_6), because repolarization (in contrast with what occurs normally) now proceeds from en-

docardium to epicardium with negative changes in front.[1,10–13,21,22] See Fig. 13-2, middle, which shows an abnormally oriented T vector with a normally located gradient.

【 】 PSEUDOPRIMARY (?) T-WAVE CHANGES, CARDIAC MEMORY, ACCUMULATION, AND DISSIPATION

Rosenbaum and coworkers[23] studied the prolonged depolarization occurring during long periods of ventricular stimulation and found two types of altered ventricular repolarization. One, corresponding to Wilson classic theory, was transient and proportional in magnitude to the QRS complex but of opposite polarity.[23,24] The other, concealed by (but occurring during) the former, required a longer time to reach maximal effect—as well as to disappear—becoming apparent only when the ventricular complexes became narrow (Fig. 13-3).[23] They appeared to be modulated by electrotonic interactions occurring during cardiac activation in such a way that repolarization is accelerated at sites where depolarization starts and delayed in sites where depolarization ends.[23] Because in a single, static ECG the T waves seem to be primary (but occur only because the QRS complexes were previously wide, thus depending on this widening), Rosenbaum and coworkers categorized them as "pseudoprimary" (see Fig. 13-3).[23,24] The concept of cardiac memory was used to categorize this form of electrophysiologic remodeling, characterized by (1) a T-wave vector having the same direction as that of the abnormally activated QRS complexes; (2) increased magnitude of this vector with repeated episodes of abnormal activation (accu-

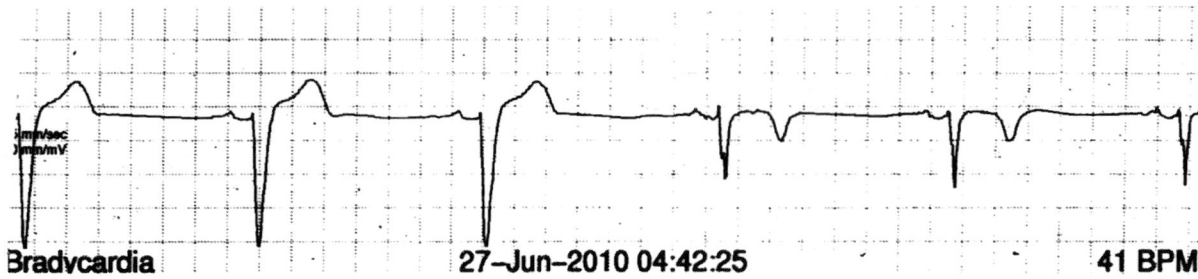

FIGURE 13-3. Rate-dependent complete left bundle-branch block (LBBB) (lead V₁). Negative T waves become manifest when the LBBB disappears in leads showing a predominant negative (S-wave) deflection. The patient has sclerodegenerative conduction system disease with no other evidence of organic heart disease. These changes are attributed to the type of long-term memory effects that become manifest after disappearance of an abnormal sequence of depolarization. BPM, beats per minute.

mulation); and (3) persistence of the abnormal T wave for variable periods (time to dissipation).[23–27]

Rosen defined the underlying mechanisms to be a likely variant on the same processes that determine memory in the central nervous system. Thus, cardiac memory can be classified as being of short, intermediate, or long-term duration.[26] These T-wave changes can be seen after disappearance of a variety of inciting events, such as complete LBBB, RV pacing, wide QRS tachycardias, and after spontaneous or radiofrequency-induced disappearance of preexcitation syndromes.[1,23–27]

THE NORMAL QT INTERVAL: THE DURATION OF DEPOLARIZATION AND REPOLARIZATION

Although this interval has been considered as a surrogate of action potential duration, it yields a limited view of the complicated electrogenesis of ventricular repolarization.[28–31] The manual method of Lepeschkin and Surawicz consists of measuring from the beginning of the q wave to the end of the T wave, defined as the return to the isoelectric, or TP, baseline.[1,29] However, there are difficulties in determining the exact moment where the T wave ends in some leads, as when they are of low amplitude or merged with U (or even P) waves. Certain T-wave morphologies can also cause great difficulties.[1] The most popular algorithm uses the so-called tangent method, which defines the end of the T wave as the point in which one tangent drawn to the steepest portion of its terminal part crosses the isoelectric line.[30,31] For simplicity, when measured manually, a lead with a large T wave (V₃ has been said to be the best) and a distinct termination can be used, but obviously multichannel recordings are more helpful.[1,30,31] Some authors believe that QT intervals still can give useful information even if the QRS complexes are wide and accompanied by the obligatory, secondary T-wave changes.[7,28] A pacing site-dependent change in ventricular activation in diffusely fibrotic hearts was able to produce varying degrees of differential prolongation of the QT intervals.[32]

The QT interval is slightly longer in women than in men, is affected by autonomic tone as well as catecholamines, and it shows circadian variations.[1,28,30] The most important aspect of this interval is its relation with heart rate.[28,32–50] A large number of formulas that have been proposed to establish a rule allowing conversion of a pair of QT and R-R durations into a standardized QTc value corresponding to a "basal" R-R interval of 1 second.

Bazett is the most commonly used (in spite of its imperfection) formula, in which:

$$QTc = k\sqrt{RR} \text{ (in seconds)}$$

The *k* value as modified is 0.397 for men and 0.415 for women. Values of 0.46 second for men and 0.47 second for women apply only when rates are within the normal range, because this formula tends to overcorrect at rapid rates and undercorrect at slower rates. Tables have been proposed by several authors with mean values ranging from 0.40 to 0.44 second at rates of 60/min and 0.31 to 0.34 second at rates of 100/min.[1,49] Whereas the uncorrected QT interval decreases with increasing rates including during exercise, the QTc first increases until reaching approximately a rate of 120/min, thereafter again decreasing.[36]

Adjustment of the QT interval to changes in rate does not occur immediately but rather gradually. A steady state is not reached until several cycles have elapsed. In *normal* subjects and even in persons with minimal myocardial abnormalities (with, mainly, conducting system disease) abrupt R-R changes do not prolong the QT interval if the pauses are short (Fig. 13–4).[28,37]

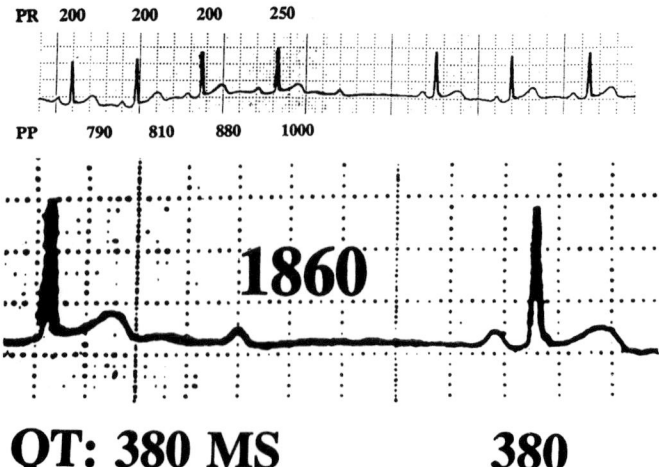

FIGURE 13-4. Vagal-induced atrioventricular nodal block in a young person without structural heart disease. All values are expressed in milliseconds (ms). The uncorrected QT interval does not increase at the end of an 1860 ms (R-R) pause. This can be caused by another form of cardiac memory, whereby the QT interval *remembers* its prepause values because of the slow adjustment to abrupt changes in cycle length as a result of cumulative effects of previous cycle lengths.

Longer pauses produce some prolongation, but restitution tends to occur in the first postpause beat (Fig. 13–5). What was said above also applies to QT interval encompassing wide QRS complexes in patients with absent or minimal myocardial disease (see Fig. 13–5).[28,37]

THE ABNORMAL QT INTERVAL

Shortening of the QT interval is discussed in the section, Electrolyte Imbalances, and congenital and acquired causes of QT shortening and prolongation are dealt with in the corresponding chapters on arrhythmias in Part 6 of this book.

ST-SEGMENT CHANGES CAUSED BY ELECTROCARDIOGRAPHIC INJURY: MECHANISMS

Physiologic acute myocardial ischemia should not be necessarily equated with *electrocardiographic* ischemia, which is simply a pattern consisting of negative T waves symmetric in shape (Fig. 13–6). Severe physiologic ischemia shortens the action potential, reduces the resting membrane potential and decreases the rate of rise of phase 0. The shortening and decreased amplitude of the action potential creates potential differences in voltage gradient between normal and ischemic regions, resulting in the currents of injury. Conventionally, ST-segment changes have been explained by the existence of diastolic and systolic currents of injury. The former implies that the ST segment, which appears to be abnormally displaced above the baseline actually reflects disappearance of the diastolic current of injury. However, the abnormal ST-segment elevation in leads facing the affected zone does not merely represent the (passive) return of the baseline to its preinjury level but reflects a true, active, positive displacement.[1,10,13,51–53] According to the systolic current of injury concept, the ST segment becomes actively elevated above and beyond the preinjury baseline because of the relative potential difference existing at the end of depolarization. Most likely, injury reflects both disappear-

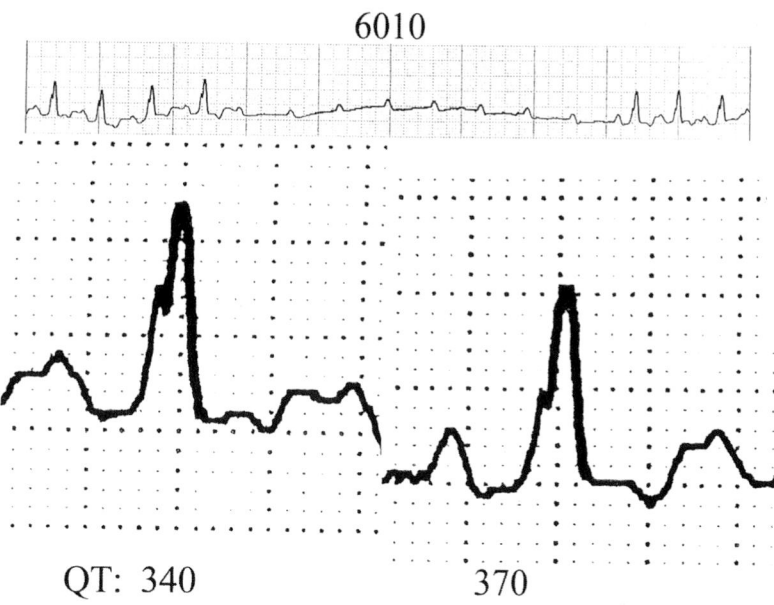

FIGURE 13–5. Lead I from a patient with complete left bundle-branch block caused by sclerodegenerative conduction system disease without myocardial involvement. Note that a pause of 6010 milliseconds (ms) caused by paroxysmal atrioventricular block produces only a relatively small increment in the QT interval (30 ms) with restitution of the preblock duration in the second postpause beat. Magnified complexes on the bottom, left, and to bottom, right, correspond to the last preblock and the first postblock beats, respectively.

ance of diastolic baseline shifts and active ST-segment elevation.[1,2,7,8,10–13] Regardless as to the underlying mechanism, one of the most important postulates in clinical ECG is that the *injury vector points toward the injured zone*: the epicardium in epicardial and transmural injury and the endocardium in subendocardial injury. Reciprocal changes occur in the (spatial) contralateral parts of the heart.

LOCALIZATION OF THE AFFECTED SITES BY ANALYSIS OF LEADS SHOWING ABNORMAL ST-SEGMENT ELEVATION

Unfortunately electrocardiographers use different leads to categorize the site where transmural (physiological) ischemia causes ST-segment elevation. ST-segment elevation in all precordial leads and I

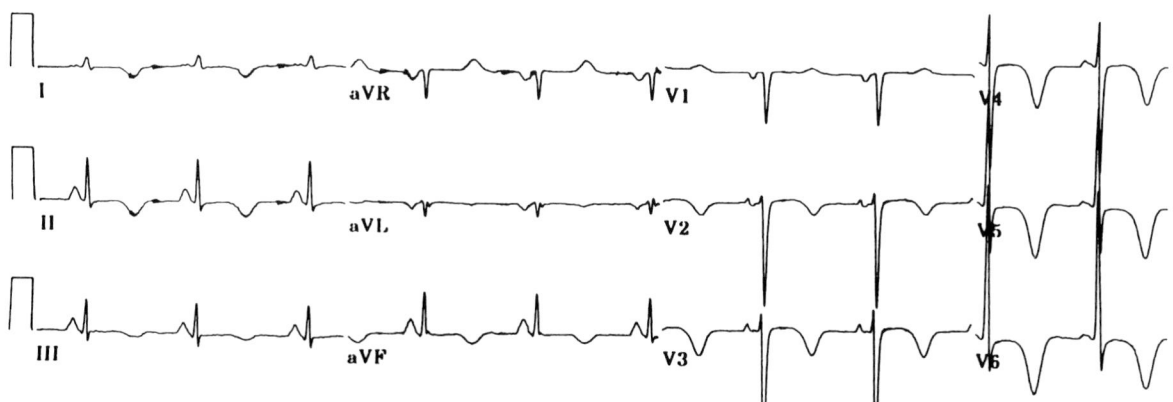

FIGURE 13–6. Pattern of electrocardiographic ischemia consisting of diffuse T-wave inversion and QT prolongation in all leads (except aV$_R$) in a patient with acute intracerebral bleeding.

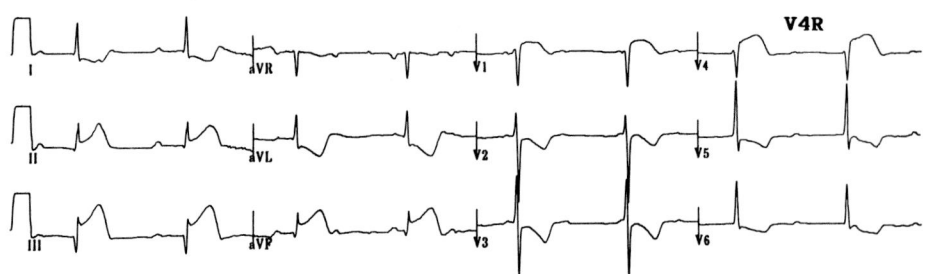

FIGURE 13-7. Acute inferior (diaphragmatic) injury showing ST-segment elevation in the inferior leads as well as in V_1 and V_{4R} (caused by right ventricular infarction). There are reciprocal changes from V_2 to V_6 as well as an atrioventricular (AV) junctional rhythm caused by complete AV block. These changes were caused by proximal right coronary artery occlusion.

and aVL have been used to indicate extensive anterior injury; in I and aVL only, high lateral injury; in V_1, V_2 and V_3, anteroseptal injury, in V_4, V_5 and V_6, apical and (or) anterolateral injury in II, III, and aVF inferior injury, right-sided precordial leads (and occasionally in V_1, V_2, and V_3) RV injury.[1,2,10,12,51,53] Likewise, ST-segment depression in anterior leads can be reciprocal to ST-segment elevation (injury) in the posterior or posterolateral wall.[1,10,12] What is really important is that the first ECG recorded from a patient with a new ST-segment elevation myocardial infarction (MI) can also give information regarding the degree, size, and site of the injury (that is, of physiologic ischemia) as well as not only of the involved coronary artery but of the more proximal or distal affected site as discussed in a limited fashion in Figs. 13–7 to 13–10.[10,11,51,53,54]

ABNORMAL Q WAVES

In general, the depth of the Q wave is proportional to wall-thickness involvement[12,13] so that a QS complex reflects transmural necrosis. The duration of the Q wave is proportioned to the extent of the area of necrosis parallel to the epicardial surface. If the latter is large enough, starts in the subendocardium, and extends toward the epicardium, the corresponding unipolar leads will record QR or Qr complexes, depending on the amount of living tissue located between dead tissue and the recording electrode. Therefore abnormal Q waves can occur in MIs that are not completely transmural.[8,13,55,56]

The following changes have been said to be equivalent to Q waves in non–Q-wave MI: R/S ratio changes, acute frontal plane right axis deviation, new left axis deviation or LBBB, initial and terminal QRS notching, and some types of "poor r-wave progression."[56,57] Abnormal Q waves also have been attributed to an intensity of cellular affectation (*injury*) severe enough to produce a significant degree of hypopolarization capable of rendering them electrically unexcitable (even though they are not anatomically, irreversibly necrotic).[8,9,55,57,58] Spontaneous recanalization of an occluded vessel, quick reversion of the ischemia or spasm, and interventions (pharmacologic or mechanical) that improve cellular metabolism and oxygenation can restore the normal polarization. If these cells become again excitable, the abnormal Q waves can disappear or vanish.[55,57] Ischemic necrosis usually takes longer to appear than the accelerated abnormal Q waves seen in most patients with Q-wave MI after successful thrombolysis or effective coronary artery angioplasty performed early in its course.[59] Because some of these Q waves also tend to disappear quickly, other authors consider that they reflect factors other than myocardial necrosis, such as reversal of regional dysmetabolism or the occurrence of transient interstitial ischemia or hemorrhage.[59,60] Profound and prolonged ischemia can cause myocardial stunning with reversible functional, metabolic, ultrastructural, and electrophysiologic abnormalities.[61] Thus transient Q waves can be the ECG counterpart (electrical stunning) of the corresponding mechanical stunning.[57,59–61] Myocardial stunning often lags behind electrical recovery.[57,62] Myocardial *stunning* should be differentiated from myocardial *hibernation*. The latter is a term used in reference to mechanical dysfunction of an ischemic area that is not transient but chronic.[62,63]

ACUTE MI

The *classic* ECG evolution of clinical acute Q wave MI has been drastically transformed by relatively recently introduced laboratory stud-

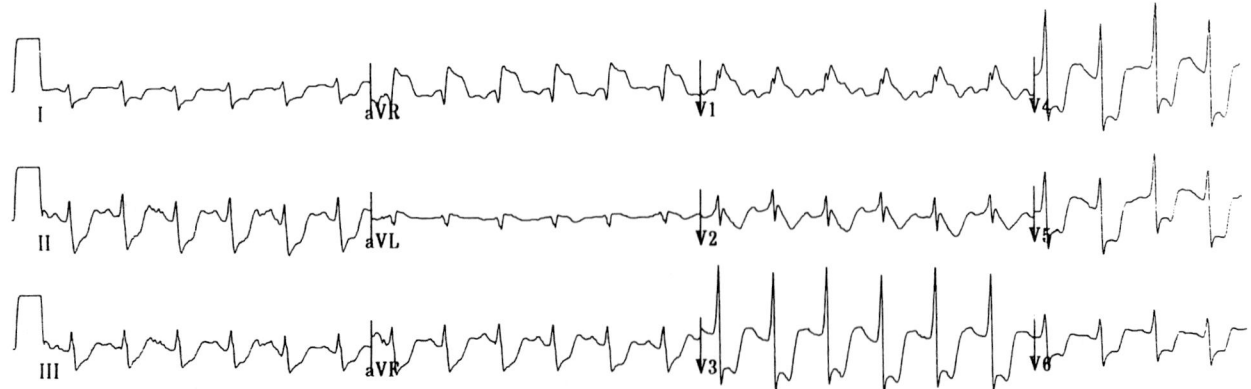

FIGURE 13-8. Changes produced by occlusion of the left main coronary artery. Note right bundle-branch block with ST-segment elevation in aVR greater than in V_1 (features of an occlusion proximal to the first septal branch). There is extensive ST-segment depression in all other leads, with an injury vector pointing superiorly and to the right, indicating predominant severe posterobasal physiologic ischemia.

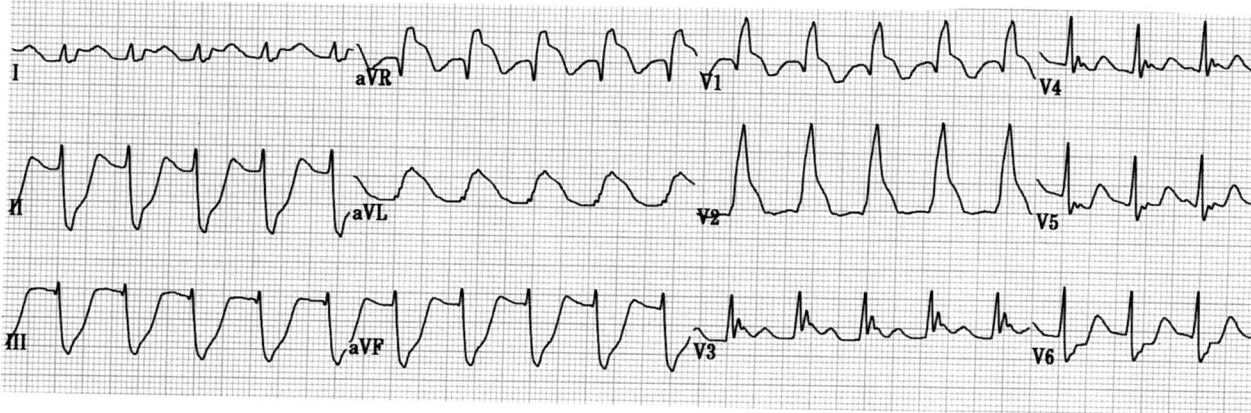

FIGURE 13–9. Changes produced by occlusion of the proximal left anterior descending coronary artery. Note right bundle-branch block (RBBB) with ST-segment elevation in aV$_R$ greater than in V$_1$. The ST segment is also elevated in leads I and aV$_L$, depressed in II, III, aV$_F$, V$_5$, and V$_6$, with an injury vector pointing superiorly and to the left.

ies, pharmacologic therapies, and interventional techniques. The typical nonintervened succession of events in what could end up as a Q wave MI is from hyperacute T waves (on occasion) to ST-segment elevation to abnormal Q waves to T-wave inversion (Fig. 13–11).[1–12,64,65] Commonly two or more of these findings appear together, depending on the timing of the first recorded static ECG. Acceleration of these phases is now common with intentional effective reperfusion.[60–67] The time course of regression of ST-segment elevation is a good predictor of reperfusion.[59] Because older 12-lead ECG studies on ST-segment evolution were based almost exclusively on static recordings obtained at fixed intervals, it became clear that continuous ECG monitoring (which falls outside the realm of this chapter) was useful in evaluating the occurrence of reperfusion (Fig. 13–12).[68,69] Some support the hypothesis that ST-segment resolution is an acceptable surrogate for tissue-level reperfusion.[59] Persistent ST-segment elevation suggests either an occluded infarct-related artery or a patent artery with failure of myocardial and microvascular reperfusion.[59]

LOCATION OF Q-WAVE MYOCARDIAL INFARCTION

The Committee on Nomenclature of Myocardial Wall Segments of the International Society of Computerized Electrocardiography

recommended adopting a 12-segment LV subdivision based on the works of Selvester and colleagues[1,11,70] The six most common locations of MI given are (1) large anterior, (2) anteroseptal, (3) anteroapical, (4) anterolateral, (5) inferior, and (6) posterior.[1,11] A recent American Heart Association (AHA)/ACC Consensus using MRI as a gold standard has reached slightly different conclusions.

RIGHT VENTRICULAR MYOCARDIAL INFARCTION

ST-segment elevation of at least 1 millimeter (mm) in lead V$_{4R}$ in patients with *acute inferior MI* had a sensitivity of 100 percent, a specificity of 87 percent, and a predictive accuracy of 92 percent for the diagnosis of RV infarction in patients with ST-segment elevation in leads II, III, and aVF (see Fig. 13–7).[71] In addition to V$_{4R}$, ST-segment elevation can be seen in leads V$_{5R}$ and V$_{6R}$ and in some cases (with decreasing amplitude) in V$_1$, V$_2$, and even V$_3$.[71]

PERICARDITIS

In pericarditis, ST segments can be elevated in all leads except aV$_R$ and, rarely, in V$_1$ (Fig. 13–13). Symmetric T-wave inversion (caused

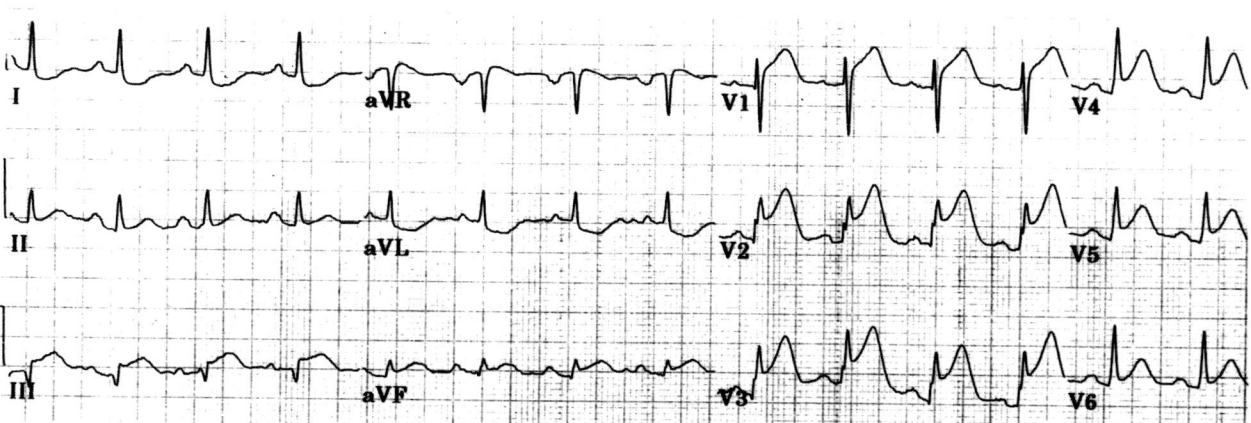

FIGURE 13–10. Changes produced by a *wrapped-up* distal left anterior descending coronary artery showing ST segment elevation in all precordial leads as well as inferior leads.

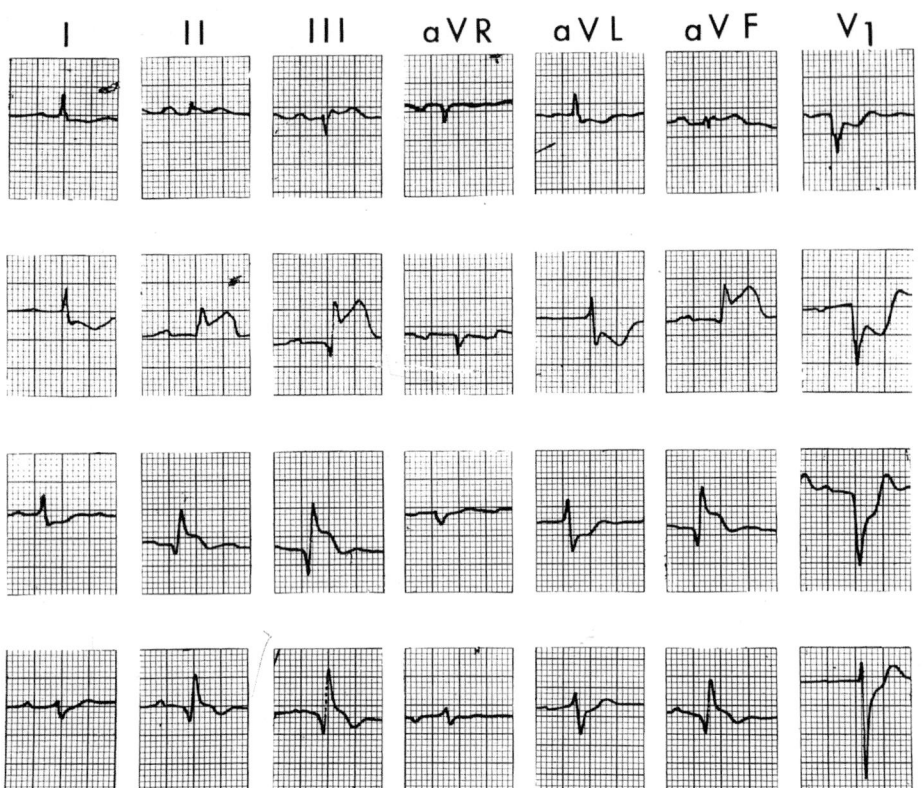

FIGURE 13–11. Spontaneous evolution of an acute inferior wall myocardial infarction in the preinterventional era varying from isolated ST-segment changes on admission (*top strip*) to the development of abnormal Q waves, slight ST elevation, and negative T waves in the bottom strip. The latter also shows slight right axis deviation, which could be caused by left posterior fascicular block.

by epicardial *ischemia*) usually develops after the ST segments have returned to the baseline (but can appear during the injury stage).[1] Neither reciprocal ST-segment changes nor abnormal Q waves are seen. In most cases of acute pericarditis, the PR segment is depressed (see Fig. 13–13). Average ECG resolution occurs in close to 2

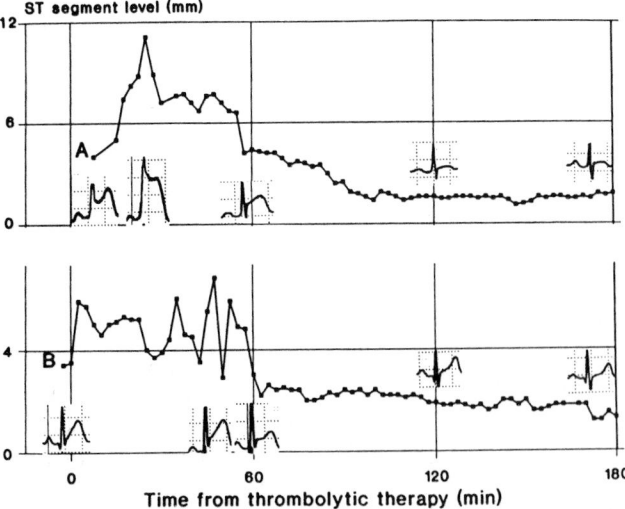

FIGURE 13–12. Plots of ST-segment levels versus time from therapy in two selected patients with patency of the infarct-related vessel at 60 minutes. Note that a 50 percent decrease in ST-segment levels within 60 minutes occurred only when measurements were made from the peak ST-segment level (highest ST-segment level measurement within the first 60 min).

weeks.[72] Sometimes acute pericarditis can be difficult to differentiate from that of the normal variant referred to as *early repolarization*.

EARLY REPOLARIZATION

In its classic form, there is J-point elevation (of no more than 3 mm) with an upwardly concave ST segment. R waves can be tall and at times have a distinct notch and slur on the downstroke (Fig. 13–14). ST-segment elevation is more frequent in chest leads but can occur in leads I and II. These dynamic ECG changes can be affected by exercise and hyperventilation. Isoproterenol reduces and propranolol increases ST-segment elevation.[73–75]

SELECTIVE NONISCHEMIC ST-SEGMENT ELEVATION IN THE RIGHT PRECORDIAL LEADS

Foremost amongst this is the Brugada syndrome, which is a familial disease causing ventricular fibrillation.[76–79] ECG abnormalities constituting the hallmark of this entity have been recently proposed by a Consensus Report.[78] They occur in absence of identifiable structural heart disease or electrolyte abnormalities. The three types of dynamic repolarization abnormalities are shown in Figs. 13–15 and 13–16A.[78] The QT interval is usually normal but can be prolonged.[78,79] Strong Na-channel blocking drugs can produce ST-segment elevations even in patients without any evidence of syncope or ventricular fibrillation.[80] The changes produced by potassium (dialyzable current of injury) are discussed in the section of hyperkalemia. Very slight ST-segment elevation with an incomplete right bundle-branch block (RBBB) pattern showing an epsilon wave has been described in arrhythmogenic RV dysplasia[81] (see Fig. 13–16). High-pass filters of electrocardiographic machines can cause ST-segment changes, which simulate those of acute anteroseptal MI.

NONSPECIFIC ST-SEGMENT– T-WAVE CHANGES

Although nonspecific (or rather, nondiagnostic) ST-segment–T-wave changes are the most commonly diagnosed ECG abnormalities, they have not been categorized adequately and represent different findings for various interpreters.[82,83] In the classic paper, Friedberg and Zager[82] considered depth of ST-segment depression and T-wave inversion as well as their contour (Fig. 13–17). When analyzed without clinical information, this diagnosis was made in 40 percent of 410 abnormal ECGs. The

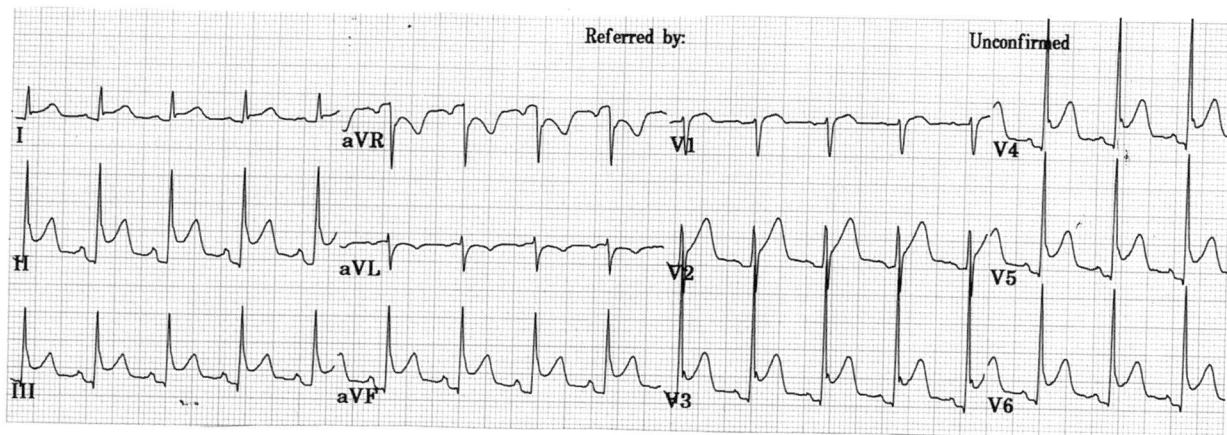

FIGURE 13-13. Acute nonspecific pericarditis showing ST-segment elevation in all leads except aVR and V_1.

number was reduced to 10 percent, however, when clinical data became available. In the absence of structural heart disease, these changes can be caused by a variety of physiologic (i.e., hyperventilation, anxiety, body position, food, neurogenic influences, and temperature), pharmacologic (i.e., antiarrhythmic and psychotropic drugs, digoxin), and extracardiac (i.e., electrolyte abnormalities, upper gastrointestinal processes, allergic reactions, etc.) factors.[82,83]

ST-SEGMENT DEPRESSION DURING SUPRAVENTRICULAR TACHYCARDIAS

These can occur during paroxysmal supraventricular tachycardias in young individuals and even children.[84] Their mechanism probably differs from that producing post-tachycardia T-wave changes, which are seen when sinus rhythm is reestablished. Fig. 13–18 is an example occurring when the rate was 214 beats/min. Lactate studies in cases similar to this showed no evidence of physiologic metabolic MI in spite of the resemblance to the changes observed in main left coronary artery disease occlusion. These changes

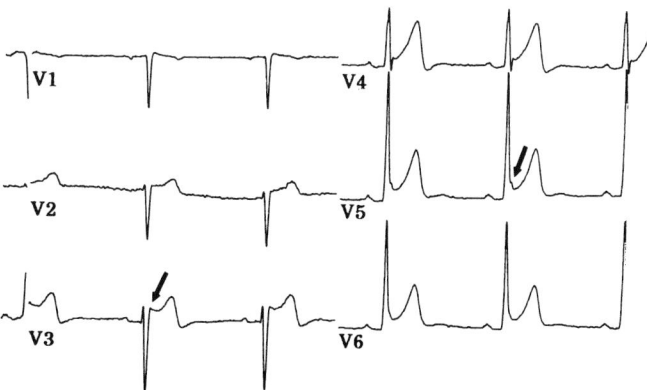

FIGURE 13-14. Early repolarization. This normal variant is characterized by narrow QRS complexes with J-point and ST-segment elevation in the chest leads. Left chest leads often show tall R waves with a distinct notch or slur in their downstroke (*arrow* in V_5), although the right chest leads can display ST segments having a *saddleback* or *humpback* shape (*arrow* in V_3).

probably reflect rapid-rate, incomplete filling–related, *pure electrical* injury caused by differences in action potential duration between subendocardium and epicardium.

FASCICULAR BLOCKS
【 】 LEFT ANTERIOR FASCICULAR BLOCK

Criteria for the diagnosis of uncomplicated left anterior fascicular block (LAFB) are given in Table 13–1 and Fig. 13–19, top. The constant feature of the axis deviation produced by LAFB is its *superior* orientation, not its superior and leftward orientation (abnormal left axis deviation).[9,58,85–89] Because of the multiple interconnections between the fascicles of the LBB system, the appearance of LAFB does not increase QRS duration by more than 0.025 second.[9] Therefore an LAFB pattern with a wider QRS complex generally indicates the presence of additional conduction disturbances such as RBBB, MI, or nonspecific intraventricular conduction delays caused by free wall fibrosis.[9,58,85–90] Other causes of abnormal left axis deviation are shown in Fig. 13–19.

【 】 LEFT ANTERIOR FASCICULAR BLOCK COEXISTING WITH MYOCARDIAL INFARCTION

The ECG changes imposed by MIs of different locations on LAFB are shown in Fig. 13–20.

【 】 LEFT POSTERIOR FASCICULAR BLOCK

In pure left posterior fascicular block (LPFB), the impulse emerges from the unblocked anterosuperior division, thus producing small q waves in leads II, III, and aV_F[9,58] (Fig. 13–21, top) thereafter moving in an inferior and rightward direction.[9,58,85] Because similar QRS changes can also occur in RV hypertrophy, pleuropulmonary disease (acute or chronic), and extremely vertical anatomic heart positions caused by a slender body build or chest wall deformities, it is evident that the diagnosis of *pure* LPFB cannot be made from the ECG alone. Additional clinical, echocardiographic, or pathologic information is required for this purpose.[9,58,85] The changes imposed in LPFB by MIs of different locations are depicted in Fig. 13–21.[9,58,85]

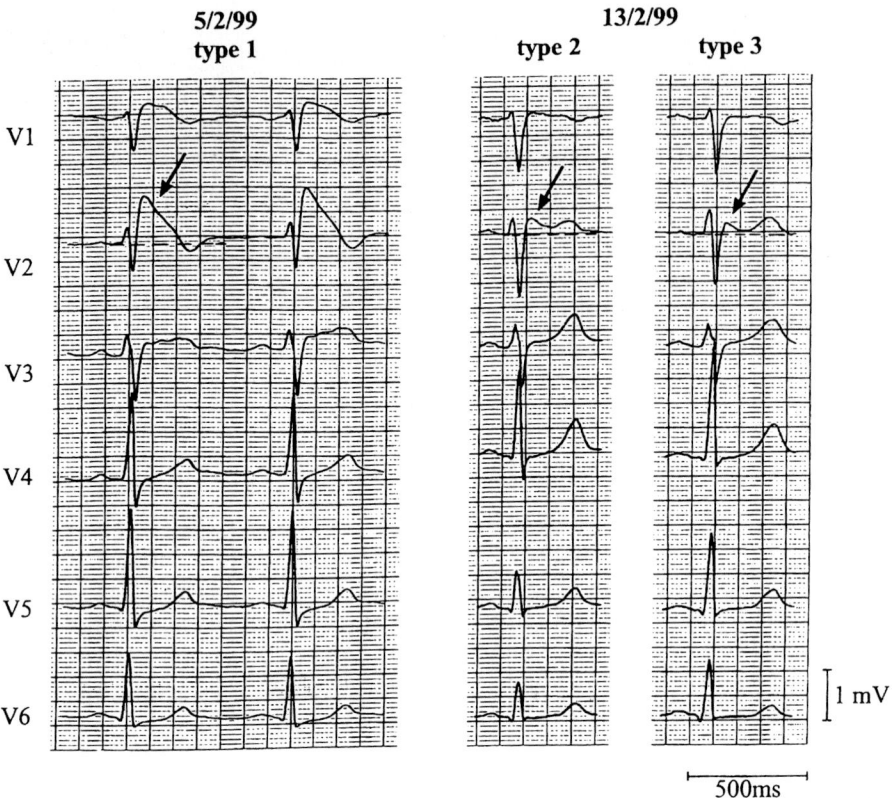

FIGURE 13–15. The three types of repolarization patterns proposed in the Consensus Report.[78] Type 1 is characterized by a prominent coved ST-segment elevation displaying a J wave or ST segment ≥2 mm at its peak followed by a negative T wave with little or no isoelectric separation. Type 2 also has a high takeoff ST elevation with J-wave amplitude ≥2 mm, giving rise to descending ST-segment elevation followed by a T wave with a saddleback configuration. Type 3 shows ST-segment elevation of <1 mm of saddleback type, coved type, or both. *Source: Wilde, Antzelevitch, Borggrefe, et al.[78] Reproduced with permission.*

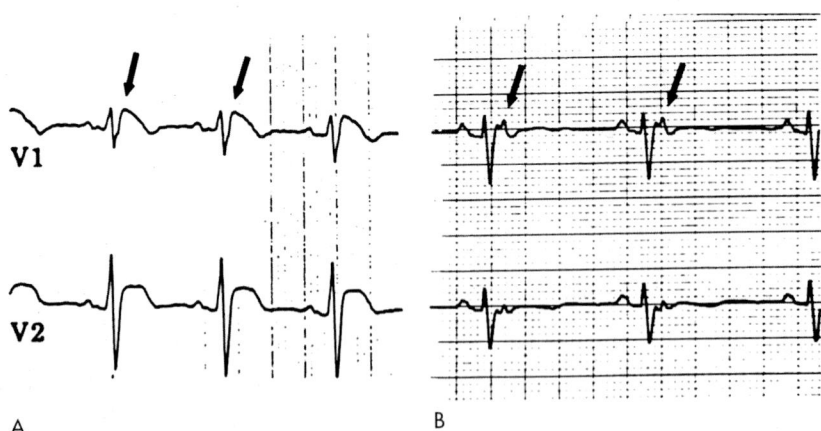

FIGURE 13–16. A. Nonischemic ST-segment elevation in the right precordial leads in a young patient with the Brugada syndrome. **B.** Epsilon wave of a patient with arrhythmogenic right ventricular dysplasia.

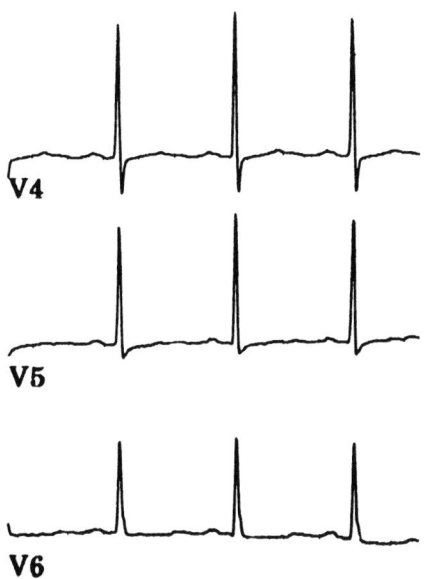

FIGURE 13–17. Nonspecific (nondiagnostic) ST-segment–T-wave changes, the most common abnormalities in ECG interpretation.

[ ] LEFT-MIDDLE (SEPTAL) FASCICULAR BLOCKS

There is no consensus regarding the ECG diagnosis of this conduction disturbance.[90,91] It is rarely discussed in books and is rarely (if ever) diagnosed in daily electrocardiographic interpretation.

NONSPECIFIC INTRAVENTRICULAR CONDUCTION DELAYS

Several names have been applied to the conduction disturbances occurring in the left-sided Purkinje-myocardial junctions, left septal surface, or free wall of the left ventricle.[9,58,92–98] The morphologies are not those of fascicular or bundle-branch blocks (Fig. 13–22, left). These conduction disturbances have different electrogenetic mechanisms. Thus the cellular *affectation* caused by acute injury resulting from coronary artery disease, hyperkalemia, drugs, and intracoronary injections of contrast material occurs within (inside)

the affected regions.[5,9,52,58] Blocks occurring in subacute or chronic MI after the appearance of abnormal Q waves (peri-infarction block) as well as those occurring in the presence of diffuse myocardial fibrosis are caused by the circuitous and irregular activation of living cells surrounding areas of fibrotic tissue.[58,93–98]

BUNDLE-BRANCH BLOCK
[ ] COMPLETE RIGHT BUNDLE-BRANCH BLOCK

In pure complete RBBB, the EA should not be deviated abnormally either to the left or to the right. These axis deviations reflect coexisting fascicular blocks or right ventricular hypertrophy (see Fig. 13–21 and Fig. 13–22, right).[9]

[ ] INCOMPLETE RIGHT BUNDLE-BRANCH BLOCK PATTERNS

Incomplete RBBB *patterns* can be produced by various mechanisms[99–103]: (1) different degrees of conduction delays through the main trunk of the right bundle branch (RBB); (2) an increased conduction time through an elongated RBB that is stretched because of a concomitant enlargement of the right septal surface; (3) a diffuse Purkinje myocardial delay caused by right ventricular stretch or dilatation; (4) surgical trauma or disease-related interruption of the major ramifications of the right branch (*distal* RBBB); or (5) congenital variations of the distribution of the major distal ramifications resulting in a slight delay in activation of the crista supraventricularis.[102,103]

[ ] COMPLETE LEFT BUNDLE-BRANCH BLOCK

The diagnostic criteria consist of prolongation of the QRS complexes (≥0.12 s) with neither a q nor an S wave in leads I, aV$_L$, and a *properly placed* V$_6$. A wide R wave with a notch on its top (*plateau*) is seen in these leads. Apparently, the EAs of most *uncomplicated* complete LBBBs usually are not located much beyond –30°.[9,58,89] Complete LBBB with abnormal left axis deviation occasionally coexists with a great degree of left Purkinje, and myocardial, disease.[1,9,58,89]

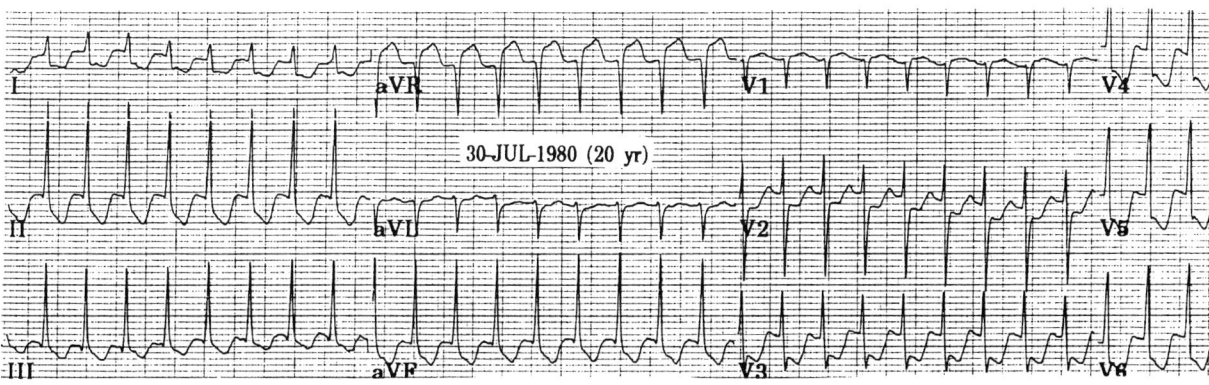

FIGURE 13–18. Paroxysmal supraventricular tachycardia. Marked ST-segment depression in an otherwise normal 20-year-old female presumably not caused by physiologic (metabolic) ischemia but by predominantly a rate-related electrocardiographic injury, which could have been produced by differential duration and morphologies of endocardial and epicardial action potentials.[84]

TABLE 13-1

Criteria for Diagnosis of Pure Left Anterior Fascicular Block

1. Abnormal left-axis deviation (usually between −45° and −60°) but right superior axis deviation can occur with atypical right bundle-branch blocks or extensive antero-lateral myocardial infarction
2. rS complexes in leads II, III, and aVF and qR complexes in leads I and aVL
3. Delayed intrinsicoid deflection in leads I and aVL
4. Peak of r wave in lead III occurring earlier than peak of r wave in lead II
5. Peak of R wave in lead aVL occurring earlier than peak of R wave in aVR
6. Exclusion of other causes of abnormal left axis deviation (Fig. 13–19)

SOURCE: Castellanos, Pina, Zaman, et al[85]; and Milliken.[88] With permission.

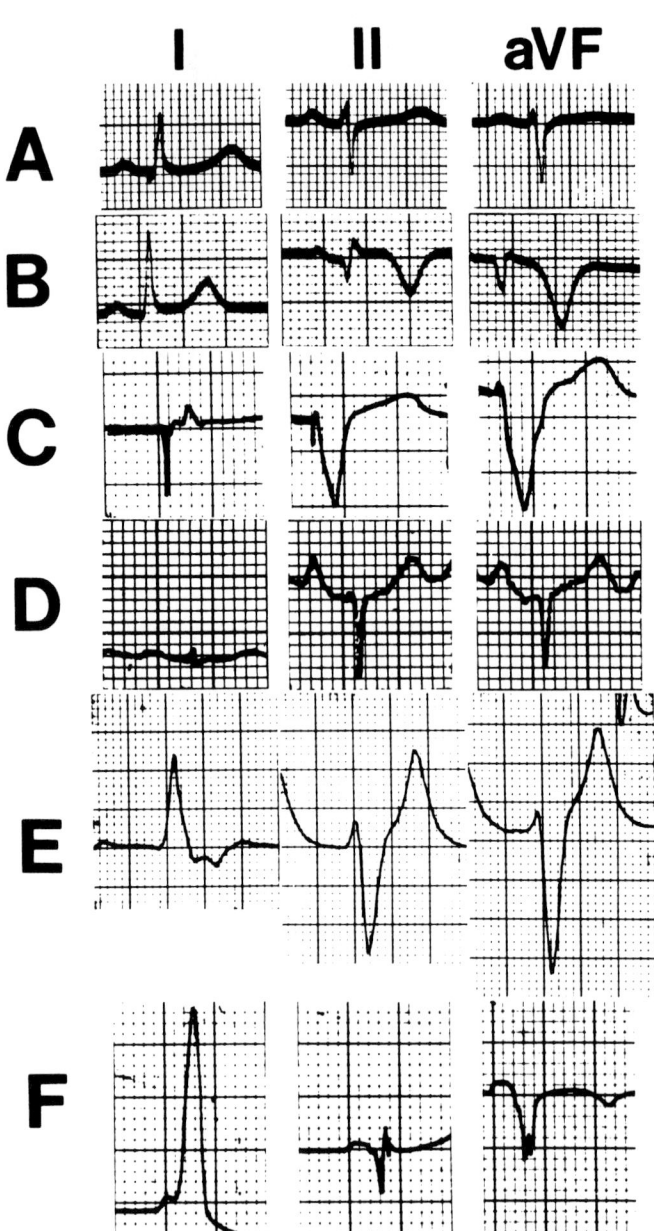

FIGURE 13–19. Causes of abnormal left axis deviation. **A.** Left anterior fascicular block. Note rS complexes in II and aV_F. **B.** Extensive inferior wall myocardial infarction (MI) showing Qr complexes in II. **C.** Pacing from the spatial inferior regions of the heart, as from the right ventricular apex and middle cardiac or inferior or posterolateral veins. **D.** Rare cases of pulmonary emphysema with very low voltage in lead I and "P pulmonale." **E.** Hyperkalemia. **F.** Ventricular preexcitation caused by posteroseptal accessory pathways.

【 】 COMPLETE LEFT BUNDLE-BRANCH BLOCK WITH ACUTE MYOCARDIAL INFARCTION

The classic QRS pattern of LBBB may not be modified by a small area of myocardial necrosis in the lateral or inferior walls. Sgarbossa[104] has suggested that ST-segment elevation of 1 mm or more concordant with QRS polarity has a high specificity and sensitivity. ST-segment elevation of 5 mm or more discordant with QRS polarity, ST-segment depression of 1 mm or more in V_1, V_2, and V_3, and (sudden) positive (primary) T waves in V_4 and V_5 have a high specificity but a low sensitivity.[104–106] Examples of LBBB complicated by acute anterior and inferior MI are shown in Figs. 13–23 and 13–24. The above-mentioned criteria also can be applied to diagnose acute MI in patients with pacemakers.[104]

【 】 COMPLETE LEFT BUNDLE-BRANCH BLOCK WITH OLD MYOCARDIAL INFARCTION

If the infarction is anteroseptal (but neither lateral or inferior), the initial vectors point toward the free wall of the right ventricle because now the RV free-wall forces are not neutralized by the normally preponderant septal and/or initial LV free-wall forces.[1,2,8,11–13,105,106] Thus a small q wave will be recorded in leads I, V_5, and V_6 (where it is not normally present in complete LBBB). Similar findings can be seen in paced beats when in lead I the spike is followed by a well-defined q wave. Late notching of S waves in V_3 through V_5 has been found to have higher to moderate specificity and moderate to low sensitivity.[106] Notching of the upstroke of the R wave in leads I, aV_1, V_5, and V_6 has a sensitivity of 21 percent and a specificity of 82 percent.[106]

【 】 COMPLETE LEFT BUNCLE-BRANCH BLOCK WITH LEFT VENTRICLE HYPERTROPHY

This is discussed under Left Ventricular Hypertrophy below.

【 】 INCOMPLETE LEFT BUNDLE-BRANCH BLOCK PATTERN

An incomplete LBBB pattern can be diagnosed if leads I and an *appropriately placed* V_6 show an R wave not preceded by a q wave but followed by a negative T wave.[8,58] There are rS or QS complexes in lead V_1 and even V_2 with a QRS duration of 0.10 and 0.12 second.

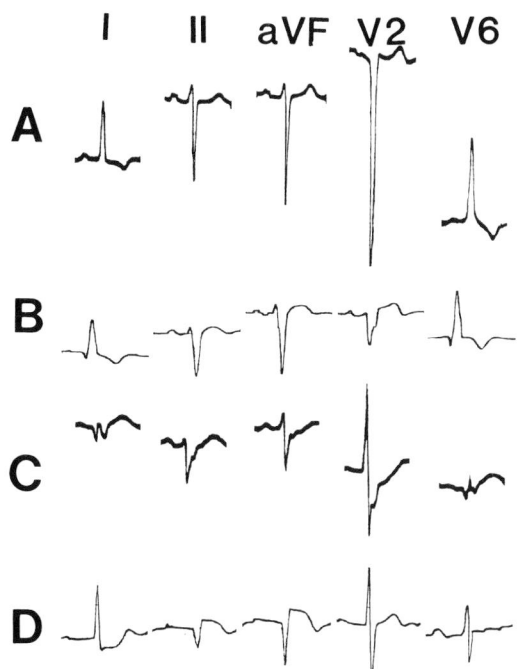

FIGURE 13–20. Diagnosis of left anterior fascicular block (LAFB) associated with myocardial infarction (MI). Diagnostic feature given in parentheses. **A.** LAFB and anteroseptal MI (QS complexes in right chest leads). **B.** LAFB and anterolateral MI (abnormal q wave in leads I and V₆). **C.** LAFB and anterolateral MI with electrical axis in the right superior quadrant (large Q waves in leads I and V₆). **D.** LAFB and inferior wall MI (QR or QS complexes and elevation of J point and ST segments in leads II and III).

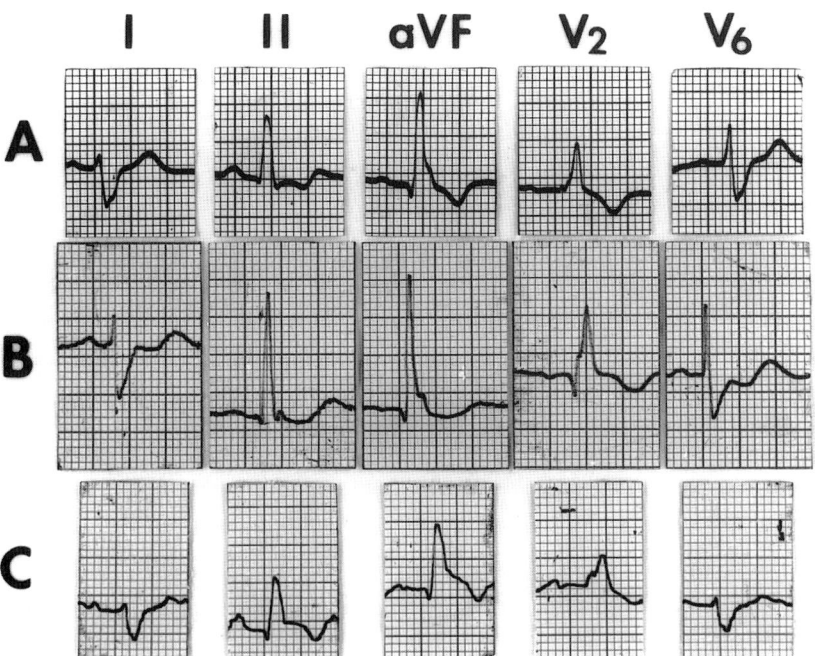

FIGURE 13–21. Left posterior fascicular block (LPFB) with right bundle-branch block (RBBB). **A.** No myocardial infarction (MI). **B.** Anteroseptal MI (note q wave in V₂). **C.** Inferior MI (note ST-segment elevation and T-wave inversion in leads II and aV_F with slight ST-segment depression in lead I). The differences in QRS complexes between **A** and **C** are not very marked because pure LPFB can produce an almost abnormal Q wave in the inferior leads.

WIDE QRS COMPLEXES CAUSED BY MANIFEST PREEXCITATION SYNDROMES

As a rule the ventricular complex ventricular complex is a fusion beat resulting from ventricular activation by two wavefronts.[107–113] The degree of preexcitation (amount of muscle activated through the accessory pathway) can be extremely variable and depends on many factors: distance between the sinus node and atrial insertion of the accessory pathway, differences in refractory period duration, and differences in conduction time through the normal pathway and the accessory pathway (Fig. 13–25A). If there is total block at the AV node or His-Purkinje system, the impulse will be conducted exclusively by means of the accessory pathway (see Fig. 13–25B).[110] Consequently the QRS complexes are different from fusion beats, although the direction of the delta wave remains the same. Moreover, the QRS complexes are as wide as (and really simulating) those produced by artificial or spontaneous beats arising in the vicinity of the ventricular end of the accessory pathway.

Near the end of the millennium, Basiouny and colleagues[112] reported that there were 41 publications dealing with methods for localizing the accessory pathways of patients with preexcitation syndrome. For the purposes of this chapter, we will first refer to the pioneer work which considered that only four segments were necessary. This appeared logical, for at the time that this method was proposed, most ablations were performed surgically.[111,112] Left free-wall accessory pathways are characterized by positive or isoelectric and rarely negative delta waves in leads I, aVL, V₅, or V₆ and right axis deviation during *maximal* preexcitation (see Fig. 13–25). Lead V₁ shows R or Rs complexes. Posteroseptal accessory pathways show negative delta waves in leads III and aVF and R waves in V₂. A QS complex in V₁ suggests a right posteroseptal pathway (Fig. 13–26), whereas R, RS, or Rs complexes in the same lead can correspond to a left posteroseptal pathway. Right free wall accessory pathways display an LBBB pattern defined, for purposes of accessory pathway localization, by an R wave greater than 0.09 second in lead I and rS complexes in leads V₁ and V₂, with an electrical axis ranging between +30 and –60°. Right anteroseptal accessory pathways show an LBBB pattern (as defined) with an electrical axis ranging between +30 and +120° (usually around +60°). A q wave can be present in lead aVL but not in leads I and V₆. Mixed patterns resulted from the existence of two separate accessory pathways.

Because accessory pathways can traverse almost any part of the atrioventricular regions, this classification is obviously insufficient when catheter ablation is contemplated. As mentioned earlier, multiple algorithms have been proposed.[112] Because the most useful are complex, clinical electrocardiographers find them difficult to memorize. They are also not completely satisfactory, because smaller degrees of preexcitation seem to limit diagnostic accuracy, and the polarity of delta waves (positive, biphasic [+ or –], negative, and isoelectric) has to be properly categorized.[113]

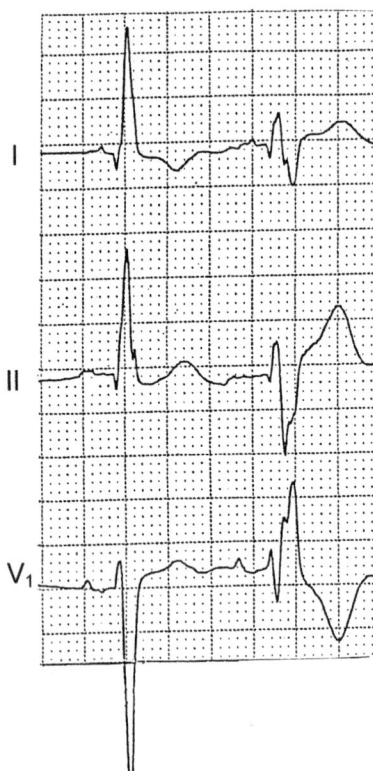

FIGURE 13–22. Nonspecific left sided intraventricular conduction delay (*left*) characterized by QRS widening (0.13 sec) and terminal notching in lead II but without the characteristics of right bundle-branch block (RBBB) or left bundle-branch block. The right-sided beat shows RBBB and left anterior fascicular block with a greater QRS duration (0.18 sec). Note that the left-sided conduction disturbance has been concealed, presumable because the bundle-branch block–related right to left transeptal delay was greater than the left-sided intraventricular delay.

Fig. 13–27 illustrates a useful (but one of many) algorithm to predict accessory pathway location from the 12-lead ECG.[113]

The currently used nomenclature for accessory pathway location was discussed extensively (and has been challenged) by experts in the field of preexcitation.[114]

WIDE QRS COMPLEXES PRODUCED BY VENTRICULAR PACING FROM DIFFERENT SITES

【 】 MONO (RIGHT) VENTRICULAR PACING

In determining the location of the stimulating electrodes it is best *not* to describe the electrically produced ventricular beats as having an RBBB or LBBB morphology, because what is relevant is the polarity of the *properly positioned* V_1 and V_2 electrodes and the direction of the EA[115,116] (Fig. 13–28). For example, endocardial or epicardial stimulation of the *anteriorly* located right ventricle at any site (apical [inferior], or mid/outflow tract [superior]) yields predominantly negative deflections in the right chest leads caused by the *posterior* spread of activation (first and second vertical rows in Fig. 13–28). The reverse (positive deflections in V_1 and V_2) occurs when the epicardial stimulation of the superior and lateral portions of the posterior left ventricle by catheter electrodes in the distal coronary sinus or great and middle cardiac veins (or by implanted electrodes in the nearby muscle) results in *anteriorly* oriented forces (third and fourth vertical rows in Fig. 13–28). RV apical pacing can produce positive deflections in V_1 in rare cases and if this lead is (mis)placed above its usual level. Conversely, *superior* deviation of the electrical axis only indicates that a spatial *inferior* ventricular site has been stimulated, regardless of whether this site is the apical portion of the RV or the inferior part of the LV, the latter being paced through the middle cardiac vein (first and fourth vertical rows in Fig. 13–28). Conversely, an *inferior* vertical axis is simply a consequence of pacing from a *superior* site, which can be the endocardium of the RV outflow tract or the epicardium of the posterosuperior and lateral portions of the left ventricle (second and third vertical rows in Fig. 13–28). The method discussed above to locate the site of impulse initiation during pacing is simpler than the more complicated ones used to determine the ventricular sites of exit from accessory pathways.

【 】 BIVENTRICULAR PACING

Although with this technique the right-sided electrode is usually in a single site, namely the endocardium of the right ventricular apex, the location of the epicardial left-sided electrode varies with the vein (or segment of the latter) in which it is placed (posterior or anterior great cardiac vein, lateral or posterolateral veins or even middle cardiac vein) depending on the preference, luck of the

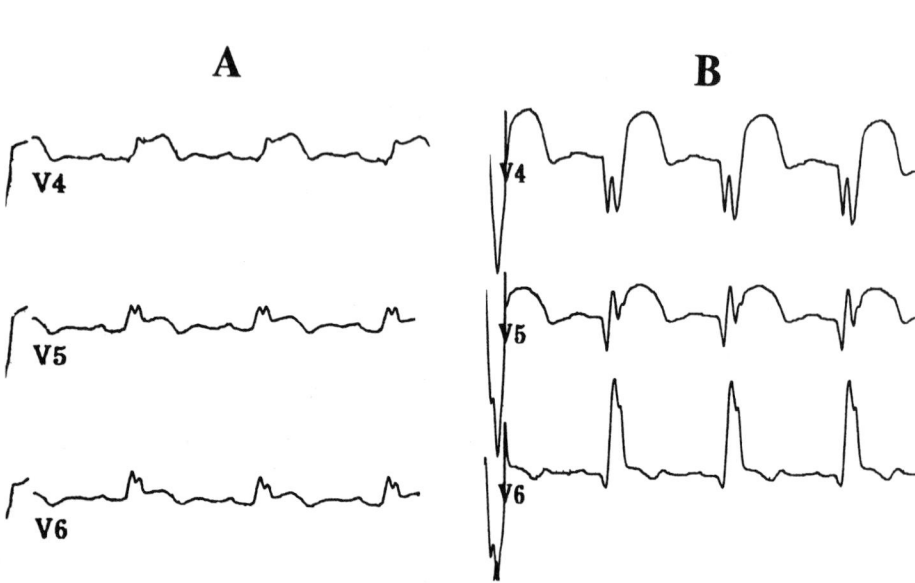

A   **B**

V4

V5

V6

FIGURE 13–23. Morphologic characteristics of complete left bundle-branch block (LBBB) complicated by acute anterior myocardial infarction (MI). **A.** Abnormal ST-segment elevation without Q waves (QRS duration: 0.14 s). **B.** Abnormal ST-segment elevation, obtained from another patient, persisted after the appearance of abnormal Q waves (QRS duration: 0.13 s).

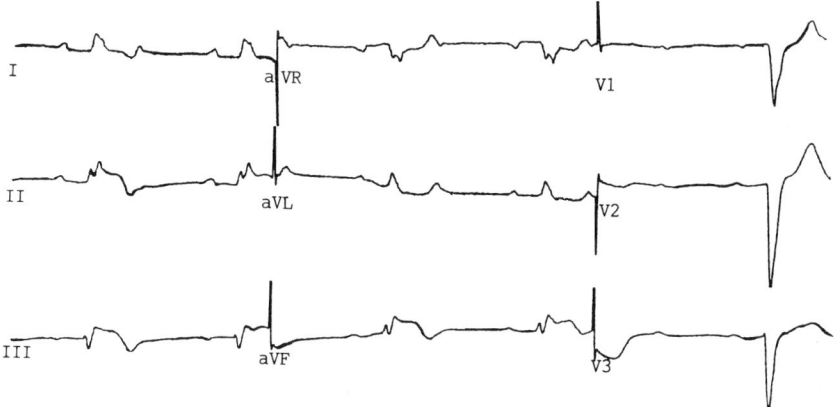

FIGURE 13–24. Morphologic features of complete left bundle-branch block (LBBB) complicated by acute inferior myocardial infarction (MI). There is abnormal ST-segment elevation in leads II, III, and aVF (QRS duration: 0.14 s). Atrioventricular (AV) block is also present.

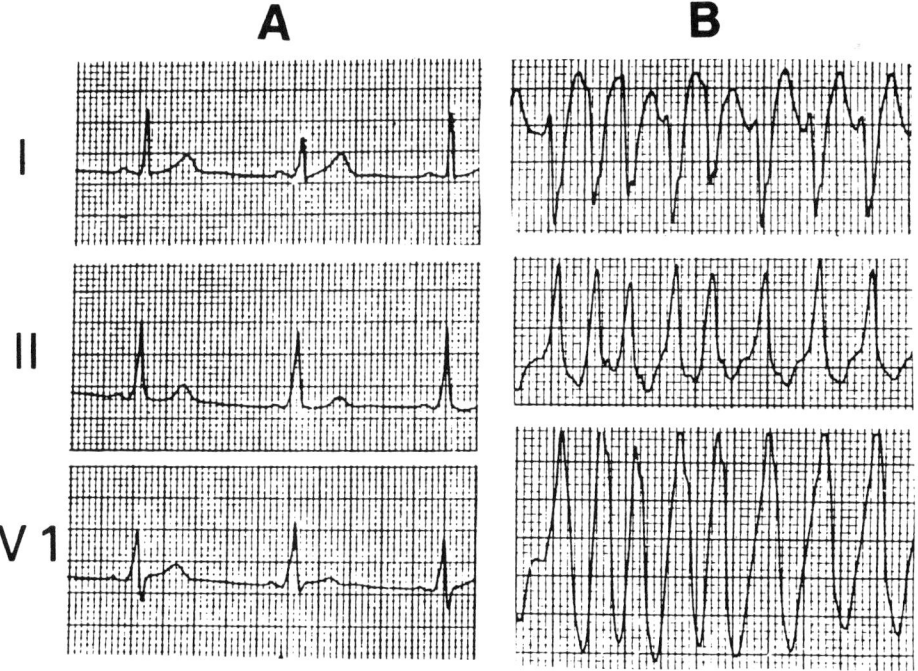

FIGURE 13–25. Wolff-Parkinson-White syndrome in a patient with a left free-wall accessory pathway. **A.** Sinus rhythm with fusion beats showing different degrees of preexcitation. **B.** Maximal preexcitation during atrial fibrillation. Note marked change in QRS duration and electrical axis which is now pointing inferiorly and to the right.

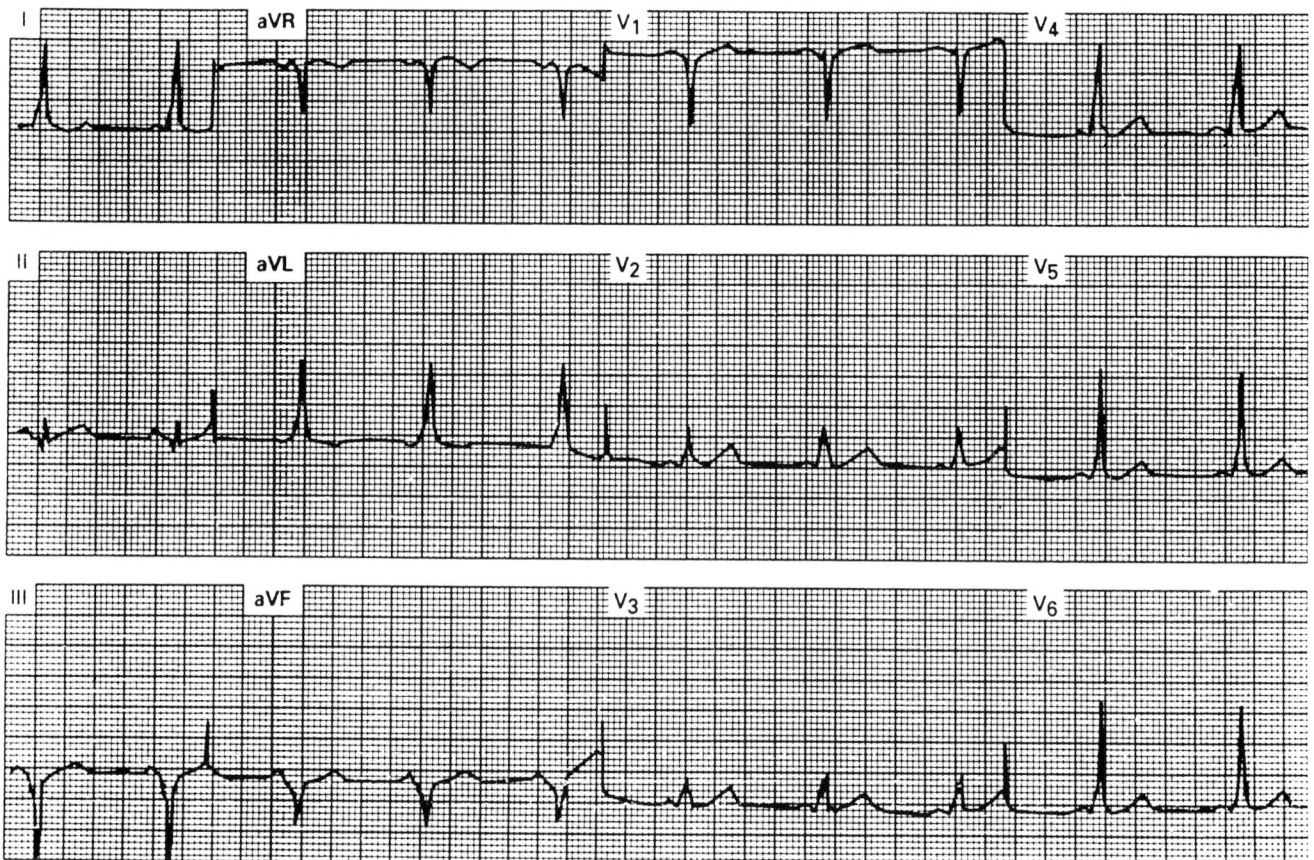

FIGURE 13–26. Wolff-Parkinson-White syndrome in a patient having a right posteroseptal accessory pathway. Note short PR intervals with negative delta waves in leads III and aVF (false pattern of inferior myocardial infarction [MI]). Lead V₁ shows all-negative QRS complexes.

implanting physician,[117–119] or normal anatomic variations of those veins (Fig. 13–29). Because of this, and because of the unevenly distributed, severe, myocardial fibrosis which these patients have, various different and difficult to interpret wide QRS patterns occur (right axis deviation with usually an RS, but also QS and, rarely, R waves in V_1; right superior axis with similar waves in the latter lead; and, infrequently, left superior axis deviation with a QS in V_1). Persons with less severe myocardial disease have narrower ventricular complexes with possibly a shorter depolarization conduction time. Consequently the QT intervals can become shorter (see Fig. 13–29).

LV HYPERTROPHY

Because the advent of other noninvasive techniques, there has been a changing role for the ECG in the diagnosis of ventricular hypertrophy.[120,121] Necropsy studies have exposed the superiority of echocardiography with respect to the electrocardiography for detecting LV hypertorphy.[121] Echocardiography is also a better method for serial followup of changes during progression or regression of LV hypertrophy.[121] Multiple criteria have been proposed to diagnose LV hypertrophy using necropsy or echocardiographic information[1,64] (Tables 13–2 and 13–3). For a more extensive discussion of the subject, see Bayes de Luna[64] and Surawicz.[121]

With echocardiography as the gold standard, several authors have postulated ECG criteria for diagnosis of LV hypertrophy in the presence of complete LBBB and LAFB[120,122] (Tables 13–4 and 13–5). The high sensitivity and specificity reported by Gertsch and coworkers[120] for diagnosis of LV hypertrophy with LAFB have not been corroborated in studies performed in our department.

PROCESSES PRODUCING OR LEADING TO RIGHT VENTRICULAR HYPERTROPHY AND ENLARGEMENT

RV hypertrophy is manifest in the ECG only when the RV forces predominate over those of the left ventricle. Because the latter has roughly three times more mass than the former, the right ventricle can double in size (when the left ventricle is normal) or triple its weight (when there is significant RV hypertrophy) and still not result in the necessary requirements to pull the electrical forces anteriorly and to the right. For these reasons, RV hypertrophy cannot be recognized easily in adult patients. Despite these limitations, the ECG manifestations of RV hypertrophy or enlargement can be subdivided into the following main types: (1) the pulmonary disease pattern (Fig. 13–30); (2) the volume overloading pattern of patients with congenital heart disease (Fig. 13–31); (3) the pattern of mitral stenosis (Fig. 13–32); and (4) the classic RV hypertrophy pattern

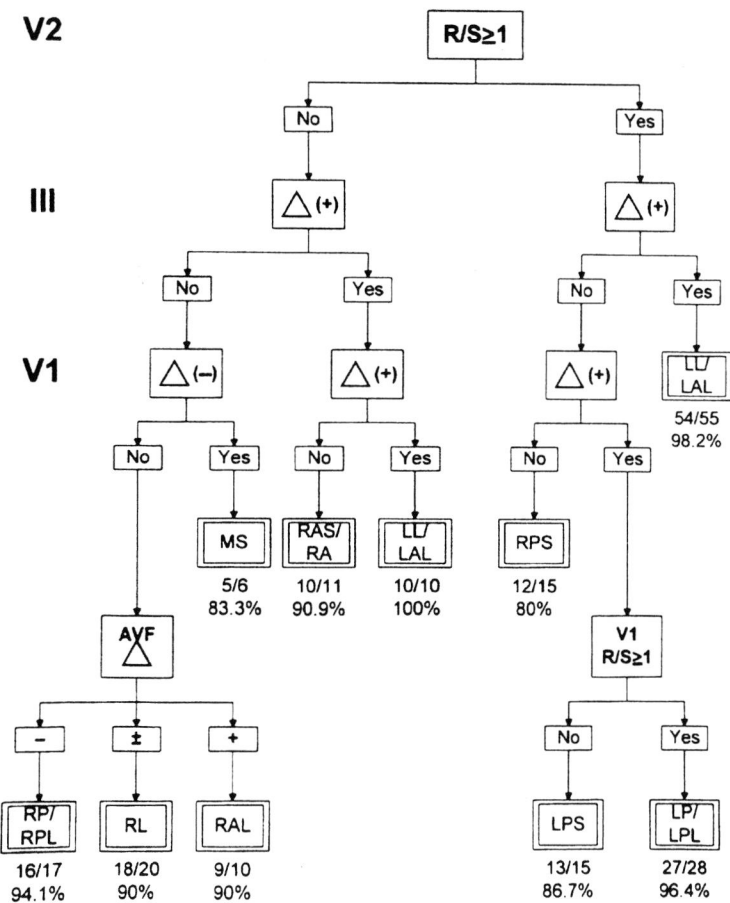

FIGURE 13–27. Useful algorithm to predict accessory pathway location from the 12-lead ECG. Step 1: Analysis of R/S ratio in V_2. Step 2: Existence of positive (+) delta wave in lead III (initial 40 ms). Step 3: Existence of positive or negative (–) delta wave in V_1 (initial 60 ms). Step 4: Delta-wave polarity in aV_F (initial 40 ms) or analysis of R/S ratio in V_1 (+ = 5 biphasic or isoelectric). The accuracy of the algorithm for each location in 187 prospective patients is also shown at the bottom. LAL, left anterolateral; LL, left lateral; LP, left posterior; LPL, left posterolateral; LPS, left posteroseptal; MS, midseptal; RA, right anterior; RAL, right anterolateral; RAS, right anteroseptal; RL, right lateral; RP, right posterior; RPL, right posterolateral; RPS, right posteroseptal. *Source: Chiang, Chen, Teo, et al.[146] Reproduced with permission from the publisher and authors.*

characteristic of pressure overloading patients (Fig. 13–33). False patterns of RV hypertrophy can occur in patients with true posterior (basal) MI, complete RBBB with LPFB, and Wolff-Parkinson-White syndrome resulting from AV conduction through left free wall or left posteroseptal accessory pathways.[1,2,58]

ELECTROLYTE IMBALANCES

In practice, the major problem with the ECG diagnosis of electrolyte imbalance is not the negative ECG with abnormal serum values but the production of similar changes by other conditions in patients with normal serum values.[123]

【 】 HYPERKALEMIA

The initial effect of acute hyperkalemia is the appearance of peaked T waves with a narrow base (Fig. 13–34A). The diagnosis is almost certain when the duration of the base is 0.20 second or less (with rates between 60 and 110 beats/min).[1,123,124] As the degree of hyperkalemia increases, the QRS complex

widens (Fig. 13–35, right), with the electrical axis usually being deviated abnormally to the left and only rarely to the right. In addition, the PR interval prolongs, and the P wave flattens until it disappears.[1] Rarely, hyperkalemia produces (in the absence of coronary artery disease) a degree of ST segment elevation in the right chest leads capable of suggesting a Brugada pattern or that of anteroseptal myocardial injury (see Fig. 13–35). The latter constitutes the previously mentioned "dialyzable current of injury in potassium intoxication" reported by Levine and colleagues.[123,124]

【 】 HYPOKALEMIA

The abnormal and delayed repolarization that occurs in hypokalemia is best expressed as QU rather than QT prolongation because at times it can be difficult to differentiate between notching of the T wave and T- and U-wave fusion.[1,30] On the basis of the previously mentioned M cells, some of these U waves are part of notched T waves, suggesting that that term be used in place of U. As the serum potassium level falls, the ST segment becomes progressively more depressed, and there is a gradual blending of the T wave into what

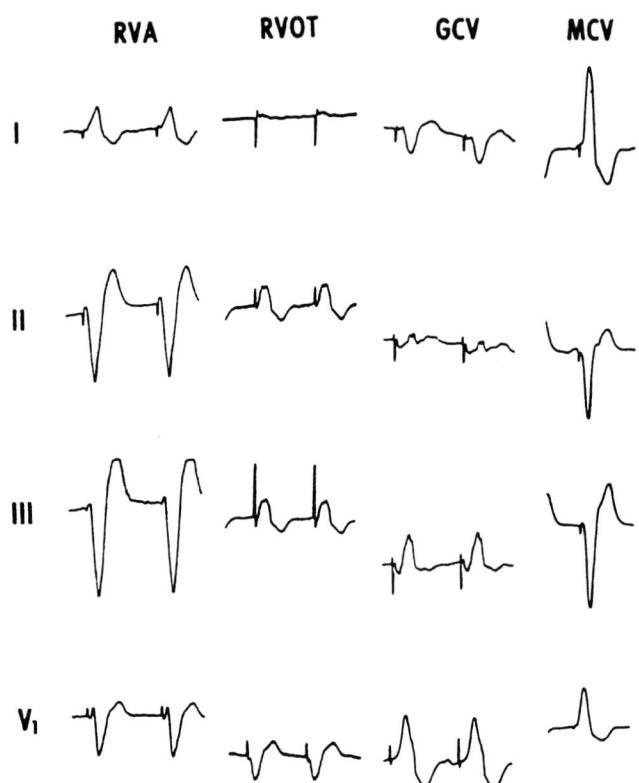

FIGURE 13–28. QRS changes (location of the electrical axis and polarity of lead V_1) produced by monoventricular pacing from right ventricular apex (RVA), right ventricular outflow tract (RVOT), great cardiac vein (GCV), and middle cardiac vein (MCV).

appears to be a tall U wave (Fig. 13–36, top).[1,123] An ECG pattern similar to that of hypokalemia can be produced by some antiarrhythmic drugs, especially quinidine and, experimentally, DL-sotalol.[15] In any case, when repolarization is greatly prolonged, ventricular arrhythmias, including torsades de pointes, can occur.[15]

HYPOMAGNESEMIA

Hypomagnesemia does not produce QU prolongation unless the coexisting hypokalemia (with which it is almost invariably associated) is severe.[125,126] Long-standing and very marked magnesium deficiency lowers the amplitude of the T wave and depresses the ST segment.[125,126] It can be difficult to differentiate the changes produced by magnesium from those produced by potassium.[124]

HYPERMAGNESEMIA

Similarly, in clinical tracings, the effects of hypermagnesemia on the ECG are difficult to identify because the changes are dominated by calcium.[127] Administration of intravenous magnesium to patients with normal ECGs can shorten the QT interval.[125–127] Other authors found no effects on ventricular refractoriness that could be reflected by changes in the QT interval.[124] Intravenous magnesium given to patients with torsades de pointes controls the arrhythmia in a high percentage without changing the prolonged QT interval significantly.[126] The calcium-blocking activity of magnesium was suggested to be one of the mechanisms responsible for this antiarrhythmic activity.[126]

HYPERCALCEMIA AND OTHER CAUSES OF SHORT QT INTERVALS

During sinus rhythm with normal rates, the QT interval is short (see Fig. 13–36, bottom) in hypercalcemia.[124] Occasionally the Q-to-apex of T intervals is also short. If factors known to modify the QT interval are not present, it has been said that a reasonably accepted correlation exists between the duration of the interval and serum calcium levels.[1,123] Occasionally, the ST segment disappears, and the T waves can become inverted in left and right chest leads. Digitalis also shortens the QT interval but produces its characteristic *effects* in leads where the R waves predominate.[1] The classic upward concavity of the ST segment is seen in the left chest leads in patients with LV hypertrophy and in leads V_1 and V_2

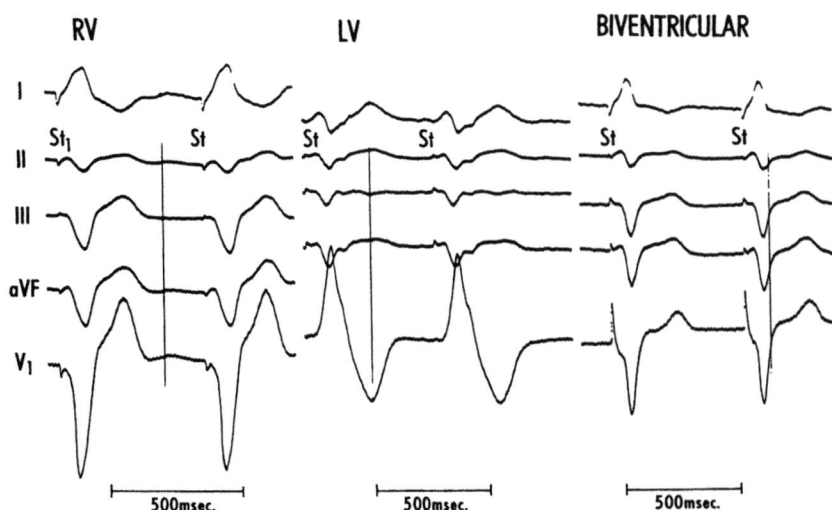

FIGURE 13–29. Simultaneous biventricular stimulation (right) compared with mono right ventricular (RV) pacing (left) and mono left ventricular (LV) pacing (center) in an individual without myocardial disease. In this case, the QRS complexes and T-wave are narrower and consequently the QT intervals shorter, when both ventricles were stimulated at the same time. Paper speed was 100 mm/sec.

TABLE 13–2

Electrocardiographic Criteria for Left Ventricular Enlargement

VOLTAGE CRITERIA	SENSITIVITY %	SPECIFICITY %	ACCURACY %
RI + S_{III} >25 mm	10.6	100	55
RVL >7.5 mm	22.5	96.5	59.5
RVL >11 mm	10.6	100	55
RVF >20 mm	1.3	99.5	50
SV_1 + RV_{5-6} ≥35 mm (Sokolow-Lyon)	42.5	95	74
SV_1 + RV_{5-6} >30 mm	55.6	89.5	73
InV_1–V_6, the tallest S + tallest R >45 mm	45	93	69
RV_{5-6} >26 mm	25	98	62
Romhilt-Estes score	60	97	78

SOURCE: From Bayes de Luna.[64] With permission.

TABLE 13–3

Romhilt-Estes Score.[64] There is Left Ventricular Enlargement if 5 or More Points Are Obtained. Left Ventricular Enlargement is Probable if the Sum is 4 Points.

A. Criteria Based on QRS Modifications
  1. Voltage criteria — 3 points
     One of the following should be present:
     • R or S in the FP ≥20 mm
     • S in V_1–V_2 ≥30 mm
     • R in V_5–V_6 ≥30 mm
  2. ÂQRS at –30° or more to the left — 2 points
  3. Intrinsicoid deflection in V_5–V_6 0.05 sec — 1 point
  4. QRS duration ≥ 0.09 sec — 1 point
B. Criteria Based on ST-T Changes
  1. ST-T vector opposite to QRS without digitalis — 3 points
  2. ST-T vector opposite to QRS with digitalis — 1 point
C. Criteria Based on P-wave Abnormalities
  1. Negative terminal P mode in V_1 ≥1 mm in depth and 0.04 sec in duration — 3 points

SOURCE: From Bayes de Luna.[64] With permission.

TABLE 13–4

Criteria for Diagnosis of Left Ventricular Hypertrophy in Presence of Complete Left Bundle-Branch Block

	SENSITIVITY %	SPECIFICITY %
1. R in aVL ≥11 mm	24	100
2. Electrical axis ≥40 (or S_2 ≥R_1)	39	100
3. SV_1 + RV_5 or RV_6 ≥40 mm	58	97
4. SV_2 ≥30 mm and SV_3 ≥25 mm	75	90

SOURCE: Kafka, Burggraf, Milliken.[122] With permission.

TABLE 13–5

Criteria for Diagnosis of Left Ventricular Hypertrophy in Presence of Left Anterior Fascicular Block[1]

STUDY	ECG CRITERIA	SENSITIVITY (%)	SPECIFICITY (%)	POSITIVE PREDICTIVE VALUE (%)	NEGATIVE PREDICTIVE VALUE (%)
Bozzi and Figini	SV_1 + (RV_5 + SV_5) ≥ 25 mm	69	92	80	73
Milliken	RaVL ≥13 mm	35	92	82	56
Milliken	SIII ≥15 mm	38	87	77	57
Gerstch et al.[120]	SIII + maximal sum of R + S in any single precordial lead	96	87	89	95
Reevaluated Gerstch criteria		80	55	78	58

[1]Left ventricular hypertrophy diagnosed by echocardiography when left ventricular mass is ≥ 124 g/m^2.
SOURCE: Used with permission from Gertsch, Theler, Foglia.[120]

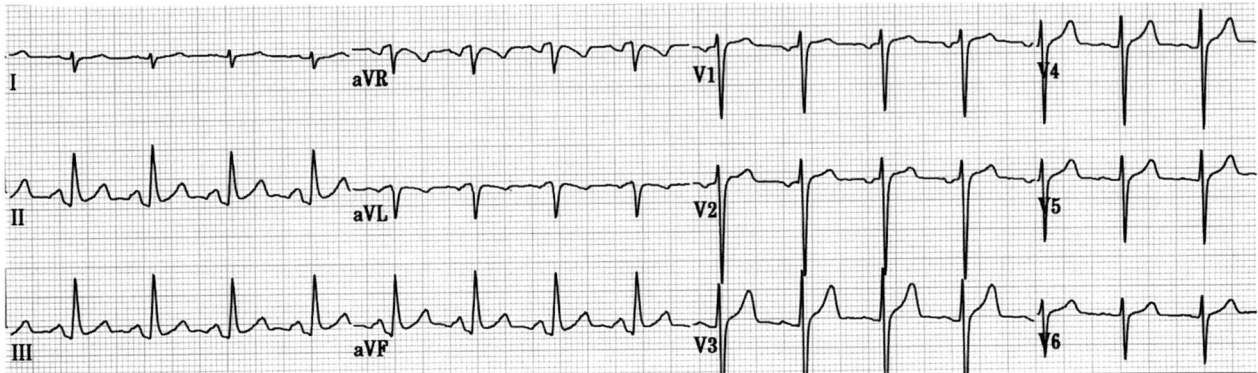

FIGURE 13–30. ECG from a patient with pulmonary emphysema showing slight right-axis deviation with small rS complexes in lead I, an electrically vertical heart position (with aVL similar to aV$_R$), overall tendency to low voltage, and rS complexes in all chest leads.

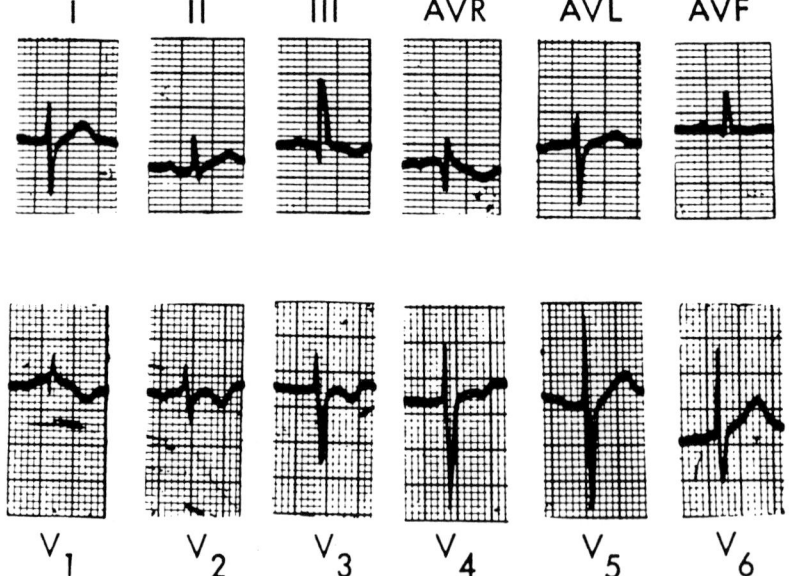

FIGURE 13–31. ECG from a patient with RV enlargement (volume overload in type) caused by a small atrial septal defect (ostium secundum). Right axis deviation was associated with an incomplete RBBB pattern (rSR' complexes in lead V$_1$). *Source: Lemberg, Castellanos.*[140] *Reproduced with permission from the publisher and authors.*

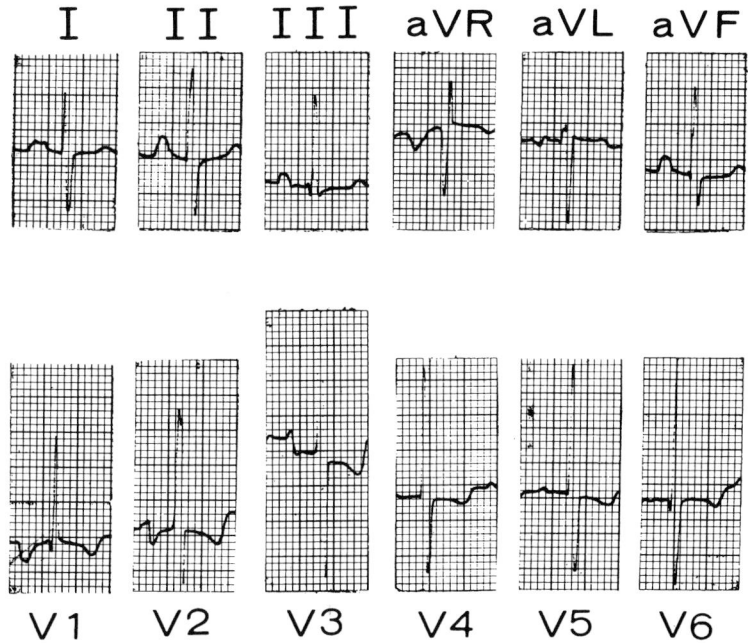

FIGURE 13–32. ECG from a patient with right ventricular (RV) hypertrophy caused by mitral stenosis showing P *mitrale*, right axis deviation, and R waves in V₁ and V₂. Negative T waves in V₅ and V₆ are caused by coexistent left ventricular hypertrophy caused by associated mitral regurgitation.

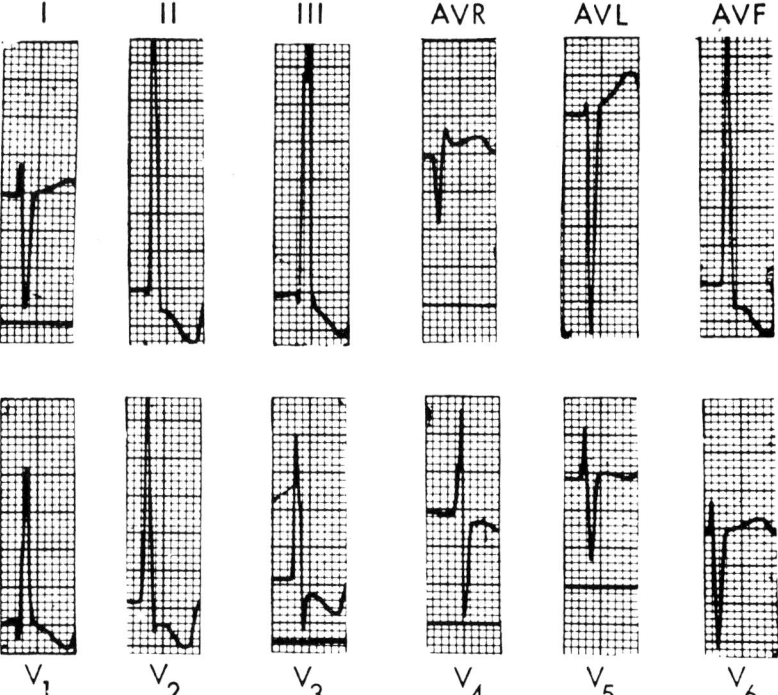

FIGURE 13–33. ECG from a 17-year-old patient who had right ventricular (RV) enlargement (pressure overloading in type) caused by severe pulmonic stenosis. Note extreme right axis deviation, overall high voltage, and qR complexes in lead V₁ without an incomplete right bundle-branch block (RBBB) pattern. *Source: Lemberg, Castellanos.*[140] *Reproduced with permission from the publisher and authors.*

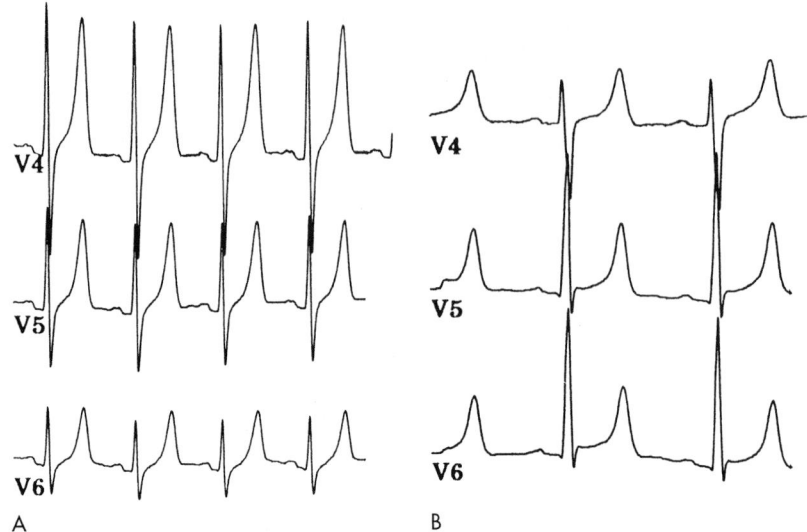

FIGURE 13-34. Electrocardiographic manifestations of early hyperkalemia. **A.** The slightly prolonged QRS complex is followed by a peaked T wave having a very narrow base. Uncorrected and corrected QT intervals of 0.32 and 0.44 second, respectively. **B.** Hyperkalemia with hypocalcemia characterized by prolongation of the QT interval at the expense of the ST segment preceding the narrow-based T wave. Uncorrected and corrected QT intervals of 0.52 and 0.53 second, respectively.

when there is RV hypertrophy (with predominantly positive deflections in these leads). In addition, short QT intervals have been reported in hyperthermia, some causes of hyperkalemia and *altered* autonomic tone. The congenital short-QT syndrome described by Gussak in 2001 is characterized by a QTc shorter than 300 milliseconds (ms) in most cases and by its association with atrial fibrillation, malignant ventricular arrhythmia, and sudden death.[128]

【 】 HYPOCALCEMIA

The typical ECG pattern of hypocalcemia consists of QT prolongation at the expense of the ST segment. The T wave is usually of normal width but can be narrow if there is coexisting (moderate)

hyperkalemia (see Fig. 13–34B).[124] A very marked injury (with the so-called hyperacute ST-T changes) can produce a similar pattern, but in such cases the T wave, although peaked, is not as narrow-based.[124] An ECG pattern similar to that of hypocalcemia can be produced by some organic abnormalities of the central nervous system and by congenitally prolonged QT intervals.[124]

HYPOTHERMIA

Subnormal temperatures of the body has been defined as a temperature below 97°F (36°C).[11] The QT interval becomes prolonged. In addition, a deflection, called an *Osborn wave*, appears

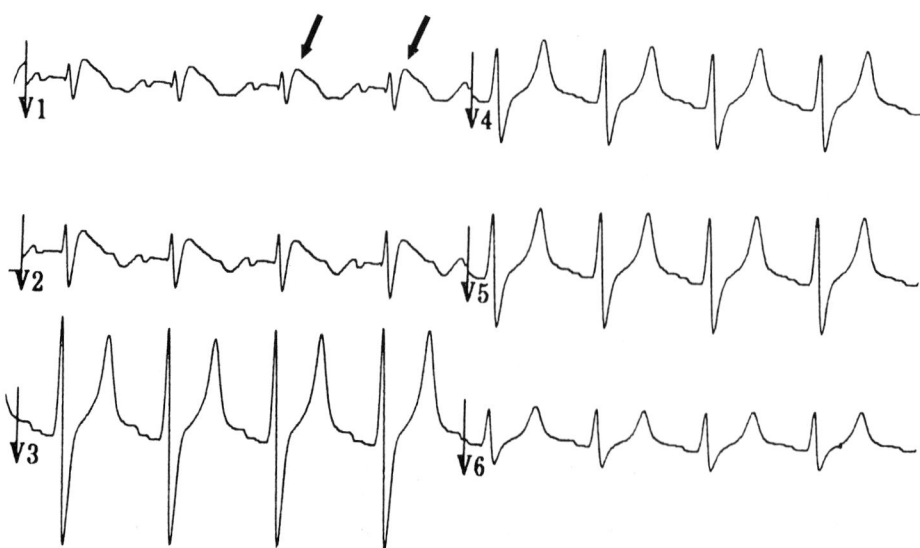

FIGURE 13-35. Advanced hyperkalemia. The wide (0.14-s) QRS complexes are followed by peaked T waves (best seen in lead V_3). The hyperkalemia-induced ST-segment elevation in lead V_1 (arrows), known as the *dialyzable current of injury*, disappeared after appropriate treatment. Note resemblance with the ST changes of the Brugada syndrome (Fig. 13–16A).

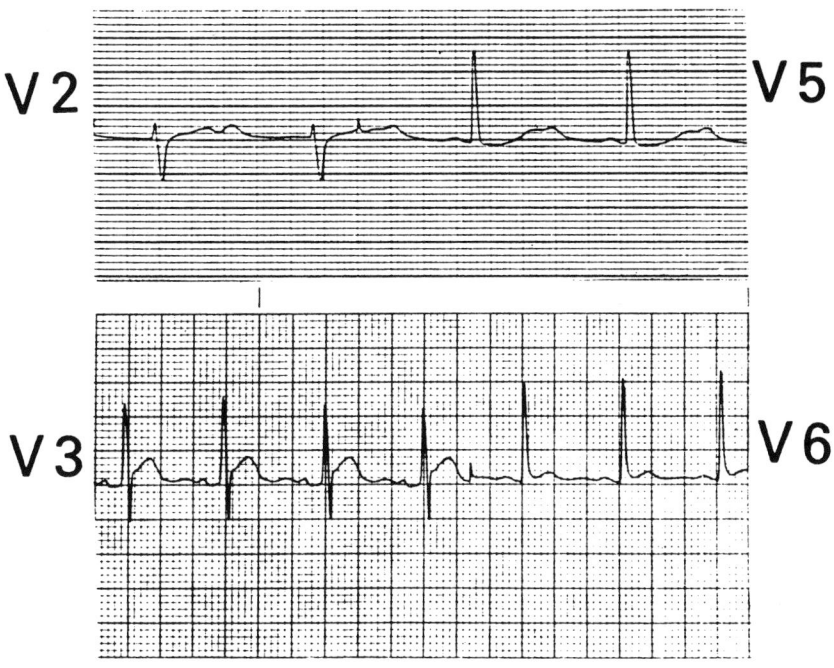

FIGURE 13–36. Electrocardiographic manifestations of hypokalemia (*upper strip*) and hypercalcemia (*lower strip*).

in a place said to be located between the end of the QRS complex and the beginning of the ST segment[1] (Fig. 13–37). This deflection has been attributed to delayed depolarization, to a current of injury, or to *early* repolarization. In leads facing the left ventricle, the deflection is positive, and its size is inversely related to body temperature. The role played by the intramyocardial M cells in its genesis has been discussed previously.[15]

ARTIFACTS

These are very important, are frequently dismissed in teaching, and cause enormous problems for computer comparison of serial

ECGs. Muscle tremor and alternating-current interference are the most common.[130] But in clinical practice, worldwide experience in ECG has shown that recordings of precordial electrodes are made with astonishingly marked neglect as to the employment of the proper chest landmarks.[131] This is a problem more common now than previously; in 1961 Simonson noted the considerable variation in chest lead placement in the same patient by different technicians and even by the same technician in several ECGs in the same patient.[131] Simonson also found that in a controlled study, placement of the V_2 electrode varied 10 cm vertically and 8 cm horizontally in 103 healthy subjects. He also observed that others found a rather large error in placement of chest electrodes (2 to 3 cm in both the horizontal and vertical directions) in repeated trials

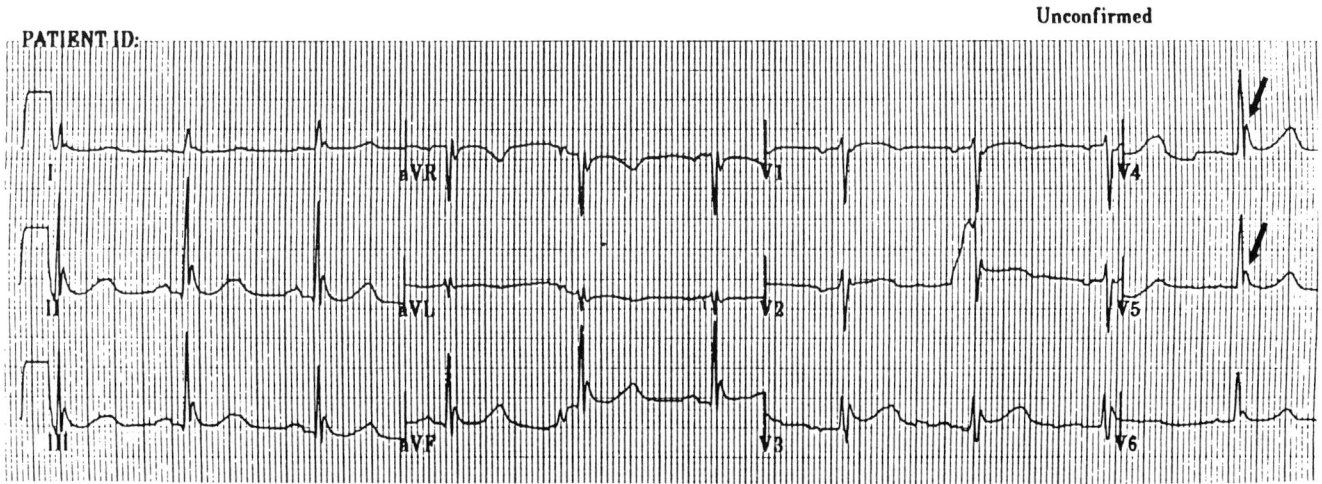

FIGURE 13–37. ECG obtained from a patient with hypothermia. The characteristic Osborn wave (*arrows*) is the terminal deflection inscribed between the slender part of the QRS complexes and the beginning of the ST segment. Note that it is not easy to determine where the ST segment starts. In addition, there is marked prolongation of the QT interval.

in the same patients by the same technicians.[131] A more recent study found that there was a superior displacement of more than 0.625 inch in V_1 and V_2, and inferior and upward displacement of more than 0.625 inch in V_4, V_5, and V_6.[130] Such a variability creates severe problems for computer interpretation of serial ECGs and considerable difficulties for the diagnosis of MI in the presence of LBBB.[130,132] In our institution the most frequent cause of "poor r-wave progression in the anteroseptal leads" (often interpreted by the computer as indication of septal or anterior MI) is misplacement of the corresponding electrodes. This is more common than switching the limb electrodes. To identify the latter, the method depicted in Fig. 13–38 based on the analysis of single extremity leads only is simpler than those starting from the bipolar (standard) lead.[1,133] Still, not uncommon is the misplacement of the right leg (ground) electrode recognized depending with what electrode it is switched by almost flat lines in leads I and II.[133] The most recently described, important artifact is cable malfunction characterized by identical morphologies in two or three left chest leads.

Finally, overshooting, overdamping, the indiscriminate use of filters, the running down of standardization battery, changing size, as well as polarity, of large unipolar pacemakers spikes and the almost microscopic size of some bipolar spikes should be taken into consideration.

[ ] PSEUDOARTIFACTS

The ECG changes produced by heart transplantation can be interpreted as artifacts. Orthotopic transplantation shows the small, barely visible P waves of the recipient's heart dissociated from the QRST complexes produced by the donor's heart. Heterotopic heart transplantation produces a unique interheart dissociation, resembling what in older Holter systems occurred when recordings were made on previously used unerased tapes (Fig. 13–39).[134]

COMPUTER APPLICATIONS

At the onset of the millennium the use of computer technology in ECG interpretation is universal.[134,135] Unfortunately (except in the case of arrhythmias) the frequent lack of value of these interpretations has received undue attention. An example is the report finding that interpretations of ECGs obtained 1 minute apart in the same patient by the same technician without changing electrodes were grossly different in 36 of 92 (39 percent) of unselected pair of tracings.[136] This only represented the findings with one instrument of one manufacturer in one institution.[136] For these, and many other multiple reasons, the findings of the ACC/AHA Task Force on Guidelines for Electrocardiography have stated that "no computer program can replace the skilled physician"; and that of the studies examining the accuracy of computer interpretations echoes the thinking of most cardiologists.[135] However, in truth, this is not a failure of technology but of the programmers and tautologic attitude of electrocardiographers themselves who have not used the technology to its maximum to maintain supremacy of human over machine for philosophical and economical reasons. Better results can be assured with appropriate greater interest, improvement of programs, and better use of technology.

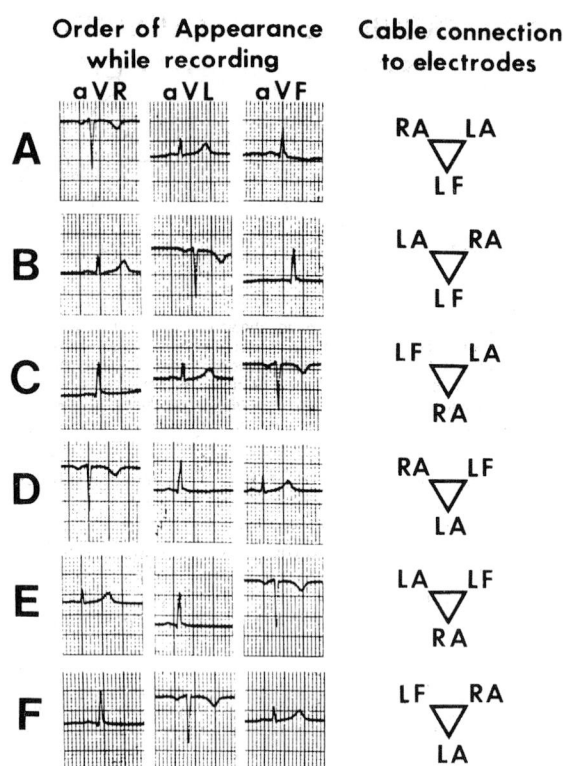

FIGURE 13–38. Identification of improper connections of the cables from the electrocardiographic machine to the corresponding electrodes placed on the patient's limbs. Note that aV_R, aV_L, and aV_F invariably refer to whatever morphology is recorded when, while the ECG is being obtained, the corresponding knobs are turned in this order (regardless of whether the cables were attached properly or improperly). Conversely, RA (*right arm*), LA (*left arm*), and LF (*left foot*) correspond to the normal morphology recorded by the cables so labeled, regardless of the limb to which they were connected. **A.** Normal. **B.** Because LA appears in aV_R and RA appears in aVL (with LF being in its normal position), the right arm and left arm cables must have been switched. **C.** Because LF appears in aV_R and RA appears in aV_F (with LA in its normal position), the right arm and left leg cables must have been switched. **D.** Because LA appears in aV_F and LF appears in aV_L (with RA in its normal position), the left arm and left leg cables must have been switched. **E.** Counterclockwise switching of all three cables. **F.** Clockwise switching of all three cables.

SPATIAL VECTORCARDIOGRAPHY
[ ] GENERALITIES

Because the ECG deals with electrical forces, it follows that very strictly speaking, all electrocardiography can be considered vectorial. However, there are multiple methods to express the vectorial concept.[8,137,138] When analyzing the vectorcardiogram (VCG), one should consider the activation of each muscle cell as producing an electrical force that can be represented by a vector depicting the spatial orientation and magnitude of this force.

If all manifest spatial vectors are diagrammatically represented as having a common point of origin and if the distal points of the vectors are joined, a single spatial loop is formed for ventricular depolarization (QRS), ventricular repolarization (ST-T), and the atrial complex (P). The VCG consists of four different loops (Figs. 13–40 and 13–41). The electrical activity of the atria is recorded as a small loop designated the *P loop*, the depolarization of the

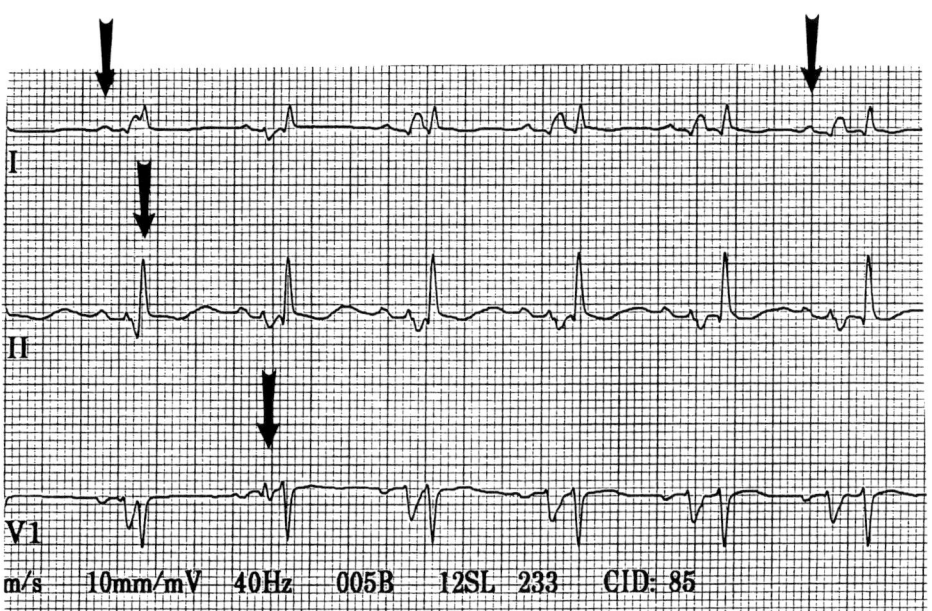

FIGURE 13–39. Pseudoartifact. Typical ECG pattern obtained after heterotopic heart transplantation. There is an "interheart" dissociation during which the ventricular activity of the recipient's heart (*arrow in lead I*) is totally independent from that of the donor's heart (*arrows in lead II*). To compound the problem, occasional ventricular ectopic beats (*arrow in lead V₁*) occasionally appear after the donor's P wave but with a shorter than normal PR interval.

their motion, has three dimensions, and positions are characterized by three numbers. The instant of an event is the fourth number. Four definite numbers correspond to every event; a definite event corresponds to any four numbers. Therefore the world of clinical events really forms a four-dimensional continuum.[139–141] Obviously what is perceived by the senses does not correlate with physical theories such as the almost Star Trekkian "string theory"; Hawking M theories (p-branes), which involve 10 or 26 dimensions; or algebraic concepts dealing with more than three dimensions.[141,142] For example, Malik correctly considers that in algebraic terms the 12-lead ECG can be represented by an algebraic path within an 8-dimensional space (in algebraic meaning).[143] This is simply an extension of the term *dimension* as used in physics into algebra, where analysis can deal with several *n* coordinates which, in turn, leads to spaces of *n* dimensions.[142,143] Future and comprehensive analysis of these concepts, which paradoxically emerged from critical analysis of QT dispersion will be discussed at the end of this chapter.

ventricles is recorded as a large loop designated the *QRS loop*, although the repolarization of the ventricles is recorded as a smaller loop designated the *ST-T loop*. Finally, at high magnifications, even a small *U loop* also can be recorded. A fundamental concept is that the term *loop* has a VCG, not an ECG, connotation.[139,140]

To obtain the spatial VCG, electrodes are placed on the body surface so as to record three leads with planes that are at right angles to each other. The true spatial VCG requires three corrected orthogonal leads with the following features[139]: (1) mutual perpendicularity, with each lead being parallel to one of the rectilinear coordinate axes of the human body. Such axes are the horizontal, *X* (left-to-right and right-to-left) axis; the vertical, *Y* (inferosuperior or superoinferior) axis; and sagittal, *Z* (anteroposterior or postero-anterior) axis; (2) equal amplitude from the vectorial viewpoint; and (3) retention of the same magnitude and direction for all points where cardiac electromotive forces are generated.

【 】 SPACE: THE FINAL FRONTIER AND MULTIPLE DIMENSIONS

The theory of the truly spatial VCG is theoretically attractive. Because the heart is a tridimensional structure (*located in space*), its electrical activity should best be recorded by a spatial method. Indeed, space, as conceived by human senses through objects and

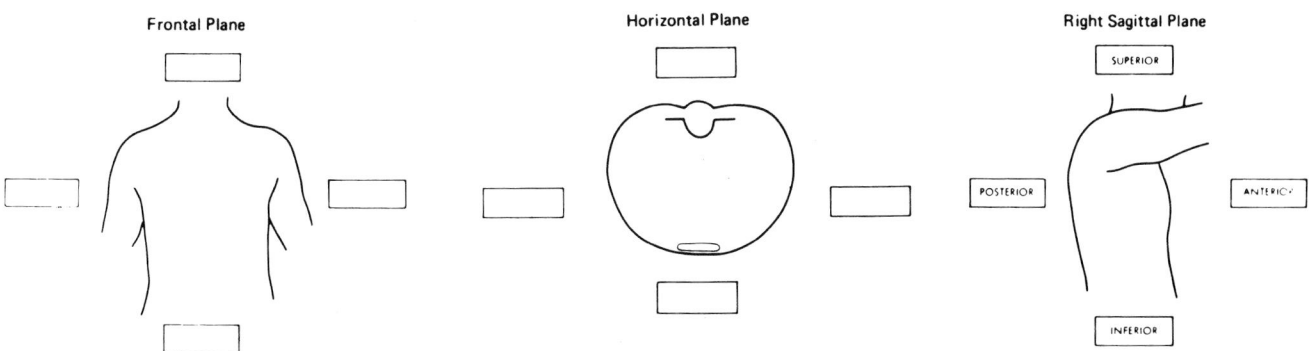

FIGURE 13–40. The spatial vectorcardiographic loops cannot be analyzed routinely in space with presently available techniques. Therefore it is customary to study their projections in three planes, seen as depicted in this figure. Note that the frontal plane conforms to Einthoven view of his equilateral triangle, the horizontal plane is seen in such a way that the anterior surfaces of the heart and sternum are displayed in the inferior portions of the paper (in contrast to other noninvasive, nonelectrical methods), and the sagittal plane is viewed from the right side of the patient. *Source: Lemberg, Castellanos.*[140] *Reproduced with permission from the publisher and authors.*

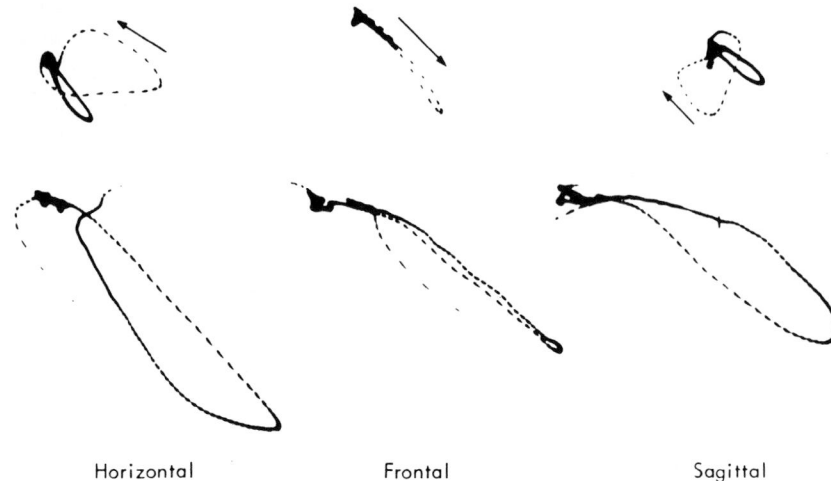

Horizontal   Frontal   Sagittal

FIGURE 13–41. Planar projections of normal spatial vectorcardiogram (VCG) obtained with the Frank method. The ST-T loops are enlarged in the bottom view. In the horizontal plane, the QRS loop shows the expected normal, counterclockwise (CCW) rotation (*arrows*). Although the narrow frontal plane QRS loop has clockwise (CW) rotation, in this plane either CCW, CW, or figure-eight rotations can be normal. In the right sagittal plane, the QRS loop displays its normal (CW) rotation. Enlargement of the ST-T loop clearly shows that its first half is inscribed more slowly. Therefore, the dashes (each representing 0.0025 s, or 2.5 ms) are closer together. The rotation of the ST-T loop is similar to the rotation of the QRS loop in all planes. *Source: Lemberg, Castellanos.[140] Reproduced with permission from the publisher and authors.*

that can be of different duration in different precordial leads.[1,12,14] In the 12-lead ECG (especially when the precordial electrodes are misplaced) however, these forces can move spatially not only in a left-to-right and anteroposterior direction but also in an inferosuperior direction, as in leads V_5 and V_6 in patients with a very superior and leftward deviation of the EA. Conversely, the theory of truly spatial vectorcardiography states that the horizontal plane and unipolar leads derived from them just record left-to-right and anteroposterior forces (see Fig. 13–40B) and that they do not record local potentials, so that any differences in the duration of such derived measurements are an illusion caused by the isoelectricity in a lead resulting from total perpendicularity of vectors. In spatial VCG electric forces moving superiorly or inferiorly cannot be reflected in the horizontal plane but only in the frontal or sagittal planes.[139,140]

QT DISPERSION AND NOVEL MODES OF REPOLARIZATION ANALYSIS

This problem is discussed after dealing with VCG because investigators have proposed the use of the previously mentioned reconstructed VCGs as improvements over this measurement. In fact, the concept of QT dispersion (differences between the longest and the shortest QT intervals of the 12-lead ECG) has received considerable attention.[30,31,146–148] Increased dispersion has been reported to be associated with QT prolongation as a result of proarrhythmic drugs, with increased mortality in epidemiologic studies and after acute myocardial infarction, as well as a marker of therapeutic efficiency in the congenital or acquired long QT syndromes.[30,31] Interestingly, more recent studies have challenged the usefulness of this measurement, which has even been considered an illusion.[30,31] Strictly speaking, if it is considered that vector loops lack nondipolar information, then the differences in QT interval in the various ECG leads simply reflect perpendicularity of vectors in some of them. This is certainly true in regard to the bipolar and unipolar extremity leads but need not apply to the precordial leads, which can record local potentials.[30] More important, Malik and Butcharov found that values are largely overlapping both between healthy and cardiac subjects as well as between patients with and without adverse outcome.[148] For these authors, QT dispersion is only a crude approximate method of determining the course of repolarization, and probably only grossly abnormal values (100 ms) that are outside measurement error have practical value.[148]

The most widely used, corrected, truly spatial VCG method probably is the one introduced by Frank.[139,140] Because the spatial loop cannot be analyzed tridimensionally, it is customary to study its planar projections (see Figs. 13–40 and 13–41). Lately there has been a revival of the VCG using methods derived or reconstructed from the ECG.[144,145] Some methods tended to duplicate the Frank system, such as the inverse Dower matrix and the Bjerle and Marquette (Marquette Electronics, Milwaukee system) methods.[144,145] It is commonly accepted that the Frank system does not record local or nondipolar components, because proximity effects do not apply.[143] Nondipolar components can be quantified from the 12-lead ECG, but whether they can be obtained from a reconstructed VCG is a subject of debate and speculation.[31,144–146] According to Malik and coworkers, this can be done in a way that requires the use of nonclinical, nonphysical, but valid mathematical terms, such as, for example, *dimension energy*.[31] Here, energy represents the variance of the projection of a vector into a dimension, whereas the latter, as previously stated, is used in reference to three spatial or eight algebraic dimensions.

【 】 DIFFERENCES BETWEEN ELECTROVECTORCARDIOGRAPHY AND SPATIAL VECTORCARDIOGRAPHY

Emphasis should be placed on the fact that the spatial VCG method is distinctly different from the various nonspatial vectorial methods of ECG interpretation, such as those proposed by Sodi-Pallares and coworkers[8] and Grant.[138] For example, the unipolar precordial leads are derived from the horizontal plane loops. Leads thus derived are different from the usual precordial ECG leads. The latter, as mentioned previously, record electrical forces moving toward or away from them, including local potentials

Some have reported that certain novel spatial modes of repolarization analysis should be more accurate and clinically useful surface-ECG markers of heterogeneity of repolarization than simple scalar intervals obtained from the ECG, such as QT dispersion. These articles,[31,146–148] although extremely original and intellectually stimulating, are complex, because they deal with semiconventional mathematical and physical concepts. More important, they interchange ECG and VCG terms and concepts. Novel descriptors include[146–148] (1) principal component analysis (essentially the ratio of the long and short axis of the three-dimensional (3D) T loop, which is equivalent to the length-to-width bidimensionally projected classical VCG concept); (2) T-loop dispersion (variation of interlead relationships); (3) normalized T-loop area (spatial area of the 3D loop projected in two dimensions [!]); and (4) the so-called TCRT, which is the vectorial deviation of R and T loops (equivalent to Wilson ventricular gradient).

Regardless of whether QT dispersion is an illusion or not, if it can be superseded by these other measurements, all of them give *global* values different from the more *regional* transmural dispersion of repolarization in single (presumably) precordial leads.[15] Experimentally, the latter is given by the time elapsing between the peak of the T wave (reflecting the end of epicardial action potentials) and its termination (reflecting the end of the action potentials of M cells).[15]

REFERENCES

1. Surawicz B, Knilans TK. *Chou's Electrocardiography in Clinical Practice*. 5th ed. Philadelphia, PA: Saunders; 2002:22, 76, 93, 451–453.
2. MacFarlane PW, Lawrie TDV, eds. *Comprehensive Electrocardiology: Theory and Practice in Health and Disease*. New York: Pergamon Press; 1989.
3. Hurst JW. Where have all the teachers of electrocardiography gone? *J Electrocardiol*. 2006;39:112.
4. Task Force Report of the American College of Cardiology and the American Heart Association. ACC/AHA Guidelines for Electrocardiography. *Circulation*. 1992;19:473–481.
5. Castellanos A, Myerburg RJ. Electrocardiography. In: Schlant RC, Alexander RW, Lipton MJ, eds. *Diagnostic Atlas of the Heart*. New York: McGraw-Hill; 1996.
6. American College of Cardiology/American Heart Association Task Force on Practice Guidelines (Committee on Pacemaker Implantation). ACC/AHA guidelines for implantation of cardiac pacemakers and antiarrhythmia devices. *J Am Coll Cardiol*. 1998;31:1175–1209.
7. Lepeschkin E. *Modern Electrocardiography*. Vol 1. Baltimore, MD: Williams & Wilkins; 1951:180–186.
8. Sodi-Pallares D, Medrano GA, Bisteni A, et al. *Deductive and Polyparametric Electrocardiography*. Mexico City: Instituto Nacional Cardiologia Mexico; 1970:36,136.
9. Rosenbaum MB, Elizari MV, Lazzari JO. *The Hemiblocks*. Oldsmar, FL: Tampa Tracings; 1970.
10. Schamroth L. *The Electrocardiology of Coronary Artery Disease*. 2nd ed. Oxford, England: Blackwell Scientific; 1984.
11. Wagner GS. Marriott's *Practical Electrocardiography*. 10th ed. Baltimore, MD: Lippincott, Williams & Wilkins; 2001.
12. Barker JM. *The Unipolar Electrocardiogram: A Clinical Interpretation*. New York: Appleton-Century-Crofts; 1952.
13. Lipman BS, Massie E, Kleiger RE. *Clinical Scalar Electrocardiography*. 6th ed. Chicago: Year Book; 1972:210–215.
14. Holland RP, Arnsdorf MF. Solid angle theory and the electrocardiogram: physiologic and quantitative interpretations. *Prog Cardiovasc Dis*. 1997;19:6:431–456.
15. Antzelevitch C, Shimizu W, Yan GX, et al. The M cell: its contribution to the ECG and to normal and abnormal electrical function of the heart. *J Cardiovasc Electrophysiol*. 1999;10:1124–1152.
16. Sejersten M, Pahlm O, Pettersson J, et al. Comparison of EASI-derived 12-lead electrocardiograms versus paramedic-acquired 12-lead electrocardiograms using Mason-Likar limb lead configuration in patients with chest pain. *J Electrocardiol*. 2006;39:13–21.
17. Task Force of the European Society of Cardiology and the North American Society of Pacing and Electrophysiology. Heart rate variability: standards of measurement, physiological interpretation, and clinical use. *Circulation*. 1996;93:1043–1065.
18. Schmidt G, Malik M, Barthel P, et al. Heart rate turbulence after ventricular premature beats as a predictor of mortality after acute myocardial infarction. *Lancet*. 1999;353:130–196.
19. Malik M, Wichtele D, Schmidt G. Heart rate turbulence. *G Ital Cardiol*. 1999;29:65–69.
20. Ceri Davies L, France DP, Ponikowski P, et al. Relation of heart rate and blood pressure turbulence following premature ventricular complexes to baroreflex sensitivity in chronic congestive heart failure. *Am J Cardiol*. 2001;87:737–742.
21. Cabrera E, Gaxiola A. *Teoria y Practica de la Electrocardiografia*. 2nd ed. Mexico City: La Prensa Medica Mexicana; 1966.
22. Wilson FN, MacLeod AG, Barker PS, et al. The determination and significance of the areas of the ventricular deflections of the electrocardiogram. *Am Heart J*. 1934;10:46–61.
23. Rosenbaum MB, Blanco HH, Elizari MV, et al. Electrotonic modulation of ventricular repolarization and cardiac memory. In: Rosenbaum MB, Elizari MV, eds. *Frontiers of Cardiac Electrophysiology*. Boston: Martinus Nijhoff; 1983:67–99.
24. Rosenbaum MB, Blanco HH, Elizari MV, et al. Electrotonic modulation of the T wave and cardiac memory. *Am J Cardiol*. 1982;50:213–222.
25. Surawicz B. Letters to the ed. *J Cardiovasc Electrophysiol*. 2001;12:390–391.
26. Rosen MR. What is cardiac memory? *J Cardiovasc Electrophysiol*. 2000;11:1289–1293.
27. Surawicz B. Transient T wave abnormalities after cessation of ventricular pre-excitation: memory of what? *J Cardiovasc Electrophysiol*. 1996;7:51–59.
28. Moleiro F, Castellanos A, Diaz JO, Myerburg RJ. Dynamics of the QT intervals encompassing secondary repolarization abnormalities during sudden but transient lengthening of the RR intervals. *Am J Cardiol*. 2003;91:7:883–885.
29. Lepeschkin E, Surawicz B. The measurement of the QT interval on the electrocardiogram. *Circulation*. 1951;6:378–384.
30. Coumel P, Maison-Blanche P, Badilini F. Dispersion of ventricular repolarization: Reality? Illusion? Significance? *Circulation*. 1998;97:2491–2493.
31. Malik M, Acar B, Gang Y, et al. QT dispersion does not represent electrocardiographic interlead heterogeneity of ventricular repolarization. *J Cardiovas Electrophysiol*. 2000;11:835–843.
32. Medina-Ravell VA, Lankipalli RS, Yan GX, et al. Effect of epicardial or biventricular pacing to prolong QT interval and increase transmural dispersion of repolarization. *Circulation*. 2003;107:740–746.
33. Rautaharju PM, Zhang Z, Prineas R, Heiss G. Assessment of prolonged QT and JT intervals in ventricular conduction defects. *Am J Cardiol*. 2004;93:1017–1021.
34. Rautaharju PM, Zhang ZM. Linearly scaled, rate-invariant normal limits for QT interval: eight decades of incorrect application of power functions. *J Cardiovasc Electrophysiol*. 2002;13:1211–1218.
35. Malik M. Is there a physiologic QT/RR relationship? *J Cardiovasc Electrophysiol*. 2002;13:1219–1221.
36. Moleiro F, Misticchio F, Torres JM, et al. Paradoxical behavior of the QT interval during exercise and recovery and its relationship with cardiac memory. *Clin Cardiol*. 1999;22:413–416.
37. Castellanos A, Moleiro F, Lopera G, et al. Dynamics of the uncorrected QT interval during vagal-induced lengthening of RR intervals. *Am J Cardiol*. 2000;86:1390–1392.
38. Boyett MR, Fedida D. Changes in the electrical activity of dog cardiac Purkinje fibers at high heart rates. *J Physiol*. 1984;350:361–391.
39. Elharrar V, Surawicz B. Cycle length effect on restitution of action potential duration in dog cardiac fibers. *Am J Physiol*. 1983;244: H782–792.
40. Coghlan JG, Madden B, Norell MN, et al. Paradoxical early lengthening and subsequent linear shortening of the QT interval in response to exercise. *Eur Heart J*. 1992;13:1325–1328.
41. Kligfield P, Kevin GL, Okin PM. QTc behavior during treadmill exercise as a function of the underlying QT heart-rate relationship. *J Electrocardiol*. 1996;28:206–210.
42. Mirvis DM. Spatial variation of QT intervals in normal persons and patients with acute myocardial infarction. *J Am Coll Cardiol*. 1985;5(3):625–631.
43. Ahvine S, Vallin H. Influence of heart rate and inhibition of autonomic tone on the QT interval. *Circulation*. 1982;65:433–435.
44. ZaZa A, Malfatto G, Schwartz PJ. Sympathetic modulation of the relation between ventricular repolarization and cycle length. *Circ Res*. 1991;68:1191–1203.
45. Cappato R, Alboni P, Pedroni P, et al. Sympathetic and vagal influences on rate-dependent changes of QT interval in healthy subjects. *Am J Cardiol*. 1991;68:1188–1193.
46. Litovsky SH, Antzelevitch C. Rate dependence of action potential duration and refractoriness in canine ventricular endocardium differs from that of epicardium: role of the transient outward current. *J Am Coll Cardiol*. 1989;14:1053–1066.

47. Coumel P, Fayn J, Maison-Blanche P, et al. Clinical relevance of assessing QT dynamicity in Holter recordings. *J Electrocardiol.* 1997;27(suppl):62–66.

48. Shvilkin A, Danilo P Jr, Wang J, et al. Evolution and resolution of long-term cardiac memory. *Circulation.* 1998;97:1810–1817.

49. The Criteria Committee of the New York Heart Association. *Nomenclature and Criteria for Diagnosis of Diseases of the Heart and Great Vessels.* 8th ed. New York: New York Heart Association; 1979:304.

50. Franz MR, Swerdlow CD, Liem LB, Schaefer J. Cycle length dependence of human action potential duration in vivo. Effects of single extrastimuli, sudden sustained rate acceleration and deceleration, and different steady-state frequencies. *J Clin Invest.* 1988;82:972–979.

51. Sclarovsky S. *Electrocardiography of Acute Myocardial Ischaemic Syndromes.* London: Martin Dunitz; 1999.

52. Holland RP, Brooks H. QT-ST segment mapping: critical review and analysis of current concepts. *Am J Cardiol.* 1977;40:110–129.

53. Birnbaum Y, Sclarovsky S. The grades of ischemia on the presenting electrocardiogram of patients with ST-segment elevation acute myocardial infarction. *J Electrocardiol.* 2001;34(suppl):17–26.

54. Kim TY, Alturk N, Shaikh N, et al. An electrocardiographic algorithm for the prediction of the culprit lesion site in acute anterior myocardial infarction. *Clin Cardiol.* 1999;22:77–83.

55. Castellanos A, Lemberg L. *A Programmed Introduction to the Electrical Axis and the Action Potential.* Oldsmar, FL: Tampa Tracings; 1974:34:114.

56. Phibbs B, Marcua F, Marriott HJC, et al. Q-wave versus non-Q-wave myocardial infarction: a meaningless distinction. *J Am Coll Cardiol.* 1999;33:576–582.

57. Barold SS, Falkoff MD, Ong LS, et al. Significance of transient electrocardiographic Q waves in coronary artery disease. *Cardiol Clin.* 1987;5:367–380.

58. Castellanos A, Myerburg RJ. *The Hemiblocks in Myocardial Infarction.* New York: Appleton-Century-Crofts; 1976.

59. de Lemos JA, Braunwald E. ST segment resolution as a tool for assessing the efficacy of reperfusion therapy. *J Am Coll Cardiol.* 2001;38:1283–1294.

60. Timmis GC. Electrocardiographic effects of reperfusion. *Cardiol Clin.* 1987;5:427–446.

61. Braunwald E, Kloner RA. The stunned myocardium: prolonged postischemic ventricular dysfunction. *Circulation.* 1982;66:1146–1149.

62. Braunwald E, Rutherford JD. Reversible ischemic left ventricular dysfunction: Evidence for the "hibernating myocardium." *J Am Coll Cardiol.* 1986;8:1467–1470.

63. Rahimtoola SH. A perspective on the three large multicenter randomized clinical trials of coronary bypass surgery for chronic stable angina. *Circulation.* 1985;72(suppl 5):123–135.

64. Bayes de Luna A. *Clinical Electrocardiography: A Textbook.* Mt. Kisco, NY: Futura; 1993:450.

65. Califf RM, Mark DB, Wagner GS. *Acute Coronary Care in the Thrombolytic Era.* Chicago: Year Book; 1988.

66. Shah PK, Zahger D, Ganz W. Streptokinase in acute myocardial infarction. In: Francis GS, Alpert JS, eds. *Coronary Care.* 2nd ed. Boston: Little, Brown; 1995:409–450.

67. Goodman S. Q wave and non-Q wave myocardial infarction after thrombolysis (letter). *J Am Coll Cardiol.* 1996;27(7):1817–1819.

68. Fernandez AR, Sequeira RF, Chakko S, et al. ST segment tracking for rapid determination of patency of the infarct-related artery in acute myocardial infarction. *J Am Coll Cardiol.* 1995;26:675–683.

69. Veldkamp RF, Simoons ML, Pope JE, et al. Continuous multilead ST segment monitoring in acute myocardial infarction. In: Clements IP, ed. *The Electrocardiogram in Acute Myocardial Infarction.* Mt. Kisco, NY: Futura; 1998.

70. Selvester RH, Wagner GE, Iderker RE. Myocardial infarction. In: MacFarlane PW, Lawrie TD, eds. *Comprehensive Electrocardiology.* New York: Pergamon; 1989.

71. Braat SH, Brugada P, den Dulk K, et al. Value of lead V_{4R} for recognition of the infarct coronary artery in acute inferior myocardial infarction. *Am J Cardiol.* 1984;53:1538–1541.

72. Marriott HJL, ed. *Practical Electrocardiography.* 8th ed. Baltimore, MD: Williams & Wilkins; 1998.

73. Wasserburger RH, Alt WJ. The normal RS-T segment elevation variant. *Am J Cardiol.* 1961;8:184–192.

74. Goldberger AL. ST segment elevation: normal variants: Benign (functional) ST segment elevation, "early repolarization variant." In: Goldberger AL, ed. *Myocardial Infarction: ECG Differential Diagnosis.* 3rd ed. St. Louis, MI: Mosby; 1984:1970–1978.

75. Morace G, Padeletti L, Porciani MC, et al. Effect of isoproterenol on the early repolarization syndrome. *Am Heart J.* 1979;97:343–347.

76. Miyazaki T, Mitamura H, Miyoshi S, et al. Autonomic and antiarrhythmic drug modulation of ST segment elevation in patients with Brugada syndrome. *J Am Coll Cardiol.* 1996;27:1061–1070.

77. Brugada P, Brugada J. Right bundle branch block, persistent ST segment elevation and sudden cardiac death: a distinct clinical and electrocardiographic syndrome. *J Am Coll Cardiol.* 1992;20:1391–1396.

78. Wilde AAM, Antzelevitch C, Borggrefe M, et al. Proposed diagnostic criteria for the Brugada syndrome. Consensus Report. *Circulation.* 2002;106:2514–2519.

79. Corrado D, Nava A, Buja G, et al. Familial cardiomyopathy underlies syndrome of right bundle branch block, ST segment elevation and sudden death. *J Am Coll Cardiol.* 1996;27:443–448.

80. Fujiki A, Usui M, Nagasawa H, et al. ST segment elevation in the right precordial leads induced with class IC antiarrhythmic drugs: Insight into the mechanism of Brugada syndrome. *J Cardiovasc Electrophysiol.* 1999;10:214–218.

81. Fontaine G, Fontaliran F, Lascault P, et al. In: Zipes DP, Jalife J, eds. *Cardiac Electrophysiology: From Cell to Bedside.* 2nd ed. Philadelphia, PA: Saunders; 1995:754–768.

82. Friedberg CK, Zager A. Nonspecific ST- and T-wave changes. *Circulation.* 1961;23:655–661.

83. Sequeira RF, Lemberg L. The electrocardiogram read as nonspecific ST-T waves. *ACC Curr J Rev.* 1995;July/August:36–40.

84. Nelson SD, Kou WH, Annesley T, et al. Significance of ST segment depression during paroxysmal supraventricular tachycardia. *J Am Coll Cardiol.* 1988;12:383–387.

85. Castellanos A, Pina IL, Zaman L, et al. Recent advances in the diagnosis of fascicular blocks. *Cardiol Clin.* 1987;5:469–488.

86. Rosenbaum MB, Corrado G, Oliveri R, et al. Right bundle branch block with left anterior hemiblock surgically induced in tetralogy of Fallot. *Am J Cardiol.* 1970;26:12–19.

87. Cohen SI, Lau SH, Stein E, et al. Variations of aberrant ventricular conduction in man: Evidence of isolated and combined block within the specialized conduction system. *Circulation.* 1968;38:899–916.

88. Milliken JA. Isolated and complicated left anterior fascicular block: a review of suggested electrocardiographic criteria. *J Electrocardiol.* 1983;16:199–211.

89. Rosenbaum MB, Elizari MV, Lazzari JO. The differential electrocardiographic manifestations of hemiblocks, bilateral bundle branch blocks and trifascicular blocks. In: Schlant RC, Hurst JW, eds. *Advances in Electrocardiography.* New York: Grune & Stratton; 1972:145–161.

90. Nakaya Y, Hiasa Y, Murayama Y, et al. Prominent anterior QRS forces as a manifestation of left septal fascicular block. *J Electrocardiol.* 1978;11:39–46.

91. Gambetta M, Childers RW. Rate-dependent right precordial Q waves: "Septal focal block." *Am J Cardiol.* 1973;32:196–201.

92. Dhala A, Gonzalez-Zuelgaray J, Deshpande S, et al. Unmasking the trifascicular left intraventricular conduction system by ablation of the right bundle branch. *Am J Cardiol.* 1996;77:706–712.

93. Grant RP. Peri-infarction block. *Progr Cardiovasc Dis.* 1959;27:237–247.

94. Oppenheimer BS, Rothschild MA. Electrocardiographic changes associated with myocardial involvement: With special reference to prognosis. *JAMA.* 1997;69:429–431.

95. Castle CH, Keane WM. Electrocardiographic "peri-infarction block": A clinical and pathologic correlation. *Circulation.* 1965;31:403–408.

96. Conte RA, Parkin TW, Brandenburg RO, et al. Peri-infarction block: postmyocardial infarction intraventricular conduction disturbance. *Am Heart J.* 1965;69:150–153.

97. First SR, Bayley RH, Bedford DR. Peri-infarction block. *Circulation.* 1950;2:31–36.

98. Wilson FN, Hill IGW, Johnston FD. The form of electrocardiogram in experimental myocardial infarction: III. The later effects produced by ligation of the anterior descending branch of the left coronary artery. *Am Heart J.* 1935;10:903–915.

99. Barker JM, Valencia F. The precordial electrocardiogram in incomplete right bundle branch block. In: Johnson FD, Lepeschkin E, eds. *Selected Papers of Dr. Frank N. Wilson.* Ann Arbor, MI: Edwards Brothers; 1954:884–914.

100. Blount SG, Munyan EA Jr, Hoffman MS. Hypertrophy of the right ventricular outflow tract: a contract of the electrocardiographic findings in atrial septal defect. *Am J Med.* 1957;22:784–790.

101. Moore EN, Hoffman BF, Patterson DF, et al. Electrocardiographic changes due to delayed activation of the wall of the right ventricle. *Am Heart J.* 1964;68:347–361.

102. Sung RJ, Tamer DM, Agha AS, et al. Etiology of the electrocardiographic pattern of "incomplete right bundle branch block" in atrial septal defect: An electrophysiologic study. *J Pediatr.* 1975;87:1182–1186.

103. Castellanos A, Ramirez AV, Mayorga-Cortes A, et al. Left fascicular blocks during right-heart catheterization using the Swan-Ganz catheter. *Circulation.* 1981;64:1271–1276.

104. Sgarbossa EB. Recent advances in the electrocardiographic diagnosis of myocardial infarction: left bundle branch block and pacing. *PACE.* 1998;21:120–131.

105. Kindwall KE, Brown JP, Josephson ME. Predictive accuracy of criteria for chronic myocardial infarction in pacing-induced left bundle branch block. *Am J Cardiol.* 1986;57:1255–1260.

106. Wackers FJT. The diagnosis of myocardial infarction in the presence of left bundle branch block. *Cardiol Clin.* 1987;5:393–401.

107. Castillo CA, Castellanos A Jr. His bundle recordings in patients with reciprocating tachycardias and Wolff-Parkinson-White syndrome. *Circulation.* 1970;42:271–285.

108. Rosenbaum FF, Hecht HH, Wilson FN, et al. The potential variations of the thorax and esophagus in anomalous atrioventricular excitation (Wolff-Parkinson-White syndrome). *Am Heart J.* 1945;29:281–326.

109. Wallace AG, Sealy WC, Gallagher JJ, et al. Ventricular excitation in Wolff-Parkinson-White syndrome. In: Wellens HJJ, Lie KI, Janse MJ, eds. *The Conduction System of the Heart: Structure, Function and Clinical Implications.* Leiden, The Netherlands: HE Stenfert Kroese; 1976:613–630.

110. Castellanos A, Agha AS, Portillo B, et al. Usefulness of vectorcardiography combined with His bundle recordings and cardiac pacing in evaluation of the preexcitation (Wolff-Parkinson-White) syndrome. *Am J Cardiol.* 1972;30:623–628.

111. Milstein S, Sharma AD, Guiraudon GM, et al. An algorithm for the electrocardiographic localization of accessory pathways in the Wolff-Parkinson-White syndrome. *PACE.* 1987;10:555–563.

112. Basiouny T, De Chillou D, Fareh S, et al. Accuracy and limitations of published algorithms using the twelve-lead electrocardiogram to localize over atrioventricular accessory pathways. *J Cardiovasc Electrophysiol.* 1999;10:1340–1349.

113. Chiang CE, Chen SA, Teo WS, et al. An accurate stepwise electrocardiographic algorithm for localization of accessory pathways in patients with Wolff-Parkinson-White syndrome from a comprehensive analysis of delta waves and r/s ratio during sinus rhythm. *Am J Cardiol.* 1995;76:40–46.

114. Cosio FG, Anderson RH, Kuck KH, et al. ESCWGA/NASPE/P experts consensus statement: living anatomy of the atrioventricular junctions. A guide to electrophysiologic mapping. *J Cardiovasc Electrophysiol.* 1999;10:1162–1170.

115. Castellanos A Jr, Ortiz JM, Pastis N, et al. The electrocardiogram in patients with pacemakers. *Prog Cardiovasc Dis.* 1970:13:190–209.

116. Castellanos A Jr, Lemberg L, Salhanick L, et al. Pacemaker vectorcardiography. *Am Heart J.* 1968;75:6–18.

117. Befeler B, Berkovits BV, Aranda JM, et al. Programmed simultaneous biventricular stimulation in man, with special reference to its use in the evaluation of intraventricular reentry. *Eur J Cardiol.* 1979;9:369–378.

118. Popovic ZB, Grimm RA, Perlic G, et al. Noninvasive assessment of cardiac resynchronization therapy for congestive heart failure using myocardial strain and left ventricular peak power as parameters of myocardial synchrony and function. *J Cardiovasc Electrophysiol.* 2002;13:1203–1208.

119. Varma C, Sharma S, Firoozi S, et al. Atriobiventricular pacing improves exercise capacity in patients with heart failure and intraventricular conduction delay. *J Am Coll Cardiol.* 2003;41:582–588.

120. Gertsch M, Theler A, Foglia E. Electrocardiographic detection of left ventricular hypertrophy in the presence of left anterior fascicular block. *Am J Cardiol.* 1988;61:1089–1101.

121. Surawicz B. Electrocardiographic diagnosis of chamber enlargement. *J Am Coll Cardiol.* 1986;8:711–724.

122. Kafka H, Burggraf GW, Milliken JA. Electrocardiographic diagnosis of left ventricular hypertrophy in the presence of left bundle branch block: an echocardiographic study. *Am J Cardiol.* 1985;55:103–106.

123. Vander Ark CR, Ballantyne F III, Reynolds EW Jr. Electrolytes and the electrocardiogram. *Cardiovasc Clin.* 1973;5:269–294.

124. Fisch C. Electrocardiography and vectorcardiography. In: Braunwald E, ed. *Heart Disease.* 4th ed. Philadelphia, PA: Saunders; 1992:116–160.

125. Kulick DL, Hong R, Ryzen E, et al. Electrophysiologic effects of intravenous magnesium in patients with normal conduction systems and no clinical evidence of significant cardiac disease. *Am Heart J.* 1988;148:367–373.

126. Tzivoni D, Keren A, Cohen AM, et al. Magnesium therapy for torsades de pointes. *Am J Cardiol.* 1984;53:528–530.

127. Mosseri M, Porath A, Ovsyshcher I, et al. Electrocardiographic manifestations of combined hypercalcemia and hypermagnesemia. *J Electrocardiol.* 1990;23:235–241.

128. Gussak I, Bjerregaard P. Short QT syndrome-5 years of progress. *J Electrocardiol.* 2005;38:375–377.

129. Osborn JJ. Experimental hypothermia: respiratory and blood pH changes in relation to cardiac function. *Am J Physiol.* 1953;175:389–398.

130. Wenger W, Kligfield P. Variability of precordial electrode placement during routine electrocardiography. *J Electrocardiol.* 1996;29(3):179–184.

131. Simonson E. *Differentiation between Normal and Abnormal in Electrocardiography.* St. Louis, MI: Mosby; 1961:262.

132. Schijvenaars BJ, Kors JA, van Herpen G, et al. Effect of electrode positioning on ECG interpretation by computer. *J Electrocardiol.* 1997;30(3):247–256.

133. Castellanos A, Saoudi NC, Schwartz A, et al. Electrocardiographic patterns resulting from improper connections of the right leg (ground) cable. *PACE.* 1985;8:364–368.

134. Proceedings of the Engineering Foundation Conference "Computerized Interpretation of the Electrocardiogram XII. XII." *J Electrocardiol.* 1987;20(suppl):preface.

135. American College of Cardiology/American Heart Association (ACC/AHA)/ACP-ASIM Task Force on Clinical Competence (ACC/AHA Committee to Develop a Clinical Competence Statement on Electrocardiography and Ambulatory Electrocardiography). Clinical Competence Statement on Electrocardiography and Ambulatory Electrocardiography. *J Am Coll Cardiol.* 2001;38(7):2091–2100.

136. Spodick DH, Bishop RL. Computer treason: intraobserver variability of an electrocardiographic computer system. *Am J Cardiol.* 1997;80:102–103.

137. Hurst JM. Methods used to interpret the 12-lead electrocardiogram: pattern memorization versus the use of vector concepts. *Clin Cardiol.* 2000;24:4–13.

138. Grant RP, Estes EH Jr. *Spatial Vector Electrocardiography.* New York: Blakiston; 1951.

139. Chou TC, Helm RA, Kaplan S. *Clinical Vectorcardiography.* 2nd ed. New York: Grune & Stratton; 1974.

140. Lemberg L, Castellanos A Jr. *Vectorcardiography.* 2nd ed. New York: Appleton-Century-Crofts; 1975.

141. Castellanos A, Myerburg RJ. The dimensions of dimensions. *J Cardiovasc Electrophysiol.* 2001;12(2):277–278.

142. Hawking S. *The Universe in a Nutshell.* New York: Bantam Books; 2001:88.

143. Malik M. Why modern electrocardiography needs mathematics. *J Cardiovasc Electrophysiol.* 2001;12(2):278–279.

144. Kors JA, van Herpen G, Sittig AC, van Bemmel JH. Reconstruction of the Frank vectorcardiogram from standard electrocardiographic leads: diagnostic comparison of different methods. *Eur Heart J.* 1990;11:1083–1092.

145. Edenbrandt L, Pahlm O. Vectorcardiogram synthesized from a 12-lead ECG. Superiority of the inverse Dower matrix. *J Electrocardiol.* 1988;21(4):361–367.

146. Malik M, Batchvarov V. The heart vector, the regional information in the electrocardiogram and QT dispersion. *Am J Cardiol.* 2002;90:1276–1277.

147. Rautaharju PM. A farewell to QT dispersion. Are the alternatives any better? *J Electrocardiol.* 2005;38:7–9.

148. Malik M, Batchvarov VN. Measurement, interpretation and clinical potential of QT dispersion. *J Am Coll Cardiol.* 2000;36:1749–1766.

CHAPTER (14)

ECG Exercise Testing

Gregory Engel / Victor F. Froelicher

Exercise testing is a noninvasive tool to evaluate the cardiovascular system's response to exercise under carefully controlled conditions. Exercise is the body's most common physiologic stress, and it places major demands on the cardiopulmonary system. Thus, exercise can be considered the most practical test of cardiac perfusion and function. The exercise test, alone and in combination with other noninvasive modalities, remains an important testing method because of its high yield of diagnostic, prognostic, and functional information.

The adaptations that occur during an exercise test allow the body to increase its resting metabolic rate up to 20 times, during which time cardiac output can increase as much as 6 times. The magnitude of these adjustments is dependent on age, gender, body size, type of exercise, fitness, and the presence or absence of heart disease. The major central and peripheral adaptations that occur from rest to maximal exercise are illustrated in Fig. 14–1. The interpretation of the exercise test requires understanding exercise physiology and pathophysiology as well as expertise in electrocardiography. Certification is extremely important because this technology has spread beyond the subspecialty of cardiology. Training and experience are re-

quired as they are for other diagnostic procedures. For these reasons, the American College of Physicians (ACP) and American College of Cardiology (ACC), and the American Heart Association (AHA) have published guidelines on clinical competence for physicians performing exercise testing (www.acc.org/qualityandscience/clinical/statements.htm, www.cardiology.org).[1,2]

BASIC PRINCIPLES

【 】 EXERCISE PHYSIOLOGY

Two basic principles of exercise physiology are important to understand in regard to exercise testing. The first is a physiologic principle: total body oxygen uptake and myocardial oxygen uptake are distinct in their determinants and in the way they are measured or estimated (Table 14–1).

Total body or ventilatory oxygen uptake (volume oxygen consumption [VO_2]) is the amount of oxygen that is extracted from inspired air as the body performs work. The determinants of VO_2 are cardiac output and the peripheral arteriovenous oxygen differ-

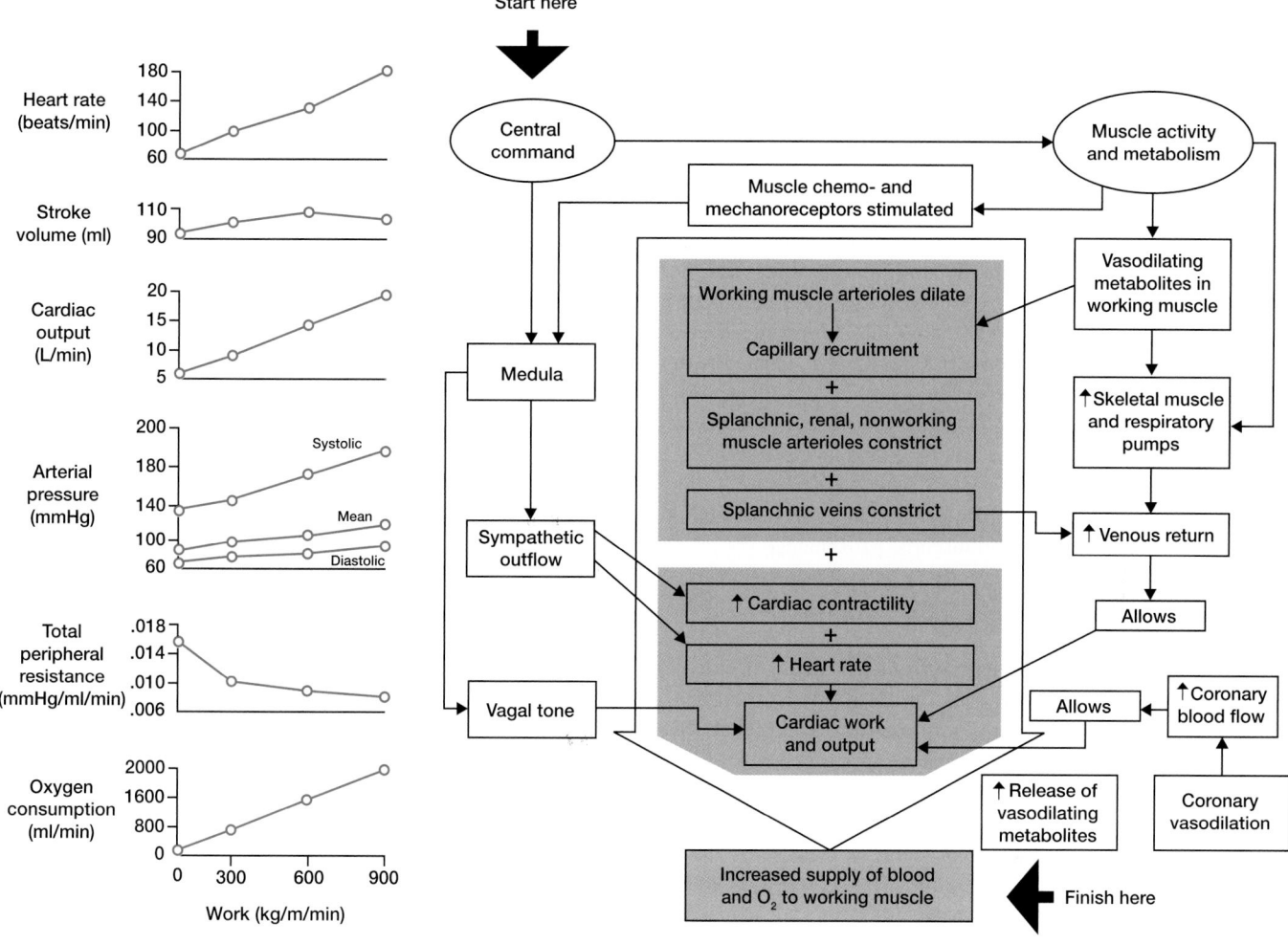

FIGURE 14–1. A. Graphs of the hemodynamic responses to dynamic exercise. **B.** Sequence of physiological responses to dynamic exercise. *Source: Cardiovascular Physiology at a Glance with permission of Blackwell Publishers, 2004.*

ence. Maximal arteriovenous difference is physiologically limited to roughly 15 to 17 mL/dL. Thus maximal arteriovenous difference behaves more or less as a constant, making maximal oxygen uptake an indirect estimate of maximal cardiac output.

Myocardial oxygen uptake is the amount of oxygen consumed by the heart muscle. The determinants of myocardial oxygen uptake include intramyocardial wall tension (left ventricular pressure and end-diastolic volume), contractility, and heart rate. It has been shown that myocardial oxygen uptake can be reasonably estimated by the product of heart rate and systolic blood pressure (double product). This information is valuable clinically because exercise-induced angina often occurs at the same myocardial oxygen demand (double product),

and the higher the double product achieved the better is myocardial perfusion and prognosis. When such is not the case, the influence of other factors should be suspected, such as a recent meal, abnormal ambient temperature, or coronary artery spasm.

The second principle is one of pathophysiology: considerable interaction takes place between the exercise test manifestations of abnormalities in myocardial perfusion and function. The electrocardiographic response and angina are closely related to myocardial ischemia (and coronary artery disease), whereas exercise capacity, systolic blood pressure, and heart rate responses to exercise can be determined by the presence of myocardial ischemia, myocardial dysfunction or responses in the periphery. Exercise-induced is-

TABLE 14–1

Two Basic Principles of Exercise Physiology

Myocardial oxygen consumption	≈ Heart rate × systolic blood pressure (determinants include wall tension ≈ left ventricular pressure × volume; contractility; and heart rate)
Ventilatory oxygen consumption (VO_2)	≈ External work performed, or cardiac output[a] × A-VO_2 difference

A-VO_2, arteriovenous oxygen difference; VO_2, volume oxygen consumption; vol%, volume percent.
[a]The arteriovenous O_2 difference is approximately 15 to 17 vol% at maximal exercise in most individuals; therefore, VO_2max generally reflects the extent to which cardiac output increases.

chemia can cause cardiac dysfunction that results in exercise impairment and an abnormal systolic blood pressure response.

[ ] METABOLIC EQUIVALENTS

Because exercise testing fundamentally involves the measurement of work, there are several concepts regarding work that are important to understand. The common biologic measure of total body work is the oxygen uptake, which is usually expressed as a rate (making it a measure of power) in liters per minute. The MET, or metabolic equivalent, is a term commonly used clinically to express the oxygen requirement of the work rate during an exercise test on a treadmill or cycle ergometer. One MET is equated with the resting metabolic rate (approximately 3.5 mL of O_2/kg/min), and a MET value achieved from an exercise test is a multiple of the resting metabolic rate, either measured directly (as oxygen uptake) or estimated from the maximal workload achieved using standardized equations.[3] Table 14–2 lists clinically meaningful METs for exercise, prognosis, and maximal performance.

[ ] ENERGY AND MUSCULAR CONTRACTION

Muscular contraction is a complex mechanism involving the interaction of multiple components of the contractile mechanism. Voluntary muscle contraction begins with electrical impulses at the myoneural junction, initiating the release of calcium ions. Calcium is released into the sarcoplasmic reticulum that surrounds the muscle filaments and binds to the troponin complex, which allows the tropomyosin molecule to be removed from its blocking position between actin and myosin. The myosin head attaches to actin, and muscular contraction occurs. Myosin and actin filaments in the muscle slide past one another as the muscle fibers shortens during contraction. Energy for this contraction is supplied by adenosine triphosphate.

The relative exercise intensity in which lactate accumulation occurs is an important determinant of endurance performance. The degree to which lactate accumulates in the blood is related to exercise intensity and the extent to which fast-twitch (Type IIB) fibers are recruited. Although lactate can contribute to fatigue by increasing ventilation and inhibiting other enzymes of glycolysis, it can also serve as an important energy source in muscles other than those in which it was formed, and it serves as an important precursor for liver glycogen during exercise.[4,5]

ACUTE CARDIOPULMONARY RESPONSE TO EXERCISE

The cardiovascular system responds to acute exercise with a series of adjustments that assure the following:

- Active muscles receive blood supply appropriate to their metabolic needs.
- Heat generated by the muscles is dissipated.
- Blood supply to the brain and heart is maintained.

This response requires a major redistribution of cardiac output along with a number of local metabolic changes. The usual measure of the capacity of the body to deliver and use oxygen is the maximal oxygen consumption (VO_2max). Thus, the limits of the cardiopulmonary system are defined by VO_2max, which can be expressed by the Fick principle:

$$VO_2\text{max} = \text{maximal cardiac output} \times \text{maximal arteriovenous oxygen difference}$$

Cardiac output must closely match ventilation in the lung to deliver oxygen to the working muscle. VO_2max is determined by the maximal amount of ventilation (volume of expired gas [V_E]) moving into and out of the lung and by the fraction of this ventilation that is extracted by the tissues:

$$VO_2 = V_E \times (FiO_2 - FeO_2)$$

where V_E is minute ventilation, and FiO_2 and FeO_2 are the fractional concentration of oxygen in the inspired and expired air, respectively. To measure VO_2 accurately, CO_2 in the expired air (carbon dioxide elimination [VCO_2]) must also be measured; the major purpose of VCO_2 in this equation is to correct for the difference in ventilation between inspired and expired air. VCO_2 is also a valuable measurement clinically for chronic heart failure patients because the rate of increase in VCO_2 relative to the work rate or ventilation parallels the severity of heart failure and is a powerful prognostic marker.

The cardiopulmonary limits (VO_2max) are therefore defined by the following:

- *A central component (cardiac output) describes the capacity of the heart to function as a pump.*
- *Peripheral factors (arteriovenous oxygen difference) describe the capacity of the lung to oxygenate the blood delivered to it as well as the capacity of the working muscle to extract this oxygen from the blood.*

[ ] CENTRAL FACTORS

Fig. 14–2 shows the central determinants of maximal ventilatory oxygen uptake.

TABLE 14–2

Clinically Significant Metabolic Equivalents for Maximum Exercise

1 MET	Resting
2 METs	Level walking at 2 mph
4 METs	Level walking at 4 mph
<5 METs	Poor prognosis; peak cost of basic activities of daily living
10 METs	Prognosis with medical therapy as good as coronary artery bypass surgery
13 METs	Excellent prognosis regardless of other exercise responses
18 METs	Elite endurance athletes
20 METs	World-class athletes

MET, metabolic equivalent, or a unit of sitting resting oxygen uptake. 1 MET = 3.5 mL/kg/min oxygen uptake. mph, miles per hour.

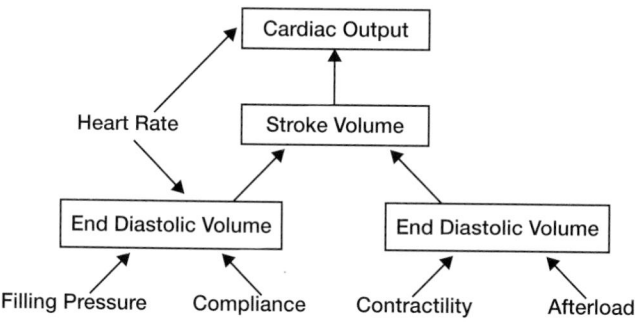

FIGURE 14–2. Central determinants of maximal oxygen uptake. *Source: Myers J, Froelicher VF. Hemodynamic determinants of exercise capacity in chronic heart failure. Ann Intern Med. 1991;115: 377–386.*

Heart Rate

Sympathetic and parasympathetic nervous system influences underlie the cardiovascular system's first response to exercise, an increase in heart rate. Vagal withdrawal is responsible for the initial 10 to 30 beats per minute change, whereas the remainder is thought to be largely caused by increased sympathetic outflow. Of the two major components of cardiac output, heart rate and stroke volume, heart rate is responsible for most of the increase in cardiac output during exercise, particularly at higher levels. Heart rate increases linearly with workload and oxygen uptake.

The heart rate response to exercise is influenced by several factors, including age, type of activity, body position, fitness, the presence of heart disease, medication use, blood volume, and environment. Of these, the most important factor is age; a significant decline in maximal heart rate occurs with increasing age. This decline appears to be a result of intrinsic cardiac changes rather than neural influences. It should be noted that there is a great deal of variability around the regression line between maximal heart rate and age; thus, age-related maximal heart rate estimates are a relatively poor index of maximal effort. Because prediction of maximal heart rate is inaccurate, exercise should be symptom-limited and not targeted on achieving a certain heart rate. Thus, a test should not be considered nondiagnostic if a percentage of age-predicted maximal heart rate (i.e., 85 percent) is not reached. Maximal heart rate is unchanged or can be slightly reduced after a program of training whereas resting heart rate is frequently reduced after training as a result of enhanced parasympathetic tone.

Stroke Volume

The product of stroke volume (the volume of blood ejected per heartbeat) and heart rate determines cardiac output. Stroke volume is equal to the difference between end-diastolic and end-systolic volume. Thus, a greater diastolic filling (preload) will increase stroke volume. Alternatively, factors that increase arterial blood pressure will resist ventricular outflow (afterload) and result in a reduced stroke volume. During exercise, stroke volume increases up to approximately 50 to 60 percent of maximal capacity, after which increases in cardiac output are caused by further increases in heart rate. The extent to which increases in stroke volume during exercise reflect an increase in end-diastolic volume or a decrease in end-systolic volume, or both, is not entirely clear but

appears to depend on ventricular function, body position, and intensity of exercise. In healthy subjects, stroke volume increases at rest and during exercise after a period of exercise training. Although the mechanisms have been debated, evidence suggests that this adaptation is caused more by increases in preload—and possibly local adaptations that reduce peripheral vascular resistance—than by increases in myocardial contractility. The end-diastolic and end-systolic responses to *acute* exercise have varied greatly in the literature, but are dependent on presence and type of disease, exercise intensity, and exercise position (supine vs. upright).

End-Systolic Volume

End-systolic volume depends on two factors: contractility and afterload.

Contractility describes the forcefulness of the heart's contraction. Increasing contractility reduces end-systolic volume, which results in a greater stroke volume and thus greater cardiac output. Contractility is commonly quantified by the ejection fraction, the percentage of blood ejected from the ventricle during systole (traditionally measured using echocardiographic, radionuclide or angiographic techniques).

Afterload is a measure of the force resisting the ejection of blood by the heart. Increased afterload (or aortic pressure, as is observed with chronic hypertension) results in a reduced ejection fraction and increased end-diastolic and end-systolic volumes. During dynamic exercise, the force resisting ejection in the periphery (total peripheral resistance) is reduced by vasodilation, owing to the effect of local metabolites on the skeletal muscle vasculature. Thus, despite even a fivefold increase in cardiac output among normal subjects during exercise, mean arterial pressure increases only moderately.

[ ] PERIPHERAL FACTORS (ARTERIOVENOUS OXYGEN DIFFERENCE)

Fig. 14–3 shows the peripheral determinants of maximal oxygen uptake. Oxygen extraction by the tissues during exercise reflects the difference between the oxygen content of the arteries (generally 18 to 20 mL O_2/100 mL at rest) and the oxygen content in the veins (generally 13 to 15 mL O_2/100 mL at rest, yielding a typical arteriovenous oxygen difference (A-VO_2) at rest of 4 to 6 mL O_2/100 mL,

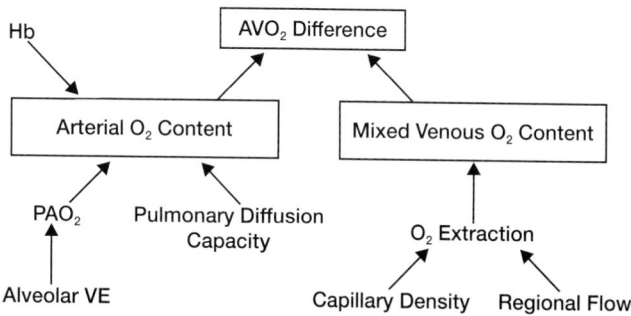

FIGURE 14–3. Peripheral determinants of maximal oxygen uptake. The A-VO_2 difference is the difference between arterial and venous oxygen. A-VO_2, arteriovenous oxygen difference; Hb, hemoglobin; PAO_2, partial pressure of alveolar oxygen; VE, minute ventilation. *Source: Myers J, Froelicher VF. Hemodynamic determinants of exercise capacity in chronic heart failure. Ann Intern Med. 1991;115: 377–386.*

approximately 23 percent extraction). During exercise, this difference widens as the working tissues extract greater amounts of oxygen; venous oxygen content reaches very low levels and A-VO$_2$ can be as high as 16 to 18 mL O$_2$/100 mL with exhaustive exercise. Some oxygenated blood always returns to the heart, however, as smaller amounts of blood continue to flow through, metabolically less active tissues do not fully extract oxygen. The A-VO$_2$ is generally considered to widen by a relatively *fixed* amount during exercise, and differences in VO$_2$max are predominantly explained by differences in cardiac output. Some patients with cardiovascular or pulmonary disease, however, exhibit reduced VO$_2$max values that can be attributed to a combination of central and peripheral factors.

Determinants of Arterial Oxygen Content

Arterial oxygen content is related to the partial pressure of arterial oxygen, which is determined in the lung by alveolar ventilation and pulmonary diffusion capacity, and in the blood by hemoglobin content. In the absence of pulmonary disease, arterial oxygen content and saturation are usually normal throughout exercise. Patients with symptomatic pulmonary disease often neither ventilate the alveoli adequately nor diffuse oxygen from the lung into the bloodstream normally, and a decrease in arterial oxygen saturation during exercise can occur. Arterial hemoglobin content is also usually normal throughout exercise.

Determinants of Venous Oxygen Content

Venous oxygen content reflects the capacity to extract oxygen from the blood as it flows through the muscle. It is determined by the amount of blood directed to the muscle (regional flow) and capillary density. Muscle blood flow increases in proportion to the increase in work rate and thus the oxygen requirement. The increase in blood flow is brought about not only by the increase in cardiac output, but also by a preferential redistribution of the cardiac output to the exercising muscle. Locally produced vasodilatory mechanisms along with possible neurogenic dilatation resulting from higher sympathetic activity reduce local vascular resistance and mediate the greater skeletal muscle blood flow. A marked increase in the number of open capillaries reduces diffusion distances, increases capillary blood volume, and increases mean transit time, facilitating oxygen delivery to the muscle.

AUTONOMIC CONTROL
【 】 NEURAL CONTROL MECHANISMS

The neural control mechanisms responsible for the cardiovascular response to exercise occur through two processes that initiate and maintain this response:

1. Central command—neural impulses, arising from the central nervous system, recruit motor units, excite medullary and spinal neuronal circuits and cause the cardiovascular changes during exercise.
2. Muscle afferents—muscle contraction stimulates afferent endings within the skeletal muscle, which in turn reflexively evoke the cardiovascular changes.

The latter mechanism called *exercise pressor reflex*, comprises all of the cardiovascular changes reflexly induced from contracting skeletal muscle that cause changes in the efferent sympathetic and parasympathetic outputs to the cardiovascular system that are in turn responsible for increases in arterial blood pressure, heart rate, myocardial contractility, cardiac output, and blood flow distribution. A specific subset of muscle afferents serve as ergo-receptors activated by either mechanical or metabolic perturbations.

As the demand for cardiac output increases, parasympathetic activity becomes attenuated, while sympathetic activity increases. The sympathetic system releases norepinephrine directly through the sympathetic trunk to the sinus node and myocardium. In addition, norepinephrine and epinephrine from the adrenal medulla act to increase heart rate and increase myocardial contractility, as well as to redirect blood flow to working muscle. By mediating peripheral vasoconstriction in relatively inactive tissues (e.g., the kidneys and gut), the sympathetic system increases venous return, and vasodilatory metabolites maintain local increased flow to active skeletal muscle. Actively contracting skeletal muscle also increases preload by acting as a venous pump and stimulating sympathetic afferent fibers within the muscle itself.

Pharmacologic blockade studies have helped elucidate the differential contributions of the two autonomic branches during exercise. Blockade of parasympathetic control with atropine reveals that most of the initial response to exercise, up to a heart rate of 100 to 120 beats per minute (i.e., a delta heart rate [HR] of 30–40 beats per minute [bpm]), is attributable to the withdrawal of tonic vagal activity. Vagal withdrawal induces a rapid increase in heart rate and cardiac output. Conversely, blockade of sympathetic control with propranolol reveals the importance of augmented sympathetic activity during moderate and heavy exercise. During light exercise, with work loads of 25 to 40 percent of VO$_2$max or while heart rate remains within 30 beats per minute over baseline, plasma norepinephrine levels do not significantly increase, confirming that the sympathetic nervous system is more important with higher levels of exercise.

【 】 AUTONOMIC MODULATION DURING IMMEDIATE RECOVERY FROM EXERCISE

Autonomic physiology during recovery from acute bouts of exercise involves reactivation of the parasympathetic system and deactivation of sympathetic activity. The decline of heart rate after cessation of exercise is the variable most commonly analyzed to assess the underlying mechanisms. A delay in heart rate recovery has been used as a marker of autonomic dysfunction and/or failure of the cardiovascular (CV) system to respond to the normal autonomic responses to exercise. This delay has been shown to be a powerful prognostic marker. Time constants have been calculated by fitting heart rate decay data to a number of mathematical models, but the simple change in heart rate from peak exercise to minute 1 or 2 of recovery appears to distinguish survival as well. Early recovery after acute bouts of exercise appears to be dominated by parasympathetic reactivation, with sympathetic withdrawal becoming more important later in recovery. In a pharmacologic blockade study, Imai and colleagues computed HR recovery decay curves using beat-to-beat data and concluded that short- and moderate-term HR recovery curves are vagally mediated, because HR decay 30 seconds and 2 minutes into recovery was prolonged with atropine and dual blockade; however, the HR decay for 2 minutes was more prolonged with dual blockade than with atropine alone, indicating that later recovery also depends on sympathetic modulation. Rather than declining, plasma norepinephrine concentrations during the first minute of recovery remain constant or even increase immediately after exercise.

METHODOLOGY OF EXERCISE TESTING

Use of proper methodology is critical for patient safety and accurate results. Updated guidelines are available from the AHA/ACC that are based on a multitude of research studies over the last 20 years and have led to greater uniformity in methods.[6,7]

[ ] SAFETY PRECAUTIONS AND EQUIPMENT

The safety precautions outlined in the guidelines are very explicit with regard to the requirements for exercise testing. Perhaps because of an expanded knowledge concerning indications, contraindications, and endpoints, maximal exercise testing appears safer today (less than 1 untoward event per 10,000 tests) than it did 20 years ago.

Besides emergency equipment, the safety and accuracy of the testing equipment should be considered. The treadmill should have front and side rails to help subjects steady themselves. It should be calibrated monthly. Some models can be greatly affected by the weight of the subject and will not deliver the appropriate workload to heavy individuals.

Although numerous clever devices have been developed to automate blood pressure measurement during exercise, none can be recommended except those that allow audible monitoring of the Korotkoff sounds and operator validation. The time-proven method of holding the subject's arm with a stethoscope placed over the brachial artery remains most reliable.

[ ] PRETEST PREPARATIONS

When the test is scheduled, the patient should be instructed not to eat, drink, or smoke at least 2 hours prior to the test and to come dressed for exercise, including proper footwear.

During the pretest evaluation, the patient's usual level of exercise activity should be established to help determine the appropriate target workload for testing. The physician should also review the patient's medical history, making note of any conditions that can increase the risk of testing. Table 14–3 lists the absolute and relative contraindications to exercise testing. Testing patients with aortic stenosis should be done with great care because they can develop severe cardiovascular complications. *Thus, a physical examination—including assessment of systolic murmurs—should be performed before all exercise tests.* If a loud systolic murmur is heard, an echocardiogram should be considered prior to testing.

Pretest standard 12-lead ECGs are necessary in both the supine and standing positions. Good skin preparation is necessary for good conductance to avoid artifacts and is especially important for elderly patients who have a higher skin resistance and tendency toward contact noise. The changes caused by exercise electrode placement can be kept to a minimum by keeping the arm electrodes off the chest and placing them on the shoulders, placing the

TABLE 14–3

Contraindications to Exercise Testing

ABSOLUTE

High-risk unstable angina
Uncontrolled cardiac arrhythmias causing symptoms or hemodynamic compromise
Symptomatic severe aortic stenosis
Uncontrolled symptomatic heart failure
Acute pulmonary embolus or pulmonary infarction
Acute myocarditis or pericarditis
Acute aortic dissection

RELATIVE[a]

Left main coronary stenosis
Moderate stenotic valvular heart disease
Electrolyte abnormalities
Severe arterial hypertension[b]
Tachyarrhythmias or bradyarrhythmias
Hypertrophic cardiomyopathy and other forms of outflow tract obstruction
Mental or physical impairment leading to inability to exercise adequately
High-degree atrioventricular block

[a]Relative contraindications can be superseded if the benefits of exercise outweigh the risks.
[b]In the absence of definitive evidence, the committee suggests systolic blood pressure of >200 mmHg and/or diastolic blood pressure of >110 mmHg.
SOURCE: Modified from Gibbons, Balady, Bricker, et al.[6]

ground (right leg) electrode on the back out of the cardiac field, placing the left leg electrodes below the umbilicus and recording the baseline ECG supine. In this situation, the modified exercise limb-lead placement can serve as the reference resting ECG prior to an exercise test.

Hyperventilation should be avoided before testing. Subjects with and without disease can exhibit ST-segment changes with hyperventilation; thus, hyperventilation to identify false-positive responders is no longer considered useful.

[ ] DURING THE TEST

Most complications can be avoided by measuring blood pressure, monitoring the ECG, questioning the patient about symptoms and levels of fatigue and assessing appearance during the test. Subjects should be reminded not to grasp the front or side rails because this decreases the work performed and creates noise in the ECG. The subject can rest his or her hands on the rails for balance but should not hang on. Hanging on the rails results in an overestimation of exercise capacity.

Target heart rates based on age should not be used because the relationship between maximal heart rate and age is poor, and a wide scatter exists around the many different recommended regression lines. Such heart-rate targets result in a submaximal test for some individuals, a maximal test for some, and an unrealistic goal for others. The absolute and relative indications for test termination are listed in Table 14–4. If none of these endpoints are

TABLE 14–4

Indications for Terminating Exercise Testing

ABSOLUTE INDICATIONS

Moderate to severe angina

Increasing nervous system symptoms (e.g., ataxia, dizziness, or near-syncope)

Signs of poor perfusion (cyanosis or pallor)

Technical difficulties in monitoring ECG or systolic blood pressure

Subject's desire to stop

Sustained ventricular tachycardia

ST-segment elevation (≥1.0 mm) in leads without diagnostic Q waves (other than V_1 or aVR)

RELATIVE INDICATIONS

Drop in systolic blood pressure of ≥10 mmHg from baseline blood pressure despite an increase in workload in the absence of other evidence of ischemia

ST or QRS changes such as excessive ST-segment depression (>2 mm of horizontal or downsloping ST-segment depression) or marked axis shift

Arrhythmias other than sustained ventricular tachycardia, including multifocal PVCs, triplets of PVCs, supraventricular tachycardia, heart block, or bradyarrhythmias

Fatigue, shortness of breath, wheezing, leg cramps, or claudication

Development of bundle branch block or intraventricular conduction delay that cannot be distinguished from ventricular tachycardia

Increasing chest pain

Hypertensive response[a]

PVC, premature ventricular contractions.

[a]In the absence of definitive evidence, the committee suggests systolic blood pressure of >250 mmHg and/or a diastolic blood pressure of >115 mmHg.

SOURCE: Modified from Gibbons, Balady, Bricker, et al.[6]

met, the test should be symptom-limited. The Borg scales are an excellent means of quantifying an individual's effort. Subjects should be monitored for perceived effort level by using the 6-to-20 Borg scale at 2-minute intervals.

To ensure the safety of exercise testing, the following list of the most dangerous circumstances in the exercise testing laboratory should be recognized:

• When patients exhibit ST-segment elevation (without baseline diagnostic Q waves), this can be associated with dangerous arrhythmias and infarction. The incidence is approximately 1 in 1000 clinical tests and usually occurs in V_2 or aVF rather than V_5.

• When a patient with an ischemic cardiomyopathy exhibits severe chest pain because of ischemia (angina pectoris), a cool-down walk is advisable.

• When a patient develops exertional hypotension accompanied by ischemia (angina or ST-segment depression) or when it occurs in a patient with a history of congestive heart failure, cardiomyopathy, or recent myocardial infarction, safety is a serious issue.

• When a patient with a history of sudden death or collapse during exercise develops premature ventricular depolarizations that become frequent, a cool-down walk is advisable.

【 】 RECOVERY AFTER EXERCISE

If maximal sensitivity is to be achieved with an exercise test, patients should be supine as soon as possible during the postexercise period (maximal wall stress). It is advisable to record approximately 10 seconds of ECG data while the patient is standing motionless but still at near-maximal heart rate and then have the patient lie down. Having the patient perform a cool-down walk after the test can delay or eliminate the appearance of ST-segment depression, while having patients lie down enhances ST-segment abnormalities in recovery.

Monitoring should continue for at least 5 minutes after exercise or until changes stabilize. An abnormal response occurring only in the recovery period is neither unusual nor necessarily suggestive of a false-positive result. The recovery period, particularly the third minute is critical for ST analysis. Noise should not be a problem, and ST depression at that time has important implications regarding the presence and severity of coronary artery disease (CAD).

A cool-down walk can be helpful in performing tests on patients with an established diagnosis undergoing testing for other than diagnostic reasons, as in testing athletes or patients with congestive heart failure (CHF), valvular heart disease, or a recent myocardial infarction (MI).

【 】 EXERCISE TEST MODALITIES

Three types of exercise can be used to stress the cardiovascular system: isometric, dynamic, and a combination of the two. *Isometric exercise,* defined as constant muscular contraction without movement (such as handgrip), imposes a disproportionate pressure load on the left ventricle relative to the body's ability to supply oxygen. *Dynamic exercise* is defined as rhythmic muscular activity resulting in movement, and it initiates a more appropriate increase in cardiac output and oxygen exchange. Chapter 14 considers only dynamic exercise testing, because a delivered workload can be calibrated accurately and the physiologic response measured easily. Isometric exercise is not recommended for routine exercise testing.

【 】 BICYCLE ERGOMETER VERSUS TREADMILL

The bicycle ergometer usually costs less, takes up less space, and makes less noise than a treadmill. Although bicycling is a dynamic exercise, most individuals perform more work on a treadmill because a greater muscle mass is involved, and most subjects are more familiar with walking than cycling. In most studies comparing exercise on an upright cycle ergometer versus a treadmill exercise, maximal heart rate values have been demonstrated to be roughly similar, whereas maximal oxygen uptake has been shown to be up to 25 percent greater during treadmill exercise.

【 】 EXERCISE PROTOCOLS

The most common protocols, their stages, and the predicted oxygen cost of each stage are illustrated in Fig. 14–4. The exercise pro-

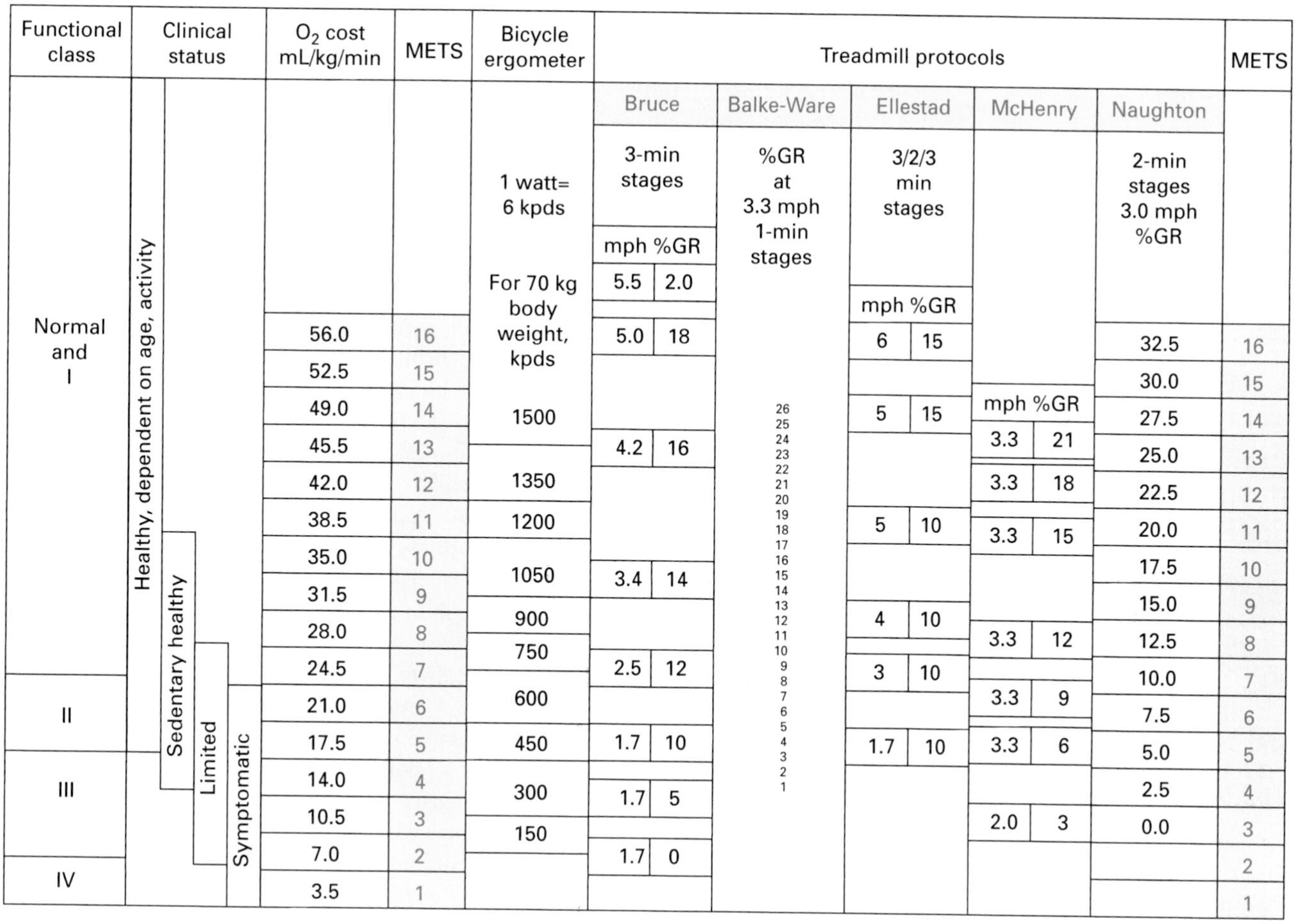

Functional class	Clinical status	O₂ cost mL/kg/min	METS	Bicycle ergometer	Bruce 3-min stages mph	%GR	Balke-Ware %GR at 3.3 mph 1-min stages	Ellestad 3/2/3 min stages mph	%GR	McHenry mph	%GR	Naughton 2-min stages 3.0 mph %GR	METS
				1 watt= 6 kpds	5.5	2.0							
		56.0	16	For 70 kg body weight, kpds	5.0	18		6	15			32.5	16
		52.5	15									30.0	15
		49.0	14	1500			26 25	5	15	3.3	21	27.5	14
		45.5	13		4.2	16	24 23 22					25.0	13
		42.0	12	1350			21 20			3.3	18	22.5	12
		38.5	11	1200			19 18 17	5	10	3.3	15	20.0	11
Normal and I	Healthy, dependent on age, activity	35.0	10	1050			16 15					17.5	10
		31.5	9		3.4	14	14 13					15.0	9
	Sedentary healthy	28.0	8	900			12 11 10	4	10	3.3	12	12.5	8
		24.5	7	750	2.5	12	9 8	3	10	3.3	9	10.0	7
II		21.0	6	600			7 6 5					7.5	6
	Limited	17.5	5	450	1.7	10	4 3	1.7	10	3.3	6	5.0	5
III	Symptomatic	14.0	4	300	1.7	5	2 1					2.5	4
		10.5	3	150						2.0	3	0.0	3
IV		7.0	2		1.7	0							2
		3.5	1										1

FIGURE 14–4. The most common protocols, their stages, and the predicted oxygen cost of each stage. GR, grade; METs, metabolic equivalents.

tocol should be progressive with even increments in speed and grade whenever possible. Smaller, even, and more frequent work increments are preferable to larger, uneven, and less frequent increases, because the former yield a more accurate estimation of exercise capacity. *Recent guidelines suggest that protocols should be individualized for each subject such that test duration is approximately 8 to 12 minutes. Because ramp testing uses small and even increments, it permits a more accurate estimation of exercise capacity and can be individualized to yield targeted test duration.*

HEMODYNAMICS

The increased demand for myocardial oxygen required by dynamic exercise is the key to the use of exercise testing as a diagnostic tool for CAD. Myocardial oxygen consumption cannot be directly measured in a practical manner, but its relative demand can be estimated from its determinants, such as heart rate, wall tension (left ventricular pressure and diastolic volume), contractility, and cardiac work. Although all of these factors increase during exercise, increased heart rate is particularly important in patients who have obstructive CAD. An increase in heart rate results in a shortening of the diastolic filling period, the time during which coronary blood flow is the greatest. In normal coronary arteries, dilation occurs. In obstructed vessels, however, dilation is limited and flow can be decreased by the shortening of the diastolic filling period. This causes inadequate blood flow and therefore insufficient oxygen supply.

Hemodynamic information, including heart rate, blood pressure, and exercise capacity, are important features of the exercise test. Because it can objectively quantify exercise capacity, exercise testing is now commonly used for disability evaluation rather than reliance on functional classifications. No questionnaire or submaximal test can provide as reliable a result as a symptom-limited exercise test.

HEART RATE

Age-predicted maximal heart rate targets are relatively useless for clinical purposes, and they should not be used for exercise testing endpoints. It is surprising how much steeper the age-related decline in maximal heart rate is in clinically referred populations as compared with age-matched normal subjects or volunteers. Nomograms greatly facilitate the description of exercise capacity relative to age and enable comparisons among patients (Fig. 14–5). However, numerous different regression equations express exercise capacity relative to gender and age.

EXERCISE CAPACITY

When expressing exercise capacity as a relative percentage of what is deemed normal, careful consideration should be given to population specificity. Exercise capacity is influenced by many factors other than age and gender, including health, activity level, body composition, and the exercise mode and protocol used. Exercise capacity should not be reported in total time but rather as the oxy-

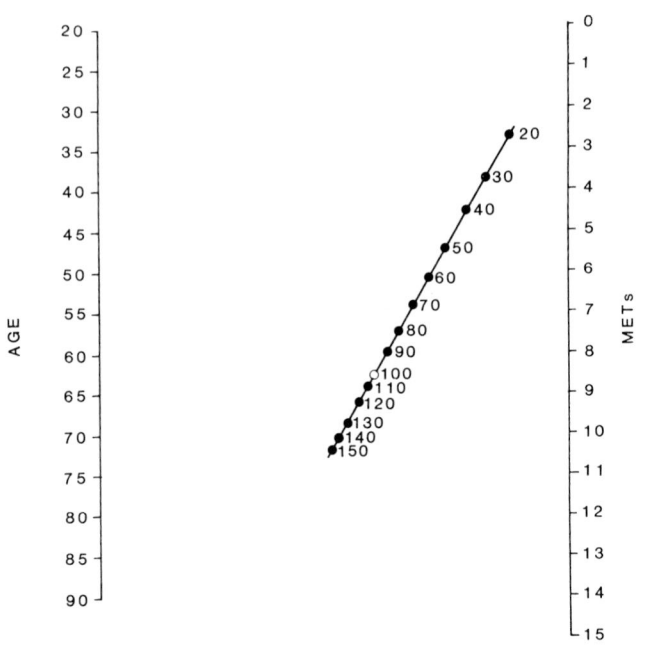

EXERCISE CAPACITY
(% of Normal In Referral Males)

FIGURE 14–5. The exercise capacity nomogram, providing a relative estimate of normal for age, with 100 percent being as expected for age in a clinical population. METs, metabolic equivalents.

gen uptake or MET equivalent of the workload achieved. This method permits the comparison of the results of many different exercise testing protocols.

【 】 BLOOD PRESSURE

Systolic blood pressure should rise with increasing treadmill workload, whereas diastolic blood pressure usually remains approximately the same or drops (Fig. 14–6). Although exertional hypotension has been defined in many different ways, it has been shown to predict severe angiographic CAD and is associated with a poor prognosis. A drop in systolic blood pressure (SBP) below preexercise values is the most ominous criterion. A failure of systolic blood pressure to adequately increase is particularly worrisome in patients who have sustained an MI.

ECG INTERPRETATION

【 】 ST-SEGMENT ANALYSIS

ST-segment depression is a representation of global subendocardial ischemia, with a direction determined largely by the placement of the heart in the chest. ST-depression does not localize coro-

nary artery lesions. ST-depression in the inferior leads (II, AVF) is most often caused by the atrial repolarization wave, which begins in the PR segment and can extend to the beginning of the ST-segment. Severe transmural ischemia, resulting in wall motion abnormalities, causes a shift of the vector in the direction of the wall motion abnormality. However, preexisting areas of wall motion abnormality (i.e., scar) usually indicated by a Q wave, also cause such a shift resulting in ST elevation without ischemia being present. When the resting ECG shows Q waves of an old MI, ST elevation is caused by ischemia or wall-motion abnormalities or both, whereas accompanying ST-depression can be caused by a second area of ischemia or reciprocal changes. When the resting ECG is normal, however, ST elevation is a result of severe ischemia (spasm or a critical lesion), although accompanying ST-depression is reciprocal. Such ST elevation is uncommon, very arrhythmogenic, and it localizes. Exercise-induced ST-depression loses its diagnostic power in patients with left bundle-branch block, Wolff-Parkinson-White (WPW) syndrome, electronic pacemakers, intraventricular conduction defects (IVCDs) with inverted T-waves and in patients with more than one millimeter of resting ST-depression. ST-segment changes isolated to the inferior leads are more likely to be false-positive responses unless profound (i.e., more than 1 mm). The various patterns of ST segment changes are illustrated in Fig. 14–7.

Precordial lead V_5 alone consistently outperforms the inferior leads or the combination of leads V_5 with II, because lead II has been shown to have a high false-positive rate. Exercise-induced ST-segment depression in inferior limb leads is a poor marker for CAD in and of itself.[8] In patients without prior myocardial infarction and normal

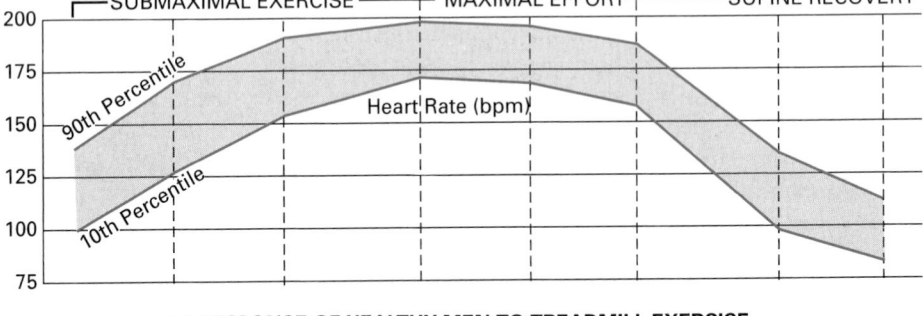

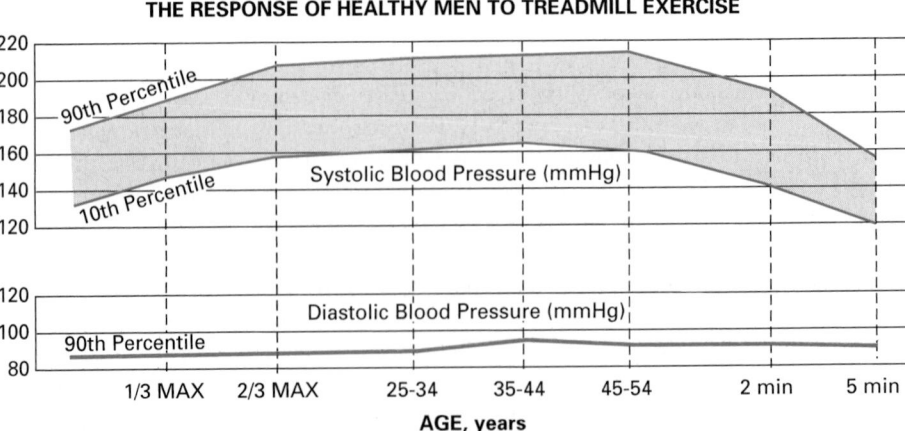

FIGURE 14–6. The results of a large number of normal individuals who underwent a progressive treadmill test show the response of heart rate and blood pressure according to age. bpm, beats per minute.

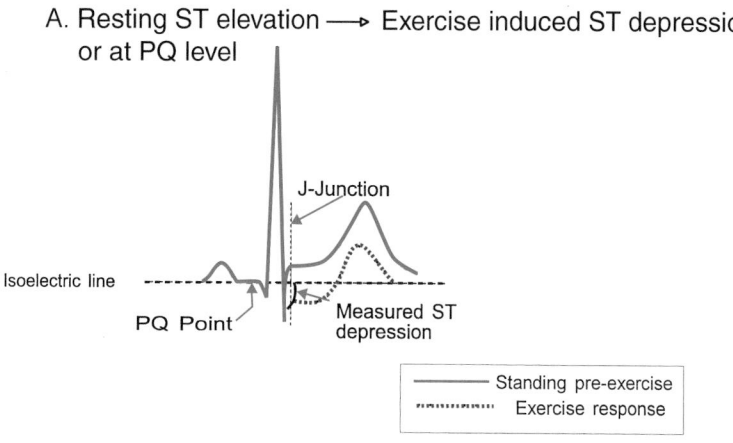

A. Resting ST elevation → Exercise induced ST depressic
or at PQ level

J-Junction

Isoelectric line

PQ Point

Measured ST
depression

——— Standing pre-exercise
·············· Exercise response

B. When the ST level begins below the isoelectric line:

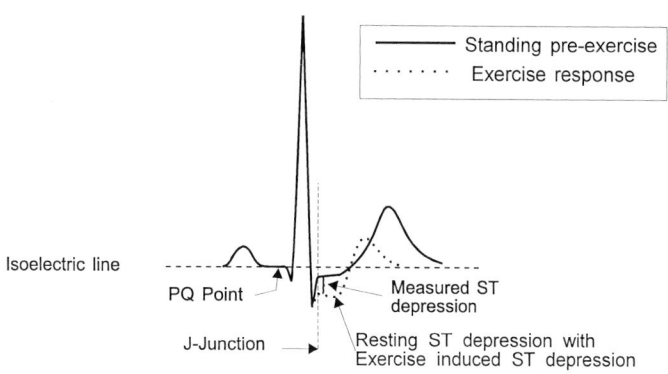

——— Standing pre-exercise
········· Exercise response

Isoelectric line

PQ Point

Measured ST
depression

J-Junction

Resting ST depression with
Exercise induced ST depression

FIGURE 14–7. The various patterns of ST-segment shift. The standard criterion for abnormal is 1 mm of horizontal or downsloping ST-segment depression below the PR isoelectric line or 1 mm further depression if there is baseline depression.

resting electrocardiograms, ST-depression in precordial lead V_5 along with V_4 and V_6 are reliable markers for coronary artery disease, and the monitoring of inferior limb leads adds little additional diagnostic information, but elevation inferiorly should not be ignored.

Exercise-induced R-wave and S-wave amplitude changes do not associate with changes in left ventricular volume, ejection fraction, or ischemia. The consensus of many studies is that such changes do not have diagnostic value. ST-segment depression limited to the recovery period does not generally represent a "false-positive" response. Inclusion of analysis during this time period increases the diagnostic yield of the exercise test. Other criteria including downsloping ST changes in recovery and prolongation of depression can improve test performance.

Computerized ST measurements should be used cautiously and require physician over-reading. Errors can be made both in the choice of isoelectric line and the beginning of the ST segment. Filtering and averaging can cause false ST depression because of distortion of the raw data.

【 】 SILENT ISCHEMIA

The evidence base for an exaggerated concern with silent ischemia is scant. Patients with silent ischemia (painless ST-depression) usually have milder forms of coronary disease and a better prognosis. The evidence base for silent ischemia being more prevalent in diabetics is not as convincing as one would think given its widespread clinical acceptance. Many physicians feel that treadmill testing should be used for routine screening of diabetics.

【 】 EXERCISE INDUCED ARRHYTHMIAS

As with resting ventricular arrhythmias, exercise-induced ventricular arrhythmias have an independent association with death in most patients with coronary disease and in asymptomatic individuals. The risk can be more delayed (more than 6 years) than that associated with ST-depression. Nonsustained ventricular tachycardia is uncommon during routine clinical treadmill testing and is usually well-tolerated. In patients with a history of syncope, sudden death, physical examination with a large heart, murmurs, ECG showing prolonged QT, preexcitation, Q waves, and heart failure (HF), then exercise-testing–induced ventricular arrhythmias are more worrisome. When healthy individuals exhibit premature ventricular contractions (PVCs) during testing, there is no need for immediate concern. Exercise-testing–induced supraventricular arrhythmias are relatively rare compared to ventricular arrhythmias and appear to be benign except for their association with the development of atrial fibrillation in the future.

DIAGNOSTIC UTILIZATION OF EXERCISE TESTING

The exercise test plays a pivotal role in diagnosis because the equipment and personnel for performing it are readily available, the testing equipment is relatively inexpensive, it can be performed in the doctor's office, and it does not require injections or exposure to radiation. Furthermore, it can determine the degree of disability and impairment to quality of life as well as be the first step in rehabilitation and altering a major risk factor (physical inactivity).

【 】 ADD-ONS TO THE EXERCISE TEST

Some of the newer add-ons or substitutes for the exercise test have the advantage of being able to localize ischemia as well as diagnose coronary disease when the baseline ECG negates ST analysis (more than one millimeter ST depression, left bundle-branch block, WPW). Nuclear perfusion scans and stress echocardiograms also provide an estimation of ventricular function. Nonexercise stress techniques also permit diagnostic assessment of patients unable to exercise. Although the newer technologies appear to have better diagnostic characteristics, this is not always the case, particularly when diagnostic scores are used that incorporate other variables in addition to the ST-segment change from the exercise test.

【 】 GUIDELINES FOR PROPER SELECTION OF PATIENTS

The ACC/AHA guidelines for the diagnostic use of the standard exercise test have stated that it is appropriate for testing of adult male or female patients (including those with complete right bundle-branch block or with less than one millimeter of resting ST depression) with an *intermediate pretest probability* of coronary artery disease based on gender, age, and symptoms (Table 14–5).

【 】 EVALUATION OF RESEARCH STUDIES ON DIAGNOSTIC TESTS

The criteria for *methodological standards* for diagnostic tests have been clearly elucidated. The purpose of these standards is to improve patient care, reduce health care costs, improve the quality of diagnostic test information, and eliminate useless tests or testing methodologies. The two most important criteria to consider when evaluating such studies are limited challenge and workup bias. Limited challenge usually results in exaggerated values for sensitivity, specificity, predictive accuracy, and receiver operating characteristic (ROC) curve area. Workup bias results in shifting cut-point performance further along the ROC curve and when removed shows that the exercise test has a high specificity in office practice. The mnemonics SnNout and SpPin help to remember the performance of a test with high values of either sensitivity or specificity. When a test has a very high sensitivity, a negative test rules out the diagnosis (SnNout); when a test has a very high specificity, a positive test rules in the diagnosis (SpPin). The ACP Journal Club has published an excellent roadmap for systematic reviews of diagnostic test evaluations.[9]

In studies that took into account the number of coronary arteries involved, all found increasing sensitivity of the test as more vessels were involved. The most false negatives have been found among patients with single-vessel disease, particularly if the diseased vessel was not the left anterior descending artery. No matter what techniques are used, there is a reciprocal relationship between sensitivity and specificity. The more specific a test is (i.e., the more able it is to determine who is disease free), the less sensi-

TABLE 14–5

Pretest Probability of Coronary Artery Disease by Symptoms, Gender, and Age

AGE[a]	GENDER	TYPICAL/ANGINA[b]	ATYPICAL/PROBABLE ANGINA	NONANGINAL CHEST PAIN	ASYMPTOMATIC
30–39	Men	Intermediate	Intermediate	Low	Very low
	Women	Intermediate	Very Low	Very low	Very low
40–49	Men	High	Intermediate	Intermediate	Low
	Women	Intermediate	Low	Very low	Very low
50–59	Men	High	Intermediate	Intermediate	Low
	Women	Intermediate	Intermediate	Low	Very low
60–69	Men	High	Intermediate	Intermediate	Low
	Women	High	Intermediate	Intermediate	Low

[a]There are no data for patients younger than 30 or older than 69, but it can be assumed that the prevalence of coronary artery disease increases with age.
[b]High = >90%, intermediate = 10%–90%, low = <10%, very low = <5%.

tive it is and vice versa. The values for adjusting the criterion can alter sensitivity and specificity for the cut point used for abnormal. For instance, when the criterion for an abnormal exercise-induced ST-segment response is altered to 0.2 mV (2 mm) depression, making it more specific for coronary artery disease, the sensitivity of the test will be reduced by half.

[ ] BETA BLOCKERS

In our most recent study of the effects of β blockade and heart rate response, we found the sensitivity and predictive accuracy of standard ST criteria for exercise-induced ST-depression significantly decreased in male patients taking β blockers and not reaching an adequate heart rate. In those who fail to reach target heart rate and are not β blocked, sensitivity and predictive accuracy were maintained. *The only way to maintain sensitivity with the standard exercise test in the β blocker group who failed to reach target heart rate was to use a treadmill score or 0.5-mm ST-depression as the criterion for abnormal.*[10] Because of a greater potential for cardiac events with the cessation of β blockers, they should not be automatically stopped prior to testing. If a patient is to be tested off β blockers, they should not be stopped abruptly but tapered off gradually under physician guidance.

[ ] WOMEN

The summary from the guidelines are clearly stated regarding testing women: concern about false-positive ST responses can be addressed by careful assessment of pretest probability and selective use of a stress imaging test before proceeding to angiography. The optimal strategy for circumventing false-positive test results for the diagnosis of coronary disease in women requires the use of scores. There is insufficient data to justify routine stress imaging tests as the initial test for women.

[ ] DIAGNOSTIC SCORES

Studies considering non-ECG data consistently demonstrate that the multivariable equations outperform simple ST diagnostic criteria. These equations generally provide a predictive accuracy of 80 percent (ROC area of 0.80). To obtain the best diagnostic characteristics with the exercise test, clinical and non-ECG test responses should be considered. We have validated simple scores for both men and women. Calculation of a *simple* exercise test score can be done using Figure 14–8[11] for men and Figure 14–9[12] for women. Diagnostic scores should be applied during every exercise test because they are easy to use and significantly improve the prediction of angiographic CAD.

[ ] EXERCISE TESTING AND ACUTE CORONARY SYNDROMES

Although the concept of acute coronary syndromes (ACS) has altered the clinical milieu, the CNR Cardiology Research group in Italy reviewed the literature to determine if evidence still supports the use of the exercise ECG as first-choice stress-testing modality for ACS.[13] They concluded that a large body of evidence supports the use of the exercise ECG as a cost-effective tool for prognostic purposes and for quality of life assessment following ACS. This is consistent with the ACC/AHA guidelines. The guidelines state that patients who are pain free, have either a normal or nondiagnostic ECG or one that is unchanged from previous tracings, and have a normal set of initial cardiac enzymes are candidates for further evaluation. If the patient is low risk and does not experience any further ischemic discomfort and a followup 12-lead ECG and cardiac marker measurements after 6 to 8 hours of observation are normal, the patient can be considered for an early exercise test to provoke ischemia. This test can be performed before discharge and should be supervised by an experienced physician. Alternatively, the patient can be discharged and return for the test as an outpatient within 3 days.

PROGNOSTIC UTILIZATION OF EXERCISE TESTING

The two principal reasons for estimating prognosis are to provide accurate answers to patients' questions regarding the probable outcome of their illnesses and to identify those patients in whom interventions might improve outcome. Exercise capacity is the primary predictor of prognosis in all categories of patients. With each decrease in the MET value achieved there is a 10 to 20 percent increase in overall mortality.

Recent studies of prognosis have provided important information focused on CV endpoints as death data is now relatively easy to obtain from death certificates whereas previously investigators had to follow the patients and contact them or review their records. Although death certificates have their limitations, in general they classify those with accidental, gastrointestinal (GI), pulmonary, and cancer deaths so that those remaining are most likely to have died of CV causes. Although all-cause mortality is a more important endpoint for intervention studies, CV mortality is more appropriate for evaluating a CV test (i.e., the exercise test).

The mathematical models for determining prognosis are usually more complex than those used for identifying severe angiographic disease. Diagnostic testing can use multivariate discriminant function analysis to determine the probability of severe angiographic disease being present or not. Prognostic testing must use survival analysis, which includes censoring for patients with uneven followup because of "lost to follow up" or other cardiac events (i.e., coronary artery bypass surgery [CABS], percutaneous coronary intervention [PCI]) and must account for time-person units of exposure. We have proposed the rules in Table 14–6 to assess prognostic studies.

There is much information supporting the use of exercise testing as the first noninvasive step after the history, physical examination, and resting ECG in the prognostic evaluation of CAD patients. It accomplishes both of the purposes of prognostic testing: to provide information regarding the patient's status and to help make recommendations for optimal management. This assessment should always include calculation of a properly designed score such as the Duke Treadmill Score or the VA Treadmill Score (Table 14–7).

CARDIOPULMONARY EXERCISE TESTING IN HEART FAILURE

Although the exercise test was once considered only a tool to diagnose coronary disease, it is now recognized that it has major appli-

Variable	Circle response	Sum
Maximal Heart Rate	Less than 100 bpm = 30	
	100 to 129 bpm = 24	
	130 to 159 bpm = 18	
	160 to 189 bpm = 12	
	190 to 220 bpm = 6	
Exercise ST Depression	1-2mm = 15	
	> 2mm = 25	
Age	>55 yrs = 20	
	40 to 55 yrs = 12	
Angina History	Definite/Typical = 5	
	Probable/atypical = 3	
	Non-cardiac pain = 1	
Hypercholesterolemia?	Yes = 5	
Diabetes?	Yes = 5	
Exercise Test Induced Angina?	Occurred = 3	
	Reason for stopping = 5	
	Total Score:	

Men

<40 = Low Probability

40-60 = Intermediate Probability

>60 = High Probability

FIGURE 14–8. Calculation of the simple score for angiographic coronary disease in men. Choose only one per group. bpm, beats per minute.

cations for assessing functional capabilities, therapeutic interventions, and estimating prognosis in HF. Numerous hemodynamic abnormalities underlie the reduced exercise capacity commonly observed in chronic heart failure, including impaired heart rate responses, inability to distribute cardiac output normally, abnormal arterial vasodilatory capacity, abnormal cellular metabolism in skeletal muscle, higher than normal systemic vascular resistance, higher than normal pulmonary pressures, and ventilatory abnormalities that increase the work of breathing and cause exertional dyspnea.[14] Intervention with angiotensin-converting enzyme (ACE)-inhibition, β blockade, cardiac resynchronization therapy (CRT), or exercise training can improve many of these abnormalities. Over the last 15 years, exercise testing with ventilatory gas exchange responses has been demonstrated to have a critical role in the risk paradigm in HF.

Directly measured VO_2 now has an established place in predicting outcomes in patients with HF. Peak VO_2 has been demonstrated in numerous studies to be an independent marker for risk of death or other endpoints and is now a recognized criterion for selecting patients who could potentially benefit from heart transplantation. Increased automation of gas-exchange systems has made these data easier to obtain, and this objective information is replacing the former dependence on subjective measures of clinical and functional status.

Peak VO_2 is influenced by age, gender, body weight, and mode of exercise, and some studies have demonstrated that peak VO_2 expressed as a percentage of the predicted value (taking these variables into account) is a more powerful predictor of outcome than absolute peak VO_2. This approach is complicated by the fact that there are many age- and gender-predicted *standards* for peak VO_2.[15]

Cardiopulmonary exercise variables other than peak VO_2 also have important prognostic value in HF. Several studies have focused on the V_E/VO_2 slope and other expressions of ventilatory efficiency, including the maximal ventilatory equivalent for CO_2, the oxygen uptake efficiency slope (OUES), various measures of oxygen kinetics, and oxygen uptake in recovery have also been shown to be strong prognostic markers. Summary reports from metabolic systems should be configured to provide both the V_E/VCO_2 slope and peak VO_2, and consideration should be given to including the V_E/VCO_2 slope in the HF and transplantation guidelines.

Variable	Circle response	Sum
Maximal Heart Rate	Less than 100 bpm = 20	
	100 to 129 bpm = 16	
	130 to 159 bpm = 12	
	160 to 189 bpm = 8	
	190 to 220 bpm = 4	
Exercise ST Depression	1-2mm = 6	
	> 2mm =10	
Age	>65 yrs = 25	
	50 to 65 yrs = 15	
Angina History	Definite/Typical = 10	
	Probable/atypical = 6	
	Non-cardiac pain = 2	
Hypercholesterolemia?	Yes = 10	
Diabetes?	Yes = 10	
Exercise Test Induced Angina?	Occurred = 9	
	Reason for stopping =15	
Estrogen Status	Positive=-5, Negative=5	
	Total Score:	

Women

<37 = Low Probability

37-57 = Intermediate Probability

>57 = High Probability

FIGURE 14–9. Calculation of the simple score for angiographic coronary disease in women. Choose only one per group.

TABLE 14-6

Proposed Criteria for Studies Assessing Prognostic Value of Clinical and Exercise Test Variables

1. *Study population:* Inclusion criteria such as catheterization should be specified. Prevalence of clinical conditions (prior myocardial infarction, Q waves on resting ECG, diabetes), and angina should be stated. Patients with heart failure and LV dysfunction in general should be considered separately.

2. *Avoidance of "workup bias":* Limited study populations such as patients referred for catheterization should be avoided, or validation studies in different populations or bootstrapping techniques should be used.

3. *Exercise testing procedures:* Protocols used and criteria for abnormal values should be well described.

4. *Clinical and exercise test variables:* Variables must be clearly defined and entered into the statistical analysis separately.

5. *Study end points:* Cardiovascular death and nonfatal myocardial infarction should be used.

6. *Avoidance of "overfitting the data":* The ratio of events to the number of variables studied should be at least 5 to 10 to ensure enough hard outcomes per given variable studied.

7. *Follow-up:* Length and completeness should be documented.

8. *Treatment of interventions:* Coronary artery bypass surgery and PCI should not be used as end points.

9. *Censoring:* Patients should be censored on interventions (coronary artery bypass surgery or PCI) and on "lost to follow up."

10. *Relationship between censored events and studied variables:* It should be determined whether censoring is random or correlated with specific clinical and exercise test markers.

11. *Multivariate survival analysis techniques:* Cox proportional hazard model or discriminant analysis should be used.

12. *Concordance with the hierarchical nature of clinical data acquisition:* Variables should be entered into multivariate analysis in an order similar to clinical practice (i.e., clinical parameters followed by exercise test variables and then invasive test variables).

13. *Interactions between variables:* Associations between variables (i.e., digoxin use and congestive heart failure or ST elevation over Q waves) should be noted and treated appropriately.

14. *Avoidance of test review bias:* Investigators should be blinded to patient characteristics and results of other diagnostic and prognostic tests.

LV, left ventricular; PCI, percutaneous coronary intervention.

TABLE 14-7

Prognostic Scores: The Duke Treadmill Score and the VA Treadmill Score

Duke Score = METs − 5 × (mm E-I ST depression) − 4 × (TM AP index)

VA Score = 5 × (CHF/Dig) + mm E-I ST depression + Change in SBP score − METs

CHF, congestive heart failure; METs, metabolic equivalents; SBP, systolic blood pressure; TM AP, treadmill angina pectoris.
TM AP score: 0 if no angina, 1 if angina occurred during test, 2 if angina was the reason for stopping.
Change in SBP score: from 0 for rise greater than 40 mmHg to 5 for drop below rest.

Recent studies have considered other exercise test responses including heart rate recovery[16] and ectopy[17] and found both to have independent prognostic power in patients with HF. These exercise test responses have not yet been combined or compared to expired gas analysis results and could improve risk stratification.

Peak VO_2 or other related measures should not be used as the only prognostic markers in heart failure. The combination of cardiopulmonary exercise data and other clinical and hemodynamic responses in multivariate scores has been shown to more powerfully stratify risk.

EXERCISE TESTING AFTER MYOCARDIAL INFARCTION

The benefits of performing an exercise test in post-MI patients are listed in Table 14–8. Submitting patients to exercise testing can expedite and optimize their discharge from the hospital. Patients' responses to exercise, their work capacity, and limiting factors at the time of discharge can be assessed by the exercise test. An exercise test prior to discharge is important for giving patients guidelines for exercise at home, reassuring them of their physical status, advising them to resume or increase their activity level, advising them on timing of return to work and determining the risk of complications. Psychologically, it can cause an improvement in the patient's self-confidence by making the patient less anxious about daily physical activities and help them to rehabilitate themselves. The test has been helpful in reassuring spouses of post-MI patients of their physical capabilities.

Exercise testing is also an important tool in exercise training as part of comprehensive cardiac rehabilitation, where it can be used to develop and modify the exercise prescription, assist in providing activity counseling, and assess the patient's response at the initiation of, and progress in, the exercise training program.

One consistent finding in the review of the post-MI exercise test studies that included a followup for cardiac end points is that patients who met whatever criteria set forth for exercise testing were at lower risk than patients not tested. From meta-analyses of multiple studies, only an abnormal SBP response or a low exercise capacity were consistently associated with a poor outcome and were more predictive of adverse cardiac events after MI than measures of exercise-induced ischemia.[18,19]

SCREENING

Screening for asymptomatic coronary artery disease has become a topic of increased interest because of the remarkable efficacy of the statins in reducing the risk of cardiac events even in asymptomatic individuals. The first step in screening asymptomatic individuals for preclinical coronary disease should be using global risk factor equations such as the Framingham score. This is available as nomograms that are easily applied by health care professionals, or it can be calculated as part of a computerized patient record. Several additional testing procedures have promise for screening including the simple ankle-brachial index (particularly in the elderly), C-reactive protein and other emerging biomarkers, carotid ultrasound measurements of intimal thickening, and the resting ECG (particularly spatial QRS-T wave angle). Despite the promotional concept of atherosclerotic burden, electron-beam computed tomography (EBCT) does not have test characteristics superior to the standard exercise test. If any screening test could be used to accurately determine the need for statin therapy and not affect insurance or occupational status, this would be extremely helpful. However, screening tests are controversial because they often generate a high rate of false positives, which can lead to unnecessary procedures, and the overall cost-benefit to society is unclear.

True demonstration of the effectiveness of a screening technique requires randomizing the target population, one-half receiving the screening technique, standardized action taken in response to the screening test results, and then outcomes assessed. For the screening technique to be effective, the screened group must have lower mortality and/or morbidity. Such a study has been completed for mammography but not for any cardiac testing modalities. The next best validation of efficacy is to demonstrate that the technique improves the discrimination of those asymptomatic individuals with higher risk for events over that possible with the available risk factors. Mathematical modeling makes it possible to determine how well a population will be classified if the characteristics of the testing method are known.

Several well-designed followup studies have improved our understanding of the application of exercise testing as a screening tool. The predictive value of the abnormal maximal exercise electrocardiogram ranges from 5 to 46 percent. The first prospective studies of exercise testing in asymptomatic individuals included angina as a cardiac disease end point. This led to a bias for individuals with abnormal tests to subsequently report angina or to be diagnosed as having angina resulting in a high predictive value being reported for the test. When only hard end points (death or MI) were used, the results were less encouraging. The test could only identify one-third of the patients with hard events, and only 5 percent of the abnormal responders developed coronary heart disease over the followup period. Thus, more than 90 percent of the abnormal responders were false positives. Overall, the exercise test's characteristics as a screening test probably lie in between the results of studies using hard or soft endpoints because some of the subjects who develop chest pain really have angina and coronary disease. The sensitivity is probably between 30 and 50 percent (at a specificity of 90 percent), but the critical limitation is the predictive value (and risk ratio), which depends on the prevalence of disease (which is low in the asymptomatic population).

The iatrogenic problems resulting from screening (i.e., morbidity from subsequent procedures, employment and insurance issues) would make using a test with a high false-positive rate unreasonable. The recent U.S. Preventive Services Task Force statement states that "false positive tests are common among asymptomatic adults, especially women, and can lead to unnecessary diagnostic testing, over treatment and labeling" (www.preventiveservices.ahrq.gov or www.guideline.gov).[20] In the majority of asymptomatic people, screening with any test or test add-on is more likely to yield false positives than true positives. This is the mathematical reality associated with all of the available tests.

If the exercise treadmill test is to be used to screen, it should be done in groups with a higher estimated prevalence of disease using the Framingham score or another predictive model. In addition, a positive test result should not immediately lead to invasive testing. In most circumstances an add-on imaging modality (echo or nuclear) should be the first choice in evaluating asymptomatic individuals with an abnormal exercise test.

Three recent studies lead to the logical conclusion that exercise testing should be part of the preventive health recommendations for screening healthy, asymptomatic individuals along with risk-factor assessment. The data from Norway (2,000 men, 26-year followup)[21], the Cooper Clinic (26,000 men, 8-year followup)[22], and Framingham (3,000 men, 18-year followup)[23] provide additional risk classification power and demonstrate incremental risk ratios for the synergistic combination of the standard exercise test and risk factors.

There are several other reasons why the exercise test should be promoted for screening. Most tests currently being promoted for screening do not have the documented favorable test characteristics of the exercise test. In addition, physical inactivity has reached epidemic proportions and what better way to make our patients conscious of their deconditioning than having them do an exercise

---

> ## TABLE 14–8
>
> ### Benefits of Exercise Testing Post-MI
>
> #### PREDISCHARGE SUBMAXIMAL TEST
>
> Optimizing discharge
> Altering medical therapy
> Triaging for intensity of followup
> First step in rehabilitation—assurance, encouragement
> Reassuring spouse
> Recognizing exercise-induced ischemia and dysrhythmias
>
> #### MAXIMAL TEST FOR RETURN TO NORMAL ACTIVITIES
>
> Determining limitations
> Prognostication
> Reassuring employers
> Determining level of disability
> Triaging for invasive studies
> Deciding on medications
> Exercise prescription
> Continued rehabilitation

TABLE 14–9

Exercise Testing Rules to Maximize Information Obtained

- The exercise protocol should be progressive, with even increments in speed and grade whenever possible.
- The treadmill protocol should be adjusted to the patient, and one protocol is not appropriate for all patients; consider using a manual or automated ramp protocol.
- Report exercise capacity in METs, not minutes of exercise.
- Hyperventilation prior to testing is not indicated.
- ST-segment measurements should be made at ST0 (J-junction), and ST-segment depression should be considered abnormal only if horizontal or downsloping.
- Raw ECG waveforms should be considered first and then supplemented by computer-enhanced (filtered and averaged) waveforms when the raw data are acceptable.
- In testing for diagnostic purposes, patients should be placed supine as soon as possible after exercise, with a cool-down walk avoided.
- The 3-minutes recovery period is critical to include in analysis of the ST-segment response.
- Measurement of systolic blood pressure during exercise is extremely important and exertional hypotension is ominous; manual blood pressure measurement techniques are preferred.
- Age-predicted heart rate targets are largely useless because of the wide scatter for any age; exercise tests should be symptom limited.
- A treadmill score should be calculated for every patient; use of multiple scores or a computerized consensus score should be considered as part of the treadmill report.

METs, metabolic equivalents; min, minute.

test that can also "clear them" for exercise? Including the exercise test in the screening process sends a strong message to our patients that we consider their exercise status as important. Each 1 MET increase in exercise capacity equates with to a 10 to 25 percent improvement in survival in all populations studied[24] as well a 5 percent decline in health care costs.[25]

If screening could be performed in a logical way with test results helping to make decisions regarding therapies rather than leading to invasive interventions, insurance or occupational problems, then the recent results summarized above should be applied to preventive medicine policy. There may be enough evidence to consider recommending a routine exercise test every five years for men older than 40 and women older than 50 years of age, especially if one of the potential benefits is the adoption of an active lifestyle.[26]

CONCLUSIONS

The exercise test complements the medical history and the physical examination, and it remains the second most commonly performed cardiologic procedure next to the routine ECG. The addition of echocardiography or myocardial perfusion imaging does not negate the importance of the ECG or clinical and hemodynamic responses

to exercise. The renewed efforts to control costs undoubtedly will support the role of the exercise test. Convincing evidence that treadmill scores enhance the diagnostic and prognostic power of the exercise test certainly has cost-efficacy implications.

Use of proper methodology is critical for safety and obtaining accurate and comparable results. The use of specific criteria for exclusion and termination, interaction with the subject, and appropriate emergency equipment is essential.

Table 14–9 lists important rules to follow for getting the most information from the standard exercise test.

The ACC/AHA guidelines for exercise testing clearly indicate the correct uses of exercise testing. Since the last guidelines, exercise testing has been extended as the first diagnostic test in women and in individuals with right bundle-branch block and resting ST-segment depression. The use of diagnostic scores and prognostic scores such as the Duke Treadmill Score increases the value of the exercise test. In fact, the use of scores results in test characteristics that approach the nuclear and echocardiographic add-ons to the exercise test.

REFERENCES

1. American College of Cardiology. COCATS guidelines: guidelines for training in adult cardiovascular medicine, Core Cardiology Training Symposium: June 27–28,1994. *J Am Coll Cardiol.* 1995;25:1–34.
2. Schlant RC, Friesinger GC, Leonard JJ. Clinical competence in exercise testing a statement for physicians from the ACP/ACC/AHA Task Force on Clinical Privileges in Cardiology. *J Am Coll Cardiol.* 1990;16:1061–1065.
3. American College of Sports Medicine. *Guidelines for Exercise Testing and Prescription.* 6th ed. Baltimore: Lippincott, Williams & Wilkins; 2000.
4. Myers J, Ashley E. Dangerous curves: a perspective on exercise, lactate, and the anaerobic threshold. *Chest.* 1997;111:787–795.
5. Brooks GA. Intra- and extra-cellular lactate shuttles. *Med Sci Sports Exerc.* 2000;32:790–799.
6. Gibbons RJ, Balady GJ, Bricker JT, et al. ACC/AHA 2002 guideline update for exercise testing: a report of the American College of Cardiology/American Heart Association Task Force on Practice Guidelines (Committee on Exercise Testing). *Circulation.* 2002;106:1883–1892.
7. Fletcher GF, Balady GJ, Amsterdam EA, et al. Exercise standards for testing and training: a statement for healthcare professionals from the American Heart Association. *Circulation.* 2001;104:1694–1740.
8. Miranda CP, Liu J, Kadar A, et al. Usefulness of exercise-induced ST-segment depression in the inferior leads during exercise testing as a marker for coronary artery disease. *Am J Cardiol.* 1992;69:303–308.
9. Pai M, McCulloch M, Enanoria W, et al. Systematic reviews of diagnostic test evaluations: What's behind the scenes? *ACP J Club.* 2004;141:A11–A13.
10. Gauri AJ, Raxwal VK, Roux L, et al. Effects of chronotropic incompetence and beta-blocker use on the exercise treadmill test in men. *Am Heart J.* 2001;142:136–141.
11. Raxwal V, Shetler K, Do D, et al. A simple treadmill score. *Chest.* 2000;113:1933–1940.
12. Morise AP, Lauer MS, Froelicher VF. Development and validation of a simple exercise test score for use in women with symptoms of suspected coronary artery disease. *Am Heart J.* 2002;144:818–825.
13. Bigi R, Cortigiani L, Desideri A. Exercise electrocardiography after acute coronary syndromes: still the first testing modality? *Clin Cardiol.* 2003;26:390–395.
14. Pina IL, Apstein CS, Balady GJ, et al. American Heart Association Committee on exercise, rehabilitation, and prevention. Exercise and heart failure: a statement from the American Heart Association Committee on exercise, rehabilitation, and prevention. *Circulation.* 2003;107:1210–1225.
15. Myers J. *Essentials of Cardiopulmonary Exercise Testing.* Champaign, IL: Human Kinetics; 1996.
16. Lipinski MJ, Vetrovec G, Gorelik D, et al. The importance of heart rate recovery in patients with heart failure or left ventricular systolic dysfunction. *J Card Fail.* 2005;11:624–630.

17. O'Neill JO, Young JB, Pothier CE, et al. Severe frequent ventricular ectopy after exercise as a predictor of death in patients with heart failure. *J Am Coll Cardiol.* 2004;44:820–826.

18. Froelicher VF, Perdue S, Pewen W, et al. Application of meta-analysis using an electronic spreadsheet to exercise testing in patients with myocardial infarction. *Am J Med.* 1987;83:1045–1054.

19. Shaw LJ, Peterson ED, Kesler K, et al. A metaanalysis of predischarge risk stratification after acute myocardial infarction with stress electrocardiographic, myocardial perfusion, and ventricular function imaging. *Am J Cardiol.* 1996;78:1327–1337.

20. U.S. Preventive Services Task Force. Screening for coronary heart disease: recommendation statement. *Ann Intern Med.* 2004;140:569–572.

21. Erikssen G, Bodegard J, Bjornholt JV, et al. Exercise testing of healthy men in a new perspective: from diagnosis to prognosis. *Eur Heart J.* 2004;25:978–986.

22. Gibbons LW, Mitchell TL, Wei M, et al. Maximal exercise test as a predictor of risk for mortality from coronary heart disease in asymptomatic men. *Am J Cardiol.* 2000;86:53–58.

23. Balady GJ, Larson MG, Vasan RS, et al. Usefulness of exercise testing in the prediction of coronary disease risk among asymptomatic persons as a function of the Framingham Risk Score. *Circulation.* 2004;110:1920–1925.

24. Myers J, Kaykha A, George S, et al. Fitness versus physical activity patterns in predicting mortality in men. *Am J Med.* 2004;117:912–918.

25. Weiss JP, Froelicher VF, Myers JN, et al. Health-care costs and exercise capacity. *Chest.* 2004;126:608–613.

26. DiPietro L, Kohl HW 3rd, Barlow CE, et al. Improvements in cardiorespiratory fitness attenuate age-related weight gain in healthy men and women: the Aerobics Center Longitudinal Study. *Int J Obes Relat Metab Disord.* 1998;22:55–62.

CHAPTER 15

Cardiac Roentgenography

Robert A. O'Rourke / Robert C. Gilkeson

As discussed in other chapters in this text (see Chaps. 16 to 23), the relatively low-cost chest roentgenogram is less commonly used as a primary diagnostic technique for determining the presence and severity of cardiac disease, even when it provides diagnostic information (e.g., pulmonary venous hypertension).

With the development of many new cardiac imaging techniques, familiarity with the altered anatomy and understanding of the underlying pathophysiology of a diseased heart are the cornerstones to appropriate interpretation of its roentgen manifestations. The conventional four-view cardiac series is tabulated in Table 15–1, and the views are illustrated in Fig. 15–1C to F.

The approach to the chest roentgenogram should be thorough and objective so that no clue is overlooked and no bias is incorporated in the process of radiographic analysis.[1–4] Rib notching (Fig. 15–1A,B) provides important clues to the diagnosis of coarctation of the aorta.[3,5] To prevent erroneous clinical information from misleading the radiographic interpretation, films should initially be interpreted without any knowledge about the patient.

A secundum atrial septal defect can be incorrectly diagnosed as mitral stenosis (MS) because of similar physical signs. The split-second sound can be misinterpreted as the opening snap (see Chap. 12). The diastolic rumble caused by the increased flow through a normal tricuspid valve can mimic the murmur of MS. The radiographic signs of the two entities, however, are quite different (Fig. 15–2B versus Fig. 15–3A). The *final* radiologic diagnosis, however, should be made only after correlating the x-ray findings with clinical information and other laboratory data.[6]

The radiologic examination for heart disease consists of five major steps. They are (1) roentgenographic examination for anatomy, (2) comparison of serial studies, (3) statistical guidance, (4) clinical correlation, and (5) conclusion (Table 15–2).

ROENTGENOGRAPHIC EXAMINATION FOR ANATOMY

【 】 AN OVERVIEW

The first step is to survey the roentgenogram and assess all the structures, searching particularly for noncardiac conditions that can reflect heart disease. For instance, a right-sided stomach with an absent image of the inferior vena cava suggests the possibility of congenital interruption of the inferior vena cava with azygos continuation[7,8] (Fig. 15–4). A narrowed anteroposterior (AP) diameter of the thorax can be the cause of an innocent murmur[9] (Fig. 15–5).

【 】 PULMONARY VASCULATURE

The lung can often reflect the underlying pathophysiology of the heart. For example, if uniform dilatation of all pulmonary vessels is present, the diagnosis of a left-to-right shunt (see Fig. 15–2B) is more likely than a left-sided obstructive lesion. The latter typically shows a cephalic pulmonary blood flow pattern (see Fig. 15–3A).

【 】 LUNG PARENCHYMA

With right heart failure, the lungs become unusually radiolucent because of decreased pulmonary blood flow (PBF). Conversely, significant left heart failure is characterized by the presence of pulmonary

TABLE 15–1

Conventional Four-View Cardiac Series

Posteroanterior (PA) view	With barium
Left lateral (lateral) view	With barium
45° Right anterior oblique (RAO) view	With barium
60° Left anterior oblique (LAO) view	Without barium

edema and/or a cephalic blood flow pattern (Fig. 15–6). Long-standing, severe pulmonary venous hypertension can lead to hemosiderosis and/or ossification of the lung.[10,11] When right heart failure results from severe left heart failure, the preexisting pulmonary congestion can improve because of the decreased PBF (Fig. 15–6B).

【 】 CARDIAC SIZE

An enlarged heart is always abnormal; however, mild cardiomegaly can reflect a higher-than-average cardiac output from a normal heart, as seen in athletes with slow heart rates. The cardiothoracic ratio remains the simplest yardstick for assessment of cardiac size;[1] the mean ratio in the upright posteroanterior (PA) view is 44 percent.

The nature of cardiomegaly can often be determined by the specific roentgen appearance. As a rule, when the PBF pattern remains normal, volume overload tends to present a greater degree of cardiomegaly than lesions with pressure overload alone. For ex-

ample, patients with aortic stenosis (AS) typically show features of left ventricular hypertrophy (LVH) without dilatation. Conversely, the left ventricle both dilates and hypertrophies in the case of aortic regurgitation (AR), producing a much larger heart even before the development of heart failure.

A smaller-than-average heart is encountered in patients with chronic obstructive pulmonary disease (see Fig. 15–7A), Addison disease, anorexia nervosa, and starvation. An abnormally small heart, however, is difficult to define except retrospectively after successful therapy.

【 】 CARDIAC CONTOUR

Any significant deviation from the normal cardiovascular contour can be a clue to the correct diagnosis. For instance, *coeur en sabot*, a "boot-shaped heart" (see Fig. 15–2C), is characteristic of tetralogy of Fallot. A bulge along the left cardiac border with a retrosternal double density is virtually diagnostic of left ventricular (LV) aneurysm (Fig. 15–8). A markedly widened right cardiac contour with a straightened left cardiac border is seen frequently in patients with severe MS leading to tricuspid regurgitation (TR) (see Fig. 15–7D).

【 】 ABNORMAL DENSITIES

Besides the familiar double density cast by an enlarged left atrium (LA), other increased densities can be found within the cardiac shadow, indicating a variety of dilated vascular structures (e.g., tor-

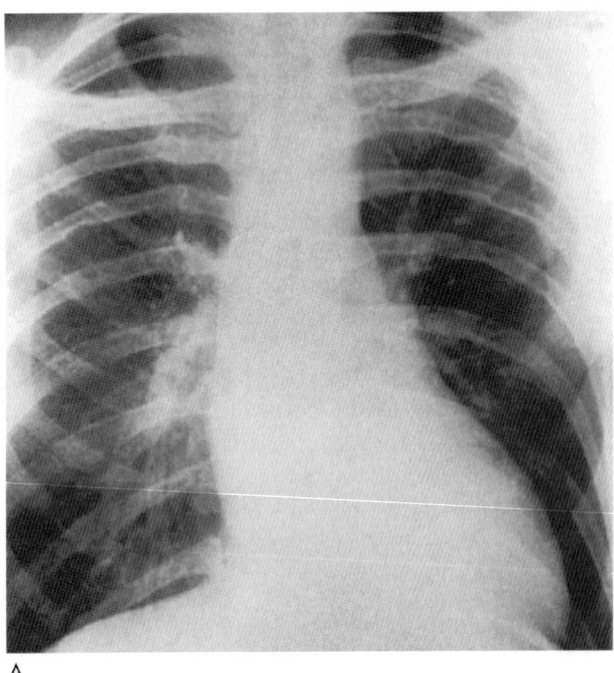

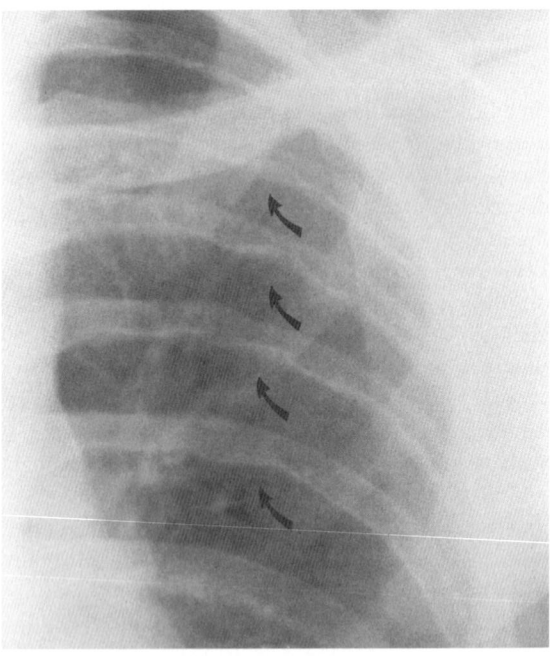

A   B

FIGURE 15–1. Practical application of four-view cardiac series. **A.** Posteroanterior (PA) view in a patient with coarctation of the aorta showing areas of rib notching bilaterally and left ventricular (LV) enlargement in the inferior and leftward direction. **B.** Magnified view of the left upper thorax of the same patient showing multiple areas of rib notching (*arrows*). **C.** PA view of another patient with aortic coarctation showing the *3 sign* of the deformed descending aorta and *E sign* on the barium-filled esophagus. The *upper arrow* points to the level of coarctation. The *lower arrow* marks the apex of the enlarged left ventricle. The *arrow* on the patient's right indicates the dilated ascending aorta. **D.** Lateral view of a third patient with the same disease showing a barium-filled esophagus to be pushed forward (*upper arrow*) by the poststenotic dilatation of the descending aorta and pushed backward (*middle arrow*) by the enlarged left atrium (LA). The very large left ventricle (*lower arrow*) simply casts a shadow behind the esophagus without displacing it. The *oblique arrow* points to the calcified stenotic bicuspid aortic valve. **E.** Right anterior oblique (RAO) view of same patient whose PA view is shown in Fig. 15–7D. Note the huge right atrium (RA) casting a triangular density (*lower horizontal arrow*) behind the esophagus without displacing it. The esophagus is deviated posteriorly by the enlarged left atrium (LA) (*upper horizontal arrow*). The upper oblique arrows indicate the direction of the enlarging pulmonary trunk and right ventricle. The *lower oblique arrow* points to the normal left ventricle with the undisturbed left costophrenic sulcus. **F.** Left anterior oblique (LAO) view of a patient with valvular aortic stenosis (AS). The dilated ascending aorta (*upper white arrow*) is immediately above the flat anterior border of normal right ventricle. The *black arrow* points to the calcified aortic valve. The *lower white arrow* marks the enlarged left ventricle.

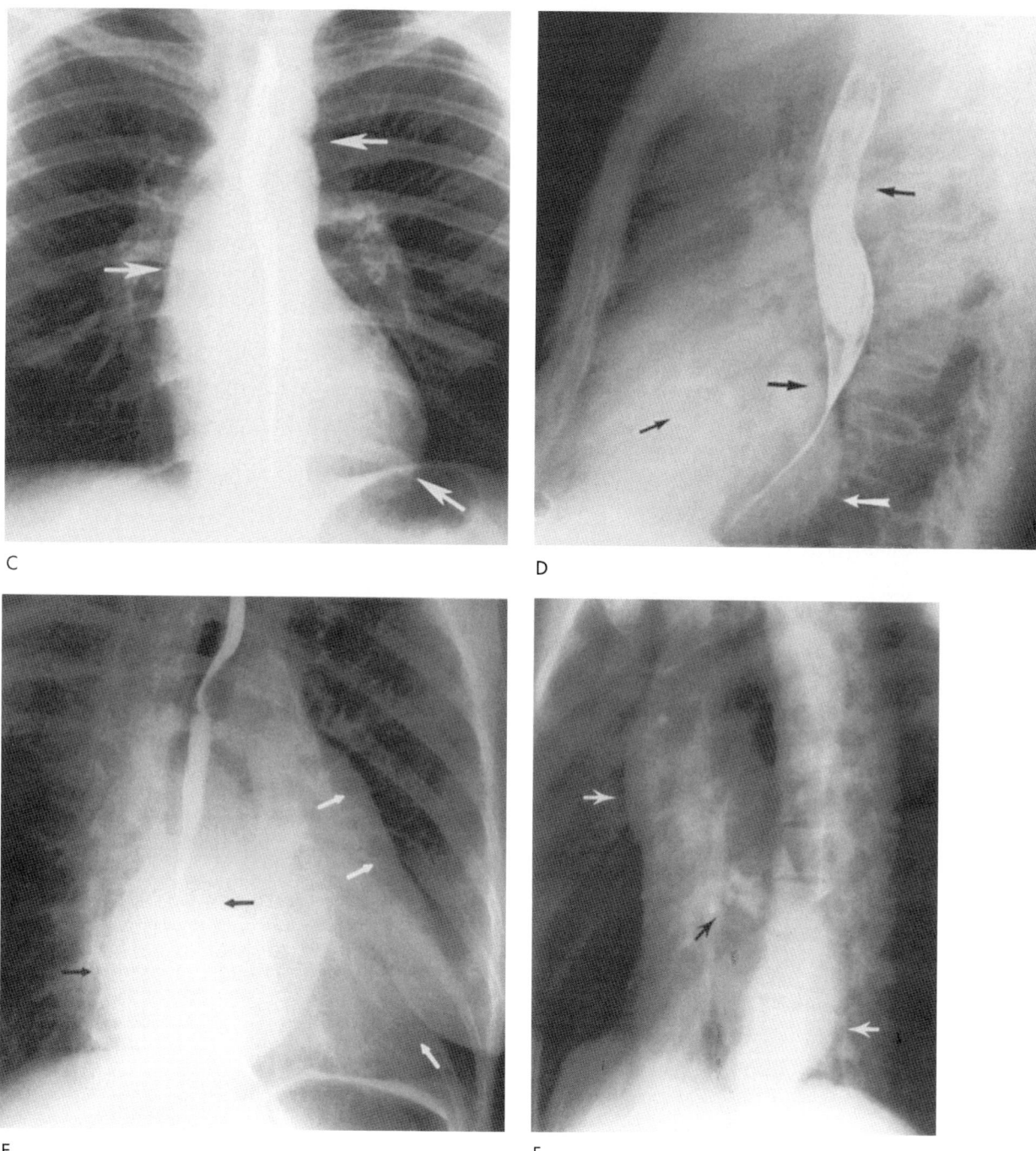

FIGURE 15–1. *(continued)*

tuous descending aorta, aortic aneurysm, coronary artery [CA] aneurysm, pulmonary varix).[2] Furthermore, large cardiac calcifications are readily seen, in lateral and oblique views. If smaller calcific deposits are suspected, they should be verified promptly, ruled out by cardiac fluoroscopy or CT (see Chap. 20). Any radiologically detectable calcification in the heart is clinically important. In general, the heavier the calcification, the more significant it becomes (see Fig. 15–1F). The extent of valvular calcification tends to be proportionate to the severity of the valve stenosis regardless of the other roentgen signs of the disease.[1,2,12,13] Calcification of the CA is almost always atherosclerotic in nature. A fluoroscopically detectable coronary calcification correlates with major vessel occlusion in 94 percent of patients *with chest pain*;[14] however, the sensitivity of the test is only 40 percent.

Recently, electron-beam CT (EBCT) scanning has proven to be a sensitive method for detection and quantifying coronary calcifications (see Chaps. 20 and 64). Although a negative result can indicate no need for further testing in asymptomatic individuals, a positive result does not necessarily denote severe obstructive coronary artery disease (CAD). The sensitivity for detecting any coronary calcifications is greater than 95 percent with a *specificity of less than 65 percent* for significant CA luminal stenosis. A calcified ascending aortic aneurysm with AR is highly suggestive of syphilitic aortitis[15] (Fig. 15–9).

ABNORMAL LUCENCY

The abnormal lucent areas in and about the heart include (1) displaced subepicardial fat stripes caused by effusion or thickening

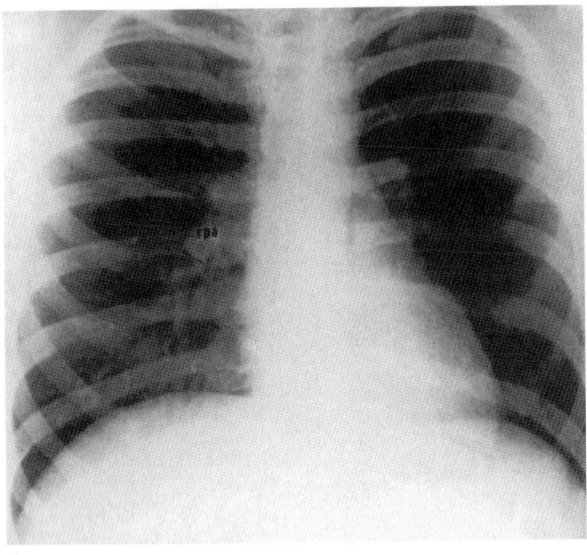

A

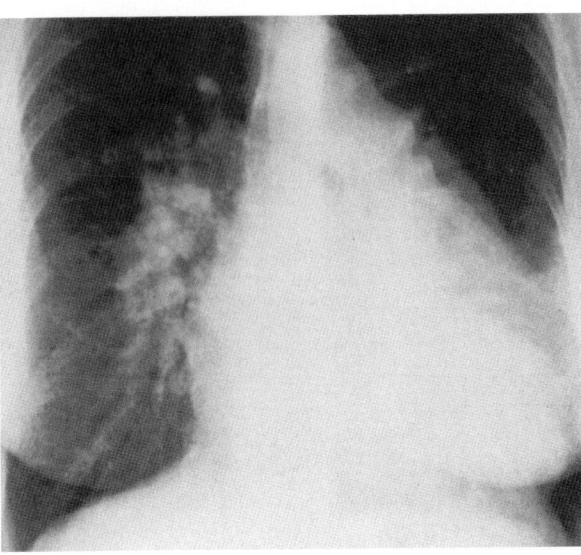

B

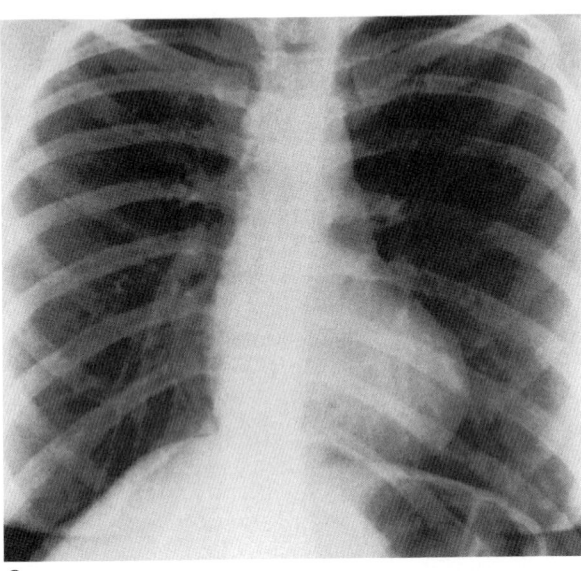

C

FIGURE 15–2. Roentgenographic assessment of the volume of pulmonary blood flow. **A.** *Normal.* There is caudalization of the pulmonary vascularity because of gravity. The right descending pulmonary artery (RPA) measures 13 mm in diameter in this young man. **B.** *Increased.* Patient with a secundum atrial septal defect showing uniform increase in pulmonary vascularity bilaterally. The right descending pulmonary artery is markedly enlarged, measuring 27 mm. **C.** *Decreased.* Patient with tetralogy of Fallot showing a boot-shaped heart and uniform decrease in pulmonary vascularity. The right descending pulmonary artery is much smaller than normal, measuring 6 mm in diameter.

FIGURE 15–3. Abnormal pulmonary blood flow patterns. **A.** *Cephalization.* Patient with severe mitral stenosis (MS) showing dilatation of the upper vessels with constriction of the lower vessels. **B.** *Centralization.* Patient with primary pulmonary hypertension (PH) showing marked dilatation of the pulmonary trunk and the central segments of both pulmonary arteries with pruning of the peripheral branches. **C.** *Lateralization.* Patient with massive pulmonary embolism obstructing the left main pulmonary artery. Note the uneven distribution of pulmonary blood flow between the two lungs in favor of the right. **D.** *Localization.* A cyanotic child showing localized vascular changes representing a large pulmonary arteriovenous fistula in the right lower lobe. **E.** *Collateralization.* A child with pseudotruncus arteriosus with cardiomegaly and a right aortic arch (*small arrow*). Note severe pulmonary oligemia with numerous small tortuous vessels (*large arrow*) in upper medial lung zones, representing bronchial arterial collaterals.

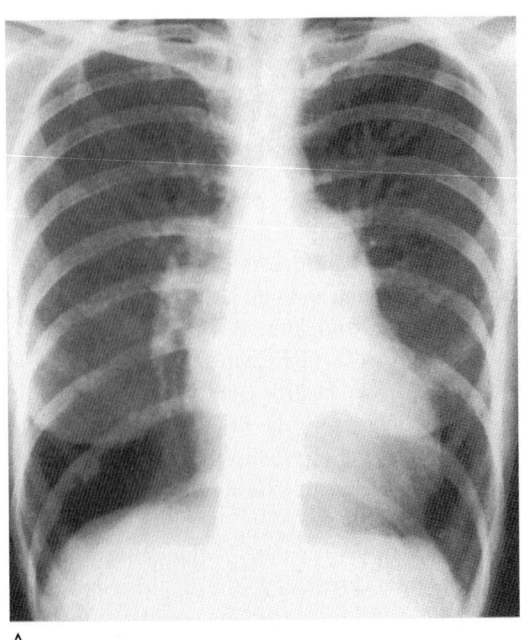

A

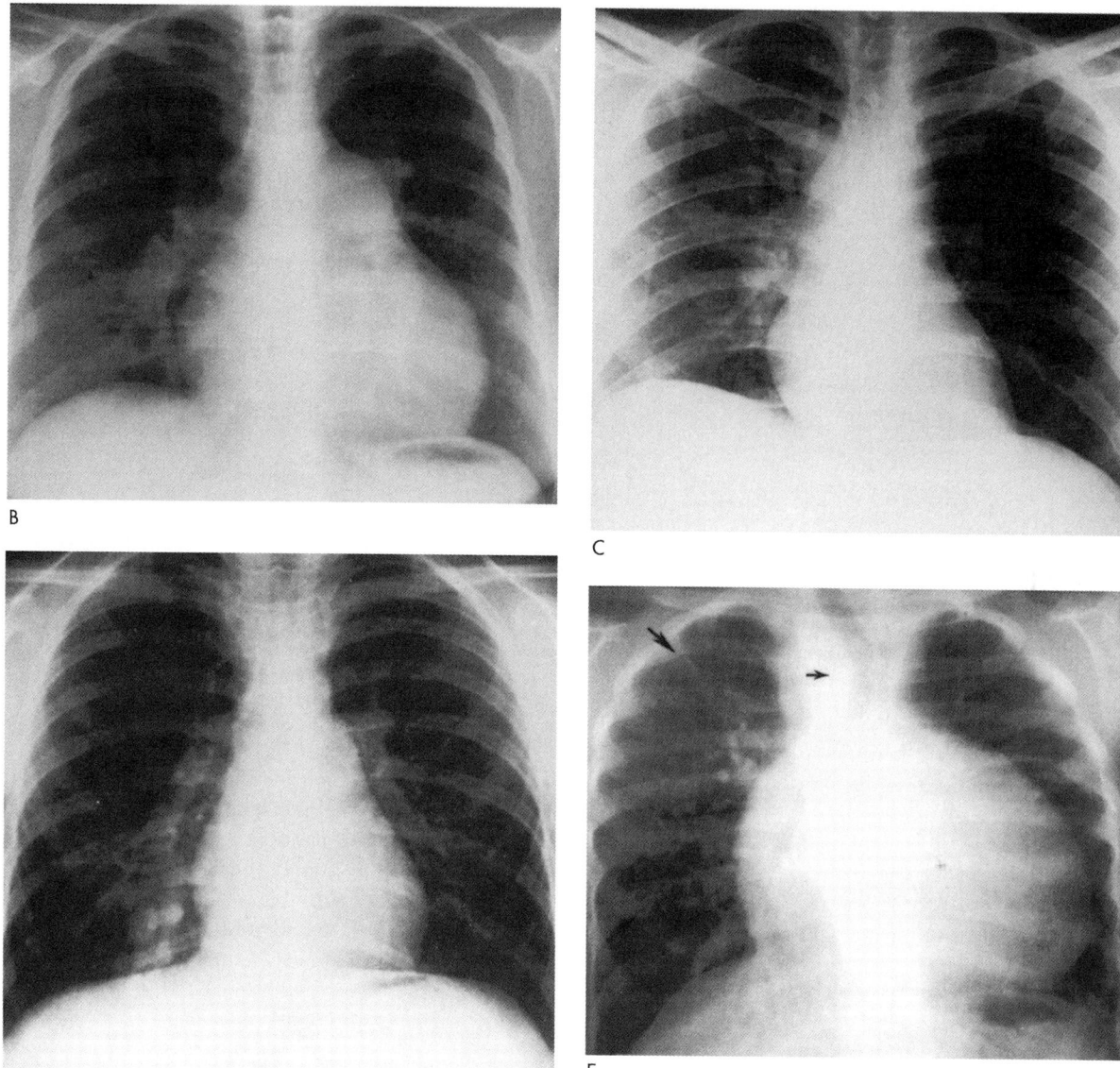

B

C

D

E

FIGURE 15–3. *(continued)*

of the pericardium (Fig. 15–10), (2) pneumopericardium (Fig. 15–11), and (3) pneumomediastinum. Pneumomediastinum is differentiated from pneumopericardium by the fact that the former shows a superior extension of the air strip beyond the confines of the pericardium.

【 】 CARDIAC MALPOSITIONS

Cardiac malpositions are diagnosed only when either the heart or the stomach is out of the normal left-sided position. This definition is crucial in distinguishing an isolated right-sided aortic arch from a cardiac malposition.[7,8]

Dextrocardia with Situs Inversus

Recently the term *dextrocardia* has been used to indicate any congenital right-sided heart regardless of the position of abdominal viscera. *Dextrocardia with situs inversus* indicates the mirror image of normal. In this situation, the incidence of congenital heart disease is only 5 percent, a ninefold increase over the general popula-

---

TABLE 15–2

Major Steps of Roentgenologic Examination

Roentgenographic examination for anatomy
  Overview, e.g., rib notching
  Pulmonary vascularity, e.g., shunt vascularity in ASD
  Lung parenchyma, e.g., ossification in critical MS
  Cardiac size, e.g., huge right heart in Ebstein anomaly
  Cardiac contour, e.g., boot-shaped heart in TOF
  Abnormal densities, e.g., calcification of LV aneurysm
  Abnormal lucency, e.g., conspicuous fat stripes in PE
  Cardiac malpositions, e.g., dextrocardia with SS
  Other abnormalities, e.g., Holt-Oram syndrome
Fluoroscopic observation for dynamics
Comparison of serial studies
Statistical guidance
Clinical correlation
Conclusion

ASD, atrial septal defect; MS, mitral stenosis; TOF, tetralogy of Fallot; LV, left ventricle; PE, pericardial effusion; SS, situs solitus.

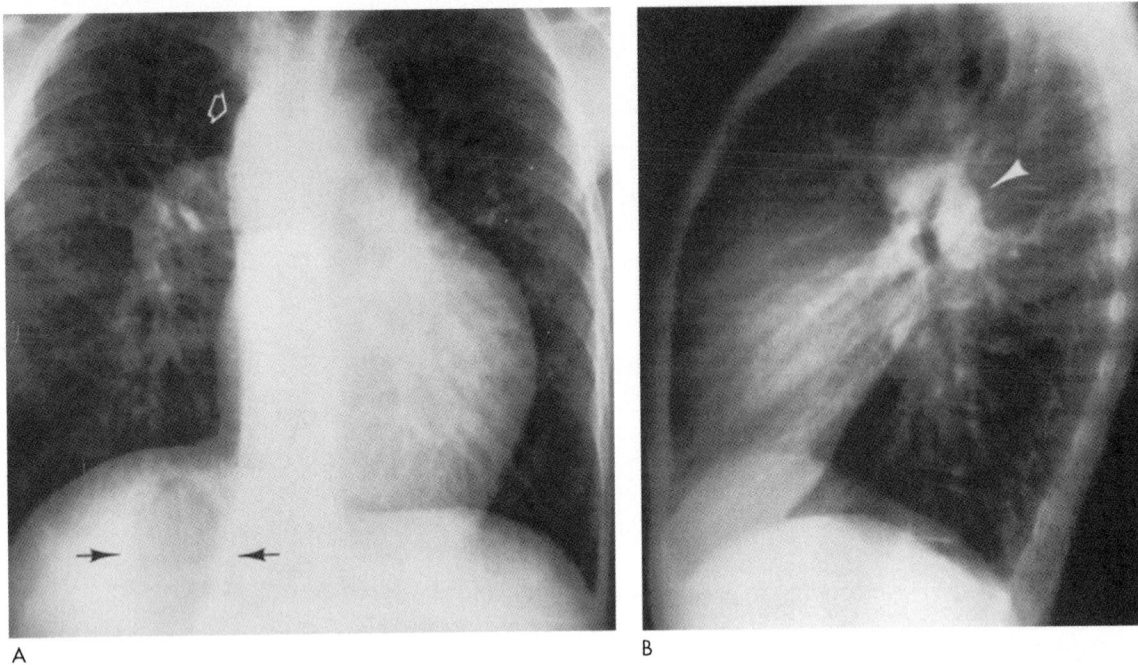

FIGURE 15–4. Patient with situs ambiguus, interruption of the inferior vena cava, ventricular septal defect, and polysplenia. **A.** Posteroanterior (PA) view shows that the aortic arch and the heart are left-sided, and the stomach (*lower arrows*) is right-sided. The azygos vein (*upper arrow*) is markedly enlarged. The heart is mildly enlarged, and there is a moderate increase in pulmonary vascularity. **B.** Lateral view shows an absent image of the inferior vena cava. The azygos arch (*arrow*) is markedly dilated.

tion. The combination of dextrocardia, sinusitis, and bronchiectasis is known as *Kartagener triad*.

Dextrocardia with Situs Solitus

This represents an anomaly with normal situs but a right-sided heart. Radiographically, normal situs (situs solitus) is a certainty when both the aortic knob and the gastric air bubble are on the left side. *Situs solitus* also means that both the abdominal viscera and the atria are in the normal position. Under these circumstances, if the ventricles fail to swing from the primitive right-sided position to the normal left-sided position, abnormal relationships between the ventricles and the rest of the cardiovascular structures are bound to develop. This entity was formerly termed *dextroversion*.

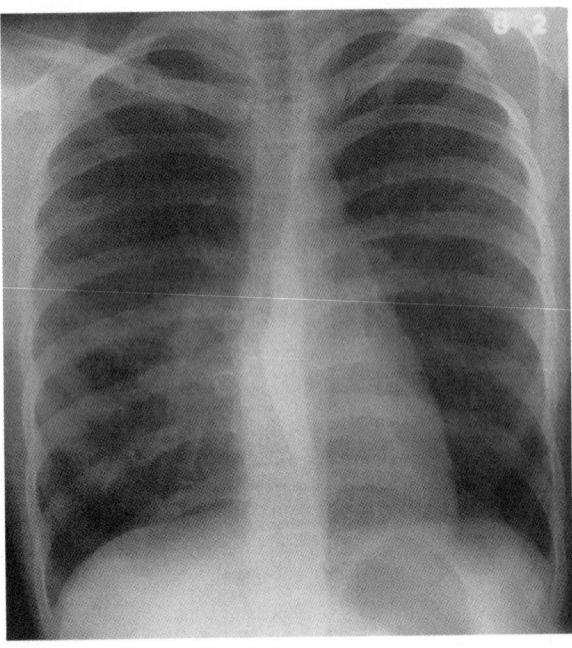
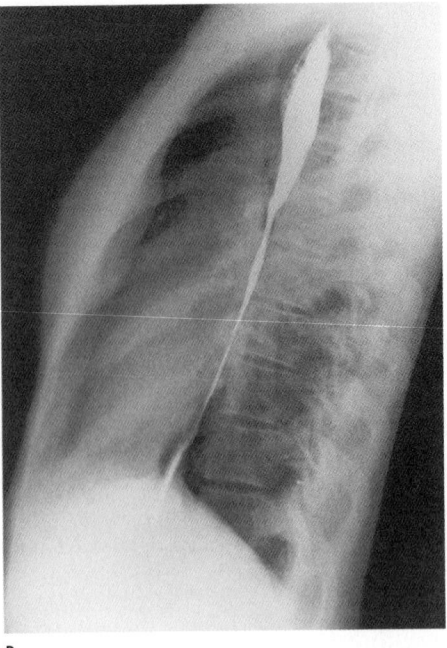

FIGURE 15–5. A 16-year-old girl with straight-back syndrome. **A.** Posteroanterior (PA) radiograph shows normal pulmonary vascularity and normal heart size. Note leftward displacement and rotation of the heart, making its left border unusually prominent. **B.** Lateral view shows that the anteroposterior (AP) diameter of the chest is extremely narrow. The heart is squeezed, creating an innocent murmur.

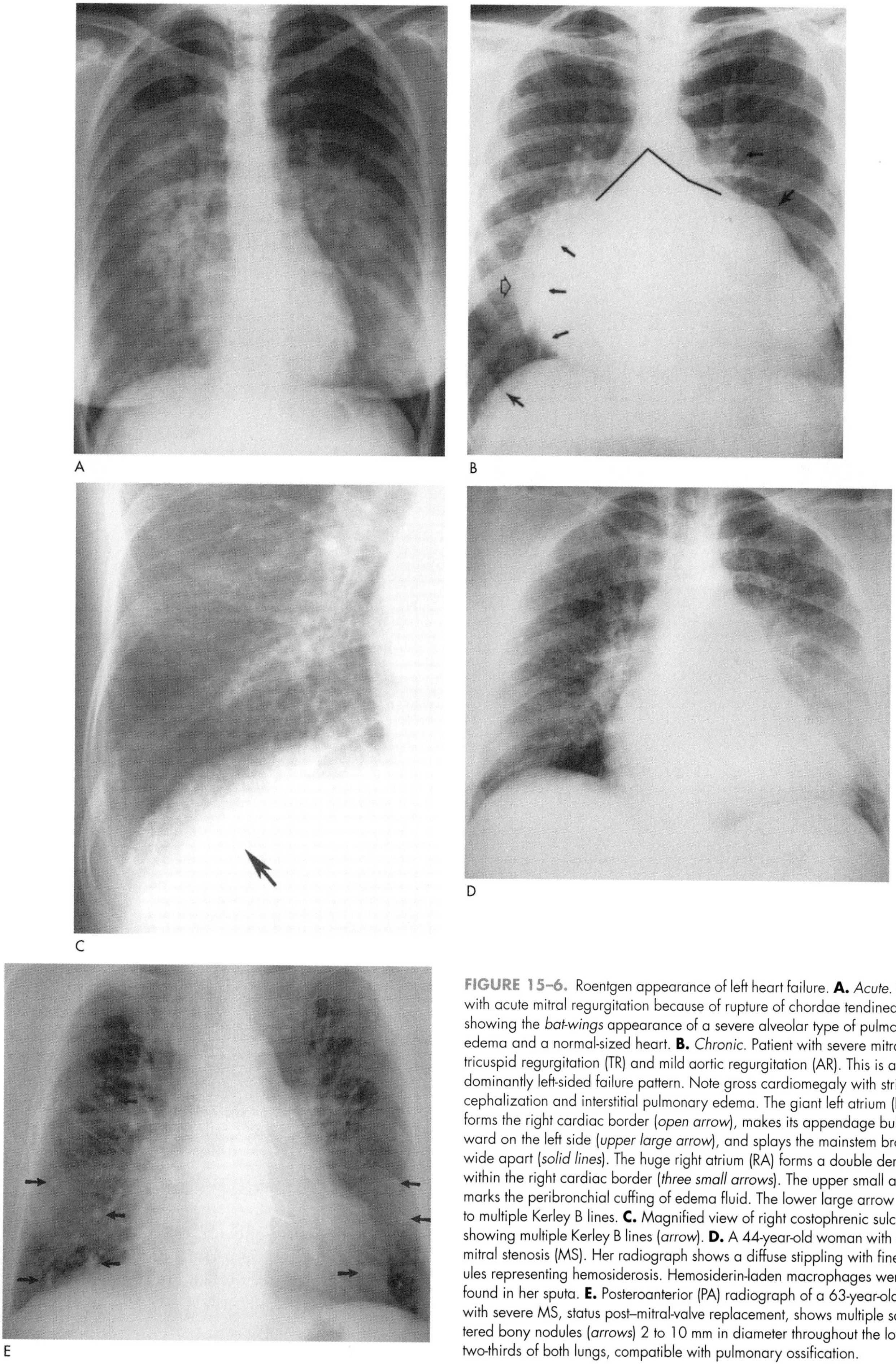

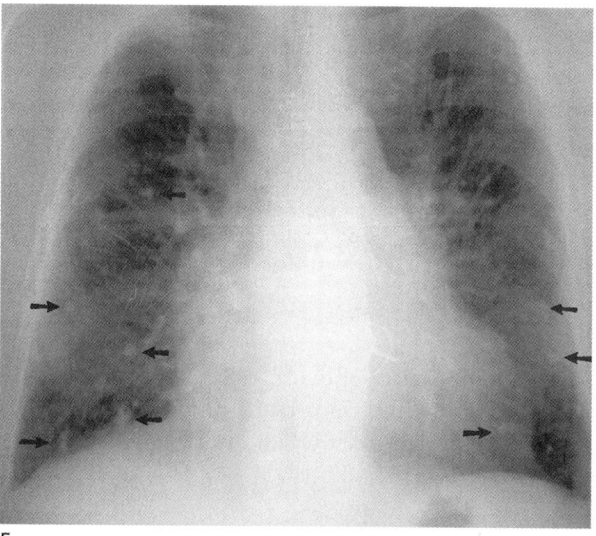

FIGURE 15–6. Roentgen appearance of left heart failure. **A.** *Acute.* Patient with acute mitral regurgitation because of rupture of chordae tendineae showing the *bat-wings* appearance of a severe alveolar type of pulmonary edema and a normal-sized heart. **B.** *Chronic.* Patient with severe mitral and tricuspid regurgitation (TR) and mild aortic regurgitation (AR). This is a predominantly left-sided failure pattern. Note gross cardiomegaly with striking cephalization and interstitial pulmonary edema. The giant left atrium (LA) forms the right cardiac border (*open arrow*), makes its appendage bulge outward on the left side (*upper large arrow*), and splays the mainstem bronchi wide apart (*solid lines*). The huge right atrium (RA) forms a double density within the right cardiac border (*three small arrows*). The upper small arrow marks the peribronchial cuffing of edema fluid. The lower large arrow points to multiple Kerley B lines. **C.** Magnified view of right costophrenic sulcus showing multiple Kerley B lines (*arrow*). **D.** A 44-year-old woman with severe mitral stenosis (MS). Her radiograph shows a diffuse stippling with fine nodules representing hemosiderosis. Hemosiderin-laden macrophages were found in her sputa. **E.** Posteroanterior (PA) radiograph of a 63-year-old man with severe MS, status post–mitral-valve replacement, shows multiple scattered bony nodules (*arrows*) 2 to 10 mm in diameter throughout the lower two-thirds of both lungs, compatible with pulmonary ossification.

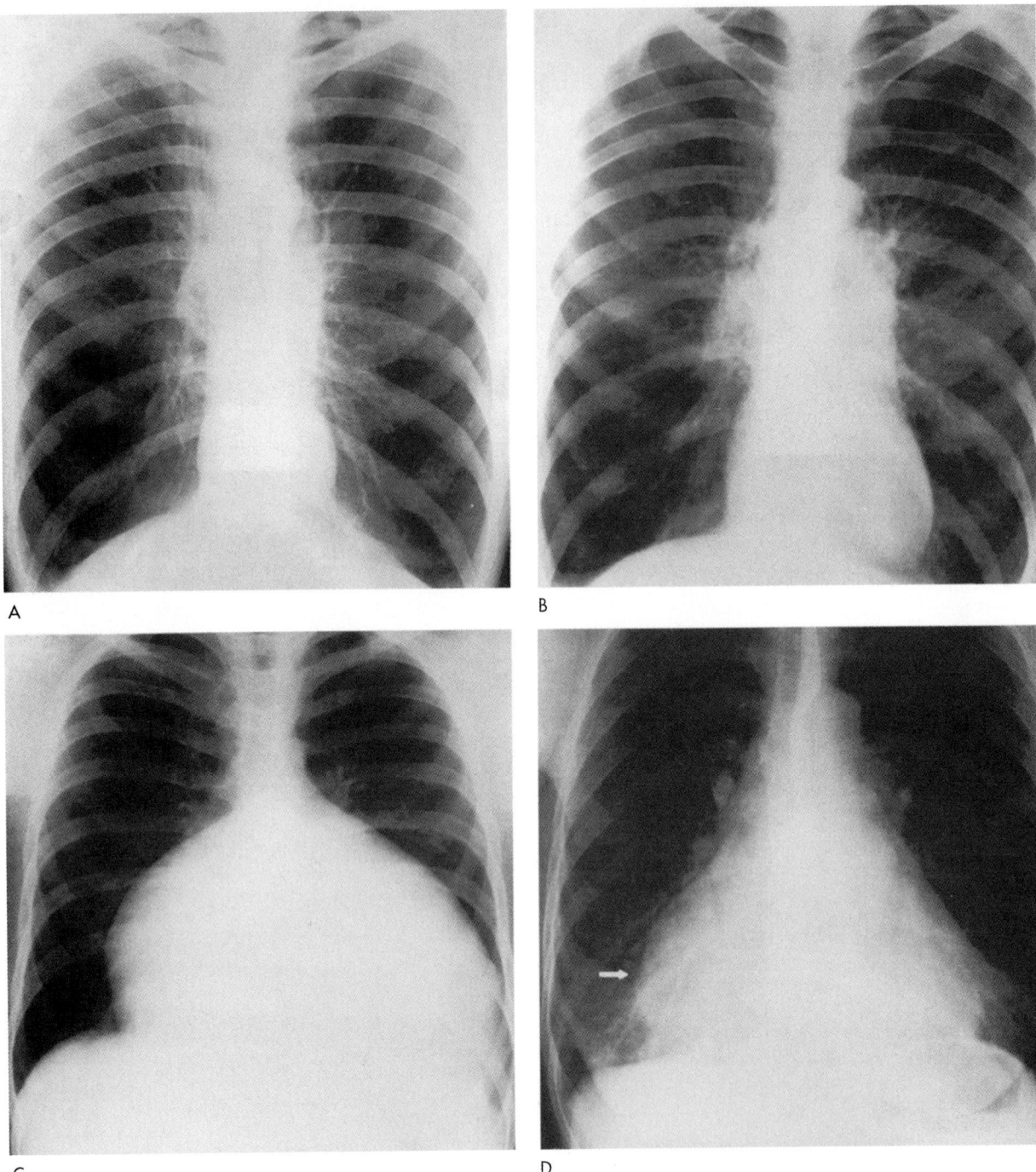

A

B

C

D

FIGURE 15–7. Roentgen appearance of right heart failure. **A.** Patient with severe obstructive emphysema showing overaeration of the lungs, centralized flow pattern, and a small heart size. **B.** Three years later, the patient was in frank right heart failure. Note that the heart got bigger as his emphysema got worse. The centralized flow pattern became more severe. **C.** Patient with Ebstein anomaly showing gross cardiomegaly with severe decrease in pulmonary vascularity. The right cardiac border represents the huge right atrium (RA), and the left cardiac border represents the giant right ventricle. **D.** Patient with mitral stenosis (MS) showing a giant RA (*arrow*) representing severe functional tricuspid regurgitation (TR) caused by unrelenting left-sided failure. The pulmonary venous congestion had improved following the onset of right-sided heart failure.

In patients with dextroversion, the incidence of congenital heart disease has been estimated at 98 percent. More than 80 percent have congenitally corrected (or L loop) transposition of great arteries. The next most commonly associated lesions are a combination of ventricular septal defect and pulmonary stenosis, a tetralogy-like pathophysiology (Fig. 15–12).

Levocardia with Situs Inversus

This is a mirror image of dextroversion, and it is associated with nearly a 100 percent incidence of cyanotic congenital cardiac lesions similar to those seen in dextroversion. This entity was formerly termed *levoversion*.

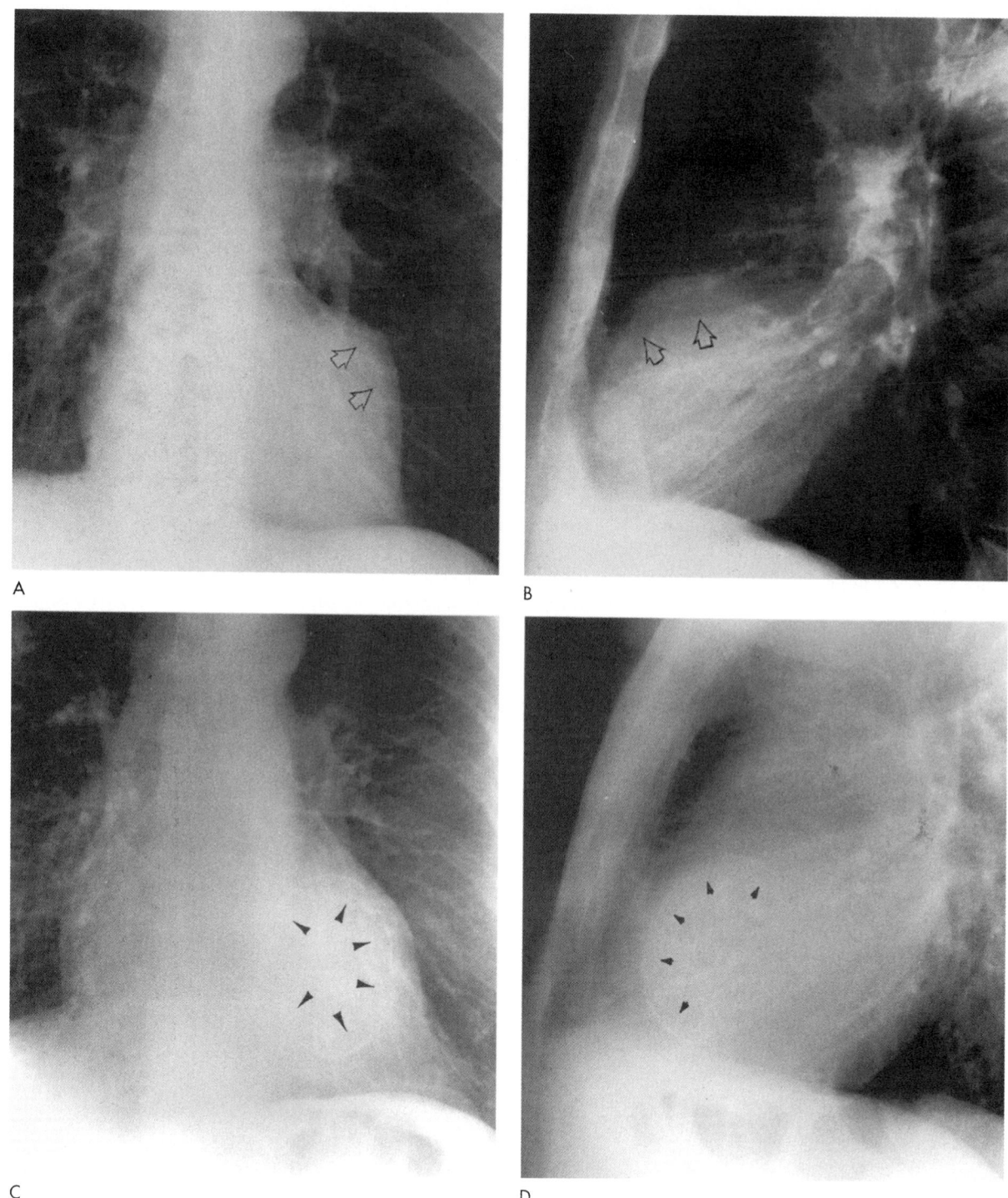

FIGURE 15–8. Left ventricular aneurysms. **A.** Posteroanterior (PA) view of patient 1 shows a localized bulge (*arrows*) along the left cardiac border representing a left ventricular aneurysm from the anterolateral wall. **B.** Lateral view shows a double density with sharp borders anteriorly and superiorly (*arrows*). This is the left ventricular aneurysm that casts a shadow on the normal right ventricle. Fluoroscopically, it is easy to confirm its origin and to separate it from the right ventricle by rotating the patient under direct vision. **C.** PA view of patient 2, a 69-year-old man, shows total calcification of an anterolateral apical left ventricular aneurysm (*arrows*). **D.** Lateral view shows the same (*arrows*).

Levocardia with Situs Solitus

This is entirely normal.

Cardiac Malpositions with Situs Ambiguus

In this group, the patient's heart can be either left- or right-sided. The site is ambiguous because the aortic arch and the stomach are not on the same side. Under these circumstances, we are dealing with either asplenia or polysplenia syndrome. Patients with polysplenia syndrome tend to be acyanotic and frequently survive into adulthood. The associated lesions are bilateral left-sidedness, interruption of the inferior vena cava with azygos continuation (see Fig. 15–4), polysplenia, and a left-to-right shunt, most frequently an atrioventricular septal defect.

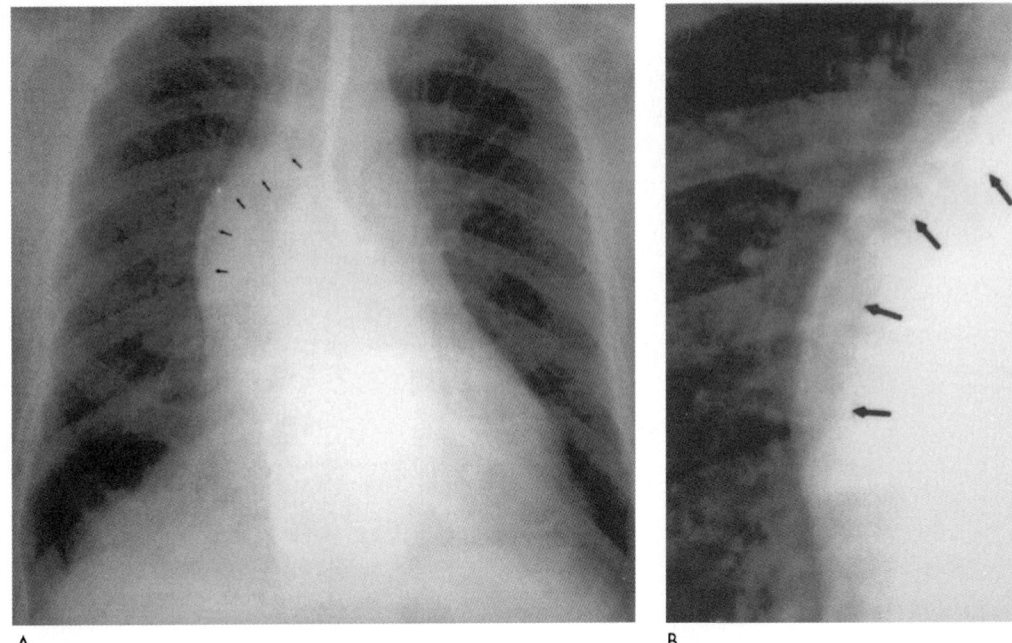

FIGURE 15–9. A 71-year-old woman with syphilitic aortitis. Her posteroanterior (PA) radiograph (**A**) shows a huge, calcified ascending aortic aneurysm (*arrows*). In addition, the entire aorta and the left ventricle are markedly dilated, compatible with severe aortic regurgitation (AR). A magnified view of the ascending aorta (**B**) shows the calcified aneurysm to better advantage. *Source: Chen.*[15] *With permission.*

Patients with asplenia tend to be cyanotic and critically ill; they die in infancy.

[ ] OTHER ABNORMALITIES

Great Vessels

The roentgen appearance of the great vessels often provides valuable information for the diagnosis of heart disease.[2,3,16,17] For example, selective dilatation of the ascending aorta is the hallmark of valvular AS (Fig. 15–13); whereas generalized dilatation of the entire thoracic aorta (Fig. 15–14) suggests AR, systemic hypertension, or both, depending on the size of the left ventricle. In

atrial septal defect and MS, the pulmonary trunk is quite large, and the aortic knob is usually small (see Fig. 15–2B). A leftward cardiac rotation occurs when an enlarged RV coexists with a normal-sized left ventricle. When the heart rotates to the left, the aorta folds on itself in the midline and becomes inconspicuous. Meanwhile, the pulmonary trunk is brought laterally and looks larger than it actually is. Aortic aneurysm (Fig. 15–15) and dissection are frequently associated with hypertensive and atherosclerotic disease.

Prominence of the pulmonary trunk is a reliable secondary sign of right ventricular (RV) enlargement (Fig. 15–16; see also Fig. 15–2B), with the following exceptions: (1) tetralogy of Fallot with

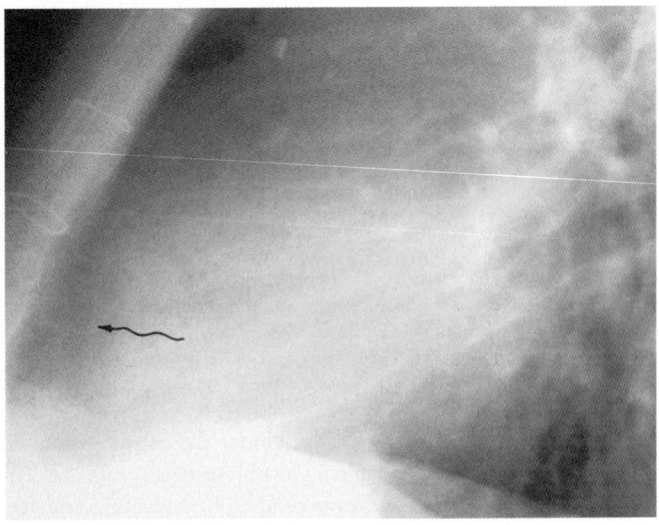

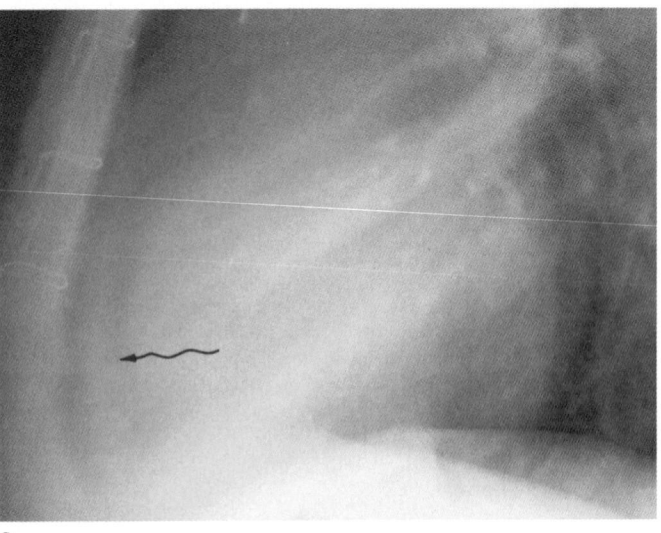

FIGURE 15–10. Developing pericardial effusion in 2 weeks. **A.** A magnified view of the retrosternal area showing the hairlike normal pericardium (*arrow*) sandwiched between the subepicardial fat stripe interiorly and the mediastinal fat stripe exteriorly. The maximal width of normal pericardium is 2 mm. **B.** The same patient 2 weeks later, with moderate pericardial effusion. The pericardial cavity now measures more than 1 cm in width (*arrow*).

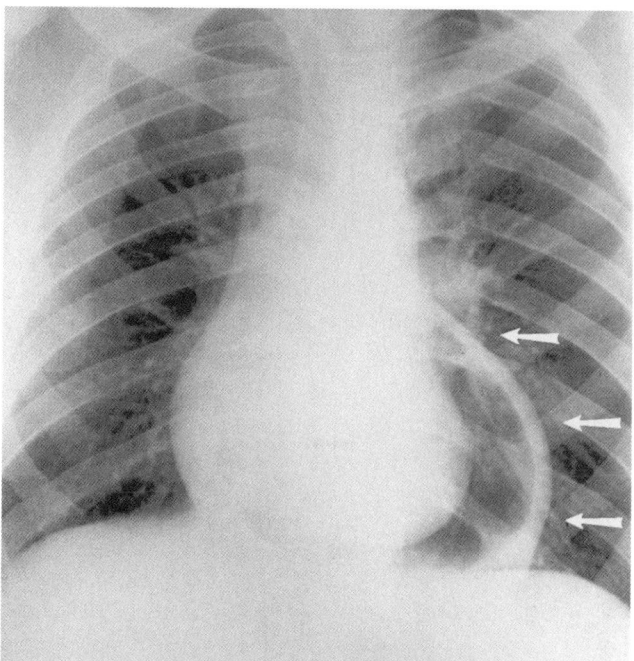

FIGURE 15–11. Traumatic constrictive-effusive pericarditis in a young man. Following emergent pericardiocentesis and injection of air, a radiograph was taken in the supine position. Air is confined to the left side of the pericardium. Note markedly thickened parietal layer (*arrows*).

RV hypertrophy but pulmonary trunk hypoplasia; (2) idiopathic dilatation of the pulmonary artery; (3) patent ductus arteriosus with dilated pulmonary trunk but normal RV; and (4) straight-back syndrome, pectus excavatum, and scoliosis with narrowed AP diameter of the chest. Under the latter conditions, the heart is

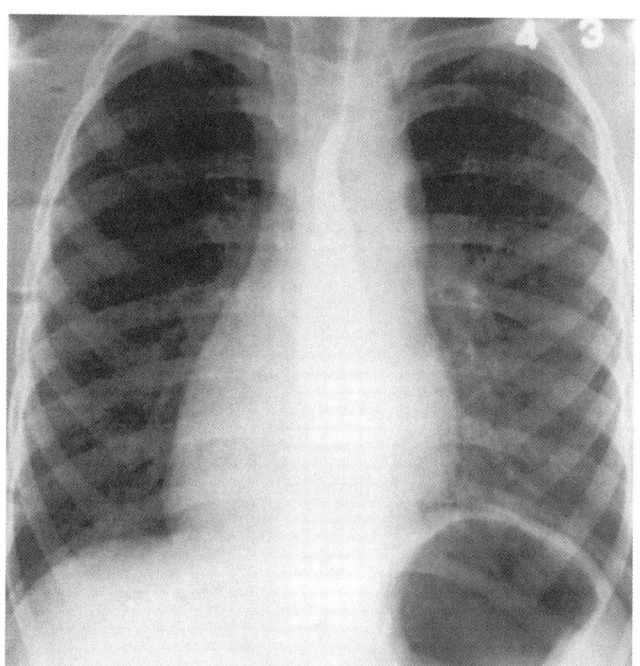

FIGURE 15–12. Posteroanterior (PA) view of a patient with dextrocardia and situs solitus. Note that the aortic arch and the stomach air bubble are both on the left (*situs solitus*) and the apex of the ventricles is pointing to the right inferiorly. According to statistics and proved by cardiac catheterization, this patient had the typical combination of congenitally corrected transposition of the great arteries, ventricular septal defect, and pulmonary stenosis. He was cyanotic. The pulmonary vascularity appears decreased.

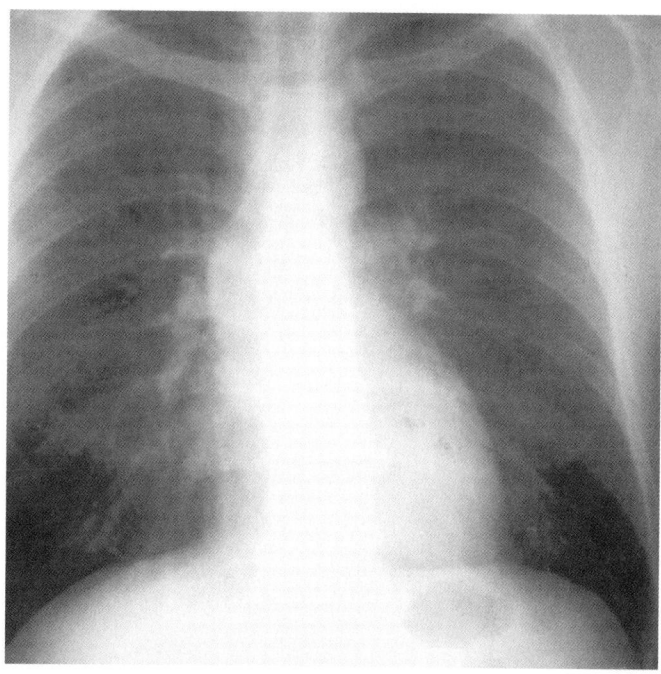

FIGURE 15–13. A 17-year-old boy with congenital aortic valve stenosis. Note dilatation of the ascending aorta, increased convexity of the left ventricle, and normal pulmonary vascularity. The systolic aortic pressure gradient was 100 mmHg.

compressed, displaced, and rotated to the left, giving rise to a falsely enlarged pulmonary artery.

In coarctation of the aorta, the engorged aortic knob and the poststenotic dilatation of the descending aorta can cause a *3 sign* on the aorta and an *E sign* on the barium-filled esophagus, both depicting the site of coarctation[7] (see Fig. 15–1C).

The abnormal size and distribution of both the pulmonary and systemic veins are important clues to the presence of certain conditions—for example, anomalous pulmonary venous connections, pulmonary arteriovenous fistulas, pulmonary varix, persistent left superior vena cava, and interruption of inferior vena cava with azygos continuation (see Fig. 15–4).

Mediastinal Structures

The mediastinal organs are frequently affected by the cardiovascular structures because of their close spatial interrelationships. An enlarged LA not only displaces the esophagus (see Fig. 15–1C to E) and the descending aorta but also elevates and compresses the left mainstem bronchus. A double aortic arch can compress both the trachea and the esophagus. Also, malignant processes can invade the heart and great vessels, causing cardiac tamponade or the superior vena cava syndrome. Usually, these mediastinal changes are evident on the chest roentgenogram and should be recognized promptly.[16–20]

Pleura

A right-sided pleural effusion is often present with left heart failure. A bilateral hydrothorax suggests bilateral heart failure or a noncardiac etiology of the effusion. Congestive heart failure is also known to be associated with a pseudotumor or *vanishing* tumor, representing an interlobar collection of pleural fluid (Fig. 15–17). As congestive heart failure improves, the *tumor* disappears.

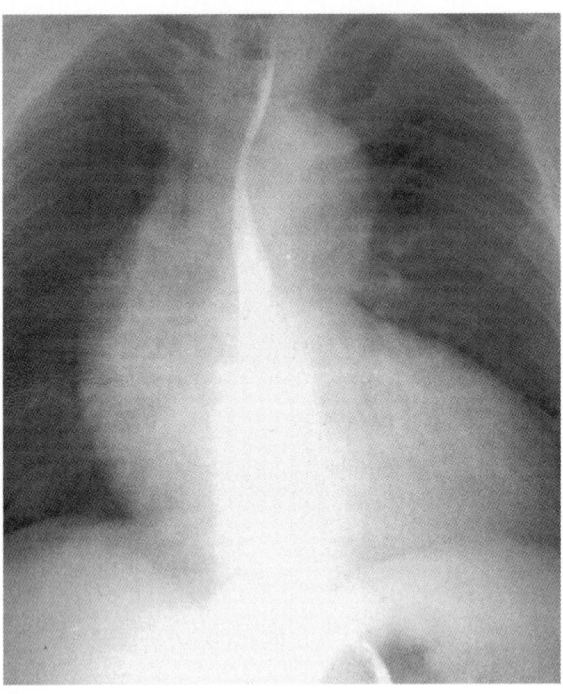
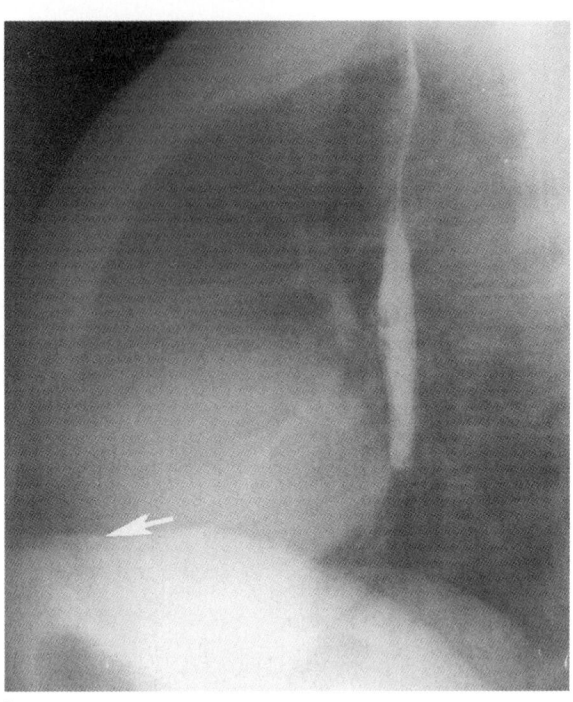

A   B

FIGURE 15–14. A 45-year-old man with Marfan syndrome, severe aortic regurgitation (AR), and proximal aortic dissection into the pericardial cavity. **A.** Posteroanterior (PA) view shows a huge left ventricle and aneurysmal dilatation of the ascending aorta. There is no sign of heart failure. **B.** Lateral view shows a small pericardial effusion (*arrow*).

Bones and Joints

Notching of the ribs has many origins. Basically, any of the three major intercostal structures can enlarge, compress, and erode the lower borders of the ribs, producing areas of notching. They are intercostal arteries, veins, and nerves. Coarctation of the aorta[7] (see Fig. 15–1A) represents the most common cause of rib notching as a result of dynamic dilatation and tortuosity of the arteries. Superior vena cava syndrome can cause a similar phenomenon of venous origin. Neurofibromatosis also can produce rib notching by numerous intercostal tumors.

Soft Tissues over the Chest

Patients with renal failure can show severe edema in the soft tissues over the chest as part of the picture of general anasarca (Fig. 15–18).

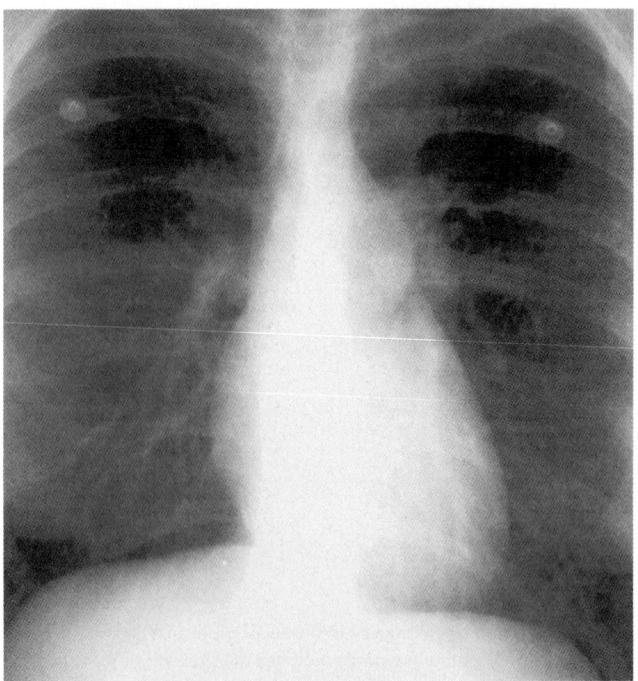

FIGURE 15–16. A 37-year-old woman with congenital valvular pulmonary stenosis. Note enlarged pulmonary trunk and left pulmonary artery versus diminished right pulmonary artery. Also note increased pulmonary blood flow on the left side and decreased pulmonary blood flow on the right side.

FIGURE 15–15. PA view of a 77-year-old man shows a huge descending aortic aneurysm (*arrows*).

Extrathoracic Structures

In Holt-Oram syndrome (Fig. 15–19 and see Chap. 12), the upper extremity abnormalities can be evident in a chest roentgenogram or on other films in the patient's radiograph folder (see Chap. 72). A large arteriovenous malformation with curvilinear calcifications may be seen in the neck, thereby providing a clue as to the etiology of the patient's heart failure.[8,9]

COMPARISON OF SERIAL STUDIES

To appreciate the acuteness or chronicity of the disease or its response to therapy, one must carefully compare serial roentgenograms. As demonstrated in Fig. 15–7B, the heart can be considered neither enlarged nor failing if the baseline study made 3 years earlier in Fig. 15–7A were not available for comparison. Similarly, an enlarging heart with normal pulmonary vascularity is highly suggestive of pericardial effusion. Conversely, a shrinking heart in the presence of normal vascularity is compatible with resolution of a pericardial effusion (Figs. 15–20A,B).

STATISTICAL GUIDANCE

Certain roentgenologic findings are diagnostic of a disease; other signs are suggestive of a diagnosis on the basis of statistics only. Nevertheless, the latter can be quite useful by virtue of their high predictive value of a particular disease or a group of similar diseases. The incidence of congenital heart disease in patients with a right-sided aortic arch increases 10- to 100-fold depending on the anatomic details of the anomaly.[18,19] There are only two types of right-sided aortic arch. The first has been called the *avian type*, implying a normal status for birds but a detrimental one for humans. The overwhelming majority of patients with this type are born with cyanotic congenital heart disease. The second can be called the *common type* because of its higher incidence in the general

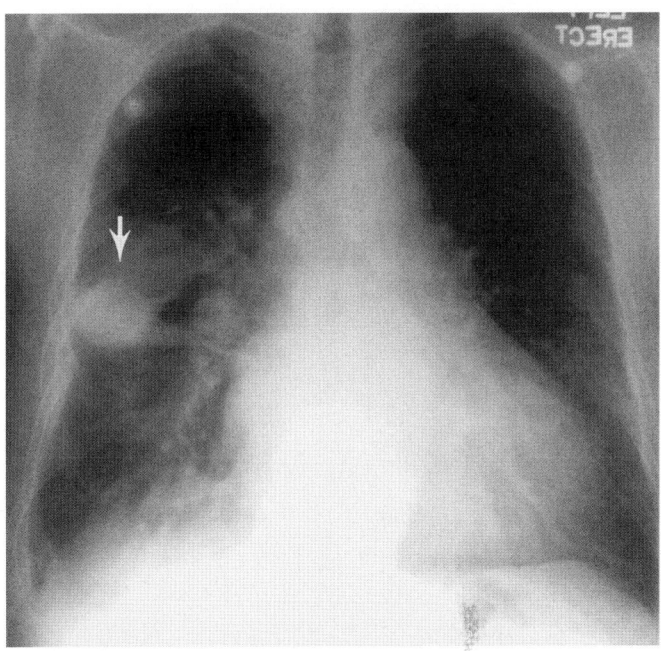

FIGURE 15–17. Patient with congestive heart failure. Note gross cardiomegaly, cephalization, interstitial pulmonary edema, and right-sided pleural effusion. Some of the fluid was loculated in the minor interlobar fissure (*arrow*), which disappeared with improved cardiac function.

population. Most patients with the common type are physiologically normal and have their anomaly incidentally diagnosed on chest radiographs or a barium meal study. The radiographic findings of the two types are similar in the PA view but quite different in the lateral view (Fig. 15–21). The incidence and list of congenital heart diseases with each type[19] are shown in Table 15–3. Only 2 percent of patients with the avian type are physiologically normal. Tetralogy of Fallot should be the diagnosis in these patients until proved otherwise.[18,19]

Patients with a double aortic arch rarely have congenital heart disease, although they tend to be symptomatic in infancy because of a compressing vascular ring.[19]

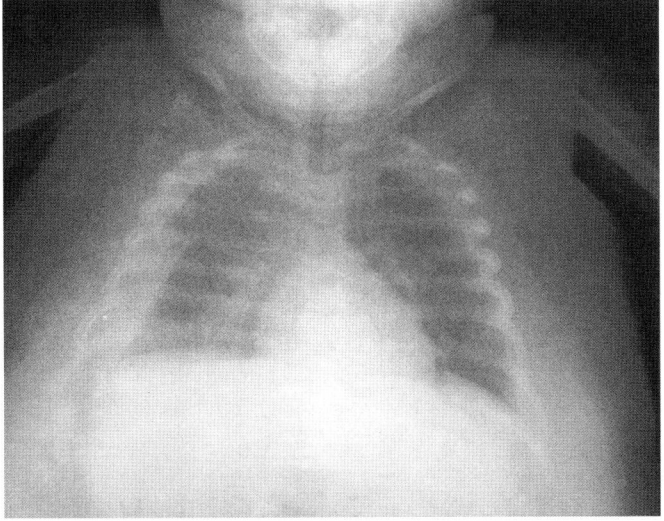

A

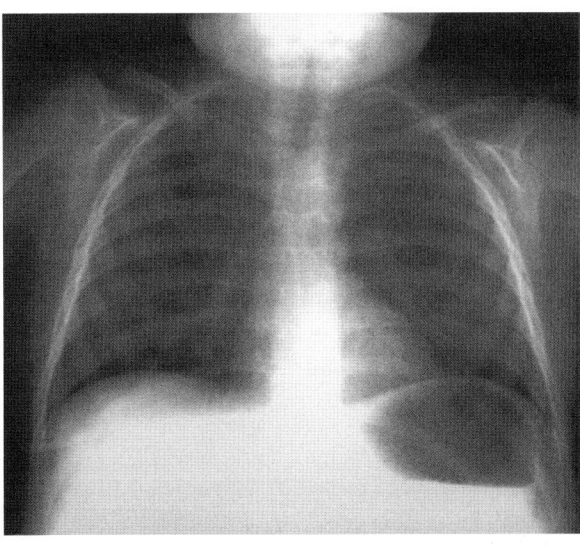

B

FIGURE 15–18. A child suffering from nephrotic syndrome, which was treated successfully. **A.** Posteroanterior (PA) view during the worst period of his disease shows general anasarca, pulmonary edema, and pleural effusion. Note considerable soft tissue edema in the chest wall. **B.** With proper treatment, everything returned to normal in 2 weeks.

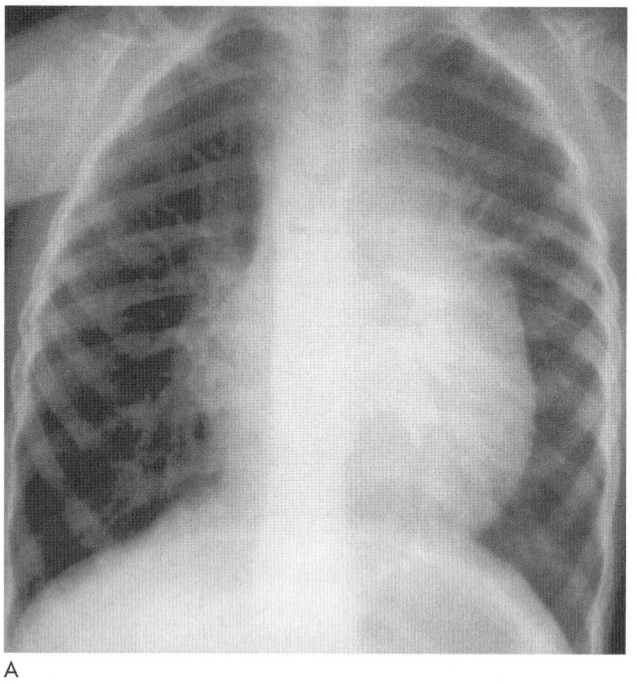

A

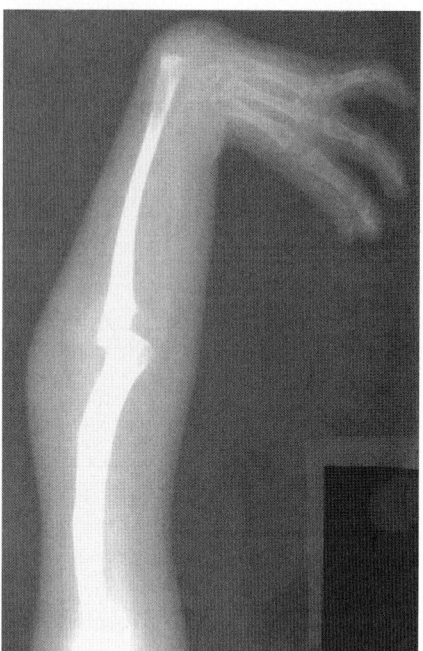

B

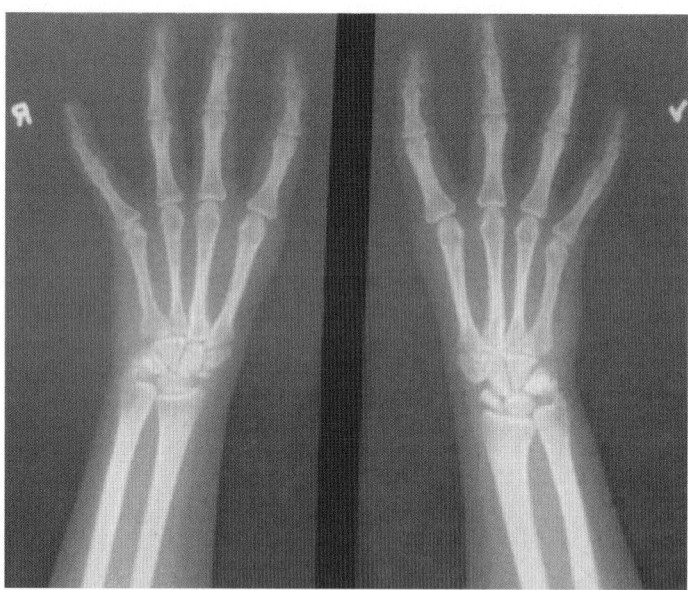

C

FIGURE 15–19. Patients with Holt-Oram syndrome. **A.** Posteroanterior (PA) view of patient 1, a 7-year-old girl, shows a globular cardiac contour with increased pulmonary blood flow. The aortic arch is on the right side. Catheterization diagnosis: secundum atrial septal defect. **B.** Her left arm shows absent radius and thumb with radial clubhand. Her right arm is a mirror image of the left (not shown). **C.** Forearms of patient 2, a 33-year-old woman with secundum atrial septal defect, show bilateral absence of thumb.

CLINICAL CORRELATION

The roentgenologic findings must be correlated with the clinical information and other laboratory parameters for a final conclusion. It can become necessary at this point to reexamine the radiograph or review the fluoroscopic observation or both. After detailed analysis of some finer points, a wrong impression can be corrected or a correct diagnosis reinforced[1] (see Table 15–2).

PULMONARY VASCULARITY

【 】 NORMAL

The normal roentgen appearance of the pulmonary vasculature of an upright human being is typified by a caudal flow pattern because of gravity. The pressure differential between the apex and the base of the lung is approximately 22 mmHg in adults in the upright position.[2,21] Therefore, more flow under higher distending pressure is expected in the lower-lobe vessels than in the upper. Normally, one sees very little vascularity above the hilum, whereas more and larger vessels are found below the hilum. Because the pulmonary resistance is normal, all vessels taper gradually in a tree-like manner from the hilum toward the periphery of the lung. The right descending pulmonary artery measures 10 to 15 mm in diameter in males and 9 to 14 mm in females[1,22] (see Fig. 15–2).

【 】 ABNORMAL

Abnormal pulmonary vascularity can be classified into two categories, either in terms of volume or in terms of distribution[2,11,23] (see Table 15–3).

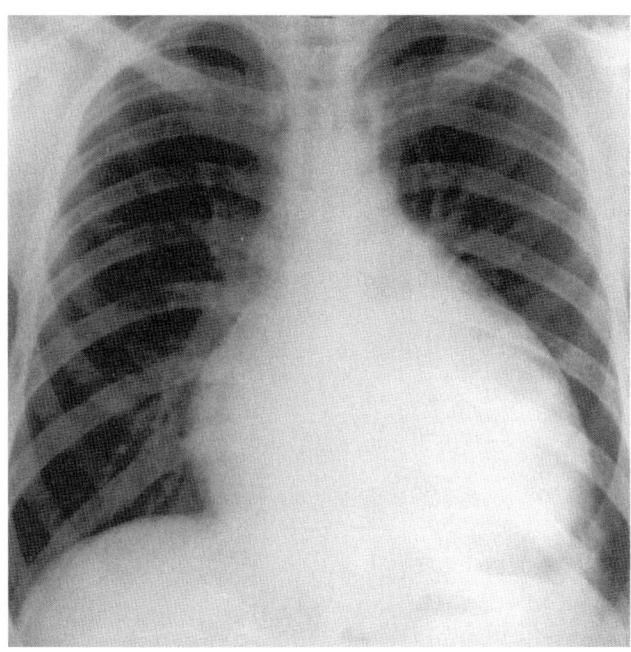
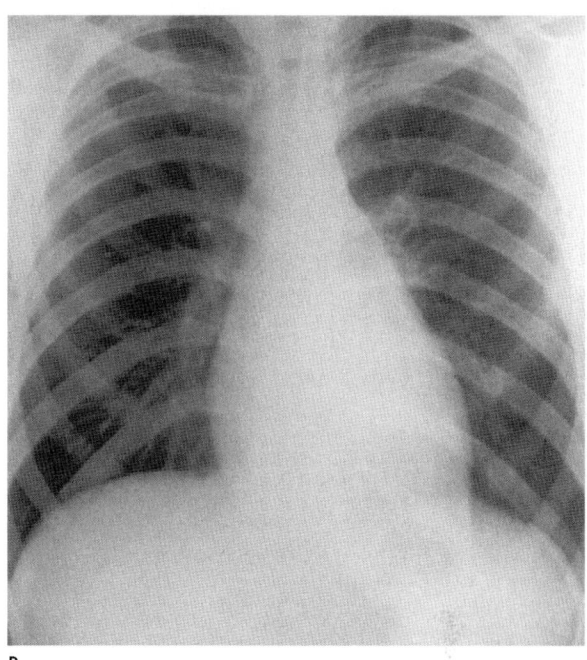

A   B

FIGURE 15–20. A young man with acute pericarditis with effusion. **A.** Posteroanterior (PA) view shows a water bottle–shaped cardiomegaly, clear lungs, and normal pulmonary vascularity. **B.** Repeat film taken 5 days later shows excellent response to therapy.

【 】 ABNORMALITIES IN VOLUME

In the evaluation of pulmonary vasculature, the caliber of the vessels is more important than the length or the number. As long as the PBF pattern remains normal, with a greater amount of flow to the bases than to the apices, the volume of the flow is proportional to the caliber of the pulmonary arteries (see Fig. 15–2). Besides measuring the

TABLE 15–3
Pulmonary Vascularity

Normal
  Caudal PBF pattern in upright position (PBF controlled by gravity)
  Gradual branching, treelike
  RDPA = 10–15 mm in males
  RDPA = 9–14 mm in females
  A/B ratio = 1
Abnormal
  Volume with normal PBF pattern (distribution)
    Increased, larger vessels, e.g., ASD
    Decreased, smaller vessels, e.g., TOF
  Distribution with abnormal PBF pattern
    Cephalic, e.g., MS
    Centralized, e.g., Eisenmenger syndrome
    Lateralized, e.g., Westermark sign
    Localized, e.g., pulmonary AV fistulas
    Collateralized, e.g., severe TOF
Combined
  Decreased volume and cephalization, e.g., critical MS
  Lateralization and localization, e.g., Scimitar syndrome

A/B, artery/bronchus; ASD, atrial septal defect; AV, arteriovenous; MS, mitral stenosis; PBF, pulmonary blood flow; RDPA, right descending pulmonary artery; TOF, tetralogy of Fallot.

right descending pulmonary artery, pulmonary blood volume can be assessed by comparing the size of the pulmonary artery with that of the accompanying bronchus where they are viewed on end. Normally, the two structures have approximately equal diameters.[2,24] When the artery-bronchus ratio is greater than unity, increased blood flow is suggested. Conversely, when the ratio is smaller than unity (see Fig. 15–2), decreased flow is likely.

Increased Pulmonary Blood Flow

In the case of mild to moderate left-to-right shunts, for example, the vessels dilate in proportion to the increased flow with no significant change in pressure, resistance, or flow pattern. This phenomenon is also called *shunt vascularity* or *equalization*. Equalization of the PBF between the upper and lower lung zones is only apparent rather than real, however; the lower lobes still receive a great deal more blood than the upper lobes, although the ratio of PBF between the two zones has changed—for example, from 5:1 to 4:1 or 3:1. A mild increase in pulmonary vascularity with slight cardiomegaly is commonly found in pregnant women and trained athletes with increased cardiac output (see Chap. 100).

Decreased Pulmonary Blood Flow

Patients with tetralogy of Fallot frequently show decreased pulmonary vascularity with smaller and shorter pulmonary arteries and veins and more radiolucent lungs (see Fig. 15–2C). Marked reduction in PBF is also encountered in patients with isolated right-sided heart failure without a right-to-left shunt (see Fig. 15–7). This is attributed to the significant decrease in cardiac output from both ventricles.

【 】 ABNORMALITIES IN DISTRIBUTION

An abnormal distribution of PBF (or an abnormal PBF pattern) always reflects a changed pulmonary vascular resistance, either locally or diffusely.

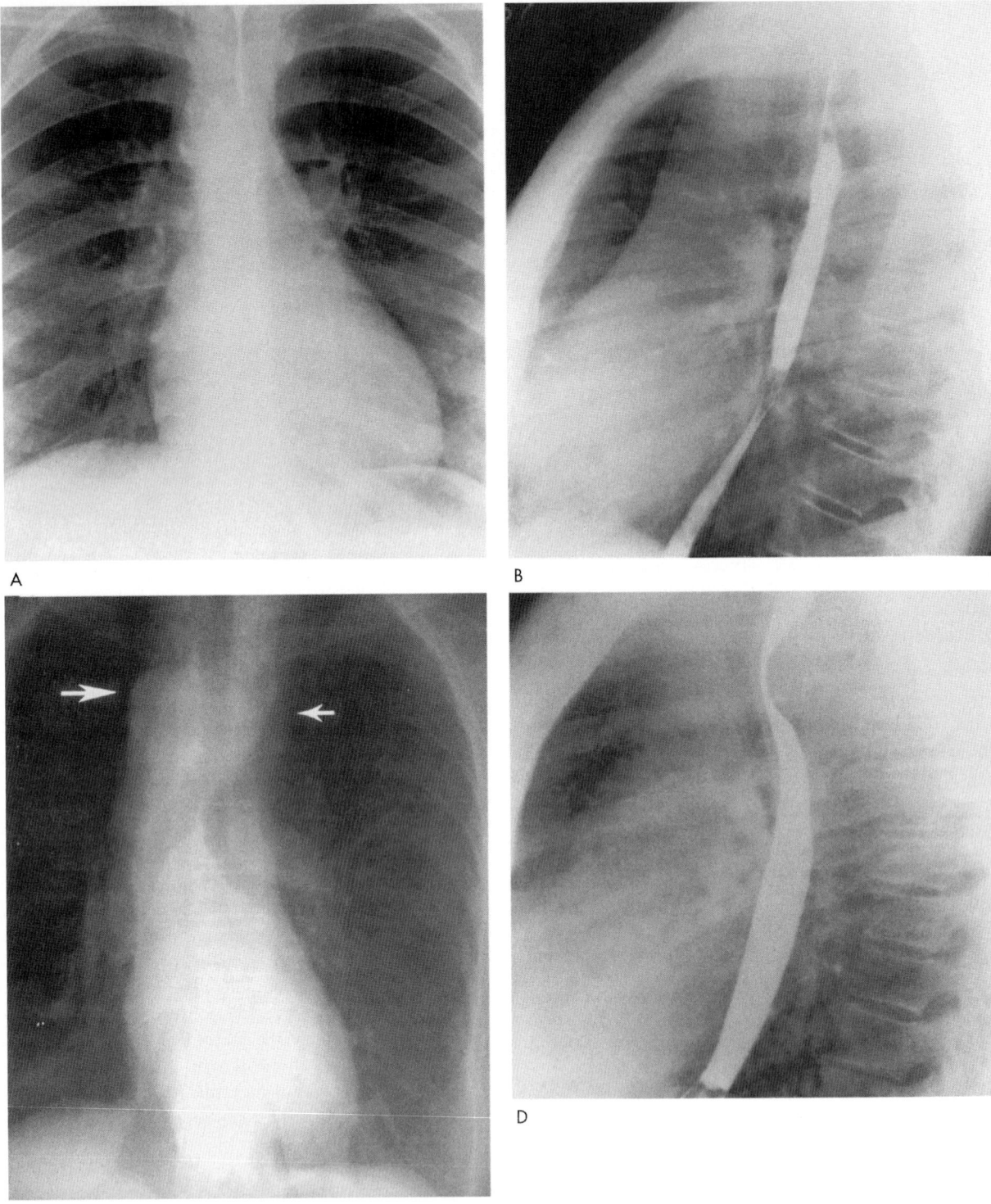

FIGURE 15–21. Statistical guidance focusing on the best diagnostic possibilities. **A.** Posteroanterior (PA) view of a patient with tetralogy of Fallot showing a right aortic arch, avian type. Note that the esophagus and trachea are deviated to the left. The cardiovascular structures are otherwise within normal limits. **B.** Lateral view of the same patient showing the aortic arch normally situated, in front of the trachea and esophagus. **C.** PA radiograph of a healthy woman shows a right aortic arch (*large arrow*) with a large aortic diverticulum (*small arrow*) that protrudes to the left of the midline. The distal segment of the trachea is deviated to the left side by the right arch. Unlike double aortic arch, the left lateral margin of the trachea is not indented because the diverticulum is posterior and not lateral in position. **D.** Lateral view of a similar patient, a healthy man. Note that both the esophagus and the trachea are markedly displaced anteriorly by a huge diverticulum, which invariably gives rise to the aberrant left subclavian artery.

Cephalization

In the presence of postcapillary pulmonary hypertension (PH), physiologic disturbances begin when the total intravascular pressure exceeds the oncotic pressure of the blood. As a result, fluid leaks out of the vessels and collects in the interstitium before filling the alveoli.

Pulmonary edema interferes with gas exchange, resulting in a state of hypoxemia. Alveolar hypoxia has a profound influence on the pulmonary vessels, causing them to constrict. Because there is greater alveolar hypoxia in the lung bases than in the apices, the basilar vessels constrict significantly, forcing the blood to flow upward. This phenomenon actually represents a reversal of the normal PBF pattern: redistribution or cephalization of the pulmonary vascularity.

Cephalization occurs in any of three conditions: (1) left-sided obstructive lesions—for example, MS[22] or AS; (2) LV failure—for example, coronary heart disease or cardiomyopathies; and (3) severe mitral regurgitation (MR) even before pump failure of the left ventricle occurs. It should be emphasized that unless there is obvious *constriction* of the lower-lobe vessels, the diagnosis of cephalization should not be made. Dilatation of the upper-lobe vessels is of secondary importance and can be found without narrowing of the basilar vessels in a number of entities, most noticeably left-to-right shunts.

Centralization

In the presence of precapillary PH, the pulmonary trunk and central pulmonary arteries dilate, whereas the distal pulmonary arteries constrict in a concentric fashion from the periphery of the lung toward the hilum. This phenomenon is called *centralization of the pulmonary vascularity*. It occurs in patients with primary PH, Eisenmenger syndrome, recurrent pulmonary thromboembolic disease, or severe obstructive emphysema (see Fig. 15–7A,B).

Lateralization

Massive unilateral pulmonary embolism can cause a lateralized PBF pattern. Because one major pulmonary artery is obstructed, the blood is forced to flow through the healthy lung only. The paucity of pulmonary vascularity in the diseased lung with the ob-

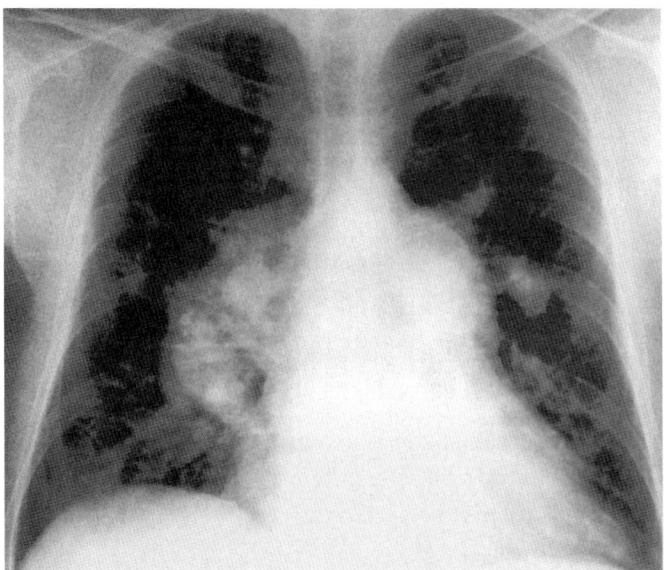

FIGURE 15–22. A 42-year-old man with Eisenmenger atrial septal defect. Note increased pulmonary blood flow with a centralized pattern.

structed pulmonary artery is termed the *Westermark sign* (see Fig. 15–3C). In the case of congenital valvular pulmonary stenosis, a jet effect from the stenotic valve can cause a lateralized PBF pattern in favor of the left side (see Fig. 15–16).

Localization

A localized abnormal flow pattern is exemplified by a congenital pulmonary arteriovenous fistula in a cyanotic child.

Collateralization

Patients with markedly decreased PBF (e.g., severe tetralogy) tend to show numerous small, tortuous bronchial arterial collaterals in the upper medial lung zones near their origin from the descending aorta. The native pulmonary arteries are extremely small, although smooth and gracefully branching.

【 】 COMBINED ABNORMALITIES

In reality, an abnormal pulmonary vascularity is often a mixed type. There is a great variety of possible combinations—for example, cephalization plus decreased flow in severe MS or centralization with increased PBF in Eisenmenger atrial septal defect (Fig. 15–22).

HEART FAILURE

In addition to specific chamber enlargement, the pulmonary vasculature uniquely portrays the underlying pathophysiology of heart failure. In the chronic setting, decreased flow with increased pulmonary lucency is the hallmark of right heart failure (see Fig. 15–7); striking cephalization of the pulmonary vasculature is typical for left-sided decompensation (see Figs. 15–3A and 15–6B).

【 】 LEFT-SIDED

Acute Left-Sided Heart Failure

The pulmonary vascular changes associated with acute LV failure are usually not discernible for two reasons: (1) the resulting severe pulmonary edema obscures the pulmonary vasculature, and (2) the redistribution of PBF secondary to acute left-sided heart failure is usually relatively mild. The combination of alveolar pulmonary edema and a normal-sized heart is the hallmark of acute left-sided heart failure[10] (see Fig. 15–6A). The edema fluid tends to distribute in a butterfly pattern.[24]

Chronic Left-Sided Heart Failure

Chronic left-sided heart failure is characterized by gross cardiomegaly, striking cephalization of the pulmonary vasculature, and interstitial pulmonary edema or fibrosis with multiple distinct Kerley B lines. Pulmonary hemosiderosis, ossification, or both can result from long-standing severe postcapillary PH (Figs. 15–6B to E).

【 】 RIGHT-SIDED

Acute Right-Sided Heart Failure

Acute right-sided heart failure most commonly results from massive pulmonary embolism. The typical radiographic signs are rapidly developing centralization of the pulmonary vasculature and dilatation of the right-sided cardiac chambers and venae cavae. In addition, the lungs can show localized or lateralized oligemia (see Fig. 15–3C). Eventually, opacities in either or both lungs can develop as a result of pulmonary infarction.

Chronic Right-Sided Heart Failure

Chronic right heart failure has many causes. The common ones include congenital pulmonary stenosis, Ebstein anomaly, severe chronic obstructive pulmonary disease, and recurrent pulmonary thromboembolic disease. Diffusely decreased pulmonary vascularity with unusually lucent lungs is seen in patients with right heart failure without PH (see Fig. 15–7C). Centralized PBF pattern is encountered when the right-sided heart failure is secondary to precapillary PH (see Fig. 15–7A,B). A cephalized flow pattern with unusually lucent lungs is found in patients with right-sided heart failure secondary to long-standing severe left heart failure (see Fig. 15–7D). The degree of right-sided chamber enlargement is proportional to the severity of TR.

[ ] COMBINED

Right heart failure is caused most often by severe left heart failure. This is exemplified by patients with severe MS leading to severe TR (see Fig. 15–7D). Other examples of bilateral heart failure are cardiac tamponade and constrictive pericarditis (see Fig. 15–20).

CARDIAC FLUOROSCOPY

Cardiac fluoroscopy explores the dynamic features of the organ that are discernible only in motion.[25] However, it has been largely displaced by other imaging techniques, particularly two-dimensional echocardiography outside the cardiac catheter laboratory.

The normal movements of cardiac valve prostheses are parallel between the two phases of the cardiac cycle. If a significant angle of tilt (more than 12 degrees) is formed between the two phases, instability of the valve with associated regurgitation is nearly always present.[1,24,26,27]

The bileaflet St. Jude valve is used in both mitral and aortic positions. The valve is difficult to see radiographically but is readily detected under the fluoroscope.[1] When the leaflets move sluggishly, thrombotic stenosis of the valve should be suspected. Rarely, one leaflet can dislodge and embolize distally, causing acute valvular regurgitation.[28]

The position of the pacemaker can be determined promptly under the fluoroscope and recorded on film.[1,28] The subepicardial fat line overlies the myocardium and underlies the pericardium. If the pacing catheter is found within the fat stripe, it may have passed through the coronary sinus and entered one of the major cardiac veins. If the tip of the catheter is seen outside the fat stripe, however, it can have perforated the myocardium and thus be lying in the pericardium or beyond.[2] Although the wires and electrodes of a transmediastinal pacemaker can look normal on the films, minor breakage can be appreciated only in ventricular systole with the aid of fluoroscopy.

REFERENCES

1. Chen JTT. *Essentials of Cardiac Imaging.* 2nd ed. Philadelphia: PA. Lippincott-Raven Press; 1997.
2. Chen JTT. The plain radiograph in the diagnosis of cardiovascular disease. In: Putman C, ed. Symposium on cardiopulmonary imaging. *Radiol Clin North Am.* 1983;21:609–621.
3. Juhl JH, Grummy AB. *Essentials of Radiologic Imaging.* 6th ed. Philadelphia, PA: Lippincott; 1993:1065–1138.
4. Meschan I, Formanek A. Roentgenology of the heart inclusive of major vessels. In: Meschan I, ed. *Roentgen Signs in Diagnostic Imaging.* 2nd ed. Philadelphia, PA: Saunders; 1987:784–925.
5. Figley M. Accessory roentgen signs of coarctation of the aorta. *Radiology.* 1954;62:671–686.
6. Durkman W, Vander Belt RJ. The chest x-ray in heart disease. In: Chissner M, ed. *Classic Teachings in Clinical Cardiology.* Washington, DC: Laennec Publishing; 1996:241–258.
7. Elliott LP, Jue KL, Amplatz K. A roentgen classification of cardiac malpositions. *Invest Radiol.* 1966;1:17–28.
8. Elliott LP, Schiebler GL. *X-ray Diagnosis of Congenital Cardiac Disease.* 2nd ed. Springfield, IL: Charles C Thomas; 1979.
9. deLeon AC, Perloff JK, Twigg HL. The straight back syndrome: clinical and cardiovascular manifestations. *Circulation.* 1965;32:193–203.
10. Chen JTT, Capp MP, Johnsrude IS, Goodrich JK, Lester RG. Roentgen appearance of pulmonary vascularity in the diagnosis of heart disease. *AJR Am J Roentgenol.* 1971;112:559–570.
11. Woodley K, Stark P. Pulmonary parenchymal manifestations of mitral valve disease. *Radiographics.* 1999;19:965–972.
12. Margolis JR, Chen JTT, Kong Y, et al. The diagnostic and prognostic significance of coronary artery calcification: a report of 800 cases. *Radiology.* 1980;137:609–616.
13. Applegate KE, Goske MJ, Pierce G, Murphy D. Situs revisited: imaging of the heterotaxy syndrome. *Radiographics.* 1999;19:837–852.
14. Meszaros WT. *Cardiac Roentgenology.* Springfield, IL: Charles C Thomas; 1969.
15. Chen JTT. The significance of cardiac calcifications. *Appl Radiol.* 1992;21:11–19.
16. Cooley RN. *Radiology of the Heart and Great Vessels.* 3rd ed. Baltimore, MD: Williams & Wilkins; 1978.
17. Swischuck LE. *Plain Film Interpretation in Congenital Heart Disease.* 2nd ed. Baltimore, MD: Williams & Wilkins; 1979.
18. Shuford WH, Sybers RG. *The Aortic Arch and Its Malformations.* Springfield, IL: Charles C Thomas; 1974:18.
19. Stewart JR, Kincaid OW, Titus JL. Right aortic arch: plain film diagnosis and significance. *AJR Am J Roentgenol.* 1966;97:377–389.
20. Fraser RG, Pare JAP, Pare PD, et al. Factors influencing pulmonary circulation. In: Fraser RG, Pare JAP, Pare PD, et al, eds. *Diagnosis of Diseases of the Chest.* 3rd ed. Vol I. Philadelphia, PA: Saunders; 1988:128–129.
21. Chen JTT, Behar VS, Morris JJ, et al. Correlation of roentgen findings with hemodynamic data in pure mitral stenosis. *AJR Am J Roentgenol.* 1968;102:280–292.
22. Milne ENC, Pistolesi M. *Reading the Chest Radiograph: A Physiologic Approach.* St. Louis, MI: Mosby; 1993:164–241,343–369.
23. Wojtowicz J. Some tomographic criteria for an evaluation of the pulmonary circulation. *Acta Radiol Diagn (Stockh).* 1964;2:215–224.
24. Chen JTT. Cardiac fluoroscopy. In: Kelley MJ, ed. Symposium on chest radiography for the cardiologist. *Cardiol Clin.* 1983;1:565–573.
25. Jeffers K, Rees S, eds. *Clinical Cardiac Radiology.* 2nd ed. London: Butterworth; 1980.
26. Chen JTT, Lester RG, Peter RH. Posterior wedging sign of mitral insufficiency. *Radiology.* 1974;113:451–453.
27. Gimenez JL, Soulen RL, Davila JC. Prosthetic valve detachment: its roentgenographic recognition: report of cases. *AJR Am J Roentgenol.* 1968;103:595–600.
28. Sorkin RP, Schuurmann BJ, Simon AB. Radiographic aspects of permanent cardiac pacemakers. *Radiology.* 1976;119:281–286.

CHAPTER (16)

Echocardiography

Anthony N. DeMaria / Daniel G. Blanchard

The term *echocardiography* refers to the evaluation of cardiac structure and function with images and recordings produced by ultrasound. In the past 30 years, it has become a fundamental component of the cardiac evaluation. Currently, echocardiography (*echo*) provides essential (and sometimes unexpected) clinical information and is the second most frequently performed diagnostic procedure.[1] A one-dimensional (1D) method performed from the precordial area to assess cardiac anatomy has evolved into a two-dimensional (2D) modality performed from either the thorax (TTE) or from within the esophagus (TEE), capable of also delineating flow and deriving hemodynamic data.[2] Newly evolving technical developments have extended the capacity of ultrasound to routine three-dimensional (3D) visualization[3] and the assessment, in conjunction with contrast agents,[4] of myocardial perfusion.

The development of echocardiography is usually credited to Elder and Hertz in 1954.[5] For nearly two additional decades, clinical echocardiography consisted primarily of 1D time-motion (M-mode) recordings, as popularized by Feigenbaum.[6] In the mid-1970s, Bom and colleagues developed a multielement linear-array scanner that could produce anatomically correct images of the beating heart.[7] 2D images of superior quality were soon achieved by mechanical sector scanners[8] and ultimately by phased-array instruments developed by Thurston and Von Ramm as the present-day standard.[9] Recently, 3D instruments capable of real-time volumetric imaging have been developed.[10] Miniaturization of ultrasound transducers has also led to their incorporation into gastroscopes and cardiac catheters to achieve transesophageal and intravascular images.[11,12]

Although efforts to use the Doppler principle to measure flow velocity by ultrasound were begun in the early 1970s by Baker,[13] clinical application of this technique did not thrive until the work of Hatle in the early 1980s.[14] Pulsed and continuous-wave Doppler recordings soon were expanded to full 2D color-flow imaging. Most recently, Doppler velocity recordings have been obtained from myocardium itself, enabling measurement of tissue velocities and the derivation of values for regional strain.

PRINCIPLES OF ECHOCARDIOGRAPHY
【 】 PHYSICS AND INSTRUMENTATION

Sound is an energy form that travels through a medium as a series of alternating compressions and rarefactions of the molecules (Fig. 16–1). It is typically characterized by its wavelength, which is the distance between any two consecutive phases of the cycle (e.g., peak compression to peak compression), and by its frequency, which is the number of wavelengths per unit time [customarily expressed as cycles per second, or hertz (Hz)]. The velocity of sound is the product of wavelength and frequency; thus, there is an inverse relationship between these two characteristics: the greater the frequency, the shorter the wavelength. Ultrasound is sonic energy with a frequency more than the audible range of the human ear (>20,000 Hz) and is useful for diagnostic imaging, because, like light, it can be directed as a beam that obeys the laws of reflection and refraction.[15,16] Thus, an ultrasound beam travels in a straight line through a homogeneous medium. If the beam meets an interface of different acoustic impedance, however, part of the energy reflects and the remaining attenuated signal is transmitted. The reflected energy, or echo, is used to construct an image (Fig. 16–2).

The transducer is responsible for both transmitting and receiving the ultrasound signal. The transducer consists of electrodes and a piezoelectric crystal, whose ionic structure results in deformation of shape when exposed to an electric current. Thus, piezoelectric crystals are composed of synthetic materials, such as barium titanate, which, when exposed to electric current from the electrodes, alternately expand and contract to create sound waves. When subjected to the mechanical energy of sound returning from a reflecting surface, the same piezoelectric element changes shape, thereby generating an electrical signal detected by the electrodes (Fig. 16–3). Thus, the transducer both produces and receives ultrasonic signals.

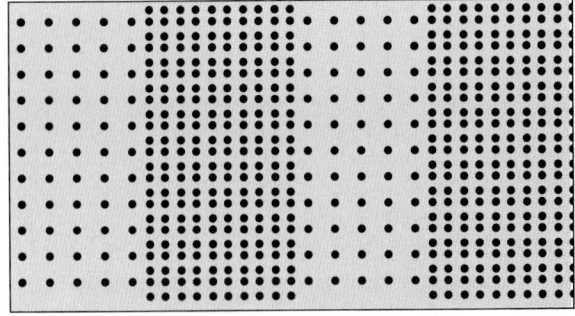

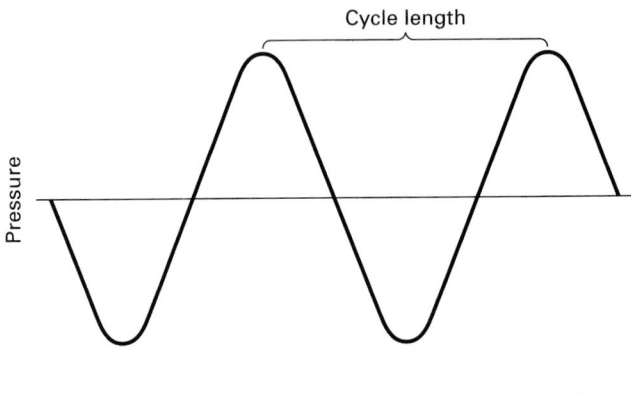

FIGURE 16–1. Sound energy results in alternating compression and rarefaction of particles in a conducting medium. This alternation, which can be plotted against time (or distance), conforms to a sine-wave pattern (*bottom panel*). *Source: Modified from Hagan AD, DeMaria AN. Clinical Applications of Two-Dimensional Echocardiography and Cardiac Doppler. Boston: Little, Brown; 1989. With permission.*

In the past echographs have both transmitted and received signals of the same frequency. Recently, *harmonic imaging* has been implemented, in which ultrasound energy is transmitted at a baseline (fundamental) frequency but then received at a higher multi-

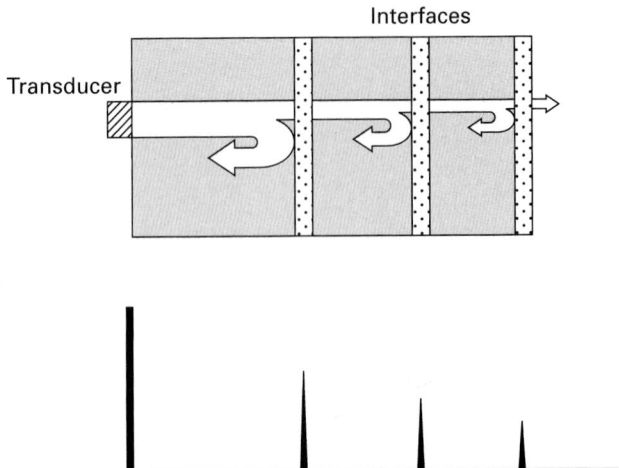

FIGURE 16–2. Upper panel: Attenuation of an ultrasound beam emitted from a transducer. There is reflection and progressive loss of energy at each interface encountered. **Lower panel:** the reflected wavefronts are recorded as signals of varying amplitudes (A mode) via the piezoelectric crystal. *Source: Upper panel modified from Hagan AD, DeMaria AN. Clinical Applications of Two-Dimensional Echocardiography and Cardiac Doppler. Boston: Little, Brown; 1989. With permission.*

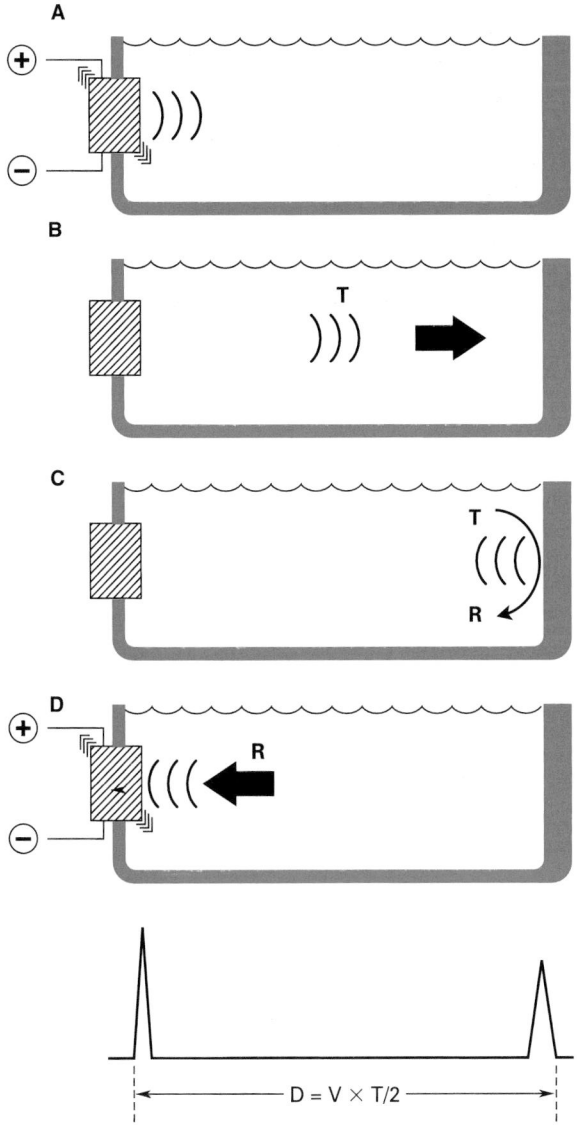

FIGURE 16–3. The basic principle of ultrasonic imaging. The piezoelectric crystal is activated, producing a transmitted pulse (T), which reflects off the interface. The reflected pulse (R) excites the crystal, producing an electric current. Because the velocity of the pulse is constant, distance can be calculated based on the transit time. (Because the pulse must travel back and forth from the interface, the time is divided by 2.) *Source: Modified from Weyman AE. Principles and Practice of Echocardiography, 2nd ed. Philadelphia: Lea & Febiger; 1994. With permission.*

ple (harmonic) of that frequency (usually the first harmonic). Harmonic imaging is based on the change in the ultrasound frequency of a transmitted wave induced by the interaction with a reflecting target. The sinusoidal waveform becomes peaked as it travels through tissue, thereby undergoing a change in frequency. Similarly, if a sound signal strikes a contrast microbubble, the periodic expansion and contraction (resonation) of the bubble changes the frequency of the wave.

A simplistic analogy of this phenomenon would be the morphologic changes seen in ocean waves as they approach the shore and are affected by the rising ocean floor. The cresting of the waves (the tops move more rapidly than the bases) and the changes in their height are analogous to the harmonic signals generated by the interaction of ultrasound and tissue. These signals take some

time (and distance) to develop. Therefore, structures close to the transducer do not generate much harmonic signal at all; and thus, near-field artifacts and reverberation artifacts are minimized.

Harmonic imaging has also been very useful in conjunction with intravascular echo contrast agents. These microbubbles demonstrate cyclic expansion and constriction during ultrasound imaging, and this resonance produces a large amount of harmonic energy.[17] In contrast, myocardial tissue does not resonate to any appreciable degree. The net effect of harmonic imaging with echocardiographic contrast is a marked enhancement of the signal from the left ventricular (LV) cavity compared to that of the myocardium.

Ultrasound presents several unique *technical difficulties.* Sound energy is poorly transmitted through air and bone, and the ability to record adequate images depends on a thoracic window that gives the interrogating beam adequate access to cardiac structures. The degree to which ultrasonic energy is reflected depends on how perpendicular the interrogating beam is to the interface. When the ultrasound beam is directed to the interface, little or no sound energy reflects to the transducer. Therefore, poor signal transmission, a nonorthogonal orientation of the ultrasound beam to the surface, and energy attenuation can cause failure to record signals from cardiac structures—a phenomenon referred to as *echo dropout.*[18] Conversely, some structures may be such strong ultrasonic reflectors, being perpendicular to the beam or extremely dense, that sufficient energy returns to the transducer to reflect and again transmit into the field. This phenomenon can lead to *reverberations,* or the reproduction of the echoes of anatomic structures at multiple locations within the image.[19] Finally, targets lying on the periphery of the ultrasound beam may be recorded and displayed as if they were located along the central scan line (Fig. 16–4). This problem may be accentuated in the setting of strong reflectors that result in the formation of *side lobes.*[20]

The construction of a cardiac image from ultrasound signals is based on computation of the distance between an anatomic structure and the transducer (see Fig. 16–3). Thus, an ultrasound beam is produced by a handheld transducer positioned on the thorax and directed into the heart. This beam travels in a straight line until it reaches an interface between structures of different acoustic impedance, such as blood and myocardium. At this point, some

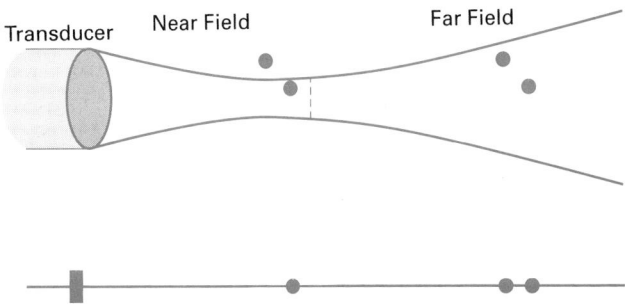

FIGURE 16–4. *Upper panel:* The transducer emits an ultrasonic beam that has a near field (where the beam is relatively focused) and a far field (where the beam width increases). *Lower panel:* B-mode diagram showing the effect of beam width. In the near field, the beam reflects off only one of two objects in close proximity to each other. In the far field, however, two similarly positioned objects are both within the beam width. Therefore, lateral resolution is compromised and the objects' positions are misrepresented.

ultrasonic energy reflects. Some scatters and some continues forward. The amplitude of the propagating signal is attenuated because of the reduction in energy at the interface (see Fig. 16–2). Electronic circuitry within the echograph measures the time interval required for the transit of the ultrasound beam from the transducer to the interface and back again. Because the velocity of sound in soft tissue is constant (approximately 1540 m/sec), the instrument can calculate the total distance traveled to and from the reflecting surface as the product of transit time and velocity of sound. Interface location is derived as one-half of the total transit distance, and a signal is depicted on an oscilloscope or video monitor at that point (see Fig. 16–3). The amplitude of ultrasonic energy re-

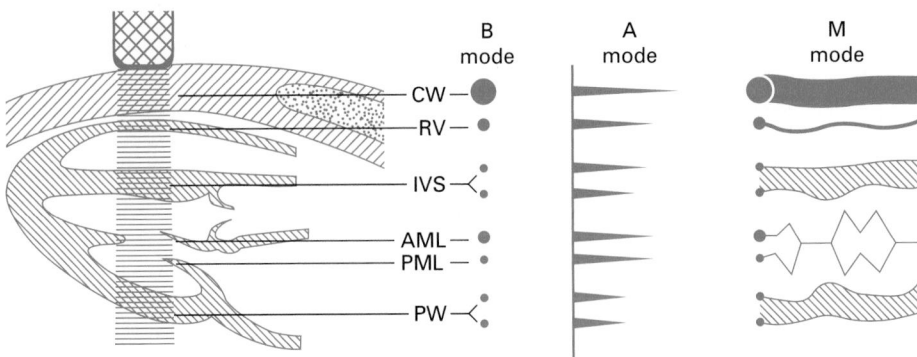

FIGURE 16–5. Formation of A-mode, B-mode, and M-mode echocardiograms. The transducer emits an ultrasound beam, which reflects at each anatomic interface. The reflected wavefronts can be represented as dots (B mode) or spikes (A mode). The dot brightness and spike magnitude vary with the amplitude of the reflected wave. If the B-mode scan is swept from left to right with time, an M-mode image is produced. AML, anterior mitral leaflet; CW, chest wall; IVS, interventricular septum; PML, posterior mitral leaflet; PW, posterior wall; RV, right ventricle. *Source: Modified from Hagan AD, DeMaria AN. Clinical Applications of Two-Dimensional Echocardiography and Cardiac Doppler. Boston: Little, Brown; 1989. With permission.*

flected from each target interface is represented by the brightness of the signal that is displayed.

In the most basic form of echocardiography, a single scan line produced by a piezoelectric crystal is passed through the heart (Fig. 16–5). At each structural interface, ultrasonic energy is reflected back and displayed at the appropriate distance as a signal, whose amplitude represents the acoustic impedance or density of the material encountered. These signals are subsequently displayed as dots, whose brightness is proportional to the amplitude of reflected ultrasonic energy. Accordingly, if repetitive B-mode scan lines are produced and swept across the screen over time, the movement of the heart can be obtained as a time-motion (or M-mode) recording, providing dynamic cardiac images (see Fig. 16–5). In clinical use, the piezoelectric crystal within the transducer is activated by alternating electric current to transmit at a rate of approximately 1000 pulses per second. This same crystal also receives the returning echo reflections and actually spends most of the time (>90 percent) in the *receive* rather than the *transmit* mode. Because the beam is confined to a single location and transmits ultrasound signals at the pulse rate of the transducer, M-mode echocardiography provides *very high temporal resolution*. Importantly, M-mode is excellent for timing cardiac events or recording high-velocity motion. As opposed to B- or M-mode recordings, 2D echocardiography provides additional information in either superoinferior or mediolateral directions.

High-quality images require optimal resolution—that is, the ability to distinguish two individual objects separated in space. Short wavelengths yield excellent resolution in echo imaging, because the shorter the cycle length, the smaller the object that will reflect the signal and be detected by the echo scanner. Because wavelength is inversely related to frequency, transducers that emit a high-frequency signal (3.5 to 7.0 MHz or greater) yield high-resolution images. Because ultrasonic beams diverge as they propagate away from the transducer, the width of the beam can become sufficiently great to encompass multiple targets and decrease resolution (see Fig. 16–4). The degree of beam divergence is less with high-frequency sonic energy than with low-frequency signals. The smaller wavelengths associated with high-frequency signals, however, are

subject to greater reflection and scattering, with substantially higher attenuation as the beam propagates through tissue. The resultant attenuation is greater and leads to decreased sensitivity. Therefore, in clinical practice, echocardiographic examinations are performed using the highest-frequency transducer capable of obtaining signals from all potential targets within the ultrasound field.

M-MODE ECHOCARDIOGRAPHY

The Standard M-Mode Examination

Despite the availability of 2D imaging, M-mode echocardiography remains a useful part of the ultrasound examination. Figures 16–6A through 16–6D show the typical views obtained when the transducer is placed at the left parasternal area and rocked through the heart from apex to base. Tissue typically reflects ultrasound at its surface (specular reflectors) and from internal inhomogenicity (backscatter), whereas blood is homogenous and does not produce reflections. At the mitral valve (MV) level (Fig. 16–6C), the cardiac structure seen closest to the transducer is the right ventricular (RV) free wall; it is followed by the RV cavity, the interventricular septum, the MV apparatus, and the LV posterior wall as the beam travels backward. At this level, MV excursion is well seen and is more easily recorded for the longer anterior leaflet. For the anterior leaflet, diastolic mitral opening is bipeaked (M shaped), with maximal opening during early diastolic filling at the E point, a subsequent reclosure downslope to the F point, and a reopening with atrial contraction at the A point before valve closure at the C point[21] (Fig. 16–7). The posterior leaflet manifests a mirror-image W-shaped pattern. When LV end-diastolic pressure is elevated, a shoulder (*B* bump) is often present between the A and C points (Fig. 16–8). If the transducer beam is directed inferolaterally from the MV level, the papillary muscles and LV apex are imaged (see Fig. 16–6A). With superior and medial angulation, the left atrium (LA), aortic valve (AoV), and aortic root (AO) are seen. The tricuspid valve (TV) can be imaged by angulating the transducer inferomedially and the pulmonic valve (PV) by angulating slightly superiorly and laterally.

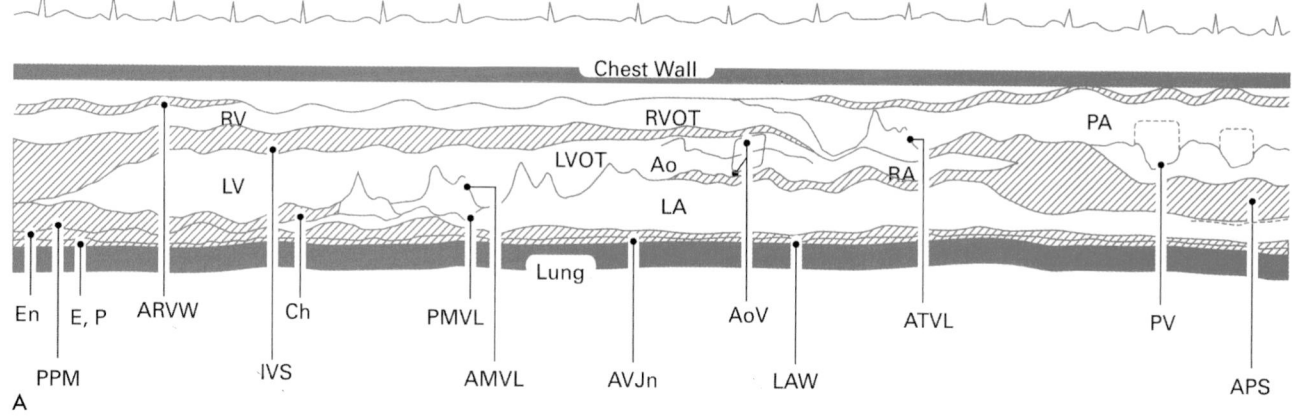

A

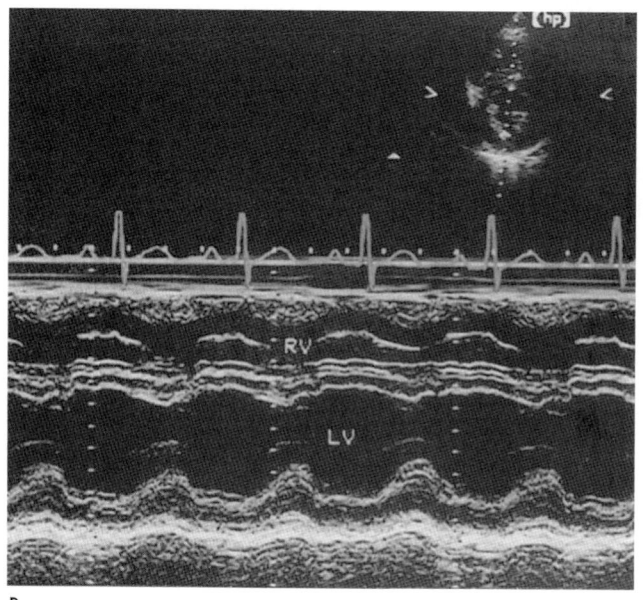

B

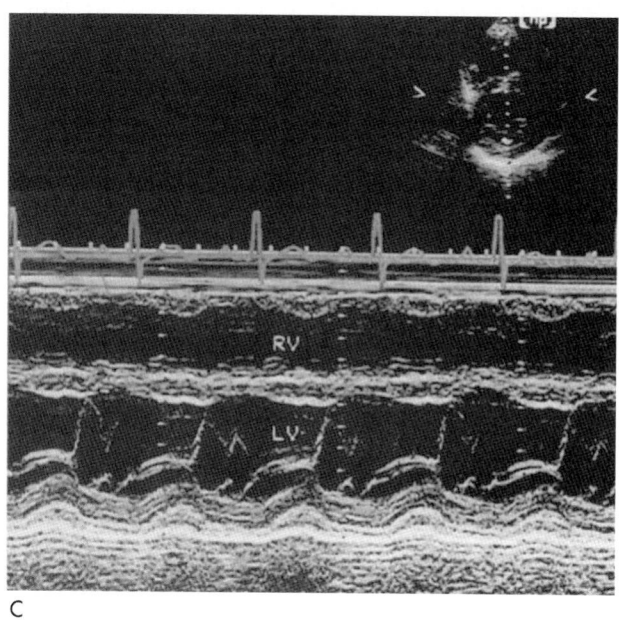

C

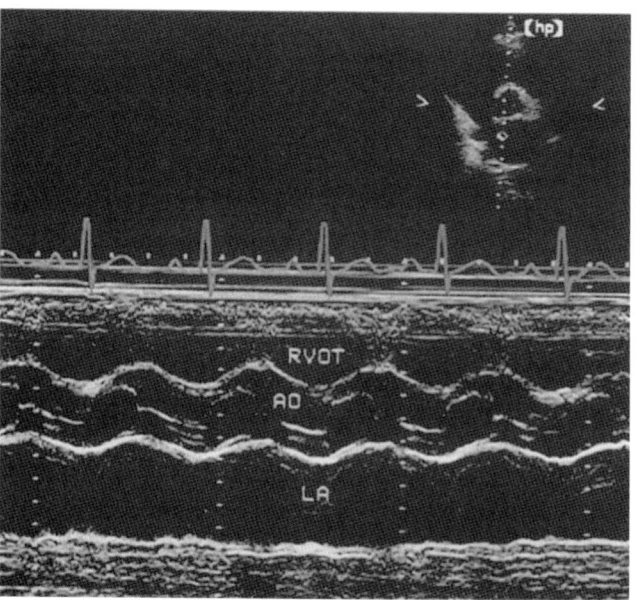

D

FIGURE 16–6. A. Diagram of an M-mode sweep from apex to base in a normal heart (parasternal view). **B** to **D.** M-mode sweep from apex to base in a normal individual. aMVL, anterior mitral valve leaflet; Ao, aorta; AoV, aortic valve; APS, atriopulmonic sulcus; ARVW, anterior right ventricular wall; ATVL, anterior tricuspid valve leaflet; AVJ, atrioventricular junction; Ch, chordae tendineae; EN, endocardium; E,P, epicardial/pericardial interface; IVS, interventricular septum; LA, left atrium; LAW, left atrial wall; LV, left ventricle; LVOT, left ventricular outflow tract; PA, pulmonary artery; PMVL, posterior mitral valve leaflet; PPM, posterior papillary muscle; PV, pulmonic valve; RA, right atrium; RV, right ventricle; RVOT, right ventricular outflow tract. *Source: A, from Felner JM, Schlant RC. Echocardiography: A Teaching Atlas. New York: Grune & Stratton; 1976. With permission.*

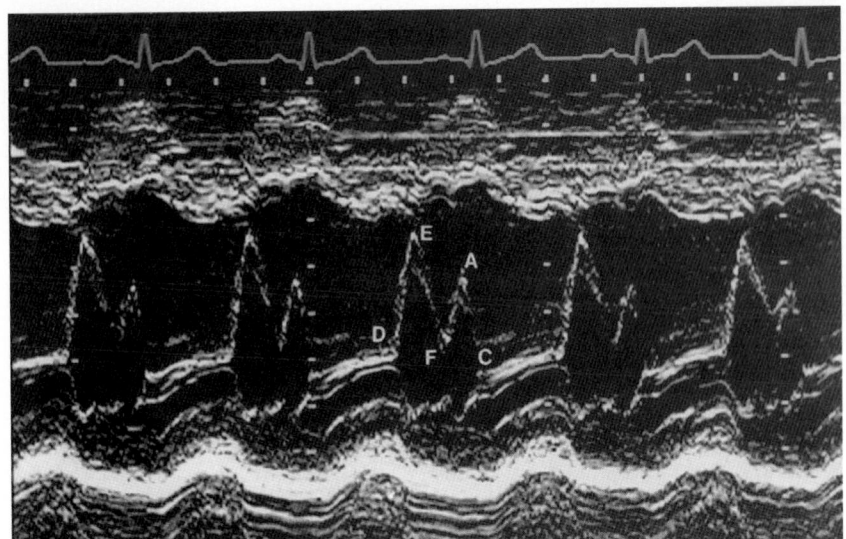

FIGURE 16-7. Standard M-mode image through the left ventricle at the level of the mitral valve. See text for discussion of nomenclature.

Assessment of Systolic Function by M-Mode Echocardiography

Measurements of the LV cavity dimension and wall thickness can be readily derived from M-mode recordings (Fig. 16–9) and are usually made according to the recommendations of the American Society of Echocardiography (ASE) at end diastole (the onset of the QRS complex) and end systole (the point of maximum upward motion of the LV posterior wall endocardium).[22] Measurements should be made from leading edge to leading edge. They are accurate if the beam is orthogonal to the long axis of the ventricle. By convention, left atrial dimension is measured at end systole, and AO diameter is recorded at end diastole at the level of the base of the heart (see Fig. 16–9). During systole, opening of the aortic leaflets appears as a parallelogram produced by motion of the right coronary and (usually) the noncoronary AoV cusps.

The M-mode LV cavity dimensions can be used to estimate ventricular volumes and ejection fraction (EF) if desired, most simply by merely cubing the value (D^3). Such calculations involve several assumptions regarding LV geometry that are not uniformly valid.[23] The fractional shortening can also be determined.[24] This value is often helpful in assessing systolic function, but it reflects the function of the LV in one chord and in one plane and can be misleading with asynchronous contraction.[25] An additional M-mode marker of systolic function is *E-point to septal separation*, or the

distance between the anterior MV leaflet at its most anterior opening excursion (the E point) and the interventricular septum. A value of 8 mm or greater is abnormal.[26] The normal M-mode measurements are seen in Table 16–1.

〖 〗 TWO-DIMENSIONAL ECHOCARDIOGRAPHY

Multiple individual B-mode scan lines can be rapidly transmitted, received, and displayed in appropriate spatial orientation to construct a 2D image of the heart. The initial approach simply used a linear array of 20 piezoelectric crystals placed side by side, each of which transmitted and received signals independently (Fig. 16–10A). The resulting scan lines were displayed simultaneously to yield rectangular images.

Current 2D scanners use B-mode scan lines that are independently transmitted and received and are directed through a wedge-shaped sector of cardiac anatomy by means of mechanical or electrical beam steering (see Fig. 16–10A and B). A variety of motorized devices are available that can mechanically direct multiple scan lines through a sector arc of the cardiovascular system. The position of the beam in space is derived by

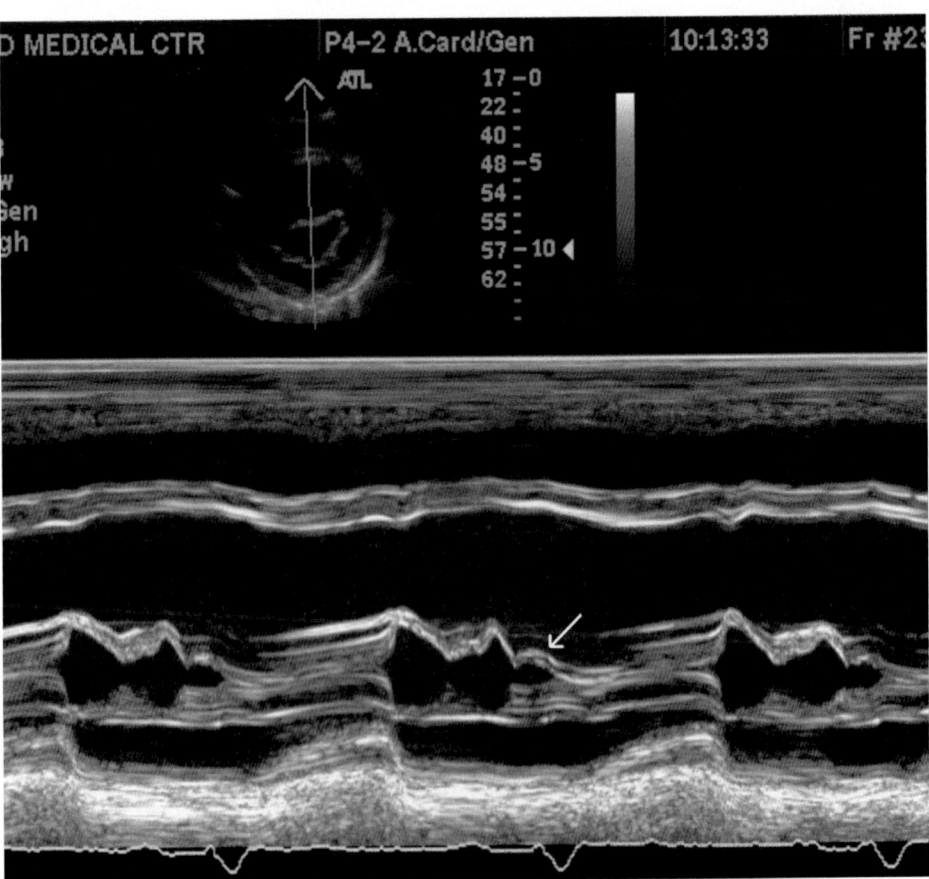

FIGURE 16-8. M-mode image through the mitral valve showing a *B bump*, suggesting high left ventricular diastolic pressure (*arrow*). The E-point septal separation is also increased. (Transducer is in the left parasternal position.)

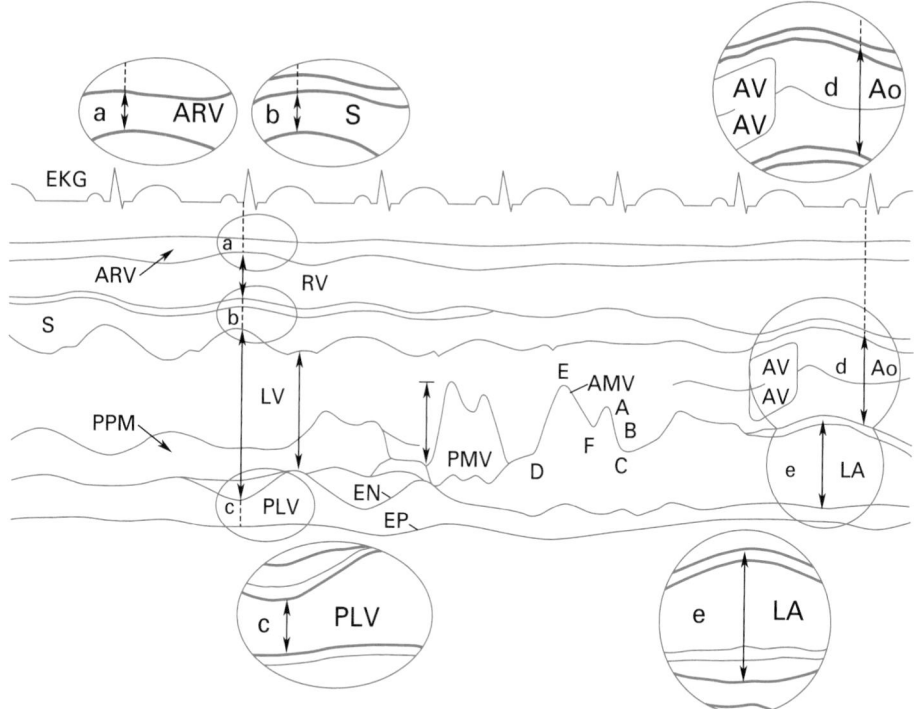

FIGURE 16–9. Recommended criteria for M-mode measurement of cardiac dimensions (see text for details). The figure and the elliptical inserts (a, b, c, d, and e) illustrate the leading-edge method. aMVL, anterior mitral valve leaflet; Ao, aorta; AoV, aortic valve; ARV, anterior right ventricular wall; EN, endocardium; EP, epicardium; LA, left atrium; LV, left ventricle; PLV, posterior left ventricular (wall); PPM, papillary muscle; PMVL, posterior mitral valve leaflet; RV, right ventricle; S, septum. *Source: Reproduced with permission from Sahn DJ, DeMaria AN, Kisslo J, Weyman AE.*[22]

determining the orientation of the piezoelectric crystal. Most current 2D scanners use a phased-array approach, where multiple ultrasonic crystals are employed in concert to create individual B-mode scan lines. The piezoelectric crystals are activated in a closely coordinated temporal sequence, so that the individual wavelets produced by each element merge to form a single beam whose direction is determined by the sequence of crystal firing (Fig. 16–11). The beam can be electrically swept throughout a 90-degree sector arc. Also, a firing sequence can be employed that results in dynamic focusing of the beam along its length to achieve minimal beam width and increased resolution. Phased-array 2D scanners employ small transducers with no moving parts that could require repair.

Originally, echocardiographic data were displayed in analogue form on a standard oscilloscope, transferred to a video monitor by a television camera, and hard-copied onto videotape or paper. Currently, computerized analogue-to-digital scan conversion is standard, so the polar signals of individual scan lines are con-

TABLE 16–1

Normal Values

	MEAN ± STANDARD DEVIATION	RANGE	MEAN ± STANDARD DEVIATION	RANGE
No. of patients	25	—	50	—
Age, years	10 ± 3	4–18	24 ± 0.6	1.10–2.53
BSA, m²	1.33 ± 0.38	0.72–2.04	1.81 ± 0.34	1.10–2.53
$LVID_d$, mm	44 ± 6	32–50	50 ± 3	42–60
$LVID_s$, mm	28 ± 7	32–50	50 ± 3	22–43
FSLV	34 ± 4	25–42	33 ± 3	28–37
IVS thickness, mm	8 ± 2	5–10	9 ± 1	7–12
IVS excursion, mm	7 ± 1	5–9	9 ± 1	7–12
PW_d thickness, mm	7 ± 2	4–9	9 ± 1	7–12
PW_s thickness, mm	12 ± 3	8–17	16 ± 2	13–20
α thickening PW	0.70 ± 0.25	0.41–0.95	0.50 ± 0.19	0.32–0.69
PW excursion, mm	9 ± 2	7–14	11 ± 2	9–17
RVD_d supine, mm	—	—	15 ± 6	7–22
RVD_d left lateral, mm	—	—	20 ± 8	10–37
$Aorta_d$ mm	23 ± 4	15–27	28 ± 5	26–36
LAD_s mm	25 ± 5	20–31	27 ± 6	12–35

BSA, Body surface area; FSLV, fractional shortening of left ventricle; IVS, interventricular septum; LAD, left atrial dimension; $LVID_d$, left ventricular internal diameter, end diastole; $LVID_s$, left ventricular internal diameter, end systole; PW, posterior wall; PWV, posterior wall velocity; RVD, right ventricular dimension.

Source: Data from Felner JM, Schlant RC. Echocardiography: A Teaching Atlas. New York: Grune & Stratton; 1976.

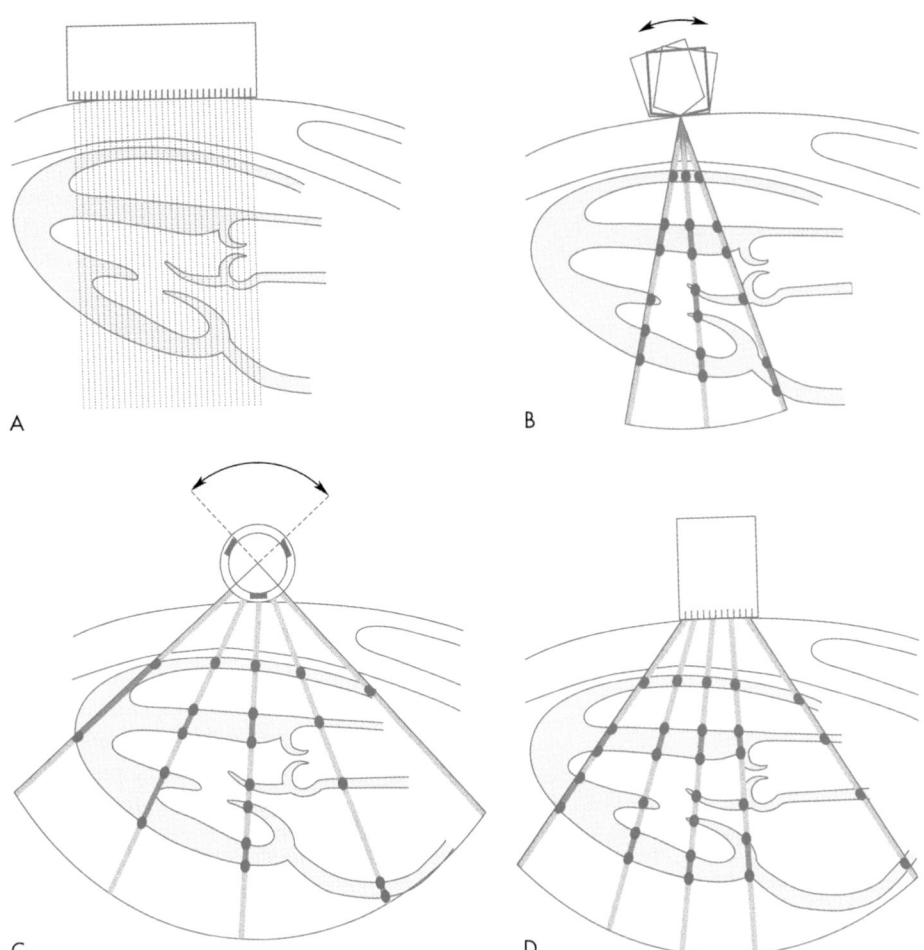

FIGURE 16–10. The four major types of ultrasonic scanners used to acquire 2D echocardiographic images. **A.** Linear-array scanner. **B.** Oscillating scanner. **C.** Rotating mechanical scanner. **D.** Phased-array scanner. *Source: From Hagan AD, DeMaria AN. Clinical Applications of Two-Dimensional Echocardiography and Cardiac Doppler. Boston: Little, Brown; 1989. With permission.*

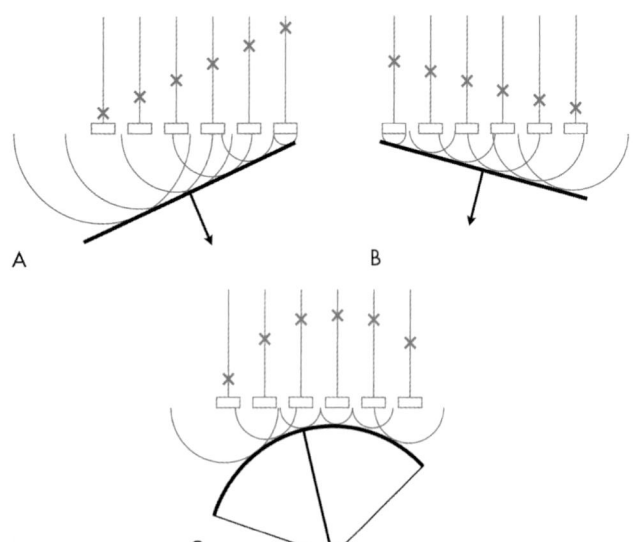

FIGURE 16–11. Electronic *steering* of a phased-array ultrasound beam. **A.** Elements are fired in sequence from left to right, resulting in a beam directed to the left. **B.** Elements are fired in sequence opposite to those in (**A**), producing a beam directed to the right. **C.** Elements are fired from the periphery toward the center, producing a beam that converges on a given focal point. *Source: From Hagan AD, DeMaria AN. Clinical Applications of Two-Dimensional Echocardiography and Cardiac Doppler. Boston: Little, Brown; 1989. With permission.*

verted to a series of numerical gray-level values for individual box-like picture elements (pixels) aligned along X-Y coordinates.[27] The ability of a digital step-gradation technique to reproduce the continuous gradation of analog methods is a function of the density of pixels in the matrix and the gray level shades available. The digital format provides the opportunity for image processing, enhancement, and quantitation. Storage in digital format can avoid the image degradation inherent in videotape, provide random access and easy comparison of studies, enable rapid image transmission, and prevent deterioration with image copying and prolonged storage. Fully digital acquisition and storage of echocardiograms will be commonplace in the near future, replacing analog videotape recordings.

The Standard Two-Dimensional Examination

To help standardize the 2D examination, the ASE recommends that cardiac imaging be performed in three orthogonal planes:

1. Long-axis (from AO to the apex)
2. Short-axis (perpendicular to long axis)
3. Four-chamber (traversing both ventricles and atria through the mitral and TVs)[28] (Fig. 16–12)

The long and short axes are those of *the heart*, not the body. These three planes can be visualized using four basic transducer

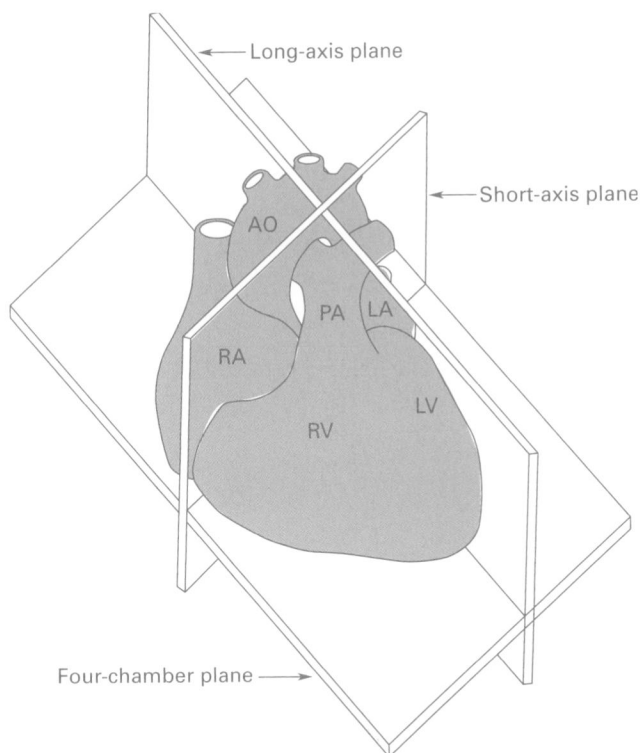

FIGURE 16–12. The three basic tomographic imaging planes used in echocardiography: long axis, short axis, and four chamber. Ao, aorta; LA, left atrium; LV, left ventricle; PA, pulmonary artery; RA, right atrium; RV, right ventricle. *Source: From Hagan AD, DeMaria AN. Clinical Applications of Two-Dimensional Echocardiography and Cardiac Doppler. Boston: Little, Brown; 1989. With permission.*

positions: parasternal, apical, subcostal, and suprasternal (Fig. 16–13A to C). The four-chamber views are obtained from the apical and subcostal positions. The ASE recommends that an image obtained within 45 degrees of a basic orthogonal plane be identified with that orthogonal plane. Table 16–2 lists the standard transducer positions and transthoracic echocardiographic (TEE) views. Anatomic drawings of the various imaging planes are seen in Fig. 16–13 through Fig. 16–20.

The echocardiographic examination is iterative and largely determined by the anatomic characteristics of the patient and manual manipulation of the transducer by the operator. Of paramount importance is the identification of a thoracic site (window) that enables transmission of the ultrasound signal to the heart. The echocardiographic examination is performed with the operator either to the patient's left or right. The patient is in the left lateral decubitus position for most of the examination, with the head of the bed elevated 20 to 30 degrees. Use of a thick foam rubber mattress (made expressly for echocardiography) with a removable section under the area of the cardiac apex may facilitate the examination.

The examination customarily begins with the transducer in the left parasternal position in the long-axis view (see Fig. 16–14). This provides excellent images of the LV, aorta, LA, and the mitral and AoVs. By angling the beam slightly rightward and inferiorly (RV inflow view), the right atrium (RA), RV, and TV are visualized (see Fig. 16–15).

A 90-degree clockwise turn of the transducer produces the parasternal short-axis view. Slight axial angulation of the transducer enables visualization of the LV at various levels of the short

axis, including the papillary muscle, mitral leaflets, and AoV (see Fig. 16–16). With angulation toward the base, the LA, right heart structures, main pulmonary artery (PA), and occasionally the LA appendage are also recorded. The apical views are best acquired with the patient in a steep left lateral decubitus position and the transducer at the point of the apical impulse. The four-chamber view is obtained by turning the transducer so that both ventricles, atrioventricular valves, and atria are visualized (see Fig. 16–17). In this view, the septal, apical, and lateral walls of the LV are visualized. Slight superior angulation of the transducer will add the AoV and proximal ascending aorta to the echocardiographic image (apical five-chamber view). From the four-chamber view, 90 degrees of counterclockwise transducer rotation produce the apical two-chamber view (see Fig. 16–18A and B). This imaging plane demonstrates the LA and the inferior, apical, and anterior wall segments of the LV (the right heart structures are absent). If the transducer is rotated slightly back toward the four-chamber plane, a three-chamber view similar to the parasternal long-axis view is produced (see Fig. 16–18C) and provides images of the posterior, apical, and anteroseptal LV wall segments as well as the LA, aorta, and mitral and AoVs.

To facilitate subcostal imaging, the patient is moved into a supine position. The subcostal four-chamber view is much like the apical four-chamber view (see Fig. 16–19), but because the ultrasound beam is now more perpendicular to the interventricular and interatrial septa, subcostal imaging is often helpful in the examination of these structures. A 90-degree rotation of the transducer will record a subcostal short-axis view. The transducer can also be angled to image the RV outflow and PA as well as the inferior vena cava (see Fig. 16–19).

The long-axis suprasternal imaging plane is shown in Fig. 16–20. In adults the LV is usually not visualized satisfactorily from the suprasternal position, but these imaging planes are well suited for examination of the thoracic aorta, PA, and great vessels. Normal values for 2D echocardiographic measurements are shown in Table 16–3.

THREE-DIMENSIONAL ECHOCARDIOGRAPHY

Several approaches exist to obtaining 3D echocardiographic images. The simplest approach is to merely move the transducer through a defined space and reconstruct an image by aligning the tomographic slices appropriately. A variety of spatial locator devices can be attached to the transducer to provide spatial orientation. Images obtained in this way can be high quality and accurate, but they require computer reconstruction and therefore cannot be displayed in *real time*. Nevertheless, these reconstructed 3D images can be valuable in quantifying cardiac volumes and EF, assessing congenital heart disease (CHD) and evaluating structures of complex geometry such as the RV.[29] A pyramid-shaped ultrasound beam was produced that could often encompass the entire heart from one transducer location and acquire an entire data set in a single cardiac cycle. Although the initial images often lacked resolution, this type of real-time 3D imaging has evolved considerably, and new software advances have improved surface rendering and endocardial border definition (see Fig. 16–20C and D). Recent studies have shown an excellent correlation between real-time 3D echo and MRI in the measurement of regional and global LV volume and time-wall mo-

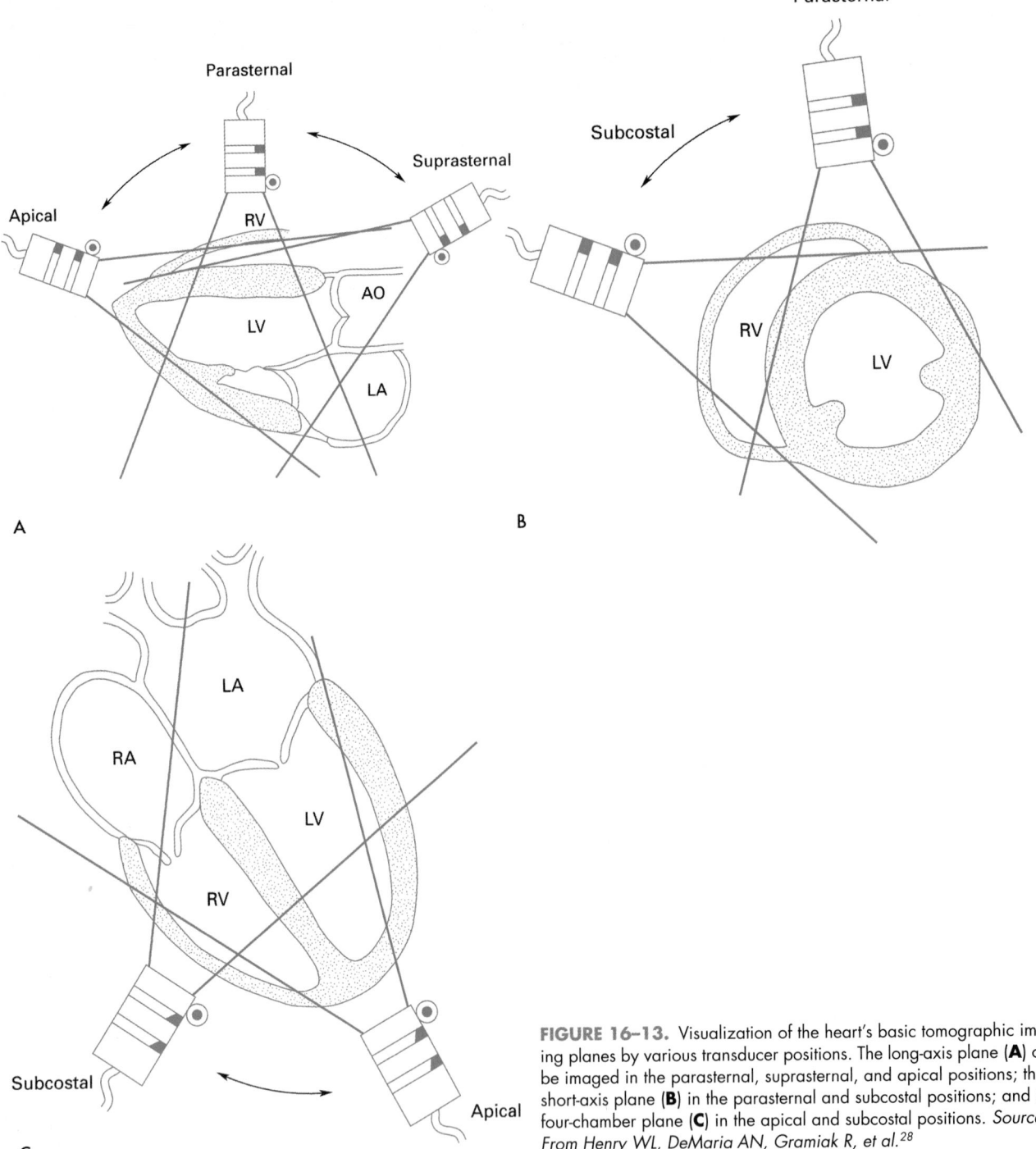

FIGURE 16-13. Visualization of the heart's basic tomographic imaging planes by various transducer positions. The long-axis plane (**A**) can be imaged in the parasternal, suprasternal, and apical positions; the short-axis plane (**B**) in the parasternal and subcostal positions; and the four-chamber plane (**C**) in the apical and subcostal positions. *Source: From Henry WL, DeMaria AN, Gramiak R, et al.*[28]

TABLE 16–2

Standard Two-Dimensional Echocardiographic Transducer Positions

Parasternal Position
Long axis
    Left ventricular long axis
    Right ventricular long
    Right ventricular outflow
Short axis
    Short axis through the plane of the
        Cardiac base
        Mitral valve
        Chordae tendineae
        Papillary muscles
        Apex

Apical Position
Four-chamber plane
Five-chamber plane
    (Four-chamber plane angled superiorly to include the aorta)
Two-chamber plane
Three-chamber plane

Subcostal Position
Four-chamber plane
Short axis through the plane of the
    Mitral valve
    Papillary muscles
    Cardiac base
Posteriorly directed planes through the venae cavae and
    atria

Suprasternal Position
Long axis (through the ascending and descending aorta)
Short axis

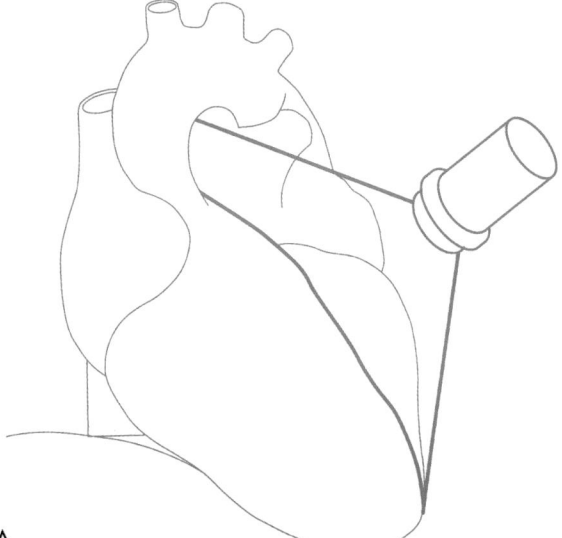

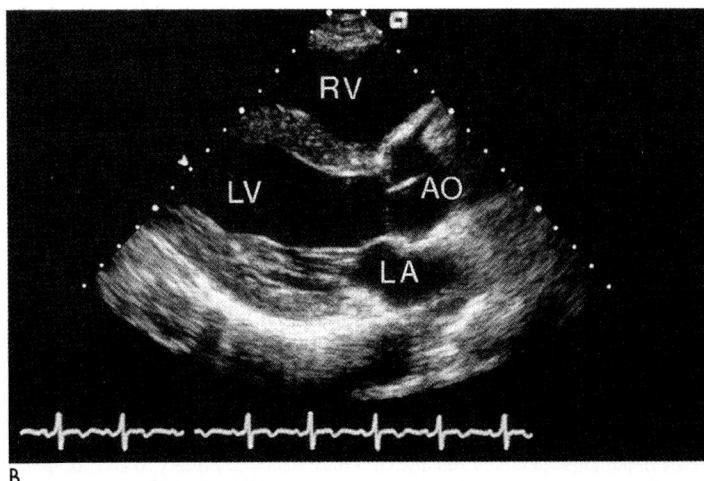

A

B

FIGURE 16–14. A. Orientation of the sector beam and transducer position for the parasternal long-axis view of the left ventricle. **B.** 2D image of the heart, parasternal long-axis view. Ao, aorta; LA, left atrium; LV, left ventricle; RV, right ventricle.

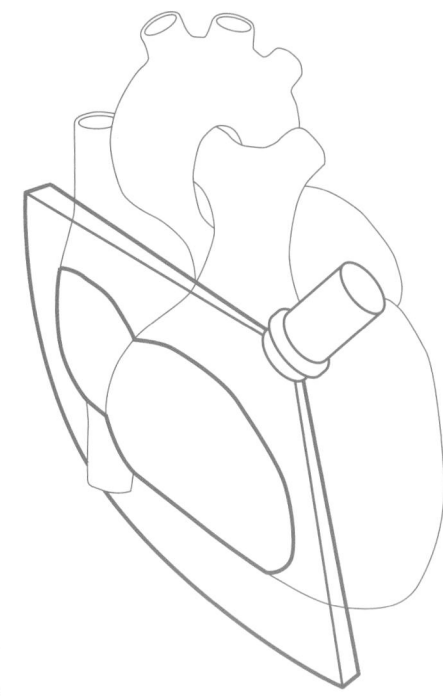

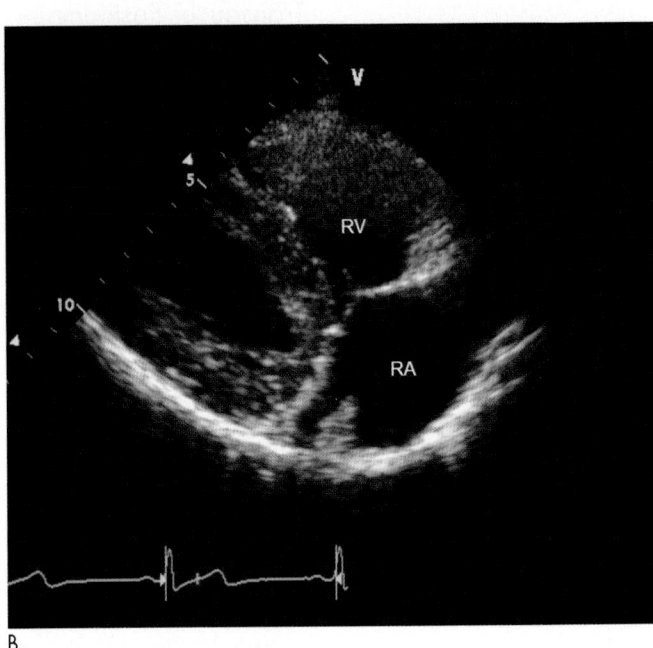

A   B

FIGURE 16–15. A. Orientation of the sector beam and transducer position for the parasternal RV inflow plane. **B.** Two-dimensional image of RV inflow plane. RA, right atrium; RV, right ventricle. *Source: A, from Hagan AD, DeMaria AN. Clinical Applications of Two-Dimensional Echocardiography and Cardiac Doppler. Boston: Little, Brown; 1989. With permission.*

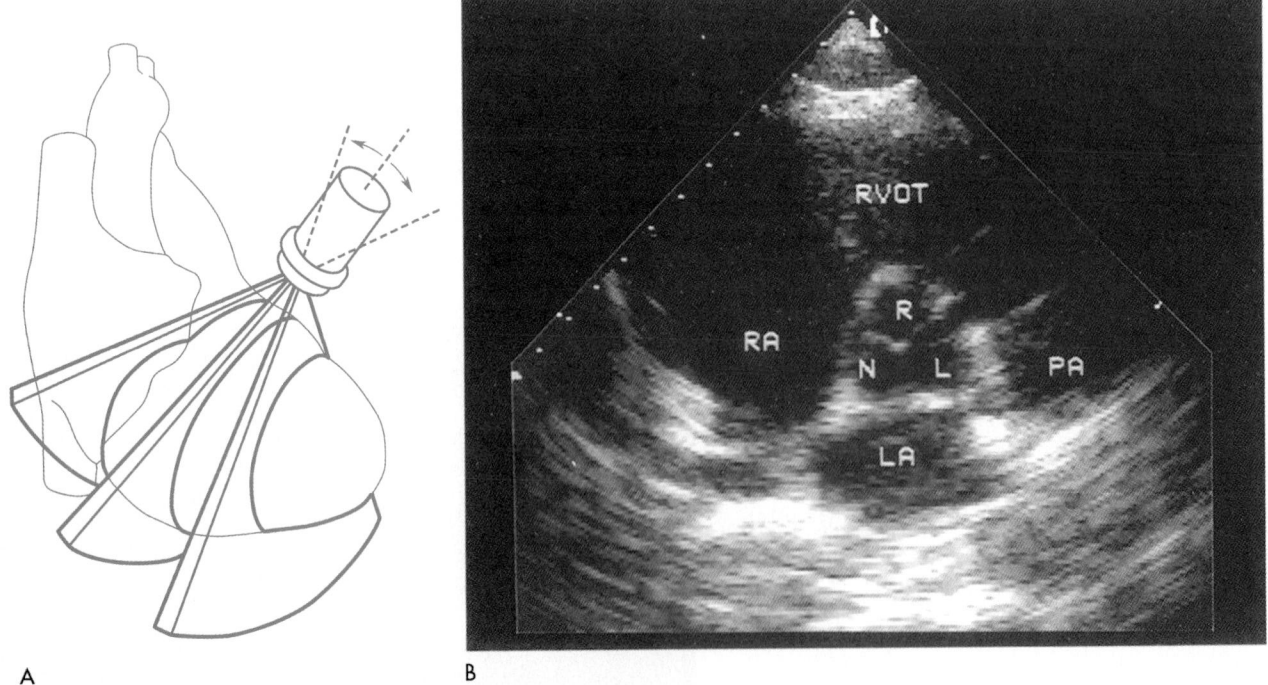

A   B

FIGURE 16–16. A. Orientation of various short-axis sector beams through the left ventricle obtained by angling the transducer in the parasternal position. **B.** Short-axis plane through the base of the heart. **C.** At the level of the mitral valve leaflets. **D.** At the papillary muscle level. **E.** Modified parasternal short axis plane through the RV outflow tract and pulmonary artery. aMVL, anterior mitral valve leaflet; L, left cusp of the aortic valve; LA, left atrium; LV, left ventricle; N, noncoronary cusp of the aortic valve, PA, pulmonary artery; PMVL, posterior mitral valve leaflet; RA, right atrium; R, right cusp of the aortic valve; RV, right ventricle; RVOT, right ventricular outflow tract. *Source: A, from Hagan AD, DeMaria AN. Clinical Applications of Two-Dimensional Echocardiography and Cardiac Doppler. Boston: Little, Brown; 1989. With permission.*

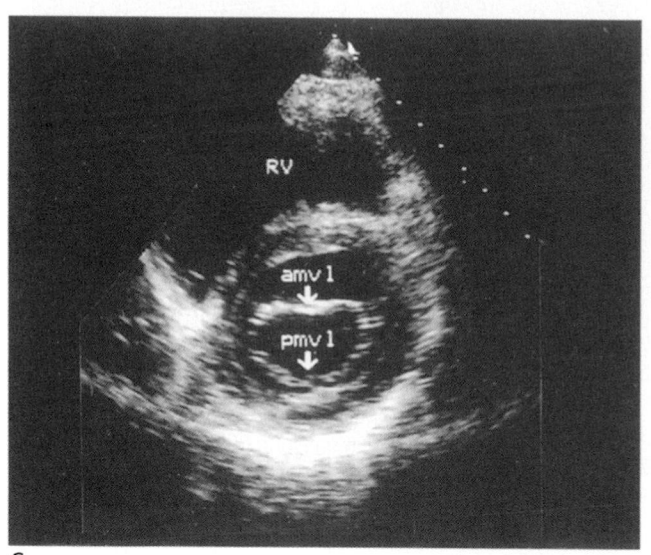

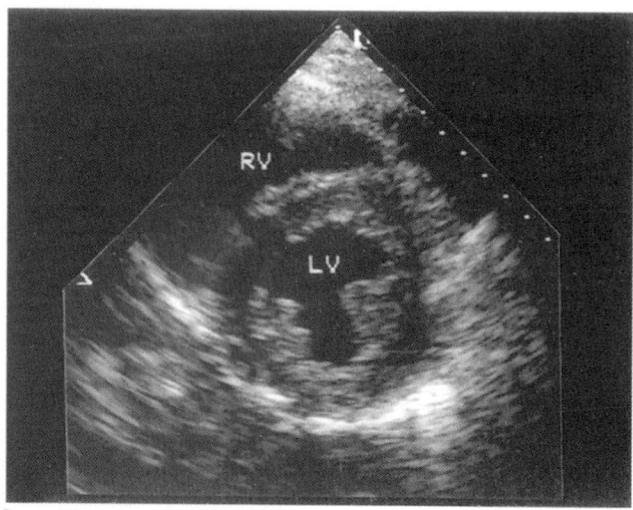

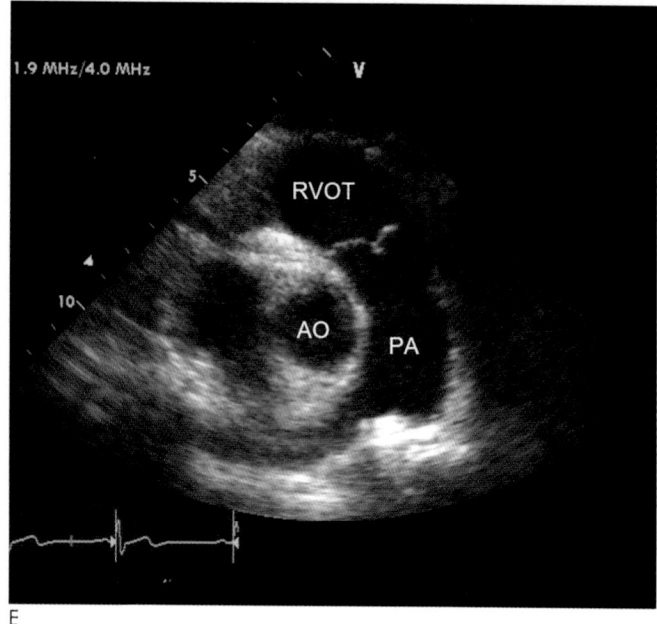

FIGURE 16–16. (continued)

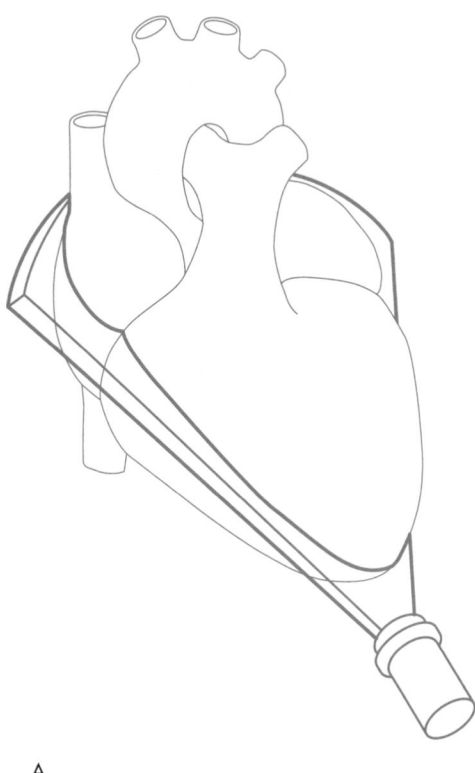

A

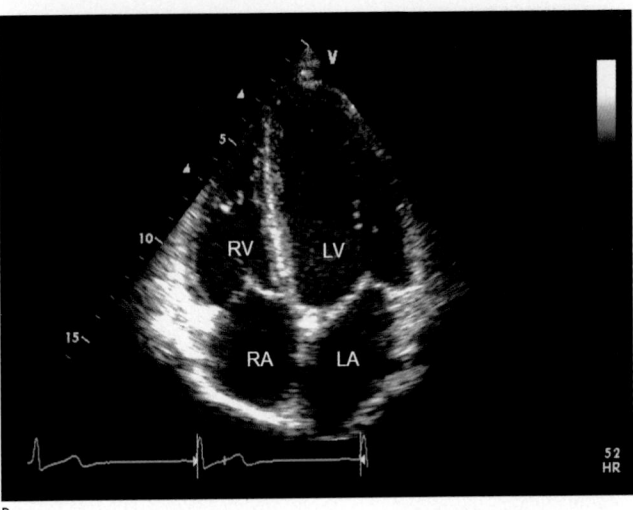

B

FIGURE 16–17. A. Orientation of the sector beam and transducer position for the apical four-chamber plane. **B.** 2D image of the apical four-chamber plane. LA, left atrium; LV, left ventricle; RA, right atrium; RV, right ventricle. *Source: A, from Hagan AD, DeMaria AN. Clinical Applications of Two-Dimensional Echocardiography and Cardiac Doppler. Boston: Little, Brown; 1989. With permission.*

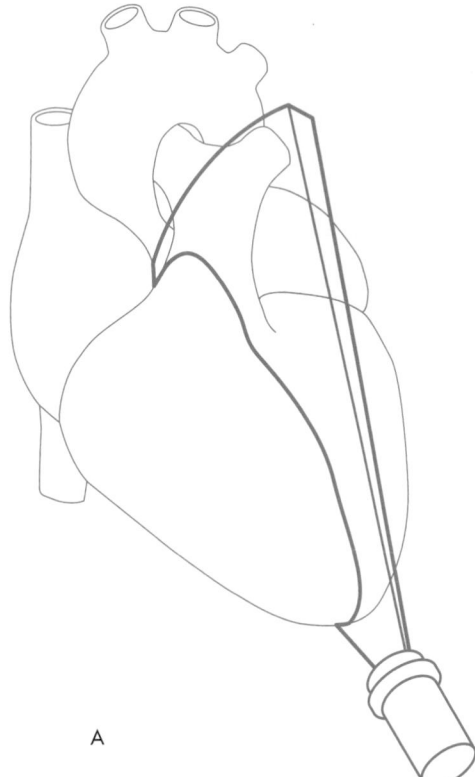

A

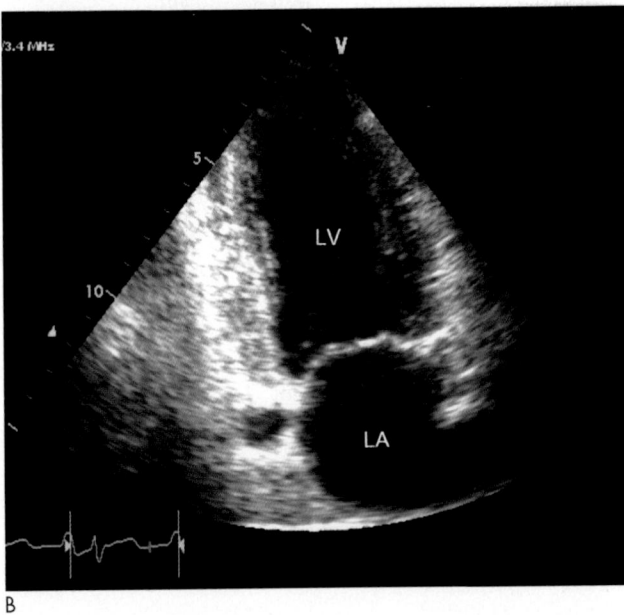

B

FIGURE 16–18. A. Orientation of the sector beam and transducer position for the apical two-chamber plane. **B.** 2D image of the apical two-chamber plane. **C.** 2D image of the apical three-chamber view. Ao, aorta; LA, atrium; LV, left ventricle. *Source: A, From Hagan AD, DeMaria AN. Clinical Applications of Two-Dimensional Echocardiography and Cardiac Doppler. Boston: Little, Brown; 1989. With permission.*

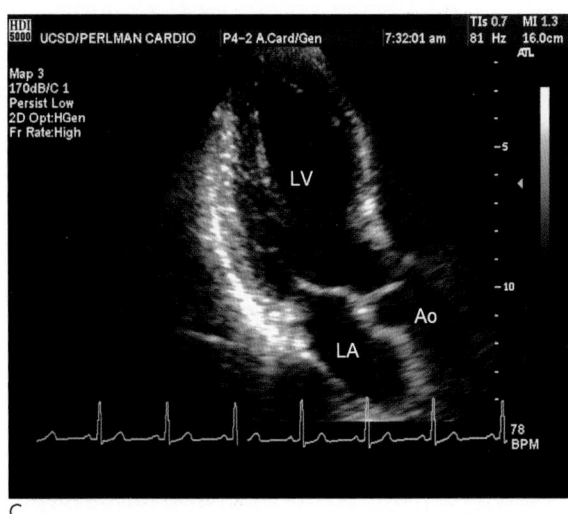

C

FIGURE 16–18. (continued)

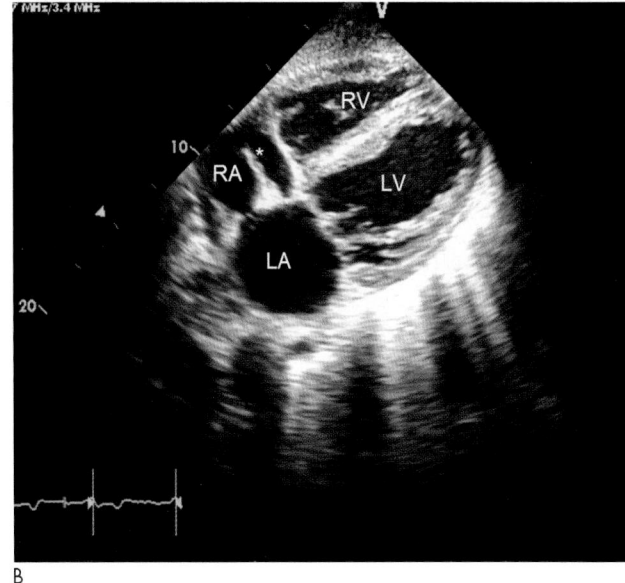

B

A

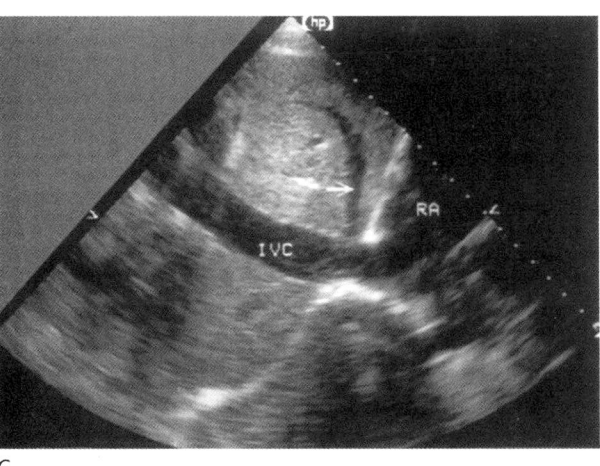

C

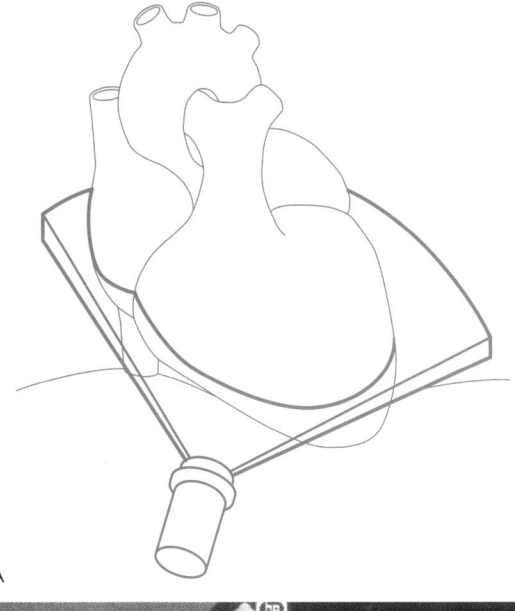

D

FIGURE 16–19. **A.** Orientation of the sector beam and transducer position for the subcostal four-chamber plane. **B.** Two-dimensional image of the subcostal four-chamber plane. **C.** Subcostal 2D image demonstrating the right atrium (RA), inferior vena cava (IVC) and hepatic vein (*arrow*). **D.** 2D image of the subcostal short-axis plane. Asterisk, a prominent eustachian valve; LA, left atrium; LV, left ventricle; RA, right atrium; RV, right ventricle. *Source: A, from Hagen AD, DeMaria AN. Clinical Applications of Two-Dimensional Echocardiography and Cardiac Doppler. Boston: Little, Brown; 1989. With permission.*

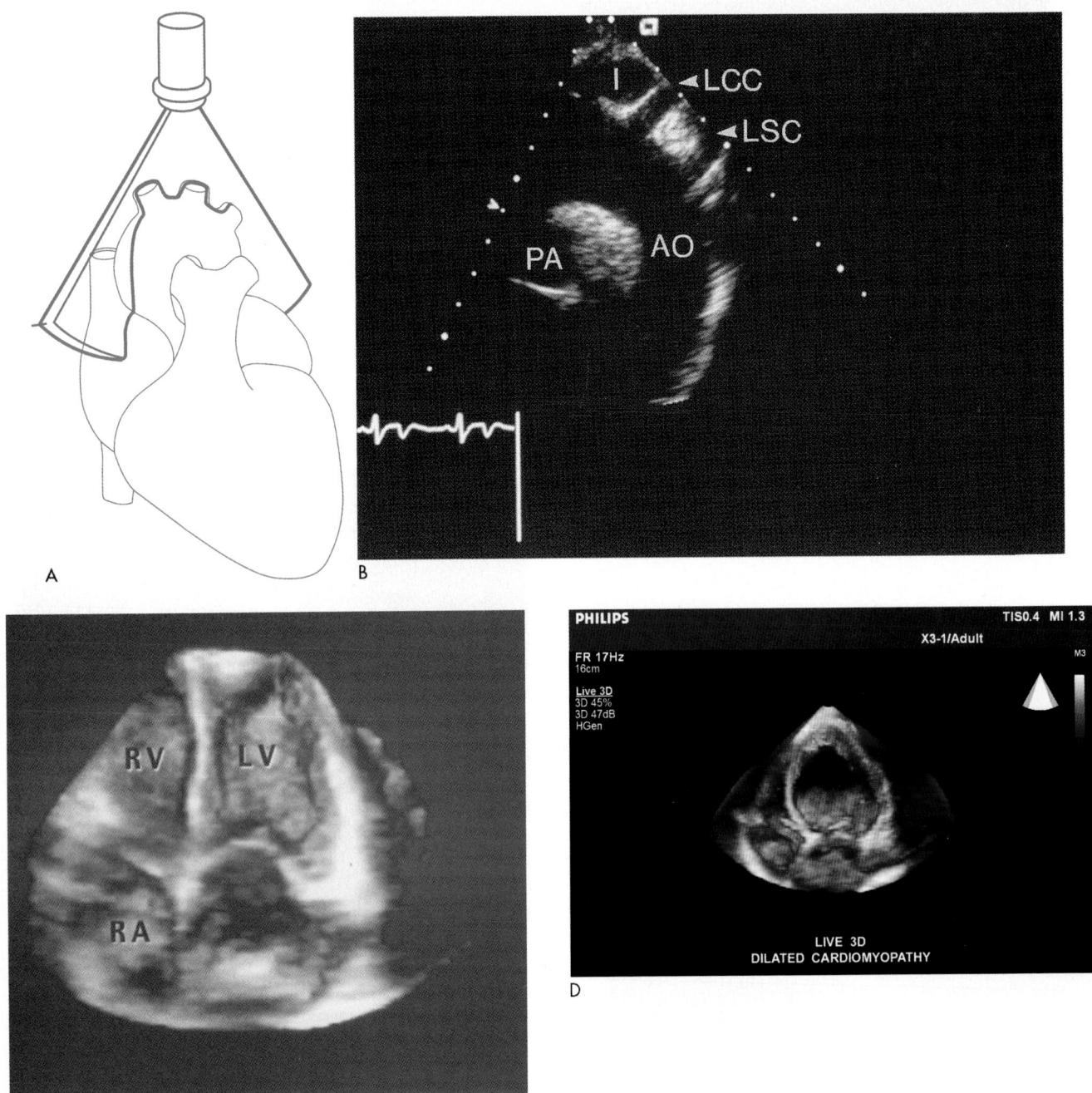

FIGURE 16–20. A. Orientation of the sector beam and transducer position for long-axis plane through the aorta from the suprasternal position. **B.** 2D image of the suprasternal long-axis view of the thoracic aorta. **C.** Real-time 3D image, apical four-chamber plane. **D.** Example of real-time 3D image in a case of dilated cardiomyopathy. Ao, aorta; I, innominate artery; LCCA, left common carotid artery; LSC, left subclavian artery; LV, left ventricle; PA, right pulmonary artery; RA, right atrium; RV, right ventricle.

tion curves.[30] Also real-time 3D echo imaging has potential for assessing regional EF and dyssynchrony (discussed in Ventricular Dyssynchrony and Cardiac Resynchronization Therapy on page 460).[31]

Assessment of Systolic Function by Two-Dimensional Echocardiography

2D echocardiography is significantly superior to M-mode approaches for the measuring cardiac chamber volumes and EF.[32–34]

Numerous algorithms have been applied to calculate LV volumes by echocardiography (Fig. 16–21). Most algorithms assumed that the LV conforms to the shape of a prolate ellipsoid and calculate volume by diameter-length or area-length formulas.[35] Multiple studies comparing LV volume calculated by area-length methods to those obtained by other techniques have yielded good correlations, with the best results obtained using biplane apical views.[36] Other algorithms have assumed an LV cavity configuration that is a combination of geometric shapes.[37] Currently, the most com-

TABLE 16–3

Cardiac Dimensions by Two-Dimensional Echocardiography

CARDIAC FEATURE	RANGE	MEAN	INDEX, CM/M²
Apical Four-Chamber View			
LV_d major	6.9–10.3 cm	8.6 cm	4.1–5.7
LV_d minor	3.3–6.1 cm	4.7 cm	2.2–3.1
LV_s minor	1.9–3.7 cm	2.8 cm	1.3–2.0
LV_d area	21.2–40.2 cm²	31.2 cm²	—
LV_s area	8.0–21.1 cm²	14.2 cm²	—
RV major	6.5–9.5 cm²	8.0 cm	3.8–5.3
RV minor	2.2–4.4 cm²	3.3–3.5 cm	1.0–2.8
RV_d area	12.0–22.2 cm²	18.6–2.1 cm²	—
RV_s area	5.4–14.6 cm²	9.9 cm²	—
LA major	4.1–6.1 cm	5.1 cm	2.3–3.5
LA minor	2.8–4.3 cm	3.5 cm	1.6–2.4
LA area	10.2–17.8 cm²	14.7 cm²	—
RA major (inf-sup)	3.5–5.5 cm	4.3–4.5 cm	2.0–3.1
RA minor	2.5–4.9 cm	3.7 cm	1.7–2.5
RA area	11.3–16.7 cm²	13.8–14 cm²	—
Apical Two-Chamber View			
LV_d major	6.8–9.4 cm	8.0 cm	—
LV_d minor	3.8–5.7 cm	4.6 cm	—
LV_d area	19.4–48.0 cm²	35.6 cm²	—
LV_s	8.9–27.0 cm	14.3 cm	—
Parasternal Long-Axis View			
LV_d	3.5–6.0 cm	4.8 cm	2.3–3.1
LV_s	2.1–4.0 cm	3.1 cm	1.4–2.1
RV	1.9–3.8 cm	2.8 cm	1.2–2.0
LA (A-P)	2.7–4.5 cm	3.6 cm	1.6–2.4
LA (S-I)	3.1–5.5 cm	4.4 cm	—
LA area	9.0–19.3 cm²	13.8 cm²	—
Ao	2.2–3.6 cm	2.9 cm	1.4–2.0
Parasternal Short-Axis View			
Ao	2.3–3.7 cm	3.0–2.3 cm	1.6–2.4
RVOT	1.9–2.2 cm	2.7 cm	—
RA	1.5–2.5 cm	1.9–2.2 cm	—
LA	2.6–4.5 cm	3.6 cm	1.6–2.4
LA area	7.2–13.0 cm²	10.8 cm²	—
LV_d (PM level)	3.5–5.8 cm	4.7 cm	2.2–3.1
LV_s (PM level)	2.2–4.0 cm	3.1 cm	1.4–2.2
LV_d area (PM level)	16.0–31.2 cm²	22.2 cm²	—
LV_s area (PM level)	5.2–13.4 cm²	8.5 cm²	—
LV_d (Ch. level)	3.5–6.2	4.8 cm	2.3–3.2
LV_s (Ch. level)	2.3–4.0	3.2 cm	1.5–2.2
LV_d area (Ch. level)	16.4–32.3 cm²	22.5 cm²	—
LV_s area (Ch. level)	6.1–16.8 cm²	10.7 cm²	—
Subcostal View			
IVC diameter		1.8 cm	—

Ao, aorta; Ch., chordal; IVC, inferior vena cava; LA, left atrium; LV, left ventricle; LV_d, left ventricle, end diastole; LV_s, left ventricle, end systole; PA, pulmonary artery; PM, papillary muscle; RA, right atrium; RV, right ventricle; RV_d, right ventricle, end diastole; RVOT, right ventricular outflow tract; RV_s, right ventricle, end systole.

SOURCE: The values shown in this table represent a compilation of data from three sources: Schnittinger I, Gordon EP, Fitzgerald PJ, et al. Standardized intracardiac measurements of two-dimensional echocardiography. J Am Coll Cardiol 1983; 5:934. Triulzi M, Weyman A. Normal cross-sectional measurements in adults. In: Weyman A, ed. Echocardiography. Philadelphia: Lea & Febiger; 1982;497. Hagan AD, DiSessa TG, Bloor CM, et al. Two-Dimensional Echocardiography: Clinical-Pathological Corrections in Adult and Congenital Heart Disease. Boston: Little, Brown; 1983;553.

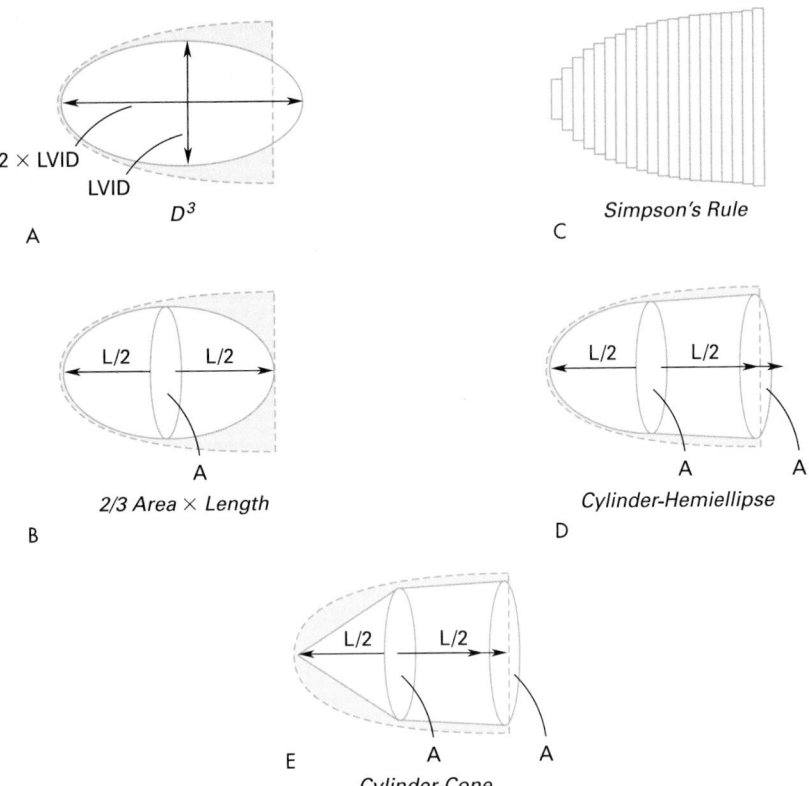

FIGURE 16–21. Various models used to estimate left ventricular volume. **A.** *D-cubed*. **B.** Two-thirds area × length. **C.** Simpson rule. **D.** Cylinder-hemiellipse. **E.** Cylinder-cone. A, cross-sectional area; L, length of left ventricle major axis; LVID, left ventricular internal dimension (minor axis).

the endocardial surface.[37] Greater enhancement of endocardial border delineation and improvement of the reliability of measures of LV size and contraction have been achieved using tissue harmonic imaging and by the injection of ultrasonic contrast agents to opacify the LV cavity.[38] A software package that provides instantaneous and automated endocardial border delineation throughout the cardiac cycle has been developed based on the display of tissue signals as backscatter rather than specular reflection.[39] This technique of automated quantitation can yield continuous measurements of LV volume throughout the cardiac cycle and can derive values for EF, ejection rate, and rate of filling during diastole (Fig. 16–22). This same technology has been used to display endocardial excursion throughout systolic contraction or diastolic expansion in a color format superimposed on the tissue image (Fig. 16–23). This technique has been valuable in the recognition of abnormalities of LV contraction and regional disturbances of LV diastolic function.[40,41] Finally, studies employing 3D echocardiography have reported better reproducibility of measurements than 2D methods.

monly used algorithm to calculate LV volumes is based on the Simpson rule, which derives measurements by dividing the LV by parallel planes into a number of small segments and then summating the area of the individual disks. Although all modifications of the Simpson rule give good results, the optimal correlations have been achieved with a modification that separately quantifies the volume of the apex as an ellipsoid.[34,36]

Accurate calculations of LV volumes by echocardiography are critically dependent on high-quality images to delineate the endocardium and image the entire LV perimeter. Echocardiographic estimates of LV volumes underestimate those calculated by other techniques and are most accurate in the absence of significant alterations of LV size and contraction. End-systolic measurements are more accurate than end diastolic, probably owing to superior endocardial definition. Nevertheless, echocardiographic calculations of LV volumes have generally yielded correlation coefficients in excess of 0.75 as compared with radionuclide angiography, cineangiography, and autopsy studies regardless of the algorithm employed.[31–36]

Images of the power spectrum of the Doppler signal produced by contraction/relaxation and colorization of the B-mode tissue image have been used to visualize

DOPPLER ECHOCARDIOGRAPHY: PRINCIPLES AND APPLICATIONS

【 】 THE DOPPLER PRINCIPLE

Using the principle first delineated by the physicist Johann Christian Doppler,[42] ultrasound can be used to determine the velocity

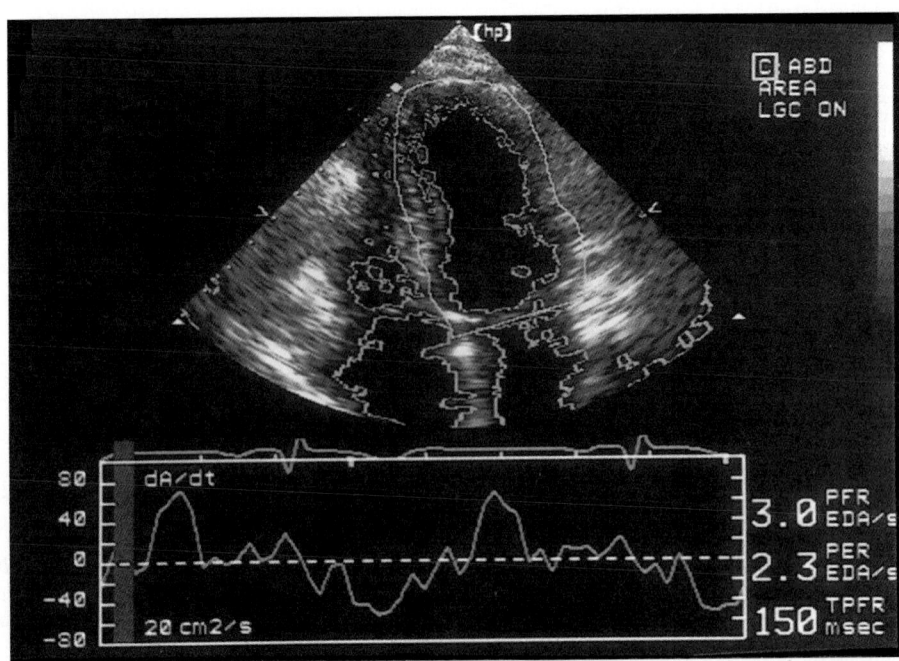

FIGURE 16–22. Example of endocardial border detection and on-line calculation of change in area over time (dA/dt).

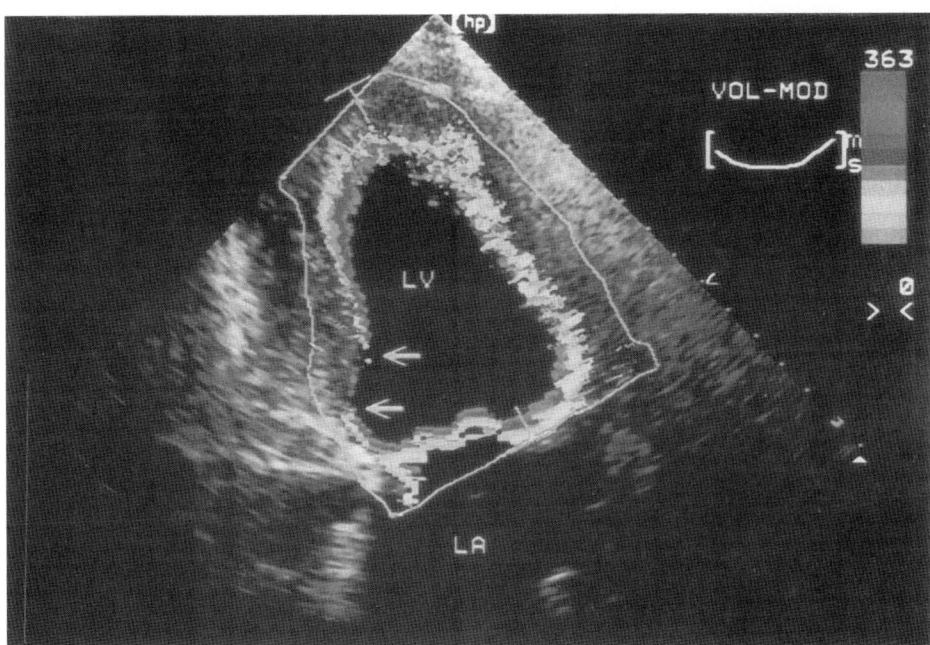

FIGURE 16–23. Color kinesis image (apical two-chamber view) from a patient with an inferobasal infarction. Systolic motion in this area (*arrows*) is markedly diminished.

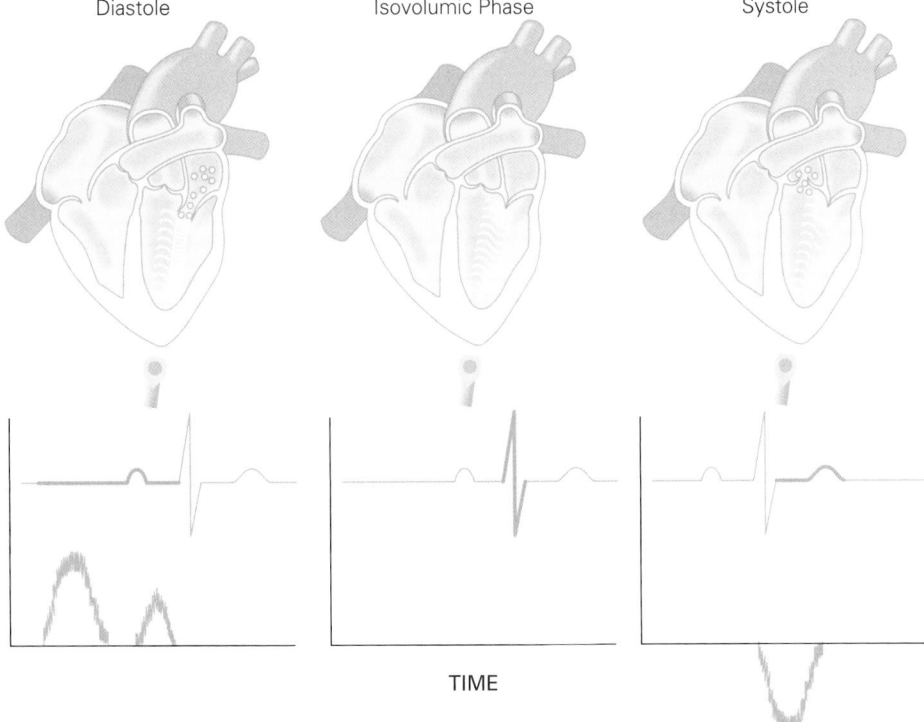

FIGURE 16–24. Basic principle of the Doppler shift. During diastole (*left panel*), an ultrasound beam directed toward the junction of the mitral and aortic annuli is reflected by red blood cells moving toward the transducer. The frequency of the received ultrasound is greater than that of the transmitted beam, and the spectral tracing is recorded above the baseline (i.e., flow is toward the transducer). During the isovolumic phase (*middle panel*), both the mitral and AoVs are closed and little flow occurs within the left ventricle. Therefore, there are no significant changes in the transmitted and received frequencies of the Doppler beam and no spectral tracing is recorded. During systole (*right panel*), the transmitted beam is reflected by red blood cells moving away from the transducer. Therefore, the frequency of the received ultrasound is lower than that of the transmitted beam, and the spectral tracing is recorded below the baseline. AoV, aortic valve.

and direction of blood flow by measuring the change in frequency produced when sound waves are reflected from red blood cells. Thus, information regarding the presence, direction, velocity, and turbulence of blood flow can be acquired by cardiac ultrasound.

The Doppler principle states that when a sound (or light) signal strikes a moving object, the frequency of that signal is altered, and the increase or decrease in frequency is proportional to the velocity and direction at which the object is moving (Fig. 16–24). If a stationary transducer at the apex emits a sound wave with a transmitted frequency of f_o and the wave is reflected by nonmoving red blood cells (RBCs) in an isovolumic phase of the cardiac cycle, the received frequency f_r will be identical to f_o. If the signal is reflected by RBCs that are moving toward the transducer, as through the MV in diastole, the returning waves will be compressed so that $f_r > f_o$. Conversely, if the target RBCs are moving away from the transducer, as in the outflow tract in systole, the returning sound waves will be elongated and the received frequency will be decreased. It is important to note that the magnitude of change in the received frequency is directly related to the velocity at which blood is flowing toward or away from the transducer.[43] If the velocity of sound and the angle θ between the direction of RBC flow and the beam path are known, then the velocity of the RBCs is described by the Doppler equation:

$$V = f_d(c) / 2f_o(cos\ \theta)$$

where f_d is the frequency shift recorded, f_o the transmitted frequency, and c the velocity of sound. Note that the denominator is doubled. By measuring Doppler shift frequencies, the velocity and direction of blood flow can be calculated, displayed, and recorded.

The angle between the direction of blood flow and the course of the sound beam is a most important factor in Doppler ultrasound (Fig. 16–25). Velocity is a vectorial entity, having magnitude and direction; and Doppler detects only those velocities parallel or near parallel to the interrogating signal. Because the relationship between velocity and the angle is a cosine function and the cosine of angles up to 20 degrees is 0.9, little

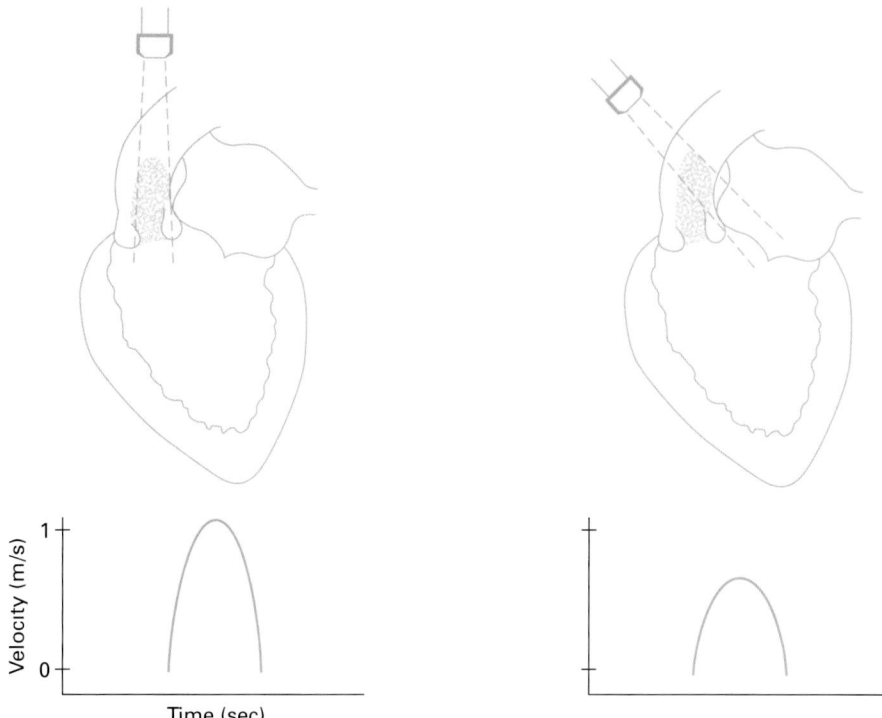

FIGURE 16–25. Effect of the angle of incidence on the velocity recorded with Doppler analysis. The true velocity is underestimated when the ultrasound beam is not parallel to the direction of blood flow. *Source: From Hagan AD, DeMaria AN. Clinical Applications of Two-Dimensional Echocardiography and Cardiac Doppler. Boston: Little, Brown; 1989. With permission.*

error is introduced within this range.[43] However, considerable errors occur when it is >20 degrees. Moreover, the angle of incidence in 3D space usually cannot be determined with certainty from 2D echocardiographic images. Therefore, it is crucial to position and direct the transducer so that the beam is as parallel to flow as possible. In clinical use the frequency of transmitted ultrasound is in the range of 2 to 7 MHz, the velocity of sound in tissue is approximately 1540 m/sec, and the Doppler shift frequency is relatively small (approximately 1 to 4 kHz) as compared with the transmitted frequency. Because the Doppler shift frequencies are in the audible range, a speaker integrated into the Doppler echocardiography system can present them as an audible signal. Normal signals are tonal or musical.

Fig. 16–26 shows the typical graphic pulsed Doppler pattern of normal systolic blood flow through the RV outflow tract into the PA, with flow velocity on the Y-axis and time on the X-axis. The location and size of the area from which Doppler recordings are derived is determined by positioning a sample volume on the echo image. The absence of flow is represented by the zero or no-flow line, termed the *baseline*. By convention, flow toward the transducer is displayed above the baseline and flow away from the transducer is displayed below the baseline. The velocities above and below baseline represent flow toward or away from the transducer, not forward or backward in the circulation. The sample volume almost invariably includes RBCs flowing at slightly different velocities. Even normal laminar blood flow in the great vessels varies in velocity across the lumen, because RBCs in the center of the vessel move at higher velocity than those exposed to viscous friction at the wall. Therefore, any returning Doppler-shifted signal contains a spectrum of velocities, each of which can be displayed

by means of fast Fourier transform analysis. The graphic output of the Doppler signal displays the range of velocities within the sample volume site at any time in gray scale and the number of RBCs moving at any velocity as relative intensity. Normal laminar flow is characterized by a uniformity of velocity and direction of individual RBCs, and therefore a narrowly dispersed signal, whereas disturbed or turbulent flow is manifest by marked variability in velocity and direction and therefore a broad signal.

Echographs have now been modified to enable recording of the low-velocity, high-amplitude Doppler signals produced by moving tissue as well as those of RBCs. The ability to assess tissue velocity provides an evaluation of transmural rate of contraction and relaxation.[44] Also, Doppler tissue recordings permit assessment of regional function and appear to be quite useful in the assessment of diastolic function (see The Standard Doppler Examination on page 379).[45] Finally, Doppler tissue recordings provide the basis for the derivation of regional strain measurements by echocardiography. Such measurements are independent of overall cardiac motion and passive motion and therefore enable the most accurate assessment of myocardial contractile performance.

【 】 CONTINUOUS- AND PULSED-WAVE DOPPLER

Time-velocity spectral recordings of blood flow are generally obtained with two types of Doppler interrogation: continuous and pulsed wave (Fig. 16–27).[46] In the continuous-wave (CW) mode, sound waves are both transmitted and received continuously. This

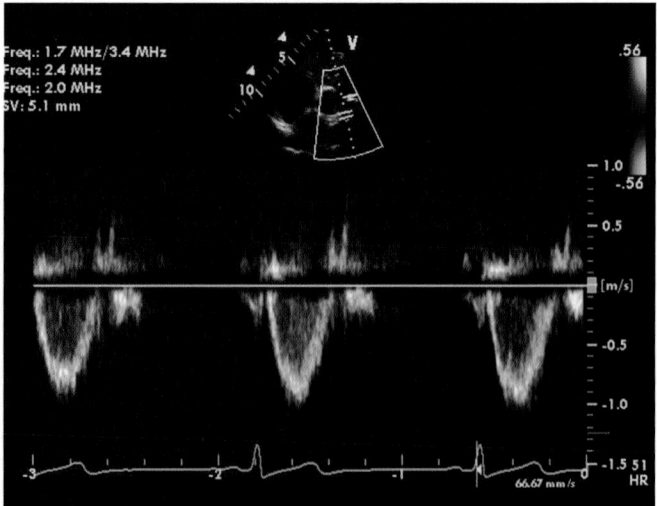

FIGURE 16–26. Doppler spectral envelope of normal blood flow through the RVOT during systole. The transducer is in the parasternal position and the sample volume is placed just proximal to the pulmonic valve. RVOT, right ventricular outflow tract.

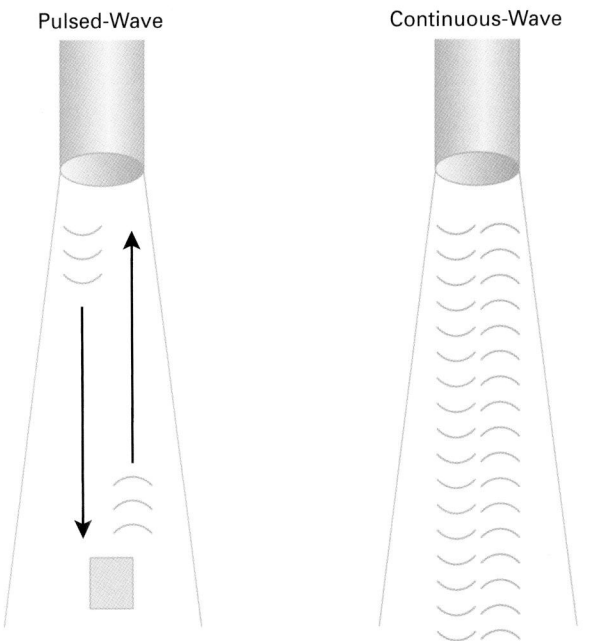

Pulsed-Wave   Continuous-Wave

FIGURE 16–27. Pulsed-wave (PW) and continuous-wave (CW) Doppler. With PW, a single pulse of ultrasound energy is emitted, and its reflection from a sample volume is received before the following pulse is transmitted. With CW, there is continuous transmission and reception of ultrasound energy.

requires two piezoelectric crystals in each transducer, one for transmitting and one for receiving. Because all flow velocities along the beam are recorded, CW Doppler cannot define individual signals at specific distances from the transducer—a problem referred to as *range ambiguity.* CW Doppler can accurately measure the direction and velocity of overall flow but cannot discern the precise site of origin of individual components within the signal (Fig. 16–28B).

The problem of range ambiguity can be overcome by pulsed-wave Doppler (PWD). Short bursts of signal are transmitted from the transducer at a given pulse repetition frequency (PRF). The instrument then receives the signal for only a brief period: an interval that corresponds to the time required for sound energy to travel and return from a specific site along the beam path. The operator selects the location at which flow is to be examined by positioning a sample volume, and the instrument determines the period during which to receive the incoming reflected frequencies. With PWD only a single piezoelectric crystal is needed and flow can be recorded in one small area within the heart or vasculature.[46] Unfortunately, pulsed Doppler techniques employ intermittent sampling and are therefore susceptible to a problem of range ambiguity referred to as *aliasing.*[47] Aliasing is the erroneous representation of flow in the direction opposite to that in which it is actually occurring. To correctly record the velocity of blood flow by pulsed Doppler, the PRF must be at least double the Doppler shift frequency, a value known as the *Nyquist limit.* If the blood flow examined is of very high velocity or far from the transducer (requiring a long transit time), it may necessitate an unobtainably high PRF. In such cases aliasing will occur as Doppler signals that depict flow at high velocity in ambiguous or opposite directions compared to actual flow (see Fig. 16–28A). An intermediate-mode, high-PRF Doppler is also available. This mode enables higher-velocity recordings to be obtained at a compromise of depicting two to four sample sites simultaneously.

COLOR-FLOW DOPPLER

The major limitation of pulsed and CW Doppler (*spectral Doppler*) is that no spatial information regarding the size, shape, and 2D direction of flow is provided. An extension of PWD techniques, color-flow Doppler (CFD), provides real-time M-mode or 2D imaging of blood flow by presenting the velocity and direction of RBC movement as shades of color superimposed on gray-level 2D tissue structure. Standard pulsed Doppler yields flow signals from a single site along a single scan line. In CFD rapid pulsed-wave interrogations are performed at multiple sites for multiple scan lines to create a spatially correct and dynamic display of moving blood within the heart and vasculature (Fig. 16–29). Doppler signals are presented as colors assigned to individual sites (Fig. 16–30). Blood flow moving toward the transducer is displayed in red, flow away from the transducer is displayed in blue, and increasing velocity is depicted in brighter shades of each color. The variance within each signal is calculated as a statistical marker of turbulence and is presented by adding green to the image (Fig. 16–31). Therefore, turbulent flow jets appear as a mosaic mix of colors. CFD also can be superimposed onto M-mode tracings (Fig. 16–32), often termed *Color M-mode imaging,* and is helpful in clarifying the timing of flow phenomena.

NORMAL AND ABNORMAL FLOW DYNAMICS

Normal flow is laminar, with all RBCs exhibiting the same velocity and direction of flow. Most pathologic conditions, with the exception of atrial septal defects, involve disturbed or turbulent flow and share a common hydrodynamic basis for the resultant flow dynamics. Specifically, nearly all circulatory disturbances (stenosis, regurgitation, shunt) involve blood flow from a high-pressure chamber to a lower-pressure chamber through a restricted orifice.[43] For example, aortic stenosis (AS) is a forward flow disturbance in which turbulent blood travels from a high-pressure LV to a lower-pressure aorta through a restricted aortic orifice in systole. Aortic regurgitation (AR) is a retrograde flow disturbance in which turbulent blood regurgitates from a high-pressure aorta to a lower-pressure left ventricle through a small regurgitant orifice in diastole. In each case, the pressure gradient results in a high-velocity jet coursing through a restricted orifice, reaching its maximal velocity at a site just distal to the orifice, designated the *vena contracta,* at which time shear forces produce vortices resulting in flow of varying direction and velocity (Fig. 16–33). In each case, the velocity of the jet is related to the pressure gradient across the orifice. On pulsed Doppler recordings, these hemodynamic abnormalities cause broadening of the spectral signal and aliasing. On CW recordings, high velocity represents the primary abnormality. By color-flow imaging, the disturbance is manifest by the increased variance and higher velocities in the signal.

THE STANDARD DOPPLER EXAMINATION

A clinical Doppler examination must be performed with full consideration of the three different Doppler modalities available, the types of information each can provide, the multiple sites for flow interrogation, and the spectrum of pathologic lesions that pro-

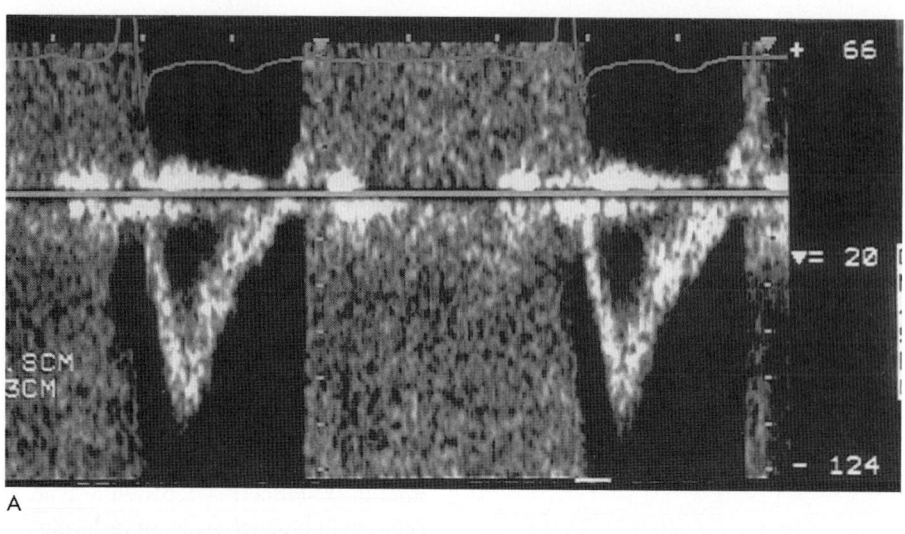

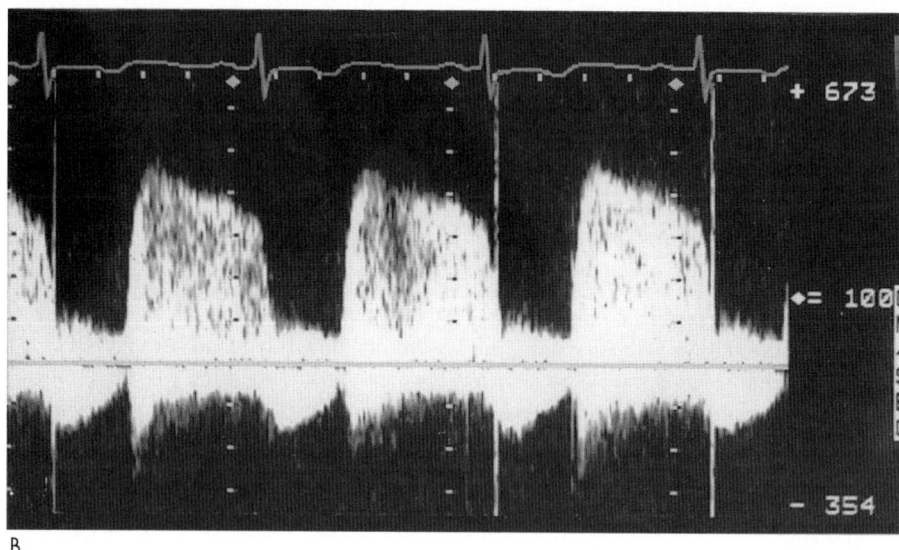

FIGURE 16–28. A. PW Doppler tracing from a patient with aortic regurgitation. The transducer is in the apical position and the sample volume is in the left ventricular outflow tract. A laminar envelope is seen during systole, whereas aliased flow is present during diastole because of high-velocity flow. **B.** CW Doppler tracing through the left ventricular outflow tract (with transducer in the apical position). The maximal velocity of the aortic regurgitation is now measurable, but all other velocities along the Doppler beam are recorded as well. CW, continuous wave; PW, pulsed wave.

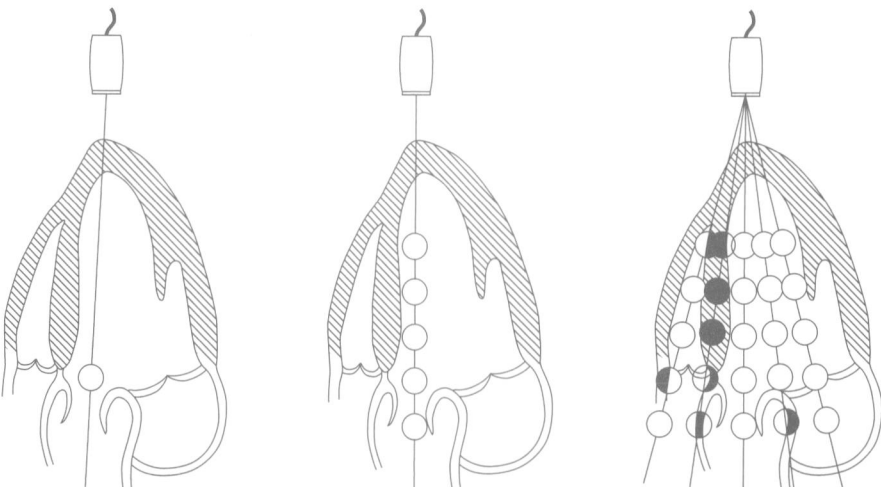

FIGURE 16–29. Simplified mechanism of color-flow Doppler imaging. Single-gate (*left*) or multiple-gate pulsed Doppler (*center*) can evaluate flow at points along a single ultrasound beam path. Color-flow imaging (*right*) assesses the velocity and direction of flow for multiple sample volumes along multiple beam paths and assigns a color indicative of velocity and direction at each sample volume site. *Source: From Hagan AD, DeMaria AN. Clinical Applications of Two-Dimensional Echocardiography and Cardiac Doppler. Boston: Little, Brown; 1989. With permission.*

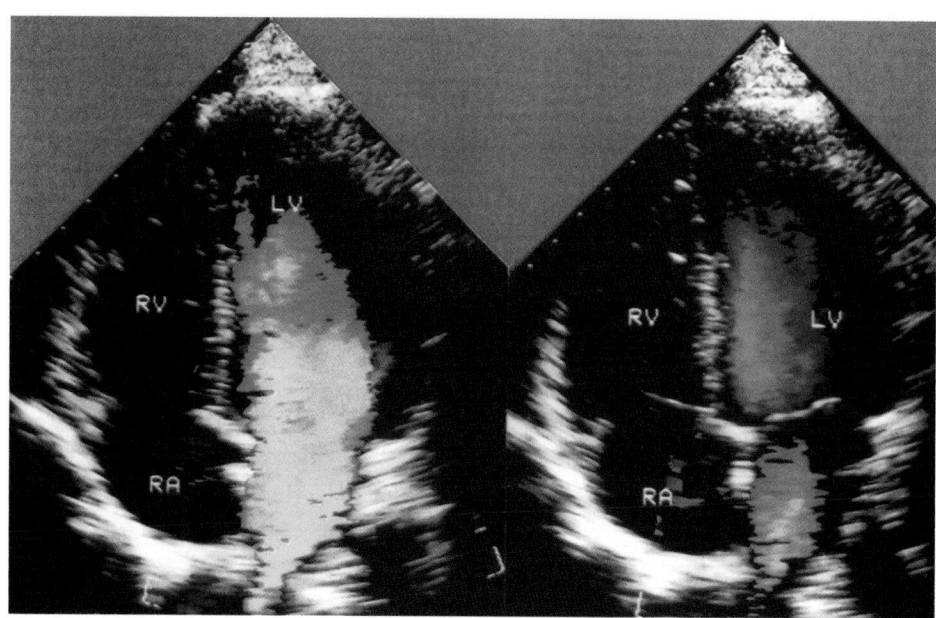

FIGURE 16–30. Apical four-chamber images with color-flow Doppler during diastole and systole. Red flow indicates movement toward the transducer (diastolic filling); blue flow indicates movement away from the transducer (systolic ejection). LV, left ventricle; RA, right atrium; RV, right ventricle.

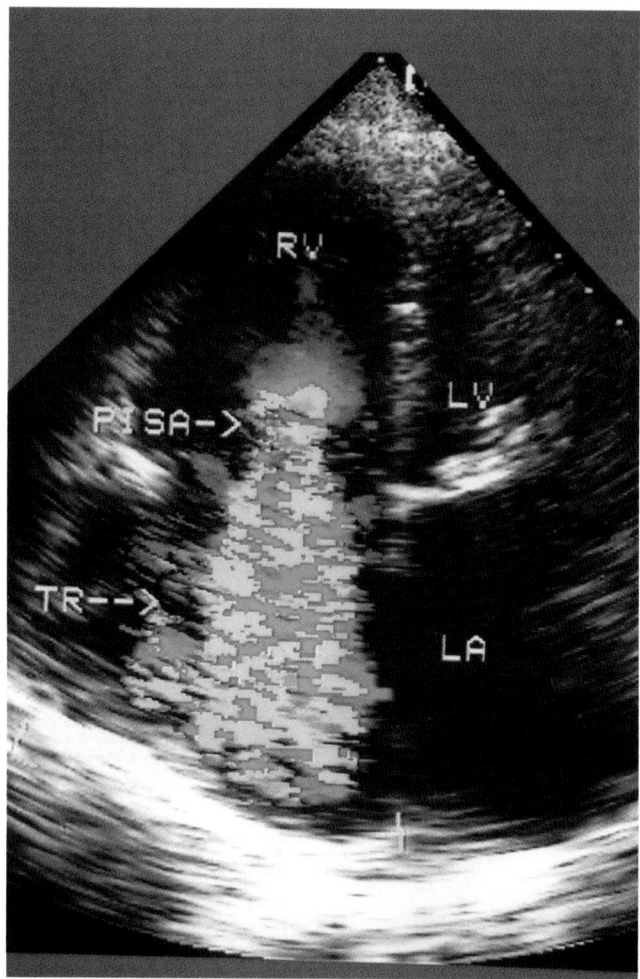

FIGURE 16–31. Apical four-chamber view of severe tricuspid regurgitation. The Doppler color jet fills the right atrium (RA). PISA, proximal isovelocity surface area; LV, left ventricle; LA, left atrium; RV, right ventricle.

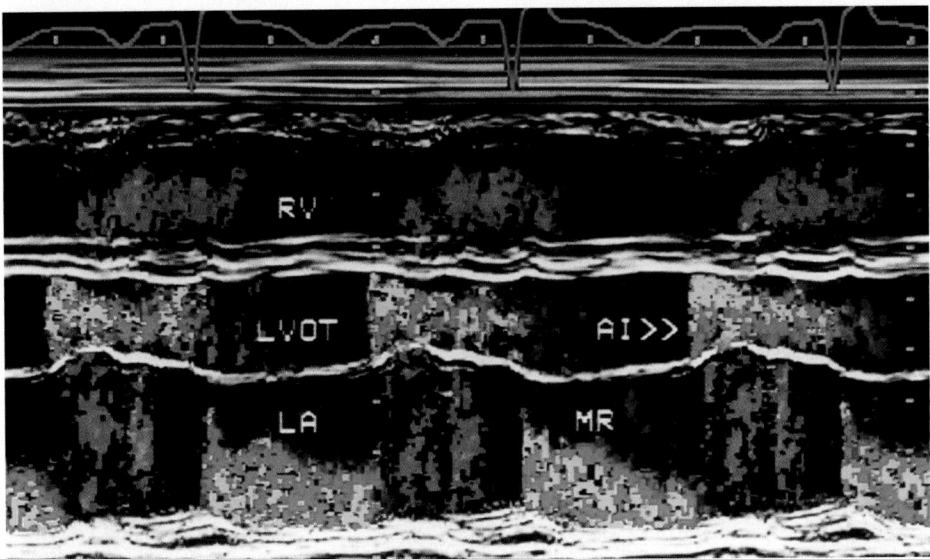

FIGURE 16–32. Color-flow Doppler superimposed on an M-mode image. The transducer is in parasternal position, and the cursor is directed through the left ventricular outflow tract (*LVOT*) and left atrium (*LA*). The patient under study has both aortic insufficiency (*AI*) and mitral regurgitation (*MR*). RV, right ventricle.

duces flow disturbances. However, most echocardiographic examinations include screening for flow disturbances by CFD. Because Doppler signals are best recorded with the ultrasound beam parallel to flow, screening is typically performed in long-axis or apical views. Any flow disturbances visualized are subsequently examined by CW spectral recordings and, in most laboratories, by PWD. Although CW examination is typically reserved for flow disturbances, PWD may also be of value in quantifying flow dynamics in the setting of laminar flow. In this regard pulsed Doppler recordings obtained at the mitral, tricuspid, and aortic valvular orifices, PA, and pulmonary veins constitute part of a standard echocardiogram in many laboratories (see Fig. 16–26 and Fig. 16–34 to Fig. 16–37).

Because the Doppler examination is usually performed with a long-axis or apical transducer orientation, diastolic filling is characteristically encoded in red and ejection in blue (see Fig. 16–30). Color aliasing is often observed at the levels of the mitral annulus and LV outflow tract as an abrupt change from bright red to bright

blue or vice versa, usually in the center of the flow stream. Pulsed Doppler recordings of transmitral flow velocities are often recorded at the level of both the leaflet tips and annulus. Velocities are higher at the tips, whereas recordings at the annulus offer the ability to calculate flow through a cross-sectional area that is relatively uniform throughout the cardiac cycle. A sample volume positioned in the right upper pulmonary vein reveals systolic (S) and diastolic (D) flow velocities of nearly equal magnitude followed by a short, low-velocity reversal of flow into the pulmonary veins following atrial contraction (A) (see Fig. 16–36). Flow in the LV outflow tract and aortic annulus area is characterized by a progressive increase of velocity peaking in early systole, followed by a more gradual deceleration of flow (see Fig. 16–35). Examinations of the tricuspid and pulmonary valves give qualitatively similar results to those of the mitral and AoVs (see Fig. 16–26 and Fig. 16–37). Normal values for forward flow velocity are given in Table 16–4. Velocity in normal individuals is highest in the aorta and is less than 2 m/sec.[48] Other common measurements include the acceleration time, from the beginning of flow to peak velocity of flow in the ascending aorta or PA; and the deceleration time, from LV inflow peak E-wave velocity extrapolated to baseline zero velocity.

DOPPLER ASSESSMENT OF DIASTOLIC FUNCTION

There has been a great deal of interest in using mitral inflow velocity patterns to evaluate LV diastolic properties.[49–52] Transmitral filling velocities reflect the pressure gradient between the LA and LV during diastole[49] (see Fig. 16–34). In early diastole pressure in the LV normally falls below that in the LA, producing an increase in velocity due to rapid transmitral inflow (E wave). Flow decelerates as the pressures equilibrate in mid-diastole. In late diastole LA contraction restores a small gradient, causing transmitral flow to accelerate to a second peak (A wave) that is of less magnitude than the E wave. In individuals in whom early LV relaxation is impaired, the

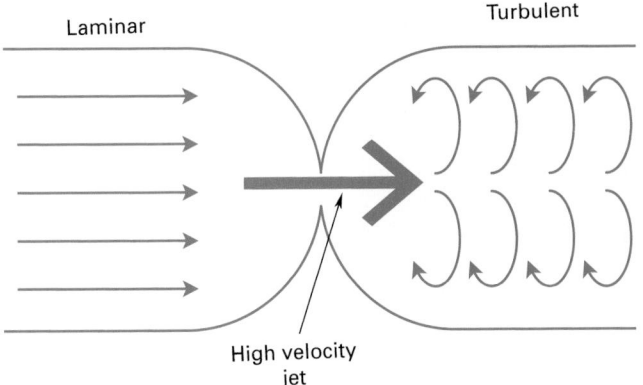

FIGURE 16–33. Flow characteristics through a stenotic orifice. Proximal to the stenosis, the flow is laminar. Near the point of maximal stenosis, the flow velocity is markedly increased. Turbulent flow is present distal to the stenosis.

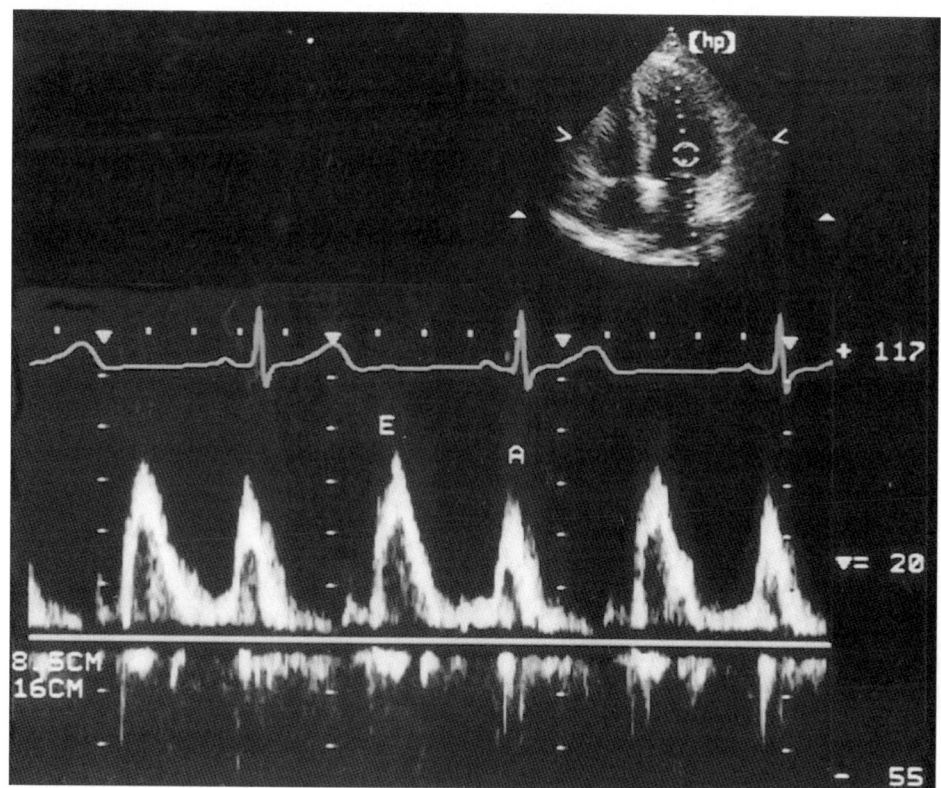

FIGURE 16–34. Normal PWD tracing from the left ventricular inflow tract, displaying the early rapid filling (*E*) and atrial contraction (*A*) phases of diastolic flow. The transducer is in the apical position and the sample volume is at the mitral leaflet tips. PWD, pulsed-wave Doppler.

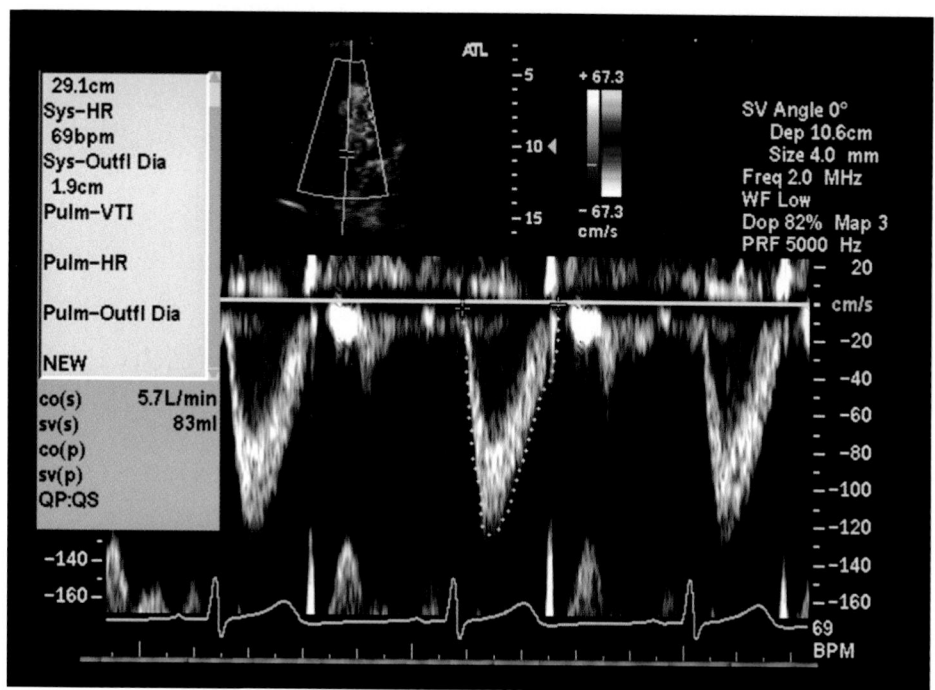

FIGURE 16–35. Normal PWD tracing with the sample volume in the left ventricular outflow tract (apical transducer position). PWD, pulsed-wave Doppler.

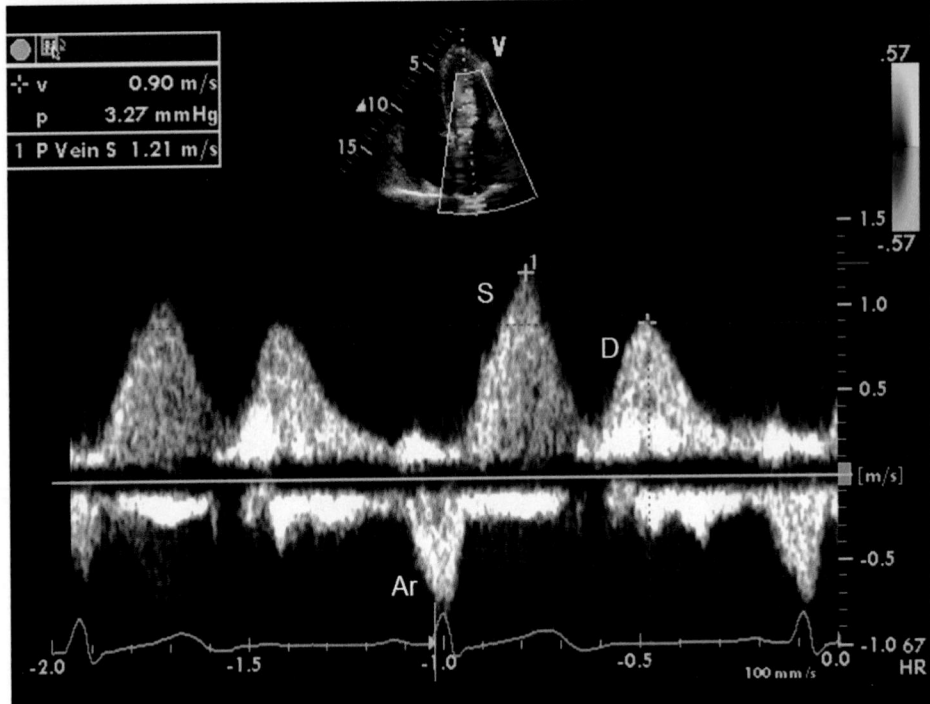

FIGURE 16–36. PWD tracing from the right upper pulmonary vein (recorded from the apical transducer position). Flow toward the heart is biphasic, with peaks in systole (*S*) and diastole (*D*). A small amount of reversed flow is seen during atrial contraction (*A*). PWD, pulsed-wave Doppler.

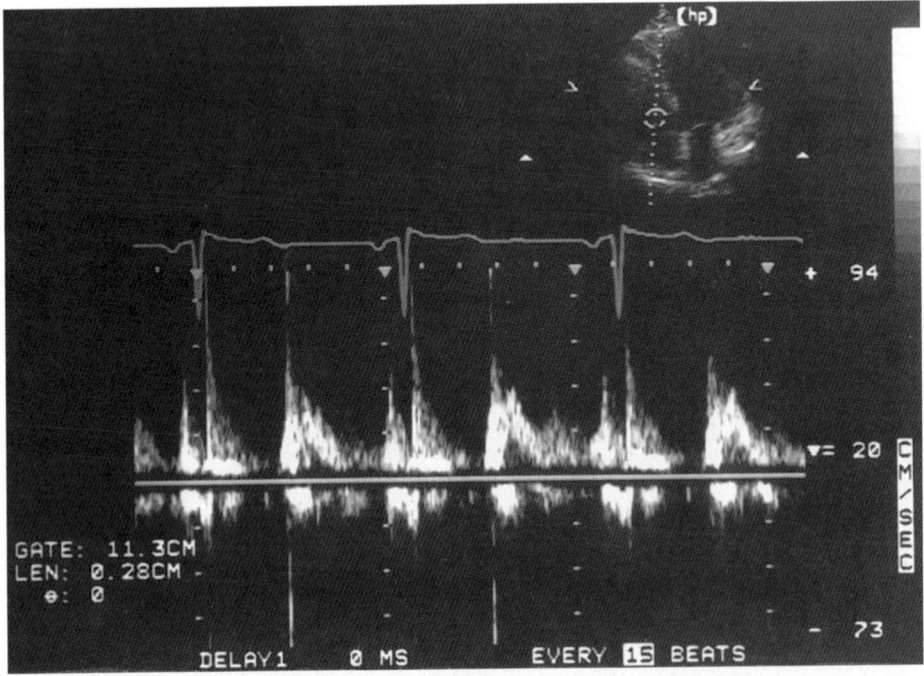

FIGURE 16–37. PWD tracing from the RV inflow tract (apical transducer position). PWD, pulsed-wave Doppler; RV, right ventricle.

TABLE 16–4

Normal Intracardiac Doppler Velocities

	VELOCITY, M/SEC
Right ventricle	
Tricuspid flow	0.3–0.7
Pulmonary artery	0.6–0.9
Left ventricle	
Mitral flow	0.6–1.3
Aorta	1.0–1.7

SOURCE: Hatle L, Angelsen B. Doppler Ultrasound in Cardiology, 2nd ed. Philadelphia: Lea & Febiger; 1985.

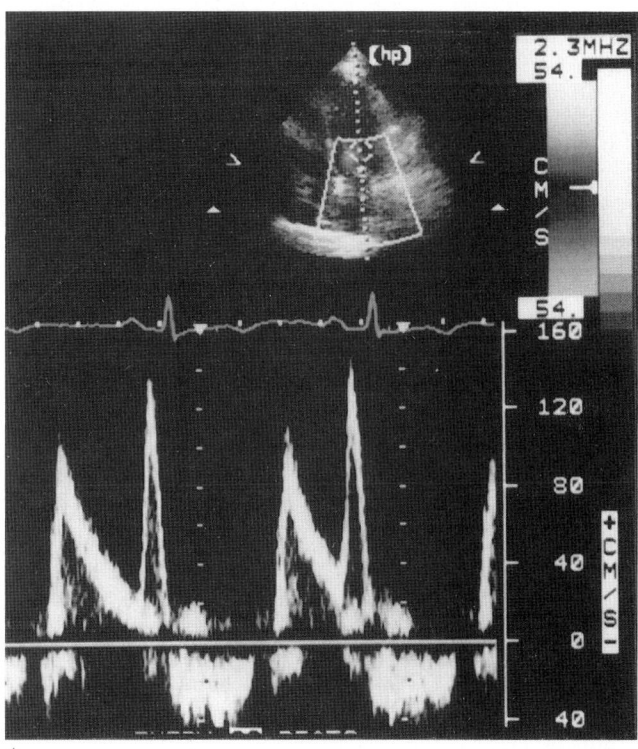
A

transmitral pressure gradient is blunted, resulting in a decrease in both the velocity of early filling and rate of E-wave deceleration[50,51] (Fig. 16–38A). Conversely, in patients with marked increases of LA pressure and LV stiffness, early diastolic filling velocities are high, deceleration is rapid, and late filling following atrial contraction is markedly reduced. This is the so-called *restrictive pattern of LV filling* (see Fig. 16–38B). Accordingly, an E-wave velocity that is substantially less than the A-wave velocity and is accompanied by a prolonged deceleration time represents evidence of impaired early diastolic relaxation by Doppler, whereas an increased E-wave velocity and decreased A-wave velocity (E/A ratio >2.5:1 or 3:1) accompanied by a diminished deceleration time (<160 ms) is indicative of a noncompliant LV with markedly elevated left atrial pressures.[51] A restrictive pattern occurs with restrictive cardiomyopathy or advanced LV dysfunction of any cause and in pericardial disease.[53]

These abnormal mitral inflow patterns can be clinically useful and, when they are markedly distorted, are generally reliable in identifying and characterizing diastolic dysfunction. Several variables other than diastolic function, however, are capable of influencing transmitral filling velocities. Transmitral Doppler filling dynamics are affected by the age of the patient, changes in heart rate,[54] respiration, and even the position of the Doppler sample volume within the MV orifice.[55] Transmitral inflow is sensitive to loading conditions, and reductions in LV preload induced by nitroglycerin and/or lower body negative pressure can induce a striking decrease in early transmitral filling velocities independent of changes in diastolic properties. The influence of LV loading on transmitral filling is most striking when an increase

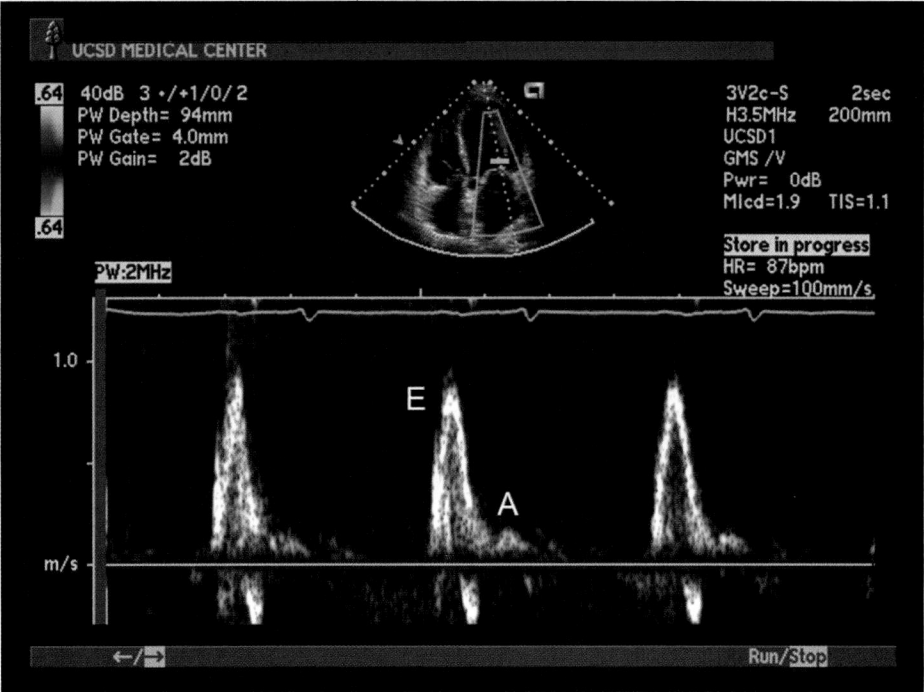
B

FIGURE 16–38. **A.** PWD tracing of diastolic relaxation abnormality (see text for details). **B.** PWD tracing of diastolic restrictive abnormality (see text for details) **C.** Tissue Doppler recording of normal lateral mitral annular motion (apical transducer position). Peak early diastolic annular velocity is 15 cm/sec. **D.** PWD recording of pulmonary venous flow in mild diastolic dysfunction (abnormal relaxation). The S wave is prominent whereas the D wave is small. **E.** Tissue Doppler image (lateral mitral annulus) in mild diastolic dysfunction. Early diastolic velocity is blunted (8 cm/sec). **F.** PWD recording of pulmonary venous flow in severe diastolic dysfunction. The S wave is small whereas the D wave is prominent. **G.** Tissue Doppler image in severe diastolic dysfunction. Both E_m and A_m velocities are abnormally low. A, atrial contraction; E, early rapid filling; PWD, pulsed-wave Doppler. *(continued)*

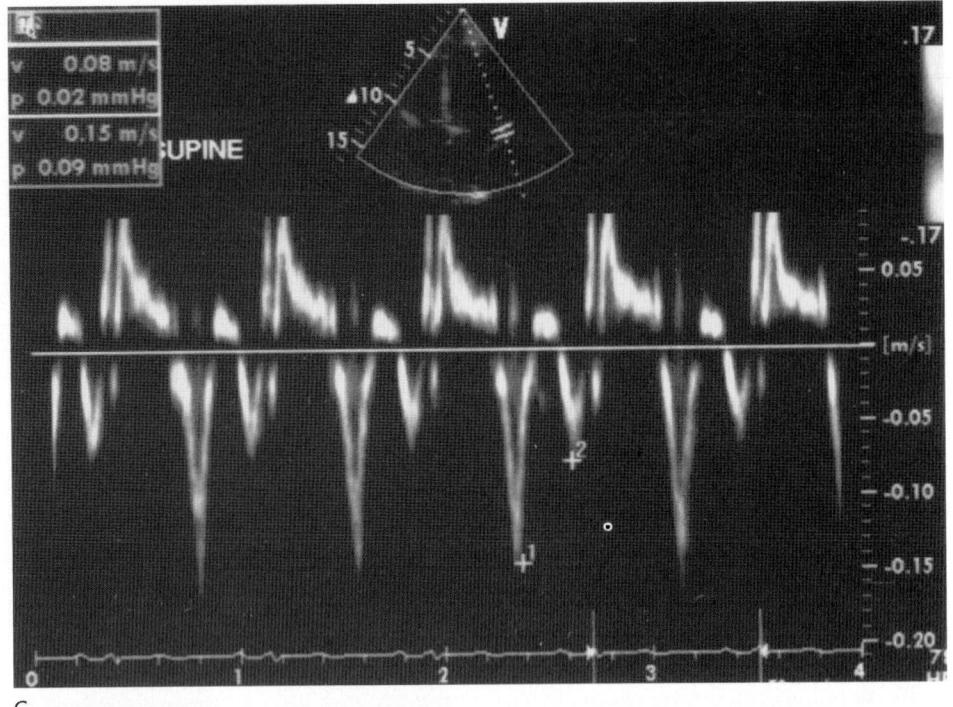

C

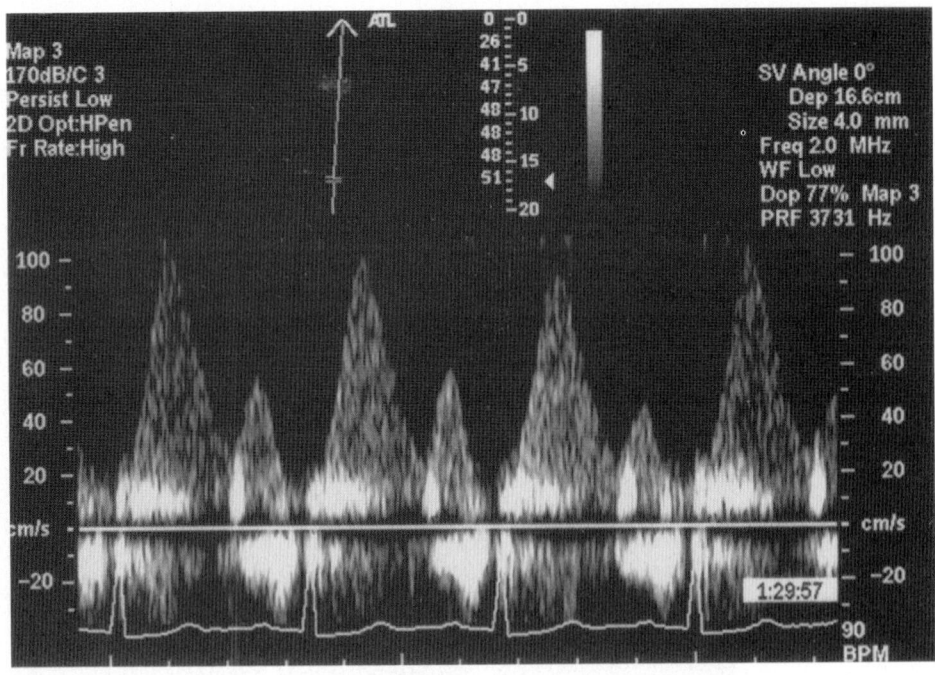

D

FIGURE 16–38. (continued)

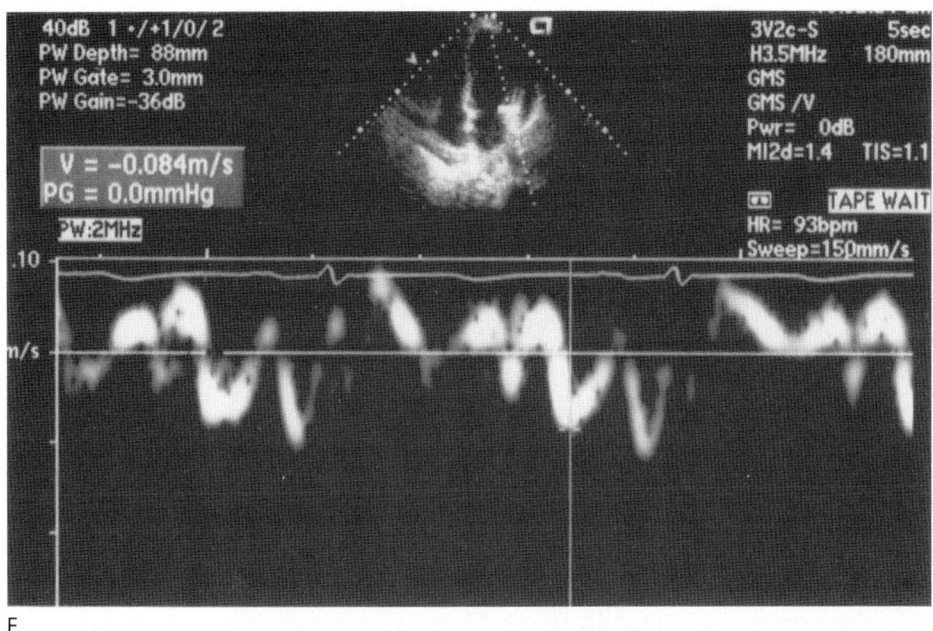

E

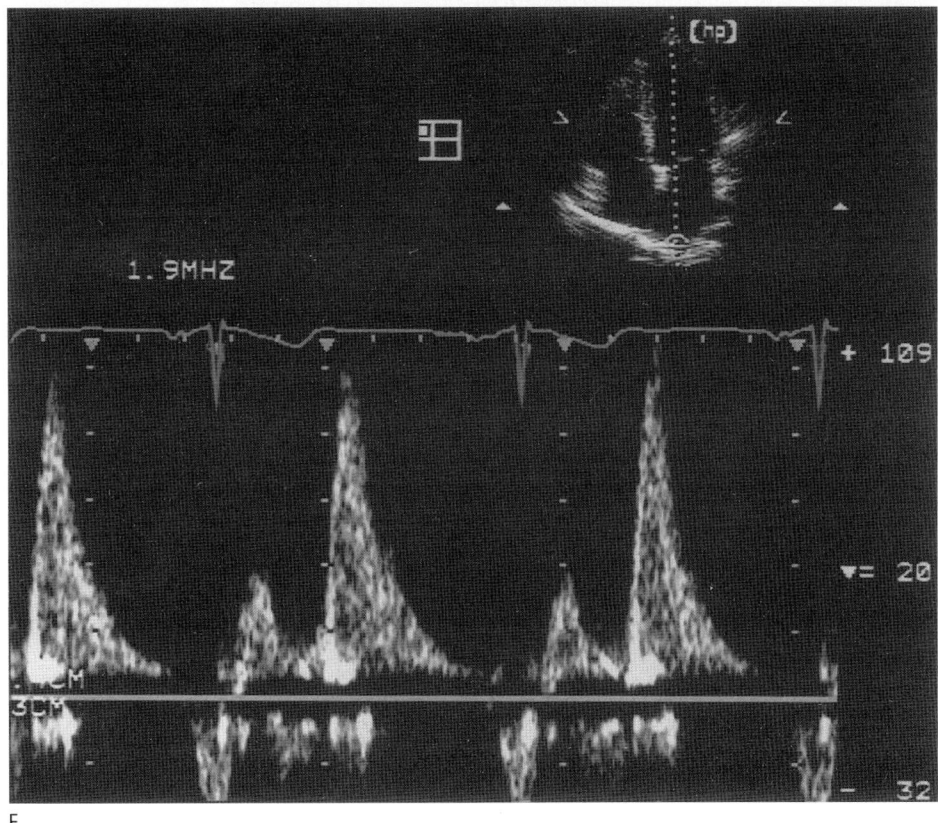

F

FIGURE 16–38. (*continued*)

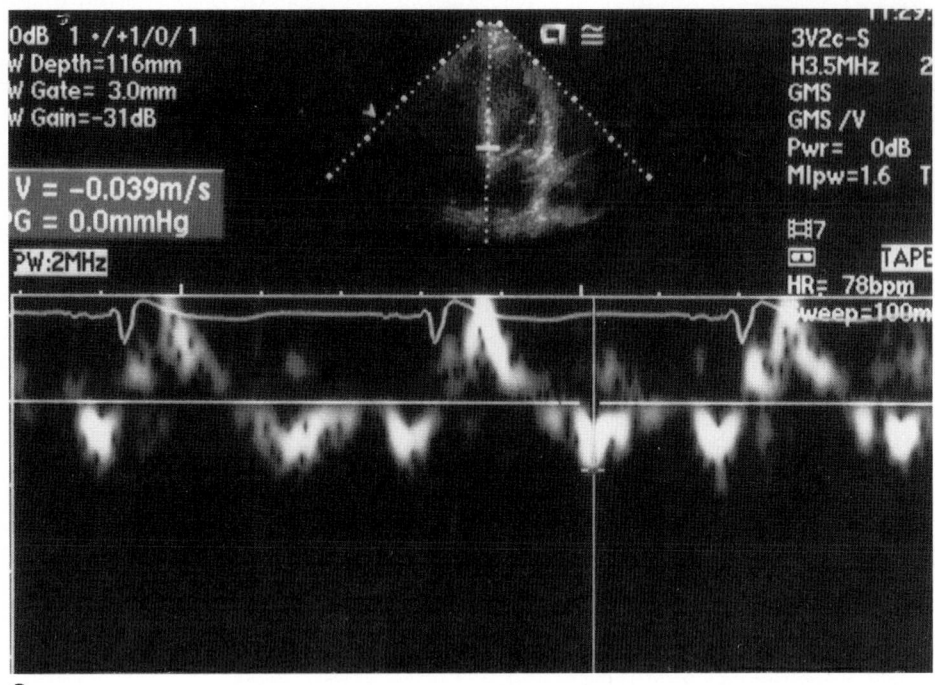

G

FIGURE 16–38. (continued)

in LA pressure caused by cardiac dysfunction restores early diastolic filling velocities and obscures impaired relaxation, thus inducing *pseudonormalization*. Therefore, because Doppler transmitral filling dynamics have many limitations in assessing diastolic function, particular filling patterns should not be interpreted as *pathognomonic* findings of diastolic dysfunction but rather as components of a complete clinical and echocardiographic evaluation.

The addition of pulsed-wave tissue Doppler imaging (TDI) into the clinical arena has significantly enhanced the noninvasive assessment of diastolic function, especially when used together with transmitral and pulmonary venous PWD. TDI measurements are obtained from the apical transducer position (four-chamber plane), with the sample volume placed on either the lateral or septal portion of the mitral annulus. Although TDI can assess systolic performance, it is most often used to measure the motion of the annulus away from the transducer during diastole. The diastolic pattern is similar to the PW transmitral flow pattern, but the velocities are considerably less and in the opposite direction. The normal velocity of the early TDI motion (E_m) is 12 cm/sec or greater at the lateral annulus and 8 cm/sec or more at the septal annulus. In addition, the ratio of transmitral E velocity to E_m is normally in the range of 8 to 15. In a young, healthy individual, the E/A ratio is generally between 1.5:1 and 2:1 (see Fig. 16–34). Because of high LV compliance, the

D velocity is greater than the S velocity in the pulmonary venous Doppler tracing (see Fig. 16–36). With age the LV compliance drops somewhat, so that by age 40 to 50 years, the S and D pulmonary venous velocities are similar. As mentioned, TDI velocity is 12 cm/sec or greater (see Fig. 16–38C). In the setting of mild diastolic dysfunction, the E/A ratio is <1, the E deceleration time is prolonged (*relaxation abnormality*, see Fig. 16–38A), and the pulmonary venous S wave is considerably larger than the D wave (S/D ratio >1) (see Fig. 16–38D). TDI shows blunting of the E_m wave with relative preservation of the later atrial component (A_m) (see Fig. 16–38E). As diastolic function worsens and LV filling pressures increase, a pseudonormal pattern occurs in the transmitral flow tracing (Fig. 16–39). Pulmonary venous and tissue Doppler imaging are especially helpful in this case: if the S/D ratio is <1 (except in the setting of a young individual), high LV filling pressure is likely present. Similarly, the presence of a low, blunted E_m velocity in the setting of a *normal* transmitral E/A ratio strongly suggests diastolic dysfunction and

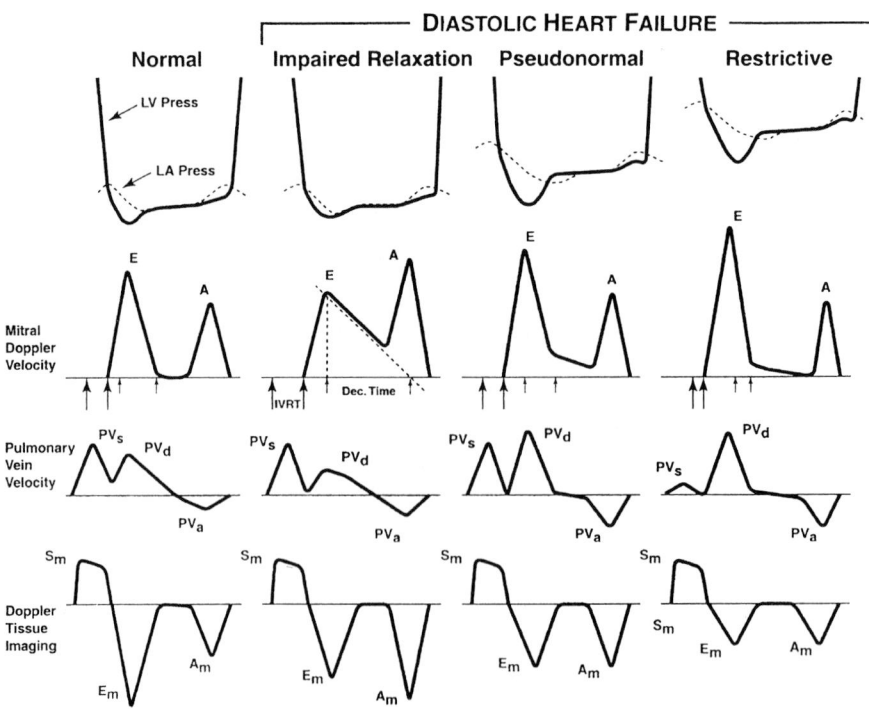

FIGURE 16–39. Doppler assessment of progressive diastolic dysfunction utilizing transmitral PWD, pulmonary venous Doppler, and mitral annular tissue Doppler imaging. A, atrial component of LV filling; A_m, myocardial velocity during LV filling produced by atrial contraction; Dec. Time, E wave deceleration time; E, early LV filling velocity; E_m, early diastolic myocardial velocity; IVRT, isovolumic relaxation time; PV_a, pulmonary vein velocity resulting from atrial contraction; PV_d, diastolic pulmonary vein velocity; PV_s, systolic pulmonary vein velocity; S_m, systolic myocardial velocity. *Source: From Zile MR, Brutsaert DL. New concepts in diastolic dysfunction and diastolic heart failure: Part I. Circulation 2002;105:1387–1393. With permission.*

elevated LV filling pressure. In fact, the ratio of the E/E_m velocities correlates reasonably well with pulmonary capillary wedge pressure, and a ratio of >15:1 reliably identifies an abnormal elevation of wedge pressure.[56] Of note, the Valsalva maneuver can be helpful in cases of pseudonormal transmitral flow patterns. In normal individuals both E and A velocities drop to a similar degree with Valsalva. In pseudonormal cases, however, the drop in preload caused by the Valsalva maneuver changes the transmitral pattern to that of mild diastolic dysfunction.

In severe diastolic dysfunction, transmitral flow demonstrates a *restrictive* pattern, with an abnormally high E/A ratio and a markedly shortened E wave deceleration time (see Fig. 16–38B). Concomitant pulmonary venous tracings show a very low S velocity and elevated D velocity (S << D) (see Fig. 16–38F). In some cases, the pulmonary venous atrial reversal wave can be prominent and prolonged. In this regard an abnormally prolonged duration of reversed pulmonary venous flow during atrial contraction accurately predicts elevated LV filling pressures.[49] TDI in severe LV diastolic dysfunction shows marked blunting of both E_m and A_m velocities (see Fig. 16–38G). An exception to this occurs in constrictive pericarditis, where early diastolic mitral annular motion is often preserved. Thus, when transmitral and pulmonary venous Doppler suggest severe diastolic dysfunction, a normal TDI pattern suggests constrictive rather than restrictive physiology.

Color M-mode imaging has been used to assess the velocity of propagation of the transmitral filling stream into the LV. This technique appears helpful in distinguishing constrictive pericarditis from restrictive cardiomyopathy.

Many recent studies have demonstrated the importance of LA enlargement in the setting of diastolic dysfunction and elevated LV filling pressure. Indeed, left atrial enlargement appears to predict adverse cardiovascular outcomes in general, not just elevated LV diastolic pressure.[57] Clearly, the E/A ratio, pulmonary venous flow pattern, and mitral annular TDI are all load dependent and can often change quickly with medical intervention. However, LA volume increases over the long term in response to elevated pressure.[58] LA volume does not change significantly with short-term fluctuations in loading conditions. LA volume can be calculated relatively easily and should be normalized to body surface area. LA volume >28 cc/m^2 is abnormal and signifies long-term diastolic dysfunction and elevated LV filling pressure.[58] An exception to this relationship occurs with atrial fibrillation: In this setting LA volume is less predictive of cardiovascular events and elevated LV filling pressure.[57]

[ ] DOPPLER ASSESSMENT OF SYSTOLIC FUNCTION AND CARDIAC OUTPUT

Doppler interrogation provides a unique and complementary noninvasive assessment of systolic function. Thus, LV systolic dysfunction often results in decreased aortic velocity and acceleration time. As discussed below, in the presence of mitral regurgitation (MR), the acceleration of the MR jet can provide information regarding contractile function.[59]

One of the most important applications of Doppler is in the *calculation of the stroke volume*.[60] The volume of flow through any orifice or tube can be calculated as the product of the cross-sectional area through which flow occurs and the velocity of that flow (Fig. 16–40).

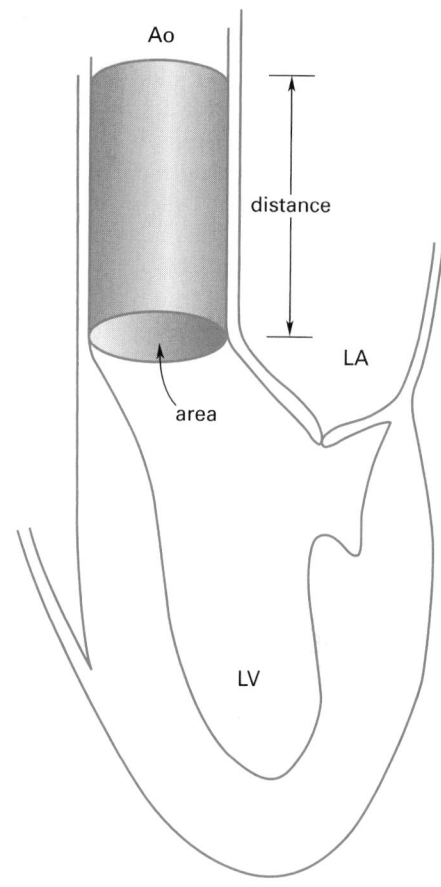

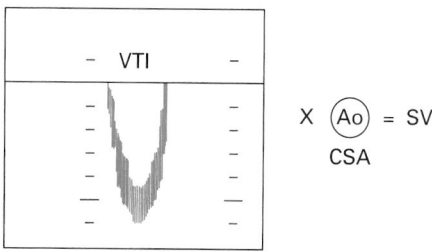

FIGURE 16–40. *Calculation of stroke volume. Multiplying the cross-sectional area (CSA) of the blood column in the ascending aorta by the distance the column moves during a single cardiac contraction yields the stroke volume (SV). The velocity-time integral (VTI), expressed in units of length, represents the stroke distance. Source: Modified from Pearlman AS. Technique of Doppler and color flow Doppler in the evaluation of cardiac disorders and function. In: Schlant RC, Alexander RW, eds. The Heart, Arteries, and Veins, 8th ed. New York: McGraw-Hill; 1994:2229. With permission.*

Measurements of anatomic cross-sectional area can be derived from echocardiographic images, while velocity can be determined by Doppler. As the annulus of the AoV is nearly circular, its cross-sectional area can be estimated from a measurement of diameter as π (diameter/2)^2. The PWD envelope also can be recorded at the same level. The mean flow velocity through the orifice is calculated by integrating velocity over time (that is, by measuring the area under the Doppler curve). This velocity-time integral, often called the *stroke distance*, is then multiplied by the cross-sectional area at the level of the Doppler interrogation to obtain the stroke volume.[60,61] The product of the stroke volume and heart rate then yields cardiac output.

Calculation of stroke volume by the Doppler method involves a number of assumptions. The orifice must be circular and constant in size, and the flow velocity must be uniform throughout the cross-sectional area. In addition, the angle between flow and the interrogating beam must be <20 degrees. Nevertheless, Doppler-derived measurements of cardiac output and stroke volume have been shown to correspond well with thermodilution, Fick, and the angiographic calculations, but the correlation is not perfect.[60,61]

Theoretically, stroke volume can be calculated at any valve annulus.[61] In clinical practice however, this is not always possible. Because the measurement of annular radius is squared in the computation of area, it is the most important source of error of Doppler stroke-volume analyses. Stroke-volume analysis through the mitral annulus is cumbersome; it is uncertain whether the mitral annulus is best described as a circle or an ellipse, and the cross-sectional area of the annulus probably changes slightly during diastole. Despite these limitations, measurements of stroke volume through the various cardiac valves are clinically useful and can be used to calculate pulmonary-to-systemic shunt ratios, regurgitant volumes,[62,63] and orifice areas of stenotic valves by the continuity equation.[64]

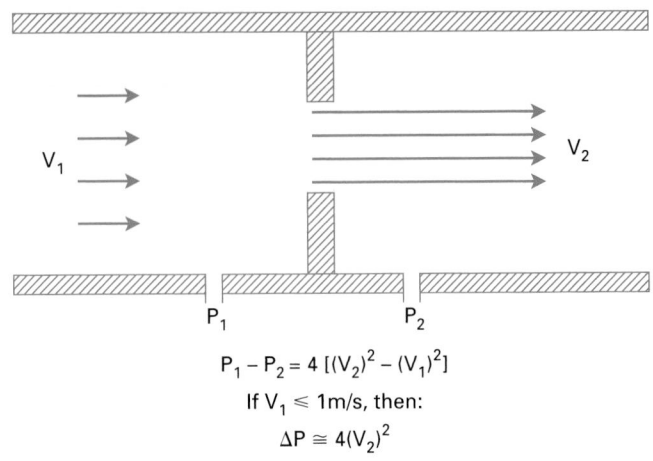

$$P_1 - P_2 = 4\,[(V_2)^2 - (V_1)^2]$$

If $V_1 \leq 1$ m/s, then:

$$\Delta P \cong 4(V_2)^2$$

FIGURE 16–41. The modified Bernoulli equation. Pressure drop across a small orifice can be estimated as four times the square of the peak velocity (if the proximal velocity is <1 m/sec). V_1 and P_1, proximal velocity and pressure; V_2 and P_2, distal velocity and pressure. *Source: Modified from Pearlman AS. Technique of Doppler and color flow Doppler in the evaluation of cardiac disorders and function. In: Schlant RC, Alexander RW, eds. The Heart, Arteries, and Veins, 8th ed. New York: McGraw-Hill; 1994:2229. With permission.*

【 】 THE BERNOULLI EQUATION

An important application of Doppler echocardiography is the calculation of pressure gradients within the cardiovascular system using a modification of the Bernoulli equation.[65] This theorem states that the pressure drop across a discrete stenosis in the heart or vasculature occurs because of energy loss caused by three processes: (1) acceleration of blood through the orifice (*convective acceleration*), (2) inertial forces (*flow acceleration*), and (3) resistance to flow at the interfaces between blood and the orifice (*viscous friction*). Therefore, the pressure drop across any orifice can be calculated as the sum of these three variables (Fig. 16–41). The pressure gradient can be calculated from the velocities of blood proximal to and at the level of an orifice:

$$\text{gradient} = 4[(\text{orifice velocity})^2 - (\text{proximal velocity})^2]$$

If the blood velocity proximal to the stenosis is low (<1.0 m/sec), this term can be ignored as well. The resulting modified equation states that the pressure gradient across a discrete orifice is equal to four times the square of the peak velocity (V) through the stenosis ($PG = 4V^2$).[65]

The modified Bernoulli equation can be used to calculate pressure gradients across any flow-limiting orifice and has been validated against invasive measurements.[66] If at least trivial valvular regurgitation is present, systolic gradients across the tricuspid and end-diastolic gradients across the PV can be calculated.[67] If the RV diastolic pressure is known (or estimated as the right atrial or central venous pressure), peak RV and PA pressure (assuming pulmonic stenosis is absent) can be computed as follows:[68]

$$\text{Peak PA pressure} = 4(\text{TR velocity})^2 + \text{RA pressure}$$

End-diastolic PA pressure (PAD) also can be calculated:

$$\text{PAD} = 4(\text{end-diastolic pulmonary regurgitation velocity})^2 + \text{RA pressure}$$

In the presence of MR, a variety of calculations can be made. With measurement of peak systolic arterial pressure, systolic left atrial pressure can be estimated:

$$\text{LA systolic pressure} = \text{systolic blood pressure} - 4(\text{MR velocity})^2$$

Further, the acceleration of the MR jet can be used to estimate LV systolic dP/dt. Thus, from the Bernoulli equation, the LA-to-LV pressure gradients at regurgitant velocities of 1 and 3 m/sec are 4 and 36 mmHg, respectively. Therefore dP/dt can be calculated as 32 mmHg divided by the time (in seconds) required for the mitral regurgitant jet to accelerate from 1 to 3 m/sec. In the case of ventricular septal defects (VSDs) or aortopulmonary shunts, measurements of the peak systolic arterial pressure and the peak Doppler velocity across the defect allows calculation of the RV (or pulmonary arterial) systolic pressure.

【 】 THE CONTINUITY EQUATION

Although transvalvular pressure gradients can be calculated from CW Doppler recordings using the modified Bernoulli equation, gradients sometimes can be misleading in the evaluation of valvular stenosis. The transvalvular gradient is determined by both the size of the stenotic orifice and the stroke volume traversing it. Severe AS and accompanying LV systolic dysfunction may produce a low transvalvular gradient despite a small valve area, whereas coexistent AR may result in a large gradient with only mild AS. The calculation of orifice area by Doppler echocardiography employs the *continuity equation*, which is derived from the law of the conservation of mass and states that the product of cross-sectional area and velocity is constant in a closed system of flow (Fig. 16–42). Thus, in the case of AS, the product of the area and velocity of the left LV outflow tract equals the product of the area and velocity of the AoV orifice. Measurements of annular diameter and integrated velocity are derived by the standard volumetric approach, whereas

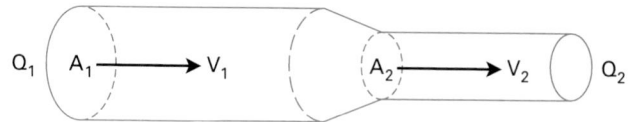

$$(A_1) = \pi r^2 = \pi \left(\frac{D}{2}\right)^2 = 0.785 \ (D^2)$$

$$(A_2)(V_2) = (A_1)(V_1) \text{ or } (A_2) = \frac{(A_1)(V_1)}{(V_2)}$$

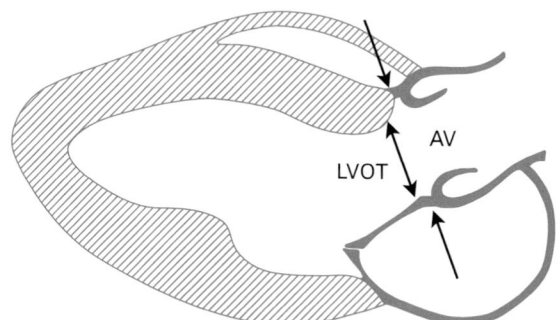

FIGURE 16–42. The continuity equation. In a closed system (*top*) with constant flow, $Q_1 = Q_2$. Therefore, $A_1 \times V_1$ must equal $A_2 \times V_2$. Determination of any three of the variables allows calculation of the fourth. Clinically (*bottom*), the area of the left ventricular outflow tract (*LVOT*) can be estimated and used to determine AoV area. AoV, aortic valve. *Source: From Hagan AD, DeMaria AN. Clinical Applications of Two-Dimensional Echocardiography and Cardiac Doppler. Boston: Little, Brown; 1989. With permission.*

the velocity across the stenotic orifice is derived by CW Doppler. The equation is then solved for the valve area.[64]

The most common pitfall is an inaccurate estimation of the cross-sectional area proximal to the stenosis. In addition, it is essential that blood velocity proximal to a stenosis be measured outside the area of flow acceleration. Finally, the continuity equation actually solves for the area of the vena contracta, which is usually just distal to the stenotic orifice.

[ ] DETERMINANTS OF THE SIZE OF FLOW DISTURBANCES

Although CFD yields primarily qualitative information, it is unique in its ability to provide measurements of the size of flow disturbances. The size of a turbulent jet should correlate with the volume of blood contained within the flow disturbance. Regardless of the lesion, however, the area of turbulence recorded by CFD has multiple determinants.[69] The pressure gradient operative in any flow disturbance is also an important determinant of the spatial distribution or *spray area* of turbulence.[69] Also, the size of a flow disturbance is in-

fluenced by the orifice through which flow occurs as well as the size and compliance of the receiving chamber.[69] Finally, a number of technical factors can influence jet size, including instrument gain, the angle of incidence of the interrogating beam, the frequency and pulse repetition rate of the transducer, and the temporal sampling rate.[70] Therefore, measurements derived from the size of the turbulent jet recorded by color Doppler, are at best semiquantitative and should not be expected to correlate with the volume of blood contained in the flow disturbance.

TRANSESOPHAGEAL ECHOCARDIOGRAPHY

Transthoracic echocardiography (TTE) usually defines cardiac anatomy and function satisfactorily, often obviating the need for further cardiac imaging. Occasionally, however, TTE does not provide complete or adequately detailed information. This is especially true in the evaluation of posterior cardiac structures (e.g., LA, LA appendage, interatrial septum, aorta distal to the root), in the assessment of prosthetic cardiac valves, and in the delineation of cardiac structures <3 mm in size (e.g., small vegetations or thrombi). Ultrasonic imaging from the esophagus is uniquely suited to these situations, because the esophagus is adjacent to the LA and the thoracic aorta for much of its course[71] and affords excellent access of the interrogating beam to these structures.

Flexible transesophageal ultrasound probes capable of multiplanar imaging of the heart have supplanted the older biplane probes.[72] The current generation of probes also provide full pulsed-wave, CW, and CFD capabilities.

Although images can be recorded from a variety of probe positions most authorities recommend three basic positions: (1) posterior to the base of the heart, (2) posterior to the LA, and (3) inferior to the heart (transgastric position) (Fig. 16–43). Fig. 16–44 to Fig. 16–47 show TEE images obtained in various planes through the heart. It must be emphasized that, with the transducer in the

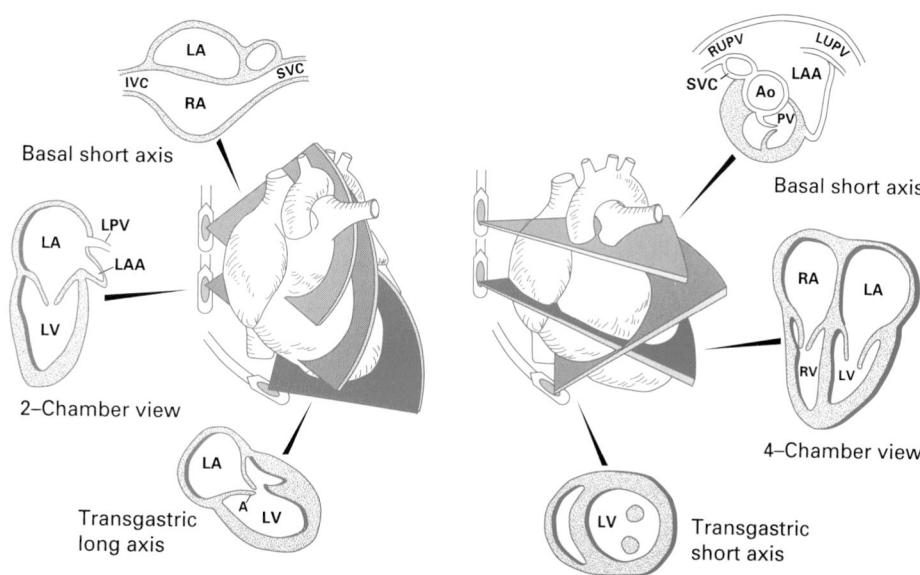

FIGURE 16–43. Standard TEE imaging planes in transverse and longitudinal axes. TEE, transesophageal echocardiography. *Source: From Fisher EA, Stahl JA, Budd JH, Goldman ME. Transesophageal echocardiography: procedures and clinical applications. J Am Coll Cardiol 1991;18:1333–1348. With permission.*

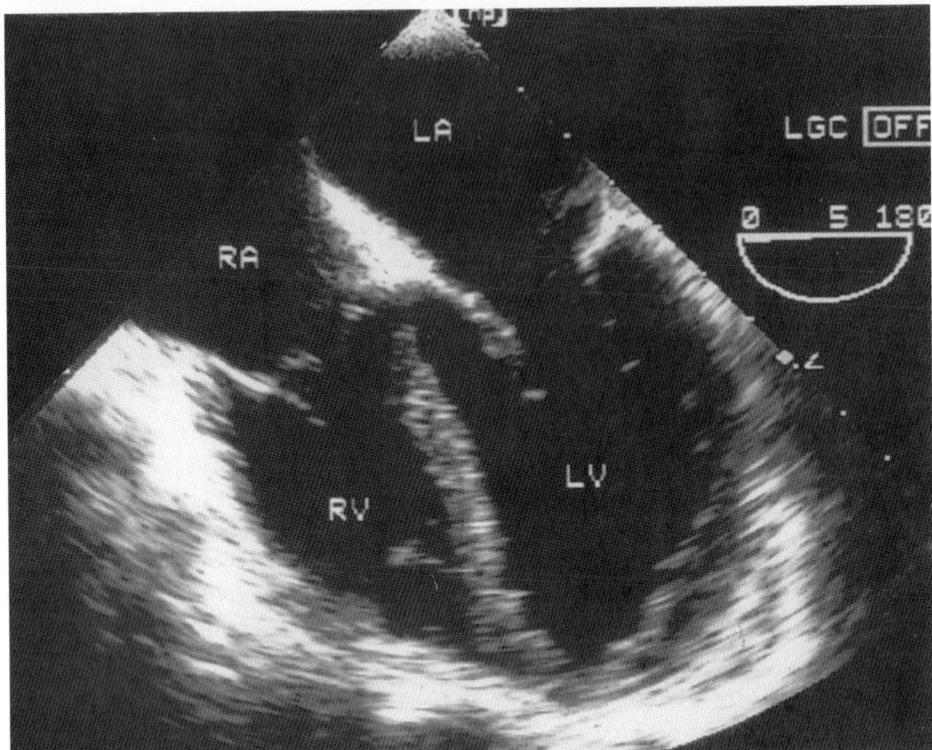

FIGURE 16–44. Transverse four-chamber TEE plane. LA, left atrium; LV, left ventricle; RA, right atrium; RV, right ventricle.

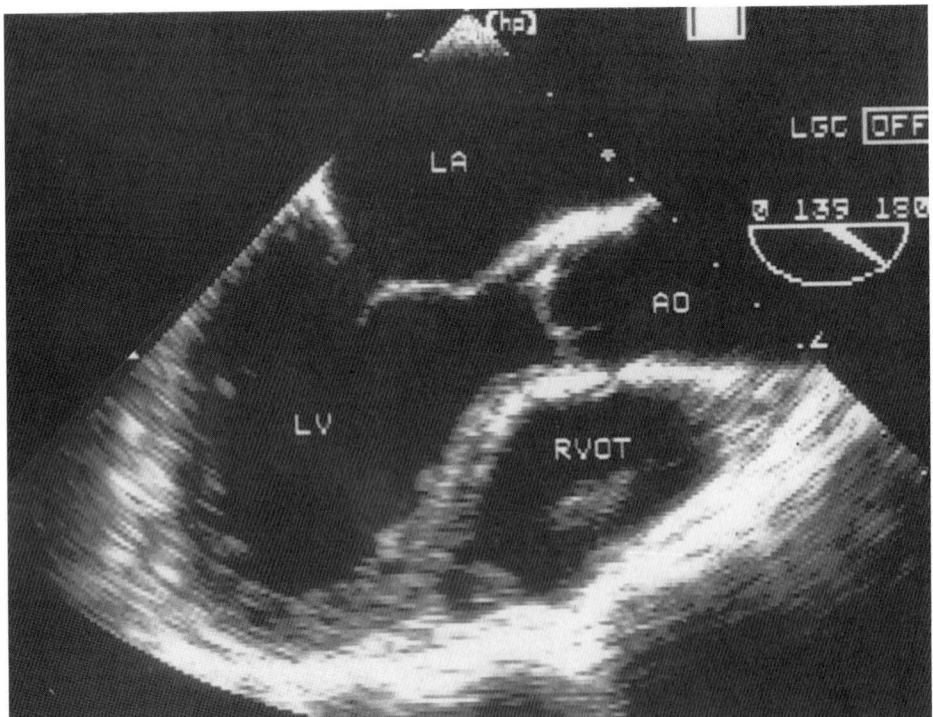

FIGURE 16–45. Modified longitudinal TEE plane (with transducer rotated to approximately 140 degrees), demonstrating a TEE apical *three-chamber* view. Ao, ascending aorta; LA, left atrium; LV, left ventricle; RVOT, right ventricular outflow tract; TEE, transesophageal echocardiography.

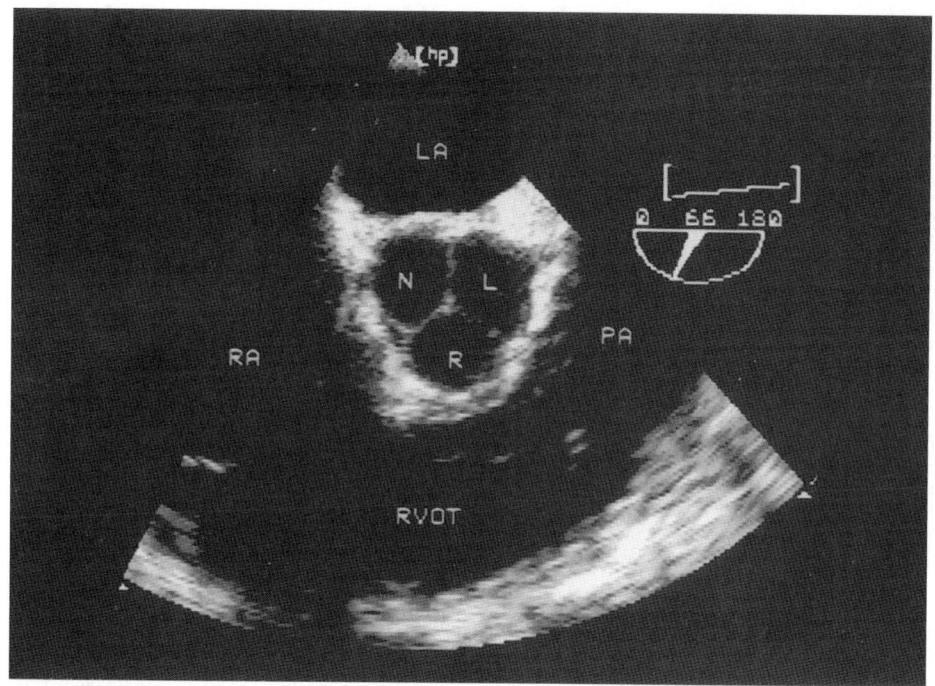

A

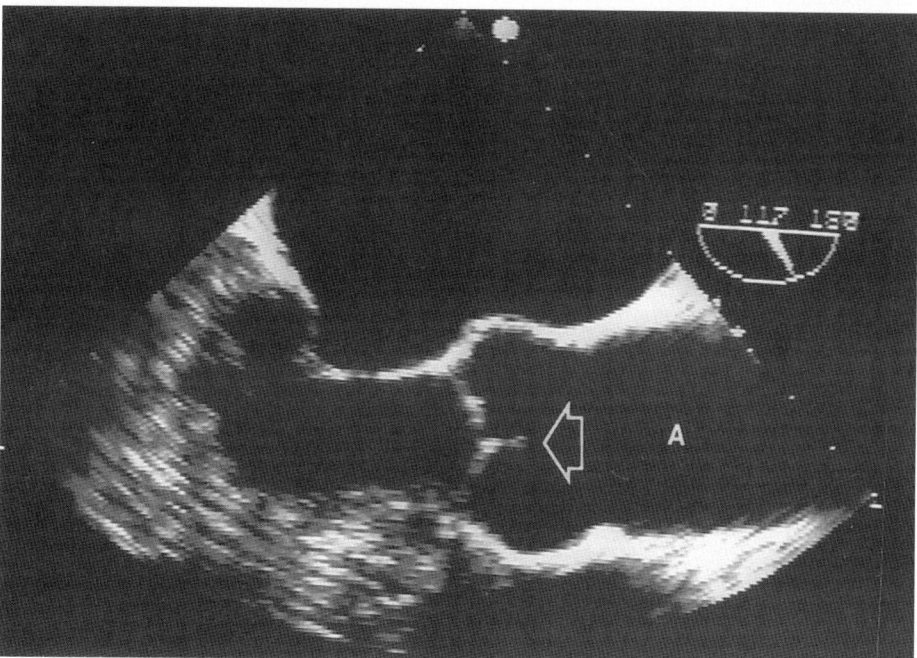

B

FIGURE 16–46. **A.** Modified short-axis view through the level of the AoV, demonstrating the left (*L*), right (*R*), and noncoronary (*N*) valvular cusps. **B.** Magnified longitudinal view of the AoV (*arrow*) showing the coaptation of the cusps and the sinuses of Valsalva. **C.** Longitudinal image at level of the aortic arch, demonstrating the transverse aorta (*A*), the brachiocephalic vein (*V*), and the main pulmonary artery (*PA*). The pulmonic valve is visible as well (*arrow*). Ao, aorta; AoV, aortic valve; LA, left atrium; PA, pulmonary artery; RA, right atrium; RVOT, right ventricular outflow tract. *Source: B, from Blanchard DG, Kimura BJ, Dittrich HC, DeMaria AN.[71] With permission.* (continued)

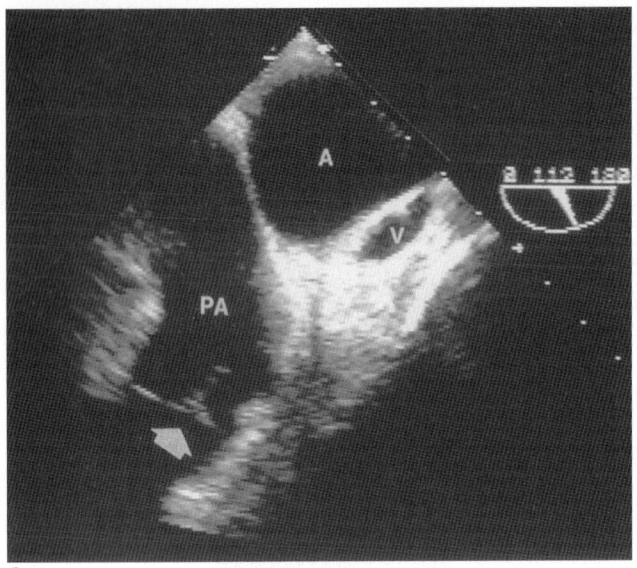

FIGURE 16–46. (continued)

esophagus, posterior structures appear at the top of the image. With the transducer in the stomach, a short-axis view is standardly obtained, with long-axis and apical views available to a variable degree. On withdrawing the transducer to the esophagus, apical-equivalent four-chamber and long-axis views, with multiple intermediate projections are usually obtained. Further withdrawal of the probe to the base yields excellent views of the atria, great vessels and semilunar valves, and pulmonary veins. Of particular value are views that delineate the LA appendage, all three leaflets of the AoV in short axis, and the transverse and descending aorta.

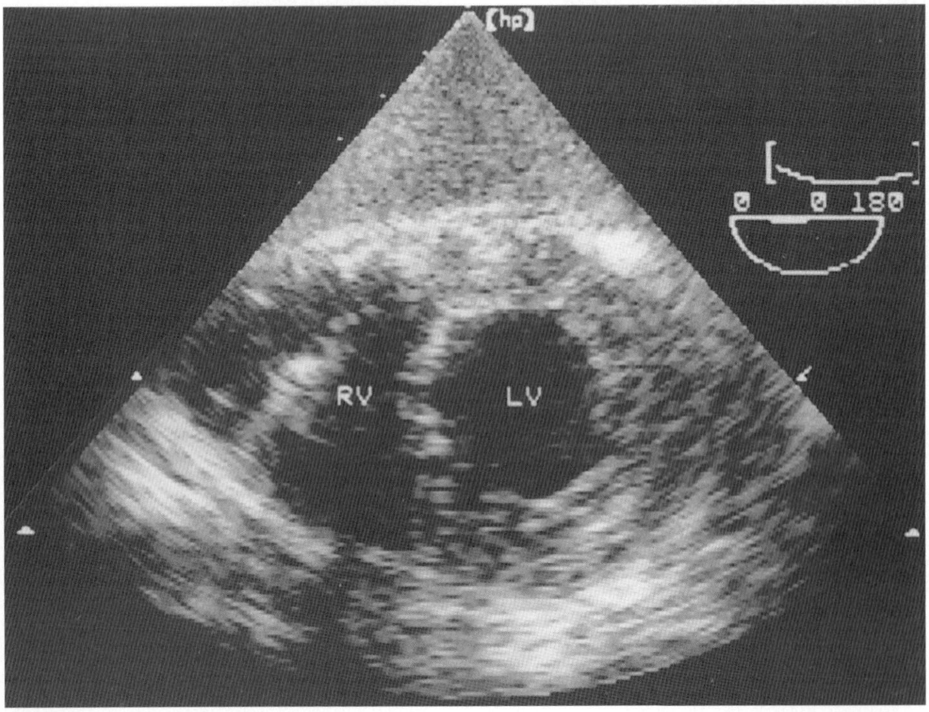

TEE is an important imaging modality for the diagnosis and management of infective endocarditis and its complications, including valvular vegetations, chordal rupture, fistulas, perivalvular abscesses, and mycotic aneurysms.[73] TEE is more accurate in detecting vegetations and abscesses than TTE[73] and provides prognostic information as well (Fig. 16–48). In addition, TEE imaging may aid in accurate quantification of valvular disease (particularly MR) if TTE is inconclusive (Fig. 16–49). TEE is especially useful for Doppler interrogation of the pulmonary veins (Fig. 16–50). Flow patterns in these vessels reflect LA pressure, and systolic reversal of pulmonary venous flow is an accurate marker of severe MR.[74] Although MR color jets are easier to see with TEE than TTE, they are usually larger, and care must be exercised not to overestimate the severity of the regurgitation. Multiplane TEE can be used to planimeter the orifice area in AS.[75] The technique is also quite helpful in detection of aortic disease, including dissection, aneurysm, congenital malformations, and atherosclerosis.[71] Because of its portability, accuracy, and short preparation and procedural times, TEE is now the recommended, preferred diagnostic study in many cases of suspected aortic dissection (Fig. 16–51).[71,76]

Thromboemboli may originate from posterior cardiac structures such as the LA and LA appendage, interatrial septum, and aorta[77]; therefore, TEE has received wide application in the evaluation of possible cardiogenic embolization. The ability of TEE to visualize the LA appendage is of particular value (Fig. 16–52). TEE can also detect spontaneous contrast signals, which appear to represent transient rouleaux formation and predispose to thromboemboli. In addition, TEE has provided unique real-time images of mobile, pedunculated, atherosclerotic *debris* in the thoracic aorta (Fig. 16–53A and B). Although the optimal therapy for this disorder is currently unknown, warfarin may be helpful and mobile or protruding aortic atheromas appear to be significant risk factors for embolic events.[78,79]

One proven application of TEE is the evaluation of prosthetic valve dysfunction, particularly mechanical valves in the mitral position.[80] The areas behind prosthetic valves are usually hidden from view when transthoracic imaging is used. TEE is clearly superior to TTE imaging for detection of prosthetic regurgitation, infection, tissue ingrowth, and thrombosis (Fig. 16–54).

TEE has also become an important intraoperative tool for the detection of cardiac ischemia, the evaluation of valve function after repair or replacement, and the delineation of CHD. Cardiac surgeons often request intraoperative TEE for evaluation of cardiac anatomy and confirmation of a success of surgical repair before closing the chest. In this regard, TEE has almost completely replaced TTE. When TTE images are inadequate, TEE helps manage critically ill patients and also can be used to

FIGURE 16–47. Short-axis TEE plane through the left ventricle from transgastric position. The inferior wall is closest to the transducer, the anterior wall farthest. The interventricular septum is to the reader's left, the lateral wall to the right. LV, left ventricle; RV, right ventricle; TEE, transesophageal echocardiography.

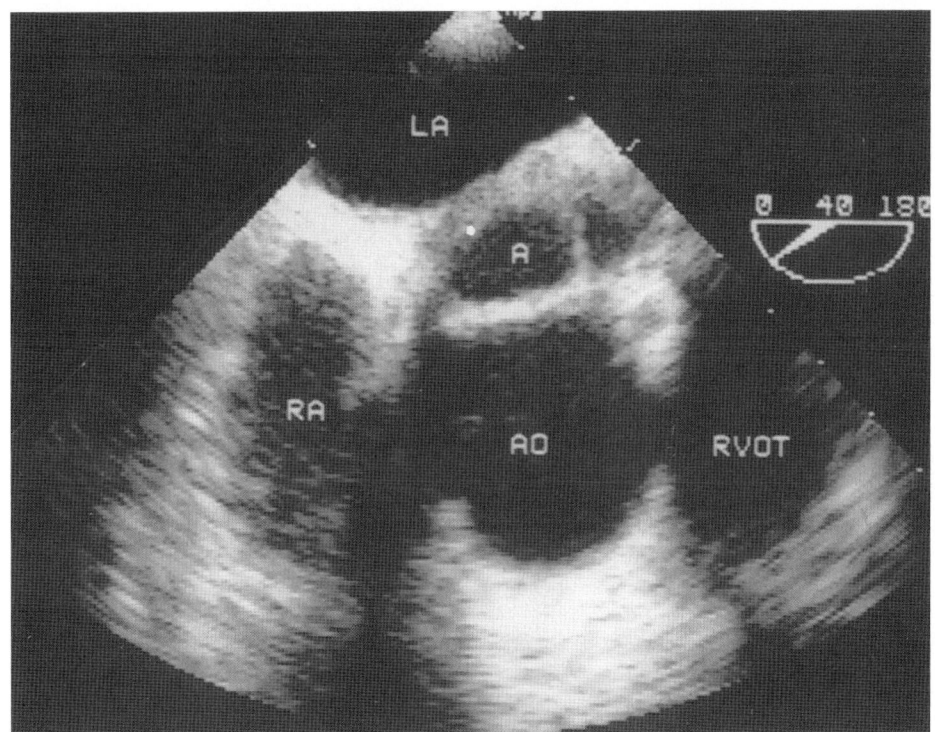

A

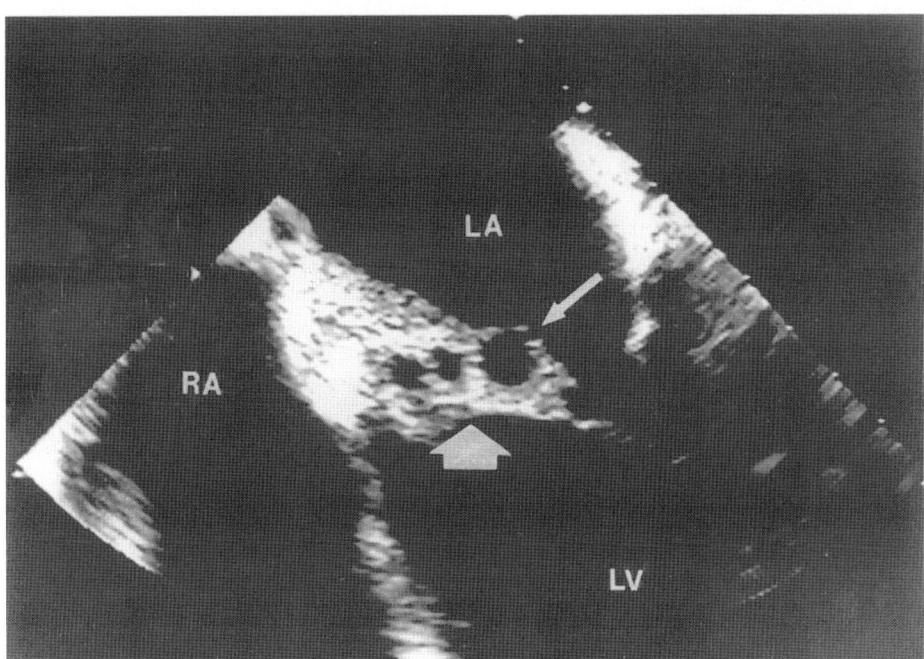

B

FIGURE 16–48. A. Short-axis TEE plane through the cardiac base. A large septated abscess cavity (*A*) is present between the aortic root (*AO*) and the left atrium (*LA*). **B.** Modified transverse four-chamber TEE plane showing a large abscess with several cavitations (*arrows*) involving the anterior mitral valve leaflet and the intervalvular fibrosa. LA, left atrium; LV, left ventricle; RA, right atrium; RVOT, right ventricular outflow tract; TEE, transesophageal echocardiography. *Source: From Sobel J, Maisel AS, Tarazi R, Blanchard DG. Gonococcal endocarditis: assessment by transesophageal echocardiography. J Am Soc Echocardiogr 1997;10:367–370. With permission.*

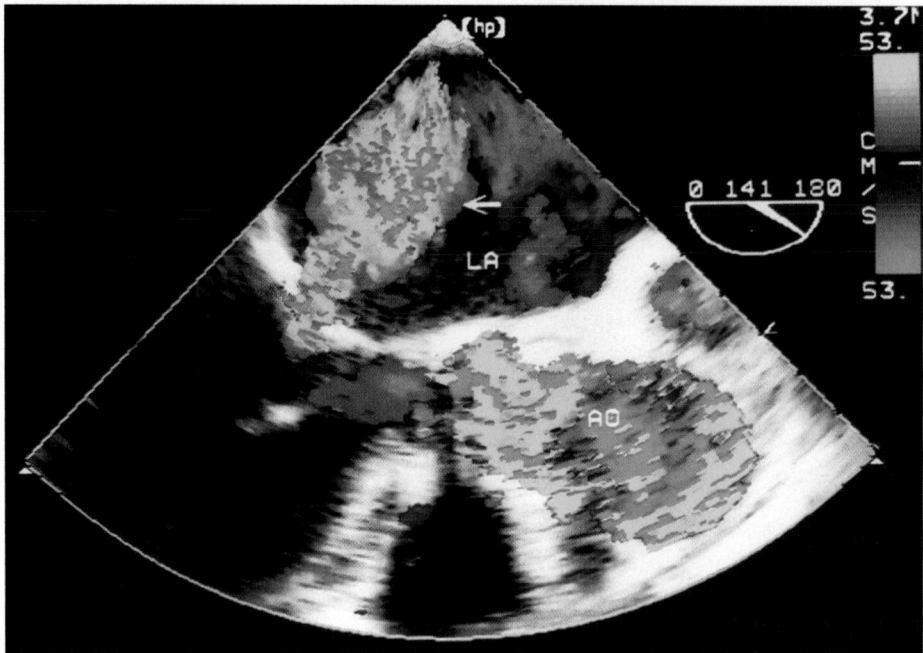

FIGURE 16–49. Transesophageal echocardiography image (three-chamber plane) demonstrating a jet of mitral regurgitation (*arrow*) in the left atrium (*LA*). Ao, aorta; LV, left ventricle.

monitor or guide interventional procedures, such as transseptal catheterization, mitral valvuloplasty, pericardiocentesis, and endomyocardial biopsy.

【 】 HANDHELD ECHOCARDIOGRAPHY

Recently, advances in electronic technology have led to production of small, relatively lightweight (5–6 lb) echocardiography units. These handheld devices can be carried to the clinic exam room or hospital bed, thereby facilitating point-of-care echo evaluation by the physician. The appropriate use of these scanners is currently controversial. Experts in the field have raised numerous questions about the merits of handheld echocardiography: There are concerns about the sonographic skills required for accurate diagnosis (because physicians, rather than sonographers, will likely perform most studies with these devices), legal ramifications of potential misdiagnosis, added time commitments during clinic visits, and overall quality control (see Chap. 13).[81]

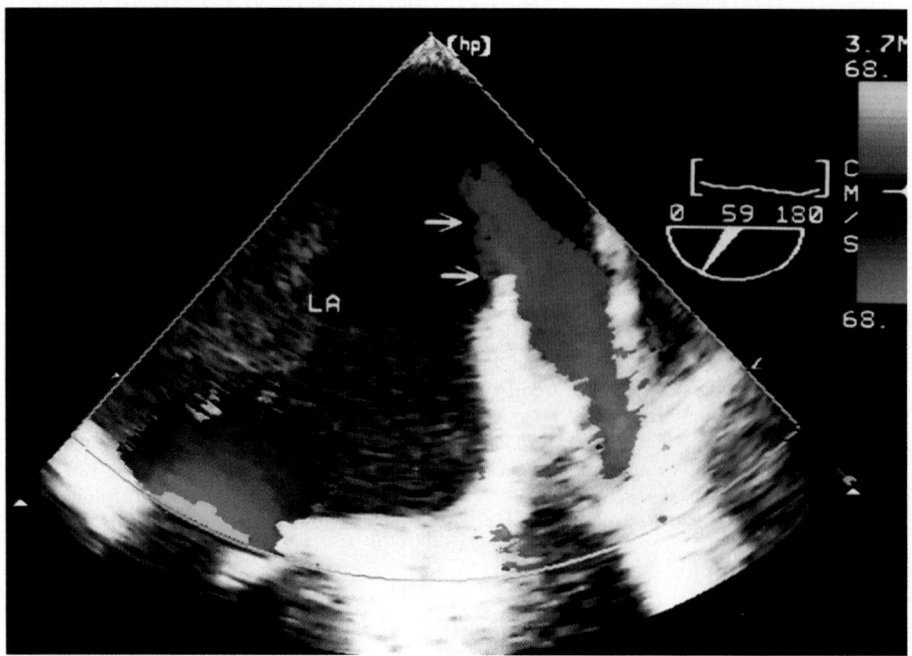

FIGURE 16–50. Transesophageal echocardiography image of pulmonary venous flow (*arrows*) entering the left atrium (*LA*) during diastole.

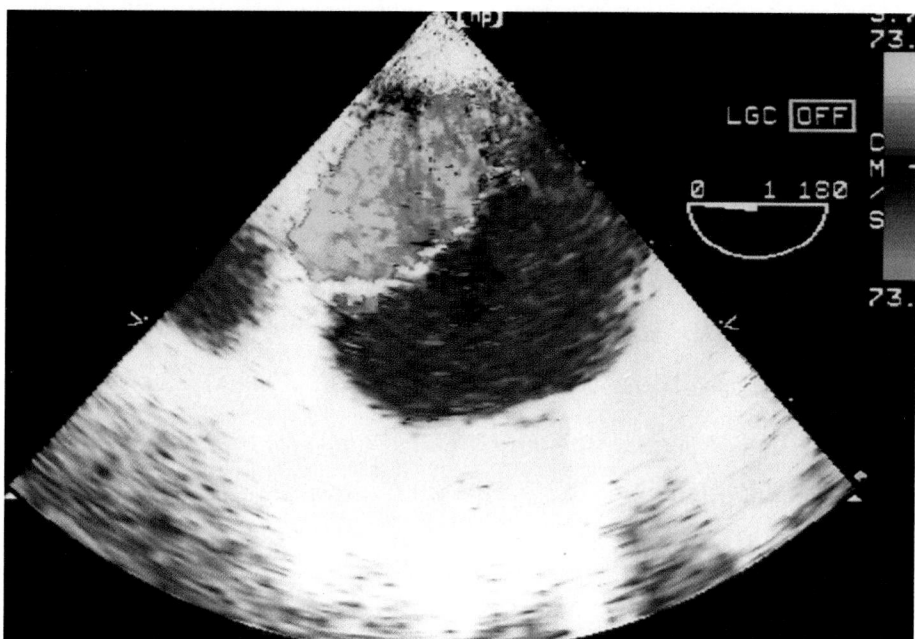

FIGURE 16–51. Transverse TEE image of a descending aortic dissection. The true lumen is color-coded orange. The false lumen is mostly devoid of flow, but a small blue jet of communication between the two channels is present. TEE, transesophageal echocardiography.

Several studies have shown benefits from handheld scanning in the detection of cardiac and aortic pathology, whereas others have shown limited utility, especially in critically ill patients. The devices must become smaller and less expensive to achieve a role in standard clinical practice. It is clear, however, that the sonographic skills of the person performing the study are critical. To ensure adequate imaging competency, the ASE currently recommends that individuals performing handheld scanning have level 2 or 3 training in echocardiography.[82]

A wide spectrum of opinion exists in this area. At present it may be best to view examinations with handheld echo devices as limited extensions of the stethoscope. Performed by a competent individual,

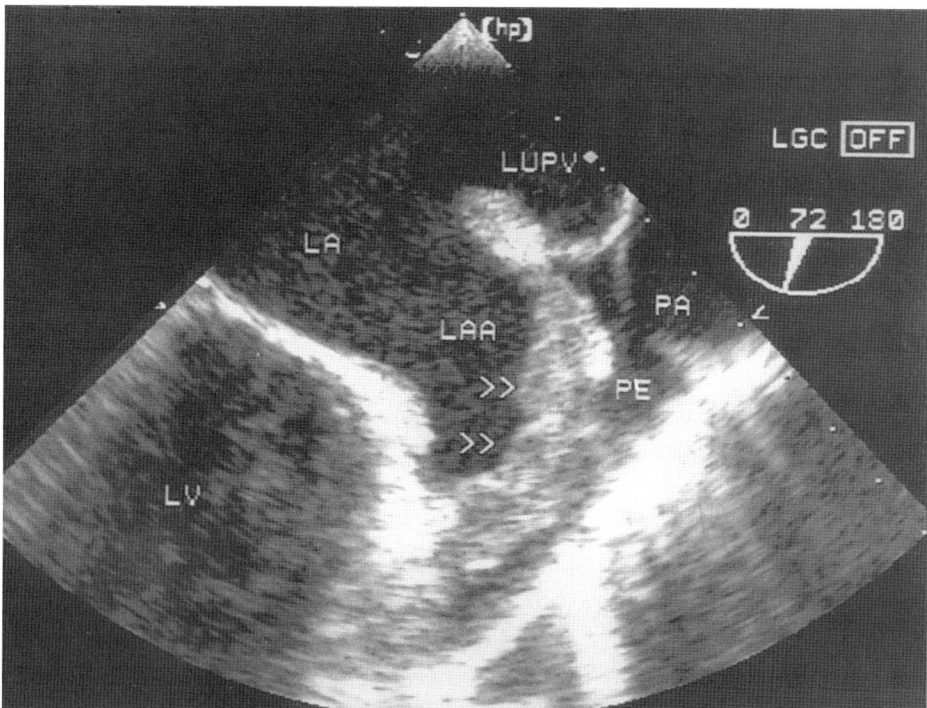

FIGURE 16–52. Transesophageal echocardiography image of a laminar thrombus (*arrows*) within the left atrial appendage (LAA). This thrombus was not visible with transthoracic echocardiography. LA, left atrium; LV, left ventricle; LUPV, left upper pulmonary vein; PA, pulmonary artery; PE, small pericardial effusion.

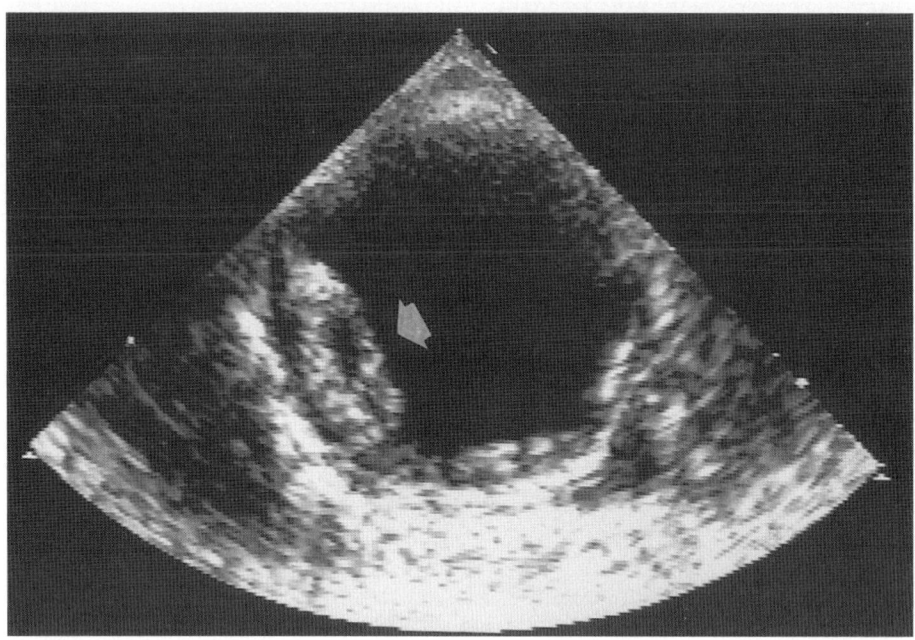

A

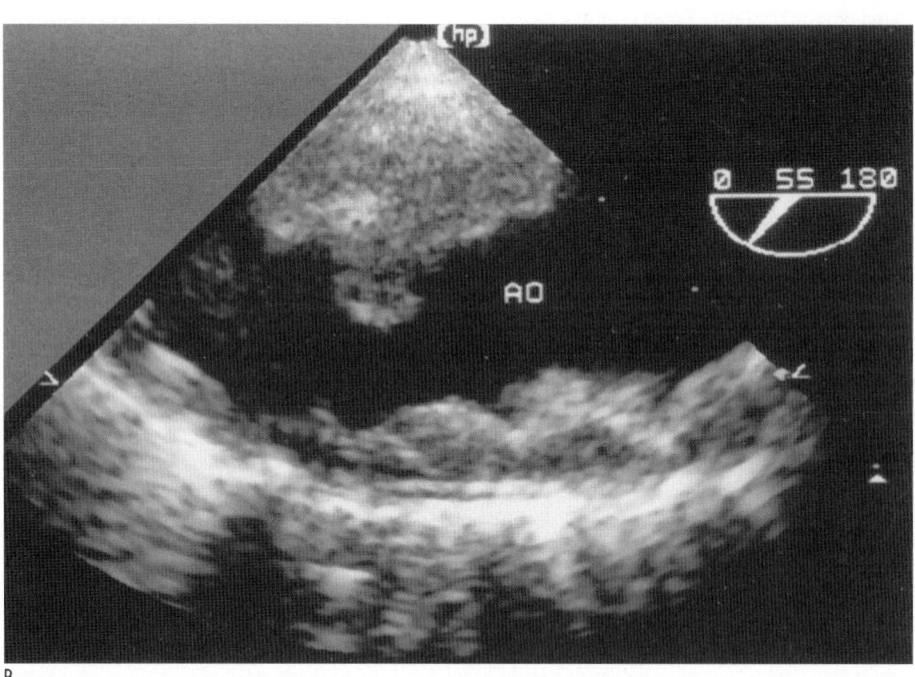

B

FIGURE 16–53. **A.** Transverse TEE image of the descending aorta, demonstrating atherosclerosis and a large atheroma (*arrow*). **B.** Longitudinal TEE image of the descending aorta, demonstrating severe, extensive atherosclerosis. TEE, transesophageal echocardiography.

the diagnostic capability of such an examination is at least equal to that of auscultation alone (see Chap. 12). Handheld ultrasound units can also provide clinically useful information by imaging the carotid arteries, the abdominal aorta, and the inferior vena cava.

CONTRAST ECHOCARDIOGRAPHY

Opacification of the right heart cavities with dense ultrasonic reflectances during intravenous contrast injection was first applied

clinically in 1968. Subsequently, it became clear that the origin of the dense intracavitary echoes were microbubbles within the injectate, and that any agitated liquid injected intravenously caused the effect. Because room-air microbubbles with the diameter of pulmonary capillaries persist intact in blood for <1 second before dissolving, agitated agents injected intravenously cannot cross the lungs and enter the left-sided cardiac chambers. Thus, the presence of echocardiographic contrast entering left heart chambers after intravenous injection of an agitated liquid indicates the presence of a right-to-left shunt.[83]

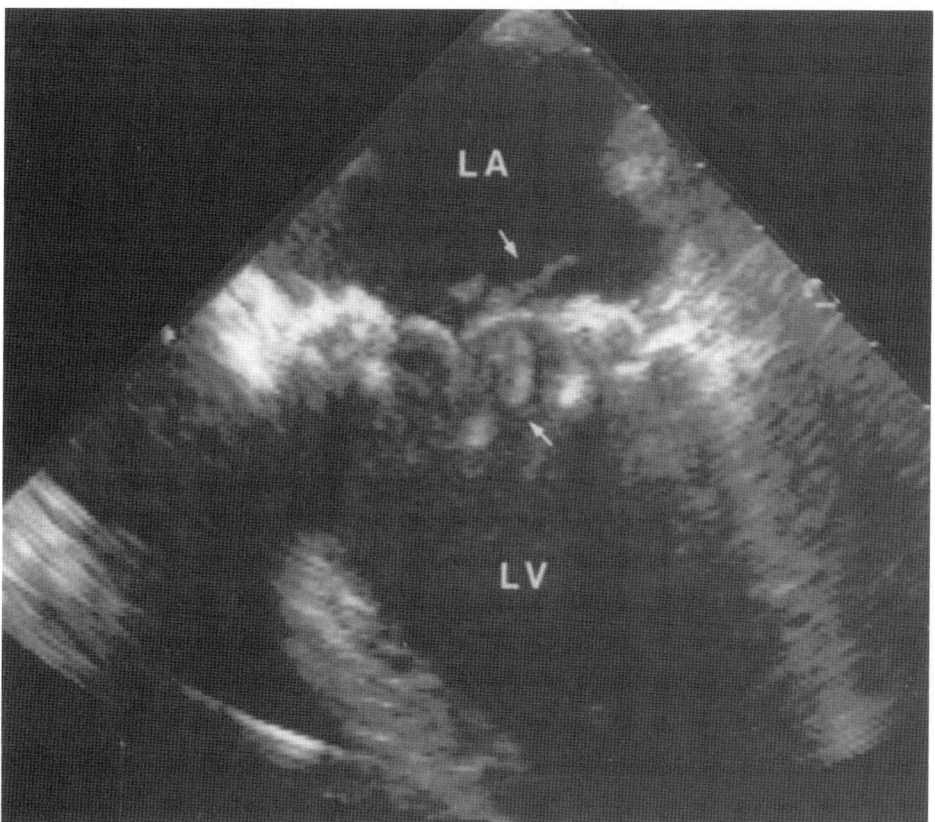

FIGURE 16–54. Transverse four-chamber TEE image of infective vegetations (*arrows*) on a porcine prosthesis in the mitral position. LA, left atrium; LV, left ventricle.

even biodegradable polymer materials, and fluorocarbon gases, which are dense and poorly soluble. These new microbubble agents are all capable of producing dense, high-intensity signals not only within the LV but also within the myocardium following intravenous injection.[85,86] Of significance, the presence of microcirculatory flow and integrity by contrast injections is a reliable predictor of viable myocardium.

Intravenous injection of stabilized solutions of microbubbles opacifies the LV in nearly all patients, thereby facilitating identification of the endomyocardial border. This capacity has found its greatest application in stress echocardiography, where detection of the endocardium is of fundamental importance in recognizing abnormal contraction produced by ischemia. Marginal Doppler spectral tracings in cases of MR, tricuspid regurgitation, and AS often improved dramatically after contrast injection, facilitating the quantitation of valvular lesions and pulmonary hypertension.[87]

In addition to new contrast agents, novel imaging technology directed to the amplification of contrast signals are also available. Harmonic imaging amplifies the ultrasonic backscatter from contrast microbubbles, which resonate in an ultrasonic field, relative to the returning signal from myocardium, which does not resonate. (Fig. 16–57). As discussed previously, tissue harmonic

Identification of intracardiac shunts, particularly patent foramen ovale in patients with unexplained cerebral ischemia (Fig. 16–55), remains a frequent indication for contrast echocardiography. Simple agitated normal saline solution remains the most commonly used contrast agent for such studies.

Echocardiographic opacification of the LV cavity and myocardium by intracardiac or intravenous injection is now easily performed.[84] Because direct injection of coronary contrast into the left heart or aorta (Fig. 16–56) is limited by its invasive nature, stabilized solutions of microbubbles have been developed, which can achieve sufficiently prolonged bubble persistence to traverse the pulmonary capillary bed in high concentration after intravenous injection. The persistence time of a bubble prior to dissolving in blood can be increased by using a shell- or surface-modifying agent that inhibits the leakage of gas across the bubble surface; or by using a dense, high-molecular-weight gas with a reduced capacity to diffuse across the bubble shell and a low saturation constant in blood, favoring return of gas back into the bubble. Therefore, the new ultrasonic contrast agents use shells made of human serum albumin, liposomes, or

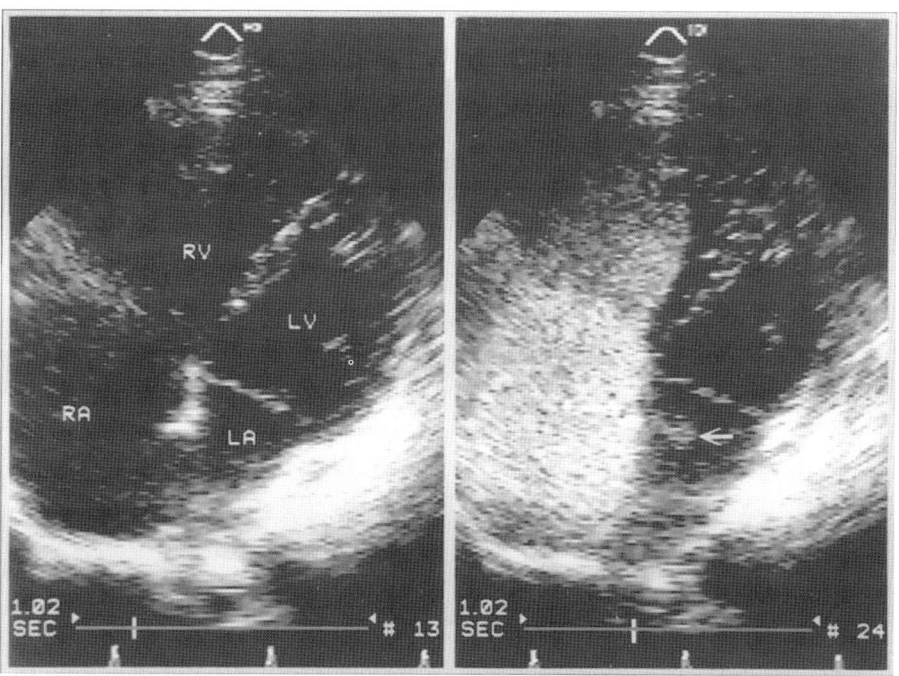

FIGURE 16–55. Contrast microbubble injection demonstrating a shunt (*arrow*) from the right atrium (*RA*) to left atrium (*LA*). LV, left ventricle; RV, right ventricle.

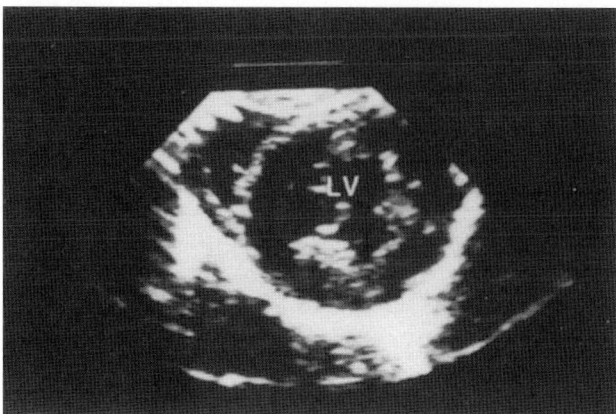
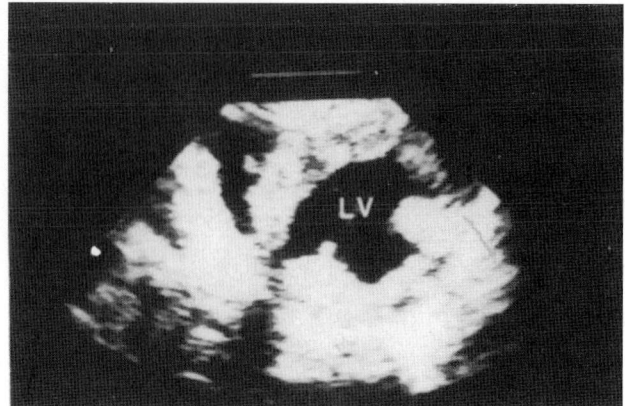

FIGURE 16–56. Short-axis plane through the left ventricle (LV) before (*left*) and after (*right*) injection of microbubbles into the aortic root. The myocardium is densely opacified on the right. *Source: From Hagan AD, DeMaria AN. Clinical Applications of Two-Dimensional Echocardiography and Cardiac Doppler. Boston: Little, Brown; 1989. With permission.*

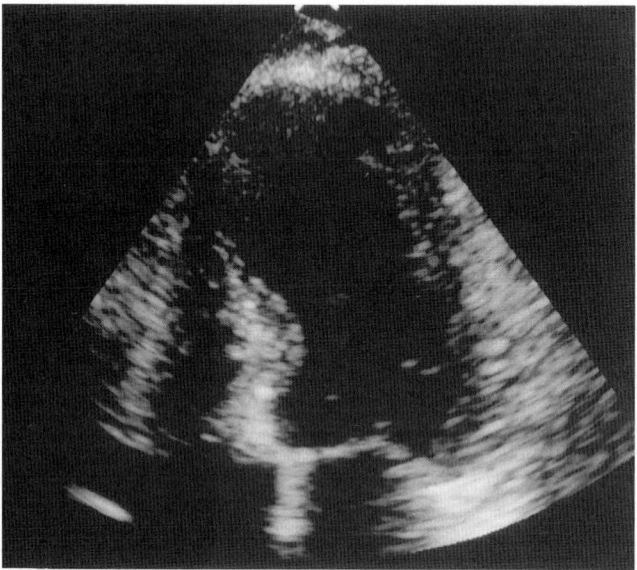

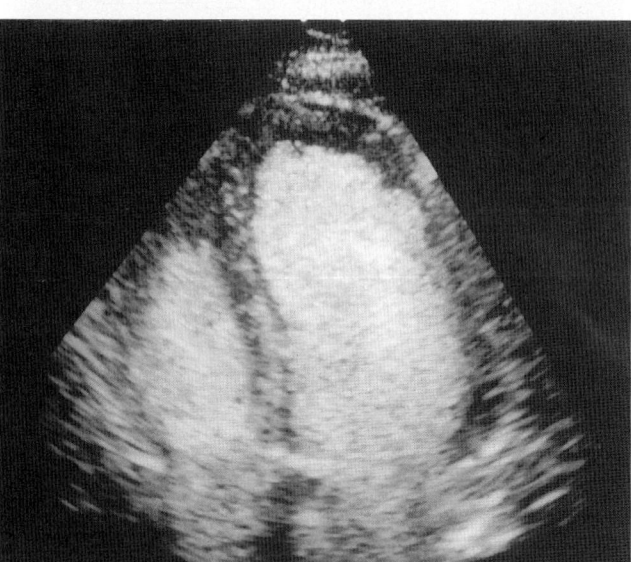

FIGURE 16–57. Harmonic imaging after intravenous injection of echocardiographic contrast. Endocardial border definition before injection is fair (*upper panel*) but is markedly improved with harmonic imaging following contrast injection (*lower panel*).

imaging can also be used to visualize cardiac structures in the absence of contrast injection: This technique decreases clutter and other artifacts, often improving endocardial definition (Fig. 16–58). Power Doppler imaging is a method that correlates signals between successively transmitted pulses to derive images of moving blood or cardiac structures. Power Doppler techniques are especially well suited to detect the changing signals produced by movement and/or dissolution of contrast microbubbles.[37]

The ability to disrupt bubbles is the basis for the quantitation of blood flow by contrast. Following destruction of all bubbles in an ultrasound field by a high energy pulse, new blood with undestroyed bubbles progressively reenters the field until it is once again filled. This refilling can be fit by the equation

$$y = A(1 - e^{-\beta t})$$

where y is the intensity at pulsing interval t; A is the plateau intensity representing myocardial blood volume, and β is the rate constant reflecting the rate of rise of mean microbubble velocity. It has been found that both flow velocity and volume are diminished in the presence of significant coronary stenoses, and that the degree of reduction is proportional to the severity of the lesion.[88] Thereby, destroy/refill phenomena from myocardial contrast echo can be used not only to diagnose coronary artery disease (CAD) but potentially to assess coronary flow reserve.

Intermittent electrocardiographic (ECG-gated) imaging rather than continuous ultrasound transmission can prolong microbubble persistence and amplify contrast signals by limiting bubble destruction but at the cost of not visualizing motion. Most recently, low-power, real-time techniques have been developed that enable imaging of myocardial opacification without the need for ECG gating and intermittent imaging. This is accomplished based on the nonlinearity of bubble behavior versus that of myocardium. When combined with the new ultrasonic contrast agents, both high-energy–triggered and low-energy–real-time imaging modalities can achieve visualization of myocardial opacification following intravenous drug administration, thereby delineating myocardial perfusion.

Recent studies indicate that 2D and 3D myocardial contrast echocardiography can yield information regarding myocardial

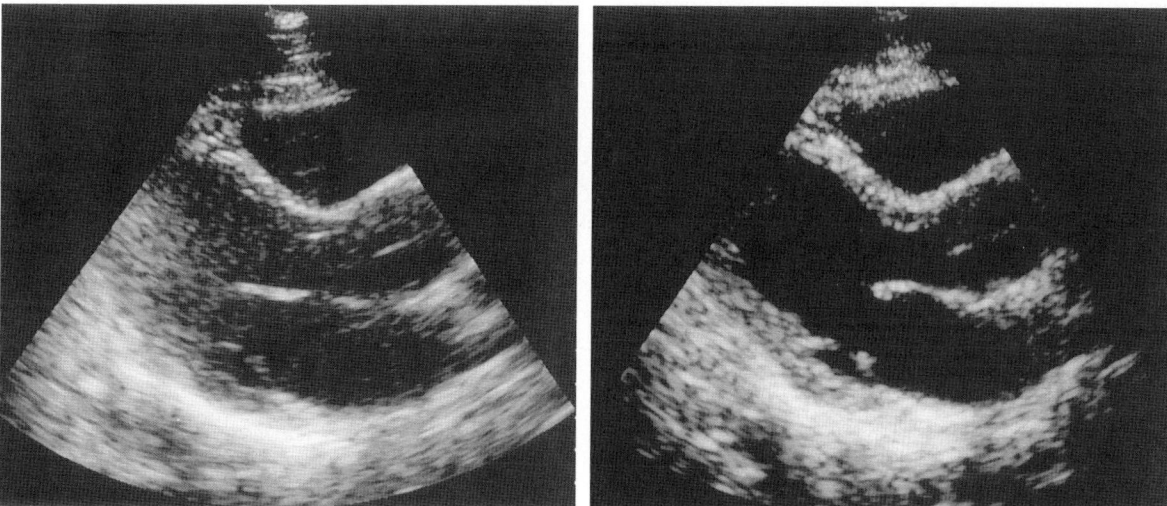

FIGURE 16–58. Tissue harmonic imaging. The *left panel* shows a parasternal long-axis new figure view obtained with standard (fundamental) imaging. Endocardial definition is poor but is markedly enhanced with tissue harmonic imaging (*right panel*).

perfusion comparable to that obtainable by radionuclide techniques and can be valuable in delineating coronary artery stenoses.[89,90] However, the ability to obtain technically high-quality images is imperfect, and no large multicenter studies have been published. Myocardial contrast echocardiography can identify infarct areas in acute myocardial infarction (MI), document the absence of microcirculatory flow after epicardial coronary reperfusion (*no-reflow* phenomenon), and predict postinfarction viability. Intravenous injection of contrast agents also permits visualization of intramyocardial vessels.[87] The ability to delineate regional myocardial perfusion is a major step forward in noninvasive imaging At the present time, it remains an investigative tool.

DISEASES OF THE AORTIC VALVE AND AORTA

【 】 AORTIC STENOSIS

The AoV is best imaged in the parasternal views.[91] The leaflets are thin, linear structures. All three can be visualized in the short-axis view and produce a triangular orifice during systolic opening. The long-axis view exhibits the right and usually the noncoronary leaflets, which normally open to the walls of the aorta. Mild thickening and reduction of mobility is often observed in the elderly (aortic sclerosis) and is associated with an increased risk of CAD. In older adults, acquired AS is manifested by markedly thickened, often calcified, immobile AoV leaflets,[92] whereas doming leaflets suggests congenital AS and is usually encountered in younger patients (Fig. 16–59). Subaortic stenosis (SAS)

may be caused by asymmetrical septal hypertrophy with systolic anterior mitral motion, a subaortic membrane, or (less commonly) a subaortic tunnel. Bicuspid valves exhibit an oval rather than triangular orifice (Fig. 16–60). Although the severity of stenosis can be assessed semiquantitatively by 2D and M-mode image echocardiography, valvular calcification may shadow the leaflets or produce reverberations and obscure their motion.[92] Therefore, attempts to measure valve area by transthoracic planimetry have been unsuccessful, but multiplane TEE has been of greater value[75]

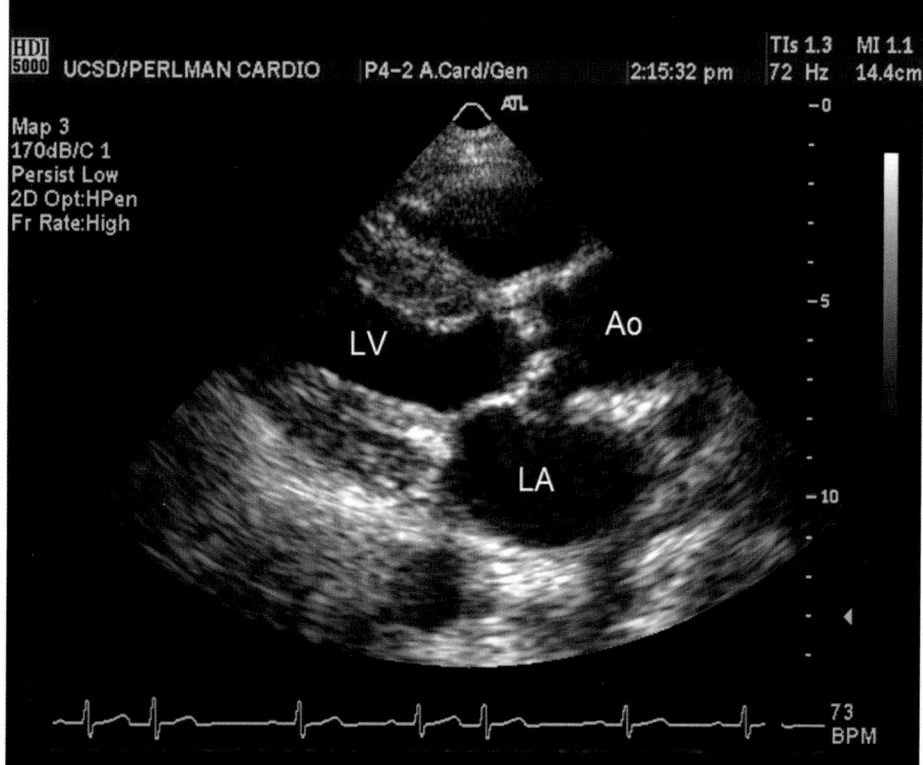

FIGURE 16–59. Parasternal long-axis plane demonstrating a thickened, stenotic AoV. Ao, aorta; AoV, aortic valve; LA, left atrium; LV, left ventricle.

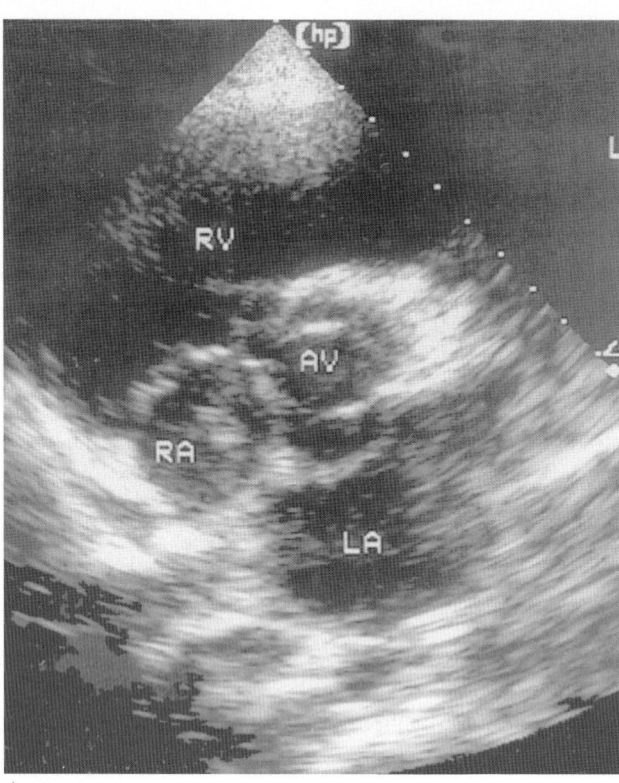

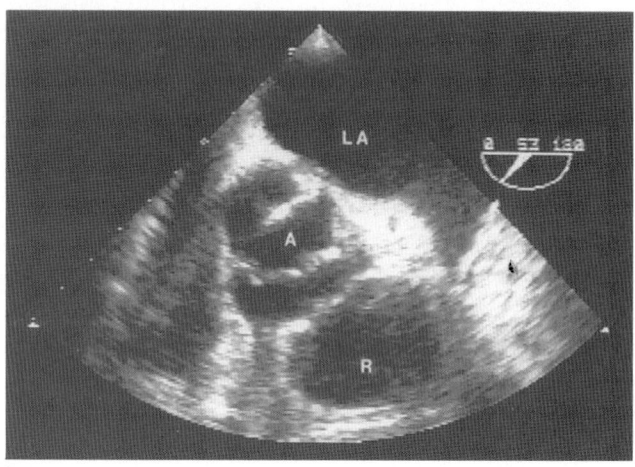

A

B

FIGURE 16-60. A. Parasternal short-axis image of a bicuspid AoV (AoV) during systole. RV, right ventricle; RA, right atrium; LA, left atrium. **B.** Transesophageal image of a bicuspid AoV (*A*). LA, left atrium, R, right ventricular outflow tract. *Source: From Blanchard DG, Kimura BJ, Dittrich HC, DeMaria AN.*[71] *With permission.*

(Fig. 16–61). Thus, 2D-echocardiographic imaging accurately detects the presence and etiology of AS but not the severity. Likewise, CFD demonstrates turbulent flow through the AoV and may guide CW interrogation but provides little quantitative data. The use of Doppler echocardiography and the modified Bernoulli and continuity equations have now made noninvasive calculation of aortic gradients and valve area routine and have affected use of cardiac catheterization in AS patients (see Chap. 75).

The cornerstone of the ultrasound evaluation of AS is CW Doppler interrogation through the AoV. The calculated gradient using the peak Doppler velocity $[4(AS\ velocity)^2]$ correlates closely with the peak instantaneous gradient measured at catheterization[65] (Fig. 16–62). The first two physiologic parameters represent simultaneous pressure differences between LV and aorta and can be measured accurately by Doppler echocardiography. The peak-to-peak gradient, commonly used in the catheterization laboratory, compares the highest pressures reached in the LV and aorta (even though not simultaneous) and is uniformly lower than the peak instanta-neous gradient recorded by Doppler. The maximal Doppler gradient does not correlate with the peak-to-peak catheterization gradient, and comparisons between the two should be avoided (see Chap. 75).

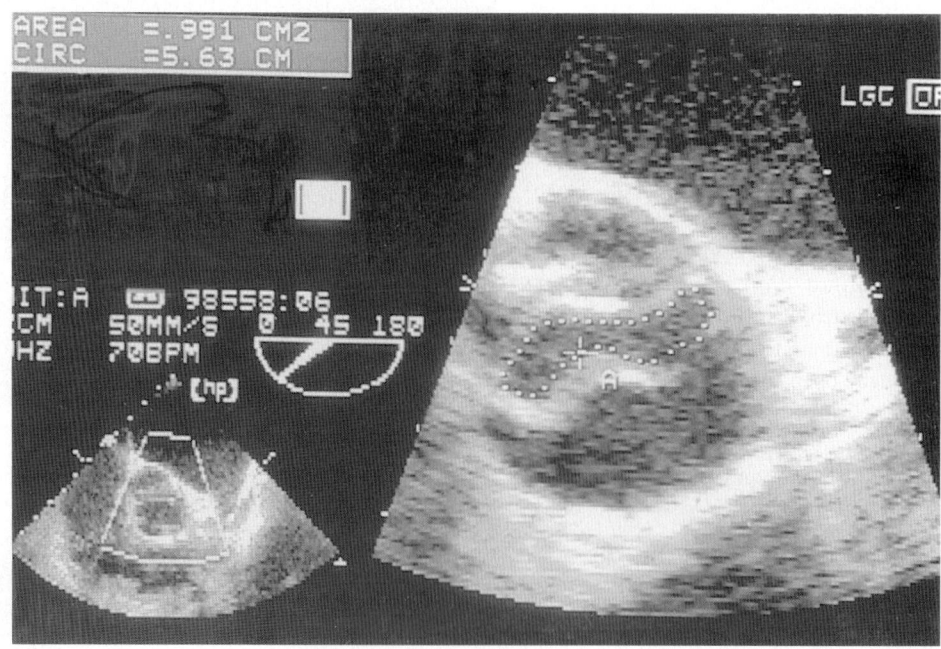

FIGURE 16-61. Transesophageal image of a stenotic bicuspid AoV (*A*) with superimposed planimetry of the valve area (approximately 1 cm²). AoV, aortic valve.

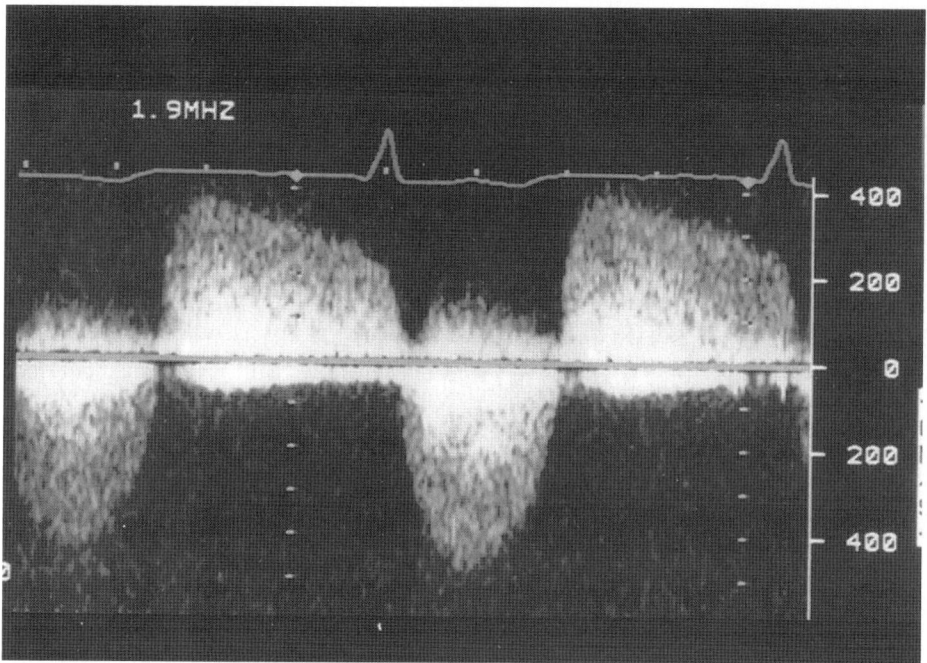

FIGURE 16–62. CW Doppler tracing (from the apical transducer position) through the AoV in a case of combined AS and insufficiency. The peak systolic velocity approaches 5 m/sec. AoV, aortic valve; CW, continuous wave.

Several potential sources of error exist in the estimation of the transvalvular aortic gradient by CW Doppler recordings. It is imperative that Doppler signals from the stenotic jet be obtained with an angle of incidence of <20 degrees. Because 2D techniques rarely reveal the precise direction of the jet, each examination must employ all possible windows and angulations. Also, one must be careful to account for the proximal flow velocity in the Bernoulli equation if it is 1.5 m/sec or greater. It is important to record CW signals as close to the aortic leaflets as possible. Values for the AoV area can be calculated using the continuity equation by measuring the velocity of the jet across the AoV with CW Doppler, the velocity in the LV outflow tract just proximal to the valve with PWD, and deriving the area of the outflow tract from the diameter of the aortic annulus. Results from the continuity equation have been found to correlate well with the area calculations based on catheterization data and the Gorlin formula.[64] CW Doppler can occasionally overestimate peak systolic pressure gradients, especially in patients with narrow AOs. Because both AS jet velocity and aortic annular radius are squared in the continuity equation, accurate determination of these parameters is essential for reliable measurements. When atrial fibrillation is present, the peak Doppler velocity still correlates with peak instantaneous gradient through the AoV, but calculations of valve area may be problematic.

In summary, a comprehensive echocardiographic examination in a patient with AS should establish both the presence and severity of disease (see Chap. 75). The continuity equation should provide reliable estimates of AoV area. In cases where the relative roles of orifice stenosis and LV dysfunction are uncertain, TEE imaging or Doppler recordings during inotropic stimulation with dobutamine may be of value.[75,93] In addition, dobutamine echocardiography is helpful in distinguishing high-risk patients with AS and severe LV dysfunction.[94]

AORTIC REGURGITATION

In contrast to AS, the AoV leaflets are often anatomically normal by echocardiography in patients with AR. 2D and M-mode echocardiography often provide indirect evidence of the presence of AR, including signs of LV volume overload, diastolic fluttering of the anterior MV leaflet, AO enlargement, and incomplete coaptation of the AoV leaflets. The important M-mode finding of premature diastolic closure of the MV prior to the onset of systole caused by LV filling by the regurgitant jet signifies acute, severe AR (Fig. 16–63) and the need for surgery (see Chap. 75).

Perhaps the most important contribution of echocardiographic tissue imaging to the assessment of AR is in identifying the etiology. Thus, thickened leaflets restricted in movement are observed in patients with acquired AS, whereas oval doming of two functional leaflets will be observed in the presence of a bicuspid AoV (see Fig. 16–60). AR caused by infectious endocarditis can be identified by the presence of valvular vegetations, whereas regurgitation caused by diseases of the aorta are manifest by anatomic changes of the vessel. Less common etiologies of AR, such as those associated with subvalvular pathology or VSD, may also be recognized by echocardiographic imaging.

Doppler interrogation is necessary to obtain direct evidence of the presence and severity of AR. Screening with CFD demonstrates turbulent flow in the LV outflow tract during diastole in

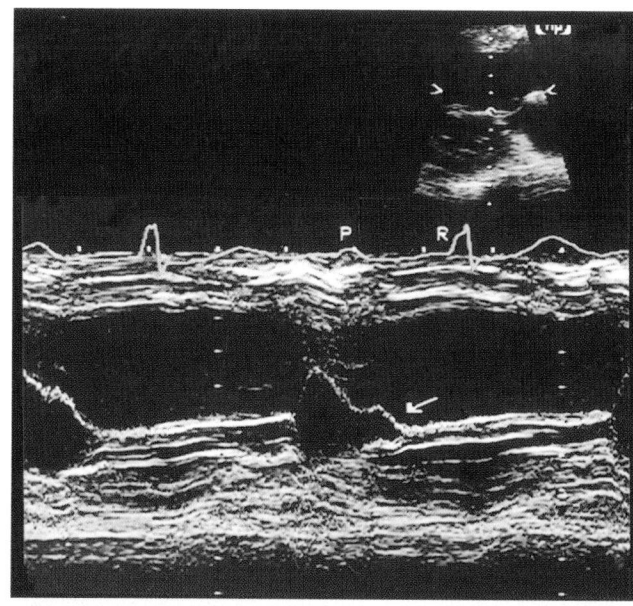

FIGURE 16–63. M-mode tracing (from the parasternal position) in a patient with acute severe aortic regurgitation. The mitral valve leaflets close (arrow) before ventricular contraction begins. P, p wave; R, QRS complex.

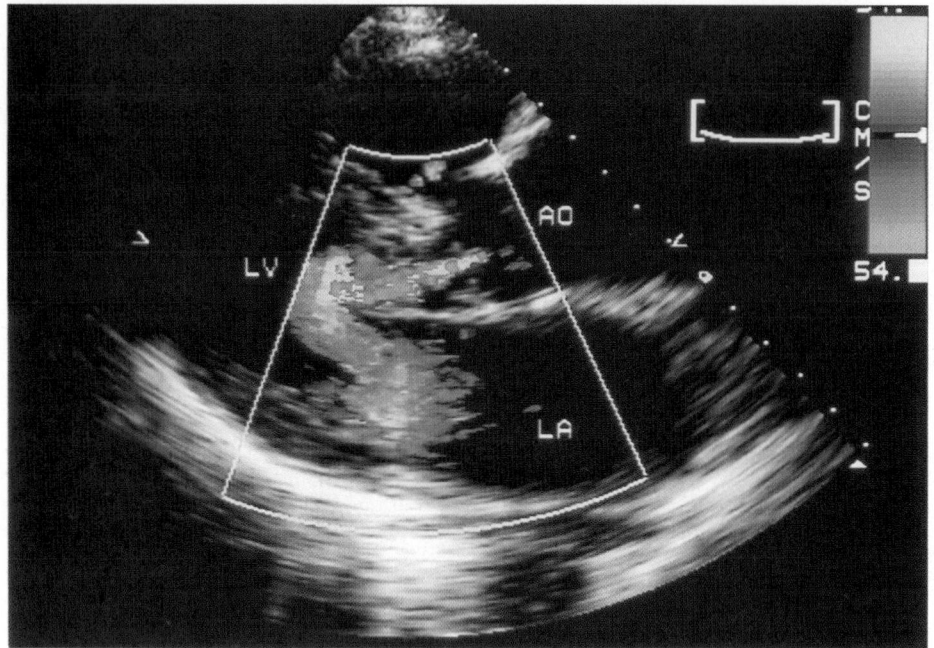

A

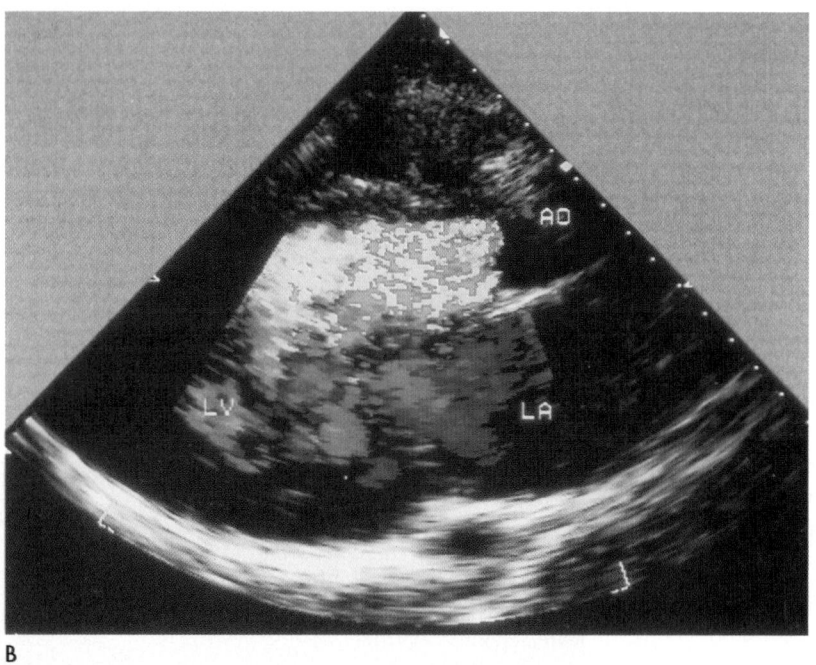

B

FIGURE 16–64. **A.** Parasternal long-axis plane showing a multicolor jet (indicating turbulent flow) of aortic regurgitation in the left ventricular outflow tract. The jet is narrow in width, suggesting mild regurgitation. **B.** Parasternal long-axis plane with color-flow Doppler imaging. The aortic regurgitant (AR) color jet is as wide as the left ventricular outflow tract, suggesting severe AR. **C.** Parasternal long-axis image of acute severe aortic regurgitation (AR). The accompanying marked elevation of LV diastolic pressure causes diastolic mitral regurgitation (MR). Ao, aorta; LA, left atrium; LV, left ventricle.

generally has a much slower deceleration, and does not have an increased velocity following atrial contraction.

Conventional echocardiographic imaging can provide evidence of the presence and extent of LV volume overload. More direct evidence of the severity of AR can be derived from the deceleration rate of the jet recorded by CW Doppler (Fig. 16–65).[96] In the presence of mild degrees of AR, the transvalvular pressure gradient is maintained throughout diastole, creating a high-velocity jet with a minimal deceleration rate. Conversely, severe AR reduces aortic pressures and increases LV pressures in diastole, eliminating the pressure gradient and creating a rapid jet deceleration to a low velocity (see Fig. 16–65). Severe, acute AR can also cause diastolic MR (see Fig. 16–64C). The most common approach to assessing the deceleration rate of the AR jet is by calculating the time required for the velocity to fall to one-half of the maximal pressure equivalent. A pressure half-time of <250 ms reliably identifies patients with severe degrees of AR. Application of the pressure half-time approach to quantifying AR must take into account that because the deceleration rate is a reflection of pressure gradient, it is determined by both the volume of AR and the LV compliance.

The estimate of severity most commonly derived from echocardiography is the size of the AR jet by CFD.[95] Conceptually, jets distributed over a small area of the LV outflow tract represent lesser degrees of AR than jets that penetrate widely and to the level of the papillary muscles. The optimal results occur when the width of the AR jet just proximal to the valve is expressed as a percentage of the width of the LV outflow tract; a jet occupying 50 percent or more of the outflow tract correlates with severe regurgitation by angiography.[95] Also, entrainment and displacement of RBCs in the LV outflow tract also influence the size of the regurgitant jet. Finally, convergence of AR with normal transmitral filling may obscure the flow disturbance. Therefore, assessment of the severity of AR by the size and shape of the flow disturbance is at best semiquantitative.

The AR volume can be estimated by comparing volumetric measurements of LV inflow and LV outflow calculated from annular velocity and cross-sectional area (derived from pulsed Doppler and 2D images, respectively).[63] This method depends on the absence of valvular stenosis and of other regurgitant lesions. In the

virtually all views[95] (Fig. 16–64A–C). The jet is typically elliptical and may be located anywhere in the LV outflow tract. CW Doppler spectral recordings from this jet yield a high-velocity diastolic signal directed toward the apex (see Fig. 16–62). Because AR jet velocity accurately reflects the diastolic pressure gradient between aorta and LV, it is maximum at the point of valve closure and decreases throughout diastole.[96] The flow pattern of AR, higher in velocity than mitral inflow, begins immediately after AoV closure,

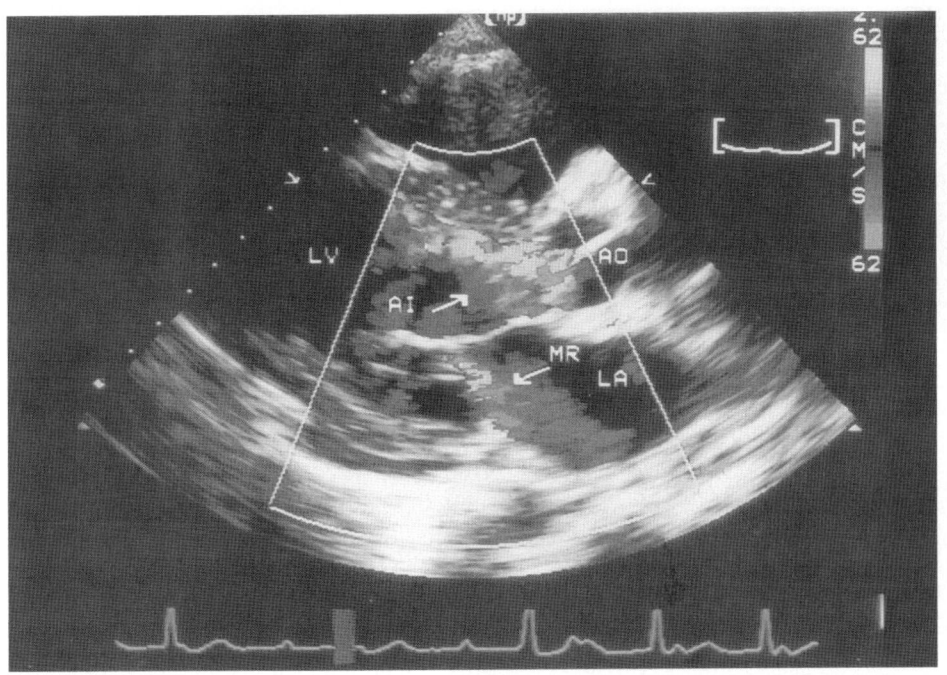

C

FIGURE 16–64. *(continued)*

setting of AR, the volume ejected through the aortic annulus represents both systemic flow and regurgitant volume, whereas the volume coursing through the mitral annulus represents only systemic flow. Thereby, LV outflow exceeds LV inflow by the amount of the regurgitant volume.[63] An alternate *quantitative approach* derives estimates of regurgitant fraction from reverse diastolic flow in the aorta.[97] Although this is somewhat imprecise, the presence of a significant flow reversal in the aorta visualized by color or spectral Doppler is a reliable marker of severe AR (Fig. 16–66).

Determination of the optimal timing of surgical intervention in patients with AR remains a difficult problem in clinical medicine (see Chap. 75). Several criteria derived from echocardiographic recordings have been proposed to guide this decision. Most prominently, an LV end-systolic dimension of 55 mm or greater with a shortening fraction of 25 percent or less have been advocated as criteria for surgical intervention in the absence of symptoms. However, no universally accepted echocardiographic criteria exist for determining the optimal role for surgical treatment.

【 】 DISEASES OF THE AORTA

The thoracic aorta is best visualized from the left and right parasternal positions and from the suprasternal notch.

The descending aorta may also be imaged from subcostal and modified apical views. Normally, short-axis images of the AO yield a circular structure, whereas long-axis images exhibit two parallel linear walls with a maximal diameter of 35 mm.[98] Although 2D imaging is used commonly, M-mode recordings of the AO facilitate precise measurement of its dimensions.

Aortic Dissection

Echocardiography has dramatically changed the diagnostic approach to aortic dissection (see Chap. 105). TTE is a convenient screening test (Fig. 16–67) and often enables accurate detection of ascending aortic dissection. The diagnostic findings include a dilated aorta with a mobile intimal flap that presents as a thin, linear signal within the lumen. Transthoracic imaging is unreliable for detection of descending aortic dissection, but it occasionally visualizes the complete length of the thoracic aorta (see Chap. 105).

Although several noninvasive methods exist to diagnose aortic dissection, TEE has become the procedure of choice in many hospitals because of its accuracy, portability, rapid procedural time,

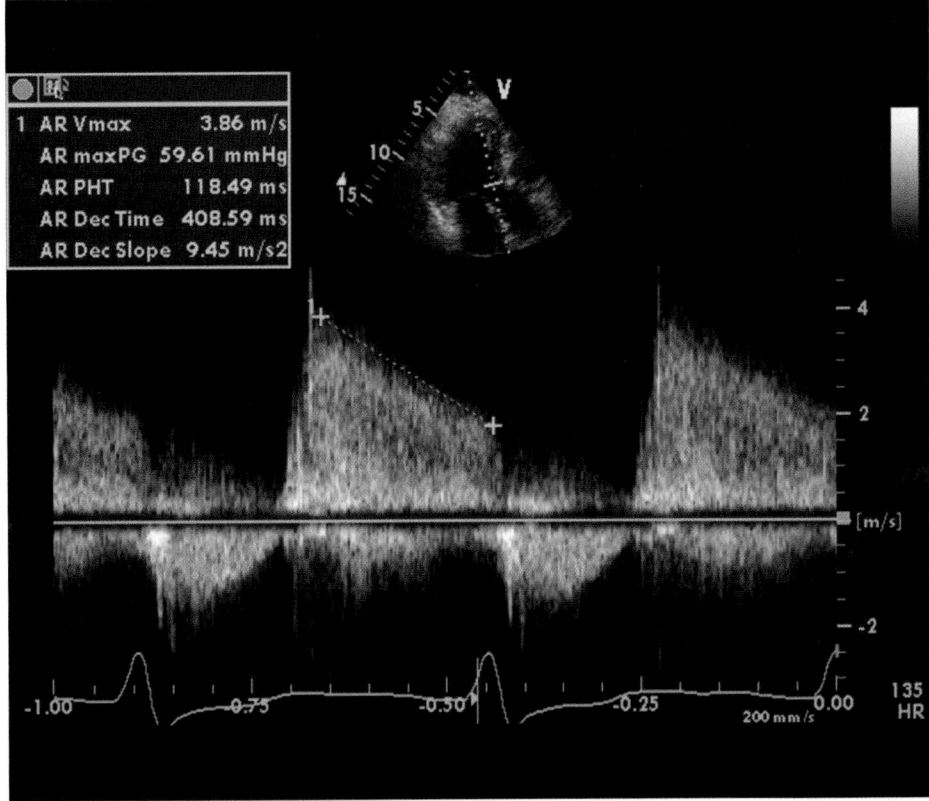

1	AR Vmax	3.86 m/s
	AR maxPG	59.61 mmHg
	AR PHT	118.49 ms
	AR Dec Time	408.59 ms
	AR Dec Slope	9.45 m/s2

FIGURE 16–65. CW Doppler tracing (from the apical transducer position) of severe AR. The pressure half-time of the AR envelope is approximately 120 ms. AR, aortic regurgitation.

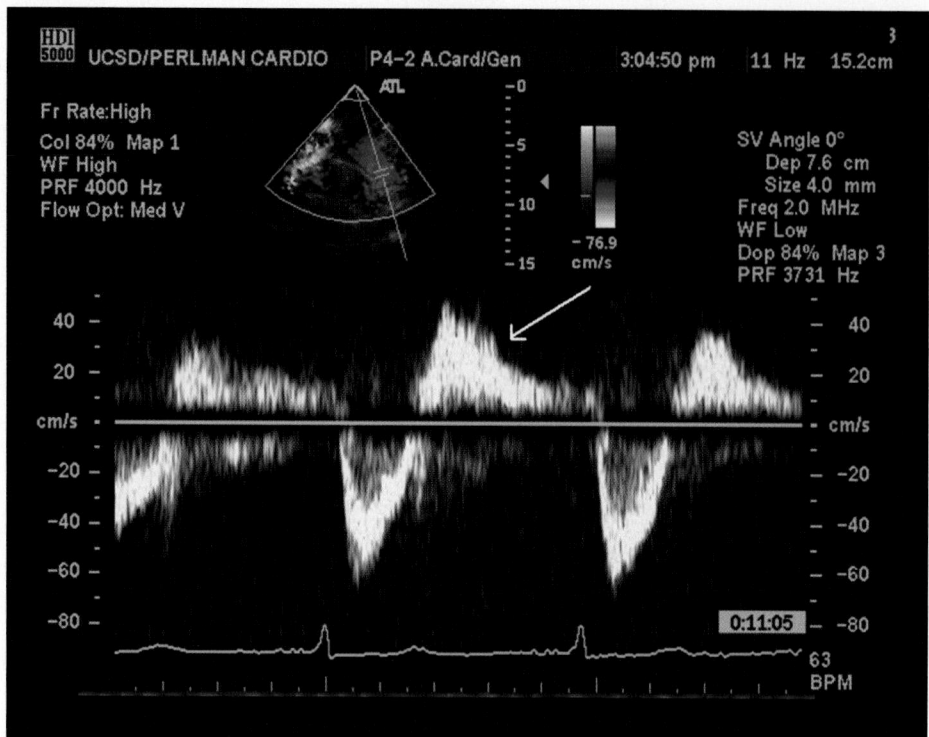

FIGURE 16-66. Pulsed-wave Doppler tracing (from the suprasternal transducer position) in a case of severe aortic regurgitation. The sample volume is in the descending thoracic aorta, and holodiastolic flow reversal (*arrow*) is present.

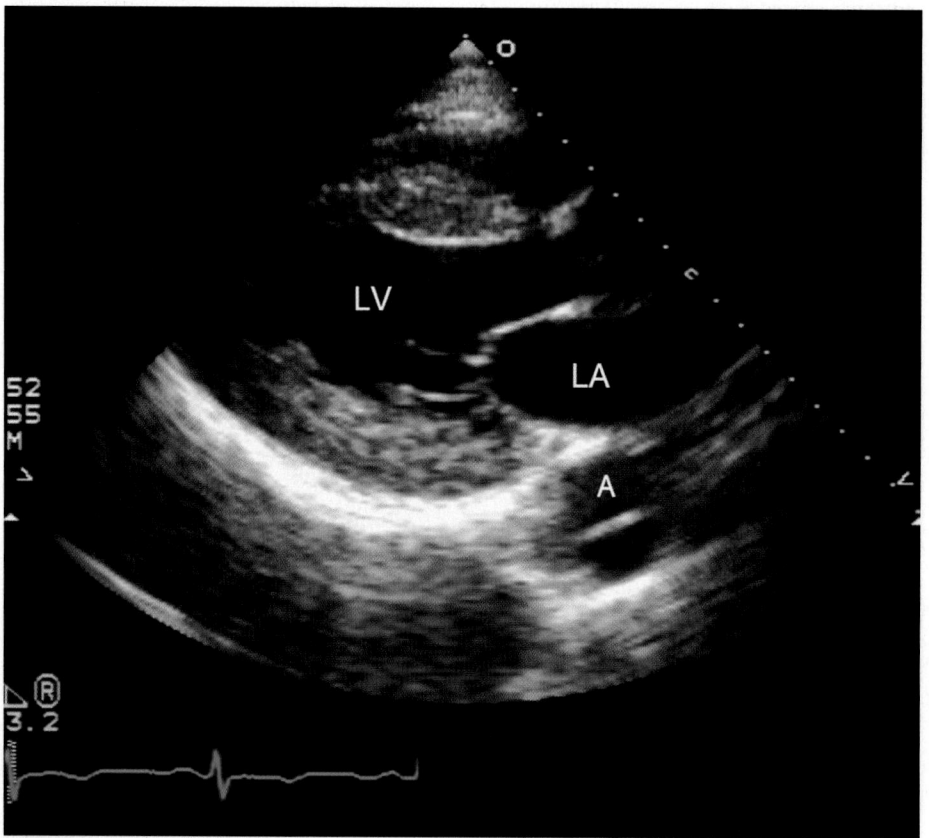

FIGURE 16-67. Transthoracic parasternal long-axis plane demonstrating a dissection of the descending thoracic aorta (*A*). Marked left ventricular hypertrophy is present, and an intimal flap is seen in the descending aorta. LA, left atrium; LV, left ventricle.

and ability to provide data regarding valvular regurgitation and LV function.[99,100] Except for a short portion of the proximal aortic arch, which is obscured by the bronchus, multiplane TEE provides excellent visualization of the entire thoracic aorta and high accuracy in detecting aortic enlargement, intimal tears, and false lumen thrombus (Fig. 16–68). CFD may reveal communications between true and false channels (see Fig. 16–51, Fig. 16–69). TEE also appears useful for the diagnosis of aortic intramural hematoma, an increasingly recognized disorder that has a clinical prognosis similar to that of classic dissection. In this disorder hemorrhage occurs within the aortic media, but an intimal tear (and a dissection flap) is absent. The finding of a curvilinear, asymmetric density within the aortic wall in a patient with typical symptoms of dissection strongly suggests a diagnosis of aortic intramural hematoma.[101]

Aortic Aneurysm

Aneurysms of the aorta may be saccular or fusiform and are recognized as localized or circumferential areas of aortic enlargement, often with thin walls. TTE is especially useful in detecting ascending aortic dilatation but can also visualize descending thoracic and abdominal aortic aneurysms.[98,102] Echocardiography has been used extensively to assess aortic pathology in patients with Marfan syndrome (see Chap. 88). The nature of the lesion is relatively specific in that there is symmetrical dilatation of the annulus, sinuses of Valsalva, and AO (Fig. 16–70A). Aortic leaflet coaptation may be compromised leading to AR. Echocardiography is helpful in determining prognosis and timing of AO replacement.

Sinus of Valsalva aneurysms are also well visualized by both TTE and TEE. These lesions cause asymmetric dilatation of the AO and seem to affect the right coronary sinus most frequently. They are prone to rupture, often into the right heart (see Fig. 16–70B). Doppler echocardiography in such settings demonstrates fluttering of the TV, a color jet crossing from the AO into the right heart, and occasionally diastolic opening of the PV.

Congenital aortic disease also can be detected with echocardiography (see Congenital Heart Disease below, and

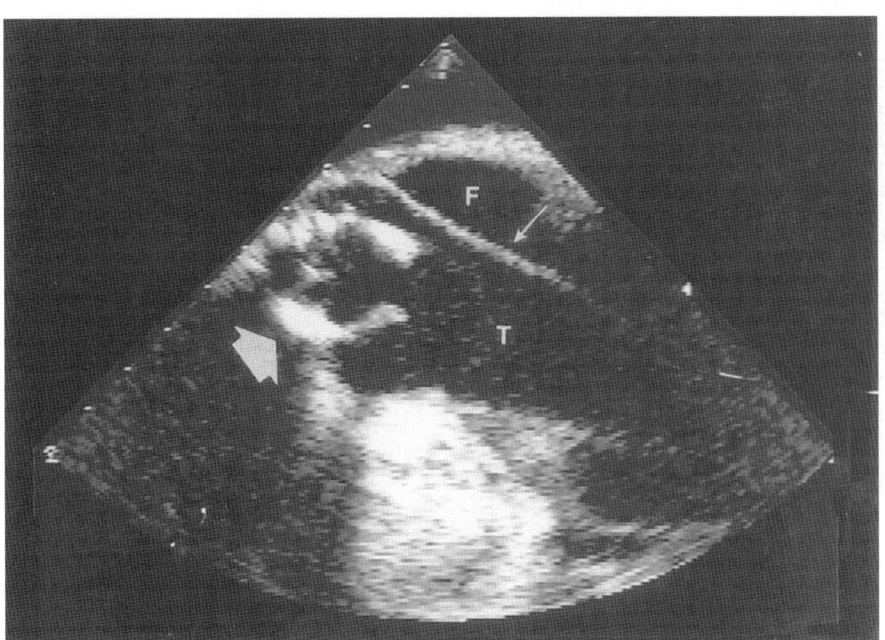

FIGURE 16–68. Longitudinal TEE view of an ascending aortic dissection in a patient with a porcine prosthetic valve in the aortic position (*large arrow*). The false (*F*) and true (*T*) lumens are separated by an intimal flap (*small arrow*). TEE, transesophageal echocardiography. *Source: From Blanchard DG, Kimura BJ, Dittrich HC, DeMaria AN.*[71]

Chaps. 82 and 83). In these conditions, suprasternal and transesophageal imaging are often helpful. SAS is recognized as an *hourglass* narrowing or a discrete fibrous ridge just distal to the leaflets, whereas coarctation presents a more localized, abrupt luminal reduction in the descending aorta or distal portion of the aortic arch.

Aortic Atherosclerosis

As mentioned in the section on TEE, recent studies suggest that aortic atherosclerosis is an important cause of stroke and embolic

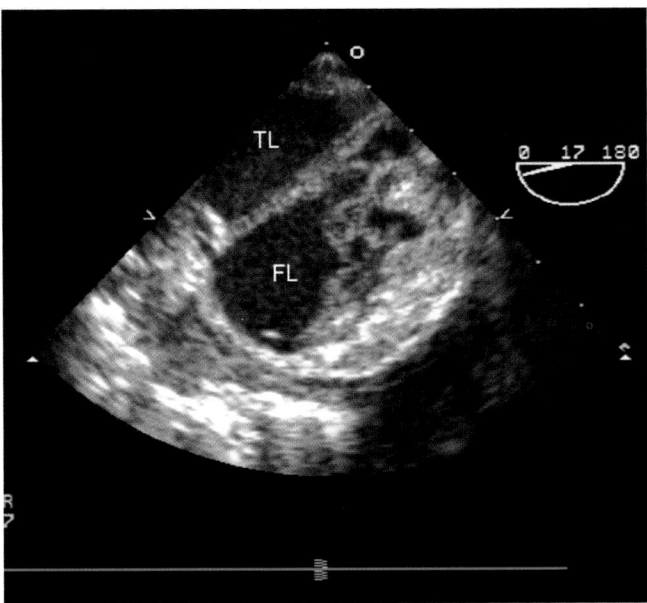

FIGURE 16–69. Transverse TEE view of an aortic dissection. The false (*FL*) and true (*TL*) lumens are separated by an intimal flap. Thrombus is present in the FL. TEE, transesophageal echocardiography.

events. Mobile and protruding intimal plaques have been detected by TEE (see Fig. 16–53) in patients with stroke, a finding not previously appreciated by other imaging techniques. Optimal treatment for extensive aortic atherosclerosis is currently unknown but warfarin appears useful.[103] When such plaques are present prior to cardiopulmonary bypass, prompt adjustment of cannula placement is indicated to avoid dislodging the aortic debris.

Penetrating aortic ulceration, which affects the descending aorta and mimics the clinical syndrome of acute aortic dissection, may also be diagnosed by TEE (Fig. 16–71). A localized defect is visualized with protrusion of the ulcer into the vessel wall. Urgent surgery is warranted to avoid aortic rupture. Aortic tears induced by trauma are also accurately detected by TEE (Fig. 16–72).

DISEASES OF THE MITRAL VALVE

MITRAL STENOSIS

Detection of *mitral stenosis* (MS) was one of the earliest clinical applications of echocardiography (see Chap. 77). In most individuals the MV leaflets are easily visualized and yield thin linear echoes that exhibit wide bipeaked excursions because they open in early and late diastole.[21] The characteristic 2D ultrasound findings of MS are seen clearly in nearly all patients with this disorder. The MV leaflets are thickened and often present bright, high-intensity reflections indicating calcification. Thickening and shortening of the chordal apparatus occur as well. There are varying degrees of commissural fusion restricting mitral leaflet separation, especially at the distal tips. This leads to diastolic *doming* or a right-angle bend of the anterior MV leaflet as high LA pressure creates a bulge in the leaflet's midportion (Fig. 16–73). The posterior leaflet actually may be pulled anteriorly during diastole because of commissural fusion with the longer anterior leaflet The LA is nearly always enlarged with MS.

The effects of stenosis on MV motion are often best demonstrated by M-mode recordings (Fig. 16–74). M-mode tracings also depict a characteristic decrease in the reclosure rate of the anterior mitral leaflet in early diastole (reduced E-F slope) caused by a persistent LA–LV pressure gradient and a slow rate of LV filling. The decrease of the E-F slope has been found to correlate grossly with the severity of MS. This finding without MS may occur whenever early diastolic filling is reduced.[21]

The entire perimeter of the MV orifice can be visualized in the 2D parasternal short-axis view, and mitral leaflet excursion normally approaches the endocardial borders of the LV at the mitral tip level. In the setting of MS, the thickened leaflets form a fishmouth orifice, which occupies only a small portion of the cross-sectional area of the LV (see Chap. 77). Measurements of orifice area, obtained by planimetry of the orifice visualized in the parasternal short-axis view, correlate well with those obtained by

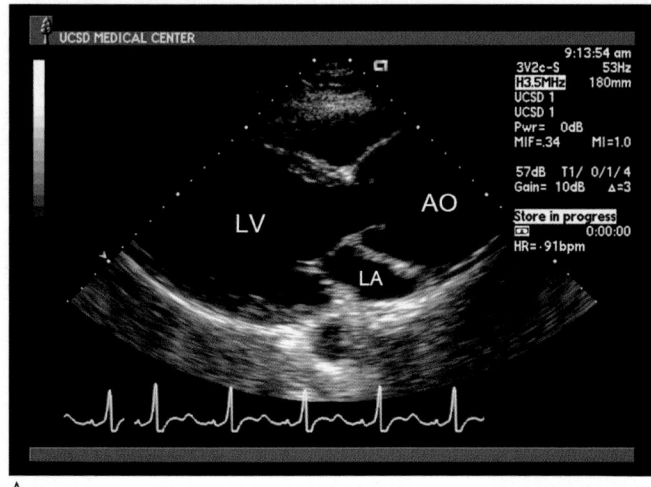

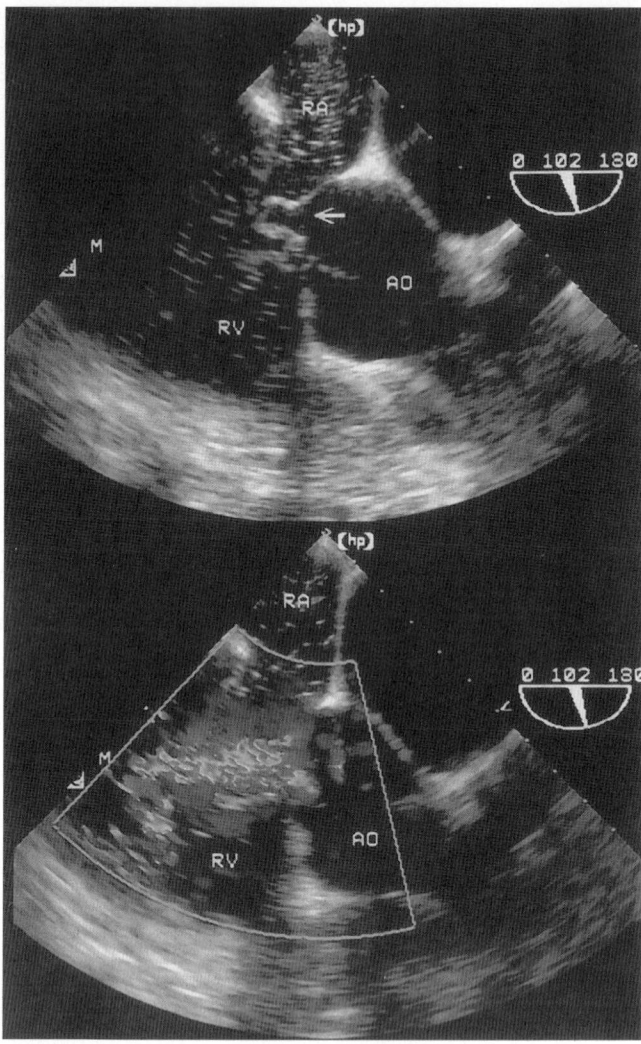

FIGURE 16–70. A. Parasternal long-axis plane demonstrating severe aortic root (AO) enlargement. **B.** TEE image of a ruptured sinus of Valsalva aneurysm. The upper image shows focal aneurysmal dilatation of the right coronary sinus with the appearance of a *windsock*. Color Doppler (*lower image*) reveals a high-velocity flow jet from the aorta into the RV. Agitated saline was injected intravenously to highlight right heart structures. LA, left atrium; LV, left ventricle; RV, right ventricle; TEE, transesophageal echocardiography.

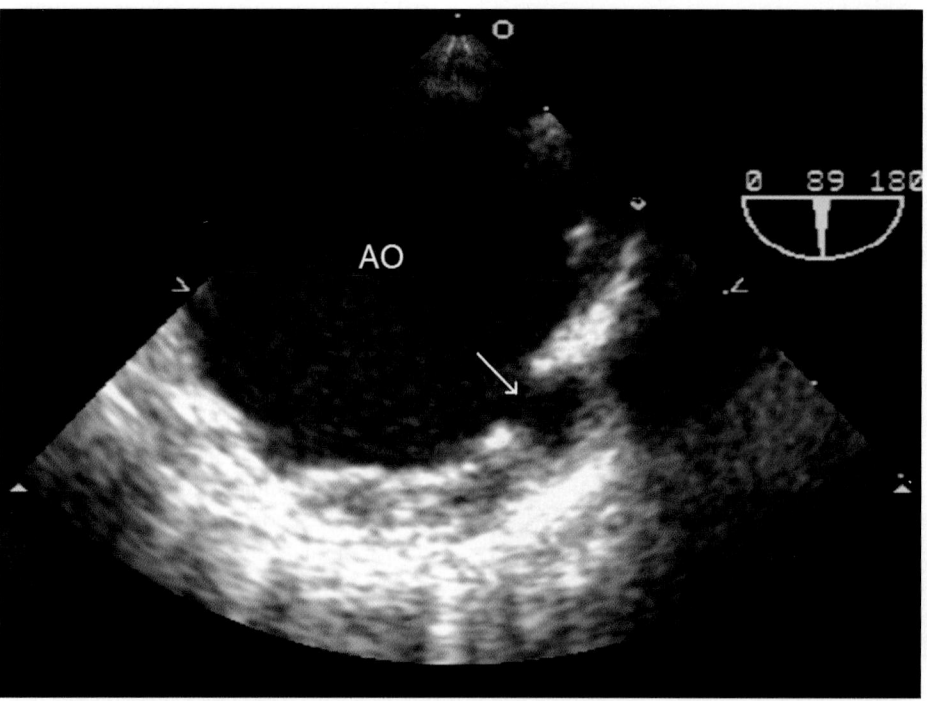

FIGURE 16–71. Transverse TEE view of penetrating ulceration in the aortic arch. The mouth of the ulcer crater is visible (*arrow*). TEE, transesophageal echocardiography.

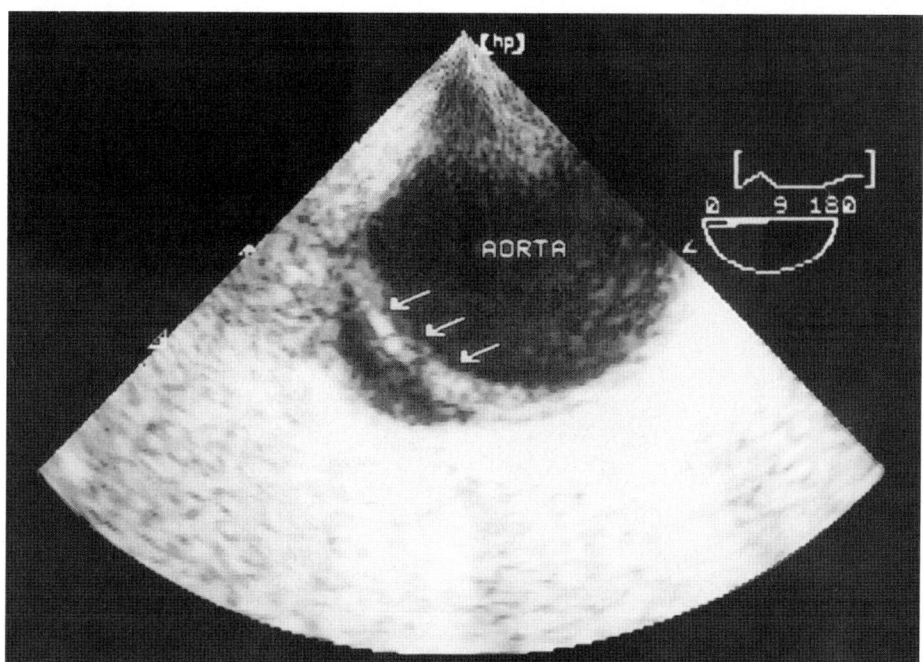

FIGURE 16–72. Transverse TEE image of traumatic aortic disruption and partial transection (*arrows*) involving the distal portion of the aortic arch. TEE, transesophageal echocardiography.

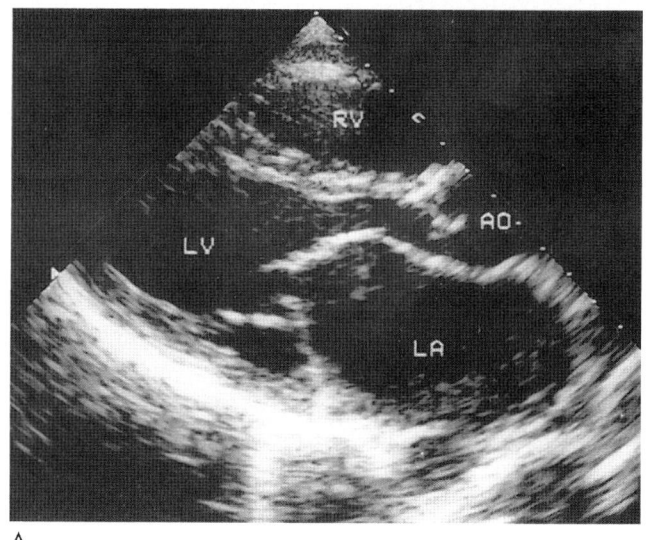

A

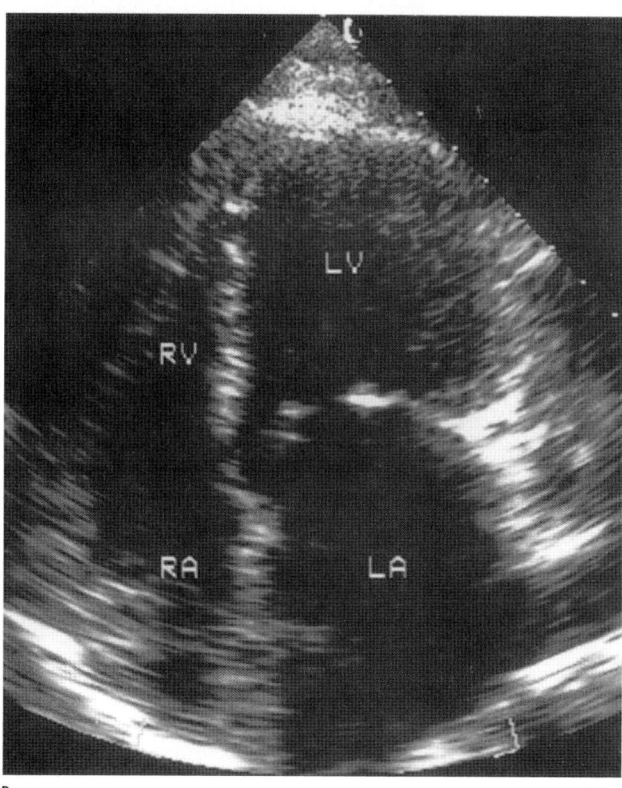

B

FIGURE 16–73. A. Parasternal long-axis view of MS. The LA is enlarged, mitral opening is limited, and *doming* of the anterior mitral leaflet is present. **B.** Apical four-chamber view in mitral stenosis. The LA is markedly dilated. **C.** Parasternal short-axis plane in mitral stenosis. **D.** Transesophageal image showing doming of the anterior mitral valve leaflet. Ao, aorta; LA, left atrium; LV, left ventricle; MS, mitral stenosis; RA, right atrium; RV, right ventricle. (*continued*)

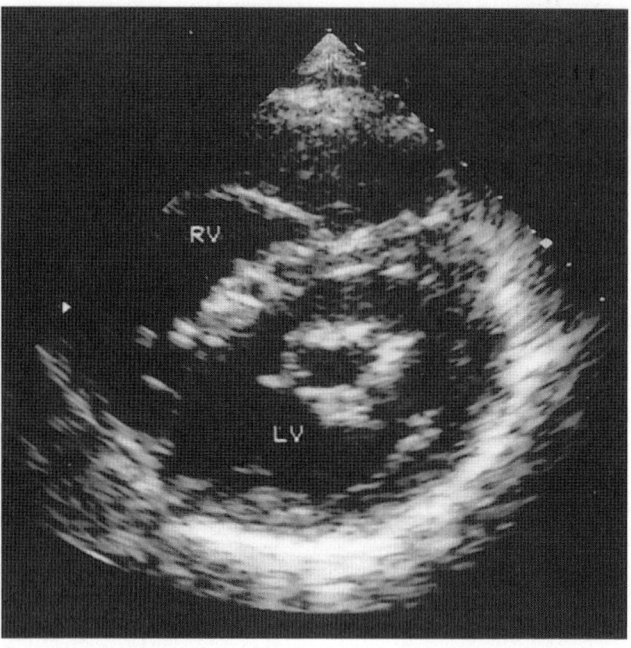

C

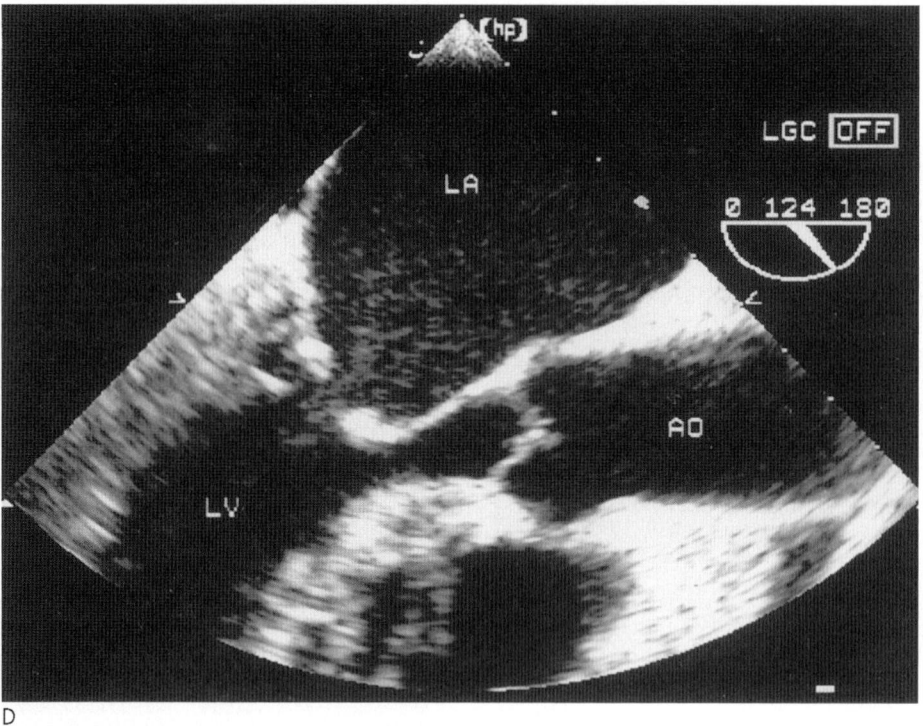

D

FIGURE 16–73. (continued)

cardiac catheterization (see Fig. 16–73). It is crucial to identify the smallest cross-sectional area and obtain recordings with orthogonal beam orientation at that point to avoid overestimation.

Doppler examination provides additional quantitation of MS (see Chap. 77). Interrogation of mitral inflow with either PW or CW modes (depending on velocity and Nyquist limit) reveals elevated diastolic velocities, with a reduction in the rate of deceleration in early diastole yielding a pattern similar to the decreased E-F slope seen with M-mode in MS (Fig. 16–75). The maximal gradient across the MV can be calculated from the peak diastolic

velocity using the Bernoulli equation. The maximal transmitral gradient is very sensitive to changes in heart rate and loading; thus, the mean transmitral gradient obtained as the average of a number of individual gradients derived throughout diastole is commonly used to assess the severity of MS. Also, the Doppler technique may provide estimates of mitral valve area (MVA) by means of the calculation of the pressure halftime. The pressure halftime represents the interval required for transmitral velocity to decelerate from its highest point (E) to a velocity that yields one-half of the pressure equivalent (see Fig. 16–75). As the severity of MS increases, the

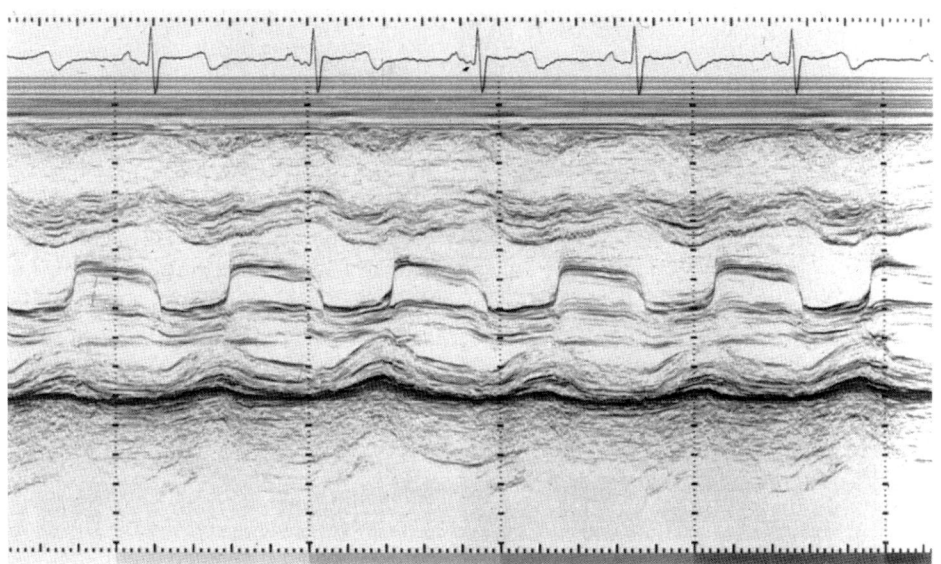

FIGURE 16–74. Parasternal M-mode image through the mitral valve in a patient with mitral stenosis. The normal rapid downslope of the anterior mitral leaflet after early rapid diastolic filling is absent.

rate of deceleration decreases, prolonging the pressure halftime. Further, dividing an empiric constant of 220 by the pressure halftime yields an estimate of MVA, which correlates with values obtained during cardiac catheterization. Doppler estimates of MVA are considered less accurate than direct measurements of MVA derived by planimetry of the MV orifice. Echocardiography can help assess the feasibility and appropriateness of percutaneous balloon mitral valvuloplasty (PBMV) to treat individual patients with MS.[104] An echocardiographic scoring system based on evaluation of mitral valvular thickening, calcification, mobility, and subvalvular involvement has been devised. Each variable is assigned a grade of 1 (minimal involvement) to 4 (severe), with a maximal score of 16. Although the prognostic capability of this method is limited, the outcome of balloon valvuloplasty in patients with higher scores, particularly >12, is less satisfactory and involves a higher risk of complications than in patients with lower scores.[104] Therefore, echocardiographic analysis is an important part of the decision-making process prior to PBMV. Preprocedural TEE is also often performed to detect left atrial thrombi. Following PBMV, echocardiography can identify complications including MR and atrial septal defect.

MITRAL REGURGITATION

Although echocardiography is extremely accurate in the detection of mitral (and aortic) regurgitation, *quantitation* is more difficult (see Chap. 76). 2D imaging alone does not provide direct evidence of MR but usually reveals the etiology of the lesion. Thus, 2D echocardiography reveals thickened, restricted leaflets in rheumatic disease, vegetations in infective endocarditis, flail mitral leaflets with torn chordae, and redundant leaflets with abnormal coaptation in MV prolapse. 2D echocardiography can also detect LA and LV abnormalities associated with MR, such as myxoma, papillary muscle dysfunction, and dilated cardiomyopathy. Enlargement of these chambers offers indirect evidence of the severity of MR. In cases of chronic, severe MR, 2D echocardiography can also discern the presence of depressed LV function and decreased EF (see Chap. 76).

Doppler echocardiography is the primary method for the detection and evaluation of MR and reveals a disturbed flow jet in the LA during systole. Spectral Doppler recordings provide several indexes of severity, which are semiquantitative. Similarly, an increase in transmitral filling velocities reflects increased forward flow and suggests a large regurgitant volume. Measurements obtainable from the envelope

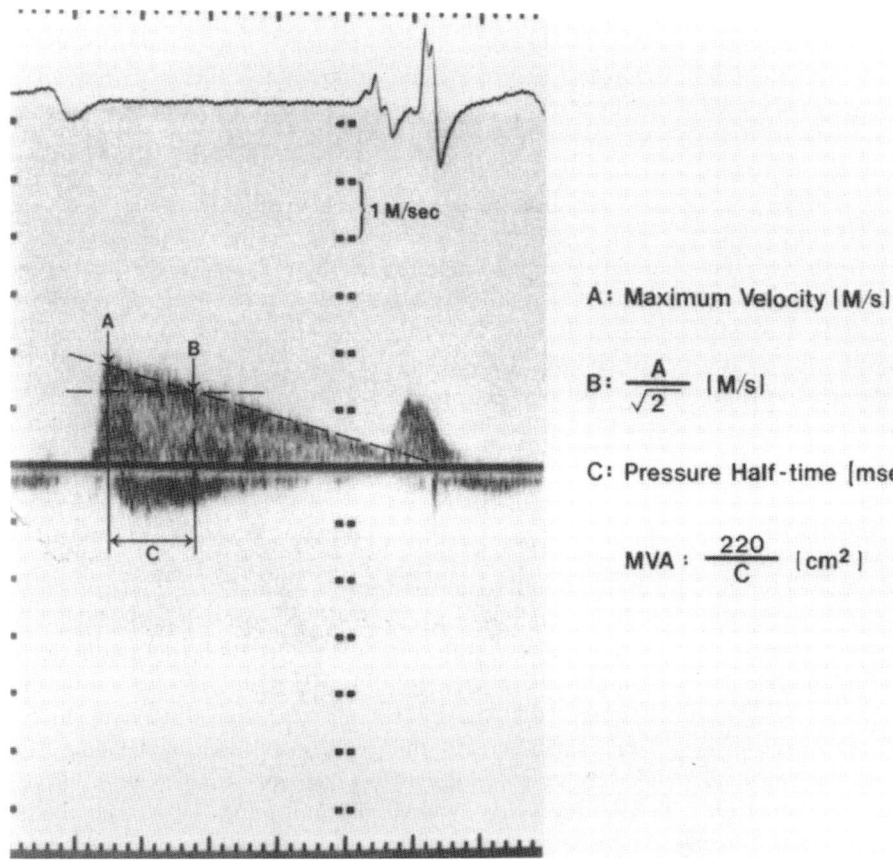

A: Maximum Velocity (M/s)

B: $\dfrac{A}{\sqrt{2}}$ (M/s)

C: Pressure Half-time (msec)

$$MVA: \dfrac{220}{C} \; (cm^2)$$

FIGURE 16–75. Pressure half-time method for calculation of mitral valve area (MVA). *Source: From Hagan AD, DeMaria AN. Clinical Applications of Two-Dimensional Echocardiography and Cardiac Doppler. Boston: Little, Brown; 1989. With permission.*

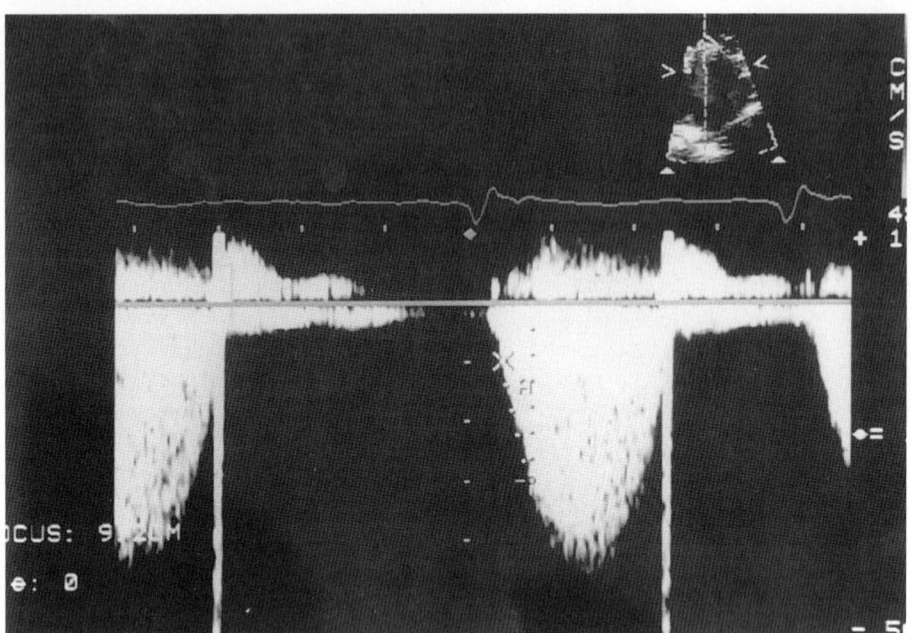

FIGURE 16–76. CW tracing of mitral regurgitation with calculation of dP/dt (apical transducer position). The time period between velocities of 1 and 3 m/sec is 0.07 sec; the calculated dP/dt is approximately 460 mmHg/sec. See text for details. CW, continuous wave.

of the CW Doppler recording of the MR jet include a slow rate of acceleration, indicative of a diminished LV dP/dt (Fig. 16–76).

As in the case of AR, volumetric calculations of LV inflow and outflow by combined pulsed Doppler and 2D echocardiographic imaging techniques can be used to derive measurements of regurgitant volume. In the case of MR, transmitral filling represents both systemic and regurgitant volume, whereas aortic outflow represents only systemic flow. Therefore, mitral filling should exceed LV ejection, and the difference will be regurgitant volume.

The most commonly applied method for the evaluation of MR is assessment of jet size by CFD. Imaging of the LA in systole reveals a turbulent, mosaic jet of varying direction, size, and configuration (Fig. 16–77A and B). Previous studies have demonstrated that a MR jet whose absolute area exceeds 8 cm^2 or fills at least 40 percent of the area of the LA is predictive of finding 3+ to 4+ MR by LV angiography. The lack of correlation between CFD jet area and regurgitant volume is attributable to the additional variables that influence the distribution of the flow disturbance, such as the pressure gradient and the volume and compliance of the LA, as well as technical limitations. The Coanda effect is of particular significance in regard to MR, because jets into the LA are often eccentric (for example, in cases of MV prolapse and torn chordae tendineae). Eccentric MR jets are drawn along the walls of the LA, resulting in cross-sectional jet areas that are smaller than centrally directed flow disturbances of comparable regurgitant volume (see Fig. 16–77 and Fig. 16–78). This effect can lead to underestimation of the severity of regurgitation.

TEE is also useful for the assessment of MR, because the close proximity of the probe and its higher-frequency interrogating beam permit imaging of regurgitant jets in greater detail than with TTE. Eccentric jets and mitral valvular anatomy are well visualized (see Fig. 16–78A and B), and rightward bulging of the interatrial septum with severe MR is also sometimes apparent. Because the regurgitant jets often appear larger with TEE than with TTE, avoid overestima-

tion of MR severity. TEE often yields Doppler interrogation of the pulmonary veins that is superior to that of TTE, and several recent studies have shown that systolic reversal of flow into the pulmonary veins is a reliable sign of severe MR[74] (Fig. 16–79).

Another color Doppler method of flow quantitation involves measurement of the zone of flow convergence proximal to the regurgitant orifice (or the *proximal isovelocity surface area* [PISA]). The mechanism for this phenomenon is derived from the hydrodynamic principle that blood flow accelerates before passing through a small orifice under high pressure. If this increase in flow velocity exceeds the Nyquist limit, color aliasing occurs and the velocity aliasing border is equal to the Nyquist limit (see Fig. 16–31, and Fig. 16–80A and B). If one assumes that the aliasing border conforms to the geometry of a hemisphere around the mitral orifice, the instantaneous flow rate of blood through the orifice can be calculated as:

$$\text{Flow} = 2\pi r^2 \, (V_r)$$

where r is the radius of the hemisphere shell (distance from alias border to orifice) and V_r is the velocity of blood at distance r (the Nyquist limit velocity). If the maximal calculated flow rate is divided by the peak regurgitant flow velocity (measured with CW Doppler), the regurgitant orifice area is then obtained.[105] The product of regurgitant orifice area and integrated velocity of the MR jet by CW yields regurgitant volume. The PISA method avoids the variables associated with jet size and the assumptions and technical limitations of volumetric calculations. Numerous studies have shown a correlation between both flow rate and regurgitant orifice area calculated by PISA and the severity of MR assessed by standard methods.[105] In addition, flow convergence calculations have been applied to other valvular lesions, including AR and MS (Fig. 16–81), VSD, and prosthetic heart valves. The proximal flow convergence assumes a hemispheric geometry for the PISA signal and that the plane of the mitral leaflets is flat, two sources of potential error.[106]

[ ] MITRAL VALVE PROLAPSE

The echocardiographic findings in mitral valve prolapse (MVP) have been controversial.[107] The classic echocardiographic findings in overt MVP consists of mid- to late-systolic bulging of one or both mitral leaflets across the plane of the MV annulus into the LA (Fig. 16–82A to C). The leaflets are often observed to be structurally abnormal, with thickening, elongation, and hooding. Mid- to late-systolic MR is sometimes present, often eccentric, and generally directed away from the prolapsing leaflet. The chordae tendineae may be thickened and elongated, the AO may be dilated, and the TV leaflets may prolapse as well. LV function is usually normal, but the LA and LV may be enlarged if MR is significant. The greater temporal resolution of M-mode over 2D

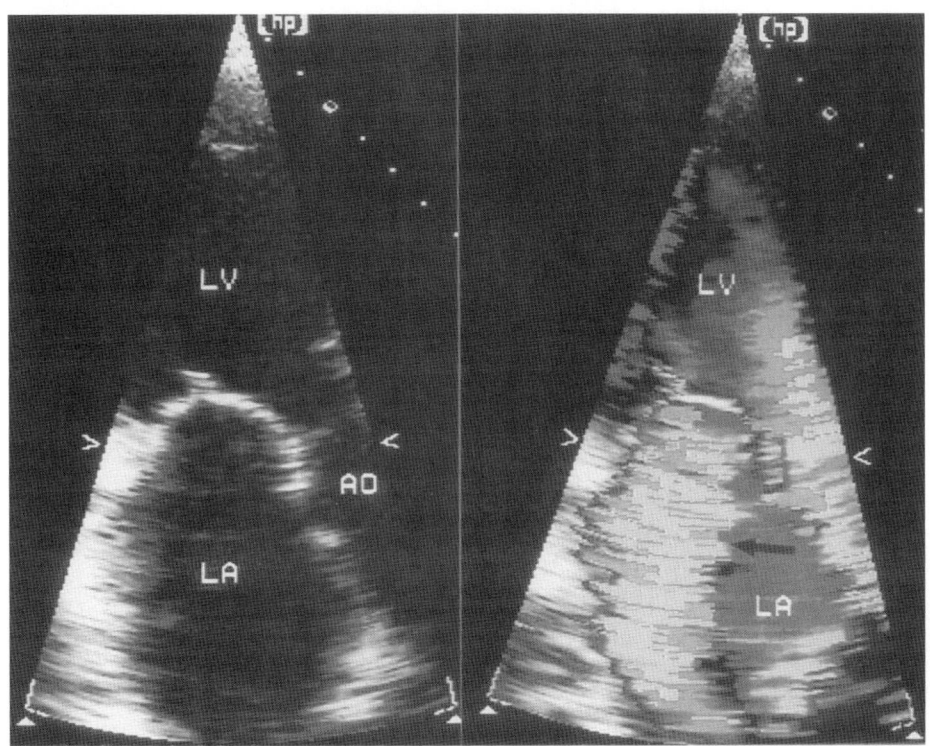

A

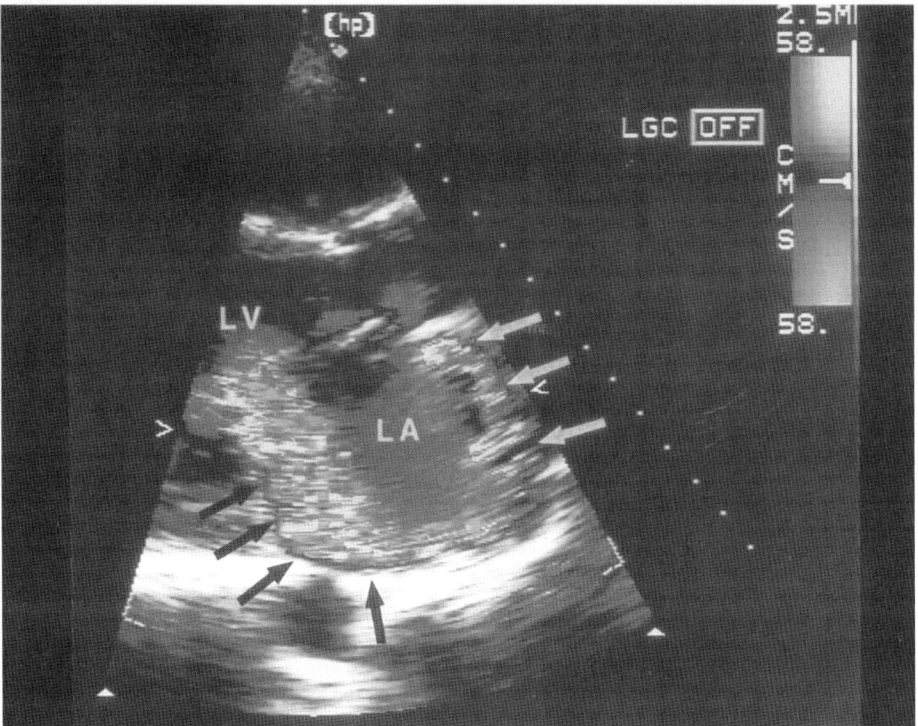

B

FIGURE 16–77. A. Mitral regurgitation. Left: apical three-chamber plane. Right: same plane with color Doppler imaging. A large jet of mitral regurgitation (*arrow*) is present. **B.** Parasternal long-axis view from a patient with angiographically proved severe mitral regurgitation. The color Doppler jet in this case is directed posteriorly and eccentric (*black arrows*). The jet hugs the wall of the LA and wraps around all the way to the aortic root (*white arrows*). Ao, aorta; LA, left atrium; LV, left ventricle.

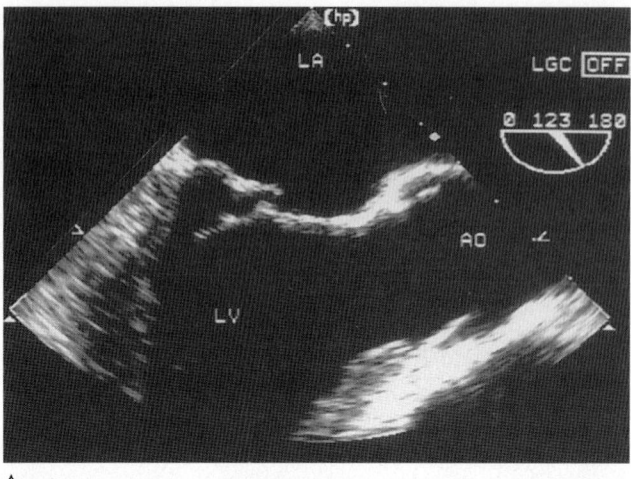

A

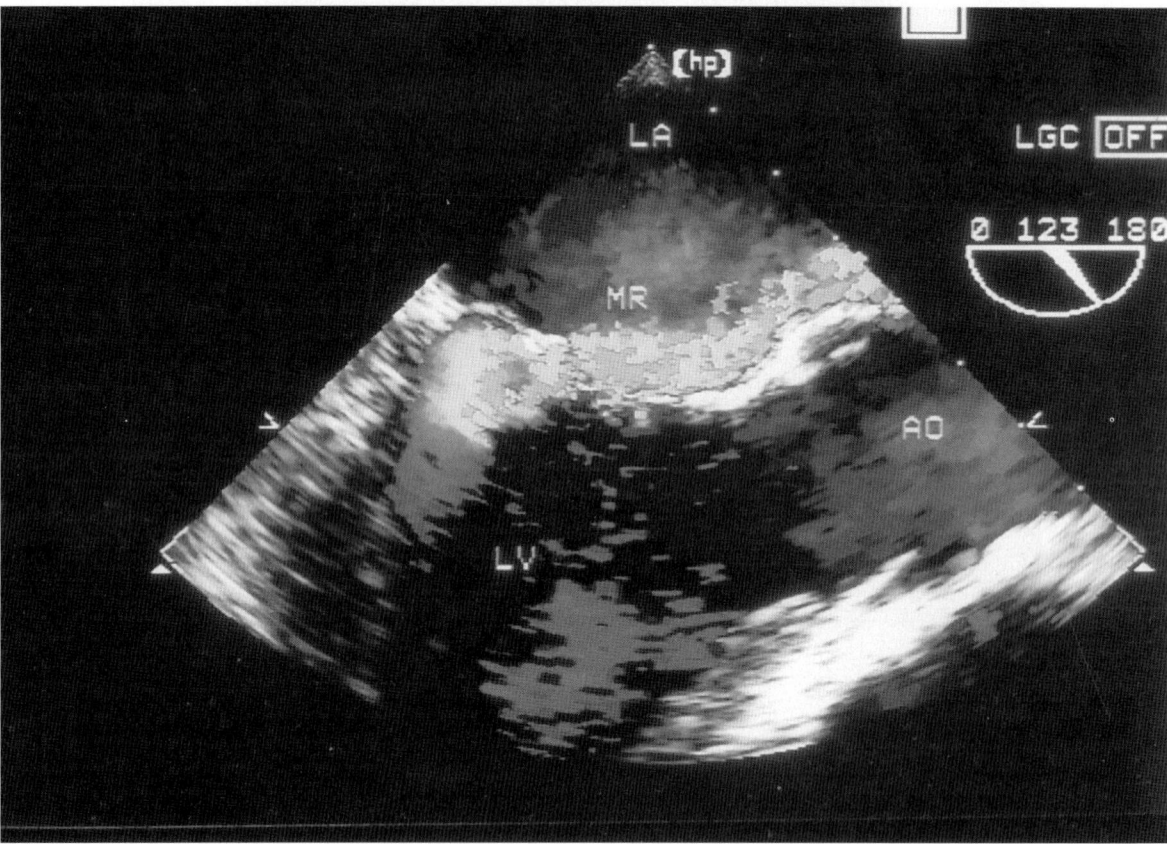

B

FIGURE 16–78. TEE images from a case of severe MR secondary to a flail posterior mitral valve leaflet. **A.** abnormal coaptation and prolapse of the posterior leaflet is apparent. **B.** Color Doppler imaging demonstrates an eccentric jet of MR directed anteriorly toward the aortic root (*AO*). LA, left atrium; LV, left ventricle; MR, mitral regurgitation.

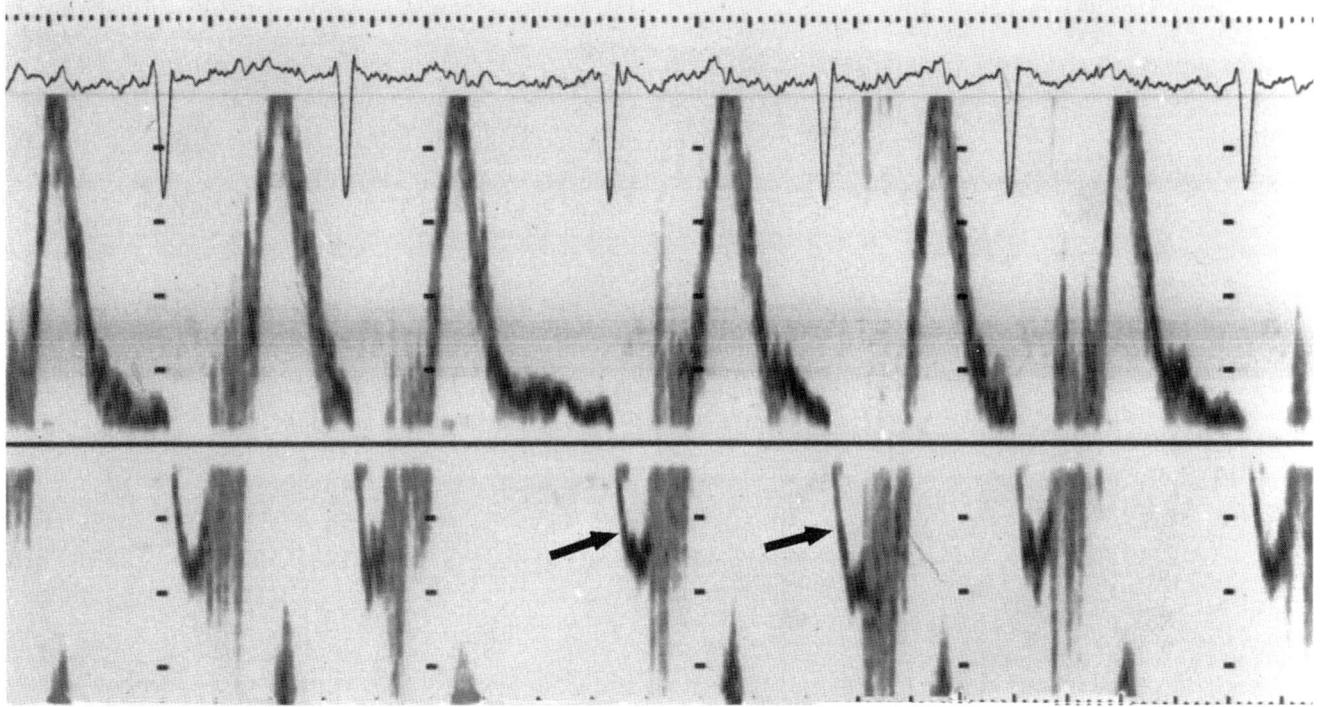

FIGURE 16–79. Pulmonary venous pulsed-wave Doppler in severe mitral regurgitation. Systolic flow reversal (i.e., systolic flow into the pulmonary vein) is present (*arrows*).

echocardiography often yields striking evidence of abrupt midsystolic posterosuperior motion of the MV leaflets in prolapse patients (see Fig. 16–82C). Although such M-mode findings, which resemble a question mark on its side, are specific for MV prolapse, patients with classic MVP occasionally may demonstrate diagnostic findings only with 2D imaging (see Chap. 76).

Although the diagnosis of classic, fully expressed MVP is straightforward by echocardiography, identification of mild prolapse is more difficult, and no absolute diagnostic criteria currently exist. For prolapse to be present, the MV leaflets must cross the plane of the MV annulus after initial systolic coaptation. The MV annulus is not flat but rather saddle-shaped, reaches its nadir in the apical four-chamber view, and even normally coapting MV leaflets may appear to prolapse in this projection. Therefore, current criteria require that MVP be diagnosed only when one or both of the mitral leaflets clearly bulge past the plane of the MV annulus in the parasternal long-axis view. Unfortunately, the degree to which the mitral leaflets must break the plane of the annulus is controversial. The greater the portion of the MV leaflets entering the LA, the more likely the diagnosis: A peak distance behind the annulus of 2 mm almost invariably establishes the presence of MVP. The diagnosis of mild MVP may be assisted by examination of the structure of the leaflets and chordae tendineae, because it has been demonstrated that patients with redundant or thickening valve leaflets (>5 mm in midleaflet) are at increased risk of complications, including severe MR and infective endocarditis (see Chap. 88).

TORN CHORDAE TENDINEAE

Rupture of chordae tendineae may occur spontaneously or in conjunction with MVP or endocarditis. This can result in a flail mitral leaflet and severe MR. Although TTE often detects these lesions, TEE is especially sensitive and accurate and often demonstrates free motion of the leaflet and ruptured chord into the LA even when TTE is equivocal (Fig. 16–83A and B). As with MVP, the MR jet in this condition is usually eccentric and directed away from the affected leaflet, often *hugging* the adjacent left atrial wall (Coanda effect). Therefore, the jet's cross-sectional area may be misleadingly small. The findings of mitral valvular anatomy on TEE may also be helpful in predicting the feasibility and success of valve repair surgery.

In the setting of ischemic heart disease, both LV enlargement and papillary muscle dysfunction (from infarction or transient ischemia) may cause MR. Both the MR and the contractile abnormality responsible for it are usually well visualized by 2D echocardiography. In rare cases, papillary muscle rupture (partial or complete) occurs in the postinfarction period.

MITRAL ANNULAR CALCIFICATION

The finding of mitral annular calcification (MAC) is fairly common in adults and occurs more frequently with advancing age. Although ultrasound cannot discern histology, calcification typically appears as thickened, extremely high-intensity (*bright*) signals (Fig. 16–84). The posterior portion of the mitral annulus is affected much more commonly and calcification often extends into the posterior mitral leaflet, sometimes restricting its motion. The abnormality, best visualized in the parasternal long- and short-axis views, is seen as a bright calcific density at the junction of the posterior mitral leaflet and the annulus. In the short-axis view, the posterior band of calcification often appears crescentic.

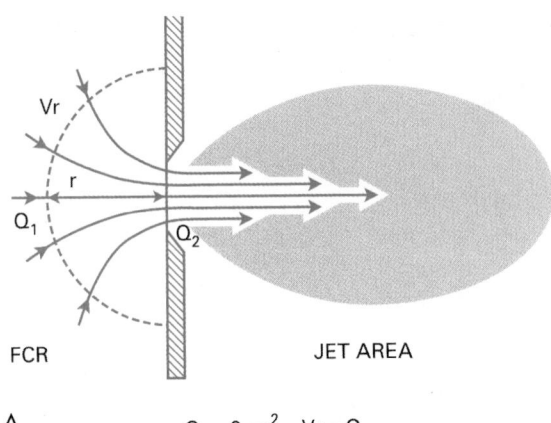

$$Q_1 = 2\,\pi r^2 \cdot Vr = Q_2$$

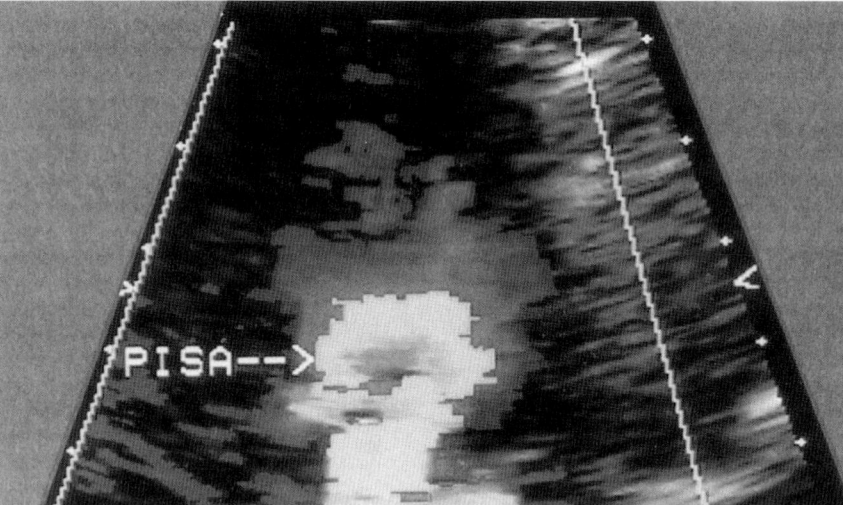

FIGURE 16–80. A. Proximal isovelocity surface area (*PISA*). See text for details. **B.** Magnified view (from the apical four-chamber plane) of mitral regurgitation (*MR*) demonstrating color Doppler flow convergence proximal to the mitral valve (PISA). FCR, flow convergence region; Q, flow; r, radius of isovelocity hemisphere; Vr, velocity of flow at distance r from the orifice. *Source: A, from Bargiggia GS, Tronconi L, Sahn DJ, et al. A new method for quantitation of mitral regurgitation based on color flow Doppler imaging of flow convergence proximal to regurgitant orifice. Circulation 1991;84:1481–1489. With permission.*

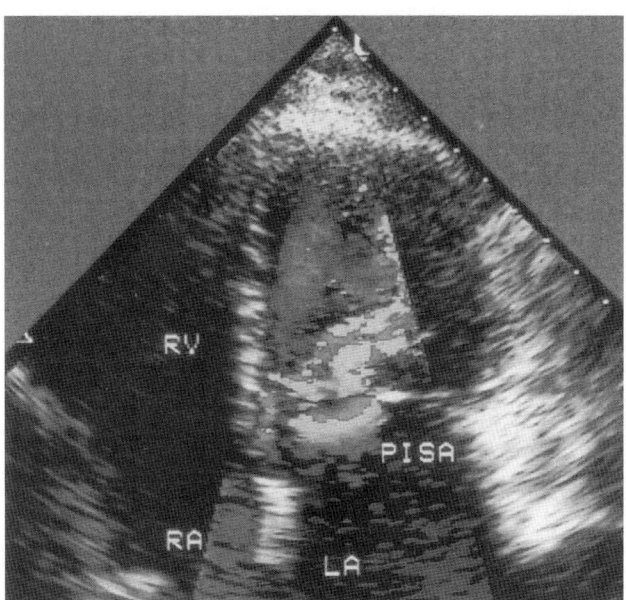

FIGURE 16–81. Apical four-chamber plane in mitral stenosis. Color flow imaging in the mitral valve region shows flow convergence (*PISA*) proximal to the valve during diastole. LA, left atrium; RA, right atrium; RV, right ventricle.

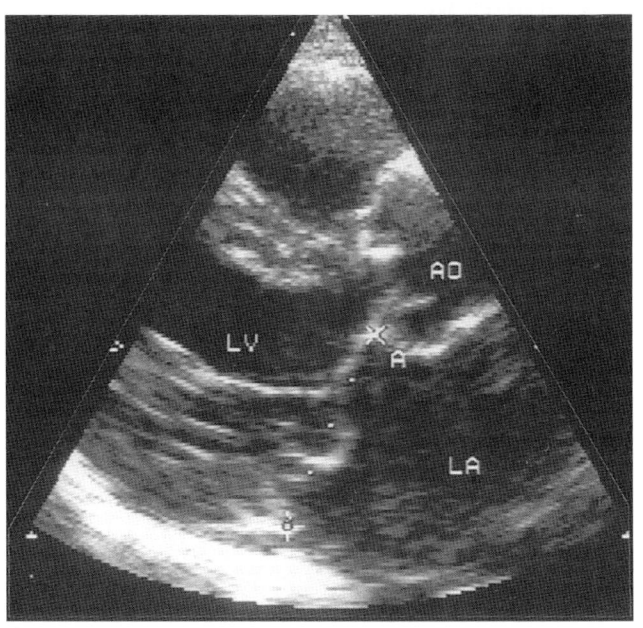

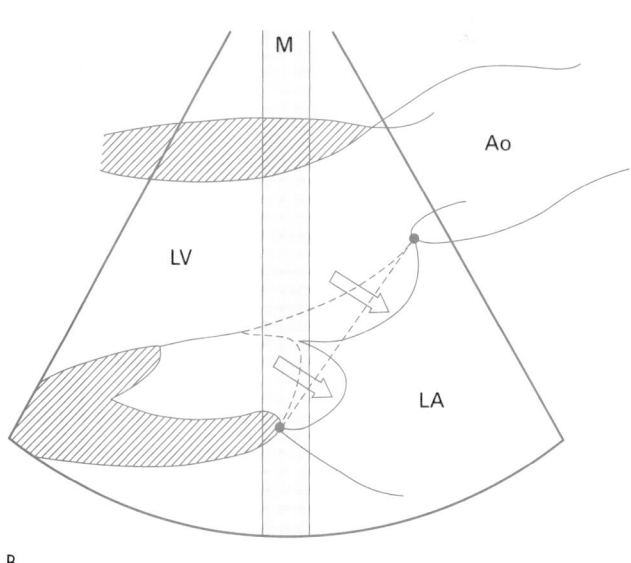

A   B

FIGURE 16–82. A. Parasternal long-axis plane through the mitral valve in late systole. The plane of the mitral annulus (*A*) is drawn in a dotted line. The posterior mitral leaflet prolapses past the level of the annulus into the LA. **B.** Diagram of true mitral valve prolapse. The mitral leaflets clearly prolapse (*arrows*) posterior to the plane of the mitral annulus (*straight dotted line*). **C.** M-mode image through the plane of the mitral valve demonstrating posterior prolapse of the leaflets during systole (*arrow*). A, atrial component; Ao, aorta; LA, left atrium; LV, left ventricle; E, early diastolic filling; M, M-mode imaging beam. *Source: From Devereux RB, Kramer-Fox R, Kligfield P. Mitral valve prolapse: causes, clinical manifestations, and management. Ann Intern Med 1989;111:305–317. With permission.* (*continued*)

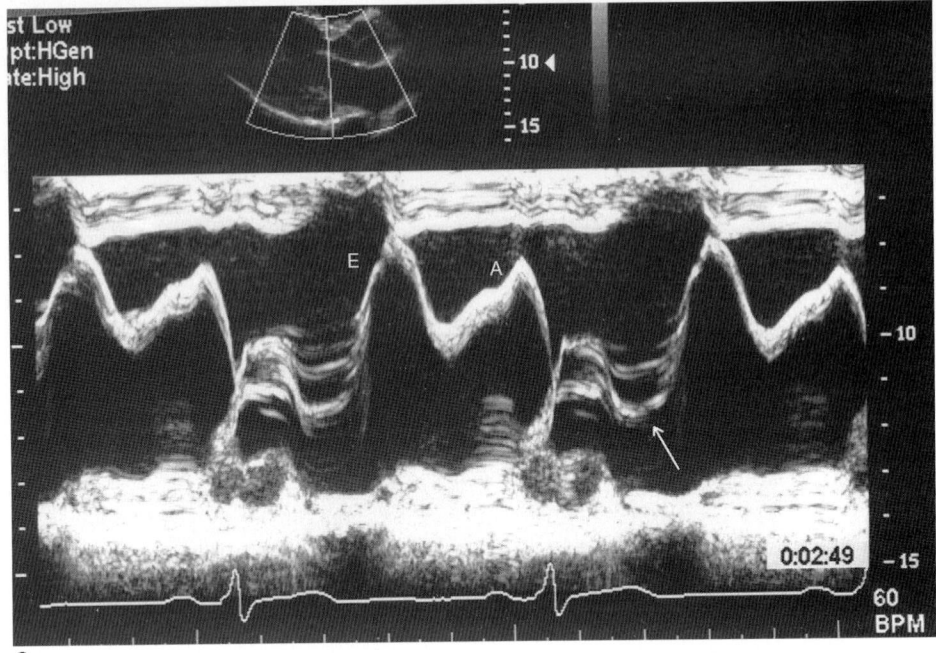

C

FIGURE 16–82. (*continued*)

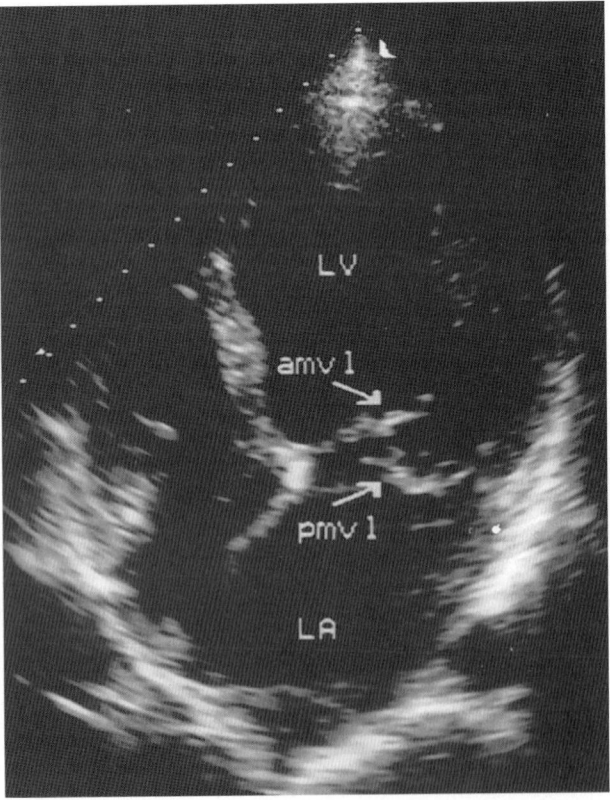

A

FIGURE 16–83. A. Apical four-chamber image of a flail posterior mitral valve leaflet (PMVL). The mitral valve is thickened and myxomatous. **B.** Transesophageal echocardiography image (transverse four-chamber plane) of a flail posterior mitral valve leaflet (*arrows*) secondary to ruptured chordae. aMVL, anterior mitral valve leaflet; LA, left atrium; RA, right atrium; LV, left ventricle.

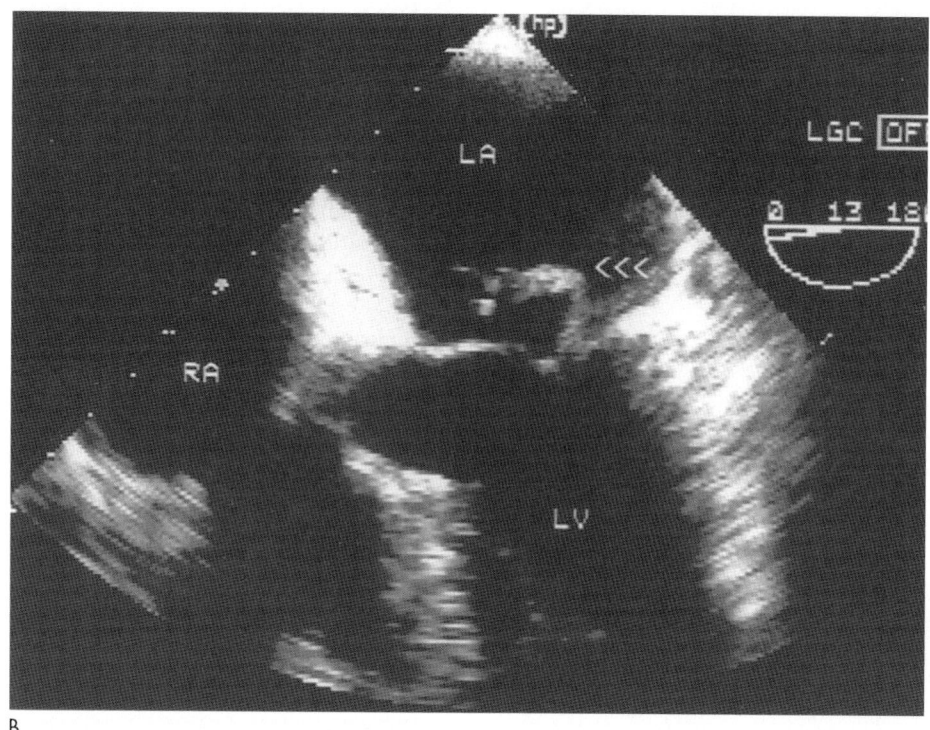

B

FIGURE 16–83. (*continued*)

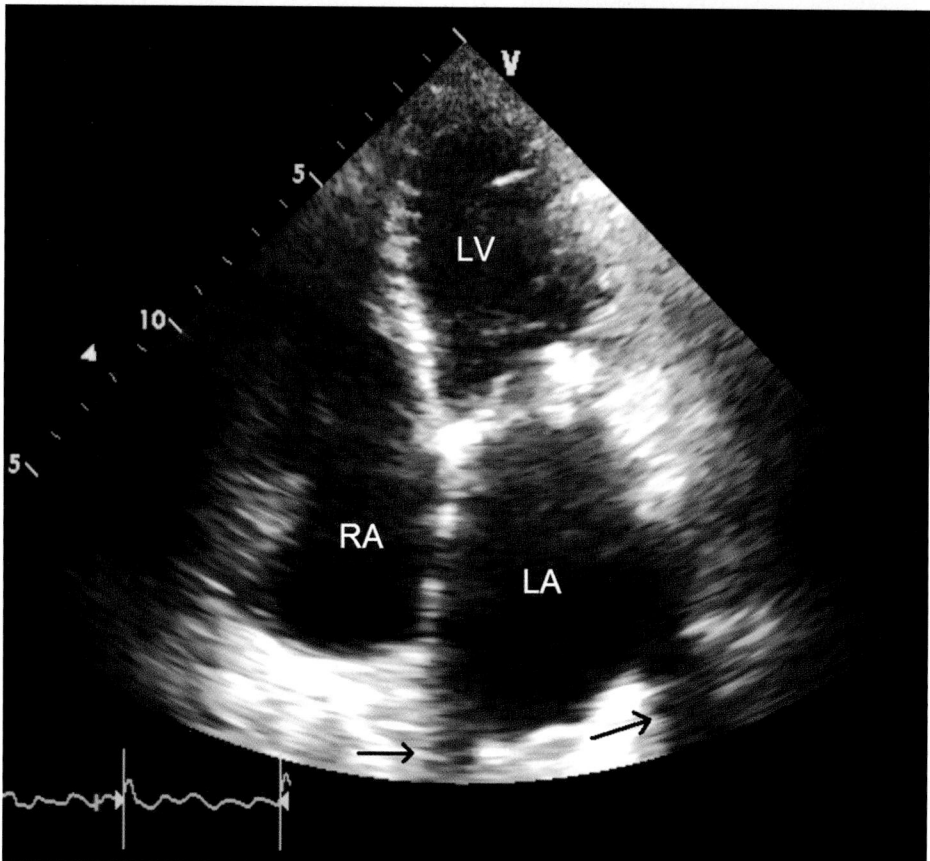

FIGURE 16–84. Apical 4-chamber plane demonstrating calcification of the mitral annulus with ultrasonic shadowing posteriorly (*black arrows*). LA, left atrium; LV, left ventricle; RA, right atrium.

RIGHT-SIDED VALVULAR DISEASE AND PULMONARY HYPERTENSION

【 】 PULMONIC VALVE

Major structural abnormalities of the PV are relatively rare. *Pulmonic stenosis* (PS) is usually congenital in origin and resembles congenital AS in many respects. The stenotic valve does not open fully and exhibits characteristic thickening and systolic doming on 2D imaging (Fig. 16–85). M-mode recordings of the PV often show a large a wave, since RV diastolic pressure is often so high and PA pressure so low that the atrial *kick* is sufficient to open the PV. Doppler interrogation reveals turbulent flow distal to the valve, and CW measurements can be used to calculate gradients and valve areas with the Bernoulli and continuity equations much as in AS.

Although severe *pulmonic regurgitation* (PR) is rare, mild PR is common and appears as a flame-shaped flow disturbance in the *RV outflow tract* (RVOT) in diastole. Many individuals have trivial PR on color Doppler examination; this is a physiologic, normal variant (Fig. 16–86). Hemodynamically significant PR is uncommon; when present, it is usually caused by CHD, valvular tumors, endocarditis, or carcinoid heart disease (see Chap. 78). The echocardiographic grading of PR is semiquantitative, based on the density of the CW envelope, area of the color Doppler jet, and width of the jet at the valve. The PR pressure half-time by CW Doppler may be shorter with more severe PR. Measurements derived from the CW Doppler recording also provide estimates of PA end-diastolic pressure (PAEDP) using the Bernoulli equation, as follows:

$$PAEDP = 4(PR\ end\text{-}diastolic\ velocity)^2 + central\ venous\ pressure\ (CVP)$$

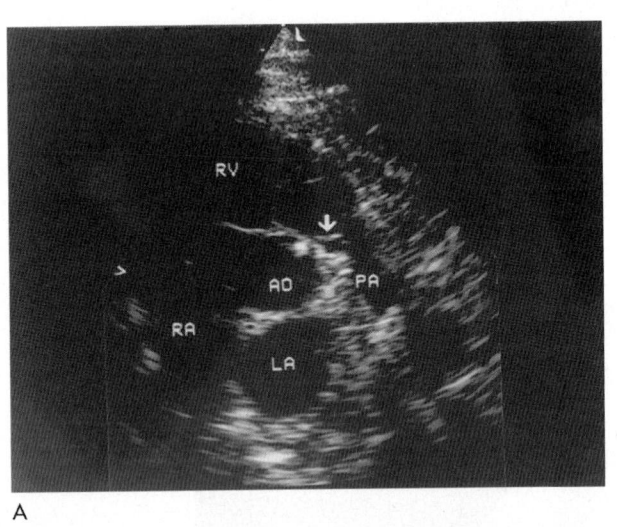

A

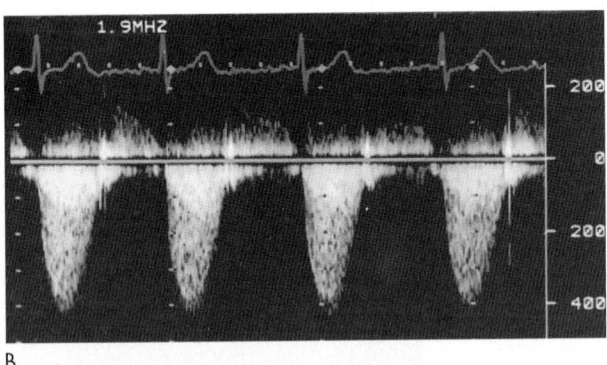

B

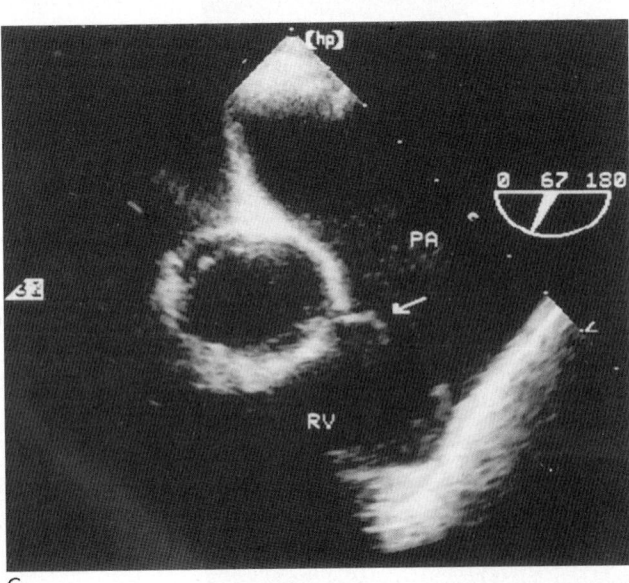

C

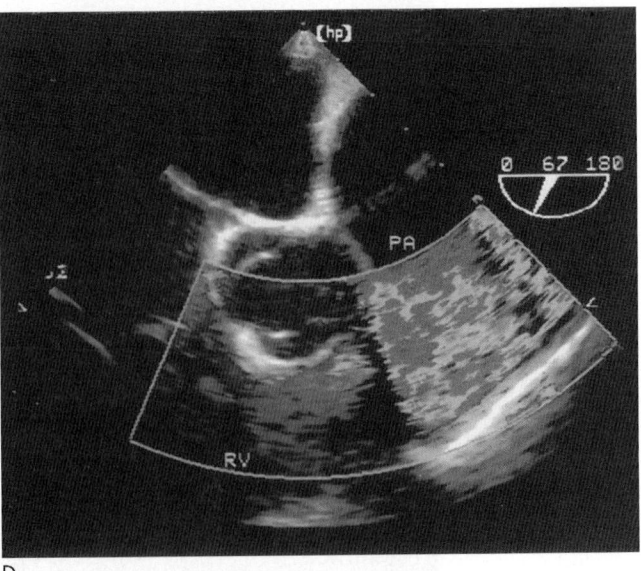

D

FIGURE 16–85. A. Pulmonic stenosis. The pulmonic valve leaflet is thickened and echo-reflective, and does not open completely during systole (*arrow*). **B.** Doppler interrogation reveals increased flow velocity (4 m/sec) through the valve orifice. **C.** Transesophageal image of pulmonic stenosis. The valve leaflets exhibit doming during systole (*arrow*). **D.** TEE image with color Doppler, showing high-velocity, turbulent flow in the main pulmonary artery. Ao, aorta; LA, left atrium; PA, pulmonary artery; RA, right atrium; RV, right ventricle; TEE, transesophageal echocardiography.

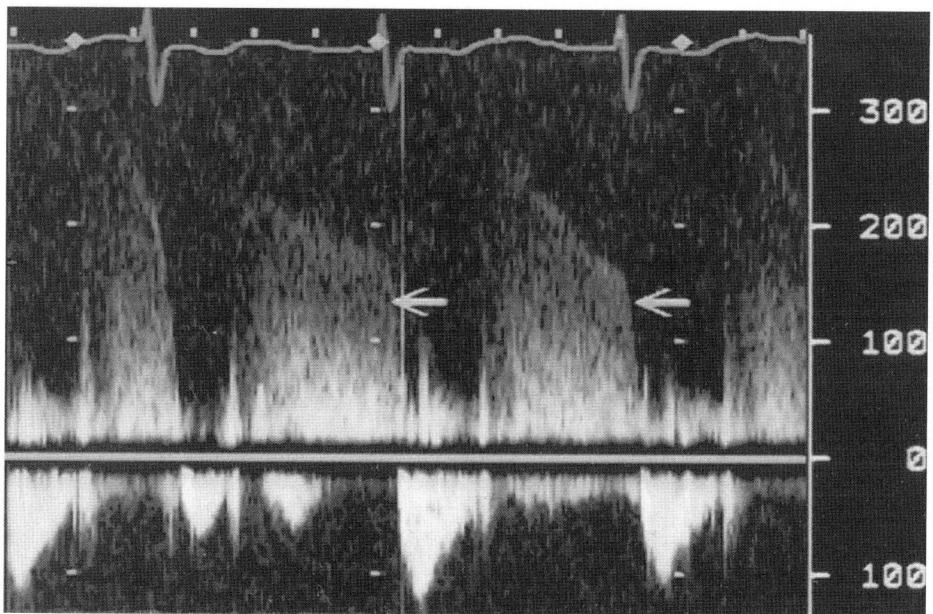

FIGURE 16–86. Continuous-wave Doppler tracing through the right ventricular outflow tract and pulmonary artery (left parasternal transducer position). Mild pulmonic regurgitation is present (*arrows*).

TRICUSPID VALVE

Tricuspid stenosis (TS) is usually rheumatic in origin, and coexistent mitral and aortic valvular disease are the rule. Congenital or acquired (nonrheumatic) causes of TS are quite uncommon. On rare occasions TS may be caused by carcinoid heart disease or by leaflet adhesions to permanent pacemaker leads. Because of the large size of the tricuspid annulus, obstruction is unlikely to cause stenosis (see Chap. 78).

Regardless of the etiology, diastolic doming of the valve leaflets suggests stenosis. CW Doppler interrogation is also helpful and mimics the findings of MS (high diastolic velocity with prolonged pressure halftime). The pressure half-time equation used to calculate the area of the MV orifice cannot be applied directly to the TV.

Tricuspid regurgitation (TR) is much more common than TS, and, like PR, is present to a mild degree in many normal individuals (see Chap. 78). Hemodynamically significant TR may be caused by endocarditis, rheumatic valvular disease, pulmonary hypertension (PH), CHD (for example, the Ebstein anomaly), carcinoid heart disease, flail TR leaflet, and TV prolapse. Echocardiographic findings in TR generally mirror those found in MR. Although 2D imaging can detect abnormalities associated with TR—such as incomplete leaflet coaptation, flail leaflet, and right-sided chamber enlargement—the technique cannot accurately quantify TR severity. Doppler echocardiography, especially color-flow mapping, is the procedure of choice to detect TR and has reasonable accuracy for semiquantitation of severity.[108] The

severity of TR can be estimated by regurgitant jet area, ratio of jet area to right atrial area, and size of proximal flow convergence zones (see Fig. 16–31). Doppler interrogation of the hepatic vein is also useful, as systolic flow reversal within the vein suggests severe TR (Fig. 16–87). Peak RV (and PA) pressure can be estimated using measurements of peak TR velocity by CW Doppler (see The Bernoulli Equation above). If necessary, intravenous echocardiographic contrast agents can be injected to accentuate the TR Doppler jet and facilitate more accurate measurements of PA pressure.

RIGHT VENTRICULAR FUNCTION AND PULMONARY HYPERTENSION

RV enlargement and PH can be diagnosed and assessed by echocardiography (Fig. 16–88A and B). Because of the asymmetric and crescentic shape of the RV, accurate volume calculations are difficult. Nonetheless, 2D imaging provides useful general information regarding RV size and function. In the apical four-chamber view, the RV should appear somewhat smaller than the LV; therefore, RV enlargement can be diagnosed qualitatively when the RV's cross-sectional area exceeds that of the LV. RV chamber area measurements in the apical four-chamber imaging plane can also be compared to standardized normal values. Measurements of RV wall thickness can be performed from the parasternal or subcostal view; a value of 5 mm is generally accepted as the upper limit of normal. Systolic motion of the RV free wall and LV lateral wall toward the interventricular septum should be similar and roughly symmetric in normal situa-

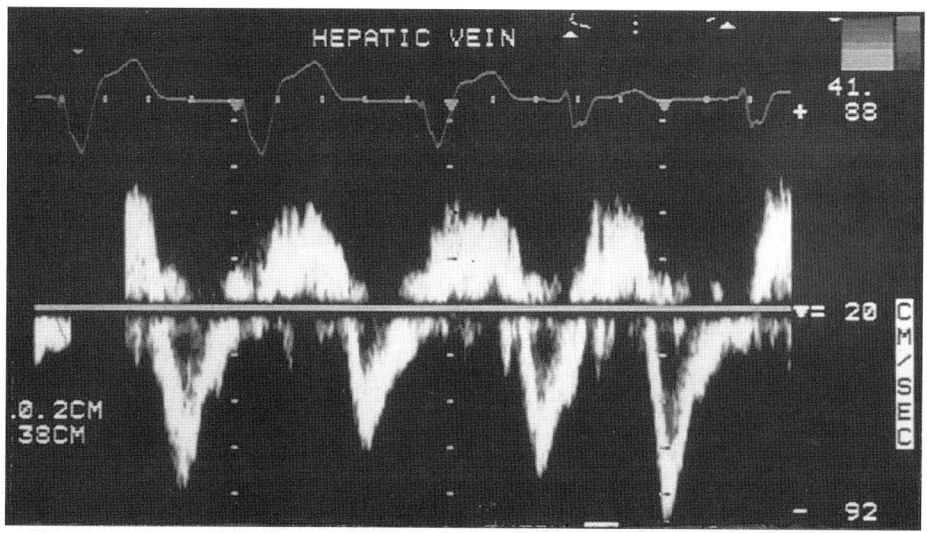

FIGURE 16–87. Pulsed-wave Doppler tracing of the hepatic vein in severe tricuspid regurgitation (TR) (subcostal transducer position). Systolic flow reversal into the hepatic vein is present.

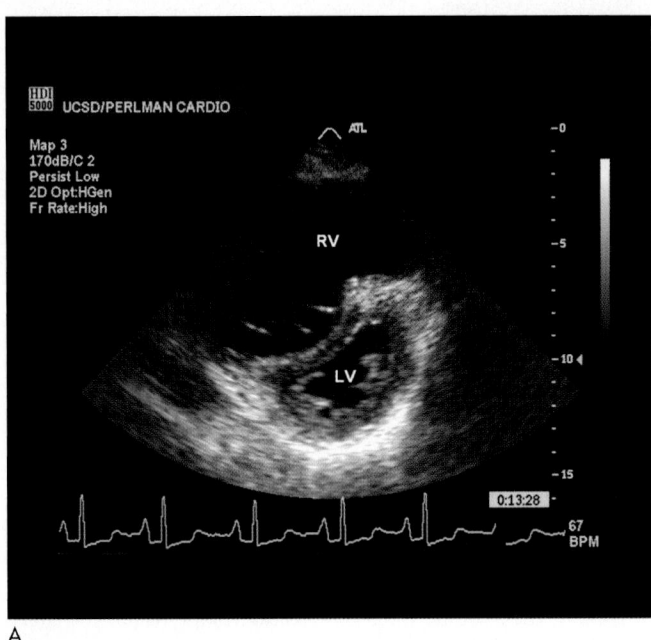

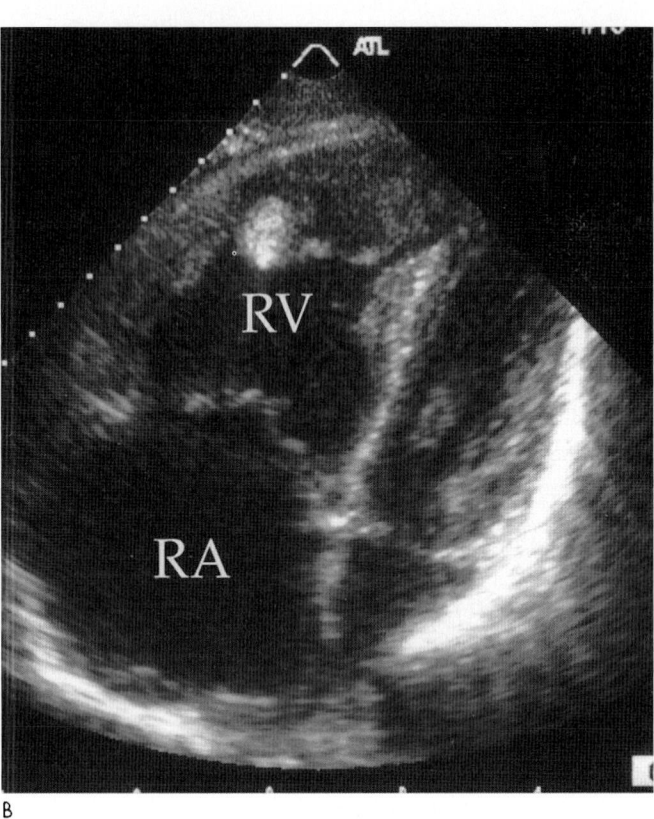

A

B

FIGURE 16–88. A. Parasternal short-axis view in severe pulmonary hypertension with marked enlargement of the right ventricle (*RV*). The left ventricle (*LV*) is small, and the interventricular septum is flattened. **B.** Apical four-chamber view in pulmonary hypertension. The right atrium (*RA*) and *RV* are much larger than the left-sided chambers.

tions. Asymmetric hypokinesis of the RV free wall indicates RV dysfunction. RV volume overload can lead to right ventricular hypertension (RVH), chamber enlargement, and, in advanced stages, depressed RV systolic function. TR can result from or cause RV overload, and the TR Doppler velocity allows estimation of the peak RV systolic pressure. The interventricular septum also becomes abnormal in RV overload and tends to flatten or even bulge toward the LV (Fig. 16–89). The pattern of septal movement can help distinguish between volume and pressure overload: In pure volume overload, the RV diastolic pressure may equal or exceed that of the LV, whereas the systolic pressure of the LV greatly exceeds that of the RV. Therefore, the interventricular septum flattens during diastole and returns to its normal curvature during systole. With RV pressure overload, however, the abnormally high RV pressures persist through the entire cardiac cycle and the interventricular septum remains deformed during both systole and diastole.

The hallmark of pulmonary hypertension by Doppler echocardiography is

a high-velocity TR jet in the absence of PS. Peak TR jet velocity can be converted to peak systolic PA pressure as follows:

$$4(\text{TR velocity})^2 + \text{CVP}$$

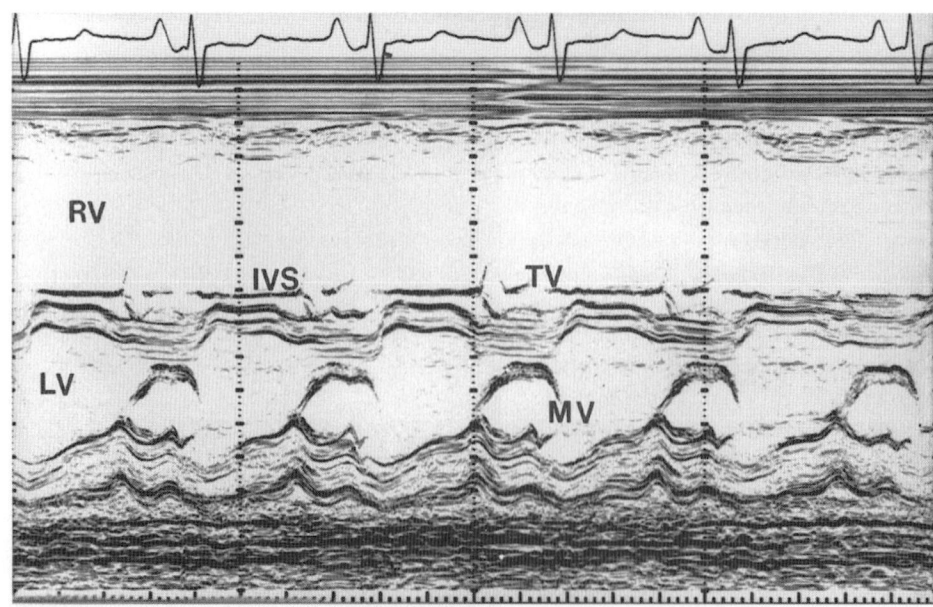

FIGURE 16–89. M-mode in severe pulmonary hypertension. The dimension of the right ventricle (*RV*) is larger than that of the left ventricle (*LV*). The interventricular septum (*IVS*) moves paradoxically (i.e., *toward* the mitral valve [*MV*] during diastole rather than away). *TV*, tricuspid valve.

where CVP = central venous pressure. In the setting of severe PH, the main PA and the inferior vena cava are often dilated. If RA pressure is elevated, the inferior vena cava (IVC) does not decrease in diameter with inspiration as normally expected. M-mode examination of the pulmonic valve in PH may show a characteristic W-shaped motion of the valve leaflet during systole[109] (Fig. 16–90) and loss of the normal a dip caused by partial opening of the valve during atrial contraction. The loss of the a wave is probably caused by resulting inability of the atrial contraction to partially open the pulmonic valve. The midsystolic closure of the valve and partial reopening in late systole (sometimes called the *flying W*) may be caused by elevated pulmonary vascular resistance and oscillation of a pressure wavefront within the PA. Characteristic PWD abnormalities in PH include a decrease in the velocity-time integral of flow through the pulmonic valve (secondary to depressed RV stroke volume) and a shortening of the acceleration time (measured from beginning of flow through the pulmonic valve to peak velocity). The acceleration time (in milliseconds) can be used to estimate the mean PA pressure as:

$$\text{Mean PA pressure} = 80 - (\text{acceleration time}/2)$$

Interestingly, RVH and severe PH affect LV diastolic filling characteristics, possibly through septal effects (or by relative underfilling of the left ventricle). Diastolic *abnormal relaxation* patterns of LV filling (E < A) are common in severe PH, and LV diastolic function often returns to normal if PH is reversed. Pulmonic regurgitation is also common in the setting of PH and is usually well recorded by pulsed Doppler.

PROSTHETIC CARDIAC VALVES

Echocardiography is a critically important tool in the evaluation and serial followup of mechanical and bioprosthetic valves. Unfortunately, the increased echo reflectivity of prosthetic valves (especially the mechanical models) causes extensive distal shadowing and reverberations that markedly limit the utility of transthoracic 2D echocardiography (Fig. 16–91 and Fig. 16–92). TTE imaging may detect partial ring dehiscence manifest as abnormal *rocking* motion of a prosthetic valve. TTE may also identify reduced movement of the valve disks or leaflets and may occasionally visualize adherent thrombi, tissue ingrowth, and vegetations. Leaflet thickening, detachment, and flail motion also may be visualized for bioprosthetic valves.

Doppler interrogation is the cornerstone of the echocardiographic assessment of prosthetic valvular stenosis and regurgitation. Color-flow imaging can document the presence, direction, and size of the forward flow stream. CFD can also detect regurgitant flow

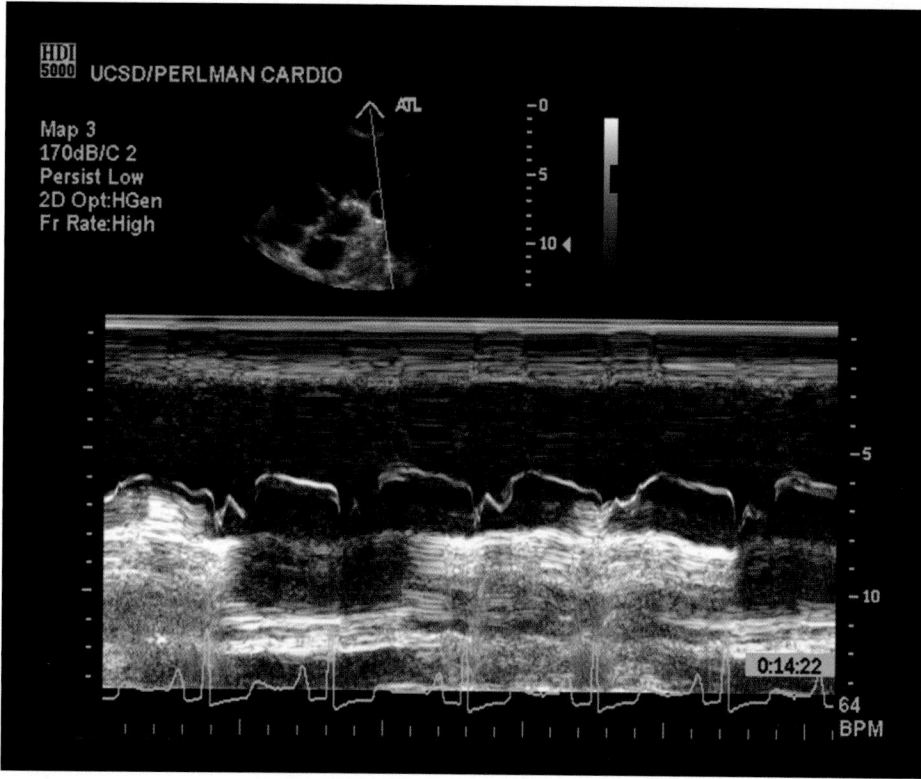

FIGURE 16–90. M-mode image of the pulmonic valve in severe pulmonary hypertension (parasternal transducer position). The A dip is absent, and a characteristic W-shaped motion of the leaflet is present during systole, indicating partial closure of the valve during midsystole followed by reopening prior to diastole.

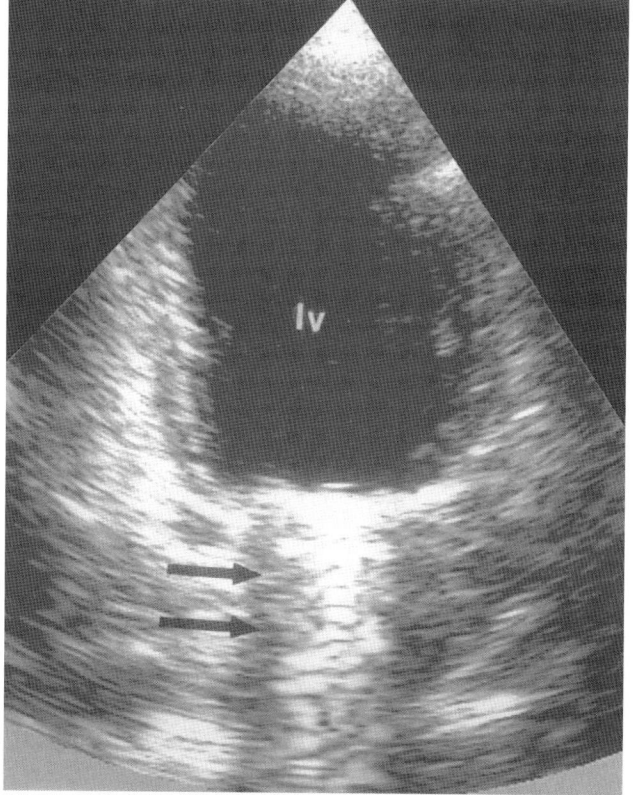

FIGURE 16–91. Apical two-chamber view of a mechanical prosthetic valve (mitral position) during systole. The LA is completely obscured by ultrasonic shadowing (*arrows*). LA, left atrium; LV, left ventricle.

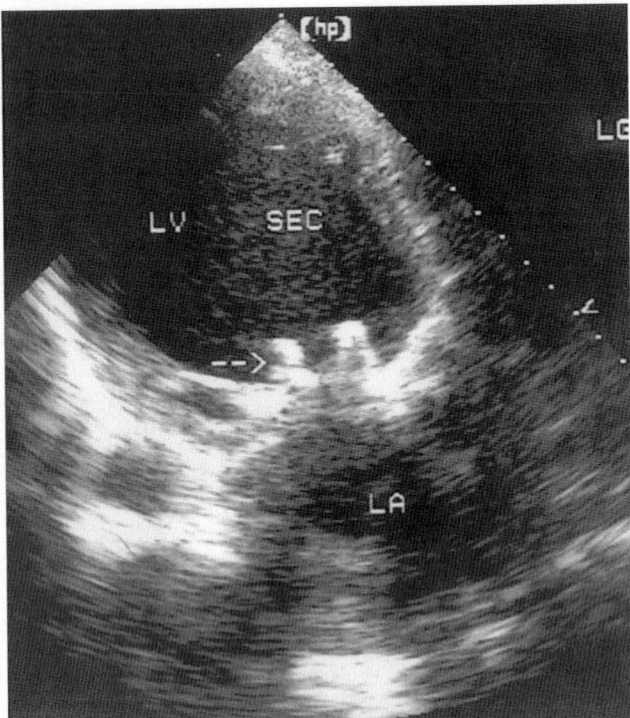

FIGURE 16–92. Apical view of a bioprosthetic valve (*arrow*) in the mitral position (two of the three prosthetic valve struts are apparent). Spontaneous echo contrast (*SEC*) is also present, secondary to systolic dysfunction and enlargement of the LV. LA, left atrium; LV, left ventricle.

jets; but like 2D imaging, it is limited by acoustic shadowing distal to the prosthesis. Doppler color jets caused by prosthetic AR can be readily visualized from the transthoracic apical view, but jets produced by prosthetic mitral and tricuspid regurgitation are often obscured. Therefore, although detection of prosthetic regurgitation by

transthoracic Doppler is usually feasible, quantitation is often difficult. A small flow signal shortly after valve closure may be observed frequently with prosthetic valves and is likely related to the blood caught behind the occluder as it closes.[110]

Doppler flow velocities and gradients through normal prosthetic valves vary depending on the type, position, and diameter of the prosthesis. The velocities and gradients across prosthetic valves are flow-dependent as well and therefore related to LV function. It is not surprising that a wide range of transvalvular gradients exists for normally functioning prosthetic valves. Nevertheless, *normal* ranges have been reported for various valve types and can be used as a guide to recognize malfunction. With AoV prostheses, peak systolic Doppler velocities may indicate higher systolic pressure gradients than those actually found during cardiac catheterization. This problem may be more prevalent with Starr-Edwards (ball-in-cage) and St. Jude (bileaflet tilting disk) valves than with Medtronic-Hall (single tilting disk) and bioprosthetic valves. Because of these variabilities, an echocardiographic examination is warranted following prosthetic valve implantation to establish its baseline Doppler characteristics. Mean transvalvular gradients calculated by Doppler correlate reasonably well with direct catheter measurements. TEE has dramatically changed the diagnostic approach to prosthetic valve dysfunction and is especially useful for assessing mitral prostheses, because it overcomes the problem of left atrial shadowing and reverberation (Fig. 16–93). TEE is extremely accurate in the detection of prosthetic regurgitation and impaired movement of the valve occluder, and it is the diagnostic procedure of choice in most cases of suspected prosthetic valve endocarditis. Small thrombi, tissue ingrowth, infected or sterile vegetations, and even sutures in the sewing ring can usually be visualized. The enhanced sensitivity of TEE requires operator experience and judgment. Nearly all mechanical prostheses *normally* exhibit a small amount of regurgitation, which should not be misinterpreted as pathologic. TEE may

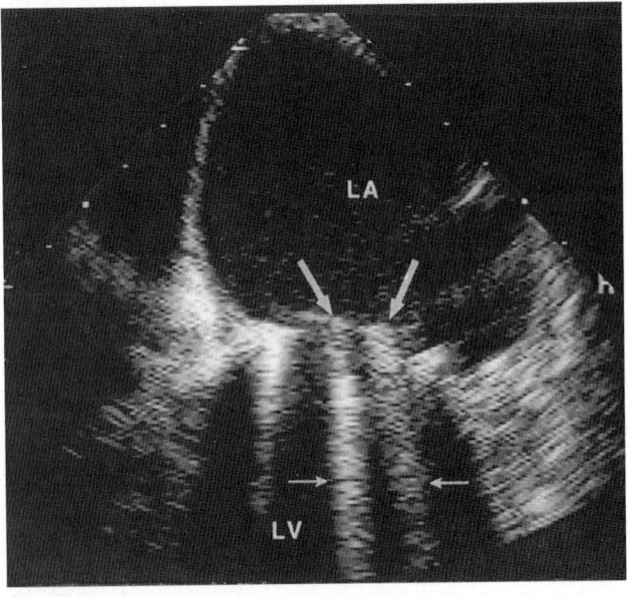

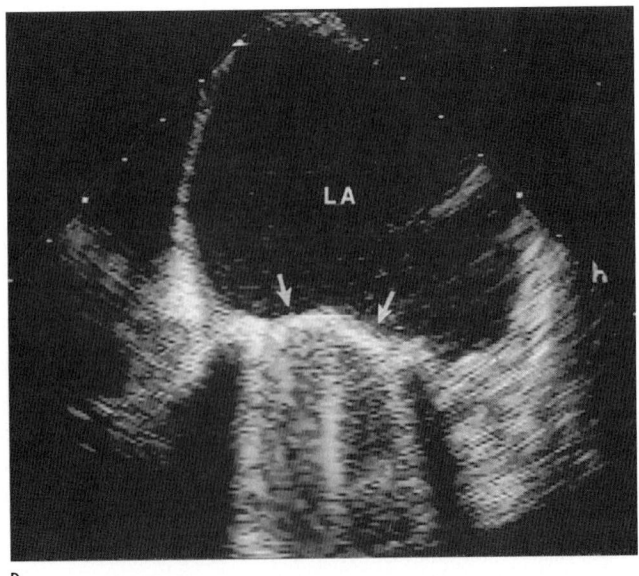

A   B

FIGURE 16–93. TEE images from a patient with a St. Jude prosthetic valve in the mitral position. **A.** Diastolic image. The two struts of the open valve are seen (*large arrows*) as well as their ultrasonic shadows (*small arrows*). **B.** Systolic image. The two prosthetic leaflets are closed (*arrows*) and cast a dense ultrasonic shadow, obscuring the *LV*. LA, left atrium; LV, left ventricle.

also visualize thin, fibrinous strands sometimes attached to prosthetic valves; these structures appear to be a potential source of cardiogenic embolization. The technique is quite accurate in the diagnosis of prosthetic valve thrombosis, a potentially fatal medical emergency, and can assist clinical decision making in this disorder.

INFECTIVE ENDOCARDITIS

Infective endocarditis remains an all too common illness, with a significant risk of morbidity and mortality (see Chap. 85). Traditionally, the diagnosis is based on either the cumulative results of blood cultures, physical examination, and laboratory findings or on pathologic proof of infected valvular vegetations at surgery or autopsy. In newer clinical algorithms,[111] however, echocardiography is important in the diagnosis of infective endocarditis, as well as detection of associated cardiac abnormalities and hemodynamic dysfunction, prognosis, and the need for surgery. Vegetations can be visualized noninvasively in many cases of endocarditis and have become the echocardiographic hallmark of this disorder.[112] Thus, even though TTE cannot exclude endocarditis, abnormal findings may strongly suggest the disorder, even in the presence of negative blood cultures. Strategies for diagnosis have been devised based on a number of criteria,[111] and definite echocardiographic vegetations are designated as a major criterion. Both TTE and TEE are valuable in the detection of perivalvular abscesses and prosthetic-valve endocarditis. Although there is considerable debate concerning the most accurate diagnostic criteria for endocarditis, echocardiography has become one of the most commonly used techniques for the evaluation of potentially affected patients. Echocardiography (both TTE and TEE) is also useful for evaluation of patients with systemic lupus erythematosus complicated by Libman-Sacks endocarditis.[113]

With 2D echocardiography, valvular vegetations typically appear as irregular, usually localized masses of varying echocardiographic density attached to valvular or perivalvular structures (Fig. 16–94 and Fig. 16–95) without significantly altering their mobility. The vegetations may be small or quite large and may attach directly to the valve leaflets or the supporting chordal apparatus.[112] Occasionally, vegetations may be attached to unusual structures, such as the atrial wall or the eustachian valve. Aggressive infections often cause perforation or distortion of the affected leaflet, leading to varying degrees of valvular regurgitation. This is distinctly different from most cases of nonbacterial thrombotic (marantic) endocarditis, where the valvular vegetations are usually nondestructive. In cases of infective endocarditis, the presence of vegetations by TTE increases the risk of heart failure, embolic events, and the ultimate necessity of valve replacement.[114] Up to 20 percent of patients with proved native-valve endocarditis have unremarkable examinations. The sensitivity of TTE in prosthetic valve endocarditis has been found to be even lower (approximately 60 percent) because of technical limitations in imaging.

TEE is significantly more sensitive than TTE for detection of infective vegetations and is extremely helpful for the diagnosis of perivalvular abscesses, mycotic diverticula, and prosthetic valve involvement. The technique is also useful for assessing valvular regurgitation, fistulas (Fig. 16–96), other hemodynamic complications of endocarditis, and risk of embolization.[115] Although a negative TEE examination cannot completely exclude infective endocarditis, it confers a relatively good prognosis in those cases where the diagnosis is eventually confirmed. The optimal use of TEE in suspected endocarditis remains controversial: Some authorities recommend routine TEE in all cases, but many do not. A reasonable approach may be to perform TTE as the first screening test in patients with suspected endocarditis. If the study is technically difficult or equivocal, or detects vegetations in patients at high risk for

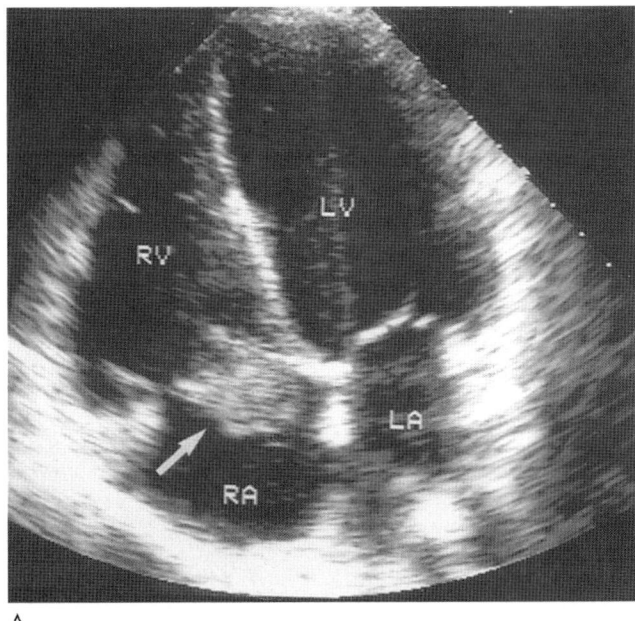

A

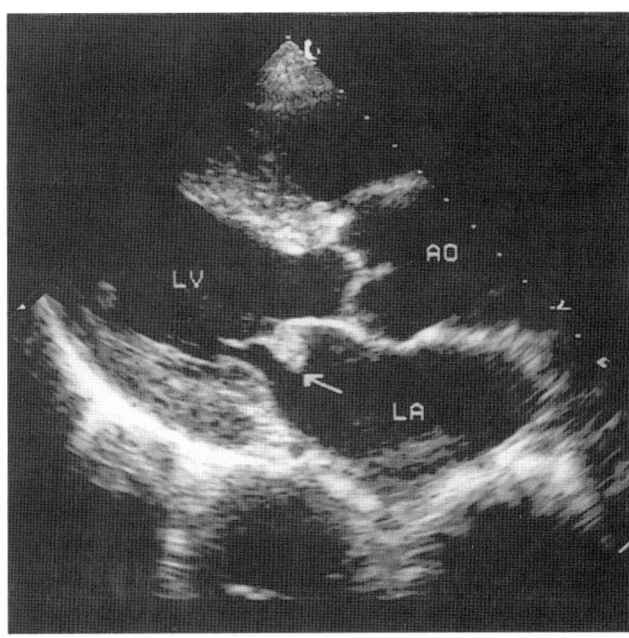

B

FIGURE 16–94. A. Apical four-chamber view demonstrating a large tricuspid valve vegetation (*arrow*). **B.** Parasternal long axis view demonstrating a vegetation (*arrow*) on the anterior valve leaflet; Ao, aorta; LA, left atrium; LV, left ventricle; RA, right atrium; RV, right ventricle.

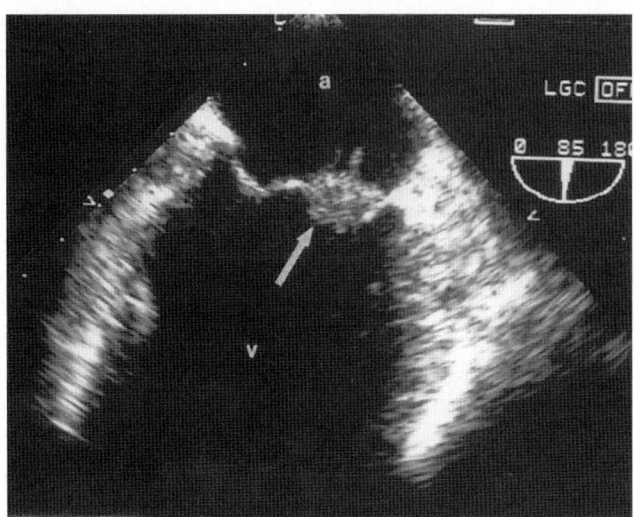

FIGURE 16–95. Longitudinal TEE view of a large mitral valve vegetation (*arrow*). *a*, left atrium; *v*, left ventricle. *Source: Courtesy of William D. Keen, Jr., MD.*

perivalvular complications or hemodynamic compromise, TEE should be performed. If TTE is unremarkable or detects vegetations in patients at low risk for complications, TEE may not be necessary.[73] In high-risk patients (i.e., with possible prosthetic valve involvement, CHD, or infection with especially virulent organisms), TEE is recommended even if TTE is normal.[73]

Echocardiographic evaluation of suspected endocarditis has some pitfalls. It may be quite difficult to detect active vegetations in patients with preexisting valvular abnormalities such as calcification, myxomatous change, rheumatic involvement, and healed vegetations. Overreliance on echocardiography may cause mistakes. Therefore, echocardiographic results should be integrated with other clinical information to diagnose this disorder accurately[116] (see Chap. 85).

ISCHEMIC HEART DISEASE

【 】 ECHOCARDIOGRAPHY IN CORONARY HEART DISEASE

Echocardiography has now become one of the most important techniques for the detection and quantitative assessment of myocardial ischemia and infarction. Cardiac ultrasound—because it is rapid, portable, noninvasive, and inexpensive—is especially well suited to the evaluation of ischemic heart disease. Although visualization of coronary artery structure and flow has been achieved by echocardiography, its application in ischemic heart disease continues to revolve primarily about the assessment of LV function. However, ongoing research with contrast

agents has shown that echocardiography can be used to assess regional myocardial perfusion.

Currently, the primary application of echocardiography in patients with coronary heart disease is based on the detection of the effects of myocardial ischemia and/or infarction on LV structure and function. Interruption of coronary flow or imposition of an oxygen demand that exceeds oxygen supply quickly leads to impaired systolic thickening and excursion of the affected myocardium. If flow is not restored, the affected myocardium may become akinetic or dyskinetic and eventually thinned and fibrotic. In addition, myocardial ischemia produces diastolic dysfunction, which may be detected by analysis of transmitral Doppler flow recordings or tissue Doppler tracings.

2D imaging is the primary technique for the examination of LV size, wall thickness, myocardial thickening, and regional wall motion, because it enables visualization of all LV wall segments. Standard echocardiographic approaches can be used to calculate LV diastolic and systolic volumes as well as EF. Digital echo analysis and 3D echocardiographic techniques can be used to enhance the accuracy of volume calculations and regional strain patterns.

The echocardiographic manifestations of CAD consist of one or more of the following:

- Reduction in systolic thickening
- Abnormal segmental wall motion during systole or diastole
- Alterations in the acoustic properties of the myocardium (usually termed *tissue characterization*)
- Diminished regional blood flow (as measured during the LV myocardial phase after intravenous echo contrast injection)

These abnormalities may be expressed as a disturbance in global LV size and function, an increase in LV volume, and a decrease in

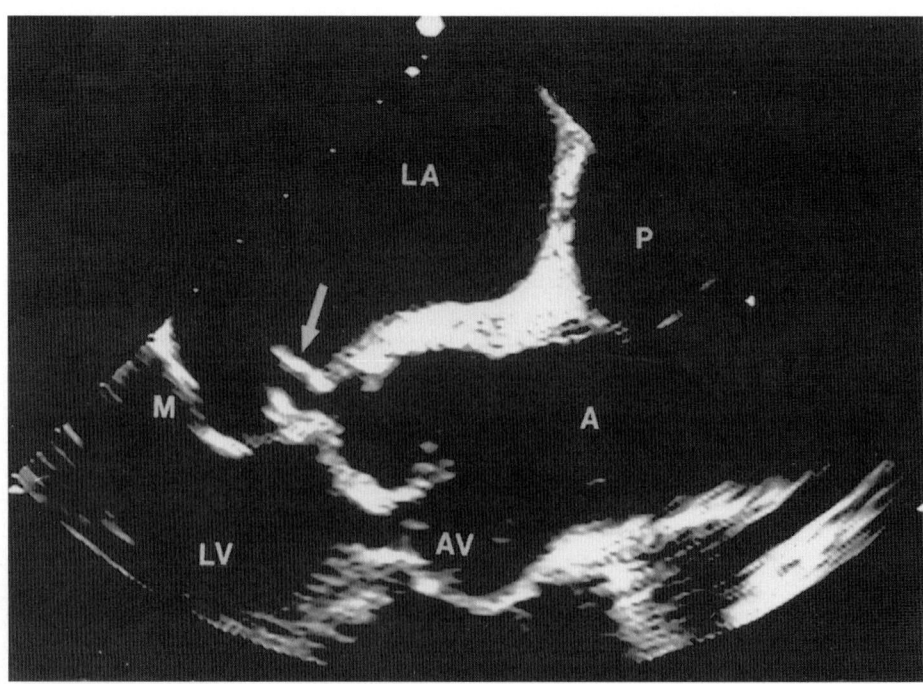

FIGURE 16–96. Longitudinal TEE image demonstrating a fistula between the aorta (*A*) and left atrium (*LA*) in a patient with endocarditis. AoV, aortic valve; LV, left ventricle; M, mitral valve; P, pulmonary artery. *Source: From Sobel J, Maisel AS, Tarazi R, Blanchard DG. Gonococcal endocarditis: assessment by transesophageal echocardiography. J Am Soc Echocardiogr 1997;10:367–370. With permission.*

LVEF calculated by standard approaches. In addition, using the standard tomographic planes, the LV can be divided into 16 wall segments according to the format recommended by the ASE (Fig. 16–97). A 17-segment format has been proposed more recently.[117,118] By grading the contraction of each of the various segments as hyperkinetic, normal, hypokinetic, akinetic, or dyskinetic, a semiquantitative wall motion score can be calculated as the mean numerical value for all segments. Wall motion scores of this kind have been used to assess prognosis in both acute myocardial infarction (AMI) and chronic CAD. When LV dysfunction is detected echocardiographically, the specific coronary artery responsible can often be inferred based on the dyssynergy region(s) (see Chaps. 59 and 60). The echocardiographic findings of akinesis with segmental myocardial thinning can also be used to distinguish CAD from dilated cardiomyopathy, which typically manifests global hypokinesis and decreased wall thickness. There is overlap in the echocardiographic findings; severe ischemic disease may cause global hypokinesis and nonischemic cardiomyopathy may sometimes cause heterogeneous dysfunction.

【 】 MYOCARDIAL INFARCTION AND POSTINFARCTION COMPLICATIONS

Cardiac ultrasound has achieved an important role in the evaluation of patients with AMI and is frequently used for diagnosis, quantitative functional assessment, risk stratification, and detection of complications (see Chap. 60). Echocardiography is valuable in *excluding* transmural infarctions, because these are almost always associated with regional akinesis or dyskinesis (Fig. 16–98 to Fig. 16–100).[119] Non-ST elevation infarctions are more difficult to diagnose with certainty. Echocardiography has been used to evaluate chest pain in the emergency department and appears to have a reasonable sensitivity and specificity in the diagnosis of MI. Myocardial contrast echocardiography and LV strain imaging (discussed below) may help detect these smaller infarctions. Also, a recent study showed that myocardial contrast echo improved early risk assessment in patients presenting with chest pain and nondiagnostic electrocardiograms.[120]

Echocardiography is now the most commonly utilized approach to assess the effects of MI on LV function. Ultrasound imaging studies of LV remodeling have demonstrated that infarct expansion occurs commonly with anterior infarctions, often beginning within the first 10 days, and conveys an adverse prognosis. Similarly, calculation of the wall motion score has identified a cohort of post-MI patients at markedly increased risk for in-hospital complications. This prognostic marker appears superior to conventional clinical criteria in predicting events.

Echocardiography is probably of greatest value in assessing complications associated with AMI. Most such complications are

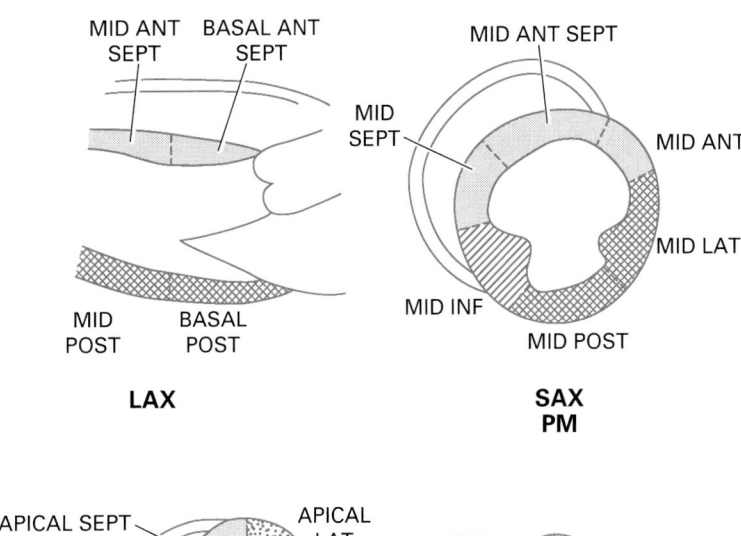

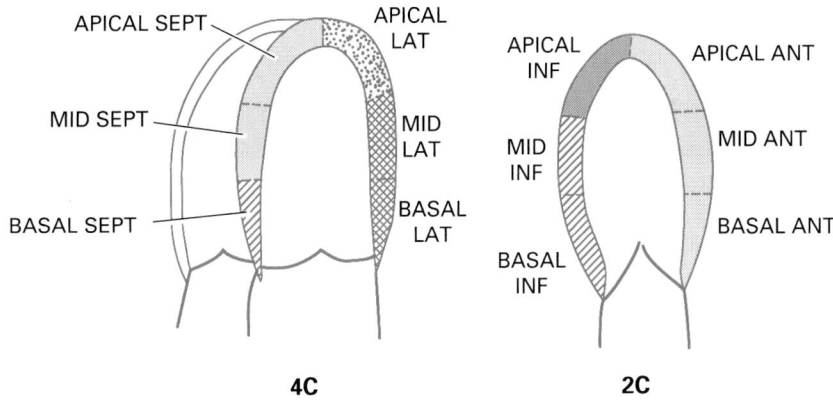

FIGURE 16–97. Sixteen-segment format for identification of left ventricular wall segments. Coronary arterial territories are also included. 2C, apical two-chamber; 4C, apical four-chamber; ANT, anterior; INF, inferior; LAT, lateral; LAX, parasternal long axis; POST, posterior; SAX PM, short axis at papillary muscle level; SEPT, septal. *Source: From Segar D, Brown S, Sawada S, et al. Dobutamine stress echocardiography: correlation with coronary lesion severity as determined by quantitative angiography. J Am Coll Cardiol 1992;19:1197. With permission.*

quickly detected by echocardiography. Severe LV dysfunction resulting in advanced heart failure or shock can be readily identified by echocardiography. In addition, aneurysm formation is usually quite apparent in ultrasonic images. By definition, postinfarction LV aneurysms are recognized as wide-mouthed, thin-walled myocardial segments that display dyskinetic expansion during systole. Aneurysms are a favored site for development of LV thrombi, which are covered in detail in the discussion of cardiac masses below. However, the presence of significant pericardial effusion on echocardiography in patients with hemodynamic compromise in the postinfarction period should suggest this condition. If a free wall rupture is sealed off by clot and pericardial inflammation, a pseudoaneurysm is formed[121] (Fig. 16–101). This lesion is distinguished from a true aneurysm by its highly localized nature and the presence of a narrow neck connecting it with the ventricle. Pseudoaneurysms frequently have multilayered thrombi within them and exhibit characteristic Doppler flow signals at the junc-

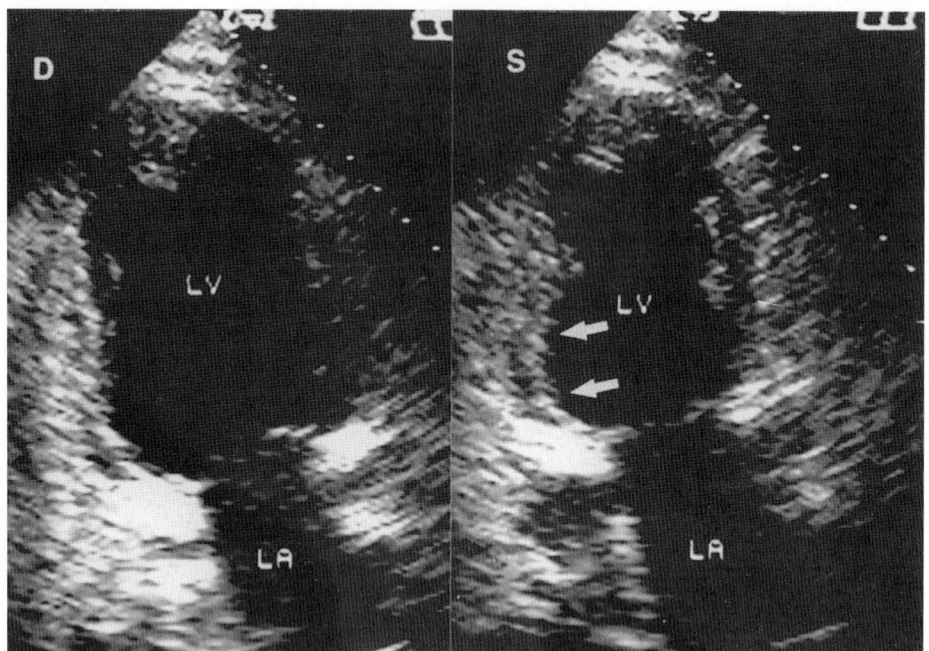

FIGURE 16–98. Diastolic (*left*) and systolic (*right*) images (apical two-chamber plane) from a patient with an inferior wall MI. The inferobasal segment is dyskinetic (*arrows*). LA, left atrium; LV, left ventricle; MI, myocardial infarction.

tion with the ventricle.[121] Because the risk of rupture is high, accurate diagnosis and prompt surgical repair of pseudoaneurysms is important.

Although postinfarction free wall rupture does not lend itself well to echocardiographic detection, acquired defects of the interventricular septum are more commonly delineated by cardiac ultrasound.[122] Acquired VSDs often consist of a latticework of tissue rather than a discrete orifice, but nevertheless echocardiographic

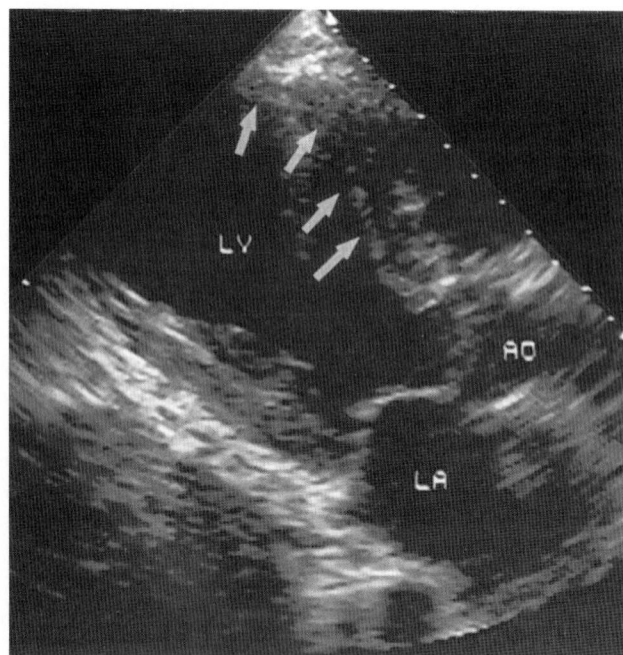

FIGURE 16–99. Parasternal long-axis view of a large anteroseptal MI, with thinning and dyskinesis of the anteroseptal wall (*arrows*). Ao, aorta; LA, left atrium; LV, left ventricle; MI, myocardial infarction.

images can depict absence of myocardium and distinct flow jets communicating between the left and right ventricles (Fig. 16–102). These color jets are typically high-velocity and aliased, coursing from the septum into the RV. The echocardiographic location of the defect and jet correlate well with the location by cineangiography, surgery, or autopsy.

MR is a common sequela of AMI; if severe, it may result in profound congestive heart failure and shock. Several mechanisms may be responsible for the occurrence of postinfarction MR including dilation of the LV cavity and mitral annulus, papillary muscle dysfunction, and partial or complete rupture of a papillary muscle (Fig. 16–103). MR from papillary dysfunction may lead to eccentric color jets within the LA. In general, the recognition and quantitation of MR occurring in the postinfarction period is no different from that of any other type of MR. TEE may play an important role in the identification and quantitative assessment of this complication, as well as in ensuring adequate operative repair.

In the setting of inferior wall infarction caused by occlusion of the proximal right coronary artery, RV MI may occur. The most specific echocardiographic sign of RV infarction is a regional wall motion abnormality, which is usually best visualized in the RV free wall (Fig. 16–104). RV infarction is typically accompanied by RV enlargement and tricuspid regurgitation; associated inferior or posterior LV wall motion abnormalities are virtually always present.

Pericarditis is a common complication of AMI, typically occurring during the acute phase of the illness and much less often in the late phases as part of the Dressler syndrome. Postinfarction pericarditis is not typically associated with marked echocardiographic abnormalities.

TEE has assumed a central role in the evaluation of patients with significant hemodynamic abnormalities in the postinfarction period. When TTE is technically suboptimal, transesophageal images can rapidly identify LV dyssynergy, valvular dysfunction, and other abnormalities associated with infarction. TEE may enable direct visualization of acquired VSDs when the lesion is not obvious or seen only as a disturbed flow stream in the RV with transthoracic imaging. Perhaps of greatest significance, TEE can provide definitive identification of a ruptured papillary muscle and a quantitative assessment of postinfarction MR.

Echocardiography has been used to evaluate the extent of reperfusion after thrombolytic or interventional therapy for AMI. Several reports have demonstrated that LV systolic function assessed by 2D imaging improved within 24 hours to 10 days of successful thrombolysis. More recently, contrast echocardiograms obtained after intravenous or direct intracoronary injection have shown that reperfusion of the infarct-related epicardial coronary artery by angiography is not necessarily accompanied by evidence of normal flow in the downstream microcirculation. In addition, this *no-*

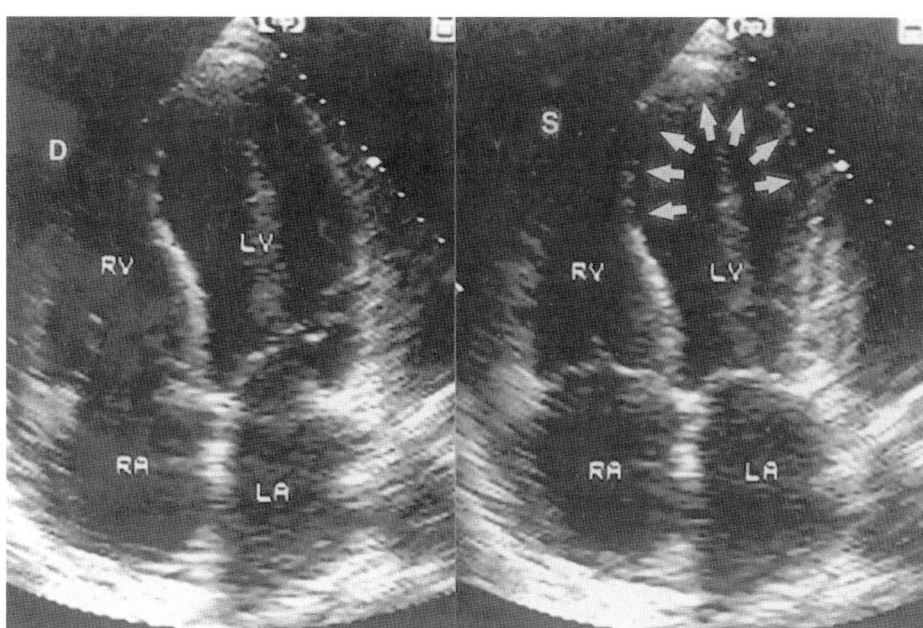

FIGURE 16–100. Apical four-chamber images of a large apical infarction. Diastole (*D*) is displayed on the left, systole (*S*) on the right. During systole, the base of the ventricle contracts, but the apex is dyskinetic (*arrows*).

reflow phenomenon on echocardiography heralds a poor prognosis, including failure of improvement of LV performance as well as increased late complications.[123]

[ ] STRESS ECHOCARDIOGRAPHY

The combination of stress testing and echocardiography (stress echocardiography) has assumed an important role in the diagnosis of CAD. The utility of this technique improved dramatically when technological advances permitted side-by-side viewing of rest and stress images together in a cine-loop format.[124] The application of stress echocardiography is based on the concept that a stress-induced imbalance in the myocardial supply-to-demand ratio will produce regional ischemia and resultant abnormalities of regional contraction, which can be readily identified by echocardiography (Fig. 16–105). The location of wall motion abnormalities may be used to predict the stenosed coronary vessel(s), whereas the ratio of dyssynergic to normal myocardium can provide a quantitative assessment of LV ischemia.

The types of stress employed fall into two basic groups: exercise and pharmacologic. Exercise testing can be performed either on a treadmill or a stationary bicycle (either upright or supine). Echo imaging usually can be accomplished only before and after treadmill exercise, however, whereas bicycle exertion facilitates the acquisition of images during the exercise protocol. Thus far, treadmill has been the preferred exercise modality. Of importance, all postexertional images should be obtained within a 1-minute window following exercise to avoid recording normal contractile function after recovery from ischemia.

Pharmacologic stress has the advantages of reducing the motion artifact of exercise, enabling continuous imaging throughout the protocol, and assessing myocardial viability.[125] Pharmacologic stress echocardiography can employ vasodilator agents such as dipyridamole or adenosine, which induce a heterogeneity of myocardial perfusion in ischemic heart disease, or inotropic agents such as dobutamine, which increase myocardial oxygen demand and directly produce ischemia.[125] As with exercise stress, diagnostic criteria include induction of regional wall motion abnormalities and LV dilatation. It is important to recognize that the normal response to exercise is hyperkinesis, and wall motion abnormalities may take the form of a lesser degree of hyperkinesis of a given segment in comparison with the rest of the LV myocardium. Dobutamine stress echocardiography appears particularly valuable in detecting myocardial viability.[124–126]

The safety and accuracy of stress echocardiography for the diagnosis of myocardial ischemia has been examined in several studies.[125,126] Both exercise and pharmacologic stress carry an extremely low risk of arrhythmia or infarction, but dobutamine can result in hypotension or *systolic anterior motion of the MV (SAM)* with resultant LV outflow obstruction. In general, stress echocardiography and nuclear scintigraphy yield similar results, although stress echocardiography may be slightly less sensitive and slightly more specific than scintigraphy.[124] The two techniques are comparable in their accuracy of detecting CAD.[124] The most common clinical application of stress echocardiography is in the diagnosis of CAD, and it appears especially useful in cases where exercise *electrocardiography* (ECG) may be inaccurate or falsely positive (e.g., abnormal baseline ECG, left ventricular hypertrophy [LVH], or chronic digitalis administration).[90,127] In this regard stress echocardiography appears especially useful for detection of ischemia in

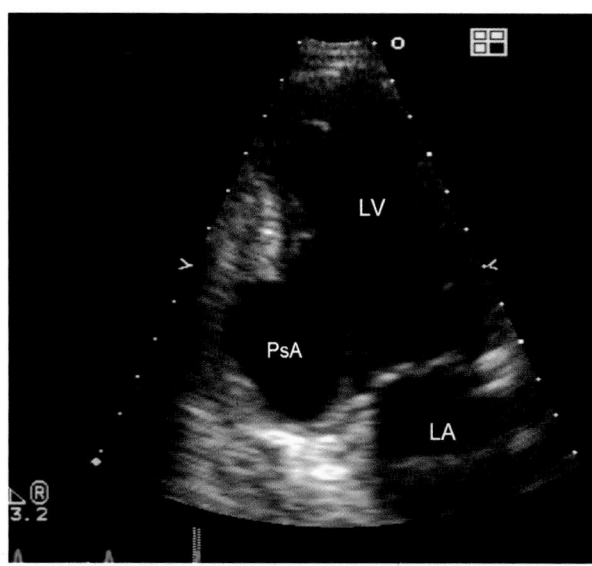

FIGURE 16–101. Apical 2-chamber view demonstrating a pseudoaneurysm (*PsA*) in the inferobasal portion of the left ventricle (*LV*). LA, left atrium. *Source: Courtesy of Thomas J. Waltman, MD.*

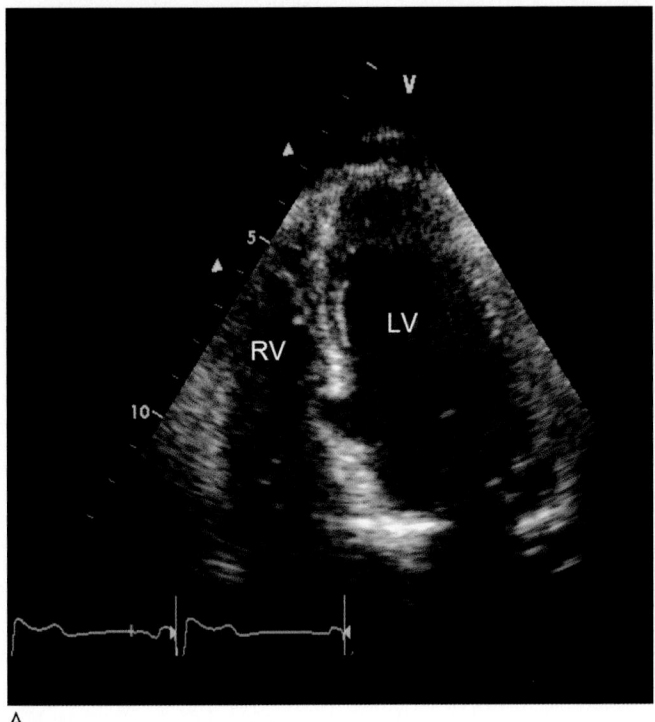
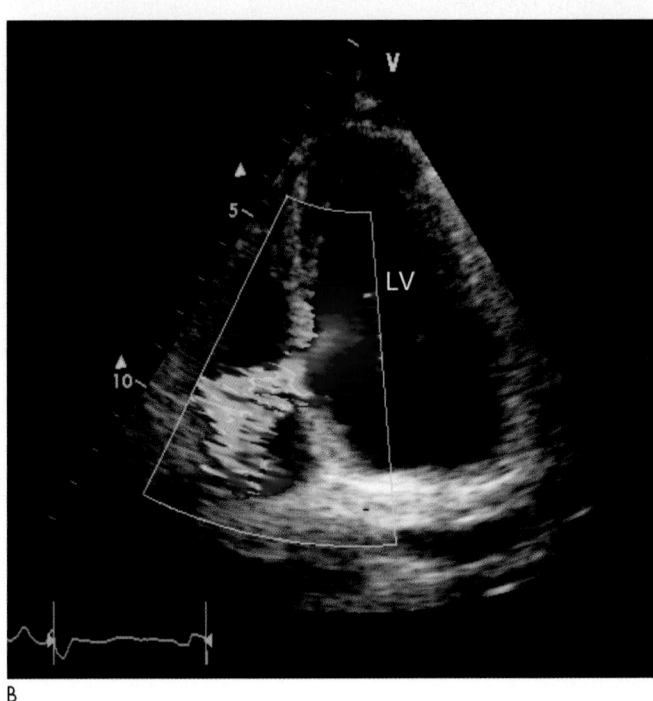

A
B

FIGURE 16–102. Modified apical four-chamber image of a ventricular septal rupture following MI. With 2D imaging (**A**) a defect is seen in the mid-septum. With color Doppler imaging (**B**) a high-velocity color jet is seen entering the right ventricle (*RV*) through the septal rupture. LV, left ventricle; MI, myocardial infarction.

women with false-positive ECG results. Stress echocardiography also adds independent prognostic information to exercise ECG, even in multivessel CAD. Dobutamine echocardiography may aid in the detection of ischemia in patients with cardiac transplantation and allograft vasculopathy (chronic rejection). In patients with known CAD, exercise echocardiography may facilitate localization and quantitation of ischemia, guide revascularization procedures, and assess the functional severity of coronary artery stenoses. Stress echocardiography can also demonstrate resolution of regional ischemia after successful coronary artery bypass surgery or angioplasty.

Stress echocardiography can play an important role in determining the prognosis of patients with CAD.[128] Both exercise and pharmacologic stress echocardiography appear superior to exercise ECG for identification of patients at high risk of recurrent ischemic events after MI. In addition, dobutamine stress echocardiography is useful in predicting perioperative ischemic complications in patients undergoing noncardiac surgery.[128] It has a strong negative predictive value.

In patients with chronic CHD, dobutamine stress echocardiography can identify hypokinetic yet viable myocardium and predicts improvement in function after successful revascularization.[126] Functional improvement in a hypokinetic segment with low-dose dobutamine infusion that then progresses to hypokinesis or akinesis with higher dobutamine dose (the so-called *biphasic*

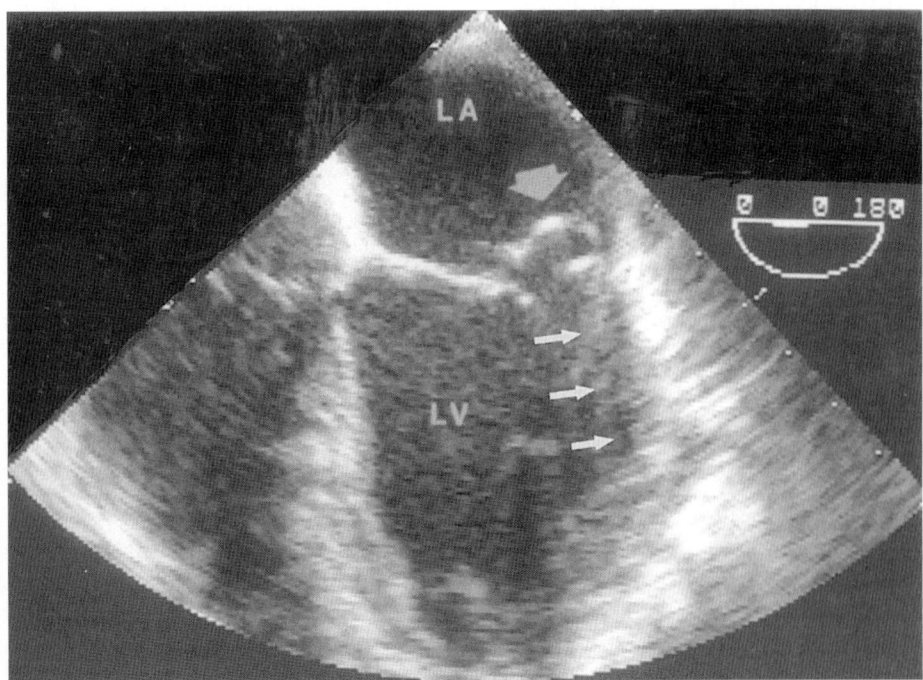

FIGURE 16–103. Transverse four-chamber TEE image of a posterolateral infarction causing posterior papillary muscle ischemia and partial rupture. The posterior mitral leaflet (*large arrow*) is poorly supported (but not actually flail) and prolapses into the left atrium (*LA*). The basal lateral wall segment (*small arrows*) of the left ventricle (LV) is dyskinetic.

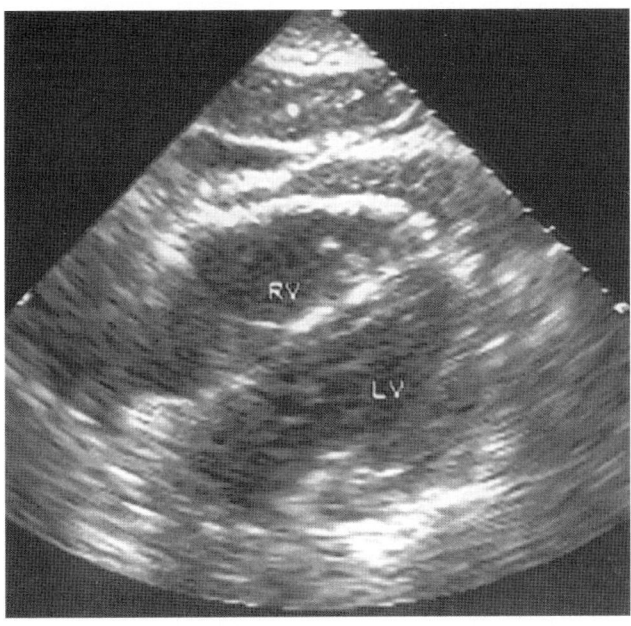
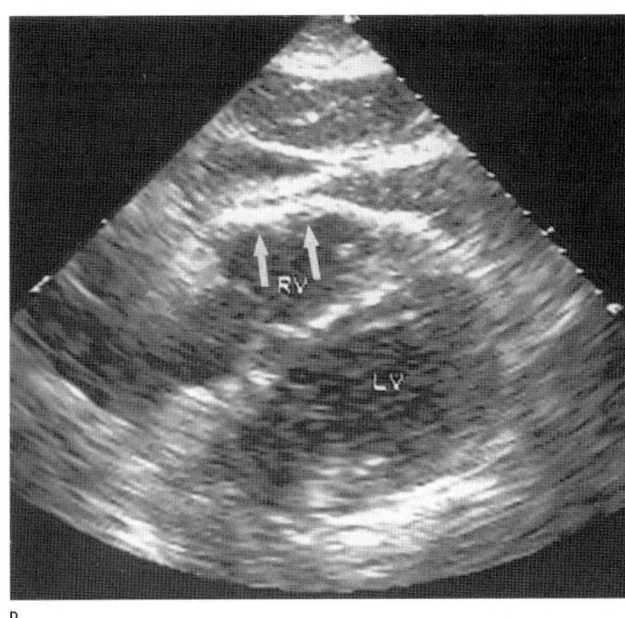

FIGURE 16–104. Diastolic (**A**) and systolic (**B**) subcostal four-chamber images of right ventricular (*RV*) myocardial infarction (MI). The RV free wall is dyskinetic (*arrows*) during systole (**B**).

response) correlates well with the presence of ischemic yet viable (*hibernating*) myocardium. Studies suggest that dobutamine stress echocardiography compares well with positron emission tomography and thallium single-photon emission computed tomography imaging in this regard. In addition, quantitation of regional myocardial blood flow using intravenous echo contrast agents may enhance the usefulness of stress echocardiography in the detection of both ischemia and viability.

There is evidence that exercise echocardiography can provide useful information regarding the hemodynamic status and functional severity of valvular heart disease.[129] Specifically, stress echocardiography has been used to assess the degree of obstruction in

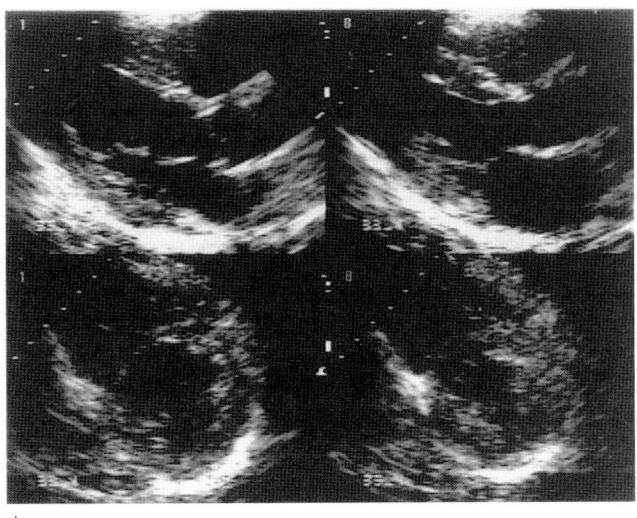
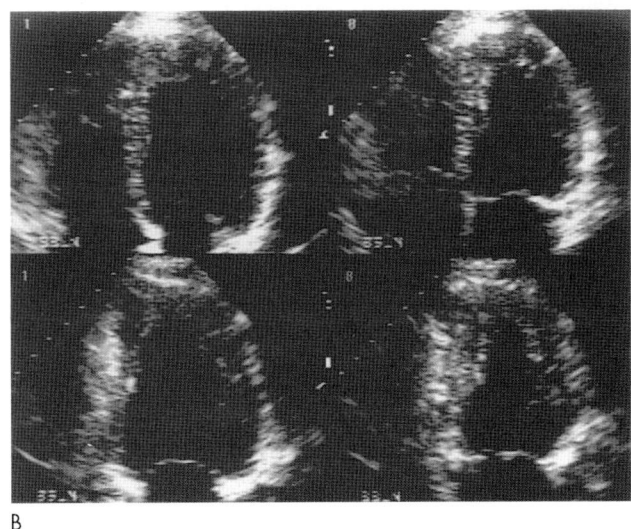

FIGURE 16–105. A. Digitized parasternal views during diastole (*left*) and systole (*right*) from a normal individual. *Upper panels*: long-axis plane; *lower panels*: short-axis plane. **B.** Digitized apical views during diastole (*left*) and systole (*right*) from a normal individual. *Upper panels*: four-chamber plane; *lower panels*: two-chamber plane. **C.** Digitized parasternal long-axis views at peak systole before (*left*) and immediately after exercise (*right*). The anteroseptal wall moves normally at rest (*arrows*) but becomes dyskinetic with exercise. **D.** Digitized apical four-chamber views at peak systole before (*left*) and immediately after exercise (*right*). The apical septal, apical, and apical lateral walls become dyskinetic with exercise, suggesting inducible ischemia in the left anterior descending artery territory. **E.** Digitized parasternal short-axis views (all recorded at peak systole) during dobutamine echocardiography in a patient with three-vessel CAD. At baseline (*upper left panel*) the left ventricular systolic function is normal. With low-dose dobutamine (5 µg/kg/min, *upper right panel*), function improves. With 10 µg/kg/min, however (*lower left panel*), function is similar to that at baseline. At 20 µg/kg/min (*lower right panel*), systolic function deteriorates and the left ventricle dilates. This response suggests global ischemia induced by dobutamine infusion. Ao, aorta; CAD, coronary artery disease; LA, left atrium; LV, left ventricle. (*continued*)

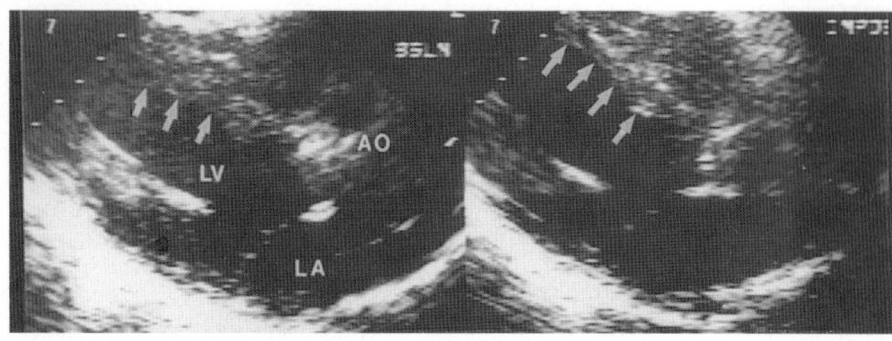

C

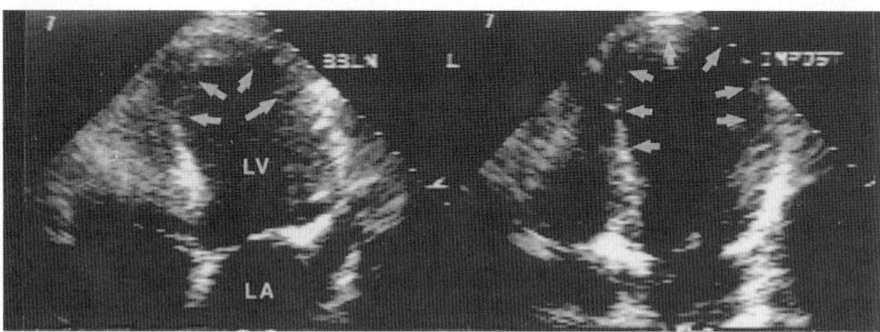

D

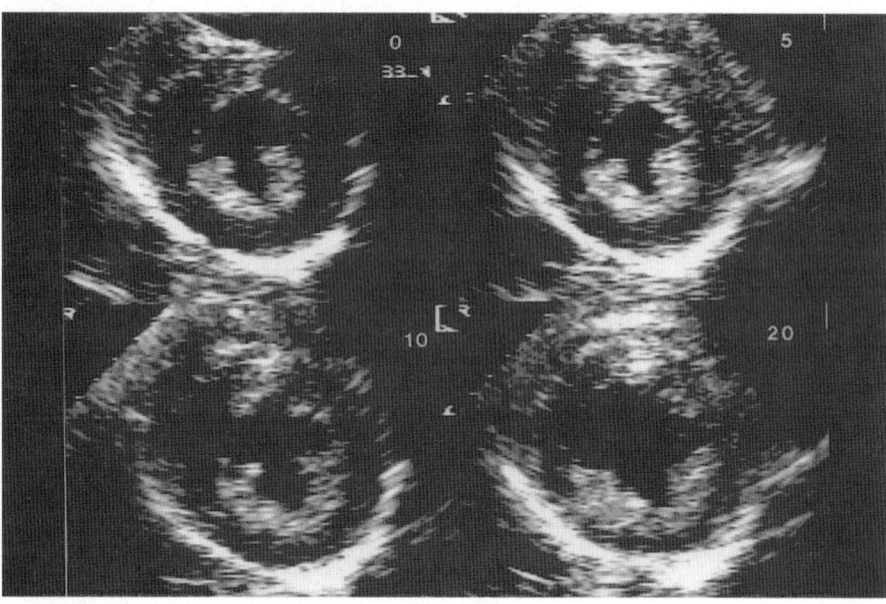

E

FIGURE 16–105. (continued)

patients with MS and the severity of AS in patients with advanced LV dysfunction.[129]

As is true of all diagnostic modalities, stress echocardiography has certain limitations. High-quality ultrasound images may be difficult to acquire in some patients. Also, considerable expertise is required to interpret stress echocardiographic images accurately. Nevertheless, stress echocardiography has many advantages over alternate diagnostic approaches such as radionuclide scintigraphy and coronary angiography. Harmonic imaging (both with and without intravenous echocardiographic contrast) has also enhanced endocardial border definition, facilitating stress echo studies in many patients with suboptimal fundamental (nonharmonic) echo images.

THE CARDIOMYOPATHIES

A diagnostic strategy has evolved that initially seeks to place patients into one of three pathophysiologic categories: dilated, hypertrophic, or restrictive; then the specific etiologies recognized as producing the individual pathophysiologic state are pursued. However, a recent classification that varies from former designations is discussed in Chap. 28. Dilated cardiomyopathies are associated with myocyte loss and necrosis, a marked increase in LV volume, thinning of the myocardium, and profound systolic dysfunction. *Hypertrophic cardiomyopathy* (HCM) (see Chap. 30) is recognized by increased myocardial thickness, particularly involving the interventricular septum, with preserved systolic function. Restrictive cardiomyopathies may be caused by infiltration of the myocardium by abnormal substances or fibrotic tissue; these cause symmetrical degrees of wall thickening with modest or no diminution of systolic function and little change in cavity size. Echocardiography is the cornerstone of such evaluations and provides data on cavity size, wall thickness, and systolic function. Thus, on echocardiogram, patients with dilated cardiomyopathy exhibit a marked increase in left LV and volume, little change in wall thickness, and severe contractile dysfunction. Patients with HCM exhibit a dramatic increase in LV wall thickness, with the septum characteristically disproportionate to the posterior wall, and often SAS induced by systolic anterior motion of the anterior MV leaflet. Patients with restrictive cardiomyopathy are identified by a symmetric increase in wall thickness accompanied by modest changes in contractile function and LV cavity size.

【 】 HYPERTROPHIC CARDIOMYOPATHY

HCM is a primary abnormality of the myocardium that exhibits myocyte disarray and unprovoked hypertrophy, often affecting the septum disproportionately (see Chap. 30). The disorder, which is often transmitted in an autosomal dominant pattern, has been linked to a number of abnormalities in genes that code for myocardial proteins. A number of classic echocardiographic findings occur in HCM (Fig. 16–106). The fundamental abnormality on

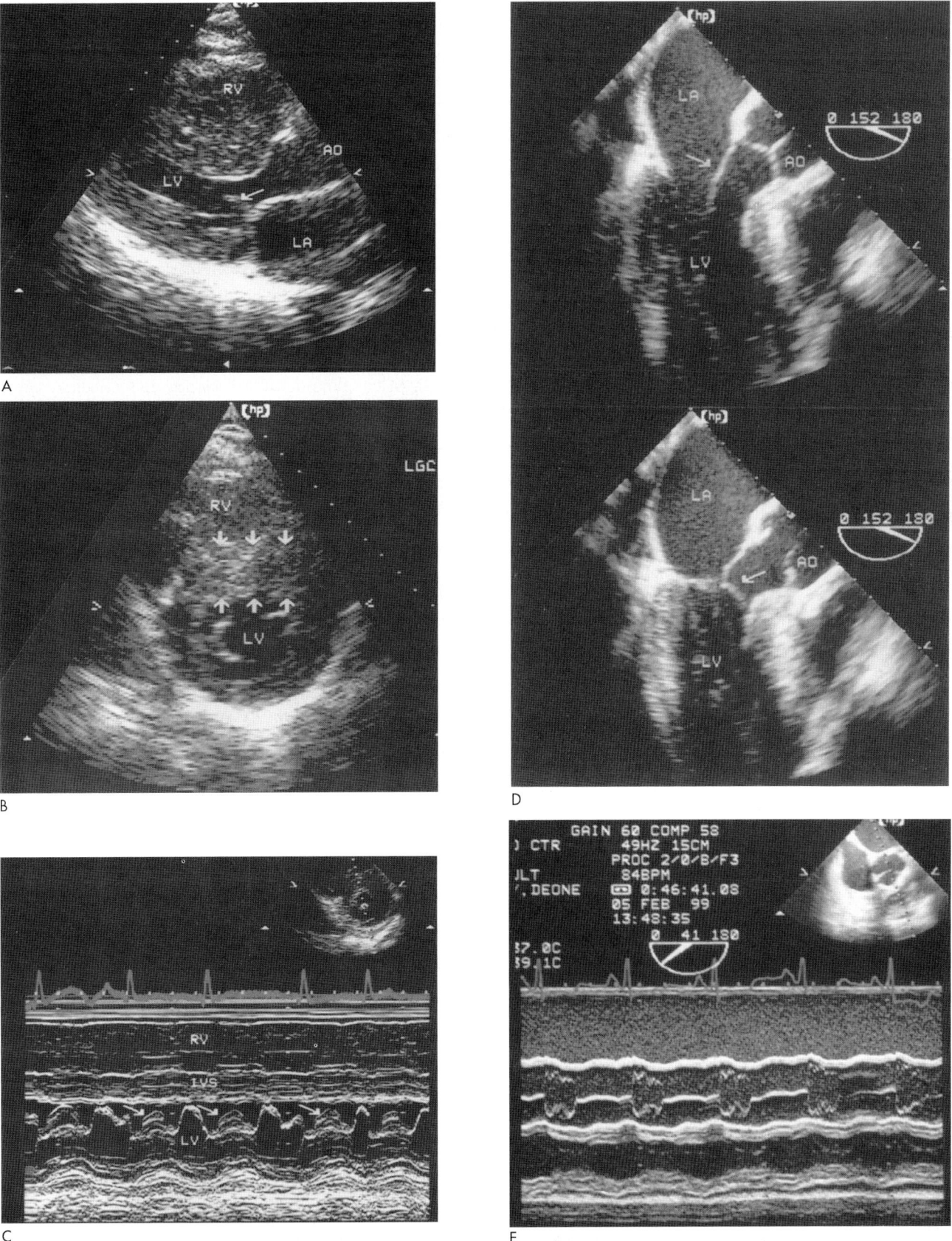

FIGURE 16–106. A. Parasternal long-axis view (during systole) of hypertrophic cardiomyopathy (HCM). Asymmetrical septal hypertrophy is present, as is systolic anterior motion of the anterior mitral valve leaflet (*arrow*). **B.** Parasternal short-axis view of HCM. Asymmetrical septal hypertrophy is present (*arrows*). **C.** Parasternal M-mode image from a patient with HCM, demonstrating systolic anterior motion of the anterior mitral valve leaflet (*arrows*). **D.** Transesophageal image of HCM. The aMVL appears normal during diastole (*upper panel*), but systolic anterior motion occurs during systole (*lower panel*). **E.** Transesophageal M-mode tracing through the AoV. Midsystolic notching and partial closure of the valve leaflets is present. aMVL, anterior mitral valve leaflet; Ao, aorta; AoV, aortic valve; IVS, interventricular septum; LA, left atrium; LV, left ventricle; RV, right ventricle.

echocardiogram in HCM is LVH, which is often severe. Although the hypertrophy may be confined to the septum, it may be concentric or involve any other portion of the LV. The customary classic finding is *asymmetric septal hypertrophy* (ASH), defined as a disproportionate thickness of the interventricular septum compared to the posterobasal wall with a ratio of >1.3:1. In some cases the entire septum is hypertrophied, whereas in others the thickening may be localized to the proximal, mid-, or distal (apical) septum. Asymmetric hypertrophy of the proximal interventricular septum may lead to dynamic LV outflow tract obstruction—*hypertrophic obstructive cardiomyopathy* (HOCM). Although ASH is almost always present in cases of dynamic LV outflow tract obstruction, it is not a specific marker for HCM and may occur in some patients with RV hypertrophy, inferior MI, and a minority with hypertensive LVH. Extent of hypertrophy does not appear to correlate well with risk of sudden death, because patients with minimal hypertrophy may still be at significant risk.[130]

The second characteristic finding of HCM is systolic anterior motion of the MV, or SAM, which usually involves the anterior MV leaflet. Encroachment of the pathologically thickened septum on the LV outflow tract creates a pressure drop by a Venturi effect, which draws the mitral leaflets toward the septum, creating dynamic LV outflow tract obstruction (see Fig. 16–106). There are also important effects from papillary muscle position and chordal tension on systolic mitral morphology and SAM. Because of distorted mitral coaptation during systole, SAM generally causes MR of variable severity. Like asymmetrical septal hypertrophy, SAM (especially systolic motion of the chordae) is not pathognomonic for HCM and can occur in other conditions such as hypovolemia, anemia, and states where LV outflow tract narrowing and hyperdynamic contraction are present.

The third manifestation of classic HCM is midsystolic closure of the AoV (see Fig. 16–106E). This finding is best seen on M-mode recordings, occurs only in the presence of outflow tract obstruction, and is probably a manifestation of the sudden pressure drop during mid- and late systole caused by SAM. As with ASH and SAM, midsystolic aortic closure is not specific for HCM and can occur in MR, AO dilatation, VSD, low cardiac-output states, and discrete SAS.

The fourth important abnormality of HCM is observed on Doppler examination of the LV outflow tract (LVOT). Normally, Doppler interrogation of this area produces a spectral tracing that peaks early in systole and has a maximum velocity of <1.7 m/sec. In many patients HCM creates a high-pressure gradient coincident with SAM, which is detected by Doppler as a high-velocity systolic jet in the LVOT. As opposed to valvular AS, however, the maximal velocity in obstructive HCM peaks later in systole, creating a characteristic *saber-tooth* pattern (Fig. 16–107A). Although the subaortic gradient can be estimated using the modified Bernoulli equation, the assumptions used in this equation may not apply to HCM. Similar Doppler patterns also may be seen occasionally within the LV in patients with HCM if systolic obliteration of the hypertrophied LV causes localized areas of high flow velocity in the more distal portions of the ventricular cavity. LV cavity obliteration produces a very late systolic rise in flow velocity (see Fig. 16–107B), and this Doppler pattern should not be mistaken for true LV outflow tract obstruction.

Diastolic dysfunction has been long recognized in HCM. Doppler interrogation of LV inflow often reveals a relaxation abnormality, with a reduced early diastolic (E) velocity, a prolonged deceleration slope of the E wave, and an increased velocity of the atrial systolic (A) component.[131] Color Doppler imaging can be used to demonstrate intraventricular flow characteristics.

DILATED CARDIOMYOPATHY

In cases of *dilated cardiomyopathy* (DCM), the heart is typically greatly enlarged and systolic function is markedly depressed (see Chap. 29). Four-chamber dilatation is a common but not uniform finding, because some patients may have relatively preserved RV size. Marked LV enlargement and generalized dysfunction can also be caused by severe ischemic heart disease, chronic alcohol abuse, various infectious myocarditides, anthracyclines and other cardiotoxic agents, nutritional deficiencies, and hereditary myopathies. Severe ischemic disease is often segmental and has been reported to spare the posterior wall frequently, whereas the LV dysfunction of DCM is usually global. The echocardiographic findings in DCM include an increased LV end-diastolic diameter and volume with decreased fractional shortening, thinning LV walls (Fig. 16–108), increased E point-septal separation, LA enlargement, and limited mitral and AoV opening (caused by low stroke volume). Intracardiac thrombi are frequently observed and are most often found in the LV apex. M-mode imaging of the mitral leaflets may demonstrate a *B bump,* or notch just before systolic valve closure, indicating elevated LV diastolic pressure (see Fig. 16–8). Mitral annular dilatation and secondary MR are common.

Doppler echocardiography often reveals an abnormally low-velocity time integral in the LV outflow or inflow tracts. Diastolic MR caused by elevated LV diastolic pressure also may be present. Diastolic dysfunction is common, and PWD interrogation of mitral inflow may show an abnormal relaxation, restrictive or pseudonormal pattern depending on LV diastolic pressures and loading conditions.[132] A restrictive pattern of mitral inflow Doppler confers a poor prognosis in patients with DCM.

RESTRICTIVE CARDIOMYOPATHY

Restrictive cardiomyopathy may be idiopathic or secondary to infiltrative diseases such as amyloidosis, hemochromatosis, hypereosinophilic syndrome and Loeffler endocarditis, sarcoidosis, radiation toxicity, glycogen storage diseases, and Gaucher disease (see Chap. 31). Typical 2D echocardiographic features of these diseases include (1) a diffuse increase of ventricular thickness in the absence of marked ventricular chamber dilation, and (2) marked biatrial enlargement (Fig. 16–109). Systolic function is often modestly decreased. Doppler examination may show a mitral inflow relaxation abnormality early in the course of restrictive cardiomyopathy; but restrictive pattern (E >> A, with shortened E deceleration time) is a more classic finding, which often evolves with time and indicates both a high LA pressure and poor prognosis. In advanced cases, tissue Doppler imaging of the mitral annulus shows marked reductions in both early and late diastolic annular velocities.

Amyloidosis is generally the most commonly encountered restrictive cardiac disease. In addition to biventricular hypertrophy,

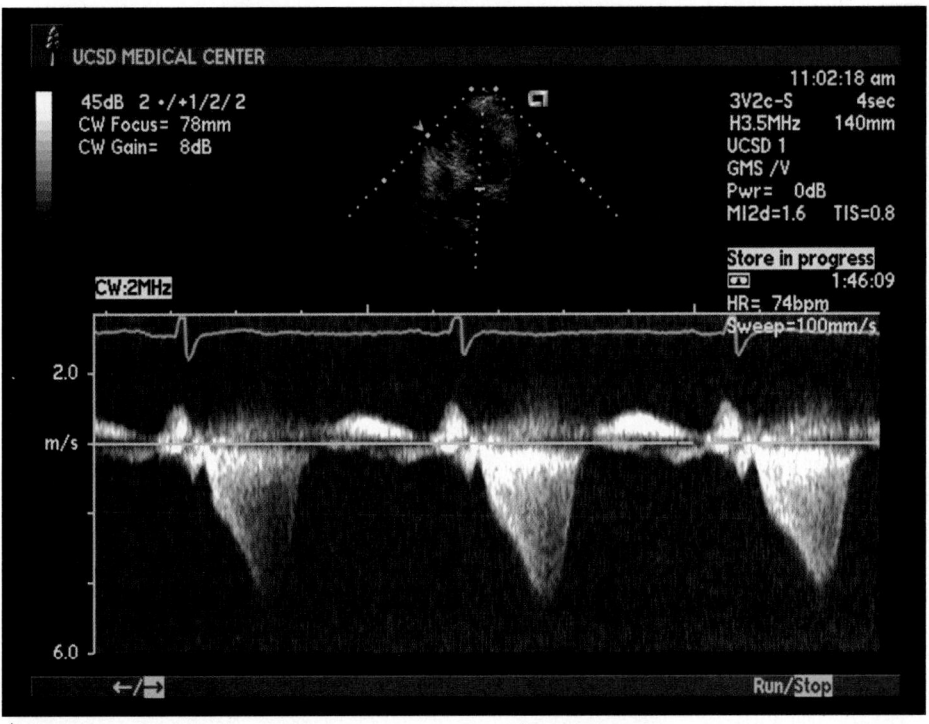

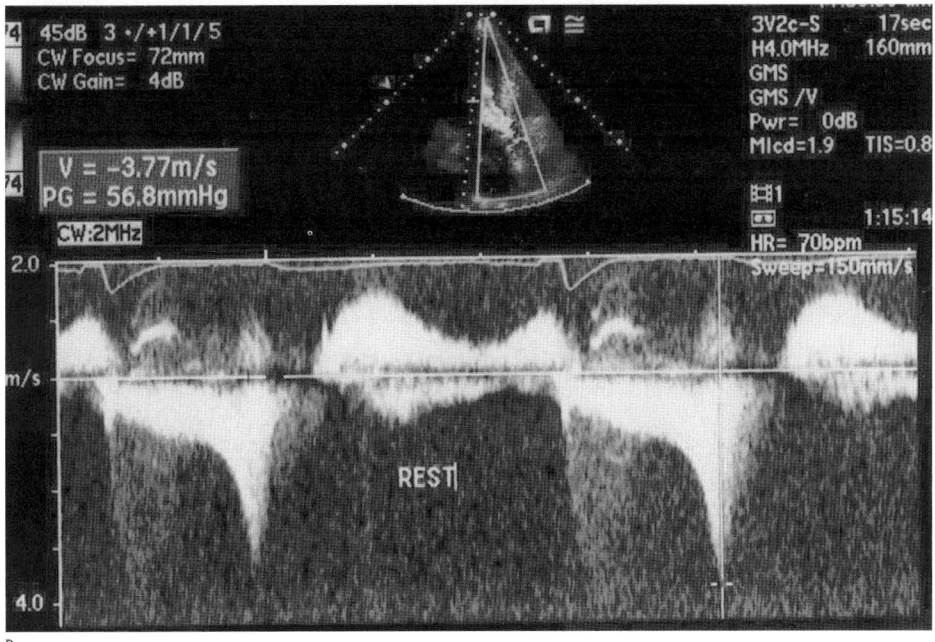

FIGURE 16–107. A. CW Doppler tracing through the LV outflow tract (from the apical transducer position) in hypertrophic obstructive cardiomyopathy. In comparison to valvular AS, the rise in velocity is delayed (reflecting dynamic rather than fixed outflow obstruction). **B.** CW Doppler tracing through the LV (from the apical transducer position) in LV hypertrophy with end-systolic LV cavity obliteration. The very late systolic rise in blood velocity is more consistent with obliteration than true LV outflow tract obstruction. AS, aortic stenosis; CW, continuous wave; LV, left ventricle.

amyloidosis is also associated with diffuse thickening of the interatrial septum and cardiac valves. In advanced disease, depressed systolic function is also common. An abnormal *speckled* pattern or *ground glass* appearance of the myocardium has been described on 2D echocardiography, but this sign is absent in many cases and therefore has minimal clinical usefulness. The finding of a restric-tive mitral inflow pattern on Doppler echocardiography is identified as a marker of advanced disease and poor prognosis. In addition to increased myocardial thickness, endocardial thickening and fibrosis as well as restricted atrioventricular leaflet motion are common features of Loeffler endocarditis and endomyocardial fibroelastosis. Intraventricular thrombi are also common in these processes.

CONGENITAL HEART DISEASE

【 】 ECHOCARDIOGRAPHIC IDENTIFICATION OF CONGENITAL CARDIAC ANOMALIES

2D and Doppler echocardiography have had a major impact on the diagnosis and management of patients with CHD (see Chaps. 81 and 82). From isolated congenital lesions to complex, extensive cardiac malformations, echocardiographic imaging (often with intravenous contrast injection) is usually sufficient to delineate cardiac anatomy. TEE is an important adjunctive technique as well; in many cases a thorough echocardiographic evaluation may obviate the need for cardiac catheterization and angiography.

The ultrasound diagnosis of a simple intracardiac shunt is usually straightforward, but the task of defining complex congenital cardiac abnormalities can be daunting. It is useful to remember a few basic anatomic rules. The venae cavae and pulmonary veins generally empty into the morphologic RA and LA, respectively. The atrioventricular valves uniformly follow their ventricles through embryologic development: A TV accompanies the morphologic RV and a MV accompanies the left. Similarly, the semilunar valves follow the great vessels. The aorta and PA can be distinguished, regardless of their position, by the bifurcation of the PA.

Several features aid identification of the morphologic right and left ventricles. The RV has a tricuspid atrioventricular valve; in comparison with the mitral annulus, the tricuspid annulus is positioned slightly closer to the cardiac apex. The RV also has a moderator band, coarser trabeculations than those in the left ventricle, and an infundibulum that separates the inlet area from the RVOT.

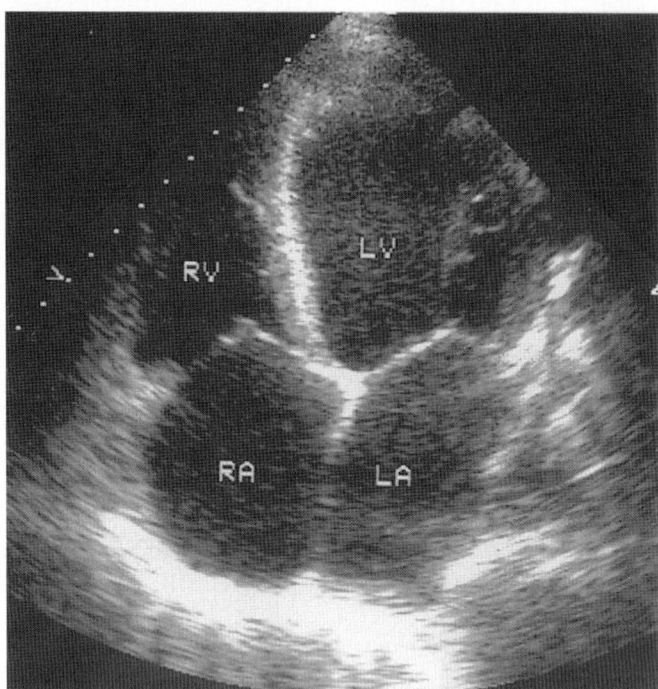

FIGURE 16–108. Apical four-chamber image of dilated cardiomyopathy. There is four-chamber enlargement as well as left ventricular (*LV*) spontaneous echo contrast. LA, left atrium; RA, right atrium; RV, right ventricle.

【 】 CARDIOVASCULAR SHUNTS

Atrial Septal Defect

Most secundum and primum *atrial septal defects* (ASDs) are easily visualized by echocardiography, but sinus venous defects are often difficult to detect without TEE. Therefore, the subcostal view provides the optimal imaging plane to detect lesions of the atrial septum.[133] Ostium secundum defects are the most common form of ASD, and 2D imaging shows a localized absence of septal tissue in the midportion of the interatrial septum (Fig. 16–110A). Lack of any interatrial septal tissue between the defect and the base of the interventricular septum characterizes an ostium primum defect (see Fig. 16–110B). Although ostium secundum defects are usually isolated, ostium primum (or partial AoV canal) defects are often accompanied by other lesions. Sinus venosus defects are strongly associated with partial anomalous pulmonary venous return (Fig. 16–111A). Rarely, the atrial septum may be completely absent (Fig. 16–112). With all but small ASDs, the RA is enlarged and RV volume overload is present, with a dilated RV and paradoxical septal motion.

Intravenous contrast injection generally demonstrates shunting across the ASD, frequently with bidirectional flow. Therefore *negative jets* of unopacified flow from the LA into the contrast-filled RA may alternate with the appearance of contrast bubbles flowing through the defect into the LA. When an ASD is present, contrast should appear within three to five heartbeats in the LA after entering the RA. Delayed appearance of contrast in the LA may indicate an intrapulmonary shunt rather than an ASD.

Color Doppler imaging can be useful for detecting flow through ASDs (see Fig. 16–110A), but the pressure drop between atria often does not produce turbulence. Color inflow from the in-

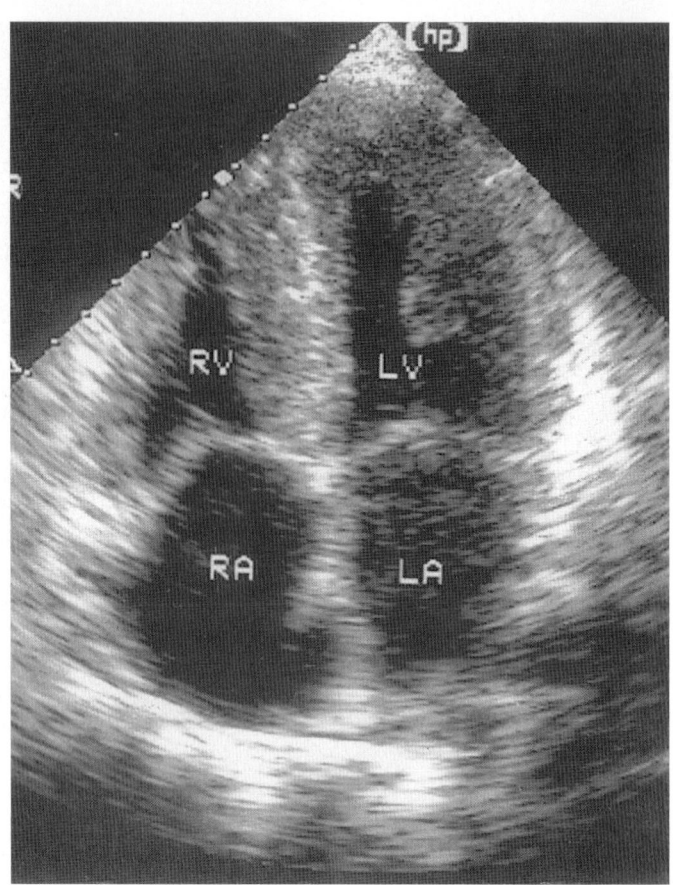

FIGURE 16–109. Apical four-chamber image of cardiac amyloid. LA, left atrium; LV, left ventricle; RA, right atrium; RV, right ventricle.

ferior vena cava and right-sided pulmonary veins may be prominent in normal subjects and should not be misinterpreted as a shunt.[134] PWD recordings through an ASD usually reveal continuous flow, which peaks in late systole. Pulmonary-to-systemic flow ratios can be estimated in ASD (and VSDs) by comparing volumetric flow measurements through the LVOT and RVOT. With the advent of umbrella or *clamshell* devices that permit percutaneous closure of ASDs, TEE has assumed an important role in defining the cross-sectional dimensions and exact position of the ASD (see Fig. 16–111B). TEE is also useful in confirming accurate placement of closure devices and subsequent correction of the interatrial shunt.

Ventricular Septal Defect

Ventricular septal defects (VSDs) may be classified as perimembranous, inlet, outlet, or trabecular. Echocardiography is quite useful for the detection and classification of VSDs.[135] The defect itself is sometimes visible with 2D imaging alone (Fig. 16–113A), but smaller VSDs are easily missed. Complete absence of the interventricular septum (single ventricle) is quite rare (see Fig. 16–113B). PWD or CW Doppler interrogation often reveals discrete areas of high-velocity flow across the interventricular septum. Measurement of the peak CW velocity through the shunt allows calculation of the interventricular pressure gradient (via the modified Bernoulli equation); subtraction of this gradient from the systolic blood pressure (in the absence of AoV disease) approximates the RV systolic pressure.

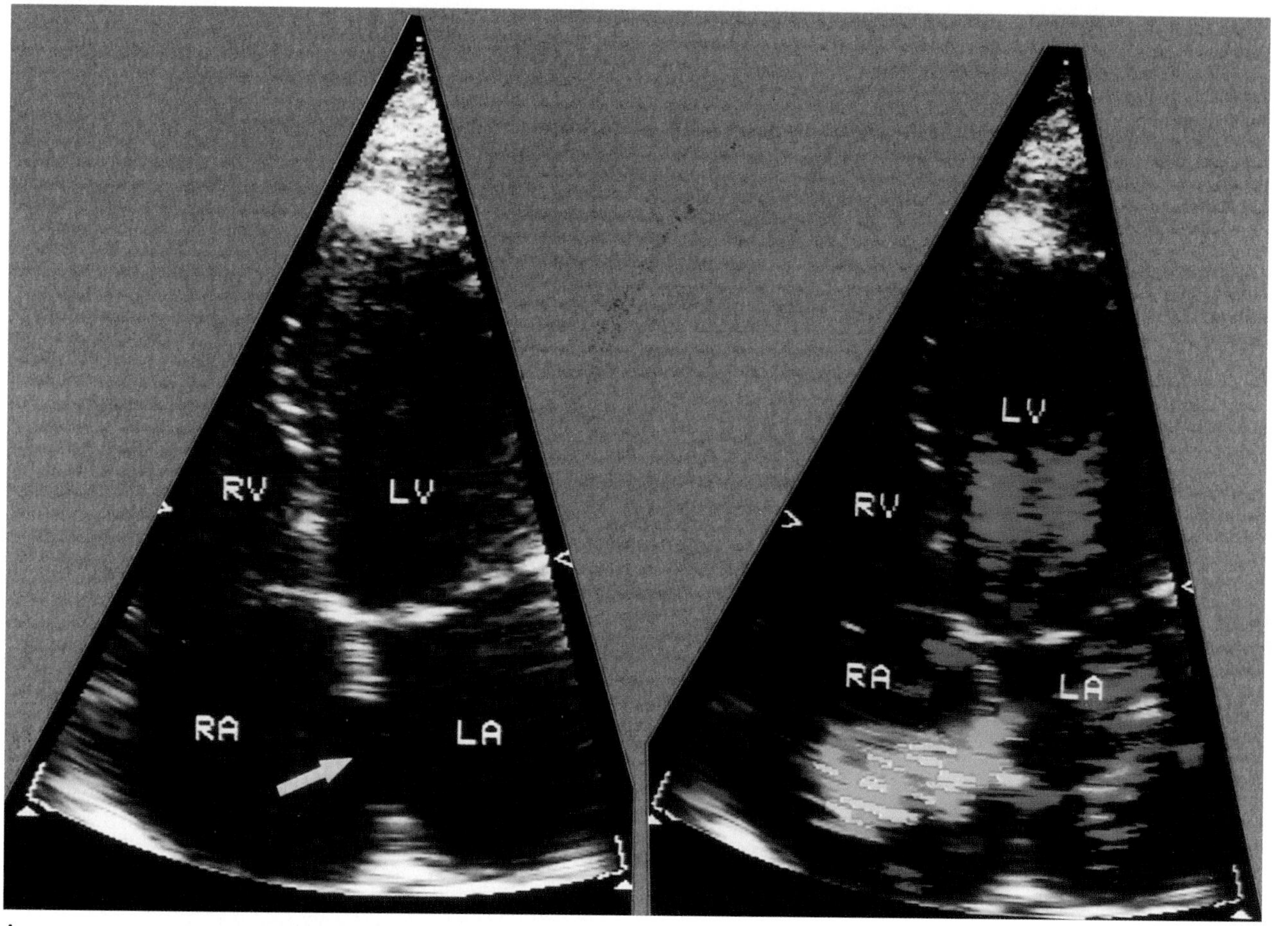

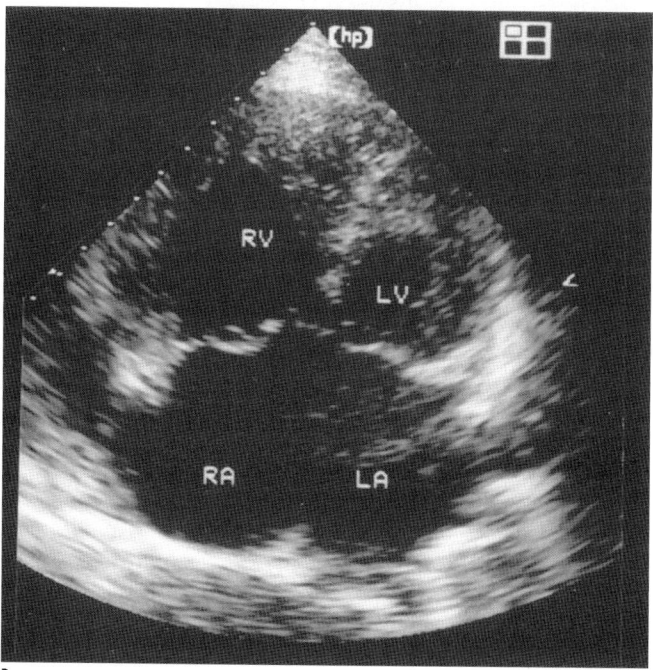

FIGURE 16–110. A. Apical four-chamber view of an ostium secundum ASD. On the left, a defect in the mid atrial septum is apparent (*arrow*). On the right, there is color flow through the shunt. **B.** Apical four-chamber view of a large ostium primum ASD (as well as an inlet VSD) in a patient with Down's syndrome. ASD, atrial septal defect; LA, left atrium; LV, left ventricle; RA, right atrium; RV, right ventricle; VSD, ventricular septal defect.

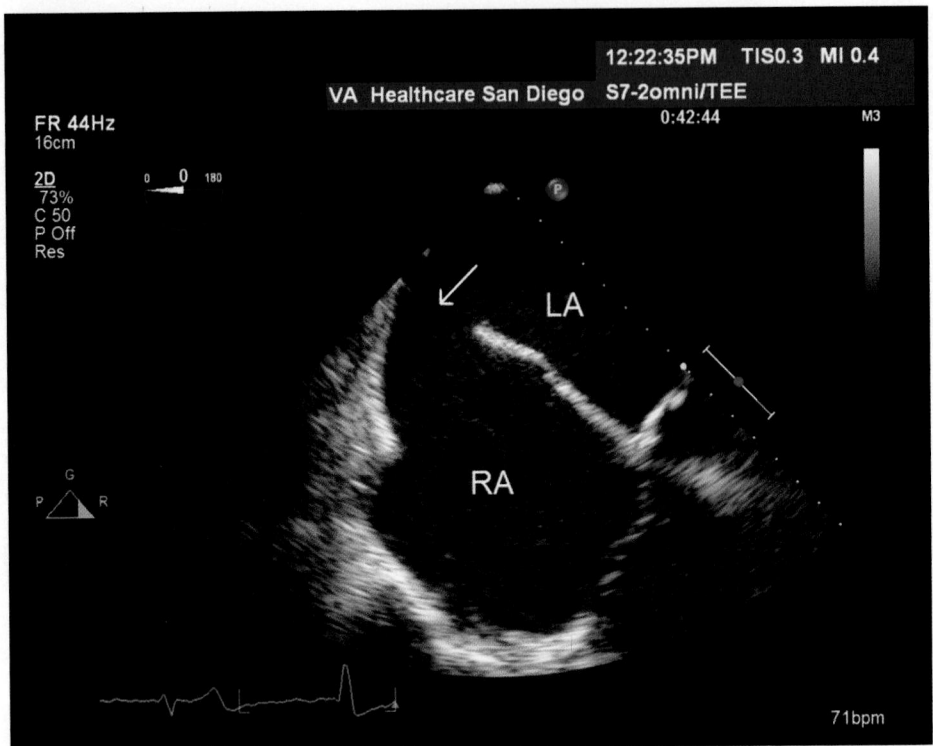

A

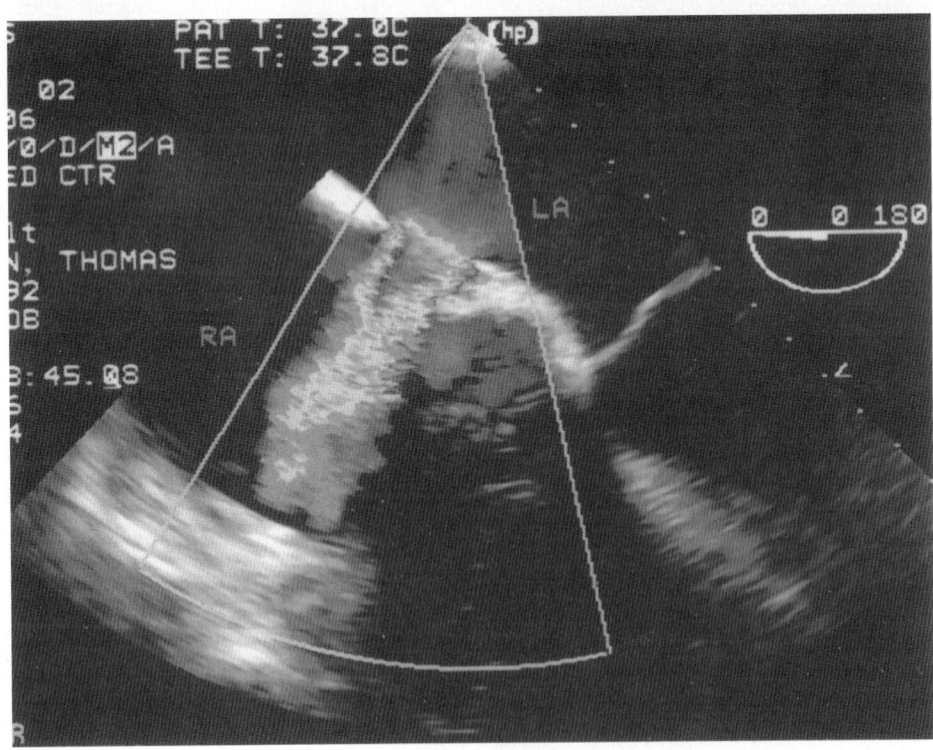

B

FIGURE 16–111. A. Transesophageal image of a sinus venosus atrial septal defect (ASD). The defect (*arrow*) is present in the superior portion of the interatrial septum. **B.** Transesophageal image of an ostium secundum ASD. Color-flow Doppler confirms a left to right shunt, and the size of the defect can be measured accurately. LA, left atrium; RA, right atrium.

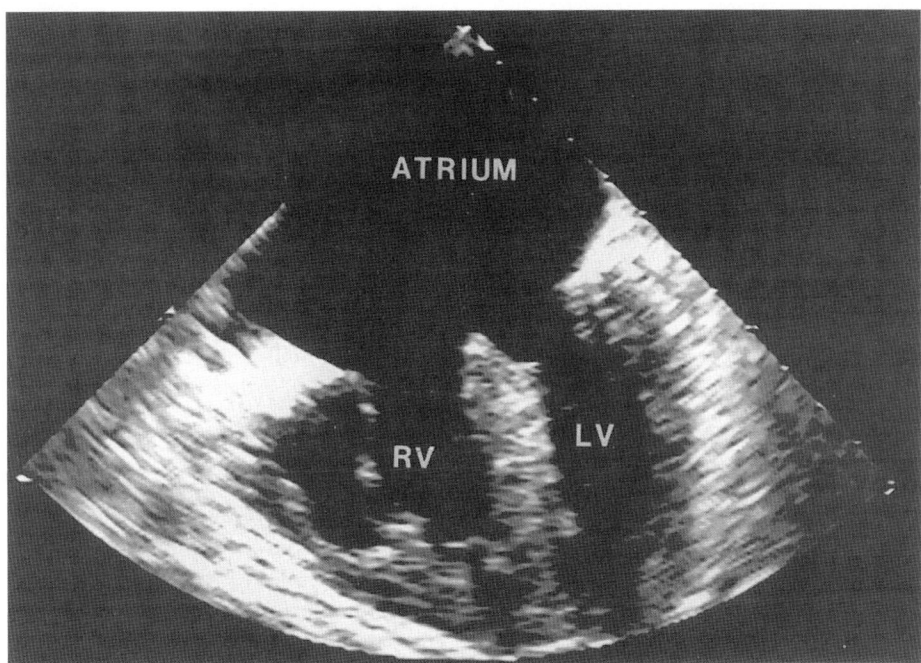

FIGURE 16–112. Transverse transesophageal image of single atrium. RV, right ventricle; LV, left ventricle. *Source: From Blanchard DG, Scott ED. Single atrium. Circulation 1997;95:273. With permission.*

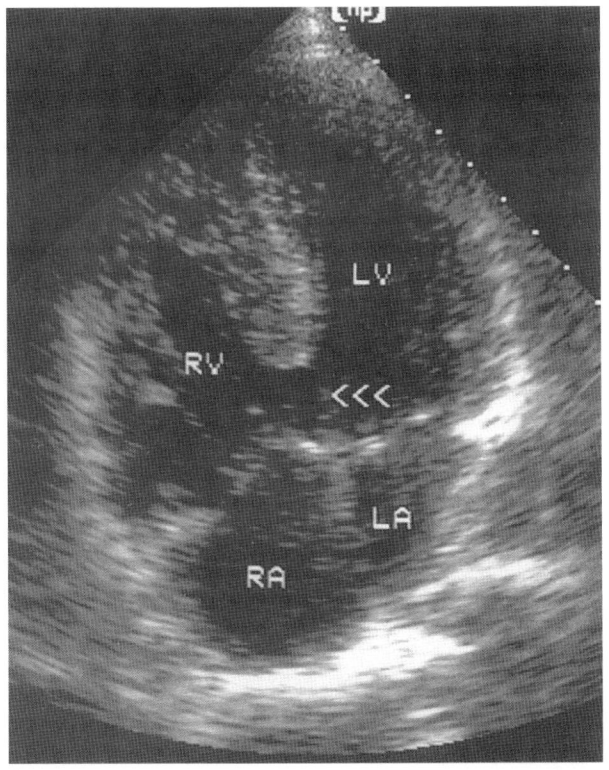

A

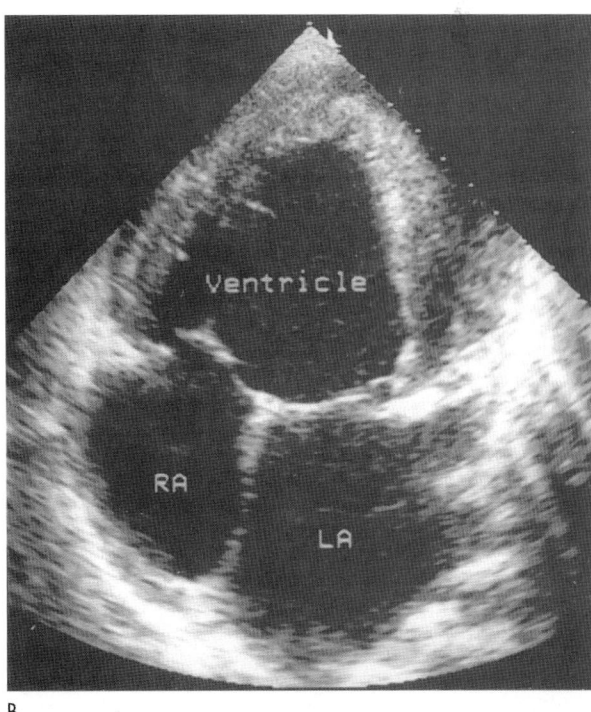

B

FIGURE 16–113. A. Apical four-chamber image of an inlet ventricular septal defect (VSD). The defect (*arrows*) is situated more inferiorly than the typical position of a perimembranous VSD. **B.** Apical image of single ventricle. LA, left atrium; LV, left ventricle; RA, right atrium; RV, right ventricle.

Overall, color-flow imaging is the most useful Doppler technique for the diagnosis of VSDs.[135] Typically, a high-velocity systolic color jet is seen traversing the interventricular septum, but the velocity is lower with large defects and in the presence of PH (Fig. 16–114). The appearance of the color jet in the standard imaging planes can be used to determine the type of VSD. Intravenous contrast injection may reveal a negative contrast jet in the RV, and contrast may cross the defect and partially opacify the left ventricle. In the absence of MR, contrast does not enter the LA, distinguishing an isolated VSD from an ASD. Accurate detection of other associated cardiac lesions (see Chap. 82) is especially critical before surgical intervention.

Patent Ductus Arteriosus

The ductus arteriosus originates just to the left of the PA bifurcation and inserts into the aorta slightly distal to and opposite from the ostium of the left subclavian artery. Given this posterior location, it is difficult to image a *patent ductus arteriosus* (PDA) itself with 2D TTE alone, and TEE is usually superior for direct visualization of the lesion (Fig. 16–115A and B). In most cases CFD reliably detects high-velocity diastolic flow within the PA in nearly all non-Eisenmenger patients.[136] The flow jet characteristically enters the distal left region of the main PA and streams anterior along the medial wall of the vessel (see Fig. 16–115B). With large shunts, volume overload and subsequent dilation of the left ventricle occurs. Aortopulmonary window is a much rarer shunt involving the great vessels which presents as a communication anteriorly between the ascending aorta and proximal PA. It is embryologically distinct from a PDA and more closely related to a truncus arteriosus defect.

VENOUS INFLOW ABNORMALITIES

Anomalous pulmonary venous return (APVR) may be partial or total. Partial APVR is present in 80 percent of sinus venosus ASD cases and is a feature of the scimitar syndrome. The usual finding on TTE is RV volume overload. TEE is quite useful in detecting these abnormal venous connections. In total APVR, the pulmonary veins may empty directly into the RA or into a common posterior chamber or vein. This structure and its connection with the RA may be visualized echocardiographically, along with the obligatory ASD.[137] In some cases, the collecting chamber posterior to the LA may mimic the appearance of *cor triatriatum,* an entity characterized by a membrane in the posterior LA which may obstruct pulmonary venous inflow, causing symptoms similar to those of MS (Fig. 16–116).

Persistent left superior vena cava occurs in 0.5 percent of the normal population. In most cases, the anomalous vein empties into the coronary sinus, which then drains into the RA (Fig. 16–117). Unless the coronary sinus is unroofed and drains into the LA, no shunting occurs. The typical echocardiographic finding is a large coronary sinus, which is especially well seen on transesophageal or parasternal trans-thoracic views. The diagnosis may be confirmed by intravenous contrast injection from the left arm, because this will opacify the coronary sinus shortly before filling the RA.

CONOTRUNCAL AND AORTIC ABNORMALITIES

Tetralogy of Fallot is one of the more common conotruncal abnormalities, and affected individuals may sometimes survive to adulthood without surgical intervention (see Chap. 82). The classic

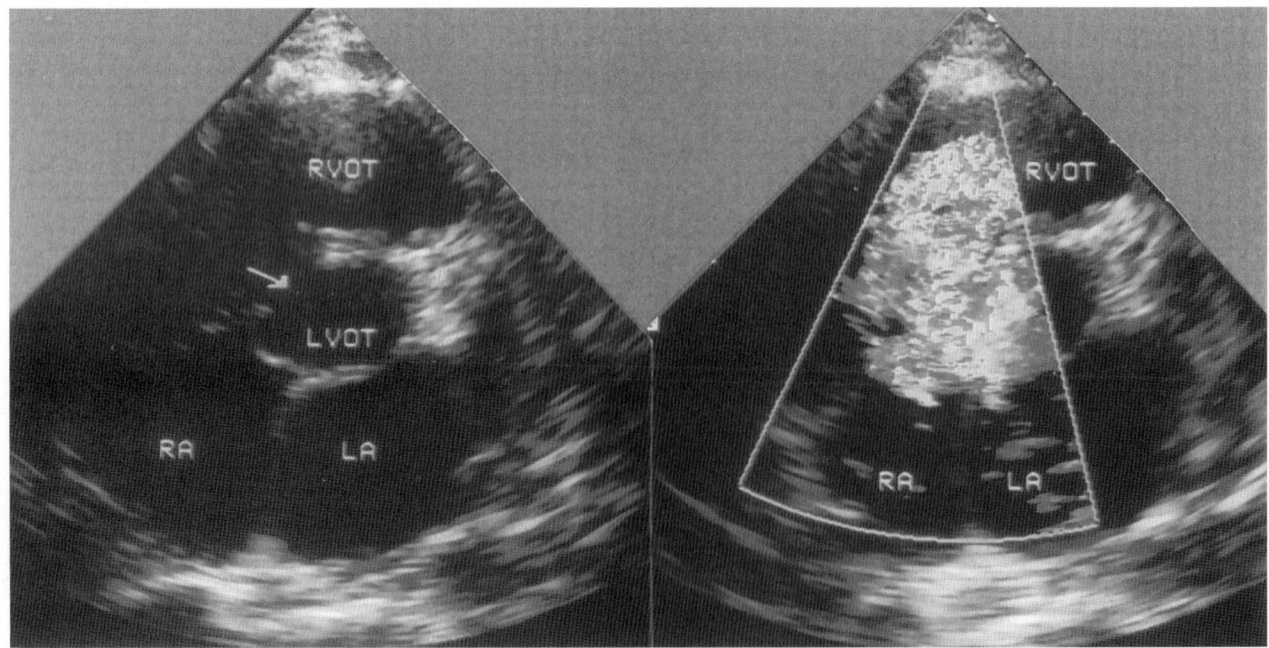

FIGURE 16–114. Parasternal short-axis images of a large perimembranous ventricular septal defect (VSD) (*arrow*) without (*left*) and with (*right*) superimposed color flow Doppler. A large, turbulent color jet crosses the VSD during systole (*right*). LA, left atrium; LVOT, left ventricular outflow tract; RA, right atrium; RVOT, right ventricular outflow tract.

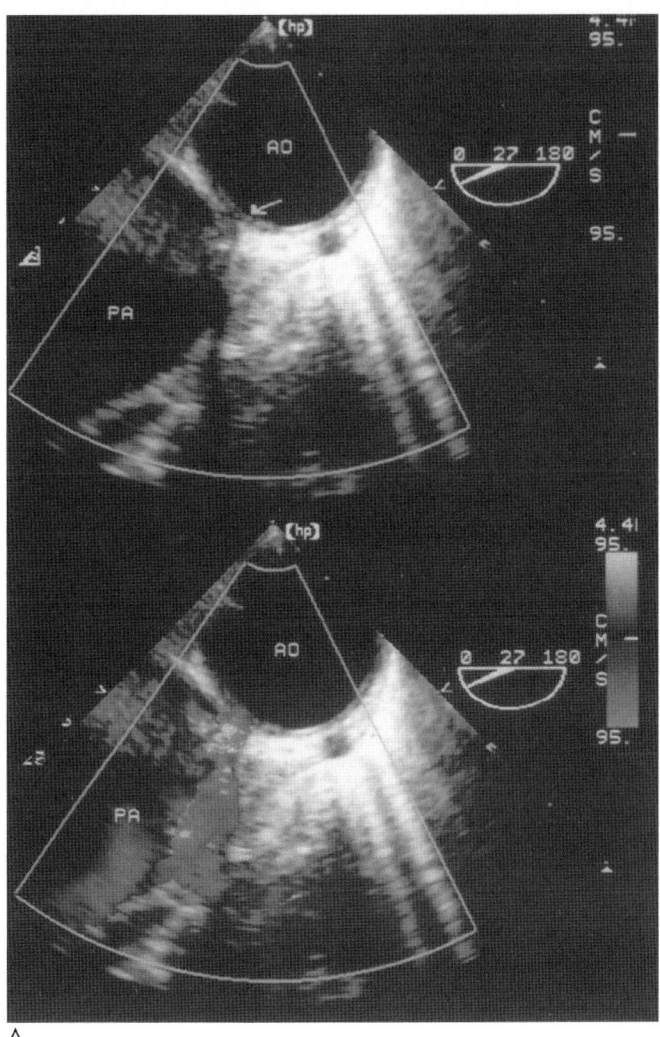

FIGURE 16–115. A. Transesophageal image of a patent ductus arteriosus (PDA). The upper panel shows a small communication (*arrow*) between the Ao and PA, which is confirmed with color-flow Doppler imaging (*lower panel*). **B.** Parasternal short-axis images at the AoV level. Color imaging reveals diastolic flow within the PA (*arrow*), consistent with a patent ductus arteriosus. Mild pulmonary regurgitation is also present. Ao, aorta; AoV, aortic valve; LA, left atrium; PA, pulmonary artery; RVOT, right ventricular outflow tract.

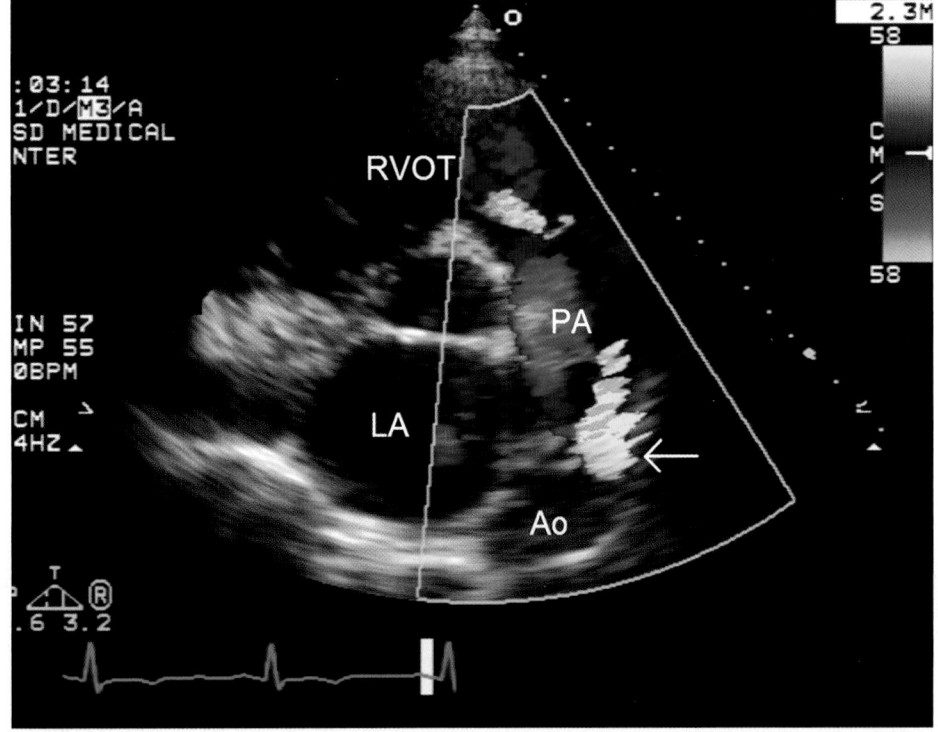

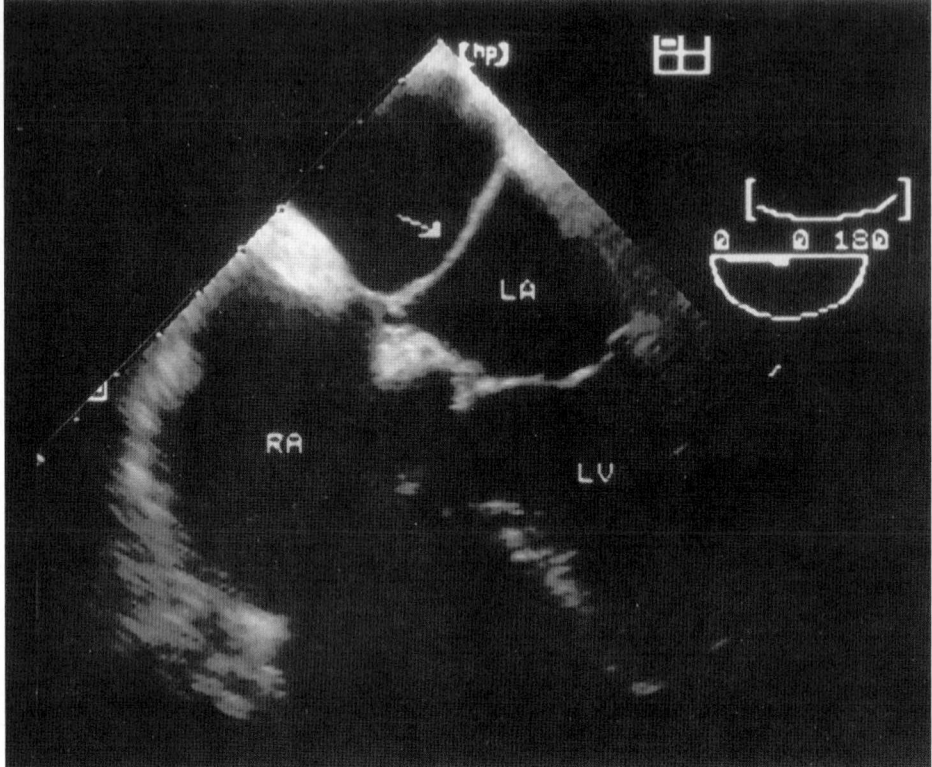

FIGURE 16–116. Transverse transesophageal image of cor triatriatum. A membrane (*arrow*) is present in the left atrium. LA, left atrium; LV, left ventricle; RA, right atrium.

well visualized in the parasternal long-axis view, whereas the RVOT and proximal PA are best seen in the parasternal short-axis view at the base of the heart. Doppler interrogation can provide evaluation of the severity of pulmonic stenosis, before and after surgery. Echocardiography may aid detection of infants with tetralogy who will require early surgical intervention. Although *double-outlet RV* (DORV) shares several clinical characteristics with tetralogy of Fallot—VSD and anterior aortic displacement are invariably present, and pulmonic valvular stenosis and ASD are common in both—it is morphologically distinct. Normal continuity of the posterior aortic wall with the anterior MV leaflet (always present in tetralogy of Fallot) is absent in DORV, and an interposed mass of fibrous tissue between the LA and the nearest great vessel is seen on 2D imaging. In addition, the great vessels may be transposed in DORV, resulting in a characteristic side-by-side appearance of the aorta and PA on parasternal short-axis images.

echocardiographic features include a large perimembranous VSD, an anteriorly displaced aorta that overrides the VSD, RV enlargement and dysfunction, and pulmonic stenosis (either infundibular, valvular, or supravalvular) (Fig. 16–118).[138] The VSD and aorta are

Echocardiography has become a valuable tool for the detection, management, and postoperative followup of patients with *transposition of the great arteries* (see Chap. 82). In D-transposition, the aorta arises from the RV, the PA arises from the LV, and one or more obligatory shunts are present. With L-transposition, the morphologic

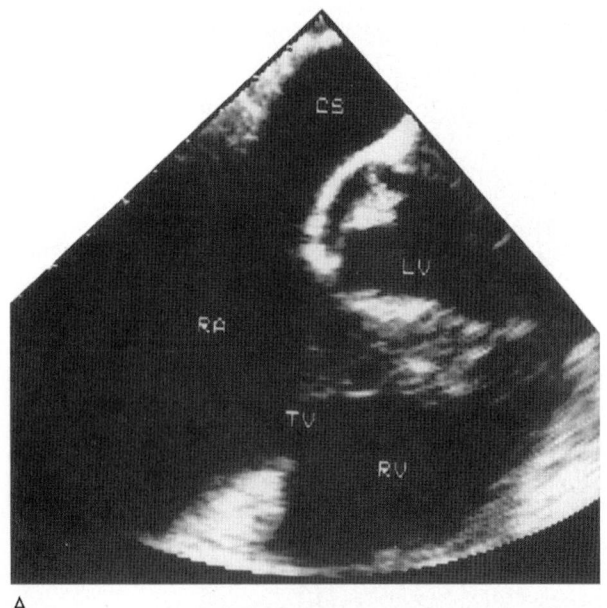

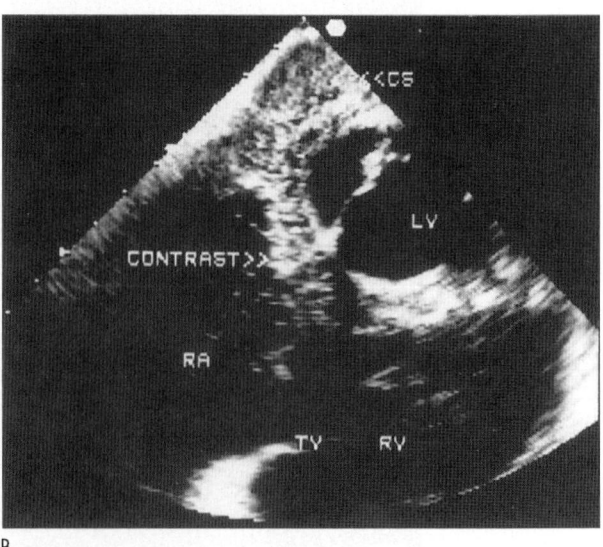

FIGURE 16–117. A. Transesophageal image (transverse plane) from a patient with persistent left superior vena cava. The coronary sinus (*CS*) is dilated. **B.** After injection of agitated saline into the left antecubital vein, contrast is seen entering the right atrium (*RA*) via the *CS*. LV, left ventricle; RV, right ventricle; TV, tricuspid valve. **C.** Transthoracic parasternal long-axis image of persistent left superior vena cava. The coronary sinus is dilated. *Source: B, from Blanchard DG, DeMaria AN. Cardiac and extracardiac masses: echocardiographic evaluation. In: Skorton DJ, Schelbert HR, Wolf GL, Brundage BH, eds. Marcus' Cardiac Imaging, 2nd ed. Philadelphia: Saunders; 1996:452–480. With permission.*

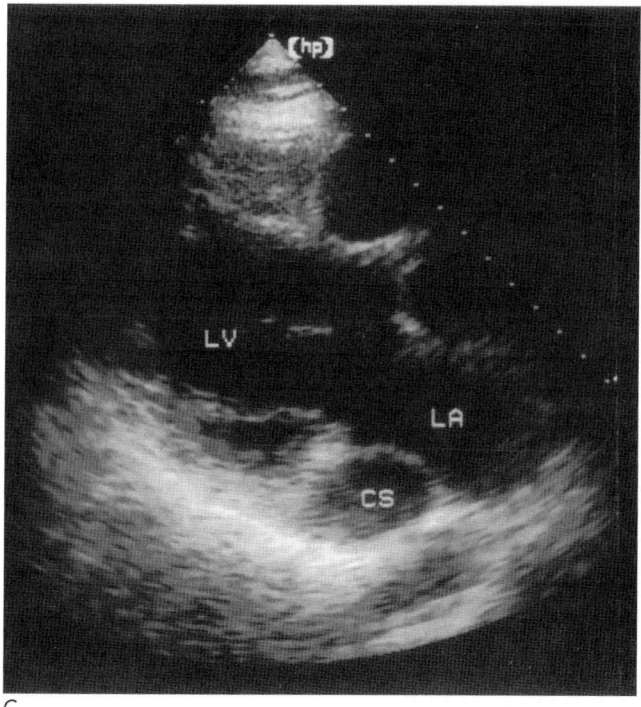

C

FIGURE 16–117. *(continued)*

right and left ventricles are switched, and associated anomalies such as VSD and pulmonic stenosis are common. In both types of transposition, the normal echocardiographic orientation of the great vessels on parasternal short-axis images (a sausage-shaped RVOT and PA draped over a circular aorta) is no longer present, and the two great vessels are typically side by side and parallel (Fig. 16–119 and Fig. 16–120). In general, the aorta is anterior and to the right of the PA in D-transposition and anterior and to the left in L-transposition. Apical displacement of the tricuspid annulus is an important sign that helps define the anatomic position of the

morphologic right ventricle. Both TTE and TEE are an important part of continuing care after surgical repair or palliation of transposition (see Fig. 16–120).[139]

Truncus arteriosus is a rare anomaly characterized by a large VSD, a single semilunar valve, and a single great vessel that divides into the ascending aorta and PA. Ultrasound imaging can determine the anatomy of the great vessels and assist in defining the various subsets of truncus arteriosus.

Coarctation of the aorta (see Chap. 82) is associated with a bicuspid AoV and is best visualized from the suprasternal position. 2D imaging may identify the site of coarctation. Clear visualization of narrowing in the proximal descending aorta with poststenotic dilatation, however, is *pathognomonic of coarctation.*[140] Doppler interrogation from the suprasternal notch demonstrates increased systolic velocity in the descending aorta and may also reveal a persistent flow gradient throughout diastole in cases of severe coarctation (Fig. 16–121A). Color imaging may display flow acceleration proximal to the site of coarctation and aliasing distal to it (see Fig. 16–121B). *Supravalvular AS,* either isolated or associated with Williams syndrome (see Chap. 12), is generally imaged best from the suprasternal and superior parasternal positions. Transesophageal imaging is also very helpful (Fig. 16–122E). Echocardiography reveals either an hourglass-shaped stenosis of the aorta above the sinuses of Valsalva, diffuse hypoplasia of the ascending aorta, or a focal fibrous ridge at the sinotubular junction (see Fig. 16–122E).

ABNORMALITIES OF THE VENTRICULAR OUTFLOW TRACTS AND SEMILUNAR VALVES

Right Ventricle

Infundibular stenosis is rare outside the setting of tetralogy of Fallot and is much less common than valvular PS. On 2D imaging, muscular hypertrophy is often visualized proximal to the PA, whereas

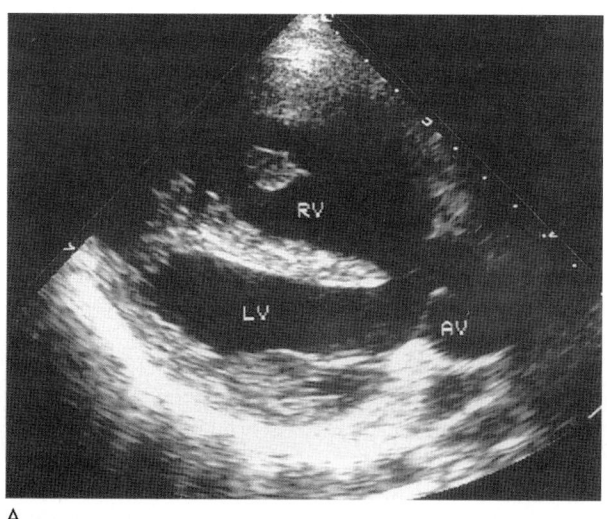

A

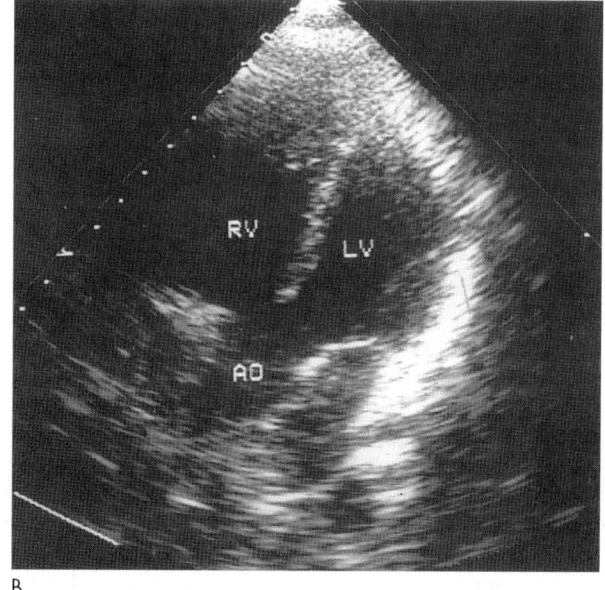

B

FIGURE 16–118. Parasternal long-axis (**A**) and apical four-chamber (**B**) images of tetralogy of Fallot. The right ventricle (*RV*) is enlarged, and a large VSD is present. The aorta (*Ao*) overrides the interventricular septum. LV, left ventricle. *Source: Courtesy of Reinaldo W. Beyer, MD.*

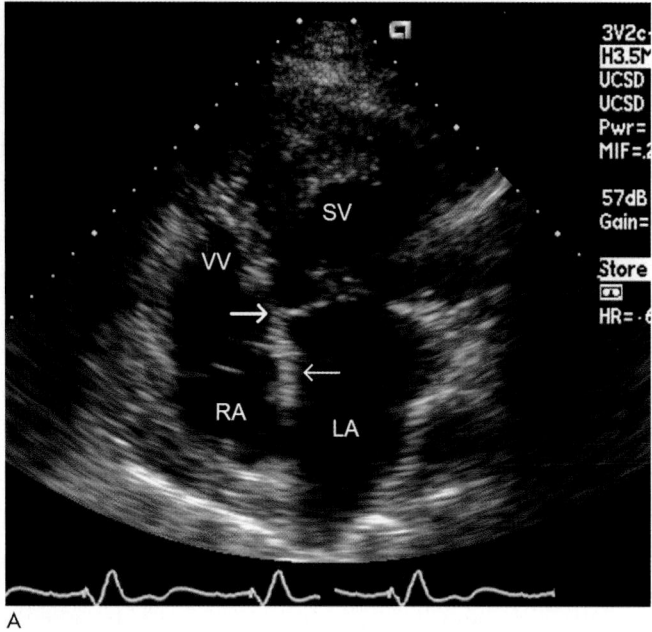

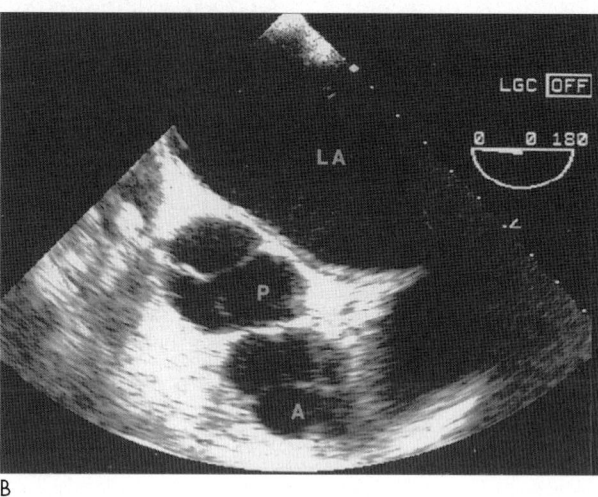

A   B

FIGURE 16–119. A. Apical 4-chamber image of ʟ-transposition (*congenitally corrected*). The morphologic *LV* and *RV* are inverted in position, whereas the atria remain intact. The bold arrow marks the annulus of the left-sided atrioventricular valve; the thin arrow marks the right-sided atrioventricular valve annulus. The left-sided annulus is displaced apically, identifying it as the tricuspid valve. Therefore, the systemic ventricle (*SV*) is a morphologic right ventricle, whereas the venous ventricle (*VV*) is a morphologic left ventricle. **B.** Transverse transesophageal image through the semilunar valves in ʟ-transposition. The aortic valve (*A*) is anterior and to the left of the pulmonic valve (*P*). LA, left atrium; LV, left ventricle; RV, right ventricle.

Doppler interrogation reveals increased flow velocities through the infundibulum. PS is reasonably common and may be either isolated or associated with other congenital lesions. Typical echocardiographic features include thickening of the leaflets, restricted leaflet motion, systolic doming of the valve, and elevated systolic flow velocity on Doppler (see Fig. 16–85). The PV is best visualized in the parasternal short-axis view through the base (or a modified parasternal view of the RVOT). In children, the subcostal position frequently provides excellent visualization of the RVOT and PV. TEE can provide detailed images of the PV. In pulmonic stenosis, the valve leaflets may calcify over time, and poststenotic dilatation of the PA (particularly the left) is often present.

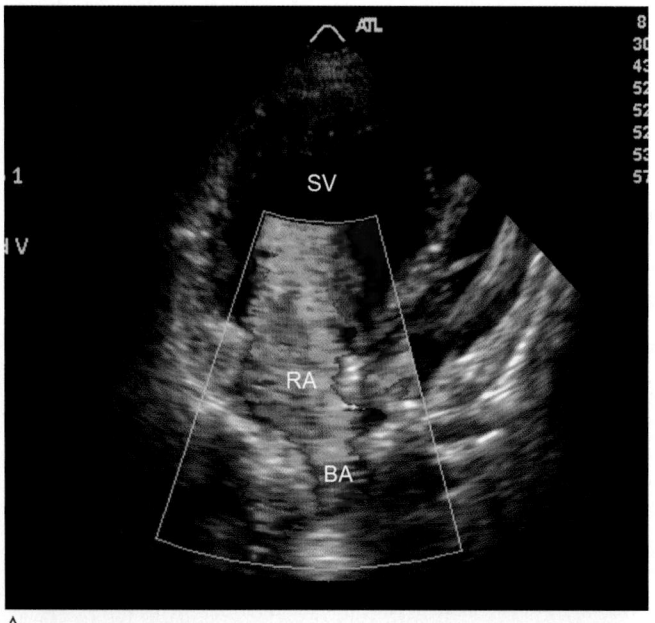

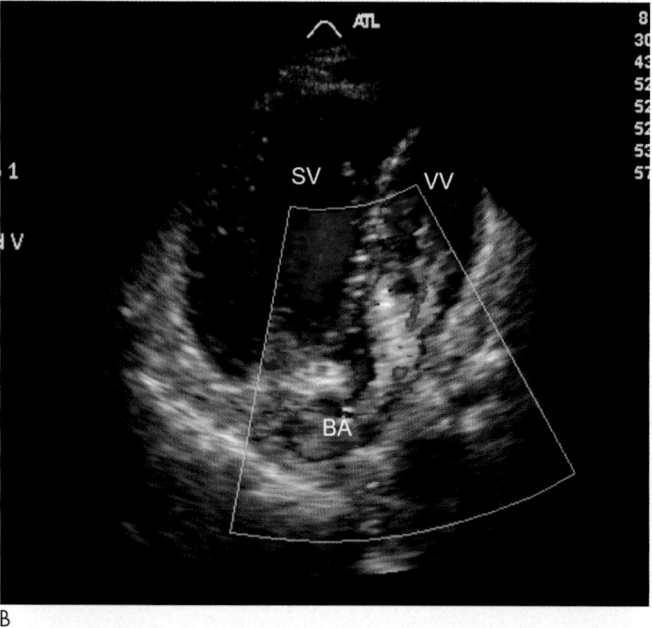

A   B

FIGURE 16–120. A. Modified apical image of ᴅ-transposition following baffle (Mustard) procedure. Pulmonary venous blood flows through a baffle (*BA*) to enter the right atrium (*RA*) and the systemic ventricle (*SV*), which is a morphologic right ventricle. The SV ejects into the aorta. There is no evidence of baffle stenosis. **B.** Modified apical image from the same patient showing vena caval blood flow through a BA into the left atrium and venous ventricle (*VV*), which is a morphologic left ventricle. The venous ventricle ejects into the pulmonary artery. Again, there is no evidence of baffle stenosis.

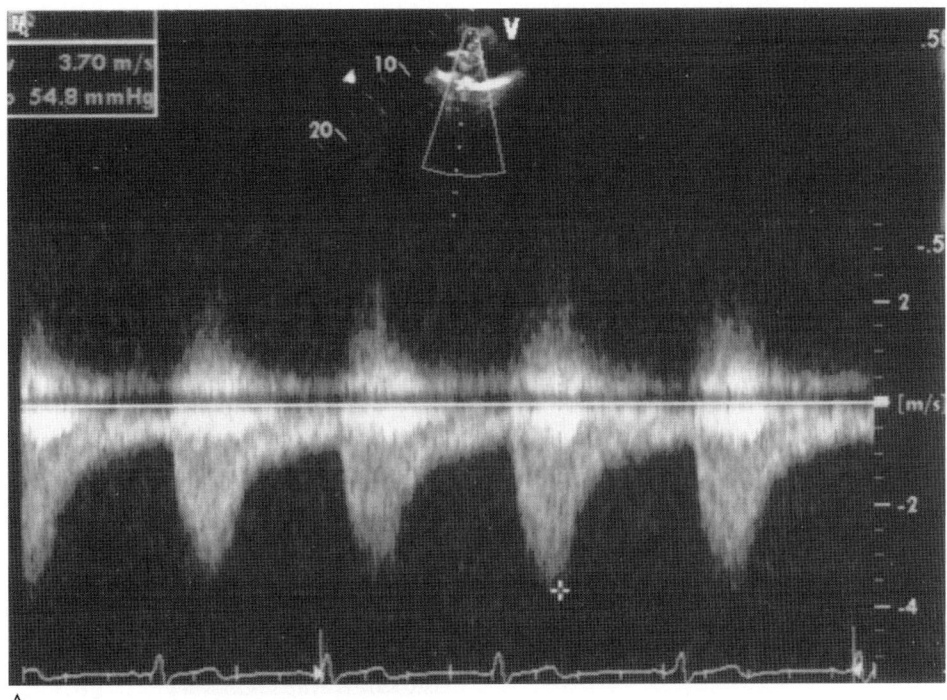

A

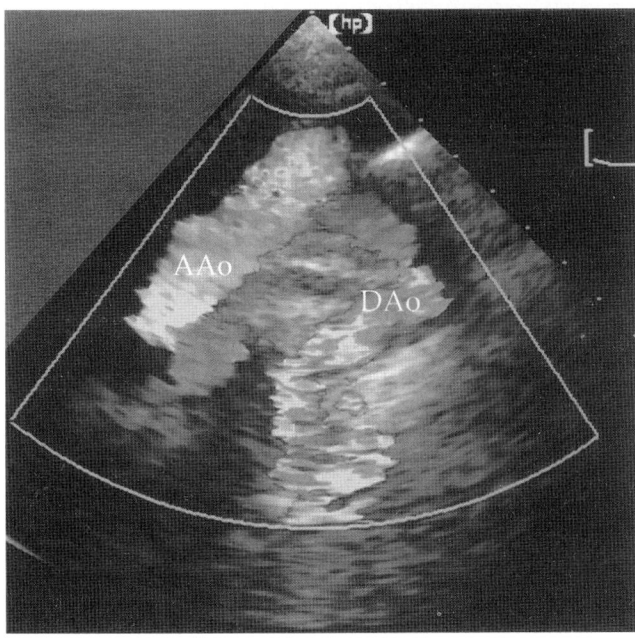

B

FIGURE 16–121. A. Continuous-wave Doppler tracing of the descending aorta (from the suprasternal position) in aortic coarctation. Peak systolic velocity is 3.7 m/sec, and there is persistent flow during diastole, suggesting severe coarctation. **B.** Suprasternal image of aortic coarctation. The descending aorta (*DAo*) is focally narrowed and tortuous, and turbulent (aliased) flow is present distal to the site of coarctation.

Left Ventricle

Subvalvular obstruction may be dynamic or fixed. HCM, which may present at any age, is discussed above. Discrete SAS may be caused by a thin membrane in the LVOT, a fibromuscular ridge, or diffuse muscular narrowing of the outflow tract (see Fig. 16–122A–D). 2D echocardiographic imaging can distinguish these various forms of discrete subvalvular stenosis, and Doppler analysis permits estimation of the systolic gradient. Color-flow imaging demonstrates increased turbulence in the LVOT as well as aortic valvular regurgitation in approximately 50 percent of cases (see Fig. 16–122D). Apical views are sometimes more useful for detecting thin subaor-

tic membranes. Subaortic fibromuscular ridges are sometimes associated with anomalous MV chordae connecting the papillary muscles or the anterior MV leaflet to the septum.

Bicuspid AoV is the most common congenital cardiac lesion in adults and is present in 1 to 2 percent of all individuals (see Chap. 82). Initially, eccentric diastolic coaptation of the aortic cusps was reported on M-mode in patients with bicuspid valves. However, M-mode findings are less accurate than 2D imaging, and the parasternal short-axis view is generally best for defining the fish-mouthed systolic aortic valvular anatomy (see Fig. 16–60 and Fig. 16–61). Bicuspid valves are best detected during systole. In equivocal cases, TEE is usually diagnostic (see Fig. 16–61).

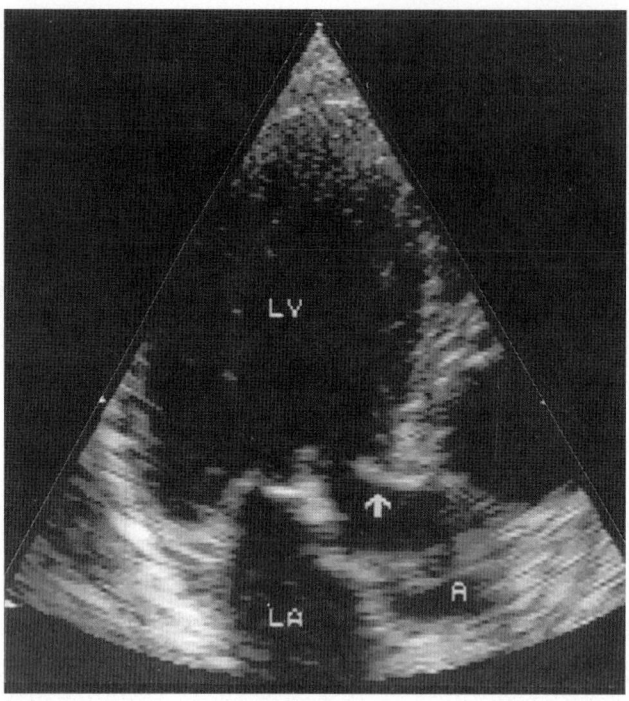

A

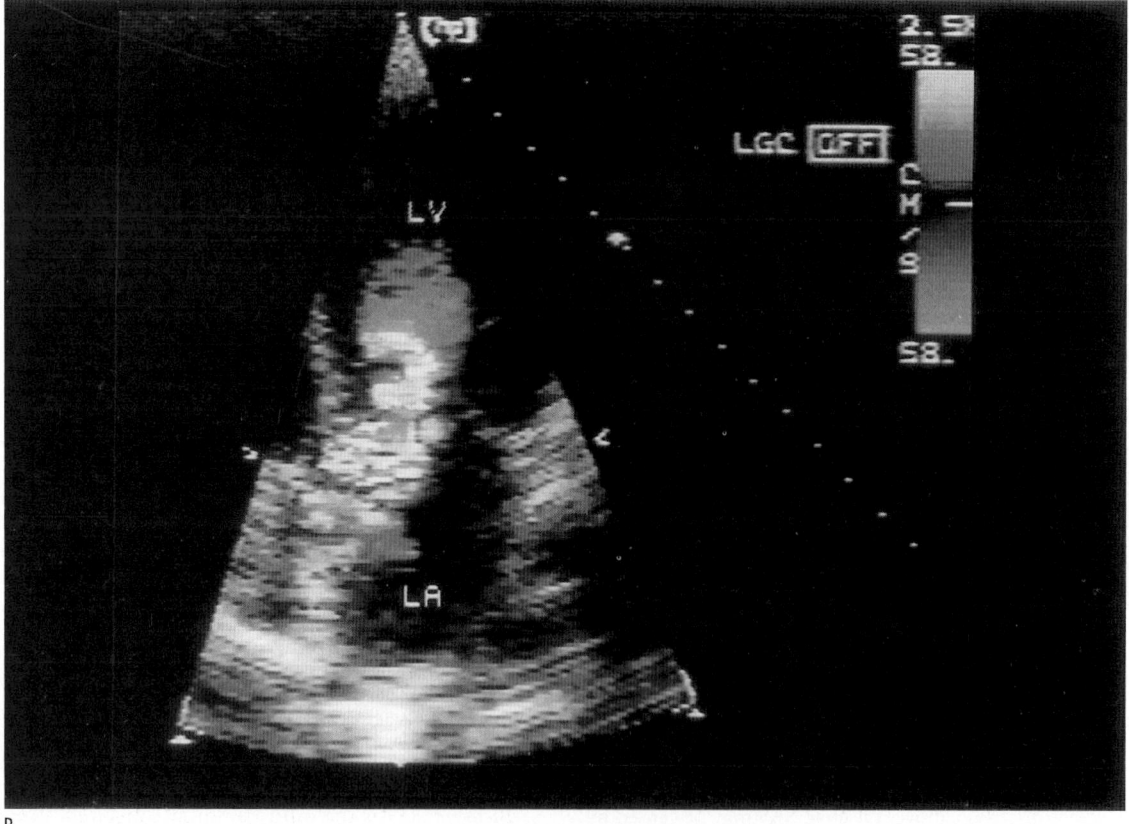

B

FIGURE 16-122. Subvalvular and supravalvular AS. **A.** Apical three-chamber view of discrete SAS. A fibromuscular ridge (*arrow*) is present in the left ventricular outflow tract. **B.** Apical five-chamber view of discrete SAS with color-flow Doppler, demonstrating aliasing and proximal flow convergence in the *LV* outflow tract. **C.** Transesophageal image of discrete SAS. A fibrous ridge in the outflow tract of the LV is present (*arrow*). **D.** Transesophageal image with color-flow Doppler, demonstrating mild aortic insufficiency associated with discrete SAS. **E.** Transesophageal image of supravalvular AS. A fibrous ridge extends into the aortic lumen just above the sinus of Valsalva. AO, aortic root; AS, aortic stenosis; LA, left atrium; LV, left ventricle; SAS, subaortic stenosis.

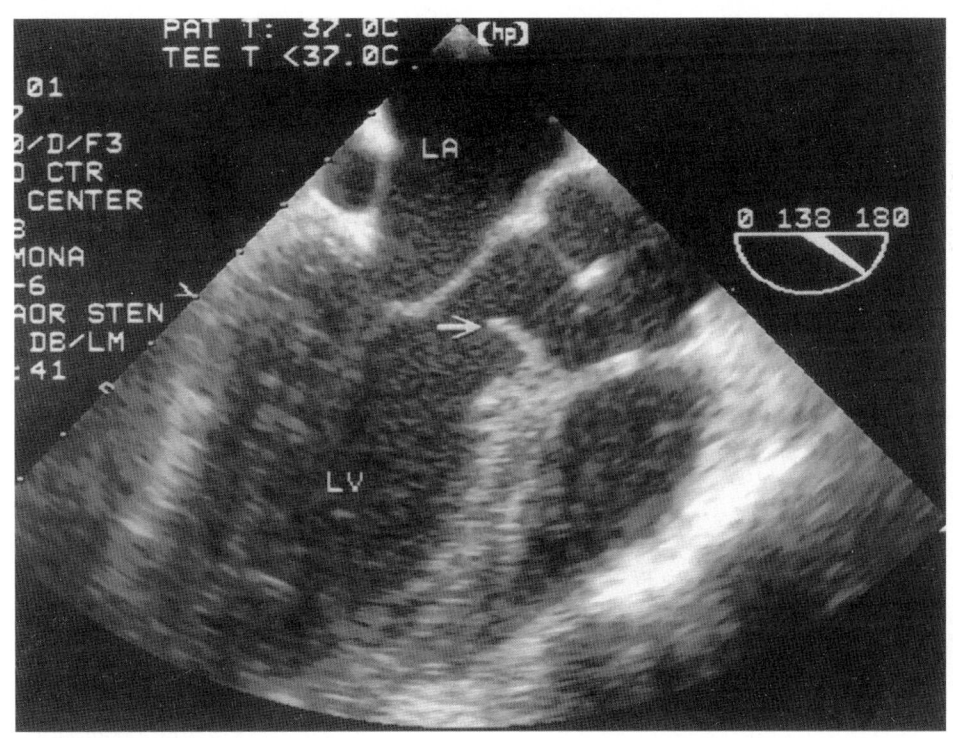

C

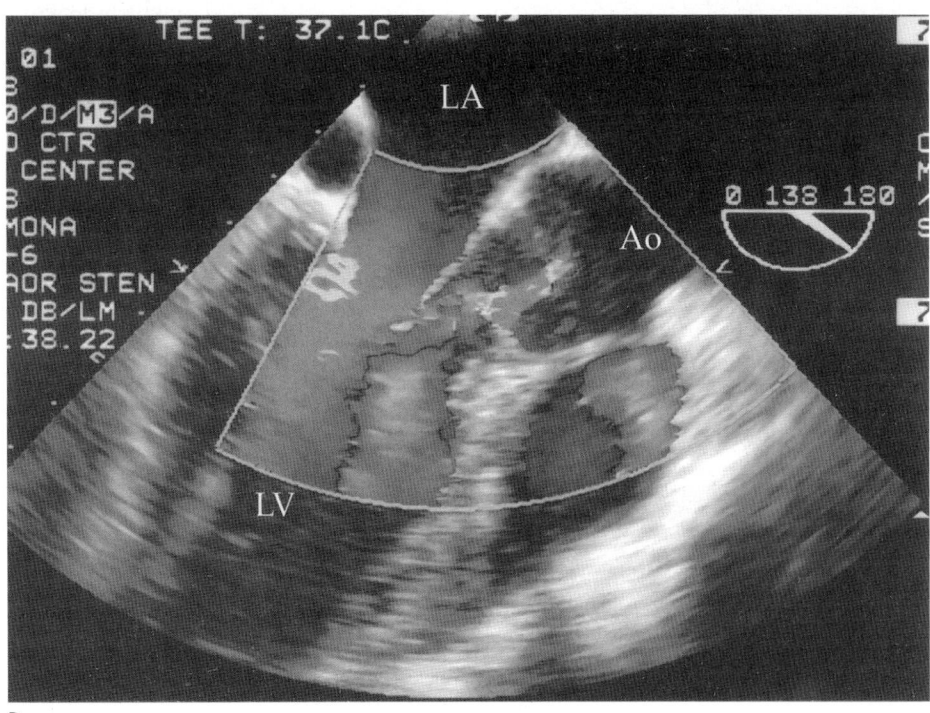

D

FIGURE 16–122. *(continued)*

【 】 ABNORMALITIES OF THE VENTRICULAR INFLOW TRACT

Ebstein anomaly is a congenital deformity of the TV in which the leaflets are displaced into the RV (see Chap. 82). Associated findings include TR, right atrial enlargement, and ASD. 2D imaging typically shows abnormal apical displacement of the septal leaflet insertion, with variable deformity of the leaflet (Fig. 16–123). The anterior leaflet originates from the tricuspid annulus but is elongated and often tethered to the RV free wall by abnormal chordal attachments. The tricuspid deformity and regurgitation are best visualized in the apical four-chamber view.[141]

Atrioventricular valvular atresia is usually accompanied by hypoplasia of the corresponding ventricle. Echocardiographic images of

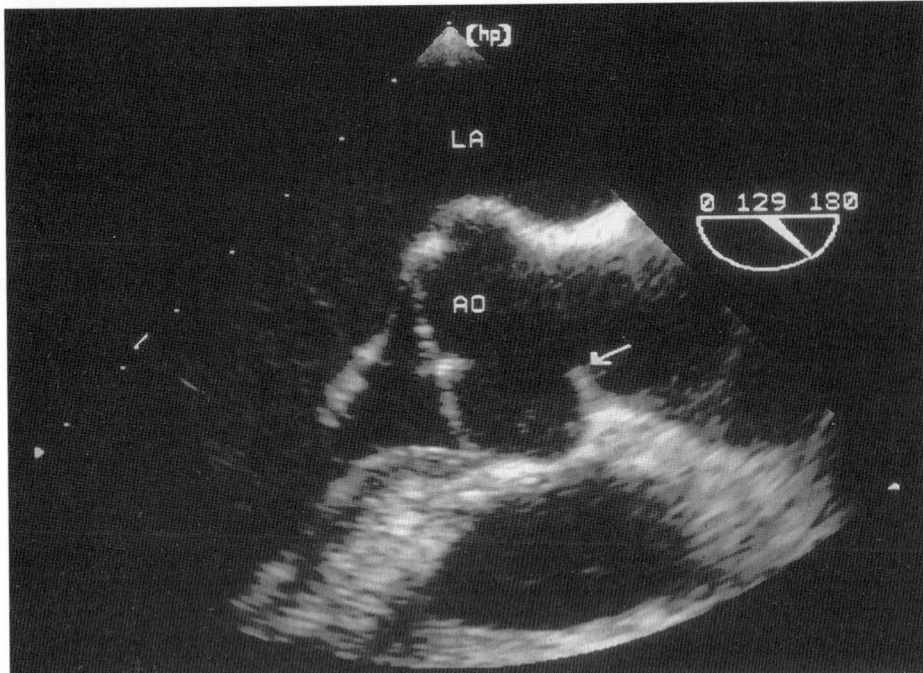

E

FIGURE 16–122. (continued)

tricuspid atresia characteristically show a small, nonfunctional RV, an interatrial communication of variable size, and a normally developed left ventricle. Echocardiography is an important tool in the management of patients with tricuspid atresia after palliation with the Fontan procedure.

[ ] FETAL ECHOCARDIOGRAPHY

The average risk for significant heart disease in the fetus is approximately 0.4 to 0.8 percent. Fetal echocardiography has evolved over the past 20 years into a sophisticated method for intrauterine detection of cardiac abnormalities (Fig. 16–124). The technique has been advocated for the preterm diagnosis of CHD, especially

in higher-risk cases. Fetal echocardiography has successfully identified a variety of congenital lesions.[142] Prenatal detection of these lesions may improve prognosis and guide therapy.

CARDIAC MASSES, THROMBI, AND TUMORS

[ ] NORMAL VARIANTS AND MASSES OF UNCERTAIN SIGNIFICANCE

When an abnormally localized accumulation of dense reflectances appears on the echocardiogram, it is said to represent a mass. Echocardiographic masses may be caused by technical artifacts or anomalous structures, but they are of greatest significance in representing true lesions of the heart such as tumors, thrombi, and vegetations. Echocardiography is the procedure of choice for the detection and evaluation of cardiac mass lesions and particularly helps delineate small lesions such as papillary fibroelastomas.

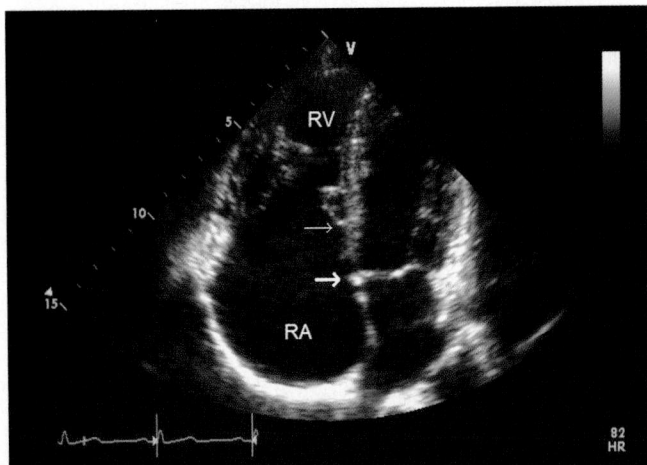

FIGURE 16–123. Ebstein anomaly, apical four-chamber view. The tricuspid valve annulus (*thin arrow*) is apically displaced in comparison to the mitral annulus (*thick arrow*). The right ventricle (*RV*) and right atrium (*RA*) are enlarged.

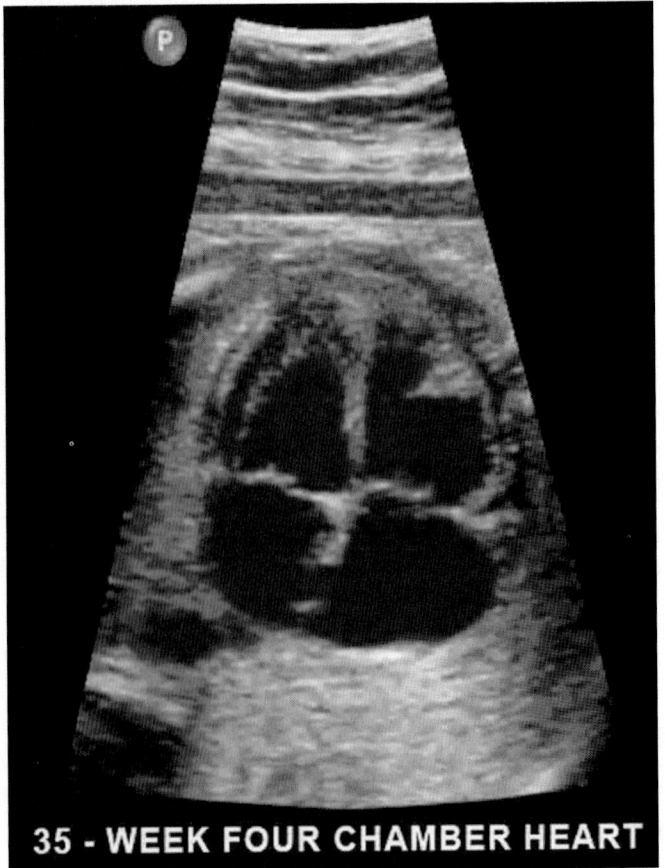

FIGURE 16–124. Fetal echocardiogram (four-chamber view, with left heart on the viewer's left).

A number of technical artifacts are capable of appearing as masses on echocardiogram. For example, side lobe signals, reverberations, and noise artifact may lead to accumulations of ultrasonic reflectance within the cavities or adjacent to the myocardium of the heart.[19,20] Such structures usually lack distinct borders, do not move appropriately through the cardiac cycle, lack identifiable attachments to endocardial surfaces, and cannot be visualized in all views and at all depth settings. In artifacts the absence of wall motion abnormalities is of particular value.[143]

Several benign normal variant findings can be observed during echocardiographic examination. Thus, many adults manifest persistence of the eustachian valve (Fig. 16–125), a thin ridge of tissue at the junction of the inferior vena cava and RA. The eustachian valve appears as a long, linear, freely mobile structure in the RA at the mouth of the inferior vena cava and is nearly always benign. An additional embryonic remnant that may be seen in the posterior RA is the Chiari network, which typically appears as a weblike mobile structure. In some individuals RVH may produce significant enlargement of the RV moderator band coursing along the interventricular septum to the apex of the RV. Similarly, false chordae tendineae ("heartstrings") can occasionally be visualized as linear structures spanning the LV cavity attached to endomyocardium at both ends (Fig. 16–126).

A variety of foreign bodies and iatrogenically induced anatomic alterations may be visualized on echocardiogram and must be distinguished from pathologic lesions. Intracardiac catheters, pacemaker leads (Fig. 16–127), prosthetic valves or patches, and atrial suture lines after cardiac transplantation can be visualized during echocardiographic examination. These structures are usually easily recognized because of the highly reflective properties of the foreign material, which result in bright echoes, reverberations, and shadowing behind the structures. Several morphologic changes involving the interatrial septum are often considered under the classification of cardiac mass lesions of uncertain significance. Aneurysms of the interatrial septum have been reported in approximately 1 percent of the population and are recognized on echocardiogram as a protrusion of the interatrial septum of at least 1.5 cm from its longitudinal plane dividing the left and RA (Fig. 16–128A). Interatrial septal aneurysms are often associated with a patent foramen ovale and have been implicated as a source of cardiogenic emboli.[144] Interatrial septal aneurysms may be detected by TTE, but they are more readily imaged by the transesophageal approach.[144] Lipomatous hypertrophy appears as a highly reflective thickening of the interatrial septum that typically spares the foramen ovale, thereby creating a characteristic dumbbell-shaped echocardiographic appearance (see Fig. 16–128B).

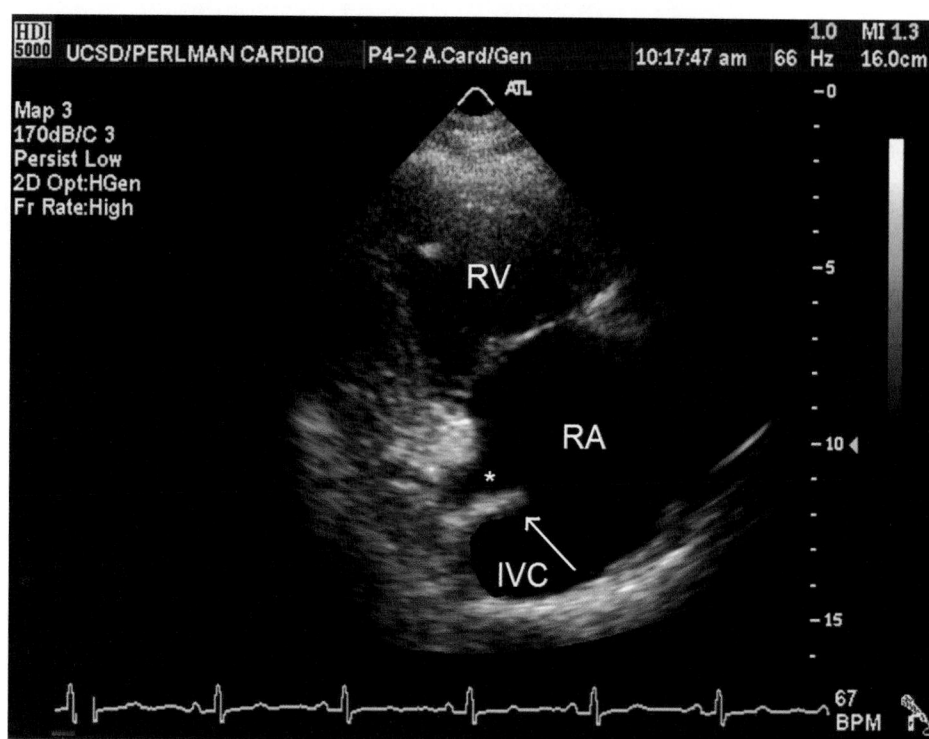

FIGURE 16–125. Right ventricular inflow view showing a prominent eustachian valve (*arrow*) at the junction of the inferior vena cava (*IVC*) and the right atrium (*RA*). Asterisk, ostium of the coronary sinus; RV, right ventricle.

【 】 INTRACARDIAC THROMBI

Intracardiac thrombi may be visualized in any chamber of the heart and frequently result in embolic events. The major predisposing factors to intracardiac thrombi include localized stasis of flow, low cardiac output, and cardiac injury. In addition, migration of venous thrombi may also result in intracardiac clots. The appearance of intracardiac thrombi may vary considerably. Thrombi typically have identifiable borders and may be layered and homogeneous or heterogeneous, with areas of central liquefaction (Fig. 16–129 and

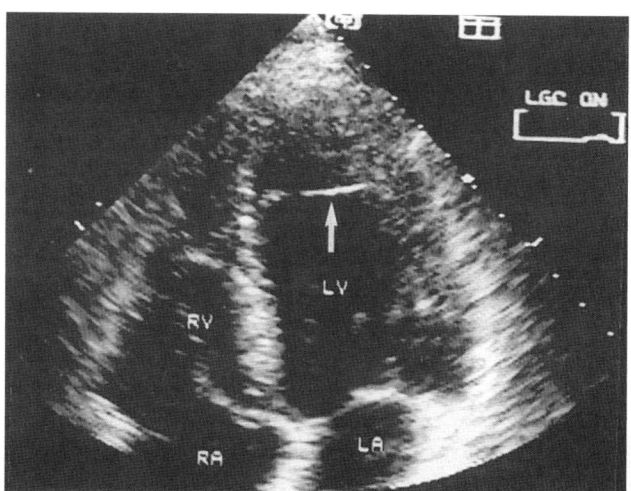

FIGURE 16–126. Apical four-chamber view demonstrating a false chord (*arrow*) within the left ventricle (*LV*). LA, left atrium; RA, right atrium; RV, right ventricle. *Source: From Blanchard DG, DeMaria AN. Cardiac and extracardiac masses: echocardiographic evaluation. In: Skorton DJ, Schelbert HR, Wolf GL, Brundage BH, eds. Marcus' Cardiac Imaging, 2nd ed. Philadelphia: Saunders; 1996:452–480. With permission.*

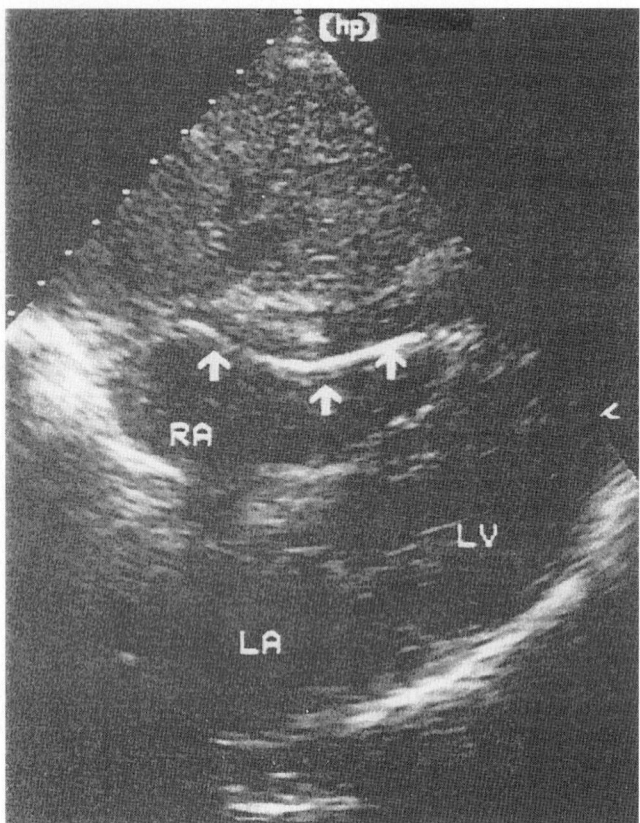

FIGURE 16–127. Subcostal four-chamber image demonstrating a pacemaker wire (*arrows*) in the right heart. LA, left atrium; LV, left ventricle; RA, right atrium.

Fig. 16–130). Contrast echocardiography may be of great value in delineating the presence of a thrombus, which cannot be visualized in the nonenhanced recording.

Right Heart

Thrombi within the right heart chambers may form locally or migrate from the venous circulation; they are found most commonly in the RA. As opposed to the laminar, relatively immobile nature of RA thrombi that form in situ, venous thromboemboli trapped in the RA tend to be serpentine and mobile. The potential for pulmonary embolism is high. Thrombi also can be seen within the main pulmonary arteries. RV thrombi are rare but may occur with RV infarction and endomyocardial fibrosis. Their appearance is similar to that of LV thrombi.

Left Atrium

Left atrial thrombi occur in the setting of low cardiac output, mitral valvular disease, atrial fibrillation, and LA enlargement. Both TTE and TEE can detect thrombi within the main cavity of the LA (Fig. 16–131A), but TEE is clearly superior for visualizing thrombi within the left atrial appendage. TEE is the diagnostic procedure of choice to detect this lesion. LA thrombi appear as discrete masses, either fixed or mobile, and are usually of homogeneous echo density (see Fig. 16–52). On TEE normal pectinate muscular ridges in the appendage must be distinguished from small thrombi. In addition, the left atrial appendage may occasionally be multilobed. Although this anatomic variant may be a risk factor for appendage

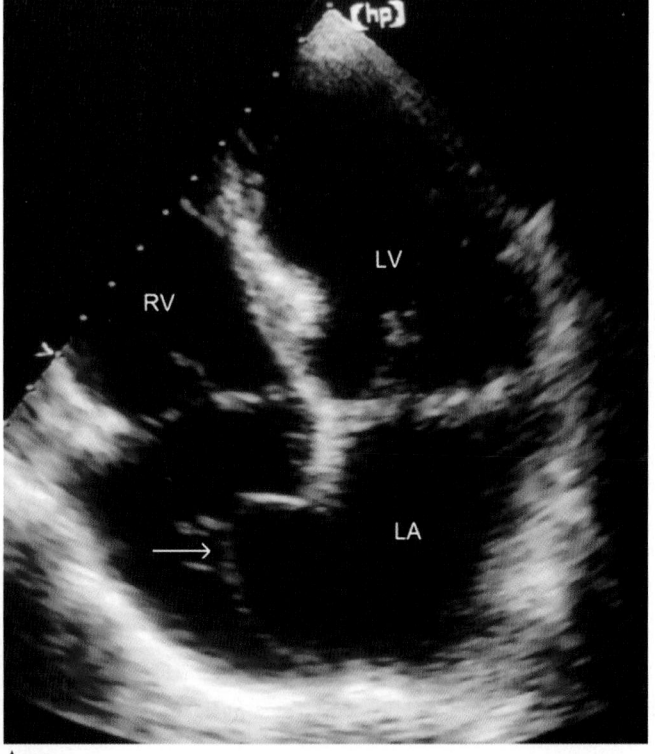

A

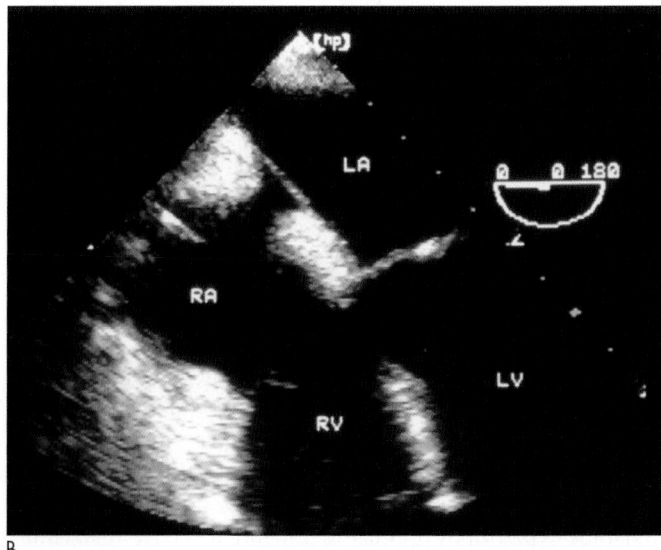

B

FIGURE 16–128. A. Apical 4-chamber image of a large interatrial septal aneurysm (arrow). **B.** Transesophageal image of lipomatous interatrial septal hypertrophy. The interatrial septum is markedly thickened, but the fossa ovalis is spared. LA, left atrium; LV, left ventricle; RA, right atrium; RV, right ventricle.

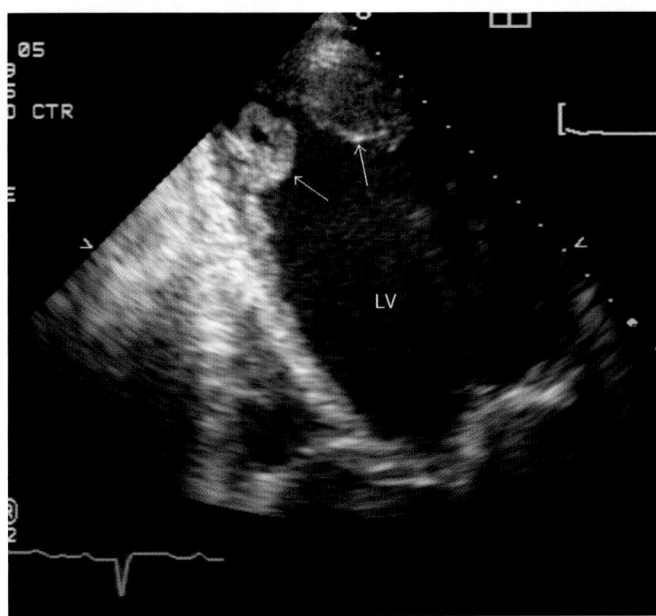

FIGURE 16–129. Magnified apical view demonstrating thrombi (*arrows*) in the apex of the left ventricle (*LV*).

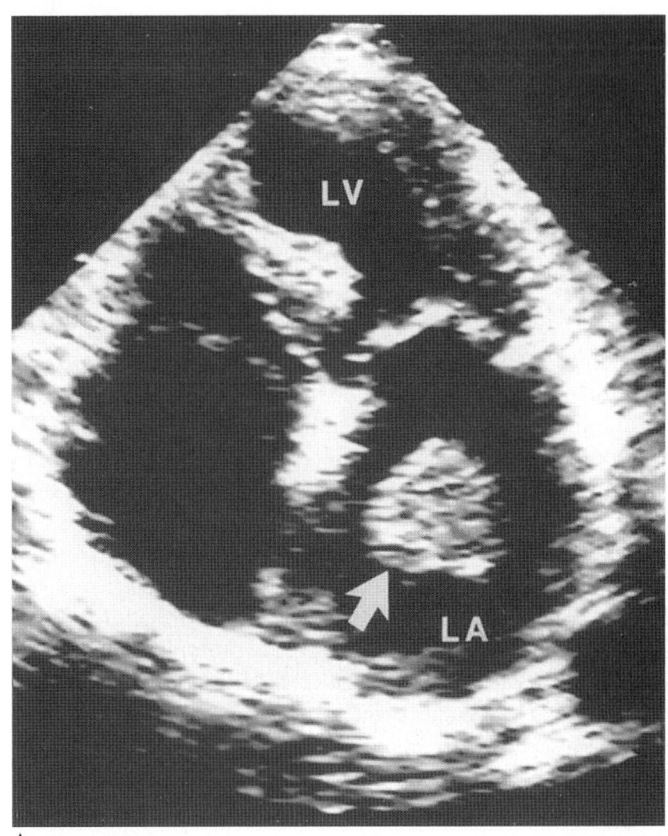

A

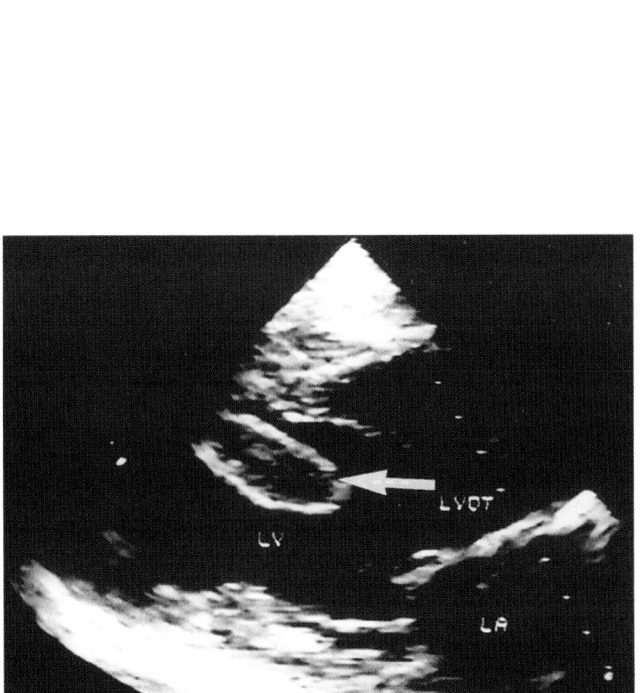

FIGURE 16–130. Parasternal long-axis view of a large mobile thrombus (*arrow*) attached to the anteroseptal segment of the left ventricle (*LV*). LA, left atrium; LVOT, left ventricular outflow tract. *Source: From Blanchard DG, DeMaria AN. Cardiac and extracardiac masses: echocardiographic evaluation. In: Skorton DJ, Schelbert HR, Wolf GL, Brundage BH, eds. Marcus' Cardiac Imaging, 2nd ed. Philadelphia: Saunders; 1996:452–480. With permission.*

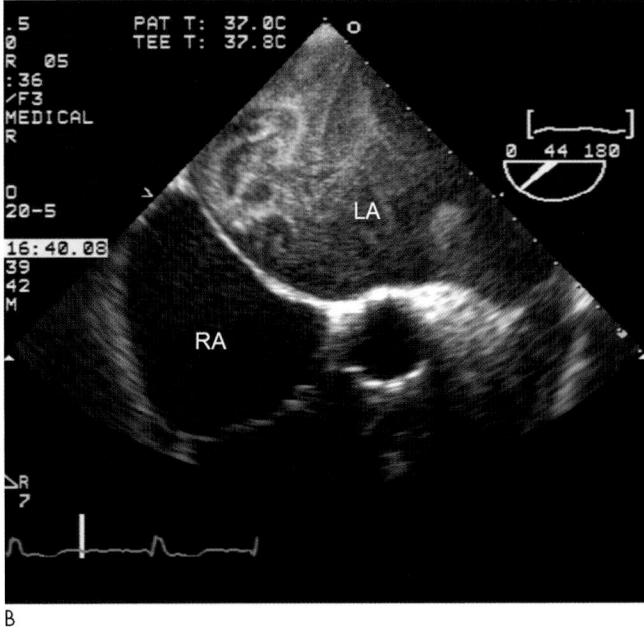

B

FIGURE 16–131. A. Apical four-chamber image of a large mobile *ball* thrombus (*arrow*) in the left atrium (*LA*). **B.** Transesophageal image of spontaneous echo contrast (*smoke*) seen in an enlarged *LA*. The spontaneous contrast swirled on real-time imaging. LV, left ventricle; RA, right atrium. *Source: A, from Blanchard DG, DeMaria AN. Cardiac and extracardiac masses: echocardiographic evaluation. In: Skorton DJ, Schelbert HR, Wolf GL, Brundage BH, eds. Marcus' Cardiac Imaging, 2nd ed. Philadelphia: Saunders; 1996:452–480. With permission.*

thrombi, the atrial tissue separating the lobes should not be mistaken for clot. Left atrial thrombi are often accompanied by spontaneous echo contrast (or *smoke*) within the LA. This finding indicates stagnant blood flow. Left atrial spontaneous echo contrast, like LA thrombus, has been associated with embolic events[145] and may be a marker of regional prothrombotic activity (see Fig. 16–131B). On 2D imaging, the contrast signals are in constant motion and can be missed if gain settings are inappropriately low.

Left Ventricle

Most LV thrombi occur in settings of abnormal systolic contraction (dilated cardiomyopathy, AMI, and chronic LV aneurysm). LV thrombi have been reported in up to one-half of patients with large MIs and occur more frequently in anterior infarctions (up to 30 to 40 percent of such patients). Most thrombi are located in the apex and thus are best visualized in the apical views (see Fig. 16–129). Although echocardiography is the procedure of choice for detecting LV thrombi, the technique's true sensitivity and specificity remains uncertain.

LV thrombi may be laminar and fixed or protruding and mobile, and they may have a heterogeneous echo density (see Fig. 16–129 and Fig. 16–130). Studies suggest that *immature* thrombi are often filamentous, with irregular borders, whereas older thrombi tend to be echodense and fixed.[143] The echocardiographic characteristics of thrombi may influence the risk of cardiogenic embolization, because irregularly shaped, mobile, and protruding thrombi are more likely to embolize than laminar, immobile clots. True LV thrombi have a density distinct from the underlying myocardium, appear in multiple imaging planes, and move concordantly with the underlying myocardium.

CARDIAC TUMORS

Although diagnosed infrequently, cardiac tumors often are included in the differential diagnosis of cardiac problems because of their protean clinical manifestations (see Chap. 89). Cardiac tumors may be intracavitary or intramural, and the location determines their echocardiographic appearance. Intracavitary tumors appear as sessile or mobile echo densities attached to the mural endocardium, whereas intramural tumors appear as localized thickening of the LV wall. The pericardium also may be involved with cardiac tumors, with or without the presence of concomitant effusion (see Chap. 89).

【 】 MYXOMAS

Myxomas are the most common primary cardiac tumors, accounting for approximately 25 percent of all such lesions (see Chap. 89).[146] Myxomas can occur in any cardiac chamber, but 75 percent are found in the LA.[146] On 2D imaging, myxomas usually appear as gelatinous, speckled, sometimes globular masses with frond-like projections (Fig. 16–132A and B). Tissue heterogeneity is common, but calcification is rare. Myxomas are usually attached to the endocardial surface by a pedicle. Typically, they are attached to the interatrial septum. Large tumors are almost always mobile to some degree, and a sizable left atrial mass that appears fixed in

position is therefore less likely to be a myxoma. Large left atrial myxomas may move back and forth into the MV annulus during the cardiac cycle, entering the orifice in diastole and the LA in systole. Accordingly, Doppler interrogation may demonstrate either obstruction of flow, valvular regurgitation, or both. Most myxomas are visible on TTE, but TEE is superior for the delineation of tumor attachments and detection of small myxomas. Recently, it has been shown that contrast injection will intensify the signals from tumors, but not from thrombi, enabling the differential diagnosis.[147] Because approximately 5 percent of myxomas are biatrial, careful evaluation of the RA is mandatory.[146]

【 】 ADDITIONAL PRIMARY TUMORS

Benign

Rhabdomyomas are rare cardiac tumors associated with tuberous sclerosis (see Chap. 89). There is a strong tendency for multiple tumors to occur within an affected heart (90 percent of cases). Fibromas are found most often in children and affect the left ventricle most frequently. The tumor may grow within the myocardium rather than expanding into a cardiac chamber. Papillary fibroelastomas are usually quite small in size (<1 cm in diameter) and often grow on cardiac valves or chordae (Fig. 16–133A). Echocardiographic differentiation from vegetations can be difficult.

Malignant

Primary malignant cardiac tumors are quite rare and confer a very poor prognosis (see Chap. 89). Angiosarcoma is the most common and occurs most often in the RA (see Fig. 16–133B). Rhabdomyosarcoma is an additional primary cardiac malignancy. Echocardiography can be useful in monitoring response to therapy: Its diagnostic utility is limited as most findings are nonspecific.

【 】 METASTATIC AND SECONDARY TUMORS OF THE HEART AND PERICARDIUM

Metastatic tumors to the pericardium and heart occur 20 to 40 times more often than primary cardiac tumors (see Chap. 89, Fig. 16–134A). Tumors that commonly involve the heart and pericardium include breast and lung carcinoma, melanoma, and lymphoma (see Fig. 16–134B and C). In these cases the tumor is often visible in the inferior vena cava and RA. Pericardial effusion is the most common echocardiographic manifestation in patients with cardiac metastases. Intracavitary and pericardial masses are easily visualized with 2D imaging, but intramural tumors are sometimes difficult to image. Echocardiographic findings are nonspecific, and metastatic tumors may be mistaken for primary cardiac neoplasms, vegetations, thrombi, or even prominent muscular trabeculations (see Chap. 89).

【 】 ADDITIONAL CARDIAC MASSES

The heart is rarely involved in echinococcal disease (<2 percent of cases), but intracardiac or intrapericardial rupture of a cyst can lead to anaphylaxis and cardiac tamponade, respectively. Echocar-

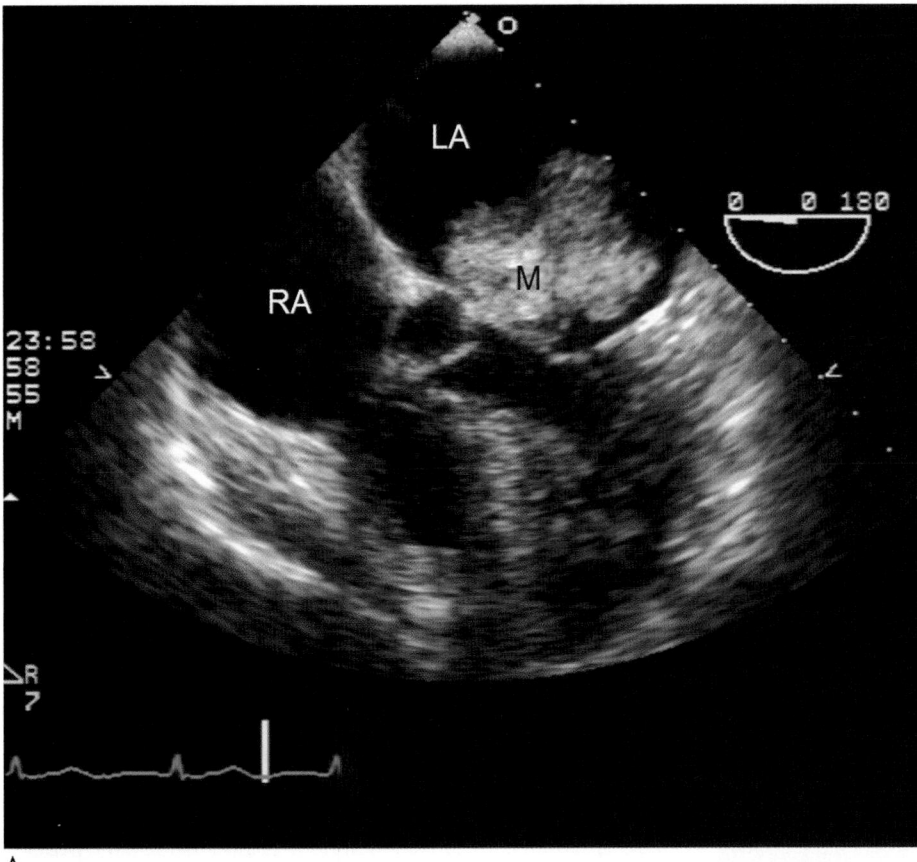

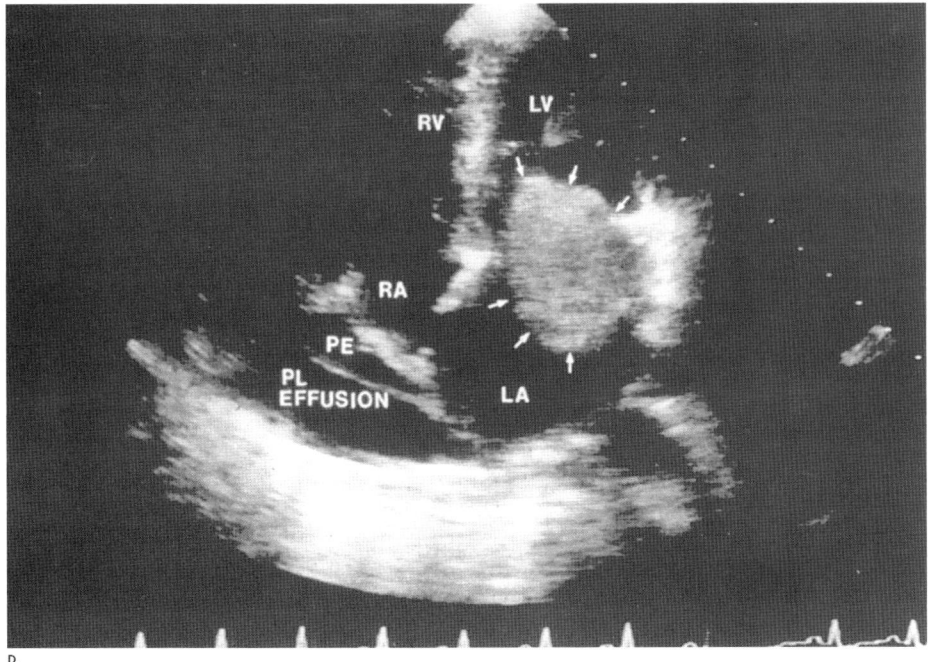

FIGURE 16–132. A. Transesophageal image of a large myxoma (*M*) in the left atrium (*LA*). **B.** Apical four-chamber image of a large left atrial myxoma (*arrows*), which is attached to the lateral wall of the atrium. LV, left ventricle; PE, pericardial effusion; PL, pleural; RA, right atrium; RV, right ventricle.

diographic detection of a multiseptated cyst in the left ventricle or interventricular septum suggests cardiac echinococcal disease. Simple pericardial cysts usually occur in the right costophrenic angle (posterior to the RA) and have a benign prognosis. The struc-

tures are nonseptated and fluid filled; they do not compress the cardiac chambers.[148]

Pericardial Disease

In normal subjects the pericardium is difficult to visualize because the pericardial cavity is only a potential space, and visceral and parietal pericardial layers appear as a single echo (see Chap. 84). In pericardial effusion, the fluid appears as a sonolucent area (or clear space) separating epicardium from pericardium. Pericarditis unaccompanied by pericardial effusion may be undetectable by echocardiography. Therefore, the evaluation of constrictive pericarditis by echocardiography primarily involves Doppler flow recordings.[149]

Pericardial Effusion

Echocardiography is the diagnostic procedure of choice for detection of pericardial fluid (Fig. 16–135), and early M-mode studies demonstrated that volumes as small as 20 to 30 mL could be detected reliably.[149] A sonolucent area between the epicardium and pericardium is diagnostic of a pericardial effusion. Although epicardial-pericardial separation may be seen during systole in normal cases, separation throughout the cardiac cycle is abnormal.

Echocardiography can be used to identify pericardial loculations, fibrous strands, and pericardial tumors as well as to assess the size of effusions (Fig. 16–136). Pericardial effusions may be concentric or loculated. Pericardial tissue reflects on itself behind the LA between the pulmonary veins (the oblique sinus), and fluid is rarely seen in this area. Small, nonloculated effusions may move depending on patient position and thus are often drawn posteriorly and inferiorly by gravity during routine imaging. A rim of pericardial fluid surrounding the heart is evidence of a moderate or large effusion, and the heart can sometimes be seen *swinging* back and forth within the pericardial space, creating the mechanism of *electrical alternans*. In general, small effusions are seen posteriorly rather than anteriorly on supine imaging. Moderate-sized (100–500 mL) nonloculated effusions are present both anterior and posterior to the heart. Large nonloculated effusions (>500 mL) are circumferential and frequently allow free motion of the heart within the fluid-filled space.

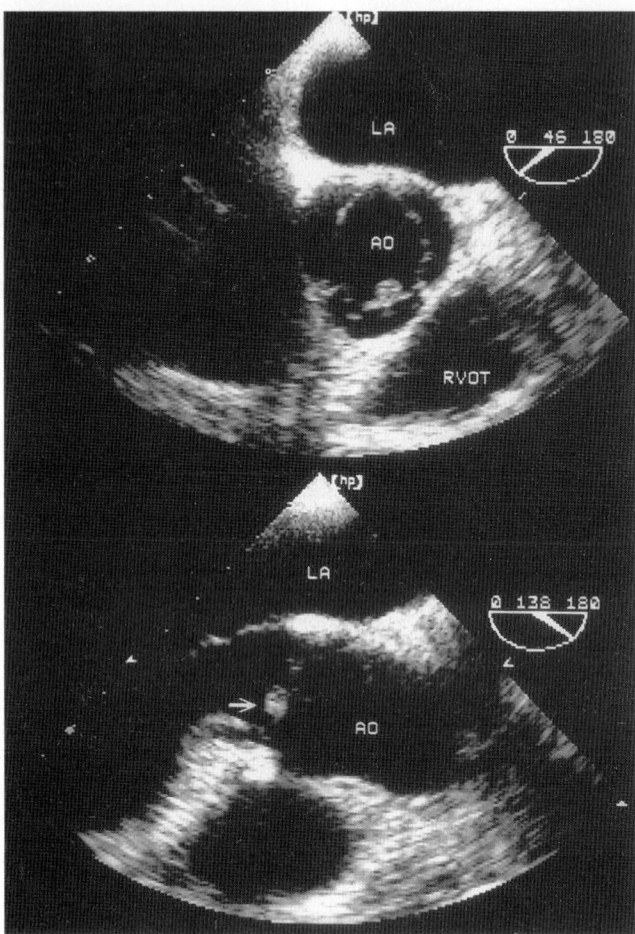

A

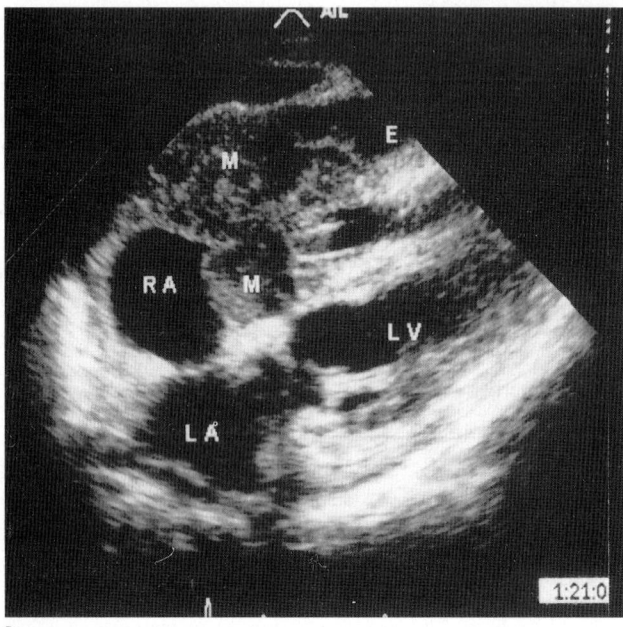

B

FIGURE 16–133. A. Transesophageal images of a surgically proven papillary fibroelastoma on the right coronary cusp of the AoV (*arrow*). The upper and lower panels show transverse and longitudinal planes through the AoV, respectively. **B.** Primary cardiac angiosarcoma (subcostal imaging plane). The tumor mass (*M*) is present in the right atrium (*RA*), and has extended through the atrial wall into the pericardial space. AoV, aortic valve; E, pericardial effusion; LA, left atrium; LV, left ventricle.

Distinguishing between pericardial and pleural effusions is occasionally difficult with echocardiography. If these conditions coexist, the pericardium usually can be identified as a linear density separating fluid in the two spaces. The parasternal long-axis view is often helpful in differentiating the disorders. The descending aorta is a mediastinal structure; therefore, pericardial effusions will often separate the heart and descending aorta, whereas pleural effusions are seen inferior and posterior to the aorta (Fig. 16–137). In cases of large pleural effusions, atelectatic lung tissue also may be present (see Fig. 16–137). Subcostal views are often valuable and may yield the only satisfactory transthoracic images in postoperative or posttraumatic cases. The inferior vena cava also can be imaged in this view; if the vessel does not display inspiratory collapse >50 percent of its maximum diameter, elevated RA pressure is present.

On parasternal images, an echolucent space is sometimes visualized anterior to the RV. Although this finding may represent pericardial fluid, it usually is caused by epicardial fat (without effusion) and has no pathologic significance.

【 】 CARDIAC TAMPONADE

Because the pericardium is a relatively noncompliant membrane that adapts slowly to volume changes, pericardial effusions (especially those that accumulate rapidly) may limit cardiac filling and cause cardiac tamponade. Echocardiography can help diagnose this condition by detecting morphologic signs of increased intrapericardial pressure as well as abnormal intracardiac flow patterns caused by tamponade and enhanced ventricular interdependence.

Because diastolic pressures are slightly lower in the right heart than the left, the RA and RV are usually the first chambers to exhibit evidence of increased intrapericardial pressure. High intrapericardial pressure can cause compression or collapse of right heart chambers. Invagination of the right atrial wall during atrial systole is a sensitive (but not specific) sign of tamponade (Fig. 16–138). Diastolic collapse or *buckling* of the RV free wall is a more specific sign of tamponade and can be visualized both on 2D and M-mode imaging (see Fig. 16–135B and C).

Doppler echocardiographic recordings in patients with tamponade have demonstrated an enhancement or exaggeration of the normal respiratory variation in ventricular inflow and outflow. Thus, transmitral and LVOT velocities decrease significantly with inspiration, most likely because of enhanced ventricular interdependence and a marked decrease in the transmitral diastolic gradient during inspiration (Fig. 16–139). The latter is caused both by high intrapericardial pressure as well as leftward motion of the interventricular septum from increased RV filling. Studies have also indicated that when echocardiography is used to direct pericardiocentesis to the site of greatest fluid accumulation, the risks associated with blind pericardial puncture are decreased.

【 】 CONSTRICTIVE PERICARDITIS

The diagnosis of constrictive pericarditis is sometimes difficult to establish, even by cardiac catheterization. 2D and M-mode echocardiography may provide evidence of thickened pericardial tissue by demonstrating increased reflectivity and multiple parallel moving echoes in the area of the pericardium (see Chap. 84). The criteria for pericardial thickening on echocardiogram are imperfect.

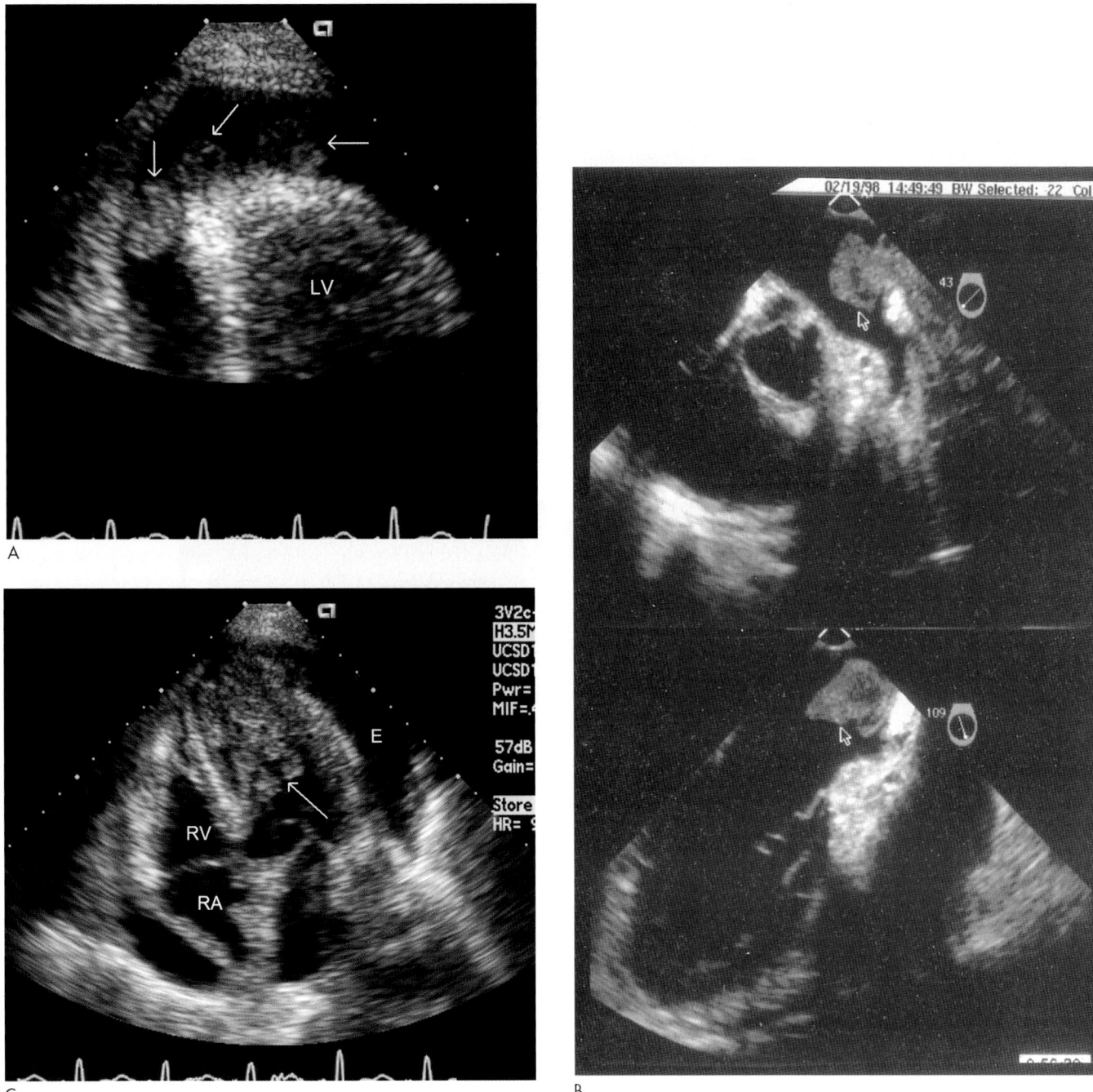

FIGURE 16–134. A. Magnified apical image showing several small metastatic tumors (*arrows*) on the epicardial surface. **B.** Transesophageal images from a case of metastatic lung carcinoma. The tumor (*arrows*) has entered the left atrium via contiguous spread through the left upper pulmonary vein. **C.** Apical 4-chamber image of metastatic melanoma, with a large tumor (*arrow*) in the left ventricle and a malignant pericardial effusion (*E*). LV, left ventricle; RA, right atrium; RV, right ventricle.

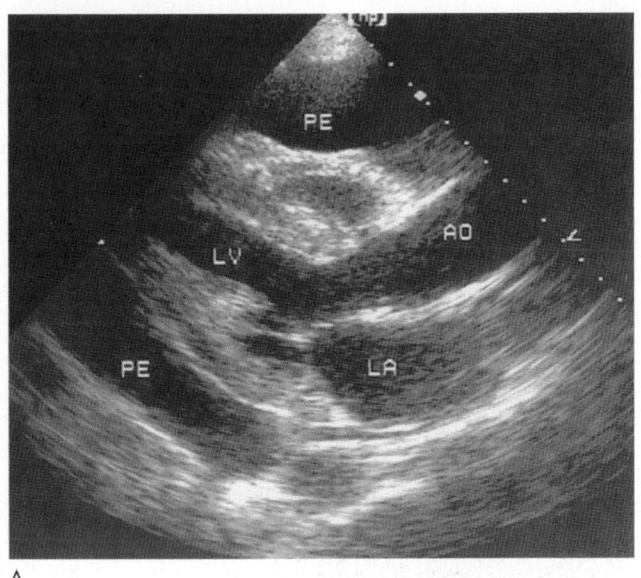

A

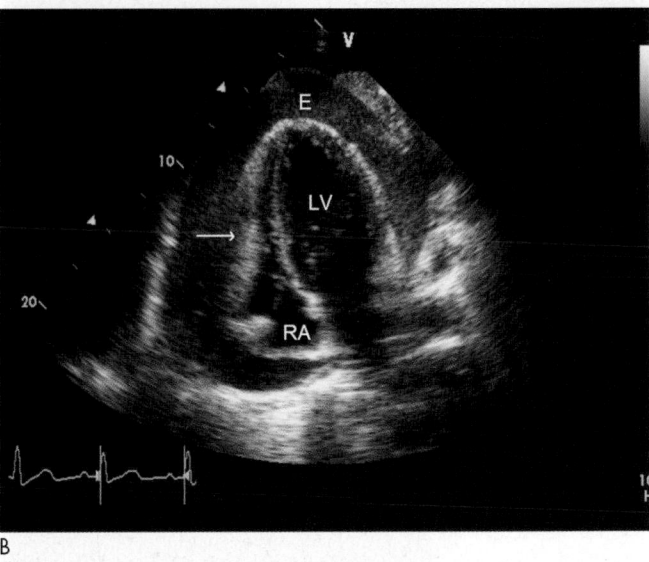

B

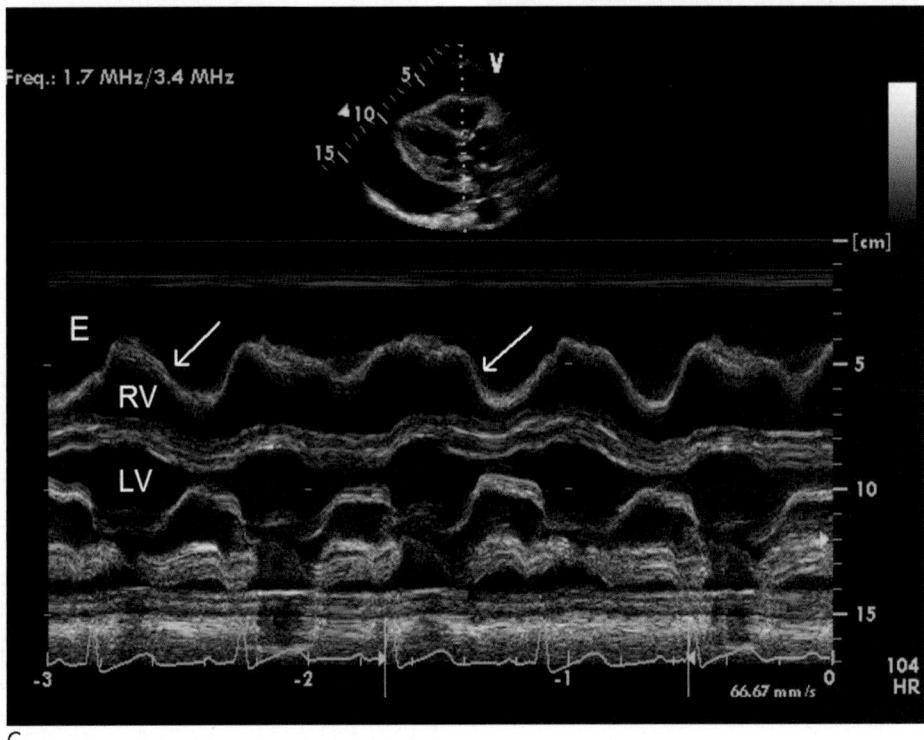

C

FIGURE 16–135. A. Large pericardial effusion (*PE*) on parasternal long-axis imaging. **B.** RV compression (*arrow*) in cardiac tamponade (apical 4-chamber plane). **C.** M-mode image of cardiac tamponade and right ventricular diastolic collapse. The *RV* free wall (*arrows*) moves posteriorly toward the interventricular septum during diastole. Ao, aorta; E, effusion; LA, left atrium; LV, left ventricle; RV, right ventricle.

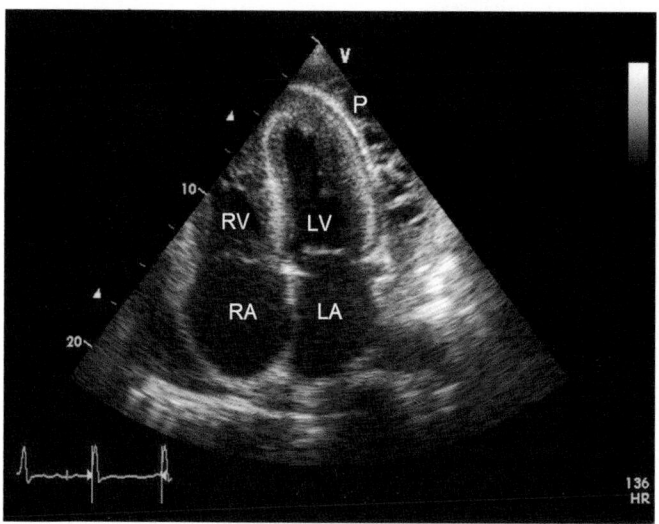

FIGURE 16–136. Apical four-chamber image in a case of malignant pericardial effusion (*P*). Numerous fibrinous strands are seen within the effusion. LA, left atrium; LV, left ventricle; RA, right atrium; RV, right ventricle.

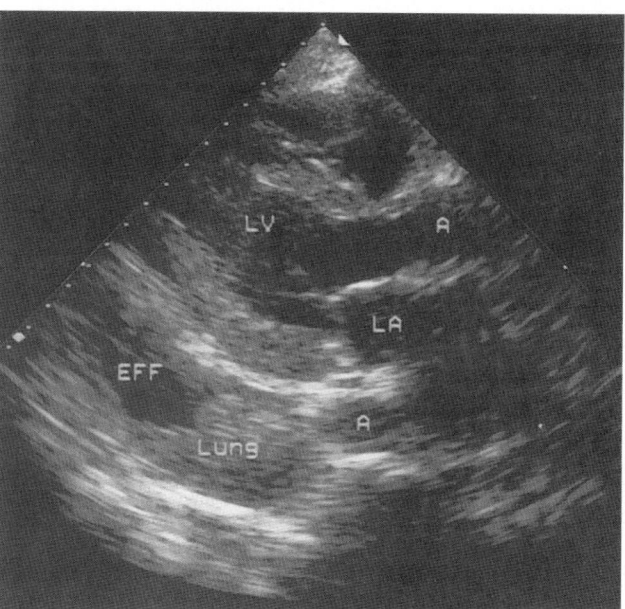

FIGURE 16–137. Parasternal long-axis view in a patient with a pleural effusion (EFF) posterior to the heart. Atelectatic lung tissue is present within the effusion. Ao, aorta; LA, left atrium; LV, left ventricle.

Paradoxical septal motion may be seen on M-mode with constriction, as can an abnormal inspiratory interventricular septal *bounce* and limited diastolic motion of the posterior LV wall.

The utility of Doppler recordings in evaluating constrictive pericarditis has been shown in several studies.[149] As with cardiac tamponade, pericardial constriction produces exaggerated respiratory variation in the isovolumic relaxation time and in flow velocities within RV and LV, pulmonary veins, and hepatic vein.[149] A respiratory variation of >20 percent in peak mitral E velocity favors the diagnosis of constriction over restrictive cardiomyopathy, whereas little respiratory variation favors restrictive physiology.[149] Unfortunately, exaggerated respiratory flow variation is not specific for pericardial constriction and also can be seen in chronic obstructive pulmonary disease and asthma. In these cases Doppler examination of superior vena cava flow is useful: Patients with asthma have increased flow toward the heart during inspiration, whereas limited forward flow is seen in constriction (the echocardiographic equivalent of Kussmaul sign). In addition, tissue Doppler imaging of the mitral annulus is useful in differentiating constrictive versus restrictive physiology. Both forms of diastolic dysfunction typically exhibit restrictive patterns on transmitral (E > A) and pulmonary venous (S < D) spectral flow recordings. In cases of pericardial constriction, however, the early diastolic velocity of the mitral annulus (E_m) remains normal. In restrictive cardiomyopathy, this velocity is abnormally low. Finally, respiratory variation in the peak velocity and duration of CW Doppler TR spectral envelopes appear to reflect accurately the enhanced ventricular interdependence seen in constrictive pericarditis.[150]

IMAGING OF THE CORONARY ARTERIES

The ability to visualize the proximal segments of the left and right coronary arteries has been demonstrated. The ability of color and spectral Doppler examination to image and record the velocity of flow from TTE and TEE approaches is established particularly with regard to the left anterior descending coronary artery. However, the resolution of the technique is at the limit of vessel size and the vessels are circuitous and move vigorously, often coursing in and out of the beam path. Yet, transthoracic imaging has proven useful for the diagnosis and follow-up of patients with Kawasaki

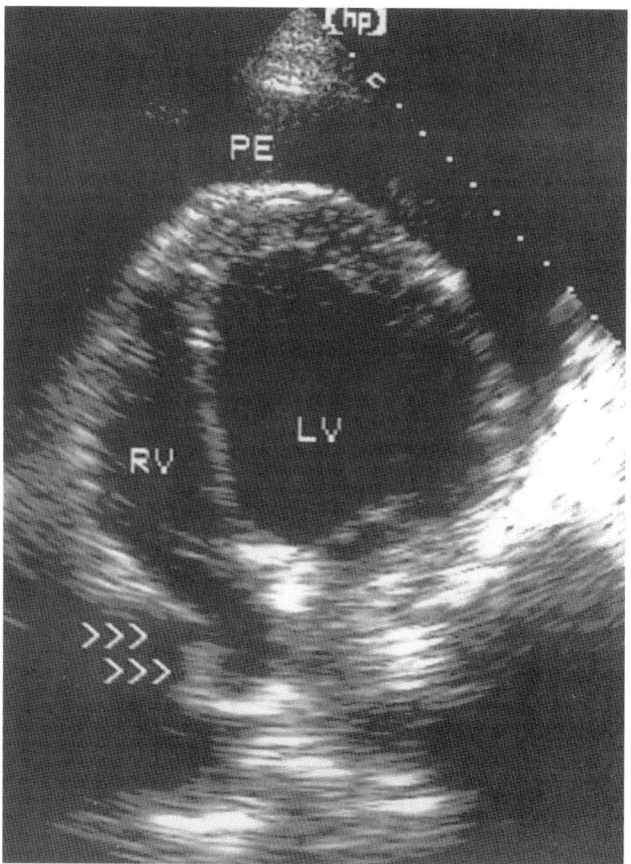

FIGURE 16–138. Right atrial collapse (*arrows*) in cardiac tamponade. LV, left ventricle; PE, pericardial effusion; RV, right ventricle.

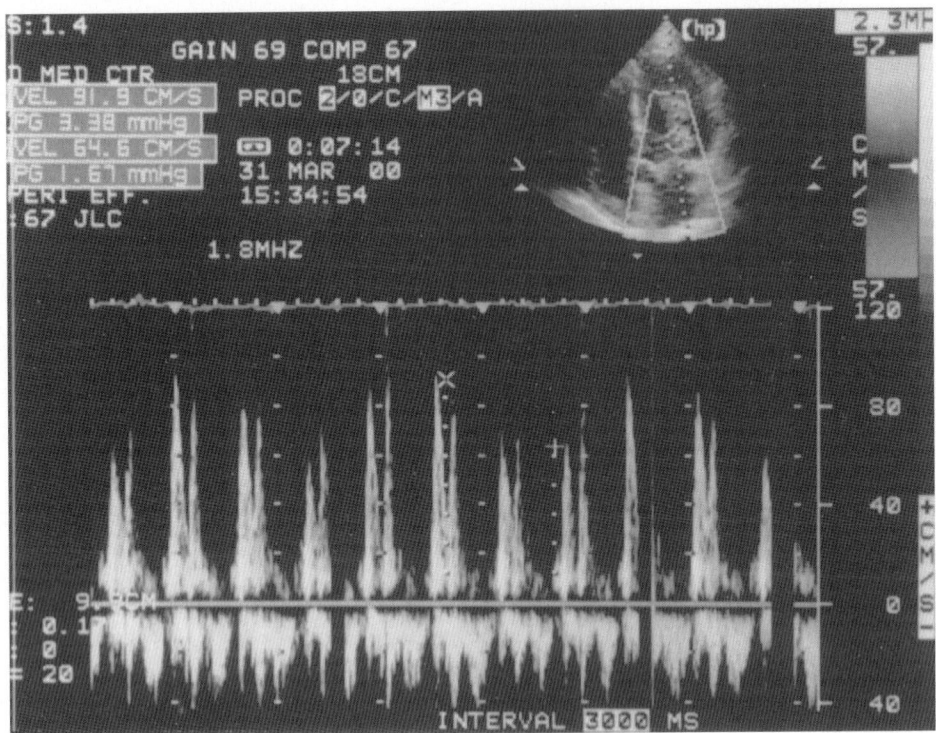

FIGURE 16–139. Pulsed-wave Doppler tracing of LV inflow in cardiac tamponade (apical transducer position). There is abnormal respiratory variation in the peak E wave velocity (which varies from 92 to 65 cm/sec).

disease and coronary involvement (Fig. 16–140) and may also help distinguish normal from atherosclerotic coronary arteries.

The coronary arteries are routinely imaged with TEE, which can detect proximal stenoses, atherosclerosis, and congenital abnormalities of the coronaries more accurately than surface imaging. Doppler TEE analysis also has been used to determine coronary flow reserve.[151]

Visualization of mid- and distal coronary arteries is problematic with both TTE and TEE. Fig. 16–141A shows color flow within a septal coronary artery. Fig. 16–141B shows a spectral Doppler recording of flow within the distal left anterior descending coronary artery (note the predominance of diastolic flow). These images were produced by an instrument using a fundamental frequency range of 5 to 7 MHz, rather than the more

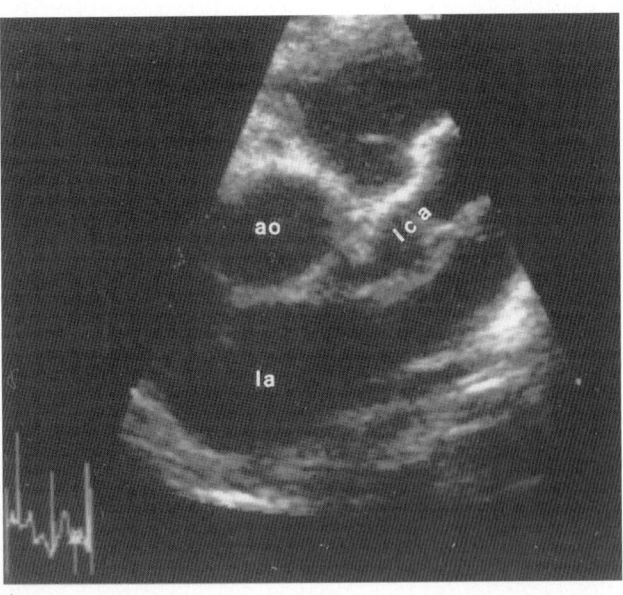

A

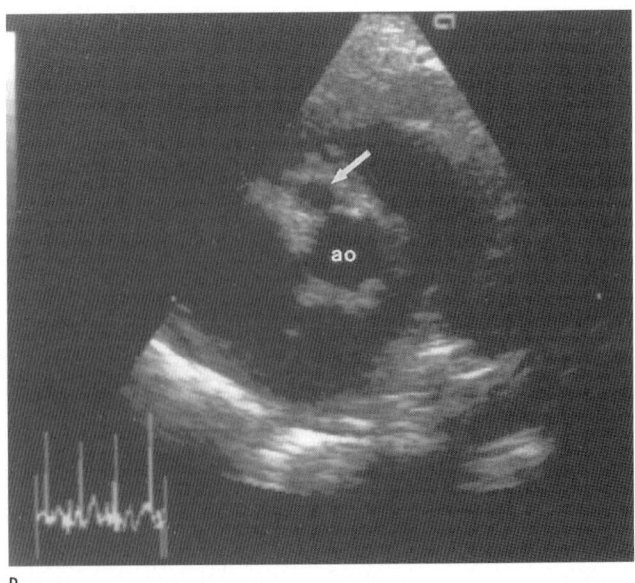

B

FIGURE 16–140. Parasternal short-axis images of coronary artery aneurysms associated with Kawasaki disease. **A.** The proximal left coronary artery (LCA) is diffusely dilated and aneurysmal. **B.** A proximal right coronary artery aneurysm (*arrow*) is shown. Ao, aorta, LA, left atrium. *Source: Courtesy of Victor Lucas, MD, and Paul Grossfeld, MD.*

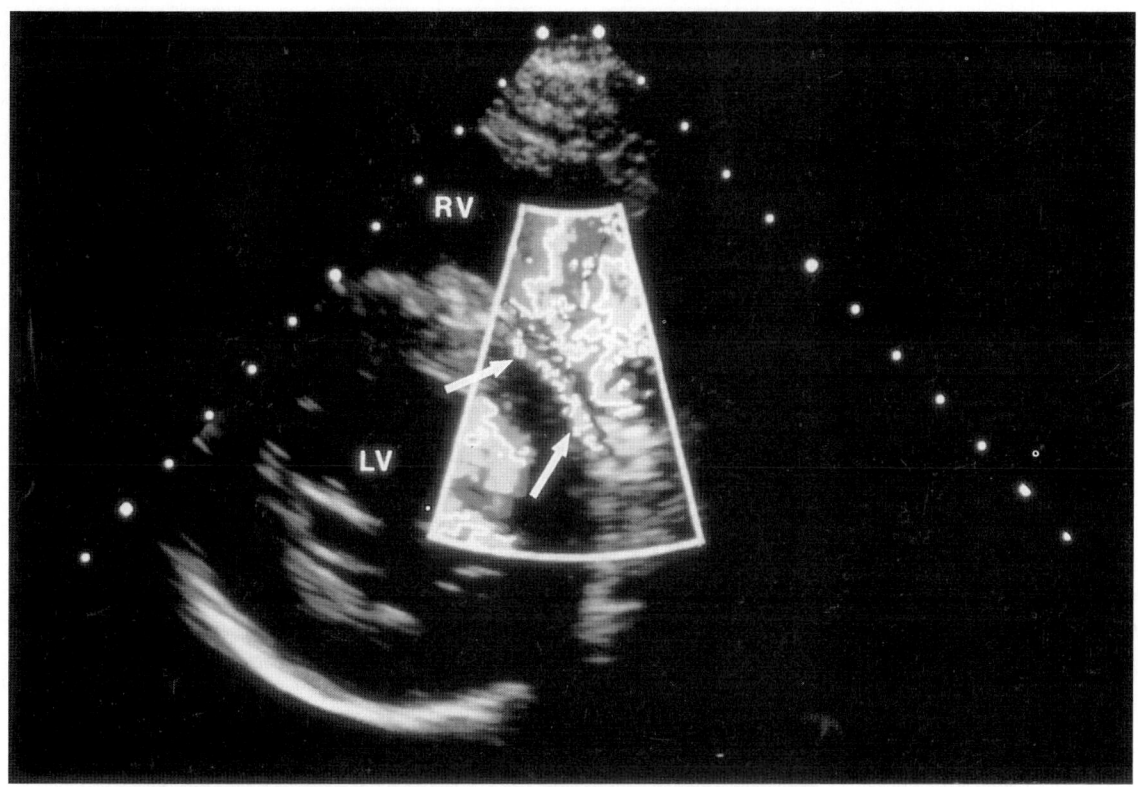

A

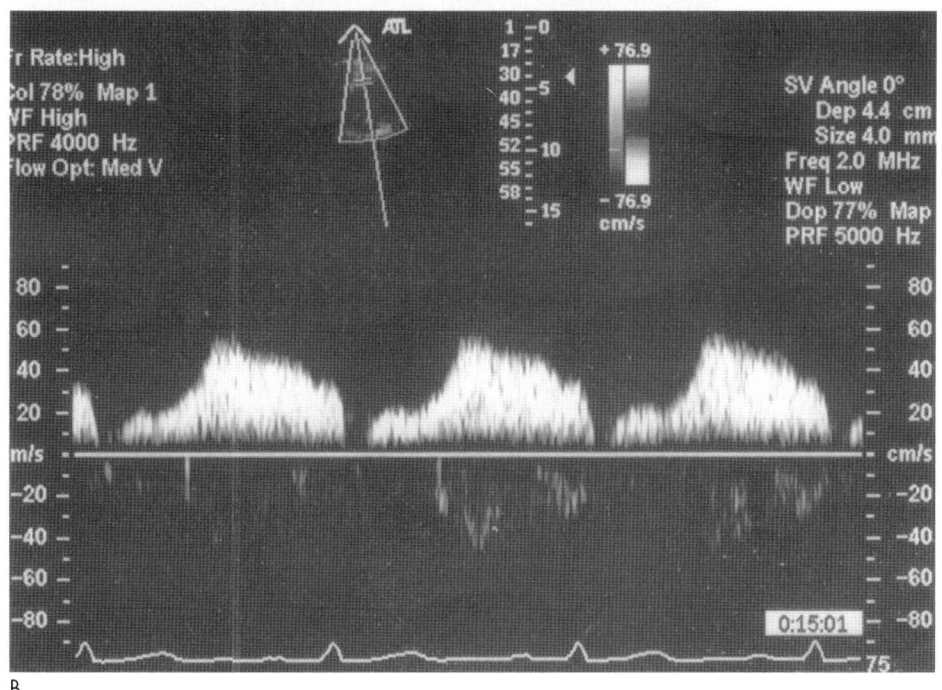

B

FIGURE 16–141. A. Transthoracic short-axis image of a coronary artery within the interventricular septum (*arrows*). **B.** Pulsed-wave spectral Doppler tracing of flow within the distal left anterior descending artery. Diastolic flow is predominant. LV, left ventricle; RV, right ventricle. *Source: Courtesy of Ajit Raisinghani, MD.*

commonly used range of 2.5 to 5.0 MHz S > D.

VENTRICULAR DYSSYNCHRONY AND CARDIAC RESYNCHRONIZATION THERAPY

Tissue Doppler imaging (TDI) enables accurate analysis of regional LV wall motion velocity. These recordings are usually performed in the apical view, so assess longitudinal myocardial velocity toward and away from the transducer. These data can be displayed graphically or parametrically as shades of color on a 2D image. If the velocities of two sites are compared not to the transducer position but instead to each other, the extent of regional deformation (i.e., change in length or strain) and the rate of deformation (i.e., strain rate) can be calculated.[152,153] Recently, tracking of intramyocardial speckle signals has enabled the assessment of strain in the radial and circumferential planes as well as the determination of ventricular torsion (Fig. 16–142).[154–156] By definition, lengthening of myocardium is a positive strain, whereas shortening is a negative strain. Strain is analogous to regional EF, whereas strain rate is analogous to regional dP/dt. These ultrasound measurements have been validated against MRI, which remains the gold standard for noninvasive assessment of LV strain. Strain and strain-rate imaging have shown promise in detecting ischemia and regional dysfunction in the setting of preserved EF[157] and, like tissue Doppler velocity, can be displayed graphically or as a 2D color-encoded parameter. Doppler-derived LV strain, however, is susceptible to artifacts; and future development of the technique is necessary to improve its reproducibility.

Recently, TDI recordings have played a major role in the selection of patients for cardiac resynchronization therapy (CRT) by biventricular pacing. Multiple studies have shown that CRT devices improve symptoms and decrease mortality,[158] but 20 to 30 percent of patients treated did not show a beneficial response. In addition, some patients without a wide QRS complex *did* respond to CRT. It is now clear that most benefit is derived by improving *intra*ventricular dyssynchrony.[159]

PWD evaluation of LV and RV ejection and M-mode imaging of the LV, initially used in the evaluation of dyssynchrony, have

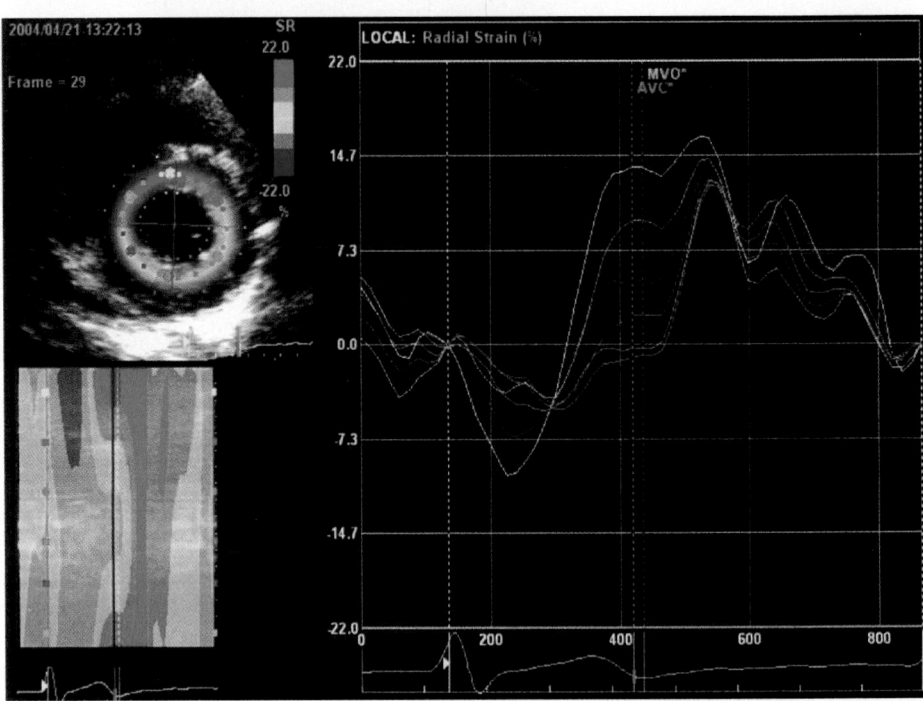

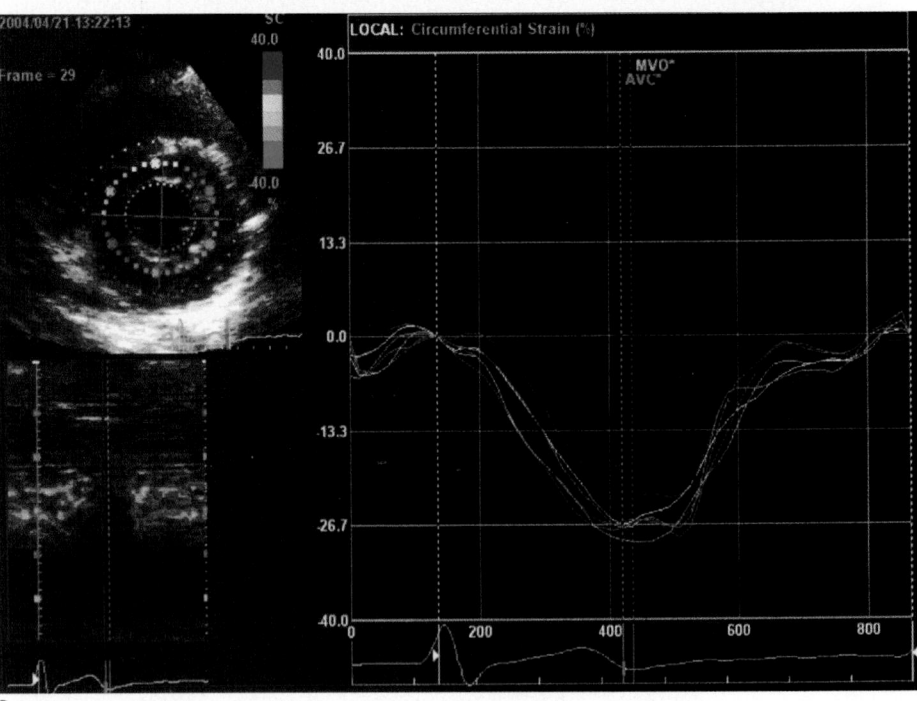

FIGURE 16–142. 2D speckle tracking with LV strain analysis in a normal case. Radial (**A**), circumferential (**B**), and longitudinal (**C**) strain can be calculated and displayed. In *A* and *C* regional strain is also displayed on a color map. Positive strain is displayed in varying shades of red; negative strain in varying shades of blue. AVC, aortic valve closure; LV, left ventricle; MVO, mitral valve opening. *Source: Courtesy of Andrew M. Kahn, MD, PhD.*

been largely supplanted by tissue Doppler imaging. One study has reported that strain rate imaging failed to predict response to CRT, whereas tissue Doppler imaging succeeded.[160]

Most studies of TDI and dyssynchrony have measured the time-to-peak systolic velocity. Bax and coworkers[161] measured time to peak systolic velocity (from QRS onset) in the basal septal, anterior, lateral, and posterior segments and found that a dif-

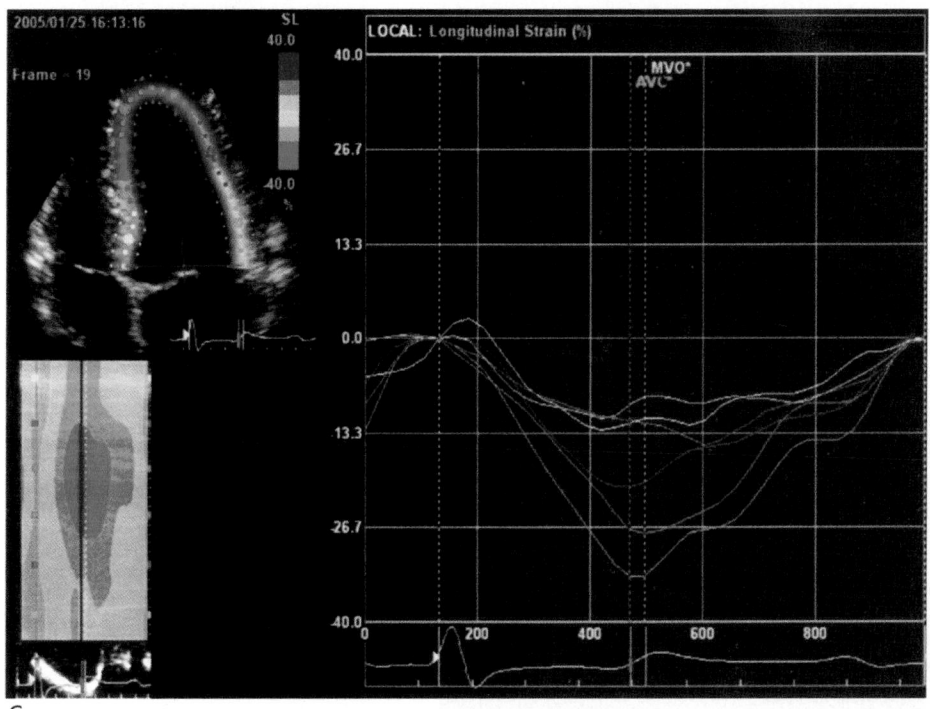

C

FIGURE 16–142. (continued)

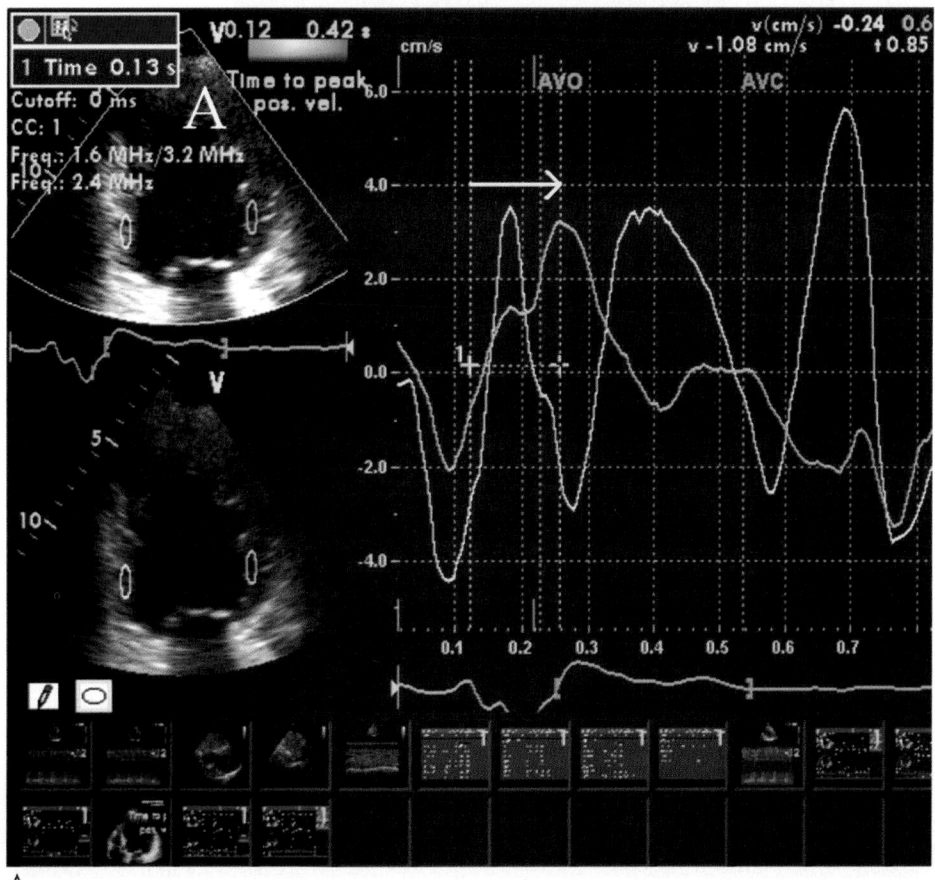

A

FIGURE 16–143. Measurement of time from QRS onset to peak systolic velocity in an apical two-chamber imaging plane. The basal anterior segmental velocity is color-coded light blue (**A**) and the basal inferior velocity yellow (**B**). Peak velocity occurs in 130 msec anteriorly and 270 msec inferiorly. The difference of 140 msec is consistent with significant dyssynchrony. (continued)

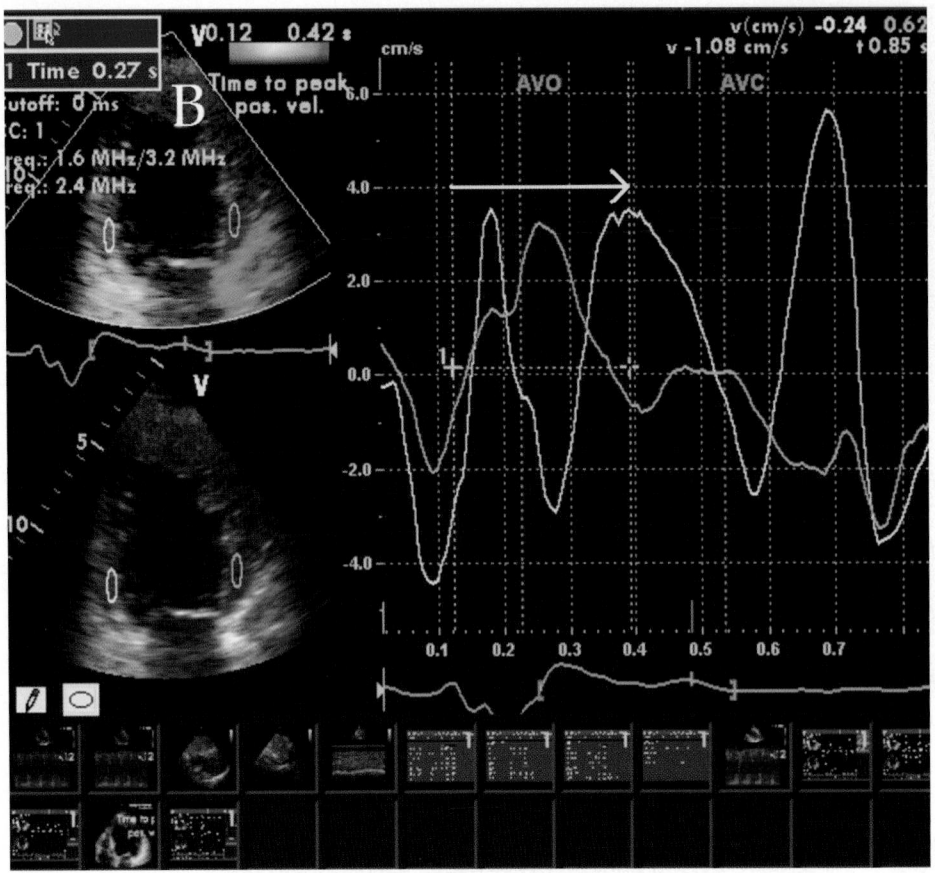

FIGURE 16–143. (continued)

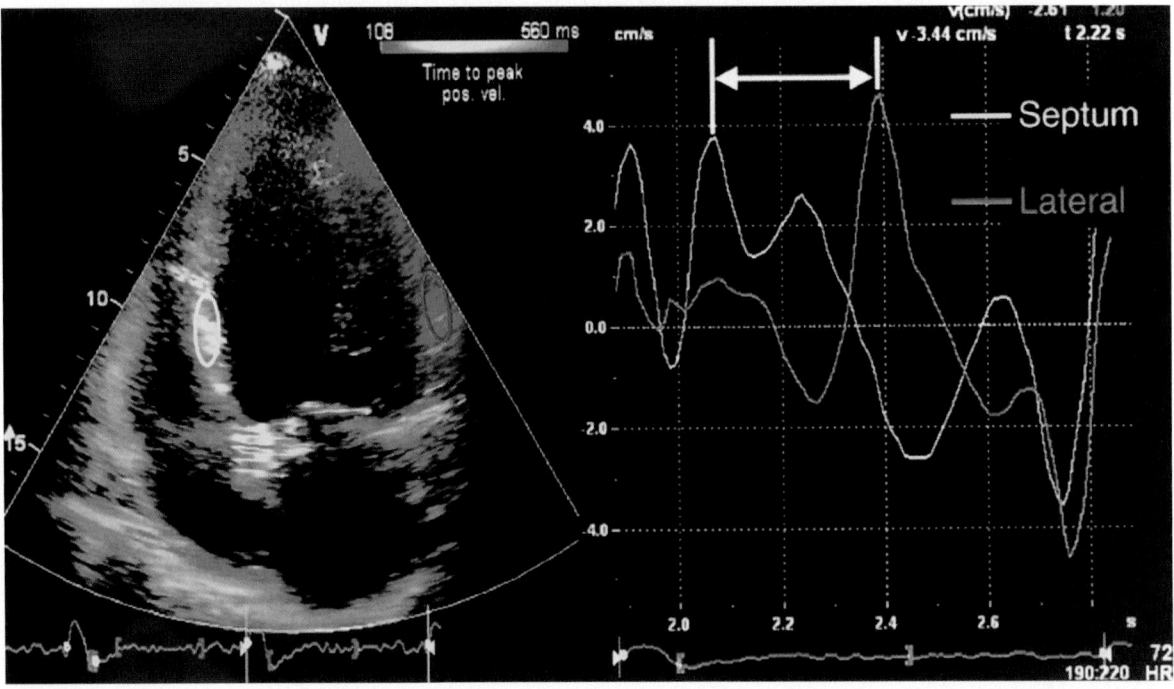

FIGURE 16–144. Tissue synchronization imaging, four-chamber view (*left*). The color represents timing: green, normal timing; red, severe delay. Color-guided visual identification of the site of latest activation facilitates sample-placement to derive the tissue Doppler imaging (*TDI*) velocity tracings. In this patient the earliest activation (*green*) is in the lateral wall, and the latest activation is in the lateral wall (*red*); the TDI velocity tracings (*right*) confirm the delay between the septum and lateral wall. *Source: From Bax JJ, Abraham T, Barold SS, et al.[159] With permission.*

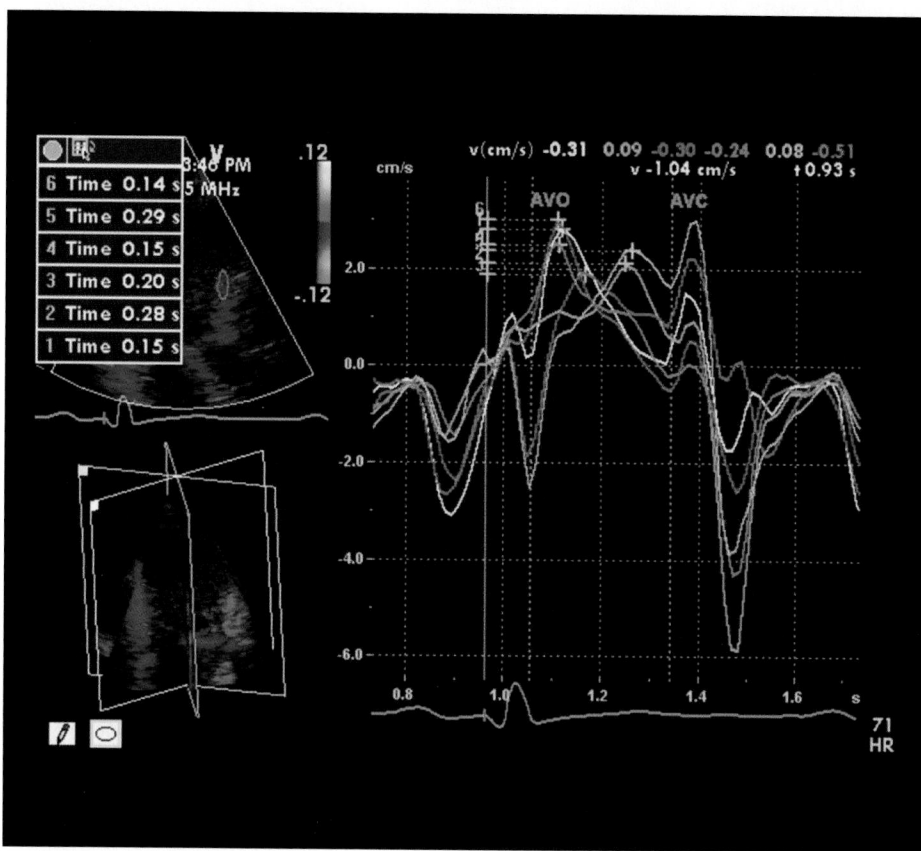

FIGURE 16–145 3D tissue velocity measurement. After a single heartbeat was captured with 3D echo, the time from QRS onset to peak systolic velocity was measured in the basal septal, anteroseptal, anterior, lateral, posterior, and inferior segments. The times to peak systolic velocity range from 140 to 290 msec, suggesting significant LV dyssynchrony. AVC, aortic valve closure; AVO, aortic valve opening; LV, left ventricle.

ference of >65 msec between two opposing walls correlated strongly with a favorable response to CRT. An example of this type of analysis is shown in Fig. 16–143. Yu and colleagues[162] used a 12-segment model and determined the mean and standard deviation of the times from QRS peak systolic velocity in each segment. A 2D *tissue tracking* program, which produces a color-coded image of time to peak velocity, has been developed and permits a visual assessment of overall LV dyssynchrony (Fig. 16–144). The presence of extensive delayed LV activation predicted subsequent improvement in LVEF with CRT. Three-dimensional echo enables regional TDI measurements to be performed on a single beat, eliminating potential beat-to-beat variations (Fig. 16–145).

REFERENCES

1. ACC/AHA Guidelines for the Clinical Application of Echocardiography: Executive Summary. A report of the American College of Cardiology/American Heart Association Task Force on Practice Guidelines (Committee on Clinical Application of Echocardiography). *J Am Coll Cardiol* 1997;29:862–879.
2. Daniel WG, Mügge A. Transesophageal echocardiography. *N Engl J Med* 1995;332:1268–1279.
3. Handschumacher MD, Lethor JP, Siu SC, et al. A new integrated system for three-dimensional echocardiographic reconstruction: development and validation for ventricular volume with application in human subjects. *J Am Coll Cardiol* 1993;21:743–753.
4. Rovai D, DeMaria AN, L'Abbate A. Myocardial contrast echo effect: the dilemma of coronary blood flow and volume. *J Am Coll Cardiol* 1995;26:12–17.
5. Elder I, Hertz CH. The use of ultrasonic reflectoscope for the continuous recording of movement of heart walls. *Clin Physiol Funct Imaging* 1954;24:40–45.
6. Feigenbaum H, Zaky A. Use of diagnostic ultrasound in clinical cardiology. *J Indiana State Med Assoc* 1966;49:140–152.
7. Bom N, Lancee CT Jr, Van Zwieten G, et al. Multiscan echocardiography: I. Technical description. *Circulation* 1973;48;1066–1073.
8. Griffith JM, Henry WL. A sector scanner for real time two-dimensional echocardiography. *Circulation* 1974;49:1147–1152.
9. VonRamm OT, Thurstone FL. Cardiac imaging using a phased array ultrasound system: I. System design. *Circulation* 1976;53:258–262.
10. Omoto R. *Color Atlas of Real-Time Two-Dimensional Doppler Echocardiography,* 2nd ed. Tokyo: Sindan-to-Chiryo, 1987.
11. Hanrath P, Kremer P, Langenstein BA, et al. Transoesophageale eckokardiographie: ein neues verfahren zur dynamischenventrikel-funktionsanalyse. *Dtsch Med Wochenschr* 1981;106:523–525.
12. Seward JB, Khanderia BK, Oh JK, et al. Transesophageal echocardiography: Technique, anatomic correlations, implementation and clinical applications. *Mayo Clin Proc* 1988;63:649–680.
13. Baker DW. Pulsed ultrasonic Doppler blood-flow sensing. *IEEE Trans Sonics Ultrasonics* 1970;SU–17(3).
14. Hatle L, Angelsen B, Tromsdal A. Noninvasive assessment of atrioventricular pressure half-time by Doppler ultrasound. *Circulation* 1979;60:1096–1104.
15. Hatle L, Angelsen BA, Tromsdal A. Noninvasive assessment of aortic stenosis by Doppler ultrasound. *Br Heart J* 1980;3:284–292.
16. Wells PNT. *Ultrasonics in Clinical Diagnosis,* 2nd ed. New York: Churchill Livingstone, 1977.
17. Main ML, Asher CR, Rubin DN, et al. Comparison of tissue harmonic imaging with contrast (sonicated albumin) echocardiography and Doppler myocardial imaging for enhancing endocardial border resolution. *Am J Cardiol* 1999;83:218–222.
18. Kremkau FW, Taylor KJW. Artifacts in ultrasound imaging. *J Ultrasound Med* 1986;15:227–237.
19. Yeh E. Reverberations in echocardiograms. *J Clin Ultrasound* 1977;5:84–86.
20. Weyman AE. Physical principles of ultrasound. In: Weyman AE, ed. *Principles and Practice of Echocardiography,* 2nd ed. Philadelphia: Lea & Febiger; 1994:3–28.
21. DeMaria AN, Miller RR, Amsterdam EA, et al. Mitral valve early diastolic closing velocity in the echocardiogram: relation to sequential diastolic flow and ventricular compliance. *Am J Cardiol* 1976;37:693–700.
22. Sahn DJ, DeMaria A, Kisslo J, Weyman AE. Recommendations regarding quantitation in M-mode echocardiography: results of a survey of echocardiographic measurements. *Circulation* 1978;58:1072–1083.
23. Teichholz LE, Kreulen T, Herman MV, Gorlin R. Problems in echocardiographic volume determinations: echocardiographic-angiographic correlations in the presence or absence of synergy. *Am J Cardiol* 1976;37:7–11.
24. McDonald IG, Feigenbaum H, Chang S. Analysis of left ventricular wall motion by reflected ultrasound: application to assessment of myocardial function. *Circulation* 1972;46:14–25.
25. Feigenbaum H. Echocardiographic examination of the left ventricle. *Circulation* 1975;51:1–7.
26. Massie BM, Schiller NB, Ratshin RA, Parmley WW. Mitral-septal separation: new echocardiographic index of left ventricular function. *Am J Cardiol* 1977;39:1008–1016.

27. Ophir J, Maklad NF. Digital scan converters in diagnostic ultrasound imaging. *Proc IEEE* 1979;67–75.

28. Henry WL, DeMaria A, Gramiak R, et al. Report of the American Society of Echocardiography: nomenclature and standards in two-dimensional echocardiography. *Circulation* 1980;62:212–217.

29. Shiota T, Jones M, Chikada M, et al. Real-time three-dimensional echocardiography for determining right ventricular stroke volume in an animal model of chronic right ventricular volume overload. *Circulation* 1998;97:1896–1900.

30. Corsi C, Lang RM, Veronesi F, et al. Volumetric quantification of global and regional left ventricular function from real-time three-dimensional echocardiographic images. *Circulation* 2005;112:1161–1170.

31. Kapetanakis S, Kearney MT, Siva A, et al. Real-time three-dimensional echocardiography: a novel technique to quantify global left ventricular mechanical dyssynchrony. *Circulation* 2005;112:992–1000.

32. Wyatt HL, Heng MK, Meerbaum S, et al. Cross-sectional echocardiography: II. Analysis of mathematic models for quantifying volume of formalin fixed left ventricle. *Circulation* 1980;61:1119–1125.

33. Wyatt HL, Meerbaum S, Heng MK, et al. Cross-sectional echocardiography: III. Analysis of mathematic models for quantifying volume of symmetric and asymmetric left ventricles. *Am Heart J* 1980;100:821–828.

34. Schiller NB, Acquatella H, Ports TA, et al. Left ventricular volume from paired biplane two-dimensional echocardiography. *Circulation* 1979;60:547–555.

35. Folland ED, Parisi AF, Moynihan PF, et al. Assessment of left ventricular ejection fraction and volumes by real-time, two-dimensional echocardiography and radionuclide techniques. *Circulation* 1979;60:760–766.

36. Stamm RB, Carabello BA, Mayers DL, Martin RP. Two-dimensional echocardiographic measurement of left ventricular ejection fraction: prospective analysis of what constitutes an adequate determination. *Am Heart J* 1982;104:136–144.

37. Becher H, Tiemann K, Schlief R, et al. Harmonic power Doppler contrast echocardiography: preliminary clinical results. *Echocardiography* 1997;14:637–642.

38. Spencer KT, Bednarz J, Rafter PG, et al. Use of harmonic imaging without echocardiographic contrast to improve two-dimensional image quality. *Am J Cardiol* 1998;82:794–799.

39. Perez JE, Waggoner AD, Barzilai B, et al. On-line assessment of ventricular function by automatic boundary detection and ultrasonic backscatter imaging. *J Am Coll Cardiol* 1992;19:313.

40. Lang RM, Vignon P, Weinert L, et al. Echocardiographic quantification of regional left ventricular wall motion with color kinesis. *Circulation* 1996;93:1877–1885.

41. Godoy IE, Mor-Avi V, Weinert L, et al. Use of color kinesis for evaluation of left ventricular filling in patients with dilated cardiomyopathy and mitral regurgitation. *J Am Coll Cardiol* 1998;31:1598–1606.

42. Doppler JC. Ueber das farbige Licht der Dopplesterne und einiger anderer Gestirne des Himmels. *Abhandlungen der Konigl, Bohmischen Gesellschaft der Wissenschaften,* 5th ser, 1842;2:465.

43. Hatle L, Angelsen B. *Doppler Ultrasound in Cardiology: Physical Principles and Clinical Applications,* 2nd ed. Philadelphia: Lea & Febiger, 1984.

44. Garcia MJ, Thomas JD, Klein AL. New Doppler echocardiographic applications for the study of diastolic function. *J Am Coll Cardiol* 1998;32:865–875.

45. Garcia MJ, Smedira NG, Greenberg NL, et al. Color M-mode Doppler flow propagation velocity is a preload insensitive index of left ventricular relaxation: Animal and human validation. *J Am Coll Cardiol* 2000;35:201–208.

46. Baker DW, Rubenstein SA, Lorch GS. Pulsed Doppler echocardiography: principles and applications. *Am J Med* 1977;63:69–80.

47. Bom K, deBoo J, Rijsterborgh H. On the aliasing problem in pulsed Doppler cardiac studies. *J Clin Ultrasound* 1984;12:559–567.

48. Feigenbaum H. Appendix: echocardiographic measurements and normal values. In: Feigenbaum H, ed. *Echocardiography,* 5th ed. Philadelphia: Lea & Febiger; 1994:658–683.

49. Nishimura RA, Housmans PR, Hatle LK, Tajik AJ. Assessment of diastolic function of the heart: background and current applications of Doppler echocardiography: part I. Physiologic and pathophysiologic features. *Mayo Clin Proc* 1989;64:71–81.

50. Nishimura RA, Hatle LK, Abel MD, Tajik AJ. Assessment of diastolic function of the heart: Background and current applications of Doppler echocardiography: part II. Clinical studies. *Mayo Clin Proc* 1989;4:181–204.

51. Oh JK, Hatle L, Tajik AJ, Little WC. Diastolic heart failure can be diagnosed by comprehensive two-dimensional and Doppler echocardiography. *J Am Coll Cardiol* 2006;47:500–506.

52. DeMaria AN, Blanchard D. The hemodynamic basis of diastology. *J Am Coll Cardiol* 1999;34:1659–1662.

53. Appleton CP, Hatle LK, Popp RL. Cardiac tamponade and pericardial effusion: respiratory variation in transvalvular flow velocities studied by Doppler echocardiography. *J Am Coll Cardiol* 1988;11:1020–1030.

54. Harrison M, Clifton G, Pennell A, DeMaria A. Effect of heart rate on left ventricular diastolic transmitral flow velocity patterns assessed by Doppler echocardiography in normal subjects. *Am J Cardiol* 1991;67:622–627.

55. Dittrich HC, Blanchard DG, Wheeler K, et al. Influence of Doppler sample location on the assessment of changes in mitral inflow velocity profiles. *J Am Soc Echocardiogr* 1990;3:303–309.

56. Dokainish H, Zoghbi WA, Lakkis NM, et al. Optimal noninvasive assessment of left ventricular filling pressures: a comparison of tissue Doppler echocardiography and B-type natriuretic peptide in patients with pulmonary artery catheters. *Circulation* 2004;109:2432–2439.

57. Tsang TSM, Abhayaratna WP, Barnes ME, et al. Prediction of cardiovascular outcomes with left atrial size: Is volume superior to area or diameter? *J Am Coll Cardiol* 2006;47:1018–23.

58. Pritchett AM, Mahoney DW, Jacobsen SJ, et al. Diastolic dysfunction and left atrial volume: a population-based study. *J Am Coll Cardiol* 2005;45:87–92.

59. Chen C, Rodriguez L, Guerrero JL, et al. Noninvasive estimation of the instantaneous first derivative of left ventricular pressure using continuous-wave Doppler echocardiography. *Circulation* 1991;83:2101–2110.

60. William GA, Labovitz AJ. Doppler estimation of cardiac output: principles and pitfalls. *Echocardiography* 1987;4:355–374.

61. Sahn DJ. Determination of cardiac output by echocardiographic Doppler methods: relative accuracy of various sites for measurement. *J Am Coll Cardiol* 1985;6:663–664.

62. Barron JV, Sahn DJ, Valdes-Cruz LM, et al. Clinical utility of two-dimensional Doppler echocardiographic techniques for estimating pulmonary to systemic flow ratios in children with left to right shunting, atrial septal defect, ventricular septal defect and patent ductus arteriosus. *J Am Coll Cardiol* 1984;3:169–178.

63. Xie G-Y, Berk MR, Smith ND, DeMaria AN. A simplified method for determining regurgitant fraction by Doppler echocardiography in patients with aortic regurgitation. *J Am Coll Cardiol* 1994;24:1041–1045.

64. Zoghbi WA, Farmer KL, Soto JG, et al. Accurate noninvasive quantitation of stenotic aortic valve area by Doppler echocardiography. *Circulation* 1986;73:452–459.

65. Currie PJ, Seward JB, Reeder GS, et al. Continuous wave Doppler echocardiographic assessment of severity of calcific aortic stenosis: a simultaneous Doppler-catheter correlative study in 100 adult patients. *Circulation* 1985;71:1162–1169.

66. Currie PJ, Hagler DJ, Seward JB, et al. Instantaneous pressure gradient: a simultaneous Doppler and dual catheter correlative study. *J Am Coll Cardiol* 1986;7:800–806.

67. Lee RT, Lord CP, Plappert T, Sutton MS. Prospective Doppler echocardiographic evaluation of pulmonary artery diastolic pressure in the medical intensive care unit. *Am J Cardiol* 1989;64:1366–1370.

68. Yock PG, Popp RL. Noninvasive estimation of right ventricular systolic pressure by Doppler ultrasound in patients with tricuspid regurgitation. *Circulation* 1984;70:657–662.

69. Simpson IA, Valdes-Cruz LM, Sahn DJ. Color Doppler flow mapping of simulated in vitro regurgitant jets: evaluation of the effects of orifice size and hemodynamic variables. *J Am Coll Cardiol* 1989;13:1195.

70. Matsumura M, Wong M, Omoto R. Assessment of Doppler color flow mapping in quantification of aortic regurgitation: correlations and influencing factors. *Jpn Circ J* 1989;53:735–746.

71. Blanchard DG, Kimura BJ, Dittrich HC, DeMaria AN. Transesophageal echocardiography of the aorta. *JAMA* 1994;272:546–551.

72. Freeman WK, Seward JB, Khanderia BK, Tajik AJ, eds. *Transesophageal Echocardiography.* Boston: Little, Brown, 1994.

73. Yvorchuk KJ, Chan K-L. Application of transthoracic and transesophageal echocardiography in the diagnosis and management of infective endocarditis. *J Am Soc Echocardiogr* 1994;14:294–308.

74. Klein AL, Obarski TP, Stewart WJ, et al. Transesophageal Doppler echocardiography of pulmonary venous flow: a new marker of mitral regurgitation severity. *J Am Coll Cardiol* 1991;18:518–526.

75. Hoffmann R, Flachskampf FA, Hanrath P. Planimetry of orifice area in aortic stenosis using multiplane transesophageal echocardiography. *J Am Coll Cardiol* 1993;22:529–534.

76. Cigarroa JE, Isselbacher EM, DeSanctis RW, Eagle KA. Diagnostic imaging in the evaluation of suspected aortic dissection. *N Engl J Med* 1993;328:35–43.

77. Manning WJ, Weintraub RM, Waksmonski CA, et al. Accuracy of transesophageal echocardiography for identifying left atrial thrombi: a prospective, intraoperative study. *Ann Intern Med* 1995;123:817–822.

78. The French Study of Aortic Plaques in Stroke Group. Atherosclerotic disease of the aortic arch as a risk factor for recurrent ischemic stroke. *N Engl J Med* 1996;334:1216–1221.

79. Dressler FA, Craig WR, Castello R, Labovitz AJ. Mobile aortic atheroma and systemic emboli: efficacy of anticoagulation and influence of plague morphology on recurrent stroke. *J Am Coll Cardiol* 1998;31:134–138.

80. Van den Brink RBA, Visser CA, Basart DCG, et al. Comparison of transthoracic and transesophageal color Doppler flow imaging in patients with mechanical prostheses in the mitral valve position. *Am J Cardiol* 1989;63:1471–1474.

81. Schiller NB. Hand-held echocardiography: Revolution or hassle? *J Am Coll Cardiol* 2001;37:2023–2024.

82. Seward JB, Douglas PS, Erbel R, et al. Hand-carried cardiac ultrasound (HCU) device: recommendations regarding new technology. A report from the echocardiography task force on new technology of the nomenclature and standards committee of the American Society of Echocardiography. *J Am Soc Echocardiogr* 2002;15:369–373.

83. Valdes-Cruz LM, Sahn DJ. Seminar on contrast two-dimensional echocardiography: applications and new developments: part II. *J Am Coll Cardiol* 1984;3:978–985.

84. DeMaria AN. Echocardiographic visualization of myocardial perfusion by left heart and intracoronary injection of echo contrast agents [abstract]. *Circulation* 1980;60(suppl 3):II–143.

85. Price RJ, Skyba DM, Kaul S, Skalak TC. Delivery of colloidal particles and red blood cells to tissue through microvessel ruptures created by targeted microbubble destruction with ultrasound. *Circulation* 1998;98:1264–1267.

86. Porter TR, Li S, Kricsfeld D, Armbruster RW. Detection of myocardial perfusion in multiple echocardiographic windows with one intravenous injection of microbubbles using transient response second harmonic imaging. *J Am Coll Cardiol* 1997;29:791–799.

87. Porter TR, Xie F, Kresfeld A, Kilzer K. Noninvasive identification of acute myocardial ischemia and reperfusion with contrast ultrasound using intravenous perfluoropropane-exposed sonicated dextrose albumin. *J Am Coll Cardiol* 1995;26:33–40.

88. Masugata H, Lafitte S, Peters B, Strachan GM, DeMaria AN. Comparison of real-time and intermittent triggered myocardial contrast echocardiography for quantification of coronary stenosis severity and transmural perfusion gradient. Circulation 2001;104:1550–1556.

89. Jeetley P, Hickman M, Kamp O, et al. Myocardial contrast echocardiography for the detection of coronary artery stenosis: a prospective multicenter study in comparison with single-photon emission computed tomography. *J Am Coll Cardiol* 2006;47:141–145.

90. Toledo E, Lang RM, Collins KA, et al. Imaging and quantification of myocardial perfusion using real-time three-dimensional echocardiography. *J Am Coll Cardiol* 2006;47:146–154.

91. Tajik AJ, Seward JB, Hagler DJ, et al. Two-dimensional real-time ultrasonic imaging of the heart and great vessels: technique, image orientation, structures, identification, and validation. *Mayo Clin Proc* 1978;53:271–303.

92. DeMaria AN, Bommer W, Joye JA, et al. Value and limitations of cross-sectional echocardiography of the aortic valve in the diagnosis and quantification of valvular aortic stenosis. *Circulation* 1980;62:304–312.

93. Quere J-P, Monin J-L, Levy F, et al. Influence of preoperative left ventricular contractile reserve on postoperative ejection fraction in low-gradient aortic stenosis. *Circulation* 2006;113:1738–1744.

94. Lange RA, Hillis D. Dobutamine stress echocardiography in patients with low-gradient aortic stenosis. *Circulation* 2006;113:1718–1720.

95. Perry GJ, Nelmcke F, Nanda NC, et al. Evaluation of aortic insufficiency by Doppler color flow mapping. *J Am Coll Cardiol* 1987;9:952–959.

96. Grayburn PA, Handshoe R, Smith MD, et al. Quantitative assessment of the hemodynamic consequences of aortic regurgitation. *J Am Coll Cardiol* 1987;10:135–141.

97. Perlman AS, Otto CM. Quantification of valvular regurgitation. *Echocardiography* 1987;4:271–287.

98. DeMaria AN, Bommer W, Newmann A, et al. Identification and localization of aneurysms of the ascending aorta by cross-sectional echocardiography. *Circulation* 1979;59:755–761.

99. Ballal RS, Nanda NC, Gatewood R, et al. Usefulness of transesophageal echocardiography in assessment of aortic dissection. *Circulation* 1991;84:1903–1914.

100. Nienaber CA, Spielman RP, von Kodolitsch Y, et al. Diagnosis of thoracic aortic dissection: magnetic resonance imaging versus transesophageal echocardiography. *Circulation* 1992;85:434–447.

101. Sawhney NS, DeMaria AN, Blanchard DG. Aortic intramural hematoma: an increasingly recognized and potentially fatal entity. *Chest* 2001;120:1340–1346.

102. Eisenberg MJ, Geraci SJ, Schiller NB. Screening for abdominal aortic aneurysms during transthoracic echocardiography. *Am Heart J* 1995;130:109–115.

103. Tunick PA, Kronzon I. Atheromas of the thoracic aorta: clinical and therapeutic update. *J Am Coll Cardiol* 2000;35:545–554.

104. Cannon CR, Nishimura RA, Reeder GS, et al. Echocardiographic assessment of commissural calcium: a simple predictor of outcome after percutaneous mitral balloon valvotomy. *J Am Coll Cardiol* 1997;29:175–180.

105. Vandervoort PM, Rivera JM, Mele D, et al. Application of color Doppler flow mapping to calculate effective regurgitant orifice area: an in vitro study and initial clinical observations. *Circulation* 1993;88:1150–1156.

106. Simpson IA, Shiota T, Gharib M, Sahn DJ. Current status of flow convergence for clinical applications: is it a leaning tower of "PISA"? *J Am Coll Cardiol* 1996;27:504–509.

107. DeMaria AN, King JF, Bogren HG, et al. The variable spectrum of echocardiographic manifestations of the mitral valve prolapse syndrome. *Circulation* 1974;50:33–41.

108. Curtius MM, Thyssen M, Breuer HWM, Loogen F. Doppler versus contrast echocardiography for diagnosis of tricuspid regurgitation. *Am J Cardiol* 1985;56:333–336.

109. Weyman AE, Dillon JC, Feigenbaum H, Chang S. Echocardiographic patterns of pulmonary valve motion with pulmonary hypertension. *Circulation* 1974;50:905–910.

110. Mahmud E, Raisinghani A, Hassankhani A, et al. Correlation of left ventricular diastolic filling characteristics with right ventricular overload and pulmonary artery pressure in chronic thromboembolic pulmonary hypertension. *J Am Coll Cardiol* 2002;40:318–324.

111. Habib G, Derumeaux G, Avierinos JF, et al. Value and limitations of the Duke criteria for the diagnosis of infective endocarditis. *J Am Coll Cardiol* 1999;33:2023–2029.

112. Wann LS, Dillon JC, Weyman AE, Feigenbaum H. Echocardiography in bacterial endocarditis. *N Engl J Med* 1976;295:135–139.

113. Roldan CA, Shively BK, Crawford MH. An echocardiographic study of valvular heart disease associated with systemic lupus erythematosus. *N Engl J Med* 1996;335:1424–1430.

114. Steckelberg JM, Murphy JG, Ballard D, et al. Emboli in infective endocarditis: the prognostic value of echocardiography. *Ann Intern Med* 1991;114:635–640.

115. Di Salvo G, Habib G, Pergola V, et al. Echocardiography predicts embolic events in infective endocarditis. *J Am Coll Cardiol* 2001;37:1069–1076.

116. Lindner JR, Case RA, Dent JM, et al. Diagnostic value of echocardiography in suspected endocarditis: an evaluation based on pretest probability of disease. *Circulation* 1996;93:730–736.

117. Cerqueira MD, Weissman NJ, Dilsizian V, et al. Standardized myocardial segmentation and nomenclature for tomographic imaging of the heart: a statement for healthcare professionals from the cardiac imaging committee of the council on clinical cardiology of the American Heart Association. *Circulation* 2002;105:539–542.

118. Lang RM, Bierig M, Devereux RB, et al. Recommendations for chamber quantification: a report from the American Society of Echocardiography's guidelines and standards committee and the chamber quantification writing group, developed in conjunction with the European Association of Echocardiography, a branch of the European Society of Cardiology. *J Am Soc Echocardiogr* 2005;18:1440–1463.

119. Weiss JL, Buckley BH, Hutchins GM, Mason SJ. Two-dimensional echocardiographic recognition of myocardial injury in man: comparison with postmortem studies. *Circulation* 1981;63:401–408.

120. Tong KL, Kaul S, Wang XQ, et al. Myocardial contrast echocardiography versus thrombolysis in myocardial infarction score in patients presenting to the emergency department with chest pain and a nondiagnostic electrocardiogram. *J Am Coll Cardiol* 2005;46:920–927.

121. Roelandt J, Sutherland GR, Yoshida K, Yoshikawa J. Improved diagnosis and characterization of left ventricular pseudoaneurysm by Doppler color imaging. *J Am Coll Cardiol* 1988;12:807–811.

122. Helmcke F, Mahan EF, Nanda NC, et al. Two-dimensional echocardiography and Doppler color flow mapping in the diagnosis and prognosis of ventricular septal rupture. *Circulation* 1990;81:1775–1783.

123. Porter TR, Li S, Oster R, Deligonul U. The clinical implications of no reflow demonstrated with intravenous perfluorocarbon containing microbubbles following restoration of Thrombolysis in Myocardial Infarction (TIMI) 3 flow in patients with acute myocardial infarction. *Am J Cardiol* 1998;82:1173–1177.

124. Quinones MA, Verani MS, Haichin RM, et al. Exercise echocardiography versus T1–201 single photon emission computerized tomography in evaluation of coronary artery disease: analysis of 292 patients. *Circulation* 1992;85:1026–1031.

125. Geleijnse ML, Floretti PM, Roelandt J. Methodology, feasibility, safety and diagnostic accuracy of dobutamine stress echocardiography. *J Am Coll Cardiol* 1997;30:595–606.

126. Afridi I, Grayburn PA, Panza JA, et al. Myocardial viability during dobutamine echocardiography predicts survival in patients with coronary artery dis-

ease and severe left ventricular systolic dysfunction. *J Am Coll Cardiol* 1998;32:921–926.

127. Marwick T, Wilemart B, D'Hondt AM, et al. Selection of the optimal non-exercise stress for the evaluation of ischemic regional myocardial dysfunction and malperfusion: comparison of dobutamine and adenosine using echocardiography and Tc-99m MIBI single photon emission computerized tomography. *Circulation* 1993;87:345–354.

128. Das MK, Pellikka PA, Mahoney DW, et al. Assessment of cardiac risk before nonvascular surgery: dobutamine stress echocardiography in 530 patients. *J Am Coll Cardiol* 2000;35:1647–1653.

129. deFilippi CR, Willett DL, Brickner ME, et al. Usefulness of dobutamine echocardiography in distinguishing severe from nonsevere valvular aortic stenosis in patients with depressed left ventricular function and low transvalvular gradients. *Am J Cardiol* 1995;75:191–194.

130. Blanchard DG, Ross J Jr. Hypertrophic cardiomyopathy: prognosis with medical or surgical therapy. *Clin Cardiol* 1991;14:11–19.

131. Spirito P, Maron BJ. Relation between extent of left ventricular hypertrophy and diastolic filling abnormalities in hypertrophic cardiomyopathy. *J Am Coll Cardiol* 1990;15:808–813.

132. Nishimura RA, Appleton CP, Redfield MM, et al. Noninvasive Doppler echocardiographic evaluation of left ventricular filling pressures in patients with cardiomyopathies: a simultaneous Doppler echocardiographic and cardiac catheterization study. *J Am Coll Cardiol* 1996;28:1226–1233.

133. Shub C, Dimopoulos IN, Seward JB, et al. Sensitivity of two-dimensional echocardiography in the direct visualization of atrial septal defect utilizing the subcostal approach: experience with 154 patients. *J Am Coll Cardiol* 1983;2:127–135.

134. Pollick C, Sullivan H, Cujec B, Wilansky S. Doppler color-flow imaging assessment of shunt size in atrial septal defect. *Circulation* 1988;78:522–528.

135. Linker DT, Rossvoll O, Chapman JV, Angelsen B. Sensitivity and speed of color Doppler flow mapping compared with continuous wave Doppler for the detection of ventricular septal defects. *Br Heart J* 1991;65:201–203.

136. Liao P-K, Su W-J, Hung J-S. Doppler echocardiographic flow characteristics of isolated patent ductus arteriosus: better delineation by Doppler color flow mapping. *J Am Coll Cardiol* 1988;12:1285–1291.

137. Smallhorn JF, Burrows P, Wilson G, et al. Two-dimensional and pulsed Doppler echocardiography in the postoperative evaluation of total anomalous pulmonary venous connection. *Circulation* 1987;76:289–305.

138. Flanagan MF, Foran RB, VanPraagh R, et al. Tetralogy of Fallot with obstruction of the ventricular septal defect: Spectrum of echocardiographic findings. *J Am Coll Cardiol* 1988;11:386–395.

139. Smallhorn J, Grow R, Freedom R, et al. Pulsed Doppler echocardiographic assessment of the pulmonary venous pathway after the Mustard or Senning procedure for transposition of the great arteries. *Circulation* 1986;73:765–774.

140. Simpson IA, Sahn DJ, Valdes-Cruz LM, et al. Color Doppler flow mapping in patients with coarctation of the aorta: new observations and improved evaluation with color flow diameter and proximal acceleration as predictors of severity. *Circulation* 1988;77:736–744.

141. Shiina A, Seward JB, Edwards WD, et al. Two-dimensional echocardiographic spectrum of Ebstein's anomaly: detailed anatomic assessment. *J Am Coll Cardiol* 1984;3:356–370.

142. Sharland GK, Chita SK, Allan LD. The use of color Doppler in fetal echocardiography. *Int J Cardiol* 1990;28:229–236.

143. DeMaria AN, Bommer W, Neumann A, et al. Left ventricular thrombi identified by cross-sectional echocardiography. *Ann Intern Med* 1979;90:14–18.

144. Hara H, Virmani R, Ladich E, et al. Patent foramen ovale: current pathology, pathophysiology, and clinical status. *J Am Coll Cardiol* 2005;46:1768–1776.

145. Daniel WG, Nellessen U, Schroder E, et al. Left atrial spontaneous echo contrast in mitral valve disease: an indicator for an increased thromboembolic risk. *J Am Coll Cardiol* 1988;11:1204–1211.

146. Reynen K. Cardiac myxomas. *N Engl J Med* 1995;1610–1617.

147. Kirkpatrick JN, Wong T, Bednarz JE. Differential diagnosis of cardiac masses using contrast echocardiographic perfusion imaging. *J Am Coll Cardiol* 2004;43:1412–1419.

148. McAllister HA Jr. Primary tumors and cysts of the heart and pericardium. *Curr Probl Cardiol* 1979;4:1–51.

149. Hatle LK, Appleton CP, Popp RL. Differentiation of constrictive pericarditis and restrictive cardiomyopathy by Doppler echocardiography. *Circulation* 1989;79:357–370.

150. Kodas E, Nishimura RA, Appleton CP, et al. Doppler evaluation of patients with constrictive pericarditis: use of tricuspid regurgitation velocity curves to determine enhanced ventricular interaction. *J Am Coll Cardiol* 1996;28:652–657.

151. Redberg RF, Sobol Y, Chou TM, et al. Adenosine-induced coronary vasodilatation during transesophageal Doppler echocardiography: rapid and safe measurement of coronary flow reserve ratio can predict significant left anterior descending coronary stenosis. *Circulation* 1995;92:190–196.

152. Weidemann F, Jamal F, Sutherland GR, et al. Myocardial function defined by strain rate and strain during alterations in inotropic states and heart rate. *Am J Physiol Heart Circ Physiol* 2002;283:H792–H799.

153. Sutherland GR, Di Salvo G, Claus P, et al. Strain and strain rate imaging: a new clinical approach to quantifying regional myocardial function. *J Am Soc Echocardiogr* 2004;17:788–802.

154. Suffoletto MS, Dohi K, Cannesson M, et al. Novel speckle-tracking radial strain from routine black-and-white echocardiographic images to quantify dyssynchrony and predict response to cardiac resynchronization therapy. *Circulation* 2006;113:960–968.

155. Amundsen BH, Helle-Valle T, Edvardsen T, et al. Noninvasive myocardial strain measurement by speckle tracking echocardiography: validation against sonomicrometry and tagged magnetic resonance imaging. *J Am Coll Cardiol* 2006;47:789–793.

156. Dohi K; Pinsky MR; Kanzaki H; Severyn D; Gorcsan J. Effects of radial left ventricular dyssynchrony on cardiac performance using quantitative tissue Doppler radial strain imaging. *J Am Soc Echocardiogr* 2006;19:475–482.

157. Kukulski T, Jamal F, Herbots L, et al. Identification of acutely ischemic myocardium using ultrasonic strain measurements: a clinical study in patients undergoing coronary angioplasty. *J Am Coll Cardiol* 2003;41:810–819.

158. Cleland JG, Daubert JC, Erdmann E, et al. The effect of cardiac resynchronization on morbidity and mortality in heart failure. *N Engl J Med* 2005;352:1539–1549.

159. Bax JJ, Abraham T, Barold SS, et al. Cardiac resynchronization therapy: part 1—issues before device implantation. *J Am Coll Cardiol* 2005;46:2153–2167.

160. Yu CM, Fung JW, Zhang Q, et al. Tissue Doppler imaging is superior to strain rate imaging and postsystolic shortening on the prediction of reverse remodeling in both ischemic and nonischemic heart failure after cardiac resynchronization therapy. *Circulation* 2004;110:66–73.

161. Bax JJ, Bleeker GB, Marwick TH, et al. Left ventricular dyssynchrony predicts response and prognosis after cardiac resynchronization therapy, *J Am Coll Cardiol* 2004;44:1834–1840.

162. Yu CM, Chau E, Sanderson JE, et al. Tissue Doppler echocardiographic evidence of reverse remodeling and improved synchronicity by simultaneously delaying regional contraction after biventricular pacing therapy in heart failure. *Circulation* 2002;105:438–45.

CHAPTER (17)

Cardiac Catheterization, Cardiac Angiography, and Coronary Blood Flow and Pressure Measurements

Morton J. Kern / Spencer B. King III

CARDIAC CATHETERIZATION   467
Indications and Contraindications / 467
Preparation of the Patient for Cardiac
    Catheterization / 468
Techniques of Vascular Access / 468
Access Site Hemostasis / 468
Equipment in the Catheterization
    Laboratory / 469
Radiographic Contrast Media / 471
Complications of Cardiac
    Catheterization / 472

CARDIAC ANGIOGRAPHY   473
Coronary Arteriography / 473
Techniques of Cannulating Coronary
    Arteries and Grafts / 473
Angiographic Views / 474
Interpretation of the Coronary
    Arteriogram / 476
Left Ventriculography / 482
Other Cardiovascular Angiographic
    Studies / 486

THE X-RAY IMAGE   486
Generation of the X-Ray Image / 486
Radiation Safety / 488

**HEMODYNAMIC DATA FROM THE
CARDIAC CATHETERIZATION
LABORATORY   488**
Pressure Measurements / 488
Computations for Hemodynamic
    Measurements / 489
Calculation of Valve Areas / 490
Cardiac Output Techniques / 492
Intracardiac Shunts / 492
Normal Hemodynamic Waveforms / 494
Pathologic Hemodynamic
    Waveforms / 495
Physiologic Maneuvers in the
    Catheterization Laboratory / 496

**SPECIAL CATHETERIZATION
TECHNIQUES   499**
Transseptal Heart Catheterization / 499
Endomyocardial Biopsy / 499
Pericardiocentesis / 499
Intraaortic Balloon Counterpulsation / 499
Cardiac Catheterization in Heart
    Transplant Patients and Adults with
    Congenital Heart Disease / 500

**CORONARY BLOOD FLOW
AND PRESSURE
MEASUREMENTS   501**
Coronary Blood Flow and Resistance / 501
Coronary Flow Velocity and Reserve / 501
Pressure-Derived Fractional Flow
    Reserve of the Myocardium / 502
Method of Sensor Guidewire Use / 503
Clinical Applications of Coronary Blood
    Flow and Pressure Measurements / 506

APPENDICES   522

CARDIAC CATHETERIZATION

In 1929 Werner Forssman, a resident surgeon at Eberswalde in Germany, inserted a urologic catheter into his right atrium from a left antecubital vein cutdown he had performed on himself using a mirror. After walking downstairs to the radiology suite, the position of the catheter tip was verified by a roentgenogram. This was the beginning of cardiac catheterization: the insertion and passage of small plastic catheters into arteries, veins, the heart, and other vascular structures. Because there have been dramatic and innovative advances in both methods and materials, catheterization has become a standard medical procedure allowing the clinician to use physiologic data to guide treatment; measure cardiovascular hemodynamics such as pressures, cardiac output, oximetry data; acquire radiographic images of coronary arteries and cardiac chambers; and examine the aorta (Ao), pulmonary veins, and peripheral vessels for diseases, anomalies, or obstructions. In the last three decades, cardiac catheterization has evolved further, from a diagnostic modality to one of a treatment through numerous catheter-based interventions (e.g., angioplasty, stenting, closure of atrial septal defects) (Table 17–1).

[ ] INDICATIONS AND CONTRAINDICATIONS

Cardiac catheterization is used to diagnose atherosclerotic artery disease, cardiomyopathy, myocardial infarction, and valvular or congenital heart abnormalities. The principal indications for cardiac catheter-

TABLE 17–1

Diagnostic and Therapeutic Interventional Procedures That May Accompany Coronary Angiography

DIAGNOSTIC PROCEDURES	COMMENT
Central venous access (femoral, internal jugular, subclavian)	Access for emergency medications or fluids, temporary pacemaker
Hemodynamic assessment	
Left heart pressures (aorta, left ventricle)	Routine for all studies
Right and left heart combined pressures	Not routine for coronary artery disease; mandatory for valvular heart disease; congestive heart failure (CHF), right ventricular dysfunction, pericardial diseases, cardiomyopathy, intracardiac shunts, congenital abnormalities
Transseptal or LV puncture	Valvular heart disease
Intracoronary pressure/flow	Coronary lesion assessment
Left ventricular angiography	Routine for all studies; may be excluded with high-risk patients, left main coronary or aortic stenosis, severe CHF, renal failure
Internal mammary artery and saphenous vein bypass graft selective angiography	Routine for coronary bypass conduit
Pharmacologic studies	
Ergonovine	Routine for suspected coronary vasospasm
IC/IV/sublingual nitroglycerin	Routine for all coronary angiography
Aortography	Routine for aortic insufficiency, aortic dissection, aortic aneurysm, with or without aortic stenosis, routine to locate bypass grafts not visualized by selective angiography
Renal and peripheral vascular angiography	For renovascular hypertension and peripheral vascular disease
Cardiac pacing and electrophysiologic studies	Arrhythmia evaluation
Therapeutic interventional procedures	
Coronary disease	Percutaneous coronary interventions (e.g., PTCA, stenting)
Valvular stenosis	Balloon catheter valvuloplasty
Atrial septal defect	Atrial septal defect closure
Hypertrophic obstructive cardiomyopathy (HOCM)	Transseptal alcohol septal ablation for HOCM
Arrhythmia	Electrophysiologic conduction tract catheter ablation
Arterial access site closure devices	Available for patients prone to access site bleeding

IC, intracardiac; LV, left ventricular; PTCA, percutaneous transluminal coronary angioplasty.
SOURCE: From Kern MJ.[1] With permission.

ization are summarized in Table 17–2. In general, cardiac catheterization is an elective diagnostic procedure and should be deferred if the patient is not prepared either psychologically or physically. For urgent procedures, especially if the patient is unstable from a suspected cardiac cause such as acute myocardial infarction, catheterization must proceed. In the event of decompensated congestive heart failure requiring cardiac catheterization for diagnosis and potential treatment, rapid medical management in the catheterization laboratory may be an expeditious option whereby endotracheal intubation, intraaortic balloon pumping, and vasopressors can be instituted rapidly before angiography and revascularization. Relative contraindications to cardiac catheterization include fever, anemia, electrolyte imbalance (especially hypokalemia predisposing to arrhythmias), or other systemic illnesses needing stabilization (Table 17–3).

[ ] PREPARATION OF THE PATIENT FOR CARDIAC CATHETERIZATION

The procedure should be explained to the patient in simple terms as to what will take place and the reason for each step of the procedure.

The operator (preferably) or the assistant, usually a physician, obtains consent. The operator should explain the risks for routine cardiac catheterization to the patient and family. The incidence of major risks of stroke, death, and myocardial infarction is approximately 0.1 percent. The minor risks of vascular injury, allergic reaction, bleeding, hematoma, and infection range from 0.04 to 5 percent and should be discussed. Certain patient groups are at higher risk for complications (Table 17–4). Patient information should be tailored to the specific individual and the associated clinical problems (Table 17–5). Patients with diabetes mellitus, renal insufficiency, or previous reported hypersensitivity to iodinated contrast media constitute groups who need special consideration. For diabetic patients the dose of neutral protamine Hagedorn (NPH) insulin should be cut by 50 percent, because overnight fast with their normal morning dose of insulin causes hypoglycemia. Patients receiving NPH insulin are also at higher risk for protamine reactions. Some diabetic patients receive an antihyperglycemic agent, such as metformin, an analogue of phenformin that is associated with a risk of lactic acidosis, particularly in patients with chronic renal failure where metformin is contraindicated. There is no evidence that withholding metformin for 48

TABLE 17–2

Indications for Cardiac Catheterization

INDICATIONS	PROCEDURES
Suspected or known coronary artery disease	
New onset angina	LV, COR
Unstable angina	LV, COR
Evaluation before a major surgical procedure	LV, COR
Silent ischemia	LV, COR
Positive ETT	LV, COR
Atypical chest pain or coronary spasm	LV, COR, ERGO
Myocardial infarction	
Unstable angina postinfarction	LV, COR
Failed thrombolysis	LV, COR, RH
Shock	LV, COR, RH
Mechanical complications (ventricular septal defect, rupture of wall, or papillary muscle)	LV, COR, RH
Sudden cardiovascular death	LV, COR, R + L
Valvular heart disease	LV, COR, R + L, AO
Congenital heart disease (before anticipated corrective surgery)	LV, COR, R + L, AO
Aortic dissection	AO, COR
Pericardial constriction or tamponade	LV, COR, R + L
Cardiomyopathy	LV, COR, R + L, BX
Initial and follow up assessment for heart transplant	LV, COR, R + L, BX

AO, aortography; BX, endomyocardial biopsy; COR, coronary angiography; ERGO, ergonovine provocation of coronary spasm; ETT, exercise tolerance test; LV, left ventriculography; RH, right heart oxygen saturations and hemodynamics (e.g., placement of Swan-Ganz catheter); R + L, right and left heart hemodynamics.
SOURCE: From Kern MJ.[1] With permission.

hours before a catheter procedure in patients with normal renal function provides any clinical benefit.

TECHNIQUES OF VASCULAR ACCESS

Vascular access is determined by the anticipated pathologic and anatomic findings relevant to the patient. Previous documentation of any difficulties, especially of vascular access, should be reviewed. Prior to a procedure, assessment of all peripheral pulses is mandatory.

Percutaneous Femoral Artery Puncture

Percutaneous femoral arterial catheterization is the most widely used technique for vascular access. In patients with claudication, chronic arterial insufficiency, diminished or absent pulses, or bruits over the iliofemoral area, alternate entry sites should be considered (Table 17–6). A detailed explanation of percutaneous femoral puncture technique can be found elsewhere.[1–3] In brief, the proposed entry site into the femoral artery (FA) can be verified by fluoroscopy using the tip of a metal clamp and placing it near the medial edge of the middle of the head of the femur (Fig. 17–1). Palpation identifies the center line of the artery and the needle is advanced at a 30-degree angle to the vessel puncturing only the front wall. The guidewire is then advanced and the needle exchanged for a valved sheath.

Percutaneous Femoral Vein Puncture

The femoral vein is located approximately 1 cm medial to the FA. The procedure for femoral vein percutaneous entry is similar to that for the FA with only minor differences. Because venous pressure is low, it may be difficult to detect backbleeding from the needle on entry. A syringe may be attached to the Seldinger needle and gently aspirated during needle advancement. Once in the vein, the remainder of the venous sheath placement is completed in the same fashion as described for the femoral arterial sheath insertion.

Radial Artery Catheterization

The radial approach has several distinct advantages[4,5]: (1) The radial artery is easily accessible in most patients and is not located near significant veins or nerves; (2) the superficial location of the radial artery makes for easy control of bleeding; (3) no significant clinical sequelae after radial artery occlusion occur in patients with a normal Allen test because of the collateral flow to the hand through the ulnar artery; (4) patient comfort is enhanced by the ability to sit up and walk immediately after the procedure; and (5) the radial artery access provides the most secure hemostasis in the fully anticoagulated patient. Patients with a normal Allen test (Table 17–7) are candidates for the radial approach with 4 to 6 Fr sheaths and catheters. Small or female patients are more likely to have spasm of the radial artery, but this can be treated effectively with the use of intraarterial nitroglycerin or verapamil. Specially coated hydrophilic sheaths reduce spasm on sheath insertion and removal. Arterial puncture using a short 20-gauge needle, a 0.025-in. guidewire, and a radial artery sheath system (24 cm) is performed in a manner similar to FA puncture. The point of puncture is over the radial artery pulsation on the wrist. After puncture, the

TABLE 17–3

Contraindications to Cardiac Catheterization

Absolute contraindications
  Inadequate equipment or catheterization facility
Relative contraindications
  Acute gastrointestinal bleeding or anemia
  Anticoagulation (or known uncontrolled bleeding diathesis)
  Electrolyte imbalance
  Infection/fever
  Medication intoxication (e.g., digitalis, phenothiazine)
  Pregnancy
  Recent carebral vascular accident (>1 mo)
  Renal failure
  Uncontrolled congestive heart failure, high blood pressure, arrhythmias
  Uncooperative patient

SOURCE: From Kern MJ.[1] With permission

TABLE 17-4

Conditions of Patients at Higher Risk for Complications of Catheterization

Acute myocardial infarction
Advanced age (>75 y)
Aortic aneurysm
Aortic stenosis
Congestive heart failure
Diabetes
Extensive three-vessel coronary artery disease
Left ventricular dysfunction (left ventricular ejection fraction <35%)
Obesity
Prior cerebral vascular accident
Renal insufficiency
Suspected or known left main coronary stenosis
Uncontrolled hypertension
Unstable angina

SOURCE: From Kern MJ.[1] With permission.

small guidewire is inserted followed by a long arterial sheath. During insertion of the arterial sheath, 5000 U of heparin, 2 mL of 1 percent lidocaine, and 200 μg of nitroglycerin are often given through the partially positioned sheath. An additional intraarteriolar vasodilator—such as diltiazem, verapamil, papaverine, or adenosine—may be necessary to minimize spasm. After vascular access has been secured, angiographic and hemodynamic data are obtained, as discussed below.

ACCESS SITE HEMOSTASIS

After the catheterization procedure has been completed and the catheters removed, the sheath is flushed. If heparin has been given, an activated clotting time is obtained; if this is >200 sec, protamine sulfate may be given before sheath removal (25 to 50 mg protamine IV reverses 10,000 U heparin). Caution should be used in giving protamine to patients receiving NPH insulin, who may have higher likelihood of a protamine reaction (Table 17–8).

To remove the FA sheath, gentle pressure is applied over the puncture site while the sheath is removed, taking care not to crush the sheath and *strip* clot into the distal artery. Firm downward pressure is applied for 15 to 30 minutes, periodically evaluating distal pulses. After manual hemostasis is achieved, an adhesive bandage is used to cover the wound. Large pressure dressings are generally ineffective to prevent bleeding and obscure the puncture site. Additional methods to secure postprocedure arterial hemostasis include mechanical pressure clamps and vascular closure devices. A variety of vascular closure devices are currently available.[6–8] These devices reduce the time to obtain hemostasis and early ambulation. These devices may be helpful in anticoagulated patients and patients with back pain or an inability to lie flat. The advantages and disadvantages are summarized in Table 17–9. All vascular closure devices should be used with caution in patients with peripheral vascular disease or low arterial puncture (at or below the femoral bifurcation). Femoral angiography with an ipsilateral ob-

lique angle reveals the puncture site and any artery disease. Patients at high risk for groin hematoma and arterial complications may need longer pressure application or may benefit with a vascular closure device are listed in Table 17–10.

For radial artery hemostasis, sheath removal uses a plastic bracelet with a pressure pad placed around the wrist. While pressing the pad over the puncture site, the sheath is gently withdrawn and the bracelet tightened. The bracelet should be tight enough to ensure hemostasis but not occlude the flow to the hand. Between 1 and 2 hours later, the patient is checked and the bracelet is loosened. The patient can be discharged 2 hours later and the bracelet removed at home.

EQUIPMENT IN THE CATHETERIZATION LABORATORY

Catheters for Angiography and Hemodynamics

Numerous shapes and sizes of catheters are available to the angiographer. Basic, routine catheters that are preshaped for normal anat-

TABLE 17-5

Conditions Requiring Special Preparations for Cardiac Catheterization

CONDITION	MANAGEMENT
Allergy	Treat potential hypersensitivity
Prior contrast studies	Contrast premedication
Iodine, fish	Contrast reaction algorithm
Premedication allergy	Hold premedication
Lidocaine	Use Marcaine (1 mg/mL)
Patients receiving anti-coagulation (INR >1.5)	Defer procedure
	Vitamin K
	Fresh frozen plasma
	Hold heparin
	Protamine for heparin
Diabetes	Hydration, urine output >50 mL/h
NPH insulin (protamine reaction)	Glucophage held 48 h
Renal function	If renal insufficiency postpone catheterization
Glucophage usage (prone to CIN)	Consider urgency and risks of lactic acidosis
Electrolyte imbalance (K⁺, Mg²⁺, or Mg⁺⁺)	Defer procedure, replenish/correct electrolytes
Arrhythmias	Defer procedure, administer anti-arrhythmics
Anemia	Defer procedure
	Control bleeding
	Transfuse
Dehydration	Hydration
Renal failure	Limit contrast
	Maintain high urine output
	Hydrate

CIN, contrast induced renal failure; NPH, neutral protamine Hagedorn.
SOURCE: From Kern MJ.[1] With permission.

TABLE 17–6

Possible Vascular Access Routes

Arterial
  Axillary
  Brachial
  Femoral
  Radial
  Subclavian—*not* used for cardiac catheterization
  Translumbar—*not* used for cardiac catheterization
Venous
  Brachial
  Femoral
  Internal jugular
  Subclavian

omy are available for both the radial and femoral approaches. There is an array of shapes and sizes to aid the angiographer when abnormal anatomy is present (Fig. 17–2).

Judkins-Type Coronary Catheters The Judkins catheters have unique preshaped curves and tapered end-hole tips. The Judkins left coronary catheter has a double curve. The length of the segment between the primary and secondary curve determines the size of the catheter (i.e., 3.5, 4.0, 5.0, or 6.0 cm). The proper size of the left Judkins catheter is selected depending on the length and width of the ascending Ao. The ingenious design of the left Jud-

kins catheter permits cannulation of the left coronary artery without any major catheter manipulation except the slow advance of the catheter under fluoroscopic control. The catheter tip follows the ascending aortic border and falls into the left main coronary ostium, often with an abrupt jump. A left 4-cm Judkins catheter is appropriate for most adult patients. When catheter size is adequate, the catheter tip is aligned with the long axis of the left main coronary trunk. A smaller, 3.5-cm catheter in the same patient will tip upward toward the anterior descending artery and a larger, 5.0-cm catheter will tip downward into the circumflex ostium.

The Judkins right coronary catheter is sized by the length of the secondary curve and comes in 3.5-, 4.0-, and 5.0-cm sizes. The 4.0-cm catheter is adequate for most cases. The right Judkins catheter is advanced into the ascending Ao (usually in the left anterior oblique [LAO] projection) with the tip directed caudally.

Amplatz-Type Catheters The left Amplatz-type catheter (see Fig. 17–2) is a preshaped half circle with the tapered tip extending perpendicular to the curve. Amplatz catheter sizes (left 1, 2, and 3 and right 1 and 2) indicate the diameter of the tip's curve. In the LAO projection, the tip is advanced into the left aortic cusp. Further advancement of the catheter causes the tip to move upward into the left main trunk. It is necessary to advance the Amplatz catheters slightly to disengage the catheter tip upward and out of the left main ostium. If the catheter is pulled instead of first being advanced, the tip moves downward and into the left main or circumflex artery. Amplatz catheters have a higher risk of coronary dissection than Judkins-style catheters. The

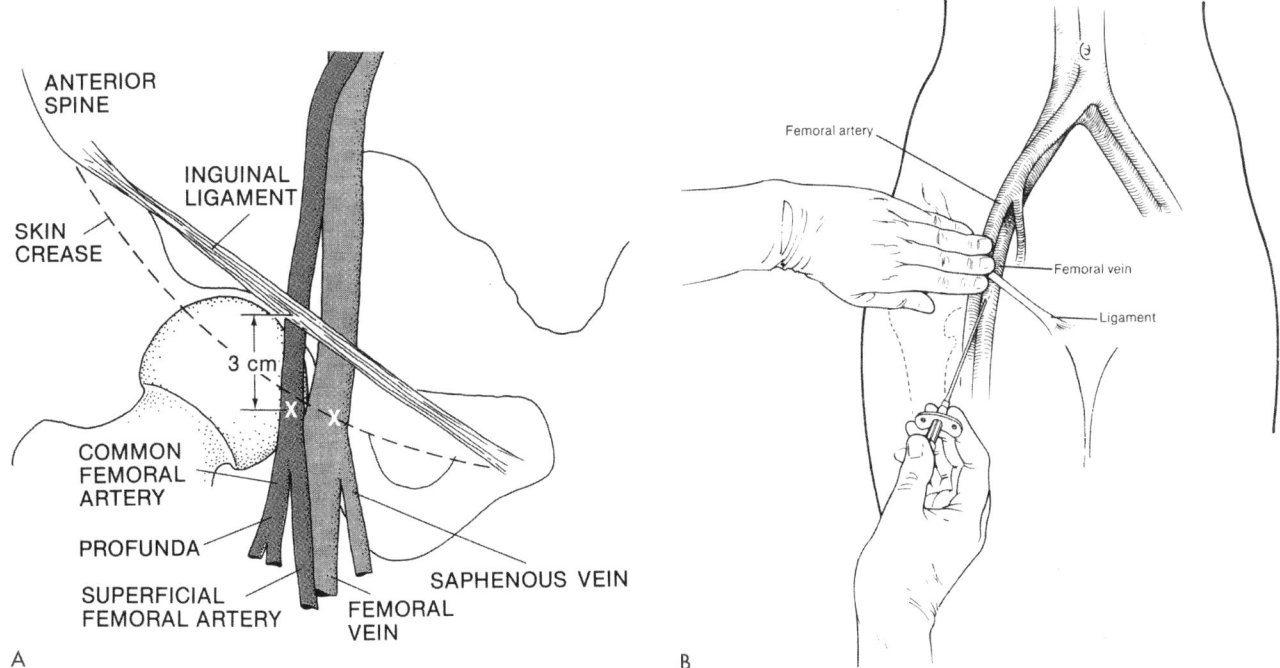

FIGURE 17–1. A. Anatomy relevant to percutaneous catheterization of the femoral artery (FA) and vein. The right FA vein pass underneath the inguinal ligament, which connects the anterior-superior iliac spine and public tubercle. The arterial skin nick (indicated by *X*) should be placed approximately 1-1/2 to 2 fingerbreadths (3 cm) below the inguinal ligament and directly over the FA pulsation. The venous skin nick should be placed at the same level, but approximately 1 fingerbreadth medial. **B.** Femoral vein puncture with the needle at a 30- to 45-degree angle aiming medially toward the umbilicus. *Sources: A, from Baim DS, Grossman W. Percutaneous approach including transseptal and apical puncture. In Baim DS, Grossman W, eds. Grossman's Cardiac Catheterization, Angiography, and Intervention, 6th ed. Baltimore: Lippincott, Williams & Wilkins; 2000. With permission. B, from Tilkian AG, Daily EK. Cardiovascular Procedures: Diagnostic Techniques and Therapeutic Procedures. St Louis: Mosby; 1986. With permission.*

TABLE 17–7

The Allen Test

The Allen test assesses the circulation of an intact palmar arterial arch.
Method:
1. The radial and ulnar arteries are simultaneously occluded while the patient makes a fist.
2. The hand is opened appearing blanched.
3. The ulnar artery is released, and the hand observed for change in color.
Satisfactory ulnar flow is present if color returns to palm in 8 to 10 sec or if pulse oximetry normalizes on release of the artery.

right Amplatz (modified) catheter has a smaller but similar hook-shaped curve. The catheter is advanced into the right coronary cusp. Like Judkins right catheters, the catheter is rotated clockwise for 45 to 90 degrees. The same maneuver is repeated at different levels until the right coronary artery is entered. After coronary injections, the catheter may be pulled, advanced, or rotated out of the coronary artery.

Multipurpose Catheters These catheters are mostly gently curved catheters with an end hole and two side holes placed close to the tapered tip. The multipurpose catheter can be used for both left and right coronary intubation and left ventriculography.

Special-Purpose Femoral Catheters for Bypass Grafts The right coronary vein graft catheter is similar to a right Judkins catheter with a wider, more open primary curve allowing cannulation of cranially oriented coronary artery vein graft. The left vein graft catheter is similar to the right Judkins catheter with a smaller diameter secondary curve, allowing easy cannulation of left anterior descending coronary artery (LAD) and left circumflex vein grafts, which usually are placed higher and more anterior than the right coronary grafts with a relatively horizontal and upward takeoff

TABLE 17–8

Characteristics and Treatment of a Protamine Reaction[a]

CHARACTERISTICS
Shaking
Flushing
Chills
Back, chest, or flank pain
Vasomotor collapse

TREATMENT
1. Morphine (2 mg IV) or meperidine (25 mg IV),
2. Diphenhydramine (25–50 mg IV)
3. Saline administration
4. Support of low blood pressure

[a]Protamine reactions are usually self-limited (<1 h).

TABLE 17–9

Advantages/Disadvantages of Vascular Closure Devices

DEVICE	MECHANISM	ADVANTAGES AND LIMITATIONS
AngioSeal	Collagen seal	Secure hemostasis; Anchor may catch on side branch
Duett	Collagen-thrombin	Stronger collagen-thrombin seal; Intraarterial injection of collagen-thrombin
Perclose	Sutures	Secure hemostasis of suture; Device failure may require surgical repair
VasoSeal	Collagen plug	No intraarterial components; Positioning wire may catch on side branch
Starclose	Nitinol Clip	No intraarterial material; Secure hemostasis of clip

from the Ao. The internal mammary artery graft catheter has a hook-shaped tip configuration that facilitates the engagement of internal mammary artery grafts.

Ventriculography Catheters The pigtail catheter has a tapered tip, preshaped to make a full circle 1 cm in diameter. Five to twelve side holes are located on the straight portion of the catheter above the curve. A pigtail catheter with an angled (145-degree) shaft is also available for horizontally oriented hearts. The multipurpose catheter is also used for ventriculography, but a high-pressure contrast jet from the end hole often produces ventricular

TABLE 17–10

Patients Who May Benefit from a Vascular Closure Device

Obese patients
Patients with hypertension
Elderly
Women
Patients with aortic regurgitation
Patients who have undergone prior arterial puncture
Patients with advanced peripheral atherosclerosis
Patients who suffer from coagulopathy or those receiving anticoagulant or antiplatelet agents

SOURCE: From Kern MJ.[1] With permission.

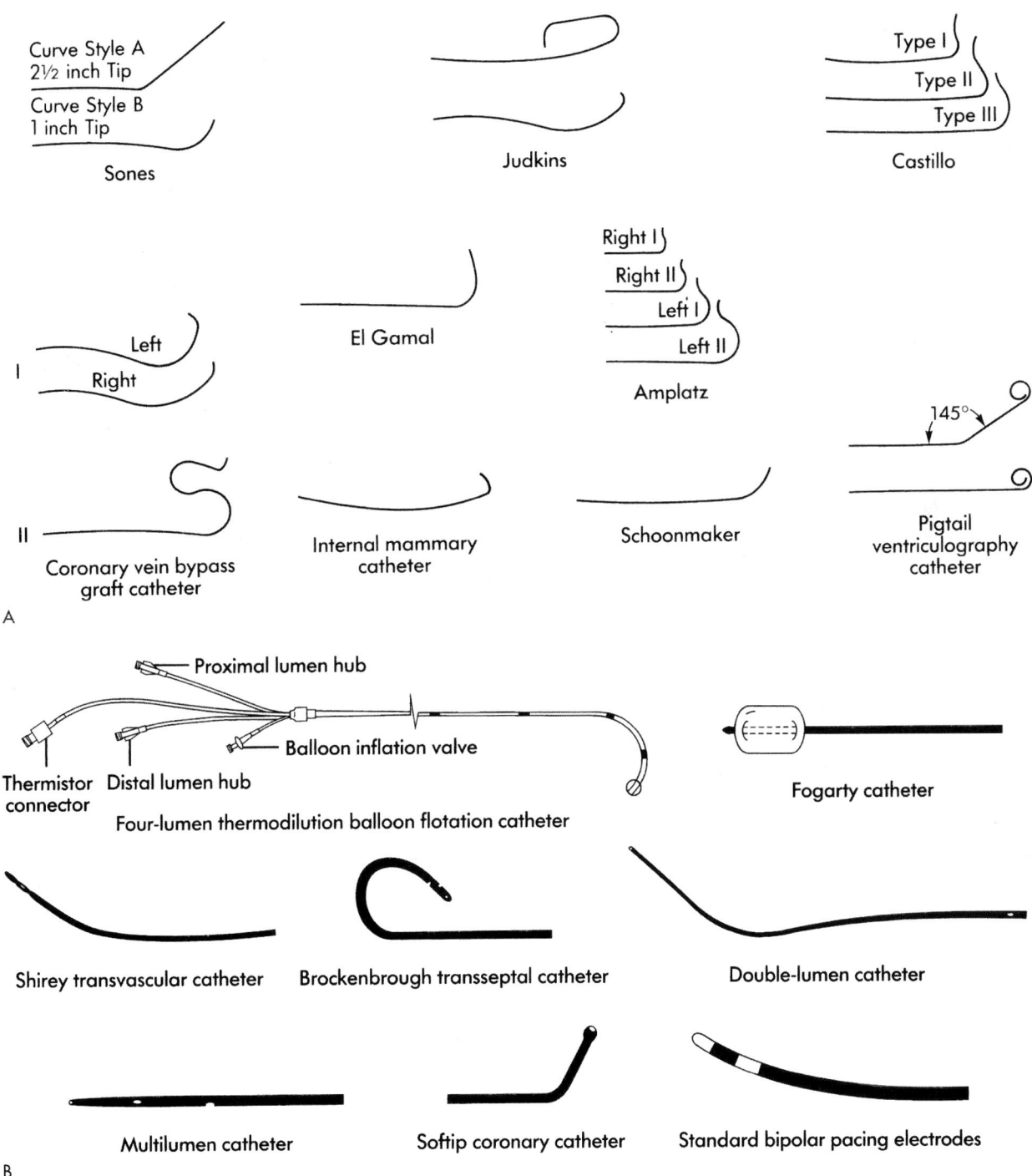

FIGURE 17–2. A. Left heart catheters in common use for selective coronary arteriography and ventriculography. **B.** Various special-purpose catheters for right and left heart catheterization. *Sources: A, from Kern MJ.[1] With permission. B, modified from Tilkian AG, Daily EK. Cardiovascular Procedures: Diagnostic Techniques and Therapeutic Procedures. St. Louis: Mosby; 1986. With permission.*

tachycardia; rarely, myocardial tissue contrast staining or perforation occurs. A comprehensive discussion of left heart catheter types and techniques can be found elsewhere.[1–3] The new operator should concentrate on mastering a few types of catheters and gain extensive experience in using them effectively.

Right Heart Catheters For right heart catheterization, a balloon-tipped flotation catheter (see Fig. 17–2), is the most widely used. The balloon tip allows the catheter to float through the right side of the heart safely and easily in most cases. The balloon *wedges* in the distal pulmonary artery (PA) to measure pressure and accurately reflects left atrial and ventricular filling pressures. Thermodilution cardiac output measurements are exclusive to this type of catheter. The balloon-tipped catheter can be introduced through any venous access route. The balloon is inflated with air. The balloon-tipped catheters do not provide good torque control, making catheterization of the PA in patients with right atrial (RA) or ventricular enlargement, pulmonary hypertension, or tricuspid regurgitation difficult from the femoral approach.

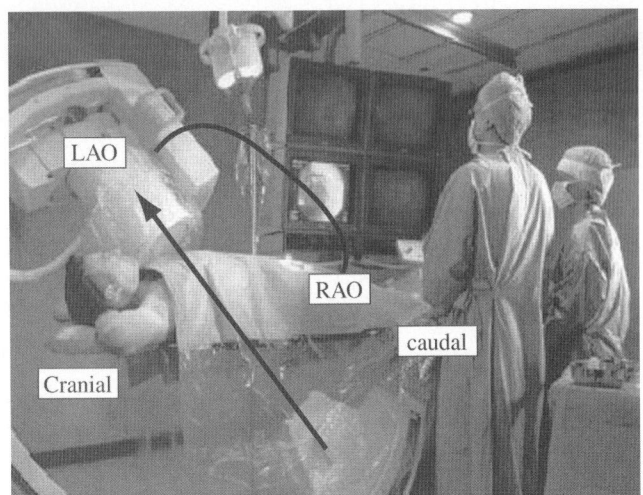

FIGURE 17–3. The cardiac catheterization laboratory. The operators stand on the patient's right side facing the fluoroscopic and hemodynamic monitors. The fluoroscope is positioned over the patient's left shoulder to produce a left anterior oblique (LAO) cranially angulated view of the heart. The image intensifier can be rotated to other positions (e.g., caudal or right anterior oblique (RAO) as well to visualize the cardiac structures from any angle.

For right heart angiography, the Berman catheter, a large-lumen, balloon-tipped angiographic catheter with side holes placed proximally to the balloon, is introduced easily into the right heart. Keeping the balloon inflated increases the catheter stability during angiography. A regular pigtail catheter, or one with a special obtuse angle (Grollman), can also be used for right ventriculography.

The Fluoroscopic Imaging System

Passage of catheters and acquisition of angiographic data requires a high-resolution image-intensifier television system with digital cineangiographic capabilities. The components are mounted on a U or C arm, which is a support with the radiograph tube beneath the patient and the image intensifier above. Rotation of the arm allows viewing over a wide range of different angles. Some laboratories have two systems perpendicular to one another (called *biplane*) and use a double monitoring system, providing simultaneous visualization of the heart from two different angles (Fig. 17–3).

The Physiologic Monitor and Recording System

During catheterization, it is necessary to monitor and record electrocardiographic and hemodynamic signals. Digital recording systems incorporate physiologic data with digital angiographic data.

Contrast Power Injector

A high-pressure contrast media injector is needed to administer a large bolus (20 to 50 mL) of contrast media into the left ventricle at a rate of 10 to 20 mL/sec, pulmonary arteries 10 to 25 mL/sec, or aortic arch 40 to 60 mL/sec. When properly set and flushed, the power injector can be used to inject contrast into the coronary arteries (at a rate of 3 to 8 mL/sec). Some injector systems also incorporate a pressure transducer and have replaced traditional manifolds with stopcocks.

Resuscitation Equipment and Defibrillator

Every cardiovascular laboratory is equipped with an emergency crash cart containing emergency drugs, oxygen, airways, suction apparatus, and other emergency equipment. A defibrillator should be charged and ready for use during a procedure.

Sterile Equipment and Supplies

The angiographer works from a sterile pack or tray that contains the various supplies needed to perform the procedure. The pack will contain syringes and needles, local anesthetic, basins for flushing solutions, small drapes and towels, clamps, scalpels, pressure manifolds and connecting tubings, and the like.

▋ ▋ RADIOGRAPHIC CONTRAST MEDIA
Characteristics of Contrast Media

All contrast media contain three iodine molecules attached to a fully substituted benzene ring. The fourth position in the standard ionic agent is taken up by sodium or methylglucamine as a cation; the remaining two positions of the benzene ring have side chains of diatrizoate, metatrizoate, or iothalamate. All media are excreted predominantly by glomerular filtration. The normal half-time of excretion is 20 minutes; biliary excretion is 1 percent. The vasodilator effect and the transient decrease in systemic vascular resistance are directly related to the degree of osmolality of the contrast medium used. Transient hypervolemia and depressed contractility are related to both osmolality and ionic charge and in part responsible for the elevation of left atrial and left ventricular (LV) end-diastolic pressure after contrast injection. To reduce the osmotic effects of contrast medium, the number of dissolved particles must be decreased or the molal concentration of iodine per particle must be increased. New-generation, nonionic, monomeric, and ionic dimeric contrast agents have approximately the same viscosity and iodine concentration but have only one-half or less of the osmolality of the ionic agents.[9–11] Ionic contrast media produce hypotension by peripheral arterial vasodilation, transient myocardial dysfunction, and decreasing circulating volume and blood pressure after osmotic diuresis. Initially, contrast media increase circulating fluid volume by osmotically shifting fluid into vascular space. The advantages of the nonionic, low-osmolar agents include less hemodynamic loading, patient discomfort, binding of ionic calcium, depression of myocardial function and blood pressure, and possibly fewer anaphylactoid reactions.[9–11] Currently, nonionic, low-osmolar agents are preferred in all patients, but especially in adults with extremely poor LV function; patients with renal disease, especially those with diabetes; and patients with a history of serious reaction to contrast media or with multiple allergies. Table 17–11 provides a summary of commonly used contrast agents for coronary and LV angiographic studies. Although thousands of studies have been performed safely with conventional high-osmolar/ionic agents, considerable data exist indicating that low-osmolar/nonionic agents may be safer and provide satisfactory diagnostic quality, especially for high-risk patients[12] (Table 17–12).

TABLE 17-11

Commonly Used Iodinated Contrast Agents in Cardiac Angiography

PRODUCT CATEGORY	PROPRIETARY NAME	GENETIC CONSTITUENT	RATIO OF IODINE TO OSMOTICALLY ACTIVE PARTICLES	CALCIUM CHELATION	ANTICOAGULATION EFFECT
High-osmolar, ionic	Renografin-76	Diatrizoate and citrate	1.5	(+)	(+++)
High-osmolar, ionic	Hypaque-76	Diatrizoate only	1.5	(−)	(+++)
Low-osmolar, ionic	Hexabrix	Ioxaglate	3.0	(−)	(+++)
Low-osmolar, nonionic	Isovue	Iopamidol	3.0	(−)	(+)
Low-osmolar, nonionic	Omnipaque	Iohexol	3.0	(−)	(+)
Low-osmolar, nonionic	Optiray	Ioversol	3.0	(−)	(+)

(+), present; (+++), strongly present; (−), absent.
SOURCE: From Peterson KL, Nicod P. Cardiac Catheterization: Methods, Diagnosis, and Therapy. Philadelphia: Saunders; 1997. With permission.

Contrast Media Reactions

There are three types of contrast allergies (Table 17–13): (1) minor cutaneous and mucosal manifestations, (2) smooth muscle and minor anaphylactoid responses, and (3) major cardiovascular and anaphylactoid responses. Major reactions involving laryngeal or pulmonary edema often are accompanied by minor or less severe reactions. Although some reactions to a pretest contrast dose may be violent (but rarely life-threatening), pretesting has been found to be of no value in determining who will have an adverse reaction. Nonionic contrast media has replaced ionic contrast media for most patients to minimize chance of allergic and other adverse contrast reactions. Patients reporting allergic reactions to contrast media should be premedicated with prednisone and diphenhydramine. The routine for the laboratories may vary; but common dosages include 60 mg prednisone the night before, and 60 mg of prednisone the morning of, along with 50 mg oral diphenhydramine given at the time of call to the catheterization laboratory. Pretreatment with corticosteroids has been found to be helpful in reducing all types of reactions except those characterized predominantly by hives. Premedication may not prevent the occurrence of adverse reactions completely. Additional routine treatment of patients with prior allergic reactions with an H_2 blocker (e.g., cimetidine) does not appear to have any benefit. Patients with known prior anaphylactic reactions to contrast dye should be pretreated with steroids and an H_1 blocker.

Contrast-Induced Renal Failure

Patients with diabetes or renal insufficiency or those who are dehydrated from any cause are at risk for contrast-induced nephropathy (CIN). Advanced preparations to limit CIN include hydration and maintenance of large-volume urine flow (>200 mL/h). These patients should be hydrated intravenously the night before the procedure. Following the contrast study, intravenous fluids should be liberally continued unless intravascular volume overload is a problem. Furosemide, mannitol, and calcium channel blockers are not helpful in reducing CIN (see Table 17–14). *N*-acetylcysteine given intravenously before the procedure are associated with reduced CIN in some studies[13–15] but not in others.[16] A decreased urine output after the procedure that is unresponsive to increased intravenous fluids indicates that renal insufficiency is probable. A consultation with a nephrologist is often helpful. All types of contrast agents (ionic, nonionic, or low-osmolar) are associated with a similar incidence of contrast-induced nephropathy.

【 】 COMPLICATIONS OF CARDIAC CATHETERIZATION

Table 17–15 lists the major and minor complications of cardiac catheterization. For diagnostic catheterization, analysis of the

TABLE 17-12

Indications for Low-Osmolar/Nonionic Contrast Agents

Unstable ischemic syndromes
Congestive heart failure
Diabetes
Renal insufficiency
Hypotension
Severe bradycardia
History of contrast allergy
Severe valvular heart disease
Use for internal mammary artery and peripheral vascular injections

TABLE 17–13

Anaphylactoid Reactions to Contrast Medium

Cutaneous and mucosal
  Angioedema
  Flushing
  Laryngeal edema
  Pruritus
  Urticaria
Smooth muscle
  Bronchospasm
  Gastrointestinal spasm
  Uterine contraction
Cardiovascular
  Arrhythmia
  Hypotension (shock)
  Vasodilatation

complications in more than 200,000 patients indicates the incidence of risks as follows: death, <0.2 percent; myocardial infarction, <0.05 percent; stroke, <0.07 percent; serious ventricular arrhythmia, <0.5 percent; and major vascular complications (thrombosis, bleeding requiring transfusion, or pseudoaneurysm), <1 percent[17–20] (Table 17–16). Vascular complications are more frequent when the brachial approach is used. Risks are higher in well-described subgroups.

Complications of Arterial Access

The most common complication from femoral catheterization is hemorrhage and local hematoma formation, increasing in frequency with the increasing size of the sheath, the amount of anticoagulation, and obesity. Other common complications (in order of decreasing frequency) include retroperitoneal hematoma, pseudoaneurysm, arteriovenous (A-V) fistula, arterial thrombosis, stroke,[19] sepsis with or without abscess formation, and cholesterol or air embolization.[20] The frequency of these complications is increased in obese patients, high-risk procedures, critically ill elderly patients with extensive atheromatous disease, patients receiving anticoagulation, antiplatelet, and fibrinolytic therapies, and concomitant interventional procedures. Compared to the femoral approach, the radial approach causes significantly fewer vascular complications. A retroperitoneal hematoma should be suspected in patients with hypotension, tachycardia, pallor, a rapidly falling hematocrit postcatheterization, lower abdominal or back pain, or neurologic changes in the leg with the puncture. This complication is associated with high femoral arterial puncture and full anticoagulation.[18] Pseudoaneurysm is a complication associated with low femoral arterial puncture (usually below the head of the femur). With ultrasound imaging techniques, the pseudoaneurysm can easily be identified and nonsurgical closure performed. Manual compression of the expansile growing mass guided by Doppler ultrasound with or without thrombin or collagen injection is an acceptable therapy for femoral pseudoaneurysm.[21]

Protamine Reactions

Protamine is sometimes used to reverse the systemic effects of heparin. Minor protamine reactions may appear as back and flank pain or flushing with peripheral vasodilation and low blood pressure. Major protamine reactions simulate anaphylaxis. Although rare, major reactions involve marked facial flushing and vasomotor collapse, which may be fatal. The incidence of major protamine reactions in NPH insulin-dependent diabetics is 27 percent, compared to 0.5 percent in patients with no history of insulin use. It is recommended that diabetics on NPH insulin and patients with allergies to fish undergoing cardiac catheterization do so without use of protamine or, when necessary, that protamine be administered cautiously in anticipation of a major reaction.

Complications of Right Heart Catheterization

Right heart catheterization may be complicated by arrhythmia caused by stimulation of the right ventricular (RV) outflow tract, which may result in atrioventricular block, or rarely, right bundle-branch block (Table 17–17). Significant but transient ventricular arrhythmias occur in 30 to 60 percent of patients undergoing right heart catheterization and are terminated when the catheter is readjusted. Sustained ventricular arrhythmias have been reported, especially in unstable patients or those with electrolyte imbalance, acidosis, or concurrent myocardial ischemia. In patients with left bundle-branch block, a temporary pacemaker may be needed if right bundle-branch block occurs during right heart catheterization.

TABLE 17–14

Summary of Contrast-Induced Renal Failure Prophylaxis Trials

BENEFICIAL	DELETERIOUS	CONFLICTING DATA	NO EFFECT
IV hydration	Furosemide (without volume replacement)	Calcium channel blockers	Hemodialysis
Forced duresis	Ionic contrast	Dopamine	Atrial natriuretic peptide
Nonionic contrast	Endothelin receptor blocker	Theophylline	Allopurinol
Acetylcysteine	Mannitol (without volume replacement)	Captopril	
PGE-1			
Fenoldopam			
Sodium Bicarbonate			

PGE, Prostaglandin E-1.
SOURCE: From McCullough PA, Mauley HS. Prediction and prevention of contrast nephropathy. J Intervent Cardiol 2001;14:547–558. With permission.

TABLE 17–15

Complications of Cardiac Catheterization

Major
  Cerebrovascular accident
  Death
  Myocardial infarction
  Ventricular tachycardia, fibrillation, or serious arrhythmia
Other
  Aortic dissection
  Cardiac perforation, tamponade
  Congestive heart failure
  Contrast reaction/anaphylaxis/nephrotoxicity
  Heart block, asystole
  Hemorrhage (local, retroperitoneal, pelvic)
  Infection
  Protamine reaction
  Supraventricular tachyarrhythmia, atrial fibrillation
  Thrombosis/embolus/air embolus
  Vascular injury, pseudoaneurysm
  Vasovagal reaction

CARDIAC ANGIOGRAPHY

In 1923, Osborn noted that the urinary bladder of luetic patients treated with oral and intravenous sodium iodide became opaque to x-rays because of the absorption of photons by iodine. Contrast medium was first injected through a rubber catheter placed in the right ventricle by Chavez in 1947. *Cineangiography* is the term used to describe the x-ray photographing of cardiac and vascular structures. This term persists even though radiographic images are now stored electronically on digital computer imaging media rather than on cine film.[22] Angiographic images are the visual representation of the vascu-

TABLE 17–16

Incidence of Major Complications of Diagnostic Catheterizations

	PERCENT
Death	0.11
Myocardial infarction	0.05
Neurologic	0.07
Arrhythmia	0.38
Vascular	0.43
Contrast	0.37
Hemodynamic	0.26
Perforation	0.03
Other	0.28
Total (patients)	1.98

SOURCE: *Modified from Noto TJ, Johnson LW, Krone R, et al. Cardiac catheterization 1990: a report of the Registry of the Society for Cardiac Angiography and Interventions (SCA&I), Cathet Cardiovasc Diagn 1991;24:75–83 and Uretzky BF, Weinert HH. Cardiac Catheterization: Concepts, Techniques, and Applications. Walden, MA: Blackwell; 1997. With permission.*

TABLE 17–17

Complications of Right Heart (Pulmonary Artery) Catheterization

	MAJOR	MINOR
Access Hemothorax	Pneumothorax	Hematoma
	Thrombosis	
	Tracheal perforation (subclavian route)	
Sepsis Intracardiac	Cellulitis	
	Right ventricular perforation	Ventricular arrhythmia
	Heart block (right bundle-branch block)	
	Pulmonary rupture	
	Pulmonary infarction	

lar conduits and networks connected to internal structures (organs) and, at times, predict cardiovascular function. Angiography begins with the positioning of the patient on the table, performing the angiographic image recording, storing the digital image data, and finally displaying the images for review and analysis. Angiography is the primary method of defining coronary anatomy in living patients, providing an anatomic map of the site, severity, shape and distribution of stenotic lesions. In addition, the following characteristics can be obtained: distal vessel size, intracoronary thrombus, diffuse atherosclerotic disease, mass of myocardium served, an approximate index of coronary flow, and identification of collateral vessels. By using provocative maneuvers, the presence of coronary spasm can be ascertained.[23] The functional significance of a coronary stenosis can be assessed by measuring coronary flow or pressure directly, using information obtained both at rest and during maximal coronary vasodilatation.[24] A full discussion of assessing the functional significance of coronary angiographic lesions is provided later in this chapter. Left ventriculography is included in nearly every coronary angiographic study. Contrast opacification of the contracting ventricle enables one to make a visual analysis of wall motion. Ventricular systolic and diastolic volume and ejection fraction can be calculated. Examination of the left ventriculogram helps identify viable myocardium. LV wall motion can be further evaluated by the addition of stress such as atrial pacing, pharmacologic agents, or exercise. Assessing viability through augmenting LV contraction by the use of nitrates, catecholamines, or postextrasystolic beats facilitate decisions for revascularization.[25–27] LV angiography also documents mitral regurgitation.

CORONARY ARTERIOGRAPHY

Sones ushered in the modern era of coronary arteriography in 1958 when he developed a safe and reliable method of selective coronary arteriography.[28] Percutaneous arterial catheterization, described in 1953 by Seldinger,[29] was first used to study the coronary arteries, as reported by Ricketts and Abrams in 1962.[30] Modification of catheters was made by Amplatz et al.[31] and by Judkins[32] in 1967.[33] The description of the performance of coronary arteriography provided herein is necessarily brief; more detailed descriptions are available.[1–3,34] Expertise in performing coronary arteriography is achieved by training in an active laboratory and performing hundreds of coronary arteriograms under close supervision. In this way the physician can gain needed skills and an appreciation of the potential hazards of coronary arteriography. The American College of Cardiology/American Heart Association (ACC/AHA) recommendations for the performance of coronary angiography[35] are provided in Appendix 17–1.

[ ] TECHNIQUES OF CANNULATING CORONARY ARTERIES AND GRAFTS

Left Coronary Artery

A short left main and separate ostia for left anterior descending and circumflex arteries can present problems for cannulation. In these cases it may be necessary to cannulate the LAD and circumflex (CX) arteries separately. An Amplatz-type catheter is especially useful to cannulate the CX artery separately but must be used with care to avoid arterial dissection. An unusually high origin of the left main coronary artery from the Ao usually can be cannulated using a multipurpose catheter or an Amplatz-type catheter (e.g., AL 2).

Right Coronary Artery

The origin of the right coronary artery shows more variation than that of the left coronary artery. A contrast injection low into the right coronary cusp will show the origin of the right coronary artery and help the angiogapher direct the catheter. If the right coronary artery is not seen with this injection, it may be totally occluded or may have an anomalous origin, anteriorly on the Ao or from the left sinus of Valsalva. In this case the orifice usually is located above the sinotubular ridge. A left Amplatz catheter or a left bypass graft catheter can be used successfully to engage the right coronary artery orifice located anteriorly or in the left cusp.

Saphenous Vein Bypass Grafts

In general, saphenous vein bypass grafts are anastomosed to the anterior wall of the ascending Ao (Fig. 17–4). The right coronary artery graft usually is anastomosed a few centimeters above and anterior to the right coronary orifice. Left anterior descending and diagonal grafts usually are anastomosed somewhat higher and slightly to the left. Obtuse marginal grafts are usually the highest and furthest left.

Internal Mammary Artery Graft Cannulation

The left internal mammary artery (IMA) originates anteriorly from the caudal wall of the subclavian artery distal to the vertebral artery origin. The left subclavian artery can be entered using a right Judkins catheter but a more sharply angled catheter tip on the mammary artery catheter is preferred. The right Judkins or IMA catheter is advanced into the aortic arch up to the level of the right brachiocephalic truncus with the tip directed caudally. Subsequently, the catheter is withdrawn slowly and rotated counterclockwise. The catheter tip is deflected cranially, usually engaging the left subclavian artery at the top of the aortic knob in the anteroposterior projection. Once the subclavian artery is engaged, the catheter is advanced over a J-tipped or flexible straight tip guidewire beyond the internal mammary orifice. After the catheter has been advanced beyond the internal mammary artery takeoff, the guidewire is withdrawn slowly and small contrast injections are given to visualize the internal mammary artery

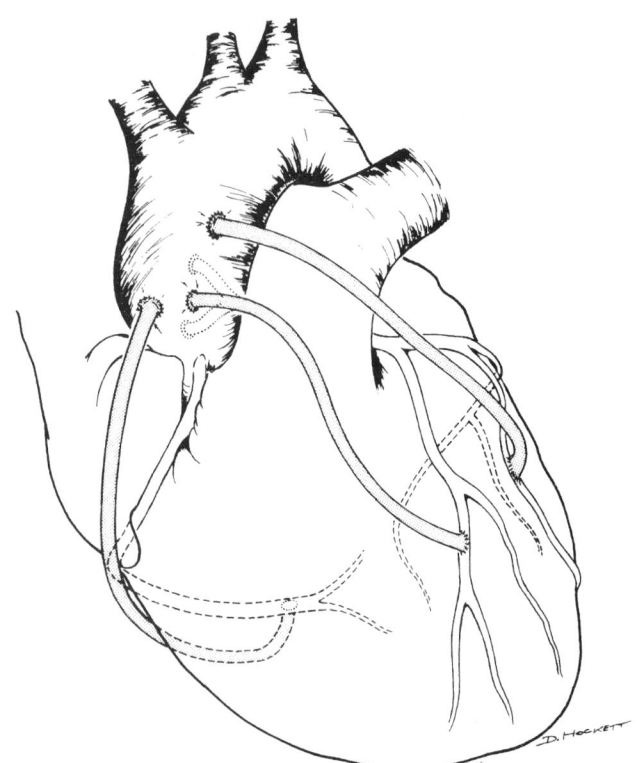

FIGURE 17–4. Usual insertion sites of vein grafts to coronary arteries. The proximal (aortic) anastomosis site of the graft to the right coronary artery is most anterior and usually the lowest. Grafts to the branches of the left coronary artery usually are inserted in a progressively higher and more posterolateral position. Variations frequently occur. *Source: From Tilkian AG, Daily EK. Cardiovascular Procedures: Diagnostic Techniques and Therapeutic Procedures. St. Louis: Mosby; 1986. With permission.*

orifice. Because of the peculiar tip configuration, the internal mammary curve catheter and especially the C-type IMA catheter usually engages into the IMA ostium without much difficulty.

Right Internal Mammary Artery Graft Cannulation

Right internal mammary artery cannulation is less common and more difficult than left internal mammary artery cannulation. The right brachiocephalic truncus is entered using a right Judkins catheter by deflecting the tip with a counterclockwise rotation at the level of the brachiocephalic truncus. The catheter is advanced into the subclavian artery. The rest of the manipulation is similar to that described for left internal mammary artery graft cannulation. In patients for whom cannulation of the internal mammary artery is not possible because of excessive tortuosity or obstructive lesions, an internal mammary artery catheter can be introduced through the ipsilateral radial artery. The catheter is advanced beyond the mammary artery orifice over a guidewire. Withdrawing it slowly and making frequent, small contrast injections engage the catheter. A technique for cannulation of the contralateral internal mammary artery from the arm approach using a Simmons catheter also has been described.

[ ] ANGIOGRAPHIC VIEWS

For all catheterization laboratories, the x-ray source is under the table and the image intensifier is directly on top of the patient (Fig. 17–5 and Table 17–18). The x-ray source and image intensi-

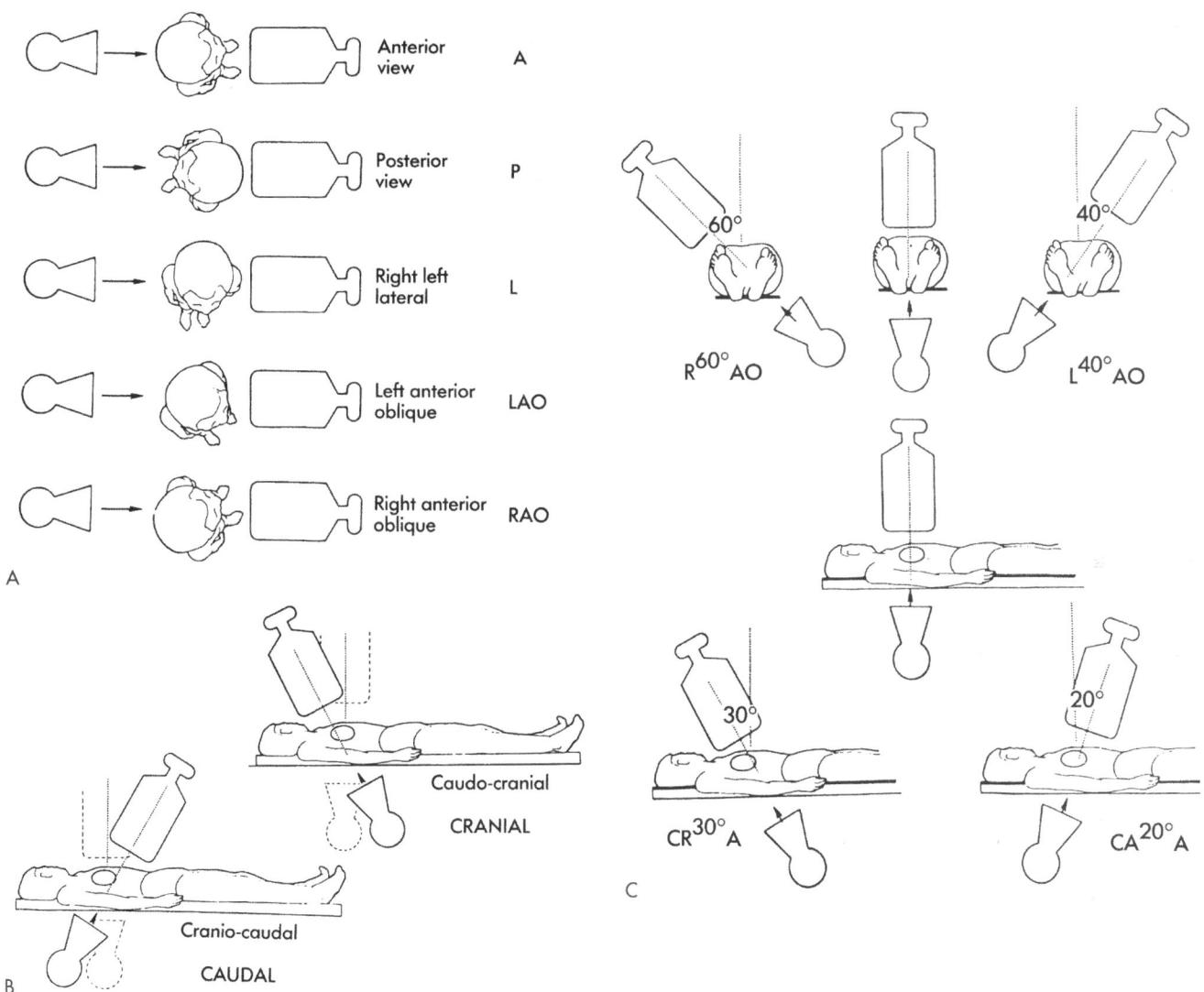

FIGURE 17-5. Nomenclature for radiographic projections. The small black arrowheads show the direction of the x-ray beam. **A.** Anterior (A), posterior (P), lateral (L), and oblique (O). **B.** If the intensifier is tilted toward the feet of the patient, a caudal (CA) view is produced. If the intensifier is tilted toward the head of the patient, a cranial (CR) view is produced. **C.** CR and CA oblique views. *Source: Redrawn from Paulin S. Terminology for radiographic projects in cardiac angiography. Cathet Cardiovasc Diagn 1981;7:341. With permission.*

fier are moved in opposite directions in an imaginary circle around the patient, who is positioned in the center of this circle. The body surface of the patient that faces the observer determines the specific view. This relationship holds true whether the patient is supine, standing, or rotated.

Anteroposterior (AP) position: The image intensifier is directly over the patient with the beam traveling perpendicular back to front, (i.e., from posterior to anterior) to the patient lying flat on the radiograph table. An oblique view is achieved by turning the left/right shoulder forward (anterior) to the camera (image intensifier) or in the cath lab, rotating the image intensifier toward the shoulder.

Right anterior oblique (RAO) position: The image intensifier is to the right side of the patient.

LAO position: The image intensifier is to the left side of the patient.

Cranial/caudal position: This nomenclature refers to image intensifier angles in relation to the patient's long axis.

Cranial: The image intensifier is tilted toward the head of the patient.

Caudal: The image intensifier is tilted toward the feet of the patient.

Cranial views are best for the left anterior descending artery; caudal views are best for the circumflex artery. Cranial and caudal views are used to *open* overlapped coronary segments that are foreshortened or obscured in regular views.

The Left Coronary Artery

The ostium of the left coronary artery originates from the left sinus of Valsalva near the sinotubular ridge. The anterior descending artery is usually best visualized in a cranially angulated RAO view. If the orientation of the anterior descending artery is unusually superior, a caudally angulated LAO view or a straight lateral view may be helpful. The circumflex coronary artery travels in the A-V groove, after its right-angle origin from the left anterior descending artery. Its course is quite variable. The artery may terminate in one or more large, obtuse marginal branches coursing over the lateral to posterolateral LV free wall. The circumflex may continue as a large artery in the interventricular groove. In 10 to 15 percent of cases, the circumflex gives rise to a posterior descending

TABLE 17-18

Angiographic Views for Specific Coronary Artery Segments

CORONARY SEGMENT	ORIGIN/ BIFURCATION	COURSE/BODY
Left main	AP	AP
	LAO cranial	LAO cranial
	LAO caudal[a]	
Proximal LAD	LAO cranial	LAO cranial
	RAO caudal	RAO caudal
Mid-LAD	LAO cranial	
	RAO cranial	
	Lateral	
Distal LAD	AP	
	RAO cranial	
	Lateral	
Diagonal	LAO cranial	RAO cranial, caudal or straight
	RAO cranial	
Proximal circumflex	RAO caudal	LAO caudal
	LAO caudal	
Intermediate	RAO caudal	RAO caudal
	LAO caudal	Lateral
Obtuse marginal	RAO caudal	RAO caudal
	LAO caudal	
	RAO cranial (distal marginals)	
Proximal RCA	LAO	
	Lateral	
Mid-RCA	LAO	LAO
	Lateral	Lateral
	RAO	RAO
Distal RCA	LAO cranial	LAO cranial
	Lateral	Lateral
PDA	LAO cranial	RAO
Posterolateral	LAD cranial	RAO
	RAO cranial	RAO cranial

AP, anteroposterior; LAD, left anterior descending artery; LAO, left anterior oblique; PDA, posterior descending artery (from RCA); RAO, right anterior oblique; RCA, right coronary artery.
[a]Horizontal hearts.

artery[36] (Fig. 17–6). The artery that supplies the major posterior descending artery is commonly referred to as the dominant artery. The circumflex artery in the A-V groove is best seen in either caudally angulated LAO or RAO views (Fig. 17–7).

The Right Coronary Artery

The right coronary artery ostium normally is located in the right sinus of Valsalva. It may be high near the sinotubular ridge or above it, in the midsinus, or occasionally low near the aortic valve. The artery commonly courses upward from the plane of the aortic valve and then travels in the right A-V groove to reach the posterior LV wall (Fig. 17–8). Along the way, several vessels arise. The conus branch and si-

nus node arteries branch first, followed by small RV branches, then a large branch that courses over the right ventricle. The right coronary continues to become the posterior descending artery before reaching the crux of the heart (junction of the interventricular and interatrial septa). The posterior descending artery sends branches at right angles into the posterior interventricular groove, providing the perforating branches to the basal and posterior one-third of the septum. A right coronary artery that supplies the major posterior descending branch has been referred to as a *dominant right coronary artery*. The posterior descending artery usually stops before reaching the apex, but it may curl around the apex in association with a short anterior descending artery. After giving rise to the posterior descending artery, the right coronary artery becomes intramyocardial at the crux, gives rise to the A-V node artery. The LV branches of the right coronary artery are variable and cover the same area as the posterolateral branches of a large circumflex system. The proximal portion of the right coronary artery is well seen in standard RAO and LAO views. However, because of its horizontal orientation, the origin and length of the posterior descending artery, well seen in the RAO view, is foreshortened in the LAO view. Thus, cranial angulation provides a better view of the patent ductus arteriosus (PDA).

【 】 INTERPRETATION OF THE CORONARY ARTERIOGRAM

The coronary arteriogram should be viewed in a systematic fashion. Because coronary anatomy can be variable, the entire LV surface and septum should be adequately supplied with vessels. No gaps should exist. If significant vessels are missing, an occluded or anomalous artery is likely. Areas of foreshortening and overlap should be examined in other orthogonal or oblique views to demonstrate the region in question. Several observers should review an arteriogram. As each segment is viewed, a systematic scoring and reporting system is helpful to maintain a consistent and dependable report.

Angiographic Assessment of Coronary Artery Narrowings

An angiographic lumen narrowing is commonly referred to as a *stenosis*, which may be caused by atherosclerosis, vasospasm, or angiographic artifact (Fig. 17–9). The evaluation of a stenosis relates the percentage reduction in the diameter of the narrowed vessel site to the adjacent unobstructed vessel. The diameter stenosis is calculated in the projection where the greatest narrowing is seen. An exact evaluation of dimensions is impossible and, in fact, the severity of stenotic lesions are roughly classified. It should be noted that the stenotic lumen is compared to a nearby unobstructed lumen, which indeed may have diffuse atherosclerotic disease and thus is *angiographically* normal but may still be diseased (Fig. 17–10). This fact explains why postmortem examinations report much more plaque than is seen on angiography.[37–39] The angiographic *normal* adjacent proximal segments may be larger than distal segments, explaining the large disparity between several observer estimates of stenosis severity.[39] Also note that area stenosis is always greater than diameter stenosis and assumes the lumen is circular whereas in reality the lumen is usually eccentric.[40] For nonquantitative reports the

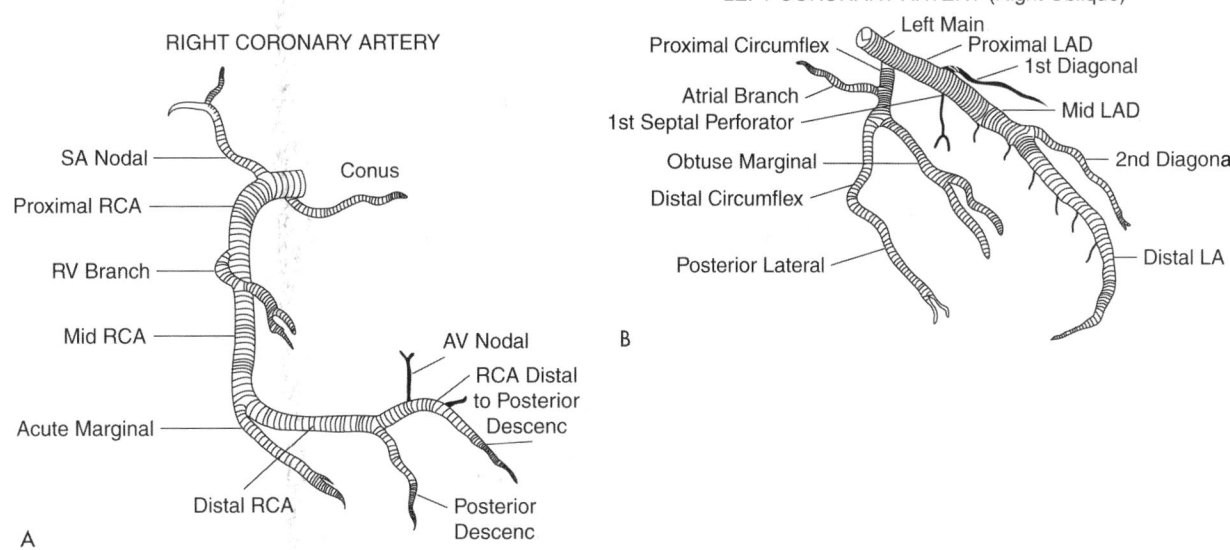

FIGURE 17–6. Diagrams of the anatomy of the right (**A**) and left (**B**) coronary circulation. AV, arteriovenous; LA, left atrium; LAD, left anterior descending coronary artery; RCA, right coronary artery; RV, right ventricular; SA, sinoatrial.

length of a stenosis may be simply mentioned (e.g., LAD proximal segment stenosis diameter 25 percent, long or short). Other features of the coronary lesion (e.g., distribution eccentricity, calcification, true length) may not be appreciated by angiography and require intravascular ultrasound imaging (Fig. 17–11). Because of the subjective nature of visual lesion assessment, there is a ± 20 percent variation between readings of two or more experienced angiographers, especially for lesions narrowed by 40 to 70 percent. Different angiographers may interpret the same angiographic image differently, and the same angiographer may render a different interpretation at a time remote from the first reading.[41,42] In addition, there may be disagreement about the number of major vessels with 70 percent stenosis approximately 30 percent of the time.[43] Angiographic narrowings of 40 to 75 percent narrowing do not always correspond to abnormal physiology and myocardial ischemia. For such lesions noninvasive or direct physiologic measurements of impaired flow validate decisions for revascularization.

Quantitative Angiographic Assessment

The degree of coronary stenosis is usually a visual estimation of the percentage of diameter narrowing using the proximal assumed normal arterial segment as a reference. The ratio of normal-to-stenosis artery diameter is widely used in clinical practice, is inadequate for a true quantitative methodology. The intraobserver variability may range between 40 and 80 percent, and there is frequently a range as wide as 20 percent on interobserver differences. Quantitative methodologies include digital calipers, automated or manual edge detection systems, or densitometric analysis with digital angiography.[44]

Intravascular Ultrasound Assessment of Coronary Artery Narrowings

Intravascular ultrasound (IVUS) generates a tomographic, cross-sectional image of the vessel and lumen. IVUS enables the operator to make measurements of luminal dimensions, such as mini-

mum and maximum diameter, cross-sectional area, vessel wall and plaque thickness. Intravascular coronary ultrasound images the soft tissues within the arterial wall enabling characterization of atheroma size, plaque distribution, and lesion composition during diagnostic or therapeutic catheterization.[45,46] The ACC/AHA recommendations for intravascular ultrasound imaging are provided in Appendix 17–2.[3]

Assessment of Coronary Spasm

Coronary spasm can appear as an angiographic narrowing, provoked by mechanical stimulation (Fig. 17–12), acetylcholine, cold pressor testing, or hyperventilation. Definitive diagnosis is demonstrated by relief of the narrowing either spontaneously or by nitrate administration. In years past, the methylergonovine provocative test was the most reliable test for coronary spasm in patients with Prinzmetal variant angina. However, this agent is no longer available. Intracoronary acetylcholine has also been used as a provocative test for coronary spasm. Its effectiveness is comparable to methylergonovine. In patients with one episode of variant angina per day, the hyperventilation provocative test is nearly as effective as methylergonovine in causing vasospasm. The end point of a pharmacologic provocative test is focal coronary narrowing, which can be reversed with intracoronary nitroglycerin. In patients with ST-segment elevation with chest pain and a normal coronary angiogram, provocative tests are unnecessary.

Angiographically Estimated Coronary Blood Flow (TIMI Flow)

Myocardial blood flow has been assessed angiographically using the thrombolysis in myocardial infarction (TIMI) score for qualitative grading of coronary flow. TIMI flow grades 0 to 3 have become a standard description of angiographic coronary blood flow in clinical trials. In acute myocardial infarction trials, TIMI grade 3 flows have been associated with improved clinical outcomes. The four grades of flow are described as follows:

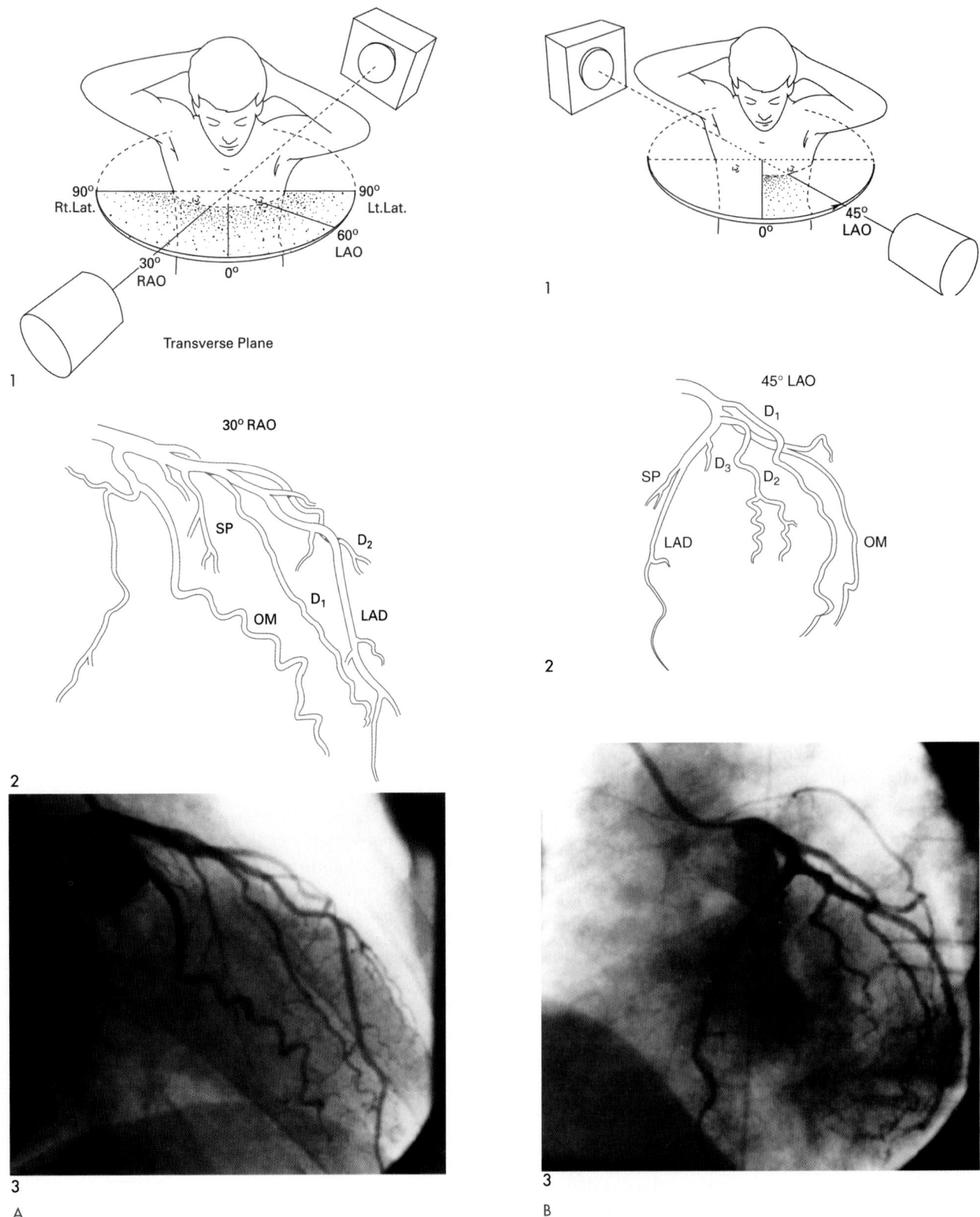

FIGURE 17–7. A. Diagrammatic representation of the standard RAO view of the left coronary angiogram, the direction of the x-ray beam, and the position of the overhead image intensifier. Most of the left coronary artery is well visualized in this projection, but there is considerable overlap of the middle left anterior descending (LAD) artery and the diagonal branches. When the left main, circumflex, and diagonal branches have a leftward initial course, the long axis of these arterial segments is projected away from the image intensifier, preventing optimal visualization from the RAO view. The image intensifier is placed anteriorly in an RAO position relative to the patient. **B.** Diagrammatic representation of the LAO left coronary angiogram and the direction of the x-ray beam in this view. The value of this view depends in large part on the orientation of the long axis of the heart. When the heart is relatively horizontal, the LAD coronary artery and diagonal branches are seen end-on throughout much of the course. In this illustration the longitudinal axis is an intermediate position and there is moderate foreshortening of the anterior descending and diagonal branches in their proximal portions. The LAO projection is frequently inadequate to visualize the proximal LAD and its branches: the left main segment, which is directed toward the image tube and therefore foreshortened, and the proximal circumflex coronary artery, which may be obscured by overlapping vessels, as in this illustration. The LAO projection is frequently used to visualize the distal LAD and its branches, the midcircumflex coronary artery in the A-V groove, and the distal right coronary artery that is filling via collaterals from the left coronary artery. (*continued*)

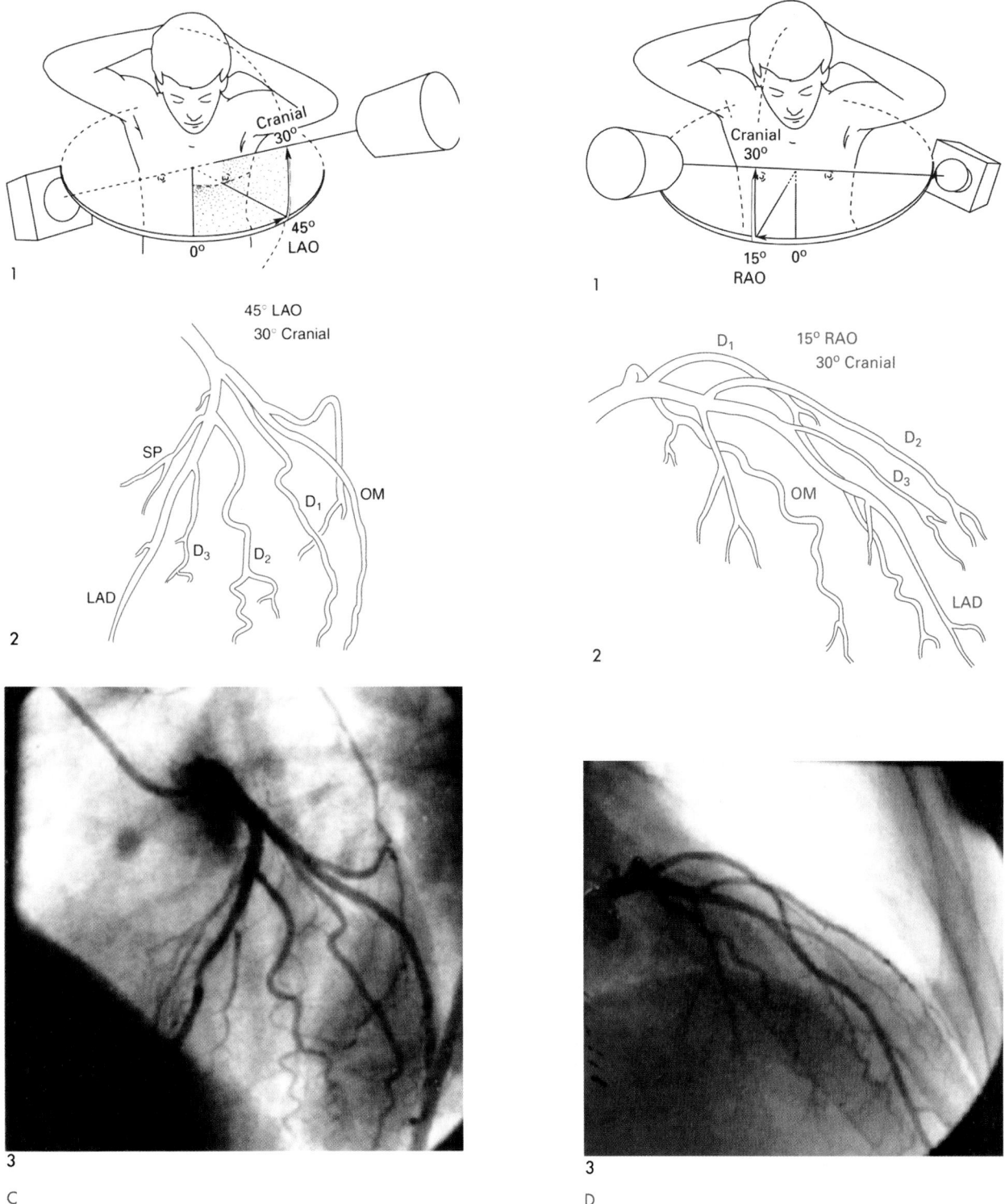

FIGURE 17–7. (*Continued*) The image intensifier is above the patient in an LAO position. **C.** Diagrammatic illustration of the left coronary angiogram in the 45-degree LAO with 30 degrees of cranial angulation and the direction of the x-ray beam used to produce this view. This is the most valuable view of the left coronary artery in most patients. Foreshortening of the left main and proximal left anterior descending and diagonal branches present in the LAO view is usually overcome by cranial angulation of the image intensifier. The proximal left coronary arterial segments are frequently visualized at an angle almost perpendicular from their long axis. The ostium of the left main coronary artery, the most proximal portion of the LAD, and the origin of the diagonal branches are usually well visualized without overlap (compare with Fig. 17–9B). Some overlap may occur with branches of the proximal circumflex coronary artery, and this is frequently overcome by using a 60-degree LAO with 30 degrees of cranial angulation. The value of the LAO with cranial angulation is considerably less when the proximal left coronary artery is superiorly directed, in which case caudal angulation of the image intensifier is frequently helpful. The direction of the x-ray beam in the 45-degree LAO with 30 degrees of angulation is demonstrated. **D.** Diagrammatic illustration of the direction of the x-ray beam and the left coronary angiogram in the 15-degree RAO with 30 degrees of cranial angulation. This view is particularly helpful in analyzing the mid–left anterior descending artery and the diagonal branch points. Overlap with diagonal branches is usually avoided. The origin of the circumflex artery may be well seen, as in this illustration. LAD, left anterior descending coronary artery; LAO, left anterior oblique; OM, obtuse marginal; RAO, right anterior oblique. *Source: From King SB, Douglas JS, Morris DC.[36] Reproduced with permission from the publisher, editor, and authors.*

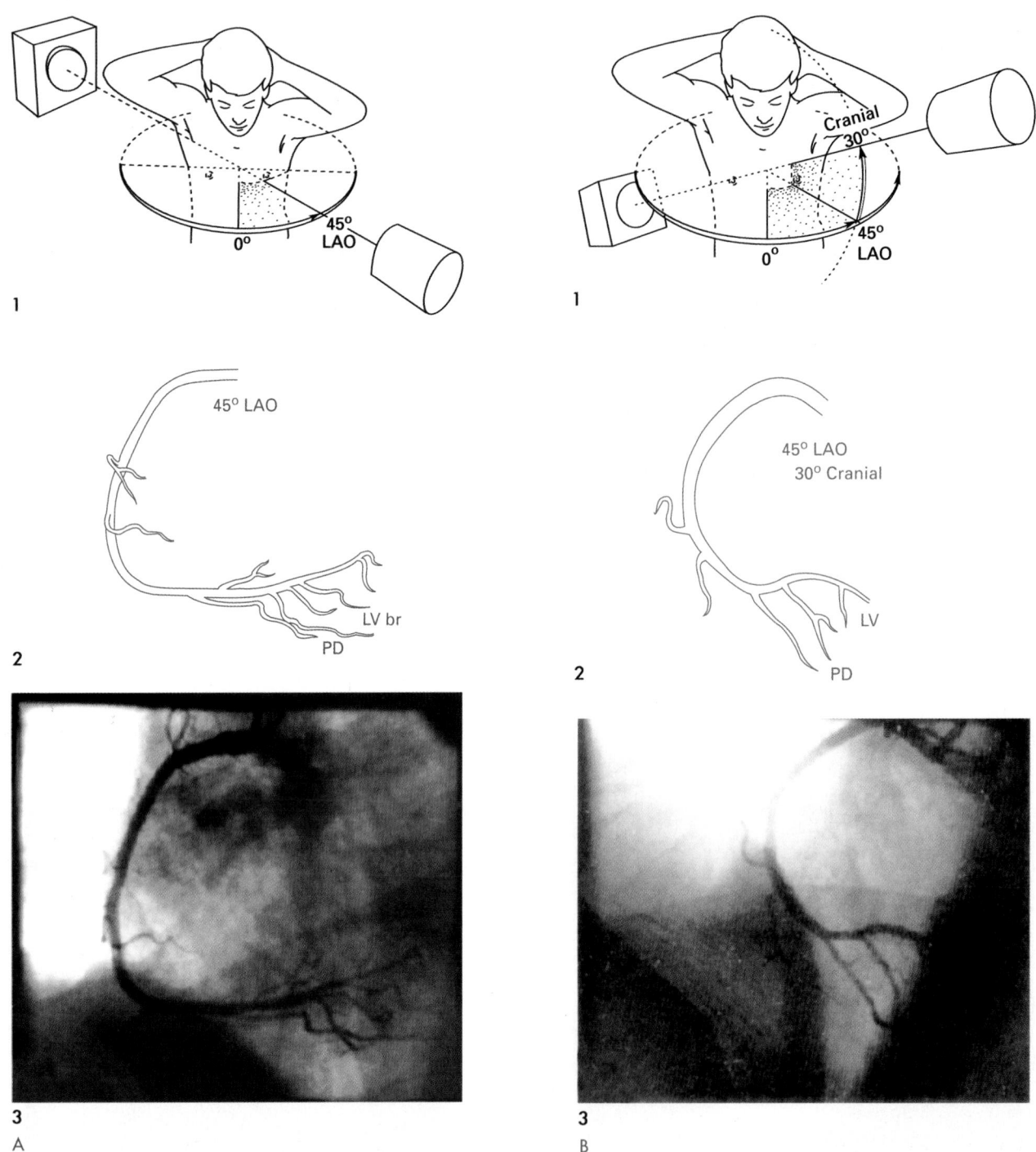

FIGURE 17–8. A. Diagrammatic illustration of the direction of the x-ray beam and the right coronary artery in the 45-degree LAO projection. This view is excellent for visualizing the proximal mid- and distal right coronary artery in the A-V groove, because the direction of the x-ray beam is perpendicular to these arterial segments. Ostial lesions of the right coronary artery are now well visualized if the proximal right coronary artery takes an anterior direction from the Ao and therefore originates in a direction parallel to the x-ray beam. This usually can be overcome by turning to a more severe left oblique projection. The posterior descending and LV branches of the right coronary artery, which pass down the posterior aspect of the heart toward the apex, are severely foreshortened because the long axis of these vessels is in the same direction as the x-ray beam. The proximal posterior descending branches can be visualized by cranial angulation of the overhead intensifier or from a right oblique view. The image intensifier is in the standard LAO position. **B.** Diagrammatic illustration of the direction of the x-ray beam and the right coronary artery in 30-degree LAO with 30 degrees cranial angulation. Cranial angulation of the image intensifier overcomes the problem of foreshortening of the posterior descending and LV branches observed in Fig. 27–27. Lesions in the posterior descending or LV branches can be well visualized in this projection. When the right coronary artery originates anteriorly from the Ao, the proximal portion of the vessel is frequently well seen in this projection. With anomalous origin of the left anterior descending artery from the right coronary artery, this view is helpful because the standard LAO view produces considerable foreshortening of the anomalous artery. The direction of x-ray beam is the same as in Fig. 17–25. Ao, aorta; A-V, arteriovenous; LAO, left anterior oblique; LV br, left ventricular branch; PD, patent ductus. *Source: From King SB, Douglas JS, Morris DC.* [36] *Reproduced with permission from the publisher, editor, and authors.*

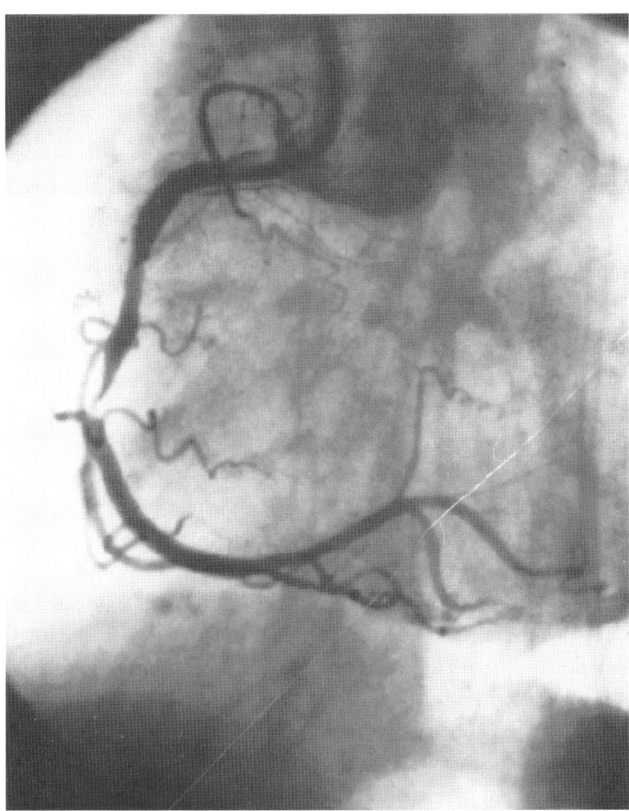

FIGURE 17-9. Left anterior oblique (LAO) view of the right coronary artery (RCA) with high-grade lesion in its midportion.

1. Flow equal to that in noninfarct arteries (TIMI-3)
2. Distal flow in the artery less than non infarct arteries (TIMI-2)
3. Filling beyond the culprit lesion but no antegrade flow (TIMI-1)
4. No flow beyond the total occlusion (TIMI-0) [47]

The quantitative method of TIMI flow uses cineangiography with 6F catheters and filming at 30 frames per second. The number of cine frames from the introduction of dye in the coronary artery to a predetermined distal landmark is counted. The TIMI frame count for each major vessel is thus standardized according to specific distal landmarks. The first frame used for TIMI frame counting is that in which the dye fully opacifies the artery origin and in which the dye extends across the width of the artery touching both borders with antegrade motion of the dye. The last frame counted is when dye enters the first distal landmark branch. Full opacification of the distal branch segment is not required. Distal landmarks used commonly in analysis are (1) for the LAD, the distal bifurcation of the left anterior descending artery; (2) for the circumflex system, the distal bifurcation of the branch segments with the longest total distance; (3) for the right coronary artery, the first branch of the posterolateral artery. The TIMI frame count can further be quantitated for the length of the left anterior descending coronary artery for comparison to the two other major arteries; this is called the corrected TIMI frame count (CTFC).[47] The average left anterior descending coronary artery is 14.7 cm long, the right 9.8 cm, and the circumflex 9.3 cm, according to Gibson and colleagues.[47] CTFC accounts for the distance the dye has to travel in the LAD relative to the other arteries. CTFC divides the absolute frame count in the LAD by 1.7 to standardize the

distance of dye travel in all three arteries. Normal TIMI frame count (TFC) for LAD is 36 ± 3 and CTFC 21 ± 2; for the circumflex (CFX), TFC = 22 ± 4; for the right coronary artery (RCA), TFC = 20 ± 3. TIMI flow grades do not correspond to measured Doppler flow velocity or the CTFC. High TFC may be associated with microvascular dysfunction despite an open artery. CTFC of <20 frames were associated with low risk for adverse events in patients following myocardial infarction. A contrast injection rate increase of ≥1 mL/sec by hand injection can decrease the TIMI frame count by two frames. The TIMI frame count method provides valuable information relative to clinical responses after coronary interventions.

Collateral Circulation

The reopacification of a totally or subtotally (99 percent) occluded vessel from antegrade or retrograde filling is defined as collateral filling. The collateral circulation is graded angiographically as follows:

Grade	Collateral Appearance
0	No collateral circulation
1	Very weak (ghostlike) reopacification
2	Reopacified segment, less dense than the feeding vessel and filling slowly
3	Reopacified segment as dense as the feeding vessel and filling rapidly

It is useful but difficult to establish the size of the recipient vessel exactly, whether the collateral circulation is ipsilateral (e.g., same side filling, proximal RCA to distal RCA collateral supply) or contralateral (e.g., opposite side filling, LAD to distal RCA collateral supply). Identification of exactly which region is affected by collateral supply will influence decisions regarding management of stenoses in the artery feeding the collateral supply. Collateral vessel evaluation is important for making decisions regarding which vessels might be protected or lost during coronary angioplasty.[48]

Pitfalls in Coronary Arteriography

There are a number of pitfalls in coronary arteriography that should be avoided.

Short Left Main or Double Left Coronary Orifices

When the left main orifice is very short or absent, selective injection of the ante-

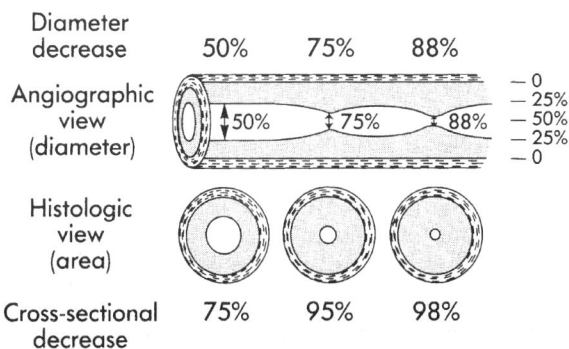

FIGURE 17-10. Diagrammatic representation of angiographic versus postmortem analysis of coronary artery stenosis. *Source: From Robert WC. Coronary heart disease: a review of abnormalities observed in the coronary arteries. Cardiovasc Med 1977;2:29–38. With permission.*

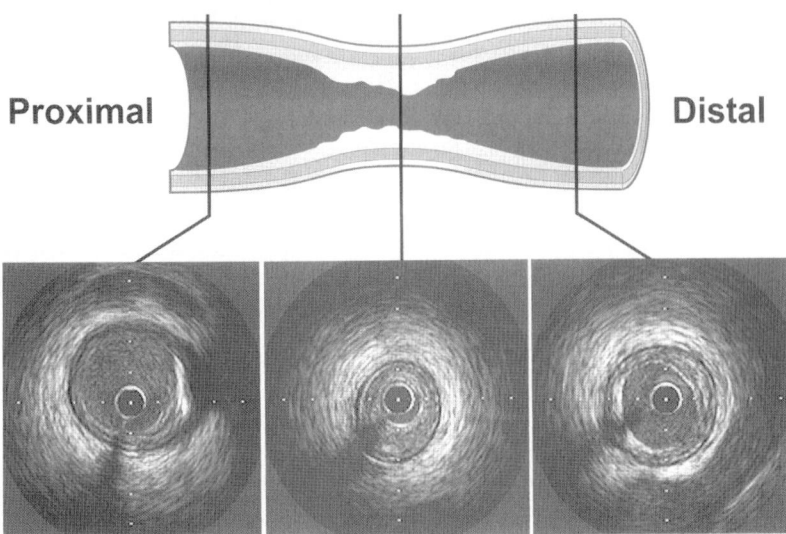

Proximal   **Distal**

FIGURE 17–11. Intravascular ultrasound (IVUS) imaging of the coronary artery.

rior descending or circumflex arteries may be done. The absence of circumflex or anterior descending artery filling, either primarily or through collaterals from the right coronary artery, may indicate that the artery was missed by subselective injection, or an anomalous location.

Ostial Lesions The left and right coronary artery orifices need to be seen on a tangent with the aortic sinuses. Some contrast reflux from the orifices is needed to fully opacify the ostium to see whether an ostial narrowing is present. Catheter pressure damping is an additional indication of an ostial stenosis.

Myocardial Bridges The anterior descending, diagonal, and marginal branches occasionally run intramyocardial. The overlying myocardium may compress the artery during systole. If the coronary artery is not viewed carefully in diastole, this bridging may give the appearance of an area of stenosis.[49]

Foreshortening Foreshortening is the viewing of a vessel in plane with its long axis. Vessels seen on end cannot display a lesion along its length. When possible, arteries that are seen coming toward or away from the image intensifier should be viewed in angulated (cranial/caudal) views. Dense opacification of segments seen end-on-end may produce the appearance of a lesion in an intervening segment.

Coronary Spasm Catheter-induced spasm may appear as a lesion (Fig. 17–12). When spasm is suspected (usually at the catheter tip in the right coronary artery), intracoronary nitroglycerin (100 to 200 μg) should be given, and the angiogram should be repeated in 1 to 2 minutes. Spontaneous coronary artery spasm may also present as an atherosclerotic narrowing. When this is suspected, an angiogram is obtained before and after administration of nitrates. If clinically indicated, provocation with ergot derivatives will identify most patients with spontaneous coronary artery spasm.

Totally Occluded Arteries or Vein Grafts Absence of vascularity in a portion of the heart may indicate total occlusion of its arterial supply. Collateral channels often permit visualization of the distal occluded artery. Vessels filled solely by collaterals are under low pressure and may appear smaller than their actual lumen size. This finding should not exclude the possibilities for surgical anastomosis.

Anomalous Coronary Arteries Coronary arteries may arise from anomalous locations, or a single coronary artery may be present.[50] Only by ensuring that the entire epicardial surface has an adequate arterial supply can one be confident that all branches have been visualized. Misdiagnosis of unsuspected anomalous origin of the coronary arteries is a potential problem for any angiographer. Because the natural history of a patient with an anomalous origin of a coronary artery may be dependent on the initial course of the anomalous vessel, it is the angiographer's responsibility to define accurately the origin and course of the vessel. It is an error to assume a vessel is occluded when in fact it has not been visualized because of an anomalous origin. It is often difficult even for experienced angiographers to delineate the true course of an anomalous vessel. For the most critical anomaly, the anomalous left main artery originating from the right cusp, a simple *dot and eye* method for determining the proximal course of anomalous artery from an RAO ventriculogram, an RAO aortogram, or selective RAO injection is proposed[51] (Table 17–19). The RAO view best separates the normally positioned Ao and PA. Placement of right-sided catheters or injection of contrast in the PA is unnecessary and often misleading. Fig. 17–13 diagrams the four common pathways of anomalous left coronary arteries. Alternative imaging modalities such as MRI angiography or CT angiography can provide information on the course of anomalous coronary arteries and their relationship to surrounding structures.

Complications of Coronary Arteriography Minor complications of coronary angiography include local arterial complications, arterial occlusion or stenosis, hematoma formation, false aneurysm, and infection. Major complications are potentially lethal and include thromboembolic events or depression of myocardial function caused by infarction or acute ischemia.

〖 〗 LEFT VENTRICULOGRAPHY

Left ventriculography is the standard method for evaluating LV function in the cardiac catheterization laboratory. The normal pattern of LV contraction is a uniform and almost concentric inward movement of all points along the endocardial surface during systole. Harrison introduced the term *asynergy,* which has been used to indicate a disturbance of the normal contraction pattern. The Ad Hoc Committee for Grading of Coronary Artery Disease of the American Heart Association[52] has recommended that five RAO segments and two LAO LV segments be defined and characterized as to wall motion (Fig. 17–14). Herman and coworkers[53] classified LV asynergy according to the severity of the contractile abnormality.

Ventricular Wall Motion Analysis

There are three distinct types of asynergy (Fig. 17–15):

1. *Hypokinesia:* a diminished but not absent motion of one part of the LV wall (also called weak or poor contraction)

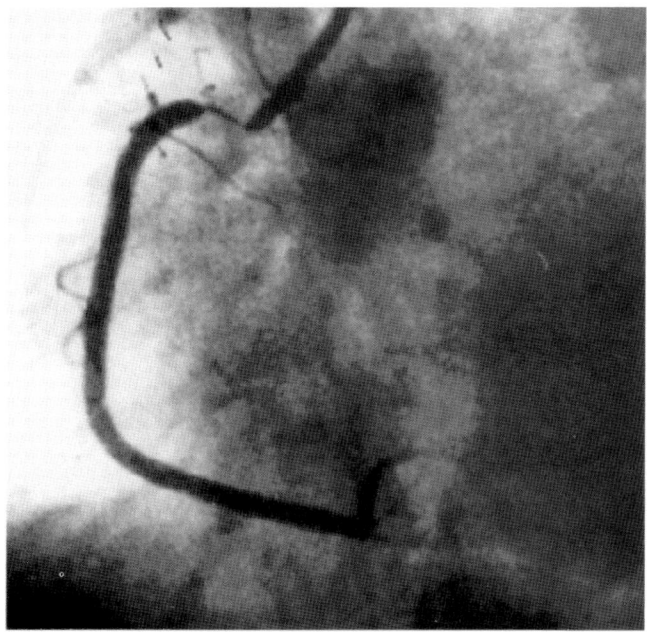

A

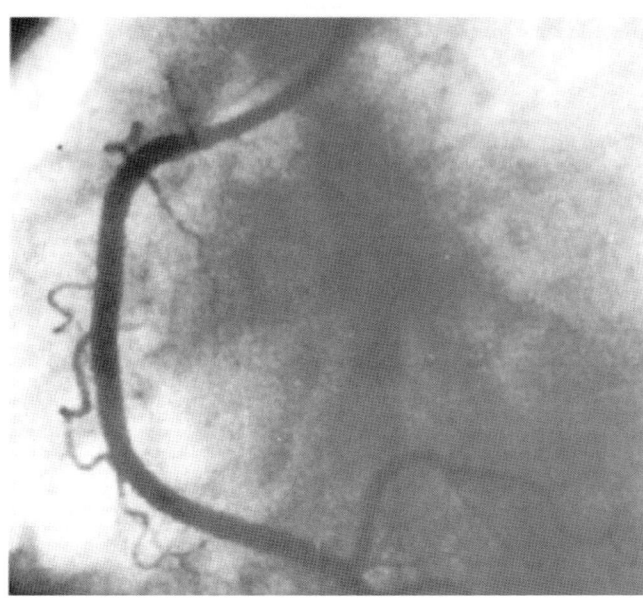

B

FIGURE 17–12. A. LAO view of right coronary injection showing pericatheter spasm. **B.** Same view following nitroglycerin, showing relief of spasm. LAO, left anterior oblique.

2. *Akinesia:* total lack of motion of a portion of the LV wall (i.e., no contraction)
3. *Dyskinesia:* paradoxical systolic motion or expansion of one part of the LV wall (i.e., an abnormal bulging outward during systole)

There are several methods for analyzing LV wall motion. A point system based on the regional severity of abnormal wall motion from the Coronary Artery Surgery Study[52] is used to produce a wall motion score reflecting overall LV function. The RAO and LAO left ventriculograms are divided into five segments. Points are assigned as follows: normal contraction = 1 point; moderate hypokinesis = 2; severe hypokinesis = 3; akinesis = 4; aneurysm-dyskinesis = 5. A normal score is 5. Higher scores indicate more severe wall motion abnormalities.

For determination of quantitative regional wall motion abnormalities, three methods have been commonly employed:

1. *Long axis method:* Determines the major long axis and division of the long axis into equal segments with perpendicular lines.
2. *Center point method:* Determines the midpoint of the major axis and division of the lines radiating out from the center point.
3. *Center line method:* A center line is established between the end-diastolic and end-systolic borders, 100 perpendicular chords are drawn, and shortening of these chords determines wall motion abnormalities. Results are corrected using a normal motion value for each chord length.

Some methods of determining regional wall motion abnormality use computer planimetry available currently on most advanced radiograph systems.

Indications for Left Ventriculography

1. Identify LV function for patients with coronary artery disease, myopathy, or valvular heart disease.
2. Identify ventricular septal defect.
3. Quantitate degree of mitral regurgitation.
4. Quantitate mass of myocardium for regression of hypertrophy or other similar research studies.

Ventriculography Techniques

Catheters The two most common ventriculography catheters are the pigtail and multipurpose sidehole catheters. The multipurpose catheter should be positioned freely in the LV chamber so that the high-pressure contrast jet does not produce ventricular tachycardia, contrast injection in the myocardial tissue (contrast staining),

TABLE 17–19

Radiographic Appearance of Anomalous Origin of the Left Main Coronary Artery from the Right Sinus of Valsalva

COURSE OF ANOMALOUS LEFT MAIN CORONARY	DOT	EYE	LAD LENGTH	SEPTAL ARISING FROM LMCA
Septal	—	+(upper CFX) (lower LMCA)	Short	Yes
Anterior	—	+(upper LMCA) (lower CFX)	Short	No
Retroaortic	+(posterior)	—	Normal	No
Interarterial	+(anterior)	—	Normal	No

+, present; –, absent (posterior and anterior are in reference to the aorta root); Ao, aorta; LAD, left anterior descending coronary artery; LMCA, left main coronary artery; CFX, circumflex coronary artery.

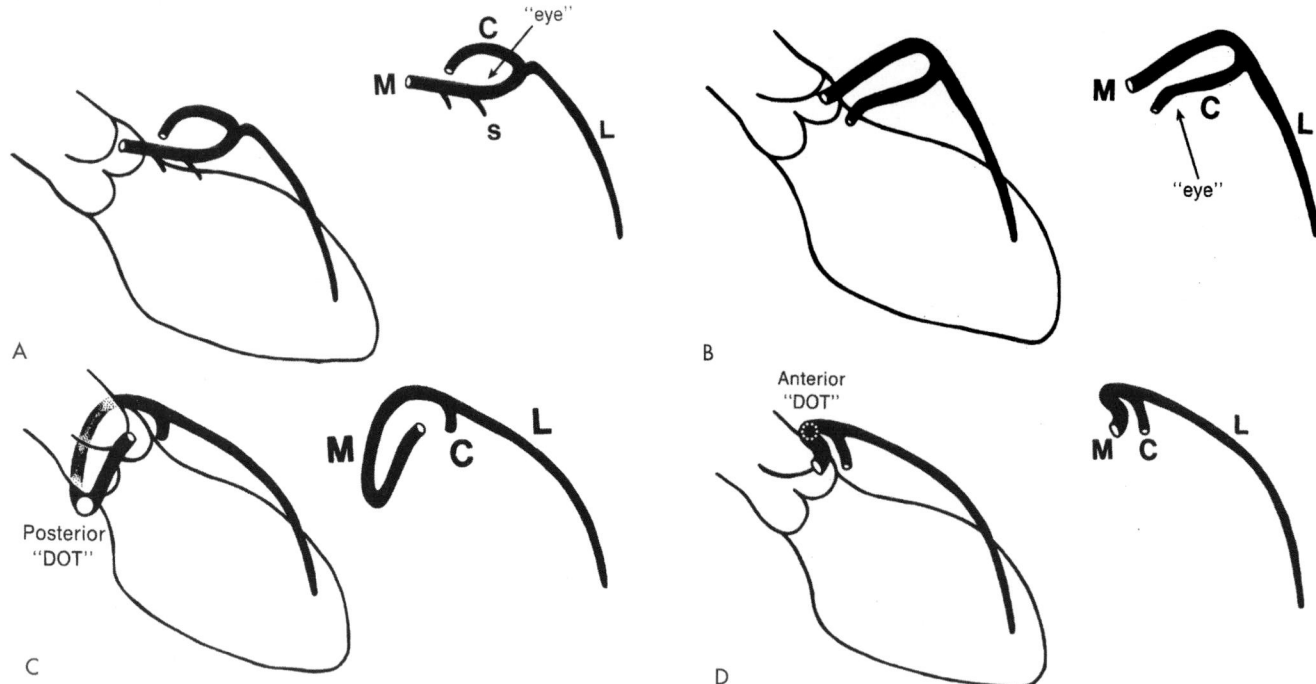

FIGURE 17-13. A. Diagram of septal course of anomalous left coronary artery. **B.** Diagram of anterior course of anomalous left coronary artery. **C.** Diagram of retroaortic course of anomalous left coronary artery. **D.** Diagram of interarterial course of left main coronary artery. C, circumflex; L, left anterior descending artery; M, left main; S, septals. *Source: From Kern MJ.[1] With permission.*

or perforation. The pigtail catheter (and halo-modified pigtail) is safer and produces less ectopy contrast staining and perforation than a multipurpose catheter.

Left Ventriculography Views

Standard left ventriculographic views are (1) a 30-degree RAO that visualizes the high lateral, anterior, apical, and inferior LV walls; and (2) a 45- to 60-degree LAO, 20 degrees of cranial angulation that best identifies the lateral and septal LV walls. The degrees of axial obliquity and cranial angulation are used as follows:

The 40-degree LAO and 30-degree cranial position (four-chamber view) outlines the posterior third of the ventricular septum, the valve plane in A-V canal defects, and the four heart chambers without superimposition.

The 60-degree LAO and 30-degree cranial position (long-axial view) outlines the anterior two-thirds of the ventricular septum, the membranous ventricular septum, and the LV outflow tract.

The LAO with cranial angulation provides a view of the interventricular septum, projected on edge and tilted downward to give the best view of ventricular septal defects and septal wall motion. An elongated RAO view, which is useful for seeing the RV infundibulum and supracristal ventricular septal defect, is obtained by a 30-degree axial RAO and 40 degrees of cranial angulation. The main PA and its bifurcation are seen in the frontal position with 30 degrees of cranial angulation; a steep LAO position with marked cranial angulation is also used.

Ventricular Volume Measurement

LV volume is estimated from the opacified image of the LV cavity. Although a single-plane mode using the frontal or RAO projec-

tion often is adequate,[54,55] biplane view image pairs including frontal and lateral, right and left anterior oblique, or half-axial left anterior oblique and conventional RAO may be more precise.[56,57] In the classic biplane technique, each image of the LV cavity is treated as an ellipse. The long axis of the ventricle (L_m) and the two mutually perpendicular short axes at its midpoint (D_a and D_l) are measured, and the volume (V) is calculated from the formula for volume of an ellipsoid (Fig. 17–16). In the single-plane method, the long axis and one short axis are measured; the second nonvisible short axis is assumed to equal the first. More often, in either the biplane or single-plane method, the short-axis dimension is derived from the measured long axis and the area (A) of the LV shadow, treated as an ellipse (area-length method of Dodge). Volume can be calculated from the measured area and long axis by substituting for D. Corrections must be made for magnification because of the divergence of the x-ray beam[56] using a calibrated grid or circular reference marker. Digital ventriculography provides rapid, computer-derived ventricular volumes. Techniques for

LEFT VENTRICULOGRAM — WALL SEGMENTS

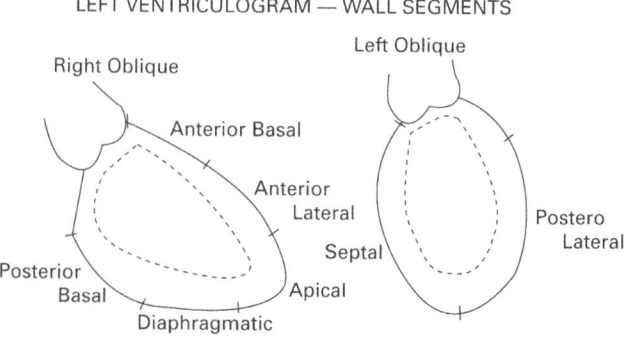

FIGURE 17-14. LV wall silhouette in RAO and LAO views. LV, left ventricular; LAO, left anterior oblique; RAO, right anterior oblique.

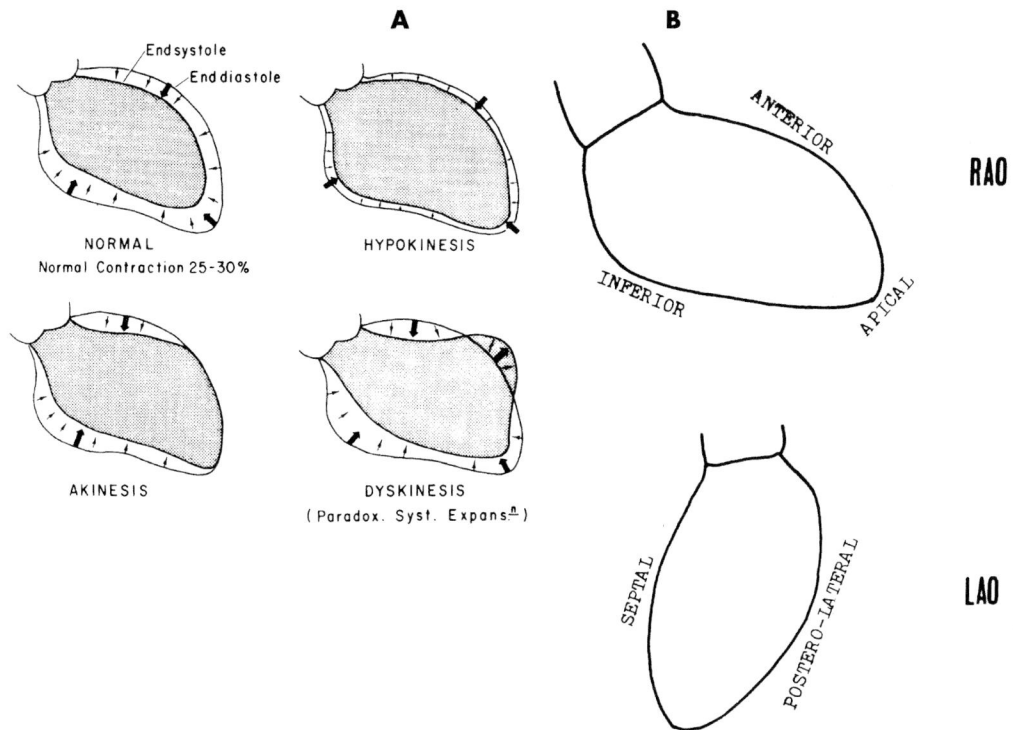

FIGURE 17–15. A. Types of ventricular asynergy. **B.** Diagrammatic representation of the zones of the left ventricular (LV) inner wall in the right anterior oblique (RAO) above and left anterior oblique (LAO) below left ventriculograms. *Sources: A, from Herman MV, Heinle RA, Klein MD.[53] With permission. B, from Yang SS. From Cardiac Catheterization Data to Hemodynamic Parameters. 3rd ed. Philadelphia: FA Davis; 1987. With permission.*

calculation of ventricular volumes have been validated using geometric and nongeometric count-based radionuclide methods as well as with magnetic resonance imaging.[57]

The methods for determination of ventricular volume by biplane ventriculography are described elsewhere.[58,59] Important parameters of LV volume measurements include LV end-diastolic volume (normally 70 ± 20 mL/m^2), the end-systolic volume (24 ± 10 mL/m^2), and the ejection fraction (0.67 ± 0.08). LV ejection fraction (EF) values below 0.55 are considered abnormal. Diastolic LV wall thickness measured by angiography is 9 mm for women and 12 mm for men, and LV wall mass is 76 g/m^2 for women and 99 g/m^2 for men.[59] The major measurements of LV contractility are the ejection fraction (EF) and stroke volume (SV). EF (percent) is calculated as follows:

$$SV = EDV - ESV$$

where EDV = end-diastolic volume; ESV = end-systolic volume; SV = stroke volume. The velocity of circumferential fiber shortening (cm/sec) is calculated as

$$VCF = \frac{\left(\dfrac{D_{ed} - D_{es}}{D_{ed}}\right)}{LVET}$$

where D_{ed} = diameter end diastole, D_{es} = diameter end systole, and $LVET$ = LV ejection time (ms).

Angiographic Assessment of Valve Regurgitation

1. LV opacification visualizes mitral but not aortic valvular regurgitation. For the aortic valve, contrast injections made low in the aortic root serve to quantify aortic regurgitation. In mild degrees of aortic regurgitation, a fine regurgitant jet or puff is noted. Opacification is limited to the LV outflow tract, clearing with each systole (grade 1), or faint, persistent, incomplete opacification of the LV cavity (grade 2) occurs. In grades 3 and 4, no distinct jet is seen, and dense complete opacification of the left ventricle occurs either progressively or in one or two diastolic cycles, and LV density exceeds aortic density in the severe case (Fig. 17–17).

2. For the mitral valve, LV injection in the RAO view detects and quantifies mitral regurgitation. The angiographic criteria for grading mitral regurgitation are highly subjective. Mild grades

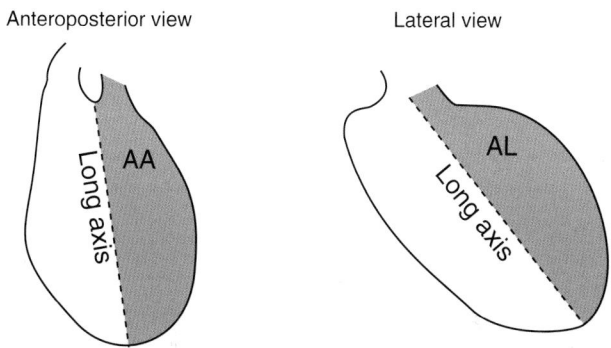

FIGURE 17–16. Dimensions of the left ventricular (LV) cavity in end-diastole used for the calculation of the ventricular volume by the area-length method, biplane technique. See text for formulas.

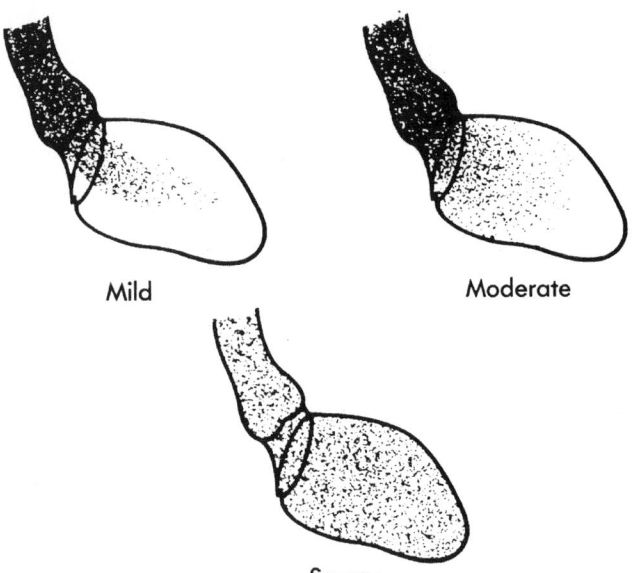

FIGURE 17-17. Angiographic evaluation of aortic regurgitation, right anterior oblique view. When the left anterior oblique view is used, overestimation of the aortic regurgitation occurs. *Source: From Pujadas G. Coronary angiography in the Medical and Surgical Treatment of Ischemic Heart Disease. New York: McGraw-Hill, 1980. With permission.*

1 and 2 mitral regurgitation have a narrow-to-moderate width regurgitant jet of slight to moderate density with minimum-to-moderate opacification of the left atrium clearing quickly. Grades 3 and 4 have no well-defined jet with intense and persistent left atrial opacification. The left atrium appears denser than the left ventricle or Ao in grade 4 mitral regurgitation. If there is associated mitral valve prolapse, shown best in a lateral projection, all or a portion of one or both leaflets balloons may appear above the mitral annulus in systole. A normal mitral valve may be transiently regurgitant if ectopic beating occurs.

Mitral regurgitation can also be quantitated by calculating a regurgitant fraction as follows: The total SV obtained by left ventriculography is used to assess the severity of mitral and aortic valve regurgitation. Total SV minus forward SV equals regurgitant SV. The regurgitant fraction equals regurgitant SV divided by total SV.

Severe valvular regurgitation has a regurgitant fraction of 0.50 or greater. The angiographic quantitation of valvular regurgitation is shown in Table 17–20.

Right Ventriculography

The RV volume is estimated by applying the Simpson rule or the area-length method to the cavity silhouettes after biplane angiography.[60] The end-diastolic volume of the right ventricle in normal persons is 81 ± 12 mL/m^2. The opacified left atrial shadow is represented as an ellipsoid, so the left atrial volume also can be calculated in the biplane mode; the normal left atrial maximal volume is 63 ± 16 mL with a mean volume of 35 ± 8.7 mL. Indications for right ventriculography include documentation of tricuspid regurgitation, RV dysplasia for arrhythmias, pulmonary stenosis, abnormalities of pulmonary outflow tract, RV-to-LV shunts.

Complications of Ventriculography

Cardiac arrhythmias, especially ventricular tachycardia and ventricular fibrillation, require immediate cardioversion. Intramyocardial *staining*, injection of contrast into the myocardium, is generally transient and of no clinical importance unless it is deep or perforating (emergency pericardiocentesis may be required). Arrhythmias and staining are more common with end-hole catheters than any pigtail catheters. Embolism from thrombi or air may occur. These events are minimized with careful catheter and injection syringe preparation, flushing, and debubbling. Contrast-related complications including allergic-type vasomotor collapse may occur during this procedure. Transient hypotension (<15–30 sec) was common with ionic contrast media.

【 】 OTHER CARDIOVASCULAR ANGIOGRAPHIC STUDIES

Ascending Aortography

Although cut film is an established radiologic method for aortography, cineangiography is acceptable in patients with suspected dissection of the Ao. Indications and contraindications are shown in Table 17–21.

TABLE 17–20

Angiographic Quantitation of Valvular Regurgitation

	MITRAL REGURGITATION		AORTIC REGURGITATION
	Mild LA opacification; clears rapidly, often jet-like	+	Small regurgitant jet only; LV ejects contrast each systole
++	Moderal LA opacification, <LV	++	Regurgitant jet faintly opacifies LV cavity; not cleared each systole
+++	Diffuse contrast Regurgitant; LA Opacification = LV; LA Significantly enlarged[a]	+++	Persistent LV Opacification = aortic root density; LV enlargement[a]
++++	LA opacification > LV, persistent; systolic pulmonary vein opacification may occur; often marked LV enlargement[a]	++++	Persistent LV Opacification > aortic root concentration; often marked LV enlargement[a]

++, mild; +++, moderate; ++++, severe; LA, left atrium; LV, left ventricle.
[a]Chronic regurgitation.

TABLE 17-21

Indications and Contraindications for Ascending Aortography

INDICATIONS

Aortic regurgitation
Nonselective coronary or bypass graft arteriography
Supravalvular aortic stenosis
Brachiocephalic or arch vessel disease
Coarctation of the aorta
Aortic to pulmonary artery or right heart (e.g., sinus of Valsalva fistula) communication
Aortic or periaortic neoplastic disease
Arterial thromboembolic disease
Arterial inflammatory disease

CONTRAINDICATIONS

Contrast media reaction
Injection into false lumen of aortic dissection
End-hole catheter malposition
Inability to tolerate additional radiographic contrast media

Radiographic Projections for Aortography *LAO or Lateral projection*: This view is excellent for identifying dissection of the ascending Ao extending up to the neck vessels; optimally delineating the aortic arch; opening the aortic curvature; and providing clear views of the innominate, common carotid artery, and left subclavian arteries. The coronary arteries at the root of the Ao are displayed in a semilateral projection.

RAO projection: The descending thoracic Ao and the ascending Ao may be superimposed across the arch in the AP or LAO projection. The RAO view is more helpful in delineating the effect of dissection on the lower thoracic Ao and intercostal arteries as well as the origin of bypass grafts to the left coronary system. There are no advantages to cranial or caudal tilts for viewing the Ao. In nonselective coronary arteriography in which aortic root angiography may help to identify a vein graft takeoff, the cranial and caudal angulation may provide some increased detail.

Abdominal Aortography

Indications for abdominal aortography are shown in Table 17–22. A lateral projection is commonly needed for anteriorly angulated aneurysm, especially if stent graft repair of abdominal aortic aneurysm is being considered. Evaluation of peripheral lower extremity disease requires identification of iliac bifurcation and common FA patency before selective injections. The contraindications of abdominal aortography are the same as thoracic aortography.

Pulmonary Angiography

Pulmonary angiography, the visualization of vascular abnormalities of the lung vessels (e.g., intraluminal defects representing pulmonary emboli, shunts, stenosis, A-V malformation, and anomalous connections), should be preceded by the measurements of right heart pressures.

Peripheral Vascular Angiography

Once the techniques of coronary angiography have been mastered, peripheral vascular angiography is not difficult. Digital subtraction angiography is the method of choice for identifying peripheral vascular disease. However, cineangiography can provide satisfactory information if the filming time, frame rates, and contrast dosages are properly established. Cine angiography is also helpful to detect the speed of vessel opacification and collateral filling. Based on clinical signs and symptoms of arterial insufficiency to the legs, suspected obstructions of vessel are often screened with noninvasive studies (i.e., ankle brachial index) before angiography is performed. Small-diameter (4–5 Fr) catheters are satisfactory. Reduced volume of contrast (10–20 mL over 1–2 sec) are injected during filming with panning down the artery, following the course to the most distal locations. Angulated views may be necessary to open bifurcations and overlying vessels that obscure the vessel origin. When possible, angiographic filming should extend at least to the ankle. Nonionic contrast agents are less painful than ionic media for peripheral angiography. The area most frequently involved in peripheral atherosclerotic disease involves the distal superficial FA at the abductor canal. The calf (tibial) and knee (popliteal) arteries are the next most commonly involved vessels after the superficial FA. Disease in the deep FA (femoral profunda) is rare. Pathways of collateralization are often rich and varied in patients with chronic distal FA disease, especially in total occlusions of the superficial FA that reconstitutes at or below the knee, close to the branching trifurcation of the tibial and deep peroneal arteries. Determining the level of reconstitution of collateralized vessels and distal runoff is crucial in determining the feasibility of revascularization.

Renal Arteriography

Selective renal arteriography evaluates the renal artery origins and vasculature. Selective arterial injections provide the most detail and are easily obtained with a JR4 catheter. For screening aortography, the renal artery origins usually arise at L1 vertebra (just below the T12 ribs). The 30-degree ipsilateral oblique projection often provides the best view of the renal artery ostia in a majority of patients. Acutely angled takeoffs of the renal artery may require specially shaped catheters or an arm approach. Atherosclerotic disease of the renal artery usually involves the proximal one-third of the renal artery and is seldom present without abdominal atherosclerotic plaques. Delayed imaging to see the nephrogram is essential to exclude accessory renal arteries and to screen for presence of

TABLE 17-22

Indications for Abdominal Aortography

Nonselective evaluation of renal arteries and mesenteric vessels
Abdominal aneurysm or dissection
Abdominal aortic atherosclerotic disease
Vascular assessment prior to IAB counterpulsation
Initial evaluation of claudication
Evaluation of cause of difficult catheter movement for coronary angiography

IAB, intraaortic balloon.

severe parenchymal disease. Measurement of a pressure gradient across ostial proximal lesion is recommended to determine the need for intervention.

THE X-RAY IMAGE
[ ] GENERATION OF THE X-RAY IMAGE

Cardiac angiography uses a complex interaction of radiographic x-ray elements, transforming energy into a visual image. The x-ray image generation chain can be simplified into three major components: (1) the x-ray generator; (2) the x-ray tube; and (3) the image intensifier. The details of x-ray equipment should be familiar to all personnel working in a catheterization laboratory.

X-Ray Generator

The generator provides the power source necessary to accelerate the electrons through the x-ray tube. The duration of x-ray exposure is similar to the shutter speed on a regular camera. During the cardiac *photographic* examination, the exposure usually is set fast enough to stop blurring as a result of heart movement. During selective coronary arteriography, the shorter the exposure time, the better the image. Exposure times of 3 to 6 msec reduce movement blur. Most modern generators are capable of delivering adequate power while providing precise and automatically adjusted exposure timing. Current generators are equipped with either multiple phase (alternating on/off) or short/long pulse widths that are automatically adjusted for correct exposure. Manual settings, which are operator selected, are limited to film frame rates (e.g., 15, 30, or 60 frames per second).

X-Ray Tubes

The function of the x-ray tube is to convert electrical energy, provided from the generator, to an x-ray beam. Electrons emitted from a heated filament (cathode) are accelerated toward a rapidly rotating disc (anode) and at contact undergo conversion to x-radiation. This process generates extreme heat. The heat capacity of an x-ray tube is a major limiting factor in the design of x-ray tubes. Only 0.2 to 0.6 percent of the electrical energy provided to the tube eventually is converted to x-rays. In addition to the exposure times (controlled by the generator system) and the size of the imaging field (controlled by the x-ray tube), two other factors of the x-ray determine the quality of x-ray for proper image exposures.

Electrical Current (mA)
The number of photons (electrical particles) generated per unit of time. The greater the electrical current the greater the number of photons, resulting in improved image resolution. If the photon volume if marginal, the resulting image may be *mottled* or have a spotty appearance. Increasing the milliamperage will improve this result, but the level of milliamperage is limited by the heat capacity of the x-ray tubes. Also, increasing the number of milliamperes markedly increases radiation exposure and scatter to patient and catheterization personnel.

The Level of Kilovoltage (kV)
The energy spectrum (wavelengths) of the x-ray beam. The higher the level of kilovoltage, the shorter the wavelength of radiation and the greater the ability of x-rays to penetrate target tissue. Increased kilovoltage is especially important in obese patients. To obtain better images through more tissue, a higher kilovolt level is required. Unfortunately, a high kilovolt level also will produce lower resolution because of wide scatter. There is also greater radiation exposure to patients and laboratory personnel. Modern radiographic equipment currently allows for variability of the amperage and voltage to attain optimal quality radiographic images. An automatic exposure control system sets exposure times to incorporate changes in voltage (kV) and amperage (mA), providing the desired images at the best exposures possible (Fig. 17–18).

Image Intensifier and Image Distortion

After the x-rays penetrate the body, the partially absorbed beams are cast in a shadow fashion on the input screen of the image intensifier. The image intensifier converts the invisible x-ray image into a visual image. Each x-ray photon hits the phosphorous covered plate of the intensifier resulting in a light particle which is detected and its position and intensity noted. The sum of all events produces an image for video and digital recording. Image intensifiers are equipped with different-sized image fields that alter the image resolution. In general, the smaller the input screen diameter, the smaller the image field size and the sharper the resolution. Smaller input screen diameters (5- to 7-in. screens) are better suited for selective coronary cineangiography because of their enhanced resolution. For more detailed work, such as percutaneous transluminal coronary angioplasty, even smaller input diameter (4-in.) screens have been particularly useful. In contrast, large-screen (or field) examinations (i.e., left ventriculography, aortogra-

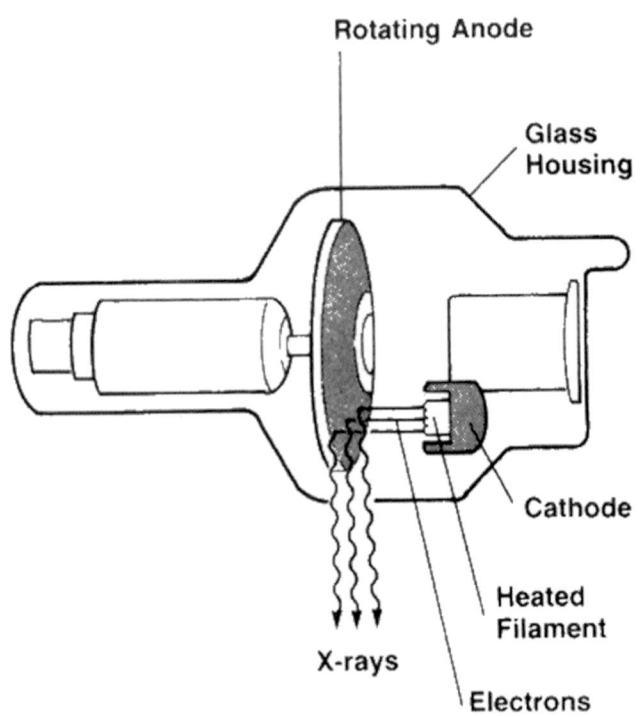

FIGURE 17–18. X-ray generation. *Source: From Baim D, Grossman W, eds. Grossman's Cardiac Catheterization, Angiography and Intervention. 6th ed. Philadelphia: Lippincott Williams & Wilkins; 2000:19. With permission.*

phy, or peripheral angiography) use input screen diameters of 9 to 11 in. The trade-off, of course, is that detailed resolution is reduced. Image distortion may be caused by magnification or foreshortening. The x-ray image casts an x-ray shadow onto the input screen of the image intensifier. The distance of the object from the screen produces an image that may be either sharp or indistinct, depending on the distance. Increasing the distance of the heart to the image intensifier also requires more kilovoltage, thereby further reducing image quality. Distortion of the object's perspective is called *foreshortening*. When the longitudinal axis is seen at an oblique angle, there is foreshortening of the length shadow; and when it is perpendicular to the x-ray beam (parallel to the film plane), there is a full and true image of the length and contour details. Because of foreshortening, arterial lesions that may appear severe in one projection may not appear at all or seem significantly less severe in other projections. For this reason multiple angulated projections are used to identify the severity of lesions within the coronary tree.

Digital Angiography Imaging

Digital angiography converts the x-ray image into a quantitative information format for storage and display on a computer. Digital angiography stores x-ray images on magnetic tapes, disks, or other electronic media rather than on x-ray film. Digital angiography permits compact storage and quantitative image analysis. Digital imaging also permits various manipulations to be performed to enhance the stored images. The contrast image can be amplified or enlarged or contrast adjusted. One image can be subtracted from another, and that image can be subtracted from a third image. Similar contrast adjustments and enlargements are not possible with film radiographs. The durability of some digital archival media has been questioned.

【 】 RADIATION SAFETY

The catheterization laboratory environment should be made as safe as possible for the staff and patient. Standards for radiation protection (from the Society for Cardiac Angiography and Intervention)[61] include four basic principles:

1. The less exposure, the less chance of absorbed energy biologic interaction.
2. No known level of ionizing radiation is a permissible dose or absolutely safe.
3. Radiation exposure is cumulative. There is no washout phenomenon.
4. All participants in the cardiac catheterization laboratory have voluntarily accepted some degree of radiation exposure, but they are obliged to minimize and reduce risks to other personnel and themselves.

The primary x-ray beam, emanating from the under table x-ray tube upward through the patient and onto the image intensifier exposes all subjects to radiation in a dose geometrically inverse to the distance from the source. Radiation scatter is increased when the angle of the x-ray tube is set obliquely. A high degree of angulation increases the amount of radiation scatter (Fig. 17–19). Acrylic shields and table-mounted lead aprons reduce exposure from x-ray scatter. Fluoroscopy generates approximately one-fifth

the x-ray exposure of cineangiography. The increased use of cineangiography for complex catheterization procedures has increased the total exposure and should be a consideration in procedures requiring extensive intracardiac manipulation, such as angioplasty, valvuloplasty, or electrophysiology studies.[62–64] Practices to ensure radiation dose limitation should be routinely employed. Although no known threshold for radiation exposure exists to define specific risks, the National Council on Radiation Protection and Measurements indicates that no dose >3 rem should be allowed over a 3-month period. The eyes, gonads, and red bone marrow have a whole-body limit of 5 rem (roentgen equivalent man) per year; any specific organ, such as the thyroid or skin, has a yearly limit of 15 rem. The maximal permissible dose, or *safe* exposure, for catheterization laboratory personnel is 100 mrem per week monitored by an unshielded left collar badge. Definitions of radiation units are provided in Table 17–23. Radiation exposure is greater during angioplasty than during diagnostic catheterization. If the protective shields are employed carefully, the radiation exposure for single- and double-vessel angioplasty as compared to diagnostic catheterization may be comparable. However, it should be

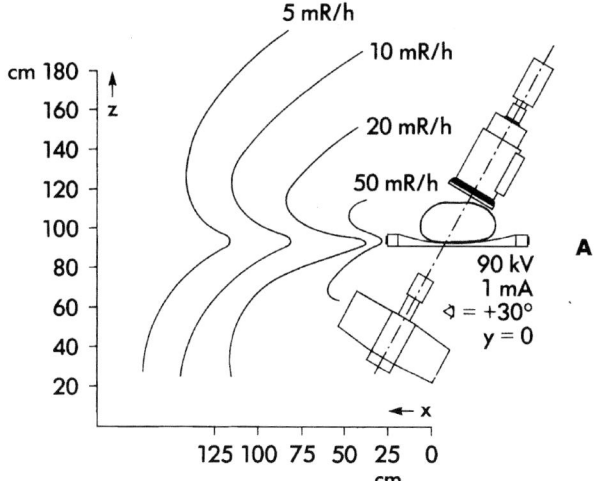

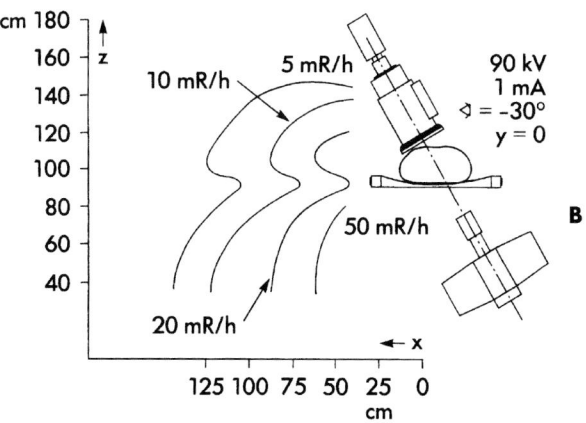

FIGURE 17–19. Isoexposure curves representing ranges of relative exposure in the position usually occupied by the operator performing an angiographic procedure from the right arm. **A.** 30-degree left anterior oblique. **B.** 30-degree right anterior oblique. *Source: From Balter S, Sones FM, Brancato R. Radiation exposure to the operator performing cardiac angiography with U-arm systems. Circulation 1978;58:925. With permission.*

TABLE 17–23

Definitions of Radiation Units

Roentgen (R) is the measure of ionization delivered to a specific point (exposure). One chest radiography equals 3 to 5 mR.

Radiation absorbed dose (rad) is the amount of radiation energy deposited per unit mass of tissue. The amount of absorbed dose per given exposure is dependent upon tissue type. For example, for soft tissue, 1 R = 1 rad; for bone, 1 R = 4 rad (i.e., greater absorption)

Radiation equivalent dose in man (rem) is used to express the biological impact of a given exposure. For x-radiation, 1 rad = 1 rem.

understood that radiation exposures are generally higher for these procedures, especially when biplane angiography is performed.

HEMODYNAMIC DATA FROM THE CARDIAC CATHETERIZATION LABORATORY

In conjunction with angiographic data gathered during the cardiac catheterization, hemodynamic information is recorded from catheters inside vascular structures. Hemodynamic data includes pressure measurements, blood flow, and blood oxygen saturation measurements. Protocols for systematic hemodynamic data collection are available elsewhere.[1-3] Clinical indications for hemodynamic studies are summarized in Table 17–1.

[ ] PRESSURE MEASUREMENTS

Pressure-Recording Systems

Blood within the heart or vessels exerts pressure. A pressure wave is created by cardiac muscular contraction and is transmitted from the vessel or chamber along a closed, fluid-filled column (catheter) to a pressure transducer, converting the mechanical pressure to an electrical signal that is displayed on a video monitor. Cardiac pressure waveforms are cyclical, repeating the pressure change from the onset of one cardiac contraction (systole) to the onset of the next contraction. The complete description of the physiology of heart function is discussed in Chap. 4. An examination of the cardiac cycle and corresponding pressures will provide an understanding of basic hemodynamics in the cardiac catheterization laboratory. The collection of hemodynamic data for cardiac catheterization is an integral part of every procedure. Even complex hemodynamic data recording can be accomplished accurately and rapidly if an efficient and consistently used methodology is established in the laboratory. A predetermined plan for data collection facilitates simultaneous pressure measurements across the heart, concentrating on the aortic and mitral valves, those that are affected most commonly by disease. Different hemodynamic measurements for specific clinical situations are necessary. In conjunction with pressure measurements, cardiac output can be measured using the thermodilution technique or by application of the Fick principle (oxygen consumption) method. To measure suspected cardiac shunts, arterial, vena caval (superior and inferior), RA

(high, middle, and low right atria), RV, RV outflow tract, and PA oxygen saturations are collected. Pressure wave fidelity depends on quality components that can transmit the pressure wave to a transducer without signal distortion. If the heart rate is 60 to 120 beats/min, the fundamental frequency of the basic wave is 1 to 2 per second. The higher frequency sine-wave components of the pressure wave then occur at frequencies of up to 10 to 20 Hz; For best results the transducer must detect these components without phase lag or amplitude distortion because their sum represents the rising and falling contours of the native pressure curve. A properly responding pressure-recording system should have a high natural frequency and optimal damping to minimize over- or undershoot of the waveform. A high natural frequency is obtained by using a bubble-free, saline solution–filled system of minimum length whose catheter and connector tubings have stiff walls and wide bores. A frequency response and damping coefficient can be obtained by introducing a square-wave pressure input to the pressure system and measuring the amplitude ratio of any two successive peak pressure amplitudes and the time interval between peaks. For clinical cardiac catheterization, a manometer system with a uniform dynamic response of greater than 20 Hz is desirable. Clinically, the zero (atmospheric) position for an external pressure transducer is set at the lateral midchest level. Specifically, hydrostatic zero is considered to be at the level of most anterior surfaces of the LV blood pool.[65] An additional limiting factor in pressure recording is the superimposition of artifacts on the pressure pulse by the accelerating and decelerating movements imparted to the fluid-filled cardiac catheter by the beating heart. Distortion of the catheter-obtained phasic pressure waveform by motion or damping artifact can be avoided with the use of a catheter-tip, side-mounted, miniature semiconductor gauge. This manometer system is required for first- or second-derivative measurements of the pressure curve and is principally a research tool.

The Femoral Artery and Left Ventricular Pressure

The most common pressure measurements include systemic pressure and LV pressure. The FA sheath is often used to compare aortic pressure (AoP) to LV pressure to assess the aortic valve. A delay in pressure transmission and overshoot of the systolic pressure compared to centrally measured AoP are characteristic of FA pressure measurements. The LV pressure should be examined for waveform characteristics to insure all side holes are beneath the aortic valve and that the catheter system is flushed to permit accurate interpretation of the diastolic LV waveform.[66] Right heart hemodynamics are easily obtained with balloon-tipped flotation catheter. Blood oxygen saturations in the inferior vena cava, right atrium and PA are collected to screen for cardiac shunts. RA, RV, PA, and pulmonary capillary wedge (PCW) pressures are measured and cardiac output estimated by thermodilution. If necessary during right heart pressure catheter pullback, the LV pressure can be compared to RV pressure to identify constrictive/restrictive physiology.

Right Heart Pressures and the Pulmonary Capillary Wedge Pressure

PCW pressure closely approximates left atrial (LA) pressure. PCW pressure overestimates LA pressure in patients with acute respiratory failure, chronic obstructive lung disease with pulmonary hypertension, pulmonary venoconstriction, or LV failure with volume overload. Discrepancies between LA and PCW may be caused, in part, by different types of catheters: balloon-tipped flotation catheters are soft with small lumens; LA pressure catheters (e.g., Brockenbrough or Mullins-type sheath) are stiff with large lumens. In most patients, the PCW is sufficient to assess LV filling pressure. However, in patients with mitral valvular disease or mitral valve prostheses, the most accurate method is direct LA pressure measurement by transeptal puncture. PCW pressure can be identified from adequate pressure waveforms and confirmed by oximetry. The best location of the PCW pressure has been questioned, but for practical purposes any of the four locations (left or right upper lobes or left or right lower lobes) within the pulmonary tree are generally acceptable. In patients with high PA pressures (>50 mmHg), an inflated balloon should not be left in place for more than 10 minutes because prolonged balloon inflation may cause pulmonary infarction or damage to the PA. Care should be taken not to inflate a balloon vigorously in distal portions of the lung, where the balloon may tear a small pulmonary vessel. Complications of PA catheterization are described in Table 17–24.

【 】 COMPUTATIONS FOR HEMODYNAMIC MEASUREMENTS

Once the hemodynamic data have been obtained, computations are made to clarify and enhance quantitation of cardiac function. The most often used computations involve quantitation of cardiac work, flow resistance, valve areas, and amount of shunting. Specific derivations and applications of these formulas can be found elsewhere.[1-3]

1. Cardiac output (CO) using the Fick principle (O_2 consumption) is calculated as follows:

$$CO = \frac{O_2 \text{ consumption (mL/min)}}{A\,Vo_2 \text{ difference(mL } O_2/100 \text{ mL blood)} \times 10}$$

In 1870, Adolph Fick expounded a theory for the measurement of flow: "The total uptake or release of a substance by an organ is the product of the blood flow to the organ and of the arteriovenous concentration of the substance." Using total oxygen consumption of 300 mL/min, arterial blood oxygen content of 19 mL/100 mL of blood, and mixed venous blood oxygen content of 14 mL/100 mL of blood, the cardiac output, in liters per minute, is equal to the oxygen consumption divided by the arteriovenous oxygen difference (A-Vo_2) multiplied by 10 (to

TABLE 17–24

Complications of Pulmonary Artery Catheterization

Complications of vascular access
Pulmonary infarction
Pulmonary artery rupture
Injury to chordae in right ventricle
Tricuspid regurgitation
Right bundle-branch block
Dislodgment of pacemaker leads

convert the latter to liters). With these data in this case, the cardiac output equals 6.0 L/min. Oxygen consumption is measured from a metabolic *hood*; it also can be estimated as 3 mLO_2/min/kg or 125 mL/min/m². A-Vo_2 is calculated from arterial–mixed venous (PA) O_2 content, where O_2 content = saturation × 1.36 × hemoglobin concentration. For example, if the arterial saturation is 95 percent, the PA saturation is 65 percent, the hemoglobin concentration is 13.0 g/dL, and the O_2 consumption is 210 mLO_2/min (70 kg × 3 mLO_2/min/kg), then the cardiac output is:

$$\frac{210}{(0.95-0.65)\times 1.36 \times 13.0 \times 10} = \frac{210}{53} = 3.96 \text{ L/min}$$

2. Cardiac index (CI, L/min/m²)

$$CI = \frac{CO(\text{mL/beat})}{BSA(m^2)}$$

where CO = cardiac output; BSA = body surface area.

3. Stroke volume (SV, mL/beat)

$$SV = \frac{CO(\text{mL/min})}{HR(\text{bpm})}$$

where HR = heart rate.

4. Stroke index (SI, mL/beat/m²)

$$SI = \frac{SV(\text{mL/beat})}{BSA(m^2)}$$

5. Stroke work (SW, g • m)

$$SW = (\text{mean LV systolic pressure} - \text{mean LV diastolic pressure}) \times SV \times 0.0144$$

6. Pulmonary arteriolar resistance (PAR, Wood units)

$$PAR = \frac{\text{mean pulmonary arterial pressure} - \text{mean LA pressure (or mean PCW)}}{CO}$$

7. Total pulmonary resistance (TPR, Wood units)

$$TPR = \frac{\text{mean pulmonary arterial pressure}}{CO}$$

8. Systemic vascular resistance (SVR, Wood units)

$$SVR = \frac{\text{mean systemic arterial pressure} - \text{mean right atrial pressure}}{CO}$$

Resistance calculations follow the form of Ohm's law, where

$$R = \Delta p / \dot{Q}$$

R = resistance; Δp = mean pressure differential across the vascular bed; $\dot{Q}$ = blood flow. Resistance units (mmHg/L/min) are also called *Hybrid resistance units* or Wood units. To convert Wood units to metric resistance (dynes × s × cm⁻⁵), multiply by 80.

【 】 CALCULATION OF VALVE AREAS

Valvular or vascular obstruction produces a pressure gradient across a stenosis or vascular conduit/chamber narrowing. A pressure gradient is defined as the pressure difference across an area of valvular or vascular obstruction (such as a stenosis or an occlusion). The pressure gradient is influenced by physiologic variables such as rate of blood flow (cardiac output, coronary blood flow, etc.), resistance to flow, proximal chamber pressure and compliance, and anatomic variables, such as shape and length of valve orifice, tortuousities of the vessels (for arterial stenosis), or multiple or serial lesions (for both cardiac valves and arterial stenosis). In addition, pressure measurements may be influenced by artifactual variables, including miscalibrated pressure transducers; pressure leaks on catheter manifold or connecting tubing; pressure tubing type, length, and connectors; air in system; catheter sizes (especially small diameters); and fluid viscosity.

Valve Area Formulas

A valve area can be calculated from standard hemodynamic data with the following formula:

$$\text{Area (cm}^2) = \frac{\text{valve flow (mL/s)}}{K \times C \times \sqrt{\text{MVG}}}$$

where MVG = mean valvular gradient (mmHg); K (44.3) = a derived constant by Gorlin and Gorlin[67,68]; C = an empiric constant that is 1 for semilunar valves and tricuspid valve and 0.85 for mitral valve; valve flow is measured in milliliters per second during the diastolic or systolic flow period.

For mitral valve flow:

$$\frac{\text{CO (mL/min)}}{\text{(diastolic filling period)(HR)}}$$

For aortic valve flow:

$$\frac{\text{CO (mL/min)}}{\text{(systolic ejection period)(HR)}}$$

Calculating Aortic Valve Area

The method of calculating aortic valve area (AVA) from data obtained at catheterization for a patient with aortic stenosis (Fig. 17–20) is as follows. Assuming CO = 4000 mL/min, HR = 60 beats/min.

1. Planimeter aortic-LV pressure gradients (area = 12.2 cm^2) and measure systolic ejection periods (SEPs = 4.1 cm). Next convert cm to time and convert planimetered area to mean systolic pressure gradient. Systolic ejection period of 4.1 cm/beat at paper speed of 100 mm/sec = 0.41 sec/beat. Mean valve gradient (MVG) = (area × scale factor)/SEP (Scale Factor: 1 cm = 19.6 mmHg [directly measured paper calibration lines of 200 mmHg])

$$\text{MVG} = 12.2 \text{ cm}^2 \times \frac{19.6 \text{ mmHg}/1 \text{ cm}}{4.1 \text{ cm}} = \frac{239}{4.1} = 58 \text{ mmHg}$$

2. Compute aortic valve flow.

$$\text{Flow} = \frac{\text{CO}}{\text{SEP} \times \text{HR}} = \frac{4000 \text{ mL/min}}{0.41 \text{ s/beat} \times 60 \text{ bpm}}$$

$$= \frac{4000}{24.6} = 126.6 \text{ mL/min}$$

3. Compute aortic valve area.

$$\text{AVA} = \frac{\text{Aortic valve flow}}{1.0 \times 44.3\sqrt{\text{MVG}}} = \frac{162.6}{44.3 \times \sqrt{58}}$$

$$= \frac{162.6}{44.3 \times 7.6} = \frac{162.6}{336.6} = 0.48 \text{ cm}^2$$

Although mean pressure is used in the Gorlin formula, peak-to-peak pressure gradients are easily measured and also used to estimate valve area. The peak-to-peak gradient is not equivalent to mean gradient for mild and moderate stenosis but often approximates mean gradient for severe stenosis. The delay in pressure

transmission and augmented pressure wave reflection from the proximal Ao to the FA artificially increases the mean gradient. Femoral pressure overshoot (amplification) reduces the true gradient. If the femoral arterial pressure is used, phase shifting of the femoral arterial pressure to the left ventricle upstroke may be important. In patients with low gradients (i.e., <35 mmHg), more accurate valve areas were obtained with unadjusted LV–Ao pressure tracings.[69] Optimally, a second catheter can be positioned directly above the aortic valve to eliminate transmission delay and pressure amplification.[70] Transseptal cardiac catheterization also can be performed to obtain LV pressure (via crossing mitral valve). Aortic valve area can also be estimated closely by a simplified formula as cardiac output divided by the square root of the LV–Ao peak-to-peak pressure difference. For example, if peak-to-peak gradient = 65 mmHg and CO = 5 L/min, then a simplified valve area[70] = 0.63 cm^2.

$$\frac{5 \text{ L/min}}{\sqrt{65}} = \frac{5 \text{ L/min}}{8} = 0.63 \text{ cm}^2$$

The simplified formula for valve area differs from the Gorlin formula by 18 ± 13 percent in patients with bradycardia (<65 beats/min) or tachycardia (>100 beats/min).[71,72] The Gorlin equation at low flow states overestimates the severity of valve stenosis. In low flow states (CO < 2.5 L/min), the Gorlin formula should be modified to employ the mean transvalvular gradient with new empirically derived constants.

Use of Valve Resistance for Aortic Stenosis

Valve resistance, a measure of valve obstruction, has recently been shown to have clinical use. Although proposed around the same time that the Gorlin valve area formula was initially reported, valve resistance has not been used because the units of dynes × s × cm^{-5} were not well related to clinical outcome. Despite obvious strengths, valve area measurements have both practical and theoretical limitations. Area is a planar measurement without consideration of the funnel-like nature of the mitral inflow or the more tubelike configuration of the aortic outlet. Valve area is based on laminar flow of a noncompressible fluid. Turbulence is not consid-

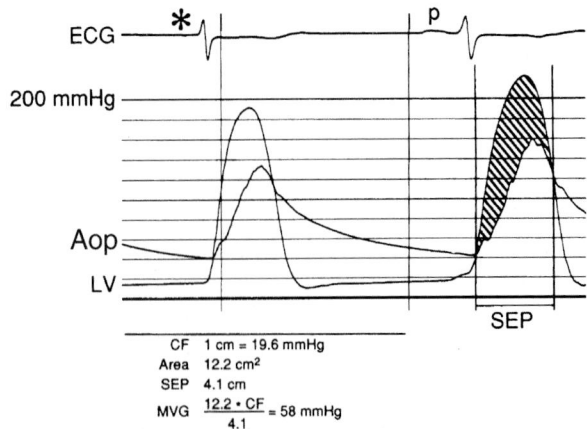

FIGURE 17–20. Aortic valve area is determined from the planimetered area of the aortic valve gradient. The aortic valve gradient area (shaded area) is bounded by the systolic ejection period (SEP). AoP, aortic pressure; LV, left ventricular pressure (scale 0–200 mmHg); CF, correction factor or scale factor; MVG, mean value gradient. See text for details. *Source: From Kern MJ.[1] With permission.*

ered. The constant in the denominator of the Gorlin formula is the square root of gravity, 2gH (acceleration of water due to gravity), and assumes that blood flow is gravity driven and nonpulsatile.[73] Valve areas <0.7 cm² are almost always associated with an important clinical syndrome, and areas >1.1 cm² are usually not associated with significant symptoms, but the areas in between remain in a gray zone. One of the most common clinical situations is found in the patient with a valve area of 0.9 to 1.0 cm², a low transvalve pressure gradient, low cardiac output, and poor LV function. There is uncertainty regarding the outcome following valve replacement with a high mortality if ventricular function does not improve following surgery. Valve resistance (R), as an alternative method to assess valve obstruction, is calculated using the same variables used for valve area measurement as:

$$R = \frac{\text{Mean gradient}}{(\text{CO}/\text{SEP}) \times \text{HR}} \times 80$$

where *CO* = cardiac output; *SEP* = systolic ejection period; *HR* = heart rate. In contrast to valve area, the mean pressure gradient is considered a linear variable rather than taken as a square root term. Thus, the contribution of pressure gradient to the magnitude of valve resistance is greater. Resistance also has been shown to be more constant under conditions of changing cardiac output than valve area. Resistance thus necessarily has a close relationship to valve area. Fig. 17–21 shows resistance and area calculated in a group of patients before and after balloon aortic valve dilatation. Resistance rises sharply below a valve area of 0.7 cm². The shoulder of this curve is between 0.7 and 1.1 cm², which is the common area of indeterminate significance of Gorlin aortic valve area. Some patients in this gray zone tend to have higher valve resistance than others. It has been shown in this setting that the patients with resistance >250 dynes × sec × cm⁻⁵ are more likely to have significant obstruction while those with resistance below 200 dynes × sec × cm⁻⁵ are less likely. There remains a gray zone using this index as well. In addition, some patients may have a resistance below 250 despite a planar valve area of 0.7 to 0.8 cm². Resistance

is a complementary index, not a replacement for valve area. Valve resistance is not expected to remain consistent. Some changes in valve area observed in a single patient under different conditions or at different times might be more acceptable when considered as changes in valve resistance than planar area. As with peripheral resistance, valve resistance is interpreted in the context of the clinical conditions under which it is measured. A peripheral resistance of 1000 dynes × sec × cm⁻⁵ has a greatly different significance in a patient with presumed sepsis than it does in a patient with LV failure. Similarly, we can expect valve resistance to vary as cardiac output changes.

Calculations for Mitral Valve Area

To calculate the most accurate valve area, use the direct LA pressure from transseptal measurement. Transseptal catheterization should be performed to confirm large pressure gradients, especially for suspected prosthetic mitral stenosis. The PCW pressure overestimates LA pressure (transseptal catheterization) in patients with prosthetic mitral valves (Fig. 17–22). Overestimation is caused, in part, by large v waves increasing the phase delay, making correction and alignment of pressure tracings difficult.[74] However, if the PCW pressure-LV pressure tracings show no significant gradients, transseptal catheterization is unnecessary. Mitral valve area from the following data is calculated below. Assuming CO = 3500 mL/min, HR = 80 beats/min.

1. Planimeter LV-PCW areas (area = 9.46 cm²) and measure diastolic filling period (DFP = 3.4 cm). Next convert cm to time and planimetered area to mean diastolic pressure gradient.

   Diastolic filling period of 3.4 cm/beat at paper speed of 100 mm/sec = 0.34 sec/beat>
   Mean valve gradient (MVG) = (area × scale factor)/DFP (Scale Factor: 1 cm = 3.9 mmHg [directly measured paper calibration lines of 40 mmHg])

   $$\text{MVG} = 9.46 \text{ cm}^2 \times \frac{3.9 \text{ mmHg}/1 \text{ cm}}{3.4 \text{ cm}} = 10.85 \text{ mmHg}$$

2. Compute mitral valve flow.
   $$\text{Flow} = \frac{\text{CO}}{\text{DFP} \times \text{HR}} = \frac{3500 \text{ mL/min}}{0.34 \text{ s/beat} \times 80 \text{ bpm}}$$
   $$= \frac{3500}{0.34 \times 80} = \frac{3500}{27.2} = 128.7 \text{ mL/min}$$

3. Compute mitral valve area.
   $$\text{MVA} = \frac{\text{Mitral valve flow}}{0.85 \times 44.3 \sqrt{10.85}} = \frac{128.7}{0.85 \times 44.3 \times 3.3}$$
   $$= \frac{128.7}{124.3} = 1.0 \text{ cm}^2$$

[ ] CARDIAC OUTPUT TECHNIQUES
Thermodilution Technique

The thermodilution technique was introduced by Fegler in 1953 to measure volume flow rate. A multiple-lumen, balloon-tipped flow-directed thermistor catheter is placed in the PA. Ten mL of room-temperature 71.6°F (22°C) 5 percent dextrose or normal saline solution is injected rapidly (<4 sec) through a second lumen into the right atrium. As the injectate blood mixture initially passes from the right ventricle, the PA blood temperature drops

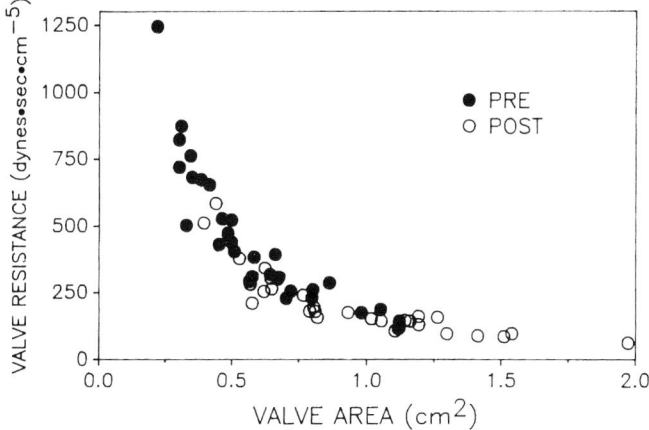

FIGURE 17–21. Comparison of valve area by Gorlin formula versus valve resistance before (*pre*) and after (*post*) aortic valvuloplasty. Valve resistance <200 dynes × sec × cm⁻⁵ is associated with minimal obstruction, >250 dynes × sec × cm² with significant obstruction. This measure complements and refines valve area decision making. *Source: From Feldman T, Ford L, Chiu YC, Carroll J. Changes in valvular resistance power dissipation and myocardial reserve with aortic valvuloplasty. J Heart Valve Dis 1992;1:55–64. With permission.*

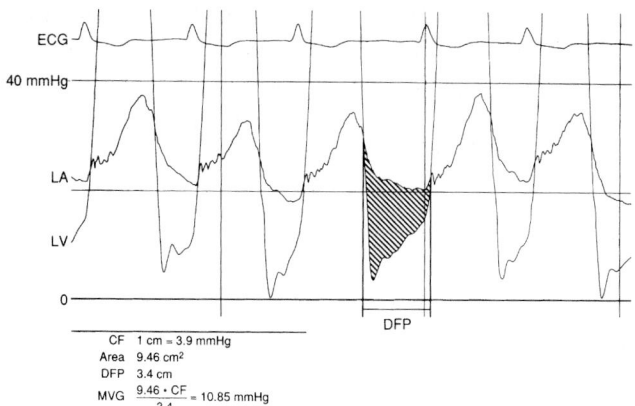

FIGURE 17–22. Hemodynamic tracing used to calculate mitral valve area. The shaded area is the diastolic mitral valve gradient surrounded by the diastolic filling period (DFP). CF, correction factor or scale factor; LA, left atrial pressure; LV, left ventricular pressure (scale 0–40 mmHg), MVG, mean value gradient. See text for details.

maximally and then progressively rises in a beat-to-beat disappearance slope as the residual injectate blood mixture is washed out of the right ventricle. The recirculation phase is negligible. The area under the time–temperature curve is electronically integrated, and the cardiac output is computed by the Stewart-Hamilton formula. Because there is no *gold standard* for cardiac output, the results have been compared with the dye-dilution and Fick techniques and have correlated well, except in low cardiac output states, where the Fick method is preferable. If severe tricuspid or pulmonary regurgitation or significant left-to-right shunting is present, the indicator (temperature loss) is attenuated and the downslope of the temperature curve is prolonged, so the thermal dilution cardiac output will be unreliable.[75–77] In general, when one uses thermal dilution, a true directional change in cardiac output is reflected by an observed change of ± 10 percent. Thermodilution is inaccurate in patients with low cardiac output. Significant variations among cardiac output techniques occur in patients with low cardiac output or in those with aortic or mitral regurgitation. In patients with mitral and aortic valve regurgitation, and low cardiac output, the dye dilution method varied by more than 20 percent from the Fick method.

The Fick Method of Cardiac Output

The Fick method most often uses an assumed oxygen consumption value or less frequently a metabolic hood to measure oxygen consumption. The Fick calculation is described above.

Angiographic Cardiac Output

Cardiac output determined angiographically is computed as the SV (end-diastolic volume minus the end-systolic volume) times the heart rate. Angiographic cardiac output provides the best estimate of cardiac output through a stenotic valve when any degree of regurgitation is present. Errors in SV computation are increased with enlarged ventricles, especially when single-plane cineangiography is employed. Angiographic cardiac output is not determined simultaneously with a transvalvular gradient; therefore, additional error may be introduced by delay in simultaneous measurements. A calibrated ventriculogram is also necessary.

[ ] INTRACARDIAC SHUNTS

A shunt is an abnormal communication between the left and right heart chambers. The direction of blood flowing through the shunt may be left to right, right to left, or sometimes bidirectional. In the absence of shunting, the pulmonary blood flow (right heart output) is equal to the systemic blood flow. Table 17–25 lists intracardiac shunt locations. A left-to-right shunt increases the amount of blood to the right heart and increases pulmonary blood flow, now equal to the sum of the systemic blood flow plus shunt flow. With a right-to-left shunt, the amount of blood shunted from the right side to the left is added to that normally ejected into the systemic circulation. Systemic blood flow is then greater than pulmonary blood flow by the amount of the shunt. Intracardiac shunts have been evaluated by four methods:

1. Oximetry
2. Indocyanine green dye dilution curves
3. Angiography
4. Radioactive tracers

Oximetry for Cardiac Shunts

An increase in the oxygen content of blood from the chambers of the right side of the heart in excess of the normal variation in oxygen content on serial sampling is used as evidence of a left-to-right shunt.[78] Oxygen content can be expressed as volumes percent (vol% = mL O_2/100 mL blood) or can be expressed from percent oxygen saturation where content is calculated from the hemoglobin concentration assuming a constant relationship for oxygen carrying capacity (1.36 mL O_2/g hemoglobin). Thus an oxygen step-up from the superior vena cava

TABLE 17–25

Shunt Locations and Oximetry Sampling Sites

LOCATION	EARLIEST STEP-UP LOCATION (FOR LEFT-TO-RIGHT SHUNTS)
Atrial septal defects	
Primum (low)	RA, RV
Secundum (mid)	RA
Sinus venosus (high)	RA
Partial anomalous pulmonary venous return (pulmonary veins entering right atrium)	RA
Ventricular septal defects	
Membranous (high)	RV
Muscular (mid)	RV
Apical (low)	RV
Aorticopulmonary window (connection of Ao to pulmonary artery)	PA
Patent ductus arteriosus (normally closed Ao–PA connection at birth)	PA

Ao, aorta; PA, pulmonary artery; RA, right atrium; RV, right ventricle.

TABLE 17–26

Oxygen Saturation Values for Shunt Detection

LEVEL OF SHUNT	SIGNIFICANT STEP-UP DIFFERENT[a] O_2 SATURATION
Atrial (SVC/IVC to right ventricle)	7
Ventricular	5
Great vessel	5

SVC, superior vena cava; IVC, inferior vena cava; PA, pulmonary artery pressure.
[a]Difference distal-proximal chamber. For example, for atrial septal defect:

$$RV - \frac{3\,SVC + 1\,IVC}{4}$$

(SVC) to the right atrium of more than 1.9 vol% indicates shunting into the right atrium; a step-up from the right atrium to the right ventricle of 0.9 vol% or more and a step up from the right ventricle to the PA of 0.5 vol% or more indicates a left-to-right shunt at the RV and PA levels, respectively. By these criteria, false-positive results are rare, but false-negative results can occur in patients with small shunts. In an anemic or polycythemic patient, the detection of shunting is best reflected by the step-up in percentage oxygen saturation rather than the step-up in volume percent, because the latter depends on the hemoglobin concentration.[79] Studies show that sensitivity in detecting left-to-right shunts is improved if numerous serial paired blood samples are withdrawn in rapid succession for oximetry. Assuming an arterial saturation of 95 percent, a 9 percent saturation increase between the SVC and the right atrium indicates a large atrial shunt, a 5 percent saturation increase between the right atrium and the right ventricle indicates a ventricular shunt, and a 3 percent saturation increase between the right ventricle and the PA indicates a PA shunt. The rise in oxygen saturation step-up for a given left-to-right shunt is related to the saturation of mixed venous blood (MVB). For example, if the MVB is 85 percent, a 5 percent step-up represents a 2:1 shunt; if MVB is 75 percent, a 10 percent step up is needed; if the MVB is 65 percent, a 15 percent step up indicates a 2:1 shunt. Left-to-right shunts of <20 percent of pulmonary flow are not detectable by oximetry. Desaturation of arterialized blood samples from the left heart chambers and Ao suggests a right-to-left shunt. In determining the site of the right-to-left shunt, sequential sampling can be made from the left atrium, left ventricle, and Ao (Table 17–26). Mixed venous blood is assumed to be fully mixed PA blood. If there is a left-to-right shunt, mixed venous blood is measured one chamber proximal to the step-up. In the case of an atrial septal defect, the mixed venous oxygen content is computed from the weighted average of vena caval blood, (i.e., as the sum of three times the superior vena cava plus one inferior vena cava oxygen content and divided by 4). When pulmonary venous blood is not collected, PVO_2 (pulmonary vein) percentage saturation is assumed to be 95 percent. The oximetric technique has some well-known limitations, which include inability to detect small shunts, poor blood oxygen mixing, and inaccuracies with high flow states.[80]

Angiography and Radionuclide Shunt Detection

Angiography is nonquantitative method used to localize either left-to-right or right-to-left shunts. The angiographic method may be useful when origin of the shunt cannot be entered. To detect the shunt, contrast media can be injected into the closest proximal chamber. The LAO view with cranial angulation puts the interatrial and interventricular septae on edge, providing an ideal view for detection of contrast passage across the atrial and ventricular septal defects. Intracardiac shunts have also been detected and quantified by indicator-dilution curves.

Shunt Calculations

The Fick or left-sided indicator dilution methods of cardiac output determination are employed to measure systemic flow. Using the Fick method, the following formulas apply:

1. Systemic flow,

$$Q_S(L/min) = \frac{O_2 \text{ consumption(mL/min)}}{(\text{arterial} - \text{mixed venous})\, O_2 \text{ content}}$$

2. Pulmonary flow, Q_P (L/min)

$$= \frac{O_2 \text{ consumption (mL/min)}}{(\text{pulmonary venous} - \text{pulmonary arterial})\, O_2 \text{ content}}$$

Thus, the effective pulmonary blood flow (EPB)

$$Q_{EPB} = \frac{O_2 \text{ consumption (mL/min)}}{(\text{pulmonary venous} - \text{mixed venous})\, O_2 \text{ content}}$$

The effective pulmonary blood flow is that volume of blood which, after returning to the right atrium, actually reaches the pulmonary capillaries.

It follows that

$$L \rightarrow R \text{ shunt} = Q_P - Q_{EPB}$$

and

$$R \rightarrow L \text{ shunt} = Q_S - Q_{EPB}$$

If arterial blood is fully saturated, then there is no $R \rightarrow L$ shunt, because arterial O_2 content is equal to pulmonary venous O_2 content and $Q_S = Q_{EPB}$.

The shunt ratio is defined as Q_P/Q_S. Shunt ratios of >1.5 are associated with anatomic defects that often require closure.

3. Example calculations for a simple left-to-right shunt in a patient with an atrial septal defect (ASD) using data obtained at catheterization are as follows:

Assume Hgb = 14.1 g/dL, O_2 consumption = 225 mL O_2/min and oxygen saturation data as follows:

Location	Oxygen Saturation (%)
Arterial	98
SVC	71
Mid-RA	71
PA	81
Pulmonary	98
IVC	70

a. Compute O_2 content.
Arterial O_2 content = 0.98×1.36 mL O_2/g $\times 14.1$ g/dL $\times 10$
= 188 mL O_2/L
Mixed venous O_2 content (Use estimate of mixed venous oxygen saturation.):

$$\frac{3SVC + 1IVC}{4} \text{ for mixed venous oxygen saturation.}):$$

$$\frac{(.71 + .71 + .71 + .70)}{4} = 0.71$$

$71 \times 1.36 \text{ mL O}_2/g \times 14.1 \text{ g/dL} \times 10 = 136 \text{ mL O}_2/L$

Pulmonary artery O$_2$ content = $(0.81 \times 1.36 \text{ mL O}_2/gm \times 14.1 \text{ g/dL} \times 10) = 155 \text{ mL O}_2/L$

Pulmonary vein O$_2$ content = $(0.98 \times 1.36 \text{ mL O}_2/g \times 14.1 \text{ g/dL} \times 10) = 188 \text{ mL O}_2/L$

b. Compute systemic flow [Equation (1)].

$$\frac{225 \text{ mL O}_2/min}{(188 - 136)\text{mL O}_2/liter} = \frac{225}{52} = Q_S = 4.3 \text{ L/min}$$

c. Compute pulmonary flow [Equation (2)].

$$\frac{225 \text{ mL O}_2/min}{(188 - 155)\text{mL O}_2/liter} = \frac{225}{33} = Q_P = 6.8$$

d. Compute,

$$\frac{Q_P}{Q_S} = \frac{6.8}{4.3} = 1.6$$

and the $L \rightarrow R$ shunt is 6.8 L/min – 4.3 L/min or 2.5 L/min

If absolute flows are not required, the Q_P/Q_S ratio can be determined using saturations only as follows:

$$\frac{Q_P}{Q_S} = \frac{SAo_2 - MVo_2}{PVo_2 - PAo_2}$$

where SAO_2 = systemic arterial O$_2$ saturation; PVO_2 = pulmonary venous O$_2$ saturation; MVo_2 = mixed venous O$_2$ saturation; PAO_2 = pulmonary artery O$_2$ saturation.

Using saturation data from the example of left-to-right shunt:

$$\frac{Q_P}{Q_S} = \frac{98 - 71}{98 - 81} = \frac{27}{17} = 1.6$$

Example calculations for a more complex, bidirectional shunt from data obtained at catheterization are as follows:

Assume Hgb = 15 g/dL, O$_2$ consumption = 195 mL O$_2$/min, and oxygen saturation data:

Location	Oxygen Saturation (%)
Arterial	89
SVC	81
RA, mid	83
RA, low	82
LA	88
PA	82
Pulmonary vein	96
IVC	70

a. Compute O$_2$ content.

Arterial = $(0.89 \times 15 \text{ g}/100 \text{ mL} \times 1.36 \text{ mL O}_2/g \times 10) = 182$ mL O$_2$/L

Mixed venous estimated mixed venous saturation =
$(.81 + .81 + .81 + .70) 4 = 0.78$

Mixed venous = $(0.78 \times 15 \text{ g/dL} \times 1.36 \text{ m O}_2/g \times 10) = 159$ mL O$_2$/L

Pulmonary arterial = $(0.82 \times 15 \text{ g/dL} \times 1.36 \text{ mL O}_2/g \times 10) = 167$ mL O$_2$/L

Pulmonary venous = $(0.96 \times 15 \text{ g/dL} \times 1.36 \text{ mL O}_2/gm \times 10) = 196$ mL O$_2$/L

b. Compute systemic flow.

$$\frac{O_2 \text{ consumption}}{(\text{arterial} - \text{mixed venous}) \text{ O}_2 \text{ content}} = \frac{195 \text{ mL O}_2/min}{(182 - 159)\text{mL O}_2/L}$$

c. Compute pulmonary blood flow.

$$\frac{O_2 \text{ consumption}}{(\text{pulmonary venous} - \text{pulmonary arterial}) \text{ O}_2 \text{ content}}$$

$$= \frac{195 \text{ mL O}_2/min}{(196 - 197) \text{ mL O}_2/L} = 6.7 \text{ L/min}$$

d. Compute effective pulmonary blood flow.
Effective pulmonary blood flow

$$= \frac{O_2 \text{ consumption}}{(\text{pulmonary venous} - \text{mixed venous}) \text{ O}_2 \text{ content}}$$

$$= \frac{195 \text{ mL O}_2/min}{(196 - 159) \text{ mL O}_2/L} = 5.3 \text{ L}$$

$$\text{Left-right shunt} = Q_P - Q_{EPB}$$

$$= 6.7 - 5.3$$

$$= 1.4 \text{ L/min}$$

$$\text{Right-to-left shunt} = Q_S - Q_{EPB}$$

$$= 8.5 - 5.3$$

$$= 3.2 \text{ L/min}$$

❚ ❩ NORMAL HEMODYNAMIC WAVEFORMS
Normal Right Heart Pressure Waves

Simultaneous RV and RA pressures (Fig. 17–23) demonstrate the correspondence of the atrial contraction *a* wave and the *v* wave (caused by venous return to the RA while the tricuspid valve is closed) to the RV pressure tracing. Following the *a*

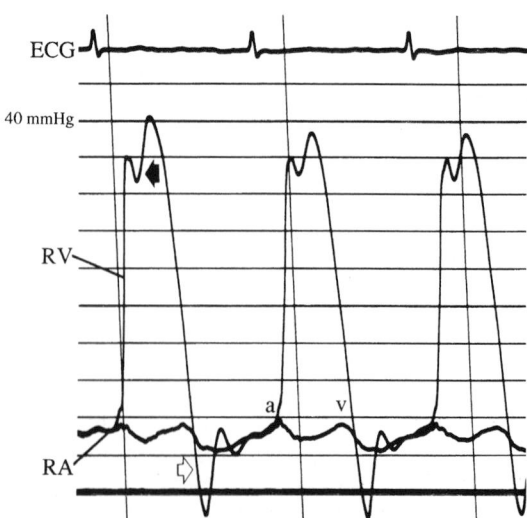

FIGURE 17–23. Right atrial (RA) and right ventricular (RV) tracings in a normal patient. Notch of ringing or overshoot on RV pressure rise (*closed arrow*). Ringing and overshoot of decline in RV pressure at early diastole (*open arrow*). a, atrial wave; v, ventricular filling wave. *Source: From Kern MJ.[1] With permission.*

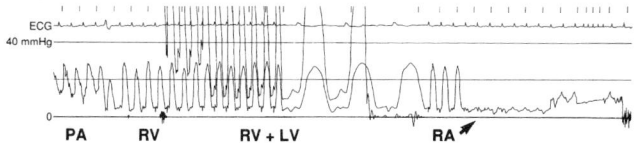

FIGURE 17–24. Continuous hemodynamic tracing during catheter pullback from the pulmonary artery (PA) to right atrium (RA). Differences in left ventricular (LV) and right ventricular (RV) pressures are shown (0–40 mmHg full scale). *Source: From Kern MJ.[1] With permission.)*

wave is the X descent and following the v wave is the normal Y descent. These features may be altered in the presence of disease or obscured in patients who have atrial arrhythmias. The notch (*closed arrow*) on the top of the RV tracing is the *ringing* (underdamping) of a fluid-filled catheter. This rebound or ringing also is evident on the early diastolic part of the pressure wave (*open arrow,* bottom of same beat). During the continuous pressure on pullback across the interatrial septum from the left atrium to the right atrium of a patient with aortic stenosis the differences between LA and RA a and v waves are seen. The v waves on the left atrium are very prominent with their corresponding X and Y descents. In the right atrium, the a and v waves are present but less striking. In general, RA a waves are bigger than v waves. In the left atrium, v waves are more prominent than a waves. RA pressure can be markedly altered by respiration. Normal right heart pressures during continuous pressure recording (using balloon-tipped PA catheter) on catheter pullback from PA to right ventricle and right atrium (0 to 40 mmHg scale) (Fig. 17–24) show the simultaneous LV and RV pressures for evaluation of constrictive or restrictive myocardial physiology. The premature ventricular contractions in RV pressure are common when catheters contact the RV outflow tract.

PCW Pressure and LA Pressure with Simultaneous Transseptal and Right Heart Catheterization

The PCW pressure measured through a 7 Fr fluid-filled balloon-tipped catheter and the LA pressure measured through a Brockenbrough catheter (Fig. 17–25) demonstrate that the LA pressure rise precedes that of the PCW pressure for every waveform by approximately 100 to 150 msec. The generally good correspondence of these two pressures permits clinical use of PCW pressure for the majority of standard hemodynamic cases (a, a′ and v, v′ are the LA and PCW pressures, respectively).

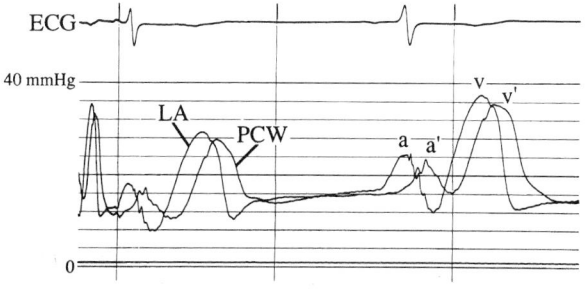

FIGURE 17–25. Simultaneous left atrial (LA) and pulmonary capillary wedge (PCW) tracings. *Source: From Kern MJ.[1] With permission.*

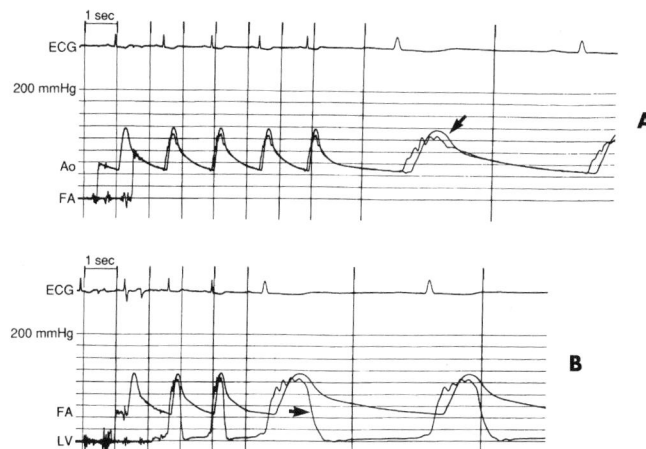

FIGURE 17–26. A. Simultaneous hemodynamic tracings of femoral artery (FA) pressure taken through the side arm of the 8 Fr sheath and central aortic pressures (AoPs). Central AoP is obtained through the 7 Fr pigtail catheter. The overshoot of the FA pressure (*arrow*) and lag in the pressure upstroke are the normal characteristics for the femoral tracings. **B.** FA and left ventricular (LV) pressure (*arrow*). *Source: From Kern MJ.[1] With permission.*

Normal Femoral Arterial and Central Aortic Pressures

The femoral arterial pressure measured through the side arm of the femoral arterial sheath (8 Fr) is matched against pressure in the pigtail catheter (7 Fr) positioned above the aortic valve (Fig. 17–26). These pressures normally correspond closely with only a slight overshoot of the more peripheral femoral artery (FA) pressure (*open arrow*). The timing of upstroke of the pressures distinguishes the central aortic (first tracing rising) from FA pressure. The mean of the two pressures is identical (*closed arrow*). Simultaneous arterial pressure with LV pressures recorded before and after crossing the aortic valve permits satisfactory assessment of most aortic valvular lesions. Note the phase lag and normal overshoot of the arterial pressure compared to the LV pressure.

【 】 PATHOLOGIC HEMODYNAMIC WAVEFORMS

Right Atrial Pressure with Tricuspid Regurgitation

Unlike the normal pattern, the RA pressure rises throughout RV systole as a result of tricuspid valvular regurgitation pushing blood back into the right atrium (Fig. 17–27). In this patient the RA pressure during diastole matches the RV pressure, indicating no tricuspid stenosis.

RA Pressure in a Patient with Atrioventricular Dissociation

Normal a waves represent atrial contraction into the ventricle with no obstruction to inflow. In an atrioventricular block, the atria are not contracting at the proper time in relation to the ventricles. Immediately after the QRS, the ventricles contract and the tricuspid and mitral valves close. If the p wave (and atrial contraction) comes after the tricuspid valve is closed, a giant C or cannon wave can be seen. When atrioventricular synchrony (normal sequence) occurs on beats 6 and 7, the a waves return, proportional in size to

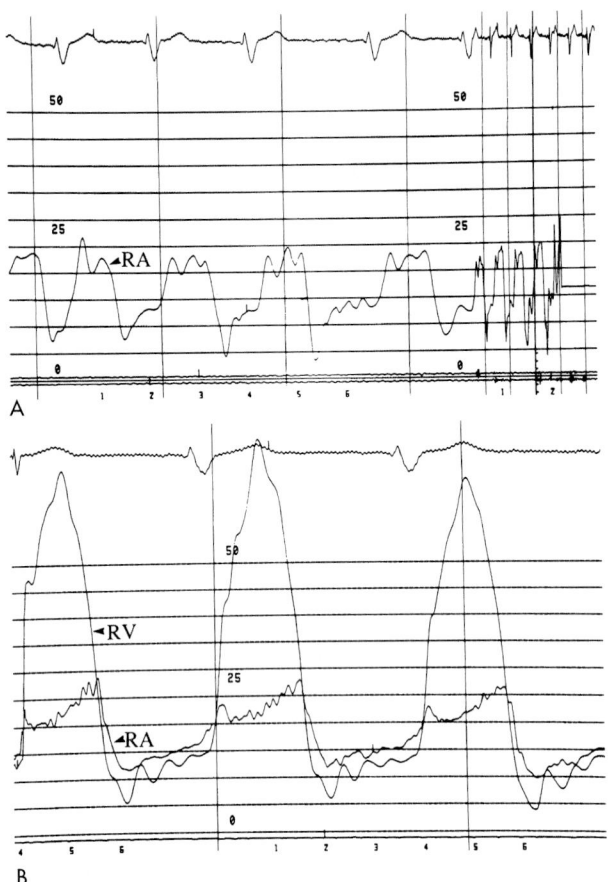

A

B

FIGURE 17–27. A. Right atrial (RA) pressure in a patient with severe tricuspid regurgitation. **B.** When paired with simultaneous right ventricular (RV) pressure, tricuspid regurgitation can now be seen associated with tricuspid stenosis as the separation (gradient) between the RA–RV pressures during diastole. *Source: From Kern MJ.¹ With permission.*

the timing of the atrial contraction, emptying blood before ventricular systole (QRS). Similar findings may be seen when the dissociation is caused by a pacemaker. Giant C waves can occur during pacing.

Large Waves on the PCW Tracing

The PCW has moderate and large v waves. On beat 2 the atrium contracts after the ventricle, resulting in a different initial upstroke of the LV pressure and a cannon wave. The v wave on a PCW pressure tracing usually is associated with significant mitral regurgitation. However, large v waves are not highly sensitive nor are they specific for mitral regurgitation. Large v waves also may be present with mitral stenosis or ventricular septal defect or any condition in which the left atrial volume [e.g., ventricular septal defect (VSD)] or left atrial pressure relationship (the stiffness or compliance) is increased (such as rheumatic heart disease, postcardiac surgery, and infiltrative heart diseases).

Aortic–Left Ventricular Gradients

The atrial contraction is important in patients with aortic stenosis (Fig. 17–28). Simultaneous aortic and LV pressure (transseptal approach) shows that atrial activity is absent in the first beat, a junctional beat (* denotes specific beat on Fig. 17–28). With atrial contraction (second beat) LV pressure increases to 225 mmHg, an

approximate 25 percent increase over the first beat. Hypertrophic cardiomyopathy is a condition in which very thick heart muscle, especially inside the LV chamber, contracts so hard that it obstructs flow out of the ventricle, and thus by its own contraction produces a pressure gradient with a normal aortic valve. Fig. 17–29 depicts simultaneous LV and AoP showing a large aortic–LV gradient (LV = 220 mmHg; Ao = 120 mmHg). On pullback of the LV catheter (multipurpose) from the distal LV to a position just beneath the aortic valve the Ao–LV gradient disappears (see the LV pressure matching with AoP) *(arrow)*.

Left Atrial–Left Ventricular Gradients

Simultaneous LV and PCW pressures demonstrate a mitral valve gradient throughout diastole. The a wave is absent in this patient in atrial fibrillation. As can be seen, mitral valve gradients are strongly influenced by heart rate. Large v waves in the PCW tracing represent LV pressure transmitted backward through an incompetent mitral valve. The v wave (up to 60 mmHg) occurs on the downstroke of the LV pressure in a patient with mitral regurgitation. Matching elevated diastolic pressures with an early dip followed by a plateau during diastole (first beat) is the characteristic pattern. Often, only during slow heart rates does the classic dip-and-plateau configuration appear. Tachycardia and respiratory effort obscure the pattern, but matching both RV–LV pressures during diastole is consistent. Dynamic respiratory variation differentiate constrictive from restrictive pathology (Fig. 17–30).

【 】 PHYSIOLOGIC MANEUVERS IN THE CATHETERIZATION LABORATORY

Exercise

Exercise evaluation of cardiac function is helpful to relate symptoms to hemodynamic changes, especially for patients with valvular heart disease (e.g., mitral stenosis). Hemodynamics are measured at rest and during peak exercise using bicycle ergometry; repeated leg or arm lifts; and, occasionally, arm bicycle ergometry. Commonly measured responses to exercise include minute ventilatory capacity, oxygen extraction, heart rate, cardiac output, ventricular volume and filling pressures, and metabolic substrate utili-

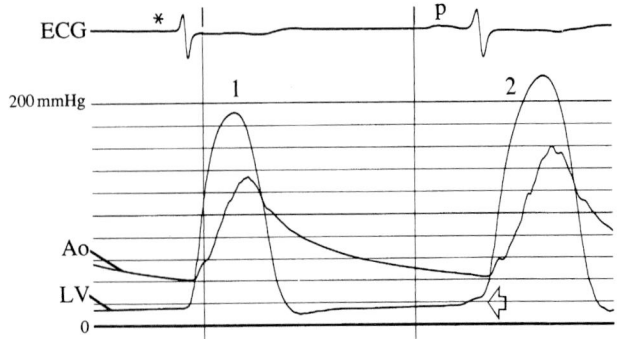

FIGURE 17–28. Simultaneous LV (obtained with transseptal technique) and AoPs from fluid-filled catheter systems. Note the contribution of atrial contraction (*arrow*) to the change in LV and systemic pressures on beat 2. The wide pulse pressure also is indicative of aortic insufficiency with mild stenosis. *, absence of p wave on this tracing; AoP, aortic pressure; LV, left ventricular; p, p wave. *Source: From Kern MJ.¹ With permission.*

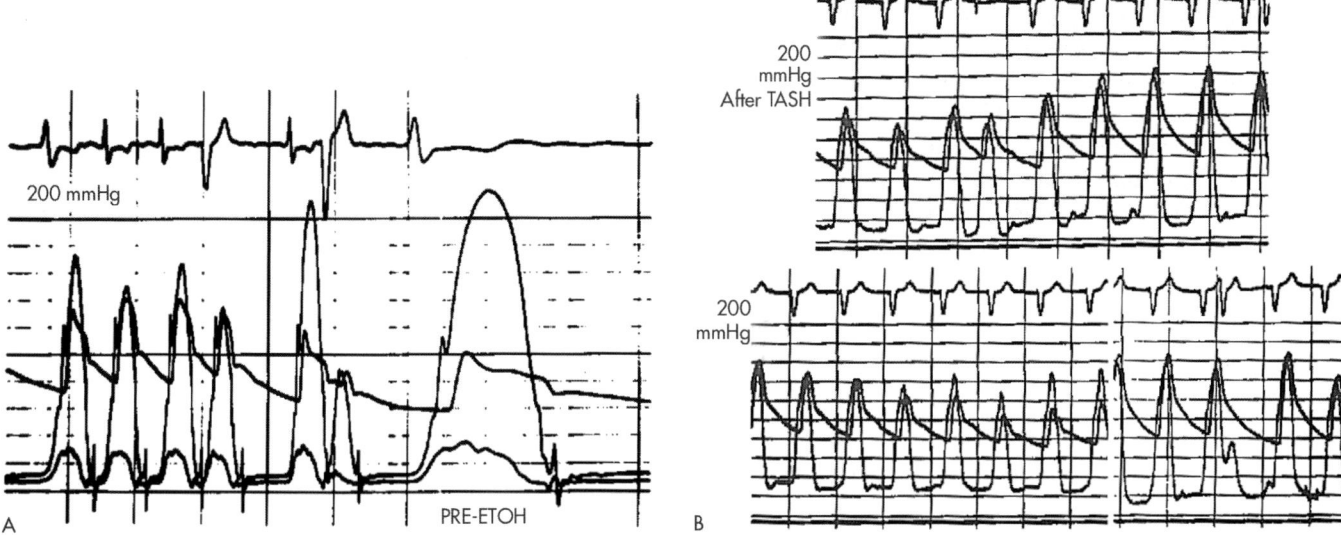

FIGURE 17–29. Hemodynamic tracings of patient with hypertrophic obstructive cardiomyopathy. **A.** Before alcohol septal ablation. **B.** Valsalva maneuver. After transluminal alcohol septal ablation (TASH). EtOH, ethyl alcohol.

zation (e.g., glucose concentration without lactate production). Exercise may be dynamic or isometric. Measurement of each type demonstrates different features of LV function. Dynamic exercise measures the ability of the cardiovascular system to supply oxygen in keeping with increased metabolic demands. Oxygen consumption and work load increases should be parallel until the maximal oxygen consumption for the patient is reached. Dynamic exercise in the cardiac catheterization laboratory requires simultaneous right and left heart pressure measurements during exercise (e.g., treadmill device mounted on the catheterization table). The patient's oxygen consumption also is measured by artery and vein oxygen saturations and is compared to the normal hemodynamic responses. Supine exercise in the catheterization laboratory differs from normal upright exercise in four ways:

1. Ventricular volumes are larger when the patient is supine rather than upright.
2. Heart rate and diastolic arterial pressure are higher when the patient is upright rather than supine.
3. Pulmonary and intracardiac filling pressures are lower when the patient is upright.
4. SV increases 100 percent with maximal exercise when the patient is upright and only 20 percent to 50 percent when the patient is supine.

It can be noted that both upright and supine exercise are normally associated with increases in LV end-diastolic volume and decreases in end-systolic volume with concomitant increase in ejection fraction. In patients with coronary artery disease, these finding may not occur. Exercise data are analyzed with respect to change in hemodynamics (valve gradients), cardiac output, and oxygen consumption. Patients may be unable to exercise because of leg weakness, depressed cardiac function, peripheral vascular disease, or severe deconditioning. These factors may preclude determination of accurate exercise results in the catheterization laboratory and should be considered before undertaking the study. Isometric exercise consists of skeletal muscle contraction without shortening. Isometric exercise commonly is performed using a

hand grip with a graded hand dynamometer. Measurements of hemodynamics and ventricular function are obtained during sustained hand grip at a predetermined range (15–50 percent of the maximal hand-grip contraction) for a period of 3 to 4 minutes. In patients with coronary artery disease, isometric exercise rarely precipitates ischemia but may induce new LV wall motion abnormalities, a decrease in LV ejection fraction, and an increase in end-systolic volume with no change in diastolic volume. SV and CO may decline during isometric exercise. In patients with congestive heart failure, heart rate and systemic pressure may rise appropriately with a fall in SV and CO resulting in increase in LV end-diastolic volume and PA pressure. Several measurements of the response to exercise are important. CO is useful measurement for studying practically all types of heart disease. Measurement of CO for the corresponding oxygen uptake allows categorization of a patient's physiologic cardiovascular response to activity. A predicted cardiac index (CI) with exercise can be determined as 2.99 + 0.0059 × (measured O_2 consumption index). The measured CI with exercise divided by the predicted CI is called the exercise (Dexter) index and expresses exercise capacity as a percentage of the normal response. An index of ≥ 0.8 indicates a normal CO response to exercise. An *exercise factor* can also be computed. For every 100 mL/min increase in O_2 consumption with exercise, the CO should increase by at least 600 mL/min. The exercise factor is calculated directly from observed changes in CO and O_2 consumption and is normalized to BSA, as follows:

$$\text{Exercise Factor} = \frac{\text{CO (mL/min)}}{O_2 \text{ consumption (mL/min)}} \geq 6$$

Appropriate increases in arterial blood pressure and heart rate should also be noted.

Valsalva, Mueller, and Other Physiologic Maneuvers

The Valsalva maneuver is performed by having the patient forcibly expire against a closed glottis and straining as if having a bowel movement. The magnitude of the Valsalva can be quantitated by measuring the pressure against which the patient must expire. The Valsalva maneuver can be performed safely and without complications by almost every type of patient. The four phases of the normal Valsalva maneuver (strain, hypotension, release, and pressure overshoot) may be absent in patients with specific cardiac diseases (congestive heart failure, coronary artery disease, and obstructive cardiomyopathy). In addition, the hemodynamics demonstrated for different types of valvular lesions may be more pronounced during the Valsalva maneuver because of changes in ventricular filling. The Mueller maneuver is performed by inspiring against a closed glottis, and it is considered the inverse or opposite of the Valsalva maneuver. The subject inhales and the force of inhalation is measured with a manometer, usually 30 to 60 mmHg for 30 seconds. Hemodynamic alterations of the Mueller maneuver include increased RV filling, increased period of diminished filling as result of the collapse of the venae cavae at thoracic inlets, increasing LV afterload with increase in LV end-diastolic and end-systolic volumes, diminished SV, reduced CO, and reduced ejection fraction. This maneuver is used to augment right-sided heart murmurs and to decrease the physical findings of obstructive cardiomyopathy by a reduction in LV outflow gradient. A reduction in the intensity of the systolic murmur in patients with echocardiographic evidence of anterior mitral valve leaflet motion also can be demonstrated with this maneuver. Pharmacologic and physiologic stress on LV performance can be obtained in the cath lab by cold pressor testing, hyperventilation, or pharmacologic stimuli such as dobutamine, nitroglycerin, or any nitrates.

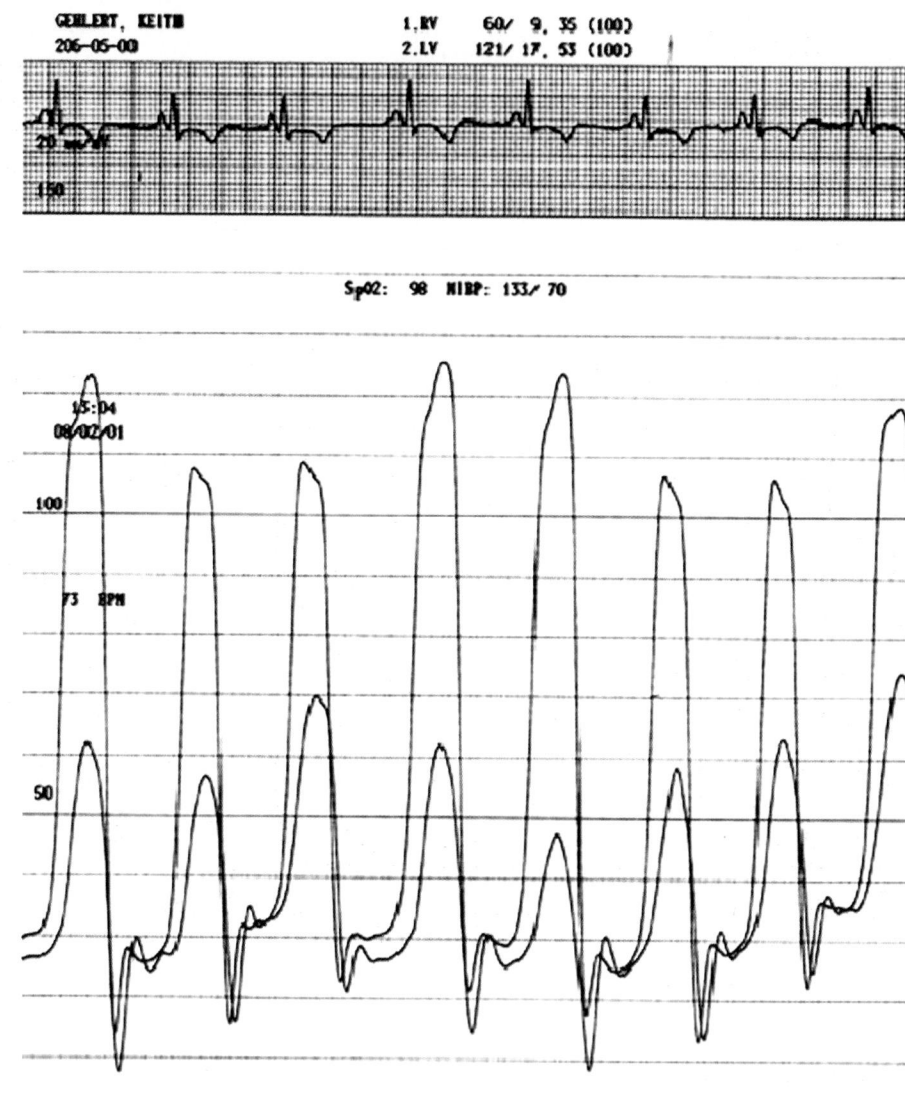

A

FIGURE 17-30 A. Hemodynamic tracings showing physiology of constrictive pericardial constraint. Simultaneous RV and LV pressures during respiration increase discordantly with LV increase and RV decreasing during expiration and vice versa. **B.** Hemodynamics of restrictive pathophysiology shows concordance of systolic pressure changes in both right and left ventricles during respiration. LV, left ventricular; RV, right ventricular.

SPECIAL CATHETERIZATION TECHNIQUES

[ ] TRANSSEPTAL HEART CATHETERIZATION

Retrograde left heart catheterization for aortic or mitral stenosis or prosthetic valve dysfunction may not be suitable or possible in all patients. Transseptal access across the thin atrial septal membrane at the fossa ovalis into the left atrium and left ventricle is an established and safe technique in experienced hands.[81-84]

Indications

Conditions that require direct LA or LV measurement of pressure (such as mitral stenosis, pulmonary venous disease, left intraventricular gradient, aortic stenosis, or hypertrophic cardiomyopathy).

Access for mitral balloon-catheter valvuloplasty.

Access for deployment of atrial septal defect closure devices.

Prosthetic aortic or mitral heart valve dysfunction. Retrograde crossing of a tilting disk-type prosthetic valve has been associated with death from entrapped catheters and should not be attempted.

Contraindications

Patients who cannot lie flat or fully cooperate

Anticoagulant therapy, low platelet count, or other hemostatic abnormalities

LA or RA thrombus

Atrial myxoma

Inferior vena cava mass or obstruction

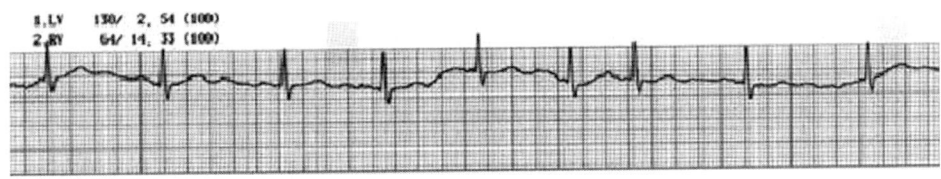

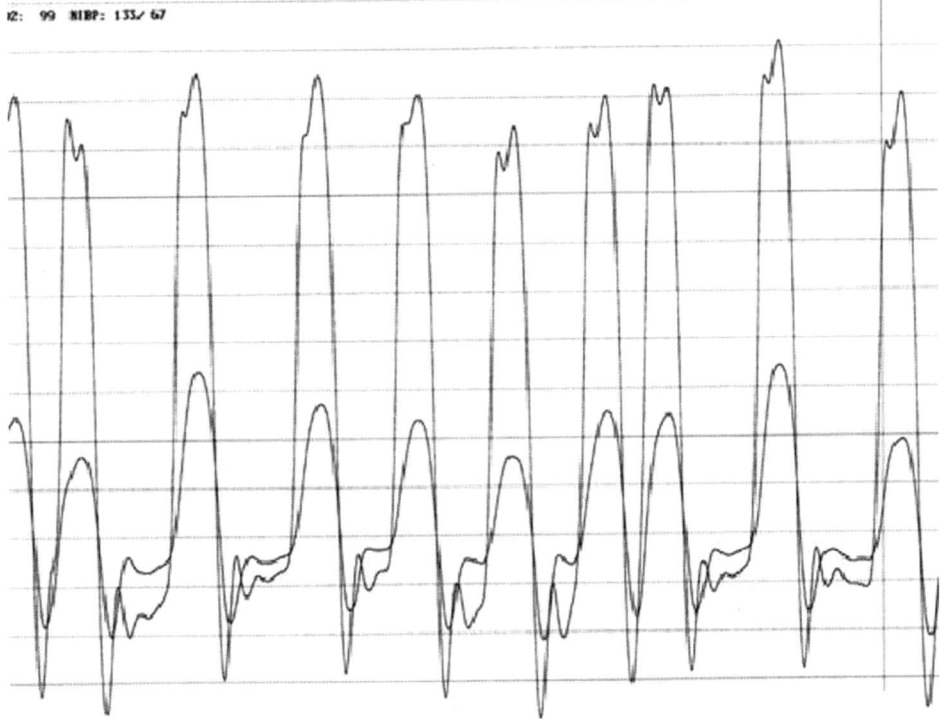

B

Timeline Interval 10 sec.

FIGURE 17–30 (continued)

Transseptal left heart catheterization should be considered carefully in patients with distorted cardiac anatomy secondary to congenital heart disease, dilated aortic root, marked atrial enlargement, or thoracic skeletal deformity.

Risks

Punctures of the aortic root, coronary sinus (CS), or the posterior free wall of the atrium are potentially lethal problems. In patients who have not been given anticoagulants, the 21-gauge tip of the transseptal needle rarely causes a problem. However, if the large transeptal catheter is advanced into these spaces, cardiac tamponade may occur. A detailed description of the transseptal technique can be found elsewhere.[81–84]

ENDOMYOCARDIAL BIOPSY

Endomyocardial biopsy is a common procedure in the catheterization laboratory. Monitoring cardiac transplant rejection and anthracycline cardiotoxicity are the two major indications for endomyocardial biopsy. Other indications include diagnosis for secondary causes of cardiomyopathy, myocarditis (when there is a history of congestive heart failure in the preceding 6 months), and differentiation between restrictive and constrictive cardiomyopathies. The two major contraindications to endomyocardial biopsy are anticoagula-

tion, anatomic abnormality precluding bioptome placement. Complications of endomyocardial biopsy include access-site–related events (3 percent), biopsy related (3 percent), arrhythmia (1 percent), conduction abnormalities (1 percent), perforation (0.7 percent), and death (0.4 percent). All complication rates are higher for patients with cardiomyopathy compared to heart transplant recipients.

PERICARDIOCENTESIS

Pericardiocentesis may be required for diagnosis and management of acute and chronic pericardial effusions. In cardiac tamponade this is a lifesaving technique. A sufficient degree of operator skill must be employed to prevent damage to the heart and pericardium. Pericardiocentesis usually is preceded by echocardiographic confirmation of pericardial fluid. However, in cases in which a large pericardial effusion is known or suspected with hemodynamic compromise in which tamponade is acute, echocardiographic assessment is not required and may be detrimental by delaying needed intervention. A Seldinger puncture technique is used from a subxyphoid approach to access the pericardial space, verify the position by echo-contrast or hemodynamics, and introduce a catheter to drain the pericardial effusion. Although monitoring of pericardial pressure is not essential for elective procedures, it is important to document evidence of cardiac tamponade and resolution of pericardial pressure restricting cardiac output.

INTRAAORTIC BALLOON COUNTERPULSATION

Mechanisms

Intraaortic balloon (IAB) counterpulsation was first introduced in 1967 by Kantrowitz and Moulopoulos, positioning a balloon in the descending Ao to improve hemodynamics. It is the most commonly used system for temporary mechanical support of patients in a wide variety of clinical settings, such as the cardiac catheterization laboratory, operating room, and the intensive care unit. IAB counterpulsation increases coronary blood flow and decreases myocardial oxygen demand.[85] Balloon inflation in diastole, at the dicrotic notch on the central arterial pressure tracing, augments aortic diastolic pressure, increasing both coronary artery pressure and flow. Balloon deflation at end-diastole, the upstroke of arterial pressure tracing, decreases aortic volume and ventricular afterload, decreasing myocardial oxygen consumption and increasing CO (Fig. 17–31). Augmented diastolic blood pressure typically produces a substantial increase in mean arterial blood pressure. LV end-diastolic pressures decrease during IAB counterpulsation with a preservation or increase in LV SV and ejection fraction. LV

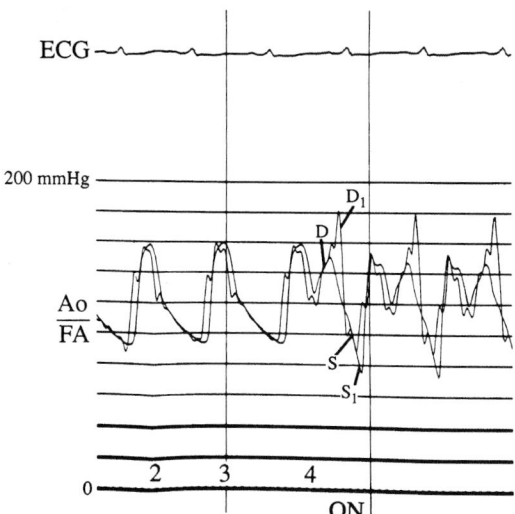

FIGURE 17–31. Hemodynamic tracings of femoral artery (FA) and central aortic pressure (AoP) during intraaortic balloon pumping, demonstrating the augmentation in diastole in the central position (D) and femoral artery position (D1) and reduction in systolic load in the central position (S) and the femoral artery position (S1). Moving the timing of inflation toward the dicrotic notch and the timing of deflation away from systolic upstroke will augment the diastolic pressure and optimally reduce systolic load. ON, the point at which the balloon pump is turned on. *Source: From Kern MJ.[1] With permission.*

work is reduced by the reduction in afterload. Coronary perfusion occurs predominantly during diastole when the balloon is inflated causing a rise in the AoP, causing the coronary perfusion pressure gradient (Aortic-LVEDP) to increase. However, coronary perfusion is determined not only by the perfusion gradient, but also by the degree of stenosis in the coronary vessels, the collateral circulation, and the duration of diastole. Kern and colleagues[86] showed that IAB counterpulsation augmented coronary flow velocity proximal but not distal to a high-grade stenosis. After a successful angioplasty of a stenotic lesion in the same vessel, the IAB augmented coronary flow velocity throughout the entire vessel. IAB increases diastolic flow velocity more in patients with a basal systolic blood pressure <90 mmHg.[87]

Indications and Contraindications

The indications and contraindications for IAB counterpulsation are listed in Table 17–27. In high-risk or unstable patients, an IAB pump (IABP) may be inserted before catheterization. During catheterization or interventional procedures, IAB counterpulsation is indicated for hypotension (not responding to volume loading or intravenous vasopressors) or refractory angina.

Technique of IAB Insertion

Before IAB catheter insertion, the patient must be assessed for iliofemoral and aortic vascular disease. Significant peripheral vascular disease is a relative contradiction. An abdominal aortogram identifies the course and disease of iliac and femoral vessels before the IAB insertion. The 8F intraaortic balloon sheath is inserted into either femoral groin artery using standard Seldinger technique. Aortic dissection may occur if the balloon has not been advanced and positioned carefully over a guidewire. Blind insertion of a counterpulsation balloon catheter without a leading guidewire is not recommended. The tip of the IABP catheter should be positioned left 1 to 2 cm below the top of

the aortic arch and then secured. After the patient has returned to the intensive care unit, IAB position is checked by chest radiograph.

Complications of IAB Counterpulsation

Complications of IAB placement most commonly result from low site of puncture, perforation of the superficial FA, or forceful arterial dissection due to advancement of the guidewire. The puncture site should be located similar to or slightly more proximal to a standard femoral puncture for diagnostic catheterization. A puncture lower than the prescribed site may involve a small superficial FA and cause leg ischemia. Assessment of the patient during IAB counterpulsation includes evaluation for infection, thrombocytopenia, hemorrhage, hemolysis, and vascular obstruction with limb ischemia. Thrombus or dissection may be present at the puncture site or proximally. Heparin administration (5000-unit bolus with 1000 units/h) is standard practice in most institutions.

[ ] CARDIAC CATHETERIZATION IN HEART TRANSPLANT PATIENTS AND ADULTS WITH CONGENITAL HEART DISEASE

Transplantation

Cardiac transplantation is a common procedure in most tertiary care centers. Routine yearly followup of the transplant patient includes cardiac catheterization, coronary angiography, and assessment of LV function, PA pressures, and endomyocardial biopsy. Cardiac transplant patients have unique problems that may include altered anatomic relationships, absence of anginal pain, con-

TABLE 17–27

Indications and Contraindications to Intraaortic Balloon Counterpulsation

INDICATIONS	CONTRAINDICATIONS
Acute myocardial infarction ± cardiogenic shock	Severe peripheral vascular disease
Refractory unstable angina	Severe aortic incompetence
Stabilization of left main disease	Active bleeding
Complications of AMI— acute MR or VSD	Patients with contraindication to anticoagulation
Weaning from cardiopulmonary bypass	Thrombocytopenia (<50,000)
High-risk cardiac percutaneous revascularization	Acute stroke
Bridge to cardiac transplantation	
High-risk noncardiac surgery in coronary patients	
Refractory arrhythmias	
Myocardial contusion	
Right ventricular failure	

AMI, acute myocardial infarction; VSD, ventricular septal defect.

trast allergic reactions, and high sensitivity to infection, all of which must be considered in the approach to this unusual patient population. Routine left and right heart catheterization is usually performed from the femoral approach. If femoral scar tissue is excessive on one side, approach from the opposite groin or arm may be necessary. If endomyocardial biopsy is considered, the internal jugular or femoral venous approach may be suitable using either fluoroscopy or echocardiographically guided biopsy. Angiography in the heart transplant patient must account for the transplanted heart that is rotated clockwise. Thus, the right coronary ostium is anterior and the left coronary ostium is located in a more posterior plane than the normal heart. In addition, a suture ridge in the lower ascending Ao at the site of the aortic anastomosis may be encountered, causing the Judkins catheter to snag or bend as it is advanced. The anterior position of the right coronary ostia may be better engaged using an AP or slightly rightward oblique view. The multipurpose angiographic catheter may be required for unusual positions of the coronary ostia. These patients are generally preload-dependent, and thus the recommended administration of intracoronary nitroglycerine before angiographic studies may result in a significant drop in blood pressure.

Congenital Heart Disease

Adults with corrected congenital heart disease are encountered with increasing frequency by the adult cardiac catheterization physician. Detailed knowledge of previous cardiac surgery, catheterization, and echocardiographic findings is necessary for the performance of a complete and accurate catheterization. Residual hemodynamic and electrophysiologic abnormalities must be identified in these patients to maintain long-term survival. Among the most commonly encountered problems are those of ventricular septal defects and conditions resulting in cyanosis. Ventricular septal defects may occur at the muscular septum or the site of an old patch in corrected hearts. Great vessel shunts may occur from collateral supply, especially in those patients with repaired cyanotic heart disease or incompletely occluded shunts. Cyanosis in these individuals may result from the following:

Persistent left SVC to left atrium shunting with or without coronary sinus or septal defect
Right pulmonary A-V fistula (Glenn anastomosis)
Acquired lung disease
A combination of the above

Careful hemodynamic and oximetric measurements are important to examine cardiac or extracardiac shunting. Both right and left pulmonary arteries must be sampled for oxygen saturations during the oximetry run. Patients with cyanosis are placed on 100 percent oxygen to identify cardiac causes of cyanosis from noncardiac causes. Large-format image intensifiers (9-in. screen) or biplane angiography may be needed to display both ventricles simultaneously. Coronary artery abnormalities may occur and contribute to ventricular dysfunction in the adult with congenital heart disease. The late natural history of coronary atherosclerosis in corrected forms of congenital heart disease is unknown. It is recommended that any patient older than age 35 years with evidence of ventricular dysfunction undergo coronary arteriography. Patients with complex congenital heart disease—such as tetralogy of Fallot with an overriding Ao, ventricular septal defect, and pulmonary stenosis or truncus arteriosus (common arterial trunk with ventricular septal defect)—may have abnormally large aortic roots requiring modified coronary catheters. Single coronary arteries or anomalous origins of the left coronary from the right coronary artery may be part of the truncus arteriosus (a common pulmonary and aortic outflow tube) and transposition of the great vessels (switching of PA and Ao).

CORONARY BLOOD FLOW AND PRESSURE MEASUREMENTS

The inability to determine the functional significance of a coronary stenosis remains a well-recognized limitation of angiography,[88,89] repeatedly demonstrated anatomically by IVUS imaging and physiologically by ischemia stress testing.[90–92] Measurements of coronary blood flow and pressure provide unique information that complements the anatomic (angiographic) evaluation and facilitates decision making regarding therapy in the catheterization laboratory.

CORONARY BLOOD FLOW AND RESISTANCE

Coronary blood flow can increase from a resting level to a maximum depending on increases in myocardial oxygen demand or in response to neurogenic or pharmacologic hyperemic stimuli. The ratio of maximal-to-basal flow is coronary flow reserve (CFR), or coronary vasodilatory reserve (CVR). Resistance to flow increase occurs at three levels: epicardial conduits (R1), precapillary arterioles (R2), and intramyocardial resistance (R3). Normally, large epicardial vessel resistance (R1) is trivial. Most coronary flow is regulated by the myocardial precapillary arteriolar resistance vessels (R2). In a normal artery supplying normal myocardium, coronary blood flow reserve can exceed 3. However, several conditions, including LV hypertrophy, myocardial ischemia, or diabetes can affect the microcirculatory resistance R3, blunting the maximal absolute increase in coronary flow. Increased R3 resistance may also be associated with increased resting flow above the expected level for myocardial oxygen demand at rest also resulting in reduced coronary flow reserve (Fig. 17–32). Significant atherosclerotic stenosis produces epicardial conduit resistance. In response to the loss of perfusion pressure and flow to the distal microcirculation bed, precapillary resistance vessels (R2) dilate to maintain satisfactory basal flow appropriate for myocardial oxygen demand. In parallel with resistance to flow, viscous friction, flow separation forces, and flow turbulence at the site of the stenosis produce energy loss at the stenosis. Energy (heat) is extracted reducing pressure distal to the stenosis, producing a pressure gradient between proximal and distal artery regions. The pressure loss increases with increasing coronary flow along an exponential pressure-flow relationship of the specific coronary stenosis resistance [93,94] (Fig. 17–33). There exists an absolute poststenotic myocardial perfusion pressure threshold below which myocardial ischemia may be easily induced. The hemodynamic significance of a given stenosis can be measured by the pressure-flow relationship using sensor angioplasty guidewires.[89]

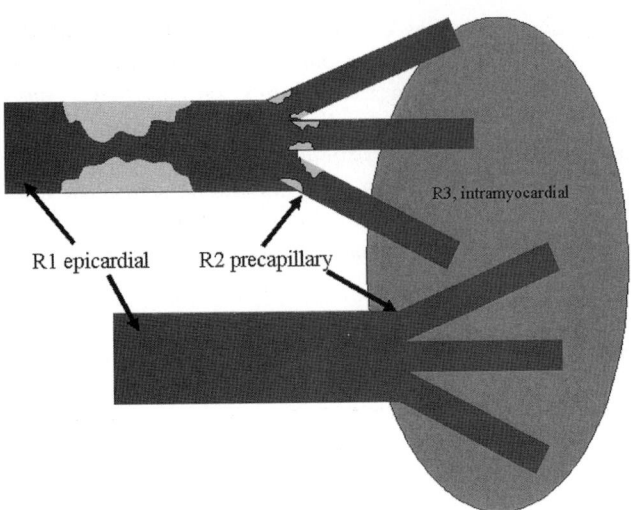

FIGURE 17–32. Coronary circulation. *R1, R2, R3,* epicardial, anteriolar, and microvascular resistance, respectively.

【 】 CORONARY FLOW VELOCITY AND RESERVE

The coronary flow velocity of red blood cells moving past the ultrasound emitter/receiver on the end of a 0.014-in. Doppler-tipped angioplasty guidewire can be determined from the frequency shift, defined by the Doppler equation as the difference between the transmitted and returning frequency:

$$V = (F_1 - F_0) \times (C)/(2F_0) \times (Cos\ \emptyset)$$

where V = velocity of blood flow; F_0 = transmitting (transducer) frequency; F_1 = returning frequency; C = constant for the speed of sound in blood; $\emptyset$ = angle of incidence. Flow velocity measurements have been validated.[89] Volumetric flow is the product of vessel area (cm²) and flow velocity (cm/sec) yielding a value in cm³/sec. Absolute Doppler flow velocities represent changes in volumetric coronary flow when the vessel cross-sectional area remains constant over the measurement period. Compared to volumetric measurements, velocity may underestimate the volumetric flow reserve in some vessels, which demonstrated intact endothelial mediated vasodilation. CVR is the ratio of maximal hyperemic-to-basal mean flow velocity in the target vessel obtained distal to the stenosis. As stenosis severity increases, hyperemic flow becomes attenuated, and CVR decreases. Absolute CVR measures the capacity of the two-component system of the R1 coronary artery resistance and the R2 vascular resistance to achieve maximal blood flow in response to a given hyperemic stimulation. Normal CVR in young patients with IVUS demonstrated normal arteries commonly exceeds 3.0.[95,96] In patients with chest pain undergoing cardiac catheterization with angiographically normal vessels, the normal absolute CVR is 2.7 ± 0.6,[95] suggesting a degree of patient to patient variability and distal microvascular disease that is beyond the threshold of angiographic detection. The values for CVR associated with nonobstructed coronary arteries in patients with chest pain syndromes, transplanted hearts, and in normal arteries in patients with obstructive coronary artery disease elsewhere are 2.8 ± 0.6, 3.1 ± 0.9, and 2.5 ± 0.95, respectively.[95] The incidence of impaired coronary vasodilatory reserve <2.0 in 450 an-

giographically normal coronary arteries from 220 patients undergoing evaluation for chest pain or cardiac transplantation follow up angiography is approximately 12 percent.[95]

Factors Influencing Coronary Flow Reserve

Coronary flow reserve (CFR or CVR) is subject to variations in hemodynamics that may alter resting flow and land limit maximal hyperemic flow. Tachycardia increases basal flow; thus, CFR is reduced by 10 percent for every 15 heartbeats.[96] Increasing mean arterial pressure reduces maximal vasodilatation; thus, reducing hyperemia with less alteration in basal flow. CFR may be reduced in patients with essential hypertension and normal coronary arteries[96–98] and in patients with aortic stenosis and normal coronary arteries.[99] In some patients with moderate coronary artery disease, the stenotic configuration and surrounding vessel segments are subject to vasomotor stimuli. Thus vasoconstrictor, neurologic, or humoral influences, endothelial dysfunction, and extracardiac vasoconstrictor stimuli may produce dynamic or episodic ischemia-related symptoms with activities of daily life such as exercise, emotional stress, or adrenergic stimulation.[100,101] The variability in CVR in unobstructed arteries may also be due to age.[102,103] The correction formula for age[103] showed that only patients with diabetes had a significant decrease of the traditional CVR and corrected CVR, whereas hypertension and current smoking had no influence on corrected CVR.[104] Table 17–28 lists pathologies associated with impairment of the microcirculation.

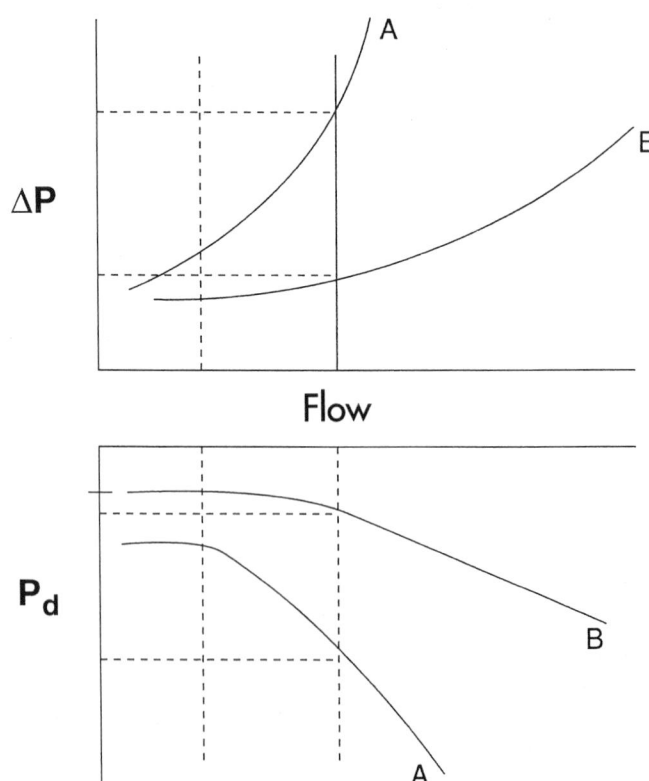

FIGURE 17–33. Coronary pressure-flow relationships for two stenoses of the same angiographic severity. **Top.** ΔP versus coronary flow. **Bottom.** Absolute distal coronary pressure P_d versus flow. Increasing flow produces marked loss of P_d as well as an increase in ΔP. The loss of P_d in absolute terms determines myocardial perfusion pressure (P_d venous pressure) and the potential for inducible ischemia. ΔP, pressure gradient (aortic-distal coronary pressure); P_d, distal coronary pressure.

TABLE 17–28

Pathologies Impairing the Microcirculation

Abnormal vascular reactivity
Abnormal myocardial metabolism
Abnormal sensitivity toward vasoactive substances
Coronary vasospasm
Myocardial infarction
Hypertrophy
Vasculitis syndromes
Hypertension
Diabetes
Recurrent ischemia

SOURCE: From Baumgart D, Haude M, Liu F, et al.[123]

Relative Coronary Flow Velocity

CVR is the summed response of the major two coronary flow resistances and, therefore, an abnormal value (e.g.,< 2.0) cannot distinguish between increased resistance at R1 epicardial level or R2 microvascular level. A relative CVR (rCVR) can be determined in a fashion similar to that defined by Gould and coworkers.[93,94] rCVR is defined as the ratio of maximal flow in the coronary with stenosis (S) to flow in a normal coronary without stenosis (N) It was shown that rCVR is independent of the AoP and rate pressure product and was well suited to assess the physiologic significance of coronary stenoses when an adjacent nondiseased coronary artery is available. For flow velocity studies, rCVR in the catheterization laboratory is defined as the ratio of CVR_{target} to CVR in an angiographically normal reference vessel ($rCVR = (QS/Q_{base})/(N/Q_{base}) = (CVR_{target}/CVR_{reference})$), and assumes basal flow in the two vessels is similar and, thus, mathematically resembles Gould's derivation. The normal range for rCVR is 0.8 to 1.0.[105,106] rCVR cannot be used in patients with three-vessel coronary disease who have no suitable reference vessel. rCVR relies on the assumption that the microvascular circulatory response is uniformly distributed among the myocardial beds; thus, rCVR is of no value in patients with myocardial infarction, with LV regional dysfunction, or in whom the microcirculatory responses are heterogeneous.

【 】 PRESSURE-DERIVED FRACTIONAL FLOW RESERVE OF THE MYOCARDIUM

Myocardial perfusion is closely linked to myocardial ischemia and is directly dependent on the coronary *driving* pressure associated with three major coronary vascular resistances. The myocardial perfusion pressure (AoP minus LV pressure or RA pressure) is reduced when an epicardial stenosis causes pressure loss distal to the stenosis. If the myocardial bed resistances are stimulated to maximal hyperemia and remain constant, the poststenotic hyperemic coronary artery pressure represents the maximal achievable perfusion available in that vessel and can be used to produce an estimate of normal coronary blood flow and an ischemic threshold. Using coronary pressure measured at constant and minimal myocardial resistances (i.e., maximal hyperemia), Pijls and colleagues[107,108] as well as De Bruyne and coworkers[109] derived an estimate of the per-

centage of normal coronary blood flow expected to go through a stenotic artery. This pressure-derived ratio is called the fractional flow reserve (FFR). FFR_{cor} is defined as the maximum coronary flow in the presence of a stenosis divided by the normal maximum flow of the artery (i.e., the maximum flow in that artery if no stenosis were present).[107] Similarly, FFR_{myo} is defined as maximum myocardial blood flow distal to an epicardial stenosis divided by its value if no epicardial stenosis were present. Stated another way, FFR represents that fraction of normal maximum flow that remains despite the presence of an epicardial lesion. FFR can be derived separately for the myocardium, epicardial coronary artery, and collateral supply. Calculations of myocardial, coronary, and collateral fraction flow reserve from pressure measurements taken during maximal arterial vasodilation (i.e. hyperemia) are as follows:

Myocardial FFR

$$(FFR_{myo}) = 1 - \Delta P/P_a - P_v = (P_d - P_v)/(P_a - P_v)$$

Coronary FFR

$$(FFR_{cor}) = 1 - \Delta P/(P_a - P_w) = (P_d - P_w)/(P_a - P_w)$$

Collateral FFR

$$(FFR_{coll}) = FFR_{myo} - FFR_{cor}$$

where P_a = mean AoP; P_d = mean distal coronary pressure; *P = mean translesional pressure gradient; Pv = mean RA pressure; Pw = mean coronary wedge pressure or distal coronary pressure during balloon inflation.[107] Because FFR_{cor} uses Pw it can be calculated only during balloon coronary angioplasty. For daily clinical practice, FFR can be easily calculated by a simplified ratio of pressures and expressed as:

$$P_d \ FFR \ *\_\_\_\_\_ \ P_a$$

The FFR is simplified to P_d/P_a assuming P_v is negligible relative to P_a. An FFR value of 0.6 means that the maximum myocardial flow across the stenosis is only 60 percent of what it should be without the stenosis. An FFR of 0.9 after percutaneous coronary intervention (PCI) means that the maximum flow to the myocardium is 90 percent of a completely normal vessel. The concept of FFR has been thoroughly examined in both experimental and clinical studies.[107–109] Unlike most other physiologic indexes, FFR has a normal value of 1.0 for every patient and every coronary artery. Despite findings in animal studies defining an effect of heart rate and arterial pressure, human studies did not show significant changes in FFR with changes in heart rate, blood pressure, or contractility.[109] FFR has a high reproducibility and low intra-individual variability. Moreover, FFR, unlike CFR, is independent of gender or coronary artery disease risk factors such as hypertension and diabetes and has less variability with common doses of adenosine.[110] Because of the necessity to know P_w, FFR_{cor} can be calculated only during percutaneous transluminal coronary angioplasty (PTCA). FFR_{myo}, however, can also be calculated during diagnostic procedures. The difference between FFR_{myo} and FFR_{cor} represents the contribution of collateral flow to total myocardial perfusion and is called *fractional collateral flow*. Because FFR_{myo} reflects both antegrade and collateral contribution to maximum myocardial perfusion, it is the most important flow index from a clinical point of

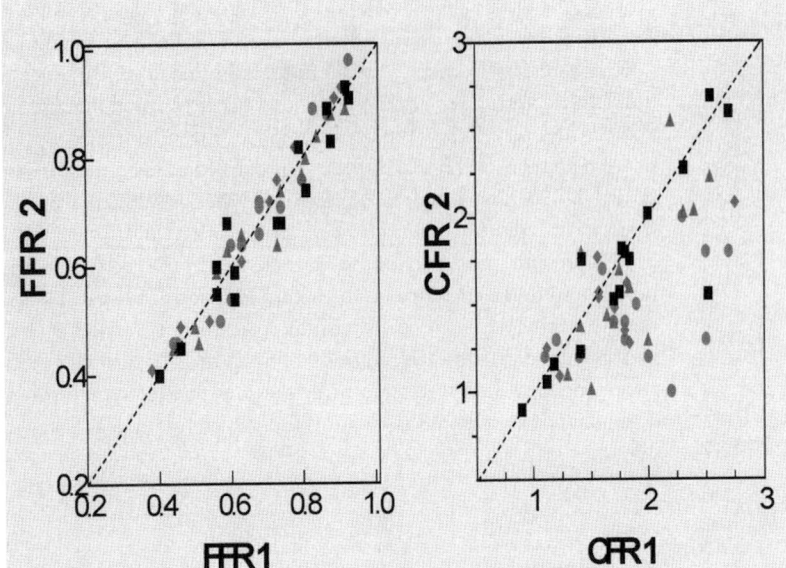

FIGURE 17–34. Reproducibility of FFR versus CVR for changing heart rate, blood pressure, and contractility. Circles, contractility; CVR, coronary vasodilatory reserve; diamond, MAP; FFR, fractional flow reserve; square, duplicate measurement; triangle, heart rate. *Source: From de Bruyne B, Bartunek J, Sys SU, et al. Circulation 1996;94:1842–1849. With permission.*

view. It describes to what extent maximum myocardial perfusion is affected by the epicardial coronary stenosis. The FFR is calculated as the ratio of the poststenotic coronary pressure to Ao pressure obtained at sustained minimal resistance (i.e., maximal hyperemia). FFR reflects both antegrade and collateral myocardial perfusion rather than merely transstenotic pressure loss (i.e., a stenosis pressure gradient). Because it is calculated only at peak hyperemia, FFR is also differentiated from CVR by being largely independent of basal flow, driving pressure, heart rate, systemic blood pressure, or status of the microcirculation[109] (Fig. 17–34). The FFR, but not the resting pressure or hyperemic pressure gradient, is strongly related to provocable myocardial ischemia demonstrated by comparisons to different clinical stress testing modalities in patients with stable angina.[108] FFR and rCVR are more specific for flow limitations caused by a stenosis than is CVR. Absolute CVR did not correlate with percent area stenosis or FFR. In patients with a nonuniform microcirculation, such as those with myocardial infarction, neither absolute CVR nor rCVR can be used for assessment of lesion severity. Even in patients with potential microcirculatory impairment, an epicardial narrowing is best assessed by FFR. In patients with an abnormal microcirculation, it can be argued that a normal FFR indicates the conduit resistance is not a major contributing factor to perfusion impairment, and that focal conduit enlargement (e.g., stenting) would not restore normal perfusion. The current physiologic criteria have not been completely examined in patients with profound microvascular disease.

[ ] METHOD OF SENSOR GUIDEWIRE USE

After diagnostic angiography or during angioplasty, the sensor guidewire is passed through an angioplasty Y connector attached to a guiding catheter. Intravenous (IV) heparin 40 to 60 units/kg

is given. Intracoronary (IC) nitroglycerin (100 to 200 μg) is also given several minutes before the guidewire is advanced into the artery. For flow velocity the sensor tip is advanced at least 5 to 10 artery-diameter lengths (>2 cm) beyond the stenosis to measure reestablished laminar flow. Resting flow velocity data are recorded. Induction of coronary hyperemia by intracoronary or intravenous adenosine is performed with continuous recording peak hyperemic flow velocity. CVR is computed as maximal hyperemic to basal average peak velocity (APV) (Fig. 17–35). Poor Doppler signal acquisition may occur in 10 to15 percent of patients even within normal arteries. As in transthoracic echo Doppler studies, the operator must adjust the guidewire's position (sample volume) to optimize the velocity signal. Several different tip orientations interrogating the maximal velocity spectra are necessary.

For FFR the guidewire is advanced in the guide catheter to the coronary ostium and the sensor pressure is matched to the guide catheter pressure. The wire is then advanced into the artery beyond the stenosis. Baseline pressure is recorded. Coronary hyperemia with intracoronary or intravenous adenosine is induced, while both guide catheter and sensor wire pressures are continuously recorded. FFR is computed as the ratio pressure$_{distal}$ to pressure$_{aorta}$ at maximal hyperemia (Fig. 17–36). Pressure signal artifacts may be reduced by careful attention to technique.[107] The safety of intracoronary sensor-wire measurements has been excellent, as reported by Qian and coworkers[110] in 906 patients. Complications included severe transient bradycardia after intracoronary adenosine (1.7 percent), coronary spasm during passage of the Doppler guidewire (1 percent), and ventricular fibrillation during the procedure (0.2 percent). All complications could easily be managed medically.

Combined Pressure and Flow Measurements

Recent advancements in technology allow a more complete evaluation of the coronary circulation with a single wire equipped with pressure and velocity sensors, or with pressure and thermodilution sensors. With combined measurements beyond a stenosis, a clinician can acquire relevant hemodynamic data regarding physiological condition of the entire coronary circulation and its clinical implications for treatment. Presently, there are two methods used for these calculations. The first method combines simultaneous measurement of the phasic pressure and Doppler velocity distal to a stenosis. These measurements permit the calculation of stenosis and microvascular resistances and have been applied clinically. Using distal pressure and velocity during hyperemic conditions, a hyperemic stenosis resistance (HSR) (by velocity, v) index is calculated as $HSR_v = \Delta P/v$, where ΔP = hyperemic pressure gradient (P_a P_d); v = average peak velocity at hyperemia.[111,112] This index purportedly provides a refined physiologic measurement quantifying the impediment to maximal flow caused exclusively by the stenosis. Like FFR, HSR_v has a normal reference value (HSR_v = 0) and is independent of basal hemodynamic conditions, with high reproducibility and low variability.[111,112] Simultaneous measurement of

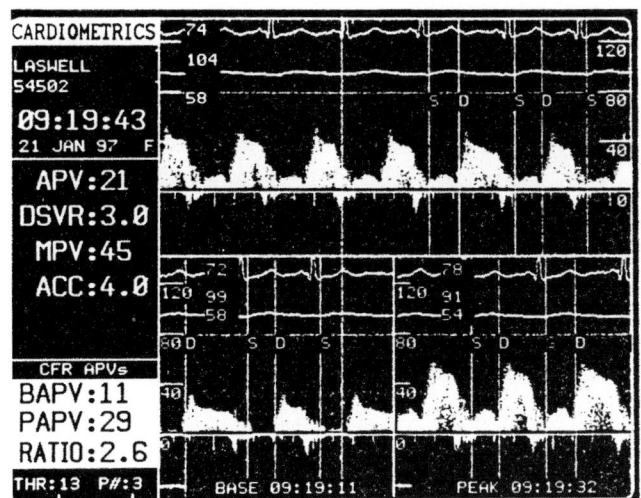
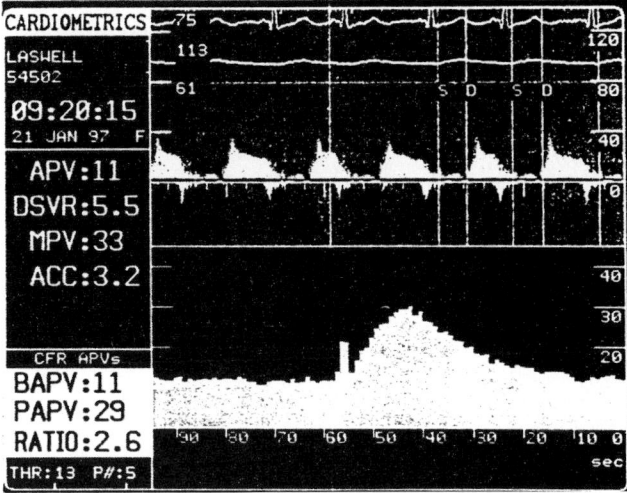

FIGURE 17-35. Left. Coronary flow velocity signals obtained in a normal circumflex artery (CFX) of a patient undergoing angioplasty of the right coronary artery. The top half represents continuous flow-velocity signals in real time. The electrocardiogram, AoP, and spectral flow signals are provided from top to bottom. The scale is 0 to 120 cm/sec. S and D periods demarcated by the electrocardiogram. **Right.** The trend plot of the continuous flow velocity measurement APV is shown in the right-hand panel on the lower tracing. After intracoronary adenosine administration, APV increased from 11 to 29 cm/sec, producing a coronary flow reserve of 2.6. The duration of hyperemia is 45 sec. The trend velocity scale is 0 to 40 cm/sec. The time base is 90 sec. AoP, aortic pressure; APV, average peak velocity; D, diastolic; S, systolic. *Source: From Kern MJ, de Bruyne B, Pijls NHJ, et al. From research to clinical practice: Current role of physiologically based decision making in the catheterization laboratory. J Am Coll Cardiol 1997;30:613–620. With permission.*

distal pressure and flow velocity also allows the separate assessment of microvascular resistance,[113, 114] and the construction of stenosis pressure gradient-velocity curves that uniquely characterize the hemodynamics of any lesion and associated physiologic responses.[112,115] The pressure drop-velocity relations are also well suited to visualize the effect of percutaneous intervention.[112] An

HSR_v value >0.8 mmHg/cm/sec is the threshold for prediction of reversible ischemia when compared to noninvasive stress testing,[111] HSR_v had a higher diagnostic accuracy than either pressure (FFR) or flow velocity (CFR) alone, especially in cases where outcomes of FFR and CFR do not agree.[116] HSR_v requires the use of both a distal pressure and flow velocity signal, which can be ob-

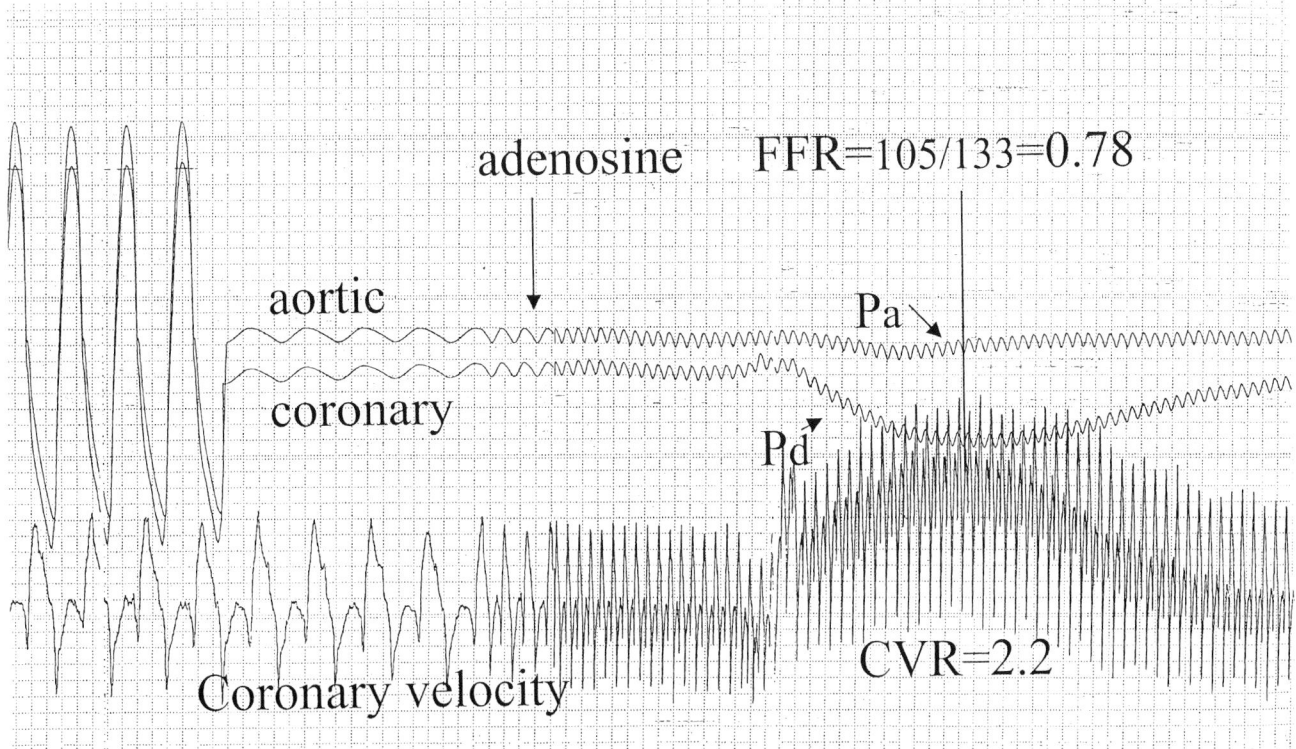

FIGURE 17-36. Hemodynamic and coronary flow velocity tracings demonstrating coronary vasodilatory reserve (CVR) and fractional flow reserve (FFR) data collection. Aortic (P_a) and distal coronary pressure (P_d) at baseline and during adenosine hyperemia (at vertical line). Coronary velocity shows a 2.2-fold increase with adenosine. FFR = 0.78.

TABLE 17–29

Characteristics of Physiologic Measurements in the Cath Lab

FFR	DOPPLER	CVR	HSR
Ischemic threshold range	0.75–0.80	<2.0	>0.8
Normal value	1.0	variable	0
Epicardial lesion specific	**yes**	**no**	**yes**
Independent of hemodynamics	yes	no	yes
Reproducibility	+++	+	++
Spatial resolution	+++	+	++
Assesses microvascular integrity	–	+++	+++
Assess both stenosis and microvasculature	–	–	+++
Pressure-flow curves	–	–	+++

FFR, fractional flow reserve; CVR, coronary velocity reserve; HSR, hyperemic stenosis resistance.

tained with a dual-sensor (pressure and Doppler velocity) guidewire.[112, 113] The second method uses distal pressure and thermodilution flow, as assessed by the inverse of the arrival (transit) time of a room temperature saline bolus to the distal coronary artery segment.[116–120] By measuring the mean transit time at rest and comparing it to the mean transit time at peak hyperemia, a thermodilution CFR can be calculated. Experimental animal and human studies have validated CFR_{thermo} against $CFR_{Doppler}$.[117–120] Although principally a research tool, the simultaneous measurement of FFR and CFR also permits a unique characterization of the epicardial and microvascular resistances. The significant features of available physiologic measurements in the cath lab are listed on Table 17–29.

Assessing Stenosis Severity with Pharmacologic Hyperemic Stimuli

Stenosis severity should always be assessed using measurements obtained during maximal hyperemia. The most widely used maximal vasodilator agents are dipyridamole (DP), papaverine, and adenosine. Intracoronary nitroglycerin (100–200 µg) should be given before flow velocity measurements to paralyze vasomotion and minimize any flow-mediated vasodilation. Intracoronary papaverine increases coronary blood flow velocity four to six times over resting values in patients with normal coronary arteries.[121] Papaverine (8–12 mg) produces a response equal to that of an intravenous infusion of DP in a dose of 0.56 to 0.84 mg/kg of body weight but can cause QT prolongation occasionally and ventricular tachycardia or fibrillation.[123] Adenosine, both intracoronary and intravenous, has a short half-life. The total duration of the hyperemic response of intracoronary adenosine is only 25 percent that of papaverine or DP.[124,125] Adenosine is benign in the appropriate dosages (20–30 µg in the right coronary artery or 40–60 µg in the left coronary artery or infused intravenously at 140 µg/kg/min). Because bolus intracoronary adenosine does not increase vessel cross-sectional area,[126] coronary flow velocity reserve can be used as a surrogate for coronary volumetric flow reserve. Jeremias and coworkers[127] found a linear relationship between the intracoronary and intravenous methods ($r = 0.978$,

$p < 0.001$). The mean measurement difference for FFR was 0.004 ± 0.03. In 8 percent of the cases, intracoronary adenosine FFR was ± 0.05 units different from intravenous FFR. Thus, in a small percentage of cases, maximal coronary hyperemia may require increased intracoronary doses of adenosine.

CLINICAL APPLICATIONS OF CORONARY BLOOD FLOW AND PRESSURE MEASUREMENTS

Physiologic Criteria

CVR alone is no longer considered useful for lesion assessment but rather widely used to understand the microvascular circulation in patients. Coronary physiologic measurements associated with several major clinical outcomes are supported by numerous studies[127] and are summarized in Table 17–30. The recommendation for use of physiologic measurements during invasive procedures is provided in Appendix 17–3.

Ischemic Stress Testing

Strong correlations exist between myocardial stress testing and FFR or CVR.[128–142] An FFR of <0.75 identified physiologically significant stenoses associated with inducible myocardial ischemia, with high sensitivity (88 percent), specificity (100 percent), positive predicted value (100 percent), and overall accuracy (93 percent). An abnormal CVR (<2.0) corresponded to reversible myocardial perfusion imaging defects with high sensitivity (86 to 92 percent), specificity (89 to 100 percent), predictive accuracy (89 to 96 percent), and positive and negative predictive values (84 to 100 percent and 77 to 95 percent, respectively). A summary of ischemic stress testing and coronary physiologic measurements is provided in Table 17–31.

Diffuse Atherosclerosis

Coronary arteries without focal stenosis are generally considered nonflow-limiting. A diffusely diseased atherosclerotic coronary ar-

TABLE 17–30

Catheter-Based Anatomic and Physiologic Criteria Associated with Clinical Outcomes

APPLICATION	IVUS	CVR	RCVR	FFR
Ischemia detection	<3–4 mm^2	<2.0	<0.8	<0.75
Deferred angioplasty	—	>2.0	—	>0.75
Endpoint of angioplasty	—	>2.0–2.5 With <35% DS	—	>0.90
Endpoint of stenting	>9 mm^2 >80 percent ref. area, full apposition	—	—	>0.94

CVR, coronary vasodilator reserve; DS, diameter stenosis; FFR, fractional flow reserve; IVUS, intravascular ultrasound; rCVR, relative coronary vasodilator reserve.

SOURCE: From Kern MJ. Coronary physiology revisited. Circ 2000;101:1344–1351. With permission.

tery can be viewed as a series of branching units diverting and gradually distributing flow and reducing pressure longitudinally along the conduit. In such a vessel, a reduced CVR is not associated with any single location of stenotic pressure loss. Thus, mechanical therapy to treat presumed *culprit* plaque would be futile. De Bruyne and coworkers[143] examined patients with coronary artery disease in nonstenotic arteries with diffuse coronary atherosclerosis. Coronary pressure and FFR were obtained in 37 arteries in 10 individuals without atherosclerosis, and from 106 nonstenotic arteries in 62 patients. FFR was normal, 0.97 ± 0.02, in group 1, with no resistance to flow in truly normal arteries but was significantly lower, 0.89 ± 0.08, in group 2, indicating significant resistance. In 57 percent of arteries in group 2, FFR was lower than the lowest value in group 1. In 8 percent of arteries in group 2, FFR was less than 0.75, well below the ischemic threshold (Fig. 17–37). Diffuse atherosclerosis on angiography was associated with a continuous pressure loss along the arterial length contributing to myocardial ischemia and a potential for ischemia, despite the absence of an epicardial focal stenosis.[143] Measuring continuous coronary pressure during wire pullback from a distal to proximal location permits assessment of both focal and diffusely diseased regions responsible for pressure loss and potential ischemia. Diffuse atherosclerosis, rather than a focal narrowing, is characterized by a continuous and gradual pressure recovery without localized abrupt increase in pressure related to an isolated stenosis. Diffuse atherosclerosis also explains a persistently abnormal distal FFR despite unobstructed proximal segments.

Deferral of Coronary Intervention

The clinical outcomes of deferring coronary intervention for intermediate stenoses with normal physiology are remarkably consistent, with clinical event rates of <10 percent over a 2-year follow-up period.[144–154] FFR can be used to determine the appropriateness of angioplasty and moderate coronary stenosis. Bech et al.[149] studied 325 patients with intermediate coronary stenosis without documented myocardial ischemia. FFR was measured. When FFR was >0.75, patients were randomly assigned to a deferral group of 91 patients or a performance group of 90 patients. If FFR was less than 0.75, PTCA was performed as planned. These patients were followed as a reference group of 144 patients. At clinical follow up of 1, 3, 6, 12, and 24 months, the event-free survival was similar between the deferral and performance groups, 92 versus 89 percent at 12 months; 89 versus 83

percent at 24 months. However, these data were significantly lower in the reference group, 80 percent at 12 months and 78 percent at 24 months. These data indicated that in patients with coronary stenosis without evidence of ischemia, coronary pressure–derived FFR identifies those patients who will benefit from PTCA and also indicates that performance of PTCA in such individuals provides no additional benefit to their outcome.

Significance of Abnormal Physiology after Percutaneous Coronary Intervention

Early in the evolution of balloon angioplasty, improvement in physiology was poorly correlated to angiography because of the inherent limitations of the angiogram as described earlier. FFR has important prognostic value but limited value to determine whether full apposition of the stent has been achieved. In cases where stenting is not possible, it is gratifying to know that a normal FFR after balloon angioplasty alone is associated with stent-like late clinical outcomes.[147] In 43 percent of patients with optimal quantitative coronary angiography, a residual diameter stenosis <35 percent and good functional (FFR > 0.90) results (26 of 60 single vessel angioplasty), had event-free survival rates which were significantly better at 6 months (92 vs. 72 percent, $p = 0.047$), 12 months (92 vs. 69 percent, $p = 0.028$), and 24 months (88 vs. 59 percent, $p = 0.014$) compared to those patients with an FFR <0.90. No improvement in clinical outcome was gained by additional stenting. Coronary pressure measurements after stenting predict adverse cardiac events at follow up. Pijls and colleagues[148] examined 750 patients with postprocedural FFR and related these findings to major adverse cardiac events at 6 months. In 76 patients (10.2 percent) one adverse event occurred. Five patients died, 19 experienced myocardial infarction, and 52 underwent at least one repeat target vessel revascularization. FFR immediately after stenting was an independent variable related to all types of events. (Fig. 17–38). The authors concluded that FFR after stenting is a strong predictor of outcome at 6 months. These data suggests that both edge stent subnormalization and diffuse disease are associated with worse long-term outcome (Fig. 17–39).

FFR for Ostial Lesions and Stented Side Branches

Koo and coworkers[155] examined the physiologic assessment of jailed side branches using FFR and compared the FFR with the quantitative coronary angiography (QCA) of stenosis severity.

TABLE 17–31

Stress Testing and Directly Measured Coronary Blood Physiology

AUTHOR	REF NO.	N	ISCHEMIC TEST	PHYSIOLOGIC THRESHOLD	SENSITIVITY	SPECIFICITY	PV+	PV–	ACCURACY
POSTSTENOTIC CVR/RCVR									
Miller	128	33	Adeno/Dipy MIBI	<2.0	82	100	100	77	89
Joye	129	30	Exercise thallium	<2.0	94	95	94	95	94
Deychak	130	17	Exercise thallium	<1.8	94	94	100	91	96
Heller	131	100	Exercise thallium	<1.8	89	92	96	89	92
Danzi	134	30	Dipy echo	<2.0	91	84	—	—	87
Schulman	136	35	Exercise ECG	<2.0	95	71	—	—	86
Donahue	137	50	Exercise/pharm thallium	<2.0	98	76	88	88	—
Duffy	138	43	Stress echo	<2.0	80	93	—	—	88
				rCVR <0.75	100	76	—	—	81
Chamuleau	139	127	Dipy MIBI	CVR <2.0,	—	—	—	—	69
				rCVR <0.75	—	—	—	—	75
El Shafei	142	53	Exercise/pharm thallium	CVR <0.20,	71	83	81	74	—
				rCVR <0.75	63	88	83	70	—
FFR									
Pijls	108	45	Four-test standard	<0.75	88	100	100	88	93
de Bruyne	132	60	Exercise ECG	<0.72	100	87	—	—	—
Bartunek	135	37	Dobu/exercise echo	<0.68	95	90	—	—	75
Chamuleau	139	127	Dipy MIBI	<0.75	—	—	—	—	75
Caymaz	140	30	Exercise thallium	<0.75	—	—	91	100	95
Fearon	141	10	Exercise thallium	<0.75	90	100	—	—	95

Adeno/Dipy MIBI, adenosine or dipyridamole sestamibi scan; CVR, coronary vasodilatory reserve; Dobu, dobutamine; FFR, fractional flow reserve; PV+, predictive value positive; PV–, predictive value negative.

514

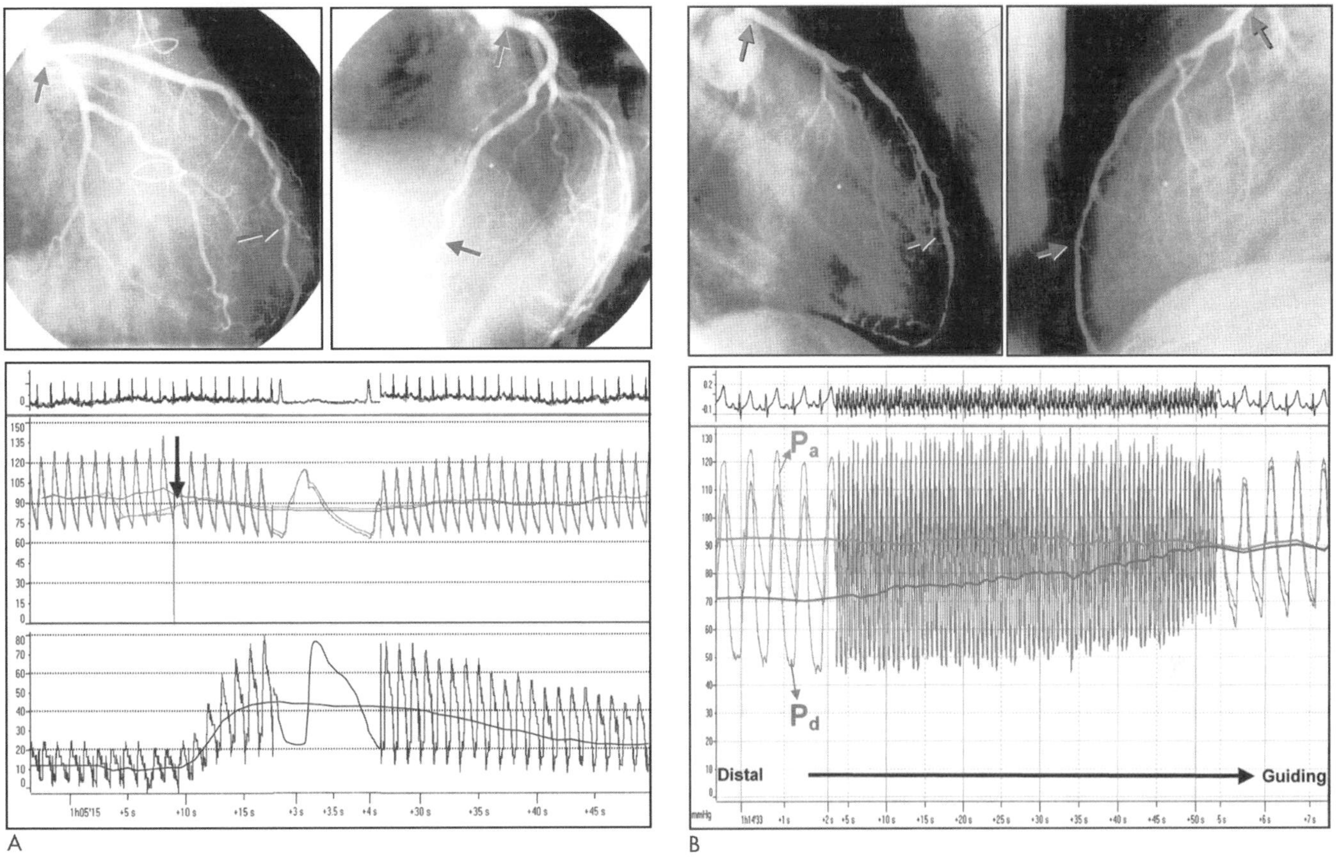

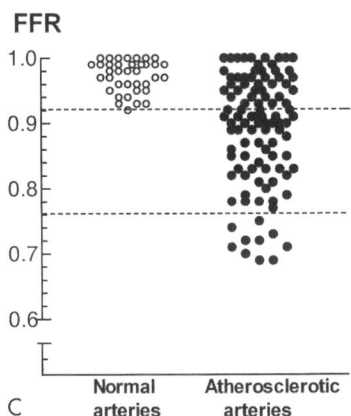

FIGURE 17–37. A. Normal coronary angiogram (*upper panels*) and simultaneous P_a and P_d and coronary flow velocity recordings (*lower pane*) in a 55-year-old patient 3 weeks after orthotopic cardiac transplantation. Even during an adenosine-induced fourfold increase in coronary blood flow velocity, no pressure gradient was measured between the proximal and distal LAD, illustrating that normal coronary arteries do not cause appreciable resistance to blood flow. The exact locations of aortic and distal coronary pressure measurements are indicated by the *arrows*, respectively. **B.** Example of a 44-year-old man with stable angina pectoris. A tight stenosis in the mid-RCA was treated by angioplasty. The coronary angiogram of the LAD (*upper panels*) did not show any focal stenosis, but luminal irregularities suggested diffuse atherosclerosis. P_a and P_d recordings (*lower pane*) during adenosine-induced maximal hyperemia show a pressure gradient of 23 mmHg (corresponding to a FFR of 0.76) when the pressure sensor is located in the distal LAD. This pressure gradient indicates that the diffusely atherosclerotic artery is responsible for approximately one-fourth of the total resistance to blood flow. When the sensor is slowly pulled back, a graded, continuous increase in P_d is observed, which indicates diffuse atherosclerosis, not focal stenosis. The exact locations of P_a and P_d measurements are indicated by the *arrows*, respectively. **C.** Graphs of individual values of FFR in normal arteries and in atherosclerotic coronary arteries without focal stenosis on arteriogram. The upper dotted line indicates the lowest value of FFR in normal coronary arteries. The lower dotted line indicates the 0.75 threshold level. FFR, fractional flow reserve; LAD, left anterior descending coronary artery; RCA, right coronary artery. P_a, aortic coronary pressure; P_d, distal coronary pressure. *Source: From De Bruyne B, Hersbach F, Pijls NHJ, et al. Abnormal epicardial coronary resistance in patients with diffuse atherosclerosis but "normal" coronary angiography. Circulation 2001;104:2401–2406. With permission.*

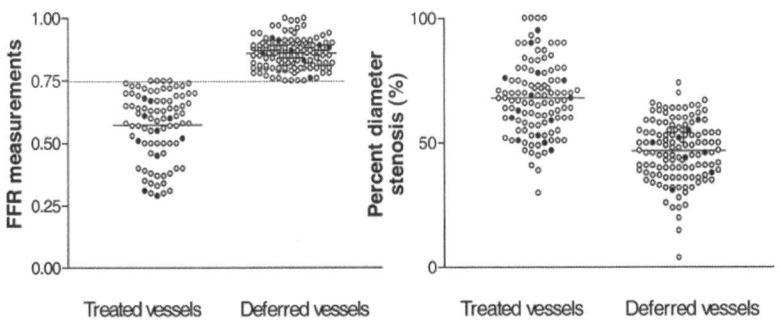

FIGURE 17–38. Individual values of fractional flow reserve (FFR) and individual values of the percent diameter stenosis in treated and deferred arteries. The black dots indicate the stenoses responsible for a major adverse cardiac event at follow-up. Mean values are shown in both groups (*bar*). The dotted line indicates the cutoff value of FFR (0.75). *Source: Berger A, Botman KJ, MacCarthy PA, Wijns W et al. Long-term clinical outcome after fractional flow reserve-guided percutaneous coronary intervention in patients with multivessel disease. J Am Coll Cardiol 2005;46:438–442.*

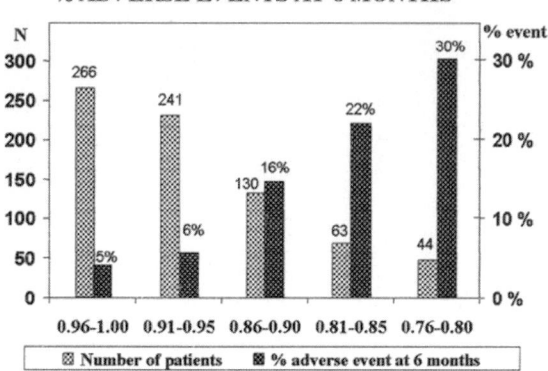

FFR-post-STENT Registry (N =750)
% ADVERSE EVENTS AT 6 MONTHS

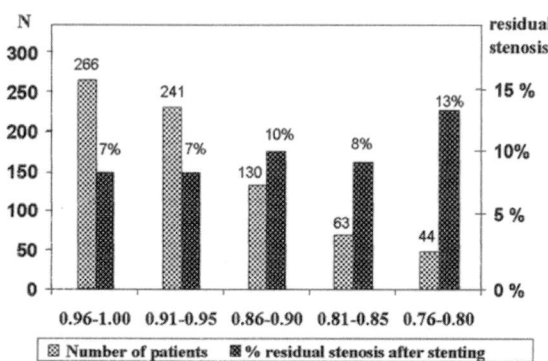

FFR-post-STENT Registry (N =750)
RESIDUAL STENOSIS AFTER STENTING

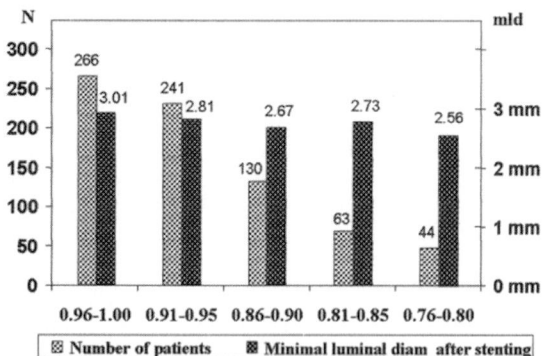

FFR-post-STENT Registry (N =750)
MLD AFTER STENTING

FIGURE 17–39. Top. Distribution of the study population over the five FFR categories. A strong inverse correlation was present between FFR after stenting and event rate at 6-month follow up. **Middle.** Distribution of percentage residual stenosis in the five FFR categories. **Bottom.** Minimal luminal diameter (mid) in the five FFR categories. FFR, fractional flow reserve. From Pijls NHJ, Klauss V, Siebert U, et al.[148] With permission.

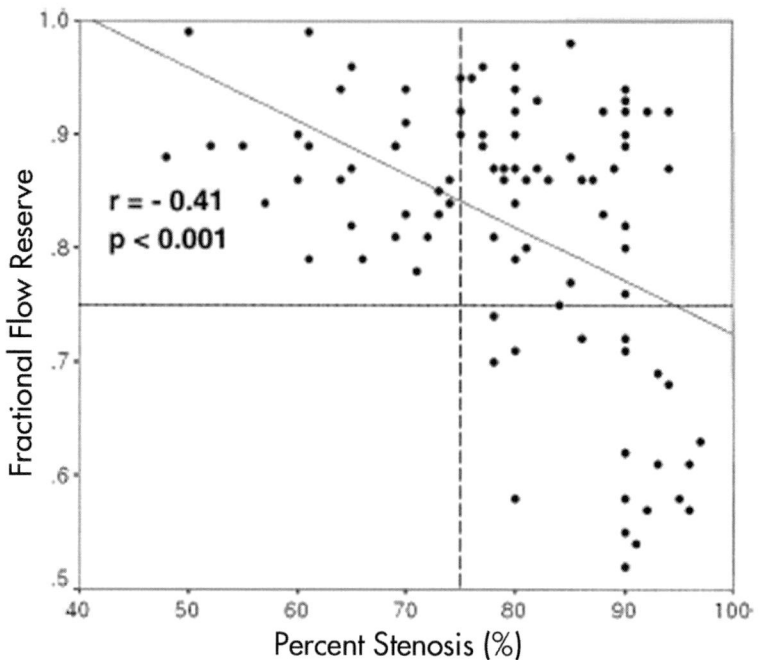

FIGURE 17–40. Comparison of percent diameter stenosis to FFR across jailed side branches. *Source: From Koo BK, Kang HJ, Youn TJ, et al.[155] With permission.*

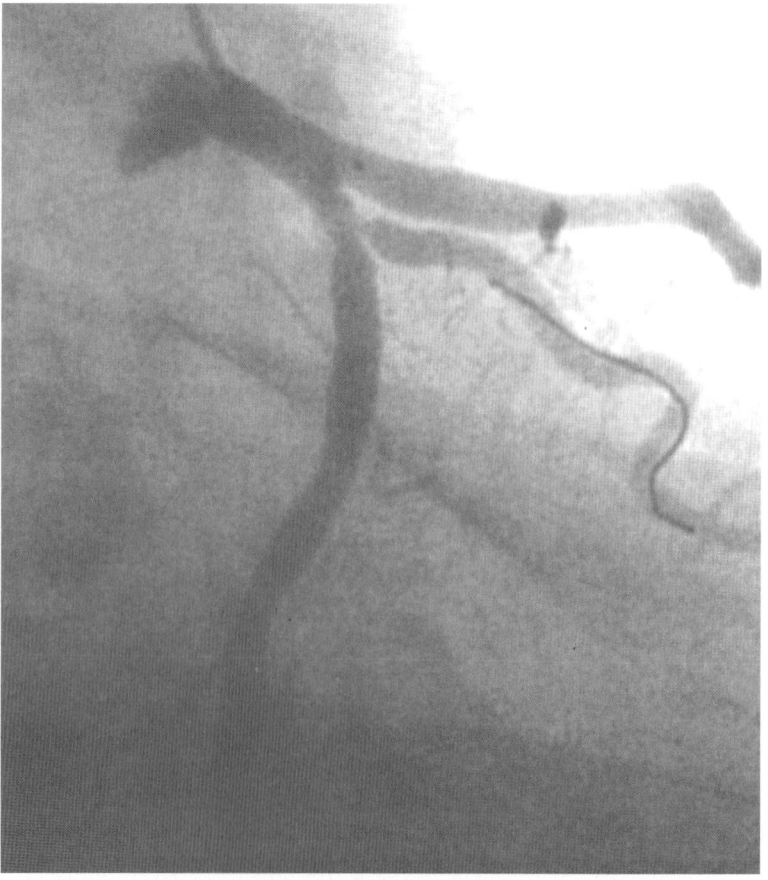

FIGURE 17–41. Cineangiographic frame demonstrating severe ostial lesion of obtuse marginal branch in the only one projection that could visualize the lesion. Coronary hemodynamic tracings demonstrating a fractional flow reserve (FFR) of 0.94, a normal value. *Source: From Ziaee A, Parham WA, Herrmann SC, Stewart RE, Lim MJ, Kern MJ.[157] With permission.*

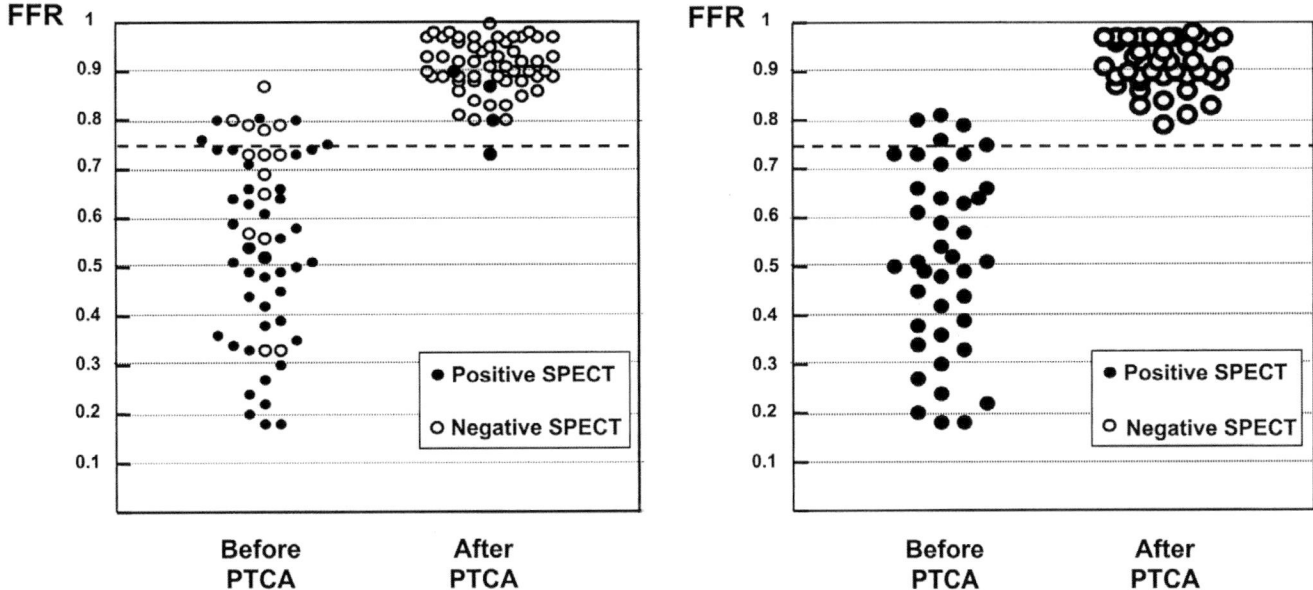

FIGURE 17–42. Values of FFR before and after angioplasty for myocardial infarction according to results of sestamibi SPECT myocardial perfusion imaging in patient population as a whole (*left*) and in patients with truly positive and truly negative SPECT imaging (*right*). FFR, fractional flow reserve; PCTA, percutaneous transluminal coronary angioplasty; SPECT, single-photon emission computed tomography. *Source: From De Bruyne B, Pijls NHJ, Bartunek J, et al.*[158] *With permission.*

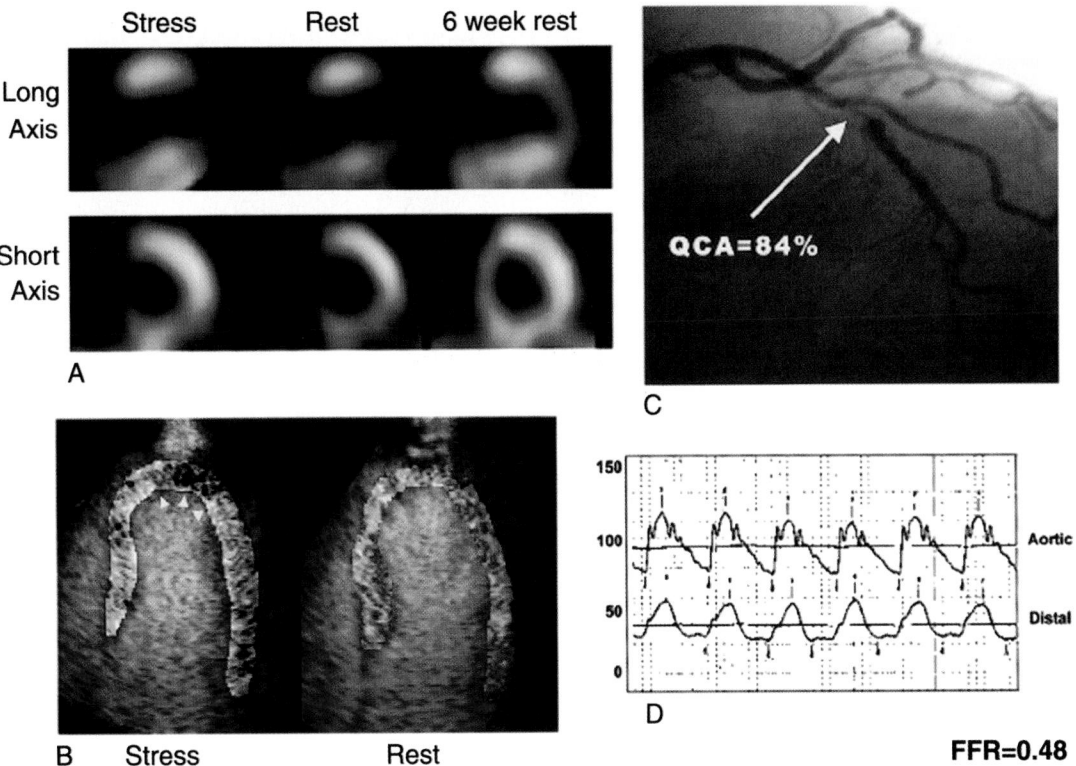

FIGURE 17–43. **A.** Baseline rest and dipyridamole (DP)-stress vertical long axis single-photon emission computed tomography (SPECT) images and 10-week follow up rest images are shown from a patient with anterior myocardial infarction who received thrombolytic therapy. When DP stress is paired with initial rest images there is a fixed perfusion defect in the anteroapical wall. When DP stress is paired with the delayed rest images, SPECT is reclassified as reversible. **B.** Rest and post-DP stress myocardial contrast echocardiography images from the apical four-chamber view of the same patient demonstrate an apical-lateral perfusion defect during DP that was not present at rest, indicating reversibility. **C.** Angiogram of the patient showing an 84 percent lesion in the left anterior descending coronary artery. **D.** Fractional flow reserve (FFR) tracings showing an FFR of 0.48. QCA, quantitative coronary angiography. *Source: From Samady H, Lepper W, Powers ER, et al.*[159] *With permission.*

Ninety-seven jailed side branch lesions in vessels >2.0 mm with a percent stenosis >50 percent by visual estimation after stent implantation underwent FFR measuring pressure 5 mm distal and proximal to the ostial side branch lesion. In 94 lesions the mean FFRs were 0.94 ± 0.04 and 0.85 ± 0.11 at the main branches and jailed side branches, respectively. There was a negative correlation between the percent stenosis and FFR ($r = 0.41$, $p < 0.001$). However, no lesion with <75 percent stenosis had FFR < 0.75. Among 73 lesions with >75 percent stenosis, only 20 lesions were functionally significant (Fig. 17–40). The authors concluded that measurement of FFR in jailed side branch lesions is both safe and feasible; and like other intermediate lesions, quantitative coronary angiography is unreliable. Moreover, the measurement of FFR suggests that most of these lesions do not have functional significance and that intervention on these nonsignificant lesions may not be necessary. Similar findings have been reported for native ostial and branch lesions during routine coronary angiography[156,157] (Fig. 17–41).

Coronary Physiology in Patients with Acute Myocardial Infarction

A normal FFR is indicative of reversal of myocardial perfusion defects in patients with prior myocardial infarction. De Bruyne et al.[158] examined FFR in 57 patients who had sustained a myocardial infarction more than 6 days prior to investigation. Sensitivity and specificity of an FFR of 0.75 to detect abnormal scintigraphic imaging were 82 and 87 percent, respectively; the concordance between FFR and scintigraphy was 85 percent ($p < 0.001$). An FFR >0.75 distinguished patients after myocardial infarction with negative scintigraphic imaging (Fig. 17–42). Similar findings relating FFR of infarct-related arteries in patients early after myocardial infarction to reversible perfusion defects by and myocardial contrast echocardiography has been reported by Samady and colleagues[159] (Fig. 17–43).

Microvascular Disease

As part of the Women's Ischemic Syndrome Evaluation (WISE) study, Reis and coworkers[160] examined 48 women with chest pain, normal coronary arteries, or minimal luminal irregularities with CVR. Sixty percent of women with CVR <2 had a hyperemic velocity of 89 percent of baseline, but no change in cross-sectional vessel area. Forty percent of women with normal microcirculation with CVR on average of 3.24 were associated with increases in coronary flow velocity and a cross-sectional area by 179 and 17 percent, respectively. A CVR of 2.2 provided a high sensitivity and specificity (90 and 89 percent, respectively) for the diagnosis of microvascular dysfunction. Failure of epicardial coronary artery to dilate at least 9 percent was also a sensitive (79 percent) and specific (79 percent) surrogate marker of microvascular dysfunction. The attenuated epicardial coronary dilatory response likely represents significant microvascular dysfunction in women with chest pain and no obstructive coronary artery disease.

Collateral Circulation

The collateral circulation can be described by intracoronary pressure and flow relationships. Ipsilateral collateral flow and contralateral arterial responses have been described in numerous studies using both pressure and flow to provide new information regarding mecha-

nisms, function, and clinical significance of collateral flow in patients[161–164] and provide new insights into coronary artery disease.[165] The reader is referred to excellent works elsewhere for details.[161–164] In summary, coronary blood flow and pressure can be determined during cardiac catheterization to provide insight into pathophysiologic mechanisms as well as unique data, which may facilitate clinical decisions regarding coronary revascularization. In the laboratory coronary physiologic measurements have a strong association with noninvasive ischemia testing. Clinical validation supports operator confidence that coronary physiology can be used to facilitate clinical decisions, especially for coronary arteries narrowed between 40 percent and 70 to 80 percent in diameter. Measurements of coronary physiology strongly complement coronary lumenography and permit exploration of the coronary microcirculation, collateral flow, myocardial infarction physiology, and mechanisms of interventions for coronary artery disease.

ACKNOWLEDGMENTS

Portions of this chapter come from Morton J. Kern, Spencer B. King III, John S. Douglas Jr., and Robert H. Franch, Chapter 17 in the 11th edition of *Hurst's The Heart*. Other portions come from M.J. Kern, ed. *The Cardiac Catheterization Handbook*, 4th ed. St. Louis: Mosby; 2004: 352–325. With permission.

REFERENCES

1. Kern MJ. *The Cardiac Catheterization Handbook.* 4th ed. St. Louis: Mosby, 2003.
2. Baim DS, Grossman W, eds. *Grossman's Cardiac Catheterization, Angiography and Intervention.* 6th ed. Baltimore: Lippincott, Williams & Wilkins, 2000.
3. Pepine CJ, Hill JA, Lambert CR. *Diagnostic and Therapeutic Cardiac Catheterization.* 3rd ed. Baltimore: Williams & Wilkins, 1998.
4. Campeau L. Percutaneous radial artery approach for coronary angiography. *Cathet Cardiovasc Diagn* 1989;16:3–7.
5. Kiemeneij F, Laarman GJ, Odekerken D, et al. A randomized comparison of percutaneous transluminal coronary angioplasty by the radial, brachial and femoral approaches: the access study. *J Am Coll Cardiol* 1997;29:1269–1275.
6. Silber S. Rapid hemostasis of arterial puncture sites with collagen in patients undergoing diagnostic and interventional cardiac catheterization. *Clin Cardiol* 1997;20:981–982.
7. Chamberlin JA, Lardi AB, McKeever LS, et al. Use of vascular sealing devices (Vasoseal and Perclose) versus assisted manual compression (Femostop) in transcatheter coronary interventions requiring abciximab (ReoPro). *Catheter Cardiovasc Interv* 1999;47:143–147.
8. Sanborn TA, Gibbs HH, Brinker JA, et al. A multicenter randomized trial comparing a percutaneous collagen hemostasis device with conventional manual compression after diagnostic angiography and angioplasty. *J Am Coll Cardiol* 1993;22:1273.
9. Kern MJ. Selection of radiocontrast media in cardiac catheterization: comparative physiology and clinical effects of nonionic and ionic dimeric formulations. *Am Heart J* 1991;122:195–201.
10. Hirshfield JW Jr. Cardiovascular effects of contrast agents. *Am J Cardiol* 1990;66(suppl):9F–17P.
11. Rihal CS, Textor SC, Grill DE, et al. Incidence and Prognostic importance of acute renal failure after percutaneous coronary intervention. *Circulation* 2002;105:2259–2264.
12. McClennan BL. Ionic and nonionic iodinated contrast media: evolution and strategies for use. *AJR Am J Roentgenol* 1990;155:225–233.
13. Tepel M, va der Geit M, Schwarzfeld C, et al. Prevention of radiographic-contrast-agent-induced reductions in renal function by acetylcysteine. *N Engl J Med* 2000;343:180–184.
14. Chu VL, Cheng JW. Fenoldopam in the prevention of contrast media-induced acute renal failure. *Ann Pharmacother* 2001;35:1278–1282.
15. Madyoon H, Crushore L, Weaver D, et al. Use of fenoldopam to prevent radiocontrast nephropathy in high-risk patients. *Catheter Cardiovasc Interv* 2002;53:341–345.
16. Stone GW, McCullough PA, Tumlin JA, et al. Fenoldopam mesylate for the prevention of contrast-induced nephropathy: a randomized controlled trial: *JAMA* 2003;290(17):2284–2291.

17. Krone RJ, Johnson L, Noto T. Five year trends in cardiac catheterization: a report from the Registry of the Society for Cardiac Angiography and Interventions. *Cathet Cardiovasc Diagn* 1996;39:31–35.

18. Trerotola SO, Kuhlman JE, Fishman EK. Bleeding complications of femoral catheterization: CT evaluation. *Radiology* 1990;174:37–40.

19. Lazar JM, Uretsky BF, Denys BG, et al. Predisposing risk factors and natural history of acute neurologic complications of left-sided cardiac catheterization. *Am J Cardiol* 1995;75:1056–1060.

20. Douglas JS Jr, King SB III. Complications of coronary arteriography: management during and following the procedure. In King SB III, Douglas JS Jr, eds. *Coronary Arteriography.* New York: McGraw-Hill, 1984:302–313.

21. Chatterjee T, Do D, Kaufmann U, et al. Ultrasound-guided repair for treatment of femoral artery pseudoaneurysm. *Cathet Cardiovasc Diagn* 1996;38:335–340.

22. Holmes DR, Wondrow MA, Bell MR, et al. Cine angiographic image replacement digital archival requirements and remaining obstacles. *Cathet Cardiovasc Diagn* 1998;44:346–356.

23. Waters DD, Szlachcic J, Bonan R. Comparative sensitivity of exercise, cold pressor and ergonovine testing in provoking attacks of variant angina in patients with active disease. *Circulation* 1983;67:310–315.

24. Donohue TJ, Kern MJ, Aguirre FV, et al. Assessing the hemodynamic significance of coronary artery stenoses: analysis of translesional pressure-flow velocity relations in patients. *J Am Coll Cardiol* 1993;22:449–458.

25. Helfant RH, Pine R, Meister SG, et al. Nitroglycerin to unmask reversible asynergy: correlation with post coronary bypass ventriculography. *Circulation* 1974;50:108–113.

26. Horn HR, Teichholz LE, Cohn PF, et al. Augmentation of left ventricular contraction pattern in coronary artery disease by inotropic catecholamine: the epinephrine ventriculogram. *Circulation* 1974;49:1063–1071.

27. Dyke SH, Cohn PF, Gorlin R, Sonnenblick EH. Detection of residual myocardial function in coronary artery disease using post extrasystolic potentiation. *Circulation* 1974;50:694–699.

28. Sones FM Jr, Shriey EK. Cine coronary arteriography. *Mod Concepts Cardiovasc Dis* 1962;31:735–738.

29. Seldinger SI. Catheter replacement of the needle in percutaneous arteriography: a new technique. *Acta Radiol* 1953;39:368–376.

30. Ricketts HJ, Abrams HL. Percutaneous selective coronary cine arteriography. *JAMA* 1962;181:620–626.

31. Amplatz K, Formanek G, Stranger P, Wilson W. Mechanics of selective coronary artery catheterization via femoral approach. *Radiology* 1967;89:1040–1047.

32. Judkins MP. Selective coronary arteriography: I. A percutaneous transfemoral technique. *Radiology* 1967;89:815–824.

33. Judkins MP, Judkins EJ. The Judkins technique. In King SB III, Douglas JS, Jr, eds. *Coronary Arteriography.* New York: McGraw-Hill, 1984:182–217.

34. King SB III, Douglas JS Jr. Catheterization techniques in coronary arteriography and left ventriculography: multipurpose techniques. In King SB III, Douglas JS Jr, eds. *Coronary Arteriography.* New York: McGraw-Hill, 1984:239–274.

35. Scanlon PJ, Faxon DP, Auden AM, et al. A Report of the American College of Cardiology/American Heart Association Task Force on Practice Guidelines (Committee on Coronary Angiography) Developed in Collaboration with the Society for Cardiac Angiography and Interventions Committee Members. ACC/AHA Guidelines for Coronary Angiography: Executive Summary and Recommendations. *Circulation* 1999;99:2345–2357.

36. King SB, Douglas JS, Morris DC. New angiographic views for coronary arteriography. In Hurst JW, ed. *The Heart, Update IV.* New York: McGraw-Hill, 1980:275–287.

37. Arnett EN, Isner JM, Redwood DR, et al. Coronary artery narrowing in coronary heart disease: comparison of cine angiographic and necropsy findings. *Ann Intern Med* 1979;91:350–356.

38. Grandin CM, Dyrda I, Pastemac A, et al. Discrepancies between cineangiographic and postmortem findings in patients with coronary artery disease and recent myocardial revascularization. *Circulation* 1974;49:703–708.

39. Roberts CS, Roberts WC. Cross-sectional area of the proximal portions of the three major epicardial coronary arteries in 98 patients with different coronary events: relationship to heart, weight, age, and sex. *Circulation* 1980;62:953–959.

40. Isner JM, Kishel J, Kent KM, et al. Inaccuracy of angiographic determination of left main coronary arterial narrowing: angiographic-histologic correlative analysis of 29 patients. *Circulation* 1979;59,60 (suppl 2):ii–161.

41. Zir LM, Miller SW, Dinsmore RE, et al. Interobserver variability in coronary arteriography. *Circulation* 1976;53:627–630.

42. DeRouen TA, Murray JA, Owen W. Variability in the analysis of coronary arteriograms. *Circulation* 1977;55:324–328.

43. Schwartz JN, King Y, Hackel DB, Bartel AG. Comparison of angiographic and postmortem findings in patients with coronary artery disease. *Am J Cardiol* 1975;36:174–178.

44. Hermiller JB, Cusma JT, Spero LA, et al. Quantitative and qualitative coronary angiographic analysis: review of methods, utility and limitations. *Cathet Cardiovasc Diagn* 1992;25:110–131.

45. Nissen SE, Yock P. Intravascular ultrasound. Novel pathophysiological insights and current clinical applications. *Circulation* 2001;103:604–616.

46. Takahashi T, Honda Y, Russo RJ, Fitzgerald PJ. Intravascular ultrasound and quantitative coronary angiography. Catheter Cardiovasc Interv 2002;55:118–128.

47. Gibson CM, Cannon CP, Daley WL, et al. TIMI frame count: a quantitative method of assessing coronary artery flow. *Circulation* 1996;93:879–888.

48. Levin DC. Pathways and functional significance of the coronary collateral circulation. *Circulation* 1974;50:831–837.

49. Kramer JR, Kitazume H, Proudfitt WL, Sones FM Jr. Clinical significance of isolated coronary bridges: benign and frequent conditions involving the left anterior descending artery. *Am Heart J* 1982;103:283–288.

50. Douglas JS Jr, Franch RH, King SB III. Coronary artery anomalies. In King SB III, Douglas JS Jr, eds. *Coronary Arteriography and Angioplasty.* New York: McGraw-Hill, 1985:33–85.

51. Serota H, Barth CW III, Seuc CA, et al. Rapid identification of the course of anomalous coronary arteries in adults: the "dot and eye" method. *Am J Cardiol* 1990;65:891–898.

52. The Principal Investigators of CASS and their Associates. The National Heart, Lung, and Blood Institute Coronary Artery Surgery Study: historical background, design, methods, the registry, the randomized trial, clinical database. *Circulation* 1981;63(suppl I):1–181.

53. Herman MV, Heinle RA, Klein MD, et al. Localized disorders in myocardial contraction: asynergy and its role in congestive heart failure. *N Engl J Med* 1967;227:225.

54. Sandler H, Dodge HT. The use of single plane angiocardiograms for the calculation of left ventricular volume in man. *Am Heart J* 1968;75:325–334.

55. Kennedy JW, Trenholme SE, Kasser IS. Left ventricular volume and mass from single plane cineangiocardiograms. *Am Heart J* 1970;80:343–352.

56. Sheehan FH, Mitten-Lewis S. Factors influencing accuracy in left ventricular volume determination. *Am J Cardiol* 1989;64:661–664.

57. Lawson MA, Blackwell GG, Doves ND, et al. Accuracy of biplane long-axis left ventricular volume determined by cine magnetic resonance imaging in patients with regional and global dysfunction. *Am J Cardiol* 1996;77:1098–1104.

58. Kennedy JW, Baxley WA, Figley MM, et al. Quantitative angiocardiography: I. The normal left ventricle in man. *Circulation* 1966;34:272–278.

59. Kennedy JW, Trenholme SE, Kasser IS. Left ventricular volume and mass from single plane cineangiocardiograms. *Am Heart J* 1970;80:343–352.

60. Shimazaki Y, Kawashima Y, Mori T, et al. Angiographic volume estimation of right ventricle. *Chest* 1980;77:390–395.

61. Johnson LW, Moore RJ, and Balter S. Review of radiation safety in the cardiac catheterization laboratory. *Cathet Cardiovasc Diagn* 1992;25:186–194.

62. Limacher ML, Douglas PS, Germano G, et al. Radiation safety in the practice of cardiology. *J Am Coll Cardiol* 1998;31:892–893.

63. Cusma JT, Bell MR, Wondrow MA, et al. Real time measurement of radiation exposure during diagnostic coronary angiography and percutaneous interventional procedures. *J Am Coll Cardiol* 1999;33:427–435.

64. Balter S. Radiation safety in the cardiac catheterization laboratory. *Catheter Cardiovasc Interv* 1999;47:347–353.

65. Courtois M, Faltal PG, Kovacs SJ, et al. Anatomically and physiologically based reference levels for measurement of intracardiac pressures. *Circulation* 1995;92:1994–2000.

66. Assey ME, Zile MR, Usher BW, et al. Effect of catheter positioning on the variability of measured gradient in aortic stenosis. *Cathet Cardiovasc Diagn* 1993;30:287–292.

67. Gorlin R, Gorlin G. Hydraulic formula for calculation of area of stenotic mitral valve, other cardiac valves and central circulatory shunts. *Am Heart J* 1951;41:1–29.

68. Cohen MV, Gorlin R. Modified orifice equation for the calculation of mitral valve area. *Am Heart J* 1972;84:839–840.

69. Folland ED, Parisi AF, Carbone C. Is peripheral arterial pressure a satisfactory substitute for ascending aortic pressure when measuring aortic valve gradients? *J Am Coll Cardiol* 1984;4:1207–1212.

70. Hays J, Lujan M, Chilton R. Aortic stenosis catheterization revisited: A long sheath single puncture technique. *J Invasive Cardiol* 2006;18:262–267.

71. Bache RJ, Jorgensen CR, Wany Y. Simplified estimation of aortic valve area. *Br Heart J* 1972;34:408–411.

72. Angel J, Soler-Soler J, Anivarro I, Domingo E. I. Hemodynamic evaluation of stenotic cardiac valves. II. Modification of the simplified formula for mitral and aortic valve area calculation. *Cathet Cardiovasc Diagn* 1985;11:127–138.

73. Voelker W, Reul H, Niehaus G, et al. Comparison of valvular resistance, stroke work loss and Gorlin valve area for quantification of aortic stenosis. *Circulation* 1995;91:1196–1204.

74. Hosenpud JD, McAnulty JH, Morton MJ. Overestimation of mitral valve gradients obtained by phasic pulmonary artery wedge pressure. *Cathet Cardiovasc Diagn* 1983;9:283–290.

75. Hamilton MA, Stevenson LW, Woo RN, et al. Effect of tricuspid regurgitation on the reliability of the thermodilution cardiac output technique in congestive heart failure. *Am J Cardiol* 1989;64:945–948.

76. Lehmann KG, Platt MS. Improved accuracy and precision of thermodilution cardiac output measurement using a dual thermistor catheter system. *J Am Coll Cardiol* 1999;33:883–891.

77. Levett JM, Replogle RL. Thermodilution cardiac output: a critical analysis and review of the literature. *J Surg Res* 1979;27:392–404.

78. Hillis DL, Firth BG, Winniford MD. Variability of right-sided cardiac oxygen saturations in adults with and without intracardiac left-to-right shunting. *Am J Cardiol* 1986;58:129–132.

79. Freed MD, Miettinen OS, Nadas AS. Oximetric detection of intracardiac left-to-right shunts. *Br Heart J* 1979;42:690–694.

80. Shepherd AP, McMahan CA. Role of oximeter error in the diagnosis of shunts. *Cathet Cardiovasc Diagn* 1996;37:435–446.

81. O'Keefe JH, Vlietstra RE, Hanley PC, Seward JB. Revival of the transseptal approach for catheterization of the left atrium and ventricle. *Mayo Clin Proc* 1985;60:790–795.

82. Mullins CE. Transseptal left heart catheterization: experience with a new technique in 520 pediatric and adults patients. *Pediatr Cardiol* 1983;4:239–246.

83. Laskey WK, Kusiak V, Untereker WJ, Hirshfeld JW. Transseptal left heart catheterization: utility of a sheath technique. *Cathet Cardiovasc Diagn* 1982;8:535–542.

84. Croft CH, Lipscomb K. Modified technique of transseptal left heart catheterization. *J Am Coll Cardiol* 1985;5:904–910.

85. Nanas JN, Moulopoulos SD. Counterpulsation: historical background, technical improvements, hemodynamic and metabolic effects. *Cardiology* 1994;84:156–167.

86. Kern MJ, Aguirre F, Bach R, et al. Augmentation of coronary blood flow by intra-aortic balloon pumping in patients after coronary angioplasty. *Circulation* 1993;87:500–511.

87. Kern MJ, Aguirre FV, Tatineni S, et al. Enhanced coronary blood flow velocity during intraaortic balloon counterpulsation in critically ill patients. *J Am Coll Cardiol* 1993;21:359–368.

88. Topol EJ, Nissen SE. Our preoccupation with coronary luminology: the dissociation between clinical and angiographic findings in ischemic heart disease. *Circulation* 1995;92:2333–2342.

89. Kern M. Curriculum in interventional cardiology: coronary pressure and flow measurements in the cardiac catheterization laboratory. *Catheter Cardiovasc Interv* 2002;54:378–400.

90. Toshihiko N, Amanullah AM, Luo H, et al. Clinical validation of intravascular ultrasound for assessment of coronary stenosis severity. *J Am Coll Cardiol* 1999;33:1870–1878.

91. White CW, Wright CB, Doty DB, et al. Does visual interpretation of the coronary arteriogram predict the physiologic importance of a coronary stenosis? *N Engl J Med* 1984;310:819–824.

92. Harrison DG, White CW, Hiratzka LF, et al. The value of lesion cross-sectional area determined by quantitative coronary angiography in assessing the physiologic significance of proximal left anterior descending coronary arterial stenoses. *Circulation* 1984;69:1111–1119.

93. Gould KL, Kirkeeide RL, Buchi M. Coronary flow reserve as a physiologic measure of stenosis severity. *J Am Coll Cardiol* 1990;15:459–474.

94. Gould KL, Lipscomb K, Hamilton GW. Physiologic basis for assessing critical coronary stenosis: Instantaneous flow response and regional distribution during coronary hyperemia as measures of coronary flow reserve. *Am J Cardiol* 1974;33:87–94.

95. Kern MJ, Bach RG, Mechem C, et al. Variations in normal coronary vasodilatory reserve stratified by artery, gender, heart transplantation and coronary artery disease. *J Am Coll Cardiol* 1996;28:1154–1160.

96. McGinn AL, White CW, Wilson RF. Interstudy variability of coronary flow reserve: Influence of heart rate, arterial pressure, and ventricular preload. *Circulation* 1990;81:1319–1330.

97. Marcus ML, Mueller TM, Gascho JA, Kerber RE. Effects of cardiac hypertrophy secondary to hypertension on the coronary circulation. *Am J Cardiol* 1979;44:1023–1031.

98. Chauhan A, Millins PA, Petch MC, Schonfeld PM. Is coronary flow velocity response really normal in syndrome X? *Circulation* 1994;89:1998–2004.

99. Marcus ML, Doty DB, Hiratzka LF, et al. Decreased coronary flow reserve: a mechanism for angina pectoris in patients with aortic stenosis and normal coronary arteries. *N Engl J Med* 1982;307:1362–1367.

100. Cobb F, McHale P, Remert J. Effects of acute cellular injury on coronary vascular reactivity in awake dogs. *Circulation* 1978;57:962–968.

101. Gould KL. Dynamic coronary stenosis. *Am J Cardiol* 1980;45:286–292.

102. Czernin J, Muller P, Chan S, et al. Influence of age and hemodynamics on myocardial blood flow and reserve. *Circulation* 1993;88:62–69.

103. Wieneke H, Haude M, Ge J, et al. Corrected coronary flow velocity reserve: a new concept for assessing coronary perfusion. *J Am Coll Cardiol* 2000;35:1713–1720.

104. Akasaka T, Yoshida K, Hozumi T, et al. Retinopathy identifies marked restriction of coronary flow reserve in patients with diabetes mellitus. *J Am Coll Cardiol* 1997;30:935–941.

105. Baumgart D, Haude M, Goerge G, et al. Improved assessment of coronary stenosis severity using the relative flow velocity reserve. *Circulation* 1998;98:40–46.

106. Kern MJ, Puri S, Bach RG, et al. Abnormal coronary flow velocity reserve after coronary artery stenting in patients: role of relative coronary reserve to assess potential mechanisms. *Circulation* 1999;100:2491–2498.

107. Pijls NH, Van Gelder B, Van der Voort P, et al. Fractional flow reserve: a useful index to evaluate the influence of an epicardial coronary stenosis on myocardial blood flow. *Circulation* 1995;92:3183–3193.

108. Pijls NH, De Bruyne B, Peels K, et al. Measurement of fractional flow reserve to assess the functional severity of coronary-artery stenoses. *N Engl J Med* 1996;334:1703–1708.

109. De Bruyne B, Bartunek J, Sys SU, et al. Simultaneous coronary pressure and flow velocity measurements in humans: feasibility, reproducibility, and hemodynamic dependence of coronary flow velocity reserve, hyperemic flow versus pressure slope index, and fractional flow reserve. *Circulation* 1996;94:1842–1849.

110. Qian J, Ge J, Baumgart D, et al. Safety of intracoronary Doppler flow measurement. *Am Heart J* 2000;140:502–510.

111. Meuwissen M, Siebes M, Chamuleau SA, et al. Hyperemic stenosis resistance index for evaluation of functional coronary lesion severity. *Circulation* 2002;106:441–446.

112. Siebes M, Verhoeff B-J, Meuwissen M, et al. Single-wire pressure and flow velocity measurement to quantify coronary stenosis hemodynamics and effects of percutaneous interventions. *Circulation* 2004;109:756–762.

113. Chamuleau SAJ, Siebes M, Meuwissen M, et al. The association between coronary lesion severity and distal microvascular resistance in patients with coronary artery disease. *Am J Physiol Heart Circ Physiol* 2003;285: H2194–H2200.

114. Verhoeff B-J, Siebes M, Meuwissen M, et al. Influence of percutaneous coronary intervention on coronary microvascular resistance index. *Circulation* 2005;111:76–82.

115. Marques KMJ, Spruijt HJ, Boer C, Westerhof N, Visser CA and Visser FC. The diastolic flow-pressure gradient relation in coronary stenoses in humans. *J Am Coll Cardiol* 2002;39:1630–1636.

116. Meuwissen M, Chamuleau SAJ, Siebes M, et al. Role of variability in microvascular resistance on fractional flow reserve and coronary blood flow velocity reserve in intermediate coronary lesions. *Circulation* 2001;103:184–187.

117. De Bruyne B, Pijls NHJ, Smith L, Wievegg, M, Heyndrickx GR. Coronary thermodilution to assess flow reserve: experimental validation. *Circulation* 2001;104:2003.

118. Pijls NH, De Bruyne B, Smith L, et al. Coronary thermodilution to assess flow reserve: validation in humans. *Circulation* 2002;105:2482–2486.

119. Fearon WF, Farouque HMO, Balsam LB, et al. Comparison of coronary thermodilution and Doppler velocity for assessing coronary flow reserve. *Circulation* 2004;108:2198–2200.

120. Barbato E, Aarnoudse W, Aengevaeren WR, et al. Validation of coronary flow reserve measurements by thermodilution in clinical practice. *Eur Heart J* 2004;25:219–223.

121. Wilson RF, Laughlin DE, Ackell PH, et al. Transluminal subselective measurement of coronary artery blood flow velocity and vasodilator reserve in man. *Circulation* 1985;72:82–92.

122. Wilson RF, White C. Serious Ventricular dysrhythmias after intracoronary papaverine. *Am J Cardiol* 1988;62:1301–1302.

123. Baumgart D, Haude M, Liu F, Ge J, Goerge G, Erbel R. Current concepts of coronary flow reserve for clinical decision making during cardiac catheterization. *Am Heart J* 1998;136:136–149.

124. Wilson RF, Wyche K, Christensen BV, et al. Effects of adenosine on human arterial circulation. *Circulation* 1990;82:1595–1606.

125. Kern MJ, Deligonul U, Tatineni S, et al. Intravenous adenosine: continuous infusion and low dose bolus administration for determination of coronary vasodilatory reserve in patients with and without coronary artery disease. *J Am Coll Cardiol* 1991;18:718–729.

126. Caracciolo EA, Wolford TL, Underwood RD, et al. Influence of intimal thickness on coronary blood flow responses in orthotopic heart transplant recipients: A combined intravascular Doppler and ultrasound imaging study. *Circulation* 1995;92:II-182–II-190.

127. Jeremias A, Whitbourn RJ, Filardo SD, et al. Adequacy of intracoronary versus intravenous adenosine-induced maximal coronary hyperemia for fractional flow reserve measurements. *Am Heart J* 2000;140:651–657.

128. Miller DD, Donohue TJ, Younis LT, et al. Correlation of pharmacologic 99mtc-sestamibi myocardial perfusion imaging with poststenotic coronary flow reserve in patients with angiographically intermediate coronary artery stenoses. *Circulation* 1994;89:2150–2160.

129. Joye JD, Schulman DS, Lasorda D, et al. Intracoronary Doppler guide wire versus stress single-photon emission computed tomographic thallium-201 imaging in assessment of intermediate coronary stenoses. *J Am Coll Cardiol* 1994;24:940–947.

130. Deychak YA, Segal J, Reiner JS, et al. Doppler guide wire flow-velocity indexes measured distal to coronary stenoses associated with reversible thallium perfusion defects. *Am Heart J* 1995;129:219–227.

131. Heller LI, Popma J, Cates C, et al. Functional assessment of stenosis severity in the cath lab: a comparison of Doppler and tl-201 imaging. *J Interven Cardiol* 1995;7:23A.

132. de Bruyne B, Bartunek J, Sys SU, Heyndrickx GR. Relation between myocardial fractional flow reserve calculated from coronary pressure measurements and exercise-induced myocardial ischemia. *Circulation* 1995;92:39–46.

133. Zilstra F, Fioretti P, Reiber J, Serruys PW. Which cineangiographically assessed anatomic variable correlates best with functional measurements of stenosis severity? A comparison of quantitative analysis of the coronary cineangiogram with measure coronary flow reserve and exercise/redistribution thallium-201 scintigraphy. *J Am Coll Cardiol* 1988;12:686–691.

134. Danzi GB, Pirelli S, Mauri L, et al. Which variable of stenosis severity best describes the significance of an isolated left anterior descending coronary artery lesion? Correlation between quantitative coronary angiography, intracoronary Doppler measurements and high dose dipyridamole echocardiography. *J Am Coll Cardiol* 1998;31:526–533.

135. Bartunek J, Van Schuerbeeck E, De Bruyne B. Comparison of exercise electrocardiography and dobutamine echocardiography with invasively assessed myocardial fractional flow reserve in evaluation of severity of coronary arterial narrowing. *Am J Cardiol* 1997;79:478–481.

136. Schulman DS, Lasorda D, Farah T, et al. Correlations between coronary flow reserve measured with a Doppler guide wire and treadmill exercise testing. *Am Heart J* 1997;134:99–104.

137. Donohue TJ, Miller DD, Bach RG, et al. Correlation of poststenotic hyperemic coronary flow velocity and pressure with abnormal stress myocardial perfusion imaging in coronary artery disease. *Am J Cardiol* 1996;77:948–954.

138. Duffy SJ, Gelman JS, Peverill RE, et al. Agreement between coronary flow velocity reserve and stress echocardiography in intermediate-severity coronary stenoses. *Catheter Cardiovasc Interv* 2001;53:29–38.

139. Chamuleau SAJ, Meuwissen M, van Eck-Smit BLF, et al. Fractional flow reserve, absolute and relative coronary blood flow velocity reserve in relation to the results of technetium-99m sestamibi single-photon emission computed tomography in patients with two-vessel coronary artery disease. *J Am Coll Cardiol* 2001;37:1316–1322.

140. Caymaz O, Fak AS, Tezcan H, et al. Correlation of myocardial fraction flow reserve with thallium-201 SPECT imaging in intermediate- severity coronary artery lesions. *J Invasive Cardiol* 2000;12:345–350.

141. Fearon WF, Takagi A, Jeremias A, et al. Use of fractional myocardial flow reserve to assess the functional significance of intermediate coronary stenosis. *Am J Cardiol* 2000;86:1013–1014.

142. El-Shafei A, Chiravuri R, Stikovac MM, et al. Comparison of relative coronary Doppler flow velocity reserve to stress myocardial perfusion imaging in patients with coronary artery disease. *Catheter Cardiovasc Interv* 2001;53:193–201.

143. De Bruyne B, Hersbach F, Pijls NHJ, et al. Abnormal epicardial coronary resistance in patients with diffuse atherosclerosis but "normal" coronary angiography. *Circulation* 2001;104:2401–2406.

144. Kern MJ, Donohue TJ, Aguirre FV, et al. Clinical outcome of deferring angioplasty in patients with normal translesional pressure-flow velocity measurements. *J Am Coll Cardiol* 1995;25:178–187.

145. Ferrari M, Schnell B, Werner GS, Figulla HR. Safety of deferring angioplasty in patients with normal coronary flow velocity reserve. *J Am Coll Cardiol* 1999;33:83–87.

146. Bech GJ, De Bruyne B, Bonnier HJRM, et al. Long-term follow-up after deferral of percutaneous transluminal coronary angioplasty of intermediate stenosis on the basis of coronary pressure measurement. *J Am Coll Cardiol* 1998;31:841–847.

147. Bech GJW, Pijls NHJ, De Bruyne B, et al. Usefulness of fractional flow reserve to predict clinical outcome after balloon angioplasty. *Circulation* 1999;99:883–888.

148. Pijls NHJ, Klauss V, Siebert U, et al. Coronary pressure measurement after stenting predicts adverse events at follow-up: a multicenter registry. *Circulation* 2002;105:2950–2954.

149. Bech GJW, De Bruyne B, Pijls NHJ, et al. Fractional flow reserve to determine the appropriateness of angioplasty in moderate coronary stenosis: a randomized trial. *Circulation* 2001;103:2928–2934.

150. Tsunoda T, Nakamura M, Wakatsuki T, et al. The pattern of alteration in flow velocity in the recanalized artery is related to left ventricular recovery in patients with acute infarction and successful direct balloon angioplasty. *J Am Coll Cardiol* 1998;32:338–344.

151. Claeys MJ, Vrints CJ, Bosmans J, et al. Coronary flow reserve during coronary angioplasty in patients with recent myocardial infarction: relation to stenosis and myocardial viability. *J Am Coll Cardiol* 1996;28:1712–1719.

152. Neumann FJ, Blasini R, Schmitt C, et al. Effect of glycoprotein IIb/IIIa receptor blockade on recovery of coronary flow and left ventricular function after the placement of coronary-artery stents in acute myocardial infarction. *Circulation* 1998;98:2695–2701.

153. Feldman LJ, Himbert D, Juliard JM, et al. Reperfusion syndrome: Relationship of coronary blood flow reserve to left ventricular function and infarct size. *J Am Coll Cardiol* 2000;35:1162–1169.

154. Gruberg L, Kapeliovich M, Roguin A, et al. Deferring angioplasty in intermediate coronary lesions based on coronary flow criteria is safe: Comparison of a deferred group to an intervention group. *Int J Cardiovasc Interv* 1999;2:35–40.

155. Koo BK, Kang HJ, Youn TJ, et al. Physiologic assessment of jailed side branch lesions using fractional flow reserve *J Am Coll Cardiol* 2005;46:633–637.

156. Lim MJ, Kern MJ. Utility of coronary physiologic hemodynamics for bifurcation, aorto-ostial and ostial branch stenoses to guide treatment decisions. *Catheter Cardiovasc Interv* 2005;65:461–468.

157. Ziaee A, Parham WA, Herrmann SC, Stewart RE, Lim MJ, Kern MJ. Lack of relationship between imaging and physiology in ostial coronary artery narrowings. *Am J Cardiol* 2004;93:1404–1407.

158. De Bruyne B, Pijls NHJ, Bartunek J, et al. Fractional flow reserve in patients with prior myocardial infarction. *Circulation* 2001;104:157–162.

159. Samady H, Lepper W, Powers ER, et al. Fractional flow reserve of infarct-related arteries identifies reversible defects on noninvasive myocardial perfusion imaging early after myocardial infarction. *J Am Coll Cardiol* 2006;47:2187–2193.

160. Reis SE, Holubkov R, Lee JS, et al for the WISE Investigators. Coronary flow velocity response to adenosine characterizes coronary microvascular function in women with chest pain and obstructive coronary disease. *J Am Coll Cardiol* 1999;33:1469–1475.

161. Seiler C, Fleisch M, Billinger M, Meier B. Simultaneous intracoronary velocity- and pressure-derived assessment of adenosine-induced collateral hemodynamics in patients with one- to two-vessel coronary artery disease. *J Am Coll Cardiol* 1999;34:1985–1994.

162. Pijls NHJ, Bech GJW, el Gamal MIH, et al. Quantification of recruitable coronary collateral blood flow in conscious humans and its potential to predict future ischemic events. *J Am Coll Cardiol* 1995;25:1522–1528.

163. Piek JJ, van Liebergen RAM, Koch KT, et al. Clinical, angiographic and hemodynamic predictors of recruitable collateral flow assessed during balloon angioplasty coronary occlusion. *J Am Coll Cardiol* 1997;29:275–282.

164. Billinger M, Kloos P, Eberli FR, et al. Physiologically assessed coronary collateral flow and adverse cardiac ischemic events: a follow-up study in 403 patients with coronary artery disease. *J Am Coll Cardiol* 2002;40:1545–1550.

165. Gruberg L, Mintz GS, Fuchs S, et al. Simultaneous assessment of coronary flow reserve and fractional flow reserve with a novel pressure-based method. *J Interv Cardiol* 2000;13:323–330.

APPENDIX 17-1

Class I Recommendations for Coronary Angiography

	LEVEL OF EVIDENCE
IN STABLE ANGINA OR ASYMPTOMATIC INDIVIDUALS	
1. CCS class III and IV angina on medical treatment	B
2. High-risk criteria on noninvasive testing regardless of anginal severity (Table 17–1)	A
3. Patients who have been successfully resuscitated from sudden cardiac death or have sustained (>30 s) monomorphic ventricular tachycardia or nonsustained (<30 s) polymorphic ventricular tachycardia	B
IN UNSTABLE CORONARY SYNDROMES	
1. High or intermediate risk for adverse outcome in patients with unstable angina (Table 17-2) refractory to initial adequate medical therapy or with recurrent symptoms after initial stabilization. Emergent catheterization is recommended.	B
2. High risk for adverse outcome in patients with unstable angina (Table 17–2). Urgent catheterization is recommended.	B
3. High- or intermediate-risk unstable angina that stabilizes after initial treatment.	A
4. Initially low short-term–risk unstable angina (Table 17–2) that is subsequently high risk on noninvasive testing (Table 17–1).	B
5. Suspected Prinzmetal variant angina.	C
DURING THE INITIAL MANAGEMENT OF ACUTE MI (MI SUSPECTED AND ST ELEVATION OR BBB PRESENT):CORONARY ANGIOGRAPHY COUPLED WITH THE INTENT TO PERFORM PRIMARY PTCA	
1. As an alternative to thrombolytic therapy in patients who can undergo angioplasty of the infarct artery within 12 h of the onset of symptoms or beyond 12 h if ischemic symptoms persist, if performed in a timely fashion[a] by individuals skilled in the procedure and supported by experienced personnel in an appropriate laboratory environment.	A
2. In patients who are within 36 h of an acute ST elevation/Q-wave or new LBBB MI who develop cardiogenic shock, are <75 years of age, and in whom revascularization can be performed within 18 h of the onset of shock.	
DURING THE RISK-STRATIFICATION PHASE OF MI (PATIENTS WITH ALL TYPES OF MI)	
Ischemia at low levels of exercise with ECG changes (1-mm ST-segment depression or other predictors of adverse outcome) (Table 17–3) and/or imaging abnormalities	B
IN PERIOPERATIVE EVALUATION BEFORE (OR AFTER) NONCARDIAC SURGERY: PATIENTS WITH SUSPECTED OR KNOWN CAD	
1. Evidence for high risk of adverse outcome based on noninvasive test results (Table 17–1)	C
2. Angina unresponsive to adequate medical therapy	C
3. Unstable angina, particularly when facing intermediate or high-risk noncardiac surgery	C
4. Equivocal noninvasive test result in a high-clinical-risk patient undergoing high-risk surgery	C
IN PATIENTS WITH VALVULAR HEART DISEASE	
1. Before valve surgery or balloon valvotomy in an adult with chest discomfort, ischemia by noninvasive imaging, or both	B
2. Before valve surgery in an adult free of chest pain but of substantial age and/or with multiple risk factors for coronary disease	C
3. Infective endocarditis with evidence of coronary embolization	C

(continued)

APPENDIX 17–1

Class I Recommendations for Coronary Angiography (continued)

	LEVEL OF EVIDENCE
IN PATIENTS WITH CHF	
1. CHF due to systolic dysfunction with angina or with regional wall motion abnormalities and/ or scintigraphic evidence of reversible myocardial ischemia when revascularization is being considered	B
2. Before cardiac transplantation	C
3. CHF secondary to postinfarction ventricular aneurysm or other mechanical complications of MI	C

BBB, bundle branch block; CCS, Canadian Cardiovascular Society; CHF, congestive heart failure; LBBB, left bundle branch block; MI, myocardial infarction; PTCA, percutaneous transluminal coronary angioplasty.
aPerformance standard: within 90 min. Individuals who perform >75 PTCA procedures per year. Centers that perform >200 PTCA procedures per year and have cardiac surgical capability.
SOURCE: Modified and reproduced with permission from the American Heart Association. Scanlon PJ, Faxon DP, Auden AM, et al. A Report of the American College of Cardiology/American Heart Association Task Force on Practice Guidelines (Committee on Coronary Angiography). Developed in collaboration with the Society for Cardiac Angiography and Interventions Committee Members. ACC/AHA Guidelines for Coronary Angiography: Executive Summary and Recommendations. Circulation 1999;99:2345–2357.

APPENDIX 17–2

ACC/AHA Recommendations for Coronary Intravascular Ultrasound

	LEVEL OF EVIDENCE
CLASS I NONE	
CLASS II A	
1. Evaluation of lesion severity at a location difficult to image by angiography in patients with a positive functional study and a suspected flow-limiting stenosis	C
2. Assessment of a suboptimal angiographic result after coronary intervention	C
3. Diagnostic and management of coronary disease after cardiac transplantation	C
4. Assessment of the adequacy of deployment of the Palmaz-Schatz coronary stent, including the extent of stent apposition and determination of the minimal luminal diameter within the stent	B
CLASS II B	
1. Determination of plaque location and circumferential distribution for guidance of directional coronary atherectomy	C
2. Further evaluation of patients with characteristic anginal symptoms and a positive functional study with no focal stenoses or mild CAD on angiography	C
3. Determination of the mechanism of stent restenosis (inadequate expansion versus neointimal proliferation) and to enable selection of appropriate therapy (plaque ablation versus repeat balloon expansion)	C
4. Preinterventional assessment of lesional characteristics as a means to select an optimal revascularization device	C

SOURCE: Reproduced with permission from the American Heart Association. Scanlon PJ, Faxon DP, Auden AM, et al. A Report of the American College of Cardiology/American Heart Association Task Force on Practice Guidelines (Committee on Coronary Angiography). Developed in collaboration with the Society for Cardiac Angiography and Interventions Committee Members. ACC/AHA Guidelines for Coronary Angiography: Executive Summary and Recommendations. Circulation 1999;99:2345–2357.

APPENDIX 17–3

Recommendations for Intracoronary Physiologic Measurements (Doppler Ultrasound, FFR)

	LEVEL OF EVIDENCE
CLASS I NONE	
CLASS II A	
1. Assessment of the physiologic effects of intermediate coronary stenosis (30 to 70 percent luminal narrowing) in patients with anginal symptoms. Coronary pressure or Doppler velocimetry may also be useful as an alternative to performing noninvasive functional testing (e.g., when the functional study is absent or ambiguous) to determine whether an intervention is warranted.	B
CLASS II B	
1. Evaluation of the success of percutaneous coronary revascularization in restoring flow reserve and to predict the risk of restenosis	C
2. Evaluation of patients with anginal symptoms without an apparent angiographic culprit lesion	C

SOURCE: From Smith SC, Jr, Dove JT, Jacobs AK, et al. ACC/AHA guidelines for percutaneous coronary intervention: a report of the American College of Cardiology/American Heart Association Task Force on Practice Guidelines (Committee to Revise the 1993 Guidelines for Percutaneous Transluminal Coronary Angioplasty). J Am Coll Cardiol 2001;37:2239i–lxvi. With permission.

CHAPTER (18)

Coronary Intravascular Ultrasound Imaging

E. Murat Tuzcu / Stephen J. Nicholls / Steven E. Nissen

After two decades of continuous development, coronary intravascular ultrasound (IVUS) has achieved general acceptance as an essential element in all contemporary catheterization laboratories. Although angiography continues to serve as the primary imaging modality used to assess the anatomy of coronary artery disease (CAD), IVUS represents an important complimentary method for examination of the coronaries during diagnostic or interventional catheterization.[1] Studies comparing angiography and IVUS have demonstrated important differences in quantitative and qualitative findings.[2] Unlike angiography, which portrays the vessel as a silhouette of the lumen, IVUS provides tomographic images that depict not only the lumen but also the deeper intramural structures within the vessel wall.

The ability of ultrasound to penetrate and image soft tissue enables direct visualization of the atheroma, providing insights into the pathophysiology of coronary disease not obtainable by any other technique. Accordingly, intraluminal ultrasound imaging is now commonly used to confirm, refute, or supplement angiographic data in patients with coronary disease.[1] Recently, because of its ability to measure atherosclerosis progression and regression, IVUS has been increasingly employed in cardiovascular clinical trials. Ongoing studies using this methodology offer the opportunity to develop new antiatherosclerotic therapies, supplementing traditional long-term morbidity and mortality trials.

RATIONALE FOR INTRAVASCULAR ULTRASOUND
【 】 LIMITATIONS OF ANGIOGRAPHY

Visual interpretation of angiograms is associated with significant observer variability, and necropsy examination is often discordant with the apparent angiographic severity of lesions.[3,4] In comparison to postmortem evaluation, angiography often significantly underestimates the extent of atherosclerosis.[3,4] Angiographic assessment of lesion severity is strikingly discordant with measurements of the physiologic effects of stenoses.[5] Angiography depicts coronary anatomy from a planar two-dimensional silhouette of the contrast-filled lumen. However, coronary lesions are often complex, with markedly distorted or eccentric luminal shapes, and mechanical interventions (other than stenting) exaggerate luminal eccentricity by fracturing or dissecting the atheroma.[6]

The traditional method for characterizing angiographic lesion severity depends on visual or computer measurements of the percentage stenosis. This process requires comparison of luminal dimensions within both the lesion and an adjacent, uninvolved *normal* reference segment. However, necropsy studies demonstrate that coronary disease is frequently diffuse and contains no truly normal reference segment.[4] In the presence of diffuse disease, calculation of percent stenosis will predictably underestimate disease severity. Diffuse, concentric, and symmetrical disease affecting the entire vessel may result in the angiographic appearance of a small but normal artery.[6] Angiography is also confounded by the phenomenon of coronary *remodeling,* observed histologically as the outward displacement of the external vessel wall in segments with atherosclerosis.[7] This adventitial enlargement attenuates lumen encroachment, thereby concealing the presence of the atheroma on angiography. Although such lesions do not restrict blood flow, clinical studies have demonstrated that these minimal, nonobstructive lesions represent an important cause of acute coronary syndromes.[8] Angiographically unrecognized disease virtually always underlies an ergonovine-positive response in symptomatic patients with a *normal* coronary angiogram.[9]

IVUS has several unique properties of theoretical value in the detection and quantitation of coronary disease.[10] The cross-sectional perspective of ultrasound permits visualization of the full 360-degree circumference of the vessel wall. Accordingly, measurement of luminal area can be determined by planimetry, independent of the radiographic projection or magnification.[6,10] The tomographic perspective of ultrasound enables evaluation of vessels difficult to assess by angiographic techniques, including diffusely diseased segments and bifurcation or ostial lesions. The ability to directly image the atheroma within the vessel wall represents a truly unique capability not possible using any other commonly available imaging modality.

IMAGING TECHNOLOGY

【 】 CATHETER DESIGN

Intracoronary ultrasound equipment consists of two major components: a catheter incorporating a miniaturized transducer and a console containing the electronics necessary to reconstruct the image. High frequencies (20–50 MHz) are employed, resulting in excellent theoretical resolution (axially <100 μm and laterally <250 μm). Two dissimilar technical approaches to transducer design exist: mechanically ro-

tated devices and multielement electronic arrays. Each design has yielded small intravascular devices suitable for coronary imaging, typically ranging in size from approximately 2.6 to 3.5 Fr (diameter of 0.86–1.17 mm). Mechanical catheters contain a single transducer mechanically rotated at 1800 rpm, equivalent to 30 revolutions per second generating 30 images per second. To facilitate subselective coronary cannulation and catheter exchanges, ultrasound catheters provide a lumen for a guidewire. In phased array systems ultrasound crystals are placed circumferentially, obviating the need for rotation. Most systems generate images at a temporal frequency of 30 frames per second for recording on videotape.

【 】 LIMITATIONS AND ARTIFACTS

IVUS devices generate artifacts that may adversely affect image quality, alter interpretation, or reduce quantitative accuracy (Fig. 18–1).[11] Ring-down artifact arises from acoustic oscillations in the piezoelectric transducer, resulting in high-amplitude signals that preclude imaging close to the transducer surface. Accordingly, the *acoustic* size of catheters is slightly larger than their physical size. Because the minimum size of current devices is approximately 0.9 mm, some severe stenoses cannot be imaged prior to intervention. Geometric distortion can result from imaging in an oblique plane (not perpendicular to the long axis of the vessel), resulting in an elliptical rather than circular imaging plane.[12]

Mechanical, but not electronic, transducers may exhibit cyclical oscillations in rotational speed, resulting in an artifact known as nonuniform rotational distortion (NURD).[11] This artifact arises from mechanical friction within the catheter drive shaft during the portions of its rotational cycle. This speed variation produces readily visible distortion, often observed as circumferential stretching of a portion of the image with compression of the contralateral vessel wall (see Fig. 18–1). NURD is most evident when the drive shaft is bent into a small radius of curvature by a tortuous vessel. Improvements in the mechanical precision of ultrasound devices have reduced the impact of the artifact, but it still remains troublesome during some examinations.

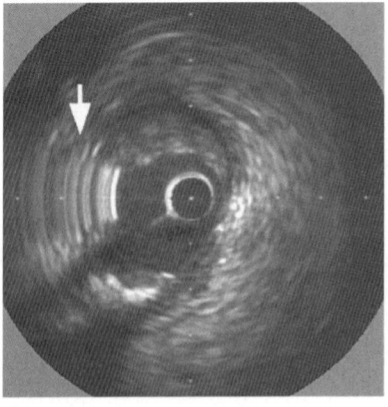 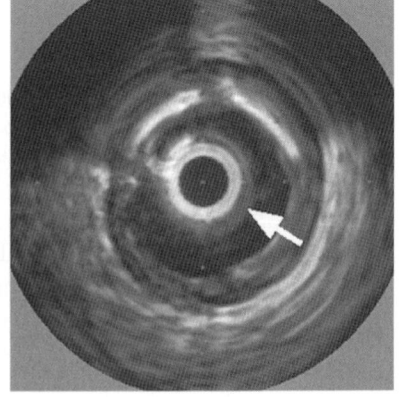

A   B

FIGURE 18–1. IVUS artifacts. In the *left panel,* there is an example of nonuniform rotational distortion (NURD) with circumferential *stretching* of the image from 8 to 10 o'clock (*arrow*). The *right panel* shows an example of ring-down artifact. IVUS, intravascular ultrasound.

CORONARY IMAGING

【 】 EXAMINATION TECHNIQUE

Standard interventional techniques for intracoronary catheter delivery are used for intraluminal ultrasound examination. Intravenous heparin and intracoronary nitroglycerin are routinely administered. Using a 6-Fr guiding catheter, the operator advances a guidewire into the target coronary artery. A stable guiding catheter position with good support is desirable, because current ultrasound catheters have less trackability and a larger profile than modern angioplasty equipment. The operator carefully advances or retracts the imaging catheter over the wire to examine the vessel in real time, recording images digitally or on other media such as videotape for subsequent quantitative or qualitative analysis. Side branches, visualized with both angiography and ultrasound, are often used as landmarks to facilitate interpretation. A motorized pullback device, which withdraws the catheter at a constant speed (between 0.25 and 1 mm/sec, but most often 0.5 mm/sec), is used to systematically assess the coronary artery. In clinical practice manual catheter movement for more prolonged and thorough examination of sites of interest is also used. However, in studies of atherosclerosis progression versus regression and in serial studies for interventional therapies, the motorized pullback is an integral feature of the investigative procedure. In this application during analysis of the motorized pullback, *slices* are selected at regular intervals (typically every 1 mm) and subsequently analyzed in a core laboratory. By comparing atheroma burden at a baseline examination with a similar study at follow up, the extent of disease progression or regression can be precisely characterized.

【 】 SAFETY OF CORONARY ULTRASOUND

Although IVUS requires intracoronary instrumentation, studies have demonstrated few serious untoward effects.[13–15] The most frequently encountered complication is focal coronary spasm, which usually responds rapidly to intracoronary nitroglycerin. Data from European centers report a 1.1 percent complication rate in 718 ultrasound examinations.[14] Another report from 28 centers (2207 studies) documents spasm in 2.9 percent and major complications, such as occlusion or dissection, judged to have a *certain relation* to instrumentation in 0.4 percent.[13] In both studies complications (spasm, vessel dissection, or guidewire entrapment) occurred in patients undergoing angioplasty rather than diagnostic imaging. In 170 cardiac transplant recipients (240 studies), there was no morbidity, but spasm occurred in 20 patients (8.3 percent) despite pretreatment with nitroglycerin.[15] Furthermore, the use of serial IVUS for the routine clinical surveillance of transplant vasculopathy does not accelerate angiographically evident transplant CAD.[16] Any intracoronary instrumentation carries the potential risk of intimal injury or vessel dissection. Accordingly, most laboratories limit credentialing for this procedure to personnel with interventional training.

【 】 NORMAL CORONARY ANATOMY

Studies performed either in vivo or using excised, pressure-distended vessels have characterized the appearance of normal coronaries by IVUS.[17,18] Important determinants of vessel wall appearance include both the normal arterial structure and the inherent properties of ultrasound. An ultrasound reflection occurs at a tissue boundary whenever there is an abrupt change in acoustic impedance. Normally, two strong acoustic interfaces are visualized by ultrasound, the leading edge of the intima (at the interface between the blood-filled lumen and the endothelium) and the outer border of the media (at the junction of media and external elastic membrane). Underlying the trailing edge of the intima, a middle sonolucent layer is usually evident, which is composed principally of the tunica media. The echodense intima and adventitia with a sonolucent medial layer often give the wall a trilaminar appearance. However, this pattern is not a universal finding; in 30 to 50 percent of normal segments, a thin intimal layer reflects ultrasound poorly, which results in a monolayer appearance (Fig. 18–2).[18] In a necropsy study, the ultrasound-derived intimal thickness in segments with three layers was significantly greater than for monolayered sites (0.24 ± 0.1 vs. 0.11 ± 0.06 mm, p <0.001). The mean age in the three-layered group was greater, 42.8 ± 9.8 vs. 27.1 ± 8.5 years (p <0.001).[19] Other studies demonstrate that a trilaminar appearance is dependent not only on the age but also on the histologic characteristics of the vessel. A three-layered appearance is consistently observed if an internal elastic membrane is present.[20] However, if an internal elastic membrane is absent, a trilaminar appearance is observed only when the collagen content of the media is low. In older *normal* subjects, intimal thickening usually results in a pattern of two distinct echogenic layers *sandwiching* a sonolucent intermediate layer. In nearly all cases, the deepest arterial layers exhibit a characteristic onionskin pattern, representing the adventitia and periadventitial tissues with an indistinct outer vessel border (see Fig. 18–2). In both normal and abnormal arteries, the lumen exhibits faint, finely textured, swirling echoes that arise from acoustic reflections from circulating blood elements. This blood *speckle* may assist image interpretation by providing a means to confirm the communication between dissection planes and the lumen. The pattern of blood speckle is dependent on the velocity of flow, showing increased intensity and a more coarse appearance when flow is reduced. In some cases the coarse blood speckle can mimic the appearance of tissue, complicating image interpretation. The physical presence of the ultrasound catheter may exacerbate this problem, particularly if there exists a stenosis with relatively severe narrowing proximal to the imaged site. In such cases the reduction of blood flow produced by partial obstruction of the proximal narrowing, may result in reduced blood flow at the imaged site, and the resulting coarse blood speckle may be misinterpreted at tissue protruding into the lumen.

CHARACTERIZATION OF ATHEROSCLEROSIS

【 】 ATHEROMA COMPOSITION

The subtle changes that occur early in the development of atherosclerosis, such as fatty streaks, are not visible using current ultrasound devices. Atherosclerotic arteries exhibit a variety of features that reflect the distribution, severity, and composition of the atheroma.[17] Sites with limited disease exhibit generalized or focal thickening of the intimal leading edge, whereas advanced lesions

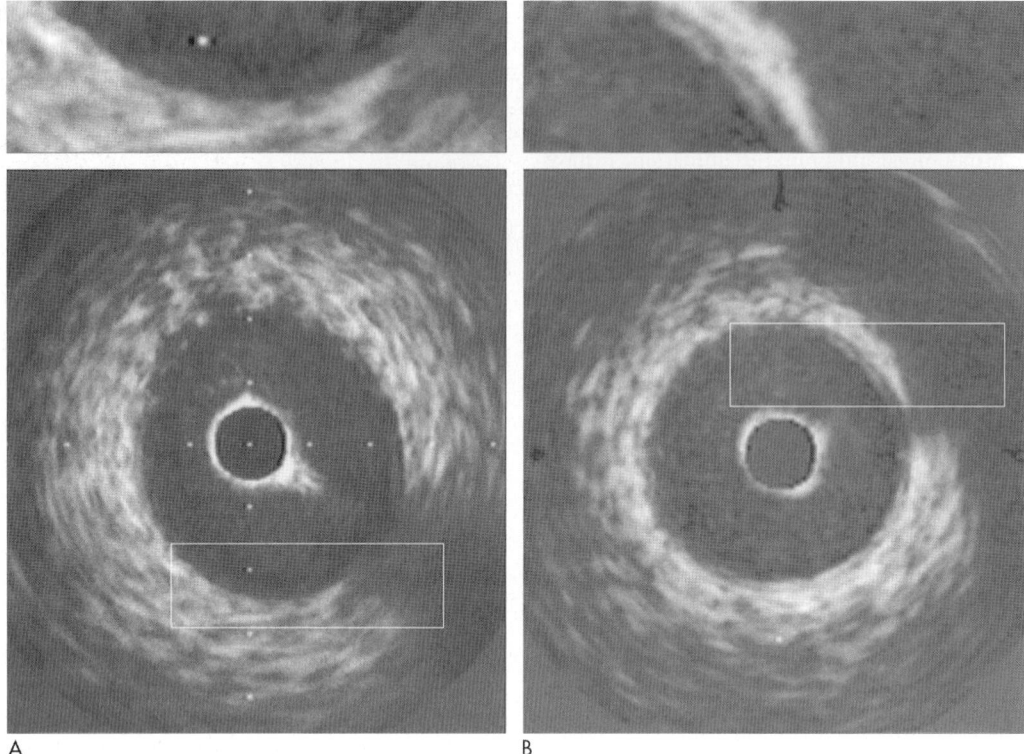

FIGURE 18–2. Two variants of normal coronary anatomy by IVUS. In both images a magnified view of the area contained within the rectangle is shown at the top. In the *left panel* there is a monolayered artery; in the *right panel* the artery has a trilaminar structure. IVUS, intravascular ultrasound.

appear as large echogenic masses encroaching on the lumen. A comparative study of ultrasound and histology in 1100 fresh necropsy sections demonstrated that lipid-laden lesions are usually hypoechoic.[17] Soft, low-intensity echoes most often represent fibromuscular lesions and very bright echoes are characteristic of dense fibrous or calcified tissues (Fig. 18–3). In highly echogenic plaques, areas of calcification are recognized by obstruction or severe attenuation of ultrasound penetration, which obscures deeper layers, a phenomenon known as *acoustic shadowing.*

The echogenicity of the plaque components is dependent not only on the acoustic properties of tissue but also on the acquisition settings (gain, compression, etc.). Accordingly, most morphologic classification schemes compare the echogenicity of the plaque to the surrounding adventitia to adjust for differences in ultrasound technique. However, in plaques containing a zone of reduced echogenicity, it is not possible to determine whether these represent areas of lipid deposition, thrombus, or necrotic degeneration, all of which can appear as zones of low density. Plaque composition was accurately predicted by ultrasound imaging in 96 percent of 112 quadrants from 21 freshly explanted human coronary arteries.[20] Fibrous and calcified plaque quadrants were correctly identified in almost all cases (100 of 103, or 97 percent), but only 7 of 9 quadrants (78 percent) with predominantly lipid deposits were correctly identified. Accordingly, some caution is warranted in the IVUS classification of atheroma composition using gray scale imaging. Although currently available devices produce detailed

views of the vessel wall, interpretation employs visual inspection of acoustic reflections to impute morphology. Different histologic features may exhibit comparable acoustic properties, and well-validated methods for objective or automated classification of atheromatous lesions do not yet exist. Thus, gray scale IVUS can delineate the thickness and echogenicity of vessel wall structures, but this technique does not provide actual histology.

More recently, sophisticated image processing techniques have been employed to classify the composition of atherosclerotic

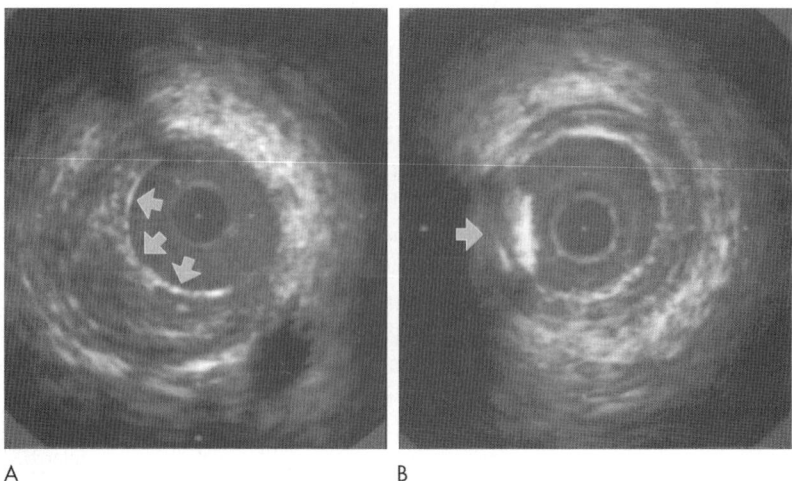

FIGURE 18–3. Atheroma morphology by IVUS. In the *left panel* a large, *soft,* lipid-laden atheroma with a thin fibrous cap is seen (*arrows*). It is eccentric, involving only approximately 50 percent of the vessel wall. The *right panel* shows a circumferential atheroma with an area of focal calcification is evident (*arrow*). IVUS, intravascular ultrasound.

plaques. The most promising methods employ analysis of raw radiofrequency data from ultrasound studies to assess the morphology of the atheroma.[21] Using necropsy specimens some recent investigations demonstrated that automated methods for characterization of atheroma morphology are more accurate and reproducible than methods based on simple visual inspection.[22] This accuracy has been further demonstrated in vivo using atheroma samples removed at the time of directional coronary atherectomy.[23] By plotting morphologic characteristics as a color overlay superimposed on the ultrasound image, such methods facilitate relatively facile image interpretation (Fig. 18–4).

Increasing application of radiofrequency analysis has been employed to investigate the vascular biology of atherosclerotic plaque in different clinical and remodeling settings. A number of groups have reported a greater proportion of lipid and necrotic core and less fibrotic tissue in patients with an acute coronary syndrome.[23,24] This is associated with a greater prevalence of lesions deemed to have thin fibrous caps.[25] Greater proportions of lipidic tissue were found in more proximal segments.[26] Further, lesions that demonstrate expansive remodeling, which are typically more often found in the setting of acute ischemic syndromes, contain greater amounts of lipidic and less fibrotic tissue.[27,28] The clinical implications of these findings require further exploration. An early report of the serial change in atheroma composition using radiofrequency analysis demonstrates a beneficial impact of statin therapy.[29] Fifty-two patients were randomized to treatment with pravastatin, atorvastatin, or diet for 6 months. Treatment with either statin was associated with a reduction in lipid core and greater fibrotic tissue compared with assessment at baseline. Further technological developments in this field provides the opportunity to assess the impact of emerging medical therapies on both the extent and composition of atherosclerotic plaque. Studies aimed at the definition of the natural history of atherosclerosis using tissue characterization are currently underway.

【 】 DETECTION OF CALCIFICATION

Ultrasound imaging is more sensitive than fluoroscopy or angiography for the detection of coronary calcification. In a series of 110 patients undergoing intervention, target lesion calcification was detected by ultrasound and fluoroscopy in 84 and 50 patients, respectively (76 vs. 14 percent, p <0.001).[30] Another retrospective study analyzed calcification by angiography and ultrasound in 183 interventional patients.[31] Assessment by the two techniques was concordant in 92 and discordant in 91 cases. Calcification was detected in 138 patients by ultrasound and 63 by fluoroscopy, showing a sensitivity and specificity for angiography of 46 and 82 percent, respectively. When calcium was detected angiographically, calcification by ultrasound often subtended >90 degrees and was superficial to the lumen in location. If no calcification could be visualized on the angiogram, the chance of detecting a large superficial arc of calcium by ultrasound was low (12 percent).

Most classification schemes quantify the extent of calcification, usually by measuring the circumferential angle subtended by calcified plaque.[30] Commonly, the axial length of the calcified portion

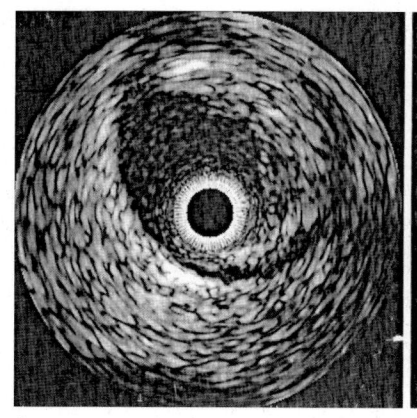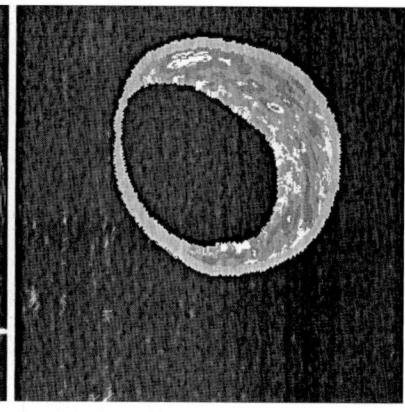

A   B

FIGURE 18–4. Ultrasonic characterization of plaque composition. The *left panel* shows a grayscale tomographic image of atherosclerotic plaque within the arterial wall. The *right panel* shows a tissue map of radiofrequency spectra from integrated backscatter analysis. The findings have been correlated with plaque components in ex vivo specimens.

of the lesion is also reported. The depth of calcification is also assessed, described as superficial when the calcium remains in contact with the luminal surface and deep if no portion of the calcium deposit is superficial. During initial development of IVUS, the extent of calcification was often utilized in the selection of interventional devices, particularly as a means to select vessels suitable for directional coronary atherectomy. However, in recent years the reduced importance of directional atherectomy and the nearly universal application of coronary stenting has lessened the importance of calcification as a determinant of the interventional approach. Accordingly, in current practice, IVUS is uncommonly performed solely as a means to detect coronary calcification.

【 】 ARTERIAL REMODELING

The term *arterial remodeling* refers to a change in arterial dimensions associated with the development of atherosclerosis. In a necropsy study of 136 human left main coronary arteries, Glagov and colleagues originally described focal arterial enlargement at atherosclerotic sites, reporting a positive correlation between external elastic membrane (EEM) area and the area occupied by atheroma (r = 0.44, p <0.001).[7] At sites with area stenosis <40 percent, the increase in arterial size *overcompensated* for the plaque deposition, leading to an increase in absolute lumen area. The conventional view has held that with more advanced lesions (area stenosis >40 percent), the degree of arterial enlargement or remodeling was blunted, resulting in a smaller lumen area. The authors hypothesized that this phenomenon represented a compensatory mechanism to preserve lumen size.

The findings of Glagov and coworkers were later confirmed in vivo by IVUS imaging (Fig. 18–5).[32] In 80 ultrasound cross sections obtained from 44 patients undergoing coronary interventions, EEM area correlated closely with plaque area (r = 0.79, p = 0.0001). In this study lumen area increased with early atherosclerosis, confirming the phenomenon of overcompensation in early stages of the disease. With more advanced atherosclerosis, there was a correlation between increasing area stenosis and decreasing lumen area (r = 0.58, p = 0.0001).[32] Enlargement has also been

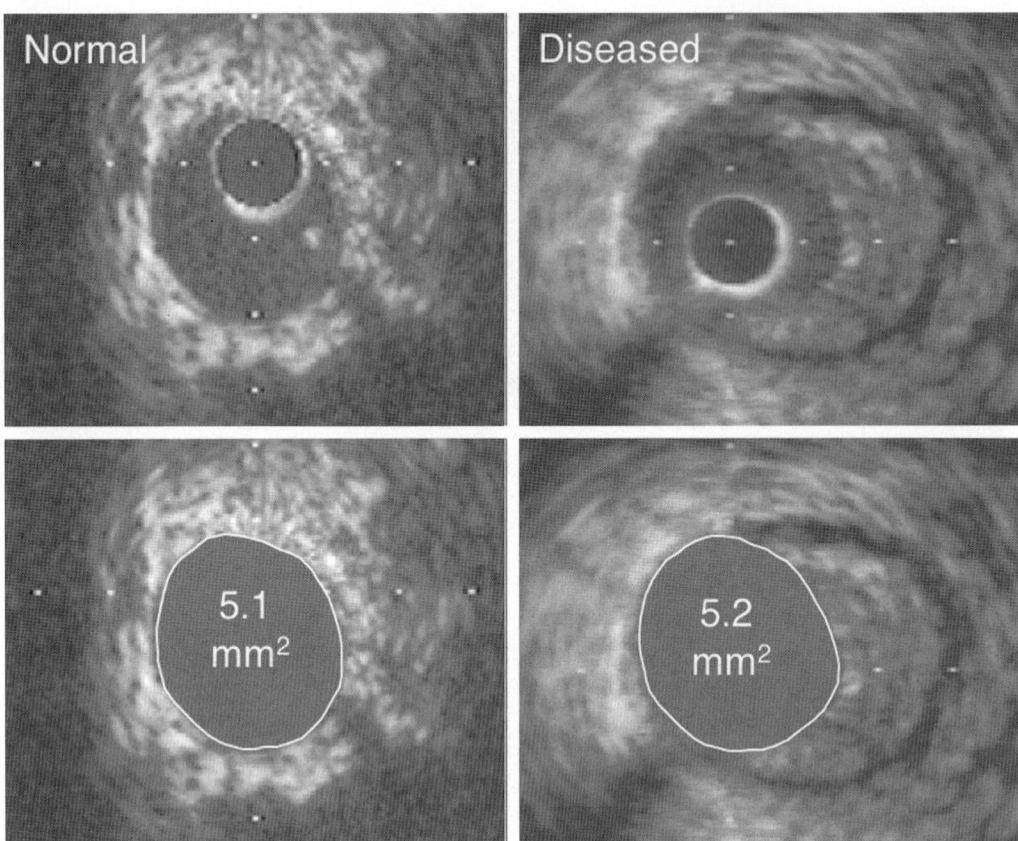

FIGURE 18-5. Example of coronary remodeling. The *left upper panel* shows a normal segment of the circumflex coronary. In the *right upper panel,* an atherosclerotic segment of the coronary a few millimeters proximal to the normal segment is shown. In the bottom two panels, measurements taken at each of the sites show very similar cross-sectional areas. The preservation of luminal area results in a coronary angiogram that is normal despite the presence of a large atherosclerotic plaque in the involved segment.

demonstrated by ultrasound in superficial femoral arteries; however, there was no difference between lesions less than and greater than 40 percent stenosis.[33] Reports have demonstrated the presence of positive remodeling beyond an area stenosis >40 percent. A review of 128 focal lesions that underwent progression in patients receiving statin therapy demonstrated that the EEM area increased with plaque area, regardless of whether the area stenosis was less than or greater than 40 percent.[34]

In recent years, ultrasound studies have demonstrated a new dimension to arterial remodeling, the phenomenon of *negative* remodeling.[35,36] At diseased sites the EEM area may actually be reduced in size, contributing to luminal narrowing, rather than compensating for it. In 51 femoral arteries, EEM area was smaller at lesions than adjacent reference sites, with a negative correlation between stenosis severity and EEM area reduction ($r = 0.62$ by histology and 0.66 by ultrasound, $p <0.001$ for both).[35] *Inadequate* remodeling, defined as an EEM area within the lesion <78 percent of a proximal reference site, has also been described in the coronaries of patients with stable angina.[36] Although 91 of 603 lesions (15 percent) fit this definition, there was a highly variable response among lesions within the same patient. However, when remodeling is defined in this fashion, there is an assumption that the reference EEM area represents the original vessel size, which may not be correct, because angiographic reference sites are frequently diseased by ultrasound.

Although the exact mechanisms of positive (expansive) or negative remodeling remain unclear, these phenomena have important clinical implications. Positive remodeling represents an important factor in the underestimation of the severity of atherosclerosis by angiography. Thus, a vessel site may contain a very large atheroma but minimal stenosis if outward remodeling of the EEM has *compensated* for the plaque accumulation. Recent evidence suggest such sites may be particularly prone to plaque rupture. Because remodeling can affect both the lesion and adjacent reference segments, remodeling may also influence the estimation of the vessel size during coronary interventions. Recently, negative remodeling has been implicated in restenosis following atherectomy and balloon angioplasty.[37]

The emerging role of serial IVUS to monitor potential regression of atherosclerosis in response to a range of medical therapies provides an opportunity to investigate vascular remodeling that accompanies reductions in atheroma volume. Several reports have described the presence of reverse remodeling in association with atheroma regression. The rapid regression of coronary atheroma that was observed in patients who received intravenous infusions of synthetic high-density lipoprotein (HDL) containing recombinant apolipoprotein A-I Milano (apoA-I Milano) was accompanied by a 4.6 percent reduction in EEM volume, without any change in lumen volume.[38] Changes in atheroma volume correlated with changes in EEM volume but not the lumen. This result was confirmed by a similar finding in 432 patients receiving lipid-lowering therapy.[39] The findings that reverse remodeling of the EEM, without any changes in lumen dimensions, in the setting of atheroma regression highlights the importance of imaging modalities that visualize the arterial wall, rather than the lumen, to assess the potential impact of medical therapies. Furthermore, this highlights one possible mechanism that contributes to the *regression paradox* in which the benefits of preventive therapies on clinical events appears to be substantially greater than their impact on angiographic abnormalities.

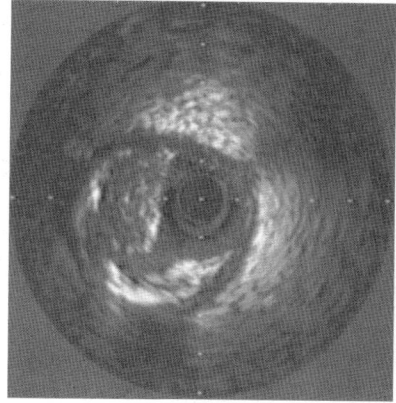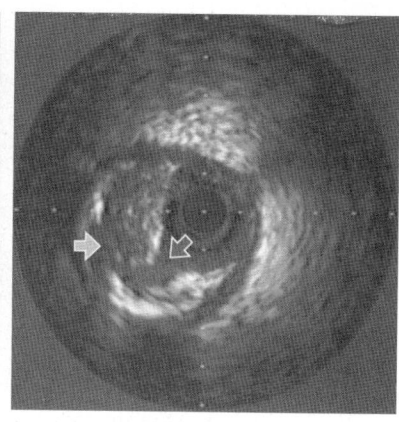

FIGURE 18–6. Ruptured coronary plaque. In these two identical images, the anatomy of a ruptured coronary plaque is seen. There is a large lipid core with a fracture of the fibrous cap (*right panel, arrow*). This image was obtained a few days after hospitalization of this patient for an unstable coronary syndrome.

【 】 UNSTABLE PLAQUE AND THROMBI

An emerging application of intracoronary ultrasound is the characterization of the atheroma associated with acute coronary syndromes (Fig. 18–6).[40–42] The typical angiographic appearance of a ruptured plaque is a stenosis with an eccentric or ulcerated lumen, often with overhanging edges (Ambrose type II lesion). However, retrospective reviews of angiograms of patients performed before an episode of unstable angina often do not reveal severe stenosis severity within the culprit lesion segment.[41] Such studies highlight the inability of angiography to identify *rupture-prone* atherosclerotic lesions. Histologic examination of unstable plaques after rupture usually reveals a lipid-laden plaque with a thin fibrous cap.[40] Based on these observations, it has been postulated that the size of the lipid pool and the thickness of the fibrous cap are more important than severity of stenosis in predicting plaque rupture.[42] Some IVUS studies have suggested the presence of an echolucent atheroma within culprit lesions in patients with acute coronary syndromes. In a very limited study of 22 stable and 43 unstable angina patients, type II eccentric lesions were detected on the angiograms in 18 percent of stable and 40 percent of unstable angina patients. Echolucent plaques were more frequently observed in patients with unstable than in those with stable angina syndromes (74 vs. 41 percent, *p* <0.01).[1] However, this finding has not been confirmed by other investigators. Several groups have reported the presence of numerous sites of plaque rupture throughout the coronary tree in patients who undergo IVUS in the setting of an acute coronary syndrome.[43] This provides further support for the concept that atherosclerosis and its complications represent a systemic process and the need for therapeutic strategies that act protect the entire arterial tree.

Recent IVUS studies have examined the relationship between remodeling and the type of clinical presentation, suggesting difference in the remodeling pattern for unstable versus stable patients.[44] The culprit lesions in 76 patients with acute coronary syndromes were compared with lesions in 40 patients with stable angina. In the unstable patients, both EEM and plaque areas were significantly larger than the corresponding measurements in the stable patients (*p* = 0.02 for both). Positive remodeling was more prevalent in the unstable group (51 vs. 18 percent, *p* = 0.002) and negative remodeling more prevalent in the stable group (58 vs. 33 percent, *p* = 0.002). In a further report of 254 patients plaque rupture sites were demonstrated to larger EEM and lumen areas, in association with a greater incidence of positive remodeling than lesions containing the smallest lumen area.[45] These findings provide further insight into the relationship between lesion severity and the likelihood of plaque rupture. Because angiographic studies suggested that minimal stenoses were associated with atheroma rupture, most investigators assumed that the culprit lesion represented a small plaque. However, the finding that rupture sites frequently exhibit positive remodeling suggests that such lesions are not particularly small plaques. Rather, the presence of remodeling enables the atheroma to reach a large size without compromising the lumen.

The formation of intraluminal thrombi at a ruptured or fissured plaque is considered the hallmark of acute coronary syndromes.[46] Angiographic criteria for diagnosis of a coronary thrombus, the presence of haziness, an intraluminal filling defect, and/or irregular lumen contour are not sensitive.[43] Small observational studies have attempted to differentiate the ultrasound appearance of thrombus, defined as hypoechoic material projecting into the lumen with a slight synchronous pulsation and a distinct acoustic interface, from more echogenic plaque (Fig. 18–7).[45] However, in vitro studies have revealed limitations in the reliability of IVUS diagnosis of thrombi (sensitivity of 57 percent and specificity of 91 percent), considerably inferior to angioscopy (sensitivity and specificity of 100 percent).[47]

Innovative new technologies targeting tissue characterization using radiofrequency and back scatter analysis have the potential to increase our understanding of all discussed issues substantially.

DIAGNOSTIC CLINICAL APPLICATIONS

【 】 QUANTITATIVE LUMINAL MEASUREMENTS

A broad spectrum of therapeutic decisions hinge on assessment of coronary luminal dimensions. Accordingly, in diagnostic and interventional practice, quantitation of vascular dimensions represents a common clinical application of IVUS. A committee of the American College of Cardiology and the European Society of Cardiology defined standards for the acquisition, measurement, and reporting of IVUS studies.[48] This standards document defines the terminology and methodology for performing IVUS measure-

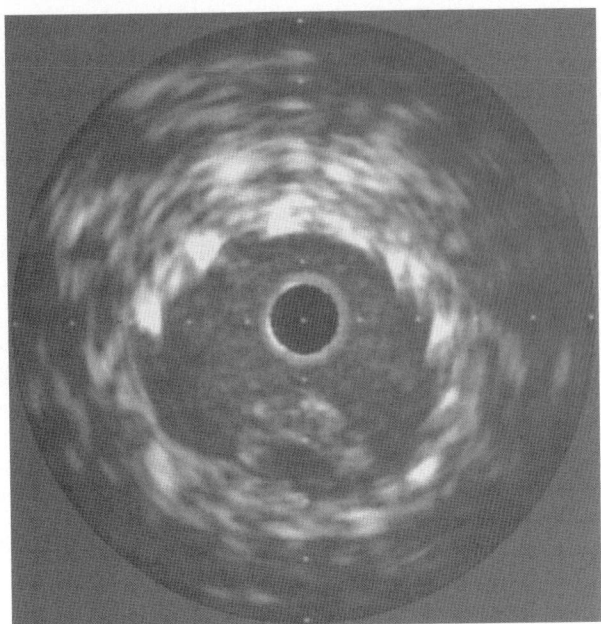

FIGURE 18-7. Thrombus within a coronary stent. In this IVUS image, a stent is well visualized. There is a globular mass projecting into the lumen at 6 o'clock; it probably represents a large thrombus. IVUS, intravascular ultrasound.

ments and constitutes the recognized standard for both clinical and research studies. The presence of standardized nomenclature and measurement methods represents a critical advance in the wider acceptance of IVUS.

Several studies have compared luminal measurements by IVUS and quantitative angiography.[1] For vessels without atherosclerosis, most studies document a relatively close correlation between angiographic and ultrasonic coronary dimensions, but a few studies suggest slightly larger measurements by ultrasound.[1] However, in patients with atherosclerotic arteries, most investigators report only a moderate correlation between ultrasonic and angiographic dimensions, with the greatest disparities in vessel segments with a noncircular lumen shape.[2] This reduced correlation is probably explained by the irregular, noncircular cross-sectional profile of diseased vessels, which cannot be adequately measured using angiography.[2]

[ ] QUANTITATION OF ATHEROSCLEROSIS

Analysis of IVUS images permits quantitative measurements of the extent and severity of coronary atherosclerosis (Fig. 18–8).[10] However, the inherent properties of ultrasound require use of different anatomic landmarks than those employed in classical histology. In all ultrasound imaging, reflections at the leading edge of any interface are located precisely at the boundary where acoustic impedance abruptly changes. However, the position of the trailing edge of any anatomic structure is determined by multiple nonanatomic factors, including ultrasound beam properties, particularly the wavelength (frequency). Thus, leading-edge measurements accurately describe the location of a boundary, whereas trailing-edge mea-

surements are unreliable. As previously noted, strong reflections are generally produced at two locations, the leading edge of the intima and the border between the media and the external elastic membrane. The position of the trailing edge of the intima is not accurately localized in IVUS images. Accordingly, quantitative measurements must calculate the atheroma's cross-sectional area by subtracting the area bounded by the intimal leading edge from the area enclosed by the external elastic membrane. This approach results in a slight overestimation of atheroma area (in comparison to histology) by including the area of the media within the calculation.

[ ] NORMAL INTIMAL THICKNESS

The threshold for abnormal intimal thickness by IVUS is controversial, particularly because the categorical classification of a continuous variable intimal thickness as normal and abnormal is inherently arbitrary. In various histologic and ultrasound studies, normal intimal thickness ranges between 0.10 and 0.35 mm, and the normal medial thickness ranges from 0.15 to 0.25 mm. In a necropsy study, normal intimal thickness not including media was age-dependent, averaging 0.21 mm in 21- to 25-year-olds, 0.22 mm in 26- to 30-year-olds, and 0.25 mm in 36- to 40-year-olds.[19] In a comparative study, IVUS measurements of the intima plus media averaged 20 percent greater than histologic measurements.[49] In a study of 262 recently transplanted patients, normal intimal thickness by IVUS was shown to be <0.3 mm in younger hearts (<40 years) and less than 0.5 mm in older hearts (>40 years).[50] Considering the histologic and ultrasound data, most clinical studies have defined threshold for coronary disease by ultrasound as a measured intimal thickness ≥0.5 mm.[51,52]

[ ] ASSESSMENT OF ATHEROMA BURDEN

The tomographic orientation of IVUS represents a problem in quantifying atherosclerosis. Since each image contains informa-

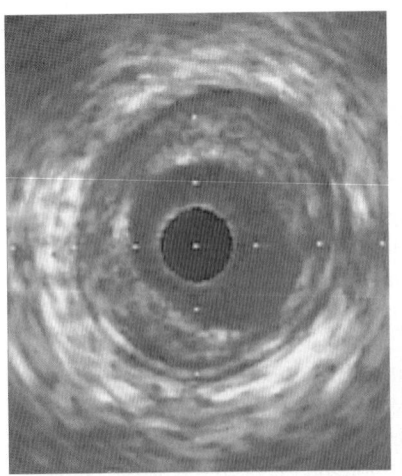 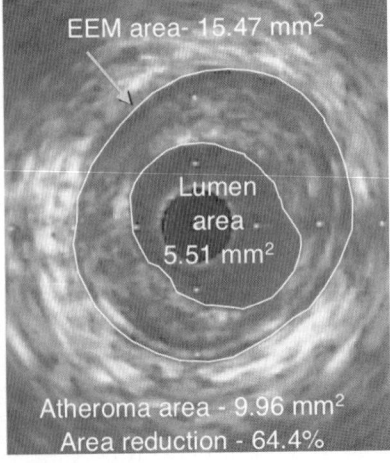

FIGURE 18-8. Boundaries for IVUS measurements. In these two identical images, an atherosclerotic plaque is well visualized. The *right panel* illustrates the planimetry typically employed to measure the extent of atherosclerotic disease. Both the lumen and external elastic membrane (EEM) are measured. The atheroma area represents the difference between the EEM and the lumen areas. The area reduction is calculated as the atheroma area divided by the EEM area multiplied by 100. IVUS, intravascular ultrasound.

tion from only a thin "slice" of the vessel, global measures of atheroma burden require the integration of multiple cross sections. One successful approach to this conundrum employs a motorized device to steadily and progressively withdraw the ultrasound catheter through the interrogated vessel, typically at 0.5 mm/sec. Since motor speed is kept constant, the operator can obtain a series of cross sections separated by a constant, recurring time interval (fixed distance from each other). A number of measures have been employed to determine the volumetric extent of atheroma (Fig. 18–9). Cross-sectional slices are individually measured and the atheroma areas summated to calculate total atheroma volume (TAV) using the Simpson rule:

$$TAV = \sum (EEM_{CSA} - Lumen_{CSA})$$

Given that evaluated segments are defined by the anatomic location of side branches, there is likely to be substantial heterogeneity in segment length between subjects. To account for this, TAV is normalized using the following formula:

$$TAV_{norm} = \sum \frac{(EEM_{CSA} - Lumen_{CSA})}{n} \times \frac{median\ number}{images\ population}$$

where n is the number of images measured in an individual pullback. Alternatively, atheroma burden can be expressed as percent atheroma volume (PAV), which is calculated as atheroma volume in proportion to the volume occupied by the external elastic membrane (EEM) using the following formula:

$$PAV = \frac{\sum (EEM_{CSA} - Lumen_{CSA})}{\sum EEM_{CSA}} \times 100$$

A number of additional measures of atheroma burden can be derived at the time of image analysis. These include the atheroma volume in the 10-mm segment containing the greatest amount of plaque at baseline and maximum plaque thickness.

ATHEROMA DISTRIBUTION

The circumferential distribution of the atheroma varies from nearly symmetrical plaques to eccentric lesions in which the entire atheroma is located on one side of the artery. Assessed by ultrasound, most plaques are eccentric, with a maximum atheroma thickness more than twice the minimum plaque thickness.[53] Studies have demonstrated a poor correlation between the apparent circumferential pattern by angiography and the actual plaque distribution revealed by ultrasound examination.[53]

ANGIOGRAPHICALLY UNRECOGNIZED DISEASE

In patients undergoing angiography for clinically suspected CAD, no angiographic evidence of narrowing is present in 10 to 15 per-

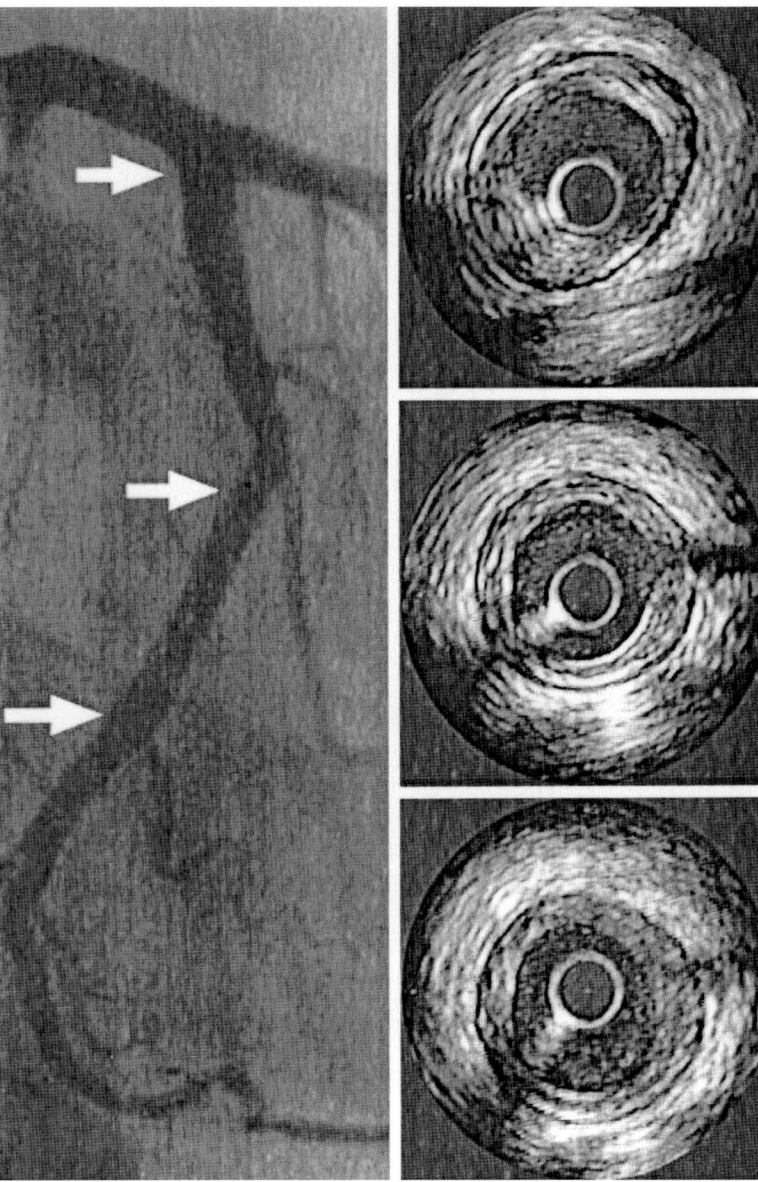

FIGURE 18–9. Measurement of atheroma volume. Withdrawal of the ultrasonic catheter through a segment of artery generates a series of tomographic images. Atheroma area is measured in images spaced precisely 1 mm apart and summated to determine atheroma volume. Monitoring the rate of plaque progression requires matching of the segment of interest at different time points. This is achieved by defining the limits of the segment by the anatomic location of a distal and proximal side branch. Upper (proximal fiduciary point), middle (midsegment), and lower (distal fiduciary point) *arrows* on the angiogram represent the corresponding tomographic ultrasound image on the right that is selected for analysis.

cent of cases. In these patients IVUS commonly detects atherosclerosis at angiographically normal sites.[6,10,54,55] Using IVUS atherosclerotic abnormalities were documented in 21 of 44 patients (48 percent) with suspected CAD and normal coronary angiograms.[54] Combining ultrasound and functional assessment (coronary flow reserve and endothelium-mediated vasodilator response), only 36 percent of patients in this cohort were completely normal. Other studies demonstrate that if any luminal irregularity is present by angiography, ultrasound usually demonstrates atherosclerosis (Fig. 18–10).[6]

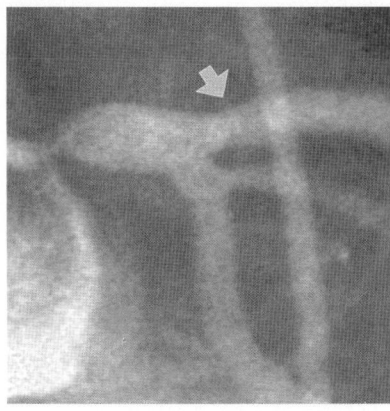
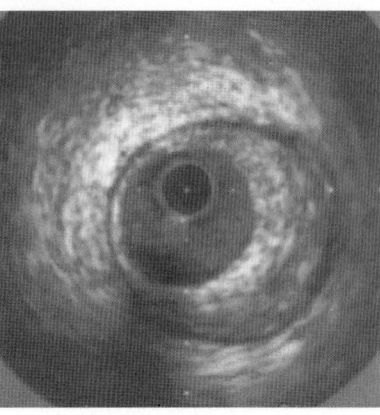

FIGURE 18–10. Underestimation of coronary atherosclerosis by angiography. In the angiogram in the left panel, a relatively minor lesion of the left anterior descending coronary is seen (*arrow*). In the right panel, this lesion is depicted by IVUS and consists of a large eccentric atherosclerotic plaque that appears much more extensive than would be suspected from the angiogram. IVUS, intravascular ultrasound.

【 】 PREVALENCE OF CORONARY ATHEROSCLEROSIS

Recent IVUS studies have demonstrated an extraordinary prevalence of coronary atherosclerosis in the general population, beginning at a relatively young age.[50] In the most thorough study, IVUS was performed in 262 transplant recipients within 31 days of transplantation to determine the prevalence of atherosclerotic disease in the donor hearts. These heart transplant donors (116 women and 146 men) had a mean age of 33 years and no known CAD. Imaging of multiple coronary segments was performed to determine the greatest and least intimal thickness in each segment for an average of 2.3 coronary arteries per patient. Assessment of 2014 sites in 1477 segments of 574 coronary arteries showed that atherosclerotic lesions, defined as an intimal thickness ≥0.5 mm, were present in 51.9 percent of donor hearts. Intimal thickness correlated with donor age with the prevalence of disease ranging from 17 percent for donors aged younger than 20 years to 85 percent in those aged at least 50 years (Fig. 18–11). For all age groups, average intimal thickness was greater in male than female donors, but similar proportions (52 and 51.7 percent) had atherosclerosis. Coronary angiography was completely normal in 92 percent of these subjects and none of the donors aged younger than 30 years had angiographic evidence of atherosclerosis.

【 】 LESIONS OF UNCERTAIN SEVERITY

Angiographers commonly encounter lesions that elude accurate characterization despite thorough examination using multiple radiographic projections. Difficult-to-assess sites include ostial or bifurcation lesions and moderate stenoses (angiographic severity ranging from 40–75 percent) in patients whose symptomatic status is difficult to evaluate. For ambiguous lesions ultrasound provides a tomographic perspective, independent of the radiographic projection, that may permit quantification of the lesion. In two prospective series,

intracoronary ultrasound changed the management strategy in approximately 20 percent of the examinations performed immediately prior to coronary intervention.[56] In both studies, however, operator selection of patients for ultrasound examination may have resulted in an overestimation of the true impact of ultrasound imaging on clinical decision making.

Functional approaches using pressure or flow measurements by Doppler wires have been employed to identify intermediate lesions of potential hemodynamic significance for intervention. Identification of lesions with a fractional flow reserve (FFR) >0.75 is typically consistent with no significant hemodynamic abnormality and favorable clinical outcome if treated medically.[57] The use of specific threshold criteria for intervention derived by IVUS measurements have not been prospectively validated with noninvasive assessments of myocardial ischemia. It appears that a minimal lumen area in the range of 3 to 4 mm^2 correlates with a significant reduction in FFR.[58,59] Different protocols to induce hyperemia and inclusion of a limited number of subjects in this intermediate range make it difficult to directly compare results from different cohorts studied. The finding that a minimal area in excess of 4 mm^2 is associated with a favorable clinical outcome has led many to regard this as the threshold for the assessment of lesions of intermediate severity on angiography.[60] Further, combination of minimal area with another parameter such as minimal lumen diameter of 1.8 mm or percent area stenosis of 70 percent might potentially be useful.[59]

Angiographic assessment of left main coronary artery (LMCA) obstruction represents a particularly vexing clinical problem. Radiographic contrast in the aortic cusp can obscure the ostium, and *streaming* of contrast from the injection vortex can result in a false impression of luminal narrowing. The LMCA is often short in length, leaving no normal reference segment. The bifurcation or trifurcation of the LMCA into daughter branches may produce vessel overlap, thereby concealing a stenosis. IVUS is commonly

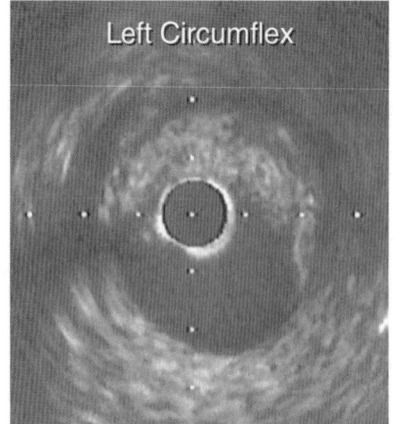
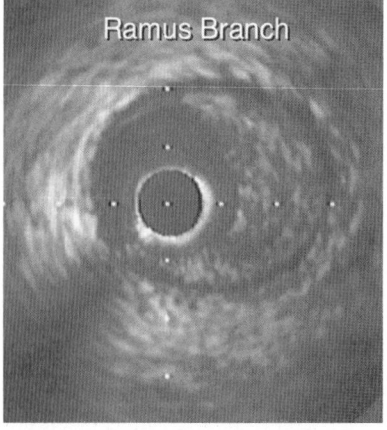

FIGURE 18–11. Atherosclerosis in a heart transplant donor. The heart was harvested from a 32-year-old woman who suffered brain death following a motor vehicle accident. In both the left circumflex coronary (*left panel*) and the ramus branch (*right panel*), there is extensive atherosclerosis.

used to quantify LMCA lesions when angiographic interpretation is uncertain.[61] The technique for examination consists of subselective placement of the ultrasound transducer in the circumflex or anterior descending, followed by slow pullback to the aorta with the guiding catheter disengaged. Although there is no consensus regarding the threshold for critical LMCA obstruction, a number of groups have attempted to address this issue. Given the larger caliber of the LMCA, different criteria are likely to be applicable compared with the remainder of the coronary tree. In a study that aimed to correlate ultrasound and hemodynamic measurements in the LMCA, it was demonstrated that a minimal lesion diameter of 2.8 mm and minimal lumen area of 5.9 mm^2 predicted a hemodynamically significant lesion.[62] This was further supported by the finding of a low clinical event rate in subjects with a minimal lumen diameter of >3 mm.[63] A recent report suggested that the threshold might be higher with a minimal area of 7.5 mm^2.[64] However, this did not correlate with any functional assessment of hemodynamic significance and was derived according to calculation of the mean and two standard deviations of minimal lumen area in a cohort of subjects with LMCA that were free of atherosclerotic disease.

CARDIAC ALLOGRAFT DISEASE

Transplant CAD is the leading cause of death beyond the first year after cardiac transplantation, with a reported incidence of 15 to 20 percent per year.[65] Although most transplant centers perform arteriograms annually for screening, these surveillance studies often fail to detect atherosclerosis prior to a clinical event.[66] Necropsy studies have demonstrated that angiography systematically underestimates coronary atherosclerosis in transplant recipients.[66] Patients may have diffuse vessel involvement that, for reasons already enumerated, conceals the atherosclerosis from the angiographer. Many active transplant centers incorporated IVUS imaging into their posttransplant surveillance, but there is no consensus on how frequent IVUS should be performed. Investigations using ultrasound to detect transplant vasculopathy report a very high incidence of abnormal intimal thickening, involving 80 percent of patients at 1 year and more than 92 percent studied 4 or more years after transplantation.[52,67]

Recent studies have revealed two pathways to transplant-associated atherosclerosis. Some patients receive atherosclerotic plaques transmitted via the donor heart, whereas others develop an immune-mediated vasculopathy.[50,52,68] In the first year after transplantation, progression occurred in 42 percent of patients.[67] The silent progression of vasculopathy in transplant recipients is associated with a poor clinical outcome. In a review of 143 patients who underwent transplantation at a single center, rapid progression of vasculopathy detected by serial IVUS was associated with a higher mortality rate.[69] The progression of vasculopathy when studied at 12 months following transplantation demonstrated higher rates of death, graft loss and nonfatal major cardiac events in a multicenter cohort of 125 patients.[70]

Serial intravascular ultrasonography has been employed to assess the potential efficacy of therapeutic strategies that target the inflammatory and proliferative events that promote the development of vasculopathy. Everolimus is an immunomodulating and antiproliferative agent of potential usefulness in heart transplanta-

tion recipients. In a randomized controlled trial, first-time transplant recipients received azathioprine 1 to 3 mg/kg or everolimus 1.5 or 3 mg daily, in combination with cyclosporine, corticosteroids, and statins. Less clinical events, including death, graft loss, retransplantation, biopsy, proven acute rejection, or rejection with hemodynamic compromise, were recorded in patients receiving either dose of everolimus compared with azathioprine. In a complimentary finding, the average increase in maximal intimal thickness and incidence of vasculopathy (increase in maximal plaque thickness greater than 0.5 mm compared with baseline) were lower in everolimus treated patients.[71]

MONITORING PROGRESSION OF ATHEROSCLEROSIS

Precise quantitation of the extent of atheroma within an arterial segment at different time points using serial IVUS provides a unique opportunity to investigate the factors that influence the natural history of atheroma progression. Early studies investigated the relationship between atherosclerotic risk factors and rate of progression of atheroma area at a single cross-sectional site.[72] These studies demonstrated that the level of low-density lipoprotein cholesterol (LDL-C) and global risk scores predicted the rate of progression of atheroma at that specific site. Technological advances have resulted in the ability to accurately quantify the volumetric extent of plaque within a segment of coronary artery and to investigate changes in atheroma volume over time. Using this approach it has recently demonstrated that individual risk factors are poor predictors of the volume of coronary atheroma.[73] Serial ultrasonography provides an exciting opportunity to monitor the rate of atheroma progression as an efficacy measure in clinical trials of emerging antiatherosclerotic therapies. Several completed studies have assessed the impact of modifying traditional risk factors and novel pathologic targets on the rate of plaque progression.

EFFECT OF INTENSIVE LIPID LOWERING

Despite the unequivocal therapeutic efficacy of lowering LDL-C with inhibitors of hydroxymethylglutaryl coenzyme A reductase (statins), considerable debate has focused on whether an incremental benefit would be obtained from intensive LDL-C lowering with high-dose statin therapy. An early study of a small cohort of patients studied the impact of LDL-C lowering with atorvastatin compared with usual care in the German Atorvastatin Intravascular Ultrasound (GAIN) study.[74] Despite a lower on-treatment level of LDL-C (86 vs. 140 mg/dL), the rate of change of atheroma volume was not reduced in atorvastatin-treated patients. However, the increase in hyperechogenicity index was greater with atorvastatin suggesting that LDL-C lowering was associated with a beneficial influence on plaque composition. In the Reversal of Atherosclerosis with Aggressive Lipid Lowering (REVERSAL) study, 502 patients with angiographically established CAD and LDL-C between 125 and 210 mg/dL were randomized to receive treatment with an intensive lipid-lowering strategy with atorvastatin 80 mg daily or a moderate lipid lowering strategy with pravastatin 40 mg daily for 18 months.[75] LDL-C levels were lowered to 110 mg/dL with pravastatin and to 79 mg/dL with atorvastatin. This was associated with a significant difference between treatment groups with regard to the rate of atheroma progression. Atheroma volume increased by 2.7 percent in pravastatin-treated patients consistent with atheroma progression. In contrast the 0.4 percent reduction in atheroma volume in atorvastatin-treated patients did not differ from the baseline value, suggesting that intensive LDL-C lowering halted progression of atherosclerosis.

Subsequent analysis revealed a direct relationship between the degree of LDL-C lowering and change in rate of atheroma volume.[75] It was further noted that this relationship differed when studied for each of the two treatment arms. Patients treated with pravastatin required an incremental lowering of LDL-C of approximately 30 mg/dL to achieve the same effect on plaque progression as patients treated with atorvastatin. This finding suggested that the difference between these therapeutic agents on plaque progression was derived from factors beyond LDL-C lowering. The subsequent finding that levels of CRP were lowered to a greater degree by atorvastatin (36 vs. 5 percent) and the direct relationship between changes in CRP and atheroma volume support the concept that some of the benefit of statin therapy may be due to in vivo anti-inflammatory properties.[76] These findings complemented the results of the Pravastatin or Atorvastatin Evaluation and Infection Therapy (PROVE-IT) study, which compared the ability of identical therapeutic regimens to reduce clinical event rates in patients with an acute coronary syndrome.[77] The greatest benefit in terms of reducing clinical events and halting atheroma progression was observed in patients who derived the greatest degree of lowering of both LDL-C and CRP.[76,78]

This beneficial effect was extended further by the report of plaque regression in response to very intensive lipid modification in A Study to Evaluate the Effect of Rosuvastatin on Intravascular Ultrasound-Derived Coronary Atheroma Burden (ASTEROID) trial.[79] Patients with angiographic CAD were treated with rosuvastatin 40 mg daily for 24 months. This resulted in lowering of LDL-C to 60.8 mg/dL and elevation of high-density lipoprotein-cholesterol (HDL-C) by 14.7 percent, with a resulting reduction in the LDL-C/HDL-C ratio by 58 percent. These lipid effects were associated with significant reductions in all measures of atheroma burden, including percent atheroma volume (0.79 percent), total atheroma volume (6.8 percent) and the atheroma volume in the 10-mm segments containing the greatest amount of plaque at baseline (5.6 mm³), consistent with unequivocal atheroma regression (Fig. 18–12). This complemented the findings of several small studies that reported atheroma regression with statin therapy. In the ESTABLISH study, 70 patients who underwent emergency percutaneous intervention in the setting of an acute coronary syndrome were randomized to treatment with atorvastatin or placebo for 6 months.[80] The 41.7 percent reduction in LDL-C was associated with a 13.1 percent reduction in atheroma volume, whereas an increased volume by 8.7 percent, consistent with plaque progression, was observed in placebo-treated patients. Similarly, a Danish study reported regression of atheroma volume by 6.3 percent that accompanied reduction in LDL-C levels by 42.6 percent in 40 males who were treated with simvastatin for 12 months.[81] In combination

these findings provide further support for the concept that in patients with established CAD, LDL-C levels should be reduced as low as can be safely achieved. Furthermore, the findings compliment the growing body of evidence that demonstrate a beneficial effect of intensive lipid lowering on clinical event rates.[82,83]

EFFECT OF INFUSING HIGH-DENSITY LIPOPROTEIN

Population[84] and animal[85] studies have established the atheroprotective properties of high-density lipoprotein cholesterol (HDL-C). The therapeutic strategies currently available for the promotion of HDL-C levels is limited. In a proof-of-concept study, infusion of synthetic HDL-C particles containing the variant apolipoprotein, apoA-I Milano, complexed with phospholipids (ETC-216), promoted rapid regression of coronary atherosclerosis.[86] Forty-seven patients within 2 weeks of an acute coronary syndrome received weekly intravenous infusions of either saline or ETC-216 containing either 15 or 45 mg/kg of protein. Follow-up ultrasonic imaging within 2 weeks of the final infusion revealed a significant 4.2 percent reduction in atheroma volume in ETC-216–treated subjects compared with baseline. Subsequent analysis demonstrated that the atheroma regression associated with administration of ETC-216 was accompanied by contraction of the EEM, without any change in lumen dimensions.[38] This further highlights the importance of employing modalities that visualize the arterial wall rather than the lumen to detect atheroma regression. The findings of this study highlight the potential importance of emerging therapies that promote HDL-C. The potential therapeutic use of directly infusing HDL-C awaits the results of larger scale clinical trials.

EFFECT OF INTENSIVE BLOOD PRESSURE LOWERING

Epidemiological studies have established that a greater cardiovascular risk is observed with increasing systolic blood pressure within the normal range.[87] Despite this, there is currently no consensus with regard to the optimal management of blood pressure in pa-

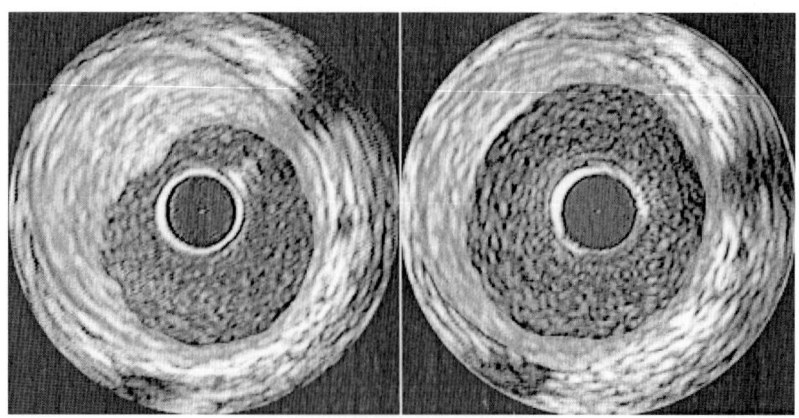

FIGURE 18–12. Atheroma regression. Matched tomographic images of coronary artery generated by IVUS with atheroma area illustrated by the shaded area. Substantial reduction in atheroma area is observed at follow up (*right panel*) compared with baseline (*left panel*) in a patient who received high-dose statin therapy. IVUS, intravascular ultrasound.

tients with CAD, who are considered to be normotensive. In the CAMELOT study, patients with CAD and a diastolic blood pressure <100 mmHg were treated with placebo or antihypertensive therapy using either amlodipine 10 mg daily or enalapril 20 mg daily.[88] Therapy with amlodipine was associated with a significant reduction in cardiovascular events.

Two hundred seventy-four patients who participated in the study underwent serial IVUS to evaluate the impact of these therapies on the rate of plaque progression.[88] Atheroma progression was observed in placebo and enalapril treated patients, but the trend just failed to meet statistical significance in the enalapril group. In contrast, there was no significant change in atheroma volume in patients treated with amlodipine consistent with halting of plaque progression. In the prespecified subgroup with baseline systolic blood pressure greater than the mean, the difference in progression rates between placebo and amlodipine treated patients was significant. A direct relationship was observed between the degree of blood pressure lowering and impact on plaque progression rates. The results suggest that in patients with established CAD, the optimal blood pressure is lower than that currently endorsed by secondary prevention guidelines.

The ability to embed serial atheroma imaging within a larger clinical event trial provides the opportunity to investigate the relationship between changes in these endpoints. It was noted that the hierarchy of treatment groups and their impact on clinical events in CAMELOT complemented the findings on atheroma progression using IVUS.

[ ] EFFECT OF INHIBITION OF INTRACELLULAR CHOLESTEROL ESTERIFICATION

Coronary ultrasonic imaging has also been applied to the assessment of therapeutic strategies that modify pathologic events within the arterial wall that contribute to atheroma formation. Intracellular cholesterol esterification, facilitated by the enzyme acyl-coenzyme A:cholesterol acyltransferase (ACAT), is a pivotal event in the formation of foam cells, the cellular hallmark of atherosclerotic plaque.[89] Experimental inhibition of ACAT has reportedly had a beneficial impact on lesion formation in a range of animal models of atherosclerosis.[89]

In the ACTIVATE study, patients with angiographic CAD received therapy with either placebo or the ACAT inhibitor pactimibe 100 mg daily.[90] There was no difference between treatment groups with regard to the change in the primary efficacy measure, percent atheroma volume. In contrast, a difference between treatment groups, favoring placebo was observed with regard to changes in secondary endpoints. The reduction in both total atheroma volume and atheroma volume in the 10-mm segments containing the greatest amount of plaque at baseline was significantly greater in placebo treated patients. This suggested that pactimibe therapy was potentially harmful with regard to its effect on atheroma progression. The result supports that of a previous report with another ACAT inhibitor, avasimibe, which resulted in an increase in LDL-C levels and had no favorable impact on the rate of atheroma progression compared with placebo.[91] These findings contrast with the benefits seen in animals, which were accompanied by a positive influence on plasma lipids.[89] The use of serial intravascular ultrasonography to demonstrate a detrimental effect of therapeutic compounds on atheroma progression highlights the pivotal role that modalities that image atherosclerotic plaque play in the translation of emerging compounds to the clinical arena.

[ ] LIMITATIONS OF REGRESSION-PROGRESSION STUDIES

Although the use of serial IVUS to monitor the impact of medical therapies on atheroma progression has provided a number of important insights into the factors that influence the natural history of atherosclerosis, a number of important limitations should be noted. These studies require an invasive catheterization procedure and therefore are currently limited to patients with established clinical CAD. As a result, the findings of these studies can only be applied to the setting of secondary prevention. Gray scale ultrasonic imaging provides a limited characterization of plaque components. It is uncertain what impact each of these medical therapies had on atheroma composition. It also remains uncertain how the impact of medical therapies on atheroma progression translates into their influence on clinical events.

INTERVENTIONAL CLINICAL APPLICATIONS

The initial development of intravascular ultrasonography was enthusiastically embraced by the interventional cardiology community, with regard to its potential routine application in guiding percutaneous interventions. Ultrasonic imaging within the coronary arteries has provided a number of pivotal insights with regard to the effect of various interventional techniques on the arterial wall. Accordingly, IVUS has played a leading role in the technological advances in the catheterization laboratory that have resulted in a declining requirement for its routine clinical use. In particular, given the low restenosis rates that accompany use of drug eluting stents, it has become difficult to justify the use of IVUS in all interventional cases. Nevertheless, there remains, an important role for the use of ultrasonic imaging in select clinical cases. The role of IVUS in the evolution of catheter based interventional techniques are reviewed.

[ ] PREINTERVENTIONAL IMAGING

Several small studies have demonstrated that ultrasound imaging of interventional target lesions may influence the approach to therapy.[92] The most common reasons cited for altering strategy included the assessment of extent and distribution of the lesion, lumen, and vessel area and diameter by ultrasound. Furthermore, in the assessment of ostial lesions, ultrasound imaging is employed to determine whether the lesion involves the *true* ostium or spares the most proximal few millimeters, which may assist optimal balloon and stent positioning. Assessment of plaque composition, such as calcification, is also an important part of preintervention evaluation. Despite promising data, reports on preinterventional imaging must be interpreted with caution. There are no prospective controlled trials demonstrating a superior outcome using preinterventional ultrasound guidance. Most importantly, previous studies suggesting a benefit for preinterventional imaging were performed in an era when techniques such as balloon angioplasty, directional atherectomy, or rotational ablation were commonly performed. The preeminence of coronary stenting has reduced the likelihood that one of these alternative revascularization approached will be performed. Accordingly, device selection using IVUS is limited to a small number of technically challenging cases. Nevertheless, it is important to review the role of IVUS in the earlier era to understand the current potential in the interventional lab.

INTRAVASCULAR ULTRASOUND AND BALLOON ANGIOPLASTY

IVUS studies improved our understanding of the mechanisms of luminal enlargement following balloon angioplasty. Prior necropsy studies in patients who expired shortly after balloon angioplasty have described plaque fracture or disruption as the most common mechanism of dilatation.[1] Most ultrasound studies have confirmed that dissection is an important mechanism of luminal enlargement, occurring in 40 to 80 percent of patients.[93] Identification of dissection or fracture is based on the visualization of blood flow in the newly created lumen, sometimes aided by injection of saline or iodinated contrast to opacify the lumen via microbubbles. Wall disruptions can be further defined by measuring the circumferential extent, length, and/or maximal depth of the dissection. Calcified lesions have been demonstrated to have a higher incidence of dissection, with a trend toward restenosis in lesions with no dissection.[49] Several alternative mechanisms for luminal enlargement have been identified using ultrasound, including arterial wall stretching and plaque compression, or *axial redistribution*.[94] The contribution of vessel stretch to lumen gain following balloon angioplasty has been validated in experimental and clinical investigations. A peripheral angioplasty study reported that plaque area was reduced by 33 percent, accounting for only 20 percent of luminal gain.[93] However, studies using automatic pullback devices have shown that *compression* actually represents redistribution of plaque along the long axis of the vessel.[94]

Ultrasound guidance of balloon sizing has been proposed as a means to improve procedural result and late clinical outcome for percutaneous transluminal coronary angioplasty.[92] Assessment of lumen diameter by ultrasound resulted in safe *upsizing* of balloon size in 34 percent of cases. Ultrasonic assessment following a *satisfactory* angiographic result was reported to reveal remodeling at the lesion and extensive plaque within the reference segment. Increasing the balloon-to-artery ratio in these regions resulted in an increase in angiographic minimal lumen diameter and lumen area on ultrasound without an increased incidence of angiographic dissection. This information maintains its importance in the evolution of drug eluting stents. A large lumen with well-apposed stent struts remains an important target for lowering restenosis and thrombosis rates.

INTRAVASCULAR ULTRASOUND AND DIRECTIONAL ATHERECTOMY

Although no longer commonly performed, directional coronary atherectomy (DCA) is an effective tool for removing of bulky plaques. Given the failure of DCA in calcified lesions, ultrasonic imaging was initially advocated for the selection of appropriate lesions for intervention. Use of IVUS in the setting of DCA has re-

vealed a number of important insights into the factors that influence outcome.[95] IVUS demonstrated that a substantial component of the luminal gain that results from DCA is derived from arterial stretching, rather than removal of atheroma. Use of IVUS in DCA provides the guidance required to achieve the largest lumen through atherectomy rather than vessel stretching, which is commonly observed following blind DCA. Many in the field believe that optimum DCA can be achieved by IVUS guidance.

INTRAVASCULAR ULTRASOUND AND CORONARY STENT DEPLOYMENT

Use of stents has become an essential component of therapeutic strategies involving percutaneous revascularization. IVUS imaging has played a pivotal role in understanding and optimizing the benefits of stent therapy.[96] A pioneering report detailing the IVUS experience of Colombo and coworkers significantly altered the understanding of optimal stent deployment and prevention of subacute thrombosis.[96] Ultrasound examination revealed a mean residual stenosis of 51 percent following angiographically guided stent deployment and a high prevalence of incomplete stent apposition (Fig. 18–13). Given their porous structures, angiographic contrast can flow outside of a partially deployed stent, resulting in the angiographic appearance of full deployment despite the presence of incomplete apposition. In the Milan study, the operators performed additional balloon inflations at higher pressures (typically 18–20 atm) or used a larger balloon (or both), reducing final ultrasound residual stenosis to 34 percent and with a subacute thrombosis rate of only 0.3 percent without a requirement for systemic antithrombotic agents, requiring antiplatelet therapy alone. It is now widely accepted that high-pressure deployment of bare metal stents dramatically reduces the incidence of subacute throm-

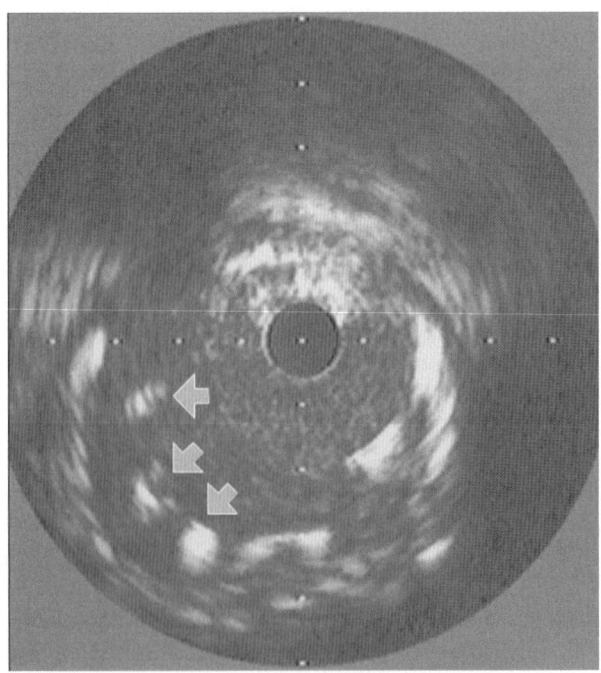

FIGURE 18–13. Underdeployed coronary stent. In this example, IVUS images show several stent struts (*arrows*) that are not in full contact with the underlying vessel wall. This process is referred to as incomplete stent apposition. IVUS, intravascular ultrasound.

bosis and obviates the need for acute and chronic administration of anticoagulant agents.[96]

Following the widespread acceptance of high-pressure postdilatation and antiplatelet regimens, the further benefit of ultrasound imaging has been debated.[97] Some investigators have suggested that despite routine use of high-pressure postdilatation, ultrasound-guided therapy could improve procedural results.[97] It is now generally accepted that after high-pressure coronary stenting, ultrasound imaging results in additional procedures in approximately 20 to 40 percent of cases.

However, it remains uncertain whether ultrasound-guided *optimal* expansion translates into better clinical outcome. Although a large number of registries and randomized trials have attempted to delineate this issue, there is no consensus that an ultrasound-guided approach results in a reduction in either death or myocardial infarction. A randomized trial in 164 patients of ultrasound-guided stenting demonstrated a 6.3 percent absolute reduction in restenosis rate, which was not statistically significant because of small sample size.[98] A nonrandomized substudy of 538 patients from the Stent Anticoagulation Regimen Study (STARS) compared the outcome of ultrasound and angiographically guided stenting. The ultrasound arm achieved a significantly larger lumen area and a 39 percent relative reduction in clinical restenosis.[99] Randomized studies have sought to clarify this issue. In the Optimization with ICUS (OPTICUS) study, ultrasound and angiographic-guided approaches resulted in similar rates of both angiographic restenosis and need for target vessel revascularization.[100] However, the finding that restenosis and target vessel revascularization rates were lower with ultrasound guidance in a cohort of subjects with long and diffuse lesions in the Thrombocyte activity evaluation and effects of Ultrasound guidance in Long Intracoronary stent Placement (TULIP) study[101] suggested that the utility of routine ultrasound guidance for stent deployment was likely to only be found in patients with a high risk for restenosis.

Several criteria for optimal stent expansion have been proposed on the basis of experience with ultrasound guidance. Colombo initially recommended achieving ≥60 percent of the average proximal and distal reference areas but later altered the definition to ≥100 percent of the distal reference lumen area.[96] Other definitions of optimal expansion include ≥90 percent of the distal reference area, ≥80 percent or ≥90 percent of the average reference area, a *lumen symmetry index* >0.7, and/or full coverage of reference-segment disease or dissections.[102] In most clinical trials, procedural endpoints are not achieved in the majority of cases. In the Optimal Stent Implantation Trial, the target of >90 percent of the average reference or >100 percent of the smaller reference area were not achieved in half the patients at an inflation pressure of 15 atm and only 60 percent of patients at 18 atm.[102] In the Angiography Versus Intravascular Ultrasound Directed stent placement (AVID) trial, the target endpoint of ≥90 percent of the distal reference area was not achieved in >70 percent of 225 patients.[103]

Other reports have questioned the clinical relevance of using the stent-to-reference ratios as target for ultrasound-guided stenting. In 165 patients target vessel revascularization was predicted by final in-stent lumen area (OR 1.4, 95 percent CI 1.1 to 1.9) and not the ratio of stent-to-reference area (OR 1.1, 95 percent CI 0.85 to 1.6).[97] Repeat revascularization was required in 30 percent of patients with a minimum in-stent lumen area <5 mm^2 but only

3 percent of cases with an area exceeding 9 mm^2. In another large cohort undergoing ultrasound-guided stenting, restenosis was inversely related to the minimum in-stent area.[104] An area of 9 mm^2 was achieved in 23 percent, but the incidence of restenosis in this subgroup was only 8 percent, compared with 29 percent in the remaining patients, p <0.0001. Thus, commonly employed ultrasound endpoints based on a predefined stent-to-reference ratio are both difficult to achieve and correlate weakly with clinical outcome.[104] The most clinically useful of all of these criteria comes from a study of 425 patients with angiographically successful stent deployment. A minimal stent area of 9 mm^2 and ratio of stent area to reference EEM area of 0.55 are the strongest predictors of freedom from restenosis. Ultrasound studies have demonstrated that the degree of in-stent neointimal hyperplasia is independent of final lumen size, which may explain the higher restenosis rates in smaller vessels and poorly expanded stents.[105] If acute lumen gain is inadequate to accommodate subsequent tissue proliferation, there is significant late loss and restenosis.

ASSESSMENT OF STENT-RELATED COMPLICATIONS

Ultrasound imaging of reference segments following stenting may help identify reference segment disease or dissections that require additional interventions. The presence of significant persistent flow-limiting lesions or dissections has been linked to higher likelihood of stent thrombosis.[106] These findings are often angiographically occult or appear as areas of indistinct haziness at the vessel border. In 201 stent patients, 31 segments with persistent angiographic haziness were detected. Ultrasound imaging revealed an angiographically inapparent obstructive lesion in 15, a persistent wall injury in 14, and mild intimal thickening in the remaining 2 segments.[107] The extent of neointimal hyperplasia at the stent margins has been linked to preexisting disease in the reference segment.[108] In stenting as a bailout for dissection, IVUS is more sensitive in detecting the extent of dissection, often revealing a greater true length than is evident from angiography, which may be helpful in guiding vessel salvage.

Many interventional cardiologists prefer to use angiography alone to guide subsequent management. However, use of ultrasound is particularly useful in a number of scenarios. When dissection is complicated by threatened acute closure, IVUS is important to ensure that the full length of dissection is covered. Coronary ultrasonic imaging is also helpful in the setting where the cause of persistent haziness is not readily discernible on angiography alone. In this scenario IVUS distinguishes patients who require further intervention to manage uncovered dissections from those who can be managed more conservatively on the basis of calcified or moderately diseased segments in the persistent region. During treatment of dissections, IVUS may be very helpful to differentiate the true lumen from the false lumen.

INTRAVASCULAR ULTRASOUND AND RESTENOSIS

Serial ultrasound examinations have shown that a late reduction in total vessel area (chronic negative remodeling) is an important mechanism of restenosis after nonstent interventional procedures.[109] Other investigators have suggested a bidirectional remodeling response following percutaneous coronary interventions: early adaptive enlargement and late shrinkage of the vessel. These observations suggest that mechanical interventions to prevent chronic recoil (such as stenting) may be more important in preventing restenosis than interventions designed to prevent intimal hyperplasia. This concept likely explains the lower restenosis rate observed in randomized multicenter studies comparing balloon angioplasty and stent implantation.[110]

Investigations employing quantitative angiography demonstrate that late lumen loss is significantly greater with stents than with balloon angioplasty. This, however, is offset by the much larger acute lumen gain, such that the net gain at follow up is significantly greater with stenting.[110] IVUS has been employed to examine the mechanism of stent restenosis. Unlike the restenotic response to other percutaneous devices, which is a mixture of arterial remodeling and neointimal growth, stent restenosis is almost exclusively caused by the neointimal proliferation.[109] In a serial study using IVUS of stented coronary segments, there was no significant change in the area bound by stent struts, indicating that stents can withstand and resist the arterial remodeling process.[111] In some cases, restenosis develops at the margins of the stent. Predictors of stent restenosis have been identified by multivariate analysis, including the smaller reference vessel and lumen size, the larger plaque burden at the reference segments, and the smaller achieved in-stent lumen area at the stent margins.[108]

[ ] INTRAVASCULAR ULTRASOUND AND BRACHYTHERAPY

Ultrasound proved useful in clarifying the mechanisms of benefit and refining the techniques used for brachytherapy.[111,112] In many cases of in stent restenosis, a small final in-stent lumen dimension is often the true culprit of restenosis. IVUS studies demonstrate that radiation inhibits neointimal proliferation within a stent. In a randomized study of 70 lesions with in-stent restenosis, at follow up, 79 percent of stents in patients who received radiation had no measurable intimal proliferation, compared to 27 percent of those randomized to the *no radiation* cohort.[111] In the nonstented segments, some studies suggest that radiation initiates a process of vessel expansion (a type of positive remodeling).[112] These effects are strongly influenced by the dose delivered to the media or adventitia, which depends on the thickness and composition of the atheroma and the position of the catheter in the lumen. Ultrasound has also demonstrated the potential for radiation to accelerate restenosis at the edges of the treatment region where the dosing falls off (*candy-wrapper* effect).[112] The efficacy of drug-eluting stents in the treatment of in-stent restenosis has resulted in brachytherapy being an obsolete therapeutic option for the management of in-stent restenosis.

[ ] INTRAVASCULAR ULTRASOUND AND DRUG-ELUTING STENTS

IVUS has proven useful in assessing the mechanism of benefit of drug-eluting stents.[113,114] Studies consistently demonstrate that drug-eluting stents have the potential to markedly reduce neointimal proliferation within the stent at 6 to 9 months follow up. In

the RAVEL trial, a subset of 95 patients underwent IVUS examination 6 months following stent implantation. The patients who received a sirolimus-eluting stent exhibited an average of only 2 mm^3 of intimal hyperplasia compared to 37 mm^3 for the control group (*p* <0001).[113] Similar, although less pronounced results were reported for a paclitaxel-eluting stent.[114] Using paclitaxel, investigators reported a dose-dependent reduction in intimal hyperplasia at 4 to 6 months from 31 mm^3 in the control arm to 18 mm^3 in a low-dose cohort to 13 mm^3 in the highest dose paclitaxel group.

Ultrasound has been an important tool in understanding the important role of underexpansion of drug-eluting stents in the subsequent development of both angiographic restenosis and subacute stent thrombosis. In studies using sirolimus-eluting stents, achieving a postdeployment minimal stent area of 5 mm^2 predicts a reduced likelihood of angiographic restenosis.[115] Despite the fact that the restenosis rate with drug-eluting stents is now less than 10 percent, the clinical usefulness of ultrasound guidance in stent deployment maintains its importance, albeit in select cases such as long segments, particularly of small vessels, bifurcation stenting, ostial lesions, treatment of in-stent restenosis and left main stenting. IVUS remains a useful adjunct in the situation where uncertainty approximately the optimal stent size exists. In the absence of a *normal* reference segment the optimal stent diameter can be estimated to be equivalent to the average of the lumen and EEM area at the least diseased site. Furthermore, given the risk of stent thrombosis and late closure, it is critical to cover any residual stenosis with a stent of adequate length and to detect any residual edge dissection. Ultrasonic imaging has demonstrated the presence of intraluminal echolucent tissue (black holes) within drug-eluting stents.[116] This is likely to represent an altered proliferative response that contributes to neointima formation. Registries and randomized trials have demonstrated the incidence of black holes in drug-eluting, but not bare metal, stents. The incidence is substantially greater in regions that have previously undergone brachytherapy. Studies in a limited number of patients showed no clinical consequence of these black holes. The application of each of these insights to clinical utility of drug eluting stents has substantially reduced the rate of restenosis and stent thrombosis. As a result, the routine use of IVUS in the guidance of drug eluting stent deployment has become obsolete.

FUTURE DIRECTIONS

IVUS is commonly but not routinely performed in the United States during coronary interventions. Approximately 5 to 10 percent of interventional procedures are currently performed with ultrasound guidance. Use in Europe is considerably less than in the United States; in Japan it is considerably higher, reflecting differing practice patterns and reimbursement rates. IVUS is more likely to be incorporated into practice algorithms in countries where its use is deemed to be cost effective. Although high-frequency probes enable better axial and lateral resolution, there are significant trade-offs in moving beyond the current 40-MHz frequency. For example, penetration is likely to be impaired in comparison with more conventional devices, and greater backscatter from blood cells at high frequencies may interfere with discrimination of the interface between lumen and vessel wall.

As previously discussed, analysis of backscattered ultrasound signals has been employed by several investigators to perform *tissue characterization*.[20,21] Intrinsic properties of the backscattered ultrasound signals—including the amplitude distribution, frequency response, and power spectrum of the signal—may convey specific information about tissue types.[20] However, the ability of computer-based analysis of the unprocessed radiofrequency backscatter to differentiate the histologic layers of the normal vessel wall remains investigational. The promise of this research is the potential to identify *vulnerable* atherosclerotic plaques, defined as lesions at high risk for plaque rupture leading to thrombosis and acute coronary syndromes.

Three-dimensional reconstruction of IVUS has been proposed as a means to facilitate understanding of the spatial relationship between the structures within different tomographic cross sections. Despite the promise of these methods, many unresolved problems remain. The algorithms applied for three-dimensional reconstruction do not consider the presence of curvatures of the vessel and assume that the catheter passes in a straight line through the center of consecutive cross sections. The systolic expansion of the coronary vessel and the movements of the catheter within the vessel during the cardiac cycle also generate artifacts. Accordingly, the reconstructed images should not be considered faithful representations of the vessel and should not be used for volumetric plaque determination.

SUMMARY

The equipment, technique, and applications for IVUS imaging continue to evolve. The insights provided by the unique ability of IVUS to directly image coronary plaques have contributed greatly to our understanding of the nature of atherosclerosis and the effects of both interventional devices and anti-atherosclerotic therapies. Current studies using IVUS to measure atherosclerosis progression and regression have expanded the utility of this important diagnostic method and now play an important role in the translation of emerging therapeutic approaches to the clinical setting.

REFERENCES

1. Nissen SE, Di Mario C, Tuzcu EM. Intravascular ultrasound, angioscopy, Doppler, and pressure measurement. In: Topol EJ, ed. *Topol Cardiovascular Medicine.* Philadelphia: Lippincott-Raven, 1997.
2. Topol EJ, Nissen SE. Our preoccupation with coronary luminology: the dissociation between clinical and angiographic findings in ischemic heart disease. *Circulation* 1995;92:2333–2342.
3. Grodin CM, Dydra I, Pastgernac A, et al. Discrepancies between cineangiographic and post-mortem findings in patients with coronary artery disease and recent myocardial revascularization. *Circulation* 1974;49:703–709.
4. Roberts WC, Jones AA. Quantitation of coronary arterial narrowing at necropsy in sudden coronary death. *Am J Cardiol* 1979;44:39–44.
5. White CW, Wright CB, Doty DB, et al. Does visual interpretation of the coronary arteriogram predict the physiologic importance of a coronary stenosis? *N Engl J Med* 1984;310:819–824.
6. Topol EJ, Nissen SE. Our preoccupation with coronary luminology: the dissociation between clinical and angiographic findings in ischemic heart disease. *Circulation* 1995;92:2333–2342.
7. Glagov S, Weisenberg E, Zarins CK, et al. Compensatory enlargement of human coronary arteries. *N Engl J Med* 1987;316:1371–1375.
8. Little WC, Constantinescu M, Applegate RJ, et al. Can arteriography predict the site of a subsequent myocardial infarction in patients with mild-to-moderate coronary artery disease? *Circulation* 1988;78:1157–1166.
9. Yamagishi M, Miyatake K, Tamai J, et al. Detection of atherosclerosis at the site of focal vasospasm in angiographically normal or minimally narrowed coronary segments by intravascular ultrasound. *J Am Coll Cardiol* 1994;23:352–357.
10. Nissen SE, DeFranco A, Tuzcu EM. Detection and quantification of atherosclerosis: the emerging role for intravascular ultrasound. In: Fuster V, ed. *Syndromes of Atherosclerosis: Correlations of Clinical Imaging and Pathology.* Armonk, New York: Futura; 1996:291.
11. TenHoff H, Korbijn A, Smit TH, et al. Image artifacts in mechanically driven ultrasound catheters. *Int J Cardiovasc Imaging* 1989;4:195–199.
12. Di Mario C, Madretsma S, Linker D, et al. The angle of incidence of the ultrasonic beam: a critical factor for the image quality in intravascular ultrasonography. *Am Heart J* 1993;125:442–448.
13. Hausmann D, Erbel R, Alibelli-Chemarin MJ, et al. The safety of intracoronary ultrasound: a multicenter survey of 2207 examinations. *Circulation* 1995;91:623–630.
14. Batkoff BW, Linker DT. Safety of intracoronary ultrasound: data from a multicenter European registry. *Cathet Cardiovasc Diagn* 1996; 38:238–241.
15. Pinto FJ, St Goar FG, Gao SZ, et al. Immediate and one-year safety of intracoronary ultrasonic imaging: evaluation with serial quantitative angiography. *Circulation* 1993;88:1709–1714.
16. Ramasubbu K, Schoenhagen P, Balghith MA, et al. Repeated intravascular ultrasound imaging in cardiac transplant recipients does not accelerate transplant coronary artery disease. *J Am Coll Cardiol* 2003;41:1739–1743.
17. Gussenhoven EJ, Essed CE, Lancee CT, et al. Arterial wall characteristics determined by intravascular ultrasound imaging: an in vitro study. *J Am Coll Cardiol* 1989;4:947–952.
18. Fitzgerald PJ, St Goar FG, Connolly AJ, et al. Intravascular ultrasound imaging of coronary arteries: are three layers the norm? *Circulation* 1992;86:154–158.
19. Velican D, Velican C. Comparative study on age-related changes and atherosclerotic involvement of the coronary arteries of male and female subjects up to 40 years of age. *Atherosclerosis* 1981;38:39–50.
20. Maheswaran B, Leung CY, Gutfinger DE, et al. Intravascular ultrasound appearance of normal and mildly diseased coronary arteries: correlation with histologic specimens. *Am Heart J* 1995;130:976–986.
21. Bridal SL, Fornes P, Bruneval P, Berger G. Parametric (integrated backscatter and attenuation) images constructed using backscattered radio frequency signals (25–56 MHz) from human aortae in vitro. *Ultrasound Med Biol* 1997;23:215–229.
22. Nair A, Kuban BD, Tuzcu EM, et al. Coronary plaque classification with intravascular ultrasound radiofrequency data analysis. *Circulation* 2002;206;106(17):2200–2202.
23. Nasu K, Tsuchikane E, Katoh O, et al. Accuracy of in vivo coronary plaque morphology assessment: a validation study of in vivo virtual histology compared with in vitro histopathology. *J Am Coll Cardiol* 2006;47:2405–2412.
24. Rodriguez-Granillo GA, McFadden EP, Valgimigli M, et al. Coronary plaque composition of nonculprit lesions, assessed by in vivo intracoronary ultrasound radio frequency data analysis, is related to clinical presentation. *Am Heart J* 2006;151:1020–1024.
25. Rodriguez-Granillo GA, Garcia-Garcia HM, Mc Fadden EP, et al. In vivo intravascular ultrasound-derived thin-cap fibroatheroma detection using ultrasound radiofrequency data analysis. *J Am Coll Cardiol* 2005;46:2038–2042.
26. Valgimigli M, Rodriguez-Granillo GA, Garcia-Garcia HM, et al. Distance from the ostium as an independent determinant of coronary plaque composition in vivo: an intravascular ultrasound study based radiofrequency data analysis in humans. *Eur Heart J* 2006;27:655–663.
27. Fujii K, Carlier SG, Mintz GS, et al. Association of plaque characterization by intravascular ultrasound virtual histology and arterial remodeling. *Am J Cardiol* 2005;96:1476–1483.
28. Rodriguez-Granillo GA, Serruys PW, Garcia-Garcia HM, et al. Coronary artery remodelling is related to plaque composition. *Heart* 2006;92:388–391.
29. Kawasaki M, Sano K, Okubo M, et al. Volumetric quantitative analysis of tissue characteristics of coronary plaques after statin therapy using three-dimensional integrated backscatter intravascular ultrasound. *J Am Coll Cardiol* 2005;45:1946–1953.
30. Mintz GS, Popma JJ, Pichard AD, et al. Patterns of calcification in coronary artery disease: A statistical analysis of intravascular ultrasound and coronary angiography in 1,155 lesions. *Circulation* 1995;91:1959–1965.
31. Tuzcu EM, Berkalp B, DeFranco AC, et al. The dilemma of diagnosing coronary calcification: angiography versus intravascular ultrasound. *J Am Coll Cardiol* 1996;27:832–838.
32. Hermiller JB, Tenaglia AN, Kisslo KB, et al. In vivo validation of compensatory enlargement of atherosclerotic coronary arteries. *Am J Cardiol* 1993;71:665–668.

33. Losordo DW, Rosenfield K, Kaufman J, et al. Focal compensatory enlargement of human arteries in response to progressive atherosclerosis: in vivo documentation using intravascular ultrasound. *Circulation* 1994;89:2570–2577.

34. Sipahi I, Tuzcu EM, Schoenhagen P, et al. Compensatory enlargement of human coronary arteries during progression of atherosclerosis is unrelated to atheroma burden: serial intravascular ultrasound observations from the REVERSAL trial. *Eur Heart J* 2006;27:1664–1670.

35. Pasterkamp G, Wensing PJ, Post MJ, et al. Paradoxical arterial wall shrinkage may contribute to luminal narrowing of human atherosclerotic femoral arteries. *Circulation* 1995;91:1444–1449.

36. Mintz GS, Kent KM, Pichard AD, et al. Contribution of inadequate arterial remodeling to the development of focal coronary artery stenoses: an intravascular ultrasound study. *Circulation* 1997;95:1791–1798.

37. Kimura T, Kaburagi S, Tamura T, et al. Remodeling of human coronary arteries undergoing coronary angioplasty or atherectomy. *Circulation* 1997;96:475–483.

38. Nicholls SJ, Tuzcu EM, Sipahi I, et al. Relationship between atheroma regression and change in lumen size after infusion of apolipoprotein A-I Milano. *J Am Coll Cardiol* 2006;47:992–997.

39. Tardif JC, Gregoire J, LíAllier PL, et al. Effect of atherosclerotic regression on total luminal size of coronary arteries as determined by intravascular ultrasound. *Am J Cardiol* 2006;98:23–27.

40. Richardson PD, Davies MJ, Born GV. Influence of plaque configuration and stress distribution on fissuring of coronary atherosclerotic plaques. *Lancet* 1989;2:941–944.

41. Ambrose JA, Winters SL, Arora RR, et al. Angiographic evolution of coronary artery morphology in unstable angina. *J Am Coll Cardiol* 1986;7:472–478.

42. Loree HM, Kamm RD, Stringfellow RG, Lee RT. Effects of fibrous cap thickness on peak circumferential stress in model atherosclerotic vessels. *Circ Res* 1992;71:850–858.

43. Schoenhagen P, Stone GW, Nissen SE, et al. Coronary plaque morphology and frequency of ulceration distant from culprit lesions in patients with unstable and stable presentation. *Arterioscler Thromb Vasc Biol* 2003;23:1895–1900.

44. Schoenhagen P, Ziada KM, Kapadia SR, et al. Extent and direction of arterial remodeling in stable versus unstable coronary syndromes: an intravascular ultrasound study. *Circulation* 2000;101:598–603.

45. Maehara A, Mintz GS, Bui AB, et al. Morphologic and angiographic features of coronary plaque rupture detected by intravascular ultrasound. *J Am Coll Cardiol* 2002;40:904–910.

46. Siegel RJ, Ariani M, Fishbein MC, et al. Histopathologic validation of angioscopy and intravascular ultrasound. *Circulation* 1991;84:109–117.

47. Bocksch W, Schartl M, Beckmann S, et al. Intravascular ultrasound imaging in patients with acute myocardial infarction. *Eur Heart J* 1995;2;16(suppl J):46–45.

48. Mintz G. Nissen SE, Anderson WD, et al. Standards for the acquisition measurement and reporting of intravascular ultrasound studies. *J Am Coll Cardiol* 2001;479;37(5):1478–1.

49. Wong M, Edelstein J, Wollman J, Bond MG. Ultrasonic-pathological comparison of the human arterial wall: verification of intima-media thickness. *Arterioscler Thromb* 1993;13:482–486.

50. Tuzcu EM, Kapadia SR, Tutar E, et al. High Prevalence of coronary atherosclerosis in asymptomatic teenagers and young adults: evidence from intravascular ultrasound. *Circulation* 2001;103:2705–2710.

51. Tuzcu EM, Hobbs H, Rincon G, et al. Occult and frequent transmission of atherosclerosis coronary disease with cardiac transplantation. *Circulation* 1995;91:1706–1713.

52. Tuzcu EM. DeFranco AC, Goormastic M, et al. Dichotomous pattern of coronary atherosclerosis 1 to 9 years after transplantation: insights from systematic intravascular ultrasound imaging. *J Am Coll Cardiol* 1996;27:839–846.

53. Mintz GS, Popma JJ, Pichard AD, et al. Limitations of angiography in the assessment of plaque distribution in coronary artery disease: a systematic study of target lesion eccentricity in 1446 lesions. *Circulation* 1996;93:924–931.

54. Erbel R, Ge J, Bockisch A, et al. Value of intracoronary ultrasound and Doppler in the differentiation of angiographically normal coronary arteries: a prospective study in patients with angina pectoris. *Eur Heart J* 1996;17:880–889.

55. Mintz GS, Painter JA, Pichard AD, et al. Atherosclerosis in angiographically "normal" coronary artery reference segments: an intravascular ultrasound study with clinical correlations. *J Am Coll Cardiol* 1995;25:1479–1485.

56. Lee DY, Eigler N, Luo H, et al. Effect of intracoronary ultrasound imaging on clinical decision making. *Am Heart J* 1995;129:1084–1093.

57. Bech GJ, De Bruyne B, Pijls NH, et al. Fractional flow reserve to determine the appropriateness of angioplasty in moderate coronary stenosis: a randomized trial. *Circulation* 2001;103:2928–2934.

58. Takagi A, Tsurumi Y, Ishii Y, et al. Clinical potential of intravascular ultrasound for physiological assessment of coronary stenosis: relationship between quantitative ultrasound tomography and pressure-derived fractional flow reserve. *Circulation* 1999;100:250–255.

59. Briguori C, Anzuini A, Airoldi F, et al. Intravascular ultrasound criteria for the assessment of the functional significance of intermediate coronary artery stenoses and comparison with fractional flow reserve. *Am J Cardiol* 2001;87:136–141.

60. Abizaid AS, Mintz GS, Mehran R, et al. Long-term follow-up after percutaneous transluminal coronary angioplasty was not performed based on intravascular ultrasound findings: importance of lumen dimensions. *Circulation* 1999;100:256–261.

61. Hermiller JB, Buller CE, Tenaglia AN, et al. Unrecognized left main coronary artery disease in patients undergoing interventional procedures. *Am J Cardiol* 1993;71:173–176.

62. Jasti V, Ivan E, Yalamanchili V, et al. Correlations between fractional flow reserve and intravascular ultrasound in patients with an ambiguous left main coronary artery stenosis. *Circulation* 2004;110:2831–2836.

63. Abizaid AS, Mintz GS, Abizaid A, et al. One-year follow-up after intravascular ultrasound assessment of moderate left main coronary artery disease in patients with ambiguous angiograms. *J Am Coll Cardiol* 1999;34:707–715.

64. Fassa AA, Wagatsuma K, Higano ST, et al. Intravascular ultrasound-guided treatment for angiographically indeterminate left main coronary artery disease: a long-term follow-up study. *J Am Coll Cardiol* 2005;45:204–211.

65. Uretsky BF, Kormos RL, Zerbe TR, et al. Cardiac events after heart transplantation: incidence and predictive value of coronary arteriography. *J Heart Transplant* 1992;11:S45–S50.

66. Johnson DE, Alderman EL, Schroeder JS, et al. Transplant coronary artery disease: histopathological correlations with angiographic morphology. *J Am Coll Cardiol* 1991;17:449–457.

67. St Goar FG, Pinto FJ, Alderman EL, et al. Detection of coronary atherosclerosis in young adult hearts using intravascular ultrasound. *Circulation* 1992;86:756–763.

68. Kapadia SR, Nissen SE, Ziada KM, et al. Development of transplant vasculopathy and progression of donor-transmitted atherosclerosis: a comparison by serial intravascular ultrasound imaging. *Circulation* 1998;8:2672–2678.

69. Tuzcu EM, Kapadia SR, Sachar R, et al. Intravascular ultrasound evidence of angiographically silent progression in coronary atherosclerosis predicts long-term morbidity and mortality after cardiac transplantation. *J Am Coll Cardiol* 2005;45:1538–1542.

70. Kobashigawa JA, Tobis JM, Starling RC, et al. Multicenter intravascular ultrasound validation study among heart transplant recipients: outcomes after five years. *J Am Coll Cardiol* 2005;45:1532–1537.

71. Eisen HJ, Tuzcu EM, Dorent R, et al. Everolimus for the prevention of allograft rejection and vasculopathy in cardiac-transplant recipients. *N Engl J Med* 2003;349:847–858.

72. von Birgelen C, Hartmann M, Mintz GS, et al. Relationship between cardiovascular risk as predicted by established risk scores versus plaque progression as measured by serial intravascular ultrasound in left main coronary arteries. *Circulation* 2004;110:1579–1585.

73. Nicholls SJ, Tuzcu EM, Crowe T, et al. Relationship between cardiovascular risk factors and atherosclerotic disease burden measured by intravascular ultrasound. *J Am Coll Cardiol* 2006;47:1967–1975.

74. Schartl M, Bocksch W, Koschyk DH, et al. Use of intravascular ultrasound to compare effects of different strategies of lipid-lowering therapy on plaque volume and composition in patients with coronary artery disease. *Circulation*, 2001;104:387–392.

75. Nissen SE, Tuzcu EM, Schoenhagen P, et al. Effect of intensive compared with moderate lipid-lowering therapy on progression of coronary atherosclerosis: a randomized controlled trial. *JAMA* 2004;291:1071–1080.

76. Nissen SE, Tuzcu EM, Schoenhagen P, et al. Statin therapy, LDL cholesterol, C-reactive protein, and coronary artery disease. *N Engl J Med* 2005;352:29–38.

77. Cannon CP, Braunwald E, McCabe CH, et al. Intensive versus moderate lipid lowering with statins after acute coronary syndromes. *N Engl J Med* 2004;350:1495–1504.

78. Ridker PM, Cannon CP, Morrow D, et al. C-reactive protein levels and outcomes after statin therapy. *N Engl J Med* 2005;352:20–28.

79. Nissen SE, Nicholls SJ, Sipahi I, et al. Effect of very high-intensity statin therapy on regression of coronary atherosclerosis: the ASTEROID trial. *JAMA* 2006;295:1556–1565.

80. Okazaki S, Yokoyama T, Miyauchi K, et al. Early statin treatment in patients with acute coronary syndrome: demonstration of the beneficial effect on atherosclerotic lesions by serial volumetric intravascular ultrasound analysis during half a year after coronary event: the ESTABLISH Study. *Circulation* 2004;110:1061–1068.

81. Jensen LO, Thayssen P, Pedersen KE, et al. Regression of coronary atherosclerosis by simvastatin: a serial intravascular ultrasound study. *Circulation* 2004;110:265–270.

82. LaRosa JC, Grundy SM, Waters DD, et al. Intensive lipid lowering with atorvastatin in patients with stable coronary disease. *N Engl J Med* 2005;352:1425–1435.

83. Pedersen TR, Faergeman O, Kastelein JJ, et al. High-dose atorvastatin vs usual-dose simvastatin for secondary prevention after myocardial infarction: the IDEAL study: a randomized controlled trial. *JAMA* 2005;294:2437–2445.

84. Gordon DJ, Probstfield JL, Garrison RJ, et al. High-density lipoprotein cholesterol and cardiovascular disease. Four prospective American studies. *Circulation* 1989;79:8–15.

85. Nicholls SJ, Cutri B, Worthley SG, et al. Impact of short-term administration of high-density lipoproteins and atorvastatin on atherosclerosis in rabbits. *Arterioscler Thromb Vasc Biol* 2005;25:2416–2421.

86. Nissen SE, Tsunoda T, Tuzcu EM, et al. Effect of recombinant ApoA-I Milano on coronary atherosclerosis in patients with acute coronary syndromes: a randomized controlled trial. *JAMA* 2003;290:2292–2300.

87. Relationship between baseline risk factors and coronary heart disease and total mortality in the Multiple Risk Factor Intervention Trial. Multiple Risk Factor Intervention Trial Research Group. *Prev Med* 1986;15:254–273.

88. Nissen SE, Tuzcu EM, Libby P, et al. Effect of antihypertensive agents on cardiovascular events in patients with coronary disease and normal blood pressure: the CAMELOT studyóa randomized controlled trial. *JAMA* 2004;292:2217–2225.

89. Rudel LL, Lee RG, Parini P. ACAT2 is a target for treatment of coronary heart disease associated with hypercholesterolemia. *Arterioscler Thromb Vasc Biol* 2005;25:1112–1118.

90. Nissen SE, Tuzcu EM, Brewer HB, et al. Effect of ACAT inhibition on the progression of coronary atherosclerosis. *N Engl J Med* 2006;354:1253–1263.

91. Tardif JC, Gregoire J, LíAllier PL, et al. Effects of the acyl coenzyme A cholesterol acyltransferase inhibitor avasimibe on human atherosclerotic lesions. *Circulation* 2004;110:3372–3377.

92. Stone GW, Hodgson JM, St Goar FG, et al. Improved procedural results of coronary angioplasty with intravascular ultrasound-guided balloon sizing: the CLOUT pilot trial—Clinical Outcomes with Ultrasound Trial (CLOUT) investigators. *Circulation* 1997;95:2044–2052.

93. Losordo DW, Rosenfield K, Pieczek A, et al. How does angioplasty work? Serial analysis of human iliac arteries using intravascular ultrasound. *Circulation* 1992;86:1845–1858.

94. Mintz GS, Pichard AD, Kent KM, et al. Axial plaque redistribution as a mechanism of percutaneous transluminal coronary angioplasty. *Am J Cardiol* 1996;77:427–430.

95. Matar FA, Mintz GS, Pinnow E, et al. Multivariate predictors of intravascular ultrasound end points after directional coronary atherectomy. *J Am Coll Cardiol* 1995;25:318–324.

96. Colombo A, Hall P, Nakamura S, et al. Intracoronary stenting without anticoagulation accomplished with intravascular ultrasound guidance. *Circulation* 1995;91:1676–1688.

97. Prati F, Gil R, Di Mario C, et al. Is quantitative angiography sufficient to guide stent implantation? A comparison with three-dimensional reconstruction of intracoronary ultrasound images. *G Ital Cardiol* 1997;27:328–336.

98. Schiele F, Meneveau N, Vuillemenot A, et al. Impact of intravascular ultrasound guidance in stent deployment on 6-month restenosis rate: a multicenter, randomized study comparing two strategies—with and without intravascular ultrasound guidance. RESIST Study Group (REStenosis after IVUS guided STenting). *J Am Coll Cardiol* 1998;32:320–328.

99. Fitzgerald PJ, Oshima A, Hayase M, et al. Final results of the Can Routine Ultrasound Influence Stent Expansion (CRUISE) study. *Circulation* 2000;102:523–530.

100. Mudra H, di Mario C, de Jaegere P, et al. Randomized comparison of coronary stent implantation under ultrasound or angiographic guidance to reduce stent restenosis (OPTICUS Study). *Circulation* 2001;104:1343–1349.

101. Oemrawsingh PV, Mintz GS, Schalij MJ, et al. Intravascular ultrasound guidance improves angiographic and clinical outcome of stent implantation for long coronary artery stenoses: final results of a randomized comparison with angiographic guidance (TULIP Study). *Circulation* 2003;107:62–67.

102. de Jaegere P, Mudra H, Figulla H, et al. Intravascular ultrasound-guided optimized stent deployment: immediate and 6 months clinical and angiographic results from the Multicenter Ultrasound Stenting in Coronaries Study (MUSIC Study). *Eur Heart J* 1998;19:1214–1223.

103. Russo RJ, Nicosia A, Teirstein PS, Investigators AVID. Angiography versus intravascular ultrasound-directed stent placement. *J Am Coll Cardiol* 1997;29:369A.

104. Kasaoka S, Tobis JM, Akiyama T, et al. Angiographic and intravascular ultrasound predictors of in-stent restenosis. *J Am Coll Cardiol* 1998;32:1630–1635.

105. Hoffmann R, Mintz GS, Pichard AD, et al. Intimal hyperplasia thickness at follow-up is independent of stent size: a serial intravascular ultrasound study. *Am J Cardiol* 1998;82:1168–1172.

106. Schuhlen H, Hadamitzky M, Walter H, et al. Major benefit from antiplatelet therapy for patients at high risk for adverse cardiac events after coronary Palmaz-Schatz stent placement: analysis of a prospective risk stratification protocol in the Intracoronary Stenting and Antithrombotic Regimen (ISAR) trial. *Circulation* 1997;95:2015–2021.

107. Ziada KM, Tuzcu EM, De Franco AC, et al. Intravascular ultrasound assessment of the prevalence and causes of angiographic "haziness" following high-pressure coronary stenting. *Am J Cardiol* 1997; 80:116–121.

108. Hoffmann R, Mintz GS, Kent KM, et al. Serial intravascular ultrasound predictors of restenosis at the margins of Palmaz-Schatz stents. *Am J Cardiol* 1997;79:951–953.

109. Mintz GS, Popma JJ, Pichard AD, et al. Arterial remodeling after coronary angioplasty: a serial intravascular ultrasound study. *Circulation* 1996;94:35–43.

110. Fischman DL, Leon MB, Baim DS, et al. A randomized comparison of coronary-stent placement and balloon angioplasty in the treatment of coronary artery disease. *N Engl J Med* 1994;331:496–501.

111. Morino Y, Limpijankit T, Honda Y, et al. Late vascular response to repeat stenting for in-stent restenosis with and without radiation: an intravascular ultrasound volumetric analysis. *Circulation* 2002; 468;105(21):2465–2462.

112. Mintz GS, Weissman NJ, Fitgerald PJ. Intravascular ultrasound assessment of the mechanisms and results of brachytherapy. *Circulation* 2001;325;104(11):1320–1321.

113. Serruys PW, Degertekin M, Tanabe K, et al. Intravascular ultrasound findings in the multicenter, randomized, double blind RAVEL trial. *Circulation* 2002;03;106(7):798–798.

114. Park SJ, Shim WH, Ho DS, et al. A paclitaxel eluting stent for the prevention of coronary restenosis. *N Engl J Med* 2003;545;348(16):1537–1545.

115. Fujii K, Mintz GS, Kobayashi Y, et al. Contribution of stent underexpansion to recurrence after sirolimus-eluting stent implantation for in-stent restenosis. *Circulation* 2004;109:1085–1088.

116. Costa MA, Sabate M, Angiolillo DJ, et al. Intravascular ultrasound characterization of the îblack holeî phenomenon after drug-eluting stent implantation. *Am J Cardiol* 2006;97:203–206.

CHAPTER (19)

Nuclear Cardiology

Daniel S. Berman / Rory Hachamovitch / Leslee J. Shaw / Sean W. Hayes / Guido Germano

OVERVIEW

Nuclear cardiology is an integral part of cardiovascular practice, with stress nuclear cardiology procedures accounting for more than one-third of all stress tests performed by cardiologists and sustaining growth rates approaching 20 percent per year. This chapter provides a synopsis of nuclear cardiology procedures and the published evidence of their role in the diagnosis and risk assessment of patients with suspected or known coronary artery disease (CAD).

❪ ❫ HISTORICAL PERSPECTIVES IN NUCLEAR CARDIOLOGY

The Anger scintillation camera, the imaging device used today for virtually all nuclear cardiology procedures except positron emis-

sion tomography (PET), became clinically available in the late 1960s. By providing dynamic images of the cardiac distribution of radioactivity, this camera marked the beginning of clinical nuclear cardiology. The commercial availability in 1976 of thallium-201 (^{201}Tl) initiated the broad application of clinical myocardial perfusion scintigraphy, which with two-dimensional planar imaging was quickly shown to be useful for detection of CAD and, in the early 1980s, was demonstrated to be highly valuable in risk stratification of the CAD patient. Also in the early 1980s, single photon emission computed tomography (SPECT), using a rotating Anger camera detector, became widely available, increasing the ability to localize and quantify regional myocardial perfusion defects. In 1990, technetium-99m (^{99m}Tc)-sestamibi was approved for use in the United States, followed shortly thereafter by another ^{99m}Tc-based agent, ^{99m}Tc-tetrofosmin. The higher myocardial count rates of the ^{99m}Tc agents made it possible to perform gated single-photon emission computed tomography (SPECT) myocardial perfusion imaging (MPI) by obtaining images from the different parts of the cardiac cycle (gated SPECT). By the late 1990s, the widespread availability of dual detector cameras and dramatic increases in speed of computer systems allowed gated SPECT MPI to become a common clinical routine.[1] By 2003 nearly 90 percent of SPECT MPI in the United States used a ^{99m}Tc MPI agent, and slightly over 90 percent employed gated SPECT, providing routine objective clinical assessments of rest and stress myocardial perfusion and function. SPECT MPI makes up >95 percent of all nuclear cardiology procedures and thus is the focus of this chapter.

Although radionuclide angiography played a prominent role in noninvasive testing in decades past, by the 1990s, the use of this modality was largely replaced by echocardiography. Some important clinical applications of this modality remain, however, and are discussed in the latter portion of this chapter. The recent American College of Cardiology/American Heart Association/American Society of Nuclear Cardiology (ACC/AHA/ASNC) Guidelines for the Clinical Use of Cardiac Radionuclide Imaging provide a useful, comprehensive review of the state of the art and current recommendations for the field of nuclear cardiology.[2]

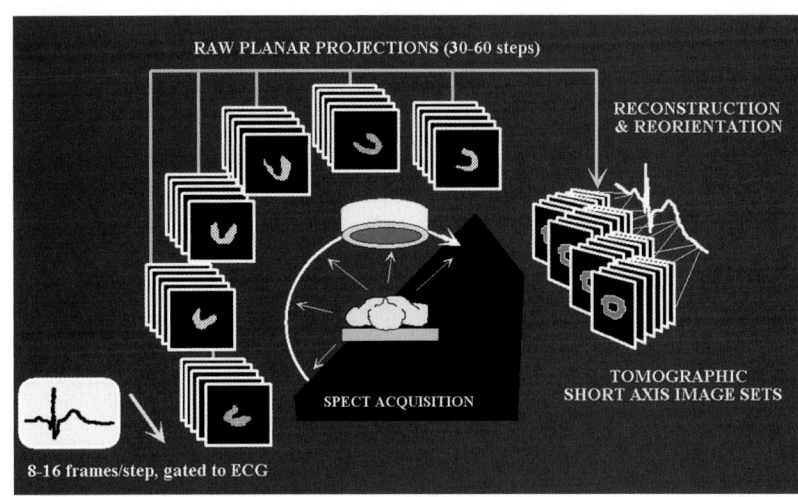

FIGURE 19–1. Schematic representation of ECG-gated perfusion SPECT acquisition and processing.

SPECT MYOCARDIAL PERFUSION IMAGING

【 】 BASIC CONCEPTS OF GATED SPECT MPI

SPECT MPI is performed using a scintillation camera and an intravenously injected radiopharmaceutical that distributes to the heart in proportion to regional myocardial perfusion. Various standardized SPECT MPI protocols are available for imaging at rest and after exercise or pharmacologic stress. For SPECT the scintillation camera detectors rotate 180 degrees around the patient in a semicircular or elliptical fashion, collecting a series of planar *projection* images at regular angular intervals. The three-dimensional (3D) distribution of radioactivity in the myocardium is then mathematically *reconstructed* from the two-dimensional projections, and the resulting data is displayed in series of slices in the short axis, vertical long axis, and horizontal long axis orientations. For gated SPECT (Fig. 19–1), the feature that distinguishes it from nongated SPECT is that the projection images are acquired in 8 to 16 phases of the cardiac cycle based on electrocardiographic (ECG) triggering (*gating*). Reconstruction of a summation of the frames is used to assess myocardial perfusion, and reconstruction of each of the separate phases is used to evaluate ventricular function.

【 】 RADIOPHARMACEUTICALS

The radiopharmaceuticals used for gated myocardial perfusion SPECT share the characteristic that they are accumulated in viable myocardium in proportion to regional myocardial blood flow (for a review of these agents, see Taillefer[3]). The concept that CAD can be detected with this approach is based on the ability to detect a reduction in myocardial perfusion in a region supplied by a stenosed vessel compared to a normal region during hyperemia. The relationship between the degree of coronary artery narrowing and the maximal hyperemic response was first elucidated by Gould in 1974.[4] Resting myocardial perfusion is normal until the luminal diameter narrowing of a coronary artery exceeds 90 to 95 percent. With maximal coronary hyperemia produced by dipyridamole, Gould demonstrated a progressive decrease in the hyperemic response associated with increasing degrees of stenosis greater than 50 percent, which implies that all forms of stress testing will be insensitive for the detection of coronary atherosclerosis until a hemodynamically significant lesion has developed. This hemodynamically significant lesion could be fixed or dynamic, such that spasm or paradoxical vasoconstriction during stress could result in a reduction of peak hyperemic perfusion even in the absence of a fixed >50 percent stenosis by angiography. The amount of the injected tracer in the myocardium at the time of imaging (net extraction) is a function of the proportion extracted by the myocardium (extraction fraction) and the amount retained at the time of imaging. With the exception of oxygen-15 water, used only for research purposes, all available SPECT or PET radiopharmaceuticals (see Chap. 23) manifest a falloff in this amount as coronary flow increases to high levels. Because mild stenoses may produce a decrease in flow only at very high flow rates, the net extraction is one of the most important characteristics of perfusion tracers (Fig. 19–2).

Thallium-201

A cyclotron-generated radionuclide with a half-life of 73 hours, ^{201}Tl emits photons at 68 to 80 keV (90 percent abundance) and at 167 keV (10 percent abundance). Owing to its relatively long half-life, the absorbed radiation dose is such that recommended injected doses are limited to 3 to 4 mCi, approximately one-tenth of those used with ^{99m}Tc agents. ^{201}Tl has excellent physiologic properties for MPI. Importantly for stress myocardial perfusion scintigraphy, a linear relationship between blood flow and ^{201}Tl uptake is maintained during exercise up to very high levels of flow (approximately

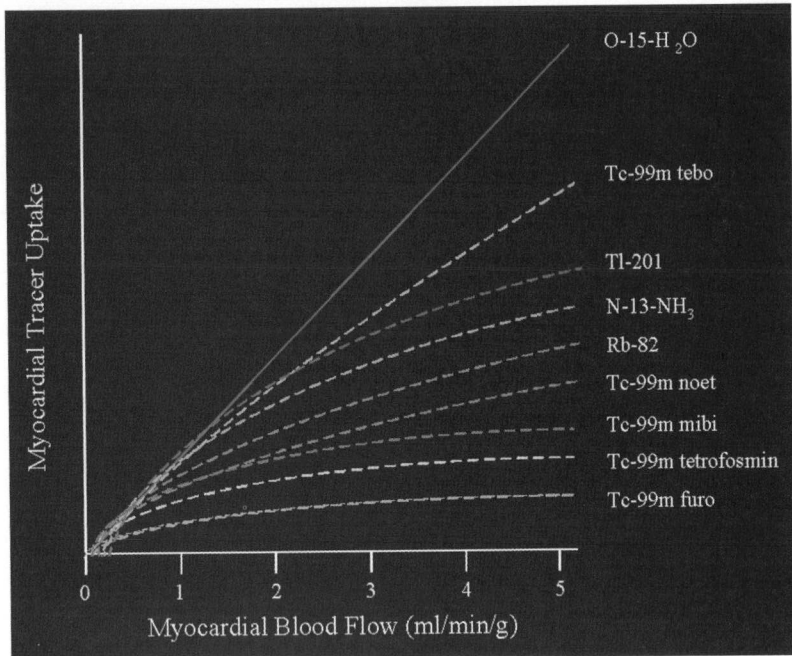

FIGURE 19–2. Relationship between tracer uptake and myocardial blood flow: theoretical considerations. N-13-NH$_2$, nitrogen-13 ammonia; tebo, teboroxime; mibi, sestamibi; furo, furofosmin; Rb, rubidium.

>3 mL/min/g) where a *roll-off* in uptake occurs[3] (see Fig. 19–2). As an unbound potassium analogue, ^{201}Tl redistributes over time[5]; its initial distribution is proportional to regional myocardial perfusion and, at equilibrium, the distribution of ^{201}Tl is proportional to the regional potassium pool, reflecting viable myocardium. The mechanisms of ^{201}Tl redistribution are differential washout rates between hypoperfused but viable myocardium and normal zones and wash-in to initially hypoperfused zones.

The washout rate of ^{201}Tl is the concentration gradient between the myocardial cell and the blood. Hyperinsulinemic states reduce blood ^{201}Tl concentrations and slow redistribution; thus fasting is recommended prior to and for 4 hours following ^{201}Tl injection.[3] An inverse relationship between the degree of coronary stenosis and subsequent redistribution of ^{201}Tl (i.e., late redistribution) has been reported.[3,6]

^{99m}Tc-Sestamibi and ^{99m}Tc-Tetrofosmin

^{99m}Tc is produced from a molybdenum-99m generator, has a half-life of 6 hours, and emits monoenergetic gamma rays at 140 keV. The whole-body radiation dose is estimated to be 16 mrad/mCi, in contrast to 240 mrad/mCi associated with ^{201}Tl, allowing greater amounts of ^{99m}Tc to be injected clinically. Following extraction from the blood, ^{99m}Tc-sestamibi and tetrofosmin are quickly bound by mitochondria, and only a limited amount of myocardial washout (or wash-in) occurs over time.[3,7] Both tracers exhibit lower myocardial uptake than thallium, and this uptake is lowest with tetrofosmin.[8] Another drawback of the ^{99m}Tc tracers is more hepatic and gastrointestinal uptake than thallium potentially interfering with inferior myocardial wall visualization.[3]

From a practical standpoint, the ^{99m}Tc agents provide greater flexibility than ^{201}Tl. Because of mitochondrial binding, they do not require that imaging commence soon after the stress injection for maximal sensitivity. In contrast, with ^{201}Tl, imaging must be performed soon after stress testing, to detect mild, reversible defects,

since such defects may demonstrate rapid redistribution. Thus, if soft tissue attenuation or patient motion compromises a study, the benefit of repeating the acquisition is questionable with ^{201}Tl. With ^{99m}Tc sestamibi or tetrofosmin, however, stress testing and tracer injection could take place at a location remote from the imaging laboratory, and image acquisition can simply be repeated (e.g., in the prone position[9]) when patient motion, soft tissue attenuation, or other artifact is considered to be responsible for the production of a perfusion defect.

^{99m}Tc-Teboroxime

^{99m}Tc-teboroxime has a higher extraction fraction than ^{201}Tl and a plateau at a higher flow rate than other agents.[10] However, very rapid myocardial washout[3] requires that initial imaging be completed within the first few minutes after injection. Although impractical with standard Anger cameras, ^{99m}Tc-teboroxime would be well suited to use with very rapid SPECT cameras that have recently been described.[11]

[ ] EXERCISE PROTOCOLS

Exercise stress is generally preferred over pharmacologic stress for use with SPECT MPI in patients who can exercise adequately, because it allows assessment of exercise capacity, heart rate (HR) and blood pressure (BP) responses, and symptoms as well as ST-segment response, providing additional clinical information that can be useful in daily clinical decision making.[2] For exercise SPECT MPI, an indwelling intravenous line is inserted preexercise, the tracer is injected at maximal stress, and exercise is continued for an additional 1 min at peak workload.

Although it is desirable for treadmill exercise to be symptom-limited, achieving 85 percent of the maximum predicted HR (220 – age) has been the traditional cutoff for an acceptable level of stress.[2] Recently, however, chronotropic incompetence, defined as a low percent of HR reserve achieved = (peak HR – rest HR)/(220 – age – rest HR) × 100, with <80 percent considered abnormal, has been shown to be a powerful predictor of cardiac death and all-cause mortality in patients undergoing exercise myocardial perfusion SPECT.[12,13] In a recent study, inability to achieve 80 percent of HR reserve was a more powerful predictor of cardiac death than failure to reach 85 percent of maximal predicted HR.[13] Also, patients with normal SPECT MPI but abnormal HR reserve achieved were at just as high a risk for overall mortality as patients with abnormal SPECT MPI but normal HR reserve achieved. Thus, physicians should not be misled that patients with normal stress SPECT MPI in the setting of an abnormal HR reserve are a low-risk group—they are at substantial risk. These considerations illustrate how the prognostic information of the exercise stress test itself must be integrated with the nuclear findings and is a benefit of performing exercise stress over pharmacologic stress. It has been suggested that when assessing HR response to exercise, the HR reserve approach should be used and should replace the traditional percent of age-predicted HR achieved.

Postexercise stress imaging routinely commences 15 minutes after stress, but with the ^{99m}Tc perfusion tracers, because of the absence of significant redistribution, imaging can begin up to a few hours after stress injection. The advantage of starting imaging earlier is that it increases the opportunity to observe stress-induced stunning during gated SPECT acquisition.[14]

【 】 PHARMACOLOGIC STRESS PROTOCOLS

Vasodilator Stress

For patients who cannot achieve an adequate level of exercise (≥ 85 percent of maximal predicted HR,[2] pharmacologic stress testing is preferred.[15] The preferred pharmacologic stress agents for SPECT MPI are coronary vasodilators: adenosine or dipyridamole. These agents provide a three- to fivefold increase in coronary flow. Dipyridamole blocks the cellular reuptake of adenosine, increasing the extracellular adenosine concentration. Increased extracellular adenosine results in coronary vasodilation. Adenosine is growing in use more than dipyridamole, predominantly because of its rapid onset and offset of peak effect. Methylxanthines, such as theophylline or caffeine, block adenosine binding and can eliminate the coronary vasodilation effects of adenosine or dipyridamole, leading to false-negative stress perfusion studies. In general, being off caffeine-containing medicines, foods, or beverages for 24 hours is recommended, because the half-life of caffeine is variable.[2] The diagnostic accuracies of SPECT MPI using exercise or pharmacologic stress are equivalent, despite the higher coronary flow rates associated with the vasodilators.[16]

Regarding the clinical and hemodynamic responses to vasodilator stress, normally there is a mild rise in HR and fall in BP with adenosine or dipyridamole infusion. However, clinical assessment and hemodynamic responses to vasodilators are not useful in identifying patients in whom the pharmacologic effects of adenosine or dipyridamole have been blocked by caffeine; failure of HR or BP to change with adenosine stress does not imply lack of myocardial perfusion response.[17] Recent data suggest that resting tachycardia and failure to mount a tachycardia in response to vasodilator stress is associated with a considerable increase in mortality risk.[18]

Dipyridamole Infusion
Dipyridamole is usually infused at 0.142 mg/kg/min for 4 minutes, but some investigators have recommended increasing the dose by 50 percent.[16] The maximal effect occurs approximately 3 to 4 minutes after end of the infusion. Mild transient side effects are common, including chest pain, shortness of breath, dizziness, and flushing. Severe side effects are rare, being noted in only 1 of 10,000 patients.[19] Side effects can usually be reversed by intravenous aminophylline, usually 75 to 125 mg. Because of the potential side effect of severe bronchospasm, dipyridamole is contraindicated for asthmatics.

Adenosine Infusion
Adenosine is infused intravenously (140 μg/kg/min), usually over 4 to 6 minutes, with radiopharmaceutical administration at 2 to 3 minutes of infusion.[16,20] Transient side effects occur more frequently than with dipyridamole,[16] but because of the duration of action of approximately 13 seconds, reversal with aminophylline is not needed. With adenosine, there is an increased incidence of ad-

vanced atrioventricular (AV) block. Adenosine is considered contraindicated for patients with greater than first-degree AV block, sick sinus syndrome, or bronchospasm.

Selective A2A Agonists
One of the limitations of current vasodilator agents is the high frequency of uncomfortable systemic side effects and the risk of bronchoconstriction in asthmatics. There are three selective A2A agonists currently being evaluated for use as vasodilator stress agents. All these agents can be administered as a bolus rather than with an infusion[21-23] and have a longer duration of activity than adenosine (Fig. 19–3). It is considered likely that the A2A agonists will become the standard vasodilator agents in the future for use in MPI studies. In general, these more specific agents result in a lower frequency of side effects.[21-23] Although theoretically these agents could be used in patients with bronchospasm, this possibility has not yet been studied.

Vasodilator Stress with Low Level Exercise
It has become increasingly common to combine vasodilator stress with low-level exercise.[24] This generally is accomplished by beginning exercise at the beginning of adenosine infusion or at the end of a dipyridamole infusion. The low-level exercise reduces splanchnic blood flow and, thereby, hepatic uptake of ^{99m}Tc sestamibi or tetrofosmin, facilitating early postinfusion imaging with these tracers (as early as 15 minutes following injection) compared to the 1-hour delay required when adjunctive exercise is not performed. Another key benefit is a marked reduction in the frequency as well as in the severity of side effects from the vasodilator stress agents, possibly caused by the increased attention to the task of walking in patients who usually cannot perform maximal exercise. Being able to perform low-level exercise also provides additional prognostic information.[25] Given all of these advantages, we perform the *adenowalk* protocol with all adenosine infusions when possible, with the exception of patients with left bundle-branch block (LBBB) or paced rhythm in whom it is preferable not to have the increased HR associated with exercise.

Left Bundle-Branch Block and Right Ventricular Pacing
With exercise stress, patients with LBBB frequently demonstrate reversible defects in the septal wall in the absence of CAD. Stress modalities that do not increase HR as markedly as exercise, such as aden-

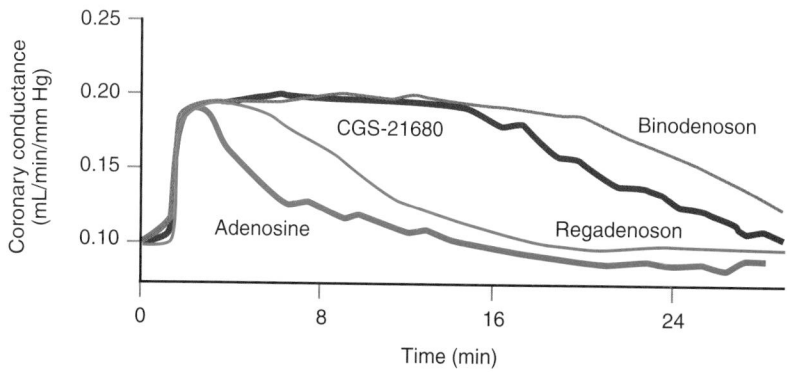

FIGURE 19–3. Time course of changes in coronary conductance caused by regadenoson (red), binodenoson (green), CGS-21680 (brown), and adenosine (blue). *Source: Reproduced with permission from Gao Z, Li Z, Baker SP, et al.[146]*

osine or dipyridamole stress without walking, are generally considered preferable in LBBB patients.[26] With exercise SPECT MPI, the perfusion defect associated with LBBB in the absence of left anterior descending CAD most commonly involves the interventricular septum with sparing of the apex of the left ventricular, a pattern that would be uncommon for left anterior descending CAD.[27] Myocardial perfusion defects in the inferior and apical walls have also been reported in the absence of CAD in patients with prolonged right ventricular (RV) pacing.[16]

Practical Tip: Because of the relationship between the increase in HR and the presence of perfusion defects without CAD in LBBB and paced ventricular rhythms, vasodilator stress is preferred over exercise in these patients; and the vasodilator stress protocols are performed without adjunctive low-level exercise.[2]

Aortic Stenosis Exercise stress testing is generally not recommended in patients with significant aortic stenosis because of safety concerns. Although exercise testing is generally safe in asymptomatic patients, studies have shown low specificity with MPI for the diagnosis of CAD. Vasodilator stress is reportedly effective in patients with moderate to severe aortic stenosis.[28] In patients with critical aortic stenosis, any form of stress testing (exercise, vasodilator, dobutamine) is considered contraindicated.

Dobutamine Stress

An alternative to vasodilator stress is inotropic stress with dobutamine. At the present time, dobutamine stress is usually reserved for patients with asthma, chronic obstructive pulmonary disease with bronchospasm, or those who have ingested caffeine. Dobutamine stress results in a lower-rate pressure product than exercise and a lower peak coronary blood flow with vasodilator stress. Side effects, including ventricular irritability, are more common than with the vasodilator stress. The protocol employed is the same as that used for dobutamine stress echocardiography. As with echocardiography, atropine is commonly used in addition if the target HR (>85 percent) is not achieved.

Patient Preparation for Stress Imaging

In general, for purposes of diagnosis or initial risk stratification, stress nuclear testing is performed with the patient off of antiischemic medications,[2] because they may limit the development of ischemia during the stress test. When feasible use of β blockers or long-acting calcium channel blockers should be discontinued at least 48 hours before and long-acting nitrates should be discontinued at least 12 hours before stress imaging.[2] Although *initial risk stratification* studies are generally performed off of cardiac active medications, potentially useful clinical information can be derived from exercise or pharmacologic SPECT MPI performed on cardiac medications.[2] Regarding pharmacologic stress testing, Sharir and colleagues[29] reported that compared to SPECT MPI performed off medications, dipyridamole SPECT MPI performed *on medications* was associated with smaller and less reversible perfusion defects and approximately a one-third lowering of overall vessel

sensitivity (62 percent vs. 92 percent). A recent study has demonstrated that acute beta blockade reduces the size of adenosine stress myocardial perfusion defects and doubles the likelihood of false negative studies (14.3 percent vs. 28.6 percent).[30] It has been shown that patients with normal exercise SPECT MPI who achieve less than 80 to 85 percent MPHR are at greater risk than those who achieve maximal workload.[31,32] Thus, recommendations are that patients be off of caffeine prior to exercise or vasodilator stress SPECT MPI.[2] If a patient fails to achieve 85 percent of maximal predicted HR (MPHR) during exercise, pharmacologic testing with adenosine or dipyridamole can then be immediately substituted prior to stress tracer injection.

【 】 IMAGING PROTOCOLS

^{201}Tl Protocols

With ^{201}Tl, a variety of SPECT protocols are available (Fig. 19–4). When ^{201}Tl is the only radiopharmaceutical, the usual protocol uses some combination of stress with redistribution and/or reinjection SPECT MPI (see Fig. 19–4A). The initially described stress/redistribution/reinjection methods required three image acquisitions and a decision to reinject. A two-acquisition sequence with stress and one reinjection/redistribution image is commonly performed, with additional 24-hour imaging if nonreversible (*fixed*) defects are found at 4-hour (see Fig. 19–4B). Sublingual nitroglycerin prior to ^{201}Tl reinjection may reduce the need for 24-hour imaging. Rest/redistribution ^{201}Tl SPECT MPI is commonly used for resting ischemia/viability testing[5] (see Fig. 19–4C). Even with rest ^{201}Tl SPECT, 24-hour imaging can result in additional redistribution compared to 4-hour imaging.[16]

With ^{201}Tl SPECT, the timing of initial poststress acquisition is important, because early ^{201}Tl redistribution can decrease sensitiv-

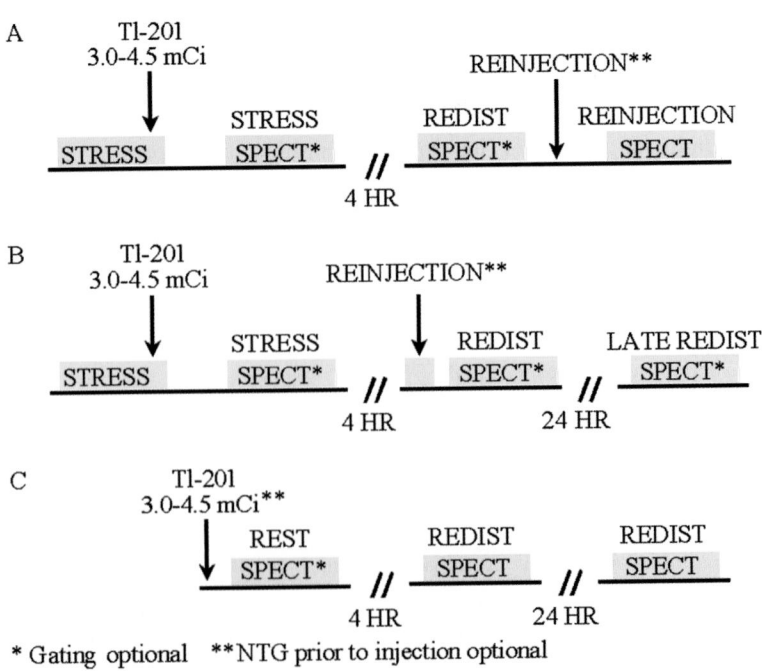

FIGURE 19–4. ^{201}Tl, protocols. **A.** Stress/redistribution (redist), reinjection. **B.** Stress/reinjection/late redistribution. **C.** Rest/redistribution. Tl-201, thallium-201.

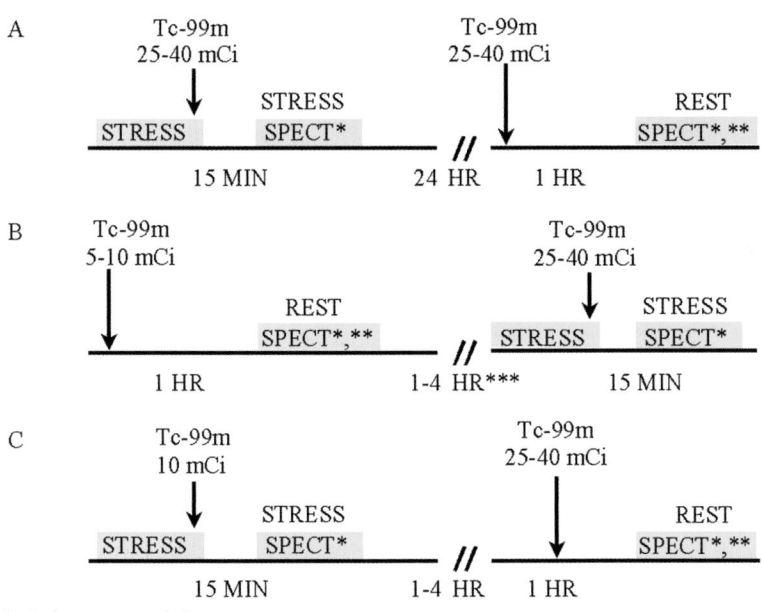

A

Tc-99m
25-40 mCi

STRESS | STRESS SPECT*

15 MIN   24 HR

Tc-99m
25-40 mCi

REST SPECT*,**

1 HR

B

Tc-99m
5-10 mCi

REST SPECT*,**

1 HR   1-4 HR***

Tc-99m
25-40 mCi

STRESS | STRESS SPECT*

15 MIN

C

Tc-99m
10 mCi

STRESS | STRESS SPECT*

15 MIN   1-4 HR

Tc-99m
25-40 mCi

REST SPECT*,**

1 HR

* Gating recommended
** NTG prior to rest injection optional
*** Delay time can be reduced by lowering rest dose and increasing stress dose

FIGURE 19–5. Two-day (**A**), same-day rest-stress (sequence interchangeable) (**B**), and same-day stress-rest (**C**), ⁹⁹ᵐTc-sestamibi or tetrofosmin protocols. NTG, nitroglycerin; SPECT, single-photon emission computed tomography; Tc-99m, technetium-99m-sestamibi or tetrofosmin.

ity for CAD if poststress imaging is delayed. With either ²⁰¹Tl or ⁹⁹ᵐTc agents, SPECT MPI should not begin <10 minutes after stress because of *upward creep of the heart*,[16] an artifact related to increased depth of respiration very early poststress, causing the heart to gradually move cephalad during the early portion of SPECT acquisition.

⁹⁹ᵐTc-Sestamibi or Tetrofosmin Protocols

Because uptake and radiation dosimetry of these compounds are similar, the recommended acquisition protocols are the same. The radiation dosimetry of these agents is better than that of ²⁰¹Tl. Because of the absence of clinically significant redistribution, separate rest and stress injections are needed with ⁹⁹ᵐTc-sestamibi or tetrofosmin SPECT (Fig. 19–5)[16] to assess reversibility of perfusion defects. With these agents, if imaging artifact is suspected on supine images, additional prone imaging can be performed to increase the specificity of SPECT MPI (Fig. 19–6).[9,16]

A variety of protocols can be used with these agents, including 2-day stress/rest, same-day rest/ stress, same-day stress/rest, and dual-isotope. From the standpoint of defect contrast and image quality, the 2-day stress/rest protocol is ideal (see Fig. 19–5A). Both stress and rest studies are obtained after injection of high doses of ⁹⁹ᵐTc-sestamibi or tetrofosmin, allowing acquisition of consistent high-count images. The drawback is its requirement for two imaging days. The most common ⁹⁹ᵐTc agent protocol is same-day low-dose rest/high-dose stress (see Fig.

19–5B).[16] Although convenient, it has the disadvantage of reduction in stress-defect contrast, as approximately 15 percent of the radioactivity observed at the time of stress imaging comes from the preexisting resting injection. The same-day low-dose stress/high-dose rest sequence (see Fig. 19–5C) has the advantage of image acquisition times the same as those used for stress ²⁰¹Tl imaging, facilitating mixing of these two protocols. The principal drawback of this approach is that the count rates associated with the stress image set are low. With either the 1- or 2-day stress/rest sequences, an advantage is the ability to perform the stress image only.[16] Viability assessment with ⁹⁹ᵐTc sestamibi or tetrofosmin may be improved by the administration of nitroglycerin prior to the rest-injection study.[16,33]

Dual Isotope Protocols

An alternative to these ⁹⁹ᵐTc-sestamibi or tetrofosmin protocols is a rest ²⁰¹Tl/stress ⁹⁹ᵐTc-sestamibi dual-isotope SPECT (Fig. 19–7),[20] taking advantage of the Anger camera's ability to collect data in different energy windows. It is usually performed with separate rest/stress acquisitions, including redistribution thallium images either before the stress study (see Fig. 19–7B) or at 24 hours (after stress) (see Fig. 19–7C) if a rest defect is present. Advantages of this approach are increased efficiency and the ability to assess resting perfusion defect reversibility (detecting resting ischemia by ²⁰¹Tl redistribution images). The separate acquisition approach does not require correction for cross-contamination between the two radioisotopes,[20] which are important for simultaneous dual-isotope approach, a potentially efficient approach not yet in general clinical use.

In any protocol using the rest/stress sequence, the resting images can be inspected prior to stress testing (Fig. 19–8), enabling the identification of patients with unexpected rest perfusion defects, usually secondary to critical CAD, in whom unnecessary stress testing can be avoided.[34]

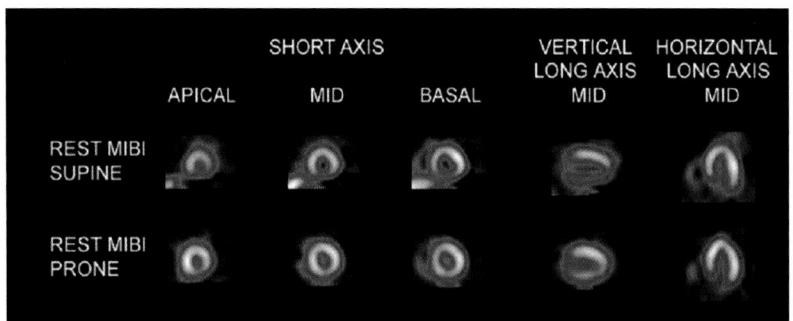

FIGURE 19–6. Rest sestamibi (MIBI) SPECT images in the supine position (*top*) and prone position (*bottom*) in a 55-year-old patient with a low likelihood of CAD. Prone images are normal, demonstrating that the apparent inferior wall perfusion defect on the supine images is secondary to soft tissue attenuation. Normal wall motion was noted on gated SPECT MPI. Gated resting MPI: EDV 55 mL, ESV 35 mL, EF 55 percent. CAD, coronary artery disease; MPI, myocardial perfusion imaging; SPECT, single-photon emission computed tomography. *Source: Reproduced with permission from Berman DS, Germano G.*[147]

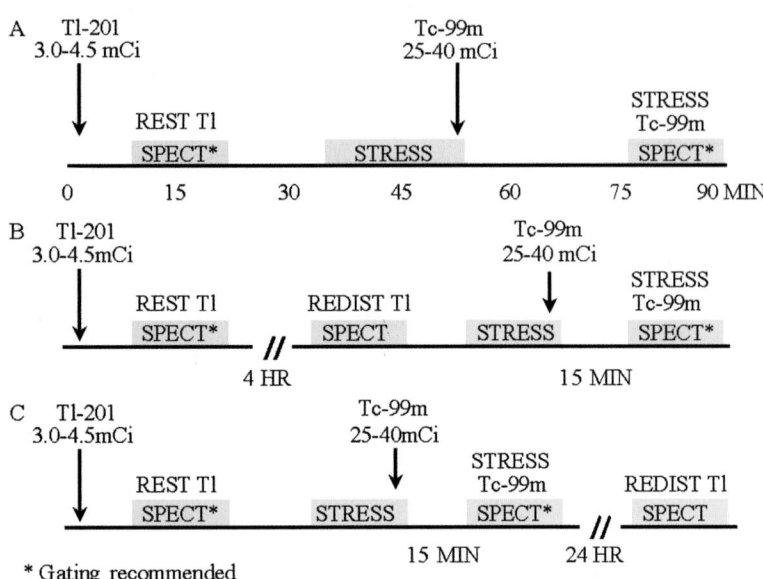

FIGURE 19–7. Variations of the resting ^{201}Tl/^{99m}Tc-sestamibi or tetrofosmin dual-isotope SPECT MPI protocol. Most commonly, only rest and stress imaging is performed (**A**). When resting defects are present, redistribution imaging is recommended and may be performed before (**B**) or 24 hours after (**C**) injection of the technetium perfusion agent. MPI, myocardial perfusion imaging; SPECT, single-photon emission computed tomography; Tc-99m, technetium-99m-sestamibi or tetrofosmin; Tl-201, thallium-201.

Prone Imaging

One of the most difficult areas of interpretation of myocardial perfusion SPECT is the differentiation of artifactual from true perfusion defects. Imaging the patient in the prone position with the nuclear detector rotating underneath the patient decreases the frequency of attenuation artifacts in the inferior wall and also decreases motion artifact (see Fig. 19–6).[35] However, prone imaging may create artifactual anteroseptal defects caused by the more pronounced sternal attenuation in this position.[16] As a consequence, combined prone and supine imaging with the sestamibi or tetrofosmin has been described. Hayes and coworkers reported that patients with inferior wall defects on supine SPECT MPI but normal prone SPECT MPI have as low a risk of subsequent cardiac events, as patients with normal supine only studies.[35] A quantitative method for computer-based interpretation of combined supine and prone sestamibi SPECT images has recently been reported.[9] With this approach, supine and prone images are compared to their respective normal databases and only regions found concordantly abnormal by both positions are considered abnormal. The combined quantitation has demonstrated an increase in the normalcy rate without a loss of sensitivity.

Attenuation Correction

Several camera manufacturers have recently provided hardware and software implementation of attenuation correction (AC) protocols. In general, these corrections are imperfect reducing but not eliminating apparent perfusion defects caused by soft tissue attenuation in normal patients.[36]

Several reports have compared the diagnostic accuracy of AC and non-AC SPECT using a variety of commercially available approaches. In general, these have demonstrated improved specificity with no change in overall sensitivity.[37,38] Despite these considerations, attenuation correction is not yet widely used, possibly because of the lack of a common approach to its commercial implementation by camera manufacturers.[36]

BASICS OF INTERPRETATION

The interpretation of SPECT MPI is performed by visual or computer-based quantitative methods.

[ ] PERFUSION DEFECTS

Perfusion defects are characterized by their type as well as their extent and severity. The various defect types are illustrated in Fig. 19–9 for stress and rest SPECT MPI and in Fig. 19–10 for rest SPECT MPI viability patterns. The distribution of SPECT abnormalities provides information regarding the location of coronary artery stenoses. Representative examples of SPECT defect locations associated with individual coronary artery stenoses are illustrated in Fig. 19–11 and Fig. 19–12.

Visual Semiquantitative Segmental Scoring

Semiquantitative perfusion scoring systems standardize the visual interpretation of scans, reduce the likelihood of overlooking significant defects, and provide global indices for overall assessment of extent and severity of perfusion abnormality. Further, they are more systematic and reproducible than simple qualitative evaluation.

17-Segment Model A 17-segment scoring system for SPECT MPI is preferred over the previously widely used 20-segment system because it more accurately represents the size of each segment (Fig. 19–13).[39] Segmental assignment is based on three

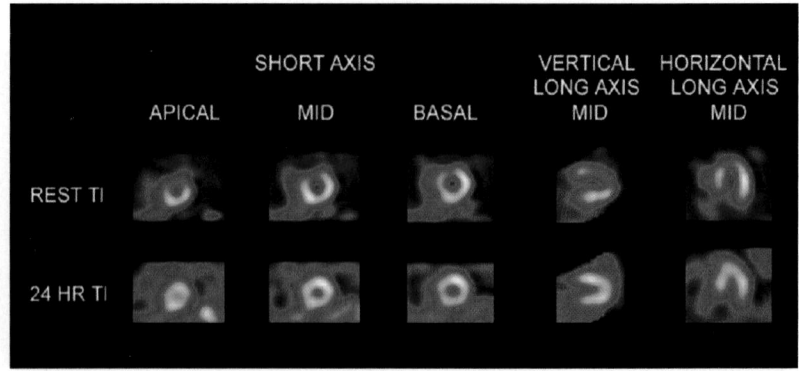

FIGURE 19–8. Rest and 24-hour redistribution ^{201}Tl SPECT MPI of a 75-year-old male with atypical angina showing a large amount of resting ischemia in the left anterior descending territory, which subsequently revealed a 95 percent proximal stenosis by coronary angiography. Of note, the LV was larger at rest than at the time of redistribution imaging. The stress SPECT MPI study was cancelled in this patient because of the unexpected perfusion defect. LV, left ventricle; MPI, myocardial perfusion imaging; SPECT, single-photon emission computed tomography.

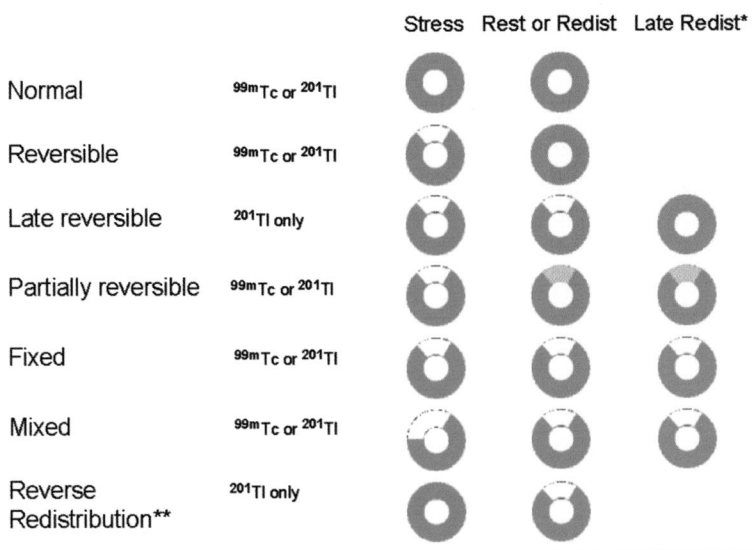

FIGURE 19–9. Patterns of stress/rest or redistribution SPECT MPI defects. *Red* represents normal tracer update; *white* represents a definite perfusion defect; *gray* represents less severe but still definite perfusion defect (seen in the partially reversible defect example). 99mTc, technetium-99m-sestamibi or tetrofosmin; 201Tl, thallium-20.

short-axis slices (4 distal [apical], 6 mid, and 6 basal) representing the entire left ventricle (LV), with the apical segments visualized in a midvertical long-axis image. Each of the 17 segments has a distinct name and is scored using a 5-point system (0 = normal; 1, 2, 3 = mild [equivocal], moderate, and severe reductions of a radioisotope; and 4 = absence of detectable tracer uptake).[2,27] Severe reversible perfusion defects with scores of 3 or 4 (see Fig. 19–11 *second row* and Fig. 19–11 *bottom row*; see Fig. 19–12 *second row* and Fig. 19–12 *bottom row*) can be reported as consistent with a critical (≥ 90 percent) coronary stenosis.[27] The differences between the 17- and 20-segment model is that with 17-segment scoring, the smaller size of the distal short-axis slice is accounted for by 4 versus 6 segments and the apex is 1 rather than 2 segments.

Summed Scores Segmental scoring systems lend themselves to the derivation of summed scores from the 17 to 20 segments (i.e., global indices of perfusion).[2,40] The overall extent and severity of perfusion defects are reflected by the summed stress score (SSS), the summed rest score (SRS), and the summed differences score (SDS), the latter defined by SSS-SRS and measuring the degree of reversibility. Risk groups may be defined using SSS categories[2,27] (Table 19–1).

More recently, we have described expressing overall perfusion defects as percent myocardium involved (percent stress, reversible, fixed) and now routinely use this approach for clinical reporting and all prognostic publications.[32] The conversion of summed scores to percent myocardium is accomplished by dividing the summed scores by the worst segmental score possible in the specific model used (68 for 17 segments, 80 for 20 segments) and multiplying by 100 (5-point scoring with 0 = normal and 4 = absent uptake). The benefits

of this approach are that it provides a measure with intuitive implications (percent myocardium hypoperfused) not possible with the unitless summed scores, that it can easily be applied with scoring systems using varying numbers of segments (e.g., 17, 20, 14, 12), and that it is applicable to quantitative methods that directly measure these abnormalities as percent myocardium. Risk groups by the percent stress abnormal, which correlate with SSS risk groups, are <5 percent (normal or minimally abnormal), 5 to 10 percent mildly abnormal, 11 to 14 percent moderately abnormal, and ≥ 15 percent severely abnormal[27,32,41] (see Table 19–1). When converted to percent myocardium abnormal, the prognostic implications of the 17 and 20 segment scoring have been shown to be equivalent (Fig. 19–14).[42]

Quantitative Analysis

A variety of commercially available software packages are available to assist in image interpretation, and the wealth of quantitative measurements they can provide are summarized in Table 19–2. With respect to myocardial perfusion assessment, these computer approaches generally operate by automatic determination of the amount of radioactivity at rest and stress within each pixel or small zone of the myocardium, scaling this amount by the maximal amount of radioactivity in the myocardium (normalization), and then comparing this scaled amount to the lower limit of normal. The change between rest and stress is usually also assessed and compared to normal, providing information approximately perfusion defect reversibility. The results are most commonly displayed using polar maps. Fig. 19–15 displays polar maps associated with the various scan abnormalities shown in Fig. 19–11 and Fig. 19–12.

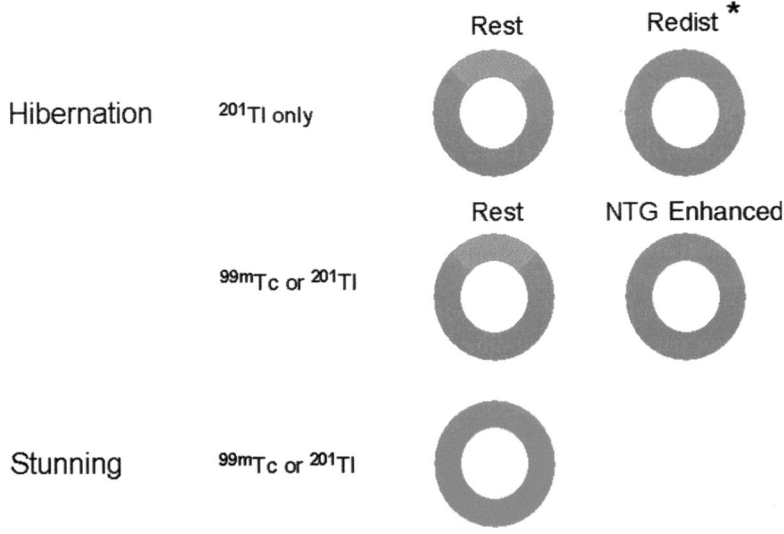

FIGURE 19–10. Patterns of myocardial viability associated with regional contractile abnormality. *Gray* represents perfusion defect. 99mTc, technetium-99m-sestamibi or tetrofosmin; 201Tl, thallium-20.

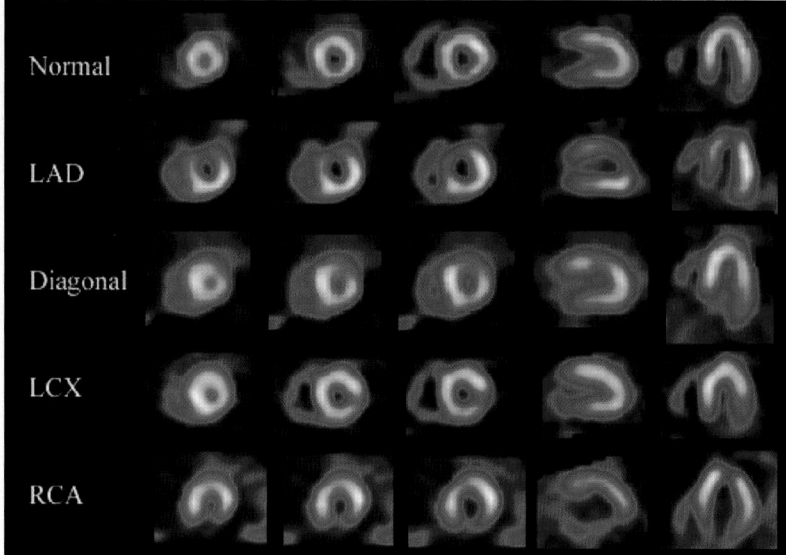

FIGURE 19–11. Examples of typical stress perfusion patterns corresponding to normal (*top*) and various single-territory abnormalities. Coronary angiographic findings in these patients were as follows: LAD (left anterior descending coronary artery) proximal 95 percent stenosis; diagonal (occluded proximal first diagonal artery); left circumflex coronary artery (LCX); occluded first marginal artery branch; right coronary artery (RCA); mid-95 percent stenosis. All patients had no evidence of myocardial infarction and normal SPECT MPI at rest. From left to right, the images represent distal short axis, mid-short axis, basal short axis, midvertical long axis, and midhorizontal long axis. These patients show the typical distributions of perfusion defects associated with the specific coronary arteries involved, as shown in Fig. 19–13.

finding of region wall motion abnormalities post-stress not seen on the resting studies.[14]

Quantitation of gated SPECT MPI can be performed by a variety of algorithms. The most common approaches are fully 3D and based on the automatic detection of endocardial and epicardial surface points.[1,45] In validation studies of LVEF by gated SPECT, published to date,[1] the agreement between gated SPECT and other standard measurements of LVEF has been shown to be very good to excellent. Although LVEF measured by the various quantitative algorithms correlate highly, the thresholds for abnormality are different depending on the method used.[46,47] With some methods, the normal threshold for the global LVEF measured by gated SPECT MPI images is slightly lower than that measured using other imaging modalities (approximately 45 percent) principally because of the use of only eight gating intervals.[1] Recently, 16-frame gating has become more common, reducing the underestimation of LVEF. Gender-based normal limits for LVEF and LV volumes and volume indices have been reported.[48] With multidetector systems, LVEF and LV volumes by gated thallium-201 SPECT MPI correlate highly with those of ^{99m}Tc-sestamibi SPECT MPI,[1] which in turn have been widely validated by comparison with a variety of other tests.[1]

Because these computer-based quantitative programs do not take into account artifacts that may be easily detected visually (such as marked breast attenuation), the final interpretation currently always includes visual verification and if necessary modification.[1,27] The results of quantitative analysis has been shown to be prognostically useful and may complement information derived from visual analysis alone.[43]

[ ] VENTRICULAR FUNCTION

With all of the SPECT protocols, whether ^{201}Tl or ^{99m}Tc tracers are used, it is currently recommended that ECG gating also be performed.[44] Gated SPECT MPI allows the assessment of a variety of ventricular function parameters. Regional wall motion or thickening is most commonly assessed by semiquantitative visual analysis, using the same segmental system employed for perfusion defect assessment. Automatic computer-based methods quantify global function parameters, including left ventricular ejection fraction (LVEF), end-diastolic volumes, end-systolic volumes (ESVs), and diastolic function. Regional LV myocardial wall motion and thickening can be quantitated from gated SPECT MPI images and is useful in the identification of hibernation, stunning, and infarction as well as distinguishing true perfusion defects from attenuation artifacts. Gating of both the rest and the poststress acquisition is currently performed in most laboratories, providing the ability to detect stress-induced stunning by

[ ] TRANSIENT ISCHEMIC DILATION AND LUNG UPTAKE

In addition to perfusion defects, several nonperfusion abnormalities can be observed with SPECT MPI, including size and shape of the LV, transient ischemic dilation (TID) of the LV,[49,50]

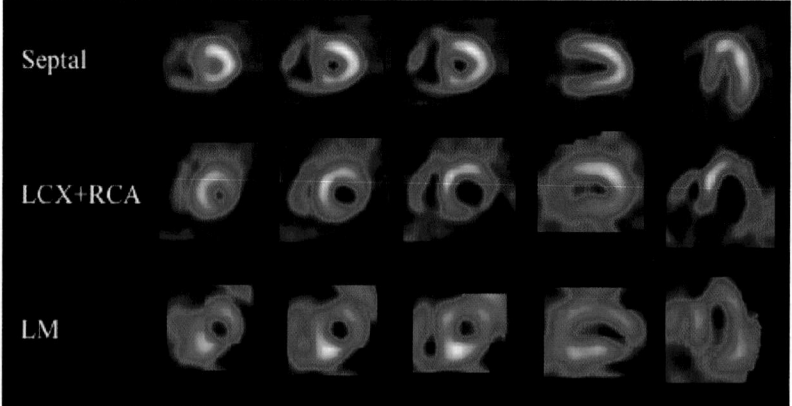

FIGURE 19–12. Stress SPECT MPI images demonstrating more complex patterns associated with known coronary lesions in patients with normal resting perfusion images and no history of prior MI. *Septal*: trapped septal perforator coronary artery (occlusion of first septal coronary artery) in a patient with critical LAD stenoses proximal and distal to the septal perforator takeoff and patent right posterior descending coronary artery, vein grafts to the left circumflex marginal coronary artery, and patent LAD internal mammary graft. *LCX plus RCA*: occlusion of proximal left circumflex and proximal right coronary arteries; left main (*LM*): subtotal left main coronary artery stenosis. LAD, left anterior descending coronary artery; LCX, left circumflex coronary artery; MI, myocardial infarction; MPI, myocardial perfusion imaging; RCA, right coronary artery; SPECT, single-photon emission computed tomography.

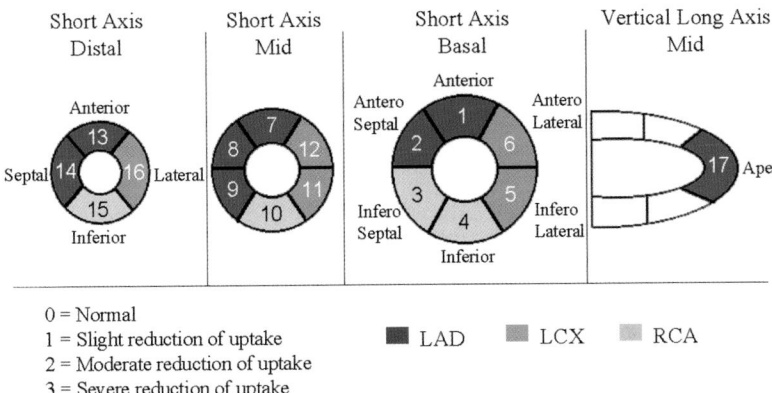

Myocardial Perfusion SPECT 17-Segment Scoring

0 = Normal
1 = Slight reduction of uptake
2 = Moderate reduction of uptake
3 = Severe reduction of uptake
4 = Absent of radioactive uptake

■ LAD   ■ LCX   ■ RCA

FIGURE 19-13. Diagrammatic representation of segmental division of the SPECT slices and assignment of the segments to the individual coronary arteries using the 17-segment model. LAD, left anterior descending coronary artery; LCX, left circumflex coronary artery; RCA, right coronary artery; SPECT, single-photon emission computed tomography.

specific for critical stenosis (>90 percent narrowing) in vessels supplying a large portion of the myocardium (i.e., proximal left anterior descending or multivessel 90 percent lesions).[49,50] Dipyridamole or adenosine-induced TID has similar implications as those associated with exercise.[52] Fig. 19–16 illustrates an example of TID on SPECT MPI from a patient with severe disease of the left anterior descending artery. TID can easily be measured by the quantitative gated SPECT algorithms. The upper limit of normal for the TID ratio with exercise SPECT MPI has been reported to be 1.22 for dual-isotope imaging, and 1.14 for 2-day ^{99m}Tc imaging. Patients who have TID of the LV (TID >1.22) are likely to have severe and extensive CAD (>90 percent stenosis of the proximal left anterior descending coronary artery [LAD] or of multiple vessels).[50] For reasons that are not known, with vasodilator stress, the upper limit of normal to consider TID to

RV myocardial uptake pattern, RV size, and abnormalities of lung uptake or other abnormal extracardiac activity. TID is considered present when the LV cavity appears to be significantly larger in the poststress images than at rest[49,50] and may actually be an apparent cavity dilation secondary to diffuse subendocardial ischemia (obscuring the endocardial border). This explains why TID may be seen for several hours following stress, when true cavity dilation is probably no longer present. The correlation between LV TID and lung uptake is weak, suggesting that there may be different pathophysiologic mechanisms for each, and their measurements may be complementary in assessing the extent and severity of CAD for risk stratification.[51] TID is considered to represent severe and extensive ischemia and has been shown to be highly

TABLE 19-1

Definitions of Summed Perfusion Scores and Percent Myocardium Hypoperfused

Summed stress score (SSS)[a]	Sum of the segmental scores at stress	Amount of infarcted, ischemic, or jeopardized myocardium
Summed rest score (SRS)[a]	Sum of the segmental scores at rest	Amount of infarcted or hibernating myocardium
Summed difference score (SDS)[a]	SSS − SRS	Amount of ischemic or jeopardized myocardium
	20-Segment	17-Segment
Percent total	= SSS × 100/80	= SSS × 100/68
Percent ischemic	= SDS × 100/80	= SDS × 100/68
Percent fixed	= SRS × 100/80	= SRS × 100/68

[a]Reflects the extent and severity of perfusion abnormality.
SOURCE: Based on data from Hachamovitch R, Hayes SW, Friedman JD, et al.[32]

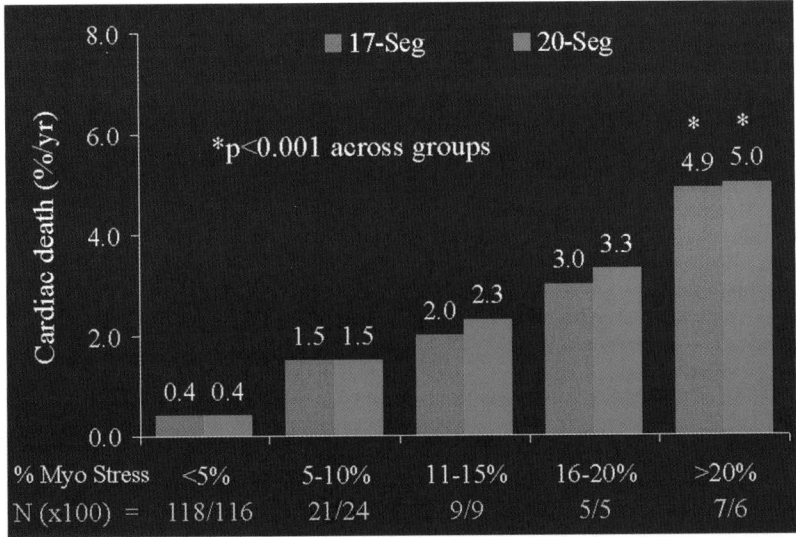

FIGURE 19-14. The prognostic value of the percent myocardium abnormal at stress (horizontal axis) is plotted versus the cardiac death rate (vertical axis) for 17 and 20 segment scoring systems. The cardiac mortality rate rises steadily with either approach, and there are no significant differences between the 17 and 20 segment systems when analyzed in this normalized summed score manner. Myo, myocardial. *Source: Based on data from Berman DS, Germano G.[147]*

TABLE 19–2

Quantitative Measurements Possible with Gated Myocardial Perfusion SPECT

TYPE	PARAMETER	COMMENT
Perfusion	Perfusion defect extent	Expressed as % of LV myocardium
	Perfusion defect severity	Related to the degree of hypoperfusion in the defect area
	Total perfusion deficit	Combines perfusion defect extent and severity; expressed as % of LV myocardial perfusion deficit
	Segmental scores and summed scores (post-stress, rest, reversibility)	Depends on specific myocardial model chosen
	Normalized summed scores	Normalized to worse possible score in chosen model, therefore model-independent
Function (Global)	LV ejection fraction	
	LV end-systolic and end-diastolic volume	
	Peak filling rate, time to PFR	LV diastolic function
Function (Regional)	Wall motion and wall thickening	
Other	LV contraction histogram	LV contraction phase/dyssynchrony
	Lung/heart ratio	Ratio of uptake in lung and LV
	Transient ischemic dilation ratio	Ratio of LV cavity volume post-stress vs. at rest
	LV myocardial mass	
	LV eccentricity, shape index	Estimates of LV shape (global or regional)

LV, left ventricle; SPECT, single-photon emission computed tomography.
SOURCE: Based on data from Germano G, Berman DS.[45]

be present is higher, approximately 1.36 with dual-isotope SPECT.[52,53]

Increased lung uptake of thallium reflects increased pulmonary capillary wedge pressure. Nonischemic causes of increased pulmonary capillary wedge pressure, such as mitral regurgitation, miral stenosis, and so on, are also associated with increased pulmonary thallium uptake. Increased thallium lung uptake after exercise has been shown to have incremental prognostic information over myocardial perfusion defect assessment.[54] Prognostic value of increased pulmonary uptake of ^{99m}Tc-sestamibi has recently been reported.[55]

【 】 SOURCES OF ARTIFACT

As with any diagnostic test, quality control is critical to clinical application of SPECT MPI. Artifactual perfusion defects have a variety of causes, most common of which are patient motion, breast and diaphragmatic attenuation, reconstruction artifacts caused by adjacent or superimposed extracardiac radioactivity, and poor count statistics.[44] With gated SPECT MPI, several technical artifacts can affect the accuracy of LVEF measurement. LVEFs can be overestimated in analyzing gated SPECT images of small hearts,[47] because of the limitations of spatial resolution with SPECT. In patients with LVH, LVEF may also be underestimated because of failure to accurately determine the endocardial border in the presence of the large muscle mass. Marked arrhythmia results in a falsely low LVEF measurement.

Assessment of Myocardial Viability

Assessment of myocardial viability with the myocardial perfusion tracers applies to segments with contractile dysfunction.[27] Viability is considered present if the degree of uptake at rest, redistribution, or following nitrate-augmented rest injection[56] is normal or nearly normal. Various patterns of myocardial viability associated with regional wall motion abnormality in these studies are shown in Fig. 19–10. A dysfunctional segment or region with severely reduced or absent uptake of radioactivity is considered to be nonviable. Areas with moderate reduction of counts in these conditions

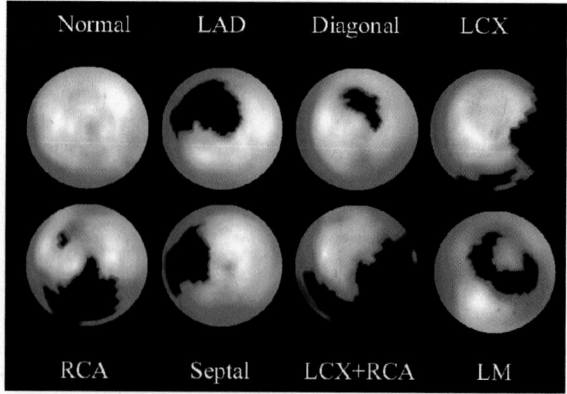

FIGURE 19–15. Quantitative stress polar maps of stress MPI in patients shown in Fig. 19–11 and Fig. 19–12 showing typical vascular perfusion patterns; black represents regions of quantitative perfusion defect when compared to normal limit files. LAD, left anterior descending coronary artery; LCX, left circumflex coronary artery; LM, left main; MPI, myocardial perfusion imaging; RCA, right coronary artery.

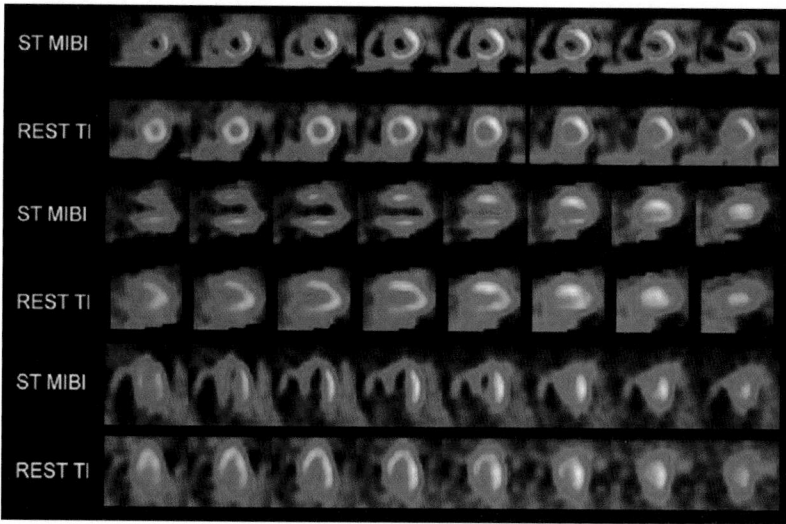

FIGURE 19–16. Exercise stress ^{99m}Tc-sestamibi (MIBI)/rest ^{201}Tl-myocardial perfusion SPECT images in an 63-year-old male with typical angina. There is evidence of a severe and extensive reversible defect throughout the LAD coronary artery and transient ischemia dilation of the LV. Angiography revealed 3-vessel disease with proximal subtotal occlusion of the LAD. ^{99m}Tc, technetium-99m-sestamibi or tetrofosmin; ^{201}Tl, thallium-20; LAD, left anterior descending coronary artery; LV, left ventricle; SPECT, single-photon emission computed tomography.

(e.g., a score 2/4 at redistribution or nitrate-augmented rest) are usually partially viable, and patients in this group have a variable response in terms of improvement after revascularization. When perfusion defects are seen at rest and not after redistribution or after separate reinjection following administration of nitroglycerin, SPECT MPI is commonly interpreted as showing *resting ischemia* and considered to represent regions of critically reduced blood flow to viable myocardium,[34] generally requiring rapid consideration of revascularization.

CLINICAL APPLICATIONS OF SPECT MPI

The principles underlying the efficient use of stress nuclear techniques and the optimal use of the test results are discussed below. The most common applications are assessing the likelihood of CAD in patients with suspected disease, assessing the likelihood that a patient with known CAD has ischemia, and assessing the magnitude of ischemia for prognostic purposes. The section that follows explores these applications and discusses the evidence for the use of SPECT MPI in specific patient populations commonly encountered in clinical cardiology settings.

【 】 SELECTING THE APPROPRIATE PATIENTS FOR TESTING

Central to appropriate patient selection for nuclear imaging and the interpretation of test results is the ability to determine an individual patient's pretest likelihood of CAD based on demographic, clinical, and historical information. The accurate evaluation of pretest likelihood of CAD allows for the appropriate selection of patients who would most likely benefit from referral

to nuclear imaging. The pretest likelihood or risk assessment may be estimated from published nomograms or by using available computerized programs (see Chap. 14, Chap. 38, and Chap. 40). Several models have been developed to predict significant and extensive CAD as well as cardiac survival.[57]

The rationale for applying SPECT MPI to noninvasive diagnostic testing is based on Bayesian theory (see Chap. 14 and Chap. 40), by which for a given test result, the posttest likelihood is a function of only three variables: The patient's pretest likelihood of disease and the test's sensitivity and specificity. The degree to which the test result alters the posttest likelihood is strongly affected by the pretest likelihood of disease. For any imperfect test, the greatest shift in posttest likelihood of disease occurs in patients with an intermediate pretest likelihood of CAD. As a benchmark, for a test with sensitivity and specificity of 90 percent, a patient with a pretest likelihood of 50 percent (e.g., a 50 year old man or a 65-year-old woman with atypical angina[58]) will have a posttest likelihood of 10 percent (*low*) with a normal test result and a 90 percent likelihood (*high*) with an abnormal test result. For purposes of assessing the posttest likelihood of CAD when using SPECT MPI, the patient's pretest likelihood takes into account all available information, including age, sex, symptoms, risk factors, the degree of coronary atherosclerosis if known (e.g., from a coronary artery calcium score), and the results of the nonnuclear stress testing components of the examination (e.g., the duration of exercise and degree of ST-segment depression).

【 】 DIAGNOSIS OF CORONARY ARTERY DISEASE

Detection of CAD is one of the most common indications for performing stress SPECT MPI. This referral is most appropriate in patients who have an intermediate likelihood of CAD. Exercise is the preferred form of stress because of the additional information derived from clinical, hemodynamic, and ECG responses to exercise. As noted above, principal exceptions to this are patients with LBBB or paced LV rhythms (Class I indication in the recent guidelines[2,59]) and patients with moderate aortic stenosis.

Diagnostic Accuracy

The accuracy of diagnostic testing for CAD is defined clinically on the basis of sensitivity and specificity for identification of angiographically significant stenoses, most commonly employing either a 50 percent or a 70 percent diameter-narrowing cutoff. Recent ACC/AHA/ASNC guidelines on cardiac radionuclide imaging report a pooled sensitivity and specificity of 87 and 73 percent for exercise SPECT MPI (based on 33 published studies) and 89 and 75 percent for vasodilator SPECT MPI (based on 17 published studies) for detection of CAD.[2] An improved predictive accuracy by nuclear testing over pretest information and ECG stress testing has been consistently documented.[60] In women, the specificity of SPECT MPI is increased with gated ^{99m}Tc-based agents compared to ungated ^{201}Tl SPECT MPI, attributed to less susceptibility to breast attenuation of gated SPECT MPI with ^{99m}Tc-based agents.[61] The ability to immediately reacquire SPECT images with ^{99m}Tc-based agents when either attenuation or motion artifact is suspected further increases specificity with these agents.[9,62] Improvements in specificity have also been reported with the use of attenuation correction algorithms.[63] The use of ECG gating attenuation correction, and combined prone and supine imaging are also considered to be associated with improvement in reader confidence.

Referral or Verification Bias

A major limitation in assessing the diagnostic accuracy of SPECT MPI for CAD is current clinical reality that the test result influences the decision to perform catheter-based coronary angiography, the *gold standard,* thereby biasing the population available for analysis of sensitivity and specificity. Using a multivariable analysis, Hachamovitch and colleagues[32] have recently demonstrated that the extent of ischemia by SPECT MPI provided 83 percent of the information appearing to determine referral for catheterization (see Fig. 19–22). Thus, in estimating the true sensitivity and specificity of noninvasive testing, this referral or workup bias must be taken into account.[64] As routine patient workup results in preferential catheterization of patients with abnormal (ischemic) test results, this referral bias leads to an overestimation of test sensitivity and a reduction in test specificity,[65] with the latter showing the most dramatic change.

Normalcy Rate

The normalcy rate has been advocated as another means of assessing test *specificity* without requiring the angiographic standard.[20] The normalcy rate is defined as the percentage of patients with normal test results in a population with a low likelihood of disease, usually employing a <5 percent criterion. The recent ACC/AHA/ASNC guidelines report a normalcy rate for SPECT MPI of 91 percent. Even in obese patients, normalcy rates >90 percent have been reported when attenuation correction or combined supine/prone imaging is employed.[9,113]

Diagnostic Testing

In general, SPECT MPI is not used as a screening test. For diagnosis, the principal application is in patients with an intermediate likelihood of CAD.[2,60,66–68] In the lower range of intermediate CAD likelihood (e.g., 0.15–0.50), many advocate the use of exercise tolerance test (ETT) alone. Although patients with pre-ETT likelihood of CAD in the 0.50 to 0.85 range could also considered candidates for ETT alone,[67] because a negative ETT would not result in a low CAD likelihood, many experts consider SPECT MPI the appropriate first test. Patients with an indeterminate CAD likelihood after ETT (e.g., intermediate-risk Duke treadmill score[2,68]) are candidates for SPECT MPI. Patients with ECG uninterpretable for ETT (e.g., left ventricular hypertrophy [LVH], digoxin, Wolff-Parkinson-White, >1-mm resting ST-depression, LBBB, permanent pacemaker, etc.) are candidates for SPECT MPI rather than ETT. As noted below,

the development CT coronary angiography may alter this approach, possibly becoming the first diagnostic test toward the lower part of the pretest likelihood spectrum.

【 】 RISK ASSESSMENT
Principles of Risk Stratification

A widely used paradigm in patient management is that of a *risk-based approach* to patients with suspected CAD in whom symptoms are nonlimiting. In patients referred directly to catheterization for any reason, pericatheterization SPECT MPI may serve to identify the culprit lesion. However, in less symptomatic patients, precatheterization risk assessment is more important. With a risk-based approach, the focus is not on predicting the presence of CAD but on identifying patients at risk for specific, potentially preventable adverse events. Subsequent management focuses on reducing the risk of these outcomes, whether cardiac death, nonfatal myocardial infarction (MI), or CAD progression. Invasive diagnostic and therapeutic procedures are limited to patients who are most likely to benefit from them. The basic concept underlying the use of nuclear testing for risk stratification is that patients known to be at high- or low-risk for events would not need risk stratification with nuclear imaging because they are already stratified.

Risk Thresholds   For the purposes of risk assessment, it has been proposed that low risk be defined as a <1 percent annual cardiac mortality rate, and intermediate risk could be defined by the range of 1 to 3 percent per year.[67] Because the mortality risk for patients undergoing revascularization is ≥1 percent (see Chap. 62 and Chap. 65), symptomatic patients with a <1 percent annual mortality rate would not appear to be candidates for revascularization to improve survival. It has been suggested that a >3 percent annual mortality rate is a threshold to identify patients with symptoms whose mortality rate can be improved by coronary artery bypass surgery (CABS).[69] SPECT MPI is most appropriate in patients with >1 percent annual mortality and intermediate or high likelihood of CAD. The exact level of these risk thresholds would vary according to the population being tested.

Physiologic Basis of Risk Assessment in SPECT MPI   Many major determinants of prognosis in CAD are assessed by measurements of stress-induced perfusion and function, including infarcted and jeopardized myocardium (supplied by vessels with hemodynamically significant stenosis) and the degree of jeopardy (tightness of the individual coronary stenosis). Of additional importance is the stability (or instability) of the CAD process, a factor that may explain an apparent paradox. Although nuclear tests in general are expected to identify only hemodynamically significant stenoses, it has been observed that most MIs occur in regions with less than 50 percent diameter narrowing.[70] Yet normal SPECT MPI, expected in patients with no or insignificant CAD, is associated with a low risk of either cardiac death or nonfatal MI. Several explanations may account for this apparent paradox. Patients with severe CAD may have more numerous mild plaques subject to potential instability and rupture than patients with no severe stenoses. Furthermore, a paradoxical vasoconstrictive response to stress caused by endothelial dysfunction with unstable mild stenoses may also contribute.[71]

Risk Stratification in Patients with Suspected or Known CAD

Stress SPECT MPI is an integral part of the evaluation of symptomatic patients for CAD and is commonly used in patients at intermediate post-ETT risk or with resting ECG abnormalities. As with diagnostic testing, if the patient's rest ECG is uninterpretable for purposes of stress testing, direct referral to SPECT MPI is effective in prognostic stratification (see Chap. 14).

Incremental Prognostic Value   The clinical value of SPECT MPI for prognostic assessment of CAD results from the incremental or added prognostic information yielded by this modality over all data available prior to the test (clinical, historical, and stress data), as first demonstrated by Ladenheim and colleagues.[72]

Event Risk after a Normal Scan   A synthesis of available data reveals that a normal scan is generally associated with a <1 percent annual risk of cardiac death or MI. A recent meta-analysis of the prognostic value of a normal stress perfusion scan (N = 29,788) reveals that the annual risk of MI or cardiac death after a normal perfusion scan is 0.5 percent (95 percent CI 0.3 to 0.7 percent).[73] This uniformly low event rate is critical in applying nuclear test information to risk stratification, because in the absence of symptoms, patients with normal perfusion scans can be managed conservatively. This approach includes follow-up for signs of clinical worsening and treatment of cardiac risk factors and related symptoms (see Chap. 40). The recent study has suggested that when inferior wall defects seen on supine imaging are not seen on prone imaging and are thus considered to be attenuation artifacts, the event rate is as low as in patients with normal supine studies.[35]

Despite the low risk associated with normal SPECT studies, a limited number of studies have reported somewhat higher levels of risk. Recently, a study examining predictors of risk and its temporal characteristics in a series of 7376 patients with normal stress SPECT MPI identified the use of pharmacologic stress and the presence of known CAD (Fig. 19–17A), diabetes mellitus (in particular, female diabetics), and advanced age as markers of increased risk and shortened time to a hard event (e.g., risk in the first year of follow up was less than in the second year).[31] Hence, a dynamic temporal component of risk was present and the existence of a *warranty* period for specific patient groups was defined (see Fig. 19–17B). This increased risk after normal SPECT in a small subset of patients is caused by the presence of comorbidities that in-

crease baseline risk of all patients (diabetes mellitus, age, inability to exercise, prior CAD, dyspnea as the presenting symptom[74]) and, in some patients, the possibility that extensive CAD was *missed* because of balanced reduction of flow. The latter would lead to a severe underestimation of the extent of ischemia by SPECT MPI. Although many patients can be detected by ancillary markers (e.g., LV transient ischemic dilation,[52] a rest to poststress fall in LVEF, or increased lung tracer uptake) in some patients with high-risk anatomic lesions, SPECT MPI will appear completely normal.

Event Risk with Abnormal Scans   The relationship of varying extent and severity of perfusion abnormalities with cardiac outcomes has been reported in a variety of patient subsets[42,60,67,75]; consistently, increasing scan abnormality is associated with an increasing risk of cardiac events. Although both reversible and fixed stress perfusion defects are predictors of prognosis, those at highest risk of cardiac events are patients with extensive stress abnormalities. Prognosis is also dependent on both the severity and extent of perfusion defects, correlates of the stenosis magnitude, and the amount of myocardium subtended by

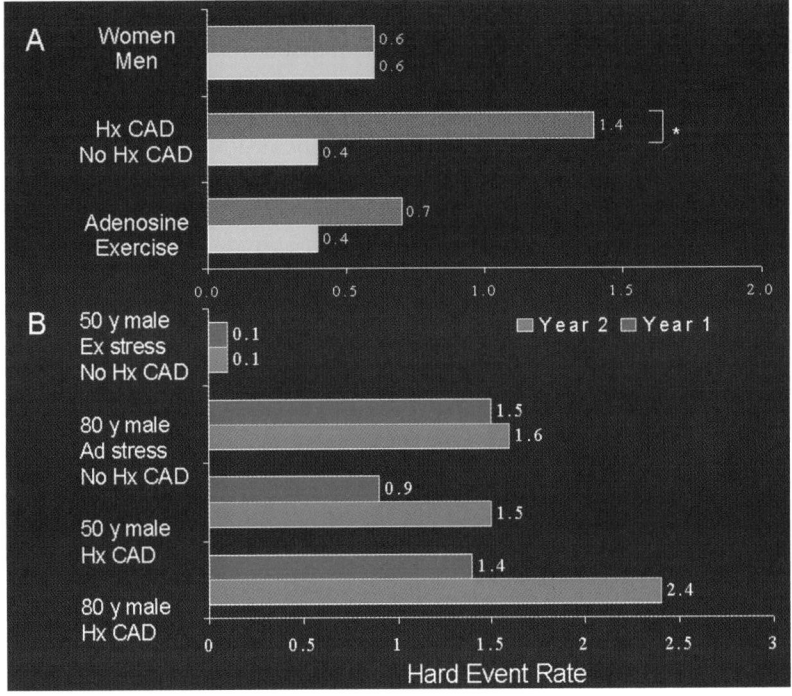

FIGURE 19–17. A. Annual rates of hard events in patients after normal SPECT MPI. The following subgroups are shown: women versus men, patients with and/without history (Hx) of CAD, and patients undergoing adenosine versus exercise stress. **B.** A significant risk is noted in the patients with Hx CAD Rates of hard events in first and second years of followup after normal SPECT MPI. Four examples are given: a 50-year-old male undergoing exercise stress with no history of CAD, an 80-year-old male undergoing adenosine stress with no history of CAD, a 50-year-old male with a history of CAD, and an 80-year-old male with a history of CAD. In patients with no history of CAD, the event rates in the first and second years after SPECT MPI are not different; however, the event rate for normal SPECT MPI goes up significantly with increased patient risk. In patients with previous CAD, the event rates in the second year after SPECT MPI were greater than in the first year, and there is additional increase in the event rate with clinical risk. Asterisk, $p < 0.001$; CAD, coronary artery disease; MPI, myocardial perfusion imaging; SPECT, single-photon emission computed tomography. *Source: Based on data from Hachamovitch R, Hayes S, Friedman JD, et al.[31]*

the stenosed vessels.[76] As these parameters worsen, risk of major cardiac outcomes increase (see Fig. 19–14). The definitions for SPECT MPI categories of abnormality are show in Table 19–1. Annual cardiac event rates have been reported to range from 0.3 to 4.2 percent for patients with normal, mild, moderate, and severely abnormal perfusion scans, with significant variability associated with each level of defect extent and severity. Similar findings have been described with ^{201}Tl and with ^{99m}Tc tetrofosmin.[73,77]

Mildly Abnormal SPECT MPI Previously, we had described patients with mildly abnormal scans to be at intermediate risk for MI but at low risk for subsequent mortality.[78] Although the overall observation holds true for groups of patients, risk assessment in an individual patient is improved by taking into account findings other than those of the scan. The presence of high-risk clinical or historical markers identifies a subset of patients at greater risk *for any level of scan abnormality*; that is, prescan data yields incremental prognostic information over SPECT MPI results (Fig. 19–18).[32,41,78,79] Hence, although patients with mildly abnormal SPECT MPI results generally are at low risk of cardiac death, the risk is higher in a variety of subgroups with significant comorbidities and presentations (e.g., advanced age, diabetes mellitus, atrial fibrillation, pharmacologic stress, reduced left ventricular function, dyspnea).[74,80]

Moderately to Severely Abnormal SPECT MPI As discussed above, this category of scan abnormality is associated with the highest levels of risk. Anticipated patient risk is greatest in patients with high risk cardiovascular comorbidities, increased left ventricular size/reduced left ventricular function, extensive scar, and so on. As discussed below, patients in this SPECT MPI category with extensive ischemia are most likely to benefit from revascularization as opposed to conservative management.

patients undergoing medical therapy when moderate to severe ischemia was present (>10 percent of the total myocardium ischemic) (Fig. 19–19).[32] This survival benefit was particularly striking in higher-risk patients (elderly, requiring adenosine stress, and women, especially diabetics). These results have been extended to incorporate gated SPECT MPI ejection fraction (EF) information.[81] Comparing the roles in risk assessment of perfusion and function data—although EF, percent myocardium ischemic and the percent myocardium fixed are all predictors of cardiac death—the former is by far the best predictor of cardiac mortality. Conversely, only inducible ischemia identified patients who would benefit from revascularization in comparison to medical therapy (Fig. 19–20). With increasing amounts of ischemia, increasing survival benefit for revascularization over medical therapy was found, irrespective of EF. However, as shown by previous RCTs, the absolute benefit to be gained from a therapeutic strategy, for any level of ischemia present, is proportional to underlying patient risk. Thus, in assessing treatment options in an individual patient, cardiac risk factors, comorbidities, and EF all have to be considered along with ischemia to determine the potential advantages of a specific therapeutic strategy.

【 】 INTEGRATING CLINICAL DATA WITH SPECT MPI RESULTS

A challenge facing clinicians attempting to apply SPECT MPI results to patient care is to distill all information reported after SPECT MPI—clinical, historical, stress test, perfusion, and function data—into an estimate of likelihood of CAD or risk of adverse events for an individual patient. Because SPECT MPI and pre-SPECT MPI data add incrementally to each other, accurate final estimates of risk must also adjust for clinical data. Further, as outlined above, post-SPECT MPI patient treatment must be con-

【 】 USING SPECT MPI FOR MEDICAL DECISION MAKING: ASSESSING RISK VERSUS ASSESSING POTENTIAL SURVIVAL BENEFIT

Beyond risk-stratification, optimal selection of patient treatment is based on reasonable estimates of potential patient benefit with one treatment option versus an alternative. To this end, a major step forward is the recently evolved paradigm indicating that rather than identify patient risk, the role of SPECT MPI in a testing strategy is the identification of patients who may accrue a *survival benefit* from revascularization as opposed to those who lack a survival benefit from this procedure and, conversely, which patients will have a superior survival with medical therapy alone. In a recent study examining 10,627 patients without prior MI or revascularization who underwent stress SPECT MPI, a survival benefit was present for patients undergoing medical therapy versus revascularization in the setting of no or mild ischemia, whereas patients undergoing revascularization had an increasing survival benefit over

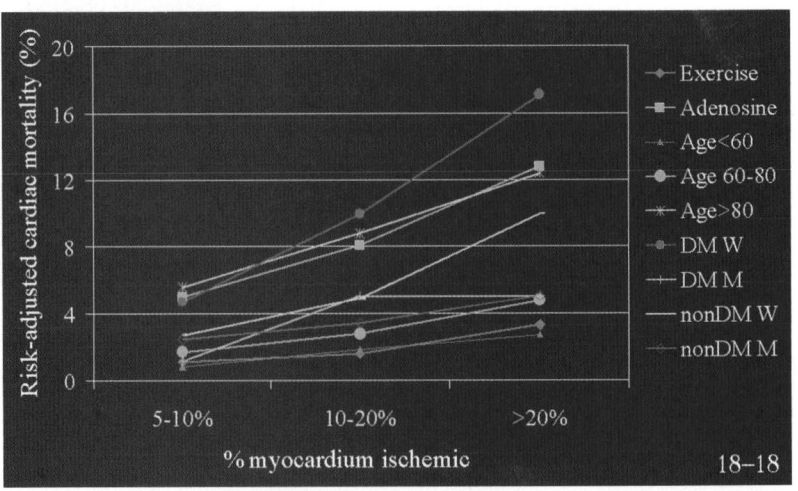

FIGURE 19–18. Rates of risk-adjusted cardiac mortality as a function of percent myocardium ischemic (5–10%, 10–20%, and >20%) in medically treated patients (exercise vs. adenosine stress; patients aged <60 y, 60–80 y, and >80 y; diabetic men vs. women; and nondiabetic men vs. women). Although predicted cardiac mortality increases with increasing percent myocardium ischemic, the rates at any level of ischemia varies widely at any level of ischemia as a function of clinical information. DM, diabetes mellitus; M, men; W, women. *Source: Based on data from Hachamovitch R, Hayes SW, Friedman JD, et al.[32]*

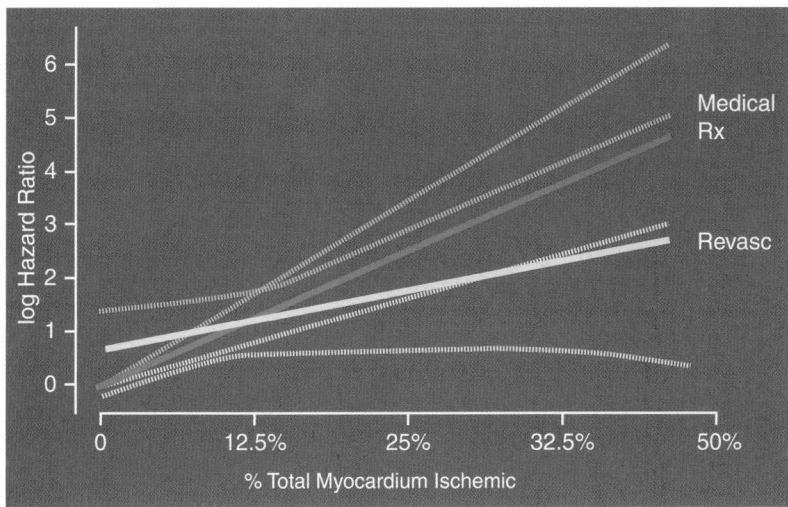

FIGURE 19-19. Relationship between percent myocardium ischemic and log of the hazard ratio in 10,647 patients treated either with medical therapy (*dashed line*) or early revascularization (< 60 days post-SPECT MPI; *solid line*) based on multivariable modeling. In the setting of little or no ischemia, medical therapy is associated with superior survival; with increasing amounts of ischemia, a progressive survival benefit with revascularization over medical therapy is present. 95 percent confidence intervals are shown by the *closely dotted lines*. MPI, myocardial perfusion imaging; revasc, revascularization; Rx, medical therapy; SPECT, single-photon emission computed tomography. *Source: Reproduced with permission from Hachamovitch R, Hayes SW, Friedman JD, et al.*[32]

sidered as well because of considerations of both treatment effect and the referral bias introduced.

Ideally, validated prognostic scores can be developed incorporating all available sources of information, including SPECT MPI results, could be incorporated into SPECT MPI reporting. Incorporating nonnuclear variables in risk assessment is particularly difficult with pharmacologic stress, because prognostically important variables used in exercise testing, such as exercise duration and exertional chest pain, are not prognostically useful components of adenosine stress testing protocols.

Recently, the first such score was developed in 5873 patients studied by adenosine stress who experienced 387 cardiac deaths on follow up (6.6 percent).[25] Using a combination of split set validation and bootstrapping techniques, the authors derived a complex score taking into account all significant variables including age, percent myocardium ischemic, percent myocardium fixed, diabetes, dyspnea as the presenting symptom, resting HR, peak HR, and ECG findings. Separate scores can be calculated for therapeutic choices of medical therapy or revascularization (Fig. 19–21). Conceptually, the major contributions of these studies examining SPECT MPI and subsequent therapeutic choices are that physicians need to focus not simply on risk but on potential benefit to maximally impact patient care, and these assessments require integration of all available information. Of course, that clinical judgment is paramount in the application of these approaches because of imperfections in the data de-

rived from populations in defining all variables that might be operative in determining the risk of an individual patient as well as limitations of the tests themselves.

【 】 GUIDING DECISIONS FOR CATHETERIZATION

Several investigators have shown that SPECT MPI results appear to heavily influence post-SPECT MPI clinical decision making. Among patients with normal scans, only a small proportion undergo early post-SPECT MPI cardiac catheterization, usually as a result of clinical symptomatology.[40] As first shown by Hachamovitch and colleagues, the extent and severity of reversible defects shown by the SPECT MPI result is the dominant factor driving subsequent resource utilization[32] (Fig. 19–22). Similar results have been shown by other authors.[78] Regarding the cost-effectiveness of this approach, Shaw and colleagues,[82] in a multicenter study of 11,249 patients, showed that a strategy of SPECT MPI with selective subsequent catheterization produced a substantial reduction (31 to 50 percent) in costs for all levels of pretest clinical risk compared to a direct catheterization approach (Fig. 19–23), with essentially identical outcomes as assessed by cardiac death and MI rates. Importantly, in the SPECT MPI strategy, rates of revascularization, cardiac cathe-

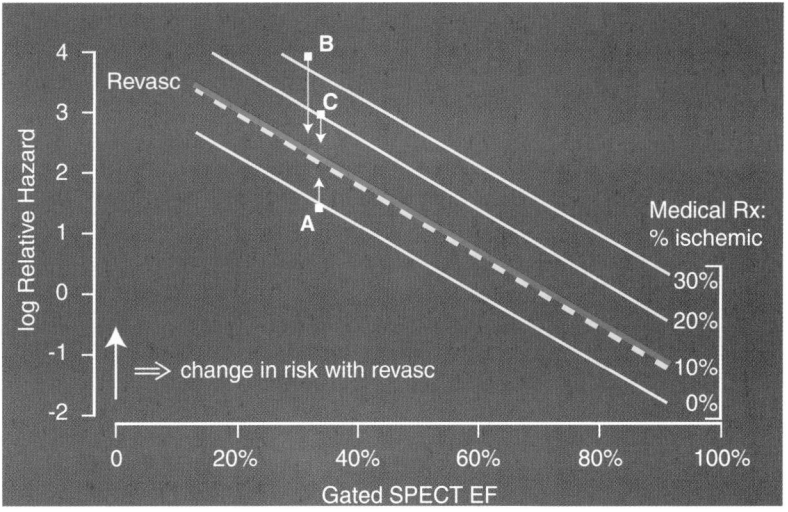

FIGURE 19-20. Relationship between gated SPECT EF and log of the hazard ratio in 5366 patients based on multivariable modeling. *Solid lines* represent predicted survival for 0 percent, 10 percent, 20 percent, and 30 percent myocardium ischemic in medically treated patients. *Dashed lines* represent predicted survival for patients treated with revascularization for all values of percent myocardium ischemic. Overall, risk increased with decreasing EF. For any value of EF, however, risk also increased as percent myocardium ischemic increased, indicating an incremental value for percent myocardium ischemic over EF. Compared to risk in patients treated medically, risk in patients undergoing early revascularization was independent of the percent myocardium ischemic present (as evidenced by a single [*dashed*] line representing survival after revascularization for all degrees of ischemia). Risk in the early revascularization patients was similar to the risk of medically treated patients with 10% myocardium ischemic, throughout the range of EF. EF, ejection fraction; revasc, revascularization; Rx, medical therapy; SPECT, single-photon emission computed tomography. *Source: Reproduced with permission from Hachamovitch R, Rozanski A, Hayes SW, et al.*[81]

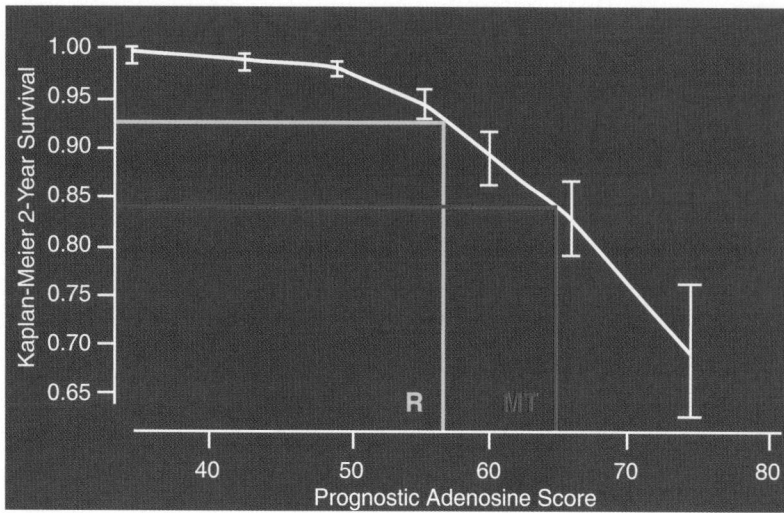

FIGURE 19–21. Relationship between prognostic adenosine score and 2-year Kaplan-Meier survival free of cardiac death. With lower scores, patient risk is relatively low with narrower confidence intervals. As scores increase, particularly >50, risk increases more rapidly and confidence intervals increase as well. The orthogonal lines represent a specific example of an 80-year-old man with exertional shortness of breath who demonstrated 30% myocardium ischemic and 0% myocardium fixed on *no-walk* adenosine MPI. Using the adenosine score, early revascularization *(R, green)* would be predicted to have a 93% 2-year survival and medical therapy *(MT, red)* an 84% survival. *Source: Reproduced with permission from Hachamovitch R, Hayes SW, Friedman JD, et al.[25]*

terization after normal SPECT MPI, and the frequency of normal coronary angiographic findings were significantly reduced.[78,82]

Estimating the True Prognostic Value of SPECT MPI and Posttest Referral Bias

Although there is compelling evidence that SPECT MPI is effective in the prognostic stratification of patients, the current data on risk stratification by SPECT MPI may underestimate the strength of this modality due to a prognostic counterpart to the diagnostic verification bias described above. Most prognostic analyses performed to date are comprised of patients undergoing medical therapy after testing, censoring revascularized patients from analyses due to the relationship between the test results and the referral to revascularization.[65] The result is a potential underestimation of the prognostic value of SPECT MPI since the highest-risk patients, with the most abnormal test results, are removed from the population being studied.[65,78,83]

A recent study quantified the reduction in observed event rates in medically treated patients with severe amounts of ischemia due to this referral bias[83] and made several important observations. First, reported event rates in observational studies limited to medically treated patients may be misleading, particularly in the absence of information regarding post-SPECT MPI referral patterns to revascularization (the latter defining the amount of potential bias). Further, if post-SPECT MPI referral to revascularization is based on one variable (e.g. ischemia) but not on a second (e.g., scar), a referral bias results in underestimation of risk associated with the first variable (blunted increase in risk as a func-

tion of ischemia); but no such finding with respect to the second variable (appropriate increase in risk as a function of increasing scar). Finally, this bias introduced by the clinical use of SPECT MPI can be overcome by statistical adjustment of observational patient data using both medically treated and revascularized patients.[25,32,65]

【 】 ADDED VALUE OF GATED SPECT MPI: INTEGRATED CLINICAL ALGORITHMS

Because gated SPECT MPI has become routine only recently, there are several reports of its incremental value over perfusion in assessing prognosis. The first report showed that poststress LVEF and LV ESV, as measured by gated SPECT, provided incremental information over the perfusion defect assessment in the prediction of cardiac death.[84] In a recent report of 6713 patients, using separate criteria for EF and ESV for men and women, Sharir and coworkers reported that perfusion (percent myocardium ischemic) and function (LVEF or ESV) provided incremental prognostic information regarding cardiac death and hard events[48] (Fig. 19–24), with particularly high event rates noted in women with reduced function and >10 percent myocardium ischemic. As noted above, a recent study has shown that in patients undergoing gated SPECT MPI, only inducible ischemia identifies patients who are likely to benefit from revascularization at all levels of E.F.[81] Further, this study confirmed previous work that perfusion and function data add incrementally to each other.[81,85,86]

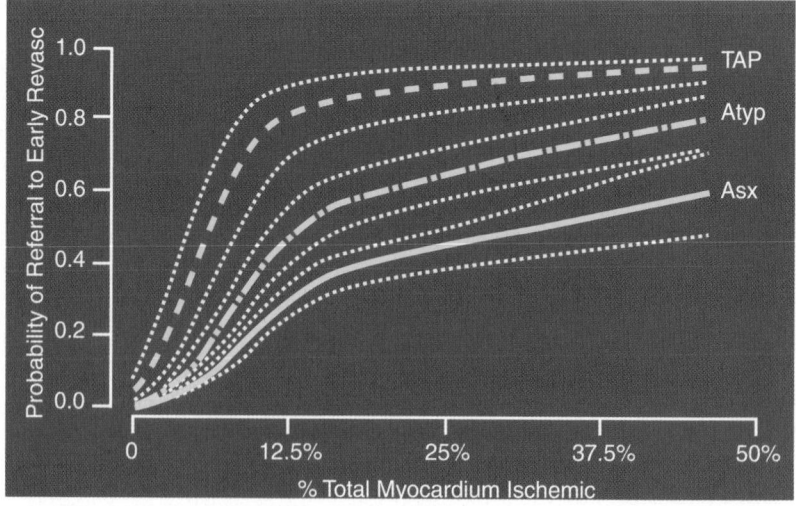

FIGURE 19–22. Relationship between percent myocardium ischemic and probability of referral to early revascularization (<60 days post-SPECT MPI). Results based on multivariable modeling in 10,647 patients. In this study percent myocardium ischemic was most strongly associated with referral to revascularization (83% of all information used for decision making). Further, patients' presenting symptoms also influenced this process as evidenced by greater likelihood of referral at any level of ischemia with typical versus atypical versus asymptomatic patients. Atyp, atypical; Asx, asymptomatic; MPI, myocardial perfusion imaging; SPECT, single-photon emission computed tomography; TAP, typical angina pectoris. *Source: Reproduced with permission from Hachamovitch R, Hayes SW, Friedman JD, et al.[25]*

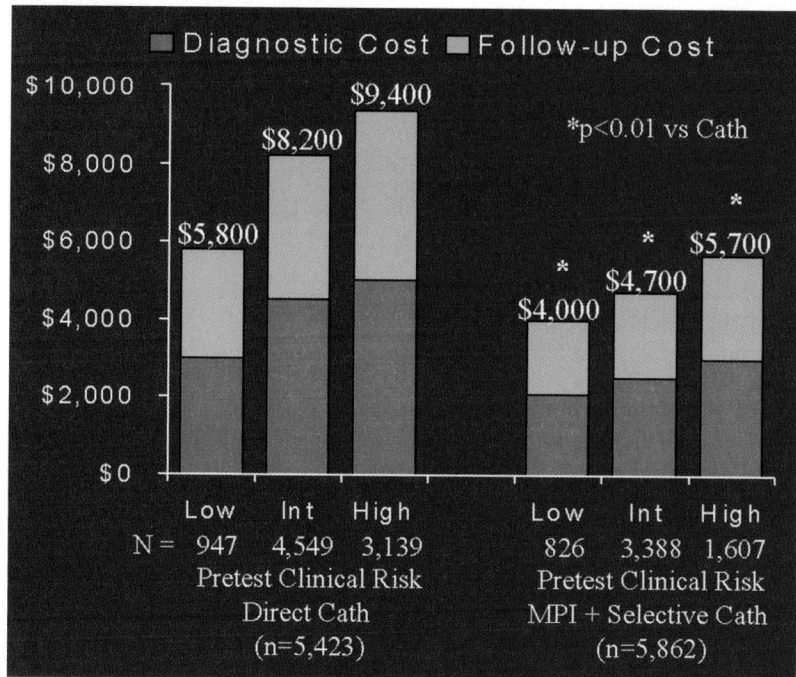

FIGURE 19–23. Comparative cost between screening strategies employing direct catheterization (Cath) and myocardial perfusion imaging (MPI) with selective Cath. Low, Int, and High represent low-, intermediate-, and high-risk subsets of the patients with stable angina. Shown are the initial diagnostic costs (*solid bars*) and follow-up costs including costs of revascularization (*gray bars*). A 30% to 41% reduction in costs was noted in each category. Hard event rates were similar with the two strategies, but the revascularization rate was twice as high in the direct cath group. *Source: Reproduced with permission from Shaw LJ, Hachamovitch R, Berman DS, et al.*[82]

In the future, complex algorithms will need to be developed that incorporate all of the information from gated SPECT MPI for purposes of guiding patient management. With this regard, it is likely that poststress EF (related predominately to the size of MI) and percent myocardium reversible (the SPECT MPI measure of ischemia) will provide the greatest complementary information.[76]

Other important information that can be derived from SPECT MPI and may be related to risk has not been widely included in the prognostic assessment (Table 19–3). The assessment of poststress wall motion abnormalities on gated SPECT MPI are a sign of exercise-induced stunning and a marker of severe CAD.[87] Transient ischemic dilation of the LV[49,50,52] and pulmonary uptake of radioactivity as determined by the measurement of lung-to-heart ratios of radioactivity have been shown to be of prognostic importance.[54] Extensive reversibility of resting defects (as determined by 24-hour ^{201}Tl imaging after rest ^{201}Tl/stress ^{99m}Tc-sestamibi SPECT MPI) has been shown to be predictive of a higher mortality rate than would be predicted by rest or stress perfusion defect abnormalities alone.[88] Finally, as noted above, inducible ischemia or viable myocardium—not EF—appears to identify patients who may benefit from revascularization.[89,90]

USE OF SPECT MPI IN SPECIFIC PATIENT POPULATIONS

A principal strength of nuclear cardiology is that large databases have been accumulated resulting in evidence documenting the effectiveness of SPECT MPI for risk stratification of appropriately selected patients, comprising the full spectrum of patients with suspected or chronic CAD. This evidence has resulted in many class I indications for the use of stress SPECT MPI.[2] Several specific lines of evidence are described below.

1. Evidence Supporting Nuclear Imaging for Patients With an Intermediate Risk or Indeterminate Treadmill Test. Several reports support nuclear testing in patients with uninterpretable or intermediate exercise ECG response.[2] An initial report from Cedars-Sinai demonstrated that SPECT MPI was most effective in risk stratification and governing management of patients with intermediate Duke treadmill score (DTS).[91] Patients with a low DTS (hard-event rate <1 percent) or high DTS (hard-event rate 7.7 percent) did not show further risk stratification with SPECT MPI. However, patients with an intermediate DTS, comprising the majority of patients studied, had an intermediate risk of hard events; patients with a normal SPECT MPI scan had very low event rates and were infrequently catheterized, those with moderately abnormal scans had intermediate rates of events and catheterization, and those with moderately to severely abnormal scans had higher rates of events and catheterization. Similar results were shown in subsequent multicenter studies reporting event rates and catheterization rates.[2]

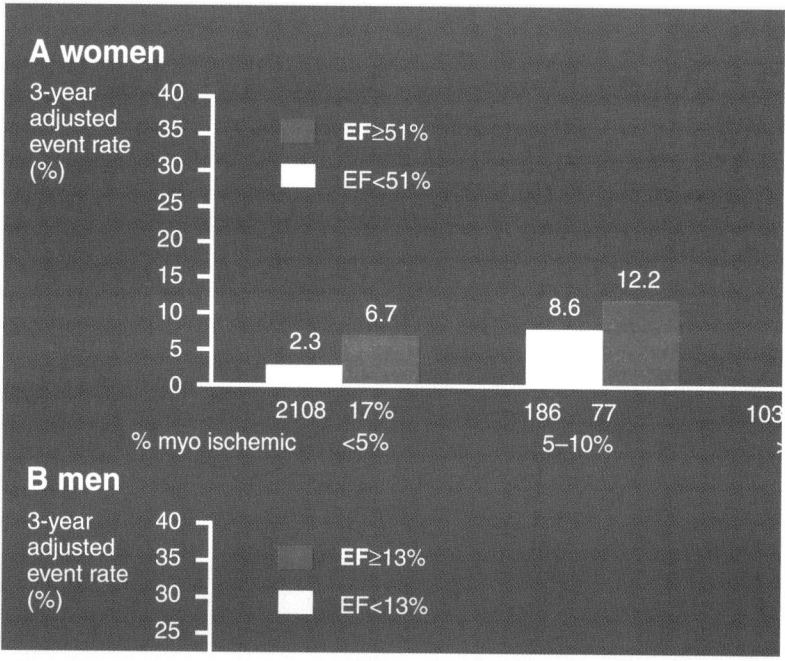

FIGURE 19–24. Three-year adjusted cardiac hard event rates in women (A) and men (B) as a function of the amount of ischemia (% myo [myocardial] ischemic) and gender-specific normal/abnormal ejection fraction (EF). *Source: Reproduced with permission from Sharir T, Kang X, Germano G, et al.*[48]

TABLE 19–3

Markers of High Risk

CLINICAL	STRESS TEST	SPECT
Diabetes mellitus (especially women) insulin dependence	Severe ST-segment depression	TID
Atrial fibrillation	Pharmacologic stress	Lung uptake
Elderly	Exercise hypotension	Stress-induced stunning
Marked resting ECG abnormalities	Blunted HR response to adenosine	Reduced EF
Dyspnea as presenting symptom	Marked hypotension with adenosine stress	Severe and/or extensive defects
Typical angina		
Unstable angina		

ECG, electrocardiogram; EF, ejection fraction; HR, heart rate; SPECT, single-photon emission computed tomography; TID, transient ischemic dilation.

2. Evidence Supporting Nuclear Imaging for Patients with Normal Resting ECG Able to Exercise. Patients with normal resting ECGs represent a large and important subgroup who are commonly encountered in clinical practice in whom the use of SPECT MPI is controversial.[72,90,92] Generally, patients with a normal resting ECG have an excellent prognosis[90] and are likely (92 to 96 percent) to have normal LV function.[93]

Several studies have examined the added value of exercise SPECT MPI over clinical and ETT data in this patient group.[72,90,92] The Mayo Clinic demonstrated that although SPECT MPI yielded incremental value over clinical and ETT data for the prediction of left main or three-vessel disease, the yield was modest and not cost effective.[92] More recently, a study of 3058 patients with normal resting ECGs showed that selective use of SPECT MPI in patients with intermediate to high post-ETT CAD likelihood yielded significant risk stratification, statistical incremental value, and cost-effectiveness in predicting hard events.[90] A subsequent study from the Mayo Clinic has shown that patients with a high clinical score (based on age, sex, prior MI, and diabetic state) are at too high pretest risk to be classified as low risk by exercise testing. The author suggests that initial stress SPECT MPI testing might be appropriate in this group.[94] Complementary findings were also recently shown in the ability of stress SPECT MPI to define a low post-SPECT risk in most patients with a high pretest likelihood of CAD.[83] Thus, although recent ACC appropriateness criteria report that it is inappropriate to refer *functionally* capable patients with a normal ECG to SPECT MPI,[59] several lines of evidence described above indicate that there are patient groups able to exercise with normal rest ECG such as those with a high pretest likelihood of CAD and the elderly in which many experts have opined that SPECT MPI may be indicated.[95]

3. Evidence Supporting Nuclear Imaging for Patients with Normal Resting ECG Unable to Exercise. In patients unable to exercise,

there is a clear consensus in support of pharmacologic stress imaging as the initial test in symptomatic male and female patients with intermediate or high pretest likelihood of CAD unable to achieve maximal exercise levels.[2,96] Consistent with other functionally disabled cohorts, the overall expected risk of major adverse cardiac events in these patients is elevated.[97] As reported by the recent AHA consensus statement on cardiac imaging in women, functionally impaired patients (e.g., <5 METs of exercise) have at least a 2 percent per year risk of congenital heart disease (CHD) death or MI; ranking them as having event rates equivalent to patients with established coronary heart disease.[96] The higher event rates than in exercising patients are driven by excessive comorbidity and risk factor burden. In multivariable models the need for pharmacologic stress (as opposed to exercise) is itself an incremental predictor of adverse outcomes[31] with event rates that are at least 50 percent higher than an exercising population. Despite the higher event rates for any test result, for patients who have a normal resting ECG and an intermediate to high likelihood of CAD but unable to exercise, vasodilator stress SPECT MPI has been shown to be effective for both CAD diagnosis and risk stratification.[25,41,79]

4. Evidence Supporting Nuclear Imaging for Asymptomatic Patients. Several studies have examined the diagnostic and prognostic value of stress SPECT MPI in asymptomatic populations. In a study examining asymptomatic siblings of patients with manifest CAD, a cohort acknowledged to be at increased risk of developing CAD, a relative risk of 4.7 for experiencing an adverse cardiac event was reported for individuals with an abnormal scan[98] and the presence of both an abnormal exercise ECG and abnormal perfusion scan yielded a relative risk of 14.5. As predicted by Bayesian principles, however, the routine use of any test for detection of CAD in a low risk/low prevalence of CAD asymptomatic population will be associated with high cost-effectiveness ratios and low positive predictive values. Nonetheless, these evaluations are often performed in patients with high-risk occupations (e.g., pilots, firefighters, etc.).[2] Further studies are warranted to determine the added value of routine testing of selected asymptomatic patients. As noted below, sequential testing with atherosclerosis imaging followed by ischemia testing only if warranted may become an appropriate model.

5. Evidence Supporting Nuclear Imaging for Patients with Diabetes Mellitus. SPECT MPI has now been reported to be effective in risk stratification of patients with diabetes.[41,78,99] In a study comparing 1271 patients with diabetes to 5862 without, SPECT MPI risk stratified patients in both groups, but risk-adjusted event-free survival was worse in patients with diabetes than in those without.[100] These findings were confirmed in a multicenter series.[99] In the latter study, diabetic women had the worst outcome for any given extent of MI. In patients with normal SPECT MPI results, survival worsened sooner in diabetic compared to nondiabetic patients, suggesting that retesting of diabetics with normal studies might be needed earlier than in nondiabetics. It has been shown that 22 percent of asymptomatic diabetic patients have ischemia by adenosine SPECT MPI.[101] Another recent, large study has shown that 59 percent of asymptomatic diabetics have abnormal stress SPECT MPI studies, including 20 percent with a *high-risk* scan.[102] A further study by this group showed that ECG Q waves and/or evidence of peripheral artery disease identified the most suitable diabetic candidates for screening with SPECT MPI.[103] Nonetheless, as

discussed below, some investigators recommend atherosclerosis testing rather than SPECT MPI as a more cost-effective approach to the initial screening tool of diabetics.[66,104]

6. Evidence Supporting Nuclear Imaging for Patients with LBBB. Current guidelines support cardiac imaging in symptomatic patients with LBBB.[2] Exercise-induced false-positive perfusion defects, more often in the interventricular septum, are observed less frequently with vasodilator stress.[2] The sensitivity for left anterior descending stenosis >50 percent was similar (on average 89 percent) with exercise and vasodilator SPECT MPI, but a higher specificity was found for vasodilator stress (81 percent) as compared to exercise (36 percent) SPECT MPI.[105] Dobutamine stress SPECT MPI has also been reported to be accurate in CAD detection in patients with LBBB, providing an alternate form of stress for patients unable to exercise if there is a contraindication to the use of the vasodilators. Vasodilator stress SPECT MPI is an excellent predictor of cardiac events in LBBB patients.[106] Patients with LBBB and normal SPECT MPI have demonstrated very low event rates over time.[106] In contrast, patients with LBBB and *high risk* perfusion findings on SPECT MPI have high event rates. Although there is less reported regarding patients with ventricular pacemakers, expert consensus is that these patients are appropriately risk-stratified by vasodilator SPECT MPI, similar to patients with LBBB.[2]

7. Evidence Supporting Nuclear Imaging for Patients with LVH or Atrial Fibrillation. In patients with LVH, exertional ST-segment depression is frequently associated without significant CAD. SPECT MPI has been shown to be similarly effective in patients with and without LVH for identifying obstructive disease and for risk stratification. In a report patients with LVH and a low-risk SPECT MPI had a <1 percent annual risk of cardiac death or MI whereas the annual cardiac death or MI rates ranged from 4.9 percent for mildly abnormal scans to 10.3 percent for those with moderate-severely abnormal SPECT MPI.[107]

In asymptomatic patients with new onset atrial fibrillation, the use of stress SPECT MPI in patients with a high pretest risk is considered appropriate[59] in view of a higher baseline clinical risk resulting in higher expected cardiac events. A recent observational report in 16,048 patients on the prognostic value of SPECT MPI in patients with atrial fibrillation showed an annual rate of cardiac death in patients with normal SPECT MPI was 1.6 percent per year for those with atrial fibrillation and 0.4 percent for the remaining cohort of nonatrial fibrillation patients ($p < 0.001$).[79] Of interest, with atrial fibrillation, even patients with only mildly abnormal SPECT MPI, were at much higher risk than those without atrial fibrillation: 6.3 percent vs. 1.2 percent per year, respectively [$p < 0.0001$]).

8. Gender-Based Differences in the Prognostic Value of SPECT MPI. Recent guidelines for cardiac imaging have been published by the AHA.[96] In women, caused by breast tissue artifact, false-positive SPECT MPI examinations are most notable in the anterior and anterolateral segments of the heart and are more common with ^{201}Tl than with the ^{99m}Tc agents.[96] Improved accuracy has been reported with use of the ^{99m}Tc agents as well with combined acquisition of gated EF and wall motion imaging, prone imaging, and with the use of validated attenuation correction algorithms,[62,96] with the resultant sensitivity and specificity being similar in women and men.

Regarding prognosis, pooled data including more than 7500 women noted annual rates of cardiac death or nonfatal MI of 0.4 per-

cent for women with low-risk or normal SPECT MPI.[108] High-risk findings elevated a woman's risk by nearly 10-fold with annual rates of major cardiac events of 6.3 percent for all women and 10.9 percent for diabetic subsets of women.[108] Separate criteria for abnormality have been recommended for ventricular function in women and men, resulting in similar prognostic content of combined perfusion and function information from gated SPECT in men and women.[48]

Endothelial dysfunction and microvascular disease have been proposed as mechanisms for false positive stress testing results in women, suggesting that some of these studies may represent true perfusion abnormalities without large vessel CAD. Recent evidence suggests that these SPECT MPI perfusion findings may be associated with increased near-term risk of major cardiac events,[109] suggesting that prognostically important coronary disease states not involving obstructive CAD occur more frequently in women than in men, and that SPECT MPI could provide a tool for detection of this process.

9. Evidence Supporting Nuclear Imaging for Elderly Patients. With recent increased longevity of the population and the increasing prevalence of CAD as a function of age, large numbers of elderly patients are requiring diagnostic and/or prognostic assessment for CAD. The DTS, useful in many patient subsets, has been reported to be less effective in risk stratification of elderly patients.[95] The Mayo Clinic group reported that exercise SPECT MPI provides effective risk stratification in elderly men and elderly women. A cohort of 247 patients 75 years of age or older, patients undergoing ^{201}Tl SPECT MPI were followed for a median of 6.4 years for cardiac death. The summed stress score from SPECT MPI was significantly associated with cardiac death, but the DTS was not. The summed stress score from SPECT MPI classified 49 percent of patients as low risk and 35 percent of patients as high risk, with annual cardiac mortality rates of 0.8 percent and 5.8 percent respectively. Long proponents of the ETT as the initial test, the Mayo group concluded that if their results can be confirmed in future studies, exercise SPECT rather than ETT may emerge as the initial exercise testing modality in both women and men aged 75 years and older, even those who are able to exercise.[95]

Pharmacologic stress testing is increasingly being applied in the elderly who frequently are unable to exercise adequately and the elderly comprise a high proportion of patients undergoing pharmacologic stress imaging. For elderly patients as well as for those with functional limitations, similar risk assessment is possible with exercise and pharmacologic stress SPECT.[75] Consistent with data on other functionally impaired patients, the prognostic value of SPECT MPI is associated with higher cardiac event rates for normal to severely abnormal test results. These results were extended to dobutamine stress.[110]

10. Evidence Supporting Nuclear Imaging for African-American and Other Ethnic Minority Patients. The rate of cardiac death or MI in African Americans with a normal SPECT MPI is approximately 2 percent per year,[2] likely a result of higher risk burden.[109] In a recent series 2-year cardiovascular death or MI were compared in 1993 African American and 464 Hispanic patients as compared with 5258 white, non-Hispanics undergoing stress ^{99m}Tc tetrofosmin SPECT MPI.[77] Moderate to severely abnormal SPECT MPI occurred more often in ethnic-minority patients. The prognostic results noted a 1.4- to 1.6-fold and 2.3- to 5.6-fold higher risk of hard events in African-American and Hispanic patients, respectively, with mild and moderate to severely abnormal SPECT MPI findings ($p < 0.0001$ vs. whites), likely caused by higher degree of comorbidity.

11. Evidence Supporting Nuclear Imaging for Obese Patients. SPECT MPI remains a highly useful test for diagnosis and prognosis in obese patients although excess soft-tissue attenuation can make scan interpretation more difficult. For obese patients the [99mTc] agents are considered preferable to [201Tl], because of the higher photon energy of [99mTc]. Recently, two studies have demonstrated that attenuation correction hardware and software, combined with quantitation and ECG gating, had significantly higher specificity and normalcy rates without loss of sensitivity for detection of CAD in obese patients when compared to studies without attenuation correction.[111,112] Without attenuation correction, by using combined supine and prone [99mTc] sestamibi stress SPECT MPI acquisitions, equally high sensitivity, specificity, and normalcy rates among normal weight, overweight, and obese patients, have been reported in a large clinical series. Furthermore, these investigators reported that when a quantitative approach to analysis of supine, prone, and combine supine/prone acquisitions was employed, the combined supine/prone approach increased the specificity in identifying CAD without significant reduction in sensitivity.[113] Most SPECT imaging tables have weight limits (often 300 lb [136.1 kg]). Although the use of planar scintigraphy is an alternative for the very obese patients, it is less accurate than SPECT and many interpreting physicians are less familiar with its interpretation. PET imaging may prove to be superior to conventional SPECT MPI in obese patients because of the robust attenuation correction and the higher photon energy associated with positrons, the source of the emissions imaged by PET (see Chap. 23).

Regarding prognosis, a recent large study has demonstrated that combined prone and supine SPECT MPI is highly effective in risk stratification across weight groups. Normal SPECT MPI studies were associated with a low risk of events in all weight categories. Interestingly, an inverse relationship between weight and risk of cardiac death, with higher event rates was observed in the patients with abnormal scans or known CAD.[114]

12. Evidence Supporting Nuclear Imaging after Coronary Calcium Screening or CT Coronary Angiography (CTA). Recent evidence supports the use of the CT-derived coronary calcium score (CCS) as a means to evaluate asymptomatic patients with multiple risk factors for detection of early, subclinical coronary atherosclerosis.[115,115a] In patients with high risk CCS, referral to SPECT MPI as a second test has been evaluated in a number of series and in a recent information statement from the ASNC.[116,117] Data from published series are consistent that when the CCS is <400, the rate of SPECT MPI abnormalities is low. When the CCS exceeds 400, the rate of an ischemic SPECT MPI is elevated and has been reported to be as high as 47 percent.[117] When ischemia is documented, catheterization is frequently recommended. When no ischemia is found, aggressive medical therapy without catheterization is recommended. The safety of medical management in patients without ischemia and having extensive coronary atherosclerosis has recently been documented.[115a] Recent consensus documents and the recent ACC appropriateness criteria support the use of SPECT MPI in patients with a high risk CCS ≥ 400.[59,117]

Although reports from unselected patient series have revealed a threshold for increased SPECT MPI abnormalities at a CCS ≥ 400, recent subset analyses have yielded a differential threshold in higher risk patients including type-2 diabetics with or without the metabolic syndrome and in those with a family history of premature CHD.[104,118,119] In these cohorts, a greater frequency of ischemic SPECT MPI was reported at a CCS ≥ 100. In patients with the metabolic syndrome, the frequency of an ischemic SPECT MPI was 15 percent for CCS 100 to 400 equivalent to patients with normal metabolic status with CCS ≥ 400.[119] From a prospective, well-controlled clinical trial, Anand and colleagues[104] enrolled 510 asymptomatic, type-2 diabetics who underwent CCS and SPECT MPI. Data from this series revealed that the rate of abnormal SPECT MPI (including both fixed and reversible defects) was 0 percent (n = 15) for CCS ≤ 10, 18 percent (n = 38) for CCS 11 to 100, 23 percent (n = 70) for CCS 101 to 400, 48 percent (n = 29) for CCS 401 to 1000, and 71 percent (n = 28) for CCS >1000, respectively. Similar results were reported for patients with a family history of premature CHD with a greater frequency of ischemic SPECT MPI when CCS is 100 or greater.[118]

In some patients it may be appropriate to perform coronary calcium scanning after SPECT MPI. Combined CT and SPECT MPI allow for an integration of anatomic and physiologic data. For example, a normal SPECT MPI does not provide information regarding subclinical coronary atherosclerosis that may merit aggressive medical therapy. In one study of 1119 patients with normal SPECT MPI findings, 25 percent, 20 percent, and 11 percent had CCS scores from 100 to 399, 400 to 999, and ≥ 1000, respectively.

CTA is increasingly used for detection and assessment of patients with suspected or known CAD. Although the diagnostic accuracy of coronary CTA is very high, borderline coronary narrowing is frequently observed, resulting in clinical uncertainty regarding the need for invasive coronary angiography and the need to consider coronary revascularization. If the results of the coronary CTA are equivocal for a proximal coronary stenosis or if the CTA is clearly abnormal but the anatomy is not *compelling* regarding the need for revascularization, referral for ischemia testing with SPECT MPI appears appropriate to determine the need to consider coronary revascularization.[66] It is noteworthy in this respect that Raff and coworkers[120] reported that even with a 64-slice scanner, the 95 percent confidence interval to predict >50 percent stenosis by invasive coronary angiography ranged from 25 percent to 75 percent (i.e., only if the coronary CTA showed <25 percent narrowing or >75 percent stenosis could the absence or presence of a >50 percent stenosis be predicted with 95 percent certainty). Because of the newness of the coronary CTA, there is little data published to support the recommendation of the use of SPECT MPI following equivocal coronary CTA findings; however, the approach is already part of appropriateness criteria.[59]

13. Evidence Supporting Nuclear Testing for Patients after Percutaneous Coronary Intervention (PCI). Post-PCI SPECT MPI can potentially play a number of roles, because SPECT MPI abnormalities post-PCI may detect restenosis, periprocedural myocardial injury, side-branch compromise, de novo disease, or functionally significant angiographic disease in nonrevascularized vessels. As part of a staged procedure, SPECT MPI can assess the remaining ischemic burden after the initial PCI. Post-PCI SPECT MPI has been extensively used for the detection of silent or minimally symptomatic restenosis. Based on reviews of the literature and a meta-analysis,[121,122] several statements can be made regarding the value of SPECT MPI. It is superior to ETT for this application. It can detect silent restenosis. However, post-PCI patients undergoing SPECT MPI have a low overall annual event rate, suggesting no need for *routine* testing, despite the predictive value of abnormal SPECT MPI for adverse events. Because of the relatively low prevalence of clinically significant silent restenosis in the era of drug-eluting stents, routine poststent SPECT MPI is not currently recommended.[2,59]

In general, however, when *symptoms* develop after PCI or in high risk subgroups, SPECT MPI can be helpful in defining the culprit vessel and assessing the extent of ischemic abnormality. The ACC/AHA 2002 Guideline Update for Exercise Testing favors selective stress imaging in patients considered to be at particularly high risk (e.g., patients with decreased LV function, multivessel CAD, proximal LAD disease, previous sudden death, diabetes mellitus, hazardous occupations, and suboptimal PCI results). Whenever moderate to severe ischemia is found by nuclear testing, consideration should be given to repeat catheterization, even in the absence of symptoms. Zellweger and colleagues found that 23 percent of patients had silent ischemia in the area of their target lesion 6 months after PCI.[123] Silent ischemia had more ominous outcomes than no ischemia, but less severe consequences than symptomatic ischemia.

14. Evidence Supporting Nuclear Testing for Patients after CABS. Nuclear testing has become central in the assessment of the post-CABS patient. It is known that >50 percent of vein grafts can be expected to be occluded by 10 years after surgery, hence an intermediate likelihood of vein graft disease.[121] Thus, a 5-year cutoff point to evaluate the post-CABS patient may be appropriate.[121,124–126] In post-CABS patients with new symptoms, SPECT MPI can identify the presence and extent of ischemia. In asymptomatic patients, SPECT MPI should be considered 5 or more years after CABS. Whenever moderate to severe ischemia is present, catheterization should be considered.[121,126]

15. Evidence Supporting Nuclear Imaging for Preoperative Risk Assessment in Noncardiac Surgery Patients. Assessment of LV function and/or jeopardized myocardium provides an accurate method to complement clinical preoperative risk assessment. A large body of literature exists documenting the effectiveness of nuclear stress testing in patients undergoing peripheral vascular surgery. Nuclear testing is best reserved for patients with an intermediate risk of a cardiac event undergoing an intermediate- to high-risk procedure (see Chap. 74). Current guidelines suggest that candidates for SPECT MPI are patients with two of three of the following: (1) intermediate clinical predictors (Canadian class I or II angina, prior MI, congestive heart failure [CHF], or diabetes mellitus), (2) poor functional capacity, or (3) high-risk surgical procedure (emergency major operation, aortic repair, peripheral vascular surgery, prolonged surgical procedure with large fluid shifts or blood loss).

16. High-Pretest Likelihood of CAD. In general, patients with *chest pain symptoms* and high-pretest CAD likelihood are appropriate candidates for SPECT MPI. The ACC appropriateness criteria support SPECT MPI in high-likelihood patients who have an interpretable or uninterpretable ECG as well as for those able or unable to exercise.[59] Relevant evidence on risk-assessment of this group with SPECT MPI has been published by Hachamovitch and coworkers.[83] In this consecutive series of 1270 patients with a high CAD likelihood (i.e., ≥0.85), the annual rate of cardiac death or MI was 1.3 percent for normal SPECT MPI, which was found in most the patients. A strategy incorporating initial testing with SPECT MPI in these patients to guide decision for coronary angiography, was shown to be cost effective.[82,83]

While coronary CTA might be considered in these symptomatic patients, if the pretest likelihood of CAD is truly high, most of the patients are likely to have abnormal coronary CTA studies; thus, the CTA result, unlike the nuclear result, is unlikely to result in a decision not to proceed to invasive coronary angiography.[11] Currently, the consensus of experts is to employ ischemia testing rather than coronary CTA in this group.

When asymptomatic high-risk patients are seen by clinicians, many consider them to have a high pretest likelihood of CAD (e.g., high Framingham risk, diabetics, peripheral arterial disease, siblings of patients with premature CAD). While the frequency of abnormal SPECT MPI studies in these patients is not unlike that observed in more symptomatic patients, the overall risk of these patients is not as great as in the symptomatic cohort. Thus, strategies employing initial CCS followed by selective SPECT MPI may prove to be most effective for detection of at-risk asymptomatic patients (as noted in section 13 above).[66,104,118] The recent ACC appropriateness criteria supports the use of SPECT MPI in patients with a high Framingham risk.

17. Assessment of Therapy: Serial Testing. In patients with no change in symptoms, the need for repeat testing and the appropriate interval for this retesting has not been fully explored. From the recent ACC/ASNC appropriateness criteria, repeat imaging 2 or more years after the index scan is acceptable. Two large, randomized trials employing serial imaging strategies in chronic CAD[128] and diabetic (i.e., Bypass Angioplasty Revascularization Investigation in Diabetics [BARI IID]) patients are nearing completion and should provide additional evidence to guide future appropriateness criteria. Nuclear substudies of these trials may provide evidence whether assessing the response to medical therapy using serial MPI testing can be useful in better selecting patients in whom revascularization is needed for purposes of improving prognosis.

There is no consensus regarding the whether serial testing should be performed with the patients on or off antianginal medications. If the purpose of repeat testing is to assess the effects of therapy on ischemic in daily life, the repeat testing can be performed with medications *on board*. In clinical trials serial imaging has been explored to determine a patient's residual ischemic burden following intercurrent treatment, whether medical therapy alone or in combination with coronary revascularization. In this testing strategy, the amount of ischemia by imaging is used as a surrogate outcome (Fig. 19–25).[129]

USE FOR ASSESSMENT OF MYOCARDIAL VIABILITY AND CONGESTIVE HEART FAILURE

Because of the high mortality rate and increasing prevalence of heart failure and the need to tailor therapy to the etiology and the stage of the condition, testing of patients with heart failure will become increasingly common. Radionuclide methods are useful in initial staging CHF (measurement of EF and ventricular volumes), ruling out CAD as an etiology, and determining the likelihood of response to interventional therapies. The recommendations of the ACC/AHA/ASNC task force regarding the general applications of radionuclide imaging[2] in patients with heart failure are summarized in Table 19–4.

DETECTING CORONARY ARTERY DISEASE AS THE ETIOLOGY OF CONGESTIVE HEART FAILURE

Because CAD represents the largest etiology of CHF and because the therapy of CAD is so distinct from that of the general management of patients with CHF from other etiologies, ruling out CAD as the cause of CHF is of clinical importance. If a patient with CHF is found to have no abnormalities of myocardial perfusion at stress (percent myocardium ischemic <5), the likeli-

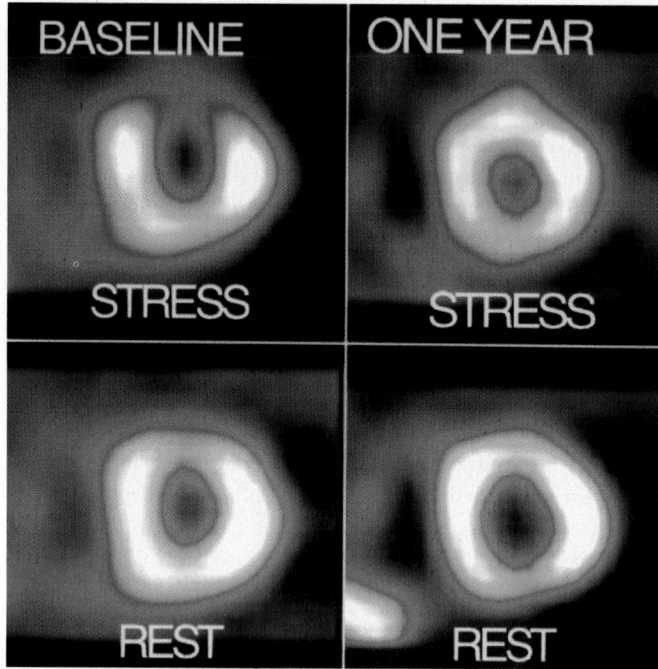

FIGURE 19-25. Case example of reversal of the stress myocardial perfusion defect with medical therapy. Baseline vasodilator stress and rest sestamibi mid–short-axis SPECT images (*left*) and repeat images 1 year after intensive medical therapy in a 50-year-old patient with baseline reversible defect in the LAD territory (*right*). One year into therapy, the stress perfusion defect is markedly improved. Baseline coronary angiography revealed an 80% mid-LAD stenosis, which improved angiographically on repeat coronary angiography at 1 year. Two years later there are no reversible imaging defects and the patient is asymptomatic. LAD, left anterior descending coronary artery; SPECT, single-photon emission computed tomography. *Source: Reproduced with permission from O'Rourke RA, Chaudhuri T, Shaw L, et al.[148]*

hood of CAD as the cause of CHF can be considered low.[2] Thus, in the appropriate setting, a normal SPECT MPI study might obviate the need for coronary angiography in a patient with CHF of unknown etiology.

【 】 IDENTIFYING HIBERNATING MYOCARDIUM

In patients with CAD and heart failure, SPECT MPI is used to distinguish viable but nonfunctioning myocardium from nonviable myocardium.[56] Myocardium subjected to acute or chronic ischemia may remain viable and demonstrate prolonged alterations in regional and global LV function that can be improved with revascularization.[56] Consequently, the distinction of ventricular dysfunction caused by fibrosis from that arising from viable myocardium has important implications for patients with low LVEF. Failure to identify patients with these potentially reversible causes of heart failure may lead to progressive cellular damage, heart failure, and death.[56]

【 】 PREDICTING RECOVERY OF LV FUNCTION AFTER REVASCULARIZATION

The clinical setting in which viability assessment is most commonly used is the evaluation of CAD patients with poor LV function in whom revascularization is being considered. Various protocols using combinations of rest, redistribution, and reinjection ^{201}Tl imaging have been validated to assess the presence of hibernating myocardium. When reversibility of defects is noted on stress/rest or stress/redistribution studies, the likelihood of postrevascularization improvement of regions with abnormal ventricular function is high. Improvement would also be expected in patients with significant angiographic CAD if normal or mildly reduced tracer uptake is noted on rest scintigraphy. When severe reduction in uptake of radioactivity is noted on redistribution ^{201}Tl imaging, the likelihood of improvement in regional ventricular function is low; a moderate defect on rest (or redistribution) has an intermediate likelihood of improvement.[56] Fluorine-18 fluorodeoxyglucose PET and/or CMRI for predicting myocardial viability are increasingly being favored over SPECT MPI and dobutamine echocardiography for prediction of functional recovery after revascularization.

【 】 PREDICTING IMPROVED PATIENT SURVIVAL

The demonstration of viable myocardium in patients with CAD and LV dysfunction appears to identify patients with enhanced survival with revascularization but with particularly poor prognosis with medical therapy. A meta-analysis of observational studies based on either radionuclide or echocardiographic assessments that dichotomize patients into groups with or without myocardial

【 】 TABLE 19-4

Use of RNI in Patients with Heart Failure: Fundamental Assessment

	INDICATION	TEST	CLASS	LEVEL OF EVIDENCE
1.	Initial assessment of LVF and RVF at rest	Rest RNA	I	A
2.	Assessment of myocardial viability for consideration of revascularization in patients with CAD and LV systolic dysfunction who do not have angina	Myocardial perfusion imaging	I	B
3.	Assessment of the co-presence of CAD in patients without angina	Myocardial perfusion imaging	IIa	B
4.	Routine serial assessment of LVF and RVF at rest	Rest RNA	IIb	B
5.	Initial or serial assessment of ventricular function with exercise	Exercise RNA	IIb	B

CAD, coronary artery disease; LV, left ventricular; LVF, left ventricular function; PET, positron emission tomography; RNA, radionuclide angiography; RNI, radionuclide imaging; RVF, right ventricular function.
Source: Klocke FJ, Baird MG, Bateman TM, et al.[2]

viability suggest that only patients with extensive myocardial viability have survival improvement with CABS compared to medical therapy[89] (Fig. 19–26).

Several technical changes could improve the use of SPECT MPI in the assessment of myocardial viability, including administration of nitroglycerin prior to rest injection and late redistribution imaging.[88] The use of combined rest-redistribution ^{201}Tl/stress ^{99m}Tc-sestamibi or tetrofosmin SPECT may be particularly effective in assessing myocardial viability, because the protocol can combine what an optimal rest SPECT MPI protocol (rest/redistribution ^{201}Tl) with a stress imaging assessment.[20] Table 19–5 illustrates conceptually the relationship between several different myocardial states associated with chronic CAD and the patterns that might be observed on SPECT MPI.

The ACC/AHA/ASNC recommendations for radionuclide techniques in assessing myocardial viability are shown in Table 19–6.

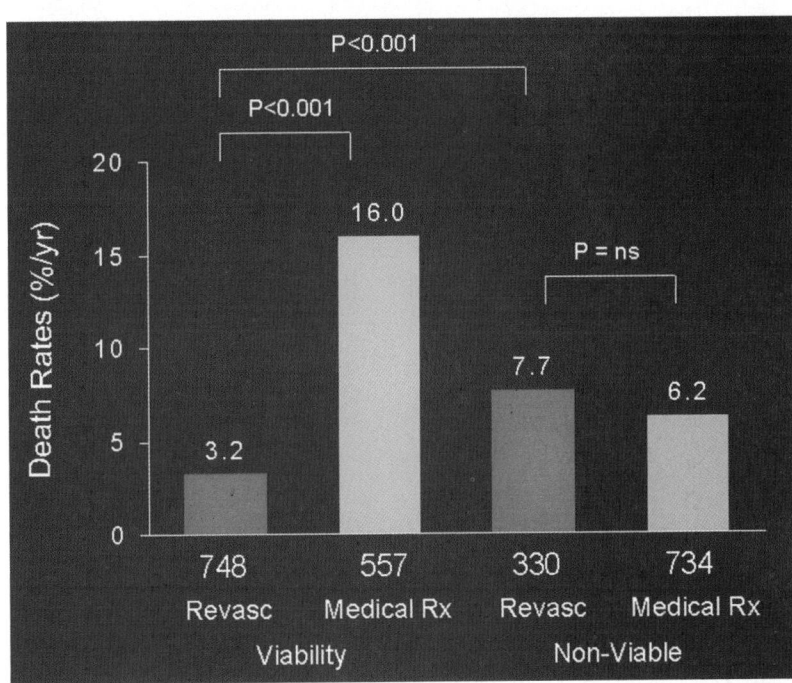

FIGURE 19–26. Meta-analysis of studies examining rates of death in patients undergoing revascularization (revasc) versus medical therapy (Rx). When viability was present by noninvasive testing, a significant reduction in cardiac death rates was present in patients undergoing revascularization compared to those undergoing medical therapy. No such difference was present in patients without viability. Further, patients with viability undergoing revascularization had a significantly lower cardiac death rate compared to patients without viability. *Source: Reproduced with permission from Allman KC, Shaw LJ, Hachamovitch R, et al.[89]*

ACUTE CORONARY ISCHEMIC SYNDROMES

〘 〙 EVALUATION OF ACUTE CHEST PAIN

Because of the relationship to closure of a coronary artery, SPECT MPI is an effective means of detecting patients with acute ischemic syndromes. Although the diagnosis of acute MI is frequently straightforward, in many patients it is not. For patients with normal or nondiagnostic initial ECGs on presentation to the emergency department (ED), an important clinical problem is to distinguish those with acute coronary syndromes requiring hospital admission from those who may be safely discharged.

Because most patients presenting with acute chest pain subsequently *rule out* for acute ischemic syndromes, chest pain units have

been instituted for the acute evaluation of chest pain patients presenting to the ED. ^{99m}Tc-sestamibi or tetrofosmin SPECT MPI, with injection during chest pain, provides an excellent opportunity to reduce clinical indecision in the acute evaluation of chest pain (Fig. 19–27). A number of studies have demonstrated a role for SPECT MPI in the initial evaluation of these patients. A normal rest ^{99m}Tc-sestamibi or tetrofosmin SPECT MPI study has a 99 percent negative predictive value.[2] A prospective, randomized, controlled multicenter trial examined whether incorporating acute rest

TABLE 19–5

Scintigraphic and Clinical Characteristics of Hypocontractile Regions According to Their Viability Status

VIABILITY STATUS	REST	REDISTRIBUTION ([201]TL)	REST REVERSIBILITY	STRESS/REST/RI REVERSIBILITY	LIKELIHOOD OF IMPROVEMENT WITH REVASC
Q MI	↓↓↓	↓↓↓	—	—	—
Non-Q MI	↓–↓↓	↓–↓↓	—	±[a]	±[a]
Hibernation	→ to ↓↓↓	→ to ↓	+	+++	+++
Stunning (with ACS)	→	→	→	±[a]	++
Stunning (with exercise)	→	→	→	+++	+++
Remodeled	→	→	→	→	→
Nonischemic CM with incidental CAD	→	→	→	→	→

ACS, acute coronary syndrome; CM, cardiomyopathy; MI, myocardial infarction; Q, Q wave; Revasc, revascularization; RI, reinjection.
[a]Depends on stenosis of IRA and the degree of transmurality of the infarct.

TABLE 19–6

Radionuclide Techniques for Assessing Myocardial Viability

INDICATION	TEST	CLASS	LEVEL OF EVIDENCE
1. Predicting improvement in regional and global LV function after revascularization	Stress/redistribution/reinjection [201]Tl	I	B
	Rest-redistribution imaging	I	B
	Perfusion plus PET FDG imaging	I	B
	Resting sestamibi imaging	I	B
	Gated SPECT sestamibi imaging	IIa	B
	Late ^{201}Tl redistribution imaging (after stress)	IIb	B
	Dobutamine RNA	IIb	C
	Postexercise RNA	IIb	C
	Postnitroglycerin RNA	IIb	C
2. Predicting improvement in heart failure symptoms after revascularization	Perfusion plus PET FDG imaging	IIa	B
3. Predicting improvement in natural history after revascularization	[201]Tl imaging (rest-redistribution and stress/ redistribution/reinjection)	I	B
	Perfusion plus PET FDG imaging	I	B

[201]Tl, thallium 201; FDG, fluorodeoxyglucose; PET, positron emission tomography; RNA, radionuclide angiography; SPECT, single-photon emission computed tomography.
SOURCE: Based on data from Klocke FJ, Baird MG, Bateman TM, et al.[2]

SPECT MPI into an emergency room evaluation strategy of patients presenting with suspected acute ischemia improved initial ER triage.[130] A significant reduction in hospitalization was noted in patients with normal SPECT MPI studies.

GUIDELINES FOR SPECT IMAGING IN THE EMERGENCY DEPARTMENT

Several considerations are important for effective application of SPECT MPI in the ED. In patients with prior MI, the studies are generally not useful, unless the results of previous SPECT MPI are immediately available for comparison. Also, combined assessment of perfusion and function should be routinely performed to minimize the false negative rate. Combined supine and prone imaging or attenuation correction is useful in reducing the false-positive rate. An abnormal rest SPECT MPI study triggers admission and therapy for an acute ischemic syndrome. Patients with normal rest studies, after negative enzymes are obtained, frequently undergo stress SPECT MPI to evaluate underlying CAD. If no stress or rest abnormality of perfusion or function is observed, patients are typically discharged from the ED. Those with evidence of ischemia (Fig. 19–28) or infarct are admitted. A randomized clinical trial comparing the effectiveness of this rest/stress SPECT MPI approach to that of 64-slice CT coronary angiography is starting in 2007 (CT-STAT).

ASSESSMENT OF THERAPY

SPECT MPI can be used effectively in patients with acute MI before and after therapy (or even simply after therapy) for examining the efficacy of a variety of therapies compared to conventional mortality endpoints.[2,131]

GUIDING MANAGEMENT DECISIONS

Many clinically low-risk MI patients are not catheterized acutely and are candidates for predischarge stress testing. Both exercise[132] and pharmacologic stress testing post-MI[133] have been shown to effectively identify patients at low and high risk of subsequent events. Although either type of stress would be recommended by guidelines, evidence that favors the use of vasodilator stress includes the following: (1) vasodilator stress does not require that the patient be able to exercise; (2) it can be easily and safely employed as early as 2 days following MI; (3) it lowers rather than raises BP, avoiding possible myocardial rupture; and (4) it produces a maximal hyperemic stimulus, thereby obviating the need for maximal exercise testing.

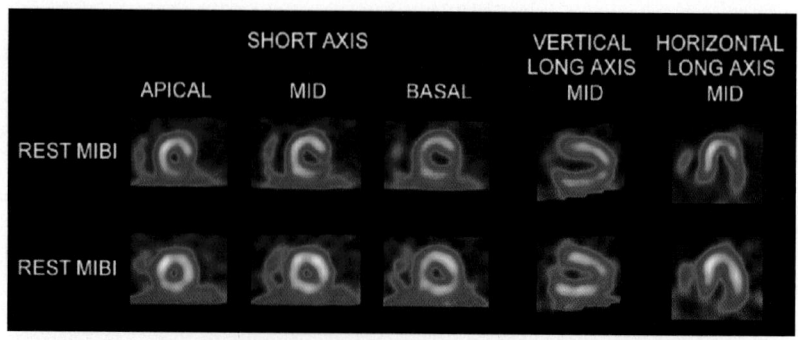

FIGURE 19–27. Resting sestamibi (MIBI) injected during chest pain in emergency department (*top*) and 3 days post-PCI of the left circumflex coronary artery (LCX) (*bottom*) in a patient with no EGG or enzyme abnormalities. Clear evidence of extensive myocardial salvage in LCX territory is shown. PCI, percutaneous coronary intervention.

Overall, high-risk SPECT MPI results (indicating the need for angiography) in the predischarge patient include reversible defects in the MI zone, a multivessel defect pattern, large nonreversible defects, transient LV dilation, increased lung uptake, and reduced LV ejection fraction.[134] Two multicenter, randomized trials have evaluated the prognostic value of SPECT MPI in the post-MI setting. Brown and coworkers compared submaximal ^{99m}Tc-sestamibi SPECT at discharge to early dipyridamole ^{99m}Tc-sestamibi SPECT performed 2 to 4 days after acute MI[133] in 451 patients presenting with first acute MI. The very early use of dipyridamole testing was associated with no adverse events, indicating the safety of this approach in appropriately selected post-MI patients. Multivariable predictors of post discharge cardiac events included the SSS, the summed difference score, the summed stress score, and anterior MI. Dipyridamole sestamibi imaging showed better risk stratification than submaximal exercise MPI. Additionally, the amount of SPECT ischemia provided incremental prognostic information over the total defect size (SSS).

Recently, the Adenosine Sestamibi SPECT Post-Infarction Evaluation (INSPIRE) trial, a prospective randomized multicenter trial evaluating SPECT MPI in assessing risk and therapeutic outcomes in post-MI survivors, was completed.[135] In this randomized trial, Mahmarian and coworkers have explored this serial imaging approach in patients after acute MI. The trial selected 205 stable survivors of an uncomplicated MI, who were randomized to medical therapy versus coronary revascularization. Patients underwent SPECT MPI 1 to 10 days after acute MI and after 4 to 8 weeks of medical therapy or coronary revascularization.[135] Entry criteria limited enrollment to patients whose index SPECT scan exhibited total perfusion defect >20 percent of the myocardium with the >10 percent of that being ischemic and an ejection fraction ≥ 35 percent. The study results revealed that for both medical therapy and coronary revascularization, total and ischemic defect size was reduced by 16 to 17 percent. In this study, total suppression of ischemia was noted in 80 percent of patients randomized to either strategy. The finding suggest that serial SPECT MPI could be used to identify a cohort responding to aggressive medical management and not requiring acute revascularization during recovery from acute MI. Whether the reduction in perfusion defect size observed with medical therapy in these patients with postinfarction jeopardized myocardium treated medically is associated with a sustained reduction in risk comparable to that achieved by revascularization has yet to be defined.

Hot-Spot Scintigraphy for Direct Imaging of Myocardial Necrosis

Hot-spot (infarct-avid) imaging methods for detecting acute MI are among the earliest techniques in nuclear cardiology. The most common of these techniques was ^{99m}Tc-pyrophosphate myocardial scintigraphy.[2] Although cardiac uptake of ^{99m}Tc-pyrophosphate usually indicates necrosis, in cardiac amyloidosis there is a characteristic pattern of diffuse, intense

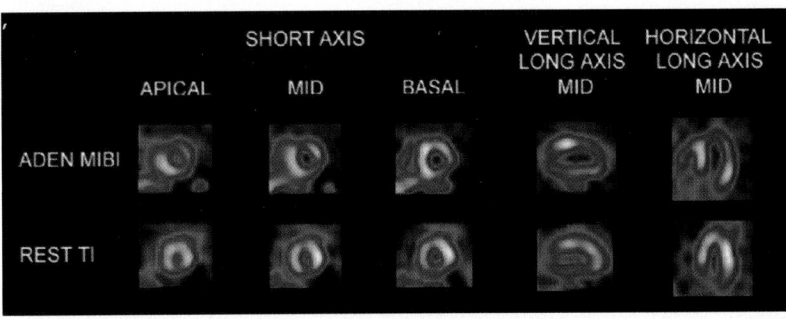

FIGURE 19–28. Normal rest ^{201}Tl SPECT (*bottom*) followed by adenosine ^{99m}Tc-sestamibi (ADEN MIBI) (*top*) in a patient with intermittent chest pain that had resolved prior to rest ^{201}Tl injection. Reversible defects are seen in the left anterior descending and left circumflex territories. Angiography revealed 50% left main, 100% left anterior descending, 90% left circumflex, and 50% right coronary artery stenoses. Aden, adenosine; mibi, sestamibi; Tl, Thallium.

myocardial uptake.[136] More recently, *hot-spot* myocardial scintigraphy has largely been replaced by delayed enhancement CMR (see Chap. 20).

RADIONUCLIDE ANGIOGRAPHY

Radionuclide angiography (RNA) can be performed by either equilibrium or first-pass methods, with assessments of LVEF, RVEF, LV regional wall motion, and LV volumes. Equilibrium RNA uses ECG-gated acquisition, in which each frame corresponds to a specific portion (interval or gate) of the cardiac cycle, identified relative to the R wave on the patient's ECG. Because of the use of a multiple gated acquisition, the term *MUGA scan* has also been applied to this technique. The cardiac cycle is divided into 16 to 64 intervals and data from multiple cardiac cycles are averaged to ensure adequate count statistics. With the equilibrium approach, a blood-pool tracer (usually ^{99m}Tc-labeled red blood cells) is used. With the first-pass approach, imaging is performed only during the initial transit of radioactivity through the central circulation. This technique is a type of dynamic acquisition that uses rapid temporal sampling (20–100 frames per second) to look at the initial transit of a radionuclide bolus through the central circulation. Both equilibrium and first-pass techniques can be performed during exercise as well as at rest.

Because of the ability to image the blood-pool radiopharmaceuticals for a substantial time period, SPECT acquisition is also practical with equilibrium radionuclide angiography. It has recently been shown that equilibrium blood-pool SPECT acquisition and processing are essentially the same as for SPECT MPI, and thus can be easily adopted in the laboratory where SPECT MPI is performed. Methods for automatically assessing LVEF from gated blood-pool SPECT have been developed and validated.[137] Because the SPECT approach avoids the overlap of cardiac chambers inherent in planar imaging, it enhances assessment of regional function and may well become the method of choice for radionuclide angiography. Techniques for assessing regional asynchrony from the gated blood-pool SPECT have been described, and may be of use in predicting the benefit from cardiac resynchronization therapy (Fig. 19–29).

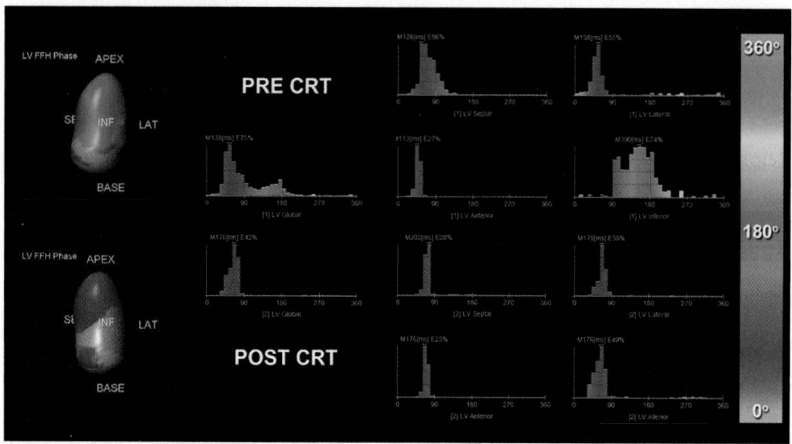

FIGURE 19–29. Phase information from blood pool SPECT studies acquired pre-CRT (*top*) and post-CRT (*bottom*) in a patient with CHF. First Fourier harmonic phase information from endocardial wall motion is mapped onto the pre- and post-CRT LV surfaces (*left*); gray indicates areas where amplitude of contraction is lower than 5% of the maximum. Global (*left*) and regional phase histograms (*middle* and *right*) are shown. The four regional histograms represent the septal (*upper left*), anterior (*lower left*), lateral (*upper right*), and inferior (*lower right*) walls of the LV. For each histogram the location of the peak is related to the timing of the onset of contraction and the width is related to intraventricular dyssynchrony). Pre-CRT, wide histograms are seen for the inferior and to a lesser extent the septal walls; and there is marked shift between the peaks of the LV regional histograms. Post-CRT, the histograms narrow and the peaks are more synchronized. Viewing with a gated display simplifies the detection of phase changes. The color scale for parametric mapping and histograms is displayed on the far right. CHF, congestive heart failure; INF, inferior; LAT, lateral; LV, left ventricle; SPECT, single-photon emission computed tomography. *Source: Data from Kriekinge SV, Berman DS, Germano G.[149]*

[ ] THE ROLE OF RNA IN CHRONIC CORONARY ARTERY DISEASE

In chronic CAD the principal application of RNA at the present time is measurement LVEF.[2] This measurement is used in a variety of settings such as defining the need for specific therapy including angiotensin-converting enzyme inhibitors, AICDs, surgical ventricular restoration, in guiding the use of cardiotoxic chemotherapy and in documenting severe reduction of LVEF prior to admission into heart failure trials.

For the detection and management of patients with CAD, exercise RNA played a prominent role in the past but is now not commonly used, predominantly because of advances in stress echocardiography and the ability of gated SPECT MPI to assess ventricular function as well as myocardial perfusion.

[ ] SPECIAL APPLICATIONS OF RNA

Assessment of Anthracycline Cardiotoxicity

RNA is commonly used for evaluating the effects of doxorubicin and other anthracyclines on LV function in patients with suspected cardiotoxicity. In an early report, Alexander and colleagues demonstrated that patients with normal LVEF that had not fallen by more than 15 points did not develop cardiotoxicity with continued doxorubicin therapy; however, once EF fell to <45 percent or by >15 percent, continued doxorubicin therapy was commonly associated with irreversible cardiac failure. In a subsequent report of a large high-risk population from the same group, guidelines were established for the use of continued doxorubicin therapy.[138]

In a group of 70 high-risk patients in whom these guidelines were strictly followed, 2.9 percent developed subsequent CHF that responded to therapy. Of 212 high-risk patients in whom the recommendations were not closely followed, 21 percent developed CHF (*p* <0.001 versus the strict-guideline group), which was usually moderate to severe.

Cardiac CT: Complementary Role with Nuclear Cardiology

Noninvasive cardiac imaging has undergone a recent resurgence with the development of new approaches for imaging coronary atherosclerosis. Noncontrast computed tomography (CT) for imaging the extent of coronary artery calcification (CAC) and contrast CT for noninvasive coronary angiography (CTA) are developments with a growing evidence base regarding risk assessment and diagnosing obstructive coronary disease (see Chap. 19). CT CAC measurement, now shown to be accurately assessed by multislice CT, is increasingly accepted as a useful noninvasive means of identifying asymptomatic patients with subclinical atherosclerosis, providing independent and incremental information over that provided by the Framingham risk score. In the last few years, dramatic changes have occurred in CT, with the widespread availability of 64-slice CT scanners with rotation times of ≤ 400 msec. Early clinical studies suggest that the sensitivity and specificity of coronary CTA is higher than that associated with all other noninvasive testing. Additionally, by allowing visualization of the coronary artery wall, the method offers promise for assessing the extent of noncalcified plaque, potentially of prognostic importance over the information regarding assessment of stenosis. To date, there is no information available regarding the ability of coronary CTA to risk stratify patients, and the technique is limited in circumstances of dense coronary calcium, arrhythmia, and with some scanners high HRs.

It is likely that the use of CAC in asymptomatic patients and the use of coronary CTA in symptomatic patients will become an increasing part of mainstream cardiovascular imaging practices. In some patients these predominantly anatomic imaging methods will result in the need for functional testing with methods such as SPECT MPI that can assess ischemia. In the case of testing for subclinical atherosclerosis using CT CAC, approximately 10 percent of patients tested have been reported to show extensive CAC, a finding associated with an elevated risk. In such individuals SPECT MPI is useful in further risk stratification and in guiding management decisions regarding the need for catheterization and consideration of revascularization.[59,66] When coronary CTA is used for symptomatic patients, coronary lesions of uncertain clinical significance result in ischemia testing with SPECT MPI for guiding the decision regarding invasive management.

Conversely, in patients with equivocal SPECT MPI findings or findings that are discordant with stress ECG or clinical findings, additional testing with coronary CTA may be helpful in determining the need for catheterization. Thus, clinical strategies are likely to emerge in which some patients (a minority) will benefit from both cardiac CT and nuclear cardiology assessments.[66]

FUTURE OF NUCLEAR CARDIOLOGY

The last decade has seen new developments in noninvasive imaging technology and improvements in existing modalities. The options for imaging in known or suspected CAD include echocardiography, CMR, multidetector CT, and PET as alternative or complementary modalities to SPECT MPI. Each modality is likely to play an important clinical role for the foreseeable future. In many patients these tests will be used in combination to most effectively guide patient management decisions. The ability of myocardial perfusion SPECT to provide standardized procedures that are not highly technologist dependent and provide objective quantization assessments of myocardial perfusion and function with equipment of only moderate expense offers a strength likely to sustain this approach for many years. Recently, this growth has been predominantly seen in a rapid upsurge in the United States of nuclear cardiology practices in cardiology offices. Over a longer time frame, cardiac echo, CT, and CMR may increasingly be used for many of the applications for which SPECT is commonly used today. During this time, however, opportunities for growth of molecular imaging methods both in SPECT and in PET are likely to be developed as growth areas for the field of nuclear cardiology. Although the basic SPECT camera has had little fundamental change over several decades, two entirely new SPECT approaches (the CardiArc system and the D-spect camera from Spectrum Dynamics) have been introduced very recently, both claiming the potential to increase both sensitivity (reducing imaging time or radiation dose) and resolution.

【 】 NEW SPECT RADIOPHARMACEUTICALS

Radionuclide imaging has an inherent advantage over other cardiac imaging techniques for assessment of myocardial metabolic and biochemical processes. Although a wider variety of biochemical processes have been examined by PET, both PET and SPECT must go through the standard FDA phase I, II, and III steps prior to commercial availability. For SPECT, two new tracers are in clinical trials using iodine-123 (^{123}I). From a radiochemistry standpoint, ^{123}I is an excellent radionuclide, because unlike the more commonly used ^{99m}Tc, it is easily incorporated into a wide variety of physiologically important compounds by a halogen exchange reaction in which the iodine replaces a methyl group. From a physical standpoint, ^{123}I has favorable half-life (13 hours), photon energy (159 KeV), and radiation exposure characteristics, all nearly as favorable as those of ^{99m}Tc for gamma camera imaging. Although none of the ^{123}I-labeled compounds is currently commercially available for routine cardiac applications in the United States, the two new SPECT radiopharmaceuticals in clinical trials—one for imaging of myocardial innervation and the other for fatty-acid imaging—are already in common use in countries outside of the United States.

Metaiodobenzylguanidine Imaging

Imaging of Myocardial Innervation
Metaiodobenzylguanidine (MIBG) is an analogue of the false nerve transmitter guanethidine developed at the University of Michigan as an imaging agent for the adrenal medulla.[139] Labeled with ^{123}I, this radiopharmaceutical is now in common clinical use in Japan and is undergoing phase III clinical trials in the United States. MIBG is taken up in myocardial sympathetic nerve endings in a manner similar to norepinephrine, but it is not metabolized. For cardiac applications this agent is imaged initially and 4 hours after injection, usually with planar imaging, and more recently also with SPECT, the latter allowing assessment regional cardiac uptake. On planar images the heart-to-mediastinum ratio is measured, with the mediastinum serving as a *background* measurement for standardization.[140] Considered to provide an objective assessment of cardiac sympathetic function, MIBG may be useful in a variety of settings, principal among which are heart failure and assessment of potential for lethal arrhythmia.[140] Normally, there is excellent visualization of the myocardium initially, and only moderate washout over 4 hours. Patients with increased circulating catecholamine levels such as associated with advanced heart failure generally show poor initial uptake and fast washout of MIBG and show a low heart-to-mediastinum ratio at both times (<1.85). In denervated myocardium, such as early following cardiac transplantation, MIBG uptake is absent, even when perfusion is normal.[140]

Impaired cardiac sympathetic innervation and function in heart failure patients can be assessed by MIBG.[140] A reduced myocardial-to-mediastinal MIBG uptake 4 hours after injection has been shown to be the most powerful predictor of cardiac death, providing incremental information over clinical variables in clinical studies including ejection fraction.[140] Furthermore, MIBG imaging may be useful in predicting the effectiveness of β blocker therapy for patients with dilated cardiomyopathies.[140] It appears that excessive norepinephrine levels result in low uptake and rapid washout of the MIBG, creating very low heart-to-mediastinal ratio on 4-hour delayed MIBG images. This finding appears to be predictive of a poor response to β blocker therapy[140] as well as a worsened prognosis. There is widespread interest in investigating the potential clinical role of MIBG in assessing patients with heart failure and patients at risk for sudden cardiac death. This application is currently being explored in the phase III trials currently being conducted in the United States.

A variety of other cardiac conditions have been explored with MIBG, chiefly in Japan. In *syndrome X* abnormal cardiac MIBG uptake has been reported in 75 percent of patients, with the abnormality out of proportion to perfusion defects supporting the cardiac origin of chest pain in this syndrome.[140] In diabetic patients assessment of myocardial MIBG uptake may be useful in defining autonomic dysfunction.[140] Abnormal MIBG uptake has been reported in idiopathic ventricular tachycardia and ventricular fibrillation.[140] Asymmetric uptake of MIBG has been shown in patients with ventricular tachycardia and no CAD[140] and potentially may be of value in determining patient subsets who may benefit from the use of ICD implantation.

Fatty Acid Imaging
Although radionuclide imaging of fatty acids has been studied for decades, it is not yet in common use with either SPECT or PET, with the exception of one SPECT radiopharmaceutical beta-methyl-iodophenyle-pentadecanoic acid (BMIPP), currently in clinical use in Japan. BMIPP is a modified branched-chain fatty acid first introduced by Knapp and coworkers.[141] This tracer appears to have *ischemic memory* properties offering unique capability for the assessment of previously severely ischemic myocardium. Discordant myocardial fatty acid uptake/perfusion findings, with less BMIPP uptake than rest ^{201}Tl, has been described in patients who have had a recent episode of severe

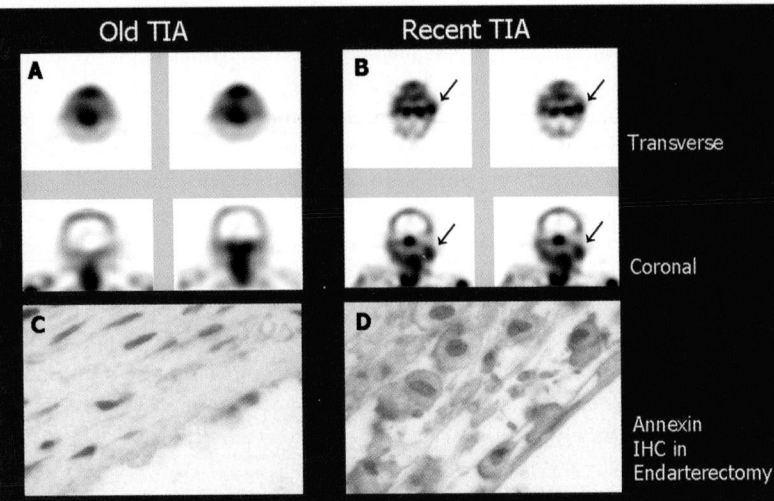

FIGURE 19-30. Images of unstable (*right*) and stable (*left*) atherosclerotic carotid artery lesions obtained with [99mTc] annexin A5. **A,** Transverse and coronal SPECT images from a patient who had a left-sided transient ischemic attack (TIA) 3 months prior to imaging and no recent symptoms. There is no evidence of uptake of [99mTc] annexin A5 in the area of the carotid arteries. **B,** Corresponding SPECT images from a patient with a left-sided TIA 3 days before imaging. Although this patient had clinically significant stenosis of both carotid arteries, uptake of radiolabeled annexin A5 is evident only on the right (*arrows*). Histopathologic analysis of an endarterectomy specimens from the two patients are shown below. In the patient with the recent TIA (**C**), polyclonal rabbit antiannexin A5 antibody, × 400 staining shows substantial infiltration of macrophages into the neointima, with extensive binding of annexin A5 (*brown*). In the patient with old TIA (**A**), histopathologic analysis of an endarterectomy specimen (polyclonal rabbit antiannexin A5 antibody, × 400) shows a lesion rich in smooth-muscle cells, with negligible binding of annexin A5. [99mTc], technetium-99m-sestamibi or tetrofosmin; ANT, anterior; IHC, immunohistochemistry. *Source: Adapted with permission from Kietselaer BL, Reutelingsperger CP, Heidendal GA, et al.[150]*

ischemia, with BMIPP representing the previously ischemic zone and the [201Tl] the infarcted zone.[142] This finding likely represents a persistent metabolic abnormality out of proportion to the perfusion abnormality at the time of injection. Dilsizian and colleagues recently reported a phase II study in which 32 patients with ischemia by exercise [201Tl] SPECT were studied by BMIPP SPECT injected with BMIPP at a mean of 6.2 hours after exercise in 21 and a mean of 24.9 hours after in 11. More than 90 percent agreement was observed between the studies for presence of abnormality. In a clinical study from Japan of 111 patients with possible acute coronary syndrome, BMIPP SPECT 1 to 5 days after pain was more sensitive for abnormality in the zone of the culprit vessel than thallium-201 (74 percent vs. 38 percent, respectively, $p < 0.05$). These findings suggest that a possible clinical application of BMIPP would be assessment of patients presenting several hours to days after a possible severe ischemic episode, potentially providing direct evidence of the recent severe ischemia at a time when perfusion had returned to normal.[143]

[ ] MOLECULAR IMAGING

The current explosion of information in cell biology has led to initial formulations of imaging agents with specific molecular targets. Perhaps the greatest future potential of the discipline of nuclear cardiology lies in molecular imaging, because of the ability of the radiotracer technique to assess minute tracer concentrations, of critical importance this field. SPECT and PET meth-

ods are thousands of times more sensitive than ultrasound, MRI, or CT methods.[140] Although most work has occurred with PET in this regard, molecular SPECT tracers have also been developed. For example, indium-111 ([111In]) antimyosin antibody,[140] is highly specific for myocardial necrosis and has been shown to be useful in the assessment of myocarditis[140] and the necrosis associated with cardiac transplant rejection.[140] The full commercialization of this molecular imaging agent, however, was not pursued. The most promising of the molecular imaging SPECT radiopharmaceuticals has been [99mTc]-annexin, an agent which allows imaging of apoptosis by specific binding to the exteriorized phosphatidylserine molecules, normally only found in the inner leaflet of the cell membrane and which become exteriorized during apoptosis.[144] Initial clinical trials with this agent demonstrated high sensitivity for MI. Other clinical settings in which the usefulness of this agent as a myocardial imaging agent could include myocarditis, transplant rejection, and possibly CHF. Provocative work has been performed using [99mTc] annexin SPECT for imaging apoptosis within atherosclerotic plaque (Fig. 19–30).

An interesting potential of these approaches is imaging of rupture-prone coronary plaques. High-resolution SPECT cameras have recently been described that may have the spatial resolution necessary to pursue this goal. In the future, by combining PET or high-resolution SPECT with CT coronary angiography and using a combination of cardiac gating, respiratory gating, and accurate image registration, nuclear techniques could have the ability to identify vulnerable coronary plaques in need of aggressive intervention,[145] one of the most elusive goals of imaging in CAD.

ACKNOWLEDGMENT

The authors gratefully acknowledge the invaluable expert assistance of Xingping Kang, MD, in all aspects of the preparation of this chapter.

REFERENCES

1. Germano G, Berman DS. Quantification of ventricular function. In: Germano G, Berman DS, eds. *Clinical Gated Cardiac SPECT.* 2nd ed. Oxford, UK: Blackwell Publishing; 2006:93–137.
2. Klocke FJ, Baird MG, Bateman TM, et al. ACC/AHA/ASNC Guidelines for the clinical use of cardiac radionuclide imaging: A report of the American 1995 guidelines for the clinical use of radionuclide imaging. *Circulation* 2003;108:1404–1418.
3. Taillefer R. Radiopharmaceuticals. In: DePuey E G, Garcia EV, Berman DS, eds. *Cardiac SPECT Imaging.* Philadelphia: PA. Lippincott Williams & Wilkins; 2001:117–152.
4. Gould KL, Lipscomb K, Hamilton GW. Physiologic basis for assessing critical coronary stenosis: instantaneous flow response and regional distribution during coronary hyperemia as measures of coronary flow reserve. *Am J Cardiol* 1974;33:87–94.
5. Pohost GM, Zir LM, Moore RH, et al. Differentiation of transiently ischemic from infarcted myocardium by serial imaging after a single dose of thallium-201. *Circulation* 1977;55:294–302.
6. Gutman J, Berman DS, Freeman M, et al. Time to completed redistribution of thallium-201 in exercise myocardial scintigraphy: relationship to the degree of coronary artery stenosis. *Am Heart J* 1983;106:989–995.

7. Sinusas AJ, Bergin JD, Edwards NC, et al. Redistribution of ^{99m}Tc-sestamibi and ^{201}Tl in the presence of a severe coronary artery stenosis. *Circulation* 1994;89:2332–2341.

8. Leppo JA, Meerdink DJ. Comparison of the myocardial uptake of a technetium-labeled isonitrile analogue and thallium. *Circ Res* 1989;65:632–639.

9. Nishina H, Slomka PJ, Abidov A, et al. Combined supine and prone quantitative myocardial perfusion SPECT: method development and clinical validation in patients with no known coronary artery disease. *J Nucl Med* 2006;47:51–58.

10. Leppo JA, Meerdink DJ. Comparative myocardial extraction of two technetium-labeled BATO derivatives (SQ30217, SQ32014) and thallium. *J Nucl Med* 1990;31:67–74.

11. Berman DS. Fourth annual Mario S. Verani, MD Memorial Lecture: noninvasive imaging in coronary artery disease: changing roles, changing players. *J Nucl Cardiol* 2006;13:457–473.

12. Lauer MS, Francis GS, Okin PM, et al. Impaired chronotropic response to exercise stress testing as a predictor of mortality. *JAMA* 1999;281:524–529.

13. Azarbal B, Hayes SW, Lewin HC, et al. The incremental prognostic value of percentage of heart rate reserve achieved over myocardial perfusion single-photon emission computed tomography in the prediction of cardiac death and all-cause mortality: superiority over 85 percent of maximal age-predicted heart rate. *J Am Coll Cardiol* 2004;44:423–430.

14. Johnson LL, Verdesca SA, Aude WY, et al. Postischemic stunning can affect left ventricular ejection fraction and regional wall motion on post-stress gated sestamibi tomograms. *J Am Coll Cardiol* 1997;30:1641–1648.

15. Verani MS, Mahmarian JJ, Hixson JB, et al. Diagnosis of coronary artery disease by controlled coronary vasodilation with adenosine and thallium-201 scintigraphy in patients unable to exercise. *Circulation* 1990;82:80–87.

16. Hayes SW, Berman DS, Guido Germano. Stress testing and imaging protocols. In: Germano G, Berman DS, eds. *Clinical Gated Cardiac SPECT*. 2nd ed. Oxford, UK: Blackwell Publishing; 2006:47–68.

17. Amanullah AM, Berman DS, Kiat H, et al. Usefulness of hemodynamic changes during adenosine infusion in predicting the diagnostic accuracy of adenosine technetium-99m sestamibi single-photon emission computed tomography (SPECT). *Am J Cardiol* 1997;79:1319–1322.

18. Abidov A, Hachamovitch, R, Hayes, SW, et al. Prognostic Impact of Hemodynamic Response to Adenosine in Patients Older Than Age 55 Years Undergoing Vasodilator Stress Myocardial Perfusion Study. *Circulation* 2003;107:2894–2899.

19. Lette J, Tatum JL, Fraser S, et al. Safety of dipyridamole testing in 73,806 patients: the Multicenter Dipyridamole Safety Study. *J Nucl Cardiol* 1995;2:3–17.

20. Berman DS, Kiat H, Friedman JD, et al. Separate acquisition rest thallium-201/stress technetium-99m sestamibi dual-isotope myocardial perfusion single-photon emission computed tomography: a clinical validation study. *J Am Coll Cardiol* 1993;22:1455–1464.

21. Glover DK, Riou LM, Ruiz M, et al. Reduction of infarct size and postischemic inflammation from ATL-146e, a highly selective adenosine A2A receptor agonist in reperfused canine myocardium. *Am J Physiol Heart Circ Physiol* 2005;288:H1851–H1858.

22. Udelson JE, Heller GV, Wackers FJ, et al. Randomized, controlled dose-ranging study of the selective adenosine A2A receptor agonist binodenoson for pharmacological stress as an adjunct to myocardial perfusion imaging. *Circulation* 2004;109:457–464.

23. Hendel RC, Bateman TM, Cerqueira MD, et al. Initial clinical experience with regadenoson, a novel selective A2A agonist for pharmacologic stress single-photon emission computed tomography myocardial perfusion imaging. *J Am Coll Cardiol* 2005;46:2069–2075.

24. Pennell DJ, Mavrogeni SI, Forbat SM, et al. Adenosine combined with dynamic exercise for myocardial perfusion imaging. *J Am Coll Cardiol* 1995;25:1300–1309.

25. Hachamovitch R, Hayes SW, Friedman JD, et al. A prognostic score for prediction of cardiac mortality risk after adenosine stress myocardial perfusion scintigraphy. *J Am Coll Cardiol* 2005;45:722–729.

26. O'Keefe JH, Jr., Bateman TM, Barnhart CS. Adenosine thallium-201 is superior to exercise thallium-201 for detecting coronary artery disease in patients with left bundle branch block. *J Am Coll Cardiol* 1993;21:1332–1338.

27. Berman DS, Germano G. Interpretation and reporting of gated myocardial perfusion SPECT. In: Germano G, Berman DS, eds. *Clinical Gated Cardiac SPECT*. 2nd ed. Oxford, UK: Blackwell Publishing; 2006:139–171.

28. Samuels B, Kiat H, Friedman JD, et al. Adenosine pharmacologic stress myocardial perfusion tomographic imaging in patients with significant aortic stenosis. Diagnostic efficacy and comparison of clinical, hemodynamic and electrocardiographic variables with 100 age-matched control subjects. *J Am Coll Cardiol* 1995;25:99–106.

29. Sharir T, Rabinowitz B, Livschitz S, et al. Underestimation of extent and severity of coronary artery disease by dipyridamole stress thallium-201 single-photon emission computed tomographic myocardial perfusion imaging in patients taking antianginal drugs. *J Am Coll Cardiol* 1998;31:1540–1546.

30. Taillefer R, Ahlberg AW, Masood Y, et al. Acute beta-blockade reduces the extent and severity of myocardial perfusion defects with dipyridamole Tc-99m sestamibi SPECT imaging. *J Am Coll Cardiol* 2003;42:1475–1483.

31. Hachamovitch R, Hayes S, Friedman JD, et al. Determinants of risk and its temporal variation in patients with normal stress myocardial perfusion scans: what is the warranty period of a normal scan? *J Am Coll Cardiol* 2003;41:1329–1340.

32. Hachamovitch R, Hayes SW, Friedman JD, et al. Comparison of the short-term survival benefit associated with revascularization compared with medical therapy in patients with no prior coronary artery disease undergoing stress myocardial perfusion single photon emission computed tomography. *Circulation* 2003;107:2900–2907.

33. Sciagra R, Bisi G, Santoro GM, et al. Comparison of baseline-nitrate technetium-99m sestamibi with rest-redistribution thallium-201 tomography in detecting viable hibernating myocardium and predicting postrevascularization recovery. *J Am Coll Cardiol* 1997;30:384–391.

34. Aboul-Enein F, Hayes SW, Matsumoto N, et al. Rest perfusion defects in patients with no history of myocardial infarction predict the presence of a critical coronary artery stenosis. *J Nucl Cardiol* 2003;10:656–662.

35. Hayes SW, De Lorenzo A, Hachamovitch R, et al. Prognostic implications of combined prone and supine acquisitions in patients with equivocal or abnormal supine myocardial perfusion SPECT. *J Nucl Med* 2003;44:1633–1640.

36. O'Connor M K, Kemp B, Anstett F, et al. A multicenter evaluation of commercial attenuation compensation techniques in cardiac SPECT using phantom models. *J Nucl Cardiol* 2002;9:361–376.

37. Heller GV, Links J, Bateman TM, et al. American Society of Nuclear Cardiology and Society of Nuclear Medicine joint position statement: attenuation correction of myocardial perfusion SPECT scintigraphy. *J Nucl Cardiol* 2004;11:229–230.

38. Masood Y, Liu YH, Depuey G, et al. Clinical validation of SPECT attenuation correction using x-ray computed tomography-derived attenuation maps: multicenter clinical trial with angiographic correlation. *J Nucl Cardiol* 2005;12:676–686.

39. Cerqueira MD, Weissman NJ, Dilsizian V, et al. Standardized myocardial segmentation and nomenclature for tomographic imaging of the heart: a statement for healthcare professionals from the Cardiac Imaging Committee of the Council on Clinical Cardiology of the American Heart Association. *Circulation* 2002;105:539–542.

40. Berman DS, Hachamovitch R, Kiat H, et al. Incremental value of prognostic testing in patients with known or suspected ischemic heart disease: a basis for optimal utilization of exercise technetium-99m sestamibi myocardial perfusion single-photon emission computed tomography. *J Am Coll Cardiol* 1995;26:639–647.

41. Berman DS, Kang X, Hayes SW, et al. Adenosine myocardial perfusion single-photon emission computed tomography in women compared with men: impact of diabetes mellitus on incremental prognostic value and effect on patient management. *J Am Coll Cardiol* 2003;41:1125–1133.

42. Berman DS, Abidov A, Kang X, et al. Prognostic validation of a 17-segment score derived from a 20-segment score for myocardial perfusion SPECT interpretation. *J Nucl Cardiol* 2004;11:414–423.

43. Leslie WD, Tully SA, Yogendran MS, et al. Prognostic value of automated quantification of ^{99m}Tc-sestamibi myocardial perfusion imaging. *J Nucl Med* 2005;46:204–211.

44. Hansen CL, Goldstein RA, Berman DS, et al. ASNC Imaging Guidelines: myocardial perfusion and function SPECT. *J Nucl Cardiol* 2006;13:e97–120.

45. Germano G, Berman DS. Digital Techniques for the acquisition, processing, and analysis of nuclear cardiology images. In: Sandler MP, Coleman RE, Patton JA, Wackers FJTh, Gottschalk A, eds. *Diagnostic Nuclear Medicine*. 4th ed. Philadelphia: PA. Lippincott Williams & Wilkins; 2003:207–222.

46. Lipke CS, Kuhl HP, Nowak B, et al. Validation of 4D-MSPECT and QGS for quantification of left ventricular volumes and ejection fraction from gated ^{99m}Tc-MIBI SPET. comparison with cardiac magnetic resonance imaging. *Eur J Nucl Med Mol Imaging* 2004;31:482–490.

47. Hambye AS, Vervaet A, Dobbeleir A. Variability of left ventricular ejection fraction and volumes with quantitative gated SPECT influence of algorithm,

pixel size and reconstruction parameters in small and normal-sized hearts. *Eur J Nucl Med Mol Imaging* 2004;31:1606–1613.

48. Sharir T, Kang X, Germano G, et al. Prognostic value of poststress left ventricular volume and ejection fraction by gated myocardial perfusion SPECT in women and men: gender-related differences in normal limits and outcomes. *J Nucl Cardiol* 2006;13:495–506.

49. Weiss AT, Berman DS, Lew AS, et al. Transient ischemic dilation of the left ventricle on stress thallium-201 scintigraphy: a marker of severe and extensive coronary artery disease. *J Am Coll Cardiol* 1987;9:752–759.

50. Mazzanti M, Germano G, Kiat H, et al. Identification of severe and extensive coronary artery disease by automatic measurement of transient ischemic dilation of the left ventricle in dual-isotope myocardial perfusion SPECT. *J Am Coll Cardiol* 1996;27:1612–1620.

51. Hansen CL, Sangrigoli R, Nkadi E, et al. Comparison of pulmonary uptake with transient cavity dilation after exercise thallium-201 perfusion imaging. *J Am Coll Cardiol* 1999;33:1323–1327.

52. Abidov A, Bax JJ, Hayes SW, et al. Transient Ischemic Dilation Ratio of the Left Ventricle Is a Significant Predictor of Future Cardiac Events in Patients with Otherwise Normal Myocardial Perfusion SPECT. *J Am Coll Cardiol* 2003;42:1818–1825.

53. Abidov A, Bax JJ, Hayes SW, et al. Integration of automatically measured transient ischemic dilation ratio into interpretation of adenosine stress myocardial perfusion SPECT for detection of severe and extensive CAD. *J Nucl Med* 2004;45:1999–2007.

54. Gill JB, Ruddy TD, Newell JB, et al. Prognostic importance of thallium uptake by the lungs during exercise in coronary artery disease. *N Engl J Med* 1987;317:1486–1489.

55. Leslie WD, Tully SA, Yogendran MS, et al. Prognostic value of lung sestamibi uptake in myocardial perfusion imaging of patients with known or suspected coronary artery disease. *J Am Coll Cardiol* 2005;45:1676–1682.

56. Travin MI, Bergmann SR. Assessment of myocardial viability. *Semin Nucl Med* 2005;35:2–16.

57. Grundy SM, Pasternak R, Greenland P, et al. Assessment of cardiovascular risk by use of multiple-risk-factor assessment equations: a statement for healthcare professionals from the American Heart Association and the American College of Cardiology. *Circulation* 1999;100:1481–1492.

58. Diamond GA, Forrester JS. Analysis of probability as an aid in the clinical diagnosis of coronary-artery disease. *N Engl J Med* 1979;300:1350–1358.

59. Brindis RG, Douglas PS, Hendel RC, et al. ACCF/ASNC appropriateness criteria for single-photon emission computed tomography myocardial perfusion imaging (SPECT MPI): a report of the American College of Cardiology Foundation Quality Strategic Directions Committee Appropriateness Criteria Working Group and the American Society of Nuclear Cardiology endorsed by the American Heart Association. *J Am Coll Cardiol* 2005;46:1587–1605.

60. Gibbons RJ, Abrams J, Chatterjee K, et al. ACC/AHA 2002 guideline update for the management of patients with chronic stable angina—summary article: a report of the American College of Cardiology/American Heart Association Task Force on practice guidelines (Committee on the Management of Patients With Chronic Stable Angina). *J Am Coll Cardiol* 2003;41:159–168.

61. Taillefer R, DePuey EG, Udelson JE, et al. Comparative diagnostic accuracy of Tl-201 and Tc-99m sestamibi SPECT imaging (perfusion and ECG-gated SPECT) in detecting coronary artery disease in women. *J Am Coll Cardiol* 1997;29:69–77.

62. Slomka PJ, Nishina H, Abidov A, et al. Combined quantitative supine-prone myocardial perfusion SPECT improves detection of coronary artery disease and normalcy rates in women. *J Nucl Cardiol* 2007;14:44–52.

63. Heller GV, Bateman TM, Johnson LL, et al. Clinical value of attenuation correction in stress-only Tc-99m sestamibi SPECT imaging. *J Nucl Cardiol* 2004;11:273–281.

64. Rozanski A, Diamond GA, Berman D, et al. The declining specificity of exercise radionuclide ventriculography. *N Engl J Med* 1983;309:518–522.

65. Hachamovitch R, Shaw L, Berman DS. Methodological considerations in the assessment of noninvasive testing using outcomes research: pitfalls and limitations. *Prog Cardiovasc Dis* 2000;43:215–230.

66. Berman DS, Hachamovitch R, Shaw LJ, et al. Roles of nuclear cardiology, cardiac computed tomography, and cardiac magnetic resonance: noninvasive risk stratification and a conceptual framework for the selection of noninvasive imaging tests in patients with known or suspected coronary artery disease. *J Nucl Med* 2006;47:1107–1118.

67. Gibbons RJ, Chatterjee K, Daley J, et al. ACC/AHA/ACP-ASIM guidelines for the management of patients with chronic stable angina: a report of the American College of Cardiology/American Heart Association Task Force on Practice Guidelines (Committee on Management of Patients With Chronic Stable Angina). *J Am Coll Cardiol* 1999;33:2092–2197.

68. Gibbons RJ, Hodge DO, Berman DS, et al. Long-term outcome of patients with intermediate-risk exercise electrocardiograms who do not have myocardial perfusion defects on radionuclide imaging. *Circulation* 1999;100:2140–2145.

69. Yusuf S, Zucker D, Peduzzi P, et al. Effect of coronary artery bypass graft surgery on survival: overview of 10-year results from randomised trials by the Coronary Artery Bypass Graft Surgery Trialists Collaboration. *Lancet* 1994;344:563.

70. Little WC, Constantinescu M, Applegate RJ, et al. Can coronary angiography predict the site of a subsequent myocardial infarction in patients with mild-to-moderate coronary artery disease? *Circulation* 1988;78:1157–1166.

71. Kinsella JP, Torielli F, Ziegler JW, et al. Dipyridamole augmentation of response to nitric oxide. *Lancet* 1995;346:647–648.

72. Ladenheim ML, Kotler TS, Pollock BH. Incremental prognostic power of clinical history, exercise electrocardiography and myocardial perfusion scintigraphy in suspected coronary artery disease. *Am J Cardiol* 1987;59:270–277.

73. Shaw LJ, Hendel R, Lauer MS, et al. Prognostic Value of Normal Exercise and Adenosine Tc-99m Tetrofosmin SPECT Imaging: Results from the Multicenter Registry in 4,728 Patients. *J Nucl Med* 2003;44:134–139.

74. Abidov A, Rozanski A, Hachamovitch R, et al. Prognostic significance of dyspnea in patients referred for cardiac stress testing. *N Engl J Med* 2005;353:1889–1898.

75. Hachamovitch R, Berman DS, Shaw LJ, et al. Incremental prognostic value of myocardial perfusion single photon emission computed tomography for the prediction of cardiac death: differential stratification for risk of cardiac death and myocardial infarction. *Circulation* 1998;97:535–543.

76. Ladenheim ML, Pollock BH, Rozanski A, et al. Extent and severity of myocardial hypoperfusion as predictors of prognosis in patients with suspected coronary artery disease. *J Am Coll Cardiol* 1986;7:464–471.

77. Shaw LJ, Hendel RC, Cerquiera M, et al. Ethnic differences in the prognostic value of stress technetium-99m tetrofosmin gated single-photon emission computed tomography myocardial perfusion imaging. *J Am Coll Cardiol* 2005;45:1494–1504.

78. Hachamovitch R, Berman DS. The use of nuclear cardiology in clinical decision making. *Semin Nucl Med* 2005;35:62–72.

79. Abidov A, Hachamovitch R, Rozanski A, et al. Prognostic implications of atrial fibrillation in patients undergoing myocardial perfusion single-photon emission computed tomography. *J Am Coll Cardiol* 2004;44:1062–1070.

80. Marwick TH. Dyspnea and risk in suspected coronary disease. *N Engl J Med* 2005;353:1963–1965.

81. Hachamovitch R, Rozanski A, Hayes SW, et al. Predicting therapeutic benefit from myocardial revascularization procedures: are measurements of resting left ventricular ejection fraction and stress-induced myocardial ischemia both necessary? *J Nucl Cardiol* 2006;13:768–778.

82. Shaw LJ, Hachamovitch R, Berman DS, et al. The economic consequences of available diagnostic and prognostic strategies for the evaluation of stable angina patients: an observational assessment of the value of precatheterization ischemia. Economics of Noninvasive Diagnosis (END) Multicenter Study Group. *J Am Coll Cardiol* 1999;33:661–669.

83. Hachamovitch R, Hayes SW, Friedman JD, et al. Stress myocardial perfusion SPECT is clinically effective and cost-effective in risk-stratification of patients with a high likelihood of CAD but no known CAD. *J Am Coll Cardiol* 2004;43:200–2008.

84. Sharir T, Germano G, Kavanagh PB, et al. Incremental prognostic value of post-stress left ventricular ejection fraction and volume by gated myocardial perfusion single photon emission computed tomography. *Circulation* 1999;100:1035–1042.

85. Thomas GS, Miyamoto MI, Morello AP III, et al. Technetium 99m sestamibi myocardial perfusion imaging predicts clinical outcome in the community outpatient setting. The Nuclear Utility in the Community (NUC) Study. *J Am Coll Cardiol* 2004;43:213–223.

86. Travin MI, Heller GV, Johnson LL, et al. The prognostic value of ECG-gated SPECT imaging in patients undergoing stress Tc-99m sestamibi myocardial perfusion imaging. *J Nucl Cardiol* 2004;11:253–262.

87. Sharir T, Bacher-Stier C, Dhar S, et al. Identification of severe and extensive coronary artery disease by postexercise regional wall motion abnormalities in Tc-99m sestamibi gated single-photon emission computed tomography. *Am J Cardiol* 2000;86:1171–1175.

88. Sharir T, Berman DS, Lewin HC, et al. Incremental prognostic value of rest-redistribution (201)Tl single-photon emission computed tomography. *Circulation* 1999;100:1964–1970.

89. Allman KC, Shaw LJ, Hachamovitch R, et al. Myocardial viability testing and impact of revascularization on prognosis in patients with coronary artery disease and left ventricular dysfunction: a meta-analysis. *J Am Coll Cardiol* 2002;39:1151–1158.

90. Hachamovitch R, Berman DS, Kiat H, et al. Value of stress myocardial perfusion single photon emission computed tomography in patients with normal resting electrocardiograms: an evaluation of incremental prognostic value and cost-effectiveness. *Circulation* 2002;105:823–829.

91. Hachamovitch R, Berman DS, Kiat H, et al. Exercise myocardial perfusion SPECT in patients without known coronary artery disease: incremental prognostic value and use in risk stratification. *Circulation* 1996;93:905–914.

92. Christian TF, Miller TD, Bailey KR, et al. Exercise tomographic thallium-201 imaging in patients with severe coronary artery disease and normal electrocardiograms. *Ann Intern Med* 1994;121:825–832.

93. O'Keefe JH, Jr., Zinsmeister AR, Gibbons RJ. Value of normal electrocardiographic findings in predicting resting left ventricular function in patients with chest pain and suspected coronary artery disease. *Am J Med* 1989;86:658–662.

94. Poornima IG, Miller TD, Christian TF, et al. Utility of myocardial perfusion imaging in patients with low-risk treadmill scores. *J Am Coll Cardiol* 2004;43:194–199.

95. Valeti US, Miller TD, Hodge DO, et al. Exercise single-photon emission computed tomography provides effective risk stratification of elderly men and elderly women. *Circulation* 2005;111:1771–1776.

96. Mieres JH, Shaw LJ, Arai A, et al. Role of noninvasive testing in the clinical evaluation of women with suspected coronary artery disease: consensus statement from the Cardiac Imaging Committee, Council on Clinical Cardiology, and the Cardiovascular Imaging and Intervention Committee, Council on Cardiovascular Radiology and Intervention, American Heart Association. *Circulation* 2005;111:682–696.

97. Shaw LJ, Olson MB, Kip K, et al. The value of estimated functional capacity in estimating outcome: results from the NHBLI-Sponsored Women's Ischemia Syndrome Evaluation (WISE) Study. *J Am Coll Cardiol* 2006;47:S36–S43.

98. Blumenthal RS, Becker DM, Moy TF, et al. Exercise thallium tomography predicts future clinically manifest coronary heart disease in a high-risk asymptomatic population. *Circulation* 1996;93:915–923.

99. Giri S, Shaw LJ, Murthy DR, et al. Impact of diabetes on the risk stratification using stress single-photon emission computed tomography myocardial perfusion imaging in patients with symptoms suggestive of coronary artery disease. *Circulation* 2002;105:32–40.

100. Kang X, Berman DS, Lewin HC, et al. Incremental prognostic value of myocardial perfusion single photon emission computed tomography in patients with diabetes mellitus. *Am Heart J* 1999;138:1025–1032.

101. Wackers FJ, Young LH, Inzucchi SE, et al. Detection of silent myocardial ischemia in asymptomatic diabetic subjects: the DIAD study. *Diabetes Care* 2004;27:1954–1961.

102. Di Carli MF, Hachamovitch R. Should we screen for occult coronary artery disease among asymptomatic patients with diabetes? *J Am Coll Cardiol* 2005;45:50–53.

103. Rajagopalan N, Miller TD, Hodge DO, et al. Identifying high-risk asymptomatic diabetic patients who are candidates for screening stress single-photon emission computed tomography imaging. *J Am Coll Cardiol* 2005;45:43–49.

104. Anand DV, Lim E, Hopkins D, et al. Risk stratification in uncomplicated type 2 diabetes: prospective evaluation of the combined use of coronary artery calcium imaging and selective myocardial perfusion scintigraphy. *Eur Heart J* 2006;27:713–721.

105. Vaduganathan P, He ZX, Raghavan C, et al. Detection of left anterior descending coronary artery stenosis in patients with left bundle branch block: exercise, adenosine or dobutamine imaging? *J Am Coll Cardiol* 1996;28:543–550.

106. Wagdy HM, Hodge D, Christian TF, et al. Prognostic value of vasodilator myocardial perfusion imaging in patients with left bundle-branch block. *Circulation* 1998;97:1563–1570.

107. Amanullah AM, Berman DS, Kang X, et al. Enhanced prognostic stratification of patients with left ventricular hypertrophy with the use of single-photon emission computed tomography. *Am Heart J* 2000;140:456–462.

108. Shaw LJ, Iskandrian AE. Prognostic value of gated myocardial perfusion SPECT. *J Nucl Cardiol* 2004;11:171–185.

109. Shaw LJ, Bairey Merz CN, Pepine CJ, et al. Insights from the NHLBI-Sponsored Women's Ischemia Syndrome Evaluation (WISE) Study: part I. gender differences in traditional and novel risk factors, symptom evaluation, and gender-optimized diagnostic strategies. *J Am Coll Cardiol* 2006;47:S4-S20.

110. Schinkel AF, Elhendy A, Biagini E, et al. Prognostic stratification using dobutamine stress 99mTc-tetrofosmin myocardial perfusion SPECT in elderly patients unable to perform exercise testing. *J Nucl Med* 2005;46:12–18.

111. Grossman GB, Garcia EV, Bateman TM, et al. Quantitative Tc-99m sestamibi attenuation-corrected SPECT. development and multicenter trial validation of myocardial perfusion stress gender-independent normal database in an obese population. *J Nucl Cardiol* 2004;11:263–272.

112. Thompson RC, Heller GV, Johnson LL, et al. Value of attenuation correction on ECG-gated SPECT myocardial perfusion imaging related to body mass index. *J Nucl Cardiol* 2005;12:195–202.

113. Berman DS, Kang X, Hayes SW, et al. Diagnostic accuracy of gated myocardial perfusion SPECT with combined supine and prone acquisitions to detect coronary artery disease in obese and nonobese patients. *J Nucl Cardiol* 2006;13:191–201.

114. Kang X, Shaw LJ, Hayes SW, et al. Impact of body mass index on cardiac mortality in patients with known or suspected coronary artery disease undergoing myocardial perfusion single-photon emission computed tomography. *J Am Coll Cardiol* 2006;47:1418–1426.

115. Greenland P, Bonow RO, Brundage BH, et al. Computed tomography: ACC/AHA writing committee to update the 2000 clinical expert consensus document on electron-beam computed tomography for the diagnosis and prognosis for coronary artery disease. *J Am Coll Cardiol* 2007;49:378–402.

115a. Rozanski A, Gransar H, Wong ND. Clinical outcomes after both coronary calcium scanning and exercise myocardial perfusion scintigraphy. *J Am Coll Cardiol* 2007;49:1352-1361.

116. Berman DS, Wong ND, Gransar H, et al. Relationship between stress-induced myocardial ischemia and atherosclerosis measured by coronary calcium tomography. *J Am Coll Cardiol* 2004;44:923–930.

117. Shaw LJ, Berman DS, Bax JJ, et al. Computed tomographic imaging within nuclear cardiology. *J Nucl Cardiol* 2005;12:131–142.

118. Blumenthal RS, Becker DM, Yanek LR, et al. Comparison of coronary calcium and stress myocardial perfusion imaging in apparently healthy siblings of individuals with premature coronary artery disease. *Am J Cardiol* 2006;97:328–333.

119. Wong ND, Rozanski A, Gransar H, et al. Metabolic syndrome and diabetes are associated with an increased likelihood of inducible myocardial ischemia among patients with subclinical atherosclerosis. *Diabetes Care* 2005;28:1445–1450.

120. Raff GL, Gallagher MJ, O'Neill WW, et al. Diagnostic accuracy of noninvasive coronary angiography using 64-slice spiral computed tomography. *J Am Coll Cardiol* 2005;46:552–557.

121. Berman DS, Zellweger MJ, Shaw LJ, et al. Evaluation of patients after intervention. In: Poshost GM, O'Rourke RA, Berman DS, Shah PM, eds. *Imaging in Cardiovascular Disease*. Philadelphia: PA. Lippincott Williams & Wilkins; 2000:543–563.

122. Garzon PP, Eisenberg MJ. Functional testing for the detection of restenosis after percutaneous transluminal coronary angioplasty: a meta-analysis. *Can J Cardiol* 2001;17:41–48.

123. Zellweger MJ, Weinbacher M, Zutter AW, et al. Long-term outcome of patients with silent versus symptomatic ischemia six months after percutaneous coronary intervention and stenting. *J Am Coll Cardiol* 2003;42:33–40.

124. Palmas W, Bingham S, Diamond GA, et al. Incremental prognostic value of exercise thallium-201 myocardial single-photon emission computed tomography late after coronary artery bypass surgery. *J Am Coll Cardiol* 1995;25:403–409.

125. Lauer MS, Lytle B, Pashkow F, et al. Prediction of death and myocardial infarction by screening with exercise-thallium testing after coronary-artery-bypass grafting. *Lancet* 1998;351:615–622.

126. Zellweger MJ, HC L, Lai S, et al. When to stress patients after coronary artery bypass surgery? Risk stratification in patients early and late post-CABG using stress myocardial perfusion SPECT. implications of appropriate clinical strategies. *J Am Coll Cardiol* 2001:144–152.

127. Blumenthal RS, Becker DM, Yanek LR, et al. Detecting occult coronary disease in a high-risk asymptomatic population. *Circulation* 2003;107:702–707.

128. Shaw LJ, Heller GV, Casperson P, et al. Gated myocardial perfusion single photon emission computed tomography in the clinical outcomes utilizing revascularization and aggressive drug evaluation (COURAGE) trial, Veterans Administration cooperative study no. 424. *J Nucl Cardiol* 2006;13:685–698.

129. Taylor A, Shaw LJ, Fayad Z, et al. Tracking atherosclerosis regression: a clinical tool in preventive cardiology. *Atherosclerosis* 2005;180:1–10.

130. Udelson JE, Beshansky JR, Ballin DS, et al. Myocardial perfusion imaging for evaluation and triage of patients with suspected acute cardiac ischemia: a randomized controlled trial. *JAMA* 2002;288:2693–2700.

131. Gibbons RJ, Valeti US, Araoz PA, et al. The quantification of infarct size. *J Am Coll Cardiol* 2004;44:1533–1542.

132. Gibson RS, Watson DD, Craddock GB, et al. Prediction of cardiac events after uncomplicated myocardial infarction: a prospective study comparing predischarge exercise thallium-201 scintigraphy and coronary angiography. *Circulation* 1983;68:321–336.

133. Brown KA, Heller GV, Landin RS, et al. Early dipyridamole (99m)Tc-sestamibi single photon emission computed tomographic imaging 2 to 4 days after acute myocardial infarction predicts in-hospital and postdischarge cardiac events: comparison with submaximal exercise imaging. *Circulation* 1999;100:2060–2066.

134. Beller GA, Zaret BL. Contributions of nuclear cardiology to diagnosis and prognosis of patients with coronary artery disease. *Circulation* 2000;101:1465–1478.

135. Mahmarian JJ, Dakik HA, Filipchuk NG, et al. A strategy of intensive medical therapy is comparable to that of coronary revascularization for suppression of myocardial ischemia in high risk but stable survivors of acute myocardial infarction. *J Am Coll Cardiol* 2006;48:2458–2467.

136. Wizenberg TA, Muz J, Sohn YH, et al. Value of positive myocardial technetium-99m-pyrophosphate scintigraphy in the noninvasive diagnosis of cardiac amyloidosis. *Am Heart J* 1982;103:468–473.

137. Van Kriekinge SD, Berman DS, Germano G. Automatic quantification of left ventricular ejection fraction from gated blood pool SPECT. *J Nucl Cardiol* 1999;6:498–506.

138. Schwartz RG, McKenzie WB, Alexander J, et al. Congestive heart failure and left ventricular dysfunction complicating doxorubicin therapy: seven-year experience using serial radionuclide angiocardiography. *Am J Med* 1987;82:1109–1118.

139. Wieland DM, Brown LE, Rogers WL, et al. Myocardial imaging with a radioiodinated norepinephrine storage analog. *J Nucl Med* 1981;22:22–31.

140. Dobrucki LW, Sinusas AJ. Cardiovascular molecular imaging. *Semin Nucl Med* 2005;35:73–81.

141. Knapp FF, Jr., Goodman MM, Callahan AP, et al. Radioiodinated 15-(p-iodophenyl)-3,3-dimethylpentadecanoic acid: a useful new agent to evaluate myocardial fatty acid uptake. *J Nucl Med* 1986;27:521–31.

142. Furutani Y, Shiigi T, Nakamura Y, et al. Quantification of area at risk in acute myocardial infarction by tomographic imaging. *J Nucl Med* 1997;38:1875–1882.

143. Dilsizian V, Bateman TM, Bergmann SR, et al. Metabolic imaging with beta-methyl-p-[(123)I]-iodophenyl-pentadecanoic acid identifies ischemic memory after demand ischemia. *Circulation* 2005;112:2169–2174.

144. Narula J, Acio ER, Narula N, et al. Annexin-V imaging for noninvasive detection of cardiac allograft rejection. *Nat Med* 2001;7:1347–1352.

145. Braunwald E. Epilogue: what do clinicians expect from imagers? *J Am Coll Cardiol* 2006;47:C101–C103.

146. Gao Z, Li Z, Baker SP, et al. Novel short-acting A2A adenosine receptor agonists for coronary vasodilation: inverse relationship between affinity and duration of action of A2A agonists. *J Pharmacol Exp Ther* 2001;298:209–218.

147. Berman DS, Germano G. Clinical applications of nuclear cardiology. In: Germano G, Berman DS, eds. *Clinical Gated Cardiac SPECT*. Armonk, NY: Futura,1999:1–71.

148. O'Rourke RA, Chaudhuri T, Shaw L, et al. Resolution of stress-induced myocardial ischemia during aggressive medical therapy as demonstrated by single photon emission computed tomography imaging. *Circulation* 2001;103:2315.

149. Kriekinge SV, Berman DS, Germano G. Quantitative gated blood pool SPECT. In: Germano G, Berman DS, eds. *Clinical Gated Cardiac SPECT*. 2nd ed. Oxford, UK: Blackwell Publishing, 2006:273–284.

150. Kietselaer BL, Reutelingsperger CP, Heidendal GA, et al. Noninvasive detection of plaque instability with use of radiolabeled annexin A5 in patients with carotid-artery atherosclerosis. *N Engl J Med* 2004;350:1472–3.

CHAPTER (20)

Computed Tomography of the Heart

Matthew J. Budoff / Michael Poon / Giuseppe Maiolino

Computed tomography (CT) is a technique that can fully evaluate both cardiac structure and function. Recent advances in imaging speed have allowed for more complete evaluation of relatively stationary structures, such as the thoracic aorta, and rapidly moving structures, such as the myocardium and coronary arteries, providing the ability to noninvasively diagnose or rule out significant epicardial coronary artery disease (CAD). When combined with electrocardiographic (ECG) gating, *freeze-frame* images of the heart can be obtained, obviating most of the blur caused by motion artifact. This is particularly important in obtaining contrast-enhanced images of the coronary arteries or quantifying coronary artery calcium. These advances in spatial and temporal resolution and image reconstruction software have also helped in the evaluation of cardiac structures including coronary veins, pulmonary veins, atria, ventricles, aorta, and thoracic arterial and venous structures, with definition of their spatial relationships for the comprehensive assessment of a variety of cardiovascular disease processes. This chapter details the current and future role of cardiac CT for the assessment of cardiovascular pathology.

TECHNICAL CONSIDERATIONS

[ ] MULTIROW DETECTOR COMPUTED TOMOGRAPHY

Advancements in CT technology have improved image acquisition speed and patient throughput. Multidetector computed tomography (MDCT) scanners produce images by rotating an x-ray tube around a circular gantry through which the patient advances on a moving couch. Increased numbers of detectors have allowed much faster throughput, essentially reducing the time to image the entire cardiac anatomy to <10 seconds. The introduction of multirow spiral CT detector systems (i.e., multislice CT) currently allow acquisition of 4 to 64 simultaneous images, with slice thickness reduced to 0.5 to 0.625 mm. Improvements in gantry rotation speeds and the development of partial reconstruction algorithms have reduced effective single-image acquisition time to <200 msec. However, image acquisition within 50 msec is required to completely avoid cardiac motion artifacts.[1,2] The coronary arteries also

577

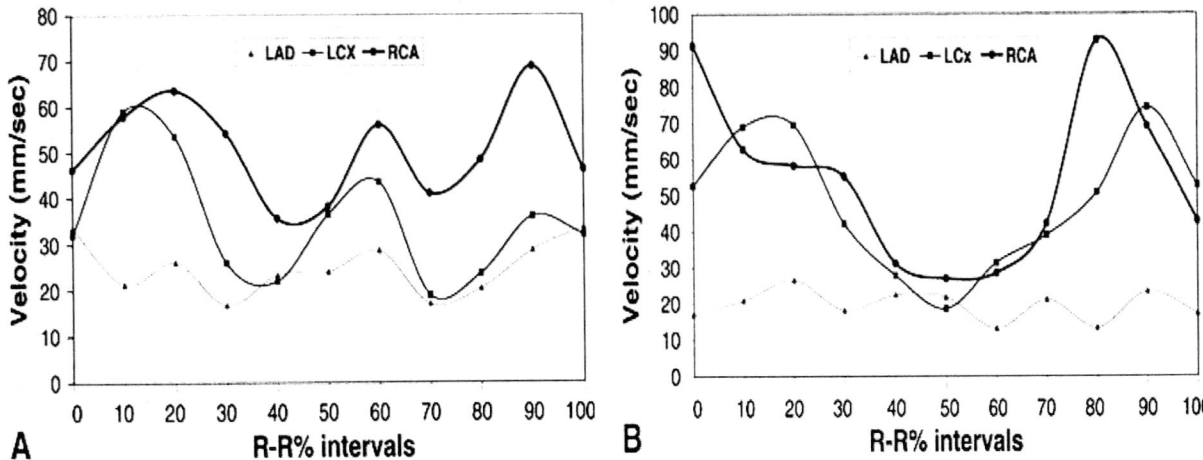

FIGURE 20–1. Coronary artery velocity varies substantially throughout the cardiac cycle, depending on whether the heart rate is relatively slow (**A,** 72 beats/min) or fast (**B,** 89 beats/min). The greatest motion occurs in the right coronary artery (RCA), followed by the left circumflex (LCX) and left anterior descending (LAD) coronary arteries. **A.** A biphasic pattern of rest is found during end-systole (at 40–50 percent of the R-R interval) and mid-diastole (at 70–80 percent of the R-R interval). **B.** A monophasic rest period pattern was found near end systole (at 40–60 percent of the R-R interval). *Source: From Lu B, Mao SS, Zhuang N, et al.[2] Reproduced with permission from the publisher and the authors.*

move independently throughout the cardiac cycle and even at slow heart rates (i.e., <70 beats/min) exhibit significant translational motion of up to 60 mm/sec for the right coronary artery (RCA) and 20 to 40 mm/sec for the left anterior descending (LAD) and circumflex coronary arteries[2,3] (Fig. 20–1).

Retrospective gating with MDCT employs acquisition of multiple images throughout each cardiac cycle. With multirow detector CT systems, temporal resolution may be further improved by selecting specific partial image sector data from different heartbeats and detector rings to reconstruct a complete 240-degree image data set. With retrospective gating, several hundred images can be acquired during a single cardiac study, allowing one to *pick and choose* images with the least amount of motion-related distortion prior to final image reconstruction. However, this oversampling leads to significant excess radiation exposure to the patient. The typical radiation exposure from an electron-beam computed tomography (EBCT) study is <1.0 rad,[4] whereas MDCT scanners using retrospective gating can increase exposure approximately 13-fold.[5] Prospective gating during either spiral or nonspiral acquisitions employs image triggering only at a specific temporal location of the cardiac cycle, thereby significantly reducing radiation exposure. Gating works relatively well at slow heart rates (i.e., <60 beats/min), where the R-R interval is >1000 msec and the fastest imaging protocols are used. However, at faster heart rates, a 200-msec acquisition effectively covers most of the cardiac cycle, thus obviating any potential benefit from gating the image acquisition.

⟦ ⟧ ELECTRON-BEAM COMPUTED TOMOGRAPHY

EBCT uses an electron beam (current 630 mA, voltage 130 kV), which is deflected via a magnetic coil and focused to strike a series of four tungsten targets located beneath the patient (Fig. 20–2). The electron beam is magnetically swept along the tungsten targets at a 210-degree arc, and each target ring is separated by a 4-mm distance. The resultant x-rays generated beneath the patient are then attenuated as they pass through the thorax and recorded by a series of two twin fixed detector arrays arranged in a semicircle above the patient. Because EBCT has no moving parts, as

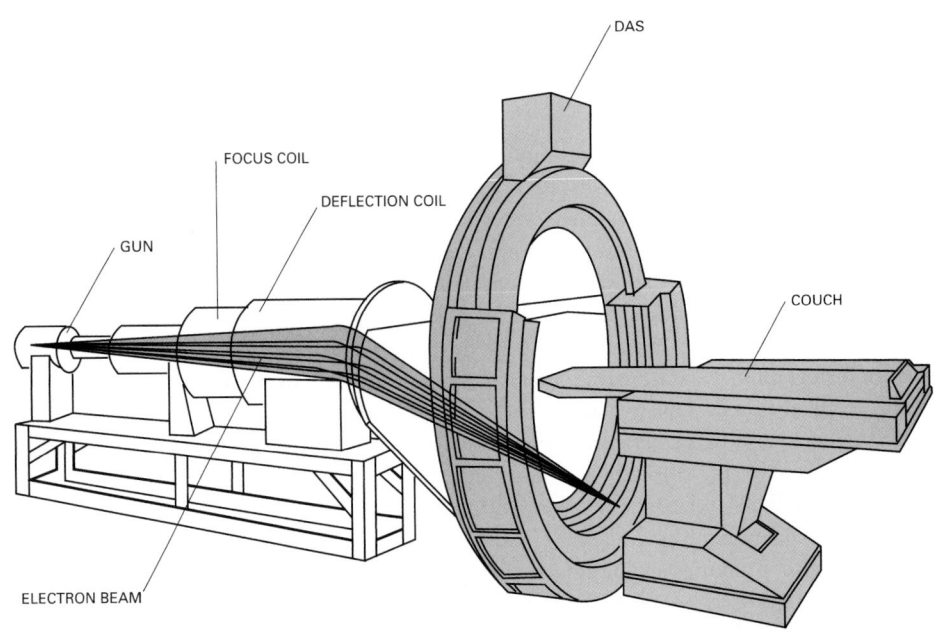

FIGURE 20–2. Diagram of the EBCT scanner. The electron beam is emitted from the electron gun and focused onto the tungsten targets by the magnetic deflection coil. DAS, immediate memory; EBCT, electron-beam computed tomography.

found in conventional and MDCT scanners, imaging time is complete within 50 msec, which is the time required for the electron beam to sweep along the tungsten targets. With a 100-msec acquisition time, a freeze-frame image of the myocardium and coronary arteries in end-diastole can be achieved with little if any motion blur.

EBCT is commonly operated using three different acquisition modes. The cine mode creates real-time, cross-sectional views of the beating heart and is commonly used to assess both global and regional right and left ventricular (LV) function (Fig. 20–3). The volume mode allows acquisition of a single image with each preselected movement of the patient couch. Up to 40 continuous slices can be obtained scanning 12 to 32 cm of anatomy, depending on the couch speed selected (Fig. 20–4). This imaging mode is commonly gated to the ECG to obtain high-resolution static images for detailed evaluation of cardiovascular anatomy, such as coronary artery calcification (CAC). The triggered (flow) mode is used to assess blood flow through specific cardiac chambers and the myocardium itself. This mode allows acquisition of some 20 to 40 consecutive scans where imaging occurs at a designated time during each cardiac cycle. From these consecutive scans, time-density curves can be constructed, which can estimate blood flow through specific cardiac chambers and within the myocardium.

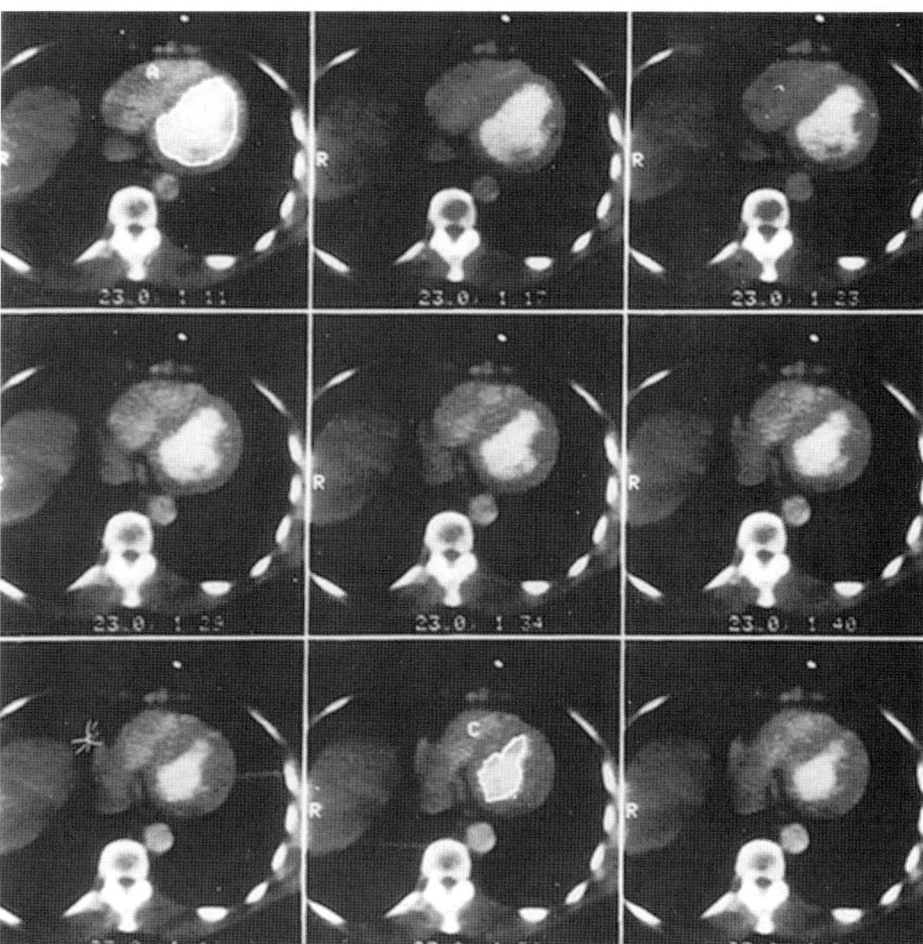

FIGURE 20–3. An 8-mm-thick CT slice of the mid–left ventricle imaged for one complete cardiac cycle at 58-msec intervals. A, end-diastole; C, end-systole.

EVALUATION OF MYOCARDIAL FUNCTION

Right and left ventricles are equally well visualized by contrast cardiac computed tomography angiography (CTA). The combination of ECG gating and image postprocessing permits the reconstruction of multiple datasets at predetermined percentages of the R-R interval throughout the entire cardiac cycle (Fig. 20–5). This multiphase image reconstruction can be displayed in cine mode as in echocardiography or cardiac magnetic resonance (CMR) imaging. Therefore, end systolic and end diastolic images can be obtained to assess ventricular volumes and function (see Fig. 20–5).

Both ventricles are well visualized by MDCT and EBCT, allowing excellent spatial separation between the two structures. Delineation of the epicardial and endocardial surfaces allows accurate and reproducible measurement of LV and right ventricular (RV) wall thickness and myocardial mass.[6] LV hypertrophy can be quantified and serially assessed.

CT can assess left and RV hemodynamics[7] as well as regional myocardial wall motion and thickening.[7,8] The cine mode is used to acquire multiple gated images of the right and left ventricles during maximal contrast enhancement.[8] This affords accurate and reproducible quantification of LV and RV end-diastolic and end-systolic volumes and ejection fraction (EF).[8] CT is comparable to first-pass radionuclide angiography for the calculation of left ventricular ejection fraction (LVEF) in patients with myocardial infarction (MI)[9] (Fig. 20–5).

Both MDCT and EBCT allow precise measurements of the LV volumes and overall function and such measurements have a close correlation with echocardiography.[6,10–13] When compared with CMR, the current gold standard for cardiac functional evaluation, MDCT is an adequate alternative.[12]

Furthermore, MDCT and EBCT are also valuable tools in estimating LV wall thickness, mass, and segmental wall motion and demonstrate good overall agreement with echocardiography and CMR.[6,11–13]

Ventricular remodeling can be assessed by CT in a fashion similar to gated blood-pool radionuclide angiography and echocardiography. CT can identify wall thinning and impaired LV thickening in an area of previous MI and delineate anterior and posterior LV aneurysms and associated mural thrombus[6,14] (Fig. 20–6).

RV volume and functional assessment by MDCT is feasible and agrees well with both radionuclide ventriculography and CMR.[6,11] Typically, the RV is not well opacified during the routine image acquisition of a coronary CTA because the timing of contrast injection and the bolus chase with normal saline is aimed at the op-

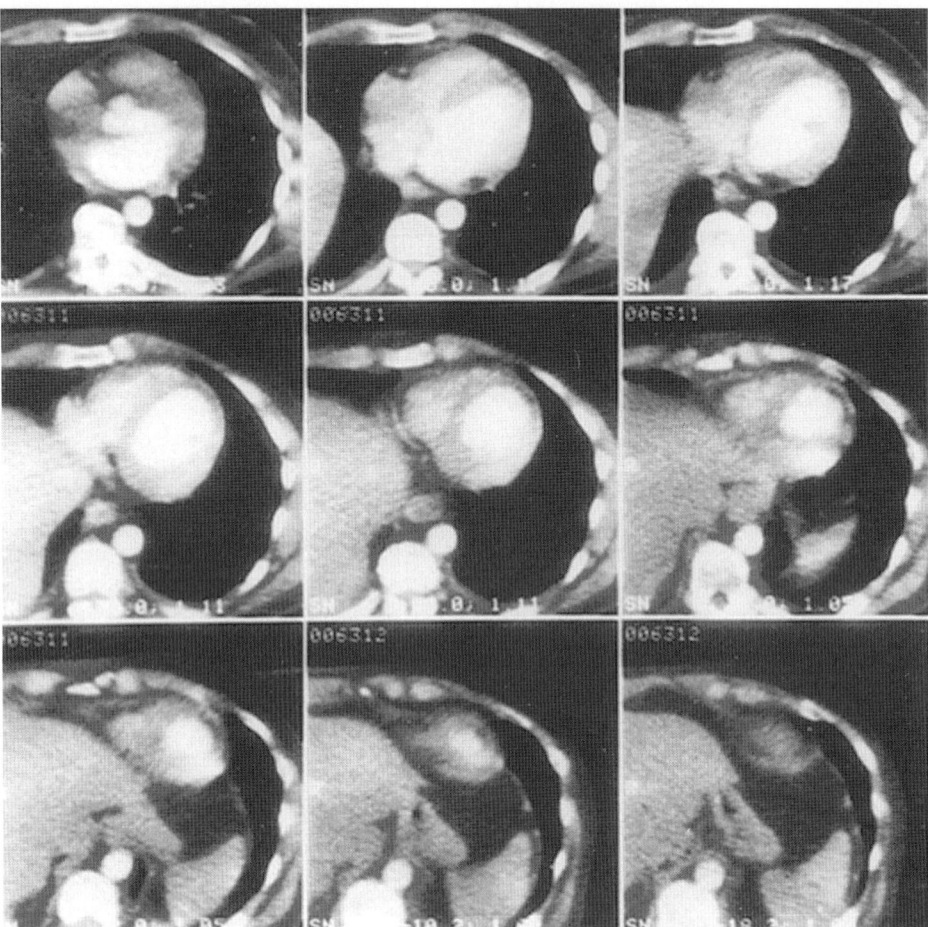

FIGURE 20–4. Fifty-millisecond contrast-enhanced EBCT images gated to end-diastole include the left ventricle from base (*top left*) to apex (*bottom right*). EBCT, electron-beam computed tomography. *Source: From Brundage BH, Chomka E. Evaluation of acute myocardial infarction by computed tomography. In: Brundage BH, ed. Comparative Cardiac Imaging. Rockville, MD: Aspen; 1990:223–229. Reproduced with permission from the publisher and the authors.*

timal opacification of the left heart and the coronaries (see Fig. 20–5 and Fig. 20–6, Fig. 20–7). Dense coronary calcification can interfere with the CT evaluation of the native coronary artery (Fig. 20–8). Hyperenhancement of the right ventricle with contrast could adversely affect the visualization of the RCA (Fig. 20–9). Our group typically uses a 65 to 80 mL bolus of contrast followed by a 50 mL mix of contrast and normal saline, usually in a ratio of 30:70, respectively, and then a 50 mL normal saline chaser. This protocol offers adequate opacification of the right ventricle and the interventricular septum for determination of RV function and LV mass.

Stress-rest EBCT imaging can detect underlying ischemic heart disease based on changes in global LVEF and regional wall motion. One small study compared semisupine bicycle exercise contrast-enhanced EBCT to technetium-99m (^{99m}Tc) single-photon emission computed tomography (SPECT) of the myocardium in patients with suspected CAD. Coronary angiography was used as the gold standard.[8] An abnormal EBCT study was defined as a <5 percent increase in LVEF during exercise. Regional LVEF was assessed by computer analysis of end-diastolic and end-systolic images. The sensitivity and specificity of exercise EBCT for detecting CAD were 81 and 76 percent, respectively, when the global LVEF

criteria for abnormalcy were used. However, these percentages improved to 88 and 100 percent when regional wall motion abnormalities were considered. EBCT was as accurate as ^{99m}Tc SPECT in the diagnosis of CAD.

When valvular surgery is considered, CT can delineate the important parameters of LV chamber size, wall thickness, and LVEF.[6,14] As with gated blood-pool radionuclide angiography, CT cannot clearly distinguish mitral from aortic regurgitation and cannot calculate the regurgitant fraction if significant right-sided valvular insufficiency is present (see CT Structure below).[6,14] Congestive heart failure or left atrial enlargement can be complicated by left atrial thrombi. One study showed greater accuracy of EBCT as compared to transthoracic echocardiography in demonstrating such thrombi[15] (see Fig. 20–7). Whether CT can detect thrombi as well as transesophageal echocardiography remains to be determined, as only limited studies are currently available. However, the superior spatial resolution of CT should allow visualization of thrombi with high accuracy.

For cardiac functional assessment, EBCT was shown to provide a highly accurate EF (±1 percent), with 50 msec image acquisition per image. Retrospective electrocardiographic gating allows for image reconstruction in any phase of the cardiac cycle.

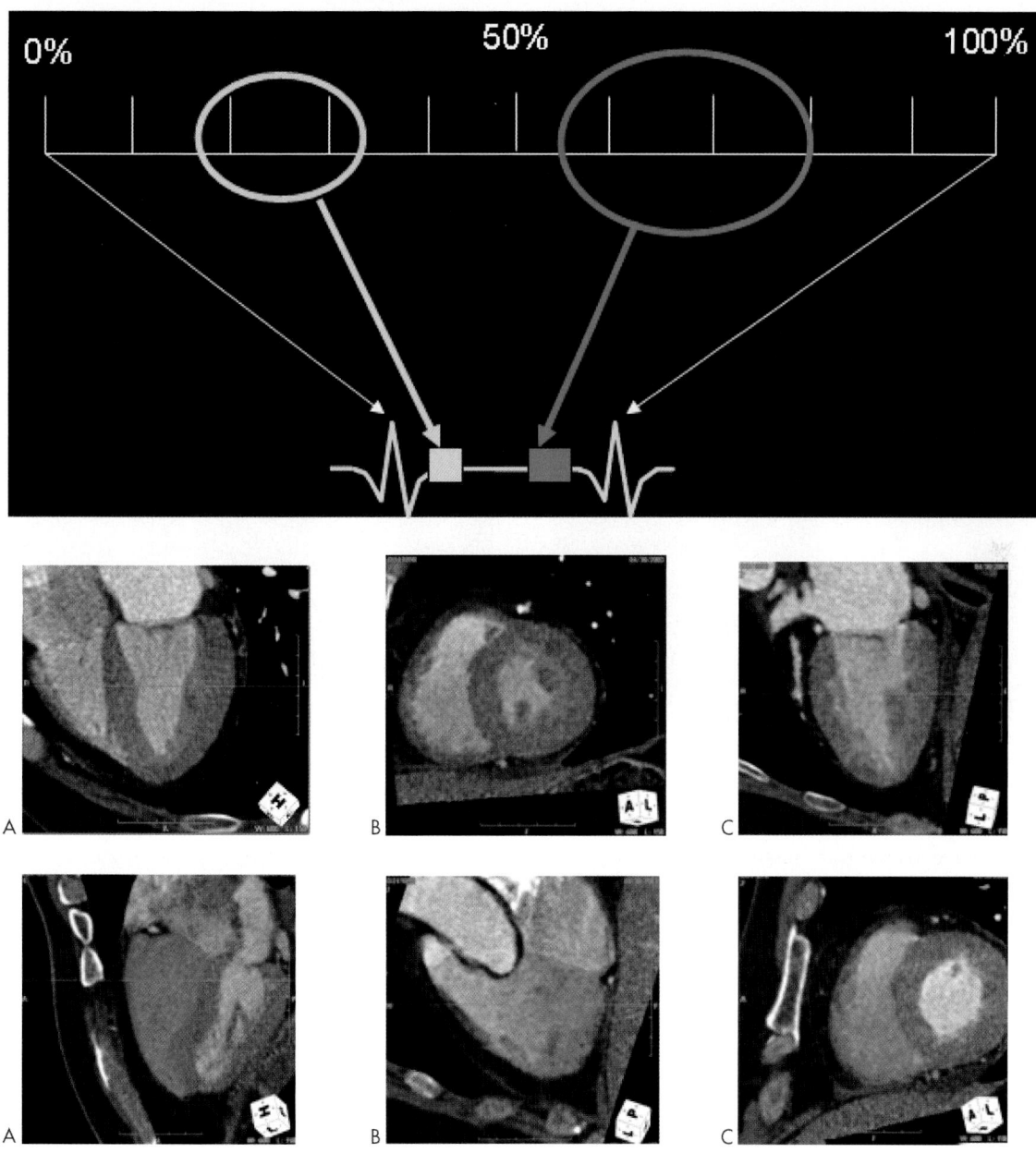

FIGURE 20–5. Evaluation of cardiac function. *Upper panel*: A diagram showing the division of the cardiac cycle into 10 percent intervals. The two ovals cover the two regions of the cardiac cycle where the motions are the most still. The *light blue oval* covers the mid- to end-systolic phase and the *red oval* covers the mid- to end-diastolic phase. *Middle panel*: Images generated by an automatic contrast and contour detection software for quantitative functional evaluation. The three views are four chamber (**A**), short axis (**B**), and 2 chamber (**C**) of the left ventricle. *Lower panel*: Images generated by the same software for RVEF calculation. The three views are four chamber (**A**), RV outflow (**B**), and short axis (**C**). RVEF, right ventricular ejection fraction.

Thus, end systolic and end diastolic images can be produced to assess ventricular volumes and function. Despite lower temporal resolution than EBCT, MDCT preserves the ability to assess EF. Functional parameters by MDCT have shown good agreement with findings on echocardiography, cineventriculography, SPECT and magnetic resonance imaging (MRI).[6] The technical development of scanner hardware along with multisegmental image reconstruction has led to rapid improvement in spatial and temporal resolution and significantly faster cardiac scans. Although the same data acquired for MDCT angiography can be used for evaluation of cardiac function, MDCT is not a first-line imaging tool for this application unless images from echocardiography are of poor quality or CMR is contraindicated. MDCT is limited by its radiation exposure, which can reach 15–20 mSv in 64-slice CT if current modulation is not used. There is limited data using a scan protocol with current modulation; however, one study showed a very good correlation of LV volumes and function between MDCT and CMR.[10] In addition, the results from MDCT were better than from echocardiography. Considering the contrast media load, radiation exposure and limited temporal resolution, MDCT solely for analysis of cardiac function parameters does not seem reasonable at the present time.

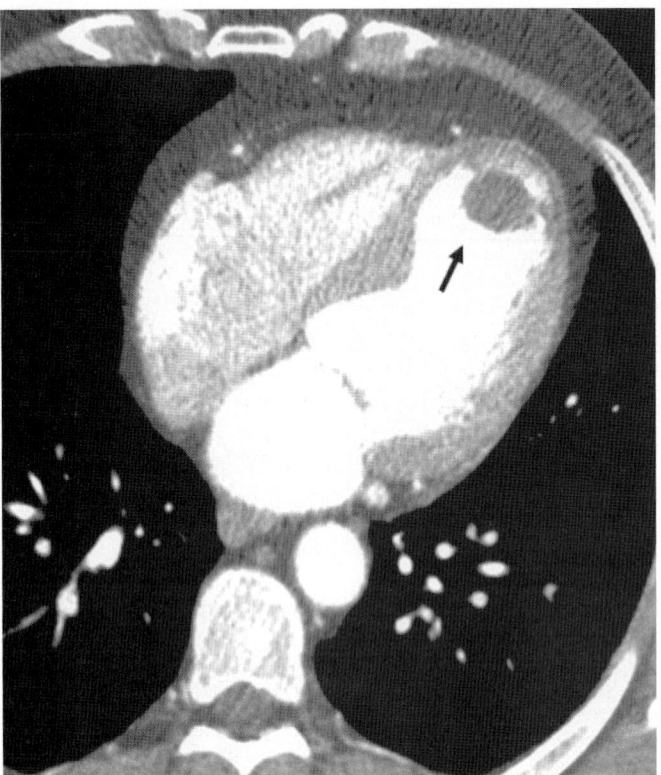

FIGURE 20–6. A single frame from a contrast-enhanced cine CT demonstrates thrombus in a left ventricular (LV) aneurysm. Also note that the wall of the aneurysm is calcified.

However, because the data is already obtained during a coronary evaluation, the combination of coronary artery imaging and assessment of cardiac function with MDCT frequently adds clinically useful information.

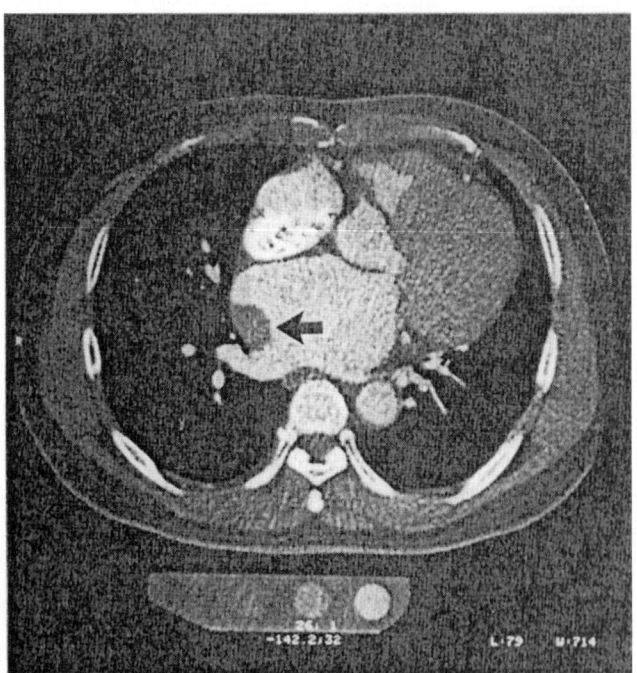

FIGURE 20–7. A left atrial thrombus (*arrow*) anterior to the right superior pulmonary vein is well described in this contrast-enhanced EBCT scan. The transthoracic echocardiogram did not detect any left atrial thrombus. EBCT, electron-beam computed tomography.

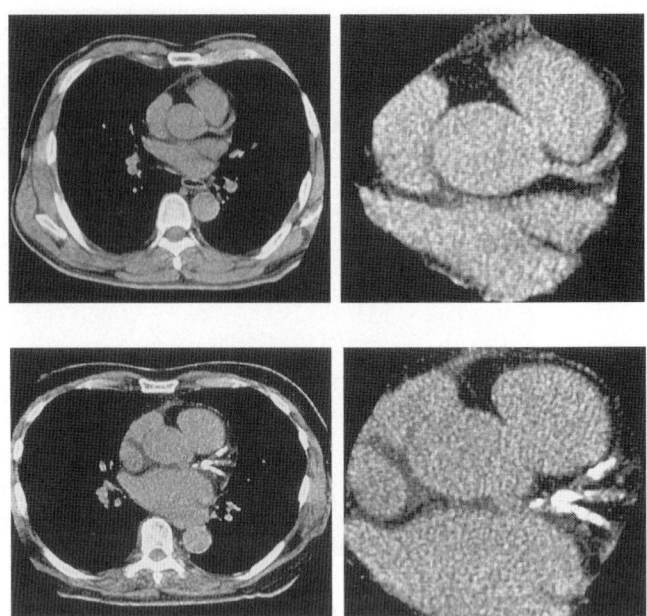

FIGURE 20–8. Single-level noncontrast EBCT scan of a normal subject (*left*) and an individual with severe CAC (*right*). Calcium is shown as intensely white areas within the coronary arteries. CAC, coronary artery calcification; EBCT, electron-beam computed tomography.

EVALUATION OF CORONARY ARTERY DISEASE

【 】 DETECTION OF CORONARY ARTERY CALCIFICATION

The standard EBCT imaging protocol is to acquire 40 consecutive 3-mm-thick images at a rate of 100 msec per image from the base of the heart to just below the carina. Images are obtained at end-inspiration, with ECG triggering typically at 80 percent of the R-R interval (end-diastole). Image pixel size using a 512×512 reconstruction matrix is 0.26 or 0.34 mm^2 based on a 26- or 30-cm field of vision, respectively.

A calcified lesion is generally defined as either two or three adjacent pixels (0.68 to 1.02 mm^2 for a 512^2 reconstruction matrix and camera field size of 30 cm) of >130 Hounsfield units (HUs). Using the traditional Agatston method, each calcified lesion is multiplied by a density factor as follows: 1 for lesions with a maximal density between 130 and 199 HU; 2 for lesions between 200 and 299 HU; 3 for lesions between 300 and 399 HU; and 4 for lesions >400 HU. The total coronary artery calcium score (CACS) is calculated as the sum of each calcified lesion in the four main coronary arteries over all the consecutive tomographic slices (see Fig. 20–8). The EBCT-derived CACS correlates well with calcified areas found in individual coronary arteries as determined by histomorphometric measurements ($r = 0.96$, $p < 0.0001$)[16] (see Fig. 20–9).

MDCT imaging protocols vary among different camera systems and manufacturers. Generally 40 consecutive 2.5- to 3-mm-thick images are acquired per cardiac study. Calcified lesions are defined as two or three adjacent pixels with a tomographic density of either >90 or >130 HU. Effective pixel size for a reconstruction matrix of 512×512 pixels with a common field of view of 26 cm is 0.26 mm^2. Calcium scoring is usually based on the traditional

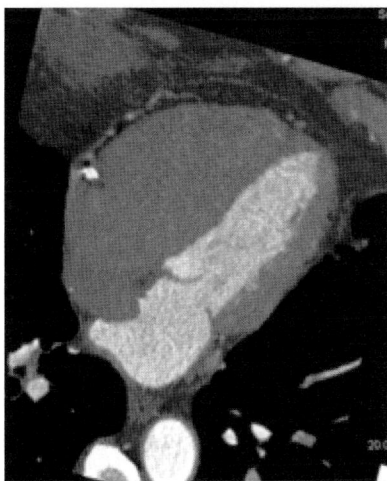

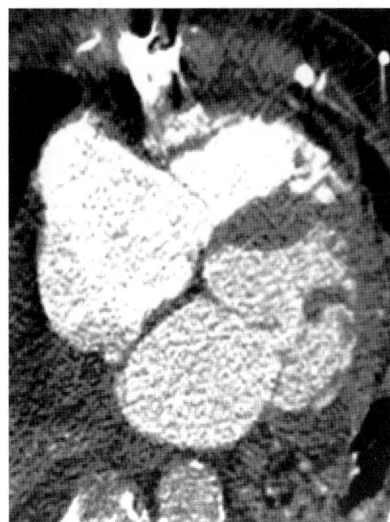

FIGURE 20–9. Evaluation of the RV function. *Upper panel*: MPR image of a four-chamber view of a heart. The study was performed with normal saline chaser. No-contrast enhancement is noted in the right ventricle allowing optimal evaluation of the RCA, intracardiac shunts, and atrial septal aneurysm (as shown in this case). *Lower panel*: MPR image of a four-chamber view of a heart. This study was performed without saline chaser and the timing of the study was suboptimal for the assessment of the left heart and coronary arteries. Over enhancement of the right ventricle with contrast leads to difficult in the assessment of the RCA. There is also significant beam hardening artifact from the sternal wire. MPR, maximum pulse rate; RCA, right coronary artery; RV, right ventricular.

Agatston method (i.e., initial density of >130 HU). As with EBCT scoring, the total CACS is calculated as the sum of each calcified plaque over all the tomographic slices.

MULTIROW DETECTOR COMPUTED TOMOGRAPHY COMPARED TO ELECTRON BEAM COMPUTED TOMOGRAPHY

The comparability of MDCT- and EBCT-derived coronary artery calcium scores has been explored in separate studies involving approximately 400 patients.[17–19] The MDCT protocols vary considerably in these studies, ranging from conventional CT to single-slice CT (with either retrospective or prospective gating) to multislice CT (Table 20–1). EBCT imaging was performed using the stan-

dard protocol conventionally used in routine clinical practice. Coronary calcification was defined as >130 HU for EBCT but varied from 90 to 130 HU for MDCT. Although high correlation coefficients were reported between EBCT and MDCT CACS, there was significant variability in individual CACS results (range 17 to 84 percent) (see Table 20–1).

A more recent study by Knez and coworkers compared MDCT to EBCT using prospective ECG gating for both techniques.[19] The CACS was calculated using the volumetric (rather than the Agatston) calcium scoring method. Variability in CACS between the two techniques ranged from 20 percent (CACS <100) to 15 percent (CACS >100), with a mean variability of 17 percent. Further research is still needed to determine which MDCT technique, imaging protocol, calcium criterion, and scoring system best approximates the values determined by EBCT, especially with the new 64-detector systems. No calcium data is yet available from these state-of-the art scanners.

CORONARY ARTERY CALCIFICATION AND ATHEROSCLEROTIC PLAQUE BURDEN

The presence of CAC is clearly indicative of coronary atherosclerosis.[25,26] Furthermore, the CACS severity, as assessed by EBCT, is directly related to the total atherosclerotic plaque burden present in the epicardial coronary arteries.[25,26] Coronary calcification is thought to begin early in life, but it progresses more rapidly in older individuals who have further advanced atherosclerotic lesions.[27] Calcification is an active, organized, and regulated process occurring during atherosclerotic plaque development where calcium phosphate in the form of hydroxyapatite precipitates in atherosclerotic coronary arteries in a similar fashion as observed in bone mineralization.[28–30] Although lack of calcification does not categorically exclude the presence of atherosclerotic plaque, calcification occurs exclusively in atherosclerotic arteries and is not found in normal coronary arteries.

The presence and extent of histologically determined plaque area has been compared to the total calcium area as assessed by EBCT in individual coronary arteries derived from autopsied hearts.[25] A strong linear correlation exists between total coronary artery plaque area and the extent of CAC as found in individual hearts ($r = 0.93$, $p < 0.001$) and in individual coronary arteries ($r = 0.90$, $p < 0.001$) (Fig. 20–10). However, the total calcium area underestimates total plaque area, with approximately five times as many noncalcified as calcified plaques.[25]

CORONARY ARTERY CALCIFICATION AND STENOSIS SEVERITY

Significant (>50 percent) coronary artery stenosis by angiography is almost universally associated with the presence of coronary artery calcium as assessed by EBCT. However, the severity of angiographic coronary artery stenosis is not directly related to the total CACS. A recent study compared calcium extent to coronary artery luminal diameter stenosis determined by morphologic examination of 723 coronary artery segments.[26] Although coronary stenosis severity increased with increasing CAC, this relationship was poor and could not be used to estimate angiographic stenosis severity on a segment-by-segment basis (Fig. 20–11). One expla-

TABLE 20–1

EBCT versus Mechanical CT[a]

AUTHOR	YEAR	NUMBER OF PATIENTS	AGE	AVERAGE CA²⁺ SCORE	MECHANICAL CT TECHNIQUE	GATING	NUMBER OF DETECTORS	CORRELATION COEFFICIENT	MEAN % DIFFERENCE
Becker[20]	1999	50	61	983	Nonspiral	No	Single	0.98	42%
Budoff[17]	2001	33	54	52	Nonspiral	No	Single	0.68	84%
Becker[21]	2000	50	62	—	Nonspiral	Prosp	Single	0.98	25%
Carr[22]	2000	36	68	432	Spiral	Retrosp	Single	0.96	17%
Goldin[23]	2001	70	48	70	Spiral	Retrosp	Single	NA	28%
Becker[24]	2001	88	63	793	Spiral	Prosp	4	0.99	32%
Knez[19b]	2002	99	60	722	Spiral	Prosp	4	0.99	17%

Ca²⁺, calcium; CT, computed tomography; EBCT, electron-beam computed tomography; prosp, prospective; retrosp, retrospective.
[a]Agatston score except as indicated.
[b]Volumetric score.

nation is that coronary artery remodeling occurs with increasing plaque burden so as to maintain luminal diameter and arterial patency.[31] Although the extent of coronary calcification does not precisely predict stenosis severity, noncalcified plaques are almost universally associated with <50 percent diameter stenosis and typically <20 percent stenosis.[26] These data indicate that lack of coronary calcification predicts a very low likelihood of obstructive CAD.

Clinical angiographic trials confirm the relationship between CACS severity and the presence of significant (≥50 percent) CAD.[32–41] Although the diagnostic accuracy of EBCT improves with age, most patients younger than 50 years with obstructive CAD also have coronary calcification (85 percent).[33,35] To date there are 15 studies evaluating EBCT with coronary angiography in which obstructive CAD was defined as >50 percent luminal diameter stenosis[32–41] (Table 20–2). In these studies, the overall sensitivity and specificity for detecting obstructive CAD were 97 and 39 percent, respectively. In the largest series, Haberl and colleagues performed EBCT within 30 days of coronary angiography in 1764 patients who had suspected CAD.[41] Only 5 of 940 patients (0.5 percent) with significant (≥50 percent) coronary artery stenosis had a normal EBCT, and four of these were younger than 45 years of age. Although differences in CACS were noted among men and women, EBCT predicted CAD equally well in both genders, based on age-specific CACS thresholds[41] (Fig. 20–12). Coronary artery calcification (CAC) assessment may also be useful for detecting CAD in heart transplant recipients.[47]

The poor specificity of coronary calcium scanning can be reconciled by the fact that the coronary calcification confirms the presence of atherosclerotic plaque but it may not necessarily be obstructive (Fig. 20–13). The CACS severity may be a better barometer of obstructive CAD than the mere presence of calcium. Budoff and coworkers observed that specificity increased with the number of calcified coronary arteries (i.e., high calcium scores).[33] Two separate reports in patients referred for coronary angiography found that a CACS >100 best predicted obstructive CAD with an equally high sensitivity and specificity of 80 percent.[48,49] There appears to be a threshold CACS above which most patients will have significant coronary artery stenosis. The accuracy for identifying significant CAD based on CACS may be further improved by incorporating age, gender,[39,41,50] and traditional risk-factor information[49,51] (Fig. 20–14). However, despite the rela-

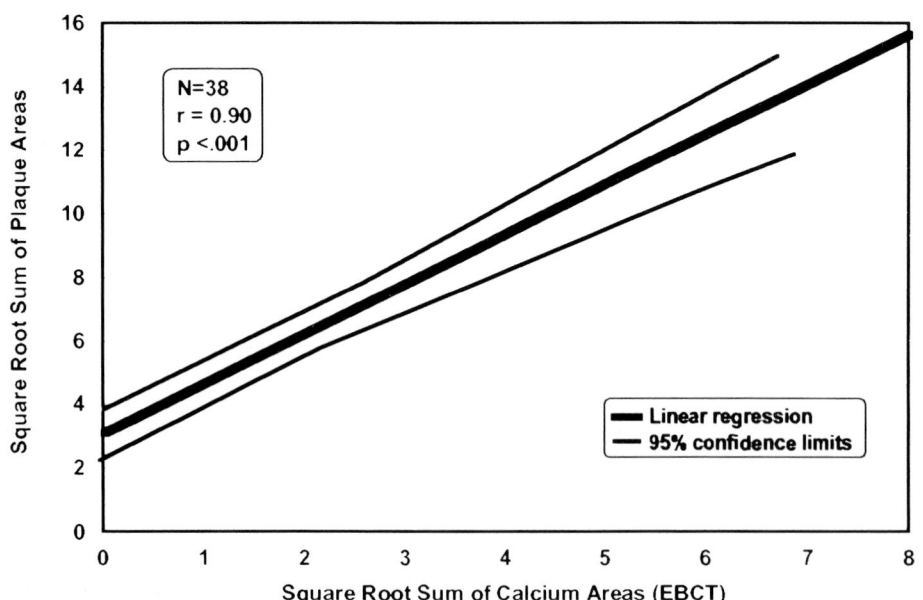

FIGURE 20-10. Comparison of the square root sum of total coronary calcium area (mm) by EBCT to actual atherosclerotic plaque area (mm) for 38 individual coronary arteries. The linear regression line and 95 percent confidence intervals are shown. EBCT, electron-beam computed tomography. *Source: From Rumberger JA, Simons DB, Fitzpatrick LA, et al.*[25]

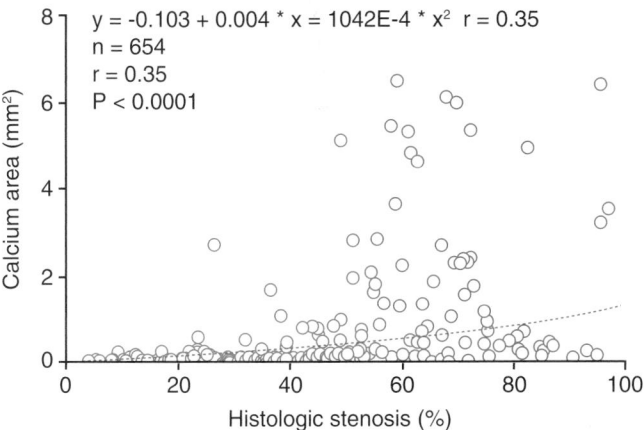

$$y = -0.103 + 0.004 * x = 1042E-4 * x^2 \quad r = 0.35$$

n = 654
r = 0.35
P < 0.0001

FIGURE 20–11. Graph showing the polynomial regression analysis of coronary calcium area (mm²) versus percent histologic stenosis for 654 coronary artery segments with calcium >0 mm². *Source: From Sangiorgi G, Rumberger JA, Severson A, et al.[26] Reproduced with permission from the publisher and authors.*

CORONARY ARTERY CALCIFICATION AND MYOCARDIAL ISCHEMIA

A recent trial explored the complementary role of EBCT and myocardial perfusion SPECT for identifying both subclinical CAD and silent myocardial ischemia in a generally asymptomatic population who had risk factors for CAD development.[52] The purpose of this study was to identify patients with subclinical CAD who might benefit from aggressive risk factor modification and are at relatively higher short-term risk for cardiac events based on the presence of silent myocardial ischemia. Among the 3895 subjects who had EBCT, 411 also underwent stress SPECT within a close temporal period (median 17 days). The mean CACS was significantly higher in the 81 subjects (20 percent) who had an abnormal (1065 ± 983) as compared to a normal (286 ± 394, *p* < 0.00001) SPECT. The likelihood of an abnormal SPECT increased dramatically with the total CACS (Fig. 20–15). Although only 1 percent of subjects with a total CACS <100 had an abnormal SPECT, this was observed in 46 percent of those with scores ≥400. Only 10 percent of all 3895 subjects scanned with EBCT had a CACS ≥400. Large ischemic perfusion defects were virtually confined to subjects who had a CACS score of 400 or higher. Patients with large ischemic perfusion defects by SPECT are known to be at high risk for subsequent cardiac events; whereas patients with small perfusion defects or those with normal scans, have an exceedingly low cardiac event rate.[53–56] Although a similar percentage of subjects had an abnormal SPECT (16.1 percent) or stress ECG (17.5 percent, *p* = NS) only the former was related to the total CACS (Fig. 20–16), further illustrating the limited predictive accuracy of treadmill ECG testing for detecting CAD in asymptomatic subjects. (Fig. 20–17 to Fig. 20–19).

tionship between obstructive CAD and CACS severity, the latter is still too imprecise in itself to be used as a definitive criterion for proceeding directly to coronary angiography. The current American College of Cardiology/American Heart Association (ACC/AHA) guidelines on coronary angiography do not recommend coronary angiography on the basis of a positive EBCT but do suggest angiography may be avoided with the finding of a negative (zero score) study.

TABLE 20–2

Accuracy of EBCT Coronary Artery Calcification in Detecting Significant (>50%) Coronary Artery Stenosis as Defined by Angiography

INVESTIGATOR	YEAR	NUMBER OF SUBJECTS	SENSITIVITY (%)	SPECIFICITY (%)	POSITIVE PREDICTIVE ACCURACY	NEGATIVE PREDICTIVE ACCURACY
Agatston[32]	1990	584	96	51	31	98
Breen[42]	1992	100	100	47	63	100
Bielak[43]	1994	160	96	45	57	93
Kaufman[44]	1995	160	93	67	81	86
Rumberger[45]	1995	139	98	39	59	97
Braun[46]	1996	102	93	73	93	73
Budoff[33]	1996	710	95	44	72	84
Detrano[34]	1996	491	95	31	51	89
Fallavollita[35]	1996	106	85	45	66	70
Baumgart[36]	1997	57	97	21	56	86
Schmermund[37]	1997	118	95	88	99	58
Kennedy[38]	1998	368	96	31	51	90
Bielak[39]	2000	213	99	39	64	98
Shavelle[40]	2000	97	96	47	80	82
Haberl[41]	2001	1764	99	30	62	98
Total		5169	97	39	61	92

EBCT, electron-beam computed tomography.

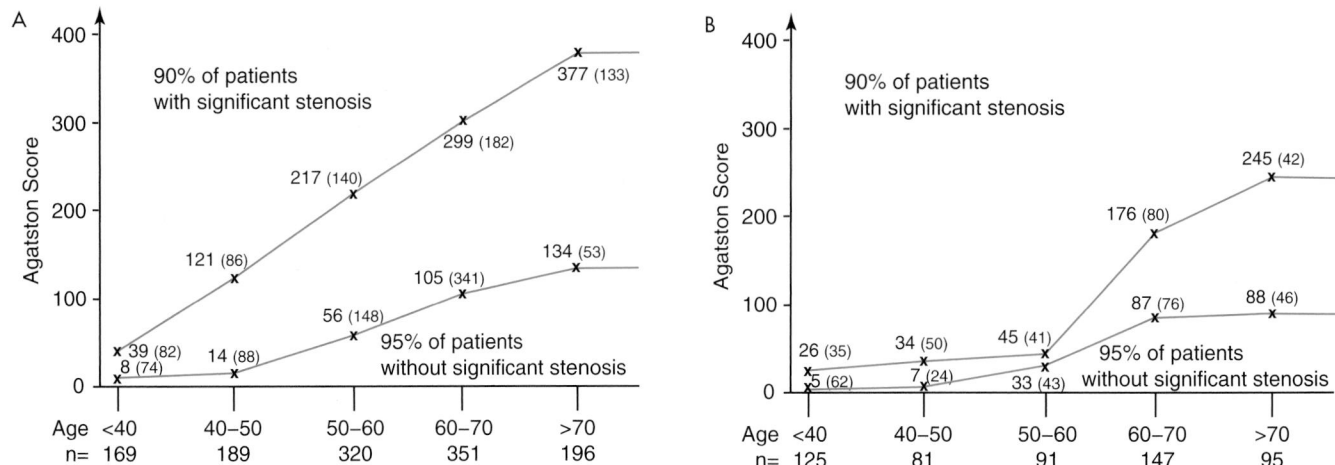

FIGURE 20-12. Diagnostic yield of calcium screening in symptomatic men (**A**) and women (**B**). The lower scores define the calcium score thresholds for the 95 percent of patients without significant stenoses. The higher scores give the calcium score thresholds for the 90 percent of patients with significant stenoses. Within the central area the diagnosis is uncertain. The numbers in parentheses give the number of patients within the area. For example, a man at the age of 50 years is probably free of coronary stenosis if his score is <56. At score values ≥217, he bears a high risk of stenosis. *Source: From Haberl R, Becker A, Leber A, et al.[41] Reproduced with permission from the publisher and the authors.*

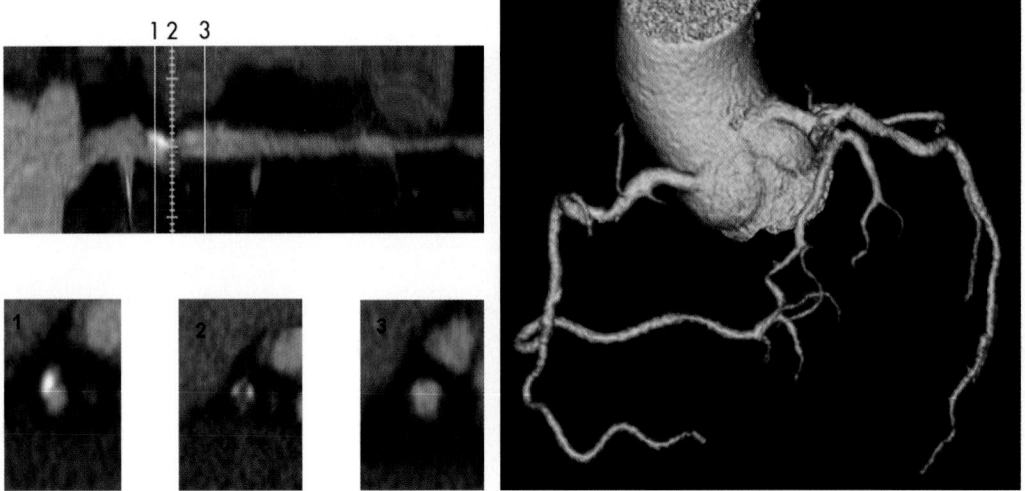

FIGURE 20-13. Four noncontrast EBCT images of a patient demonstrating calcification in all 3 major coronary arteries (*left*). Circles define regions of coronary calcification. The total CACS is moderate at 271 and highest in the RCA (176). Coronary arteriogram demonstrates a nonobstructive plaque in the mid–RCA (*right*). The LAD and LCX coronary arteries were normal. The patient also had a normal exercise myocardial perfusion scan. EBCT, electron-beam computed tomography; LAD, left anterior descending; LCX, left circumflex; RCA, right coronary artery.

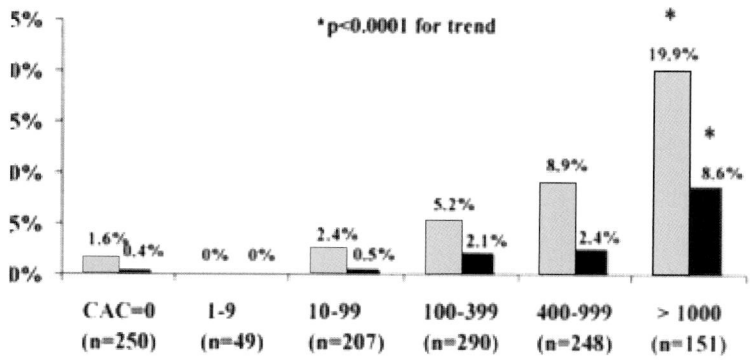

FIGURE 20–14. Single photon emission computed tomography (SPECT) results based on total coronary artery calcium score (CACS). Increasing calcium scores were associated with a higher likelihood of abnormal SPECT Scan (white bars represent >5 percent ischemic segment; black bars represent >10 percent ischemia present). *Source: From He et al.[62] Reproduced with permission from the publisher and authors.*

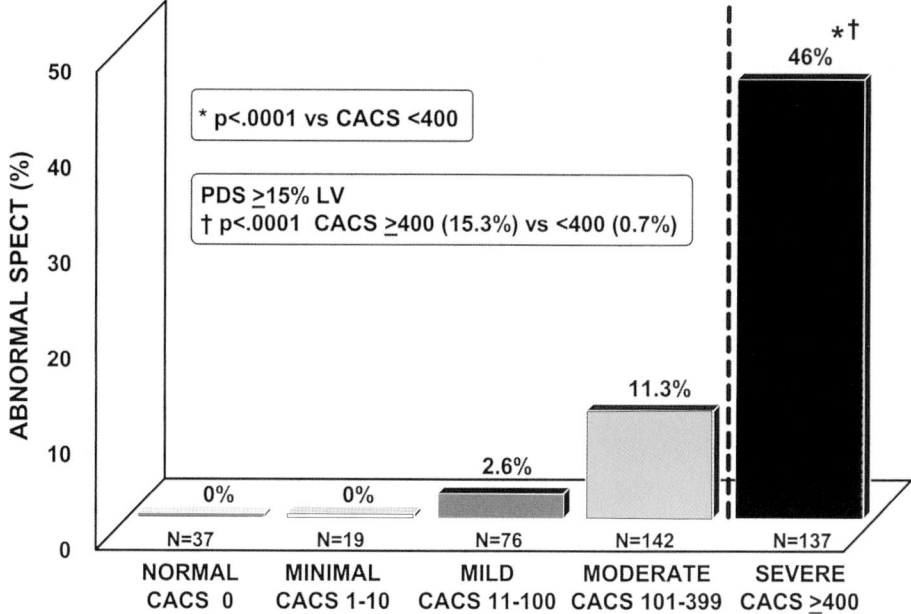

FIGURE 20–15. Single-photon emission computed tomography (SPECT) results based on total coronary artery calcium score (CACS). Few subjects with CACS <400 had abnormal SPECT (6.6 percent) and most (99.3 percent) had only a small (<15 percent) perfusion defect size (PDS). LV, left ventricle. *Source: From He ZX, Hedrick TD, Pratt CM, et al.[52] Reproduced with permission from the publisher and authors.*

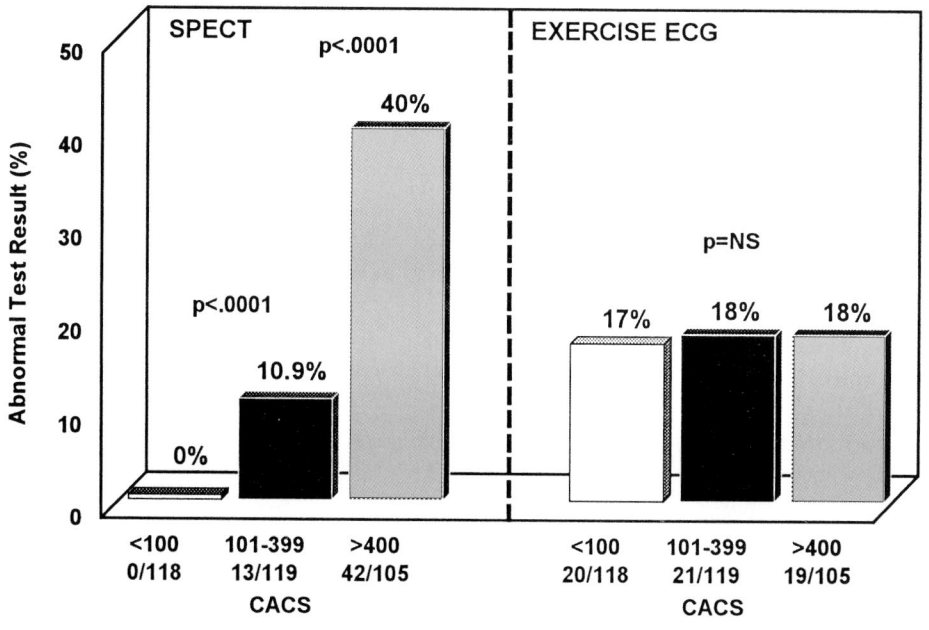

FIGURE 20–16. The frequency of an ischemic myocardial perfusion single photon emission computed tomography (>5 percent ischemic) (stippled bars) and of a moderate to severe ischemia (>10 percent ischemic) (black bars) for patients divided into six coronary artery calcium (CAC) score groupings. *Source: From He ZX, Hedrick TD, Pratt CM, et al.[52] Reproduced with permission of the publisher.*

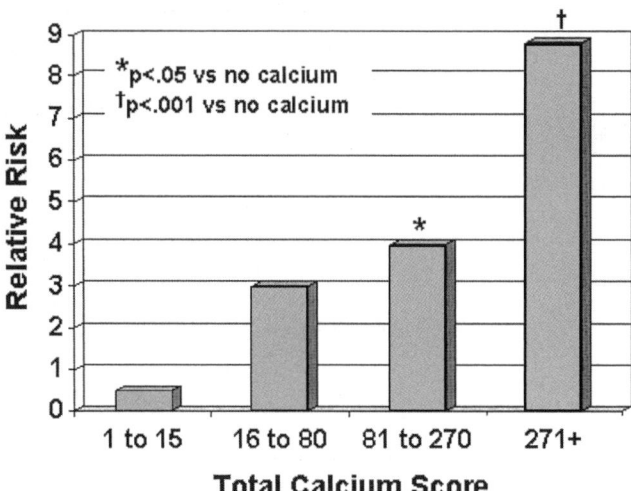

FIGURE 20–17. Relative risks for total cardiovascular events in patients at various total calcium score quartiles versus those without calcium, adjusting for age, gender, hypertension, hyperlipidemia, smoking history, and diabetes. *Source: Redrawn from Wong ND, Hsu JC, Detrano RC, et al.[70]*

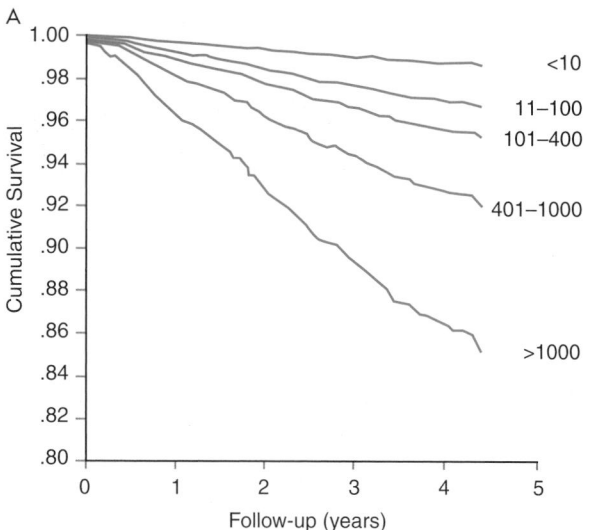

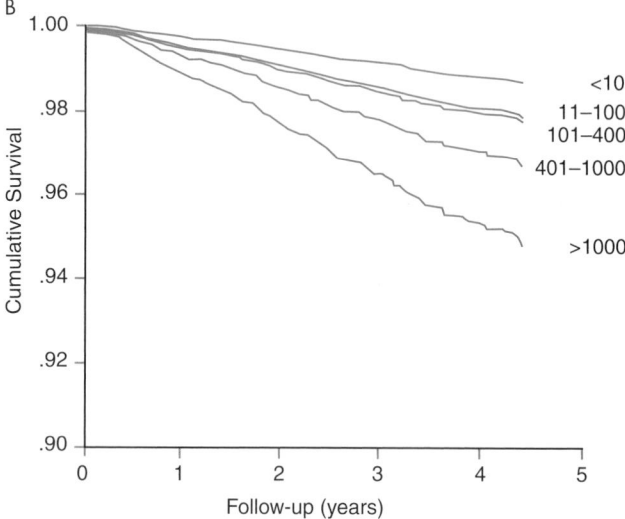

FIGURE 20–18. Risk factor–unadjusted (**A**) and risk factor–adjusted (**B**) cumulative survival curves in 10,377 asymptomatic individuals based on EBCT-derived coronary artery calcium score results. EBCT, electron-beam computed tomography. *Source: Shaw LJ, Raggi P, Schisterman E, et al.[75] Reproduced with permission from the publisher and the authors.*

A recent study of 1195 patients who underwent CAC measurement with EBCT and myocardial perfusion SPECT (MPS) assessment demonstrated that CAC was often present in the absence of myocardial perfusion SPECT abnormalities (normal nuclear test), and that <2 percent of all patients with CAC <100 had positive MPS studies.[57] This is supported by the other published reports and is synthesized in a recent appropriateness guideline from the American Society of Nuclear Cardiology (ASNC) and the ACC.[58] Because calcified plaque may be present in nonobstructive lesions, the presence of CAC in asymptomatic persons does not provide rationale for revascularization but rather risk factor modification and possible further functional assessment. Clinicians must understand a positive calcium scan indicates atherosclerosis, but most often, no significant stenosis. The absence of coronary calcium is most often associated with a normal nuclear test and no obstructive disease on angiography. The ACC/ASNC appropriateness criteria suggest that a low score precludes the need for MPS assessment, and a high score would warrant further assessment. A person with an Agatston score >400 may benefit from functional testing to detect occult ischemia.

Detection of Subclinical CAD and Stress Testing

Noninvasive techniques, such as exercise treadmill testing and myocardial perfusion imaging, can identify patients with coronary atherosclerosis. However, unlike EBCT, which can detect coronary atherosclerosis at its earliest stages, these techniques can identify only patients with advanced CAD who manifest myocardial ischemia. Although the presence and extent of ischemia can accurately identify asymptomatic individuals at high risk for cardiac events[53,54,59] (Fig. 20–20), the very low prevalence of a positive test result (<5 percent) precludes the use of these methodologies as primary screening tests for the early detection and treatment of CAD.

Coronary Artery Calcification and Ischemic Burden

Recent studies emphasize the effectiveness of selectively combining stress myocardial perfusion imaging with EBCT in the anticipated small (10 percent) number of asymptomatic subjects who will have a high (≥400) CACS so as to specifically identify those with silent myocardial ischemia[52,58] (Fig. 20–21). This testing strategy may prove to be optimal based on the known prognostic value of perfusion imaging and the superior sensitivity of EBCT over the former for detecting preclinical CAD. Appropriateness criteria for nuclear testing considers a calcium score >400 in an asymptomatic person to be a generally appropriate indication for MPS testing.[58]

【 】 CORONARY ARTERY CALCIFICATION: PROGNOSTIC IMPLICATIONS

The likelihood of plaque rupture and the development of acute cardiovascular events is related to the total atherosclerotic plaque

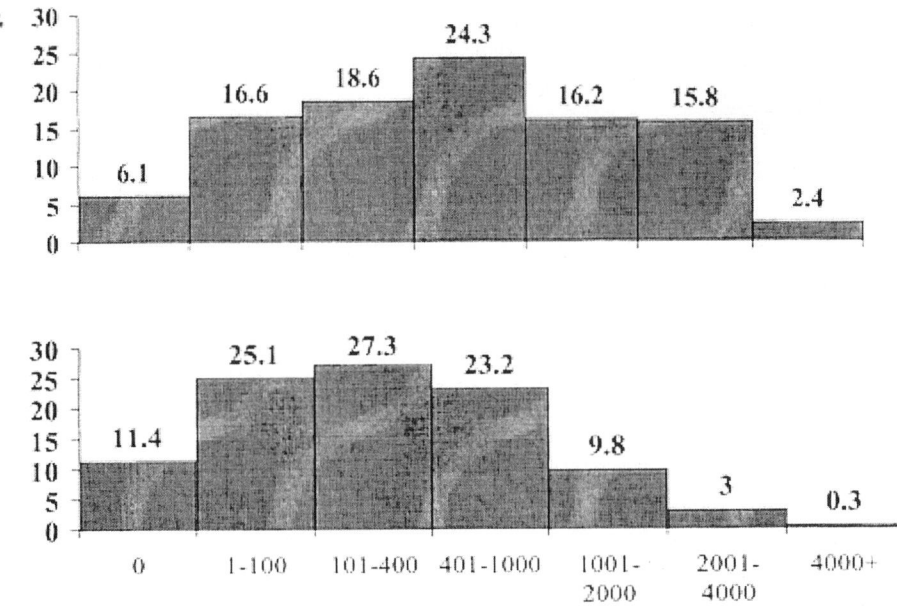

Coronary Artery Calcification Score

FIGURE 20–19. Distribution of the coronary artery calcification (CAC) score in elderly men (*top*) and women (*bottom*). *Source: From Newman AB, Naydeck BL, Sutton-Tyrrell K, et al.[86] Reproduced with permission from the publisher and the authors.*

burden.[60–62] Although controversy exists as to whether calcified or noncalcified plaques are more prone to rupture,[63,64] extensive calcification indicates the presence of both plaque morphologies.[25,26] There is a direct relationship between the CACS severity, the extent of atherosclerotic plaque, and the presence of silent myocar-

dial ischemia. Many studies have now demonstrated an increased risk for cardiac events in asymptomatic patients who have extensive silent myocardial ischemia.[53,54,59,65] Therefore, the CACS could be useful for risk assessment of asymptomatic individuals and potentially guide therapeutics.

Several recent trials in both symptomatic[66,67] and asymptomatic[68–73] patients have studied whether the extent of CAC as assessed by EBCT can predict subsequent patient outcome. In 422 symptomatic patients followed for 30 ± 12 months[66] cardiac events were 10-fold higher in patients with a CACS above the 75th percentile for age (9.5 percent) versus those below the 25th percentile (0.9 percent). Another study of 288 symptomatic patients referred for coronary angiography[67] showed that patients with a CACS >100 had a 3.2-fold higher relative risk of death or MI than those with a lower CACS (95 percent confidence limit: 1.17–8.71).

In the longest study of EBCT scanning of the coronary arteries, the South Bay Heart Watch study, 1196 asymptomatic patients were followed (median = 7.0 years) and it was demonstrated that the CACS score added predictive power beyond that of standard coronary risk factors and C reactive protein.[68]

Among 1173 asymptomatic patients followed for 3.6 years after an initial screening EBCT,[69] no events occurred in patients with a normal study and the negative predictive value was 99.8 percent in patients with a CACS <100. These results show a 5, 7, and 13 percent hard cardiac event rate in individuals with a CACS ≥80, ≥160, and ≥600, respectively.[69] The CACS remained the best single predictor of risk after adjustment (Table 20–3). Wong and colleagues also showed that the CACS severity predicted subsequent events independent of age, gender, and patient risk-factor profile[70] (see Fig. 20–17).

Raggi and coworkers reported on 172 patients who had EBCT within 60 days of an unheralded MI and on 632 asymptomatic patients who were referred for a screening EBCT and then followed for 32 ± 7 months.[71] Ninety-six percent of all patients with infarction were abnormal by EBCT, and the CACS was ≥100 in 62 percent and ≥400 in 47 percent of patients. Both the absolute CACS and the relative CACS percentiles adjusted

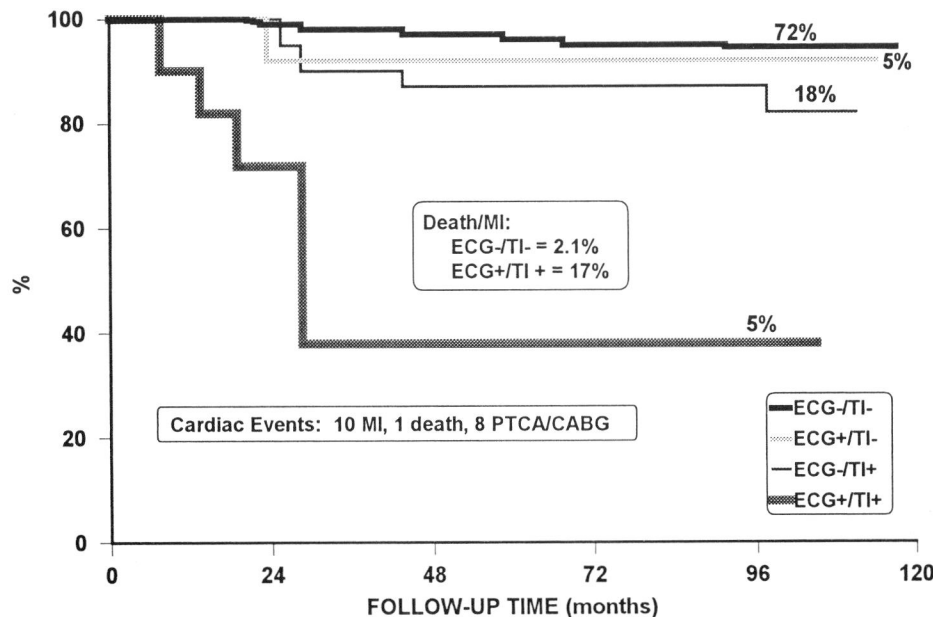

FIGURE 20–20. Kaplan-Meier survival curves based on exercise ECG and thallium-201 (²⁰¹Tl) scan results. The highest event rate is observed in patients with ischemia (+) by both tests. The percentage of patients with each test combination are shown above the curves. CABG, coronary artery bypass grafting; MI, myocardial infarction; PTCA, percutaneous transluminal coronary angioplasty. *Source: From Blumenthal RS, Becker DM, Moy TF, et al.[53] Reproduced with permission from the publisher and the authors.*

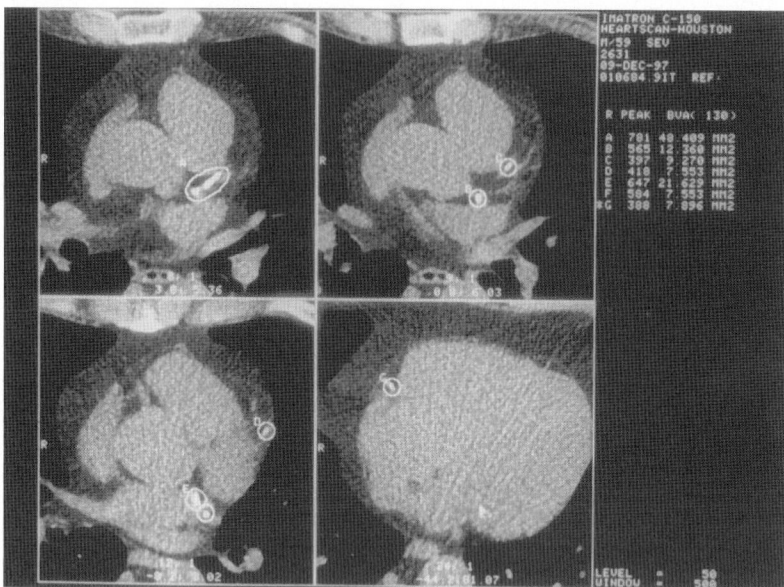

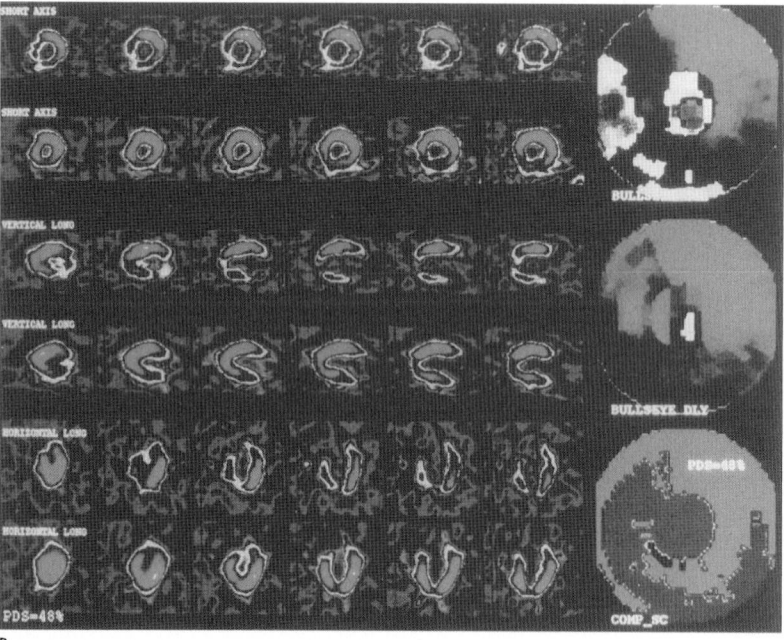

FIGURE 20–21. EBCT (**A**) and SPECT (**B**) images of asymptomatic subject who had a high-risk CACS of 937. Circles define regions of coronary calcification. The treadmill test was terminated at 9.0 min because of patient fatigue. SPECT demonstrated a large, reversible 48 percent perfusion defect within the distribution of all three major coronary arteries (COMP-SC) (**B**). This patient had severe three-vessel disease on angiography and underwent CABG. CACS, coronary artery calcium score; EBCT, electron-beam computed tomography; PDS, perfusion defect size; SPECT, single-photon emission computed tomography. *Source: From He ZX, Hedrick TD, Pratt CM, et al.[52] Reproduced with permission from the publisher and authors.*

for age and gender predicted subsequent death and nonfatal MI. Hard cardiac events occurred in only 0.3 percent of subjects with a normal EBCT, but this increased to 13 percent in those with a CACS >400. A very high CACS ≥1000 may portend a particularly high risk of death or MI (i.e., 25 percent per year).[72]

Larger trials have been reported, demonstrating approximately 10-fold increased risk with the presence of CAC.[73, 74] In one of the largest observational trials to date, Shaw and colleagues re-

ported all-cause mortality among 10,377 asymptomatic patients (4191 women and 6186 men) who had a baseline EBCT and were then followed for 5.0 ± 3.5 years.[75] Most subjects had cardiac risk factors including a family history of CAD (69 percent), hyperlipidemia (62 percent), hypertension (44 percent), and current cigarette smoking (40 percent). The CACS was a strong independent predictor of mortality (x^2 = 36.6, $p < 0.00001$) with 43 percent additional predictive value contained within the CACS beyond risk factors alone. Mortality significantly increased with increasing CACS (see Fig. 20–18).

Similarly, in a younger cohort of asymptomatic persons[76] the 3 year mean follow up in 2000 participants (mean age 43 years) showed that coronary calcium was associated with an 11.8-fold increased risk for incident coronary heart disease (CHD) ($p < 0.002$) in a Cox model controlling for the Framingham risk score. The Rotterdam Heart Study[77] investigated 1795 asymptomatic participants (mean age 71 years) who had CAC and measured risk factors. During a mean follow up of 3.3 years, the multivariate-adjusted relative risk of coronary events was 3.1 (95 percent CI, 1.2–7.9) for calcium scores of 101 to 400, 4.6 (95 percent CI, 1.8–11.8) for calcium scores of 401 to 1000, and 8.3 (95 percent CI, 3.3–21.1) for calcium scores >1000 compared with calcium scores of 0 to 100.

The Cooper Clinic Study[78] included 10,746 adults who were 22 to 96 years of age and free of known CHD. During a mean follow up of 3.5 years, 81 hard events (CHD death, nonfatal MI) occurred. Age-adjusted rates (per 1000 person-years) of hard events were computed according to four CAC categories: no detectable CAC and incremental sex-specific thirds of detectable CAC; these rates were, respectively, 0.4, 1.5, 4.8, and 8.7 (trend $p < 0.0001$) for men and 0.7, 2.3, 3.1, and 6.3 (trend $p < 0.02$) for women. The association between CAC and CHD events remained significant after adjustment for CHD risk factors. A Munich Study determined the extent of CAC by MDCT in 924 patients (443 men, 481 women, aged 59.4 ± 18.7 years).[79] During the 3-year follow-up period, the event rates for coronary revascularization (5.4 %/y vs. 2.9 %/y), MI (3.8 %/y vs. 1.8 %/y), and cardiac death (2.1 %/y vs. 1.0 %/y) in patients with volume scores above the 75th percentile were significantly higher compared to the total study group and no cardiovascular events occurred in patients with scores of zero. Receiver operating characteristic (ROC) analysis demonstrated it outperformed both PROCAM and Framingham models ($p < 0.0001$), where 36 percent and 34 percent of MIs occurred in the high risk cohorts, respectively.

A study demonstrated the risk stratification in uncomplicated type 2 diabetes in a prospective evaluation of CAC and MPS.[80] Risk factors and CAC scores were prospectively measured in 510 asymptomatic type 2 diabetic subjects (mean age 53 ± 8 years, 61 percent males) without prior cardiovascular disease with a median

TABLE 20–3

Multivariate Analyses of the Association of Coronary Artery Calcium Scores and Self-Reported Traditional Coronary Disease Risk Factors with All Events[a]

	VARIABLE	ODDS RATIO (95% CI)
Independent of EBC	Elevated cholesterol	3.9 (1.3–11.7)
	Hypertension	2.8 (1.2–6.5)
	Diabetes	5.4 (2.0–14.9)
With EBCT CACS ≥80	CACS >80	14.3 (4.9–42.3)
	Age >55 y	3.3 (1.3–8.4)
	Elevated cholesterol	4.0 (1.3–12.2)
	Hypertension	2.6 (1.1–6.1)
	Diabetes	4.8 (1.6–13.9)
With EBCT CACS ≥160	CACS >160	19.7 (6.9–56.4)
	Age >55 y	4.5 (1.6–12.2)
	Elevated cholesterol	3.7 (1.2–11.5)
	Hypertension	3.0 (1.2–7.4)
	Diabetes	5.8 (2.1–19.7)
With EBCT CACS ≥600	CACS >600	20.2 (7.3–55.8)
	Age >55 y	2.9 (1.1–7.9)
	Elevated cholesterol	3.5 (1.1–10.8)
	Hypertension	2.9 (1.2–7.3)
	Diabetes	4.4 (1.4–13.7)

CI, confidence interval; EBCT, electron-beam computed tomography.
[a]Analyses were performed with and without the coronary artery calcium scores (CACS).
SOURCE: Reprinted from Arad Y, Spadaro LA, Goodman K, et al.[69] With permission.

follow up of 2.2 years. In the multivariable model, the CAC score and extent of myocardial ischaemia were the only independent predictors of outcome ($p < 0.0001$). ROC analysis demonstrated that CAC predicted cardiovascular events with the best area under the curve (0.92), significantly better than the United Kingdom Prospective Diabetes Study Risk Score (0.74) and Framingham Score (0.60, $p < 0.0001$). The relative risk to predict a cardiovascular event for a CAC score of 101 to 400 was 10.13, and increased to 58.05 for scores >1000 ($p < 0.0001$). No cardiac events or perfusion abnormalities occurred in subjects with CAC ≤10 Agatston units up until 2 years of follow up.

The CAC score appears to provide complementary prognostic information to that obtained by the Framingham risk model.[75–80] Combining EBCT results with biochemical markers, such as C-reactive protein, may more precisely define risk than either test alone[75–81] (Table 20–4). More data is needed in different ethnic groups prior to widespread application.[82]

Risk-Factor Analysis

Traditional risk-factor analysis is commonly used to identify individuals who are at increased risk for developing cardiovascular disease based on standard clinical criteria.[83,84] Because the development of symptomatic cardiovascular disease occurs almost exclusively in patients with atherosclerosis, it seems advantageous in risk assessment to use a technique that directly measures the presence and severity of atherosclerotic burden rather than estimating its presence through indirect measures. For example, although there is a clear relationship between the number of cardiac risk factors and the presence and extent of CAC, 40 percent of men and 30 percent of women without risk factors in one recent series had CAC, whereas 26 percent of men and 36 percent of

TABLE 20–4

Characteristics and Risk Ratio for Follow-Up Studies Using EBCT

AUTHOR	NUMBER	MEAN AGE (Y)	FOLLOW-UP DURATION (Y)	CALCIUM SCORE CUTOFF	COMPARATIVE GROUP FOR R-R CALCULATION	RELATIVE RISK RATIO
Greenland[68]	1312	66	7.0	CAC >300	No CAC	3.9
Arad[69]	1173	53	3.6	CAC >160	CAC <160	20.2
Wong[70]	926	54	3.3	Top quartile	First score quartile	8.8
Raggi[71]	632	52	2.7	Top quartile	Lowest quartile	13
Kondos[73]	5635	51	3.1	CAC	No CAC	3.86 (men) 1.53 (women)
Arad[74]	4613	59	4.3	CAC ≥100	CAC <100	9.2
Shaw[75]	10,377	53	5	CAC 401–1000	CAC ≤10	6.2
Taylor[76]	2000	43	3	CAC	No CAC	11.8
Vliegenthart[77]	1795	71	3.3	>1000	0–100	8.1
Lamonte[78]	10,746	54	3.5	CAC top third	No CAC	8.7 (men) 6.3 (women)
Becker[79]	924	60	3	Top quartile (75th percentile)	Total study group	7.3

CAC, coronary artery calcification.

women with more than three traditional risk factors did not.[85] Likewise, Newman and colleagues showed great heterogeneity in the EBCT-derived CACS even among elderly men and women, which was only weakly associated with the presence of cardiac risk factors.[86] In this series, 9 percent of patients had a normal EBCT and 31 percent had a CACS <100 (see Fig. 20–19). Increasing age and tobacco use were significantly associated with increasing CACS in both men and women, whereas hypertension, diabetes, and hyperlipidemia were not.

Hecht and coworkers demonstrated that 76 percent of asymptomatic subjects with an abnormal EBCT had a low-density lipoprotein (LDL) cholesterol <160 mg/dL and therefore would not meet National Cholesterol Education Program (NCEP) II guidelines for lipid-lowering therapy.[87] Conversely, 52 percent of patients with an LDL cholesterol <130 mg/dL and 46 percent with an LDL <100 mg/dL had an abnormal EBCT. Similarly, in the Healthy Women Study, risk-factor analysis was imprecise at predicting coronary calcification in postmenopausal women.[88] Although the combination of a high LDL cholesterol, a low high-density lipoprotein (HDL) cholesterol, and a history of cigarette smoking was a strong predictor of CAC, this risk-factor profile was observed in only 6 percent of all women studied. Furthermore, only 6 of 21 women with the highest calcium scores (>101) had this risk-factor profile. Conversely, 20 percent of women in the lowest risk profile (i.e., nonsmokers, LDL cholesterol <130 mg/dL, and HDL cholesterol >60 mg/dL) had calcium by EBCT. Hecht and colleagues likewise showed that 42 percent of women aged ≤55 and 48 percent aged older than 55 years who were at low risk based on NCEP II guidelines (i.e., LDL cholesterol <130 and HDL ≥35 mg/dL) had evidence of coronary atherosclerosis based on an abnormal EBCT study.[89]

TRACKING CHANGES IN CORONARY ARTERY CALCIFICATION

Much interest has been directed at using CAC to measure plaque burden, and then remeasuring at some point in time to assess for progression of disease. Callister and coworkers[90] was one of the first studies to demonstrate a relationship between cholesterol control and atherosclerosis progression. There was a significant net increase in mean calcium-volume score among individuals not treated with cholesterol-reducing medications (mean change: 52 ± 36 percent, $p < 0.001$). There was a graded response depending on the LDL reduction with statin therapy, with those treated to LDL <120 mg/dL demonstrating an average diminution of coronary calcium (7 ± 23 percent) and those individuals treated less aggressively (LDL >120 mg/dL) showed a calcium-volume score increase of 25 ± 22 percent ($p < 0.001$ for comparison with aggressively treated subjects).

A study by Budoff and colleagues evaluated 299 patients who underwent two consecutive scans at least 12 months apart.[91] The average change in the calcium score (Agatston method) for the entire group was 33.2 ± 9.2 percent per year. Those patients reporting use of a statin had an annual rate of progression of 15 percent, compared with 39 percent annual increase in EBCT score for nonstatin users.

Prospective studies demonstrating a link between CAC progression and coronary events have recently been reported. The first

study demonstrated in 817 persons for whom EBCT-measured progression was the strongest predictor of cardiac events.[92] This observational study suggests that continued accumulation of CAC in asymptomatic individuals is associated with increased risk of MI. A second study measured the change in CAC in 495 asymptomatic subjects submitted to sequential EBCT scanning.[93] Statins were started after the initial EBCT scan. On average, MI subjects demonstrated a CAC change of 42 ± 23 percent yearly; event-free subjects showed a 17 ± 25 percent yearly change ($p = 0.0001$). *Relative risk of having an MI in the presence of CAC progression was 17-fold (95 percent CI: 4.1 to 71.2) higher than without CAC progression ($p < 0.0001$).*

A prospective study using EBCT to measure progression of CACP evaluated 4613 asymptomatic persons aged 50 to 70 at baseline and again at 2 years with clinical follow-up for 4.3 years.[74] The median (interquartile range) calcium score increased by 4 (0, 38) units from baseline to the year two scan in subjects who did not sustain a coronary event at any time during the study. In contrast, median (interquartile range) calcium score increased by 247 (40, 471) units in 49 subjects who experienced a first coronary disease event after the year 2 scan ($p < 0.0001$). Multiple logistic regression demonstrated only age ($p = 0.03$), male gender ($p = 0.04$), LDL cholesterol ($p = 0.01$), HDL cholesterol ($p = 0.04$), and 2-year change in calcium score ($p < 0.0001$) were significantly associated with subsequent CAD events. Increasing calcium scores were most strongly related to coronary events in this clinical study, similar to observational studies reported.

The Multi-Ethnic Study of Atherosclerosis will measure baseline CAC scores and repeat this measurement after 3.5 years in 6814 patients. Interim events, within the 3.5 years, will be measured. Future events in the subsequent 3.5 years (total 7 years follow up) will be measured.[94]

Coronary Artery Calcification Reproducibility

The reproducibility of CAC has been evaluated using the traditional Agatston scoring system and more recent volumetric and area methods. With the Agatston method, good inter- and intraobserver reproducibility is reported for recalculating the CACS on a single scan.[32,95] However, early studies showed significant variability when the results of two separate studies on the same patient were compared.[18,43,96–110] Over the years technical advances and improvements in calcium scoring methodologies have reduced interscan variability. Achenbach and coworkers, using *state-of-the-art* EBCT imaging, reported an interscan variability of only 19.9 ± 36 percent with a median Agatston score variability of 7.8 percent.[99] As in previous studies, there was a strong inverse relationship between the initial CACS value and interscan reproducibility, with the largest percent variation occurring in patients with the lowest CACS (Table 20–5). The variability for a CACS ≥100 was minimal at 10.5 ± 10.4 percent, with a median variability of only 7.1 percent.

The traditional Agatston scoring system has been challenged by more recently proposed area[99–101] and volumetric scoring methods.[102] The volumetric method uses isotropic interpolation to calculate the volume of calcified plaque area with a density of ≥130 HU,[102] rather than generating a CACS based on an arbitrary maximal plaque attenuation coefficient (i.e., Agatston method).[32] The calcified-area method directly measures and sums the area (in

TABLE 20-5

Comparison of Interscan Variability for the Agatston and Volumetric Scores Depending on Severity of Initial Coronary Artery Calcium Score

AGATSTON SCORE	NUMBER OF PATIENTS	AGATSTON SCORE VARIABILITY (PERCENT)	VOLUMETRIC SCORE VARIABILITY (PERCENT)
≥0	120	19.9 ± 36.0 (7.8)	16.2 ± 29.6 (5.7)
≥0.1	102	23.5 ± 39.5 (10.3)	19.9 ± 31.2 (8.3)
≥10	87	16.5 ± 22.7 (8.8)	18.0 ± 24.6 (9.1)
≥50	70	11.5 ± 11.1 (7.5)	11.6 ± 11.2 (6.6)
≥100	62	10.5 ± 10.4 (7.1)	11.4 ± 11.0 (6.6)
≥400	31	9.5 ± 9.1[a] (7.3)	7.3 ± 8.8.0[a] (4.9)
≥1000	11	8.3 ± 6.9 (6.2)	6.1 ± 4.9 (5.9)

[a]Volumetric score variability significantly lower than Agatston score variability. Values are expressed as mean ± SD (median).
SOURCE: From Achenbach S, Ropers D, Mohlenkamp S, et al.[99] With permission.

mm²) of all coronary artery lesions. The volumetric and calcified-area methods are more reproducible than the Agatston method,[99,101,102] probably because of a reduction in partial volume effects and image noise on scan results.

In the largest series to date, Bielak and colleagues defined the reproducibility of sequential EBCT imaging in 1376 patients where scanning was performed minutes apart.[100] This data set is the first to allow calculation of 95 percent confidence intervals for individual changes in sequential scores for calcified areas ranging as low as 5 mm² to more than 1000 mm² (Table 20–6).

TABLE 20-6

Predicted Calcific Area in 1376 Asymptomatic Patients

MEAN CALCIFIC AREA IN DUAL-SCAN RUNS	CALCIFIC AREA AT > LIMIT OF AGREEMENT[a]	
	UPPER 95%	LOWER 95%
5	8	1
10	14	5
20	25	14
50	60	41
75	88	63
100	117	85
150	174	130
200	231	174
250	288	219
300	346	263
400	460	352
500	575	441
750	861	663
1000	1147	885

[a]Data are rounded to nearest whole number.
SOURCE: From Bielak LF, Sheedy PF, Peyser PA.[100] With permission.

Despite improvements in image acquisition and processing, cardiac motion still remains an important source of scan variability. The optimization of ECG triggering when cardiac motion is at a nadir may further improve reproducibility.[101]

The current reproducibility of CT with the area or volumetric methods appears adequate to track temporal changes in coronary atherosclerosis and assess the effects of pharmacologic therapy on plaque progression. In asymptomatic subjects with an abnormal EBCT, CACS progression is approximately 30 percent per year, which is significantly greater than the inherent variability in CAC score measurements.[103,104]

【 】 DISTINGUISHING ISCHEMIC FROM NONISCHEMIC CONDITIONS WITH COMPUTED TOMOGRAPHY

The presence or absence of CAC by CT may help to distinguish patients with ischemic versus nonischemic dilated cardiomyopathy.[105,106] Importantly, 44 of 45 patients with a normal EBCT had nonischemic dilated cardiomyopathy (98 percent negative predictive value). The total CACS increased with the extent and severity of underlying CAD (see Fig. 20–20 and Fig. 20–21, Fig. 20–22 and Fig. 20–23). The differentiation of ischemic from nonischemic dilated cardiomyopathy has also been demonstrated with MDCT.[106]

EBCT can distinguish ischemic from nonischemic chest pain in patients presenting to the emergency department with nondiagnostic ECGs and also predict subsequent cardiac risk for future events.[107–109] Two recent series comprising 239 patients showed a 0 percent cardiac event rate over 1[107] and 4[108] months in those with a normal EBCT. A third study in 192 patients showed 100

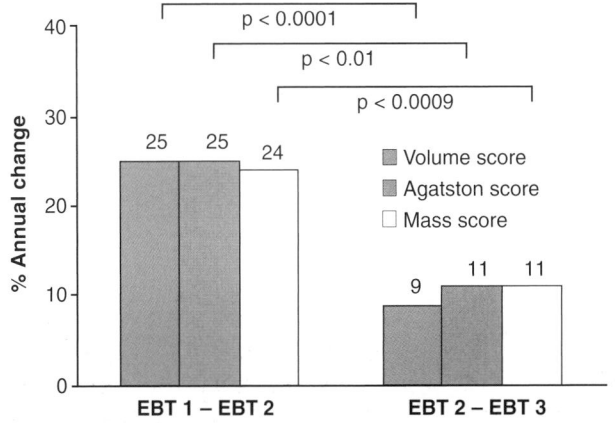

FIGURE 20-22. Median annualized relative increase in volume, Agatston, and mass scores during the untreated period (EBT1 to EBT2) and following statin treatment (EBT2 to EBT3). EBT, electron-beam tomography. *Source:* Redrawn from Achenbach S, Ropers D, Pohle K, et al. Influence of lipid-lowering therapy on the progression of coronary artery calcification: a prospective evaluation. *Circulation* 2002;106:1077–1082.

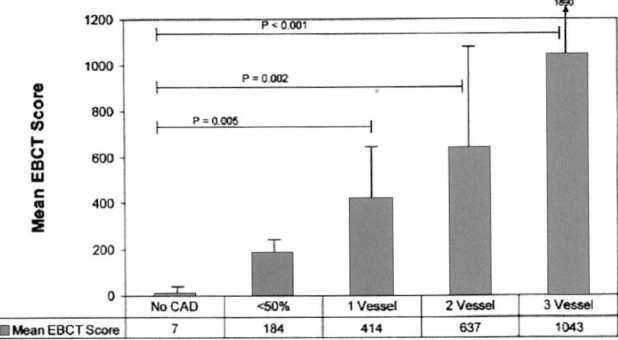

FIGURE 20–23. Mean EBCT CACS based on the presence and extent of angiographic CAD in patients with cardiomyopathy. CACS, coronary artery calcium score; CAD, coronary artery disease; EBCT, electron-beam computed tomography. *Source: From Budoff MJ, Shavelle DM, Lamont DH, et al.[105] Reproduced with permission from the publisher and authors.*

percent infarct-free survival over 50 ± 10 months of followup in patients with a normal EBCT.[109] The cardiac event rate increased significantly with the CACS (Fig. 20–24). The high negative predictive value of EBCT may improve triage of patients with questionable ischemic symptoms.

In three recent reports, most asymptomatic patients who had a subsequent first acute MI had coronary calcification by EBCT (96 percent).[64,74,110] Because many acute MIs occur following rupture of nonobstructive plaques, it is not surprising that the CACS were mild (<100) in a large percentage (34 percent) of patients and severe (>400) in relatively few (27 percent).[71] In one study evaluating survivors of a first MI with MDCT, 19 percent lacked CAC.[111] This higher percentage of normal studies may reflect the lower sensitivity of earlier generation MDCT scanners as compared to EBCT for detecting calcium. Patients without calcium are generally younger in age and tend to be active smokers.[71,112] With the exception of young smokers, a normal EBCT defines a population at low likelihood for significant CAD and subsequent acute cardiac events. Larger prospective trials in patients with acute coronary syndromes are needed to further delineate the role of EBCT in this population.

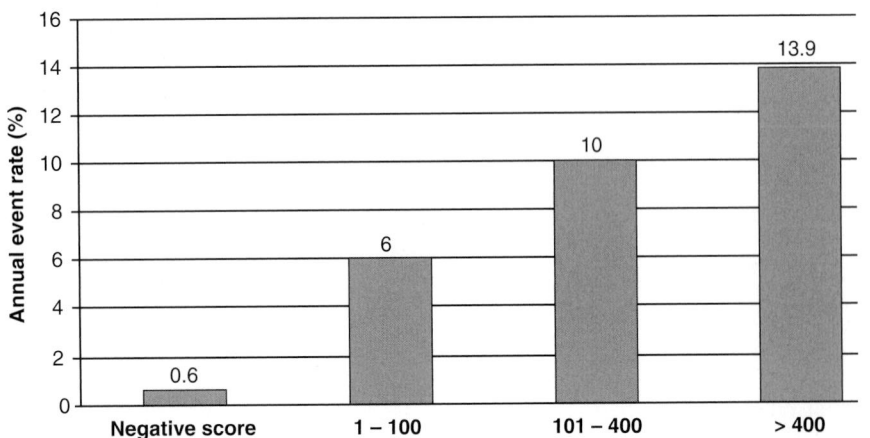

FIGURE 20–24. Annualized rates for future cardiovascular events by Cox proportional hazards regression. Patients with scores >400 had a significantly higher annualized event rate (13.9 percent) than those with scores of zero (0.6 percent) (p < 0.001). *Source: From Georgiou D, Budoff MJ, Kaufer E, et al.[109] Reproduced with permission from the publisher and authors.*

COMPUTED TOMOGRAPHY ANGIOGRAPHY

【 】 ASSESSMENT OF DISEASE OF NATIVE CORONARY ARTERIES

Noninvasive detection of CAD is one of the most interesting but most challenging applications of coronary CT angiography.[113] Invasive coronary angiography carries procedural risk as well as high procedural cost.[114] It was estimated that approximately 20 to 27 percent of patients who undergo coronary angiography have normal angiograms,[115] and many patients with significant CAD do not require revascularization procedures.[116,117]

Studies demonstrate that 16-slice MDCT scanners made by different vendors achieve evaluative images in close to 95 percent of subjects, after exclusion of small diameter vessels (usually <2 mm).[113] In spite of the improved temporal resolution with the latest technology (gantry rotation speed between 330–400 msec per rotation), 64-MDCT is incapable of freezing the motion at heart rates greater than 70 beats/min; and as such, a small proportion of patients (0–7 percent) still have nondiagnostic scans in spite of careful patient selection and administration of heart rate–lowering agents (Fig. 20–25).[118–126] The velocity of coronary artery motion increases significantly with rising heart rate.[127] The effort to reduce and maintain heart rate to below 65 beats/min with either blockers or calcium channel blockers, is still the critical element in achieving good overall image quality. For those individuals without contraindication to blockade, these drugs are still the medication of choice because they not only decrease the heart rate through the reduction of sympathetic tone, but they may also reduce the number of premature atrial or ventricular beats, which adversely affect the overall quality of the images. Another crucial element for obtaining high-quality coronary images is to maximally dilate coronary vessels with nitroglycerin using one or two sublingual tablets or a sublingual spray (Fig. 20–26). Most centers prefers the use of sublingual nitroglycerin (400 μg) right before the acquisition of the topogram. Despite those limitations, results of trials with 64-MDCT scanners are encouraging with a per-patient sensitivity of 88 to 100 percent, specificity of 79 to 100 percent, a positive predictive value of 86 to 100 percent, and a negative predictive value of 86 percent to 100 percent.[113,118,120–126]

Because of its high negative predictive value, the consensus among many imaging experts is that MDCT may be used as a reliable filter before invasive coronary angiography in the assessment of symptomatic patients with intermediate risk of CAD and in patients with uninterpretable or equivocal stress tests.[128] A recent scientific statement from the American Heart Association on Cardiac CT concluded, "CT coronary angiography is reasonable for the assessment of obstructive disease in symptomatic patients (Class IIa, Level of Evidence B)."[113] Other important clinical roles of MDCT (discussed below) include the assessment

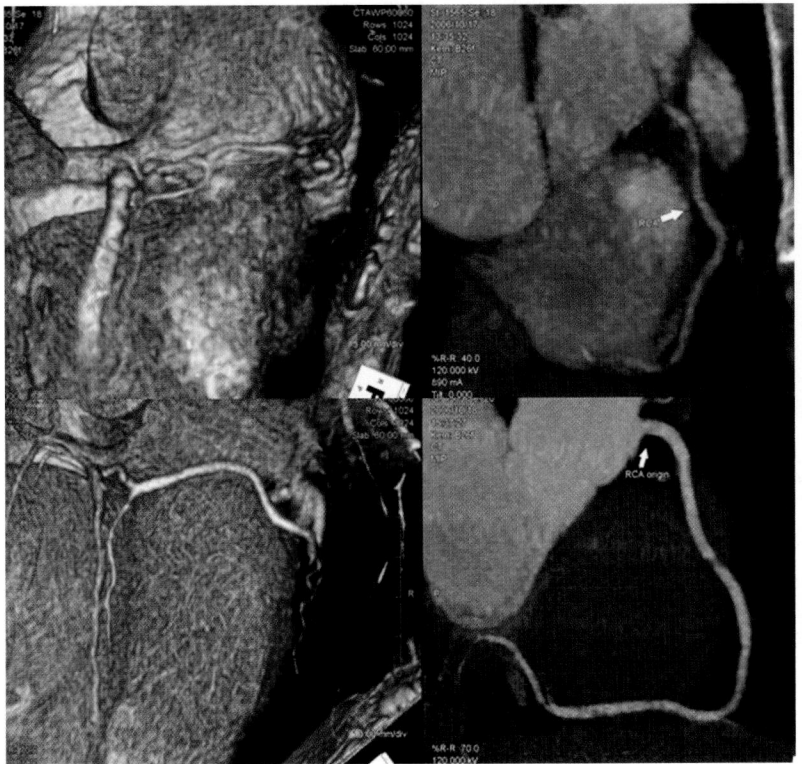

FIGURE 20–25. Cardiac motion artifact. *Top left panel*: 3D rendering image of a heart with significant motion artifact affecting the interpretation of the distal RCA. This patient was scanned with a dual source CT (temporal resolution of 83 msec) and the heart rate in the time of the scan was 105 beats/min. *Top right panel*: Maximum-intensity projection (MIP) image of the same patient showing significant transitional motion artifact in the proximal and mid-RCA. *Bottom left panel*: 3D rendering image of a heart without motion artifact showing the distal RCA. The heart rate was 75 beats/min and the patient was scanned with a dual source CT. *Bottom right panel*: MIP image of the same patient showing only slight transitional motion artifact in the mid-RCA. RCA, right coronary artery.

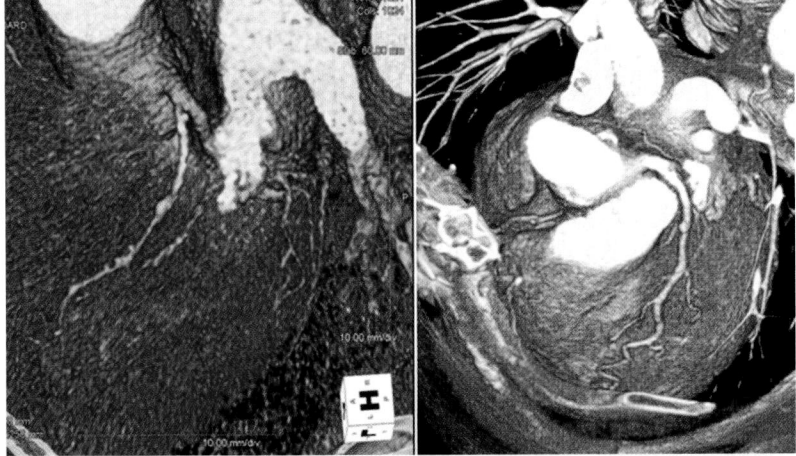

FIGURE 20–26. Effect of optimal coronary vasodilation with nitroglycerin. *Left panel*: 3D rendering image showing only portion of the LAD with evidence of calcified plaques in mid LAD. The study was performed without nitroglycerin. *Right panel*: 3D rendering image of the same patient who was given an oral sublingual nitroglycerin prior to the scan. In contrast to the image on the left panel, a significant improvement of the LAD with clear showing of all the side branches and the mid to distal portion of the vessel. LAD, left anterior descending (coronary artery).

of complex congenital heart disease, suspected coronary anomalies, and ruling out significant CAD as a cause of new onset clinical heart failure.[113,128]

Careful selection of patients is crucial to increase the diagnostic yield of coronary CTA using MDCT. Three major limitations of spiral coronary CT angiography are relatively fast heart rate (i.e., more than 70 beats/min), irregular heart rhythm, and extensive CAC. Heavy calcification does not affect the negative predictive value of MDCT on a segment-based analysis[121] and the newer generation of MDCT technology with even faster gantry rotation may further reduce the blooming artifact associated with coronary calcification (Fig. 20–27). Moreover, MDCT remained highly accurate in mildly overweight individuals, but significant obesity (body mass index >30 kg/m²) reduced the specificity from 91 to 86 percent and the negative predictive value from 100 to 86 percent. For this reason, the recent appropriateness criteria for coronary CT angiography do not endorse the use of coronary CTA in the evaluation of patients with BMI >40 kg/m².[128]

[ ] ASSESSMENT OF DISEASE OF CORONARY BYPASS GRAFTS

Coronary CT angiography demonstrated good diagnostic accuracy for evaluating graft stenosis with a sensitivity of 69 to 98 percent and a specificity of 89 to 100 percent.[129–133] Despite these promising preliminary results, the assessment of bypass graft stenosis has several important limitations, namely the image artifacts caused by surgical clips and the presence of extensive coronary calcification in the native coronary arteries (Fig. 20–28).

Furthermore, the severity of CAD in patients post-coronary bypass grafting is usually very extensive; and thus the number of noninterpretable segments is usually high, such as 31 percent in the study by Stauder and coworkers,[130] which considered the whole native coronary arterial tree, with a 92 percent sensitivity and 77 percent specificity. This high percentage of unevaluative segments of native coronary vessels may be less relevant in the clinical decision-making process because the most extensively calcified vessel, therefore not assessable, are often bypassed. Presently, coronary CTA may be used for the evaluation of coronary bypass grafts and coronary anatomy in symptomatic patients.[128] In the case of reoperation, coronary CTA may provide critically important information on the status and anatomy of the bypass grafts (Fig. 20–29). The AHA Scientific Statement on Cardiac CT states, "It might be reasonable in most cases to not only assess the patency of bypass graft but also the presence of coronary stenoses in the course of the bypass graft or at the anastomotic site as well as in the native coronary artery system (Class IIb, Level of Evidence: C)."[113] In summary, coronary CTA using MDCT may be appropriate in properly selected pa-

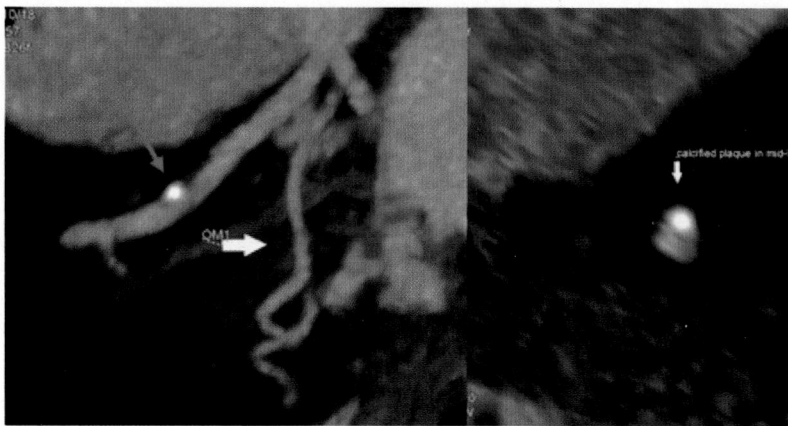

FIGURE 20–27. Evaluation of coronary atherosclerosis. *Left panel*: Longitudinal MIP view of the mid LAD showing a calcified nonobstructive plaque. The image was obtained using a dual source CT scanner. *Right panel*: Axial MPR view of the same plaque. LAD, left anterior descending (coronary artery); MIP, maximum-intensity projection; MPR, myocardial perfusion reserve.

tients by providing useful information on the overall status and the patency of the bypass grafts without exposing them to an invasive diagnostic approach (Fig. 20–30).

[ ] ASSESSMENT OF IN-STENT RESTENOSIS

Despite promising results, assessment of symptomatic patients with implanted coronary stents using current CT technology is one of the uncertain areas in terms of its overall clinical utility.[128] To date, four prospective studies on 16-MDCT[134–137] and one on 40-MDCT,[138] were published focusing on the accuracy in the diagnosis of in-stent restenosis using MDCT. Two studies used EBCT for this purpose.[139,140] Sensitivity and specificity data range between 64 and 100 percent and 88 and 100 percent, respectively,

with an unassessable rate of stented segments that could reach 36 percent. The problems that current imaging technology is facing are mostly related to the partial volume effect caused by the metallic stents with or without the coexistence of coronary calcification. Such artifact limits the overall visibility of the inner lumen of a deployed stent. Similar to native coronary CTA imaging, the location of the stents in the coronary system is equally important with most interpretable results found in stents that were deployed in the left median (LM) and the LAD following by the left circumflex coronary artery (LCX) and the RCA. Studies with more advanced CT technologies, such as the 64-slice MDCT, are not currently available. Early results using in vitro models suggest some improvement in the visibility of the stent lumen.[141] However, the expert consensus thus far does not advocate the routine use of MDCT in ruling out in-stent restenosis except for highly selected cases (Fig. 20–31, see Fig. 20–7).[128]

[ ] EVALUATION OF CARDIAC STRUCTURE

Although echocardiography is generally used to assess native and prosthetic valvular heart disease, CT is an alternative but limited to patients with poor acoustic windows and who cannot undergo CMR or transesophageal echocardiography.[128] Cardiac CT has been used to evaluate mitral and aortic valve calcification, bicuspid aortic valves, as well as other structures such as the atrial and ventricular septum. MDCT has good sensitivity and specificity, 90 and 100 percent, respectively, in detecting tricuspid regurgitation.[142] In patients with mitral or aortic regurgitation, EBCT can accurately determine left and RV stroke volumes and thereby calculate valvular regurgitant fractions.[14] As with gated blood-pool radionuclide angiography, MDCT cannot distinguish mitral from aortic regurgitation and cannot calculate the regurgitant fraction if significant right-sided valvular insufficiency is present.[6] Furthermore, MDCT has a positive predictive value of 95 percent and a negative predictive value of 70 percent in detecting aortic insufficiency using the central valvular leakage area, which correlated with the severity of aortic regurgitation by transthoracic echocardiography.[143] In addition, MDCT has a positive predictive value of 97 percent, and a negative predictive value of 100 percent in detecting the presence of aortic stenosis, but only fair correlation with mean transvalvular pressure gradients by transthoracic[144] and transesophageal echocardiography.[145]

[ ] EVALUATION OF CORONARY ANOMALIES

Anomalies of the coronary arteries are reported in 0.3 to 1 percent of healthy individuals[146,147] and, despite usually being benign, they can be hemodynamically significant and some lead to abnormalities of myocardial perfusion and/or sudden death.[148] The coronary anomalies that may be associated with significant clinical symptoms or adverse outcomes including sudden

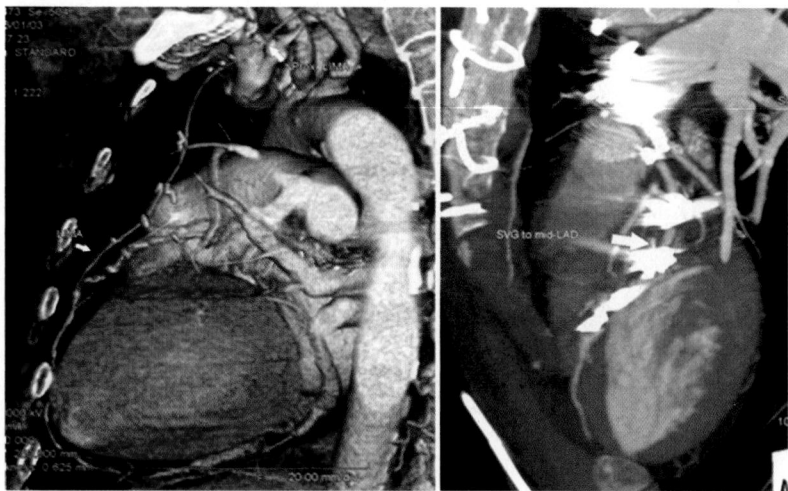

FIGURE 20–28. Evaluation of coronary bypass grafts. *Left panel*: 3D rendering image showing minimal surgical clip artifact along the path of the LIMA that is anastomosed to the distal LAD. *Right panel*: MIP image of a patient who also had a coronary bypass graft from the LIMA to the distal LAD. However, significant surgical clip artifact precludes the accessibility of the bypass graft. LAD, left anterior descending (coronary artery); LIMA, left internal mammary artery; MIP, maximum-intensity projection.

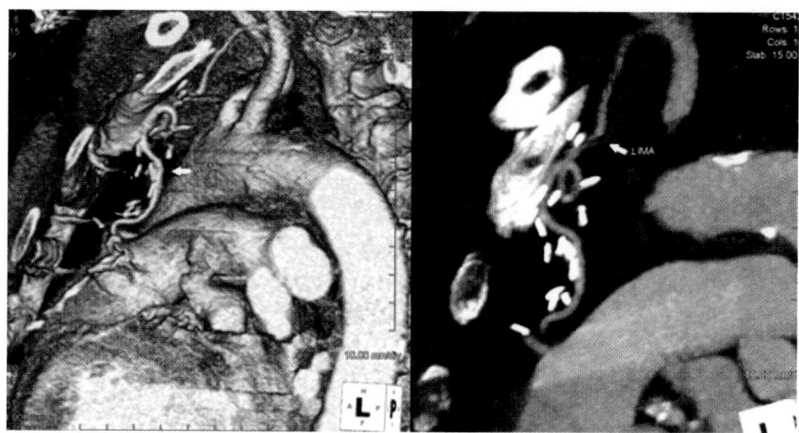

FIGURE 20-29. Preoperative evaluation of a patient who is going for a reoperation CABG. *Left panel*: 3D rendering image showing the adhesion of the mid-portion of the LIMA graft to the sternum. *Right panel*: MIP image showing the proximal origin of the LIMA graft and the overall tortuosity of the graft and the adhesion of the body of the LIMA graft to the sternum. CABG, coronary artery bypass graft; LIMA, left internal mammary artery; MIP, maximum-intensity projection.

of pericardial calcium makes its detection relatively easy. The three-dimensional (3D) representation of anatomy by CT provides the surgeon with precise detail of the extent of calcification and the degree of myocardial invasion. CT scanning can be useful particularly when visualization of the pericardium is suboptimal with echocardiography. CT scanning can readily detect pericardial effusion and can help determine the characteristics of the fluid based on CT density.[155]

CT scanning is useful in accurately diagnosing constrictive pericarditis and distinguishing it from similar conditions, such as restrictive myopathy.[153] Based on the presence of pericardial thickening (see Fig. 20–30) or calcification (see Fig. 20–31), CT can assess both the anatomic and functional abnormalities associated with pericardial constriction.[154] A pericardial thickness of more than 4 mm in a patient with typical abnormal rapid early LV diastolic filling is diagnostic of pericardial constriction.

death are those that course between the pulmonary artery and the aorta.

Until recently, invasive coronary artery angiography has been the gold standard for the detection of such anomalies. However, advances in CT technology have helped make cardiac CTA a better diagnostic alternative.[146] In two recent studies comparing CT and invasive coronary angiography, the latter was able to detect 80 percent of the anomalous origins but only 53 percent of the anomalous coronary courses[149] and to make a precise anatomic diagnosis in only 55 percent of patients.[150] Furthermore, based on a multicenter coronary artery CT registry, cardiac CTA was able to unequivocally demonstrate the origin and the course of the anomalous artery in all patients referred for such procedure as a result of equivocal findings from invasive coronary angiography.[151] Up to 50 percent of patients who had invasive coronary angiography had inconclusive demonstration of the course of the anomalous coronary artery that could be a crucial piece of information in determining the proper therapeutic option (see Fig. 20–30).

Coronary CTA is considered the preferred imaging modality in patients with suspected coronary artery anomalies and in patients in whom an invasive diagnostic procedure was inconclusive.[128]

EVALUATION OF PERICARDIAL DISEASE

CT scanning provides excellent visualization of the pericardium and associated mediastinal structures.[152–154] CT is aided by the fact that epicardial and extrapericardial fat often outline the normal pericardium. Fat, being of very low density, serves as a natural contrast agent. Therefore, even minimal pericardial thickening (4–5 mm) is well recognized by cardiac CT. The high density

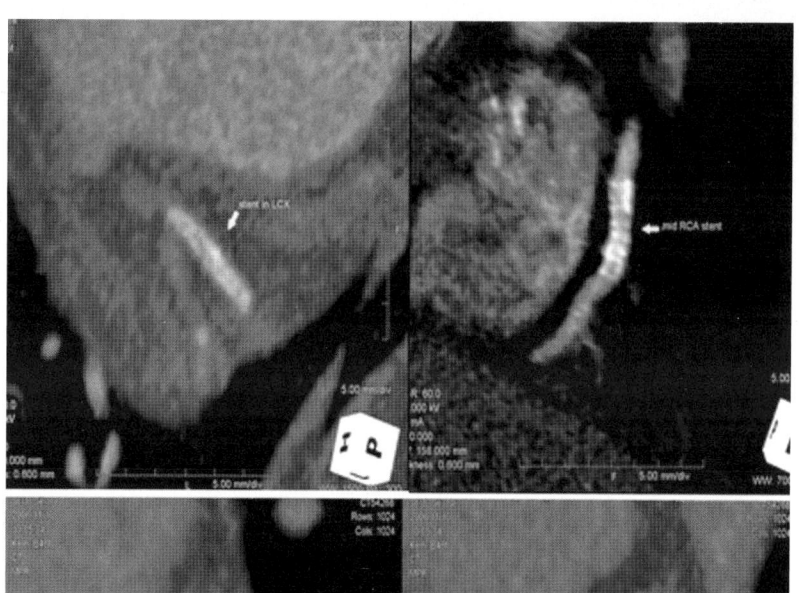
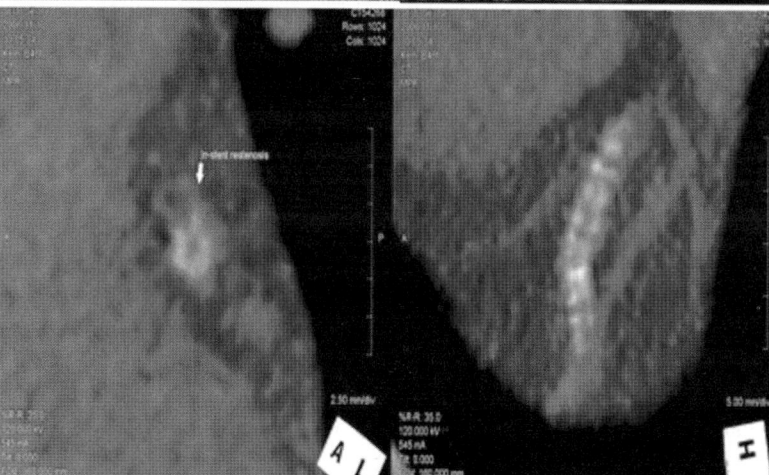

FIGURE 20-30. Evaluation of coronary stents. *Upper left panel*: MPR image of an occluded stent with no contrast at either the proximal or the distal end of the stent. *Upper right panel*: MPR image of a patent stent with good overall contrast enhancement on both ends and the body of the stent. *Lower left panel*: MPR axial image of a stent with evidence of in-stent restenosis showing an area of hypoenhancement along the luminal aspect of the stent. *Lower right panel*: MPR longitudinal image of the same stent as shown on the lower left panel showing areas of hypoenhancement in the proximal and mid portion of the stent. MPR, myocardial perfusion reserve.

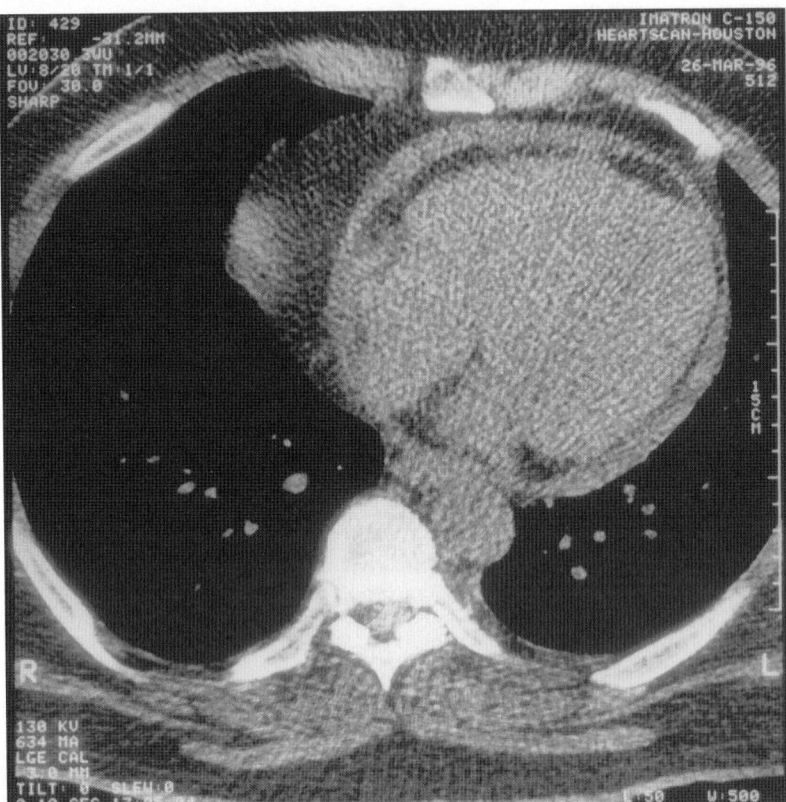

FIGURE 20–31. Diffuse pericardial thickening surrounding the entire heart in a patient with pericardial constriction. *Source: From Brundage BH, Mao SS. In: Schlant RC et al, eds. Diagnostic Atlas of the Heart. New York: McGraw-Hill; 1996:243. Reproduced with permission from the publisher and authors.*

CT scanning can assess congenital abnormalities such as absence of the pericardium[156] or pericardial cyst.[157] CT scanning is currently one of the best techniques for defining the location and extent of mediastinal tumors and in diagnosing metastatic involvement of the pericardium.[157,158] In addition to providing an excellent description of the anatomy of pericardial constriction, EBCT also defines the degree of hemodynamic abnormality by describing diastolic filling from ventricular volume measurements. Cine mode images of the right atrium and RV can also detect diastolic collapse when pericardial tamponade is present. Enlargement of the superior and inferior vena cavae can also be identified when either constriction or tamponade is present.

EVALUATION OF CONGENITAL HEART DISEASE

Cardiac CT has been used increasingly for the assessment of congenital heart disease (Fig. 20–32), as has CMR. Both modalities can be rendered into 3D images that are useful in clarifying the often complex anatomic relationships in patients with congenital heart disease. CMR may be of limited use in critically ill patients because of its relatively long scan time, and it is contraindicated in patients with history of severe claustrophobia and with metallic implants. However, CMR is still preferred more than CTA because it does not involve ionizing radiation or nephrotoxic contrast agents, and it allows the precise quantification of flows and

better tissue characterization. Advances in CT image quality, decreases in radiation dose, and the provision of accurate functional information have helped make CT a viable alternative for assessment of these patients. Furthermore, MRI most often requires significant sedation in children (often necessitating intubation), which is not necessary with the very fast study times of CT.

Anomalies of the aortic arch, septal defects, tetralogy of Fallot, Ebstein anomaly, and abnormal arteriovenous connections can all be carefully evaluated with cardiac CTA[159,160] (see Fig. 20–32). CT, because of its high spatial resolution, can also evaluate the atrioventricular valves in conditions such as tricuspid and mitral valve atresia.[161–163] CT can also be used to accurately quantify intracardiac shunts[161,163–168] as well as masses.[169] An increasingly popular application of cardiac CTA is the evaluation of septal defects. Both atrial and ventricular septal defects can be detected and analyzed with contrast enhanced cardiac CTA.[163–168] CT evaluation has been used prior to closure device implantation.[168] Other abnormalities of the ventricle, such as LV pseudoaneurysm, can be visualized. The high spatial and temporal resolution of cardiac CT (compared with MRI) make this an attractive option for assessment of a multitude of congenital heart defects. Limited data exist for evaluation of congenital heart defects at this time, but early studies have revealed a high sensitivity and specificity for these abnormalities. The development of four-dimensional (4D) capability has accelerated over the last few years.

The heart is a dynamic organ best understood when studied throughout the cardiac cycle. Hence, the development of 4D CT cineangiography (time being the fourth dimension) is a milestone in the clinical application of this technology. It is ideally suited for the complex dynamic dilemmas frequently encountered in congenital heart disease.[161] This application has recently been included in the appropriateness criteria for CT and MR.[128]

RV dysplasia is accurately diagnosed based on the characteristic CT findings of an enlarged right ventricle, with a scalloped appearance, trabeculations with low attenuation characteristics, and abundant epicardial adipose tissue.[170,171]

In conclusion, the application of CT in evaluating congenital heart disease is feasible and appropriate. In selected cases, CT may be a valuable alternative to CMR for both structural and functional delineation of the anatomic abnormality.

EVALUATION OF CARDIAC TUMORS

The presence and extent of intracardiac tumors can be well defined with either conventional CT or EBCT. CT scanning can also delineate metastatic tumor within the myocardial wall. Intracardiac tumors are readily detected by noninvasive two-dimensional echocardiography. Tumors such as myxomas, however, are also well visualized by EBCT, particularly when imaging is performed following intravenous contrast enhancement[169] (Fig. 20–33).

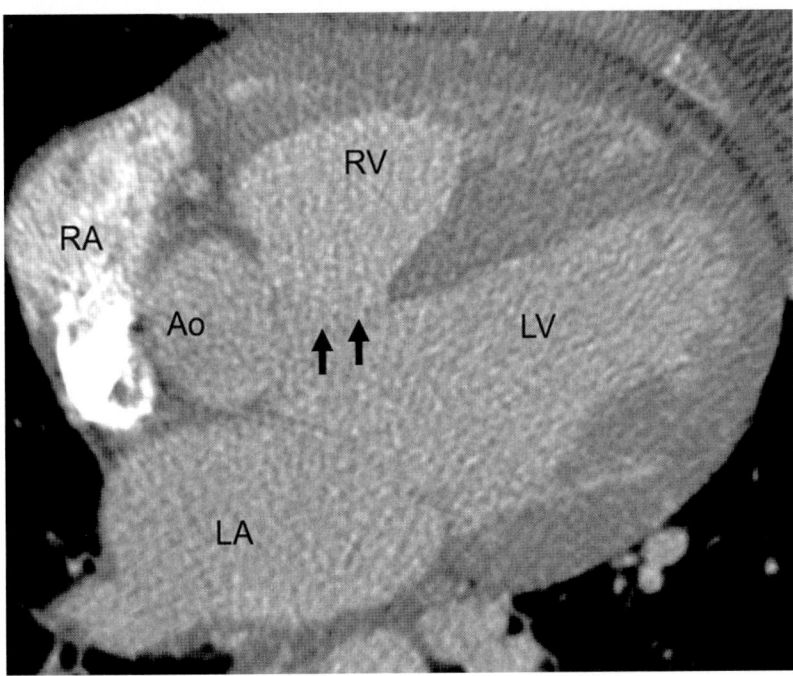

FIGURE 20–32. A patient with tetrology of Fallot with large ventricular septal defect (*black arrows*), overriding aorta (Ao) and thickened right ventricle (RV). Cardiac CT is very helpful with all forms of congenital heart disease in defining the anatomy. Ao, aorta; LA, left atrium; LV, left ventricle; RA, right atrium; RV, right ventricle.

DISEASES OF THE GREAT VESSELS

Conventional CT scanning is widely used for diagnosing thoracic aortic aneurysms and dissections.[172–173] With the introduction of MDCT scanners, hundreds of images of approximately 0.625 to 2.5-mm thickness can be acquired within a single breathhold. A complete study of the thoracic aorta can be completed in only 10 to 15 seconds. Following scan acquisition, three-dimensional reconstructions are readily produced, which can be rotated in multiple views. EBCT can also acquire rapid CT images with elimination of aortic pulsation as a cause of potential artifact.[174]

Aortic dissection is readily diagnosed with CT angiography with >90 percent accuracy. In a recent study comparing MDCT, magnetic resonance imaging, and 2D echocardiography, CT and magnetic resonance imaging were shown to be superior to echocardiography in diagnostic accuracy.[173] CT scanning is also an effective method for diagnosing aortic aneurysm, defining its maximal diameter, and monitoring its expansion over time[174] (Fig. 20–34). CT scanning can diagnose traumatic aneurysms of the thoracic aorta,[172] sinus of Valsalva aneurysms, and coarctation of the aorta (Fig. 20–35). In patients undergoing *redo* coronary artery bypass surgery, CT scanning has several advantages. CT angiography may guide the surgical approach by defining the position of the sternum to the right ventricle, existing grafts and aorta and thereby avoid unnecessary bleeding.[175] CT is an excellent modality to evaluate the aorta for plaque and atherosclerotic disease, allowing the surgeon to plan an arterial revascularization rather than depending on saphenous vein grafting.

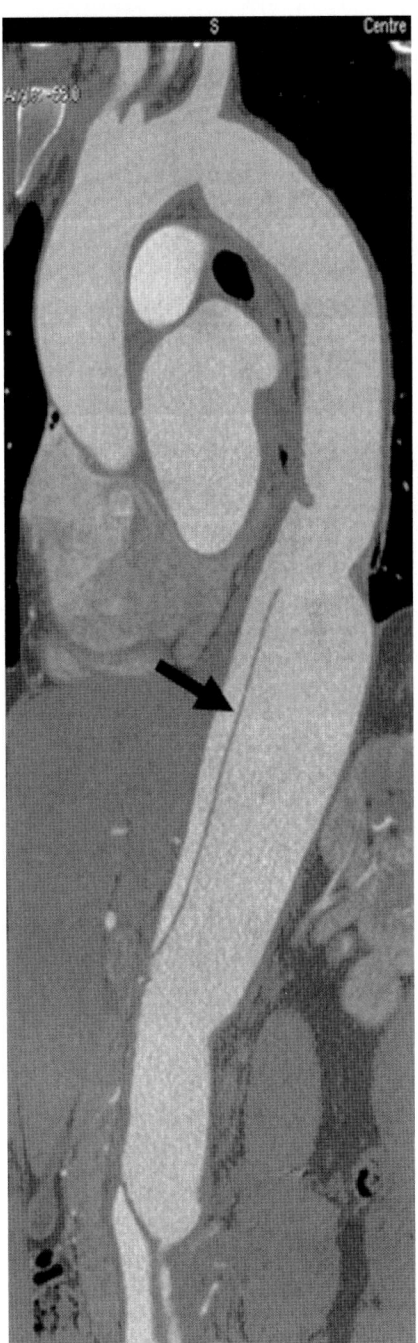

FIGURE 20–33. An aortic dissection starting in the descending thoracic aorta and extending down to right iliac artery. Black arrow demonstrates the coarctation on a sagittal image.

Both MDCT[176,177] and EBCT[178] can diagnose acute and chronic pulmonary thromboembolism (Fig. 20–36). CT angiography of the pulmonary arteries may be particularly useful in the diagnosis of acute pulmonary embolism, replacing the nuclear ventilation perfusion scan in many centers.[177,179,180] The cross-sectional view of the main and proximal right and left pulmonary arteries provides clear delineation of the proximal extent of the thrombi, which is essential for successful surgical treatment.[181] Accurate measurement of pulmonary artery size may also help to estimate the severity of pulmonary hypertension.[182]

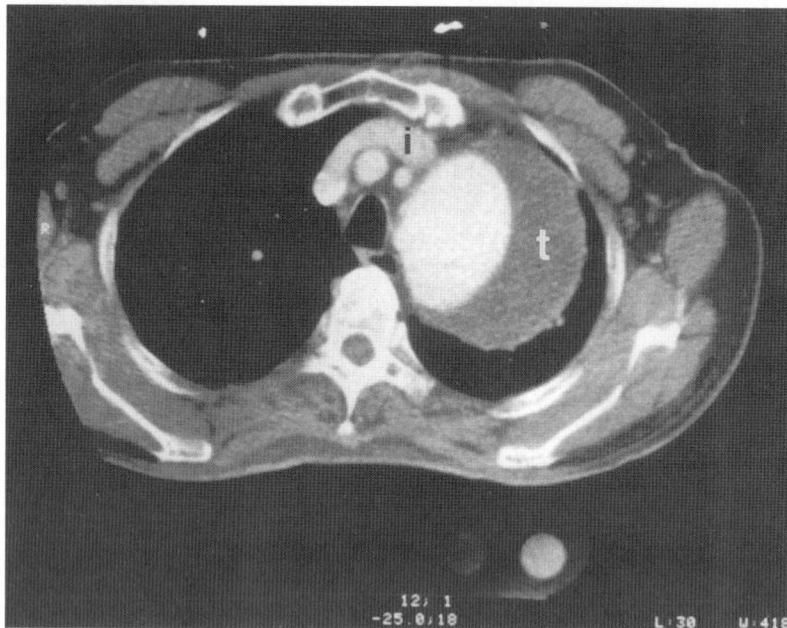

FIGURE 20–34. A large thrombus (*t*)-filled aneurysm of the aortic arch occupies most of the upper left thoracic cavity. The innominate vein (*i*) courses anterior to the innominate and left common carotid artery.

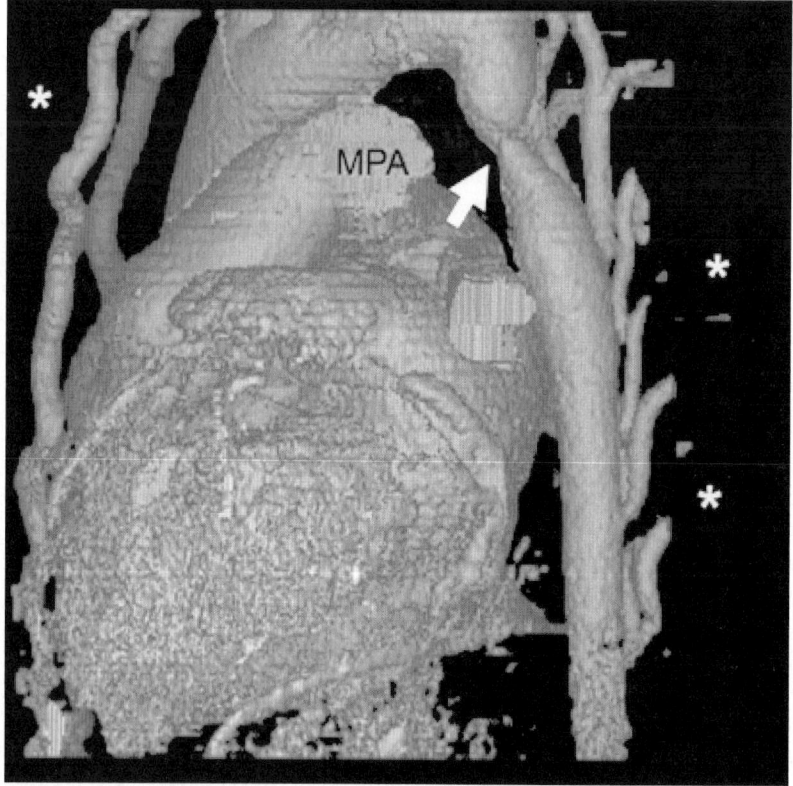

FIGURE 20–35. Coarctation of the aorta in the descending aorta (*white arrow*) with *asterisks* demonstrating the collaterals from the vertebral arteries filling the descending aorta. MPA, main pulmonary artery.

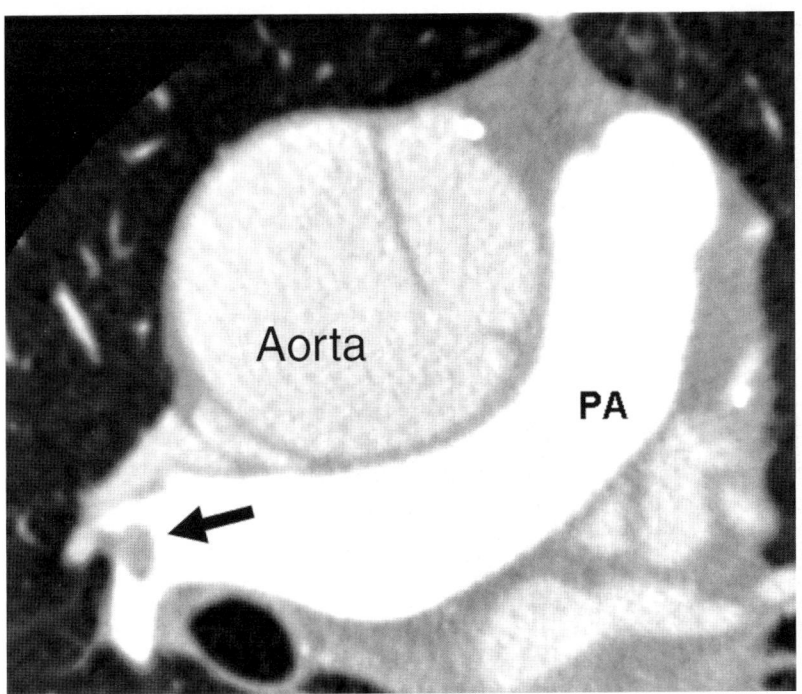

FIGURE 20–36. Patient with both an aortic dissection evidenced in a dilated aorta and a small pulmonary embolism (*black arrow*) in the left pulmonary artery (PA).

leagues observed a sensitivity and specificity of 4-slice MSCT to detect MI with invasive ventriculography serving as standard of reference to be 85 and 91 percent, respectively.[183] Moreover, the authors have demonstrated the ability of MSCT to differentiate old and recent MI on the basis of the tissue density expressed in HU, old infarctions having lower CT densities compared to recently infarcted areas (44 ± 17 HU vs. 63 ± 19 HU; p = 0.0465).[163] Because of high spatial resolution of MSCT, the differentiation of subendocardial and transmural infarctions is possible, which may have additional prognostic information. Wada and coworkers have demonstrated poor recovery of regional and global systolic LV function in patients having transmural infarction at 6 months after the onset of acute MI, whereas the subendocardial infarction group exhibited good recovery of LV function.[184] Mahnken and colleagues evaluated myocardial perfusion with 16-slice MSCT in the early phase of the contrast bolus and 15 minutes after contrast injection. An excellent agreement was demonstrated between the infarct size on late enhancement of MRI and late enhancement of MSCT (Fig. 20–37).[185] Further evaluation is necessary to define the clinical role of myocardial perfusion assessment with MSCT.

【 】 VIABILITY AND PERFUSION IMAGING WITH CT

Assessment of LV function with multislice spiral computed tomography (MSCT) is only possible at rest, because repeated scanning during stress and resting conditions is not justifiable because of the high radiation dose. For LV perfusion analysis, the density of the hypoperfused and normally perfused myocardial areas is assessed and expressed in HU. The hypoperfused areas may be quantitatively assessed with the use of available software. Perfusion abnormalities at rest may be observed in the early phase of the contrast bolus. Several reports have evaluated the diagnostic performance of MSCT in the diagnosis of the MI. Nikolaou and col-

SUMMARY

The training standards for practitioners and interpreters of cardiac imaging with CT and MRI have recently been published by the American College of Cardiology Foundation/American Heart Association/American College of Physicians Task Force on Clinical Competence and Training.[186] Calcium artery scanning is a valuable tool for diagnosis of CAD, allowing assessment of risk for future cardiac events. Current applications for CAC should be focused on risk stratification for intermediate-risk patients and ruling out obstructive disease in the symptomatic patient with low probability of

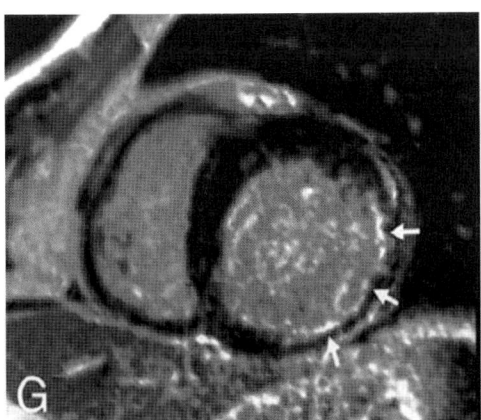
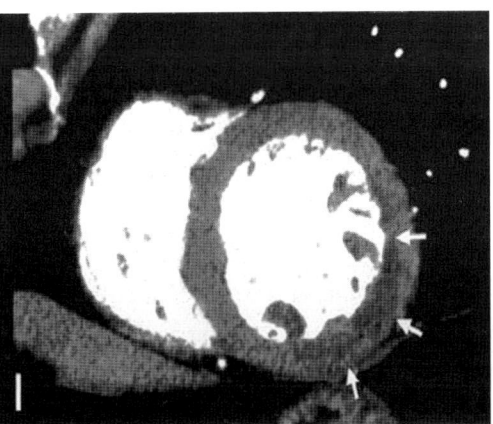

FIGURE 20–37. There was an excellent agreement between delayed-enhancement MRI (**G**) and multidetector CT (**I**). *Source: From Mahnken AH, Koos R, Katoh M, et al.[185] Reproduced with permission from the publisher and the authors.*

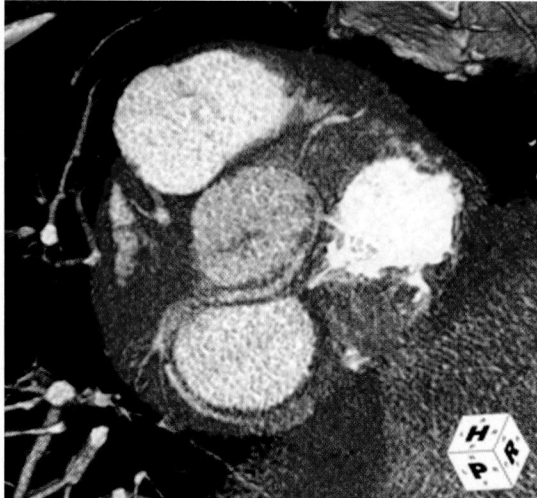

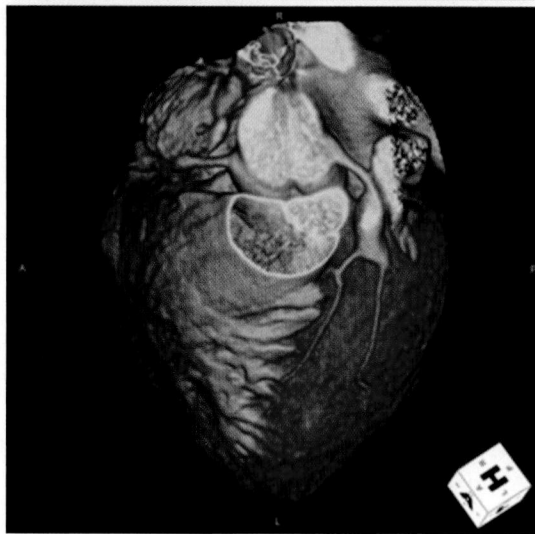

FIGURE 20–38. Evaluation of coronary anomaly. *Upper panel*: 3D rendering image showing an anomalous left circumflex arising from the right coronary sinus and it courses between the aorta and the left atrium. *Lower panel*: 3D rendering image showing a coronary aneurysm involving the LM, the proximal LAD, and a diagonal branch. LAD, left anterior descending (coronary artery); LM, left main.

disease. Computed tomography, particularly CTA with detection of both luminal stenosis and calcified and noncalcific plaque, should significantly aid in improving risk stratification and diagnoses. Computed tomographic angiography is likely to become an initial test in the symptomatic patient with a low to intermediate probability of obstructive CAD. Given a consistent negative predictive power >97 percent in multiple studies, CTA is unlikely to misclassify a patient at risk for CAD. It affords significant clinical information but must be used in context of other tests and in specific clinical situations, because the current radiation dose and contrast requirements preclude its use as a screening test. The course of anomalous coronary arteries are very easily visualized with cardiac CT (Fig. 20–38), as are structural abnormalities such as valve calcification, septal defects, and pulmonary veins (Fig. 20–39). The applications of cardiac CT, although robust, must be used in context of other imaging modalities and the appropriate patient settings. EBCT is best suited for calcium scoring, with virtually all validation work being done with this modality, and MDCT better applied to CT angiography, due to the higher spatial resolution.

REFERENCES

1. Boyd DP, Lipton MJ. Cardiac computed tomography. *Proc IEEE Nucl Sci* 1983;71:298–307.
2. Lu B, Mao SS, Zhuang N, et al. Coronary artery motion during the cardiac cycle and optimal ECG triggering for coronary artery imaging. *Invest Radiol* 2001;36:250–256.
3. Achenbach S, Ropers D, Holle J, et al. In-plane coronary arterial motion velocity. Measurement with electron-beam CT. *Radiology* 2000;216:457–463.
4. McCollough CH, Zink FE, Morin RL. Radiation dosimetry for electron beam CT. *Radiology* 1994;192:637–642.
5. Horiguchi J, Nakanishi T, Ito K. Quantification of coronary artery calcium using multidetector CT and a retrospective ECG-gating reconstruction algorithm. *AJR Am J Roentgenol* 2001;177:1429–1435.
6. Orakzai SH, Orakzai RH, Nasir K, Budoff MJ. Assessment of cardiac function using multidetector row computed tomography. *J Comput Assist Tomogr* 2006;30(4):555–563.
7. Roig E, Chomka EV, Castaner A, et al. Exercise ultrafast computed tomography for the detection of coronary artery disease. *J Am Coll Cardiol* 1989;13:1073–1081.
8. Budoff MJ, Gillespie R, Georgiou D, et al. Comparison of exercise electron beam computed tomography and sestamibi in the evaluation of coronary artery disease. *Am J Cardiol* 1998;81:682–687.

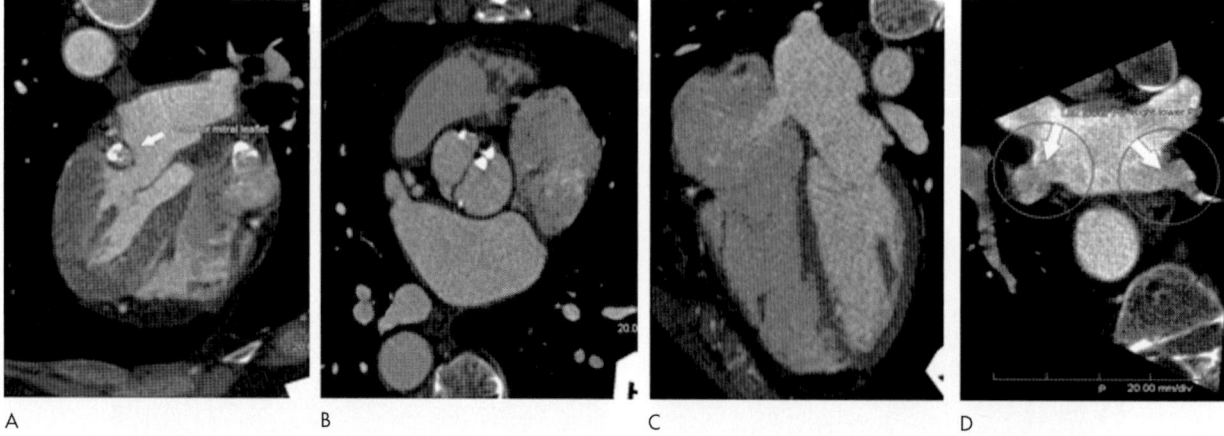

FIGURE 20–39. Evaluation of cardiac structure. **A.** MPR image of a heart with significant mitral annular calcification. **B.** MPR image of a bicuspid aortic valve. **C.** MPR image showing a jet of dye going from the left atrium to the right atrium indicating the presence of a left to right shunt caused by a large secundum atrial septal defect. **D.** MPR image of the left atrium and its associated pulmonary veins. This patient had previous radiofrequency ablation and the image shows mild left inferior PV narrowing at the ostium. MPR, myocardial perfusion reserve.

9. Gerber TC, Behrenbeck T, Allison T, et al. Comparison of measurement of left ventricular ejection fraction by Tc-99m sestamibi first-pass angiography with electron beam computed tomography in patients with anterior wall acute myocardial infarction. *Am J Cardiol* 1999;83:1022–1026.

10. Heuschmid M, Rothfuss JK, Schroeder S, Fenchel M, Stauder N, Burgstahler C, et al. Assessment of left ventricular myocardial function using 16-slice multidetector-row computed tomography: comparison with magnetic resonance imaging and echocardiography. *Eur Radiol* 2006;16(3):551–555.

11. Henneman MM, Bax JJ, Schuijf JD, et al. Global and regional left ventricular function: a comparison between gated SPECT, 2D echocardiography and multi-slice computed tomography. *Eur J Nucl Med Mol Imaging* 2006;33(12):1452–1460. Epub July 25, 2006.

12. Belge B, Coche E, Pasquet A, Vanoverschelde JL, Gerber BL. Accurate estimation of global and regional cardiac function by retrospectively gated multidetector row computed tomography: comparison with cine magnetic resonance imaging. *Eur Radiol* 2006;16(7):1424–1433.

13. Raman SV, Shah M, McCarthy B, Garcia A, Ferketich AK. Multi-detector row cardiac computed tomography accurately quantifies right and left ventricular size and function compared with cardiac magnetic resonance. *Am Heart J* 2006;151(3):736–744.

14. Reiter SJ, Rumberger JA, Stanford W, et al. Quantitative determination of aortic regurgitant volume in dogs by ultrafast computed tomography. *Circulation* 1987;76:728–735.

15. Helgason CM, Chomka E, Louie E, et al. The potential role for ultrafast cardiac computed tomography in patients with stroke. *Stroke* 1989;20:465–472.

16. Mautner GC, Mautner SL, Froehlich J, et al. Coronary artery calcification: assessment with electron beam CT and histomorphometric correlation. *Radiology* 1994;192:619–623.

17. Budoff MJ, Mao S, Zalace CP, et al. Comparison of spiral and electron beam tomography in the evaluation of coronary calcification in asymptomatic persons. *Int J Cardiol* 2001;77:181–188.

18. Becker CR, Kleffel T, Crispin A, et al. Coronary artery calcium measurement: agreement of multirow detector and electron beam CT. *AJR Am J Roentgenol* 2001;176:1295–1298.

19. Knez A, Becker C, Becker A, et al. Determination of coronary calcium with multi-slice spiral computed tomography: a comparative study with electron-beam CT. *Int J Cardiovasc Imaging* 2002;18:295–303.

20. Becker CR, Knez A, Jakobs TF, et al. Detection and quantification of coronary artery calcification with electron-beam and conventional CT. *Eur Radiol* 1999;9:620–624.

21. Becker CR, Jakobs TF, Aydemir S, et al. Helical and single-slice conventional CT versus electron beam CT for the quantification of coronary artery calcification. *AJR Am J Roentgenol* 2000;174:543–547.

22. Carr JJ, Crouse JR III, Goff DC Jr, et al. Evaluation of subsecond gated helical CT for quantification of coronary artery calcium and comparison with electron beam CT. *AJR Am J Roentgenol* 2000;174:915–921.

23. Goldin JG, Yoon HC, Greaser LE III, et al. Spiral versus electron-beam CT for coronary artery calcium scoring. *Radiology* 2001;221:213–221.

24. Becker CR, Kleffel T, Crispin A, et al. Coronary artery calcium measurement: Agreement of multirow detector and electron beam CT. *AJR Am J Roentgenol* 2001;176:1295–1298.

25. Rumberger JA, Simons DB, Fitzpatrick LA, et al. Coronary artery calcium area by electron-beam computed tomography and coronary atherosclerotic plaque area: a histopathologic correlative study. *Circulation* 1995;92:2157–2162.

26. Sangiorgi G, Rumberger JA, Severson A, et al. Arterial calcification and not lumen stenosis is highly correlated with atherosclerotic plaque burden in humans: a histologic study of 723 coronary artery segments using nondecalcifying methodology. *J Am Coll Cardiol* 1998;31:126–133.

27. Janowitz WR, Agatston AS, Kaplan G, et al. Differences in prevalence and extent of coronary artery calcium detected by ultrafast computed tomography in asymptomatic men and women: Relation to age and risk factors. *Am J Cardiol* 1993;72:247–254.

28. Ikeda T Shirasawa T, Esaki Y, et al. Osteopontin mRNA is expressed by smooth muscle-derived foam cells in human atherosclerotic lesions of the aorta. *J Clin Invest* 1993;92:2814–2820.

29. Fitzpatrick LA, Severson A, Edwards WD, et al. Diffuse calcification in human coronary arteries: association of osteopontin with atherosclerosis. *J Clin Invest* 1994;94:1597–1604.

30. Hirota S, Imakita M, Kohri K, et al. Expression of osteopontin messenger RNA by macrophages in atherosclerotic plaques: a possible association with calcification. *Am J Pathol* 1993;143:1003–1008.

31. Glagov S, Weisenberg BA, Zarins CK, et al. Compensatory enlargement of human atherosclerotic coronary arteries. *N Engl J Med* 1987;316:1371–1375.

32. Agatston AS, Janowitz WR, Hildner FJ, et al. Quantification of coronary artery calcium using ultrafast computed tomography. *J Am Coll Cardiol* 1990;15:827–832.

33. Budoff MJ, Georgiou D, Brody A, et al. Ultrafast computed tomography as a diagnostic modality in the detection of coronary artery disease: a multicenter study. *Circulation* 1996;93:898–904.

34. Detrano R, Hsiai T, Wang S, et al. Prognostic value of coronary calcification and angiographic stenoses in patients undergoing coronary angiography. *J Am Coll Cardiol* 1996;27:285–290.

35. Fallavollita JA, Brody AS, Bunnell IL, et al. Fast computed tomography detection of coronary calcification in the diagnosis of coronary artery disease: comparison with angiography in patients <50 years old. *Circulation* 1994;89:285–290.

36. Baumgart D, Schmermund A, George G, et al. Comparison of electron beam computed tomography with intracoronary ultrasound and coronary angiography for detection of coronary atherosclerosis. *J Am Coll Cardiol* 1997;30:57–64.

37. Schmermund A, Baumgart D, Gorge D, et al. Coronary artery calcium in acute coronary syndromes: a comparative study of electron-beam computed tomography, coronary angiography, and intracoronary ultrasound in survivors of acute myocardial infarction and unstable angina. *Circulation* 1997;96:1461–1469.

38. Kennedy J, Shavelle R, Wang S, et al. Coronary calcium and standard risk factors in symptomatic patients referred for coronary angiography. *Am Heart J* 1998;135:696–702.

39. Bielak LF, Rumberger JA, Sheedy PF, et al. Probabilistic model for prediction of angiographically defined obstructive coronary artery disease using electron beam computed tomography calcium score strata. *Circulation* 2000;102:380–385.

40. Shavelle DM, Budoff MJ, LaMont DH, et al. Exercise testing and electron beam computed tomography in the evaluation of coronary artery disease. *J Am Coll Cardiol* 2000;36:32–38.

41. Haberl R, Becker A, Leber A, et al. Correlation of coronary calcification and angiographically documented stenoses in patients with suspected coronary artery disease: results of 1,764 patients. *J Am Coll Cardiol* 2001;37:451–457.

42. Breen JF, Sheedy PF, Schwartz RS, et al. Coronary artery calcification detected with ultrafast CT as an indication of coronary artery disease. *Radiology* 1992;185:435–439.

43. Bielak LF, Kaufmann RB, Moll PP, et al. Small lesions in the heart identified at electron beam CT. Calcification or noise? *Radiology* 1994;192:631–636.

44. Kaufmann RB, Sheedy PF, Maher JE, et al. Quantity of coronary artery calcium detected by electron beam computed tomography in asymptomatic subjects and angiographically studied patients. *Mayo Clin Proc* 1995;70:223–232.

45. Rumberger JA, Sheedy PF, Breen JF, et al. Coronary calcium, as determined by electron beam computed tomography, and coronary disease on arteriogram: effect of patient's sex on diagnosis. *Circulation* 1995;91:1363–1367.

46. Braun J, Oldendorf M, Moshage W, et al. Electron beam computed tomography in the evaluation of cardiac calcification in chronic dialysis patients. *Am J Kidney Dis* 1996;27:394–401.

47. Knollmann FD, Bocksch W, Spiegelsberger S, et al. Electron-beam computed tomography in the assessment of coronary artery disease after heart transplantation. *Circulation* 2000;101:2078–2082.

48. Rumberger JA, Sheedy PF, Breen JF, et al. Electron beam computed tomographic coronary calcium score cutpoints and severity of associated angiographic lumen stenosis. *J Am Coll Cardiol* 1997;29:1542–1548.

49. Guerci AD, Spadaro LA, Goodman KJ, et al. Comparison of electron beam computed tomography scanning and conventional risk factor assessment for the prediction of angiographic coronary artery disease. *J Am Coll Cardiol* 1998;32:673–679.

50. Budoff MJ, Diamond GA, Raggi P, et al. Continuous probabilistic prediction of angiographically significant coronary artery disease using electron beam tomography. *Circulation* 2002;105:1791–1796.

51. Schmermund A, Bailey KR, Rumberger JA, et al. An algorithm for noninvasive identification of angiographic three-vessel and/or left main coronary artery disease in symptomatic patients on the basis of cardiac risk and electron-beam computed tomographic calcium scores. *J Am Coll Cardiol* 1999;33:444–452.

52. He ZX, Hedrick TD, Pratt CM, et al. Severity of coronary artery calcification by electron beam computed tomography predicts silent myocardial ischemia. *Circulation* 2000;101:244–251.

53. Blumenthal RS, Becker DM, Moy TF, et al. Exercise thallium tomography predicts future clinically manifest coronary heart disease in a high-risk asymptomatic population. *Circulation* 1996;93:915–923.

54. Fleg JL, Gerstenblith G, Zonderman AB, et al. Prevalence and prognostic significance of exercise-induced silent myocardial ischemia detected by thal-

lium scintigraphy and electrocardiography in asymptomatic volunteers. *Circulation* 1990;81:428–436.

55. Iskandrian AS, Chae SC, Heo J, et al. Independent and incremental prognostic value of exercise single-photon emission computed tomographic (SPECT) thallium imaging in coronary artery disease. *J Am Coll Cardiol* 1993;22:665–670.

56. Hachamovitch R, Berman DS, Kiat H, et al. Exercise myocardial perfusion SPECT in patients without known coronary artery disease: incremental prognostic value and use in risk stratification. *Circulation* 1996;93:905–914.

57. Berman DS, Wong ND, Gransar H, et al. Relationship between stress-induced myocardial ischemia and atherosclerosis measured by coronary calcium tomography. *J Am Coll Cardiol* 2004;44(4):923–930.

58. Brindis RG, Douglas PS, Hendel RC, et al. ACCF/ASNC appropriateness criteria for single-photon emission computed tomography myocardial perfusion imaging (SPECT MPI): a report of the American College of Cardiology Foundation Quality Strategic Directions Committee Appropriateness Criteria Working Group and the American Society of Nuclear Cardiology endorsed by the American Heart Association. *J Am Coll Cardiol* 2005;46:1587–1605.

59. Ekelund L-G, Suchindran CM, McMahon RP, et al. Coronary heart disease morbidity and mortality in hypercholesterolemic men predicted from an exercise test: The Lipid Research Clinics Coronary Primary Prevention Trial. *J Am Coll Cardiol* 1989;14:556–563.

60. Gibbons RJ, Abrams J, Chatterjee K, et al. ACC/AHA 2002 guideline update for the management of patients with chronic stable angina—summary article: a report of the American College of Cardiology/American Heart Association Task Force on Practice Guidelines (Committee on the Management of Patients With Chronic Stable Angina). *J Am Coll Cardiol* 2003;41:159–168.

61. Emond M, Mock MB, David KR, et al. Long-term survival of medically treated patients in the Coronary Artery Surgery Study (CASS) Registry. *Circulation* 1994;90:2645–2657.

62. Goldstein JA, Demetriou D, Grines CL, et al. Multiple complex coronary plaques in patients with acute myocardial infarction. *N Engl J Med* 2000;343:915–922.

63. Huang H, Virmani R, Younis H, et al. The impact of calcification on the biomechanical stability of atherosclerotic plaques. *Circulation* 2001;103:1051–1056.

64. Mascola A, Ko J, Bakhsheshi H, et al. Electron beam tomography comparison of culprit and nonculprit coronary arteries in patients with acute myocardial infarction. *Am J Cardiol* 2000;85:1357–1359.

65. Heller LI, Tresgallo M, Sciacca RR, et al. Prognostic significance of silent myocardial ischemia on a thallium stress test. *Am J Cardiol* 1990;65:718–721.

66. Detrano R, Hsiai T, Wang S, et al. Prognostic value of coronary calcification and angiographic stenoses in patients undergoing coronary angiography. *J Am Coll Cardiol* 1996;27:285–290.

67. Keelan PC, Bielak LF, Ashai K, et al. Long-term prognostic value of coronary calcification detected by electron-beam computed tomography in patients undergoing coronary angiography. *Circulation* 2001;104:412–417.

68. Greenland P, LaBree L, Azen SP, et al. Coronary artery calcium score combined with Framingham score for risk prediction in asymptomatic individuals. *JAMA* 2004;291:210–215.

69. Arad Y, Spadaro LA, Goodman K, et al. Prediction of coronary events with electron beam computed tomography. *J Am Coll Cardiol* 2000;36:1253–1260.

70. Wong ND, Hsu JC, Detrano RC, et al. Coronary artery calcium evaluation by electron beam computed tomography and its relation to new cardiovascular events. *Am J Cardiol* 2000;86:495–498.

71. Raggi P, Callister TQ, Cooil B, et al. Identification of patients at increased risk of first unheralded acute myocardial infarction by electron-beam computed tomography. *Circulation* 2000;101:850–855.

72. Wayhs R, Zelinger A, Raggi P. High coronary artery calcium scores pose an extremely elevated risk for hard events. *J Am Coll Cardiol* 2002;39:225–230.

73. Kondos GT, Hoff JA, Sevrukov A, et al. Electron-beam tomography coronary artery calcium and cardiac events: a 37-month follow-up of 5635 initially asymptomatic low- to intermediate-risk adults. *Circulation* 2003;107:2571–2576.

74. Arad Y, Roth M, Newstein D, et al. Coronary calcification, coronary risk factors, and atherosclerotic cardiovascular disease events. The St. Francis Heart Study. *J Am Coll Cardiol* 2005;46:158–165.

75. Shaw LJ, Raggi P, Schisterman E, et al. Prognostic value of cardiac risk factors and coronary artery calcium screening for all-cause mortality. *Radiology* 2003;28:826–833.

76. Taylor AJ, Bindeman J, Feuerstein I, Cao F, Brazaitis M, O'Malley PG. Coronary calcium independently predicts incident premature coronary heart disease over measured cardiovascular risk factors. *J Am Coll Cardiol* 2005;46:807–814.

77. Vliegenthart R, Oudkerk M, Hofman A, et al. Coronary calcification improves cardiovascular risk prediction in the elderly. *Circulation* July 26, 2005;112(4):572–577.

78. LaMonte MJ, FitzGerald SJ, Church TS, et al. Coronary artery calcium score and coronary heart disease events in a large cohort of asymptomatic men and women. *Am J Epidemiol* 2005;162:1–9.

79. Becker A, Knez A, Becker C, et al. Prediction of serious cardiovascular events by determining coronary artery calcification measured by multi-slice computed tomography. *Dtsch Med Wochenschr* October 28, 2005130(43):2433–2438.

80. Anand DV, Lim E, Hopkins D, et al. Risk stratification in uncomplicated type 2 diabetes: prospective evaluation of the combined use of coronary artery calcium imaging and selective myocardial perfusion scintigraphy. *Eur Heart J* March 1, 2006;27(6):713–721. Epub Feb 23, 2006.

81. Park R, Detrano R, Xiang M, et al. Combined use of computed tomography coronary calcium scores and C-reactive protein levels in predicting cardiovascular events in nondiabetic individuals. *Circulation* 2002;106:2073–2077.

82. Budoff MJ, Yang TP, Shavelle RM, et al. Ethnic differences in coronary atherosclerosis. *J Am Coll Cardiol* 2002;39:408–412.

83. Califf RM, Armstrong PW, Carver JR, et al. Task Force 5. Stratification of patients into high, medium and low risk subgroups for purposes of risk factor management. *J Am Coll Cardiol* 1996;27:1007–1019.

84. Wilson PWF, D'Agostino RB, Levy D, et al. Prediction of coronary heart disease using risk factor categories. *Circulation* 1998;97:1837–1847.

85. Wong ND, Kouwabunpat D, Vo AN, et al. Coronary calcium and atherosclerosis by ultrafast computed tomography in asymptomatic men and women: relation to age and risk factors. *Am Heart J* 1994;127:422–430.

86. Newman AB, Naydeck BL, Sutton-Tyrrell K, et al. Coronary artery calcification in older adults to age 99: prevalence and risk factors. *Circulation* 2001;104:2679–2684.

87. Hecht HS, Superko HR, Smith LK, et al. Relation of coronary artery calcium identified by electron beam tomography to serum lipoprotein levels and implications for treatment. *Am J Cardiol* 2001;87:406–412.

88. Kuller LH, Matthews KA, Sutton-Tyrrell K, et al. Coronary and aortic calcification among women 8 years after menopause and their premenopausal risk factors: the healthy women study. *Arterioscler Thromb Vasc Biol* 1999;19:2189–2198.

89. Hecht HS, Superko HR. Electron beam tomography and national cholesterol education program guidelines in asymptomatic women. *J Am Coll Cardiol* 2001;37:1506–1511.

90. Callister TQ, Raggi P, Cooil B, Lippolis NJ, Russo DJ. Effect of HMG-CoA reductase inhibitors on coronary artery disease as assessed by electron beam computed tomography. *N Engl J Med* 1998;339:1972–1978.

91. Budoff MJ, Lane KL, Bakhsheshi H, et al. Rates of progression of coronary calcification by electron beam computed tomography. *Am J Cardiol* July 1, 2000;1;86(1):8–1.

92. Raggi P, Cooil B, Shaw L, et al. Progression of coronary calcification on serial electron beam tomography scanning is greater in patients with future myocardial infarction. *Am J Cardiol* 2003;92:827–829.

93. Raggi P, Callister TQ, Shaw LJ. Progression of coronary artery calcium and risk of first myocardial infarction in patients receiving cholesterol-lowering therapy. *Arterioscler Thromb Vasc Biol* July 2004;24(7):1272–1774.

94. Bild DE, Bluemke DA, Burke GL, et al. Multi-ethnic study of atherosclerosis: objectives and design. *Am J Epidemiol* 2002;156:871–881.

95. Kajinami K, Seki H, Takekoshi N, et al. Quantification of coronary artery calcification using ultrafast computed tomography: reproducibility of measurements. *Coron Artery Dis* 1993;4:1103–1108.

96. Devries S, Wolfkiel C, Shah V, et al. Reproducibility of the measurement of coronary calcium with ultrafast computed tomography. *Am J Cardiol* 1995;75:973–975.

97. Yoon HC, Goldin JG, Greaser LE III, et al. Interscan variation in coronary artery calcium quantification in a large asymptomatic patient population. *AJR Am J Roentgenol* 2000;174:803–809.

98. Wang S, Detrano RC, Secci A, et al. Detection of coronary calcification with electron-beam computed tomography: Evaluation of interexamination reproducibility and comparison of three image-acquisition protocols. *Am Heart J* 1996;132:550–558.

99. Achenbach S, Ropers D, Mohlenkamp S, et al. Variability of repeated coronary artery calcium measurements by electron beam tomography. *Am J Cardiol* 2001;87:210–213.

100. Bielak LF, Sheedy PF, Peyser PA. Coronary artery calcification measured at electron-beam CT. Agreement in dual scan runs and change over time. *Radiology* 2001;218:224–229.

101. Mao S, Budoff MJ, Bakhsheshi H, et al. Improved reproducibility of coronary artery calcium scoring by electron beam tomography with a new electrocardiographic trigger method. *Invest Radiol* 2001;36:363–367.

102. Callister TQ, Cooil B, Raya SP, et al. Coronary artery disease: improved reproducibility of calcium scoring with an electron-beam CT volumetric method. *Radiology* 1998;208:807–814.

103. Budoff MJ, Lane KL, Bakhsheshi H, et al. Rates of progression of coronary calcium by electron beam tomography. *Am J Cardiol* 2000;86:8–11.

104. Maher JE, Bielak LF, Raz JA, et al. Progression of coronary artery calcification: a pilot study. *Mayo Clin Proc* 1999;74:347–355.

105. Budoff MJ, Shavelle DM, Lamont DH, et al. Usefulness of electron beam computed tomography scanning for distinguishing ischemic from nonischemic cardiomyopathy. *J Am Coll Cardiol* 1998;32:1173–1178.

106. Shemesh J, Tenenbaum A, Fisman EZ, et al. Coronary calcium as a reliable tool for differentiating ischemic from nonischemic cardiomyopathy. *Am J Cardiol* 1996;77:191–194.

107. McLaughlin VV, Balogh T, Rich S. Utility of electron beam computed tomography to stratify patients presenting to the emergency room with chest pain. *Am J Cardiol* 1999;84:327–328.

108. Laudon DA, Vukov LF, Breen JF, et al. Use of electron-beam computed tomography in the evaluation of chest pain patients in the emergency department. *Ann Emerg Med* 1999;33:15–21.

109. Georgiou D, Budoff MJ, Kaufer E, et al. Screening patients with chest pain in the emergency department using electron beam tomography: a follow-up study. *J Am Coll Cardiol* 2001;38:105–110.

110. Schmermund A, Baumgart D, Gorge D, et al. Coronary artery calcium in acute coronary syndromes: a comparative study of electron-beam computed tomography, coronary angiography, and intracoronary ultrasound in survivors of acute myocardial infarction and unstable angina. *Circulation* 1997;96:1461–1469.

111. Shemesh J, Stroh CI, Tenenbaum A, et al. Comparison of coronary calcium in stable angina pectoris and in first acute myocardial infarction utilizing double helical computerized tomography. *Am J Cardiol* 1998;81:271–275.

112. Schmermund A, Baumgart D, Adamzik M, et al. Comparison of electron-beam computed tomography and intracoronary ultrasound in detecting calcified and noncalcified plaques in patients with acute coronary syndromes and no or minimal to moderate angiographic coronary artery disease. *Am J Cardiol* 1998;81:141–146.

113. Budoff MJ, Achenbach S, Blumenthal RS, et al. Assessment of coronary artery disease by cardiac computed tomography, a scientific statement from the American Heart Association Committee on Cardiovascular Imaging and Intervention, Council on Cardiovascular Radiology and Intervention, and Committee on Cardiac Imaging, Council on Clinical Cardiology. *Circulation* 2006;114(16):1761–1791.

114. Noto TJ Jr, Johnson LW, Krone R, et al. Cardiac catheterization 1990: a report of the Registry of the Society for Cardiac Angiography and Interventions. *Cathet Cardiovasc Diagn* 1991;24(2):75–83.

115. Bashore TM, Bates ER, Berger PB, et al. American College of Cardiology/Society for Cardiac Angiography and Interventions Clinical Expert Consensus Document on cardiac catheterization laboratory standards. A report of the American College of Cardiology Task Force on Clinical Expert Consensus Documents. *J Am Coll Cardiol* 2001;37(8):2170–2214.

116. Coronary angioplasty versus medical therapy for angina: the second Randomised Intervention Treatment of Angina (RITA-2) trial. RITA-2 trial participants. *Lancet* 1997;350(9076):461–468.

117. Pitt B, Waters D, Brown WV, et al. Aggressive lipid-lowering therapy compared with angioplasty in stable coronary artery disease: Atorvastatin versus Revascularization Treatment Investigators. *N Engl J Med* 1999;341(2):70–76.

118. Ehara M, Surmely JF, Kawai M, et al. Diagnostic accuracy of 64-slice computed tomography for detecting angiographically significant coronary artery stenosis in an unselected consecutive patient population: comparison with conventional invasive angiography. *Circ J* 2006;70(5):564–571.

119. Leber AW, Knez A, von Ziegler F, et al. Quantification of obstructive and nonobstructive coronary lesions by 64-slice computed tomography: a comparative study with quantitative coronary angiography and intravascular ultrasound. *J Am Coll Cardiol* 2005;46(1):147–154.

120. Leschka S, Alkadhi H, Plass A, et al. Accuracy of MSCT coronary angiography with 64-slice technology: first experience. *Eur Heart J* 2005;26(149):1482–1487.

121. Mollet NR, Cademartiri F, van Mieghem CA, et al. High-resolution spiral computed tomography coronary angiography in patients referred for diagnostic conventional coronary angiography. *Circulation* 2005;112(149):2318–2323.

122. Nikolaou K, Knez A, Rist C, et al. Accuracy of 64-MDCT in the diagnosis of ischemic heart disease. *AJR Am J Roentgenol* 2006;187(1):111–117.

123. Pugliese F, Mollet NR, Runza G, et al. Diagnostic accuracy of noninvasive 64-slice CT coronary angiography in patients with stable angina pectoris. *Eur Radiol* 2006;16(3):575–582.

124. Raff GL, Gallagher MJ, O'Neill WW, Goldstein JA. Diagnostic accuracy of noninvasive coronary angiography using 64-slice spiral computed tomography. *J Am Coll Cardiol* 2005;46(3):552–557.

125. Ropers D, Rixe J, Anders K, et al. Usefulness of multidetector row spiral computed tomography with 64- x 0.6-mm collimation and 330-ms rotation for the noninvasive detection of significant coronary artery stenoses. *Am J Cardiol* 2006;97(3):343–348.

126. Schuijf JD, Pundziute G, Jukema JW, et al. Diagnostic accuracy of 64-slice multislice computed tomography in the noninvasive evaluation of significant coronary artery disease. *Am J Cardiol* 2006;98(2):145–148.

127. Lu B, Mao SS, Zhuang N, et al. Coronary artery motion during the cardiac cycle and optimal ECG triggering for coronary artery imaging. *Invest Radiol* 2001;36(5):250–256.

128. Hendel RC, Patel MR, Kramer CM, et al. ACCF/ACR/SCCT/SCMR/ASNC/NASCI/SCAI/SIR 2006 appropriateness criteria for cardiac computed tomography and cardiac magnetic resonance imaging: a report of the American College of Cardiology Foundation Quality Strategic Directions Committee Appropriateness Criteria Working Group, American College of Radiology, Society of Cardiovascular Computed Tomography, Society for Cardiovascular Magnetic Resonance, American Society of Nuclear Cardiology, North American Society for Cardiac Imaging, Society for Cardiovascular Angiography and Interventions, and Society of Interventional Radiology. *J Am Coll Cardiol* 2006;48(7):1475–1497.

129. Anders K, Baum U, Schmid M, et al. Coronary artery bypass graft (CABG) patency: assessment with high-resolution submillimeter 16-slice multidetector-row computed tomography (MDCT) versus coronary angiography. *Eur J Radiol* 2006;57(3):336–344.

130. Stauder NI, Kuttner A, Schroder S, et al. Coronary artery bypass grafts: assessment of graft patency and native coronary artery lesions using 16-slice MDCT. *Eur Radiol* 2006;16(11):2512–2520.

131. Pache G, Saueressig U, Frydrychowicz A, et al. Initial experience with 64-slice cardiac CT: noninvasive visualization of coronary artery bypass grafts. *Eur Heart J* 2006;27(8):976–980.

132. Martuscelli E, Romagnoli A, D'Eliseo A, et al. Evaluation of venous and arterial conduit patency by 16-slice spiral computed tomography. *Circulation* 2004;110(20):3234–3238.

133. Chiurlia E, Menozzi M, Ratti C, Romagnoli R, Modena MG. Follow-up of coronary artery bypass graft patency by multislice computed tomography. *Am J Cardiol* 2005;95(9):1094–1097.

134. Kefer JM, Coche E, Vanoverschelde JL, Gerber BL. Diagnostic accuracy of 16-slice multidetector-row CT for detection of in-stent restenosis vs detection of stenosis in nonstented coronary arteries. *Eur Radiol* January 2007;17(1):87–96. Epub May 30, 2006.

135. Kitagawa T, Fujii T, Tomohiro Y, et al. Noninvasive assessment of coronary stents in patients by 16-slice computed tomography. *Int J Cardiol* 2006;109(2):188–194.

136. Ohnuki K, Yoshida S, Ohta M, et al. New diagnostic technique in multi-slice computed tomography for in-stent restenosis: pixel count method. *Int J Cardiol* 2006;108(2):251–258.

137. Gilard M, Cornily JC, Pennec PY, et al. Assessment of coronary artery stents by 16 slice computed tomography. *Heart* 2006;92(1):58–61.

138. Gaspar T, Halon DA, Lewis BS, et al. Diagnosis of coronary in-stent restenosis with multidetector row spiral computed tomography. *J Am Coll Cardiol* 2005;46(8):1573–1579.

139. Pump H, Mohlenkamp S, Sehnert CA, et al. A coronary arterial stent patency: assessment with electron-beam CT. *Radiology* February 2000;214(2):447–452.

140. Lu B, Dai RP, Bai H, et al. Detection and analysis of intracoronary artery stent after PTCA using contrast-enhanced three-dimensional electron beam tomography. *J Invasive Cardiol* 2000;12:1–6.

141. Mahnken AH, Muhlenbruch G, Seyfarth T, et al. 64-slice computed tomography assessment of coronary artery stents: a phantom study. *Acta Radiol* 2006;47(1):36–42.

142. Groves AM, Win T, Charman SC, Wisbey C, Pepke-Zaba J, Coulden RA. Semi-quantitative assessment of tricuspid regurgitation on contrast-enhanced multidetector CT. *Clin Radiol* 2004;59(8):715–719.

143. Feuchtner GM, Dichtl W, Schachner T, et al. Diagnostic performance of MDCT for detecting aortic valve regurgitation. *AJR Am J Roentgenol* 2006;186(6):1676–1681.

144. Feuchtner GM, Dichtl W, Friedrich GJ, et al. Multislice computed tomography for detection of patients with aortic valve stenosis and quantification of severity. *J Am Coll Cardiol* 2006;47(7):1410–1417.

145. Alkadhi H, Wildermuth S, Plass A, et al. Aortic stenosis: comparative evaluation of 16-detector row CT and echocardiography. *Radiology* 2006;240(1):47–55.

146. Budoff MJ, Ahmed V, Gul KM, Mao SS, Gopal A. Coronary anomalies by cardiac computed tomographic angiography. *Clin Cardiol* 2006;29:489–493.

147. Angelini P, Velasco JA, Flamm S. Coronary anomalies: incidence, pathophysiology, and clinical relevance. *Circulation* 2002;105(20):2449–2454.

148. Eckart RE, Scoville SL, Campbell CL, et al. Sudden death in young adults: a 25-year review of autopsies in military recruits. *Ann Intern Med* 2004;141(11):829–834.

149. Shi H, Aschoff AJ, Brambs HJ, Hoffmann MH. Multislice CT imaging of anomalous coronary arteries. *Eur Radiol* 2004;14(12):2172–2181.

150. Schmitt R, Froehner S, Brunn J, et al. Congenital anomalies of the coronary arteries: imaging with contrast-enhanced, multidetector computed tomography. *Eur Radiol* 2005; 15(6):1110–1121.

151. Datta J, White CS, Gilkeson RC, et al. Anomalous coronary arteries in adults: depiction at multi-detector row CT angiography. *Radiology* 2005;235(3):812–818.

152. Ling LH, Oh JK, Tei C, et al. Pericardial thickness measured with transesophageal echocardiography: feasibility and potential clinical usefulness. *J Am Coll Cardiol* 1997;29:1317–1323.

153. Oren RM, Grover-McKay M, Stanford W, et al. Accurate preoperative diagnosis of pericardial constriction using cine computed tomography. *J Am Coll Cardiol* 1993;22:832–838.

154. Doppman JL, Rienmuller R, Lissner J, et al. Computed tomography in constrictive pericardial disease. *J Comput Assist Tomogr* 1981;5:1–11.

155. Tomoda H, Hoshiai M, Furuya H, et al. Evaluation of pericardial effusion with computed tomography. *Am Heart J* 1980;99:701–706.

156. Baim RS, MacDonald IL, Wise DJ, et al. Computed tomography of absent left pericardium. *Radiology* 1980;135:127–128.

157. Moncada R, Baker M, Salinas M, et al. Diagnostic role of computed tomography in pericardial heart disease: congenital defects, thickening, neoplasms and effusions. *Am Heart J* 1982;103:263–282.

158. Glazer GM, Gross BH, Oringer MB, et al. Computed tomography of pericardial masses. *J Comput Assist Tomogr* 1984;8:895–899.

159. Farmer DW, Lipton MJ, Webb WR, et al. Computed tomography in congenital heart disease. *J Comput Assist Tomogr* 1984;8:677–687.

160. Webb WR, Gansu G, Speckman G, et al. CT demonstration of mediastinal aortic arch anomalies. *J Comput Assist Tomogr* 1982;6:445–451.

161. Aboulhosn J, Oudiz RJ. Congenital heart disease and computed tomography. In: Budoff M, Shinbane J, eds. *Cardiac CT Imaging: Diagnosis of Cardiovascular Disease,* 1st ed. London, UK: Springer, 2006.

162. Gilkeson RC, Ciancibello L, Zahka K. Pictorial essay: multidetector CT evaluation of congenital heart disease in pediatric and adult patients. *AJR Am J Roentgenol* 2003;180(4):973–980.

163. Bean MJ, Pannu H, Fishman EK. Three-dimensional computed tomographic imaging of complex congenital cardiovascular abnormalities. *J Comput Assist Tomogr* 2005;29(6):721–724.

164. Rius T, Goyenechea M, Poon M. Combined cardiac congenital anomalies assessed by multi-slice spiral computed tomography. *Eur Heart J* 2006; 98;27(6):637.

165. MacMillan RM, Shakriari A, Sumithisena F, et al. Contrast enhanced cine computed tomography for the diagnosis of right coronary to coronary sinus arteriovenous fistulae. *Am J Cardiol* 1985;56:997–999.

166. MacMillan RM, Rees MR, Eldredge WJ, et al. Quantitation of shunting at the atrial level using rapid acquisition computed tomography with comparison to cardiac catheterization. *J Am Coll Cardiol* 1986;7:946–948.

167. Skotvicki R, Maranhao V, Clark D, et al. Detection of atrial septal defect by cine CT scanning. *Cathet Cardiovasc Diagn* 1986;12:103–106.

168. Aboulhosn J, Shavelle DM, Matthews R, French WJ, Buljubasic N, Budoff MJ. Images in cardiology: electron beam angiography of percutaneous atrial septal defect closure. *Clin Cardiol* 2004;27:702.

169. Bateman TM, Sethna DH, Whiting JS, et al. Comprehensive noninvasive evaluation of left atrial myxoma using cardiac cine-computed tomography. *J Am Coll Cardiol* 1987;9:1180–1183.

170. Tada H, Shimizu W, Ohe T, et al. Usefulness of electron-beam computed tomography in arrhythmogenic right ventricular dysplasia: relationship to electrophysiological abnormalities and left ventricular involvement. *Circulation* 1996;94:437–444.

171. Shinbane JS, Budoff MJ. CT imaging: cardiac electrophysiologic applications. In: Budoff M, Shinbane J, eds. *Cardiac CT Imaging: Diagnosis of Cardiovascular Disease,* 1st ed. London, UK: Springer, 2006.

172. Nienaber CA, von Kodolitsch Y, Nicolas V. The diagnosis of thoracic aortic dissection by noninvasive imaging procedures. *N Engl J Med* 1993;328:1–9.

173. Sommer T, Fehske W, Holzknecht N, et al. Aortic dissection: a comparative study of diagnosis with spiral CT, multiplanar transesophageal echocardiography, and MR imaging. *Radiology* 1996;199:347–352.

174. Stanford W. Ultrafast computed tomography in the diagnosis of aortic aneurysms and dissections. *J Thorac Imaging* 1990;5:32–39.

175. Cremer J, Teebken OE, Simon A, et al. Thoracic computed tomography prior to redo coronary surgery. *Eur J Cardiothorac Surg* 1998;13:650–654.

176. Remy-Jardin M, Remy J, Deschildre F, et al. Diagnosis of pulmonary embolism with spiral CT: comparison with pulmonary angiography and scintigraphy. *Radiology* 1996;200:699–706.

177. Mayo JR, Remy-Jardin M, Muller NL, et al. Pulmonary embolism: prospective comparison of spiral CT with ventilation perfusion scintigraphy. *Radiology* 1997;205:447–452.

178. Teigen CL, Maus TP, Sheedy PF, et al. Pulmonary embolism diagnosis with contrast-enhanced electron-beam CT and comparison with pulmonary angiography. *Radiology* 1995;194:313–319.

179. Galvin JR, Gingrich RD, Hoffman E, Kao SC, Stern EJ, Stanford W. Ultrafast computed tomography of the chest. *Radiol Clin North Am* 1994;32:775–793.

180. Stanford W, Reiners TJ, Thompson BH, et al. Contrast enhanced thin slice ultrafast computed tomography for the detection of small pulmonary emboli in the pig. *Invest Radiol* 1994;29:184–187.

181. Moser KM, Auger WR, Fedullo PF. Chronic major-vessel thromboembolic pulmonary hypertension. *Circulation* 1990;81:1735.

182. Kuriyama K, Gamsu G Stern RG, et al. CT determined pulmonary artery diameters in predicting pulmonary hypertension. *Invest Radiol* 1984;19:16.

183. Nikolaou K, Knez A, Sagmeister S, et al. Assessment of myocardial infarctions using multidetector-row computed tomography. *J Comput Assist Tomogr* 2004;28(2), 286–292.

184. Wada H, Kobayashi Y, Yasu T, et al. Multi-detector computed tomography for imaging of subendocardial infarction: prediction of wall motion recovery after reperfused anterior myocardial infarction. *Circ J* 185;68(5):512–515.

185. Mahnken AH, Koos R, Katoh M, et al. Assessment of myocardial viability in reperfused acute myocardial infarction using 16-slice computed tomography in comparison to magnetic resonance imaging. *J Am Coll Cardiol* 186;45(12): 2042–2042.

186. Budoff MJ, Cohen MC, Garcia MJ, et al. ACCF/AHA clinical competence statement on cardiac imaging with computed tomography and magnetic resonance: A report of the American College of Cardiology Foundation/American Heart Association/American College of Physicians Task Force on Clinical Competence and Training. *J Am Coll Cardiol* 2005;46:383–402.

CHAPTER (21)

Magnetic Resonance Imaging of the Heart

Han W. Kim / Wolfgang G. Rehwald /
James A. White / Raymond J. Kim

In the last decade, cardiovascular magnetic resonance (CMR) imaging has changed dramatically. Technical and clinical advances have expanded CMR imaging from primarily a tomographic imaging modality, providing static images of morphology, to one that is dynamic, allowing the rapid, high-resolution imaging of ventricular function, valvular motion, and myocardial perfusion. Moreover, CMR is now considered the gold standard for the assessment of regional and global systolic function, myocardial infarction and viability, and the assessment of congenital heart disease. The aims of this chapter are to provide an introduction to the technical aspects of CMR imaging and to provide an overview of the clinical applications that are available to clinicians today.

BASIC PRINCIPLES

Similar to other medical imagining techniques, magnetic resonance imaging (MRI) acquires images through the transmission and receiving of energy. However, unlike other modalities, MRI offers the capability to modulate both the emitted and received signals so that a multitude of tissue characteristics can be examined and differentiated without the need to change scanner hardware. As a result, from a single imaging session, one could obtain cardiac function and morphology, myocardial perfusion and viability, hemodynamics, large vessel anatomy, and so forth. This information, however, is gathered not from a single long acquisition, but rather from multiple short acquisitions, each requiring different pulse sequences (software programs that drive

the scanner) with specific operational parameters and optimal settings. Additionally, magnetic resonance (MR) vendors may use proprietary names for these pulse sequences and settings.[1,2] Thus the goal of this section will be to clarify these issues and to provide a simple framework of the technical aspects of MRI.

[ ] MAGNETIC RESONANCE PHYSICS

It is important to recognize that an MRI scanner is not a single device, but rather consists of multiple separate components. A schematic of these components is shown in Fig. 21–1. A detailed explanation of each of these components is beyond the scope of this chapter, however, a basic understanding is useful. For instance, poor image quality can arise from a variety of problems, and the ability to quickly distinguish those that are complex (e.g., hardware malfunction that requires servicing) from those that are simple (e.g., motion artifact that can be immediately resolved by better communication with the patient) will be highly valuable.

An MRI scanner performs three basic operations (Fig. 21–2): (1) the generation of a static magnetic field, (2) the transmission of energy within the radiofrequency (RF) range to the patient, and (3) the reception of the MR signal following the transmission of RF energy. Most clinical CMR imaging scanners today have a static magnetic field strength (B_0) of 1.5 tesla (T), which is 30,000 times stronger than the earth's magnetic field. This high magnetic-field strength is generated by a superconducting magnet that is housed within the MRI scanner itself. When a patient is placed within the bore of the scanner, hydrogen

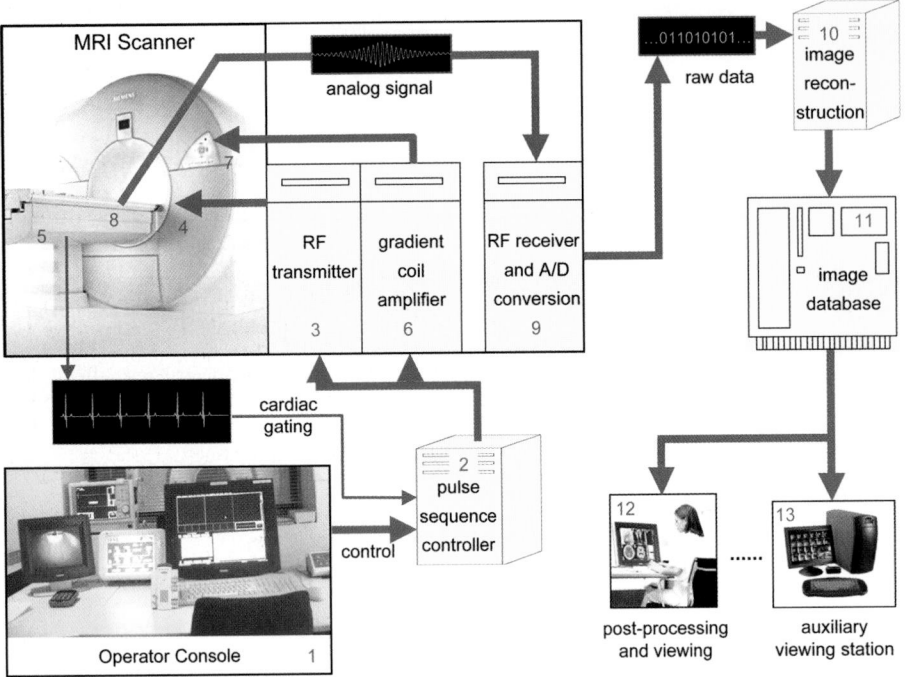

FIGURE 21–1. Components of the MRI scanner. For a cardiovascular magnetic resonance (CMR) imaging study, the operator defines the type of examination and manipulates the imaging parameters from a control computer console using a graphical user interface (*1*). Software, known as a pulse sequence, is selected from a menu to acquire images that are appropriate for the diagnostic question. The precisely timed radiofrequency (RF) pulses, used to stimulate tissues, are generated by the pulse sequence controller (*2*), RF transmitter (*3*), and RF coil (*4*). For CMR imaging, the electrocardiogram signal (*5*) from the patient is often used for timing. Spatial image information is encoded by the gradient coil amplifier (*6*) and gradient coil (*7*), which alter the net magnetic field (B_0) of the MRI scanner. The magnetic resonance (MR) signal from the body is detected from fixed receiver coil arrays (*8*) that are built into the patient table and from flexible arrays that can be placed on top of the patient. These received signals, which are usually analog, are processed and digitized by an analog-digital converter (*9*) and then passed to a computer dedicated to image reconstruction (*10*). The final images are then stored in a image database or picture archiving and communication system (PACS) (*11*) and can undergo post-processing at a workstation (*12*) and interpretation at auxiliary viewing stations (*13*). A/D, analog-to-digital.

protons within the patient's body align parallel or antiparallel to the static magnetic field. More protons align parallel to the field than against the field, leading to a small net magnetization vector (see Fig. 21–2A). The equilibrium distribution of parallel and antiparallel protons is predicted by the classical Boltzmann distribution. While aligned in the magnetic field, these protons rotate or precess about the field (in the same way a spinning top precesses in a gravitational field) at a rate known as the *Larmor frequency*. This frequency (ω_o) depends on magnetic field strength (B_0) and a nuclei specific physical constant, known as the gyromagnetic ratio (γ), by the formula, $\omega_o = \gamma B_0$. For hydrogen protons precessing in a 1.5 T magnetic field, the Larmor frequency is 63.9 MHz, which is in the radiofrequency range.

The next step toward image generation is the transmission of energy to the region of interest. Importantly, transmission of energy to the precessing hydrogen protons is only possible when the frequency is equal to the Larmor frequency (i.e., on resonance). With the absorption of the energy from the RF pulse, the net magnetization vector is tilted from its equilibrium orientation parallel to the static magnetic field (longitudinal direction) into the transverse plane. The angle of displacement of the net magnetization vector is known as the *flip angle* (see Fig. 21–2B) and can be varied depending on the pulse sequence. Rotation of the precessing net magnetization vector into the transverse plane results in the creation of a time-varying magnetic field. This vary-

ing magnetic field induces an alternating current in the receiver coil arrays in the same manner that a spinning electromagnetic generator produces electricity. The signal created from a single RF excitation is illustrated in Fig. 21–2C and is known as a *free induction decay* (FID).

Following the RF excitation, two independent relaxation processes return the net magnetization vector to its thermal equilibrium (realigned with the static magnetic field; Fig. 21–3). The first process, known as longitudinal or spin-lattice relaxation, describes the regrowth of the magnetization vector parallel to the static magnetic field (see Fig. 21–3A). Longitudinal relaxation time (T1) results from the transfer of energy from the excited protons to surrounding molecules in the local environment. The time constant, T1, describes the exponential regrowth of longitudinal magnetization. The second process, known as *transverse* or *spin-spin relaxation*, describes the decay of the magnetization vector in the transverse (X-Y) plane (see Fig. 21–3B). Transverse relaxation time (T2) can take place with or without energy dissipation. For example, the transfer of energy leading to longitudinal relaxation also results in transverse relaxation. Additionally, processes that simply cause proton spins to lose phase coherence without energy dissipation lead to transverse relaxation as well. The latter mechanism most commonly results from static or slowly fluctuating vari-

ations in the magnetic field within the imaged sample. The time constant, T2, describes the exponential decay of transverse magnetization. The T1 and T2 are intrinsic properties of any given tissue. Pulse sequences use differences in T1 and T2 to generate image contrast between tissues.

IMAGE ACQUISITION AND SIGNAL PROCESSING

The MR signals following RF excitation are localized in three-dimensional space by the use of magnetic fields generated by three sets of gradient coils (Fig. 21–4). These gradient coils alter the strength of the static magnetic field as a linear function of distance from the isocenter of the magnet in each of three orthogonal directions (X-, Y-, or Z-axes). The variation in field strengths across space produces differences in proton precessional frequencies along each axis. Specifically, to form a two-dimensional image, the gradients allow the selection of the slice of interest (e.g., slice encoding direction) and also modulate the MR signals to provide in-plane spatial information along the frequency encoding direction and the phase encoding direction. For slice selection, the slice-encoding gradient (Z-axis gradient for a transaxial slice) is played during RF excitation (see Fig. 21–4B). Because energy deposition

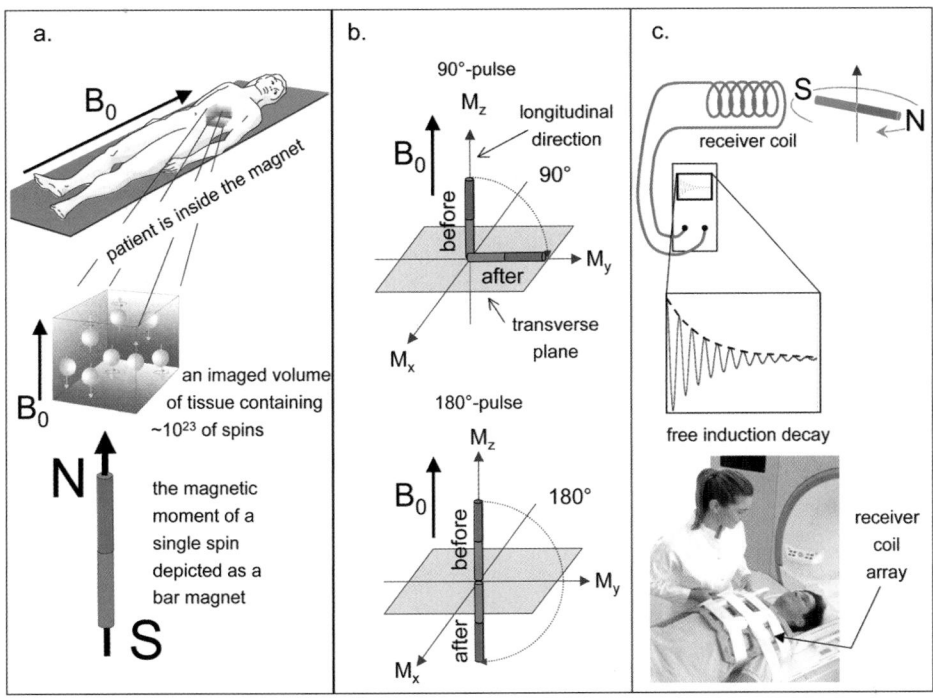

FIGURE 21–2. Basic operations of the MRI scanner. **A.** The static magnetic field (B_0). The protons align parallel or antiparallel to the static magnetic field creating a small net magnetization vector. While aligned to the magnetic field, the protons precess at the Larmor frequency. **B.** Transmission of radiofrequency (RF) energy. Energy is transmitted to the rotating protons by a RF pulse at the Larmor frequency. RF pulses that result in a flip angle of 90° and 180° are shown (*top and bottom, respectively*). The figures are presented in the rotating frame of reference, where the X-Y axes are rotating at the Larmor frequency and thus appear stationary. **C.** Generation of the magnetic resonance (MR) signal. Rotation of the net magnetization vector into the transverse plane results in the creation of a time-varying magnetic field, which in turn induces an alternating current in the receiver coil array, which is the MR signal.

is only possible on-resonance, altering the center frequency of the RF pulse varies the slice location. Increasing or decreasing the bandwidth of frequencies in the transmitted RF pulse increases or decreases the thickness of the imaged slice. For spatial localization in the frequency encoding direction, the X-axis gradient (for a transaxial slice) is played during MR signal receive (see Fig. 21–4C). As a result, specific frequency components of the MR signal arise directly from specific spatial locations along the X-axis. Spatial localization in the phase encoding direction is more difficult conceptually. The Y-axis gradient (for a transaxial slice) is played for a finite time before MR signal receive. This results in a phase shift in the precessing protons that varies with location along the Y-axis. Importantly, each image is the result of multiple MR signal readouts, each of which were preceded by a phase encoding gradient step with slight differences in the strength (amplitude) of the Y-axis gradient. After all the phase encoding steps are completed, the raw data from the scanner consists of a two-dimensional grid of data (also known as *k-space*), which is converted to an MR image by an inverse two-dimensional Fourier transform by the image reconstruction computer (see Fig. 21–1).

FIGURE 21–3. Longitudinal recovery and transverse decay following a 90° flip angle excitation. **A.** Longitudinal magnetization recovery (T1 relaxation). The green growth curve demonstrates the exponential regrowth of the longitudinal component of the net magnetization vector. **B.** Transverse magnetization decay (T2 relaxation). The red decay curve illustrates the exponential decline of the transverse component of the net magnetization vector. **C.** The net magnetization vector. The vector sum of the longitudinal and transverse components that comprise the net magnetization vector is shown.

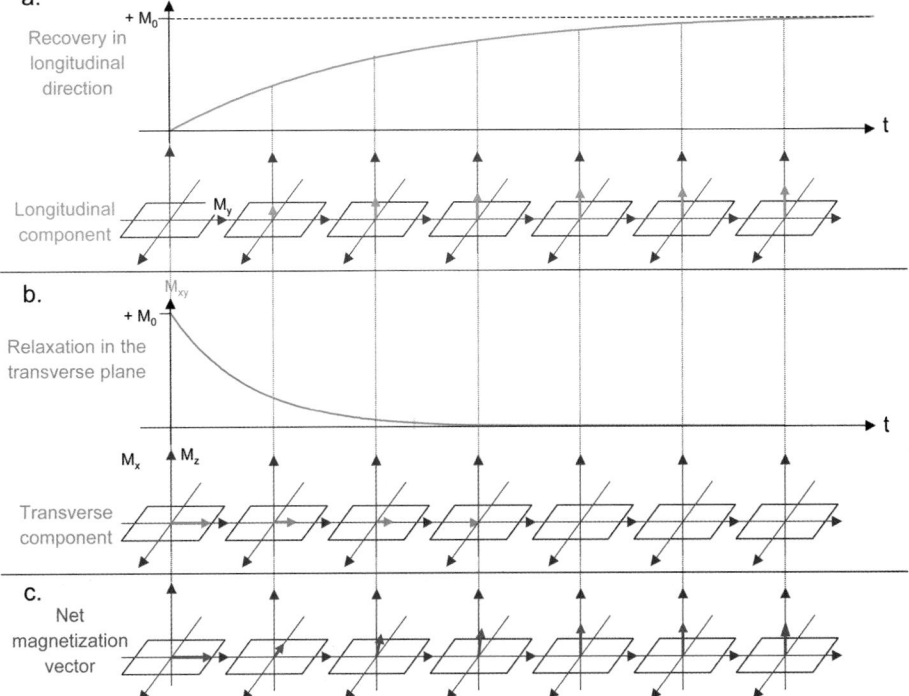

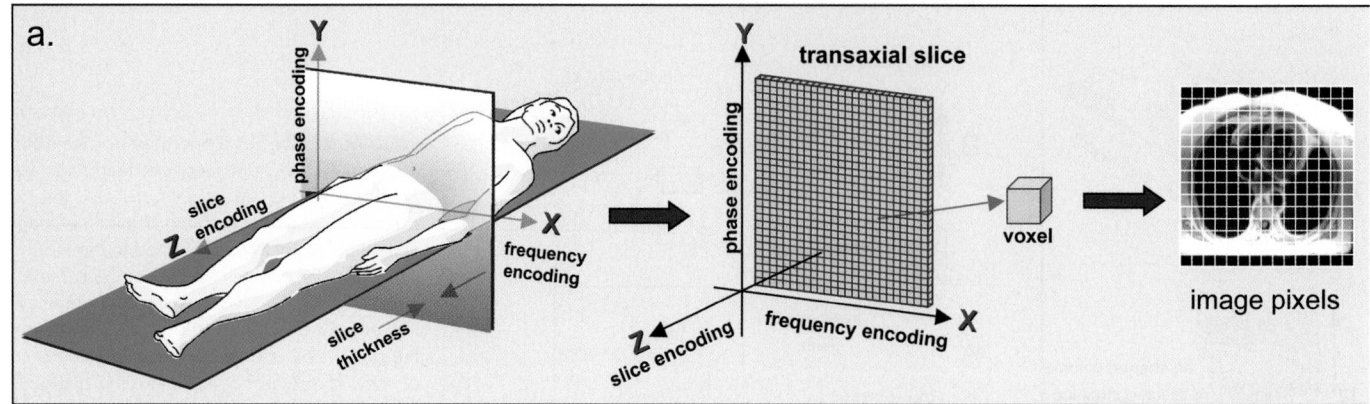

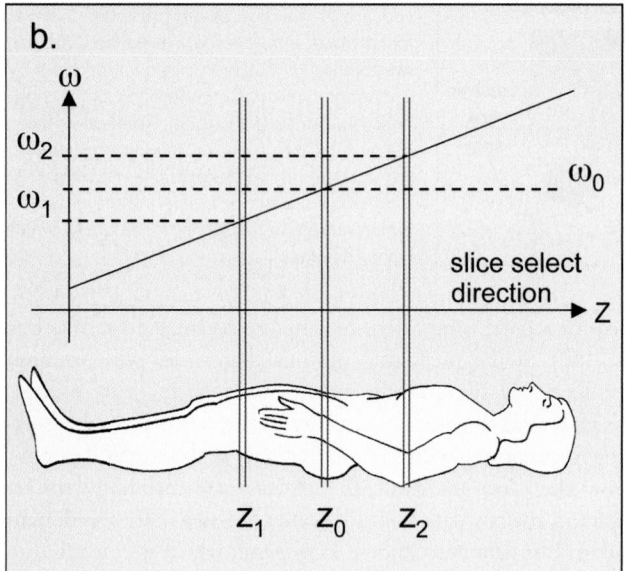

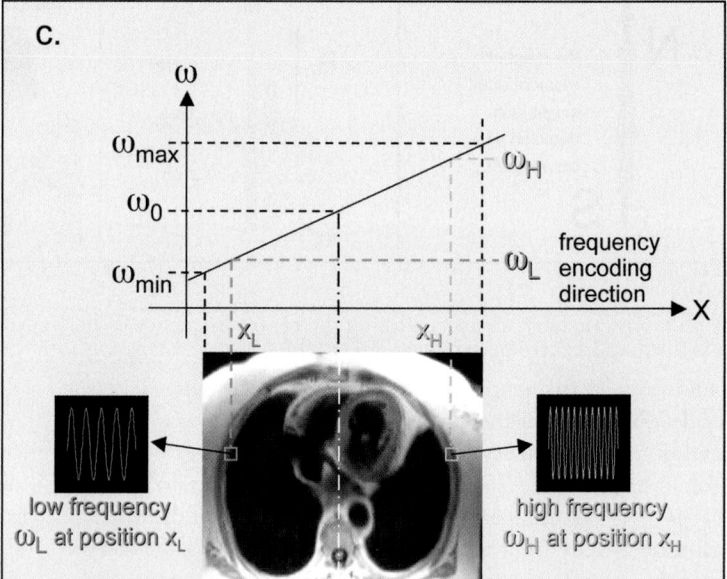

FIGURE 21–4. Spatial localization of the magnetic resonance (MR) signal. **A.** Orthogonal magnetic field gradients are used to localize the MR signal. The gradients are shown oriented for a transaxial imaging plane, however, the axes can be oriented orthogonally in any arbitrary direction. **B.** Slice selection. The radiofrequency (RF) pulse with center frequency ω_o excites proton spins located at position z_0 along the direction of the gradient when applied in the presence of the linear-slice select magnetic-field gradient. Changing the RF pulse center frequency to ω_1 or ω_2 shifts the location of the imaging slice to z_1 or z_2, respectively. **C.** Frequency encoding. During MR signal receive, the frequency encoding gradient alters the frequency of the MR signal depending on its position along the direction of the gradient. The MR signal from any given position has a unique frequency. In the example shown, frequency ω_L (or ω_H) is an MR signal from position X_L (or X_H).

【 】 CREATING CONTRAST IN MAGNETIC RESONANCE IMAGES

One of the important advantages of MRI is the ability to generate substantial soft-tissue contrast by the use of pulse sequences and the administration of contrast media. In general, pulse sequences are adjusted to emphasize differences in tissue T1 and T2, which can be inherent or altered by the presence of contrast media. For instance, on pulse sequences that are T1 weighted, tissues with short T1, such as fat, appear bright. Traditionally, T1 weighting is accomplished by imaging with short-RF repetition times (TR), which magnify differences in longitudinal recovery between tissues. Newer sequences use magnetization preparation pulses, such as saturation or inversion pulses to create improved T1 contrast (Fig. 21–5). An inversion (180°) compared with saturation (90°) prepulse provides greater T1 weighting, but the sequence is more prone to artifacts when gating is irregular (either because of ECG artifact or arrhythmia). T2-weighted pulse sequences are traditionally created using relatively long echo times (TEs). With long TE (on the order of tissue T2),

there is increased separation of different T2 relaxation curves, which translates into larger differences in image intensity.

The administration of intravenous contrast agents can also be used to affect image contrast by altering tissue T1 and/or T2. The magnitude of T1 and/or T2 change depends on the specific relaxivities of the contrast media, the distribution characteristics (i.e., intravascular, extracellular, or targeted to a specific tissue) and tissue perfusion. Gadolinium-based contrast media is commonly used in CMR imaging. Gadolinium is a lanthanide metal with seven unpaired electrons, making it strongly paramagnetic. When administered, it primarily shortens the T1 in the tissues where it is distributed (Fig. 21–6).

【 】 CARDIOVASCULAR MAGNETIC RESONANCE IMAGING SAFETY

The CMR imaging environment has the potential to pose serious risks to patients and facility staff in several ways. Injuries

a.

Saturation Recovery

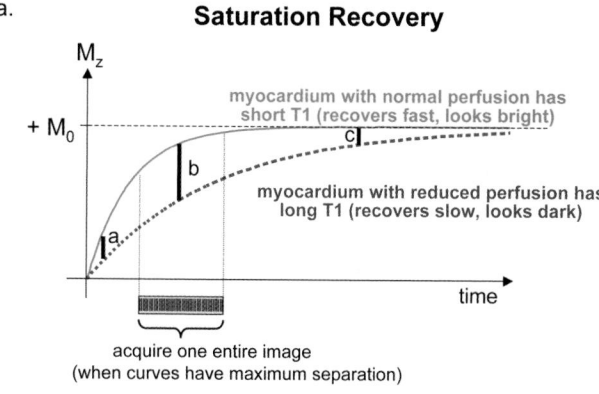

b.

Inversion Recovery

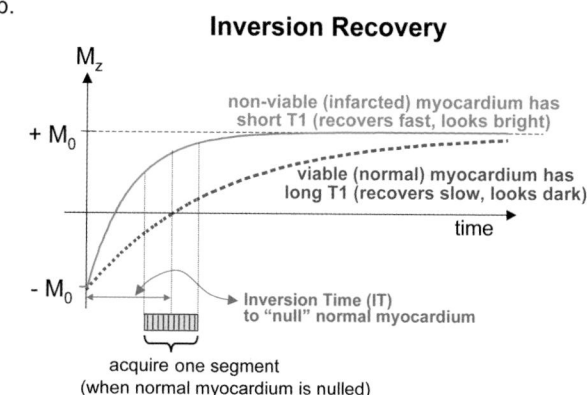

FIGURE 21–5. Magnetization preparation pulses to create T1 contrast. **A.** Saturation recovery. A 90° radiofrequency (RF) pulse followed by strong gradient spoilers reduces the net magnetization to zero. Magnetization recovers depending on tissue T1. For instance, immediately following intravenous bolus administration of gadolinium contrast, myocardium with normal perfusion has substantial uptake of gadolinium, thus has short T1, and appears bright on saturation recovery perfusion MRI. In comparison, myocardium with reduced perfusion has diminished uptake of gadolinium, longer T1, and appears dark. Ideally, data readout should follow the saturation pulse at a specific time (timepoint *b* rather than timepoint *a* or *c* to achieve maximum separation between the T1 relaxation curves of normal and abnormal myocardium. **B.** Inversion recovery. An 180° RF pulse inverts the longitudinal magnetization from the +z-axis to the –z-axis. Often used in infarct imaging, the time between the inversion pulse and the center of data readout (inversion time) is selected to accentuate the differences of gadolinium uptake in normal and infarcted myocardium. Specifically, the inversion time is chosen so that the center of image readout (for linear k-space acquisition) occurs when the T1 curve of normal myocardium crosses zero (e.g., nulled). Note that with this inversion time, the T1 curve of infarcted myocardium is above the zero crossing and infarcted tissue is bright.

can result from the static magnetic field (projectile impact injuries), very rapid gradient-field switching (induction of electric currents leading to peripheral nerve stimulation), RF-energy deposition (heating of the imaged portion of the body), and acoustic noise. The risks of projectile injuries from the static magnetic field are minimized by the institution of policies that strictly limit access to the magnet room. For instance, patients are extensively screened prior to imaging, and all facility personnel undergo dedicated training in MR safety. The use of *MR-safe* or compatible equipment (stethoscopes, wheelchairs, gurneys, oxygen tanks, infusion pumps, monitors, etc.) with clear labeling of such in the scanner area reduces this risk further. The Food and Drug Administration (FDA) has placed limits on the

rate of change of gradient magnetic fields (e.g., the slew rate) and the amount of RF energy (e.g., specific absorption rate [SAR]) that can be transmitted to patients. All scanners monitor the slew rate and calculate the SAR to help prevent nerve stimulation and heating. Acoustic noise of 100 dB or more are generated from the vibration or motion of the gradient coils during image acquisition. The use of protective hearing devices, such as headphones or earplugs, reduces noise to levels that do not result in hearing impairment or patient discomfort. In practice, continuous communication with the patient throughout the examination is important for patent comfort and safety.

Patients with medical devices or implants can face additional potential hazards, including device heating, movement, or malfunction. For example, ferromagnetic aneurysm clips or electronic medical devices (e.g., neural stimulators, insulin pumps) are strict contraindications to MRI. However, there is a specific subset of patients with a metallic implants or devices that can safely undergo MRI. A comprehensive list of devices and implants that are compatible with undergoing MRI scanning can be found elsewhere.[3,4] Regarding cardiac devices, it is important to note that prosthetic valves and coronary artery stents are now considered safe for MRI scanning.[3-5] Indeed, recently, the FDA approved the use of MRI immediately after the implantation of paclitaxel and sirolimus drug-eluting stents. At most institutions, MRI scans are not performed in patients with implanted pacemakers or defibrillators because of the potential risk of device malfunction, excessive device or lead heating, or induction of currents within the leads. Recently, however, a few preliminary reports have emerged, suggesting that MRI can be possible in patients with modern pacemakers and defibrillators in whom the benefits are deemed greater than the risks.[6-8] In patients in whom devices have been extracted, but with the leads remaining (both transvenous or epicardial), MRI is contraindicated as the risk of heating or induction of currents can be higher.

Recently, in several small case series, it has been reported that a small subset of patients with end-stage renal disease, receiving gadolinium contrast, may be at risk for developing nephrogenic systemic fibrosis (NSF).[145] NSF is characterized by an increased tissue deposition of collagen, often resulting in thickening and tightening of the skin and predominantly involving the distal extremities. Additionally, fibrosis may affect other organs, including skeletal muscles, lungs, pulmonary vasculature, heart, and diaphragm. Although a definitive causal link with gadolinium contrast agents has yet to be established, gadolinium contrast agents should be utilized cautiously (and alternative tests considered) in patients with severe renal disease, particularly those undergoing peritoneal dialysis or hemodialysis, or with acute renal failure. A policy statement regarding the use of gadolinium contrast agents in the setting of renal disease has been published by the American College of Radiology.[145]

THE CARDIOVASCULAR EXAMINATION

【 】 PULSE SEQUENCE STRUCTURE

Although a comprehensive review of pulse sequences is beyond the scope of this chapter, a brief discussion is presented to facilitate understanding of the basic framework of the CMR imaging exam-

T1-weighted T2-weighted

before contrast agent administration

normal (T1 ~ 880 ms) infarcted (T1 = 970 ms) normal (T2 ~ 75 ms) infarcted (T2 ~ 85 ms)

after contrast agent administration

normal (T1 ~ 430 ms) infarcted (T1 = 130 ms) normal (T2 ~ 70 ms) infarcted (T2 ~ 80 ms)

FIGURE 21–6. The effect of gadolinium contrast on T1- and T2-weighted imaging. Prior to contrast administration, there are minimal differences in inherent tissue T1 and T2 between normal and infarcted myocardium, thus infarction is poorly delineated (*top panel*). After gadolinium administration, the T1 of infarction (although not T2) is markedly shortened leading to clear delineation on the T1-weighted image (*bottom panel*). T1-weighted images were acquired using an inversion recovery gradient echo sequence. T2-weighted images were acquired using a dark blood turbo spin echo sequence.

FIGURE 21–7. MRI pulse-sequence structure. The MRI pulse sequence is composed of two separate elements: the *imaging engine* and *modifiers*. Typical images using different imaging engines and modifiers are shown (*bottom*). All images are of the same short-axis spatial location. See text for further information. FFE, fast-field echo; LV, left ventricular. *Source: Modified from Shaw DJ, Judd RM, Kim RJ,[9] with permission.*

IMAGING ENGINE

TYPE

Spin echo (SE)
- The first pulse sequence used to image the heart.
- Only a variant, turbo spin-echo (**TSE**), is used today. Used primarily to delineate morphology.

Gradient-recalled echo (GRE)
- Common work-horse sequence used for cine imaging (produces movies similar to echocardiography), dynamic perfusion imaging, vascular imaging, and delayed-enhancement imaging (**DE-MRI**), among others.

Echo-planar imaging (EPI)
- Rapid form of imaging usually combined with GRE.
- Often used for dynamic perfusion imaging.

Steady-state free precession (SSFP)
- The most recent technique. Also known as TrueFISP, FIESTA, Balanced FFE.
- The current gold standard technique for imaging ventricular morphology and function.
- Provides high signal-to-noise. Becoming a ubiquitous choice for cardiovascular imaging. Used for coronary, vascular, perfusion, and delayed-enhancement imaging, among others.

MODE

Single-shot
- Entire dataset for one image is acquired in a single continuous stream.
- Allows "real-time" or "snap-shot" imaging during free-breathing.
- Example includes half Fourier single-shot TSE (**HASTE**) for rapid morphologic imaging.

Segmented
- Dataset for one image is acquired piecemeal over several heartbeats.
- Allows imaging with high spatial resolution and high temporal resolution (a narrow window within the cardiac cycle).

EXAMPLE IMAGES

GRE **SSFP**

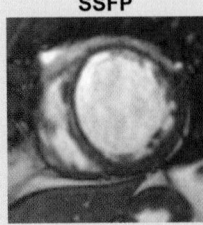

MODIFIERS

Black-blood
- Vascular structures (or cardiac chambers) with fast moving blood appear black.
- Slow flowing blood can be bright and hard to distinguish from cardiac or vascular structures (e.g. LV apex, false lumen of aortic dissection, etc).

Fat suppression
- Useful for diagnosis of cardiac and pericardial masses, right ventricular dysplasia, and to distinguish epicardial contrast hyperenhancement from fat.

Inversion prepulse
- Used to produce high levels of T1-weighting. Important component of delayed-enhancement imaging.

Saturation prepulse
- Also used for T1-weighting. Commonly used for dynamic perfusion imaging.

Tagging
- A saturation prepulse variant that labels the heart muscle with a dark grid. Useful to demonstrate intramural rotation, contraction, and strain.

Velocity-encoded
- Similar to echo Doppler techniques. Used for quantification of cardiac output, shunts, and valvular dysfunction.

Parallel imaging
- Recent method used to speed imaging at the cost of signal-to-noise. Can be combined with nearly all forms of cardiovascular imaging.
- Multiple variants are in use (e.g. SENSE, SMASH, etc).

EXAMPLE IMAGES

Black-blood **Inversion prepulse**

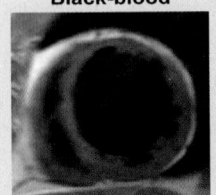

Tagging

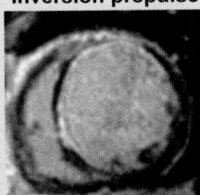

ination. An individual pulse sequence is a combination of radiofrequency pulses, magnetic gradient-field switches, and timed-data acquisitions, all applied in a precise order, that results in either accentuation or suppression of specific biological parameters. A simple way to conceptualize pulse sequences is to consider them as consisting of two separate elements: the *imaging engine* and associated *modifiers*.[9] The *imaging engine* is a required component that provides information regarding the spatial relationship of objects within the imaging field (i.e., the imaging engine is the main component that produces the image). *Modifiers* are optional components that can be added to the imaging engine either individually or in combination to provide specific information regarding tissue characteristics or to speed imaging. Fig. 21–7 lists some of the more commonly used imaging engines and modifiers in CMR imaging.

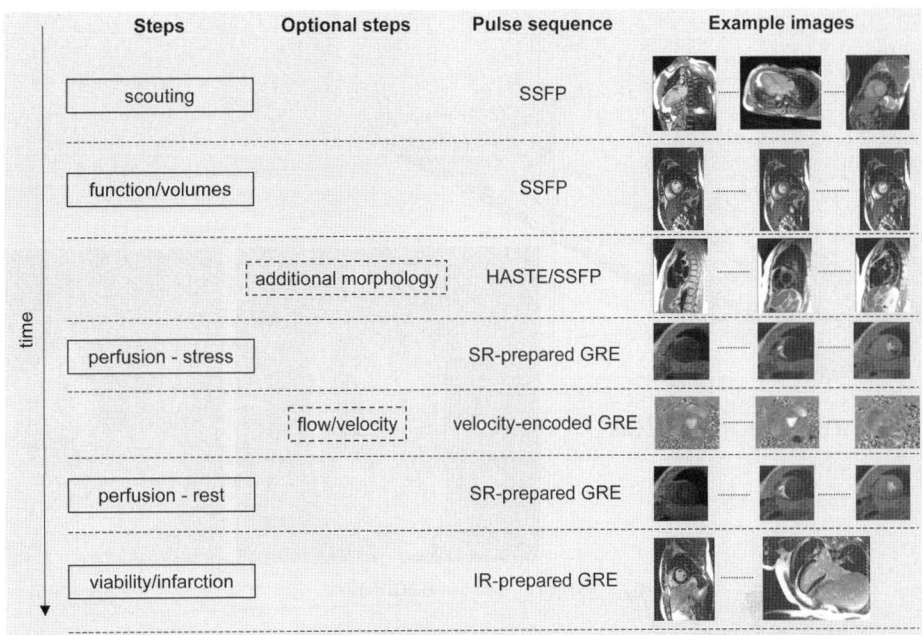

FIGURE 21–8. Typical cardiovascular magnetic resonance (CMR) imaging core examination with stress-testing. The protocol steps, associated pulse sequences, and the timeline of a typical core cardiovascular examination that includes stress-testing are depicted with example images. GRE, gradient-recall echo; HASTE, half-Fourier acquisition single-shot turbo spin-echo; SSFP, steady-state free precession.

【 】 THE CORE EXAMINATION

Fig. 21–8 depicts the protocol steps, associated pulse sequences, and the timeline of a typical core examination that includes stress-testing. Depending on the CMR-imaging study indications and the findings during the course of the examination, additional elements can be added to fully investigate the clinical question.

Scouting

Scouting is the first and simplest procedure to perform. The goal of scouting is to establish the short- and long-axis views of the heart. Because of patient anatomic variation both the short- and long-axis cardiac views lie at arbitrary angles with respect to scanner coordinates and are therefore referred to as *double oblique* planes. To obtain these views, a standard procedure should be followed (Fig. 21–9). Scout images are acquired using a single-shot imaging engine (steady-state free precession [SSFP] or half-Fourier acquisition single-shot turbo spin-echo [HASTE]) during free breathing.

Function and Volumes

The assessment of cardiac function and volumes is a fundamental component of the core examination. CineMRI, using a gradient recall echo (GRE)- or SSFP-imaging engine, has been shown to be highly accurate and reproducible in the measurement of ejection fraction, ventricular volumes, and cardiac mass.[10] In recent years, cineMRI has become widely accepted as the gold standard for the measurement of these parameters.[10] Moreover, it is also increasingly used as an endpoint in studies of left ventricular (LV) remodeling[11–13] and as a reference standard for other imaging techniques.[14,15]

The *goal* of cine imaging is to capture a movie of the beating heart to visualize its contractile function. Typically, between 20 and 25 cine frames are acquired per cardiac cycle with each frame comprising 35 to 45 milliseconds (ms). CineMRI can be acquired in either a *real-time* single-shot mode or by means of a segmented k-space data acquisition approach (see Fig. 21–7). Real-time cineMRI can be performed during free breathing and with minimal patient cooperation, making it ideal for children or patients who have difficulty following breathing instructions. Segmented cineMRI is performed during a breathhold and offers substantial improvement in image quality with superior spatial and temporal resolution compared to real-time imaging. Thus, in clinical practice, segmented imaging is usually preferred.[16,17] In segmented acquisition, data is collected over multiple, consecutive heartbeats (typically 5–10). During each heartbeat, blocks of data (segments) are acquired with reference to ECG timing, which represent the separate phases or frames of the cardiac cycle. Following the full acquisition, data from a given phase, collected from the multiple heartbeats, are combined to form the complete image of the particular cine frame.

Currently, the most common imaging engine for cineMRI is SSFP. The advantages over other sequences such as GRE include intrinsically high signal-to-noise ratio and excellent blood-myocardium contrast that facilitates the identification of the endocardial border.[18] For the core examination, a short-axis stack from the mitral-valve plane through the apex and two-, three-, and four-chamber long-axis views are obtained. In general, the slice thickness is 5 to 6 mm.

Perfusion at Stress and Rest

With recent technical and protocol advances, adenosine stress-perfusion MRI has changed status from a promising research tool to an everyday clinical test.[19] In part because of

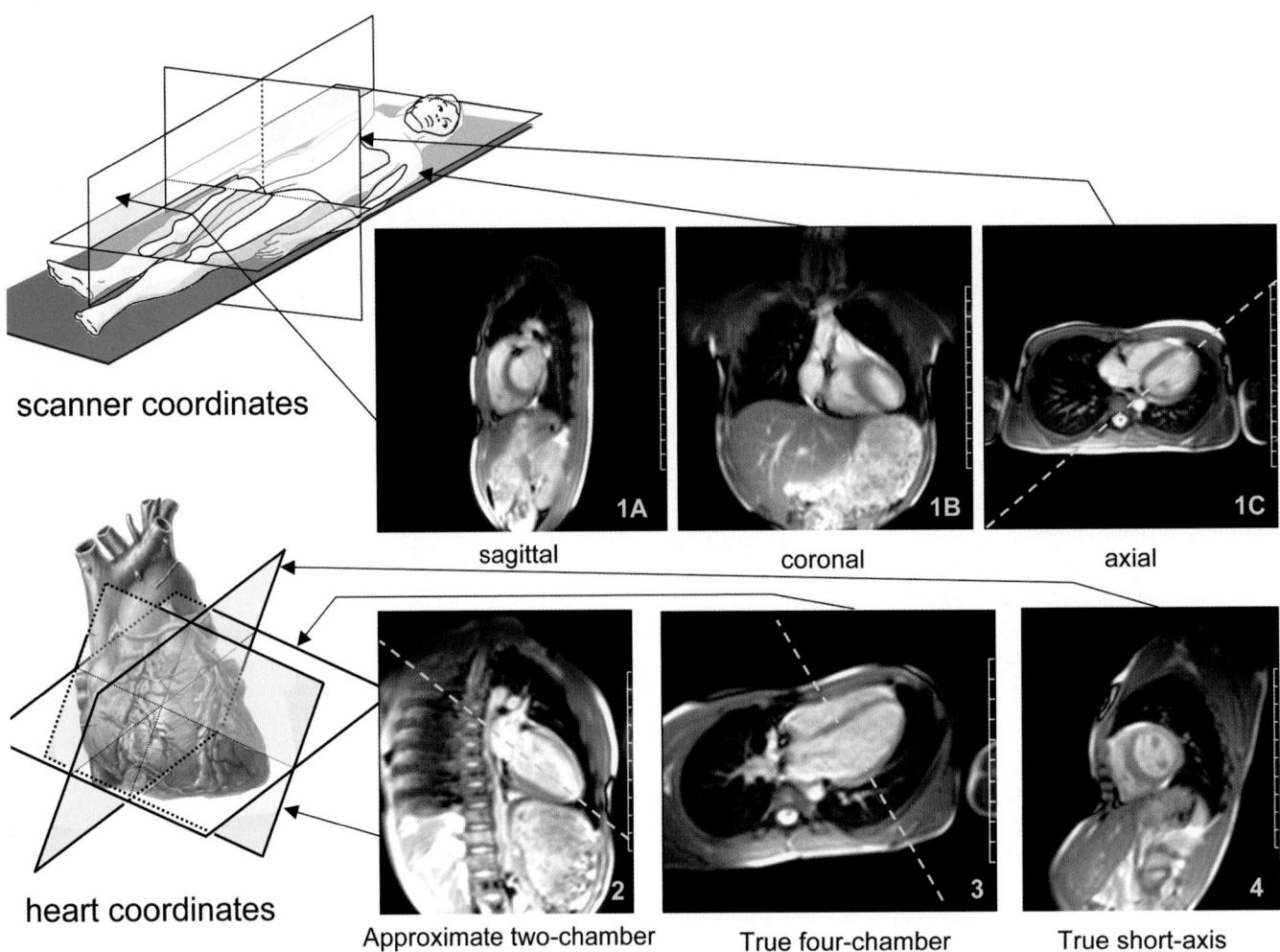

scanner coordinates

1A   sagittal

1B   coronal

1C   axial

heart coordinates

2   Approximate two-chamber

3   True four-chamber

4   True short-axis

FIGURE 21–9. Procedure for scouting. To establish the short- and long-axis planes of the heart, the following steps are followed. Step 1: Images are obtained along the scanner axes (sagittal, coronal, and axial; panels **1A**, **1B**, and **1C**, respectively). Step 2: From a pseudo–four-chamber, long-axis view (usually from the axial image), one prescribes a perpendicular plane through the approximate apex, which results in an approximate two-chamber view. Step 3: Another perpendicular plane is prescribed through the apex, which results in a true long-axis view (usually four-chamber). Step 4: A perpendicular plane, *breadloafing* the heart, delivers the true short-axis plane.

this transition, CMR imaging itself has changed from a modality that was used nearly exclusively for boutique indications such as cardiac neoplasms and arrhythmogenic right ventricular (RV) cardiomyopathy to one that is now considered a competitive first-line test for the most common indications including the assessment of ischemic heart disease.[20] Currently, in dedicated CMR-imaging clinical centers, perfusion stress-testing is often the fastest growing component of the clinical volume and can comprise nearly half of all referrals.[21] For these reasons, we have incorporated perfusion stress testing into the core examination.

The goal of perfusion imaging is to create a movie of the transit of contrast media (typically gadolinium based) with the blood during its initial pass through the LV myocardium (*first-pass contrast-enhancement*). Usually four to five short-axis views are obtained every heartbeat with a total of 40 to 60 heartbeats consisting of the entire first-pass (Fig. 21–10). Although more views could be obtained every two heartbeats, this is not recommended unless tachycardia is present, because clinically, the benefit of improving LV coverage does not outweigh the detri-

ment of halving the sampling frequency of the dynamic first-pass process.

A variety of pulse sequences are in use today for perfusion MRI, and the pace of development is rapid. Common *imaging engines* are SSFP, GRE, and GRE–echo-planar imaging (EPI) hybrid sequences (see Fig. 21–7). Virtually all sequences include a saturation prepulse modifier to provide T1 weighting and to accentuate regional differences in myocardial gadolinium concentration (see Fig. 21–5A). Because images are acquired in single-shot mode, a parallel imaging[22,23] *modifier* is essential to speed imaging and allow adequate LV coverage as well as reduced motion artifacts.[24] In general, image readout times more than 120 to 130 ms can lead to substantial motion artifacts in images acquired during periods of the cardiac cycle in which there is rapid LV motion.

The timeline for a comprehensive CMR-imaging stress test is displayed in Fig. 21–11. After scout and cine imaging, the patient table is pulled out partially to allow direct observation of the patient and full access; adenosine (140 μg kg⁻¹ • min⁻¹) is then infused under continuous electrocardiography and blood

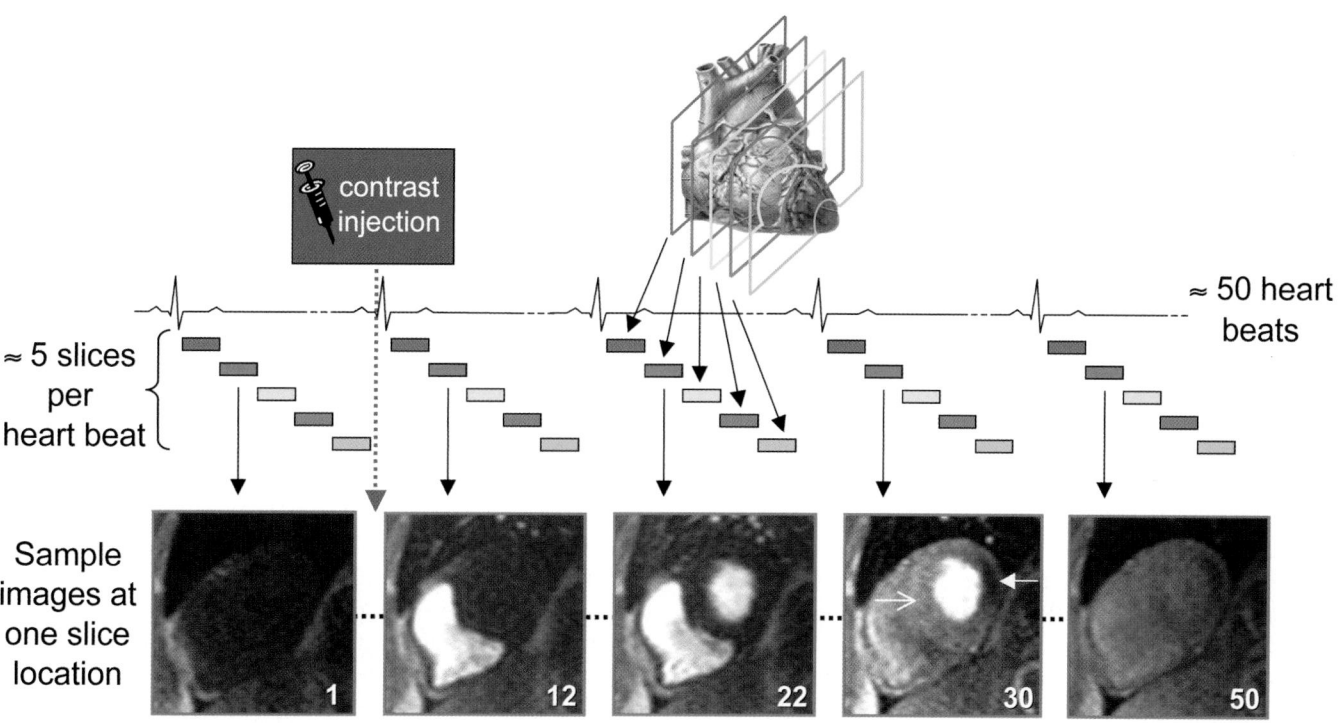

FIGURE 21–10. First-pass perfusion MRI acquisition. Images are acquired serially at multiple slice locations (usually four to five short-axis views for left ventricular coverage) every heartbeat to depict the passage of a compact contrast bolus as it transits the heart. Example images of one slice location are shown at several representative timepoints: before arrival of contrast (*frame 1*); contrast in right ventricular (RV) cavity (*frame 12*); contrast in left ventricular (LV) cavity (*frame 22*); peak contrast in LV myocardium (*frame 30*), showing normal perfusion in the septum (*open arrowhead*) and abnormal perfusion in the inferolateral wall (*solid arrowhead*); and the contrast wash-out phase (*frame 50*).

pressure monitoring for at least 2 minutes prior to the initiation of perfusion imaging. The perfusion sequence is then applied by the scanner operator, resulting in automatic recentering of the patient back in the scanner bore and commencement of imaging. Gadolinium contrast (0.075 to 0.10 mmol/kg body weight) is then administered followed by a saline flush (≈50 mL) at a rate of at least 3 mL/s by means of an antecubital vein. On the console, the perfusion images are observed as they are acquired, with breath-holding starting from the appearance of contrast in the RV cavity. If the scanner software does not provide real-time image display, breath-holding should be started no more than 5 to 6 seconds after beginning gadolinium injection. Breath-holding is performed to ensure the best possible image quality (i.e., no artifacts because of respiratory motion) during the initial wash-in of contrast into the LV myocardium. Once the contrast bolus has transited the LV myocardium, adenosine is stopped, and imaging is completed 5 to 10 seconds

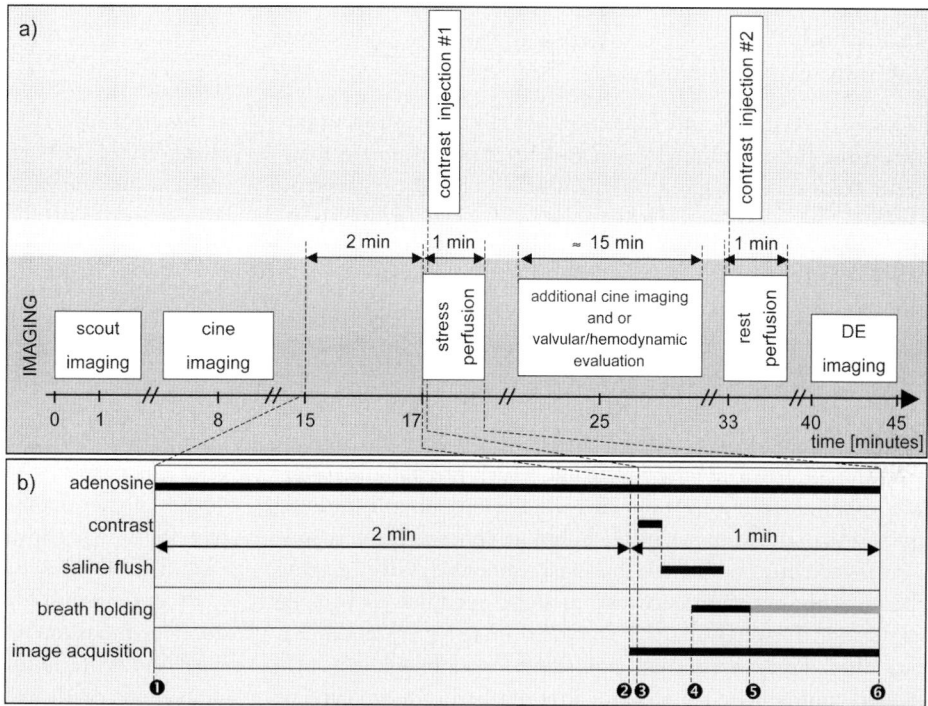

FIGURE 21–11. Timeline for the comprehensive cardiovascular magnetic resonance (CMR) imaging stress test. DE, delayed enhancement MRI.

later. Typically, the total imaging time is 40 to 50 seconds, and the total time of adenosine infusion is 3 to 3.5 minutes.

Prior to the rest perfusion scan, a waiting period of approximately 15 minutes is required for gadolinium to sufficiently clear from the blood pool. During this time, additional cine scans and or velocity/flow imaging for valvular or hemodynamic evaluation can be performed. For the rest perfusion scan an additional dose of 0.075 to 0.10 mmol/kg gadolinium is given, and the imaging parameters are identical to the stress scan. Approximately 5 minutes after rest perfusion, delayed enhancement imaging (see next section, Viability and Infarction) can be performed. The total scan time for a comprehensive CMR-imaging stress test, including cine imaging, stress and rest perfusion, and delayed enhancement is usually well under 45 minutes.

Unlike vasodilator radionuclide imaging in which adenosine is typically infused for 6 minutes (tracer injection at 3 minutes), stress-perfusion MRI is performed using an abbreviated adenosine protocol (~3 minutes) because the requirements for imaging are different.[19] With radionuclide imaging, maintaining a vasodilated state for 2 to 3 minutes after tracer injection is necessary to allow time for tracer uptake into myocytes. In contradistinction, with MRI, currently available gadolinium media are inert, extracellular agents that do not cross sarcolemmal membranes,[25] and vasodilation needs to be maintained only for the initial first-pass through the myocardium. Although severe reactions to adenosine are rare, a shortened protocol is relevant because moderate reactions that affect patient tolerability are relatively commonplace.[26] A minimum 2-minute infusion duration was chosen on the basis of physiologic studies in humans demonstrating that maximum coronary blood flow is reached, on average, 1 minute after the start of intravenous adenosine infusion (140 µg kg^{-1} • min^{-1}) and in nearly everyone by 2 minutes.[27]

Viability and Infarction

Myocardial viability and infarction are simultaneously examined using the technique known as delayed enhancement magnetic resonance imaging (DEMRI).[28–32] In the literature, DEMRI is used interchangeably with late gadolinium-enhancement CMR imaging or delayed hyperenhancement imaging. Although at first glance, the utility of DEMRI appears to be limited to those with coronary artery disease, new applications are steadily arising over a wide range of cardiovascular disorders. Thus, DEMRI is an essential component of the core examination.

The goal of DEMRI is to create images with high contrast between abnormal myocardial tissue, which generally accumulates excess gadolinium (following intravenous administration), and normal tissue in which gadolinium concentration is low. This is currently best achieved using a segmented, GRE imaging engine with inversion recovery prepulse modifier to provide very strong T1 weighting.[28–32] A parallel imaging[22,23] modifier is also often used to shorten acquisition time. Imaging is performed approximately 5 minutes after rest perfusion-imaging or 10 to 15 minutes after a one-time intravenous gadolinium dose of 0.15 to 0.20 mmol/kg if stress-rest perfusion imaging is not

performed. Short- and long-axis views in the identical planes used for cine imaging are obtained during repeated 6- to 10-second breath-holds. Data acquisition (readout period) is timed with the ECG in mid-diastole to minimize cardiac motion. Only every other heartbeat is used for data collection to allow for adequate recovery of longitudinal relaxation between inversion pulses (if bradycardia is present, imaging can occur every heartbeat).[33]

Following an intravenous bolus, gadolinium distributes throughout the intravascular and interstitial space, while simultaneously being cleared by the kidneys. In normal myocardium, where the myocytes are densely packed, tissue volume is predominately intracellular (~75–80 percent of the water space).[34] Because gadolinium is unable to penetrate intact sarcolemmal membranes,[25] the volume of distribution is small, and one can consider viable myocytes as actively excluding gadolinium media. In acute myocardial infarction, myocyte membranes are ruptured, allowing gadolinium to passively diffuse into the intracellular space. This results in an increased gadolinium volume of distribution, and thus increased tissue concentration compared with normal myocardium.[35–37] Similarly in chronic infarction, as necrotic tissue is replaced by collagenous scar, the interstitial space is expanded, and gadolinium tissue concentration is increased.[37]

Higher tissue concentrations of gadolinium lead to shortened T1 relaxation. Thus, when parameters are set properly, T1-weighted sequences such as used for DEMRI can depict infarcted regions as bright or *hyperenhanced* whereas viable regions appear black or *nulled* (see Fig. 21–6). One of the most important parameters to set correctly for DEMRI is the time between the inversion prepulse and data readout, known as the inversion time. The acronym commonly used is "*TI*", but to avoid confusion with T1 (longitudinal relaxation time) we prefer the use of "*IT*." Fig. 21–5B demonstrates that to maximize contrast between infarcted and viable myocardium, IT should be set to when the T1 curve of viable myocardium crosses zero. In general, once the optimal IT has been determined, no adjustment is necessary if DEMRI is completed in approximately 5 minutes. However, it is important to keep in mind that gadolinium gradually washes out of viable myocardium, and IT will need to be adjusted upwards if DEMRI is performed at multiple time points after contrast administration.[33]

Compared with other imaging techniques that are currently used to assess myocardial viability, an important advantage of DEMRI is the high spatial resolution. With a standard implementation, a group of 10 hyperenhanced pixels (voxel resolution ~1.9 × 1.4 × 6 mm) in a DEMRI image would represent an infarction of 0.16 gram, or a region one-thousandth of the left ventricular mass.[32] This level of resolution, which is more than 40-fold higher than single-photon emission computed tomography (SPECT), allows visualization of even microinfarcts that cannot be detected by other imaging methods.[31,38]

Recently an ultrafast, real-time version of DEMRI has been developed that can acquire snap-shot images during free-breathing.[39,40] This technique uses an SSFP imaging engine in single-shot mode with parallel-imaging acceleration, and provides complete LV coverage in less than 30 seconds. This technique could be considered the preferred approach in patients more acutely ill, unable to breath-hold, or with irregular heart rhythm. However, compared with standard, segmented DEMRI, sensitivity for detecting myocardial infarction is mildly reduced, and the transmural extent of infarction can be underestimated.[40]

Additional Imaging

Morphology Occasionally, additional structural/anatomic information is necessary to fully investigate the clinical question, such as in the setting of congenital heart disease, cardiac masses, or patients with aortic root dilation on initial three-chamber cineMRI. In general, a *morphology* scan consists of a series of parallel slices, which *bread-loaf* the anatomic region of interest (Figure 21–27A). Although any orientation can be imaged, usually axial, sagittal, or coronal planes (or all three) are chosen first.

Morphology imaging is primarily performed in single-shot mode using either an SSFP or turbo-spin echo (TSE) imaging engine. In its native form (without additional modifiers), SSFP produces images in which blood in the cardiac chambers and vasculature appear bright; thus it is known as a *bright-blood* technique. To first order, SSFP images are T2/T1 weighted.[30] In contrast, spin-echo based sequences such as TSE produce images in which flowing blood is dark; thus, these are known as *black-blood* techniques. However, blood signal suppression can be incomplete, and a black-blood modifier, which consists of a double-inversion prepulse,[41] is often added to improve blood nulling. A single-shot version of TSE that is commonly used in cardiovascular imaging is black-blood HASTE.

With SSFP or HASTE morphologic imaging, the entire thorax can be imaged in multiple orthogonal views in less than 2 minutes without breathholding. The choice between SSFP and HASTE is made depending on the clinical question and whether bright- or black-blood contrast is desired. Occasionally, small structures can be obscured on SSFP imaging by bright signal from the blood. Conversely, stagnant blood flow by virtue of incomplete suppression can be mistaken as tissue on HASTE imaging. Accordingly, both techniques should be performed when images from one are inconclusive, because the time cost is minimal. If higher spatial resolution is desired for certain key views, segmented cineMRI or segmented TSE can be performed during a breath-hold. Black-blood sequences should be performed before gadolinium administration because shortening blood T1 will impair the suppression of blood signal. SSFP sequences can be performed either before or after gadolinium administration.

Flow/Velocity Depending on the clinical question, the core examination can include velocity-encoded cineMRI (VENC MRI) to measure blood velocities and flows in arteries and veins, and across valves and shunts. Also known as phase-contrast velocity mapping, the underlying principle is that signal from moving blood or tissue will undergo a phase shift relative to stationary tissue, if a magnetic-field gradient is applied in the direction of motion.

The goal of VENC MRI is to produce a cine loop across the cardiac cycle, where on any given frame, pixel intensity is proportional to blood velocity. Generally displayed using a grey scale, white corresponds to maximum flow in one direction, black to maximum flow in the opposite direction, and mid-grey indicates

that flow is absent (Fig. 21–12). Although blood velocity can be measured in any arbitrary direction, it is usually assessed in reference to the imaging plane. Encoding velocity in the slice gradient direction allows measurement of *through-plane* velocities, and encoding in either the frequency or phase-encode gradient directions allows *in-plane* measurement of velocity components directed either vertically or horizontally within the image plane.

VENC MRI is commonly performed using a segmented GRE imaging engine during a patient breathhold. The sequence, however, is modified to measure the effects of a magnetic-field gradient on the precessing protons within flowing blood. The precise details of VENC MRI are complex and are considered more comprehensively elsewhere.[42–44] However, optimizing the maximum velocity that can be measured—which is inversely related to gradient strength (for a constant application time)—is important. Setting the maximum velocity too low will lead to aliasing, whereas setting it too high will lead to more noise or inaccuracy in the velocity measurement. Retrospective rather than prospective ECG gating is preferred to allow data collection throughout the entire cardiac cycle including end-diastole.

Although VENC MRI appears analogous to Doppler echocardiography, there are important differences (Table 21–1). For instance, an advantage of VENC MRI is that blood flow through an orifice is directly measured on an en-face image of the orifice with *through-plane* velocity encoding. With echocardiography there are two limitations. First, the blood flow profile is not directly measured but assumed to be flat (i.e., velocity in the center of the orifice is the same as near the edges) so that, hopefully, one sampling velocity would indicate average velocity. Second, the cross-sectional area of the orifice is estimated from a diameter measurement of the orifice at a different time from when Doppler velocity was recorded using a different examination (M-mode or two-dimensional imaging). Conversely, VENC MRI has some disadvantages. Perhaps most importantly, VENC MRI is not performed in real time and requires breathholding to minimize artifacts from respiratory motion. One consequence is that it is difficult to measure changes in flow that occur with respiration.

CLINICAL APPLICATIONS

【 】 CORONARY ARTERY DISEASE AND ISCHEMIA

A number of CMR approaches exist for the detection of coronary artery disease (CAD). Each of these techniques exploits specific anatomic or physiologic properties that occur as a result of CAD (Table 21–2). However, clinically, the most widespread approach for evaluating CAD is stress-testing with imaging of either myocardial contraction or perfusion.

Dobutamine-Stress Cine Magnetic Resonance Imaging

Analogous to echocardiography, cineMRI during dobutamine stimulation can be used to detect ischemia-induced wall-motion abnormalities (Table 21–2). Dobutamine cineMRI can yield higher diagnostic accuracy than dobutamine echocardiography[45] and can be effective in patients not suited for echocardiography

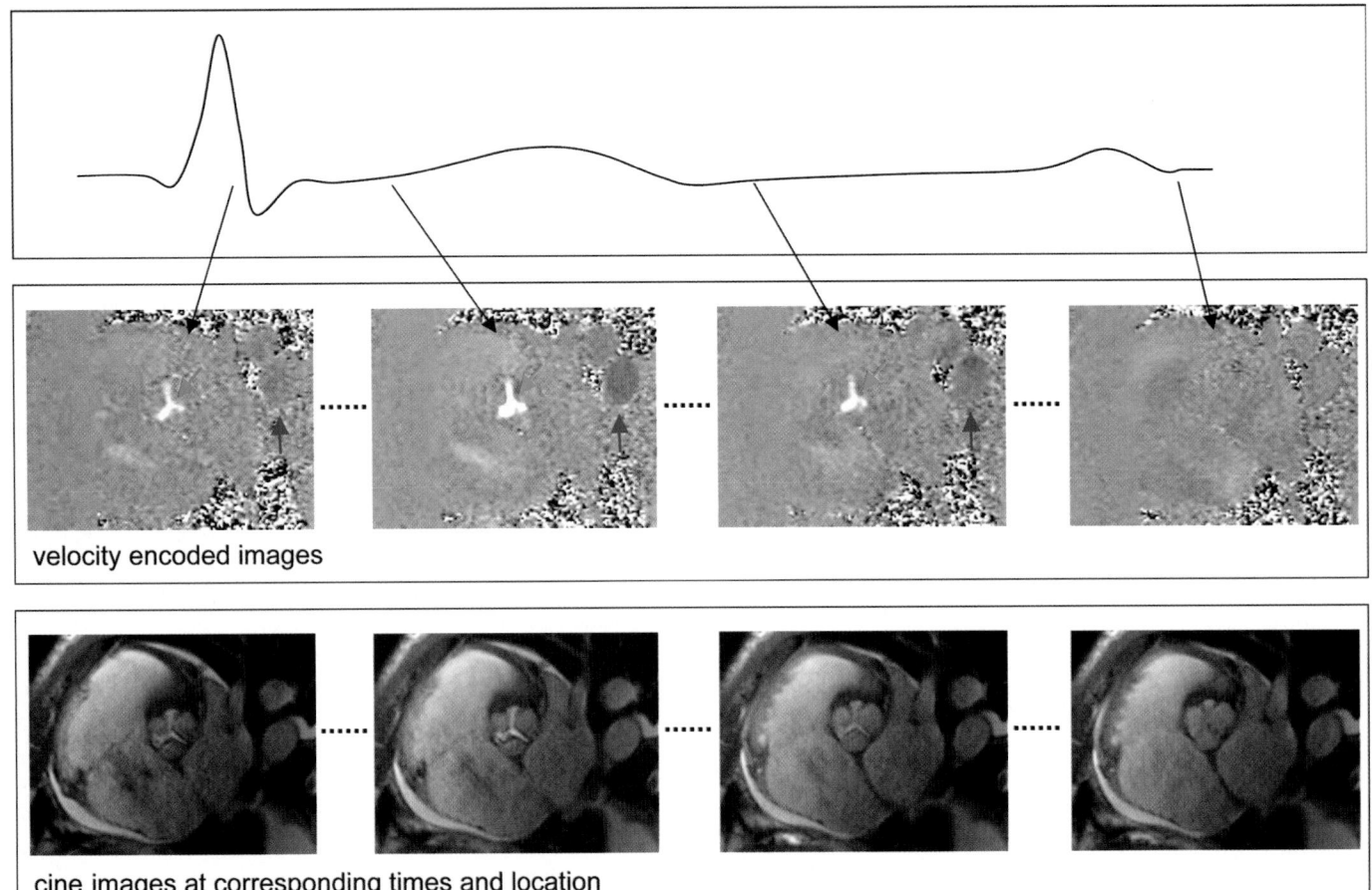

FIGURE 21–12. ECG-gated velocity-encoding MRI. Analogous to cine imaging, each velocity-encoded image (*top row of images*) corresponds to a cardiac phase, and gating to the electrocardiogram is necessary. On the images, white represents maximal velocity (in this case across the aortic valve, *red arrow*). Black represents flow in the opposite direction (in the descending thoracic aorta, *blue arrow*). Grey represents no flow. The *bottom row* demonstrates the corresponding cineMRI images.

because of poor acoustic windows.[46] Recent data suggests that the presence of inducible ischemia by this technique predicts subsequent cardiac mortality.[47] Nonetheless, a major practical issue is the need to administer dobutamine while the patient is inside the magnet. Inotropic stimulation in patients with ischemic heart disease is intrinsically associated with the risk of eliciting an ischemic event, and the position of the patient within the magnet impairs physician-patient interaction. In addition, the diagnostic utility of the ECG is diminished during imaging because the shape of the ECG waveform is directly altered by the magnetic field. Perhaps in part, because of these issues, only a few centers worldwide routinely perform this technique.

Adenosine Stress-Perfusion Magnetic Resonance Imaging

First-pass perfusion MRI during adenosine vasodilation is rapidly becoming the stress test of choice in clinical CMR-imaging centers. Perfusion MRI is promising for several reasons. Decreased perfusion is the first step in the ischemic cascade. There-

TABLE 21–1

Comparison of Velocity-Encoded MRI and Doppler Echocardiography

IMAGING CHARACTERISTIC	VELOCITY-ENCODING MRI	DOPPLER ECHOCARDIOGRAPHY
Imaging during free breathing	Limited	Yes
Imaging during arryth-mias	Limited	Yes
Temporal resolution	~50 ms[a]	<10 ms
Peak velocity location	Yes	Location ambiguity (CW Doppler)
Angle dependence	Yes, 20 degrees	Yes, 20 degrees
Imaging planes	Any	Echocardiographic windows
Blood flow profile	Directly measured	Flat profile assumed
Flow quantification	En face	In-plane[b]

[a]Given temporal resolution is for breathhold imaging. Temporal resolution may be significantly improved for nonbreathhold imaging, but artifacts caused by respiratory motion artifact may be prominent.
[b]Conduit cross-sectional area is estimated from diameter measurement.

TABLE 21-2

Cardiovascular Magnetic Resonance Techniques for the Detection of Coronary Artery Disease

PHYSIOLOGIC SUBSTRATE	CMR TECHNIQUE	STRESS TEST[a]	CLINICAL APPLICATION
Coronary anatomy and morphology	Coronary MRA	None	+[b]
Coronary artery blood flow/velocity	Velocity Encoding MRI	Adenosine/Dypiridamole	−[c]
Deoxygenated hemoglobin content	BOLD MRI	Adenosine/Dypiridamole	−
Phosphocreatinine/ATP content	31P-Spectroscopy	Handgrip exercise	−
Ventricular function	Multi-phase cineMRI	Dobutamine	++
Myocardial perfusion	Dynamic first pass perfusion contrast-enhanced MRI	Adenosine/Dypiridamole	++

ATP, adenosine triphosphate; BOLD, blood oxygenation level-dependent; CMR, cardiovascular magnetic resonance; MRA, magnetic resonance angiography; MRI, magnetic resonance imaging.
[a]Rest studies alone may provide some information regarding the presence of coronary artery disease.
[b]For assessment of coronary anomalies and patency of coronary bypass grafts.
[c]Recent studies suggest potential utility for assessment of coronary bypass patency and in-stent restenosis.

fore, techniques that assess perfusion have the potential to be more sensitive than techniques that assess later steps.[48–52] Logistically, as discussed earlier (see Fig. 21–11), stress-perfusion imaging is quick and simple. The duration of adenosine infusion is short (~3 minutes), and direct access to the patient is limited only during imaging of the first pass (~45 seconds). Compared with competing technologies such as radionuclide imaging, perfusion MRI has many potential advantages: more than an order of magnitude improvement in spatial resolution (typical voxel dimensions, MRI $3.0 \times 1.8 \times 8$ mm = 43 mm³ versus SPECT $10 \times 10 \times 10$ mm = 1000 mm³; Fig. 21–13); the ability to identify regional differences in flow over the full range of coronary vasodilation (i.e., no plateau in signal at high-flow rates, as seen with radionuclide tracers[53,54]; Fig. 21–14); the lack of ionizing radiation; and an examination time of 30 to 45 minutes versus 2 to 3 hours.

The diagnostic performance of stress-perfusion MRI has been evaluated in a number of studies in humans.[19,55–72] Overall, these studies have shown good correlations with radionuclide imaging and x-ray coronary angiography, although there have been some variable results. Table 21–3 summarizes the published stress perfusion MRI studies in humans with coronary angiography comparison. A total of 20 studies have been completed, consisting of 1086 patients with known or suspected coronary artery disease (CAD). On average, the sensitivity and specificity of perfusion MRI for detecting obstructive

CAD were 83 percent (range, 44–93 percent) and 82 percent (range, 60–100 percent), respectively. Likely on the basis of these studies, the most recent consensus report on clinical indications for CMR imaging classified perfusion imaging as a Class II indication for the assessment of CAD (provides clinically relevant information and is frequently useful).[10]

Despite the mostly favorable results of these studies, a number of issues should be considered. Some studies are of limited clinical applicability because they required central venous catheters,[59] imaged only one slice per heartbeat,[59,63] or excluded patients with di-

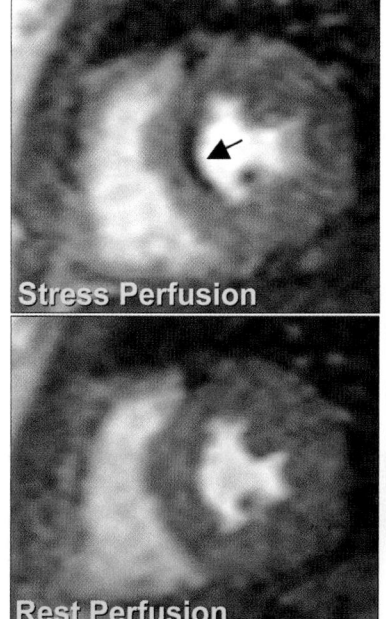
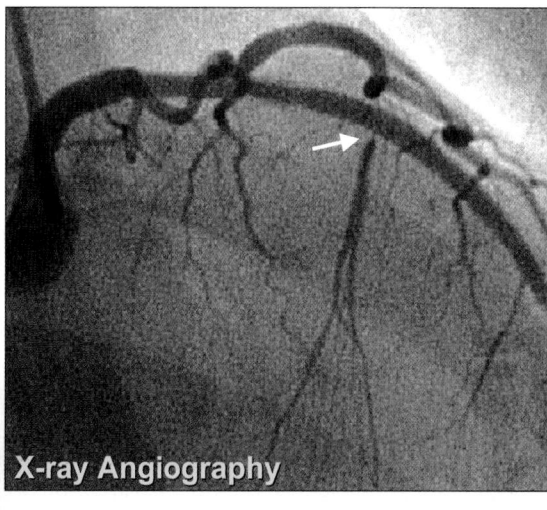

FIGURE 21–13. Importance of spatial resolution in stress-perfusion imaging. Patient has an inducible perfusion defect limited to the subendocardial portion of the septal wall (*black arrow*) caused by an ostial stenosis (*white arrow*) of a septal branch of the left anterior descending coronary artery.

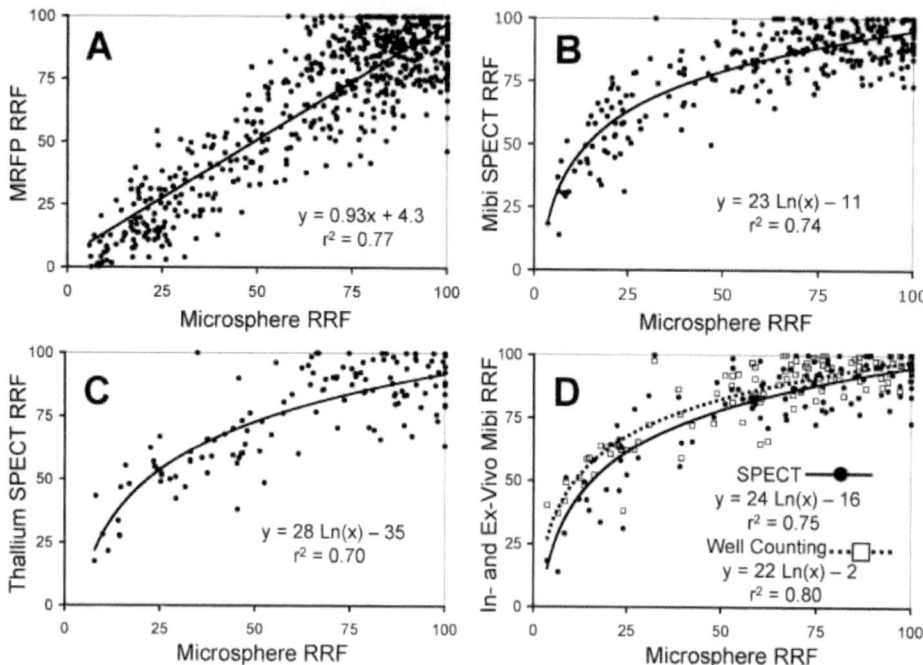

FIGURE 21–14. Comparisons of perfusion MRI, radionuclide, and microsphere flows. MRI signal intensity–time curves were linearly related to reference microsphere flows over the full range of vasodilation. Relationships between technetium-99m sestamibi single-photon emission (^{99m}Tc-sestamibi) and ^{201}thallium (Tl) activity and microsphere flows were curvilinear, plateauing as flows increased. Data suggest that perfusion MRI, unlike radionuclide imaging, has the potential for detecting stenoses producing only moderate limitations in flow reserve. **A.** Normalized magnetic resonance first-pass perfusion (MRFP) imaging and full-thickness microsphere relative regional flows (RRF). **B.** Normalized ^{99m}Tc-sestamibi and full-thickness microsphere RRFs. **C.** Normalized ^{201}Tl and full-thickness microsphere RRFs. **D.** In-vivo single-photon emission computed tomography (SPECT) and ex-vivo well counting values of ^{99m}Tc-sestamibi versus microsphere RRFs. *Source: Lee, Simonetti, Harris, et al.*[52] *Used with permission.*

abetes.[68] Many studies had small sample sizes—8 had 30 or fewer patients. Most included patients already known to have CAD or known to have prior myocardial infarction. In these studies there is pretest referral or *spectrum* bias, which can artificially raise test sensitivity and/or specificity.[73,74]

Two practical issues also limit clinical applicability when evaluating these studies. First, there is no consensus regarding the optimal pulse sequence or imaging protocol. The studies in Table 21–3 are very heterogeneous in terms of the techniques and methods employed. For example, the dose of gadolinium contrast administered varied sixfold, with doses over a wide range (0.025 to 0.15 mmol/kg). The inconsistent results likely reflect the lack of a standard method for performing perfusion MRI. Second, many of the studies used a quantitative approach (i.e., regions of interest are drawn on the images, and image intensities are measured) for diagnostic assessment. Although a quantitative approach has the potential advantage of allowing the measurement of absolute blood flow, the approach requires extensive interactive postprocessing. At present, a quantitative approach is not feasible for everyday clinical use.

In contrast, image interpretation by simple visual assessment would be a realistic approach for a clinical CMR practice. Unfortunately the results in the literature regarding visual assessment of perfusion MRI are mixed, generally demonstrating adequate sensitivity but relatively poor specificity for the detection of CAD. In large part, image artifacts are responsible for reduced specificity. However, there is no reason to interpret the

stress perfusion images in isolation. The "core" exam is a multicomponent protocol that includes cine and delayed-enhancement imaging in addition to stress and rest perfusion. In this context, it is noteworthy that recently an interpretation algorithm that combines data from perfusion MRI and DEMRI has been introduced that substantially improves the specificity and accuracy of rapid visual assessment for the detection of CAD (Fig. 21–15).[19]

The algorithm is based on two simple principles. First, with perfusion MRI and DEMRI, we have independent methods to obtain information regarding the presence or absence of myocardial infarction (MI). Thus, one method could be used to confirm the results of the other. Second, DEMRI image quality (e.g., signal-to-noise ratio) is far better than perfusion MRI because it is less demanding in terms of scanner hardware (DEMRI images can be built up over several seconds rather than in 0.1 seconds as is required for first-pass perfusion).[75] Thus, DEMRI should be more accurate for the diagnosis of MI.[75] Conceptually, it then follows that perfusion defects that have similar intensity and extent during both stress and rest (*matched defect*) but do not have infarction on DEMRI are artifactual and should not be considered positive for CAD. Conversely, the presence of infarction on DEMRI favors the diagnosis of CAD even if the results of perfusion imaging are equivocal.

Coronary Magnetic Resonance Angiography

Coronary magnetic resonance angiography (MRA) can be used to directly visualize coronary anatomy and morphology. However, coronary MRA is technically demanding for several reasons. The coronary arteries are small (3–5 mm) and tortuous compared with other vascular beds that are imaged by MRA, and there is nearly constant motion during both the respiratory and cardiac cycles. Thus, precise assessment of stenosis severity and visualization of distal segments are difficult, leading to intermediate sensitivity and specificity values for the detection of CAD in validation studies.[76] Currently, the only clinical indication that is considered appropriate for coronary MRA is the evaluation of patients with suspected coronary anomalies.[20] Coronary MRA is discussed further in Chap. 22.

【 】 VIABILITY AND INFARCTION

Although a variety of MRI techniques have been utilized to assess myocardial viability, currently only dobutamine cineMRI and

TABLE 21–3

Stress Perfusion MRI Studies in Humans with Coronary Angiography Comparison

YEAR	AUTHOR	REFERENCE	N	PTS WITH KNOWN CAD EXCLUDED	MRI PERFUSION PROTOCOL[b]	GADOLINIUM DOSE (MMOL/KG)	PULSE-SEQUENCE	X-RAY ANGIOGRAPHY (CAD DEFINITION)	ANALYSIS METHOD[c]	SENSITIVITY	SPECIFICITY
1993	Klein	AJR 161:257	5	no	Stress alone	0.05	IR-GRE	>50	prospective	81[a]	100[a]
1994	Harnell	AJR 163:1061	18	no	Rest/Stress	0.04	IR-GRE	≥70	prospective	83	100
1994	Eichenberger	JMRI 4:425	10	no	Rest/Stress	0.05	GRE	>75	retrospective	44[a]	80[a]
2000	Al-Saadi	Circ 101:1379	34	yes	Rest/Stress	0.025	IR-GRE	≥75	prospective[d]	90	83
2001	Bertschinger	JMRI 14:556	14	no	Stress alone	0.1	SR-EPI	≥50	retrospective	85	81
2001	Schwitter	Circ 103:2230	48	yes	Stress alone	0.1	SR-GRE-EPI hybrid	≥50	retrospective	87	85
2001	Panting	JMRI 13:192	22	no	Rest/Stress	0.05	IR Spin Echo-EPI	>50	retrospective	79	83
2002	Sensky	Int J CV Imaging 18:373	30	no	Rest/Stress	0.025	IR-GRE	>50	prospective	93[a]	60[a]
2002	Ibrahim	JACC 39:864	25	no	Rest/Stress	0.05	SR-GRE-EPI hybrid	>75	retrospective	69[a]	89[a]
2003	Chiu	Radiology 226:717	13	no[e]	Rest/Stress	0.05	IR-SSFP	>50	NS	92[a]	92[a]
2003	Ishida	Radiology 229:209	104	no	Stress/Rest	0.075	SR-GRE-EPI hybrid	≥70	prospective	90	85
2003	Nagel	Circ 108:432	84	no	Rest/Stress	0.025	SR-GRE-EPI hybrid	≥75	retrospective	88	90
2003	Doyle	JCMR 5:475	138	no	Rest/Stress	0.04	SR-GRE	≥70	prospective[d]	57	85
2004	Wolff	Circ 110:732	75	no	Stress/Rest	0.05–0.15	SR-GRE-EPI hybrid	≥70	prospective[f]	93	75
2004	Giang	EHJ 25:1657	80	no	Stress alone	0.05–0.15	SR-GRE-EPI hybrid	≥50	retrospective[f]	93	75
2004	Paetsch	Circ 110:835	79	no	Stress/Rest	0.05	SR-GRE-EPI hybrid	>50	prospective	91	62
2004	Plein	JACC 44:2173	68	no[e]	Rest/Stress	0.05	SR-GRE[g]	≥70	prospective	88	83
2005	Plein	Radiology 235:423	92	no	Rest/Stress	0.05	SR-GRE[g]	>70	retrospective	88	82
2006	Klem	JACC 47:1630	100	yes	Stress/Rest	0.063	SR-GRE[g]	≥70	prospective	84[h]	58[h]
2006	Cury	Radiology 240:39	47	no	Stress/Rest	0.1	SR-GRE-EPI hybrid	≥70	prospective	81[i]	87[i]
Total	20		1086								
Average										83	82

CAD, coronary artery disease; DEMRI, delayed enhancement MRI; EPI, echoplanar imaging; GRE, gradient-recalled echo; IR, inversion recovery prepulse; MRI, magnetic resonance imaging; NS, not stated; SR, saturation recovery prepulse; SSFP, steady-state free precession.

[a]Numbers based on a regional rather than per patient analysis

[b]When both rest and stress imaging were performed in the order listed

[c]Prospective studies were those in which the criteria for test abnormality were prespecified before data analysis

[d]Pilot study performed first to determine the best threshold for test abnormality

[e]At enrollment all patients has the clinical diagnosis of non-ST elevation MI or acute coronary syndrome

[f]Reported sensitivity and specificity are from a fraction of the total cohort, a subgroup with the best results

[g]With parallel imaging acceleration

[h]Sensitivity/specificity were higher after incorporating DEMRI (89% and 87%, respectively)

[i]Sensitivity/specificity were higher after incorporating DEMRI (87% and 89%, respectively)

a. Interpretation Algorithm

b. Examples

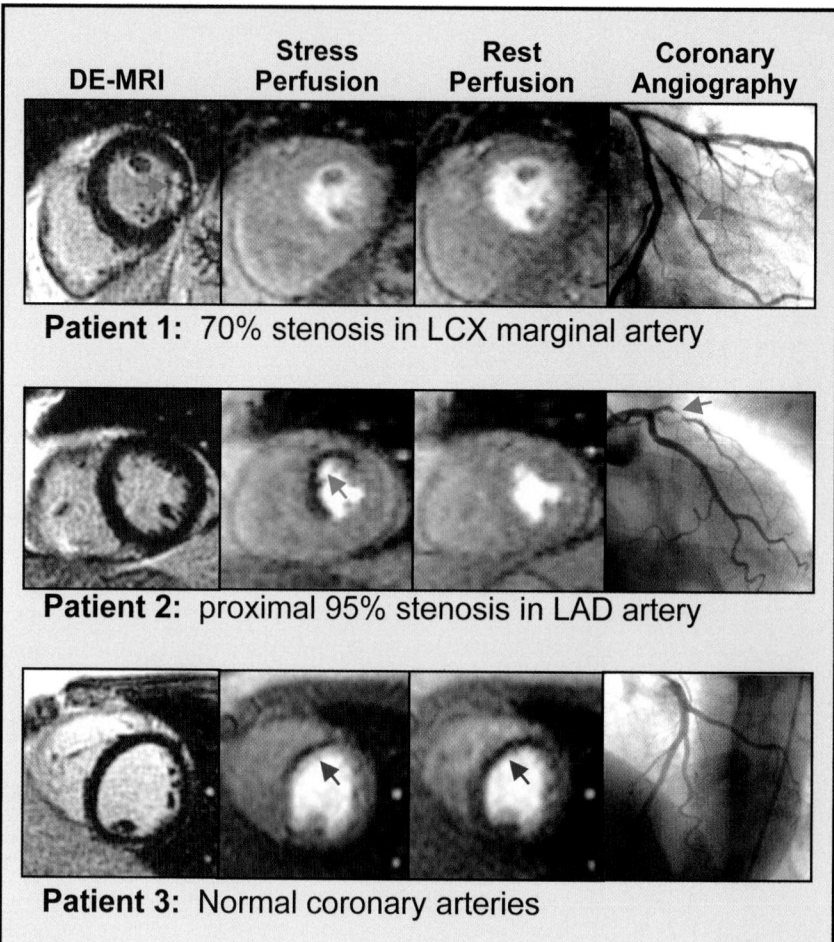

FIGURE 21–15. Interpretation algorithm for incorporating delayed enhancement imaging (DEMRI) with stress- and rest-perfusion MRI for the detection of coronary disease. **A.** Schema of the interpretation algorithm. First is the positive DEMRI study: Hyperenhanced myocardium consistent with a prior myocardial infarction (MI) is detected. Does not include isolated midwall or epicardial hyperenhancement, which can occur in nonischemic disorders. Second, standard negative stress study: No evidence of prior MI or inducible perfusion defects. Third, standard positive stress study: No evidence of prior MI, but perfusion defects are present with adenosine that are absent or reduced at rest. Fourth, artifactual perfusion defect: Matched stress- and rest-perfusion defects without evidence of prior MI on DEMRI. **B.** Patient examples. (*top row*) Patient with a positive DEMRI study demonstrating an infarct in the inferolateral wall (*red arrow*) although perfusion-MRI is negative. The interpretation algorithm (step 1) classified this patient as positive for coronary artery disease (CAD). Coronary angiography verified disease in a circumflex marginal artery. Cine cardiovascular magnetic resonance (CMR) imaging demonstrated normal contractility. (*middle row*) Patient with a negative DEMRI study but with a prominent reversible defect in the anteroseptal wall on perfusion-MRI (*red arrow*). The interpretation algorithm (step 3) classified this patient as positive for CAD. Coronary angiography demonstrated a proximal 95 percent left anterior descending (LAD) stenosis. (*bottom row*) Patient with a matched stress-rest perfusion defect (*blue arrows*) but without evidence of prior MI on DE-CMR imaging. The interpretation algorithm (step 4) classified the perfusion defects as artifactual. Coronary angiography demonstrated normal coronary arteries. LCX, left circumflex coronary artery. *Source: Klem I, Heitner JF, Shah DJ, et al, with permission.*[19]

DEMRI are used clinically. In general, DEMRI is preferred over dobutamine cineMRI, since DEMRI may be performed without the use of inotropic agents or special monitoring equipment.[80] Thus, we will focus the following discussion on DEMRI.

Validation Studies

There is an abundance of validation data in animal models in which DEMRI has been directly compared to the histopathology.[28,29,37] These data demonstrate a nearly exact relationship between the size and shape of infarcted myocardium by DEMRI to that by histopathology (Fig. 21–16). Human studies demonstrate that DEMRI is effective in identifying the presence, location, and

extent of MI in both the acute and chronic settings.[30,32] Typical DEMRI images in patients with large and small myocardial infarction are shown in Fig. 21–17. Moreover, DEMRI provides scar size measurements that are closely correlated with positron emission tomography (PET) in patients with ischemic cardiomyopathy,[81] and provides results superior to SPECT in patients with subendocardial infarctions.[31]

DEMRI also permits assessment of gradations of injury within acute myocardial infarction. For instance, rather than simply identifying a region of acute infarction as nonviable, DEMRI can distinguish between acute infarcts with only necrotic myocytes and acute infarcts with necrotic myocytes and damaged microvasculature. The latter, termed the *no-reflow phenomenon*, indicates the

TTC MRI

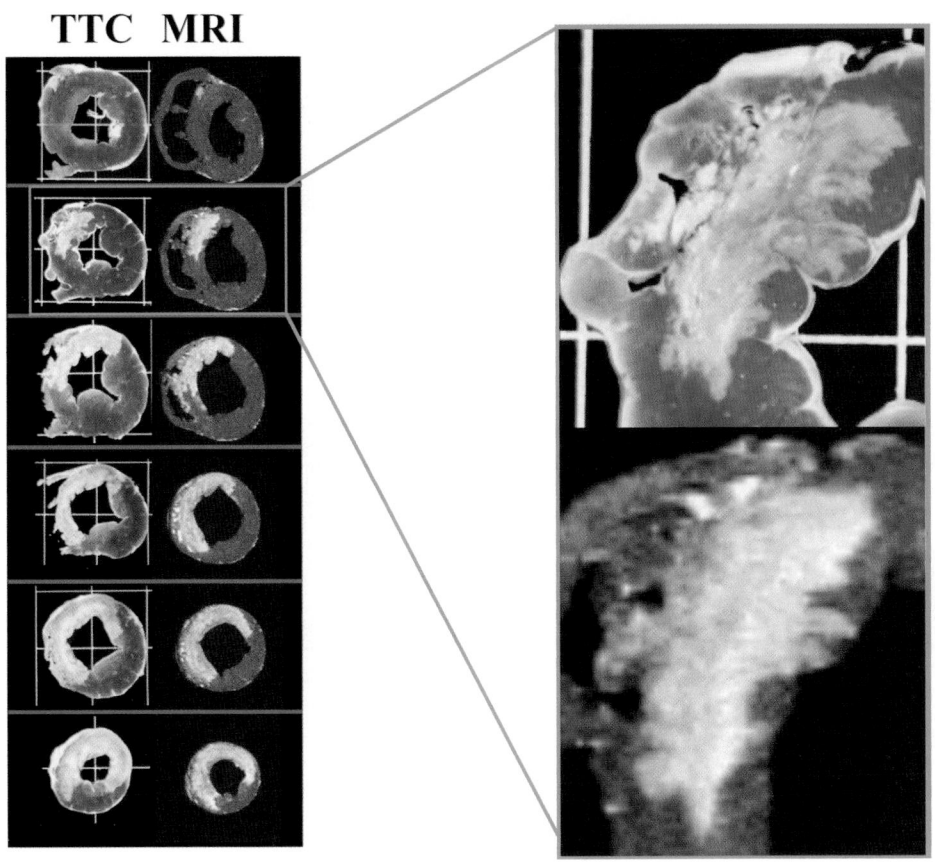

FIGURE 21–16. Comparison of ex-vivo, high-resolution delayed enhancement magnetic resonance (MR) images with acute myocardial necrosis defined histologically by triphenyltetrazolium chloride (TTC) staining. Note that the size and shape of the infarcted region (*yellowish-white region*) defined histologically by TTC staining is nearly exactly matched by the size and shape of the hyperenhanced (*bright*) region on the delayed enhancement image. *Modified from Kim, Fieno, Parrish, et al.[29] Used with permission.*

presence of compromised tissue perfusion despite epicardial artery patency.[91] No-reflow regions appear as hypoenhanced (dark) areas completely encompassed by hyperenhanced myocardium and the LV cavity (Fig. 21–20). Importantly, if imaging is repeated over time, no-reflow regions can gradually become hyperenhanced, as contrast slowly accumulates in these regions. The incidence and extent of early no-reflow appears to be associated with worse LV remodeling and outcome.[92] Although initial MR studies of no-reflow used single-shot perfusion sequences 1 to 2 minutes after contrast injection,[93] DEMRI performed 5 to 10 minutes after contrast provides higher image quality and delineates regions with more profound microvascular injury.[91, 94]

Clinical Interpretation

A straightforward clinical application of DEMRI is to differentiate patients with potentially reversible ventricular dysfunction from those with irrevers-

Large Myocardial Infarction

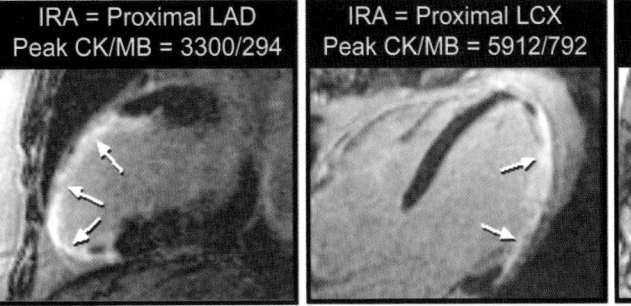

| IRA = Proximal LAD Peak CK/MB = 3300/294 | IRA = Proximal LCX Peak CK/MB = 5912/792 | IRA = Proximal RCA Peak CK/MB = 3352/389 |

Small Myocardial Infarction

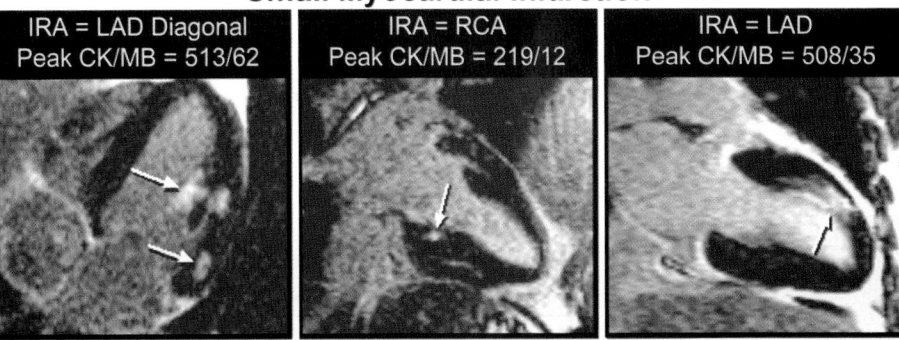

| IRA = LAD Diagonal Peak CK/MB = 513/62 | IRA = RCA Peak CK/MB = 219/12 | IRA = LAD Peak CK/MB = 508/35 |

FIGURE 21–17. Representative delayed enhancement magnetic resonance imaging (DEMRI) images in patients with chronic myocardial infarction. Both large (*top*) and small (*bottom*) infarcts are shown. CK, creatine kinase; IRA, infarct related artery; LAD, left anterior descending coronary artery; LCX, left circumflex coronary artery; MI, myocardial infarction; MB, creatine kinase MB isoenzyme; RCA, right coronary artery. *Source: Modified from Wu, Judd, Vargas, et al.[32] Used with permission.*

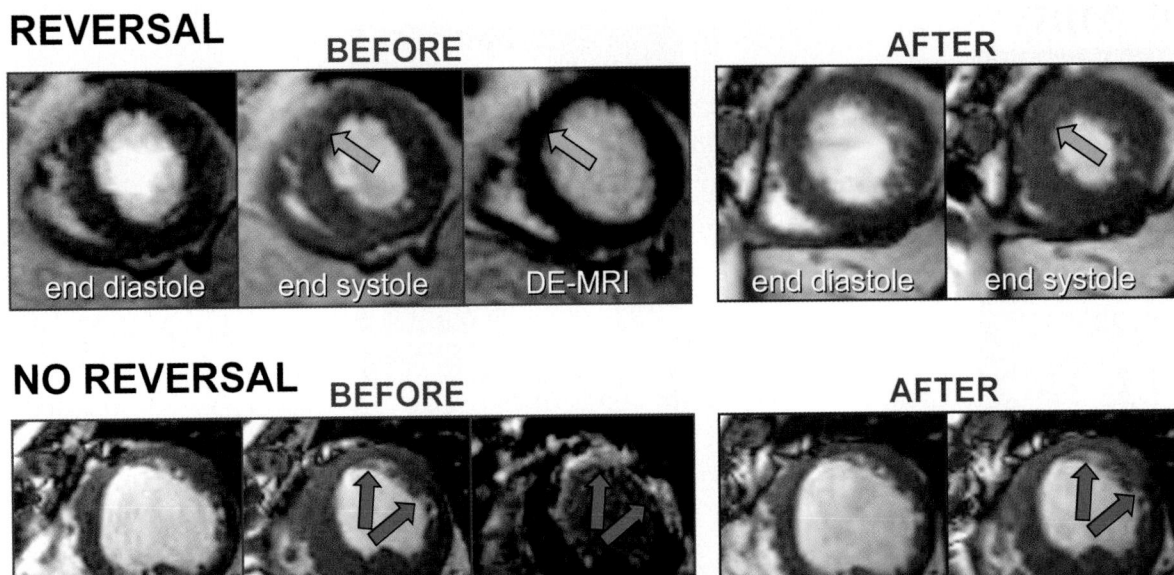

FIGURE 21–18. Representative cine and delayed enhancement images from one patient with reversible ventricular dysfunction and one with irreversible dysfunction. The patient with reversible dysfunction initially had severe hypokinesia of the anteroseptum (*orange arrows*). This area was not hyperenhanced prior to revascularization, and contractility improved after revascularization. The patient with irreversible dysfunction had akinesia of the anterolateral wall (*red arrows*). This area was hyperenhanced prior to revascularization, and contractility did not improve after revascularization. DEMRI, delayed enhancement magnetic resonance imaging. *Source: Kim, Wu, Rafael, et al.*[82] *Used with permission.*

ible dysfunction. In the setting of ischemic heart disease, it is primarily the former group that will benefit from coronary revascularization. Kim and coworkers published the initial study demonstrating that DEMRI done before coronary revascularization could be used to predict functional improvement after revascularization.[82] Fig.

21–18 shows representative cine and DEMRI images from two patients in the study. Regional wall-motion analysis demonstrated that the likelihood of functional improvement was inversely related in a progressive stepwise fashion to the transmural extent of hyperenhancement (infarction). For instance, in all dysfunctional segments,

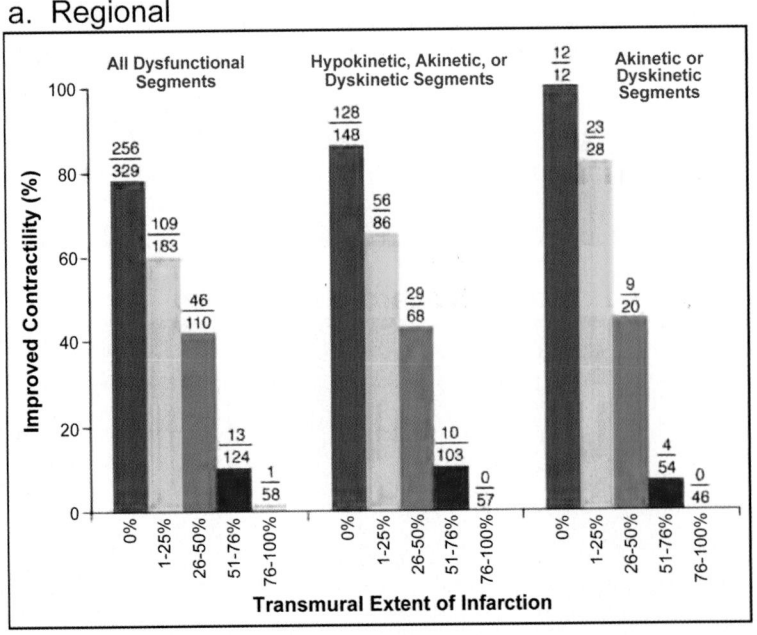
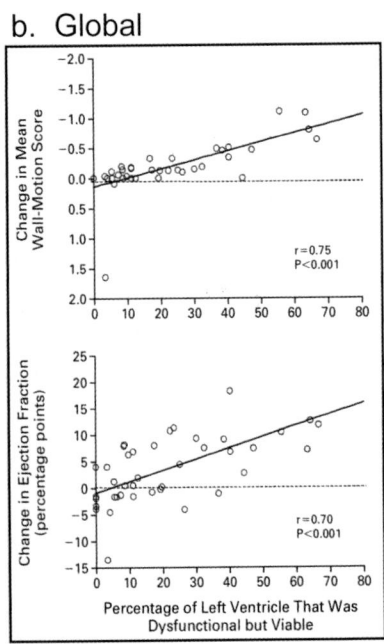

FIGURE 21–19. Prediction of improvement in regional and global systolic function by delayed enhancement MRI. **A.** Relation between the transmural extent of hyperenhancement (infarction) before revascularization and the likelihood of improved contractility after revascularization. **B.** Relation between amount of dysfunctional but viable left ventricle before revascularization and improvement in global function after revascularization. Decreases in wall-motion scores indicate increases in contractility. *Source: Kim, Wu, Rafael, et al.*[82] *Used with permission.*

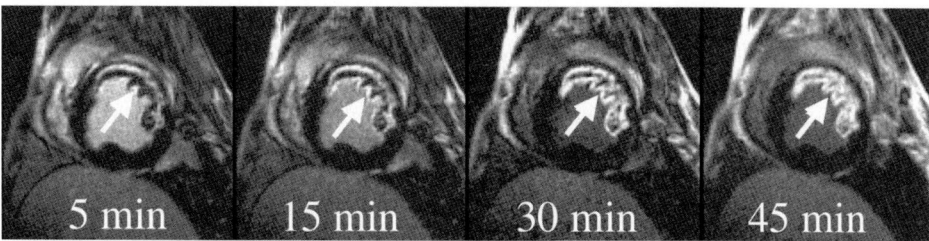

FIGURE 21–20. The *no reflow* phenomenon visualized by delayed enhancement MRI. Labels refer to time after administration of gadolinium contrast. The subendocardial black zone surrounded by hyperenhancement corresponds to the region of no reflow (*white arrows*). This region can be distinguished from normal myocardium because it is encompassed in three-dimensional space by hyperenhanced myocardium or the left ventricular (LV) cavity, and by the fact that it slowly becomes hyperenhanced over time. *Source: Kim, Choi, Judd, et al.*[94] *Reproduced with permission from the BMJ Publishing group.*

78 percent with no hyperenhancement improved, whereas only 2 percent with more than 75 percent hyperenhancement improved (Fig. 21–19A). Interestingly, the relationship was even steeper for segments with worse baseline dysfunction. In segments with akinesia or dyskinesia, 100 percent with no hyperenhancement improved, compared with 0 percent in those with more than 75 percent hyperenhancement. When the volume of dysfunctional but viable myocardium was calculated on a patient basis, this parameter predicted the magnitude of improvement in global function after revascularization as measured by mean LV wall motion score and left ventricular ejection fraction (LVEF) (Fig. 21–19B). Recently, Schvartzman and colleagues demonstrated similar findings in a patient cohort with more severe baseline cardiomyopathy (ejection fraction [EF], 28 ± 10 percent).[83]

In the setting of acute myocardial infarction, early reperfusion with primary angioplasty or thrombolysis has been shown to result in salvage of ischemic, but viable myocardium and long-term improvement in LVEF and survival.[84–88] However, in the immediate postinfarction setting, it is difficult to distinguish whether myocardial dysfunction is caused by necrosis and thus is permanent, or is caused by stunning and will eventually improve. A number of studies have demonstrated the utility of DEMRI in differentiating infarcted from viable myocardium soon after acute myocardial infarction and reperfusion therapy.[89,90] Similar to the findings in the chronic setting, the transmural extent of infarction (TEI) measured by DEMRI was inversely related to improvement in segmental function in a stepwise fashion.[89] In addition to predicting improvement in regional function, DEMRI also provided the best predictor of improvement in global function: the percentage of the left ventricle that was dysfunctional but viable (i.e., ≤ 25 percent TEI) was directly related to future changes in the LV wall thickening score (r = 0.87, p < 0.0001) and LVEF (r = 0.65, p = 0.002).[89]

Physiologic Insights

The ability of DEMRI to directly visualize the transmural extent of both viable and nonviable myocardium has led to some recent observations that appear to refute certain traditional concepts regarding cardiac pathophysiology. When only viable myocardium can be visualized (as is the case with nuclear scintigraphy), the *percentage of viability* in a given segment is assessed indirectly and generally refers to the amount of viability in the segment normalized to the segment with the maximum amount of viability, or to data from a gender-specific database of controls. Conversely, when both viable and infarcted myocardium can be visualized, the percentage of viability can be assessed directly and expressed as the amount of viability in the segment normalized to the amount of viability plus infarction in the same segment (Fig. 21–21A).[75,95] These differences in the way in which viability is measured can alter clinical interpretation. Fig. 21–21B demonstrates MR images in a patient with chronic coronary disease and an akinetic anterior wall. Although the anterior wall is thinned, only a small subendocardial portion of the anterior wall is infarcted. In this case, an indirect method would show that the anterior wall is only 39 percent viable (compared to the remote region), whereas a direct method would show that the anterior wall is 70 percent viable. The indirect method would predict absence of wall motion recovery after revascularization, whereas the direct method would predict recovery. The postrevascularization images (see Fig. 21–21B) demonstrate in this patient that the direct method is correct.

This case runs counter to presently accepted clinical dogma. Prior reports have concluded that in patients with CAD and ventricular dysfunction regions with thinned myocardium represent scar tissue and cannot improve in contractile function after revascularization.[96] However, this patient case along with data from an ongoing pilot study,[97] indicate that thinning should not be equated with the absence of viability, and that in some patients, these regions can improve after revascularization. Additional studies will be needed to elucidate these provocative initial findings.

Prognostic Value

Because DEMRI is a relatively new technique, there is a paucity of data regarding the prognostic importance of myocardial infarction or scarring detected by this technique. However, this is an area of intense investigation, and the literature is growing rapidly. Recently in a single-center study, Kwong and coworkers demonstrated that the presence of unrecognized myocardial scarring detected by DEMRI was associated with poor outcomes, even after accounting for common clinical, angiographic, and functional predictors.[98] Results from a large multicenter study have recently been presented and demonstrate that the extent of scarring by DEMRI in patients referred for clinical CMR imaging is a predictor of all-cause mortality, independent of LVEF.[99] Although these data are provocative, both are retrospective studies. Additional investigation is needed—preferably in a broad range of patients enrolled prospectively—to determine the full prognostic significance of DEMRI findings.

【 】 HEART FAILURE AND CARDIOMYOPATHIES

Approach to Determining Etiology with Dynamic Enhanced Magnetic Resonance Imaging

In patients with heart failure, it is important to determine the etiology of heart failure to appropriately plan therapy and provide prog-

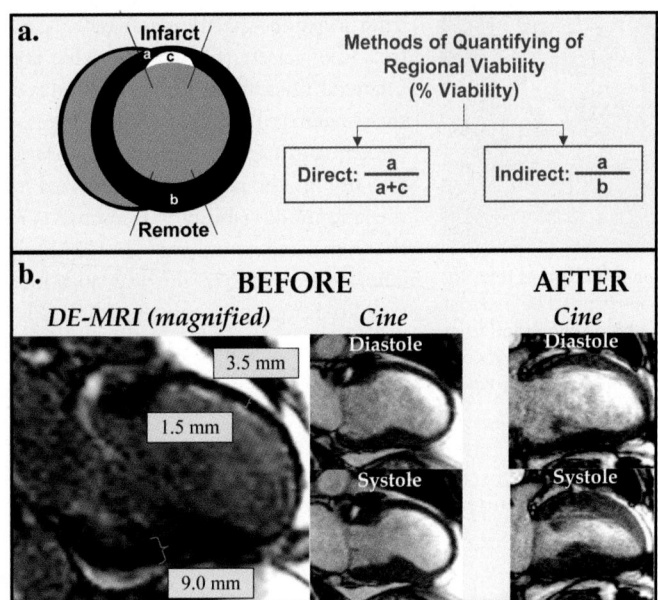

FIGURE 21–21. A. Cartoon highlighting differences between direct and indirect method of quantifying regional viability. Viable myocardium is black, and infarct is white. *Remote* zone represents segment with maximum amount of viability. **B.** Long-axis images of patient before and 2 months after revascularization. Although akinetic anterior wall is *thinned* (diastolic wall thickness 5 mm; remote zone 9 mm), DEMRI demonstrates that there is only subendocardial infarction (1.5 mm thick). Direct assessment of viability would show that anterior wall is predominately viable (3.5/5 mm = 70 percent viable), whereas indirect method would show that anterior wall is predominately nonviable (3.5/9 mm = 39 percent viable). Cine views after revascularization demonstrate recovery of wall motion and diastolic wall thickness. Cine, cineangiocardiographic; DEMRI, delayed enhancement magnetic resonance imaging. *Source: Modified from Kim, Shah.[95] Used with permission.*

nostic information.[100] Even in asymptomatic patients in whom systolic dysfunction is not yet evident, early diagnosis can allow preventive measures that can change the natural history of the disease and can trigger family-screening procedures in genetic disorders. Unfortunately, the etiology of cardiomyopathy is often difficult to ascertain, and standard noninvasive imaging may not be definitive.

The importance of assessing myocardial viability is readily evident in patients with ischemic heart failure who undergo coronary revascularization. The assessment of viability, or conversely, the detection of prior infarction or scarring, however, can be important in many patients in whom coronary revascularization is not an issue. Viability assessment may not be considered in these patients because of assumptions derived from experience with traditional imaging modalities. With its ability to directly visualize both viable and nonviable myocardium with high spatial resolution, DEMRI provides new information for the clinician. Correspondingly, the clinical role of DEMRI can be greater than first expected over a wide range of cardiovascular disorders. For instance, DEMRI is useful not only for detecting acute and chronic MI, and predicting functional improvement after revascularization but also for characterizing an extensive array of cardiomyopathies. Table 21–4 lists many of the important DEMRI studies that have been performed in humans since the initial study in 2000.[82]

The utility of DEMRI in the setting of cardiomyopathy is based on the understanding that rather than simply measuring viability,

the presence and pattern of hyperenhancement (nonviable myocardium) holds additional information. Recently, a systematic approach to interpreting DEMRI images in patients with heart failure or cardiomyopathy has been proposed.[79,101] This approach is based on the following three steps: (Step 1) The presence or absence of hyperenhancement is determined. In the subset of patients with longstanding severe ischemic cardiomyopathy, the data indicate that virtually all patients have prior MI.[102] The implication is that in patients with severe cardiomyopathy but without hyperenhancement, the diagnosis of idiopathic dilated cardiomyopathy should be strongly considered. (Step 2) If hyperenhancement is present, the location and distribution of hyperenhancement should be classified as a CAD or non-CAD pattern. For this determination, the concept that ischemic injury progresses as a *wavefront* from the subendocardium to the epicardium is crucial.[103] Correspondingly, hyperenhancement patterns that spare the subendocardium and are limited to the middle or epicardial portion of the LV wall are clearly in a non-CAD pattern. (Step 3) If hyperenhancement is present in a non-CAD pattern, further classification should be considered. There is emerging data that suggest certain nonischemic cardiomyopathies have predilection for specific scar patterns. For example, in the setting of LV hypertrophy, the presence of midwall hyperenhancement in one or both junctions of the interventricular septum and RV (RV) free wall is highly suggestive of hypertrophic cardiomyopathy, whereas midwall or epicardial hyperenhancement in the inferolateral wall is consistent with Anderson-Fabry disease. Moreover, instead of there being an infinite variety of hyperenhancement patterns, it appears that a broad stratification is possible into a limited number of common DEMRI phenotypes. Fig. 21–22 illustrates potential hyperenhancement patterns that can be encountered in clinical practice along with a partial list of their differential diagnoses.

Dilated Cardiomyopathy

The clinical presentation of ischemic and nonischemic dilated cardiomyopathy (DCM) can be indistinguishable. However, gross pathologic evaluation demonstrates distinct differences. In chronic ischemic cardiomyopathy, autopsy studies have demonstrated that myocardial scarring consistent with prior infarcts is present in virtually all patients, even those without clinical history of MI, angina, or electrocardiographic Q-waves.[102–104] Conversely, prior infarction in DCM is uncommon. Roberts and colleagues observed myocardial scars indistinguishable from prior MI at cardiac necropsy in only 14 percent (22:152) of patients with idiopathic DCM.[105] Uretsky and coworkers evaluated chronic heart failure patients at autopsy and found old infarcts in 12 percent of patients without CAD.[106] A number of mechanisms can be responsible for infarcts in patients without CAD, including coronary vasospasm, thrombosis with spontaneous lysis superimposed on minimal atherosclerosis, or coronary emboli.

DEMRI studies have demonstrated similar findings. Bello and colleagues evaluated 45 patients with heart failure and systolic dysfunction.[107] Whereas 100 percent of patients with ischemic cardiomyopathy had hyperenhancement consistent with prior MI, only 12 percent of patients with idiopathic DCM had hyperenhancement. Indeed, DEMRI hyperenhancement was the best clinical parameter in noninvasively discriminating ischemic from nonis-

TABLE 21–4

Human Studies Using DEMRI in Major Clinical Journals[a]

YEAR	AUTHOR	N[a]	REFERENCE	COMMENTS
Acute Ischemic Disease				
2001	Simonetti	18	*Radiology* 218:215–223	Original description of DEMRI using segmented IR-FGE
2001	Choi	24	*Circulation* 104:1101–1107	Prediction of functional improvement after acute MI
2001	Ricciardi	14	*Circulation* 103:2780–2783	Detection of post PCI microinfarction
2002	Gerber	20	*Circulation* 106:1083–1089	Prediction of functional improvement after acute MI
2003	Britten	28	*Circulation* 108:2212–2218	Infarct remodeling after progenitor cells treatment in acute MI
2003	Beek	30	*J Am Coll Cardiol* 42:895–901	Prediction of functional improvement after acute MI
2003	Kwong	161	*Circulation* 107:531–537	Detection of acute coronary syndrome
2003	Kitagawa	22	*Radiology* 226:138–144	Comparison to SPECT for predicting functional improvement
2003	Chiu	13	*Radiology* 226:717–722	Comparison with first-pass perfusion and XRA in NSTEMI
2004	Abdel-Aty	73	*Circulation* 109:2411–2416	Differentiation between acute and chronic MI
2004	Ingkanisorn	33	*J Am Coll Cardiol* 43:2253–2259	Correlation with acute and chronic indices of infarct size
2004	Lund	60	*Radiology* 232:49–57	Comparison to SPECT for infarct size
2005	Ibrahim	33	*J Am Coll Cardiol* 45:544–552	Comparison to SPECT for infarct size
2005	Selvanayagam	50	*Circulation* 111:1027–1032	Post PCI microinfarction, comparison with troponin I
2005	Baks	22	*Eur Heart J* 26:1070–1077	Prediction of functional recovery post primary PCI
2006	Klem	100	*J Am Coll Card* 47:1630–1638	Improved detection of CAD by stress perfusion with DEMRI
2006	Yan	144	*Circulation* 114:32–39	Peri-infarct zone characteristics for prediction of post-MI mortality
2006	Porto	52	*Circulation* 114:662–669	Post PCI infarction and relation to plaque morphology
Chronic Ischemic Disease				
2000	Kim	50	*N Engl J Med* 343:1445–1453	Initial use of DEMRI to predict functional improvement
2001	Wu	82	*Lancet* 357:21–28	Detection of Q-wave and non Q-wave chronic MI
2002	Mahrholdt	20	*Circulation* 106:2322–2327	Comparison to SPECT for chronic MI size reproducibility
2002	Klein	31	*Circulation* 105:162–167	Comparison to PET for viability assessment
2002	Perin	15	*Circulation* 106:957–961	Comparison to electromechanical mapping for viability
2002	Mollet	57	*Circulation* 106:2873–2876	Comparison to cineMRI and echo for LV thrombus detection
2002	Plein	10	*Radiology* 225:300–307	Part of comprehensive protocol for detection of CAD
2003	Wagner	91	*Lancet* 361:374–379	Comparison to SPECT for detection of subendocardial MI
2003	Knuesel	19	*Circulation* 108:1095–1100	Comparison to PET for viability assessment
2003	Kuhl	26	*J Am Coll Cardiol* 41:1341–1348	Comparison to PET for viability assessment
2003	Schvartzman	29	*Am Heart J* 146:535–541	Prediction of functional improvement in severe dysfunction
2004	Lee	20	*Radiology* 230:191–197	Comparison to SPECT for viability assessment

(continued)

TABLE 21-4

Human Studies Using DEMRI in Major Clinical Journals[a] *(continued)*

YEAR	AUTHOR	N[a]	REFERENCE	COMMENTS
2004	Selvanayagam	60	*Circulation* 109:345–350	Monitoring injury after off-pump versus on-pump CABG
2004	Nelson	60	*J Am Coll Cardiol* 43:1248–1256	Comparison with DSE and SPECT
2004	Wellnhofer	29	*Circulation* 109:2172–2174	Comparison to dobutamine MRI for functional improvement
2004	Moon	100	*J Am Coll Cardiol* 44:554–560	Transmural extent of Q-wave and non-Q-wave chronic MI
2004	Selvanayagam	52	*Circulation* 110:1535–1541	Predicting improvement after on- or off-pump CABG
2005	Bello	48	*J Am Coll Cardiol* 45:1104–1108	Identifying substrate for sustained ventricular tachycardia
2006	Bleeker	40	*Circulation* 113:969–976	Effect of posterolateral wall scar on response to CRT
2006	Baks	27	*J Am Coll Cardiol* 47:721–725	Prediction of functional recovery post PCI for CTO
2006	Kwong	195	*Circulation* 113:2733–2743	Unrecognized MI and impact on cardiovascular events
2006	White	28	*J Am Coll Cardiol* 48:1953–1960	Prediction of response to CRT by detection of scar
Nonischemic Heart Disease				
2002	Choudhury	21	*J Am Coll Cardiol* 40:2156–2164	Initial description of scar patterns in HCM
2003	Moon	53	*J Am Coll Cardiol* 41:1561–1567	Assessment of clinical risk in HCM
2003	McCrohon	90	*Circulation* 108:54–59	Differentiation of ischemic from nonischemic heart failure
2003	Moon	26	*Eur Heart J* 24:2151–2155	Initial description of scar oatterns in Anderson-Fabry disease
2004	van Dockum	24	*J Am Coll Cardiol* 43:27–34	Assessment of septal MI from ethanol infusion in HCM
2004	Mahrholdt	32	*Circulation* 109:1250–1258	Hyperenchantment patterns in myocarditis
2004	Moon	1	*J Am Coll Cardiol* 43:2260–2264	HCM case report with histology assessment of explanted heart
2005	Maceira	30	*Circulation* 111:195–202	Initial description of hyperenchantment in amyloidosis
2005	Tandri	30	*J Am Coll Cardiol* 45:98–103	Detection of fibrosis in Arrhythmogenic RV Cardiomyopathy
2005	Soriano	71	*J Am Coll Cardiol* 45:743–748	Differentiation of ischemic from nonischemic heart failure
2005	Smedema	58	*J Am Coll Cardiol* 45:1683–1690	Accuracy in the diagnosis of cardiac sarcoidosis
2005	Laissy	55	*Radiology* 237:75–82	Differentiation of AMI from myocarditis using DEMRI & CMR stress
2005	Soriano	71	*J Am Coll Card* 45:743–748	Identification of underlying CAD in undifferentiated heart failure
2005	Nazarian	26	*Circulation* 112:2821–2825	Prediction of inducible arrythmias in dilated cardiomyopathy
2005	Rochitte	51	*J Am Coll Cardiol* 46:1553–1558	Assessment of disease activity in Chagas' disease
2006	De Cobelli	23	*J Am Coll Cardiol* 47:1649–1654	Identification of myocardial injury in chronic myocarditis

CABG, coronary artery bypass grafting; CRT, cardiac resynchronization therapy; CTO, chronic total occlusion; DEMRI, delayed enhancement MRI; DSE, dobutamine stress echocardiography; HCM, hypertrophic cardiomyopathy; IR-FGE, inversion-recovery fast gradient-echo; MI, myocardial infarction; NSTEMI, non-ST elevation MI; PCI, percutaneous coronary intervention; PET, positron emission tomography; RV, right ventricular; SPECT, single-photon emission computed tomography; XRA, coronary x-ray angiography.
[a]The listed studies include a total of 2648 patients who have been studied with segmented inversion-recovery DEMRI.

chemic cardiomyopathy. It should be noted, however, that in this study only hyperenhancement patterns consistent with prior MI were tallied; linear mid-wall striae with increased image intensity were not scored as hyperenhanced regions.

More recently, McCrohon and co-workers performed DEMRI in 90 patients with heart failure including 63 with idiopathic DCM.[108] Similar to the findings by Bello and colleagues, 13 percent of patients with DCM had hyperenhancement consistent with prior MI. McCrohon and coworkers, however, also found that an additional 28 percent had hyperenhancement in an unusual pattern, primarily involving the ventricular mid-wall with subendocardial sparing. As discussed in the previous section, this type of hyperenhancement is consistent with a *non-CAD* pattern of scarring. A cartoon illustration of this pattern is shown in Fig. 21–22, and a typical patient example is demonstrated in Fig. 21–23.

Hypertrophic Cardiomyopathy

CMR imaging is proving to be increasingly valuable in the clinical evaluation of hypertrophic cardiomyopathy (HCM). For example, Rickers reported that in 6 percent of patients with suspected or known HCM, cineMRI established the diagnosis of HCM, while no hypertrophy was seen on the echocardiography.[109] Moreover, echocardiography appeared to underestimate the magnitude of hypertrophy in comparison with cineMRI. This finding may be of clinical relevance since extreme hypertrophy (wall thickness of ≥30 mm) is recognized as an important risk factor for sudden death.

Myocardial tissue characterization by DEMRI appears to offer additional diagnostic and perhaps prognostic information.[110,111] Choudhury and colleagues first reported that myocardial scarring is common in HCM patients that are asymptomatic or minimally symptomatic. Scars were visible in 81 percent of patients, although scar size was usually limited (8 ± 9 percent of LV mass). The pattern of scarring was peculiar: scarring occurred only in hypertrophied regions, predominantly involving the middle third of the ventricular wall in a patchy, multifocal distribution (see Fig. 21–22). Interestingly, all patients with scarring had involvement in one or both junctions of the interventricular septum and the RV free wall. Despite the scarring, LV ejection fraction was normal (70 ± 11 percent). Similar findings have been reported by others who have included HCM patients with heart failure (scarring in 79 percent)[111] and patients with HCM caused by mutations in troponin-I (scarring in 80 percent of patients with LV hypertrophy).[112]

The mechanism of scarring in HCM is unknown, however, autopsy studies have demonstrated a high proportion of abnormal intramural arteries within regions of scar, suggesting that localized ischemia can be playing a central role.[113] The clinical importance of detecting scar by DEMRI in HCM patients is currently being investigated by several groups. The presence of scarring can be helpful in distinguishing LV hypertrophy because of HCM from hypertension or physiologic hypertrophy. In the latter, unless there is coexisting CAD, scarring is usually absent. Because scarring is observed in the majority of patients with HCM, the simple pres-

CAD

A. Subendocardial Infarct

B. Transmural Infarct

Non-CAD

A. Mid-wall HE

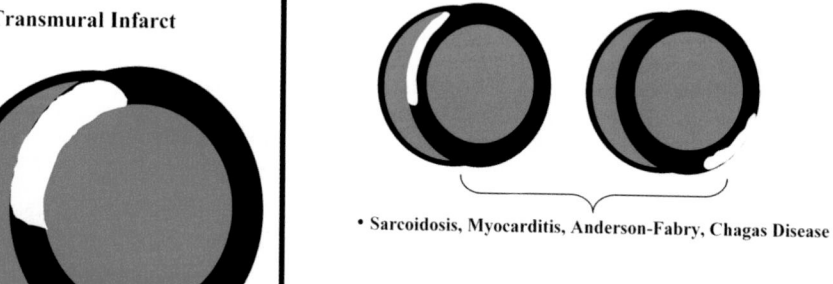

- Dilated Cardiomyopathy
- Myocarditis

- Hypertrophic Cardiomyopathy
- Right ventricular pressure overload (e.g. congenital heart disease, pulmonary HTN)

- Sarcoidosis
- Myocarditis
- Anderson-Fabry
- Chagas Disease

B. Epicardial HE

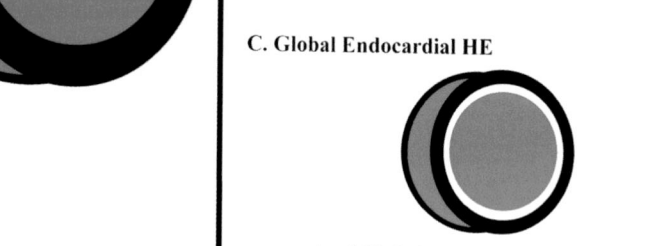

- Sarcoidosis, Myocarditis, Anderson-Fabry, Chagas Disease

C. Global Endocardial HE

- Amyloidosis, Systemic Sclerosis, Post cardiac transplantation

FIGURE 21–22. Hyperenhancement patterns that can be encountered in clinical practice. Because myocardial necrosis caused by coronary artery disease (CAD) progresses as a *wavefront* from the subendocardium to the epicardium, hyperenhancement (if present) should always involve the subendocardium in patients with ischemic disease. Isolated mid-wall or epicardial hyperenhancement strongly suggests a *nonischemic* etiology. Additionally, endocardial hyperenhancement that occurs globally (i.e., throughout the left ventricle) is uncommon even with diffuse CAD and therefore a nonischemic etiology should be considered. HE, hyperenhancement; HTN, hypertension. *Source: Shah, Kim.[79] Used with permission.*

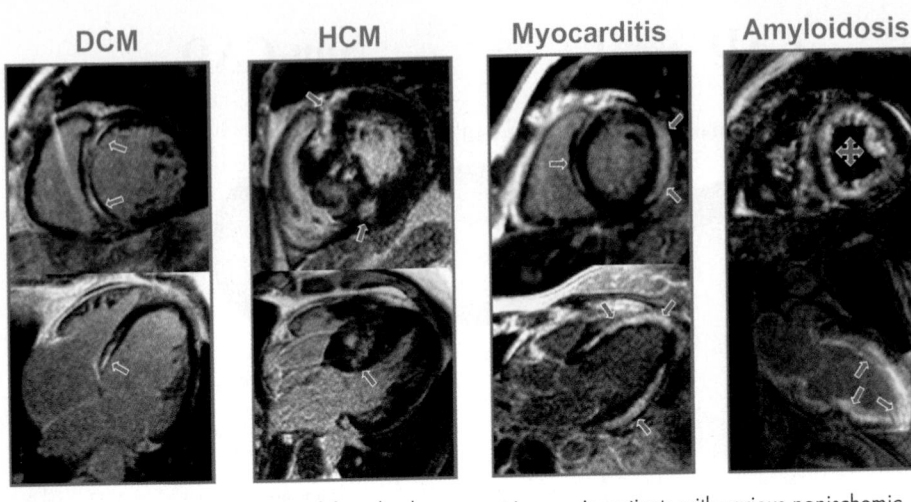

FIGURE 21–23. Representative delayed enhancement images in patients with various nonischemic cardiomyopathies. The hyperenhancement patterns in all patients are distinctly *non-CAD* type. Dilated cardiomyopathy (**DCM**): *Arrows* point to a linear stripe of hyperenhancement that is limited to the mid-wall of the interventricular septum. Hypertrophic cardiomyopathy (**HCM**): *Arrows* point to multiple foci of hyperenhancement, which are predominantly mid-myocardial in location and occur in the hypertrophied septum and not in the lateral left ventricular (LV) free wall. The junctions of the right ventricular (RV) free wall and interventricular septum are commonly involved. **Myocarditis**: *Arrows* point to two separate regions of hyperenhancement, a linear mid-wall stripe in the interventricular septum, and a large confluent region affecting the epicardial half of the LV lateral wall. **Amyloidosis.** *Arrows* point to hyperenhancement affecting the subendocardial half of the myocardial wall diffusely throughout the entire left ventricle.

secutive patients with biopsy proven systemic sarcoidosis.[118] In this pilot study, a twofold higher rate of cardiac involvement was diagnosed by CMR imaging compared with a standard clinical evaluation using Japanese Ministry of Health criteria. Frequently, hyperenhancement was found isolated to the mid-myocardial wall or epicardium, indicative of a non-CAD pattern. However, subendocardial or transmural hyperenhancement was also observed, mimicking the pattern of myocardial infarction.

Amyloidosis

Cardiac amyloidosis is a common cause of restrictive cardiomyopathy and is associated with poor prognosis. DEMRI can demonstrate diffuse LV hyperenhancement in these patients (see Fig. 21–23).[119] Although the subendocardium is preferentially involved, hyperenhancement is clearly in a non-CAD pattern because the distribution often is global and does not match any specific coronary artery perfusion territory. It is believed that amyloid deposition causes an expansion of myocardial interstitial space resulting in an increased gadolinium volume of distribution and hyperenhancement.[119] From an imaging point of view, the presence of diffuse myocardial involvement can make setting the parameters for DEMRI problematic. Specifically, it can be difficult to determine the optimal inversion time that will null normal myocardium, as there can be few areas that are completely normal. In this situation, it is helpful to acquire multiple images of the same view using a range of inversion times. We have found empirically that if a large portion of LV myocardium (i.e., >50 percent) goes through the null point earlier than the LV cavity blood pool and this region is not in an obvious coronary artery distribution, infiltrative involvement of the myocardium is highly likely. This method is useful when the disease is advanced and diffusely involves the myocardium, reducing the post-contrast of T1 of the abnormal myocardium below that of blood. Currently, the best way in which to perform and interpret DEMRI for identifying mild forms of cardiac amyloidosis is unknown.

Myocarditis

Several CMR imaging pulse sequences have been used to evaluate patients with suspected acute myocarditis. Friedrich and coworkers were the first to systematically evaluate myocardial contrast enhancement in patients with myocarditis.[120] In 19 patients with serologic evidence for acute viral infection, normal coronary arteries, LV dysfunction, and biomarker evidence of myocardial necrosis, the authors demonstrated that contrast enhancement evolves from a focal to a disseminated process during the first 2 weeks after onset of symptoms. However, the magnitude of hyperenhancement was modest (on average only 50–100 percent higher than normal regions), most likely because a traditional spin-echo sequence was used, which has limited T1-

ence of scar in itself may not necessarily be indicative of an adverse prognosis (because most patients with HCM have a benign clinical course). However, it is possible that the *amount* of scarring can be an important prognostic determinant.[114] This hypothesis remains to be tested.

Anderson-Fabry Disease

Unlike patients with classical systemic Fabry disease, who present with multiple organ involvement, patients with the cardiac variant can manifest few or no symptoms and present only with idiopathic LV hypertrophy. In these patients, the cardiac phenotype is similar to that seen in HCM, and the diagnosis can be difficult. Recent data suggest that the prevalence of Fabry disease in a typical HCM referral population can be as high as 5 percent.[115] Moon and coworkers. reported that 50 percent of patients with genetically confirmed Fabry disease have myocardial hyperenhancement.[116] In these patients, hyperenhancement was most frequently observed in the basal inferolateral wall, and often the subendocardium was spared. Histologically, hyperenhanced regions appear to correspond to areas of replacement of viable myocardium with collagenous scar.[117]

Sarcoidosis

Autopsy studies have shown that cardiac involvement is found in 20 to 30 percent of patients with sarcoidosis. However, in vivo, cardiac involvement is recognized in less than 10 percent of patients, as current diagnostic tools are insensitive. Under-recognition of cardiac involvement can be important clinically because sudden cardiac death is one of the most common causes of mortality in sarcoid patients. Recently, Patel and colleagues performed DEMRI in 58 con-

weighting. Given that newer DEMRI techniques provide an order of magnitude improvement in signal-to-noise ratio and contrast-to-noise ratio (CNR) for detecting necrotic myocardium compared with older spin-echo techniques, Mahrholdt and colleagues performed segmented inversion-recovery DEMRI in 32 patients meeting clinical criteria for acute myocarditis.[121] Hyperenhancement was a frequent finding, occurring in 28 patients (88 percent). Additionally, hyperenhanced regions had a predilection for the epicardial half of the lateral free wall (see Fig. 21–23), and on average, 9 ± 11 percent of LV mass was involved. Repeat imaging 3 months later demonstrated substantial shrinkage of hyperenhanced regions (3 ± 4 percent of LV mass). Although some investigators have interpreted this finding as evidence that hyperenhancement in the setting of acute myocarditis can represent viable myocardium, the more likely explanation is that hyperenhanced regions decrease in size because the volume of nonviable myocardium shrinks. As part of the normal healing process, necrotic regions undergo involution as they remodel and are replaced by dense collagenous scar.[121]

Chagas Disease

Chagas disease is an inflammatory disease caused by the protozoan, *Trypanosoma cruzi*. Although most patients survive the acute phase of the disease and remain asymptomatic for many years, 20 percent eventually develop chronic heart failure. Rochitte and coworkers studied 51 patients with Chagas disease.[122] DEMRI demonstrated that the prevalence of myocardial scarring progressively increased from 20 percent in asymptomatic patients without structural heart disease by echocardiography to 100 percent in patients with left ventricular dysfunction and ventricular tachycardia. Scarring occurred most commonly in the LV apex and inferolateral wall. Both non-CAD (isolated epicardial or mid-wall involvement) and CAD type (indistinguishable from prior MI) scar patterns were observed.

Arrhythmogenic Right Ventricular Cardiomyopathy

Traditionally, a major focus in the evaluation of arrhythmogenic right ventricular cardiomyopathy (ARVC) by CMR has been to identify fatty infiltration of RV myocardium using spin-echo sequences.[123–125] However, there is growing realization that this focus can be misplaced because of technical as well as physiologic reasons.[126] Older spin-echo sequences, which take several minutes to acquire, can have substantial motion artifacts as well as partial volume effects because free-breathing occurs throughout image acquisition. Newer TSE sequences are faster and can provide an image during a single breath-hold, however, the amount of cardiac motion that can occur during image acquisition (even when gated to mid-diastole) can be substantial when considering that the RV free wall is normally only 2 to 3 mm thick.[127] Additionally, necropsy studies have demonstrated that intramyocardial fat is frequently seen in normal hearts and that fat infiltration per se should not be considered synonymous with ARVC.[127]

The primary goal of the CMR-imaging examination should be to determine global and regional RV morphology and function. cine imaging should be performed, with high spatial (<2 mm in-plane, ≤6 mm slice thickness) and temporal resolution (≤40 msec per phase), and complete anatomic coverage including the RV outflow tract. In addition to standard cardiac views, two-chamber, long-axis

RV views are often helpful. Although assessment of RV function is more reproducible and specific than fat infiltration,[128] scans can still be overinterpreted because the right ventricle has substantial normal variations including highly variable trabeculation and small outward bulges near the insertion of the moderator band.

More recently, data suggest a potential role for DEMRI in the CMR imaging protocol. Tandri and colleagues reported that hyperenhancement consistent with RV fibrosis was found in 8 of 12 patients (67 percent) that met Task Force criteria for ARVC.[129] Moreover, there was an excellent correlation with histopathology, and DEMRI findings were strongly associated with inducible ventricular tachycardia (VT) on programmed electrical stimulation.

Prognostic and Therapeutic Implications

The hyperenhancement patterns detected by DEMRI can have clinical significance beyond that of simply aiding diagnosis, as there can be prognostic implications. Scarred myocardium is an established anatomic and electrophysiologic substrate for the occurrence of ventricular tachyarrhythmias and sudden death in patients with ischemic heart disease.[130] Additionally, there is reason to believe that scar tissue can serve as substrate for malignant ventricular tachyarrhythmias in patients with nonischemic disorders as well.[131]

[ ] HEMODYNAMICS

CMR examinations often include hemodynamic assessment, which may range from a straightforward evaluation of a single valvular lesion to a complex evaluation involving multiple shunts and baffle leaks in a patient with congenital heart disease. Similar to other CMR protocols, hemodynamic assessment may comprise one or several pulse sequences, depending on the physiologic parameters that are appraised. For example, in valvular stenosis, morphologic characteristics (e.g., leaflet structure and mobility, etc.) and quantitative measurements, such as aortic valve area, can be directly assessed from the cineMRI images. Signal voids, which results from the dephasing of spins that occur with turbulent flow, can be used to qualitatively assess valvular regurgitation. First-pass perfusion imaging can be used to follow the transit of contrast media to determine the presence of intracardiac shunts in a manner analogous to a bubble study in echocardiography. Velocity encoding MRI (VENC MRI) can be used to estimate pressure gradients and blood flow across and orifice. A few select pathophysiologic conditions will be discussed briefly as working examples.

Atrial Septal Defect

CMR-imaging evaluation of atrial septal defect (ASD) has focused on hemodynamic severity as measured indirectly by VENC MRI of the pulmonary artery and aorta (i.e., Qp/Qs). Although this type of approach provides results comparable to invasive oximetry,[132] patient management depends on several additional factors. For instance, the suitability of percutaneous closure using an occluder device depends on the type, size, shape, and location of the defect, in addition to ASD hemodynamic severity. Although these parameters are routinely assessed noninvasively by transthoracic and transesophageal echocardiography, the multiplanar capability of CMR imaging offers the additional advantage of imaging the ASD *en face* (i.e., viewing the ASD

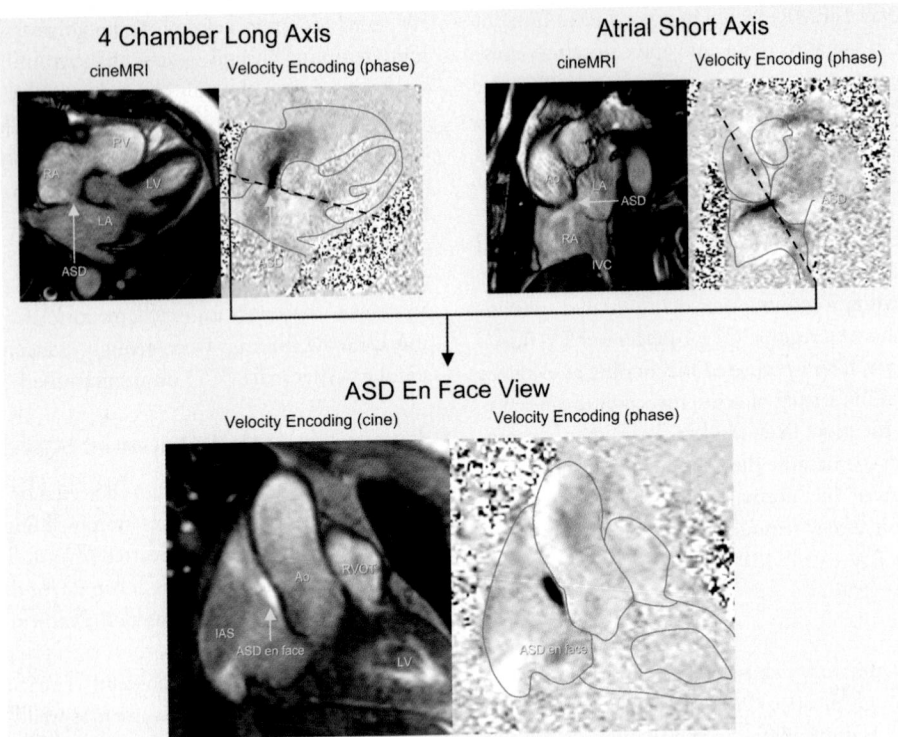

4 Chamber Long Axis

cineMRI   Velocity Encoding (phase)

Atrial Short Axis

cineMRI   Velocity Encoding (phase)

ASD En Face View

Velocity Encoding (cine)   Velocity Encoding (phase)

FIGURE 21–24. Approach to visualization and evaluation of secundum atrial septal defects (ASD) by cardiovascular magnetic resonance (CMR) imaging. *Top:* The approximate plane of the ASD is initially found on long- and short-axis cineangiocardiographic (cine) MRI views of the atria. In-plane velocity-encoding MRI is used to visualize the direction of ASD flow. An en face view of the ASD is prescribed as a plane orthogonal to the direction of ASD flow in both the long- and short-axis planes (*dashed black line*). *Bottom:* ASD flow can be directly measured from the en face view using through-plane velocity-encoding MRI. Adding the en face ASD flow to aortic flow and dividing the sum by aortic flow can calculate the shunt fraction. Also, note the minimal retro-aortic rim that precluded percutaneous closure in this patient. Ao, Aorta; ASD, atrial septal defect; IAS, interatrial septum; IVC, inferior vena cava; LA, left atrium; LV, left ventricle; RA, right atrium; RV, right ventricle.

in the plane of the interatrial septum). From the en face view, the rim of tissue separating the ASD from the base of the aorta (retro-aortic rim), tricuspid valve, vena cavae, and coronary sinus can be viewed from a single image plane[133] (Fig. 21–24). Moreover, from this plane, the anterior-posterior and cranial-caudal diameter of the ASD can be accurately measured, both of which can be important to assess because many defects are irregularly shaped. Flow across the ASD can also be measured directly from the en face view by VENC MRI (see Fig. 21–24). Although earlier literature has suggested that direct en face measurement of flow to determine ASD severity is less accurate than measuring flow in the pulmonary artery and aorta,[132] these studies may have failed to capture the optimal en face imaging plane by not taking into account the double-oblique nature of the interatrial septum, cardiac cycle interatrial septal motion, and ASD flow direction.[134]

Aortic Stenosis

Several validation studies have demonstrated good agreement of aortic valve area by planimetry on cineMRI with measures derived using transesophageal and transthoracic echocardiography, and invasive hemodynamic measurements during cardiac catheterization.[135–137] Ad-

ditionally, peak velocity measurements by VENC MRI appear to correlate well with Doppler echocardiography.[138,139] For both planimetry measurements on cineMRI and velocity measurements on VENC MRI, it is important to image in the correct short-axis plane across the leaflet tips. The correct plane is determined by first, obtaining at least two orthogonal long-axis views of the high velocity jet across the valve (by either cineMRI or VENC MRI). Then, the short-axis plane is placed at the origin of the jet, and the plane is positioned to be orthogonal to the direction of the jet on all the long-axis views. Importantly, a stack of consecutive, parallel short-axis images (at least three) is obtained to make sure that the plane with the highest peak velocity and the smallest peak systolic opening is not missed. Planimetry for valve area is performed on cineMRI with higher spatial and temporal resolution than usual for standard imaging. Planimetry on VENC MRI is not recommended as this usually leads to overestimation of valve area. Pulmonic and mitral valve stenosis are evaluated using a similar approach.

Regurgitant Valvular Lesions

On cineMRI, regurgitant jets appear as signal voids because of intravoxel dephasing of proton spins associated with nonlaminar flow (turbulence, acceleration, etc.). Similar to echocardiography, the size and extent of the regurgitant jet can be used to semiquantitatively grade the severity of regurgitation. An advantage compared with echocardiography is that any imaging plane that is desired can be obtained. A disadvantage is that technical settings such as the TE time (time to echo) and type of pulse sequence can also affect the size of the signal void. Thus, when serial examinations are performed, it is important to use the same sequence with the same settings. Although it has been reported that cine imaging with a spoiled GRE sequence and long TE can be more sensitive to small regurgitant jets than standard SSFP imaging, we have not found this to be clinically significant, perhaps because SSFP imaging has higher signal-to-noise ratio and better image quality.

For quantitative assessment of regurgitation, the regurgitation fraction (ReF) can be calculated from data derived from VENC MRI sometimes in combination with cineMRI. When peak velocities are not that high (< 3 m/s) and flow is not that turbulent, such as often is the case in the setting of pulmonic insufficiency, both forward and regurgitant volume can be directly measured from a single through-plane VENC MRI of the valve in cross-section, and thus ReF calculated. With regurgitant lesions that have higher peak velocities and more turbulent flow (e.g. mitral or aortic regurgitation), the calculation of regurgitant volume and ReF is more complex. Similar to cineMRI, turbulent flow leads to dephasing, and signal loss in VENC MRI. The consequence of signal loss in VENC MRI is an underestimation in flow. Thus, the regurgitant volume is best measured indirectly for both mitral (MR) and aortic (AR) regurgitation. For example, with MR the regurgitant volume can be obtained by subtracting the effective forward flow across the proximal ascending aorta from the diastolic inflow across the mitral valve from two separate through-plane VENC MRI acquisitions. Another approach would be to subtract systolic flow in the proximal ascending aorta measured by VENC MRI from LV stroke volume measured by volumetric quantification of a stack of cineMRI

images. For all VENC MRI acquisitions, TE should be minimized to reduce dephasing and signal loss.

【 】 PERICARDIAL DISEASE AND CARDIAC MASSES

Constrictive Pericarditis

Most of the literature regarding the evaluation of the pericardium has focused on morphologic characterization using older spin-echo (SE) sequences. Using these sequences, pericardial thicknesses of >4 mm were considered abnormal,[140] whereas thicknesses <2 mm were normal. These thresholds were helpful in confirming a diagnosis of constrictive pericarditis,[140] particularly when pericardial thickening was found to be extreme (>5 mm). However, it is important to note the limitations of SE imaging and these threshold values. These older SE sequences were usually gated to the ECG, but because of long acquisition times (several minutes), imaging was performed during free-breathing. Thus, because of respiratory motion, effective in-plane pixel resolution may have been on the order of ≥4 mm. More recently, with the use of faster sequences with image acquisition during breathholding, in-plane resolution is routinely <2 mm, and more subtle pericardial thickening can be appreciated. However, the published literature with regards to normal physiologic values does not yet reflect these technical advancements.

Currently, pericardial constriction is best assessed using a combination of TSE morphology and SSFP cine imaging (Fig. 21–25). The key advantage of TSE over conventional SE sequences is that acquisition time is substantially shorter, allowing an image to be acquired during a single breath. Importantly, however, to minimize motion artifacts and motion-related blurring, imaging should be gated to mid-diastole during relative cardiac standstill (<100 ms in length). SSFP cineMRI is also useful in evaluating the pericardium as it can provide both high spatial resolution and dynamic functional information. In addition to conventional cine imaging, tagged cine-

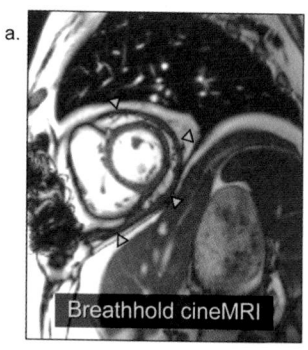
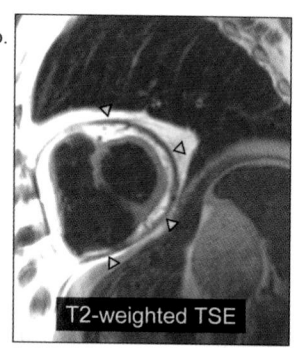
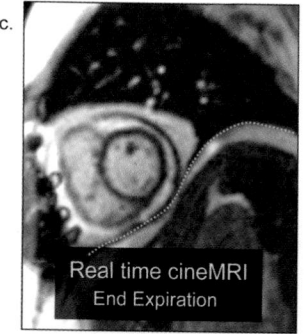
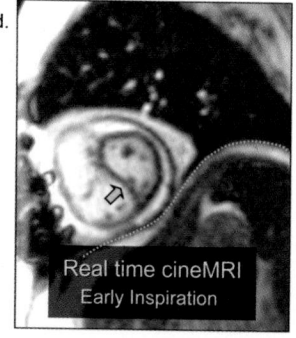
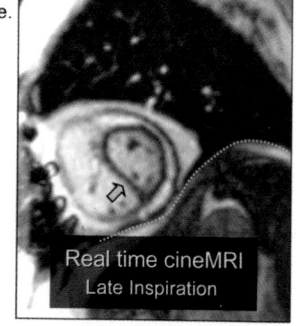

FIGURE 21–25. Representative images from a patient with pericardial constriction. Breathhold cineMRI (single phase shown) and transverse relaxation time (T2)-weighted turbo spin echo imaging shows marked pericardial thickening (*orange arrowheads*). Real-time cineMRI demonstrates displacement of the interventricular septum (*orange arrows*) toward the left ventricle during early inspiration, consistent with ventricular interdependence. The *dotted orange line* highlights the movement of the diaphragm.

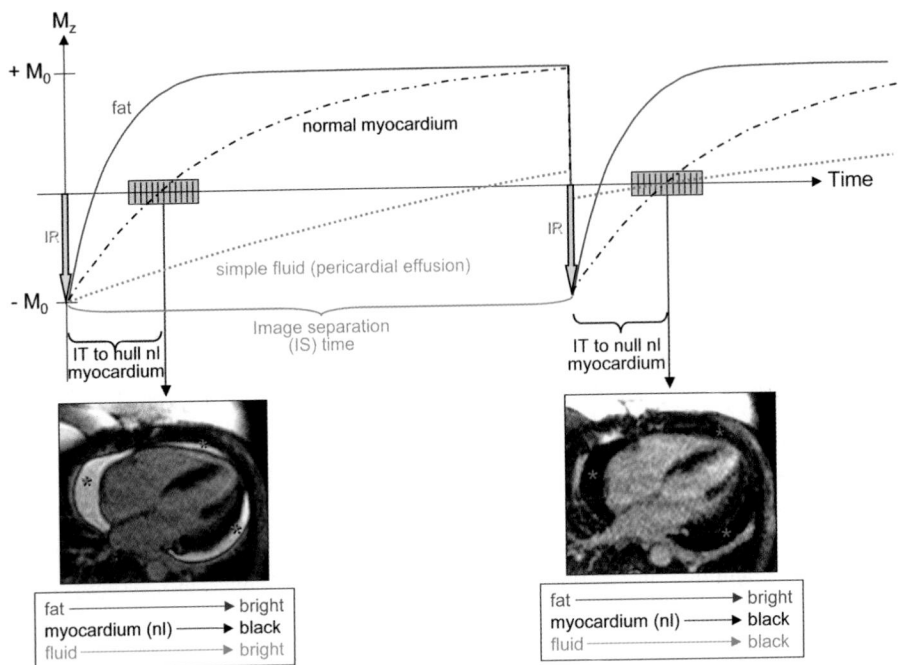

FIGURE 21–26. Evaluation of pericardial effusion using a novel single-shot, steady-state free precession implementation of delayed enhancement MRI (DEMRI). Simple (transudate) effusions exhibit a long longitudinal relaxation time (T1) recovery time that is unchanged by the intravenous administration of gadolinium contrast because gadolinium does not typically penetrate into the pericardial space. With DEMRI, this principle is exploited by obtaining two consecutive images with prespecified timing. Initially, an image is obtained with an inversion time set to null normal myocardium (i.e., conventional DEMRI settings). Fat and fluid will appear bright as these tissues are above and below, respectively, the zero crossing on their T1 relaxation curves. A second image is obtained exactly 2 seconds later with the identical settings. This timing is chosen for two reasons: first, structures with blood perfusion such as myocardium or inherently short T1 such as fat will have recovered magnetization back to baseline; second, pericardial fluid will be near its zero crossing. Thus, on the second image, pericardial fluid will have changed in image intensity from white to black, whereas all other structures will have the same image intensity as on the first image. When the two images are placed in a cine loop for rapid image interpretation, pericardial fluid will *blink* or flicker from white to black continuously. Complex pericardial effusion can be diagnosed if the image separation time that is needed to produce blinking is significantly less than 2 seconds (<1.5 s). Pleural effusion or other fluid collections will demonstrate similar behavior. IR, inversion recovery preparation prepulse; IS, image separation time; IT, inversion time; M_0, baseline magnetization; nl, normal.

MRI and real-time cineMRI can provide supplementary information. With cardiac tagging, discrete tissue points can be tracked throughout the cardiac cycle. This is accomplished using radiofrequency prepulses to label tissue (usually at end-diastole) with a dark grid pattern (see Fig. 21–7). Normally, gridlines at the interface between pericardium and epicardium (actually between parietal and visceral pericardium, as the latter is attached to the epicardium) should shear during systole because the two surfaces move independently and slide during contraction. Conversely, in the setting of pericardial adhesions, gridlines at the interface should remain intact, as motion of the two surfaces would be concordant.

Real-time cineMRI can be used to demonstrate increased ventricular interdependence, a hemodynamic hallmark of pericardial constriction.[141] Specifically, abnormal ventricular septal motion toward the left ventricle in early diastole is seen during the onset of inspiration (see Fig. 21–25). Although the number of patients that have been studied is quite small, this finding appears helpful in distinguishing between constrictive pericarditis and restrictive cardiomyopathy.[141]

Pericardial Effusion

Both loculated and circumferential pericardial effusions are readily identified by CMR imaging. Simple (transudate) effusions typically appear bright and homogenous on T2-weighted images and dark on T1-weighted images. On SSFP cineMRI, which exhibits T2/T1 weighing, simple effusions appear bright with the same or even higher image intensity than epicardial fat. Complex effusions can appear heterogeneous and darker on T2 and SSFP imaging. Additionally, unlike simple effusions, complex effusions can demonstrate increased image intensity on T1-weighted imaging after administration of gadolinium-contrast media. We have found that a novel version of delayed enhancement MRI post–gadolinium contrast can be particularly helpful in detecting even minute amounts of pericardial effusion and distinguishing effusion from other nearby structures (Fig. 21–26).

Masses

There is a large body of literature that addresses the utility of CMR imaging for the evaluation of cardiac masses. Much of this

Morphology (a)   Motion (b)   Perfusion (c)   Delayed Enhancement (d)

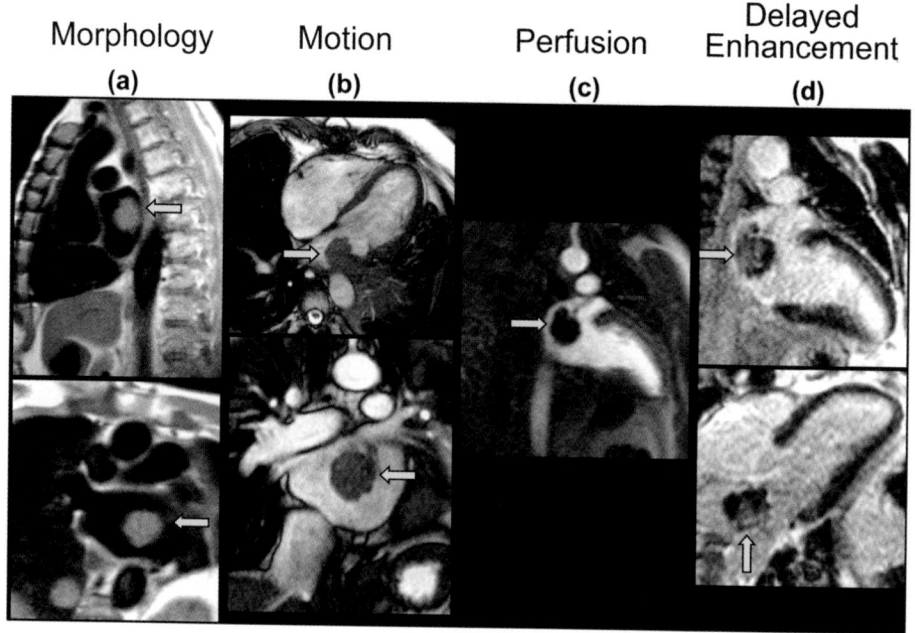

FIGURE 21-27. Evaluation of a cardiac mass. **A.** The protocol consists of one or more stacks of single-shot imaging that combines rapid image acquisition with comprehensive anatomic coverage to quickly delineate morphology. **B.** Cine imaging to view motion during the cardiac cycle. **C.** First-pass perfusion imaging during the transit of an intravenous bolus of gadolinium contrast. **D.** Postcontrast delayed enhancement magnetic resonance imaging (DEMRI), which accentuates differences in contrast uptake between the mass and normal myocardium and between different regions of the mass. In this patient with a left atrial mass (*arrows*), biopsy demonstrated recurrent invasive thymoma (note several extracardiac masses are also present). Perfusion is reduced compared with left ventricular (LV) myocardium. Hyperenhancement is present in a heterogeneous fashion. *Source: Fuster, Kim.[75] Used with permission.*

literature involved attempts to characterize different tissues by comparing image intensities on T1-, T2-, and proton-density weighted images. Differentiating between benign and malignant masses by image intensities, however, was usually poor.[142] This approach to cardiac masses, which relied primarily on older SE sequences, should no longer be used in clinical practice. Instead, at present, a typical protocol for the evaluation of a cardiac mass should consist of multiple pulse sequences where the aim is to assess morphology, motion, perfusion, and delayed enhancement, in addition to inherent differences in T1 and T2 (see Fig. 21–27). This comprehensive protocol identifies both normal variants often mistaken for cardiac masses (e.g., eustachian valve, lipomatous septal hypertrophy, Coumadin ridge) and abnormal physiological characteristics of masses, which can point to a specific diagnosis. For instance, perfusion MRI can demonstrate increased vascularity, which can be prominent in malignancies such as angiosarcoma; DEMRI can identify areas of tissue necrosis within the core of a malignant tumor, which appear as areas of hyperenhancement. Other sequences can also be helpful. Fat can be verified by imaging first without and then with fat saturation techniques. Simple cysts can be identified by characteristic high image intensity on SSFP sequences or by DEMRI in a manner similar to that used to detect pericardial fluid. Finally,

other morphologic characteristics such as tissue invasion or compression, flow obstruction, and associated pericardial effusion are imaged by this protocol (Fig. 21–28).

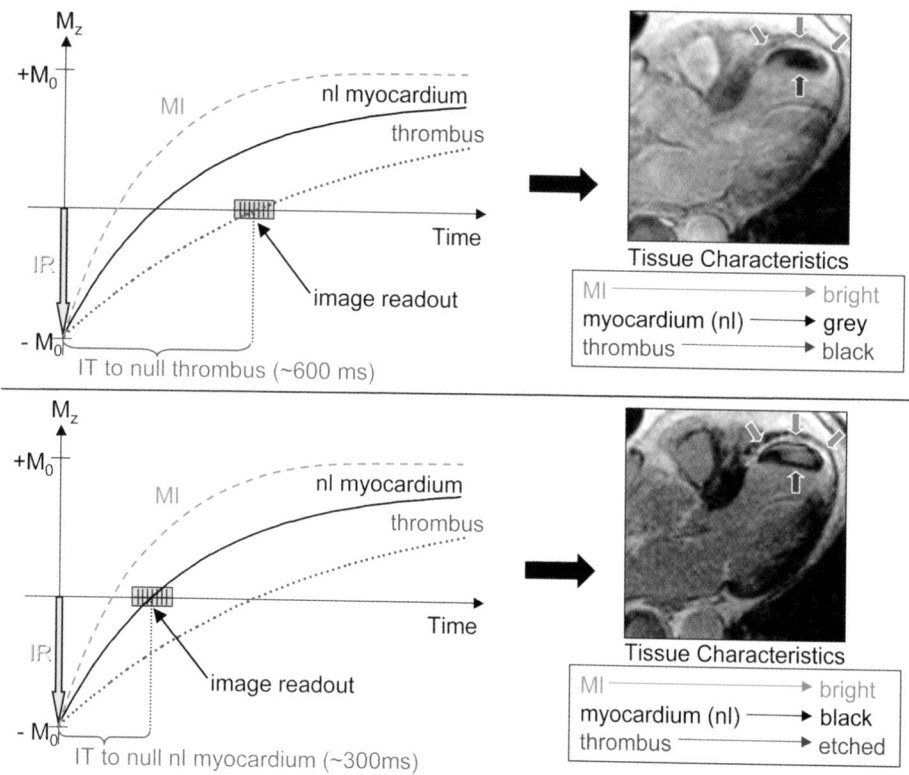

FIGURE 21-28. Evaluation of left ventricular thrombus using delayed enhancement MRI. Following gadolinium administration, the longitudinal relaxation time (T1) relaxation time for thrombus is longer than normal myocardium. When an inversion time (~600 ms) is used to null thrombus, thrombus (*blue arrows*) appears black, whereas normal myocardium appears grey and infarction bright (*red arrows*). When an inversion time to null normal myocardium (~300 ms) is used, thrombus will appear "etched" (grey in center surrounded by dark ring) because of partial volume effects at the periphery. IT, inversion time; nl, normal; MI, myocardial infarction; ms, milliseconds.

Left Ventricular Thrombus

LV thrombus represents an important subset of cardiac masses. Although most common in the LV apex, thrombus can occur elsewhere, with predilection for locations with stagnant blood flow such as adjacent to akinetic, infarcted myocardium. The presence of LV thrombus can be apparent on cineMRI, if the thrombus is clearly intracavitary. However, layered mural thrombus can be difficult to detect because image intensity differences between thrombus and myocardium are minimal.[143,144] Recent studies suggest that delayed enhancement MRI (DEMRI) following contrast administration can be an improved method for detecting LV thrombus (Figure 21–28). The basic principle utilized is that thrombus is avascular and has essentially no contrast uptake. Thus, it should be easily distinguished as a non-enhancing defect surrounded by bright ventricular blood pool and contrast-enhanced myocardium. In separate reports, Mollet[143] and Srichair[144] reported that DEMRI was superior to cineMRI and echocardiography for detection of LV thrombus, respectively. In the latter study, where the truth standard for the presence of thrombus was direct visualization of the LV cavity during surgery or histopathology from resected specimens, DEMRI had markedly higher sensitivity (88 percent) than either transthoracic (23 percent) or transesophageal (40 percent) echocardiography. All three imaging tests had high specificity for LV thrombus (≥96 percent). Based on these data, DEMRI may represent an emerging gold standard for the diagnosis of LV thrombus.

CONCLUSION

Cardiovascular magnetic resonance provides a multifaceted approach to cardiac diagnosis by enabling the assessment of morphology, function, perfusion, viability, tissue characterization, and blood flow during a single comprehensive examination. Establishing standard protocols for image acquisition and interpretation will facilitate widespread adoption as a routine part of clinical practice. Although undoubtedly technical advances will continue, a major goal of future investigation should be to validate a range of currently available clinical applications in large, multi-center trials.

REFERENCES

1. Brown MA, Semelka RC. MR imaging abbreviations, definitions, and descriptions: a review. *Radiology.* 1999;213:647–662.
2. Gibby WA. Basic principles of magnetic resonance imaging. *Neurosurg Clin N Am.* 2005;16:1–64.
3. Shellock FG, Kanal E. *Magnetic Resonance: Bioeffects, Safety, and Patient Management.* New York: Raven Press; 1994.
4. Shellock FG. *Reference Manual for Magnetic Resonance Safety, Implants, and Devices.* 2006 ed. Los Angeles, CA: Biomedical Research Publishing Group; 2006.
5. Patel MR, Albert TS, Kandzari DE, et al. Acute myocardial infarction: safety of cardiac MR imaging after percutaneous revascularization with stents. *Radiology.* 2006;240:674–680.
6. Roguin A, Zviman MM, Meininger GR, et al. Modern pacemaker and implantable cardioverter/defibrillator systems can be magnetic resonance imaging safe: in vitro and in vivo assessment of safety and function at 1.5 T. *Circulation.* 2004;110:475–482.
7. Roguin A, Donahue JK, Bomma CS, et al. Cardiac magnetic resonance imaging in a patient with implantable cardioverter-defibrillator. *Pacing Clin Electrophysiol.* 2005;28:336–338.
8. Nazarian S, Roguin A, Zviman MM, et al. Clinical utility and safety of a protocol for noncardiac and cardiac magnetic resonance imaging of patients with permanent pacemakers and implantable-cardioverter defibrillators at 1.5 tesla. *Circulation.* 2006;114:1277–1284.
9. Shah DJ, Judd RM, Kim RJ. Technology insight: MRI of the myocardium. *Nat Clin Pract Cardiovasc Med.* 2005;2:597–605.
10. Pennell DJ, Sechtem UP, Higgins CB, et al. Clinical indications for cardiovascular magnetic resonance (CMR): consensus panel report. *Eur Heart J.* 2004;25:1940–1965.
11. Bellenger NG, Davies LC, Francis JM, et al. Reduction in sample size for studies of remodeling in heart failure by the use of cardiovascular magnetic resonance. *J Cardiovasc Magn Reson.* 2000;2:271–278.
12. Osterziel KJ, Strohm O, Schuler J, et al. Randomised, double-blind, placebo-controlled trial of human recombinant growth hormone in patients with chronic heart failure because of dilated cardiomyopathy. *Lancet.* 1998;351:1233–1237.
13. Bellenger NG, Rajappan K, Rahman SL, et al. Effects of carvedilol on left ventricular remodelling in chronic stable heart failure: a cardiovascular magnetic resonance study. *Heart.* 2004;90:760–764.
14. Ioannidis JP, Trikalinos TA, Danias PG. Electrocardiogram-gated single-photon emission computed tomography versus cardiac magnetic resonance imaging for the assessment of left ventricular volumes and ejection fraction: a meta-analysis. *J Am Coll Cardiol.* 2002;39:2059–2068.
15. Corsi C, Lang RM, Veronesi F, et al. Volumetric quantification of global and regional left ventricular function from real-time three-dimensional echocardiographic images. *Circulation.* 2005;112:1161–1170.
16. Schulen V, Schick F, Loichat J, et al. Evaluation of K-space segmented cine sequences for fast functional cardiac imaging. *Invest Radiol.* 1996;31:512–522.
17. Atkinson DJ, Edelman RR. Cineangiography of the heart in a single breath hold with a segmented turboFLASH sequence. *Radiology.* 1991;178:357–360.
18. Barkhausen J, Ruehm SG, Goyen M, et al. MR evaluation of ventricular function: true fast imaging with steady-state precession versus fast low-angle shot cine MR imaging: feasibility study. *Radiology.* 2001;219:264–269.
19. Klem I, Heitner JF, Shah DJ, et al. Improved detection of coronary artery disease by stress perfusion cardiovascular magnetic resonance with the use of delayed enhancement infarction imaging. *J Am Coll Cardiol.* 2006;47:1630–1638.
20. Hendel RC, Patel MR, Kramer CM, et al. ACCF/ACR/SCCT/SCMR/ ASNC/NASCI/SCAI/SIR 2006 appropriateness criteria for cardiac computed tomography and cardiac magnetic resonance imaging: a report of the American College of Cardiology Foundation Quality Strategic Directions Committee Appropriateness Criteria Working Group. *J Am Coll Cardiol.* 2006;48:1475–1497.
21. Rehwald WG, Wagner A, Albert TSE, et al. Clinical CMR imaging techniques. In: Manning WJ, Pennell DJ, eds. *Cardiovascular Magnetic Resonance.* New York: Churchill Livingstone; in press.
22. Sodickson DK, Manning WJ. Simultaneous acquisition of spatial harmonics (SMASH): fast imaging with radiofrequency coil arrays. *Magn Reson Med.* 1997;38:591–603.
23. Pruessmann KP, Weiger M, Scheidegger MB, et al. SENSE. sensitivity encoding for fast MRI. *Magn Reson Med.* 1999;42:952–962.
24. Storey P, Chen Q, Li W, et al. Band artifacts due to bulk motion. *Magn Reson Med.* 2002;48:1028–1036.
25. Weinmann HJ, Brasch RC, Press WR, et al. Characteristics of gadolinium-DTPA complex: a potential NMR contrast agent. *AJR Am J Roentgenol.* 1984;142:619–624.
26. Cerqueira MD, Verani MS, Schwaiger M, et al. Safety profile of adenosine stress perfusion imaging: results from the Adenoscan Multicenter Trial Registry. *J Am Coll Cardiol.* 1994;23:384–389.
27. Rossen JD, Quillen JE, Lopez AG, et al. Comparison of coronary vasodilation with intravenous dipyridamole and adenosine. *J Am Coll Cardiol.* 1991;18:485–491.
28. Fieno DS, Kim RJ, Chen EL, et al. Contrast-enhanced magnetic resonance imaging of myocardium at risk: distinction between reversible and irreversible injury throughout infarct healing. *J Am Coll Cardiol.* 2000;36:1985–1991.
29. Kim RJ, Fieno DS, Parrish TB, et al. Relationship of MRI delayed contrast enhancement to irreversible injury, infarct age, and contractile function. *Circulation.* 1999;100:1992–2002.
30. Simonetti OP, Kim RJ, Fieno DS, et al. An improved MR imaging technique for the visualization of myocardial infarction. *Radiology.* 2001;218:215–223.
31. Wagner A, Mahrholdt H, Holly TA, et al. Contrast-enhanced MRI and routine single photon emission computed tomography (SPECT) perfusion imaging for detection of subendocardial myocardial infarcts: an imaging study. *Lancet.* 2003;361:374–379.

32. Wu E, Judd RM, Vargas JD, et al. Visualisation of presence, location, and transmural extent of healed Q-wave and non-Q-wave myocardial infarction. *Lancet.* 2001;357:21–28.

33. Kim RJ, Shah DJ, Judd RM. How we perform delayed enhancement imaging. *J Cardiovasc Magn Reson.* 2003;5:505–514.

34. Polimeni PI. Extracellular space and ionic distribution in rat ventricle. *Am J Physiol.* 1974;227:676–683.

35. Judd RM, Lugo-Olivieri CH, Arai M, et al. Physiological basis of myocardial contrast enhancement in fast magnetic resonance images of 2-day-old reperfused canine infarcts. *Circulation.* 1995;92:1902–1910.

36. Judd RM, Wagner A, Rehwald WG, et al. Technology insight: assessment of myocardial viability by delayed-enhancement magnetic resonance imaging. *Nat Clin Pract Cardiovasc Med.* 2005;2:150–158.

37. Rehwald WG, Fieno DS, Chen EL, et al. Myocardial magnetic resonance imaging contrast agent concentrations after reversible and irreversible ischemic injury. *Circulation.* 2002;105:224–229.

38. Ricciardi MJ, Wu E, Davidson CJ, et al. Visualization of discrete microinfarction after percutaneous coronary intervention associated with mild creatine kinase-MB elevation. *Circulation.* 2001;103:2780–2783.

39. Li W, Li BS, Polzin JA, et al. Myocardial delayed enhancement imaging using inversion recovery single-shot steady-state free precession: initial experience. *J Magn Reson Imaging.* 2004;20:327–330.

40. Sievers B, Elliott MD, Hurwitz LM, et al. Rapid detection of myocardial infarction by sub-second, free breathing delayed contrast-enhanced cardiovascular magnetic resonance. *Circulation.* In press.

41. Edelman RR, Chien D, Kim D. Fast selective black blood MR imaging. *Radiology.* 1991;181:655–660.

42. Debatin JF, Ting RH, Wegmuller H, et al. Renal artery blood flow: quantitation with phase-contrast MR imaging with and without breath holding. *Radiology.* 1994;190:371–378.

43. Pelc LR, Pelc NJ, Rayhill SC, et al. Arterial and venous blood flow: noninvasive quantitation with MR imaging. *Radiology.* 1992;185:809–812.

44. Saloner D. Flow and motion. *Magn Reson Imaging Clin N Am.* 1999;7:699–715.

45. Nagel E, Lehmkuhl HB, Bocksch W, et al. Noninvasive diagnosis of ischemia-induced wall motion abnormalities with the use of high-dose dobutamine stress MRI. comparison with dobutamine stress echocardiography. *Circulation.* 1999;99:763–770.

46. Hundley WG, Hamilton CA, Thomas MS, et al. Utility of fast cine magnetic resonance imaging and display for the detection of myocardial ischemia in patients not well suited for second harmonic stress echocardiography. *Circulation.* 1999;100:1697–1702.

47. Hundley WG, Morgan TM, Neagle CM, et al. Magnetic resonance imaging determination of cardiac prognosis. *Circulation.* 2002;106:2328–2333.

48. Wilke N, Jerosch-Herold M, Wang Y, et al. Myocardial perfusion reserve: assessment with multisection, quantitative, first-pass MR imaging. *Radiology.* 1997;204:373–384.

49. Epstein FH, London JF, Peters DC, et al. Multislice first-pass cardiac perfusion MRI. validation in a model of myocardial infarction. *Magn Reson Med.* 2002;47:482–491.

50. Klocke FJ, Simonetti OP, Judd RM, et al. Limits of detection of regional differences in vasodilated flow in viable myocardium by first-pass magnetic resonance perfusion imaging. *Circulation.* 2001;104:2412–2416.

51. Christian TF, Rettmann DW, Aletras AH, et al. Absolute myocardial perfusion in canines measured by using dual-bolus first-pass MR imaging. *Radiology.* 2004;232:677–684.

52. Lee DC, Simonetti OP, Harris KR, et al. Magnetic resonance versus radionuclide pharmacological stress perfusion imaging for flow-limiting stenoses of varying severity. *Circulation.* 2004;110:58–65.

53. Beller GA, Holzgrefe HH, Watson DD. Effects of dipyridamole-induced vasodilation on myocardial uptake and clearance kinetics of thallium-201. *Circulation.* 1983;68:1328–1338.

54. Glover DK, Okada RD. Myocardial kinetics of Tc-MIBI in canine myocardium after dipyridamole. *Circulation.* 1990;81:628–637.

55. Plein S, Greenwood JP, Ridgway JP, et al. Assessment of non-ST-segment elevation acute coronary syndromes with cardiac magnetic resonance imaging. *J Am Coll Cardiol.* 2004;44:2173–2181.

56. Plein S, Radjenovic A, Ridgway JP, et al. Coronary artery disease: myocardial perfusion MR imaging with sensitivity encoding versus conventional angiography. *Radiology.* 2005;235:423–430.

57. Klein MA, Collier BD, Hellman RS, et al. Detection of chronic coronary artery disease: value of pharmacologically stressed, dynamically enhanced turbo-fast low-angle shot MR images. *AJR Am J Roentgenol.* 1993;161:257–263.

58. Hartnell G, Cerel A, Kamalesh M, et al. Detection of myocardial ischemia: value of combined myocardial perfusion and cineangiographic MR imaging. *AJR Am J Roentgenol.* 1994;163:1061–1067.

59. Al-Saadi N, Nagel E, Gross M, et al. Noninvasive detection of myocardial ischemia from perfusion reserve based on cardiovascular magnetic resonance. *Circulation.* 2000;101:1379–1383.

60. Eichenberger AC, Schuiki E, Kochli VD, et al. Ischemic heart disease: assessment with gadolinium-enhanced ultrafast MR imaging and dipyridamole stress. *J Magn Reson Imaging.* 1994;4:425–431.

61. Bertschinger KM, Nanz D, Buechi M, et al. Magnetic resonance myocardial first-pass perfusion imaging: parameter optimization for signal response and cardiac coverage. *J Magn Reson Imaging.* 2001;14:556–562.

62. Schwitter J, Nanz D, Kneifel S, et al. Assessment of myocardial perfusion in coronary artery disease by magnetic resonance: a comparison with positron emission tomography and coronary angiography. *Circulation.* 2001;103:2230–2235.

63. Panting JR, Gatehouse PD, Yang GZ, et al. Echo-planar magnetic resonance myocardial perfusion imaging: parametric map analysis and comparison with thallium SPECT. *J Magn Reson Imaging.* 2001;13:192–200.

64. Sensky PR, Samani NJ, Reek C, et al. Magnetic resonance perfusion imaging in patients with coronary artery disease: a qualitative approach. *Int J Cardiovasc Imaging.* 2002;18:373–383.

65. Ibrahim T, Nekolla SG, Schreiber K, et al. Assessment of coronary flow reserve: comparison between contrast-enhanced magnetic resonance imaging and positron emission tomography. *J Am Coll Cardiol.* 2002;39:864–870.

66. Chiu CW, So NM, Lam WW, et al. Combined first-pass perfusion and viability study at MR imaging in patients with non-ST segment-elevation acute coronary syndromes: feasibility study. *Radiology.* 2003;226:717–722.

67. Ishida N, Sakuma H, Motoyasu M, et al. Noninfarcted myocardium: correlation between dynamic first-pass contrast-enhanced myocardial MR imaging and quantitative coronary angiography. *Radiology.* 2003;229:209–216.

68. Nagel E, Klein C, Paetsch I, et al. Magnetic resonance perfusion measurements for the noninvasive detection of coronary artery disease. *Circulation.* 2003;108:432–437.

69. Doyle M, Fuisz A, Kortright E, et al. The impact of myocardial flow reserve on the detection of coronary artery disease by perfusion imaging methods: an NHLBI WISE study. *J Cardiovasc Magn Reson.* 2003;5:475–485.

70. Wolff SD, Schwitter J, Coulden R, et al. Myocardial first-pass perfusion magnetic resonance imaging: a multicenter dose-ranging study. *Circulation.* 2004;110:732–737.

71. Giang TH, Nanz D, Coulden R, et al. Detection of coronary artery disease by magnetic resonance myocardial perfusion imaging with various contrast medium doses: first European multi-centre experience. *Eur Heart J.* 2004;25:1657–1665.

72. Paetsch I, Jahnke C, Wahl A, et al. Comparison of dobutamine stress magnetic resonance, adenosine stress magnetic resonance, and adenosine stress magnetic resonance perfusion. *Circulation.* 2004;110:835–842.

73. Cecil MP, Kosinski AS, Jones MT, et al. The importance of work-up (verification) bias correction in assessing the accuracy of SPECT thallium-201 testing for the diagnosis of coronary artery disease. *J Clin Epidemiol.* 1996;49:735–742.

74. Detrano R, Janosi A, Lyons KP, et al. Factors affecting sensitivity and specificity of a diagnostic test: the exercise thallium scintigram. *Am J Med.* 1988;84:699–710.

75. Fuster V, Kim RJ. Frontiers in cardiovascular magnetic resonance. *Circulation.* 2005;112:135–144.

76. Kim WY, Danias PG, Stuber M, et al. Coronary magnetic resonance angiography for the detection of coronary stenoses. *N Engl J Med.* 2001;345:1863–1869.

77. Fieno DS, Shea SM, Li Y, et al. Myocardial perfusion imaging based on the blood oxygen level-dependent effect using T2-prepared steady-state free-precession magnetic resonance imaging. *Circulation.* 2004;110:1284–1290.

78. Wacker CM, Hartlep AW, Pfleger S, et al. Susceptibility-sensitive magnetic resonance imaging detects human myocardium supplied by a stenotic coronary artery without a contrast agent. *J Am Coll Cardiol.* 2003;41:834–840.

79. Shah DJ, Kim RJ. Magnetic resonance of myocardial viability. In: Edelman RR, ed. *Clinical Magnetic Resonance Imaging.* 3rd ed. New York: Elsevier; 2005.

80. Kim RJ, Manning WJ. Viability assessment by delayed enhancement cardiovascular magnetic resonance: will low-dose dobutamine dull the shine? *Circulation.* 2004;109:2476–2479.

81. Klein C, Nekolla SG, Bengel FM, et al. Assessment of myocardial viability with contrast-enhanced magnetic resonance imaging: comparison with positron emission tomography. *Circulation.* 2002;105:162–167.

82. Kim RJ, Wu E, Rafael A, et al. The use of contrast-enhanced magnetic resonance imaging to identify reversible myocardial dysfunction. *N Engl J Med.* 2000;343:1445–1453.

83. Schvartzman PR, Srichai MB, Grimm RA, et al. Nonstress delayed-enhancement magnetic resonance imaging of the myocardium predicts improvement of function after revascularization for chronic ischemic heart disease with left ventricular dysfunction. *Am Heart J.* 2003;146:535–541.

84. Christian TF, Gibbons RJ, Gersh BJ. Effect of infarct location on myocardial salvage assessed by technetium-99m isonitrile. *J Am Coll Cardiol.* 1991;17:1303–1308.

85. Gruppo Italiano per lo Studio della Streptochinasi nell'Infarto Miocardico (GISSI). Effectiveness of intravenous thrombolytic treatment in acute myocardial infarction.. *Lancet.* 1986;1:397–402.

86. Randomised trial of intravenous streptokinase, oral aspirin, both, or neither among 17,187 cases of suspected acute myocardial infarction: ISIS-2. Second International Study of Infarct Survival Collaborative Group. *Lancet.* 1988;2:349–360.

87. Grines CL, Browne KF, Marco J, et al. A comparison of immediate angioplasty with thrombolytic therapy for acute myocardial infarction. The Primary Angioplasty in Myocardial Infarction Study Group. *N Engl J Med.* 1993;328:673–679.

88. Zijlstra F, de Boer MJ, Hoorntje JC, et al. A comparison of immediate coronary angioplasty with intravenous streptokinase in acute myocardial infarction. *N Engl J Med.* 1993;328:680–684.

89. Choi KM, Kim RJ, Gubernikoff G, et al. Transmural extent of acute myocardial infarction predicts long-term improvement in contractile function. *Circulation.* 2001;104:1101–1107.

90. Gerber BL, Garot J, Bluemke DA, et al. Accuracy of contrast-enhanced magnetic resonance imaging in predicting improvement of regional myocardial function in patients after acute myocardial infarction. *Circulation.* 2002;106:1083–1089.

91. Albert TS, Kim RJ, Judd RM. Assessment of no-reflow regions using cardiac MRI. *Basic Res Cardiol.* 2006;101:383–390.

92. Wu KC, Zerhouni EA, Judd RM, et al. Prognostic significance of microvascular obstruction by magnetic resonance imaging in patients with acute myocardial infarction. *Circulation.* 1998;97:765–772.

93. Lima JA, Judd RM, Bazille A, et al. Regional heterogeneity of human myocardial infarcts demonstrated by contrast-enhanced MRI. Potential mechanisms. *Circulation.* 1995;92:1117–1125.

94. Kim RJ, Choi KM, Judd RM. Assessment of myocardial viability by contrast enhancement. In: Higgins CB, Roos AD, eds. Cardiovascular MRI and MRA. Philadelphia, PA: Lippincott Williams & Wilkins; 2003:209–237.

95. Kim RJ, Shah DJ. Fundamental concepts in myocardial viability assessment revisited: when knowing how much is "alive" is not enough. *Heart.* 2004;90:137–140.

96. Cwajg JM, Cwajg E, Nagueh SF, et al. End-diastolic wall thickness as a predictor of recovery of function in myocardial hibernation: relation to rest-redistribution T1–201 tomography and dobutamine stress echocardiography. *J Am Coll Cardiol.* 2000;35:1152–1161.

97. Shah DJ, Kim HW, Elliott M, et al. Contrast MRI predicts reverse remodeling and contractile improvement in akinetic thinned myocardium. *Circulation.* 2003;108:IV-697.

98. Kwong RY, Chan AK, Brown KA, et al. Impact of unrecognized myocardial scar detected by cardiac magnetic resonance imaging on event-free survival in patients presenting with signs or symptoms of coronary artery disease. *Circulation.* 2006;113:2733–2743.

99. Klem I, Shah DJ, White RD, et al. Prognostic value of cardiovascular magnetic resonance assessment of LV function and scar—a multicenter study. *Eur Heart J.* 2006;47:1630–1638.

100. Felker GM, Thompson RE, Hare JM, et al. Underlying causes and long-term survival in patients with initially unexplained cardiomyopathy. *N Engl J Med.* 2000;342:1077–1084.

101. Mahrholdt H, Wagner A, Judd RM, et al. Delayed enhancement cardiovascular magnetic resonance assessment of non-ischaemic cardiomyopathies. *Eur Heart J.* 2005;26:1461–1474.

102. Schuster EH, Bulkley BH. Ischemic cardiomyopathy: a clinicopathologic study of fourteen patients. *Am Heart J.* 1980;100:506–512.

103. Reimer KA, Jennings RB. The "wavefront phenomenon" of myocardial ischemic cell death. II. Transmural progression of necrosis within the framework of ischemic bed size (myocardium at risk) and collateral flow. *Lab Invest.* 1979;40:633–644.

104. Boucher CA, Fallon JT, Johnson RA, et al. Cardiomyopathic syndrome caused by coronary artery disease. III. Prospective clinicopathological study of its prevalence among patients with clinically unexplained chronic heart failure. *Br Heart J.* 1979;41:613–620.

105. Roberts WC, Siegel RJ, McManus BM. Idiopathic dilated cardiomyopathy: analysis of 152 necropsy patients. *Am J Cardiol.* 1987;60:1340–1355.

106. Uretsky BF, Thygesen K, Armstrong PW, et al. Acute coronary findings at autopsy in heart failure patients with sudden death: results from the assessment of treatment with lisinopril and survival (ATLAS) trial. *Circulation.* 2000;102:611–616.

107. Bello D, Shah DJ, Farah GM, et al. Gadolinium cardiovascular magnetic resonance predicts reversible myocardial dysfunction and remodeling in patients with heart failure undergoing beta-blocker therapy. *Circulation.* 2003;108:1945–1953.

108. McCrohon JA, Moon JC, Prasad SK, et al. Differentiation of heart failure related to dilated cardiomyopathy and coronary artery disease using gadolinium-enhanced cardiovascular magnetic resonance. *Circulation.* 2003;108:54–59.

109. Rickers C, Wilke NM, Jerosch-Herold M, et al. Utility of cardiac magnetic resonance imaging in the diagnosis of hypertrophic cardiomyopathy. *Circulation.* 2005;112:855–861.

110. Choudhury L, Mahrholdt H, Wagner A, et al. Myocardial scarring in asymptomatic or mildly symptomatic patients with hypertrophic cardiomyopathy. *J Am Coll Cardiol.* 2002;40:2156–2164.

111. Moon JC, McKenna WJ, McCrohon JA, et al. Toward clinical risk assessment in hypertrophic cardiomyopathy with gadolinium cardiovascular magnetic resonance. *J Am Coll Cardiol.* 2003;41:1561–1567.

112. Moon JC, Mogensen J, Elliott PM, et al. Myocardial late gadolinium enhancement cardiovascular magnetic resonance in hypertrophic cardiomyopathy caused by mutations in troponin I. *Heart.* 2005;91:1036–1040.

113. Maron BJ, Wolfson JK, Epstein SE, et al. Intramural ("small vessel") coronary artery disease in hypertrophic cardiomyopathy. *J Am Coll Cardiol.* 1986;8:545–557.

114. Mahrholdt H, Choudhury L, Wagner A. Relation of myocardial scarring to clinical risk factors for sudden cardiac death in hypertrophic cardiomyopathy. *Circulation.* 2002;106:652.

115. Sachdev B, Takenaka T, Teraguchi H, et al. Prevalence of Anderson-Fabry disease in male patients with late onset hypertrophic cardiomyopathy. *Circulation.* 2002;105:1407–1411.

116. Moon JC, Sachdev B, Elkington AG, et al. Gadolinium enhanced cardiovascular magnetic resonance in Anderson-Fabry disease. Evidence for a disease specific abnormality of the myocardial interstitium. *Eur Heart J.* 2003;24:2151–2155.

117. Moon JC, Sheppard M, Reed E, et al. The histological basis of late gadolinium enhancement cardiovascular magnetic resonance in a patient with Anderson-Fabry disease. *J Cardiovasc Magn Reson.* 2006;8:479–482.

118. Patel MR, Crawley PJ, Heitner JF. Improved diagnostic sensitivity of contrast enhanced cardiac MRI for cardiac sarcoidosis. *Circulation.* 2004;2004:645.

119. Maceira AM, Joshi J, Prasad SK, et al. Cardiovascular magnetic resonance in cardiac amyloidosis. *Circulation.* 2005;111:186–193.

120. Friedrich MG, Strohm O, Schulz-Menger J, et al. Contrast media-enhanced magnetic resonance imaging visualizes myocardial changes in the course of viral myocarditis. *Circulation.* 1998;97:1802–1809.

121. Mahrholdt H, Goedecke C, Wagner A, et al. Cardiovascular magnetic resonance assessment of human myocarditis: a comparison to histology and molecular pathology. *Circulation.* 2004;109:1250–1258.

122. Rochitte CE, Oliveira PF, Andrade JM, et al. Myocardial delayed enhancement by magnetic resonance imaging in patients with Chagas' disease: a marker of disease severity. *J Am Coll Cardiol.* 2005;46:1553–1558.

123. Blake LM, Scheinman MM, Higgins CB. MR features of arrhythmogenic right ventricular dysplasia. *AJR Am J Roentgenol.* 1994;162:809–812.

124. Midiri M, Finazzo M, Brancato M, et al. Arrhythmogenic right ventricular dysplasia: MR features. *Eur Radiol.* 1997;7:307–312.

125. Ricci C, Longo R, Pagnan L, et al. Magnetic resonance imaging in right ventricular dysplasia. *Am J Cardiol.* 1992;70:1589–1595.

126. Bluemke DA, Krupinski EA, Ovitt T, et al. MR Imaging of arrhythmogenic right ventricular cardiomyopathy: morphologic findings and interobserver reliability. *Cardiology.* 2003;99:153–162.

127. Burke AP, Farb A, Tashko G, et al. Arrhythmogenic right ventricular cardiomyopathy and fatty replacement of the right ventricular myocardium: are they different diseases? *Circulation.* 1998;97:1571–1580.

128. Tandri H, Castillo E, Ferrari VA, et al. Magnetic resonance imaging of arrhythmogenic right ventricular dysplasia: sensitivity, specificity, and observer variability of fat detection versus functional analysis of the right ventricle. *J Am Coll Cardiol.* 2006;48:2277–2284.

129. Tandri H, Saranathan M, Rodriguez ER, et al. Noninvasive detection of myocardial fibrosis in arrhythmogenic right ventricular cardiomyopathy using delayed-enhancement magnetic resonance imaging. *J Am Coll Cardiol.* 2005;45:98–103.

130. Hurwitz JL, Josephson ME. Sudden cardiac death in patients with chronic coronary heart disease. *Circulation.* 1992;85:143–49.

131. Kim RJ, Judd RM. Gadolinium-enhanced magnetic resonance imaging in hypertrophic cardiomyopathy: in vivo imaging of the pathologic substrate for premature cardiac death? *J Am Coll Cardiol.* 2003;41:1568–1572.

132. Beerbaum P, Korperich H, Barth P, et al. Noninvasive quantification of left-to-right shunt in pediatric patients: phase-contrast cine magnetic resonance imaging compared with invasive oximetry. *Circulation.* 2001;103:2476–2482.

133. Beerbaum P, Korperich H, Esdorn H, et al. Atrial septal defects in pediatric patients: noninvasive sizing with cardiovascular MR imaging. *Radiology.* 2003;228:361–369.

134. Crowley AL, Thomson LEJ, Heitner JF, et al. Direct en face assessment of atrial septal defects by velocity-encoded cardiac magnetic resonance alters clinical management. *Circulation.* 2004;110:497.

135. John AS, Dill T, Brandt RR, et al. Magnetic resonance to assess the aortic valve area in aortic stenosis: how does it compare to current diagnostic standards? *J Am Coll Cardiol.* 2003;42:519–526.

136. Friedrich MG, Schulz-Menger J, Poetsch T, et al. Quantification of valvular aortic stenosis by magnetic resonance imaging. *Am Heart J.* 2002;144:329–334.

137. Kupfahl C, Honold M, Meinhardt G, et al. Evaluation of aortic stenosis by cardiovascular magnetic resonance imaging: comparison with established routine clinical techniques. *Heart.* 2004;90:893–901.

138. Caruthers SD, Lin SJ, Brown P, et al. Practical value of cardiac magnetic resonance imaging for clinical quantification of aortic valve stenosis: comparison with echocardiography. *Circulation.* 2003;108:2236–2243.

139. Kilner PJ, Manzara CC, Mohiaddin RH, et al. Magnetic resonance jet velocity mapping in mitral and aortic valve stenosis. *Circulation.* 1993;87:1239–1248.

140. Masui T, Finck S, Higgins CB. Constrictive pericarditis and restrictive cardiomyopathy: evaluation with MR imaging. *Radiology.* 1992;182:369–373.

141. Francone M, Dymarkowski S, Kalantzi M, et al. Assessment of ventricular coupling with real-time cineMRI and its value to differentiate constrictive pericarditis from restrictive cardiomyopathy. *Eur Radiol.* 2006;16:944–951.

142. Hoffmann U, Globits S, Schima W, et al. Usefulness of magnetic resonance imaging of cardiac and paracardiac masses. *Am J Cardiol.* 2003;92:890–895.

143. Mollet NR, Dymarkowski S, Volders W, et al. Visualization of ventricular thrombi with contrast-enhanced magnetic resonance imaging in patients with ischemic heart disease. *Circulation.* 2002;106:2873–2876.

144. Srichai MB, Junor C, Rodriguez LL, et al. Clinical, imaging, and pathological characteristics of left ventricular thrombus: a comparison of contrast-enhanced magnetic resonance imaging, transthoracic echocardiography, and transesophageal echocardiography with surgical or pathological validation. *Am Heart J.* 2006;152:75–84.

145. Kanal E, Barkovich AJ, Bell C, et al. ACR Guidance Document for Safe MR practices: 2007. *Am J Radiology.* 2007;188:1–27.

CHAPTER (22)

Magnetic Resonance Imaging and Computed Tomography of the Vascular System

Jean-Christophe Cornilly / Valentin Fuster / Zahi A. Fayad

IMAGING OF THE VASCULATURE WITH MAGNETIC RESONANCE IMAGING AND COMPUTED TOMOGRAPHY

【 】 BACKGROUND

Imaging of the vasculature has evolved greatly in the past 15 years. Although the perceived current gold standard is the time-honored but invasive method of x-ray angiography, noninvasive modalities such as magnetic resonance imaging (MRI) and computed tomography (CT) are becoming routine in the diagnostic examination of patients with vascular diseases. In many instances, either MRI or multislice spiral computed tomography (MSCT) has replaced x-ray angiography as the imaging modality of choice, owing to the ever-increasing quality of the images, the noninvasive application of these modalities, the ease and comfort of the patients, and the clinical versatility of both CT and MRI.

【 】 MAGNETIC RESONANCE ANGIOGRAPHY

Magnetic resonance angiography (MRA) has evolved rapidly since its introduction more than 20 years ago. Initially, non–contrast-enhanced MRA techniques found their way into clinical routine for imaging vascular morphology. These early approaches can in principle be divided into two subgroups, that is, *black-blood* and *bright-blood* sequences. Although black-blood techniques based on signal voids within vessels containing flowing spins can confirm vessel patency, they remain of limited use in the assessment of vascular morphology. They are currently gaining acceptance for the evaluation of the vascular wall.[1,2] Bright-blood MRA techniques are generally divided into those influenced by the effect of blood flow on the signal amplitude (time of flight [TOF]) and those based on the effect of blood flow on phase contrast. Phase-contrast angiography derives image contrast from the differences in the phases accumulated by stationary and moving spins in a magnetic-field gradient. The amount of phase accumulated is directly proportional to the flow velocity, allowing quantitative measurements of flow velocities and the discrimination of flow direction. Spins moving in the direction of the magnetic-field gradient accumulate positive phase, whereas spins moving in the opposite direction accumulate negative phase. Hence, the magnitude of the phase determines the velocity whereas the sign of the accumulated phase determines flow direction. The flow dependence and associated artefacts inherent to these techniques have restricted the clinical use of these MRA techniques primarily to the extra- and intracranial arterial system and the portal venous system. With the advent of high-performance gradient systems, a new MRA strategy has been developed: contrast-enhanced MRA (CEMRA) initially using gadolinium chelates and then other gadolinium-based contrast agents such as blood-pool contrast agents.[3] CEMRA is based on a combination of rapid three-dimensional (3D) imaging and the longitudinal relaxation time (T1)-shortening effect of intravenously infused paramagnetic contrast agent. These techniques have been proven to give an extensive and diagnostically accurate evaluation of intra-[4] and extracranial, thoracic, abdominal, and peripheral vessels. In most centers, 3D CEMRA has replaced conventional x-ray angiography for the clarification of pathologies in arterial vessels. The challenge today is to reduce MRI acquisition time conserving high image quality. Magnetic resonance (MR) scanners at high field strength (≥ 3 tesla [T]) have been introduced in expectation of a larger signal-to-noise ratio, which can decrease the length of scan time and improve the spatial resolution. In some indications such as intracranial arteries assessment, TOF MRA at 3.0 tesla imaging has been shown to provide diagnostic improvement compared to 1.5 T.[4,5]

【 】 WHOLE BODY MAGNETIC RESONANCE ANGIOGRAPHY

Technical improvements including the availability of different high image quality MR sequences, the remote movement of the imaging table and the use of specialized surface coils have rendered whole-body screening with MRI a feasible proposition. Whole-body MRA of patients suspected of having systemic atherosclerotic disease has been shown to be feasible and accurate for evaluation of arteries from the carotid arteries to the lower arteries.[6,7] It usually excludes the intracranial and coronary arteries for which a dedicated examination is still required (Fig. 22–1). Nevertheless, some teams associate vascular examination with MR imaging of the brain and the heart.[8] Compared with digital substraction angiography, its sensitivity for the detection of significant plaques is 96 percent and its specificity 95 to 96 percent;[6,8] those data are comparable to the values for single-station MRA. The contrast-agent dose is comparable to that used for single-station MRA also. In some studies, paramagnetic contrast agent with some degree of albumin binding resulting in high intravascular relaxivity have been employed.[9] Bolus scan time is approximately 60 seconds providing images with high signal-to-noise ratio and contrast-to-noise ratio, whereas total in-room time is 15 to 55 minutes in cases of associated brain or heart imaging.[8,9] Whole-body MRA can also be performed with a standard clinical scanner, but motion artefacts and

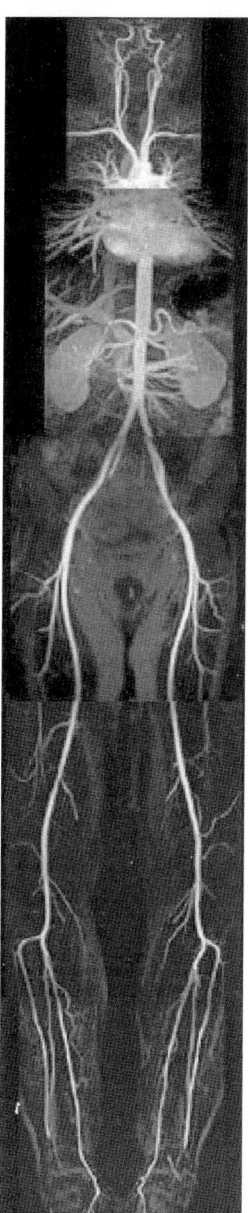

FIGURE 22–1. Coronal three-dimensional, T1-weighted, gradient-recalled-echo, fast low-angle shot, whole-body magnetic resonance (MR) angiograms obtained with a rolling table platform and five contiguous stations in a 31-year-old volunteer. The arterial signal is improved with venous compression. *Source: Modified from Herborn CU, Ajaj W, Goyen M, et al. Peripheral vasculature: whole-body MR angiography with midfemoral venous compression—initial experience. Radiology. 2004;230:872–878.*

timing of the contrast agent through the different segments are still problems to be solved.[10] The total body 3D-MRA permits a comprehensive evaluation of the arterial system in patients with atherosclerosis and does indeed have an impact on patient management in patients with peripheral arterial occlusive disease.[11]

【 】 COMPUTED TOMOGRAPHY ANGIOGRAPHY

Single-spiral (i.e., helical) CT became part of routine diagnostic imaging in the early 1990s; CT as a whole has matured into a volume-scanning modality. 3D-postprocessing methods such as volume-rendering techniques were clinically successful because of the availability of continuous volume data from spiral scanning. However, in practice, the spiral data sets suffered from a considerable mismatch between the transverse (in-plane) and the longitudinal (out-of-plane) spatial resolution. Similarly, many practical limitations still remained that prevented the scanning protocol from being fully adapted to the diagnostic needs of routine practice. The advent in the late 1990s of multidetector CT (MDCT) systems was the first real quantum leap in CT since the introduction of CT. Since, the capabilities of spiral CT have been expanded in several ways allowing the ability to scan anatomic volumes with standard techniques at significantly reduced scan times, to scan larger volumes previously not feasible within the practical limits of scan time or to scan anatomic volumes with high axial resolution (to obtain voxels of $0.35–0.4mm^3$ for 64-MDCT scanners) for excellent 3D-postprocessing and diagnosis.

In addition, the faster gantry rotation time of the new MDCT systems of 330 milliseconds (ms) or less revolutionized the CT application for diagnosis of moving organs. Cardiac CT combines *partial scans* techniques with ECG triggering to freeze heart motion. Multislice spiral scans of the heart with ECG gating provide continuous 3D–data sets during diastole. In combination with dedicated spiral reconstruction algorithms, which are optimized for a high temporal resolution (<100 ms for 64-MDCT scanners), cardiac and coronary CT have became a routine clinical examination with high performances.[12–14] Besides cardiac CT, the advantages of MDCT for assessing the vasculature in general are substantial. MDCT allows reduction of the dose of iodinated contrast agent, improves spatial resolution, and shows fewer pulsation artefacts and greater coverage than single-spiral CT. MDCT technology has substantially improved CT angiography of cerebral, thoracic, abdominal, pulmonary, and peripheral vasculature.

[ ] ELECTRON-BEAM COMPUTED TOMOGRAPHY

Another technique specially designed for cardiac imaging is electron-beam computed tomography (EBCT). EBCT has mainly been used for accurate quantification of coronary calcium from scans of the entire heart in a single breath-hold from rapid (50 to 100 ms) tomographic scans done in synchrony with the heart cycle. Recent MDCT improvement even in calcium scoring showed its superiority on EBCT in term of reproducibility.[15] EBCT is not recommended for risk prediction in asymptomatic patients.[16] The overall role of EBCT in other vascular territories is also limited.

CAROTID ARTERIES

[ ] BACKGROUND

Atherosclerosis of the carotid arteries results in a significant morbidity and mortality. The multicenter North American Symptomatic Carotid Endarterectomy Trial (NASCET) has shown the benefit of carotid endarterectomy for patients with significant and nonsignificant carotid artery stenoses (see Chap. 106). Other studies have also provided convincing evidence that a decision regarding therapy should be based on the degree of stenosis.[17] Congruity in the measurement of carotid stenosis is desirable because patient management can otherwise differ substantially.[18]

X-ray angiography has been the gold standard for diagnosis of carotid bulb disease. However, this modality provides injection images of the carotid bulb, which leads to variation in the measurement of the percent stenosis depending on the observer or the projection. The associated direct and indirect costs and increased procedural risks have prompted the development of other less invasive techniques. Noninvasive imaging tools of extracranial carotid disease include Doppler ultrasound, MRA, and computed tomography angiography (CTA). These modalities have become standard in the preoperative evaluation of carotid artery stenosis. MRA and CTA allow the rapid acquisition of data that can be reconstructed into two-dimensional (2D) and 3D images. High-resolution axial images can provide a cross-sectional view of the carotid vessel and atherosclerotic plaques. Maximum-intensity projection (MIP) allows data to be reconstructed into images that closely resemble conventional x-ray angiograms and can be rotated 360 degrees to be viewed from many angles. With both modalities, by using both axial and MIP images, extensive informations regarding the carotid bifurcation and plaque characteristics can be obtained. A current question is the evaluation of the cost-effectiveness of diagnostic strategies comparing the feasible associations of MRA, CTA, and Doppler ultrasound.[19,20]

[ ] MAGNETIC RESONANCE ANGIOGRAPHY OF THE CAROTID ARTERIES

MRA of the carotid arteries was initially implemented using 2D and 3D TOF techniques; good results for the detection of extracerebral arterial disease were reported.[21] 2D TOF probably offers the best edge definition and sensitivity to slow flow, but its utility is limited because of high incidence of flow voids and susceptibility to artifactual lesions resulting from patient movements. It remains a useful tool for the determination of carotid patency but has generally been replaced by 3D TOF and contrast-enhanced MRA (CEMRA) for routine imaging because these 3D techniques give better spatial resolution and create fewer artefacts.

CEMRA has become the state of the art technique for imaging the carotid circulation. Using gadolinium-enhanced MRA, the external carotid can be imaged in 10 to 20 seconds versus approximately 10 minutes with standard TOF techniques (Fig. 22–2). Several studies have shown CEMRA has high sensitivities and specificities in revealing carotid artery stenosis (Table 22–1). It is now feasible to visualize the entire carotid circulation, including the circle of Willis and aortic branch vessels, in a single study. In addition, breath-holding is not mandatory because these vessels are unaffected by respiratory motion. Differentiation of high-grade stenoses and total vessel occlusions from MRAs of the carotid arteries can be difficult, as the flow characteristics of high-grade stenoses can lead to a signal void in the area of stenoses and might mimic total vessel occlusion. Early venous enhancement in the carotid circulation can interfere with the visualization of the arterial system unless the contrast bolus is accurately timed to the short true arterial phase.

Time-resolved 3D contrast-enhanced MR acquisitions are complementary MRA sequences that enable the visualization of contrast flow dynamics in various types of neurovascular disorders.[32] The short acquisition time allows a selective visualization of the internal carotid arteries without degradation from venous enhancement.[33] The comparatively low spatial resolution is their major limitation.

Other new acquisition techniques alter the method of selecting the information from k-space to enhance spatial resolution while suppressing venous overlap at the same time. Elliptic-centric acquisition acquires the high-contrast elements within k-space prior to venous enhancement, which result in a relative suppression of venous signal intensity.

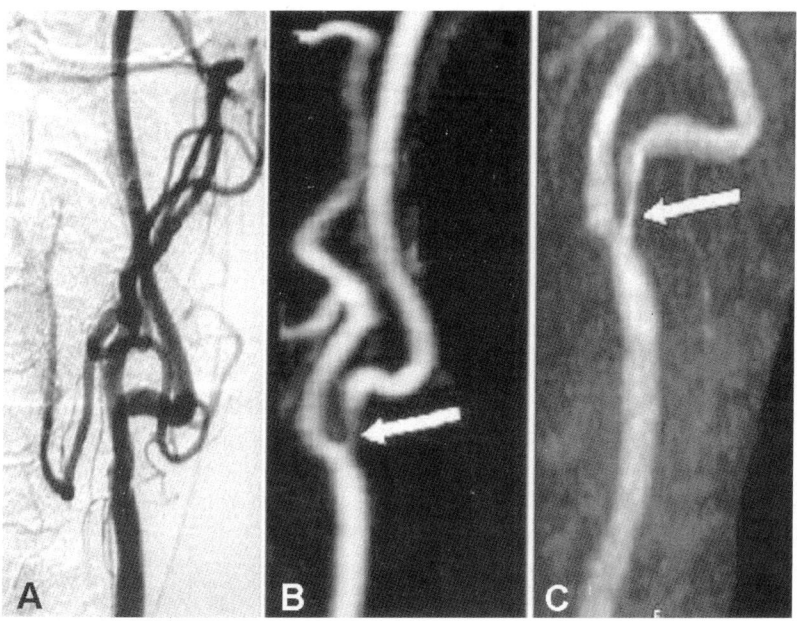

FIGURE 22–2. Images of a 72-year-old man show severe stenosis (*arrows*) of left internal carotid artery at contrast-enhanced magnetic resonance angiography (MRA) (**B**) and three-dimensional, time-of-flight magnetic resonance angiography (**C**). **A.** Stenosis was not visible at conventional digital substraction angiography in this projection. *Source: Modified from Anzalone, Scomazzoni, Castellano, et al.*[22]

and imaging is not dependent on flow characteristics. Thus, severely stenotic but patent vessels can be visualized accurately. Axial images can be magnified to examine plaque morphology and avoid artefacts created by intense calcifications. Single-slice helical CT systems were limited in temporal and spatial resolution, but diagnostic accuracy approaching 90 percent has been reported.[34] The advantages of 4–dynamic computed tomography (DCT) were significant. The next generation of 16-DCT showed further improvements. Studies using 64-DCT have not been reported yet. A scan range of 30 centimeters (cm) can now be covered in an acquisition time of less than 10 seconds, allowing for imaging the whole length of the carotid artery from the aortic arch to the circle of Willis in a true arterial phase (Fig. 22–3). The voxel size can be reduced to 0.3 mm^3 with 16-DCT. The potential of this technique to replace conventional x-ray angiography of the carotid arteries has been demonstrated.[27] The simple calcium score in the cervical carotid arteries can represent an independent marker for luminal stenoses and ischemic symptoms.[35] For intracranial stenoses and occlusion, CTA seems to have a higher sensitivity and specificity than TOF MRA.[36] Using adapted contrast-injection protocols, a comprehensive evaluation of the extra- and intracranial arterial system and of the cerebral veins is feasible in a single CT scan. Extensive strong calcification can still be a limitation because of the overestimation inherent in the CT technique, but the improvement in spatial resolution using 16- and 64-DCT will improve the delineation of calcified plaques. Table 22–1 gives an overview of recent clinical studies on the value of CTA for the detection of significant stenoses of the carotid arteries.

Using the modern imaging approaches described above, isotropic submillimeter voxel sizes can be achieved, covering the complete carotid vasculature in a short acquisition time for true arterial contrast.

【 】 COMPUTED TOMOGRAPHY ANGIOGRAPHY OF THE CAROTID ARTERIES

Besides MRA, CTA has been introduced as a noninvasive procedure for the detection of significant carotid artery stenoses. Intravenous application of iodine contrast agent is required,

TABLE 22–1

Magnetic Resonance Angiography and Computed Tomography Angiography of the Carotid Arteries[a]

REFERENCE	TECHNIQUE	CAROTIDS (N)	SENSITIVITY (%)	SPECIFICITY (%)
Anzalone et al, 2005[22]	MRA	98	100	90
Fellner et al, 2005[23]	MRA	21	100	96.7
Johnson et al, 2000[24]	MRA	76	94	95
Serfaty et al, 2000[25]	MRA	63	94	85
Sardanelli et al, 2000[26]	MRA	56	100	100
Barlett et al, 2006[27]	CTA	268	88.2	92.4
Anderson et al, 2000[28]	CTA	80	77	92
Leclerc et al, 1999[29]	CTA	44	100	97
Marcus et al, 1999[30]	CTA	46	93	97
Verhoek et al, 1999[31]	CTA	38	100	100

[a]Sensitivity and specificity of magnetic resonance angiography (MRA) and computed tomography angiography (CTA) for the detection of significant carotid artery stenoses (>75 percent). Results of a selection of clinical trials as compared to conventional angiography.

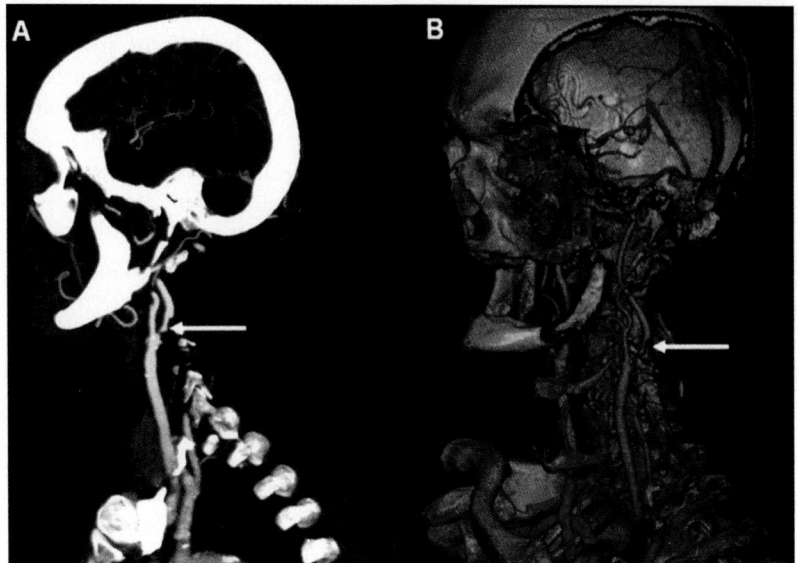

FIGURE 22–3. Contrast-enhanced 16-detector-row computed tomogram of the supra-aortal and intracranial vessels, acquiring a caudocranial scan range of 30 cm in a total of just 12 seconds acquisition time with 0.75-mm thickness. Maximum-intensity projection (MIP) (**A**) and volume-rendering technique (VRT) (**B**) both reveal a complex ulcerated plaque in the proximal right internal carotid artery associated with a high-grade stenosis (arrows). Source: Ertl-Wagner B, Hoffmann RT, Bruning R, et al. [CT-angiographic evaluation of intracranial aneurysms—a review of the literature and first experiences with 4- and 16-slice multi-detector CT scanners.] Radiologe. 2002;42:892–897. Courtesy of B Ertl-Wagner, Ludwig-Maximilians-University, Munich, Germany.

AORTA

█] AORTIC DISSECTION

Acute aortic dissection is a challenging clinical emergency that can have mortal consequences if it is not diagnosed and treated promptly (see Chap. 105). There are 10 to 20 cases per million population per year; if they are not treated, 36 to 72 percent of patients die within 48 hours of diagnosis and 62 to 91 percent within a week.[37] Recent technical advances in noninvasive imaging have greatly improved early diagnosis and treatment planning. 3D CEMRA has become established as a safe and reliable technique for evaluation of the thoracic aorta and major aortic branch arteries. Aortic dissection is potentially life threatening and has routinely been evaluated with modalities highly available in emergency and with rapid examination times: initially x-ray angiography and more recently transesophageal echocardiography and CTA. In the past, emergency MR evaluation for aortic injury or disease was impractical and unsafe because of prolonged examination times. The choice of imaging technique is still controversial and most patients require at least two tests.[38] Most contemporary diagnostic algorithms have placed less emphasis on the role of aortography (sensitivity, 88 percent; specificity, 94 percent).[39] The sensitivity of transesophageal echocardiography has been reported to be as high as 98 percent, and the specificity ranged from 63 to 96 percent.[40] Chest and abdominal dynamic, contrast-enhanced fine-cut CT scanning has a reported sensitivity of 83 to 95 percent and a specificity of 87 to 100 percent for the diagnosis of acute dissection.[41] Each imaging modality has certain advantages and disadvantages. MDCT is now available in most hospitals, usually on an emergency basis. 3D CT scan reconstructions can aid in

treatment planning, but axial imaging affords the best opportunity to detect topographic relationships of the true and false lumens and potential aortic branch compromise. It is unable to provide hemodynamic informations and relies on the use of nephrotoxic contrast agents. Conversely, MRI offers improved anatomic delineation of the aorta and can provide high-quality images in several planes, including a left anterior oblique view that displays the entire thoracic aorta (Fig. 22–4). It does not require the use of nephrotoxic contrast agent but is relatively expensive and not as readily available as conventional CT. Moreover it can be inappropriate in hemodynamically unstable patients, who can be intubated and receiving intravenous medication with continuous arterial pressure monitoring. Total examination time for a complete assessment of the aorta has been reported to be between 10 and 45 minutes; with the recent combination of steady-state gradient echo techniques and advanced gradient hardware, a family of high-speed pulse sequences with very favorable vascular imaging properties has been introduced. Imaging of the aorta can be achieved in a significantly shorter time with adequate image-quality modality, and the imaging time can be reduced to less than 4 minutes. Aortic motion artefacts are frequently seen on thoracic MDCT, especially in patients with low heart rates. If aortic disease is suspected, then measures to reduce motion artefacts, such as ECG-gating should be considered.

█] AORTIC INTRAMURAL HEMATOMA

Aortic intramural hematoma, a variant form of classic aortic dissection, has been accepted as an increasingly recognized and potentially fatal entity of acute aortic syndromes. In CT, demonstration of continuous, usually crescentic, high-attenuation areas along the aortic wall without intimal flap is characteristic before contrast injection, which fails to be enhanced after injection of contrast medium. MRI also very easily detects crescentic aortic wall thickening without intimal flap or tear. As normal thickness of aorta is less than 3 mm by any imaging modality, a wall thickness ≥ 5 mm is sufficient for the diagnosis of intramural hematoma in patients with typical clinical symptoms suggesting acute aortic syndrome.[42,43]

█] AORTIC ANEURYSM
Thoracic Aortic Aneurysm

Although thoracic aortic aneurysms expand at a slower rare than abdominal aortic aneurysm, surgical repair is contemplated when thoracic aneurysm reach a diameter of 5 to 6 cm, depending on their shape and etiology (see Chap. 105). Aneurysm of the thoracic aorta can be classified according to their localization (sinus of Valsalva, ascending aorta, aortic arch, descending aorta), their etiology (congenital, atherosclerotic, luetic, mycotic, traumatic, inflammatory) or their shape (saccular, fusiform, dissecting). For the thoracic aorta, a diameter exceeding 4 cm is generally considered

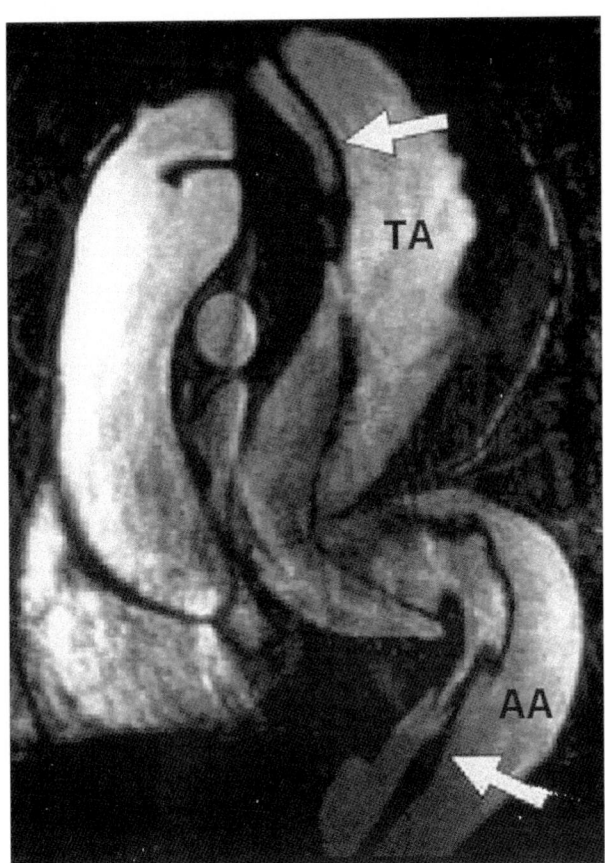

FIGURE 22–4. Contrast-enhanced magnetic resonance angiograms of a 32-year-old patient suffering from Marfan syndrome. The oblique multiplanar reconstruction (MPR) shows an aneurysm of the aorta, extending from the thoracic to the abdominal aorta with extensive elongation and kinking in the course of the complete descending aorta. A dissecting membrane extending from the aortic arch to the distal abdominal aorta (*arrows*) is depicted. AA, abdominal aorta; TA, thoracic aorta. *Source: Huber A, Matzko M, Wintersperger BJ, et al. [Reconstruction methods in postprocessing of CT- and MR-angiography of the aorta]. Radiologe. 2001;41:689–694. Courtesy of A Huber, Ludwig-Maximilians-University, Munich, Germany.*

aneurysmal. When fusiform aneurysms exceed 6 cm in diameter, the risk of rupture is increased, and surgical repair is recommended for patients who can tolerate major surgery. For those who cannot tolerate surgery, endoluminal stenting can be considered. Saccular aneurysms, mycotic aneurysms, and aneurysms that are rapidly increasing in size at a rate exceeding 1 cm per year are also thought to be at increased risk for rupture.[44]

Magnetic Resonance Angiography of Thoracic Aneurysms 3D contrast-enhanced MRA provides a comprehensive overview of the thoracic vascular anatomy, particularly the relationship of aortic aneurysm to branch-vessel origin. Both true and false aneurysms are equally well depicted. A study correlating 3D CEMRA with conventional angiography and surgical exploration demonstrated a diagnostic accuracy of 100 percent for accessing the size and extent of the aneurysm and its relationship to aortic branches.[45] By evaluating the entire aorta, 3D MRA clearly delineates the number of aneurysms present. Arterial phase MRA, however, contains little information about the morphology of the aortic wall. It displays the lumen but can fail to show the full extend

of aneurysm, such as an area that is partially thrombosed. 3D MRA should therefore be complemented by postcontrast acquisitions. The remaining contrast within the blood permits easy differentiation between flowing blood and thrombus. The aortic wall can also be assessed. Enhancement of the aortic wall and surrounding soft tissues is indicative of an inflammatory process, as found in mycotic aneurysm or aortitis. Involvement of the aortic valve should always be considered in the presence of an aneurysm affecting the ascending aorta. Here, the acquisition of cineangiocardiographic (CINE) steady-state free precession (SSFP) sequences in a plane along the axis of the aortic outflow tract can determine whether aortic stenosis and/or regurgitation are present. MRA appears to be effective and reliable for use as the sole imaging method before endovascular repair of aortic aneurysms in patients with renal impairement.[46] The preoperative detection of the artery of Adamkiewicz can also be performed accurately with MRA techniques to avoid spinal complications during surgery.[47]

Abdominal Aortic Aneurysm

Background Abdominal aortic aneurysms (AAAs) are characteristically fusiform in configuration, although occasionally a saccular aneurysm can be seen. Evaluation of patients with abdominal aortic aneurysm should include a systematic description of the following morphologic details: (1) the relationship of the aneurysm to the main and accessory renal, iliac, superior, and inferior mesenteric arteries; (2) the extension of the aneurysm into the common, external, or internal iliac arteries to determine the type and length of prosthetic graft used; and (3) evaluation of coexistent iliac or renal occlusive disease. Conventional x-ray aortography has traditionally been the imaging modality of choice prior to resection of AAAs. Yet, the advantages of cross-sectional imaging provided by MR or CT over x-ray angiography are well established. CT angiography has been the preferred modality for cross-sectional imaging of the abdominal aorta. 3D CEMRA, however, has overcome limitations inherent to conventional MR techniques including long imaging times and reduced vessel-to-background contrast in regions of slow flow (Fig. 22–5).

Magnetic Resonance Angiography of Abdominal Aortic Aneurysms Previously, the use of MRI in the assessment of patients with AAAs has been limited. Noncontrasted bright-blood and black-blood, gradient-echo and spin-echo MRA techniques depend on flow effects to create contrast between vessels and background tissues. The complex and frequently slow-flow patterns typically seen within AAAs result in signal loss and can lead to difficulties in distinguishing between slow flow and thrombus. To prevent saturation effects, images must be acquired in a plane perpendicular to the vessels, resulting in long imaging times with consequent image degradation because of respiratory artefacts and patient motion. Contrast-enhanced MRA techniques are essentially flow-independent. Imaging can be performed in any plane, allowing rapid acquisitions covering a large field of view during a single breath-hold. Analysis of an aneurysmal aorta should always be based on both arterial phase 3D contrast-enhanced MRA, displaying the aortic lumen, in combination with delayed postcontrast scans, depicting the thrombosed portions of the lumen.[48] These delayed scans also evaluate enhancement of the aortic wall

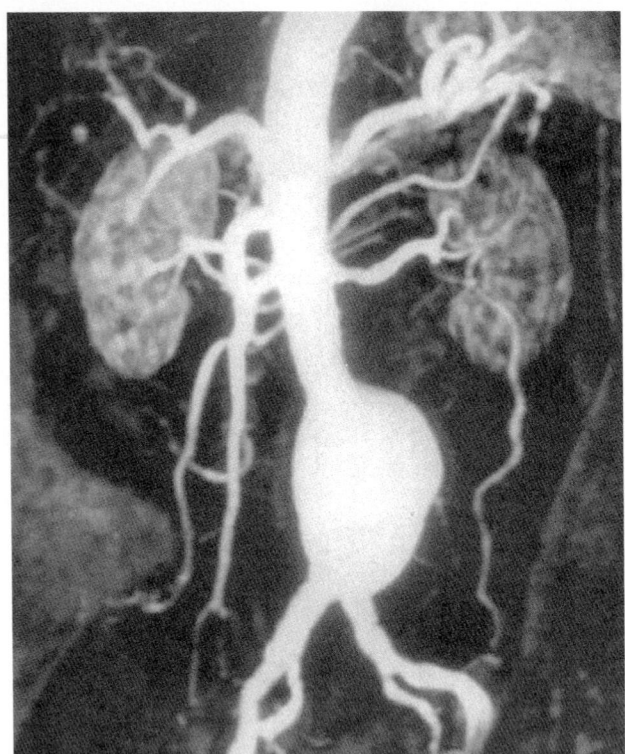

FIGURE 22–5. A 79-year-old man with infra-renal aortic abdominal aneurysm. Contrast-enhanced three-dimensional maximum-intensity-projection magnetic resonance angiographic image shows abdominal aorta and its major branches. *Source: Modified from Atar, Belenky, Hadad, et al.*[46]

and surrounding tissues in inflammatory or mycotic aneurysms. With contrast-enhanced MRA, all details of the aneurysmal morphology are well depicted. The large coronal field-of-view reveals extension of the aneurysm into the iliac arteries. Multiplanar reformations help unfold even reformations, the exact dimensions of the aneurysm can be determined prior to any surgical or percutaneous intervention. MRA is also effective in demonstrating the status of renal arterial origins and their relationship to the aortic aneurysm (see Fig. 22–5). High diagnostic accuracy of 3D CEMRA regarding morphologic analysis of AAAs has been confirmed by several clinical studies.[49,50]

Computed Tomography Angiography of Abdominal Aortic Aneurysms CT has been advocated in the preoperative evaluation of AAAs.[51] It is noninvasive, more accurate than conventional angiography for predicting the size of an AAA, and superior to angiography in its ability to demonstrate mural thrombus within an aneurysm, inflammatory aneurysms, perianeurysmal blood caused by contained rupture, and coexistent nonvascular abdominal disease. Single-slice spiral CT has been shown to enable an accurate depiction of the aneurysmal neck relative to aortic branch vessels as well as an evaluation of the aortic branch vessels themselves. Juxta- and suprarenal extension of an AAA can be missed on x-ray angiography because of the presence of mural thrombus and atheroma at the proximal neck. The ability of CTA to identify renal artery stenoses in the presence of AAAs has been reported with a 94 percent sensitivity and 96 percent specificity for significant stenoses (>50 percent). The introduction of MDCT with adapted contrast-injection protocols has further increased image quality

and diagnostic accuracy. MDCT provides the same information regarding aneurysmal size and extent of mural thrombus available with single-slice helical CT; however, the volumetric acquisition of thinner slices allows multiplanar and 3D renderings to be generated perpendicular to the long axis of the aneurysm, resulting in greater accuracy of the aneurysmal size measurements. Additionally, the improved quality of the dataset available for 3D-image reconstruction and manipulation makes possible the routine display, in considerable detail, of the mesenteric vasculature (Fig. 22–6).

PERIPHERAL VESSELS

【 】 MAGNETIC RESONANCE ANGIOGRAPHY OF THE PERIPHERAL VESSELS

Successful surgical and endovascular arterial revascularization depends on accurate and detailed imaging of the location and degree of the occlusive arterial lesion (see Chaps. 108 and 109). X-ray angiography has been considered the imaging standard in evaluating peripheral arteries and planning treatment of lower limb ischemia. However x-ray angiography has been questioned as the gold standard because it can fail to reveal patent infrapopliteal vessels in patients with multisegmental occlusive lesions and low inflow pressure. Furthermore, a noninvasive alternative to x-ray is attractive because of the small but significant risk of serious complications of 2 to 3 percent using the transfemoral technique. Initially, lower extremity MRA was approached using a TOF technique.[52,53] MRA and conventional angiography were found to be of nearly equivalent accuracy; however, TOF MRA is time consuming and prone to artefacts particularly in the evaluation of vessels in the pelvis. Thus, CEMRA has supplanted TOF MRA for lower extremity arterial imaging. Meta-analyses consistently demonstrated greater accuracy of CEMRA compared with TOF MRA; they suggested a pooled sensitivity rate of 96 to 98 percent and a specificity rate of 96 percent for CEMRA for the detection of significant stenoses.[54] The high degree of agreement between MRA and conventional angiography has lead to surgical planning on the basis of MRA alone (see Fig. 22–6). CEMRA is also suitable for the evaluation of lower extremity bypass grafts and has been found to be 100 percent sensitive and specific for this purpose.[55] Ongoing technical advances in MR such as continuously moving tables, integration of sensitivity encoding (SENSE) strategies,[56,57] will continue to yield higher resolution images. Promising work suggests that MRA with flow-spoiled gradient echo pulses can be used for fresh-blood imaging, thus eliminating the need for contrast while maintaining the short acquisition time and improved spatial resolution of CEMRA.

At present, no single method has emerged as the preferred option, each having different strengths and weaknesses. In various evaluations of lower extremity arterial disease clinical studies, CEMRA was found to be superior to duplex ultrasound and highly accurate compared to conventional angiography, with pooled values of sensitivity of 81 to 100 percent and specificities of 83 to 99 percent (Table 22–2). The agreement between x-ray angiography and CEMRA in patients facing vascular reconstruction is good, and CEMRA is proving to be a noninvasive alternative to x-ray angiography in presurgical evaluation.

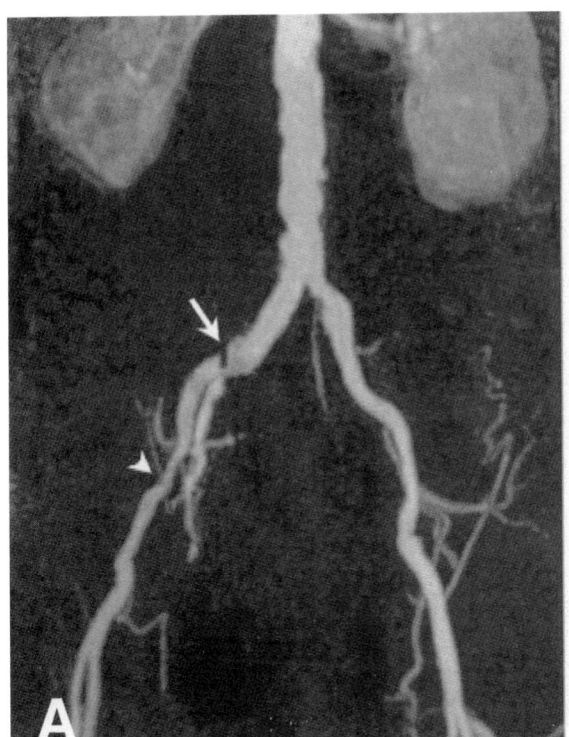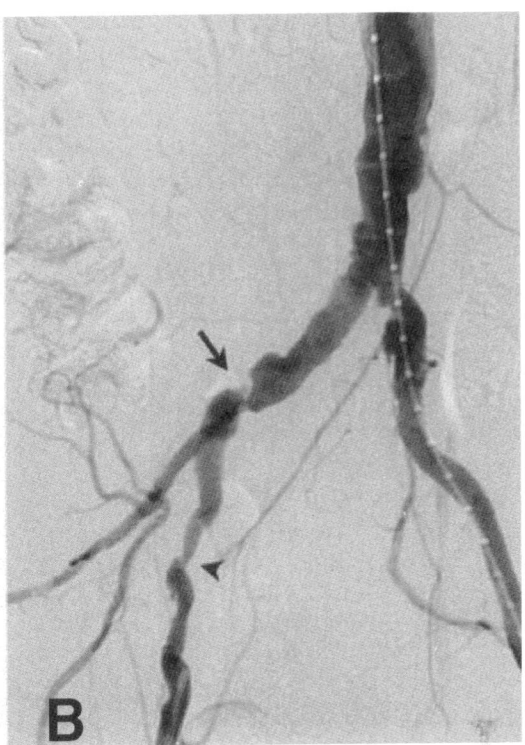

FIGURE 22–6. A 67-year-old male patient suffering from intermittent claudication. Both contrast-enhanced magnetic resonance angiography (**A**) and digital substraction angiography (**B**) show significant stenosis in the right common iliac artery (*arrow*) and in the right external iliac artery (*arrowhead*). *Source: Modified from de Vries M, de Koning PJ, de Haan MW, et al. Accuracy of semiautomated analysis of 3D contrast-enhanced magnetic resonance angiography for detection and quantification of aortoiliac stenoses. Invest Radiol. 2005;40:495–503.*

The early detection of renovascular disease has been previously hampered by the lack of an adequate noninvasive diagnostic modality. CTA and above all CEMRA were found to be significantly more accurate than ultrasound scanning or captopril renal scintigraphy for diagnosis of renal artery stenosis.[66] Sensitivity and specificity rates for the diagnosis of renal artery stenosis with CEMRA have ranged from 82 to 100 percent and 64 to 100 percent respectively. MRA also provides functional information. With phase-contrast MRA, a time-resolved velocity profile of renal arterial flow can be obtained. An abnormal flow corresponds closely to critical renal artery stenosis.[67]

TOF MRA has been validated for imaging of the proximal portions of splanchnic vessels,[68] but it is technically limited by long scan times and flow-dependent signal loss from in-plane and turbulent flow. The advent of CEMRA has provided greater spatial resolution with greater signal-to-noise ratio. Sensitivity and specificity rates for the visualization of the celiac and superior mesenteric arteries and their major branches is 94 to 100 percent.[50,69]

【 】 COMPUTED TOMOGRAPHY ANGIOGRAPHY OF THE PERIPHERAL VESSELS

Until the relatively recent introduction of MDCT, CT angiography was limited to not more than 40 cm of craniocaudal coverage dur-

TABLE 22–2

Magnetic Resonance Angiography and Computed Tomography Angiography of the Peripheral Arteries[a]

REFERENCE	TECHNIQUE	PATIENTS (N)	SENSITIVITY (%)	SPECIFICITY (%)
Hentsch et al, 2003[58]	MRA	203	93	90
Ruehm et al, 2000[59]	MRA	61	92	98
Huber et al, 2000[60]	MRA	24	100	98
Sueyoshi et al, 1999[61]	MRA	23	97	99
Willmann et al, 2005[62]	MDCT (16)	39	96	97
Martin et al, 2003[63]	MDCTA (4)	41	98	97
Ofer et al, 2003[64]	MDCTA (4)	18	91	92
Rieker et al, 1997[65]	SCTA	30	93	99

(4), four detector rows; (16), sixteen detector rows; MDCTA, multidetector CTA; SCTA, spiral CTA.
[a]Sensitivity and specificity of magnetic resonance angiography (MRA) and computed tomography angiography (CTA) for the detection of significant stenoses of peripheral arteries (>75 percent). Results of a selection of clinical trials as compared to conventional angiography.

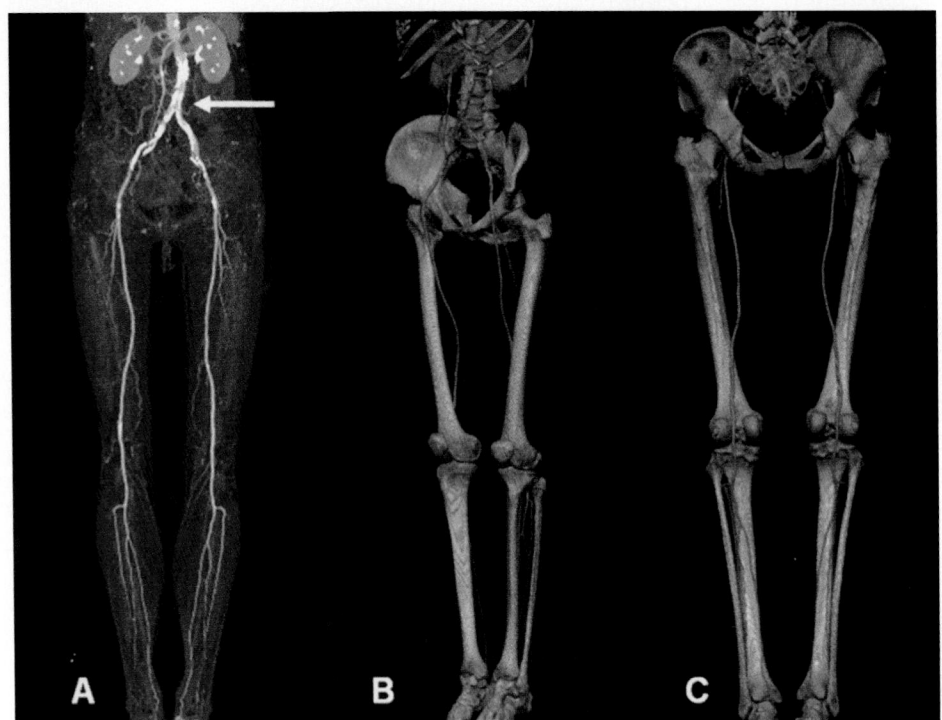

FIGURE 22–7. A 16-DCT angiogram of the peripheral vasculature in a 74-year-old male patient, acquiring 1500 images in an acquisition time of less than 40 seconds; 0.75-mm slice thickness. For maximum-intensity-projections (MIP) (**A**), bony structures have to be segmented manually for a clear visualization of the peripheral vessels. Significant calcifications are demonstrated in the abdominal aorta (*arrow*), but patent arteries are depicted down to the ankle joints on both sides. Using volume-rendering-techniques (VRT) (**B,C**) three-dimensional reconstruction is fast and easy, but bony structures are still visible, so various rotational views have to be obtained for full delineation of the peripheral vessels. *Source: Wintersperger BJ, Herzog P, Jakobs T, et al. Initial experience with the clinical use of a 16-detector row CT system. Crit Rev Comput Tomogr. 2002;43:283–316. Courtesy of BJ Wintersperger, Ludwig-Maximilians-University, Munich, Germany.*

ing a single intravenous contrast injection. Although this distance was sufficient for imaging the majority of systemic arteries, it was insufficient for studying the arterial inflow and runoff of the lower extremities. MDCT with four channels of simultaneous acquisition has eliminated this limitation. This modality is now able to assess lower extremity arterial inflow and runoff offering shorter acquisition times, lower dose of contrast medium, and improved spatial resolution for assessing smaller arterial branches.[70] The 16-DCT systems are able to cover a range of up to 150 cm in less than 40 seconds with a 0.75-mm slice thickness, acquiring approximately 1500 axial images in total (Fig. 22–7). Data on the 64-DCT systems haven't been published yet. Several clinical studies on the implementation of spiral and MDCT for the assessment of peripheral disease have been published, reporting sensitivities of 91 to 98 percent for significant stenoses >75 percent (see Table 22–2). Severe diffuse calcifications can lead to misinterpretation by CT, leading to both false-positive and false-negative results. The inability of conventional angiography to show calf vessels in patients with proximal occlusions is well documented, and it has been indicated that MDCT angiography can allow better visualization of calf vessels in these patients, because a systemic contrast bolus is used and because image quality is largely unaffected by patient motion. The high level of interobserver agreement in the published clinical trials so far indicates that the results as determined by MDCT angiography are highly reproducible. An important consideration in the implementation of CT is that of radiation dose. In the first clinical study on peripheral

MDCT angiography, the calculated radiation dose was 3.9 times lower than that with x-ray angiography.[70] As MDCT angiography continues to improve, technique must be refined further to minimize radiation exposure without compromising image quality. MDCT has improved imaging of the arteries in the lower extremities. The main advantage of this still novel technology are the exceptionally fast scan times, high spatial resolution, increase anatomic coverage, and capability to generate high-quality multiplanar reformations and 3D renderings from raw data that can be reprocessed easily and quickly. The application of MDCT in imaging the lower extremities are multiple and varied, including the evaluation of peripheral arterial occlusive and aneurysmal disease, the patency and integrity of bypass grafts, and arterial injury owing to trauma.[71,72]

MDCTA has been successfully used for the assessment of atherosclerotic renal and mesenteric artery stenoses (see Fig. 22–7). Its diagnostic accuracy is high and similar to that of CEMRA.[66] Nevertheless, a recent study by Vasbinder and colleagues concludes that CTA (sensitivity: 61 to 69 percent, and specificity: 89 to 97 percent) and MRA (sensitivity: 57 to 67 percent, and specificity: 77 to 90 percent) are not reproducible or sensitive enough to rule out renal artery stenosis in hypertensive patients. Therefore, digital subtraction angiography (DSA) remains the diagnostic method of choice.[73]

PULMONARY ARTERIES

【 】 BACKGROUND

The diagnosis of pulmonary embolism (PE) remains difficult because clinical findings are nonspecific, and all available objective tests have practical or clinical limitations (see Chaps. 71 and 72). Pulmonary x-ray angiography remains the gold standard diagnostic test, but it is invasive, can give false-positive results and is not readily available in many centers. Various combinations of noninvasive aids to diagnosis, including assessment of clinical probability of PE, plasma D-dimer concentration, lung scintigraphy (ventilation/perfusion [VQ]), and venous-compression ultrasonography of the legs have been developed and validated to reduce the need for pulmonary angiography. Nevertheless, this procedure is still sometimes necessary in patients with regard to whom the clinical suspicion for PE is high, even after a combination of all the available noninvasive diagnostic tests have been used. In addition to being an invasive test, conventional x-ray angiography carries a risk of major complications of 1 percent and a mortality risk of 0.5 percent.[74] In the last decade, MRA and especially spiral CT have become viable alternatives to conventional angiography in the diagnosis of acute and chronic pulmonary embolism.[75]

【 】 MAGNETIC RESONANCE ANGIOGRAPHY OF THE PULMONARY ARTERIES

Contrast-enhanced MR imaging uses safer contrast agents (i.e., gadolinium chelates) than CT and does not involve radiation exposure. This diagnostic technique is improving constantly. Several methods can be employed to perform MRA, ranging from TOF angiography to gadolinium-enhanced 3D MRA or the use of new blood-pool contrast agents. TOF MRA was applied with some success for imaging of the central pulmonary arteries; however, several problems were identified, including a lack of spatial resolution, insensitivity to slow flow, motion sensitivity, and field-distortion artefacts. The introduction of higher gradient strength systems and the development of short repetition time (TR) 3D-gradient echo sequences allowed the development of single breath-hold 3D contrast-enhanced MRA (Fig. 22–8). The use of shorter scan times allows the investigation even of severely breathless patients. The diagnostic accuracy of time-resolved protocols seems promising.[76] In contrast-enhanced MRA with the use of parallel acquisition techniques, the breath-hold duration of monophasic protocols might be reduced at constant spatial resolution, or the spatial resolution of time-resolved imaging protocols might be improved at fixed breath-hold duration.[77] In addition, MRI allows for the depiction of functional aspects such as perfusion and ventilation, which can further aid in the differential diagnosis of PE and thus facilitate appropriate patient care and treatment. A number of clinical studies have reported high sensitivities and specificities for the detection of pulmonary emboli as compared to conventional pulmonary angiography (Table 22–3). A combined "one-stop-shopping" MRI approach for PE and deep venous thrombosis seems to be feasible and accurate.[86] MRI is more than a promising diagnostic tool that can offer a fast, reliable test for the diagnosis of PE. Management studies will need to demonstrate the additional value of MRA, especially in terms of cost-effectiveness.

Differentiation between different forms of pulmonary hypertension is essential for correct disease management. High spatial-resolution MRA and time-resolved MRA enables the differentiation of primary pulmonary hypertension from chronic thromboembolic pulmonary arterial hypertension with high accuracy.[87,88]

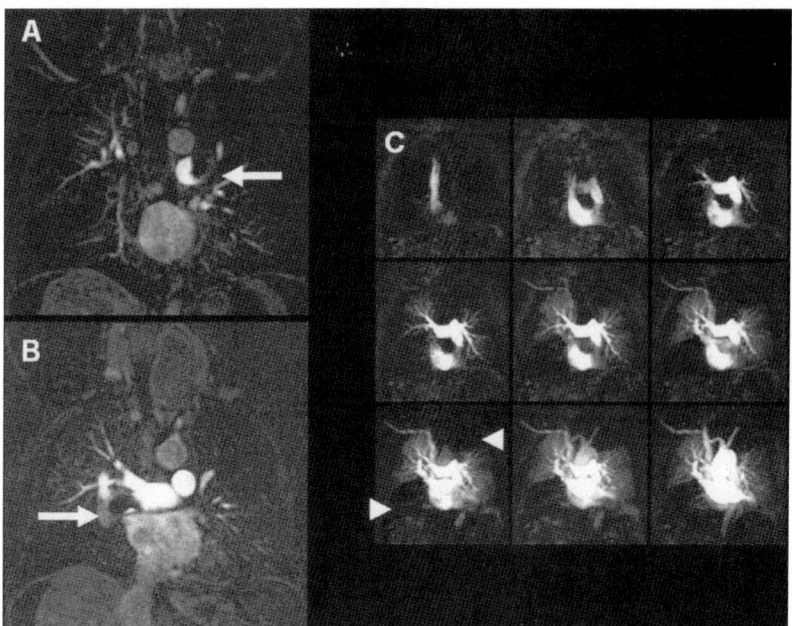

FIGURE 22–8. Three-dimensional, contrast-enhanced, high-resolution magnetic resonance angiography (MRA) of the pulmonary vasculature in a 55-year-old patient (**A,B**) revealing large thromboembolic clots in the central pulmonary artery tree on both sides (*arrows*). Using time-resolved MRA perfusion techniques and acquiring one data set every 1.1 seconds, significant perfusion defects in the upper and right lower lobe become visible (*arrowheads*) (**C**). Time-resolved, contrast-enhanced, high-resolution MRA of the pulmonary vasculature in a 33-year-old patient with Eisenmenger syndrome caused by large membranous ventricular septal defect. The left anterior oblique view of the MRA shows spontaneous contrast filling of both the main pulmonary artery (*black arrow*) and the aorta (*white arrow*) as a result of the right-to-left shunt. *Courtesy of K Nikolaou, Ludwig-Maximilians-University, Munich, Germany.*

TABLE 22–3

Magnetic Resonance Angiography and Computed Tomography Angiography of the Pulmonary Arteries[a]

REFERENCE	TECHNIQUE	PATIENTS (N)	SENSITIVITY (%)	SPECIFICITY (%)
Pleszewski et al, 2006[78]	MRA	48	82	100
Ohno et al, 2004[76]	MRA	48	83	97
Oudkerk et al, 2002[79]	MRA	118	77	98
Gupta et al, 1999[80]	MRA	36	85	96
Meanney et al, 1997[69]	MRA	30	100	95
Stein et al, 2006[81]	CTA	824	83	96
Stone et al, 2003[82]	CTA	25	57	94
Perrier et al, 2001[83]	CTA	299	70	91
Blachere et al, 2000[84]	CTA	179	94	95
Remy-Jardin et al, 2000[85]	CTA	370	96	100

[a]Sensitivity and specificity of magnetic resonance angiography (MRA) and computed tomography angiography (CTA) for the detection of thromboembolic events in the pulmonary vasculature. Results of a selection of clinical trials as compared to conventional angiography.

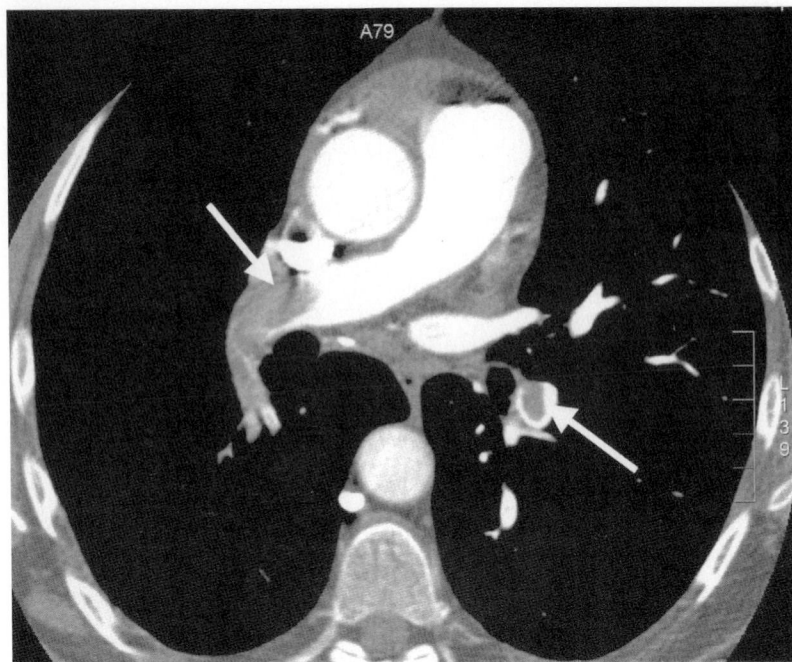

FIGURE 22–9. A 16-dynamic computed tomography (DCT) pulmonary angiography in a 61-year-old female patient with a high clinical probability of pulmonary embolism (PE). CT reveals large thromboembolic clots on both sides confirming a massive PE. *Courtesy of G Le Gal, University Hospital, Brest, France.*

【 】 COMPUTED TOMOGRAPHY ANGIOGRAPHY OF THE PULMONARY ARTERIES

Conventional x-ray angiography has in most institutions been replaced by spiral CT, which is more readily available and yields lower procedure-associated risks. The sensitivity of spiral CT is on the order of 90 percent for central, lobar, or segmental pulmonary emboli (see Table 22–3). The advent of MDCT has enabled better visualization of subsegmental pulmonary arteries also, whereas subsegmental PE is of uncertain clinical significance.[89] CTA has been proven to be an accurate, safe, noninvasive, easily and rapidly performed, widely accepted, and cost-effective technique for direct detection and demonstration of intraluminal PE (Fig. 22–9).[90] The follow-up studies have shown that CT pulmonary angiography can be used in combination with investigation for deep vein thrombosis to exclude PE.[91] CT venography of the pelvis and lower extremities is sometimes incorporated into the CT protocol to identify or exclude concurrent deep venous thrombosis.[92] This strategy seems to have minimal additional benefit.[93] Nowadays, spiral CT pulmonary angiography should be considered the initial imaging modality of choice, particularly in subgroups known for a high rate of nondiagnostic VQ scintigraphy scans, such as hospitalized patients, patients with a history of cardiopulmonary disease, or those with abnormal chest x-rays. Perrier and coworkers showed the potential clinical use of a diagnostic strategy for ruling out PE on the basis of D-dimer testing and multidetector-row CT without lower limb ultrasonography.[94]

CORONARY ARTERIES
【 】 BACKGROUND

The small size and fast motion of the coronary arteries puts any noninvasive diagnostic imaging modality to the test. So far, no cross-sectional imaging modality has proven to be capable of depicting the coronary arteries with a sufficiently high temporal and spatial resolution for a consistent and adequate image quality as good as that of x-ray angiography. Alternative modalities such as EBCT, MRI, and 4-, 16-, and 64-DCT systems have all been tested for their ability to reliably detect significant coronary artery stenoses, with varying results and conclusions but with a constant improvement. In most of the early reports, the pictures were quite impressive but the number of vessel segments or patients excluded because of nonassessability as a direct result of the limitations in image quality were quite high (ranging from 5 to 30 percent.[95] In addition, the assessment was usually limited to the proximal and middle segments of the vessels. Active research and development to overcome the technical barriers of EBCT and MRI is ongoing. At present both MR and EBCT are outperformed by the last generation of CT (64 detector rows, 83 ms temporal resolution, 0.35 mm isotropic voxel spatial resolution). For the first time, a noninvasive procedure has arrived as a robust and reliable noninvasive imaging modality that is capable of producing consistent, high-quality images of the coronary arteries in most patients.

【 】 MAGNETIC RESONANCE ANGIOGRAPHY OF THE CORONARY ARTERIES

Although several imaging modalities have been tested clinically for the detection of coronary artery lesions, MRI deserves special attention. MRI can deliver high-resolution images with superb contrast characteristics in any desired orientation; it is therefore especially suited to studies of the coronary anatomy. Functional parameters such as myocardial function or perfusion under rest and pharmacological stress can be used to complement the evaluation of suspected coronary artery lesions. Coronary arteries are surrounded by epicardial fat; thus, using bright-blood techniques, fat suppression is essential for adequate visualization of the vessel. Further improvements to enhance contrast from the coronary artery to the myocardium include additional preparatory pulses such as magnetization transfer and transverse relaxation time (T2) preparation, which are likely to improve the image quality overall.

Since the first clinical result in 1993,[96] noninvasive coronary MRA has undergone numerous technical improvements and innovations. MRA of the coronary arteries (MRCA) is still an area of active research. The major challenges for MRCA include spatial resolution and coverage, compensation of cardiac and respiratory motion, and signal-to-noise limitations. Many imaging techniques are available: 2D breath-hold MRCA scans,[96] 3D respiratory-gated MRCA scans[97] that provide greater signal-to-noise ratio (Fig. 22–10), and breath-hold 3D MRCA scans.[98] A multicenter study using a 3D respiratory navigator approach reported an acceptable overall sensitivity of 82 percent for detecting significant stenoses (>50 percent) in proximal and middle vessel segments.[99] Still, after more than 10 years of preclinical trials using different MRCA techniques, none has yet emerged as superior to provide a sensitivity and specificity for coronary lesion detection that can compare with that of conventional x-ray angiography.[100]

MRI methods continue to improve. Advanced new generation noncontrast-enhanced and contrast-enhanced 3D or four-dimensional (4D) breath-hold techniques appear to be fast and easy to use. These and other various new MRCA techniques await further clinical trials to determine their effectiveness. The majority of manufacturers now offer dedicated MRI cardiac scanners with strong imaging gradients (>30 mT/m) and fast rise times (>150 mT/m) optimized for a smaller effective imaging field of view to provide higher speed and a better signal-to-noise ratio. Improved quantitative and qualitative coronary MRA image measurement has been achieved using adiabatic T2 preparation at 3 teslas.[101] Introduction of parallel MRI acquisition techniques, such as simultaneous acquisition of special harmonics (SMASH) [102] and sensitivity encoding (SENSE)[103] provide additional speed enhancement that is required to shorten imaging time.

New intravascular contrast agents can provide the long-awaited boost for reliable MRCA. First studies on animals[104–106] or in healthy volunteers[107] have shown promising results. Fibrin-binding molecular MR contrast agents have shown their ability in detecting coronary thrombus and in-stent-thrombosis.[108,109]

Today, established clinical applications include the evaluation of the patency of coronary artery bypass grafts (see Noninvasive Imaging of Bypass Grafts below) and the imaging of anomalous coronary arteries.[110] MRA is also a reliable tool for coronary artery aneurysm identification in patients with Kawasaki disease.[111] The capability to detect reliably significant coronary artery stenoses in proximal and middle-vessel segments with an acceptable sensitivity using any of the techniques available today is still being discussed, with significant differences of opinion. As the MR technique continues to improve, the long-term value of MRCA cannot be underestimated in spite of the advent of MDCT coronary angiography.

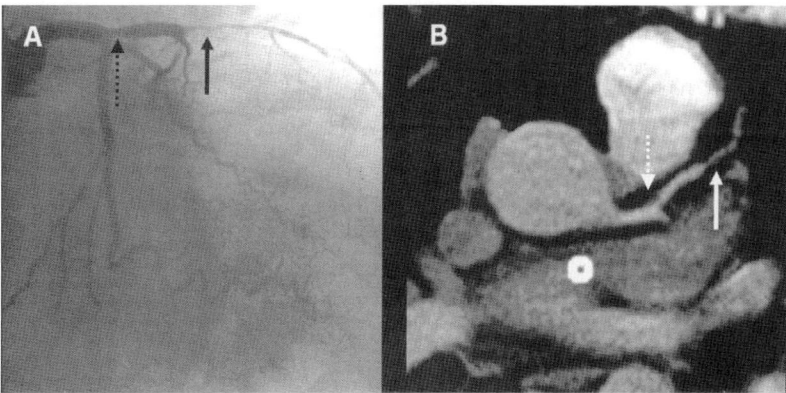

FIGURE 22–10. Conventional coronary x-ray angiograms of a 60-year-old male patient show a nonsignificant plaque at the ostium of the proximal left anterior descending coronary artery (LAD) (*black dotted arrow*) and a high-grade extended stenosis beginning in the middle part of the proximal lad (*black arrow*) (**A**). A maximum intensity projection (MIP) of a three-dimensional, noncontrast-enhanced, navigator-gated, time-of-flight magnetic resonance angiogram shows a signal loss in the corresponding vessel segments (*white dotted arrow and white arrow*) (**B**). *Source: Modified from Nikolaou, Huber, Knez, et al.*[95]

【 】 COMPUTED TOMOGRAPHY ANGIOGRAPHY OF THE CORONARY ARTERIES

The introduction of 4-DCT in 1998 had a major impact on non-invasive imaging of the coronary arteries.[65] The introduction of its immediate successor, the 16-DCT system in 2002 has extended the dominant role of CT in noninvasive coronary imaging today. The 64-DCT era makes CT routine practice for coronary artery imaging.

The gantry rotation time in 16-DCT for cardiac investigations was 420 ms allowing for 210-ms exposure time up to a rate of 65 per minute. This was a 20 percent gain in temporal resolution over that of a 4-channel detector system. The special resolution along the Z axis improved by 25 percent to reach 0.75 mm versus 1.0 mm on a 4-DCT system. In-plane resolution had remained the same, but still, using 16-DCT, almost isotropic voxels were acquired with a voxel size of approximately $0.6 \times 0.6 \times 0.75$. The depiction and delineation of calcified and noncalcified plaques were improved. The complete heart, on a 16-DCT scanner, could be depicted in a significantly shorter breath-hold time of less than 20 seconds compared to 35 to 40 seconds breath-hold on a 4-DCT. This resulted in a considerable reduction in motion artefacts. The

continuous data acquisition of a coronary MDCT data set allows slice reconstruction at different time positions within the cardiac cycle. These scans are typically reviewed on the basis of cross-sectional images in combination with 3D reconstructions.[112] The increase in dosage comparing 4-DCT to 16-DCT coronary angiography was not significant at approximately 4 millisievert (mSv) for 4-DCT and 8 to 5 mSv for 16-DCT if prospective tube current modulation is used.[113] β blocker preparation in patients with heart rates >65 beats per minute was mandatory to ensure motion-free image quality. Using 16-DCT, with shorter image-acquisition times, contrast timing was more accurate, so that less contrast agent was needed (80 mL of contrast agent in comparison to 120 to 160 mL for 4-DCT).[112]

The vendors introduced the 64-DCT in the fall of 2004. All the technical parameters were improved once again, although the clinical implications are not all defined yet. Spatial resolution reaches 0.35 mm isotropic voxels. Tube rotation time has been increased to 330 ms, allowing temporal resolution of 83 ms compared with 40 to 66 ms for conventional angiography.[114] Scan time has fallen to less than 12 seconds.[14] In the same time, ECG-gating techniques and image analysis software has also been improved.

Clinical studies using 4-DCT scanners have reported sensitivities and specificities for significant coronary artery stenoses (>75 percent) of 78 to 85 percent and 76 to 98 percent, respectively (Table 22–4). Up to 30 percent of the proximal and middle coronary segments were interpretable because of insufficient image quality. The studies on 16-DCT report high sensitivities and specificities of 92 to 95 percent and 86 to 93 percent. The number of poorly assessable segments was lower (6 to 21 percent), indicating the robustness of the technique. Nevertheless, some recent studies are less optimistic and show a high rate of false positives.[125] The studies on 64-DCT report even higher sensitivities and specificities of 86 to 94 percent and 95 to 97 percent respectively with a low rate of nonassessable segments (0 to 12 percent).

Nevertheless, major limitations remain. Severe calcifications are still causing partial volume beaming artefacts in spite of the improvement in spatial resolution, producing false positive results

TABLE 22–4

Magnetic Resonance Angiography and Computed Tomography Angiography of the Coronary Arteries[a]

REFERENCE	TECHNIQUE	PATIENTS (N)	SENSITIVITY (%)	SPECIFICITY (%)
Klem et al, 2006[115]	MRA	100	89	87
Ishida et al, 2005[116]	MRA	49	88	87
Regenfus et al, 2003[117]	MRA	61	85	90
Plein et al, 2003[118]	MRA	40	74	88
Watanabe et al, 2002[119]	MRA	22	80	85
Leber et al, 2005[120]	MDCTA (64)	59	80	97
Raff et al, 2005[121]	MDCTA (64)	70	95	90
Leschka et al, 2005[14]	MDCTA (64)	47	95	95
Ropers et al, 2003[122]	MDCTA (16)	77	92	93
Nieman et al, 2001[123]	MDCTA (4)	35	81	97
Nikolaou et al, 2002[95]	EBCTA	20	85	77
Budoff et al, 1999[124]	EBCTA	52	78	91

(4), four detector rows; (16), sixteen detector rows; MDCTA, multidetector CTA; SCTA, spiral CTA.
[a]Sensitivity and specificity of magnetic resonance angiography (MRA) and computed tomography angiography (CTA) for the detection of significant coronary arteries stenoses (>75 percent). Results of a selection of clinical trials as compared to conventional angiography.

compared to cardiac x-ray angiography. In segments with extensive calcifications, significant coronary artery stenoses can neither be concluded nor ruled out. The one major disadvantage of increasing the number of slices of data obtained and reducing the slice collimation (thickness) is an increase in the radiation dose to the patient. Recent MDCT studies show a substantial increase in dose to 11 to 21 mSv.[14,126] ECG-gated tube current modulation reduces the dose by up to 50 percent but at the expense of inability to reconstruct end-systolic images and greater sensibility to arrhythmia. Zanzonico and colleagues estimate that the higher dose exposure yields lifetimes risks of 0.07 percent (MDCT) and 0.02 percent(conventional x-ray angiography) of inducing a fatal cancer in the general population, but, combining radiogenic and non-radiogenic risks of both procedures, it yields a 0.13 percent overall risk of mortality from conventional angiography (nearly twofold higher than that for MDCT angiography [0.07 percent]).[127]

The main advantage of 64-DCT angiography of the coronary artery system seems to be the increased number of investigations with sufficiently good image quality. This improvement in clinical application is also a consequence of shorter breath-holding time, improved spatial and temporal resolution, and the decreasing need of blockers for heart rate control. Although there are not any guidelines about the clinical use of MDCT, its high negative predictive value indicates that it can be an ideal tool to rule out coronary artery disease (CAD) in low-prevalence populations, as in symptomatic patients with atypical chest pain. Cordeiro and coworkers show that MDCT could be a good tool to assess stenoses severity in patients with known severe CAD and high calcification level;[128] nevertheless, MDCT appears not yet to be suited to determine disease severity or progression in CAD patients. These patients would still best be approached by conventional x-ray angiography, which would also allow percutaneous interventions in the same session. MDCT has been eval-

uated with good results in heart transplant patients and allows to avoid conventional coronary angiography as far as patients have strictly normal MDCT at followup.[129] MDCT showed its accuracy, also, in the preoperative assessment of CAD in patients with aortic valve stenosis (Fig. 22–11) and in the detection of CAD in elderly and obese patients.[130–132]

Coronary stents can now be well visualized using 16- and 64-DCT. The patency of the stent lumen can be confirmed or excluded in most patients, and the degree of in-stent stenoses can be estimated (Fig. 22–12).[133]

Another technique for cardiac imaging and coronary angiography is EBCT. EBCT has mainly been used for accurate quantification of coronary artery calcium, scanning the entire heart in a single breath-hold from rapid (100 ms) tomographic scans done in synchrony with the heart cycle. It can be effective for detection of stenotic lesions and occlusions in the proximal and middle segments of coronary arteries.[134] Sensitivities range from 74 percent

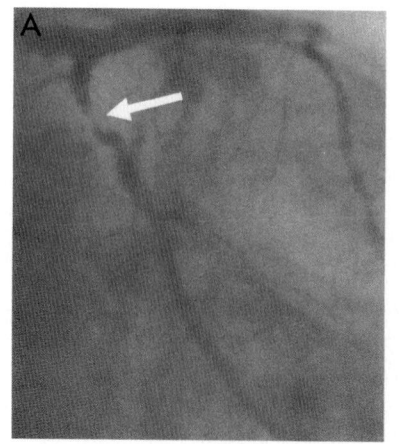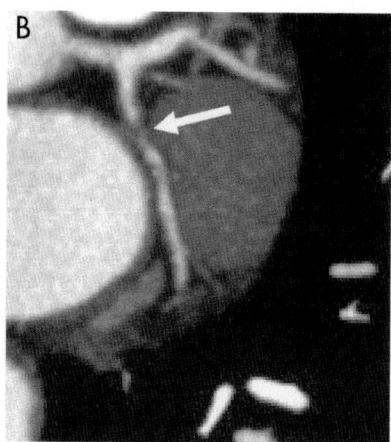

FIGURE 22–11. Images of a 78-year-old man undergoing presurgical testing before aortic valve replacement (aortic valve degenerative stenosis). Angiogram (**A**) and 16-dynamic computed tomography (DCT) (**B**) show a suboccluded left circumflex artery. *Gilard, Cornilly, Pennec, et al.[130] Courtesy of M Gilard, University Hospital, Brest, France.*

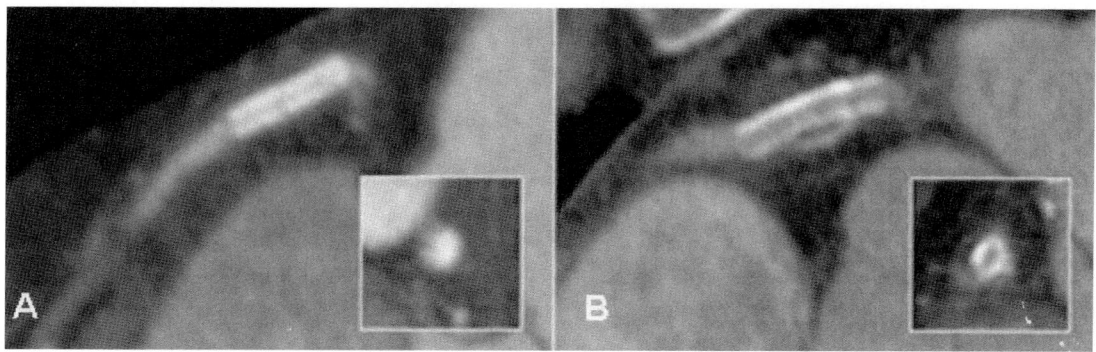

FIGURE 22–12. Right coronary artery stents. **A.** Stent of 2.5 mm diameter with a noninterpretable lumen. **B.** Stent of 3.5 mm diameter with an interpretable lumen. *Source: Gilard, Cornilly, Pennec, et al.*[133] *Courtesy of M. Gilard, University Hospital, Brest, France.*

to 92 percent, and specificities range from 66 to 94 percent.[95] One limitation has consistently been that a substantial number of coronary artery segments cannot be evaluated for stenoses because of a poor image quality (11 to 28 percent of the segments).[134] Calcifications within the coronary arteries can also be assessed by EBCT without contrast enhancement. The presence of coronary artery calcium detected by EBCT in asymptomatic individuals has a high predictive value for cardiac events and overall mortality during the following 3 to 5 years.[135,136]

【 】 NONINVASIVE IMAGING OF BYPASS GRAFTS

Background

Coronary artery bypass graft surgery is still a frequently performed revascularization procedure in patients with multivessel CAD. The clinical outcome after bypass surgery depends on the status of the grafts postoperatively. Initially most patients are free of angina, but patients can develop chest pain as a result of acute occlusion early after surgery or gradual progression of atherosclerosis in the long term. Coronary angiography is the gold standard to evaluate the status of graft patency, but this is an invasive procedure with a small risk of potentially serious complications. These disadvantages make the use of coronary angiography less attractive as a diagnostic screening tool for patients with bypass grafts who present with postoperative angina. The need for alternative noninvasive method is apparent.

Magnetic Resonance Imaging of Bypass Grafts

MR imaging is a noninvasive alternative that allows direct visualization of coronary artery bypass grafts. Previously, 2D spin-echo and gradient-echo MR techniques and 3D breath-hold contrast-enhanced MR angiography techniques have enabled the evaluation of graft patency, but these techniques as a whole could only differentiate between patency and occlusion. Visualization of different graft segments and detection of graft stenosis remain difficult. MRI with flow mapping and high-resolution navigator-gated 3D MRA allows good differentiation between patent and occluded but also the assessment of vein graft disease with a fair diagnostic accuracy. These approaches offer perspective as a noninvasive diagnostic tool for patients with recurrent chest pain after vein graft surgery.[137,138]

Computed Tomography Imaging of Bypass Grafts

With the faster speed of 16- and 64-DCT systems, CTA of bypasses can now be performed with thin collimations and has become a useful tool in clinical practice. Depicting a range from the aortic arch or the subclavian artery to the base of the heart now takes 15 to 30 seconds. Using ECG gating, high quality angiograms become feasible. Several clinical studies on the assessment of mammary and venous bypass grafts using MDCT have been published. Graft patency has been accurately evaluated with 4- and 16- DCT (sensitivity: 97 to 100 percent; specificity: 98 percent).[139,140] Evaluation of stenosed segments is more challenging, and published results are not all concordant. Sensitivity and specificity to detect significant stenosis on a per-segment basis are 80 to 98.5 percent and 85 to 93.9 percent respectively.[140–142] However patient-based analysis reveals that only a relatively small number of patients (*negative* and completely evaluatable graft-CTA) truly profits from noninvasive workup and could be spared invasive angiography.[143]

ATHEROSCLEROTIC PLAQUE

【 】 MAGNETIC RESONANCE PLAQUE IMAGING

Conventional x-ray angiography is an excellent tool to determine the degree and extent of luminal narrowing, but it cannot detect early lesion development when the luminal area is maintained by positive vascular remodelling. This is an important limitation of angiography in that high-grade coronary stenoses are more likely to produce stable ischemia, but lesions with positive remodelling are often the lesions that cause myocardial infarction or sudden death. MR imaging allows for 3D evaluation of vascular structures and outstanding depiction of various components of the atherosclerotic plaque, including lipid, fibrous tissue, calcium and thrombus formation.[143,144] Combining MRI with cellular and molecular targeting can provide important data on the biological activity of potentially vulnerable lesions (i.e., cap thickness, lipid content, presence of activated macrophages, microvessels density, tissues factors, etc.). MRI has been used to determine plaque size and composition in aortas and carotid arteries (Fig. 22–13). In-vivo coronary artery plaque imaging is much more challenging; preliminary studies in a pig model show that the difficulties of coronary wall imaging result from a combina-

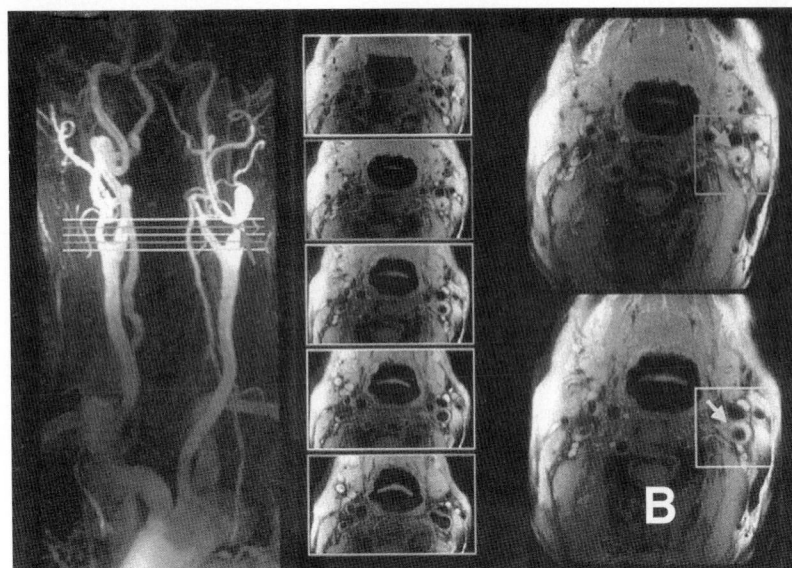

FIGURE 22–13. Carotid magnetic resonance (MR) angiograms (*left panel*) showing severe stenosis in the left internal carotid artery (*arrow, left panel*). MR angiogram was obtained with a contrast-enhanced, three-dimensional, fast gradient-echo and carotid-aortic-arch–phased array coil. Cross-sectional MR black-blood images of carotid arteries are shown in the *middle* and *right panels*. Display of MR slice positions are shown in *left panels* (*lines*). Magnified views of some carotid are shown in the *right panel*. Arrows indicate carotid plaques. *Source: Fayad ZA, Fuster V. Clinical imaging of the high-risk or vulnerable atherosclerotic plaque. Circ Res. 2001;89:305–316. Courtesy of ZA Fayad, Mount Sinai School of Medicine, New York.*

tion of cardiac and respiratory motion artefacts, nonlinear course, small size, and location.[145] Human in-vivo data have been published, but future studies are still needed to further explore these advanced imaging techniques (Fig. 22–14).[146] The role of MRI for the assessment of plaque morphology has been demonstrated in several investigations: discrimination between medial and adventitial layers,[147] between collagenous cap, lipid core, and calcifications,[1] determination of the presence of necrotic core and recent haemorrhage.[148,149] MRI has been used also to diagnose and follow the development of in-vivo atherosclerotic lesions either in animals[150] or humans.[151,152] An extensive area of MRI research has been the use of noninvasive MRI techniques for molecular and targeted contrast imaging. Conventional gadolinium-containing contrast agent can improve detection of plaque[153,154] or identify plaque with increased vascularity.[154] Gadolinium-based agents can enhance lipid-rich plaque;[155] ultrasmall particles of iron oxide are present in 75 percent of the aorta vulnerable plaques but only 7 percent of the stable plaques[156] and are a marker of macrophage rich plaques.[157] Many specific contrast agents have been or are tested with different targets: thrombus recombinant HDL-like nanoparticles, agents targeting $\alpha_n\beta_3$ integrin, metalloproteinase inhibitors, and so forth.

COMPUTED TOMOGRAPHY PLAQUE IMAGING

Primary requisites for the assessment of atherosclerotic calcified and noncalcified plaques are similar to the requirements for a high-quality CTA of the arteries, es-

pecially the coronary arteries, that is, achieving both high spatial and high temporal resolution at the same time. Compared to low pressure arterial systems, such as the pulmonary arteries where calcifications are absent, and the injection rate can be increased to visualize the smallest arterial branches, in coronary arteries the opacification must not exceed approximately 300 Hounsfield units (HU) for a reliable depiction and judgement of calcifications. Optimization of the vessel contrast-to-noise ratio is also mandatory for sufficient visualization of noncalcified plaques. Methods to enhance the contrast-to-noise ratio in the vessel wall include either the use of a test bolus setting or a bolus tracking. Because nonenhanced blood and noncalcified plaques have a similar attenuation on CT (50 to 70 HU), this type of lesion can be detected only after the administration of contrast media. Therefore, vessel enhancement significantly above the CT values of noncalcified plaques (150 HU) must be achieved to allow for reliable detection of noncalcified plaques. With this vessel enhancement, calcified coronary lesions remain detectable because their attenuation is significantly higher. CT has become an established method for noninvasive and highly sensitive detection of coronary artery calcifications. It has the potential to identify early, noncalcified plaques in vivo even in the coronary arteries. MDCT sensitivity for detection of calcified plaques is high, 94 to 95 percent, but it drops to 53 to 78 percent for the detection of exclusively noncalcified plaques.[158,159] Although some authors reported a high diagnostic accuracy for detection of vulnerable lesions when compared to intravascular ultrasonography,[160] others reported difficulties in differentiating between fibrous-rich and lipid-rich plaques either in vivo in

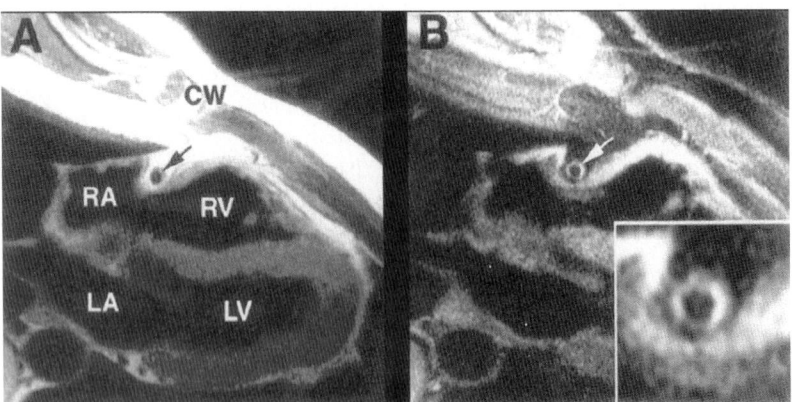

FIGURE 22–14. In-vivo, cross-sectional black-blood MRIs of lumen (**A**) and wall (**B**) of the right coronary artery (RCA) from a 45-year-old male patient with ecstatic atherosclerotic coronary arteries and a thickened coronary wall. The luminal image (**A**) is obtained without fat saturation; the wall image (**B**) is obtained with fat saturation to better delineate the coronary artery wall. Blood flow in the coronary artery lumen is suppressed with velocity-selective inversion preparatory pulses. Maximum wall thickness is 3.3 mm. The BB-magnetic resonance (MR) cross-sectional luminal image reveals a circular lumen and anterior plaque (*arrow*) (**A**). The cross-sectional image of the wall clearly reveals a variably thick proximal RCA, with the wall being thinner at approximately the 6 o'clock position and thicker in other sectors (**B**). B, Inset, Magnified view. LA, left atrium; LV, left ventricle; RA, right atrium; RV, right ventricle. *Source: Fayad, Fuster, Fallon, et al.[146] Courtesy of ZA Fayad, Mount Sinai School of Medicine, New York.*

animals[161] or under ex-vivo conditions.[162] More recently, using a 64-DCT system, Leber and coworkers showed an overall sensitivity and specificity to detect nonsignificant coronary plaques of 84 percent and 91 percent respectively[120] and encouraging results to detect different types of coronary plaques in the proximal coronary system.[12] These different studies determine soft plaques (14 to 51 HU), intermediate plaques (71 to 116 HU), and calcified plaques (391 to 715 HU).[159,161,163] Acute intravascular thrombi can also be detected in vivo; the appearance of the irregular thrombus is typical with low attenuation numbers in the range of 20 to 30 HU. The precise characterization of plaque with CT is still not accessible with current techniques. Moreover, the quantification of wall thickness is also limited.[12]

CONCLUSION

In conclusion, in the very near future and for most vascular territories, it will be possible to perform diagnostic angiography using noninvasive methods such as MRA or CTA. Both modalities offer significant advantages for certain vascular territories but with significant drawbacks inherent to both. In the peripheral circulation, MRA might be the imaging procedure of choice. CTA plays a major role in pulmonary and coronary imaging. MRA is more suited for elective diagnosis rather than clinical emergencies. Both noninvasive imaging technologies are improving by leaps and bounds. Thus it is difficult to predict which will dominate future clinical applications and indications, as both are undergoing rapid evolution in hardware, principal acquisition techniques, postprocessing tools, and specific contrast agents. It is safer to conclude that the future of catheter-based x-ray angiography will generally be downgraded to an adjunctive role in the diagnosis of various vascular diseases or primarily as a conduit to the rising number of catheter-based cardiovascular interventions.

REFERENCES

1. Quick HH, Debatin JF, Ladd ME. MR imaging of the vessel wall. *Eur Radiol* 2002;12:889–900.
2. Toussaint JF, Lamuraglia GM, Southern JF, et al. Magnetic resonance images lipid, fibrous, calcified, hemorrhagic, and thrombotic components of human atherosclerosis in vivo. *Circulation* 1996;94:932–938.
3. Saeed M, Wendland MF, Higgins CB. Blood pool MR contrast agents for cardiovascular imaging. *J Magn Reson Imaging* 2000;12:890–898.
4. Majoie CB, Sprengers ME, van Rooij WJ, et al. MR angiography at 3t versus digital subtraction angiography in the follow-up of intracranial aneurysms treated with detachable coils. *AJNR Am J Neuroradiol* 2005;26:1349–1356.
5. Willinek WA, Born M, Simon B, et al. Time-of-flight MR angiography: comparison of 3.0-t imaging and 1.5-t imaging—initial experience. *Radiology* 2003;229:913–920.
6. Fenchel M, Requardt M, Tomaschko K, et al. Whole-body MR angiography using a novel 32-receiving-channel MR system with surface coil technology: first clinical experience. *J Magn Reson Imaging* 2005;21:596–603.
7. Brennan DD, Johnston C, O'Brien J, et al. Contrast-enhanced bolus-chased whole-body MR angiography using a moving tabletop and quadrature body coil acquisition. *AJR Am J Roentgenol* 2005;185:750–755.
8. Fenchel M, Scheule AM, Stauder NI, et al. Atherosclerotic disease: whole-body cardiovascular imaging with MR system with 32 receiver channels and total-body surface coil technology—initial clinical results. *Radiology* 2006;238:280–291.
9. Ruehm SG, Goehde SC, Goyen M. Whole body MR angiography screening. *Int J Cardiovasc Imaging* 2004;20:587–591.
10. Hansen T, Wikstrom J, Eriksson MO, et al. Whole-body magnetic resonance angiography of patients using a standard clinical scanner. *Eur Radiol* 2006;16:147–153.
11. Goyen M, Herborn CU, Kroger K, et al. Total-body 3D magnetic resonance angiography influences the management of patients with peripheral arterial occlusive disease. *Eur Radiol* 2006;16:685–691.
12. Leber AW, Becker A, Knez A, et al. Accuracy of 64-slice computed tomography to classify and quantify plaque volumes in the proximal coronary system: a comparative study using intravascular ultrasound. *J Am Coll Cardiol* 2006;47:672–677.
13. Ropers D, Rixe J, Anders K, et al. Usefulness of multidetector row spiral computed tomography with 64- × 0.6-mm collimation and 330-ms rotation for the noninvasive detection of significant coronary artery stenoses. *Am J Cardiol* 2006;97:343–348.
14. Leschka S, Alkadhi H, Plass A, et al. Accuracy of MSCT coronary angiography with 64-slice technology: first experience. *Eur Heart J* 2005.
15. Ulzheimer S, Kalender WA. Assessment of calcium scoring performance in cardiac computed tomography. *Eur Radiol* 2003;13:484–497.
16. O'Rourke RA, Brundage BH, Froelicher VF, et al. American College of Cardiology/American Heart Association expert consensus document on electron-beam computed tomography for the diagnosis and prognosis of coronary artery disease. *J Am Coll Cardiol* 2000;36:326–340.
17. Rothwell PM, Gutnikov SA, Warlow CP. Reanalysis of the final results of the European carotid surgery trial. *Stroke* 2003;34:514–523.
18. U-King-Im, JM, Trivedi RA, Cross JJ, et al. Measuring carotid stenosis on contrast-enhanced magnetic resonance angiography: diagnostic performance and reproducibility of 3 different methods. *Stroke* 2004;35:2083–2088.
19. Nonent M, Serfaty JM, Nighoghossian N, et al. Concordance rate differences of 3 noninvasive imaging techniques to measure carotid stenosis in clinical routine practice: results of the CARMEDAS multicenter study. *Stroke* 2004;35:682–686.
20. Buskens E, Nederkoorn PJ, Buijs-van der Woude T, et al. Imaging of carotid arteries in symptomatic patients: cost-effectiveness of diagnostic strategies. *Radiology* 2004;233:101–112.
21. Carriero A, Scarabino T, Magarelli N, et al. High-resolution magnetic resonance angiography of the internal carotid artery: 2d vs 3d tof in stenotic disease. *Eur Radiol* 1998;8:1370–1372.
22. Anzalone N, Scomazzoni F, Castellano R, et al. Carotid artery stenosis: intraindividual correlations of 3D time-of-flight MR angiography, contrast-enhanced MR angiography, conventional DSA, and rotational angiography for detection and grading. *Radiology* 2005;236:204–213.
23. Fellner C, Lang W, Janka r, et al. Magnetic resonance angiography of the carotid arteries using three different techniques: accuracy compared with intra-arterial x-ray angiography and endarterectomy specimens. *J Magn Reson Imaging* 2005;21:424–431.
24. Johnson MB, Wilkinson ID, Wattam J, et al. Comparison of Doppler ultrasound, magnetic resonance angiographic techniques and catheter angiography in evaluation of carotid stenosis. *Clin Radiol* 2000;55:912–920.
25. Serfaty JM, Chirossel P, Chevallier JM, et al. Accuracy of three-dimensional gadolinium-enhanced MR angiography in the assessment of extracranial carotid artery disease. *AJR Am J Roentgenol* 2000;175:455–463.
26. Sardanelli F, Molinari G, Zandrino F, et al. Three-dimensional, navigator-echo MR coronary angiography in detecting stenoses of the major epicardial vessels, with conventional coronary angiography as the standard of reference. *Radiology* 2000;214:808–814.
27. Bartlett ES, Walters TD, Symons SP, et al. Quantification of carotid stenosis on CT angiography. *AJNR Am J Neuroradiol* 2006;27:13–19.
28. Anderson GB, Ashforth R, Steinke DE, et al. CT angiography for the detection and characterization of carotid artery bifurcation disease. *Stroke* 2000;31:2168–2174.
29. Leclerc X, Godefroy O, Lucas C, et al. Internal carotid arterial stenosis: CT angiography with volume rendering. *Radiology* 1999;210:673–682.
30. Marcus CD, Ladam-Marcus VJ, Bigot JL, et al. Carotid arterial stenosis: evaluation at CT angiography with the volume-rendering technique. *Radiology* 1999;211:775–780.
31. Verhoek G, Costello P, Khoo EW, et al. Carotid bifurcation CT angiography: assessment of interactive volume rendering. *J Comput Assist Tomogr* 1999;23:590–596.
32. Meckel S, Mekle R, Taschner C, et al. Time-resolved 3D contrast-enhanced MRA with grappa on a 1.5-t system for imaging of craniocervical vascular disease: initial experience. *Neuroradiology* 2006.
33. Lenhart M, Framme N, Volk M, et al. Time-resolved contrast-enhanced magnetic resonance angiography of the carotid arteries: diagnostic accuracy and

inter-observer variability compared with selective catheter angiography. *Invest Radiol* 2002;37:535–541.

34. Schwartz RB, Jones KM, Chernoff DM, et al. Common carotid artery bifurcation: evaluation with spiral CT: work in progress. *Radiology* 1992;185:513–519.

35. Nandalur KR, Baskurt E, Hagspiel KD, et al. Carotid artery calcification on CT may independently predict stroke risk. *AJR Am J Roentgenol* 2006;186:547–552.

36. Bash S, Villablanca JP, Jahan R, et al. Intracranial vascular stenosis and occlusive disease: evaluation with CT angiography, MR angiography, and digital subtraction angiography. *AJNR Am J Neuroradiol* 2005;26:1012–1021.

37. Prendergast BD, Boon NA, Buckenham T. Aortic dissection: advances in imaging and endoluminal repair. *Cardiovasc Intervent Radiol* 2002;25:85–97.

38. Moore AG, Eagle KA, Bruckman D, et al. Choice of computed tomography, transesophageal echocardiography, magnetic resonance imaging, and aortography in acute aortic dissection: international registry of acute aortic dissection (IRAD). *Am J Cardiol* 2002;89:1235–1238.

39. Petasnick JP. Radiologic evaluation of aortic dissection. *Radiology* 1991;180:297–305.

40. Hartnell G, Costello P. The diagnosis of thoracic aortic dissection by noninvasive imaging procedures. *N Engl J Med* 1993;328:1637; author reply 1638.

41. Lepage MA, Quint LE, Sonnad SS, et al. Aortic dissection: CT features that distinguish true lumen from false lumen. *AJR Am J Roentgenol* 2001;177:207–211.

42. Song JK. Diagnosis of aortic intramural haematoma. *Heart* 2004;90:368–371.

43. Song JM, Kim HS, Song JK, et al. Usefulness of the initial noninvasive imaging study to predict the adverse outcomes in the medical treatment of acute type a aortic intramural hematoma. *Circulation* 2003;2002;108(suppl 1):ii324–328.

44. Elefteriades JA. Natural history of thoracic aortic aneurysms: indications for surgery, and surgical versus nonsurgical risks. *Ann Thorac Surg* 74:s1877–1880; discussion s1892–1898.

45. Prince MR, Narasimham DL, Jacoby WT, et al. Three-dimensional gadolinium-enhanced MR angiography of the thoracic aorta. *AJR Am J Roentgenol* 1996;166:1387–1397.

46. Atar E, Belenky A, Hadad M, et al. MR angiography for abdominal and thoracic aortic aneurysms: assessment before endovascular repair in patients with impaired renal function. *AJR Am J Roentgenol* 2006;186:386–393.

47. Hyodoh H, Kawaharada N, Akiba H, et al. Usefulness of preoperative detection of artery of Adamkiewicz with dynamic contrast-enhanced MR angiography. *Radiology* 2005;236:1004–1009.

48. Ludman CN, Yusuf SW, Whitaker SC, et al. Feasibility of using dynamic contrast-enhanced magnetic resonance angiography as the sole imaging modality prior to endovascular repair of abdominal aortic aneurysms. *Eur J Vasc Endovasc Surg* 2000;19:524–530.

49. Hany TF, Debatin JF, Leung DA, et al. Evaluation of the aortoiliac and renal arteries: comparison of breath-hold, contrast-enhanced, three-dimensional MR angiography with conventional catheter angiography. *Radiology* 1997;204:357–362.

50. Prince MR, Narasimham DL, Stanley JC, et al. Breath-hold gadolinium-enhanced MR angiography of the abdominal aorta and its major branches. *Radiology* 1995;197:785–792.

51. Papanicolaou N, Wittenberg J, Ferrucci JT Jr, et al. Preoperative evaluation of abdominal aortic aneurysms by computed tomography. *AJR Am J Roentgenol* 1986;146:711–715.

52. Owen RS, Carpenter JP, Baum RA, et al. Magnetic resonance imaging of angiographically occult runoff vessels in peripheral arterial occlusive disease. *N Engl J Med* 1992;326:1577–1581.

53. Baum RA, Rutter CM, Sunshine JH, et al. Multicenter trial to evaluate vascular magnetic resonance angiography of the lower extremity. American College of Radiology Rapid Technology Assessment Group. *JAMA* 1995;274:875–880.

54. Eiberg JP, Lundorf E, Thomsen C, et al. Peripheral vascular surgery and magnetic resonance arteriography—a review. *Eur J Vasc Endovasc Surg* 2001;22:396–402.

55. Bertschinger K, Cassina PC, Debatin JF, et al. Surveillance of peripheral arterial bypass grafts with three-dimensional MR angiography: comparison with digital subtraction angiography. *AJR Am J Roentgenol* 2001;176:215–220.

56. Hu HH, Madhuranthakam AJ, Kruger DG, et al. Continuously moving table MRI with sense. application in peripheral contrast enhanced MR angiography. *Magn Reson Med* 2005;54:1025–1031.

57. Maki JH, Wilson GJ, Eubank WB, et al. Utilizing sense to achieve lower station sub-millimeter isotropic resolution and minimal venous enhancement in peripheral MR angiography. *J Magn Reson Imaging* 2002;15:484–491.

58. Hentsch A, Aschauer MA, Balzer JO, et al. Gadobutrol-enhanced moving-table magnetic resonance angiography in patients with peripheral vascular disease: a prospective, multi-centre blinded comparison with digital subtraction angiography. *Eur Radiol* 2003;13:2103–2114.

59. Ruehm SG, Hany TF, Pfammatter T, et al. Pelvic and lower extremity arterial imaging: diagnostic performance of three-dimensional contrast-enhanced MR angiography. *AJR Am J Roentgenol* 2000;174:1127–1135.

60. Huber A, Heuck A, Baur A, et al. Dynamic contrast-enhanced MR angiography from the distal aorta to the ankle joint with a step-by-step technique. *AJR Am J Roentgenol* 2000;175:1291–1298.

61. Sueyoshi E, Sakamoto I, Matsuoka Y, et al. Aortoiliac and lower extremity arteries: comparison of three-dimensional dynamic contrast-enhanced subtraction MR angiography and conventional angiography. *Radiology* 1999;210:683–688.

62. Willmann JK, Baumert B, Schertler T, et al. Aortoiliac and lower extremity arteries assessed with 16-detector row CT angiography: prospective comparison with digital subtraction angiography. *Radiology* 2005;236:1083–1093.

63. Martin ML, Tay KH, Flak B, et al. Multidetector CT angiography of the aortoiliac system and lower extremities: a prospective comparison with digital subtraction angiography. *AJR Am J Roentgenol* 2003;180:1085–1091.

64. Ofer A, Nitecki SS, Linn S, et al. Multidetector CT angiography of peripheral vascular disease: a prospective comparison with intraarterial digital subtraction angiography. *AJR Am J Roentgenol* 2003;180:719–724.

65. Rieker O, Duber C, Neufang A, et al. CT angiography versus intraarterial digital subtraction angiography for assessment of aortoiliac occlusive disease. *AJR Am J Roentgenol* 1997;169:1133–1138.

66. Vasbinder GB, Nelemans PJ, Kessels AG, et al. Diagnostic tests for renal artery stenosis in patients suspected of having renovascular hypertension: a meta-analysis. *Ann Intern Med* 2001;135:401–411.

67. Schoenberg SO, Knopp MV, Londy F, et al. Morphologic and functional magnetic resonance imaging of renal artery stenosis: a multireader tricenter study. *J Am Soc Nephrol* 2002;13:158–169.

68. Miyazaki T, Yamashita Y, Shinzato J, et al. Two-dimensional time-of-flight magnetic resonance angiography in the coronal plane for abdominal disease: its usefulness and comparison with conventional angiography. *Br J Radiol* 1995;68:351–357.

69. Meaney JF, Prince MR, Nostrant TT, et al. Gadolinium-enhanced MR angiography of visceral arteries in patients with suspected chronic mesenteric ischemia. *J Magn Reson Imaging* 1997;7:171–6.

70. Rubin GD, Schmidt AJ, Logan LJ, et al. Multi-detector row CT angiography of lower extremity arterial inflow and runoff: initial experience. *Radiology* 2001;221:146–158.

71. Keller D, Wildermuth S, Boehm T, et al. CT angiography of peripheral arterial bypass grafts: accuracy and time-effectiveness of quantitative image analysis with an automated software tool. *Acad Radiol* 2006;13:610–620.

72. Inaba K, Potzman J, Munera F, et al. Multi-slice CT angiography for arterial evaluation in the injured lower extremity. *J Trauma* 2006;60:502–506; discussion 506–507.

73. Vasbinder GB, Nelemans PJ, Kessels AG, et al. Accuracy of computed tomographic angiography and magnetic resonance angiography for diagnosing renal artery stenosis. *Ann Intern Med* 2004;141:674–682; discussion 682.

74. Stein PD, Athanasoulis C, Alavi A, et al. Complications and validity of pulmonary angiography in acute pulmonary embolism. *Circulation* 1992;85:462–468.

75. Haage P, Piroth W, Krombach G, et al. Pulmonary embolism: comparison of angiography with spiral computed tomography, magnetic resonance angiography, and real-time magnetic resonance imaging. *Am J Respir Crit Care Med* 2003;167:729–734.

76. Ohno Y, Higashino T, Takenaka D, et al. MR angiography with sensitivity encoding (sense) for suspected pulmonary embolism: comparison with MDCT and ventilation-perfusion scintigraphy. *AJR Am J Roentgenol* 2004;183:91–98.

77. van Beek EJ, Wild JM, Fink C, et al. MRI for the diagnosis of pulmonary embolism. *J Magn Reson Imaging* 2003;18:627–640.

78. Pleszewski B, Chartrand-Lefebvre C, Qanadli SD, et al. Gadolinium-enhanced pulmonary magnetic resonance angiography in the diagnosis of acute pulmonary embolism: a prospective study on 48 patients. *Clin Imaging* 2006;30:166–172.

79. Oudkerk M, Van Beek EJ, Wielopolski P, et al. Comparison of contrast-enhanced magnetic resonance angiography and conventional pulmonary angiography for the diagnosis of pulmonary embolism: a prospective study. *Lancet* 2002;359:1643–1647.

80. Gupta A, Frazer CK, Ferguson JM, et al. Acute pulmonary embolism: diagnosis with MR angiography. *Radiology* 1999;210:353–359.

81. Stein PD, Fowler SE, Goodman LR, et al. Multidetector computed tomography for acute pulmonary embolism. *N Engl J Med* 2006;354:2317–2327.

82. Stone E, Roach P, Bernard E, et al. Use of computed tomography pulmonary angiography in the diagnosis of pulmonary embolism in patients with an intermediate probability ventilation/perfusion scan. *Intern Med J* 2003;33:74–78.

83. Perrier A, Howarth N, Didier D, et al. Performance of helical computed tomography in unselected outpatients with suspected pulmonary embolism. *Ann Intern Med* 2001;135:88–97.

84. Blachere H, Latrabe V, Montaudon M, et al. Pulmonary embolism revealed on helical CT angiography: comparison with ventilation-perfusion radionuclide lung scanning. *AJR Am J Roentgenol* 2000;174:1041–1047.

85. Remy-Jardin M, Remy J, Baghaie F, et al. Clinical value of thin collimation in the diagnostic workup of pulmonary embolism. *AJR Am J Roentgenol* 2000;175:407–411.

86. Kluge a, Mueller C, Strunk J, et al. Experience in 207 combined MRI examinations for acute pulmonary embolism and deep vein thrombosis. *AJR Am J Roentgenol* 2006;186:1686–1696.

87. Nikolaou K, Schoenberg SO, Attenberger U, et al. Pulmonary arterial hypertension: diagnosis with fast perfusion MR imaging and high-spatial-resolution MR angiography—preliminary experience. *Radiology* 2005;236:694–703.

88. Ley S, Fink C, Zaporozhan J, et al. Value of high spatial and high temporal resolution magnetic resonance angiography for differentiation between idiopathic and thromboembolic pulmonary hypertension: initial results. *Eur Radiol* 2005;15:2256–2263.

89. Le Gal G, Righini M, Parent F, et al. Diagnosis and management of subsegmental pulmonary embolism. *J Thromb Haemost* 2006;4:724–731.

90. Ghaye B, Remy J, Remy-Jardin M. Non-traumatic thoracic emergencies: CT diagnosis of acute pulmonary embolism: the first 10 years. *Eur Radiol* 2002;12:1886–1905.

91. Hogg K, Brown G, Dunning J, et al. Diagnosis of pulmonary embolism with CT pulmonary angiography: a systematic review. *Emerg Med J* 2006;23:172–178.

92. Kanne JP, Lalani TA. Role of computed tomography and magnetic resonance imaging for deep venous thrombosis and pulmonary embolism. *Circulation* 2004;109:i15–21.

93. Johnson JC, Brown MD, Mccullough N, et al. CT lower extremity venography in suspected pulmonary embolism in the ED. *Emerg Radiol* 2006.

94. Perrier A, Roy PM, Sanchez O, et al. Multidetector-row computed tomography in suspected pulmonary embolism. *N Engl J Med* 2005;352:1760–1768.

95. Nikolaou K, Huber A, Knez , et al. Intraindividual comparison of contrast-enhanced electron-beam computed tomography and navigator-echo-based magnetic resonance imaging for noninvasive coronary artery angiography. *Eur Radiol* 2002;12:1663–1671.

96. Manning WJ, Li W, Edelman RR. A preliminary report comparing magnetic resonance coronary angiography with conventional angiography. *N Engl J Med* 1993;328:828–832.

97. Huber A, Nikolaou K, Gonschior P, et al. Navigator echo-based respiratory gating for three-dimensional MR coronary angiography: results from healthy volunteers and patients with proximal coronary artery stenoses. *AJR Am J Roentgenol* 1999;173:95–101.

98. Regenfus M, Ropers D, Achenbach S, et al. Noninvasive detection of coronary artery stenosis using contrast-enhanced three-dimensional breath-hold magnetic resonance coronary angiography. *J Am Coll Cardiol* 2000;36:44–50.

99. Kim WY, Danias PG, Stuber M, et al. Coronary magnetic resonance angiography for the detection of coronary stenoses. *N Engl J Med* 2001;345:1863–1869.

100. Danias PG, Roussakis A, Ioannidis JP. Diagnostic performance of coronary magnetic resonance angiography as compared against conventional x-ray angiography: a meta-analysis. *J Am Coll Cardiol* 2004;44:1867–1876.

101. Nezafat R, Stuber M, Ouwerkerk R, et al. B1-insensitive T2 preparation for improved coronary magnetic resonance angiography at 3 T. *Magn Reson Med* 2006;55:858–864.

102. Sodickson DK, Mckenzie CA, Li W, et al. Contrast-enhanced 3D MR angiography with simultaneous acquisition of spatial harmonics: a pilot study. *Radiology* 2000;217:284–289.

103. Pruessmann K.P, Weiger M, Scheidegger Mb, et al. Sense. Sensitivity encoding for fast MRI. *Magn Reson Med* 1999;42:952–962.

104. Li D, Zheng J, Weinmann HJ. Contrast-enhanced MR imaging of coronary arteries: comparison of intra- and extravascular contrast agents in swine. *Radiology* 2001;218:670–678.

105. Deshpande VS, Cavagna F, Maggioni F, et al. Comparison of gradient-echo and steady-state free precession for coronary artery magnetic resonance angiography using a gadolinium-based intravascular contrast agent. *Invest Radiol* 2006;41:292–298.

106. Ringgaard S, Pedersen M, Rickers J, et al. Spiral coronary angiography using a blood pool agent. *J Magn Reson Imaging* 2005;22:213–218.

107. Sandstede JJ, Pabst T, Wacker C, et al. Breath-hold 3D MR coronary angiography with a new intravascular contrast agent (feruglose)—first clinical experiences. *Magn Reson Imaging* 2001;19:201–205.

108. Botnar RM, Buecker A, Wiethoff AJ, et al. In vivo magnetic resonance imaging of coronary thrombosis using a fibrin-binding molecular magnetic resonance contrast agent. *Circulation* 2004;110:1463–1466.

109. Botnar RM, Perez AS, Witte S, et al. In vivo molecular imaging of acute and subacute thrombosis using a fibrin-binding magnetic resonance imaging contrast agent. *Circulation* 2004;109:2023–2029.

110. Taylor AM, Thorne SA, Rubens MB, et al. Coronary artery imaging in grown up congenital heart disease: complementary role of magnetic resonance and x-ray coronary angiography. *Circulation* 2000;101:1670–1678.

111. Mavrogeni S, Papadopoulos G., Douskou M, et al. Magnetic resonance angiography is equivalent to x-ray coronary angiography for the evaluation of coronary arteries in Kawasaki disease. *J Am Coll Cardiol* 2004;43:649–652.

112. Vogl TJ, Abolmaali ND, Diebold T, et al. Techniques for the detection of coronary atherosclerosis: multi-detector row CT coronary angiography. *Radiology* 2002;223:212–220.

113. Jakobs TF, Becker CR, Ohnesorge B, et al. Multislice helical CT of the heart with retrospective ECG gating: reduction of radiation exposure by ECG-controlled tube current modulation. *Eur Radiol* 2002;12:1081–1086.

114. Peebles C. Computed tomographic coronary angiography: how many slices do you need? *Heart* 2006;92:582–584.

115. Klem I, Heitner JF, Shah DJ, et al. Improved detection of coronary artery disease by stress perfusion cardiovascular magnetic resonance with the use of delayed enhancement infarction imaging. *J Am Coll Cardiol* 2006;47:1630–1638.

116. Ishida M, Sakuma H, Kato N, et al. Contrast-enhanced MR imaging for evaluation of coronary artery disease before elective repair of aortic aneurysm. *Radiology* 2005;237:458–464.

117. Regenfus M, Ropers D, Achenbach S, et al. Diagnostic value of maximum intensity projections versus source images for assessment of contrast-enhanced three-dimensional breath-hold magnetic resonance coronary angiography. *Invest Radiol* 2003;38:200–206.

118. Plein S, Jones TR, Ridgway JP, et al. Three-dimensional coronary MR angiography performed with subject-specific cardiac acquisition windows and motion-adapted respiratory gating. *AJR Am J Roentgenol* 2003;180:505–512.

119. Watanabe Y, Nagayama M, Amoh Y, et al. High-resolution selective three-dimensional magnetic resonance coronary angiography with navigator-echo technique: segment-by-segment evaluation of coronary artery stenosis. *J Magn Reson Imaging* 2002;16:238–245.

120. Leber AW, Knez A, Von Ziegler F, et al. Quantification of obstructive and non-obstructive coronary lesions by 64-slice computed tomography: a comparative study with quantitative coronary angiography and intravascular ultrasound. *J Am Coll Cardiol* 2005;46:147–154.

121. Raff GL, Gallagher MJ, O'Neill WW, et al. Diagnostic accuracy of noninvasive coronary angiography using 64-slice spiral computed tomography. *J Am Coll Cardiol* 2005;46:552–557.

122. Ropers D, Baum U, Pohle K, et al. Detection of coronary artery stenoses with thin-slice multi-detector row spiral computed tomography and multiplanar reconstruction. *Circulation* 2003;107:664–666.

123. Nieman K, Oudkerk M, Rensing BJ, et al. Coronary angiography with multi-slice computed tomography. *Lancet* 2001;357:599–603.

124. Budoff MJ, Oudiz RJ, Zalace CP, et al. Intravenous three-dimensional coronary angiography using contrast enhanced electron beam computed tomography. *Am J Cardiol* 1999;83:840–845.

125. Garcia MJ, Lessick J, Hoffmann MH. Accuracy of 16-row multidetector computed tomography for the assessment of coronary artery stenosis. *JAMA* 2006;296:403–411.

126. Hausleiter J, Meyer T, Hadamitzky M, et al. Radiation dose estimates from cardiac multislice computed tomography in daily practice: impact of different scanning protocols on effective dose estimates. *Circulation* 2006;113:1305–1310.

127. Zanzonico P, Rothenberg LN, Strauss HW. Radiation exposure of computed tomography and direct intracoronary angiography: risk has its reward. *J Am Coll Cardiol* 2006;47:1846–1849.

128. Cordeiro MA, Miller JM, Schmidt A, et al. Non-invasive half millimetre 32-detector row computed tomography angiography accurately excludes significant stenoses in patients with advanced coronary artery disease and high calcium scores. *Heart* 2006;92:589–597.

129. Romeo G, Houyel L, Angel CY, et al. Coronary stenosis detection by 16-slice computed tomography in heart transplant patients: comparison with conven-

tional angiography and impact on clinical management. *J Am Coll Cardiol* 2005;45:1826–1831.

130. Gilard M, Cornily JC, Pennec PY, et al. Accuracy of multislice computed tomography in the preoperative assessment of coronary disease in patients with aortic valve stenosis. *J Am Coll Cardiol* 2006;47:2020–2024.

131. Burgstahler C, Beck T, Kuettner A, et al. Image quality and diagnostic accuracy of 16-slice multidetector computed tomography for the detection of coronary artery disease in obese patients. *Int J Obes (Lond)* 2005.

132. Burgstahler C, Beck T, Kuettner A, et al. Image quality and diagnostic accuracy of 16-slice multidetector spiral computed tomography for the detection of coronary artery disease in elderly patients. *J Comput Assist Tomogr* 2005;29:734–738.

133. Gilard M, Cornily JC, Pennec PY, et al. Assessment of coronary artery stents by 16-slice computed tomography. *Heart* 2006;92:58–61.

134. Achenbach S, Hoffmann U, Ferencik M, et al. Tomographic coronary angiography by EBCT and MDCT. *Prog Cardiovasc Dis* 2003;46:185–195.

135. Kondos GT, Hoff JA, Sevrukov A, et al. Electron-beam tomography coronary artery calcium and cardiac events: a 37-month follow-up of 5635 initially asymptomatic low- to intermediate-risk adults. *Circulation* 2003;107:2571–2576.

136. Shaw LJ, Raggi P, Schisterman E, et al. Prognostic value of cardiac risk factors and coronary artery calcium screening for all-cause mortality. *Radiology* 2003;228:826–833.

137. Langerak SE, Vliegen HW, De Roos A, et al. Detection of vein graft disease using high-resolution magnetic resonance angiography. *Circulation* 2002;105:328–333.

138. Langerak SE, Vliegen HW, Jukema JW, et al. Value of magnetic resonance imaging for the noninvasive detection of stenosis in coronary artery bypass grafts and recipient coronary arteries. *Circulation* 2003;107:1502–1508.

139. Ropers D, Ulzheimer S, Wenkel E, et al. Investigation of aortocoronary artery bypass grafts by multislice spiral computed tomography with electrocardiographic-gated image reconstruction. *Am J Cardiol* 2001;88:792–795.

140. Anders K, Baum U, Schmid M, et al. Coronary artery bypass graft (CABG) patency: assessment with high-resolution submillimeter 16-slice multidetector-row computed tomography (MDCT) versus coronary angiography. *Eur J Radiol* 2006;57:336–344.

141. Stauder NI, Kuttner A, Schroder S, et al. Coronary artery bypass grafts: assessment of graft patency and native coronary artery lesions using 16-slice MDCT. *Eur Radiol* 2006.

142. Pache G, Saueressig U, Frydrychowicz A, et al. Initial experience with 64-slice cardiac CT noninvasive visualization of coronary artery bypass grafts. *Eur Heart J* 2006;27:976–980.

143. Fuster V, Corti R, Fayad ZA, et al. Integration of vascular biology and magnetic resonance imaging in the understanding of atherothrombosis and acute coronary syndromes. *J Thromb Haemost* 2003;1:1410–1421.

144. Wilensky RL, Song HK, Ferrari VA. Role of magnetic resonance and intravascular magnetic resonance in the detection of vulnerable plaques. *J Am Coll Cardiol* 2006;47:c48–56.

145. Worthley SG, Helft G, Fuster V, et al. Noninvasive in vivo magnetic resonance imaging of experimental coronary artery lesions in a porcine model. *Circulation* 2000;101:2956–2961.

146. Fayad ZA, Fuster V, Fallon JT, et al. Noninvasive in vivo human coronary artery lumen and wall imaging using black-blood magnetic resonance imaging. *Circulation* 2000;102:506–510.

147. Martin AJ, Gotlieb AI, Henkelman RM. High-resolution MR imaging of human arteries. *J Magn Reson Imaging* 1995;5:93–100.

148. Yuan C, Mitsumori LM, Beach KW, et al. Carotid atherosclerotic plaque: noninvasive MR characterization and identification of vulnerable lesions. *Radiology* 2001;221:285–299.

149. Kampschulte A, Ferguson MS, Kerwin WS, et al. Differentiation of intraplaque versus juxtaluminal hemorrhage/thrombus in advanced human carotid atherosclerotic lesions by in vivo magnetic resonance imaging. *Circulation* 2004;110:3239–3244.

150. Helft G, Worthley SG, Fuster V, et al. Progression and regression of atherosclerotic lesions: monitoring with serial noninvasive magnetic resonance imaging. *Circulation* 2002;105:993–998.

151. Corti R, Osende JI, Fallon JT, et al. The selective peroxisomal proliferator-activated receptor-gamma agonist has an additive effect on plaque regression in combination with simvastatin in experimental atherosclerosis: in vivo study by high-resolution magnetic resonance imaging. *J Am Coll Cardiol* 2004;43:464–473.

152. Corti R, Fayad ZA, Fuster V, et al. Effects of lipid-lowering by simvastatin on human atherosclerotic lesions: a longitudinal study by high-resolution, noninvasive magnetic resonance imaging. *Circulation* 2001;104:249–252.

153. Yuan C, Kerwin WS, Ferguson MS, et al. Contrast-enhanced high resolution MRI for atherosclerotic carotid artery tissue characterization. *J Magn Reson Imaging* 2002;15:62–67.

154. Kramer CM, Cerilli LA, Hagspiel K, et al. Magnetic resonance imaging identifies the fibrous cap in atherosclerotic abdominal aortic aneurysm. *Circulation* 2004;109:1016–1021.

155. Sirol M, Itskovich VV, Mani V, et al. Lipid-rich atherosclerotic plaques detected by gadofluorine-enhanced in vivo magnetic resonance imaging. *Circulation* 2004;109:2890–2896.

156. Kooi ME, Cappendijk VC, Cleutjens KB, et al. Accumulation of ultrasmall superparamagnetic particles of iron oxide in human atherosclerotic plaques can be detected by in vivo magnetic resonance imaging. *Circulation* 2003;107:2453–2458.

157. Hyafil F, Laissy JP, Mazighi M, et al. Ferumoxtran-10-enhanced MRI of the hypercholesterolemic rabbit aorta relationship between signal loss and macrophage infiltration. *Arterioscler Thromb Vasc Biol* 2005.

158. Achenbach S, Moselewski F, Ropers D, et al. Detection of calcified and noncalcified coronary atherosclerotic plaque by contrast-enhanced, submillimeter multidetector spiral computed tomography: a segment-based comparison with intravascular ultrasound. *Circulation* 2004;109:14–17.

159. Leber AW, Knez A, Becker A, et al. Accuracy of multidetector spiral computed tomography in identifying and differentiating the composition of coronary atherosclerotic plaques: a comparative study with intracoronary ultrasound. *J Am Coll Cardiol* 2004;43:1241–1247.

160. Caussin C, Ohanessian A, Ghostine S, et al. Characterization of vulnerable nonstenotic plaque with 16-slice computed tomography compared with intravascular ultrasound. *Am J Cardiol* 2004;94:99–104.

161. Viles-Gonzalez JF, Poon M, Sanz j, et al. In vivo 16-slice, multidetector-row computed tomography for the assessment of experimental atherosclerosis: comparison with magnetic resonance imaging and histopathology. *Circulation* 2004;110:1467–1472.

162. Schroeder S, Kuettner A, Wojak t, et al. Non-invasive evaluation of atherosclerosis with contrast enhanced 16-slice spiral computed tomography: results of ex vivo investigations. *Heart* 2004;90:1471–1475.

163. Schroeder S, Kuettner A, Leitritz M, et al. Reliability of differentiating human coronary plaque morphology using contrast-enhanced multislice spiral computed tomography: a comparison with histology. *J Comput Assist Tomogr* 2004;28:449–454.

CHAPTER (23)

Positron Emission Tomography for the Noninvasive Study and Quantitation of Myocardial Blood Flow and Metabolism in Cardiovascular Disease

Heinrich R. Schelbert

The study of the human heart with conventional radionuclide techniques is largely confined to assessments of the relative distributions of regional myocardial blood flow and of global and regional myocardial contractile function. Positron emission tomography (PET) extends these capabilities because it offers assays for probing and defining regional functional processes that span from blood flow to biochemical reaction rates, substrate fluxes, membrane receptor density and function, and neuronal activity. Newly developed assays, still in the investigational stage, can target the expression of transfected and endogenous genes, visualize cell trafficking, or probe molecular processes. There are many positron-emitting biologically active tracers that can be quantitated in vivo. The recent addition of structural imaging with PET/CT hybrid systems will further refine the regional, functional, and biochemical processes to be more accurately localized and related to structure. Novel insights into the function of the human heart become possible. The clinical use of these techniques can impact decisively on patient diagnosis and management.

TOOLS FOR PROBING MYOCARDIAL TISSUE FUNCTION

Fundamental to PET are (1) quantitative imaging and high temporal resolution, (2) in-vivo application of tracer kinetic principles, and (3) availability of many physiologically active radiotracers.

IMAGING WITH POSITRON EMITTING RADIOPHARMACEUTICALS

Dedicated Positron Emission Tomography Systems

The quantitative imaging capability of PET results from physical properties unique to positrons. After losing their kinetic energy, positrons combine with an electron and *annihilate* each other. The annihilation represents the conversion of mass into energy. The combined mass of the positron and electron converts into two 511 kiloelectron volt (keV) photons that leave the site of the annihilation in diametrically opposed directions. If both strike at the same time two scintillation detectors connected by coincidence circuitry, an annihilation event is registered. Its location in space can be defined by circular arrays of scintillation detectors. Tomographic reconstruction algorithms analogous to those used with x-ray computed tomography are used. Accordingly, the spatial resolution throughout the image plane is rather homogeneous, which differs from that obtainable with conventional, single-photon emission computed tomography (SPECT) approaches where the spatial resolution declines as the distance of the imaged object to the scintillation detectors increases. By acquiring

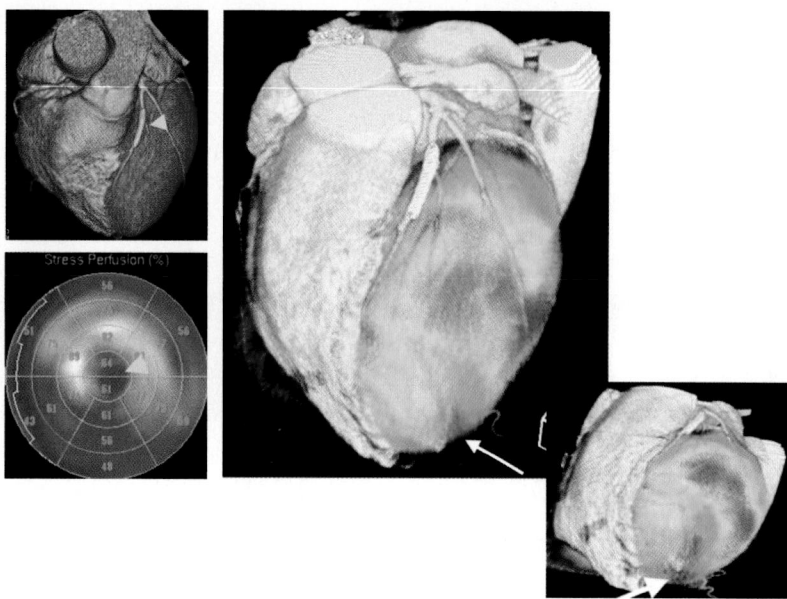

FIGURE 23–1. Merging function and structure with positron emission tomography (PET)/CT. The CT-coronary angiogram (*upper left panel*) reveals an in-stent stenosis of the left anterior descending coronary artery. After coregistering the coronary angiogram with a three-dimensional display of stress myocardial perfusion images, the coronary stenosis is associated with a downstream stress-induced perfusion defect (*indicated in blue and green*). *Courtesy of P. Kaufmann, University of Zurich, Zurich, Switzerland.*

transmission images with external rotating or circular sources of positron-emitting isotopes or, with CT for in-line PET/CT systems, and thus, measuring the photon attenuation, the images of the tracer tissue concentrations (*emission images*) are corrected for photon attenuation so that the resulting tomographic images represent accurately the true regional radioactivity concentrations (millicurie [mCi] or megabecquerel [MBq]/cm³). State-of-the-art PET systems offer intrinsic spatial resolutions as high as 4 to 5 millimeter (mm) full-width at half maximum (FWHM). Because the circular imaging gantry is stationary, serial images can be acquired at sampling rates in the range of seconds so that rapidly changing radiotracer tissue concentrations can be measured.

Positron Emission Tomography Combined with Computed Tomography

A more recent development combines PET with CT as an imaging device, which is referred to as *in-line PET/CT*. Designed primarily for oncological applications, the CT component of the system measures the photon attenuation and its anatomic distribution and, thus, shortens total imaging times. The CT component visualizes the anatomy so that this imaging system is ideally suited for fusing functional with structural information (Fig. 23–1). In-line PET/CT holds considerable promise for merging functional information (i.e., myocardial blood flow, vascular inflammation, or apoptosis) with structural information (i.e., coronary calcifications, CT coronary angiog-

raphy, arterial plaques, or regional or global left ventricular (LV) contractile function; see Fig. 23–1).

【 】 TRACER KINETIC PRINCIPLES

Positron-emitting isotopes of elements that constitute major parts of living matter such as carbon-11 (^{11}C), nitrogen-13 (^{13}N), and oxygen-15 (^{15}O) can be inserted into molecules without disturbing their physiologic properties. Their high specific activity (radioactivity per mass) permits administration in tracer quantities that do not exert a mass effect and perturb the process to be studied. As their physiologic half-life is short, functional processes can be measured repeatedly or within the same study session. The radioactivity concentrations of these tracers in tissues such as arterial blood and myocardium and their changes over time are determined noninvasively. Time-activity curves derived from serially acquired tomographic images at sampling rates of 1 to 10 seconds are fitted with equations that are based on tracer kinetic models and yield quantitative estimates of regional functional processes.

Tracer compartment models describe the distribution of the tracer radiolabel in tissue and its time dependent changes (Fig. 23–2). These models relate the externally derived signal to the metabolic fate of the tracer label and its relationship to the functional process under study. Such tracer kinetic models typically consist of functional rather than anatomic compartments that contain the radiotracer or its metabolites (see Fig. 23–2). Exchange of radiotracers between compartments is described usually by first-order rate constants. Flux of a radiotracer through a given compartment depends on the flux rate of the tracer or of its metabolite as well as on the size of the compartment. Estimates of regional functional processes are derived in absolute units.

【 】 POSITRON-EMITTING TRACERS OF MYOCARDIAL TISSUE FUNCTION

Blood Volume and Tissue Characterization

Blood can readily be radiolabeled with small quantities of either ^{15}O or ^{11}C carbon monoxide (CO). Once inhaled, the radiolabeled CO binds to hemoglobin thereby tagging red blood cells.

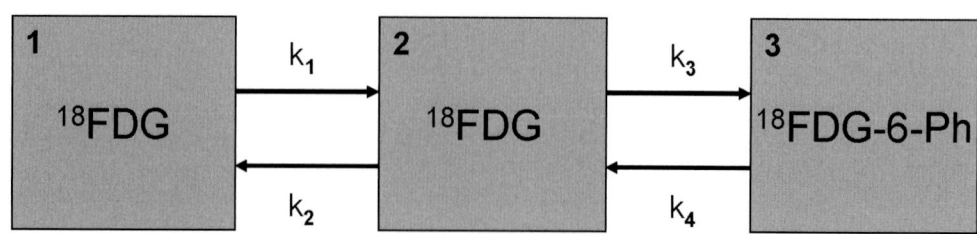

FIGURE 23–2. Tracer Compartment Model: Compartment 1 describes the radiotracer activity in the vascular space, compartment 2 in tissue, and compartment 3 the metabolized radiotracer in tissue. Exchange of radiotracer between compartments is described by first order rate constants (k; in this particular configuration k_1 describes the rate of exchange from blood into tissue, and k_2 a return of tracer from the extravascular space into blood. k_3 describes the rate constant for the metabolic reaction that traps the radiotracer.

The latter serves to define the components of the myocardium in terms of vascular space, viable and normal myocytes, and scar tissue. One such characterization assumes that only living myocytes exchange water rapidly.[1] The approach employs transmission images representing the densities of the various tissues in the chest. They resemble low spatial resolution x-ray CT images and delineate, for example, the volume of the myocardium together with the blood in its cavities. The true extravascular volume can then be obtained by subtracting blood-pool images from the transmission images. The fraction of the extravascular volume that exchanges water rapidly is estimated with [15]O labeled water and is referred to as *water perfusable tissue index*" (PTI). If all of the extravascular volume does indeed rapidly exchange water, then the PTI approaches unity.[1] If conversely, as is the case in patients with prior myocardial infarction, a portion of the myocardium has been injured irreversibly and scar tissue has formed, this fraction becomes less than unity.[2,3] The PTI was found to be inversely correlated with the fractional amount of fibrosis and scar tissue in animal experimental studies.[4] The PTI will also be reduced in instances of diffuse interstitial fibrosis. Clinical investigations demonstrated that the fraction of irreversibly injured myocardium or of regional scar tissue formation can be measured and predicts whether an impairment in regional contractile function is irreversible or whether a postrevascularization improvement is likely.[2] In this regard, the PTI provides information analogous to that obtained with delayed contrast-enhanced magnetic resonance imaging (MRI).[5,6] If, however, functionally compromised but viable myocardium exchanges water as rapidly as normal myocardium, this might limit the predictive value of the PTI for it does not distinguish between normal and *ischemically compromised* myocardium. A reduced PTI was found to be highly predictive of the irreversibility of contractile function, whereas a near normal PTI was less accurate than ^{18}F-fluoro-2-deoxy-D-glucose (^{18}F-FDG) in predicting a postrevascularization improvement in contractile function.[7] The sum of viable and normal myocytes in a given myocardial segment can be used as a reference to which transmural estimates of blood flow or substrate metabolism can be related.[8]

Myocardial Blood Flow

Several approaches exist for the evaluation of the relative distribution of and regional myocardial blood flow (MBF) in absolute units. Tracers such as [82]rubidium or ^{13}N-ammonia are retained in myocardium in proportion to blood flow so that images of their regional activity concentrations in the myocardium depict the relative distribution of blood flow in the myocardium at the time of tracer injection. [82]Rubidium is available through a generator-based push-button operated infusion system and, hence, is easy to use clinically. Its physical half-life is 75 seconds so that perfusion imaging can be repeated at time intervals of as little as 10 minutes. The short physical half-life produces low counts and, thus, noisy images. Modern three-dimensional (3D) PET systems can overcome this limitation and even allow gated acquisition of [82]rubidium-perfusion images.[9] The longer (9.8 minutes) physical half-life of ^{13}N-ammonia produces images of higher count rates and thus of higher diagnostic quality but requires 40 to 50 minute time intervals between studies and, importantly, an on-site cyclotron for production.

Common to most diffusible flow tracers is their nonlinear myocardial uptake in relation to increases in blood flow because of a flow-dependent curvilinear decline of the first pass extraction fraction. Tracer compartment models compensate for the nonlinear tissue response so that noninvasive quantitative estimates of blood flow linearly trace changes in blood flow. Such compensation is not needed for ^{15}O-water because capillary and sarcolemmal membranes exert little if any barrier effect on the exchange of ^{15}O-water so that the extraction fraction is largely flow-independent, and radiotracer tracer net uptakes increase linearly with higher flows. Hence, ^{15}O-water, at least in theory, is most ideally suited for measurements of blood flow.[10] The tracer is also metabolically inert whereas uptake and retention of ^{13}N-ammonia or of [82]rubidium are potentially susceptible to alterations in regional myocardial metabolism although such effects were shown in animal experiments to be negligible.[11,12] Current research focuses on the development and validation of additional positron-emitting tracers of MBF. Most promising are potential flow tracers labeled with the more widely available fluorine-18 (^{18}F) isotope that can be used without an on-site cyclotron and without a generator system. These tracers appear to provide exquisite high quality myocardial perfusion images.[13]

Measurements of Myocardial Blood Flow

Current PET approaches with different tracers of flow and/or different tracer compartment models yield comparable estimates of blood flow in human myocardium both at rest and during pharmacologically induced hyperemia.[14–23] Interstudy differences in reported MBF are likely related to methodology and patient-related factors as well as to differences in study conditions at the time of measurement. Blood flow in normal myocardium depends largely on oxygen demand and, thus, on cardiac work.[24] Accordingly, individual flow measurements should be interpreted within the context of the rate pressure product as a measure of cardiac work.[25] Differences might also be related to gender. In one study for example, women were found to have higher blood flows both at rest and during hyperemia when compared to age-matched males, a finding the authors attributed to higher high-density lipoprotein (HDL) cholesterol and lower triglyceride plasma levels in females.[26]

Important for measurements of MBF is their reproducibility. Repeat studies in normal volunteers report a 10 ± 11 percent reproducibility (average percent difference of flows normalized to the rate pressure product) for rest blood flow and of 12 ± 9 percent for hyperemic blood flows.[27] Other studies report similar values for both, ^{13}N-ammonia and for ^{15}O-water.[28–30] Noninvasive measurements of blood flow have been validated in animals against independently measured microsphere MBFs[14,19,31–33] and in humans against measurements of hyperemic flow responses by intracoronary flow velocity probes.[34]

In normal volunteers, stimulation of hyperemia with vascular smooth muscle dilating agents such as dipyridamole, adenosine, or adenosine triphosphate has been shown to produce interindividually variable hyperemic flow responses but induce on average three- to fivefold increases in blood flow.[14,15,17,35] Several factors can account for this variability. They include (1) the coronary driving pressure, best reflected by the mean arterial blood pressure;

(2) extravascular resistive forces as a function of wall tension and tension development, which in turn depend on the diastolic volume and the myocardium's contractile state; (3) β- and especially α-adrenergic control of the basal vasomotor tone[36]; (4) endothelium-related contributions to vasomotion[37]; (5) pharmacologic effects on smooth muscle relaxation; and (6) age and gender.

Dipyridamole (at a dose of 0.56 mg • kg^{-1} over 4 min) and adenosine (140 μg • min^{-1} • kg^{-1}, using a standard infusion time of 6 min) produce comparable levels of hyperemic blood flows[18]; the vasodilator effect of these agents can however be modified by antagonists such as caffeine or theophylline-containing agents[38] so that it is imperative that patients refrain from these substances for at least 24 hours prior to pharmacologic stress testing. Higher doses of dipyridamole (by 50 percent) failed to stimulate higher flows, nor did they reduce the interpatient variability in flow responses.[39]

Hyperemic MBFs and, especially, myocardial flow reserves decline with age.[40–42] Possible contributing factors include an age-dependent decline in the vasodilator capacity as well as an age-dependent increase in baseline blood flow because of a progressive increase in the rate pressure product as a major determinant of blood flow at rest. Changes in vascular compliance can further contribute to the age-dependent decline.

It is important to note that the vasodilator reserve as determined pharmacologically may not necessarily reflect the myocardium's true ability to increase flow during physical exercise. For example, levels of vasodilator-stimulated hyperemic MBFs in normal volunteers were unrelated to their exercise capacity,[43] or, further, as observed in patients with hypertrophic cardiomyopathy, MBF failed to increase or even declined with supine bicycle exercise despite some residual flow reserve as demonstrated with dipyridamole-stimulation.[44]

Positive inotropic agents as for example dobutamine are also employed for stress interventions. This predominantly β$_2$-adreno-receptor agonist increases MBF in proportion to increases in cardiac work.[45] In one study, for example, intravenous infusion of dobutamine in normal volunteers at a rate of 40 μg • min^{-1} • kg^{-1} body weight produced a 2-fold increase in rate pressure product that was paralleled by a 2.25-fold increase in MBF.[45–47] To augment the flow response to dobutamine, mostly through further increases in heart rate, some laboratories supplement the infusion of dobutamine with intravenous atropine (typically 0.5 mg).[48]

Myocardial Substrate Metabolism

The major components of the myocardial substrate metabolism are illustrated in Fig. 23–3. According to this simplified depiction, the myocardium chooses between various substrates; foremost are free fatty acid, glucose, lactate, and ketone bodies. Selection of a fuel substrate depends largely on its concentration in plasma and the overall hormonal milieu.[49,50] These in turn are governed by the dietary state, the level of physical activity and, further, plasma concentrations of catecholamine, insulin, and glucagon. In the fasting state, for example, circulating free fatty acid levels are

high, and insulin levels are low so that as much as 70 to 80 percent of the myocardium's oxygen consumption can be accounted for by oxidation of free fatty acid.[51] Oral glucose raises plasma glucose and, in response, insulin levels and lowers free fatty acid levels so that myocardium shifts its fuel selection to glucose.[50] Strenuous physical exercise increases release of lactate from skeletal muscle. Plasma levels therefore increase, and lactate becomes the major fuel substrate.[52,53] In fact, as much as 60 percent of the oxygen consumption has been accounted for by oxidation of lactate during strenuous exercise. Other determinants of substrate selection include catecholamines, which accelerate lipolysis so that circulating free fatty acid levels increase, associated with a shift in the heart's substrate selection to free fatty acid.

Glucose enters the cell by means of facilitated transport systems, the largely insulin-independent glucose-transport protein 1(GLUT-1) and the insulin-dependent glucose-transport protein 4 (GLUT-4). The hexokinase reaction phosphorylates glucose to glucose-6-phosphate. The reaction product can be synthesized to glycogen or, alternatively, enters glycolysis with pyruvate as the end product. Converted to lactate, it can leave the myocardium or, if activated to acetyl-coenzyme A (CoA), enters the tricarboxylic acid (TCA) cycle as the final oxidative pathway shared by most fuel substrates. Exogenous lactate can be converted by means of nicotinamide adenine dinucleotidase (NAD+) to pyruvate, which after esterification to acyl-CoA enters the TCA cycle. Free fatty acid can enter like glucose by two different metabolic pathways. On entering the cells, it is esterified by the thiokinase reaction to acetyl-CoA. This compound can then enter an endogenous lipid pool, consisting mostly of glycerides and phospholipids or proceed by means of the carnitine shuttle to the inner mitochondrial membrane. It is there where β-oxidation cleaves the long chain acyl-CoA units into 2-carbon fragments, which then engage in the TCA cycle. The TCA cycle metabolizes the 2-carbon units into CO_2 and H_2O. The rate of flux through the TCA cycle is coupled closely to oxidative phosphorylation where the energy resulting

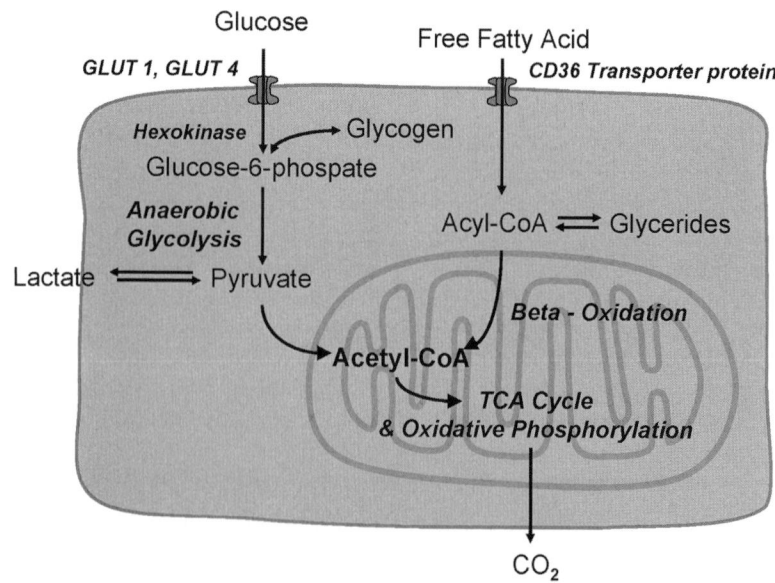

FIGURE 23–3. Highly simplified depiction of the myocardium's substrate metabolism. GLUT-1, glucose transporter 1; GLUT-4, glucose transporter 4; TCA, tricarboxylic acid.

from the synthesis of oxygen and hydrogen ions is stored in the high energy phosphate bonds of adenosine triphosphate (ATP). The latter is shuttled into the cytosol with transfer of energy to the high energy phosphate bond of creatine phosphate as a readily available source of energy. Other sites of high energy production include glycolysis. Energy yields in terms of ATP relative to oxygen differ between the various substrates. For example, for one mole of oxygen, glucose yields 6.3 moles ATP, lactate 6 moles ATP, and free fatty acid 5.7 moles ATP.[54]

Myocardial Glucose Utilization

As shown schematically in Fig. 23–3, the initial metabolic step of exogenous glucose metabolism can be evaluated and quantified with ^{18}F-FDG. This radiolabeled glucose analog exchanges across the capillary and sarcolemmal membranes in proportion to glucose with which it then competes for hexokinase for phosphorylation to ^{18}F-FDG phosphate (see also Fig. 23–2).[55,56] Unlike its natural counterpart, the phosphorylated glucose analog is a poor substrate for glycogen formation, glycolysis, and the fructose-pentose shunt; its rate of dephosphorylation is low in myocardium, and it is relatively impermeable to the cell membrane. The phosphorylated tracer thus becomes trapped in the cell so that images of the myocardial ^{18}F activity concentrations acquired approximately 40 to 60 minutes after tracer injection reflect the relative distribution of exogenous glucose utilization rates. Because the compound traces only the initial steps of glucose utilization (up to the branch point between glycogen synthesis and glycolysis; (see Fig. 23–3), it offers no direct information on glycolytic rates, glucose oxidation, or glycogen synthesis. Yet, in states of glycogen depletion, as for example during ischemia, exogenous glucose serves as the major source of glycolytic flux so that ^{18}F-FDG can offer an estimate of the rate of glycolysis.

The tissue kinetics of ^{18}F-FDG have been described by a unidirectional transport model,[55,56] which affords the quantification of regional rates of myocardial glucose utilization through relatively simple, rapid, and computationally efficient analysis approaches.[47,57] Typical values for exogenous glucose utilization under different dietary conditions and as reported from several laboratories are approximately 0.10 to 0.24 μmol/min/g in the fasting state, approximately 0.69 μmol/min/g after oral glucose loading, and approximately 74 μmol/min/g during hyperinsulinemic-euglycemic clamping.[58–60] To adjust for differences in the affinity of glucose and the glucose analog tracer for the hexokinase reaction and for differences in the transmembrane exchange, a so-called *lumped constant* (LC) is used. The value used most frequently is 0.7 as derived for canine myocardium.[56] However, the LC may not truly be constant but depend on study conditions.[61–63] This can be related to changes in the affinity of ^{18}F-FDG for transmembrane exchange in hexokinase and hence in the LC but, at the same time, suggest that the LC can be derived individually from the morphology of the myocardial ^{18}F time activity curve.[64]

A more recently developed approach to measurements of myocardial glucose metabolism entails the use of ^{11}C-glucose. Accumulation and clearance of radiotracer in the myocardium are estimated from serially acquired PET images. Using estimates of the myocardial extraction of ^{11}C-glucose, of MBF as determined with ^{15}O-water and the arterial blood glucose concentration, the myocardial consumption of glucose can be measured.[65–68] Different

from the ^{18}F-FDG approach, the ^{11}C-glucose method potentially allows a more comprehensive evaluation of glucose metabolism. ^{18}F-FDG traces only the initial metabolic step of exogenously derived glucose whereas an assessment of the fractional distribution of glucose between glycogen synthesis and glycolysis and oxidation appears feasible with the ^{11}C labeled compound.

Myocardial Fatty Acid Metabolism

This particular substrate pathway can be evaluated with 1-[^{11}C] palmitate. The labeled long-chain fatty acid participates fully in the metabolic fate of its natural counterpart (see Fig. 23–3). Once esterified to acyl-CoA, a fraction of tracer label proceeds by means of the carnitine shuttle into mitochondria where β-oxidation catabolizes the long-chain fatty acid into 2-carbon fragments that are then oxidized by means of the tricarboxylic acid (TCA) cycle. The label is released from the myocardium in the form of [11]CO_2. The remaining fraction of the initially extracted and activated tracer enters intracellular lipid pools, consisting mostly of di- and triglycerides and phospholipids. The biexponential morphology of the myocardial tissue time-activity curve reflects the metabolic fate of the tracer. The slow turnover rate of the intracellular lipid pools accounts for the slow clearance phase, whereas the relative size and slope of the rapid clearance curve component correspond to the fraction of tracer that has entered oxidative pathways and its rate of oxidation. Ischemia reduces the rate of fatty acid oxidation and of TCA cycle activity. Accordingly, size and rate of the rapid clearance curve component on the ^{11}C myocardial time-activity curve typically decline.[69,70] A disproportionately greater fraction of tracer label is then shunted into slow turnover, endogenous lipid pools. However, enhanced back diffusion of nonmetabolized tracer can complicate the evaluation of fatty acid oxidation in acutely ischemic myocardium as demonstrated in canine experiments.[71] Used mostly as a tracer for the qualitative evaluation of regional myocardial fatty acid metabolism, recent studies indicate the possibility of quantitating myocardial fatty acid oxidation in milliequivalent (mEq) free fatty acid per gram myocardium per minute.[65–68]

Another, more recently introduced approach for estimating the myocardial uptake of free fatty acid entails a radio-fluorinated fatty acid analogue, [^{18}F]fluoro-6-thia-heptadecanoic acid ([18]FTHA). The compound is thought to selectively trace oxidation and, analogous to ^{18}F-FDG, becomes metabolically trapped in the myocardium. Rates of myocardial free fatty acid utilization, derived from serially acquired PET images after intravenous administration of [18]FTHA are comparable to those obtained invasively with the Fick method and further, are similar to those derived with ^{11}C-palmitate.[72–74]

Preferential utilization of a fuel substrate, as for example glucose, lactate, or free fatty acid, depends on its concentration in arterial blood, which in turn depends on the dietary state, serum levels, or insulin resistance or on physical stress.[75] Changes in the myocardium's preferential substrate utilization can be demonstrated with either ^{11}C-palmitate and ^{18}F-FDG or both[75,76] (Figs. 23–4 and 23–5). In the presence of high free fatty acid and low glucose and insulin levels, use of free fatty acid as the preferred substrate is reflected on the ^{11}C-palmitate curve by the large relative size of the rapid clearance phase and its steep slope (both corresponding to increased fatty acid oxidation) and the low or even undetectable ^{18}F-FDG uptake. Carbohydrate ingestion raises plasma glucose levels, stimulates insu-

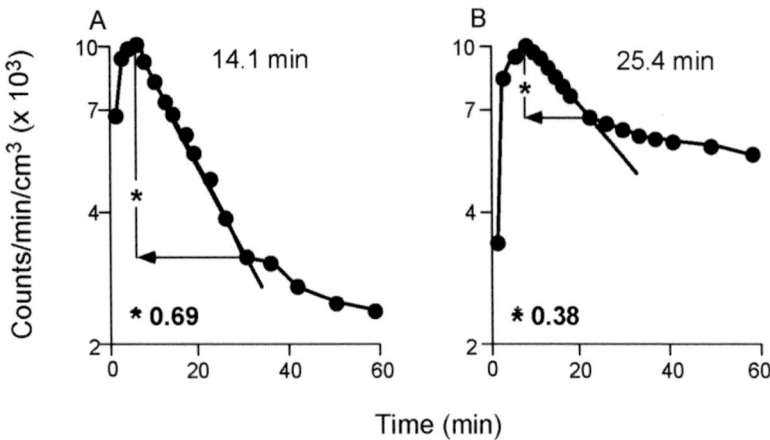

FIGURE 23–4. Whole body images of ¹⁸F-FDG uptake in a patient after overnight fasting (*left panel*) and 1 hour after oral glucose loading (*right panel*). Note the ¹⁸F-FDG uptake by brain under both conditions and the absence of ¹⁸F-FDG uptake by myocardium after an overnight fasting implicating free fatty acid as a preferred fuel substrate with little glucose utilization. However, in response to oral glucose loading there is a marked increase in ¹⁸F-FDG uptake by myocardium, suggesting a change in substrate metabolism and utilization of glucose.

lin secretion, and depresses free fatty acid levels. The corresponding shift in myocardial glucose utilization is reflected by a decline in the size and slope of the rapid clearance phase of ¹¹C-palmitate and by an increase in myocardial ¹⁸F-FDG uptake.

Myocardial Oxygen Consumption

Molecular ¹⁵O-oxygen, administered by inhalation, affords measurements of the myocardial oxygen consumption. The myocardial extraction of labeled oxygen is determined by PET first and, when multiplied by MBF,[77,78] the mass of oxygen consumed per minute per gram myocardium can be estimated. A more widely applied assay of myocardial oxidative metabolism and thus, of oxygen employs ¹¹C labeled acetate. The radiotracer clears rapidly from blood into myocardium and produces high signal-to-background images.[79–81] It directly traces the rate of substrate flux through the TCA cycle as the final oxidative pathway shared by most fuel substrates. The rate of clearance of ¹¹C activity from the myocardium as derived from serially acquired images, corresponds to the TCA cycle activity and, because of its close coupling to oxidative phosphorylation, to oxidative metabolism and myocardial oxygen consumption. It should be emphasized, however, that the tracer does not yield mass fluxes but only rate constants that can be converted into units of O_2 per minute per gram myocardium. Unlike ¹¹C-palmitate or ¹⁸F-FDG , the clearance rate of ¹¹C-acetate from myocardium is relatively insensitive to changes in myocardial preferential substrate utilization.[79] A tracer compartment model, based on biochemical assays of the tracer tissue kinetics of carbon-14 (¹⁴C)-acetate in isolated rat hearts[82] forms the base for estimating myocardial oxygen consumption in absolute units in the human heart and, at the same time, of regional MBFs.[83,84] Both, the ¹⁵O-oxygen and the ¹¹C-acetate technique yield similar estimates of the myocardial oxygen consumption in the normal human myocardium.[85]

However, values in regions with reduced blood flow have been found to differ, mostly because of methodological differences where the ¹¹C-acetate approach yields average transmural values whereas the ¹⁵O-water approach renders estimates selectively for the water perfusable tissue fraction.

CLINICAL APPLICATIONS IN CARDIOVASCULAR DISEASE

Identification of coronary artery disease, assessment of its extent and severity and risk stratification of patients together with the assessment of myocardial viability have been and continue to be major clinical applications of PET in cardiology. Myocardial perfusion imaging has been defined as a class 1 indication that is especially useful in patients with equivocal or nondiagnostic SPECT myocardial perfusion studies.[86] Recent developments indicate additional diagnostic benefits including more accurate estimates of the extent of coronary disease and identification of preclinical coronary atherosclerosis. PET/CT hybrid devices offer additional possibilities as for example, the combined assessment of function and morphology of the coronary arteries. Other developments that can prove to be clinically useful include the characterization of potentially vulnerable plaques. Assessment of myocardial

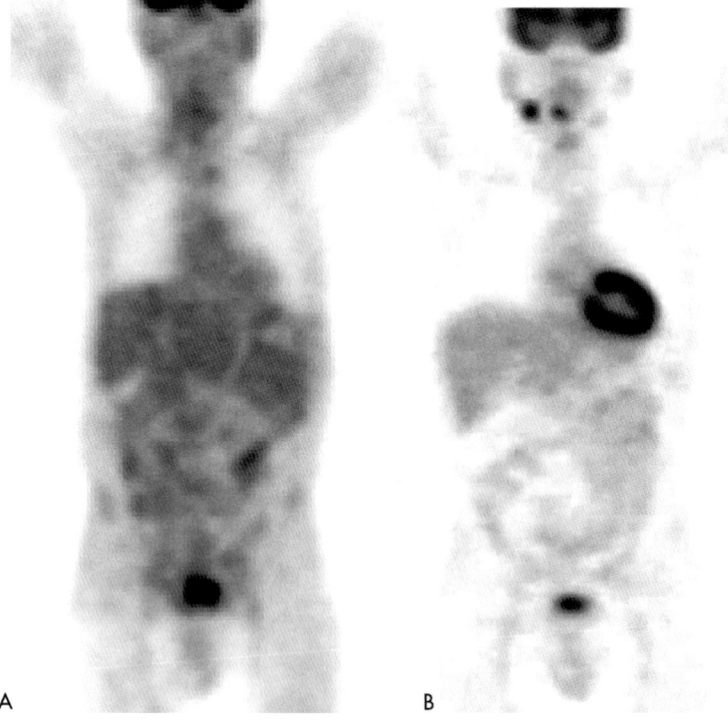

FIGURE 23–5. Effects of substrate availability on myocardial fatty-acid metabolism. Panels **A** and **B** depict myocardial time activity curves for ¹¹C-palmitate derived from serial positron emission tomography (PET) images. As seen on the time activity curves, the radiotracer clears from myocardium in a biexponential fashion; the slow clearance phase corresponds to the radiotracer in the lipid pool, whereas the rapid clearance phase reflects the fraction of radiotracer that undergoes oxidation. In the fasting state (**A**), a large fraction of radiotracer becomes immediately oxidized as reflected by the large size of the rapid clearance phase. This fraction declines however after oral glucose administration (**B**) when plasma free fatty acid levels decline and glucose and insulin levels increase and myocardium shifts from free fatty acid to glucose utilization.

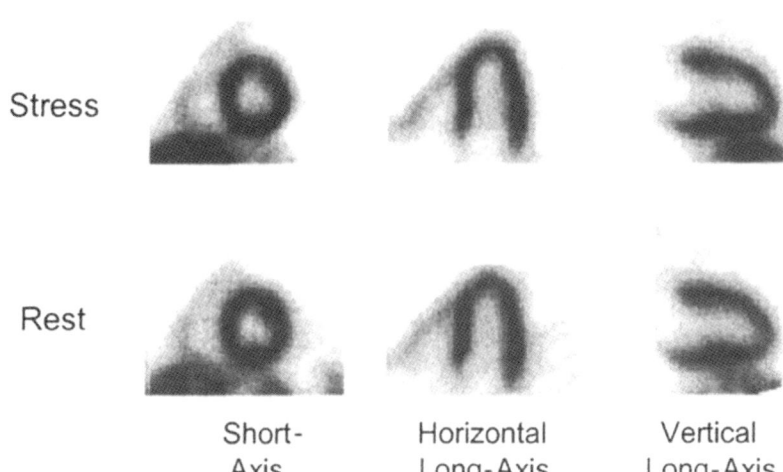

Stress

Rest

Short-Axis   Horizontal Long-Axis   Vertical Long-Axis

FIGURE 23–6. Nitrogen-13 (^{13}N)-ammonia images of myocardial perfusion in a normal volunteer obtained during adenosine stress (*upper panel*) and at rest (*lower panel*). Note the homogenous distribution of tracer throughout the myocardium as seen on the short axis and the horizontal and vertical lung axis images.

viability as the second major clinical use of PET advantageously employs radiotracers of myocardial perfusion and substrate metabolism and employs metabolic criteria for identifying potentially reversible impairments in regional contractile function.

[ ] IDENTIFICATION AND CHARACTERIZATION OF CORONARY ARTERY DISEASE

General Considerations

PET studies of MBF have generally focused on three aspects of coronary atherosclerosis and coronary artery disease: (1) detection of obstructive coronary artery disease and characterization of its extent and severity; (2) determination of fluid-dynamic consequences of obstructive coronary stenoses on regional MBF in terms of absolute units of blood flow; and, (3) assessment of coronary vasomotor function and its alterations in individuals at risk for coronary artery disease.

Detection of Coronary Artery Disease

For the detection of coronary artery disease (CAD), the relative distribution of MBF is initially examined at rest and then during stress. PET investigations almost invariably employ pharmacologic stress with adenosine, dipyridamole, or adenosine triphosphate because of the short physical half-life of the positron emitting flow tracers ^{82}rubidium and ^{13}N-ammonia and the requirement for maintaining patients in exactly the same position for acquisition of the emission and the transmission images. Both ^{82}rubidium and ^{13}N-ammonia are retained in myocardium in proportion to blood flow so that the resulting images depict the relative distribution of MBF at rest and during hyperemia. The approach identifies resting flow defects as well as attenuated responses of regional blood flow to hyperemia as a consequence of a coronary stenosis (Figs. 23–6 and 23–7). Images of rest and hyperemic perfusion are analyzed by visual inspection and by quantitative analysis where re-

gional tracer activity concentrations are compared to a database of normal and are displayed in the form of standardized polar maps, or as surface-rendered 3D images of the LV myocardium.

Clinical investigations have confirmed PET's high diagnostic performance for the detection of CAD.[87–93] Sensitivities range from 87 to 97 percent and specificities from 78 to 100 percent. Most studies compared the findings with stress-rest perfusion imaging to coronary angiographic findings where fluid-dynamically significant stenoses were defined by 50 or 70 percent luminal narrowing. Gould and coworkers[94] and, subsequently, Demer colleagues[89] graded stenosis severity by estimating the coronary flow reserve from quantitative angiograms. PET correctly identified 94 percent of vessels with moderate to severe, 49 percent of vessels with intermediate, and 5 percent of vessels with minimal stenosis.

Comparison of Positron Emission Tomography and Single-Photon Emission Computed Tomography Myocardial Perfusion Imaging

Comparisons have found PET to be more sensitive than SPECT.[89,95] Moderate to severe coronary stenoses were detected with a 95 percent sensitivity by PET and a 72 percent sensitivity by ^{201}T1 SPECT, and intermediate stenoses with a 49 percent sensitivity by PET whereas none was detected by SPECT.

Other investigations compared the diagnostic accuracies of PET and SPECT in the same patients.[90,91] PET and SPECT exhibited comparable sensitivities whereas the specificity was higher for PET than for SPECT. There were no differences in diagnostic accuracies between patients submitted to treadmill stress testing and patients with pharmacologically induced hyperemia.

A recent comparative study provided further support for the high diagnostic accuracy of PET stress-rest myocardial perfusion imaging

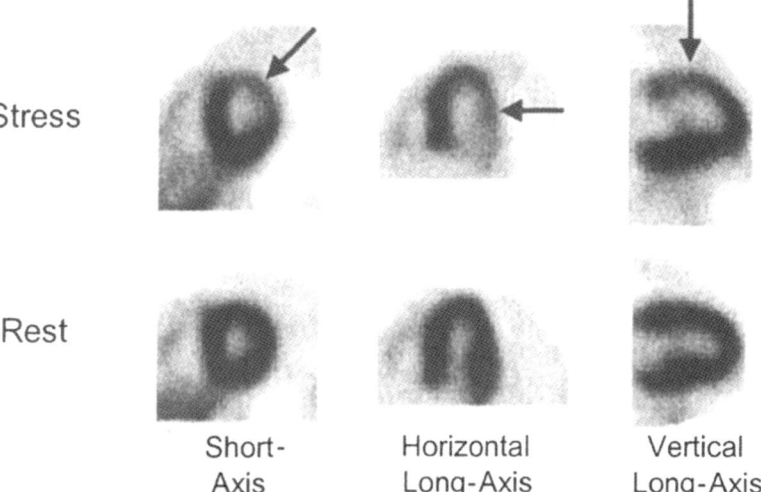

Stress

Rest

Short-Axis   Horizontal Long-Axis   Vertical Long-Axis

FIGURE 23–7. Myocardial perfusion images obtained with nitrogen-13 (^{13}N)-ammonia during adenosine stress and at rest in a patient with coronary artery disease. Note the extensive perfusion defect on the stress images (*arrows*) with normalization of myocardial perfusion during rest.

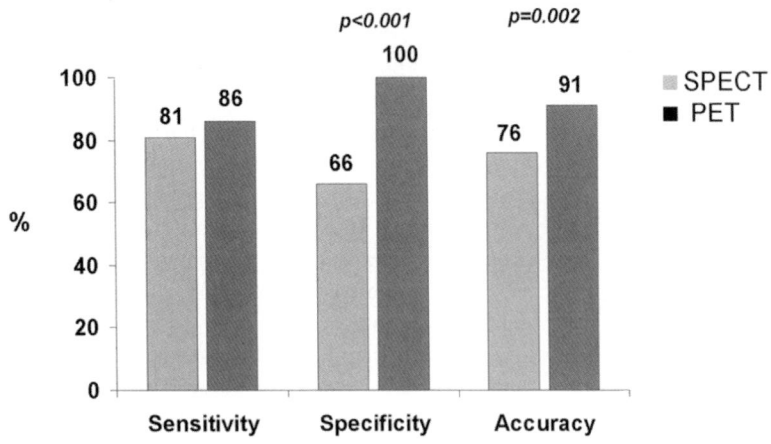

FIGURE 23–8. Comparative sensitivities, specificities, and diagnostic accuracies for single-photon emission computed tomography (SPECT) and positron emission tomography (PET) stress myocardial perfusion imaging. *Source: Adapted from Bateman, Heller, McGhie, et al.[9]*

and explored reasons for its superior diagnostic performance.[9] The higher diagnostic performance of PET was because of a significantly higher specificity whereas the gain in sensitivity was only marginal and statistically insignificant (Fig. 23–8). PET also proved more accurate than SPECT in identifying the number of stenosed coronary vessels and, thus, the extent of coronary artery disease. The greater proportion of "high quality" images, of images without photon attenuation artifacts, and without activity cross-contamination between liver and bowels and the LV myocardium were thought to account for the higher diagnostic performance and higher interpretive certainty of PET.

Two other developments promise additional improvements in diagnostic accuracy, especially for assessing disease extent and severity. One relates to measurements of MBF, whereas the second one results from the ability to measure LV function at the time of peak vasodilator stress. Conventional myocardial perfusion imaging delineates the relative distribution of MBF. Myocardial regions with the highest radiotracer uptake are considered *normal* and serve as reference for regions with reduced tracer activity. This *reference* approach is however limited in triple vessel disease when the flow response to pharmacologic vasodilation in such normal regions is also diminished, although less in regions tended by less severely stenosed coronary vessels. However, the diminished vasodilator response in the referenced myocardial regions can be identified by quantitative flow estimates.[96] A second development includes measurements of the left ventricular ejection fraction (LVEF) from gated [82]rubidium myocardial perfusion images during peak vasodilator stress.[97,98] Larger clinical trials, especially in previously undiagnosed patients with normal blood flow and normal wall motion at baseline are needed for defining more clearly the diagnostic gain achievable with PET.[99]

Prognostic Implications of Positron Emission Tomography Rest-Stress Perfusion Imaging

Few investigations have explored the prognostic value of PET stress and rest perfusion imaging. One preliminary survey of 108 patients with a relatively low pretest likelihood of

CAD found a zero cardiac morbidity or mortality for 2 years after a normal PET study.[100] When PET was employed in a population with strongly suspected or known CAD, the prognostic value of PET was maintained.[101] PET's value for assessing the preoperative risk in patients scheduled for aortic, carotid, and femoral artery surgery has been explored.[102]

Another more recent investigation explored the prognostic value of [82]rubidium rest-stress perfusion imaging with PET in a more diverse study population with known coronary artery disease.[103] The annual cardiac event rates were directly related to the severity of the stress perfusion scores (Fig. 23–9). A normal study was associated with an annual rate of hard events (death and nonfatal myocardial infarctions) of 0.4 percent for patients with normal stress perfusion images and of 2.3 percent and 7.0 percent for patients

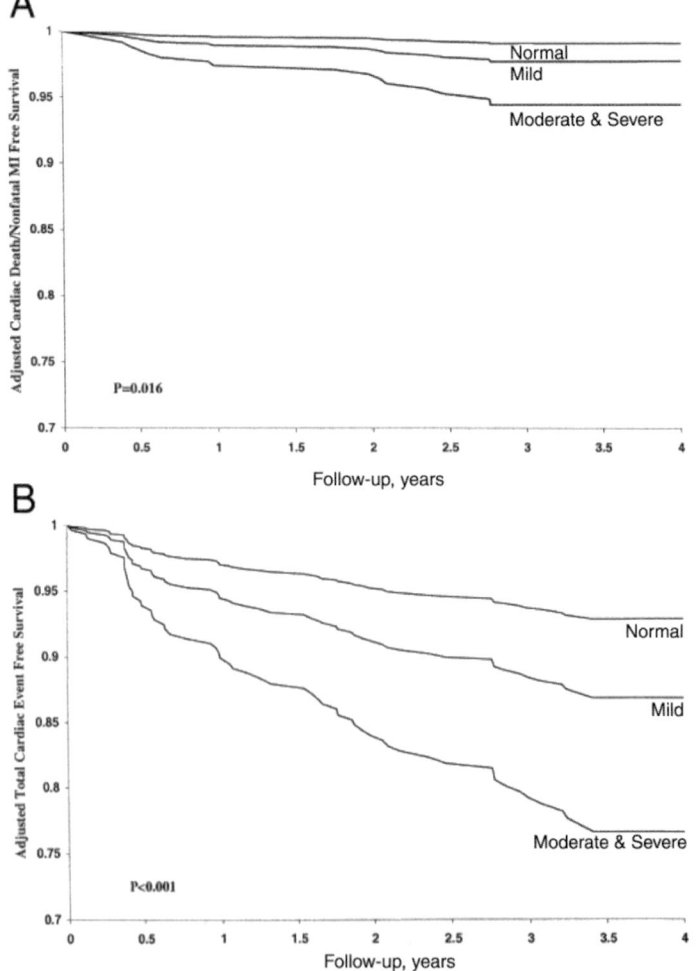

FIGURE 23–9. Predictive value of positron emission tomography (PET) [82]rubidium stress-rest myocardial perfusion imaging. **A.** Risk-adjusted survival, free from hard cardiac events (cardiac deaths and nonfatal myocardial infarction) as a function of the summed stress score; and **B**, risk-adjusted survival, free from any (total cardiac events as a function of the summed stress score; see text). *Source: Reproduced from Yoshinaga, Chow, Williams, et al.[103] Used with permission.*

with mildly, and with moderately to severely abnormal stress perfusion images.

Clinical Use of Positron Emission Tomography for Perfusion Imaging

As ^{13}N-ammonia and, especially, as [82]rubidium have become more widely available and as PET is now widely used in clinical nuclear medicine, it has become more accessible to the cardiac patient. Perfusion imaging with PET has been approved and is reimbursed by CMS and most insurance carriers. As many laboratories equipped with PET also use SPECT for myocardial perfusion imaging, there is a need for identifying those patients who are likely to benefit specifically from PET perfusion imaging. The recently revised practice guidelines for nuclear cardiology have classified PET perfusion imaging as a level 1 indication, that is, as a well established and clinical useful diagnostic approach.[86]

Myocardial perfusion imaging with PET appears to be especially useful in the following conditions and individuals:

1. Equivocal or nondiagnostic SPECT stress-rest perfusion images
2. Findings on SPECT perfusion images that are inconsistent with clinical findings
3. Patients expected to have suboptimal SPECT perfusion images, for example, low count densities or attenuation artifacts as is the case in obese patients or frequently in females
4. Patients anticipated to have only mild coronary artery disease but possibly detectable with higher spatial and contrast resolution of PET imaging
5. Patients with extensive and severe coronary artery disease including left main or balanced coronary artery disease.

Fluid-Dynamic Consequences of Coronary Stenoses

PET's quantitative capability for measurements of MBF has been used to explore the relationship between the angiographic stenosis severity, the hyperemic flow responses, and the vasodilator capacity.[104–106] Statistically significant correlations between the anatomic stenosis severity and the attenuation of the hyperemic response to pharmacologic vasodilation have been found. Similar correlations between MBF and coronary stenosis severity were noted for flow responses to inotropic stimulation with dobutamine.[107]

The inverse, nonlinear correlation between the cross-sectional area reduction of the stenosis and the flow reserve in the stenosis-dependent myocardium as reported in one of these investigations (Fig. 23–10)[106] resembles Gould's now classic nonlinear flow-stenosis relationship in experimental animals. This flow-stenosis relationship was observed after exclusion of confounding factors such as stenosis-in-series or stenosis-dependent myocardium supplied also by collateral vessels. There was considerable scatter of the data, which can reflect method-related inaccuracies, variability of the hyperemic, differences in patients' age, and baseline hemodynamic states or anatomic and functional properties of human coronary artery stenosis.

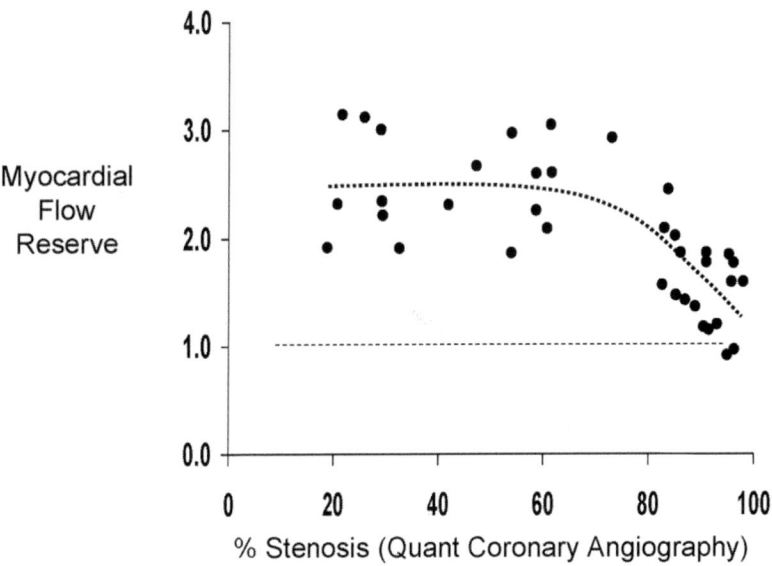

FIGURE 23–10. Myocardial flow reserve and coronary artery stenosis severity by quantitative angiography. Note the curvilinear relationship between the myocardial flow reserve as determined quantitatively from hyperemic and rest myocardial blood flow (MBF) measurements with nitrogen-13 (^{13}N)-ammonia. *Source: Reproduced with permission of the American Heart Association, Di Carli, Czernin, Hoh, et al.*[106]

Hybrid Imaging with Positron Emission Tomograph and Computed Tomography in Coronary Artery Disease

Current developments indicate exciting possibilities for the detection and characterization of coronary artery disease with PET-CT hybrid imaging. Near simultaneous acquisition of attenuation maps, available within seconds with current 64-multidetector CT not only shortens the study time but reduces the occurrence of misalignments between emission and transmission images and thus of image artifacts. Fusion of myocardial perfusion, both relative and absolute, with the coronary anatomy allows an assessment of the functional consequences of coronary stenoses (Fig. 23–11; see also Fig. 23–1). Impairments in regional contractile function detected on the gated perfusion or the contrast CT angiographic images can be related to regional perfusion and its reserve, and further, to anatomic alterations of the coronary vessels.[108]

Multidetector CT coronary angiography will likely impact the use of myocardial perfusion imaging. Given the high specificity of a normal CT coronary angiogram, assuming that the investigation is not limited by coronary calcifications, the need for an additional stress-rest perfusion imaging study will likely diminish in such patients.[109,110] High-grade stenoses on CT angiography can also lessen the need for perfusion imaging because such lesions usually correlate well with high-grade stenoses on conventional angiograms or with findings on myocardial perfusion imaging.[111–114] The need for complementary myocardial perfusion imaging studies can increase in patients with CT angiographically intermediate. For CT angiographic lesions of intermediate severity, defined as 50 percent or greater luminal narrowing, stress-rest myocardial perfusion imaging indicated that only 30 to 50 percent of such lesions were fluid-dynamically significant.[111–114]

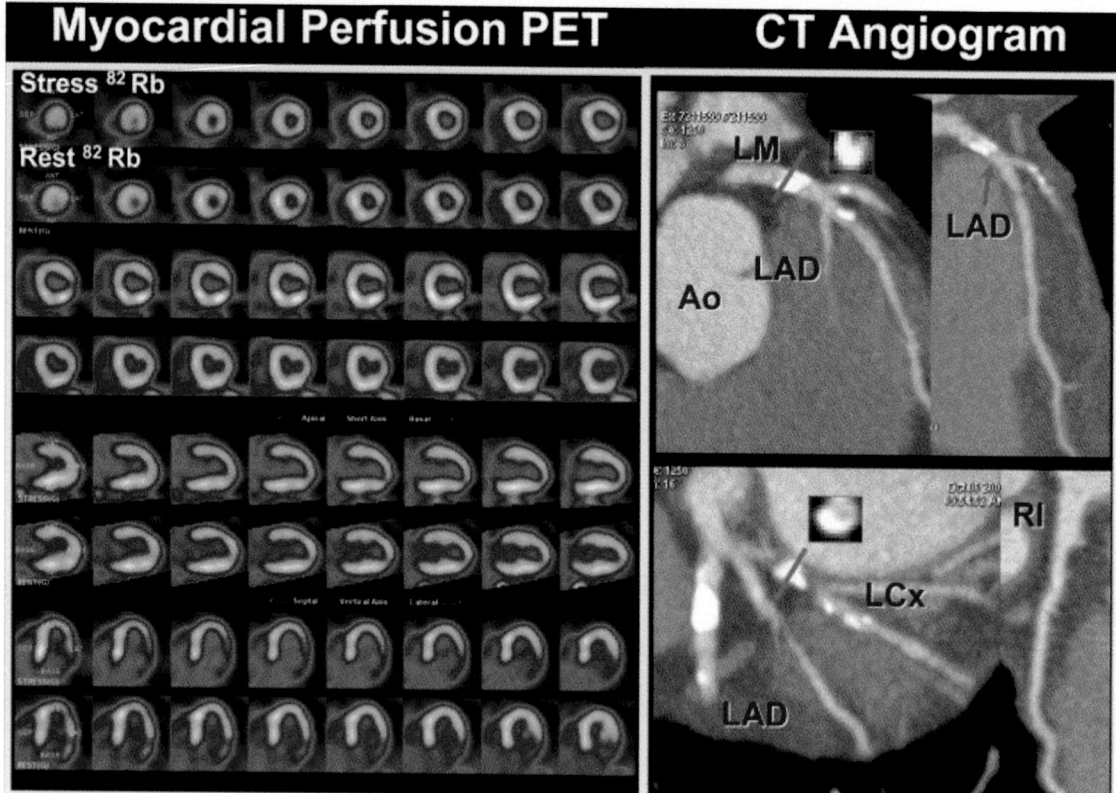

FIGURE 23–11. ^{82}Rubidium stress-rest perfusion imaging and coronary anatomy by CT angiography. The stress-rest myocardial perfusion images obtained with positron emission tomography (PET) demonstrate a small sized, but severe perfusion defect in the lateral wall of the left ventricular myocardium, which is not completely reversible. The coronary angiogram demonstrates severe luminal narrowing of the proximal left anterior descending and the left circumflex coronary artery. The combined CT and PET perfusion findings indicate that only the left circumflex coronary artery stenosis is fluid dynamically significant. *Source: Reproduced from Di Carli MF, Dorbala S, Hachamovitch R. Integrated cardiac PET-CT for the diagnosis and management of CAD. J Nucl Cardiol. 2006;13(2):139–144.*

Coronary Vasomotion and Preclinical Coronary Artery Disease

Noninvasive measurements of regional MBF offer the intriguing possibility of uncovering functional abnormalities of the human coronary circulation. Several indices of coronary circulatory function can be derived noninvasively through measurements of MBF. One is the pharmacologically-stimulated hyperemic MBF. It reflects the total integrated vasodilator capacity of the coronary circulation and depends on the function of both vascular smooth muscle and endothelium. A second one is the flow response to sympathetic stimulation with, for example, cold-pressor testing; it predominantly depends on and thus reflects endothelial function. A third measure of coronary function is a heterogeneity of blood flow in the base-to-apex direction of the LV myocardium; it is related to an impairment of the flow-mediated, endothelium-dependent vasodilation of the epicardial coronary conduit vessels and thus to endothelium dysfunction.

Pharmacologically-Stimulated Hyperemia and Myocardial Perfusion Reserve

Numerous investigations with PET measurements of MBF have examined effects of traditional coronary risk factors on the total vasodilator capacity and the myocardial flow reserve (as the ratio of hyperemic over baseline blood flows). Studies in asymptomatic individuals with hypercholesteremia revealed an approximately 32 percent reduction in myocardial perfusion reserve or an approximately 18 percent reduction in adenosine-stimulated flows.[115–119] Attenuated hyperemic flows were found in patients with diabetes.[120–123]

Invasive studies of the human coronary circulation have emphasized the central role of endothelial dysfunction early in the atherosclerotic process.[124,125] These invasive approaches probe endothelial function at two sites of the coronary circulation, the large epicardial conduit and the coronary resistance vessels. Observations with PET measurements of MBF appear to differ from those made by invasive techniques where the predominantly vascular smooth muscle mediated vasodilator response to intracoronary papaverine or adenosine was frequently fully preserved even in the presence of coronary risk factors, whereas primarily endothelium-mediated responses were markedly abnormal.[126] The major resistance to flow through the coronary circulation resides at the 100 to 400 μ diameter vessels.[127] If flow increases exert shear stresses on the endothelium of the 400 μ vessels, then primarily flow- (endothelium) dependent mechanisms augment the flow response to predominantly vascular smooth muscle vasodilators. Consistent with such augmentation are observations with measurements of forearm blood flow and with PET of MBF.[37,128]

Responses of Myocardial Blood Flow to Cold Pressor Testing

Sympathetic stimulation with cold-pressor testing evokes coronary flow responses that are modulated by a complex interaction between vascular smooth muscle and endothelium and where vasodilator forces are balanced by vasoconstrictor forces. Exposure to cold prompts an increase in heart rate and systolic blood pressure and thus, in cardiac work, which in turn leads to a metabolically mediated decrease in coronary resistance and thus an increase in coronary blood flow. Effects of high flow velocity related shear stress on the endothelium, possibly together with direct adrenergic stimulation, lead to an endothelium-dependent vasodilation, whereas direct, α-adrenergic vascular smooth muscle stimulation leads to vasoconstriction. In this interplay between opposing forces, vasoconstrictor effects prevail if endothelial function is impaired and attenuate the flow responses to cold stimulation.

The observed paradoxical decrease rather than increase in luminal diameter of mildly diseased epicardial coronary artery as well as an increase rather than decrease in coronary resistance to cold-pressor testing lends support to the preponderance of vasoconstrictor forces at the level of the coronary conduit and the resistance vessels when endothelial dysfunction is present.[129-131] Cold-induced responses of MBF measured with PET were found to correlate with changes in the conduit vessel diameter, demonstrated by quantitative angiography.[132] In patients with angiographically normal coronary arteries, changes in the epicardial coronary artery diameter as an index of endothelium-related coronary vasomotion were found to be correlated strongly with cold-induced changes in MBF (Fig. 23–12).

Observations in normal individuals but with long-term smoking as the only well-defined coronary risk factor further confirmed such possibility. The dipyridamole-stimulated hyperemic flow response was fully preserved, whereas cold stimulation produced only modest and statistically insignificant increases in MBF.[133] These observations with PET measurements of MBF are consistent with those by invasive techniques.[124,131,134] Cold-induced increases in rate pressure product in these studies were associated with proportional increases in MBF in nonsmokers but not in the smokers. A similar uncoupling of flow responses from cardiac work has also been observed in patients with risk factors for coronary artery disease or with type II diabetes.[135,136]

Other investigations explored the utility of cold-pressor testing combined with PET measurements of MBF for the identification of coronary vasomotor abnormalities in a number of different conditions including insulin resistance, obesity, and dyslipidemias.[120,133,137-139] In postmenopausal women for example, MBF responses were found to be significantly diminished in comparison to young women studied at midmenstrual cycle.[140]

Critical to the use of cold-pressor testing for monitoring responses to drug interventions and to risk-factor modification, is the reproducibility of the flow measurements. Studies in normal individuals with and without risk factors for coronary ar-

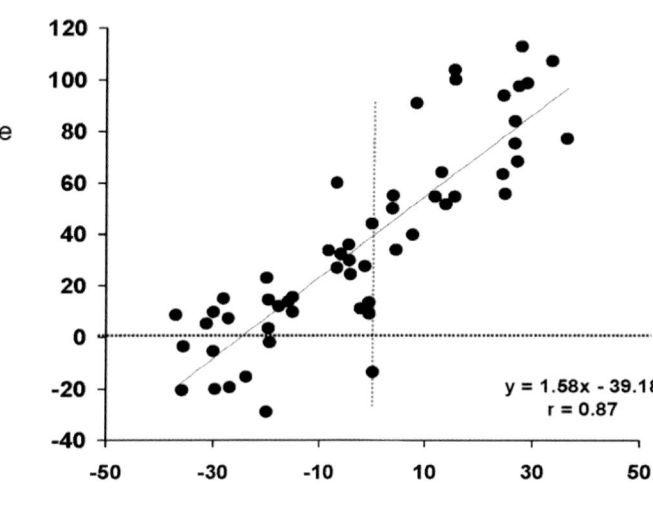

FIGURE 23–12. Correlation between cold-pressor induced changes in the luminal diameter of the epicardial coronary arteries (determined by quantitative coronary angiography) and myocardial blood flow (measured with nitrogen-13 [^{13}N]-ammonia and positron emission tomography [PET]). *Source: Adapted from Schindler, Nitzsche, Olschewski, et al.[132]*

tery disease have indeed established the reproducibility of such measurements.[141]

Longitudinal, Base-to-Apex Myocardial Perfusion Gradient

A potentially attractive approach for identifying noninvasively endothelium-related functional alterations of the coronary epicardial conduit vessels, is the concept of a decline in the "longitudinal, base-to-apex myocardial perfusion gradient."[142] The normal epicardial conduit vessels exert little if any resistance to flow so that the intracoronary pressure is fully maintained over the length of the conduit vessel, and myocardial perfusion is homogenous. Diffuse luminal narrowing of the epicardial coronary arteries, however, even in the absence of discrete coronary stenosis, raises the resistance to especially high velocity flows so that the intracoronary pressure progressively declines from proximal to distal leading to a progressive decline in tissue perfusion from the base to the apex of the LV myocardium.[143] In coronary vessels free of angiographic disease in patients with coronary artery disease, intracoronary pressures were found to decrease from proximal to distal by approximately 5 mmHg at rest and by 10 mmHg during pharmacologically induced hyperemia. This intracoronary pressure decrease was significantly greater than that observed in normal individuals.

Measurements of MBF in normal individuals with normal stress myocardial perfusion images but with coronary risk factors revealed a perfusion gradient during pharmacologically stimulated hyperemia (Fig. 23–13).[144,145] Although diffuse luminal narrowing of the epicardial conduit vessels or other structural changes such as increases in intima-media thickness cannot be excluded entirely as explanation, more likely is a functional alteration of the endothelium in these young healthy volunteers in whom a smoking-related impairment in endothelial function accounted for an inadequate adjustment of the coronary diameter to higher velocity blood flows.[146]

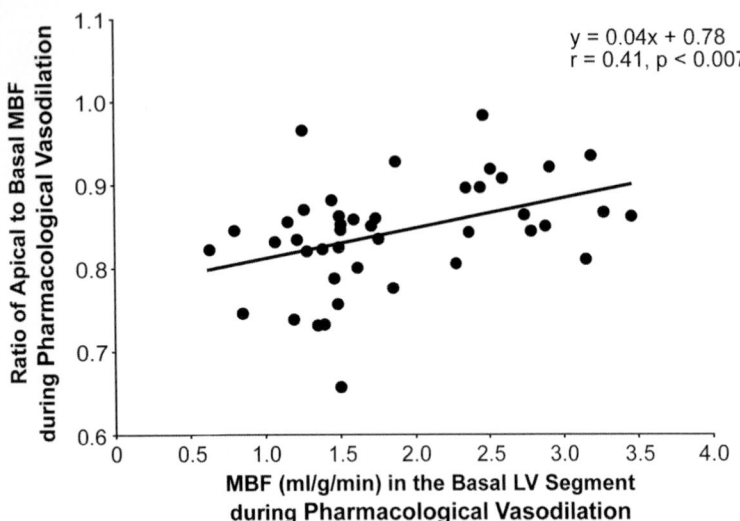

FIGURE 23-13. Relationship between the base-to-apex myocardial perfusion gradient and hyperemic myocardial blood flows (see text). *Source: Reproduced from Schindler, Facta, Prior, et al.[145]*

Coronary Vasomotor Abnormalities and Prediction of Adverse Events

Standard stress-rest myocardial perfusion imaging with SPECT, and as mentioned above, more recently with PET offers important predictive information on future adverse coronary events. The predictive value of these imaging approaches exceeds that available through anatomic angiographic findings, because an addition to information on functional consequences of anatomic alterations it also contains direct information on endothelium and vascular smooth muscle related functional derangements.[149–151]

Measurements of MBF with PET have been shown to contain predictive information. In 72 individuals with angiographically normal coronary arteries but an abnormal flow response to cold-pressor testing, the incidence of cardiovascular events during the 66-month followup period was significantly greater than in individuals with a normal flow response to cold-pressor testing (Fig. 23–15). Cardiovascular events included cardiovascular death,

Characterization of Coronary Vasomotor Abnormalities

The combined assessment of flow responses to cold stimulation and to vasodilator stress with adenosine or dipyridamole can allow a more comprehensive characterization of the coronary circulatory function. Observations with PET measurements of MBF in one investigation in insulin-resistant individuals suggested that the severity of vasomotor abnormalities parallels the severity of the insulin resistance.[147] The flow response to cold was defined as the difference in MBF between cold stimulation and rest and was expressed in units of mL/min/g myocardium (delta MBF).[147,148] Pharmacologically stimulated hyperemic MBFs were fully maintained in individuals with normoglycemic insulin resistance and with impaired glucose tolerance and thus, in less severe states of insulin resistance (Fig. 23–14). Hyperemic flows were diminished in individuals with type II diabetes with and without hypertension as more advanced states of insulin resistance. Flow responses to cold were already attenuated in individuals with normoglycemic insulin resistance and tended to progressively worsen with more severe states of insulin resistance. The observation implies a progressive deterioration of coronary circulatory function that initially affects only the endothelium and subsequently extends to the vascular smooth muscle function. The effects of insulin resistance alone on the endothelium, hypercholesterolemia, hypertriglyceridemia and hyperglycemia-related oxidative stress can exert a cumulative effect on the function of both, endothelium and vascular smooth muscle,[125,134] and account for the progressive impairment of coronary vasomotor function.

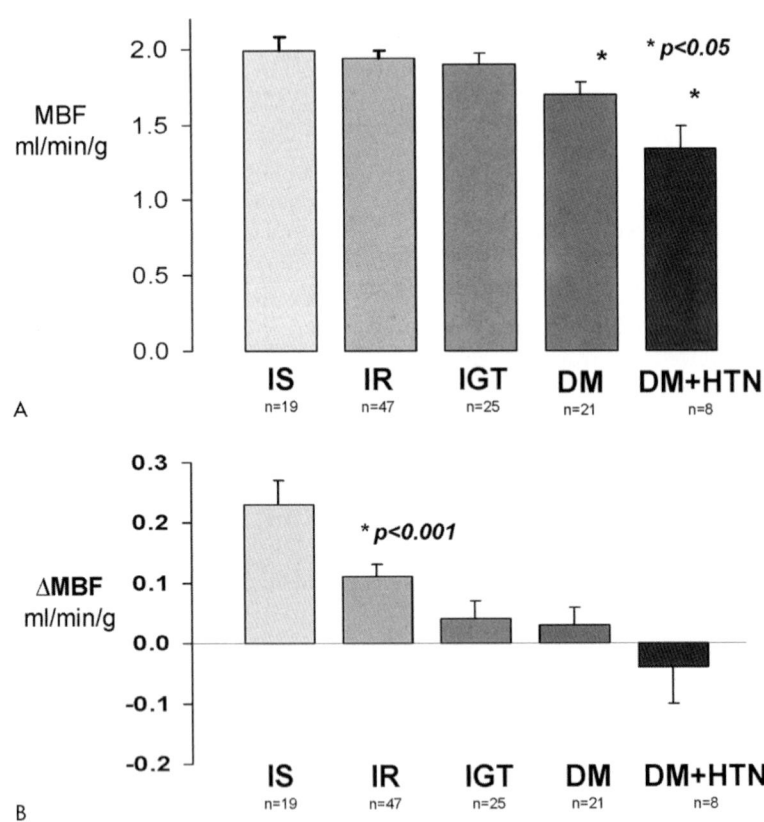

FIGURE 23-14. Coronary circulatory function in states of insulin resistance of increasing severity. Myocardial blood flow was measured during pharmacologically induced hyperemia (**A**) and in response to cold-pressor testing in 19 normal, insulin-sensitive individuals (IS), in 47 normoglycemic insulin-resistant individuals (IR), in 25 individuals with impaired glucose tolerance (IGT), in 21 patients with type II diabetes mellitus (DM), and in 8 patients with type II diabetes mellitus and hypertension. As shown in **A**, hyperemic myocardial blood flows were significantly attenuated only in patients with diabetes mellitus whereas, as shown in **B**, the flow response to cold-pressor testing (defined as the change in myocardial blood flow, delta myocardial blood flow [MBF]) from rest to cold-pressor testing, was already attenuated in normoglycemic insulin-resistant individuals. *Source: Adapted from Prior, Quinones, Hernandez-Pampaloni, et al.[147]*

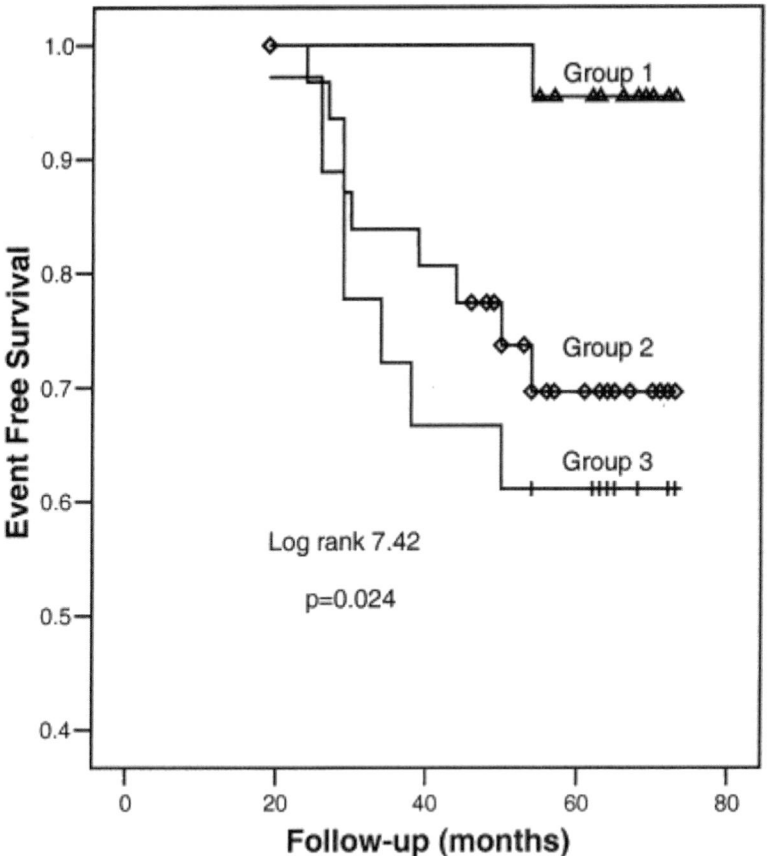

FIGURE 23–15. Predictive value of the flow response to cold-pressor testing as determined with positron emission tomography. In this study, individuals were grouped by the flow response to cold-pressor testing where in Group 1 individuals, blood flow increased by more than 40 percent from rest, whereas flow increases in Group 2 individuals were reduced (<20 percent) and were absent or paradoxical in Group 3 individuals. *Source: Reproduced from Schindler, Hornig, Buser, et al.[139] Used with permission.*

acute coronary syndrome, myocardial infarction, percutaneous transluminal coronary angioplasty, and coronary artery bypass grafting, ischemic stroke, or peripheral revascularization.

These PET findings appear to be inconsistent with those from stress-rest perfusion imaging of the relative distribution of MBF, where only regional perfusion defects are predictive of future cardiovascular events. In contrast, participants in the cold-pressor study had angiographically normal coronary vessels so that their stress-rest perfusion images were expected to be normal and thus, be predictive of a low incidence of adverse cardiovascular events. However, different from the conventional stress-rest perfusion imaging that is highly predictive of the first 2-year cardiovascular events, adverse events in the cold-pressor studies occurred only after a longer latent period, that is, after approximately 2 years. This then suggests that functional alterations can be an earlier predictor of future cardiovascular events, and further such functional alterations progress to anatomic (structural changes as identified by conventional stress-rest perfusion imaging).

Monitoring Responses to Risk-Factor Modification

PET measurements of MBF are equally suited for monitoring responses in coronary vasomotion to pharmacologic interventions as well as to risk-factor modification as initially demonstrated in pa-

tients participating in a short (6 week) cardiovascular conditioning program.[152] Rigorous life-style and risk-factor modification have previously been shown with PET to result in smaller and less severe stress-induced perfusion defects.[153,154]

Other studies with PET measurements of MBF have demonstrated beneficial effects of risk-factor modification and drug interventions on coronary vasomotor function.[155–159] Glucose control in type II diabetic patients is associated with higher levels of hyperemic blood flows.[160] Other studies have demonstrated improvements in cold-pressor flows and, thus, in endothelial function in response to long-term antioxidant treatment,[161] to treatment with insulin-sensitizing agents for 3 months,[162] and to glucose lowering in type II diabetes patients.[163]

【 】 IMAGING OF ATHEROSCLEROTIC VASCULAR PLAQUES

PET holds considerable promise for the noninvasive characterization of the potentially vulnerable atherosclerotic plaque. This is especially true when imaging is combined with multidetector CT or with high-resolution MRI. These high spatial resolution imaging techniques have been shown to visualize noninvasively the large arteries and the coronary vessels in exquisite anatomic detail.[164,165] Detailed morphologic information on vascular remodeling and on atherosclerotic plaques becomes available with measurements of size and volume of atherosclerotic plaques and, to some extent, composition. Key features of the potentially vulnerable plaque includes its size, the large lipid core, massive macrophage infiltration, apoptosis of macrophages, expression of proteolytic enzymes (i.e., macrophage-derived matrix metalloproteinase), and the thin fibrous cap.[166] Plaques visualized on CT angiograms are classified by radiographic density as calcified, noncalcified (or soft), and mixed (consisting of calcified and noncalcified regions). Radiographically soft plaques are thought to be associated with potential plaque instability. However, a more detailed assessment of the composition of plaques in terms of lipid, cells, and fibrous tissue content remains limited, largely because of method-related variations in radiographic densities (Hounsfield units) within the plaque.[164]

Studies with radiolabeled molecular probes in animal models of atherosclerosis have demonstrated the feasibility of specifically targeting components of the vulnerable plaque, as for example, expression of matrix metalloproteinases,[167] proliferation of vascular smooth muscle cells,[168,169] of the lipid pool,[170] of macrophages infiltration,[171–173] and macrophage apoptosis. Relatively low target-to-background ratios of these radiolabeled molecular probes together with the small spatial dimension of the thin arterial wall pose considerable challenges to the in-vivo application of these radiolabeled molecular probes in large-animal experimental models, and even more so, in humans. Most promising has been the use of ^{18}F-FDG, a positron emitting tracer that is widely available and is extensively used in the clinic for tumor imaging and staging with PET. The radiolabeled compound traces the transmembranous ex-

PET   Contrast CT   Fusion

Right

Left

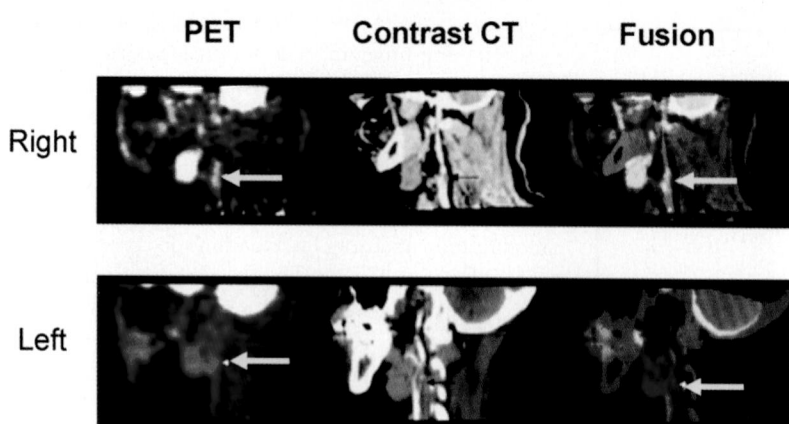

FIGURE 23–16. Focally increased uptake of ^{18}F-FDG in the right carotid artery (arrow) in a patient with a recent cerebrovascular event. *Source: Reproduced from Rudd, Warburton, Fryer, et al.[182] Used with permission of the American Heart Association.*

change of glucose and its initial hexokinase-mediated phosphorylation to glucose-6-phosphate. The phosphorylated radiotracer is retained in the cell so that its externally imaged accumulation reflects the rate of cellular exogenous glucose utilization. Polymorphous leukocytes, monocytes, and macrophages have been shown to accumulate ^{18}F-FDG.[174] Invasion of the arterial wall by these inflammatory cells can therefore be visualized noninvasively with ^{18}F-FDG and PET, as several investigations in patients with giant cell arteritis or Takayasu disease have shown, demonstrating the feasibility of delineating and identifying cellular processes even in the thin walled or small sized arterial wall.[175,176]

Different from the diffuse vascular ^{18}F-FDG uptake in arteritis patients, atherosclerosis is characteristically associated with focal increases of ^{18}F-FDG- uptake as noted in several studies in patients undergoing whole-body PET for tumor detection and staging.[177–181] Focal increases in ^{18}F-FDG uptake were found to be frequently associated with multiple arterial calcific lesions and were more prevalent in patients with than without risk factors for coronary artery disease or with coronary artery disease. These focal increases in vascular ^{18}F-FDG uptake in the large arteries are usually separate in location from calcified lesions; they are located adjacent to or remote from vascular calcium deposits.

The intensity of the focal arterial ^{18}F-FDG -uptake appears to reflect the degree of plaque inflammation and thus, its potential vulnerability. In patients with carotid artery stenoses, ^{18}F-FDG uptake in the symptomatic carotid artery was found to be consistently higher than in the contralateral, nonsymptomatic carotid artery (Fig. 23–16).[182] Histopathology and autoradiography of endarterectomy specimens in these patients revealed colocalization of ^{18}F-FDG with macrophages, suggesting a quantitative relationship between the intensity of ^{18}F-FDG–uptake and the degree of macrophage invasion. Moreover, studies in animal models of atherosclerosis revealed statistically significant correlations between radiotracer concentrations in atherosclerotic arterial segments and the number of macrophages or the macrophage content as identified by rabbit macrophage-specific monoclonal antibody, RAM-11, histochemical-staining techniques.[172,173,183] Subsequent studies have confirmed the validity of the animal experi-

mental findings in human atherosclerotic disease. The findings implicate the vascular ^{18}F-FDG concentration as a measure of macrophage invasion and hence, of the degree of plaque inflammation. When considered within the context of histopathologic findings in potentially vulnerable coronary arterial plaques in patients with fatal myocardial infarctions, the ^{18}F-FDG concentration can indeed contain independent predictive information on plaque instability.[184] When plaques in the carotid artery study were grouped by percent CD68 staining as a measure of plaque vulnerability, then plaques with greater than 15 percent CD68 staining and considered histopathologically as unstable, exhibited significantly higher ^{18}F-FDG concentrations than plaques considered stable by histopathologic criteria (Fig. 23–17).[185]

Lipid-lowering therapy with hydroxymethylglutaryl coenzyme A (HMG-CoA) reductase inhibitors has been shown to exert an antiinflammatory effect on human atherosclerosis[186] that can also be demonstrated noninvasively by imaging the vascular ^{18}F-FDG uptake.[187]

The majority of investigations on the vascular ^{18}F-FDG uptake have thus far focused on the carotid arteries and the thoracic and the abdominal aorta. Evaluation of atherosclerotic plaques in the coronary vessels has remained challenging and thus far has been reported in only one investigation. Difficulties relate to cardiac and respiratory motion, the small size of the coronary vessels and, the uptake of ^{18}F-FDG in the myocardium that obscures the uptake of ^{18}F-FDG in the coronary vessels.[179] In these patients, foci of increased ^{18}F-FDG uptake were found to be located mostly in the proximal epicardial vessels. These metabolic foci frequently coexisted with coronary calcifications but rarely overlapped or were superimposed.

Evaluation of atherosclerotic plaques located in the coronary arteries will remain challenging. It requires development of study approaches and protocols for suppression of myocardial ^{18}F-FDG

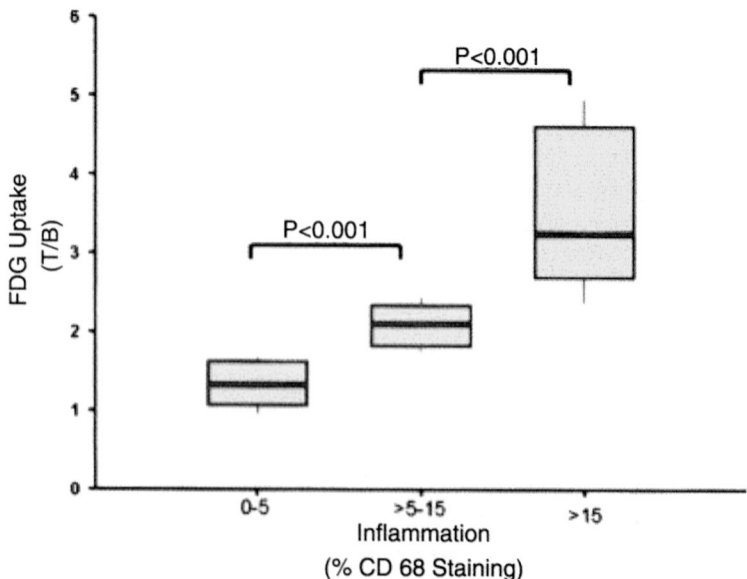

FIGURE 23–17. ^{18}F-FDG uptake in atherosclerotic regions of the carotid artery (by positron emission tomography [PET]) and severity of inflammation by immunohistochemistry (see text). *Source: Reproduced from Tawakol, Migrino, Bashian, et al.[185]*

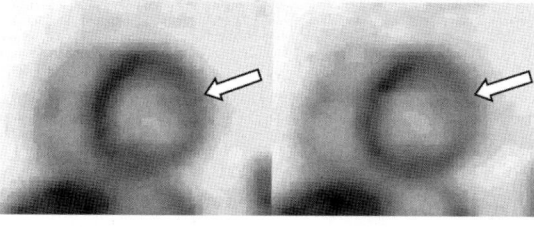

Perfusion
^{13}NH$_3$

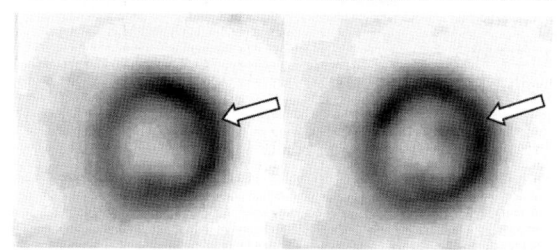

Metabolism
^{18}FDG

FIGURE 23–18. Myocardial blood flow metabolism mismatch: The upper panel demonstrates two contiguous short-axis myocardial perfusion images with a moderate decrease in perfusion in the anterior and anterolateral wall (arrows). On the ^{18}F-FDG metabolism images as shown in the bottom panel, glucose utilization is enhanced in the hypoperfused myocardium consistent with a perfusion metabolism mismatch.

uptake. Imaging of the coronary arteries will also require synchronization of the image data acquisition with cardiac and respiratory motion, which is available with acquisition of image data in list-mode and subsequent re-binning of the image data. Finally, instrumentation-related improvements in spatial resolution are likely to provide for better visualization of coronary artery lesions; yet, given the small size of the vessels, full evaluation of the entire coronary artery can remain incomplete. Evaluation of only the proximal portions of the coronary circulation can suffice, because most atherosclerotic plaques of possible clinical consequence are located in the most proximal segments of the coronary artery.

【 】 ASSESSMENT OF MYOCARDIAL VIABILITY

Myocardial viability pertains to an impairment of contractile myocardial function that is potentially reversible. Distinction of such potentially reversible from an irreversible impairment of contractile function is of considerable clinical importance but remains diagnostically challenging. This is because both types of tissue injury share several features as for example similar degrees of abnormal systolic wall motion, reduced blood flow, and electrocardiographic abnormalities. However, persistence of metabolic activity for sustaining vital, energy-requiring processes including cellular homeostasis, which in turn depends on some residual blood flow for removal of inhibitory metabolites as well as for supply of fuel substrates. Hence, key features of viable myocardium include the following:

- Impairment of systolic wall motion at rest
- Normal or reduced but not absent blood flow
- Preservation of cellular homeostasis
- Persistent metabolic activity for high energy phosphate production
- Recruitable contractile reserve

General Considerations

Findings in experimental animals provided the base for the detection of myocardial viability. Initial investigations had indicated that known alterations in substrate metabolism during acute myocardial ischemia could indeed be demonstrated noninvasively with positron emitting tracers of myocardial substrate metabolism.[188] Consistent with an impaired fatty acid oxidation was the diminished initial uptake of ^{11}C-palmitate and its delayed subsequent rate of clearance from the myocardium.[70,75] Additionally, the known increase in glucose extraction and glucose utilization was reflected by a regional increase in ^{18}F-FDG uptake.[189] Initial studies in patients with clinical evidence of acute myocardial ischemia revealed blood flow and glucose metabolism patterns that were virtually identical to those found in animals with mild stress induced ischemia, e.g., enhanced ^{18}F-FDG uptake in hypoperfused dysfunctional myocardial regions. Unexpected was however the existence of the same pattern in patients with chronic CAD but without clinical signs of acute ischemia (Fig. 23–18). This then raised the question as to whether the blood flow metabolism pattern as observed on PET was indeed unique to acute ischemia or whether it represented a more general metabolic pattern in chronically dysfunctional and hypoperfused myocardium. No less intriguing were observations in other CAD patients with a segmentally reduced ^{18}F-FDG uptake, which paralleled the reduction in regional MBF (Fig. 23–19).[190] A more systematic exploration of these findings in patients scheduled for coronary artery bypass grafting confirmed the working hypothesis that the regionally enhanced ^{18}F-FDG uptake, in contrast to a reduction, reflected sustained glucose utilization and, thus, metabolic activity as evidence of viability in myocardium with complete or partial loss of contractile function.[191] Restoration of tissue perfusion was followed by an improvement of contractile function in myocardium with persistent glucose metabolic activity.

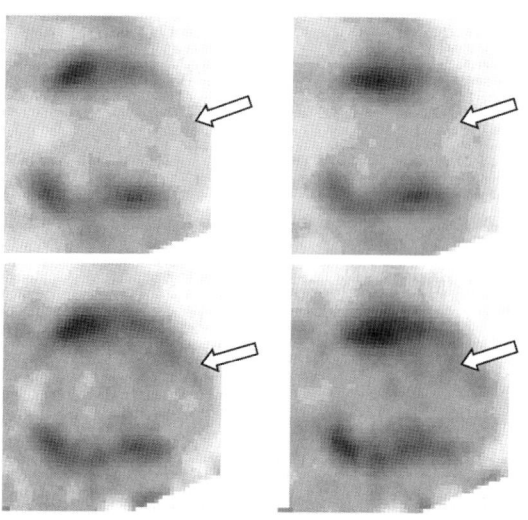

Perfusion
^{13}NH$_3$

Metabolism
^{18}FDG

FIGURE 23–19. Myocardial blood flow metabolism match: The upper panel depicts two contiguous vertical long-axis images of myocardial perfusion obtained with nitrogen-13 (^{13}N)-ammonia, the lower panel the corresponding vertical long-axis cuts on the ^{18}F-FDG images. Note the concordant reductions in ^{18}F-FDG uptake and myocardial perfusion, consistent with the pattern of a perfusion metabolism match.

Possible Mechanisms of the Blood Flow Metabolism Pattern

The above observations established the clinical utility of PET findings although the underlying mechanisms remained uncertain. Patients with CAD undergoing supine bicycle exercise revealed in myocardium with stress-induced flow defects an augmented ^{18}F-FDG uptake when the radiotracer was administered 20 to 30 minutes after exercise and after the stress-induced flow defect had resolved (Fig. 23–20).[192] This then implied that the enhanced tracer uptake might indeed represent *stunned myocardium*, a possibility supported by observations in experimental animals and in patients with unstable angina.[193–195] These studies also demonstrated the evolution of a blood flow metabolism pattern in chronically reperfused myocardium: An immediate postreperfusion decrease in glucose uptake was followed by an increase that subsequently declined to normal as contractile function returned.[194] The enhanced ^{18}F-FDG uptake was attributed to increased lactate release and, thus, to anaerobic glycolysis that persisted even after blood flow had been restored.[196] The evolution of such metabolic pattern might pertain also to early postinfarction patients,[197] but does not fully explain the flow metabolism observations in patients with chronic CAD. Another possibility is *repetitive stunning*[198] as an explanation of the persistent increase in ^{18}F-FDG uptake in dysfunctional myocardium. An impairment in contractile function associated with enhanced glucose utilization was noted in collateral dependent myocardium only if the flow reserve was markedly restricted.[195] The coronary circulation is then unable to appropriately respond to increases in oxygen demand during daily life, leading to transient ischemic episodes, each followed by stunning and preventing recovery of contractile function. Consistent with this concept are findings during dobutamine stimulation where development of wall motion abnormalities depended on the residual perfusion reserve and, in turn, on the angiographic coronary stenosis severity.[199,200]

Myocardial *hibernation* serves as another possible explanation.[201] The postulated down-regulation of contractile function in response to diminished rest blood flow is thought to be associated with an alteration of the myocardium's substrate metabolism with a dominant role for the more oxygen-efficient glucose. Hibernation in its truest sense then implies that the downregulated energy requirements match the available energy supply. A new supply demand imbalance is established but at a lower level. Such new balance would however be a precarious one because even moderate increases in demand or decreases in supply could disturb the steady state and cause ischemia. It is thus possible and likely that both, hibernation and stunning coexist to varying extents in many patients. Observations in experimental animals suggest that sustained reductions in both blood flow and contractile function can be maintained for some time without significant necrosis although structural alterations develop that resemble those in patients with chronic CAD[202–205] and that provide an animal experimental underpinning for the concept of hibernation.

Both concepts, repetitive *stunning* and *hibernation* can, in their purest form, represent the two ends of a spectrum. This spectrum begins with a reduction in myocardial flow reserve when increases in demand can no longer be fully met by appropriate increases in supply and ends with a complete loss of the myocardial flow re-

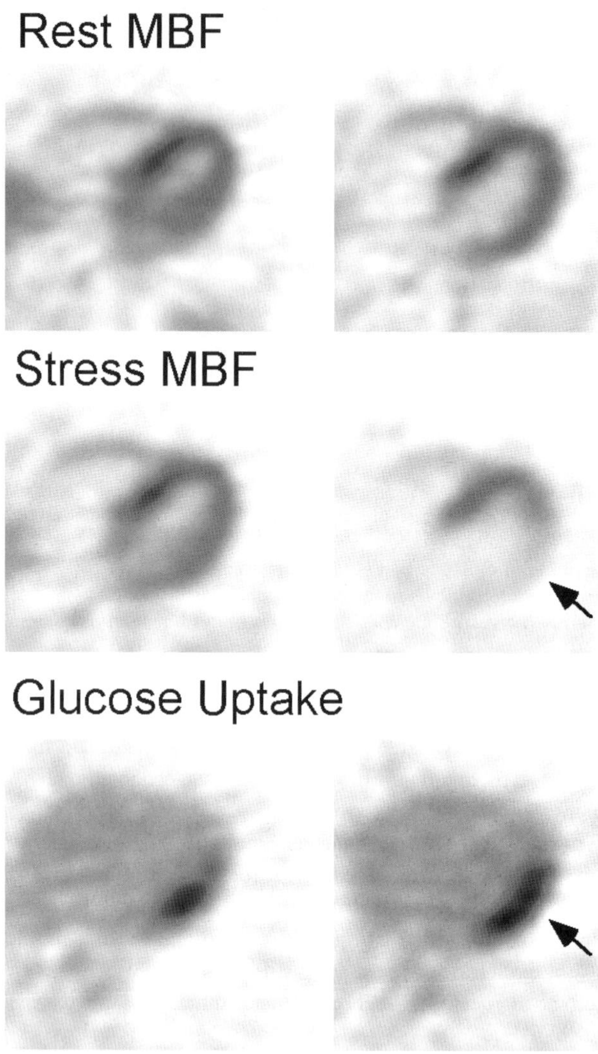

FIGURE 23–20. Rest and stress myocardial perfusion images (myocardial blood flow [MBF]) and rest ^{18}F-FDG images (glucose uptake) in a patient with coronary artery disease. Note on the horizontal long-axis images the homogenous myocardial perfusion at rest but the segmentally increased ^{18}F-FDG uptake in the posterior lateral wall. On the stress myocardial perfusion images, a perfusion defect is noted in the same area. The perfusion metabolism pattern in this patient most likely reflects *myocardial stunning*.

serve and a reduction in regional MBF at rest, associated with a downregulation of contractile function and adaptation of substrate metabolism. The spectrum could also represent a temporal progression in coronary stenosis severity. Recent findings in chronically instrumented animals with a progressive decline and ultimately loss of regional flow reserve associated with a decrease in rest blood flow support such a scenario.[204–207] Conversely, reductions in flow can also occur rapidly in view of the high incidence of blood flow metabolism mismatches in early postinfarction patients.[190,197,208] As acute animal experimental studies have demonstrated, sudden moderate reductions of regional blood flow are initially associated with evidence of acute ischemia as for example release of lactate and enhanced glucose uptake. An apparent *resetting* or *adjustment* of demand occurs thereafter when lactate release converts to uptake and high energy phosphate stores are replenished and a new supply demand balance seems to have returned.[202,209,210] Some debate has focused on the issue whether blood flow at rest can indeed be chronically reduced.[211] This was because hibernating myocardium no longer demonstrated the postulated perfusion contraction match. To some extent, this can be because of the admixture or coexistence of scar tissue or replacement fibrosis but also because of ultrastructural changes of myocytes including loss of contractile proteins, that is neither specific to repetitive stunning nor to myocardial hibernation.[212–216] Nevertheless, findings in chronic animal experiments as well as substantial improvements in resting blood flow following surgical revascularization argue in favor of the possibility of a true chronic regional hypoperfusion.[205–207,217,218]

Viability Assessment in the Clinical Setting

The classic and now most widely applied approach entails evaluation of the relative distribution of blood flow and of exogenous glucose utilization with ^{18}F-FDG. Three distinct patterns of perfusion metabolism in dysfunctional myocardium are found (Fig. 23–21):

1. Normal blood flow and normal or enhanced glucose uptake
2. Reduced blood flow with glucose uptake in excess of blood flow (*mismatch*)
3. Reduced blood flow and proportionately reduced glucose uptake (*match*)[191]

Although these terms are purely operational, they infer, at least to some extent, the underlying pathophysiology accounting for the contractile dysfunction. Normal flow and/or metabolism might represent *stunned* whereas the classic *mismatch* might be consistent with *hibernating* myocardium. Both patterns predict a postrevascularization improvement in contractile function whereas the concordant reduction in blood flow and metabolism predicts that function will not improve.[191,219,220] Regional flow reductions in both matches and mismatches, can vary considerably in severity. Mild to modest concordant reductions in both blood flow and ^{18}F-FDG uptake can reflect a prior nontransmural infarction as compared to a more severe reduction or even absence of both in transmural infarctions. Also, flow reductions in mismatches can vary considerably as a reflection of varying degrees of transmural involvement and of the amount of scar tissue.

The observed correlations between tissue fibrosis and relative flow-tracer concentrations indicate that regional MBF alone can serve as a measure of reversibility of contractile dysfunction.[221,222] Severe reductions to less than 25 percent of normal or complete absence of blood flow reflect complete or nearly complete transmural scar tissue formation and, hence, nonreversiblity.[223] According to another study, flow reductions of more than 60 percent were highly accurate in predicting nonreversibility of contractile dysfunction.[224] Conversely, normal or only mildly reduced (<20 percent) flow in dysfunctional myocardium argue against the presence of significant amounts of tissue fibrosis; it possibly reflects myocardial stunning and thus indicates functional reversibility.[225] Intermediate flow reductions are less reliable discriminators; for example, a nontransmural infarction can lead to a mild to moderate flow reduction; if the remainder of the transmural segment consists of normal myocardium, then the regional ^{18}F-FDG uptake will be reduced in proportion to flow and contractile function would be unlikely to improve.[226] Conversely, if glucose uptake were increased, it would indicate the coexistence of reversibly dysfunctional myocardium with scar tissue and be predictive of a postrevascularization improvement in contractile function.

Similar considerations apply to the assessment of myocardial viability with late contrast-enhanced MRI.[5] The transmural extent of hyperenhancement reflects the transmural extent of scar tissue and, thus, the fraction of myocardium with irreversible loss of contractile function. As postrevascularization studies of regional contractile function have indicated, a more than 75 percent transmural contrast enhancement accurately predicts nonreversibility of contractile function whereas a less than 25 percent transmural contrast enhancement is highly predictive of a postrevascularization improvement. However less reliably, intermediate extents of hyperenhancement distinguish potential reversibility from irreversibility of contractile function. For example, transmural hyperenhancements ranging from 26 to 50 percent in dysfunctional myocardial segments predicted with a less than 50 percent accuracy a postrevascularization improvement in contractile function.

The hyperenhancement reflects the presence of scar tissue. Because myocardial perfusion at rest declines in inverse proportion to the amount of scar tissue, segments with intermediate degrees

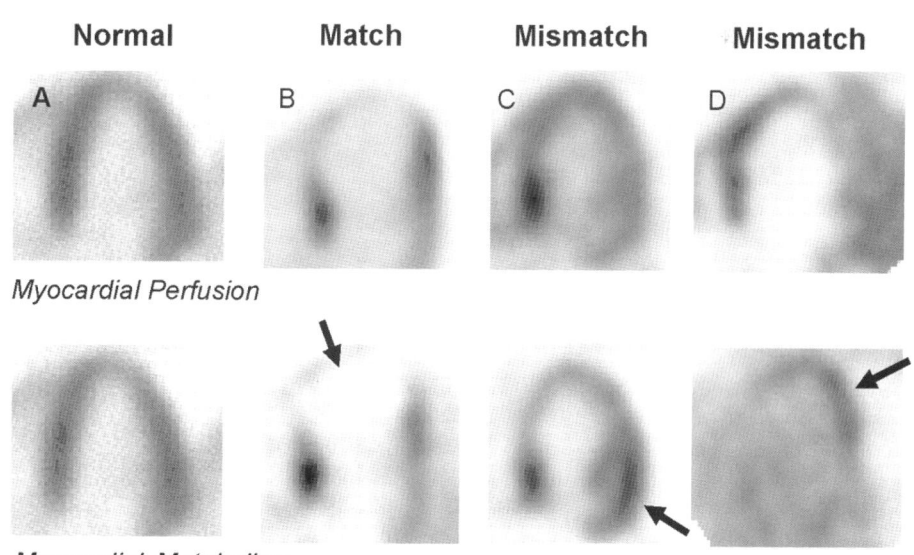

Normal A | **Match** B | **Mismatch** C | **Mismatch** D

Myocardial Perfusion

Myocardial Metabolism

FIGURE 23–21. Patterns of myocardial perfusion (*upper panel*) and metabolism (with ^{18}F-FDG; *lower panel*). **A.** Normal myocardial perfusion and metabolism. **B.** Severely reduced myocardial perfusion in the anterior wall associated with a concordant reduction in ^{18}F-FDG uptake (*arrow*), corresponding to a match. **C.** Mildly reduced perfusion in the lateral and posterior lateral wall associated with a segmental increase in glucose metabolism (mismatch). **D.** Severely reduced myocardial perfusion in the lateral wall with a segmental increase in ^{18}F-FDG uptake (*arrow*), reflecting a perfusion metabolism mismatch.

of hyperenhancement are therefore associated with intermediate reductions in myocardial perfusion which, as mentioned above, are of limited accuracy in distinguishing between viability and nonviability. Comparison studies between late contrast MRI and PET myocardial perfusion metabolism imaging in patients with diminished LV function have emphasized the close agreement between late contrast enhancement and regional myocardial ^{18}F-FDG concentrations.[227] Importantly however, the majority of segments evaluated in this comparison studies were associated with perfusion metabolism matches so that the concordance of regional ^{18}F-FDG uptake with the amount of segmental *viable myocardium* would be expected.

Identification of reversible contractile dysfunction can also be possible with ^{18}F-FDG alone. This approach derives from comparative studies with gated MRI and PET and assumes that regional reductions in ^{18}F-FDG greater than 50 percent relative to remote myocardium represent irreversible contractile function, whereas mildly reduced or normal uptake indicates the presence of reversible dysfunction.[228,229] While used for some time as a measure for defining the accuracy of thallium-201 (^{201}Tl)-based techniques for assessing myocardial viability,[228] only recent studies have tested the validity of this particular approach against the postrevascularization outcome in regional contractile function.[230] ECG-gated image acquisition affords simultaneous evaluation of regional function and metabolism and thus can further augment the predictive accuracy of the ^{18}F-FDG stand-alone approach.[231,232] The utility of measurements of exogenous glucose utilization in absolute units has also been explored. A threshold value of 0.25 µmol/min/g yielded a 93 percent positive and a 95 percent negative predictive accuracy for the improvement of contractile dysfunction.[233] Nevertheless, limitations with this approach remain, especially when glucose utilization and, hence, ^{18}F-FDG uptake cannot be sufficiently controlled. Because of this, another study pointed out the limited value of quantitative glucose uptake measurements for identifying myocardial viability.[234] Further, use of ^{18}F-FDG alone can prove unreliable for identifying normal myocardium. ^{18}F-FDG uptake can be markedly diminished or even absent when myocardium preferentially uses free fatty acid so that normal myocardium will be difficult to distinguish from scar tissue. However, scar tissue can readily be identified and distinguished from scar tissue by evaluating the distribution of regional MBF.[235]

Alternate Approaches to Blood Flow and Glucose Metabolism Imaging

Several institutions successfully use SPECT myocardial perfusion imaging with either ^{201}Tl or technetium-99m (^{99m}Tc)-sestamibi and metabolic imaging with ^{18}F-FDG with dedicated PET systems. These institutions report predictive accuracies for changes in segmental and global LV function that approach those obtained with dedicated PET systems.[236] Nevertheless, such combined PET/SPECT approaches present at times with diagnostic limitations, especially because of considerable differences in contrast and spatial resolutions as well as artifactual reductions in tracer concentrations because of photon attenuation.[237] This then can limit the ability to accurately estimate the extent of a blood flow metabolism mismatch which, as discussed below, can be useful for predicting the magnitude of changes in global LV function and con-

gestive heart failure-related symptoms. Other approaches rely solely on the use of multipurpose SPECT-like systems, equipped with ultrahigh photon energy general purpose collimators. Studies with SPECT ^{201}Tl or ^{99m}Tc labeled flow tracers and with SPECT ^{18}F-FDG imaging report predictive accuracies that are comparable to those reported with dedicated PET systems.[238, 239]

^{201}Tl rest-redistribution imaging has been useful for identifying myocardial viability and for predicting the postsurgical outcome of ischemic cardiomyopathy although with a somewhat lower predictive accuracy. While the concept of ^{201}Tl redistribution for evaluation of blood flow and the myocardial potassium pool as an indicator of the cell membrane integrity is clearly a scientifically sound one, it suffers from instrumentation-related shortcomings especially in patients with poor LV function and, consequently, poor signal-to-noise ratios. ^{201}Tl offers a negative signal (reduced tracer uptake) as compared to ^{18}F-FDG with a positive signal (enhanced tracer uptake), which is more readily accessible to visual analysis.[235] Consistent with this are findings in patients with severely depressed LV function. One study for example reports that ^{18}F-FDG and PET identified myocardial viability in 18 of 20 patients with an average ejection fraction of 23 percent and only fixed ^{201}Tl defects on SPECT,[240] which is similar to another report on viability by ^{18}F-FDG in 17 of 33 patients (LVEF <35 percent) with fixed or minimally redistributing ^{201}Tl defects.[241] Further, in a comparison study of ^{201}Tl and ^{18}F-FDG SPECT, there was generally an excellent agreement between both approaches.[242] However, disparities occurred in patients with severely depressed LV function where ^{18}F-FDG revealed more viable myocardial segments than ^{201}Tl SPECT.

In synthesizing the currently available information, it appears that ultimately the total fraction of scar tissue in a given myocardial segment determines largely whether or not contractile function will improve. Because of the linear correlation between scar tissue and relative blood flow,[222,243] evaluation or even quantitation of regional blood flow offers information on potential reversibility. Conversely, if in viable although functionally compromised myocardium blood flow is also reduced, then the augmented glucose utilization as evidenced by the enhanced ^{18}F-FDG uptake offers additional and critical information. This has prompted some investigators to predict the functional outcome from a combined assessment of blood flow and ^{18}F-FDG uptake.[244,245] Further, the temporal recovery of contractile function after revascularization appears to depend on the degree of ultrastructural changes of myocytes as well as the fractional distribution between myocytes with only mild and with severe ultrastructural changes.[244] If, as postulated, only mild structural changes are associated with a full functional recovery within 3 months, more severe structural changes can require substantially longer time periods and, further, can account for the persistence of increased ^{18}F-FDG uptake even for many months following revascularization.[246]

[ ] CLINICAL ROLE OF POSITRON EMISSION TOMOGRAPHY VIABILITY ASSESSMENT

Conclusions reached from a meta-analysis of 24 clinical investigations including 3088 patients with coronary artery disease, reduced LVEF (average 32 ± 8 percent) and congestive heart failure systems (average NYHA functional class 2.8) highlight the importance of myocardial viability.[247] All patients had been examined for the presence of viable myocardium, using either low-dose dobutamine stress (8 investigations), ^{201}Tl rest-redistribution scintigraphy (6 investigations) or blood flow metabolism imaging with ^{18}F-FDG (11 investigations). During the 25 ± 10 months followup period, 375 cardiac deaths occurred. Grouping patients by presence or absence of myocardial viability and further by treatment (medically and revascularization) revealed significant intergroup differences in cardiac mortality. Patients without myocardial viability revealed an annual mortality rate of 6.2 percent on medical treatment as compared to a 7.7 percent ($p = 0.23$, not significant) when treated by revascularization. Importantly, the annual mortality for patients with myocardial viability was 16 percent on medical treatment but only 3.2 percent when treated surgically ($p < 0.0001$). They suggest that the search for viable myocardium can identify patients at an especially high risk of cardiac death and, further, that such risk can be reduced by coronary revascularization. Thus, in addition to identifying patients with ischemic cardiomyopathy who are likely to benefit most from therapeutic revascularization, the assessment of myocardial viability also provides prospective information on other clinically relevant questions including the amount of viable myocardium or the extent of scar tissue needed for a postrevascularization change in LV function, and, possibly congestive heart failure-related symptoms as well as an assessment of the risk to benefit ratio of the surgical procedure. Finally, the assessment of myocardial viability can also aid in identifying the leading cause of poor LV function and thus distinguish between an intrinsic myopathic process and CAD.

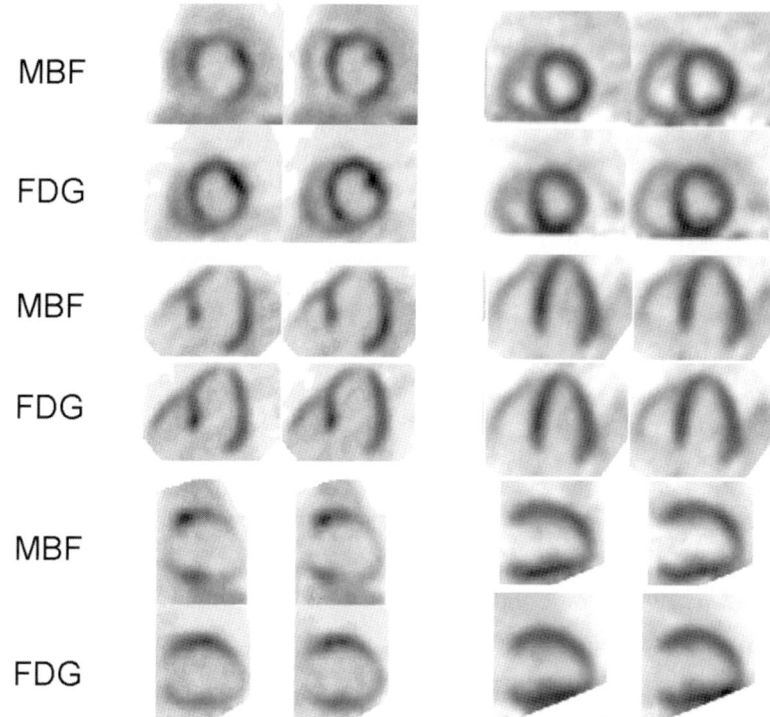

FIGURE 23–22. Perfusion and metabolism patterns in a patient with ischemic cardiomyopathy (*left panel*) and with idiopathic dilated cardiomyopathy (*right panel*). Short-axis (*top*), horizontal (*middle*), and vertical long-axis (*bottom*), images of myocardial perfusion (myocardial blood flow [MBF]) and glucose metabolism ([^{18}F]fluoro-2-deoxy-D-glucose [FDG]) are shown. Note the segmentally reduced perfusion and glucose metabolism in the anterior wall in the patient with ischemic cardiomyopathy and the homogenous perfusion and metabolism in the patient with idiopathic dilated cardiomyopathy.

Ischemic versus Idiopathic Dilated Cardiomyopathy

In addition to heart failure symptoms, ischemic cardiomyopathy shares several other features with idiopathic dilated cardiomyopathy as for example LV enlargement, frequently diffuse hypokinesis, low LVEF and, frequently, mitral regurgitation. Conduction abnormalities often limit the accuracy of electrocardiographic criteria to distinguish between both entities. An intrinsic myopathic process including LV remodeling can exist in patients with CAD so that the leading cause of the poor LV function can remain unknown or difficult to elucidate.

Both disease entities reveal remarkably different patterns of blood flow and substrate metabolism on PET. A comparison study in patients with ischemic cardiomyopathy and with idiopathic dilated cardiomyopathy found the distribution of MBF to be characteristically homogeneous in idiopathic cardiomyopathy as compared to distinct flow reductions clearly corresponding in ischemic cardiomyopathy to the coronary vascular territories.[248] Similarly, uptake of ^{18}F-FDG was noted to be homogeneous in dilated cardiomyopathy, whereas matches and/or mismatches between blood flow and ^{18}F-FDG uptake were present in ischemic cardiomyopathy (Fig. 23–22). Combined imaging of blood flow and glucose metabolism distinguished with an overall accuracy of 85 percent

between both disease entities. This value exceeded the diagnostic accuracy of electrocardiographic criteria, regional wall motion abnormalities, or right ventricular enlargement.

Prediction of the Outcome in Global Left Ventricular Function

Numerous clinical investigations have reported the high accuracy of ^{18}F-FDG imaging with PET in predicting the postrevascularization outcome in regional LV wall motion.[191,219,220,229,230,236,246,249,250] Even though some of these investigations employed permutations of the initially described blood flow metabolism approach or relied only on the evaluation of regional ^{18}F-FDG uptake in dysfunctional myocardium,[229,230] the predictive accuracy both positive and negative, remained high. These studies focused on segmental contractile function to prove the concept of blood flow metabolism patterns as accurate predictors of the outcome of regional wall motion after restoration of MBF. However, more relevant in the clinical setting is whether blood flow metabolism patterns can predict the postrevascularization outcome in global LV function.

Initial semiquantitative studies demonstrated some correlation between the extent of the blood-flow metabolism mismatch and the postrevascularization gain in LVEF.[191] Patients with blood-flow metabolism mismatches that occupied at least two or more of a total of seven myocardial segments revealed a statistically significant increase in the LVEF following coronary bypass grafting.[191] No such im-

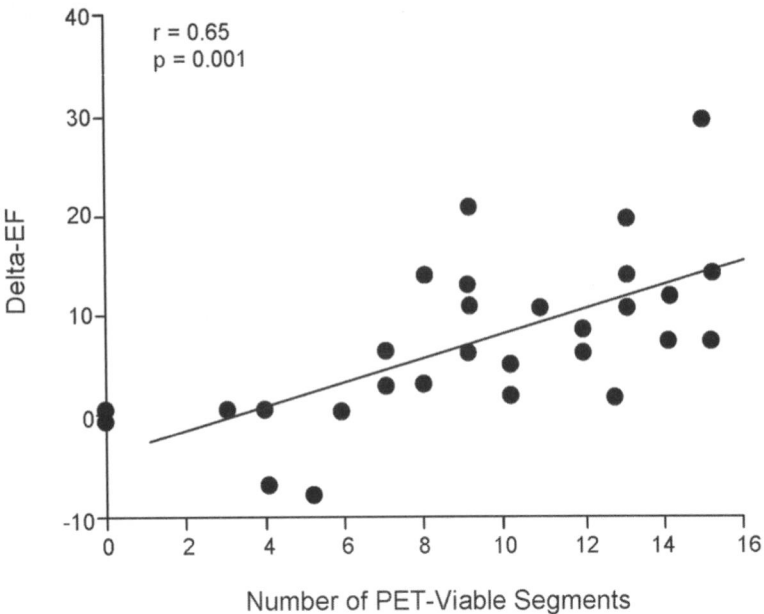

FIGURE 23–23. Postrevascularization improvement in left ventricular ejection fraction (LVEF) as a function of the number of viable myocardial segments as determined by positron emission tomography (PET). *Source: Reproduced with permission Pagano, Townend, Littler, et al.[263]*

provement was observed in patients with only one mismatch segment or with only matches. Subsequent studies confirmed these initial observations and reported significant gains in LV function in patients with blood-flow metabolism mismatches as compared to no improvement in those patients without metabolic evidence of viability.[216,217,220,222,236,238,241,243,251–262] Several investigations report statistically significant correlations between the percentage of the LV with a blood-flow metabolism mismatch and the postrevascularization increase in the LVEF. Accordingly, the extent of a blood-flow metabolism mismatch contains predictive value on the postsurgical gain in global LV performance (Fig. 23–23).[260,263,264] A mismatch of at least 20 to 25 percent of the LV myocardium appears necessary for achieving a significant postrevascularization gain in LVEF (≥ 5 percent).

Some investigations fail to report a significant postrevascularization improvement in the LVEF at rest, despite the presence of "blood flow metabolism mismatches." It appears however that this difference is related to a laboratory-unique image and analysis approach.[251] MBF is evaluated with [82]rubidium at rest and during pharmacologic stress. The distribution of MBF during stress is compared to the myocardial glucose uptake at rest. The approach therefore identifies both stress-induced ischemia and "viable myocardium" at rest. Hence, blood flow and, possibly, wall motion at rest can be normal in some patients so that revascularization predominantly improves the capacity of the LV to more appropriately respond to exercise [251] and thus to improve the quality of life even though no significant correlations between mismatch size and changes in congestive heart failure (CHF) functional class were observed.[264,265] The magnitude of an improvement in LV function following surgical revascularization depends further on the fraction of irreversibly injured myocardium or scar tissue. In evaluating the outcome of LV function following coronary artery bypass grafting in 82 patients with a LVEF of <35 percent, the fraction of scar as identified at baseline by PET ^{18}F-FDG and by PET ^{13}N-ammonia or SPECT ^{99m}Tc-tetrofosmin rest-perfusion imaging was

found to be an independent predictor of a change in the LVEF.[266]

An improvement in regional and especially global LV function may not occur immediately but slowly although progressively following revascularization.[267] Clinical observations suggest a correlation between severity of the mismatch and the rate and completeness of recovery of contractile function. Wall motion recovered faster and more completely in segments with normal blood flow as compared to segments with reduced flow and possibly, more severe structural alterations.[225] The slow recovery of contractile function can be related to rebuilding of the contractile machinery.[244] Finally, in addition to a slow recovery of contractile function in reversibly dysfunctional myocardium other studies describe an associated decline in end-diastolic and end-systolic volumes suggesting the possibility of a reversal of LV remodeling.[268, 269]

Effect on Congestive Heart Failure–Related Symptoms

A related question is whether such functional improvement is also associated with relief or amelioration of CHF symptoms. Several retrospective studies do in fact indicate such possible symptomatic improvement.[270,271]

The amount of viable myocardium as determined by perfusion and ^{18}F-FDG imaging with PET contains information on the magnitude of the postrevascularization improvement in CHF symptoms (Fig. 23–24).[272,273] As seen in Fig. 23–23, there was a statistically significant correlation between the improvement in functional status and the anatomic extent of the blood-flow metabolism mismatch.

Impact on Long-Term Survival

Several studies examined the long-term fate of patients after being evaluated for MBF and metabolism with PET.[262,270,271,274–276] These studies presented compelling evidence for the notion of an increased incidence of cardiac events in patients with blood-flow metabolism mismatches and on medical treatment. They also implied that revascularization of blood flow metabolism mismatches might avert future nonfatal and fatal cardiac events.

Despite this general agreement, important differences emerged from these studies. One study in 129 chronic CAD patients followed clinically for an average time period of 17 ± 19 months found the presence of mismatches in the absence of revascularization to be independent predictors of the 17 nonfatal ischemic events.[275] In another investigation in patients with more homogeneously depressed LV function, the predictive value of a low ejection fraction applied equally to all groups.[271] As shown in Fig. 23–25, the cumulative long-term survival was lowest in the patient subgroup with blood-flow metabolism mismatches who were on medical treatment. LVEF was without significant predictive value, whereas by Cox Model analysis, the extent of a mismatch had a significant negative effect on survival ($p < 0.02$), and revascularization of mismatch patients had a significant positive effect on survival ($p < 0.04$).[270,271] Among the patient groups with and without mismatches, the subgroup of patients with mismatches demon-

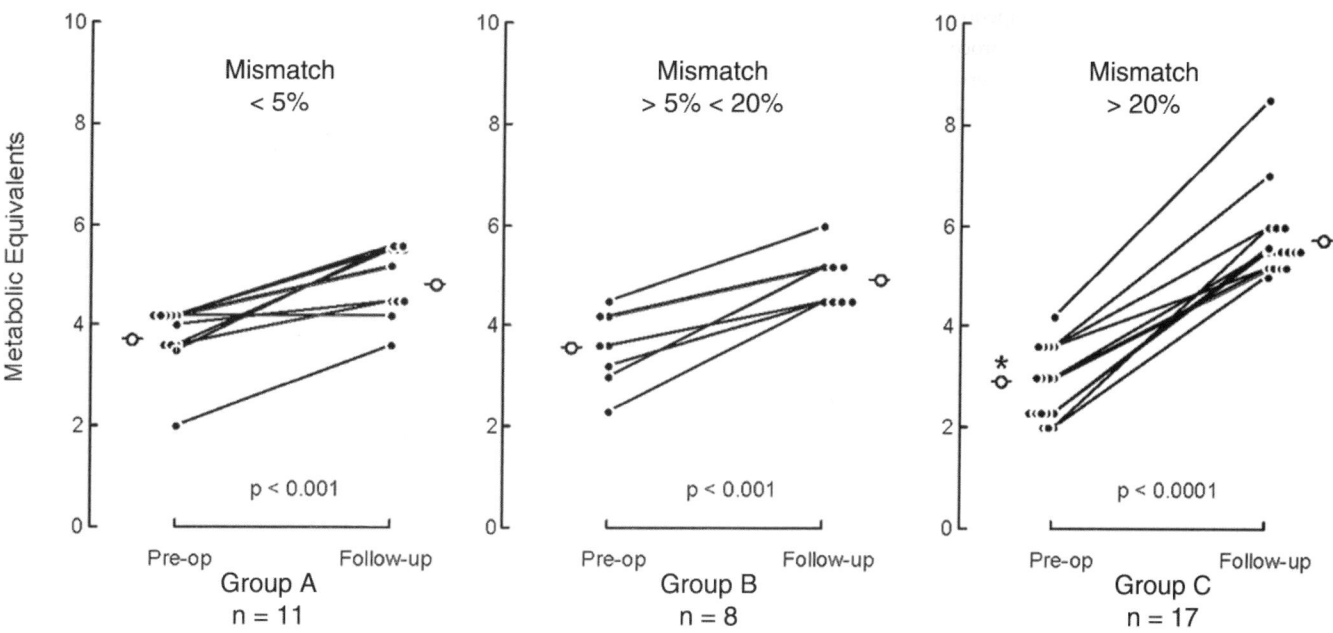

FIGURE 23–24. Correlation between extent of blood-flow metabolism mismatch and postsurgical improvement in physical activity as defined on a specific activity scale (SAS) and expressed in metabolic units (METS). *Source: Reproduced with permission from Di Carli, Asgarzadie, Schelbert, et al.[272]*

strated a 33 percent incidence of cardiac death during the 12-month followup period as compared to an only 4 percent mortality in patients with mismatches undergoing revascularization.

Assessment of Perioperative Risk

Critical for planning surgical revascularization of patients with ischemic cardiomyopathy is the high perioperative mortality and morbidity. This then raises the question whether imaging of blood flow and glucose metabolism with PET can contribute to predicting the surgical risk. Two investigations have explored the contribution of PET to the surgical risk assessment.[255,277] Although these reports include relatively few patients or are retrospective, further confirmation of such short-term benefits seems warranted.

If confirmed, PET evaluations of patients with ischemic cardiomyopathies would then offer important and possibly critical prognostic information on the immediate and long-term risks of cardiovascular surgery in patients with severe ischemic cardiomyopathy.

In summary, these observations imply that the presence of blood-flow metabolism mismatches identify patients who are at high risk for a nonfatal cardiac event and, in instances of severely depressed LV function, for sudden cardiac death. The observations further suggest that revascularization can significantly lower the cardiac risk and improve long-term survival. If large enough, a mismatch further contains predictive information on the postrevascularization improvement in CHF-related symptoms and further, on the outcome in global LV function. Blood-flow metabolism imaging therefore can decisively impact the risk to benefit ratio of surgical revascularization

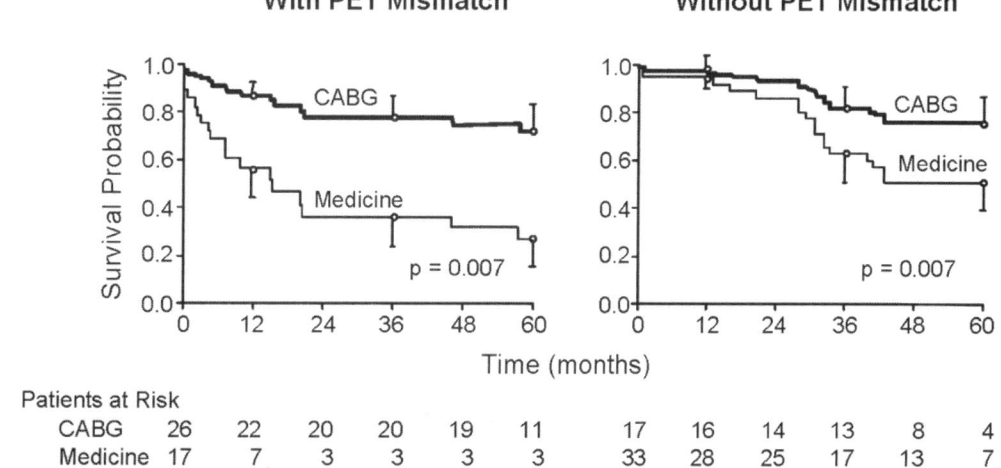

Patients at Risk											
CABG	26	22	20	20	19	11	17	16	14	13	8	4
Medicine	17	7	3	3	3	3	33	28	25	17	13	7

FIGURE 23–25. Estimated survival probabilities by Kaplan-Meier analysis for patients with left ventricular (LV) function treated medically (medicine) and with surgical revascularization (coronary artery bypass graft [CABG]) based on the absence or presence of viability as determined by positron emission tomography (PET) blood flow-metabolism imaging. *Source: Reproduced with permission from Di Carli, Maddahi, Rokhsar, et al.[274]*

and thus more generally affect therapeutic strategies. The absence of viability can affirm the decision to proceed with medical management or cardiac transplantation. Conversely, in the presence of large amounts of viable myocardium, interventional revascularization represents a true and effective alternative. In fact, the prevalence of substantial amounts of reversibly dysfunctional myocardium is substantial. A survey of 283 patients with ischemic cardiomyopathy revealed a 55 percent prevalence of blood flow and glucose metabolism mismatches.[278] In approximately half of the patients with mismatches, the mismatch extent involved 25 percent or more of the LV myocardium, which is predictive of significant gains in LV function and clinical symptoms after revascularization. Although considered a possible substrate of potential lethal arrhythmias, small-perfusion metabolism mismatches have been found not to be associated with an increased long-term cardiac morbidity and mortality.[279] In the setting of ischemic cardiomyopathy, inclusion of PET in the diagnostic algorithm can be cost effective and, at the same time, cost saving.[280,281] Clinical criteria for deciding on coronary artery bypass grafting in patients with ischemic cardiomyopathy have already been developed.[282] In addition to the diastolic dimension, the LVEF and suitable target vessels the criteria include the presence of viable myocardium affecting at least 15 to 20 percent of the LV myocardium.

SUMMARY AND CONCLUSIONS

Imaging with positron emitting tracers has provided novel and important information on the cardiovascular physiology and, specifically, on functional alterations of the human coronary circulation associated with evolving or established CAD as well as on consequences of severe and endstage CAD, especially in patients with ischemic cardiomyopathy. Observations with PET have raised numerous mechanistic questions in regard to hibernation and stunning. At the same time, assessment of these entities in the clinical setting with radiotracers of blood flow and of glucose metabolism has emerged as a gold standard for determining myocardial viability. Other radiotracers again have remained in the domain of investigations and await clinical applications in the future. Importantly, instrumentation-related developments and wider availability of radiotracers of metabolism have rapidly expanded the clinical availability of imaging positron emitting radiotracers. This in turn has resulted in a rapid dissemination of this new technology into the clinical setting. Although the now more widespread use of positron imaging focuses mostly on diagnostic and management issues in oncology, it is likely to be associated with a greater use for cardiovascular diseases in the clinical setting.

REFERENCES

1. Iida H, Rhodes C, de Silva R, Yamamoto Y, Araujo L, Maseri A, et al. Myocardial tissue fraction—correction for partial volume effects and measure of tissue viability. *J Nucl Med.* 1991;32:2169–175.
2. Yamamoto Y, De Silva R, Rhodes C, Araujo L, Iida H, Rechavia E, et al. A new strategy for the assessment of viable myocardium and regional myocardial blood flow using ^{15}O-water and dynamic positron emission tomography. *Circulation.* 1992;86(1):167–178.
3. de Silva R, Yamamoto Y, Rhodes CG, Iida H, Nihoyannopoulos P, Davies GJ, et al. Preoperative prediction of the outcome of coronary revascularization using positron emission tomography. *Circulation.* 1992;86:1738–1742.
4. Iida H, Tamura Y, Kitamura K, Bloomfield PM, Eberl S, Ono Y. Histochemical correlates of (15)O-water-perfusable tissue fraction in experimental canine studies of old myocardial infarction. *J Nucl Med.* 2000;41(10):1737–1745.
5. Kim RJ, Wu E, Rafael A, Chen EL, Parker MA, Simonetti O, et al. The use of contrast-enhanced magnetic resonance imaging to identify reversible myocardial dysfunction. *N Engl J Med.* 2000;343(20):1445–1453.
6. Wagner A, Mahrholdt H, Holly TA, Elliott MD, Regenfus M, Parker M, et al. Contrast-enhanced MRI and routine single photon emission computed tomography (SPECT) perfusion imaging for detection of subendocardial myocardial infarcts: an imaging study. *Lancet.* 2003;361(9355):374–379.
7. Bax JJ, Fath-Ordoubadi F, Boersma E, Wijns W, Camici PG. Accuracy of PET in predicting functional recovery after revascularization in patients with chronic ischaemic dysfunction: head-to-head comparison between blood flow, glucose utilisation and water-perfusable tissue fraction. *Eur J Nucl Med. Mol Imaging* 2002;29(6):721–727.
8. Marinho N KB, Costa D, Lammertsma A, Ell P, Camici P. Pathophysiology of chronic left ventricular dysfunction. *Circulation.* 1996;93:737–744.
9. Bateman TM, Heller GV, McGhie AI, Friedman JD, Case JA, Bryngelson JR, et al. Diagnostic accuracy of rest/stress ECG-gated Rb-82 myocardial perfusion PET. comparison with ECG-gated Tc-99m sestamibi SPECT. *J Nucl Cardiol.* 2006;13(1):24–33.
10. Bergmann SR, Fox KA, Rand AL, McElvany KD, Welch MJ, Markham J, et al. Quantification of regional myocardial blood flow in vivo with H215O. *Circulation.* 1984;70(4):724–733.
11. Schelbert HR, Phelps ME, Huang SC, MacDonald NS, Hansen H, Selin C, Kuhl DE. N-13 ammonia as an indicator of myocardial blood flow. *Circulation.* 1981;63(6):1259–1272.
12. Goldstein RA, Mullani NA, Marani SK, Fisher DJ, Gould KL, O'Brien HA, Jr. Myocardial perfusion with rubidium-82. II. Effects of metabolic and pharmacologic interventions. *J Nucl Med.* 1983;24(10):907–915.
13. Madar I, Ravert HT, Du Y, Hilton J, Volokh L, Dannals RF, et al. Characterization of uptake of the new PET imaging compound 18F-fluorobenzyl triphenyl phosphonium in dog myocardium. *J Nucl Med.* 2006;47(8):1359–1366.
14. Bergmann SR, Herrero P, Markham J, Weinheimer CJ, Walsh MN. Noninvasive quantitation of myocardial blood flow in human subjects with oxygen-15-labeled water and positron emission tomography. *J Am Coll Cardiol.* 1989;14(3):639–652.
15. Araujo L, Lammertsma A, Rhodes C, McFalls E, Iida H, Rechavia E, et al. Noninvasive quantification of regional myocardial blood flow in coronary artery disease with oxygen-15-labeled carbon dioxide inhalation and positron emission tomography. *Circulation.* 1991;83:875–885.
16. Krivokapich J, Smith GT, Huang SC, Hoffman EJ, Ratib O, Phelps ME, et al. ^{13}N ammonia myocardial imaging at rest and with exercise in normal volunteers. Quantification of absolute myocardial perfusion with dynamic positron emission tomography [see comments]. *Circulation.* 1989;80(5):1328–1337.
17. Hutchins GD, Schwaiger M, Rosenspire KC, Krivokapich J, Schelbert H, Kuhl DE. Noninvasive quantification of regional blood flow in the human heart using N-13 ammonia and dynamic positron emission tomographic imaging. *J Am Coll Cardiol.* 1990;15(5):1032–1042.
18. Chan SY, Brunken RC, Czernin J, Porenta G, Kuhle W, Krivokapich J, et al. Comparison of maximal myocardial blood flow during adenosine infusion with that of intravenous dipyridamole in normal men. *J Am Coll Cardiol.* 1992;20(4):979–985.
19. Bellina CR, Parodi O, Camici P, Salvadori PA, Taddei L, Fusani L, et al. Simultaneous in vitro and in vivo validation of nitrogen-13-ammonia for the assessment of regional myocardial blood flow. *J Nucl Med.* 1990;31(8):1335–1343.
20. Nitzsche EU, Choi Y, Czernin J, Hoh CK, Huang SC, Schelbert HR. Noninvasive quantification of myocardial blood flow in humans. A direct comparison of the [^{13}N]ammonia and the [^{15}O]water techniques. *Circulation.* 1996;93(11):2000–2006.
21. deKemp RA, Ruddy TD, Hewitt T, Dalipaj MM, Beanlands RS. Detection of serial changes in absolute myocardial perfusion with 82Rb PET. *J Nucl Med.* 2000;41(8):1426–1435.
22. Chow BJ, Ruddy TD, Dalipaj MM, de Kemp RA, Nadeau C, Ukkonen H, et al. Feasibility of exercise rubidium-82 positron emission tomography myocardial perfusion imaging. *J Am Coll Cardiol.* 2003;41(6 suppl B):428.
23. El Fakhri G, Sitek A, Guerin B, Kijewski MF, Di Carli MF, Moore SC. Quantitative dynamic cardiac 82Rb PET using generalized factor and compartment analyses. *J Nucl Med.* 2005;46(8):1264–1271.
24. Holmberg S, Serzysko W, Varnauskas E. Coronary circulation during heavy exercise in control subjects and patients with coronary heart disease. *Acta Med Scand.* 1971;190:465–480.

25. Brunken R CJ, Chan S, Chan A, Müller P, Schelbert H. Can the myocardial blood flow response to pharmacologic vasodilation be predicted by systemic hemodynamic changes? *J Am Coll Cardiol.* 1993;21(57A).

26. Duvernoy CS, Meyer C, Seifert-Klauss V, Dayanikli F, Matsunari I, Rattenhuber J, et al. Gender differences in myocardial blood flow dynamics: lipid profile and hemodynamic effects. *J Am Coll Cardiol.* 1999;33(2):463–470.

27. Nagamachi S, Czernin J, Kim AS, Sun KT, Böttcher M, Phelps ME, et al. Reproducibility of measurements of regional resting and hyperemic myocardial blood flow assessed with PET. *J Nucl Med.* 1996;37(10):1626–1631.

28. Sawada S, Muzik O, Beanlands RS, Wolfe E, Hutchins GD, Schwaiger M. Interobserver and interstudy variability of myocardial blood flow and flow-reserve measurements with nitrogen 13 ammonia-labeled positron emission tomography. *J Nucl Cardiol.* 1995;2(5):413–422.

29. Kaufmann PA, Gnecchi-Ruscone T, Yap JT, Rimoldi O, Camici PG. Assessment of the reproducibility of baseline and hyperemic myocardial blood flow measurements with 15O-labeled water and PET. *J Nucl Med.* 1999;40(11):1848–1856.

30. Wyss CA KP, Mikolajczyk K, Burger C, Von Schulthess GK, Kaufmann PA. Bicycle exercise stress in PET for assessment of coronary flow reserve: repeatability and comparison with adenosine stress. *J Nucl Med.* 2003;44:146–154.

31. Kuhle WG, Porenta G, Huang SC, Buxton D, Gambhir SS, Hansen H, et al. Quantification of regional myocardial blood flow using ¹³N-ammonia and reoriented dynamic positron emission tomographic imaging. *Circulation.* 1992;86(3):1004–1017.

32. Bol A, Melin JA, Vanoverschelde JL, Baudhuin T, Vogelaers D, De Pauw M, et al. Direct comparison of [¹³N]ammonia and [¹⁵O]water estimates of perfusion with quantification of regional myocardial blood flow by microspheres. *Circulation.* 1993;87(2):512–525.

33. Muzik O, Beanlands RS, Hutchins GD, Mangner TJ, Nguyen N, Schwaiger M. Validation of nitrogen-13-ammonia tracer kinetic model for quantification of myocardial blood flow using PET. *J Nucl Med.* 1993;34(1):83–91.

34. Merlet P MB, Hittinger L, Valette H, Saal J, Bendriem B, Crozatier B, et al. Assessment of coronary reserve in man: comparison between positron emission tomography with oxygen-15-labeled water and intracoronary Doppler technique. *J Nucl Med.* 1993;34:1899–1904.

35. Chan SY, Kobashigawa J, Stevenson LW, Brownfield E, Brunken RC, Schelbert HR. Myocardial blood flow at rest and during pharmacological vasodilation in cardiac transplants during and after successful treatment of rejection. *Circulation.* 1994;90(1):204–212.

36. Czernin J, Sun K, Brunken R, Bottcher M, Phelps M, Schelbert H. Effect of acute and long-term smoking on myocardial blood flow and flow reserve. *Circulation.* 1995;91(12):2891–2897.

37. Buus NH, Bottcher M, Hermansen F, Sander M, Nielsen TT, Mulvany MJ. Influence of nitric oxide synthase and adrenergic inhibition on adenosine-induced myocardial hyperemia. *Circulation.* 2001;104(19):2305–2310.

38. Böttcher M, Czernin J, Sun KT, Phelps ME, Schelbert HR. Effect of caffeine on myocardial blood flow at rest and during pharmacological vasodilation. *J Nucl Med.* 1995;36(11):2016–2021.

39. Czernin J, Auerbach M, Sun KT, Phelps M, Schelbert HR. Effects of modified pharmacologic stress approaches on hyperemic myocardial blood flow. *J Nucl Med.* 1995;36(4):575–580.

40. Czernin J, Müller P, Chan S, Brunken RC, Porenta G, Krivokapich J, et al. Influence of age and hemodynamics on myocardial blood flow and flow reserve. *Circulation.* 1993;88(1):62–69.

41. Senneff MJ, Geltman EM, Bergmann SR. Noninvasive delineation of the effects of moderate aging on myocardial perfusion [published erratum appears in *J Nucl Med.* 1992 Feb;33(2):201] [see comments]. *J Nucl Med.* 1991;32(11):2037–2042.

42. Uren NG, Camici PG, Melin JA, Bol A, de Bruyne B, Radvan J, et al. Effect of aging on myocardial perfusion reserve. *J Nucl Med.* 1995;36(11):2032–2036.

43. Raitakari OT, Toikka JO, Laine H, Ahotupa M, Iida H, Viikari JS, et al. Reduced myocardial flow reserve relates to increased carotid intima-media thickness in healthy young men. *Atherosclerosis.* 2001;156(2):469–475.

44. Nienaber CA, Gambhir SS, Mody FV, Ratib O, Huang SC, Phelps ME, et al. Regional myocardial blood flow and glucose utilization in symptomatic patients with hypertrophic cardiomyopathy. *Circulation.* 1993;87(5):1580–1590.

45. Krivokapich J, Huang SC, Schelbert HR. Assessment of the effects of dobutamine on myocardial blood flow and oxidative metabolism in normal human subjects using nitrogen-13 ammonia and carbon-11 acetate. *Am J Cardiol.* 1993;71(15):1351–1356.

46. Choi Y, Huang SC, Hawkins RA, Kuhle WG, Dahlbom M, Hoh CK, et al. A simplified method for quantification of myocardial blood flow using nitro-gen-13-ammonia and dynamic PET [see comments]. *J Nucl Med.* 1993;34(3):488–497.

47. Choi Y, Hawkins RA, Huang SC, Gambhir SS, Brunken RC, Phelps ME, et al. Parametric images of myocardial metabolic rate of glucose generated from dynamic cardiac PET and 2-[18F]fluoro-2-deoxy-d-glucose studies. *J Nucl Med.* 1991;32(4):733–738.

48. Tadamura E, Iida H, Matsumoto K, Mamede M, Kubo S, Toyoda H, et al. Comparison of myocardial blood flow during dobutamine-atropine infusion with that after dipyridamole administration in normal men. *J Am Coll Cardiol.* 2001;37(1):130–136.

49. Opie LH. Metabolism of the heart in health and disease. I. *Am Heart J.* 1968;76(5):685–698.

50. Liedtke AJ. Alterations of carbohydrate and lipid metabolism in the acutely ischemic heart. *Prog Cardiovasc Dis.* 1981;23(5):321–336.

51. Bing RJ. The metabolism of the heart. *Harvey Lecture Series.* New York: Academic Press; 1954:27–70.

52. Keul J, Doll E, Steim H, Fleer U, Reindell H. Über den Stoffwechsel des menschlichen Herzens. III. Der oxidative Stoffwechsel des menschlichen Herzens unter verschiedened Arbeitsbedingungen II. *Pflugers Arch Gesamte Physiol Menschen Tiere.* 1965;282:43–53.

53. Keul J, Doll E, Steim H, Homburger H, Kern H, Reindell H. Uber den Stoffwechsel des menschlichen Herzens. I. Substratversorgung des gesunden Herzens in Ruhe, während und nach körperlicher Arbeit. *Pflugers Arch Gesamte Physiol Menschen Tiere.* 1965;282:1–27.

54. Taegtmeyer H. Myocardial metabolism. In: Phelps M, Mazziotta J, Schelbert H, eds. *Positron Emission Tomography and Autoradiography: Principles and Applications for the Brain and Heart.* New York: Raven Press; 1986:149–195.

55. Sokoloff L, Reivich M, Kennedy C, Des Rosiers MH, Patlak CS, Pettigrew KD, et al. The [14C]-deoxyglucose method for the measurement of local cerebral glucose utilization: theory, procedure and normal values in the conscious and anesthetized albino rat. *J Neurochem.* 1977;28:897–916.

56. Ratib O, Phelps ME, Huang SC, Henze E, Selin CE, Schelbert HR. Positron tomography with deoxyglucose for estimating local myocardial glucose metabolism. *J Nucl Med.* 1982;23(7):577–586.

57. Gambhir SS, Schwaiger M, Huang SC, Krivokapich J, Schelbert HR, Nienaber CA, et al. Simple noninvasive quantification method for measuring myocardial glucose utilization in humans employing positron emission tomography and fluorine-18 deoxyglucose. *J Nucl Med.* 1989;30(3):359–366.

58. Hicks R, von Dahl J, Lee K, Herman W, Kalff V, Schwaiger M. Insulin-glucose clamp for standardization of metabolic conditions during F-18 fluoro-deoxyglucose PET imaging. *J Am Coll Cardiol.* 1991;17(2):381A.

59. vom Dahl J, Hicks R, Lee K, Eitzman D, Al-Aouar Z, Schwaiger M. Positron emission tomography myocardial viability studies in patients with diabetes mellitus. *J Am Coll Cardiol.* 1991;17(2):121A.

60. Knuuti M, Nuutila P, Ruotsalainen U, Saraste M, Härkönen R, Ahonen A, et al. Euglycemic hyperinsulinemic clamp and oral glucose load in stimulating myocardial glucose utilization during positron emission tomography. *J Nucl Med.* 1992;33:1255–1262.

61. Hariharan R, Bray M, Ganim R, Doenst T, Goodwin GW, Taegtmeyer H. Fundamental limitations of [F-18]2-deoxy-2-fluoro-D-glucose for assessing myocardial glucose uptake. *Circulation.* 1995;V91(N9):2435–2444.

62. Doenst T, Taegtmeyer H. Complexities underlying the quantitative determination of myocardial glucose uptake with 2-deoxyglucose. *J Mol Cell Cardiol.* 1998;V30(N8):1595–1604.

63. Depre C, Vanoverschelde JL, Taegtmeyer H. Glucose for the heart. *Circulation.* 1999;99(4):578–588.

64. Botker HE, Goodwin GW, Holden JE, Doenst T, Gjedde A, Taegtmeyer H. Myocardial glucose uptake measured with fluorodeoxyglucose: a prospect method to account for variable lumped constants. *J Nucl Med.* 1999;V40(N7):1186–1196.

65. Peterson LR, Herrero P, Schechtman KB, Racette SB, Waggoner AD, Kisrieva-Ware Z, et al. Effect of obesity and insulin resistance on myocardial substrate metabolism and efficiency in young women. *Circulation.* 2004;109(18):2191–2196.

66. de las Fuentes L, Herrero P, Peterson LR, Kelly DP, Gropler RJ, Davila-Roman VG. Myocardial fatty acid metabolism: independent predictor of left ventricular mass in hypertensive heart disease. *Hypertension.* 2003;41(1):83–87.

67. Davila-Roman VG, Vedala G, Herrero P, de las Fuentes L, Rogers JG, Kelly DP, et al. Altered myocardial fatty acid and glucose metabolism in idiopathic dilated cardiomyopathy. *J Am Coll Cardiol.* 2002;40(2):271–277.

68. Peterson LR, Eyster D, Davila-Roman VG, Stephens AL, Schechtman KB, Herrero P, et al. Short-term oral estrogen replacement therapy does not aug-

ment endothelium-independent myocardial perfusion in postmenopausal women. *Am Heart J.* 2001;142(4):641–647.

69. Schelbert HR, Henze E, Schon HR, Keen R, Hansen H, Selin C, et al. C-11 palmitate for the noninvasive evaluation of regional myocardial fatty acid metabolism with positron computed tomography. III. In vivo demonstration of the effects of substrate availability on myocardial metabolism. *Am Heart J.* 1983;105(3):492–504.

70. Schön HR, Schelbert HR, Najafi A, Hansen H, Huang H, Barrio J, et al. C-11 labeled palmitic acid for the noninvasive evaluation of regional myocardial fatty acid metabolism with positron-computed tomography. II. Kinetics of C- 11 palmitic acid in acutely ischemic myocardium. *Am Heart J.* 1982;103(4 pt 1):548–561.

71. Fox KA, Abendschein DR, Ambos HD, Sobel BE, Bergmann SR. Efflux of metabolized and nonmetabolized fatty acid from canine myocardium. Implications for quantifying myocardial metabolism tomographically. *Circ Res.* 1985;57(2):232–243.

72. Mäki MT, Haaparanta M, Nuutila P, Oikonen V, Luotolahti M, Eskola O, et al. Free fatty acid uptake in the myocardium and skeletal muscle using fluorine-18-fluoro-6-thia-heptadecanoic acid. *J Nucl Med.* 1998;39(8):1320–1327.

73. Stone CK, Pooley RA, DeGrado TR, Renstrom B, Nickles RJ, Nellis SH, et al. Myocardial uptake of the fatty acid analog 14-fluorine-18-fluoro-6-thia-heptadecanoic acid in comparison to beta-oxidation rates by tritiated palmitate. *J Nucl Med.* 1998;39(10):1690–1696.

74. Takala TO, Nuutila P, Pulkki K, Oikonen V, Gronroos T, Savunen T, et al. 14(R,S)-[^{18}F]Fluoro-6-thia-heptadecanoic acid as a tracer of free fatty acid uptake and oxidation in myocardium and skeletal muscle. *Eur J Nucl Med Mol Imaging.* 2002;29(12):1617–1622.

75. Schelbert HR, Henze E, Keen R, Schon HR, Hansen H, Selin C, et al. C-11 palmitate for the noninvasive evaluation of regional myocardial fatty acid metabolism with positron-computed tomography. IV. In vivo evaluation of acute demand-induced ischemia in dogs. *Am Heart J.* 1983;106(4 pt 1):736–750.

76. Choi Y, Brunken RC, Hawkins RA, Huang SC, Buxton DB, Hoh CK, et al. Factors affecting myocardial 2-[F-18]fluoro-2-deoxy-D-glucose uptake in positron emission tomography studies of normal humans. *European J Nucl Med.* 1993;20(4):308–318.

77. Iida H, Rhodes CG, Araujo LI, Yamamoto Y, de Silva R, Maseri A, et al. Noninvasive quantification of regional myocardial metabolic rate for oxygen by use of 15O2 inhalation and positron emission tomography. Theory, error analysis, and application in humans. *Circulation.* 1996;94(4):792–807.

78. Yamamoto Y, de Silva R, Rhodes CG, Iida H, Lammertsma AA, Jones T, et al. Noninvasive quantification of regional myocardial metabolic rate of oxygen by 15O2 inhalation and positron emission tomography. Experimental validation. *Circulation.* 1996;94(4):808–816.

79. Buxton DB, Nienaber CA, Luxen A, Ratib O, Hansen H, Phelps ME, et al. Noninvasive quantitation of regional myocardial oxygen consumption in vivo with [1-11C]acetate and dynamic positron emission tomography. *Circulation.* 1989;79(1):134–142.

80. Armbrecht JJ, Buxton DB, Brunken RC, Phelps ME, Schelbert HR. Regional myocardial oxygen consumption determined noninvasively in humans with [1-11C]acetate and dynamic positron tomography. *Circulation.* 1989;80(4):863–872.

81. Henes CG, Bergmann SR, Walsh MN, Sobel BE, Geltman EM. Assessment of myocardial oxidative metabolic reserve with positron emission tomography and carbon-11 acetate. *J Nucl Med.* 1989;30(9):1489–1499.

82. Ng CK, Huang SC, Schelbert HR, Buxton DB. Validation of a model for [1-11C]acetate as a tracer of cardiac oxidative metabolism. *Am J Physiol.* 1994;266(4 pt 2):H1304–1315.

83. Sun KT, Chen K, Huang SC, Buxton DB, Hansen HW, Kim AS, et al. Compartment model for measuring myocardial oxygen consumption using [1-11C]acetate. *J Nucl Med.* 1997;38(3):459–466.

84. Sun KT, Yeatman LA, Buxton DB, Chen K, Johnson JA, Huang SC, et al. Simultaneous measurement of myocardial oxygen consumption and blood flow using [1-carbon-11]acetate. *J Nucl Med.* 1998;39(2):272–280.

85. Ukkonen H, Knuuti J, Katoh C, Iida H, Sipila H, Lehikoinen P, et al. Use of [11C]acetate and [15O]O2 PET for the assessment of myocardial oxygen utilization in patients with chronic myocardial infarction. *Eur J Nucl Med.* 2001;28(3):334–339.

86. Klocke FJ, Baird MG, Lorell BH, Bateman TM, Messer JV, Berman DS, et al. ACC/AHA/ASNC guidelines for the clinical use of cardiac radionuclide imaging—executive summary: a report of the American College of Cardiology/American Heart Association Task Force on Practice Guidelines (ACC/ AHA/ASNC Committee to Revise the 1995 Guidelines for the Clinical Use of Cardiac Radionuclide Imaging). *J Am Coll Cardiol.* 2003;42(7):1318–1333.

87. Schelbert HR, Wisenberg G, Phelps ME, Gould KL, Henze E, Hoffman EJ, et al. Noninvasive assessment of coronary stenoses by myocardial imaging during pharmacologic coronary vasodilation. VI. Detection of coronary artery disease in human beings with intravenous N-13 ammonia and positron computed tomography. *Am J Cardiol.* 1982;49(5):1197–1207.

88. Tamaki N, Yonekura Y, Senda M, Yamashita K, Koide H, Saji H, et al. Value and limitation of stress thallium-201 single photon emission computed tomography: comparison with nitrogen-13 ammonia positron tomography. *J Nucl Med.* 1988;29(7):1181–1188.

89. Demer LL, Gould KL, Goldstein RA, Kirkeeide RL, Mullani NA, Smalling RW, et al. Assessment of coronary artery disease severity by positron emission tomography. Comparison with quantitative arteriography in 193 patients. *Circulation.* 1989;79:825–835.

90. Go RT, Marwick TH, MacIntyre WJ, Saha GB, Neumann DR, Underwood DA, et al. A prospective comparison of rubidium-82 PET and thallium-201 SPECT myocardial perfusion imaging utilizing a single dipyridamole stress in the diagnosis of coronary artery disease [see comments]. *J Nucl Med.* 1990;31(12):1899–1905.

91. Stewart R, Schwaiger M, Molina E, Popma J, Gacioch G, Kalus M, et al. Comparison of rubidium-82 positron emission tomography and thallium-201 SPECT imaging for detection of coronary artery disease. *Am J Cardiol.* 1991;67:1303–1310.

92. Simone G, Mullani N, Page D, Anderson B Sr. Utilization statistics and diagnostic accuracy of a nonhospital-based positron emission tomography center for the detection of coronary artery disease using rubidium-82. *Am J Physiol Imaging.* 1992;7:203–209.

93. Williams B, Millani N, Jansen D, Anderson B. A retrospective study of the diagnostic accuracy of a community hospital-based PET center for the detection of coronary artery disease using rubidium-82. *J Nucl Med.* 1994;35:1586–1592.

94. Gould KL, Goldstein RA, Mullani NA, Kirkeeide RL, Wong WH, Tewson TJ, et al. Noninvasive assessment of coronary stenoses by myocardial perfusion imaging during pharmacologic coronary vasodilation. VIII. Clinical feasibility of positron cardiac imaging without a cyclotron using generator-produced rubidium-82. *J Am Coll Cardiol.* 1986;7:775–789.

95. Zijlstra F, Fioretti P, Reiber JH, Serruys PW. Which cineangiographically assessed anatomic variable correlates best with functional measurements of stenosis severity? A comparison of quantitative analysis of the coronary cineangiogram with measured coronary flow reserve and exercise/redistribution thallium-201 scintigraphy. *J Am Coll Cardiol.* 1988;12(3):686–691.

96. Parkash R, deKemp RA, Ruddy TD, Kitsikis A, Hart R, Beauchesne L, et al. Potential utility of rubidium 82 PET quantification in patients with 3-vessel coronary artery disease. *J Nucl Cardiol.* 2004;11(4):440–449.

97. Dorbala S, Limaye A, Sampson U, et al. Normal and abnormal responses of left ventricular ejection fraction during vasodilator stress rubidium 82 positron emission tomography (PET/CT). *J Nucl Med.* 2005;46:268P.

98. Dorbala S, Sampson U, Limaye A, et al. Diagnostic value of changes in left ventricular ejection fraction during peak vasodilator stress gated cardiac PET/CT: correlation with the extent of angiographic coronary artery disease. *Circulation.* 2005;112:II–365.

99. Merhige ME, Houston T, Shalton V, Kay J, Stern G, Oliverio J, et al. PET myocardial perfusion imaging reduces the cost of coronary disease management by eliminating unnecessary invasive diagnostic and therapeutic procedures. *Circulation.* 1999;100(suppl I):I–26.

100. Flamm SD, Khanna S, Dicarli M, Phelps M, Schelbert HR, Maddahi J. Prognostic significance of normal adenosine stress myocardial perfusion PET study in patients presenting with chest pain. *J Nucl Med.* 1994;35(5 suppl):60P.

101. Marwick TH, Shan K, Patel S, Go RT, Lauer MS. Incremental value of rubidium-82 positron emission tomography for prognostic assessment of known or suspected coronary artery disease. *Am J Cardiol.* 1997;80(7):865–870.

102. Marwick TH, Shan K, Go RT, MacIntyre WJ, Lauer MS. Use of positron emission tomography for prediction of perioperative and late cardiac events before vascular surgery. *Am Heart J.* 1995;130(6):1196–1202.

103. Yoshinaga K, Chow BJ, Williams K, Chen L, deKemp RA, Garrard L, et al. What is the prognostic value of myocardial perfusion imaging using rubidium-82 positron emission tomography? *J Am Coll Cardiol.* 2006;48(5):1029–1039.

104. Uren NG, Melin JA, De Bruyne B, Wijns W, Baudhuin T, et al. Relation between myocardial blood flow and the severity of coronary-artery stenosis. *N Engl J Med.* 1994;330(25):1782–1788.

105. Beanlands RS, Muzik O, Melon P, Sutor R, Sawada S, Muller D, et al. Non-invasive quantification of regional myocardial flow reserve in patients with coronary atherosclerosis using nitrogen-13 ammonia positron emission tomography. Determination of extent of altered vascular reactivity. *J Am Coll Cardiol.* 1995;26(6):1465–1475.

106. Di Carli M, Czernin J, Hoh CK, Gerbaudo VH, Brunken RC, Huang SC, et al. Relation among stenosis severity, myocardial blood flow, and flow reserve in patients with coronary artery disease. *Circulation.* 1995;91(7):1944–1951.

107. Krivokapich J, Czernin J, Schelbert HR. Dobutamine positron emission tomography: absolute quantitation of rest and dobutamine myocardial blood flow and correlation with cardiac work and percent diameter stenosis in patients with and without coronary artery disease. *J Am Coll Cardiol.* 1996;28(3):565–572.

108. Schwaiger M, Ziegler S, Nekolla SG. PET/CT: challenge for nuclear cardiology. *J Nucl Med.* 2005;46(10):1664–1678.

109. Leber AW, Knez A, von Ziegler F, Becker A, Nikolaou K, Paul S, et al. Quantification of obstructive and nonobstructive coronary lesions by 64-slice computed tomography: a comparative study with quantitative coronary angiography and intravascular ultrasound. *J Am Coll Cardiol.* 2005;46(1):147–154.

110. Leschka S, Alkadhi H, Plass A, Desbiolles L, Grunenfelder J, Marincek B, et al. Accuracy of MSCT coronary angiography with 64-slice technology: first experience. *Eur Heart J.* 2005;26(15):1482–1487.

111. Di Carli M, Dorbala S, Limaye A, et al. Clinical value of hybrid PET/CT cardiac imaging complementary roles of multi-detector CT coronary angiography and stress PET perfusion imaging (abstr) *J Am Coll Cardiol.* 2006;47:111 (abstract).

112. Hacker M, Jakobs T, Hack N, Nikolaou K, Becker C, von Ziegler F, et al. Sixty-four slice spiral CT angiography does not predict the functional relevance of coronary artery stenoses in patients with stable angina. *Eur J Nucl Med Mol Imaging.* 2007;34(1):4–10.

113. Hacker M, Jakobs T, Matthiesen F, Vollmar C, Nikolaou K, Becker C, et al. Comparison of spiral multidetector CT angiography and myocardial perfusion imaging in the noninvasive detection of functionally relevant coronary artery lesions: first clinical experiences. *J Nucl Med.* 2005;46(8):1294–1300.

114. Schuijf JD, Wijns W, Jukema JW, Atsma DE, de Roos A, Lamb HJ, et al. Relationship between noninvasive coronary angiography with multi-slice computed tomography and myocardial perfusion imaging. *J Am Coll Cardiol.* 2006;48(12):2508–2514.

115. Dayanikli F, Grambow D, Muzik O, Mosca L, Rubenfire M, Schwaiger M. Early detection of abnormal coronary flow reserve in asymptomatic men at high risk for coronary artery disease using positron emission tomography. *Circulation.* 1994;90(2):808–817.

116. Pitkänen OP, Nuutila P, Raitakari OT, Porkka K, Iida H, Nuotio I, et al. Coronary flow reserve in young men with familial combined hyperlipidemia. *Circulation.* 1999;99(13):1678–1684.

117. Pitkänen OP, Raitakari OT, Niinikoski H, Nuutila P, Iida H, Voipio-Pulkki LM, et al. Coronary flow reserve is impaired in young men with familial hypercholesterolemia. *J Am Coll Cardiol.* 1996;28(7):1705–1711.

118. Yokoyama I, Murakami T, Ohtake T, Momomura S, Nishikawa J, Sasaki Y, et al. Reduced coronary flow reserve in familial hypercholesterolemia. *J Nucl Med.* 1996;37(12):1937–1942.

119. Yokoyama I, Ohtake T, Momomura S, Nishikawa J, Sasaki Y, Omata M. Reduced coronary flow reserve in hypercholesterolemic patients without overt coronary stenosis. *Circulation.* 1996;94(12):3232–3238.

120. Di Carli MF, Bianco-Batlles D, Landa ME, Kazmers A, Groehn H, Muzik O, Grunberger G. Effects of autonomic neuropathy on coronary blood flow in patients with diabetes mellitus. *Circulation.* 1999;100(8):813–819.

121. Pitkänen OP, Nuutila P, Raitakari OT, Rönnemaa T, Koskinen PJ, Iida H, et al. Coronary flow reserve is reduced in young men with IDDM. *Diabetes.*1998;47(2):248–254.

122. Yokoyama I, Momomura S, Ohtake T, Yonekura K, Nishikawa J, Sasaki Y, et al. Reduced myocardial flow reserve in non-insulin-dependent diabetes mellitus [see comments]. *J Am Coll Cardiol.* 1997;30(6):1472–1477.

123. Yokoyama I, Ohtake T, Momomura S, Yonekura K, Woo-Soo S, Nishikawa J, et al. Hyperglycemia rather than insulin resistance is related to reduced coronary flow reserve in NIDDM. *Diabetes.* 1998;47(1):119-124.

124. Egashira K, Inou T, Hirooka Y, Yamada A, Urabe Y, Takeshita A. Evidence of impaired endothelium-dependent coronary vasodilatation in patients with angina pectoris and normal coronary angiograms [see comments]. *N Engl J Med.* 1993;328(23):1659–1664.

125. Zeiher AM, Drexler H, Wollschlager H, Just H. Modulation of coronary vasomotor tone in humans. Progressive endothelial dysfunction with differ-ent early stages of coronary atherosclerosis. *Circulation.* 1991;83(2):391–401.

126. Reddy K NR, Sheehan H, Hodgson JM. Evidence that selective endothelial dysfunction may occur in the absence of angiographic or ultrasound atherosclerosis in patients with risk factors for atherosclerosis. . *J Am Coll Cardiol.* 1994;23:833–843.

127. Bache RJ. Vasodilator reserve: a functional assessment of coronary health [editorial; comment]. *Circulation.* 1998;98(13):1257–1260.

128. Smits P, Williams S, Lipson D, Banitt P, Rongen G, Creager M. Endothelial release of nitric oxide contributes to the vasodilator effect of adenosine in humans. *Circulation.* 1995;92(8):2135–2141.

129. Nabel EG, Ganz P, Gordon JB, Alexander RW, Selwyn AP. Dilation of normal and constriction of atherosclerotic coronary arteries caused by the cold pressor test. *Circulation.* 1988;77(1):43–52.

130. Nabel EG, Selwyn AP, Ganz P. Large coronary arteries in humans are responsive to changing blood flow: an endothelium-dependent mechanism that fails in patients with atherosclerosis. *J Am Coll Cardiol.* 1990;16(2):349–356.

131. Zeiher AM, Drexler H. Coronary hemodynamic determinants of epicardial artery vasomotor responses during sympathetic stimulation in humans. *Basic Res Cardiol.* 1991;2006;86(suppl 2):203–213.

132. Schindler TH, Nitzsche EU, Olschewski M, Brink I, Mix M, Prior J, et al. PET-measured responses of MBF to cold pressor testing correlate with indices of coronary vasomotion on quantitative coronary angiography. *J Nucl Med.* 2004;45(3):419–428.

133. Campisi R, Czernin J, Schöder H, Sayre JW, Marengo FD, Phelps ME, et al. Effects of long-term smoking on myocardial blood flow, coronary vasomotion, and vasodilator capacity. *Circulation.* 1998;98(2):119–125.

134. Zeiher AM, Drexler H, Saurbier B, Just H. Endothelium-mediated coronary blood flow modulation in humans. Effects of age, atherosclerosis, hypercholesterolemia, and hypertension. *J Clin Invest.* 1993;92(2):652–662.

135. Nitenberg A, Ledoux S, Valensi P, Sachs R, Attali JR, Antony I. Impairment of coronary microvascular dilation in response to cold pressor–induced sympathetic stimulation in type 2 diabetic patients with abnormal stress thallium imaging. *Diabetes.* 2001;50(5):1180–1185.

136. Nitenberg A, Valensi P, Sachs R, Dali M, Aptecar E, Attali JR. Impairment of coronary vascular reserve and ACh-induced coronary vasodilation in diabetic patients with angiographically normal coronary arteries and normal left ventricular systolic function. *Diabetes.* 1993;42(7):1017–1025.

137. Di Carli MF, Tobes MC, Mangner T, Levine AB, Muzik O, Chakroborty P, et al. Effects of cardiac sympathetic innervation on coronary blood flow. *N Engl J Med.* 1997;336(17):1208–1215.

138. Pop-Busui R, Kirkwood I, Schmid H, Marinescu V, Schroeder J, Larkin D, et al. Sympathetic dysfunction in type 1 diabetes: association with impaired myocardial blood flow reserve and diastolic dysfunction. *J Am Coll Cardiol.* 2004;44(12):2368–2374.

139. Schindler TH, Hornig B, Buser PT, Olschewski M, Magosaki N, Pfisterer M, et al. Prognostic value of abnormal vasoreactivity of epicardial coronary arteries to sympathetic stimulation in patients with normal coronary angiograms. *Arterioscler Thromb Vasc Biol.* 2003;23(3):495–501.

140. Campisi R, Nathan L, Pampaloni MH, Schoder H, Sayre JW, Chaudhuri G, et al. Noninvasive assessment of coronary microcirculatory function in postmenopausal women and effects of short-term and long-term estrogen administration. *Circulation.* 2002;105(4):425–430.

141. Schindler TH, Zhang X, Cadenas J, Sayre JW, Dahlbom M, Schelbert HR. Assessment of intra- and interobserver reproducibility of rest and cold-pressor-test stimulated myocardial blood flow with ^{13}N-ammonia and PET. *Eur J Nucl Med Mol Imaging.* 2007; ahead of print, available online only at http://www.springerlink.com.

142. Gould KL, Nakagawa Y, Nakagawa K, Sdringola S, Hess MJ, Haynie M, et al. Frequency and clinical implications of fluid dynamically significant diffuse coronary artery disease manifest as graded, longitudinal, base-to-apex myocardial perfusion abnormalities by noninvasive positron emission tomography. *Circulation.* 2000;101(16):1931–1939.

143. De Bruyne B HF, Pijls NH, Bartunek J, Bech JW, Heyndrickx GR, Gould KL, et al. Abnormal epicardial coronary resistance in patients with diffuse atherosclerosis but "Normal" coronary angiography. *Circulation.* 2001;104:2401–2406.

144. Hernandez-Pampaloni M, Keng FYY, Kudo T, Sayre JS, Schelbert HR. Abnormal longitudinal base to apex myocardial perfusion gradient by quantitative blood flow measurements in patients with coronary risk factors. *Circulation.* 2001;in press.

145. Schindler TH, Facta AD, Prior JO, Campisi R, Inubushi M, Kreissl MC, et al. PET-measured heterogeneity in longitudinal myocardial blood flow in response to sympathetic and pharmacologic stress as a non-invasive probe of

epicardial vasomotor dysfunction. *Eur J Nucl Med Mol Imaging.* 2006;33(10):1140–1149.

146. Tuzcu EM, Kapadia SR, Tutar E, Ziada KM, Hobbs RE, McCarthy PM, et al. High prevalence of coronary atherosclerosis in asymptomatic teenagers and young adults: evidence from intravascular ultrasound. *Circulation.* 2001;103(22):2705–2710.

147. Prior JO, Quinones MJ, Hernandez-Pampaloni M, Facta AD, Schindler TH, Sayre JW, et al. Coronary circulatory dysfunction in insulin resistance, impaired glucose tolerance, and type 2 diabetes mellitus. *Circulation.* 2005;111(18):2291–2298.

148. Prior JO, Schindler TH, Facta AD, Hernandez-Pampaloni M, Campisi R, Dahlbom M, et al. Determinants of myocardial blood flow response to cold pressor testing and pharmacologic vasodilation in healthy humans. *Eur J Nucl Med Mol Imaging.* 2007;34(1):20–27.

149. Halcox JP, Schenke WH, Zalos G, Mincemoyer R, Prasad A, Waclawiw MA, et al. Prognostic value of coronary vascular endothelial dysfunction. *Circulation.* 2002;106(6):653–658.

150. Schachinger V, Britten MB, Zeiher AM. Prognostic impact of coronary vasodilator dysfunction on adverse long-term outcome of coronary heart disease. *Circulation.* 2000;101(16):1899–1906.

151. Suwaidi JA, Hamasaki S, Higano ST, Nishimura RA, Holmes DR Jr, Lerman A. Long-term follow-up of patients with mild coronary artery disease and endothelial dysfunction. *Circulation.* 2000;101(9):948–954.

152. Czernin J, Barnard RJ, Sun KT, Krivokapich J, Nitzsche E, Dorsey D, et al. Effect of short-term cardiovascular conditioning and low-fat diet on myocardial blood flow and flow reserve. *Circulation.* 1995;92(2):197–204.

153. Gould KL. Reversal of coronary atherosclerosis. Clinical promise as the basis for noninvasive management of coronary artery disease. *Circulation.* 1994;90(3):1558-1571.

154. Gould KL, Ornish D, Scherwitz L, Brown S, Edens RP, Hess MJ, et al. Changes in myocardial perfusion abnormalities by positron emission tomography after long-term, intense risk factor modification [see comments]. *JAMA.* 1995;274(11):894–901.

155. Baller D, Notohamiprodjo G, Gleichmann U, Holzinger J, Weise R, Lehmann J. Improvement in coronary flow reserve determined by positron emission tomography after 6 months of cholesterol-lowering therapy in patients with early stages of coronary atherosclerosis. *Circulation.* 1999;99(22):2871–2875.

156. Guethlin M, Kasel AM, Coppenrath K, Ziegler S, Delius W, Schwaiger M. Delayed response of myocardial flow reserve to lipid-lowering therapy with fluvastatin. *Circulation.* 1999;99(4):475–481.

157. Huggins GS, Pasternak RC, Alpert NM, Fischman AJ, Gewirtz H. Effects of short-term treatment of hyperlipidemia on coronary vasodilator function and myocardial perfusion in regions having substantial impairment of baseline dilator reserve. *Circulation.* 1998;98(13):1291–1296.

158. Janatuinen T, Laaksonen R, Vesalainen R, Raitakari O, Lehtimaki T, Nuutila P, et al. Effect of lipid-lowering therapy with pravastatin on myocardial blood flow in young mildly hypercholesterolemic adults. *J Cardiovasc Pharmacol.* 2001;38(4):561–568.

159. Yokoyama I, Yonekura K, Inoue Y, Ohtomo K, Nagai R. Long-term effect of simvastatin on the improvement of impaired myocardial flow reserve in patients with familial hypercholesterolemia without gender variance. *J Nucl Cardiol.* 2001;8(4):445–451.

160. Yokoyama I, Yonekura K, Ohtake T, Yang W, Shin WS, Yamada N, et al. Coronary microangiopathy in type 2 diabetic patients: relation to glycemic control, sex, and microvascular angina rather than to coronary artery disease. *J Nucl Med.* 2000;41(6):978–985.

161. Schindler TH, Nitzsche EU, Munzel T, Olschewski M, Brink I, Jeserich M, et al. Coronary vasoregulation in patients with various risk factors in response to cold pressor testing: contrasting myocardial blood flow responses to short- and long-term vitamin C administration. *J Am Coll Cardiol.* 2003;42(5):814–822.

162. Quinones MJ, Hernandez-Pampaloni M, Schelbert H, Bulnes-Enriquez I, Jimenez X, Hernandez G, et al. Coronary vasomotor abnormalities in insulin-resistant individuals. *Ann Intern Med.* 2004;140(9):700–708.

163. Schindler TH, Facta AD, Prior JO, Cadenas J, Hsueh W, Quinones M, et al. Improvement of coronary vascular dysfunction in type 2 diabetic patients with euglycemic control. *Heart.* 2007;93(3):345–349.

164. Achenbach S. Computed tomography coronary angiography. *J Am Coll Cardiol.* 2006;48(10):1919–1928.

165. Fuster V, Fayad ZA, Moreno PR, Poon M, Corti R, Badimon JJ. Atherothrombosis and high-risk plaque: part II. Approaches by noninvasive computed tomographic/magnetic resonance imaging. *J Am Coll Cardiol.* 2005;46(7):1209–1218.

166. Kolodgie FD, Petrov A, Virmani R, Narula N, Verjans JW, Weber DK, et al. Targeting of apoptotic macrophages and experimental atheroma with radiolabeled annexin V. A technique with potential for noninvasive imaging of vulnerable plaque. *Circulation.* 2003;108(25):3134–3139.

167. Schafers M, Riemann B, Kopka K, Breyholz HJ, Wagner S, Schafers KP, et al. Scintigraphic imaging of matrix metalloproteinase activity in the arterial wall in vivo. *Circulation.* 2004;109(21):2554–2559.

168. Carrio I, Pieri PL, Narula J, Prat L, Riva P, Pedrini L, et al. Noninvasive localization of human atherosclerotic lesions with indium 111-labeled monoclonal Z2D3 antibody specific for proliferating smooth muscle cells. *J Nucl Cardiol.* 1998;5(6):551–557.

169. Johnson LL, Schofield LM, Weber DK, Kolodgie F, Virmani R, Khaw BA. Uptake of 111In-Z2D3 on SPECT imaging in a swine model of coronary stent restenosis correlated with cell proliferation. *J Nucl Med.* 2004;45(2):294–299.

170. Matter CM, Wyss MT, Meier P, Spath N, von Lukowicz T, Lohmann C, et al. 18F-choline images murine atherosclerotic plaques ex vivo. *Arterioscler Thromb Vasc Biol.* 2006;26(3):584–589.

171. Elmaleh DR, Fischman AJ, Tawakol A, Zhu A, Shoup TM, Hoffmann U, et al. Detection of inflamed atherosclerotic lesions with diadenosine-5',5'''-P1,P4-tetraphosphate (Ap4A) and positron-emission tomography. *Proc Natl Acad Sci U S A.* 2006;103(43):15992–15996.

172. Ogawa M, Ishino S, Mukai T, Asano D, Teramoto N, Watabe H, et al. (18)F-FDG accumulation in atherosclerotic plaques: immunohistochemical and PET imaging study. *J Nucl Med.* 2004;45(7):1245–1250.

173. Tawakol A, Migrino RQ, Hoffmann U, Abbara S, Houser S, Gewirtz H, et al. Noninvasive in vivo measurement of vascular inflammation with F-18 fluorodeoxyglucose positron emission tomography. *J Nucl Cardiol.* 2005;12(3):294–301.

174. Kubota R, Yamada S, Kubota K, Ishiwata K, Tamahashi N, Ido T. Intratumoral distribution of fluorine-18-fluorodeoxyglucose in vivo: high accumulation in macrophages and granulation tissues studied by microautoradiography. *J Nucl Med.* 1992;33(11):1972–1980.

175. Belhocine T, Blockmans D, Hustinx R, Vandevivere J, Mortelmans L. Imaging of large vessel vasculitis with (18)FDG PET. Illusion or reality? A critical review of the literature data. *Eur J Nucl Med Mol Imaging.* 2003;30(9):1305–1313.

176. Kobayashi Y, Ishii K, Oda K, Nariai T, Tanaka Y, Ishiwata K, et al. Aortic wall inflammation due to Takayasu arteritis imaged with 18F-FDG PET coregistered with enhanced CT. *J Nucl Med.* 2005;46(6):917–922.

177. Ben-Haim S, Kupzov E, Tamir A, Frenkel A, Israel O. Changing patterns of abnormal vascular wall F-18 fluorodeoxyglucose uptake on follow-up PET/CT studies. *J Nucl Cardiol.* 2006;13(6):791–800.

178. Ben-Haim S, Kupzov E, Tamir A, Israel O. Evaluation of 18F-FDG uptake and arterial wall calcifications using 18F-FDG PET/CT. *J Nucl Med.* 2004;45(11):1816–1821.

179. Dunphy MP, Freiman A, Larson SM, Strauss HW. Association of vascular 18F-FDG uptake with vascular calcification. *J Nucl Med.* 2005;46(8):1278–1284.

180. Tatsumi M, Cohade C, Nakamoto Y, Wahl RL. Fluorodeoxyglucose uptake in the aortic wall at PET/CT: possible finding for active atherosclerosis. *Radiology.* 2003;229(3):831–837.

181. Yun M, Jang S, Cucchiara A, Newberg AB, Alavi A. 18F FDG uptake in the large arteries: a correlation study with the atherogenic risk factors. *Semin Nucl Med.* 2002;32(1):70–76.

182. Rudd JH, Warburton EA, Fryer TD, Jones HA, Clark JC, Antoun N, et al. Imaging atherosclerotic plaque inflammation with [18F]-fluorodeoxyglucose positron emission tomography. *Circulation.* 2002;105(23):2708–2711.

183. Zhang Z, Machac J, Helft G, Worthley SG, Tang C, Zaman AG, et al. Noninvasive imaging of atherosclerotic plaque macrophage in a rabbit model with F-18 FDG PET. A histopathological correlation. *BMC Nucl Med.* 2006;6:3.

184. Falk E, Shah PK, Fuster V. Coronary plaque disruption. *Circulation.* 1995;92(3):657–671.

185. Tawakol A, Migrino RQ, Bashian GG, Bedri S, Vermylen D, Cury RC, et al. In vivo 18F-fluorodeoxyglucose positron emission tomography imaging provides a noninvasive measure of carotid plaque inflammation in patients. *J Am Coll Cardiol.* 2006;48(9):1818–1824.

186. Crisby M, Nordin-Fredriksson G, Shah PK, Yano J, Zhu J, Nilsson J. Pravastatin treatment increases collagen content and decreases lipid content, inflammation, metalloproteinases, and cell death in human carotid plaques: implications for plaque stabilization. *Circulation.* 2001;103(7):926–933.

187. Tahara N, Kai H, Ishibashi M, Nakaura H, Kaida H, Baba K, et al. Simvastatin attenuates plaque inflammation: evaluation by fluorodeoxyglucose positron emission tomography. *J Am Coll Cardiol.* 2006;48(9):1825-1831.

188. Opie LH, Owen P, Riemersma RA. Relative rates of oxidation of glucose and free fatty acids by ischemic and non-ischemic myocardium after coronary artery ligation in the dog. *Eur J Clin Invest.* 1973;3:419–435.

189. Schelbert HR, Phelps ME, Selin C, Marshall RC, Hoffman EJ, Kuhl DE. Regional myocardial ischemia assessed by ^{18}fluoro-2-deoxyglucose and positron emission computed tomography. In: Kreuzer H, Parmley WW, Rentrop P, Heiss HW, eds. *Quantification of Myocardial Ischemia.* Vol I. New York: Gehard Witzstrock Publishing House; 1980:437–447.

190. Marshall RC, Tillisch JH, Phelps ME, Huang SC, Carson R, Henze E, et al. Identification and differentiation of resting myocardial ischemia and infarction in man with positron computed tomography, 18F-labeled fluorodeoxyglucose and N-13 ammonia. *Circulation.* 1983;67(4):766–778.

191. Tillisch J, Brunken R, Marshall R, Schwaiger M, Mandelkern M, Phelps M, et al. Reversibility of cardiac wall-motion abnormalities predicted by positron tomography. *N Engl J Med.* 1986;314(14):884–888.

192. Camici P, Araujo LI, Spinks T, Lammertsma AA, Kaski JC, Shea MJ, et al. Increased uptake of ^{18}F-fluorodeoxyglucose in postischemic myocardium of patients with exercise-induced angina. *Circulation.* 1986;74:81–88.

193. Gerber BL, Wijns W, Vanoverschelde JL, Heyndrickx GR, De Bruyne B, Bartunek J, et al. Myocardial perfusion and oxygen consumption in reperfused noninfarcted dysfunctional myocardium after unstable angina: direct evidence for myocardial stunning in humans. *J Am Coll Cardiol.* 1999;34(7):1939–1946.

194. Schwaiger M, Schelbert HR, Ellison D, Hansen H, Yeatman L, Vinten-Johansen J, et al. Sustained regional abnormalities in cardiac metabolism after transient ischemia in the chronic dog model. *J Am Coll Cardiol.* 1985;6(2):336–347.

195. Vanoverschelde JL, Wijns W, Depré C, Essamri B, Heyndrickx GR, Borgers M, et al. Mechanisms of chronic regional postischemic dysfunction in humans. New insights from the study of noninfarcted collateral-dependent myocardium [see comments]. *Circulation.* 1993;87(5):1513–1523.

196. Schwaiger M, Neese RA, Araujo L, Wyns W, Wisneski JA, Sochor H, et al. Sustained nonoxidative glucose utilization and depletion of glycogen in reperfused canine myocardium. *J Am Coll Cardiol.* 1989;13(3):745–754.

197. Schwaiger M, Brunken R, Grover-McKay M, Krivokapich J, Child J, Tillisch JH, et al. Regional myocardial metabolism in patients with acute myocardial infarction assessed by positron emission tomography. *J Am Coll Cardiol.* 1986;8(4):800–808.

198. Bolli R. Myocardial "stunning" in man. *Circulation.* 1992;86(6):1671–1691.

199. Barnes E, Baker CS, Dutka DP, Rimoldi O, Rinaldi CA, Nihoyannopoulos P, et al. Prolonged left ventricular dysfunction occurs in patients with coronary artery disease after both dobutamine and exercise induced myocardial ischaemia. *Heart.* 2000;83(3):283–289.

200. Barnes E, Camici PG. Prevalence of hibernating myocardium in patients with severely impaired ischaemic left ventricles [letter]. *Heart.* 1999;82(4):535.

201. Rahimtoola SH. The hibernating myocardium. *Am Heart J.* 1989;117:211–221.

202. Schulz R, Rose J, Martin C, Brodde O-E, Heusch G. Development of short-term myocardial hibernation—its limitation by the severity of ischemia and inotropic stimulation. *Circulation.* 1993;88:684–695.

203. Chen C GL, Chen L, Knibb D, Knight D, Waters D. Temporal hierarchy in functional and ultrastructural recoveries between short-term and chronic hibernating myocardium after reperfusion:. *Circulation.* 1995;92:I-552.

204. Fallavollita J, Bryan P, Cantry J. ^{18}F-2-deoxyglucose deposition and regional flow in pigs with chronically dysfunctional myocardium: evidence for transmural variations in chronic hibernating myocardium. *Circulation.* 1997;95:1900–1909.

205. Fallavollita JA, Canty JM, Jr. Differential 18F-2-deoxyglucose uptake in viable dysfunctional myocardium with normal resting perfusion: evidence for chronic stunning in pigs. *Circulation.* 1999;99(21):2798–2805.

206. Shivalkar B, Flameng W, Szilard M, Pislaru S, Borgers M, Vanhaecke J. Repeated stunning precedes myocardial hibernation in progressive multiple coronary artery obstruction. *J Am Coll Cardiol.* 1999;V34(N7):2126–2136.

207. Lim H, Fallavollita JA, Hard R, Kerr CW, Canty Jr JM. Profound apoptosis-mediated regional myocyte loss and compensatory hypertrophy in pigs with hibernating myocardium. *Circulation.* 1999;100:2380–2386.

208. Fragasso G, Chierchia S, Lucignani G, Landoni C, Conversano A, Gilardi M, et al. Time dependence of residual tissue viability after myocardial infarction assessed by [18F] fluorodeoxyglucose and positron emission tomography. *Am J Cardiol.* 1993;72:131G–139G.

209. Fedele FA, Gewortz J, Capone RJ, Sharaf B, Most AS. Metabolic response to prolonged reduction of myocardial blood flow distal to a severe coronary artery stenosis. *Circulation.* 1988;78:729–735.

210. Schaefer S, Schwartz G, Wisneski J, Trocha S, Christoph I, Steinman S, et al. Response of high-energy phosphates and lactate release during prolonged regional ischemia in vivo. *Circulation.* 1992;85:342–349.

211. Camici PG, Wijns W, Borgers M, De Silva R, Ferrari R, Knuuti J, et al. Pathophysiological mechanisms of chronic reversible left ventricular dysfunction due to coronary artery disease (hibernating myocardium). *Circulation.* 1997;96(9):3205–3214.

212. Borgers M, Ausma J. Structural aspects of the chronic hibernating myocardium in man. *Basic Res Cardiol.* 1995;90:44–46.

213. Elsässer A, Schlepper M, Kleovekorn WP, Cai WJ, Zimmermann R, Meuller KD, et al. Hibernating myocardium: an incomplete adaptation to ischemia. *Circulation.* 1997;96(9):2920–2931.

214. Flameng W, Suy R, Schwarz F, Borgers M, Piessens J, Thone F, et al. Ultrastructural correlates of left ventricular contraction abnormalities in patients with chronic ischemic heart disease: determinants of reversible segmental asynergy post-revascularization surgery. *Am Heart J.* 1981;102:846–857.

215. Schwarz E, Schaper J, vom Dahl J, Altehoefer C, Buell U, Schoendube F, et al. Myocardial hibernation is not sufficient to prevent morphological disarrangements with ischemic cell alterations and increased fibrosis. *Circulation.* 1994;90:I–378.

216. Schwarz ER, Schaper J, vom Dahl J, Altehoefer C, Grohmann B, Schoendube F, et al. Myocyte degeneration and cell death in hibernating human myocardium. *J Am Coll Cardiol.* 1996;27(7):1577–1585.

217. Maes A, Flameng W, Borgers M, Nuyts J, Ausma J, Bormans G, et al. Regional myocardial blood flow, glucose utilization and contractile function before and after revascularization and ultrastructural findings in patients with chronic coronary artery disease. *European J Nucl Med.* 1995;22(11):1299–1305.

218. Wolpers HG, Burchert W, van den Hoff J, Weinhardt R, Meyer GJ, Lichtlen PR. Assessment of myocardial viability by use of 11C-acetate and positron emission tomography. Threshold criteria of reversible dysfunction. *Circulation.* 1997;95(6):1417–1424.

219. Tamaki N, Yonekura Y, Yamashita K, Saji H, Magata Y, Senda M, et al. Positron emission tomography using fluorine-18 deoxyglucose in evaluation of coronary artery bypass grafting. *Am J Cardiol.* 1989;64:860–865.

220. Carrel T, Jenni R, Haubold-Reuter S, Von Schulthess G, Pasic M, Turina M. Improvement of severely reduced left ventricular function after surgical revascularization in patients with preoperative myocardial infarction. *Eur J Cardiothorac Surg.* 1992;6:479–484.

221. Depré C, Vanoverschelde JL, Gerber B, Borgers M, Melin JA, Dion R. Correlation of functional recovery with myocardial blood flow, glucose uptake, and morphologic features in patients with chronic left ventricular ischemic dysfunction undergoing coronary artery bypass grafting. *J Thorac Cardiovasc Surg.* 1997;113(2):371–378.

222. Depré C, Vanoverschelde JL, Melin JA, Borgers M, Bol A, Ausma J, et al. Structural and metabolic correlates of the reversibility of chronic left ventricular ischemic dysfunction in humans. *Am J Physiol.* 1995;268(3 pt 2):H1265–1275.

223. Gewirtz H, Fischman A, Abraham S, Gilson M, Strauss H, Alpert N. Positron Emission tomographic measurements of absolute regional myocardial blood flow permits identification of nonviable myocardium in patients with chronic myocardial infarction. *J Am Coll Cardiol.* 1994;23:851–859.

224. Duvernoy CS, vom Dahl J, Laubenbacher C, Schwaiger M. The role of nitrogen 13 ammonia positron emission tomography in predicting functional outcome after coronary revascularization. *J Nucl Cardiol.* 1995;2(6):499–506.

225. Haas F, Augustin N, Holper K, Wottke M, Haehnel C, Nekolla S, et al. Time course and extent of improvement of dysfunctioning myocardium in patients with coronary artery disease and severely depressed left ventricular function after revascularization: correlation with positron emission tomographic findings. *J Am Coll Cardiol.* 2000;36(6):1927–1934.

226. Bax JJ, Visser FC, Elhendy A, Poldermans D, Cornel JH, van Lingen A, et al. Prediction of improvement of regional left ventricular function after revascularization using different perfusion-metabolism criteria. *J Nucl Med.* 1999;40(11):1866–1873.

227. Klein C, Nekolla SG, Bengel FM, Momose M, Sammer A, Haas F, et al. Assessment of myocardial viability with contrast-enhanced magnetic resonance imaging: comparison with positron emission tomography. *Circulation.* 2002;105(2):162–167.

228. Bonow RO, Dilsizian V, Cuocolo A, Bacharach SL. Identification of viable myocardium in patients with chronic coronary artery disease and left ventricular dysfunction. Comparison of thallium scintigraphy with reinjection and PET imaging with 18F-fluorodeoxyglucose [see comments]. *Circulation.* 1991;83(1):26–37.

229. Knuuti M, Saraste M, Nuutila P, Härkönen R, Wegelius U, Haapanen A. Myocardial viability: fluorine-18-deoxyglucose positron emission tomography in prediction of wall motion recovery after revascularization. *Am Heart J.* 1994;127:785–796.

230. Baer FM, Voth E, Deutsch HJ, Schneider CA, Horst M, de Vivie ER, et al. Predictive value of low dose dobutamine transesophageal echocardiography and fluorine-18 fluorodeoxyglucose positron emission tomography for recovery of regional left ventricular function after successful revascularization. *J Am Coll Cardiol.* 1996;28(1):60–69.

231. Buvat I, Bartlett M, Srinivasan G, Jousse F, Kitsiou A, Carson J, et al. Can gated FDG PET assess LV function as well as gated bloodpool SPECT? *J Nucl Med.* 1996;37:39P.

232. Buvat I, Kitsiou A, Srinivasan G, Dilsizian V, Bacharach S. Relationship between metabolism and function in CAD patients using gated FDG PET. *J Nucl Med.* 1996;37:161P.

233. Fath-Ordoubadi F, Beatt KJ, Spyrou N, Camici PG. Efficacy of coronary angioplasty for the treatment of hibernating myocardium. *Heart.* 1999;82(2):210–216.

234. Gerber BL, Ordoubadi FF, Wijns W, Vanoverschelde JL, Knuuti MJ, Janier M, et al. Positron emission tomography using (18)F-fluoro-deoxyglucose and euglycaemic hyperinsulinaemic glucose clamp: optimal criteria for the prediction of recovery of post-ischaemic left ventricular dysfunction. Results from the European Community Concerted Action Multicenter study on use of(18)F-fluoro-deoxyglucose positron emission tomography for the detection of myocardial viability. *Eur Heart J.* 2001;22(18):1691–1701.

235. DePuey EG, Ghesani M, Schwartz M, Friedman M, Nichols K, Salensky H. Comparative performance of gated perfusion SPECT wall thickening, delayed thallium uptake, and F-18 fluorodeoxyglucose SPECT in detecting myocardial viability. *J Nucl Cardiol.* 1999;6(4):418–428.

236. Lucignani G, Paolini G, Landoni C, Zuccari M, Paganelli G, Galli L, et al. Presurgical identification of hibernating myocardium by combined use of technetium-99m hexakis 2-methoxyisobutylisonitrile single photon emission tomography and fluorine-18 fluoro-2-deoxy-D-glucose positron emission tomography in patients with coronary artery disease. *Eur J Nucl Med.* 1992;19:874–881.

237. Sawada SG, Allman KC, Muzik O, Beanlands RS, Wolfe ER Jr, Gross M, et al. Positron emission tomography detects evidence of viability in rest technetium-99m sestamibi defects. *J Am Coll Cardiol.* 1994;23(1):92–98.

238. Bax JJ, Cornel JH, Visser FC, Fioretti PM, Huitink JM, van Lingen A, et al. F18-fluorodeoxyglucose single-photon emission computed tomography predicts functional outcome of dyssynergic myocardium after surgical revascularization. *J Nucl Cardiol.* 1997;4(4):302–308.

239. Bax JJ, Valkema R, Visser FC, Poldermans D, Cornel JH, van Lingen A, et al. Detection of myocardial viability with F-18-fluorodeoxyglucose and single photon emission computed tomography [editorial]. *G Ital Cardiol.* 1997;27(11):1181–1186.

240. Dreyfus GD, Duboc D, Blasco A, Vigoni F, Dubois C, Brodaty D, et al. Myocardial viability assessment in ischemic cardiomyopathy: benefits of coronary revascularization. *Ann Thorac Surg.* 1994;57(6):1402–1407; discussion 1407–1408.

241. Akinboboye OO, Idris O, Cannon PJ, Bergmann SR. Usefulness of positron emission tomography in defining myocardial viability in patients referred for cardiac transplantation. *Am J Cardiol.* 1999;83(8):1271–1274, A1279.

242. Srinivasan G, Kitsiou AN, Bacharach SL, Bartlett ML, Miller-Davis C, Dilsizian V. [18F]fluorodeoxyglucose single photon emission computed tomography: can it replace PET and thallium SPECT for the assessment of myocardial viability? *Circulation.* 1998;97(9):843–850.

243. Maes A, Flameng W, Nuyts J, Borgers M, Shivalkar B, Ausma J, et al. Histological alterations in chronically hypoperfused myocardium. Correlation with PET findings. *Circulation.* 1994;90(2):735–745.

244. Shivalkar B, Maes A, Borgers M, Ausma J, Scheys I, Nuyts J, et al. Only hibernating myocardium invariably shows early recovery after coronary revascularization. *Circulation.* 1996;94(3):308–315.

245. Grandin C, Wijns W, Melin JA, Bol A, Robert AR, Heyndrickx GR, et al. Delineation of myocardial viability with PET. *J Nucl Med.* 1995;36(9):1543–1552.

246. Marwick TH, MacIntyre WJ, Lafont A, Nemec JJ, Salcedo EE. Metabolic responses of hibernating and infarcted myocardium to revascularization. A follow-up study of regional perfusion, function, and metabolism. *Circulation.* 1992;85(4):1347–1353.

247. Allman KC, Shaw LJ, Hachamovitch R, Udelson JE. Myocardial viability testing and impact of revascularization on prognosis in patients with coronary artery disease and left ventricular dysfunction: a meta-analysis. *J Am Coll Cardiol.* 2002;39(7):1151–1158.

248. Vaghaiwalla Mody F, Brunken R, Warner-Stevenson L, Nienaber C, Phelps M, Schelbert H. Differentiating cardiomyopathy of coronary artery disease from non-ischemic dilated cardiomyopathy utilizing positron tomography. *J Am Coll Cardiol.* 1991;17:373–383.

249. Tamaki N, Yonekura Y, Yamashita K, Ohtani H, Hirata K, Ban T, et al. Prediction of reversible ischemia after coronary artery bypass grafting by positron emission tomography. *J Cardiol.* 1991;21(2):193–201.

250. Gropler RJ, Bergmann SR. Flow and metabolic determinants of myocardial viability assessed by positron-emission tomography. *Coron Artery Dis.* 1993;4(6):495–504.

251. Marwick T, Nemec J, Lafont A, Salcedo E, MacIntyre W. Prediction by postexercise fluoro-18 deoxyglucose positron emission tomography of improvement in exercise capacity after revascularization. *Am J Cardiol.* 1992;69:854–859.

252. Paolini G, Lucignani G, Zuccari M, Landoni C, Vanoli G, Di Credico G, et al. Identification and revascularization of hibernating myocardium in angina-free patients with left ventricular dysfunction. *Eur J Cardiothorac Surg.* 1994;8(3):139–144.

253. vom Dahl J, Eitzman D, Al-Aouar A, Kanter H, Hicks R, Deeb G, et al. Relation of regional function, perfusion, and metabolism in patients with advanced coronary artery disease undergoing surgical revascularization. *Circulation.* 1994;90:2356–2366.

254. vom Dahl J, Altehoefer C, Sheehan F, Buechin P, Uebis R, Messmer B, et al. Recovery of regional left ventricular dysfunction after coronary revascularization: Impact of myocardial viability assessed by nuclear imaging and vessel patency at follow-up angiography. *J Am Coll Cardiol.* 1996;28:948–958.

255. Haas F, Haehnel CJ, Picker W, Nekolla S, Martinoff S, Meisner H, et al. Preoperative positron emission tomographic viability assessment and perioperative and postoperative risk in patients with advanced ischemic heart disease [see comments]. *J Am Coll Cardiol.* 1997;30(7):1693–1700.

256. Flameng WJ, Shivalkar B, Spiessens B, Maes A, Nuyts J, VanHaecke J, et al. PET scan predicts recovery of left ventricular function after coronary artery bypass operation. *Ann Thorac Surg.* 1997;64(6):1694–1701.

257. Fath-Ordoubadi F, Pagano D, Marinho NV, Keogh BE, Bonser RS, Camici PG. Coronary revascularization in the treatment of moderate and severe postischemic left ventricular dysfunction. *Am J Cardiol.* 1998;82(1):26–31.

258. Pagano D, Bonser RS, Townend JN, Ordoubadi F, Lorenzoni R, Camici PG. Predictive value of dobutamine echocardiography and positron emission tomography in identifying hibernating myocardium in patients with postischaemic heart failure. *Heart.* 1998;79(3):281–288.

259. Beanlands RS, Hendry PJ, Masters RG, deKemp RA, Woodend K, Ruddy TD. Delay in revascularization is associated with increased mortality rate in patients with severe left ventricular dysfunction and viable myocardium on fluorine 18–fluorodeoxyglucose positron emission tomography imaging. *Circulation.* 1998;98(19 suppl):II51–56.

260. Schöder H, Campisi R, Ohtake T, Hoh CK, Moon DH, Czernin J, et al. Blood flow-metabolism imaging with positron emission tomography in patients with diabetes mellitus for the assessment of reversible left ventricular contractile dysfunction. *J Am Coll Cardiol.* 1999;33(5):1328–1337.

261. Bax JJ, Visser FC, Poldermans D, Elhendy A, Cornel JH, Boersma E, et al. Relationship between preoperative viability and postoperative improvement in LVEF and heart failure symptoms. *J Nucl Med.* 2001;42(1):79–86.

262. Zhang X, Liu XJ, Wu Q, Shi R, Gao R, Liu Y, et al. Clinical outcome of patients with previous myocardial infarction and left ventricular dysfunction assessed with myocardial (99m)Tc-MIBI SPECT and (18)F-FDG PET. *J Nucl Med.* 2001;42(8):1166–1173.

263. Pagano D, Townend JN, Littler WA, Horton R, Camici PG, Bonser RS. Coronary artery bypass surgery as treatment for ischemic heart failure: the predictive value of viability assessment with quantitative positron emission tomography for symptomatic and functional outcome. *J Thorac Cardiovasc Surg.* 1998;115(4):791–799.

264. Pasquet A, Lauer MS, Williams MJ, Secknus MA, Lytle B, Marwick TH. Prediction of global left ventricular function after bypass surgery in patients with severe left ventricular dysfunction. Impact of pre-operative myocardial function, perfusion, and metabolism [see comments]. *Eur Heart J.* 2000;21(2):125–136.

265. Pasquet A, Robert A, D'Hondt AM, Dion R, Melin JA, Vanoverschelde JL. Prognostic value of myocardial ischemia and viability in patients with chronic left ventricular ischemic dysfunction. *Circulation.* 1999;100(2):141–148.

266. Beanlands RS, Ruddy TD, deKemp RA, Iwanochko RM, Coates G, Freeman M, et al. Positron emission tomography and recovery following revascularization (PARR-1): the importance of scar and the development of a

prediction rule for the degree of recovery of left ventricular function. *J Am Coll Cardiol.* 2002;40(10):1735–1743.

267. Nienaber CA, Brunken RC, Sherman CT, Yeatman LA, Gambhir SS, Krivokapich J, et al. Metabolic and functional recovery of ischemic human myocardium after coronary angioplasty [see comments]. *J Am Coll Cardiol.* 1991;18(4):966–978.

268. Vanoverschelde JL, Janier MF, Bakke JE, Marshall DR, Bergmann SR. Rate of glycolysis during ischemia determines extent of ischemic injury and functional recovery after reperfusion. *Am J Physiol.* 1994;267(5 pt 2):H1785–1794.

269. Vanoverschelde JL, Melin JA. The pathophysiology of myocardial hibernation: current controversies and future directions. *Prog Cardiovasc Dis.* 2001;43(5):387–398.

270. Eitzman D, Al-Aouar Z, Vom Dahl J, Kirsh M, Schwaiger M. Clinical outcome of patients with advanced coronary artery disease after viability studies with positron emission tomography. *J Am Coll Cardiol.* 1992;20(3):559–565.

271. Di Carli M, Davidson M, Little R, Khanna S, Mody F, Brunken R, et al. Value of metabolic imaging with POSITRON EMISSION TOMOGRAPHY for evaluating prognosis in patients with coronary artery disease and left ventricular dysfunction. *Am J Cardiol.* 1994;73(8):527–533.

272. Di Carli MF, Asgarzadie F, Schelbert HR, Brunken RC, Laks H, Phelps ME, et al. Quantitative relation between myocardial viability and improvement in heart failure symptoms after revascularization in patients with ischemic cardiomyopathy. *Circulation.* 1995;92(12):3436–3444.

273. Goldman L, Hashimoto B, Cook E, Loscalzo A. Comparative reproducibility and validity of systems for assessing cardiovascular functional class: advantages of a new specific activity scale. *Circulation.* 1981;64:1227–1234.

274. Di Carli MF, Maddahi J, Rokhsar S, Schelbert HR, Bianco-Batlles D, Brunken RC, et al. Long-term survival of patients with coronary artery disease and left ventricular dysfunction: implications for the role of myocardial viability assessment in management decisions. *J Thorac Cardiovasc Surg.* 1998;116(6):997–1004.

275. Lee KS, Marwick TH, Cook SA, Go RT, Fix JS, James KB, et al. Prognosis of patients with left ventricular dysfunction, with and without viable myocardium after myocardial infarction. Relative efficacy of medical therapy and revascularization. *Circulation.* 1994;90(6):2687–2694.

276. Tamaki N, Kawamoto M, Takahashi N, Yonekura Y, Magata Y, Nohara R, et al. Prognostic value of an increase in fluorine-18 deoxyglucose uptake in patients with myocardial infarction: comparison with stress thallium imaging. *J Am Coll Cardiol.* 1993;22(6):1621–1627.

277. Landoni C, Lucignani G, Paolini G, Zuccari M, Galli L, Di Credico G, et al. Assessment of CABG-related risk in patients with CAD and LVD. Contribution of PET with [18F]FDG to the assessment of myocardial viability. *J Cardiovasc Surg.* 1999;40(3):363–372.

278. Auerbach MA, Schöder H, Hoh C, Gambhir SS, Yaghoubi S, Sayre JW, et al. Prevalence of myocardial viability as detected by positron emission tomography in patients with ischemic cardiomyopathy. *Circulation.* 1999;99(22):2921–2926.

279. Desideri A, Cortigiani L, Christen AI, Coscarelli S, Gregori D, Zanco P, Komorovsky R, Bax JJ. The extent of perfusion-F18-fluorodeoxyglucose positron emission tomography mismatch determines mortality in medically treated patients with chronic ischemic left ventricular dysfunction. *J Am Coll Cardiol.* 2005;46(7):1264–1269.

280. Duong T, Hendi P, Fonarow G, Asgarzadie F, Stevenson L, Di Carli M, et al. Role of positron emission tomographic assessment of myocardial viability in the management of patients who are referred for cardiac transplantation. *Circulation.* 1995;92:I-123.

281. Duong T, Fonarow G, Laks H, Hendi P, Czernin J, Phelps M, et al. Cost effectiveness of positron emission tomography (PET) in the management of ischemic cardiomyopathy patients who are referred for cardiac transplantation. *J Am Coll Cardiol.* 1996;27:144A.

282. Louie HW, Laks H, Milgalter E, Drinkwater DC Jr, Hamilton MA, Brunken RC, et al. Ischemic cardiomyopathy. Criteria for coronary revascularization and cardiac transplantation. *Circulation.* 1991;84(5 suppl):III290–295.

PART 4 Heart Failure

CHAPTER 24

Pathophysiology of Heart Failure

Gary S. Francis / Edmund H. Sonnenblick /
W. H. Wilson Tang / Philip Poole-Wilson

Heart failure is a complex clinical syndrome in which the typical symptoms of shortness of breath and fatigue are associated with functional or structural damage to the heart. The diagnosis usually portends an early death preceded by unpleasant symptoms limiting the quality of life. Heart failure is common and becoming more common as the population ages and as patients survive myocardial infarction with consequent persistent damage to the muscle of the heart. The entity of heart failure is easily recognized by the experienced physician, can be detected in the community, and treatment reduces both morbidity and mortality. Although the molecular biology and integrated physiology of heart failure remain incompletely understood, several concepts and principles have evolved over the past decades. The key feature of heart failure is the impaired ability of the heart to act as a pump. But many body responses, which are secondary adaptive responses maintaining short-term circulatory function, eventually become maladaptive and contribute substantially to the long-term progression of heart failure. These numerous adaptations in response to the onset of heart failure occur in the peripheral circulation, the kidney, skeletal muscle, and almost all organs of the body. The changes contribute to the overall clinical syndrome and phenotype of heart failure. An understanding of how these changes occur provides insight into the pathophysiology of the syndrome and explains why some are therapeutic targets.

DEFINING HEART FAILURE AND CARDIAC DYSFUNCTION

A widely known definition of heart failure is "a pathophysiological state in which an abnormality of cardiac function is responsible for the failure of the heart to pump blood at a rate commensurate with the requirements of the metabolizing tissues."[1] This definition places the emphasis on the physiology of the circulation. More recent definitions have taken a more pragmatic and clinically useful approach. One American definition is "Heart failure is a complex clinical syndrome that can result from any structural or functional cardiac disorder that impairs the ability of the ventricle to fill with or eject blood. The cardinal manifestations of heart failure are dyspnea and fatigue, which may limit exercise tolerance, and fluid retention, which may lead to pulmonary congestion and peripheral edema."[2] A recent European definition is similar: "Heart failure is a complex syndrome that can result from any structural or functional cardiac disorder that impairs the ability of the heart to function as a pump to support a physiological circulation. The syndrome of heart failure is characterized by symptoms such as breathlessness and fatigue, and signs such as fluid retention."[3]

Congestive heart failure denotes the clinical syndrome with the features of dyspnea, increased fatigue, and fluid accumulation (jugular venous distention, dependent edema, enlarged liver, and pulmonary edema). Congestive heart failure should be distinguished from cardiac dysfunction, which is a structural definition based on imaging techniques and characterized by abnormal contractility (systolic) or relaxation (diastolic), often accompanied by *compensatory* ventricular hypertrophy and/or dilatation (so-called *cardiac remodeling*). The term *cardiomyopathy* is often used to describe any condition with evidence of structural abnormalities of the myocardium. The classification of cardiomyopathy can be found in Chap. 28. The nomenclature of heart failure can be con-

fusing because many adjectives are used to emphasize one or another feature (Table 24–1). The extent and progression of ventricular damage (ventricular hypertrophy or dilation) and the impact on body organs is, in general, related to the neurohumoral/cytokine systemic response. Ventricular performance, in general and when expressed as the left ventricular ejection fraction (LVEF), does not correlate with either the peripheral changes or the ability to exercise. That is largely because the ejection fraction (EF) is more a measure of ventricular size at end-diastole than a measure of the mechanical function or reserve of the heart.

TABLE 24–1

Classifications and Definitions of Some Common Types of Heart Failure

Definitions of Heart Failure
A pathophysiological state in which an abnormality of cardiac function is responsible for the failure of the heart to pump blood at a rate commensurate with the requirements of the metabolizing tissues.[1]

Heart failure is a complex clinical syndrome that can result from any structural or functional cardiac disorder that impairs the ability of the ventricle to fill with or eject blood. The cardinal manifestations of heart failure are dyspnea and fatigue, which can limit exercise tolerance, and fluid retention, which can lead to pulmonary congestion and peripheral edema.[2]

Heart failure is a complex syndrome that can result from any structural or functional cardiac disorder that impairs the ability of the heart to function as a pump to support a physiological circulation. The syndrome of heart failure is characterized by symptoms such as breathlessness and fatigue, and signs such as fluid retention.[3]

Congestive Heart Failure
Similar to the above but with features of circulatory congestion (fluid retention) such as jugular venous distension, rales, peripheral edema, and ascites. Adjectives such as chronic, overt, treated, untreated, undulating, worsening and compensated can precede the phrase.

Noncardiac Circulatory Failure
A syndrome that is clinically indistinguishable from congestive heart failure where there is no reason to ascribe the condition to structural heart disease. There must be a noncardiac cause such as acute renal failure. This entity includes so-called *high output heart failure*; a better terminology is *circulatory failure* because in these conditions the heart is usually not abnormal.

Systolic Heart Failure
A clinical syndrome with classic symptoms of breathlessness, fatigue, and exercise intolerance whereby the dominant cardiac feature is a large, dilated heart and impaired systolic performance. There may or may not be concomitant valvular disease.

Diastolic Heart Failure
This term is used when the ejection fraction at rest is normal or near normal. An alternative phrase is *preserved ejection fraction*. The features of heart failure are present, and the heart is small or normal in size. There is often left ventricular (LV) hypertrophy and impaired filling of the heart caused by altered LV stiffness or other evidence of diastolic dysfunction. Severe systemic hypertension and/or valvular disease such as mitral regurgitation can be present. This form of heart failure can coexist with systolic heart failure, particularly on exercise.

Right-Sided Heart Failure
A clinical syndrome characterized by tissue congestion including jugular venous distention, peripheral edema, ascites, and abdominal organ engorgement. There is marked impairment of right ventricular systolic performance, usually with right ventricular dilatation and severe tricuspid regurgitation. There are multiple causes of this syndrome, including severe left-sided heart failure (the commonest cause), severe lung disease with chronic hypoxemia and pulmonary hypertension (*cor pulmonale*), right ventricular myocardial infarction, primary pulmonary hypertension and congenital abnormalities of the heart.

Left-Sided Heart Failure
A clinical syndrome where the dominant feature is fluid congestion in the lung (pulmonary edema) rather than in the systemic circulation.

Acute Heart Failure
Some physicians limit this term to a serious medical emergency synonymous with acute pulmonary edema. In recent years the meaning of the phrase has been extended to include new onset heart failure and worsening heart failure on a background of chronic heart failure.

ACUTE VERSUS CHRONIC HEART FAILURE

The spectrum of biological processes involved depends on the nature and temporal sequence of alterations leading to the clinical presentation. The acute heart failure syndrome (or *acute decompensated heart failure*, or simply *acute heart failure* commonly characterized by pulmonary edema) is defined as a short term or rapid change in heart failure signs and symptoms resulting in a need for urgent therapy.[4] These symptoms can develop in a progressive manner over a short period of time, sometimes with a defining event such as during acute ischemia of the ventricle (e.g., a myocardial infarction), recent onset of atrial fibrillation, other arrhythmias, or sudden loss of valve function such as that caused by rupture of a papillary muscle or chordae tendinea. An acute shift of blood volume from the systemic to the pulmonary circulation (sometimes referred to as *flash pulmonary edema*) can even occur before significant salt or water retention has ensued. Acute heart failure is distinguished from chronic heart failure, which refers to a relatively more stable but symptomatic condition, in many cases being considered as compensated heart failure. Specific factors involved in converting from a compensated to a decompensated state in any individual patient with heart failure can vary, are not well understood, and can take place over days to weeks. In chronic heart failure, fatigue can occur because of a limited cardiac output and neurological signals from underperfused and damaged skeletal muscle. Fluid accumulation can occur leading to pulmonary congestion and peripheral edema, that is, congestive heart failure.

SYSTOLIC VERSUS DIASTOLIC HEART FAILURE

A more contemporary distinction in patients with heart failure is to characterize the particular structural abnormalities with cardiac imaging techniques, and the majority of clinical studies in heart failure have used this phenotyping. Systolic dysfunction describes a large, dilated, and often eccentrically hypertrophied ventricle in which output is limited by impaired ejection during systole, whereas diastolic dysfunction refers to a thickened, small cavity ventricle in which filling is limited because of abnormalities during diastole (Table 24–2). These terms are most appropriately defined in terms of altered ventricular performance and geometry rather than systemic hemodynamics or overt symptoms as they can manifest with almost identical symptomatology. It is also clear that systolic and diastolic dysfunction frequently coexist in patients with heart failure because systolic dysfunction, notably on exercise, can directly influence diastolic function. Systemic symptoms may not correlate with the degree of ventricular dysfunction as assessed by contraction during systole at rest.

LEFT VERSUS RIGHT HEART FAILURE

Because both sides of the heart are part of a circuit in series, one side of the circulation cannot pump significantly more blood than the other for any length of time in the absence of abnormal shunts, communications, or regurgitation. In most situations, the expression *left heart failure* (or *pump failure*) is used clinically in reference to symptoms and signs of elevated pressure and congestion in the pulmonary veins and capillaries, whereas the term *right heart failure* refers to symptoms and signs of elevated pressure and

TABLE 24–2

The Differential Diagnosis of Systolic Heart Failure and Heart Failure with Normal Systolic Function (Diastolic Heart Failure)

SYSTOLIC HEART FAILURE	DIASTOLIC HEART FAILURE
Large, dilated heart	Small LV cavity, concentric LV hypertrophy
Normal or low blood pressure	Systemic hypertension
Broad age group; more common in men	Elderly women more common
Low ejection fraction	Normal or increased ejection fraction
S_3 gallop	S_4 gallop
Systolic and diastolic impairment by echo	Diastolic impairment by various echo measurements
Treatment well established	Treatment not well established
Poor prognosis	Prognosis not as poor
Role of myocardial ischemia important in selected cases	Myocardial ischemia common

LV, left ventricular; S_3, third heart sound; S_4, fourth heart sound.

congestion in the systemic veins and capillaries characterized by jugular vein engorgement and hepatic congestion. Abnormal function of the left ventricle with impaired forward flow not only overloads the right ventricle from augmented pulmonary pressures (the old fashioned term was *backward heart failure*), but also can affect the right ventricle by means of the shared septum. Therefore, right-sided heart failure commonly follows left-sided heart failure. However, significant amounts of sodium and water retention, with subsequent peripheral edema formation, can occur with pure left-sided heart failure without hemodynamic evidence of right-sided heart failure. This occurs because reduced perfusion of the kidney leads to salt and water retention (old fashioned *forward failure*). An increase in the diastolic pressure in either ventricle can increase the diastolic pressure or decrease the distensibility of the contralateral ventricle, especially if the pericardium is intact; the biochemistry and hemodynamics of the contralateral ventricle can also be abnormal even in "pure" one-sided failure.

PATHOPHYSIOLOGIC CONCEPTS OF HEART FAILURE

INDEX EVENTS AND HEART FAILURE ETIOLOGY

The causes of heart failure are classified into six main categories: (1) failure related to an abnormality of the myocardium. This can be caused by loss of myocytes (e.g., myocardial infarction), incoordinate contraction (e.g., left bundle-branch block), reduced contractile force (e.g., cardiomyopathy or cardiotoxicity) or disorientation of cells (e.g., hypertrophic); (2) failure primarily related to external work overload (e.g., hypertension); (3) failure related to valve abnormalities; (4) failure caused by an abnormal cardiac rhythm (e.g., tachycardia); (5) failure caused by pericardial abnormalities or a pericardial effusion (tamponade); and (6) congenital deformities of the heart. Because any form of heart disease can lead to heart failure, there is no single causative mechanism. Likewise at the organ and the cellular level, there is no single mechanism that accounts for malfunction of heart muscle although identification of fundamental mechanisms remains an area of very active investigation. Multiple subsequent alterations in organ and cellular physiology contribute to the syndrome of heart failure under various circumstances and at different points in time (Table 24–3). For example, with myocardial failure, ventricular dilation can occur (Starling effect) maintaining stroke volume. This dilation can lead to failure of the mitral valves to close completely, resulting in mitral regurgitation. This then creates a secondary functional volume load for the already compromised left ventricle. Adaptive processes in the periphery occur that can adversely affect the myocardium, kidneys, smooth and skeletal muscles, endothelium, peripheral vasculature, and multiple reflex control mechanisms, adding to the complexity of the syndrome (Table 24–4). The schema of the sequence of events in heart failure is daunting. Distinguishing primary etio-

TABLE 24–3

Possible Mechanisms of Myocardial Failure

Loss of myocytes
Hypertrophy of remaining myocytes
Energy production and utilization
  Oxygen and energy supply
  Substrate utilization and energy storage
  Inadequate mitochondria mass and function
Ventricular remodeling
Contractile proteins
  Abnormal myofibrillar or myosin ATPase
  Abnormal myocardial proteins
  Defective protein synthesis
  Nonuniformity of contraction and function
Activation of contractile elements
  Membrane Na^+,K^+-ATPase defects
  Abnormal sarcoplasmic reticulum function
    Abnormal Ca^{2+} release
    Abnormal Ca^{2+} uptake
Abnormal myocardial receptor function
  Downregulation of β adrenoreceptors
  Decreased $β_1$ receptors
  Decreased Gs protein
  Increased G1 protein
Autonomic nervous system
  Abnormal myocardial norepinephrine function or kinetics
  Abnormal baroreceptor function
Increased myocardial fibroblast growth and collagen synthesis
Aging changes, presbycardia
Sustained tachycardia
Miscellaneous

ATPase, adenosine triphosphate; Ca^{2+}, calcium; Na^+,K^+-ATPase, sodium-potassium adenosine triphosphate.

TABLE 24–4

Compensatory Mechanisms in Heart Failure

Autonomic nervous system
  Heart
    Increased heart rate
    Increased myocardial contractile stimulation
    Increased rate of relaxation
  Peripheral circulation
    Arterial vasoconstriction (increased afterload)
    Venous vasoconstriction (increased preload)
  Kidney (renin-angiotensin-aldosterone)
    Arterial vasoconstriction (increased afterload)
    Venous vasoconstriction (increased preload)
    Sodium and water retention (increased preload and afterload)
    Increased myocardial contractile stimulation
Endothelin-1 (increased preload and afterload)
Arginine vasopressin (increased preload and afterload)
Atrial and brain natriuretic peptides (decreased afterload)
Prostaglandins
Peptides
Frank-Starling law of the heart
  Increased end-diastolic fiber length, volume, and pressure (increased preload)
Hypertrophy
Stem cell maturation replacing lost myocardium
Peripheral oxygen delivery
  Redistribution of cardiac output
  Altered oxygen-hemoglobin dissociation
  Increased oxygen extraction by tissues
Anaerobic metabolism

logic forces from secondary epiphenomena is difficult. Identification of the precise mechanisms whereby heart failure evolves and quantifying the contributions of individual components such as a primary decrease in capacity of myocytes to shorten adequately (e.g., decreased contractility) or loss of myocytes (e.g., apoptosis) has remained elusive. Indeed, loss of myocytes with compensatory dilation of the ventricle can lead to further loss of myocytes. What triggers the early activation of the sympathetic nervous system and withdrawal of vagal tone, or how spontaneous resolution of heart failure occurs remains unclear. Nevertheless, enough information has accrued to construct a reasonably coherent working hypothesis.

MOLECULAR ADAPTATIONS AND MALADAPTATIONS: ALTERED CELLULAR PROTEINS

The growth of genetics and molecular cardiology has provided important insights into the pathophysiology of heart failure (see Chaps. 6, 9, and 10). However, because the cause and progression of heart failure is complex, both environment and genetics play important roles. Thus, there is no single cause or unifying mechanism of heart failure, and current therapeutic strategies target multiple pathophysiologic processes.

Alterations are found in the failing heart in numerous contractile proteins, especially in heredity-based idiopathic dilated cardiomyopathies. In the latter situation, these alterations can interact with abnormal loading conditions to cause heart failure. Such alterations have been found in the proteins of the cytoskeleton, myosin, troponin T, and actin, and likely contribute to diminished myocardial performance. In animal models of various overloads can result in heart failure, whether from systolic loads (hypertension), loss of myocardium (infarction), or inflammation, and so forth. Further, in human failing hearts, etiology can be modified from that in animal models. In the human failing heart, many changes in gene expression at the mRNA or protein level have been found in failing hearts harvested at the time of cardiac transplantation. However, these are often hearts with end-stage myocardial disease in which many factors (such as receiving multiple inotropic drugs) can obscure initial pathogenesis.

β-Myosin Heavy Chain

More than half of the volume of cardiac myocytes contains contractile proteins. Myosin comprises the thick filament that hydrolyzes adenosine triphosphate (ATP), interacts with the thin filaments, actin, to produce force and shortening. Two myosin heavy chain (MHC) isoforms are present in mammalian heart, α- and β-MHC. The α-MHC is cardiac-specific and is more enzymatically active. The less active β-MHC is present in the heart and also in slow-twitch skeletal muscle. The distribution of α- and β-MHC is developmentally and hormonally regulated. Mechanical stress, such as pressure overload, induces a α- to β-MHC transition in the ventricles of experimental animals, thus imparting a slower but more economical type of work for the overloaded heart. Either way, myosin remains a principal structural and contractile unit of muscle fiber.

There is a general agreement that myofibrillar function is depressed in the human failing heart, but its causal role remains controversial. Downregulation of α-MHC and upregulation of β-MHC using mRNA measurements from right ventricular endomyocardial biopsies from nonfailing hearts and failing human hearts has been demonstrated,[5] and their sequential changes can be observed with recovery of cardiac performance.[6] This alteration, if translated into protein expression, would decrease myosin adenosine triphosphatase (ATPase) enzyme velocity and slow the speed of contraction. Although such adaptive changes could be viewed to have an *economical* survival advantage in the face of increased load, slower contraction and relaxation could also contribute to diastolic dysfunction. In addition, isoform changes involving both the heavy and the light chains, as been suggested, can play a role in heart failure. In contrast to smaller mammalian species such as mouse, rat, and rabbit, the normal human ventricle contains at least 90 percent slow β-MHC, so an isoform shift to increase the large amount of β-MHC already in the cell is unlikely to be extensive.

Ion Channels and Calcium Flux Proteins

Plasma membrane ion channels initiate excitation-contraction by generating and then propagating the action potentials that depolarize the myocardium. These ion channels are complex and contain several subunits that surround the ion-selective pore. The intracellular calcium (Ca^{2+}) release channels are in the sarcoplasmic reticulum (SR), and are quite different from those of the plasma membrane. The SR Ca^{2+} release channels are referred to as ryanodine receptors and interact with the ligand inositol triphosphate (IP_3). The Ca^{2+} pump ATPases are found in both the plasma membrane and SR. Both calcium pumps are activated by cytosolic Ca^{2+}. The sodium-calcium exchanger (NCX) transports calcium out of the cytosol into the extracellular space, using the osmotic energy of the sodium gradient across the plasma membrane to generate active transport. The sodium-potassium ($Na,^+K^+$)-ATPase pump uses energy derived from ATP hydrolysis to exchange sodium that enters the cell for potassium lost from the cytosol during repolarization. There are also calcium-binding storage proteins (e.g., calsequestrin) that maintain a calcium store that can be readily used during excitation-contraction coupling. The heart's voltage-gated ion channels (especially sodium channels) can be altered in the failing heart,[7] as are potassium channels (see Chap. 32).[8] Of course, arrhythmias and sudden death are common in heart failure and occur in the form of both bradyarrhythmias and tachyarrhythmias. Although multiple mechanisms, including excessive catecholamines, scar tissue, and electrolyte abnormalities contribute to sudden death in heart failure, it is plausible that perturbations in ion channels and ion-exchange mechanisms are in part responsible for many of these arrhythmias.

Excitation-Contraction Coupling Proteins

Excitation-contraction coupling links plasma membrane depolarization to the release of calcium into the cytosol, where it binds to troponin C permitting the force-generating interaction between myosin and actin. Relaxation is also an energy-dependent process, but is not simply a reversal of the steps in excitation-contraction coupling. During relaxation, calcium is actively transported out of the cytosol by entirely different structures. The basic mechanism of cardiac excitation-contraction coupling involves calcium (Ca^{2+}) entry from the extracellular fluid by means of the voltage-dependent L-type calcium channel to produce a trigger in increasing $[Ca^{2+}]_i$ and opening of the intracellular SR Ca^{2+} release channel or *ryanodine receptor* (RyR). Defects in sarcolemma Ca^{2+} uptake (sarcolemmal transport via $Na,^+K^+$-ATPase) and release by the SR are present in heart failure, especially at later stages,[9] whereas uptake of calcium by the SR can remain intact. These alterations in calcium transport can be secondary to quantitative alterations of gene expression of SR calcium transport proteins, especially the sarcoplasmic-endoplasmic reticulum calcium ATPase (SERCA) and phospholamban, a reversible inhibitor of cardiac SR Ca^{2+}-ATPase activity. Other calcium-cycling proteins such as Na^+-Ca^{2+} exchanger proteins[10] also can be altered in heart failure. Phosphokinase A hyperphosphorylation of RyR has recently been shown to alter calcium signaling from the SR by depleting calcium stores and reducing calcium transients that can impair contractility in the failing myocardium.[11] Several of these alterations can occur concurrently, and can vary from model to model and may not always be relative to failing human hearts. Nevertheless, it is likely that heart failure is characterized by reduced myofilament activation and decreased calcium available for activation as well as heightened cytosolic calcium levels in diastole. Some studies have shown increased myofibrillar calcium sensitivity[12] and altered calcium kinetics. These abnormalities of calcium metabolism can be of primary importance in some types of heart failure, and they can be secondary or epiphenomena in other types. Most abnormalities of myocardial contractile activation have been demonstrated only in the late stages of heart failure and therefore can be the result of maladaptive hypertrophy rather than a primary cause of ventricular dysfunction. Molecular and cellular mechanisms for pathologic cardiac hypertrophy and failure are reviewed in detail in Chap. 6.

【 】 METABOLIC ADAPTATIONS AND MALADAPTATIONS

Energy Production and Use

High energy phosphate levels are reduced in both animal models of heart failure[13] and failing human hearts.[14] Levels of phosphocreatine (PC) are more depressed than ATP. Reduced phosphocreatine levels impairs the *shuttle* that normally transfers energy from the mitochondria to the cytosol. The abnormal pattern of energy production in the failing heart resembles that of the fetal heart. This is also true of abnormalities in excitation-contraction coupling, myocyte contraction, and myocyte relaxation. In essence, the failing (and fetal) heart is less reliant on the more efficient pathways of mitochondrial ATP production. There are less high-energy phosphates available to meet the increased work demands of the failing heart. Even a small reduction in the phosphorylation potential impairs ATP-dependent reactions, as the heart has only a small phosphorylation *reserve* capacity. Moreover, decreased PC levels reflect more PC use and not a lack of adequate PC.

Oxygen deprivation, which is most often caused by coronary artery disease, results in impaired relaxation and weakened contraction, as can be seen in transient angina pectoris. That is readily reversible. With prolonged ischemia, decreased contraction (dyskinesis) can persist for hours beyond return of blood flow (stunning). If coronary blood flow is chronically reduced, myocardium can fail to contract normally (hibernation), even if necrosis does not ensue (see Chap. 54). With more serious loss of flow, infarction can occur. All these stages can produce substantial dyskinesia for which the remaining myocardium must sustain this load. The result is hypertrophy of the nonischemic portion of the ventricle; if this is inadequate, an increase in ventricular volume occurs using the Frank-Starling mechanism to sustain stroke volume. Whether there is a true limitation of energy supply or its use in the failing myocardium remains controversial.

In patients with heart failure, the total oxygen requirement of the heart can be increased significantly because of the increased total mass, the increase in myocardial systolic wall tension because of the Laplace relationship, and perhaps some wasted contractile energy. This increase can result in the extraction of a greater amount of oxygen from each unit of coronary blood flow and a widening of the coronary arteriovenous oxygen difference. Many patients with heart failure are able to increase coronary blood flow during exercise; however, some patients with a dilated ventricle that increases in diameter during exercise can have a further widening of the coronary arteriovenous oxygen difference during exercise and a decrease in coronary blood flow reserve (see Chaps. 3 and 37). In the presence of severe left ventricular (LV) hypertrophy, coronary blood flow per unit mass of myocardium is usually normal at rest.

Conversely, the capacity of the coronary vascular bed to dilate during reactive hyperemia, which is normally four- to fivefold, is reduced in the presence of severe hypertrophy where filling pressures are elevated. Tachycardia, such as can occur with atrial fibrillation, can reduce diastolic time for coronary perfusion, producing ischemic ventricular failure. Although reduced perfusion is probably common in end-stage heart failure, a deficit in coronary blood flow or oxygen delivery has not been clearly demonstrated to be a primary cause of heart failure associated with hypertrophy, except in the presence of obstructive coronary disease (see below).

Substrate Use and Energy Storage

Although the myocardial uptake of fatty acids and glucose per 100 grams of myocardium is normal in heart failure, there is conflicting evidence on whether or not there is a primary decrease in energy liberation by mitochondrial oxidative phosphorylation. The reductions in stores of myocardial high-energy phosphate, creatine phosphate, and/or ATP generally found in heart failure are thought to be secondary. This can be a consequence of the failure rather than the primary cause of the failure. There can also be reduced levels of creatine kinase and changes in the isoenzymes of creatine kinase in heart failure.

The major consequences of the state of energy starvation that is observed in failing hearts are caused by attenuation of important allosteric (regulatory) effects of ATP rather than reduction in the supply of substrate for the many energy-consuming reactions involved in contraction, relaxation, and excitation-contraction coupling. By facilitating the many calcium fluxes involved in excitation-contraction coupling and relaxation, these allosteric or regulatory effects of ATP exert both inotropic and lusitropic effects.

Mitochondrial Mass and Function

There are conflicting data on whether or not there is a significant decrease in the mass of mitochondria relative to the mass of myofibrils that occurs in experimental cardiac hypertrophy. It is possible that this is one of the limitations of severe hypertrophy. Defects in mitochondrial oxidative phosphorylation and in mitochondrial calcium metabolism also can be associated with myocardial failure. Except in circumstances where coronary flow is limited, such as with large vessel obstructive disease (see Chap. 40) or purported microvascular obstructive or vasospastic disease, a primary role of energy limitation in the evolution of heart failure has yet to be demonstrated. It is possible that it can play a role during periods of higher metabolic demand, such as tachycardia, as noted previously.[15] Further, mitochondrial dysfunction can produce increased reactive oxygen species that can produce additional damage and death of myocytes.

Hibernation and Stunned Myocardium

Systolic ventricular dysfunction as a result of focal loss of contraction can be dynamic and transient as can occur with acute ischemia. With restoration of metabolic requirements of an ischemic segment of myocardium, either from restoring adequate coronary flow or reducing oxygen requirements, myocardial contraction can be restored. Sometimes restoration is delayed, so-called *stunning*. Chronically reduced coronary flow can be inadequate to preserve contraction, but adequate for myocardial survival. Such persistent depressed myocardium has been termed *hibernation* and with reperfusion can recover contractility over a period of time (see Chap. 54).

PHYSIOLOGIC ADAPTATIONS AND MALADAPTATIONS

Autonomic Nervous System Dysfunction

Heart failure is characterized by many abnormal reflex control mechanisms. Peripheral vascular resistance is increased; there is defective cardiac parasympathetic control, an abnormal response to upright tilt, altered baroreceptor function,[16,17] and reduced cardiac sympathetic activity in response to a variety of stimuli.[18–20] Indeed, an early sign of heart failure is increased sympathetic tone accompanied by reduced vagal tone resulting in a modest increased heart rate even at rest.

An increase in systemic vascular resistance is generally observed in well-established heart failure. It is likely caused by a combination of locally active heightened vasoconstrictors (norepinephrine, angiotensin II, endothelin, vasopressin, neuropeptide Y) and by structural changes in blood vessels from fluid retention and reduced endothelial-dependent vasodilation. These later changes are closely associated with limitations of exercise in heart failure. Early in heart failure there can be a fall in cardiac output, arterial pressure, and baroreceptor activity, leading to an *adaptive* increase in excessive neuroendocrine drive. The sympathetic nervous system is activated early, followed by the renin-angiotensin-aldosterone system (RAAS). Arginine vasopressin is released. Sodium and water retention occur, hypervolemia restores cardiac output and arterial pressure, and neuroendocrine activity can reach a steady state. However, as heart failure progresses, there is impaired cardiosensory activity that fails to reduce neuroendocrine drive. For unclear reasons, cardiac afferent activity to the central nervous system is reduced, leading to unhindered, efferent excitatory responses from the brain to the periphery. Reflex vasoconstrictor responses to unloading the heart are paradoxically blunted.[20] There are abnormal vascular responses to postural change. Some of these changes lead to alterations in regional blood flow that accompany heart failure. Parasympathetic (vagal) tone is decreased, and heart rate variability is markedly reduced, a hallmark of congestive failure. Further, decreased heart rate variability can provide independent prognostic value in the identification of patients at risk for premature death.[21]

Although the genesis of these abnormal reflex control mechanisms is poorly understood, the changes can be more functional than structural. Heart transplantation reverses cardiopulmonary baroreflex control mechanisms to some extent, but this is inconsistent. The role that abnormal reflex control mechanisms plays in the progression of heart failure, like other neuroendocrine alterations, has been difficult to quantitate. Nevertheless, it is now increasingly clear that the sympathetic nervous system and the RAAS greatly influence the progression and natural history of heart failure with very important therapeutic implications.

Myocardial Receptor Dysfunction

The failing heart commonly demonstrates a decreased response to inotropic stimuli. Although no single mechanism accounts for this, the reduction in myocardial β-adrenergic receptors and the subsequent second messenger cyclic adenosine monophosphate (cAMP) can play an important role.[22] β-Adrenergic stimulation contributes importantly to the cardiac response to exercise, and β-adrenergic desensitization and uncoupling can be at least partially responsible for the reduced chronotropic and inotropic response to peak exercise commonly found in patients with heart failure. The β-adrenergic receptor abnormalities in heart failure appear to be caused by desensitization and uncoupling of the β_1 receptor produced by local and not systemic alterations in catecholamines. In severe heart failure, the norepinephrine (NE) stores in sympathetic nerve endings are depleted. In a sense, the failing myocardium becomes functionally denervated. cAMP responses are reduced by approximately 30 to 35 percent, leading to further contractile dysfunction. Despite downregulation of the β_1 receptor, a relatively high proportion of β_2 receptors remain to mediate chronotropic and inotropic responses.[23] However, there is some uncoupling of the β_2 receptor from its G protein and a modest upregulation of the $G\alpha_i$ subunit, further contributing to a depressed response to chronotropic and inotropic stimuli.[24] There is also a profound decrease in cardiac β-adrenergic responsiveness with aging,[25] which has clinical implications because heart failure is heavily concentrated in the aging population.

The desensitization and uncoupling of β-adrenergic receptors that occurs early with mild to moderate ventricular dysfunction is related to the degree of heart failure and is associated with a very reduced response to β-adrenergic stimulation with drugs such as dobutamine. Long-term stimulation of β-adrenergic receptors can enhance myocardial β-adrenergic receptor kinase (β-ARK) activity,[26] leading to further desensitization and uncoupling of the β-adrenergic receptor.

Of great therapeutic interest, β-adrenergic blockade with metoprolol, a relatively cardioselective β_1 blocker, upregulates the β_1 receptor, whereas carvedilol, a nonselective β_1 and β_2 blocker with additional α_1 blocking activity, does not increase β_1 receptor density.[27] Both drugs improve LV function substantially in approximately two-thirds of patients. The ventricular improvement seen with chronic β blocker use may not be caused by upregulation of β-adrenergic receptors, and the beneficial effects of β-adrenergic receptor blockade in heart failure remains unexplained. Moreover, high plasma norepinephrine levels do not predict benefit from carvedilol,[28] suggesting that there is not a simple relation between activation of the sympathetic nervous system and response to β-adrenergic blocking drugs in patients with heart failure.

Force-Frequency Response to Heart Failure

The failing human myocardium is characterized by an abnormal force-frequency response that parallels the severity of heart failure. Normally, an increase in frequency of stimulation is accompanied by an increased rate of force development, a decrease duration of contraction, and an enhanced rate of relaxation (Bowditch effect). This tends to preserve or increase contractile force while preserving diastolic time. The later effect is important in the tachycardic intact heart in preserving time in diastole to prevent ventricular filling and coronary blood flow. In isolated failing heart muscle, an increase in heart rate has been accompanied by a decrease in myocardial performance. Some impairment of systolic function in response to increased heart rate can also be related to impaired LV filling, although a negative inotropic effect as shown in isolated muscle has been related to alterations in intracellular Ca^{2+} handling. A reduced force of contraction and lack of shortening of contractile activity can contribute importantly to impairment of cardiac function during exercise.[29,30]

Hemodynamic Perturbations: The Hemodynamic Hypothesis

The term *heart failure* implies structural heart disease, and the central problem of heart failure remains impaired cardiac performance, although many of the secondary *adaptive* responses become maladaptive and contribute substantially to progression of heart failure. An understanding of how these changes occur can provide insight into the pathophysiology over the course of the syndrome.

In patients with mild heart failure, the ventricular end-diastolic pressure (EDP) and the cardiac output can be normal at rest, but the former can become elevated to abnormal levels during stress such as exercise with increased cardiac output or an increase in afterload as the blood pressure rises. The ability to increase the cardiac output in response to the increase in oxygen consumption is also reduced (see below and Chap. 3). In patients with more severe systolic dysfunction, the EDP can be elevated even at rest. As diastolic volume is increased, so is the end-systolic volume. This results in reduced elastic recoil of the ventricle during relaxation and is reflected in loss of rapid early diastolic ventricular filling (as revealed by a reduced E wave of the echocardiogram). This helps increase the mean diastolic pressure further. The elevated LV diastolic pressure increases pulmonary venous and capillary pressures and contributes to increased dyspnea as a result of changes in pulmonary compliance because of pulmonary congestion and edema. Before one reaches this stage of clinical heart failure, the body has used many compensatory mechanisms, but compensatory mechanisms eventually have failed.

Myocardial failure can develop from many causes of *overload*. In pressure overload, myocytes hypertrophy to meet the demands of the load. Hypertrophied cells contract and relax more slowly and can be subject to metabolic limitations. In addition, hypertrophied myocardial cells can have a shortened life span. This is of considerable prognostic importance because cardiac myocytes appear to have a reduced capacity to proliferate. When age-related myocyte loss is added to the picture, particularly in association with a late decrease in myocyte contractile activity, diastolic failure can ensue. As the process continues, ventricular dilatation can occur with systolic failure as well. Loss of myocytes—whether segmental, as in acute myocardial infarction, or diffuse, as in myocarditis—sets up a vicious cycle that leads to reactive hypertrophy in remaining myocytes. As compensatory hypertrophy becomes more marked in some disease states, the contractility unit of the myocardium often declines because of molecular changes in the heart's contractile proteins and ac-

tivation system. This is especially likely to occur in response to pressure overload, as in systemic arterial hypertension or aortic stenosis, but also ensues when myocytes are lost from any mechanism.

As ventricular function becomes impaired, the Frank-Starling law of the heart becomes operative (Fig. 24–1). Inadequate emptying of the ventricle leads to increased end-diastolic volumes (EDVs). This is referred to as *increased preload,* and it produces an increase in stroke volume (SV) during the next contraction. The Frank-Starling law simply states that the increase in contractile force (i.e., contractility) is related to sarcomere lengthening (up to 2.2 μm). For any given amount of Ca^{2+} released into the myocyte, there is increased crossbridge formation and enhanced sensitivity of the myofilament to Ca^{2+} as the sarcomeres lengthen.

In the failing ventricle, the extent of shortening for a given diastolic fiber length and load (afterload) is reduced. The ventricle can maintain a normal or near-normal SV with an increased end-diastolic volume and thus maintain end-diastolic fiber length for a period of time. Eventually, the filling pressure rises inordinately, limiting this compensation. Further, the clinically dilated ventricle tends to *give* like an overstretched elastic band, and end-diastolic volume can increase somewhat with no increase in LV end-diastolic pressure, reflecting a shift in the passive pressure-volume curve to the right. An obligatory

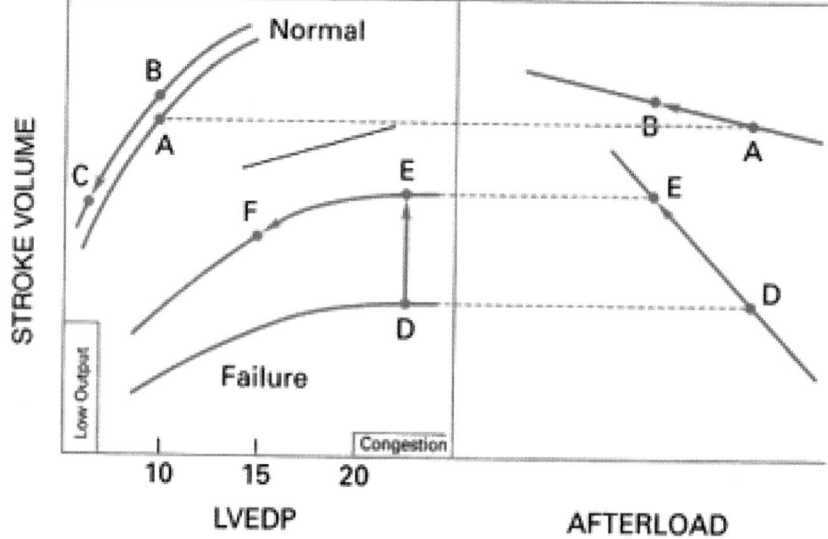

FIGURE 24–1. Relationship between stroke volume and left ventricular (LV) end-diastolic pressure (LVEDP) (*left*) and afterload (*right*). Normally, the ventricle operates on a sharply rising Frank-Starling curve with an LVEDP less than 12 mmHg (*point A*), where small changes in filling pressure yield large changes in stroke volume. Further, stroke volume is largely independent of the afterload. When failure occurs, ventricular function is characterized by a shift of the curve relating stroke volume to LVEDP to the right and downward. Low output can ensue if the curve is sufficiently depressed, whereas pulmonary congestion occurs as the LVEDP is increased. At the same time, this failing ventricle is now highly afterload-dependent, in that small changes in afterload produce large changes in stroke volume. When afterload is reduced in the normal heart (*point A to point B, right*), stroke volume rises very slightly. If, at the same time, venodilation reduces filling pressure, stroke volume falls to point C (*left*). The net result is a decrease in cardiac output. On the contrary, when afterload is reduced in the presence of severe ventricular failure, stroke volume is increased (*point D to point E, right*). Because the Frank-Starling curve is relatively flattened, a simultaneous decrease in filling pressure leads to a decrease in LVEDP with only a small decrease in stroke volume (*point E to point F, left*). The net result of these opposing consequences can be an increase in stroke volume. These results are observed clinically when a vasodilator is administered along with a diuretic in treating the failing ventricle.

reduction in EF occurs when stroke volume is maintained in the face of a large end-diastolic volume (EF = SV/EDV; normal EF = 0.62 + 0.12). Eventually, further increases in end-diastolic pressure produce little change in end-diastolic volume, thus flattening the SV-EDP curve (see Fig. 24–1). There is no true descending limb to Starling curve because increasing preload indefinitely will ultimately lead to mitral regurgitation, displacing the increased load created by the Laplace relation. As the heart dilates, the increase in wall stress according to the Laplace relationship will also increase afterload, which can account for any observed reduction in SV as the heart dilates further (i.e., the perception of a descending limb) (see Fig. 24–1). It is important to keep in mind that LV performance depends not only on systolic pump function but also on active relaxation, diastolic elastic recoil, passive diastolic properties, and vascular loading conditions. It is likely that at high LV end-diastolic pressure, valvular incompetence (mitral regurgitation) is a major cause of a decrease in cardiac output. Thus, in end-stage heart failure in the intact circulation, the Starling curve flattens out. It is possible under certain experimental conditions that the severely failing heart is able to use the Frank-Starling mechanism, but a hallmark of heart failure is the inability of the chamber to respond robustly to an increase in preload.

Loading Conditions and the Concept of the Laplace Relation A characteristic feature of the dilated, failing heart is that it gradually becomes less sensitive to preload (end-diastolic volume and fiber length) and more sensitive to afterload stress. At very high LV filling pressures (>30 mmHg) when the sarcomeres are fully extended and the preload reserve is exhausted, the SV becomes exquisitely sensitive to alterations in the afterload. The impedance to ejection includes blood viscosity, vascular resistance, vascular distensibility, and myocardial wall tension. The afterload is the total load that the heart must work against during contraction. Much of the afterload is made up of ventricular myocardial wall tension. In the ventricle, the tension on the walls increases as ventricular chamber volume increases, even if intraventricular pressure remains constant. As the ventricle empties, tension is reduced, even as pressure rises. Calculations of myocardial wall tension are defined by the Laplace equation and are expressed in terms of tension, T, per unit of cross-sectional area (dynes per centimeter [dyn/cm]).

Within a cylinder, the law of Laplace states that wall tension is equal to the pressure within the cylinder times the radius of curvature of the wall:

$$T = P \times R$$

where T is wall tension (dyn/cm), P is pressure (dyn/cm^2), and R is the radius (cm). Basically, wall tension is proportional to radius. Because the heart has thick ventricular walls, wall tension is distributed over a large number of muscle fibers, thereby reducing tension on each. The equation for a thick-walled cylinder such as the heart is:

$$T = (P \times R)/h$$

where h is wall thickness. The equation is sometimes stated as:

$$T = \frac{P \times R}{2h}$$

Because the geometry of the ventricles is more complex than a cylinder, ventricular wall tension cannot be measured with precision. Wall stress, the force distributed across an area, is actually more correct but is seldom measured.

There are two fundamental principles that stem from the relationship between the geometry of the ventricular cavity and the tension on its muscular walls:

1. *Dilation of the ventricles leads directly to an increase in tension on each muscle fiber.*
2. *An increase in wall thickness reduces the tension on any individual muscle fiber. Therefore, ventricular hypertrophy reduces afterload by distributing tension among more muscle fibers.*

The wall tension is highest in the inner surface of the heart. The endocardial surfaces must do more work and therefore are also more vulnerable to reductions in coronary blood flow. Dilatation of the heart decreases cardiac efficiency, unless hypertrophy is sufficient to normalize wall stress. In heart failure, wall tension (or stress) is high, and thus afterload is increased. The energetic consequences of the law of Laplace can have some role in progressive deterioration of energy-starved cardiac myocytes in the failing heart.

Another major disadvantage of the dilated ventricle is the inability to decrease the average radius during contraction. In the normal heart, wall tension falls during ventricular ejection as the volume decreases, even though pressure is rising. In heart failure, given the dilated heart with reduced ejection, the average tension in the myocardial fibers actually can continue to increase from the beginning of the ejection until peak systolic pressure is reached, adding additional afterload during ejection. The rate of myocardial fiber shortening is reduced, further contributing to diminished myocardial performance. It is difficult to overstate the importance of the law of Laplace when considering the syndrome of heart failure. This contrast is apparent in mitral insufficiency. With preserved contractility and a relatively small end-diastolic volume, mitral insufficiency leads to rapid unloading of volume and reduced tension. When ventricular dilatation occurs with decreased ventricular contractility, ejection is reduced, and tension remains high during systole, leading to an unsteady state that cannot be maintained for long.

Ventricular dilatation, although initially adaptive as an attempt to sustain SV, eventually becomes a substantial disadvantage and contributes importantly to impaired myocardial performance. As the left and right ventricles dilate, functional mitral and tricuspid regurgitation can occur, adding to circulatory congestion. Stretched myocardial cells can induce programmed cell death (apoptosis), thereby contributing to further disease progression.[31] Any treatment that slows progressive dilatation of the heart, such as angiotensin-converting enzyme (ACE) inhibitors or β-adrenergic blockers, will likely have a powerful role in the treatment of heart failure. The plasticity of progressive dilatation is now more apparent, with remarkable reversal of dilatation observed in response to ACE inhibitors and β-adrenergic blockers, cessation of alcohol use in patients with alcoholic cardiomyopathy and spontaneous improvement in patients with inflammatory myocarditis.

Myocyte Response to Altered Loading Conditions In response to increased load, whether created by increased pressure or loss of myocytes, hypertrophy occurs and tends to normalize the load per cell. With an increased volume load, myocytes elongate and to a small extent may undergo division.[32,33] Hyperplasia and apoptosis of myocytes occur with abnormal loading but involves less than 1 percent of the cardiac myocytes. Reprogramming of the cardiac myocytes occurs, resulting in a more fetallike state. More B-type natriuretic peptide is synthesized. Metabolism begins to favor glucose over free fatty acids. The myocytes enlarge presumably rendering a short-term structural and functional advantage.[34] The reprogramming requires altered signals, both mechanical and *chemical*, to reach the nucleus of the cardiac myocyte to set into motion *new* gene transcription.[35] Contractile proteins are altered and gain an economic advantage. Ultimately, there is a transition from hypertrophy to heart failure,[36] that has been recognized for more than 100 years but is still not well understood.[37] In a sense, this *unnatural growth response* of myocyte hypertrophy leads to the structural changes of LV remodeling, thus creating a large, dilated, and poorly functioning heart. The processes of cellular remodeling and subsequent architectural changes in cell and chamber size and shape are highly complex[35] and include many components other than myocardial cell hypertrophy. Myocardial fibrosis and cell dropout occurs, and perhaps myocyte slippage can occur, increasing dilatation. As cardiac output falls, multiple neurohormones including renin and norepinephrine are *released* in an attempt to protect blood pressure and organ perfusion,[38] while atavistic counter-regulatory natriuretic peptides are *released* in an attempt to offset vasoconstriction, hypertrophy, and volume conservation.[39] The story is undoubtedly much more complex than this,[40] and includes a cornucopia of molecular mechanisms,[35,41] some of which primarily affect the cardiac interstitium and others the cardiac myocytes.

Maladaptive remodeling of cardiac myocyte size and shape begins long before clinical heart failure begins.[42–45] Alterations in myocyte proteins and mitochondria size and as well as changes in myocardial interstitium and collagen content/architecture are seen in response to a variety of *injuries* including pressure overload,[46–48] volume overload, and myocardial ischemia.[49] Additional phenotypic changes in heart failure include apoptosis.[50,51] It is important to recognize that much of the neuroendocrine activation that occurs in a primordial attempt to conserve organ perfusion appears to facilitate this myriad of pathologic change in the heart at the cellular level, thereby possibly contributing to the success of neuroendocrine blockers as therapy for heart failure. Lastly, there is no single phenotypic change, protein expression, or signal-transduction pathway that is dominant. Rather, there is extraordinary redundancy in these mechanisms. This observation has important implications for therapy. For example, blocking one neuroendocrine system can lead to enhanced overactivity of other neuroendocrine systems. Blocking one signal-transduction pathway can lead the cell to hypertrophy through alternative pathways.

Noncardiac Adaptations: The Neurohumoral Hypothesis

A large number of neurohormones have been found to circulate in abnormal quantities in heart failure (Table 24–5). The natriuretic peptides, in particular, atrial natriuretic peptide (ANP) and B-type natriuretic peptide (BNP), are considered counter-regulatory because they tend to reduce right atrial pressure, systemic vascular resistance, aldosterone secretion, sympathetic nerve stimulation, and hypertrophy of cells and can enhance sodium excretion.[39,52] The predominant consequence of most neurohormone *release* in heart failure, however, is vasoconstriction coupled with salt and water

TABLE 24–5

Neurohormonal Changes in Heart Failure

Increased sympathetic nervous system activity (increased norepinephrine, epinephrine)
Increased endothelin
Increased arginine vasopressin
Increased renin and angiotensin II
Increased aldosterone
Increased neuropeptide Y
Increased atrial and B-type natriuretic peptides
Increased
  Insulin
  Cortisol
  Growth hormone (decreased insulinlike growth factor 1 [IGF-1])
  Tumor necrosis factor α (TNF-α)
  Interleukin-6
  Vasoactive intestinal peptide (VIP)
  Adrenomedullin
  Urodilantin
  Urotensin-II
  Cardiotrophin-I
Increased dopamine
Increased prostaglandins (PGI2, PGE2)
Increased vasodilator peptides (e.g., bradykinin)

PGE2, prostaglandin E_2; PGI2, prostaglandin I_2.
Note: Measurements in individual patients vary significantly and changes may not always be present.

retention. The regulation of body fluid volume is complex but has a primitive relation to many of the neurohormones and their propensity to facilitate retention of sodium and water while at the same time protecting perfusion pressure. The integrity of the arterial circulation as a function of cardiac output and systemic vascular resistance (SVR) is also determined by flexibility in renal sodium and water excretion.[53] Underfilling of the arterial bed by low cardiac output or vasodilation activates neuroendocrine reflexes that stimulate sodium and water retention. Sodium and water retention cease to be major problems after heart transplantation, indicating that there is no intrinsic renal dysfunction in heart failure. The kidney responds to a perceived reduction in arterial filling in an appropriate manner by retaining volume.

Decreases in blood pressure, stroke volume (pulse pressure), and perfusion (flow) in heart failure are sensed by mechanoreceptors in the left ventricle, carotid sinus, aortic arch, and renal afferent arterioles. When there is diminished activation of these receptors, as in heart failure, there is augmentation of sympathetic outflow, activation of the RAAS, and nonosmotic release of arginine vasopressin (AVP).[53] Heightened peripheral vasoconstriction occurs along with increased blood volume, thereby *restoring* circulatory integrity and perfusion pressure. Of course, neuroendocrine activation has many important actions at the cellular level, including facilitation of myocyte hypertrophy[35] and collagen synthesis.[54] Activation of the sympathetic nervous system contributes to tachycardia and arrhythmias and can be directly toxic to the myocardium.[55,56] In this sense, heart failure begins with pathological changes in the heart itself that may or may not produce symptoms. With increased sympathetic tone in heart failure, increased phosphorylation of the ryanodine component of the L calcium channel can occur, leading to abnormalities of Ca^{2+} activation.

As heart failure persists, there are important changes in the peripheral circulation with downregulation of the nitric oxide (NO) system. Under normal conditions, NO permits peripheral arteriole dilation and increased peripheral blood flow in response to exercise. As this system downregulates, peripheral dilation does not occur with exercise, the lack of appropriate blood flow limits exercise and decreased functional capacity. With exercise training, this system can be restored, and clinical status improved, even with no alteration of the heart.

Cardiac myocyte necrosis also occurs in response to low levels of angiotensin II.[57] Although neuroendocrine responses are not the primary cause of heart failure under most circumstances, they clearly contribute to the progression of the syndrome[58] (Fig. 24–2). The overly simplistic view that neurohormones in heart failure are a response to perceived *hypovolemia* is clearly incorrect.[59] Neuroendocrine mechanisms are now the targets of several important and successful therapeutic interventions in heart failure and hypertension[60] and have a key role in determining prognosis.[61] ACE inhibitors, β-adrenergic blockers, and aldosterone antagonists now have a prominent role in the treatment of heart failure, and new, more innovative neuroendocrine-blocking agents are being rapidly developed, adding strong support to the neurohumoral hypothesis.[58]

Norepinephrine It has long been recognized that patients with heart failure manifest signs and symptoms of a hyperadrenergic state. Vascular constriction, tachycardia, diaphoresis, and oliguria are manifestations of increased sympathetic drive. Starling's observations in 1897,[62] amplified in the early 1960s, predicted increased plasma NE levels in patients with heart failure.[63] Myocardial stores of NE were found to be depleted, but later studies by various investigators using the more sensitive radioenzymatic technique of plasma NE described a correlation with functional class[64] and extent of hemodynamic dysfunction.[65]

Norepinephrine synthesis begins in the body of the neuron with the synthesis of enzymes necessary to change from tyrosine to NE. The enzymes are transported down the neuron to the dendrites of the cell, where the actual synthetic steps take place. Dopamine

is synthesized and transported into storage vesicles, where the final synthetic steps occur. These storage vesicles are both large and small, the large vesicles containing additional peptides such as neuropeptide Y. Following discharge of an axonal action potential, exocytosis occurs, allowing the vesicle contents to be released into the synaptic cleft. The vast majority of the NE is then taken back up into the cell for storage and rerelease (uptake 1). Some NE is taken up by effector organs and metabolized (uptake 2), and only a small quantity is released into the plasma (≈ 5 percent), where it circulates as plasma NE. There are now microneurographic techniques than can be used to directly measure sympathetic traffic direction[66] and *spillover* techniques using tritiated norepinephrine, that can measure specific organ sympathetic activity.[67] In the course of heart failure, increased cardiac sympathetic traffic precedes more generalized sympathetic activation. Plasma NE level has served as a useful research and prognostic guide for the study of patients with heart failure. It is overly simplistic to consider NE to be *good* or *bad* for patients with heart failure. Those with severe New York Heart Association (NYHA) class IV heart failure can be

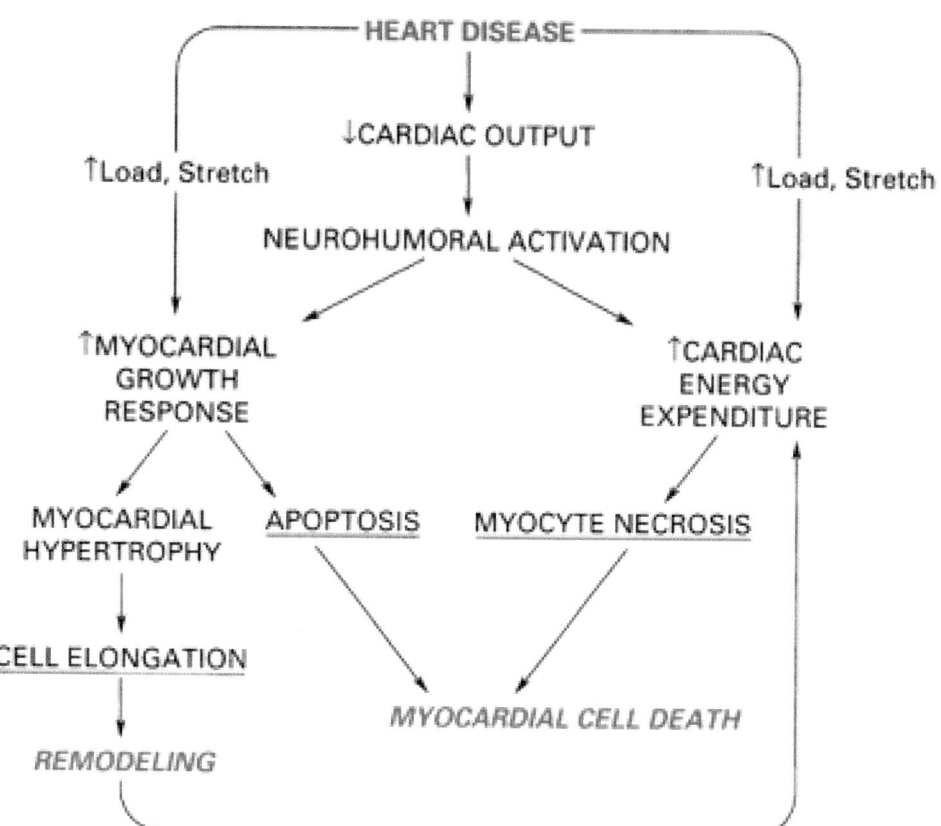

FIGURE 24–2. Possible mechanisms by which overloading can cause progressive deterioration of the heart (*cardiomyopathy of overload*). Several mechanisms, including myocyte stretch, activate a growth response that initiates myocardial hypertrophy in the overloaded heart (*left*). The same growth response can also activate signal transduction systems that cause programmed cell death (apoptosis). The hypertrophic response to overload, by causing sarcomeres to be added in series, can also lead to cell elongation and so accelerate remodeling; the resulting increase in wall tension, along with the overload itself (*right*), increases cardiac energy expenditure that, in the overloaded heart, can accelerate myocyte necrosis. Reduced cardiac output activates neurohumoral responses (*center*), which, by increasing afterload and β-adrenergic stimulation of the heart, also increase cardiac energy expenditure. Because many mediators of the neurohumoral response to a fall in cardiac output promote myocardial cell growth, neurohumoral activation can also accelerate both apoptosis and remodeling.

quite dependent on catecholamine support and sometimes require a continuous dobutamine infusion to maintain suitable organ perfusion prior to heart transplantation. However, there is no question that NE is toxic to the myocardium and is responsible in part for progressive LV remodeling.[68,69] NE is thus a double-edged sword in heart failure (Table 24–6).

The Renin-Angiotensin-Aldosterone System The RAAS plays an important role in the pathogenesis of heart failure (Fig. 24–3), and consistent benefit has been derived from ACE-inhibitor therapy in patients with heart failure. The mechanisms responsible for the release of renin from the renal cortex have been exhaustively studied[70] and include sympathetic drive to the kidneys, hyponatremic perfusate to the macula densa of the kidney, and use of diuretics and a low sodium diet, which tends to promote a relative volume contraction. Renin proteolytic enzyme has little biologic activity, but it interacts with angiotensinogen to split off two amino acids to form angiotensin I. This is then cleaved by ACE (distributed widely in the vascular system, especially the lungs) to produce angiotensin II, a peptide with a vast range of biologic activities. Angiotensin II in turn stimulates release of aldosterone from the adrenal cortex, which also has an array of biologic effects, including sodium and water retention, kaliuresis, and enhanced collagen turnover and organ remodeling (Fig. 24–4).

There now are at least four recognized angiotensin II receptors, but much of the activity is subserved by the AT_1 receptor. The AT_1 actions include arterial vasoconstriction, cell growth (hypertrophy), apoptosis in myocytes, polydipsia, NE release, sensitization of blood vessels to NE, AVP release, and aldosterone release. The AT_2 receptor appears to subserve somewhat counter-regulatory effects, including antigrowth/anti-remodeling, apoptosis, vasodilation, and activation of the kinin–nitric oxide–cyclic 3',5'-guanosine monophosphate (cGMP) system.[71] Because AT_1 receptor-blocking drugs (so-called *angiotensin II receptor blockers* [*ARBs*]) increase angiotensin II levels, they can indirectly activate unoccupied AT_2 receptor activity. Angiotensin II levels tend to *escape* the pharmacologic effects of chronic ACE inhibition irrespective of dosage,[72] and can stimulate AT_2 and AT_2 receptor activity. It is also now clear that the RAAS is not solely a classic endocrine system but has autocrine and

paracrine activity that can be particularly important in cardiovascular, brain, and renal tissue. With our current knowledge that ACE inhibitors remarkably reduce all cardiovascular events and even limit the onset of new diabetes mellitus in patients with cardiovascular disease,[73] it is difficult to overstate the role of the RAAS in the pathogenesis of heart and vascular disease, including progressive heart failure.[74–76]

Arginine Vasopressin Patients with heart failure sometimes have water retention in excess of sodium retention, leading to hyponatremia. The hyponatremia is caused in part by nonosmotic release of AVP, which acts on the kidney to reduce of free water clearance. Release of AVP in heart failure probably occurs by means of activation of carotid baroreceptors.[53] Plasma AVP levels are often but not always increased in patients with LV dysfunction[77] and heart failure.[78] AVP acts on the V_2 receptors in the collecting duct of the kidney via adenylate cyclase to translocate aquaporin-2 water channels from cytoplasmic vesicles to the apical surface of the collecting duct. AVP also increases aquaporin-2 synthesis. Activation of V_1 receptors in vascular tissue contributes to heightened vascular resistance and myocardial dysfunction in heart failure.[79] Indeed, hyponatremia is associated with a worsened outcome in heart failure. It will be of interest if these vasopressin antagonists can reduce hyponatremia and benefit outcome. Recognition of the role of AVP in the pathogenesis of heart failure has led to the development and investigation of selective V_2 and dual V_1-V_2 receptor blockers (such as conivaptan and tolvaptan) as potential adjunctive treatment.

Natriuretic Peptides A family of natriuretic peptides including ANP, BNP, and C-type natriuretic peptide (CNP) is encoded by separate genes, each with a tissue-specific distribution, regulation, and biologic activity.[52] These natriuretic peptides are often increased in patients with heart failure. ANP is a 28-amino-acid peptide that is normally synthesized and stored in the atria and to some extent in the ventricles. It is released into the circulation during atrial distention. BNP is synthesized mainly by the ventricles and is released in LV dysfunction or early heart failure, following cleavage (presumably by a serine protease, corrin) from the propeptide to BNP and NT-proBNP (both can be detected by commercial assays). For the most part, these peptides act via guanylate cyclase receptors to promote vasodilation (ANP, BNP, CNP) and natriuresis (ANP, BNP). They also can attenuate NE release, RAAS activity, and the growth/hypertrophy of target cells—hence the term *counter-regulatory hormones*.

Patients with heart failure are relatively resistant to the natriuretic effects of these peptides when they are administered exogenously, perhaps because of decreased sodium delivery to the collecting duct as a result of diminished glomerular filtration or increased sodium reabsorption in the proximal tubule.[53] Nevertheless, BNP infusion has a beneficial hemodynamic effect in heart failure,[80] and drugs designed to inhibit degradation of natriuretic peptides (so-called *neutral endopeptidase inhibitors*, or vasopeptidase inhibitors such as omapatrilat) have been combined with ACE-inhibitor activity as potential therapy for hypertension and heart failure.

Endothelin Endothelins are a family of vasoconstrictor peptides produced by vascular endothelial cells.[81] Their physiologic function is as yet unclear. Although blood levels are increased in patients with heart failure,[82] endothelin-1 (ET-1) is more of a paracrine than an

---

TABLE 24–6

Favorable and Detrimental Effects of Sympathetic Drive in Patients with Heart Failure

Favorable	
↑ HR, improved cardiac output ↑ contractility, improved cardiac output maintenance of perfusion pressure	NYHA class IV
Detrimental	
Progressive LV remodeling	NYHA class I–III
LV hypertrophy → failure	
↑ myocardial $M\dot{V}_{O_2}$ arrhythmias	
↑SVR → ↑ afterload	
Na$^+$ and H$_2$O retention, facilitation of renin release, oliguria	

LV, left ventricular; $M\dot{V}_{O_2}$, myocardial oxygen consumption; Na$^+$, sodium; SVR, systemic vascular resistance.

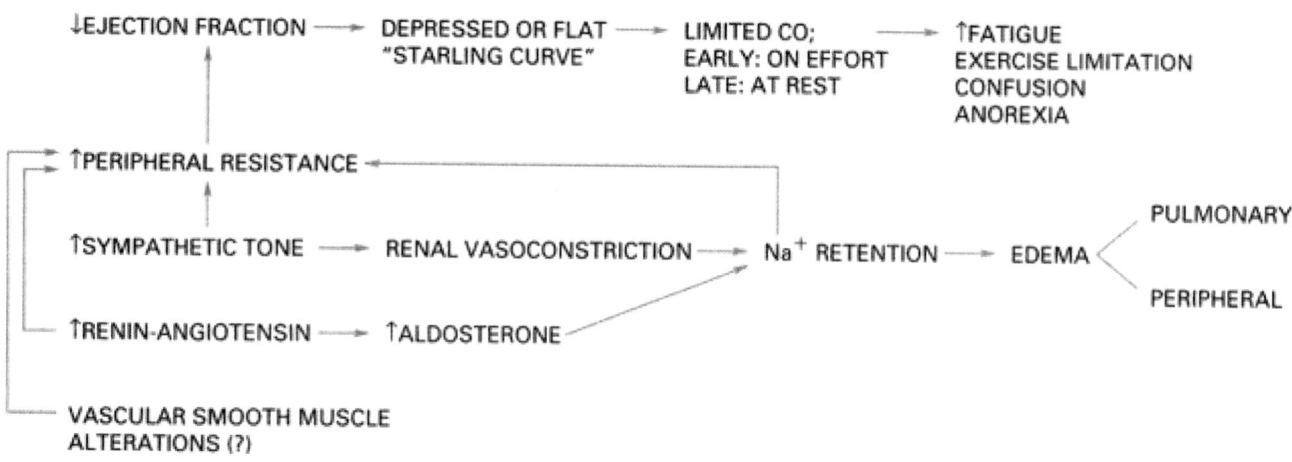

FIGURE 24–3. Schema of events in congestive heart failure leading to symptoms. Note that fatigue and other symptoms of limited cardiac output are primarily related to decreased ejection, whereas peripheral and pulmonary edema are related to sodium and water retention from increased sympathetic tone and increased renin-angiotensin-aldosterone. See text for details. CO, cardiac output; Na⁺, sodium.

endocrine hormone. In heart failure, myocardial tissue ET-1 levels are increased, possibly more as a result of decreased clearance by the lungs than of increased synthesis. Endothelial cells synthesize ET-1 rapidly and convert so-called *big endothelin-1* into endothelin by an endothelin-converting enzyme. The synthesis of ET-1 is enhanced by

angiotensin II, NE, growth factors, insulin, hypoxia, oxidized low-density lipoproteins (oxLDLs), shear stress, and thrombin.[83] Its synthesis is antagonized by ANP and prostaglandins.

Endothelin acts on at least two types of G protein-coupled receptors, A and B. The ET-A receptor subserves smooth muscle vasocon-

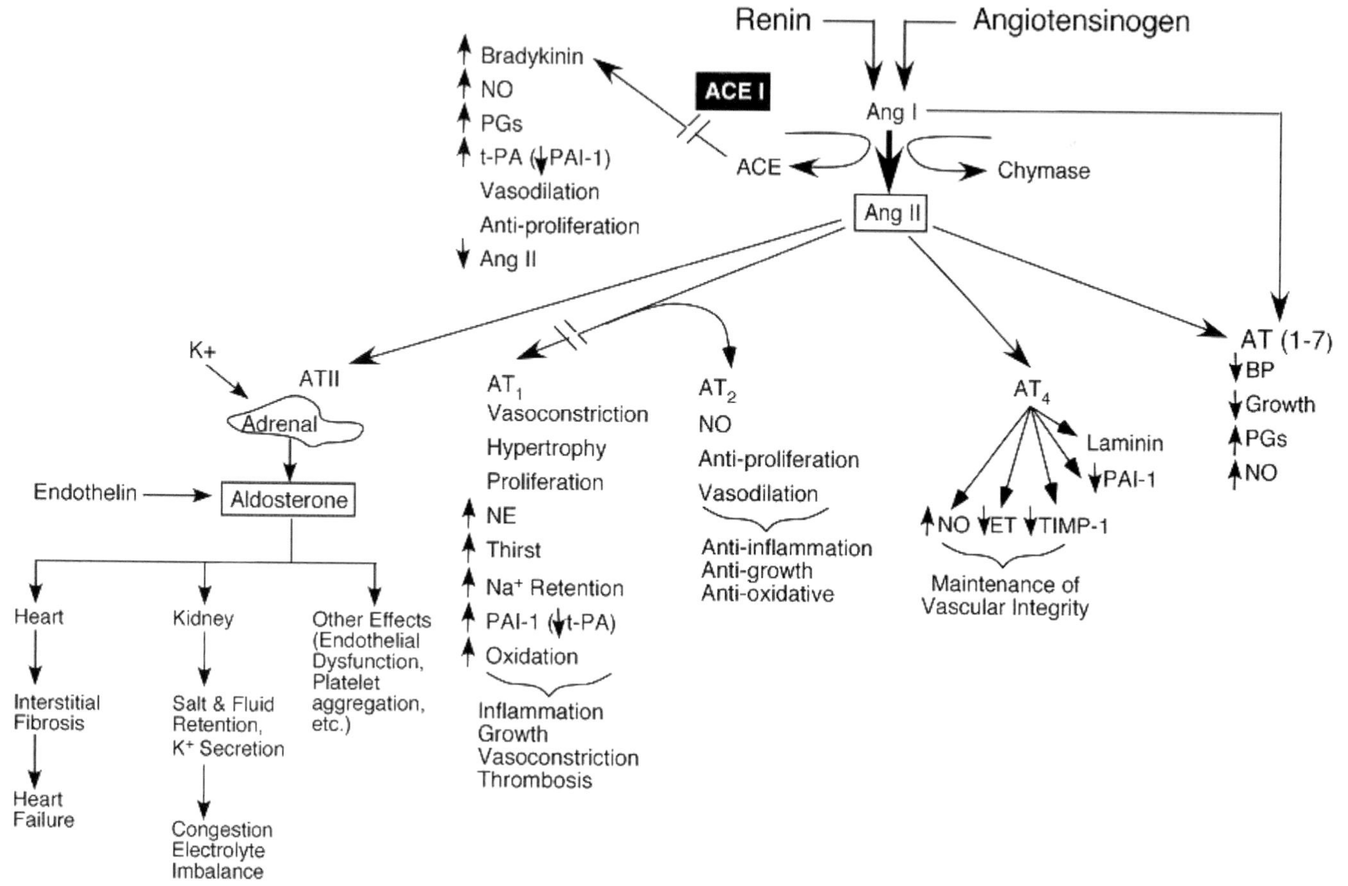

FIGURE 24–4. The Renin-Angiotensin-Aldosterone System. Ang II, angiotensin II; AT₁, angiotensin II receptor-1; AT₂, angiotensin II receptor-2; AT₄, angiotensin II receptor-4; BP, blood pressure; ET, endothelin; K⁺, potassium; Na⁺, sodium; NE, norepinephrine NO, nitric oxide; PAI-1, plasminogen activator inhibitor type 1; PGs, prostaglandins; TIMP-1, tissue inhibitor of metalloproteinase; t-PA, tissue plasminogen activator. *Source: From Kalidindi SR, Tang WW, Francis GS. Drug Insight: Aldosterone-receptor antagonist in heart failure—the journey continues. Nat Clin Pract Cardiovasc Med 2007;4(7):368–378. Reproduced with permission from the publisher and author.*

striction and cell proliferation/hypertrophy and mainly resides on vascular smooth muscle cells. The ET-B receptor, which is mainly endothelial, subserves vasodilation that is probably mediated by a variety of mechanisms including increased production of nitric oxide and prostaglandins and activation of potassium channels. ET-1 also can act on the heart to cause hypertrophy, on the adrenal gland to release aldosterone, and on the kidney to promote sodium and water retention.[83] The importance of ET-1 in the pathogenesis of heart failure is highlighted by the development and clinical testing of several new endothelin antagonists. Bosentan, a dual ET_A-ET_B receptor blocker, failed to demonstrate a survival benefit in patients with heart failure, but is marketed for the treatment of primary pulmonary hypertension.

Other Neurohormones

Other neurohormones that can play a role in the pathogenesis of heart failure, include neuropeptide Y, vasointestinal peptide, bradykinin, prostaglandins, adrenomedullin, urodilatin, cardiotropin-1, and urotensin-II, and some of them can emerge as *systems* to block or enhance in heart failure, depending on their primary function.

Inflammatory Responses: The Inflammatory Hypothesis

Cellular Responses

In recent years, it has been widely recognized that there is a strong association between inflammation and cardiac diseases. Erythrocyte sedimentation rate (ESR),[84] C-reactive protein,[85] tumor necrosis factor alpha (TNF-α), and interleukin 6 (IL-6) have all been demonstrated to *predict* heart failure.[86] Often, these inflammatory markers are said to be "significant predictors of heart failure independent of established risk factors." Circulating levels of TNF-α are increased in cachetic patients with chronic heart failure, and this elevation is associated with marked activation of the RAAS.[87] When TNF-α is overexpressed in mice, posttranslational processing of the TNF promotes adverse cardiac remodeling.[88] When patients with heart failure and severe mitral regurgitation have mitral valve repair, TNF-α expression is reversed and there is less LV remodeling.[89] Although TNF-α is primarily produced by macrophages and leukocytes, it is also produced by cardiac myocytes and fibroblasts. A substantial body of experimental literature supports a role for inflammation in the pathogenesis of heart failure, remodeling, and cachexia. Until we have treatment that we understand how to use in this syndrome, the inflammatory hypothesis will be difficult to test.

Cytokines

Circulating TNF-α, a proinflammatory cytokine, is increased in cachetic patients with chronic heart failure.[87] Proinflammatory cytokines such as circulating TNF-α can play an important role in modulating abnormal myocardial structure and function in late stages of heart failure.[90] This group of proinflammatory cytokines also includes interleukin 1 (IL-1) and interleukin 6 (IL-6), proteins which are largely products of macrophages and lymphocytes, and can, under some circumstances, be expressed by myocardial tissue. Each of these cytokines can influence the expression of the other two, and each can modulate cardiovascular performance when expressed in sufficiently high levels. A continuous infusion of circulating TNF-α leads to time-dependent depression in LV function in an animal model[91] and provokes a hypertrophic growth response in adult cardiac myocytes.[92] When synthesized in large quantities, circulating TNF-α spills over into the circulation and acts as an endocrine *hormone* leading to meta-bolic wasting and cachexia.[93] Overexpression of circulating TNF-α in a transgenic mouse model leads to a phenotype consistent with cardiomyopathy.[94] Circulating TNF-α acts by means of two different membrane receptors. The transduction signal pathways are not fully understood, but in the heart they can mediate cell growth, negative inotropy, and apoptosis. Thus far, inhibitors of circulating TNF-α have not been shown to alter the outcome of heart failure in man, despite the beneficial effects in animal studies.

Nitric Oxide, Endothelial Dysfunction, and Oxidative Stress

The balance between antioxidant and prooxidant systems establishes the *redox state* in cells that is intricately balanced and is used in all physiologic processes. Although reactive oxygen species (ROS) can modulate cell function, receptor signaling, and immune responses under physiological conditions, when generated in excess, appear to serve as central mediators of progressive cellular injury (*oxidative stress hypothesis*[95]). Prolonged exposure of ROS can lead to activation of specific pathways of oxidant stress with available substrates (such as NO), leading to enzyme activation/deactivation, DNA breakage, and lipid peroxidation, which are ultimately responsible for subsequent myocyte apoptosis and pathological remodeling seen in the heart failure phenotype.[96] However, the specific pathways implicating ROS in the pathophysiology of heart failure is still under investigation.[97]

Over the past decades, evidence has supported the role for heightened oxidative stress in the pathophysiology of heart failure.[98] Biomarkers of oxidative stress, albeit nonspecific, were often elevated in patients with established heart failure.[99] The levels of oxidative stress and severity of heart failure were often correlated and irrespectively of the underlying etiology.[98] However, the precise mechanisms contributing to oxidative stress in heart failure is multifactorial. Catecholamines and angiotensin II promote prooxidant activities within the myocardium, including enhanced superoxide (O_2^-) formation and generation of NO-derived oxidants as a necessary consequence of increased myocardial oxygen consumption. Several recent studies also observed an association between insulin resistance and heart failure in the absence of overt diabetes.[100,101] The role of insulin resistance in heart failure remains unclear, although subclinical ischemia caused by endothelial dysfunction can play an important role, and can explain why the presence of insulin resistance has found to be an independent prognostic factor.

Animal and human studies indicate that endothelium-dependent vasodilation is abnormal in a number of disease states, including atherosclerosis, hypertension, heart failure, hyperhomocysteinemia, insulin resistance, and hypercholesterolemia. Endothelial dysfunction has been demonstrated in experimental animals[102] and in patients with heart failure.[103] As already discussed briefly, such endothelial dysfunction in heart failure (i.e., failure to vasodilate in response to a specific endothelial-dependent vasodilator) can be caused by a reduced release of nitric oxide during stimulation. The basal release of nitric oxide can be preserved or even enhanced in heart failure[104] and can be compensatory by antagonizing neuroendocrine vasoconstrictor forces. However, impairment of endothelium-dependent peripheral vasodilation can be a factor contributing to exercise intolerance in patients with chronic heart failure, perhaps by limiting nutritive skeletal muscle flow during exercise.[105] This dysfunction of the endothelium can be related to deconditioning in later stages of heart failure, and with training, it is largely reversible. Further, abnormal endothelium-dependent responses in heart failure are reversible following heart transplantation.[106]

The roles of nitric oxide and nitric oxide synthase in the failing heart are much more complex and new data are beginning to emerge.[107,108] Nitric oxide has been considered to be present as a freely diffusible molecule, which inhibits the positive inotropic response to β-adrenergic stimulation in the failing heart.[109,110] Smaller physiologic amounts of nitric oxide produced by constitutive nitric oxide synthase (cNOS, or nitrous oxide synthase [NOS3]) are necessary for normal function and have an antioxidant effect that can protect cells. The inducible isoform of nitric oxide synthase (iNOS or NOS2) is overexpressed in human heart failure[111] and therefore can contribute to worsening heart failure, as high levels of nitric oxide in the heart can exert proapoptotic and cytotoxic effects. Although there is decreased myocardial nitric oxide synthesis during decompensation of experimental heart failure,[112] direct inhibition of nitric oxide synthase can be beneficial in the setting of cardiogenic shock.[113] Thus the roles of nitric oxide are quite variable, very important, and depend on conditions.

Nitric oxide can act in subcellular signaling compartments or modules.[114] Furthermore, covalent modification of cysteine thiol moieties of proteins (S-nitrosylation[115]) can be an important second messenger signaling process, working in parallel ROS and nitrogen species. Therefore, disruption of this cyclic GMP signaling process can be caused by either increased formation of ROS or decreased production of reactive nitrogen species (so-called *nitroso-redox imbalance*).[116] Heart failure is thus a composite term that encompasses several distinct syndromes, some of which coexist in the same patient.

▌ ❚ STRUCTURAL ADAPTATIONS AND MALADAPTATIONS: THE REMODELING HYPOTHESIS

Heart failure is often preceded by a substantial period of *myocardial* dysfunction during which cardiac pumping function and cardiac output (at least while at rest) can be maintained by compensatory mechanisms that include myocardial hypertrophy and ventricular dilatation. For this reason, in the early stages, patients can have little or no limitations or symptoms. Initially, the cardiac output can be within the normal range at rest but fails to increase or can even decline during exercise or stress. Ultimately, the cardiac output is decreased even at rest. Associated changes include an increase in SVR at rest and a failure of the SVR to decrease with increased metabolic needs.

When one portion of the ventricle is disabled, an increase in intraventricular volume slowly occurs. This involves increased myocyte length, with the limit being at the level of the sarcomere at 2.2 μm. With systolic overload, compensatory hypertrophy occurs with the addition of sarcomeres in parallel, leading to a lateral thickening of the myocyte, although sarcomere length does not change.

Acute ventricular dilatation is limited by the fixed length of the sarcomere, which at 2.2 μm attains maximum force. Beyond this point, stiffness of the sarcomere and the myocardium becomes very large, and resting tension rises to high levels. Such acute dilatation can lead to relative *side-to-side* slippage of myocytes. When distending forces become chronic, addition of new sarcomeres in series also occurs. Dilatation of the ventricle also adds to the load by means of the Laplace relation. Tension in the wall rises with increased volume at the same pressure. This results in some lateral growth of myocytes, although elongation is the major alteration. Whether new myocytes are also formed from stem cells has been suggested, replacing divid-

ing cells, but this is very controversial. In addition, functional mitral regurgitation can result from excessive ventricular volume that prevents valve closure, and this adds to the volume overload. When increased systolic tension occurs, myocyte hypertrophy that occurs by the laying down of sarcomeres in parallel is accomplished by biochemical alterations in both the contractile proteins and activating membrane systems (see Chap. 5). The regulation of sarcomere assembly is not well understood, but clearly mechanical forces must be sensed which in turn alter gene transcription by means of complex stretch-activated pathways.[117]

Although overstretch of sarcomeres can rarely be present very transiently, it does not appear to be an important primary mechanism of chronic heart failure. There is evidence, however, that excessive stretch of myocytes can lead to myocyte death, apparently by the process of local activation of angiotensin resulting in apoptosis (programmed cell death), which can lead to further heart failure.[50,118] The effects of the law of Laplace with ventricular dilatation were noted earlier. Nonuniformity of myocardial contraction and functional mitral regurgitation also contribute to heart failure. The discoordinated contraction is particularly troublesome for patients with underlying cardiac dysfunction. Resynchronization by pacing the left ventricle improves mechanic-energetic efficiency and systolic function and reduces systolic wall stress (see Chap. 23).[119,120]

Myocardial Hypertrophy

Hypertrophy of myocardial myocytes occurs to meet the demand of increased rate of use of mechanical energy. It is basically a response to sustained hemodynamic overloading of the heart, be it a volume or pressure overload or a combination of the two. Ischemic heart disease leads to a reduction of contractile tissue, ventricular dilatation, and a volume overload on the remaining viable myocytes. In this sense, it is a form of volume overload hypertrophy. Up to a point, the increased mass of cardiac muscle is beneficial in terms of normalizing wall stress and providing for a larger number of contractile elements (sarcomeres).

The heart demonstrates remarkable plasticity in response to a variety of growth factors and hemodynamic loads.[35] Isolated cell deformation is a sufficient stimulus for induction of hypertrophic growth, but the modulating role of angiotensin II, norepinephrine, altered membrane ion channels, and numerous growth factors is of obvious importance. Changing loading conditions appear to be the primary driving force behind myocardial hypertrophy in heart failure, and other factors likely act as modulators or facilitators of the process. Hyperplasia, or an increase in new myocardial cells, can occur to some extent under conditions of excessive loading or myocyte loss.[121] However, the capacity for new cardiac myocytes to form is limited, and whether they are functionally useful is unknown. Rather, the primary response to altered load is the assembly of new working units or sarcomeres per myocardial cell. In general, pressure overload results in replication of sarcomeres in parallel, whereas volume overload leads to new sarcomeres both in parallel and in series. There is hyperplasia of fibroblasts,[54,122–125] which outnumber cardiac myocytes by 3:1 to 4:1. It is the fibroblasts that are the major source of the reparative and replacement collagen when myocytes are lost in the evolution of heart failure.

Other changes in the myocardium are occurring simultaneously, and hypertrophy is only one important factor. Biochemical changes, phenotypic changes in protein synthesis, altered excitation-contraction, slower velocity of shortening caused by a slower myosin, and reduced β-adrenergic receptor density are all occurring simultaneously. Reduced velocity of contraction, delayed time to peak tension, and slower relaxation are observed in the myocardium of failing hearts. All these factors likely converge to produce clinical decompensation. Delayed ventricular relaxation can limit filling, leading to heightened filling pressure, pulmonary congestion, and shortness of breath. Force development and shortening capacity remain intact in the face of hypertrophy, and only in very late failure does contractility or contractile force decline. What ultimately happens to the patient can depend on the acuteness or chronicity of the load, the extent of hypertrophy and fibrosis, the amount of myocyte loss, the heart rate, synchrony of atrioventricular contraction and a host of invisible perturbations occurring at the level of the cell.

Diastole is usually divided into several mechanical phases (Fig. 24–5). Investigation of patients with heart failure and normal systolic function, usually by echo, often indicates LV hypertrophy and abnor-

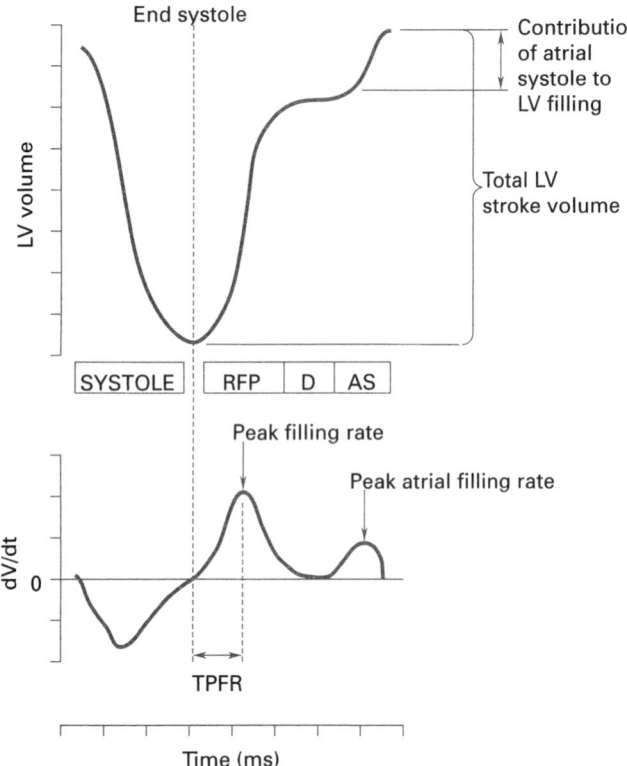

FIGURE 24–5. Idealized plot of left ventricular (LV) volume versus time (*top*) and the rate of change of volume (*dV/dt*) versus time (*bottom*), such as might be obtained from contrast or radionuclide ventriculographic studies. The representative cardiac cycle begins at end-diastole. Subsequent events, as depicted by the bars in the center of the figure, are (*1*) systole, during which LV volume decreases to a minimum and *dV/dt* reaches its maximum, and (*2*) diastole, the beginning of which is signaled by the opening of the mitral valve and the onset of LV filling. Diastole has three distinct phases in normal individuals: (1) the rapid filling phase (RFP), during which the left ventricle fills rapidly but passively, and the peak filling rate occurs; (2) diastasis (D), during which relatively little left ventricular volume change occurs; and (3) atrial systole (AS), in which active atrial contraction fills the left ventricle to its end-diastolic volume. The diastolic parameters that have been derived from such analysis are the peak filling rate, the time to peak filling rate (TPFR), the percent contribution of atrial systole, and the first third filling fraction. *Source: Labovitz AJ, Pearson AC. Evaluation of left ventricular diastolic function: clinical relevance and recent Doppler echocardiographic insights. Am Heart J. 1987;114:836–849. Reproduced with permission from the publisher and authors.*

mal diastolic function, with concomitant left atrial enlargement. However, there is no agreement as to what constitutes abnormal diastolic function. Disturbances include alterations in relaxation (reduced rate of decline in wall tension), an upward shift of the LV diastolic pressure-volume relationship (a decrease in LV diastolic distensibility) (Fig. 24–6), discordant wall motion during isovolumic relaxation, and altered ventricular inflow velocity. These measurements are influenced by loading conditions, ischemia, heart rate, and age, making it difficult to determine the actual contribution of diastolic dysfunction to heart failure. This is why some prefer the phrase "heart failure with intact or normal systolic function." Nevertheless, disturbances in diastolic function are common in patients with heart failure and are multifactorial. Diastolic impairment is frequently symptomatic in patients with LV hypertrophy, coronary artery disease, and diabetes mellitus. There also can be impairment of diastolic function because of an infiltrative process such as amyloid or restrictive cardiomyopathy. For any given end-diastolic volume, there is often a higher LV end-diastolic pressure, indicating increased chamber stiffness and a smaller LV cavity size. With atrial dilatation, atrial fibrillation can develop, resulting in a rapid heart rate and reduced diastolic ventricular filling time, and this can result in resultant acute pulmonary edema in such patients.

The Cardiac Interstitium

Collagen and the interstitium are normally in a steady state but increase during hypertrophy and following loss of myocytes because of myocardial injury. In heart failure, the interstitial space includes reparative and interstitial fibrosis. Contrary to previous concepts, the interstitium is a very dynamic structure, with both matrix removal and synthesis occurring simultaneously. Connective tissue remodeling, either physiologic or pathologic, is in most cases a homeostatic process between collagen synthesis and collagen degradation by matrix metalloprotease (MMP). The matrix of the heart is a very complex scaffolding composed of fibrillar and ground substance proteins (collagen) that pattern around and between myocytes in a very precise and organized pattern. The matrix likely plays a very important role in maintaining an ideal ventricular shape.[123] Changes in the cardiac *skeleton* can contribute to impairment of both diastolic and systolic function.[126] In the failing human heart resulting from advanced coronary disease (so-called *ischemic cardiomyopathy*), fibrosis is the major part of LV remodeling. Infarct scars can account for 30 percent of fibrosis, whereas microscopic fibrosis remote from the infarct can account for 70 percent of the total fibrous tissue found in the ventricles.[122] In general, interstitial loci of fibrosis are the *tombstones* of lost myocytes. It is likely that increased MMPs contribute to ventricular dilatation in heart failure.[127] Tissue inhibitors of MMPs (TIMPs) exist in the myocardium and are regulated independently of MMPs,[127] an observation with potentially important therapeutic implications. Enhanced protease activity in heart failure contributes to fibrillar collagen degradation, setting the stage for weakened connective tissue and disrupted organ integrity, and ventricular remodeling.

The growth of the interstitium in response to pressure and volume overload is highly complex and involves fibroblasts and their ability to sense altered mechanical forces. Hormones, including the RAAS[54] and endothelin,[128] also facilitate the production of collagen through their interaction with fibroblasts. Once abnormal loading conditions are removed, connective tissue hypertrophy regresses more slowly than myocyte hypertrophy. The importance of this once-considered inert ground substance has emerged over the past 15 years and is now clear that the

SYSTOLIC FAILURE

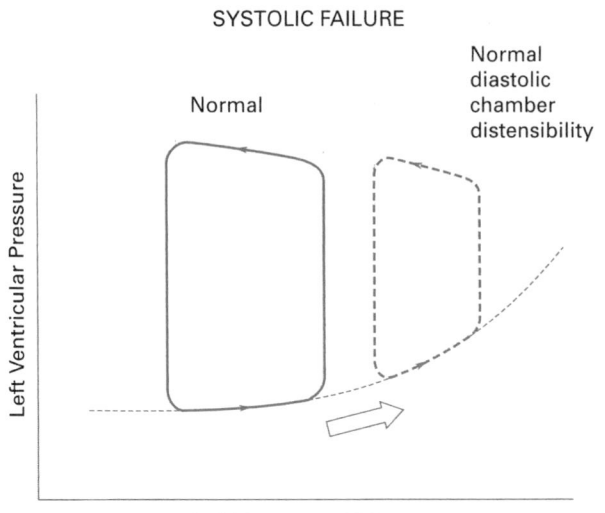

DIASTOLIC FAILURE

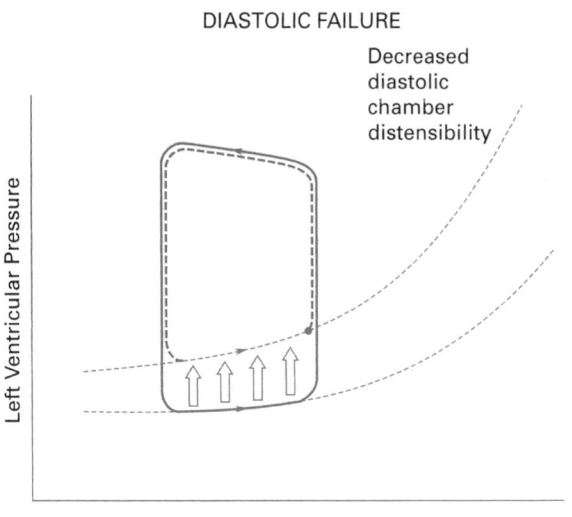

FIGURE 24–6. The left panel shows a schematized left ventricular (LV) pressure-volume loop from a patient with primary systolic failure. A normal LV pressure-volume loop (*solid loop*) is shown on the left portion of the curve; the transition to inotropic failure (*dashed loop*) is shown on the right. Systolic failure is manifest as an increase in LV end-systolic volume and as a reduction in the extent of shortening (stroke volume). LV end-diastolic pressure (LVEDP) is increased because LV volume is increased. As indicated by the arrow, the diastolic portion of the pressure-volume loop has simply shifted to the right, along the same diastolic pressure-volume relationship; thus no change in the distensibility of the left ventricle has occurred. The right panel shows an LV pressure-volume loop from a patient with primary diastolic failure (*dashed loop*). Note that the LVEDP is the same as that in the patient with primary inotropic failure, as denoted by the heavy dot on both pressure-volume loops. In the right panel, however, this is caused by an upward shift of the LV diastolic pressure-volume relationship (*arrows*), which indicates a decrease in LV diastolic distensibility such that a higher diastolic pressure is required to achieve the same diastolic volume. In this patient, no change in end-diastolic volume or systolic shortening has occurred. *Source: Lorell BH. Left ventricular diastolic pressure-volume relations: understanding and managing congestive heart failure. Heart Failure 1988;4:206–223. Reproduced with permission from the publisher and author.*

cardiac interstitium is very important in the syndrome of heart failure, contributing in many ways to the structural and functional alterations.

INTEGRATIVE PATHOPHYSIOLOGY WITH OTHER ORGAN SYSTEMS

【 】 CARDIOPULMONARY CONNECTIONS

Dyspnea, Orthopnea, and Paroxysmal Nocturnal Dyspnea

Pulmonary dysfunction is common in patients with heart failure and also can contribute to exercise intolerance. The amount of intrathoracic space available for ventilation can be decreased by alveolar and interstitial edema, by pleural effusions, or by an increase in blood volume. Increased pulmonary vascular congestion decreases lung compliance and increases the work of breathing. Excessive ventilation including an increased $V_E/\dot{V}_{O_2}$ slope during exercise is a hallmark of heart failure and has important prognostic implications.[129] Acute reduction in pulmonary capillary wedge pressure has no effect on the augmented ventilatory response, and the extent of excessive ventilation does not relate to either resting or exercise pulmonary capillary wedge pressure.

Exercise Intolerance

Many factors limit increased cardiac output during exercise in patients with heart failure, including a reduced myocardial force-frequency response, inability to fully use the Starling effect, and chronotropic incompetence. These limitations of cardiac performance are combined with endothelial dysfunction in the peripheral arterioles,

leading to impaired vasodilation and reduced nutritive skeletal muscle blood flow. Disuse atrophy of skeletal muscles also occurs. The latter effects appear to be excessively dependent on a glycolytic metabolism,[130] in part because of reduced metabolic efficiency in performing external work. Additional mechanisms include changes in muscle fiber recruitment, selective atrophy of oxidative fibers, and physical deconditioning. The mitochondrial content of skeletal muscle is reduced in heart failure.[131] Increased expression of the inducible isoform of nitric oxide synthase in skeletal muscle is correlated with reduced mitochondrial creatine kinase expression and exercise intolerance.[132] Apoptosis is frequently found in skeletal muscle of patients with heart failure and is also associated with exercise impairment.[133] Of importance, exercise capacity and EF are very poorly correlated in heart failure, suggesting that impairment in limited cardiac output is not the dominant reason for exercise intolerance.

Potential mechanisms responsible for exercise intolerance in heart failure are numerous. Exertional symptoms generally correlate with reduced maximal exercise capacity,[134] although exertional symptoms frequently underestimate the severity of functional disability. It is important to note that left ventricular ejection fraction does not correlate well with exercise tolerance; the latter can be better related to blood flow to the muscles.

【 】 CARDIORENAL CONNECTIONS

Salt and Water Retention

Renal retention of sodium and water, resulting in signs and symptoms of fluid retention, has long been a hallmark of heart failure. The precise mechanism whereby the heart signals the kidney in the early stages of heart failure to retain sodium and water is still unknown, although in the late stages reduced cardiac output and impaired renal blood flow are likely playing a major role.

In early heart failure, when normal cardiac output is maintained by means of compensatory mechanisms and renal blood flow is not reduced, some sodium retention still occurs. Curiously, some patients with advanced heart failure may not demonstrate peripheral edema or ascites. This suggests that in some cases, counter-regulatory natriuretic peptides can be acting to maintain natriuresis. Perhaps release of ANP and BNP in the early stages of heart failure can offset the tendency to retain sodium. Salt and water retention usually becomes evident in heart failure as peripheral vasoconstriction occurs in the face of a falling cardiac output. This is associated with activation of the RAAS. Angiotensin II preserves glomerular filtration rate in patients with heart failure even when renal perfusion is severely compromised, independent of its propensity to support systemic blood pressure.[135] Intraglomerular hydraulic pressure and therefore glomerular filtration are preserved by the constriction of glomerular efferent arterioles through angiotensin II.[136] Increased intrarenal formation of angiotensin II during a reduction in renal artery pressure maintains efferent arteriolar tone and, consequently, the effective filtration pressure.[137] The resulting high level of filtration fraction favors changes in the postglomerular circulation that promote avid proximal fluid reabsorption by means of elevated peritubular capillary oncotic pressure.[136] Increased aldosterone acts principally on the cortical collecting tubules to conserve sodium, with a concomitant loss of potassium. Because the plasma volume and blood pressure vary considerably from day to day, there is no consistent relation between the RAAS and fluid retention.

The mechanisms of sodium and water retention in heart failure are multiple and complex (Table 24–7). Sympathetic nervous system traffic to the kidney favors sodium retention. Increased AVP activity diminishes free water clearance. The prostaglandins normally dilate afferent glomerular arterioles to enhance intraglomerular flow and pressure, and their inhibition by nonsteroidal antiinflammatory agents (NSAIDs) can lead to a marked reduction in filtration and sodium retention. Enhanced sodium reabsorption of heart failure also occurs in the ascending loop of Henle, as well as in the cortical and medullary collecting ducts. Eventually, plasma volume expansion occurs, but at the expense of circulatory and tissue congestion.

❚ ❳ CARDIONEURAL CONNECTIONS

Sleep Apnea

Severe untreated sleep-disordered breathing can further impair LV function, leading to arterial oxyhemoglobin desaturation and arrhythmias.[138] Central sleep apnea can occur in as many as 40 percent of patients with heart failure, and 10 percent suffer from obstructive sleep apnea.[139] Obstructive sleep apnea increases afterload and heart rate during sleep but is responsive to continuous positive airway pressure.[140]

Cheyne-Stokes Respiration

Periodic breathing (Cheyne-Stokes) is common in patients with severe heart failure and is associated with a poor prognosis.[141] It can be caused by lung edema, which can excite carbon dioxide responses through vagal reflexes. Enhanced sensitivity to carbon dioxide can predispose some patients with heart failure to the development of central sleep apnea.[142] Successful treatment of Cheyne-Stokes respi-

ration with nocturnal nasal oxygen improves sleep, exercise tolerance, and cognitive function in patients with heart failure.[143]

❚ ❳ CARDIOMETABOLIC CONNECTIONS: CARDIAC CACHEXIA

Obesity is a known risk factor for cardiovascular disease, and for the development of chronic heart failure.[144] However, recent data suggest that increased body mass index (BMI) is associated with a more favorable prognosis once heart failure is established.[145–147] Negative energy balance and subsequent weight loss can be of importance. Adipose tissue secretes a number of cytokines, including adiponectin. Elevated adiponectin level is associated with increased mortality,[148] probably as a marker or wasting. Moreover, low rather than high cholesterol levels are associated with a poor outcome in patients with chronic heart failure. Once wasting occurs, it is a strong independent risk factor for mortality in chronic heart failure.[149] Cachexia has been defined as a nonintentional documented weight loss of at least 7.5 percent of a previously normal weight. In heart failure, whole-body protein synthesis seems to be suppressed, and breakdown of myofibrillar protein, principally leg skeletal muscle is increased. A significant decrease in LV mass also occurs in patients with cardiac cachexia.[150]

❚ TABLE 24–7

Compensatory Mechanisms Initiated by Low Cardiac Output[a]

MECHANISM	SHORT-TERM ADAPTIVE RESPONSE	LONG-TERM MALADAPTIVE RESPONSE
Salt and water retention	↑ Preload, ↑ cardiac output[b]	Edema, anasarca, pulmonary congestion
Vasoconstriction	↑ Afterload maintained blood pressure	↓ Cardiac output, ↓ cardiac energy expenditure cell death[b]
↑ Cardiac, adrenergic drive	↑ Contractility, ↑ relax-action, ↑ heart rate, ↑ cardiac output[b]	Arrhythmias, ↑ cardiac energy expenditure cell death[b]
Transcription factor activation, cell growth	Adaptive hypertrophy	Maladaptive hypertrophy
	↑ Sarcomere number	Apoptosis, mitochondrial DNA abnormalities, cell death[b]
	↑ Cardiac output[b]	

[a]The compensatory mechanisms initiated by a short-term fall in cardiac output, as occurs following hemorrhage, generate an adaptive response. However, when sustained, as in the chronically overloaded heart, these same mechanisms cause maladaptive responses that further reduce cardiac output, exacerbate symptoms, and appear to accelerate cell death.
[b]Secondary responses.
SOURCE: *Adapted with permission from Katz AM. The cardiomyopathy of overload: an unnatural growth response in the hypertrophied heart. Ann Intern Med 1994;121(5):363–371.*

【 】 MYOCYTE REGENERATION

The heart of a normal human weighs approximately 300 grams and contains approximately 2×10^{10} myocytes. Until recently the accepted understanding was that myocyte cell division in the human heart ceased a few weeks after birth.[151] Thereafter enlargement of the heart was as a result of cell hypertrophy or the laying down of collagen in the extracellular space. That view was based on the observations that cancer in the heart is extremely rare, DNA turnover is almost undetectable except in pathological states, and pathologists disputed whether mitotic figures of myocytes had ever been seen. Approximately 20 percent of myocytes in the human heart have two nuclei, so that cell separation, rather than mitosis, could bring about a small increase in the total cell number. The precise mechanism for the suppression of cell division in the human heart is unknown. What is established is that damage to human heart muscle results in fibrosis and any repair process, were it to exist, is insufficient to overcome the rate of loss of cells. In some species such as the salamander and zebra fish, damage to myocardium is repaired by the generation of new myocardial cells, and the process is under genetic control. If the major problem in the worsening of heart failure is the continuing loss of myocytes then a new approach is to either inhibit the loss of cells, through the processes of apoptosis or necrosis, or to promote the growth of new cells. Much research at present has the objective of increasing the number of myocytes in human myocardium either by introducing other cells (such as skeletal myoblasts, cells derived from bone marrow or other sources), which are intended to transform into cardiac myocytes, or by the stimulation of resident primitive cells within cardiac muscle.

【 】 EVOLUTIONARY ASPECTS

The pathophysiology of heart failure and the body response to damage to the heart is now quite well described. What is much less clear is the nature of the stimuli that initiate and maintain the body response to malfunction of the heart. At present at least five ideas are being considered: (1) The damaged heart can itself release cytokines, which activate systems elsewhere in the body. (2) The continued stimulation of the sympathetic system possibly by neural pathways from receptors in skeletal muscle can in the long-term account for cytokine activation. (3) Tissue hypoxia can contribute. (4) Imbalance of the autonomic nervous system modifies the function of the immune system. (5) Bacteria or endotoxins can gain access to the circulation and stimulate monocytes to generate cytokines.

The maintenance of the circulation is critical to survival of the species. The reflexes and responses, which are activated in heart failure are identical to those which occur during severe exercise.[152] These are ancient reflexes honed by evolutionary development over the ages. Their key purpose is to maintain the blood pressure, prevent hemorrhage, and to exclude infectious agents from the body. These are the systems that are activated in heart failure.

CONCLUSIONS

Heart failure is readily recognized at the bedside or in clinic, but is difficult to define and has a highly variable course. It is a heterogeneous mix of a number of clinical syndromes. The pathophysiology is complex, and our understanding of it still emerging. Heart failure is fundamentally caused by structural and functional abnormalities of the heart. The consequences are impaired filling, impaired emptying, and arrhythmias. The peripheral vasculature is also involved, and changes here can be responsible for impaired nutritive blood flow to multiple organs and reduced exercise intolerance. Treatment for heart failure has improved over the years but is not curative. There is no question that prevention of heart failure must be given a higher priority. We now know that most coronary heat disease can be prevented by control of coronary risk factors. Because 60 to 65 percent of all heart failure in Western civilization is associated with advanced coronary disease, it is clear that controlling blood pressure, reducing plasma lipids, maintaining ideal weight (and thus reducing the chances of developing diabetes mellitus), staying physically fit, and avoiding cigarettes can have a substantial prevention effect on the development of heart failure. The ability to alter genetically induced cardiomyopathy can come later. Effective prevention would tower over our current pharmacologic and device treatments. An improved understanding of the pathophysiology of heart failure can allow us to identify early biomarkers of pre-heart failure, thus allowing for a rational aggressive and cost-effective prevention strategy before patients reach the late stages of the syndrome.

REFERENCES

1. Braunwald E. *Heart Disease: A Textbook of Cardiovascular Medicine.* Philadelphia, PA: W. B. Saunders; 1980.
2. Hunt SA, Abraham WT, Chin MH, et al. ACC/AHA 2005 guideline update for the diagnosis and management of chronic heart failure in the adult: a report of the American College of Cardiology/American Heart Association Task Force on Practice Guidelines (Writing Committee to Update the 2001 Guidelines for the Evaluation and Management of Heart Failure): developed in collaboration with the American College of Chest Physicians and the International Society for Heart and Lung Transplantation: endorsed by the Heart Rhythm Society. *Circulation.* 2005;112(12):e154–235.
3. National Collaborating Centre for Chronic Conditions. *Chronic heart failure. National clinical guideline for diagnosis and management in primary and secondary care.* London: National Institute for Clinical Excellence (NICE); 2003:1–163. (Clinical Guideline 5.)
4. Gheorghiade M, Zannad F, Sopko G, et al. Acute heart failure syndromes: current state and framework for future research. *Circulation.* 2005;112(25):3958–3968.
5. Lowes BD, Minobe W, Abraham WT, et al. Changes in gene expression in the intact human heart. Downregulation of alpha-myosin heavy chain in hypertrophied, failing ventricular myocardium. *J Clin Invest.* 1997;100(9):2315–2324.
6. Lowes BD, Zolty R, Minobe WA, et al. Serial gene expression profiling in the intact human heart. *J Heart Lung Transplant.* 2006;25(5):579–588.
7. George AL Jr. Inherited disorders of voltage-gated sodium channels. *J Clin Invest.* 2005;115(8):1990–1999.
8. Priori SG, Napolitano C. Cardiac and skeletal muscle disorders caused by mutations in the intracellular Ca^{2+} release channels. *J Clin Invest.* 2005;115(8):2033–2038.
9. Meyer M, Schillinger W, Pieske B, et al. Alterations of sarcoplasmic reticulum proteins in failing human dilated cardiomyopathy. *Circulation.* 1995;92(4):778–784.
10. Hasenfuss G, Schillinger W, Lehnart SE, et al. Relationship between Na^+-Ca^{2+}-exchanger protein levels and diastolic function of failing human myocardium. *Circulation.* 1999;99(5):641–648.
11. Reiken S, Gaburjakova M, Guatimosim S, et al. Protein kinase A phosphorylation of the cardiac calcium release channel (ryanodine receptor) in normal and failing hearts. *J Biol Chem.* 2003;278(1):444–453.
12. Wolff MR, Buck SH, Stoker SW, Greaser ML, Mentzer RM. Myofibrillar calcium sensitivity of isometric tension is increased in human dilated cardi-

omyopathies: role of altered beta-adrenergically mediated protein phosphorylation. *J Clin Invest.* 1996;98(1):167–176.

13. Liao R, Nascimben L, Friedrich J, Gwathmey JK, Ingwall JS. Decreased energy reserve in an animal model of dilated cardiomyopathy. Relationship to contractile performance. *Circ Res.* 1996;78(5):893–902.

14. Neubauer S, Horn M, Pabst T, et al. Cardiac high-energy phosphate metabolism in patients with aortic valve disease assessed by 31P-magnetic resonance spectroscopy. *J Investig Med.* 1997;45(8):453–462.

15. Scheuer J. Metabolic factors in myocardial failure. *Circulation.* 1993;87(suppl VII):VII54-VII7.

16. Thames MD, Kinugawa T, Smith ML, Dibner-Dunlap ME. Abnormalities of baroreflex control in heart failure. *J Am Coll Cardiol.* 1993;22(4 suppl A):56A-60A.

17. Zucker H, Wang W, Brandle M. Baroreflex abnormalities in congestive heart failure. *NIPS.* 1993;8:87–90.

18. Dibner-Dunlap ME, Thames MD. Control of sympathetic nerve activity by vagal mechanoreflexes is blunted in heart failure. *Circulation.* 1992;86(6):1929–1934.

19. Grassi G, Seravalle G, Cattaneo BM, et al. Sympathetic activation and loss of reflex sympathetic control in mild congestive heart failure. *Circulation.* 1995;92(11):3206–3211.

20. Newton GE, Parker JD. Cardiac sympathetic responses to acute vasodilation. Normal ventricular function versus congestive heart failure. *Circulation.* 1996;94(12):3161–3167.

21. Brouwer J, van Veldhuisen DJ, Man in 't Veld AJ, et al. Prognostic value of heart rate variability during long-term follow-up in patients with mild to moderate heart failure. The Dutch Ibopamine Multicenter Trial Study Group. *J Am Coll Cardiol.* 1996;28(5):1183–1189.

22. Bristow MR, Ginsburg R, Minobe W, et al. Decreased catecholamine sensitivity and beta-adrenergic-receptor density in failing human hearts. *N Engl J Med.* 1982;307(4):205–211.

23. Bristow MR, Ginsburg R, Umans V, et al. Beta 1- and beta 2-adrenergic-receptor subpopulations in nonfailing and failing human ventricular myocardium: coupling of both receptor subtypes to muscle contraction and selective beta 1-receptor down- regulation in heart failure. *Circ Res.* 1986;59(3):297–309.

24. Vatner DE, Sato N, Galper JB, Vatner SF. Physiological and biochemical evidence for coordinate increases in muscarinic receptors and Gi during pacing-induced heart failure. *Circulation.* 1996;94(1):102–107.

25. White M, Roden R, Minobe W, et al. Age-related changes in beta-adrenergic neuroeffector systems in the human heart. *Circulation.* 1994;90(3):1225–1238.

26. Iaccarino G, Tomhave ED, Lefkowitz RJ, Koch WJ. Reciprocal in vivo regulation of myocardial G protein-coupled receptor kinase expression by beta-adrenergic receptor stimulation and blockade. *Circulation.* 1998;98(17):1783–1789.

27. Gilbert EM, Abraham WT, Olsen S, et al. Comparative hemodynamic, left ventricular functional, and antiadrenergic effects of chronic treatment with metoprolol versus carvedilol in the failing heart. *Circulation.* 1996;94(11):2817–2825.

28. Richards AM, Doughty R, Nicholls MG, et al. Neurohumoral prediction of benefit from carvedilol in ischemic left ventricular dysfunction. Australia-New Zealand Heart Failure Group. *Circulation.* 1999;99(6):786–792.

29. Bhargava V, Shabetai R, Mathiasen RA, Dalton N, Hunter JJ, Ross J Jr. Loss of adrenergic control of the force-frequency relation in heart failure secondary to idiopathic or ischemic cardiomyopathy. *Am J Cardiol.* 1998;81(9):1130–1137.

30. Hajjar RJ, DiSalvo TG, Schmidt U, et al. Clinical correlates of the myocardial force-frequency relationship in patients with end-stage heart failure. *J Heart Lung Transplant.* 1997;16(11):1157–1167.

31. Cheng W, Li B, Kajstura J, et al. Stretch-induced programmed myocyte cell death. *J Clin Invest.* 1995;96(5):2247–2259.

32. Anversa P, Kajstura J. Ventricular myocytes are not terminally differentiated in the adult mammalian heart. *Circ Res.* 1998;83(1):1–14.

33. Kajstura J, Leri A, Finato N, Di Loreto C, Beltrami CA, Anversa P. Myocyte proliferation in end-stage cardiac failure in humans. *Proc Natl Acad Sci U S A.* 1998;95(15):8801–8805.

34. Gerdes AM, Kellerman SE, Moore JA, et al. Structural remodeling of cardiac myocytes in patients with ischemic cardiomyopathy. *Circulation.* 1992;86(2):426–430.

35. Hunter JJ, Chien KR. Signaling pathways for cardiac hypertrophy and failure. *N Engl J Med.* 1999;341(17):1276–1283.

36. Lorell BH. Transition from hypertrophy to failure. *Circulation.* 1997;96(11):3824–3827.

37. Katz AM. The cardiomyopathy of overload: an unnatural growth response in the hypertrophied heart. *Ann Intern Med.* 1994;121(5):363–371.

38. Harris P. Congestive cardiac failure: central role of the arterial blood pressure. *Br Heart J.* 1987;58(3):190–203.

39. de Bold AJ. Atrial natriuretic factor: a hormone produced by the heart. *Science.* 1985;230(4727):767–770.

40. Francis GS. Changing the remodeling process in heart failure: basic mechanisms and laboratory results. *Curr Opin Cardiol.* 1998;13(3):156–161.

41. Swynghedauw B. Molecular mechanisms of myocardial remodeling. *Physiol Rev.* 1999;79(1):215–262.

42. Francis GS, Carlyle WC. Hypothetical pathways of cardiac myocyte hypertrophy: response to myocardial injury. *Eur Heart J.* 1993;14(suppl J):49–56.

43. Francis GS, McDonald KM. Left ventricular hypertrophy: an initial response to myocardial injury. *Am J Cardiol.* 1992;69(18):3G-7G.

44. Francis GS, McDonald KM, Cohn JN. Neurohumoral activation in preclinical heart failure. Remodeling and the potential for intervention. *Circulation.* 1993;87(5 suppl):IV90–96.

45. Onodera T, Tamura T, Said S, McCune SA, Gerdes AM. Maladaptive remodeling of cardiac myocyte shape begins long before failure in hypertension. *Hypertension.* 1998;32(4):753–757.

46. Gerdes AM, Onodera T, Wang X, McCune SA. Myocyte remodeling during the progression to failure in rats with hypertension. *Hypertension.* 1996;28(4):609–614.

47. Tamura T, Onodera T, Said S, Gerdes AM. Correlation of myocyte lengthening to chamber dilation in the spontaneously hypertensive heart failure (SHHF) rat. *J Mol Cell Cardiol.* 1998;30(11):2175–2181.

48. Wang X, Li F, Gerdes AM. Chronic pressure overload cardiac hypertrophy and failure in guinea pigs: I. Regional hemodynamics and myocyte remodeling. *J Mol Cell Cardiol.* 1999;31(2):307–317.

49. Anversa P, Li P, Zhang X, Olivetti G, Capasso JM. Ischaemic myocardial injury and ventricular remodelling. *Cardiovasc Res.* 1993;27(2):145–157.

50. Olivetti G, Abbi R, Quaini F, et al. Apoptosis in the failing human heart. *N Engl J Med.* 1997;336(16):1131–1141.

51. Williams RS. Apoptosis and heart failure. *N Engl J Med.* 1999;341(10):759–760.

52. Levin ER, Gardner DG, Samson WK. Natriuretic peptides. *N Engl J Med.* 1998;339(5):321–328.

53. Schrier RW, Abraham WT. Hormones and hemodynamics in heart failure. *N Engl J Med.* 1999;341(8):577–585.

54. Weber KT, Brilla CG. Pathological hypertrophy and cardiac interstitium. Fibrosis and renin-angiotensin-aldosterone system. *Circulation.* 1991;83(6):1849–1865.

55. Mann DL, Kent RL, Parsons B, Cooper Gt. Adrenergic effects on the biology of the adult mammalian cardiocyte. *Circulation.* 1992;85(2):790–804.

56. Rona G. Catecholamine cardiotoxicity. *J Mol Cell Cardiol.* 1985;17(4):291–306.

57. Tan LB, Jalil JE, Pick R, Janicki JS, Weber KT. Cardiac myocyte necrosis induced by angiotensin II. *Circ Res.* 1991;69(5):1185–1195.

58. Francis GS, Goldsmith SR, Levine TB, Olivari MT, Cohn JN. The neurohumoral axis in congestive heart failure. *Ann Intern Med.* 1984;101(3):370–377.

59. Packer M. Neurohormonal interactions and adaptations in congestive heart failure. *Circulation.* 1988;77(4):721–730.

60. Packer M. The neurohormonal hypothesis: a theory to explain the mechanism of disease progression in heart failure. *J Am Coll Cardiol.* 1992;20(1):248–254.

61. Packer M, Lee WH, Kessler PD, Gottlieb SS, Bernstein JL, Kukin ML. Role of neurohormonal mechanisms in determining survival in patients with severe chronic heart failure. *Circulation.* 1987;75(5 Pt 2):IV80–92.

62. Starling EH. Points on pathology of heart disease. *Lancet.* 1897;1:569–572.

63. Chidsey CA, Harrison DC, Braunwald E. Augmentation of the plasma norepinephrine response to exercise in patients with congestive heart failure. *N Engl J Med.* 1962;267:650–654.

64. Thomas JA, Marks BH. Plasma norepinephrine in congestive heart failure. *Am J Cardiol.* 1978;41(2):233–243.

65. Levine TB, Francis GS, Goldsmith SR, Simon AB, Cohn JN. Activity of the sympathetic nervous system and renin-angiotensin system assessed by plasma hormone levels and their relation to hemodynamic abnormalities in congestive heart failure. *Am J Cardiol.* 1982;49(7):1659–1666.

66. Leimbach WN Jr, Wallin BG, Victor RG, Aylward PE, Sundlof G, Mark AL. Direct evidence from intraneural recordings for increased central sympathetic outflow in patients with heart failure. *Circulation.* 1986;73(5):913–919.

67. Hasking GJ, Esler MD, Jennings GL, Burton D, Johns JA, Korner PI. Norepinephrine spillover to plasma in patients with congestive heart failure: evi-

dence of increased overall and cardiorenal sympathetic nervous activity. *Circulation.* 1986;73(4):615–621.

68. Eichhorn EJ, Bristow MR. Medical therapy can improve the biological properties of the chronically failing heart. A new era in the treatment of heart failure. *Circulation.* 1996;94(9):2285–2296.

69. Hall SA, Cigarroa CG, Marcoux L, Risser RC, Grayburn PA, Eichhorn EJ. Time course of improvement in left ventricular function, mass and geometry in patients with congestive heart failure treated with beta-adrenergic blockade. *J Am Coll Cardiol.* 1995;25(5):1154–1161.

70. Keeton TK, Campbell WB. The pharmacologic alteration of renin release. *Pharmacol Rev.* 1981;31:81–227.

71. Matsubara H. Pathophysiological role of angiotensin II type 2 receptor in cardiovascular and renal diseases. *Circ Res.* 1998;83(12):1182–1191.

72. Tang WH, Vagelos RH, Yee YG, et al. Neurohormonal and clinical responses to high- versus low-dose enalapril therapy in chronic heart failure. *J Am Coll Cardiol.* 2002;39(1):70–78.

73. Yusuf S, Sleight P, Pogue J, Bosch J, Davies R, Dagenais G. Effects of an angiotensin-converting-enzyme inhibitor, ramipril, on cardiovascular events in high-risk patients. The Heart Outcomes Prevention Evaluation Study Investigators. *N Engl J Med.* 2000;342(3):145–153.

74. Francis GS. The renin-angiotensin system. In: Parmley W, Chatterjee K, eds. *Cardiology.* New York: Lippincott-Raven; 1997:1–16.

75. Gibbons GH, Pfeffer MA. The role of angiotensin in cardiovascular disease: pathophysiologic insights and therapeutic implications. In: Topol EJ, ed. *Textbook of Cardiovascular Medicine.* New York: Lippincott-Raven; 1998:1–12.

76. Pitt B, Zannad F, Remme WJ, et al. The effect of spironolactone on morbidity and mortality in patients with severe heart failure. Randomized Aldactone Evaluation Study Investigators. *N Engl J Med.* 1999;341(10):709–717.

77. Francis GS, Benedict C, Johnstone DE, et al. Comparison of neuroendocrine activation in patients with left ventricular dysfunction with and without congestive heart failure. A substudy of the Studies of Left Ventricular Dysfunction (SOLVD). *Circulation.* 1990;82(5):1724–1749.

78. Goldsmith SR, Francis GS, Cowley AW Jr, Levine TB, Cohn JN. Increased plasma arginine vasopressin levels in patients with congestive heart failure. *J Am Coll Cardiol.* 1983;1(6):1385–1390.

79. Goldsmith SR, Francis GS, Cowley AW, Jr., Goldenberg IF, Cohn JN. Hemodynamic effects of infused arginine vasopressin in congestive heart failure. *J Am Coll Cardiol.* 1986;8(4):779–783.

80. Young JB. Intravenous nesiritide vs nitroglycerin for treatment of decompensated congestive heart failure: a randomized controlled trial. *JAMA.* 2002;287(12):1531–1540.

81. Yanagisawa M, Kurihara H, Kimura S, et al. A novel potent vasoconstrictor peptide produced by vascular endothelial cells. *Nature.* 1988;332(6163):411–415.

82. McMurray JJ, Ray SG, Abdullah I, Dargie HJ, Morton JJ. Plasma endothelin in chronic heart failure. *Circulation.* 1992;85(4):1374–1379.

83. Levin ER. Endothelins. *N Engl J Med.* 1995;333(6):356–363.

84. Ingelsson E, Arnlov J, Sundstrom J, Lind L. Inflammation, as measured by the erythrocyte sedimentation rate, is an independent predictor for the development of heart failure. *J Am Coll Cardiol.* 2005;45(11):1802–1806.

85. Shah SJ, Marcus GM, Gerber IL, et al. High-sensitivity C-reactive protein and parameters of left ventricular dysfunction. *J Card Fail.* 2006;12(1):61–65.

86. Vasan RS, Sullivan LM, Roubenoff R, et al. Inflammatory markers and risk of heart failure in elderly subjects without prior myocardial infarction: the Framingham Heart Study. *Circulation.* 2003;107(11):1486–1491.

87. Levine B, Kalman J, Mayer L, Fillit HM, Packer M. Elevated circulating levels of tumor necrosis factor in severe chronic heart failure. *N Engl J Med.* 1990;323(4):236–241.

88. Diwan A, Dibbs Z, Nemoto S, et al. Targeted overexpression of noncleavable and secreted forms of tumor necrosis factor provokes disparate cardiac phenotypes. *Circulation.* 2004;109(2):262–268.

89. Oral H, Sivasubramanian N, Dyke DB, et al. Myocardial proinflammatory cytokine expression and left ventricular remodeling in patients with chronic mitral regurgitation. *Circulation.* 2003;107(6):831–837.

90. Torre-Amione G, Kapadia S, Lee J, et al. Tumor necrosis factor-alpha and tumor necrosis factor receptors in the failing human heart. *Circulation.* 1996;93(4):704–711.

91. Bozkurt B, Kribbs SB, Clubb FJ, Jr, et al. Pathophysiologically relevant concentrations of tumor necrosis factor-alpha promote progressive left ventricular dysfunction and remodeling in rats. *Circulation.* 1998;97(14):1382–1391.

92. Yokoyama T, Nakano M, Bednarczyk JL, McIntyre BW, Entman M, Mann DL. Tumor necrosis factor-alpha provokes a hypertrophic growth response in adult cardiac myocytes. *Circulation.* 1997;95(5):1247–1252.

93. Anker SD, Chua TP, Ponikowski P, et al. Hormonal changes and catabolic/anabolic imbalance in chronic heart failure and their importance for cardiac cachexia. *Circulation.* 1997;96(2):526–534.

94. Bryant D, Becker L, Richardson J, et al. Cardiac failure in transgenic mice with myocardial expression of tumor necrosis factor-alpha. *Circulation.* 1998;97(14):1375–1381.

95. Mak S, Newton GE. The oxidative stress hypothesis of congestive heart failure: radical thoughts. *Chest.* 2001;120(6):2035–2046.

96. Hare JM. Oxidative stress and apoptosis in heart failure progression. *Circ Res.* 2001;89(3):198–200.

97. Giordano FJ. Oxygen, oxidative stress, hypoxia, and heart failure. *J Clin Invest.* 2005;115(3):500–508.

98. White M, Ducharme A, Ibrahim R, et al. Increased systemic inflammation and oxidative stress in patients with worsening congestive heart failure: improvement after short-term inotropic support. *Clin Sci (Lond).* 2006;110(4):483–489.

99. Nakamura K, Kusano KF, Matsubara H, et al. Relationship between oxidative stress and systolic dysfunction in patients with hypertrophic cardiomyopathy. *J Card Fail.* 2005;11(2):117–123.

100. Witteles RM, Tang WH, Jamali AH, Chu JW, Reaven GM, Fowler MB. Insulin resistance in idiopathic dilated cardiomyopathy: a possible etiologic link. *J Am Coll Cardiol.* 2004;44(1):78–81.

101. Ingelsson E, Sundstrom J, Arnlov J, Zethelius B, Lind L. Insulin resistance and risk of congestive heart failure. *JAMA.* 2005;294(3):334–341.

102. Drexler H, Lu W. Endothelial dysfunction of hindquarter resistance vessels in experimental heart failure. *Am J Physiol.* 1992;262(6 pt 2):H1640–H1645.

103. Kubo SH, Rector TS, Bank AJ, Williams RE, Heifetz SM. Endothelium-dependent vasodilation is attenuated in patients with heart failure. *Circulation.* 1991;84(4):1589–1596.

104. Winlaw DS, Smythe GA, Keogh AM, Schyvens CG, Spratt PM, Macdonald PS. Increased nitric oxide production in heart failure. *Lancet.* 1994;344(8919):373–374.

105. Katz SD, Schwarz M, Yuen J, LeJemtel TH. Impaired acetylcholine-mediated vasodilation in patients with congestive heart failure: role of endothelium-derived vasodilating and vasoconstrictive factors. *Circulation.* 1993;88:55–61.

106. Kubo SH, Rector TS, Bank AJ, et al. Effects of cardiac transplantation on endothelium-dependent dilation of the peripheral vasculature in congestive heart failure. *Am J Cardiol.* 1993;71(1):88–93.

107. Drexler H. Nitric oxide synthases in the failing human heart: a doubled-edged sword? *Circulation.* 1999;99(23):2972–2975.

108. Saraiva RM, Hare JM. Nitric oxide signaling in the cardiovascular system: implications for heart failure. *Curr Opin Cardiol.* 2006;21(3):221–228.

109. Hare JM, Givertz MM, Creager MA, Colucci WS. Increased sensitivity to nitric oxide synthase inhibition in patients with heart failure: potentiation of beta-adrenergic inotropic responsiveness. *Circulation.* 1998;97(2):161–166.

110. Hare JM, Loh E, Creager MA, Colucci WS. Nitric oxide inhibits the positive inotropic response to beta-adrenergic stimulation in humans with left ventricular dysfunction. *Circulation.* 1995;92(8):2198–2203.

111. Haywood GA, Tsao PS, von der Leyen HE, et al. Expression of inducible nitric oxide synthase in human heart failure. *Circulation.* 1996;93(6):1087–1094.

112. Recchia FA, McConnell PI, Bernstein RD, Vogel TR, Xu X, Hintze TH. Reduced nitric oxide production and altered myocardial metabolism during the decompensation of pacing-induced heart failure in the conscious dog. *Circ Res.* 1998;83(10):969–979.

113. Cotter G, Kaluski E, Blatt A, et al. L-NMMA (a nitric oxide synthase inhibitor) is effective in the treatment of cardiogenic shock. *Circulation.* 2000;101(12):1358–1361.

114. Champion HC, Skaf MW, Hare JM. Role of nitric oxide in the pathophysiology of heart failure. *Heart Fail Rev.* 2003;8(1):35–46.

115. Badorff C, Fichtlscherer B, Rhoads RE, et al. Nitric oxide inhibits dystrophin proteolysis by coxsackieviral protease 2A through S-nitrosylation: a protective mechanism against enteroviral cardiomyopathy. *Circulation.* 2000;102(18):2276–2281.

116. Hare JM. Nitroso-redox balance in the cardiovascular system. *N Engl J Med.* 2004;351(20):2112–2114.

117. Force T, Michael A, Kilter H, Haq S. Stretch-activated pathways in left ventricular remodeling. *J Card Fail.* 2002;8(6 suppl):S351–S358.

118. Steenbergen C, Afshari CA, Petranka JG, et al. Alterations in apoptotic signaling in human idiopathic cardiomyopathic hearts in failure. *Am J Physiol Heart Circ Physiol.* 2003;284(1):H268–276.

119. Auricchio A, Spinelli JC, Trautmann SI, Kloss M. Effect of cardiac resynchronization therapy on ventricular remodeling. *J Card Fail.* 2002;8(6 suppl):S549–S555.

120. Ukkonen H, Beanlands RS, Burwash IG, et al. Effect of cardiac resynchronization on myocardial efficiency and regional oxidative metabolism. *Circulation*. 2003;107(1):28–31.

121. Anversa P, Capasso JM, Olivetti G, Sonnenblick EH. Cellular basis of ventricular remodeling in hypertensive cardiomyopathy. *Am J Hypertens*. 1992;5(10):758–770.

122. Weber KT. Monitoring tissue repair and fibrosis from a distance. *Circulation*. 1997;96(8):2488–2492.

123. Weber KT, Brilla CG, Janicki JS. Myocardial fibrosis: functional significance and regulatory factors. *Cardiovasc Res*. 1993;27(3):341–348.

124. Weber KT, Pick R, Silver MA, et al. Fibrillar collagen and remodeling of dilated canine left ventricle. *Circulation*. 1990;82(4):1387–1401.

125. Zhao MJ, Zhang H, Robinson TF, Factor SM, Sonnenblick EH, Eng C. Profound structural alterations of the extracellular collagen matrix in postischemic dysfunctional ("stunned") but viable myocardium. *J Am Coll Cardiol*. 1987;10(6):1322–1334.

126. Weber KT. Cardiac interstitium in health and disease: the fibrillar collagen network. *J Am Coll Cardiol*. 1989;13(7):1637–1652.

127. Thomas CV, Coker ML, Zellner JL, Handy JR, Crumbley AJ 3rd, Spinale FG. Increased matrix metalloproteinase activity and selective upregulation in LV myocardium from patients with end-stage dilated cardiomyopathy. *Circulation*. 1998;97(17):1708–1715.

128. Harada M, Itoh H, Nakagawa O, et al. Significance of ventricular myocytes and nonmyocytes interaction during cardiocyte hypertrophy: evidence for endothelin-1 as a paracrine hypertrophic factor from cardiac nonmyocytes. *Circulation*. 1997;96(10):3737–3744.

129. Robbins M, Francis G, Pashkow FJ, et al. Ventilatory and heart rate responses to exercise: better predictors of heart failure mortality than peak oxygen consumption. *Circulation*. 1999;100(24):2411–2417.

130. Massie BM. Exercise tolerance in congestive heart failure. Role of cardiac function, peripheral blood flow, and muscle metabolism and effect of treatment. *Am J Med*. 1988;84(3A):75–82.

131. Massie BM, Simonini A, Sahgal P, Wells L, Dudley GA. Relation of systemic and local muscle exercise capacity to skeletal muscle characteristics in men with congestive heart failure. *J Am Coll Cardiol*. 1996;27(1):140–145.

132. Hambrecht R, Adams V, Gielen S, et al. Exercise intolerance in patients with chronic heart failure and increased expression of inducible nitric oxide synthase in the skeletal muscle. *J Am Coll Cardiol*. 1999;33(1):174–179.

133. Adams V, Jiang H, Yu J, et al. Apoptosis in skeletal myocytes of patients with chronic heart failure is associated with exercise intolerance. *J Am Coll Cardiol*. 1999;33(4):959–965.

134. Wilson JR, Hanamanthu S, Chomsky DB, Davis SF. Relationship between exertional symptoms and functional capacity in patients with heart failure. *J Am Coll Cardiol*. 1999;33(7):1943–1947.

135. Packer M, Lee WH, Kessler PD. Preservation of glomerular filtration rate in human heart failure by activation of the renin-angiotensin system. *Circulation*. 1986;74(4):766–774.

136. Ichikawa I, Yoshioka T, Fogo A, Kon V. Role of angiotensin II in altered glomerular hemodynamics in congestive heart failure. *Kidney Int Suppl*. 1990;30:S123–126.

137. Hall JE, Guyton AC, Jackson TE, Coleman TG, Lohmeier TE, Trippodo NC. Control of glomerular filtration rate by renin-angiotensin system. *Am J Physiol*. 1977;233(5):F366–372.

138. Javaheri S, Parker TJ, Wexler L, et al. Occult sleep-disordered breathing in stable congestive heart failure. *Ann Intern Med*. 1995;122(7):487–492.

139. Javaheri S, Parker TJ, Liming JD, et al. Sleep apnea in 81 ambulatory male patients with stable heart failure. Types and their prevalences, consequences, and presentations. *Circulation*. 1998;98(21):2154–2159.

140. Tkacova R, Rankin F, Fitzgerald FS, Floras JS, Bradley TD. Effects of continuous positive airway pressure on obstructive sleep apnea and left ventricular afterload in patients with heart failure. *Circulation*. 1998;98(21):2269–2275.

141. Lanfranchi PA, Braghiroli A, Bosimini E, et al. Prognostic value of nocturnal Cheyne-Stokes respiration in chronic heart failure. *Circulation*. 1999;99(11):1435–1440.

142. Javaheri S. A mechanism of central sleep apnea in patients with heart failure. *N Engl J Med*. 1999;341(13):949–954.

143. Andreas S, Clemens C, Sandholzer H, Figulla HR, Kreuzer H. Improvement of exercise capacity with treatment of Cheyne-Stokes respiration in patients with congestive heart failure. *J Am Coll Cardiol*. 1996;27(6):1486–1490.

144. Kenchaiah S, Evans JC, Levy D, et al. Obesity and the risk of heart failure. *N Engl J Med*. 2002;347(5):305–313.

145. Lavie CJ, Osman AF, Milani RV, Mehra MR. Body composition and prognosis in chronic systolic heart failure: the obesity paradox. *Am J Cardiol*. 2003;91(7):891–894.

146. Davos CH, Doehner W, Rauchhaus M, et al. Body mass and survival in patients with chronic heart failure without cachexia: the importance of obesity. *J Card Fail*. 2003;9(1):29–35.

147. Horwich TB, Fonarow GC, Hamilton MA, MacLellan WR, Woo MA, Tillisch JH. The relationship between obesity and mortality in patients with heart failure. *J Am Coll Cardiol*. 2001;38(3):789–795.

148. Kistorp C, Faber J, Galatius S, et al. Plasma adiponectin, body mass index, and mortality in patients with chronic heart failure. *Circulation*. 2005;112(12):1756–1762.

149. Anker SD, Ponikowski P, Varney S, et al. Wasting as independent risk factor for mortality in chronic heart failure. *Lancet*. 1997;349(9058):1050–1053.

150. Florea VG, Moon J, Pennell DJ, Doehner W, Coats AJ, Anker SD. Wasting of the left ventricle in patients with cardiac cachexia: a cardiovascular magnetic resonance study. *Int J Cardiol*. 2004;97(1):15–20.

151. von Harsdorf R, Poole-Wilson PA, Dietz R. Regenerative capacity of the myocardium: implications for treatment of heart failure. *Lancet*. 2004;363(9417):1306–1313.

152. Harris P. Evolution and the cardiac patient. *Cardiovasc Res*. 1983;17:313–9,73–78,437–445.

CHAPTER 25

The Epidemiology and Diagnosis of Heart Failure

Owais Dar / Martin R. Cowie

INTRODUCTION

In recent years much has been published on the clinical epidemiology of heart failure, including the secular trends in incidence, prevalence, etiology, and prognosis. A clear definition of any condition under study is essential but has proven difficult for heart failure, with no generally accepted gold standard. As a consequence comparison between studies and countries, and over time, is difficult. A full discussion of the diagnostic tests and strategies that can be employed in making a diagnosis of heart failure is described in Chap. 26, but an overview of the approaches used in population-based studies is provided here.

Unquestionably heart failure is an important healthcare issue. Developed countries spend 1 to 2 percent of their healthcare budget on patients with this condition, and heart failure is the single most common diagnostic related group for admissions to U.S. hospitals. Hospital readmission rates are high, particularly where chronic disease monitoring is poor, and admissions tend to be long, particularly in Europe. Much effort has been expended in improving the standards of care for patients with heart failure, with the publication of international guidelines and the development of chronic disease management programs key to the implementation of these guidelines.

Epidemiologic studies have provided a wealth of information about who is at risk of developing heart failure and how they fare after diagnosis. They also allow predictions to be made about the likely future burden of disease.

Most of the published data has come from studies in developed countries, initially North America, but more recently Europe. Much more limited information is available from the developing world. With epidemiological transition, it is likely that the epidemiology of heart failure will become increasingly similar across the world, driven by the major etiological forces of coronary artery disease, hypertension, and diabetes mellitus. Even now, cardiovascular disease is overtaking infectious disease as the leading cause of death worldwide.

Before describing the epidemiology of heart failure, it is important to appreciate the challenge of defining heart failure in a robust but practical manner suitable for population-based studies.

THE DIAGNOSIS OF HEART FAILURE IN EPIDEMIOLOGIC STUDIES

Heart failure is not a complete diagnosis in itself; this requires characterization of the syndrome in terms of its severity, the underlying cardiac abnormality, its etiology, and the manner in which the whole body has adjusted to the pump dysfunction. The advent of high-resolution noninvasive imaging, particularly echocardiography, has helped confirm underlying structural or functional cardiac abnormalities in patients with symptoms and signs suggestive of heart failure. Problems remain in determining what is outside normality, particularly in the aging heart.

The definition of heart failure has evolved over time. There is no currently widely-accepted gold standard based on an objective test. Different definitions are employed in epidemiologic studies, clinical trials, and in clinical practice, making comparisons difficult.[1,2] Recent population studies have attempted to apply more clinically-based definitions, but are labor intensive.

Heart failure has been defined as a "syndrome that develops as a consequence of cardiac disease and is recognized clinically by a constellation of symptoms and signs produced by complex circulatory and neurohormonal responses to cardiac dysfunction."[3] Although accurate, this definition does not lend itself to use in an epidemiologic study.

The European Society of Cardiology guideline on the diagnosis and treatment of heart failure suggests that symptoms should be present, either at rest or on exercise, with objective evidence of cardiac dysfunction provided preferably by echocardiography. Where an element of doubt persists, response to therapy directed toward heart failure can help confirm or refute the diagnosis.[4] The most recent guidelines from the Heart Failure Society of America advocate a similar approach, with a careful history supplemented by physical examination and tests to assess cardiac structure and function.[5] In both guidelines, the measurement of the plasma concentration of B-type natriuretic peptide is recommended to help make or rule out a diagnosis in patients where there remains uncertainty.[4,5] Such a clinical approach to diagnosis is time consuming, but has recently been adopted in population-based studies, tending to replace the older approach of using scoring systems, such as the Framingham Heart Study score, which is discussed below.

[ ] SIGNS AND SYMPTOMS OF HEART FAILURE

Heart failure can manifest as a wide range of symptoms and signs. Few are specific for heart failure, and the sensitivity can be low and reduced further by cardioactive medication. Table 25–1 shows the sensitivity and specificity of various symptoms and signs. Although orthopnea and paroxysmal nocturnal dyspnea are relatively specific for heart failure, they are not sensitive for a diagnosis of heart failure. Many persons with the syndrome will not demonstrate these features in the history. Similarly, a raised jugular venous pressure is highly specific, but is insensitive and requires clinical expertise for reliable detection.[6]

Clinical examination can help determine the underlying cardiac abnormality, such as significant valve disease but cannot be used reliably to distinguish systolic from isolated diastolic abnormalities (Table 25–2).[7]

Patients admitted to the hospital with heart failure, understandably, have severe symptoms and breathlessness predominates. Within the Acute Decompensated Heart Failure National Registry (ADHERE) registry of patients admitted to hospitals in the United States with acute heart failure, 34 percent presented with dyspnea at rest, 68 percent had lung rales, and 66 percent had signs of peripheral edema.[8] Those presenting in the community are likely to have less severe symptoms and fewer clinical signs.

[ ] ACUTE OR CHRONIC HEART FAILURE?

Heart failure is commonly referred to as either acute or chronic, the former either being acute *de novo* heart failure or acute decompensation of chronic heart failure. Acute heart failure constitutes 5 percent of adult emergency medical admissions in the United Kingdom.[9] Two surveys of such acute admissions have been devised: the ongoing ADHERE program in the United States[8] and a series of

---

TABLE 25–1

Sensitivity and Specificity of Signs and Symptoms of Heart Failure, as Defined as an Ejection Fraction <40 Percent in a Series of 1306 Patients with Coronary Artery Disease Undergoing Cardiac Catheterization

	SENSITIVITY (%)	SPECIFICITY (%)	POSITIVE PREDICTIVE VALUE (%)
Medical history			
Shortness of breath	66	52	23
Orthopnea	21	81	2
Nocturnal dyspnea	33	76	26
Edema by history	23	80	22
Physical examination			
Tachycardia	7	99	6
Rales	13	99	6
Edema on examination	10	93	3
Ventricular gallop sound (S_3)	31	95	61
Neck vein distension	10	97	2
Chest radiograph			
Cardiomegaly	62	67	32

S_3, third heart sound.
SOURCE: Harlan WR, Obermann A, Grimm R, et al.[6]

TABLE 25–2

Prevalence of Specific Symptoms and Signs in Systolic and Diastolic Heart Failure, Expressed as Percentage of Patients in Each Group with the Listed Symptom or Sign of Heart Failure[a]

	DIASTOLIC HEART FAILURE (EF >50%)	SYSTOLIC HEART FAILURE (EF <50%)
Symptoms		
Dyspnea on exertion	85	96
Paroxysmal nocturnal dyspnea	55	50
Orthopnea	60	73
Physical examination		
Jugular venous distension	35	46
Rales	72	70
Displaced apical impulse	50	60
S_3	45	65
S_4	45	66
Hepatomegaly	15	16
Edema	30	40
Chest radiograph		
Cardiomegaly	90	96
Pulmonary venous hypertension	75	80

EF, ejection fraction; S_3, third heart sound; S_4, fourth heart sound.
[a]There are no statistically significant differences between the two groups.
SOURCE: Modified from Zile MR, Brutsaert DL.[7]

snapshot surveys across Europe, under the auspices of the European Society of Cardiology.[10] The characteristics of the patients identified in the two geographical areas are remarkably similar (Table 25–3).

SYSTOLIC OR DIASTOLIC HEART FAILURE

The underlying abnormality of cardiac function in an individual with heart failure can also be used to describe more fully the nature of the heart failure. Most trials of drug therapy have enrolled patients with obvious underlying systolic dysfunction of the left ventricle, often termed *systolic heart failure*. A cut-point is usually chosen for ejection fraction, below which the heart is said to have systolic dysfunction. Typically an ejection fraction of 35 or 40 percent (large heart) has been accepted. In some patients, however, heart failure occurs in the presence of good left ventricular systolic function. This has been termed *heart failure with preserved systolic function* or *diastolic heart failure* but is a heterogenous group, including valve dysfunction, arrhythmia, pericardial disease, right ventricular dysfunction, or a stiff and noncompliant left ventricle. The latter abnormality is usually termed *isolated diastolic heart failure* but is used in different senses by different authors. Strictly speaking, the most rigorous definition would demand convincing evidence of good systolic function of both ventricles at rest and on exercise, no arrhythmia or valve disease, and a proven abnormality of diastolic function on pressure-volume loop calculation at the time of cardiac catheterization. Rarely is this strict definition used, mainly for pragmatic reasons, and the label of *diastolic heart failure* is applied to a patient with a clinical diagnosis of heart failure and normal systolic function (or at least a near normal calculated ejection fraction or a

small- or normal-sized heart) on echocardiography. It is thus a diagnosis of exclusion, and such a nonspecific approach can lead to many patients being given a diagnosis of heart failure incorrectly. Much controversy has arisen around the best noninvasive methods of identifying heart failure caused by isolated diastolic dysfunction, with European guidelines suggesting that to make this diagnosis there should be signs or symptoms of heart failure, and normal (or only mildly abnormal) left ventricular systolic function, and evidence of abnormal left ventricular relaxation, filling, diastolic distensibility, or diastolic stiffness.[11] Such a definition has proven difficult to use in clinical practice.

Vasan and colleagues have shied away from this strict definition and have suggested dividing the diagnosis of diastolic heart failure (HF) by the likely probability of the diagnosis being correct (definite, probable, or possible). Individuals are categorized depending on the presence or absence of symptoms and signs of HF, evidence of normal systolic function (ejection fraction [EF] >50 percent) during a heart failure event, and evidence of diastolic dysfunction chiefly from echocardiography.[12] Such an approach has been endorsed by the current American College of Cardiology/American Heart Association (ACC/AHA) Task Force on Practice Guidelines,[13] with the pragmatic suggestion that the term *heart failure with preserved systolic function* would be a more accurate description in many cases.

Heart failure with preserved systolic function was not considered to be common in many population-based studies, but recent reports from Olmsted County (Rochester Epidemiology Project) and a small nested case-control study from the Framingham Heart Study in North America suggest this can be as common as systolic dysfunction, particularly if the diagnosis of heart failure is based on accepting the clinician's opinion or using the Framingham criteria, and relying on echocardiography at any point during a hospitalization period.[14–18] Most of the studies suggest that the probability of the systolic function of the left ventricle being *preserved* in a patient with heart failure is higher in the elderly, in women, and in the obese.[16,17] In Europe, half of patients admitted to hospital with heart failure have a preserved EF (≥40 percent) at the time of measurement.[10] It has been suggested that misdiagnosis of heart failure is common in the group of patients labelled as *preserved systolic function heart failure*.[19,20] Data from case-by-case expert review in population-based studies in the United Kingdom conducted by the author suggest preserved systolic function is found in a lower proportion of new cases of heart failure—approximately 10 to 15 percent.[21,22]

INVESTIGATIONS USED TO CONFIRM OR REFUTE THE DIAGNOSIS OF HEART FAILURE

CHEST RADIOGRAPH

The main role for a chest radiograph is to exclude other causes for dyspnea—such as pleural effusion, pneumothorax, lung

TABLE 25–3

Demographic and Clinical Characteristics of Patients Admitted to Hospital with Heart Failure (Either Acute De Novo or Acute Decompensation of Chronic Heart Failure) in the EuroHeart Survey and ADHERE Programmes

CHARACTERISTIC	EURO-HF 2000–2001 (N = 11,327)	ADHERE 2002–2004 (N = 105,388)
Average age (years)	71	72
Male (%)	53	49
Dyspnea at rest (%)	40	34
Rales (%)	N/A	68
Peripheral edema (%)	23 (bilateral)	66
Prior evidence of HF (%)	65	74
Diabetes (%)	27	44
Chronic renal failure (%)	17	29
Respiratory disease (%)	32	30
BP >140 mmHg (%)	29	50
HF with preserved systolic function	55%	50%
HF admission to ITU (%)	N/A	20%
Length of stay in intensive or coronary care unit (median, days)	N/A	2.6 days
Total length of stay (median, days)	11	4.6
Requiring inotropes (%)	N/A	13
Inhospital mortality (%)	6.9	3.8
Postdischarge mortality	13% at 3 months	N/A
Postdischarge readmission rate	24% within 90 days	N/A

ADHERE, Acute Decompensated Heart Failure National Registry.
SOURCE: *Cleland JG, Swedberg K, Follath F, et al. for the Study Group on Diagnosis of the Working Group on Heart Failure of the European Society of Cardiology;[10] Yancy, Lopatin, Stevenson, De Marco, Fonarow for the ADHERE Scientific Advisory Committee and Investigators.[8]*

carcinoma, or pneumonia. Pulmonary edema supports a diagnosis of heart failure, although the reliability of identifying upper lobe venous blood diversion is poor. Cardiothoracic ratio is only of moderate value in identifying heart failure as the cause of breathlessness.[23] Echocardiography has replaced chest radiography as the method of determining cardiac chamber dimensions.

[ ] ELECTROCARDIOGRAM

In clinical practice, the ECG is used to detect arrhythmia, and can provide evidence suggestive of previous myocardial infarction or ventricular hypertrophy. Many studies have suggested that a completely normal ECG is very unlikely in a person with heart failure, but its positive predictive value is low in the elderly where ECG abnormality is common.[24]

[ ] PLASMA B-TYPE NATRIURETIC PEPTIDE

B-type natriuretic peptide (BNP) is secreted by the heart, and the plasma concentration is elevated in left ventricular hypertrophy or dysfunction (systolic or diastolic), and particularly in those with heart failure. Several studies have confirmed its value as a *rule-out* test for heart failure in patients presenting with new symptoms in either primary or secondary care settings.[23,24,25] Raised plasma concentration can occur in other conditions, such as acute myocardial infarction, pulmonary embolism, and renal failure; and normal values are higher in the elderly and in women.[26] The current European and North American heart failure guidelines[4,5,13] suggest that the measurement of the plasma concentration of BNPs can be useful in confirming or refuting a diagnosis of heart failure, particularly at the time of first presentation in the acute setting.

[ ] ECHOCARDIOGRAPHY

Transthoracic echocardiography is a simple, safe, and effective method for assessing cardiac structure and function. It is the main imaging method used in cardiology and lends itself to population-based studies. Interpretation of normality can be difficult, particularly for those with poor images because of obesity or chronic airways disease, but satisfactory images should be obtainable in 80 to 90 percent of free-living subjects.[27]

[ ] MAGNETIC RESONANCE IMAGING

Magnetic resonance imaging provides high-resolution images of cardiac structure and ventricular function. Contrast agents such as gadolinium can provide information on inflammation, fibrosis and myocardial perfusion. Valve function can also be assessed, although with less reliability than myocardial structure and function. Although becoming mainstream in large hospitals, the expense of the equipment and its lack of portability makes it of limited use in population-based studies.

[ ] CARDIAC CATHETERIZATION

Cardiac catheterization allows measurement of intracardiac pressures, estimation of cardiac output, detection of valve abnormalities, quantification of left ventricular ejection fraction, and the detection of epicardial coronary artery disease. Diastolic function can be assessed in detail. Its use in epidemiological studies is limited by the invasive nature of the procedures and the consequent risk to study participants. It has been used in a population-based study of incident (new) heart failure in England, where it demonstrated that the presence and importance of coronary artery disease is underestimated by noninvasive assessment methods.[22]

[ ] EPIDEMIOLOGIC METHODS

The modern clinical approach to the diagnosis of heart failure contrasts with the methods used in many early epidemiological studies. The first large study to address heart failure was the Framingham Heart Study. A cohort of a little more than 5000 individuals was examined every 2 years from the study inception in 1948. Heart failure was considered present if on examination there were two "major" or one "major" and two "minor" criteria fulfilled[28] (Table 25–4). Between 1949 and 1988, 652 new cases of heart failure were identified—giving an incidence of 2.3 cases per 1000 per year in men, and 1.4 cases per 1000 per year in women, and a steep rise with age in both genders (Fig. 25–1).[29] The Framingham Score has been used in several other studies in North America, including the Rochester Epidemiology Project.[17]

Although these criteria are not used in clinical practise to diagnose heart failure, the advantage of the Framingham Heart Study is that the same criteria for heart failure have been applied for many decades, making possible conclusions on secular trends in incidence and prognosis.

Other scoring-based systems have been devised.[30] These have not been used widely, and more recent studies in Europe have adopted a more clinical approach, with review of symptoms, signs, and results of chest radiograph and echocardiography by a consensus expert panel. This method appears reproducible[21,22] and has been used in several studies in England and the Netherlands.[31]

Another approach has been to assess cardiac structure and function within a random sample of the population, typically by echocardiography, and simultaneously collect information on symptoms (and occasionally also clinical signs). Abnormality of valves or left ventricular systolic function are relatively easily identified, and patients with symptoms of breathlessness or fluid retention that could not be explained by lung disease or renal dysfunction are labelled as having heart failure.[32,33] Correctly identifying isolated abnormality of diastolic function of the left ventricle and establishing a causal link with symptoms can be challenging in this setting.

INCIDENCE OF HEART FAILURE

Reliable estimates of the incidence of heart failure are available from studies such as the Framingham Heart Study in the United States,[29] and the Hillingdon and Bromley Heart Failure Studies in London, England.[21,22] The former employed set criteria at biennial examination of a cohort of individuals initially free of heart failure. More recently the cohort has been enriched by offspring of the original members. The London studies employed an expert panel approach that reviewed all the available data for those with a new diagnosis of heart failure within a geographically defined population, using a systematic method of assessment that included

TABLE 25–4

The Criteria for the Diagnosis of Heart Failure in the Framingham Heart Study

MAJOR	MINOR	MAJOR OR MINOR
Bilateral moist rales	Ankle edema	Weight loss of ≥4.5 kg in 5 days with treatment
Paroxysmal nocturnal dyspnea and/or orthopnea	Pleural effusion	
Pulmonary edema by radiography	Hepatomegaly	
Neck vein distention in the semirecumbent position	Tachycardia (≥120 beats per minute)	
Enlarging heart by radiography S₃ gallop Hepatojugular reflux	Dyspnea on exertion Night cough 33.3% decrease in vital capacity	
Peripheral venous pressure >16 cm H₂O Arm-to-tongue circulation time ≥25 seconds		

SOURCE: McKee PA, Castelli WP, McNamara PM, Kannel WB.[28]

imaging of the heart by Doppler echocardiography. Table 25–5 summarizes the results of these and other key incident studies.

The crude incidence rate in the general population ranges from 1 to 5 cases per 1000 population per year, with a steep increase with advancing age (see Fig. 25–1). The median age at first presentation in most recent studies has been in the mid-70s, with a higher incidence in men than in women at all ages.[34]

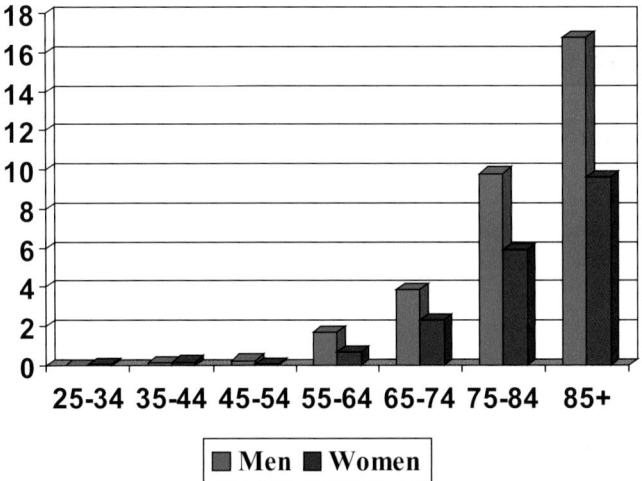

FIGURE 25–1. Incidence of heart failure by age group and gender in the Hillingdon Heart Failure Study, London, 1995 to 1997 (cases per 1000 population per year). *Source: Modified from Cowie MR, Wood DA, Coats AJ, et al.[21]*

TABLE 25–5

Incidence of Heart Failure in a Selection of Population-Based Studies

STUDY		INCIDENCE (PER 1000 POPULATION PER YEAR)		
		MEN	WOMEN	TOTAL
Cowie et al, Hillingdon, London, 1995–1996	Age			
	25–34	0	0.04	0.02
	35–44	0.2	0.2	0.2
	45–54	0.3	0.1	0.2
	55–64	1.7	0.7	1.2
	65–74	3.9	2.3	3.0
	75–84	9.8	5.9	7.4
	85+	16.8	9.6	11.6
Framingham, USA 1948–1988	Age			
	50–59	3	2	
	60–69	7	5	
	70–79	12	8	
	80–89	27	22	
Rochester, USA	1979–1984	3.6	2.8	
	1985–1990	3.9	2.9	
	1991–1995	3.8	2.6	
	1996–2000	3.8	3.2	
Framingham, USA	1950–1969	6.3	4.2	
	1970–1979	5.6	3.1	
	1980–1989	5.4	3.0	
	1990–1999	5.6	3.3	

SOURCE: Modified from Cowie MR, Mosterd A, Wood DA, et al.[2]

PREVALENCE OF HEART FAILURE

Studies from both Europe and North America suggest that the prevalence of heart failure is approximately 2 percent of the adult population, with a steep rise with age. Few adults aged younger than 40 years of age have heart failure.

Early studies used a range of methods to estimate prevalence, with quite marked differences in published results. Methodologies used included medical record/chart reviews supplemented by direct questioning and/or examination of individuals within the general population, drug prescription data analysis, monitoring of general practice activity, and appropriately sampled cohorts from the general population. The results of some key studies are shown in Table 25–6.

The first population-based study to use two-dimensional (2D) Doppler echocardiography was in Glasgow, Scotland. The prevalence of heart failure was reported as 1.5 percent of 1647 participants 25 to 74 years of age.[32] The definition of heart failure required a left ventricular EF less than 30 percent and cardiac shortness of breath on questionnaire or use of a loop diuretic. Asymptomatic left ventricular systolic dysfunction was almost as common as heart failure, at 1.4 percent of this population.

A population-based study in Rotterdam, The Netherlands, reported a prevalence of heart failure of 0.7 percent in those 55 to 64 years of age, 2.7 percent at 65 to 74 years of age, 13 percent at 75 to 84 years of age, and over 10 percent in those 85 years of age or older.[35] A trained nonmedical interviewer administered a standardized questionnaire, a clinician detected pulmonary rales and ankle edema in a subsample of individuals, and an ECG and echocardiogram were recorded. Heart failure was considered present if the individual did not have chronic pulmonary disease but evidence of cardiac disease and at least two of the following three characteristics: history of dyspnea, ankle edema, or pulmonary rales.

Definite heart failure, defined as individuals who were breathless on exertion and who had objective evidence of underlying cardiac dysfunction such as EF <40 percent, atrial fibrillation, or moderate-to-severe valve disease, was reported to be present in 2.3 percent of the general population 45 years of age and older in Birmingham, England.[36] *Probable* heart failure was reported in a further 0.8 percent.

In North America, several studies have reported similar figures, including the Cardiovascular Health Study[37] and the National Health and Nutrition Examination Survey.[38] In Olmsted County, Redfield and colleagues recently reported a prevalence of 2.2 percent in the population aged 45 years or older, applying the Framingham criteria to data in community and hospital-based medical records.[39] Of the 45 participants with a validated diagnosis of heart failure, 20 (44 percent) had an EF higher than 50 percent. The prevalence of heart failure increased steeply with age: 0.7 percent for those 45 to 54 years of age; 1.3 percent in those 55 to 64 years of age; 1.5 percent in those 65 to 74 years of age; and 8.4 percent for those 75 years of age or older.

On the basis of these studies, a conservative estimate of the burden of heart failure would be 4 million Americans and 6 million Europeans living with heart failure, out of a total population of 300 and 460 million, respectively.

TABLE 25-6

Prevalence of Heart Failure in a Selection of Population-Based Studies

STUDY	AGE	PREVALENCE (%)		
		MALE	FEMALE	TOTAL
Davies et al, West Midlands, UK, 1995–1999	45–54	0.3	0	0.2
	55–64	2.7	0.9	1.8
HF defined by ESC criteria	65–74	4.2	1.7	2.9
	75–84	7.3	6.6	6.9
	≥85	21.7	11.6	15.2
	Total	3	1.7	2.3
McDonagh et al. Glasgow, UK 1992	25–34	0	0	
	35–44	0	0	
HF defined as symptomatic left ventricular systolic dysfunction EF <30%	45–54	1.4	1.2	
	55–64	2.5	2	
	65–74	3.2	3.6	
Framingham, Massachusetts, 1948–1988	50–59	0.8	0.8	
	60–69	2.3	2.3	
HF defined by Framingham criteria	70–79	5.1	4.2	
	80–89	6.6	7.9	
Rochester, Minnesota, 1981	10–44	0	0	
	45–49	0.7	0.7	
HF defined by Framingham criteria	50–54	0.8	0.8	
	55–59	7.3	3.2	
	60–64	12	7.2	
	65–69	26.0	11.3	
	70–74	27.7	27.4	

SOURCE: *Modified from Cowie MR, Mosterd A, Wood DA, et al.*[2]

ETIOLOGY OF HEART FAILURE

Heart failure can be caused by any disease process that damages the pumping ability of the heart. The relative frequency of each pathology varies from one study to another, reflecting the population studied and the method of ascertaining etiology.

In many epidemiological studies the use of imaging (noninvasive or invasive) has been very limited. In a population-based study in South London, United Kingdom, the percentage of heart failure with unknown cause in those younger than 75 years of age declined from 42 to 10 percent after nuclear scintigraphy and cardiac catheterization, whereas the percentage of patients with coronary heart disease allocated as the etiology increased from 29 to 52 percent[22] (Fig. 25–2). In most series from the developed world, the single most common cause in the developed world is coronary heart disease. A history of hypertension is common but, at least in Europe, is rarely the sole cause of the cardiac damage leading to heart failure.[21,22] Data from the Framingham Heart Study suggest that both hypertension and valvular disease have declined in importance as the primary cause of heart failure.[40,41,42] The reported decline in the role of hypertension can have been partly related to the entirely noninvasive assessment of etiology in the early decades of the study, and consequent under-ascertainment of clinically important coronary artery disease. However, studies that do not have access to previous blood pressure readings can underestimate the importance of hypertension, as it can have *burnt out* by the time of development of heart failure.

Senile degeneration of the aortic valve is the most common valvular cause of heart failure in the developed world.[21,22] The situation in developing countries is quite different—there, acute and

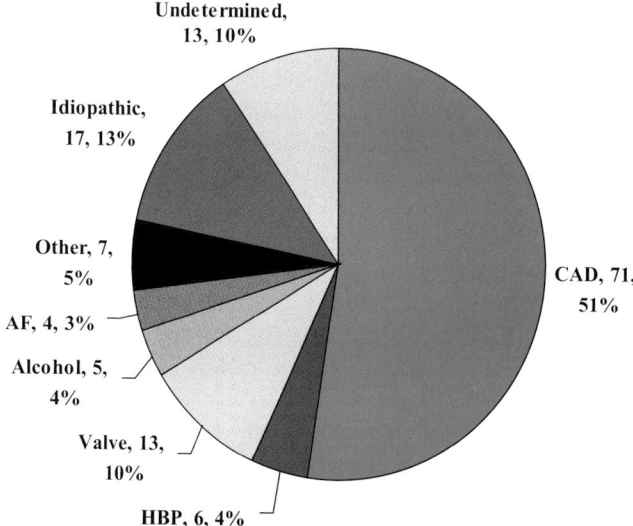

FIGURE 25-2. Etiology of heart failure in a study of incident (new) cases in Bromley, South London, for cases younger than 75 years of age, based on full investigation including nuclear scintigraphy and cardiac catheterization. AF, atrial fibrillation; CAD, coronary artery disease; HBP, high blood pressure. *Source: Modified from Fox KF, Cowie MR, Wood DA, et al.*[22]

chronic valvular damage caused by rheumatic fever is not uncommon.[43] With epidemiologic transition in the developing world, it is likely that the relative importance of the various etiologies of heart failure will become similar to that in the developed world—but currently hypertension in sub-Saharan Africa and rheumatic disease in the Far East remain very important.[43] Chagas disease is confined to the distribution of the *Trypanosoma cruzi* parasite in Central and South America, where it is a frequent cause of admission to hospital with heart failure caused by heart muscle disease in the chronic phase of the condition.[44]

RISK FACTORS FOR THE DEVELOPMENT OF HEART FAILURE

Based on observations from the Framingham Heart Study, the estimated life-time risk of developing heart failure is 1 in 5.[45] The presence of cardiovascular disease is, not surprisingly, associated with a greatly increased risk of heart failure. In the Framingham Heart Study almost 20 percent of those suffering a myocardial infarction developed heart failure within 6 years.[46] Heart failure during an acute admission with acute coronary syndrome is common.[47]

Hypertension is associated with an increased risk of heart failure, although the relative risk is lower than for myocardial infarction.[42] However, because the prevalence of hypertension is much higher than myocardial infarction, the proportion of cases of heart failure in the population that might be attributed to hypertension is higher.[42]

Other population-based studies have addressed risk factors for the development of heart failure, including the National Health and Nutrition Examination Survey,[48] "Men Born in 1913" Study from Göteborg, Sweden,[49] The Cardiovascular Health Study,[50] and other cohort studies.[51] Male gender, older age, physical inactivity, overweight, diabetes mellitus, hypertension, valvular heart disease, and coronary heart disease are consistently reported as being associated with the risk of developing heart failure.

Diabetes mellitus is associated with an increased risk of heart failure, particularly in women and after myocardial infarction.[52] Only part of this risk can be attributed to concomitant hypertension, obesity, and dyslipidemia. Diabetes can induce structural and functional changes in the myocardium that increase the risk of heart failure.[53]

Obesity is an independent risk factor for heart failure, approximately doubling the risk of heart failure.[49,52,54] Cigarette smoking also increases the risk, although the effect weakens with age.[49] The mechanism is presumably through acceleration of coronary artery disease.

There are many pathophysiological markers of underlying cardiac damage that have been reported to be associated with an increased risk of heart failure, including left ventricular hypertrophy (either by ECG or echocardiographic criteria), increased heart volume on chest radiograph, T wave abnormalities on the ECG, and a reduced expiratory flow rate.[2]

The importance of these risk factors lies in the ability to identify those individuals at particularly high risk of heart failure. Early modification of such risk factors can prevent, or at least postpone, the onset of heart failure. The most recent ACC/AHA guidelines draw attention to individuals with these risk factors, and labels

them as *Stage A* (high risk, no symptoms) or *Stage B* (structural heart disease but no symptoms) heart failure.[13] In Europe, the diagnosis of heart failure is only attached to those who at least initially have symptoms, with *asymptomatic cardiac dysfunction* being the term preferred to Stage B heart failure.

Interestingly, once heart failure develops, several conventional cardiovascular risk factors appear to be associated with a reduced risk of mortality: hypertension, obesity, and hypercholesterolemia. This has been termed *reverse epidemiology*.[55] It can be explained, at least partially, by reverse causation, where the ability to maintain such levels of a risk factor is a marker of less severe pump failure (or better adaptation to the pump failure) and hence a better prognosis.

PROGNOSIS OF HEART FAILURE

Despite current life-prolonging therapies, such as angiotensin-converting enzyme inhibitors and blockers, a new diagnosis of heart failure in England carries a prognosis similar to bowel cancer but worse than breast cancer.[56,57] The comparative survival from heart failure and a variety of malignancies in the United States is shown in Fig. 25–3.[58,59]

Fig. 25–4 shows the long-term survival in a cohort of 552 new cases of heart failure identified in the London Heart Failure Studies in 1995 to 1998. The survival of incident cases was similar in the Rotterdam Study (The Netherlands), with 1-, 2-, and 5-year survival rates of 63, 51, and 35 percent, respectively.[60] The most recent data from the Framingham Heart Study shows a similar picture but with evidence of improvement in prognosis in the past 30 years (Fig. 25–5).[61] Mortality is particularly high in the 3 months after diagnosis.

Factors associated with a poorer prognosis include male gender, advanced age, more severe symptoms (higher New York Heart Association class), coronary artery disease—particularly acute coronary syndrome, hypotension, impaired renal function, hyponatremia, and elevated plasma BNP concentration.[56,62-64]

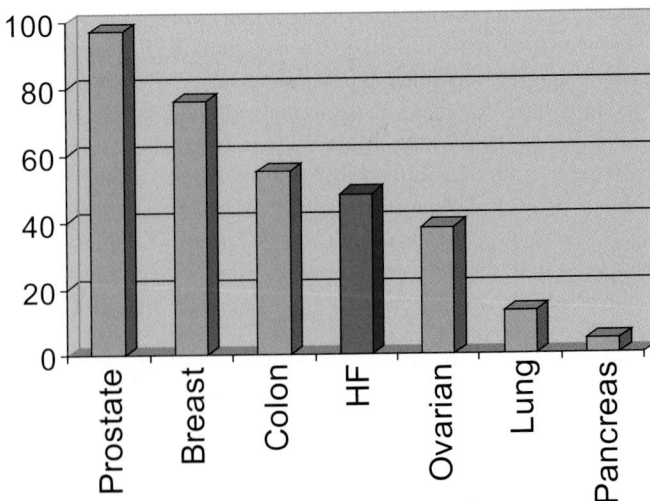

FIGURE 25–3. Comparative 5-year survival (percent) from heart failure and a number of malignant conditions in the United States, 1990 to 2000. *Source: Ries LAG, Harkins D, Krapcho M, et al, eds*[58]; *and Thom T, Haase N, Rosamond W, et al for the American Heart Association Statistics Committee and Stroke Statistics Subcommittee.*[59]

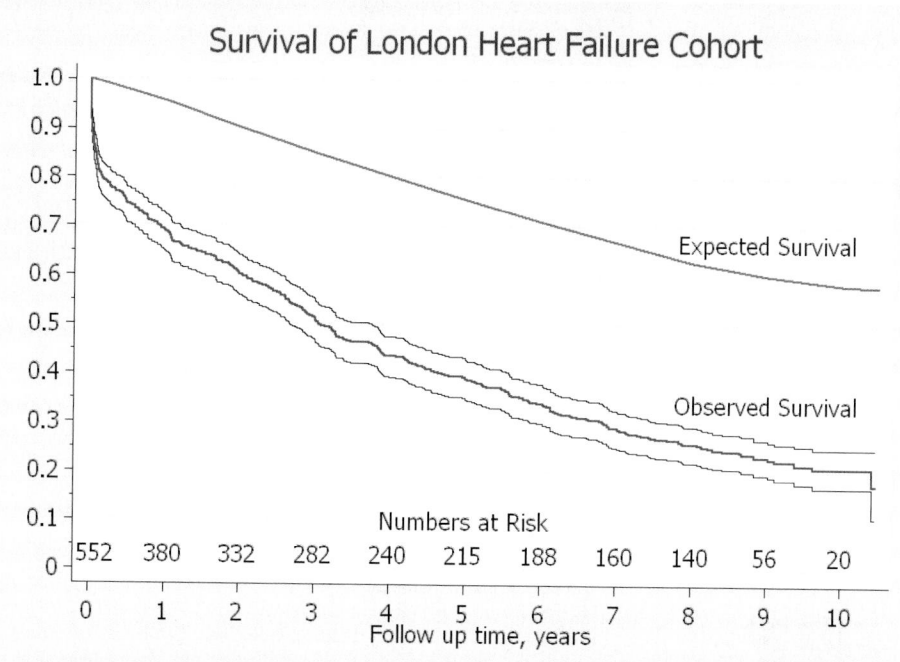

FIGURE 25–4. Cumulative survival of the 552 individuals with incident (new) heart failure identified in the Hillingdon and Bromley (London) Heart Failure Studies 1995 to 1998. Expected survival is that of the age- and gender-matched UK population. Observed survival is shown with its 95 percent confidence interval. *Source: Author's own data.*

SECULAR TRENDS IN HEART FAILURE

The literature is limited and inconsistent on whether the incidence of heart failure has changed in the past decades. The Framingham Heart Study reported no change in the period 1950 to 1999 for men, but a small decrease in the early stage of that period for women.[61] Data from Olmsted County, Minnesota reported no change from 1979 through 2000.[65,66] Less robust data from the very large Kaiser Permanente database in the Pacific Northwest of the United States suggest an increase of 14 percent in the incidence rate over the two decades from 1970 to 1974.[67] There are no reliable published data from Europe.

There is, however, good evidence that the survival from heart failure has improved in the past 30 years, for both men and women in the Framingham Heart Study[61] and in the Olmsted County Rochester Epidemiology Project.[66] Recent epidemiological data from the United Kingdom confirm these findings.[68]

The rapid aging of the population in developed countries, the lack of a fall in incidence, and an improving prognosis all act to increase the number of people living with chronic heart failure—with no likely decrease anticipated in the near future. In 2002, 12.6 percent of the population was older than 65 years of age in the United States. This is expected to rise to 16.3 percent in 2020, 19.6 percent in 2030, and 22.4 percent in 2040.[69] Similar population projections have been made for Europe.[70]

HEALTHCARE BURDEN OF HEART FAILURE

In the United States, heart failure continues to be the most common cause of hospitalization in people older than 65 years of age,[71] with a reported 174 percent rise in hospital discharge rates from 399,000 in 1979 to 1,093,000 in 2003. In Europe, 5 percent of adult internal medicine and geriatric hospitalizations are as a result of heart failure—a larger proportion than those as a result of

myocardial infarction.[72] The age-adjusted rates for hospitalization may have peaked.[73] The duration of hospitalization for heart failure, particularly in Europe, are long with a median duration in the Euroheart Heart Failure survey of 11 days.[10] The typical duration of hospitalization in the United States is closer to 5 days.[8,74]

The readmission rate is also high, with one-third to one-half of patients being readmitted within 6 months in the United States[71] or 12 months in Europe.[72,75] Mortality after hospitalization is also high, with 13 percent dying within 12 weeks in Europe.[10] Not all admissions are as a result of heart failure, but of the emergency readmissions 20 to 50 percent of them are likely to be so,[75,76] with some patients being readmitted multiple times.

The number of hospitalizations drives the costs of heart failure to the health economies. Approximately 60 percent of the total direct costs of heart failure relate to hospitalization, and this ranges from between 1 and 2 percent of the total healthcare budget in many developed countries.[76,77] Added to the direct healthcare costs are the economic consequences to the patient and their families: The total (direct and indirect) cost of heart failure is estimated to be $29.6 billion in the United States for 2006.[59]

CONCLUSIONS

Heart failure affects 2 percent of the population in the developed world, and the absolute number of people living with the syndrome is set to increase steeply in the next decades because of an improving prognosis and a rapidly aging population. The typical patient is elderly, as likely to be female as male, and will be suffering from considerable comorbidity. The direct cost to the healthcare system is substantial and is largely driven by hospitalization costs. The epidemiology suggests that efforts to prevent and treat hypertension and the other risk factors for coronary artery disease (including obesity, diabetes, hyperlipidemia, and cigarette smoking) will at least delay, if not prevent, the de-

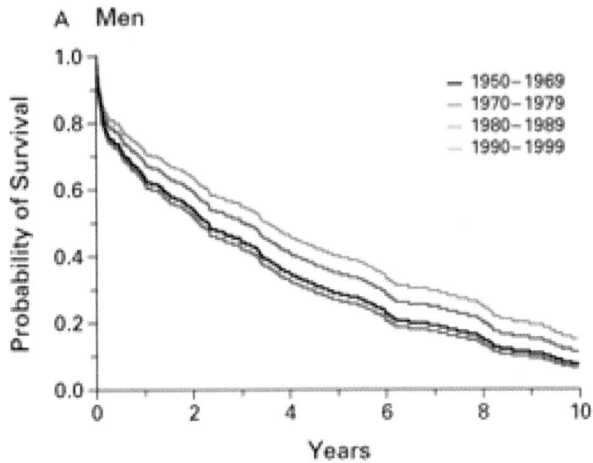

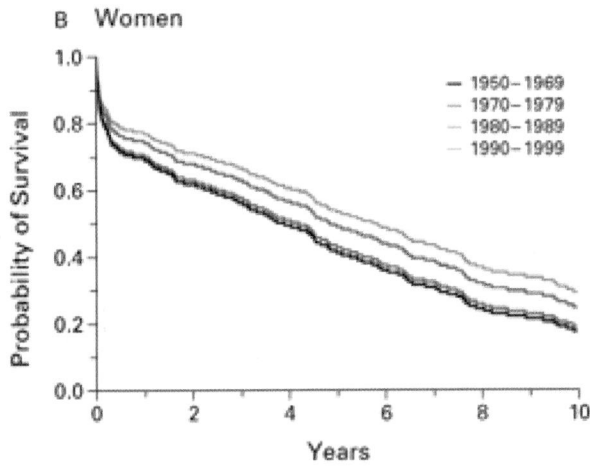

FIGURE 25–5. Secular trends in survival of incident (new) heart failure in the Framingham Heart Study. *Source: Used with permission from Levy D, Kenchaiah S, Larson MG, et al.[61]*

velopment of heart failure. Once the syndrome develops, the prognosis is poor, particularly in the first months after diagnosis, but has improved substantially in the past decades—presumably as a result of better diagnosis and therapy with angiotensin-converting enzyme inhibitors and β blockers. The epidemic of heart failure is already on us and will be a challenge for all healthcare settings for the foreseeable future.

REFERENCES

1. Marantz PR, Alderman MH, Tobin JN. Diagnostic heterogeneity in clinical trials for congestive heart failure. *Ann Intern Med.* 1988;109:55–61.
2. Cowie MR, Mosterd A, Wood DA, et al. The epidemiology of heart failure. *Eur Heart J.* 1997;18:208–225.
3. Poole-Wilson PA. Chronic heart failure: cause, pathophysiology, prognosis, clinical manifestations, investigations. In: Julian DG, Camm AJ, Fox KF, Hall RJC, Poole-Wilson PA, eds. *Diseases of the Heart.* London: Balliere-Tindall; 1989:24–36.
4. Swedberg K, Cleland J, Dargie H, et al. Guidelines for the diagnosis and treatment of chronic heart failure: executive summary (update 2005): the Task Force for the Diagnosis and Treatment of Chronic Heart Failure of the European Society of Cardiology. *Eur Heart J.* 2005;26:1115–1140.
5. Adams KF, Lindenfeld J, Arnold JMO, et al. HFSA 2006 comprehensive heart failure practice guideline. *J Cardiac Fail.* 2006;12:e1–e122.
6. Harlan WR, Obermann A, Grimm R, Rosati RA. Chronic congestive heart failure in coronary artery disease: clinical criteria. *Ann Intern Med.* 1977;86:133–138.
7. Zile MR, Brutsaert DL. New concepts in diastolic dysfunction and diastolic heart failure. Part I: diagnosis, prognosis, and measurements of diastolic function. *Circulation.* 2002;105:1387–1393.
8. Yancy CW, Lopatin M, Stevenson LW, De Marco T, Fonarow GC for the ADHERE Scientific Advisory Committee and Investigators. Clinical presentation, management, and in-hospital outcomes of patients admitted with acute decompensated heart failure with preserved systolic function: a report from the Acute Decompensated Heart Failure National Registry (ADHERE) Database. *J Am Coll Cardiol.* 2006;47:76–84. Erratum in: *J Am Coll Cardiol.* 2006;47:1502.
9. McMurray J, McDonagh T, Morrison CE, et al. Trends in hospitalization for heart failure in Scotland 1980–1990. *Eur Heart J.* 1993;14:1158–1162.
10. Cleland JG, Swedberg K, Follath F, et al for the Study Group on Diagnosis of the Working Group on Heart Failure of the European Society of Cardiology. The EuroHeart Failure survey programme—a survey on the quality of care among patients with heart failure in Europe. Part 1: patient characteristics and diagnosis. *Eur Heart J.* 2003;24:442–463.
11. European Study Group on Diastolic Heart Failure. How to diagnose diastolic heart failure. *Eur Heart J.* 1998;19:990–1003.
12. Vasan RS. Defining diastolic heart failure: a call for standardized diagnostic criteria. *Circulation.* 2000;101:2118–2121.
13. Hunt SA, American College of Cardiology (ACC), American Heart Association (AHA)Task Force on Practice Guidelines (Writing Committee to Update the 2001 Guidelines for the Evaluation and Management of Heart Failure). ACC/AHA 2005 guideline update for the diagnosis and management of chronic heart failure in the adult: a report. *J Am Coll Cardiol.* 2005;46: e1–82. Erratum in: *J Am Coll Cardiol.* 2006;47:1503–1505.
14. Chen HH, Lainchbury JG, Senni M, Bailey KR, Redfield MM. Diastolic heart failure in the community: clinical profile, natural history, therapy, and impact of proposed diagnostic criteria. *J Card Fail.* 2002;8:279–287.
15. Senni M, Tribouilloy CM, Rodeheffer RJ, et al. Congestive heart failure in the community: a study of all incident cases in Olmsted County, Minnesota in 1991. *Circulation.* 1998;98:2282–2289.
16. Senni M, Redfield MM. Heart failure with preserved systolic function. A different natural history? *J Am Coll Cardiol.* 2001;38:1277–1282.
17. Owan TE, Hodge DO, Herges RM, Jacobsen SJ, Roger VL, Redfield MM. Trends in prevalence and outcome of heart failure with preserved ejection fraction. *N Engl J Med.* 2006;355:251–259.
18. Vasan RS, Larson MG, Benjamin EJ, Evans JC, Reiss CK, Levy D. Congestive heart failure in subjects with normal versus reduced left ventricular ejection fraction: prevalence and mortality in a population-based cohort. *J Am Coll Cardiol.* 1999;33:1948–1955.
19. Banerjee P, Banerjee T, Khand A, Clark AL, Cleland JG. Diastolic heart failure: neglected or misdiagnosed? *J Am Coll Cardiol.* 2002;39:138–141.
20. Caruana L, Petrie MC, Davie AP, McMurray JJ. Do patients with suspected heart failure and preserved left ventricular systolic function suffer from "diastolic heart failure" or from misdiagnosis? A prospective descriptive study. *BMJ.* 2000;321:215–218.
21. Cowie MR, Wood DA, Coats AJ, et al. Incidence and aetiology of heart failure; a population-based study. *Eur Heart J.* 1999;20:421–428.
22. Fox KF, Cowie MR, Wood DA, et al. Coronary artery disease as the cause of incident heart failure in the population. *Eur Heart J.* 2001;22:228–236.
23. Cowie MR, Struthers AD, Wood DA, et al. Value of natriuretic peptides in assessment of patients with possible new heart failure in primary care. *Lancet.* 1997;350:1349–1353.
24. Zaphiriou A, Robb S, Murray-Thomas T, et al. The diagnostic accuracy of plasma BNP and NT-proBNP in patients referred from primary care with suspected heart failure: results of the UK natriuretic peptide study. *Eur J Heart Fail.* 2005;7:537–41.
25. McCullough PA, Nowak RM, McCord J, et al. B-type natriuretic peptide and clinical judgment in emergency diagnosis of heart failure: analysis from Breathing Not Properly (BNP) Multinational Study. *Circulation.* 2002;106:416–422.
26. Cowie MR, Jourdain P, Maisel A, et al. Clinical applications of B-type natriuretic peptide (BNP) testing. *Eur Heart J.* 2003;24:1710–1718.
27. Devereux RB, Roman MJ, Liu JE, et al. An appraisal of echocardiography as an epidemiological tool. The Strong Heart Study. *Ann Epidemiol.* 2003;13:238–244.
28. McKee PA, Castelli WP, McNamara PM, Kannel WB. The natural history of congestive heart failure: the Framingham study. *N Engl J Med.* 1971;285:1441–1446.

29. Ho KK, Anderson KM, Kannel WB, Grossman W, Levy D. Survival after the onset of congestive heart failure in Framingham Heart Study subjects. *Circulation.* 1993;88:107–115.

30. Cowie MR, Mosterd A, Wood DA, et al. The epidemiology of heart failure. *Eur Heart J.* 1997;18:208–225.

31. Rutten FH, Moons KG, Cramer MJ, et al. Recognising heart failure in elderly patients with stable chronic obstructive pulmonary disease in primary care: cross sectional diagnostic study. *BMJ.* 2005;331:1379.

32. McDonagh TA, Morrison CE, Lawrence A, et al. Symptomatic and asymptomatic left-ventricular systolic dysfunction in an urban population. *Lancet.* 1997;350:829–833.

33. Fischer M, Baessler A, Holmer SR, et al. Epidemiology of left ventricular systolic dysfunction in the general population of Germany: results of an echocardiographic study of a large population-based sample. *Z Kardiol.* 2003;92:294–302.

34. Mehta PA, Cowie MR. Gender and heart failure: a population perspective. *Heart.* 2006;92(suppl 3): iii14–18.

35. Mosterd A, Hoes AW, de Bruyne MC, et al. Prevalence of heart failure and left ventricular dysfunction in the general population; the Rotterdam Study. *Eur Heart J.* 1999;20:447–455.

36. Davies M, Hobbs F, Davis R, et al. Prevalence of left-ventricular systolic dysfunction and heart failure in the Echocardiographic Heart of England Screening study: a population based study. *Lancet.* 2001;358:439–444.

37. Mittelmark MB, Psaty BM, Rautaharju PM, et al. Prevalence of cardiovascular diseases among older adults. The Cardiovascular Health Study. *Am J Epidemiol.* 1993;137:311–317.

38. Schocken DD, Arrieta MI, Leaverton PE, Ross EA. Prevalence and mortality rate of congestive heart failure in the United States. *J Am Coll Cardiol.* 1992;20:301–306.

39. Redfield MM, Jacobsen SJ, Burnett JC Jr, Mahoney DW, Bailey KR, Rodeheffer RJ. Burden of systolic and diastolic ventricular dysfunction in the community: appreciating the scope of the heart failure epidemic. *JAMA.* 2003;289:194–202.

40. Kannel WB, Ho K, Thom T. Changing epidemiological features of cardiac failure. *Br Heart J.* 1994;72(2 suppl):S3–9.

41. McMurray JJ, Stewart S. Epidemiology, aetiology, and prognosis of heart failure. *Heart.* 2000;83:596–602.

42. Levy D, Larson MG, Vasan RS, Kannel WB, Ho KK. The progression from hypertension to congestive heart failure. *JAMA.* 1996;275:1557–1562.

43. Mendez GF, Cowie MR. The epidemiological features of heart failure in developing countries: a review of the literature. *Int J Cardiol.* 2001;80:213–219.

44. Rassi A Jr, Rassi A, Little WC. Chagas' heart disease. *Clin Cardiol.* 2000;23:883–889.

45. Lloyd-Jones DM, Larson MG, Leip EP, et al for the Framingham Heart Study. Lifetime risk for developing congestive heart failure: the Framingham Heart Study. *Circulation.* 2002;106:3068–3072.

46. Kannel WB. Epidemiology and prevention of cardiac failure: Framingham Study insights. *Eur Heart J.* 1987;8(suppl F):23–26.

47. Haim M, Battler A, Behar S, et al. Acute coronary syndromes complicated by symptomatic and asymptomatic heart failure: does current treatment comply with guidelines? *Am Heart J.* 2004;147:859–864. Erratum in: *Am Heart J.* 2004;148:325.

48. He J, Ogden LG, Bazzano LA, Vupputuri S, Loria C, Whelton PK. Risk factors for congestive heart failure in U.S. men and women: NHANES I epidemiologic follow-up study. *Arch Intern Med.* 2001;161:996–1002.

49. Eriksson H, Svardsudd K, Larsson B, et al. Risk factors for heart failure in the general population: the study of men born in 1913. *Eur Heart J.* 1989;10:647–656.

50. Gottdiener JS, Arnold AM, Aurigemma GP, et al. Predictors of congestive heart failure in the elderly: the Cardiovascular Health Study. *J Am Coll Cardiol.* 2000;35:1628–1637.

51. Chen YT, Vaccarino V, Williams CS, Butler J, Berkman LF, Krumholz HM. Risk factors for heart failure in the elderly: a prospective community-based study. *Am J Med.* 1999;106:605–612.

52. Ho KK, Pinsky JL, Kannel WB, Levy D. The epidemiology of heart failure: the Framingham Study. *J Am Coll Cardiol.* 1993;22 (suppl A):6A-13A.

53. Taegtmeyer H, McNulty P, Young ME. Adaptation and maladaptation of the heart in diabetes. Part I: general concepts. *Circulation.* 2002;105:1727–1733.

54. Kenchaiah S, Evans JC, Levy D, et al. Obesity and the risk of heart failure. *N Engl J Med.* 2002;347:305–313.

55. Kalantar-Zadeh K, Block G, Horwich T, Fonarow GC. Reverse epidemiology of conventional cardiovascular risk factors in patients with chronic heart failure. *J Am Coll Cardiol.* 2004;43:1439–1444.

56. Cowie MR, Wood DA, Coats AJ, et al. Survival of patients with a new diagnosis of heart failure: a population based study. *Heart.* 2000;83:505–510.

57. Quinn M, Babb P, Brock A, Kirby L, Jones J. *Cancer Trends in England and Wales 1950–1999.* London: The Stationery Office, Office for National Statistics; 2001.

58. Ries LAG, Harkins D, Krapcho M, et al, eds. SEER Cancer Statistics Review, 1975–2003, National Cancer Institute. Bethesda, MD. Available at: http://seer.cancer.gov/csr/1975_2003/; based on November 2005 SEER data submission, posted to the SEER Web site. Accessed September 17,2006.

59. Thom T, Haase N, Rosamond W, et al for the American Heart Association Statistics Committee and Stroke Statistics Subcommittee. Heart disease and stroke statistics—2006 update: a report. *Circulation.* 2006;113:e85–151. Erratum in: Circulation. 2006;113:e696.

60. Bleumink GS, Knetsch AM, Sturkenboom MC, et al. Quantifying the heart failure epidemic: prevalence, incidence rate, lifetime risk and prognosis of heart failure the Rotterdam Study. *Eur Heart J.* 2004;25:1614–1619.

61. Levy D, Kenchaiah S, Larson MG, et al. Long-term trends in the incidence of and survival with heart failure. *N Engl J Med.* 2002;347:1397–1402.

62. Cowburn PJ, Cleland JG, Coats AJ, Komajda M. Risk stratification in chronic heart failure. *Eur Heart J.* 1998;19:696–710.

63. Cowie MR, Jourdain P, Maisel A, et al. Clinical applications of B-type natriuretic peptide (BNP) testing. *Eur Heart J.* 2003;24:1710–1718.

64. Lloyd-Jones DM. The risk of congestive heart failure: sobering lessons from the Framingham Heart Study. *Curr Cardiol Rep.* 2001;3:184–190.

65. Senni M, Tribouilloy CM, Rodeheffer RJ, et al. Congestive heart failure in the community: trends in incidence and survival in a 10-year period. *Arch Intern Med.* 1999;159:29–34.

66. Roger VL, Weston SA, Redfield MM, et al. Trends in heart failure incidence and survival in a community-based population. *JAMA.* 2004;292:344–350.

67. Barker WH, Mullooly JP, Getchell W. Changing incidence and survival for heart failure in a well-defined older population, 1970–1974 and 1990–1994. *Circulation.* 2006;113:799–805.

68. Mehta PA, Dubrey SW, McIntyre HF, et al. Improved survival for patients with incident heart failure in the UK population. World Congress of Cardiology, Barcelona, September 2006 (poster 516).

69. United States Census Bureau. *Current Population Reports Series P25–1104. Population Projections of the United States by Age, Sex, Race and Hispanic Origin: 1993–2050.* Washington, DC: United States Census Bureau; 2001.

70. Eurostat. Long-term population projections at the national level; issue number 3/2006. Available at http://epp.eurostat.ec.europa.eu/cache/ITY_OFFPUB/KS-NK-06-003-EN.pdf. Accessed September 17, 2006).

71. Haldeman GA, Croft JB, Giles WH, Rashidee A. Hospitalization of patients with heart failure: National Hospital Discharge Survey, 1985 to 1995. *Am Heart J.* 1999;137:352–360.

72. McMurray J, McDonagh T, Morrison CE, Dargie HJ. Trends in hospitalization for heart failure in Scotland 1980–1990. *Eur Heart J.* 1993;14:1158–1162.

73. Stewart S, MacIntyre K, MacLeod MM, Bailey AE, Capewell S, McMurray JJ. Trends in hospitalization for heart failure in Scotland, 1990–1996. An epidemic that has reached its peak? *Eur Heart J.* 2001;22:209–217.

74. Krumholz HM, Parent EM, Tu N, et al. Readmission after hospitalization for congestive heart failure among Medicare beneficiaries. *Arch Intern Med.* 1997;157:99–104.

75. Cowie MR, Fox KF, Wood DA, et al. Hospitalization of patients with heart failure: a population-based study. *Eur Heart J.* 2002;23:877–885.

76. McMurray JJ, Petrie MC, Murdoch DR, Davie AP. Clinical epidemiology of heart failure: public and private health burden. *Eur Heart J.* 1998;19(suppl P):P9–16.

77. Berry C, Murdoch DR, McMurray JJ. Economics of chronic heart failure. *Eur J Heart Fail.* 2001;3:283–291.

CHAPTER (26)

Diagnosis and Management of Heart Failure

William T. Abraham / Ayesha Hasan /
Philip Poole-Wilson

In the classic text *Diseases of the Heart* published in 1933,[1] Sir Thomas Lewis identified the diagnosis and management of chronic heart failure as the cardinal problem in clinical cardiology. This observation is relevant today, because heart failure represents one of the most rapidly growing and costly forms of cardiovascular disease. As discussed in Chap. 25, both the incidence and prevalence of heart failure are substantial and rising, because heart failure remains a principal complication of virtually every form of heart disease. Moreover, heart failure is associated with high rates of morbidity, mortality, and economic cost. For example, it is estimated that at any time 30 to 40 percent of heart failure patients are judged to be in New York Heart Association (NYHA) functional class III or IV, indicating an advanced degree of disability.[2] Readmission rates for heart failure remain high, and 5-year mortality ranges from 15 percent for those with asymptomatic disease to more than 50 percent in patients with advanced heart failure.[3-6] A sound understanding of the pathophysiology of the disease (as reviewed in Chap. 24) along with a systematic approach to the evaluation and management of heart failure (presented in this chapter) results in improved patient outcomes.

The current evaluation and management of patients with chronic systolic heart failure has a large evidence base. Recommendations for its treatment are supported by numerous randomized controlled trials or by substantial clinical and observational experience. Several national and international guidelines directing the evaluation and management of chronic systolic heart failure in adults have been published.[7-10] In contrast, the treatment of diastolic heart failure remains largely empirical and is directed toward controlling symptoms by reducing ventricular filling pressures without reducing cardiac output. The treatment of acute, worsening, or rapidly decompensated heart failure has been inadequately studied. Although published guidelines address the management of decompensated heart failure, recommendations are generally based on consensus expert opinion rather than randomized controlled trials.[7-11]

GENERAL PRINCIPLES OF MANAGEMENT

Heart failure should be prevented through the early treatment of risk factors and, when present, asymptomatic left ventricular (LV) dysfunction. The first revision to the 1995 American College of Cardiology/American Heart Association Guideline for the Evaluation and Management of Heart Failure developed a framework for heart failure prevention.[12] This guideline, published in November 2001[12] and updated in September 2005,[7] views heart failure as a continuum beginning with risk factors and culminating in end-stage or refractory disease. According to these guidelines, there are known risk factors and structural prerequisites leading to the development of LV systolic and/or diastolic dysfunction and the clinical syndrome of heart failure.

The guideline proposes four stages describing the progression of heart failure (Table 26–1).[7] Stage A describes patients who exhibit one or more risk factors for the development of heart failure. If inadequately treated, these risk factors, such as hypertension, diabetes, and coronary artery disease, frequently lead to the development of a structural abnormality of the heart. Stage B is defined by the development of such a structural abnormality of the heart but no symptoms of heart failure. This is the true asymptomatic or *never been symptomatic* stage of cardiovascular disease progression to heart failure. Examples of progression from stage A to stage B include the development of LV hypertrophy in the hypertensive subject or the onset of a LV wall motion abnormality and reduced ejection fraction (EF) in the coronary artery disease patient following myocardial infarction (MI). Stage C is heralded by the onset of symptoms related to heart failure, including shortness of breath, fatigue, and exercise intolerance. By definition, stage C patients have current or prior symptoms of heart failure. Thus, even if made asymptomatic with treatment, stage C patients are not considered to have regressed to stage B. Finally, stage D defines the patient with marked heart failure symptoms at rest despite maximal medical therapy. These patients are generally in need of heroic measures, such as cardiac transplantation or mechanical assistance, or referral into a program focused on end-of-life care.

TABLE 26–1

American College of Cardiology/American Heart Association Stages of Heart Failure

STAGE	DEFINITION	PATIENT DESCRIPTION
A	High risk for developing heart failure (HF)	• Hypertension • Coronary artery disease • Diabetes mellitus • Family history of cardiomyopathy
B	Asymptomatic HF	• Previous MI • LV hypertrophy or systolic dysfunction • Asymptomatic valvular disease
C	Symptomatic HF	• Known structural heart disease • Shortness of breath and fatigue • Reduced exercise tolerance
D	Refractory end-stage HF	• Marked symptoms at rest despite maximal medical therapy (e.g., those who are recurrently hospitalized or cannot be safely discharged from the hospital without specialized interventions

LV, left ventricular; MI, myocardial infarction.

The treatment of patients with risk factors (stage A) and asymptomatic LV dysfunction (stage B) is extensively reviewed elsewhere in this textbook and briefly in this chapter. Once LV dysfunction and symptomatic heart failure ensue (stages C and D), treatment should ideally be directed at improving the function of the heart as a pump. This both increases cardiac output and decreases venous hypertension, improving both the low-output and congestive signs and symptoms of the disease. The goal of improving the functional performance of the heart as a pump is often difficult to accomplish. Moreover, the chronic use of positive inotropic agents to improve contractility consistently increases mortality when compared to standard heart failure therapy.[13–15] At the present time, standard pharmacologic management of heart failure is aimed at reducing ventricular preload and afterload and at diminishing, inhibiting, and/or antagonizing neurohormonal vasoconstrictor activation, rather than directly increasing cardiac contractility.

PREVENTION OF HEART FAILURE

Typically, stage A and B patients have one or more of the following risk factors for the development of heart failure: advanced age, hypertension, diabetes mellitus, obesity, metabolic syndrome, coronary artery disease, prior MI, and LV hypertrophy.[16,17] Other risks for heart failure include anemia, dyslipidemia, sleep disordered breathing, valvular heart disease, family history of cardiomyopathy, exposure to various cardiotoxins (e.g., anthracyclines), skeletal myopathies, and other less common disorders (Table 26–2).

Advancing age is one of the most prominent risk factors for heart failure. Data from the Framingham Study indicate that heart failure is present in approximately 1 percent of adults in their 50s and in as many as 10 percent of those in their 80s.[16] This association between advanced age and heart failure is most likely the result of decades of inadequate treatment of underlying risk factors, rather than to aging alone. Obesity acts directly or indirectly by being associated with dyslipidemia, hypertension, insulin resistance, diabetes, and LV hypertrophy, thus promoting heart failure.[18] In this regard the metabolic syndrome may represent one of the most prevalent unifying risk factors for heart failure. Obesity may also contribute to the prevalence of obstructive sleep apnea,

TABLE 26–2

Risk Factors for the Development of Heart Failure

Hypertension	Rheumatic fever
Diabetes	Mediastinal irradiation
Dyslipidemia	Sleep disordered breathing
Coronary artery disease	Collagen vascular disease
Valvular heart disease	Anemia
Obesity	Nutritional deficiencies
Metabolic syndrome	Skeletal myopathies
Excessive alcohol consumption	Exposure to cardiotoxic agents
Smoking	Thyroid disorders
Aging	Family history of cardiomyopathy

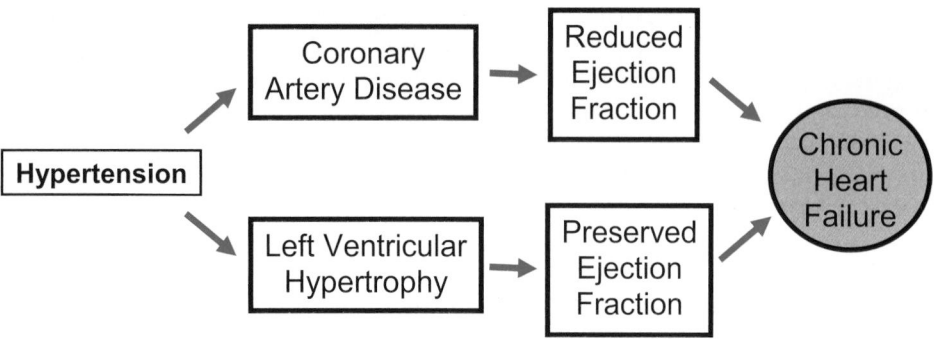

FIGURE 26–1. In general, hypertension may lead to heart failure via one of two major pathways, coronary artery disease leading to a reduced EF or LV hypertrophy resulting in heart failure with a preserved EF. EF, ejection fraction; LV, left ventricular.

another independent risk factor for the development of hypertension and heart failure.[19,20]

【 】 HYPERTENSION AS A RISK FACTOR FOR HEART FAILURE

As noted in Chap. 68, approximately 25 percent of the U.S. population is hypertensive, and the lifetime risk of developing hypertension among Americans exceeds 75 percent.[21] Elevated levels of systolic and/or diastolic blood pressure are major risk factors for the development of heart failure.[22,23] Information from the Framingham Study suggests that hypertension precedes the onset of heart failure in 91 percent of cases.[22] Thus, it is not surprising that long-term treatment of both systolic and diastolic hypertension has been shown to reduce the risk of heart failure.[24,25] Numerous randomized, controlled trials have consistently demonstrated that optimal blood pressure control decreases the risk of new-onset heart failure by approximately half.[26] In other populations hypertension is a less common cause of heart failure and usually associated with coronary heart disease.

Hypertension may lead to structural heart disease and cardiac failure through at least two pathways, first the development of LV hypertrophy resulting in heart failure associated with a preserved LV ejection fraction (LVEF) and second MI usually resulting in a regional wall motion abnormality and reduced LVEF (Fig. 26–1). LV hypertrophy is a strong and independent risk factor for heart failure.[27] However, in most instances, heart failure associated with a history of hypertension is mediated by atherosclerotic coronary artery disease rather than or in addition to LV hypertrophy. In this circumstance, hypertension may be seen as a contributor to rather than a direct cause of the LV dysfunction, which may be primarily attributed to myocardial ischemia/infarction. However, the role of hypertension leading to heart failure in post-MI subjects should not be underestimated, because the benefits of treating hypertension in heart attack survivors are dramatic with an 81 percent reduction in the incidence of heart failure.[24]

To prevent heart failure and other cardiovascular events in hypertensive subjects, both systolic and diastolic blood pressure should be lowered using evidence-based therapies recommended in guidelines. Recommendations for the treatment of hypertension are reviewed in Chap. 70 and in the current version of the guideline from the Joint National Committee on Prevention, Detection, Evaluation, and Treatment of High Blood Pressure.[28] Goal blood pressure and the selection of an antihypertensive regimen depend, in part, on the absence or presence of comorbidity. Data support a lower ideal or target blood pressure goal in patients with associated major cardiovascular risk factors, particularly those with diabetes mellitus.[29–31] Although treatment to target blood pressure should remain the primary goal of antihypertensive treatment, the choice of specific agent(s) may be determined by the particular comorbidity present (e.g., diabetes, coronary artery disease, or LV dysfunction).

Various antihypertensive agents reduce the incidence of heart failure, including diuretics, angiotensin-converting enzyme (ACE) inhibitors, and β blockers.[28,32–34] Calcium channel blockers and α blockers appear to be less effective in preventing the onset of heart failure. In the Antihypertensive and Lipid-lowering Treatment to Prevent Heart Attack Trial (ALLHAT), the α-receptor blocking agent doxazosin was associated with an increase in the incidence of new-onset heart failure.[35] Although the mechanism of increased heart failure risk with α-receptor blockade remains unknown, unopposed stimulation of β-adrenergic receptors is a likely possibility. In any event, α blockade should be discouraged in the treatment of hypertension, unless in combination with other agents, particularly β blockers. Finally, as noted in the European Society of Cardiology heart failure guideline,[9] the applicability of ALLHAT to the European community is uncertain because the trial enrolled a substantial number of African Americans.

Like ACE inhibitors, angiotensin receptor blockers (ARBs) significantly reduce the incidence of heart failure. In this regard, ARBs have been most well-studied in diabetic hypertensives.[36,37] However, recent controversy has arisen regarding a so-called *ARB paradox* describing an apparent increase in MI risk associated with ARB treatment.[38,39] While this debate plays out, the totality of currently available data support the safety and efficacy of ARBs in the treatment of hypertension.

Most hypertensive subjects require treatment with two or more agents, to achieve target blood pressure control. With this in mind, the authors of the American College of Cardiology/American Heart Association (ACC/AHA) heart failure guidelines recommend the use of agents proven to be useful for the treatment of hypertension and heart failure, particularly diuretics, ACE inhibitors, and β blockers, for the treatment of stage A and stage B hypertensive subjects.[7] Likewise, the European Society of Cardiology endorses the use of ACE inhibitors, ARBs, diuretics, and β blockers in the prevention of heart failure.[9] Finally, the guideline from the Heart Failure Society of America emphasizes the use of an ACE inhibitor in stage A patients and the addition of a β blocker in stage B subjects, particularly those with a prior MI.[8]

【 】 OBESITY, DIABETES, AND THE METABOLIC SYNDROME AS RISK FACTORS FOR HEART FAILURE

Obesity and insulin resistance are powerful risk factors for the development of heart failure.[40,41] Obesity alone has been shown to be an independent risk factor for incident heart failure.[41] There are many ways by which obesity may contribute to the development of structural heart disease and heart failure. Many of these mechanisms seem to be mediated by the proliferative milieu associated with insulin resistance/hyperinsulinemia and diabetes. Thus, the metabolic syndrome may also play a major role in increasing the risk of heart failure.[42] Approximately 40 percent of the U.S. population older than age 40 years meets the criteria for the diagnosis of the metabolic syndrome.[43] Moreover, roughly 21 percent of U.S. adults are obese as defined by a body mass index (BMI) of at least 30.[44] This includes 20.8 percent of adult women and 21 percent of adult men for a total of 44.3 million obese adult Americans. Since 1991 the percentage of overweight adults (defined as a BMI ≥ 25) increased from 45 percent to 58 percent,[44] so that more than one-half of the U.S. adult population is now considered overweight. In other developed societies such as those in Europe, the prevalence of obesity is also on the rise. Thus, the contribution of obesity, diabetes, and the metabolic syndrome to the incidence of heart failure is likely to increase worldwide.

The presence of diabetes mellitus substantially increases the risk of heart failure in patients without preexisting structural heart disease.[45] Diabetes only modestly increases the risk of heart failure in men but substantially increases the chance of heart failure in women.[22] Although diabetes is a risk factor for coronary heart disease, many diabetic patients and especially female diabetics with or without hypertension exhibit angiographically normal epicardial coronary arteries in association with dilated cardiomyopathy. This observation has lead to the proposal of a *diabetic cardiomyopathy*. The exact nature of this form of heart muscle disease is unknown, but small vessel coronary disease and/or endothelial dysfunction may play a role. Alternatively, hyperinsulinemia, hyperglycemia, and other growth-promoting hormones may mediate pathologic myocyte remodeling subsequently leading to cardiomyopathy in these patients.

The management of diabetes and the metabolic syndrome/obesity in the prevention of cardiovascular disease is discussed in Chaps. 90 and 91, respectively. In general, treatment of the metabolic syndrome is limited by the poor success associated with available weight loss therapies and programs. A downward trend in physical activity over decades associated with an upward trend in caloric consumption and the lack of truly effective drug therapies challenge progress in effectively reversing the obesity epidemic.[46] When successful, however, weight loss can effectively reduce the risk of diabetes in obese subjects. In the Diabetes Prevention Program (DPP), intensive lifestyle change, defined as a 7 percent reduction in body weight and at least 150 minutes of exercise weekly, was more effective than placebo or drug therapy with metformin in reducing the onset of diabetes mellitus.[47] Lifestyle intervention decreased the incidence of diabetes by 58 percent compared to placebo, whereas metformin diminished the chance of diabetes by 31 percent.

In patients with overt diabetes, every effort should be made to control hyperglycemia, but such control has not yet been shown to reduce the subsequent risk of heart failure. Of note, thiazolidinediones (TZDs), commonly prescribed for the treatment of diabetes, have been associated with increased peripheral edema and new-onset heart failure in patients with underlying risk factors or known cardiovascular disease.[48] The risk of developing edema with TZDs is dose related and higher in diabetic patients on concomitant insulin therapy. Thus, these agents should be used with caution in at-risk patients, and such patients should be monitored closely for fluid retention.

CORONARY ARTERY DISEASE AS A RISK FACTOR FOR HEART FAILURE

Coronary artery disease appears to account for 60 percent to 70 percent of the incidence of systolic heart failure. Annually in the United States, approximately 1.1 million individuals suffer a MI and approximately 40 percent of them may be left with a reduced LVEF.[49] Data from the Studies of Left Ventricular Dysfunction (SOLVD) Registry, which enrolled subjects in the United States and Canada, provide the following breakdown on the etiology of heart failure: ischemic heart disease, 68.5 percent; idiopathic heart disease, 12.9 percent; hypertension, 7.2 percent; and other causes, 11.3 percent.[50] This observation is supported by findings from randomized controlled trials of systolic heart failure that also demonstrate a preponderance of ischemic heart failure. However, these studies generally enrolled mostly middle-aged white men and may not have been representative of the broader heart failure population, including women and minorities. In this context, a recent trial of African-American subjects (approximately half women) with systolic heart failure demonstrated a very different distribution of risk factors for heart failure, with only a minority of patients having ischemic heart disease and most exhibiting nonischemic heart failure in association with hypertension, diabetes, and obesity.[51]

The Acute Decompensated Heart Failure National Registry (ADHERE), which includes unselected patients admitted to the hospital with worsening heart failure, evaluated the prevalence of risk factors in more than 100,000 cases.[52] Half of the cases were women. The following predominant risk factors were noted: coronary artery disease, 57 percent; prior MI, 35 percent; hypertension, 73 percent; dyslipidemia, 36 percent; chronic renal insufficiency, 30 percent; and diabetes mellitus, 44 percent.[52] It is important to note that approximately 46 percent of ADHERE cases are comprised of patients with preserved LV systolic function (i.e., EF > 40 percent). However, even in patients with reduced LVEF, multiple comorbidities are common and ischemic heart disease is listed as the primary cause of the heart failure in approximately 60 percent of cases.

MI is a common cause of heart failure. Following a MI, the development of LV systolic dysfunction and dilation are the most potent predictors of subsequent heart failure and all-cause mortality.[53-55] Once LV injury has occurred, progressive LV dysfunction and dilation ensues unless attenuated by medical and/or surgical therapy.

The pathophysiology and management of coronary artery disease is extensively reviewed in Part 8 of this textbook. A consensus statement on preventing atherosclerotic heart disease provides additional guidelines for management.[56] In this context, ACE inhibitors play a major role in the prevention of cardiovascular events and heart failure in subjects with established atherosclerotic vascular disease based on the results of randomized controlled trials.[32] Revascularization strategies, either percutaneous or surgical, may also reduce the incidence of heart failure in such patients, but this is less well-studied in contemporary large-scale randomized controlled trials. Coronary revascularization can relieve symptoms of myocardial ischemia, and coronary artery bypass surgery has been shown to lessen angina and reduce the risk of death in patients who have multivessel disease, reduced

LVEFs, and stable angina.[57] Whether or not surgical revascularization improves the natural history of ischemic heart failure is under evaluation in the National Institutes of Health sponsored Surgical Therapies for Ischemic Heart Failure (STICH) trial.

【 】 OTHER PREVENTIVE MEASURES IN HEART FAILURE

Other primary and secondary preventive strategies have also been shown to reduce the risk of incident heart failure. For example, lipid lowering therapy results in a significant reduction in new-onset heart failure.[58,59] In a large-scale trial, the administration of a lipid-lowering agent to patients with hypercholesterolemia and a prior MI reduced all-cause mortality and the risk of developing HF.[59] The role of other therapies such as continuous positive airway pressure breathing in obstructive sleep apnea to prevent new-onset heart failure remains to be fully elucidated. Other therapies resulting in reverse remodeling in patients with established (stage C) heart failure (e.g., cardiac resynchronization therapy) are being evaluated in asymptomatic or minimally symptomatic patients, as preventive measures. In this regard, pathological LV remodeling has become a major target for heart failure intervention in stages B through D of the heart failure continuum.

【 】 PATHOLOGIC REMODELING AS A TARGET FOR HEART FAILURE PREVENTION

As noted in practice guidelines, in the stage B patient preventive therapies should be directed at improving LV structure and function. Typically, adverse or pathological remodeling is defined in the context of LV dilation and systolic dysfunction as an increase in ventricular volumes (both systolic and diastolic), a decrease in EF, a loss of the normal elliptical geometry of the ventricle, and the onset of functional mitral regurgitation. LV hypertrophy should also be considered as a form of pathological ventricular remodeling and as a target for preventive intervention. The regression of LV hypertrophy in hypertensive subjects appears to improve outcomes.[60,61] Thus, therapies that promote either regression of LV hypertrophy or reverse remodeling of the dilated failing heart may be viewed as essential in the prevention or attenuation of heart failure in stage B.

Pathological ventricular remodeling within the heart can be considered as ventricular, cellular, or molecular. Ventricular remodeling is defined above. Cellular remodeling may take one of two predominant forms, involving either concentric or eccentric hypertrophy of the myocyte.[62] (Figure 26–2). In the case of concentric myocyte remodeling, the heart cells have thickened but not increased in length so that the longitudinal to transverse ratio of the cell is diminished. With eccentric hypertrophy, the cell is elongated and the longitudinal to transverse ratio is increased. Other cellular changes accompanying pathological remodeling include changes in constituent cardiac proteins, an increase in the amount of cytoskeletal elements (these are disorganized), an increase in the number of nonmyocytes (many are activated [e.g., fibroblasts] or dysfunctional [e.g., endothelium]), and an increase in the volume and structure of the extracellular matrix. At the molecular level, there is a general reversion to the fetal pattern of gene expression in the dilated failing human heart.[63,64] These changes appear to be related to increased wall stress and mediated by a variety of mechanisms, including increases in local and circulating neurohormones.[65]

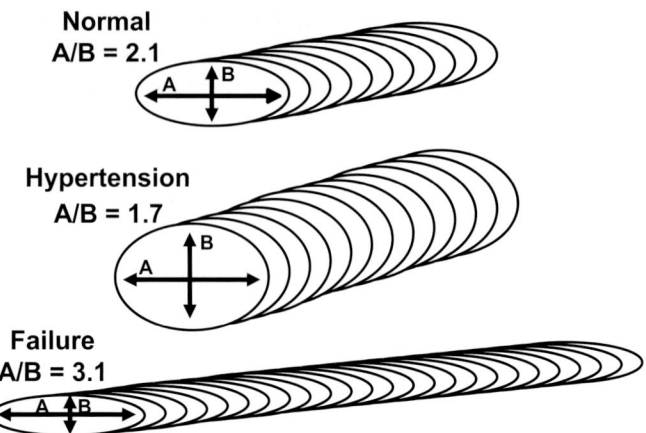

FIGURE 26–2. Cartoon of myocyte cellular remodeling in response to pressure overload (hypertension) leading to concentric remodeling of the heart cell and cardiac failure resulting in eccentric myocyte remodeling. A, length of cell; B, width of cell. *Source: From Wang X, Li F, Gerdes AM.[62] With permission.*

Many drug therapies and some device-base treatments promote an improvement in cardiac structure and function. Most antihypertensive medications promote regression of LV hypertrophy, but some appear more potent than others when indexed to the degree of blood pressure lowering.[66] In subjects with asymptomatic LV systolic dysfunction, the use of ACE inhibitors and β blockers has been shown to be particularly effective in promoting reverse remodeling and attenuating clinical events.[67,68] ARBs and aldosterone antagonists may also be useful, in this regard. These two classes of drugs have largely been studied in symptomatic patients with reduced EFs and in patients after MI.[69,70] Despite the lack of randomized controlled trials evaluating ARBs or aldosterone antagonists in truly asymptomatic LV dysfunction, ARBs represent acceptable alternatives in ACE inhibitor–intolerant patients, and the addition of an aldosterone antagonist to an ACE inhibitor/β-blocker–based regimen may optimize the reverse remodeling process. As mentioned above, mechanical interventions such as coronary revascularization following MI, cardiac resynchronization therapy or LV assist devices may also improve heart function and thus attenuate heart failure.

In summary, the prevention of heart failure is best achieved by an aggressive approach to the treatment of major risk factors, including hypertension, diabetes, obesity, metabolic syndrome, and coronary artery disease, according to published guidelines. The treatment of other comorbid risk factors, such as dyslipidemia, should not be neglected as incremental reduction in heart failure risk may be seen. Once these risk factors progress to LV hypertrophy or dysfunction, risk factor modification should continue and therapies that promote regression of LV hypertrophy or reverse remodeling of the dilated failing heart should be employed, if not already prescribed.

EVALUATION AND MANAGEMENT OF SYMPTOMATIC HEART FAILURE

【 】 EVALUATION OF CHRONIC HEART FAILURE

Tables 26–3 and 26–4, taken from the European Society of Cardiology heart failure guideline,[9] recommends a routine assessment to establish the diagnosis and likely cause of heart failure. Once the diagnosis of heart failure has been made, the first step in evaluating heart failure is to determine the severity and type of cardiac dysfunction, by measuring EF through two-dimensional echocardiography and/or radionuclide ventriculography. Measurement of EF is the gold standard for differentiating between the two forms of heart failure, systolic and diastolic, and is particularly important given that the approaches to therapy for each syndrome somewhat differ. The history and physical examination should include assessment of symptoms, functional capacity, and fluid retention. Common symptoms of heart failure are dyspnea on exertion, orthopnea, paroxysmal nocturnal dyspnea, lower extremity edema, cough (usually worse at night), abdominal complaints (nausea, vomiting, right upper quadrant pain, abdominal swelling), fatigue, nocturia, sleep disorders, and anorexia. Common physical findings include elevated jugular venous pressure, hepatojugular reflux, pulmonary crackles, sustained and displaced apical impulse, S_3 gallop, hepatomegaly, ascites, and peripheral edema.

Functional capacity is assessed from the clinical history or preferably measured by an exercise test.[71,72] Analysis of expired air during exercise offers a precise measure of the patient's physical limitations. This test is not commonly performed outside of cardiac transplant centers. The NYHA has classified heart failure into four functional classes that may be determined by history taking:[73]

Class I: no limitations of physical activity, no symptoms with ordinary activities
Class II: slight limitation, symptoms with ordinary activities
Class III: marked limitation, symptoms with less than ordinary activities
Class IV: severe limitation, symptoms of heart failure at rest

For example, patients who can walk several blocks without symptoms but have difficulty climbing two flights of stairs may have class II heart failure, whereas those who cannot walk several blocks easily or become winded while walking up a short flight of stairs might be considered class III. The NYHA functional classification should not be confused with the aforementioned stages of heart failure described in the ACC/AHA heart failure guidelines. The NYHA classification describes functional limitation and is applicable to stages B through D patients, whereas the staging system describes disease progression somewhat independently of functional status.

Assessment of fluid retention through measurement of jugular venous pressure, auscultation of the lungs, and examination for peripheral edema is central to the physical examination of heart failure patients. The physical examination alone, however, is relatively insensitive for measuring extracellular fluid volume excess.[74,75] A thorough appraisal of symptoms is essential. Even in the absence of perceptible volume excess by physical examination, mild congestive symptoms can indicate volume excess. In addition, the chest radiograph, particularly in a patient with relatively new onset heart failure, is a relatively sensitive measure of volume overload but in the setting of chronic heart failure, the chest radiograph may not reliably help to estimate ventricular filling pressure.[76]

Given the limitations of physical signs and symptoms in evaluating heart failure clinical status, a number of noninvasive and invasive tools are under development for the assessment of heart failure. One such tool that has proven useful in determining the diagnosis and prognosis of heart failure is the measurement of plasma B-type natriuretic peptide (BNP) levels. Multiple studies, including the Breathing Not Properly Multinational Study,[77] demonstrate the usefulness of BNP measurement in the diagnosis of heart failure. In this study 1586 patients who came to the emergency department with acute dyspnea underwent bedside mea-

TABLE 26–3

Assessments to Be Performed Routinely to Establish the Presence and Likely Cause of Heart Failure

ASSESSMENTS	DIAGNOSIS OF HEART FAILURE			SUGGESTS ALTERNATIVE OR ADDITIONAL DIAGNOSIS
	NECESSARY FOR	SUPPORTS	OPPOSES	
Appropriate symptoms	+++		+++ (If absent)	
Appropriate signs		+++	+ (If absent)	
Cardiac dysfunction on imaging (usually echocardiography)	+++		+++ (If absent)	
Response of symptoms or signs to therapy		+++	+++ (If absent)	
ECG			+++ (If normal)	
Chest x-ray		If pulmonary congestion or cardiomegaly	+ (If normal)	Pulmonary disease
Full blood count				Anemia/secondary polycythemia
Biochemistry and urinalysis				Renal or hepatic disease/diabetes
Plasma concentration of natriuretic peptides in untreated patients (where available)		+ (If elevated)	+++ (If normal)	Can be normal in treated patients

+, of some importance; +++, of great importance.

TABLE 26–4

Additional Tests to Be Considered to Support the Diagnosis of Heart Failure or Suggest an Alternative Diagnosis

TESTS	DIAGNOSIS OF HEART FAILURE		SUGGESTS ALTERNATIVE OR ADDITIONAL DIAGNOSES
	SUPPORTS	OPPOSES	
Exercise test	+ (If impaired)	+++ (If normal)	
Pulmonary function tests			Pulmonary disease
Thyroid function tests			Thyroid disease
Invasive investigation and angiography			Coronary artery disease, ischemia
Cardiac output	+++ (If depressed at rest)	+++ (If normal; especially during exercise)	
Left atrial pressure (pulmonary capillary wedge pressure)	+++ (If elevated at rest)	+++ (If normal; in absence of therapy)	

+, of some importance; +++, of great importance.

surement of plasma BNP concentration. The clinical diagnosis of congestive heart failure was adjudicated by two independent cardiologists, who were blinded to the results of the BNP assay. The final diagnosis was dyspnea caused by worsening heart failure in 744 patients (47 percent), dyspnea caused by noncardiac causes in 72 patients with a history of LV dysfunction (5 percent), and no finding of congestive heart failure in 770 patients (49 percent). BNP levels by themselves were more accurate than any historical or physical findings or laboratory values in identifying worsening heart failure as the cause of dyspnea. The diagnostic accuracy of BNP at a cutoff of 100 pg/mL was 83.4 percent. The negative predictive value of BNP was excellent. At levels of less than 50 pg/mL, the negative predictive value of the assay was 96 percent.

In the B-Type Natriuretic Peptide for Acute Shortness of Breath Evaluation study, from Mueller and coworkers,[78] patients presenting to the emergency department with acute dyspnea were randomly assigned to undergo either a single measurement of BNP or not. Based largely on the findings of the BNP Multinational Study, clinicians were advised that a plasma BNP concentration <100 pg/mL made the diagnosis of congestive heart failure unlikely, whereas a level >500 pg/mL made it highly likely. For BNP levels between 100 pg/mL and 500 pg/mL, the use of clinical judgment and additional testing was encouraged. In this single-blind trial of 452 patients, measurement of BNP in the emergency department resulted in a 10 percent decrease in the rate of hospital admission. Moreover, the median length of stay was reduced by three days and the mean total cost of treatment by approximately $1800. These reductions in rate of hospitalization, length of stay, and cost did not result in any negative effects on mortality or the rate of subsequent hospitalization.

Additionally, plasma BNP is useful in predicting prognosis in heart failure patients. However, serial measurement of plasma BNP as a guide to heart failure management has not yet been proven useful in the management of acute or chronic heart failure. The recommended role of BNP testing at the various stages of heart failure differs a bit among the major heart failure guidelines. The ACC/AHA heart failure guideline suggests that "measurement of BNP can be useful in the evaluation of patients presenting in the urgent care setting in whom the diagnosis of heart failure is

uncertain."[7] Although the Heart Failure Society of America guideline discourages the use of BNP testing in *at risk* patients, it more strongly recommends "that BNP or N-terminal-proBNP (NT-proBNP) be assessed in *all patients* suspected of having heart failure when the diagnosis is not certain"[8] (emphasis added). The heart failure guideline from the European Society of Cardiology emphasizes the use of BNP or NT-pro-BNP "as 'rule out' tests to exclude significant cardiac disease," particularly in primary care but also in settings such as the emergency department.[9]

APPROACH TO SYSTOLIC HEART FAILURE

Table 26–5 presents a general approach to evaluating and managing patients with current or prior symptoms of heart failure and

TABLE 26–5

General Therapeutic Approach to Chronic Heart Failure

Determine the etiology
Look for precipitating factors and correct them
Nonpharmacologic treatment
    Sodium restriction ($\leq$2 g/d)
    Aerobic exercise
    Weight loss in obese patients
Treat hypertension and other comorbidities vigorously
Pharmacologic treatment
    Angiotensin-converting enzyme inhibitors
    Angiotensin receptor blockers
    Aldosterone antagonists
    β Blockers
    Vasodilators (long-acting nitrates and hydralazine)
    Diuretics
    Digoxin
Device therapies
    Cardiac resynchronization therapy
    Implantable cardioverter defibrillators
    Left ventricular assist devices (discussed in Chap. 26)

chronic LV systolic dysfunction. This schema is consistent with published clinical practice guidelines.[7–10] In addition to pharmacologic and device-based approaches to treatment, these guidelines stress the importance of dietary counseling, patient education, lifestyle changes, and other nonpharmacologic strategies for the treatment of chronic heart failure. Many of these nonpharmacologic strategies recommended for the management of systolic heart failure also are applicable to the treatment of heart failure associated with a preserved LVEF.

When a patient presents with symptomatic heart failure, it is important to determine the underlying cause as some forms of heart failure may be reversible. It is also essential to understand those factors precipitating the transition from stage B to stage C heart failure, as well as subsequent episodes of decompensation. Therapy may then logically follow from an understanding of these factors and an appreciation for evidence-based, guidelines-recommended treatments.

Determine the Etiology of the Heart Failure

All patients presenting with new heart failure should be rigorously evaluated to determine the etiology of the disease. Routinely performing such an evaluation is important because there are several surgically correctable forms of heart failure and some potentially reversible forms of inflammatory heart disease and cardiomyopathy associated with systemic diseases or cardiotoxins. For example, some patients with heart failure caused by ischemic heart disease may realize an improvement in the LV dysfunction and chronic heart failure following revascularization with either angioplasty or coronary artery bypass surgery.[79–86] This may be the case in as much as 20 percent of patients with heart failure in the context of ischaemia, and as mentioned above, is being prospectively evaluated in the STICH trial. The presence or absence of obstructive coronary artery disease should be determined in heart failure patients and, in general, myocardial viability should be assessed in patients with ischemic cardiomyopathy. Viable myocardium and the presence of adequate target vessels for bypass predict a favorable outcome following revascularization for ischemic heart failure, so serious consideration should be given to surgical intervention in such cases.

Perhaps the most classic examples of surgically correctable heart failure are those associated with valvular heart disease. For instance, patients with critical aortic stenosis may exhibit severe LV dysfunction and advanced signs and symptoms of chronic heart failure, which may be completely reversible on replacement of the stenotic aortic valve. Severe mitral stenosis is also a cause of acutely reversible heart failure where percutaneous balloon valvuloplasty now represents a feasible and, in many cases, preferred approach to therapy.[87] Severe mitral regurgitation is another valvular etiology of left heart failure. Although early mitral valve repair or replacement may prevent the development of chronic heart failure, the presence of advanced LV dilation and severe LV dysfunction at the time of presentation often precludes surgical intervention. Newer, percutaneous approaches to mitral valve repair may represent a viable alternative to ongoing medical therapy in such patients.

The treatment of myocarditis remains controversial. Anecdotal experience suggests that some patients may benefit from therapy directed at the immune system. However, controlled trials of immunosuppressant therapy, immune globulin, and other forms of immunomodulatory therapy in myocarditis have been disappointing.[88,89] Thus, current guidelines do not recommend the routine use of immune-based drug therapies for myocarditis. Despite these recommendations many heart failure experts recommend immunosuppressant drug therapy (usually consisting of corticosteroids) for biopsy-proven myocarditis associated with rapidly worsening heart failure signs and symptoms and/or LV function. In this regard the role of endomyocardial biopsy in the evaluation of heart failure remains controversial. None of the guidelines recommend the routine use of heart biopsies in the diagnosis of new or worsening heart failure. However, in suspected cases of myocarditis, endomyocardial biopsy can provide useful information establishing the diagnosis and distinguishing lymphocytic from eosinophilic and giant cell myocarditis. This is important because eosinophilic myocarditis is often exquisitely sensitive to treatment with corticosteroids, whereas giant cell myocarditis seems resistant to immunosuppressant treatment exhibiting a relapsing course despite such medications.

Cardiomyopathies related to alcohol or cocaine abuse may respond to discontinuation of the offending agent.[90,91] Heart muscle disease associated with chemotherapeutic agents may respond to or be prevented by treatment with ACE inhibitors and/or β blockers.[92,93] Heart failure related to systemic illness such as hypothyroidism may respond to treatment of the underlying disease. Although few specific therapies exist, the diagnosis of an infiltrative cardiomyopathy may influence subsequent evaluation for systemic disease and inform the natural history of the disease. A further discussion of these less common causes of cardiomyopathy is included in Chaps. 30 and 31.

Look for Factors Precipitating Symptoms and Correct Them

One of the most important strategies for reducing morbidity and mortality in chronic heart failure is understanding and correcting the precipitating causes of clinical worsening and disease progression (Table 26–6). Dietary and/or pharmacologic noncompliance appear

TABLE 26–6

Precipitating Causes of Worsening Heart Failure

Dietary and/or Pharmacologic Noncompliance
Negative inotropes
    Antiarrhythmics
    First-generation calcium channel antagonists
Increased renal salt and water retention and/or worsening renal function
    Nonsteroidal antiinflammatory drugs
Further damage to the myocardium
    Adriamycin
    Alcohol and/or cocaine
    Myocardial infarction
    Myocarditis
Increased myocardial workload
    Anemia
    Hypoxia
    Infection
    Pulmonary embolism
Worsened valvular dysfunction
Arrhythmias

to be major causes of decompensation in patients with chronic heart failure. Thus, dietary counseling and patient education represent two major goals in the management of chronic heart failure. This may be accomplished through referral to the Dietitian, distribution of patient education materials, office or hospital-based patient education programs, heart failure telemanagement, and home health cardiac specialists. While a great first step, it is clear that education delivered in the hospital alone is inadequate and this educational message must be reinforced on an outpatient basis.

The prescription of negative inotropes, such as most antiarrhythmics and the first-generation calcium channel antagonists, may also precipitate symptomatic or worsening heart failure and probably worsen outcome in chronic heart failure patients. Because renal perfusion in heart failure patients is largely dependent on vasodilating prostaglandins, the prescription or over-the-counter use of nonsteroidal antiinflammatory drugs may result in worsening renal function and increased renal sodium and water retention.[94] In addition, the onset of acute anuric renal failure may occur following the administration of nonsteroidal antiinflammatory drugs to patients with advanced heart failure.[95] Thus, some patients may make the transition from stage B to stage C heart failure as a consequence of inappropriate drug therapy.

Anything that further damages the myocardium—such as a new MI—or places an increased workload on the heart—such as hypoxia, anemia, pulmonary embolism, or infection—may result in worsening of heart failure. Finally, worsened valvular dysfunction and arrhythmias are occasionally implicated as precipitants of symptomatic heart failure.

Nonpharmacologic Treatment of Chronic Heart Failure

The nonpharmacologic management of heart failure includes reduced sodium intake, reduced physical (particularly isometric) exertion, and weight loss in obese patients. In general, sodium intake should be limited to approximately 2 g/d. In advanced heart failure, further dietary sodium restriction may be necessary to attenuate expansion of extracellular fluid volume and the development of edema. Hyponatremia should not discourage compliance with a restricted sodium diet, because the hyponatremia is usually dilutional and associated with total body sodium and water excess. Sodium repletion therefore should only be considered in overt cases of severe excessive diuresis or dehydration. Salt substitutes may be used to improve the palatability of food. However, some agents substitute potassium chloride for sodium chloride and should be used in moderation given the potential risk of hyperkalemia, especially in patients treated with ACE inhibitors, ARBs, and/or aldosterone antagonists. Although dietary sodium restriction may attenuate the development of edema, it cannot prevent it because the kidneys are capable of reducing urinary sodium excretion to less than 10 mmol/d. Thus, diuretics (discussed below) play a key role in the management of symptomatic heart failure.

Although vigorous isometric exercise has been poorly evaluated in chronic heart failure, it is currently discouraged in symptomatic patients given the marked increase in myocardial work seen with weight training. Increased LV wall stress during isometric exercise would be expected to have an unfavorable influence on ventricular remodeling. On the other hand, a role

has emerged for monitored cardiac rehabilitation and aerobic exercise in patients with stable compensated chronic heart failure. In these patients, aerobic exercise training has been shown to consistently improve functional capacity while inconsistently improving LV function, suggesting that the benefits of aerobic training in chronic heart failure are mostly peripheral.[96–101] The effect of such training on heart failure outcomes is being evaluated in a large multinational National Institutes of Health randomized controlled trial. All patients with heart failure should receive flu immunization each year.

Treat Hypertension and Other Comorbidities Vigorously

Although many patients with chronic heart failure have normal or low blood pressures, a large subset of patients remains hypertensive. Because blood pressure is a component of ventricular afterload and it increases the workload of the heart, it should be treated vigorously in patients with chronic heart failure. Some patients with cardiomyopathy on the basis of hypertensive heart disease may recognize a marked improvement with treatment of hypertension alone. This may be accomplished with standard heart failure treatment such as an ACE inhibitor or with various antihypertensive therapies, which appear to be safe to use in patients with LV systolic dysfunction (e.g., vascular-selective calcium channel blockers). Other comorbidities, such as those mentioned earlier in this chapter, should also be treated and may modify disease progression as discussed above.

【 】 PHARMACOLOGIC TREATMENT OF CHRONIC SYSTOLIC HEART FAILURE

The current standard pharmacologic treatment of chronic systolic heart failure utilizes a diuretic or combination of diuretics, an ACE inhibitor or ARB, and a β blocker.

Diuretics

In patients with heart failure, diuretics decrease end-diastolic volume and modestly increase stroke volume and cardiac output. Clinically, diuretics improve exercise capacity and diminish symptoms caused by pulmonary and peripheral edema. Fig. 26–3 shows the tubular sites of action of commonly used diuretics and Table 26–7 reviews usual dosage recommendations for these agents.

Sites of Action of Commonly Used Diuretics

Proximal Tubular Diuretics Diuretics that act primarily to decrease proximal tubular sodium reabsorption include osmotic diuretics such as mannitol, carbonic anhydrase inhibitors including acetazolamide, and probably the organomercurials. Except for organomercurials, the proximal tubular diuretics are not very effective when administered alone. Although 50 to 70 percent of the glomerular filtrate is reabsorbed isosmotically in the proximal tubule, the distal nephron (particularly the ascending limb of the Henle loop) has the capacity to substantially increase its rate of sodium reabsorption.[102] Therefore, an increase in glomerular filtration or decrease in proximal tubular reabsorption alone may not be associated with a significant diuresis, because the increased distal sodium and fluid delivery may be reabsorbed at more distal nephron sites. Thus, these

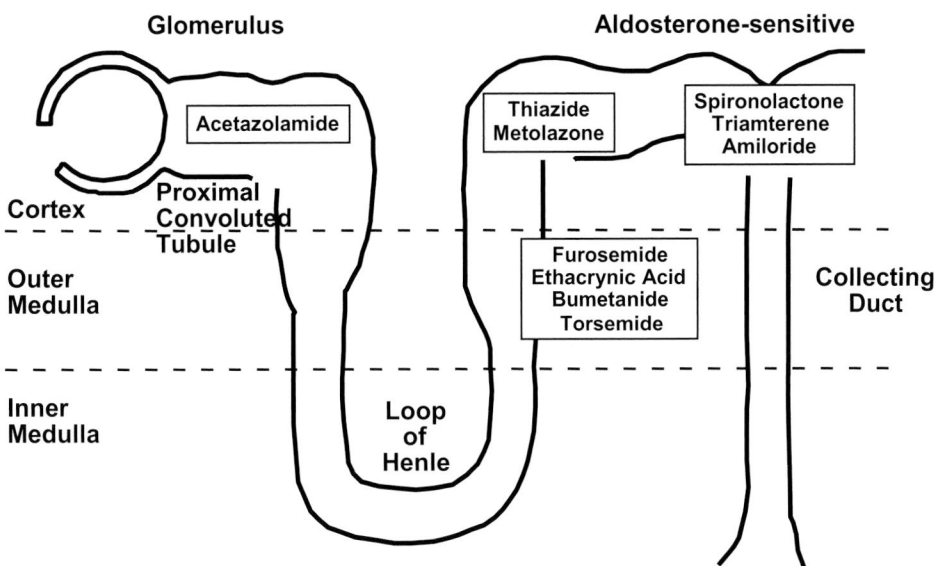

Glomerulus   **Aldosterone-sensitive**

Acetazolamide

Thiazide Metolazone

Spironolactone Triamterene Amiloride

Cortex — Proximal Convoluted Tubule

Outer Medulla

Furosemide Ethacrynic Acid Bumetanide Torsemide

Collecting Duct

Inner Medulla   Loop of Henle

FIGURE 26–3. Tubular sites of action of the major diuretics used in clinical medicine.

diuretic effects. They inhibit only urinary diluting capacity and not concentrating capacity, because these distal tubular diuretics decrease sodium reabsorption in the cortical, but not medullary, segment of the ascending limb of the Henle loop and the distal convoluted tubule. These distal tubular diuretics act proximal to the distal site of potassium secretion and, thus, are associated with an increase in urinary potassium excretion. This increase in potassium excretion appears to be caused by an increase in distal sodium delivery, which may modulate potassium reabsorption in the collecting duct.[103] This is also the likely explanation for the potassium-losing effects of the loop diuretics.

Clinically available potassium-sparing diuretics include triamterene; amiloride; and the specific aldosterone antagonists, spironolactone, and eplerenone. The action of these latter potassium-conserving diuretics depends on the presence of the adrenal cortex and circulating aldosterone. In contrast, the ability of triamterene and amiloride to block potassium secretion is independent of adrenal function. Usually, these diuretics are insufficiently potent when used alone, but they may be used to avoid the potassium-losing effects of diuretics that act at more proximal nephron sites.

agents are rarely used in clinical medicine and almost never used in the management of chronic heart failure.

Loop of Henle Diuretics Currently, available loop diuretics include furosemide, bumetanide, torsemide, and ethacrynic acid. These are the most potent diuretic agents available for use in clinical medicine. Inhibition by these agents of active sodium chloride transport in the medullary ascending limb of the Henle loop exceeds the rate-limited sodium chloride reabsorption in the more distal nephron, producing a maximal diuretic effect equivalent to 20 to 25 percent of the filtered sodium load. Accordingly, loop diuretics are most commonly used in the management of fluid retention in heart failure.

Distal Tubular Diuretics Distal tubular diuretics are broadly classified into two groups: the potassium-wasting and the potassium-sparing diuretics. Commonly used potassium-wasting distal tubular diuretics include the thiazide diuretics, chlorthalidone, and metolazone. These agents are chemically different but have similar

Collecting Duct Diuretics In contrast to the saluretic agents mentioned above, two currently available diuretics, demeclocycline and lithium, act at the level of the collecting duct and induce a water diuresis. These agents impair the ability of arginine vasopressin (AVP) to increase the water permeability of the renal collecting duct epithelium, thereby antagonizing the hydro-osmotic effect of AVP. Such agents are theoretically useful in managing the dilutional hyponatremia of heart failure; however, both agents produce significant adverse effects, which preclude their use in heart failure management. Renal or V_2 receptor AVP antagonists,

TABLE 26–7

Diuretics Used in the Management of Heart Failure

AGENT	SITE OF ACTION	TOTAL DAILY DOSE (MG)	FREQUENCY
Acetazolamide	Proximal tubule	250–375	Every day or every other day
Amiloride	Distal tubule (potassium sparing)	5–20	Once or twice daily
Bumetanide	Loop of Henle	0.5–10	Once to thrice daily
Chlorothiazide	Distal tubule (potassium wasting)	500–1500	Once or twice daily
Ethacrynic acid	Loop of Henle	50–200	Once or twice daily
Furosemide	Loop of Henle	20–500	Once to thrice daily
Hydrochlorothiazide	Distal tubule (potassium wasting)	25–100	Once or twice daily
Metolazone	Distal tubule (potassium wasting)	2.5–20	Once or twice daily
Spironolactone	Distal tubule (potassium sparing)	25–200	Once to thrice daily
Torsemide	Loop of Henle	10–200	Once or twice daily
Triamterene	Distal tubule (potassium sparing)	100–300	Once or twice daily

which directly antagonize the renal effects of AVP in the kidney, offer a promising alternative to these agents and are currently undergoing human investigation.

Potency of Commonly Used Diuretics

With optimal dosing, all thiazide-like agents have generally comparable effects on solute and water excretion with the exception of metolazone, which is more potent than the other agents. Thiazide diuretics differ from each other primarily in duration of action. In general, the loop diuretics are six to eight times more potent than the thiazides. This is not surprising, because several times more sodium chloride is reabsorbed in the loop of Henle than in the distal convoluted tubule. Because of their potency, the loop diuretics and metolazone are generally effective in patients with advanced renal insufficiency (i.e., with glomerular filtration rates <25 mL/min). This is in contrast to the thiazide diuretics, which become ineffective as the glomerular filtration rate falls <25 to 30 mL/min.

Hemodynamic and Clinical Effects of Commonly Used Diuretics

During chronic administration, diuretic therapy results in favorable effects on both cardiac preload and perhaps afterload with an associated improvement in LV performance. Wilson and colleagues[104] administered oral furosemide, with or without a thiazide, to 13 patients with hemodynamically decompensated heart failure. Right heart hemodynamics were determined at baseline and following 8 days of diuretic therapy. All patients exhibited a substantial decrease in LV filling pressure, which was generally associated with an improvement in cardiac performance measured by increases in stroke volume. Clinically, the favorable hemodynamic effects observed during chronic diuretic administration are associated with an improvement in functional capacity determined by treadmill exercise time. In a study from Bayliss and associates,[105] the administration of furosemide 40 mg plus amiloride 5 mg each daily for 1 month produced a nearly two-fold improvement in submaximal treadmill exercise time.

Neurohormonal Effects of Commonly Used Diuretics

Chronic oral diuretic therapy has been shown to increase plasma renin activity, plasma angiotensin II concentration, plasma aldosterone, and plasma norepinephrine in the setting of acute and chronic heart failure.[105,106] In addition to this diuretic-mediated increase in neurohormonal vasoconstrictor activation, chronic diuretic use also diminishes circulating concentrations of the vasodilating natriuretic peptides.[106] This is important because natriuretic peptides are known to suppress the renin-angiotensin-aldosterone system and improve renal hemodynamics. Moreover, during chronic diuretic therapy, further activation of vasoconstrictor/antinatriuretic forces and diminution of vasodilating/natriuretic plasma hormone concentrations may explain, in part, the development of progressive diuretic resistance, which is common in chronic heart failure.

Adverse Effects of Chronic Diuretic Therapy

Volume depletion and potassium depletion are the most common complications of diuretic therapy. Thiazide diuretics, metolazone, and loop diuretics commonly cause these complications. Volume depletion may result in hypotension and/or hypoperfusion of vital organs such as the brain, heart, or liver. Diminished renal perfusion also may oc-

cur, as evidenced by a rise in blood urea nitrogen and serum creatinine concentrations, despite ongoing hypervolemia. Generally, one-third of patients undergoing treatment for acutely decompensated heart failure experience a worsening of renal function.[107] Severe renal hypoperfusion may lead to the evolution of acute intrinsic renal failure (i.e., acute tubular necrosis), in addition to the development of severe prerenal azotemia. Hypokalemia may predispose heart failure patients to life-threatening ventricular arrhythmias, particularly during treatment with cardiac glycosides, or other positive inotropes.

Hyponatremia may result from the impaired water excretion associated with chronic heart failure. In addition, the saluretic effect of commonly prescribed diuretics may produce or exacerbate hyponatremia, especially in patients with advanced heart failure permitted ad-libitum fluid intake. Symptomatic hyponatremia is better treated by water restriction than by cessation of diuretic therapy, unless over-diuresis or dehydration has occurred. Metabolic acidosis is a complication of the use of carbonic anhydrase inhibition, because these agents block hydrogen ion secretion. The use of thiazide and loop diuretics may also cause metabolic alkalosis. This is usually caused by the excretion of sodium, chloride, and potassium without bicarbonate, which leads to a rise in serum bicarbonate concentration. Other adverse effects of diuretics include carbohydrate intolerance, hyperuricemia (gout), hypersensitivity reactions (interstitial nephritis, skin rashes, hematological disorders), and acute pancreatitis. Deafness, which is generally reversible on cessation of diuretic administration, may be associated with the use of ethacrynic acid or furosemide especially if given intravenously, rapidly, and in the presence of other ototoxic drugs. Some cases of diuretic-induced deafness are irreversible. Finally, one of the most perplexing and challenging adverse effects of diuretics is the development of diuretic resistance. Although no generally consensual definition exists, diuretic resistance is generally manifest as worsening renal function during diuresis or a diminishing/inadequate response to diuretic administration. This clinical situation has also been described as a part of the so-called *cardio-renal syndrome*. Importantly, diuretic resistance or the cardio-renal syndrome has been associated with worse outcomes (increased morbidity and mortality) in both chronic and acutely decompensated heart failure.[108–110]

Diuretic Resistance

The mechanisms leading to diuretic resistance are multiple. Some degree of renal insufficiency is usually present in patients with chronic heart failure. This insufficiency is related to renal hypoperfusion, which affects the amount of diuretic delivered to the tubular lumen of the kidney. With a decreased level of diuretic being delivered to its site of action, a decrease in drug potency is present. Additionally, although loop diuretics are used in various stages of renal insufficiency, thiazide diuretics have a much narrower window of efficacy with worsening renal function as mentioned above.[111] Also, inadequate dosing of diuretics can affect their efficacy. For example, the duration of action of furosemide is approximately 6 to 7 hours. Thus, a prolonged period for *compensatory* sodium retention occurs during the balance of the 24-hour period, when this diuretic is administered on a once-daily regimen. Dietary control of sodium intake is essential in mitigating this effect.[112]

The chronic use of loop diuretics can also lead to a *braking phenomenon*, which stimulates anatomical and functional alterations of the distal tubule. The resultant hypertrophy of these segments leads to an increased reabsorptive ability of the tubules and overall decreased natriuresis.[113]

Patients with advanced heart failure often develop fluid deposition in a number of varying body sites, including the gastrointestinal tract. Gut edema can often prevent the proper absorption of orally administered diuretic agents, thereby delaying the time to achieve a peak dose effect. As previously mentioned, a lack of dietary control, namely with salt intake, can result in a net positive sodium balance, despite increasing diuretic doses.[114] The use of nonsteroidal antiinflammatory drugs can also be linked to diuretic resistance. Also as mentioned previously, inhibition of cyclooxygenase by these agents results in decreased renal prostaglandin synthesis. Prostaglandins play a crucial role in not only off-setting the systemic increase of vasoconstrictors induced by heart failure but by also promoting natriuresis.[115] Use of these agents can thereby decrease the effectiveness of administered diuretics and also potentially contribute to a nephrotoxic state.

Finally, diuretic therapy itself via several of the aforementioned mechanisms may initiate an iatrogenic cardio-renal syndrome leading to worse heart failure outcomes (Fig. 26–4).

Management of Diuretic Resistance
Before a patient can be deemed diuretic resistant, a number of factors should be taken into account. Chief among them should be drug compliance, because this would be the first area of concern if any resistant state should be questioned. If compliance with medications is not an issue, sodium and fluid restriction should also be closely monitored, because this area is also notoriously difficult to successfully manage in the outpatient heart failure setting. Concomitant medications, such as nonsteroidal antiinflammatory drugs, should have their use curtailed or stopped if possible. Additionally, medications that serve to antagonize the hormonal cascade induced by the renin-angiotensin-aldosterone and adrenergic nervous systems, such as ACE inhibitors and β blockers, should be optimized to their fullest extent.

Once these factors are thoroughly evaluated and adjusted, the alteration of diuretic administration can be attempted. A common method to address an inadequate diuretic response in a patient on an oral loop diuretic is to increase the amount of diuretic dosage. As mentioned, decreased renal perfusion can diminish the secretion of loop diuretic into the renal tubule; thus, the use of an increased dose of a loop diuretic is a relatively easy way to increase the amount of drug delivered to the nephron.[116] Another variation is to increase the frequency of diuretic dosing, as this approach minimizes the compensatory postdiuretic salt retention that commonly occurs after loop diuretic administration, given the relatively short half-lives of these agents.

Loop diuretics only target specific areas of the nephron, and are thus unable to alter sodium reabsorption elsewhere in the renal circuit. Indeed, their long-term use can facilitate increased distal tubular sodium and water reabsorption. Combination therapy with other classes of diuretics can be an additional method of maximizing diuresis, through the blockade of multiple tubular sites of sodium reabsorption. Although proximally acting diuretics such as acetazolamide and potassium-sparing diuretics such as spironolactone can be used for this purpose, their chronic use brings into play a number of safety issues (e.g., metabolic acidosis and hyperkalemia, respectively). Spironolactone has established itself as a valued medi-

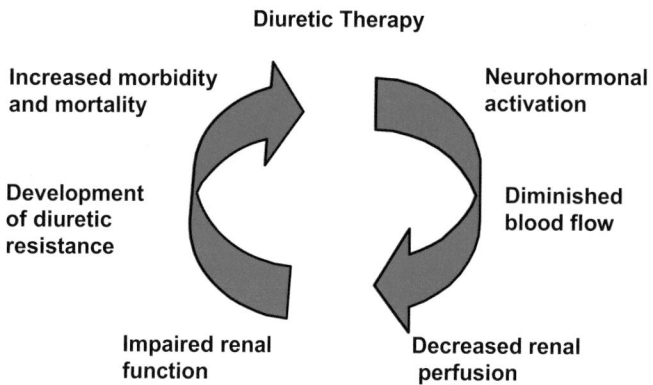

Diuretic Therapy

Increased morbidity and mortality

Neurohormonal activation

Development of diuretic resistance

Diminished blood flow

Impaired renal function

Decreased renal perfusion

FIGURE 26–4. The iatrogenic cardio-renal of heart failure. Diuretics further activate neurohormonal vasoconstrictor systems resulting in an impairment in renal function and diuretic resistance by the mechanism shown. Diuretic resistance has been associated with poor outcomes in acute and chronic heart failure. See text for details.

cation for chronic heart failure use, but this is based more on its antagonism of aldosterone as opposed to its diuretic potency. Thiazide diuretics, conversely, have emerged as viable additions to loop diuretic therapy. This approach to sequentially block sodium reabsorption at numerous sites of the nephron has proven to be effective, although signs of over-diuresis and electrolyte depletion should be carefully monitored.[117,118] Metolazone, a thiazide-like diuretic, received an initial push as the agent of choice to increase diuresis in resistant patients taking a loop diuretic because of its greater potency than other thiazides. However, hypokalemia and rapid volume depletion are real risks of this approach; alternatively, hydrochlorothiazide therapy is quite effective and carries with it less risk of producing these untoward effects.[119–120]

Recommendations for the Use of Diuretics in Chronic Heart Failure
Diuretic therapy should be initiated with a loop or thiazide-type diuretic, based on the severity of the heart failure. For severe heart failure with overt volume overload (i.e., pulmonary and/or peripheral edema) the more potent loop diuretics (i.e., furosemide, ethacrynic acid, bumetanide, and torsemide) should be used. If a loop diuretic given twice daily in doses equivalent to furosemide 100 to 200 mg/d is inadequate for diuresis, a thiazide diuretic or metolazone may be added. This often results in a synergistic effect on solute and water excretion, as noted above. Because this combination also results in substantial renal potassium wasting, an increased need for potassium supplementation should be anticipated. To conserve potassium and/or to further enhance the diuresis, a potassium-sparing diuretic may be added. However, triamterene should not be combined with furosemide because triamterene blocks the tubular secretion of furosemide thus inhibiting furosemide effect.[121] The goal of diuretic therapy in heart failure is resolution of the signs and symptoms caused by pulmonary and/or peripheral edema. Thus, once this goal has been achieved, the diuretic dose should be adjusted to maintain a euvolemic state. With specific tailored guidelines, patients may be instructed to alter their diuretic regimen on an *as needed* basis to alleviate signs and symptoms of extracellular fluid volume excess. Combinations of diuretics are usually needed in patients with heart failure of severity greater than NYHA II and are to be favored before large doses of loop diuretics are prescribed.

Angiotensin-Converting Enzyme Inhibitors

Angiotensin-converting enzyme inhibitors are part of the standard treatment of heart failure usually prescribed with diuretics. In patients with chronic heart failure, ACE inhibition improves hemodynamics and functional status (i.e., lessens symptoms and improves exercise tolerance), reduces hospitalizations for heart failure, and prolongs life.

Hemodynamic Effects of Angiotensin-Converting Enzyme Inhibition ACE inhibition exerts a number of beneficial hemodynamic effects in patients with chronic heart failure. These include decreases in systemic vascular resistance, pulmonary capillary wedge pressure, right atrial pressure, and end-diastolic and end-systolic dimensions and improvements in cardiac performance as evidenced by increased cardiac output and stoke volume and by improved fractional shortening determined by echocardiography. The acute and chronic hemodynamic effects of ACE inhibition in heart failure were first described in the early 1980s. LeJemtel and coworkers[122] examined the acute hemodynamic response to a single oral 25-mg dose of the ACE inhibitor captopril in patients with established heart failure. At baseline, these patients exhibited severely decompensated heart failure with an average systemic vascular resistance of nearly 2000 dynes × sec/cm⁵, pulmonary capillary wedge pressure of almost 30 mmHg, and cardiac index of just 2.00 L/min/m². Following the administration of the ACE inhibitor, both systemic vascular resistance and pulmonary capillary wedge pressure fell significantly. This was associated with a marked improvement in the cardiac index.

DiCarlo and colleagues[123] investigated the acute and chronic hemodynamic effects of ACE inhibition in patients with chronic heart failure. Patients were given the oral ACE inhibitor enalapril at a dose of 10 mg twice daily. Hemodynamics were assessed prior to treatment, following the initial 10 mg dose, and after 30 days of chronic therapy. Both the acute and chronic administration of the ACE inhibitor improved hemodynamics, with significant decreases in systemic vascular resistance and pulmonary capillary wedge pressure and increases in cardiac index.

Chronic ACE inhibition improves LV dimensions and function in patients with chronic heart failure. This was demonstrated in 1982 by Awan and associates,[124] who examined the effects of ACE inhibition on measures of LV size and performance determined by echocardiography in nine patients with chronic heart failure. LV end-diastolic and end-systolic dimensions and shortening fraction were determined at baseline and after 1 week, 8 weeks, and 6 months of chronic ACE inhibition. Through 8 weeks of therapy, there was a progressive decrease in LV dimensions and a statistically significant improvement in shortening fraction, evident at 1 week and maintained through 6 months of therapy.

Effects of Angiotensin-Converting Enzyme Inhibitors on Symptoms and on Exercise Capacity The effects of ACE inhibition on symptoms and on exercise capacity in chronic heart failure include improvements in symptoms of heart failure determined by patients' subjective impressions (e.g., quality of life, patient global assessments), NYHA functional class ranking, and increased exercise tolerance times. Thus, ACE inhibitors improve both subjective and objective measures of functional capacity in chronic heart failure.

In 1984 Sharpe and coworkers[125] examined the effect of chronic ACE inhibition on heart failure symptoms as reported by the patient. A total of 30 patients were randomized to receive either the ACE inhibitor enalapril (10 mg twice daily) or a matching placebo for 3 months. All 16 patients randomized to the ACE inhibitor reported feeling "much better" at follow up. In contrast, only 3 of 14 placebo-treated patients reported feeling "much better." In the placebo group, 5 patients report feeling "little better," 2 patients reported "no change." 3 patients reported feeling "little worse," and 1 patient reported feeling "much worse." Four patients in the placebo group died prior to the end-of-study assessment. Numerous other trials in chronic heart failure have also demonstrated improvement in symptoms and in NYHA functional class ranking in patients randomized to ACE inhibitors.[126–133] For example, the Captopril Multicenter Research Group examined the effect of chronic ACE inhibition on NYHA functional classification in a 12-week, double-blind, placebo-controlled evaluation of 74 patients with established heart failure.[132] Although 61 percent of the 46 ACE inhibitor-treated patients demonstrated improvement in NYHA functional class ranking, only 24 percent of placebo-treated patients exhibited functional class improvement. This ability of chronic ACE inhibition to improve NYHA functional class ranking was seen at the end of 2 weeks of study, was progressive to 8 weeks of therapy, and then maintained throughout the remainder of the 12-week period of study.

The beneficial effects of chronic ACE inhibition on exercise capacity in patients with chronic heart failure are also well established.[132,134,135] In the aforementioned Captopril Multicenter Research Group trial, treadmill exercise time was significantly and progressively improved throughout the 12 weeks of study in patients randomized to the ACE inhibitor.[132] There was a 24 percent improvement in exercise duration in the ACE inhibitor group, and virtually no change in the placebo group. Chalmers and colleagues[135] demonstrated similar findings using bicycle exercise testing and another ACE inhibitor, lisinopril. In this randomized, double-blind, placebo-controlled investigation, a significant 200-second improvement in bicycle exercise time was seen by 4 weeks of study and maintained through the end of study (week 12) in patients randomized to the ACE inhibitor.

Effects of Angiotensin-Converting Enzyme Inhibitors on Survival ACE inhibition has been shown to 1) prolong survival in advanced, NYHA class IV, heart failure; 2) prolong survival in mild to moderate, NYHA class II and III, heart failure; and, 3) prolong survival in patient with asymptomatic LV dysfunction following a MI and when heart failure complicates an acute MI. ACE inhibition in post-MI patients is discussed in Chapter 61.

The first survival trial of ACE inhibition in chronic heart failure was the CONSENSUS, or Cooperative North Scandinavian Enalapril Survival Study, published in 1987.[136] In this double-blinded clinical trial, 253 patients with advanced heart failure were randomized to receive either placebo or the ACE inhibitor enalapril. The average enalapril dose was 18.5 mg/d or approximately 10 mg given twice daily. ACE inhibition produced a highly significant reduction in mortality throughout the 1-year period of follow up. Following the CONSENSUS trial, the Studies of Left Ventricular Dysfunction (SOLVD) investigators examined the survival benefit of ACE inhibition in patients with mild to moderate chronic heart failure.[137] More than 2500 patients were randomized in this double-blinded, placebo-controlled trial of enalapril. During the 4-year period of followup, there was a highly significant 16 percent reduction in mortality observed in the ACE inhibitor group. These proven effects of ACE inhibition to prolong survival in NYHA class II through IV patients support their use as first-line agents in the pharmacologic management of chronic heart failure.

Recommendations for the Use of Angiotensin-Converting Enzyme Inhibitors

All three heart failure guidelines strongly endorse the use of ACE inhibitors as first-line agents in the management of all NYHA classes of chronic systolic heart failure. In the absence of fluid retention, these agents should be initiated first in the management of systolic heart failure, and in the case of those with fluid retention, an ACE inhibitor should be started concomitantly with a diuretic. ACE inhibitors should be initiated at a low dose and slowly titrated to doses proven to be effective in randomized controlled trials. Virtually all ACE inhibitors evaluated in heart failure have proven effective; Table 26–8 lists the evidence-based ACE inhibitors used in heart failure, including their starting and target doses. Carefully monitor patients for the major side effects of ACE inhibition including hypotension, prerenal azotemia, hyperkalemia, and cough. Cough in a heart failure patient taking an ACE inhibitor should not immediately be presumed related to the medication, as elevated LV filling pressure may commonly cause coughing. In this instance, the patient may need an increase in the diuretic dose or an increase in rather than a discontinuation of the ACE inhibitor. Finally, angioedema is a rare adverse effect of ACE inhibitor therapy.

Angiotensin Receptor Blockers

Angiotensin receptor blockers have been evaluated for use as either alternatives to ACE inhibitors or as additive therapy to an ACE inhibitor and β-blocker–based heart failure drug regimen. The concept of enhanced blockade of the renin-angiotensin system with the addition of an angiotensin II receptor type 1 (AT_1) blocking agent is conceptionally appealing and has been evaluated in multiple randomized controlled trials. Theoretically, blockade of the AT_1 receptor should result in more complete antagonism of the renin-angiotensin system and act independently of non-ACE pathways for angiotensin II production. Alternatively, blocking the effects of angiotensin II at the receptor level rather than inhibiting its production via ACE inhibition could act to preserve the postulated benefits of AT2-receptor agonism. Conversely, ACE inhibition affects not only the renin-angiotensin pathway but also the degradation of the vasodilator, bradykinin. Specifically, ACE inhibition results in decreased bradykinin degradation and thus increased circulating levels of bradykinin. Hence, the mechanisms of action of ACE inhibitors versus ARBs are complex and can be used to argue for the theoretical superiority of either agent over the other.

Effects of Angiotensin Receptor Blockers on Physiologic and Functional Endpoints

The effects of ARBs on symptoms, exercise capacity, and systemic hemodynamics in heart failure appear to be similar to those observed with ACE inhibitors.[138–140] Angiotensin II receptor blockers are extremely well tolerated and do not cause cough. Some early studies suggested that angiotensin II receptor blockers maintain or improve glomerular filtration, in contrast to the decrease in glomerular filtration commonly seen with ACE inhibitors.[140–142] This proposed effect of angiotensin II receptor antagonists may be attributable to their lack of effect on the vasodilator bradykinin.[142] However, as noted below, a differing effect between ACE inhibitors and ARBs on renal function has been difficult to demonstrate in clinical trials.

The Evaluation of Losartan in the Elderly (ELITE-I) trial hypothesized that the ARB, losartan, would be equally efficacious and associated with the development of less prerenal azotemia, when compared to the ACE inhibitor, captopril.[141] In fact, the incidence of worsening renal function defined by an increase in serum creatinine of at least 0.3 mg/dL was the same in both groups. Although ELITE-I failed to meet its primary renal function endpoint, it suggested the potential superiority of the ARB over the ACE inhibitor on the combined secondary endpoint of hospitalizations or mortality and on mortality alone. However, the ELITE-I trial was not prospectively designed or powered to assess morbidity or mortality, and at best, it may be viewed as hypothesis generating.

Effects of Angiotensin Receptor Blockers on Survival

Like ACE inhibitors, ARBs improve survival in heart failure when compared to placebo. The comparative efficacy of ACE inhibitors and ARBs on survival has been a topic of great interest over the past decade. The Losartan Heart Failure Survival Study (ELITE II) was designed to compare the efficacy of an ARB and an ACE inhibitor

TABLE 26–8

Angiotensin-Converting Enzyme Inhibitors Used in the Treatment of Heart Failure

AGENT	TOTAL DAILY DOSE (MG)	ROUTE OF ADMINISTRATION	FREQUENCY
Captopril	75–150	Oral	Thrice daily
Enalapril	10–40	Oral	Twice daily
Enalaprilat	2.5–20	Intravenous	Every 6 hours
Fosinopril	10–40	Oral	Once daily
Lisinopril	10–40	Oral	Once daily
Quinapril	10–40	Oral	Once or twice daily
Ramipril	2.5–20	Oral	Once or twice daily
Trandolapril	1–4	Oral	Once daily

(again, losartan and captopril, respectively) in elderly subjects with symptomatic heart failure caused by LV systolic dysfunction (LVEF <40 percent).[143] This study, designed as a followup to ELITE-I, evaluated all-cause mortality as its primary endpoint. There was no difference between these agents in all-cause mortality, thus failing to confirm any superiority of ARBs in the treatment of heart failure. Moreover, this trial was not statistically powered to determine the equivalency of the two agents, leaving the role of ARBs in the treatment of heart failure somewhat uncertain. More recently, a trial in patients with LV dysfunction following acute MI demonstrated the noninferiority of the ARB, valsartan, when compared to the ACE inhibitor, captopril.[69] However, there was no incremental reduction in morbidity or mortality when the two agents were used in combination.

The use of ACE inhibitors and ARBs together in patients with chronic mild or moderate heart failure has been evaluated in two large-scale randomized controlled trials. The Valsartan Heart Failure Trial (Val-HeFT) enrolled 5010 to determine the effects of valsartan (target dose 160 mg twice a day) versus placebo added to an ACE inhibitor in patients with NYHA Class II or III heart failure.[144] This study demonstrated a slight but statistically significant reduction in a clinical composite endpoint (all-cause mortality plus heart failure hospitalization) favoring the addition of the ARB. In addition, valsartan improved LVEF and decreased LV dimensions as measured by echocardiography. A posthoc subgroup analysis of 1610 patients on β blocker and ACE inhibitor therapy at baseline, however, suggested an increase in mortality with the addition of valsartan (valsartan, 16.4 percent versus placebo, 12.5 percent; $p = 0.018$) raising concerns about the combination of ARB, ACE inhibitor, and β blocker.

The Candesartan in Heart Failure Assessment of Reduction in Mortality and Morbidity (CHARM) trial addressed this issue further by prospectively analyzing the effect of candesartan (target dose of 32 mg/d) versus placebo in 4576 patients with reduced LVEFs and mild or moderate heart failure.[145] A separate cohort of patients with preserved LV systolic function was also evaluated in the CHARM study program. This study reported a statistically significant but small reduction in the combined endpoint of cardiovascular morbidity and mortality when candesartan was combined with an ACE inhibitor or an ACE inhibitor plus a β blocker. The explanation for the disparity between Val-HeFT and CHARM in the *triple therapy* group (ACE inhibitor, ARB, and β-blocker–treated patients) is unclear but could be related to differences between the two ARBs, different dosing strategies, or merely chance.[146] In CHARM, the assessment of triple therapy was a prespecified endpoint, making this the more valid assessment of triple neurohormonal therapy with an ACE inhibitor, ARB, and β blocker.

Thus, results from Val-HeFT and CHARM support the concept of a clinical benefit to more complete antagonism of the renin-angiotensin system. The magnitude of benefit is relatively small, approximately a 10 percent to 15 percent reduction in the combined endpoint of all-cause mortality and heart failure hospitalization. In both studies, the reduction in mortality alone with the addition of an ARB was less than 10 percent and was not statistically different than placebo. Finally, both trials identified a highly significant survival advantage of ARB administration in patients intolerant to an ACE inhibitor.

Recommendations for the Use of Angiotensin Receptor Blockers Angiotensin receptor blockers are strongly recommended for patients with chronic systolic heart failure, who cannot tolerate an ACE inhibitor. Angiotensin receptor blockers may also be considered first-line therapy instead of an ACE inhibitor, given similar efficacy. According to the ACC/AHA heart failure guideline, this latter option may be especially attractive in patients who are already taking an ARB for other indications. Finally, the addition of an ARB to an ACE inhibitor and β-blocker–based drug regimen may be considered in persistently symptomatic subjects. The substitution of an ARB for an ACE inhibitor caused by angioedema should be done with great caution because angioedema has been reported rarely with ARBs. Moreover, ARBs are not different than ACE inhibitors regarding the side effects of hypotension, renal insufficiency, and hyperkalemia. Generally, all precautions taken during ACE inhibitor use are relevant to ARB use. With combined ACE inhibitor and ARB therapy, the adverse effects of hypotension, renal insufficiency, and hyperkalemia are seen more frequently than with the use of either agent alone. Finally, the use of an aldosterone antagonist in combination with an ACE inhibitor and ARB is discouraged because of the lack of clinical trials data supporting such a regimen and to the likely magnified risk of hyperkalemia. Although candesartan and valsartan represent evidence-based ARBs for the treatment of heart failure, other agents have proven effective in earlier stages of cardiovascular disease progression including eprosartan, irbesartan, losartan, olmesartan, and telmisartan.

Aldosterone Antagonists

As noted in Chap. 24, aldosterone may produce deleterious effects in LV dysfunction and heart failure via multiple mechanisms, including sodium and water retention, abnormal electrolyte homeostasis (e.g., hypomagnesium and hypokalemia), myocardial hypertrophy and fibrosis, vascular remodeling, and endothelial cell dysfunction.[147] In patients with heart failure, aldosterone levels increase primarily in response to angiotensin II, but other factors may also be important. Aldosterone antagonists have been evaluated in patients with LV dysfunction following acute MI complicated by heart failure or accompanied by major risk factors (notably, diabetes) and in patients with advanced chronic systolic heart failure. These agents conserve potassium and magnesium via the kidneys, promote reverse remodeling of the failing ventricle, and, in the aforementioned cohorts, reduce morbidity and mortality.

Two large-scale randomized controlled trials direct the use of aldosterone antagonists in heart failure. The Randomized Aldactone Evaluation Study (RALES) enrolled 1663 patients with severe heart failure (NYHA class IV at or recently preceding randomization) and LV systolic dysfunction to receive either spironolactone or placebo in combination with ACE inhibition and diuretics.[148] Of note, only 11 percent of subjects randomized in RALES were receiving a β blocker at the time of enrollment. The dose of spironolactone used was low, 12.5 mg or 25 mg daily. The study was stopped early because of a highly significant 30 percent reduction in all-cause mortality in patients receiving spironolactone. Significant reductions were seen in both pump failure deaths as well as sudden cardiac death. Benefit was also observed in the relatively small subgroup of patients receiving β blockers. Not surprisingly, a significant number of men on spironolactone experienced gynecomastia or breast pain. Although significant hyperkalemia with spironolactone therapy was uncommonly observed, subjects were rigorously monitored throughout the trial. In the *real world* of clinical practice, the incidence of hyperkalemia appears to be substantially higher than that seen in the RALES trial. An observational study from Ontario, Canada, identified a marked increase in hospitalization rates for hyperkalemia paralleling an increase in the number of spironolactone prescriptions for heart failure management, in a community setting.[149]

The Eplerenone Post Acute Myocardial Infarction Heart Failure Efficacy and Survival Study (EPHESUS) enrolled 6632 patients with LV systolic dysfunction (LVEF ≤ 40 percent; average 33 percent) with or without clinical heart failure following an acute MI.[70] Patients were randomized to receive either eplerenone 25 mg to 50 mg daily or placebo, on top of standard post-MI and heart failure medications. In contrast to the RALES trial, most patients (75 percent) in EPHESUS also received β blockers, in addition to ACE inhibitors and diuretics. In EPHESUS, the selective aldosterone antagonist, eplerenone, improved survival and reduced cardiovascular hospitalization compared to the control group. The magnitude of benefit (a 15 percent reduction in all-cause mortality) was smaller than that seen in RALES but was highly statistically significant. Given the selective mineralocorticoid-receptor blocking properties of eplerenone, which does not interfere with androgen or progesterone receptors, the troublesome side effect of gynecomastia and breast pain was not encountered in the actively treated patients in the EPHESUS trial.

Recommendations for the Use of Aldosterone Antagonists Low-dose aldosterone antagonist therapy is recommended in stage C and D heart failure patients receiving standard heart failure medications (generally, an ACE inhibitor or ARB and a β blocker), when symptoms are advanced and patients can be closely monitored for hyperkalemia. In addition, patients with LV systolic dysfunction following an acute MI are also candidates for an aldosterone antagonist, if they have either heart failure (newly stage C) or additional major risk factors (stage B). To date, the role of aldosterone antagonists in mild and moderate heart failure remains poorly defined. The various heart failure guidelines differ somewhat on their enthusiasm for aldosterone antagonists in this latter group of patients. By consensus (because clinical trials evidence is lacking), the guidelines generally suggest that it is reasonable to consider an aldosterone antagonist in this population; none mandate the use of this class of agents in mild or moderate heart failure.

The decision to initiate an aldosterone antagonist must balance the potential for a reduction in mortality and morbidity with the known risk of life-threatening hyperkalemia. The dose of aldosterone antagonist should be started low and, if tolerated, increased to target dosing, which is 25 mg once a day of spironolactone and 50 mg once a day of eplerenone. Recognition of the patient at risk for hyperkalemia is the key to the safe introduction and maintenance of this treatment. Although patients with serum creatinine levels as high as 2.4 mg/dL were allowed in RALES and EPHESUS, the risk of hyperkalemia increases substantially when the serum creatinine exceeds 1.6 mg/dL, particularly in the elderly in whom creatinine may not ade-

quately reflect glomerular filtration rate. Extreme caution should be used in initiating aldosterone antagonism, if serum creatinine exceeds 2.0 mg/dL or if baseline serum potassium exceeds 5.0 mmol/L. Diabetics are also at increased risk of developing hyperkalemia, when exposed to an aldosterone antagonist. This risk factor for hyperkalemia is likely independent of serum creatinine. Thus, frequent monitoring of renal function and serum potassium is necessary after introduction of therapy, particularly if moderate to high doses of an ACE inhibitor or ARB are being used. Any changes in diuretic dose, ARB, or ACE inhibitor dose should also prompt laboratory evaluation of electrolytes and renal function. Patients should be cautioned regarding potassium intake, and all medications, including nonprescription drugs, should be reviewed prior to initiating the aldosterone antagonist. As previously noted, the combined use of ACE inhibitor, ARB, and aldosterone antagonist should generally be avoided.

β Blockers

Over the past decade, the results of numerous randomized controlled clinical trials have demonstrated that β blockade both improves the symptoms of systolic heart failure and, most importantly, attenuates disease progression when added to conventional therapy usually consisting of an ACE inhibitor, diuretic, and digoxin. Long-term (≥ 3 months) use of β blockers consistently and significantly increases LV function, as measured by EF,[150–154] and reduces the incidence of hospitalization in patients with a broad range of clinical symptoms.[150,155–158] Moreover, chronic β blockade improves survival in all NYHA class of systolic heart failure. β blockade is thus the third pillar of the standard treatment of heart failure.

Classification of β Blockers β-Adrenergic receptor blockers may be classified into three groups, or generations, depending on their β receptor selectivity (β_1 versus β_2) and the presence or absence of desirable ancillary cardiovascular properties.[159] The first-generation agents are nonselective and possess no beneficial ancillary cardiovascular properties. Examples of first-generation β-adrenergic receptor blockers are propranolol and timolol. Second-generation β blockers such as metoprolol, atenolol, and bisoprolol are selective for the cardiac or β_1 receptor and also exhibit no ancillary cardiovascular benefits. Third-generation agents are either selective or nonselective β blockers and possess desirable ancillary cardiovascular properties, such as peripheral vasodilation and antioxidant effects. Third-generation β blockers include carvedilol and nebivolol and some investigational agents (e.g., bucindolol). In general, the first-generation agents are poorly tolerated in the setting of systolic heart failure. In contrast, second- and third-generation β blockers are tolerated by greater than 90 percent of patients with chronic heart failure and no fluid volume overload, and four agents (metoprolol CR/XL, bisoprolol, carvedilol, and nebivolol) have proven effective in the treatment of heart failure.

Early Trials of β Blockade in Heart Failure The Metoprolol in Dilated Cardiomyopathy (MDC) trial randomized 383 patients with idiopathic dilated cardiomyopathy to receive either placebo or the second-generation β-adrenergic receptor blocker metoprolol tartrate for 12 to 18 months.[152] After initiation at a very low dose and subsequent titration, metoprolol was dosed in a target range of 50 mg to 75 mg twice daily. The average daily dose of metoprolol achieved was 108 mg. The average followup in the MDC trial was approximately 1 year. At 6 months metoprolol produced highly significant favorable effects on all hemodynamic parameters. There was a nearly significant ($p = 0.06$) improvement in the primary outcome parameter, the combined endpoint of need for cardiac transplantation and mortality. However, the entire risk reduction associated with metoprolol was attributable to a decrease in the need for cardiac transplantation, a somewhat *soft* endpoint. There was no significant reduction in all-cause mortality alone; and numerically, there were more instances of sudden death in metoprolol-treated patients compared to the control group. Although the MDC trial was technically a negative study, it established the possibility that β blockade could be useful in the treatment of heart failure.

The Cardiac Insufficiency Bisoprolol Survival (CIBIS) trial examined the effect of the $β_1$-selective adrenergic receptor blocker bisoprolol on survival in 641 patients with ischemic and nonischemic heart failure and reduced EFs.[154] As in the MDC and subsequent trials, the β blocker was initiated at a low dose and titrated slowly to a target dose, if tolerated. The target dose of bisoprolol in the CIBIS trial was 5 mg daily, and an average daily dose of 3.8 mg was achieved. Average followup was 1.9 years. An insignificant trend toward lower mortality (20 percent) and 30 percent fewer hospital admissions for worsening heart failure were observed in the bisoprolol group. Although there was no statistically significant survival benefit associated with bisoprolol in this study, CIBIS was viewed as supporting the need for larger and more definitive trials of β blockade in heart failure.

Landmark Trials of β Blockade in Heart Failure The U.S. Carvedilol Heart Failure Trials Program randomized 1094 patients to either placebo or to the third-generation vasodilating β blocker, carvedilol, in four parallel randomized controlled trials.[157] Patients with stable heart failure and LVEFs of 35 percent or less treated with standard therapy consisting of ACE inhibitors and diuretics with or without digoxin were eligible for this clinical trials program. Although none of the four component trials alone was prospectively designed or powered to assess survival differences compared to placebo, a 65 percent reduction in all-cause mortality was observed in carvedilol-treated patients in the overall clinical trials program, in a prospectively planned pooled mortality analysis.

One of these carvedilol trials, the Multicenter Oral Carvedilol Heart Failure Assessment (MOCHA), suggested that the mortality reduction observed with carvedilol was dose-related (Figure 26–5).[160] In this trial 345 subjects with mild to moderate heart failure were randomized to one of three doses of carvedilol (6.25 mg, 12.5 mg, or 25 mg twice daily) or to placebo. A significant linear doses response was seen for improvement in LVEF and reductions in cardiovascular hospitalization and mortality. In another component study of the U.S. Carvedilol Heart Failure Trials Program, Colucci and colleagues[155] administered carvedilol or placebo to 366 patients with mild symptoms of heart failure.

During an average treatment period of 6.5 months, addition of carvedilol to the standard regimen of diuretics and an ACE inhibitor with or without digoxin resulted in a 48 percent reduction in clinical disease progression ($p = 0.008$ versus placebo), defined as death caused by heart failure, hospitalization for heart failure, or the need for a sustained increase in heart failure medications. Several *secondary endpoints* showed improvement as well. As in earlier studies, carvedilol significantly increased the LVEF.[161-163] Carvedilol also improved various indices of clinical status, including NYHA functional classification and heart failure symptom score. Significantly, for each of these clinical indices, carvedilol reduced the percentage of patients whose condition worsened over the course of the trial, further indicating that the addition of carvedilol to the standard regimen impeded disease progression.

The Metoprolol CR/XL Randomized Intervention Trial in Congestive Heart Failure (MERIT-HF) study enrolled 3991 patients, most with NYHA class II (41 percent) and class III (55 percent) systolic heart failure, with a mean EF of 28 percent.[164] Patients received standard background therapy with an ACE inhibitor or ARB, diuretics, and digoxin. Patients were randomized to receive either placebo or metoprolol succinate (metoprolol CR/XL) with a target dose of 200 mg a day. The average dose of metoprolol CR/XL in MERIT-HF was 159 mg. This trial was stopped after a mean followup of only 1 year because of a highly significant survival benefit in the metoprolol group (relative risk reduction for mortality was 34 percent, $p = 0.0062$). A beneficial response to metoprolol succinate was also observed re-

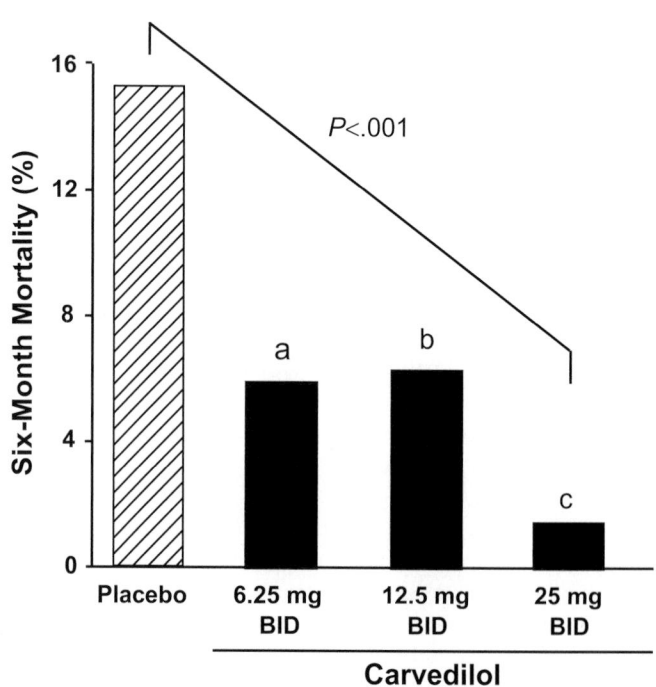

FIGURE 26–5. Dose-response effects of carvedilol in the Multicenter Oral Carvedilol Heart Failure Assessment (MOCHA) trial. Patients were receiving diuretics and ACE inhibitors, with or without digoxin; follow up 6 months. ACE, angiotensin-converting enzyme. Placebo (*n* = 84), carvedilol (*n* = 261). a, *p* < .07 vs. placebo; b, *p* < .07 vs. placebo; c, *p* < .001 vs. placebo. *Source: From Bristow MR, Gilbert EM, Abraham WT, et al, for the MOCHA Investigators.*[160] *With permission.*

garding sudden death, heart failure hospitalizations, and functional classification.

The second CIBIS trial (CIBIS II) was designed as a followup study to CIBIS. CIBIS II differed from the first CIBIS trial in that it was adequately powered to assess the effects of bisoprolol on all-cause mortality as a primary endpoint. Moreover, the target dose of bisoprolol was doubled to 10 mg daily (average dose achieved was 7.5 mg daily), in CIBIS II. Among 2647 randomized patients with moderate to severe symptoms of systolic heart failure, bisoprolol produced a 34 percent reduction in overall mortality ($p = 0.0001$), a 44 percent reduction in sudden deaths ($p = 0.0011$), a 36 percent reduction in hospitalization for heart failure ($p = 0.0001$), and a 20 percent reduction in all-cause hospitalization ($p = 0.0006$) compared with placebo during an average treatment period of 1.4 years.[158]

While the U.S. Carvedilol Heart Failure Trials Program, MERIT-HF, and CIBIS II enrolled patients with mainly mild and moderate heart failure, the Carvedilol Prospective Randomized Cumulative Survival (COPERNICUS) study was designed to assess β blockade in a more severely symptomatic group of patients.[165] In COPERNICUS, patients had symptoms at rest or with minimal activity despite treatment with standard heart failure therapies. In the trial a total of 2289 patients were randomized at 334 centers to receive either placebo or carvedilol. A low dose of carvedilol (3.125 mg twice daily) was initiated and doubled every 2 weeks until the target dose (25 mg twice daily) was reached. Patients were followed up for 24 months (average duration of follow up 10.4 months). The primary end point of all-cause mortality occurred at a rate of 19.7 percent and 12.8 percent for placebo and carvedilol, respectively, resulting in a 35 percent reduction in risk of death with carvedilol treatment ($p = 0.00013$). In addition, one secondary end point, all-cause mortality and hospitalization for any reason, was reduced in carvedilol-treated patients by 24 percent ($p = 0.00004$), whereas another secondary endpoint, all-cause mortality and hospitalization for heart failure, was reduced by 31 percent ($p = 0.000004$). Importantly, carvedilol was very well tolerated in this group of patients with advanced heart failure, and the reductions in morbidity and mortality were manifest early in the course of treatment. Thus, COPERNICUS demonstrates the safety and efficacy of β blockade in advanced heart failure. Taken together, the aforementioned carvedilol trials, MERIT-HF, CIBIS II, and COPERNICUS support the use of β blockade across all symptomatic classes (NYHA classes II, III, and IV) of stage C heart failure. The role of β blockade in stage B heart failure and in new-onset stage C heart failure following a MI was subsequently evaluated in the Carvedilol Post-Infarct Survival Controlled Evaluation (CAPRICORN) trial.

Results from the CAPRICORN trial expand the indications for β blockade to patients with asymptomatic and symptomatic LV dysfunction following an acute MI.[166] In CAPRICORN, 1959 subjects with LVEFs of ≤40 percent receiving standard medical and interventional therapies and enrolled within the early convalescent phase (3–21 days) following MI were randomized to either carvedilol or placebo. The starting dose of carvedilol was 6.25 mg twice daily, rather than the 3.125 mg twice daily used in trials of chronic heart failure. By using the definition of no current or prior symptoms of heart failure post-MI, 1023 CAPRICORN patients were considered asymptomatic. In the entire cohort (symptomatic and asymptomatic), carvedilol reduced all-cause mortality significantly by 23 percent. In the group of patients with asymptomatic post-MI LV dysfunction, carvedilol decreased all-cause mortality by 31 percent. Several other measures of efficacy were likewise improved including combined morbidity and mortality endpoints and endpoints evaluating reinfarction rates, both fatal and nonfatal. As in COPERNICUS and other carvedilol trials, the β blocker was safe and well tolerated.

Although several trials of β blockade have demonstrated the benefits of metoprolol succinate, bisoprolol, and carvedilol in the treatment of post-MI LV dysfunction and chronic heart failure, trials of other β blocking agents have been negative. For example, the β blocker xamoterol, which exhibits intrinsic sympathomimetic activity, increased mortality in a randomized controlled trial in heart failure patients.[167] In another large-scale trial (2708 patients randomized to either bucindolol or placebo), the Beta-Blocker Evaluation of Survival Trial (BEST), it was found that bucindolol did not significantly reduce mortality (relative risk reduction of 10 percent; p-value insignificant) and actually seemed to increase mortality in an African-American subset of patients.[168] Interestingly, a recent subgroup analysis in 1040 patients participating in a DNA sub-study of BEST, suggests that the response to this third-generation vasodilating β blocker may depend on variations in the β_1-adrenergic receptor genotype.[169] In this analysis, no outcome was associated with genotype in the placebo group, indicating little impact of genotype on the natural course of heart failure. However, the [389]arginine homozygotes treated with bucindolol had an age, sex, and race adjusted 38 percent reduction in mortality ($p = 0.03$) and 34 percent reduction in mortality or hospitalization ($p = 0.004$) versus placebo. In contrast, [389]glycine carriers had no clinical response to bucindolol compared to placebo. Finally, the Study of Effects of Nebivolol Intervention on Outcomes and Rehospitalization in Seniors with Heart Failure (SENIORS) trial demonstrated a reduction in the combined endpoint of all cause mortality and cardiovascular hospitalization.[170] In this randomized controlled trial of 2128 patients (all older than 70 years) with heart failure, regardless of EF, nebivolol reduced all-cause mortality (a secondary endpoint) by 12 percent (p-value insignificant) but by 38 percent in those younger than 75 years of age, which was the mean age. Thus, β blocker appear to be effective in the elderly, irrespective of the EF.

Further evidence for clinical differences among β-blocking agents may be found in the results of the Carvedilol or Metoprolol European Trial (COMET).[171,172] This study of more than 3000 patients with moderate heart failure randomized patients to metoprolol tartrate (immediate-acting metoprolol) at a dose of 50 mg twice a day or carvedilol at a target dose of 25 mg twice a day plus standard heart failure therapy. A significant 17 percent survival advantage was seen in those patients receiving carvedilol. This study seems to underscore differences between carvedilol and metoprolol tartrate, but controversy continues regarding the exact interpretation of these data. In addition, COMET should not be used to draw any firm conclusion about the relative efficacy of carvedilol versus metoprolol succinate (the long-acting formulation of metoprolol that was used in MERIT II).

Recommendations for the Use of β Blockers

Based on the totality of available information, a class effect cannot be presumed for β blockers in heart failure. Accordingly, all three major heart failure guidelines strongly recommend the use of evidence-based β blockers (metoprolol succinate, bisoprolol, and carvedilol) for the treatment of heart failure (Nebivolol is licensed in Europe for heart failure in the elderly). The ACC/AHA heart failure guideline also states that patients treated for hypertension or angina with a β blocker that is not based on evidence of heart failure should be switched to an evidence-based agent at the onset of clinical heart failure. A published algorithm may help guide switching between β-blocking agents.[173]

Institution of an evidence-based β blocker is recommended in virtually all stages and NYHA classes of heart failure. β-Blocker therapy should be considered as soon as LV dysfunction is identified (i.e., beginning in stage B). In the past the initiation and titration of β-blocker therapy was often delayed and commenced with great trepidation because of concerns of worsening heart failure and hypotension in moderately ill and decompensated patients. It is now clear that these agents can be started early and perhaps even during hospitalization for decompensated heart failure, once adequate diuresis has been achieved.[174] Starting with very low doses and titrating slowly is strongly recommended. Carvedilol should generally be started at 3.125 mg twice a day and titrated to a target dose of 25 mg twice a day. Metoprolol succinate is begun at 25 mg once a day and increased over several weeks to a target dose of 200 mg/d. Bisoprolol is started at a dose of 1.25 mg daily and titrated to 10 mg daily.

No longer are comorbid conditions such as chronic obstructive pulmonary disease (COPD), peripheral arterial disease, or diabetes mellitus absolute contraindications to β-blocker use. Although patients with significant bronchospasm and COPD, or those with a remote history of asthma, may not tolerate β_2-receptor blockade with carvedilol, selective β_1-blockade with moderate doses of metoprolol succinate may be successful. Patients with substantive metabolic derangement related to diabetes may better tolerate carvedilol because of its α-antagonist and antioxidant properties.[175]

Vasodilators

Nitrates and Hydralazine

The beneficial effects of long-acting nitrates used alone or in conjunction with hydralazine in heart failure include increased exercise capacity, improved hemodynamics, decreased mitral regurgitation,[176] improved endothelium-dependent vasodilation,[177] modestly increased LVEF, and prolonged survival. These latter two effects have only been observed when long-acting nitrates are used in combination with hydralazine and particularly in African-American subjects.[51,178,179] When used alone or together, these agents decrease ventricular preload and afterload, improve cardiac output, and increase exercise capacity in patients with heart failure.[51,178–181]

The effect of long-acting nitrates plus hydralazine on survival was evaluated in the First Veterans Heart Failure Trial (V-HeFT-I).[179] In this study, 642 men with mild to moderate heart failure

who were taking digoxin and a diuretic were randomized to receive either placebo or prazosin, 20 mg/d, or the combination of isosorbide dinitrate, 160 mg/d, plus hydralazine, 300 mg/d (all in divided doses). Compared to placebo, the mortality-risk reduction in the group treated with isosorbide dinitrate plus hydralazine was 36 percent by 3 years. In contrast, the mortality in the prazosin group was the same as that seen in the placebo-treated patients. Moreover, LVEF rose significantly at 8 weeks and at 1 year in the group treated with isosorbide dinitrate plus hydralazine but not in the prazosin or placebo groups. However, a contemporary re-evaluation of the V-HeFT-I trial questioned the statistical significance of the results and demonstrated most benefit in the African-American subgroup of V-HeFT.

The V-HeFT-II trial directly compared the combination of isosorbide dinitrate plus hydralazine with enalapril in patients with predominantly NYHA classes II and III heart failure.[178] The investigators followed 804 men randomized to one of these two therapeutic regimens for an average of 2.5 years. The study demonstrated the superiority of the ACE inhibitor in reducing cumulative mortality in these patients with mild to moderate heart failure. Mortality at 2 years was significantly lower in the enalapril group than in the isosorbide dinitrate plus hydralazine group (18 percent versus 25 percent; $P = 0.016$; relative reduction in mortality, 28 percent). In contrast, the combination of nitrates and hydralazine produced more favorable effects on LVEF and exercise capacity determined by peak oxygen consumption.

The African-American Heart Failure Trial (A-HeFT)[51] tested the hypothesis that a fixed-dose combination of isosorbide dinitrate and hydralazine (BiDil) could improve outcomes in African Americans with systolic heart failure treated with standard heart failure medications. In A-HeFT, 1050 African-American subjects with NYHA class III or IV heart failure were randomized to the fixed-dose combination or placebo. BiDil significantly improved the primary endpoint, a composite response including morbidity, mortality, and quality of life. Most impressively, a 43 percent reduction in all-cause mortality was seen in the treatment group (Fig. 26–6). The results of this study led the U.S. Food and Drug Administration (FDA) to approve BiDil for African-American patients with NYHA class III or IV heart failure and reduced EFs.

Recommendations for Nitrates and Hydralazine

Nitrates plus hydralazine may be recommended for patients who are intolerant to ACE inhibitors and ARBs. In the African-American heart failure population, this combination of vasodilators may be recommended as adjunctive therapy to ACE inhibitors (or ARBs) and β blockers to further reduce mortality. Whether this therapy is effective in other racial or ethnic groups or in patients with less severe heart failure remains to be determined. Furthermore, this vasodilator combination is not recommended as first-line treatment for those that are ACE inhibitor or β-blocker naive.

Nitrate therapy alone for heart failure management has not been extensively studied but may be effective for relief of symptoms such as exertional dyspnea or paroxysmal nocturnal dyspnea. Isosorbide dinitrate is a potent venodilator but may also reduce afterload when systemic vascular resistance is severely elevated. Targeted therapy based on specific symptoms in the individual patient may be effective.

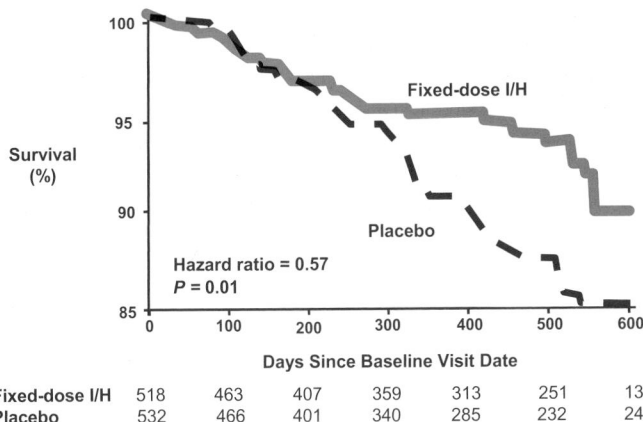

FIGURE 26–6. Kaplan-Meier estimates of time to key secondary endpoint of death from any cause in A-HeFT. The fixed-dose combination of isosorbide dinitrate and hydralazine reduced the risk of death by approximately 43 percent. A-HeFT, African-American Heart Failure Trial; I/H, fixed-dose isosorbide dinitrate and hydralazine group; placebo, optimal medical therapy group. *Source: From Taylor AL, Ziesche S, Yancy C, et al.[51] With permission.*

Digoxin

In some trials digoxin has been shown to reduce heart failure symptoms, improve NYHA functional class ranking, increase maximal treadmill exercise time, modestly increase LVEF, enhance cardiac performance (e.g., increased cardiac output and stroke work index), and to reduce slightly heart failure hospitalizations. Despite these findings digoxin does not improve survival in congestive heart failure (CHF)[182] and in the large Digitalis Investigation Group (DIG) trial did not improve symptoms or exercise capacity. The clinical benefits of digoxin in heart failure may be caused by its mildly positive inotropic effect, its apparent ability to diminish sympathetic activation in heart failure, or a combination of these and other mechanisms. The positive inotropic effect of digoxin has usually been attributed to the inhibition of sodium/potassium-adenosine triphosphate, whereas the sympathoinhibitory effect of the drug appears to result from sensitization of high-pressure baroreceptors which reduces central sympathetic outflow.[183,184]

Digoxin has been used in the treatment of heart failure for more than 200 years. In an early investigation of digoxin in patients with heart failure, the withdrawal of digoxin led to clinical deterioration in a majority of subjects studied.[185] However, the number of patients evaluated was small and the study was uncontrolled. In 1982, Lee and coworkers[186] examined the clinical efficacy of digoxin in patients with heart failure and normal sinus rhythm. Improvements in symptoms and in the cardiothoracic ratio were observed in 14 of 16 patients with decreased EFs and therapeutic digoxin levels during therapy. In these patients, the presence of an audible third heart sound was found to be the best correlate of a favorable response to digoxin. Other predictors of clinical efficacy included longer duration or greater severity of heart failure, greater LV dilation, and more severe depression of LVEF. These early observations of the clinical efficacy of digoxin in heart failure have been confirmed in more recent randomized controlled trials.[182,187,188] For example, one clinical investigation demonstrated that the withdrawal of digoxin from patients who were clinically stable on digoxin, di-

uretics, and an ACE inhibitor increased the probability of worsening heart failure during the subsequent 3 months from 5 percent to nearly 30 percent.[188] A recent analysis of digoxin withdrawal trials supports the superiority of triple drug therapy with digoxin, diuretics, and an ACE inhibitor in patients with mild or moderate heart failure,[189] but the limitations of withdrawal studies have also been documented.

The DIG trial evaluated the effect of digoxin on survival in patients with heart failure.[182] This multicenter study, which was conducted in the United States and Canada, randomized 7788 patients with symptomatic heart failure to receive either digoxin or placebo in addition to an ACE inhibitor and diuretic. The doses of digoxin used were 0.125 mg to 0.5 mg and were selected on the basis of body weight. Compared to placebo, the addition of digoxin to an ACE inhibitor and diuretic significantly reduced heart failure hospitalizations, insignificantly lowered the number of deaths attributable to progressive heart failure, and produced no difference in all-cause mortality. Of some concern, digoxin therapy was associated with a trend toward an increased incidence of sudden (presumed arrhythmic) death. A posthoc analysis of this later observation suggested a relationship between mortality and plasma digoxin concentration.[190] Specifically, digoxin concentrations >1.0 ng/mL were associated with increased mortality risk. In the subgroup of patients with lower plasma concentrations benefit has been claimed. Symptoms and exercise capacity were not improved in a substudy of the DIG trial.

Recommendations for the Use of Digoxin in Heart Failure Given the survival benefits of ACE inhibitors, ARBs, aldosterone antagonists, β blockers, nitrates and hydralazine (in African Americans), and device therapies (discussed below), digoxin now receives less priority in the treatment of heart failure and has fallen far down the list of recommended drugs. Digoxin should be considered for patients with heart failure who remain symptomatic on an ACE inhibitor (or ARB), β blocker, and diuretic and for those who are recurrently hospitalized with decompensation. Digoxin plasma concentration should be maintained in the low-therapeutic range between 0.5 and 1.1 ng/mL, given the posthoc analysis of the DIG trial.

Ancillary Drug Therapies

Antiarrhythmic Drug Therapies Ventricular ectopic activity is common in patients with systolic heart failure. Sudden cardiac death, frequently caused by ventricular tachyarrhythmias, accounts for 40 to 50 percent of the mortality associated with this disease syndrome,[191–195] but empirical antiarrhythmic drug therapy is of no proven benefit in heart failure patients. Moreover, antiarrhythmic drug therapy is less effective and has been associated with a higher incidence of proarrhythmic complications in patients with LV systolic dysfunction.[196,197] Of the antiarrhythmics studied to date in heart failure patients, only amiodarone appears to be generally safe. However, its efficacy is limited particularly in the primary prevention of death in heart failure patients (discussed below, along with implantable cardioverter defibrillators).

Antiarrhythmic drug therapy should probably be reserved for heart failure patients with documented hemodynamically destabilizing ventricular tachycardia, ventricular fibrillation, or a history of sudden cardiac death, where suppression of frequent ventricular arrhythmias is necessary to avoid excessive defibrillator shocks or in those patients who are not candidates for an implantable cardioverter defibrillator (ICD). The suppression of nonsustained ventricular tachycardia or frequent ventricular ectopic activity in heart failure patients is not advised and requires further study.

Anticoagulant Therapy

Although the exact event rate remains unclear, a retrospective analysis of major heart failure clinical trials indicates that arterial thromboembolism is common, ranging from 0.9 to 5.5 events per 100 patient years.[198] Significantly, clinical embolic phenomena appear to be more frequent in patients with very low LVEFs.[199,200] Despite the risk of arterial thromboembolism (especially stroke), the routine use of anticoagulant therapy for LV systolic dysfunction is disputed. This controversy exists because there have been no randomized controlled trials of chronic anticoagulation in heart failure demonstrating convincing benefit and there are obvious risks to anticoagulant therapy. All clinical practice guidelines agree that heart failure patients with chronic atrial fibrillation, a history of systemic or pulmonary embolism, or a documented mobile LV thrombus should receive chronic anticoagulant therapy. Although the practice guidelines acknowledge the frequent use of warfarin to prevent systemic embolization in patients with heart failure on the basis of low EF alone, none recommend it routinely.

Device Therapies in Chronic Systolic Heart Failure

Three types of devices have been shown to reduce morbidity and mortality in selected heart failure patients. This includes cardiac resynchronization therapy (CRT) devices, ICDs, and LV assist devices (LVADs). The use of LVADs in advanced heart failure is discussed in Chap. 27.

Implantable Cardioverter Defibrillators

Early ICD mortality trials compared device therapy to antiarrhythmic drug therapy with amiodarone or sotalol. These early trials evaluated the role of ICDs as secondary prevention in patients who either had documented ventricular arrhythmias or cardiac arrest or were post-MI but without advanced heart failure.[201–203] Subsequent trials focused on primary prevention in the heart failure population. Numerous clinical trials to date have established the efficacy of ICD therapy as primary prevention in heart failure patients with or without documented ventricular arrhythmias.[204–207]

Primary Prevention of Sudden Death

Early randomized controlled trials were small in enrollment and did not find a mortality benefit in patients with idiopathic dilated cardiomyopathy and reduced EFs.[208,209] The Cardiomyopathy Trial (CAT) and the Amiodarone Versus Implantable Cardioverter-Defibrillator (AMIOVIRT) trial enrolled 104 and 103 patients, respectively, with ICD versus placebo in CAT and ICD compared to amiodarone in AMIOVIRT. In addition to the small size of these trials, the latter study was also limited by the absence of a placebo group. The definitive landmark trials of primary prevention ICDs in heart failure include the second Multicenter Automatic Defibrillator Implantation Trials (MADIT II), the Defibrillators in Non-Ischemic Cardiomyopathy Treatment Evaluation (DEFINITE), and the Sudden Cardiac Death-Heart Failure Trial (SCD-HeFT).

MADIT I and MADIT II Clinical Trials

The MADIT trials evaluated prophylactic use of an ICD as primary prevention in high risk patients with coronary artery disease. MADIT I enrolled patients who were more than 3 weeks post-MI, with EFs ≤35 percent, documented asymptomatic nonsustained ventricular tachycardia (from 3–30 beats), and inducible, nonsuppressible sustained ventricular tachycardia on electrophysiology (EP) study.[210] Patients were treated with conventional medical therapy, which included antiarrhythmics at the physician's discretion (usually amiodarone) or were assigned to an ICD in addition to conventional medical therapy. A total of 196 patients were followed for 27 months, with a significant survival benefit noted in the ICD group (HR 0.46, 95 percent CI 0.26–0.82, $p = 0.009$). Although MADIT I evaluated ICD prophylaxis in post-MI patients, 37 percent of patients exhibited NYHA Class II and III heart failure. Subsequent subgroup analysis revealed ICD prophylaxis in higher risk heart failure patients (defined as an EF <26 percent, heart failure requiring therapy, and QRS ≥120 msec) independently predicted improved survival, with survival benefit proportional to the number of risk factors.[211] Criticism of this trial was aimed at the inclusion criteria of sustained ventricular tachycardia during EP study that was not suppressible by procainamide, questioning whether patients in the drug therapy arm were likely to respond to pharmacologic therapy.

MADIT II was a much larger trial enrolling 1232 patients and addressed one of the major limitations of MADIT I by including patients without a history of ventricular arrhythmias.[204] Therefore, patients were not required to have a documented history of nonsustained ventricular tachycardia nor was an EP study performed; the risk of ventricular arrhythmias was based on the patient's history of MI and cardiac dysfunction, with an EF ≤30 percent. Patients were required to be at least 40 days post-MI. The ICD group was compared to a control group of conventional medical therapy, with similar and high percentages of patients taking standard medical therapy in both groups, at the last follow-up visit.

Follow up was prematurely discontinued at 20 months because of a highly significant 31 percent reduction in all-cause mortality in the ICD group ($p = 0.016$), which was subsequently found to be entirely caused by a reduction in sudden cardiac death.[212] Sudden cardiac death occurred in 10 percent of the conventional medical therapy group compared to 3.8 percent of the ICD group ($p < 0.01$). There was no difference noted in nonsudden death in both groups.

Of note, the survival benefit after ICD prophylaxis was not seen until 9 months postimplantation of the device in MADIT II compared to the first few months in MADIT I. Explanations for this observation include a greater proportion of patients on standard medical therapy in both groups and the decision to avoid arrhythmia risk stratification in MADIT II. There was a trend toward an increased incidence of heart failure hospitalization in the ICD group, possibly related to worsening LV function from right ventricular pacing, detrimental effects of ICD shocks on the myocardium, or improved survival in such patients allowing time to develop more severe pump failure.

DEFINITE Trial

Although MADIT II exclusively enrolled patients with an ischemic cause of heart failure, DEFINITE attempted to evaluate the role of primary prevention ICDs in patients with a nonischemic etiology.[207] The EF cut-off for this trial was slightly higher than in MADIT II at ≤35 percent. Although ICD prophy-laxis resulted in significantly reduced arrhythmic death and a trend toward reduction in the primary endpoint of all-cause mortality, the study was underpowered with a lower than expected mortality rate of 14.1 percent in the control arm of conventional medical therapy. The inclusion of Class I patients, comprising 22 percent of total enrolled patients, might also have contributed to the lower mortality rate.

SCD-HeFT Trial Patients enrolled in SCD-HeFT were in NYHA class II or III with ischemic or nonischemic cardiomyopathy and LVEFs of ≤35 percent; 2520 patients were randomized to standard medical therapy plus placebo or amiodarone or an ICD.[206] Thus, SCD-HeFT was designed to answer at least two important questions in heart failure management:

1. Does amiodarone when added to a standard heart failure drug regimen reduce mortality?
2. Does the use of a primary prevention ICD when added to standard heart failure medications reduce mortality in general and in patients with either ischemic or nonischemic heart failure?

The primary endpoint of all-cause mortality was not improved by amiodarone. In contrast, the prophylactic ICD produced a significant 23 percent relative risk reduction and 7.2 percent absolute risk reduction in all-cause mortality at 5 years, compared to the placebo group (Fig. 26–7). As noted, an important aspect of this trial was the inclusion of both ischemic and nonischemic heart failure patients, with 52 percent of patients exhibiting an ischemic etiology and 48 percent a nonischemic etiology of heart failure. The study demonstrated that ICD prophylaxis was effective in the primary prevention of mortality, regardless of heart failure etiology.

Recommendations for Implantable Cardioverter Defibrillators

All three heart failure guideline endorse the use of an ICD as primary prevention of all-cause mortality in well-treated NYHA Class II and III patients with LVEFs of less than or equal to 30 percent and either ischemic or nonischemic cardiomyopathy. There is generally a weaker recommendation for such patients with EFs of 31 to 35 percent. The reasoning behind this stems from the fact that MADIT II and SCD-HeFT used different EF criteria for enrollment. In any event patients with moderate to severe LV systolic dysfunction and NYHA Class II or III heart failure should receive an ICD, unless they have a poor chance of survival related to some comorbidity or a con-traindication to the implantation or use of this device. Implantable cardioverter defibrillators are also strongly recommended in patients with hemodynamically destabilizing ventricular tachycardia, ventricular fibrillation, and resuscitated cardiac arrest, for the secondary prevention of mortality.

Cardiac Resynchronization Therapy

Cardiac resynchronization therapy has emerged as another evidence-based device treatment for heart failure. Biventricular pacing is accomplished through simultaneous pacing of both the left and right ventricles, with standard right sided transvenous lead placement as in dual-chamber and defibrillator lead implantation. Transvenous implantation of the LV lead involves cannulation of the coronary sinus and lead placement in a lateral or posterior branch, with appropriate capture threshold and avoidance of diaphragmatic stimulation. Early CRT systems required epicardial LV lead placement but usually with higher capture thresholds and often suboptimal (anterior) location. With greater expertise in the transvenous approach, and given the risk of anesthesia and a lateral thoracotomy, the epicardial technique is reserved for patients with suboptimal target vessels.

The rationale for CRT is based on the presence of ventricular dyssynchrony. Dyssynchrony may occur between the left and right ventricles and within the left ventricle, impairing the ability of the heart to function as a pump.[213] Although a left bundle-branch block or prolongation of the QRS duration ≥120 msec has been used as a measure of dyssynchrony in clinical tri-

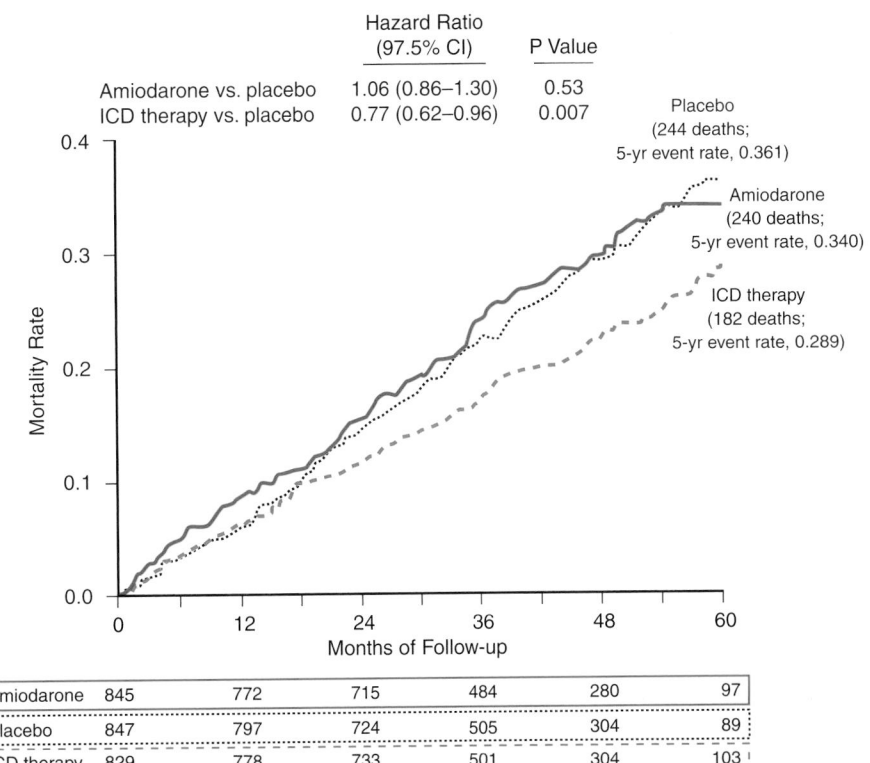

	Hazard Ratio (97.5% CI)	P Value
Amiodarone vs. placebo	1.06 (0.86–1.30)	0.53
ICD therapy vs. placebo	0.77 (0.62–0.96)	0.007

Placebo (244 deaths; 5-yr event rate, 0.361)

Amiodarone (240 deaths; 5-yr event rate, 0.340)

ICD therapy (182 deaths; 5-yr event rate, 0.289)

No. at Risk						
Amiodarone	845	772	715	484	280	97
Placebo	847	797	724	505	304	89
ICD therapy	829	778	733	501	304	103

FIGURE 26–7. Kaplan-Meier estimates of all-cause mortality in SCD-HeFT. Although the empirical use of amiodarone had no affect on outcome, the primary prevention ICD reduced the risk of the primary endpoint by approximately 23 percent. CI, confidence interval; ICD, implantable cardioverter-defibrillator. *Source: From Bardy GH, Lee KL, Mark DB, et al.[206] With permission.*

als, LV mechanical dyssynchrony as evidenced by echocardiographic parameters (predominantly tissue Doppler imaging) measuring inter- and intraventricular conduction delays has been shown to predict cardiac events in heart failure independent of QRS duration.[214–215] By such parameters, nearly half of heart failure patients with a normal QRS duration have evidence of mechanical dyssynchrony whereas one in five patients with an EF of ≤35 percent and QRS ≥150 msec do not exhibit dyssynchrony, suggesting that electrical evidence of conduction delay with QRS duration may not be the most reliable marker of ventricular dyssynchrony.[215]

Interventricular dyssynchrony refers to the time delay between contraction of the right and left ventricles, and is calculated as the difference between systolic flow in the pulmonic and aortic outflow tracts.[216] A delay of 40 msec or more suggests the need for biventricular pacing. In contrast, intraventricular dyssynchrony refers to the abnormal segmental contraction within the left ventricle itself, usually with the longest delay between the septum and lateral-posterior segments. In a typical left bundle-branch block (present in approximately one-third of heart failure patients), the septum is activated earlier than the lateral or posterior walls, resulting in paradoxical septal motion. Approaches to assess intraventricular dyssynchrony include M-mode echocardiography in the parasternal long axis view to assess the septum and posterior walls, tissue Doppler imaging of the LV segments to assess peak systolic velocities and differences in timing, and tissue strain and strain rate analysis. Newer approaches include color coding segmental contraction in tissue synchronization imaging and three-dimensional echocardiography, which also evaluate timing of segmental motion.

Dyssynchronous or abnormal contraction patterns increase LV end-systolic and end-diastolic volumes and reduce diastolic filling. Onset of LV contraction is delayed in a dyssynchronous ventricle, a finding also occurring in prolonged atrioventricular (AV) interval delay. In both circumstances, a delayed LV contraction occurs simultaneously with atrial contraction, represented by the E (passive filling of the left ventricle) and A (atrial contribution) waves coinciding on transmitral Doppler echocardiography and truncation of the A wave (suboptimal atrial contribution to diastolic filling). Both reduction in passive LV filling and suboptimal atrial contribution reduce preload in these patients. Acute CRT hemodynamic benefits are consistent with improved LV systolic function through increased slope of dP/dt and increased stroke volume.[217,218] Chronic benefits include reverse remodeling with a reduction in LV end-systolic and end-diastolic volumes, which is associated with an improvement in EF.[219,220] Atrial-synchronized, biventricular pacing restores earlier activation of the left ventricle and increases filling time, thereby increasing stroke volume.

Delayed LV contraction from dyssynchrony also contributes to systolic mitral regurgitation through inadequate leaflet closure as a result of segmental wall motion abnormalities and papillary muscle dysfunction. Dilation of the left ventricle also tethers the papillary muscles, impairing complete leaflet coaptation in systole. Both interventricular conduction delay and a prolonged AV interval contribute to diastolic (presystolic) mitral regurgitation through incomplete mitral valve closure. By restoring normal mitral valve timing with resynchronized AV activation, mitral regurgitation is reduced or possibly eliminated. In addition to timing benefits, the reduction in mitral regurgitation severity correlates with improved LV systolic function and transmitral pressure gradients, producing earlier and more effective mitral leaflet closure.[221] In addition to the immediate reduction in mitral regurgitation, further intermediate and long-term improvement has been observed and is likely related to reverse remodeling. Reverse remodeling has been noted within 3 months of CRT.[219] A progressive deterioration in such parameters was found after discontinuation of biventricular pacing in these patients. Large randomized controlled trials have consistently confirmed the long-term benefit of CRT on ventricular reverse remodeling.

Clinical Trials of Cardiac Resynchronization Therapy

The first randomized controlled CRT trials were done in the 1990s, and established the safety of implanting a transvenous coronary sinus lead for LV pacing.[217,222,223] To date, eight landmark randomized controlled trials have enrolled more than 4000 patients (Table 26–9) and have established both clinical and survival benefits of CRT in advanced heart failure, with or without an implantable cardioverter-defibrillator.[205,217,222–232]

Pacing Therapies in Congestive Heart Failure Trial

The Pacing Therapies in Congestive Heart Failure (PATH-CHF) trial was the earliest randomized CRT trial; LV and biventricular pacing produced significant acute hemodynamic benefits when compared to right ventricular pacing.[217,222] PATH-CHF was a smaller trial and evaluated immediate and short-term effects of CRT. Later trials were larger and studied intermediate- and long-term effects.

Multisite Stimulation in Cardiomyopathy Study

The Multisite Stimulation in Cardiomyopathy (MUSTIC) study was a single-blind randomized crossover study conducted in the 1990s and consisted of two arms, sinus rhythm (SR) and atrial fibrillation (AF).[223,226,227] The study evaluated the safety and efficacy of CRT in moderate heart failure. Patents with NYHA class III heart failure and QRS >150 msec were enrolled in either arm, based on their underlying rhythm, and assigned to biventricular pacing or the control of inactive pacing (right ventricular pacing in the VVIR mode or ventricular inhibited pacing at a rate of 40 beats/min). Patients were randomized to 3 months of biventricular pacing or the control, followed by a 3-month crossover period, and final programming at 6 months to their preference. MUSTIC-SR enrolled 58 patients and MUSTIC-AF had 41 patients. The primary endpoint of exercise capacity (distance walked in 6 minutes and peak oxygen consumption or VO$_2$) was significantly improved in both the sinus rhythm and the AF groups with active CRT, although to a smaller degree in those with AF. Secondary endpoints of quality of life and NYHA functional class ranking were also significantly improved. All patients in MUSTIC-SR and the majority in MUSTIC-AF preferred biventricular pacing. Both groups had fewer hospitalizations with biventricular pacing during a 12-month follow-up period and maintained clinical benefit during this time.[226] This was the first randomized study to find favorable one-year results with CRT; it was not designed as a mortality trial.

TABLE 26–9

Major Clinical Trials of Cardiac Resynchronization and Enrollment Criteria[a]

STUDY (N RANDOMIZED)	NYHA CLASS	QRS	SINUS	ICD?
MIRACLE (524)	III, IV	≥130	normal	no
MUSTIC SR (58)	III	>150	normal	no
MUSTIC AF (43)	III	>200	AF	no
PATH CHF (42)	III, IV	≥120	normal	no
CONTAK CD (581)	III–IV	≥120	normal	yes
MIRACLE ICD(362)	III–IV	≥130	normal	yes
PATH CHF II (89)	III, IV	≥120	normal	no
COMPANION (1520)	III, IV	≥120	normal	no
MIRACLE ICD II (186)	II	≥130	normal	yes
CARE HF (813)	III, IV	≥120[b]	normal	no

AF, atrial fibrillation; EF, ejection fraction; ICD, implantable cardioverter-defibrillator; LV, left ventricular; NYHA, New York Heart Association.
[a]All trials required an EF ≤ 35 percent and dilated LV dimensions.
[b]Echocardiographic evidence of dyssynchrony if QRS between 120 and 150 msec.

The Multicenter InSync Randomized Clinical Evaluation Trials Completed in 2000, the Multicenter InSync Randomized Clinical Evaluation (MIRACLE) trial was the first prospective double-blind randomized controlled trial evaluating CRT.[224,225] Enrollment was much greater than MUSTIC and PATH-CHF combined with 453 patients randomized in MIRACLE. Patients with NYHA class III and ambulatory class IV heart failure on optimal medical therapy, with QRS durations ≥130 msec, and sinus rhythm were assigned to 6 months of biventricular pacing or the control arm of medical therapy alone (no pacing). Primary endpoints were clinical parameters of quality of life, NYHA class, and the 6-minute hall walk distance, all of which improved significantly, compared to control patients. CRT patients also had significant improvement in their treadmill peak VO$_2$, EF, and exercise duration.

A significant reduction in heart failure morbidity was observed in the group with active biventricular pacing, with fewer heart failure hospitalizations ($p = 0.02$) and a reduced need for IV medications for treating worsening heart failure ($p = 0.004$). In terms of survival benefit, the study was not powered to evaluate mortality as a single endpoint. The InSync device used in this trial was approved by the FDA in August 2001, making it the first such device approved in the U.S. With experience, rates of successful CRT implantation were rising, as evident by the 92 percent implant success rate in the MIRACLE trial.

The MIRACLE-ICD trial was designed to evaluate the safety and efficacy of combining CRT devices with an ICD.[232] Patients with an active defibrillator and no biventricular pacing ($n = 182$) were compared to those with active CRT pacing and defibrillator therapies ($n = 187$). In terms of the clinical benefits of active CRT pacing, results were similar to the MIRACLE trial with significantly improved quality of life and NYHA functional class at 6 months. Survival at 6 months did not differ between the two groups and along with no observed proarrhythmic effect, supported the safety and efficacy of combining CRT with an ICD.

Comparison of Medical Therapy, Pacing, and Defibrillation in Heart Failure Trial The Comparison of Medical Therapy, Pacing, and Defibrillation in Heart Failure (COMPANION) trial was a prospective multicenter randomized controlled clinical trial designed to evaluate CRT effects on the risk of death and hospitalization in advanced heart failure.[205,229] Biventricular pacing was performed with and without defibrillator therapy to address the issues of prophylactic ICD therapy in advanced heart failure and if any benefit would be additive to those of CRT in this setting. Because COMPANION results were available prior to SCD-HeFT, this trial also addressed whether prophylactic ICD therapy would be beneficial in nonischemic cardiomyopathy, because almost half of those randomized had a nonischemic etiology. Inclusion criteria consisted of NYHA class III and IV heart failure on optimal medical therapy, LVEF ≤35 percent, QRS duration ≥120 msec, and no secondary prevention indication for ICD placement (no history of ventricular tachycardia or ventricular fibrillation and no history of sudden cardiac death). Patients were randomized in a 1:2:2 ratio into three groups. The control group ($n = 308$) received optimal medical therapy only, group 2 ($n = 617$) received optimal medical therapy and a biventricular pacing device without defibrillator capabilities, and group 3 ($n = 595$) received optimal medical therapy and a biventricular pacing device with ICD function.

The combined endpoint of all-cause mortality and all-cause hospitalization was significantly reduced by 20 percent in both CRT groups compared to the control group (Fig. 26–8). The secondary endpoint of all-cause mortality alone was reduced by 36 percent in patients receiving CRT plus an ICD ($p < 0.003$) and trended toward a significant reduction of 24 percent in those receiving CRT alone ($p = 0.06$), compared to control subjects. Subgroup analysis of the mortality benefit in the combined CRT-ICD group revealed a significantly lower risk of death in nonischemic cardiomyopathy patients compared to controls (HR of 0.50, 95 percent CI, 0.29–0.88, $p = 0.015$), forecasting the subsequent results of SCD-HeFT, which demonstrated the

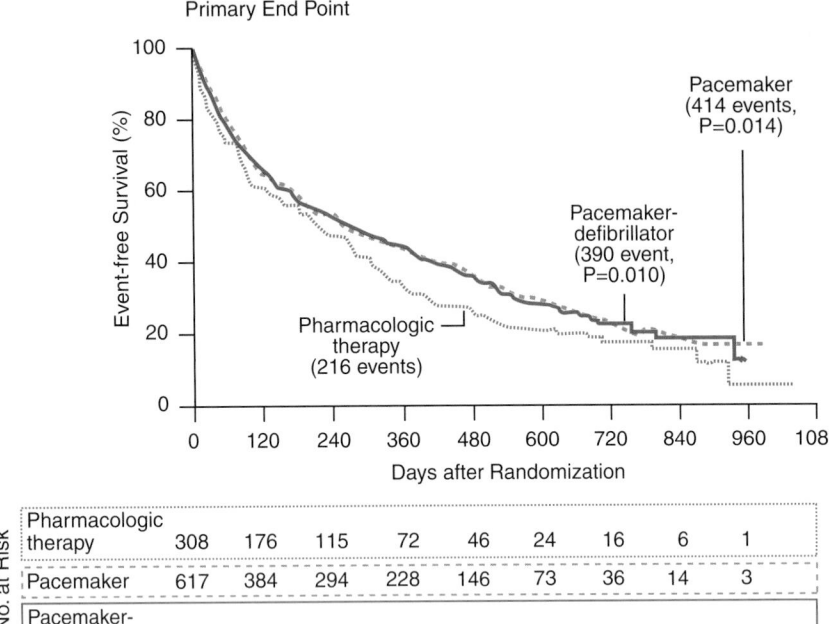

FIGURE 26–8. Kaplan-Meier estimates of time to primary endpoint of death from or hospitalization from any cause in the COMPANION (Comparison of Medical Therapy, Pacing and Defibrillation in Chronic Heart Failure) trial. *Source: From Bristow MR, Saxon LA, Boehmer J, et al.[205] With permission.*

benefit of a prophylactic ICD in this population. The reduction in the composite primary endpoint with CRT did not vary when comparing ischemic and nonischemic subgroups. This trial confirmed previous trial results by demonstrating the benefits of CRT in advanced heart failure. The COMPANION trial also demonstrated for the first time the survival benefit of combined CRT and defibrillator therapies.

Cardiac Resynchronization Heart Failure Trial COMPANION showed that CRT alone or in combination with a defibrillator reduced the composite endpoint of all-cause mortality and hospitalization; however, uncertainty about the effect of CRT alone on the risk of death remained. The Cardiac Resynchronization Heart Failure (CARE-HF) trial was a multicenter randomized unblinded study, designed as a morbidity and mortality trial to evaluate the effects of CRT without a defibrillator on the risk of complications and death in advanced heart failure (NYHA class III and IV).[230,231] It was also the first randomized CRT trial to incorporate echocardiographic evidence of ventricular dyssynchrony into the inclusion criteria. Patients with EFs ≤35 percent were enrolled if (1) QRS duration was ≥150 msec or (2) QRS duration was between 120 and 150 msec with two of three additional echocardiographic criteria for dyssynchrony: interventricular mechanical delay >40 msec, aortic preejection delay >140 msec, or delayed posterolateral activation. Those receiving optimal medical therapy (n = 404) were compared to those with biventricular pacing on optimal medical therapy and without a defibrillator (n = 409). Control patients did not receive a device to assess the entire effect of CRT, including risk from the implantation procedure and technique.

In CARE-HF, most patients had NYHA Class III heart failure (94 percent of the total enrolled) and 62 percent had nonis-

chemic etiologies of their heart failure. Patients were followed for an average of 29.4 months. The primary endpoint was a composite of death from any cause or unplanned hospitalization for a major cardiac event; the key secondary endpoint was death from any cause. A significant reduction in the primary endpoint was found with a 37 percent decrease in the CRT group (p < 0.001) compared to the control group. The main secondary endpoint of all-cause mortality was reduced by 36 percent in the treatment group (p < 0.002) (Fig. 26–9), with an absolute mortality rate of 20 percent in the CRT group (n = 82 deaths) versus 30 percent in the control group (n = 120 deaths). CARE-HF also showed that CRT significantly reduced the secondary endpoints of all-cause mortality combined with heart failure hospitalization by 46 percent and heart failure hospitalization alone by 52 percent.

The mortality reduction in CARE-HF with CRT alone is similar to the reduction in all-cause mortality noted in the COMPANION trial in the CRT-plus-defibrillator group. In the absence of a direct and adequately powered comparison of CRT versus CRT plus an ICD, conclusions cannot be drawn from this observation. However, in CARE-HF the survival benefit in the CRT group was largely attributed to a reduction in deaths from worsening heart failure, with a lesser reduction in sudden death. These differences can be explained by improved pump function with CRT and suggest that an ICD may further reduce the risk of total mortality by reducing the risk of sudden death.

Cardiac Resynchronization Therapy Device and Procedure Complications Early trials implanted an epicardial LV lead through a limited lateral thoracotomy; however, epicardial placement is associated with higher capture thresholds and often suboptimal position for resynchronization, in addition to the risk associated with general anesthesia in a higher risk patient population. With practice leading to higher success rates in the transvenous approach, epicardial placement has thus been reserved for difficult transvenous cases and those with poor targets. The transvenous technique for LV lead placement is performed in the same manner used for standard dual chamber pacing or defibrillator leads; access to a lateral or posterior branch of the coronary sinus is obtained for LV stimulation. Success rates for LV lead placement have improved and generally range from 88 to 92 percent in most clinical trials, with the most recent trials exhibiting a success rate in excess of 95 percent.

Unsuccessful implants can be caused by difficulty in cannulating the coronary sinus, often related to tortuosity of the coronary sinus or distortion of the ostium in dilated cardiomyopathy and right atrial enlargement. Deflectable electrophysiology catheters aid in mapping the coronary sinus ostium, whereas adjustment in the radiographic projection, usually left anterior oblique but sometimes right anterior oblique, aids in an uncommon takeoff of the ostium. Compared to the older stylet guided delivery of leads, the over-the-wire technique maintains more lead stability when targeting smaller, tortuous vessels. The conventional stylet technique is more appropriate for larger, nontortuous veins. Fixation of LV leads is passive, often with preshaped curves at the tip of the lead. Regardless of techniques for lead delivery, individual patient variability in venous anatomy often make suitable lead placement difficult or impossible.

Coronary sinus dissection or perforation occurs in approximately 0.4 to 4 percent of patients during LV lead placement but usually does not require further intervention, because this is a low-pressure system. Other complications during CRT implantation are similar to those seen in standard dual-chamber pacemaker placement, such as lead dislodgement, device infection, pneumothorax, and pocket erosion. Lead dislodgement with LV leads depends on the angle of the coronary sinus ostium, position of the lead, stenosis in tributaries of the coronary sinus, and operator experience. Lead dislodgments can either be evident on chest radiographs or as microdislodgments, noted only by changes in capture thresholds. Case reports have used coronary stents in stenotic tributaries of the coronary sinus to stabilize LV leads; however, the effects of stenting on long-term safety and the impact on lead extraction is unknown.[233]

High left pacing capture thresholds and diaphragmatic pacing from phrenic nerve stimulation should be avoided. The phrenic nerve runs parallel to the lateral LV free wall, making this an important consideration for lead placement. Changes in body position may contribute to a later development of phrenic nerve stimulation despite the absence of stimulation during implantation. Solutions involve changing the pacing configuration to lower capture thresholds or avoid diaphragmatic stimulation but, if unsuccessful, ultimately require lead repositioning.

Nonresponders to Cardiac Resynchronization Therapy Approximately one-quarter to one-third of patients receiving CRT devices have been defined as nonresponders, meaning they have no significant clinical or functional improvement after device implantation measured in clinical trials.[234] With the exception of CARE-HF, major landmark CRT trials enrolled patients based on electrical evidence of conduction delay; but as previously mentioned, not all patients with prolonged QRS durations exhibit mechanical dyssynchrony on echocardiography. Yu and colleagues[235] found 75 percent of heart failure patients with QRS >120 msec in duration had associated tissue Doppler findings of dyssynchrony. Lack of response to CRT in such patients may be at least partly attributed to the absence of mechanical dyssynchrony. Trials are underway to prospectively determine if echocardiographic parameters of dyssynchrony will predict response to CRT. The recently enrolled Predictors of Response to Cardiac Resynchronization Therapy (PROSPECT) trial is the first large-scale study to evaluate such echocardiographic predictors of response.[236]

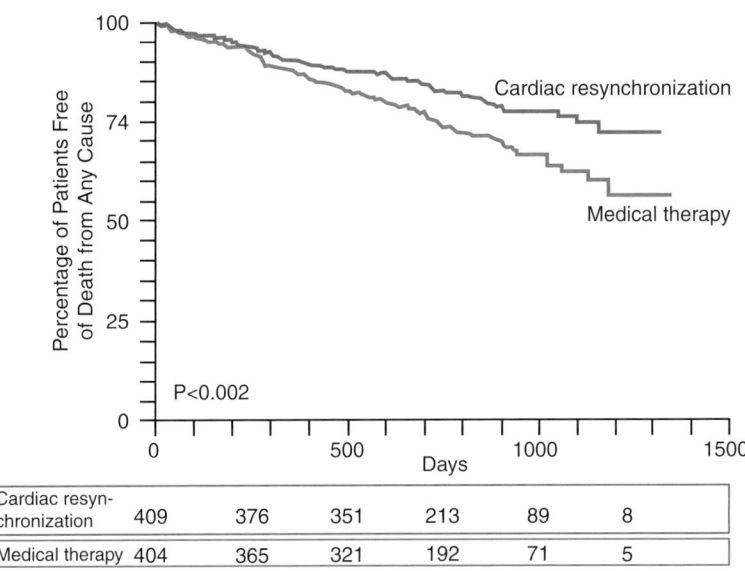

FIGURE 26–9. Kaplan-Meier estimates of time to key secondary endpoint of death from any cause in the CARE-HF (Cardiac Resynchronization Heart Failure) trial. *Source: From Cleland J, Daubert JC, Erdmann E, et al.[231] With permission.*

Suboptimal lead placement in a region that is not dyssynchronous or is anterior in location can lead to a less than favorable response. Anterior LV lead placement has been associated with worsening hemodynamics, because it usually is a region of early activation; therefore, pacing the anterior wall exacerbates intraventricular dyssynchrony.[237] Biventricular pacing should be maintained in all patients and might not be present in nonresponders, secondary to high LV capture thresholds, lead dislodgement, a long AV interval, atrial arrhythmias with rapid ventricular response, or frequent premature ventricular contractions.[238] Other explanations include placement of a lead in nonviable or scarred myocardium and suboptimal AV and ventricular-ventricular (VV) timing. *Out of the box* AV delays are usually short, in the 100 to 120 msec range and can reduce atrial contribution to LV filling. Initially, individually optimizing pacing delays in biventricular devices was considered in *nonresponders* only but should likely be performed in all CRT patients given the clear acute hemodynamic benefits noted in early studies.[239–241] Moreover, a recent randomized controlled trial demonstrated an increase in the CRT responder rate with optimization of ventricular–ventricular timing.[242]

Optimization of Atrioventricular and Interventricular Delays With newer CRT devices, adjustment of the AV and VV delays allows determination of the *optimal* duration in timing of atrial to ventricular pacing and ventricular to ventricular pacing. The optimal AV interval is based on lengthening the duration of LV filling without compromising atrial contribution and has been found to correlate with immediate improvement in hemodynamics, defined as a rise in aortic pulse pressure and the maximum rate of LV *dP/dt*.[243] This interval is determined echocardiographically either by diastolic filling patterns or systolic parameters that indirectly measure cardiac output. Recording the mitral inflow pattern allows visualization of diastolic patterns with the E and A wave relationship. Adjustment of the AV delay should allow separation of these waves with the end of the A wave occurring with the onset of systole (closure of the mitral valve), thus avoiding LV systolic contraction after suboptimal filling. Systolic parameters measure aortic outflow velocity-time integral (VTI) as a surrogate for cardiac output, and result in improved three month clinical outcomes of NYHA class and quality of life score compared to standard nonoptimized AV settings.[244] The optimal AV delay is defined by the maximum aortic VTI (indicating the maximum stroke volume).

New-generation CRT devices enable adjustment of interventricular or VV delay also. Right ventricular and LV pacing can be performed in a simultaneous manner or either the right or left ventricle can be preactivated. Individual variation in delayed left or right ventricular contraction results in longer aortic preejection time despite improved hemodynamics with AV optimization and simultaneous biventricular pacing. Early studies of sequential ventricular activation have found an even greater improvement in hemodynamics measured both invasively and noninvasively when compared to simultaneous pacing.[245,246] Sogaard and colleagues[245] reported immediate reductions in LV dyssynchrony achieved by tissue tracking and longer diastolic filling times in sequential pacing, which correlated with a more significant increase in EF compared to simultaneous pacing. The InSync III Marquis trial is the first large study demonstrating an incremental improvement in functional status with optimized VV delay compared to simultaneous VV pacing.[242]

Recommendations for Cardiac Resynchronization Therapy
Heart failure guidelines recommend CRT for patients with LVEFs less than or equal to 35 percent, normal sinus rhythm, and NYHA functional Class III or ambulatory Class IV symptoms despite recommended optimal medical therapy, who have ventricular dyssynchrony, unless contraindicated. This is based on the entry criteria to the relevant trials and not on the actual baseline measurements in the trials. Currently, guidelines define ventricular dyssynchrony as a QRS duration of at least 120 msec. However, echocardiography appears to be a promising way to define ventricular dyssynchrony in the future, so that a newer definition of ventricular dyssynchrony may one day prevail. Echocardiography and the assessment of ventricular dyssynchrony are covered elsewhere in this textbook.

Combining Cardiac Resynchronization Therapy and Implantable Cardioverter Defibrillator Therapies
The MIRACLE ICD, CONTAK-CD, and COMPANION trials evaluated the use of combined CRT and ICD devices in the treatment of heart failure. While no adequately powered comparison of CRT alone versus CRT plus a defibrillator guides current recommendations, the heart failure guidelines support the use of combined devices in patients who have indications for both an ICD and a CRT device. In addition, based on the results of the COMPANION trial, it is considered reasonable to implant a combined CRT-ICD device in ambulatory NYHA class IV patients.

Cost Effectiveness of Implantable Device Therapies
Although device therapy is expensive, the cost effectiveness of such ther-

apy, meaning the health benefits rather than the cost of the device, make therapy feasible. Generally, in the United States a value of $50,000 to $100,000 is considered cost-effective if therapy can extend life expectancy by an additional year (quality-adjusted life-years [QALYs]). A combined CRT-ICD device costs around $30,000 in the United States, but additional costs in the future arise from generator change, possible lead revisions, and other complications, such as infection and possible device or lead extraction. However, health benefits must also be considered in determining long-term costs, in terms of reduced hospitalizations and emergency visits and improved quality of life, functional capacity, and survival. Reviews of ICD trials found a projected additional 1 to 3 QALYs with an estimated cost benefit per quality-adjusted life year of $34,900 in MADIT and $70,200 in SCD-HeFT. In COMPANION, CRT alone was estimated to have an incremental cost-effectiveness ratio of $19,600 per QALY and $43,000 for combined CRT-ICD relative to optimal medical therapy alone.[247]

Future Directions in Cardiac Resynchronization Therapy
Because morbidity and mortality have improved in more severely symptomatic heart failure patients treated with CRT, the question of preventing heart failure progression in patients with milder heart failure and extending the indication for CRT to other heart failure populations has arisen. Focus has turned to mild heart failure (NYHA class I and II), narrow-QRS patients with echocardiographic evidence of mechanical dyssynchrony, and patients with indications for chronic right ventricular pacing.

To evaluate CRT benefits in preventing heart failure progression, the MIRACLE-ICD II trial was a pilot study in NYHA class II heart failure.[248] Although exercise capacity was not altered, likely related to a baseline functional status that is not as severely impaired as Class III and IV heart failure, reverse remodeling was evident with improved volumes and EFs. The impact of CRT on asymptomatic and mild heart failure will be addressed in two clinical trials: the Resynchronization Reverses Remodeling in Systolic Left Ventricular Dysfunction (REVERSE) trial, which has completed enrolling patients with NYHA class I or II heart failure, EFs ≤40 percent and QRS durations of ≥120 msec[249]; and MADIT-CRT, which is enrolling similar patients and assessing the primary endpoint of all-cause mortality and heart failure events. Other trials are evaluating the various populations described above, so the next few years should provide substantial additional information regarding the application of CRT in heart failure.

【 】 DIASTOLIC HEART FAILURE

Randomized clinical studies of the treatment of diastolic heart failure are lacking. Recommended strategies for treating heart failure in the presence of preserved systolic function are based primarily on empirical data. First, congestive symptoms, when present, should be managed by reducing ventricular filling pressures without compromising cardiac output. Second, as with systolic heart failure, treating the underlying or aggravating disorder is an important therapeutic strategy. For example, older patients in whom either systolic or diastolic hypertension is present may benefit from aggressive management of hypertension. For patients with LV hypertrophy (often resulting from hypertension), administration of antihypertensive agents that regress hypertrophy (e.g., β blockers, calcium channel blockers, ACE inhibitors, or diuretics) is advised. In addition, revascularization or aggressive antiischemic medical therapy is recommended for patients with coronary artery disease where ischemia may play a role in the diastolic dysfunction. Third, empiric pharmacologic therapy of diastolic heart failure may be considered.

Current guidelines for the management of diastolic heart failure recommend the use of diuretic agents and nitrates, while carefully avoiding hypotension, to alleviate congestive signs and symptoms. Some calcium channel blockers and most β blockers may improve diastolic filling by slowing the heart rate, thus prolonging diastolic filling time. These agents do not acutely improve ventricular relaxation or compliance but theoretically may do so chronically via regression of ventricular hypertrophy. In this regard, ACE inhibitors may also be of benefit. Angiotensin receptor blockers may also be useful. The previously mentioned CHARM trial included an additional study of diastolic heart failure and demonstrated a modest improvement in outcome.[250] Positive inotropic agents are not indicated in diastolic heart failure; but curiously, they may improve cardiac lusitropy. Agents that suppress AV conduction to control ventricular rate in patients with atrial fibrillation and anticoagulants in patients with atrial fibrillation or previous systemic or pulmonary embolization are often employed. Anticoagulants may also be employed in patients with intracardiac thrombus usually related to apical infarction.

ACUTELY DECOMPENSATED HEART FAILURE

Invariably, patients with chronic heart failure will at one time or another develop worsening congestive symptoms and or a low cardiac output syndrome, necessitating admission to the hospital for IV diuretic and/or vasoactive therapies. Like diastolic heart failure, there are few randomized controlled trials guiding the management of acutely decompensated heart failure. The only guideline devoted to the evaluation and management of acutely decompensated heart failure comes from the European Society of Cardiology,[11] but the ACC/AHA and Heart Failure Society of America heart failure guidelines also cover the topic.[7,8] As noted in Chap. 25, hospitalizations for heart failure are increasing and management of episodes of decompensation is the major contributor to the cost of heart failure care.

Paramount to treating acutely decompensated heart failure is the recognition that approximately 90 percent of patients admitted to the hospital with worsening heart failure exhibit an excess in total body fluid volume.[52,251] Only approximately 10 percent of admitted patients suffer from a strictly low output syndrome. Thus, the management of decompensated heart failure largely involves the management of extracellular fluid volume. Because the increase in fluid volume results in both hemodynamic and clinical congestion, both hemodynamic and clinical targets of therapy have been defined. In general, the goals for the treatment of decompensated heart failure include

alleviating symptoms, reducing extracellular fluid volume excess, improving hemodynamics (particularly ventricular filling pressures), and maintaining perfusion to vital organs. Identification of factors leading to decompensation is also important, and given the *teachable moment* of hospitalization, patient education should be a part of any inpatient algorithm for acutely decompensated heart failure.

General Approach to Acutely Decompensated Heart Failure

The approach to the patient with acutely decompensated heart failure begins with appropriate triage, prompt stabilization of respiratory and hemodynamic status, and rapid exclusion or treatment of immediately reversible problems. Simultaneous evaluation and empirical therapy begin with supplemental oxygen, cardiac monitoring, IV access, and a 12-lead electrocardiogram. Patients with signs of exhaustion, poor respiratory effort, or cyanosis despite supplemental oxygen require aggressive management and should not be allowed to progress to respiratory arrest. Patients with hypotension, obtundation, cool extremities, or other signs of poor perfusion should be presumed to be in or near cardiogenic shock and managed accordingly. Patients with electrocardiographic evidence of acute ischemia or infarction should be considered for emergent coronary reperfusion. For patients with end-stage renal disease and severe volume overload, hemodialysis may be emergently required. Once initial resuscitation is underway, further efforts can be made to identify the underlying cause of decompensation, if not readily apparent.

Precipitating factors should be sought and treated aggressively. Cardiovascular precipitants, such as arrhythmia, high-grade heart block, severe valvular dysfunction, or hypertensive crisis are usually apparent on initial evaluation. Coronary insufficiency should always be considered, even in the absence of characteristic electrocardiographic changes. Decompensated heart failure may also arise as a complication of another pathophysiologic state, such as sepsis, anemia, or hyperthyroidism. The prevalence of specific precipitants varies among different populations. Overall, ischemia or infarction, uncontrolled hypertension, and noncompliance with medications or dietary restrictions are the most common causes of clinical decompensation.[252–256]

Patients presenting with mild or nonspecific symptoms often pose a diagnostic challenge. Older patients in particular are difficult to evaluate because they frequently lack the typical signs and symptoms of heart failure.[257] These signs and symptoms may be obscured by the aging process itself or by the presence of coexisting medical conditions. Among patients who present to the emergency department with undifferentiated dyspnea, the diagnosis of heart failure can easily be overlooked.[258] In particular, distinguishing between cardiac and pulmonary causes of dyspnea remains a fundamental clinical challenge. In patients with heart failure, nonspecific symptoms such as weakness, lethargy, fatigue, anorexia, or lightheadedness may be a manifestation of decreased cardiac output, and occult shock is probably underappreciated.[259] Classic physical signs have limited reliability for assessing LV filling pressure and cardiac output.[260] The role of BNP or N-terminal (NT)-proBNP testing in the diagnosis of worsening heart failure has been discussed earlier in this chapter.

Pharmacologic Management

The general approach to the management of decompensated heart failure includes one or more of the following drug strategies:

IV diuretics to reduce extracellular fluid volume excess

IV vasodilators to reduce ventricular filling pressures and systemic vascular resistance

IV positive inotropic agents to improve cardiac output in low-flow states

In acute heart failure (synonymous with severe pulmonary edema) the treatment is to sit the patient up (usually patients spontaneously adopt that posture), provide oxygen, give diuretics (usually an IV bolus of a loop diuretic, such as furosemide, infused over more than 10 minutes), and an intramuscular or IV injection of morphine with an antiemetic. Noninvasive ventilation can be helpful. IV nitrates are often used in less severely ill patients.

Intravenous Diuretic Administration

The most common treatment used in the inpatient management of worsening heart failure is an IV diuretic. Usually, an IV loop diuretic is used, given its greater potency compared to other agents. The method by which this therapy is best delivered is still somewhat controversial. Traditional bolus dosing of loop diuretics, when compared to a continuous infusion, has been shown to be related to higher rates of ototoxicity, presumably caused by the higher immediate plasma level achieved with this dosing regimen.[261] Additionally, the use of a continuous diuretic infusion prevents the postdiuretic phase of sodium reabsorption seen with intermittent bolus dosing by providing a constant rate of drug delivery to the nephron.[261–263] Although no firm guidelines exist regarding the proper approach to IV diuretic dosing, a recent review by Salvador and coworkers provides evidence to support the safety and effectiveness of a continuous diuretic infusion, compared to intermittent bolus administration.[264]

Although it is widely believed that the beneficial effects are the result of rapid diuresis, evidence from many in vitro and in vivo experiments suggest that direct vascular actions of furosemide contribute in large part to the acute clinical effects, at least in patients with new acute heart failure.[265–270] However, in patients with decompensated chronic heart failure in the absence of other vasoactive drugs, some effects of acute furosemide administration may actually be detrimental. By activating the sympathetic and renin-angiotensin systems, acute furosemide may cause vasoconstriction, potentially impairing LV function and acutely/transiently worsening the degree of decompensation.[271,272] Thus, the administration of such agents should always be monitored carefully.

When congestion fails to improve in response to diuretic therapy, options include increasing the dose of loop diuretic, switching to a continuous infusion if bolus dosing has been used, adding a second type of diuretic as discussed previously,

or resorting to ultrafiltration. Recent studies employing an ultrafiltration device designed for use in heart failure management suggest a role for this therapy in diuretic resistant patients and perhaps in those with gross fluid overload.[273–276] For rapid symptom relief, diuretics may be combined with IV vasodilators, and IV vasodilators should be considered in patients who have persistent severe heart failure despite diuretic therapy.

Vasodilators

The European Society of Cardiology acute heart failure guideline emphasizes the use of nitroglycerin, whereas the Heart Failure Society of America guideline suggests that the natriuretic peptide nesiritide may be considered along with nitroglycerin and nitroprusside, in the management of decompensated heart failure.

Nitrates Nitrates are recommended as vasodilator therapy for acutely decompensated heart failure of both ischemic and nonischemic origin. A number of studies have compared the acute effects of nitrates and diuretics in acutely decompensated heart failure. As compared with furosemide, IV nitrates appear to have a more balanced hemodynamic profile, reducing both preload and afterload, and maintaining or improving cardiac output.[277–279] In head-to-head comparison, a regimen of high-dose nitrates with low-dose diuretic provided more consistent clinical improvement than a regimen of high-dose diuretic with low-dose nitrates, and was associated with lower rates of mechanical ventilation and MI.[280] Because many patients in these studies had underlying coronary artery disease, it is difficult to separate out the potentially beneficial antiischemic effects of nitrates in this setting.

With the possible exception of nesiritide, no other group of agents improves the symptoms of congestion as rapidly as nitrates. Treatment with sublingual nitroglycerin (tablets or spray) results in noticeable hemodynamic and clinical improvement within 5 minutes.[281–283] Single doses of 0.4 to 0.6 mg can be given repeatedly every 5 to 10 minutes if the patient has stable blood pressure. In the hospital setting, continuous IV administration of nitroglycerin is generally more convenient and allows for more careful titration to specific clinical or hemodynamic end-points compared to sublingual nitroglycerine or to nitroprusside. Unfortunately, tolerance to the effects of IV nitrates may develop within 24 to 48 hours, limiting their usefulness.[284] Nitroglycerin can be started at 0.3 to 0.5 µg/kg/min so long as the blood pressure is above 95 to 100 mmHg.

Sodium Nitroprusside Sodium nitroprusside is recommended for patients with marked systemic hypertension, severe mitral or aortic valvular regurgitation, or pulmonary edema not responsive to standard nitrate therapy. Nitroprusside directly dilates resistance vessels, rapidly reducing blood pressure and afterload.[285] Typically, nitroprusside is started at a dose of 0.1 to 0.2 µg/kg/min and advanced as needed to improve clinical and hemodynamic status, using a systolic pressure of 85 to 90 mmHg as a lower limit for dose titration, provided that adequate systemic perfusion is maintained. Because of the risk of severe hypotension during nitroprusside infusion, invasive monitoring of arterial blood pressure is generally recommended.

Natriuretic Peptides The natriuretic peptides are a family of endogenous hormones that have diverse actions on cardiovascular, renal, and endocrine homeostasis and one agent (human BNP or nesiritide) is used therapeutically in the setting of acutely decompensated heart failure.[286-288] For patients hospitalized with decompensated congestive heart failure, IV nesiritide significantly improves hemodynamic function and clinical status.[287,288] In a randomized controlled trial of acute decompensation of chronic heart failure, nesiritide provided significant hemodynamic and clinical benefits. The Vasodilation in the Management of Acute Congestive Heart Failure (VMAC) trial was a randomized, double-blind, placebo-controlled comparison of nesiritide and nitroglycerin (in addition to standard therapy) in patients with acutely decompensated heart failure.[288] Reductions in pulmonary capillary wedge pressure were significantly greater with nesiritide than with nitroglycerin, starting with the first measurement at 15 minutes and persisting throughout the first day, with no evidence of attenuation of effect. In addition, when compared with placebo, nesiritide, but not nitroglycerin, significantly lowered systemic vascular resistance and increased cardiac index at 1 hour and significantly reduced dyspnea within 3 hours after initiation of therapy. Finally, nesiritide produced a trend toward improvement in global clinical status at 24 hours relative to nitroglycerin.

Positive Inotropic Agents

Although the role of long-term positive inotropic therapy for chronic heart failure is controversial, short-term therapy with positive inotropes is likely to benefit selected patients with acutely decompensated heart failure. Classically, inotropic agents have been reserved for the treatment of cardiogenic shock or impending shock. This is likely appropriate, because a large-scale randomized controlled trial of milrinone and an analysis of a large heart failure registry both suggest worse outcomes when decompensated heart failure patients are treated with positive inotropic agents.[289,290] Conversely, short-term inotropic therapy clearly produces improvement in contractile performance and may be necessary when cardiac output is particularly low.

Low output cardiac failure is typically treated with either a β agonist (dobutamine, dopamine) or a phosphodiesterase inhibitor (milrinone, enoximone). In the presence of increased ventricular filling pressures and elevated systemic vascular resistance, the latter agents (also called *inodilators*) may be preferred because of their marked ability to lower cardiac preload and afterload. In Europe and elsewhere outside of the United States, newer positive inotropic agents such as levosimendan may also be used. In head-to-head comparison, there appears to be more consistent short-term hemodynamic improvement with milrinone than with dobutamine.[291] There are also theoretical advantages to phosphodiesterase inhibitors (such as milrinone) over β agonists (such as dobutamine), particularly with patients who are felt to have chronically down-regulated β recep-

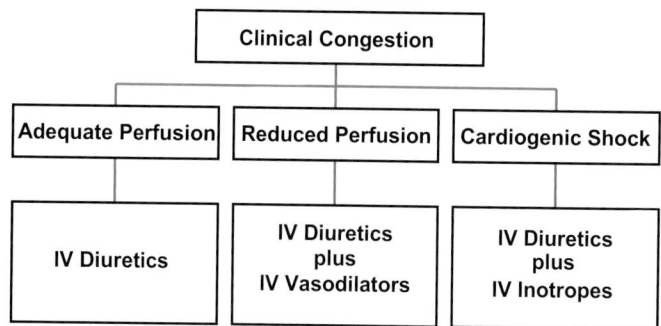

```
                    ┌─────────────────────┐
                    │ Clinical Congestion │
                    └─────────────────────┘
         ┌───────────────────┼───────────────────┐
┌──────────────────┐ ┌──────────────────┐ ┌──────────────────┐
│Adequate Perfusion│ │Reduced Perfusion │ │ Cardiogenic Shock│
└──────────────────┘ └──────────────────┘ └──────────────────┘
         │                   │                   │
┌──────────────────┐ ┌──────────────────┐ ┌──────────────────┐
│                  │ │   IV Diuretics   │ │   IV Diuretics   │
│   IV Diuretics   │ │       plus       │ │       plus       │
│                  │ │ IV Vasodilators  │ │   IV Inotropes   │
└──────────────────┘ └──────────────────┘ └──────────────────┘
```

FIGURE 26–10. Approach to treating patients with acutely decompensated heart failure. Patients presenting with clinical congestion may be grouped according to the adequacy of their peripheral perfusion into one of three groups, as shown. Because all patients are *wet* (according to this algorithm), an IV diuretic is required for all three subgroups. Patients with adequate perfusion or a normal cardiac index (≥2.5 L/min/m^2) usually require treatment with an IV diuretic and continuation of oral heart failure therapies. Those with a reduced perfusion (generally in the cardiac index range of 1.5–2.4 L/min/m^2) often require an IV vasoactive agent. Because of a better safety profile, vasodilators rather than positive inotropic agents are preferred in this group. Patients in cardiogenic shock or with a very low cardiac index (≥1.4 L/min/m^2) generally need an inotropic agent to improve perfusion to vital organs.

tors and patients treated with β-blocker therapy. This latter notion has been confirmed in a recent comparative trial of dobutamine versus milrinone in patients treated chronically with the β blocker, carvedilol.[292]

It is important to understand the effects and limitations of the various inotropic agents and set clear goals for therapy. Placement of a pulmonary artery catheter provides objective data to guide therapy, but a randomized controlled trial evaluating the use of such catheters demonstrated no benefit on outcomes.[293] It should be recognized that most inotropic agents have multiple pharmacologic actions, some of which may be adverse. The use of inotropic therapy may be limited by excessive tachycardia, arrhythmogenesis, or ischemia resulting from increased myocardial oxygen consumption.

A simple approach to the pharmacological treatment of the congested patient with acutely decompensated heart failure is presented in Fig. 26–10.

SUMMARY

Although the past has been dominated by pharmacological therapies and the present by further honing of drug therapies with the addition of devices, the future of heart failure management may reside in cellular- and molecular-based therapies. Such therapies are already under investigation, largely in proof of concept studies. The notion that we may one day replace damaged or dysfunctional heart tissue through such cellular approaches promises to move us from palliation to cure in the management of heart failure. Until that time much may be achieved by the proper application of current knowledge since there is strong evidence that adherence to guidelines results in improved outcomes. Monitoring of patients by use of miniature devices or by direct communication with patients in their homes will become more widespread and improve treatment delivery. This will be aided by advances in information technology and nanotechnology.

REFERENCES

1. Lewis T. *Diseases of the Heart Described For Practitioners and Students*. New York: Macmillan, 1933.

2. O'Connell JB. The economic burden of heart failure. *Clin Cardiol* 2000;23:III6–III10.

3. Levy D, Kenchaiah S, Larson MG, et al. Long-term trends in the incidence of and survival with heart failure. *N Engl J Med* 2002;347:1397–1402.

4. Krumholz HM, Parent EM, Tu N, et al. Readmission after hospitalization for congestive heart failure among Medicare beneficiaries. *Arch Intern Med* 1997;157:99–104.

5. Vinson JM, Rich MW, Sperry JC, Shah AS, McNamara T. Early readmission of elderly patients with congestive heart failure. *J Am Geriatr Soc* 1990;38:1290–1295.

6. Jong P, Vowinckel E, Liu PP, Gong Y, Tu JV. Prognosis and determinants of survival in patients newly hospitalized for heart failure: a population-based study. *Arch Intern Med* 2002;162:1689–1694.

7. Hunt SA, Abraham WT, Chin MH, et al. ACC/AHA 2005 guideline update for the diagnosis and management of chronic heart failure in the adult: summary article. A report of the American College of Cardiology/American Heart Association Task Force on Practice Guidelines (Committee to revise the 2001 Guidelines for the Evaluation and Management of Heart Failure). *J Am Coll Cardiol* 2005;46:1116–1143.

8. Adams KF Jr, Lindenfeld J, Arnold JM, et al. Executive summary: HFSA 2006 comprehensive heart failure practice guideline. *J Card Fail* 2006;12:10–38.

9. Swedberg K, Cleland J, Dargie H, et al. Guidelines for the diagnosis and treatment of chronic heart failure: executive summary (update 2005). The Task Force for the Diagnosis and Treatment of Chronic Heart Failure of the European Society of Cardiology. *Eur Heart J* 2005;26:1115–1140.

10. Camm J, Cleland J, Cammage M, et al. NICE Guideline No. 5: Chronic heart failure: national clinical guideline for diagnosis and management in primary and secondary care. Royal College of Physicians of London 2003;1–163.

11. Nieminen MS, Böhm M, Cowie MR, et al. Executive summary of the guidelines on the diagnosis and treatment of acute heart failure. The Task Force of Acute Heart Failure of the European Society of Cardiology. *Eur Heart J* 2005;26:384–416.

12. Hunt SA, Baker DW, Chin MH, et al. ACC/AHA guidelines for the evaluation and management of chronic heart failure in the adult: executive summary. A report of the American College of Cardiology/American Heart Association Task Force on Practice Guidelines (Committee to Revise the 1995 Guidelines for the Evaluation and Management of Heart Failure). *J Am Coll Cardiol* 2001;38:2101–2113.

13. Packer M, Carver JR, Rodeheffer RJ, et al. Effect of oral milrinone on mortality in severe chronic heart failure. *N Engl J Med* 1991;325:1468–1475.

14. Uretsky BF, Jessup M, Konstam MA, et al. Multicenter trial of oral enoximone in patients with moderate to moderately severe congestive heart failure: lack of benefit compared with placebo. Enoximone Multicenter Trial Group. *Circulation* 1990;82:774–780.

15. Cohn JN, Goldstein SO, Greenberg BH, et al. A dose-dependent increase in mortality with vesnarinone among patients with severe heart failure. Vesnarinone Trial Investigators. *N Engl J Med* 1998;339:1810–1816.

16. Kannel WB, Belanger AJ. Epidemiology of heart failure. *Am Heart J* 1991;121:951–957.

17. Kannel WB, Ho K, Thom T. Changing epidemiological features of cardiac failure. *Br Heart J* 1994;72:S3–S9.

18. U.S. Department of Health and Human Services. NHLBI Report of the Task Force on Research in Heart Failure. Springfield, VA: U.S. Department of Health and Human Services, 1994.

19. Nieto FJ, Young TB, Lind BK, et al. Association of sleep-disordered breathing, sleep apnea, and hypertension in a large community-based study. Sleep Heart Health Study. *JAMA* 2000;283:1829–1836.

20. Shahar E, Whitney CW, Redline S, et al. Sleep-disordered breathing and cardiovascular disease: cross-section results of the Sleep Heart Health Study. *Am J Respir Crit Care Med* 2001;163:19–25.

21. Vasan RS, Beiser A, Seshadri S, et al. Residual lifetime risk for developing hypertension in middle-aged women and men: the Framingham Heart Study. *JAMA* 2002;287:1003–1010.

22. Levy D, Larson MG, Vasan RS, Kannel WB, Ho KK. The progression from hypertension to congestive heart failure. *JAMA* 1996;275:1557–1562.

23. Wilhelmsen L, Rosengren A, Eriksson H, Lappas G. Heart failure in the general population of men—morbidity, risk factors and prognosis. *J Intern Med* 2001;249:253–261.

24. Kostis JB, Davis BR, Cutler J, et al. Prevention of heart failure by antihypertensive drug treatment in older persons with isolated systolic hypertension. SHEP Cooperative Research Group. *JAMA* 1997;278:212–216.

25. Izzo JL Jr, Gradman AH. Mechanisms and management of hypertensive heart disease: from left ventricular hypertrophy to heart failure. *Med Clin North Am* 2004;88:1257–1271.

26. Baker DW. Prevention of heart failure. *J Card Fail* 2002;8:333–346.

27. Vakili BA, Okin PM, Devereux RB. Prognostic implications of left ventricular hypertrophy. *Am Heart J* 2001;141:334–341.

28. Chobanian AV, Bakris GL, Black HR, et al. Seventh report of the Joint National Committee on Prevention, Detection, Evaluation, and Treatment of High Blood Pressure. *Hypertension* 2003;42:1206–1252.

29. UK Prospective Diabetes Study Group. Tight blood pressure control and risk of macrovascular and microvascular complications in type 2 diabetes: UKPDS 38. *BMJ* 1998;317:703–713.

30. Hansson L, Zanchetti A, Carruthers SG, et al. Effects of intensive blood-pressure lowering and low-dose aspirin in patients with hypertension: principal results of the Hypertension Optimal Treatment (HOT) randomised trial. HOT Study Group. *Lancet* 1998;351:1755–1762.

31. Estacio RO, Jeffers BW, Hiatt WR, Biggerstaff SL, Gifford N, Schrier RW. The effect of nisoldipine as compared with enalapril on cardiovascular outcomes in patients with noninsulin-dependent diabetes and hypertension. *N Engl J Med* 1998;338:645–652.

32. Yusuf S, Sleight P, Pogue J, Bosch J, Davies R, Dagenais G. Effects of an angiotensin-converting-enzyme inhibitor, ramipril, on cardiovascular events in high-risk patients. The Heart Outcomes Prevention Evaluation Study Investigators. *N Engl J Med* 2000;342:145–153.

33. Fox KM. Efficacy of perindopril in reduction of cardiovascular events among patients with stable coronary artery disease: randomised, double-blind, placebo-controlled, multicentre trial (the EUROPA study). *Lancet* 2003;362:782–788.

34. Staessen JA, Wang JG, Thijs L. Cardiovascular protection and blood pressure reduction: a meta-analysis. *Lancet* 2001;358:1305–1315.

35. Major outcomes in high-risk hypertensive patients randomized to angiotensin-converting enzyme inhibitor or calcium channel blocker vs diuretic: the Antihypertensive and Lipid-Lowering Treatment to Prevent Heart Attack Trial (ALLHAT). *JAMA* 2002;288:2981–2997.

36. Brenner BM, Cooper ME, de Zeeuw D, et al. Effects of losartan on renal and cardiovascular outcomes in patients with type 2 diabetes and nephropathy. *N Engl J Med* 2001;345:861–869.

37. Berl T, Hunsicker LG, Lewis JB, et al. Cardiovascular outcomes in the Irbesartan Diabetic Nephropathy Trial of patients with type 2 diabetes and overt nephropathy. *Ann Intern Med* 2003;138:542–549.

38. Strauss MH, Hall AS. Angiotensin receptor blockers may increase risk of myocardial infarction: unraveling the ARB-MI paradox. *Circulation* 2006;114:838–854.

39. Tsuyuki RT, McDonald MA. Angiotensin receptor blockers do not increase risk of myocardial infarction. *Circulation* 2006;114:855–860.

40. Taegtmeyer H, McNulty P, Young ME. Adaptation and maladaptation of the heart in diabetes: Part I. General concepts. *Circulation* 2002;105:1727–1733.

41. Kenchaiah S, Evans JC, Levy D, et al. Obesity and the risk of heart failure. *N Engl J Med* 2002;347:305–313.

42. Wilson PW, Grundy SM. The metabolic syndrome: practical guide to origins and treatment: part I. *Circulation* 2003;108:1422–1424.

43. Kereiakes DJ, Willerson JT. Metabolic syndrome epidemic. *Circulation* 2003;108:1552–1553.

44. Mokdad AH, Ford ES, Bowman BA, et al. Prevalence of obesity, diabetes, and obesity-related health risk factors, 2001. *JAMA* 2003;289:76–79.

45. He J, Ogden LG, Bazzano LA, Vupputuri S, Loria C, Whelton PK. Risk factors for congestive heart failure in US men and women: NHANES I epidemiologic follow-up study. *Arch Intern Med* 2001;161:996–1002.

46. Cooper R, Cutler J, Desvigne-Nickens P, et al. Trends and disparities in coronary heart disease, stroke, and other cardiovascular diseases in the United States: findings of the national conference on cardiovascular disease prevention. *Circulation* 2000;102:3137–3147.

47. Knowler WC, Barrett-Connor E, Fowler SE, et al, for the Diabetes Prevention Program (DPP) Research Group. Reduction in the incidence of type 2 diabetes with lifestyle intervention or metformin. *N Engl J Med* 2002;246:393–403.

48. Nesto RW, Bell D, Bonow RO, et al. Thiazolidinedione use, fluid retention, and congestive heart failure: a consensus statement from the American Heart Association and American Diabetes Association. *Circulation* 2003;108:2941–2948.

49. American Heart Association. *Heart Disease and Stroke Statistics.* 2005 Update, 2005.

50. Bourassa MG, Gurne O Bangdiwala SI, et al. Natural history and patterns of current practice in heart failure: the Studies of Left Ventricular Dysfunction (SOLVD) Investigators. *J Am Coll Cardiol* 1993;22:14A–19A.

51. Taylor AL, Ziesche S, Yancy C, et al. Combination of isosorbide dinitrate and hydralazine in blacks with heart failure. *N Engl J Med* 2004;351:2049–2057.

52. Adams KF, Fonarow GC, Emerman CL, et al, for the ADHERE Scientific Advisory Committee and Investigators. Characteristics and outcomes of patients hospitalized for heart failure in the United States: rationale, design, and preliminary observations from the first 100,000 cases in the Acute Decompensated Heart Failure National Registry (ADHERE). *Am Heart J* 2005;149:209–216.

53. Hammermeister KE, DeRouen TA, Dodge HT. Variables predictive of survival in patients with coronary disease. Selection by univariate and multivariate analyses from the clinical, electrocardiographic, exercise, arteriographic, and quantitative angiographic evaluations. *Circulation* 1979;59:421–430.

54. St. John Sutton M, Pfeffer MA, Plappert T, et al. Quantitative two-dimensional echocardiographic measurements are major predictors of adverse cardiovascular events after acute myocardial infarction. The protective effects of captopril. *Circulation* 1994;89:68–75.

55. Migrino RQ, Young JB, Ellis SG, et al. End-systolic volume index at 90 to 180 minutes into reperfusion therapy for acute myocardial infarction is a strong predictor of early and late mortality. The Global Utilization of Streptokinase and t-PA for Occluded Coronary Arteries (GUSTO)-I Angiographic Investigators. *Circulation* 1997;96:116–121.

56. Smith SC, Jr, Blair SN, Bonow RO, et al. AHA/ACC Scientific Statement: AHA/ACC guidelines for preventing heart attack and death in patients with atherosclerotic cardiovascular disease—2001 update. A statement for healthcare professionals from the American Heart Association and the American College of Cardiology. *Circulation* 2001;104:1577–1579.

57. Passamani E, Davis KB, Gillespie MJ, Killip T. A randomized trial of coronary artery bypass surgery: survival of patients with a low ejection fraction. *N Engl J Med* 1985;312:1665–1671.

58. Grundy SM, Cleeman JI, Merz CN, et al. Implications of recent clinical trials for the National Cholesterol Education Program Adult Treatment Panel III Guidelines. *J Am Coll Cardiol* 2004;44:720–732.

59. Randomised trial of cholesterol lowering in 4444 patients with coronary heart disease: the Scandinavian Simvastatin Survival Study (4S). *Lancet* 1994;344:1383–1389.

60. Devereux RB, Wachtell K, Gerts E, et al. Prognostic significance of left ventricular mass change during treatment of hypertension. *JAMA* 2004;292:2350–2356.

61. Okin PM, Devereux RB, Jern S, et al. Regression of electrocardiographic left ventricular hypertrophy during antihypertensive treatment and the prediction of major cardiovascular events. *JAMA* 2004;292:2343–2349.

62. Wang X, Li F, Gerdes AM. Chronic pressure overload cardiac hypertrophy and failure in guinea pigs: I. Regional hemodynamics and myocyte remodeling. *J Mol Cell Cardiol* 1999;31:307–317.

63. Lowes BD, Gilbert EM, Abraham WT, et al. Myocardial gene expression in dilated cardiomyopathy treated with beta-blocking agents. *N Engl J Med* 2002;346:1357–1365.

64. Abraham WT, Gilbert EM, Lowes BD, et al. Coordinate changes in myosin heavy chain isoform gene expression are selectively associated with alterations in dilated cardiomyopathy phenotype. *Mol Med* 2002;8:750–760.

65. Mann DL. Basic mechanisms of left ventricular remodeling: the contribution of wall stress. *J Card Fail* 2004;10(suppl 6):S202–S206.

66. Dahlof B. Regression of left ventricular hypertrophy: are there differences between antihypertensive agents? *Cardiology* 1992;81:307–315.

67. The SOLVD Investigators. Effect of enalapril on mortality and the development of heart failure in asymptomatic patients with reduced left ventricular ejection fractions. *N Engl J Med* 1992;327:685–691.

68. The CAPRICORN Investigators. Effect of carvedilol on outcome after myocardial infarction in patients with left-ventricular dysfunction: the CAPRICORN randomized trial. *Lancet* 2001;357:1385–1390.

69. Pfeffer MA, McMurray JJV, Velazquez EJ, et al, for the Valsartan in Acute Myocardial Infarction Trial Investigators. Valsartan, captopril, or both in myocardial infarction complicated by heart failure, left ventricular dysfunction, or both. *N Engl J Med* 2003;349:1893–1906.

70. Pitt B, Remme W, Zannand F, et al. Eplerenone, a selective aldosterone blocker in patients with left ventricular dysfunction after myocardial infarction. *N Engl J Med* 2003;348:1309–1321.

71. Guyatt GH, Sullivan MJ, Thompson PJ, et al. The 6-minute walk: a new measure of exercise capacity in patients with chronic heart failure. *Can Med Assoc J* 1985;132:919–923.

72. Weber KT, Janicki JS, McElroy PA, Maskin CS. Cardiopulmonary exercise testing in clinical practice. *Cardiology* 1987;74:62–70.

73. Criteria Committee of the New York Heart Association. *Nomenclature and Criteria for Diagnosis of Diseases of the Heart and Great Vessels.* 7th ed. Boston: Little, Brown; 1973:286.

74. Chakko S, Woska D, Martinez H, et al. Clinical, radiographic, and hemodynamic correlations in chronic congestive heart failure: conflicting results may lead to inappropriate care. *Am J Med* 1991;90:353–359.

75. Butman SM, Ewy GA, Standen JR, Kern KB, Hahn E. Bedside cardiovascular examination in patients with severe chronic heart failure: importance of rest or inducible jugular venous distension. *J Am Coll Cardiol* 1993;22:968–974.

76. Collins SP, Lindsell CJ, Storrow AB, Abraham WT. Prevalence of negative chest radiography in the emergency department patient with decompensated heart failure. *Ann Emerg Med* 2006;47:13–18.

77. Maisel AS, Krishnaswamy P, Nowak RM, et al, for the Breathing Not Properly Multinational Investigators. Rapid measurement of B-type natriuretic peptide in the emergency diagnosis of heart failure. *N Engl J Med* 2002;347:161–167.

78. Mueller C, Laule-Kilian K, Schindler C, et al. Cost-effectiveness of B-type natriuretic peptide testing in patients with acute dyspnea. *Arch Intern Med* 2006;166:1081–1087.

79. Alderman EL, Fisher LD, Litwin P, et al. Results of coronary artery surgery in patients with poor left ventricular function (CASS). *Circulation* 1983;68:785–795.

80. Baker DW, Jones R, Hodges J, Massie BM, Konstam MA, Rose EA. Management of heart failure: the role of revascularization in the treatment of patients with moderate or severe left ventricular systolic dysfunction. *JAMA* 1994;272:1528–1534.

81. Bounous EP, Mark DB, Pollock BG, et al. Surgical survival benefits for coronary disease patients with left-ventricular dysfunction. *Circulation* 1988;78;I-151–I-157.

82. Cohen M, Charney R, Hershman R, Fuster V, Gorlin R. Reversal of chronic ischemic myocardial dysfunction after transluminal coronary angioplasty. *J Am Coll Cardiol* 1988;12:1193–1198.

83. Elefteriades JA, Tolis G Jr, Levi E, Mills LK, Zaret BL. Coronary artery bypass grafting in severe left ventricular dysfunction: excellent survival with improved ejection fraction and functional state. *J Am Coll Cardiol* 1993;22:1411–1417.

84. Faulkner SL, Stoney WS, Alford WC, Thomas CS, Burrus GR, Frist RA. Ischemic cardiomyopathy: medical versus surgical treatment. *J Thorac Cardiovasc Surg* 1977;74;77–82.

85. Reinfeld HB, Samet P, Hildner FJ. Resolution of congestive failure, mitral regurgitation, and angina after percutaneous transluminal coronary angioplasty of triple vessel disease. *Cathet Cardiovasc Diagn* 1985;11:273–277.

86. Spencer FC, Green GE, Tice DA, Walsh E, Mills NL, Glassman E. Coronary artery bypass grafts for congestive heart failure: a report of experiences with 40 patients. *J Thorac Cardiovasc Surg* 1971;62:529–542.

87. Kim MJ, Song JK, Song JM, et al. Long-term outcomes of significant mitral regurgitation after percutaneous mitral valvuloplasty. *Circulation* 2006;114:2815–2822.

88. Mason JW, O'Connell JB, Herskowitz A, et al, and the Myocarditis Treatment Trial Investigators. A clinical trial of immunosuppressive therapy for myocarditis. *N Engl J Med* 1995;333:269–275.

89. McNamara DM, Holubkov R, Starling RC, et al. Controlled trial of intravenous immune globulin in recent-onset dilated cardiomyopathy. *Circulation* 2001;103:2254–2259.

90. Demakis JG, Proskey A, Rahimtoola SH, et al. The natural course of alcoholic cardiomyopathy. *Ann Intern Med* 1974;80:293–297.

91. Mølgaard H, Kristensen BÖ, Baandrup U. Importance of abstention from alcohol in alcoholic heart disease. *Int J Cardiol* 1990;26:373–375.

92. Cardinale D, Colombo A, Sandri MT, et al. Prevention of high-dose chemotherapy-induced cardiotoxicity in high-risk patients by angiotensin-converting enzyme inhibition. *Circulation* 2006;114:2474–2481.

93. Kalay N, Basar E, Ozdogru I, et al. Protective effects of carvedilol against anthracycline-induced cardiomyopathy. *J Am Coll Cardiol* 2006;48:2258–2262.

94. Riegger GA, Kahles HW, Elsner D, Kromer EP, Kochsiek K. Effects of acetylsalicylic acid on renal function in patients with chronic heart failure. *Am J Med* 1991;90:571–575.

95. Walshe JJ, Venuto RC. Acute oliguric renal failure induced by indomethacin: possible mechanism. *Ann Intern Med* 1979;91:47–49.

96. Coats AJ, Adamopoulos S, Meyer TE, Conway J, Sleight P. Effects of physical training in chronic heart failure. *Lancet* 1990;335:63–66.

97. Coats AJ, Adamopoulos S, Radaelli A, et al. Controlled trial of physical training in chronic heart failure: exercise performance, hemodynamics, ventilation, and autonomic function. *Circulation* 1992;85:2119–2131.

98. Dubach P, Froelicher VF. Cardiac rehabilitation for heart failure patients. *Cardiology* 1989;76:368–373.

99. Kellermann JJ, Shemesh J, Fisman EZ, et al. Arm exercise training in the rehabilitation of patients with impaired ventricular function and heart failure. *Cardiology* 1990;77:130–138.

100. Sullivan MJ, Higginbotham MB, Cobb FR. Exercise training in patients with chronic heart failure delays ventilatory anaerobic threshold and improves submaximal exercise performance. *Circulation* 1989;79:324–329.

101. Sullivan MJ, Higginbotham MB, Cobb FR. Exercise training in patients with severe left-ventricular dysfunction: hemodynamic and metabolic effects. *Circulation* 1988;78:506–515.

102. Morgan T, Berliner RW. A study by continuous microperfusion of water and electrolyte movements in the loop of Henle and distal tubule of the rat. *Nephron* 1969;6:388–405.

103. Giebisch G. Renal potassium excretion. In: Rouiller C, Muller AF, eds. *The Kidney: Morphology, Biochemistry, Physiology.* Vol. 3. New York: Academic; 1971:329–382.

104. Wilson JR, Reichek N, Dunkman WB, Goldberg S. Effect of diuresis on the performance of the failing left ventricle in man. *Am J Med* 1981;70:234–239.

105. Bayliss J, Norell M, Canepa-Anson R, Sutton G, Poole-Wilson P. Untreated heart failure: clinical and neuroendocrine effects of introducing diuretics. *Br Heart J* 1987;57:17–22.

106. Hensen J, Abraham WT, Dürr J, Schrier RW. Aldosterone in congestive heart failure patients: analysis of determinants and role in sodium retention. *Am J Nephrol* 1991;11:441–446.

107. Butler J, Forman DE, Abraham WT, et al. Relationship between heart failure treatment and development of worsening renal function among hospitalized patients. *Am Heart J* 2004;147:331–338.

108. Forman DE, Butler J, Wang Y, et al. Incidence, predictors and impact of worsening renal function among patients hospitalized with heart failure. *J Am Coll Card* 2004;43:61–67.

109. Hillege HL, Nitsch D, Pfeffer MA, et al. Renal function as a predictor of outcome in a broad spectrum of patients with heart failure. *Circulation* 2006;113:671–678.

110. Smith GL, Lichtman JH, Bracken MB, et al. Renal impairment and outcomes in heart failure: systematic review and meta-analysis. *J Am Coll Cardiol* 2006;47:1987–1996.

111. Brater DC. Diuretic therapy. *N Engl J Med* 1998;339:387–395.

112. Ellison DH. Diuretic resistance: physiology and therapeutics. *Semin Nephrol* 1999;19:581–597.

113. Opie LH. Diuretics. In: Opie LH, Kaplan NM, Pool-Wilson P, eds. *Drugs for the Heart.* 5th ed. Philadelphia: WB Saunders; 2001:84–106.

114. Gradual NA, Galloe AM, Garred P. Effects of sodium restriction on blood pressure, renin, aldosterone, catecholamines, cholesterols, and triglycerides. *JAMA* 1998;279:1383–1391.

115. Dzau VJ, Packer M, Lilly LS, et al. Prostaglandins in severe congestive heart failure. Relation to activation of the renin-angiotensin system and hyponatremia. *N Engl J Med* 1984;310:347–352.

116. Gerlag PGG, van Meijel JJM. High-dose furosemide in the treatment of refractory congestive heart failure. *Arch Intern Med* 1988;148:286–291.

117. Wollam GL, Tarazi RC, Bravo EL, et al. Diuretic potency of combined hydrochlorothiazide and furosemide therapy in patients with azotemia. *Am J Med* 1982;72:929–938.

118. Dormans TP, Gerlag PG. Combination of high-dose furosemide and hydrochlorothiazide in the treatment of refractory congestive heart failure. *Eur Heart J* 1996;17:1867–1874.

119. Kiyingi A, Field MJ, Pawsey CC, et al. Metolazone in treatment of severe refractory congestive cardiac failure. *Lancet* 1990;335:29–31.

120. Channer KS, McLean KA, Lawson-Matthew P, et al. Combination diuretic treatment in severe heart failure: a randomized controlled trial. *Br Heart J* 1994;71:146–150.

121. Funke Kupper A, Fintelman H, Hurge MC, Koolen JJ, Lien KL, Lustermans FA. Crossover comparison of the fixed combination of furosemide and triamterene and the free combination of furosemide and triamterene in the maintenance treatment of congestive heart failure. *Eur J Clin Pharmacol* 1986;30:341–343.

122. LeJemtel TH, Keung E, Frishman WH, Ribner HS. Hemodynamic effects of captopril in patients with severe heart failure. *Am J Cardiol* 1982;49:1484–1488.

123. DiCarlo L, Chatterjee K, Parmley WW, et al. Enalapril: a new angiotensin-converting enzyme inhibitor in chronic heart failure—acute and chronic hemodynamic evaluations. *J Am Coll Cardiol* 1983;2:865–871.

124. Awan NA, Amsterdam EA, Hermanovich J, Bommer WJ, Needham KE, Mason DT. Long-term hemodynamic and clinical efficacy of captopril therapy in ambulatory management of chronic congestive heart failure. *Am Heart J* 1982;103:474–479.

125. Sharpe DN, Murphy J, Coxon R, Hannan SF. Enalapril in patients with chronic heart failure: a placebo-controlled, randomized, double-blind study. *Circulation* 1984;70:271–278.

126. Franciosa JA, Wilen MM, Jordan RA. Effects of enalapril, a new angiotensin-converting enzyme inhibitor in a controlled trial in heart failure. *J Am Coll Cardiol* 1985;5:101–107.

127. Jennings G, Kiat H, Nelson L, Kelly MJ, Kalff V, Johns J. Enalapril for severe congestive heart failure: a double-blind study. *Med J Aust* 1984;141:723–726.

128. Lewis GR. Comparison of lisinopril versus placebo for congestive heart failure. *Am J Cardiol* 1989;63:12D–16D.

129. Magnani B, Magelli C. Captopril in mild heart failure: preliminary observations of a long-term, double-blind, placebo-controlled multicentre trial. *Postgrad Med J* 1986;62(suppl 1):153–158.

130. McGrath BP, Arnolda L, Matthews PG, et al. Controlled trial of enalapril in congestive cardiac failure. *Br Heart J* 1985;54:405–414.

131. Remes J, Nikander P, Rehnberg S, et al. Enalapril in chronic heart failure, a double-blind placebo-controlled study. *Ann Clin Res* 1986;18:124–128.

132. The Captopril Multicenter Research Group. A placebo-controlled trial of captopril in refractory chronic congestive heart failure. *J Am Coll Cardiol* 1983;2:755–763.

133. The Captopril-Digoxin Multicenter Research Group. Comparative effects of therapy with captopril and digoxin in patients with mild to moderate heart failure. *JAMA* 1988;259:539–544.

134. Riegger GA. The effects of ACE inhibitors on exercise capacity in the treatment of congestive heart failure. *J Cardiovasc Pharmacol* 1990;15(suppl 2):S41–S46.

135. Chalmers JP, West MJ, Cyran J, et al. Placebo-controlled study of lisinopril in congestive heart failure: a multicentre study. *J Cardiovasc Pharmacol* 1987;9(suppl 3):S89–S97.

136. CONSENSUS Trial Study Group. Effects of enalapril on mortality in severe congestive heart failure. *N Engl J Med* 1987;316:1429–1435.

137. SOLVD Investigators. Effect of enalapril on survival in patients with reduced left-ventricular ejection fractions and congestive heart failure. *N Engl J Med* 1991;325:293–302.

138. Gottlieb S, Dickstein K, Fleck E, et al. Hemodynamic and neurohormonal effects of the angiotensin II antagonist losartan in patients with congestive heart failure. *Circulation* 1993;88;1602–1609.

139. Crozier I, Ikram H, Awan N, et al, for the Losartan Hemodynamic Study Group. Losartan in heart failure: hemodynamic effects and tolerability. *Circulation* 1995;91:691–697.

140. Dickstein K, Chang P, Willenheimer R, et al. Comparison of the effects of losartan and enalapril on clinical status and exercise performance in patients with moderate or severe chronic heart failure. *J Am Coll Cardiol* 1995;26:438–445.

141. Pitt B, Segal R, Martinez FA, et al. Randomized trial of losartan versus captopril in patients over 65 with heart failure (Evaluation of Losartan in the Elderly Study, ELITE). *Lancet* 1997;349:747–752.

142. Kon V, Fogo A, Ichikawa I. Bradykinin causes selective efferent arteriolar dilation during angiotensin I converting enzyme inhibition. *Kidney Int* 1993;44:545–550.

143. Pitt B, Poole-Wilson PA, Segal R, et al. Effect of losartan compared with captopril on mortality in patients with symptomatic heart failure: randomized trial—the Losartan Heart Failure Survival study (ELITE II). *Lancet* 2000;355:1582–1587.

144. Cohn JN, Tognoni G, for the Valsartan Heart Failure Investigators. A randomized trial of the angiotensin receptor blocker valsartan in chronic heart failure. *N Engl J Med* 2001;345:1667–1675.

145. Young JB, Dunlap ME, Pfeffer MA, et al. Mortality and morbidity reduction with candesartan in patients with chronic heart failure and left ventricular systolic dysfunction: results of the CHARM low-left ventricular ejection fraction trials. *Circulation* 2004;110:2618–2626.

146. Young JB, Levine TB. Heart failure resulting from left ventricular systolic dysfunction. *Cardiol Rev* 2005;22:7–16.

147. Weber KT. Efficacy of aldosterone receptor antagonism in heart failure: potential mechanisms. *Curr Heart Fail Rep* 2004;1(2):51–56.

148. Pitt B, Zannad F, Remme WJ, et al. The effect of spironolactone on morbidity and mortality in patients with severe heart failure. Randomized Aldactone Evaluation Study Investigators. *N Engl J Med* 1999;341:709–717.

149. Juurlink DN, Mamdani MM, Lee DS, et al. Rates of hyperkalemia after publication of the Randomized Aldactone Evaluation Study. *N Engl J Med* 2004;351:543–551.

150. Cohn JN, Fowler MB, Bristow MR, et al. Safety and efficacy of carvedilol in severe heart failure. The U.S. Carvedilol Heart Failure Study Group. *J Card Fail* 1997;3:173–179.

151. Doughty RN, Whalley GA, Gamble, G, et al. Left ventricular remodeling with carvedilol in patients with congestive heart failure due to ischemic heart disease. Australia-New Zealand Heart Failure Research Collaborative Group. *J Am Coll Cardiol* 1997;29:1060–1066.

152. Waagstein F, Bristow MR, Swedberg K, et al. Beneficial effects of metoprolol in idiopathic dilated cardiomyopathy. Metoprolol in Dilated Cardiomyopathy (MDC) Trial Study Group. *Lancet* 1993;342:1441–1446.

153. Bristow MR, O'Connell JB, Gilbert EM, et al, for the Bucindolol Investigators. Dose-response of chronic beta-blocker treatment in heart failure from either idiopathic dilated or ischemic cardiomyopathy. *Circulation* 1994;89:1632–1642.

154. CIBIS Investigators and Committees. A randomized trial of beta-blockade in heart failure. The Cardiac Insufficiency Bisoprolol Study (CIBIS). *Circulation* 1994;90:1765–1773.

155. Colucci WS, Packer M, Bristow MR, et al, for the US Carvedilol Heart Failure Study Group. Carvedilol inhibits clinical progression in patients with mild symptoms of heart failure. *Circulation* 1996;94:2800–2806.

156. Packer M, Colucci WS, Sackner-Bernstein JD, et al. Double-blind, placebo-controlled study of the effects of carvedilol in patients with moderate to severe heart failure. The PRECISE Trial (Prospective Randomized Evaluation of Carvedilol on Symptoms and Exercise). *Circulation* 1996;94:2793–2799.

157. Packer M, Bristow MR, Cohn JN, et al. The effect of carvedilol on morbidity and mortality in patients with chronic heart failure. *N Engl J Med* 1996;334:1349–1355.

158. CIBIS-II Investigators and Committees. The Cardiac Insufficiency Bisoprolol Study II (CIBIS-II): a randomized trial. *Lancet* 1999;353:9–13.

159. Bristow MR, Abraham WT, Yoshikawa T, et al. Second and third generation beta-blocking drugs in chronic heart failure. *Cardiovasc Drugs Ther* 1997;11(suppl 1):291–296.

160. Bristow MR, Gilbert EM, Abraham WT, et al, for the MOCHA Investigators. The third-generation β-blocking agent carvedilol produces dose-related improvements in left ventricular function and survival in subjects with chronic heart failure. *Circulation* 1996;94:2807–2816.

161. Metra M, Nardi M, Giubbini R, Dei Cas L. Effects of short- and long-term carvedilol administration on rest and exercise hemodynamic variables, exercise capacity and clinical conditions in patients with idiopathic dilated cardiomyopathy. *J Am Coll Cardiol* 1994;24:1678–1687.

162. Krum H, Sackner-Bernstein JD, Goldsmith RL, et al. Double-blind, placebo-controlled study of the long-term efficacy of carvedilol in patients with severe chronic heart failure. *Circulation* 1995;92:1499–1506.

163. Olsen SL, Gilbert EM, Renlund DG, et al. Carvedilol improves left ventricular function and symptoms in chronic heart failure: a double-blind randomized study. *J Am Coll Cardiol* 1995;25:1225–1231.

164. MERIT HF Study Group. Effect of metoprolol CR/XL in chronic heart failure: Metoprolol CR/XL Randomised Intervention Trial in Congestive Heart Failure (MERIT-HF). *Lancet* 1999;353:2001–2007.

165. Packer M, Coats A, Fowler MB, et al. Effect of carvedilol on survival in severe chronic heart failure. *N Engl J Med* 2001;344:1651–1658.

166. The Capricorn Investigators. Effect of carvedilol on outcome after myocardial infarction in patients with left-ventricular dysfunction: the CAPRICORN randomized trial. *Lancet* 2001;357:1385–1390.

167. The Xamoterol in Severe Heart Failure Study Group. Xamoterol in severe heart failure. *Lancet* 1990;336:1–6.

168. Beta-Blocker Evaluation of Survival Trial (BEST) Investigators. A trial of the beta blocker bucindolol in patients with advanced chronic heart failure. *N Engl J Med* 2001;344:1659–1667.

169. Liggett SB, Mialet-Perez J, Thaneemit-Chen S, et al. A polymorphism within a conserved β₁-adrenergic receptor motif alters cardiac function and β-blocker response in human heart failure. *Proc Natl Acad Sci* 2006;103:11288–11293.

170. Flather MD, Shibata MC, Coats AJS, et al. Randomized trial to determine the effect of nebivolol on mortality and cardiovascular hospital admission in elderly patients with heart failure. *Eur Heart J* 2005;26:215–225.

171. Poole-Wilson PA, Swedberg K, Cleland JG, et al. Comparison of carvedilol and metoprolol on clinical outcomes in patients with chronic heart failure in the Carvedilol Or Metoprolol European Trial (COMET): randomized controlled trial. *Lancet* 2003;362:7–13.

172. Packer M. Do beta blockers prolong survival in heart failure only by inhibiting the beta 1-receptor? A perspective on the results of the COMET Trial. *J Card Fail* 2003;9:429–442.

173. Abraham WT. Switching between β-blockers in heart failure patients: rationale and practical considerations. *Congest Heart Fail* 2003;9:271–278.

174. Gattis WA, O'Connor CM, Gallup DS, et al. Initiation management predischarge process for assessment of carvedilol therapy for heart failure (IMPACT-HF). *J Am Coll Cardiol* 2004;43:1534–1541.

175. Bakris GL, Fonseca V, Katholi RE, et al. Metabolic effects of carvedilol vs metoprolol in patients with type 2 diabetes mellitus and hypertension: a randomized controlled trial. *JAMA* 2004;292:2227–2236.

176. Elkayam U, Roth A, Kumar A, et al. Hemodynamic and volumetric effects of venodilation with nitroglycerin in chronic mitral regurgitation. *Am J Cardiol* 1987;60:1106–1111.

177. Schwarz M, Katz SD, Demopoulos L, et al. Enhancement of endothelium-dependent vasodilation by low-dose nitroglycerin in patients with congestive heart failure. *Circulation* 1994;89:1609–1614.

178. Cohn JN, Johnson G, Ziesche S, et al. A comparison of enalapril with hydralazine-isosorbide dinitrate in the treatment of chronic congestive heart failure. *N Engl J Med* 1991;325:303–310.

179. Cohn JN, Archibald DG, Ziesche S, et al. Effect of vasodilator therapy on mortality in chronic congestive heart failure: results of a Veterans Administration Cooperative Study. *N Engl J Med* 1986;314:1547–1552.

180. Leier CV, Huss P, Magorien RD, Unverfderth DV. Improved exercise capacity and differing arterial and venous tolerance during chronic isosorbide dinitrate therapy for congestive heart failure. *Circulation* 1983;67:817–822.

181. Goldsmith SR, Cohn JN. Contrasting immediate and long-term effects of isosorbide dinitrate on exercise capacity in congestive heart failure. *Am J Med* 1980;69:559–560.

182. The Digitalis Investigation Group. The effect of digoxin on mortality and morbidity in patients with heart failure. *N Engl J Med* 1997;336:525–533.

183. Ribner HS, Plucinski DA, Hsieh A-M, et al. Acute effects of digoxin on total SVR in congestive heart failure due to dilated cardiomyopathy: a hemodynamic-hormonal study. *Am J Cardiol* 1985;56:896–904.

184. Ferguson DW, Berg WJ, Sanders JS, et al. Sympathoinhibitory responses to digitalis glycosides in heart failure patients. *Circulation* 1989;80:65–77.

185. Arnold SB, Byrd RC, Meister W, et al. Long-term digitalis therapy improves left ventricular function in heart failure. *N Engl J Med* 1980;303:1443–1448.

186. Lee DCS, Johnson RA, Bingham JB, et al. Heart failure in outpatients: a randomized trial of digoxin versus placebo. *N Engl J Med* 1982;306:699–705.

187. Uretsky BF, Young JB, Shahidi FE, et al, on behalf of the PROVED Investigative Group. Randomized study assessing the effect of digoxin withdrawal in patients with mild to moderate chronic congestive heart failure: results of the PROVED trial. *J Am Coll Cardiol* 1993;22:955–962.

188. Packer M, Gheorghiade M, Young D, et al, for the Radiance Study. Withdrawal of digoxin from patients with chronic heart failure treated with angiotensin-converting enzyme inhibitors. *N Engl J Med* 1993;329:1–7.

189. Young JB, Gheorghiade M, Uretsky BF, et al. Superiority of "triple" drug therapy in heart failure: insights from the PROVED and RADIANCE trials. *J Am Coll Cardiol* 1998;32:636–692.

190. Rathore SS, Curtis JP, Wang Y, et al. Association of serum digoxin concentration and outcomes in patients with heart failure. *JAMA* 2003;289:871–878.

191. Francis GS. Development of arrhythmias in the patient with congestive heart failure: pathophysiology, prevalence, and prognosis. *Am J Cardiol* 1986;57:3–7.

192. Chakko CS, Gheorghiade M. Ventricular arrhythmias in severe heart failure: incidence, significance, and effectiveness of antiarrhythmic therapy. *Am Heart J* 1985;109:497–504.

193. Tamburro P, Wilber D. Sudden death in idiopathic dilated cardiomyopathy. *Am Heart J* 1992;124:1035–1045.

194. Chakko S, DeMarchena E, Kessler KM, Myerburg RJ. Electrophysiology, pacing, and arrhythmia: ventricular arrhythmias in congestive heart failure. *Clin Cardiol* 1989;12:525–530.

195. Stambler BS, Wood MA, Ellenbogen KA. Sudden death in patients with congestive heart failure: future directions. *Pacing Clin Electrophysiol* 1992;15:451–470.

196. Hohnloser SH, Raeder EA, Podrid PJ, et al. Predictors of antiarrhythmic drug efficacy in patients with malignant ventricular tachyarrhythmias. *Am Heart J* 1987;114:1–7.

197. Podrid PJ, Lampert S, Graboys TB, et al. Aggravation of arrhythmia by antiarrhythmic drugs—incidence and predictors. *Am J Cardiol* 1987;59:38–44.

198. Baker DW, Wright RF. Management of heart failure. IV anticoagulation for patients with heart failure due to left ventricular systolic dysfunction. *JAMA* 1994;272:1614–1618.

199. Meltzer RS, Visser CA, Fuster V. Intracardiac thrombi and systemic embolization. *Ann Intern Med* 1986;104:689–698.

200. Dunkman WB, Johnson GR, Carson PE, et al. Incidence of thromboembolic events in congestive heart failure. The V-HeFT VA Cooperative Studies Group. *Circulation* 1993;87:V94–V101.

201. The Antiarrhythmics versus Implantable Defibrillators (AVID) Investigators. A comparison of antiarrhythmic-drug therapy with implantable defibrillators in patients resuscitated from near-fatal ventricular arrhythmias. *N Engl J Med* 1997;337:1576–1584.

202. Connolly, SJ, Gent M, Roberts RS, et al. Canadian Implantable Defibrillator Study (CIDS): a randomized trial of the implantable cardioverter-defibrillator against amiodarone. *Circulation* 2000;101:1297–1302.

203. Kuck KH, Cappato R, Seibels J, et al. Randomized comparison of antiarrhythmic drug therapy with implantable defibrillators in patients resuscitated from cardiac arrest: the Cardiac Arrest Study Hamburg (CASH). *Circulation* 2000;102:748–754.

204. Moss AJ, Zareba W, Hall WJ, et al. Prophylactic implantation of a defibrillator in patients with myocardial infarction and reduced ejection fraction. *N Engl J Med* 2002;346:877–883.

205. Bristow MR, Saxon LA, Boehmer J, et al. Cardiac-Resynchronization Therapy With or Without an Implantable Defibrillator in Advanced Chronic Heart Failure (COMPANION). *N Engl J Med* 2004;350:2140–2150.

206. Bardy GH, Lee KL, Mark DB, et al. Amiodarone or an Implantable Cardioverter-Defibrillator for Congestive Heart Failure (SCD-HeFT). *N Engl J Med* 2005;352:225–237.

207. Kadish A, Dyer A, Daubert JP, et al. Prophylactic defibrillator implantation in patients with nonischemic dilated cardiomyopathy. *N Engl J Med* 2004;350:2151–2158.

208. Bansch D, Antiz M, Boczor S, et al. Primary prevention of sudden cardiac death in idiopathic dilated cardiomyopathy: the cardiomyopathy trial (CAT). *Circulation* 2002;105:1453–1458.

209. Strickberger SA, Hummel JD, Bartlett TG, et al. Amiodarone versus implantable cardioverter defibrillator: randomized trial in patients with nonischemic dilated cardiomyopathy and asymptomatic nonsustained ventricular tachycardia (AMIOVIRT). *J Am Coll Cardiol* 2003;41:1707–1712.

210. Moss AJ, Hall WJ, Cannom DS, et al. Improved survival with an implantable defibrillator in patients with coronary disease at high risk for ventricular arrhythmia: multicenter automatic defibrillator implantation trial investigators. *N Engl J Med* 1996;335:1933–1940.

211. Moss AJ, Fadl Y, Zarebl W, et al. Survival benefit with an implantable defibrillator in relation to mortality risk in chronic coronary heart disease. *Am J Cardiol* 2001;88:516–520.

212. Greenberg H, Case RB, Moss AJ, et al. Analysis of mortality events in the Multicenter Automatic Defibrillator Implantation Trial (MADIT-II). *J Am Coll Cardiol* 2004;43:1459–1465.

213. Auricchio A, Abraham WT. Cardiac resynchronization therapy: current state of the art—cost versus benefit. *Circulation* 2004;109:300–307.

214. Bader H, Garrigue S, Lafitte S, et al. Intra-left ventricular electromechanical asynchrony: a new independent predictor of severe cardiac events in heart failure patients. *J Am Coll Cardiol* 2004;43:248–256.

215. Cho GY, Song JK, Park WJ, et al. Mechanical dyssynchrony assessed by tissue Doppler imaging is a powerful predictor of mortality in congestive heart failure with normal QRS duration. *J Am Coll Cardiol* 2005;46:2237–2243.

216. Flachskampf FA, Voigt JU. Echocardiographic methods to select candidates for cardiac resynchronization therapy. *Heart* 2006;92:424–429.

217. Auricchio A, Stellbrink C, Block M, et al. Effect of pacing chamber and atrioventricular delay on acute systolic function of paced patients with congestive heart failure. *Circulation* 1999;99:2993–3001.

218. Kass DA, Chen CH, Curry C, et al. Improved left ventricular mechanics from acute VDD pacing in patients with dilated cardiomyopathy and ventricular conduction delay. *Circulation* 1999;99:1567–1573.

219. Yu CM, Chau E, Sanderson JE, et al. Tissue Doppler echocardiographic evidence of reverse remodeling and improved synchronicity by simultaneously delaying regional contraction after biventricular pacing therapy in heart failure. *Circulation* 2002;105:438–445.

220. St. John-Sutton MG, Plappert T, Abraham WT, et al. Effect of cardiac resynchronization therapy on left ventricular size and function in chronic heart failure. *Circulation* 2003;107:1985–1990.

221. Breithardt OA, Sinha AM, Schwammenthal E, et al. Acute effects of cardiac resynchronization therapy on functional mitral regurgitation in advanced systolic heart failure. *J Am Coll Cardiol* 2003;41:765–770.

222. Auricchio A, Stellbrink C, Sack S, et al. The Pacing Therapies for Congestive Heart Failure (PATH-CHF) study: rationale, design, and endpoints of a prospective randomized multicenter study. *Am J Cardiol* 1999;83:130D–135D.

223. Cazeau S, Leclercq C, Lavergne T, et al, for the Multisite Stimulation in Cardiomyopathies (MUSTIC) study investigators. Effects of multisite biventricular pacing in patients with heart failure and intraventricular conduction delay. *N Engl J Med* 2001;344:873–880.

224. Abraham WT, on behalf of the Multisite Insync Randomized Clinical Evaluation (MIRACLE) investigators and coordinators. Rationale and design of a randomized clinical trial to assess the safety and efficacy of cardiac resynchronization therapy in patients with advanced heart failure: the Multicenter Insync Randomized Clinical Evaluation (MIRACLE). *J Card Fail* 2000;6:369–380.

225. Abraham WT, Fisher WG, Smith AL, et al, for the Multisite Insync Randomized Clinical Evaluation (MIRACLE) investigators and coordinators. Double-blind, randomized controlled trial of cardiac resynchronization in chronic heart failure. *N Engl J Med* 2002;346:1845–1853.

226. Linde C, Leclercq C, Rex S, et al, on behalf of the Multisite Stimulation in Cardiomyopathies (MUSTIC) study group. Long-term benefits of biventricular pacing in congestive heart failure: results form the Multisite Stimulation in Cardiomyopathy (MUSTIC) study. *J Am Coll Cardiol* 2002;40:111–118.

227. Leclercq C, Walker S, Linde C, et al. Comparative effects of permanent biventricular and right-ventricular pacing in heart failure patients with chronic atrial fibrillation. *Eur Heart J* 2002;23:1780–1787.

228. Higgins SL, Hummel JD, Niazi IK, et al. Cardiac resynchronization therapy for the treatment of heart failure in patients with intraventricular conduction delay and malignant ventricular tachyarrhythmias. *J Am Coll Cardiol* 2003;42:1454–1459.

229. Bristow MR, Feldman AM, Saxon LA, for the COMPANION steering committee and COMPANION clinical investigators. Heart failure management using implantable devices for ventricular resynchronization: Comparison of Medical Therapy, Pacing, and Defibrillation in Chronic Heart Failure (COMPANION) trial. *J Card Fail* 2000;6:276–285.

230. Cleland JGF, Daubert JC, Erdmann E, et al. The CARE-HF study (Cardiac Resynchronization in Heart Failure study): rationale, design, and end-points. *Eur J Heart Fail* 2001;3:481–489.

231. Cleland J, Daubert JC, Erdmann E, et al. The effect of cardiac resynchronization on morbidity and mortality in heart failure. *N Engl J Med* 2005;352:1539–1549.

232. Young JB, Abraham WT, Smith AL, et al. Safety and efficacy of combined cardiac resynchronization therapy and implantable cardioversion defibrillation in patients with advanced chronic heart failure: the Multicenter Insync ICD Randomized Clinical Evaluation (MIRACLE-ICD) trial. *JAMA* 2003;289:2685–2694.

233. Cesario DA, Shenoda M, Brar R, et al. Left ventricular lead stabilization utilizing a coronary stent. *Pacing Clin Electrophysiol* 2006;29:427–428.

234. Fox DJ, Fitzpatrick AP, Davidson NC. Optimisation of cardiac resynchronization therapy: addressing the problem of "nonresponders." *Heart* 2005;91:1000–1002.

235. Yu CM, Lin H, Zhang Q, et al. High prevalence of left ventricular systolic and diastolic asynchrony in patients with congestive heart failure and normal QRS duration. *Heart* 2003;89:54–60.

236. Yu CM, Abraham WT, Bax JJ, et al. Predictor of Response to Cardiac Resynchronization Therapy (PROSPECT): study design. *Am Heart J* 2005;149:600–605.

237. Butter C, Auricchio A, Stellbrink C, et al, on behalf of the Pacing Therapy for Chronic Heart Failure II (PATH-CHF II) study group. Effect of resynchronization therapy site on the systolic function of heart failure patients. *Circulation* 2001;104:3026–3029.

238. Wang PL, Kramer A, Estes NAM, et al. Timing cycles for biventricular pacing. *Pacing Clin Electrophysiol* 2002;25:62–75.

239. Porciani MC, Dondina C, Macioce R, et al. Echocardiographic examination of atrioventricular and interventricular delay optimization in cardiac resynchronization therapy. *Am J Cardiol* 2005;95:1108–1110.

240. Jansen AHM, Bracke FA, van Dantzig JM, et al. Correlation of echo-Doppler optimization of atrioventricular delay in cardiac resynchronization therapy with invasive hemodynamics in patients with heart failure secondary to ischemic or idiopathic dilated cardiomyopathy. *Am J Cardiol* 2006;97:552–557.

241. Kerlan JE, Sawhney NS, Waggoner AD, et al. Prospective comparison of echocardiographic atrioventricular delay optimization methods for cardiac resynchronization therapy. *Heart Rhythm* 2006;3:148–154.

242. Abraham WT, León AR, St. John Sutton MG, et al. A randomized double-blinded evaluation of optimized sequential versus simultaneous ventricular stimulation during cardiac resynchronization therapy in patients with advanced heart failure. (Submitted).

243. Auricchio A, Ding J, Spinelli JC, et al. Cardiac resynchronization therapy restores optimal atrioventricular mechanical timing in heart failure patients with ventricular conduction delay. *J Am Coll Cardiol* 2002;39:1163–1169.

244. Sawhney NS, Waggoner AD, Garhwal S, et al. Randomized prospective trial of atrioventricular delay programming for cardiac resynchronization therapy. *Heart Rhythm* 2004;1:562–567.

245. Sogaard P, Egebald H, Pedersen AK, et al. Sequential versus simultaneous biventricular resynchronization for severe heart failure. *Circulation* 2002;106:2078–2084.

246. van Gelder BM, Bracke FA, Meijer A, et al. Effect of optimizing the VV interval on left ventricular contractility in cardiac resynchronization therapy. *Am J Cardiol* 2004;93:1500–1503.

247. Feldman AM, de Lissovoy G, Bristow MR, et al. Cost effectiveness of cardiac resynchronization therapy in the Comparison of Medical Therapy, Pacing, and Defibrillation in Heart Failure (COMPANION) trial. *J Am Coll Cardiol* 2005;46:2311–2321.

248. Abraham WT, Young JB, Leon AR, et al. Effects of cardiac resynchronization on disease progression in patients with left ventricular systolic dysfunction, an indication for an implantable cardioverter defibrillator, and mildly symptomatic chronic heart failure. *Circulation* 2004;110:2864–2868.

249. Linde C, Gold M, Abraham WT, Daubert JC. Rationale and design of a randomized controlled trial to assess the safety and efficacy of cardiac resynchronization therapy in patients with asymptomatic left ventricular dysfunction with previous symptoms or mild heart failure: the Resynchronization Reverses Remodeling in Systolic Left Ventricular Dysfunction (REVERSE) study. *Am Heart J* 2006;151:288–294.

250. Yusuf S, Pfeffer MA, Swedberg K, et al, for the CHARM investigators and committees. Effects of candesartan in patients with chronic heart failure and preserved left-ventricular ejection fraction: the CHARM-Preserved Trial. *Lancet* 2003;362:777–781.

251. Fonarow GC, Abraham WT, Albert NM, et al. Organized Program to Initiate Lifesaving Treatment in Hospitalized Patients with Heart Failure (OPTIMIZE-HF): rationale and design. *Am Heart J* 2004;148:43–51.

252. Goldberger J, Peled H, Stroh J, Cohen M, Frishman W. Prognostic factors in acute pulmonary edema. *Arch Int Med* 1986;146:489–493.

253. Ghali JK, Kadakia S, Cooper R. Ferlinz J. Precipitating factors leading to decompensation of heart failure: traits among urban blacks. *Arch Intern Med* 1988;148:2013–2016.

254. Chin MH, Goldman L. Factors contributing to the hospitalization of patients with congestive heart failure. *Am J Pub Health* 1997;87:643–648.

255. Bennett SJ, Huster GA, Baker SL, et al. Characterization of the precipitants of hospitalization for heart failure decompensation. *Am J Crit Care* 1998;7:168–174.

256. Edoute Y, Roguin A, Behar D, Reisner SA. Prospective evaluation of pulmonary edema. *Crit Care Med* 2000;28:330–335.

257. Tresch DD. The clinical diagnosis of heart failure in older patients. *J Am Geriatr Soc* 1997;45:1128–1133.

258. Marantz PR, Kaplan MC, Alderman MH. Clinical diagnosis of congestive heart failure in patients with acute dyspnea. *Chest* 1990;97:776–781.

259. Ander DS, Jaggi M, Rivers E, et al. Undetected cardiogenic shock in patients with congestive heart failure presenting to the emergency department. *Am J Cardiol* 1998;82:888–891.

260. Stevenson LW, Perloff JK. The limited reliability of physical signs for estimating hemodynamics in chronic heart failure. *JAMA* 1989;261:884–888.

261. Dormans TP, van Meyel JJ, Gerlag PG, et al. Diuretic efficacy of high dose furosemide in severe heart failure: bolus injection versus continuous infusion. *J Am Coll Cardiol* 1996;28:376–382.

262. Lahav M, Regev A, Ra'anani P, et al. Intermittent administration of furosemide vs. continuous infusion preceded by a loading dose for congestive heart failure. *Chest* 1992;102:725–731.

263. Van Meijel JJ, Smits P, Dormans T, et al. Continuous infusion of furosemide in the treatment of patients with congestive heart failure and diuretic resistance. *J Intern Med* 1994;235:329–334.

264. Salvador D, Rey N, Ramos G, et al. Continuous infusion versus bolus injection of loop diuretics in congestive heart failure. *Cochrane Database Syst Rev* 2004;1:CD003178.

265. Dikshit K, Vyden JK, Forrester JS, Chatterjee K, Prakash R, Swan HJ. Renal and extrarenal hemodynamic effects of furosemide in congestive heart failure after acute myocardial infarction. *N Engl J Med* 1973;288:1087–1090.

266. Biddle TL, Yu PN. Effect of furosemide on hemodynamics and lung water in acute pulmonary edema secondary to myocardial infarction. *Am J Cardiol* 1979;43:86–90.

267. Baltopoulos G, Zakynthinos S, Dimopoulos A, Roussos C. Effects of furosemide on pulmonary shunts. *Chest* 1989;96:494–498.

268. Pickkers P, Dormans TP, Russel FG, et al. Direct vascular effects of furosemide in humans. *Circulation* 1997;96:1847–1852.

269. Dormans TP, Pickkers P, Russel FG, Smits P. Vascular effects of loop diuretics. *Cardiovasc Res* 1996;32:988–997.

270. Abraham WT, Schrier RW. Use of furosemide in the treatment of congestive heart failure. In: *Aspects of Diuretic Therapy with Furosemide: An Update—International Clinical Practice Series.* Kent: Wells Medical; 1993:23–33.

271. Francis GS, Siegel RM, Goldsmith SR, Olivari MT, Levine TB, Cohn JN. Acute vasoconstrictor response to intravenous furosemide in patients with chronic congestive heart failure: activation of the neurohumoral axis. *Ann Intern Med* 1985;103:1–6.

272. Kraus PA, Lipman J, Becker PJ. Acute preload effects of furosemide. *Chest* 1990;98:124–128.

273. Jaski BE, Ha J, Denys B, Lamba S, Trupp RJ, Abraham WT. Peripherally inserted veno-venous ultrafiltration for rapid treatment of volume overloaded patients. *J Card Fail* 2003;9:227–231.

274. Bart BA, Boyle A, Bank AJ, et al. Ultrafiltration versus usual care for hospitalized patients with heart failure: the Relief for Acutely Fluid-Overloaded Patients with Decompensated Congestive Heart Failure (RAPID-CHF) Trial. *J Am Coll Cardiol* 2005;46:2043–2046.

275. Costanzo MR, Saltzberg M, O'Sullivan J, Sobotka P. Early ultrafiltration in patients with decompensated heart failure and diuretic resistance. *J Am Coll Cardiol* 2005;46:2047–2051.

276. Costanzo MR, Guglin ME, Saltzberg MT, et. Al. Ultrafiltration versus intravenous diuretics for patients hospitalized for acute decompensated heart failure. *J Am Coll Cardiol* 2007;49(6):675–683.

277. Franciosa JA, Silverstein SR. Hemodynamic effects of nitroprusside and furosemide in left ventricular failure. *Clin Pharmacol Ther* 1982;32:62–69.

278. Nelson GI, Silke B, Ahuja RC, et al. Haemodynamic advantages of isosorbide dinitrate over furosemide in acute heart-failure following myocardial infarction. *Lancet* 1983;1:730–733.

279. Verma SP, Silke B, Hussain M, et al. First-line treatment of left ventricular failure complicating acute myocardial infarction: a randomised evaluation of immediate effects of diuretic, venodilator, arteriodilator, and positive inotropic drugs on left ventricular function. *J Cardiovasc Pharmacol* 1987;10:38–46.

280. Cotter G, Metzkor E, Kaluski E, et al. Randomised trial of high-dose isosorbide dinitrate plus low-dose furosemide versus high-dose furosemide plus low-dose isosorbide dinitrate in severe pulmonary edema. *Lancet* 1998;351:389–393.

281. Bussmann WD, Kaltenbach M. Sublingual nitroglycerin in the treatment of left ventricular failure and pulmonary edema. *Eur J Cardiol* 1976;4:327–333.

282. Bussmann WD, Schupp D. Effect of sublingual nitroglycerin in emergency treatment of severe pulmonary edema. *Am J Cardiol* 1978;41:931–936.

283. Edwards JD, Grant PT, Plunkett P, Nightingale P. The haemodynamic effects of sublingual nitroglycerin spray in severe left ventricular failure. *Intensive Care Med* 1989;15:247–249.

284. Packer M, Lee WH, Kessler PD, Gottlieb SS, Medina N, Yushak M. Prevention and reversal of nitrate tolerance in patients with congestive heart failure. *N Engl J Med* 1987;317:799–804.

285. Leier CV, Binkley PF. Parenteral inotropic support for advanced congestive heart failure. *Prog Cardiovasc Dis* 1998;41:207–224.

286. Wilkins MR, Redondo J, Brown LA. The natriuretic-peptide family. *Lancet* 1997;349:1307–1310.

287. Colucci WS, Elkayam U, Horton DP, et al, for the Nesiritide Study Group. Intravenous nesiritide, a natriuretic peptide in the treatment of decompensated congestive heart failure. *N Engl J Med* 2000;343:246–253.

288. Young J, Abraham WT, Stevenson LW, Horton DP, Elkayam U, Bourge RC. Intravenous nesiritide vs. nitroglycerin for treatment of decompensated congestive heart failure: a randomized controlled trial. *JAMA* 2002;287:1531–1540.

289. Cuffe MS, Califf RM, Adams KFJ, et al. Short-term intravenous milrinone for acute exacerbation of chronic heart failure: a randomized controlled trial. *JAMA* 2002;287:1541–1547.

290. Abraham WT, Adams KF, Fonarow GC, Costanzo MR, Berkowitz RL, LeJemtel TH, the ADHERE Scientific Advisory Committee and Investigators and the ADHERE Study Group. In-hospital mortality in patients with acute decompensated heart failure treated with intravenous vasoactive medications: an analysis from the Acute Decompensated Heart Failure National Registry (ADHERE). *J Am Coll Cardiol* 2005;46:57–64.

291. Karlsberg RP, DeWood MA, DeMaria AN, Berk MR, Lasher KP. Comparative efficacy of short-term intravenous infusions of milrinone and dobutamine in acute congestive heart failure following acute myocardial infarction. Milrinone-Dobutamine Study Group. *Clin Cardiol* 1996;19:21–30.

292. Lowes BD, Tsvetkova T, Eichhorn EJ, Gilbert EM, Bristow MR. Milrinone versus dobutamine in heart failure subjects treated chronically with carvedilol. *Int J Cardiol* 2001;81:141–149.

293. Binanay C, Califf RM, Hasselblad V, et al, for the ESCAPE Investigators and Study Coordinators. Evaluation study of congestive heart failure and pulmonary artery catheterization effectiveness: the ESCAPE trial. *JAMA* 2005;294:1625–1633.

CHAPTER (27)

Surgical Treatment of Heart Failure, Cardiac Transplantation, and Mechanical Ventricular Support

Michael X. Pham / Jonathan M. Chen / Gerald J. Berry / Eric A. Rose / John S. Schroeder

HISTORY AND OVERVIEW OF CARDIAC TRANSPLANTATION

Despite major advances in the treatment of severe myocardial failure, a sizable number of patients with terminal or progressive myocardial dysfunction are fated to die or be severely limited by symptoms. In these patients biological replacement of the heart (human transplantation) has become stan*f*dard therapy; it is widely accepted as a modality for prolonging life and improving its quality in carefully selected patients. As technological, molecular, and engineering advances occur, support or replacement of the heart by mechanical devices and xenotransplantation (transplantation of animal organs) may become alternative or complementary modalities for the treatment of such patients.

Interest in developing surgical techniques to interpose a functioning heart into a recipient's circulation dates back at least to the early part of the twentieth century. In 1905 Carrel and Guthrie[1]

described the heterotopic transplantation of a functioning donor heart into the neck of a dog. The heart in that model functioned together with the recipient's heart in the circulation and was incapable of supporting the circulation. Although the exact anatomic connections were not described in detail, this apparently nonworking model of heterotopic transplantation beat regularly for approximately 2 hours before the blood clotted in all the chambers. Carrel and his colleague Guthrie developed innovative surgical techniques for vascular anastomosis at the University of Chicago, and those advances set the stage for anastomosis leading to organ transplantation.[2] Carrel was awarded the Nobel Prize for medicine and physiology in 1912 partially because of this work.

It was not until 1933 that Mann and coworkers from the Mayo Clinic published their seminal report of a technique for heterotopic heart transplantation with circulatory loading of the right ventricle (RV).[3] Because this was a working model, the chambers did not clot immediately, and the hearts in their dogs beat for a mean of 4 days. Mann perceived several important surgical points, including the importance of avoiding ventricular distension and air embolism, and the prevention of thrombosis by heparin. His most incisive observation was that failure of a transplanted heart was not always caused by faulty surgical technique "but to some biologic factor which is probably identical to that which prevents survival of other homotransplanted tissues and organs." In what was undoubtedly the first description of acute allograft rejection, Mann recounts, "When the heart was removed just before it became quiescent . . . the surface of the heart was covered with mottled areas of ecchymoses . . . histologically the heart was completely infiltrated by large mononuclears and polymorphonuclears."[3] It took another 30 years to understand and manipulate the "biologic factor," which Mann had described as limiting the survival of allograft organs. In 1960 Lower and Shumway performed orthotopic heart transplants in dogs using cardiopulmonary bypass and topical hypothermia for donor heart preservation.[4] The dogs survived between 6 and 21 days, but died when the hearts were rejected. Lower and Shumway also recognized that "if the immunologic mechanisms of the host were prevented from destroying the graft, in all likelihood it would continue to function adequately for the normal lifespan of the animal." Their technique, involving anastomoses at the midatrial level and at the supravalvular level in the great vessels, remained the basis of cardiac transplant technique in the 1990s.

In the early 1960s, the concept of pharmacologic immunosuppression was introduced; it ushered in the marriage of surgical and medical knowledge that is known today as the field of organ transplantation. Immunosuppression was, of course, seen as a means to mitigate the "biologic factor" that otherwise limited organ graft survival. The first clinical transplants were of the kidney, a logical choice because hemodialysis was then available as a backup treatment if the graft failed, and the field has flourished since the early 1960s.[5]

The first human heart allograft procedure was performed in South Africa in 1967,[6] followed shortly by the first U.S. transplant by Shumway at Stanford in 1968 and subsequently by a flurry of transplant activity in many centers. This initial enthusiasm subsided as it became evident that postoperative survival was limited by a variety of complex medical problems, including opportunistic infections and graft rejection. Most major centers discontinued heart transplantation in the early 1970s, and it was not until the introduction of cyclosporine-based immunosuppression in 1980 and the demonstration of the attendant improvement in survival rates[7] that the procedure re-emerged as a widely accepted therapy for end-stage heart disease. In the 1990s many tertiary care centers provided programs for heart transplantation; and most medical care payers in the United States, including the federal government, provided coverage for such care. Since that time the

number of heart transplants performed worldwide has plateaued at slightly more than 4000 procedures annually, a level that is currently limited by donor availability (Fig. 27–1).[8] The progressive decline observed in the transplant volume since the late 1990s is thought to reflect a combination of underreporting by non-U.S. transplant centers and a decrease in volume from countries with mandatory reporting.

RECIPIENT SELECTION AND MANAGEMENT

【 】 INDICATIONS

Cardiac transplantation remains the treatment of choice for patients with end-stage cardiac disease with severe functional limitation (usually New York Heart Association [NYHA] functional class III or IV), whose symptoms are refractory to management with medications, and in some cases with cardiac resynchronization therapy, and surgical intervention. Table 27–1 lists the currently accepted indications for transplantation. The primary indication for adult heart transplantation today continues to be equally divided between coronary artery disease and nonischemic cardiomyopathy, and this has not changed appreciably over the past 10 years (Fig. 27–2).[8]

Although the indications for cardiac transplantation are generally well accepted, identifying the subgroup of patients most likely to derive a benefit from transplantation can be challenging. Advances in medical and device therapy for heart failure over the past decade, including the judicious use of β blockers in severe heart failure patients, the introduction of aldosterone antagonists, and the increasing use of implantable defibrillators and cardiac resynchronization therapy, have resulted in significant improvements in the 1-year survival rates of patients with advanced heart failure (NYHA Functional Class III–IV).[9–12] Patients treated with aggressive medical and device therapy have 1-year survival rates approaching 90 percent and are comparable to 1-year survival rates following transplantation.[8,12] Addition-

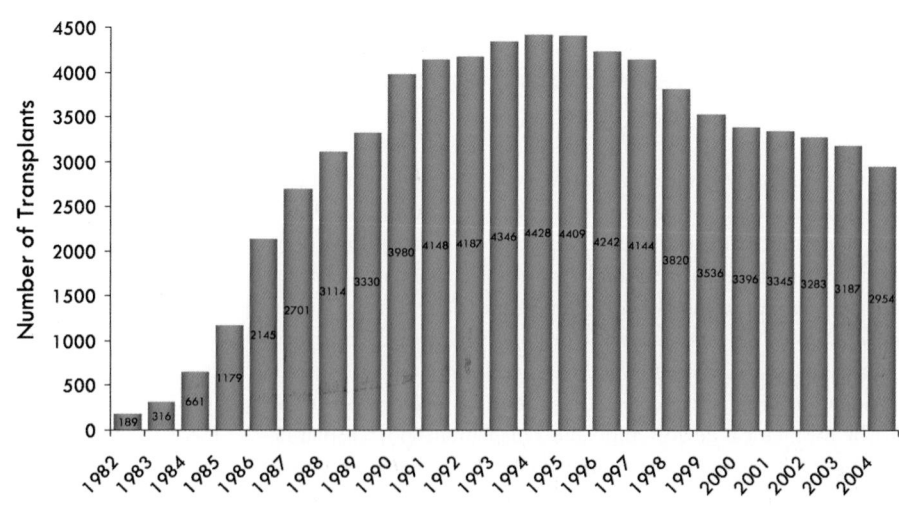

FIGURE 27–1. Number of heart transplants performed worldwide. The numbers reflect only those transplants that are reported to the ISHLT Transplant Registry. *Source: From Taylor DO, Edward LB, Boucek MM, et al.[8] Used with permission.*

TABLE 27–1

Commonly Accepted Indications for Cardiac Transplantation

Systolic heart failure (defined by LVEF <35%) with severe functional limitations and/or refractory symptoms despite maximal medical therapy
- New York Heart Association Functional Class III–IV
- Maximal oxygen uptake ($\dot{V}O_2$ max) of ≤12–14 mL/kg/min exercise testing

Cardiogenic shock not expected to recover

Ischemic heart disease with intractable angina not amenable to surgical or percutaneous revascularization and refractory to maximal medical therapy

Intractable ventricular arrhythmias, uncontrolled with standard antiarrhythmic therapy, device therapy, and/or ablative therapy

Severe symptomatic hypertrophic or restrictive cardiomyopathy

Congenital heart disease in which severe fixed pulmonary hypertension is not a complication

Cardiac tumors with low likelihood of metastasis

LVEF, left ventricular ejection fraction; $\dot{V}O_2$, peak oxygen consumption.
SOURCE: Adapted from Steinman TI, Becker BN, Frost AE, et al. Guidelines for the referral and management of patients eligible for solid organ transplantation. Transplantation. May 15 2001;71(9):1189–1204.

ally, a small percentage of patients exhibit improvements in their left ventricular systolic function and exercise tolerance following mitral valve surgery or high-risk coronary bypass surgery aimed at restoring blood flow to areas of hibernating myocardium. Electrophysiological mapping and ablative therapy can provide control of incessant ventricular arrhythmias in a subset of patients that have failed or cannot tolerate anti-arrhythmic therapy. Finally, it is important to identify potentially reversible causes of cardiomyopathy as summarized in Table 27–2. Cessation of excessive alcohol intake or slowing of the ventricular rate with drugs or atrioventricular (AV) nodal ablation in patients with rapid heart rates occasionally results in a dramatic reversal of the heart failure.[13] Although more controversial, some centers continue to treat biopsy-proven acute lymphocytic myocarditis

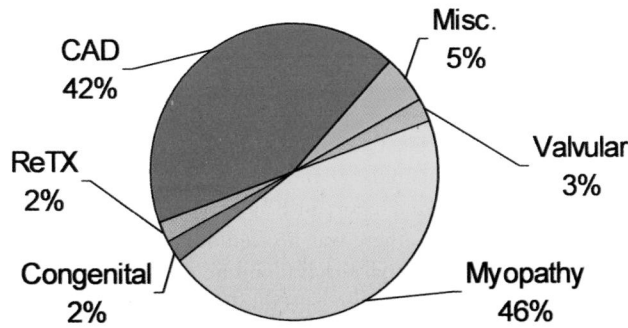

FIGURE 27–2. Primary indication for adult heart transplantation between January 1, 2001, and June 6, 2005. CAD, coronary artery disease; ReTx, retransplantation. *Source: From Taylor DO, Edward LB, Boucek MM, et al.[8] Used with permission.*

TABLE 27–2

Potentially Reversible Causes of Heart Failure

Ischemic left ventricular dysfunction with presence of hibernating myocardium
Cardiomyopathy secondary to
- Lymphocytic myocarditis
- Sarcoidosis
- Tachycardia
- Alcohol

with high-dose steroids and giant-cell myocarditis with immunosuppression. This approach is also used for sarcoid cardiomyopathy. Thus, many transplant centers have found that as many as 30 to 50 percent of patients referred for heart transplants can be stabilized by an aggressive, multidisciplinary approach, such that transplantation can be avoided or delayed. As a result, most heart transplant centers have evolved into centers for heart failure management in addition to providing the opportunity for transplantation.

Role of Exercise Testing

In patients undergoing transplant evaluation, measurement of peak oxygen consumption ($\dot{V}O_2$) during cardiopulmonary exercise testing provides an objective assessment of functional capacity and is more useful than NYHA classification, ejection fraction, or other markers of heart failure severity, for assessing prognosis and determining the optimal timing of listing for transplantation. Patients with a peak $\dot{V}O_2$ of more than 14 mL/kg/min have 1- and 2-year survival rates that are comparable or better than those achieved with transplantation, and patients should be medically managed and undergo serial exercise testing.[14] Patients with a peak $\dot{V}O_2$ between 10 and 14 mL/kg/min constitute an intermediate risk group in which continued medical therapy may offer a survival benefit similar to heart transplantation among selected patients that are able to tolerate β blockers, have low-risk Heart Failure Survival Scores (HFSS's), and have the protection of an internal defibrillator.[15,16] The HFSS is a predictive model calculated from seven prognostic variables that are commonly obtained during the transplant evaluation process (Table 27–3).[16] In patients tolerating β blockers, a peak $\dot{V}O_2$ of <12 mL/kg/min has been suggested as an appropriate threshold to identify individuals that are likely to derive a survival benefit from transplantation.[17] Patients with a peak $\dot{V}O_2$ of ≤ 10 mL/kg/min, regardless of β blocker use, have significantly reduced survival rates with medical therapy compared to cardiac transplantation, and these patients should be listed for transplantation.[14,18] The International Society for Heart and Lung Transplantation (ISHLT) has recently published guidelines that address the use of cardiopulmonary stress testing results to guide transplant listing (Table 27–4).[19]

CONTRAINDICATIONS

Appropriate candidates for cardiac transplantation should have severe functional limitations and limited life expectancy from their heart disease and should be free of established contraindications (Table 27–5). As many of the exclusion criteria are relative con-

● TABLE 27–3

Heart Failure Survival Score

VARIABLE	COEFFICIENT
Ischemic cardiomyopathy (1 = yes, 0 = no)	+0.6931
Resting heart rate (beats/min)	+0.0216
Left ventricular ejection fraction (%)	−0.0464
Mean blood pressure (mmHg)	−0.0255
IVCD (QRS ≥ 120 msec) (1 = yes, 0 = no)	+0.6083
Peak $\dot{V}O_2$ (mL/kg/min)	−0.0546
Serum sodium (mEq/L)	−0.0470

IVCD, intraventricular conduction delay.
The Heart Failure Survival Score (HFSS) is calculated by taking the sums of the products of each component variable's value and its model coefficient. Patients are categorized into low (≥ 8.10), medium (7.20–8.09), and high-risk strata (<7.20) on the basis of their total score. One-year transplant-free survival rates in the original validation sample were 88%, 60%, and 35% for low-, medium-, and high-risk HFSS strata.

● TABLE 27–4

ISHLT Guidelines for Use of Cardiopulmonary Stress Testing to Guide Transplant Listing

Class I:
1. A maximal cardiopulmonary exercise (CPX) test is defined as one with a respiratory exchange ratio (RER) >1.05 and achievement of an anaerobic threshold on optimal pharmacologic therapy (level of evidence: B).
2. In patients intolerant of a β blocker, a cutoff for peak $\dot{V}O_2$ of ≤14 mL/kg/min should be used to guide listing (level of evidence: B).
3. In the presence of a β-blocker, a cutoff for peak $\dot{V}O_2$ of ≤12 mL/kg/min should be used to guide listing level of evidence: B).

Class IIa:
1. In young patients (<50 y) and women, it is reasonable to consider using alternate standards in conjunction with peak $\dot{V}O_2$ to guide listing, including percent of predicted (≤50 percent) peak $\dot{V}O_2$ (level of evidence: B).

Class IIb:
1. In the presence of a submaximal CPX test (RER <1.05), use of ventilation equivalent of carbon dioxide (V_E/VCO_2) slope of >35 as a determinant in listing for transplantation may be considered (level of evidence: C).
2. In obese (body mass index [BMI] >30 kg/m²) patients, adjusting peak $\dot{V}O_2$ to lean body mass may be considered. A lean body mass–adjusted peak $\dot{V}O_2$ of <19 mL/kg/min can serve as an optimal threshold to guide prognosis (level of evidence: B).

Class III:
1. Listing patients based solely on the criterion of a peak oxygen consumption ($\dot{V}O_2$) measurement should not be performed (level of evidence: C).

ISHL, International Society for Heart and Lung Transplantation; V_E, volume of expired gas; VCO_2, carbon dioxide elimination.
SOURCE: From Mehra MR, Kobashigawa J, Starling R, et al.[19]

● TABLE 27–5

Contraindications to Cardiac Transplantation

Irreversible severe pulmonary arterial hypertension
- Pulmonary vascular resistance (PVR) >5 Wood units
- Pulmonary vascular resistance index (PVRI) >6
- Transpulmonary gradient >16–20 mmHg
- PA systolic pressure >50–60 mmHg or >50% of systemic pressures

Advanced age (>70 years)
Active systemic infection
Active malignancy or recent malignancy with high risk of recurrence
Diabetes mellitus with:
- End-organ damage (neuropathy, nephropathy, proliferative retinopathy)
- Poor glycemic control (HbA1c >7.5)

Marked obesity (BMI >30 kg/m² or >140% of ideal body weight)
Severe peripheral arterial disease not amenable to revascularization
Systemic process with high probability of recurrence in the transplanted heart
- Amyloidosis
- Sarcoidosis
- Hemochromatosis

Irreversible severe renal,[a] hepatic,[a] or pulmonary disease
Recent or unresolved pulmonary infarction
Psychosocial factors that may impact on patient's ability to comply with complex medical regimen
- History of poor medical compliance
- Lack of adequate support system
- Uncontrolled psychiatric illness (anxiety, depression, psychosis)
- Active or recent substance abuse (alcohol, tobacco, or illicit drugs)

BMI, body mass index; HBA1C, glycosated hemoglobin; PA, pulmonary artery.
[a]Unless combined heart-kidney or heart-liver transplant is considered.

traindications, the degree to which they are interpreted and applied may vary considerably among different transplant programs.

Advanced Age

The upper age limit for cardiac transplant recipients has expanded considerably over the past decade, with many centers advancing their official chronological age limits to 65 years and considering highly selected patients older than age 65 on a case-by-case basis. In a recent single-center report of 881 patients transplanted between 1992 and 2002, there was no significant difference in the 1-, 5-, and 10-year actuarial survival and no significant difference in the incidence of infection or rejection among the 63 recipients (7.2 percent) who were older than age 65 years at the time of their transplant, compared to a matched group of patients younger than age 65.[20] There is also limited data to suggest that carefully selected patients 70 years of age or older also have acceptable outcomes following heart transplantation, with 1- and 4-year survival rates of 93 percent and 74 percent.[21] It is now recognized that physiological age may be more important than chronological age with respect to survival and rehabilitation potential. As a result many programs are now moving away from fixed upper age limits and instead focus on a patient's functional status, integrity of major organ systems, and presence of comorbidities that might impact survival, rehabilitation potential, and quality of life. In addition to these considerations, the selection of appropriate transplant candidates must also take into consideration the optimal allocation of scare resources. In their recently published guidelines for selection of appropriate cardiac transplant candidates, the ISHLT has recommended that patients younger than 70 years of age should be considered for cardiac transplantation (class I recommendation, level of evidence C). Carefully selected patients older than 70 years of age may be considered for cardiac transplantation, but use of an alternative-type program (i.e., use of suboptimal organs that would traditionally be rejected) should be pursued in these patients (class IIb recommendation, level of evidence C).[19] Examples of organs allocated to alternative list recipients include organs from older donors, donors with positive hepatitis serology, as well as organs with coronary artery disease, left ventricular dysfunction, or hypertrophy.

Irreversible Pulmonary Hypertension

Pulmonary hypertension from chronic elevations of left ventricular end-diastolic pressure and neurohormonal activation is a common complication of longstanding heart failure and can result in irreversible changes to the pulmonary vasculature over time if left unrecognized and untreated. Early in the years of clinical experience with heart transplantation, it was found that a normal donor RV is unable to increase its external workload acutely to overcome elevated pulmonary vascular resistance (PVR), resulting in acute RV failure and cardiogenic shock postoperatively. Elevated PVR remains a strong risk factor for RV failure and early postoperative mortality in the modern era. Potential heart transplant candidates must undergo measurements of pulmonary artery pressures and calculation of PVR in the cardiac catheterization laboratory or in the intensive care unit as part of their initial transplant evaluation. A pulmonary artery systolic pressure >50 to 60 mmHg, a PVR value of >5 Wood units (approximately 400 dynes $\cdot$ s/cm^5), a PVR index of >6, or a transpulmonary gradient >15 to 20 mmHg is usually considered prohibitive of successful heart transplantation unless the pulmonary artery pressures and PVR can be reduced to acceptable levels while maintaining a systolic blood pressure >85 mmHg.[19] Pharmacologic interventions for reducing PVR include administration of IV nitroprusside, prostaglandin E$_1$, nesiritide, inhaled nitric oxide and positive inotropic and vasodilator agents such as milrinone or dobutamine. Reversibility of pulmonary artery pressures is usually documented in the cardiac catheterization laboratory at the time of the initial hemodynamic measurements, but some patients require treatment with inotropic agents, IV vasodilators, and/or inhaled nitric oxide for a period of 24 to 48 hours prior to achieving acceptable hemodynamic parameters prior to transplantation. Occasionally, mechanical support with an intraaortic balloon pump and/or left ventricular assist device (LVAD) has been used as a bridge to transplantation in patients

with severe, refractory pulmonary hypertension. The ISHLT guidelines recommend that diagnostic right heart catheterization be performed near the time of listing for cardiac transplantation and at 3- to 6-month intervals in patients who are listed (class I recommendation, level of evidence C).[19]

Active Infection and Malignancy

Patients must be free of active infection and malignancy prior to transplantation because both processes can be exacerbated by the immunosuppression that is required posttransplant to prevent rejection. The presence of an active systemic infection or severe localized infection is often considered a temporary contraindication to transplantation. Patients with a history of infection should not be activated or re-activated on the transplant waiting list until there is sufficient evidence that the infection is resolved or under control, as demonstrated by absence of fevers for a minimum of 72 hours on appropriate antibiotics, negative blood cultures, and resolving signs or symptoms of infection.

The evaluation of patients with chronic viral infections such as hepatitis B, hepatitis C, or HIV remains controversial. Although most transplant centers accept candidates that are hepatitis C–antibody positive, asymptomatic patients with evidence of hepatitis B surface antigenemia have a high risk of developing subsequent clinical liver disease with the institution of immunosuppression and are considered poor transplant candidates by many centers.[22,23] Although HIV infection was once considered an absolute contraindication to transplantation because of concerns that immunosuppressive therapy may hasten the progression of HIV disease and increase the risk of opportunistic infections or malignancy, these concerns have not been validated to date. It has now been suggested that the presence of HIV infection in itself should not serve as a contraindication for heart transplantation but that HIV infected patients should be carefully evaluated for extent of disease and presence of opportunistic infections.[24] Although some heart transplant centers have now successfully transplanted a few patients with HIV infection, the overall experience with this group remains limited.[25]

In general, patients with active malignancies, with the exception of nonmelanoma cutaneous cancers, primary cardiac tumors restricted to the heart, and low-grade neoplasms of the prostate, should be excluded from cardiac transplantation. However, preexisting neoplasms are diverse with respect to their response to therapy and risk of recurrence. Consultation with an oncologist should be obtained for any patient with a history of previous or active malignancy to assess their risk of tumor recurrence. The ISHLT guidelines recommend that cardiac transplantation should be considered when tumor recurrence is low based on tumor type, response to therapy, and negative metastatic workup. The specific amount of time to wait before transplantation after neoplasm remission depends on the aforementioned factors, and no arbitrary time period for observation should be used (class I recommendation, level of evidence C).[19]

Coexisting Conditions

Potential cardiac transplant recipients are screened for the existence of other conditions or systemic diseases that may independently limit their survival or rehabilitation potential. *Obesity* has been associated with an increased risk of infection, wound healing complications, metabolic derangements, rejection, cardiac allograft vasculopathy, and mortality following heart transplantation.[26–28] Furthermore, the need for corticosteroids and frequent further weight gain after transplantation compound these problems.[29] In severely obese patients, it is reasonable to recommend weight loss to achieve a body mass index (BMI) of <30 kg/m^2 or percent ideal body weight of <140 percent prior to listing for cardiac transplantation (class IIa recommendation, Level of Evidence C).[19]

The presence of preexisting insulin-requiring *diabetes mellitus* was once considered a relative contraindication to heart transplantation because of concern over decreased survival, increased infection rates, and worsening glycemic control with the initiation of corticosteroid immunosuppression. In recent years, several reports have demonstrated similar short- and long-term survival among diabetic and nondiabetic patients, as well as similar rates of infection, rejection, renal function, and cardiac allograft vasculopathy.[30–32] Although the safety and efficacy of heart transplantation in very carefully selected patients has been documented, most transplant programs continue to consider the presence of diabetes with end-organ damage (proliferative retinopathy, neuropathy, or nephropathy) a relative contraindication to transplantation. Because corticosteroid therapy may worsen glycemic control in patients with preexisting diabetes, the presence of poorly controlled diabetes, as manifested by a hemoglobin A1c value of >7.5 despite aggressive diabetic education and management, is also considered a relative contraindication for transplantation.

Other comorbid conditions must be considered on an individual basis, but irreversible organ dysfunction such as *pulmonary fibrosis,* severe *emphysema,* and *hepatic* or *renal dysfunction* out of proportion to that predicted as a consequence of severe heart failure are strong relative contraindications. Selected patients with irreversible renal or hepatic dysfunction may undergo combined heart and kidney or heart and liver transplantation.[33,34]

Advanced noncardiac *vascular disease,* in the form of symptomatic cerebrovascular disease or peripheral vascular disease that is not amenable to revascularization, is considered a relative contraindication to transplantation if the condition is expected to limit survival or impair rehabilitation following transplantation.

Experience has shown that *pulmonary infarcts* have a high probability of becoming pulmonary abscesses after the institution of immunosuppression. For this reason potential recipients who sustain a pulmonary infarction usually are temporarily removed from the waiting list until the infarct resolves radiographically.

Psychosocial Factors

All cardiac transplant candidates should undergo a careful psychosocial assessment with emphasis on current and previous substance abuse history, compliance with medical therapy and follow up, comprehension of and ability to follow a complex medical regimen, and adequacy of social support. Patients should also be screened for psychiatric conditions that may affect the aforementioned factors. Active substance abuse, including tobacco, excessive alcohol, and illicit drug use, is widely accepted as a contraindication for heart transplantation. Many transplant centers require documented abstinence from substance abuse for a period of 6 to 12 months prior to transplantation. In addition, patients may be

required to complete a structured rehabilitation program prior to being eligible for transplantation.

DONOR SELECTION AND MANAGEMENT

Acceptance of the concept of irreversible brain death, both legally and medically, has been central to the emergence of organ transplantation in the modern era. The most widely accepted set of guidelines for the determination of brain death was set out in the President's Commission Report in 1980 and are summarized in Table 27–6.[35] The most common causes of brain death include intracranial hemorrhage, blunt traumatic injury to the head, penetrating traumatic injury, and anoxic brain injury. Patients with irreversible brain injury accompanied by the intent to withdraw life support are considered to be potential organ donors.

DONOR EVALUATION

Once a potential donor is identified, the procurement process is initiated by contacting the local, or *host,* organ procurement organization (OPO). The host OPO is responsible for obtaining consent for organ donation, verifying pronouncement of death, evaluating and managing the donor, and equitably allocating the donor organs. The process of donor evaluation begins with a detailed history and physical examination, focusing on cause of death, past medical history, donor height and weight, and clinical course. Basic laboratory studies, including a complete blood count, metabolic panel, ABO blood typing, and viral serologies (hepatitis B and C, HIV, human T-cell lymphotropic virus, Ebstein-Barr virus [EBV], and cytomegalovirus [CMV]) are ordered. Additional studies include a chest x-ray, 12-lead ECG, and echocardiogram. To be considered suitable donors

TABLE 27–6

Criteria for Determining Brain Death

Clinical Evaluation
Mechanism of brain injury is sufficient to account for irreversible loss of brain function
Absence of reversible causes of CNS depression
- CNS depressant drugs
- Hypothermia (<32°C [85°F])
- Hypotension (MAP <55 mmHg)
Absence of neuromuscular blocking drugs that may confound the results of the neurologic exam
No spontaneous movements, motor responses, or posturing
No gag or cough reflexes
No corneal or pupillary light reflexes
No oculovestibular reflex (cold calorics)
Confirmatory Tests
Apnea test for minimum of five minutes showing:
- No respiratory movements
- P_{CO_2} >55 mmHg
- pH <7.40
No intracranial blood flow

CNS, central nervous system; MAP, mean aortic pressure.

for cardiac transplantation, brain-dead individuals must meet certain minimum criteria (Table 27–7). In more recent years, these criteria have been liberalized because of an increasing organ demand and severe shortage of available donors. Newer criteria for donor selection permit use of marginal donors, particularly when used for higher-risk patients such as those with higher than expected mortality while awaiting transplantation or those with comorbid conditions such as advanced age or positive hepatitis serology.[36] Most cardiac donors are younger than age 55, but older donors may be used selectively in critically ill recipients or allocated to alternative list recipients. There should be no evidence of severe cardiothoracic trauma or cardiac puncture. An initial echocardiogram is performed to identify significant structural heart disease such as left ventricular hypertrophy or dysfunction, occlusive coronary artery disease, valvular dysfunction, or congenital lesions. Donors with these conditions are typically excluded, but selected marginal organs can also be allocated to higher-risk recipients. Angiography is performed to exclude significant coronary artery disease (CAD) in male donors older than age 45 and in female donors older than age 50 but may also be performed in younger patients with multiple traditional risk factors for CAD. Patients with active malignancy (excluding non-melanocytic skin cancers and certain isolated brain tumors) or severe systemic infections are typically excluded. Finally, donors routinely are screened serologically for HIV and hepatitis B and C. Although the HIV-positivity remains an exclusion criterion for organ donation, hepatitis B and C positive donors may be allocated to selected higher-risk patients or matched to seropositive recipients.

TABLE 27–7

Donor Selection Criteria

Age <55 y
Absence of significant structural abnormalities
- Left ventricular hypertrophy (wall thickness >13 mm by echocardiography)
- Significant valvular dysfunction
- Significant congenital cardiac abnormality
- Significant coronary artery disease
Adequate physiologic function of donor heart
- Left ventricular ejection fraction (LVEF) ≥45% or
- Achievement of target hemodynamic criteria after hormonal resuscitation and hemodynamic management
  - Mean arterial pressure (MAP) >60 mmHg
  - Pulmonary capillary wedge pressure (PCWP) 8–12 mmHg
  - Cardiac index >2.4 L/min × m²
  - Central venous pressure 4–12 mmHg
  - Systemic vascular resistance 800–1200 dyne/sec•cm⁵
  - Dopamine or dobutamine requirement <10 mg/kg/min
Negative hepatitis C antibody, hepatitis B surface antigen, and HIV serologies
Absence of active malignancy[a] or overwhelming infection

[a]Except in the case of nonmelanoma skin cancers and certain primary brain tumors.

DONOR MANAGEMENT

Once brain death has been determined and the patient has been identified as a potential organ donor, the main goals of organ donor management are to ensure optimal organ function by providing volume resuscitation, optimizing cardiac output, normalizing systemic vascular resistance, maintaining adequate oxygenation, correcting anemia, acid base, and electrolyte abnormalities, and correcting hormonal imbalances that occur after brain death and that can impair circulatory function. Standardized algorithms incorporating early use of invasive hemodynamic monitoring along with aggressive hemodynamic management and hormonal resuscitation with insulin, corticosteroids, triiodothyronine, and arginine vasopressin have been proposed to improve cardiac donor management and maximize organ use, particularly in patients with a left ventricular ejection fraction of <45 percent on initial echocardiography.[36]

Currently, most donor hearts are harvested from the donor by a transplant donor team from the transplantation center and transported back to the center for implantation. A cold ischemic period of 4 to 6 hours in adult hearts is generally considered safe. This requirement for short ischemic times leads to the rationale for geographic subdivision into OPOs for cardiac allografts despite the drive for a national list for other organs.

Currently, <50 percent of potential organ donors in the United States become actual donors.[37] Despite ongoing efforts to increase the identification of potential donors, to increase the consent rate among eligible donors, to expand donor selection criteria, and to maximize potential donor organ function, heart transplantation will likely remain a donor-limited field for the foreseeable future.

ORGAN MATCHING AND ALLOCATION

Donor-recipient matching is performed on the basis of ABO blood group compatibility and overall body size comparability within 20 percent of body weight. Although the benefit of matching donor organs and recipients with respect to human leukocyte antigens (HLAs) has been well established in renal transplantation, HLA prospective crossmatching is reserved for presensitized heart transplant recipients, or those with >10 to 20 percent reactivity to a standard panel of common donor antigens, because of shorter tolerated ischemic times in explanted hearts. Although most transplant centers obtain routine retrospective crossmatching, the association between the degree of HLA mismatch and the risk of subsequent rejection and patient survival remains controversial. Some studies demonstrate a modest effect of HLA mismatch on patient outcomes,[38,39] whereas others show no correlation between the two.[40]

Allocation of thoracic organs in the United States is made according to the recipient's priority on the United Network for Organ Sharing (UNOS) waiting list and geographic distance from the donor. Priority on the recipient waiting list is determined by a recipient's assigned status code and time accrued within a status code. In general, patients with the highest medical urgency and lowest expected short-term survival are assigned a higher status code (Table 27–8).

Donor hearts are first offered to local status 1 patients and then extended to status 1 patients within a 500-mile radius of the donor

TABLE 27-8

Recipient Prioritization for Heart Transplantation

Status 1A
- Mechanical circulatory support
  - Ventricular assist device until clinically stable or up to 30 days[a]
  - Total artificial heart
  - Intraaortic balloon pump
  - Extracorporeal membrane oxygenator (ECMO)
- Mechanical ventilation
- Continuous infusion of single high-dose inotrope or multiple inotropes, in addition to continuous hemodynamic monitoring of left ventricular filling pressures
- Exceptional provision for patients with medical urgency not meeting above criteria

Status 1B
- Ventricular assist device beyond 30 days
- Continuous infusion of intravenous inotropes

Status 2
- Any candidate not meeting criteria for Status 1A or 1B

[a]Prioritization may be extended beyond 30 days for patients with objective medical evidence of significant device-related complications such as thromboembolism, device infection, mechanical failure, and/or life-threatening ventricular arrhythmias.

hospital (zone A). If no eligible recipients are identified, the organ is offered to local status 2 patients. This process repeats in a sequence of *zones* delineated by subsequent concentric circles of 1000, and 1500 mile radii from the donor hospital.

SURGICAL TECHNIQUE

The donor heart is explanted, or *harvested* by a surgical team at a hospital usually remote from the transplant center, and this surgery must be coordinated with the requirements of other surgical teams procuring nonthoracic organs for transplantation. The donor heart is first arrested with cardioplegic solution. The original surgical technique for orthotopic heart transplantation, or *biatrial* technique, was originally described by Lower and Shumway in 1960.[4] In this procedure both the donor and recipient hearts are removed by transecting the atria at the midatrial level, leaving the multiple pulmonary venous connections to the left atrium (LA) intact in the posterior wall of the LA and then transecting the aorta and pulmonary artery just above their respective semilunar valves. The explanted heart is topically cooled in an iced preservation solution; it is then placed in a secure con-

tainer and transported expeditiously to the transplant center. Ischemic times average 3 to 4 hours.

Implantation of the heart in the orthotopic position begins with reanastomosis at the midatrial level, beginning with the atrial septum (Fig. 27–3). Efforts are made to include a generous cuff of donor right atrium so that the sinoatrial node will be included. The great vessels are connected just above the semilunar valves. In recent years there has been a move to alter the original bicaval technique by leaving the donor atria intact and making anastomoses at the level of the superior and inferior vena cavae and pulmonary veins.[41,42] This *bicaval* technique (Fig. 27–4) results in less distortion of atrioventricular geometry, resulting in improved atrial and ventricular function, less AV valve regurgitation, decreased incidence of atrial arrhythmias, and decreased incidence of donor sinus node dysfunction and heart block requiring permanent pacemaker implantation.[43–45] Disadvantages of the bicaval technique include slightly prolonged ischemic time and development of symptomatic superior vena caval anastomotic stenosis, a rare complication occurring in 2.4 percent of cases in a single-center study.[46]

Immediate postoperative care differs little from that after more routine heart surgery except for the institution of immunosuppression (described below) and the need for chronotropic support of the donor sinoatrial node for the first 2 to 3 postoperative days, usually with temporary pacemaker support but occasionally with infusions of isoproterenol or dopamine. Postoperative bradycardia usually results from sinus node dysfunction from surgical trauma, ischemia to the sinus node, or pretransplant use of amiodarone.[47] Most cases resolve within weeks to months, and theophylline has been shown to increase the heart rate and facilitate withdrawal of

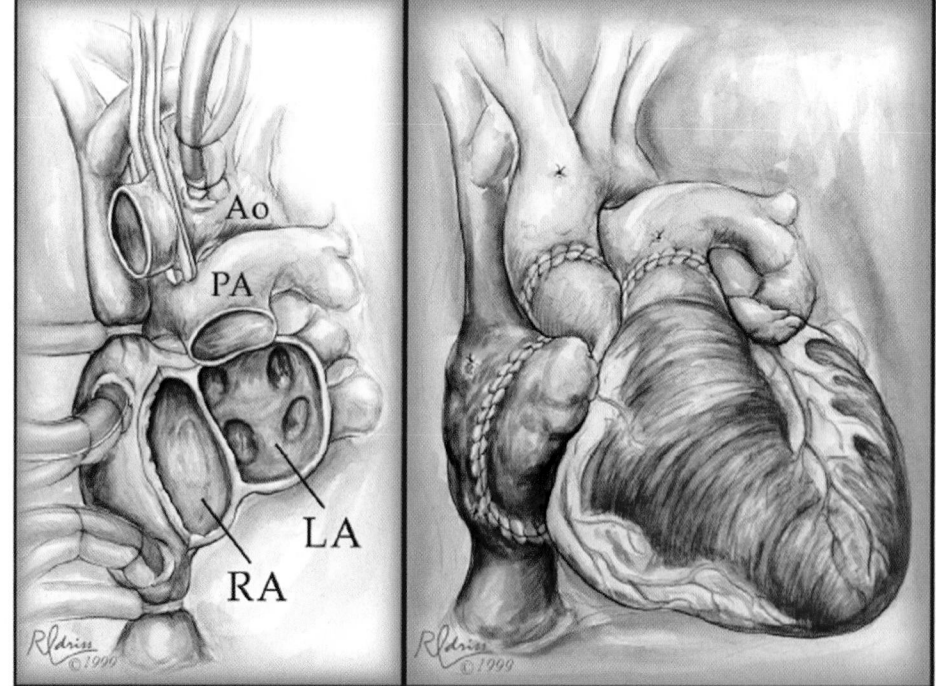

FIGURE 27-3. Original biatrial technique for orthotopic heart transplantation. The *left panel* shows the completed recipient cardiectomy with the recipient atria transected at the midatrial level. The *right panel* shows the completed reanastomosis of the donor heart. Ao, aorta; LA, left atrium; PA, pulmonary artery; RA, right atrium. *Source: Used with permission from Rachid Idriss.*

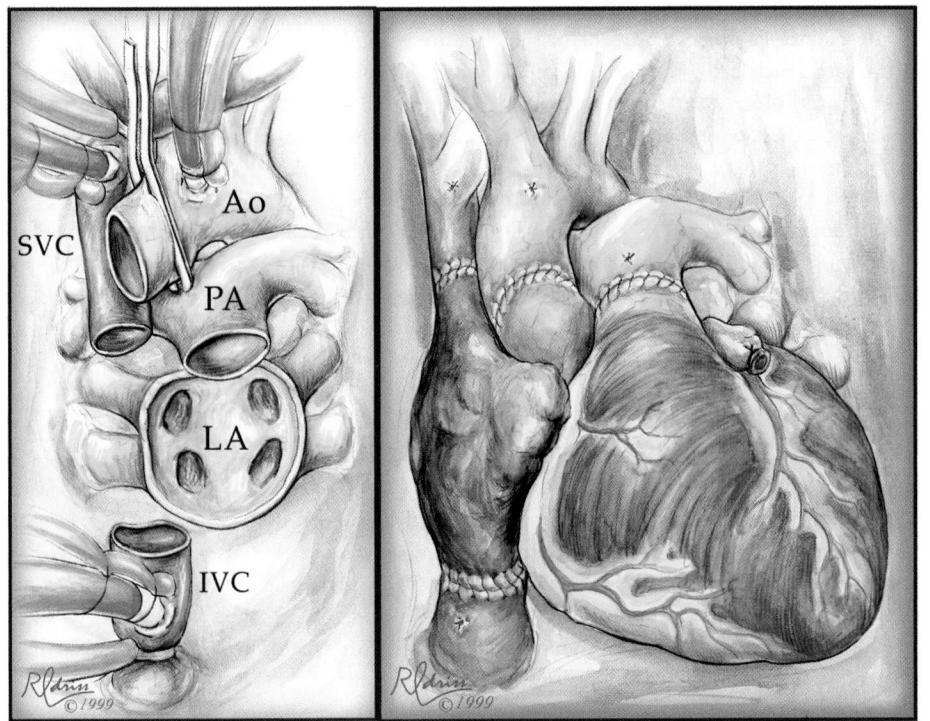

FIGURE 27–4. Bicaval technique for orthotopic heart transplantation. The *left panel* shows the completed recipient cardiectomy. The recipient atria are completed removed except for except for a cuff of tissue around the pulmonary vein orifices. The SVC and IVC are transected at their junction with the RA. The *right panel* shows the completed anastomoses of the donor heart at the level of the SVC, IVC and pulmonary veins. Ao, aorta; IVC, inferior vena cava; LA, left atrium; PA, pulmonary artery; SVC, superior vena cava. *Source: Used with permission from Rachid Idriss.*

chronotropic support in many patients.[48] The incidence of refractory bradycardia requiring permanent pacemaker implantation is between 10 and 20 percent with the bicaval technique and less than 10 percent with the bicaval technique.[44] Uncomplicated patients are discharged from the hospital as early as 7 to 10 days, postoperatively.

PHYSIOLOGY OF THE TRANSPLANTED HEART

The transplanted heart is initially completely denervated. Following recovery of donor sinus node function within the first 2 to 3 postoperative days, the denervated donor heart exhibits a faster resting heart rate (usually between 95 to 110 beats/min) caused by the intrinsic tachycardic rate of the sinus node and absence of the counter-regulatory effects of the parasympathetic system. Cardiac denervation has several important clinical manifestations. First, the cardiac allograft is slower to increase its heart rate in response to exercise and exhibits a slower heart rate recovery. At the onset of exercise, an increase in venous return results in a an increased stroke volume in accordance with the Frank-Starling principle, in which increased stretch or tension on cardiac muscle results in an increased force of contraction. Later in exercise circulating peripheral catecholamines provide chronotropic support. Second, many heart transplant patients will not experience angina with ischemia of the cardiac allograft and may present instead with congestive heart failure caused by graft dysfunction, myocardial infarction, or sudden death. Third, drugs that act primarily through the auto-

nomic nervous system will have little to no effect on the denervated heart. For example, atropine works via a vagolytic mechanism to increase heart rate and is ineffective when used to increase heart rate in the transplanted heart. Isoproterenol is better suited for this purpose because of its direct effect on β receptors, causing both increased chronotropy and inotropy. Reinnervation of the cardiac allograft is felt to occur after the first year, but the timing and degree of reinnervation is highly variable.

POSTOPERATIVE MANAGEMENT

IMMUNOSUPPRESSION

General Principles

Most clinically used immunosuppressive regimens consist of a combination of several agents used concurrently and use several general principles. The first general principle is that immune reactivity and tendency toward graft rejection are highest early (within the first 3–6 months) after graft implantation and decrease with time. Thus, most regimens employ the highest levels of immunosuppression immediately after surgery and decrease those levels over the first year, eventually settling on the lowest maintenance levels of suppression that are compatible with preventing graft rejection and minimizing drug toxicities. The second general principle is to use low doses of several drugs without overlapping toxicities in preference to higher (and more toxic) doses of fewer drugs whenever feasible. The third principle is that too much or too intense immunosuppression is undesirable because it leads to a myriad of undesirable effects, such as susceptibility to infection and malignancy. Finding the right balance between over- and under-immunosuppression in an individual patient is truly an art that uses science.

Induction Therapy

Currently, approximately 50 percent of transplant programs employ a strategy of augmented immunosuppression, or *induction* therapy, with antilymphocyte antibodies during the early postoperative period. The goal of induction therapy is to provide intense immunosuppression when the risk of allograft rejection is highest. Additionally, induction therapy allows delayed initiation of nephrotoxic immunosuppressive drugs in patients with compromised renal function following surgery. Agents used for induction therapy include cytolytic agents such as the murine monoclonal antibody ornithine-ketoacid transaminase (OKT3) or polyclonal antithymocyte or antilymphocyte agents (Atgam, Thymoglobulin). These agents may reduce the risk of early rejection but have been associated with an increased risk of infection.[49,50] In recent years, the use of anti-interleukin-2 (IL-2) receptor antagonists such as daclizumab or basiliximab has increased. These agents exhibit their immunosuppressive effects by inhibiting IL-2–mediated proliferation of activated T-lymphocytes. In a multicenter, placebo-controlled randomized trial, use of daclizumab reduced the rate of moderate or severe cellular rejection among heart transplant patients treated with standard immunosuppression (cyclosporine, mycophenolate mofetil, and corticosteroids) without increasing the incidence of opportunistic infection or cancer at 1 year. However, among patients receiving daclizumab induction, there was an increased risk of fatal infection when cytolytic therapy was concomitantly used.[51]

Maintenance Immunosuppression

Most maintenance immunosuppressive protocols employ a three-drug regimen consisting of a calcineurin-inhibitor (cyclosporine or tacrolimus), an antiproliferative agent (mycophenolate mofetil or azathioprine), and corticosteroids. The calcineurin inhibitors exert their immunosuppressive effects by blocking calcium dependent signal transduction via calcineurin and inhibiting IL-2 production, therefore preventing T-cell differentiation and proliferation. Cyclosporine and tacrolimus inhibit calcineurin by forming complexes with different binding proteins. Since the introduction of cyclosporine in the early 1980s, the calcineurin inhibitors have remained the cornerstone of maintenance immunosuppressive therapy in solid organ transplantation. In recent years the use of tacrolimus (Prograf) in heart transplantation has increased. Initial experience with this agent in two randomized, multicenter clinical trials in the United States and Europe demonstrated that this drug has similar efficacy to cyclosporine in preventing cardiac allograft rejection when used in combination with azathioprine and corticosteroids. However, the calcineurin-inhibitor associated metabolic derangements appear to be significantly attenuated with tacrolimus use. Patients on tacrolimus, compared to cyclosporine, have less hypertension, less hyperlipidemia, and similar incidences of renal dysfunction, posttransplant diabetes mellitus, and infection.[52,53] In a more recent multicenter randomized trial comparing the use of tacrolimus plus mycophenolate mofetil, tacrolimus plus sirolimus, and cyclosporine plus mycophenolate mofetil in de novo cardiac transplant recipients, there was no significant difference among the three groups with respect to the primary endpoint of 6-month incidence of moderate or severe cellular rejection or hemodynamic compromising rejection requiring treatment. However, patients in both tacrolimus groups had a lower probability of experiencing any treated rejection within the first year.[54] Among patients reported to the ISHLT registry, the use of a tacrolimus-based immunosuppressive regimen was also associated with a decreased incidence of treatable rejection and a decreased number of rejection episodes within the first year.[8]

Mycophenolate mofetil (CellCept) has replaced azathioprine (Imuran) as the preferred antiproliferative agent in recent years. It exerts its immunosuppressive effects by blocking purine synthesis and inhibiting proliferation of both T- and B-lymphocytes. In a multicenter, active-controlled, randomized trial, mycophenolate mofetil was compared with azathioprine when used in conjunction with cyclosporine and corticosteroids in de novo heart transplant recipients. Because an IV form of the study drug (myco-

phenolate mofetil) was unavailable at the time of the trial, 11 percent of the patients withdrew before receiving the drug. Survival and rejection were similar in both groups when analyzed in an intention-to-treatment manner. However, among treated patients, mycophenolate mofetil was associated with a significant reduction in both mortality and incidence of treatable rejection at 1 year.[55] In a retrospective analysis of the ISHLT registry, the use of mycophenolate mofetil in patients on a cyclosporine-based immunosuppression protocol was also associated with an actuarial survival benefit at 1 and 3 years when compared with azathioprine.[56]

In recent years, a new class of drugs called *mammalian target of rapamycin (mTOR) inhibitors* has been approved for use in renal transplantation. This new class of drugs, which includes sirolimus (Rapamune) and everolimus (Certican), blocks growth-factor-mediated IL-2 and IL-15-driven proliferation of human T-cells, B-cells, and vascular smooth muscle cells by inhibiting activation of p70S6 kinase and arresting the cell cycle at the G1 to S phase.[57] Compared to azathioprine, both sirolimus and everolimus have been shown to reduce the incidence of acute rejection and to prevent the development of cardiac allograft vasculopathy (CAV) when used in conjunction with cyclosporine and prednisone in de novo heart transplant recipients.[58,59] The mTOR inhibitors have also been used in lieu of either the calcineurin inhibitors or antiproliferative agents in heart transplant recipients with established CAV and in those with moderate to severe renal dysfunction. In patients with CAV, use of sirolimus has been shown to slow disease progression and reduce the incidence of clinically significant cardiac events.[60] Finally, in heart transplant recipients with significant renal impairment, the use of sirolimus allows for minimization or complete withdrawal of the calcineurin inhibitors and results in marked improvement in renal function without an associated increase in the risk of rejection.[61–63] Although the effects of sirolimus on CAV and renal dysfunction are encouraging, the high incidence of side effects requiring drug discontinuation (Table 27–9) is preventing more widespread use of this agent in clinical practice. Everolimus has not yet been approved for clinical use in the United States, but two multicenter, phase III randomized trials are currently underway to assess the efficacy and safety of this drug when used with reduced levels of cyclosporine in de novo heart transplantation.

Most programs also employ glucocorticoids as one of the three immunosuppressive agents, usually in relatively high doses in the early postoperative period and then tapering to low doses or discontinuing the drug after the first 6 to 12 months. The commonly used drugs and their toxicities are outlined in Table 27–9. Recent trends in the use of these drugs are presented in Fig. 27–5. In 2005, the calcineurin inhibitors cyclosporine and tacrolimus were used in equal proportions at one year postoperatively while mycophenolate mofetil remained the predominant cell-cycle agent in use. The mTOR inhibitor sirolimus was used by 13 percent of patients, and 67 percent of patients were still on prednisone at the time of their one year follow-up.[8]

In managing patients on immunosuppressive drug therapy, it is important to be aware of the potential for drug interactions when other agents are added to or deleted from the patient's regimen. A list of the most common and clinically important drug interactions is shown in Table 27–10. Drugs that decrease the metabolism of cyclosporine or tacrolimus increase their drug levels and can potentiate their nephrotoxic effects. Drugs such as the lipid-lowering agents lovastatin, atorvastatin, and simvastatin have decreased clearance and increased drug concentrations when used concurrently with the calcineurin inhibitors, and use of higher doses of these agents in this setting may lead to an increased risk of myopathy and/or rhabdomyolysis. Finally, it is important to keep in mind the potential for changing immunosuppressive drug concentrations when intercurrent renal or hepatic dysfunction exists.

COMPLICATIONS OF IMMUNOSUPPRESSION

The major toxicities associated with each of the immunosuppressive agents used in heart transplantation are listed in Table 27–9. Hypertension, hyperlipidemia, and the development of posttransplant diabetes mellitus are the most common metabolic complications associated with calcineurin-inhibitor use (Table 27–11). Renal dysfunction occurs in up to one-third of individuals and is related to the direct effects of the calcineurin inhibitors on the kidney tubules and from calcineurin-inhibitor mediated vasoconstriction of the afferent arteriole, leading to decreased kidney perfusion. In addition to experiencing drug- and class-specific toxicities, heart transplant patients have a higher risk of developing opportunistic infections and malignancy compared to the general population.

Infection

Infections are the major cause of death during the first postoperative year and remain a threat throughout the life of a chronically immunosuppressed patient. Infections in the first postoperative month are commonly bacterial and typically related to indwelling catheters and wound infections. They involve nosocomial organisms such as *Legionella*, *Staphylococcus*, *Pseudomonas*, *Proteus*, *Klebsiella*, and *Escherichia coli*. These infections typically present in the form of pneumonias, urinary tract infection, sternal wound infections and mediastinitis, and bacteremia. Late infections (those that occur 2 months to 1 year following transplantation) are more diverse. In additional to typical pathogens, transplant patients are susceptible to viruses (particularly cyto-

TABLE 27–9

Immunosuppressive Agents Used in Heart Transplantation

DRUG	TYPICAL DOSE	MAJOR TOXICITIES
Calcineurin Inhibitors		
Cyclosporine	4–8 mg/kg/d in 2 divided doses, titrated to keep therapeutic 12-h trough levels	Renal dysfunction Hypertension Dyslipidemia Hypokalemia and hypomagnesemia Hyperuricemia Neurotoxicity (encephalopathy, seizures, tremors, neuropathy) Gingival hyperplasia Hirsutism
Tacrolimus	0.05–0.1 mg/kg/d in 2 divided doses, titrated to keep therapeutic 12-h trough levels	Renal dysfunction Hypertension Hyperglycemia and diabetes mellitus Dyslipidemia Hyperkalemia Hypomagnesemia Neurotoxicity (tremors, headaches)
Antiproliferative Agents		
Azathioprine	1.5–3.0 mg/kg/d	Bone marrow suppression Hepatitis (rare) Pancreatitis Malignancy
Mycophenolate mofetil	1000–3000 mg/d in 2 divided doses	Gastrointestinal disturbances (nausea, diarrhea) Leukopenia
mTOR Inhibitors		
Sirolimus	1–3 mg/d, titrated to keep therapeutic 24-h trough levels	Oral ulcerations Hypercholesterolemia and hypertriglyceridemia Poor wound healing Lower extremity edema Interstitial pneumonitis Leukopenia, anemia, and thrombocytopenia Nephrotoxicity when used concurrently with calcineurin-inhibitor
Everolimus[a]	1.5–3.0 mg/d in 2 divided doses	Similar to sirolimus
Corticosteroids		
Prednisone	1 mg/kg/d in 2 divided doses, tapered to 0–0.05 mg/kg/d by 6–12 mo	Weight gain Hypertension Hyperlipidemia Osteopenia Hyperglycemia Poor wound healing Salt and water retention Proximal myopathy Cataracts Peptic ulcer disease Growth retardation

mTOR, mammalian target of rapamycin.
[a]Not approved for use in the United States.

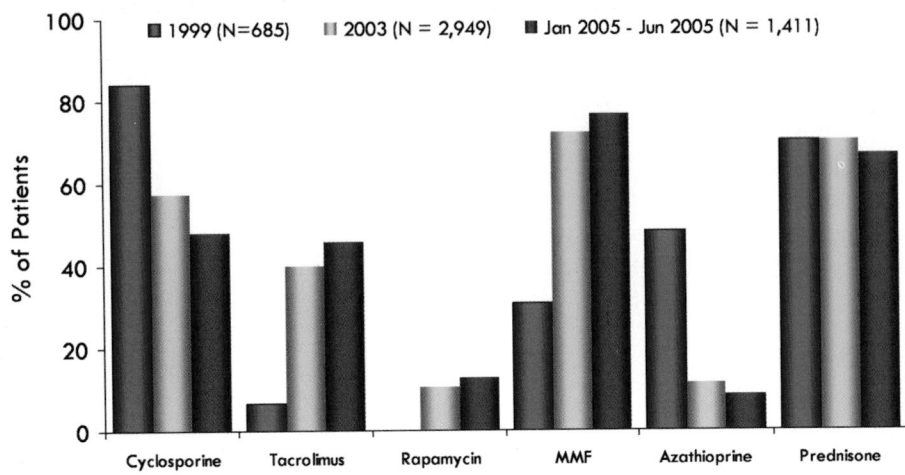

FIGURE 27–5. Trends in maintenance immunosuppression at one year in adult heart transplant recipients. MMF, mycophenolate mofetil. *Source: From Taylor DO, Edward LB, Boucek MM, et al.[8] Used with permission.*

megalovirus), fungi (*Aspergillus, Candida,* and *Pneumocystis*), *Mycobacterium, Nocardia,* and *Toxoplasma.* Effective therapy requires an extremely aggressive approach to obtaining a specific diagnosis and a background of experience in recognizing the more common clinical presentations of cytomegalovirus, *Aspergillus,* and other opportunistic infectious agents. Infection surveillance is mainly clinical, but routine chest radiography often detects infections, especially fungal and mycobacterial pulmonary infections that may be at an early and asymptomatic stage.

Malignancy

Recipients of solid organ transplants have an increased lifetime risk of cancer over the general population due to the requirement for chronic immunosuppression. The risk of neoplasm is typically related to the intensity and duration of immunosuppression. According to the most recent ISHLT registry report, the prevalence of any malignancy at 1, 5, and 10 years after heart transplantation was 3 percent, 16 percent, and 35 percent, respectively.[8] Malignancy constitutes the second most common cause of death, following cardiac allograft vasculopathy and graft failure, among patients surviving to 5 years and continues to limit long-term survival following cardiac transplantation. Among 5-year survivors, skin cancers accounted for the majority (67 percent) of malignancies reported, followed by lymphomas (10 percent). There does not appear to be an increase in the incidence of prostate, lung, bladder, breast, cervical, and colon cancers above the frequency observed in the general population; however, these cancers may behave more aggressively in an immunocompromised patient. Age-appropriate cancer screening, including dermatologic examination, screening colonoscopy for patients older than the age of 50 years, mammography and Papanicolaou testing for women, and prostate-specific antigen (PSA) level measurements for men over the age of 40, should be undertaken according to published guidelines.[64]

The most common noncutaneous malignancies in organ transplant recipients are a heterogeneous group of lymphoproliferative malignancies collectively known as posttransplant lymphoproliferative disorder (PTLD). There is convincing evidence that most cases of PTLD are related to infection (either primary or reactivation) with

EBV.[65,66] They frequently present as localized or disseminated B-cell proliferations and tend to occur in unusual, extranodal locations. Some are polyclonal while many others are monoclonal and resemble nodal malignant lymphomas. Treatment involves reduction of immunosuppression, administration of standard chemotherapy, and use of the anti-CD20 monoclonal antibody rituximab.[67–69] PTLDs are usually quite radiosensitive, and both radiotherapy and surgical resection can play a major role in therapy when there is a single lesion.

【 】 RECOGNITION AND TREATMENT OF ACUTE REJECTION

Classification

Cardiac allograft rejection is classified as hyperacute, acute cellular, acute antibody-mediated (humoral), or chronic. Hyperacute rejection is rare but may occur in the setting of circulating preformed antibodies to the ABO blood group (in cases of ABO blood group incompatibility) or to major histocompatability antigens in the donor. Possible risk factors include presensitization following multiple blood transfusions, multiparity, and previous organ grafts.[70] Hyperacute rejection manifests as severe graft failure within the first few minutes to hours after transplantation. Without inotropic and mechanical circulatory support, plasmapheresis, and emergent retransplantation, the recipient usually does not survive.

Acute cellular rejection (ACR) is the most common form of rejection and occurs in 30 to 50 percent of heart transplant recipients in the first year following transplantation.[51] Most episodes occur within the first 3 to 6 months. This type of rejection is primarily mediated by T-lymphocytes and is identified by examining histologic findings in surveillance right ventricular endomyocardial biopsies. The principle histopathologic features are the distribution and extent of inflammation and the presence or absence of myocyte damage. The severity of the rejection process reflects these features along a morphologic continuum. A uniform and standardized grading scheme for grading of ACR was developed by the ISHLT in 1990 and recently revised in 2004 (Table 27–12 and Fig. 27–6).[71] Inflammatory infiltrates and myocyte injury can be seen in conditions other than cellular rejection. These include reperfusion/ischemic injury in the early post transplant period or as a late complication of transplant associated vasculopathy, Quilty effect, infectious myocarditis, previous biopsy site, and PTLD.

Acute antibody-mediated rejection (AMR) is mediated by B-lymphocytes and is characterized by immunoglobulin deposition on the cardiac allograft microvasculature, complement activation, and graft dysfunction. It is more likely to be associated with hemodynamic instability compared with ACR, carries a worse prognosis, and is a strong risk factor for the early development of cardiac allograft vasculopathy.[72,73] The prevalence of AMR has been reported to be between 15–20 percent, and it can occur independently of or in combination with cellular rejection.[74] When occurring independently of cellular rejection, AMR is suspected when

TABLE 27–10

Important Drug Interactions

Drugs and Other Factors That Increase the Levels of Cyclosporine, Tacrolimus, and Sirolimus

Calcium channel blockers
- Diltiazem
- Nifedipine
- Nicardipine
- Verapamil

Antifungal drugs
- Itraconazole
- Fluconazole
- Ketoconazole
- Voriconazole

Macrolide antibiotics
- Erythromycin
- Clarithromycin
- Azithromycin

Amiodarone
Metoclopramide
HIV-protease inhibitors
Grapefruit juice

Drugs That Decrease the Levels of Cyclosporine, Tacrolimus, and Sirolimus

Rifampin
Phenytoin
Phenobarbital
Octreotide
St. John's wort

Drugs with Synergistic Nephrotoxicity When Used with Cyclosporine or Tacrolimus

Aminoglycoside antibiotics
NSAIDs
Colchicine
Amphotericin B
Trimethoprim/sulfamethoxazole

Drugs whose Concentrations Are Increased When Used with Cyclosporin or Tacrolimus

Lovastatin
Simvastatin
Atorvastatin
Ezetimibe

---

there is evidence of severe allograft dysfunction in the absence of a significant cellular infiltrate on the biopsy, or in the presence of interstitial edema, prominent endothelial cells lining the microvasculature and intravascular histiocytes (Fig. 27–7). More recently, diagnostic criteria for AMR have been suggested and include a combination of clinical, histologic, and immunopathologic findings, in addition to demonstration of circulating donor specific antibodies in the serum (Table 27–13).[75] Risk factors for AMR include a history of pretransplant sensitization to HLA antigens, positive pretransplant cytotoxicity crossmatch, female gender, cytomegalovirus seropositivity, prior sensitization to OKT3, multiparity, retransplantation, and a previous history of AMR.[72, 76]

Chronic rejection occurs months to years after transplantation and is typically manifested as cardiac allograft vasculopathy and late graft failure. The mechanisms of chronic rejection are incompletely understood but may involve a proliferative response to both immunologically and nonimmunologically mediated endothelial injury with progressive intimal thickening within the coronary vessels.

Diagnosis

The signs and symptoms of rejection are nonspecific and may only manifest in the late stages of rejection. Patients may present with fatigue, low-grade fevers, symptoms of heart failure, or hypotension. Occasionally, rejection manifests itself in the form atrial arrhythmias or new pericardial effusions. On examination, patients may have an elevated jugular venous pressure or a new S_3 gallop. Most patients with acute rejection are asymptomatic and have no clinical findings of allograft dysfunction. Close surveillance of heart transplant recipients for acute rejection is critical. Patients are typically monitored for rejection using a combination of clinical assessment, imaging and/or quantification of allograft function (echocardiography, multiple gated acquisition scan, and right heart catheterization), in addition to endomyocardial biopsy (EMB).

Despite its limitations (sampling error and interobserver variability of interpretation among pathologists), the EMB has remained the gold standard for the diagnosis of acute allograft rejection. It is performed via the right internal jugular vein or femoral vein by introducing a bioptome into the RV and obtaining 3 to 5 pieces of endomyocardium, typically from the right ventricular septum (Fig. 27–8). More recently, use of a blood test that measures the expression of certain genes involved in immune activation and trafficking has been proposed as a noninvasive method of detecting allograft rejection. In a multicenter observational study, the test was able to accurately detect the absence of moderate to severe cellular rejection and thus identify a state of *quiescence* in the allograft.[77] The safety and efficacy of this test, when used as part of a noninvasive protocol for rejection surveillance, is currently under clinical investigation. Protocols for the timing of rejection surveillance generally are chosen to match the observed frequency of rejection episodes, which is clearly highest in the early postoperative period. Most programs perform surveillance biopsies on a weekly basis for the first 4 to 6 postoperative weeks and then with diminishing frequency in a stable patient but at a minimum of every 3 months for the first postoperative year. The need for continued surveillance biopsies after the first year in clinically stable patients has been questioned,[78,79] but most centers continue to perform them on an every 4 to 6 months schedule during the first 5 years following transplantation.

Treatment

Rejection episodes are treated with augmented immunosuppression, the intensity of which is matched to the histologic grade and hemodynamic consequence of the episode. Mild cellular rejection (grade 1R) without associated hemodynamic compromise (defined as a decrease in left ventricular systolic function, decrease in cardiac output, or signs of hypoperfusion) typically do not require treatment. Moderate to severe cellular rejection (grades 2R and 3R) without

TABLE 27–11

Incidence of Post-Heart Transplant Morbidity

OUTCOME	WITHIN 1 YEAR (%)	WITHIN 5 YEARS (%)	WITHIN 8 YEARS (%)
Hypertension	76	94	97
Renal dysfunction	32	33	36
Abnormal creatinine <2.5mg/dL	22	21	21
Creatinine >2.5 mg/dL	7	9	10
Chronic dialysis	2	3	4
Renal transplant	0.4	0.5	1
Hyperlipidemia	69	86	91
Diabetes	31	34	37
Cardiac allograft vasculopathy	8	32	44

SOURCE: Taylor DO, Edward LB, Boucek MM, et al.[8]

hemodynamic compromise is treated with high-dose (500–1000 mg) methylprednisolone given intravenously for 3 days with or without cytolytic antibody therapy in the form of either polyclonal antithymocyte globulin (commonly of rabbit or equine origin) or

TABLE 27–12

ISHLT Standardized Cardiac Biopsy Grading

OLD (1990) GRADE	REVISED (2004) GRADE	DESCRIPTION
ACUTE CELLULAR REJECTION		
0	0R	No rejection
1A		Interstitial and/or perivascular mononuclear cell infiltrate with up to 1 focus of myocyte damage
	1R (mild)	
1B		
2		
3A	2R (moderate)	Two or more foci of mononuclear cell infiltrate with associated myocyte damage
3B		Diffuse mononuclear and/or mixed inflammatory cell infiltrates with multiple foci of myocyte damage, with or without edema, hemorrhage, or vasculitis
	3R (severe)	
4		
ANTIBODY-MEDIATED REJECTION		
AMR 0		Negative for acute antibody-mediated rejection
AMR 1		Histologic features of AMR Positive immunofluorescence or immunoperoxidase staining for AMR (positive CD68, C4d).

AMR, antibody-mediated rejection; ISHLT, International Society for Heart and Lung Transplantation; R, revised grade.
SOURCE: Adapted from Stewart S, Winters GL, Fishbein MC, et al.[71]

the murine monoclonal anti-CD3 preparation OKT3.[80,81] Cellular rejection with associated hemodynamic compromise is typically treated with IV pulse corticosteroids in addition to cytolytic therapy. Treatment of AMR typically consists of a combination of high-dose corticosteroids, plasmapheresis, IV immunoglobulin, cytolytic agents, and/or adjuvant therapy with the anti-CD20 monoclonal antibody rituximab.[82–84] Any rejection episode should prompt an investigation for precipitating causes such as CMV infection, non-compliance, or drug interactions resulting in subtherapeutic immunosuppressive drug levels. A biopsy should be repeated in 2 weeks to document resolution of the rejection episode.

Several strategies are employed as adjunctive therapy for repetitive or recalcitrant rejection episodes. They include the use of two modalities with proven efficacy in therapy for autoimmune disease: total lymphoid irradiation and low-dose methotrexate. Both have been shown to benefit patients with frequent or difficult-to-treat cardiac allograft rejection.[85–89] If all these strategies fail and severe graft dysfunction supervenes, retransplantation is the only remaining option and is offered by some centers. The results of retransplantation in this setting are poor with significantly decreased survival at 1 year compared to patients undergoing retransplantation for cardiac allograft vasculopathy (30–40 percent vs. 80–90 percent).[90,91]

[ ] CARDIAC ALLOGRAFT VASCULOPATHY

Cardiac allograft vasculopathy (CAV) is a major cause of late graft failure and death in patients following heart transplantation. It is demonstrated angiographically in approximately 10 percent of cardiac transplant recipients by the first postoperative year and in 30 to 50 percent of patients by 5 years postoperatively (see Table 27–11).[8] Despite improvements in immunosuppression over the past 2 decades, the incidence of CAV has not significantly decreased, and its development continues to limit long-term survival in patients undergoing cardiac transplantation.

Morphologic Features

In CAV the major epicardial vessels, their branches, and often the intramyocardial divisions display uniform diffuse involve-

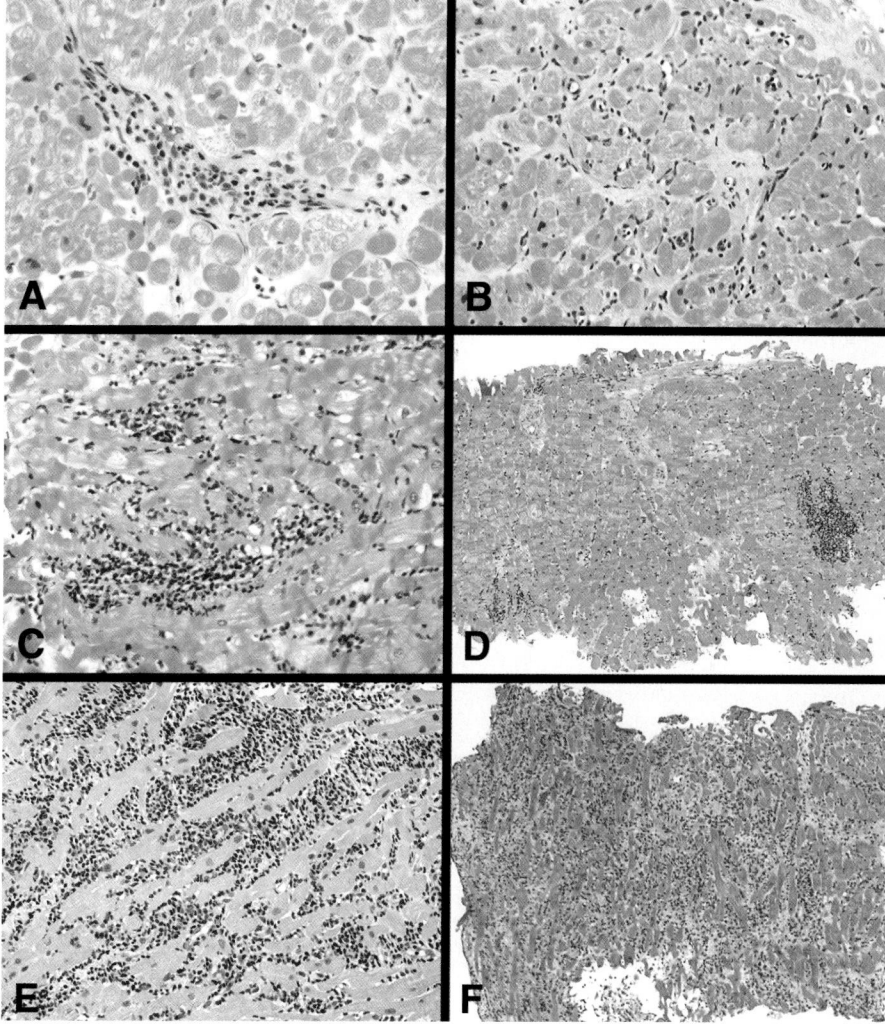

FIGURE 27-6. 2004 ISHLT Acute Cellular Rejection Grading Scheme. **A.** Mild acute rejection characterized by a perivascular cuff of mononuclear inflammatory cells without myocyte damage. This corresponds to focal mild/grade 1A in the 1990 ISHLT formulation. **B.** Mild acute rejection characterized by a diffuse interstitial pattern. This corresponds to diffuse mild/grade 1B in the 1990 ISHLT formulation. **C.** Mild acute rejection characterized by a solitary focus of mononuclear cells with rare myocyte damage. This corresponds to focal moderate/grade 2 in the 1990 ISHLT formulation. **D.** Moderate acute rejection characterized by multiple foci of inflammation and myocyte damage. This corresponds to multifocal moderate/grade 3A in the 1990 ISHLT formulation. **E.** Severe acute rejection shoeing dense interstitial infiltrates and myocyte damage. This corresponds to diffuse moderate/borderline severe/grade 3B in the 1990 ISHLT formulation. **F.** Severe acute rejection corresponding to Grade 4 rejection in 1990 ISHLT formulation. ISHLT, International Society for Heart and Lung Transplantation.

ment extending along their entire length (Fig. 27–9). The arteries are cordlike in texture. The asymmetric and calcified plaques or lesions composed of cholesterol that are characteristic of conventional atherosclerosis are not found in uncomplicated lesions of vessels affected by transplant vasculopathy. Histopathologic sections show a concentrically thickened intimal layer composed of modified smooth muscle cells, foamy macrophages, and variable numbers of histiocytes and lymphocytes within a connective tissue matrix that ranges from loose, edematous, and myxoid in early lesions to densely hyalinized and fibrotic in older lesions.[92] The internal elastic membrane is generally preserved, with only focal interruptions and reduplications. The medial layer is intact but may show atrophy in advanced lesions. Intraluminal thrombosis is uncommon.

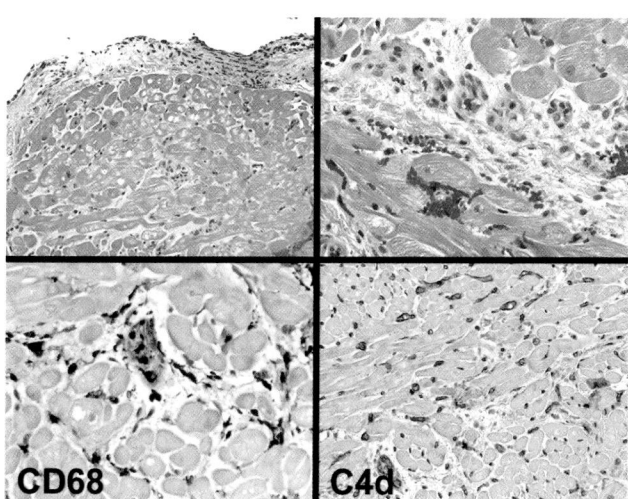

FIGURE 27-7. Acute Antibody Mediated (Humoral) Rejection. **Upper Left Panel:** Scanning magnification of endomyocardial biopsy specimen showing a mononuclear cell infiltrate within the endocardium. In the central part of the figure the small vessel displays prominent endothelial cells. **Upper Right Panel:** High power magnification showing endothelial cell hyperplasia and perivascular edema. **Lower Left Panel:** CD68 staining of interstitial and intravascular histiocytes. **Lower Right Panel:** Strong uniform staining of the microvascular for C4d, a marker of complement activation and deposition.

TABLE 27–13

Diagnostic Criteria for Acute Antibody-Mediated Rejection

Clinical evidence of acute graft dysfunction
Histologic evidence of acute capillary injury (first 2 criteria are required)
- Capillary endothelial changes: swelling or denudation with congestion
- Macrophages in capillaries
- Neutrophils in capillaries (more severe cases)
- Interstitial edema and/or hemorrhage (more severe cases)

Immunopathologic evidence for antibody-mediated injury
- IgG, IgM, and/or IgA + C3d and/or C4d or C1q (equivalent staining diffusely in capillaries, 2–3+), demonstrated by immunofluorescence
- CD68 positivity for macrophages in capillaries (identified using CD31 or CD34), and/or C4d staining of capillaries with 2–3+ intensity by paraffin immunohistochemistry
- Fibrin in vessels (more severe cases)

Serologic evidence of anti-HLA class I and/or class II antibodies or other antidonor antibody (e.g., non-HLA antibody, ABO) at the time of biopsy.

HLA, human leucocyte antigen.
SOURCE: From Reed EF, Demetris AJ, Hammond E., et al.[75]

Diagnosis

Because most cardiac transplant recipients have a persistent state of both afferent and efferent cardiac denervation, most are incapable of experiencing the subjective sensation of angina pectoris. Clinical presentations of ischemia in this patient population are typically related to sequelae of the ischemia, such as arrhythmias, myocardial infarction, or left ventricular dysfunction and symptoms of heart failure. It has been convincingly shown, however, that some cardiac transplant recipients do have physiologic evidence of reinnervation[93,94] and may experience angina pectoris.[95]

Surveillance testing is typically performed with coronary angiography, but the diffuse and concentric nature of the disease process makes it difficult to detect and easy to underestimate angiographically. In recent years the use of intravascular ultrasound (IVUS) has gained acceptance as a sensitive and early detector of the intimal thickening that characterizes CAV.[96] IVUS measurements of the degree and progression of coronary intimal thickening at 1 year posttransplantation have prognostic significance with respect to future death, graft loss, and nonfatal major adverse cardiac events;[97] these measurements now serve as surrogate endpoints for the prevention of CAV in several recent trials of new immunosuppressive agents.[59,98]

Most standard noninvasive stress tests are insensitive for detecting CAV because many of these tests are designed to detect uneven myocardial perfusion caused by focal lesions and are less effective in detecting the global ischemia of diffuse obliterative disease.[99] Several reports suggest that dobutamine stress echocardiography (DSE) may be the one noninvasive technique that offers reason-

able sensitivity and specificity, as well as prognostic value in screening for this disease.[100–103] Thus, DSE offers an attractive alternative to the usual annual coronary angiography performed in these patients.

Prognosis

The prognosis for survival once significant graft vasculopathy is detected angiographically is generally poor. In one study the 1- and 2-year survival rates after the detection of any 40 percent or more coronary artery stenosis were 67 and 44 percent, respectively. After an ischemic event such as congestive heart failure or myocardial infarction, 1-year survival was only 18 to 20 percent in this study.[104]

Prevention and Treatment

Several approaches to the prevention of CAV have been proposed. These include protecting against endothelial injury prior to and during transplantation through decreased ischemic time as well as prevention of early rejection, traditional cardiac risk factor modification, and pharmacologic therapy. Several randomized studies have shown some a decrease in the incidence and sequelae of CAV with the use of the calcium channel blocker diltiazem and the lipid-lowering agents pravastatin and simvastatin.[105–107] Additionally, the mTOR inhibitors Sirolimus and Everolimus have also shown promise in preventing the development of CAV.[58,59]

The choice of treatment for established CAV is often difficult and controversial. The diffuse nature of CAV involvement makes the dis-

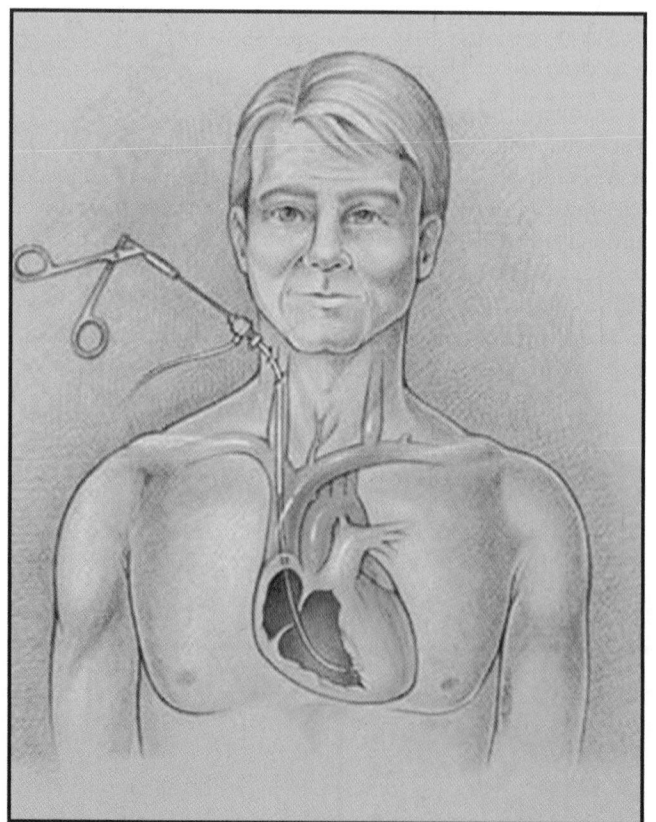

FIGURE 27–8. Endomyocardial biopsy via the right internal jugular vein.

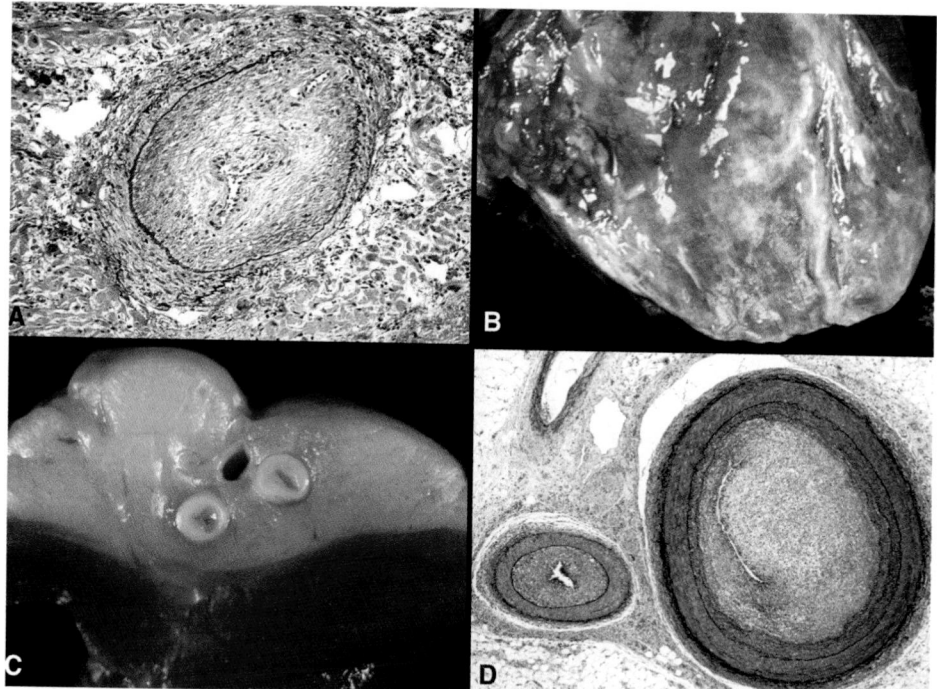

FIGURE 27–9. Cardiac allograft vasculopathy (CAV). **A.** Sinoatrial node artery in a transplant recipient from 1969 who survived for 3 months. Luminal obliteration by classic CAV is noted. **B.** Diffuse involvement of LAD artery by CAV in transplant recipient from 1971 who survived 4 months. **C.** Cross-section of epicardial arteries showing concentric narrowing with abundant yellowish lipid within the expanded intimal layer. **D.** Low-power magnification showing slit-like lumens of CAV in the epicardial artery and its small branch vessel. Preservation of the medial layer and internal elastic membrane is shown. LAD, left anterior descending.

published in the journal of that society. Since 1994, the registry has been administered by the U.S. donor allocation organization, UNOS; but the registry includes data on the vast majority of non-U.S. programs as well as all U.S. programs. The most recent registry report,[8] includes data on more than 73,000 hearts transplants performed worldwide since the registry's inception in 1982 and documents overall patient survival rates of 81, 74, and 68 percent, at 1, 3, and 5 years, respectively (Fig. 27–10). After an initial steep fall in survival during the first 6 months, there is a linear attrition rate of 3 to 4 percent per year to a survival of approximately 50 percent at 10 years. Survival during the first 6 to 12 months has slowly improved with each successive 5- to 6-year era since 1982, but the long-term attrition rate has remained unchanged. Improvements in early survival have occurred despite a trend toward accepting older organ donors, more high-risk recipients, and tolerating longer graft ischemic times. Deaths within the first 30 days posttransplant are related primarily to graft failure, multiorgan failure, and infection. Within the first year, infection accounts for the leading cause of death, followed by graft failure and infection. After 5 years cardiac allograft vasculopathy and malignancy account for the majority of deaths.[8]

Despite the requirement for long-term immunosuppression, the inherent long-term toxicities of these drug regimens, and the need for ongoing medical follow-up, most patients report an improvement in their qualify of life after transplantation. Studies have reported good quality of life, satisfaction with the outcome of the transplant surgery, and a high level of wellbeing among long-term heart transplant recipients.[111–114] At 1 year posttransplant, heart transplant recipients in one study reported that they were most satisfied with social interactions (religious faith; health care; and relationships with friends, spouses, and

ease only infrequently amenable to otherwise standard revascularization procedures such as percutaneous coronary interventions (PCIs) and coronary artery bypass grafting (CABG). In a recent report of 40 heart transplant patients undergoing PCI with stents for progressive asymptomatic CAV (45 percent), angina (12.5 percent), acute myocardial infarction (10 percent), and congestive heart failure (15 percent), the primary success rates, defined as <50 percent residual stenosis, were high and similar to those of nontransplanted patients. However, the observed in-stent and vessel restenosis rates at 6 months (48 and 65 percent) were higher compared to those historically reported in PCI of native vessels; but there was a trend toward less restenosis with the use of drug-eluting stents.[108] Outcomes following CABG have been extremely poor, with a reported 33 percent operative mortality rate and 50 percent mortality rate at 2 months in one registry.[109]

The most definitive form of therapy for graft failure resulting from severe vasculopathy is retransplantation for highly selected patients with advanced CAV but otherwise good organ function. Historically, posttransplant survival rates have been significantly lower in retransplant patients compared with primary transplants;[110] however, survival rates after retransplantation have improved significantly in the current era and are now comparable to those after primary transplantation, averaging 85 percent at 1 year in the most recent ISHLT registry report.[8]

POSTTRANSPLANT OUTCOMES

The most accurate data on volume sund outcomes of thoracic organ transplantation are provided by the Registry of the International Society for Heart and Lung Transplantation and are updated yearly and

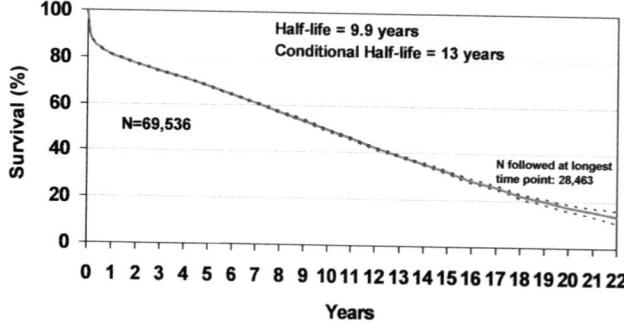

FIGURE 27–10. Actuarial survival for adult and pediatric heart transplants patients performed between January 1982 and June 2004. The half-life is the time at which 50 percent of those transplanted remain alive, and the conditional half-life is the time to 50 percent survival for those recipients surviving the first year post-transplantation. *Source: From Taylor DO, Edward LB, Boucek MM, et al.[8] Used with permission.*

children) and least satisfied with their sex lives, financial independence, and energy for daily activities.[113] Despite cardiac denervation, most heart transplant patients report no functional limitations, and some patients are able of achieving athletic performances. Data from the ISHLT registry shows that 90 percent of patients reported no activity limitations at 1 and 7 years posttransplant.[8]

SURGICAL TREATMENT FOR HEART FAILURE

Although cardiac transplantation remains the *gold standard* treatment for heart failure, the prevalence of the disease and the limited donor organs available render this sole strategy epidemiologically nonviable. Accordingly, surgical management of heart failure continues to represent one of the fastest growing aspects of adult cardiothoracic surgery.

The heart failure state may be the result of ischemic changes causing myocardial dysfunction (and thus dilatation and often valvular dysfunction), or may begin first with ventricular chamber distension and remodeling causing increased wall tension and subendocardial ischemia. Thus, apart from ventricular assist devices (described below), the major surgical approaches to heart failure can be categorized by their mode of therapeutic benefit: (a) coronary revascularization, (b) repair of valvular defects resulting in pressure and volume overload and (c) anatomic ventricular restoration. In all cases, it is imperative to determine preoperatively whether the given patient is also a transplant candidate, so as to prepare for the possible eventuality of postcardiotomy assist device bridging to transplantation.

[ ] HIGH-RISK REVASCULARIZATION

Coronary revascularization may be pursued in the setting of a low overall ejection fraction with the presumption that recruitment of ischemic, but viable, myocardium may offset the risk of (re)operation. The specific large series to support these strategies are discussed in Chap. 65. The techniques of surgical revascularization of the patient with end-stage heart failure do not differ significantly from other patients. Some surgeons prefer the use of warm-induction cardioplegia in such patient cohorts, based on the presumption of improved myocardial preservation. In contrast, off-pump coronary bypass grafting can be particularly challenging in these patients because of the large heart size and often concomitant valvular regurgitation, which may prestage hemodynamic instability with positioning and stabilization of the heart, particularly for left circumflex coronary artery revascularization.

[ ] MITRAL VALVE PROCEDURES

Mitral valve dysfunction in end-stage heart disease may be the result of degenerative valvular damage, ischemic mitral insufficiency, or a combination of both. Ischemic mitral insufficiency affects both the valvular and subvalvular apparatus by causing ventricular dilatation and papillary muscle ischemia. Thus, in the early stages of ischemic mitral regurgitation, myocardial revascularization may be sufficient to reverse the pathologic process. If permanent damage has been sustained, or if irreversible ventricular/annular dilatation has occurred, some form of mitral valve repair or replacement is necessary.

Bolling and others have demonstrated success with the use of a substantially downsized mitral annuloplasty ring to correct ischemic

mitral regurgitation in patients with dilated cardiomyopathy.[115,116] Reduction of central valvular regurgitation from annular dilatation in this setting is intuitively appealing and also represents the basis on which emerging technology has based several minimally invasive techniques, including splint-type devices placed through the coronary sinus or transmyocardially. The Coapsys device (Coapsys, Myocor, Maple Grove, Minnesota) represents such a device in which a single, flexible cord is placed from the anterior septum to the lateral wall and shortened to allow for better coaptation of valve leaflets while potentially avoiding the use of cardiopulmonary bypass.

If mitral valve repair is not possible and significant mitral insufficiency persists intraoperatively, it is essential that mitral valve replacement be performed, preferably with preservation of the subchordal attachments to help maintain ventricular geometry and function.[117–119]

[ ] VENTRICULAR RESTORATION/REMODELING

Described initially in 1996, the Batista procedure of partial left ventriculotomy involves resection of left ventricular muscle (not scar tissue) between the anterior and posterior papillary muscles (the territory of the first marginal branch of the circumflex coronary artery) in conjunction with mitral valve repair in an effort to restore ventricular geometry (Fig. 27–11).[120] The resection approximates the interpapillary distance and can result in chordal lengthening (and thus regurgitation); thus, in the original description, all patients underwent a concomitant *Alfieri-type* single suture to approximate the anterior and posterior leaflets of the mitral valve. The reduction in overall ventricular diameter caused by this resection was postulated to reduce overall wall stress, and thereby improve systolic performance and reduce subendocardial ischemia. Poor long-term followup of Batista's original Brazilian series, in conjunction with significant morbidity and postprocedure ventricular assist device implantation demonstrated in later American series, have lessened enthusiasm for the procedure. Although the Batista procedure is now essentially obsolete, its somewhat radical concept of ventricular excision to restore ventricular elliptical geometry has been applied in related techniques, especially those with left ventricular aneurysms.[121]

Left ventricular aneurysms are characterized by anatomic thinning of the ventricular wall from transmural infarction, with resultant paradoxical motion of the aneurysmal segment.[122] This paradoxical motion of both this segment and often also the interventricular septum results in volume overloading and distension of the already impaired myocardium (because the stroke volume must be increased additionally to fill the aneurysm while maintaining forward output). Moreover, the paradoxical motion serves to disturb the normal geometry of the ventricle by carrying the adjacent normal free wall away from the septum with ongoing distension.

Early surgical approaches, first described by Cooley, involved linear closure of the aneurysmal segment, and demonstrated only marginally acceptable outcomes.[123] Although this strategy did eliminate the paradoxical motion and the source of regurgitant volume, it did not eliminate paradoxical motion of the border zone or septal myocardium, nor did it necessarily address the distortions of ventricular geometry. Both the Jatene and Dor techniques of aneurysmorrhaphy attempt to address these additional concerns.

In the Jatene technique, the aneurysm is resected, and the aneurysmal portion of the septum imbricated, thereby stabilizing it against normally contracting myocardium. In addition, the base of

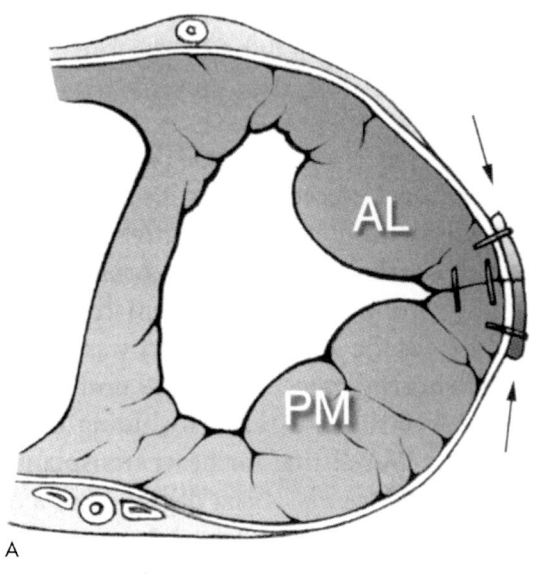

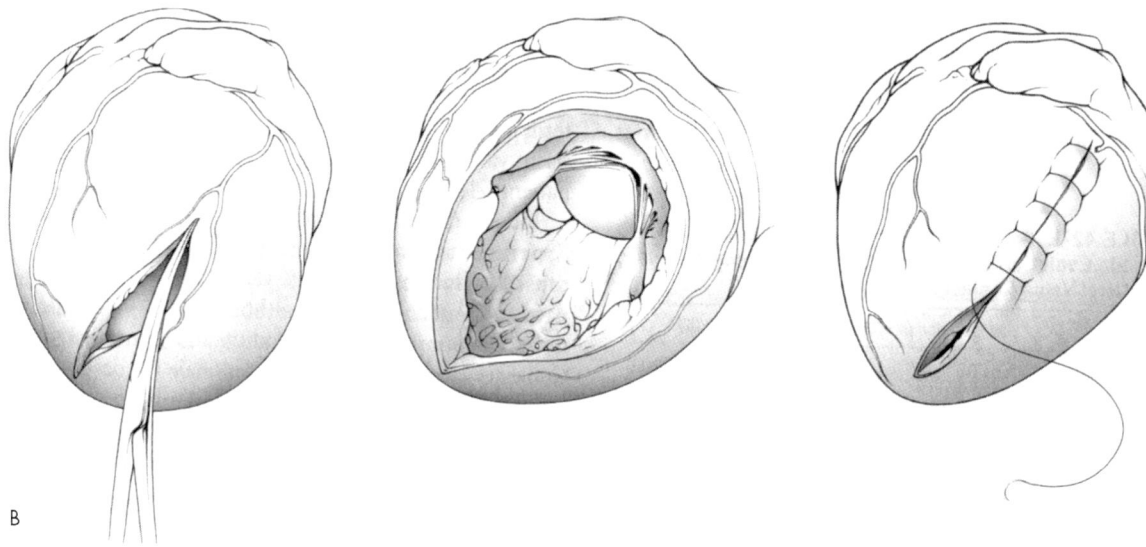

FIGURE 27–11. The Batista procedure (left ventriculectomy). The initial incision is placed between the base of the anterolateral and posteromedial papillary muscles; a bow-tie mitral valve repair stitch (not shown) is performed and the ventricle closed in layers. *Source: From Buxton B, Frazier OH, Westaby S, et al. Ischemic Heart Disease Surgical Management. Philadelphia: Mosby; 1999. With permission.*

the resected aneurysm is reapproximated with a pursestring suture, thereby drawing the free wall back to the septum, and recreating *normal* ventricular geometry.[124] In the Dor technique, the aneurysmal segment is not resected but rather is excluded from the ventricle with a Dacron patch after a pursestring suture is placed at the base of the aneurysmal segment (Fig. 27–12).[125]

Several large series have demonstrated durability of the Dor procedure with and without adjunctive mitral valve operations. Early mortality has been estimated to be less than 10 percent and long-term survival at 5 to 10 years is between 65 percent and 80 percent.[126,127] A continuum within these patient cohorts of those with akinesis or dyskinesis of the aneurysm segment has made data comparison difficult. In addition, true uniformity of technique has been limited, such as how to *size* the remaining ventricular cavity. In the original Dor technique, sizing balloons are used to estimate objectively the size of the ventricular cavity. Others have maintained that in most cases a transition zone between *normal* myocardium and the thin-walled, fibrotic segment to be excised is clearly evident, and defines easily the borders of the repair.[126] Other points of contention include whether to perform the procedure with cardioplegic arrest, how much septoplasty is required,

and the degree to which cryoablation should be applied to prevent malignant ventricular arrhythmias.

An international group of investigators referred to as the Reconstructive Endoventricular Surgery returning Torsion Original Radius Elliptical shape to the left ventricle (RESTORE) investigators assembled to review the role of anterior ventricular restoration in the treatment of postinfarction ventricular dilatation. Recent results from the RESTORE registry demonstrated improved ventricular function and functional status in 1198 post-anterior infarction patients with chronic heart failure (CHF) who were treated with surgical anterior ventricular restoration (SAVR) in addition to concomitant CABG (95 percent), mitral valve repair (22 percent), or mitral valve replacement (1 percent). In this registry 5-year survival was 69 percent, and 5-year freedom from hospital readmission for CHF was 78 percent.[128] The RESTORE registry has been criticized for its lack of a control group,[129] but the favorable short- and long-term outcomes in this group of patients suggested the need for a randomized comparison of SAVR with medical therapy or with coronary artery revascularization.[130]

The Surgical Treatment for Ischemic Heart Failure (STICH) multicenter prospective randomized trial was created to address the popu-

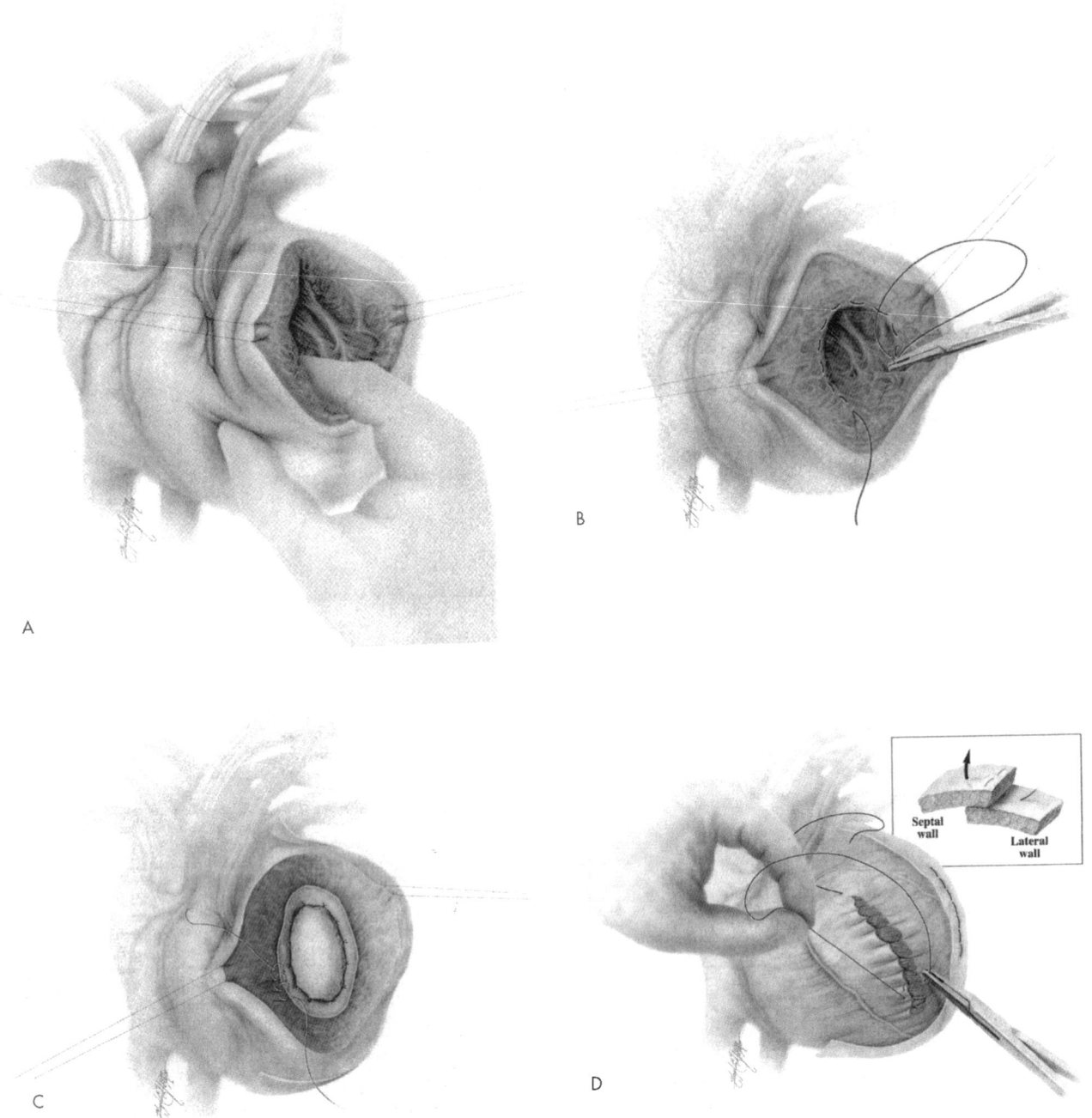

FIGURE 27–12. The Dor procedure with modifications. The anterior akinetic scar is opened and its edges palpated. An encircling suture then is used to delineate the margin and provide a substrate for the later Dacron patch. Ultimately, the scar is reapproximated over the patch. *Source: From Athanasuleas CL, Stanley AW Jr, Buckberg GD, et al. J Am Coll Cardiol 27:1199–1209. With permission.*

lation of patients with heart failure and left ventricular dysfunction who have surgically remediable coronary artery disease. In the study revascularization was compared with maximal medical therapy alone, and in addition, those undergoing revascularization were compared to those undergoing additional surgical restorative procedures.

The STICH trial seeks to enroll 1800 patients from 100 centers. Inclusion criteria include an ejection fraction less than 35 percent and coronary anatomy amenable to revascularization. Exclusion criteria are the need for aortic valve surgery, preoperative intraaortic balloon pump support, candidacy for percutaneous interventions, acute myocardial infarction, more than one prior coronary bypass procedure, or noncardiac illness that imposes either substantial operative mortality or limited life expectancy. The presumption is that coro-

nary bypass alone will confer a 20 percent reduction in mortality compared with maximal medical therapy, and that ventricular restoration may confer improvement in hospital-free survival by 20 percent when compared with coronary revascularization alone.[131]

Patients whose left ventricular end-systolic volume index exceeds 60 mL/m^2 comprise the cohort undergoing surgical ventricular restoration. Those with lower volumes comprise the cohort who will be randomized between maximal medical management and coronary revascularization. Perhaps unsurprisingly, recruitment in the latter cohort has been somewhat limited, because some previous studies have demonstrated a survival benefit to coronary bypass grafting in appropriate candidates with heart failure, making referring cardiologists less likely to enroll their patients for

Myosplint Concept

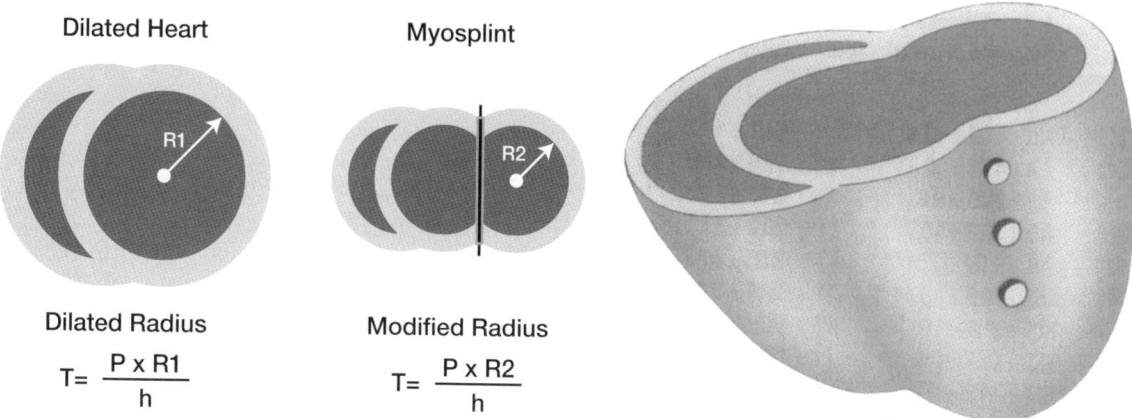

FIGURE 27–13. The Myosplint concept and illustration of the device, where the reduction in wall stress is evident in the bilobed shape produced by the device. Three transventricular splints are placed perpendicular to the long-axis of the ventricle and epicardial pads secured and used to tighten the device. *Source: From McCarthy DM, Takagaki M, Ochiai Y, et al. J Thorac Cardiovasc Surg 2001;122:482–490. With permission.*

fear of randomization to medical therapy alone.[129] Critics of the STICH trial highlight uncertainty regarding the degree of asynergy and compensatory muscle potential, and the means of measurement of ventricular volume.[132]

▌ ▌ CARDIAC SUPPORT DEVICES

Recent enthusiasm in the concept of ventricular geometric restoration has promoted the development of several cardiac support devices that attempt to limit or reverse ventricular remodeling. Some acutely alter ventricular shape and geometry, but others provide a more gradual reverse remodeling through a reduction in wall stress.

The Myosplint device (Myocor, Maple Grove, MN) is composed of three polyethylene braided splints coated with expanded polytetrafluoroethylene and a thermoplastic epicardial splint on each end covered with polyester fabric.[133] The three splints are placed via echocardiographic guidance through the left ventricle perpendicular to its long axis (Fig. 27–13). The epicardial pads are attached and tightened to a desired length, thereby causing the left ventricle to assume a bilobar geometry with a subsequent decrease in wall stress. Limited human applications have demonstrated safety, and chronic animal studies have shown an immediate and 1-month increase in ejection fraction and a decrease in wall stress and left ventricular end-systolic volume.[133,134]

The CorCap cardiac support device (CSD) (Acorn Cardiovascular, St. Paul, MN) provides wall-stress diminution through different means. The CorCap CSD is a circumferential mesh constructed from a multifilamentous yarn that provides high strength and fatigue characteristics to its diastolic support while maintaining flexibility (and thus not causing constriction). It is positioned around the ventricles (similar to a vest), where it is sewn just adjacent to the atrioventricular groove (Fig. 27–14). The device is then adjusted gradually to reduce the circumference of the heart and thereby decrease wall stress. Once this is accomplished, it is secured with several anterior stay sutures; its use does not preclude concomitant coronary or valve surgery.

Promising early data from Europe suggests that the CorCap CSD may provide a durable decrease in ventricular volumes and increase

in ejection fraction in medium-term follow-up studies.[135] Animal studies have suggested that the CorCap CSD may also help to prevent infarction extension and resultant heart failure, implying that its efficacy may be of additional benefit to impede the process of ventricular remodeling after a large myocardial infarction.[136]

▌ ▌ COMPOSITE STRATEGIES

A recent subcohort analysis from the Acorn clinical trial (CorCap device) comparing patients undergoing mitral valve surgery alone versus mitral valve surgery in conjunction with the CorCap device demonstrated additional benefit in left ventricular end-

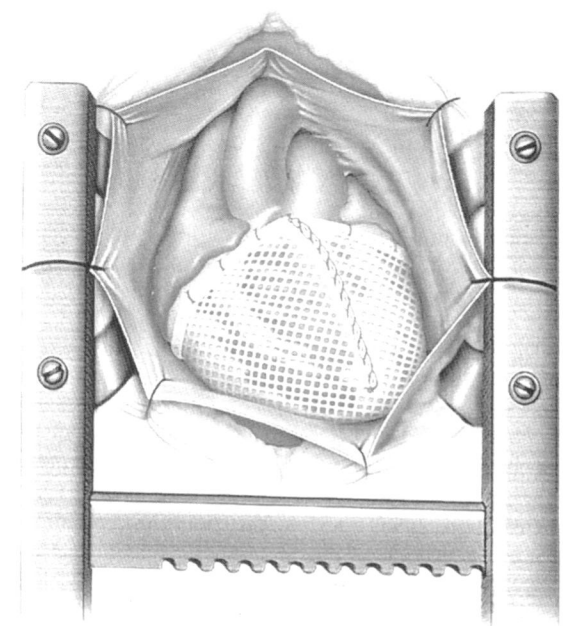

FIGURE 27–14. The CorCap device in place. The *hemline* is secured to the atrioventricular groove with several interrupted sutures. The anterior seam is created to tighten the device to the proper fit. *Source: From Oz MC, Konertz WF, Kleber FX, et al. J Thorac Cardiovasc Surg 2003; 126:983–991. With permission.*

diastolic and end-systolic volumes at 18 months follow up.[137] In this subcohort, the majority (84 percent) of patients underwent mitral valve repair with an undersized ring; the remainder underwent mitral valve replacement. Notably, the reduction in mitral regurgitation in both repair and replacement cohorts was durable at 18 months follow up, as were findings of improvement in quality of life. Both findings were additionally enhanced when mitral valve surgery was performed in conjunction with application of the CorCap CSD.[137]

The results of this recent subcohort analysis are compelling for several reasons, including the favorable results of mitral valve surgery in this group of patients with low ejection fractions where perioperative mortality was less than 2 percent. However, perhaps most intriguing is the validation of a composite strategy toward the application of surgery for end-stage heart disease. As experience with adjunctive devices and operations grows, it is perhaps logical that the specific cohorts for whom each is most beneficial will be refined. Thus, for the patient with a pure dilated cardiomyopathy and mitral valve regurgitation, the approach of restraint device *and* mitral valve surgery may be best. If that patient additionally has a ventricular aneurysm and no valvular pathology, ventricular restoration with or without coronary revascularization may be the solution. Problematically, such composite operations render survival analysis and comparison with other technique, or with medical therapy, nearly impossible. Nonetheless, surgeons involved with operations for end-stage heart failure as alternatives to transplantation should avail themselves of the full armamentarium of therapeutic options to obtain optimal outcomes.

VENTRICULAR ASSIST DEVICES

Since their inception in the late 1960s, mechanical circulatory assist devices have evolved substantially. With this evolution, we have developed a better understanding of the technological drawbacks limiting current device design as well as the appropriate indications for insertion of these devices. The dream of a completely implantable device, a total artificial heart, or a device whose design specifications allow for its use for neonates, infants, and children is likely not only attainable, but expected to enjoy clinical trials in the near future.

The clinical application of ventricular assist devices (VADs) grew from experience with their application in the operating room. Unlike the intraaortic balloon pump, VADs function to reduce myocardial work by completely unloading the ventricle while maintaining its output. They may be employed for right ventricular, left ventricular, or biventricular support for short- (<1 week) or longer-term support, or for permanent (*destination therapy*) use. The device may be completely extracorporeal, paracorporeal, implantable with percutaneous power support, or totally implantable, and it may provide continuous or pulsatile flow.

There are essentially four groups of patients for whom support with different types of VADs is appropriate. The first are those in whom reversibility of ventricular insult is anticipated, the so-called *bridge-to-recovery* group. Here, patients who may be experiencing postcardiotomy shock despite reasonable preoperative myocardial reserve or suffer from a potentially reversible process (e.g., acute myocarditis) benefit from short- to medium-term device support. The *bridge-to-bridge* cohort describes patients who experience acute cardiogenic shock at a center that does not offer transplanta-

tion or long-term VADs. In these patients the efficacious institution of short-term assistance and rapid transfer to a center specialized in ventricular assist support is warranted. Patients in the *bridge-to-transplant* cohort are those who meet criteria for transplantation and undergo VAD insertion to improve their overall transplant candidacy and stabilize their hemodynamics while awaiting transplantation.[138–141] Finally, selected patients may benefit from permanent VAD implantation and represent *destination therapy* candidates.[142]

Important clinical issues to consider when choosing a device include the expected duration of support, the need for biventricular support, cost, device-related risks (such as the need for anticoagulation and device failure rates), patient characteristics (especially the size and blood type of the patient), and UNOS classification rules.

SHORT-TERM DEVICES

Centrifugal pumps were first introduced as alternatives to roller pumps for cardiopulmonary bypass and have been available since the late 1970s for use as short-term cardiac support. These pumps are widely available, relatively inexpensive, and simple; but they require systemic anticoagulation. They are versatile and may be used as an RVAD (from right atrium or RV to pulmonary artery), as an LVAD (from left atrium or left ventricular apex to aorta), or as part of an extracorporeal membrane oxygenation (ECMO) circuit.

ECMO provides mechanical cardiac support as well as pulmonary support. Although its success has been extensively documented in the neonatal and infant population, the outcomes of its use for adults have been less promising.[143,144] The main indications for ECMO are the need for mechanical assistance in the face of combined pulmonary failure, or pure respiratory failure. ECMO's benefits include potential peripheral cannulation and implementation for both cardiac and pulmonary support in areas outside the operating room. Major limitations, however, include a requirement for sedation/paralysis to effect immobilization as well as systemic heparinization. As with the centrifugal pumps, full-time trained personnel are also necessary to manage the ECMO circuit continuously. Complications are common, including leg ischemia, renal failure, bleeding, and oxygenation failure.

The Abiomed BVS (Abiomed Cardiovascular Inc., Danvers, MA) is a short-term uni- or biventricular support system comprised of two 100 mL polyurethane blood sacs, the inlet and outlet portions of which are guarded by polyurethane valves (Fig. 27–15).[145,146] The inflow to the device is via atrial or apical cannulae with outflow Dacron grafts sutured to either pulmonary artery or aorta. The device fills passively, and a pneumatically driven console adjusts the duration of systole and diastole to maintain a stroke volume of approximately 80mL.[147]

One advantage that has made the BVS system popular is the ease of insertion and simplicity in operation, obviating the need for a full-time perfusionist at the bedside. The system functions reliably for several days to weeks. However, the BVS does commit a patient to systemic anticoagulation for the duration of support, limit mobility compared to intracorporeal devices, and generally requires ICU monitoring and management.

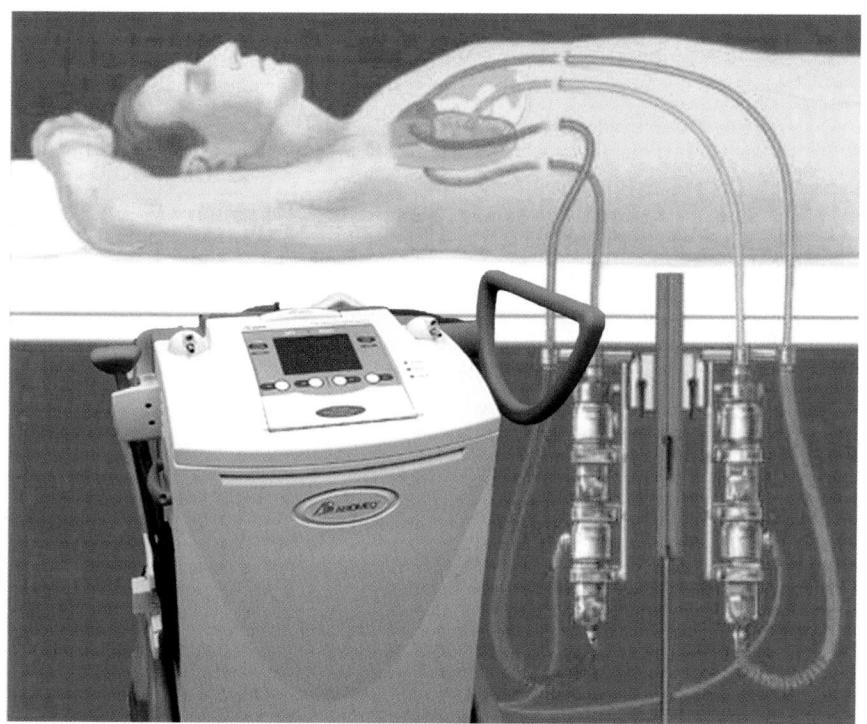

FIGURE 27–15. The Abiomed BVS 5000i. *Source: Courtesy of Abiomed, Inc. With permission.*

【 】 PULSATILE DEVICES

The HeartMate LVAD (Thoratec Corporation, Pleasanton, CA) has a titanium-alloy external housing, with inflow and outflow conduits that use porcine xenograft valves (25 mm) (Fig. 27–16). The unique characteristic of the device is its internal blood-contacting surface, which is made of textured titanium that results in the development of a pseudo-neointima on which thrombus formation is greatly reduced, thereby decreasing the need for anticoagulation. Patients with these devices take aspirin (for antiinflammation but not primarily for anticoagulation) with a remarkably low rate of thromboembolic complications and without the need for warfarin sodium (Coumadin).

The device has a pumping capacity in excess of 9 L/min, a maximal stroke volume of 83 mL, and pulsatile flow is created using a pusher-plate system. The device is inserted into the left upper quadrant of the abdomen either pre- or intraperitoneally (patients must have a body surface area [BSA] >1.5 m²). The driveline, consisting of an air vent and power cables, is tunneled subcutaneously and brought out percutaneously. Small battery units, worn in a harness, are connected to the cables; in case of an emergency, a portable hand pump can activate the device.

The Novacor (World Heart Corp., Ottawa, ON, Canada) left ventricular assist system (LVAS) is similar to the overall design of the HeartMate. However, unlike the HeartMate system, Novacor LVAS patients require anticoagulation with warfarin to avoid embolic events. Recently, a new inflow cannula made with Gore-Tex was introduced with the hope that it will reduce the rate of cerebrovascular events. Preliminary reports suggest that the Vascutek inflow conduit reduced embolic events to 12 percent (compared with historical rates between 27 percent and 41 percent).[148,149]

The Thoratec paracorporeal VAD (Thoratec Laboratories Corp., Pleasanton, CA) is a commonly used system for paracor-

poreal biventricular support (Fig. 27–17).[150] Because the actual pump chamber is outside of the body, this device can be used on patients with body sizes too small to house the HeartMate or Novacor devices (i.e., <1.5 m²). The pump consists of a prosthetic ventricle with a maximum stroke volume of 65 mL and cannulae for ventricular or atrial inflow as well as arterial outflow. Pneumatic drivers provide alternating air pressure to fill and empty the blood pump, and the pump flow rate ranges from 1.3 to 7.2 L/min. Anticoagulation with warfarin is necessary, as for patients with mechanical valves.

Like the Abiomed BVS the biggest advantage of this system is its versatility. It is easy to place with less surgical dissection; can be used for patients of various sizes; can be attached to either the atrium or ventricle; and can be used for right, left, or biventricular heart support. However, its paracorporeal location potentially limits the patient's activity and thus its use as a permanent device. The Abiomed AB5000 (Abiomed, Danvers, MA) is quite similar in design to the Thoratec paracorporeal device. It uses the same cannulae as the BVS; and in fact, patients supported with the BVS can be *transitioned* to the AB5000 relatively easily, should longer-term support be required.[151]

The Thoratec Intracorporeal VAD (Thoratec Laboratories Corp., Pleasanton, CA) is the same size as the external system but

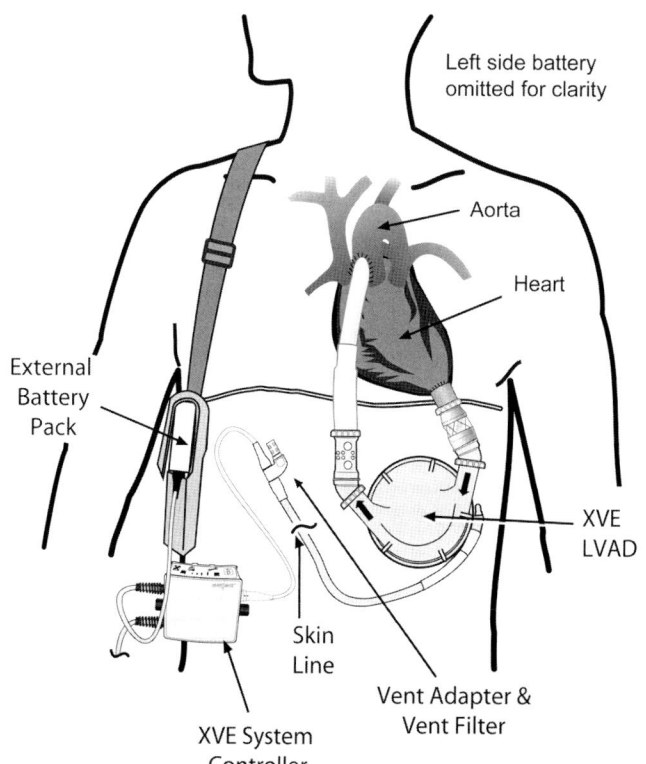

FIGURE 27–16. The HeartMate left ventricular assist device (LVAD). *Source: Courtesy of Thoratec, Inc. With permission.*

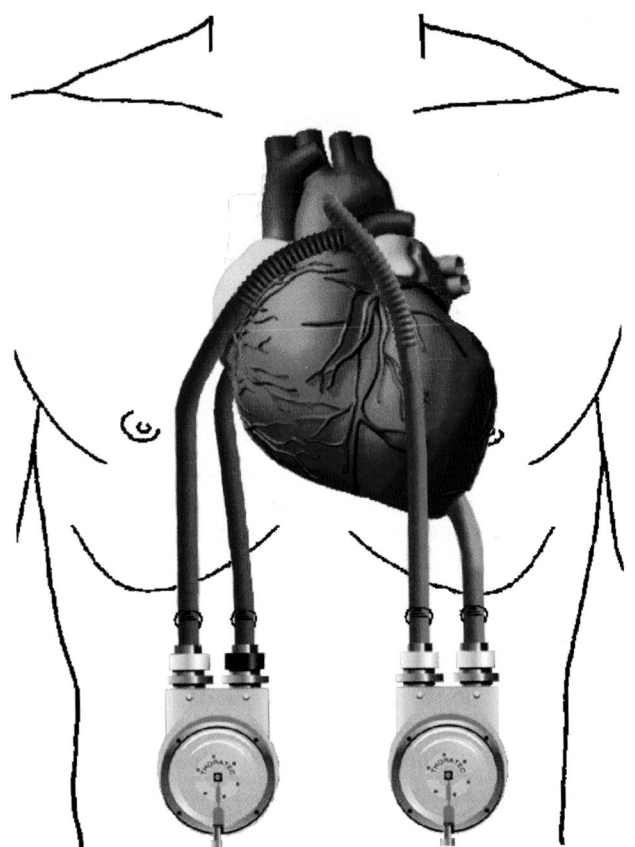

FIGURE 27–17. The Thoratec paracorporeal ventricular assist devices (VAD). *Source: Courtesy of Thoratec, Inc. With permission.*

is encased in a titanium alloy housing and its pumps can be placed intracorporeally (not paracorporeally); two drivelines still exit the skin. The advantages of this system are its small size; reliability; implantable right, left, and biventricular support; and similar technology based on the currently used Thoratec system.

[ ] AXIAL FLOW PUMPS

Axial flow pumps represent one of the newest generations of assist devices. They can provide full cardiac support with a much smaller pump, using fewer moving parts and a smaller blood-contacting surface than pusher-plate devices. Furthermore, their small size allows implantation into smaller patients compared to most pulsatile pumps. Although axial flow pumps provide nonpulsatile flow, many patients maintain some native cardiac function during axial pump support and therefore continue to have pulsatile patterns of blood flow unlike with many of the pumps previously described (which can completely unload the ventricle). Many axial flow pumps generate such continuous negative pressure that there is a potential risk of collapsing the ventricle and causing transient pump cessation (and therefore thrombus formation), or air entrainment (and therefore air emboli). Because of this phenomenon, both ventricular preload and cannula placement are of paramount importance with these pumps.

The Micromed-Debakey VAD (Micromed Inc., Houston, TX) is 3.0 cm in diameter, 7.6 cm long, and weighs 95 g. It is made of titanium casing with an impeller/inducer capable of pumping 10 L/min. The inflow cannula is inserted into the left ventricular apex, and the outflow graft is sutured to the ascending or descending aorta (a percutaneous cable connects the device to a wearable battery/control console).[152] Patients require chronic anticoagulation with warfarin and an anti-platelet agent. The major complications of this device have been either late bleeding or thrombosis.

The HeartMate II (Thoratec Inc., Pleasanton, CA) is a 124 mL titanium axial-flow rotary LVAD with a rotor capable of producing flow rates greater than 10 L/min (Fig. 27–18). Similar to the DeBakey VAD, the inflow cannula is joined to the apex of the left ventricle with the outflow graft connected to the ascending aorta.[153] Anticoagulation is at present required to keep the international normalized ratio between 1.5 and 2.5, and both power and control are supplied by a percutaneous lead that attaches to either a power base unit or to portable rechargeable batteries.

The titanium Flowmaker (formerly Jarvik 2000) pump (Jarvik Heart, Inc., NY) measures 2.4 cm in diameter, 5.5 cm in length, and weighs 85 g.[154,155] Unlike the DeBakey VAD or the HeartMate II, this pump is positioned inside the ventricle with the outflow graft sutured to the descending aorta. Unlike most other systems, which require a sternotomy, the Flowmaker may be implanted through a left thoracotomy incision. The pump is mainly used as a partial decompression device, allowing the aortic valve to open. However, if full decompression is achieved (and the aortic valve remains closed), because the outflow graft is sutured to the descending aorta, thrombus can form in areas of stagnation in the ascending aorta more proximally.

[ ] TOTAL ARTIFICIAL HEART

The CardioWest total artificial heart (TAH) (Syncardia, Tucson, AZ) is a pneumatic, biventricular, orthotopically implanted total artificial heart with an externalized driveline to its console.[138] It consists of two spherical polyurethane chambers with polyurethane diaphragms. Inflow and outflow conduits are constructed of

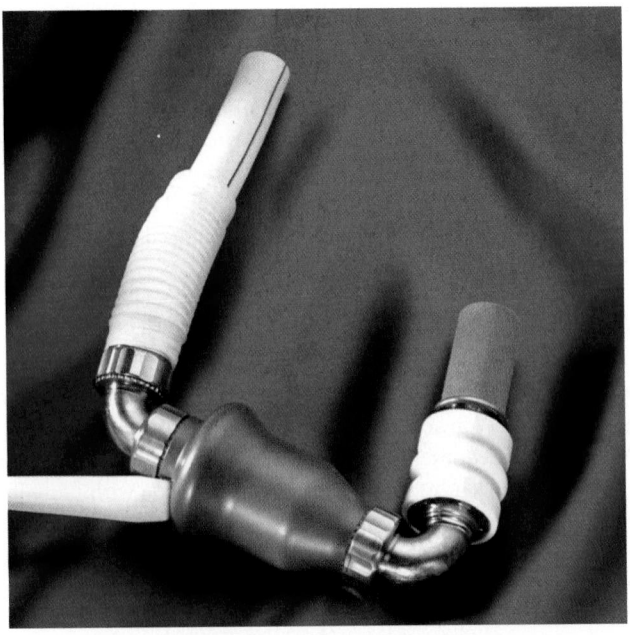

FIGURE 27–18. The HeartMate II axial flow pump. *Source: Courtesy of Thoratec, Inc. With permission.*

Dacron and contain Medtronic-Hall (Medtronic, Inc., Minneapolis, MN) valves.

The AbioCor TAH (Abiomed Cardiovascular Inc. Danvers, MA) is an electrohydraulically actuated device. The pump chambers are sutured to atrial tissue and to the great vessels by textured Dacron (E.I. du Pont de Nemours, Wilmington, DE) atrial cuffs and grafts. A centrifugal pump moves hydraulic fluid between the ventricles, providing alternate left and right ventricular pulsatile flow. Anticoagulation is maintained with warfarin and clopidogrel (Plavix, Bristol-Meyers Squibb, NY).

TAHs benefit from the ability to provide complete support and, unlike the other devices, obviate the presence of the native heart. This is particularly useful in situations where leaving the native heart in place would be detrimental or impossible (e.g., cardiac tumors). However, adequate intrathoracic space is required to accommodate the TAH: Fitting criteria include a BSA >1.7 m^2, cardiothoracic ratio >0.5, LV diastolic dimension greater than 66 mm, anterior-posterior distance greater than 10 cm, and combined ventricular volume greater than 1500 mL. In addition to size requirements, strict anticoagulation with warfarin, aspirin, and pentoxifylline is also mandatory.

[ ] BRIDGE TO RECOVERY OR TRANSPLANTATION

The profound ventricular unloading provided by LVAD support can lead to *reverse remodeling* evident at genetic, biochemical, and histological levels.[156–158] Long-term LVAD explantation is considered only if there is significant myocardial recovery as evidenced by improvement of parameters on an exercise testing protocol.[157] Experience has demonstrated that only a minority of patients can be successfully weaned from their devices.[158,159] The question of which patients are suitable for bridge-to-recovery and device explantation requires further clinical evaluation.

For patients bridged to transplantation, several analyses throughout the evolution of LVAD use, both in the acute and chronic settings, have repeatedly demonstrated a comparable posttransplant survival for patients bridged with VADs, when compared with all others undergoing transplantation.[160,161] In most cases, the rates of survival-*to*-transplantation approach or exceed 80 percent.[160]

Immunological Perturbations

Itescu and colleagues have extensively analyzed the immunological interaction of patients with the HeartMate LVAD and demonstrated several important findings.[162–164] The results of these studies suggest both a progressive defect in cellular immunity (and thus an increased risk of infection) as well as an increased rate of allosensitization. Few comparable studies have been performed with recipients of other types of devices, but some have described comparable HLA sensitization in the Novacor device.[165] However, immunologic evaluation of the patient-device interaction with some axial flow pumps, which do not promote a neointimal layer, have demonstrated an initial finding of increased markers of apoptosis.[166]

LVAD implantation may therefore be associated with an increased risk of developing circulating anti-HLA class I and II antibodies (sensitization) causing as many as 66 percent of patients with an LVAD to be sensitized prior to transplantation.[163] This increased antibody level is associated with a significant risk for early graft failure and poorer patient survival as a result of complement-mediated humoral rejection. If the patient becomes sensitized, donor-specific cross-matching is mandatory prior to transplantation, resulting in increased waiting time in those patients. However, recent studies have demonstrated that pretransplantation immunomodulatory therapy with intravenously administered cyclophosphamide, together with intravenous immunoglobulin, successfully diminishes serum alloreactivity and reduces waiting list times and the risk of acute rejection in many LVAD recipients.[164,166]

[ ] DESTINATION THERAPY

Because of the constant shortage of available donor organs, the large group of patients who would benefit from circulatory assistance, and the encouraging results from the use of current LVADs as long-term support, a randomized multicenter trial (REMATCH) was conducted to evaluate the use of LVADs as permanent devices in the treatment of heart failure. REMATCH demonstrated a 48 percent reduction in the risk of death in the group treated with LVADs as compared to the medically treated group, with superior quality of life measurements demonstrated in the LVAD treatment group.[142] Comparable preliminary results have been reported from a similar destination study using the Novacor device (the INTREPID trial).

REMATCH patients with VADs were more than twice as likely to develop an adverse event, and had a higher median number of days spent in and out of the hospital.[142] Further analysis of the REMATCH data after study completion has demonstrated improved outcomes across several *eras* of the study.[167] Notably, survival in the LVAD cohort was significantly higher for those enrolled after 2000, and 2-year survival demonstrated incremental improvement despite little change in the optimal medical management cohort.

[ ] FUTURE DEVELOPMENTS

Certainly, with the advent of more durable devices, other design improvements, and greater clinical experience, the survival benefit conferred by long-term or destination LVAD therapy is likely only to improve further. The obstacles of thrombogenicity (and embolization), device infection, and immunologic sensitization remain a target of ongoing research for the currently available VADs. Additionally, the increasing desire to miniaturize pump design to allow for complete implant ability or pediatric applications continues to drive development (Table 27–14).

Children with end-stage heart failure are at particular risk of dying while awaiting transplantation, owing to the relative unavailability of donor organs in pediatric size ranges. Most clinical experience to date with isolated ventricular assistance has been with children >6 kg; the largest experience in smaller children and neonates has been with ECMO. Several specific requirements for a pediatric assist device make its development difficult.

Worldwide, only the Berlin Heart EXCOR (Berlin Heart AG, Berlin, Germany) and the Medos (Medos AG, Langenselbold, Germany) pumps have enjoyed significant application in children (Fig. 27–19). Both are essentially miniaturized versions of the Pierce-Donachy paracorporeal biventricular assist device (similar to the Thoratec).[168,169] However, a recent directive from the NHLBI has been issued to address this need, with expectations of clinical trials in 5 years.

TABLE 27–14

Specific Design Requirements That Complicate the Development of a Pediatric Assist Device

Available across several sizes of recipient

Versatility (biventricular, single-ventricle support)

Allows the addition of an oxygenator for pulmonary support

Cannulae small enough to allow ventricular decompression without generating excessive negative pressure (and air entrainment)

Small enough to be implantable in larger children

Able to run at flows considered *low* by adult standards but will fully support children (e.g., 0.5–1.5 L/min).

Mechanical circulatory assistance has evolved over the past 20 years from an investigational strategy for the moribund, to a standard therapy supporting patients in cardiogenic shock and decompensated heart failure. Indeed, the consistent results with VAD use in this setting have advanced beyond those of pharmacotherapy to the point at which randomization for trials between VAD use and medical therapy alone have been questioned as ethically inappropriate.

It is evident now that far fewer patients are being enrolled in destination therapy trials than initially anticipated. Certainly, some of this discrepancy is likely because of reluctance on the part of referring physicians to view VAD support for nontransplant candidates as anything but supportive end-of-life care. If the prior lessons of the 1990s may be applied to the current arena, earlier implantation of VADs as destination therapy in healthier patients will likely provide superior outcomes with regard both to long-term morbidity and mortality. Thus, just as VAD implantation evolved from a form of support available only to those dying from cardiogenic shock, so too now must destination therapy be viewed as a modality available to heart failure patients other than those for whom medical therapy has reached its limits.

Only with the persistent introduction and trial of new ventricular assist devices with sufficient registries to document efficacy, adverse events, and quality-of-life measures, will innovative therapies continue to develop. The dream of the ideal device—completely implantable, requiring no anticoagulation, available across a wide variety of patient sizes, and endlessly durable—continues to evade current technology but remains a target of design for the future.

REFERENCES

1. Carrel A, Guthrie CC. The transplantation of veins and organs. *Am J Med* 1905;10:1101.
2. Edwards WS, Edwards PD. *Alexis Carrel: Visionary Surgeon.* Springfield, IL: Charles C Thomas; 1974.
3. Mann FC, Priestly JT, Markowitz J, Yater WM. Transplantation of the intact mammalian heart. *Arch Surg* 1933;26:219–224.
4. Lower RR, Shumway NE. Studies on orthotopic homotransplantation of the canine heart. *Surg Forum* 1960;11:18–19.
5. Starzl TE, Marchioro TL, Waddell WR. The reversal of rejection in human renal homografts with subsequent development of homograft tolerance. *Surg Gynecol Obstet* October 1963;117:385–395.
6. Barnard CN. The operation: a human cardiac transplant—an interim report of a successful operation performed at Groote Schuur Hospital, Cape Town. *S Afr Med J* December 30, 1967;41(48):1271–1274.
7. Reitz BA, Bieber CP, Raney AA, et al. Orthotopic heart and combined heart and lung transplantation with cyclosporin-A immune suppression. *Transplant Proc* March 1981;13(1 pt 1):393–396.
8. Taylor DO, Edwards LB, Boucek MM, et al. Registry of the International Society for Heart and Lung Transplantation: twenty-third official adult heart transplantation report—2006. *J Heart Lung Transplant* August 2006;25(8):869–879.
9. Pitt B, Zannad F, Remme WJ, et al. The effect of spironolactone on morbidity and mortality in patients with severe heart failure. Randomized Aldactone Evaluation Study Investigators. *N Engl J Med* September 2, 1999;341(10):709–717.
10. Packer M, Coats AJ, Fowler MB, et al. Effect of carvedilol on survival in severe chronic heart failure. *N Engl J Med* May 31, 2001;344(22):1651–1658.
11. Bardy GH, Lee KL, Mark DB, et al. Amiodarone or an implantable cardioverter-defibrillator for congestive heart failure. *N Engl J Med* January 20, 2005;352(3):225–237.
12. Cleland JG, Daubert JC, Erdmann E, et al. The effect of cardiac resynchronization on morbidity and mortality in heart failure. *N Engl J Med* April 14, 2005;352(15):1539–1549.
13. Packer DL, Bardy GH, Worley SJ, et al. Tachycardia-induced cardiomyopathy: a reversible form of left ventricular dysfunction. *Am J Cardiol* March 1, 1986;57(8):563–570.
14. Mancini DM, Eisen H, Kussmaul W, Mull R, Edmunds LH Jr, Wilson JR. Value of peak exercise oxygen consumption for optimal timing of cardiac transplantation in ambulatory patients with heart failure. *Circulation* March 1991;83(3):778–786.
15. Butler J, Khadim G, Paul KM, et al. Selection of patients for heart transplantation in the current era of heart failure therapy. *J Am Coll Cardiol* March 3, 2004;43(5):787–793.
16. Aaronson KD, Schwartz JS, Chen TM, Wong KL, Goin JE, Mancini DM. Development and prospective validation of a clinical

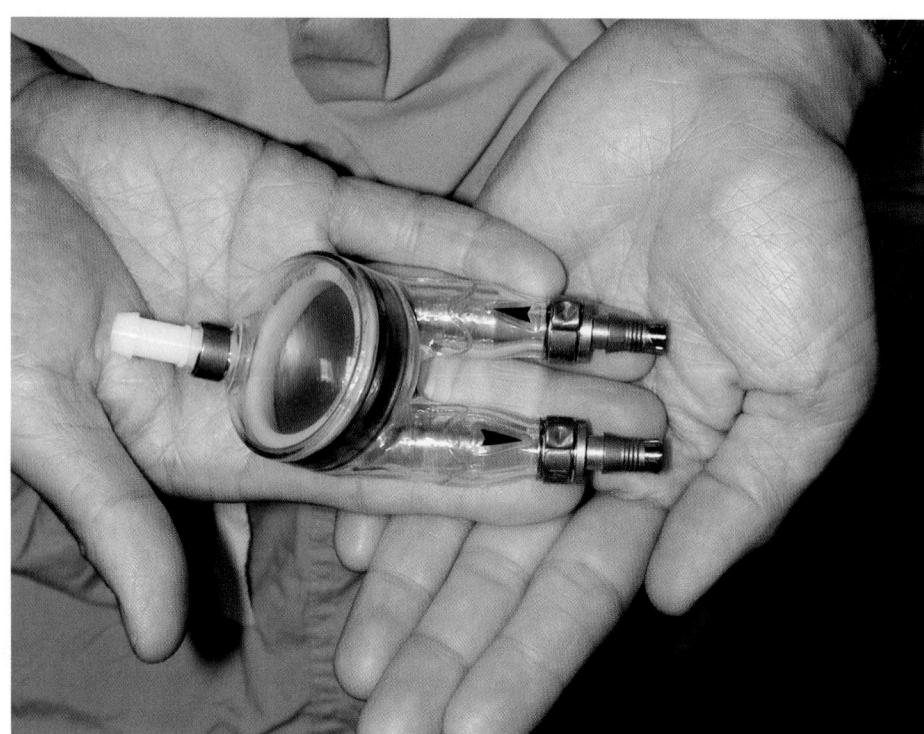

FIGURE 27–19. The Berlin Heart EXCOR pediatric ventricular assist device.

index to predict survival in ambulatory patients referred for cardiac transplant evaluation. *Circulation* June 17, 1997;95(12):2660–2667.

17. Peterson LR, Schechtman KB, Ewald GA, et al. Timing of cardiac transplantation in patients with heart failure receiving beta-adrenergic blockers. *J Heart Lung Transplant* October 2003;22(10):1141–1148.

18. O'Neill JO, Young JB, Pothier CE, Lauer MS. Peak oxygen consumption as a predictor of death in patients with heart failure receiving beta-blockers. *Circulation* May 10, 2005;111(18):2313–2318.

19. Mehra MR, Kobashigawa J, Starling R, et al. Listing criteria for heart transplantation: International Society for Heart and Lung Transplantation guidelines for the care of cardiac transplant candidates—2006. *J Heart Lung Transplant* September 2006;25(9):1024–1042.

20. Morgan JA, John R, Weinberg AD, et al. Long-term results of cardiac transplantation in patients 65 years of age and older: a comparative analysis. *Ann Thorac Surg* December 2003;76(6):1982–1987.

21. Blanche C, Blanche DA, Kearney B, et al. Heart transplantation in patients seventy years of age and older: a comparative analysis of outcome. *J Thorac Cardiovasc Surg* March 2001;121(3):532–541.

22. Lake KD, Smith CI, LaForest SK, Allen J, Pritzker MR, Emery RW. Policies regarding the transplantation of hepatitis C-positive candidates and donor organs. *J Heart Lung Transplant* September 1997;16(9):917–921.

23. Hosenpud JD, Pamidi SR, Fiol BS, Cinquegrani MP, Keck BM. Outcomes in patients who are hepatitis B surface antigen-positive before transplantation: an analysis and study using the joint ISHLT/UNOS thoracic registry. *J Heart Lung Transplant* August 2000;19(8):781–785.

24. Halpern SD, Ubel PA, Caplan AL. Solid-organ transplantation in HIV-infected patients. *N Engl J Med* July 25, 2002;347(4):284–287.

25. Bisleri G, Morgan JA, Deng MC, Mancini DM, Oz MC. Should HIV-positive recipients undergo heart transplantation? *J Thorac Cardiovasc Surg* November 2003;126(5):1639–1640.

26. Lietz K, John R, Burke EA, et al. Pretransplant cachexia and morbid obesity are predictors of increased mortality after heart transplantation. *Transplantation* July 27, 2001;72(2):277–283.

27. Grady KL, White-Williams C, Naftel D, et al. Are preoperative obesity and cachexia risk factors for post heart transplant morbidity and mortality: a multi-institutional study of preoperative weight-height indices. Cardiac Transplant Research Database (CTRD) Group. *J Heart Lung Transplant* August 1999;18(8):750–763.

28. Winters GL, Kendall TJ, Radio SJ, et al. Posttransplant obesity and hyperlipidemia: major predictors of severity of coronary arteriopathy in failed human heart allografts. *J Heart Transplant* July–August 1990;9(4):364–371.

29. Williams JJ, Lund LH, LaManca J, et al. Excessive weight gain in cardiac transplant recipients. *J Heart Lung Transplant* January 2006;25(1):36–41.

30. Munoz E, Lonquist JL, Radovancevic B, et al. Long-term results in diabetic patients undergoing heart transplantation. *J Heart Lung Transplant* September–October 1992;11(5):943–949.

31. Morgan JA, John R, Weinberg AD, Colletti NJ, Mancini DM, Edwards NM. Heart transplantation in diabetic recipients: a decade review of 161 patients at Columbia Presbyterian. *J Thorac Cardiovasc Surg* May 2004;127(5):1486–1492.

32. Ladowski JS, Kormos RL, Uretsky BF, Griffith BP, Armitage JM, Hardesty RL. Heart transplantation in diabetic recipients. *Transplantation* February 1990;49(2):303–305.

33. Porrett PM, Desai SS, Timmins KJ, Twomey CR, Sonnad SS, Olthoff KM. Combined orthotopic heart and liver transplantation: the need for exception status listing. *Liver Transpl* December 2004;10(12):1539–1544.

34. Wang SS, Chou NK, Chi NH, et al. Simultaneous heart and kidney transplantation for combined cardiac and renal failure. *Transplant Proc* September 2006;38(7):2135–2137.

35. Guidelines for the determination of death. Report of the medical consultants on the diagnosis of death to the President's Commission for the Study of Ethical Problems in Medicine and Biomedical and Behavioral Research. *JAMA* November 13, 1981;246(19):2184–2186.

36. Zaroff JG, Rosengard BR, Armstrong WF, et al. Consensus conference report: maximizing use of organs recovered from the cadaver donor: cardiac recommendations, March 28–29, 2001, Crystal City, Va. *Circulation* August 13, 2002;106(7):836–841.

37. Sheehy E, Conrad SL, Brigham LE, et al. Estimating the number of potential organ donors in the United States. *N Engl J Med* August 14, 2003;349(7):667–674.

38. Hosenpud JD, Edwards EB, Lin HM, Daily OP. Influence of HLA matching on thoracic transplant outcomes: an analysis from the UNOS/ISHLT Thoracic Registry. *Circulation* July 15, 1996;94(2):170–174.

39. Quantz MA, Bennett LE, Meyer DM, Novick RJ. Does human leukocyte antigen matching influence the outcome of lung transplantation? An analysis of 3,549 lung transplantations. *J Heart Lung Transplant* May 2000;19(5):473–479.

40. Almenar L, Maeso ML, Martinez-Dolz L, et al. Influence of HLA matching on survival in heart transplantation. *Transplant Proc* November 2005;37(9):4001–4005.

41. Dreyfus G, Jebara V, Mihaileanu S, Carpentier AF. Total orthotopic heart transplantation: an alternative to the standard technique. *Ann Thorac Surg* November 1991;52(5):1181–1184.

42. El-Gamel A, Deiraniya AK, Rahman AN, Campbell CS, Yonan NA. Orthotopic heart transplantation hemodynamics: does atrial preservation improve cardiac output after transplantation? *J Heart Lung Transplant* June 1996;15(6):564–571.

43. Traversi E, Pozzoli M, Grande A, et al. The bicaval anastomosis technique for orthotopic heart transplantation yields better atrial function than the standard technique: an echocardiographic automatic boundary detection study. *J Heart Lung Transplant* November 1998;17(11):1065–1074.

44. Meyer SR, Modry DL, Bainey K, et al. Declining need for permanent pacemaker insertion with the bicaval technique of orthotopic heart transplantation. *Can J Cardiol* February 2005;21(2):159–163.

45. Parry G, Holt ND, Dark JH, McComb JM. Declining need for pacemaker implantation after cardiac transplantation. *Pacing Clin Electrophysiol* November 1998;21(11 pt 2):2350–2352.

46. Sze DY, Robbins RC, Semba CP, Razavi MK, Dake MD. Superior vena cava syndrome after heart transplantation: percutaneous treatment of a complication of bicaval anastomoses. *J Thorac Cardiovasc Surg* August 1998;116(2):253–261.

47. Goldstein DR, Coffey CS, Benza RL, Nanda NC, Bourge RC. Relative perioperative bradycardia does not lead to adverse outcomes after cardiac transplantation. *Am J Transplant* April 2003;3(4):484–491.

48. Bertolet BD, Eagle DA, Conti JB, Mills RM, Belardinelli L. Bradycardia after heart transplantation: reversal with theophylline. *J Am Coll Cardiol* August 1996;28(2):396–399.

49. Smart FW, Naftel DC, Costanzo MR, et al. Risk factors for early, cumulative, and fatal infections after heart transplantation: a multiinstitutional study. *J Heart Lung Transplant* April 1996;15(4):329–341.

50. Miller LW, Naftel DC, Bourge RC, et al. Infection after heart transplantation: a multiinstitutional study. Cardiac Transplant Research Database Group. *J Heart Lung Transplant* May–June 1994;13(3):381–392; discussion 393.

51. Hershberger RE, Starling RC, Eisen HJ, et al. Daclizumab to prevent rejection after cardiac transplantation. *N Engl J Med* June 30, 2005;352(26):2705–2713.

52. Taylor DO, Barr ML, Radovancevic B, et al. A randomized, multicenter comparison of tacrolimus and cyclosporine immunosuppressive regimens in cardiac transplantation: decreased hyperlipidemia and hypertension with tacrolimus. *J Heart Lung Transplant* April 1999;18(4):336–345.

53. Reichart B, Meiser B, Vigano M, et al. European Multicenter Tacrolimus (FK506) Heart Pilot Study: one-year results—European Tacrolimus Multicenter Heart Study Group. *J Heart Lung Transplant* August 1998;17(8):775–781.

54. Kobashigawa JA, Miller LW, Russell SD, et al. Tacrolimus with mycophenolate mofetil (MMF) or sirolimus vs. cyclosporine with MMF in cardiac transplant patients: 1-year report. *Am J Transplant* June 2006;6(6):1377–1386.

55. Kobashigawa J, Miller L, Renlund D, et al. A randomized active-controlled trial of mycophenolate mofetil in heart transplant recipients. Mycophenolate Mofetil Investigators. *Transplantation* August 27, 1998;66(4):507–515.

56. Hosenpud JD, Bennett LE. Mycophenolate mofetil versus azathioprine in patients surviving the initial cardiac transplant hospitalization: an analysis of the Joint UNOS/ISHLT Thoracic Registry. *Transplantation* November 27, 2001;72(10):1662–1665.

57. Lorber MI, Basadonna GP, Friedman AL, et al. The evolving role of tor inhibitors for individualizing posttransplant immunosuppression. *Transplant Proc* November–December 2001;33(7–8):3075–3077.

58. Keogh A, Richardson M, Ruygrok P, et al. Sirolimus in de novo heart transplant recipients reduces acute rejection and prevents coronary artery disease at 2 years: a randomized clinical trial. *Circulation* October 26, 2004;110(17):2694–2700.

59. Eisen HJ, Tuzcu EM, Dorent R, et al. Everolimus for the prevention of allograft rejection and vasculopathy in cardiac-transplant recipients. *N Engl J Med* August 28, 2003;349(9):847–858.

60. Mancini D, Pinney S, Burkhoff D, et al. Use of rapamycin slows progression of cardiac transplantation vasculopathy. *Circulation* July 8, 2003;108(1):48–53.

61. Cabezon S, Lage E, Hinojosa R, Ordonez A, Campos A. Sirolimus improves renal function in cardiac transplantation. *Transplant Proc* April 2005;37(3):1546–1547.

62. Fernandez-Valls M, Gonzalez-Vilchez F, de Prada JA, Ruano J, Ruisanchez C, Martin-Duran R. Sirolimus as an alternative to anticalcineurin therapy in heart transplantation: experience of a single center. *Transplant Proc* November 2005;37(9):4021–4023.

63. Bestetti R, Theodoropoulos TA, Burdmann EA, Filho MA, Cordeiro JA, Villafanha D. Switch from calcineurin inhibitors to sirolimus-induced renal recovery in heart transplant recipients in the midterm follow-up. *Transplantation* March 15, 2006;81(5):692–696.

64. Smith RA, Cokkinides V, Eyre HJ. American Cancer Society guidelines for the early detection of cancer, 2006. *CA Cancer J Clin* January–February 2006;56(1):11–25; quiz 49–50.

65. Young L, Alfieri C, Hennessy K, et al. Expression of Epstein-Barr virus transformation-associated genes in tissues of patients with EBV lymphoproliferative disease. *N Engl J Med* October 19, 1989;321(16):1080–1085.

66. Hanto DW, Frizzera G, Gajl-Peczalska J, et al. The Epstein-Barr virus (EBV) in the pathogenesis of posttransplant lymphoma. *Transplant Proc* March 1981;13(1 pt 2):756–760.

67. Starzl TE, Nalesnik MA, Porter KA, et al. Reversibility of lymphomas and lymphoproliferative lesions developing under cyclosporin-steroid therapy. *Lancet* March 17, 1984;1(8377):583–587.

68. Jain AB, Marcos A, Pokharna R, et al. Rituximab (chimeric anti-CD20 antibody) for posttransplant lymphoproliferative disorder after solid organ transplantation in adults: long-term experience from a single center. *Transplantation* December 27, 2005;80(12):1692–1698.

69. Blaes AH, Peterson BA, Bartlett N, Dunn DL, Morrison VA. Rituximab therapy is effective for posttransplant lymphoproliferative disorders after solid organ transplantation: results of a phase II trial. *Cancer* October 15, 2005;104(8):1661–1667.

70. Kemnitz J, Cremer J, Restrepo-Specht I, et al. Hyperacute rejection in heart allografts. Case studies. *Pathol Res Pract* January 1991;187(1):23–29.

71. Stewart S, Winters GL, Fishbein MC, et al. Revision of the 1990 working formulation for the standardization of nomenclature in the diagnosis of heart rejection. *J Heart Lung Transplant* November 2005;24(11):1710–1720.

72. Michaels PJ, Espejo ML, Kobashigawa J, et al. Humoral rejection in cardiac transplantation: risk factors, hemodynamic consequences and relationship to transplant coronary artery disease. *J Heart Lung Transplant* January 2003;22(1):58–69.

73. Hammond EH, Yowell RL, Nunoda S, et al. Vascular (humoral) rejection in heart transplantation: pathologic observations and clinical implications. *J Heart Transplant* November–December 1989;8(6):430–443.

74. Subherwal S, Kobashigawa JA, Cogert G, Patel J, Espejo M, Oeser B. Incidence of acute cellular rejection and noncellular rejection in cardiac transplantation. *Transplant Proc* December 2004;36(10):3171–3172.

75. Reed EF, Demetris AJ, Hammond E, et al. Acute antibody-mediated rejection of cardiac transplants. *J Heart Lung Transplant.* February 2006;25(2):153–159.

76. Taylor DO, Yowell RL, Kfoury AG, Hammond EH, Renlund DG. Allograft coronary artery disease: clinical correlations with circulating anti-HLA antibodies and the immunohistopathologic pattern of vascular rejection. *J Heart Lung Transplant* June 2000;19(6):518–521.

77. Deng MC, Eisen HJ, Mehra MR, et al. Noninvasive discrimination of rejection in cardiac allograft recipients using gene expression profiling. *Am J Transplant* January 2006;6(1):150–160.

78. Sethi GK, Kosaraju S, Arabia FA, Roasdo LJ, McCarthy MS, Copeland JG. Is it necessary to perform surveillance endomyocardial biopsies in heart transplant recipients? *J Heart Lung Transplant* November–December 1995;14(6 pt 1):1047–1051.

79. White JA, Guiraudon C, Pflugfelder PW, Kostuk WJ. Routine surveillance myocardial biopsies are unnecessary beyond one year after heart transplantation. *J Heart Lung Transplant* November–December 1995;14(6 pt 1):1052–1056.

80. First MR, Schroeder TJ, Hurtubise PE, et al. Successful retreatment of allograft rejection with OKT3. *Transplantation* January 1989;47(1):88–91.

81. Cantarovich M, Latter DA, Loertscher R. Treatment of steroid-resistant and recurrent acute cardiac transplant rejection with a short course of antibody therapy. *Clin Transplant* August 1997;11(4):316–321.

82. Keren A, Hayes HM, O'Driscoll G. Late humoral rejection in a cardiac transplant recipient treated with the anti-CD20 monoclonal antibody rituximab. *Transplant Proc* June 2006;38(5):1520–1522.

83. Garrett HE Jr, Duvall-Seaman D, Helsley B, Groshart K. Treatment of vascular rejection with rituximab in cardiac transplantation. *J Heart Lung Transplant* September 2005;24(9):1337–1342.

84. Crespo-Leiro MG, Veiga-Barreiro A, Domenech N, et al. Humoral heart rejection (severe allograft dysfunction with no signs of cellular rejection or ischemia): incidence, management, and the value of C4d for diagnosis. *Am J Transplant* October 2005;5(10):2560–2564.

85. Weinblatt ME. Methotrexate for chronic diseases in adults. *N Engl J Med* February 2, 1995;332(5):330–331.

86. Hunt SA, Strober S, Hoppe RT, Stinson EB. Total lymphoid irradiation for treatment of intractable cardiac allograft rejection. *J Heart Lung Transplant* March–April 1991;10(2):211–216.

87. Levin B, Bohannon L, Warvariv V, Bry W, Collins G. Total lymphoid irradiation (TLI) in the cyclosporine era—use of TLI in resistant cardiac allograft rejection. *Transplant Proc* February 1989;21(1 pt 2):1793–1795.

88. Costanzo-Nordin MR, Grusk BB, Silver MA, et al. Reversal of recalcitrant cardiac allograft rejection with methotrexate. *Circulation.* November 1988;78(5 pt 2):III47–III57.

89. Bouchart F, Gundry SR, Van Schaack-Gonzales J, et al. Methotrexate as rescue/adjunctive immunotherapy in infant and adult heart transplantation. *J Heart Lung Transplant* May–June 1993;12(3):427–433.

90. Dein JR, Oyer PE, Stinson EB, Starnes VA, Shumway NE. Cardiac retransplantation in the cyclosporine era. *Ann Thorac Surg* September 1989;48(3):350–355.

91. Radovancevic B, McGiffin DC, Kobashigawa JA, et al. Retransplantation in 7,290 primary transplant patients: a 10-year multi-institutional study. *J Heart Lung Transplant* August 2003;22(8):862–868.

92. Pucci AM, Forbes RD, Billingham ME. Pathologic features in long-term cardiac allografts. *J Heart Transplant* July–August 1990;9(4):339–345.

93. Kaye DM, Esler M, Kingwell B, McPherson G, Esmore D, Jennings G. Functional and neurochemical evidence for partial cardiac sympathetic reinnervation after cardiac transplantation in humans. *Circulation* September 1993;88(3):1110–1118.

94. Bernardi L, Bianchini B, Spadacini G, et al. Demonstrable cardiac reinnervation after human heart transplantation by carotid baroreflex modulation of RR interval. *Circulation* November 15, 1995;92(10):2895–2903.

95. Stark RP, McGinn AL, Wilson RF. Chest pain in cardiac-transplant recipients. Evidence of sensory reinnervation after cardiac transplantation. *N Engl J Med* June 20, 1991;324(25):1791–1794.

96. Rickenbacher PR, Pinto FJ, Lewis NP, et al. Prognostic importance of intimal thickness as measured by intracoronary ultrasound after cardiac transplantation. *Circulation.* December 15, 1995;92(12):3445–3452.

97. Kobashigawa JA, Tobis JM, Starling RC, et al. Multicenter intravascular ultrasound validation study among heart transplant recipients: outcomes after five years. *J Am Coll Cardiol* May 3, 2005;45(9):1532–1537.

98. Kobashigawa JA, Tobis JM, Mentzer RM, et al. Mycophenolate mofetil reduces intimal thickness by intravascular ultrasound after heart transplant: reanalysis of the multicenter trial. *Am J Transplant* May 2006;6(5 pt 1):993–997.

99. Smart FW, Ballantyne CM, Cocanougher B, et al. Insensitivity of noninvasive tests to detect coronary artery vasculopathy after heart transplant. *Am J Cardiol* February 1, 1991;67(4):243–247.

100. Akosah KO, Mohanty PK, Funai JT, et al. Noninvasive detection of transplant coronary artery disease by dobutamine stress echocardiography. *J Heart Lung Transplant* November-December 1994;13(6):1024–1038.

101. Derumeaux G, Redonnet M, Mouton-Schleifer D, et al. Dobutamine stress echocardiography in orthotopic heart transplant recipients. VACOMED Research Group. *J Am Coll Cardiol* June 1995;25(7):1665–1672.

102. Spes CH, Klauss V, Mudra H, et al. Diagnostic and prognostic value of serial dobutamine stress echocardiography for noninvasive assessment of cardiac allograft vasculopathy: a comparison with coronary angiography and intravascular ultrasound. *Circulation.* August 3, 1999;100(5):509–515.

103. Bacal F, Moreira L, Souza G, et al. Dobutamine stress echocardiography predicts cardiac events or death in asymptomatic patients long-term after heart transplantation: 4-year prospective evaluation. *J Heart Lung Transplant* November 2004;23(11):1238–1244.

104. Keogh AM, Valantine HA, Hunt SA, et al. Impact of proximal or midvessel discrete coronary artery stenoses on survival after heart transplantation. *J Heart Lung Transplant* September–October 1992;11(5):892–901.

105. Schroeder JS, Gao SZ, Alderman EL, et al. A preliminary study of diltiazem in the prevention of coronary artery disease in heart-transplant recipients. *N Engl J Med* January 21, 1993;328(3):164–170.

106. Kobashigawa JA, Katznelson S, Laks H, et al. Effect of pravastatin on outcomes after cardiac transplantation. *N Engl J Med* September 7, 1995;333(10):621–627.

107. Wenke K, Meiser B, Thiery J, et al. Simvastatin reduces graft vessel disease and mortality after heart transplantation: a four-year randomized trial. *Circulation* September 2, 1997;96(5):1398–1402.

108. Bader FM, Kfoury AG, Gilbert EM, et al. Percutaneous coronary interventions with stents in cardiac transplant recipients. *J Heart Lung Transplant* March 2006;25(3):298–301.

109. Halle AA III, DiSciascio G, Massin EK, et al. Coronary angioplasty, atherectomy and bypass surgery in cardiac transplant recipients. *J Am Coll Cardiol* July 1995;26(1):120–128.

110. Topkara VK, Dang NC, John R, et al. A decade experience of cardiac retransplantation in adult recipients. *J Heart Lung Transplant* November 2005;24(11):1745–1750.

111. Angermann CE, Bullinger M, Spes CH, Zellner M, Kemkes BM, Theisen K. Quality of life in long-term survivors of orthotopic heart transplantation. *Z Kardiol* August 1992;81(8):411–417.

112. Jones BM, Taylor F, Downs K, Spratt P. Longitudinal study of quality of life and psychological adjustment after cardiac transplantation. *Med J Aust* July 6, 1992;157(1):24–26.

113. Grady KL, Jalowiec A, White-Williams C. Predictors of quality of life in patients at one year after heart transplantation. *J Heart Lung Transplant* March 1999;18(3):202–210.

114. Salyer J, Flattery MP, Joyner PL, Elswick RK. Lifestyle and quality of life in long-term cardiac transplant recipients. *J Heart Lung Transplant* March 2003;22(3):309–321.

115. Bolling SF, Pagani FD, Deeb GM, Bach DS. Intermediate-term outcome of mitral reconstruction in cardiomyopathy. *J Thorac Cardiovasc Surg* February 1998;115(2):381–386; discussion 387–388.

116. Bishay ES, McCarthy PM, Cosgrove DM, et al. Mitral valve surgery in patients with severe left ventricular dysfunction. *Eur J Cardiothorac Surg* March 2000;17(3):213–221.

117. Calafiore AM, Gallina S, Di Mauro M, et al. Mitral valve procedure in dilated cardiomyopathy: repair or replacement? *Ann Thorac Surg* April 2001;71(4):1146–1152; discussion 1152–1143.

118. Bitran D, Merin O, Klutstein MW, Od-Allah S, Shapira N, Silberman S. Mitral valve repair in severe ischemic cardiomyopathy. *J Card Surg* January–February 2001;16(1):79–82.

119. Sarris GE, Cahill PD, Hansen DE, Derby GC, Miller DC. Restoration of left ventricular systolic performance after reattachment of the mitral chordae tendineae: the importance of valvular-ventricular interaction. *J Thorac Cardiovasc Surg* June 1988;95(6):969–979.

120. Batista RJ, Santos JL, Takeshita N, Bocchino L, Lima PN, Cunha MA. Partial left ventriculectomy to improve left ventricular function in end-stage heart disease. *J Card Surg* March–April 1996;11(2):96–97; discussion 98.

121. McCarthy JF, McCarthy PM, Starling RC, et al. Partial left ventriculectomy and mitral valve repair for end-stage congestive heart failure. *Eur J Cardiothorac Surg* April 1998;13(4):337–343.

122. Cox JL. Left ventricular aneurysms: pathophysiologic observations and standard resection. *Semin Thorac Cardiovasc Surg* April 1997;9(2):113–122.

123. Cooley DA, Collins HA, Morris GC Jr, Chapman DW. Ventricular aneurysm after myocardial infarction; surgical excision with use of temporary cardiopulmonary bypass. *JAMA* May 31, 1958;167(5):557–560.

124. Jatene AD. Left ventricular aneurysmectomy: resection or reconstruction. *J Thorac Cardiovasc Surg* March 1985;89(3):321–331.

125. Dor V, Saab M, Coste P, Kornaszewska M, Montiglio F. Left ventricular aneurysm: a new surgical approach. *Thorac Cardiovasc Surg* February 1989;37(1):11–19.

126. Sartipy U, Albage A, Lindblom D. The Dor procedure for left ventricular reconstruction. Ten-year clinical experience. *Eur J Cardiothorac Surg* June 2005;27(6):1005–1010.

127. Dor V. The endoventricular circular patch plasty ("Dor procedure") in ischemic akinetic dilated ventricles. *Heart Fail Rev* September 2001;6(3):187–193.

128. Athanasuleas CL, Buckberg GD, Stanley AW, et al. Surgical ventricular restoration in the treatment of congestive heart failure due to post-infarction ventricular dilation. *J Am Coll Cardiol* October 6, 2004;44(7):1439–1445.

129. Doenst T, Velazquez EJ, Beyersdorf F, et al. To STICH or not to STICH. We know the answer, but do we understand the question? *J Thorac Cardiovasc Surg* February 2005;129(2):246–249.

130. Jones RH. Is it time for a randomized trial of surgical treatment of ischemic heart failure? *J Am Coll Cardiol* April 2001;37(5):1210–1213.

131. Joyce D, Loebe M, Noon GP, et al. Revascularization and ventricular restoration in patients with ischemic heart failure: the STICH trial. *Curr Opin Cardiol* November 2003;18(6):454–457.

132. Buckberg GD. Questions and answers approximately the STICH trial: a different perspective. *J Thorac Cardiovasc Surg* August 2005;130(2):245–249.

133. McCarthy PM. Mechanical assist devices. *J Card Surg* May–June 2001;16(3):177.

134. Schenk S, Reichenspurner H, Boehm DH, et al. Myosplint implant and shape-change procedure: intra- and peri-operative safety and feasibility. *J Heart Lung Transplant* June 2002;21(6):680–686.

135. Starling RC, Jessup M. Worldwide clinical experience with the CorCap Cardiac Support Device. *J Card Fail* December 2004;10(6 suppl):S225–S233.

136. Blom AS, Mukherjee R, Pilla JJ, et al. Cardiac support device modifies left ventricular geometry and myocardial structure after myocardial infarction. *Circulation* August 30, 2005;112(9):1274–1283.

137. Acker MA, Bolling S, Shemin R, et al. Mitral valve surgery in heart failure: insights from the Acorn Clinical Trial. *J Thorac Cardiovasc Surg* September 2006;132(3):568–577, e561–e564.

138. Copeland JG, Smith RG, Arabia FA, Nolan PE, Banchy ME. The CardioWest total artificial heart as a bridge to transplantation. *Semin Thorac Cardiovasc Surg* July 2000;12(3):238–242.

139. Chen JM, Spanier TB, Gonzalez JJ, et al. Improved survival in patients with acute myocarditis using external pulsatile mechanical ventricular assistance. *J Heart Lung Transplant* April 1999;18(4):351–357.

140. Marelli D, Laks H, Amsel B, et al. Temporary mechanical support with the BVS 5000 assist device during treatment of acute myocarditis. *J Card Surg* January–February 1997;12(1):55–59.

141. Minami K, el-Banayosy A, Posival H, et al. Improvement of survival rate in patients with cardiogenic shock by using nonpulsatile and pulsatile ventricular assist device. *Int J Artif Organs* December 1992;15(12):715–721.

142. Rose EA, Gelijns AC, Moskowitz AJ, et al. Long-term mechanical left ventricular assistance for end-stage heart failure. *N Engl J Med* November 15, 2001;345(20):1435–1443.

143. Levi D, Marelli D, Plunkett M, et al. Use of assist devices and ECMO to bridge pediatric patients with cardiomyopathy to transplantation. *J Heart Lung Transplant* July 2002;21(7):760–770.

144. Smedira NG, Moazami N, Golding CM, et al. Clinical experience with 202 adults receiving extracorporeal membrane oxygenation for cardiac failure: survival at five years. *J Thorac Cardiovasc Surg* July 2001;122(1):92–102.

145. Morgan JA, Stewart AS, Lee BJ, Oz MC, Naka Y. Role of the Abiomed BVS 5000 device for short-term support and bridge to transplantation. *ASAIO J* July–August 2004;50(4):360–363.

146. Jett GK. ABIOMED BVS 5000: experience and potential advantages. *Ann Thorac Surg* January 1996;61(1):301–304; discussion 311–303.

147. Sun BC, Catanese KA, Spanier TB, et al. 100 long-term implantable left ventricular assist devices: the Columbia Presbyterian interim experience. *Ann Thorac Surg* August 1999;68(2):688–694.

148. Pasque MK, Rogers JG. Adverse events in the use of HeartMate vented electric and Novacor left ventricular assist devices: comparing apples and oranges. *J Thorac Cardiovasc Surg* December 2002;124(6):1063–1067.

149. Strauch JT, Spielvogel D, Haldenwang PL, et al. Recent improvements in outcome with the Novacor left ventricular assist device. *J Heart Lung Transplant* June 2003;22(6):674–680.

150. Farrar DJ. The Thoratec ventricular assist device: a paracorporeal pump for treating acute and chronic heart failure. *Semin Thorac Cardiovasc Surg* July 2000;12(3):243–250.

151. Samuels LE, Holmes EC, Garwood P, Ferdinand F. Initial experience with the Abiomed AB5000 ventricular assist device system. *Ann Thorac Surg* July 2005;80(1):309–312.

152. Noon GP, Morley DL, Irwin S, Abdelsayed SV, Benkowski RJ, Lynch BE. Clinical experience with the MicroMed DeBakey ventricular assist device. *Ann Thorac Surg* March 2001;71(3 suppl):S133–138; discussion S144–136.

153. Griffith BP, Kormos RL, Borovetz HS, et al. HeartMate II left ventricular assist system: from concept to first clinical use. *Ann Thorac Surg* March 2001;71(3 suppl):S116–S120; discussion S114–S116.

154. Frazier OH, Shah NA, Myers TJ, Robertson KD, Gregoric ID, Delgado R. Use of the Flowmaker (Jarvik 2000) left ventricular assist device for destination therapy and bridging to transplantation. *Cardiology* 2004;101(1–3):111–116.

155. Frazier OH, Myers TJ, Westaby S, Gregoric ID. Use of the Jarvik 2000 left ventricular assist system as a bridge to heart transplantation or as destination therapy for patients with chronic heart failure. *Ann Surg* May 2003;237(5):631–636; discussion 636–637.

156. Levin HR, Oz MC, Chen JM, Packer M, Rose EA, Burkhoff D. Reversal of chronic ventricular dilation in patients with end-stage cardiomyopathy by prolonged mechanical unloading. *Circulation* June 1, 1995;91(11):2717–2720.

157. Frazier OH, Benedict CR, Radovancevic B, et al. Improved left ventricular function after chronic left ventricular unloading. *Ann Thorac Surg* September 1996;62(3):675–681; discussion 681–672.

158. Mueller J, Wallukat G, Weng Y, et al. Predictive factors for weaning from a cardiac assist device: an analysis of clinical, gene expression, and protein data. *J Heart Lung Transplant* February 2001;20(2):202.

159. Mancini DM, Beniaminovitz A, Levin H, et al. Low incidence of myocardial recovery after left ventricular assist device implantation in patients with chronic heart failure. *Circulation* December 1, 1998;98(22):2383–2389.

160. Dang NC, Topkara VK, Kim BT, Mercando ML, Kay J, Naka Y. Clinical outcomes in patients with chronic congestive heart failure who undergo left ventricular assist device implantation. *J Thorac Cardiovasc Surg* November 2005;130(5):1302–1309.

161. Morgan JA, Park Y, Kherani AR, et al. Does bridging to transplantation with a left ventricular assist device adversely affect posttransplantation survival? A comparative analysis of mechanical versus inotropic support. *J Thorac Cardiovasc Surg* October 2003;126(4):1188–1190.

162. John R, Lietz K, Schuster M, et al. Immunologic sensitization in recipients of left ventricular assist devices. *J Thorac Cardiovasc Surg* March 2003;125(3):578–591.

163. Itescu S, Schuster M, Burke E, et al. Immunobiologic consequences of assist devices. *Cardiol Clin* February 2003;21(1):119–133, ix–x.

164. Itescu S, John R. Interactions between the recipient immune system and the left ventricular assist device surface: immunological and clinical implications. *Ann Thorac Surg* June 2003;75(6 suppl):S58–65.

165. Kumpati GS, Cook DJ, Blackstone EH, et al. HLA sensitization in ventricular assist device recipients: does type of device make a difference? *J Thorac Cardiovasc Surg* June 2004;127(6):1800–1807.

166. Ankersmit HJ, Tugulea S, Spanier T, et al. Activation-induced T-cell death and immune dysfunction after implantation of left-ventricular assist device. *Lancet* August 14, 1999;354(9178):550–555.

167. Park SJ, Tector A, Piccioni W, et al. Left ventricular assist devices as destination therapy: a new look at survival. *J Thorac Cardiovasc Surg* January 2005;129(1):9–17.

168. Konertz W, Reul H. Mechanical circulatory support in children. *Int J Artif Organs* December 1997;20(12):657–658.

169. Warnecke H, Berdjis F, Hennig E, et al. Mechanical left ventricular support as a bridge to cardiac transplantation in childhood. *Eur J Cardiothorac Surg* 1991;5(6):330–333.

PART 5 Cardiomyopathy and Specific Heart Muscle Diseases

CHAPTER 28

Classification of Cardiomyopathies*

Barry J. Maron / Gaetano Thiene

Cardiomyopathies are an important and heterogeneous group of diseases for which an understanding in both the public and medical community has historically been impaired by confusion surrounding definitions and nomenclature. Classification schemes, of which there have been many,[1–8] help define and draw relationships or distinctions between these complex diseases for the purpose of promoting greater clarity. Indeed, the precise language attached to these diseases is profoundly important.

However, many classifications in the literature are to some degree contradictory in design, and indeed none of the proposed schemes can be regarded as ideal (including the most recent and contemporary one presented here). This dilemma is largely caused by the heterogeneity in the presentation of this diverse group of diseases. In 1995 a prominent classification of cardiomyopathies was represented in a brief document under the auspices of the World Health Organization (WHO).[1] However, with the identification of new diseases over the past decade, and dramatic advances in cardiovascular diagnosis and knowledge regarding etiology, some disease definitions have become outdated and the WHO classification rendered essentially obsolete. Indeed, the past several years has witnessed a rapid evolution in the molecular genetics of cardiology.[9–14] In particular, ion channelopathies have emerged as conditions predisposing to potentially lethal ventricular tachyarrhythmias, caused by mutations in proteins leading to dysfunctional sodium, potassium, calcium, and other ion channels.

Recently, under the auspices of the American Heart Association, a contemporary classification of cardiomyopathies has been presented,[15] relying substantially on recent advances in the characterization of diseases affecting the myocardium.[16–18] This new classification scheme affords a large measure of clarity to this area of investigation and facilitates interaction among the clinical and research communities in assessing the diagnosis, prognosis, and management of these complex diseases. This classification takes the place of the WHO document; but as new data emerges, it also will undoubtedly require further review and revision in the future.

The contemporary definitions of cardiomyopathies presented here are in concert with the molecular era of cardiovascular disease and have direct clinical applications and implications for cardiac diagnosis. However, by its very nature the classification is a scientific presentation that does not provide methodologies or strategies for clinical diagnosis, nor is it directly applicable to management decisions for patients.

GENERAL CONSIDERATIONS
HISTORICAL CONTEXT

The definition and classification of heart muscle diseases has seen a notable and evolving history. For example, chronic myocarditis was the only recognized cause of heart muscle disease in the 1850s.[2] In 1900 the designation of primary myocardial disease was first introduced. However, it was not until 1957 that the term *cardiomyopathy* was used for the first time. Over

*Adapted from Maron BJ, Towbin JA, Thiene G, et al. Contemporary definitions and classification of the cardiomyopathies: an American Heart Association Scientific Statement from the Council on Clinical Cardiology, Heart Failure and Transplantation Committee; Quality of Care and Outcomes Research and Functional Genomics and Translational Biology Interdisciplinary Working Groups; and Council on Epidemiology and Prevention. *Circulation* 2006;113:1807–1816. With permission of the American Heart Association and Lippincott Williams and Wilkins.

the next 25 years, a number of definitions for cardiomyopathies were advanced in concert with an increasing awareness of the nature of these diseases. Indeed, in the original WHO classification[3] cardiomyopathies were defined only as "heart muscle diseases of unknown cause," which seems primitive by today's standards and reflects the paucity of information available regarding etiology and basic disease mechanisms. The WHO most recently defined cardiomyopathies in 1995[1] as "diseases of myocardium associated with cardiac dysfunction," and included newly recognized arrhythmogenic right ventricular cardiomyopathy/arrhythmogenic right ventricular dysplasia (ARVC/ARVD) and primary restrictive cardiomyopathy for the first time and, among unclassified cardiomyopathies, noncompacted left ventricular (LV) myocardium.

【 】 PITFALLS

The diverse cardiomyopathy classifications presented through the years have been designed for either clinicians or biomedical scientists, based on a variety of premises, including etiology, anatomy, physiology, primary treatments, method of diagnosis, biopsy histopathology, and symptomatic state of patients. Although the objective is a classification scheme appreciated by (and can be of use to) all interested parties and disciplines, it is acknowledged that each of the proposed definition and classification constructs have shortcomings. Indeed, no past, present, or future classification of cardiomyopathies is likely to satisfy the purposes of all interested parties.

In particular, the popular *hypertrophic-dilated-restrictive cardiomyopathies* classification has major limitations by virtue of mixing anatomic designations (i.e., hypertrophic and dilated) with a functional one (i.e., restrictive). Consequently, confusion frequently arises when the same disease could legitimately appear in two or even three categories. Furthermore, such a classification fails to consider the heterogeneous clinical expression and course now recognized for many of these diseases. For example, hypertrophic cardiomyopathy (HCM), as well as infiltrative and storage cardiomyopathies are characterized by substantial LV hypertrophy with increased wall thickness in the absence of ventricular dilatation. These conditions are also frequently associated with restriction to diastolic filling, but purely restrictive forms of cardiomyopathy (without LV hypertrophy) are exceedingly rare. Investigation into the genetic basis of HCM and other cardiomyopathies has led to the identification of some individuals with a disease-causing mutation, who are without evidence of LV hypertrophy nevertheless (i.e., HCM without hypertrophy). Dilated forms of cardiomyopathy show a considerably increased cardiac mass (i.e., weight) with myocyte enlargement indicative of cardiac hypertrophy, but absolute LV wall thicknesses are normal. The end-stage phase of HCM may incorporate hypertrophic and dilated as well as restrictive components.

Some diseases do not have a uniformly static expression and may evolve from one category to another as a consequence of remodeling during their natural clinical course; for example, HCM, amyloid, and other infiltrative myocardial conditions may progress from a nondilated (often hyperdynamic) state with ventricular stiffness to a dilated form with systolic dys-

function and heart failure. Finally, because quantitative assessments of ventricular size represent a continuum and patients may widely vary in the degree of chamber enlargement (and dimensional cutoff values are arbitrary), it is often difficult to definitively distinguish dilated from nondilated forms of cardiomyopathy. This ambiguity may also apply to some rare, or newly identified, cardiac diseases in young patients for which little quantitative cardiac dimensional data are currently available. Indeed, as new cardiomyopathies have been defined in a contemporary fashion (often by genomics), and knowledge of pathologic disease spectrums has evolved, the *dilated-hypertrophic-restrictive* classification has become untenable and probably should be abandoned.

Etiologic classifications of cardiomyopathies are also problematic, given that diseases with the same (or similar) phenotypes can harbor diverse etiologies and mechanisms. For example, dilated cardiomyopathy may have genetic, infectious, autoimmune, and toxic causes (and in some cases are still designated as *idiopathic*), all leading, however, to the final common pathway of ventricular dilatation with systolic dysfunction. Alternatively, functional (i.e., physiologic) classifications with potential relevance to treatment considerations and theoretically most useful to clinicians are also flawed and of limited value because management strategies for these diseases constantly evolve.

PROPOSED CONTEMPORARY DEFINITIONS AND CLASSIFICATION (2006)

【 】 DEFINITIONS

The proposed definition of cardiomyopathies is as follows:

> *A heterogeneous group of diseases of the myocardium associated with mechanical and/or electrical dysfunction, which usually (but not invariably) exhibit inappropriate ventricular hypertrophy or dilatation, and are due to a variety of etiologies that frequently are genetic. Cardiomyopathies are either confined to the heart or are part of generalized systemic disorders, often leading to cardiovascular death or progressive heart failure-related disability.[15]*

Within this broad definition, cardiomyopathies are usually associated with failure of myocardial performance, which may be mechanical (e.g., diastolic or systolic dysfunction) or as a primary electrical disease prone to life-threatening arrhythmias. The ion channelopathies (e.g., long and short QT, Brugada syndrome, and catecholaminergic polymorphic ventricular tachycardia) are primary electrical diseases without gross or histopathologic abnormalities in which the functional and structural myocardial abnormalities responsible for arrhythmogenesis are at the molecular level in the cell or sarcoplasmic membranes themselves. The basic pathologic abnormality in these diseases is unidentifiable by either conventional noninvasive imaging or myocardial biopsy during life, or even by electron microscopic or autopsy examination of tissue. The ion-channelopathies are included in this classification of cardiomyopathies based on the scientifically reasonable (but largely hypothetical) assertion that ion channel mutations are responsible for altering biophysical properties and protein structure of the cardiomyocyte, thereby creating structurally abnormal ion channel interfaces and architecture. Consequently, the classification represents a distinct and major departure from prior efforts and is predicated on the view that causative mutations in genes encoding proteins regulating the transport of ions such as sodium, potassium, and calcium across the cell membrane are ultimately responsible for a structural disease state which triggers primary life-threatening ventricular tachyarrhythmias.

Although the present classification relies substantially on contemporary molecular biology, it is probably premature and inadvisable at this time to formulate a classification entirely dependent on genomics. The molecular genetics of myocardial disease is not yet completely developed, and more complex genotype–phenotype relationships will continue to emerge for these diseases. For example, several sarcomeric gene mutations are now known to cause both dilated cardiomyopathy (DCM) and HCM. Furthermore, troponin I mutations have been reported to cause both HCM and a purely restrictive form of cardiomyopathy.[19]

It is also important to specify disease entities that have *not* been included as cardiomyopathies in the present contemporary classification. We refer to pathologic myocardial processes, which are a direct consequence of other cardiovascular abnormalities such as occur with valvular heart disease, systemic hypertension, congenital heart disease, as well as atherosclerotic coronary artery disease producing ischemic myocardial damage secondary to impaired coronary flow. Therefore, the commonly-used term *ischemic cardiomyopathy* referring to myocardial ischemia and infarction is irrelevant to this classification. The following conditions have also been excluded from the cardiomyopathy classification: metastatic and primary intracavitary or intramyocardial cardiac tumors, diseases affecting endocardium with little or no myocardial involvement, as well as the imprecisely defined entity of hypertensive hypertrophic cardiomyopathy.

Classification

Cardiomyopathies are divided into two major groups based on predominant organ involvement: *Primary* cardiomyopathies (genetic, nongenetic, acquired) are those solely or predominantly confined to heart muscle, and are relatively few in number. *Secondary* cardiomyopathies show pathologic myocardial involvement as part of a large number and variety of generalized systemic (multiorgan) disorders. These systemic diseases associated with secondary forms of cardiomyopathies have previously been referred to as *specific cardiomyopathies*[1] or *specific heart muscle diseases*[3] in prior classifications, but that nomenclature has been abandoned here. The frequency and degree of secondary myocardial involvement varies considerably among cardiomyopathies, some of which are exceedingly uncommon, and for which the evidence of myocardial pathology may be sparse and reported in only a few patients. Because many cardiomyopathies may predominantly involve the heart but are not necessarily confined to that organ, some distinctions between primary and secondary cardiomyopathy made here are necessarily arbitrary and inevitably rely on judgment regarding the clinical importance and consequences of the myocardial process.

Based on all these considerations, the recommendation[15] was that cardiomyopathies can be most effectively classified as follows (Fig. 28–1):

- Primary genetic
- Primary mixed (genetic and nongenetic)
- Primary acquired
- Secondary

PRIMARY CARDIOMYOPATHIES

GENETIC

Hypertrophic Cardiomyopathy

HCM is a clinically heterogeneous but relatively common form of genetic heart disease transmitted as an autosomal dominant trait (1:500 of the general population for the disease phenotype recognized by echocardiography), and probably the most frequently occurring cardiomyopathy.[9] HCM is the most common cause of sudden cardiac death in the young as well as in trained athletes (in the United States) and is also an important substrate for heart failure disability at any age.

HCM is characterized morphologically by virtue of an otherwise unexplained hypertrophied and nondilated LV in the absence of another cardiac or systemic disease capable of producing the magnitude of wall thickening evident (e.g., systemic hypertension, aortic valve stenosis), independent of whether obstruction to LV outflow is present. Clinical diagnosis is customarily made with two-dimensional echocardiography or, alternatively, with cardiac magnetic resonance (CMR) imaging.

When LV wall thickness is mild, differential diagnosis with physiologic athlete's heart may arise. Furthermore, individuals harboring a genetic defect for HCM do not necessarily express clinical markers of their disease at all times during life, such as LV hypertrophy on echocardiogram, ECG abnormalities, or symptoms. Indeed, ECG alterations can precede the appearance of hypertrophy on echocardiography. Also, virtually any absolute LV wall thickness, even when within normal limits, is consistent with the presence of a HCM-causing mutant gene. When hypertrophy is absent, definitive diagnosis can only be made by laboratory-DNA analysis. Furthermore, recognition of LV hypertrophy may be age related with incomplete penetrance and initial appearance delayed in onset well into adulthood (adult morphologic conversion). Most HCM patients have the propensity to develop dynamic obstruction to LV outflow under resting or physiologically provocable (exercise) conditions produced by systolic anterior motion of the mitral valve and ventricular septal contact.

HCM demonstrates extreme genetic heterogeneity and is caused by a variety of mutations encoding protein components of the cardiac sarcomere.[14] Of 11 mutated sarcomeric genes presently associated with HCM, the most common are β-myosin heavy chain (the first identified) and myosin-binding protein C. The other nine genes seem to account for far fewer cases of HCM and include troponin T and I, regulatory and essential myosin light chains, titin, α-tropomyosin, α-actin, α-myosin heavy chain, and muscle LIM protein. This intergenetic diversity displayed in

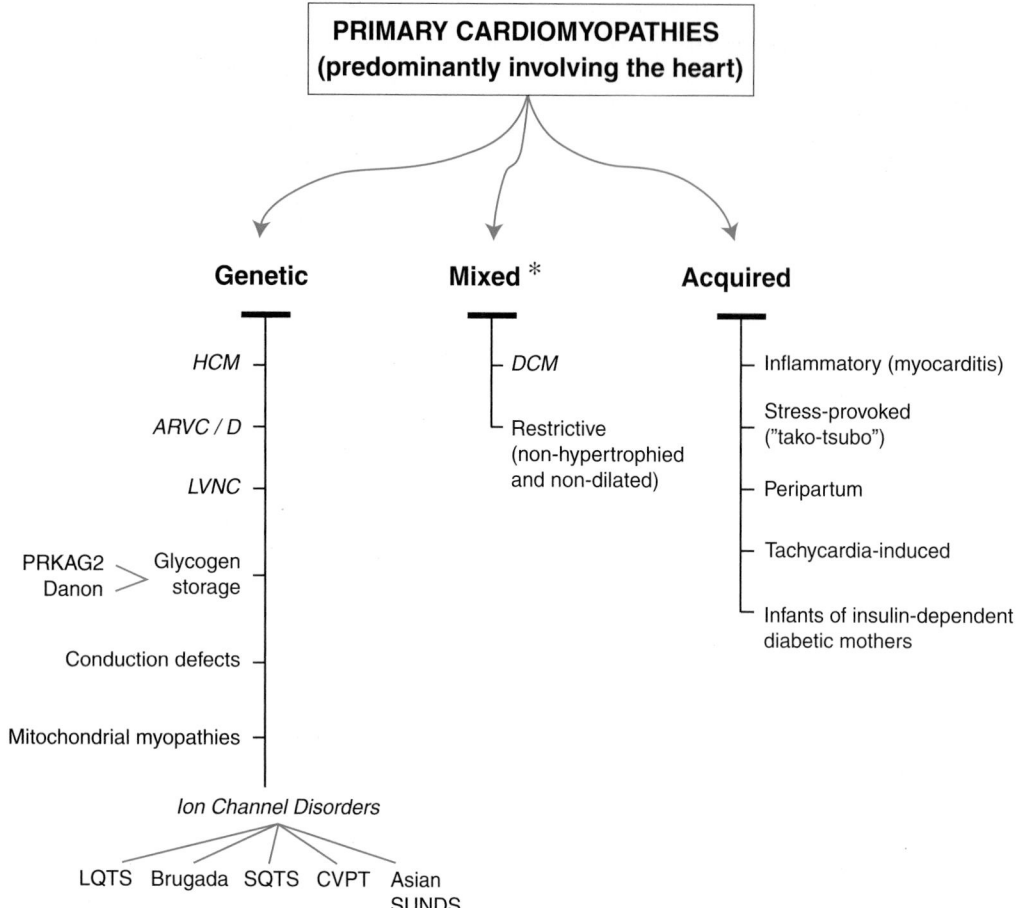

FIGURE 28–1. Primary cardiomyopathies in which the clinically relevant disease processes are solely or predominantly confined to the working myocardium. The conditions have been segregated according to their known genetic or nongenetic etiologies. *At present, familial disease with a genetic etiology reported in a minority of cases. ARVC, arrhythmogenic right ventricular cardiomyopathy; ARVD, arrhythmogenic right ventricular dysplasia; CVPT, catecholaminergic polymorphic ventricular tachycardia; DCM, dilated cardiomyopathy; LQTS, long QT syndrome; LVNC, left ventricular noncompaction; SQTS, short QT syndrome; SUNDS, sudden unexplained nocturnal death syndrome. *Source: From Maron BJ, Towbin JA, Thiene G, et al.[15]*

HCM is compounded by considerable intragenetic heterogeneity, with multiple different mutations identified in each gene ($n \geq 400$ total individual mutations now). These are most commonly missense mutations altering only a single nucleotide (such as with β-myosin heavy chain and α-tropomyosin), but other mutations cause protein truncation (e.g., myosin-binding protein C and troponin T). The characteristic diversity of the HCM phenotype is attributable to the disease-causing mutations but probably also to the influence of modifier genes and environmental factors.

In addition, nonsarcomeric protein mutations in two genes involved in cardiac metabolism have recently been reported to be responsible for primary cardiac glycogen cardiomyopathies in older children and adults with a clinical presentation mimicking (or indistinguishable from) that of sarcomeric HCM. One condition involves the gene encoding the γ_2-regulatory subunit of the AMP-activated protein kinase (PRKAG2), associated with variable degrees of LV hypertrophy and ventricular preexcitation.[20] The other involves the gene encoding lysosome-associated membrane protein 2 (LAMP-2), resulting in Danon-type storage disease.[21] Clinical manifestations are largely limited to the heart, usually with massive degrees of LV hypertrophy and also ventricular preexcitation. These disorders are now part of a subgroup of previously described infiltrative forms of LV hy-

pertrophy such as Pompe disease, a glycogen disease caused by use of α-1,4 glycosidase (acid maltase deficiency) in infants and Fabry disease, a X-linked recessive disorder of glycosphingolipid metabolism due to a deficiency of the lysosomal enzyme α-galactosidase A, resulting in intracellular accumulation of glycosphingolipids. The latter should be grouped among secondary forms of HCM.

Neither the number of HCM disease genes nor the number of HCM-causing mutations that can occur in each is known. Undoubtedly, many other mutations causing cardiac hypertrophy by disrupting sarcomere, metabolic, and other genes remain to be identified. A number of other diseases associated with LV hypertrophy involve prominent thickening of the LV wall, occurring mostly in infants and children younger than 4 years of age, which may resemble or mimic typical HCM caused by sarcomere protein mutations. These cardiomyopathies also include secondary forms such as Noonan syndrome, an autosomal-dominant cardiofacial condition associated with a variety of cardiac defects (most commonly, dysplastic pulmonary valve stenosis and atrial septal defect) caused by mutations in PTPN11, a gene encoding the nonreceptor protein tyrosine phosphatase SHP-2 genes.[22]

Other diseases in this category are mitochondrial myopathies caused by mutations encoding mitochondrial DNA (including Kearns-Sayre syndrome), or mitochondrial proteins associated with adenosine triphosphate (ATP) electron transport chain enzyme defects, which alter mitochondrial morphology.[23] Also included in these considerations are metabolic myopathies representing ATP production and use defects involving abnormalities of fatty acid oxidation (acyl-coenzyme A dehydrogenase deficiencies) and carnitine deficiency; as well as infiltrative myopathies such as glycogen storage diseases (type II; autosomal recessive Pompe disease); Hunter and Hurler diseases; and also the transient and nonfamilial cardiomyopathy as part of generalized organomegaly, recognized in infants of insulin-dependent diabetic mothers. In older patients several systemic diseases have been associated with hypertrophic forms of cardiomyopathy, including Friedreich ataxia, pheochromocytoma, neurofibromatosis, lentiginosis, and tuberous sclerosis, as well as several others.

Arrhythmogenic Right Ventricular Cardiomyopathy/Arrhythmogenic Right Ventricular Dysplasia

ARVC/ARVD is an uncommon form of inheritable heart muscle disease (estimated 1:5,000), relatively recent in its description only approximately 20 years ago.[24,25] It is mostly characterized by myocardial electrical instability and risk for life-threatening ventricular arrhythmias. ARVC/ARVD predominantly involves the right ventricle with progressive loss of myocytes and fibrofatty tissue replacement, resulting in regional (segmental) or global abnormalities. Aneurysms of the right ventricle in the triangle of dysplasia (inflow, apex, outflow) are a specific feature.[24] Apoptosis has been demonstrated as a mode of ongoing myocytes death. Although frequently associated with myocarditis (enterovirus or adenovirus), ARVC/ARVD is not considered a primary inflammatory cardiomyopathy. In addition, evidence of LV involvement with fibrofatty replacement, chamber enlargement, and myocarditis is also reported in up to 50 to 75 percent of patients.[26]

ARVC/ARVD has a broad clinical spectrum, usually presenting clinically with ventricular tachyarrhythmias (e.g., monomorphic ventricular tachycardia) and left bundle-branch block morphology. It is a recognized cause of sudden cardiac death in the young and in Italy is the most common cause of sudden death in competitive athletes.[25] Very different patterns of disease have been recognized: concealed phase, when sudden death may be the first manifestation; overt arrhythmic disorder with life-threatening tachyarrhythmias and palpitations; and congestive heart failure, with right- or biventricular pump failure. Ventricular arrhythmias are caused by re-entrant mechanism caused by slow conduction within the myocytes embedded in fibrofatty tissue. Noninvasive and invasive clinical identification is often confounding without an easily obtained, definitively diagnostic single test or finding, often necessitating an integrated assessment of electrical, functional, and anatomic abnormalities. Indeed, diagnosis often requires a high index of suspicion frequently triggered by presentation with arrhythmias, syncope, or cardiac arrest as well as global or segmental chamber dilatation or wall motion abnormalities.

Noninvasive tests used for ARVC/ARVD diagnosis, in addition to personal and family history, include 12-lead ECG, signal-average ECG, echocardiography, right ventricular angiography, CMR imaging, CT, and electroanatomic mapping of the right ventricle. Endomyocardial biopsy from the right ventricular free wall is a sensitive diagnostic marker when transmural fibrofatty infiltration is associated with surviving strands of myocytes. ECGs most commonly show abnormal repolarization with T-wave inversion in leads V_1 to V_3, as well as small amplitude potentials at the end of the QRS complex (epsilon wave). Brugada syndrome-like right bundle-branch block and right precordial ST-segment elevation accompanied by polymorphic ventricular tachycardia have also been reported in a small subset of ARVC/ARVD patients. Treatment includes lifestyle alterations (i.e., avoiding intense physical activity), antiarrhythmic drugs, and implantable cardioverter-defibrillators in high-risk patients. In case of end-stage congestive heart failure, cardiac transplantation is the final option.

In most cases ARVC/ARVD shows autosomal dominant inheritance, albeit often with incomplete penetrance. Dominant ARVC/ARVD has been mapped to eight chromosomal loci, with mutations identified thus far in five genes. These include the cardiac ryanodine receptor RyR2, which is also responsible for familial catecholaminergic polymorphic ventricular tachycardia (CPVT)[27]; desmoplakin[28]; plakophilin 2[29]; and desmoglein[30]; as well as mutations altering regulatory sequences of the transforming growth factor beta 3 gene.[31] Two recessive forms have been described in conjunction with palmoplantar keratoderma and woolly hair (Naxos disease),[32] and Carvajal syndrome,[33] caused by mutations in junctional plakoglobin and desmoplakin, respectively. In terms of genomic background, ARVC/ARVD may be considered a cell junction disease or a desmosomal cardiomyopathy. Although the function of desmosomal proteins to anchor intermediate filaments to desmosomes implicates ARVC/ARVD as a primary structural abnormality, there is also a link to ion channel dysfunction.

Left Ventricular Noncompaction

Noncompaction of ventricular myocardium is a recently recognized congenital cardiomyopathy, characterized by a distinctive (*spongy*) morphologic appearance of LV myocardium. Noncompaction predominantly involves the distal (apical) portion of the LV chamber with deep intertrabecular recesses (sinusoids) in communication with the ventricular cavity, resulting from an arrest in the normal embryogenesis. Left ventricular noncompaction (LVNC) may be an isolated finding or associated with other congenital heart anomalies such as complex cyanotic congenital heart disease.

Diagnosis is made with two-dimensional echocardiography or CMR, as well as LV angiography. The natural history of LVNC is largely unresolved but includes LV systolic dysfunction and heart failure (and some cases of heart transplantation), thromboemboli, arrhythmias and sudden death, as well as diverse forms of remodeling during the clinical course. Both familial and nonfamilial cases have been described. In the isolated form of LVNC, *ZASP* (Z-line) and mitochondrial mutations and X-linked inheritance caused by mutations in the *G4.5* gene encoding tafazzin (including associations with Barth syndrome in neonates) have been reported.[34] Noncompaction associated with congenital heart disease has been shown to result from mutations in the α-dystrobrevin gene and transcription factor *NKX2.5*.[35]

Conduction System Disease

Lenègre disease, also known as *progressive cardiac conduction defect* (PCCD), is characterized by primary progressive development of cardiac conduction defects in the His-Purkinje system leading to widening of the QRS complex and atrioventricular (AV) block with long pauses and bradycardia that may trigger syncope. Sick sinus syndrome is phenotypically similar to PCCD. Familial occurrence of both syndromes has been reported with an autosomal dominant pattern of inheritance. An ion channelopathy, in the form of SCN5A mutations, is thought to contribute to these conduction system defects.[36] It can be regarded as a cardiomyopathy of the conducting tissues. Wolff-Parkinson-White is familial in some cases, but information regarding the genetic causes is unknown.

Ion Channelopathies

There is a growing list of uncommon inherited and congenital arrhythmia disorders caused by mutations in genes encoding defective ionic channel proteins governing cell and sarcoplasmic reticulum membrane transit of sodium, potassium and calcium ions. These ion channel disorders include long QT syndrome (LQTS),[37] short QT syndrome (SQTS),[38] Brugada syndrome,[39] and CPVT. Sudden unexplained nocturnal death syndrome (SUNDS) and Brugada syndrome in young Southeast Asian males are based on a similar clinical and genetic profile.[40] A small proportion (5–10 percent) of sudden infant deaths may also be linked to ion channelopathies, including LQTS, SQTS, CPVT, and Brugada syndrome.[41] Clinical diagnosis of the ion channelopathies can often be made by identification of the disease phenotype on standard 12-lead ECG. Some cases were previously classified as idiopathic ventricular fibrillation (IVF), a description that persists for a syndrome in which mechanistic understanding is lacking.

Long QT Syndrome   LQTS is probably the most common of the ion channelopathies, characterized by prolongation of ventricular repolarization and QT interval (corrected for heart rate) on the standard 12-lead ECG, a specific form of polymorphic ventricular tachycardia (torsade de pointes),[37] and a risk for syncope and sudden cardiac death. Phenotypic expression (on the ECG) varies considerably and approximately 25 to 50 percent of affected family members may show borderline or even normal QT intervals.

Two patterns of inheritance have been described in LQTS: (1) a rare autosomal recessive disease associated with deafness (Jervell and Lange-Nielsen syndrome) and caused by two genes that encode for the slowly activating delayed rectifier potassium channel (KCNQ1 and KCNE1 [minK]); and (2) the much more common autosomal dominant disease unassociated with deafness (Romano-Ward syndrome), which is caused by mutations in eight different genes: KCNQ1 (KvLQT1; LQT1), KCNH2 (HERG; LQT2), SCN5A (Na1.5; LQT3), ANKB (LQT4), KCNE1 (minK; LQT5), KCNE2 (MiRP1; LQT6), KCNJ2 (Kir2.1; LQT7; Andersen syndrome), and CACNA1C (Ca1.2; LQT8; Timothy syndrome). Of the eight genes, six encode for cardiac potassium channels, one for the sodium channel (SCN5A; LQT3), and one for the protein ankyrin, which is involved in anchoring ion channels to the cellular membrane (ANKB).

Brugada Syndrome   Brugada syndrome is a relatively new clinical entity associated with sudden cardiac death in young people. First described in 1992,[42] the syndrome is identified by a distinctive ECG pattern consisting of right bundle-branch block and coved ST-segment elevation in the anterior precordial leads (V$_1$–V$_3$). The characteristic ECG pattern is often concealed and may be unmasked with the administration of sodium channel blockers, including ajmaline, flecainide, procainamide, or pilsicainide. Familial autosomal dominant and sporadic forms have been linked to mutations in an α-subunit of the cardiac sodium channel gene SCN5A (the same gene responsible for LQT3) in 20 percent of patients with the Brugada syndrome.[43] Another locus has been reported on the short arm of chromosome 3, but no gene has been identified so far.

Sudden Unexplained Nocturnal Death Syndrome   Found predominantly in young Southeast Asian males (i.e., Thailand, Japan, Philippines, and Cambodia), sudden unexplained nocturnal death syndrome is a disorder causing sudden death during sleep because of ventricular tachycardia/fibrillation. Some cases of sudden unexplained nocturnal death syndrome caused by SCN5A gene mutations and Brugada syndrome have been shown to be phenotypically, genetically, and functionally the same disorder.[44]

Catecholaminergic Polymorphic Ventricular Tachycardia   CPVT, a disease first described by Coumel and coworkers in 1978,[45] is characterized by syncope, sudden death and polymorphic ventricular tachycardia triggered by vigorous physical exertion or acute emotion (usually in children and adolescents), a normal resting ECG, and the absence of structural cardiac disease. Family history of one or multiple sudden cardiac deaths is evident in 30 percent of cases.[46] The resting ECG is unremarkable with the exception of sinus bradycardia and prominent U waves in some patients. The most typical arrhythmia of CPVT is bidirectional ventricular tachycardia presenting with an alternating QRS axis, triggered by effort when cardiac rhythm exceeds 120 to 125 beats/min threshold. The autosomal dominant form of the disease has been linked to the RyR2 gene encoding for the cardiac ryanodine receptor, a large protein that forms the calcium release channel in the sarcoplasmic reticulum, essential for regulation of excitation-contraction coupling and intracellular calcium levels.[27,47] An autosomal recessive form has been linked to CASQ2, a gene that encodes for calsequestrin, a protein that serves as a major calcium-binding protein in the terminal cisternae of the sarcoplasmic reticulum.[48] Calsequestrin is bound to the ryanodine receptor and participates in the control of excitation-contraction coupling.

Short QT Syndrome   SQTS, first described in 2000,[38] is characterized by short QT interval (<330 msec) on ECG and a high incidence of sudden cardiac death caused by ventricular tachycardia/fibrillation. Another distinctive ECG feature of SQTS is the appearance of tall peaked T waves, similar to those encountered with hyperkalemia. The syndrome has been linked to gain of function mutations in KCNH2 (HERG; SQT1), KCNQ1 (KvLQT1; SQT2), and KCNJ2 (Kir2.1; SQT3), causing an increase in the intensity of IKr, Iks, and Ikl, respectively.[49]

Idiopathic Ventricular Fibrillation   Idiopathic ventricular fibrillation is a subgroup of patients with sudden death, which appears in the literature with the designation idiopathic ventricular fibrillation. It is likely that idiopathic ventricular fibrillation is not an independent disease entity, however, but rather a conglomeration of conditions with normal gross and microscopic findings in which arrhythmic risk undoubtedly derives from molecular abnormalities, most likely ion channel mutations. At present, there is insufficient data available to permit the classification of idiopathic ventricular fibrillation as a distinct cardiomyopathy.

[ ] MIXED GENETIC AND NONGENETIC
Dilated Cardiomyopathy

Dilated forms of cardiomyopathy are characterized by ventricular chamber enlargement and systolic dysfunction, with normal LV wall thickness; diagnosis is usually made with two-dimensional echocardiography. DCM leads to progressive heart failure and decline in LV contractile function, ventricular and supraventricular arrhythmias, conduction system abnormalities, thromboembolism, and sudden or heart failure–related death. Indeed, DCM is a common and largely irreversible form of heart muscle disease with an estimated prevalence of 1:2500 people; it is the third most common cause of heart failure and the most frequent indication of heart transplantation. DCM may clinically manifest at a wide range of ages (most commonly in the third or fourth decade but also in young children) and is usually identified when associated with severe limiting symptoms and disability. In family screening studies with echocardiography, asymptomatic or mildly symptomatic patients may be identified.

The DCM phenotype with sporadic occurrence may derive from a particularly broad range of primary (and secondary) etiologies including infectious agents, particularly viruses, often producing myocarditis (cardiotropic viruses like coxsackievirus, adenovirus, parvovirus, HIV); but also bacterial; fungal rickettsial; mycobacterial; and parasitic (e.g., Chagas disease caused by trypanosome cruzi infection) agents. Other causes include toxins; chronic excessive consumption of alcohol, chemotherapeutic agents (anthracyclines such as doxorubicin and daunorubicin), and metals and other compounds (cobalt, lead, mercury, and arsenic); autoimmune and systemic disorders (including collagen vascular disorders); pheochromocytoma; neuromuscular disorders such as Duchenne/Becker and Emery-Dreifuss muscular dystrophies; and mitochondrial, metabolic, endocrine, and nutritional disorders (e.g., carnitine, selenium deficiencies). In addition, a substantial proportion of cases aggregate in families or remain designated as idiopathic.

Approximately 20 to 35 percent of DCM cases have been reported as familial, but with incomplete and age dependent penetrance, and linked to a diverse group of more than 20 loci and genes. Although genetically heterogeneous, the predominant mode of inheritance for DCM is autosomal dominant, with X-linked autosomal recessive and mitochondrial inheritance less frequent. Several the mutant genes linked to autosomal dominant DCM encode the same contractile sarcomeric proteins responsible for HCM, including α-cardiac actin; α-tropomyosin; cardiac troponin T, I and C; β- and α-myosin heavy chain; myosin binding protein C; and Z-disc protein-encoding genes including muscle LIM protein, α-actinin-2, ZASP, and titin have also been identified.[14]

DCM is also caused by a number of mutations in other genes encoding cytoskeletal/sarcolemmal, nuclear envelope, sarcomere, and transcriptional coactivator proteins. The most common is probably the lamin A/C gene, also associated with conduction system disease, which encodes a nuclear envelope intermediate filament protein. Mutations in this gene also cause Emery-Dreifuss muscular dystrophy (EDMD). The X-linked gene responsible for EDMD, emerin (another nuclear lamin protein) also causes similar clinical cardiac features. Other DCM genes of this type include desmin, caveolin, and α- and β-sarcoglycan as well as the mitochondrial respiratory chain gene. X-linked DCM is caused by the Duchenne muscular dystrophy (dystrophin) gene, whereas G4.5 (tafazzin), a mitochondrial protein of unknown function, causes Barth syndrome, an X-linked cardioskeletal myopathy in infants.[10]

Primary Restrictive (Nonhypertrophied) Cardiomyopathy

Primary restrictive cardiomyopathy as defined here is a rare form of nonhypertrophied, nondilated heart muscle disease and a cause of heart failure, characterized by normal or decreased volume of both ventricles associated with biatrial enlargement, normal LV wall thickness and AV valves, impaired ventricular filling with restrictive physiology, and normal (or near normal) systolic function. Both sporadic and familial forms have been described and in one family a troponin I mutation was responsible for both restrictive cardiomyopathy and HCM.[19]

[ ] ACQUIRED
Myocarditis (Inflammatory Cardiomyopathy)

Myocarditis is an acute or chronic inflammatory process affecting the myocardium produced by a wide variety of toxins and drugs (e.g., cocaine, interleukin-2) or infectious agents. The most common include viral (coxsackie, adenovirus, parvovirus HIV); bacterial (diphtheria, meningococcus, psittacosis, streptococcus); rickettsial (typhus, Rocky Mountain Spotted Fever); fungal (aspergillosis, candidiasis); and parasitic (Chagas disease, toxoplasmosis), as well as Whipple disease (intestinal lipodystrophy) and immune (giant cell myocarditis) and hypersensitivity reactions to drugs such as antibiotics, sulfonamides, anticonvulsants and antiinflammatories. Endocardial fibroelastosis is a dilated cardiomyopathy in infants and children, as a consequence of viral myocarditis in utero (mumps).[50]

Myocarditis typically evolves through active, healing, and healed stages characterized progressively by inflammatory cell infiltrates leading to interstitial edema and focal myocyte necrosis and ultimately replacement fibrosis. These pathologic processes create an electrically unstable substrate potentially predisposing to the development of ventricular tachyarrhythmias and even sudden death. In some instances an episode of viral myocarditis (frequently subclinical) can trigger an autoimmune reaction that causes immunologic damage to the myocardium or cytoskeletal disruption, culminating in DCM with LV dysfunction. Evidence for the evolution of myocarditis to DCM comes from several sources including animal models, the finding of inflammatory infiltrates and persistence of viral RNA-DNA in endomyocardial biopsies from patients with DCM, and the natural history of patients with selected conditions such as Chagas disease. The list of agents responsible for inflammatory myocarditis overlaps with that of the infectious etiology of DCM, thereby underscoring the potential interrelationship between the two conditions.

Myocarditis can be diagnosed by established histopathologic, histochemical, or molecular criteria but is challenging to identify clinically. Suspicion may be raised by chest pain, exertional dyspnea, fatigue, syncope, palpitations, ventricular tachyarrhythmias, and conduction abnormalities or by acute congestive heart failure or cardiogenic shock associated with LV dilatation and/or segmental wall motion abnormalities and ST-T changes on ECG. When myocarditis is suspected based on the clinical profile, an endomyocardial biopsy may resolve an otherwise ambiguous situation, by virtue of diagnostic inflammatory (leukocyte) infiltrate and necrosis (i.e., the Dallas criteria),[51] but is also limited by insensitivity and false-negative histologic results. The diagnostic yield of myocardial biopsies can be enhanced substantially by molecular analysis with DNA-RNA extraction and PCR amplification of the viral genome.[52] In addition to the inflammatory process, viral genome–encoded proteases seem to disrupt the cytoskeletal-sarcomeric linkages of cardiomyocytes.[53]

plete or near-complete recovery within 6 months in approximately 50 percent of cases but may also result in progressive clinical deterioration and heart failure, death, or transplantation.

An under-recognized and reversible dilated cardiomyopathy with LV contractile dysfunction occurs secondary to prolonged periods of supraventricular or ventricular tachycardia (tachycardia-induced cardiomyopathy) and may be ascribed to stunned myocardium.[57] Systolic function normalizes without residual impairment on cessation of the tachycardia. Dilated cardiomyopathy associated with excessive alcohol consumption is also potentially reversible on cessation of alcohol intake.

SECONDARY CARDIOMYOPATHIES

The most important secondary cardiomyopathies are provided in Table 28–1. This list is not intended to represent an exhaustive and complete tabulation of the vast number of systemic conditions reported to involve the myocardium, however, but is limited

Stress (*Tako-Tsubo*) Cardiomyopathy

Stress cardiomyopathy, first reported in Japan as *tako-tsubo*, is a recently described clinical entity characterized by acute but rapidly reversible LV systolic dysfunction in the absence of atherosclerotic coronary artery disease and triggered by profound psychological stress.[54,55] This distinctive form of ventricular stunning typically affects older women and preferentially involves the distal portion of LV chamber (*apical ballooning*), with the basal LV hypercontractile. Although presentation often mimics ST-segment elevation myocardial infarction, outcome is favorable with appropriate medical therapy.

Others Peripartum (postpartum) cardiomyopathy is a rare and dilated form associated with LV systolic dysfunction and heart failure of unknown etiology that manifests clinically in the third trimester of pregnancy or the first 5 months postpartum, requiring a high index of suspicion for diagnosis. Inflammatory, noninfectious cardiomyopathy may be associated as well.[56] It is regarded as a distinct clinical entity, separate from preexisting cardiomyopathies that may be adversely affected by the stress of pregnancy. Peripartum cardiomyopathy most frequently occurs in obese, multiparous women older than 30 years of age with preeclampsia. This unusual cardiomyopathy is associated with com-

TABLE 28–1

Secondary Cardiomyopathies

Infiltrative[a]	Cardiofacial
• Amyloidosis primary (AL), Familial autosomal dominant	• Noonan syndrome[b]
• (AF)[b]; Senile (SSA), Secondary (AA) forms	• Lentiginosis[b]
• Gaucher disease[b]	Neuromuscular/neurologic
• Hurler disease[b]	• Friedreich ataxia[b]
• Hunter disease[b]	• Duchenne-Becker muscular dystrophy[b]
Storage[c]	• Emery-Dreifuss muscular dystrophy (EDMD)[b]
• Hemochromatosis	• Myotonic dystrophy[b]
• Fabry disease[b]	• Neurofibromatosis[b]
• Glycogen storage disease[b] (type II; Pompe)	• Tuberous sclerosis[b]
• Niemann-Pick disease[b]	Nutritional deficiencies
Toxicity	• Beriberi (thiamine), pellagra, scurvy, selenium, carnitine, kwashiorkor
• Drugs, heavy metals, chemical agents	Autoimmune/collagen
• Endomyocardial	• Systemic lupus erythematosus
• Endomyocardial fibrosis (EMF)	• Dermatomyositis
• Hypereosinophilic syndrome	• Rheumatoid arthritis
• (Löffler endocarditis)	• Scleroderma
Inflammatory (granulomatous)	• Polyarteritis nodosa
• Sarcoidosis	Electrolyte imbalance
Endocrine	Consequence of cancer therapy
• Diabetes mellitus[b]	• Anthracyclines
• Hyperthyroidism	• Doxorubicin (Adriamycin)
• Hypothyroidism	• Daunorubicin
• Hyperparathyroidism	• Cyclophosphamide
• Pheochromocytoma	• Radiation
• Acromegaly	

[a]Accumulation of abnormal substances *between* myocytes.
[b]Genetic (familial) etiology.
[c]Accumulation of abnormal substances *within* myocytes.

to the most common of these diseases frequently associated with a cardiomyopathy.

REFERENCES

1. Richardson P, McKenna W, Bristow M, et al. Report of the 1995 World Health Organization/International Society and Federation of Cardiology Task Force on the Definition and Classification of Cardiomyopathies. *Circulation* 1996;93:841–842.

2. Abelmann WH. Classification and natural history of primary myocardial disease. *Prog Cardiovasc Dis* 1984;27:73–94.

3. Brandenbourg RO, Chazov E, Cherian G, et al. Report of the WHO/ISFC task force on the definition and classification of cardiomyopathies. *Br Heart J* 1980;44:672–673.

4. Mason JW. Classification of cardiomyopathies. In: Fuster V, Alexander RW, O'Rourke RA, eds. *Hurst's the Heart, Arteries and Veins*. 10th ed. New York: McGraw-Hill; 2001:1941–1946.

5. Wynne J, Braunwald E. The cardiomyopathies. In: Zipes DP, Libby P, Bonow RO, Braunwald ED, eds. *Braunwald's Heart Disease*. 7th ed. Philadelphia: Elsevier Saunders; 2005:1659–1696.

6. Thiene G, Angelini A, Basso C, et al. The new definition and classification of cardiomyopathies. *Adv Clin Path* 2000;4:53–57.

7. Thiene G, Corrado D, Basso C. Cardiomyopathies: is it time for a molecular classification? *Eur Heart J* 2004;25:1772–1775.

8. Keren A, Popp RL. Assignment of patients into the classification of cardiomyopathies. *Circulation* 1992;80:1622–1633.

9. Maron BJ, McKenna WJ, Danielson GK, et al. American College of Cardiology/European Society of Cardiology Clinical Expert Consensus Document on Hypertrophic Cardiomyopathy. A report of the American College of Cardiology Task Force on Clinical Expert Consensus Documents and the European Society of Cardiology Committee for Practice Guidelines Committee to Develop an Expert Consensus Document on Hypertrophic Cardiomyopathy. *J Am Coll Cardiol* 2003;42:1687–1713.

10. Towbin JA, Bowles NE. The failing heart. *Nature* 2002;415:227–233.

11. Antzelevitch C. Molecular genetics of arrhythmias and cardiovascular conditions associated with arrhythmias. *Heart Rhythm* 2004;1(5C):42C–56C.

12. Antzelevitch C, Brugada P, Borggrefe M, et al. Brugada syndrome: Report of the Second Consensus Conference—endorsed by the Heart Rhythm Society and the European Heart Rhythm Association. *Circulation* 2005;17:111:659–670.

13. Burkett EL, Hershberger RE. Clinical and genetic issues in familial dilated cardiomyopathy. *J Am Coll Cardiol* 2005;45:969–981.

14. Chien KR. Genotype, phenotype: upstairs, downstairs in the family of cardiomyopathies. *J Clin Invest* 2003;111:175–178.

15. Maron BJ, Towbin JA, Thiene G, et al. Contemporary definitions and classification of the cardiomyopathies. An American Heart Association Scientific Statement from the Council of Clinical Cardiology, Heart Failure and Transplantation Committee; Quality of Care and Outcomes Research and Functional Genomics and Translational Biology Interdisciplinary Working Groups; and Council on Epidemiology and Prevention. *Circulation* 2006;113:1807–1816.

16. Hunt SA, Abraham WT, Chin MH, et al. ACC/AHA 2005 guideline update for diagnosis and management of chronic heart failure in the adult: summary article—a report of the American College of Cardiology/American Heart Association Task Force on Practice Guidelines (Writing Committee to Update the 2001 Guidelines for the Evaluation and Management of Heart Failure). *Circulation* 2005;112:1825–1852.

17. Strickberger SA, Conti J, Daoud EG, et al. AHA Science Advisory: Patient selection for cardiac resynchronization therapy from the Clinical Cardiology Subcommittee on Electrocardiography and Arrhythmias and the Quality of Care and Outcomes Research Interdisciplinary Working Group in collaboration with the Heart Rhythm Society. *Circulation* 2005;111:2146–2150.

18. Gregoratos G, Abrams J, Epstein AE, et al. ACC/AHA/NASPE 2002 guideline update for implantation of cardiac pacemakers and antiarrhythmia devices: summary article: a report of the American College of Cardiology/American Heart Association Task Force on Practice Guidelines (ACC/AHA/NASPE Committee to Update the 1998 Pacemaker Guidelines). *Circulation* 2002;106:2145–2161.

19. Mogensen J, Kubo T, Duque M, et al. Idiopathic restrictive cardiomyopathy is part of the clinical expression of cardiac troponin I mutations. *J Clin Invest* 2003;111:209–216.

20. Gollob MH, Green, MS, Tang AS, et al. Identification of a gene responsible for familial Wolff-Parkinson-White syndrome. *N Engl J Med* 2001;344:1823–1831.

21. Horvath J, Ketelsen UP, Geibel-Zehender A, et al. Identification of a novel *LAMP2* mutation responsible for X-chromosomal dominant Danon disease. *Neuropediatrics* 2003;34:270–273.

22. Tartaglia M, Mehler EL, Goldberg R, et al. Mutations in *PTPN11*, encoding the protein tyrosine phosphatase SHP-2, cause Noonan syndrome. *Nat Genet* 2001;29:465–468.

23. Finsterer J. Mitochondriopathies. *Eur J Neurol* 2004;11:163–186.

24. Marcus FI, Fontaine G, Guiraudon G, et al. Right ventricular dysplasia: a report of 24 adult cases. *Circulation* 1982;65:384–398.

25. Thiene G, Nava A, Corrado D, et al. Right ventricular cardiomyopathy and sudden death in young people. *N Engl J Med* 1988;318:129–133.

26. Basso C, Thiene G, Corrado D, et al. Arrhythmogenic right ventricular cardiomyopathy: dysplasia, dystrophy or myocarditis. *Circulation* 1996;94:983–991.

27. Tiso N, Stephan DA, Nava A, et al. Identification of mutations in the cardiac ryanodine receptor gene in families affected with arrhythmogenic right ventricular cardiomyopathy type 2 (ARVD2). *Hum Mol Genet* 2001;10:189–194.

28. Rampazzo A, Nava A, Malacrida A, et al. Mutation in human desmoplakin domain binding to plakoglobin causes a dominant form of arrhythmogenic right ventricular cardiomyopathy. *Am J Hum Genet* 2002;71:1200–1206.

29. Gerull B, Heuser A, Wichter T, et al. Mutations in the desmosomal protein plakophilin-2 are common in arrhythmogenic right ventricular cardiomyopathy. *Nat Genet* 2004;36:1162–1164.

30. Pilichou K, Nava A, Basso C, et al. Mutations in desmoglein-2 gene are associated to arrhythmogenic right ventricular cardiomyopathy. *Circulation* 2006;113:1171–1179.

31. Beffagna G, Occhi G, Nava A, et al. Regulatory mutations in transforming growth factor-β3 gene causes arrhythmogenic right ventricular cardiomyopathy type 1. *Cardiovasc Res* 2005;65:366–373.

32. McKoy G, Protonotarios N, Crosby A, et al. Identification of a deletion of plakoglobin in arrhythmogenic right ventricular cardiomyopathy with palmoplantar keratoderma and wooly hair (Naxos disease) *Lancet* 2000;335:2219–2224.

33. Norgett EE, Hatsell SJ, Carvajal-Huerta L, et al. Recessive mutation in desmoplakin disrupts desmoplakin-intermediate filament interactions and causes dilated cardiomyopathy, woolly hair and keratoderma. *Hum Mol Genet* 2000;9:2761–2766.

34. Vatta M, Mohapatra B, Jimenez S, et al. Mutations in Cypher/*ZASP* in patients with dilated cardiomyopathy and left ventricular noncompaction. *J Am Coll Cardiol* 2003;42:2014–2027.

35. Ichida F, Tsubata S, Bowles KR, et al. Novel gene mutations in patients with left ventricular noncompaction or Barth syndrome. *Circulation* 2001;103:1256–1263.

36. Schott JJ, Alshinawi C, Kyndt F, et al. Cardiac conduction defects associate with mutations in SCN5A. *Nat Genet* 1999;23:20–21.

37. Priori SG, Schwartz PJ, Napolitano C, et al. Risk stratification in the long-QT syndrome. *N Engl J Med* 2003;348:1866–1874.

38. Gussak I, Brugada P, Brugada J, et al. Idiopathic short QT interval: a new clinical syndrome? *Cardiology* 2000;94:99–102.

39. Brugada P, Brugada J. Right bundle-branch block, persistent ST-segment elevation and sudden cardiac death: a distinct clinical and electrocardiographic syndrome. A multicenter report. *J Am Coll Cardiol* 1992;20:1391–1396.

40. Baron RC, Thacker SB, Gorelkin L, et al. Sudden death among Southeast Asian refugees: an unexplained nocturnal phenomenon. *JAMA* 1983;250:2947–2951.

41. Ackerman MJ, Siu SB, Turner Q, et al. Postmortem molecular analysis of *SCN5A* defects in sudden infant death syndrome. *JAMA* 2001;286:2264–2269.

42. Martini B, Nava A, Thiene G, et al. Ventricular fibrillation without apparent heart disease: description of six cases. *Am Heart J* 1989;118:1203–1209.

43. Chen Q, Kirsch GE, Zhang D, et al. Genetic basis and molecular mechanisms for idiopathic ventricular fibrillation. *Nature* 1998;392:293–296.

44. Vatta M, Dumaine R, Varghese G, et al. Genetic and biophysical basis of sudden unexplained nocturnal death syndrome (SUNDS), a disease allelic to Brugada syndrome. *Hum Mol Genet* 2002;11:337–345.

45. Coumel P, Leenhardt A, Hadda G, et al. Exercise ECG: prognostic implications of exercise induced arrhythmias. *Pacing Clin Electrophysiol* 1994;17:417–427.

46. Bauce B, Rampazzo A, Basso C, et al. Screening for ryanodine receptor type 2 mutations in families with effort-induced polymorphic ventricular arrhythmias and sudden death: early diagnosis of asymptomatic carriers. *J Am Coll Cardiol* 2002;40:341–349.

47. Priori S, Napolitano C, Tiso N, et al. Mutations in the cardiac ryanodine receptor gene (hRyR2) underlie catecholaminergic polymorphic ventricular tachycardia. *Circulation* 2001;103:196–200.

48. Lahti H, Prias E, Olen Der T, et al. A missense mutations in a highly conserved region of CASQ2 is associated with autosomal recessive catecholamine-induced polymorphic ventricular tachycardia in Bedouin families form Israel. *Am J Hum Genet* 2001;69:1378–1384.

49. Brugada R, Hong K, Dumaine R, et al. Sudden death associated with short-QT syndrome linked to mutations in HERG. *Circulation* 2004;109:30–35.

50. Ni J, Bowles NE, Kim YH, et al. Viral infection of the myocardium in endocardial fibroelastosis: molecular evidence for the role of mumps virus as an etiologic agent. *Circulation* 1997;95:133–139.

51. Aretz HT. Myocarditis: the Dallas Criteria. *Hum Pathol* 1987;18:619–624

52. Calabrese F, Thiene G. Myocarditis and inflammatory cardiomyopathy: microbiological and molecular biological aspects. *Cardiovasc Res* 2003;60:11–25.

53. Badorff C, Berkely N, Mehrotra S, et al. Enteroviral protease 2A directly cleaves dystrophin and is inhibited by a dystrophin-based substrate analogue. *J Biol Chem* 2000;275: 11191–11197.

54. Sharkey SW, Lesser JR, Zenovich AG, et al. Acute and reversible cardiomyopathy provoked by stress in women from the United States. *Circulation* 2005;111:472–479.

55. Wittstein IS, Thiemann DR, Lima JA, et al. Neurohumoral features of myocardial stunning due to sudden emotional stress. *N Engl J Med* 2005;352:539–548.

56. Ro A, Frishman WH. Peripartum cardiomyopathy. *Cardiol Rev* 2006;14:35–42.

57. Shinbane JS, Wood MA, Jensen DN, et al. Tachycardia-induced cardiomyopathy: a review of animal models and clinical studies. *J Am Coll Cardiol* 1997;29:709–715.

CHAPTER 29

Dilated Cardiomyopathies

Luisa Mestroni / Edward M. Gilbert / Brian D. Lowes /
Michael R. Bristow

BACKGROUND AND HISTORICAL PERSPECTIVE

This chapter describes the phenotypic and clinical characteristics of the primary and secondary dilated cardiomyopathies, the most common cause of the clinical syndrome of chronic heart failure.[1] Heart failure is an enormously important clinical problem, which, if not contained or solved, may ultimately overwhelm health care resources.[2] The clinical syndrome of heart failure is a complex process where the primary pathophysiology is quickly obscured by a variety of superimposed secondary adaptive, maladaptive, and counterregulatory processes (see also Chap. 24). Heart failure is best understood and approached from the vantage point of *myocardial failure,* most commonly associated with a dilated cardiomyopathy phenotype.[3] As an indication of their importance, the cardiomyopathies have recently been reclassified by an expert consensus panel under the auspices of the American Heart Association (AHA)[4] (see also Chap. 11).

IMPORTANCE OF HEART FAILURE

Because of its high prevalence (1–1.5 percent of the adult population) and high morbidity, including frequent hospitalizations, the clinical syndrome of heart failure is among the most costly medical problems in the United States.[2] Despite improvements in the treatment of heart failure introduced in the last 10 years,

including the general availability of cardiac transplantation and better medical treatment, clinical outcome following the onset of symptoms has not changed substantially. The mortality remains high (median survival of 1.7 years for men and 3.2 years for women), the natural history progressive, the cost excessive, and disability and morbidity among the highest of any disease or disease syndrome.[1,2,5]

RELATIONSHIP OF MYOCARDIAL FAILURE AND DILATED CARDIOMYOPATHIES TO THE CLINICAL SYNDROME OF HEART FAILURE

Most cases of heart failure are caused by heart muscle disease (cardiomyopathy). Within the classification of cardiomyopathies (Table 29–1),[4,6] the most common cause of the clinical syndrome of heart failure is a *secondary* (ischemic, valvular, hypertensive, etc.) or a *primary* (genetic, nongenetic, acquired) *dilated cardiomyopathy,* defined as a ventricular chamber exhibiting increased diastolic and systolic volumes and a low (<45 percent) ejection fraction.[7] The natural history of the clinical syndrome of heart failure depends on the course of myocardial failure, because (1) the most powerful single predictor of outcome is the degree of left ventricular (LV) dysfunction as assessed by the LV ejection fraction[8]; (2) treatment that improves intrinsic ventricular function improves the natural history of heart failure[3,9]; and (3) treatment that ultimately worsens intrinsic func-

TABLE 29-1

The Classification of the Cardiomyopathies

CATEGORY	DEFINITION
Genetic	
I. Hypertrophic (HCM)	↑↑ septal and ↑ posterior wall thickness, myofibrillar disarray
	Mutation in sarcomeric protein, autosomal dominant inheritance
II. Arrhythmogenic RV (ARVC/ARVD)	Fibrofatty replacement of RV myocardium
III. LV noncompaction	*Spongy* LV cavity (apex)
IV. Glycogen storage diseases	Danon disease, PRKAG2
V. Ion channelopathies	Conduction defects, LQTS, Brugada, SQTS, CPVT, Asian SUNDS
Mixed	
I. Dilated (DCM)	↑ EDV, ↑ ESV; low EF
II. Restrictive (RCM)	↑ EDV, ↔ ESV; ↑ FP, ↔ EF
Acquired	
I. Myocarditis	Inflammatory process
II. Stress provoked (*tako-tsubo*)	Reversible LV dysfunction
III. Peripartum	Third trimester or 5 months after pregnancy
IV. Tachycardia induced	Following prolonged periods of SVT or VT
V. Infants of insulin-dependent diabetic mothers	

ARVC, arrhythmogenic right ventricular cardiomyopathy; ARVD, arrhythmogenic right ventricular dysplasia; CM, cardiomyopathy; CPVT, catecholaminergic polymorphic ventricular tachycardia; EDV, end-diastolic volume; ESV, end-systolic volume; EF, LV ejection fraction; FP, LV filling pressure; HCM, hypertrophic cardiomyopathy; LQTS, long QT syndrome; LV, left ventricular; RV, right ventricular; SQTS, short QT syndrome; SVT, supraventricular tachycardia; SUNDS, sudden unexplained death syndrome; VT, ventricular tachycardia.

tion, such as many types of positive inotropic agents, is associated with an adverse effect on outcome.[9]

THE CLASSIFICATION OF CARDIOMYOPATHIES

The 1995 World Health Organization/International Society and Federation of Cardiology (WHO/ISFC) classification of cardiomyopathies[6] was recently revised to accommodate several rapidly emerging realities, in particular the identification of new disease entities, advances in diagnosis, and knowledge of etiology of previously unknown types of heart muscle disease.[4] The classification of cardiomyopathies is discussed in detail in Chaps. 11 and 28.

The old and new classification of cardiomyopathies are compared in Table 29–1, the WHO/ISFC classification of cardiomyopathy was mainly based on the global anatomic description of chamber dimensions in systole and diastole. Thus, the dilated and restrictive categories had definitions based on LV dimensions or volume, which also define function via calculated ejection fraction. The justification for this is that these two groups have distinct natural histories and respond distinctly differently to medical treatment. The novel AHA Scientific Statement emphasizes the genetic determinants of cardiomyopathies. Thus, dilated and restrictive cardiomyopathies are defined as *mixed* cardiomyopathies (predominantly nongenetic); however, hypertrophic cardi-

omyopathy (HCM), caused by mutations in contractile proteins, and other rare forms of cardiomyopathy including arrhythmogenic right ventricular cardiomyopathy/arrhythmogenic right ventricular dysplasia (ARVC/ARVD) and left ventricular noncompaction (LVNC), which also turned out to be completely genetic in basis, are defined *genetic* cardiomyopathies. The third category concerns *acquired* cardiomyopathies, such as peripartum and tachycardia induced cardiomyopathies. Conversely, genetic cardiomyopathies without unique phenotypes and involvement of a generalized multiorgan disorder, such as the dilated cardiomyopathy of Becker-Duchenne, are defined as *secondary* cardiomyopathies. This distinction is arbitrary and may inevitably cause significant overlap between primary and secondary cardiomyopathies.

Finally, the novel classification suggests abandoning the term *specific* cardiomyopathies and excludes valvular, hypertensive, and ischemic cardiomyopathy from the classification; but many mechanisms responsible for the natural history of myocardial dysfunction are qualitatively similar in primary versus these specific dilated cardiomyopathies,[10] which accurately predicted a qualitatively similar response to treatment targeted at these mechanisms.[11,12] In particular this is the case of *ischemic dilated cardiomyopathy* related to previous myocardial infarction (MI) and the subsequent remodeling process, or *hypertensive dilated* (or *restrictive* depending on the chamber dimensions) *cardiomyopathy*, definitions that are still widely used in the clinical practice in the literature.

【 】 MOLECULAR MECHANISMS IN CARDIOMYOPATHIES AND MYOCARDIAL FAILURE: DISEASE PHENOTYPE PRODUCED BY ALTERATIONS IN GENE EXPRESSION

As shown in Table 29–2, there are three general categories of mechanisms whereby altered gene expression can lead to a phenotypic change in cardiac myocytes:[13]

1. A single gene defect, such as lamin A/C gene mutations or α-myosin heavy chain[14–16]
2. Polymorphic variation in modifier genes, such as is present in many components of the renin-angiotensin,[17–19] adrenergic,[20–23] and endothelin systems[24]
3. Maladaptive regulated expression of completely normal genes, such as for the mechanisms responsible for progressive myocardial dysfunction and remodeling in secondary dilated cardiomyopathies[3,13]

Genetic Causes of Dilated Cardiomyopathies in Humans and Animal Models

The ability to genetically manipulate the cardiovascular system has made it possible to investigate the role of a number of genes in the

TABLE 29–2

Three General Mechanisms by which Alterations in Gene Expression Can Influence the Development or Progression of a Dilated Cardiomyopathy

TYPE OF PROCESS	EXAMPLES
Gene mutation	• Cytoskeletal/sarcolemmal/ nuclear envelope genes • Sarcomeric genes • Signaling pathway genes • Ion channels • Desmosomal genes
Polymorphic variation in modifier genes	Angiotensin-converting enzyme (ACE), α- and β-adrenergic receptors, endothelin type A receptor
Altered expression of a completely normal, wild-type gene (fetal gene program)	Decreased expression: β_1-adrenergic receptors, α-MYHC, SERCA2 Increased expression: ANP, β-MYHC, ACE, TNF-α, endothelin, *BARK*

ANP, atrial natriuretic peptide; *BARK*, beta adrenergic receptor kinase; MYHC, heavy chain cardiac myosin; SERCA2, sarcoplasmic reticulum Ca^{2+} adenosine triphosphatase; TNF-α, tumor necrosis factor-α.

developing and adult mouse heart (for a review, see Ross[25]). The discovery that mutations in sarcomeric proteins lead to HCM has made it possible to generate animal models for this disease.[26,27] In the case of myosin mutations, a single genetic defect initiates a pathway that ultimately leads to hypertrophy and then, in males, may result in late decompensation and ventricular dilatation.[26] Multiple gene mutations have now been associated causally with familial dilated cardiomyopathies, as discussed further on in this chapter.

A serendipitous genetic model of dilated cardiomyopathy and heart failure (*myf 5* mice) was generated by activation of a skeletal muscle genetic program in the heart.[28] These mice have a dilated cardiomyopathy phenotype characterized by progressive myocardial dysfunction and dilatation. They develop the clinical syndrome of heart failure, and they have an extraordinarily high (>90 percent at 260 days) heart failure–related mortality. Another serendipitous genetic model of dilated cardiomyopathy is the muscle LIM protein (MLP) knockout mouse.[29] MLP is a positive regulator of muscle differentiation, which is ordinarily expressed at high levels in the heart and may be involved in myofibrillar protein assembly along the actin-based cytoskeleton. MLP knockout mice exhibit typical features of dilated cardiomyopathy, including decreased systolic and diastolic function and β-adrenergic receptor pathway desensitization.[29]

These characteristics make this model useful in assessing the mechanisms that lead to the development and progression of myocardial failure. Thus, in transgenic mouse models, both altered expression of contractile proteins and perturbation of myocyte cytoarchitecture can lead to the dilated cardiomyopathy phenotype.

There are several additional transgenic mouse models of cardiomyopathy that may be more relevant to the production of a dilated phenotype in humans. Several of them involve overexpression of components of the adrenergic receptor pathway, the heterodimeric G-protein α_s subunit $(G\alpha_q)^{30}$; the α_2-,[31] β_1-,[32,33]

and β_2-adrenergic receptors[34]; and protein kinase A.[35] These β-adrenergic pathway transgenic mouse models exhibit similar histopathology, consisting of myocyte hypertrophy and increased fibrosis, evidence of apoptosis, systolic and diastolic dysfunction, and ultimately development of LV dilatation.[30–34,36] Other transgenic mice that ultimately develop a dilated phenotype include those with cardiac restricted overexpression of activated MEK5,[37] CaM kinase IV,[38] activated calcineurin,[39] and calsequestrin.[40] Yet another mouse model of dilated cardiomyopathy includes mitochondrial transcription factor A gene knockout.[41]

Several transgenic models of concentric or symmetric LV hypertrophy have been reported, including overexpression of *ras*,[42] *myc*,[43] α_1-adrenergic receptors,[44] the heterodimeric G-protein α_q subunit $(G\alpha_q)$,[45] and the protein kinase C (PKC).[46] The mechanisms for the induction of increased ventricular wall thickness are diverse, inasmuch as the *ras*, α_1-receptor, $G\alpha_q$, and PKC overexpressors exhibit true cellular hypertrophy with an increase in cell size,[42,44–46] whereas the *myc* animal exhibits cardiac myocyte hyperplasia.[43] The HCM phenotypes discussed earlier illustrate the principle that apparently diverse signals can culminate in the same phenotype, presumably by converging on final common pathways.

Multiple gene defects have been identified that can produce a dilated cardiomyopathy in humans, as discussed in more detail in the section on familial forms of dilated cardiomyopathy. As listed in Table 29–2 and Table 29–3, these include mutations in genes encoding proteins of the cytoskeleton, such as dystrophin[47,48]; nuclear envelope, such as lamin A/C[14,15]; sarcomere, such as cardiac β-myosin heavy chain (β-MHC) and α-myosin heavy chain (α-MHC)[16,49]; ion channels, like SCN5A[50,51]; desmosome[52]; and signaling pathways, such transcriptional and Ca^{2+}-cycling regulators.[53,54] Likewise, cytoskeletal and sarcomeric gene mutations may cause the naturally occurring dilated cardiomyopathy in animals: in the Syrian hamster, the disease is caused by mutations in the delta-sarcoglycan gene,[55] whereas in turkeys, it is caused by mutations in cardiac troponin T.[56]

Polymorphic Variation in Modifier Genes

Genes exhibit polymorphic variation; for example, normal variants of genes exist in the population that are of slightly different size or sequence.[57] Some gene polymorphisms are associated with differences in function of the expressed protein gene product, and some differences in function likely account for the *biological variation* routinely encountered in population studies of disease susceptibility or clinical response to treatment.

Examples of modifier genes that may have an impact on the natural history of a dilated cardiomyopathy (see Table 29–2) include the angiotensin-converting enzyme (ACE) *DD* genotype,[17–19] where individuals are homozygous for the *deletion* variant, which is associated with increased circulating[17] and cardiac tissue[58] ACE activity. The *DD* genotype appears to be a risk factor for early remodeling after MI[59] and for the development of end-stage ischemic and idiopathic dilated cardiomyopathy.[18,19] Other potentially important polymorphic variants that may influence the natural history of a cardiomyopathy involve the angiotensin AT_1 receptor,[60] β_2-adrenergic receptors,[20] the α_{2C}-adrenergic receptor with or without a β_1-receptor polymorphism,[21] and the endothelin receptor type A.[24]

TABLE 29–3

Known Familial DCM Genes, Loci, and Their OMIM

PHENOTYPE	ESTIMATED FREQUENCY[120] (%)	CHROMOSOMAL LOCATION	LOCUS	OMIM	GENE SYMBOL	GENE
Autosomal dominant familial DCM	56	1q32	CMD1D	191045	TNNT2	Cardiac troponin T
		3p21.1		191040	TNNC1	
		2q31	CMD1G	188840	TTN	Cardiac troponin C
		2q35	CMD1I	125660	DES	
		6q12–q16	CMD1K	172405	PLN	Titin
		9	CMD1B	600884		Desmin
		10q21–q23	CMD1C	193065	VCL	Phospholamban
		11p11		600958	MYBPC3	
						Metavinculin
		11p15.1	CMD1M	600824	CSRP3	Myosin-binding protein C
		12q22	CMD1T	188380	LAP2	
		14q12	CMD1A	160760	MYH7	Cysteine-glycine–rich protein 3
		14q12		160710	MYH6	Thymopoietin
		15q14	CMD1A	102540	ACTC	Cardiac β-myosin heavy chain
		15q22.1		191010	TPM1	
		17q12	CMD1N	604488	TCAP	Cardiac α-myosin heavy chain
		10q23.2		605906	LDB3	
		12p12.1		601439	ABCC9	
						Cardiac actin
						α-tropomyosin
						Tinin-cap (teletonin)
						Cypher/ZASP
						Regulatory SUR2A subunit of cardiac K_{ATP} channel
Autosomal recessive familial DCM	16	19q13.42		191044	TNNI3	Cardiac troponin I
		unknown		212110		
X-linked DCM	10	Xp21	XLCM	300377	DMD	Dystrophin
		Xq24		300257	LAMP2	Lysosome-associated membrane protein-2
Autosomal dominant familial DCM with skeletal muscle disease	7.7	1q11–q23	LGMD1B	150330	LMNA	Lamin A/C
		5q33–34	LGMD2F	601411	SGCD	δ-sarcoglycan
		4q11	LGMD2E	600900	SGCB	β-sarcoglycan
		6q23	CMD1F	602067		
Autosomal dominant familial DCM with conduction defects	2.6	1q1–q1	CMD1A	150330	LMNA	Lamin A/C
		2q14–q22	CMD1H	604288		
		3p22.2	CMD1E	600163	SCN5A	Na channel, voltage-gated, type V, α-polypeptide
Rare familial DCM	7.7					
Left ventricular non-compaction		Xq28		300069	TAZ	G4.5 (tafazzin)
		18q12.1–q12.2		601239	DTNA	α-dystrobrevin
		10q23.2		605906	LDB3	Cypher/ZASP
		6q23-q24	CMD1J	605362	EYA4	Transcriptional coactivator EYA4

TABLE 29–3

Known Familial DCM Genes, Loci, and Their OMIM *(continued)*

PHENOTYPE	ESTIMATED FREQUENCY[120] (%)	CHROMOSOMAL LOCATION	LOCUS	OMIM	GENE SYMBOL	GENE
Autosomal recessive with retinitis pigmentosa and deafness		6p24		125647	*DSP*	Desmoplakin
Autosomal recessive with wooly hair and keratoderma						
X-linked congenital DCM		Xq28		300069	*TAZ*	G4.5 (tafazzin)
Mitochondrial DCM		mtDNA		510000		

DCM, dilated cardiomyopathy; mtDNA, mitochondrial DNA; OMIM, Online Mendelian Inheritance in Man.
SOURCE: Modified from Taylor MRG, Carniel E, Mestroni L.[140]

Finally, recent pharmacogenomic studies have shown that polymorphic variations can influence the response to medications. Patients with the DD genotype, who were found to have a worse prognosis, at the same time appeared to respond significantly better to beta-blocker therapy compared to the other genotypes (*II* and *ID*).[19] Similarly, a polymorphism within a conserved region of the β_1-adrenergic receptor ([389]Arginine) increases the response to isotropic therapy (isoproterenol) and is associated with a reduction of mortality in patients treated with the β-blocker bucindolol.[23]

Altered, Maladaptive Expression of a Completely Normal Gene

The third way for altered gene expression to contribute to the development of a cardiomyopathy is altered, maladaptive expression of a completely normal *wild-type* gene.[13] This occurs most commonly in the context of progression of heart muscle disease and myocardial failure, which is the natural history of virtually all cardiomyopathies once they are established. Examples in this category (see Table 29–2) include downregulation of β_1-adrenergic receptors,[10] α-MHC,[61,62] and the *SERCA2* (sarcoplasmic reticulum [SR] Ca^{2+} adenosine triphosphatase [ATPase])[63] genes and upregulation in the atrial natriuretic peptide (*ANP*),[64] β-*MHC*,[61] *ACE*,[65,66] tumor necrosis factor alpha (*TNF-α*),[67] endothelin,[68] and beta-adrenergic receptor kinase (*BARK*)[69] genes. These concepts are discussed further below.

Recent data have shown that in patients who respond to treatment by increasing LV ejection fraction, β-blocker therapy may restore some aspects of altered gene expression, increasing the expression of sarcoplasmic-reticulum calcium ATPase and of α-MHC, and decreasing β-MHC.[70]

Pathophysiologic Processes Involved in Myocardial Dysfunction/Remodeling and Their Progression

Tissue preparations and myocytes isolated from failing human hearts exhibit evidence of decreased contractile function. Assuming that loading conditions and ischemia are not adversely affect-

ing cardiac myocyte function, in the setting of chronic systolic dysfunction from a dilated cardiomyopathy, progressive myocardial failure is most likely caused by myocardial cell loss or changes in the gene expression of proteins that regulate or produce muscle contraction. Fig. 29–1 and Fig. 29–2 summarize these general points and emphasize the central roles of the renin-angiotensin system (RAS) and adrenergic nervous system (ANS) in promoting cell loss, growth and remodeling, and altered gene expression.[3]

Myocardial Dysfunction and Remodeling Due to Altered Expression of Contractility-Regulating Genes and Changes in Sarcomeric Assembly

Gene expression can be defined broadly as the expression of a fully or normally functioning protein gene product or, more narrowly

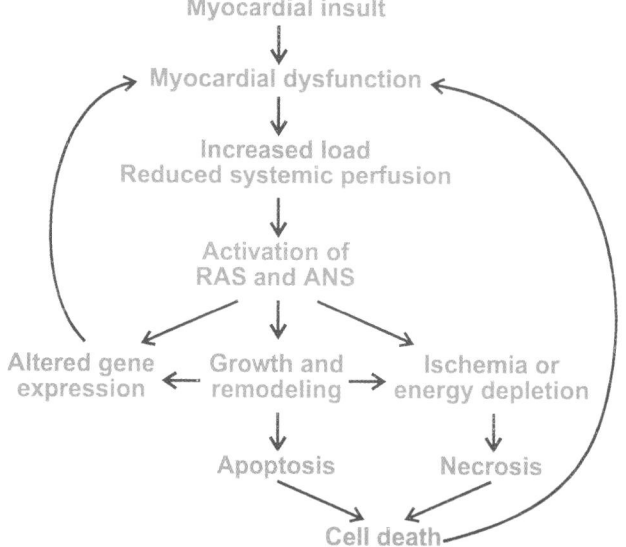

FIGURE 29–1. Relationship of neurohormonal activation and production of cardiac myocyte loss caused by apoptosis and necrosis and altered gene expression. Cell loss and altered gene expression result in more myocardial dysfunction, and a vicious cycle is established. RAS, renin-angiotensin system; ANS, adrenergic nervous system.

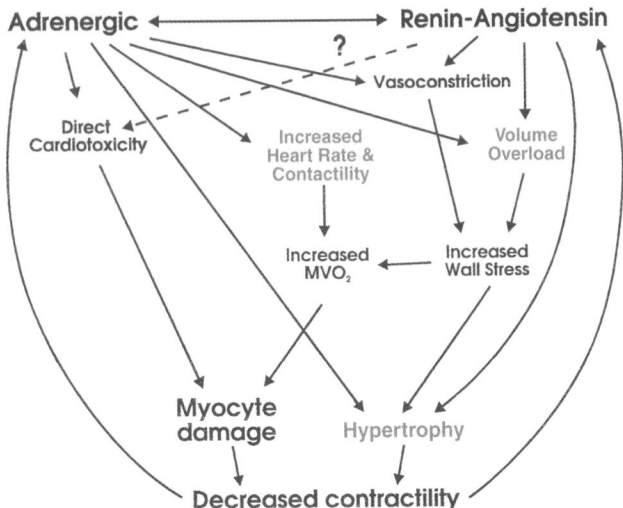

FIGURE 29–2. Heart failure compensatory mechanisms that are activated to support the failing heart. Light-colored areas indicate physiologic mechanisms that stabilize pump function.

(and commonly), as the steady-state abundance of a gene's mRNA transcript. Using either definition, numerous abnormalities of gene expression of normal, wild-type genes have been demonstrated in the failing human heart as discussed earlier, with examples listed in Table 29–2. To characterize the abnormalities that may account for progressive myocardial dysfunction and remodeling, it is useful to subdivide them into two general categories,[71] as shown in Table 29–4. The first category encompasses mechanisms that subserve *intrinsic function,* or the mechanisms responsible for contraction and relaxation of the heart in the basal or resting state. Intrinsic function is defined as myocardial contraction and relaxation in the absence of extrinsic influences, such as neurotransmitters or hormones. The second general category is *modulated function,* which comprises the mechanisms responsible for the remarkable ability of the heart to increase or decrease its performance dramatically (by 2- to 10-fold) and rapidly in response to various physiologic or physical stimuli. Other critical organs such as the brain, kidney, and liver do not exhibit this quality. Modulated function is defined as stimulation or inhibition of myocardial contraction or relaxation by endogenous bioactive compounds, including neurotransmitters, cytokines, autocrine/paracrine substances, and hormones.

In the failing human heart, changes are present in the expression of genes potentially responsible for both general types of myocardial function depicted in Table 29–4.[9,71] Abnormalities of intrinsic function include the factors responsible for an altered length–tension relation,[72,73] a blunted force–frequency response,[74] and/or the signals responsible for abnormal cellular and chamber remodeling.[3,75] In the case of the abnormal force–frequency and length–tension responses, the evidence favors abnormal contractile function of individual cardiac myocytes. As shown in Table 29–4, these abnormalities likely reside in the contractile proteins or their regulatory elements,[61,62] mechanisms involved in excitation-contraction coupling,[63] or the cytoskeleton.[29,76] However, within these possibilities for altered intrin-

sic function, currently there is not a consensus as to which specific abnormalities are present in dilated cardiomyopathy (DCM), the most common form of heart failure studied in humans. For cellular remodeling in both human ventricles[77] and animal models,[78,79] the assembly of sarcomeres in series leads to a myocyte that is markedly increased in length but not in diameter, which contributes to remodeling at the chamber level. Such remodeling places the chamber and the myocyte at an energetic disadvantage because of the attendant increase in wall stress,[80] which is one major determinant of myocardial oxygen consumption. Inadequate myocyte energy production, particularly associated with key subcellular ion flux mechanisms or the myosin ATPase cycle,[81] in turn contribute to myocyte contractile dysfunction. Moreover, the hypertrophy process itself leads to a qualitative change in contractile protein gene expression (induction of a *fetal* gene program), which reduces contractile function.[13,61,62] Conversely, cardiac myocyte contractile dysfunction likely plays a role in the remodeling process inasmuch as medical treatment, which improves intrinsic myocardial function can reverse remodeling.[3,70] Thus, contractile dysfunction and remodeling at the cellular level are intimately related to the progressive contractile dysfunction and chamber enlargement that define the natural history of myocardial failure. These concepts are summarized in Fig. 29–3.

In contrast to abnormalities of intrinsic function, a consensus has been reached on several specific abnormalities in the stimulation component of modulated function. Most changes concern β-adrenergic signal transduction.[10,12,71] The ability of β-adrenergic stimulation to increase heart rate and contractility is markedly attenuated in the failing heart caused by multiple changes at the level of receptors, G proteins, and adenylyl cyclase. This produces a major abnormality in the stimulation component of modulated function. In addition, the inhibition component of modulated function is also abnormal in the failing heart because of a reduction in parasympathetic drive.[82]

There is obviously overlap between the two major subdivisions of myocardial function. Even in the absence of adrenergic stimulation, β-adrenergic receptors have intrinsic activity.[83–85] That is, a small percentage of receptors are in an activated state without agonist occupancy and, as such, can support intrinsic myocardial function.[84,85] Thus overexpression of human β_2-adrenergic receptors can markedly increase intrinsic myocardial function,[84] as can

---

TABLE 29–4	
General Categorization of Myocardial Function	
INTRINSIC (*function in the absence of neural or hormonal influence*)	**MODULATED** (*function that may be stimulated or inhibited by extrinsic factors including neurotransmitters, cytokines, or hormones*)
• Contractile proteins • EC coupling mechanisms • R-G-adenylyl cyclase pathways • Bioenergetics • Cytoskeleton • Sarcomere and cell remodeling	• R-G-adenylyl cyclase pathways • R-G-phospholipase C pathways

EC, excitation-contraction.

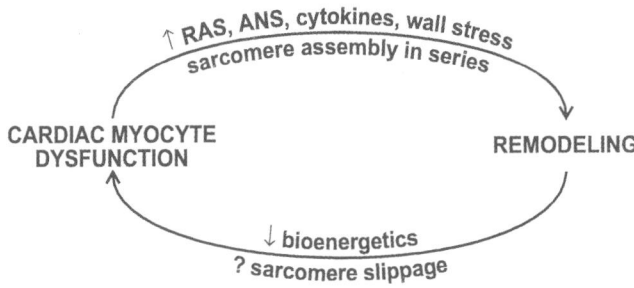

FIGURE 29–3. Relationship between progressive myocardial dysfunction and remodeling. RAS, renin-angiotensin system; ANS, adrenergic nervous system.

enhancement of SR calcium uptake and release by genetic ablation of the phospholamban gene.[86] The realization that active-state, agonist-unoccupied β-adrenergic receptors can modulate intrinsic myocardial function is the reason why the *R-G-adenylyl cyclase* mechanism appears in both categories in Table 29–4.

Progressive Myocardial Dysfunction and Remodeling Due to Loss of Cardiac Myocytes

The second general mechanism by which myocardial function may be adversely affected is by loss of cardiac myocytes, which may also play a role in the progression of ventricular dysfunction in dilated cardiomyopathies. Cardiac myocyte loss can occur via toxic mechanisms producing necrosis, or by *programmed cell death,* producing apoptosis. Apoptosis, which is likely caused by a combination of growth signaling and cell cycle dysregulation, has been described in end-stage DCM[87] as well as in the β_1-adrenergic receptor,[32] the $G\alpha_s$-overexpressor transgenic mice,[36] and in models of hypertrophy.[88] However, data from human studies refer to a very late stage of DCM or ischemic dilated cardiomyopathy, treated with multiple powerful intravenous inotropic medications; therefore, it is unclear whether apoptosis plays a significant role in remodeling and/or chamber systolic dysfunction before this point is reached in the natural history of the dilated cardiomyopathies.

[ ] IMPORTANCE OF *COMPENSATORY* MECHANISMS IN THE PROGRESSION OF MYOCARDIAL FAILURE

As depicted in Fig. 29–1 and Fig. 29–2, there is now a large body of information supporting the idea that *activation of the adrenergic nervous system and RAS compensatory mechanisms contributes to, or is responsible for, the progressive nature of both myocardial failure and the natural history of the heart failure clinical syndrome.*[9] This evidence includes the observations that activation of both systems is associated with progression of myocardial dysfunction and the heart failure syndrome, and clinical trial data that consistently demonstrate that inhibition of these systems can prevent deterioration in or improve myocardial function as well as reduce mortality.[9,12] Although we now know that chronic activation of the ANS and RAS contributes to the progressive nature of myocardial dysfunction in human heart failure, we know virtually nothing approximately how these systems adversely affect the biology of the cardiac myocyte. What we do know is that mechanisms within both general categories

outlined in Table 29–3 must be involved in the adverse myocardial effects mediated by the ANS and RAS. This is so because modulated function may be improved by treatment with ACE inhibitors or β-blocking agents. Progressive myocardial dysfunction and remodeling are attenuated by both β-blocking agents and ACE inhibitors, in cardiomyopathies intrinsic myocardial function is improved and remodeling is reversed by chronic treatment with β-blocking agents.[9,70] Additionally, mortality in chronic heart failure is directly related to activation of the ANS[89,90] and RAS[91] and may be related to the activation of other neurohormonal or autocrine/paracrine systems as well.

Regardless of the type or cause of dilated cardiomyopathy, an initial myocardial insult resulting in this phenotype exhibits common pathophysiologic features that are summarized in Fig. 29–1. That is, a myocardial insult that produces systolic dysfunction is followed by the initiation of processes designed to temporarily stabilize pump function. The possible mechanisms available for such stabilization are limited. As shown in Fig. 29–2, in chronological order of their action, they are an increase in heart rate and contractility mediated by an increase in cardiac β-adrenergic signaling (produced within seconds of the onset of pump dysfunction), volume expansion to use the Frank-Starling mechanism to increase stroke volume (evident within hours of the onset of pump dysfunction), and cardiac myocyte hypertrophy to increase the number of contractile elements (evident within days or weeks of the onset of pump dysfunction). As shown in Fig. 29–2, these compensatory adjustments are largely accomplished by activation of the RAS and adrenergic nervous ANS systems. However, despite the short-term (days to months) stability achieved via these mechanisms, they ultimately prove harmful.[9] The best evidence that chronic, continued activation of the RAS and ANS contributes to progressive myocardial dysfunction and remodeling comes from clinical trials where both inhibitors of the RAS (ACE inhibitors) and ANS (β-adrenergic receptor–blocking agents) prevent these two phenomena; and β-blocking agents actually may reverse remodeling and progressive systolic dysfunction.[3,9]

Much current work is focused on the precise pathophysiologic mechanisms by which activation of the RAS and adrenergic nervous system produces remodeling and adverse effects on myocardial function. Some possibilities are given in Fig. 29–1; they include an exacerbation of ischemia and/or energy depletion, leading to cell loss via necrosis, cell loss by programmed cell death, direct promotion of hypertrophy and remodeling through stimulation of cell growth, and alterations in cardiac myocyte gene expression.[3] A key feature of the schema shown in Fig. 29–1 is the process of remodeling, which is discussed in more detail in Chap. 24. Virtually all dilated cardiomyopathies undergo this process, which is characterized by progressive dilatation, progressive myocardial systolic dysfunction in viable segments, and a change in chamber shape whereby the ventricle becomes less elliptical and more round.[3,9,75] As shown in Fig. 29–3, this places the ventricle at an energetic disadvantage, which likely contributes to further myocardial dysfunction, which then contributes to progressive remodeling. The latter observation is based on data with β-adrenergic blocking agents, which produce an improvement in systolic dysfunction that can be detected prior to a reversal in remodeling.[9] As emphasized by Fig.

TABLE 29–5

Types of Dilated Cardiomyopathies

Ischemic insult (*ischemic cardiomyopathy*)
Valvular disease (mitral regurgitation, aortic regurgitation, aortic stenosis); (*valvular cardiomyopathy*)
Chronic hypertension (*hypertensive cardiomyopathy*)
Tachyarrhythmias (supraventricular, ventricular, atrial flutter)
Familial (autosomal dominant, autosomal recessive, X-linked, matrilinear)
Idiopathic
Toxins
  Ethanol
  Chemotherapeutic agents (anthracyclines such as doxorubicin and daunorubicin)
  Cobalt
  Antiretroviral agents (zidovudine, didanosine, zalcitabine)
  Phenothiazines
  Carbon monoxide
  Lithium
  Lead
  Cocaine
  Mercury
Metabolic abnormalities
  Nutritional deficiencies (thiamine, selenium, carnitine, protein)
  Endocrinologic disorders (hypothyroidism, acromegaly, thyrotoxicosis, Cushing disease, pheochromocytoma, catecholamines, diabetes mellitus)
  Electrolyte disturbances (hypocalcemia, hypophosphatemia)
Infectious
  Viral (coxsackievirus, cytomegalovirus, HIV, adenovirus, HSV)
  Rickettsial
  Bacterial
  Mycobacterial
  Spirochetal
  Fungal
  Parasitic (toxoplasmosis, trichinosis, Chagas disease)

Autoimmune/collagen disorders
  Systemic lupus erythematosus
Juvenile rheumatoid arthritis
  Polyarteritis nodosa
  Kawasaki disease
  Collagen vascular disorders (scleroderma, lupus erythematosus, dermatomyositis)
Infiltrative disorders
  Hemochromatosis
Amyloidosis
  Sarcoidosis
Endomyocardial disorders
  Hypereosinophilic syndrome (Löffler endocarditis)
  Endomyocardial fibrosis
Hypersensitivity myocarditis
Peri-/postpartum dysfunction
  Arrhythmogenic right ventricular dysplasia or cardiomyopathy
Infantile histiocytoid
Neuromuscular dystrophies
  Becker or Duchenne muscular dystrophy, X-linked cardioskeletal myopathy
Facioscapulohumeral muscular dystrophy
  Erb limb-girdle dystrophy
  Myotonic dystrophy
Friedreich ataxia
  Emery-Dreifuss muscular dystrophy
Inborn errors of metabolism
Mitochondrial cardiomyopathies
Keshan cardiomyopathy

HSV, herpes simplex virus.

29–3, each myocardial degenerative process likely begets the other, leading to an inexorably progressive deterioration in myocardial performance and clinical condition.

SCOPE OF DILATED CARDIOMYOPATHIES

The number of cardiac or systemic processes that can produce a dilated cardiomyopathy or are associated with it is plentiful and remarkably varied, as shown in Table 29–5. The dilated phenotype is by far the most common form of cardiomyopathy, comprising more than 90 percent of subjects referred to specialized centers.[92] In the United States the most common dilated cardiomyopathy is ischemic dilated cardiomyopathy,[1] or the cardiomyopathy that follows MI. Other common secondary dilated cardiomyopathies are hypertensive and valvular dilated cardiomyopathies, both produced in part by chronically increased wall stress. The primary car-

diomyopathy, DCM, is another relatively common dilated phenotype,[93,94] as discussed in the following section.

【 】 SELECTED COMMON TYPES OF DILATED CARDIOMYOPATHIES

Ischemic Cardiomyopathy

Definition/Diagnosis *Ischemic cardiomyopathy* is commonly defined as a dilated cardiomyopathy in a subject with a history of MI or evidence of clinically significant (i.e., ≥ 70 percent narrowing of a major epicardial artery) coronary artery disease, in whom the degree of myocardial dysfunction and ventricular dilatation is not explained solely by the extent of previous infarction or the degree of ongoing ischemia. In other words, *an ischemic dilated cardiomyopathy is present when a post-MI left ventricle experiences remodeling and a drop in ejection fraction.*

Distinct Pathophysiology Dilatation of the left ventricle and a decrease in ejection fraction occurs in 15 to 40 percent of subjects within 12 to 24 months following an anterior MI[95,96] and in a smaller percentage of subjects following an inferior MI.[96] Based on limited data,[59] it is tempting to speculate that the subjects who undergo the remodeling process and develop an ischemic dilated cardiomyopathy are individuals with particularly heightened compensatory mechanisms (see Fig. 29–1 and Fig. 29–2), perhaps as a result in polymorphic variation in these systems.[18] As discussed above, the remodeling process is an attempt of the compromised ventricle to increase its performance by increasing stroke volume; but ultimately, it correlates with an adverse outcome[3] in the long term.

The gross pathology of ischemic cardiomyopathy includes transmural or subendocardial scarring, representing old MIs, that may comprise up to 50 percent of the LV chamber. The histopathology of the noninfarcted regions is similar to changes which occur in DCM,[97] as discussed below.

Prognosis Several studies conclude that patients with ischemic cardiomyopathy have a worse prognosis than subjects with a *nonischemic* dilated cardiomyopathy,[98–100] probably because the risk of ischemic events is added to the risk of having a dilated cardiomyopathy.

Treatment The treatment of ischemic dilated cardiomyopathy and chronic heart failure is covered in detail in Chap. 26. In general, treatment consists of the use of (1) ACE inhibitors in asymptomatic or symptomatic patients, (2) β blockers in symptomatic patients, (3) diuretics in volume-overloaded subjects, (4) spironolactone in advanced patients, and (5) digoxin in symptomatic patients.[101] Recent data have demonstrated the effectiveness of devices in treating ischemic dilated cardiomyopathies, including implantable cardioverters/defibrillators (ICDs) for patients without intraventricular conduction defects (IVCDs),[102] and biventricular pacing plus ICD for patients with IVCDs.[103–105] Additionally, adjunctive therapy includes anticoagulation in subjects with lower LV ejection fraction to prevent thromboembolic complications, amiodarone to treat symptomatic arrhythmias, maintenance of potassium levels in the high normal (4.3 to 5.0 meq/L) range to prevent sudden death, keeping digoxin levels ≤1.0 ng/mL,[106] frequent clinic visits to adjust medications, and an aggressive approach to treating ischemia, including revascularization.

Hypertensive Cardiomyopathy

Definition/Diagnosis A *hypertensive dilated cardiomyopathy* is diagnosed when myocardial systolic function is depressed out of proportion to the increase in wall stress. In other words, a subject presenting in heart failure with a hypertensive crisis would not carry this diagnosis unless ventricular dilatation and depressed systolic function remained after correction of the hypertension. In addition to producing a *pure* form of hypertensive cardiomyopathy, hypertension is a major risk factor for heart failure from any cause.[107] Within the 1995 WHO/ISFC classification, *hypertensive heart disease* may present in the *dilated, restrictive,* or *unclassified* categories.[6] However, the 2006 AHA Scientific Statement has not included the hypertensive myocardial disease in the formal classification of cardiomyopathies.[4]

Distinct Pathophysiology The most important pathophysiologic element in hypertension with dilated cardiomyopathy is a sustained increase in systolic wall stress. Interestingly, in both systolic pressure-overloaded right and left ventricles, phenotypic expression is qualitatively variable[108,109] and can include dilation and systolic dysfunction without increased wall thickness, concentric hypertrophy with or without systolic dysfunction, and systolic dysfunction without concentric hypertrophy. Other contributors to the pathophysiology of hypertensive cardiomyopathies are local neurohormonal mechanisms.[110]

Prognosis The prognosis depends on the presence of other comorbid conditions such as diabetes mellitus and coronary artery disease as well as the extent of control of afterload. Compared to other forms of cardiomyopathy, in the absence of comorbid conditions, the prognosis of hypertensive cardiomyopathy in subjects whose afterload is controlled is probably better than for most other types of dilated cardiomyopathy.[100,111]

Treatment The treatment is as for ischemic dilated cardiomyopathy except that afterload must be vigorously controlled.[110] This consists of the addition of pure antihypertensive vasodilators such as amlodipine, hydralazine, nitrates or even α-blocking agents to standard heart failure therapy.

Valvular Cardiomyopathy

Definition/Diagnosis A *valvular cardiomyopathy* occurs when a valvular abnormality is present and myocardial systolic function is depressed out of proportion to the increase in wall stress. This most commonly occurs with left-sided regurgitant lesions (mitral regurgitation and aortic regurgitation), less commonly with aortic stenosis, and never as a consequence of pure mitral stenosis.

Distinct Pathophysiology The classic explanation for the typical phenotypes observed in valvular cardiomyopathies relates to exposure to different types of wall stress.[112] Within this construct, the pattern of eccentric hypertrophy derives from increased diastolic wall stress. Thus, long-standing mitral regurgitation most commonly results in compensated eccentric hypertrophy that can progress to a dilated failing phenotype. Aortic regurgitation is a particularly poorly tolerated hemodynamic insult because wall stress is increased in both systole and diastole[112]; and when decompensation occurs, ventricular volume increases with or without increased wall thickness. Aortic stenosis classically results in compensated concentric hypertrophy; but when decompensation occurs, a variety of phenotypes can be observed that are similar to hypertensive cardiomyopathies. A disturbing and fairly commonly observed phenomenon is the development of a dilated cardiomyopathy after surgical correction of mitral and sometimes aortic valve disease in subjects who preoperatively had only mild LV dysfunction. These cases are likely caused by the superimposition of myocardial damage resulting from open heart surgery and/or underlying dysfunction that was likely greater than may have been appreciated preoperatively.

Prognosis The prognosis is variable and depends on the number of associated conditions; the nature and extent of the valvular abnormality; and most important, the severity of the cardiomyopathy at the time of surgical correction (see below). In general, *severely depressed myocardial function will not improve much with surgical repair of aortic regurgitation or mitral regurgitation, but the prognosis is likely to be improved because of elimination of some of the hemodynamic insult.* Replacement of the mitral valve should not be attempted in most subjects with severe mitral regurgitation and LV ejection fraction <25 percent because of prohibitively high operative/perioperative mortality rates. Conversely, there is no impairment of LV systolic function severe enough to preclude valve replacement of severe aortic stenosis, because function invariably improves on relief of the hemodynamic insult and the prognosis is relatively good.

Treatment The treatment of a valvular dilated cardiomyopathy is surgical valve replacement or repair as soon as the cardiomyopathy is detected. Catheter valvuloplasty may be an option for patients with severe aortic stenosis who are not good surgical candidates for reasons other than heart failure.[113] Medical treatment may be the only option in subjects with aortic insufficiency or mitral regurgitation whose LV function is severely impaired. The medical treatment of either disorder should be as above for ischemic cardiomyopathy plus aggressive afterload reduction, usually hydralazine/nitrates on top of ACE inhibitors. The calcium channel blocker amlodipine is another option for afterload reduction,[114] particularly for aortic insufficiency, where calcium blocker therapy has been shown to improve survival.[115]

Idiopathic Dilated Cardiomyopathy, Including Familial Forms

Definition/Diagnosis DCM is diagnosed by excluding significant coronary artery disease, valvular abnormalities, and other causes. DCM is a relatively common cause of heart failure, with an estimated prevalence rate of 0.04 percent;[116] incidence rates vary from 0.005 to 0.006 percent.[93,94] The true incidence of DCM is undoubtedly higher owing to the fact that subjects may remain asymptomatic until marked ventricular dysfunction has occurred. The incidence of DCM increases with age and males are affected at a higher rate than females.[116] As discussed below, histologic features are nonspecific and consist of myocardial cell hypertrophy and varying amounts of increased interstitial fibrosis. Although the diagnosis is not difficult, problems arise when an apparent DCM presents in someone with a history of hypertension or excessive alcohol intake. In such cases it is best to reassign the etiology to alcohol only when the intake has exceeded 80 g/day for males and 40 g/day for females for >5 years and to hypertensive heart disease when blood pressure has been uncontrolled and high (>160/100 mmHg), as well as sustained (for years). All subjects with an unexplained dilated cardiomyopathy need a thyroid-stimulating hormone level done to exclude hypo- or hyperthyroidism, and subjects with diastolic dysfunction need to have an infiltrative process excluded. As discussed below, this is best done by performing an endomyocardial biopsy.

Distinct Pathophysiology DCM may be familial in as many as 35 to 50 percent of the cases when first-degree relatives are carefully screened.[117–119] The analysis of the phenotype identifies a wide range of clinical and pathologic forms indicating genetic heterogeneity. Accordingly, several chromosomal assignments for gene location have been made and recently, as shown in Table 29–2 and Table 29–3, several genes have been identified. Most familial patients present with autosomal dominant inheritance and a phenotype characterized by low and age-related penetrance (which is the proportion of carriers who manifest the disease).[120] It is estimated that only 20 percent of gene carriers younger than the age of 20 display the disease phenotype.[120]

Molecular genetic studies have shown that familial dilated cardiomyopathy can be caused by mutations of a large number of genes involved in various myocardial functions including the *sarcomere,* the *cytoskeleton/sarcolemma/nuclear envelope, ion channels,* the *desmosome,* and *signaling pathways.* Specific characteristics of the phenotype can help in the identification of the disease gene. The detection of an altered creatine kinase (CK) level can indicate the existence of a subclinical skeletal muscle disease. In these patients an X-linked inheritance suggests mutations in the dystrophin gene that maps on the X chromosome,[48,121–123] Skeletal muscle and endomyocardial biopsy shows abnormalities of dystrophin protein expression by immunocytochemistry.[124] An autosomal dominant transmission and the presence of conduction defects, arrhythmia, and increased CK levels suggest mutations in the lamin A/C gene.[14,15,125,126] In *laminopathies* the phenotype of the affected relatives can be very variable, from a pure DCM to a mild Emery-Dreifuss–like or limb-girdle–like muscle dystrophy.[15,125] An autosomal recessive transmission of dilated cardiomyopathy may occur in mutations of sarcoglycan genes, which encode for dystrophin complex–associated proteins.[127] Other structural proteins, such as *desmosomal* proteins, can cause a DCM phenotype. This is the case of the *desmoplakin* gene that causes Carvajal syndrome (DCM, woolly hair, and keratoderma).[52]

However, as previously seen in animal models,[26,28,128,129] it became evident that abnormalities in sarcomeric proteins—such as cardiac α-actin,[130] titin,[131] myosin-binding protein C,[132] cardiac β-myosin heavy chain,[49] cardiac α-myosin heavy chain,[16] and cardiac troponin T[49]—can also produce a dilated phenotype. Phospholamban gene mutations[54,133] have been found to cause familial dilated cardiomyopathy, confirming the hypothesis from animal studies that the disease can also be caused by other mechanisms, such as altered signal transduction and calcium dysregulation.[30,32,133]

In children X-linked familial DCM suggests mutation in the *G4.5* or *tafazzin* gene, particularly if associated with certain other signs (such as endocardial fibroelastosis, neutropenia, short stature, or skeletal muscle abnormalities).[134] Recent studies have shown that tafazzin is an acyltransferase, a mitochondrial membrane protein involved in the respiratory chain and cardiolipin metabolism.[135] Likewise, mitochondrial DNA (mtDNA) mutations can cause myocardial dysfunction, which is usually associated with multiorgan involvement (encephalopathy, lactic acidosis, skeletal muscle abnormalities, retinitis pigmentosa, etc.).[136] It has been reported that mtDNA mutations can lead to an isolated DCM phenotype in adults.[137]

Finally, a series of recent studies has shown that mutations in ion channels, the alpha subunit of the sodium channel (encoded by the *SCN5A* gene)[50,51] and the adenosine triphosphate (ATP)–sensitive potassium channel (encoded by the *ABCC9* gene),[138] can cause DCM.

Although still incomplete, new knowledge on the genetics of DCM has important clinical implications. The frequency of familial forms indicates the need for family screening in DCM,[7,139,140] which can allow genetic counseling, an early detection of the disease, and early therapeutic interventions in affected relatives. The complexity of the phenotype requires an accurate skeletal muscle investigation, which can direct the diagnosis toward a specific type of familial myopathy. Family investigations require more sensitive diagnostic criteria[7] that are able to detect minor cardiac abnormalities as initial signs of the disease. These include initial dilatation without marked systolic dysfunction, arrhythmia, segmental wall hypokinesis, and other abnormalities.[7,119] Finally, the systematic screening of genes causing DCM can identify those genes or mutations that are more prevalent and predictive of a worse outcome, so that carriers of such genes can be clinically tested. This is the case of lamin A/C gene, which is frequently mutated in patients with conduction delays[125,126] and associated with high mortality and morbidity.[125]

The major morphologic feature of DCM on postmortem examination is dilatation of the cardiac chambers.[141] One ventricle (usually the left) may be more dilated than the other. The weight of the heart is increased in DCM, with a mean cardiac weight of 551 grams for women and 632 grams for men.[141] Although there is an increase in muscle mass and myocyte cell volume in DCM, LV wall thickness is usually not increased because of the marked dilatation of the ventricular cavities. Grossly visible scars may be present in either ventricle; and although most scars are small, some may be large and transmural. Scarring occurs in the absence of significant narrowing of the epicardial coronary arteries. In most cases, the degree of fibrosis does not seem extensive enough to cause changes in systolic or diastolic function. Intracardiac thrombi and mural endocardial plaques (from the organization of thrombi) are present at necropsy in more than 50 percent of patients with DCM.[141] The effect of anticoagulation on the incidence of thrombi has not been carefully studied, but systemic and pulmonary emboli are more frequent in patients with ventricular thrombi or plaques.[142]

The characteristic findings of DCM on microscopy are marked myocyte hypertrophy, very large, bizarrely shaped nuclei,[143–145] (Fig. 29–4), increased interstitial fibrosis (see Fig. 29–4), myocyte atrophy, and myofilament loss.[141,146] In isolated cardiac myocytes, the major cellular phenotypic change is a marked increase in cell length without a concomitant increase in diameter.[77] As described earlier this cellular lengthening or remodeling contributes to the chamber remodeling/dilatation that characterizes DCM and other cardiomyopathies. These morphologic changes in DCM are not specific and are generally found in secondary cardiomyopathies such as in the noninfarcted regions of ischemic dilated cardiomyopathy.[97] Also, the morphometric changes in DCM do not correlate with the severity of illness.[145,146] Ultrastructural abnormalities such as mitochondrial changes, T-tubular dilatation, and intracellular lipid droplets may be observed in DCM but can also be seen in other forms of heart disease.[145] There may be interstitial parenchymal and perivascular focal infiltrates of small lymphocytes.[145–147]

The lymphocytic infiltrates that are present on histologic examination in DCM are not associated with adjacent myocyte damage, in contrast to myocarditis where adjacent myocyte necrosis is observed. Fibrosis is nearly always present in DCM[145–147]; and its pattern is quite variable, from a fine perimyocytic distribution to coarse scars indistinguishable from those present in chronic ischemia. However, small intramural arteries and capillaries are structurally normal in DCM.[145]

Several immune regulatory abnormalities have been identified in DCM, including humoral[148] and cellular autoimmune reactivity against myocytes,[149] decreased natural killer cell activity,[150] and abnormal suppressor cell activity.[151] It is likely that many antibodies detected in DCM and other myocardial diseases do not have pathogenic relevance but rather are secondary to the primary degenerative process. However, it is possible that certain antibodies present in DCM may have important functional implications.[152] For example, anti–β_1-adrenergic receptor antibodies could modify β-adrenergic receptor activity and produce chronic increases in signal transduction that are harmful to the failing heart.[153] Disturbed energy metabolism from antibodies to the adenosine diphosphate/ATP carrier of the inner mitochondrial membrane is another potential pathogenetic autoimmune mechanism.[154]

Human leukocyte antigens (HLAs) associations have also been identified in DCM; the frequency of HLA-B27, HLA-A2, HLA-DR4, and HLA-DQ4 is increased compared to controls; and the frequency of HLA-DRw6 is decreased compared to controls.[155] The association of DCM with specific HLAs suggests a possible immunologic etiology for this disease. However, these specific HLAs are present in <50 percent of patients with DCM, and the heterogeneity of these antigens does not point to a unique site for a putative disease-associated gene. Thus, although the autoimmune hypothesis is an attractive candidate for the etiology of some cases of DCM, it remains unproved.

A clinical and pathologic syndrome that is similar to DCM may develop after resolution of viral myocarditis in animal models and biopsy-proven myocarditis in human subjects.[156] This has led to

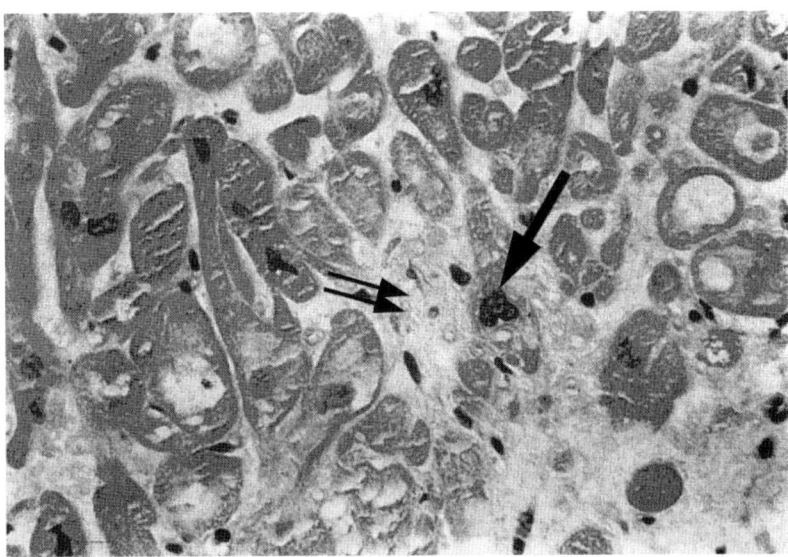

FIGURE 29–4. Right ventricular endomyocardial biopsy from a subject with DCM. Note the increased nuclear size (*large arrow*) and the increased interstitial fibrosis.

speculation that DCM may develop in some individuals as a result of subclinical viral myocarditis. Theoretically, an episode of myocarditis could initiate a variety of autoimmune reactions that injure the myocardium and ultimately result in the development of DCM. The abnormalities in immune regulation and the variety of antimyocardial antibodies present in DCM are consistent with this hypothesis. However, generally it is impossible to isolate an infectious virus or to demonstrate the presence of viral antigens in the myocardium of patients with DCM. Enteroviral RNA sequences may be found in heart biopsy samples in DCM but with a very variable frequency (0–30 percent).[157,158] Furthermore, mechanisms of inflammation in DCM have been uncertain, and in controlled trials corticosteroid therapy of patients with DCM does not result in significant clinical improvements.[159] More recent experimental data have shown in vitro and in vivo that the enteroviral protease 2A is able to cleave dystrophin and disrupt the cytoskeleton in cardiac myocytes, providing a potential link between viral infection and a genetic model of the disease.[160] Furthermore, analysis of human viruses other than enteroviruses suggests that adenoviruses, herpes, and cytomegalovirus can also cause myocarditis and potentially DCM, particularly in children and young subjects.[161,162]

As also discussed in Chap. 32, endomyocardial biopsy may be a valuable diagnostic adjunct for diagnosing specific myocardial processes that can produce a dilated phenotype, such as myocarditis and infiltrative cardiomyopathies. Because several other dilated cardiomyopathies may have specific treatments and/or a different prognosis than DCM, endomyocardial biopsy may be warranted in selected individuals presenting with a dilated cardiomyopathy. Biopsy may be used to identify abnormal gene or protein expression.[61,70] Because special staining, electron microscopy, or molecular analysis of the biopsy material may be necessary, endomyocardial biopsy should be performed in specialized cardiomyopathy/heart failure centers.

Prognosis Several studies of the natural history of DCM have been conducted.[100,163,164] The prognosis is generally better than for ischemic cardiomyopathy[100]; prior to the routine use of ACE inhibitors, the survival was approximately 50 percent in 5 years.[163] The prognosis has been substantially improved since then,[100] inasmuch as ACE inhibition,[165] β-adrenergic blockade,[12] cardiac resynchronization with biventricular pacing,[104] implantable cardioverter-defibrillator,[166] and cardiac transplantation (in the high-risk group)[167,168] are all effective treatments in this condition. Among genetic causes of DCM, *laminopathies* (caused by mutations in the lamin A/C gene) have been associated with worse prognosis, high mortality for congestive heart failure or sudden death, and need of transplant, making molecular genetic testing an important tool in the clinical management of these patients.[125,169,170]

Treatment The treatment of DCM is similar to that discussed above for ischemic cardiomyopathy except there is no issue of revascularization.[140] The risk of thromboembolic complications may be higher than in ischemic cardiomyopathy, resulting in a lower threshold for anticoagulation. β-Adrenergic blockade produces a quantitatively greater degree of improvement in LV function compared to ischemic cardiomyopathy,[171] either because there is a greater degree of adrenergic activation[10] or

there is more viable myocardium to work with in DCM. Approximately 10 percent of DCM subjects treated with β-adrenergic blockade normalize their myocardial function, and this form of treatment should be offered to all DCM subjects who do not have a contraindication before cardiac transplantation is considered.[172]

SELECTED SECONDARY DILATED CARDIOMYOPATHIES WITH UNIQUE MANAGEMENT ISSUES

【 】 ANTHRACYCLINE CARDIOMYOPATHY

Definition/Diagnosis

The commonly used and highly efficacious anthracycline antibiotic anticancer agents doxorubicin and daunorubicin produce a dose-related cardiomyopathy[173–176] that may limit their clinical application. Within the WHO/ISFC classification, an anthracycline cardiomyopathy would most likely be in the *dilated* category, because the extent of dilatation may initially be minimal (see below). The cardiomyopathy produced by these agents depends on the total cumulative dose; for the more widely used compound doxorubicin (Adriamycin), the incidence of heart failure caused by cardiomyopathy dramatically increases above total cumulative doses of 450 mg/m² in subjects without underlying cardiac problems or other risk factors.[177] *Prior mediastinal radiation involving the heart is a powerful risk factor for anthracycline cardiomyopathy,*[174] and the risk is also evident if radiation treatment follows chemotherapy.[176,178] In subjects with risk factors, anthracycline cardiomyopathy can present at lower cumulative doses than 450 mg/m².[174,175,178]

Although the diagnosis of anthracycline cardiomyopathy can be made clinically, the definitive diagnosis depends on the demonstration of a substantial number of cardiac myocytes exhibiting the characteristic anthracycline effect.[173–175,178] Tissue sampling is best done by endomyocardial biopsy, which allows for thin-section electron microscopic processing of the sample and more definitive resolution of the anthracycline effect with light microscopy.[173–175,178]

Distinct Pathophysiology

In the absence of a tissue diagnosis, anthracycline cardiomyopathy may be diagnosed clinically by exclusion of other causes of cardiomyopathy in a subject who has had at least 350 mg/m² of doxorubicin or the equivalent amount of another anthracycline. As shown in Fig. 29–5, the anthracycline cardiac myocytic lesion consists of cell vacuolization progressing to cell dropout; and myocardial dysfunction results when 16 to 25 percent of the total number of sampled cells exhibit this morphology.[173]

There are some distinguishing clinical features of anthracycline cardiomyopathy that may relate to its pathophysiology. These include a relative absence of hypertrophy and dilatation and a higher heart rate (110–130 beats/min) than is usually encountered in ambulatory heart failure. The reasons for these features are that the onset of symptoms may be relatively acute (remodeling takes time to develop) and the anthracycline inhibits contractile protein synthesis,[179] thus reducing the amount of compensatory dilatation and remodeling. In this situation the only option available for sta-

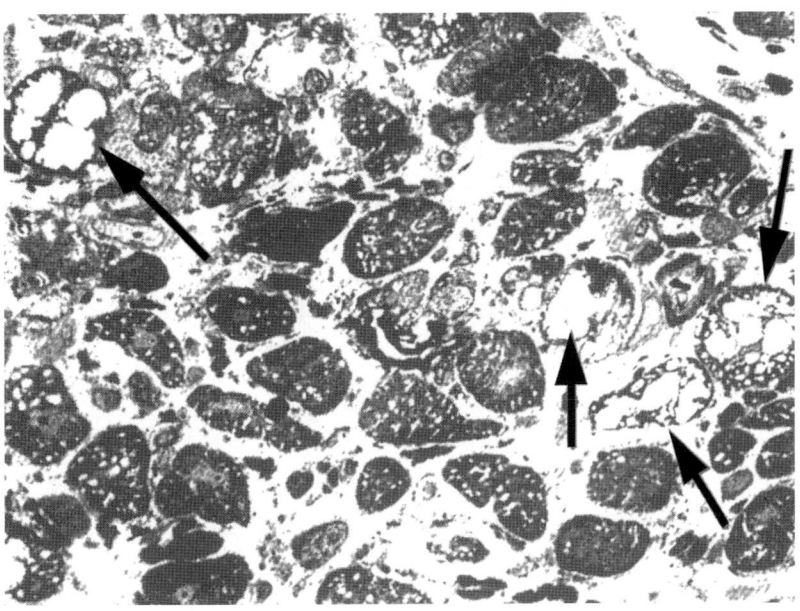

FIGURE 29-5. Cardiac myocyte vacuolization in cases of Adriamycin cardiomyopathy classified on endomyocardial biopsy as grade 3 by the Billingham classification.[174,175,184]

bilizing cardiac output is increasing the heart rate, because increasing stroke volume via a larger end-diastolic volume (ESV) has been precluded. The increased heart rate is produced by a greater than expected hyperadrenergic state; therefore these subjects may be exceptionally dependent on adrenergic support.

Prognosis

The prognosis of anthracycline cardiomyopathy is poor[100] and depends on numerous factors, including the age and underlying prechemotherapy cardiac status of the patient and the time of presentation relative to the last dose of drug. Subjects who present late (several months) or very late (years) after the last dose have a better prognosis because the anthracycline myocardial effect takes at least 60 days to become fully manifest.[180] That is, subjects who develop heart failure within a few days of the last dose of drug have an additional cardiomyopathic burden to face, because the last one to two doses produce their full morphologic effect over the next 1 to 2 months.

Treatment/Prevention

Subjects who develop anthracycline cardiomyopathy should be aggressively treated with conventional heart failure treatment, because some degree of reversibility is likely. Conventional treatment consists of ACE inhibitors, digoxin, and diuretics. β-Adrenergic blockade, in particular carvedilol,[181] has a beneficial effect and has been used successfully in some subjects[182,183]; but because of the high adrenergic drive, it may be difficult to administer. Conversely, the heightened adrenergic mechanism may produce a commensurate amount of adverse effect on the myocardium, so the potential for a favorable response may be even greater than in other kinds of cardiomyopathy. In severe refractory cases, cardiac transplantation may be performed provided that the patient's cancer is in complete remission and is not likely to recur (approximately 70 percent chance of cure).

Several strategies have been shown to lower the risk of developing anthracycline cardiomyopathy without compromising the che-

motherapy response rate. These include using endomyocardial biopsy and right-sided catheterization with exercise to assess risk, which virtually eliminates clinical cardiomyopathy and allows more anthracycline to be administered to less susceptible subjects[184]; using serial cardiac imaging techniques such as radionuclide angiography with[185] or without[186] exercise as a monitoring strategy, which may be somewhat helpful but because of a low specificity reduces the total amount of chemotherapy that can safely be administered to some subjects[184,185]; giving the agents at low doses weekly[187] or as 48- to 72-hour infusions[188] rather than as boluses every 3 to 4 weeks; using a liposomal formulation[189]; or concomitantly administering a second agent that reduces toxicity.[190] Unfortunately, none of these strategies completely eliminates the risk of developing a clinical cardiomyopathy. Recent studies have shown the potential benefit of cardioprotective agents, scavengers of free radicals produced by anthracycline, when administered in conjunction with the anthracycline therapy.[191]

【 】 POSTPARTUM CARDIOMYOPATHY

Definition/Diagnosis

Postpartum or *peripartum cardiomyopathy* is defined as the presentation of systolic dysfunction and clinical heart failure during the last trimester of pregnancy or within 6 months of delivery.[192] Given the extreme hemodynamic load produced by pregnancy, it is perhaps surprising that postpartum cardiomyopathy is not more common.

Distinct Pathophysiology

Postpartum cardiomyopathy will most likely be classified within the *dilated* WHO/ISFC category, but occasionally dilatation and remodeling have not had time to occur. Postpartum cardiomyopathy is likely a heterogeneous group of disorders, consisting of the addition of the hemodynamic load of pregnancy to a variety of underlying myocardial processes including hypertension, genetic factors, viral and autoimmune myocarditis, stress activated cytokines, increased myocyte apoptosis, and excessive prolactin production.[193]

Prognosis

Postpartum cardiomyopathy has a better prognosis than other causes of dilated cardiomyopathy.[100] Up to half of subjects who develop postpartum cardiomyopathy will recover completely,[194,195] and most of the rest will improve. Subjects who have developed a postpartum cardiomyopathy should receive appropriate family-planning counseling and should never become pregnant again, even if myocardial function has recovered fully.[193,196]

Treatment

Treatment should be aggressive, as for idiopathic dilated cardiomyopathy. Cardiac transplantation may be required in severely compromised patients who do not improve.

ALCOHOL CARDIOMYOPATHY

Definition/Diagnosis

An *alcohol cardiomyopathy* is said to be present when other causes of a dilated cardiomyopathy have been excluded and there is a history of heavy, sustained alcohol intake. The requirement in terms of alcohol amount is 80 g of alcohol per day for males and 40 g for females,[197] typically over several years. However, in susceptible individuals it is likely that lower amounts of intake can produce a cardiomyopathy. The histologic features of alcohol cardiomyopathy are nonspecific and do not differ from DCM. Other than history the only potentially distinguishing feature between DCM and alcohol cardiomyopathy is that the latter may present with a relatively high cardiac output.

Distinct Pathophysiology

The pathophysiology of alcohol cardiomyopathy is thought to be related to the toxic effects of alcohol, plus, in some subjects, nutritional components such as thiamine deficiency. Genetic factors may predispose to alcoholic cardiomyopathy, like the ACE DD polymorphism.[198]

Prognosis

The prognosis depends on the degree of impairment of myocardial function and the extent of abstinence from alcohol and, in an extremely compromised patient, the administration of thiamine. There is evidence that the prognosis is somewhat better for alcohol cardiomyopathy than for DCM.[199]

Treatment

The treatment of alcohol cardiomyopathy does not differ from that of DCM except for the need for total abstinence from alcohol. Obviously, these subjects are not good candidates for cardiac transplantation because of their high relapse rate to alcoholism.

CHAGAS CARDIOMYOPATHY

Definition/Diagnosis

Chagas disease is discussed in Chap. 32 as a cause of myocarditis. In addition, Chagas disease is the most common cause of nonischemic cardiomyopathy in South and Central America, with over 10 million people affected.[200] It is caused by a parasite, the leishmanial or tissue form of the protozoan *Trypanosoma cruzi*. Although in the United States the vector (*Triatoma*, or kissing bug) is found only in the Southwest, Chagas disease may be transmitted by blood transfusions; as a result it could become relatively more important in this country. The natural history consists of an initial myocarditis most commonly presenting in childhood, associated with acute myocardial infection followed by recovery, and, in some individuals, the development of a dilated cardiomyopathy 10 to 30 years later.

The diagnosis of Chagas cardiomyopathy is based on clinical (history, LV functional, and electrocardiographic) criteria and a positive serologic test for *T.*

cruzi.[201] Electrocardiographic abnormalities consist of bundle branch or hemiblocks (indeed, hemiblocks were first described by Rosenbaum and coworkers[202] in Chagas afflicted hearts with discrete foci of involvement), LV hypertrophy, and first- or second-degree atrioventricular block.[203,204] Recently, Doppler tissue imaging has been presented as a more sensitive technique for the study of diastolic function in Chagas disease than conventional Doppler echocardiography.[204,205] The histologic lesion of chronic Chagas consists of mononuclear infiltrates, fibrosis, and, as shown in Fig. 29–6, foci of the leishmanial form of *T. cruzi* in myocardial fibers. The LV functional abnormalities may initially be segmental and may include an apical aneurysm; later they become more global.[201,203]

Distinct Pathophysiology

The basis for Chagas cardiomyopathy is unknown but may be immunologic, whereby antibodies generated against *T. cruzi* crossreact with cardiac myocyte antigens including myosin.[206]

Prognosis

The prognosis is relatively good for a dilated cardiomyopathy and similar to that for DCM; the 5-year survival in Chagas cardiomyopathy with heart failure is approximately 50 percent.[207] Compared to DCM, death likely occurs more commonly caused by an arrhythmic mechanism.[201] However, as for DCM and most other dilated cardiomyopathies, mortality risk depends directly on the degrees of ventricular dysfunction and exercise intolerance.[201]

Treatment

There is no definitive treatment for Chagas cardiomyopathy; nonspecific treatment includes pacemaker implantation for heart block and heart failure treatment as for DCM. Verapamil has been recently demonstrated to attenuate the extent of myocardial injury in murine models of chronic *T. cruzi* infection.[208] Also, amiodarone seems particularly effective in treating arrhythmias associated with Chagas car-

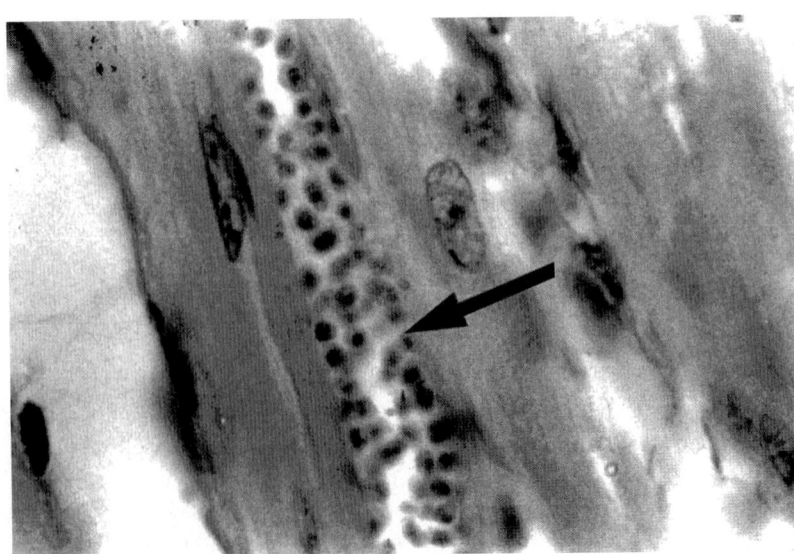

FIGURE 29–6. Leishmanial forms of *T. cruzi* within the swollen cytoplasm of a cardiac myocyte (Chagas cardiomyopathy; H&E stain, ×250). *Source: Courtesy of Dr. Elmer Koneman.*

diomyopathy; in one study it reduced mortality compared to standard treatment.[209] The role of cardiac transplantation is still somewhat uncertain; but it can be done at acceptable risk,[210] especially when coupled with trypanocidal agents.[211,212]

SUMMARY

Dilated cardiomyopathies are important because they are the most common cause of heart failure, which is the single most costly medical problem in the adult U.S. population. Cardiomyopathies in general are a heterogeneous group of diseases, but they can be classified under the WHO/ISFC and the newer AHA classification system, which although imperfect should be of great value in standardizing the terminology and encouraging systematic investigative and clinical approaches to diagnosis and treatment. Within this classification system, primary and secondary dilated cardiomyopathies comprise the single largest and most important group. Current diagnosis and treatment of dilated cardiomyopathies varies somewhat among the various types, but the cornerstones of medical management are similar in most cases.

Genetic causes and influences on the natural history of dilated cardiomyopathies are the new frontier in this field, and their elucidation is almost certain to lead to new therapeutic and diagnostic approaches. In the near future, molecular genetic testing will be routinely done for many cardiomyopathies that may have a single gene defect as the cause. As we learn more about the influence of polymorphic genetic variation on the natural history and selection of specific medical therapy, genetic testing will be performed in most patients with cardiomyopathies.

REFERENCES

1. Ho KKL, Anderson KM, Kannel WB, Grossman W, Levy D. Survival after the onset of congestive heart failure in Framingham Heart Study subjects. *Circulation* 1993;88:107–115.
2. O'Connell JB, Bristow MR. Economic impact of heart failure in the United States: time for a different approach. *J Heart Lung Transplant* 1994;13:S107–S112.
3. Mann DL, Bristow MR. Mechanisms and models in heart failure: the biomedical model and beyond. *Circulation* 2005;111:2837–2849.
4. Maron BJ, Towbin JA, Thiene G, et al. Contemporary definitions and classification of the cardiomyopathies. *Circulation* 2006;113:1807–1816.
5. Association AH. *Heart Disease and Stroke Statistics: 2005 Update.* Dallas, Texas: American Heart Association; 2005.
6. World Health Organization/International Society and Federation of Cardiology. Report of the 1995 World Health Organization/International Society and Federation of Cardiology Task Force on the Definition and Classification of Cardiomyopathies. *Circulation* 1996;93:841–842.
7. Mestroni L, Maisch B, McKenna WJ, et al. Guidelines for the study of familial dilated cardiomyopathies. *Eur Heart J* 1999;20:93–102.
8. Cohn JN, Johnson GR, Shabetai R, et al. Ejection fraction, peak exercise oxygen consumption, cardiothoracic ratio, ventricular arrhythmias, and plasma norepinephrine as determinants of prognosis in heart failure. *Circulation* 1993;87(suppl VI)]:VI5–VI16.
9. Eichhorn EJ, Bristow MR. Medical therapy can improve the biologic properties of the chronically failing heart: a new era in the treatment of heart failure. *Circulation* 1996;94:2285–2296.
10. Bristow MR, Anderson FL, Port JD, et al. Differences in β-adrenergic neuroeffector mechanisms in ischemic versus idiopathic dilated cardiomyopathy. *Circulation* 1991;84:1024–1039.
11. Packer M, Bristow MR, Cohn JN, et al. The effect of carvedilol on morbidity and mortality in patients with chronic heart failure. U.S. Carvedilol Heart Failure Study Group. *N Engl J Med* 1996;334:1349–1355.
12. Bristow MR. β-Adrenergic receptor blockade in chronic heart failure. *Circulation* 2000;101:558–569.
13. Bristow MR. Why does the myocardium fail? New insights from basic science. *Lancet* 1998;352 (suppl):8–14.
14. Fatkin D, MacRae C, Sasaki T, et al. Missense mutations in the rod domain of the lamin A/C gene as causes of dilated cardiomyopathy and conduction-system disease. *N Engl J Med* 1999;341:1715–24.
15. Brodsky GL, Muntoni F, Miocic S, Sinagra G, Sewry C, Mestroni L. A lamin A/C gene mutation associated with dilated cardiomyopathy with variable skeletal muscle involvement. *Circulation* 2000;101:473–476.
16. Carniel E, Taylor MRG, Sinagra G, et al. α-Myosin heavy chain: a sarcomeric gene associated with dilated and hypertrophic phenotypes. *Circulation* 2005;112:54–59.
17. Tiret L, Rigat B, Visvikis S, et al. Evidence, from combined segregation and linkage analysis, that a variant of the angiotensin I-converting enzyme (ACE) gene controls plasma ACE levels. *Am J Hum Genet* 1992;51:197–205.
18. Raynolds MV, Bristow MR, Bush EW, et al. Angiotensin-converting enzyme DD genotype in patients with ischaemic or idiopathic cardiomyopathy. *Lancet* 1993;342:1073–1075.
19. McNamara DM, Holubkov R, Janosko K, et al. Pharmacogenetic interactions between beta-blocker therapy and the angiotensin-converting enzyme deletion polymorphism in patients with congestive heart failure. *Circulation* 2001;103:1644–1648.
20. Liggett SB, Wagoner LE, Craft LL, et al. The Ile164 beta2-adrenergic receptor polymorphism adversely affects the outcome of congestive heart failure. *J Clin Invest* 1998;102:1534–1539.
21. Small KM, Wagoner LE, Levin AM, Kardia SLR, Liggett SB. Synergistic polymorphism of b_1- and a_{2C}-adrenergic receptors and the risk of congestive heart failure. *N Engl J Med* 2002;347:1135–1142.
22. Taylor MR, Bristow MR. The emerging pharmacogenomics of the beta-adrenergic receptors. *Congest Heart Fail* 2004;10:281–288.
23. Liggett SB, Mialet-Perez J, Thaneemit-Chen S, et al. A polymorphism within a conserved beta(1)-adrenergic receptor motif alters cardiac function and beta-blocker response in human heart failure. *Proc Natl Acad Sci U S A* 2006;103:11288–11293.
24. Charron P, Tesson F, Poirier O, et al. Identification of a genetic risk factor for idiopathic dilated cardiomyopathy: involvement of a polymorphism in the endothelin receptor type A gene—CARDIGENE group. *Eur Heart J* 1999;20:1587–1591.
25. Ross JJ. Dilated cardiomyopathy: concepts derived from gene deficient and transgenic animal models. *Circ J* 2002;66:219–224.
26. Vikstrom KL, Facxtor SM, Leinwand LA. Mice expressing mutant myosin heavy chains are model for familial hypertrophic cardiomyopathy. *Mol Med Today* 1996;2:556–567.
27. Geisterfer-Lawrence AA, Christe M, Conner DA, Ingwall JS, Seidman CE, Seidman JG. A mouse model of familial hypertrophic cardiomyopathy. *Science* 1996;272:731–735.
28. Edwards JG, Lyons GE, Micales BK, Malhotra A, Factor S, Leinwand LA. Cardiomyopathy in transgenic myf5 mice. *Circ Res* 1996;78:379–387.
29. Arber S, Hunter JJ, Ross JJ, et al. MLP-deficient mouse exhibit a disruption of cardiac cytoarchitectural organization, dilated cardiomyopathy and heart failure. *Cell* 1997;88:393–403.
30. Iwase M, Uechi M, Vatner DE, Asai K, Shannon RP, Kudej RK. Dilated cardiomyopathy induced by cardiac Gs-alpha overexpression. *Circulation* 1996;94:I–16.
31. Hein L, Altman JD, Kobilka KB. Two functionally distinct a2-adrenergic receptors regulate sympathetic neurotransmission. *Nature* 1999;402:181–184.
32. Bisognano JD, Weinberger HD, Knudson OA, et al. Myocardial directed over-expressing the human beta(1)-adrenergic receptor in transgenic mice. *J Mol Cell Cardiol* 2000;32:817–830.
33. Engelhardt S, Hein L, Wiesman F, Lohse MJ. Progressive hypertrophy and heart failure in b1-adrenergic receptor transgenic mice. *Proc Natl Acad Sci U S A* 1999;96:7059–7064.
34. Liggett SB, Tepe NM, Lorenz JN, et al. Early and delayed consequences of $β_2$-adrenergic receptor overexpression in mouse hearts: critical role for expression level. *Circulation* 2000;101:1707–1714.
35. Antos CL, Frey N, Marx SO, et al. Dilated cardiomyopathy and sudden death resulting from constitutive activation of protein kinase A. *Circ Res* 2001;89:997–1004.
36. Geng Y-J, Ishikawa Y, Vatner DE, et al. Apoptosis of cardiac myocytes in Gs alpha transgenic mice. *Circ Res* 1999;84:34–42.
37. Nicol RL, Frey N, Pearson G, Cobb M, Richardson J, Olson EN. Activated MEK5 induces serial assembly of sarcomeres and eccentric cardiac hypertrophy. *EMBO J* 2001;20:2757–2767.
38. Passier R, Zeng H, Frey N, et al. CaM kinase signaling induces cardiac hypertrophy and activates the MEF2 transcription factor in vivo. *J Clin Invest* 2000;105:1395–1406.

39. Molkentin JD, Lu JR, Antos CL, et al. A calcineurin-dependent transcriptional pathway for cardiac hypertrophy. *Cell* 1998;93:215–228.

40. Cho MC, Rapacciuolo A, Koch WJ, Kobayashi Y, Jones LR, Rockman HA. Defective beta-adrenergic receptor signaling precedes the development of dilated cardiomyopathy in transgenic mice with calsequestrin overexpression. *J Biol Chem* 1999;274:22251–22256.

41. Li H, Wang J, Wilhelmsson H, et al. Genetic modification of survival in tissue-specific knockout mice with mitochondrial cardiomyopathy. *Proc Natl Acad Sci U S A* 2000;97:3467–3472.

42. Hunter JJ, Tanaka N, Rockman HA, Ross J, Chien KR. Ventricular expression of a MLC-2v-ras fusion gene induces cardiac hypertrophy and selective diastolic dysfunction in transgenic mice. *J Biol Chem* 1995;270:23173–23178.

43. Robbins RJ, Swain JL. C-myc protooncogene modulates cardiac hypertrophic growth in transgenic mice. *Am J Physiol* 1992;62:H590–H597.

44. Milano CA, Dolber PC, Rockman HA, Bond RA, Venable ME, Allen LF. Myocardial expression of a constitutively active a_{1B}-adrenergic receptor in transgenic mice induces cardiac hypertrophy. *Proc Natl Acad Sci U S A* 1994;91:10109–10113.

45. D'Angelo DD, Sakata Y, Lorenz JN, et al. Transgenic G_{aq} overexpression induces cardiac contractile failure in mice. *Proc Natl Acad Sci U S A* 1997;94:8121–8126.

46. Wakasaki H, Koya D, Schoen FJ, et al. Targeted overexpression of protein kinase C beta2 isoform in myocardium causes cardiomyopathy. *Proc Natl Acad Sci U S A* 1997;94:9320–9325.

47. Towbin JA, Hejtmancik F, Brink P, et al. X-linked cardiomyopathy (XLCM): molecular genetic evidence of linkage to the Duchenne muscular dystrophy (dystrophin) gene at the Xp21 locus. *Circulation* 1993;87:1854–1865.

48. Muntoni F, Cau M, Ganau A, et al. Deletion of the dystrophin muscle-promoter region associated with X-linked dilated cardiomyopathy. *N Engl J Med* 1993;329:921–925.

49. Kamisago M, Sharma SD, DePalma SR, et al. Mutations in sarcomere protein genes as a cause of dilated cardiomyopathy. *N Engl J Med* 2000;343:1688–1696.

50. McNair WP, Ku L, Taylor MRG, et al. A SCN5A mutation associated with dilated cardiomyopathy, conduction disorder and arrhythmia. *Circulation* 2004;110:2163–2167.

51. Olson TM, Michels VV, Ballew JD, et al. Sodium channel mutations and susceptibility to heart failure and atrial fibrillation. *JAMA* 2005;293:447–454.

52. Norgett EE, Hatsell SJ, Carvajal-Huerta L, et al. Recessive mutations in desmoplakin disrupts desmoplakin-intermediate filament interactions and causes dilated cardiomyopathy, woolly hair and keratoderma. *Hum Genet* 2000;9:2761–2666.

53. Schönberger J, Wang L, Shin JT, et al. Mutations in the transcriptional coactivator *EYA4* causes dilated cardiomyopathy and sensorineural hearing loss. *Nat Genet* 2005;37:418–422.

54. Schmitt JP, Kamisago M, Asahi M, et al. Dilated cardiomyopathy and heart failure caused by a mutation in phospholamban. *Science* 2003;299:1410–1413.

55. Nigro V, Okazaki Y, Belsito A, et al. Identification of the Syrian Hamster cardiomyopathy gene. *Hum Mol Genet* 1997;6:601–607.

56. Biesiadecki BJ, Jin JP. Exon skipping in cardiac troponin T of turkeys with inherited cardiomyopathy. *J Biol Chem* 2002;277:18459–18468.

57. Lander E, Kruglyak L. Genetic dissection of complex traits: guidelines for interpreting and reporting linkage results. *Nat Genet* 1995;11:241–247.

58. Jan Danser AH, Maarten ADH, Schalekamp MD, et al. Angiotensin-converting enzyme in the human heart: effect of the deletion/insertion polymorphism. *Circulation* 1995;92:1387–1388.

59. Pinto YM, van Gilst WH, Kingma JH, Schunkert H, for the Captopril Thrombolysis Study Investigators. Deletion-type allele of the angiotensin-converting enzyme gene is associated with progressive ventricular dilatation after anterior myocardial infarction. *J Am Coll Cardiol* 1995;25:1622–1626.

60. Bonnardeaux A, Davies E, Jeunemaitre X, et al. Angiotensin II type 1 receptor gene polymorphisms in human essential hypertension. *Hypertension* 1994;24:63–69.

61. Lowes BD, Minobe WA, Abraham WT, et al. Changes in gene expression in the intact human heart: down-regulation of a-myosin heavy chain in hypertrophied, failing ventricular myocardium. *J Clin Invest* 1997;100:2315–2324.

62. Miyata S, Minobe WA, Bristow MR, Leinwand LA. Myosin isoform expression in the failing and nonfailing human heart. *Circ Res* 2000;86:386–390.

63. Mercadier JJ, Lompre AM, Duc P, et al. Altered sarcoplasmic reticulum Ca-ATPase gene expression in the human ventricle during end-stage heart failure. *J Clin Invest* 1990;85:305–309.

64. Feldman AM, Ray PE, Silan CM, Mercer JA, Minobe WA, Bristow MR. Selective gene expression in failing human heart: quantification of steady-state levels of messenger RNA in endomyocardial biopsies using the polymerase chain reaction. *Circulation* 1991;83:1866–1872.

65. Studer R, Reinecke H, Muler B, Holtz J, Just H, Drexler H. Increased angiotensin-I converting enzyme gene expression in the failing human heart. Quantification by competitive RNA polymerase chain reaction. *J Clin Invest* 1994;94:301–310.

66. Zisman LS, Asano K, Dutcher DL, et al. Differential regulation of cardiac angiotensin converting enzyme binding sites and AT1 receptor density in the failing human heart. *Circulation* 1998;98:1735–1741.

67. Torre-Amione G, Kapadia S, Lee J, et al. Tumor necrosis factor-a and tumor necrosis factor receptors in the failing human heart. *Circulation* 1996;93:704–711.

68. Zolk O, Quattek J, Sitzler G, et al. Expression of endothelin-1 endothelin-converting enzyme, and endothelin receptors in chronic heart failure. *Circulation* 1999;99:2118–23.

69. Ungerer M, Böhm M, Elce JS, Erdmann E, Lohse MJ. Altered expression of β-adrenergic receptor kinase and $β_1$-adrenergic receptors in the failing human heart. *Circulation* 1993;87:454–463.

70. Lowes BD, Gilbert EM, Abraham WT, et al. Myocardial gene expression in dilated cardiomyopathy treated with beta-blocking agents. *N Engl J Med* 2002;346:1357–1365.

71. Bristow MR, Gilbert EM. Improvement in cardiac myocyte function by biologic effects of medical therapy: a new concept in the treatment of heart failure. *Eur Heart J* 1995;16(suppl F):20–31.

72. Ross J, Braunwald E. Studies on Starling's Law of the Heart IX: the effects of impeding venous return on performance of the normal and failing ventricle. *Circulation* 1964;30:719–727.

73. Holubarsch C, Thorsten R, Goldstein DJ, et al. Existence of the Frank-Starling mechanism in the failing human heart: investigations on the organ, tissue, and sarcomere levels. *Circulation* 1996;94:683–689.

74. Muleiri LA, Hasenfuss G, Leavitt B, Allen PD, Alpert NR. Altered myocardial force-frequency relationship in the human heart failure. *Circulation* 1992;85:1743–1750.

75. Cohn JN. Structural basis for heart failure: ventricular remodeling and its pharmacological inhibition. *Circulation* 1995;91:2504–2507.

76. Vatta M, Stetson SJ, Perez-Verdia A, et al. Molecular remodelling of dystrophin in patients with end-stage cardiomyopathies and reversal in patients on assistance-device therapy. *Lancet* 2002;359:936–941.

77. Gerdes AM, Kellerman SE, Schocken DD. Implications of cardiomyocyte remodeling in heart dysfunction. In: Dhalla NS, RE Beamish, N Takeda, N Nagano, eds. *The Failing Heart.* New York: Raven Press; 1995:197–205.

78. Gerdes AM, Odera T, Wang X, McCune SA. Myocyte remodeling during progression to failure in rats with hypertension. *Hypertension* 1996;28:609–614.

79. Gerdes AM, Capasso JM. Structural remodeling and mechanical dysfunction of cardiac myocytes in heart failure. *J Mol Cell Cardiol* 1995;27:849–856.

80. Zhang J, McDonald KM. Bioenergetic consequences of left ventricular remodeling. *Circulation* 1995;92:1011–1019.

81. Sata M, Sugiura S, Yamashita H, Momomura S, Serizawa T. Coupling between myosin ATPase cycle and creatine kinase cycle facilitates cardiac actomyosin sliding in vitro: a clue to mechanical dysfunction during myocardial ischemia. *Circulation* 1996;93:310–317.

82. Binkley PF, Nunziata E, Haas GH, Nelson SD, Cody RJ. Parasympathetic withdrawal is an integral component of autonomic imbalance in congestive heart failure: demonstration in human subjects and verification in a paced canine model of ventricular failure. *J Am Coll Cardiol* 1991;18:464–472.

83. Mewes T, Dutz S, Ravens U, Jakobs KH. Activation of calcium currents in cardiac myocytes by empty β-adrenoceptors. *Circulation* 1993;88:2916–2922.

84. Milano CA, Allen LF, Rockman HA, et al. Enhanced myocardial function in transgenic mice overexpressing the $β_2$-adrenergic receptor. *Science* 1994;264:562–566.

85. Bond RA, Leff P, Johnson TD, et al. Physiological effects of inverse agonists in transgenic mice with myocardial overexpression of the $β_2$-adrenoceptor. *Nature* 1995;374:272–276.

86. Luo W, Grupp IL, Harrer J, et al. Targeted ablation of the phospholamban gene is associated with markedly enhanced myocardial contractility and loss of β-agonist stimulation. *Circ Res* 1994;75:401–409.

87. Narula J, Haider N, Virmani R, et al. Apoptosis in myocytes in end-stage heart failure. *N Engl J Med* 1996;335:1182–1189.

88. Teiger E, Than VD, Richard L, et al. Apoptosis in pressure overload-induced heart hypertrophy in the rat. *J Clin Invest* 1996;97:2891–2897.

89. Cohn JN, Levine TB, Olivari MT, et al. Plasma norepinephrine as a guide to prognosis in patients with chronic congestive heart failure. *N Engl J Med* 1984;311:819–823.

90. Kaye DM, Lefkovits J, Jennings GL, Bergin P, Broughton A, Esler D. Adverse consequences of high sympathetic nervous activity in the failing human heart. *J Am Coll Cardiol* 1995;26:1257–1263.

91. Swedberg K, Eneroth P, Kjekshus J, Wilhelmsen L. Hormones regulating cardiovascular function in patients with severe congestive heart failure and their relation to mortality. *Circulation* 1990;82:1730–1736.

92. Bristow MR, O'Connell JB, Mestroni L. Myocardial diseases. In: *Kelley's Textbook of Internal Medicine.* 4th ed. Philadelphia: Lippincott Williams and Wilkins; 2000:464–474.

93. Codd MB, Sugrue DD, Gersh BJ, Melton LJ. Epidemiology of idiopathic dilated and hypertrophic cardiomyopathy: a population-based study in Olmsted County, Minnesota, 1975–1984. *Circulation* 1989;80:564–572.

94. Rakar S, Sinagra G, Di Lenarda A, et al. Epidemiology of dilated cardiomyopathy: a prospective post-mortem study of 5252 necropsies. *Eur Heart J* 1997;18(1):117–123.

95. McKay RG, Pfeffer MA, Pasternak RC, et al. Left ventricular remodeling after myocardial infarction: a corollary to infarct expansion. *Circulation* 1986;74:693–702.

96. Mitchell GF, Lamas GA, Vaughan DE, Pfeffer MA. Left ventricular remodeling in the year after myocardial infarction: a quantitative analysis of contractile segment lengths and ventricular shape. *J Am Coll Cardiol* 1992;19:1136–1144.

97. Gerdes AM, Kellerman SE, Moore JA, et al. Structural remodeling of cardiac myocytes from patients with chronic ischemic heart disease. *Circulation* 1992;86:426–430.

98. Franciosa JA, Willen M, Ziesche S, Cohn JN. Survival in men with severe chronic left ventricular failure due to either coronary heart disease or idiopathic dilated cardiomyopathy. *Am J Cardiol* 1983;51:831–836.

99. Likoff MJ, Chandler SL, Kay HR. Clinical determinants of mortality in chronic congestive heart failure secondary to idiopathic dilated or to ischemic cardiomyopathy. *Am J Cardiol* 1987;59:634–638.

100. Felker GM, Thompson RE, Hare JM, et al. Underlying causes and long term survival in patients with initially unexplained cardiomyopathy. *N Engl J Med* 2000;342:1077–1084.

101. Hunt SA, Abraham WT, Chin MH, et al. ACC/AHA 2005 Guideline Update for the Diagnosis and Management of Chronic Heart Failure in the Adult. *Circulation* 2005;112:e154–e235.

102. Moss AJ, Zareba W, Hall WJ, et al, Multicenter Automatic Defibrillator Implantation Trial II Investigators. Prophylactic implantation of a defibrillator in patients with myocardial infarction and reduced ejection fraction. *N Engl J Med* 2002;346:877–883.

103. Jarcho JA. Biventricular pacing. *N Engl J Med* 2006;355:288–294.

104. Bristow MR, Saxon LA, Boehmer J, et al. Cardiac-resynchronization therapy with or without an implantable defibrillator in advanced chronic heart failure. *N Engl J Med* 2004;350:2140–2150.

105. Strickberger SA, Conti J, Daoud EG, et al. Patient selection for cardiac resynchronization therapy: from the Council on Clinical Cardiology Subcommittee on Electrocardiography and Arrhythmias and the Quality of Care and Outcomes Research Interdisciplinary Working Group, in collaboration with the Heart Rhythm Society. *Circulation* 2005;111:2146–2150.

106. Rathore SS, Curtis JP, Wang Y, Bristow MR, Krumholz HM. Association of serum digoxin concentration and outcomes in patients with heart failure. *JAMA* 2003;289:871–878.

107. Levy D, Larson MG, Vasan RS, Kannel WB, Ho KK. The progression from hypertension to congestive heart failure. *JAMA* 1996;275:1557–1562.

108. Quaife RA, Lynch D, Badesch DB, et al. Right ventricular phenotypic characteristics in subjects with primary pulmonary hypertension or idiopathic dilated cardiomyopathy. *J Card Fail* 1999;5:46–54.

109. Devereux RB, Roman MJ. Left ventricular hypertrophy in hypertension: stimuli, patterns, and consequences. *Hypertens Res* 1999;22:1–9.

110. Bristow MR. Mechanisms of development of heart failure in the hypertensive patient. *Cardiology* 1999;92:3–6.

111. Himmelmann A. Hypertension: an important precursor of heart failure. *Blood Press* 1999;8:253–260.

112. Grossman W. Cardiac hypertrophy: useful adaptation or pathologic process. *Am J Med* 1980;69:576–584.

113. Moreno PR, Jang IK, Block PC, Palacios IF. The role of percutaneous balloon valvuloplasty in patients with cardiogenic shock. *Am J Med* 1994;23:1071–1075.

114. Packer M, O'Conner CM, Ghali JK, et al. Effect of Amlodipine on morbidity and mortality in severe chronic heart failure. *N Engl J Med* 1996;335:1107–1114.

115. Scognamiglio R, Rahimtoola SH, Fasoli G, Nistri S, Dalla Volta S. Nifedipine in asymptomatic patients with severe aortic regurgitation and normal left ventricular function. *N Engl J Med* 1994;331:689–694.

116. Codd MB, Sugrue DD, Gersh BJ, Melton LJ. Epidemiology of idiopathic dilated and hypertrophic cardiomyopathy: a population based study in Olmstead County, MN 1975–1984. *Circulation* 1989;80:564–572.

117. Gregori D, Rocco C, Miocic S, Mestroni L. Estimating the frequency of familial dilated cardiomyopathy in the presence of misclassification errors. *J Appl Statistics* 2001;28:53–62.

118. Grünig E, Tasman JA, Kucherer H, Franz W, Kubler W, Katus HA. Frequency and phenotypes of familial dilated cardiomyopathy. *J Am Coll Cardiol* 1998;31:186–194.

119. Baig MK, Goldman JH, Caforio ALP, Coonar AS, Keeling PJ, McKenna WJ. Familial dilated cardiomyopathy: cardiac abnormalities are common in asymptomatic relatives and may represent early disease. *J Am Coll Cardiol* 1998;31:195–201.

120. Mestroni L, Rocco C, Gregori D, et al. Familial dilated cardiomyopathy: evidence for genetic and phenotypic heterogeneity. *J Am Coll Cardiol* 1999;34:181–190.

121. Muntoni F, Di Lenarda A, Porcu M, et al. Dystrophin gene abnormalities in two patients with idiopathic dilated cardiomyopathy. *Heart* 1997;78:608–612.

122. Milasin J, Muntoni F, Severini GM, et al. A point mutation in the 5 splice site of the dystrophin gene first intron responsible for X-linked dilated cardiomyopathy. *Hum Mol Genet* 1996;5:73–79.

123. Ortiz-Lopez R, Li H, Su J, Goytia V, Towbin JA. Evidence for a dystrophin missense mutation as a cause of X-linked dilated cardiomyopathy (XLCM). *Circulation* 1997;95:2434–2440.

124. Maeda M, Holder E, Lowes BD, Valent S, Bies RD. Dilated cardiomyopathy associated with deficiency of the cytoskeletal protein metavinculin. *Circulation* 1997;95:17–20.

125. Taylor MRG, Fain P, Sinagra G, et al. Natural history of dilated cardiomyopathy due to lamin A/C gene mutations. *J Am Coll Cardiol* 2003;41:771–780.

126. Arbustini E, Pilotto A, Repetto A, et al. Autosomal dominant dilated cardiomyopathy with atrioventricular block: a lamin A/C defect-related disease. *J Am Coll Cardiol* 2002;39:981–990.

127. Melacini P, Fanin M, Duggan DJ, et al. Heart involvement in muscular dystrophies due to sarcoglycan gene mutations. *Muscle Nerve* 1999;22:473–479.

128. Fatkin D, Christe ME, Aristizabal O, et al. Neonatal cardiomyopathy in mice homozygous for the Arg403Gln mutant in the α-cardiac myosin heavy chain gene. *J Clin Invest* 1999;103:147–153.

129. McConnell BK, Jones KA, Fatkin D, et al. Dilated cardiomyopathy in homozygous myosin-binding protein-C mutant mice. *J Clin Invest* 1999;104:1235–1244.

130. Olson TM, Michels VV, Thibodeau SN, Tai Y, Keating MT. Actin mutation in dilated cardiomyopathy, a heritable form of heart failure. *Science* 1998;280:750–752.

131. Gerull B, Gramlich M, Atherton J, et al. Mutations of TTN, encoding the giant muscle filament titin, cause familial dilated cardiomyopathy. *Nat Genet* 2002;30:201–204.

132. Daehmlow S, Erdmann J, Knueppel T, et al. Novel mutations in sarcomeric protein genes in dilated cardiomyopathy. *Biochem Biophys Res Commun* 2002;298:116–120.

133. Haghighi K, Kolokathis F, Gramolini AO, et al. A mutation in the human phospholamban gene, deleting arginine 14 results in lethal, hereditary cardiomyopathy. *Proc Natl Acad Sci U S A* 2006;103:1388–1393.

134. D'Adamo P, Fassone L, Gedeon A, et al. The X-linked gene G4.5 is responsible for different infantile dilated cardiomyopathies. *Am J Hum Genet* 1997;61:862–867.

135. Xu Y, Condell M, Plesken H, et al. A Drosophila model of Barth syndrome. *Proc Natl Acad Sci U S A* 2006;103:11584–11588.

136. Mariotti C, Tiranti V, Carrara F, Dallapiccola B, DiDonato S, Zeviani M. Defective respiratory capacity and mitochondrial protein synthesis in transformant cybrids harboring the tRNA(Leu(UUR)) mutation associated with maternally inherited myopathy and cardiomyopathy. *J Clin Invest* 1994;93:1102–1107.

137. Grasso M, Diegoli M, Brega A, Campana C, Tavazzi L, Arbustini E. The mitochondrial DNA mutation T12297C affects a highly conserved nucleotide of tRNA (Leu(CUN)) and is associated with dilated cardiomyopathy. *Eur J Hum Genet* 2001;9:311–315.

138. Bienengraeber M, Olson TM, Selivanon VA, et al. ABCC9 mutations identified in human dilated cardiomyopathy disrupt catalytic K_{ATP} channel gating. *Nat Genet* 2004;36:382–387.

139. Crispell KA, Wray A, Ni H, Nauman DJ, Hershberger RE. Clinical profiles of four large pedigrees with familial dilated cardiomyopathy: preliminary recommendations for clinical practice. *J Am Coll Cardiol* 1999;34:837–847.

140. Taylor MRG, Carniel E, Mestroni L. Cardiomyopathy, familial dilated. *Orphanet J Rare Dis* 2006;1:27.

141. Roberts WC, Siegel RJ, McManus BM. Idiopathic dilated cardiomyopathy: Analysis of 152 necropsy patients. *Am J Cardiol* 1987;60:1340–1355.

142. Falk RH, Foster E, Coats MH. Ventricular thrombi and thromboembolism in dilated cardiomyopathy. *Am Heart J* 1992;123:136–142.

143. Rowan R, Maesk MA, Billingham ME. Ultrastructural morphometric analysis of endomyocardial biopsies. *Am J Cardiovasc Pathol* 1988;2:137–144.

144. Baandrup U, Olsen EG. Critical analysis of endomyocardial biopsies from patients suspected of having cardiomyopathy. *Br Heart J* 1981;45:475–86.

145. Arbustini E, Pucci R, Pozzi R, Grasso M, Graziano G, Campani C. Ultrastructural changes in myocarditis and dilated cardiomyopathy. In: Baroldi G, F Camerini, JF Goodwin, eds. *Advances in Cardiomyopathies.* Berlin: Springer Verlag, 1990:274–289.

146. Schwarz F, Mall G, Zebe H, et al. Determinants of survival in patients with congestive cardiomyopathy: quantitative morphologic findings and left ventricular hemodynamics. *Circulation* 1984;70:923–928.

147. Hammond EH, Anderson JL, Menlove RL. Diagnostic and prognostic value of immunofluorescence and electron microscopic findings in idiopathic dilated cardiomyopathy. In: Baroldi G, F Camerini, JF Goodwin, eds. *Advances in Cardiomyopathies.* 1st ed. Berlin: Springer Verlag, 1990:290–301.

148. Caforio ALP, Keeling PJ, Zachara E, et al. Evidence from family studies for autoimmunity in dilated cardiomyopathy. *Lancet* 1994;344:773–777.

149. Kawai C, Takatsu T. Clinical and experimental studies on cardiomyopathy. *N Engl J Med* 1975;293:592–597.

150. Anderson JL, Carlquist JF, Hammond EH. Deficient natural killer cell activity in patients with idiopathic dilated cardiomyopathy. *Lancet* 1982;2:1124–1127.

151. Fowles RE, Bieker CP, Stinson EB. Defective in vitro suppressor cell function in idiopathic congestive cardiomyopathy. *Circulation* 1979;59:483–491.

152. Baba A, Yoshikawa T, Iwata M, et al. Antigen-specific effects of autoantibodies against sarcolemmal Na-K-ATPase pump in immunized cardiomyopathic rabbits. *Int J Cardiol* 2006;112:15–20.

153. Magnusson Y, Wallukat G, Waagstein F, Hjalmarson A, Hoebeke J. Autoimmunity in idiopathic dilated cardiomyopathy: characterization of antibodies against the beta 1-adrenoceptor with positive chronotropic effect. *Circulation* 1994;89:2760–2767.

154. Schultheiss HP. Disturbance of the myocardial energy metabolism in dilated cardiomyopathy due to autoimmunological mechanisms. *Circulation* 1993;87(suppl IV):43–48.

155. Carlquist JF, Menlove RL, Murray MB, O'Connell JB, Anderson JL. HLA class II (DR and DQ) antigen associations in idiopathic dilated cardiomyopathy: validation study and meta-analysis of published HLA association studies. *Circulation* 1991;83:515–522.

156. Gilbert EM, Mason JW. Immunosuppressive therapy of myocarditis. In: Engelmeier RS, JB O'Connell, eds. *Drug Therapy in Dilated Cardiomyopathy and Myocarditis.* New York: Marcel Dekker, 1987:233–263.

157. Bowles NE, Richardson PJ, Olsen ECJ, Archard LC. Detection of Coxsackie-B virus specific RNA sequences in myocardial biopsy samples from patients with myocarditis and dilated cardiomyopathy. *Lancet* 1986;1:1120–1128.

158. Giacca M, Severini GM, Mestroni L, et al. Low frequency of detection by nested polymerase chain reaction of enterovirus ribonucleic acid in endomyocardial tissue of patients with idiopathic dilated cardiomyopathy. *J Am Coll Cardiol* 1994;24:1033–1040.

159. Parrillo JE, Cunnion RE, Epstein SE, et al. A prospective, randomized, controlled trial of prednisone for dilated cardiomyopathy. *N Engl J Med* 1989;321:1061–1067.

160. Badorff C, Lee GH, Lamphear BJ, et al. Enteroviral protease 2A cleaves dystrophin: evidence of cytoskeletal disruption in an acquired cardiomyopathy. *Nat Med* 1999;5:320–326.

161. Martin AB, Webber S, Fricker FJ, et al. Acute myocarditis: rapid diagnosis by PCR in children. *Circulation* 1994;90:330–339.

162. Pauschinger M, Doerner A, Kuehl U, et al. Enteroviral RNA replication in the myocardium of patients with left ventricular dysfunction and clinically suspected myocarditis. *Circulation* 1999;99:889–895.

163. Fuster V, Gersh BJ, Giuliani ER, Tajik AJ, Brandenburg RO, Frye RL. The natural history of idiopathic dilated cardiomyopathy. *Am J Cardiol* 1981;47:525–531.

164. Redfield MM, Gersh BJ, Bailey KR, Ballard DJ, Rodeheffer RJ. Natural history of idiopathic dilated cardiomyopathy: effect of referral bias and secular trend. *J Am Coll Cardiol* 1993;22:1921–1926.

165. The SOLVD Investigators. Effect of angiotensin converting enzyme inhibition with enalapril on survival in patients with reduced left ventricular ejection fraction and congestive heart failure: Results of the treatment trial of the Studies of Left Ventricular Dysfunction (SOLVD)—a randomized double blind trial. *N Engl J Med* 1991;325:293–302.

166. Bardy GH, Lee KL, Mark DB, et al. Amiodarone or an implantable cardioverter-defibrillator for congestive heart failure. *N Engl J Med* 2005;352:225–237.

167. Deng MC, De Meester JM, Smits JM, Heinecke J, Scheld HH. Effect of receiving a heart transplant: analysis of a national cohort entered on to a waiting list, stratified by heart failure severity. *Br Med J* 2000;321:540–545.

168. Hosenpud JD, Novick RJ, Bennett LE, Keck BM, Fiol B, Daily OP. The registry of the International Society for Heart and Lung Transplantation: thirteenth official report—1996. *J Heart Lung Transplant* 1996;15:655–674.

169. Perrot A, Sigusch HH, Nagele H, et al. Genetic and phenotypic analysis of dilated cardiomyopathy with conduction system disease: demand for strategies in the management of presymptomatic lamin A/C mutant carriers. *Eur J Heart Fail* 2006;8:484–93.

170. van Berlo JH, de Voogt WG, van der Kooi AJ, et al. Meta-analysis of clinical characteristics of 299 carriers of LMNA gene mutations: do lamin A/C mutations portend a high risk of sudden death? *J Mol Med* 2005;83:79–83.

171. Woodley SL, Gilbert EM, Anderson JL, et al. β-Blockade with bucindolol in heart failure due to ischemic vs idiopathic dilated cardiomyopathy. *Circulation* 1991;84:2426–2441.

172. Waagstein F, Bristow MR, Swedberg K, et al. Beneficial effects of metoprolol in idiopathic dilated cardiomyopathy: Metoprolol in Dilated Cardiomyopathy (MDC) Trial Study Group. *Lancet* 1993;342:1441–1446.

173. Bristow MR, Mason JW, Billingham ME, Daniels JR. Doxorubicin cardiomyopathy: evaluation by phonocardiography, endomyocardial biopsy, and cardiac catheterization. *Ann Intern Med* 1978;88:168–175.

174. Bristow MR, Mason JW, Billingham ME, Daniels JR. Dose-effect and structure function relationships in doxorubicin cardiomyopathy. *Am Heart J* 1981;102:709–718.

175. Bristow MR, Billingham ME, Mason JW, Daniels JR. The clinical spectrum of anthracycline antibiotic cardiotoxicity. *Cancer Treat Rep* 1978;62:873–879.

176. Kantrowitz NE, Bristow MR. Cardiotoxicity of antitumor agents. *Prog Cardiovasc Dis* 1984;27:195–200.

177. Von Hoff DD, Layard MW, Basa P, et al. Risk factors for doxorubicin-induced congestive heart failure. *Ann Intern Med* 1979;91:710–717.

178. Billingham ME, Bristow MR, Glatstein J, Mason JW, Masek MA, Daniels JR. Adriamycin cardiotoxicity endomyocardial biopsy evidence of enhancement by irradiation. *Am J Surg Path* 1977;1:17–23.

179. Lewis W, Kleinerman J, Puszkin S. Interaction of Adriamycin in vitro with myofibrillar proteins. *Circ Res* 1982;50:547–553.

180. Jaenke RS. Delayed and progressive myocardial lesions after Adriamycin administration in rabbits. *Cancer* 1976;36:2958–2966.

181. Armstrong SC. Anti-oxidants and apoptosis: attenuation of doxorubicin induced cardiomyopathy by carvedilol. *J Mol Cell Cardiol* 2004;37:817–821.

182. Shaddy RE, Olsen SL, Bristow MR, et al. Efficacy and safety of metoprolol in the treatment of doxorubicin-induced cardiomyopathy in pediatric patients. *Am Heart J* 1995;129:197–199.

183. Shaddy RE, Tani LY, Gidding SS, et al. Beta-blocker treatment of dilated cardiomyopathy with congestive heart failure in children: a multi-institutional experience. *J Heart Lung Transplant* 1999;18:269–274.

184. Bristow MR, Lopez MB, Mason JW, Billingham ME, Winchester MA. Efficacy and cost of cardiac monitoring in patients receiving doxorubicin. *Cancer* 1982;50:32–41.

185. McKillop JH, Bristow MR, Goris ML, Billingham ME, Bockemuehl K. Sensitivity and specificity of radionuclide ejection fractions in doxorubicin cardiotoxicity. *Am Heart J* 1983;105:1048–1056.

186. Alexander J, Dainiak N, Berger HJ, et al. Serial assessment of doxorubicin cardiotoxicity with quantitative radionuclide angiocardiography. *N Engl J Med* 1979;300:278–283.

187. Torti FM, Bristow MR, Howes AE, et al. Endomyocardial biopsy evidence of reduced cardiotoxicity of doxorubicin delivered on a weekly schedule. *Ann Intern Med* 1983;99:745–749.

188. Legha SS, Benjamin RS, Mackay B, et al. Reduction of doxorubicin cardiotoxicity by prolonged continuous intravenous infusion. *Ann Intern Med* 1982;96:133–139.

189. Rahman A, More N, Schein PS. Doxorubicin-induced chronic cardiotoxicity and its prevention by liposomal administration. *Cancer* 1982;42:1817–1825.

190. Speyer JL, Green MD, Kramer E, et al. Protective effect of the bispiperazinedione ICRF-187 against doxorubicin-induced cardiac toxicity in women with advanced breast cancer. *N Engl J Med* 1988;319:745–752.

191. Iarussi D, Indolfi P, Casale F, Coppolino P, Tedesco MA, DiTullio MT. Recent advances in the prevention of anthracycline cardiotoxicity in childhood. *Curr Med Chem* November 2001;8(13):1649–1660. Review.

192. Pearson GD, Veille JC, Rahimtoola S, et al. Peripartum cardiomyopathy: National Heart, Lung, and Blood Institute and Office of Rare Diseases (National Institutes of Health) workshop recommendations and review. *JAMA* 2000;283:1183–1188.

193. Sliwa K, Fett J, Elkayam U. Peripartum cardiomyopathy. *Lancet* 2006;368:687–693.
194. O'Connell JB, Costanzo-Nordin MR, Subramanian R, et al. Peripartum cardiomyopathy: clinical, hemodynamic histologic and prognostic characteristics. *J Am Coll Cardiol* 1986;8:52–56.
195. Fett JD, Christie LG, Carraway RD, Murphy JG. Five-year prospective study of the incidence and prognosis of peripartum cardiomyopathy at a single institution. *Mayo Clin Proc* 2005;80:1602–1606.
196. Elkayam U, Tummala PP, Rao K, et al. Maternal and fetal outcomes of subsequent pregnancies in women with peripartum cardiomyopathy. *N Engl J Med* 2001;344:1567–1571.
197. Maisch B. Alcohol and the heart. *Herz* 1996;21:207–212.
198. Fernandez-Sola J, Nicolas JM, Oriola J, et al. Angiotensin-converting enzyme gene polymorphism is associated with vulnerability to alcoholic cardiomyopathy. *Ann Intern Med* 2002;137:321–326.
199. Prazak P, Pfisterer M, Osswald S, Buser P, Burkart F. Differences of disease progression in congestive heart failure due to alcoholic as compared to idiopathic dilated cardiomyopathy. *Eur Heart J* 1996;17:251–257.
200. World Health Organization Expert Committee. Chagas' disease. *World Health Organ Tech Rep Ser* 1984:50–55.
201. Mady C, Cardoso RHA, Barretto ACP, da Luz PL, Bellotti G, Pileggi F. Survival and predictors of survival in patients with congestive heart failure due to Chagas' cardiomyopathy. *Circulation* 1994;90:3098–3102.
202. Rosenbaum MB. The hemiblocks: diagnostic criteria and clinical significance. *Mod Concepts Cardiovasc Dis* 1970;39:141–146.
203. Laranja FS, Dias E, Nobrega G, Miranda A. Chagas' disease: a clinical, epidemiological, and pathological study. *Circulation* 1956;14:1035–1060.
204. Barros MV, Rocha MO, Ribeiro AL, Machado FS. Doppler tissue imaging to evaluate early myocardium damage in patients with undetermined form of Chagas' disease and normal echocardiogram. *Echocardiography* 2001;18:131–136.
205. Barros MV, Rocha MO, Ribeiro AL, Machado FS. Tissue Doppler imaging in the evaluation of the regional diastolic function in Chagas' disease. *J Am Soc Echocardiogr* 2001;14:353–359.
206. Tibbetts RS, McCormick TS, Rowland EC, Miller SD, Engman DM. Cardiac antigen-specific autoantibody production is associated with cardiomyopathy in Trypanosoma cruzi-infected mice. *J Immunol* 1994;152:1493–1299.
207. Bestetti RM, Muccillo G. Clinical course of Chagas' heart disease: a comparison with dilated cardiomyopathy. *Int J Cardiol* 1997;60:187–193.
208. Chandra M, Shirani J, Shtutin M, et al. Cardioprotective effects of verapamil on myocardial structure and function in a murine model of chronic Trypanosoma cruzi infection (Brazil Strain): an echocardiographic study. *Int J Parasit* 2002;32:207–215.
209. Nul DR, Grancelli HO, Perrone SV, Bortman GR, Curiel R. Randomised trial of low-dose amiodarone in severe congestive heart failure. *Lancet* 1994;344:493–498.
210. Bocchi EA, Bellotti G, Mocelin AO, et al. Heart Transplantation for Chronic Chagas' Heart Disease. *Ann Thorac Surg* 1996;61:1727–33.
211. Blanche C, Aleksic I, Takkenberg JJM, Czer C, Fishbein MC, Trento A. Heart transplantation for Chagas' cardiomyopathy. *Ann Thorac Surg* 1995;60:1406–1409.
212. McKusick VA. Online Mendelian Inheritance in Man, OMIM (TM). In: McKusick-Nathans Institute for Genetic Medicine, Johns Hopkins University (Baltimore, MD) and National Center for Biotechnology Information, National Library of Medicine (Bethesda, MD); 2000.

CHAPTER 30

Hypertrophic Cardiomyopathy

Steve R. Ommen / Rick A. Nishimura / A. Jamil Tajik

INTRODUCTION

Hypertrophic cardiomyopathy (HCM) usually is defined as an autosomal dominant disease of the heart muscle, with an overall prevalence of 1:500 to 1:1000, characterized by a small left ventricular cavity and marked hypertrophy of the myocardium with myofibril disarray.[1-8]

The basis of HCM has been ascribed to multiple etiologies[9,10]; however, in 1989 investigators first mapped a genetic mutation for HCM to chromosome 14.[11,12] This mutation later was shown to effect the encoding of β-myosin heavy chain protein, which is a major component of the cardiac sarcomere.[13,14] Subsequently, hundreds mutations have been found in HCM patients; most mutations involve the myofilaments of the cardiac sarcomere, however, there is increasing awareness of nonsarcomeric mutations as well.[15,16] Thus, HCM, in its most common manifestation, is felt to be a disease of the myofilaments, whose alteration in structure and/or function underlie the pathology and pathophysiology in affected individuals.[17-27]

HCM is a highly heterogeneous disease, with a diverse pathology and clinical course.[4-7] Some patients may present with severe limiting symptoms of dyspnea, angina, and syncope; yet, other patients remain completely asymptomatic throughout life. HCM is the most common cause of sudden cardiac death in young people, including trained athletes.[28-34] Yet, the overall prognosis of HCM patients is comparable to that of an age- and sex-matched control population.[4,35-41] Therefore, treatment may vary from reassurance, to implantation of a defibrillator, to creation of a localized myocardial infarction.

HISTORICAL PERSPECTIVE

The first anatomic description of HCM was by Teare in 1958, when he reported the pathologic findings in eight young patients, seven of whom had died suddenly.[42] He found massive hypertrophy of the ventricular septum with microscopic evidence of myocardial disarray of the individual muscle fibers, which was speculated to be caused by either a benign tumor or hamartoma. At the same time, Brock reported on patients with functional subvalvular left ventricular outflow (LVO) tract gradients confirmed by pressure gradients.[43] Braunwald and colleagues in the 1960s defined the specific disease process, in which asymmetric septal hypertrophy, myofibril disarray, and a dynamic subvalvular pressure gradient was documented.[44,45] This entity was considered to be a primary process with no known cause; however, a genetic connection was suggested when a familial link was shown to be associated with this entity in an autosomal dominant fashion.[46]

Since these initial descriptions, the disease process has come to be known by many names: asymmetric septal hypertrophy (ASH), idiopathic hypertrophic subaortic stenosis (IHSS), muscle subaortic stenosis, and hypertrophic obstructive cardiomyopathy (HOCM). The World Health Organization has designated the term *hypertrophic cardiomyopathy* to describe this unique process of primary muscle hypertrophy, which may exist with or without a dynamic LVO tract gradient.[47,48]

The evolution of echocardiography provided a noninvasive diagnostic tool to identify patients with HCM.[49–51] Echocardiography showed that hypertrophy in HCM patients could involve areas other than the ventricular septum and further led to the understanding of the complex pathophysiology of HCM. It is now recognized that severity and distribution of hypertrophy may be highly variable and some patients with HCM may have only mild hypertrophy yet still be at risk for disease complications such as sudden death.[33,52,53]

Early descriptions of HCM patients, which originated from several large referral centers, suggested that there were high mortality rates (3–7 percent annually) including many sudden deaths.[3–5,54–56] These studies were comprised of selected younger patients who were referred because they were judged to have either a high-risk status or severe symptoms requiring highly specialized care. More recent reports from nontertiary centers with less selected, regional, or community base cohorts have revealed that the overall mortality of HCM is similar to control populations.[4,35–41] It is now well accepted that although there still remains a select group of patients who are identified at high risk for sudden catastrophic events, most HCM patients live an uneventful, asymptomatic life.[4]

ETIOLOGY

Investigators now believe that HCM is the most common genetic cardiovascular disease. Hundreds of mutations have been associated with clinical HCM with the vast majority encoding proteins of the cardiac sarcomere myofilaments (Fig. 30–1).[17–20,24,27] Affected genes include β-myosin heavy chain, myosin-binding protein C, cardiac troponin T and I, α-tropomyosin, actin, titin, and myosin light chains.[52,53,57–70] These known mutations are inherited in an autosomal dominant manner. Importantly, mutations in other genes outside of the sarcomeric myofilaments have recently been implicated in HCM.[71] Another genetic locus has been mapped to chromosome 7 in patients with cardiac hypertrophy and electrophysiologic abnormalities such as Wolff-Parkinson-White syndrome.[72–74] This gene encodes the y2 regulatory subunit (*PRKAG2*) of adenosine monophosphate–activated protein kinase, an enzyme that modulates glucose metabolism. Histopathologic and biochemical studies of the myocardium have shown myocyte enlargement with glycogen-filled vacuoles, suggesting that patients diagnosed with HCM in the past may have a different disease process similar to a glycogen storage disease.

Several types of mutations have been identified in these genes, including deletions, insertions, missense, and splice site mutations.[26,27] Mutant peptides that are encoded affect function of the contractile unit of the myofilaments by becoming incorporated into the sarcomere itself.[17,18,75] The different mutations may result in a different biophysical consequence. Some defects may alter the actin-myosin crossbridge formation and others may affect the movement and force generation of the thick and thin filaments. It

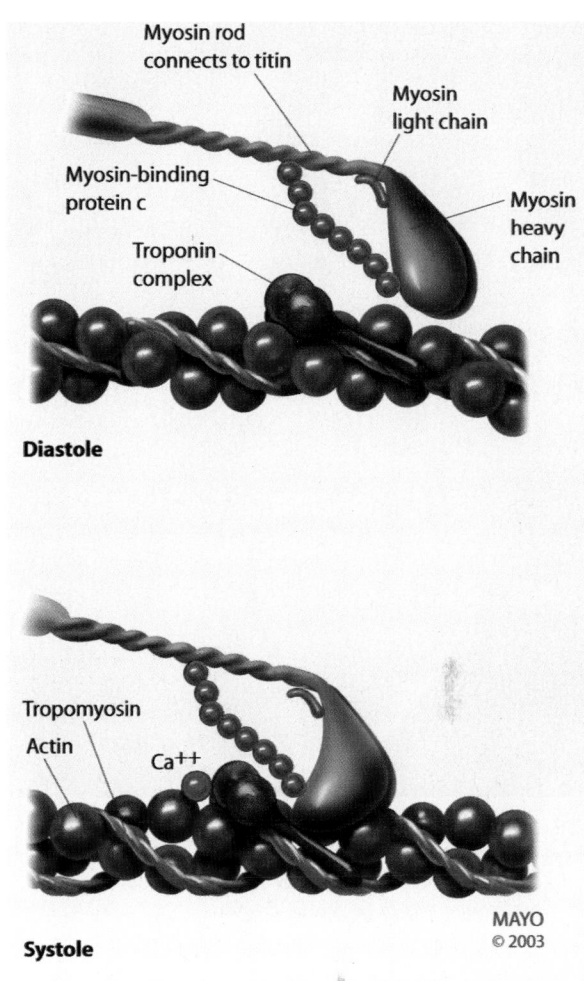

FIGURE 30–1. Schematic diagram of the sarcomere. Hypertrophic cardiomyopathy is a disease of the sarcomere, with mutations found of at least 10 genes coding for various parts of the sarcomere.

has been hypothesized that the sarcomeric dysfunction can lead to *compensatory* myocardial hypertrophy, but the precise impetus for hypertrophy has not yet been identified.[17,18,75–77] As evidenced by the large number of both sarcomeric and nonsarcomeric related mutations and the lack of a clearly identified final common pathway, there appears to be an important role for other genetic and/or environmental modifiers.[78–81] Ultimately, there may be a large number of genes that influence the phenotypic expression of HCM. While the role of specific mutations is not uniformly agreed on, the specific morphologic features of the hypertrophy appear to be different among those patients whose disease is based on the presence of mutations in the sarcomeric myofilaments as compared to those who do not harbor such a mutation.[82]

PATHOLOGY

Gross examination of the heart in HCM demonstrates asymmetric septal hypertrophy with a small left ventricular cavity[83–85] (Fig. 30–2). The mural endocardium may be thickened by fibrous tissue and, if LVO tract obstruction is present, there is often a plaque located on the upper septal area where the mitral valve has been opposed to the

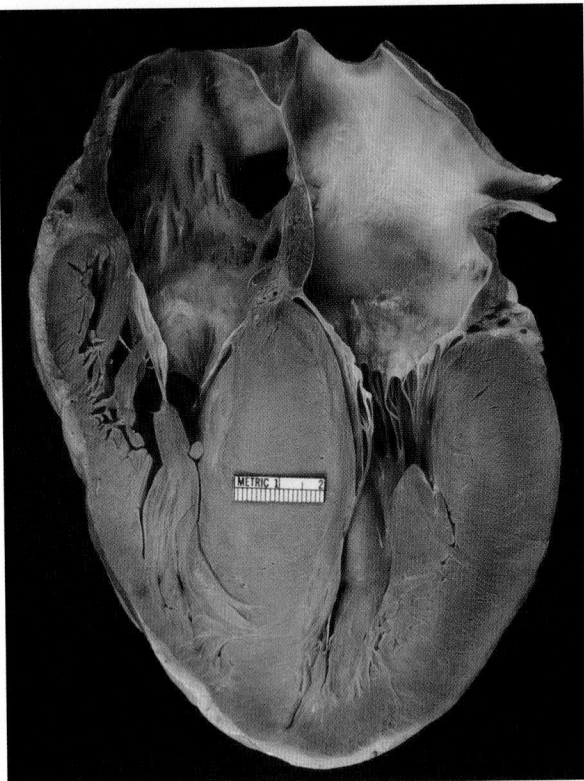

FIGURE 30–2. Pathologic specimen of a patient who died suddenly with hypertrophic cardiomyopathy. There is massive hypertrophy of the myocardium and a small left ventricular cavity. The left atrium is enlarged. *Source: Courtesy of Dr. W. D. Edwards.*

septum during systole. The mitral valve itself may be intrinsically normal; however, there may be elongation of the mitral chordae and anterior displacement of hypertrophied papillary muscles. Abnormal attachments of the mitral valve chordal apparatus to the septum and attachments of the papillary muscle head directly into the leaflets may be found. The left atrium is usually dilated at autopsy. Although the epicardial coronary arteries are normal, the intramural coronary arterioles in the septum are small because of intimal hyperplasia and increased in number.[86,87]

The original report by Teare[42] described bizarre arrangements of the muscle fiber bundles separated by clefts lined with endothelin. The myocardial disarray consists of short runs of severely hypertrophied fibers interrupted by connective tissue. There are large and bizarre nuclei and fibrosis present, with degenerating muscle fibers. This disorganization results in a *whorling* of muscle fibers that is characteristic of HCM (Fig. 30–3). Disarray can be observed throughout the myocardium, is not specific to HCM, and can be seen in any pressure-overloaded ventricle; but the proportion of myocardial disarray is much greater in HCM patients.[88,89]

PATHOPHYSIOLOGY

The pathophysiology of HCM is complex and consists of multiple interrelated abnormalities including diastolic dysfunction, LVO tract obstruction, mitral regurgitation, myocardial ischemia, and arrhythmias.[1,2,4,6,7]

【 】 DIASTOLIC DYSFUNCTION

A major pathophysiologic abnormality in HCM is diastolic dysfunction arising from multiple factors, which ultimately affect both ventricular relaxation and chamber stiffness[1,2,90–92] (Fig. 30–4). An impairment of ventricular relaxation results from the high systolic contraction load caused by an outflow tract obstruction, nonuniformity of ventricular contraction and relaxation, as well as delayed inactivation caused by abnormal intracellular calcium reuptake. The severe hypertrophy of the myocardium results in an increase in chamber stiffness. Diffuse myocardial ischemia may further affect both relaxation and chamber stiffness. Associated with these alterations is a compensatory increase in the contribution of late diastolic filling during atrial systole. With exercise or any other type of catecholamine stimulation, the decrease in diastolic filling period as well as myocardial ischemia will further lead to severe abnormalities of diastolic filling of the heart, with an increase in pulmonary venous pressure causing symptoms of dyspnea.

【 】 LEFT VENTRICULAR OUTFLOW TRACT OBSTRUCTION

The original observations by Brock and Braunwald emphasized the functional subvalvular LVO tract gradient, which was highly influenced by alterations in the load and contractility of the left ventricle (LV)[43,44] (Fig. 30–5). The clinical significance of the out-

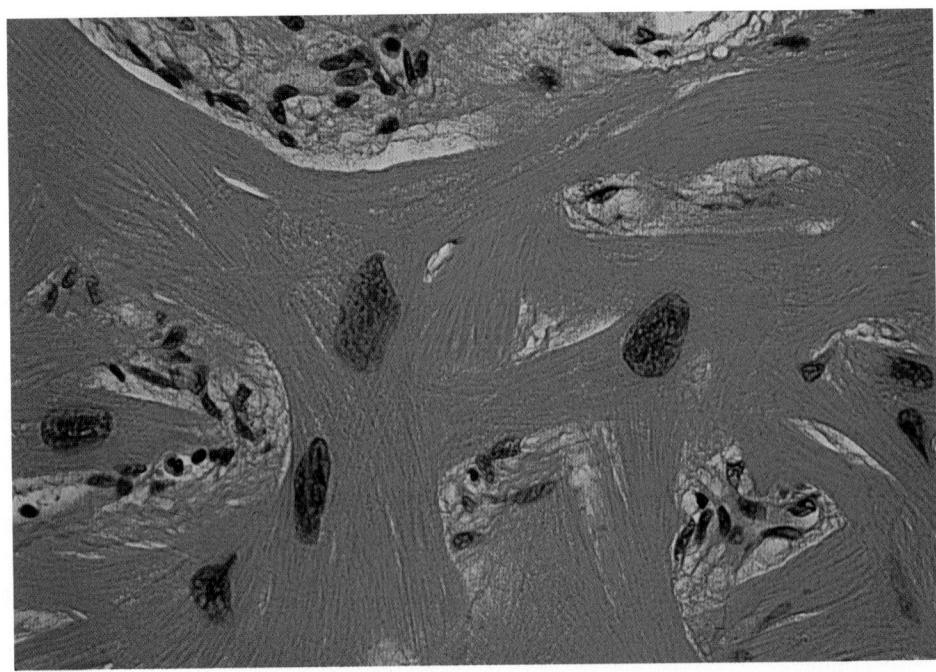

FIGURE 30–3. Microscopic section of the myocardium from a patient with hypertrophic cardiomyopathy. There is myofiber disarray present.

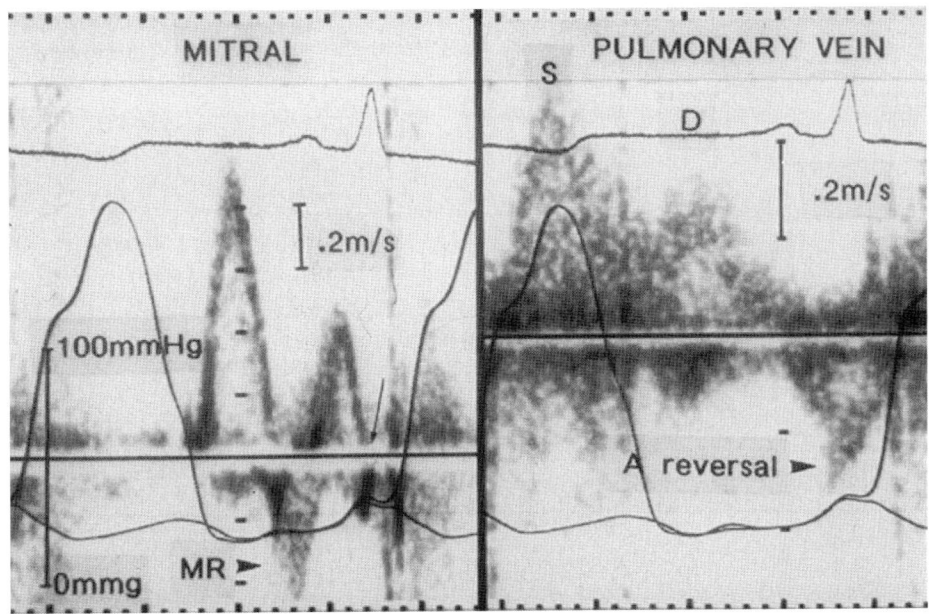

FIGURE 30-4. Evidence of severe diastolic dysfunction in a patient with hypertrophic cardiomyopathy. The left ventricular and left atrial (LA) pressures are shown in both the left and right panels. The mean LA pressure is severely elevated to 30 mm of mercury. *Left:* The mitral flow velocity curve is shown, demonstrating a high E:A ratio and a short deceleration time. Diastolic mitral regurgitation (MR) is present. There is abrupt cessation of the "a" duration (*arrow*). *Right:* The pulmonary vein velocity curve is shown, with a high velocity at atrial reversal of long duration. The systolic forward flow (S) and diastolic forward flow (D) is shown.

tractility of the ventricle[44,102] (Fig. 30–6). Increased myocardial contractility, decreased ventricular volume, or decreased afterload increases the degree of subaortic obstruction. Patients may have little or no obstruction to LVO at rest but can generate large LVO tract gradients under conditions such as exercise, the strain phase of the Valsalva maneuver, or during pharmacologic provocation. It has been well established that this dynamic LVO tract obstruction contributes in part to the debilitating symptoms that may occur in these patients and is an important determinant of outcome in HCM.[103]

MYOCARDIAL ISCHEMIA

Severe myocardial ischemia and even infarction may occur in HCM.[86,104,105] The myocardial ischemia is frequently unrelated to the atherosclerotic epicardial coronary artery disease but caused by supply–demand mismatch. Patients with HCM have increased oxygen demand

flow tract gradient has been controversial, but careful studies have shown definitively that true obstruction does exist.[1,2,93–95] The obstruction causes an increase in left ventricular systolic pressure, which leads to a complex interplay of abnormalities including prolongation of ventricular relaxation, elevation of left ventricular diastolic pressure, mitral regurgitation, myocardial ischemia, and a decrease in forward cardiac output.[1,2]

The mechanism of obstruction is multifactorial. The obstruction was initially thought to be caused by systolic contraction of the hypertrophied basal ventricular septum, which would then encroach into the LVO tract with a resultant suction, or Venturi force, that would pull the mitral valve leaflets into the LVO tract and produce further obstruction.[1,2,96] Elegant studies emphasize that during ventricular systole, flow against the abnormally positioned mitral valve apparatus results in a drag force on a portion of the mitral valve leaflets and actually *push* the leaflets into the outflow tract.[97–100] Obstruction can also be present in the midcavitary region because of hypertrophied papillary muscles abutting against the septum.[101]

The obstruction to LVO is dynamic, varying with loading conditions and con-

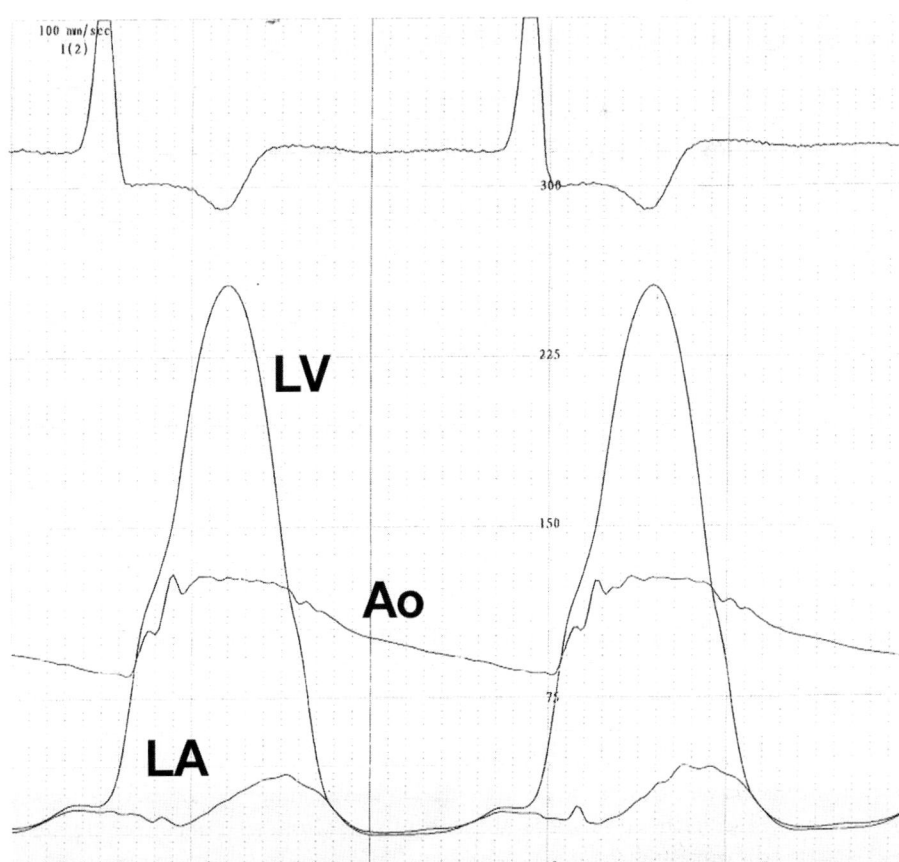

FIGURE 30-5. Cardiac catheterization pressure curves showing a severe left ventricular outflow tract obstruction. The gradient between the left ventricle (LV) and aorta (Ao) is nearly 100 mm of mercury. The left atrial (LA) pressure is also elevated. There is a *spike and dome* pattern on the aortic pressure curve.

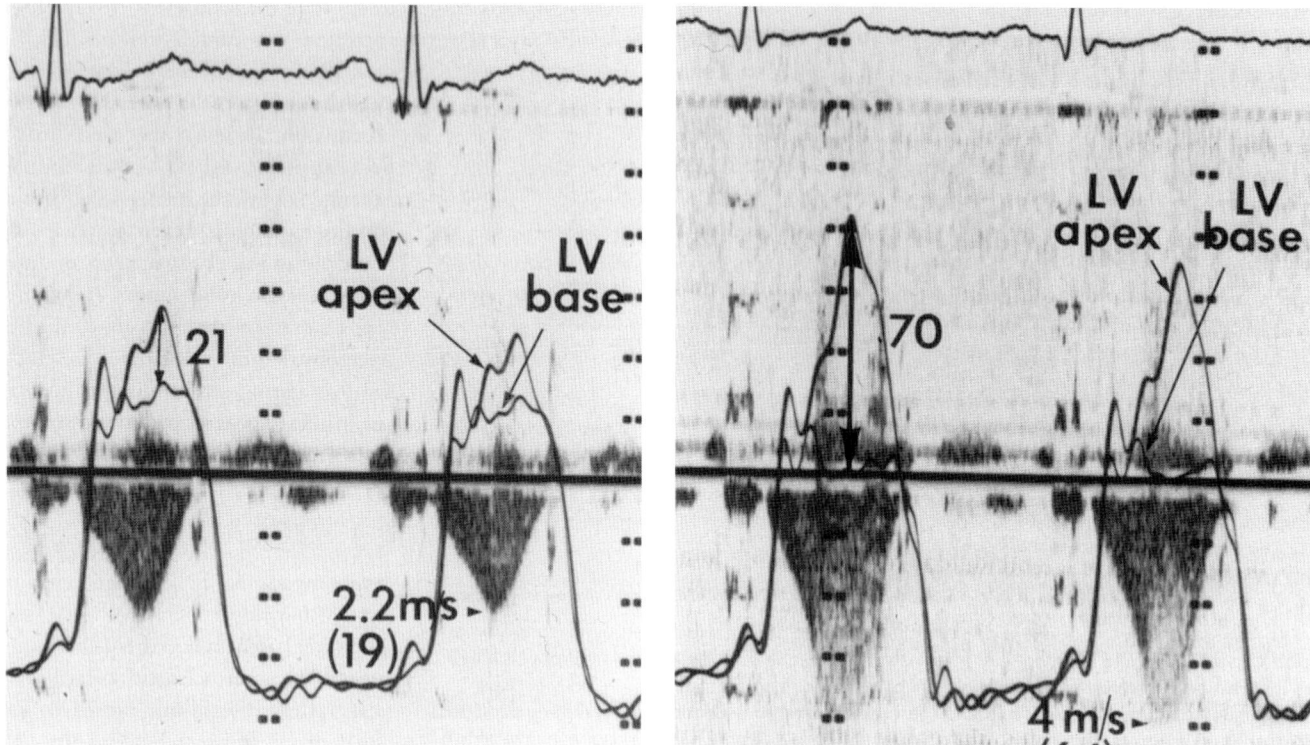

FIGURE 30–6. The dynamic nature of the left ventricular outflow (LVO) tract obstruction is shown by simultaneous Doppler echocardiography and cardiac catheterization. The cardiac catheterization is performed with a pressure measurement of the left ventricular apex and left ventricular base. The gradient occurs during systole between the left ventricular apex and left ventricular base. The continuous wave Doppler velocities through the LVO tract are shown. The calculated gradient from the Doppler echocardiogram is shown in parenthesis. *Left:* The gradient in the baseline state is 21 mm of mercury as assessed by both cardiac catheterization and Doppler echocardiography. *Right:* During inhalation of amyl nitrite, the gradient increases to 70 mm of mercury.

caused by the hypertrophy and adverse loading conditions but also have compromised coronary blood flow to the left ventricular myocardium because of abnormally small and partially obliterated intramural coronary arteries.[86,87,104,106]

[ ] AUTONOMIC DYSFUNCTION

During exercise approximately 25 percent of HCM patients have an abnormal blood pressure response defined by either a failure of systolic blood pressure to rise >20 mmHg or a fall in systolic blood pressure.[107,108] The presence of this finding is associated with a poorer prognosis.[108,109] This inability to augment and sustain systolic blood pressure occurs despite an appropriate rise in cardiac output and is caused by systemic vasodilatation during exercise. It is speculated that there is a high degree of abnormal autonomic tone in HCM.

[ ] MITRAL REGURGITATION

Mitral regurgitation is common in patients with LVO tract obstruction and may play a primary role in producing symptoms of dyspnea.[1,2,110] The temporal sequence of events of *eject-obstruct-leak* supports the concept that the mitral regurgitation in most patients is a secondary phenomenon.[1,2,110] The mitral regurgitation is usually caused by the distortion of the mitral valve apparatus from the systolic anterior motion secondary to the LVO tract obstruction. The jet of mitral regurgitation is directed laterally and

posteriorly and predominates during mid- and late systole (see Fig. 30–6); the severity is proportional to the LVO tract obstruction. Changes in ventricular load and contractility that affect the severity of outflow tract obstruction similarly affect the degree of mitral regurgitation. It is important to identify patients with additional intrinsic disease of the mitral valve apparatus (prolapse or flail), because this finding influences subsequent treatment options.[111]

CLINICAL PRESENTATION

There is a wide variability in the clinical presentation of HCM patients.[3,4] Most patients with HCM are asymptomatic, with the disease diagnosed on the basis of abnormal electrocardiogram, heart murmur, or screening echocardiogram. When symptoms are present, dyspnea, angina, and/or syncope are the most common. Additionally, sudden death may occur, particularly in the young population.

Dyspnea occurs in up to 90 percent of symptomatic HCM patients. The stiff, noncompliant hypertrophied ventricle and abnormal relaxation cause elevated left ventricular filling pressures; a situation exacerbated with exercise. The diastolic filling abnormalities are augmented by the occurrence of a dynamic LVO tract obstruction or concomitant mitral regurgitation.[1,2] However, dyspnea may occur in the absence of outflow tract obstruction or mitral regurgitation, if there is severe diastolic dysfunction.

Angina occurs in 70 to 80 percent of patients with symptomatic HCM, and 15 percent of all patients at autopsy have associated myocardial infarction.[86] The angina may frequently occur in the absence of epicardial coronary disease, related to a number of mechanisms including small artery narrowing, intramural compression of small arteries from myocardial hypertrophy, abnormal diastolic filling, oxygen supply demand mismatch, and abnormal coronary flow reserve.

Syncope occurs in approximately 20 percent and presyncope occurs in more than half of HCM patients. Syncope can be caused by either a hemodynamic or rhythm abnormality. It has been speculated that activation of left ventricular baroreceptors results in a reflex vasodilatation, and that mechanism may be worsened by a dynamic LVO tract gradient. The syncope in this case occurs either during or immediately after exercise.

Patients with HCM often describe an increase in symptoms during hot humid weather, presumably because of fluid loss and vasodilation resulting in decreases in both preload and afterload. Similarly, symptoms also may be more prominent after eating a large meal or after drinking alcohol. Other concomitant problems such as anemia or fever may exacerbate symptoms.

Older patients may present differently than younger patients.[4,5,112–115] Many patients have a history of hypertension, thus presenting on medications, such as diuretics and vasodilators, which exacerbate outflow tract obstruction. Atrial fibrillation occurs commonly in older patients (up to 25–30 percent) and may herald systemic embolism and further clinical deterioration.[4,35,39] These older patients may also have manifestations of other concomitant cardiac disease, such as coronary artery disease, degenerative valvular aortic stenosis and mitral annular calcification.

PHYSICAL EXAMINATION

The classic physical findings of HCM apply to patients with a LVO tract gradient. The HCM patients who do not have an outflow tract obstruction should have findings of left ventricular hypertrophy on physical examination.

CAROTID PULSE

The classic carotid pulsation is brisk with a *spike and dome* pattern, characterized by a rapid rise (percussion wave) followed by a midsystolic drop that is in turn followed by a secondary wave (tidal wave). The midsystolic drop in amplitude of the carotid pulse contour is caused by premature closure of the aortic valve and coincides with systolic anterior motion of the mitral valve. The late peak is caused by relief of the outflow tract gradient as the mitral valve leaflet returns to its original position. In the presence of pronounced obstruction, there is a longer ejection time. The carotid pulsation with dynamic LVO tract obstruction differs from that of a fixed obstruction, such as seen with valvular or discrete subvalvular aortic stenosis where there is a decrease in both the rate of rise and in amplitude of the pulsation.

JUGULAR VENOUS PULSE

The jugular venous pressure is normal in most HCM patients. However, the *a* wave may be prominent indicating a decrease in compliance ventricle caused by the hypertrophy of the right ventricular free wall or septum, pulmonary hypertension from left sided diastolic pressure elevation, or right ventricular outflow obstruction.

APICAL IMPULSE

The apical impulse is almost always abnormal in patients with HCM and reflects the myocardial hypertrophy. The apical impulse is a sustained systolic thrust, which continues throughout most of systole. There is frequently a bifid impulse caused by a forceful atrial systole. There may be a *triple ripple* with a third component occurring near the end of systole if outflow tract obstruction is present. A systolic thrill may be palpable at apex from severe mitral regurgitation or the lower left sternal border from outflow tract obstruction.

CARDIAC SOUNDS

Auscultation usually reveals a normal or loud first heart sound. The second heart sound is usually split physiologically, but approximately 20 percent of patients may have a paradoxical split caused by either a concomitant left bundle-branch block or severe LVO tract obstruction. A fourth heart sound is usually present, especially if there is severe hypertrophy. In young patients an early diastolic filling sound is frequently heard, indicating early rapid filling. In the presence of severe concomitant mitral regurgitation, the excess flow across the mitral valve may result in a diastolic flow rumble.

MURMURS

The classic murmur from LVO tract obstruction is a crescendo–decrescendo murmur located primarily at the left sternal border. The murmur usually ends before the second heart sound. The murmur can radiate to the base of the heart as well as to the apex but as opposed to valvular aortic stenosis, there is seldom radiation to the carotid arteries. Mitral regurgitation may be a separate murmur audible at the apex and is more holosystolic in nature. The presence of an aortic diastolic decrescendo murmur should suggest another disease, such as aortic valve disease or a discrete subvalvular stenosis.

Dynamic auscultation should be performed to differentiate the murmur of HCM from that of valvular aortic stenosis and mitral regurgitation. Maneuvers that decrease preload increase the dynamic gradient and increase the intensity of the murmur (Fig. 30–7). Although the change in murmur intensity during the strain phase of the Valsalva maneuver has been proposed as a method to diagnose the dynamic murmur of HCM, this classic response may not occur in all patients. The most reliable method for diagnosing a dynamic LVO tract obstruction is the response of the murmur to the stand-squat-stand position. From the standing position to a prompt squat, the murmur markedly decreases in intensity, because of increases in afterload and preload. From the squatting to standing position, there is an increase in intensity of the murmur immediately as afterload is reduced. A progressive increase in intensity of the murmur continues for the next four to five beats as preload to the left side of the heart is reduced. Simple exercise, such as ambulation or climbing stairs can be used to assess for augmentation of the murmur as well. Other maneuvers that are used to change the intensity of the murmur include leg-raising to increase preload or the inhalation of amyl nitrite to decrease afterload and increase heart rate.

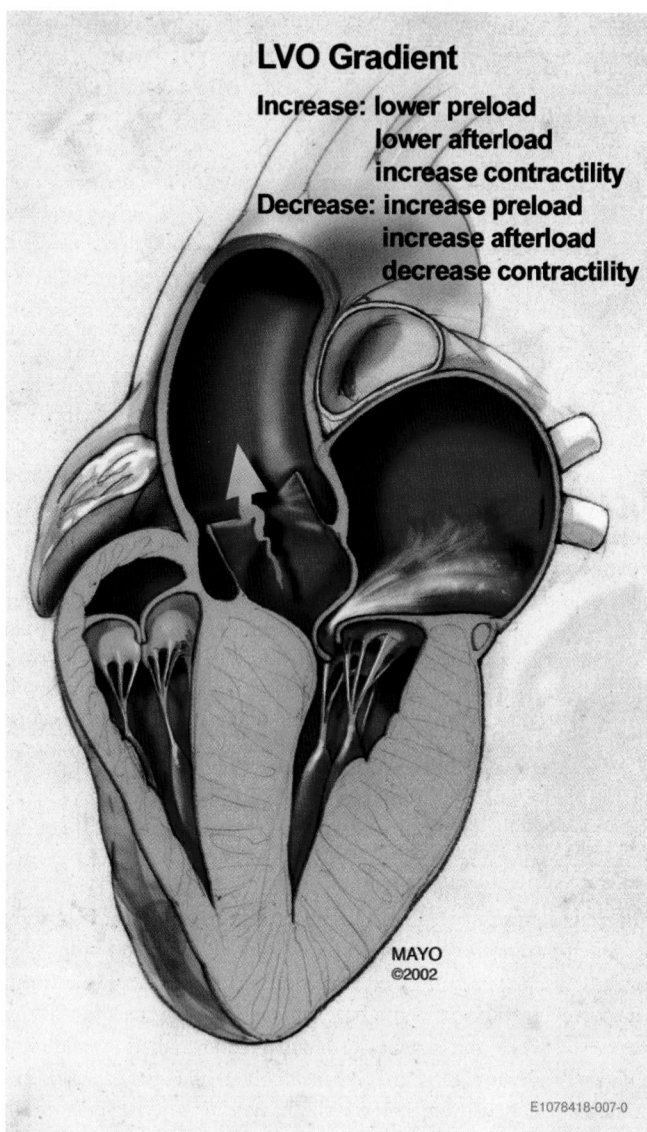

LVO Gradient

Increase: lower preload
lower afterload
increase contractility
Decrease: increase preload
increase afterload
decrease contractility

MAYO
©2002

E1078418-007-0

FIGURE 30–7. Schematic diagram of the left ventricle in hypertrophic cardiomyopathy during systole. There is projection of the basal septum into the outflow tract with systolic anterior motion of the mitral valve, which results in left ventricular outflow (LVO) tract obstruction. The obstruction is dynamic and dependent on the preload, afterload, and contractility of the heart.

The response of the intensity of the murmur after premature ventricular contraction or following any long pause is useful. Left ventricular contractility increases and afterload decreases for the beat after a long pause. Thus, intensity of the systolic murmur in obstructive HCM increases while the murmur of organic mitral regurgitation remains unchanged or decreases in intensity.

DIAGNOSTIC TESTING

【 】 ELECTROCARDIOGRAM AND HOLTER MONITORING

The electrocardiogram is abnormal in most HCM patients.[45] A normal axis is present in 60 to 70 percent of patients and a left axis in 30 percent, whereas 70 to 80 percent of patients demonstrate left ventricular hypertrophy on the resting 12-lead electrocardio-

gram (Fig. 30–8). Abnormal Q waves simulating myocardial infarction, caused by a disturbance of activation of ventricular septum, are seen in 25 percent and may appear any lead. The electrocardiogram in patients with a variant of HCM involving primarily the apex (apical HCM) may show a distinctive pattern of diffuse symmetric T wave inversions across the precordium (Fig. 30–9).

The basic rhythm in most patients is normal sinus rhythm, but ambulatory monitoring demonstrates a high incidence of supraventricular tachycardia (46 percent), premature ventricular contractions (43 percent), and nonsustained ventricular tachycardia (26 percent).[116–118] Atrial fibrillation may occur in up to 25 to 30 percent of the older population. Preexcitation has also been associated with HCM.

【 】 CHEST X-RAY

The chest x-ray usually shows mild to moderate enlargement of the cardiac silhouette. The left ventricular contour is rounded consistent with concentric left ventricular hypertrophy. There is usually enlargement of the left atrium and the right-sided chambers are usually normal. The presence of aortic valvular calcification or a dilated ascending aorta (Ao) should raise the question of aortic valvular disease.

【 】 ECHOCARDIOGRAPHY

Two-dimensional and Doppler echocardiography have become the gold standard for the diagnosis of HCM.[1,2] The finding of increased wall thickness in the absence of another etiology is the basis for the diagnosis of HCM (Fig. 30–10). The hypertrophy can be distributed throughout the myocardium in any pattern but commonly involves the entire ventricular septum (Fig. 30–11). No phenotypic expression can be considered *classic* or particularly typical of this disease. The average maximal left ventricular wall thickness in a population of HCM patients is usually 20 to 22 mm; however, 5 to 10 percent of patients have maximal wall thickness in excess of 30 mm.

The pattern of hypertrophy has been described as morphologically different in the younger versus the older patients.[112] In the young population, there is classically diffuse hypertrophy of the entire septum, with a convex septal contour. In the older population, there is the appearance of a *sigmoid* septum, in which the hypertrophy is localized to the mid- and basal septum. The remaining septum is concave in contour and there is also a sharper angle of the septum with the long axis of the Ao. These differences are likely determined by the underlying genetic substrate. Patients younger than 50 years of age at the time of diagnosis are much more likely to have myofilament mutations than older individuals.[119–121] Whether there are clinical, environmental, or other unique, nonmyofilament genetic abnormalities that are responsible for the sigmoid septal contour remains to be fully understood.

Genetic studies examining HCM patients with specific myofilament mutations have shown that the phenotype is not always expressed as severe thickening of the LV.[52,53,69,70,122] These findings may be related to the variability in the degree and age of penetrance. There are some genotype-affected patients who may only show a mild increase of 15 to 18 mm. There are other genotype-

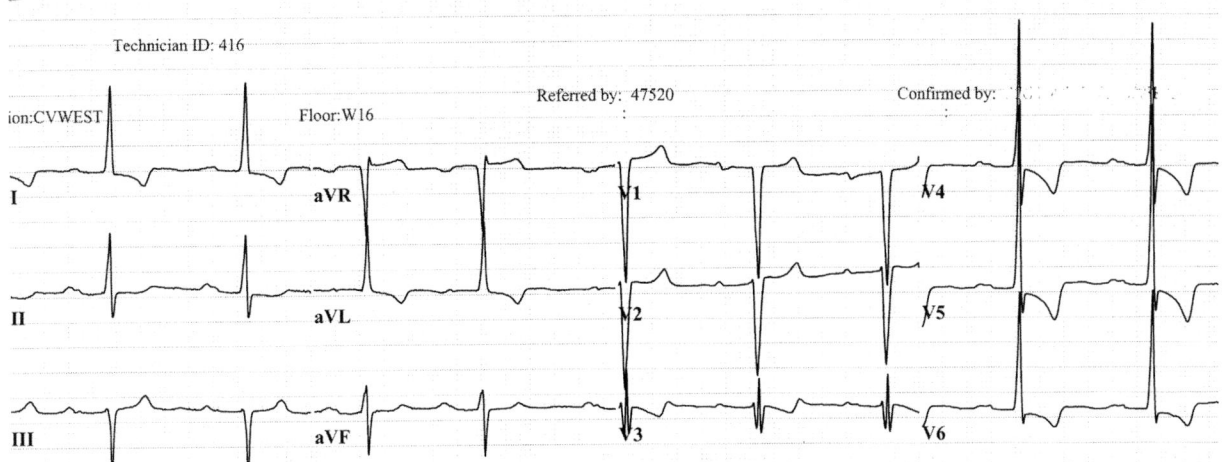

FIGURE 30–8. 12-lead electrocardiogram from a patient with hypertrophic cardiomyopathy. There is severe left ventricular hypertrophy present. There is high voltage as well as secondary ST–T wave abnormalities. aVF, augmented voltage unipolar left foot lead; aVL, augmented voltage unipolar left arm lead; aVR, augmented voltage unipolar right arm lead.

affected individuals who have been observed with normal wall thickness of <12 mm. There are some gene mutations, such as the myosin-binding protein C mutation, in which the phenotypic expression of hypertrophy may not appear until the fifth or sixth decade of life.[52,53,69,70,122] Although these genotype–phenotype correlations are intriguing, it is important to acknowledge that there are numerous and important exceptions.

The finding of increased wall thickness on echocardiography can be seen in other abnormalities that must be considered in the differential diagnosis. Increased afterload on the LV from either hypertension or valvular aortic stenosis may cause an increase in the left ventricular wall thickness. Patients with chronic renal failure, especially those on dialysis, also present with increased wall thickness on echocardiography. Infiltrative and glycogen storage diseases such as cardiac amyloidosis, Fabry disease, and Friedreich ataxia may present with increased wall thickness and thus mimic HCM on echocardiography.[123–125] It is important to correlate the findings of increased left ventricular wall thickness on echocardio-

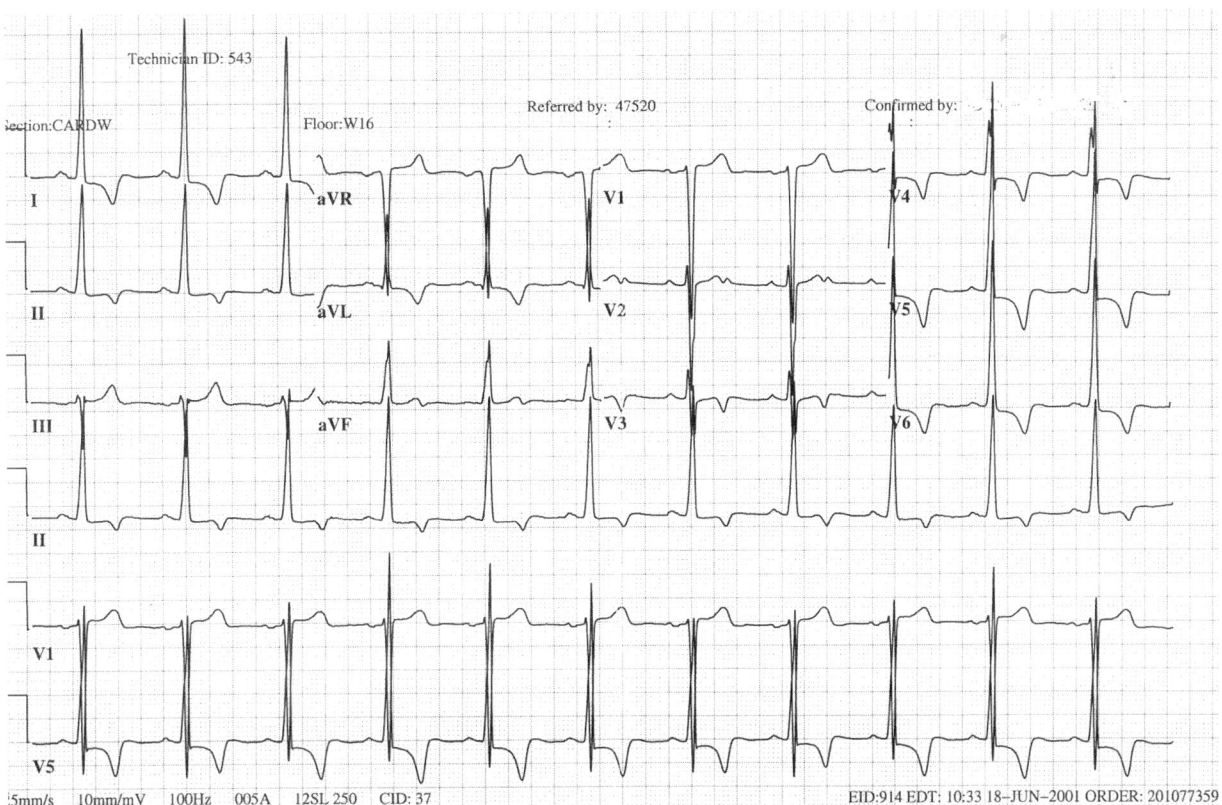

FIGURE 30–9. 12-lead electrocardiogram from a patient with the apical variant of hypertrophic cardiomyopathy. There are diffuse T-wave inversions across the precordium as well as left ventricular hypertrophy by voltage. aVF, augmented voltage unipolar left foot lead; aVL, augmented voltage unipolar left arm lead; aVR, augmented voltage unipolar right arm lead.

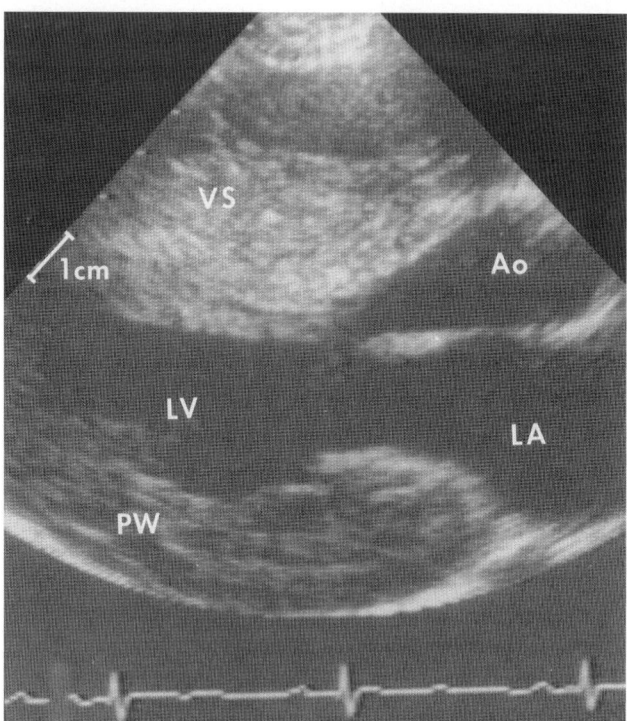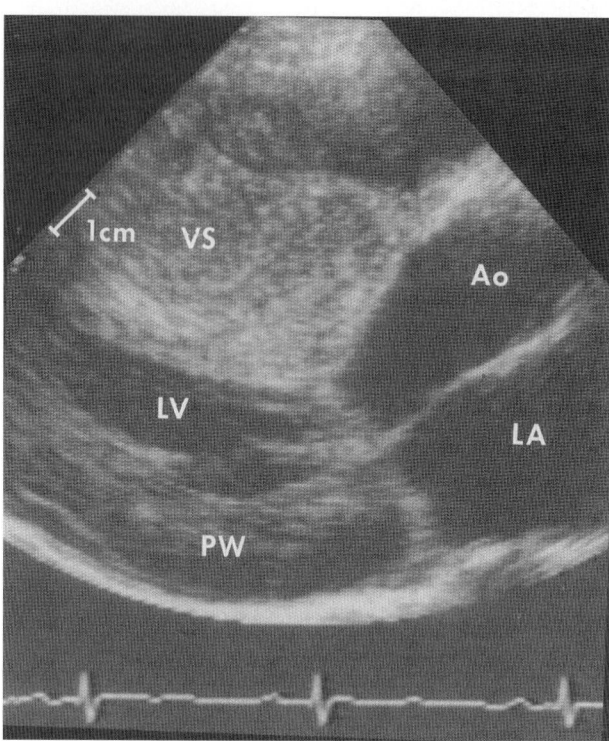

FIGURE 30–10. Two-dimensional echocardiogram from a patient with severe hypertrophic cardiomyopathy. There is a severe increase in left ventricular wall thickness, with a much greater increase in thickness of the ventricular septum (*VS*). The ratio of ventricular septal thickness to posterior wall (*PW*) thickness is 2.5:1. *Left*: Parasternal long axis view during diastole. *Right*: Parasternal long axis view during systole. There is systolic anterior motion of the mitral valve causing LVO tract obstruction. Ao, aorta; LA, left atrium; LV, left ventricular; LVO, left ventricular outflow.

graphy with the electrocardiogram. If there are relatively low voltages on the 12-lead electrocardiogram in the presence of increased wall thickness, suspicion of an infiltrative disorder (amyloidosis) should be raised (Fig. 30–12).

In young athletes a physiologic form of left ventricular hypertrophy may occur which is a physiologic adaptation to intense training that may be difficult to differentiate from HCM.[126,127] Elite athletes who have a dilated ventricular cavity with septal thickness <14 to 15 mm most likely have *athlete's heart,* but the combination of these findings may not always be present. A reduction in wall thickness after cessation of training is useful to identify the *athletic heart* but may not be practical in all patients.[126,127] Future investigation with Doppler tissue imaging, myocardial strain, and cardiac magnetic resonance imaging may provide insight into this difficult diagnostic challenge.[128,129]

Two-dimensional echocardiography is also the primary tool for defining the presence and severity of LVO tract obstruction.[130,131] If true dynamic obstruction is present, there is systolic anterior

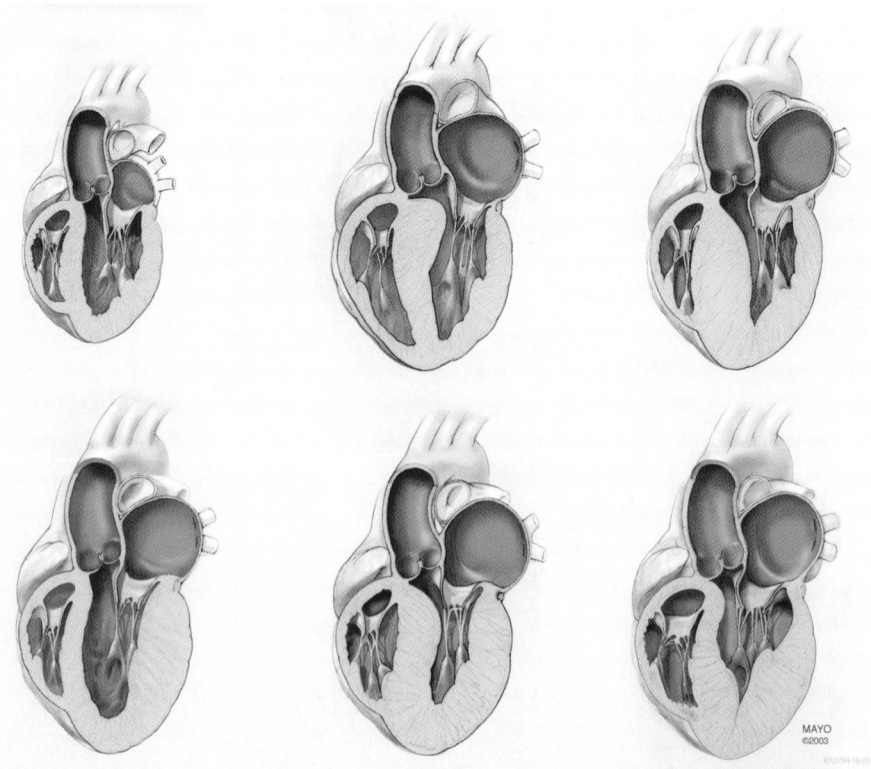

FIGURE 30–11. Schematic diagram of the different variants of hypertrophic cardiomyopathy. Upper left is the normal heart for comparison. Shown are variants of the location and degree of hypertrophy.

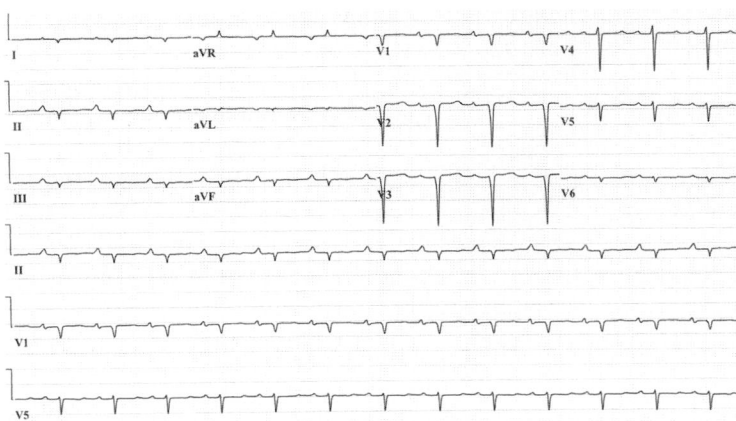

FIGURE 30–12. 12-lead electrocardiogram from a patient with amyloid heart disease. The two-dimensional echocardiogram in this patient showed a severe increase in left ventricular wall thickness, simulating hypertrophic cardiomyopathy. However, the low voltage and loss of forces on the electrocardiogram indicates that an infiltrative disease is responsible for the increased left ventricular wall thickness. aVF, augmented voltage unipolar left foot lead; aVL, augmented voltage unipolar left arm lead; aVR, augmented voltage unipolar right arm lead.

motion (SAM) of the mitral valve apparatus. Most patients have SAM of the anterior leaflet, but this may also occur with the posterior leaflet.[132] There are frequently additional abnormalities of the mitral valve supporting structures.[130,133] The exact site of the obstruction may be determined by visualizing the region of the SAM-septal contact.[134] In the classic form of obstructive HCM, the obstruction occurs at the most basal portion of the septum as it projects into the LVO tract. However, the obstruction may also extend into the LV from SAM of the chordal apparatus. There may be patients with midventricular obstruction in whom a hypertrophied papillary muscle abuts against the ventricular septum.[101] Two-dimensional echocardiography is useful for ruling out other causes of LVO tract obstruction such as discrete subaortic stenosis or tunnel subaortic stenosis.[135]

Doppler echocardiography can be used to define the pathophysiologic processes that are present in HCM. In the presence of a dynamic LVO tract obstruction, there is a high velocity *dagger-shaped* signal on continuous wave Doppler interrogation of the LVO tract[136] (Fig. 30–13). In patients with low outflow tract velocities (<3 m/sec), provocation with the Valsalva maneuver, inhalation of amyl nitrite, or exercise should be performed during the Doppler study to determine if there is a labile or latent obstruction.

Doppler color flow imaging can be used to determine the presence and severity of mitral regurgitation (Fig. 30–14).[137] If the mitral regurgitation is secondary to distortion of the mitral valve apparatus from the SAM, the color jet is directed laterally and posteriorly. In addition, the regurgitation predominates in mid- to late systole. If there is a holosystolic signal of mitral regurgitation directed centrally or anteriorly, a primary abnormality of the mitral valve apparatus should be suspected. The mitral regurgitation signal by continuous wave Doppler may contaminate the outflow tract velocity signal and care must be taken to differentiate the true outflow tract velocity from the mitral regurgitation jet (Fig. 30–15).

Diastolic function can be assessed noninvasively by Doppler echocardiography. The transmitral flow velocity curves cannot be

used alone because of the complex interplay of relaxation and compliance abnormalities present in HCM.[138] However, pulmonary vein flows and Doppler tissue imaging together with the transmitral flow velocity curves can improve the accuracy of estimates of left ventricular filling pressures.[139]

Doppler tissue imaging of the mitral annular motion helps evaluate longitudinal contraction of the myocardium, which is abnormal in HCM patients despite normal or supranormal ejection fraction. Abnormally low annular velocities may help detect subclinical disease, for example patients who carry an HCM-associated genetic abnormality but may not yet have developed the phenotypic expression of increased wall thickness.[140–142] It may also help distinguish HCM from the physiologic increase in wall thickness observed in some athletes, who would have preserved or enhanced annular velocities.[129]

Transesophageal echocardiography is usually unnecessary in the evaluation of the patient with HCM. In most patients the clinically necessary anatomic and hemodynamic information can be obtained by transthoracic echocardiography. However, patients in whom discrete subvalvular stenosis or a primary abnormality of the mitral valve is suspected may benefit from transesophageal echocardiography.

Cardiovascular magnetic resonance (CMR) imaging provides high-resolution moving images of the myocardium and accurately determines the site and extent of hypertrophy. This can be extremely important in patients with equivocal hypertrophy and/or

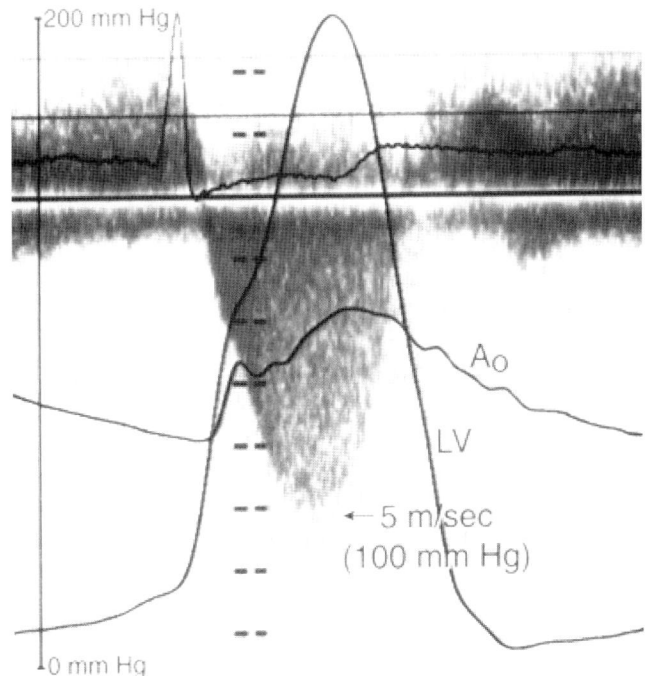

FIGURE 30–13. Simultaneous Doppler echocardiogram and cardiac catheterization demonstrating the presence of severe LVO tract obstruction. The gradient between the left ventricle (LV) and aorta (Ao) at catheterization is 100 mm of mercury. A continuous wave Doppler across the left ventricular outflow (LVO) tract reveals a peak velocity of 5 m/sec, which is consistent with a calculated LVO tract gradient of 100 mm of mercury.

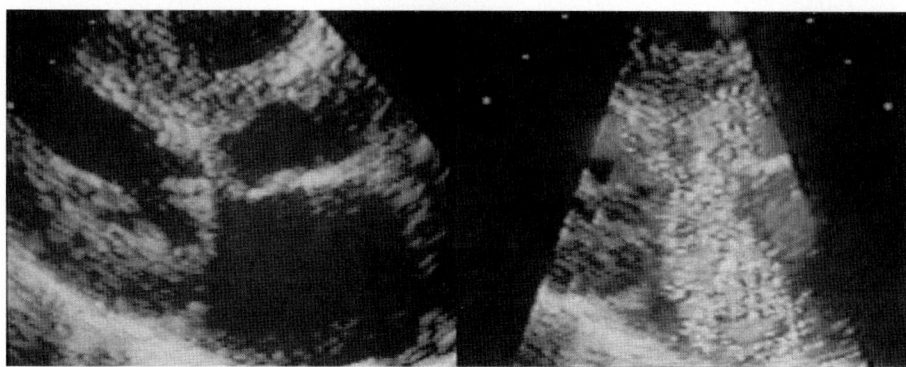

FIGURE 30–14. Color flow Doppler imaging of a patient with hypertrophic cardiomyopathy, severe systolic anterior motion of the mitral valve, and secondary mitral regurgitation. *Left*: A still frame two-dimensional echocardiogram from the parasternal view showing systolic anterior motion of the mitral valve. *Right*: Color flow imaging demonstrating a large mosaic jet of mitral regurgitation directed posteriorly.

difficult echocardiographic images. SAM of the mitral valve, LVO tract flow turbulence, mitral regurgitation, perfusion abnormalities, and intramyocardial fibrosis or scarring can also be visualized with CMR.[143,144]

[ ] CARDIAC CATHETERIZATION

Cardiac catheterization is not required in most HCM patients, because the diagnosis and determination of outflow tract obstruction can usually be made by echocardiography. In uncommon circumstances in which there is a discrepancy between the echocardiogram and the clinical presentation, cardiac catheterization may be of benefit in demonstrating the presence and severity of a LVO tract obstruction.

The outflow tract obstruction has been assessed by a *pull-back* pressure tracing, placing an end-hole catheter at the left ventricular apex, pulling back to the base and then into the Ao. The systolic gradient will be between the apex and base (Fig. 30–16). However, because of the small left ventricular cavity with hyperdynamic systolic function, cavity obliteration and catheter *entrapment* may occur, resulting in a falsely increased left ventricular systolic pressure. The gradient is ideally assessed by a simultaneous left ventricular inflow and LVO (or aortic) pressure.[1,2] The left ventricular inflow position avoids the problem of catheter entrapment and is best obtained by a transseptal approach.

When there is little resting obstruction, provocation using the Valsalva maneuver or infusion of isoproterenol should be performed in the catheterization laboratory. The Brockenbrough phenomenon helps determine the presence of a latent obstruction (Fig. 30–17). After a premature contraction, the contractility of the ventricle increases, resulting in a marked increase in the degree of dynamic obstruction. Thus, there is an increase in gradient as well as a decrease in the aortic pulse pressure after the pause. This is in contradistinction to a fixed obstruction in which there is increased gradient from the

increase in stroke volume but increased aortic pulse pressure also occurs.

Left ventriculography usually reveals a small left ventricular cavity size with hypertrophied papillary muscles further impinging into the cavity. Hyperdynamic systolic function causes complete obliteration of the mid- and apical cavity in systole (Fig. 30–18). In the apical variant of HCM, there is a fixed obliteration of the apex by the hypertrophied muscle, causing a *spade-like* configuration. There may be an apical akinetic or dyskinetic pouch with *aneurysm* formation with midventricular obstruction.

Coronary angiography may be indicated if there are symptoms of angina out of proportion to the degree of obstruction or other symptoms. Epicardial coronary disease is seen in up to 25 percent of older patients.[145] The combination of the epicardial disease and the high myocardial oxygen demand from the hypertrophied muscle may result in significant symptoms of angina and may alter outcome.[146,147] Myocardial bridging is frequent, particularly in younger patients with severe hypertrophy; however, the impact of bridging on outcome is controversial.[148,149]

[ ] STRESS TESTING

Stress testing is of limited value for the diagnosis of epicardial coronary disease in patients with HCM. The combination of the myocardial oxygen supply–demand mismatch and the small coronary arteriolar disease results in findings of myocardial ischemia on electrocardiography and nuclear imaging, even in the absence of epicardial coronary disease. Exercise testing, however, is of value in patients with HCM. Important, adverse prognostic factors include a drop in blood pressure with exercise and/or the appearance of ventricular arrhythmias.[107,150] In addition, exercise testing helps obtain an objective measurement of exercise tolerance.[151] Exercise

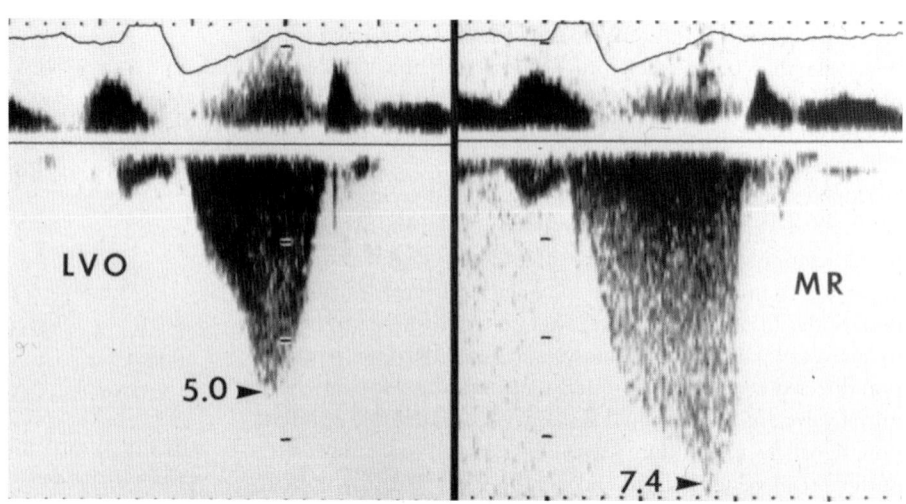

FIGURE 30–15. Continuous wave Doppler echocardiogram from a patient with both left ventricular outflow (LVO) tract obstruction and mitral regurgitation. The continuous wave Doppler jet has a similar contour for both the LVO tract velocity (*LVO*) (*left panel*) and the mitral regurgitation (*MR*) (*right panel*) jet. The mitral regurgitation signal is of higher velocity and the signal is holosystolic.

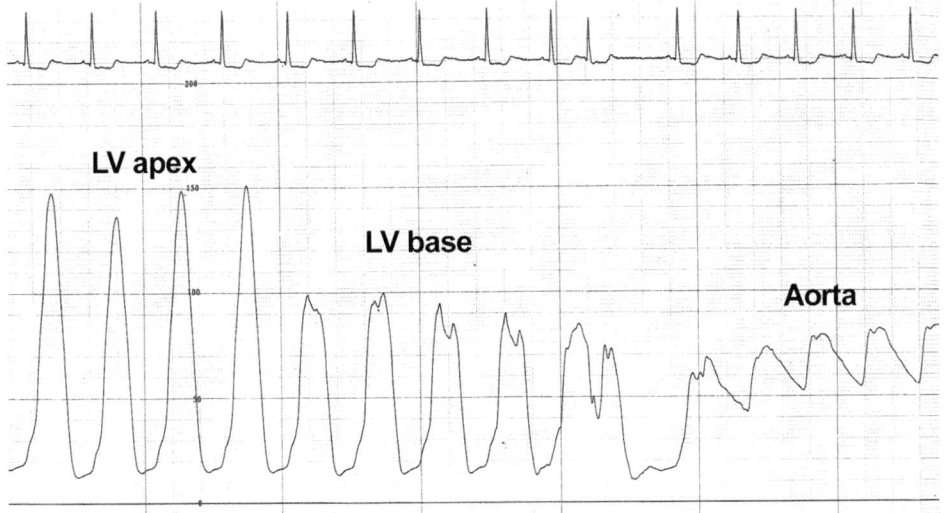

FIGURE 30–16. Cardiac catheterization traces from a patient with hypertrophic cardiomyopathy. An end-hole catheter is placed in the left ventricular apex, pulled back to the left ventricular base and finally into the ascending aorta (Ao). The systolic gradient of 50 mm of mercury is between the left ventricular apex and left ventricular base. Note the marked decrease in pulse pressure on the first beat after the catheter has been pulled into the Ao, which is a beat following a premature contraction. There is a *spike and dome* pattern on the aortic pressure curve.

is the most physiologic form of provocation to attempt to detect latent LVO tract obstruction.

NATURAL HISTORY

The natural history of HCM patients is highly variable.[3,4,6,7] The early literature describing a poor prognosis with high incidence of sudden death was influenced by significant referral biases.[54,55,118,152] These studies have been refuted by more recently reported mortality rates (approximately 1 percent per year) from unselected regional populations.[4,35–41] Indeed, HCM in the elderly has been shown to have mortality similar to control populations.[114]

Nonetheless, there are clearly patient subgroups at high risk for death.[3–5] Death can be sudden, unexpected, and may be the first manifestation of HCM, particularly in the young patients.[28,30,153,154] Sudden cardiac death (SCD) usually occurs in patients who have no or mild symptoms. SCD is most frequent in young adults but may also occur in the older population.[40] Reports of SCD in infants and very young children are extremely rare. A substantial proportion of patients die during or just after vigorous physical activity, and HCM has been shown to be the most common of sudden death among young competitive athletes.[28,29,31,32,155,156] Thus, young athletes with HCM should be advised against participating in competitive sports.[157–159]

The mechanisms of SCD, principally ventricular tachycardia and fibrillation, have been surmised from patients experiencing implantable defibrillator discharges.[160–162] However, other mechanisms including asystole, rapid atrial fibrillation, and electrical mechanical dissociation may also play a role.

There are several variables that have been associated with an increased risk of SCD:[30,55,56,116,117,153,154,163]

- A prior cardiac arrest or sustained ventricular tachycardia

- A family history of premature SCD caused by HCM
- Repetitive nonsustained ventricular tachycardia
- Massive ventricular hypertrophy (wall thickness >30 mm
- Hypotensive response to exercise

Electrophysiologic studies have not been shown to be of benefit and risk stratification in these patients.[164,165]

Other complications of HCM include infective endocarditis, systemic embolism, and atrial fibrillation. Infective endocarditis may occur in 4 to 5 percent of patients with HCM.[45,166] The lesions are usually located at the point of opposition of the mitral valve against the septum but can involve the mitral valve and less often the aortic valve. Atrial fibrillation occurs in up to 30 percent of older patients.[39,167] It usually indicates advanced disease and is associated with

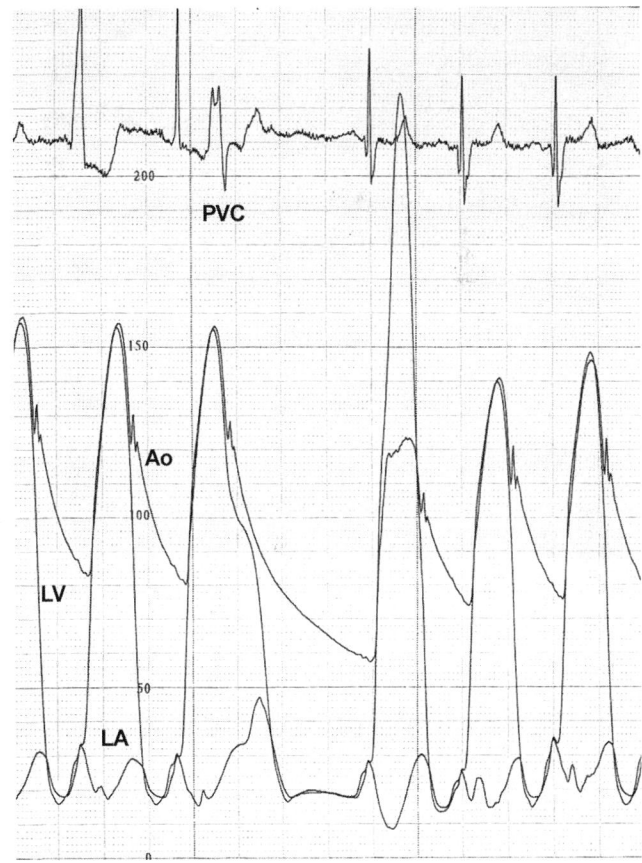

FIGURE 30–17. Cardiac catheterization from a patient with no resting LVO tract obstruction. However, following a premature ventricular contraction (PVC), there is a LVO tract gradient of near 100 mm of mercury. The pulse pressure of the ascending aorta (Ao) is decreased on the beat following the premature ventricular contraction. This phenomenon is termed the *Brockenbrough phenomenon.* LA, left atrium; LV, left ventricle; LVO, left ventricular outflow.

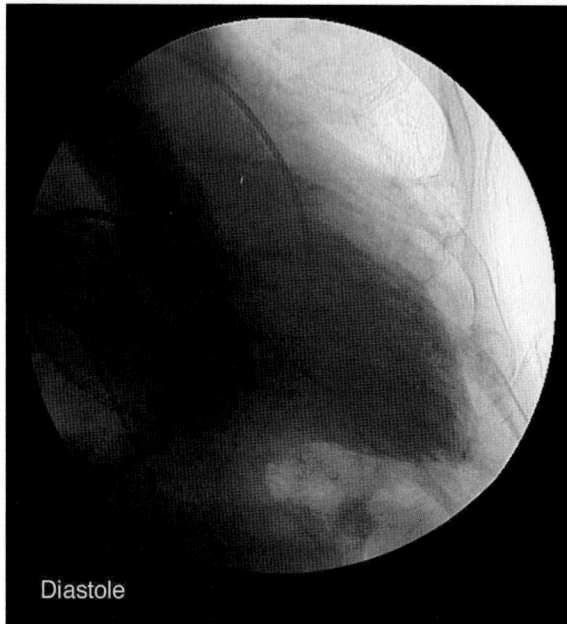

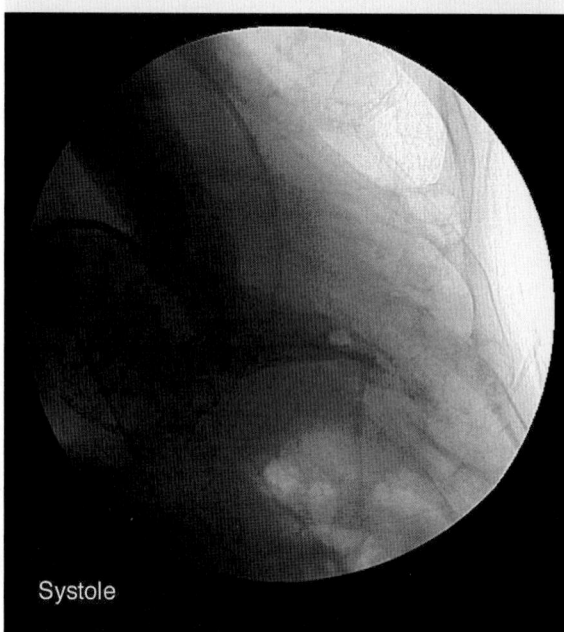

FIGURE 30–18. Left ventriculography from a patient with hypertrophic cardiomyopathy. There is near complete systolic obliteration of the left ventricular cavity.

clinical deterioration. Acute atrial fibrillation can result in prompt hemodynamic deterioration and immediate cardioversion to normal sinus rhythm is indicated. Systemic embolism occurs in 6 percent of patients and is usually associated with atrial fibrillation. Anticoagulation is recommended for patients with atrial fibrillation and HCM but will not fully eliminate the risk of stroke.

Less than 5 percent of HCM patients in a referral-based population will develop an *end-stage* phase of HCM.[168–170] In these patients there are progressive congestive heart failure symptoms with a significant limitation of exercise tolerance and atrial arrhythmias. The left ventricular cavity will enlarge and the dynamic outflow tract gradient will disappear. Eventu-

ally, the morphologic appearance of the ventricle will be similar to that of a dilated cardiomyopathy. These patients have a poor outlook with a high risk of death due to heart failure or arrhythmias.

TREATMENT

Treatment (Table 30–1) of HCM has been challenging because of the relatively small number of patients with this disease. There are no randomized trials for analysis of treatment regimens and data have been derived from retrospective observational studies of a small number of patients.

Treatment has been mainly directed at patients with obstructive HCM and there has been little to offer to patients who are symptomatic in the absence of obstruction. Although outflow tract obstruction under resting conditions is present in only 30 to 40 percent of patients, an additional 30 to 40 percent will have latent obstruction that must be carefully elucidated during the evaluation.

【 】 GENERAL GUIDELINES FOR THERAPY

General guidelines should be prescribed for all patients with HCM. Screening all first-degree relatives is recommended, because HCM is caused by an autosomal dominant gene disorder. Most commonly, echocardiography (or other imaging modality) is used as the screening tool. Using this strategy, screening of first-degree relatives should be performed every 12 to 18 months for children and anyone participating in competitive athletics. Adults who are no longer engaged in competitive athletics should be screened every 5 years. Clinical genetic testing is now available and may be useful for screening. If a mutation is identified in an affected patient, the family may be screened using targeted DNA analysis for that specific mutation. However, because many HCM patients do not have mutations detectable by current test panels, if no mutation is identified in the affected patient, the family screening must use the imaging strategy. All HCM patients should be counseled against engaging in competitive athletics.[157–159] Low to moderate levels of aerobic exercise are permitted as part of a healthy lifestyle. Patients with a dynamic LVO tract obstruction should be given infective endocarditis prophylaxis.[166] Patients should be instructed to maintain hydration at all times.

【 】 MEDICAL THERAPY

Medical therapy should be considered the initial therapeutic approach to relieving symptoms of patients with obstructive HCM. β-adrenergic blocking agents are the initial drug of choice.[6,7,45,152,241–243] Theoretic advantages of β blockers include (1) decreased heart rate response to exercise, (2) decreased outflow tract gradient with exercise, (3) relief of angina by a decrease in myocardial oxygen demand, and (4) improvement in diastolic filling. Acute hemodynamic studies have shown that β-blocking agents block the increase in gradient that occurs with exercise (or isoproterenol) but have no effect on the resting gradient. Clinical studies suggest an improvement in angina, exercise tolerance, and syncope in 60 to 80 percent of patients. However, only approximately 40 percent of patients continue to have sustained symptomatic im-

TABLE 30–1

Treatment of Hypertrophic Cardiomyopathy

REF	AUTHOR	YEAR	NUMBER OF PATIENTS	LENGTH OF FOLLOWUP	GRADIENT 1	GRADIENT 2	NYHA 1	NYHA 2	COMPLICATIONS	MORTALITY	COMMENT
Dual Chamber Pacing											
171	McDonald et al.	1988	9	3–24 mo	—	—	3	1.5	—	—	Improved exercise capacity
172	Jeanrenaud et al.	1992		82 mo	47	3			—	—	
173	Cannon et al.	1994	12	4 mo	—	—	3.3	—	—	8%	Symptoms improved by 1–2 classes
174	Fananapazir et al.	1994	84	28 mo	96	27	3.2	1.6	—	—	
175	Posma et al.	1996	6	3 mo	65	19	3.5	2	—	—	Improved homogeneity of perfusion with pacing
176	Slade et al.	1996	56	11 mo	78	36	2.75	1.69	—	—	Only patients responding to temporary pacing were entered
177	Gadler et al.	1997	19 (<40 mmHg) 22 (>40 mmHg)	6 mo	22 / 86	— / 26	3 / 2.8	1.9 / 1.8	—	0%	Comparison of outcome of minimal versus significant resting gradient
178	Kappenberger et al.	1997	83	3 mo AAI / 3 mo DDD	59 / 59	33 / 30	2.6 / 2.6	2.4 / 1.7	36%	0%	Randomized crossover
179	Nishimura et al.	1997	21	3 mo DDD / 3 mo AAI	76 / 76	55 / 83	2.9	2.4 / 2.6	—	—	Double-blind crossover study demonstrating placebo effect to AAI pacing
180	Rishi et al.	1997	10	23 mo	53	16	—		—	—	Pediatric-aged patients
181	Gadler et al.	1999	80	3 mo DDD 3 mo AAI 12 mo			2.54	1.7 2.2 1.62	—	—	Randomized crossover with 1 year of followup in preferred mode
182	Linde et al.	1999	81	3 mo DDD / 3 mo AAI	70 / 71	33 / 52	2.6 / 2.5	1.7 / 2.2	—	—	Subjective symptom reporting disproportionate to objective parameters in inactive pacing mode (PIC)

(continued)

TABLE 30-1

Treatment of Hypertrophic Cardiomyopathy (continued)

REF	AUTHOR	YEAR	NUMBER OF PATIENTS	LENGTH OF FOLLOWUP	GRADIENT 1	GRADIENT 2	NYHA 1	NYHA 2	COMPLICATIONS	MORTALITY	COMMENT
183	Maron et al.	1999	48	3 mo DDD / 3 mo AAI / 6 mo unblinded	82 82 82	48 76 48	—	—	—	—	Double-blind crossover with 6 additional months of active pacing—objective exercise data obtained
184	Pavin et al.	1999	23	16 mo	93	31	2.9	1.6	—	—	Mitral regurgitation significantly improved with pacing
185	Megevand et al.	2005	32	49 mo	82	32	2.4	1.8			
Surgery											
186	Tajik et al.	1974	43	84 mo	77		3	1.7		16%	
187	Morrow et al.	1975	83	72 mo	96	0	3.3	1.5	10%	7%	
188	Cooley et al.	1976	27	8–61 mo	74	7	—	72% improved	10%	4%	Mitral valve replacement
189	Agnew et al.	1977	49	89 mo	85	<10	2.8	1.4	10%	4%	
190	Maron et al.	1978	124	62 mo	73	23	3	1.7	—	8%	
191	Redwood et al.	1979	41	6 mo	37–118	—	—	—	5%	—	Improved cardiac output and hemodynamics
192	Maron et al.	1983	240	60 mo	—	—	≥3	70% improved	—	8%	
193	Cooper et al.	1987	11 HCM +CAD / 41 HCM no CAD	54 mo	65 95	3 17	3.2	1.9	—	27% 8%	All patients age >65
194	Cannon et al.	1989	20	6 mo	64	4	≥3	—	—	—	Improved O_2 supply–demand
195	Krajcer et al.	1989	127 Myectomy / 58 Mitral valve replacement	118 mo	69 75	10 10	3.2 3.4	2.1 2.2	3% 3%	5% 7%	
196	McIntosh et al.	1989	58	6 mo	66	4	3.1	1.8	~20%	9%	
197	Mohr et al.	1989	115	61 mo	70	9	2.3	1.4	11%	5%	Mitral valve replacement

(continued)

Ref	Author	Year	N	Follow-up							Comments
198	Mohr et al.	1989	47	60 mo	70	10	1.9	1.3	13%	0%	Mean age 21.5 y; range 0–38 y
199	Siegman et al.	1989	28	58 mo	86	3	3.3	2	21%	14%	HCM and CAD
200	Cohn et al.	1992	31	78 mo	96	5	3.1	1.7	6%	0	
201	Diodati et al.	1992	30	6 mo	79	15	—	—	—	—	Improved exercise capacity
202	McIntosh et al.	1992	36	6–12 mo	81	16	2.9	1.8	—	3%	Myectomy plus mitral valve plication
203	Schulte et al.	1993	364	98 mo	54	9	3	1.6		5%	
204	Schoendube et al.	1994	58	84	85	—	91% Class III–IV	23% Class III–IV	21%	0%	
205	ten Berg et al.	1994	38	82 mo	72	6	3	1.5	5%	0	Myectomy
206	Heric et al.	1995	178	44 mo	93	21	2.8	1.4		6%	
207	Schoendube et al.	1995	58	84 mo	79	5	3.1	1.8	7%	0	Myectomy
208	Kofflard et al.	1996	8		95	18	2.6	1	0	0	Myectomy + mitral leaflet extension
209	McCully et al.	1996	12 / 65	20 mo	87 / 73	23 / 9	2.8 / 3.2	1.7 / 1.6	0 / 6	0 / 4.6	Myectomy alone; 0% mortality in isolated myectomy
210	Robbins et al.	1996	158	72 mo	64	10	2.8			3.2	0% mortality in patients <60 y; 95% of patients with improved symptoms
211	Theodoro et al.	1996	25	77 mo	100	14	2.2	1.1	4%	0	Pediatric-age patients
212	Merrill et al.	2000	22	79 mo	78	12	—	—	9%	0	
213	Yu et al.	2000	104	5 d							Mitral regurgitation related to severity of obstruction and relieved with myectomy
214	Ommen et al.	2002	73		57	4	2.6		[a]	0	29% of patients developed transient postoperative atrial fibrillation
215	Ommen et al.	2002	256		68	10	2.7		1%	0	Intraoperative transesophageal echocardiography detected secondary cardiac anomalies
216	Woo et al.	2005	338	7.7 y	66	<15			[a]	0.8	30% of patients developed postoperative atrial fibrillation, 6% complete heart block

TABLE 30-1

Treatment of Hypertrophic Cardiomyopathy (continued)

REF	AUTHOR	YEAR	NUMBER OF PATIENTS	LENGTH OF FOLLOWUP	GRADIENT 1	GRADIENT 2	NYHA 1	NYHA 2	COMPLICATIONS	MORTALITY	COMMENT
217	Ommen et al.	2005	289	5.8 y	67	3	2.9	1.5	1.8	0.8	Long-term survival after myectomy is not different from the age-matched general population
Ablation											
218	Sigwart	1995	3	3 mo	27	8	—	—	—	4.40%	
219	Knight et al.	1997	18	3 mo	67	22	2.6	1.1	11%	0	
220	Kuhn et al.	1997									
221	Faber et al.	1998	91	3 mo	74	15	2.8	1.1	15%	1%	
222	Seggewiss et al.	1998	25	3 mo	62	18	2.8	1.2	28%	4%	
223	Gietzen et al.	1999	37	7 mo	45	5	3	1.7	38%	4%	
224	Henein et al.	1999	20	6 mo	60	22	—	—	—	—	
225	Kim et al.	1999	20	3 mo	58	14	2.7	1.6	10%	0	Improved exercise capacity
226	Kuhn et al.	1999	62	6 mo	54	6	—	—	—	—	
139	Nagueh et al.	1999	29	6 mo	54	6	3.1	1.2	—	—	Improved parameters of diastolic function following ablation
227	Faber et al.	2000	25	3 mo	60	20	2.8	1.4	20%	4%	3 patients required repeat ablation
				12 mo	60	9	2.8	1.4			
				30 mo	60	3	2.8	1.2			
228	Faber et al.	2000	162	3 mo	77	12	2.8	1.3	9%	2%	Use of echocardiographic myocardial contrast
229	Lakkis et al.	2000	50	12 mo	74	6	3	1.1	22%	4%	Improved exercise capacity
230	Ruzyllo et al.	2000	25	3 mo	85	36	2.8	—	28%	0	
				6 mo	85	32	2.8	1.2			
231	Boekstegers et al.	2001	50	4–6 mo	80	18	2.8	1.9	10%	0	
				12–18 mo	80	17	2.8	—			
232	Flores-Ramirez et al.	2001	30	6 mo	66	12	—	—	—	—	
233	Mazur et al.	2001	26	24 mo	36	0	3	1	27%	0	LVH regression demonstrated
234	Fernandes et al.	2005	137	3.6 y	74	4	3	1.2	[a]	1.5	13% developed complete heart block, 4% developed coronary dissection
235	Faber et al.	2005	242	4.9 mo	57	20	2.8	1.7		1.2	

Comparisons

236	Ommen et al.	1999	19 Pacing	3 mo	77	55	2.9	2.4	—	—	Exercise time and oxygen consumption better in surgical group
			20 Myectomy	14 mo	76	9	2.8	1.3	—	—	
237	Nagueh et al.	2001	41 Ablation	12 mo	76	8	3.4	1.1	22%	2%	9 new pacemakers, 1 death
			41 Myectomy	13 mo	78	4	3.1	1.2		0	1 new pacemaker, 8 transient AF, 0 deaths
238	Qin et al.	2001	25 Ablation	3 mo	64	24	3.5	1.9	24%	0	Similar outcomes between the two procedures
			26 Myectomy		62	11	3.3	1.5	7%	0	
239	Firoozi et al.	2002	20 Ablation		91	21	2.3	1.6	15%	5%	Surgical patients with better objective measures of exercise capacity
			24 Myectomy		83	12	2.4	1.5	4%	5%	
240	Ralph-Edwards et al.	2005	48 Myectomy		64	5	1.2	1.2	0	0	Long-term survival was better in the myectomy group
			54 Ablation		74	15	1.7	1.7		0	

AAI, atrial inhibited; CAD, coronary artery disease; DDD, dual-chamber pacemaker; HCM, hypertrophic cardiomyopathy; LVH, left ventricular hypertrophy; NYHA, New York Heart Association; PIC, pacing in cardiomyopathy.
aUnless otherwise noted.

provement.[241,242,244] There has been no proven reduction in the incidence of SCD with β blockade. The dosage of β blocker should be titrated to obtain a resting heart rate of 60 beats/min and may require up to 400 mg equivalent of metoprolol.

Calcium channel blockers, specifically verapamil and diltiazem, are also of value in the treatment of HCM.[90,245–250] Experimental work with calcium blockers as modifiers of ischemia-induced diastolic abnormalities prompted investigation of their use in HCM. By preventing calcium influx, theoretically they not only decrease inotropy and chronotropy but also improve abnormal diastolic relaxation.[90,248–250] Verapamil has been the calcium channel blocker used most frequently because of its minimal effect on afterload. Clinical studies show a decrease in both basal and provoked gradients during acute drug intervention with verapamil. In contrast to β-blocking drugs, an improvement in diastolic filling occurred with verapamil as judged by radionuclide angiographic studies.[90,248–250] Verapamil has been shown to improve exercise tolerance by 20 to 30 percent in short-term follow up. Calcium channel blockers may improve angina to a greater degree than β blockers. As with β blockers, verapamil results in sustained symptomatic improvement in <50 percent of patients. The dosage of verapamil should be titrated to obtain a resting heart rate of 60 beats/min and may require up to 480 mg/d.

A subset of patients undergo hemodynamic deterioration with calcium channel blocking agents, presumably caused by a lowering of the afterload.[251] This deterioration particularly occurs in the presence of severe outflow tract gradients and high diastolic filling pressures. Death from pulmonary edema has been reported after therapy with verapamil. Diltiazem has also been used to treat symptoms related to HCM; however, it has more theoretic vasodilating properties. Dihydropyridine-class calcium channel blockers should be avoided in patients with LVO obstruction because these pure vasodilators increase the severity of the outflow tract by reducing afterload.

Disopyramide has also been used to treat patients with obstructive HCM.[252–256] The negative inotropic effect decreases the gradient and improve symptoms. Concomitant β blockade may be important to prevent rapid atrioventricular node conduction, particularly during exercise or with coexistent atrial fibrillation.[256] Between 300 and 600 mg/d of disopyramide are required to produce symptomatic benefit. The corrected QT interval must be monitored at the initiation of this medication. The anticholinergic side effects of this approach may limit the efficacy of disopyramide in older patients.

The standard clinical practice for patients with symptomatic obstructive HCM is to start β blockade as the initial therapy. The β blocker should be gradually increased to optimal dosages. If patients cannot tolerate β blockers because of side effects, a calcium channel blocker, usually verapamil, should then be started. If there is a severe outflow tract obstruction and symptoms, the calcium blocker should be started under monitored condition in the hospital. If a patient does tolerate large dosages of either a β blocker or calcium channel blocker and continues to be severely symptomatic, there are no data to show that the combination of two drugs is better than one drug alone. Disopyramide may be added to either the β blocker or verapamil if symptoms persist. For patients in whom medical therapy is ineffective, other treatment options, such as septal myectomy, dual-chamber pacing, or septal ablation should be considered.

【 】 SEPTAL MYECTOMY

Surgical septal myectomy for HCM has been performed for more than 4 decades.[187,257] This operation is now established as a proven approach for relieving the outflow tract obstruction and has become the *gold standard* therapy for patients with obstruction and severe drug refractory symptoms.[200,203,205,209,212,258–263]

This procedure consists of a transaortic resection of a small amount of muscle from the proximal to midseptal region. This enlarges the LVO tract and significantly decreases or totally abolishes the LVO tract obstruction. In patients with concomitant mitral regurgitation secondary to SAM of the mitral valve, the mitral regurgitation also disappears as a result of the myectomy.[195,213] In some institutions, a more extensive myectomy procedure is performed in which the septal resection is wide and extended to the level of the papillary muscles.[264,265] In patients with abnormalities of the papillary muscle, dissection and reduction of the anomalous papillary muscle apparatus may also be performed at the time.[204,266] Mitral valvuloplasty or plication in combination with myectomy has been proposed for some patients with deformed or elongated mitral valve leaflets.[202,207,208]

Mitral valve replacement was recommended in patients with HCM on the assumption that the anterior leaflet of the mitral valve contributes to the outflow tract obstruction.[188] However, this should be performed only when there is associated severe and unrepairable organic disease of the mitral valve. It is highly unusual that a carefully performed septal myectomy cannot be done in patients with severe obstruction, even when there is only a modest increase in septal thickness (16–19 mm).

The operative mortality for septal myectomy over the past decade is now <1 percent.[214,216] The risk is higher in elderly patients who require other procedures, such as aortic valve replacement, mitral valve repair, or coronary artery bypass grafting. Complications (heart block, ventricular septal defect, and aortic regurgitation) of the surgery are rare. However, with increasing experience and newer surgical techniques, these complications occur in <1 percent of patients undergoing operation. These results are dependent not only on surgical expertise but also to the use of intraoperative transesophageal echocardiography.[215,267,268]

The results of an adequately performed septal myectomy are complete abolition of gradient, reduction in secondary mitral regurgitation, and a marked improvement in symptomatology. Many patients can achieve near normal exercise capacity and return to a normal lifestyle. Long-term follow up over several decades is now available for patients who have had septal myectomy.[195,200,203,207,212,216,217,261,269,270] Patients who undergo myectomy have been shown to maintain long-lasting improvement in symptoms and exercise capacity. There is some evidence from cohort studies that mortality may be improved after septal myectomy, particularly in younger patients with severe outflow tract obstruction.[198] More recently, a large cohort study has shown that survival following myectomy is equivalent to age and sex-matched expected survival in the general population and superior to that observed in a contemporary cohort of patients with outflow obstruction who did not undergo myectomy.[217] These data suggest that myectomy may influence long-term survival but are not sufficient to recommend changing the indications for operation or other interventions.

DUAL-CHAMBER PACING

Implantation of a dual-chamber pacemaker has been proposed as a less invasive therapeutic modality for treatment of symptomatic HCM patients.[271-273] Pacing the right ventricular apex in a subset of patients can decrease the outflow tract gradient, presumably because of ventricular contraction alteration with a decrease in systolic projection of the basal septum into the LVO tract. There may also be a chronic remodeling effect during continuous pacing with enlargement of the left ventricular cavity and further decrease in outflow tract obstruction.

There are technical considerations when using pacemaker therapy for treatment of patients with HCM.[271-273] Pacing or sensing atrium in addition to pacing the ventricle is necessary to maintain the important hemodynamic contribution of atrial contraction. There is an optimal atrioventricular delay for optimal hemodynamic performance[274,275] (Fig. 30–19). Too short an atrioventricular interval increases left atrial (LA) pressure and reduces preload. Too long an atrioventricular delay results in incomplete preexcitation of the right ventricle with suboptimal reduction in gradient. It is necessary to have the pacemaker tip placed in the apex of the right ventricle to achieve the greatest reduction in gradient.

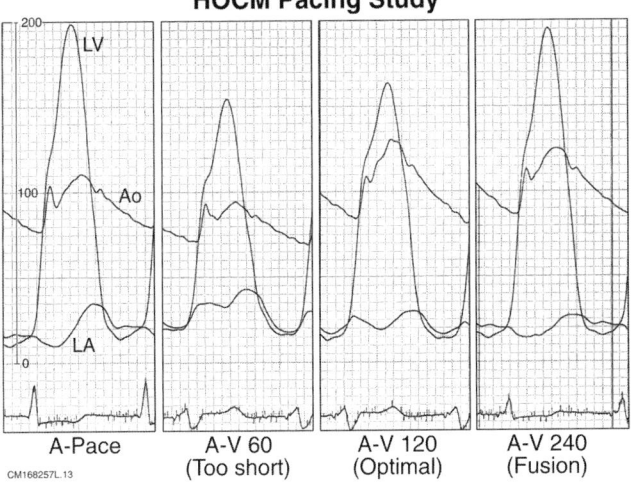

HOCM Pacing Study

A-Pace | A-V 60 (Too short) | A-V 120 (Optimal) | A-V 240 (Fusion)

CM168257L.13

FIGURE 30–19. Cardiac catheterization study during atrioventricular sequential pacing in a patient with hypertrophic obstructive cardiomyopathy, demonstrating the effect of the differing atrioventricular (AV) intervals. The left ventricular (LV) pressure, aortic pressure (Ao), and left atrial (LA) pressures are shown. In the baseline state (*A pace*) the patient is undergoing atrial pacing with native antegrade atrioventricular conduction. There is a left ventricular outflow (LVO) tract obstruction of 100 mm of mercury. *Left center panel*: The patient is undergoing atrioventricular pacing with an atrioventricular interval of 60 msec. This interval is too short, because atrial contraction is occurring on top of a closed mitral valve, causing an elevation of LA pressure. Although the gradient is decreased, there is also a drop in Ao caused by the decreased preload in the LV. *Right center panel*: This is the optimal atrioventricular interval of 120 msec. The gradient has been decreased to 35 mm of mercury. *Right panel*: The atrioventricular delay is 240 msec. There is fusion between the antegrade conduction and the paced QRS complex with incomplete preexcitation. The gradient across the LVO tract is 60 mm of mercury.

There was initial enthusiasm for dual-chamber pacing in HCM when several cohort trials emerged, which demonstrated improvement in gradient and relief of symptoms in >90 percent of patients.[174,276] However, subsequent more rigorous studies have shown that dual-chamber pacing is less efficacious than in the prior observational studies.[176–179,181–183,277] In randomized trials symptomatic improvement assessed by quality of life score was reported with a similar frequency by patients after a period of pacing versus a period of no pacing. Likewise, objective measurements of exercise capacity did not differ significantly during the periods with continuous pacing versus without continuous pacing. Although an overall decrease in outflow tract gradient did occur during pacing, the reduction was 25 to 40 percent of baseline, compared to 80 to 90 percent with septal myectomy. Thus, the average outflow tract gradient after continuous pacing in many studies remains at or over 50 mmHg.

Despite the less-than-optimal results, a subset of patients respond to dual chamber pacing. Approximately 40 percent of patients have continued symptomatic improvement with dual-chamber (DDD) pacing.[177,271] The degree of symptomatic improvement is significantly less than that achieved with other therapeutic invasive modalities.[278] Approximately 10 to 20 percent of patients achieve a combination of symptomatic improvement, a decrease in outflow tract gradient, and an objective improvement in exercise tolerance.[183] However, there are no known parameters that can identify patients who uniformly respond to dual-chamber pacing. Thus, the role of dual-chamber pacing should be limited to patients at high risk for other therapeutic modalities. Candidates for dual-chamber pacing might also include those who have significant bradycardia in which pacing may allow an increased dosage of medication or patients who need an automatic defibrillator as a primary treatment.

SEPTAL ABLATION

Alcohol septal ablation is a newer therapeutic modality in which alcohol is infused in the septal perforator arteries, producing a controlled myocardial infarction of the proximal septum.[218,219,279–284] The subsequent wall thinning and remodeling of the basal septum region induced by the infarction result in reduction of the outflow tract obstruction (Fig. 30–20 and Fig. 30–21).

The initial results from several centers have reported successful short-term outcomes following septal ablation.[219–221,223,226–229,285–292] The outflow tract gradient is reduced from a mean of 60 to 70 mm of mercury often to <20 mm of mercury. Most (80–85 percent) patients are improved from the symptomatic standpoint. There have also been documented significant increases in objective measurements of exercise tolerance.[286,290]

The major complication of septal ablation has been complete heart block. In the early experience, heart block occurred in 30 to 40 percent of patients undergoing septal ablation. However, as the procedure evolved, using smaller doses of alcohol more selectively and guidance by myocardial contrast echocardiography, the complication of complete heart block has decreased.[221,293,294] In some studies the incidence of complete heart block requiring permanent pacemaker has dropped to <10 percent. Patients are more likely to experience complete heart block if left bundle-branch block was present prior to the ablation procedure.[295,296]

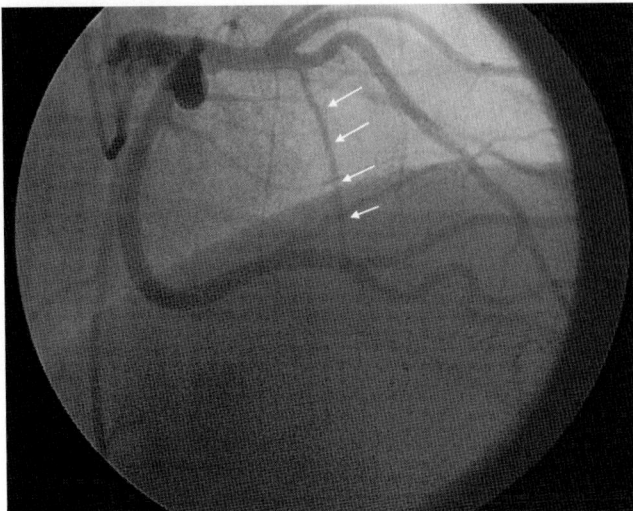 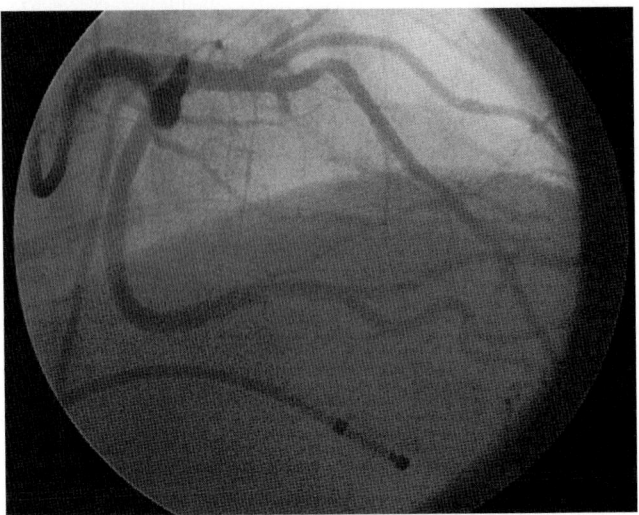

FIGURE 30–20. Coronary angiogram of a patient undergoing septal ablation. A large first septal perforator artery is shown by the *white arrows*. Following the septal ablation, there has been complete cessation of flow in the first septal perforator artery (*right panel*).

Other complications of septal ablation include coronary dissections, large myocardial infarctions from alcohol *leakage* into other coronary arteries, ventricular septal defects, and myocardial perforations. Intractable ventricular fibrillation has occurred during the time of the procedure. The true incidence of these complications is unknown, because most septal ablations are likely performed in centers that have not had the large experience or high volumes and thus are not reported in the literature.

Although septal ablation has been an attractive catheter-based alternative to septal myectomy, the ultimate role of this procedure in the treatment of HCM is unclear.[4,284,295-298] There is controversy over whether the results of septal ablation are comparable to septal myectomy.[237,239,240,299,300] Overall, septal ablation is not as efficacious as septal myectomy in eliminating the outflow tract obstruction because its results depend on the presence of a septal artery that directly supplies the region of the mitral valve–septal contact. There has been the concern that the production of a myocardial infarction may have detrimental long-term outcome. The residual scar that results from the septal ablation procedure is usually transmural and comprises 5 to 10 percent of the ventricular muscle mass.[301] These HCM patients are already prone to ventricular arrhythmias and whether a myocardial infarction may increase the susceptibility to arrhythmia is unclear. In addition, adverse ventricular remodeling after myocardial infarction is another potential concern. There is now limited followup of <8 years, which may not be long enough for long-term detrimental effects to emerge.

There is also concern that septal ablation is being performed sporadically at centers that do not have extensive knowledge of this complex, underlying disease process. Patients presenting for consideration of septal ablation may have other anatomic or pathophysiologic abnormalities that would make them unsuitable for the procedure, such as fixed subaortic stenosis, concomitant primary mitral valve disease, or anomalous papillary muscle apparatus. The large number of procedures that have been performed in recent years has raised concerns that the threshold for intervention has been lowered as a result of the less invasive nature of sep-

tal ablation. There are no data confirming that this procedure should be performed for any indication other than severe symptoms unresponsive to optimal medical management. Current guidelines support the use of septal ablation as an alternative to septal myectomy for patients with severe, medication-refractory symptoms, in whom the risk of surgical septal myectomy is felt to be increased because of comorbidities.[263]

TREATMENT OF NONOBSTRUCTIVE CARDIOMYOPATHY

Less is known about treatment of patients without obstruction, in whom the major pathophysiologic abnormality is severe diastolic dysfunction. Diuretics are used to decrease elevated filling pressures. Both β blockers and calcium channel blockers have been used to improve diastolic filling. Verapamil may have a greater effect on improving relaxation abnormalities. Cardiac transplantation remains the only therapy for patients who have severe symptoms unresponsive to conventional treatments. Promising new therapies with angiotensin-converting enzyme inhibitors, angiotensin II receptor blockers, statins, and calcium blockers may be of benefit based on animal models of HCM and await human trials.[17,18,20,26,27,302,303]

PREGNANCY

All HCM patients who wish to become pregnant should be given prenatal counseling about the risk of transmission of disease to their offspring and be followed at a tertiary center with expertise in high-risk pregnancies and cardiac disease. Patients with HCM usually tolerate pregnancy well, if they are not severely symptomatic prior to conception. This is in part because of the increase in blood volume that occurs during pregnancy. If patients have been on treatment with β blockers or calcium blockers, these drugs should be continued throughout the pregnancy. Additional low-dose diuretics may be required if pulmonary congestion occurs. There is no evidence that pregnancy increases the risk of SCD. La-

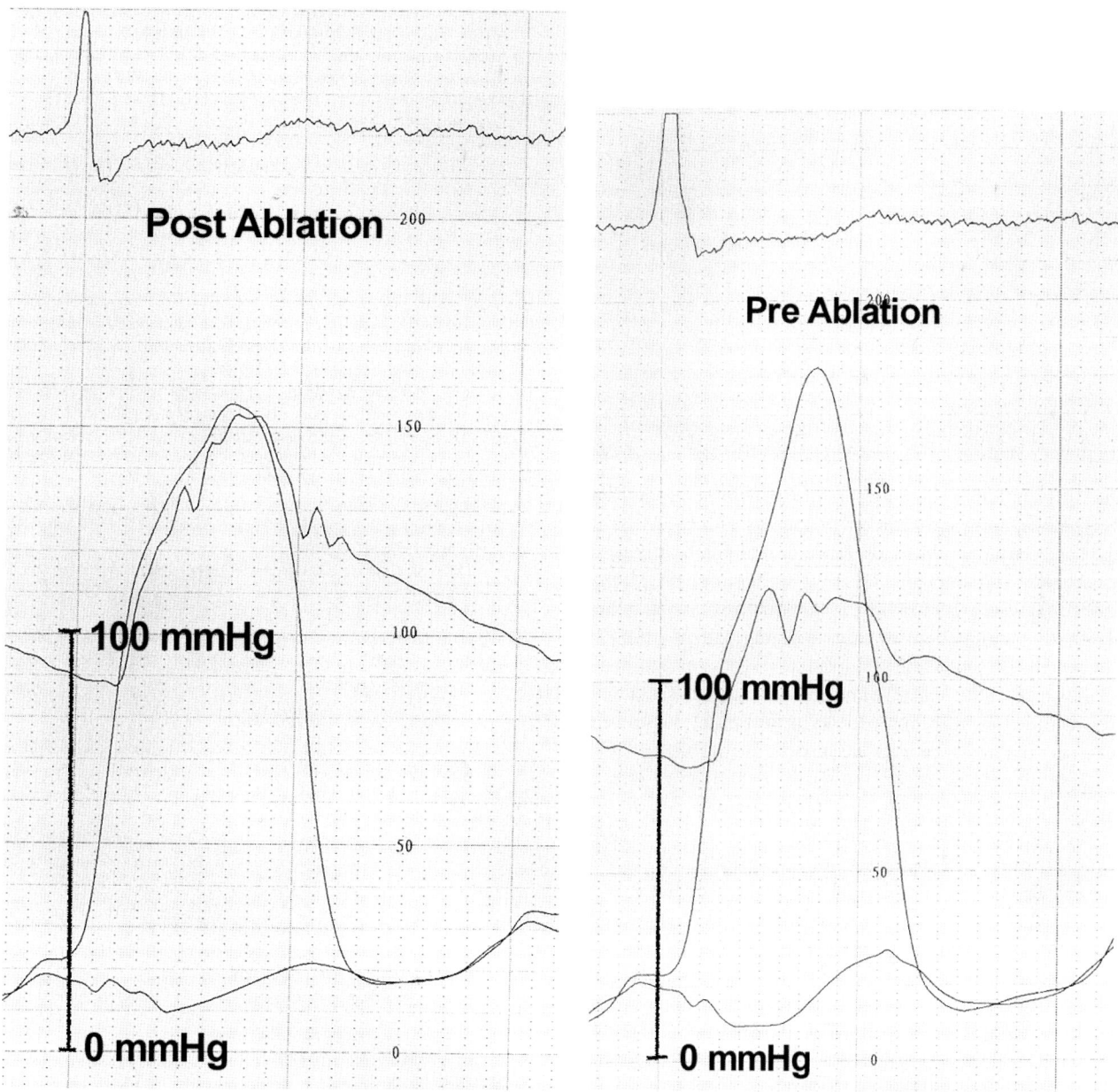

FIGURE 30–21. *Left*: Cardiac catheterization before ablation, demonstrating left ventricular outflow (LVO) tract obstruction of 60 mm of mercury. *Right*: Following the septal ablation, there has been complete obliteration of the gradient across the LVO tract.

bor and delivery should be done in a high-risk center with meticulous attention to the cardiac disease throughout, given the fluid shifts that occur.

【 】 PREVENTION OF SUDDEN DEATH

SCD is the most devastating complication of HCM.[4–7,28–34, 55,56,116,118,155,156,304,305] SCD occurs most frequently in the asymptomatic or mildly symptomatic patient and mainly in the young population. However, patients prone to SCD constitute only a few in the overall disease population. Therefore, a major focus of investigation has been to identify patients at high risk for SCD.

There are several clinical features are associated with a high risk for SCD in patients with HCM[4,6,7,55,56,116–118,153,154,163,306–308] (Table 30–2). Patients who have had a prior cardiac arrest or sponta-

neous sustained ventricular tachycardia are at highest risk. A family history of premature SCD in a patient with HCM portends a high risk, particularly if there are multiple occurrences. Other parameters include unexplained syncope, nonsustained ventricular tachycardia, abnormal blood pressure response to exercise, and extreme left ventricular hypertrophy (>30 mm). Delayed gadolinium enhancement demonstrated using cardiac magnetic resonance may also help identify higher-risk patients.[143,144]

It has been proposed that genotype analysis might used as a stratifying marker for prognosis, particularly because specific mutations have been shown to convey either favorable or adverse prognosis.[17,18,20,309–312] However, these studies are based on a relatively small number of genotyped families. Extrapolating these conclusions about risk based on genotype to an overall HCM population is not proven.[313–315]

TABLE 30–2

Clinical Features Associated with SCD

Major Risk Factors
- Prior personal history of sudden cardiac death or out-of-hospital cardiac arrest
- Spontaneous sustained ventricular tachycardia or ventricular fibrillation

Other Risk Factors
- Family history of sudden cardiac death
- Extreme left ventricular hypertrophy (>30 mm)
- Nonsustained ventricular tachycardia
- Abnormal blood pressure response to exercise
- Repetitive syncope
- Delayed gadolinium enhancement on cardiac MRI

At the present time, there are no antiarrhythmic agents that have been shown to improve survival in patients with HCM. Amiodarone has been shown in retrospective nonrandomized trials to be associated with improved survival in young HCM patients.[316,317] However, because of the potential toxicity of taking amiodarone for long periods of time in young patients, the risk may outweigh the benefit.[318] Implantation of an automatic defibrillator is the most effective and reliable treatment option at the present time for protecting patients against SCD due to ventricular arrhythmias.[162] Patients deemed at high risk for SCD should have placement of an automatic defibrillator. This is strongly warranted for patients with prior cardiac arrest or sustained spontaneous ventricular tachycardia. In other patients clinical judgment must be made for an individual patient, taking into consideration the overall clinical profile and other risk factors.

SUMMARY

HCM is a fascinating disease entity that has intrigued cardiologists for decades. It is a highly heterogeneous disease, with a diverse pathology, pathophysiology, and clinical course. Therapies have been introduced for treatment of obstruction, and the long-term follow up of each of these is required to determine the optimal therapy for individual patients. The genetic discoveries have raised important questions approximately the diagnosis and prognosis of these patients. Genetic models have provided the opportunity to identify therapies to inhibit the growth factor or its signaling pathways and attenuate the extent of hypertrophy and fibrosis. The extension of the results of these animal models to human therapy and ultimately the ability to manipulate the abnormal genome are the basis of future therapy.[17,18,20,26,27,302,303]

REFERENCES

1. Wigle ED, Sasson Z, Henderson MA, et al. Hypertrophic cardiomyopathy: the importance of the site and the extent of hypertrophy—a review. *Prog Cardiovasc Dis* 1985;28:1–83.
2. Wigle ED, Rakowski H, Kimball B, Williams WG. Hypertrophic cardiomyopathy: clinical spectrum and treatment. *Circulation* 1995;92:1680–1692.
3. Spirito P, Seidman CE, McKenna WJ, Maron BJ. The management of hypertrophic cardiomyopathy. *N Engl J Med* 1997;336:775–785.
4. Maron BJ. Hypertrophic cardiomyopathy: a systematic review. *JAMA* 2002;287:1308–1320.
5. Maron BJ. Hypertrophic cardiomyopathy. *Lancet* 1997;350:127–133.
6. Maron BJ, Bonow RO, Cannon RO III, Leon MB, Epstein SE. Hypertrophic cardiomyopathy: interrelations of clinical manifestations, pathophysiology, and therapy. *N Engl J Med* 1987;316:780–789.
7. Maron BJ, Bonow RO, Canon RO III, Leon MB, Epstein S. Hypertrophic cardiomyopathy: interrelations of clinical manifestations, pathophysiology, and therapy. *N Engl J Med* 1987;316:844–852.
8. Maron BJ, Gardin JM, Flack JM, Gidding SS, Kurosaki TT, Bild DE. Prevalence of hypertrophic cardiomyopathy in a general population of young adults: echocardiographic analysis of 4111 subjects in the CARDIA Study—Coronary Artery Risk Development in (Young) Adults. *Circulation* 1995;92:785–789.
9. Goodwin JF. ?IHSS. ?HOCM. ?ASH: a plea for unity. *Am Heart J* 1975;89:269–277.
10. Goodwin JF. The frontiers of cardiomyopathy. *Br Heart J* 1982;48:1–18.
11. Hejtmancik JF, Brink PA, Towbin J, et al. Localization of gene for familial hypertrophic cardiomyopathy to chromosome 14q1 in a diverse US population. *Circulation* 1991;83:1592–1597.
12. Jarcho JA, McKenna W, Pare JA, et al. Mapping a gene for familial hypertrophic cardiomyopathy to chromosome 14q1. *N Engl J Med* 1989;321:1372–1378.
13. Geisterfer-Lowrance AA, Kass S, Tanigawa G, et al. A molecular basis for familial hypertrophic cardiomyopathy: a beta cardiac myosin heavy chair gene missense mutation. *Cell* 1990;62:999–1006.
14. Rosenzweig A, Watkins H, Hwang DS, et al. Preclinical diagnosis of familial hypertrophic cardiomyopathy by genetic analysis of blood lymphocytes. *N Engl J Med* 1991;325:1753–1760.
15. Van Driest SL, Ommen SR, Tajik AJ, Gersh BJ, Ackerman MJ. Sarcomeric genotyping in hypertrophic cardiomyopathy. *Mayo Clin Proc* 2005;80:463–469.
16. Van Driest SL, Ommen SR, Tajik AJ, Gersh BJ, Ackerman MJ. Yield of genetic testing in hypertrophic cardiomyopathy. *Mayo Clin Proc* 2005;80:739–744.
17. Roberts R, Sigwart U. New concepts in hypertrophic cardiomyopathies, part I. *Circulation* 2001;104:2113–2116.
18. Roberts R, Sigwart U. New concepts in hypertrophic cardiomyopathies, part II. *Circulation* 2001;104:2249–2252.
19. Marian AJ, Roberts R. Molecular genetics of hypertrophic cardiomyopathy. *Annu Rev Med* 1995;46:213–222.
20. Marian AJ, Roberts R. Recent advances in the molecular genetics of hypertrophic cardiomyopathy. *Circulation* 1995;92:1336–1347.
21. Marian AJ, Yu QT, Mares A Jr, Hill R, Roberts R, Perryman MB. Detection of a new mutation in the beta-myosin heavy chain gene in an individual with hypertrophic cardiomyopathy. *J Clin Invest* 1992;90:2156–2165.
22. Marian AJ. Pathogenesis of diverse clinical and pathological phenotypes in hypertrophic cardiomyopathy. *Lancet* 2000;355:58–60.
23. Marian AJ, Roberts R. The molecular genetic basis for hypertrophic cardiomyopathy. *J Mol Cell Cardiol* 2001;33:655–670.
24. Watkins H, Rosenzweig A, Hwang DS, et al. Characteristics and prognostic implications of myosin missense mutations in familial hypertrophic cardiomyopathy. *N Engl J Med* 1992;326:1108–1114.
25. Watkins H, Thierfelder L, Hwang DS, McKenna W, Seidman JG, Seidman CE. Sporadic hypertrophic cardiomyopathy due to de novo myosin mutations. *J Clin Invest* 1992;90:1666–1671.
26. Seidman JG, Seidman C. The genetic basis for cardiomyopathy: from mutation identification to mechanistic paradigms. *Cell* 2001;104:557–567.
27. Seidman C. Genetic causes of inherited cardiac hypertrophy: Robert L. Frye lecture. *Mayo Clin Proc* 2002;77:1315–1319.
28. Maron BJ, Roberts WC, Epstein SE. Sudden death in hypertrophic cardiomyopathy: a profile of 78 patients. *Circulation* 1982;65:1388–1394.
29. Maron BJ, Roberts WC, McAllister HA, Rosing DR, Epstein SE. Sudden death in young athletes. *Circulation* 1980;62:218–229.
30. Maron BJ, Roberts WC, Edwards JE, McAllister HA Jr, Foley DD, Epstein SE. Sudden death in patients with hypertrophic cardiomyopathy: characterization of 26 patients with functional limitation. *Am J Cardiol* 1978;41:803–810.
31. Maron BJ, Shirani J, Poliac LC, Mathenge R, Roberts WC, Mueller FO. Sudden death in young competitive athletes: clinical, demographic, and pathological profiles. *JAMA* 1996;276:199–204.
32. Maron BJ, Klues HG. Surviving competitive athletics with hypertrophic cardiomyopathy. *Am J Cardiol* 1994;73:1098–1104.
33. Maron BJ, Kragel AH, Roberts WC. Sudden death in hypertrophic cardiomyopathy with normal left ventricular mass. *Br Heart J* 1990;63:308–310.
34. Maron BJ. Cardiovascular risks to young persons on the athletic field. *Ann Intern Med* 1998;129:379–386.
35. Maron BJ, Casey SA, Poliac LC, Gohman TE, Almquist AK, Aeppli DM. Clinical course of hypertrophic cardiomyopathy in a regional United States cohort. *JAMA* 1999;281:650–655.

36. Maron BJ, Mathenge R, Casey SA, Poliac LC, Longe TF. Clinical profile of hypertrophic cardiomyopathy identified de novo in rural communities. *J Am Coll Cardiol* 1999;33:1590–1595.

37. Spirito P, Chiarella F, Carratino L, Berisso MZ, Bellotti P, Vecchio C. Clinical course and prognosis of hypertrophic cardiomyopathy in an outpatient population. *N Engl J Med* 1989;320:749–755.

38. Cannan CR, Reeder GS, Bailey KR, Melton LJ III, Gersh BJ. Natural history of hypertrophic cardiomyopathy: a population-based study, 1976 through 1990. *Circulation* 1995;92:2488–2495.

39. Cecchi F, Olivotto I, Montereggi A, Santoro G, Dolara A, Maron BJ. Hypertrophic cardiomyopathy in Tuscany: clinical course and outcome in an unselected regional population. *J Am Coll Cardiol* 1995;26:1529–1536.

40. Maron BJ, Olivotto I, Spirito P, et al. Epidemiology of hypertrophic cardiomyopathy-related death: revised in a large non-referral-based patient population. *Circulation* 2000;102:858–864.

41. Maron BJ, Spirito P. Impact of patient selection biases on the perception of hypertrophic cardiomyopathy and its natural history. *Am J Cardiol* 1993;72:970–972.

42. Teare D. Asymmetrical hypertrophy of the heart in young adults. *Br Heart J* 1958;20:1–18.

43. Brock RC. Functional obstruction of the left ventricle. *Guys Hosp Rep* 1957;106:221–238.

44. Braunwald E, Lambrew CD, Rockoff SD, Ross J Jr, Morrow AG. Idiopathic hypertrophic subaortic stenosis: I. A description of the disease based on an analysis of 64 patients. *Circulation* 1964;30:3–217.

45. Frank S, Braunwald E. Idiopathic hypertrophic subaortic stenosis: clinical analysis of 126 patients with emphasis on the natural history. *Circulation* 1968;37:759–788.

46. Clark CE, Henry WL, Epstein SE. Familial prevalence and genetic transmission of idiopathic hypertrophic subaortic stenosis. *N Engl J Med* 1973;289:709–714.

47. Brandenburg RO, Chazov E, Cherian G. Report of the WHO/ISFC task force on definition and classification of cardiomyopathies. *Circulation* 1981;64:437a–438a.

48. Richardson P, McKenna W, Bristow M, et al. Report of the 1995 World Health Organization International Society and Federation of Cardiology Task Force on the definition and classification of cardiomyopathies. *Circulation* 1996;93:841–842.

49. Henry WL, Clark CE, Epstein SE. Asymmetric septal hypertrophy: echocardiographic identification of the pathognomonic anatomic abnormality of IHSS. *Circulation* 1973;47:225–233.

50. Menge H, Brandenburg RO, Brown Jr A. The clinical, hemodynamic, and pathologic diagnosis of muscular subvalvular aortic stenosis. *Circulation* 1961;24:1126–1136.

51. Shah PM, Gramiak R, Kramer DH. Ultrasound localization of left ventricular outflow obstruction in hypertrophic obstructive cardiomyopathy. *Circulation* 1969;40:3–11.

52. Charron P, Dubourg O, Desnos M, et al. Clinical features and prognostic implications of familial hypertrophic cardiomyopathy related to the cardiac myosin-binding protein C gene. *Circulation* 1998;97:2230–2236.

53. Charron P, Dubourg O, Desnos M, et al. Diagnostic value of electrocardiography and echocardiography for familial hypertrophic cardiomyopathy in genotyped children. *Eur Heart J* 1998;19:1377–1382.

54. Shah PM, Adelman AG, Wigle ED, et al. The natural (and unnatural) history of hypertrophic obstructive cardiomyopathy. *Circ Res* 1974:179–195.

55. McKenna W, Deanfield J, Faruqui A, England D, Oakley C, Goodwin J. Prognosis in hypertrophic cardiomyopathy: role of age and clinical, electrocardiographic and hemodynamic features. *Am J Cardiol* 1981;47:532–538.

56. McKenna WJ, Deanfield JE. Hypertrophic cardiomyopathy: an important cause of sudden death. *Arch Dis Child* 1984;59:971–975.

57. Yu B, French JA, Carrier L, et al. Molecular pathology of familial hypertrophic cardiomyopathy caused by mutations in the cardiac myosin binding protein C gene. *Eur J Med Genet* 1998;35:205–210.

58. Watkins H, Conner D, Thierfelder L, et al. Mutations in the cardiac myosin binding protein-C gene on chromosome 11 cause familial hypertrophic cardiomyopathy. *Nat Genet* 1995;11:434–437.

59. Watkins H, McKenna WJ, Thierfelder L, et al. Mutations in the genes for cardiac troponin T and alpha-tropomyosin in hypertrophic cardiomyopathy. *N Engl J Med* 1995;332:1058–1064.

60. Thierfelder L, Watkins H, MacRae C, et al. Alpha-tropomyosin and cardiac troponin T mutations cause familial hypertrophic cardiomyopathy: a disease of the sarcomere. *Cell* 1994;77:701–712.

61. Charron P, Dubourg O, Desnos M, et al. Diagnostic value of electrocardiography and echocardiography for familial hypertrophic cardiomyopathy in a genotyped adult population. *Circulation* 1997;96:214–219.

62. Kimura A, Harada H, Park JE, et al. Mutations in the cardiac troponin I gene associated with hypertrophic cardiomyopathy. *Nat Genet* 1997;16:379–382.

63. Karibe A, Tobacman LS, Strand J, et al. Hypertrophic cardiomyopathy caused by a novel alpha-tropomyosin mutation (V95A) is associated with mild cardiac phenotype, abnormal calcium binding to troponin, abnormal myosin cycling, and poor prognosis. *Circulation* 2001;103:65–71.

64. Ho CY, Lever HM, DeSanctis R, Farver CF, Seidman JG, Seidman CE. Homozygous mutation in cardiac troponin T: implication for hypertrophic cardiomyopathy. *Circulation* 2000;102:1950–1955.

65. Flavigny J, Richard P, Isnard R, et al. Identification of two novel mutations in the ventricular regulatory myosin light chain gene (MYL2) associated with familial and classical forms of hypertrophic cardiomyopathy. *J Mol Med* 1998;76:208–214.

66. Erdmann J, Raible J, Maki-Abadi J, et al. Spectrum of clinical phenotypes and gene variants in cardiac myosin-binding protein C mutation carriers with hypertrophic cardiomyopathy. *J Am Coll Cardiol* 2001;38:322–330.

67. Mogensen J, Klausen IC, Pedersen AK, et al. Alpha-cardiac actin is a novel disease gene in familial hypertrophic cardiomyopathy. *J Clin Invest* 1999;103:R39–R43.

68. Moolman JC, Corfield VA, Posen B, et al. Sudden death due to troponin T mutations. *J Am Coll Cardiol* 1997;29:549–555.

69. Niimura H, Patton KK, McKenna WJ, et al. Sarcomere protein gene mutations in hypertrophic cardiomyopathy of the elderly. *Circulation* 2002;105:446–451.

70. Niimura H, Bachinski LL, Sangwatanaroj S, et al. Mutations in the gene for cardiac myosin-binding protein C and late-onset familial hypertrophic cardiomyopathy. *N Engl J Med* 1998;338:1248–1257.

71. Bos J, Poley R, Ny M, et al. Genotype-phenotype relationships involving hypertrophic cardiomyopathy-associated mutations in titin, muscle LIM protein, and telethonin. *Mol Genet Metab* 2006;88:78–85.

72. Gollob MH, Green MS, Tang AS, et al. Identification of a gene responsible for familial Wolff-Parkinson-White syndrome. *N Engl J Med* 2001;344:1823–1831.

73. Blair E, Redwood C, Ashrafian H, et al. Mutations in the gamma(2) subunit of AMP-activated protein kinase cause familial hypertrophic cardiomyopathy: evidence for the central role of energy compromise in disease pathogenesis. *Hum Mol Genet* 2001;10:1215–1220.

74. Arad M, Benson DW, Perez-Atayde AR, et al. Constitutively active AMP kinase mutations cause glycogen storage disease mimicking hypertrophic cardiomyopathy. *J Clin Invest* 2002;109:357–362.

75. Marian AJ, Yu QT, Mann DL, Graham FL, Roberts R. Expression of a mutation causing hypertrophic cardiomyopathy disrupts sarcomere assembly in adult feline cardiac myocytes. *Circ Res* 1995;77:98–106.

76. Perryman MB, Yu QT, Marian AJ, et al. Expression of a missense mutation in the messenger RNA for beta-myosin heavy chain in myocardial tissue in hypertrophic cardiomyopathy. *J Clin Invest* 1992;90:271–277.

77. Marian AJ, Zhao G, Seta Y, Roberts R, Yu QT. Expression of a mutant (Arg92Gln) human cardiac troponin T, known to cause hypertrophic cardiomyopathy, impairs adult cardiac myocyte contractility. *Circ Res* 1997;81:76–85.

78. Marian AJ, Yu QT, Workman R, Greve G, Roberts R. Angiotensin-converting enzyme polymorphism in hypertrophic cardiomyopathy and sudden cardiac death. *Lancet* 1993;342:1085–1086.

79. Osterop AP, Kofflard MJ, Sandkuijl LA, et al. AT1 receptor A/C1166 polymorphism contributes to cardiac hypertrophy in subjects with hypertrophic cardiomyopathy. *Hypertension* 1998;32:825–830.

80. Lechin M, Quinones MA, Omran A, et al. Angiotensin-I converting enzyme genotypes and left ventricular hypertrophy in patients with hypertrophic cardiomyopathy. *Circulation* 1995;92:1808–1812.

81. Perkins MJ, Van Driest SL, Ellsworth EG, et al. Gene-specific modifying effects of pro-LVH polymorphisms involving the renin-angiotensin-aldosterone system among 389 unrelated patients with hypertrophic cardiomyopathy. *Eur Heart J* 2005;26:2457–2462.

82. Binder J, Ommen SR, Gersh BJ, et al. Echocardiography-guided genetic testing in hypertrophic cardiomyopathy: septal morphological features predict the presence of myofilament mutations. *Mayo Clin Proc* 2006;81:459–467.

83. Davies MJ, Pomerance A, Teare RD. Pathological features of hypertrophic obstructive cardiomyopathy. *J Clin Pathol* 1974;27:529–535.

84. Olsen EG. The pathology of cardiomyopathies: a critical analysis. *Am Heart J* 1979;98:385–392.

85. Davies MJ, McKenna WJ. Hypertrophic cardiomyopathy-pathology and pathogenesis. *Histopathology* 1995;26:493–500.

86. Maron BJ, Epstein SE, Roberts WC. Hypertrophic cardiomyopathy and transmural myocardial infarction without significant atherosclerosis of the extramural coronary arteries. *Am J Cardiol* 1979;43:1086–1102.

87. Maron BJ, Wolfson JK, Epstein SE, Roberts WC. Intramural ("small vessel") coronary artery disease in hypertrophic cardiomyopathy. *J Am Coll Cardiol* 1986;8:545–557.

88. Maron BJ, Roberts WC. Quantitative analysis of cardiac muscle cell disorganization in the ventricular septum of patients with hypertrophic cardiomyopathy. *Circulation* 1979;59:689–706.

89. Maron BJ, Anan TJ, Roberts WC. Quantitative analysis of the distribution of cardiac muscle cell disorganization in the left ventricular wall of patients with hypertrophic cardiomyopathy. *Circulation* 1981;63:882–894.

90. Bonow RO, Dilsizian V, Rosing DR, Maron BJ, Bacharach SL, Green MV. Verapamil-induced improvement in left ventricular diastolic filling and increased exercise tolerance in patients with hypertrophic cardiomyopathy: short- and long-term effects. *Circulation* 1985;72:853–864.

91. Bonow RO, Vitale DF, Maron BJ, Bacharach SL, Frederick TM, Green MV. Regional left ventricular asynchrony and impaired global left ventricular filling in hypertrophic cardiomyopathy: effect of verapamil. *J Am Coll Cardiol* 1987;9:1108–1116.

92. Nihoyannopoulos P, Karatasakis G, Frenneaux M, McKenna WJ, Oakley CM. Diastolic function in hypertrophic cardiomyopathy: relation to exercise capacity. *J Am Coll Cardiol* 1992;19:536–540.

93. Criley JM, Siegel RJ. Has "obstruction" hindered our understanding of hypertrophic cardiomyopathy? *Circulation* 1985;72:1148–1154.

94. Criley JM, Siegel RJ. Obstruction is unimportant in the pathophysiology of hypertrophic cardiomyopathy. *Postgrad Med J* 1986;62:515–529.

95. Criley JM. Unobstructed thinking (and terminology) is called for in the understanding and management of hypertrophic cardiomyopathy. *J Am Coll Cardiol* 1997;29:741–743.

96. Shah PM, Taylor RD, Wong M. Abnormal mitral valve coaptation in hypertrophic obstructive cardiomyopathy: proposed role in systolic anterior motion of mitral valve. *Am J Cardiol* 1981;48:258–262.

97. Jiang L, Levine RA, King ME, Weyman AE. An integrated mechanism for systolic anterior motion of the mitral valve in hypertrophic cardiomyopathy based on echocardiographic observations. *Am Heart J* 1987;113:633–644.

98. Sherrid MV, Chu CK, Delia E, Mogtader A, Dwyer EM Jr. An echocardiographic study of the fluid mechanics of obstruction in hypertrophic cardiomyopathy. *J Am Coll Cardiol* 1993;22:816–825.

99. Sherrid MV. Dynamic left ventricular outflow obstruction in hypertrophic cardiomyopathy revisited: significance, pathogenesis, and treatment. *Cardiol Rev* 1998;6:135–145.

100. Sherrid MV, Gunsburg DZ, Moldenhauer S, Pearle G. Systolic anterior motion begins at low left ventricular outflow tract velocity in obstructive hypertrophic cardiomyopathy. *J Am Coll Cardiol* 2000;36:1344–1354.

101. Falicov RE, Resnekov L, Bharati S, Lev M. Mid-ventricular obstruction: a variant of obstructive cardiomyopathy. *Am J Cardiol* 1976;37:432–437.

102. Kizilbash AM, Heinle SK, Grayburn PA. Spontaneous variability of left ventricular outflow tract gradient in hypertrophic obstructive cardiomyopathy. *Circulation* 1998;97:461–466.

103. Maron M, Olivotto I, Betocchi S, et al. Effect of left ventricular outflow tract obstruction on clinical outcome in hypertrophic cardiomyopathy. *N Engl J Med* 2003;348:295–303.

104. Cannon RO, III, Rosing DR, Maron BJ, et al. Myocardial ischemia in patients with hypertrophic cardiomyopathy: contribution of inadequate vasodilator reserve and elevated left ventricular filling pressures. *Circulation* 1985;71:234–243.

105. Cannon RO, III, Schenke WH, Maron BJ, et al. Differences in coronary flow and myocardial metabolism at rest and during pace between patients with obstructive and patients with nonobstructive hypertrophic cardiomyopathy. *J Am Coll Cardiol* 1987;10:53–62.

106. Tanaka M, Fujiwara H, Onodera T, et al. Quantitative analysis of narrowings of intramyocardial small arteries in normal hearts, hypertensive hearts, and hearts with hypertrophic cardiomyopathy. *Circulation* 1987;75:1130–1139.

107. Frenneaux MP, Counihan PJ, Caforio AL, Chikamori T, McKenna WJ. Abnormal blood pressure response during exercise in hypertrophic cardiomyopathy. *Circulation* 1990;82:1995–2002.

108. Sadoul N, Prasad K, Elliott PM, Bannerjee S, Frenneaux MP, McKenna WJ. Prospective prognostic assessment of blood pressure response during exercise in patients with hypertrophic cardiomyopathy. *Circulation* 1997;96:2987–2991.

109. Olivotto I, Maron BJ, Montereggi A, Mazzuoli F, Dolara C, Cecchi F. Prognostic value of systemic blood pressure response during exercise in a community-based patient population with hypertrophic cardiomyopathy. *J Am Coll Cardiol* 1999;33:2044–2051.

110. Wigle ED, Adelman AG, Auger P, Marquis Y. Mitral regurgitation in muscular subaortic stenosis. *Am J Cardiol* 1969;24:698–706.

111. Zhu WX, Oh JK, Kopecky SL, Schaff HV, Tajik AJ. Mitral regurgitation due to ruptured chordae tendineae in patients with hypertrophic obstructive cardiomyopathy. *J Am Coll Cardiol* 1992;20:242–247.

112. Lever HM, Karam RF, Currie PJ, Healy BP. Hypertrophic cardiomyopathy in the elderly: distinctions from the young based on cardiac shape. *Circulation* 1989;79:580–589.

113. Lewis JF, Maron BJ. Elderly patients with hypertrophic cardiomyopathy: a subset with distinctive left ventricular morphology and progressive clinical course late in life. *J Am Coll Cardiol* 1989;13:36–45.

114. Fay WP, Taliercio CP, Ilstrup DM, Tajik AJ, Gersh BJ. Natural history of hypertrophic cardiomyopathy in the elderly. *J Am Coll Cardiol* 1990;16:821–826.

115. Lewis JF, Maron BJ. Clinical and morphologic expression of hypertrophic cardiomyopathy in patients greater than 65 years of age. *Am J Cardiol* 1994;73:1105–1111.

116. McKenna WJ, Chetty S, Oakley CM, Goodwin JF. Arrhythmia in hypertrophic cardiomyopathy: exercise and 48 hour ambulatory electrocardiographic assessment with and without beta adrenergic blocking therapy. *Am J Cardiol* 1980;45:1–5.

117. McKenna WJ, England D, Doi YL, Deanfield JE, Oakley C, Goodwin JF. Arrhythmia in hypertrophic cardiomyopathy. I. influence on prognosis. *Br Heart J* 1981;46:168–172.

118. McKenna WJ, Franklin RC, Nihoyannopoulos P, Robinson KC, Deanfield JE. Arrhythmia and prognosis in infants, children and adolescents with hypertrophic cardiomyopathy. *J Am Coll Cardiol* 1988;11:147–153.

119. Shapiro LM, McKenna WJ. Distribution of left ventricular hypertrophy in hypertrophic cardiomyopathy: a two-dimensional echocardiographic study. *J Am Coll Cardiol* 1983;2:437–444.

120. Klues HG, Schiffers A, Maron BJ. Phenotypic spectrum and patterns of left ventricular hypertrophy in hypertrophic cardiomyopathy: morphologic observations and significance as assessed by two-dimensional echocardiography in 600 patients. *J Am Coll Cardiol* 1995;26:1699–1708.

121. Binder J, Ommen SR, Gersh BJ, et al. Echocardiography-guided genetic testing in hypertrophic cardiomyopathy: septal morphology predicts the presence of myofilament mutations. *Mayo Clin Proc* April 2006;81(4):459–467.

122. Maron BJ, Niimura H, Casey SA, et al. Development of left ventricular hypertrophy in adults in hypertrophic cardiomyopathy caused by cardiac myosin-binding protein C gene mutations. *J Am Coll Cardiol* 2001;38:315–321.

123. Alboliras ET, Shub C, Gomez MR, et al. Spectrum of cardiac involvement in Friedreich's ataxia: clinical, electrocardiographic and echocardiographic observations. *Am J Cardiol* 1986;58:518–524.

124. Chandrasekaran K, Aylward PE, Fleagle SR, et al. Feasibility of identifying amyloid and hypertrophic cardiomyopathy with the use of computerized quantitative texture analysis of clinical echocardiographic data. *J Am Coll Cardiol* 1989;13:832–840.

125. Sachdev B, Takenaka T, Teraguchi H, et al. Prevalence of Anderson-Fabry disease in male patients with late onset hypertrophic cardiomyopathy. *Circulation* 2002;105:1407–1411.

126. Pelliccia A, Maron BJ, Spataro A, Proschan MA, Spirito P. The upper limit of physiologic cardiac hypertrophy in highly trained elite athletes. *N Engl J Med* 1991;324:295–301.

127. Pelliccia A, Maron BJ, De Luca R, Di Paolo FM, Spataro A, Culasso F. Remodeling of left ventricular hypertrophy in elite athletes after long-term deconditioning. *Circulation* 2002;105:944–949.

128. Palka P, Lange A, Fleming AD, et al. Differences in myocardial velocity gradient measured throughout the cardiac cycle in patients with hypertrophic cardiomyopathy, athletes and patients with left ventricular hypertrophy due to hypertension. *J Am Coll Cardiol* 1997;30:760–768.

129. Pela G, Bruschi G, Montagna L, Manara M, Manca C. Left and right ventricular adaptation assessed by Doppler tissue echocardiography in athletes. *J Am Soc Echocardiogr* 2004;17:205–211.

130. Klues HG, Maron BJ, Dollar AL, Roberts WC. Diversity of structural mitral valve alterations in hypertrophic cardiomyopathy. *Circulation* 1992;85:1651–1660.

131. Klues HG, Roberts WC, Maron BJ. Morphological determinants of echocardiographic patterns of mitral valve systolic anterior motion in obstructive hypertrophic cardiomyopathy. *Circulation* 1993;87:1570–1579.

132. Maron BJ, Harding AM, Spirito P, Roberts WC, Waller BF. Systolic anterior motion of the posterior mitral leaflet: a previously unrecognized cause of dynamic subaortic obstruction in patients with hypertrophic cardiomyopathy. *Circulation* 1983;68:282–293.

133. Klues HG, Roberts WC, Maron BJ. Anomalous insertion of papillary muscle directly into anterior mitral leaflet in hypertrophic cardiomyopathy: significance in producing left ventricular outflow obstruction. *Circulation* 1991;84:1188–1197.

134. Schwammenthal E, Block M, Schwartzkopff B, et al. Prediction of the site and severity of obstruction in hypertrophic cardiomyopathy by color flow mapping and continuous wave Doppler echocardiography. *J Am Coll Cardiol* 1992;20:964–972.

135. Bruce CJ, Nishimura RA, Tajik AJ, Schaff HV, Danielson GK. Fixed left ventricular outflow tract obstruction in presumed hypertrophic obstructive cardiomyopathy: implications for therapy. *Ann Thorac Surg* 1999;68:100–104.

136. Sasson Z, Yock PG, Hatle LK, Alderman EL, Popp RL. Doppler echocardiographic determination of the pressure gradient in hypertrophic cardiomyopathy. *J Am Coll Cardiol* 1988;11:752–756.

137. Nishimura RA, Tajik AJ, Reeder GS, Seward JB. Evaluation of hypertrophic cardiomyopathy by Doppler color flow imaging: initial observations. *Mayo Clin Proc* 1986;61:631–639.

138. Nishimura RA, Appleton CP, Redfield MM, Ilstrup DM, Holmes DR Jr, Tajik AJ. Noninvasive Doppler echocardiographic evaluation of left ventricular filling pressures in patients with cardiomyopathies: a simultaneous Doppler echocardiographic and cardiac catheterization study. *J Am Coll Cardiol* 1996;28:1226–1233.

139. Nagueh SF, Lakkis NM, Middleton KJ, et al. Changes in left ventricular diastolic function 6 months after nonsurgical septal reduction therapy for hypertrophic obstructive cardiomyopathy. *Circulation* 1999;99:344–347.

140. Nagueh SF, Bachinski LL, Meyer D, et al. Tissue Doppler imaging consistently detects myocardial abnormalities in patients with hypertrophic cardiomyopathy and provides a novel means for an early diagnosis before and independently of hypertrophy. *Circulation* 2001;104:128–130.

141. Nagueh S, McFalls J, Meyer D, et al. Tissue Doppler imaging predicts the development of hypertrophic cardiomyopathy in subjects with subclinical disease. *Circulation* 2003;108:395–398.

142. Ho CY, Sweitzer NK, McDonough B, et al. Assessment of diastolic function with Doppler tissue imaging to predict genotype in preclinical hypertrophic cardiomyopathy. *Circulation* 2002;105:2997.

143. Moon J, McKenna W, McCrohon J, Elliott P, Smith G, Pennell D. Toward clinical risk assessment in hypertrophic cardiomyopathy with gadolinium cardiovascular magnetic resonance. *J Am Coll Cardiol* 2003;41:1561–1567.

144. Kim R, Judd R. Gadolinium-enhanced magnetic resonance imaging in hypertrophic cardiomyopathy: in vivo imaging of the pathologic substrate for premature cardiac death? *J Am Coll Cardiol* 2003;41:1568–1572.

145. Stewart S, Schreiner B. Coexisting idiopathic hypertrophic subaortic stenosis and coronary artery disease: clinical implication and operative management. *J Thorac Cardiovasc Surg* 1981;82:278–280.

146. Sorajja P, Ommen SR, Nishimura RA, Gersh BJ, Berger PB, Tajik AJ. Adverse prognosis of patients with hypertrophic cardiomyopathy who have epicardial coronary artery disease. *Circulation* 2003;108:2342–2348.

147. Sorajja P, Chareonthaitawee P, Ommen SR, Miller TD, Hodge DO, Gibbons RJ. Prognostic utility of single-photon emission computed tomography in adult patients with hypertrophic cardiomyopathy. *Am Heart J* 2006;151:426–435.

148. Yetman AT, McCrindle BW, MacDonald C, Freedom RM, Gow R. Myocardial bridging in children with hypertrophic cardiomyopathy: a risk factor for sudden death. *N Engl J Med* 1998;339:1201–1209.

149. Sorajja P, Ommen SR, Nishimura RA, Gersh BJ, Tajik AJ, Holmes DJ. Myocardial bridging in adult patients with hypertrophic cardiomyopathy. *J Am Coll Cardiol* 2003;42:889–894.

150. Frenneaux MP, Porter A, Caforio AL, Odawara H, Counihan PJ, McKenna WJ. Determinants of exercise capacity in hypertrophic cardiomyopathy. *J Am Coll Cardiol* 1989;13:1521–1526.

151. Sharma S, Elliott P, Whyte G, et al. Utility of cardiopulmonary exercise in the assessment of clinical determinants of functional capacity in hypertrophic cardiomyopathy. *Am J Cardiol* 2000;86:162–168.

152. Frank MJ, Abdulla AM, Canedo MI, Saylors RE. Long-term medical management of hypertrophic obstructive cardiomyopathy. *Am J Cardiol* 1978;42:993–1001.

153. Elliott PM, Gimeno B Jr, Mahon NG, Poloniecki JD, McKenna WJ. Relation between severity of left ventricular hypertrophy and prognosis in patients with hypertrophic cardiomyopathy. *Lancet* 2001;357:420–424.

154. Elliott PM, Poloniecki J, Dickie S, et al. Sudden death in hypertrophic cardiomyopathy: identification of high risk patients. *J Am Coll Cardiol* 2000;36:2212–2218.

155. Maron BJ, Epstein SE, Roberts WC. Causes of sudden death in competitive athletes. *J Am Coll Cardiol* 1986;7:204–214.

156. Maron BJ, Pelliccia A, Spirito P. Cardiac disease in young trained athletes: insights into methods for distinguishing athlete's heart from structural heart disease, with particular emphasis on hypertrophic cardiomyopathy. *Circulation* 1995;91:1596–1601.

157. Maron BJ, Isner JM, McKenna WJ. 26th Bethesda conference: recommendations for determining eligibility for competition in athletes with cardiovascular abnormalities. Task force 3: hypertrophic cardiomyopathy, myocarditis and other myopericardial diseases and mitral valve prolapse. *J Am Coll Cardiol* 1994;24:880–885.

158. Maron BJ, Chaitman BR, Ackerman MJ, et al. Recommendations for physical activity and recreational sports participation for young patients with genetic cardiovascular diseases. *Circulation* 2004;109:2807–2816.

159. Maron BJ, Ackerman MJ, Nishimura RA, Pyeritz RE, Towbin JA, Udelson JE. Task Force 4: HCM and other cardiomyopathies, mitral valve prolapse, myocarditis, and Marfan syndrome. *J Am Coll Cardiol* 2005;45:1340–1345.

160. Silka MJ, Kron J, Dunnigan A, Dick M. Sudden cardiac death and the use of implantable cardioverter-defibrillators in pediatric patients: the pediatric electrophysiology society. *Circulation* 1993;87:800–807.

161. Elliott PM, Sharma S, Varnava A, Poloniecki J, Rowland E, McKenna WJ. Survival after cardiac arrest or sustained ventricular tachycardia in patients with hypertrophic cardiomyopathy. *J Am Coll Cardiol* 1999;33:1596–1601.

162. Maron BJ, Shen WK, Link MS, et al. Efficacy of implantable cardioverter-defibrillators for the prevention of sudden death in patients with hypertrophic cardiomyopathy. *N Engl J Med* 2000;342:365–673.

163. Spirito P, Bellone P, Harris KM, Bruzzi P, Maron BJ. Magnitude of left ventricular hypertrophy and risk of sudden death in hypertrophic cardiomyopathy. *N Engl J Med* 2000;342:1778–1785.

164. Fananapazir L, Tracy CM, Leon MB, et al. Electrophysiologic abnormalities in patients with hypertrophic cardiomyopathy: a consecutive analysis in 155 patients. *Circulation* 1989;80:1259–1268.

165. Fananapazir L, Chang AC, Epstein SE, McAreavey D. Prognostic determinants in hypertrophic cardiomyopathy: prospective evaluation of a therapeutic strategy based on clinical, Holter, hemodynamic, and electrophysiological findings. *Circulation* 1992;86:730–740.

166. Spirito P, Rapezzi C, Bellone P, et al. Infective endocarditis in hypertrophic cardiomyopathy: prevalence, incidence, and indications for antibiotic prophylaxis. *Circulation* 1999;99:2132–2137.

167. Olivotto I, Cecchi F, Casey SA, Dolara A, Traverse JH, Maron BJ. Impact of atrial fibrillation on the clinical course of hypertrophic cardiomyopathy. *Circulation* 2001;104:2517–2524.

168. Ten Cate FJ, Roelandt J. Progression to left ventricular dilatation in patients with hypertrophic obstructive cardiomyopathy. *Am Heart J* 1979;97:762–765.

169. Spirito P, Maron BJ, Bonow RO, Epstein SE. Occurrence and significance of progressive left ventricular wall thinning and relative cavity dilatation in hypertrophic cardiomyopathy. *Am J Cardiol* 1987;60:123–129.

170. Biagini E, Coccolo F, Ferlito M, et al. Dilated-hypokinetic evolution of hypertrophic cardiomyopathy: prevalence, incidence, risk factors, and prognostic implications in pediatric and adult patients [see comment]. *J Am Coll Cardiol* 2005;46:1543–1550.

171. McDonald K, McWilliams E, O'Keefe B, Maurer B. Functional assessment of patients treated with permanent dual chamber pacing as a primary treatment for hypertrophic cardiomyopathy. *Eur Heart J* 1988;9:893–898.

172. Jeanrenaud X, Goy JJ, Kappenberger L. Effects of dual-chamber pacing in hypertrophic obstructive cardiomyopathy. *Lancet* 1992;339:1318–1323.

173. Cannon RO, III, Tripodi D, Dilsizian V, Panza JA, Fananapazir L. Results of permanent dual-chamber pacing in symptomatic nonobstructive hypertrophic cardiomyopathy. *Am J Cardiol* 1994;73:571–576.

174. Fananapazir L, Epstein ND, Curiel RV, Panza JA, Tripodi D, McAreavey D. Long-term results of dual-chamber (DDD) pacing in obstructive hypertrophic cardiomyopathy: evidence for progressive symptomatic and hemodynamic improvement and reduction of left ventricular hypertrophy. *Circulation* 1994;90:2731–2742.

175. Posma JL, Blanksma PK, Van Der Wall EE, Vaalburg W, Crijns HJ, Lie KI. Effects of permanent dual-chamber pacing on myocardial perfusion in symptomatic hypertrophic cardiomyopathy. *Heart* 1996;76:358–362.

176. Slade AK, Sadoul N, Shapiro L, et al. DDD pacing in hypertrophic cardiomyopathy: a multicentre clinical experience. *Heart* 1996;75:44–49.

177. Gadler F, Linde C, Juhlin-Dannfelt A, Ribeiro A, Ryden L. Long-term effects of dual chamber pacing in patients with hypertrophic cardiomyopathy without outflow tract obstruction at rest. *Eur Heart J* 1997;18:636–642.

178. Kappenberger L, Linde C, Daubert C, et al. Pacing in hypertrophic obstructive cardiomyopathy: a randomized crossover study. PIC study group. *Eur Heart J* 1997;18:1249–1256.

179. Nishimura RA, Trusty JM, Hayes DL, et al. Dual-chamber pacing for hypertrophic cardiomyopathy: a randomized, double-blind, crossover trial. *J Am Coll Cardiol* 1997;29:435–441.

180. Rishi F, Hulse JE, Auld DO, et al. Effects of dual-chamber pacing for pediatric patients with hypertrophic obstructive cardiomyopathy. *J Am Coll Cardiol* 1997;29:734–740.

181. Gadler F, Linde C, Daubert C, et al. Significant improvement of quality of life following atrioventricular synchronous pacing in patients with hyper-

trophic obstructive cardiomyopathy: data from 1 year of follow-up: PIC study group—Pacing in Cardiomyopathy. *Eur Heart J* 1999;20:1044–1050.

182. Linde C, Gadler F, Kappenberger L, Ryden L. Placebo effect of pacemaker implantation in obstructive hypertrophic cardiomyopathy: PIC study group—Pacing in Cardiomyopathy. *Am J Cardiol* 1999;83:903–907.

183. Maron BJ, Nishimura RA, McKenna WJ, Rakowski H, Josephson ME, Kieval RS. Assessment of permanent dual-chamber pacing as a treatment for drug-refractory symptomatic patients with obstructive hypertrophic cardiomyopathy: a randomized, double-blind, crossover study (M-PATHY). *Circulation* 1999;99:2927–2933.

184. Pavin D, De Place C, Le Breton H, et al. Effects of permanent dual-chamber pacing on mitral regurgitation in hypertrophic obstructive cardiomyopathy. *Eur Heart J* 1999;20:203–210.

185. Megevand A, Ingles J, Richmond DR, Semsarian C. Long-term follow-up of patients with obstructive hypertrophic cardiomyopathy treated with dual-chamber pacing. *Am J Cardiol* 2005;95:991–993.

186. Tajik AJ, Giuliani ER, Weidman WH, Brandenburg RO, McGoon DC. Idiopathic hypertrophic subaortic stenosis: long-term surgical follow-up. *Am J Cardiol* 1974;34:815–822.

187. Morrow AG, Reitz BA, Epstein SE, et al. Operative treatment in hypertrophic subaortic stenosis: techniques, and the results of pre and postoperative assessments in 83 patients. *Circulation* 1975;52:88–102.

188. Cooley DA, Wukasch DC, Leachman RD. Mitral valve replacement for idiopathic subaortic stenosis: results in 27 patients. *J Cardiovasc Surg (Torino)* 1976;17:380–387.

189. Agnew TM, Barratt-Boyes BG, Brandt PW, Roche AH, Lowe JB, O'Brien KP. Surgical resection in idiopathic hypertrophic subaortic stenosis with a combined approach through aorta and left ventricle. *J Thorac Cardiovasc Surg* 1977;74:307–316.

190. Maron BJ, Merrill WH, Freier PA, Kent KM, Epstein SE, Morrow AG. Long-term clinical course and symptomatic status of patients after operation for hypertrophic subaortic stenosis. *Circulation* 1978;57:1205–1213.

191. Redwood DR, Goldstein RE, Hirshfeld J, et al. Exercise performance after septal myotomy and myectomy in patients with obstructive hypertrophic cardiomyopathy. *Am J Cardiol* 1979;44:215–220.

192. Maron BJ, Epstein SE, Morrow AG. Symptomatic status and prognosis of patients after operation for hypertrophic obstructive cardiomyopathy: efficacy of ventricular septal myotomy and myectomy. *Eur Heart J* 1983;4:175–185.

193. Cooper MM, McIntosh CL, Tucker E, Clark RE. Operation for hypertrophic subaortic stenosis in the aged. *Ann Thorac Surg* 1987;44:370–378.

194. Cannon RO III, McIntosh CL, Schenke WH, Maron BJ, Bonow RO, Epstein SE. Effect of surgical reduction of left ventricular outflow obstruction on hemodynamics, coronary flow, and myocardial metabolism in hypertrophic cardiomyopathy. *Circulation* 1989;79:766–775.

195. Krajcer Z, Leachman RD, Cooley DA, Coronado R. Septal myotomy-myomectomy versus mitral valve replacement in hypertrophic cardiomyopathy: ten-year follow-up in 185 patients. *Circulation* 1989;80:157–164.

196. McIntosh CL, Greenberg GJ, Maron BJ, Leon MB, Cannon RO III, Clark RE. Clinical and hemodynamic results after mitral valve replacement in patients with obstructive hypertrophic cardiomyopathy. *Ann Thorac Surg* 1989;47:236–246.

197. Mohr R, Schaff HV, Danielson GK, Puga FJ, Pluth JR, Tajik AJ. The outcome of surgical treatment of hypertrophic obstructive cardiomyopathy: experience over 15 years. *J Thorac Cardiovasc Surg* 1989;97:666–74.

198. Mohr R, Schaff HV, Puga FJ, Danielson GK. Results of operation for hypertrophic obstructive cardiomyopathy in children and adults less than 40 years of age. *Circulation* 1989;80:II91–II96.

199. Siegman IL, Maron BJ, Permut LC, McIntosh CL, Clark RE. Results of operation for coexistent obstructive hypertrophic cardiomyopathy and coronary artery disease. *J Am Coll Cardiol* 1989;13:1527–1533.

200. Cohn LH, Trehan H, Collins JJ Jr. Long-term follow-up of patients undergoing myotomy/myectomy for obstructive hypertrophic cardiomyopathy. *Am J Cardiol* 1992;70:657–660.

201. Diodati JG, Schenke WH, Waclawiw MA, McIntosh CL, Cannon RO III. Predictors of exercise benefit after operative relief of left ventricular outflow obstruction by the myotomy-myectomy procedure in hypertrophic cardiomyopathy. *Am J Cardiol* 1992;69:1617–1622.

202. McIntosh CL, Maron BJ, Cannon RO III, Klues HG. Initial results of combined anterior mitral leaflet plication and ventricular septal myotomy-myectomy for relief of left ventricular outflow tract obstruction in patients with hypertrophic cardiomyopathy. *Circulation* 1992;86:II60–II67.

203. Schulte HD, Bircks WH, Loesse B, Godehardt EA, Schwartzkopff B. Prognosis of patients with hypertrophic obstructive cardiomyopathy after trans-

204. Schoendube FA, Klues HG, Reith S, Messmer BJ. Surgical correction of hypertrophic obstructive cardiomyopathy with combined myectomy, mobilisation and partial excision of the papillary muscles. *Eur J Cardiothorac Surg* 1994;8:603–608.

205. ten Berg JM, Suttorp MJ, Knaepen PJ, Ernst SM, Vermeulen FE, Jaarsma W. Hypertrophic obstructive cardiomyopathy: initial results and long-term follow-up after Morrow septal myectomy. *Circulation* 1994;90:1781–1785.

206. Heric B, Lytle BW, Miller DP, Rosenkranz ER, Lever HM, Cosgrove DM. Surgical management of hypertrophic obstructive cardiomyopathy: early and late results. *J Thorac Cardiovasc Surg* 1995;110:195–206.

207. Schoendube FA, Klues HG, Reith S, Flachskampf FA, Hanrath P, Messmer BJ. Long-term clinical and echocardiographic follow-up after surgical correction of hypertrophic obstructive cardiomyopathy with extended myectomy and reconstruction of the subvalvular mitral apparatus. *Circulation* 1995;92:II122–II127.

208. Kofflard MJ, van Herwerden LA, Waldstein DJ, et al. Initial results of combined anterior mitral leaflet extension and myectomy in patients with obstructive hypertrophic cardiomyopathy. *J Am Coll Cardiol* 1996;28:197–202.

209. McCully RB, Nishimura RA, Tajik AJ, Schaff HV, Danielson GK. Extent of clinical improvement after surgical treatment of hypertrophic obstructive cardiomyopathy. *Circulation* 1996;94:467–471.

210. Robbins RC, Stinson EB. Long-term results of left ventricular myotomy and myectomy for obstructive hypertrophic cardiomyopathy. *J Thorac Cardiovasc Surg* 1996;111:586–594.

211. Theodoro DA, Danielson GK, Feldt RH, Anderson BJ. Hypertrophic obstructive cardiomyopathy in pediatric patients: results of surgical treatment. *J Thorac Cardiovasc Surg* 1996;112:1589–1597.

212. Merrill WH, Friesinger GC, Graham TP Jr, et al. Long-lasting improvement after septal myectomy for hypertrophic obstructive cardiomyopathy. *Ann Thorac Surg* 2000;69:1732–1735, 1735–1736 [discussion].

213. Yu EH, Omran AS, Wigle ED, Williams WG, Siu SC, Rakowski H. Mitral regurgitation in hypertrophic obstructive cardiomyopathy: relationship to obstruction and relief with myectomy. *J Am Coll Cardiol* 2000;36:2219–2225.

214. Ommen SR, Thomson HL, Nishimura RA, Tajik AJ, Schaff HV, Danielson GK. Clinical predictors and consequences of atrial fibrillation after surgical myectomy for obstructive hypertrophic cardiomyopathy. *Am J Cardiol* 2002;89:242–244.

215. Ommen SR, Park SH, Click RL, Freeman WK, Schaff HV, Tajik AJ. Impact of intraoperative transesophageal echocardiography in the surgical management of hypertrophic cardiomyopathy. *Am J Cardiol* 2002;90:1022–1024.

216. Woo A, Williams WG, Choi R, et al. Clinical and echocardiographic determinants of long-term survival after surgical myectomy in obstructive hypertrophic cardiomyopathy [see comment]. *Circulation* 2005;111:2033–2041.

217. Ommen SR, Maron BJ, Olivotto I, et al. Long-term effects of surgical septal myectomy on survival in patients with obstructive hypertrophic cardiomyopathy [see comment]. *J Am Coll Cardiol* 2005;46:470–476.

218. Sigwart U. Non-surgical myocardial reduction for hypertrophic obstructive cardiomyopathy. *Lancet* 1995;346:211–214.

219. Knight C, Kurbaan AS, Seggewiss H, et al. Nonsurgical septal reduction for hypertrophic obstructive cardiomyopathy: outcome in the first series of patients. *Circulation* 1997;95:2075–2081.

220. Kuhn H, Gietzen F, Leuner C, Gerenkamp T. Induction of subaortic septal ischaemia to reduce obstruction in hypertrophic obstructive cardiomyopathy: studies to develop a new catheter-based concept of treatment. *Eur Heart J* 1997;18:846–851.

221. Faber L, Seggewiss H, Gleichmann U. Percutaneous transluminal septal myocardial ablation in hypertrophic obstructive cardiomyopathy: results with respect to intraprocedural myocardial contrast echocardiography. *Circulation* 1998;98:2415–2421.

222. Seggewiss H, Gleichmann U, Faber L, Fassbender D, Schmidt HK, Strick S. Percutaneous transluminal septal myocardial ablation in hypertrophic obstructive cardiomyopathy: acute results and three-month follow-up in 25 patients. *J Am Coll Cardiol* 1998;31:252–258.

223. Gietzen FH, Leuner CJ, Raute-Kreinsen U, et al. Acute and long-term results after transcoronary ablation of septal hypertrophy (TASH): catheter interventional treatment for hypertrophic obstructive cardiomyopathy. *Eur Heart J* 1999;20:1342–1354.

224. Henein MY, O'Sullivan CA, Ramzy IS, Sigwart U, Gibson DG. Electromechanical left ventricular behavior after nonsurgical septal reduction in patients with hypertrophic obstructive cardiomyopathy. *J Am Coll Cardiol* 1999;34:1117–1122.

225. Kim JJ, Lee CW, Park SW, et al. Improvement in exercise capacity and exercise blood pressure response after transcoronary alcohol ablation therapy of septal hypertrophy in hypertrophic cardiomyopathy. *Am J Cardiol* 1999;83:1220–1223.

204. Schoendube FA, Klues HG, Reith S, Messmer BJ. Surgical correction of hypertrophic obstructive cardiomyopathy with combined myectomy, mobilisation and partial excision of the papillary muscles. aortic myectomy: late results up to twenty-five years. *J Thorac Cardiovasc Surg* 1993;106:709–717.

226. Kuhn H, Gietzen FH, Schafers M, et al. Changes in the left ventricular outflow tract after transcoronary ablation of septal hypertrophy (TASH) for hypertrophic obstructive cardiomyopathy as assessed by transesophageal echocardiography and by measuring myocardial glucose utilization and perfusion. *Eur Heart J* 1999;20:1808–1817.

227. Faber L, Meissner A, Ziemssen P, Seggewiss H. Percutaneous transluminal septal myocardial ablation for hypertrophic obstructive cardiomyopathy: long term follow up of the first series of 25 patients. *Heart* 2000;83:326–31.

228. Faber L, Ziemssen P, Seggewiss H. Targeting percutaneous transluminal septal ablation for hypertrophic obstructive cardiomyopathy by intraprocedural echocardiographic monitoring. *J Am Soc Echocardiogr* 2000;13:1074–1079.

229. Lakkis NM, Nagueh SF, Dunn JK, Killip D, Spencer WH III. Nonsurgical septal reduction therapy for hypertrophic obstructive cardiomyopathy: one-year follow-up. *J Am Coll Cardiol* 2000;36:852–855.

230. Ruzyllo W, Chojnowska L, Demkow M, et al. Left ventricular outflow tract gradient decrease with non-surgical myocardial reduction improves exercise capacity in patients with hypertrophic obstructive cardiomyopathy. *Eur Heart J* 2000;21:770–777.

231. Boekstegers P, Steinbigler P, Molnar A, et al. Pressure-guided nonsurgical myocardial reduction induced by small septal infarctions in hypertrophic obstructive cardiomyopathy. *J Am Coll Cardiol* 2001;38:846–853.

232. Flores-Ramirez R, Lakkis NM, Middleton KJ, Killip D, Spencer WH III, Nagueh SF. Echocardiographic insights into the mechanisms of relief of left ventricular outflow tract obstruction after nonsurgical septal reduction therapy in patients with hypertrophic obstructive cardiomyopathy. *J Am Coll Cardiol* 2001;37:208–214.

233. Mazur W, Nagueh SF, Lakkis NM, et al. Regression of left ventricular hypertrophy after nonsurgical septal reduction therapy for hypertrophic obstructive cardiomyopathy. *Circulation* 2001;103:1492–1496.

234. Fernandes VL, Nagueh SF, Wang W, Roberts R, Spencer WH III. A prospective follow-up of alcohol septal ablation for symptomatic hypertrophic obstructive cardiomyopathy: the Baylor experience (1996–2002). *Clin Cardiol* 2005;28:124–130.

235. Faber L, Seggewiss H, Gietzen FH, et al. Catheter-based septal ablation for symptomatic hypertrophic obstructive cardiomyopathy: follow-up results of the TASH-registry of the German Cardiac Society. *Z Kardiol* 2005;94:516–523.

236. Ommen SR, Nishimura RA, Squires RW, Schaff HV, Danielson GK, Tajik AJ. Comparison of dual-chamber pacing versus septal myectomy for the treatment of patients with hypertrophic obstructive cardiomyopathy: a comparison of objective hemodynamic and exercise end point. *J Am Coll Cardiol* 1999;34:191–196.

237. Nagueh SF, Ommen SR, Lakkis NM, et al. Comparison of ethanol septal reduction therapy with surgical myectomy for the treatment of hypertrophic obstructive cardiomyopathy. *J Am Coll Cardiol* 2001;38:1701–1706.

238. Qin JX, Shiota T, Lever HM, et al. Outcome of patients with hypertrophic obstructive cardiomyopathy after percutaneous transluminal septal myocardial ablation and septal myectomy surgery. *J Am Coll Cardiol* 2001;38:1994–2000.

239. Firoozi S, Elliott PM, Sharma S, et al. Septal myotomy-myectomy and transcoronary septal alcohol ablation in hypertrophic obstructive cardiomyopathy: a comparison of clinical, haemodynamic and exercise outcomes. *Eur Heart J* 2002;23:1617–1624.

240. Ralph-Edwards A, Woo A, McCrindle BW, et al. Hypertrophic obstructive cardiomyopathy: comparison of outcomes after myectomy or alcohol ablation adjusted by propensity score. *J Thorac Cardiovasc Surg* 2005;129:351–358.

241. Flamm MD, Harrison DC, Handock EW. Muscular subaortic stenosis: prevention of outflow obstruction with propranolol. *Circulation* 1968;38:846–858.

242. Adelman AG, Shah PM, Gramiak R, Wigle ED. Long-term propranolol therapy in muscular subaortic stenosis. *Br Heart J* 1970;32:804–811.

243. Shah PM, Gramiak R, Adelman AG, Wigle ED. Echocardiographic assessment of the effects of surgery and propranolol on the dynamics of outflow obstruction in hypertrophic subaortic stenosis. *Circulation* 1972;45:516–521.

244. Kaltenbach M, Hopf R, Kober G, Bussmann WD, Keller M, Petersen Y. Treatment of hypertrophic obstructive cardiomyopathy with verapamil. *Br Heart J* 1979;42:35–42.

245. Rosing DR, Kent KM, Borer JS, Seides SF, Maron BJ, Epstein SE. Verapamil therapy: a new approach to the pharmacologic treatment of hypertrophic cardiomyopathy. I. Hemodynamic effects. *Circulation* 1979;60:1201–1207.

246. Rosing DR, Kent KM, Maron BJ, Epstein SE. Verapamil therapy: a new approach to the pharmacologic treatment of hypertrophic cardiomyopathy. II. Effects on exercise capacity and symptomatic status. *Circulation* 1979;60:1208–1213.

247. Rosing DR, Condit JR, Maron BJ, et al. Verapamil therapy: a new approach to the pharmacologic treatment of hypertrophic cardiomyopathy: III. Effects of long-term administration. *Am J Cardiol* 1981;48:545–553.

248. Bonow RO, Rosing DR, Bacharach SL, et al. Effects of verapamil on left ventricular systolic function and diastolic filling in patients with hypertrophic cardiomyopathy. *Circulation* 1981;64:787–796.

249. Bonow RO, Frederick TM, Bacharach SL, et al. Atrial systole and left ventricular filling in hypertrophic cardiomyopathy: effect of verapamil. *Am J Cardiol* 1983;51:1386–1391.

250. Bonow RO, Ostrow HG, Rosing DR, et al. Effects of verapamil on left ventricular systolic and diastolic function in patients with hypertrophic cardiomyopathy: pressure-volume analysis with a nonimaging scintillation probe. *Circulation* 1983;68:1062–1073.

251. Epstein SE, Rosing DR. Verapamil: its potential for causing serious complications in patients with hypertrophic cardiomyopathy. *Circulation* 1981;64:437–441.

252. Pollick C. Muscular subaortic stenosis: Hemodynamic and clinical improvement after disopyramide. *N Engl J Med* 1982;307:997–999.

253. Pollick C, Kimball B, Henderson M, Wigle ED. Disopyramide in hypertrophic cardiomyopathy. I. Hemodynamic assessment after intravenous administration. *Am J Cardiol* 1988;62:1248–1251.

254. Sherrid M, Delia E, Dwyer E. Oral disopyramide therapy for obstructive hypertrophic cardiomyopathy. *Am J Cardiol* 1988;62:1085–1088.

255. Matsubara H, Nakatani S, Nagata S, et al. Salutary effect of disopyramide on left ventricular diastolic function in hypertrophic obstructive cardiomyopathy. *J Am Coll Cardiol* 1995;26:768–775.

256. Sherrid MV, Barac I, McKenna WJ, et al. Multicenter study of the efficacy and safety of disopyramide in obstructive hypertrophic cardiomyopathy. *J Am Coll Cardiol* 2005;45:1251–1258.

257. Morrow AG. Operative methods utilized to relieve left ventricular outflow obstruction. *J Thorac Cardiovasc Surg* 1978;76:423–430.

258. Williams WG, Wigle ED, Rakowski H, Smallhorn J, LeBlanc J, Trusler GA. Results of surgery for hypertrophic obstructive cardiomyopathy. *Circulation* 1987;76:V104–V108.

259. McIntosh CL, Maron BJ. Current operative treatment of obstructive hypertrophic cardiomyopathy. *Circulation* 1988;78:487–495.

260. McCully RB, Nishimura RA, Bailey KR, Schaff HV, Danielson GK, Tajik AJ. Hypertrophic obstructive cardiomyopathy: preoperative echocardiographic predictors of outcome after septal myectomy. *J Am Coll Cardiol* 1996;27:1491–1496.

261. Schulte HD, Borisov K, Gams E, Gramsch-Zabel H, Losse B, Schwartzkopff B. Management of symptomatic hypertrophic obstructive cardiomyopathy—long-term results after surgical therapy. *Thorac Cardiovasc Surg* 1999;47:213–218.

262. Havndrup O, Pettersson G, Kjeldsen K, Bundgaard H. Outcome of septal myectomy in patients with hypertrophic obstructive cardiomyopathy. *Scand Cardiovasc J* 2000;34:564–569.

263. Maron BJ, McKenna W, Danielson GK, et al. ACC/ESC clinical expert consensus document on hypertrophic cardiomyopathy: a report of the American College of Cardiology Task Force on Clinical Expert Consensus Documents and the European Society of Cardiology Committee for Practice Guidelines (Committee to Develop an Expert Consensus Document on Hypertrophic Cardiomyopathy). *J Am Coll Cardiol* 2003;42:1687–1713.

264. Dearani JA, Danielson GK. Septal myectomy for obstructive hypertrophic cardiomyopathy. *Semin Thorac Cardiovasc Surg Pediatr Card* 2005:86–91.

265. Minakata K, Dearani JA, Nishimura RA, Maron BJ, Danielson GK. Extended septal myectomy for hypertrophic obstructive cardiomyopathy with anomalous mitral papillary muscles or chordae. *J Thorac Cardiovasc Surg* 2004;127:481–489.

266. Maron BJ, Nishimura RA, Danielson GK. Pitfalls in clinical recognition and a novel operative approach for hypertrophic cardiomyopathy with severe outflow obstruction due to anomalous papillary muscle. *Circulation* 1998;98:2505–2508.

267. Grigg LE, Wigle ED, Williams WG, Daniel LB, Rakowski H. Transesophageal Doppler echocardiography in obstructive hypertrophic cardiomyopathy: clarification of pathophysiology and importance in intraoperative decision making. *J Am Coll Cardiol* 1992;20:42–52.

268. Marwick TH, Stewart WJ, Lever HM, et al. Benefits of intraoperative echocardiography in the surgical management of hypertrophic cardiomyopathy. *J Am Coll Cardiol* 1992;20:1066–1072.

269. Beahrs MM, Tajik AJ, Seward JB, Giuliani ER, McGoon DC. Hypertrophic obstructive cardiomyopathy: ten- to 21-year follow-up after partial septal myectomy. *Am J Cardiol* 1983;51:1160–1166.

270. Mohr R, Schaff HV, Danielson GK, Puga FJ, Tajik AJ. The outcome of surgical treatment of hypertrophic obstructive cardiomyopathy: experience over 15 years. *J Thorac Cardiovasc Surg* 1989;97:666–674.

271. Erwin JP, 3rd, Nishimura RA, Lloyd MA, Tajik AJ. Dual chamber pacing for patients with hypertrophic obstructive cardiomyopathy: a clinical perspective in 2000. *Mayo Clin Proc* 2000;75:173–80.

272. Nishimura RA, Symanski JD, Hurrell DG, Trusty JM, Hayes DL, Tajik AJ. Dual-chamber pacing for cardiomyopathies: a 1996 clinical perspective. *Mayo Clin Proc* 1996;71:1077–1087.

273. Symanski JD, Nishimura RA. The use of pacemakers in the treatment of cardiomyopathies. *Curr Probl Cardiol* 1996;21:385–443.

274. Nishimura RA, Hayes DL, Ilstrup DM, Holmes DR Jr, Tajik AJ. Effect of dual-chamber pacing on systolic and diastolic function in patients with hypertrophic cardiomyopathy: acute Doppler echocardiographic and catheterization hemodynamic study. *J Am Coll Cardiol* 1996;27:421–430.

275. Betocchi S, Losi MA, Piscione F, et al. Effects of dual-chamber pacing in hypertrophic cardiomyopathy on left ventricular outflow tract obstruction and on diastolic function. *Am J Cardiol* 1996;77:498–502.

276. Fananapazir L, Cannon RO III, Tripodi D, Panza JA. Impact of dual-chamber permanent pacing in patients with obstructive hypertrophic cardiomyopathy with symptoms refractory to verapamil and beta-adrenergic blocker therapy. *Circulation* 1992;85:2149–2161.

277. Kappenberger LJ, Linde C, Jeanrenaud X, et al. Clinical progress after randomized on/off pacemaker treatment for hypertrophic obstructive cardiomyopathy: Pacing in Cardiomyopathy (PIC) study group. *Europace* 1999;1:77–84.

278. Ommen SR, Nishimura RA, Squires RW, Schaff HV, Danielson GK, Tajik AJ. Comparison of dual-chamber pacing versus septal myectomy for the treatment of patients with hypertropic obstructive cardiomyopathy: a comparison of objective hemodynamic and exercise end points. *J Am Coll Cardiol* 1999;34:191–196.

279. Braunwald E. A new treatment for hypertrophic cardiomyopathy? *Eur Heart J* 1997;18:709–710.

280. Braunwald E. Induced septal infarction: a new therapeutic strategy for hypertrophic obstructive cardiomyopathy. *Circulation* 1997;95:1981–1982.

281. Braunwald E. Hypertrophic cardiomyopathy: the benefits of a multidisciplinary approach. *N Engl J Med* 2002;347:1306–1307.

282. Braunwald E, Seidman CE, Sigwart U. Contemporary evaluation and management of hypertrophic cardiomyopathy. *Circulation* 2002;106:1312–1316.

283. Seggewiss H, Gleichmann U, Faber L, Fassbender D, Schmidt HK, Strick S. Percutaneous transluminal septal myocardial ablation in hypertrophic obstructive cardiomyopathy: acute results and 3-month follow-up in 25 patients. *J Am Coll Cardiol* 1998;31:252–258.

284. Wigle ED, Schwartz L, Woo A, Rakowski H. To ablate or operate? That is the question [editorial]. *J Am Coll Cardiol* 2001;15:1707–1710.

285. Faber L, Seggewiss H, Ziemssen P, Gleichmann U. Intraprocedural myocardial contrast echocardiography as a routine procedure in percutaneous transluminal septal myocardial ablation: detection of threatening myocardial necrosis distant from the septal target area. *Catheter Cardiovasc Interv* 1999;47:462–466.

286. Gietzen FH, Leuner CJ, Obergassel L, Strunk-Mueller C, Kuhn H. Role of transcoronary ablation of septal hypertrophy in patients with hypertrophic cardiomyopathy, New York Heart Association functional class III or IV, and outflow obstruction only under provocable conditions. *Circulation* 2002;106:454–459.

287. Knight CJ. Five years of percutaneous transluminal septal myocardial ablation. *Heart* 2000;83:255–256.

288. Kuhn H. Transcoronary ablation of septal hypertrophy (TASH): a 5-year experience*. *Z Kardiol* 2000;89:559–564.

289. Kuhn H, Gietzen FH, Leuner C, et al. Transcoronary ablation of septal hypertrophy (TASH): a new treatment option for hypertrophic obstructive cardiomyopathy. *Z Kardiol* 2000;89:IV41–IV54.

290. Lakkis N, Plana JC, Nagueh S, Killip D, Roberts R, Spencer WH III. Efficacy of nonsurgical septal reduction therapy in symptomatic patients with obstructive hypertrophic cardiomyopathy and provocable gradients. *Am J Cardiol* 2001;88:583–586.

291. Lakkis N. New treatment methods for patients with hypertrophic obstructive cardiomyopathy. *Curr Opin Cardiol* 2000;15:172–177.

292. Shamim W, Yousufuddin M, Wang D, et al. Nonsurgical reduction of the interventricular septum in patients with hypertrophic cardiomyopathy. *N Engl J Med* 2002;347:1326–1333.

293. Lakkis NM, Nagueh SF, Kleinman NS, et al. Echocardiography-guided ethanol for hypertrophic obstructive cardiomyopathy. *Circulation* 1998;98:1750–1755.

294. Nagueh SF, Lakkis NM, He ZX, et al. Role of myocardial contrast echocardiography during nonsurgical septal reduction therapy for hypertrophic obstructive cardiomyopathy. *J Am Coll Cardiol* 1998;32:225–229.

295. Qin JX, Shiota T, Lever HM, et al. Conduction system abnormalities in patients with obstructive hypertrophic cardiomyopathy following septal reduction interventions. *Am J Cardiol* 2004;93:171–175.

296. Talreja DR, Nishimura RA, Edwards WD, et al. Alcohol septal ablation versus surgical septal myectomy: comparison of effects on atrioventricular conduction tissue. *J Am Coll Cardiol* 2004;44:2329–2332.

297. Spirito P, Rubartelli P. Alcohol septal ablation in the management of obstructive hypertrophic cardiomyopathy. *Ital Heart J* 2000;1:721–725.

298. Maron BJ. Role of alcohol septal ablation in treatment of obstructive hypertrophic cardiomyopathy. *Lancet* 2000;355:425–426.

299. Qin JX, Shiota T, Lever HM, et al. Outcome of patients with hypertrophic obstructive cardiomyopathy after percutaneous transluminal septal myocardial ablation and septal myectomy surgery. *J Am Coll Cardiol* 2001;38:1994–2000.

300. Maron BJ, Dearani JA, Ommen SR, et al. The case for surgery in obstructive hypertrophic cardiomyopathy. *J Am Coll Cardiol* 2005;44:2044–2053.

301. Valeti US, Nishimura RA, Holmes DR, et al. Comparison of surgical septal myectomy and alcohol septal ablation with cardiac magnetic resonance imaging in patients with hypertrophic obstructive cardiomyopathy. *J Am Coll Cardiol* January 23, 2007;49(3):358–360.

302. Patel R, Nagueh SF, Tsyboulева N, et al. Simvastatin induces regression of cardiac hypertrophy and fibrosis and improves cardiac function in a transgenic rabbit model of human hypertrophic cardiomyopathy. *Circulation* 2001;104:317–324.

303. Roberts R. A perspective: the new millennium dawns on a new paradigm for cardiology—molecular genetics. *J Am Coll Cardiol* 2000;36:661–667.

304. Maron BJ. Hypertrophic cardiomyopathy and sudden death: new perspectives on risk stratification and prevention with the implantable cardioverter-defibrillator. *Eur Heart J* 2000;21:1979–1983.

305. Maron BJ, Lipson LC, Roberts WC, Savage DD, Epstein SE. "Malignant" hypertrophic cardiomyopathy: identification of a subgroup of families with unusually frequent premature death. *Am J Cardiol* 1978;41:1133–1140.

306. Spirito P, Maron BJ. Relation between extent of left ventricular hypertrophy and occurrence of sudden cardiac death in hypertrophic cardiomyopathy. *J Am Coll Cardiol* 1990;15:1521–1526.

307. Maron BJ, Cecchi F, McKenna WJ. Risk factors and stratification for sudden cardiac death in patients with hypertrophic cardiomyopathy. *Br Heart J* 1994;72:S13–S18.

308. Maron BJ, Savage DD, Wolfson JK, Epstein SE. Prognostic significance of 24 hour ambulatory electrocardiographic monitoring in patients with hypertrophic cardiomyopathy: a prospective study. *Am J Cardiol* 1981;48:252–257.

309. Watkins H. Sudden death in hypertrophic cardiomyopathy. *N Engl J Med* 2000;342:422–424.

310. Anan R, Greve G, Thierfelder L, et al. Prognostic implications of novel beta cardiac myosin heavy chain gene mutations that cause familial hypertrophic cardiomyopathy. *J Clin Invest* 1994;93:280–285.

311. Anan R, Shono H, Kisanuki A, Arima S, Nakao S, Tanaka H. Patients with familial hypertrophic cardiomyopathy caused by a Phe110IIe missense mutation in the cardiac troponin T gene have variable cardiac morphologies and a favorable prognosis. *Circulation* 1998;98:391–397.

312. Marian AJ, Mares A Jr, Kelly DP, et al. Sudden cardiac death in hypertrophic cardiomyopathy: variability in phenotypic expression of beta-myosin heavy chain mutations. *Eur Heart J* 1995;16:368–376.

313. Ackerman MJ, VanDriest SL, Ommen SR, et al. Prevalence and age-dependence of malignant mutations in the beta-myosin heavy chain and troponin T genes in hypertrophic cardiomyopathy: a comprehensive outpatient perspective. *J Am Coll Cardiol* 2002;39:2042–2048.

314. Van Driest SL, Ackerman MJ, Ommen SR, et al. Prevalence and severity of "benign" mutations in the beta-myosin heavy chain, cardiac troponin T, and alpha-tropomyosin genes in hypertrophic cardiomyopathy. *Circulation* 2002;106:3085–3090.

315. Ackerman MJ. Genetic testing for risk stratification in hypertrophic cardiomyopathy and long QT syndrome: fact or fiction? *Curr Opin Cardiol* 2005;20:175–181.

316. McKenna WJ, Harris L, Rowland E, et al. Amiodarone for long-term management of patients with hypertrophic cardiomyopathy. *Am J Cardiol* 1984;54:802–810.

317. McKenna WJ, Oakley CM, Krikler DM, Goodwin JF. Improved survival with amiodarone in patients with hypertrophic cardiomyopathy and ventricular tachycardia. *Br Heart J* 1985;53:412–416.

318. Cecchi F, Olivotto I, Montereggi A, Squillatini G, Dolara A, Maron BJ. Prognostic value of non-sustained ventricular tachycardia and the potential role of amiodarone treatment in hypertrophic cardiomyopathy assessment in an unselected non-referral based patient population. *Heart* 1998;79:331–336.

CHAPTER (31)

Restrictive, Obliterative, and Infiltrative Cardiomyopathies

Brian D. Hoit / Sanjaya Gupta

RESTRICTIVE CARDIOMYOPATHY

〖 〗 DEFINITION OF RESTRICTIVE CARDIOMYOPATHY

A recent American Heart Association consensus document proposed that cardiomyopathies be classified as either primary (i.e., predominantly confined to the heart) or secondary (i.e., as part of a generalized systemic disorder), and this classification is now preferred.[1] An earlier report from the 1995 World Health Organization/International Society and Federation of Cardiology (WHO/IFSFC) Task Force classified cardiomyopathies by dominant pathophysiology or, whenever possible, by etiologic and pathogenetic factors.[2] However, there are several limitations with this earlier approach: (1) the clinical expression of the various cardiomyopathies demonstrates considerable overlap (e.g., hypertrophic, infiltrative, and storage diseases are characterized by increased wall thickness and absence of dilation); (2) the anatomic and pathophysiologic expressions of the cardiomyopathies are not static because of cardiac remodeling and the vicissitudes of natural history (e.g., amyloidosis and hypertrophic cardiomyopathy can progress from a nondilated to a dilated left ventricular [LV] with systolic dysfunction); (3) the confusion and apparent contradictions that result from a failure to account for recent genetic insights into etiology (e.g., troponin I mutations can produce hypertrophic or restrictive cardiomyopathy) and pathophysiology (e.g., some individuals carrying a disease-causing gene mutation fail to express a phenotype or express only a subtle clinical manifestation); and (4) the ambiguities that exist when attempting to categorize heterogeneous disorders by etiology (e.g., a myopathic phenotype can have toxic, metabolic, ischemic, or genetic origins).[1]

Restrictive cardiomyopathy refers to either an idiopathic or systemic myocardial disorder characterized by restrictive filling, normal or reduced LV and right ventricular (RV) volumes, and normal or nearly normal systolic (LV and RV) function. Except for primary nonhypertrophic cardiomyopathy and a few infiltrative diseases (see below), restrictive cardiomyopathies are secondary. These can be noninfiltrative or infiltrative and occur with or without obliteration; infiltration can be interstitial (e.g., amyloidosis, sarcoidosis) or cellular (e.g., hemochromatosis).

〖 〗 CLINICAL FEATURES OF RESTRICTIVE CARDIOMYOPATHY

Involvement of the myocardium (or endomyocardium) and ventricular obliteration can occur either in isolation or in the setting of systemic or iatrogenic disease (Table 31–1). Irrespective of the etiology, terminology, or nature of the myocardial process, the ventricles are small (generally <110 mL/m²), and stiff, restricting ventricular filling. Despite normal (or near normal) systolic function at rest, ventricular diastolic, jugular, and pulmonary venous pressures are increased. Elevated atrial pressures produce symptoms of systemic and pulmonary venous congestion (dyspnea, orthopnea, edema, abdominal discom-

TABLE 31–1

Classification of the Restrictive Cardiomyopathies

Myocardial
1. Noninfiltrative cardiomyopathies
   Idiopathic
   Familial
   Pseudoxanthoma elasticum
   Scleroderma
2. Infiltrative cardiomyopathies
   Amyloidosis
   Sarcoidosis
   Gaucher disease
3. Storage disease
   Hemochromatosis
   Fabry disease
   Glycogen storage diseases
Endomyocardial
1. Obliterative
   Endomyocardial fibrosis
   Hypereosinophilic syndrome
2. Nonobliterative
   Carcinoid
   Malignant infiltration
   Iatrogenic (radiation, drugs)

fort), and underfilled ventricles result in reduced cardiac output and fatigue. In patients with restrictive cardiomyopathy as part of a systemic disorder, cardiac symptoms can dominate or overshadow symptoms referable to other organ systems.

【 】 PHYSICAL FINDINGS

Patients with advanced restrictive cardiomyopathy present with signs and symptoms suggestive of heart failure in the absence of cardiomegaly. Physical examination reflects the elevated systemic and pulmonary venous pressure. Striking elevation of the jugular venous pulse and prominent X and especially Y descents are characteristic. A low pulse volume, owing to a reduced stroke volume and tachycardia, can be seen in severe cases. The apical impulse is not displaced, and systolic murmurs of atrioventricular regurgitation and filling sounds marking the abrupt cessation of rapid early diastolic filling can be present; a fourth heart sound (S_4) can also be present. Hepatomegaly, ascites, and peripheral edema are also common clinical findings.

【 】 DIAGNOSTIC/IMAGING STUDIES

Electrocardiographic abnormalities such as abnormal voltage, atrial and ventricu-

lar arrhythmias, and conduction disturbances are frequent, particularly in infiltrative disease; when restrictive cardiomyopathy is caused by amyloid infiltration, low voltage is usual (Fig. 31–1). Atrial fibrillation is common in idiopathic restrictive cardiomyopathy and cardiac amyloidosis.

The chest radiograph usually reveals normal-sized ventricles, although atrial enlargement and pericardial effusion can produce an enlarged cardiac silhouette. Pleural effusions and signs of pulmonary congestion can also be present.

Echocardiographic findings are nonspecific but in many cases are useful to exculpate other, more common causes of heart failure. Although ventricular systolic function at rest is usually preserved, abnormal diastolic function that progresses through the patterns of abnormal relaxation to a restrictive filling can be identified.

Cardiac MRI can help distinguish between the cardiomyopathies. For example, the cardiomyopathy associated with hemochromatosis produces very low signal intensity because of deposition of iron. MRI is also excellent for differentiating between restrictive and constrictive disease.[3]

Endomyocardial biopsy is occasionally useful in patients with severe constrictive/restrictive physiology as it can identify the subset of patients with specific forms of restrictive cardiomyopathy in whom thoracotomy should be avoided.

DIFFERENTIATION FROM CONSTRICTIVE PERICARDITIS

The differentiation of restrictive cardiomyopathy and constrictive pericarditis remains a challenge. It is important to make the distinction as the treatments differ considerably. Constrictive pericarditis often requires surgical treatment and is usually curable, whereas restrictive cardiomyopathy is treated medically

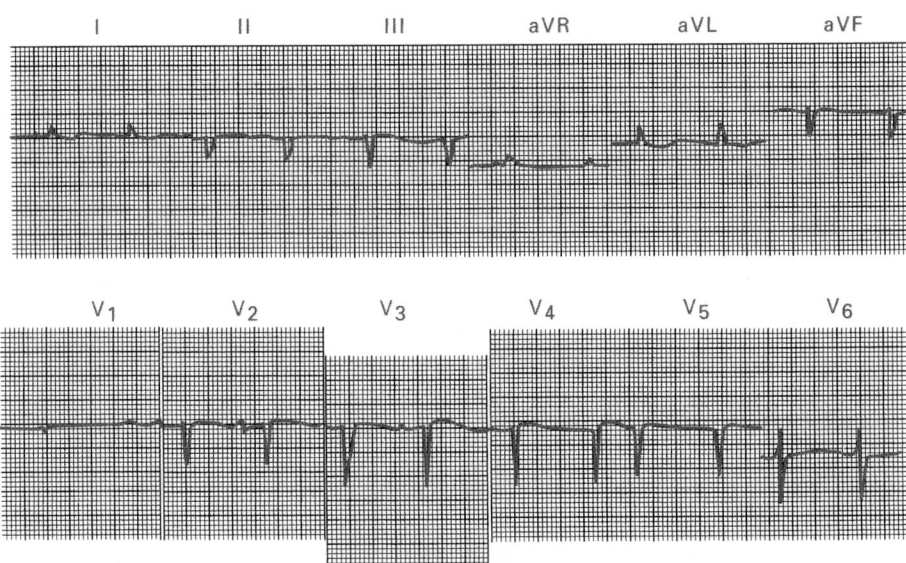

FIGURE 31–1. Electrocardiogram of a patient with amyloidosis. Note the low voltage, which is in striking contrast to the increased left ventricular wall thickness shown echocardiographically. *Source: Shabetai R. Restrictive, obliterative, and infiltrative cardiomyopathies. In: Alexander WA, Schlant R, Fuster V, et al, eds. Hurst's the Heart. 9th ed. New York: McGraw-Hill; 1998:2077. Reproduced with permission.*

TABLE 31–2

Clinical and Hemodynamic Features That Help Distinguish Restrictive Cardiomyopathy from Constrictive Pericarditis

	RESTRICTIVE CARDIOMYOPATHY	CONSTRICTIVE PERICARDITIS
History	Systemic disease that involves the myocardium, multiple myeloma, amyloidosis, cardiac transplant	Acute pericarditis, cardiac surgery, radiation therapy, chest trauma, systemic disease involving the pericardium
Chest radiogram	Absence of calcification, massive atrial enlargement	Helpful when calcification persists, moderate atrial enlargement
ECG	Bundle branch blocks, AV block	Abnormal repolarization
CT/MRI	Normal pericardium	Helpful if thickened (>4 mm) pericardium
Hemodynamics	Helpful if unequal diastolic pressures; concordant effect of respiration on diastolic pressures	Diastolic equilibration dip and plateau
Biopsy	Fibrosis, hypertrophy, infiltration	Normal

AV, atrioventricular.

and is incurable without cardiac transplantation. Although several clinical, imaging, and hemodynamic features are helpful in distinguishing restrictive cardiomyopathy from constrictive pericarditis (Table 31–2), considerable overlap and diagnostic confusion exist.

Although motion mode (M-mode) and two-dimensional (2D) echocardiographic findings of constrictive pericarditis (see Chap. 16) can help differentiate these two conditions, Doppler techniques (spectral Doppler, color M-mode, and Doppler tissue imaging) have assumed an important role in characterizing the nature of transvalvular filling and in clinically distinguishing between constrictive pericarditis and restrictive cardiomyopathy. These Doppler flow patterns and the associated respiratory changes are illustrated in Fig. 31–2. In the patient with *restrictive cardiomyopathy*, mitral valve flow shows an increased E/A wave ratio (≥2) with a short (<150 ms) deceleration time and a short (<70 msec) isovolumic relaxation time (a *restrictive* pattern of filling) without respiratory variation. The tricuspid valve flow shows an increased E/A wave ratio without respiratory variation, a shortened deceleration time, and a short isovolumic relaxation time that shortens further with inspiration. The systolic/diastolic (S/D) ratio of pulmonary venous flow is <1, atrial reversals are increased (not shown in Fig. 31–2), and there is little respiratory variation. The S/D ratio of hepatic venous flow is <1, and prominent reversals are seen during inspiration. Doppler tissue imaging shows a striking decrease in E$_a$ (<8 cm/s), and the propagation velocity on color M-mode is <45 cm/s.

MRI and CT are useful for accurately assessing pericardial thickness (Fig. 31–3); a pericardium >4.0 mm thick can distinguish the two entities. Ventricular coupling, quantified by the respiratory changes in septal excursion on real-time CINE MRI, can differentiate patients with histologically-proven constrictive pericarditis (large septal excursions) from restrictive cardiomyopathy (small septal excursions).[3]

B-type natriuretic peptide (BNP) levels are markedly elevated in patients with restrictive cardiomyopathy compared to constrictive pericarditis and appear to be a useful noninvasive biomarker to distinguish these conditions.[4] Invasive hemodynamics can be helpful (see below), and occasionally a histologic diagnosis is necessary.

It is important to remember that clinical and laboratory testing, including imaging and pathologic studies, can produce results consistent with mixed constrictive pericarditis and restrictive cardiomyopathy; indeed, the two entities can coexist (e.g., after mediastinal irradiation or after coronary artery bypass grafting [CABG]). In these cases, a decision to treat conservatively or surgically explore a patient requires experienced clinical judgment.

CARDIAC CATHETERIZATION

Most patients in whom restrictive cardiomyopathy is a serious consideration should undergo right- and left-sided heart catheterization to document the diagnosis, assess severity, and, in some patients, establish the etiology by means of endomyocardial biopsy. The venous pressure is elevated, and the deep and rapid fall of the right atrial Y descent is striking. During inspiration, the descent of the V wave in the right atrium becomes deeper, steeper, and more pointed, whereas the other waves of the venous pulse and the mean atrial pressure do not vary throughout the respiratory cycle. Patients with constrictive pericarditis generally have lower a RV systolic pressure and an RV end-diastolic pressure greater than one-third of the RV systolic pressure, as opposed to patients with restrictive cardiomyopathy, but these differences are far from absolute. The early portion of diastole is characterized by a deep, sharp dip followed by a plateau, during which no further increase in RV pressure occurs (Fig. 31–4). These hemodynamic features are identical to those of constrictive pericarditis and can cause diagnostic confusion; a higher LV than RV filling pressure strongly favors the diagnosis of restrictive cardiomyopathy rather than constrictive pericarditis. LV systolic pressure is normal, whereas the LV diastolic pressure tracing shows the same abnormalities as those of the RV (see Fig. 31–4).

Left ventriculography usually shows a normal ejection fraction and the absence of major regional wall motion abnormalities. Endomyocardial biopsy is an integral part of the workup of many patients with restrictive cardiomyopathy. When distinction from constrictive pericarditis is particularly difficult, the biopsy can furnish proof of myocardial disease and establish the cause of restrictive cardiomyopathy (e.g., amyloidosis), or (by virtue of unremarkable histology) suggest the need for surgical exploration, even in the absence of a thickened pericardium.

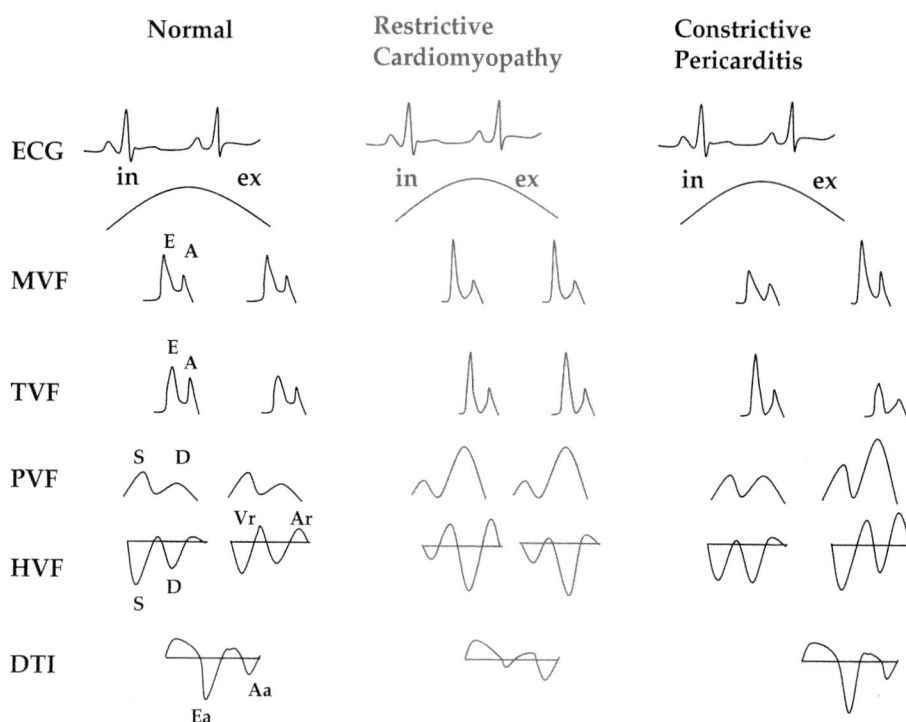

FIGURE 31–2. Schematic of Doppler flows during inspiration (*in*) and expiration (*ex*) in normals, restrictive cardiomyopathy, and constrictive pericarditis. See text for details. A, atrial systolic filling; Aa, late diastolic tissue velocities; Ar, atrial systolic reversals; D, diastolic flow; DTI, Doppler tissue imaging; E, early diastolic filling; Ea, early diastolic tissue velocities; HVF, hepatic venous flow; MVF, mitral valve flow; PVF, pulmonary venous flow; S, systolic flow; TVF, tricuspid valve flow; Vr, V-wave reversals. *Source: Hoit BD. Restrictive cardiomyopathy. In: Pohost G, O'Rourke R, Shah P, Berman D, eds. Imaging in Cardiovascular Disease. New York: Lippincott Williams & Wilkins; 2000:60–70. Reproduced with permission.*

TREATMENT OF RESTRICTIVE CARDIOMYOPATHY (GENERAL CONSIDERATIONS)

Except in certain instances described below (see Specific Restrictive Cardiomyopathic Diseases), the treatment of restrictive cardiomyopathy is empiric and directed toward the treatment of diastolic heart failure. Reduction in the elevated ventricular diastolic pressures produces substantial improvement in pulmonary and systemic congestion, but judicious use of diuretics is warranted in view of the steep pressure-volume relation of the ventricles and the need to maintain a relatively high filling pressure. Vasodilators can also jeopardize ventricular filling and should be used cautiously. Calcium channel blockers are used by some because of their beneficial effect in hypertrophic cardiomyopathies, but improvement in ventricular compliance with their use has not been demonstrated in restrictive cardiomyopathy. Low dose angiotensin-converting enzyme inhibition can be useful, but orthostatic hypotension, particularly in patients with autonomic nervous system involvement, can be limiting.[5] Atrial fibrillation potentially worsens ventricular filling and therefore maintenance of normal sinus rhythm is essential; however, digoxin should be used with caution because of its potential arrhythmogenicity, especially in amyloidosis. β Blockers are useful in the early stages of disease and control the ventricular response in atrial fibrillation but can exacerbate symptoms later.[5] Antico-

agulation with warfarin can be indicated in patients with atrial fibrillation, valvular regurgitation, and low cardiac output, because of the high incidence of thromboembolic complications. The majority of children with restrictive cardiomyopathy require transplantation.[6]

SPECIFIC RESTRICTIVE CARDIOMYOPATHIC DISEASES

A useful classification of the restrictive cardiomyopathies is shown in Table 31–1. This scheme is based on the cardiac compartment predominantly involved (i.e., myocardial versus endomyocardial); the myocardial diseases are divided into the noninfiltrative, infiltrative, and the storage diseases, and the endomyocardial diseases are divided into obliterative (i.e., endomyocardial fibrosis and the hypereosinophilic syndrome), and the nonobliterative (carcinoid, infiltrative, and iatrogenic).

【 】 MYOCARDIAL DISEASES

Noninfiltrative Cardiomyopathies

Idiopathic and Familial Restrictive Cardiomyopathy Although idiopathic restrictive cardiomyopathy is not generally recognized to have a familial predisposition, several small families have been

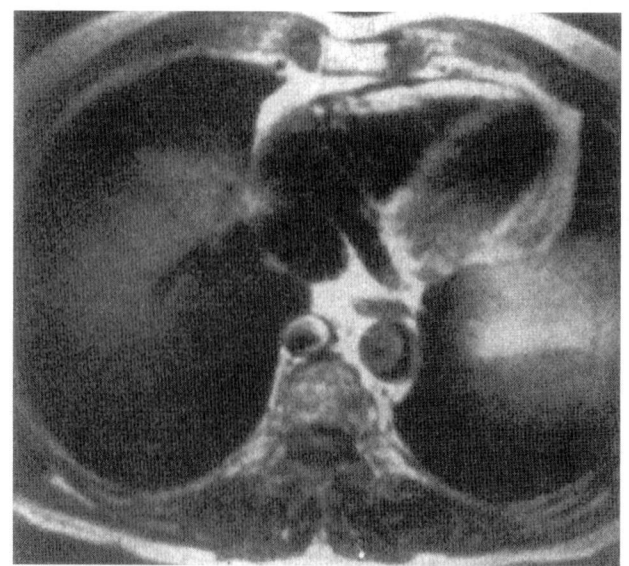

FIGURE 31–3. Magnetic resonance image showing normal pericardium as a low-intensity (*black*) line anterior to the right ventricle between high-intensity (*white*) epicardial and mediastinal fat. *Source: Hoit BD. Imaging the pericardium. Cardiol Clin 1990;8:588. Reproduced with permission.*

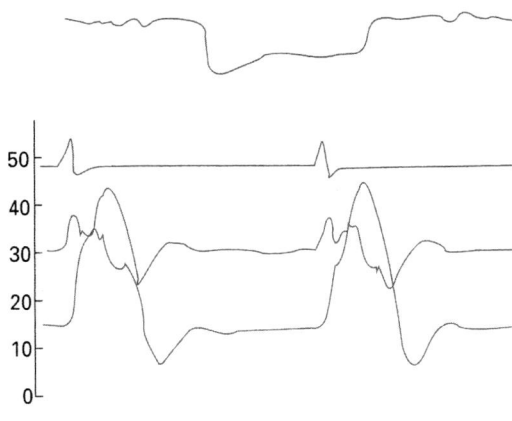

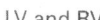

LV and RV

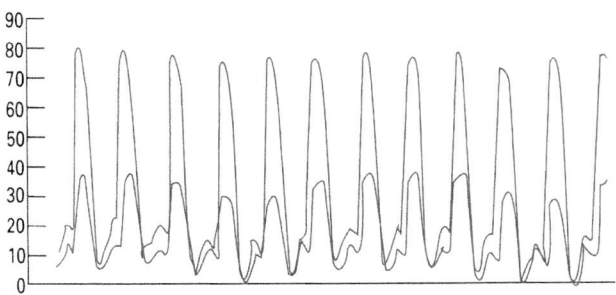

FIGURE 31–4. Top: Right-sided heart hemodynamic data from a patient with amyloidosis recorded with a high-fidelity catheter. From the top tracing down is a respirometer, electrocardiogram, right ventricular (RV) *dP/dt*, and RV pressure. Note the characteristic dip-and-plateau configuration. *Bottom:* Simultaneous RV and left ventricular (LV) pressure tracings from another patient with cardiac amyloidosis. In this patient, the typical dip-and-plateau pattern was not present, but during inspiration LV and RV diastolic pressures equilibrated. Source: From Shabetai R. Restrictive, obliterative, and infiltrative cardiomyopathies. In: Alexander WA, Schlant R, Fuster V, et al, eds. Hurst's the Heart. 9th ed. New York: McGraw-Hill; 1998:2079. Reproduced with permission.

reported.[7,8] The phenotypes have been variable with both autosomal dominant and recessive patterns of inheritance. Several missense mutations in human cardiac troponin I (one of the genetic causes of hypertrophic cardiomyopathy) have been reported to cause restrictive cardiomyopathy.[7–9] In addition, a heterogeneous group of autosomal dominant disorders are causally related to the desmin gene (*DES*, located on chromosome 2q35); these *desmin-related myopathies* are characterized by skeletal myopathy and cardiac conduction abnormalities with accumulation of desmin deposits in skeletal and cardiac muscle.[8,10] Restrictive cardiomyopathy is a relatively uncommon manifestation of desmin-related myopathy; mutations in the *DES* gene can also cause a dilated cardiomyopathy.[8]

Myocyte hypertrophy and fibrosis on endomyocardial biopsy characterize idiopathic restrictive cardiomyopathy, and the absence of myocyte disarray is an important pathologic distinction from hypertrophic cardiomyopathy. However, overlap syndromes characterized by physiologic evidence of restriction and myocyte hypertrophy but without myocyte disarray or LV hypertrophy on echocardiography are reported. Moreover, primary restrictive and hypertrophic cardiomyopathies can represent different phenotypic expressions of the same genetic disease.[9]

Doppler and 2D echocardiography are reliable, noninvasive techniques for diagnosing primary restrictive cardiomyopathy. An echocardiographic feature distinguishing primary restrictive cardiomyopathy from cardiac amyloidosis (in addition to the associated clinical features) is the increased LV wall thickness in the latter. In both disorders (and restrictive cardiomyopathies in general), ventricular dimensions are normal or reduced, systolic function is variable, and atrial dimensions are increased. A dominant mitral early diastolic *E* velocity, an increased pulmonary venous atrial systolic *A* reversal velocity and duration, and shortened mitral deceleration time are present in both children and adults with primary restrictive cardiomyopathy (Fig. 31–5). On CT or MRI scans, evidence of restrictive filling (e.g., right atrial and caval enlargement) is common in both restrictive cardiomyopathy and constrictive pericarditis. MRI can differentiate primary restrictive cardiomyopathy from amyloidosis based on tissue characterization.[11]

The prognosis of true idiopathic restrictive cardiomyopathy is difficult to establish because prior studies have included patients with hypertension, coronary artery disease, and ventricular enlargement and hypertrophy.[12] Although idiopathic restrictive cardiomyopathy initially can have a protracted course, the prognosis is poor in older patients (particularly males) with increasing signs of systemic and pulmonary venous congestion, atrial fibrillation, and marked left atrial enlargement (>60 mm); in that group, the Kaplan-Meier 5-year survival is 64 percent, compared with the expected 85 percent survival.[12]

Pseudoxanthoma Elasticum Pseudoxanthoma elasticum is a rare, genetically heterogeneous disorder characterized by fragmentation and calcification of elastic fibers involving the skin, eyes, and gastrointestinal and cardiovascular systems. Although endocardial fibroelastosis uncommonly causes restrictive cardiomyopathy (Fig. 31–6), coronary artery disease with premature death is a major problem in these patients.

Progressive Systemic Sclerosis Myocardial fibrosis, which can have a patchy distribution and be present in both ventricles, is found in the majority of patients with scleroderma at autopsy. On echocardiography, LV wall thickening in the absence of hypertension and evidence of LV dysfunction can be seen, but heart failure caused by either restrictive or dilated cardiomyopathy is rare. Pericardial involvement and electrocardiographic abnormalities (heart block, supraventricular and ventricular tachycardia, and pseudoinfarction patterns) are common. Pulmonary hypertension is a leading cause of morbidity and mortality in patients with scleroderma.

Infiltrative Cardiomyopathies

Amyloidosis Amyloidosis is a systemic disorder characterized by interstitial deposition of linear, rigid, nonbranching amyloid protein fibrils in multiple organs (e.g., heart, kidney, liver, nerve); amino acid substitutions in prefibrillar protein lead to protein instability, which in turn, causes these proteins to precipitate out of the extracellular matrix as amyloid.[13] Currently five subtypes of amyloidosis are described, based on the underlying disease:[14] (1) cardiac involvement is most common in **immuno-**

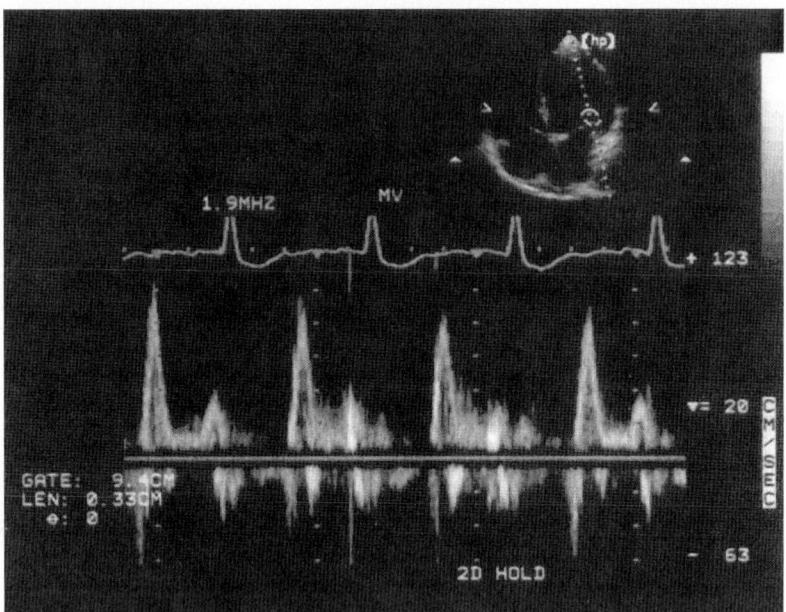

FIGURE 31–5. Doppler record of mitral inflow velocity from a patient with idiopathic restrictive cardiomyopathy. Note the dominant early diastolic wave. *Source: Shabetai R. Restrictive, obliterative, and infiltrative cardiomyopathies. In: Alexander WA, Schlant R, Fuster V, et al, eds. Hurst's the Heart. 9th ed. New York: McGraw-Hill; 1998:2077. Reproduced with permission.*

globulin amyloidosis (AL type), which is caused by plasma cell production of immunoglobulin light chains; cardiac manifestations develop in approximately one-half of patients. The initial cardiac manifestation is often a ventricular filling pattern of abnormal ventricular relaxation that gradually advances to a restrictive pattern that is accompanied by clinical signs and symptoms of right-sided heart failure. Most patients die of heart failure or arrhythmia. Atrial fibrillation and conduction abnormalities are common; infra-His prolongation is an independent predictor of sudden cardiac death.[15] AL amyloidosis is caused by several conditions, including primary amyloidosis (a plasma cell disorder in which 5–10 percent of bone marrow plasma cells have clonal dominance of a light-chain isotype, usually lambda II), multiple myeloma, and other plasma cell dyscrasias. Multiple myeloma is also reported to cause diastolic heart failure in the absence of amyloidosis. The majority of patients with primary amyloidosis and cardiac involvement have obstructive intramural coronary amyloidosis and microscopic changes of myocardial ischemia.[16] (2) Mutations of the protein transthyretin (formerly called prealbumin) are usually inherited as an autosomal dominant trait (**familial amyloidosis**) and produce peripheral and autonomic neuropathy in addition to cardiac disease; more than 80 mutations have been described.[14] Cardiac involvement occurs late in the disease and,

although present in less than one-third of cases, it is responsible for over half of the deaths.[15] The pattern of myocardial involvement, the susceptibility to cardiac amyloid deposition, the incidence of heart failure, and the prognosis is related to the specific transthyretin mutation. For example, a transthyretin mutation at isoleucine 122 is a cause of late-onset cardiac amyloidosis in African Americans.[17] (3) **Senile systemic amyloidosis** can affect one-quarter of patients older than 80 years of age. This subtype is derived from normal transthyretin and typically involves the atria. Rarely, the entire heart or the aorta can be involved. This condition is not always benign (although it carries the most favorable prognosis) and can result in atrial fibrillation, conduction disturbances heart failure, and cardiac death. (4) Cardiac deposition of amyloid protein (protein A, a nonimmunoglobin) can also occur in **secondary (AA) amyloidosis**, which is caused by chronic infections (such as tuberculosis) or autoimmune disease (such as rheumatoid arthritis). Cardiac disease is less common than the other subtypes, but when present, carries an unfavorable prognosis. (5) **Hemodialysis-associated (β_2) amyloidosis** is characterized by β_2 microglobulin amyloid fibril subunit deposition in the bones and joints of patients on chronic hemodialysis; cardiac involvement is uncommon.[14]

Clinical Features Amyloid deposits can be interstitial and widespread, resulting in restrictive cardiomyopathy, or localized to (1) conduction tissue, resulting in heart block and ventricular arrhythmias (especially familial amyloid); (2) the cardiac valves,

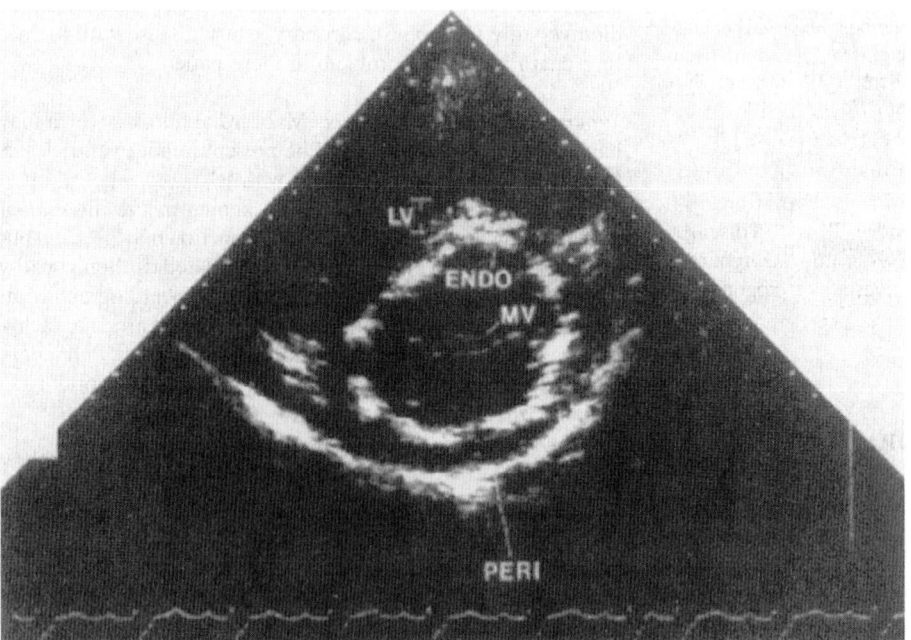

FIGURE 31–6. Short-axis view of the left ventricle at the mitral valve level in a patient with pseudoxanthoma elasticum. Note the calcified endomyocardium and echodense pericardium. The endocardial calcification was clearly visible by fluoroscopy. ENDO, endomyocardium; LV, left ventricle; MV, mitral valve; PERI, pericardium. *Source: Shabetai R. Restrictive, obliterative, and infiltrative cardiomyopathies. In: Alexander WA, Schlant R, Fuster V, et al, eds. Hurst's the Heart. 9th ed. New York: McGraw-Hill; 1998:2085. Reproduced with permission.*

causing valvular regurgitation; (3) the pericardium, producing constriction; (4) the coronary arteries, resulting in ischemia, and (5) the pulmonary vasculature causing pulmonary hypertension and cor pulmonale. Amyloid can be isolated to the subendocardium in senile amyloid and amyloid secondary to chronic disease. Deposition of amyloid and atrial natriuretic factor (ANF) in the atria is frequent in aged hearts.[18] Despite sinus rhythm, atrial mechanical failure and thrombus formation can result because of electromechanical dissociation. In some cases, the clinical picture is dominated by autonomic neuropathy (orthostatic hypotension, syncope, diarrhea, lack of sweating, and impotence), and nephropathy and cardiac involvement are unrecognized. Cardiac manifestations define a spectrum, often progressive through stages of severity, from the asymptomatic to biventricular failure.

Diagnostic/Imaging Studies The cardiac silhouette on the chest radiograph can be normal or moderately enlarged. The ECG typically shows decreased voltage, a pseudoinfarction pattern, left axis deviation; arrhythmias and conduction disturbances can predominate the clinical course.

The M-mode echocardiogram can reveal symmetrical wall thickness involving the right and left ventricles, a small or normal LV cavity, variable (but often depressed) systolic function, left atrial enlargement, and a small pericardial effusion (Fig. 31–7). 2D echocardiographic findings include thickening of the ventricular myocardium, the interatrial septum and valves (especially the atrioventricular [AV] valves), enlarged papillary muscles, and dilated atria and inferior vena cava (Fig. 31–8). LV wall thickness is an important prognostic variable; in one study, patients with biopsy-proven amyloidosis having a mean wall thickness ≥15 mm had a median survival of 0.4 years, whereas patients with a mean wall thickness ≤12 mm had a median survival of 2.4 years.[19] Highly reflective echoes producing a granular or sparkling appearance and occurring in a patchy distribution are characteristic echocardiographic findings but are neither sensitive nor specific; concentric hypertrophy, as occurs in hypertension or aortic stenosis, can produce a uniformly speckled or echolucent appearance of the myocardium; and idiopathic hypertrophic cardiomyopathy can display a patchy, granular sparkling. Amyloid cardiomyopathy can exist despite the absence of echocardiographic evidence of infiltration.

Doppler studies can show the restrictive pattern of LV filling (see Fig. 31–7) and the RV filling pattern is often abnormal. The systolic-to-diastolic pulmonary venous flow ratio is <1 and atrial reversals increase with inspiration in the pulmonary and hepatic veins. However, the *earliest sign* of amyloid cardiomyopathy is impaired LV relaxation, manifest by an E/A ratio <1, and increased isovolumic relaxation and transmitral diastolic deceleration times. In addition, Doppler has shown utility in prognosis; a deceleration time <150 msec and an increased E/A transmitral ratio are strong predictors of cardiac death.[20]

Abnormalities of LV filling are also demonstrated with the LV time-activity curve from radionuclide ventriculography. Moreover, radionuclide imaging using technetium-99m pyrophosphate or indium-111 antimyosin can be useful in diagnosis. The infiltrative pathology associated with amyloidosis can be detected by tissue characterization using MRI. In a recent study, qualitative global and subendocardial gadolinium enhancement of the myocardium, associated with faster gadolinium clearance from the blood pool,

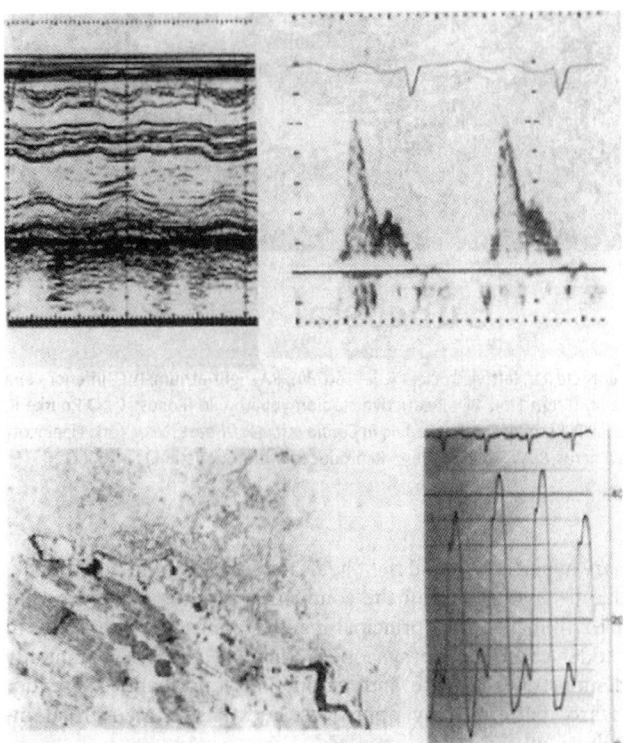

FIGURE 31–7. Amyloidosis. *Top left*: M-mode echocardiogram showing increased thickness of the left ventricular myocardium (calibration mark = 1 cm). *Top right*: Doppler tracing of mitral inflow velocity. Note that the atrial contribution to mitral blood flow velocity is markedly reduced (calibration mark = 20 cm/s). *Bottom left*: Electromicrograph showing extensive replacement of myocardium by amyloid. *Bottom right*: Right ventricular pressure tracing. A diastolic dip-plateau pattern is absent because of tachycardia. Source: Shabetai R. Restrictive, obliterative, and infiltrative cardiomyopathies. In: Alexander WA, Schlant R, Fuster V, et al, eds. Hurst's the Heart. 9th ed. New York: McGraw-Hill; 1998:2085. Reproduced with permission.

was higher in patients with cardiac amyloidosis than that in hypertensive controls, suggesting that cardiac MRI can have value in diagnosis and treatment followup.[21]

The variable clinical, diagnostic, and prognostic features reflect the location, nature, and extent of amyloid deposition and the temporal course of the disease. Serum and urine protein electrophoresis is diagnostic in most cases of primarily amyloidosis, but monoclonal protein is not secreted in 10 percent of cases.[15] Endomyocardial biopsy of the RV (most helpful if an abdominal fat aspirate is negative) provides the diagnosis, establishes the histochemistry, and quantifies myocardial damage and atrophy.[22]

Treatment and Prognosis of Amyloidosis The treatment of amyloidosis is unrewarding and symptomatic therapy is fraught with hazard; patients are sensitive to digoxin and calcium channel blockers, and hypotension with vasodilators and diuretics is a threat because of the steep LV pressure-volume relation. Angiotensin-converting enzyme inhibitors have been used with varying response rates. Amiodarone and ibutilide are effective drugs for patients with atrial fibrillation. For patients with symptomatic bradycardia or high-grade conduction system disease, a pacemaker should be implanted.[14]

Immunosuppressive therapy with melphalan and prednisone is the established treatment regimen for primary (AL) amyloido-

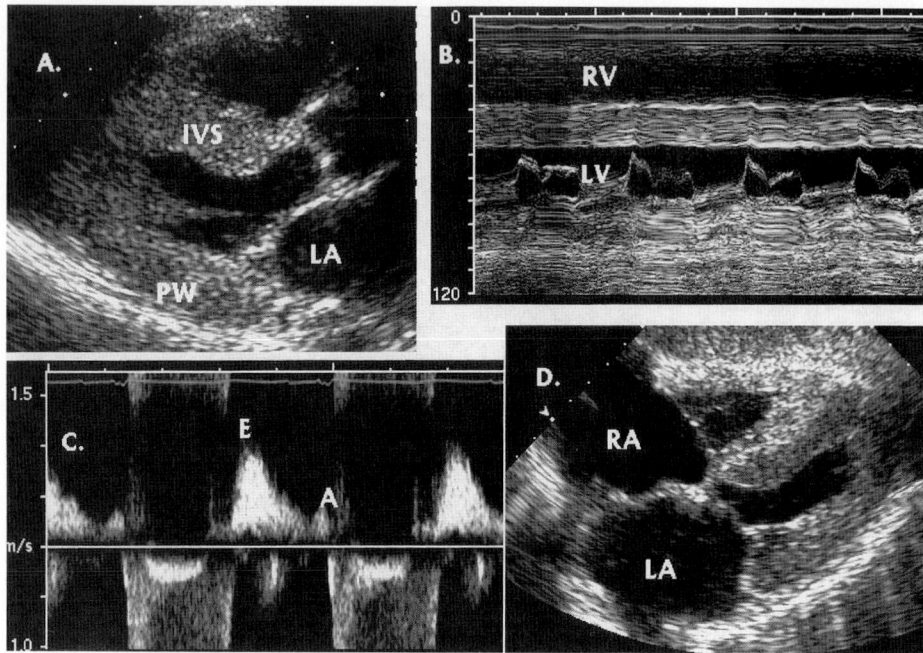

FIGURE 31–8. M-mode two-dimensional and Doppler echocardiograms from a patient with biopsy-proven amyloidosis causing hemodynamic restriction. Left ventricular systolic function is mildly impaired, wall thickness is increased, and there is biatrial enlargement. **A.** Parasternal long axis view. **B.** M-mode through the thickened mitral valve. **C.** Doppler of restrictive diastolic mitral inflow and systolic mitral regurgitation. **D.** Subcostal four-chamber view. A, late diastolic transmitral velocity; E, early diastolic transmitral velocity; IVS, interventricular septum; LA, left atrium; LV, left ventricle; PW, left ventricular posterior wall; RA, right atrium; RV, right ventricle.

sis.[23] Autologous stem-cell infusion reduces the monoclonal gammopathy but has little effect on existing infiltrative amyloid. Orthotopic cardiac transplantation is generally not recommended because of the systemic nature of amyloidosis and the possibility of recurrence in the transplant, but successful cases have been reported.[24] Liver transplantation can be lifesaving in patients with familial amyloidosis because the liver is the site of transthyretin production.

It is important to distinguish between familial and primary amyloidosis because the former carries a better prognosis (median survival of 5.8 years) than the latter (median survival of 13 months).[14] The thickness of the left ventricular wall is directly proportional to the severity of heart failure and is inversely proportional to prognosis. Syncope is an ominous sign and tends to be a precursor to sudden cardiac death. Shorter median survival times are seen with elevations of troponin I and T at the time of diagnosis and predict survival better than symptomatic heart failure or echocardiography.[14]

Sarcoidosis Sarcoidosis is a disorder of unknown etiology characterized by the presence of noncaseating granulomas that involve many organs (e.g., lung, skin, lymph nodes, liver, spleen). Granulomas involve the heart in sarcoidosis in as many as 25 percent of patients but are frequently subclinical. Nevertheless, in approximately half of the fatalities, cardiac involvement is responsible. Rarely, sarcoid is confined to the heart. The combination of extracardiac manifestations and cardiac abnormalities favors a presumptive diagnosis of sarcoidosis without biopsy. It is important to suspect cardiac sarcoidosis early, as aggressive treatment improves the prognosis. Interstitial granulomatous inflam-

mation initially produces diastolic dysfunction, but later, when the disease is more extensive, it can produce systolic (at times focal) abnormalities. Localized thinning and dilation of the basilar LV resembling ischemic heart disease are characteristic. Restrictive cardiomyopathy is uncommon. However, sarcoid pulmonary involvement is frequent and produces echo and Doppler findings of pulmonary hypertension and right heart failure. High-grade AV block, a result of involvement of the conduction system, and ventricular arrhythmias are the principal manifestations and can result in sudden cardiac death; syncope is common. The ECG commonly demonstrates T-wave and conduction abnormalities. Pseudoinfarct patterns can appear with extensive myocardial involvement.

Echocardiographic findings include evidence of systolic and diastolic LV dysfunction, LV aneurysm formation, abnormal ventricular wall thickness, pericardial effusion, regional wall motion abnormalities in the basal septum with apical sparing, and evidence of cor pulmonale. Thallium 201 has been used to indicate areas of myocardial involvement although the defects are relatively nonspecific for sarcoidosis. Patients with gallium-67 uptake have been shown to respond better to corticosteroids.[25] MRI can detect mass lesions because of sarcoid granuloma or scar. Endomyocardial biopsy is useful but can be falsely negative. An important entity in the differential diagnosis is giant-cell myocarditis, which is characterized by a more aggressive and fatal course than cardiac sarcoid. Treatment with prednisone for symptomatic patients is warranted in highly suspicious or proven cases because the cardiac granuloma can be sensitive. High-grade AV nodal block usually requires a permanent pacemaker, and in patients at high risk for sudden cardiac death, an automatic implantable cardioverter-defibrillator (AICD) is appropriate. Calcium channel blockers can ameliorate diastolic dysfunction in patients with restrictive cardiomyopathy; patients with dilated cardiomyopathy are treated for congestive heart failure. Cardiac transplantation is an appropriate consideration for intractable heart failure or arrhythmia.[26]

Gaucher Disease Gaucher disease is the most common lysosomal storage disease. It is caused by an inherited deficiency of the enzyme β-glucocerebroside, which results in accumulation of cerebroside in the reticuloendothelial system, brain, and heart. Diffuse interstitial infiltration of the left ventricle occurs, with reduced LV wall compliance and cardiac output, but is often subclinical. LV and left-sided valvular thickening and pericardial effusion are seen on echo. Enzyme replacement therapy with alglucerase (the placental derivative) and imiglucerase (the recombinant form) has revolutionized the treatment of Gaucher disease but its high cost still limits its availability in many countries.[27]

Storage Diseases

Hemochromatosis Type I or hereditary hemochromatosis is an autosomal recessive iron-storage disease caused by mutations in the HLA-linked *HFE* gene (the first hemochromatosis gene identified). It is seen mostly in men and almost entirely in people of northern European descent. Type II or juvenile hemochromatosis is a rare, autosomal recessive disease caused by an unidentified locus on chromosome 1q. Type III is autosomal recessive and is caused by mutations in TFR2 (which encodes a transferring receptor isoform). Type IV is autosomal dominant, with mutations in the gene, *ferroportin-1*, which encodes an intestinal iron transport molecule. Type V is also autosomal dominant, with mutations in the H subunit of the iron storage molecule ferritin.[28]

The clinical features of hemochromatosis are caused by accumulation of iron in the heart, pancreas, skin, liver, anterior pituitary, and gonads. Myocardial iron deposition in hemochromatosis, either primary or secondary (e.g., resulting from multiple transfusions, ineffective erythropoiesis), usually produces dilated cardiomyopathy but can cause restrictive cardiomyopathy. Arrhythmia and conduction disturbances are common; indeed, congestive heart failure, conduction abnormalities, and supraventricular and ventricular arrhythmias occur in one-third of patients. Interstitial fibrosis is variable and unrelated to the extent of iron deposition, which occurs in the myocyte; secondarily, myocardial fibrosis can develop. Bronze diabetes and hepatic dysfunction, reflecting iron deposition in the skin, pancreas and liver are frequent associated manifestations.

Findings consistent with either dilated or restrictive cardiomyopathy can be seen; the presence of systolic dysfunction indicates a poor prognosis (Fig. 31–9). Granular sparkling and atrial enlargement can be observed, but these are nonspecific signs. Quantitative ultrasonic analysis of integrated backscatter has been used experimentally to detect changes in the echo reflectivity of the myocardium because of iron deposition in thalassemia major. CT and MRI can demonstrate subclinical cardiac involvement, and tissue characterization can be possible with MRI. Endomyocardial biopsy is confirmatory; in selected instances, it can be useful in excluding the diagnosis.

Repeated phlebotomy is recommended for primary hemochromatosis, and the chelating agent desferrioxamine is often beneficial in secondary hemochromatosis; combinations with the orally active chelator deferiprone have been used successfully in Europe.[29] Cardiac transplantation (with or without liver transplantation) can be considered in selected cases.

Fabry Disease Fabry disease is an X-linked, genetically heterogeneous disorder of glycosphingolipid metabolism caused by lysosomal ceramide (α-galactosidase) deficiency that leads to accumulation of glycolipid in the heart, skin, and kidneys. Glycolipid

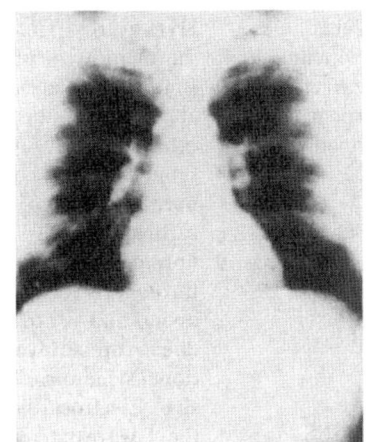
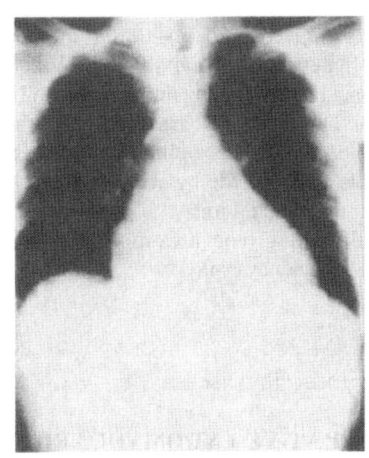
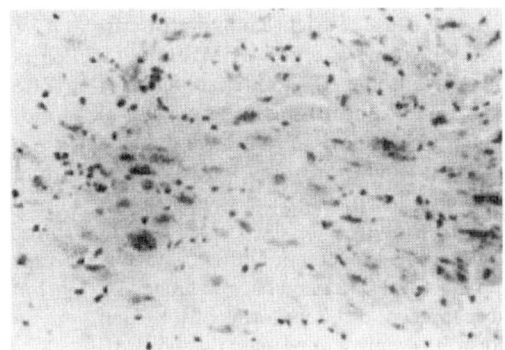

FIGURE 31–9. Chest radiograph of a patient with cardiac hemochromatosis before (*top right*) and after (*top left*) several months of treatment with phlebotomy. *Bottom*: Endomyocardial biopsy that established the diagnosis. *Source: Shabetai R. Restrictive, obliterative, and infiltrative cardiomyopathies. In: Alexander WA, Schlant R, Fuster V, et al, eds. Hurst's the Heart. 9th ed. New York: McGraw-Hill; 1998:2085. Reproduced with permission.*

accumulation in the myocardium and vascular and valvular endothelium can present with a restrictive, hypertrophic, or dilated cardiomyopathy, mitral regurgitation, ischemic heart disease, or aortic degeneration. Echocardiographic findings in restrictive cardiomyopathy mimic those seen in amyloid, and LV mass correlates with the severity of disease. Hypertension, mitral valve prolapse, and heart failure are common clinical presentations. Definitive diagnosis can require endomyocardial biopsy. Enzyme replacement therapy has proven effective but is limited by cost and the availability of the enzyme.[30]

Pompe Disease Pompe disease (glycogen storage type II) is caused by an inherited (autosomal recessive) metabolic abnormality as a result of acid maltase deficiency that causes massive amounts of glycogen deposition in the heart and skeletal muscles. A hypertrophied, hypokinetic LV in an infant with muscle hypotonia, hyperreflexia, and failure to thrive are characteristic findings. The echocardiographic manifestations can be indistinguishable from hypertrophic obstructive cardiomyopathy. The diagnosis can be made by absence of α-1,4-glucosidase activity on skeletal muscle biopsy. Adults with glycogen storage type III disease (debranching enzyme deficiency) can have marked left ventricular hypertrophy (LVH) on echocardiography.

Two new disorders belonging to the subgroup of infiltrative forms of LVH that includes Pompe and Fabry disease have clinical manifestations predominantly limited to the heart. The nonsarcomeric protein mutations in two genes involved in cardiac metabolism (the γ-2-regulatory subunit of the AMP-activated protein kinase and lysosome-associated membrane protein-2) are reported to be responsible for primary cardiac glycogen storage diseases in older children and adults; the clinical presentation resembles hypertrophic cardiomyopathy.[2]

ENDOMYOCARDIAL DISEASES

Obliterative Endomyocardial Disease

Endomyocardial Fibrosis and Hypereosinophilic Syndrome

Endomyocardial diseases that cause restrictive obliterative cardiomyopathies include endomyocardial fibrosis (EMF) and hypereosinophilic (Loeffler) syndrome. The former accounts for 10 to 20 percent of deaths because of heart disease in equatorial Africa but is seen throughout the world. In contrast, Loeffler endocarditis is seen mainly in countries with a temperate climate. Although it shares similar pathologic features with EMF, it affects mainly men; is usually related to parasitic infections, leukemia, and immunologic reactions; and is characterized by intense eosinophilia and thromboembolic phenomena. The endemic variety EMF can be related to high levels of cerium and low levels of magnesium.[31]

Cardiac involvement occurs in the majority of patients with the hypereosinophilic syndrome (unexplained eosinophilia exceeding 1500 eosinophils per cubic milliliter for at least 6 months and symptoms of organ involvement) and often has a biventricular distribution. Cardiotoxic eosinophils (abnormal cells containing vacuoles and having fewer than the normal number of granules) are central to the pathogenesis. The disease is characterized by organ damage from eosinophilic infiltration and mediator release. The cardiac pathology consists of an acute eosinophilic myocarditis, fibrinoid myocarditis, fibrinoid vasculitis of the intramural coronary arteries, mural thrombosis formation along damaged endocardium (often with eosinophils), fibrotic endocardial thickening and ultimately, endomyocardial fibrosis with ventricular obliteration. In addition to symptoms caused by cardiac involvement, patients have skin rash and constitutional symptoms. The disease is aggressive and rapidly progressive. ECG abnormalities (especially involving the T wave) are common but nonspecific. Hemodynamic findings are typical of restrictive cardiomyopathy.

ENDOMYOCARDIAL FIBROSIS

In contrast to Loeffler syndrome, EMF has a more insidious onset, has no gender predilection, and most often affects children and young adults. The disease is more indolent than Loeffler, and biventricular involvement occurs in only approximately one-half of the cases. LV involvement produces symptoms as a result of pulmonary congestion, whereas the less common isolated RV involvement (approximately 10 percent) can

simulate constrictive pericarditis. AV regurgitation and embolic episodes are frequent complications, and atrial fibrillation is common.

ECHOCARDIOGRAPHIC FEATURES

Echocardiography can be normal in the acute necrotic stage and endomyocardial biopsy can be needed to make the diagnosis if cardiac disease is suspected. Endomyocardial disease is characterized by endocardial fibrosis of the apex and subvalvular regions of one or both ventricles, resulting in restriction to inflow to the affected ventricle. Although their clinical presentations differ, the pathology, and therefore the cardiac imaging studies, are generally similar in the endomyocardial diseases; typically, apical obliteration of the right and/or left ventricle, apical thrombus, preservation of ventricular systolic function with thickening of the posterior atrioventricular valve apparatus and posterobasal LV wall, echo densities in the endocardium, and small ventricular and large atrial cavities are noted (Fig. 31–10). Involvement of the posterior mitral and tricuspid valve leaflets results in mitral and tricuspid regurgitation; less commonly, restricted motion can produce stenosis. Sparing of the outflow tracts is characteristic. Doppler interrogation yields typical patterns of restriction (increased E/A, decreased isovolumic relaxation time [IVRT]; decreased deceleration time), mitral and tricuspid regurgitation, and, less often, stenosis. Not surprisingly, the location, extent, and severity of involvement determine the clinical picture.

TREATMENT OF THE OBLITERATIVE RESTRICTIVE CARDIOMYOPATHIES

Medical therapy of Loeffler syndrome is often ineffective and frustrating. Treatment consists of symptomatic relief, anticoagulants,

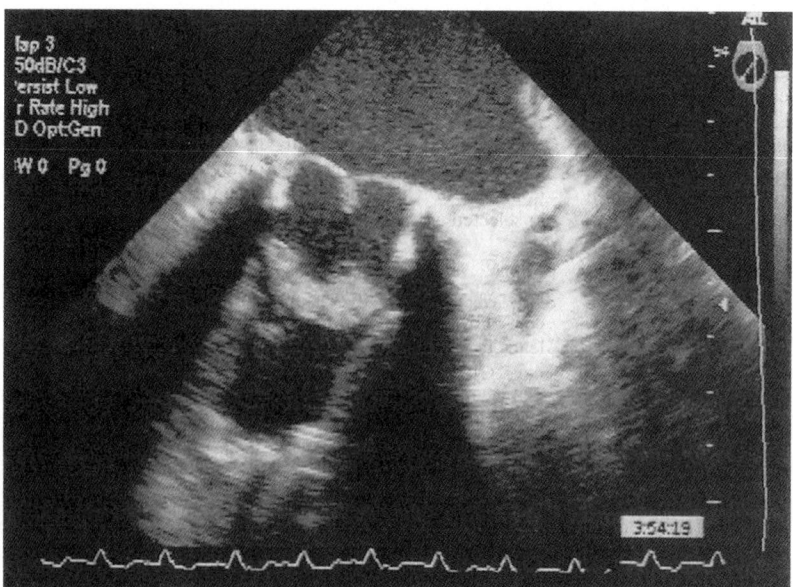

FIGURE 31–10. Transesophageal echocardiogram from a patient with eosinophilic endocarditis and prosthetic mitral valve replacement. Thrombus is noted below the valve struts, which at the time of surgery was found to be adherent to the posterior left ventricular (LV) wall. Note the apical obliteration and the apical endocardial thickening and calcification.

corticosteroids, hydroxyurea, and most recently, interferon alfa, and palliative surgery in the late, fibrotic stage.[32] Surgical excision of fibrotic endocardium and valve replacement can offer symptomatic improvement, but at the expense of high (15 to 25 percent) operative mortality; thrombosis of mechanical valves can occur despite adequate anticoagulation. The prognosis of advanced disease is grim (50 percent 2-year mortality), but it is considerably better in those with milder disease.

[ ] NONOBLITERATIVE ENDOMYOCARDIAL DISEASES

Carcinoid Syndrome

Carcinoid syndrome results from metastatic carcinoid tumors (most commonly arising in the small bowel and appendix but also the bronchus and other sites) and consists of cutaneous flushing, diarrhea, and bronchoconstriction; involvement of the heart occurs as a late complication of carcinoid syndrome in approximately 50 percent of patients. Hepatic metastases produce serotonin, bradykinin, and other substances that affect right heart structures. As these substances are inactivated in the lungs, LV involvement is distinctly uncommon and when present, suggests a right-to-left intracardiac shunt. Fibrous endocardial plaque comprising smooth muscle cells in a stroma of collagen and acid mucopolysaccharide on the tricuspid and pulmonic valves and right heart endocardium is characteristic. Although tricuspid and pulmonic stenosis and regurgitation dominate the clinical picture, restrictive cardiomyopathy can occur.

The chest radiograph is often normal, but cardiomegaly, pleural effusions, and nodules can be evident; unlike the case with congenital pulmonic stenosis, poststenotic dilation of the pulmonary artery trunk does not occur.[33] Electrocardiographic abnormalities are common, but nonspecific; a low-voltage QRS complex can be seen in advanced disease. 2D echocardiography reveals thickened, retracted, immobile tricuspid and pulmonic valves, and right atrial and ventricular enlargement; right atrial wall thickening can be seen on transesophageal echocardiography. Pulmonary outflow tract obstruction can occur as a result of pulmonary annular constriction. Low-velocity tricuspid and pulmonic regurgitation on Doppler indicates normal pulmonary arterial pressures, which is typical of carcinoid heart disease. Echocardiographic findings are detected in approximately two-thirds of patients with carcinoid. In one study, cardiac involvement was associated with a reduced 3-year survival rate as compared with those without cardiac involvement.[33] Metastatic carcinoid tumor to the heart is uncommon, intramyocardial, occurring with roughly equal frequency in the right and left ventricles, and can be recognized on echocardiography if the tumor size is at least 1 centimeter.[34] Cardiac MRI can provide additional information.[35] Catheterization findings are usually those of tricuspid regurgitation and/or pulmonic stenosis.

Therapy is symptomatic, usually with a somatostatin analog such as octreotide. Despite a decrease in 5-hydroxyindoleacetic acid (HIAA) excretion, the valvular lesions do not regress. Valvular replacement (usually mechanical) or repair is warranted in patients with severe valve dysfunction. Premature degeneration of a bioprosthetic valve can be caused by the carcinoid process.

[ ] MALIGNANT INFILTRATION

Infiltrating tumors of the heart are generally metastatic (lung, breast, melanoma, lymphoma, leukemia) and rarely produce restriction to ventricular filling unless the pericardium is involved. Infiltration on echocardiography is suggested by a localized increase in wall thickness, often associated with abnormal wall motion and pericardial effusion. CT and MRI scans are also useful.

Iatrogenic Disease

Pericardial disease frequently complicates radiation therapy to the chest and can produce constrictive pericarditis; however, endo- and myocardial involvement can produce restrictive cardiomyopathy, at times presenting years after radiation therapy has been completed. Anthracyclines and methysergide can cause endomyocardial fibrosis. Finally, a restrictive pattern of LV filling is common soon after orthotopic cardiac transplantation and can persist for at least 1 year in as many as 15 percent of cases.

REFERENCES

1. Maron BJ, Towbin JA, Thiene G, et al; American Heart Association; Council on Clinical Cardiology, Heart Failure and Transplantation Committee; Quality of Care and Outcomes Research and Functional Genomics and Translational Biology Interdisciplinary Working Groups; Council on Epidemiology and Prevention. Contemporary definitions and classification of the cardiomyopathies: an American Heart Association Scientific Statement from the Council on Clinical Cardiology, Heart Failure and Transplantation Committee; Quality of Care and Outcomes Research and Functional Genomics and Translational Biology Interdisciplinary Working Groups; and Council on Epidemiology and Prevention. *Circulation.* 2006;113:1807–1816.
2. WHO/ISFC Task Force. Richardson P (chairman). Report of the 1995 World Health Organization/International Society and Federation of Cardiology Task Force on the Definition and Classification of Cardiomyopathies. *Circulation.* 1996;93:841–842.
3. Francone M, Dymarkowski S, Kalantzi M, et al. Assessment of ventricular coupling with real-time cine MRI and its value to differentiate constrictive pericarditis from restrictive cardiomyopathy. *Eur Radiol.* 2006;16:944–951.
4. Leya FS, Arab D, Joyal D, et al. The efficacy of brain natriuretic peptide levels in differentiating constrictive pericarditis from restrictive cardiomyopathy. *J Am Coll Cardiol.* 2005;45:1900–1902.
5. Parikh S, deLemos JA. Current therapeutic strategies in cardiac amyloidosis. *Curr Treat Options Cardiovasc Med.* 2005;7:443–448.
6. Fenton MJ, Chubb H, McMahon AM, et al. Heart and heart-lung transplantation for idiopathic restrictive cardiomyopathy in children. *Heart.* 2006;92:85–89.
7. Kushuwaha SS, Fallon JT, Fuster V. Restrictive cardiomyopathy. *N Engl J Med.* 1997;336(4):267–276.
8. Fatkin D, Graham RM. Molecular mechanisms of inherited cardiomyopathies. *Physiol Rev.* 2002;82:945–980.
9. Mogensen J, Kubo T, Duque M, et al. Idiopathic restrictive cardiomyopathy is part of the clinical expression of cardiac troponin I mutations. *J Clin Invest.* 2003;111:209–216.
10. Dalakas MC, Park K, Semina-mora C, et al. Desmin myopathy: a skeletal myopathy with cardiomyopathy caused by mutations in the desmin gene. *N Engl J Med.* 2000;342:770–780.
11. Celetti F, Fattori R, Napoli G, et al. Assessment of restrictive cardiomyopathy of amyloid or idiopathic etiology by magnetic resonance imaging. *Am J Cardiol.* 1999;83:798–801.
12. Ammash NM, Seward JB, Bailey KR, et al. Clinical profile and outcome of idiopathic restrictive cardiomyopathy. *Circulation.* 2000;101:2490–2496.
13. Ikeda S. Cardiac amyloidosis: heterogeneous pathogenic backgrounds. *Intern Med.* 2004;43:1107–1114.
14. Hassan W, Al-Sergani H, Mourad W, Tabaa R. Amyloid heart disease: new frontiers and insights in pathophysiology, diagnosis and management. *Tex Heart Inst J.* 2005;32:178–184.
15. Kyle RA. Amyloidosis. *Circulation.* 1995;91:1269–1271.

16. Neben-Wittich MA, Wittich CM, Mueller PS, Larson DR, Gertz MA, Edwards WD. Obstructive intramural coronary amyloidosis and myocardial ischemia are common in primary amyloidosis. *Am J Med.* 2005;118:1287.

17. Jacobson DR, Pastore RD, Yaghoubian R, et al. Variant-sequence transthyretin (isoleucine 122) in late-onset cardiac amyloidosis in black Americans. *N Engl J Med.* 1997;336:466–473.

18. Kawamura S, Takahashi M, Ishihara T, et al. Incidence and distribution of isolated atrial amyloid: histologic and immunohistochemical studies of 100 aging hearts. *Pathol Int.* 1995;45:335–342.

19. Cueto-Garcia L, Reeder G, Kyle R, et al. Echocardiographic findings in systemic amyloidosis: spectrum of cardiac involvement and relation to survival. *J Am Coll Cardiol.* 1985;6:737–743.

20. Klein AL, Hatle LK, Taliercio CP, et al. Prognostic significance of Doppler measures of diastolic function in cardiac amyloidosis: a Doppler echocardiography study. *Circulation.* 1991;83:808–816.

21. Maceira AM, Joshi J, Prasad SK, et al. Cardiovascular magnetic resonance in cardiac amyloidosis. *Circulation.* 2005;111:186–193.

22. Arbustini E, Merlini G, Gavazzi A, et al. Cardiac immunocyte-derived (al) amyloidosis: an endomyocardial biopsy study in 11 patients. *Am Heart J.* 1995;130:528–536.

23. Gertz MA, Lacy MQ, Lust JA, et al. Prospective randomized trial of melphalan and prednisone versus vincristine, carmustine, melphalan, cyclophosphamide, and prednisone in the treatment of primary systemic amyloidosis. *J Clin Oncol.* 1999;17:262–267.

24. Pelosi F JR, Capehart J, Roberts WC. Effectiveness of cardiac transplantation for primary (al) cardiac amyloidosis. *Am J Cardiol.* 1997;79:532–535.

25. Okayama K, Kurata C, Tawarchara K, et al. Diagnostic and prognostic value of myocardial scintigraphy with thallium-201 and gallium-67 in cardiac sarcoidosis. *Chest.* 1995;107:330–334.

26. Shabetai R. Sarcoidosis and the heart. *Curr Treat Opt Cardiovasc Med.* 2000;2:385–398.

27. Elstein D, Abrahamov A, Hadas-Halpern I, et al. Gaucher's disease. *Lancet.* 2001;358:324–327.

28. Bomford A. Genetics of haemachromatosis. *Lancet.* 2002;360:1673–1681.

29. Kontoghiorghes GJ. Future chelation monotherapy and combination therapy strategies in thalassemia and other conditions. comparison of deferiprone, deferoxamine, ICL670, GT56–252, L1NAll and starch deferoxamine polymers. *Hemoglobin.* 2006;30:329–347.

30. Peters FPJ, Vermeulen A, Kho TL. Anderson-Fabry's disease: α-galactosidase deficiency. *Lancet.* 2001;357:138–140.

31. Shaper A. What's new in endomyocardial fibrosis? *Lancet.* 1993;342:255–256.

32. Baratta L, Afeltra A, Delfino M, et al. Favorable response to high-dose interferon-alpha in idiopathic hypereosinophilic syndrome with restrictive cardiomyopathy—case report and literature review. *Angiology.* 2002;53:465–470.

33. Pellikka P, Tajik A, Khandheria B, et al. Carcinoid heart disease: clinical and echocardiographic spectrum in 74 patients. *Circulation.* 1993;87:1188–1196.

34. Pandya UH, Pellika PA, Enriquez-Sarano M, et al. Metastatic carcinoid tumor to the heart: echocardiographic-pathologic study of 11 patients. *J Am Coll Cardiol.* 2002;40:1328–1332.

35. Bastarrika G, Cao MG, Cano D, Barba J, de Buruaga JD. Magnetic resonance imaging diagnosis of carcinoid heart disease. *J Comput Assis Tomogr.* 2005;29:756–759.

CHAPTER 32

Myocarditis and Specific Cardiomyopathies

Sean P. Pinney / Donna M. Mancini

The diagnosis of cardiomyopathy encompasses a wide spectrum of diseases with widely divergent pathogenic mechanisms that have as their final common pathway the syndrome of congestive heart failure. A list of etiologies associated with the development of cardiomyopathy is presented in Fig. 32–1.

Coronary artery disease, hypertension, valvular heart disease, and cardiomyopathy are the most common causes of heart failure for both sexes. Comparison of the Framingham[1] and Study of Left Ventricular Dysfunction (SOLVD)[2] registries demonstrates a shift in the predominant etiology of heart failure from hypertension to ischemic heart disease. This probably reflects recent intensified efforts to control high blood pressure.

Inflammatory cardiomyopathies, particularly viral myocarditis, have served as a model to understand the development of heart failure. More than 70 different specific cardiomyopathies associated with general systemic disease, neuromuscular disorders, hypersensitivity and toxic reactions, and the peripartum state have been described. When they are considered as a group, these disorders are infrequent; considered individually, they are rare.

Cardiomyopathy associated with HIV disease is considered in Chap. 92.

MYOCARDITIS

⟦ ⟧ INFECTIVE

Viral

In its most literal sense, *myocarditis* means inflammation of the myocardium. As early as 1806, a relationship between infection (diphtheria) and chronic heart disease was postulated, but it was not until the 1970s, with the advent of endomyocardial biopsy, that the diagnosis of myocarditis could be established during life. Multiple infectious etiologies (Table 32–1)[3] have been implicated as the cause of myocarditis, the most common being viral, specifically, the enterovirus coxsackie B. In the majority of patients, active myocarditis remains unsuspected because the cardiac dysfunction is subclinical and self-limited. The discovery of myocarditis in 1 to 9 percent of routine postmortem examinations suggests that myocarditis is a major cause of sudden, unexpected death.[4]

Pathogenesis Infection by cardiotropic viruses prompted the initial hypothesis that the viral infection was responsible for myocardial injury. However, several investigators noted that cardiac dysfunction increased after the eradication of the infective agent

TABLE 32–1

Causes of Myocarditis

Infectious
Viruses
　Coxsackievirus, echovirus, HIV, Epstein-Barr virus, influenza, cytomegalovirus, adenovirus, hepatitis (A and B), mumps, poliovirus, rabies, respiratory syncytial virus, rubella, vaccinia, varicella zoster, arbovirus
Bacteria
　Corynebacterium diphtheriae, Streptococcus pyogenes, Staphylococcus aureus, Haemophilus pneumoniae, Salmonella spp., *Neisseria gonorrhoeae, Leptospira, Borrelia burgdorferi, Treponema pallidum, Brucella, Mycobacterium tuberculosis, Actinomyces, Chlamydia* spp., *Coxiella brunetti, Mycoplasma pneumoniae, Rickettsia* spp.
Fungi
　Candida spp., *Aspergillus* spp., *Histoplasma, Blastomyces, Cryptococcus, Coccidioidomycosis*
Parasites
　Trypanosoma cruzii, Toxoplasma, Schistosoma, Trichina
Noninfectious
Drugs causing hypersensitivity reactions
　Antibiotics: sulfonamides, penicillins, chloramphenicol, amphotericin B, tetracycline, streptomycin
　Antituberculous: isoniazid, para-aminosalicylic acid
　Anticonvulsants: phenindione, phenytoin, carbamazepine
　Antiinflammatories: indomethacin, phenylbutazone
　Diuretics: acetazolamide, chlorthalidone, hydrochlorothiazide, spironolactone
　Others: amitriptyline, methyldopa, sulfonylureas
Drugs not causing hypersensitivity reactions
　Cocaine, cyclophosphamide, lithium, interferon alpha
Nondrug causes
　Radiation, giant-cell myocarditis

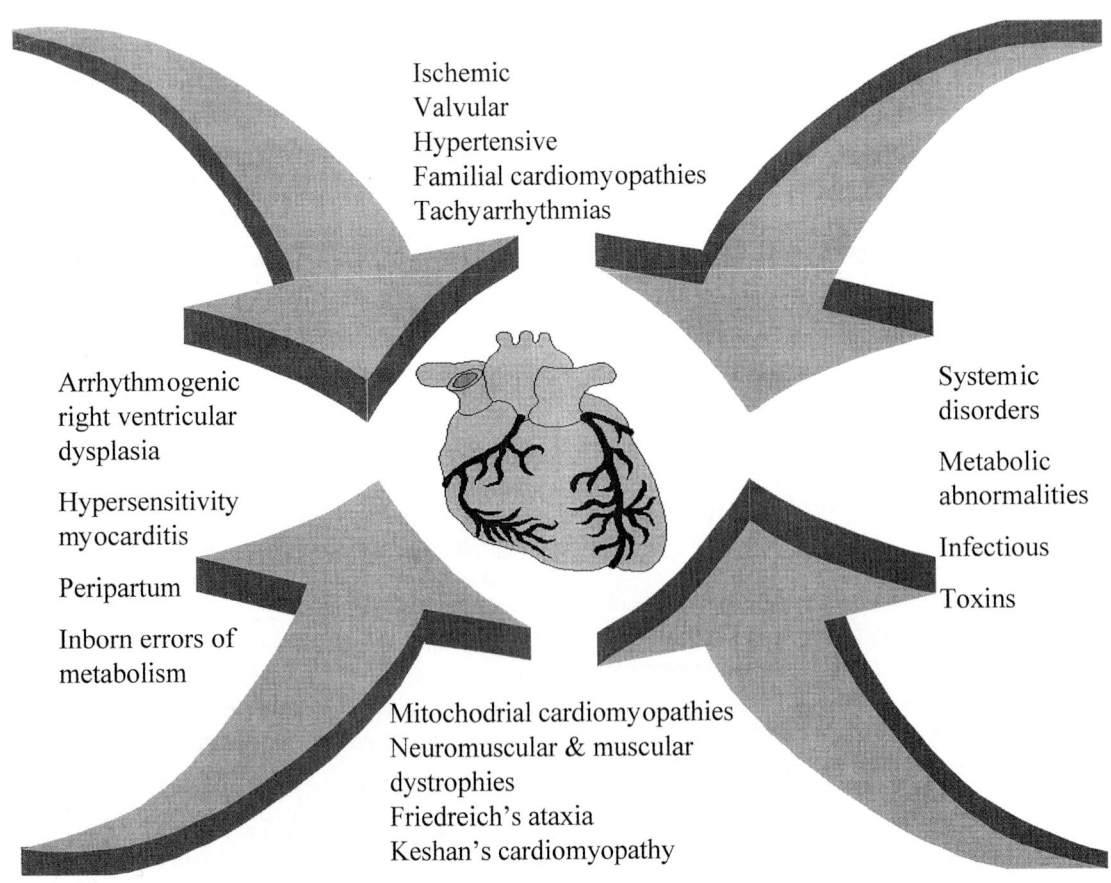

FIGURE 32–1. Various etiologies that can lead to cardiomyopathy.

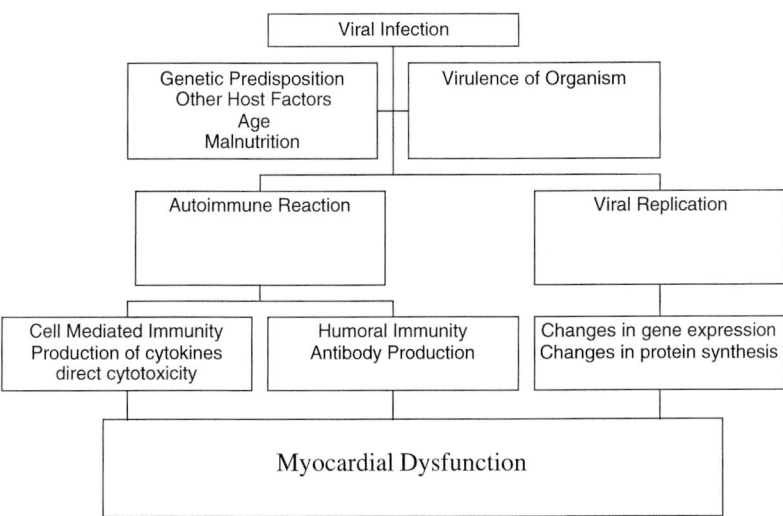

FIGURE 32–2. Flow diagram illustrating various factors that contribute to the development of myocardial dysfunction after viral infection.

and speculated that the pathogenesis of myocarditis can be caused by two distinct phases of myocardial cell damage—the first caused by direct viral infection and the second caused by the host's immune response (Fig. 32–2). Support for this theory comes initially from the work of Woodruff, who noted that the histologic evidence of cardiac injury in coxsackie B infection appeared only after the virus was no longer detectable in the myocardium.[5] Subsequently, demonstration of T-lymphocyte and macrophage infiltration, perforin granules, and a variety of cytokines known to depress myocardial contractility in endomyocardial biopsies of patients with active carditis strengthened the concept of immune-mediated injury.

Our understanding of the specific immune responses that lead to myocardial injury is derived largely from animal models of myocarditis induced by cardiotropic viruses.[6] A time-line for experimental viral myocarditis is shown in Fig. 32–3. After gaining entry to the body from the gastrointestinal tract (enterovirus) or through the respiratory tract (adenovirus and enterovirus), these cardiotropic viruses bind to the coxsackie-adenoviral receptor (CAR), which in turn allows for the incorporation of the viral genome into the myocyte.[7] In the acute phase of viral myocarditis (days 0 to 3), mice injected with coxsackievirus show evidence of direct viral cytotoxicity, with myocyte necrosis in the absence of an inflammatory cell infiltrate. Activated macrophages begin to express interleukin (IL)-1β, IL-2, tumor necrosis factor alpha (TNF-α), and interferon gamma (IFN-γ).[8]

This ushers in the second or subacute phase (days 4 to 14) of myocarditis, which is characterized by the infiltration of natural killer (NK) cells,

production of neutralizing antibody, and cell-mediated immune pathogenicity. The first wave of infiltrating cells consists mainly of NK cells that play a dual role.[6] By limiting viral replication, NK cells can be protective. However, NK cells release perforin and granzymes, which form circular pore lesions on the membrane surface of virus-infected cells.[9] Although this activity produces cardiomyocyte damage, uninfected cells are spared from injury.

Cytokines are a major mediator of immune activation and its maintenance.[10] Circulating levels of IL-1, IL-2, and IL-6 are elevated in patients with acute myocarditis, as is TNF-α mRNA and protein expression. In animal models, overexpression of TNF-α produces florid myocarditis,[11] whereas mice deficient in the TNF p55 receptor (TNF-R1$^{-/-}$) experience milder autoimmune myocarditis.[12] However, a recent study by Wada and colleagues suggests that TNF-α can actually play a protective role in the acute stage of viral myocarditis.[13] The observed full recovery of some patients with severe left ventricular dysfunction can be the result of short-term exposure to these inflammatory cytokines.[10] Host resistance to virus-mediated damage occurs through the combined actions of NK cells, infiltrating mononuclear cells, and the expression of neutralizing antibody. After invading the myocardium, coxsackievirus increases its expression, becoming maximal on day 4. Almost no neutralizing antibody is present until day 4, after which titers quickly rise, becoming maximal on day 14. The rise in antibody titer is closely related to the elimination of virus from the heart. Infiltrating mononuclear cells appear in the myocardium between 5 and 10 days following viral infection.[5] In combination with neutralizing antibodies, these mononuclear cells help to suppress viral infection and limit cardiomyocyte damage.

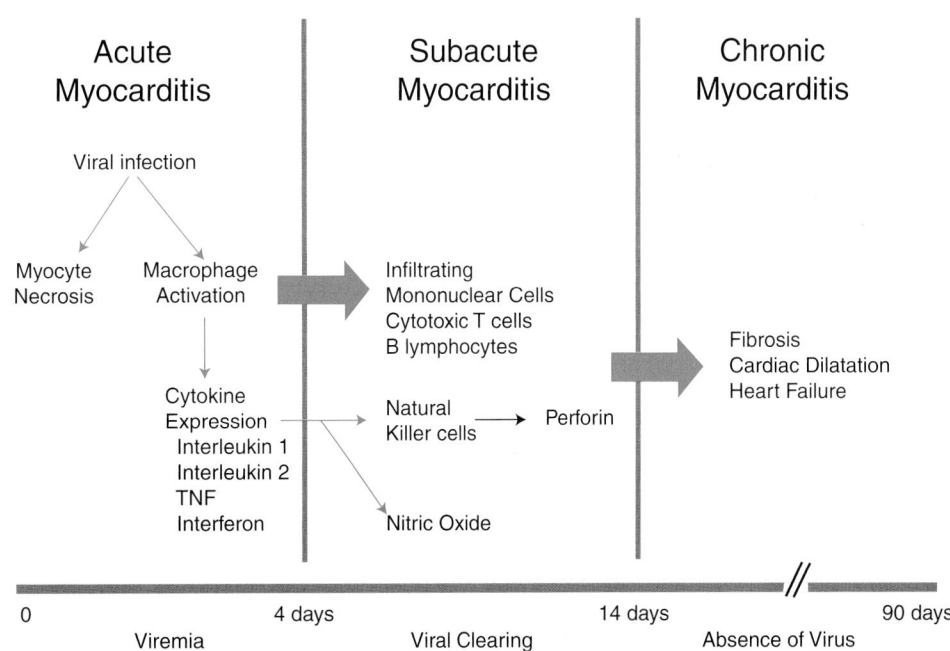

FIGURE 32–3. Time-line of viral myocarditis. TNF, tumor necrosis factor. *Source: Modified from Kawai C.[6] Used with permission.*

T lymphocytes are attracted to the myocardium through classic cell-mediated immunity. Within the cytoplasm of infected myocytes, viral particles are broken down into peptide fragments and then placed on the cell surface in association with major histocompatibility-complex class 1 antigen. Through their T-cell receptor (TCR), cytotoxic T-cells recognize virus-infected cells and destroy them by either cytokine production or perforin-mediated cell cytolysis.[6] In spite of the damage done to the myocardium in the process of eliminating infected cells, cell-mediated immunity in combination with neutralizing antibodies and NK cells limit viral replication. Indeed, when host defense mechanisms are inadequate, chronic viral infection produces widespread cardiac damage and eventual cardiac dilation and failure.[14] Conversely, continuous exuberant T-cell activation can be equally destructive. This occurs when antigens intrinsic to the myocardium cross-react with viral peptides, leading to sustained T-cell activation (so called molecular mimicry), which can ultimately lead to dilated cardiomyopathy.[10]

A third or chronic phase of viral myocarditis (days 15 to 90) occurs following the elimination of virus and is typified by insidious ongoing myocardial damage.[6] Hearts from infected mice are hypertrophied and myocardial fibrosis is prominent. Inflammatory cells are no longer seen. The mechanisms involved in the transition from this stage to the development of dilated cardiomyopathy are not fully understood, but three mechanisms seem likely—persistent viral infection, ongoing autoimmune destruction, and apoptosis.

Attempts to culture virus from human myocardial tissue have generally been unsuccessful. However, identification of viral genomic fragments in myocardial samples by in situ hybridization and polymerase chain reaction from patients with myocarditis and dilated cardiomyopathy has been reported.[15] These genomic fragments may not be capable of replicating as intact cardiotropic virus but probably serve as a persistent source of antigen to drive the deleterious immune responses. Persistence of viral genomes in the myocardium of patients with left ventricular (LV) dysfunction has been associated with a progressive impairment of ventricular function, whereas spontaneous resolution has been associated with improvement in the LV ejection fraction.[16]

Autoimmune-mediated heart disease results from a process of molecular mimicry whereby antibodies to viral proteins cross-react with structural elements of the heart. For example, injection of myosin into susceptible mice produces active myocarditis.[17] One reason for this can lie in the fact that myosin shares approximately 40 percent identity with the amino acid sequence of Coxsackie virus CVB3 capsid protein. Several other circulating heart-specific autoantibodies have been identified, including antisarcolemma antibody, which also exhibits cross-reactivity with CVB3 capsid protein.[18] Further investigation with this virus-free model of myocarditis will help in elucidating the pathogenesis of molecular mimicry.

Apoptosis, or programmed cell death, can be a third pathogenic mechanism leading from myocarditis to dilated cardiomyopathy. Although this association is currently speculative, certain viruses have been identified as triggers of apoptosis.[19] Cytokines can activate death-domain sequences or ceramide-mediated signaling pathways as part of the remodeling process.[20] Although animal models of myocarditis can progress to dilated cardiomyopathy, as can patients with clinically suspected or biopsy-proven

myocarditis, the percentage of patients with idiopathic dilated cardiomyopathy representing the end stage of an active myocarditis is unknown.

Clinical Presentation The clinical manifestations of myocarditis are variable, ranging from an asymptomatic or self-limited disease in some to profound cardiogenic shock in others. Cardiac involvement typically occurs 7 to 10 days following a systemic illness. The most obvious symptom suggesting myocarditis is an antecedent viral syndrome with fever, myalgias, and malaise. The majority of patients have no specific cardiovascular complaints but can have ST-segment and T-wave abnormalities on the ECG suggesting myocarditis. Chest pain can occur in up to 35 percent of patients and can be typically ischemic, somewhat atypical, or pericardial in character. Chest pain usually reflects associated pericarditis but occasionally can result from myocardial ischemia.[21]

Acute dilated cardiomyopathy from lymphocytic myocarditis can produce mild, moderate, or fulminant heart failure. The vast majority of patients with mild symptoms have spontaneous recovery in ventricular function and normalization of heart size. Patients with New York Heart Association (NYHA) class III or IV heart failure typically have greater degrees of ventricular dilation and dysfunction. Although some recover spontaneously, it is estimated that one-half will be left with residual myocardial dysfunction and one-quarter will either die or require cardiac transplantation.[21] Biopsy-proven relapses have occurred in some patients, and recurrent myocarditis should be suspected if ventricular function subsequently deteriorates.[22] Fulminant myocarditis is often dramatic and accompanied by a rapid onset of symptoms.[23] Patients are severely ill, with circulatory collapse and evidence of end-organ dysfunction. They frequently have fever, severe global myocardial dysfunction, and a minimal increase in LV end-diastolic dimension. Mechanical circulatory support can be required, as a bridge to either cardiac transplantation or recovery.

Occasionally patients will present with a clinical syndrome identical to an acute myocardial infarction, with ischemic chest pain and ST-segment elevations on the ECG (Fig. 32–4). LV dysfunction, when present, tends to be diffuse rather than segmental.[24] At autopsy, the coronary arteries are usually widely patent, although viral coronary arteritis has been reported.[25] Coronary vasospasm has also been associated with acute myocarditis.

Patients can present with syncope or palpitations from atrioventricular (AV) block or ventricular arrhythmia. Complete AV block is common, with some patients presenting with Stokes-Adams attacks. Sudden cardiac death can be the initial presentation of myocarditis in some patients, presumably from complete heart block or ventricular tachycardia. In a 25-year review of sudden death among military recruits, 20 percent had myocarditis documented at autopsy.[26] In some patients with refractory ventricular arrhythmias, endomyocardial biopsy or autopsy has revealed myocarditis.

Diagnosis Laboratory findings are generally not diagnostic. Leukocytosis, eosinophilia, and an elevated erythrocyte sedimentation rate are sometimes present, as are elevated titers to cardiotropic viruses. A fourfold rise in immunoglobulin G (IgG) titer over a 4- to 6-week period is required to document acute infection. Elevated immunoglobulin M (IgM) antibody titer can denote an acute infection more specifically than a rise in IgG anti-

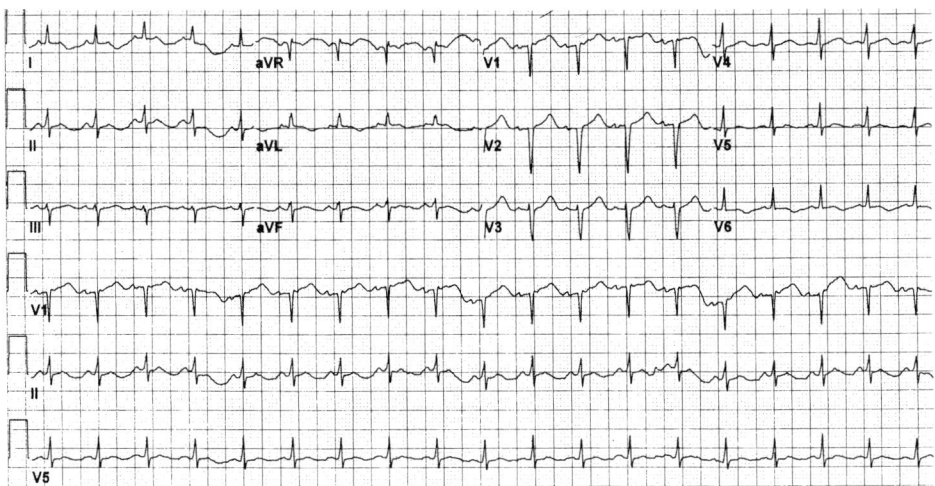

FIGURE 32–4. Electrocardiographic tracing consistent with an anteroseptal myocardial infarction and lateral ischemia in a patient with acute myocarditis and normal coronary arteries.

body titer. Unfortunately, a rise in antibody titer documents only the response to a recent viral infection and does not indicate active myocarditis. Abnormalities in peripheral T- and B-lymphocyte counts have been reported, but these findings have not been consistent and cannot be used as diagnostic adjuncts. An increase in the myocardial band (MB) of creatine phosphokinase (CPK) is observed in approximately 10 percent of patients, but newer troponin assays are proving to be more sensitive for detecting myocardial injury in suspected myocarditis.[27] The classic clinical triad of preceding viral illness, pericarditis, and associated laboratory abnormalities used to diagnose Coxsackie B–induced myocarditis is present in fewer than 10 percent of histologically proven cases.[22]

The ECG most frequently shows sinus tachycardia. Diffuse ST-T-wave changes, prolongation of the QTc, conduction delay, low voltage, and even an acute myocardial infarct pattern have been noted in patients with myocarditis. Cardiac arrhythmias are frequently observed, including complete heart block, ventricular tachycardia, and supraventricular arrhythmias—especially in the presence of congestive heart failure or pericardial inflammation.

Echocardiography can reveal LV systolic dysfunction in patients with a normal-sized LV cavity. Segmental wall-motion abnormalities can be observed. Wall thickness can be increased, particularly early in the course of the disease, when inflammation is fulminant. Echocardiographic findings in active myocarditis can mimic restrictive, hypertrophic, or dilated cardiomyopathy.

Endomyocardial biopsy is the critical test to confirm the diagnosis. Endomyocardial biopsy techniques enable the repetitive sampling of the human myocardium with minimal discomfort, minor morbidity, and a mortality rate of 0.2 percent.[28] Right ventricular myocardial specimens can be obtained by accessing the right internal jugular or femoral vein. Intravascular biopsy of the left ventricle is infrequently performed because of the higher morbidity associated with this approach. The right ventricular bioptome is positioned under fluoroscopy or echocardiography to sample the interventricular septum. As myocarditis can be focal, a minimum of four to six fragments are obtained. Diagnoses that can be made or confirmed by endomyocardial biopsy are listed in Table 32–2.

Several investigators have performed endomyocardial biopsies in patients with unexplained congestive heart failure and/or ventricular arrhythmia.[4,22,28] The percentage of patients with biopsies interpreted as myocarditis varied widely, primarily owing to the different diagnostic criteria for active myocarditis used by the investigators. This variability of endomyocardial biopsy criteria prompted a meeting of cardiac pathologists to reach a consensus on the pathologic definition of myocarditis, now known as the *Dallas criteria*.[29] These criteria separate initial biopsies into myocarditis, borderline myocarditis, or no myocarditis. Active myocarditis was defined as "an inflammatory infiltrate of the myocardium with necrosis and/or degeneration of adjacent myocytes not typical of the ischemic damage associated with coronary artery disease" (Fig. 32–5). The term *borderline* myocarditis is applied when the inflammatory infiltrate is too sparse or myocyte injury is not demonstrated. Repeat biopsy is then suggested. A high frequency of active myocarditis is confirmed by repeat biopsy in patients whose initial histologic samples demonstrated borderline myocarditis. When right ventricular endomyocardial biopsy has failed to establish the diagnosis, sampling the left ventricle can improve diagnostic yield.

TABLE 32–2

Diagnoses That Can Be Made by Endomyocardial Biopsy

1. Myocarditis
   Giant-cell myocarditis
   Cytomegalovirus
   Toxoplasmosis
   Chagas
   Rheumatic
   Lyme
2. Infiltrative
   Amyloid
   Sarcoid
   Hemochromatosis
   Carcinoid
   Hypereosinophilic
   Glycogen storage
   Cardiac tumors
3. Toxins
   Doxorubicin
   Chloroquine
   Radiation injury
4. Genetic
   Fabry
   Kearns-Sayre syndrome
   Right ventricular dysplasia

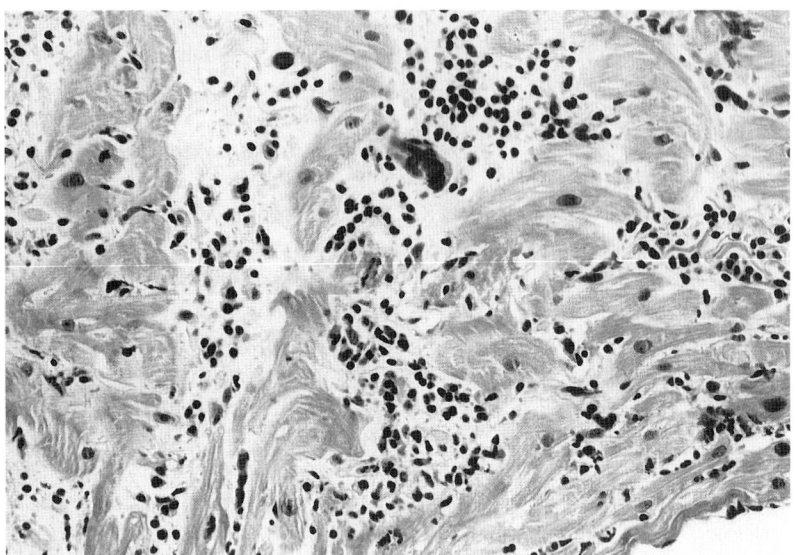

FIGURE 32–5. Photomicrograph showing extensive interstitial infiltrates of lymphocytes and myocytes with focal myocyte necrosis. (H&E, ×40.)

has been documented within 4 days of initial biopsy, with progressive clearing over several weeks on serial biopsy.[32]

Noninvasive Studies Tissue alterations associated with myocarditis can be identifiable using MRI. On the basis of several small observational studies it is believed that myocardial inflammation induces abnormal signal intensity of the myocardial walls. Use of transverse relaxation time (T2)-weighted images to visualize tissue edema has been described in several case reports of patients with active myocarditis. More recently, contrast–enhanced MRI has been used to characterize myocardial changes in myocarditis.[33] Gadolinium increases the signal of longitudinal relaxation time (T1)-weighted images. Mahrholdt and coworkers[34] used contrast-enhanced MRI to identify areas of active inflammation in patients with clinically diagnosed myocarditis. Histopathologic analysis of endomyocardial biopsy samples taken from areas of enhancement revealed active myocarditis in 19 of 21 patients. Foci of inflammation were more frequently located on the lateral wall of the left ventricle. Conversely, only 1 of 11 biopsy samples taken from regions lacking enhancement showed active myocarditis. Employing this strategy can help identify those patients who should undergo endomyocardial biopsy.

Treatment The cornerstone of therapy for patients with acute myocarditis is supportive care. Diuretics, angiotensin-converting enzyme inhibitors, β blockers, and aldosterone antagonists should be given in the proper clinical context. Digoxin can increase the expression of inflammatory cytokines, and should be used cautiously at a low dose.

When acute myocarditis presents with profound hemodynamic collapse, mechanical circulatory support devices can be used to

Although the Dallas criteria standardize the description of biopsy samples, histopathology alone can be inadequate to identify the presence of active myocarditis.[30] Alternative classification schemes have been proposed, including one that combines histopathologic and clinical criteria.[31] Myocarditis is divided into four subgroups—fulminant, acute, chronic active, and chronic persistent. These categories provide prognostic information and suggest which patients can or cannot benefit from immunosuppressive therapy (Table 32–3). Additionally, use of immunohistologic markers of inflammation, such as upregulation of histocompatibility leukocyte antigens (HLAs) on myocytes or detection of autoantibodies, can aid diagnosis as these changes are generalized and not focal.

Endomyocardial biopsy must be applied as quickly as possible to maximize the diagnostic yield. Resolution of active myocarditis

TABLE 32–3

Clinicopathologic Classification of Myocarditis

	FULMINANT	ACUTE	CHRONIC ACTIVE	CHRONIC PERSISTENT
Symptom onset	Distinct	Indistinct CHF, LV dysfunction	Indistinct CHF, LV dysfunction	Indistinct
Clinical presentation	Cardiogenic shock, severe LV dysfunction			Non-CHF symptoms, normal LV function
Initial biopsy	Multifoci of active myocarditis	Active or borderline myocarditis	Active or borderline myocarditis	Active or borderline myocarditis
Clinical natural history	Complete recovery or death	Incomplete recovery or dilated CM	Dilated CM	Non-CHF symptoms, normal LV function
Histologic natural history	Complete resolution of myocarditis	Complete resolution of myocarditis	Ongoing or resolving myocarditis, fibrosis	Ongoing or resolving myocarditis
Immunosuppressive therapy	No benefit	Sometimes beneficial	No benefit	No benefit

CHF, congestive heart failure; CM, cardiomyopathy; LV, left ventricular.
SOURCE: Modified from Lieberman EB, Hutchins GM, Rose NR, et al.[31] Used with permission.

bridge patients either to cardiac transplantation or to recovery. Although improvement in cardiac function has been reported to parallel the clearance of the inflammatory infiltrate, the duration of necessary device support has ranged from 7 to 70 days.[35] Serial endomyocardial biopsy, echocardiography, right heart catheterization, and exercise testing with simultaneous hemodynamic and echocardiographic measurements are all employed to determine native cardiac reserve and the suitability for device explantation.

Acceptance of the hypothesis of immune-mediated injury has led many to question whether antiinflammatory therapy could provide additional clinical benefit to patients with inflammatory-dilated cardiomyopathy treated with conventional heart failure regimens. Parillo studied 102 patients with dilated cardiomyopathy and classified them as being "reactive," with endomyocardial or laboratory evidence of ongoing inflammation, or "nonreactive."[36] The study's primary end point was an increase in LV ejection fraction equal to or greater than 5 percent. At 3 months followup, 67 percent of reactive patients receiving prednisone reached this end point, as compared to only 28 percent in the reactive control group. After 9 months of follow-up, the prednisone-induced improvement in LV ejection fraction was no longer present. Nonreactive patients did not improve with prednisone. In spite of these negative results, the authors concluded that prednisone therapy could provide modest improvements in clinical end points, but only in certain reactive subpopulations.

Anecdotal success with immunosuppression in active viral myocarditis led to the large multicenter Myocarditis Treatment Trial.[37] In this study, 111 patients with biopsy-proven myocarditis and LV ejection fraction less than 45 percent were randomized to receive conventional therapy alone versus immunosuppressive therapy with prednisone in combination with either azathioprine or cyclosporine. The primary end point of the study was change in ejection fraction over 28 weeks. For all patients, the average increase in ejection fraction over baseline was 9 percent. Treatment did not improve LV ejection fraction, attenuation of clinical disease, or mortality (Fig. 32–6).

A more recent study examined the selected use of immunosuppressive therapy in patients with dilated cardiomyopathy and immunohistochemical evidence of inflammation.[38] Eighty-four patients with dilated cardiomyopathy for at least 6 months who had increased HLA expression on endomyocardial biopsy specimens were randomized to receive standard heart-failure therapy alone or in combination with prednisone and azathioprine. After 2 years of followup, there was no difference in the composite primary end point of death, transplantation, or hospital readmission. Those patients treated with immunosuppressive therapy, however, experienced a significant increase in ejection fraction at 3 and 24 months.

High-dose intravenous immune globulin (IVIG) has both immune modulatory and antiviral effects. A small open-label study was performed in 10 adult patients with new-onset heart failure showed significant improvement in LV function in 9 of 10 patients treated with IVIG.[39] When IVIG was tested in a prospective placebo-controlled trial in 62 patients with recent-onset dilated cardiomyopathy and LV ejection fraction less than 40 percent, the results were disappointing.[40] Although ejection fraction improved by 16 percent at 1 year in the IVIG-treated group, this increase was essentially equaled by those taking placebo. Thus no benefit of immunomodulation could be demonstrated.

Taken as a whole, these trials do not support the routine use of immunosuppressive therapy in myocarditis. However, present data

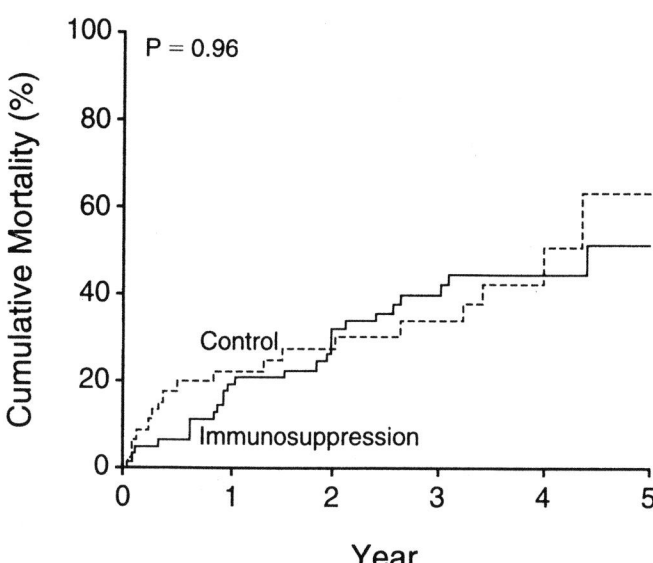

FIGURE 32–6. Actuarial mortality curves from the Myocarditis Treatment Trial illustrating no difference in survival between the treatment groups. *Source: Mason JW, O'Connell JB, Herskowitz A, et al.[37] Used with permission.*

suggest that subgroups with ongoing myocarditis can be more likely to benefit from immunosuppression, although no uniform methodology yet exists to identify them.

Prognosis Approximately one-third of those who present with clinical carditis and recover will be left with some cardiac abnormality, ranging from mild changes on ECG to significant heart failure. Approximately 40 percent of all patients will completely recover.[22] Currently there are no clinical criteria that reliably predict who will recover, although the vast majority of patients with mild reductions in LV ejection fraction and NYHA class I or II heart failure recover completely. In one study, a pulmonary capillary wedge pressure greater than 15 mmHg was a univariate predictor of death or need for cardiac transplantation.[41] In multivariate analysis, pulmonary capillary wedge pressure and histopathology of lymphocytic, granulomatous or giant-cell myocarditis each significantly predicted mortality or transplant. Paradoxically, patients with fulminant myocarditis have an excellent long-term prognosis despite their experience of circulatory collapse. In one study, long-term transplant-free survival was 93 percent, as compared to only 45 percent for those with acute myocarditis.[23] Elevated levels of IL-10 can identify a subgroup of patients with fulminant myocarditis who are at higher risk of developing cardiogenic shock with the need for mechanical circulatory support and those at higher risk of mortality.[42]

The prognosis of myocarditis depends to some extent on the causative agent, but for patients with histopathologic confirmation of myocarditis the 1 year survival is approximately 80 percent, and 5-year survival is in the range of 50 to 60 percent.[41] Chronic inflammation, viral persistence, or both can affect disease progression and prognosis. Future therapies will need to identify the predominant factor to target treatment and hopefully improve survival.

Nonviral

Chagas Disease American trypanosomiasis, or Chagas disease, is the most common cause of congestive heart failure in rural

South and Central America. This condition results from the bite of the reduviid bug, leading to infection with *Trypanosoma cruzi*. The pathogenesis of chronic chagasic cardiomyopathy is controversial because the parasite is rarely present in the myocardium. As in the viral cardiomyopathy model, the cardiac injury is thought to be immunologically mediated. Both cellular and humoral immune responses have been implicated in the myocardial injury.

Clinical Presentation This parasitic disease has an acute phase, where hematogenous spread of the parasite leads to invasion of various tissues and organ systems. The invasion is accompanied by an intense inflammatory reaction with mononuclear cells and is characterized by fever, sweating, myalgias, myocarditis, hepatosplenomegaly, and a case fatality rate of approximately 5 percent. Survivors enter an asymptomatic latent phase, but 20 to 30 percent will develop a chronic form of the disease up to 20 years after the initial infection.

The chronic stage is a result of gradual tissue destruction. The gastrointestinal tract and heart are the most common sites of involvement, with the primary cause of death being cardiac failure. In the gut, the destruction of the *myenteric plexus* is responsible for the development of megaesophagus and megacolon. In the heart, the myofibrils and the Purkinje fibers are replaced by fibrous tissue, leading to cardiomegaly, congestive heart failure, heart block, and arrhythmia.

Diagnosis of the acute disease depends on the discovery of trypomastigotes in the blood of the infected individual. In chronic infection, direct diagnosis is less useful because there are fewer circulating trypomastigotes. Xenodiagnosis (where the patient is bitten by reduviid bugs bred in the laboratory, and the parasite is subsequently identified in the intestine of the insect) is the most useful test, which will detect infection in approximately one-half of the patients. The complement-fixation test (Machado-Guerreiro test) also has high sensitivity and specificity for identification of chronic Chagas disease. In the other lab tests, it is necessary to rely on positive serologic tests (such as the indirect immunofluorescent antibody, enzyme-linked immunosorbent assay, and hemagglutination tests) together with symptoms and signs compatible with Chagas disease.

Endomyocardial biopsy can show active myocarditis using the Dallas criteria. Noninvasive assessment commonly shows segmental wall motion abnormalities, specifically apical aneurysms. ECG findings include complete heart block, atrioventricular block, or right bundle-branch block with or without fascicular block. Ventricular arrhythmias can require antiarrhythmic drugs.

The treatment of chronic Chagas disease is symptomatic and includes a pacemaker for complete heart block, an implantable cardioverter-defibrillator for recurrent ventricular arrhythmia, and standard therapy for congestive heart failure as outlined for other forms of myocarditis. Antiparasitic agents such as nifurtimox and benzimidazole eradicate parasitemia during the acute phase and are typically curative. They should be administered if the disease has not previously been treated and can be used as prophylaxis if there is a high likelihood of recurrence, such as following immunosuppressive therapy. The role of immunosuppression therapy for chagasic myocarditis is controversial, and heart transplantation is effective for end-stage refractory cardiac disease.

A prognostic scoring system based on six clinical risk factors has recently been published.[43] These include NYHA class III or IV, cardiomegaly by radiography, LV wall-motion abnormalities, nonsustained ventricular tachycardia detected by Holter monitoring, low QRS voltage, and male sex. Ten-year mortality was 9, 37, and 85 percent for those at low, intermediate, and high risk, respectively. The use of this prognostic scoring system can aid in directing resources to those patients at highest risk especially in regions of the world where access to care can be limited.

Lyme Carditis Lyme disease results from infection with the spirochete *Borrelia burgdorferi*, introduced by a tick bite. The initial presenting symptom in patients with the disease who progress to cardiac involvement is frequently complete heart block. Endomyocardial biopsy can show active myocarditis. Rarely are spirochetes seen on biopsy. Corticosteroid administration is helpful in treating Lyme carditis following therapy with tetracycline.

Other Infectious Causes of Cardiomyopathy Among other infectious etiologies is *Toxoplasma gondii*, which is curable by pyrimethamine and sulfadiazine and occurs most commonly in the immune-deficient host. Leptospirosis is another common cause in fatal cases of myocarditis. Fifty percent of cases have ST- and T-wave changes on the ECG.

Rheumatic Carditis Acute rheumatic fever can occur in children and young adults. It generally follows a group A streptococcal pharyngitis, but only indirect evidence linking the two has been found. Rheumatic carditis can result from a direct toxic effect of some streptococcal product versus an immunologic mechanism.[44] Group A streptococci have a number of structural components similar to those of human tissue. Antibodies to streptococci cross-react with the glycoproteins of heart valves. The serum of patients with rheumatic fever contains autoantibodies to myosin and sarcolemma. The Aschoff body, pathognomic for this disorder, represents persistent focal inflammatory lesions in the myocardium. These can persist for years after an acute attack. Macrophages containing myosin have been identified in these nodules.

Clinical diagnosis is made using the Jones criteria.[45] The major manifestations are carditis, polyarthritis, chorea, erythema marginatum, subcutaneous nodules, and evidence of preceding streptococcal infection (i.e., positive throat culture, history of scarlet fever, elevated antistreptolysin titers). Minor criteria are nonspecific findings such as fever, arthralgia, previous rheumatic fever or rheumatic heart disease, elevated erythrocyte sedimentation rate (ESR) or C-reactive protein, and prolonged P-R interval. Diagnosis is made by the presence of two major criteria or one major and two minor criteria.

Two-thirds of patients present with an antecedent pharyngitis, followed by the symptoms of rheumatic fever in 1 to 5 weeks, with a mean presentation of 18.6 days. Severe carditis resulting in death can occur but is unusual. Congestive heart failure (CHF) is observed in only 5 to 10 percent of cases. Usually the carditis is mild, with scarring of the heart valves more typically predominant. Physical examination is notable for fever and heart murmurs, reflecting the acute valvulitis. The mitral valve is involved three times as frequently as the aortic valve; therefore mitral murmurs are more common. Mitral regurgitation is the most common finding. A middiastolic murmur over the apical area can frequently be heard. This is called the Carey Coombs murmur, and its presence almost certainly confirms mitral valvulitis. Aortic insufficiency can be auscultated with aortic valvulitis.

There are no characteristic ECG findings, though P-R prolongation and nonspecific ST-T-wave changes are frequently described. Endomyocardial biopsy demonstrates the Aschoff body as well as a diffuse cellular interstitial infiltrate including lymphocytes, polymorphonuclear cells, histiocytes, and eosinophils. Laboratory tests suggestive of rheumatic fever include antibodies to antistreptolysin O and anti-DNAse B, an elevated ESR, and elevated C-reactive protein. Extracardiac manifestations generally include an acute migratory polyarthritis of the large joints.

Aspirin and penicillin are the mainstays of therapy. Corticosteroids can also provide symptomatic relief. Treatment with IVIG produces no detectable clinical or echocardiographic improvements.[46] Mitral valve repair during acute carditis is associated with an increased mortality risk and should be undertaken only when heart failure is refractory to optimal antiinflammatory therapy.

Once rheumatic fever is diagnosed, antibiotic prophylaxis is required to prevent recurrent episodes. The most effective method is a single monthly intramuscular injection of 1.2 million units of benzathine penicillin G until age 21.

【 】 NONINFECTIVE

Hypersensitivity

Hypersensitivity myocarditis is an example of the early phase of eosinophilic myocarditis and is thought to be caused by an allergic reaction to a variety of drugs (Table 32–4). Methyldopa, the penicillins, sulfonamides, tetracycline, and the antituberculous drugs are the pharmaceuticals most commonly associated with this entity. It is characterized by peripheral eosinophilia and infiltration into the myocardium by eosinophils, multinucleated giant cells, and leukocytes (Fig. 32–7).[47] The major basic protein of the eosinophil granule can be detected in the presence of acute necrotizing myocarditis, suggesting toxicity of the granule contents. Good success has been reported with stopping the offending agent and treatment with corticosteroids. Unfortunately, the presence of this condition often goes unnoticed, and sometimes the first manifestation of cardiac involvement is sudden death caused by arrhythmia.

Giant Cell Myocarditis

Giant cell myocarditis is an extremely rare but aggressive form of myocarditis, typically progressive and unresponsive to medical therapy.[48] This disease is most prevalent in young adults, with a mean age at onset of 42 years (and a range of 16 to 69 years). Association with other autoimmune disorders is reported in approximately 20 percent of cases. Diagnosis is made by endomyocardial biopsy. Widespread or multifocal necrosis with a mixed inflammatory infiltrate including lymphocytes and histiocytes is required for histologic diagnosis. Eosinophils are frequently noted, as are multinucleated giant cells in the absence of granuloma (Fig. 32–8). Immunophenotyping of the cellular infiltrate has shown lymphocyte populations composed of T-helper or in some cases T-suppressor cells.

TABLE 32–4

Drugs Causing Eosinophilic Myocarditis

Acetazolamide	Oxyphenylbutazone
Amitriptyline	Para-aminosalicylic acid
Amphotericin B	Penicillin
Ampicillin	Phenindione
Carbamazepine	Phenobarbital
Cefaclor	Phenylbutazone
Chloramphenicol	Phenytoin
Chlorthalidone	Spironolactone
Desipramine	Streptomycin
Hydrochlorothiazide	Sulfadiazine
Indomethacin	Sulfisoxazole
Interleukin-4	Sulfonylureas
Isoniazid	Tetanus toxoid
Methyldopa	Tetracycline

The clinical course is usually characterized by progressive CHF and is frequently associated with refractory ventricular arrhythmia. This condition is almost uniformly and rapidly fatal. Comparison of survival of patients with giant cell myocarditis with that of patients with lymphocytic myocarditis demonstrates significantly worse survival in those patients with giant cell disease (Fig. 32–9). Case reports and the Giant-cell Myocarditis Registry suggest that treatment with certain immunosuppressive regimens, but not steroids alone, can extend transplant-free survival by a few months.[49] Some patients can require mechanical circulatory support as a bridge to transplant. Rare cases of complete recovery have been described; for example, one patient treated with OKT3 and high-dose steroids had complete resolution of giant-cell myocarditis and was able to be successfully weaned off a biventricular support device.[50] However, cardiac transplantation represents the best treatment option despite the possibility of recurrence in the transplanted heart.[48] Giant cells

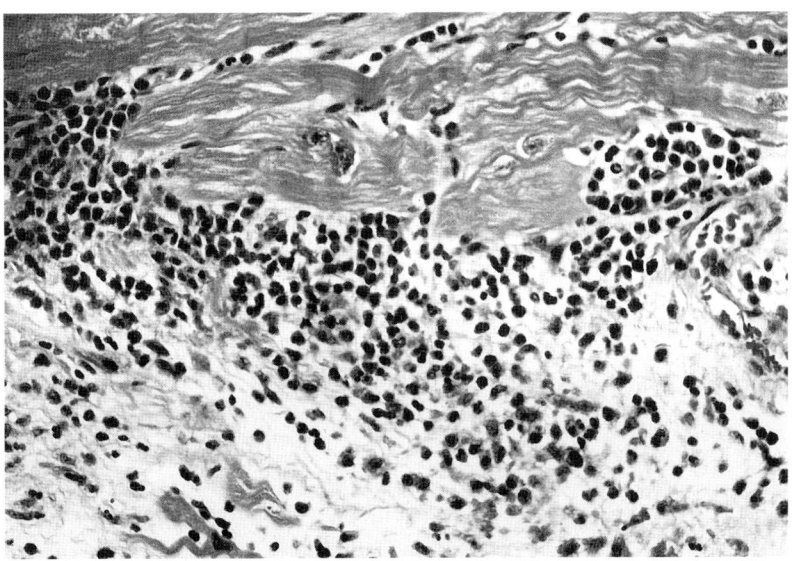

FIGURE 32–7. Photomicrograph showing interstitial infiltrates rich in eosinophils. (H&E, ×40.)

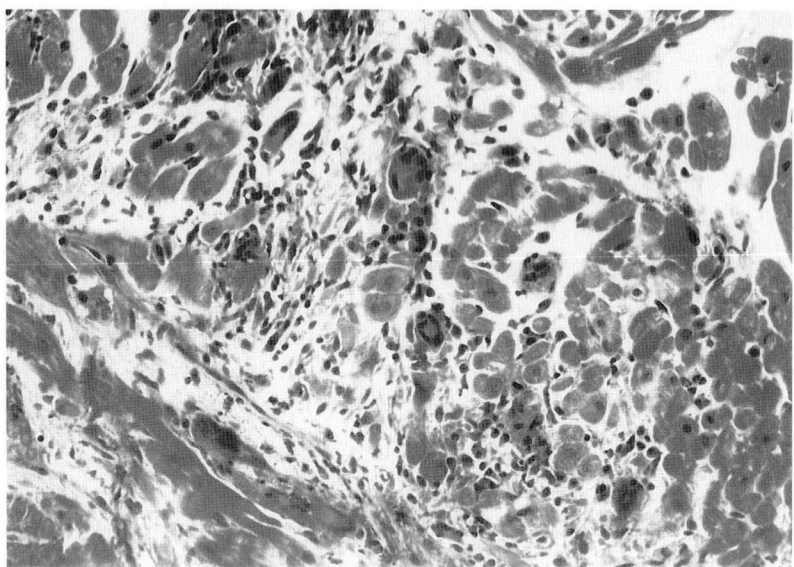

FIGURE 32–8. Photomicrograph showing extensive myocyte damage and infiltrates of mononuclear cells and numerous multinucleated giant cells. (H&E, ×60.)

can be detected on routine surveillance biopsies up to 9 years posttransplant. This cellular infiltrate can respond to an increase in immunosuppressive therapy.

PERIPARTUM CARDIOMYOPATHY

Peripartum cardiomyopathy is an uncommon form of CHF first described by Virchow in 1870. Estimates of its incidence vary from 1 in 3000 to 1 in 15,000 pregnancies in the United States. A much higher incidence is observed in Africa (1 in 3000) and Haiti (1 in 350). The disease occurs more commonly in obese multiparous black females older than 30 years of age. Twin pregnancies, preeclampsia, and long-term use of tocolytic agents are other predisposing factors. Patients present with heart failure in the last trimester of pregnancy or in the first 5 months postpartum. Absence of a demonstrable cause of heart failure and structural heart disease is required to make the diagnosis. Indeed, the hemodynamic stress of pregnancy can frequently unmask previously unknown cardiac disease. A recent report describes and contrasts the clinical characteristics of those patients presenting with cardiomyopathy prior to the last month of gestation.[51] Of 123 women diagnosed with peripartum cardiomyopathy, 23 had early symptoms. The only significant differences between the early and traditional postpartum cardiomyopathies were a higher incidence of twin gestations with shorter pregnancy duration and lower birth weights. Maternal outcome, rate of recovery, and ejection fraction at diagnosis were comparable.

PATHOGENESIS

The etiology of this disorder is unclear. Proposed mechanisms include nutritional deficiencies, genetic disorders, viral or autoimmune etiologies, hormonal problems, volume overload, alcohol, physiologic stress of pregnancy, or unmasking of latent id-

iopathic dilated cardiomyopathy. Several lines of evidence suggest that peripartum cardiomyopathy can be the result of myocarditis caused by a viral illness or an autoimmune etiology.[52] Given the relatively immunosuppressed state of pregnancy, susceptibility to cardiotropic viruses is higher. Additionally, several studies have demonstrated histologic evidence of myocarditis on endomyocardial biopsy samples obtained from patients with peripartum cardiomyopathy.[28,52] Molecular analysis of endomyocardial biopsy samples revealed viral genomes in 31 percent of patients associated with inflammatory changes.[53] Other investigators have postulated an autoimmune etiology to peripartum cardiomyopathy, specifically immunologic responses to fetal and endometrial antigens that cross-react with the patient's myocytes. In one case report, a patient with peripartum cardiomyopathy had antibodies to smooth muscle and actin produced in response to actin and myosin released during uterine degeneration after delivery. These antibodies later cross-reacted with the myocardium and induced cardiomyopathy.[54]

CLINICAL PRESENTATION

Symptoms include shortness of breath, dyspnea on exertion, edema, palpitations, syncope, sudden death, and thromboembolic phenomena. The incidence of thromboembolism is high because of the hypercoagulability of pregnancy. Physical findings are notable for third heart sound (S_3), fourth heart sound (S_4), tricuspid or mitral insufficiency murmurs, edema, rales, ascites, hepatomegaly, jugular venous distension. The ECG frequently shows LV hypertrophy. Echocardiographic findings can range from single-chamber LV enlargement to four-chamber dilation. Endomyocardial biopsy can reveal myocarditis in as many as 50 percent of these women, but generally the findings are nonspecific.[28] Biopsies in patients with peripartum cardiomyopathy have the highest yield when performed early after onset of symptoms.

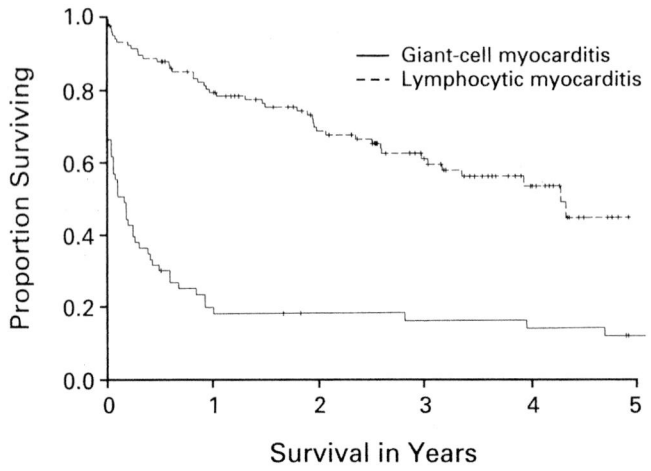

FIGURE 32–9. Kaplan-Meier survival curves for patients with giant-cell myocarditis versus lymphocytic myocarditis. *Source: Cooper LT Jr., Berry GJ, Shabetai R.[48] Used with permission.*

PROGNOSIS AND TREATMENT

Too few patients with peripartum cardiomyopathy have been studied to fully analyze the natural history of the disease. In a small series of 27 patients, LV size was analyzed at 6 months; 14 patients (50 percent) had normal dimensions. None of these patients died of CHF—compared with 85 percent of those patients with persistent cardiomegaly, who died from CHF within 5 years.[55] The authors concluded, therefore, that if the congestive cardiomyopathy persists for more than 6 months, it is likely to be irreversible and associated with a worse prognosis. Similar findings were published in another series by O'Connell and colleagues.[56] These authors noted that those patients with higher ejection fractions and smaller ventricular diastolic dimensions at the time of diagnosis have a better long-term prognosis. A fractional shortening on echocardiography less than 20 percent and a LV end diastolic dimension greater than or equal to 6 cm was associated with a threefold increase in persistent LV dysfunction.[57] Recovery of LV function correlates with resolution of myocarditis with or without immunosuppressive therapy.[52] The use of corticosteroids in the treatment of this disorder is controversial and should be reserved for patients with endomyocardial evidence of myocarditis and persistent ventricular dysfunction.[28,52] Use of pentoxifylline to inhibit proinflammatory cytokines has been shown to improve outcome in one small trial of patients with postpartum cardiomyopathy.[58] Patients with refractory heart failure referred for transplant have a posttransplant survival comparable with that of patients with idiopathic dilated cardiomyopathy, although higher early rejection rates are noted.

Questions still remain regarding the safety of subsequent pregnancy for patients with stable heart failure or recovery of LV function. There are several case reports of women with this diagnosis who went on to subsequent pregnancies. The outcomes of these patients are variable, with a few having uneventful pregnancies and others developing an exacerbation or recurrence of fulminant heart failure. Dobutamine echocardiography has detected impaired contractile reserve in some women with peripartum cardiomyopathy who apparently had recovered normal ventricular function.[59] Subsequent pregnancy should be viewed as posing a high risk, and all patients with this disorder should be counseled about birth control and contraceptive methods.

NEUROMUSCULAR DISEASES

Several heritable neuromuscular dystrophies can be associated with cardiomyopathy. Included in this category are diseases such as Becker, Duchenne, and X-linked cardioskeletal myopathy, myotonic dystrophy (Steinert disease), congenital myotonic dystrophy, limb-girdle muscular dystrophy (Erb disease), familial centronuclear myopathy, Kugelberg-Welander syndrome, Friedreich ataxia, and Barth syndrome. The myocardial involvement, natural history, and prognosis of each of these disorders are variable.

Duchenne dystrophy is an X-linked disease with proximal muscle weakness and cardiomyopathy. A dystrophin gene mutation is responsible. Death usually results from respiratory and/or cardiorespiratory failure. Patients with myotonic dystrophy present between age 20 and 50 years, usually with arrhythmias.

Several mitochondrial myopathies have also been described.[60] Mitochondria are essential cellular organelles that convert oxygen to biochemically useful energy. Additionally, mitochondria function as calcium storage sites and modulators of cellular pH. As such, mitochondrial function affects muscle and ventricular function. Mitochondria are unique organelles with their own maternally inherited DNA, which encodes several respiratory chain proteins. Genetic defects in the mitochondrial respiratory chain enzymes—specifically complexes I, III, and IV—have been recognized as the cause in some cardiomyopathies. The presentation in mitochondrial myopathies is extremely heterogeneous, as each cell will contain a mixture of normal and mutant DNA. Deletion mutations in DNA can occur and are frequently observed in these myopathies. Mitochondrial myopathies include such disorders as Kearns-Sayre syndrome, chronic ophthalmoplegia, myoclonic epilepsy, ragged-red-fiber disease, and mitochondrial encephalomyopathy. The MELAS syndrome (mitochondrial encephalopathy, lactic acidosis, and strokelike episodes) is associated with cardiomyopathy and generalized microangiopathy. Kearns-Sayre syndrome results from a deletion mutation in mitochondrial DNA. This ocular myopathic disease is associated with dilated or hypertrophic cardiomyopathy with cardiac conduction defects. Defects in transport of molecules from the cytoplasm into the mitochondria have also been associated with cardiac and skeletal myopathy.

CARDIOMYOPATHY CAUSED BY ENDOCRINE DISORDERS

THYROID

Thyroid hormone has long been recognized to affect the heart and the peripheral vasculature. Changes in cardiac function are mediated by triiodothyronine (T3) regulation of cardiac-specific genes.[61] Thyroid hormone metabolism is frequently abnormal in patients with CHF. In a study of 84 patients with advanced heart failure, T3 levels were found to be low.[62] Low conversion to T3 is postulated to be an adaptive mechanism to decreased catabolism. In a subsequent study, Hamilton and coworkers studied the effects of intravenous T3 infusion in patients with class III or IV heart failure.[63] Cardiac output increased without a change in LV ejection fraction or filling pressures. This was thought to be secondary to the effects of T3, causing vascular smooth muscle dilation and therefore peripheral vasodilatation. In another study of thyroid hormone replacement in heart failure, 20 patients with class II and III idiopathic dilated cardiomyopathy were given L-thyroxine orally.[64] Cardiac output improved, peripheral vascular resistance decreased, and exercise performance increased.

Like thyroid deficiency, thyroid toxicity can lead to the development of both high- and low-output cardiac failure. A prolonged tachycardia and high-output state caused by thyrotoxicosis is thought eventually to produce LV dilation. A consequent progressive decline in systolic function leads to low-output heart failure. This process can often be reversed by reduction of excess hormone levels. In a study of seven patients with a dilated cardiomyopathy and hyperthyroidism, Umpierrez and coworkers demonstrated echocardiographic normalization of LV function after treatment with propylthiouracil or methimazole.[65]

【 】 PHEOCHROMOCYTOMA

Hypertension and its sequelae are the major cardiovascular manifestations of pheochromocytoma. However, there have been reports of a specific catecholamine-induced myocarditis and/or cardiomyopathy.[66] Degenerative and fibrotic myocardial changes have been described in autopsy specimens of patients dying of suprarenal tumors. Although progression to cardiac involvement is unusual, when the presentation of the tumor is aggressive, pheochromocytoma patients typically die of cardiovascular causes, most commonly congestive heart failure or malignant ventricular arrhythmias. In the largest series, 15 of the 26 patients with proven pheochromocytomas had a pathologic diagnosis of myocarditis at autopsy.[66] Hemodynamic stabilization is generally obtained with α and β blockers, and prompt adrenalectomy is required to eliminate catecholamine-induced cardiotoxicity. The cardiac abnormalities can be reversed with tumor resection.

【 】 ACROMEGALY

Acromegalic cardiomyopathy appears to be a specific entity independent of the hypertension, noninsulin dependent diabetes, hyperlipidemia, and/or atherosclerosis associated with excess growth hormone. Ten to twenty percent of patients with acromegaly develop CHF. The initial increased cardiac output and decreased total peripheral resistance triggered by increased growth hormone levels over time result in myocyte hypertrophy with fibrosis leading to impaired diastolic function and finally systolic dysfunction.[67,68] The CHF that develops in these patients is particularly resistant to conventional therapy owing to higher collagen content in the acromegalic heart. Histopathologically, the myocytes display cellular hypertrophy, patchy fibrosis, and myofibrillar degeneration. A 500-fold increase in apoptosis of myocytes has been observed. Inflammatory and degenerative damage to the sinoatrial and AV nodes can lead to sudden death. Pituitary surgery and irradiation remain the mainstays of therapy, but often the cardiopathic manifestations persist despite a fall in growth hormone levels. Treatment of acromegalic patients without clinical heart failure decreases LV mass and improves diastolic function.[69] Young patients with short disease duration were more likely to reverse the acromegalic cardiac changes after 1 year of treatment with the long-acting somatostatin analogue octreotide than middle-aged patients with more prolonged disease.

【 】 DIABETES

Analysis of the Framingham data shows that the risk of developing heart failure is substantially increased among diabetic patients. Even after exclusion of patients with prior coronary or rheumatic disease and controlling for age, hypertension, obesity, and hypercholesterolemia, diabetic patients have a fivefold increased risk of developing CHF.[70] This increased incidence suggests that the metabolic abnormalities associated with diabetes affect myocyte structure and function leading to a cardiomyopathy. Hyperlipidemia with increased triglycerides and nonesterified fatty acids, hyperinsulinemia, hyperglycemia, and alterations in adipocytokines (leptin, adiponectin) are all involved in the cardiovascular pathophysiology of diabetes. Nonesterified fatty acids trigger insulin

resistance as well as myocardial contractile dysfunction and apoptosis. Hyperinsulinemia can cause cardiac hypertrophy. Hyperglycemia mediates tissue injury through the generation of reactive oxygen species and thus increases oxidative stress.[71] Histologically, this cardiomyopathy shows no evidence of epicardial atherosclerotic disease or abnormalities in myocardial capillary basal lamina. Typically, interstitial fibrosis and arteriolar hyalinization are present. Clinically both systolic and diastolic dysfunction can occur, and the severity of the dysfunction is related to the degree of metabolic control (see Chap. 86).[72]

TOXINS

【 】 ALCOHOL

Chronic alcohol abuse is a major risk factor for the development of congestive cardiomyopathy, accounting for up to 45 percent of all dilated cardiomyopathies. In one observational study completed over a 5-year period, 20 percent of chronic alcoholic women and 26 percent of chronic alcoholic men developed dilated cardiomyopathy.[73] As an estimated 10 percent of the adult population are heavy alcohol users, cardiac toxicity from alcohol is a major problem.

Pathogenesis

The cardiodepressant effects of alcohol have been demonstrated following acute and chronic ingestion in animal models and in normal and alcoholic human subjects. Chronic excessive alcohol use can result in CHF, hypertension, and arrhythmias. Cardiac damage results from direct toxic effects of alcohol or one of its metabolites. Nutritional deficiencies, toxic cofactors, sympathetic stimulation, or coexistent hypertension can also contribute to disease development.

Orally ingested alcohol is converted in the liver to acetaldehyde by the alcohol dehydrogenase enzyme system. Alcohol and acetaldehyde are both potent vasodilators. Additionally, acetaldehyde results in marked catecholamine release. Both alcohol and acetaldehyde interfere with a variety of cellular metabolic functions, including calcium transport and binding, lipid metabolism and fatty acid composition of the sarcolemma, protein synthesis, myofibrillar adenosine triphosphatase (ATPase), and mitochondrial respiration.[74] Using a transgenic mouse model that increased alcohol dehydrogenase (ADH) activity 40-fold to significantly increase cardiac exposure to acetaldehyde, researchers assessed for the development of cardiomyopathy after alcohol ingestion. Acute and chronic alcohol exposure in the ADH transgene mouse resulted in significantly greater cardiac depression compared to the wild type mouse, supporting the central role of acetaldehyde. In contrast, overexpression of acetaldehyde dehydrogenase, which facilitates removal of acetaldehyde by converting it to acetate, attenuates oxidative stress and apoptosis in human umbilical vein endothelial cells and in human cardiac myocytes.[75] Although ethanol can interfere with a number of myocardial metabolic steps, no predominant factor has been identified. Recently a nonoxidative pathway for the metabolism of alcohol in several organ systems including the heart has been described.[76] Nonesterified fatty acids are esterified with ethanol to produce fatty acid ethyl esters

(FAEE). These molecules can accumulate in mitochondria and impair cellular function. Fatty acid ethyl esters are synthesized at high rates in the heart owing to the lack of oxidative ethanol metabolism in this organ. Other studies have demonstrated interference with lipid metabolism leading to triglyceride accumulation and alteration of the fatty acid composition of the sarcolemma. Increased levels of acyl-coenzyme A (acyl-CoA) from enhanced glycerol acyltransferase activity can lead to triglyceride accumulation. The cellular membrane changes result in decreased calcium uptake by the sarcolemma. Alcohol also is found to be an inhibitor of the sodium-potassium ATPase.

For many years, alcoholic cardiomyopathy was believed to be caused by nutritional deficiencies. Indeed, subjects with heavy beer consumption could develop thiamine deficiency. As beer contains no thiamine, the consumption of this high-calorie, high-carbohydrate beverage can exhaust existing thiamine stores, particularly in the presence of a deficient diet.

In the 1960s, a new variant of alcoholic cardiomyopathy was described. Patients presented with massive pericardial effusion, low cardiac output, elevated venous pressure, and polycythemia. After considerable medical detective work, the syndrome was linked to cobaltous chloride that was added to the beer as a foaming agent. Removal of the additive resulted in the resolution of this miniepidemic. The important role of zinc in the regulation of myocardial fibrosis frequently seen in alcoholic cardiomyopathy was demonstrated recently by Wang and coworkers using a metallothionein-null mouse model.[77] Metallothionein is a small protein that binds seven atoms of zinc. Oxidative stress releases zinc, a key element involved in fibrillar collagen metabolism and deposition. The metallothionein deficient mice have a relative zinc deficiency in the presence of alcohol base diet leading to myocyte hypertrophy and fibrosis. Zinc supplementation prevented this fibrotic effect.[77]

Clinical Presentation

The disease is observed most frequently in males age 30 to 55 years with a greater than 10-year history of heavy alcohol use and is extremely rare in premenopausal women. The amount and duration of alcohol use is frequently difficult to establish. Criteria used to define heavy chronic alcohol use have included such estimates as the use of 125 mL/day of alcohol and/or 30 to 50 percent of daily calories derived from alcohol for a minimum of 10 years. Other definitions include ingestion of greater than 90 grams of alcohol daily (7 to 8 drinks/day) for greater than 5 years. Presenting symptoms include dyspnea on exertion, orthopnea, paroxysmal nocturnal dyspnea, fatigue, weakness, arrhythmias, or embolic phenomena. Atrial fibrillation is extremely common, followed by atrial flutter and ventricular premature contractions. Sudden death can be the initial presentation.

Several histologic changes have been described on endomyocardial biopsies in alcoholic cardiomyopathy, but none of these changes are pathognomonic. Changes include myocyte loss, increased fibrosis, loss of sarcolemmal integrity, myofibrillar degeneration, mitochondrial swelling, and intercellular edema.[78] Electron microscopy shows mitochondrial swelling with dense intramitochondrial inclusions, swollen vesiculated sarcoplasmic reticulum, and myofibrillar disruption.

Treatment

The mainstay of treatment is abstinence from alcohol. Alcohol withdrawal can have a remarkable impact on disease manifestation and progression, especially in the milder forms of the disease. In animal models, following cessation of alcohol use, the hearts recover. In humans, the duration and extent of abuse is correlated with outcome. Prognosis is extremely poor in those patients who continue to drink in excess of 100 grams of ethanol daily compared with patients who moderate their alcohol consumption.[79] In 1 year of followup, men with alcoholic cardiomyopathy who became abstinent or curtailed their drinking to 60 grams of ethanol per day experienced an average improvement in ejection fraction of approximately 13 percent, with sustained improvement over 4 years. In contrast, those who continued to drink heavily suffered a progressive deterioration in cardiac function.

Although abstinence can result in recovery early in the disease process, there is a point at which cessation of alcohol is no longer effective, and this correlates with the development of structural histologic abnormalities. Survival of patients with alcoholic dilated cardiomyopathy who become abstinent was believed to be significantly better than the long-term survival of patients with a comparable class of CHF because of idiopathic cardiomyopathy. A recent study of 338 men with dilated cardiomyopathy treated with angiotensin-converting enzyme (ACE) inhibitors found that 7-year transplant-free survival was greatest in the group with idiopathic dilated cardiomyopathy and poorest for those with alcoholic cardiomyopathy who continued to drink heavily.[80] Patients with alcoholic cardiomyopathy who abstained from alcohol had a significant improvement in ejection fraction and 7-year survival, which paralleled that of the idiopathic dilated cardiomyopathy group.

█] COCAINE

Myocardial ischemia, infarction, coronary spasm, cardiac arrhythmias, sudden death, myocarditis, and dilated cardiomyopathy are all reported cardiovascular complications of cocaine abuse. The pharmacologic effects of cocaine on the heart partly explain its toxic effects.[81] By blocking the reuptake of norepinephrine, cocaine induces tachycardia, vasoconstriction, hypertension, cardiomyopathy, and ventricular arrhythmias. Cardiomyopathy can then result from secondary changes in the heart caused by tachycardia or sustained increased ventricular afterload.

There are no clinical or histologic features specific for cocaine-induced myocardial damage. Endomyocardial biopsy and autopsy studies confirm the presence of myocyte necrosis and a diffuse inflammatory cellular infiltrate in cocaine users.[82] *Contraction-band necrosis* has been seen in a patient presenting with a clinical course similar to that of catecholamine cardiomyopathy, but this is not characteristic.[83] Although eosinophilic infiltrates can be seen, cocaine is not included in the list of typical drugs associated with a hypersensitivity syndrome. Thus the diagnosis is usually presumptive and is one of exclusion. The treatment of cocaine-related myocarditis and cardiomyopathy is nonspecific and focuses on abstinence and heart failure therapy. Use of β blockers is typically avoided.

【 】 CHEMOTHERAPEUTIC AGENTS

Several chemotherapeutic agents can cause an acute and/or chronic cardiomyopathy. Among them, the anthracycline group (doxorubicin) and cyclophosphamide are the most common agents associated with heart failure.

Doxorubicin has been used as single or combination therapy for treatment of many different tumors including breast and esophageal tumors as well as sarcomas and lymphomas. Its use is limited by its cardiotoxicity. The cause of the cardiotoxicity is unknown, but it is suspected to be caused by increased oxidative stress from the generation of free radicals. Moreover, endogenous antioxidants are reduced by treatment with doxorubicin. Doxorubicin can be associated with early or late cardiotoxicity. Risk factors for the development of doxorubicin cardiomyopathy include age older than 70 years, combination chemotherapy (cyclophosphamide, paclitaxel, docetaxel), mediastinal irradiation, prior cardiac disease, hypertension, and liver disease. The early or acute cardiotoxicity manifests as a pericarditis-myocarditis syndrome and is not dose-related.[84] Left ventricular dysfunction is rarely seen, but arrhythmias, abnormalities of conduction, decreased QRS voltage, and nonspecific ST-segment and T-wave abnormalities are commonly observed. The prognosis is good, with quick resolution of the abnormalities on discontinuation of therapy.

In contrast, late or chronic cardiotoxicity is caused by the development of a dose-dependent degenerative cardiomyopathy (Fig. 32–10). This syndrome generally occurs at cumulative doses above 550 mg/m². Serial assessment of nuclear ejection fractions is used clinically to monitor for adverse effects. More recently troponin T and B-type natriuretic peptide (BNP) levels have been used with varying success as biomarkers of cardiac dysfunction. However, histopathologic grading is most useful in delineating the safety of continued doxorubicin administration. Cardiotoxicity can occur during therapy, within a year of the last dose of anthracycline, or as late as 6 to 20 years after its cessation. Therefore a course of this chemotherapy commits patients to prolonged cardiac surveillance.

The best management of anthracycline cardiotoxicity is prevention by limiting dosage. Lowering the peak blood levels of the drug by giving a continuous rather than bolus infusion also appears to significantly decrease drug-related damage.[84] Coadministration of doxorubicin with agents that would block free radical formation and not decrease its antineoplastic effects has been studied. Dexrazoxane, an iron chelating agent, has been used in clinical trials of patients with breast cancer or small-cell lung cancer to limit the cardiotoxicity of doxorubicin.[85] The incidence of heart failure and the decrement in ejection fraction is lower in those patients receiving combined therapy. Unfortunately, dexrazoxane is a potent myelosuppressive agent and can also interfere with cancer therapy. Studies with probucol, an alternative antioxidant, are ongoing. Recent animal data suggests that prophylactic treatment with sildenafil attenuates the cardiac myocyte apoptosis and LV dysfunction associated with doxorubicin.[86]

Liposomal formulations of anthracyclines have been developed to limit cardiotoxicity. Liposomes are preferentially absorbed by tissues with extensive reticuloendothelial cell networks. A retrospective analysis of 8 Phase I and II trials using pegylated liposomal doxorubicin revealed that none of the 41 studied patients developed heart failure.[87] Heart failure caused by doxorubicin has

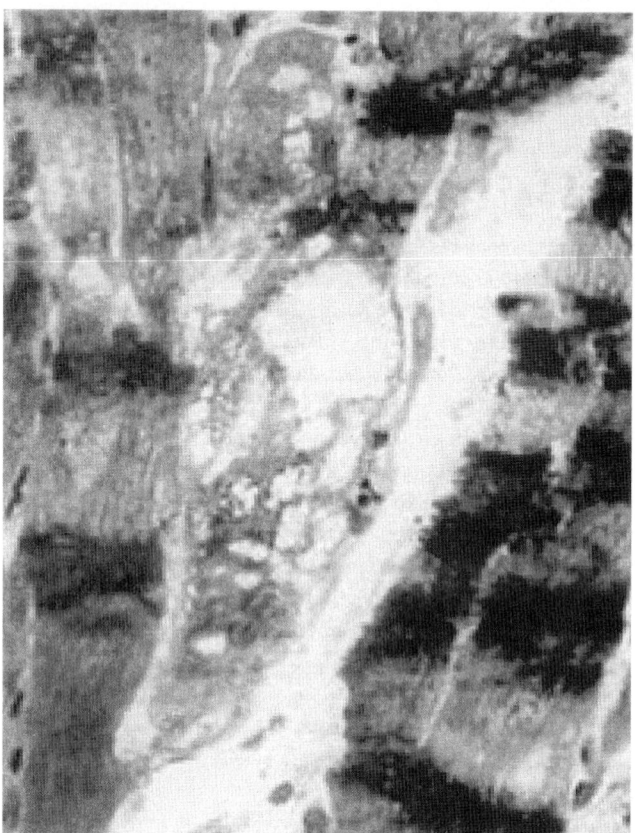

FIGURE 32–10. Loss of myofibrils and vacuolization of cytoplasm (toluidine blue stain, ×40) in a patient with doxorubicin cardiotoxicity. *Source: Singal P, Iliskovic N.[84] Used with permission.*

been very difficult to treat and is typically refractory to conventional therapy. In children with doxorubicin-induced cardiomyopathy, recent reports have described diminished symptoms and improved LV function after treatment with β blockers. Further studies on the use of these agents are needed.

In contrast to the anthracyclines, cyclophosphamide leads to an acute cardiotoxicity that is not related to cumulative dose. Pericarditis, systolic dysfunction, arrhythmias, and myocardial edema make up the spectrum of cardiac abnormalities. Prior LV dysfunction is a risk factor for development of significant cardiomyopathy with cyclophosphamide. Although mortality is not trivial, survivors exhibit no residual cardiac abnormalities.[88]

Trastuzumab is a monoclonal antibody directed against the human epidermal growth receptor 2 (HER-2) receptor protein on breast cancer cells that is associated with an increased risk of heart failure. In one study using trastuzumab as a single agent, 7 percent of women developed heart failure.[89] In contrast, the incidence rises to 28 percent when trastuzumab is used in association with anthracyclines and cyclophosphamide.

【 】 PSYCHOTHERAPEUTIC DRUGS

An increased incidence of cardiac complications including myocarditis, pericarditis, and cardiomyopathy has recently been reported with the atypical neuroleptic agent clozapine used in the treatment of schizophrenia.[90] Four-chamber dilation can occur and can be reversible with discontinuation of the drug. The duration of therapy with clozapine prior to the development of cardiomyopathy ranges from 2 weeks to 7 years with a median duration of 9 months. Of the 178 cases reported by the drug manufacturer 18 percent were fatal. The etiology can be a direct cardiotoxic effect or the result of a clozapine-induced myocarditis. There are no parameters to predict the risk of developing adverse cardiac effects or guidelines for monitoring cardiac function in clozapine treated patients.

CHEMICAL TOXINS

A variety of compounds can lead to a spectrum of cardiotoxicity, including cardiomyopathy. They include interferon alpha (IFN-α), IL-2, phenothiazines, emetine, methysergide, chloroquine, lithium, hydrocarbons, lead, and carbon monoxide. A summary of the cardiotoxicity seen with each compound is outlined in Table 32–5.

CARDIOMYOPATHIES ASSOCIATED WITH NUTRITIONAL DEFICIENCIES

VITAMINS

Thiamine deficiency, or beriberi, produces a clinical syndrome characterized by high-output cardiac failure and severe lactic acidosis. Dramatic hemodynamic improvements are seen after bolus

TABLE 32–5

Major Cardiovascular Complications of Chemical Toxins

AGENT	CARDIAC TOXICITY
Cobalt	Congestive heart failure
Cocaine	Coronary abnormalities, arrhythmias, myocarditis, myocardial depression
Interferon alpha	Arrhythmias, dilated cardiomyopathy, congestive heart failure
Interleukin-2	Myocardial ischemia/infarct, arrhythmias, eosinophilic myocarditis
Phenothiazines	Electrocardiographic changes, arrhythmias, sudden death
Emetine	Mononuclear and histiocyte infiltration, electrocardiographic abnormalities
Methysergide	Left-sided valvular lesions, fibrotic endocardial and pericardial lesions, restriction and constriction
Chloroquine	Arrhythmias, cardiac dysfunction
Lithium	Arrhythmias, cardiac dilatation with myofibrillar degeneration
Hydrocarbons	Electrocardiographic changes, arrhythmias, and cardiomegaly
Lead	Electrocardiographic changes, arrhythmias, and congestive heart failure
Carbon monoxide	Arrhythmias and transient biventricular dysfunction

infusion of thiamine. Untreated, beriberi can be fatal. Vitamin D deficiency, or rickets, and vitamin D excess are associated with cardiovascular morbidity and mortality. There are approximately 25 reported cases of hypocalcemic cardiomyopathy in the adult population caused mostly by idiopathic hypoparathyroidism.[91] Similarly in children, cardiomyopathy has been documented in cases of hypocalcemia caused by vitamin D deficiency rickets.[92] Excess doses of vitamin D in humans have been associated with calcium deposition in the heart and QT shortening but not frank cardiomyopathy.

SELENIUM

Cardiomyopathy associated with inadequate dietary intake of selenium is termed Keshan disease. This syndrome was discovered in regions of China with a low soil content of selenium.[93] Whether the cardiomyopathy results from the actual selenium deficiency or the selenium deficiency increases susceptibility to cardiotropic viruses is unclear. Coxsackievirus B3 (CVB 3/0), which causes no pathology in hearts of selenium-adequate mice, induces extensive myocarditis in selenium-deficient mice. Furthermore, coxsackievirus B3 recovered from the hearts of selenium-deficient mice and inoculated into selenium-adequate mice induced significant heart damage, suggesting mutation of the virus to a virulent genotype.[94] These findings can underlie the seasonal variation characteristic of Keshan disease.

Both acute and chronic forms of Keshan disease exist.[95] In the acute form, cardiogenic shock, severe arrhythmias, and pulmonary edema are the manifestations of the systolic impairment. The chronic type shows a moderate to severe heart enlargement with varying degrees of cardiac insufficiency; often patients are asymptomatic. Its incidence is dramatically reduced with supplementation of sodium selenite.

Other than Keshan disease, circumstantial evidence supports an association between selenium deficiency and cardiomyopathy. Congestive cardiomyopathy with low selenium levels has been reported in patients receiving total parenteral nutrition.[96] Patients with congestive cardiomyopathy have significantly lower serum selenium concentrations than healthy control subjects. LV ejection fraction is positively correlated with the selenium concentration in patients with cardiomyopathies.[96]

CARNITINE

L-Carnitine is an essential compound in the transport of long chain fatty acids into mitochondria, where they undergo β oxidation. Because the normal heart obtains approximately 60 percent of its total energy production from fatty acid oxidation, it is believed that adequate levels of carnitine are required for normal energy metabolism and contractile function of the heart.[97] Interestingly, not all patients with carnitine deficiency exhibit cardiomyopathy.

Deficiencies of carnitine can be either primary or secondary. Primary deficiencies arise from several genetic disorders involving carnitine synthesis or handling. These rare conditions are severe and are associated with muscle and plasma carnitine levels as low as 10 percent of normal (Fig. 32–11). Several case reports have established that primary carnitine deficiency is associated with car-

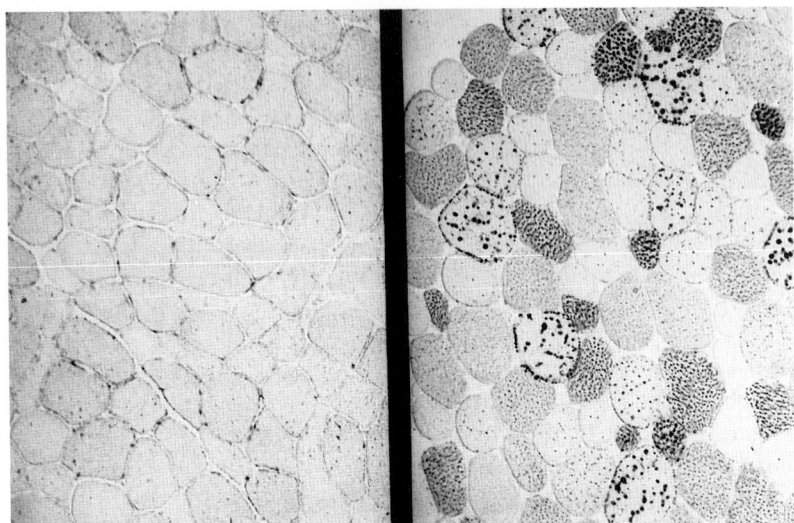

FIGURE 32-11. Photomicrograph of oil red O stain demonstrating lipid deposits in type I and II fibers in normal (*right*) and carnitine-deficient (*left*) skeletal muscle.

diomyopathy.[98] The cardiomyopathy that ensues presents within 3 to 4 years of birth and is profound; clinically, however, it responds to carnitine supplementation.

Secondary carnitine deficiencies are much more common and arise from a large number of genetic diseases associated with defects in acyl-CoA metabolism. In patients with long-chain or short-chain acyl-CoA dehydrogenase deficiency, carnitine levels are reduced to 25 to 50 percent of normal and a depression in cardiac contractile performance has been found.[99] Secondary carnitine deficiencies can also be acquired as a result of liver disease, renal disease (Fanconi syndrome, renal tubular acidosis), dietary insufficiencies (chronic total parenteral nutrition, malabsorption), diabetes mellitus, and heart failure. Many of these types of secondary carnitine deficiency are often associated with cardiomyopathy. In cases of secondary carnitine deficiency, however, it has been difficult to determine whether the symptoms are caused by carnitine deficiency or by the underlying genetic metabolic disorder. Based on this observation and the inconsistent reports of cardiomyopathy with these secondary deficiencies, it appears that a clear and strong association can be made only between cardiomyopathy and primary carnitine deficiency.

CARDIOMYOPATHIES ASSOCIATED WITH ALTERED METABOLISM

〘 〙 HYPEROXALURIA

Both primary and secondary oxalosis are characterized by excessive deposition of calcium oxalate crystals in various body tissues, including the heart.[100] Oxalate crystals are frequently deposited in the conduction system, leading to heart block, and occasionally in the myocardium and the coronary arteries. Variable degrees of cellular reaction—including fibrosis, necrosis, and mononuclear cell infiltration—can be seen histologically, along with foreign-body giant cells and myocardial granulomas. Cases of primary oxalosis can be reversed after combined kidney/liver transplantation.[101]

〘 〙 HYPERURICEMIA

Atherosclerosis and coronary artery disease are the most common cardiac manifestations associated with gout, but heart muscle disease is uncommon. Uric acid crystals can be found in the blood vessel walls, in the myocardial interstitium, along the valve surfaces, and in the pericardium and can lead to a granulomatous response with the formation of multinucleated giant cells.

TAKO-TSUBO CARDIOMYOPATHY

Initially described in the 1990s in Japan, this reversible cardiomyopathy is characterized by a distinctive shape observed on left ventriculography described as apical ballooning.[102–104] This shape is similar to a Japanese *tako-subo* pot with a narrow neck and round bottom used by fishermen to trap octopus. The clinical presentation is that of acute coronary ischemia generally preceded by a stressful emotional, physical, or psychological event such as the death of a loved one. This accounts for this syndrome's other clinical titles, that is, *broken heart syndrome* or *stress cardiomyopathy*. Symptoms include chest pain, dyspnea, and, in rare cases, syncope. Cardiac enzymes are elevated, as is BNP. The most common ECG finding is anterior ST elevations, but ST depression and T wave inversions are also observed. Echocardiography reveals mildly to severely decreased LV function with anteroapical akinesis or dyskinesis. Mitral regurgitation caused by systolic anterior wall motion of the mitral valve, LV outflow tract obstruction, and thrombus formation can also be observed. MRI shows mid to apical LV dyskinesis without delayed gadolinium hyperenhancement consistent with myocardial viability. Coronary angiography is normal. Endomyocardial biopsy is nondiagnostic. Atrial and ventricular arrhythmias have been observed. Recovery of LV function occurs over a period of days to weeks.

The etiology of this disorder is unknown but may be related to adrenergic stimulation. Differences in the density of β-adrenergic receptors in the apex and base of the heart can account for the unusual apical ballooning. Other potential etiologies include multivessel spasm, microvascular dysfunction, transient LV outflow obstruction and/or localized myocarditis. Four criteria have been proposed to diagnose this syndrome:

1. Transient mid to apical LV akinesis or dyskinesis in areas involving more than a single coronary artery
2. Absence of coronary artery disease
3. Acute ECG changes including ST-segment elevation or depression
4. No recent head trauma, intracranial hemorrhage, pheochromocytoma, myocarditis, or hypertrophic cardiomyopathy

NONCOMPACTION CARDIOMYOPATHY

Left ventricular noncompaction cardiomyopathy is an unclassified cardiomyopathy initially described in 1990. It is a genetically heterogenous disorder that may or may not be associated with other congenital abnormalities. In the absence of coexistent congenital defects, this disorder is called *isolated noncompaction of the left ventricle*. The underlying mechanism is postulated to be caused by intrauterine arrest of myocardial development with lack of compaction of the loose meshwork of ventricular trabeculae. This arrested development leads to the characteristic pathology with diffuse prominent deep trabeculations in hypertrophied and hypokinetic segments predominantly in the left ventricle. Approximately 50 percent of cases can also involve the right ventricle. Distinct genetic mutations have been described.[105] Patients can be asymptomatic or have heart failure, arrhythmias, and embolic events.[106,107] Approximately two-thirds of patients have heart failure. Diastolic dysfunction can occur from both abnormal relaxation and restricted filling from the prominent trabeculae. Subendomyocardial ischemia is not uncommon. Diagnosis is made by echocardiography combined with Doppler imaging, which show multiple prominent ventricular trabeculations with deep recesses and blood flow through these crevices in continuity with the LV cavity. CT and MRI have also been used for diagnosis. Anticoagulation to prevent embolization and close monitoring for arrhythmias with early use of implantable defibrillators are key aspects of patient management.

IDIOPATHIC CARDIOMYOPATHY

Idiopathic cardiomyopathy (IDC) is the term used to describe a group of myocardial diseases of unknown cause. Idiopathic dilated cardiomyopathy probably represents the end result of a number of disease processes involving myocyte dysfunction, myocyte loss, myocyte hypertrophy, and fibrosis. It is a diagnosis of exclusion. The prevalence of IDC is estimated to be between 7 and 13 percent of all patients with systolic dysfunction.[1,2] In 1278 patients with a dilated cardiomyopathy referred to a large tertiary care center, extensive diagnostic testing including endomyocardial biopsy failed to identify any clear etiology in 51 percent of the patients.

TABLE 32–6

Potentially Reversible Dilated Cardiomyopathies

Ischemic with viable myocardium	Endocrine Hyperthyroidism
Valvular without surgically correctable lesion	Pheochromocytoma Metabolic
Inflammatory	Hypocalcemia
CMV	Hypophosphatemia
Toxoplasmosis	Uremia
Mycoplasma	Carnitine
Lyme	Nutritional
Toxic	Selenium
Alcohol	Thiamine
Cocaine	Infiltrative
Cobalt	Hemochromatosis
	Sarcoidosis
	Hypersensitivity

CMV, Cytomegalovirus.

Myocarditis and occult coronary artery disease were the most frequently identified causes. As discussed earlier in this chapter, an idiopathic dilated cardiomyopathy can be the end result of an infectious myocarditis. Endocardial biopsy in patients with dilated cardiomyopathy can reveal an inflammatory infiltrate. Surreptitious alcohol use as well as undiagnosed and untreated hypertension probably represent other etiologies of cardiomyopathy in many of these cases. Familial factors have generally been more predominant in hypertrophic cardiomyopathies than in dilated congestive cardiomyopathy. However, accumulating data suggest that genetic factors contribute to these cases as well. When one is making the diagnosis of idiopathic dilated cardiomyopathy, it is most important to exclude potentially reversible etiologies (Table 32–6).

Several studies of the natural history of IDC have concluded that the prognosis for this condition is better than that for ischemic cardiomyopathy. The clinical response to β blockade in IDC, as gauged by improvement in ventricular function, is greater than that for the ischemic group.[108] Approximately 10 percent of patients with IDC will normalize their ejection fraction on β blockade.[109] Therefore, if tolerated, this therapy is warranted before consideration of cardiac transplantation.

REFERENCES

1. Ho K, Pinsky J, Kannel W, et al. The epidemiology of heart failure: The Framingham study. *J Am Coll Cardiol.* 1993;22:6.
2. Bourassa MG, Gurne O, Bangdiwala, et al. Natural history and patterns of current practice in heart failure. *J Am Coll Cardiol.* 1993;22:14A.
3. Brodison A, Swann J. Myocarditis: A review. *J Infect.* 1998;3:99.
4. Feldman AM, McNamara D. Myocarditis. *N Engl J Med.* 2000;343:1388.
5. Woodruff J. Viral myocarditis: a review. *Am J Pathol.* 1980;101:427.
6. Kawai C. From myocarditis to cardiomyopathy: mechanisms of inflammation and cell death: learning from the past for the future. *Circulation.* 1999;99:1091.
7. Bergelson JM, Cunningham JA, Droguett G, et al. Isolation of a common receptor for Coxsackie B viruses and adenoviruses 2 and 5. *Science.* 1997;275:1320.
8. Shioi T, Matsumori A, Sasayama S. Persistent expression of cytokine in the chronic stage of viral myocarditis in mice. *Circulation.* 1996;94:2930.
9. Gebhard JR, Perry CM, Harkins S, et al. Coxsackie B3-induced myocarditis: perforin exacerbates disease, but plays no detectable role in virus clearance. *Am J Pathol.* 1998;153:417.
10. Liu PP, Mason JW. Advances in the understanding of myocarditis. *Circulation.* 2001;104:1076.
11. Bryant D, Becker L, Richardson J, et al. Cardiac failure in transgenic mice with myocardial expression of tumor necrosis factor-α (TNF-α). *Circulation.* 1998;97:1375.
12. Bachmaier K, Pummerer C, Kozieradzki I, et al. Low-molecular weight tumor necrosis factor receptor p55 controls induction of autoimmune heart disease. *Circulation.* 1997;95:655.
13. Wada H, Saito K, Kanda T, et al. Tumor necrosis factor-α (TNF-α) plays a protective role in acute viral myocarditis in mice: A study using mice lacking TNF-α. *Circulation.* 2001;103:743.
14. Andreoletti L, Hober D, Becquart P, et al. Experimental CVB3-induced chronic myocarditis in two murine strains: Evidence of interrelationships between virus replication and myocardial damage in persistent cardiac infection. *J Med Virol.* 1997;52:206.
15. Fujioka S, Koide H, Kitaura Y, et al. Molecular detection and differentiation of enteroviruses in endomyocardial biopsies and pericardial effusions from dilated cardiomyopathy and myocarditis. *Am Heart J.* 1996;131:760.
16. Kuhl U, Pauschinger M, Seeberg B, et al. Viral persistence in the myocardium is associated with progressive cardiac dysfunction. *Circulation.* 2005;112:1965.
17. Neu N, Rose NR, Beisel KW, et al. Cardiac myosin induces myocarditis in genetically predisposed mice. *J Immunol.* 1987;139:3630.
18. Wolfgram LL, Beisel KW, Rose NR. Heart-specific autoantibodies following murine coxsackievirus B3 myocarditis. *J Exp Med.* 1985;161:1112.

19. Rao I, Debbas M, Sabbatini P, et al. The adenovirus EIA proteins induce apoptosis, which is inhibited by the EIB 19-kDa and Bcl-2 proteins. *Proc Natl Acad Sci U S A.* 1992;89:7742.

20. Liu P, Sole MJ. What is the relevance of apoptosis to the myocardium? *Can J Cardiol.* 1999;15:8B.

21. Dec GW. Introduction to clinical myocarditis. In: Cooper LT, ed. *Myocarditis: From Bench to Bedside.* Totowa, NJ: Humana Press; 2003:257–281.

22. Magnani JW, Dec GW. Myocarditis: current trends in diagnosis and treatment. *Circulation.* 2006;113:876.

23. McCarthy RE III, Boehmer JP, Hruban RH, et al. Long-term outcome of fulminant myocarditis as compared with acute (nonfulminant) myocarditis. *N Engl J Med.* 2000;342:690.

24. Dec GW Jr, Waldman H, Southern J, et al. Viral myocarditis mimicking acute myocardial infarction. *J Am Coll Cardiol.* 1992;20:85.

25. Burch G, Shewey L. Viral coronary arteritis and myocardial infarction. *Am Heart J.* 1976;92:11.

26. Eckart RE, Scoville SL, Campbell CL, et al. Sudden death in young adults: a 25-year review of autopsies in military recruits. *Ann Intern Med.* 2004;141:829.

27. Smith SC, Ladenson JH, Mason JW, et al. Elevations of cardiac troponin I associated with myocarditis: Experimental and clinical correlates. *Circulation.* 1997;95:163.

28. Felker GM, Hu W, Hare JM, et al. The spectrum of dilated cardiomyopathy: the Johns Hopkins experience with 1,278 patients. *Medicine.* 1999;78:270.

29. Aretz HT, Billingham ME, Edwards WD, et al. Myocarditis: a histopathologic definition and classification. *Am J Cardiovasc Pathol.* 1987;1:3.

30. Baughman KL. Diagnosis of myocarditis: death of Dallas criteria. *Circulation.* 2006;113:593.

31. Lieberman EB, Hutchins GM, Rose NR, et al. Clinicopathologic description of myocarditis. *J Am Coll Cardiol.* 1991;18:1617.

32. Keogh A, Billingham M, Schroeder J. Rapid histological changes in endomyocardial biopsy specimens after myocarditis. *Br Heart J.* 1990;64:406.

33. Abdel-Aty H, Boye P, Zagrosek A, et al. Diagnostic performance of cardiovascular magnetic resonance in patients with suspected acute myocarditis: comparison of different approaches. *J Am Coll Cardiol.* 2005;45:1815.

34. Mahrholdt H, Goedecke C, Wagner A, et al. Cardiovascular magnetic resonance assessment of human myocarditis: a comparison to histology and molecular pathology. *Circulation.* 2004;109:1250.

35. Holman WL, Bourge RC, Kirklin JK. Case report: circulatory support for seventy days with resolution of acute heart failure. *J Thorac Cardiovasc Surg.* 1991;102:932.

36. Parillo JE, Cunnion RE, Epstein SE, et al. A prospective, randomized, controlled trial of prednisone for dilated cardiomyopathy. *N Engl J Med.* 1989;321:1061.

37. Mason JW, O'Connell JB, Herskowitz A, et al. A clinical trial of immunosuppressive therapy for myocarditis. *N Engl J Med.* 1995;333:269.

38. Wojnicz R, Nowalany-Kozielska E, Wojciechowska C, et al. Randomized, placebo-controlled study for immunosuppressive treatment of inflammatory dilated cardiomyopathy: two-year follow-up results. *Circulation.* 2001;104:39.

39. McNamara DM, Rosenblum WD, Janosko KM, et al. Intravenous immune globulin in the therapy of myocarditis and acute cardiomyopathy. *Circulation.* 1997;95:2476.

40. McNamara DM, Holubkov R, Starling RC, et al. Controlled trial of intravenous immune globulin in recent-onset dilated cardiomyopathy. *Circulation.* 2001;103:2254.

41. Magnani JW, Danik HJ, Dec GW Jr, et al. Survival in biopsy-proven myocarditis: a long-term retrospective analysis of the histopathologic, clinical and hemodynamic predictors. *Am Heart J.* 2006;151:463.

42. Nishii M, Inomata T, Takehana H, et al. Serum levels of interleukin-10 on admission as a prognostic predictor of human fulminant myocarditis. *J Am Coll Cardiol.* 2004;44:1292.

43. Rassi A Jr., Rassi A, Little WC, et al. Development and validation of a risk score for predicting death in Chagas heart disease. *N Engl J Med.* 2006;355:799.

44. Krisher K, Cunningham M. Myosin: A link between streptococci and heart. *Science.* 1985;227:413.

45. Dajani AS, Ayoub E, Bierman FZ, et al, Special Writing Group of the Committee on Rheumatic Fever, Endocarditis and Kawasaki disease of the Council of Cardiovascular Disease in the Young of the American Heart Association. Guidelines for the diagnosis of rheumatic fever: Jones criteria: 1992 update. *JAMA.* 1992;268:2069.

46. Voss LM, Wilson NJ, Neutze JM, et al. Intravenous immunoglobulin in acute rheumatic fever: A randomized controlled trial. *Circulation.* 2001;103:401.

47. Kounis N, Zavras G, Soufas G, et al. Hypersensitivity myocarditis. *Ann Allergy.* 1989;62:71.

48. Cooper LT Jr, Berry GJ, Shabetai R. Idiopathic giant-cell myocarditis—natural history and treatment. Multicenter Giant Cell Myocarditis Study Group Investigators. *N Engl J Med.* 1997;336:1860.

49. Cooper LT Jr. Idiopathic giant cell myocarditis. In: Cooper LT, ed. *Myocarditis: From Bench to Bedside.* Totowa, NJ: Humana Press; 2003:405–420.

50. Pinderski LJ, Fonarow GC, Hamilton M, et al. Giant cell myocarditis in a young man responsive to T-lymphocyte cytolytic therapy. *J Heart Lung Transplant.* 2002;21:818.

51. Elkayam U, Akhter M, Singh H, et al. Pregnancy associated cardiomyopathy. *Circulation.* 2005;111:2050.

52. Midei MG, DeMent SH, Feldman AM, et al. Peripartum myocarditis and cardiomyopathy. *Circulation.* 1990;81:922.

53. Bultmann BD, Klingel K, Nabauer M, et al. High prevalence of viral genomes and inflammation in peripartum cardiomyopathy. *Am J Obstet Gynecol.* 2005;193:363.

54. Knobel B, Melamud E, Kishon Y. Peripartum cardiomyopathy. *Isr J Med Sci.* 1984;20:1061.

55. Demakis JG, Rahimtoola SH, Sutton GC, et al. Natural course of peripartum cardiomyopathy. *Circulation.* 1971;44:1053.

56. O'Connell JB, Costanza-Nordin MR, Subramanian R, et al. Peripartum cardiomyopathy: clinical hemodynamic and prognostic characteristics. *J Am Coll Cardiol.* 1986;8:52.

57. Chapa JB, Heiberger HB, Weinert L, et al. Prognostic value of echocardiography in peripartum cardiomyopathy. *Obstet Gynecol.* 2005;105:1303.

58. Sliwa K, Woodiwiss A, Kone V, et al. The addition of pentoxifylline to conventional therapy improves outcome in patients with peripartum cardiomyopathy. *Eur Heart J.* 2002;4:305.

59. Lambert MB, Weinert L, Hibbard J, et al. Contractile reserve in patients with peripartum cardiomyopathy and recovered left ventricular function. *Am J Obstet Gynecol.* 1997;176:189.

60. Hirano M, Davidson M, DiMauro S. Mitochondria and the heart. *Curr Opin Cardiol.* 2001;16:201.

61. Dillman W. Biochemical basis of thyroid hormone action in the heart. *Am J Med.* 1990;88:626.

62. Hamilton M, Stevenson L, Luu M, et al. Altered thyroid hormone metabolism in advanced heart failure. *J Am Coll Cardiol.* 1990;16:91.

63. Hamilton M, Stevenson L. Thyroid hormone abnormalities in heart failure: possibilities for therapy. *Thyroid.* 1996;6:527.

64. Moruzzi P, Doria E, Agostoni P, et al. Usefulness of L-thyroxine to improve cardiac and exercise performance in idiopathic dilated cardiomyopathy. *Am J Cardiol.* 1994;73:374.

65. Umpierrez G, Challapalli S, Patterson C. Congestive heart failure due to reversible cardiomyopathy in patients with hyperthyroidism. *Am J Med Sci.* 1995;310:99.

66. Imperato-McGinley J, Cautier T, Ehlers K, et al. Reversibility of catecholamine-induced dilated cardiomyopathy in a child with a pheochromocytoma. *N Engl J Med.* 1987;316:793.

67. Clayton RN. Cardiovascular function in acromegaly. *Endocr Rev.* 2003;24:272.

68. Matta MP, Caron P. Acromegalic cardiomyopathy: a review of the literature. *Pituitary.* 2003;6:203.

69. Vianna CB, Vieira ML, Mady C, et al. Treatment of acromegaly improves myocardial abnormalities. *Am Heart J.* 2002;143:873.

70. Abbott R, Donahue R, Kannel W, et al. The impact of diabetes on survival following myocardial infarction in men vs women. The Framingham Study. *JAMA.* 1988;260:3456.

71. Poornima I, Parikh P, Shannon R. Diabetic cardiomyopathy-the search for a unifying hypothesis. *Circ Res.* 2006;98:596.

72. Raman M, Nesto RW. Heart disease in diabetes mellitus. *Endocrinol Metab Clin North Am.* 1996;25:425.

73. Fernandez-Sola J, Estruch R, Nicolas JM, et al. Comparison of alcoholic cardiomyopathy in women versus men. *Am J Cardiol.* 1997;80:481.

74. Richardson P, Patel V, Preedy V. Alcohol and the myocardium. *Novartis Found Symp.* 1998;216:35.

75. Zhang X, Li S, Brown R, et al. Ethanol and acetaldehyde in alcoholic cardiomyopathy: from bad to ugly en route to oxidative stress. *Alcohol.* 2004;32:175.

76. Beckemeier M, Bora P. Fatty acid ethyl esters: Potentially toxic products of myocardial ethanol metabolism. *J Mol Cell Cardiol.* 1998;30:2487.

77. Wang L, Zhou Z, Saari J, et al. Alcohol-induced myocardial fibrosis in metal-lothionein-null mice-prevention by zinc supplementation. *Am J Pathol.* 2005;167:337.

78. Spies CD, Sander M, Stangl K, et al. Effects of alcohol on the heart. *Curr Opin Crit Care.* 2001;7:337.

79. Nicolas JM, Fernandez-Sola J, Estruch R, et al. The effect of controlled drinking in alcoholic cardiomyopathy. *Ann Intern Med.* 2002;136:192.

80. Gavazzi A, De Maria R, Parolini M, et al. Alcohol abuse and dilated cardiomyopathy in men. *Am J Cardiol.* 2000;85:1114.

81. Lange RA, Hillis D. Cardiovascular complications of cocaine use. *N Engl J Med.* 2001;345:351.

82. Virmani R, Robinowitz M, Smialek J, et al. Cardiovascular effects of cocaine: an autopsy study of 40 patients. *Am Heart J.* 1988;115:1068.

83. Chokshi S, Moore R, Pandian N, et al. Reversible cardiomyopathy associated with cocaine intoxication. *Ann Intern Med.* 1989;111:1039.

84. Singal P, Iliskovic N. Current concepts: Doxorubicin-induced cardiomyopathy. *N Engl J Med.* 1998;339:900.

85. Lipshultz S, Rifai N, Dalton V, et al. The effect of dexrazoxane on myocardial injury in doxorubicin-treated children with acute lymphoblastic leukemia. *N Engl J Med.* 2004;351:145.

86. Fischer P, Salloum F, Das A, et al. Phosphodiesterase-5 inhibition with sildenafil attenuates cardiomyocyte apoptosis and left ventricular dysfunction in a chronic model of doxorubicin cardiotoxicity. *Circulation.* 2005;111:1601.

87. Schimmel K, Richel D, van den Brink R, et al. Cardiotoxicity of cytotoxic drugs. *Cancer Treat Rev.* 2004;30:181.

88. Gottdiener J, Applebaum F, Ferrans V, et al. Cardiotoxicity associated with high dose cyclophosphamide therapy. *Arch Intern Med.* 1981;141:758.

89. Feldman A, Lorell B, Reis S. Trastuzumab in the treatment of metastatic breast cancer. Anticancer therapy versus cardiotoxicity. *Circulation.* 2000;102:272.

90. Merrill D, Dec W, Goff D. Adverse cardiac effects associated with clozapine. *J Clin Psychopharmacol.* 2005;25:32.

91. Kudoh C, Tanaka S, Marusaki S, et al. Hypocalcemic cardiomyopathy in a patient with idiopathic hypoparathyroidism. *Intern Med.* 1992;31:561.

92. Mustafa A, Birgas J-L, McCrindle B. Dilated cardiomyopathy as a first sign of nutritional vitamin D deficiency rickets in infancy. *Can J Cardiol.* 1999;15:699.

93. Yang G. Keshan disease: an endemic selenium-related deficiency disease. In: Chandara R, ed. *Trace Elements in Nutrition of Children.* New York: Raven Press; 1985.

94. Beck M, Shi Q, Morris V, et al. Rapid genomic evolution of a non-virulent Coxsackievirus B3 in selenium-deficient mice results in selection of identical virulent isolates. *Nat Med.* 1995;1:433.

95. Huttunen J. Selenium and cardiovascular disease—an update. *Biomed Environ Sci.* 1997;10:220.

96. Oster O, Prellwitz W. Selenium and cardiovascular disease. *Biol Trace Elem Res.* 1990;24:91.

97. Paulson D. Carnitine deficiency-induced cardiomyopathy. *Mol Cell Biochem.* 1998;180:33.

98. Famularo G, De Simone C. A new era for carnitine. *Immunol Today.* 1995;16:211.

99. Bennett M, Hale D, Pollitt R, et al. Endocardial fibroelastosis and primary carnitine deficiency due to a defect in the plasma membrane carnitine transport (clinical conference). *Clin Cardiol.* 1996;19:243.

100. Cochat P. Primary hyperoxaluria type 1. *Kidney Int.* 1999;55:2533.

101. Fyfe B, Israel D, Quish A, et al. Reversal of primary hyperoxaluria cardiomyopathy after combined liver and renal transplantation. *Am J Cardiol.* 1995;75:210.

102. Wittstein I, Thiemann D, Lima J, et al. Neurohumoral features of myocardial stunning due to sudden emotional stress. *N Engl J Med.* 2005;352:539.

103. Guttormsen B, Nee L, Makielski J, et al. Transient left ventricular apical ballooning: a review of the literature. *WMJ.* 2006;105:49.

104. Shah D, Sugeng L, Goonewardena S, et al. Takotsubo cardiomyopathy. *Circulation.* 2006;113:e762.

105. Klaassen S, Probst S, Gerull B, et al. Novel gene locus for autosomal dominant left ventricular noncompaction maps to chromosome 11p15. *Circulation.* 2004;109:2720.

106. Ichida F, Hamamichi Y, Miyawaki T, et al. Clinical features of isolated noncompaction of the ventricular myocardium: long-term clinical course, hemodynamic properties, and genetic background. *J Am Coll Cardiol.* 1999;34:233.

107. Oechslin E, Attenhofer C, Rojas, J, et al. Long-term follow up of 34 adults with isolated left ventricular noncompaction: a distinct cardiomyopathy with poor prognosis. *J Am Coll Cardiol.* 2000;36:493.

108. Woodley S, Gilbert E, Anderson J, et al. β-blockade with bucindolol in heart failure due to ischemic vs idiopathic dilated cardiomyopathy. *Circulation.* 1991;84:2426.

109. Waagstein F, Bristow M, Swedberg K, et al. Beneficial effects of metoprolol in idiopathic dilated cardiomyopathy. *Lancet.* 1993;342:1441.

PART 6 Rhythm and Conduction Disorders

CHAPTER 33

Genetics of Channelopathies and Clinical Implications

Silvia G. Priori / Carlo Napolitano

INHERITED ARRHYTHMOGENIC DISEASES AND SUDDEN DEATH IN THE POPULATION

Ischemic heart disease and heart failure are the most common substrate for sudden cardiac death.[1] Data from patients resuscitated from cardiac arrest and from autopsies indicate that there is no evidence of structural heart disease in approximately 5 to 8 percent of victims of sudden death.[2] At least part of these deaths is caused by the so-called *inherited arrhythmogenic diseases* that manifest with life-threatening arrhythmias in children and young adults.

In the last decade, molecular biology has greatly contributed to understand the pathophysiology of several inherited disorders and has allowed identifying many genes that can alter cardiac excitability (Fig. 33–1).

Chap. 33 reviews the clinical features, the genetic bases, and the main therapeutic strategies of the most common inherited arrhythmogenic syndromes.

GENETIC BASES OF ION CHANNEL DISORDERS AND RELATED PHENOTYPES

【 】 LONG QT SYNDROME

Definition

The long QT syndrome (LQTS) is characterized by prolonged ventricular repolarization (prolonged QT interval), abnormal T waves, and life-threatening ventricular arrhythmias manifesting as syncope and/or sudden death (Fig. 33–2).[3]

Genetic Bases and Pathophysiology

LQTS can be transmitted as an autosomal dominant (Romano Ward syndrome) or, rarely, as an autosomal recessive trait (Jervell and Lange-Nielsen syndrome, [JLN]). Both variants share an identical cardiac phenotype (see above), but JLN syndrome also presents with sensineural deafness.

Recently, additional rare variants combining a LQTS cardiac phenotype with extracardiac manifestations (dysmorphic features, paralysis, congenital heart defects, developmental disorders), namely Andersen syndrome and Timothy syndrome, have been genetically characterized. The genes involved in these latter forms of LQTS are expressed in noncardiac tissues where they play important physiologic functions, thus explaining systemic manifestations.

Currently, ten LQTS-related genes (Table 33–1; see Fig. 33–1) and hundreds of different mutations have been reported. Despite such remarkable genetic heterogeneity, more than 90 percent of the genotyped LQTS patients harbor a mutation on three genes: *KCNQ1* (LQT1), *KCNH2* (LQT2), *SCN5A* (LQT3)[4] (see also: www.fsm.it/cardmoc).[5] These genes encode for the α subunits (i.e., the main pore-forming proteins) of the I_{Ks} and I_{Kr} potassium channels and the cardiac sodium channel conducting I_{Na} current, respectively.

Mutations less represented among genotyped LQTS patients[5] are found in the *KCNE1* (LQT5) and *KCNE2* (LQT6) genes that

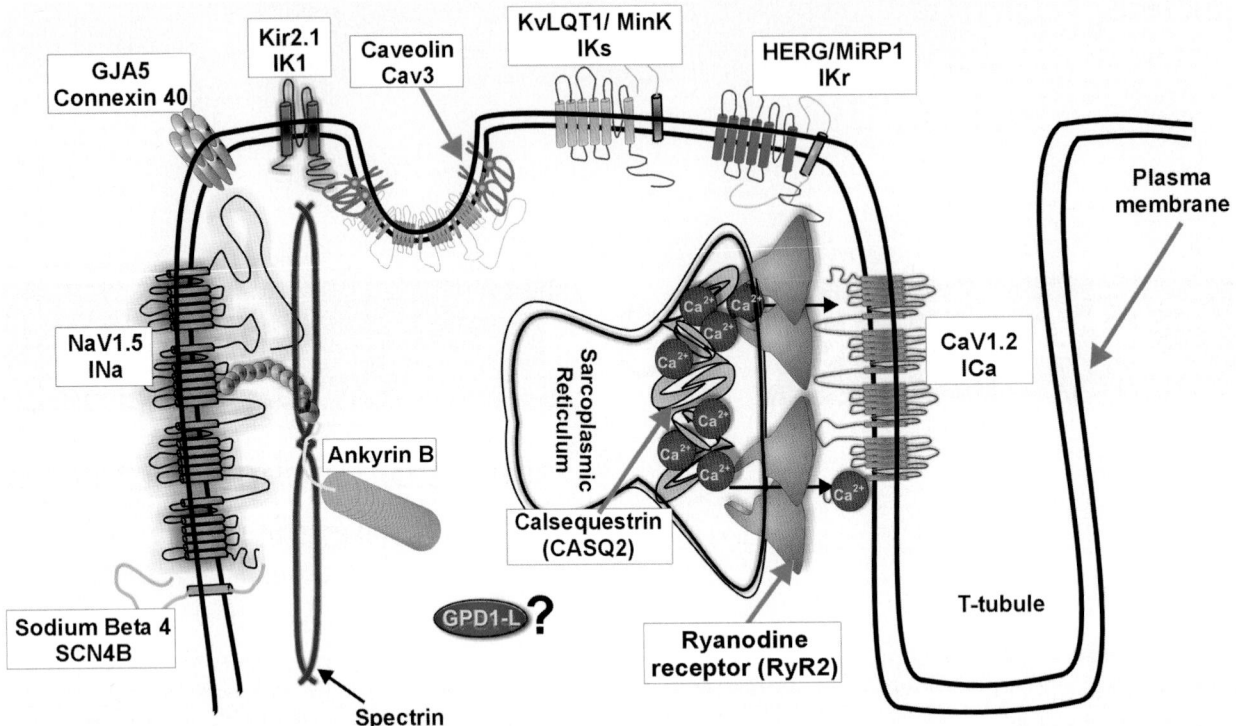

FIGURE 33-1. Proteins involved in inherited arrhythmogenic disorders. Cartoon showing the intracellular localization of the proteins involved in the pathogenesis of inherited arrhythmogenic syndromes. Each protein can be involved in more than one disease. The localization and the function of GPD1-L involved in Brugada syndrome is still unknown. (See text and tables for details and proteins' symbols). *Source: Data from Priori, Schwartz, Napolitano, et al.[12]*

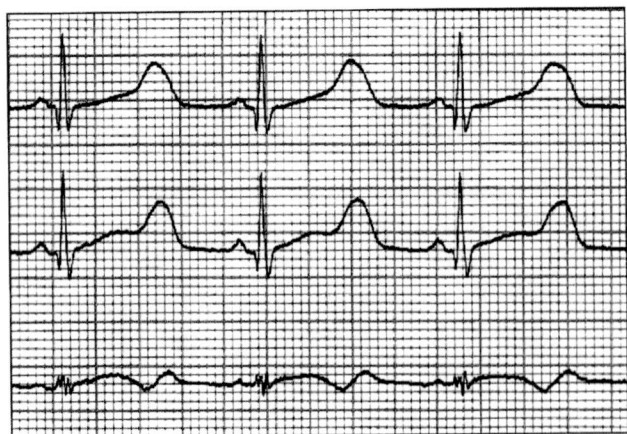

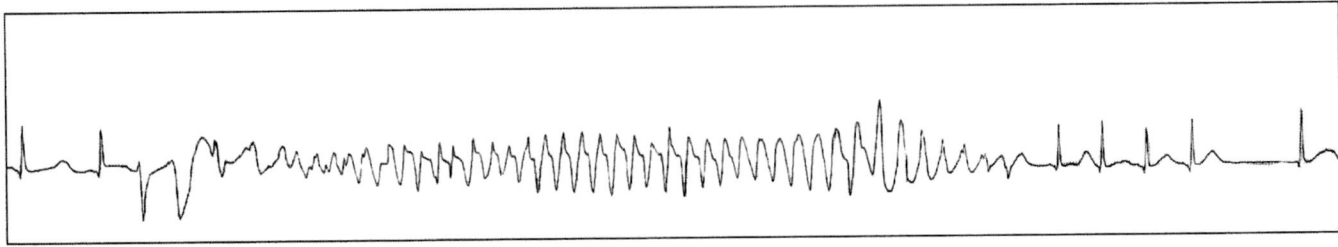

FIGURE 33-2. ECG in LQTS. *Upper panel:* typical ECG of a LQTS patient (leads D_1–D_3) with markedly abnormal repolarization (QTc 618 ms and ST-T wave abnormalities). *Lower panel:* example of a self-limiting polymorphic VT with torsade de pointes morphology in a LQTS patient.

TABLE 33–1

Genes Involved in Long QT Syndrome

VARIANT	GENE	PROTEIN	EFFECT OF MUTATIONS
LQT1	KCNQ1	KvLQT1 (potassium channel α subunit)	Reduced I_{Ks}
LQT2	KCNH2	HERG (potassium channel α subunit)	Reduced I_{Kr}
LQT3	SCN5A	Nav1.5 (sodium channel α subunit)	Increased I_{Na}
LQT4	ANK2	Ankyrin B, anchoring protein	Reduced membrane expression of Na^+ and Ca^{2+} channels
LQT5	KCNE1	MinK (potassium channel β subunit)	Reduced I_{Ks}
LQT6	KCNE2	MiRP (potassium channel β subunit)	Reduced I_{Kr}
LQT7, Andersen syndrome	KCNJ2	Kir2.1 (potassium channel α subunit)	Reduced outward I_{K1}
LQT8, Timothy syndrome	CACNA1c	Cav1.2 (L-type calcium channel α subunit)	Increased I_{Ca}
LQT9	CAV3	Cardiac caveolin gene	Increased I_{Na} due to altered gating kinetic
LQT10	SCN4B	Sodium channel $β_4$ subunit	Reduced subunit expression causing increased I_{Na}

I_{Ca}, calcium current; I_{Kl}, I_{Kr}, I_{Ks}, potassium currents; I_{Na}, sodium current; LQT, long QT.

encode for the β subunits of the channels that conduct I_{Ks} and I_{Kr} currents (these gene products coassemble with the α subunits encoded by the *KCNQ1* and *KCNH2* genes).

KCNQ1 and *KCNE1* mutations found in LQTS lead to impaired I_{Ks} current and prolong action potential duration. Heterozygous mutations of these genes cause Romano-Ward syndrome, whereas homozygous or compound heterozygous mutations cause JLN syndrome.[6]

KCNH2 loss of function mutations and *KCNE2* loss of function mutations cause a reduction of I_{Kr} current, thus prolonging the action potential. Mutations can alter different biophysical properties of the channel,[6] and they can also cause intracellular processing abnormalities (trafficking defects) of the mutant proteins.

SCN5A mutations found in LQT3 patients cause a gain of function leading to an increased I_{Na}.[6] This final effect can originate from altered current kinetic (delayed inactivation) or single channel abnormalities (disperse reopenings, bursting). In both cases the increased inward current leads to action potential prolongation.

The following are other genes accounting for a minority of LQTS cases (see also Table 33–1):

- *ANK2* (LQT4): encoding for an intracellular protein called *ankyrin*, a chaperone molecule involved in ion channels localization and anchoring to the cellular membrane.[7]
- *KCNJ2* (Andersen syndrome or LQT7), encoding for I_{K1} potassium channel, and it is characterized by QT prolongation, prominent U waves, and, inconstantly, facial dimorphisms and periodic paralysis. *KCNJ2* mutations lead to a reduced I_{K1} current.[8]
- *CACNA1c* (Timothy syndrome or LQT8): encoding for the voltage-dependent L-type calcium channel (CaV1.2). This LQTS variant presents a severe cardiac phenotype, syndactyly, congenital heart defects, and developmental disorders.[9]
- *Cav3 (LQT9):* encoding for caveolin, a protein involved in the formation of caveolae, small invaginations of the plasma membrane, with a flasklike shape that appears to control the localization of ion channels.[10]

- *SCN4B (LQT10):* encoding for the β-4 subunit of the cardiac sodium channel. Mutations in this gene appear to cause an increased I_{Na} and a LQT3-like phenotype.[11]

Overall the genes causing LQTS are directly or indirectly involved in the control of cardiac excitability and prolonged action potential duration. Unless there are clinical reasons to guide the screening (e.g. extracardiac phenotypes), the genetic testing routinely performed by analyzing the five major genes (*KCNQ1*, *KCNH2*, *SCN5A*, *KCNE1*, *KCNE2*). This approach yields up to 75 percent of successfully genotyped patients.[5]

Clinical Presentation and Diagnosis

The diagnosis of LQTS is based on the evaluation of the ECG and on the measurement of the QT interval. QTc values exceeding 440 msec (in males) and 460 msec (in females) are considered abnormal. Albeit QTc assessment is the most important step for diagnosis of LQTS, ST-T wave abnormalities (notches on the descending limb, biphasic T waves) are often evident and can support the clinical diagnosis.

Syncope is often triggered by the onset of rapid polymorphic ventricular tachycardia (VT) (torsades de pointes) that can degenerate into ventricular fibrillation and cause sudden death. The mean age of onset of symptoms is 12 years, and earlier onset is usually associated with a more severe form of the disease. Severity is also correlated with the duration of QT interval[12,13] (Fig. 33–3). In LQTS cardiac arrhythmias are often precipitated by physical or emotional stress although in 10 to 15 percent of patients, cardiac events occur at rest.

Therapy

Already in the mid-1970s, the evidences of an adrenergic trigger suggested the use of β blockers[14] to prevent cardiac arrhythmias, and the effectiveness of this approach has been constantly confirmed thereafter.[15,16] Therefore all LQTS patients with a history of syncope and asymptomatic individuals with definite QT prolongation should be treated with β blockers (Table 33–2). The most fre-

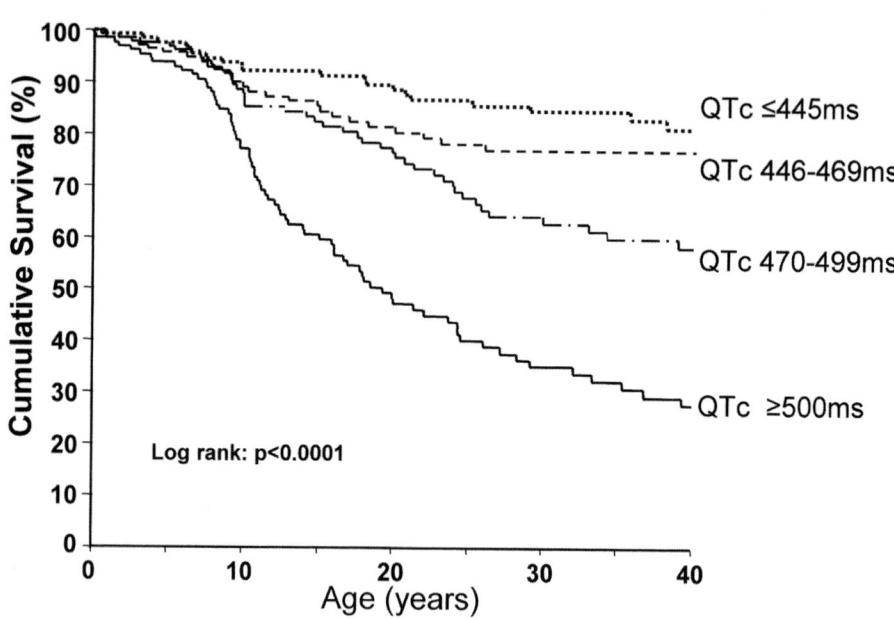

FIGURE 33–3. Cardiac events and QTc in LQTS. Kaplan-Meier analysis of the occurrence of a first cardiac event (syncope or cardiac arrest) without therapy from birth to age 40 years, according to QTc interval duration. QTc groups refer to QTc quartiles in genotyped LQTS population. *Source: Data from Priori, Schwartz, Napolitano, et al.*[12]

quently used drugs are nadolol (1–2.5 mg/kg/day) or propranolol (2–4 mg/kg/day). Life-style changes aimed at avoiding conditions that can precipitate arrhythmias are also indicated. Specifically LQTS patients should avoid competitive sports, QT prolonging drugs, and lowered potassium plasma levels (for example during diarrhea and vomiting).

For the 20 to 30 percent of patients who can have a recurrence of syncope despite β blockade, the prophylactic implant of an implantable cardioverter-defibrillator (ICD) should be considered. Obviously the ICD is indicated in all patients surviving cardiac arrest (secondary prevention). For primary prevention of cardiac arrest ICD should be adopted in patients not adequately protected by β blockers (recurrence of syncope while on therapy) and in patients with high risk genotype (see below). In all instances, β blockers should be continued after ICD implant to reduce risk cardiac arrest and shocks from the device.

TABLE 33–2

Suggested Therapy for Inherited Arrhythmogenic Diseases

CONDITION	CATEGORY	THERAPY
LQTS	Class I	Lifestyle modification is recommended for patients with an LQTS diagnosis (clinical and/or molecular). *(Level of evidence: B)*
		β Blockers are recommended for patients with an LQTS clinical diagnosis (i.e., in the presence of prolonged QT interval). *(Level of evidence: B)*
		Implantation of an ICD along with use of β blockers is recommended for LQTS patients with previous cardiac arrest and who have reasonable expectation of survival with a good functional status for more than 1 year.
		Pregnant women developing hemodynamically unstable VT or VF should be electrically cardioverted or defibrillated *(Level of evidence: B)*
		In pregnant women with the LQTS who have had symptoms it is reasonable to continue β blocker medications throughout pregnancy and afterwards, unless there are definite contraindications. *(Level of evidence: C)*
	Class IIa	β Blockers can be effective to reduce SCD in patients with a molecular LQTS analysis and normal QT interval. *(Level of evidence: B)*
		Implantation of an ICD with continued use of β blockers can be effective to reduce SCD in LQTS patients experiencing syncope and/or VT while receiving β blockers and who have reasonable expectation of survival with a good functional status for more than 1 year. *(Level of evidence: B)*
	Class IIb	LCSD can be considered for LQTS patients with syncope, torsades de pointes, or cardiac arrest while receiving β blockers. *(Level of evidence: B)*
		Implantation of an ICD with use of β blockers may be considered for prophylaxis of SCD for patients in categories possibly associated with higher risk of cardiac arrest (such as LQT2 and LQT3, QTc >500 msec) and who have reasonable expectation of survival with a good functional status for more than 1 year. *(Level of evidence: B)*

(continued)

TABLE 33–2

Suggested Therapy for Inherited Arrhythmogenic Diseases *(continued)*

CONDITION	CATEGORY	THERAPY
CPVT	Class I	β Blockers are indicated for patients who are clinically diagnosed with CPVT based on the presence of spontaneous or documented stress induced ventricular arrhythmias. *(Level of evidence: C)* Implantation of an ICD with use of β blockers is indicated for patients with CPVT who are survivors of cardiac arrest and who have reasonable expectation of survival with a good functional status for more than 1 year. *(Level of evidence: C)*
	Class IIa	β Blockers can be effective in patients without clinical manifestations when the diagnosis of CPVT is established during childhood based on genetic analysis. *(Level of evidence: C)* Implantation of an ICD with use of beta–blockers can be effective for affected patients with CPVT with syncope and/or documented sustained VT while receiving β blockers and who have reasonable expectation of survival with a good functional status for more than 1 year. *(Level of evidence: C)*
	Class IIb	β Blockers can be considered for patients with CPVT who were genetically diagnosed in adulthood and never manifested clinical symptoms of tachyarrhythmias. *(Level of evidence: C)*
BrS	Class I	An ICD is indicated for Brugada syndrome patients with previous cardiac arrest receiving chronic optimal medical therapy and who have reasonable expectation of survival with a good functional status for more than 1 year. *(Level of evidence: C)*
	Class IIa	An ICD is reasonable for Brugada syndrome patients with spontaneous ST-segment elevation in V_1, V_2, or V_3 who have had syncope with or without mutations demonstrated in the *SCN5A* gene and who have reasonable expectation of survival with a good functional status for more than 1 year. *(Level of evidence: C)* Clinical monitoring for the development of a spontaneous ST-segment elevation pattern is reasonable for the management of patients with ST-segment elevation induced only with provocative pharmacological challenge with or without symptoms. *(Level of evidence: C)* An ICD is reasonable for BrS patients with documented VT that has not resulted in cardiac arrest and who have reasonable expectation of survival with a good functional status for more than 1 year. *(Level of evidence: C)* Isoproterenol should be used to treat an electrical storm in the BrS. *(Level of evidence: C)*
	Class IIb	EP testing can be considered for risk stratification in asymptomatic BrS patients with spontaneous ST elevation with or without a mutation in the *SCN5A* gene. *(Level of evidence: C)* Quinidine might be reasonable for the treatment of electrical storm in patients with BrS. *(Level of evidence: C)*

BrS, Brugada syndrome; CPVT, catecholaminergic polymorphic ventricular tachycardia; Ep, electrophysiology; ICD, intracardia cardioverter defibrillator; LCSD, left cardiac sympathetic denervation; LQTS, long QT syndrome; SCD, sudden cardiac death; VF, ventricular fibrillation; VT, ventricular tachycardia.
Source: ACC/AHA/ESC.[18]

Left cardiac sympathetic denervation has also been suggested as a treatment able to reduce cardiac events in patients with recurrence of cardiac events on β blockers.[17] Management strategies for LQTS patients are shown in Table 33–2.[18]

Genotype-Phenotype Correlation and Clinical Management

Gene-specific ECG features were initially described by Moss and colleagues and subsequently refined by Zhang and coworkers (Fig. 33–4).[19] Schwartz and colleagues[20] have provided evidence that LQT1 patients present 97 percent of cardiac events during physical activity as opposed to LQT3 patients who present the majority of cardiac events at rest. Furthermore, it has been proposed that auditory stimuli and arousal are a specific trigger for LQT2 patients whereas swimming is a predisposing setting for cardiac events in LQT1 patients.[21,22]

LQT2 and LQT3 patients have a worse long-term prognosis as compared with LQT1 patients, and the QT interval, duration, and gender are the three most important variables that influence natural

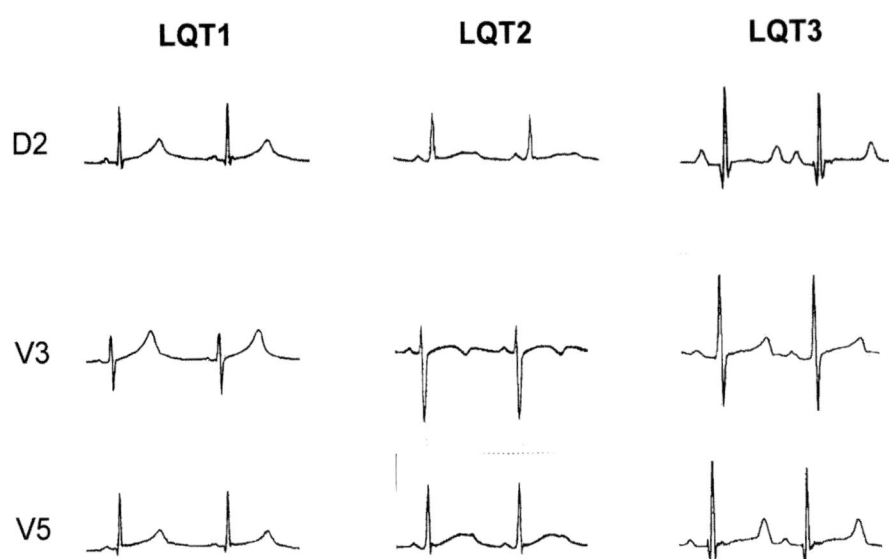

FIGURE 33–4. T wave morphology and genotype in long QT syndrome (LQTS). Leads D$_2$, V$_3$, and V$_5$ showing: LQT1 with smooth broad-based T wave (*left panel*), LQT2 notched, biphasic and low voltage T waves (*middle panel*), and LQT3 prolonged ST segment and small-peaked T wave. (*right panel*).

history of LQTS patients.[12] QTc values exceeding 500 msec are associated with worse prognosis. However, when adjusting for QTc duration, LQT1 patients have a better outcome than LQT2 and LQT3 patients with similar QTc. Furthermore a higher risk of becoming symptomatic for cardiac arrhythmias between birth and age 40 is evident among LQT2 females and LQT3 males[12] (Fig. 33–5).

The response to β-blocker therapy is highest among LQT1 patients, whereas it is significantly lower among LQT2 and LQT3 patients.[16] Three independent predictors of recurrence of cardiac events on β blockers have been identified: LQT2 or LQT3 genotype, QTc >500 msec, the occurrence of the first syncope in early childhood (younger than 7 years of age). Based on these data it was concluded that ICD implant for primary prevention of cardiac arrest could be considered for LQT2 and LQT3 patients with markedly prolonged QT interval and early onset of syncope. Therapies have been able to shorten the QT interval, but definite proof of their effectiveness on cardiac events is still lacking (see review[23]) (Table 33–3).

Low Penetrance and Variable Expressivity in LQTS

LQTS is characterized by genetic heterogeneity and variable penetrance that translates into a range of possible phenotypes including subclinical forms with borderline of QT interval and no arrhythmias or syncope.[5,24,25] The evidence of incomplete penetrance in LQTS led to the speculation that carriers of concealed genetic ab-

normalities can be prone to develop arrhythmias when exposed to precipitating factors such as drugs with potential QT prolonging effect (for more information see www.QTdrugs.org).[26–28]

Interestingly the attempt to link clinical manifestations to specific mutations has met with little success because carriers of the same mutation often present different phenotypes. The genetic or epigenetic causes of such variable penetrance are yet to be elucidated, but recent data suggest that genetic polymorphisms can influence the QT interval duration[29] and can affect the probability of the development of arrhythmias.[30,31]

CATECHOLAMINERGIC POLYMORPHIC VENTRICULAR TACHYCARDIA

DEFINITION

Catecholaminergic polymorphic ventricular tachycardia (CPVT) is a disorder of intracellular calcium handling causing adrenergic-dependent arrhythmias and sudden death in otherwise healthy individuals.[32] CPVT patients display an unremarkable resting ECG but they develop a typical pattern of bi-directional or polymorphic ventricular tachycardia that can be reproducibly elicited during exercise or catecholamine infusion (Fig. 33–6). CPVT patients have a structurally intact heart.

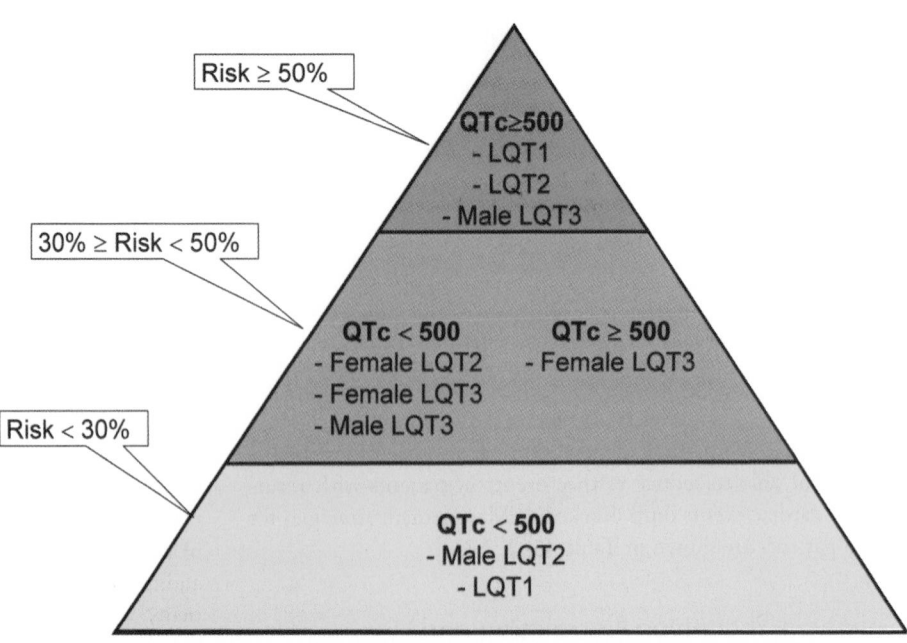

FIGURE 33–5. Risk stratification in long QT syndrome (LQTS). Risk categories in LQTS according to QTc duration, genotype and gender. Percentages on the left outside indicate the risk of a first cardiac event (syncope or cardiac arrest) younger than 40 years of age in the absence of any LQTS active treatment.

TABLE 33-3

Gene-Specific Therapy for Inherited Arrhythmias

DISEASE	GENE	EFFECT	TREATMENT
LQT2	KCNH2	Reduced I_{Kr}	Increase I_{Kr}: potassium supplements Rescue of trafficking: fexofenadine, thapsigargin
LQT3	SCN5A	Increase of I_{Na}	Block of I_{Na}: **mexiletine**
BrS	SCN5A	Reduction of I_{Na}	Block of I_{To}: **quinidine**, tedisamil, cilostazol Rescue of trafficking-defective mutants: mexiletine
SQTS	KNCH2	Increased I_{Kr}	Block of I_{Kr}: **quinidine**
CPVT (Autosomal dominant)	RYR2	Intracellular Ca^{2+} overload	Recover of FKBP12.6 binding: JTV519

BrS, Brugada syndrome; CPVT, catecholaminergic polymorphic ventricular tachycardia; I_{Kr}, potassium current; I_{Na}, sodium current; LQTS2, LQT3, long QT; SQTS, short QT syndrome.
NOTE: Bold drug names indicate the ones already used in the clinical setting with some evidence of effectiveness.

[ ] GENETIC BASES AND PATHOPHYSIOLOGY

Autosomal Dominant Catecholaminergic Polymorphic VT

On the basis of linkage mapping data[33] mutations were identified in the human *RyR2* gene encoding for the cardiac ryanodine receptor in four CPVT families with an autosomal dominant pattern of inheritance[34] (Table 33–4). CPVT-associated ryanodine receptor's mutations have subsequently been reported by other authors.[35] To date, it is clear that *RyR2* is a major CPVT gene, accounting for approximately 50 to 60 percent of clinically affected individuals (www.fsm.it/cardmoc/).

Autosomal Recessive Catecholaminergic Polymorphic VT

In 2001 Lahat and coworkers[36] mapped an autosomal recessive CPVT trait to chromosome 1p13–21 in a large Bedouin family with a high degree of consanguinity. Subsequently the same group[37] identified a missense mutation in a highly conserved region of the calsequestrin 2 gene (*CASQ2*) as the cause of this variant (CPVT2). Other mutations were reported thereafter confirming that *CASQ2* is the gene for a recessive form of CPVT. Data from our large cohort of genotyped CPVT patients suggest that *CASQ2* mutations account for a 3 to 5 percent of all genotyped CPVT patients (Priori SG, personal communication).

Mechanisms for Arrhythmogenesis

The cardiac ryanodine receptor is a tetrameric intracellular Ca^{2+} release channel spanning the membrane of the sarcoplasmic reticulum (SR) that is required for cardiac excitation-contraction coupling (see Fig. 33–1). The hypothesis that arrhythmias are initiated by delayed afterdepolarizations (DADs) and triggered activity was advanced based on the observation that the bidirectional VT observed in CPVT patients closely resembles DADs-mediated digitalis-induced arrhythmias.[32,34]

Experimental studies in vitro first and in vivo more recently, progressively substantiated the hypothesis that arrhythmias are initiated by triggered activity.[38–42] Viatchenko-Karpinski and colleagues[41] observed that CASQ2 D307H mutation impairs SR Ca^{2+} storing and reduces the CASQ2 buffering capability. More recently the same group of investigators[40] reported that *CASQ2* mutants can also disrupt the CASQ2-RyR2 interaction and impaired regulation of RyR2 by luminal Ca^{2+}. Finally, we recently reported the first CPVT patient with compound heterozygous mutations in the *CASQ2* gene: in vitro characterization of the mutations implicated DADs once more in the pathogenesis of arrhythmias.[42]

[ ] CLINICAL PRESENTATION

CPVT patients were initially described by Reid in 1975[43] and Coumel and coworkers in 1978[32] whereas the first extensive and systematic description of the disease was reported in 1995.[44]

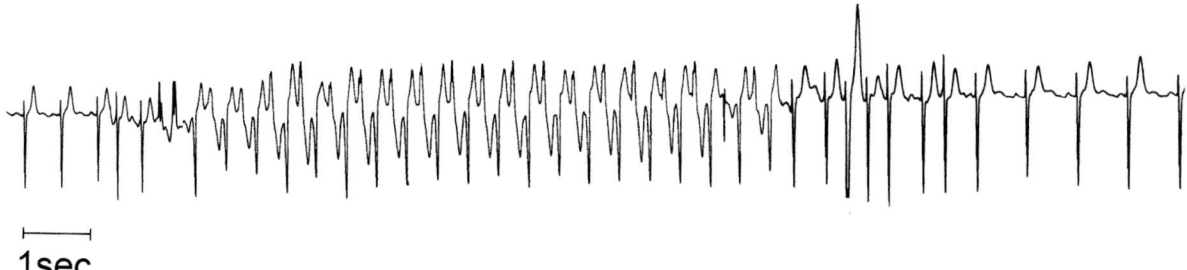

1sec

FIGURE 33–6. Exercise stress test in CPVT. ECG strip recorded in a CPVT patient during exercise stress testing showing the onset of typical bidirectional VT and repetitive supraventricular extrasystoles before and after VT.

TABLE 33–4

Genes Involved in Inherited Arrhythmias

Brugada syndrome	BrS1	SCN5A	Cardiac sodium channel alpha subunit (Nav1.5)	Loss of function—reduced outward Na+ current
	BrS2	GPD1-L	Glycerol-6-phosphate-dehydrogenase	Loss of function—reduced outward Na+ current
Catecholaminergic VT	CPVT1	RyR2	Cardiac ryanodine receptor (RyR2)	Gain of function – diastolic Ca2+ release form SR
	CPVT2	CASQ2	Cardiac calsequestrin (CASQ2)	Loss of SR Ca2+ buffering capacity
Short QT syndrome	SQTS1	KCNH2	I_{Kr} potassium channel alpha subunit (HERG)	Gain of function—increased outward K+ current
	SQTS2	KCNQ1	I_{Ks} potassium channel α subunit (KvLQT1)	Gain of function—increased outward K+ current
	SQTS3	KCNJ2	I_{K1} potassium channel (Kir2.1)	Gain of function—increased outward K+ current
Atrial fibrillation	ATFIB1	KCNQ1	I_{Ks} potassium channel α subunit (KvLQT1)	Gain of function—increased K+ outward current
	ATFIB2	KCNE2	I_{Kr} potassium channel β subunit (MiRP)	Gain of function – increased K+ outward current
	ATFIB3	KCNJ2	IK1 potassium channel (Kir2.1)	Gain of function—increased K+ outward current
	ATFIB4	GJA5	Gap-junction protein connexin 40	Impaired conduction

SR, sarcoplasmic reticulum; VT, ventricular tachycardia.

At rest CPVT patients have normal ECGs with the exception of sinus bradycardia and prominent "U" wave reported in some cases.[44,45] The development of arrhythmias during exercise stress test is highly reproducible. Isolated single premature ventricular contractions arise at a heart rate threshold of 110 to 120 beats per minute, followed by brief runs of nonsustained VT. If the patients continue to exercise, the duration of VT progressively increases, and it can become sustained. An alternating 180 degree QRS axis on a beat-to-beat basis, the so-called *bidirectional ventricular tachycardia*, is the typical pattern of CPVT-related arrhythmias (Fig. 33–6), although CPVT patients can also present with irregular, polymorphic VT.[33,46] Supraventricular arrhythmias (nonsustained supraventricular tachycardia) is a relatively common finding among CPVT patients (Fig. 33–6).[44]

The mean age of onset of symptoms in CPVT patients is 8 years of age. Syncope, triggered by exercise or acute emotion, is the typical manifestation of the disease even if sudden death can be the first manifestation in some patients.[44,46] In these latter cases, the lack of structural abnormalities of the heart could lead to the diagnosis of idiopathic ventricular fibrillation (IVF).[46] Indeed clinical data suggest that CPVT may be a rather frequent cause of IVF.[47,48] A remarkable high incidence of juvenile sudden death is often detected when collecting family history in CPVT probands. Indeed, approximately 30 percent of families present with one or multiple premature sudden deaths that usually occur during childhood even if later events can also occur (older than 20 years of age) death.[34,44,46] As compared to other inherited arrhythmogenic syndromes, CPVT appears have higher number of sporadic cases.[46] This can be the consequence of high mortality at young age that limits the transmission of the disease to offspring.

Our data showed that 75 to 80 percent of patient experience at least one life-threatening event younger than 40 years of age when left untreated.[49]

THERAPY

Treatment with β-blocking agents is the mainstay of treatment in CPVT (see Table 33–2).[44,46,50] The most widely used drug is nadolol at dosages from 1.5 to 3 mg/kg/day, and the dose should be always titrated with exercise stress testing. An ICD can be indicated when sustained or poorly tolerated VTs develop despite regular intake of the maximally tolerated β-blocker dosage. In our study, 50 percent of patients implanted with an ICD because of incomplete protection from VTs with β blockers, received an appropriate shock at followup.[46]

Preliminary data have suggested that amiodarone and class I antiarrhythmic agents can be ineffective in CPVT patients.[51,52] Verapamil may partially reduce arrhythmias in CPVT patients.[51,53,54] At present however, verapamil appears to be indicated not as an alternative to β blockers but as an adjunctive treatment.

BRUGADA SYNDROME

DEFINITION

Brugada syndrome (BrS) is an arrhythmogenic disorder presenting with a typical electrocardiographic pattern of ST segment elevation in leads V_1 to V_3, and incomplete or complete right bundle branch block[55] (Fig. 33–7). Besides such ECG abnormalities, full

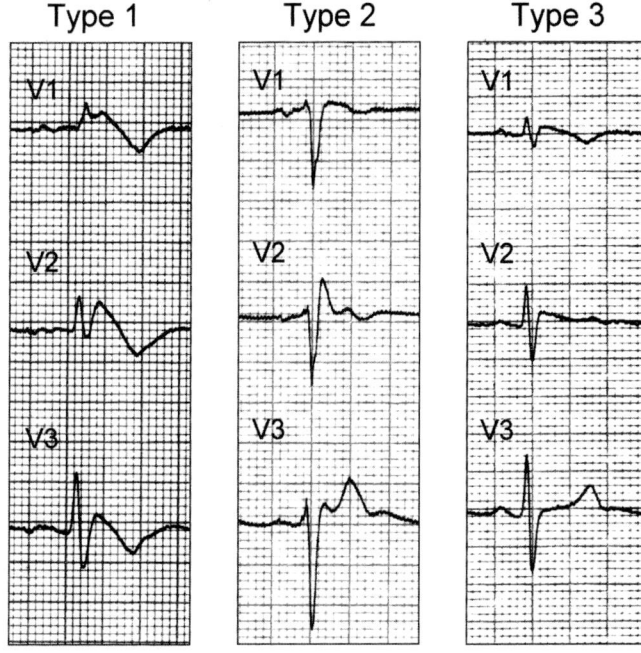

Type 1   **Type 2**   **Type 3**

FIGURE 33–7. ECG patterns in Brugada syndrome (BrS). Only type 1 ST-segment elevation either spontaneously present or induced by ajmaline/flecainide test is considered diagnostic for BrS. Types 2 and 3 may lead to suspect the presence of BrS but drug challenge is required for diagnosis. The ECGs in the right and left panels are from the same patient before (*right panel*, type III) and after (*left panel*, type I) intravenous administration of 1 mg/kg of ajmaline in 10 minutes.

blown BrS also manifests with syncope and sudden death. Typically cardiac events occur at rest and during sleep, and they can also be triggered by hyperpyrexia, large meals, and excessive alcohol consumption.

GENETIC BASES AND PATHOPHYSIOLOGY

Mutations in the cardiac sodium channel gene, SCN5A, on chromosome 3p21–23, were identified for the first time by Chen in 1998.[56] This gene encodes for the α subunit of the cardiac sodium channel protein (identified as Nav1.5), which is the most important factor in determining phase 0 of the cardiac action potential (see Fig. 33–1).

Interestingly, BrS is not the only phenotype linked to SCN5A mutations: allelic disorders are the LQT3 variant of long QT syndrome, progressive cardiac conduction defect, sick sinus syndrome (see below).[57–59] Furthermore, recent findings also suggest that SCN5A mutations may be present in patients with typical BrS ECG and myocardial abnormalities similar to those observed in arrhythmogenic right ventricular cardiomyopathy (ARVC)[60] and in families with dilated cardiomyopathy (DCM).[61,62] Approximately 65 percent of mutations identified in SCN5A gene (see www.fsm.it/cardmoc), are associated with a BrS phenotype and these mutations are located throughout the entire coding region.

In vitro expression of mutant SCN5A proteins showed that BrS mutations invariably cause a loss of sodium channel function.[56] A haplotype block of six polymorphisms in the SCN5A promoter has been identified and functionally linked to a reduced expression of the sodium current.[63] Interestingly, this variant was found among subjects of Asian origin (allelic frequency 0.22), and it

could play a role in modulating the expression of BrS in far-East countries where the disease appears to be particularly frequent.[64]

The second, recently identified BrS gene is called GPD1-L, encoding for the glycerol-3-phosphate-dehydrogenase 1-like protein (Table 33–4). A mutation was reported to cosegregate with the BrS phenotype in a single large family.[65] The function of GPD1-L is poorly known at present, but preliminary in vitro data suggest that it controls the membrane expression of the sodium channels and that the mutation identified in the family with BrS reduces the expression of the sodium channel. We have recently shown that mutations in this gene accounts for not more than 1% of Brugada syndrome cases (Priori SG, personal communication). The yield of genetic screening in BrS patients is less than 30 percent. Nonetheless, molecular diagnosis still has clinical value and helps identifying carriers of the mutation before they manifest the phenotype (incomplete and variable penetrance).[66,67]

DIAGNOSIS AND CLINICAL PRESENTATION OF BRUGADA SYNDROME

Diagnosis

According to the international consensus conference on BrS the electrocardiographic criteria that should be met for diagnosis consist of an ST-segment elevation ≥ 2 mm in at least two of the three right precordial leads (V1–V3), with a coved morphology (see Fig. 33–7) associated with incomplete or complete right bundle-branch block.[68] This pattern can be spontaneously evident, or it can be induced by provocative pharmacological testing with sodium channel blockers (ajmaline, flecainide, or procainamide).[68,69] It is important to recognize that the sensitivity of these criteria in the identification of affected individuals is still undefined, and it is certainly lower than 100 percent. One study showed that the response to a provocative test has a sensitivity of 77 percent.[70]

Clinical Presentation

Brugada syndrome manifests with syncope and cardiac arrest occurring at rest or during sleep: The first manifestation typically occurs in the third and fourth decade of life. Few patients manifest symptoms during childhood, however early manifestation (diagnostic ECG and syncope) can indicate an aggressive form of the disease. Albeit initially the incidence of life-threatening events in BrS patients was thought to be very high, the most recent figures suggest that the percentage of clinically affected patients with at least one cardiac arrest before age 60 is 10 to 15 percent thus the majority of BrS cases do not manifest life-threatening events.[64,71,72]

Therapy of Brugada Syndrome (The Role of Risk Stratification)

An ICD is the only effective treatment to abate mortality in BrS. Cardiac-arrest survivors have a class I indication for an ICD. However, the challenge for the clinician is to define which patients require the prophylactic implant of a device (primary prevention).

Agreement exists to support the implant of an ICD in patients presenting with both history of syncope and a spontaneously abnormal ECG (i.e., a diagnostic ECG without the need to perform a drug

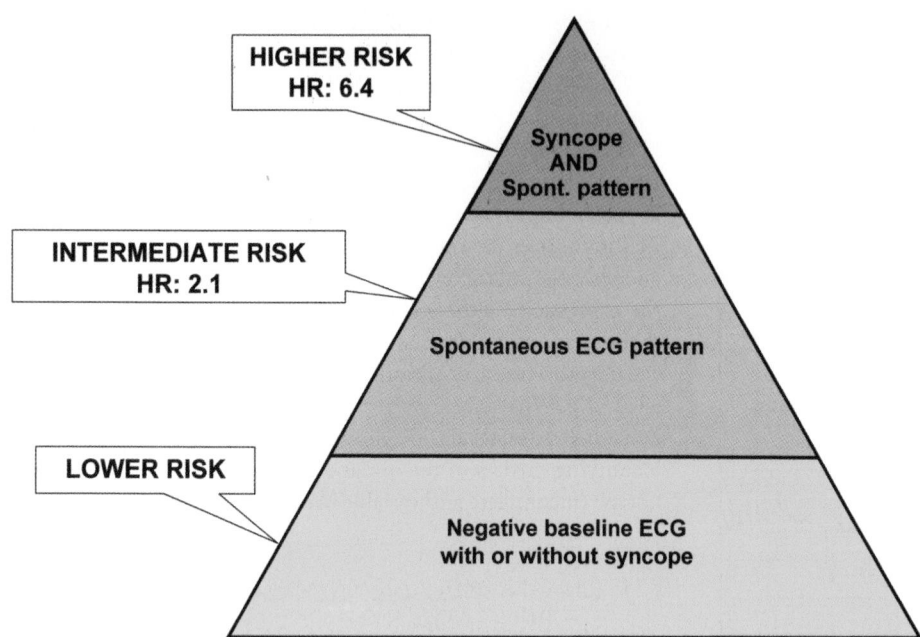

FIGURE 33–8. Risk stratification in Brugada syndrome. Categories of risk in BrS according to the presence or the absence of spontaneously abnormal ECG, history of syncope, or both. Hazard ratios (HR) quantify the risk of a cardiac arrest younger than 60 years of age using the lowest risk category (patients diagnosed only on class Ic drug challenge) as reference.

challenge) (see Table 33–2).[73,74] These patients have approximately a sixfold increased risk of cardiac arrest as compared to patients showing a coved type (type I) ECG only after provocative testing.[71]

When the diagnosis is established only after drug testing or when the diagnosis is made only on the identification of a pathogenetic mutation (nonpenetrant mutation carriers) the risk of cardiac events is significantly lower. These subjects can be reassured with the only indication to perform regular followup to monitor the possible development of a spontaneous pattern over time.

The most difficult scenario for the clinician is represented by the patients with a spontaneous type I ECG pattern without history of syncope. The risk of a life-threatening event younger than 60 years of age in these patients is intermediate between the high-risk group and the low-risk group (Fig. 33–8). Approximately 40 percent of patients diagnosed as affected by Brugada syndrome at our center fall within this group (see Fig. 33–8). A family history of sudden death at young age and the presence of a *SCN5A* mutation are not significant predictors of events.[71] Some authors suggested that the detection of late potential at signal-averaged ECG is associated with an increased risk of events, but this finding awaits confirmation.[75]

The value of induction of ventricular fibrillation during programmed electrical stimulation is controversial.[71–73,76–79] Unfortunately, the management of asymptomatic patients with spontaneously abnormal ECG remains empirical (see Fig. 33–7 and Table 33–2).

Modulation of Phenotype, Triggers, and Pharmacologic Therapy of Brugada Syndrome

Intravenous administration of isoproterenol attenuates whereas acetylcholine accentuates the ECG abnormalities in affected individuals.[80] These findings are in agreement with the fact that the majority of events occur at rest and during sleep and put forth the

rationale of performing Holter monitoring to assess ST-segment elevation at nighttime for diagnostic purposes.

Several drugs have been reported to exacerbate the ECG pattern and to trigger arrhythmias,[23] and they should be obviously avoided: local anesthetics (bupivacaine), cocaine, α-adrenergic agonists (methoxamine), β blockers, potassium channel activators (pinacidil), tricyclic antidepressants, opioid analgesics (propoxyphene), lithium, propofol.

Furthermore hyperpyrexia has been consistently reported as a trigger for fatal events,[81–83] and therefore lowering of body temperature during febrile illnesses by appropriate pharmacological means is recommended in all patients.

Quinidine, a nonspecific blocker of cardiac transient outward current (I_{to}), could restore the equilibrium between inward (constitutively reduced in Brugada syndrome) and outward currents.[84] Data show that quinidine prevents arrhythmia inducibility at programmed electrical stimulation (PES) in up to 76 percent of BrS patients[85,86] and suggest a positive long-term effect in preventing the occurrence of spontaneous arrhythmias.[86] Quinidine can be regarded as an adjunctive therapy for patients at higher risk and to reduce the number of ICD shock in patients with multiple recurrences (see Table 33–2).

SHORT QT SYNDROME

【 】 DEFINITION

Short QT syndrome (SQTS) is a rare genetically determined disorder causing arrhythmias and sudden death in the setting of an abnormally short QT interval and structurally normal heart. Three genes have been associated with the pathogenesis of SQTS (see Table 33–4), but the clinical features, the genotype-phenotype correlation, and the therapeutic strategies are still only roughly defined.

【 】 GENETIC BASES AND PATHOPHYSIOLOGY

All the three genetic forms of SQTS are characterized by abnormally short action potential and refractory period.[87–89] The gene (SQTS3) *KCNJ2*, identified by Priori and coworkers[89] causes abnormally short ventricular repolarization with a peculiar T-wave morphology (extremely fast terminal limb and a quasi-normal ST segment and ascending T-wave phase).

【 】 CLINICAL PRESENTATION AND MANAGEMENT OF SHORT QT SYNDROME

The hallmark of SQTS is a short QT interval. QT intervals of <300 ms[90,91] were initially reported, recently, patients with *KCNJ2* mutation had a QTc up to 320 ms.[89]

It is still unclear whether the diagnosis of SQTS should be based on QT or QTc, and the sensitivity and specificity of different QT/QTc cut-off values are not known. What seems established is that SQTS can be suspected in patients with a QT <350 msec (measured at resting heart rate). It has been also suggested that QT interval measurements should be made at heart rates below 80/min.[92] Several SQTS patients present morphological abnormalities of repolarization such as tall and peaked T waves (hyperkalemic-like pattern) or asymmetrical T waves with a normal ascending phase and a very rapid descending limb.

Besides ventricular fibrillation leading to sudden death, SQTS patients can also present with atrial fibrillation. Up to now only 23 cases of SQTS from six different families have been reported,[16,93] and the present experience suggests that the disease can be highly lethal. No information is available on whether specific triggers can precipitate cardiac events, and cardiac arrest occurs both at rest and under stress. Finally, ventricular fibrillation can be induced in most of the patients (90 percent) during PES, but whether it is a predictor of sudden death is unknown.

Needless to say ICD is indicated for secondary prevention of ventricular fibrillation. Furthermore, with the high risk of sudden death and the lack of drugs with documented efficacy, some authors[92,94] suggest the use of ICD also for the primary prevention of ventricular fibrillation in all affected patients.

Limited experience exists with antiarrhythmic drug therapy. Sotalol, ibutilide, and flecainide were ineffective, but encouraging results have been obtained with quinidine (see Table 33–3) as it can normalize the QT interval and prolong ventricular refractory period. More data is required to define if quinidine can impact mortality in SQTS.

OTHER INHERITED ARRHYTHMIAS

ATRIAL FIBRILLATION

Occasionally, atrial fibrillation (AF) occurs in families. A number of candidate genes have been analyzed, and four have been implicated in AF pathogenesis (see Table 33–4 and Fig. 33–1). In 2003 Chen and colleagues[95] identified in one family a missense mutation of *KCNQ1* causing a gain-of-function effect on the I_{Ks} channel. Subsequently, one AF-related *KCNE2* mutation has been reported in 2:28 probands.[96] In 2005 the same group also reported a gain of function *KCNJ2* mutation in 1:30 families with AF.[89]

Very recently Gollob and coworkers[97] have reported mutations of the connexin-40 gene (*GJA5*) in 4:15 patients with lone atrial fibrillation. Interestingly three of these patients were shown to harbor the genetic defect in atrial specimens but not in the lymphocyte-derived DNA, indicating a somatic source of the genetic defect. Functional expression revealed impaired electrical conduction in the atria. Overall these data suggest that genetic determinants of atrial fibrillation are very heterogeneous and span from cardiac ion channel mutations to defects in cell-to-cell electrical coupling.

SINUS NODE DYSFUNCTION AND CONDUCTION DEFECTS

It has been speculated some idiopathic forms of sinus node dysfunction might be genetically determined. The cardiac pacemaker current (I_f) encoding gene (*HCN4*) has been considered a strong candidate. Indeed, three *HCN4* mutations have been so far associated with sinus node dysfunction,[98–100] all of them causing loss of function (reduced spontaneous diastolic depolarization).

Sick sinus syndrome is often associated with conduction defects especially in the elderly. In 1999 Schott and coworkers[58] described two families with a *SCN5A* mutations cosegregating with progressive conduction defects. Subsequently, Benson and colleagues[59] showed that compound heterozygosity (two different mutations one from paternal and one from maternal origin) of *SCN5A* mutations can cause sick sinus syndrome with subclinical conduction disease and first-degree atrioventricular (AV) block.

Overall, functional studies showed that *SCN5A* mutations associated with sick sinus syndrome are loss of function mutations (see www.fsm.it/cardmoc). Thus, *SCN5A* mutations causing this phenotype are functionally similar to *SCN5A* mutations identified in Brugada syndrome, which is also characterized by intraventricular conduction delay. A recent study has further elaborated on this concept by suggesting that the more frequent phenotype associated with loss of function mutations of the *SCN5A* gene is indeed conduction defect.[101]

REFERENCES

1. Priori SG, Aliot E, Blomstrom-Lundqvist C, et al. Update of the guidelines on sudden cardiac death of the European Society of Cardiology. *Eur Heart J.* 2003;24:13.
2. Joint Steering Committees of the Unexplained Cardiac Arrest Registry of Europe and of the Idiopathic Ventricular Fibrillation Registry of the United States. Consensus Statement: survivors of out-of-hospital cardiac arrest with apparently normal heart. Need for definition and standardized clinical evaluation. *Circulation.* 1997;95:265.
3. Schwartz PJ, Priori SG. Long QT syndrome—phenotype genotype considerations. In: Zipes DP, Jalife J, eds. *Cardiac Electrophysiology.* 4th ed. Philadelphia, PA: Elsevier; 2004:651.
4. Splawski I, Shen J, Timothy KW, et al. Spectrum of mutations in long-QT syndrome genes: KVLQT1 HERG, SCN5A, KCNE1 and KCNE2. *Circulation.* 2000;102:1178.
5. Napolitano C, Priori SG, Schwartz PJ, et al. Genetic testing in the long QT syndrome: development and validation of an efficient approach to genotyping in clinical practice. *JAMA.* 2005;294:2975.
6. Priori SG, Rivolta I, Napolitano C. Genetics of long QT, Brugada and other Channelopathies. In: Zipes DP, Jalife J, eds. *Cardiac Electrophysiology.* 4th ed. Philadelphia, PA: Elsevier; 2003:462.
7. Mohler PJ, Schott JJ, Gramolini AO, et al. Ankyrin-B mutation causes type 4 long-QT cardiac arrhythmia and sudden cardiac death. *Nature.* 2003;421:634.
8. Plaster NM, Tawil R, Tristani-Firouzi M, et al. Mutations in Kir2.1 cause the developmental and episodic electrical phenotypes of Andersen's syndrome. *Cell.* 2001;105:511.
9. Splawski I, Timothy KW, Sharpe LM, et al. Ca(V)1.2 calcium channel dysfunction causes a multisystem disorder including arrhythmia and autism. *Cell.* 2004;119:19.
10. Ye B, Tester DJ, Vatta M, et al. Molecular and functional characterization of novel CAV3-encoded caveolin-3 mutations in congenital long QT syndrome (abstract). *Heart Rhythm.* 2006;3:S66.
11. Domingo AM, Kaku T, Tester DJ, et al. Sodium channel B4 subunit mutation causes congenital long QT syndrome (abstract). *Heart Rhythm.* 2006;3:S34.
12. Priori SG, Schwartz PJ, Napolitano C, et al. Risk stratification in the long-QT syndrome. *N Engl J Med.* 2003;348:1866.
13. Moss AJ, Schwartz PJ, Crampton RS, et al. The long QT syndrome. Prospective longitudinal study of 328 families. *Circulation.* 1991;84:1136.
14. Schwartz PJ, Periti M, Malliani A. The long Q-T syndrome. *Am Heart J.* 1975;89:378.
15. Moss AJ, Zareba W, Hall WJ, et al. Effectiveness and limitations of beta-blocker therapy in congenital long-QT syndrome. *Circulation.* 2000;101:616.
16. Priori SG, Napolitano C, Schwartz PJ, et al. Association of long QT syndrome loci and cardiac events among patients treated with beta-blockers. *JAMA.* 2004;292:1341.

17. Schwartz PJ, Priori SG, Cerrone M, et al. Left cardiac sympathetic denervation in the management of high-risk patients affected by the long-QT syndrome. *Circulation.* 2004;109:1826.

18. American College of Cardiology/American Heart Association/European Society of Cardiology. ACC/AHA/ESC 2006 guidelines for the management of patients with ventricular arrhythmias and the prevention of sudden cardiac death. *Eur Heart J.* 2006;2099.

19. Zhang L, Timothy KW, Vincent GM, et al. Spectrum of ST-T-wave patterns and repolarization parameters in congenital long-QT syndrome: ECG findings identify genotypes. *Circulation.* 2000;102:2849.

20. Schwartz PJ, Priori SG, Spazzolini C, et al. Genotype-phenotype correlation in the long-QT syndrome: gene-specific triggers for life-threatening arrhythmias. *Circulation.* 2001;103:89.

21. Moss AJ, Robinson JL, Gessman L, et al. Comparison of clinical and genetic variables of cardiac events associated with loud noise versus swimming among subjects with the long QT syndrome. *Am J Cardiol.* 1999;84:876.

22. Ackerman MJ, Tester DJ, Porter CJ. Swimming, a gene-specific arrhythmogenic trigger for inherited long QT syndrome. *Mayo Clin Proc.* 1999;74:1088.

23. Priori SG, Napolitano C, Cerrone M. Experimental therapy of genetic arrhythmias: disease-specific pharmacology. *Handb Exp Pharmacol.* 2006;171:267.

24. Vincent GM, Timothy KW, Leppert M, et al. The spectrum of symptoms and QT intervals in carriers of the gene for the long-QT syndrome. *N Engl J Med.* 1992;327:846.

25. Priori SG, Napolitano C, Schwartz PJ. Low penetrance in the long-QT syndrome: clinical impact. *Circulation.* 1999;99:529.

26. Yang P, Kanki H, Drolet B, et al. Allelic variants in long-QT disease genes in patients with drug-associated torsades de pointes. *Circulation.* 2002;105:1943.

27. Sesti F, Abbott GW, Wei J, et al. A common polymorphism associated with antibiotic-induced cardiac arrhythmia. *Proc Natl Acad Sci U S A.* 2000;97:10613.

28. Napolitano C, Schwartz PJ, Brown AM, et al. Evidence for a cardiac ion channel mutation underlying drug-induced QT prolongation and life-threatening arrhythmias. *J Cardiovasc Electrophysiol.* 2000;11:691.

29. Arking DE, Pfeufer A, Post W, et al. A common genetic variant in the NOS1 regulator NOS1AP modulates cardiac repolarization. *Nat Genet.* 2006;38:644.

30. Viswanathan PC, Benson DW, Balser JR. A common SCN5A polymorphism modulates the biophysical effects of an SCN5A mutation. *J Clin Invest.* 2003;111:341.

31. Splawski I, Timothy KW, Tateyama M, et al. Variant of SCN5A sodium channel implicated in risk of cardiac arrhythmia. *Science.* 2002;297:1333.

32. Coumel P, Fidelle J, Lucet V, et al. Catecholaminergic-induced severe ventricular arrhythmias with Adams-Stokes syndrome in children: report of four cases. *Br Heart J.* 1978;40:28.

33. Swan H, Piippo K, Viitasalo M, et al. Arrhythmic disorder mapped to chromosome 1q42-q43 causes malignant polymorphic ventricular tachycardia in structurally normal hearts. *J Am Coll Cardiol.* 1999;34:2035.

34. Priori SG, Napolitano C, Tiso N, et al. Mutations in the cardiac ryanodine receptor gene (hRyR2) underlie catecholaminergic polymorphic ventricular tachycardia. *Circulation.* 2001;103:196.

35. Laitinen PJ, Brown KM, Piippo K, et al. Mutations of the cardiac ryanodine receptor (RyR2) gene in familial polymorphic ventricular tachycardia. *Circulation.* 2001;103:485.

36. Lahat H, Eldar M, Levy-Nissenbaum E, et al. Autosomal recessive catecholamine- or exercise-induced polymorphic ventricular tachycardia. *Circulation.* 2001;103:2822.

37. Lahat H, Pras E, Olender T, et al. A missense mutation in a highly conserved region of CASQ2 is associated with autosomal recessive catecholamine-induced polymorphic ventricular tachycardia in Bedouin families from Israel. *Am J Hum Genet.* 2001;69:1378.

38. Cerrone M, Colombi B, Santoro M, et al. Bidirectional ventricular tachycardia and fibrillation elicited in a knock-in mouse model carrier of a mutation in the cardiac ryanodine receptor (RyR2). *Circ Res.* 2005;96:e77–e82.

39. Liu N, Colombi B, Memmi M, et al. Arrhythmogenesis in catecholaminergic polymorphic ventricular tachycardia. Insights from a RyR2 R4496C knock-in mouse model. *Circ Res.* 2006;99:292.

40. Terentyev D, Nori A, Santoro M, et al. Abnormal interactions of calsequestrin with the ryanodine receptor calcium release channel complex linked to exercise-induced sudden cardiac death. *Circ Res.* 2006;98:1151.

41. Viatchenko-Karpinski S, Terentyev D, Gyorke I, et al. Abnormal calcium signaling and sudden cardiac death associated with mutation of calsequestrin. *Circ Res.* 2004;94:471.

42. Raffaele di Barletta M, Viatchenko-Karpinski S, Nori A, et al. Clinical phenotype and functional characterization of CASQ2 mutations associated with

43. Reid DS, Tynan M, Braidwood L, et al. Bidirectional tachycardia in a child. A study using His bundle electrography. *Br Heart J.* 1975;37:339.

44. Leenhardt A, Lucet V, Denjoy I, et al. Catecholaminergic polymorphic ventricular tachycardia in children. A 7-year follow-up of 21 patients. *Circulation.* 1995;91:1512.

45. Postma AV, Denjoy I, Kamblock J, et al. Catecholaminergic polymorphic ventricular tachycardia: RYR2 mutations, bradycardia, and follow up of the patients. *J Med Genet.* 2005;42:863.

46. Priori SG, Napolitano C, Memmi M, et al. Clinical and molecular characterization of patients with catecholaminergic polymorphic ventricular tachycardia. *Circulation.* 2002;106:69.

47. Krahn AD, Gollob M, Yee R, et al. Diagnosis of unexplained cardiac arrest: role of adrenaline and procainamide infusion. *Circulation.*. 2005;112:2228.

48. Tester DJ, Spoon DB, Valdivia HH, et al. Targeted mutational analysis of the RyR2-encoded cardiac ryanodine receptor in sudden unexplained death: a molecular autopsy of 49 medical examiner/coroner's cases. *Mayo Clin Proc.* 2004;79:1380.

49. Cerrone M, Colombi B, Bloise R, et al. Clinical and molecular characterization of a large cohort of patients affected with catecholaminergic polymorphic ventricular tachycardia (abstract). *Circulation.* 2004;110(suppl II):552.

50. Sumitomo N, Harada K, Nagashima M, et al. Catecholaminergic polymorphic ventricular tachycardia: electrocardiographic characteristics and optimal therapeutic strategies to prevent sudden death. *Heart.* 2003;89:66.

51. Ibid.

52. Kontula K, Laitinen PJ, Lehtonen A, et al. Catecholaminergic polymorphic ventricular tachycardia: recent mechanistic insights. *Cardiovasc Res.* 2005;67:379.

53. Valdivia HH, Valdivia C, Ma J, et al. Direct binding of verapamil to the ryanodine receptor channel of sarcoplasmic reticulum. *Biophys J.* 1990;58:471.

54. Swan H, Laitinen P, Kontula K, et al. Calcium channel antagonism reduces exercise-induced ventricular arrhythmias in catecholaminergic polymorphic ventricular tachycardia patients with RyR2 mutations. *J Cardiovasc Electrophysiol.* 2005;16:162.

55. Brugada P, Brugada J. Right bundle branch block, persistent ST-segment elevation and sudden cardiac death: a distinct clinical and electrocardiographic syndrome. A multicenter report. *J Am Coll Cardiol.* 1992;20:1391.

56. Chen Q, Kirsch GE, Zhang D, et al. Genetic basis and molecular mechanism for idiopathic ventricular fibrillation. *Nature.* 1998;392:293.

57. Kyndt F, Probst V, Potet F, et al. Novel SCN5A mutation leading either to isolated cardiac conduction defect or Brugada syndrome in a large french family. *Circulation.* 2001;104:3081.

58. Schott JJ, Alshinawi C, Kyndt F, et al. Cardiac conduction defects associate with mutations in SCN5A. *Nat Genet.* 1999;23:20.

59. Benson DW, Wang DW, Dyment M, et al. Congenital sick sinus syndrome caused by recessive mutations in the cardiac sodium channel gene (SCN5A). *J Clin Invest.* 2003;112:1019.

60. Frustaci A, Priori SG, Pieroni M, et al. Cardiac histological substrate in patients with clinical phenotype of Brugada syndrome. *Circulation.* 2005;112:3680.

61. Olson TM, Michels VV, Ballew JD, et al. Sodium channel mutations and susceptibility to heart failure and atrial fibrillation. *JAMA.* 2005;293:447.

62. McNair WP, Ku L, Taylor MR, et al. SCN5A mutation associated with dilated cardiomyopathy, conduction disorder, and arrhythmia. *Circulation.* 2004;110:2163.

63. Bezzina CR, Shimizu W, Yang P, et al. Common sodium channel promoter haplotype in Asian subjects underlies variability in cardiac conduction. *Circulation.* 2006;113:338.

64. Ito H, Yano K, Chen R, et al. The prevalence and prognosis of a Brugada-type electrocardiogram in a population of middle-aged Japanese-American men with follow-up of three decades. *Am J Med Sci.* 2006;331:25.

65. London B, Sshamarendra S, Michalec, et al. A mutation in the glycerol-3-phosphate dehydrogenase 1-like gene (GPD1L) causes Brugada syndrome (abstract). *Heart Rhythm.* 2006;S32.

66. Priori SG, Napolitano C, Grillo M. Concealed arrhythmogenic syndromes: the hidden substrate of idiopathic ventricular fibrillation? *Cardiovasc Res.* 2001;50:218.

67. Priori SG, Bloise R, Napolitano C, et al. Clinical characterization of the genetic variant of Brugada syndrome associated with SCN5A mutations. *Circulation.* 2001;104(suppl II): 461.

68. Antzelevitch C, Brugada P, Borggrefe M, et al. Brugada syndrome. Report of the Second Consensus Conference. Endorsed by the Heart Rhythm Society and the European Heart Rhythm Association. *Circulation.* 2005;111:659.

69. Brugada R, Brugada J, Antzelevitch C, et al. Sodium channel blockers identify risk for sudden death in patients with ST-segment elevation and right bundle branch block but structurally normal hearts. *Circulation.* 2000;101:510.

70. Meregalli PG, Ruijter JM, Hofman N, et al. Diagnostic value of flecainide testing in unmasking SCN5A-related Brugada syndrome. *J Cardiovasc Electrophysiol.* 2006;17:1.

71. Priori SG, Napolitano C, Gasparini M, et al. Natural history of Brugada syndrome. Insights for risk stratification and management. *Circulation.* 2002;105:1342.

72. Eckardt L, Probst V, Smits JPP, et al. Long-term prognosis of individuals with right precordial ST-segment-elevation Brugada syndrome. *Circulation.* 2005;111:257.

73. Priori SG, Napolitano C. Should patients with an asymptomatic Brugada electrocardiogram undergo pharmacological and electrophysiological testing? *Circulation.* 2005;112:279.

74. Brugada J, Brugada R, Brugada P. Determinants of sudden cardiac death in individuals with the electrocardiographic pattern of Brugada syndrome and no previous cardiac arrest. *Circulation.* 2003;108:3092.

75. Ikeda T, Sakurada H, Sakabe K, et al. Assessment of noninvasive markers in identifying patients at risk in the Brugada syndrome: insight into risk stratification. *J Am Coll Cardiol.* 2001;37:1628.

76. Brugada P, Geelen P, Brugada R, et al. Prognostic value of electrophysiologic investigations in Brugada syndrome. *J Cardiovasc Electrophysiol.* 2001;12:1004.

77. Gehi AK, Duong TD, Metz LD, et al. Risk stratification of individuals with the Brugada electrocardiogram: a meta-analysis. *J Cardiovasc Electrophysiol.* 2006;17:577.

78. Eckardt L, Kirchhof P, Schulze-Bahr E, et al. Electrophysiologic investigation in Brugada syndrome; yield of programmed ventricular stimulation at two ventricular sites with up to three premature beats. *Eur Heart J.* 2002;23:1394.

79. Gasparini M, Priori SG, Mantica M, et al. Programmed electrical stimulation in Brugada syndrome: how reproducible are the results? *J Cardiovasc Electrophysiol.* 2002;13:880.

80. Miyazaki T, Mitamura H, Miyoshi S, et al. Autonomic and antiarrhythmic drug modulation of ST segment elevation in patients with Brugada syndrome. *J Am Coll Cardiol.* 1996;27:1061.

81. Ortega-Carnicer J, Benezet J, Ceres F. Fever-induced ST-segment elevation and T-wave alternans in a patient with Brugada syndrome. *Resuscitation.* 2003;57:315.

82. Mok NS, Priori SG, Napolitano C, et al. A newly characterized SCN5A mutation underlying Brugada syndrome unmasked by hyperthermia. *J Cardiovasc Electrophysiol.* 2003;14:407.

83. Saura D, Garcia-Alberola A, Carrillo P, et al. Brugada-like electrocardiographic pattern induced by fever. *Pacing Clin Electrophysiol.* 2002;25:856.

84. Yan GX, Antzelevitch C. Cellular basis for the Brugada syndrome and other mechanisms of arrhythmogenesis associated with ST-segment elevation. *Circulation.* 1999;100:1660.

85. Hermida JS, Denjoy I, Clerc J, et al. Hydroquinidine therapy in Brugada syndrome. *J Am Coll Cardiol.* 2004;43:1853.

86. Belhassen B, Glick A, Viskin S. Efficacy of quinidine in high-risk patients with Brugada syndrome. *Circulation.* 2004;110:1731.

87. Brugada R, Hong K, Dumaine R, et al. Sudden death associated with short-QT syndrome linked to mutations in HERG. *Circulation.* 2004;109:30.

88. Bellocq C, van Ginneken AC, Bezzina CR, et al. Mutation in the KCNQ1 gene leading to the short QT-interval syndrome. *Circulation.* 2004;109:2394.

89. Priori SG, Pandit SV, Rivolta I, et al. A novel form of short QT syndrome (SQT3) is caused by a mutation in the KCNJ2 gene. *Circ Res.* 2005;96:800.

90. Gussak I, Brugada P, Brugada J, et al. Idiopathic short QT interval: a new clinical syndrome? *Cardiology.* 2000;94:99.

91. Gaita F, Giustetto C, Bianchi F, et al. Short QT syndrome: a familial cause of sudden death. *Circulation.* 2003;108:965.

92. Schimpf R, Wolpert C, Gaita F, et al. Short QT syndrome. *Cardiovasc Res.* 2005;67:357.

93. Bettini R, Caselli G, D'andrea L, et al. Protocolli cardiologici per il giudizio di idoneità allo sport agonistico 2003. *Giornale Italiano di Cardiologia Pratica* 2005;(suppl 1):1.

94. Bjerregaard P, Gussak I. Short QT syndrome: mechanisms, diagnosis and treatment. *Nat Clin Pract.* 2005;2:84.

95. Chen YH, Xu SJ, Bendahhou S, et al. KCNQ1 gain-of-function mutation in familial atrial fibrillation. *Science.* 2003;299:251.

96. Yang G, Xia M, Jin Q, et al. Identification of a KCNE2 gain-of-function mutation in patients with familial atrial fibrillation. *Am J Hum Genet.* 2004;75:899.

97. Gollob MH, Jones DL, Krahn AD, et al. Somatic mutations in the connexin 40 gene (GJA5) in atrial fibrillation. *N Engl J Med.* 2006;354:2677.

98. Milanesi R, Baruscotti M, Gnecchi-Ruscone T, et al. Familial sinus bradycardia associated with a mutation in the cardiac pacemaker channel. *N Engl J Med.* 2006;354:151.

99. Schulze-Bahr E, Neu A, Friederich P, et al. Pacemaker channel dysfunction in a patient with sinus node disease. *J Clin Invest.* 2003;111:1537.

100. Ueda K, Nakamura K, Hayashi T, et al. Functional characterization of a trafficking-defective HCN4 mutation, D553N, associated with cardiac arrhythmia. *J Biol Chem.* 2004;279:27194.

101. Probst V, Allouis M, Sacher F, et al. Progressive cardiac conduction defect is the prevailing phenotype in carriers of a Brugada syndrome SCN5A mutation. *J Cardiovasc Electrophysiol.* 2006;17:270.

CHAPTER 34

Anatomy of Electrophysiology

Siew Yen Ho / Anton E. Becker

INTRODUCTION

Rapid advances have been made in electrophysiologic mapping, imaging, use of catheter ablations for drug refractory arrhythmias, and transcatheter implantation of pacing leads. A better understanding of cardiac anatomy is essential to make further progress, especially in fine-tuning interventional techniques and in developing computer models of arrhythmias. To this end, describing cardiac structures in attitudinal perspective[1] is much more useful to the clinical electrophysiologist than the *conventional* approach[2] of describing the heart as if it is standing on its apex and rotated with right and left heart chambers side-by-side. This chapter on cardiac anatomy highlights features of particular relevance to electrophysiologists.

THE HEART IN THE CHEST

For the clinician the heart must be viewed in the context of its location and relationship to surrounding structures. The frontal silhouette of the heart is nearly trapezoidal. The right border of the heart is more or less a vertical line just to the right of the sternum. It is formed exclusively by the right atrium, with the superior and inferior caval veins joining at its upper and lower margins. The inferior border lying horizontally on the diaphragm is marked by the right ventricle. The sloping left border is made up of the left ventricle and, as it merges with the upper border, the silhouette is formed by the pulmonary trunk. The upper border of the silhouette is made by the arterial trunks with the pulmonary valve leftward and superiorly situated relative to the aortic valve. On the frontal silhouette, the left atrium is barely seen; only its appendage curling around the edge of the pulmonary trunk is visible. Thus, the left atrium is the most posteriorly situated cardiac chamber. When viewed *in situ*, the proximity of the esophagus to the posterior wall of the left atrium is clear (Fig. 34–1). This spatial relationship is crucial to ablationists to reduce the risk of the postprocedural complication of atrioesophageal fistula.[3,4]

The heart itself is enclosed in a fibrous sac, the pericardium, which separates the surface of the heart from adjacent structures. The mediastinal pleura is the outermost lining of the fibrous pericardium. Within the fibrous pericardium there is a thinner double-layered membrane, the serous pericardium. One layer of the serous pericardium is fused to the inner surface of the fibrous pericardium whereas the other layer lines the outer surface of the heart as the epicardium. The pericardial cavity then is the space between the layers of the serous pericardium. Two recesses are found within the pericardial cavity. One is the transverse sinus lying between the back of the arterial trunks and the front of the atrial chambers. Another is the oblique sinus lying behind the left atrium and is limited by the right pulmonary veins and the inferior caval vein to the right side and by the left pulmonary veins to the left side.[5,6] Understanding the topography of surrounding structures is important also for those using intrapericardial catheter techniques. For instance, the descending aorta close to the left inferior pulmonary vein is at risk of damage.

On the surface of the pericardial sac descends the phrenic nerves and their accompanying pericardiophrenic arteries, which are branches from the internal mammary artery. The right phrenic nerve descends vertically along the right anterolateral surface of the superior caval vein to be related to the right aspect of the intercaval atrial

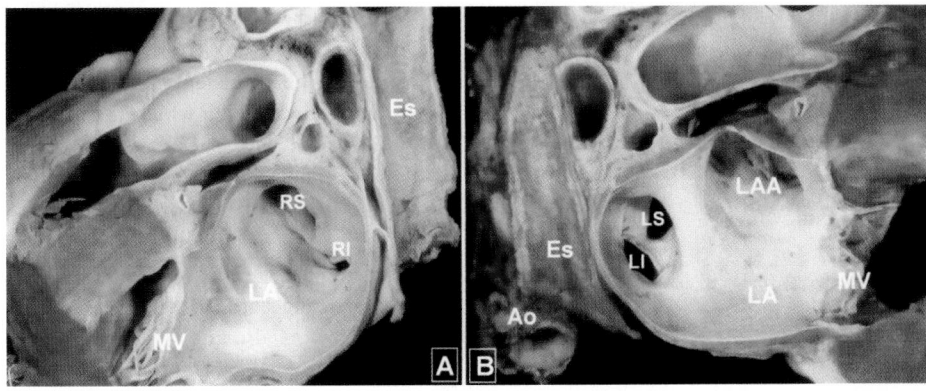

FIGURE 34–1. Two halves of the same specimen bisected longitudinally to show the relationship between the posterior wall of the left atrium and the esophagus. Ao, aorta; Es, esophagus; LA, left atrium; LAA, left atrial appendage; LI, left inferior pulmonary vein; LS, left superior pulmonary vein; MV, mitral valve; RI, right inferior pulmonary vein; RS, right superior pulmonary vein.

wall, and in front of the root of the lung, to reach the diaphragm adjacent to the lateral border of the entrance of the inferior caval vein.[7] Along the way, the right phrenic nerve can be less than 2 millimeters (mm) from the anterior wall of the right superior pulmonary vein (Fig. 34–2A).[7] The left phrenic nerve descends on the left side close to the aortic arch and onto the pericardium over the left atrial appendage and the left ventricle. It takes one of two courses over the left ventricle that takes it either over the anterior surface or leftward over the obtuse margin. The latter course is close to the lateral vein or left obtuse marginal vein (Fig. 34–2B).[7]

LOCATION OF ATRIUMS

Viewed from the front, the cavity of the right atrium is right and anterior, whereas the left atrium is situated to the left and mainly posteriorly. The anterior wall of the left atrium lies just behind the transverse pericardial sinus, whereas its posterior wall is just in front of the tracheal bifurcation and the esophagus. In humans, the right superior pulmonary vein passes posterior to the superior caval vein, with the right inferior vein posterior to the venous sinus of the right atrium (Fig. 34–3A).

The atrial septum, best appreciated in transverse section, runs obliquely from the front extending backwards and to the right. The posterior part of the left atrium receives the pulmonary veins. The orifices of the left pulmonary veins are more superiorly located than those of the right pulmonary veins. In humans it is most common to find two orifices on each side. Sometimes two veins of one, or both, sides are united prior to their entry to the atrium.[8] In others, an additional vein is found, more frequently on the right side. Related posteriorly and inferiorly to the left atrium is the coronary sinus, which is the continuation of the great cardiac vein (Fig. 34–3B). The oblique vein (of Marshall) passes from superiorly between the left atrial appendage and the left superior pulmonary vein along the posteroinferior atrial wall to join the coronary sinus. This vein is obliterated in the majority of individuals.

【 】 THE RIGHT ATRIUM

The right atrium is best considered in terms of three components—the appendage, the venous part, the vestibule.[9] A fourth

component, the septum, is shared by the two atriums and will be discussed in a separate section. From the epicardial aspect, the right atrium is dominated by its large, triangular-shaped appendage that extends anteriorly and laterally. Usually, a fat-filled groove (*sulcus terminalis*) corresponding internally to the terminal crest (*crista terminalis*) can be seen along the lateral wall demarcating the junction between appendage and venous components. The sinus node is located subepicardially in this groove, close to the superior cavoatrial junction.[10,11] Right atrial musculature often extends a short distance onto the adventitial/epicardial side of the wall of the superior caval vein (Fig. 34–4), but muscular extension surrounding the entrance of the inferior caval vein is less common.

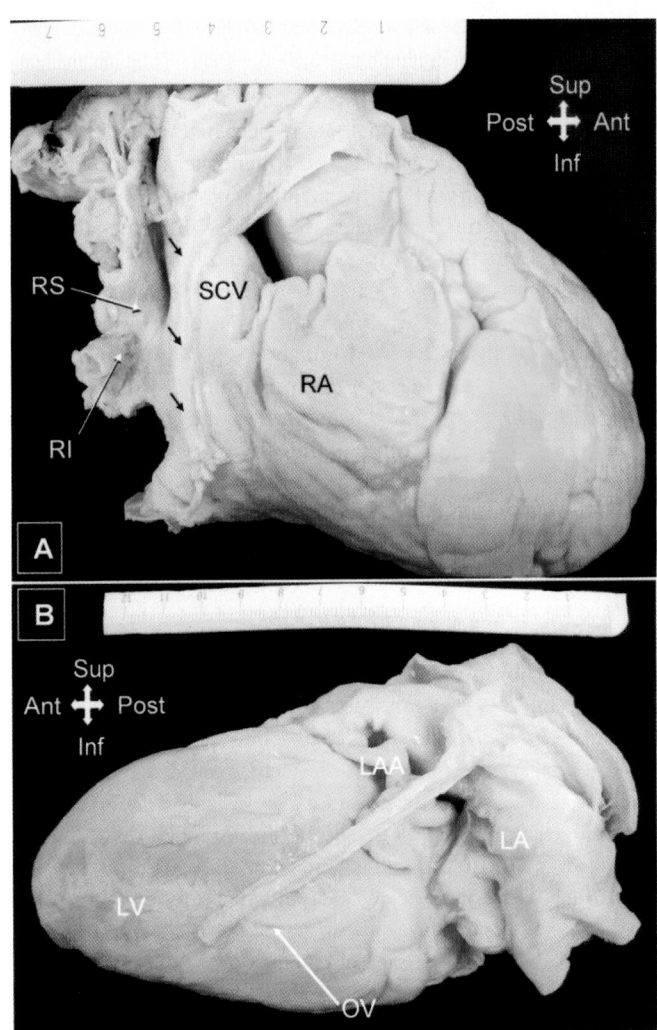

FIGURE 34–2. A. The right phrenic nerve (*arrows*) descends along the pericardium, in close proximity to the right pulmonary veins as they enter the left atrium. **B.** The descent of the left phrenic nerve is either related to the great cardiac vein and anterior descending coronary artery or, as in this specimen, over the course of the obtuse marginal vein. OV, obtuse vein; RA, right atrium; RI, right inferior pulmonary vein; RS, right superior pulmonary vein; SCV, superior caval vein.

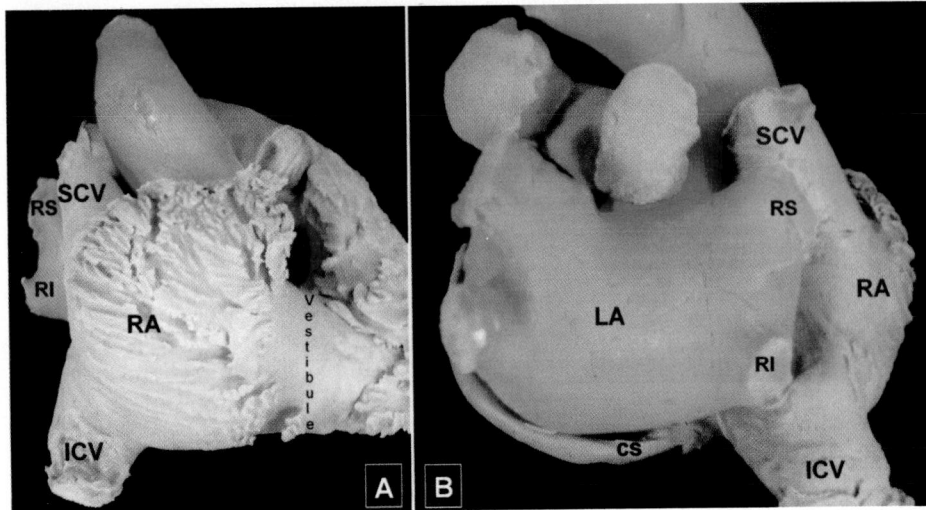

FIGURE 34–3. A. This view from the right shows the characteristically extensive pectinate muscles of the right atrial wall contrasting with the smooth vestibule. The right superior pulmonary vein is posterior to the superior caval vein. **B.** Viewed from the back the figure shows the right pulmonary veins passing behind the superior caval vein and the intercaval area. The coronary sinus is inferior to the left atrium. CS, coronary sinus; ICV, inferior caval vein; LA, left atrium; RA, right atrium; RI, right inferior pulmonary vein; RS, right superior pulmonary vein; SCV, superior caval vein.

Arising from the terminal crest, pectinate muscles spread throughout the entire wall of the appendage, reaching to the lateral and inferior walls of the atrium (Fig. 34–5). In between the ridges of pectinate muscles, the atrial wall is very thin, almost parchment like in cases. On the endocardial aspect, the branching and overlapping arrangement of the pectinate muscles is clearly visible. This arrangement can play a role in initiating intra-atrial reentry.[12] Although extensively arranged, the pectinate muscles never reach the orifice of the tricuspid valve. Always, a smooth muscular rim, the vestibule, surrounds the valvar orifice, with the musculature inserting into the valvar leaflets (see Fig. 34–5).

The venous component is also characterized by smooth walls. The division between venous and rough zones is marked by the terminal crest. This muscular bundle begins on the upper part of the medial wall and turns laterally in front of the orifice of the superior caval vein to descend obliquely along the lateral wall. Its terminal portion is indistinct, as it divides into a variable number of smaller bundles that continue toward the vestibule and the orifice of the inferior caval vein, feeding into the area of the *flutter* (cavo-tricuspid) isthmus.[13] The Eustachian valve that guards the entrance of the inferior caval vein is also variably developed. Usually it is a triangular flap of fibrous or fibromuscular tissue that inserts medially to the Eustachian ridge, or sinus septum, which is the border between the oval fossa and the coronary sinus (Fig. 34–6). In some cases, the valve is particular large and muscular, posing an obstacle to passage of catheters from the inferior caval vein to the inferior part of the right atrium. Occasionally, the valve is perforated, or even takes the form of a delicate filigree sometimes described as a *Chiari network*. The free border of the Eustachian valve continues as a tendon that runs in the musculature of the sinus septum (Eustachian ridge).[14] It is one of the borders of the triangle (of Koch) that is the right atrial landmark for determining the location of the atrioventricular node (see Fig. 34–6).[11,15,16] The anterior border of the Koch triangle is marked

by the hinge of the septal leaflet of the tricuspid valve. Superiorly, marking the apex of the triangle, is the central fibrous body through which the conduction system penetrates as the bundle of His. The inferior border of the triangle is the orifice of the coronary sinus together with the vestibule immediately anterior to it. This vestibular portion between the coronary sinus os and tricuspid valve, also known as the paraseptal isthmus (see Fig. 34–6), is the area often targeted for ablation of the slow pathway in atrioventricular nodal reentrant tachycardia. Inferior extensions of the atrioventricular node have been observed in this area (see Fig. 34–6). The so-called *fast pathway* corresponds to the area of musculature close to the apex of the triangle of Koch.[17,18]

A small crescentic flap, the thebesian valve, usually guards the orifice of the coronary sinus.[19] Frequently, the crescentic valve is fenestrated. Occasionally, the orifice is totally covered by a fenestrated valve, but an imperforate valve is very rare.[20] The atrial wall inferior to the orifice of the coronary sinus is usually pouchlike, and is often described as the sinus of Keith, or the sub-Eustachian sinus. The area between the inferior caval vein and

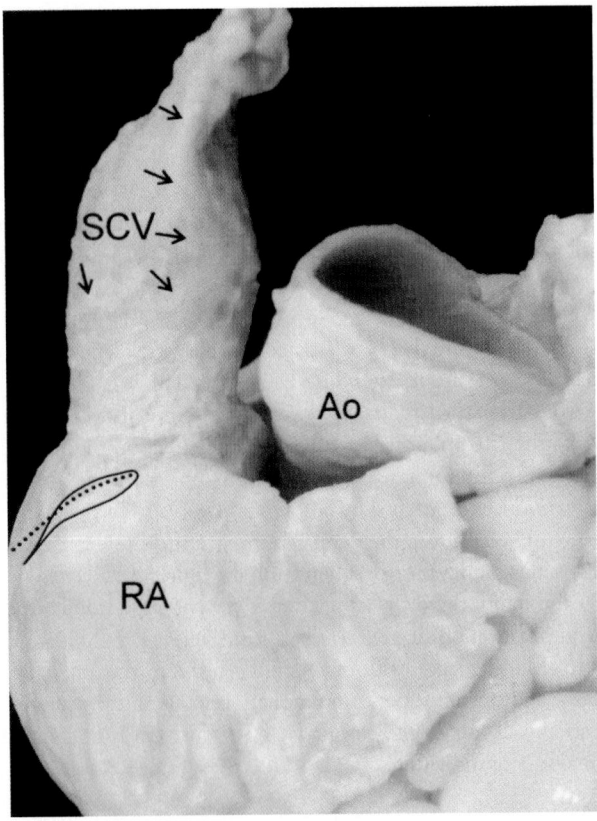

FIGURE 34–4. This anterior view of the superior cavo-atrial junction shows the location of the sinus node (*shape*) in the terminal groove (*dotted line*), and muscular extension around the outside of the venous wall (*arrows*). Ao, aorta; RA, right atrium; SCV, superior caval vein.

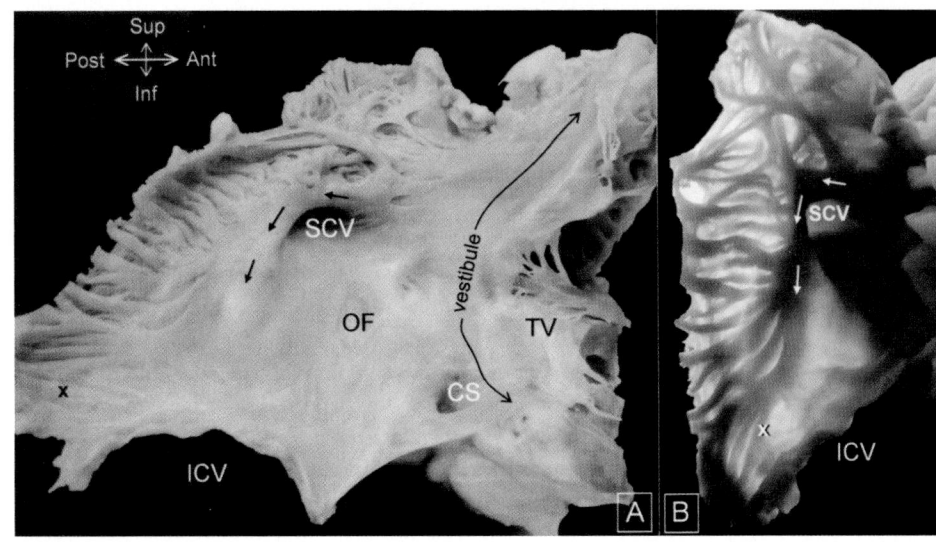

FIGURE 34–5. **A.** The parietal wall of the right atrium has been cut and deflected posteriorly to show the terminal crest (*arrows*). *X* indicates the distal ramifications of the terminal crest that lead into the flutter (cavo-tricuspid) isthmus. **B.** A similar display with transillumination reveals the thin areas in between the pectinate muscles, at the inferior isthmus, and the posteroinferior part of the intercaval atrial wall. CS, coronary sinus; ICV, inferior caval vein; OF, oval foramen; SCV, superior caval vein; TV, tricuspid valve.

the tricuspid valve (see Fig. 34–6) corresponds to the isthmus of slow conduction in the circuit of common (typical) atrial flutter and is also described as the *cavotricuspid isthmus*.[12,21] This quadrilateral-shaped isthmus has three morphologic components bordered anteriorly by the hinge of the tricuspid valve and posteriorly by the Eustachian valve.[13] The posterior component is mainly fibrous, whereas the anterior component is the musculature of the atrial vestibule and has a smooth endocardial surface. In the middle is a zone of muscular trabeculations representing the distal ramifications of the terminal crest, which are separated by variable extents of thin atrial wall composed mainly of fibrous tissue (see Fig. 34–5). Compared to the inferolateral and paraseptal isthmuses (see Fig. 34–6), the inferior isthmus (also called the central isthmus) appears most appropriate for ablationists to target on account of it being further from the compact atrioventricular node and is shorter than the inferolateral isthmus.[22]

❲ ❳ THE ATRIAL SEPTUM AND INTERATRIAL CONNECTIONS

Accessing the left atrium from the right requires an appreciation of the extent of the true atrial septum (see Fig. 34–6). Although a right anterior oblique view of the septal aspect as seen from the right atrium suggests an extensive area to be septal, this is not the case if the septum is defined as a partition that separates one cardiac chamber from another, and crossing it will not go outside the heart. The musculature that

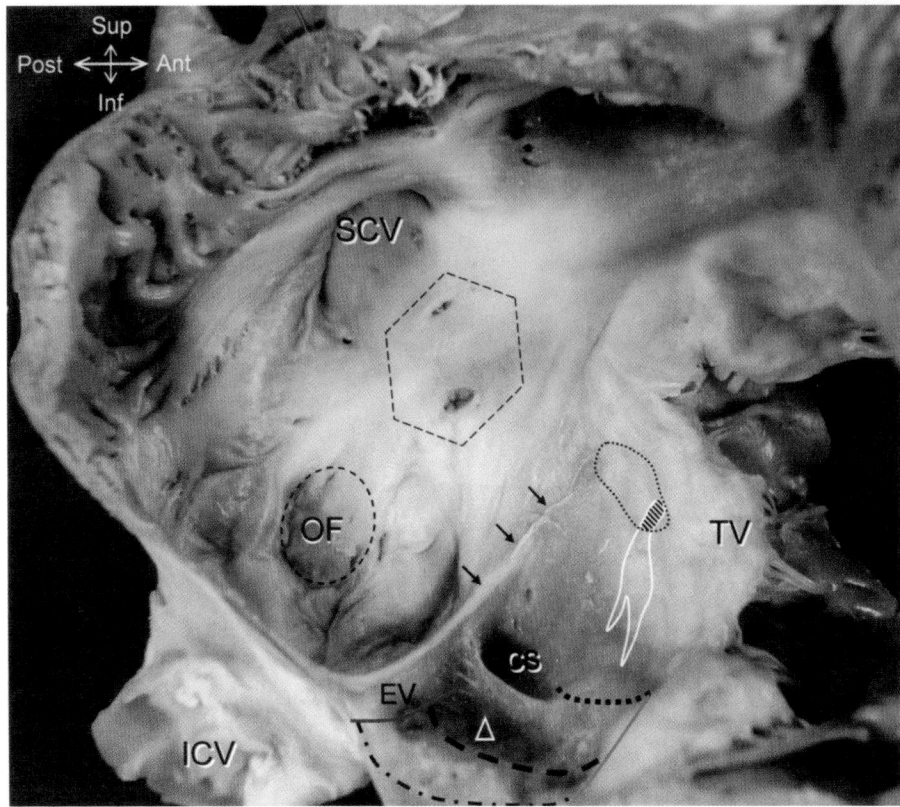

FIGURE 34–6. Simulating a right anterior oblique projection, the right atrium is opened to show the septal aspect that appears extensive, but the area marked by the hexagon is not septal. Termed the *aortic mound*, it is the anterior wall of the right atrium that abuts the non- and right coronary aortic sinuses. The true septum is limited to the valve of the oval foramen and its immediate muscular rim. The triangle of Koch is delineated posteriorly by the tendon of Todaro (*arrows*) running in the Eustachian ridge, anteriorly by the hinge line of the septal leaflet of the tricuspid valve, and inferiorly by the coronary sinus. The apex of the triangle is marked by the central fibrous body (*dotted shape*) through which the atrioventricular conduction bundle penetrates (*hatched*). The atrioventricular node and its inferior extensions are depicted by the white shape. The cavo-tricuspid isthmus is bordered posteriorly by the Eustachian valve (*blue line*) and anteriorly by the tricuspid valve (*red line*). Within this area are marked three isthmuses: paraseptal isthmus (*dots*), inferior or central flutter isthmus (*dashes*), and inferolateral isthmus (*dots and dashes*). The inferior isthmus passes through the sinus of Keith (*triangle*). The coronary sinus is guarded by a crescentic thebesian valve. CS, coronary sinus; ER, Eustachian ridge; EV, Eustachian valve; ICV, inferior caval vein; OF, oval foramen; SCV, superior caval vein; TV, tricuspid valve.

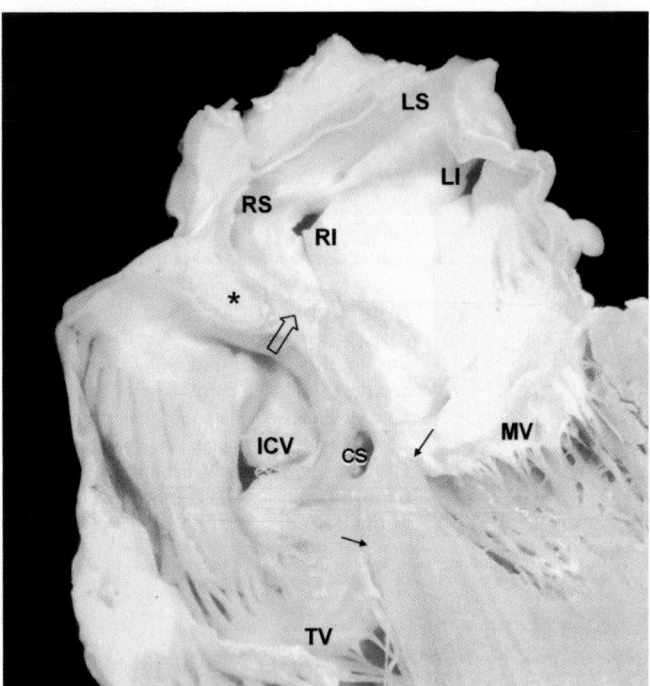

FIGURE 34–7. This long-axis section through the heart profiles the cardiac septum to show the thin valve of the oval foramen (*open arrow*) on the left atrial side and the muscular rim on the right atrial side. This cut reveals the infolding of the right atrial wall at the superior rim that is filled with epicardial fat (*asterisk*) to form the interatrial groove. At the ventricular septum, the leaflets of the tricuspid and mitral valves are hinged at different levels (*small arrows*) producing offset between the right and left atrioventricular junctions. Thus, the vestibule of the right atrium overlies the ventricular septum. CS, coronary sinus; ICV, inferior caval vein; LI, left inferior pulmonary vein; LS, left superior pulmonary vein; MV, mitral valve; RI, right inferior pulmonary vein; RS, right superior pulmonary vein; TV, tricuspid valve.

gives the impression of an extensive anterior septal wall is the anteromedial wall of the atrium lying behind the aorta through the transverse pericardial sinus (see Fig. 34–6). The superior rim as demonstrated in a *four-chamber* section is then the infolded wall between the superior caval vein and the right pulmonary veins (Fig. 34–7). Significantly, the folded rim is not a septal area. Enclosed within the fold is epicardial fat. The left aspect of the atrial septum lacks the crater like feature of the right side. The valve itself is usually fibromuscular. From the right atrium, the leftward part of the muscular fold apposing the valve continues into the musculature of the left atrial wall (see Fig. 34–7).

The true septum that interventionalists can cross safely is limited to the flap valve of the oval fossa and the immediate muscular rim that surrounds it on the right atrial aspect (see Fig. 34–7). The valve of the oval foramen can be perforated or crossed without risk of exiting the heart or damaging the arterial supply to the sinus node. Most hearts have a well-defined muscular rim on the right atrial aspect allowing the operator to *feel* the *jump* from firm muscular rim to tenting of the thin valve with the catheter for safe trans-septal puncture. Importantly, nearly one-fifth of hearts have little change in contour, and the valve is thicker making it difficult to identify the fossa.[23]

In approximately one-fourth of the normal population, there is probe patency of the oval fossa, even though on the left atrial side the valve is large enough to overlap the rim. This is because the adhesion of the valve to the rim is incomplete, leaving a gap usually in the anterosuperior margin corresponding to a C-shaped mark in the left atrial side just behind the anterior atrial wall (Fig. 34–8). The gap in adhesion allows a probe, or catheter, in the right atrium to slip between the rim and the valve into the left atrial chamber. A catheter lodged in this crevice will have its tip directed toward the anterior wall of the left atrium. This part of the wall, just inferior to the Bachmann bundle, can be very thin (see Fig. 34–8; Fig. 34–9). Exiting the heart here leads to the transverse pericardial sinus and, anteriorly, the aortic root.

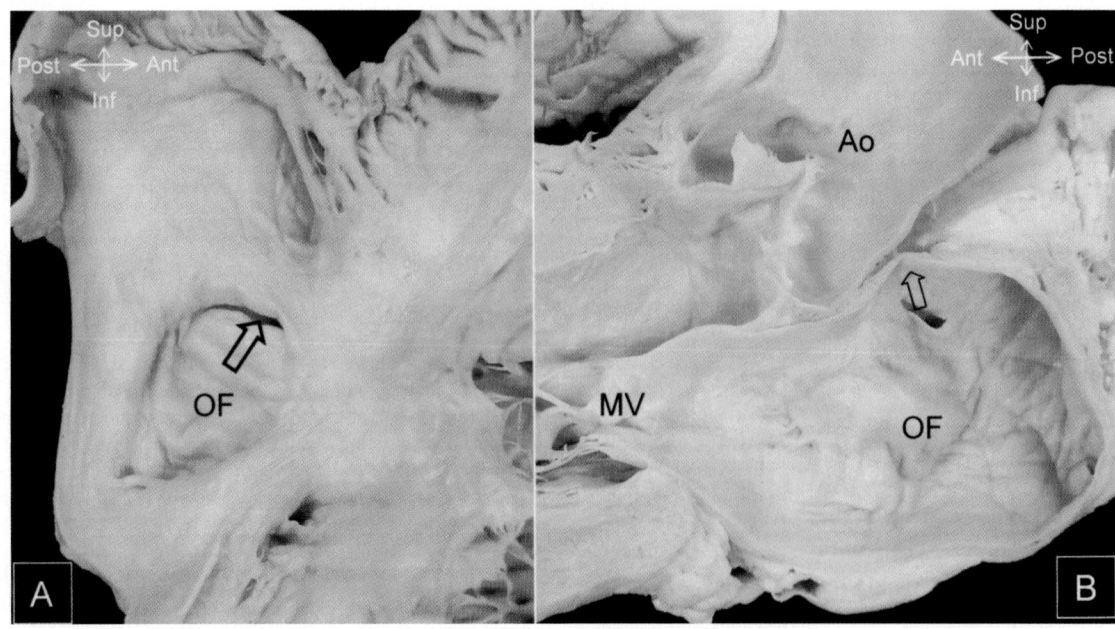

FIGURE 34–8. A. Displayed in right anterior oblique view, the anterior-cephalad margin (*open arrow*) of this oval foramen will allow a probe to pass into the left atrium behind. **B.** The left atrial view of the same heart shows the crevice through which the probe will exit and its proximity to the thin part of the left atrial wall anteriorly (*open arrow*). Ao, aorta; OF, oval foramen; MV, mitral valve.

Muscular continuity between atriums peripheral to the septum is frequently found as bridges in the subepicardium.[8,9] The most prominent interatrial bridge is the Bachmann bundle (see Fig. 34–9). This is a broad muscular band that runs in the subepicardium connecting the anterior right atrial wall of the superior cavoatrial junction with the anterior wall of the left atrium. The muscular fibers in the Bachmann bundle, as in the terminal crest, are well aligned. Multiple smaller interatrial bridges are frequently present, giving the potential for macroreentry. Some connect the muscular sleeves of the right pulmonary veins to the right atrium, and some connect the superior caval vein to the left atrium.[8,9] Posterior and inferior bridges joining the left atrium to the intercaval area on the right provide the potential for posterior breakthrough of sinus impulse (see Fig. 34–9).[24] Inferiorly, further muscular bridges from the left atrial wall often overlie and run into the wall of the coronary sinus.[8] Fine bridges connecting the remnant of the vein of Marshall to the left atrium have also been demonstrated.[25]

【 】 THE LEFT ATRIUM

As with the right atrium, the left atrium has three components and shares its septum. The atrial appendage is characteristically a small fingerlike cul-de-sac in human hearts where thrombi can form.[26] Owing to its tubular shape, its junction with the left atrium is narrow and fairly well defined. Virtually all the pectinate muscles in the left atrium are confined within the appendage. The lumen of the appendage is lined by a complicated network of muscular ridges and intervening membranes that form its wall. Its tip can be directed anteriorly overlying the pulmonary trunk, superiorly behind the arterial pedicle, or posteriorly. When its tip is directed anteriorly, the body of the appendage usually also overlies the main stem of the left coronary artery. The remnant of the vein of Marshall runs on the lateral epicardial aspect of the neck of the appendage, anterior to the left pulmonary veins (Fig. 34–10). The course of the coronary sinus is related to the inferior aspect of the left atrial wall, but it is not immediately adjacent to the hinge line of the leaflets of the mitral valve. In the adult heart, it courses some 6 to 10 mm or more proximally.

The venous component receives the pulmonary veins and the vestibular component leads to the mitral valve. There are no surface anatomical landmarks to separate the vestibule from the pulmonary venous component although frequently a few pits or crevices are seen in the inferior wall at the border zone. These have very thin walls and can be encountered when constructing ablation lines along the so-called *left atrial isthmus* (see Fig. 34–10) to link the orifice of the left inferior pulmonary vein to the mitral annulus.[27,28] Seemingly uniform, the left atrial walls are composed of one to three or more overlapping *layers* of differently aligned myocardial fibers with marked regional variations in thickness.[8,29,30] The area of the anterior wall just behind the aorta is usually thin, whereas the superior wall, or dome, and the interpulmonary wall are thicker but tend to become thinner toward the left pulmonary veins.

The orifices of the right pulmonary veins are directly adjacent to the plane of the atrial septum (see Fig. 34–7). The venous orifices are oval shaped with a longer superoinferior diameter than anteroposterior diameter. On the endocardial surface, the transition between atrium and vein is smooth. The venoatrial junction is obvious when the shape of the vein entering the atrium is cylin-

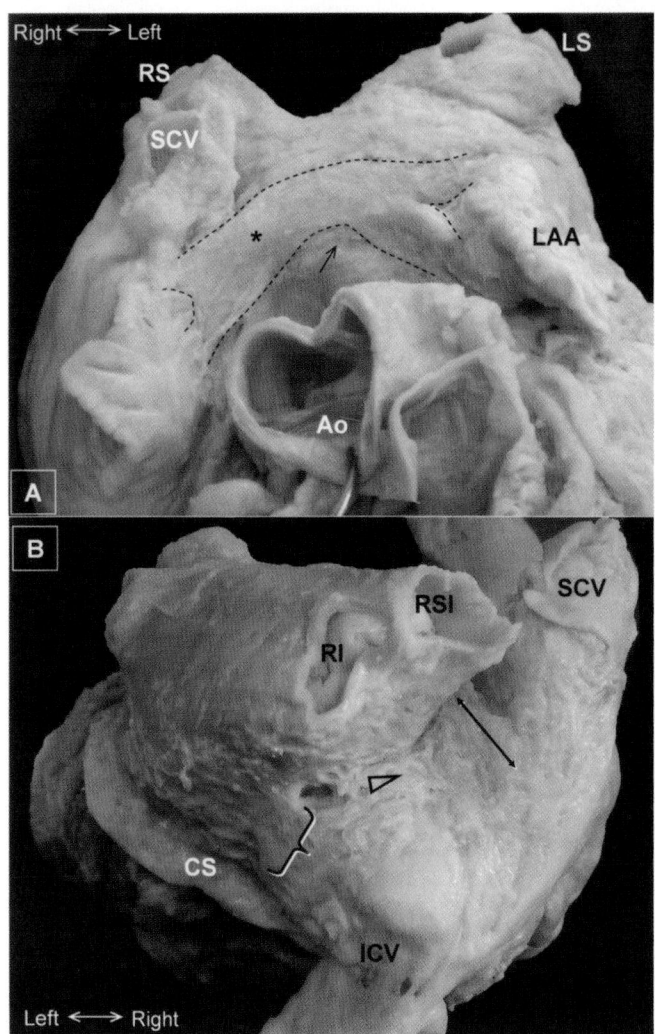

FIGURE 34–9. A. The aortic root is retracted forward to show the anterior wall of the atriums. The Bachmann bundle (*between broken lines*) is displayed crossing the anterior aspect of the interatrial groove (*asterisk*). The *arrow* indicates a thin area of the anterior left atrial wall that is frequently found inferior to the Bachmann bundle. This site corresponds to the thin area indicated on Fig. 34–8B. **B.** A heart tilted forward and viewed from the back shows muscle bridges in addition to the Bachmann bundle. A muscle bundle (*double-headed arrow*) connects the anterior wall of the left atrium with the posterior right atrial wall inferior to the superior caval vein. Further bridges are present posteriorly and inferiorly (*triangle and brace*). Ao, aorta; CS, coronary sinus; ICV, inferior caval vein; LAA, left atrial appendage; LS, left superior pulmonary vein; RI, right inferior pulmonary vein; RS, right superior pulmonary vein; SCV, superior caval vein.

drical (see Fig. 34–10B) but is less clear when the vein enters like a funnel. Musculature of the atrial wall extends into the veins to varying lengths, with the longest sleeves along the upper veins[8,31–35] (Fig. 34–11). Close to the venous insertions, the sleeves are thicker and completely surround the epicardial aspect of the vein. The distal margins of the sleeves, however, are usually thinner and irregular as the musculature fades out. Our studies[8,33] have shown mainly circularly oriented myocardial fibers with interdigitating longitudinally and obliquely oriented fibers in the sleeves. Although electrical activity in this region has long been recognized,[36,37] it is only in fairly recent years that focuses of ectopic activity have been the target of ablative procedures for treatment of paroxysmal atrial fibrillation.[38]

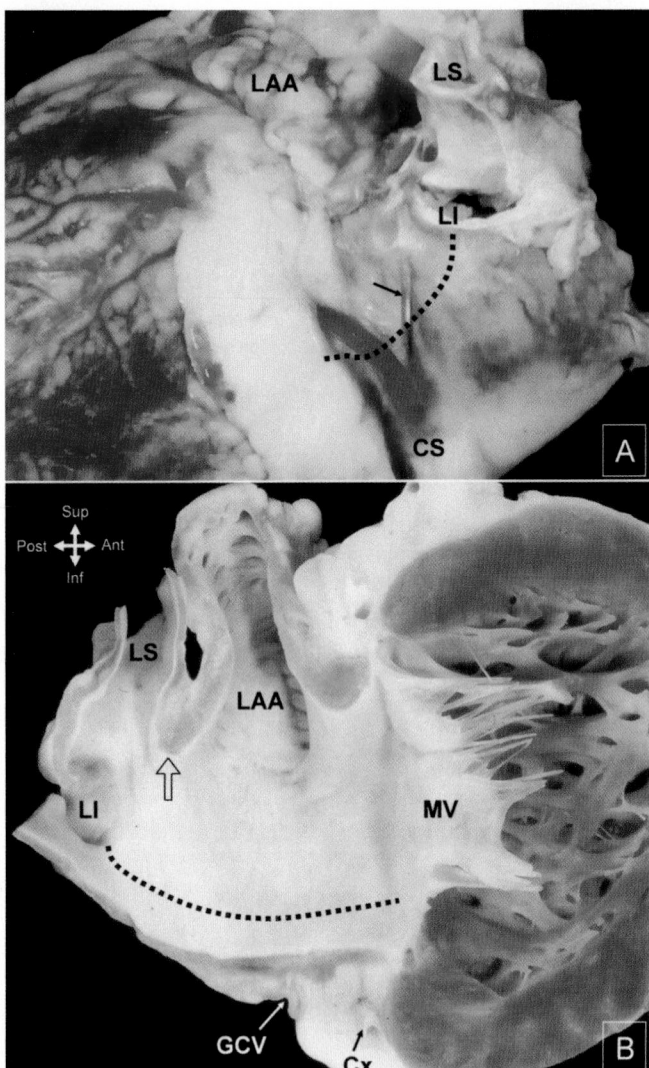

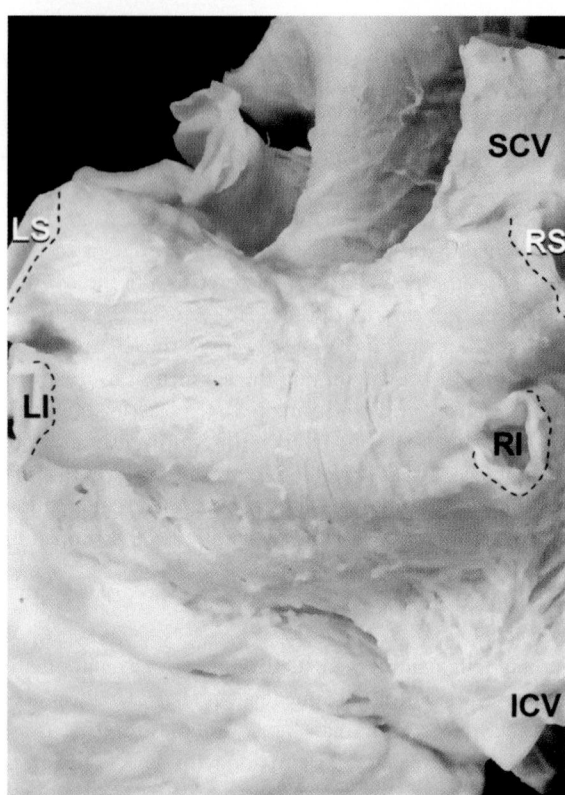

FIGURE 34-11. This view of the epicardial aspect of the left atrium from the back shows the musculature of the atrial wall extending over the pulmonary veins. The broken lines mark the transition from muscular sleeve to bare venous wall. ICV, inferior caval vein; LI, left inferior pulmonary vein; RI, right inferior pulmonary vein; RS, right superior pulmonary vein; SCV, superior caval vein.

FIGURE 34-10. A. This heart viewed from the left and inferior aspect shows a small remnant of the vein of Marshall (*arrow*) descending along the atrial wall in between the left atrial appendage and the left pulmonary veins to enter the coronary sinus. The left atrial isthmus between the left inferior pulmonary vein and the mitral valve is indicated by the *dotted line*. **B.** This long-axis cut through the left atrium and left ventricle shows the orifices of the left pulmonary veins and the left atrial isthmus (*dotted line*). Note the narrow fold (*arrow*) between the os of the left atrial appendage and the orifice of the left superior pulmonary vein in this heart. It can be challenging to keep the ablation catheter stable along this narrow fold without dropping inadvertently into the vein or the appendage. CS, coronary sinus; Cx, circumflex artery; GCV, great cardiac vein; LAA, left atrial appendage; LI, left inferior pulmonary vein; LS, left superior pulmonary vein; MV, mitral valve.

THE ATRIOVENTRICULAR JUNCTIONS

At the atrioventricular junctions the walls of the atriums and ventricles are contiguous and without myocardial continuity except at the site of the penetrating bundle of the atrioventricular conduction tissues. Anomalous muscular atrioventricular connections at the atrioventricular junctions produce the Wolff-Parkinson-White variant of ventricular preexcitation.[39] In describing the location of the accessory bundles, attitudinal terminology is desirable.[1] The

true septal component is limited to the area of the central fibrous body and immediate environs. The so-called *anterior septum* is contiguous with part of the supraventricular crest of the right ventricle, whereas the *posterior septum* is formed by the muscular floor of the coronary sinus overlying the diverging posterior walls of the ventricular mass, and the vestibule of the right atrium overlapping ventricular myocardium. Anatomically, the atrioventricular junction can be described as comprising extensive right and left parietal junctions that meet with a small septal component (Fig. 34–12). The right parietal junction is relatively circular and occupies a near vertical plane in the heart marked by the course of the right coronary artery in the atrioventricular groove. On the endocardial surface, the tricuspid vestibule overlies the ventricular wall. The superior and most medial part of the junction abuts directly on the membranous septum.

The left parietal junction surrounds the orifice of the mitral valve and part of it is the area of fibrous continuity between mitral and aortic valves (see Fig. 34–12). The potential for accessory atrioventricular connections is mainly limited to the junction supporting the hinge line of the mural leaflet of the mitral valve. This runs from posterosuperior to posterior and inferior when the heart is viewed in left-anterior oblique projection. The inferior area harbors the coronary sinus and its tributary, the great cardiac vein (see Fig. 34–10A). The inferior paraseptal region, so-called *posterior septum*, is the inferior pyramidal space, which contains epicardial

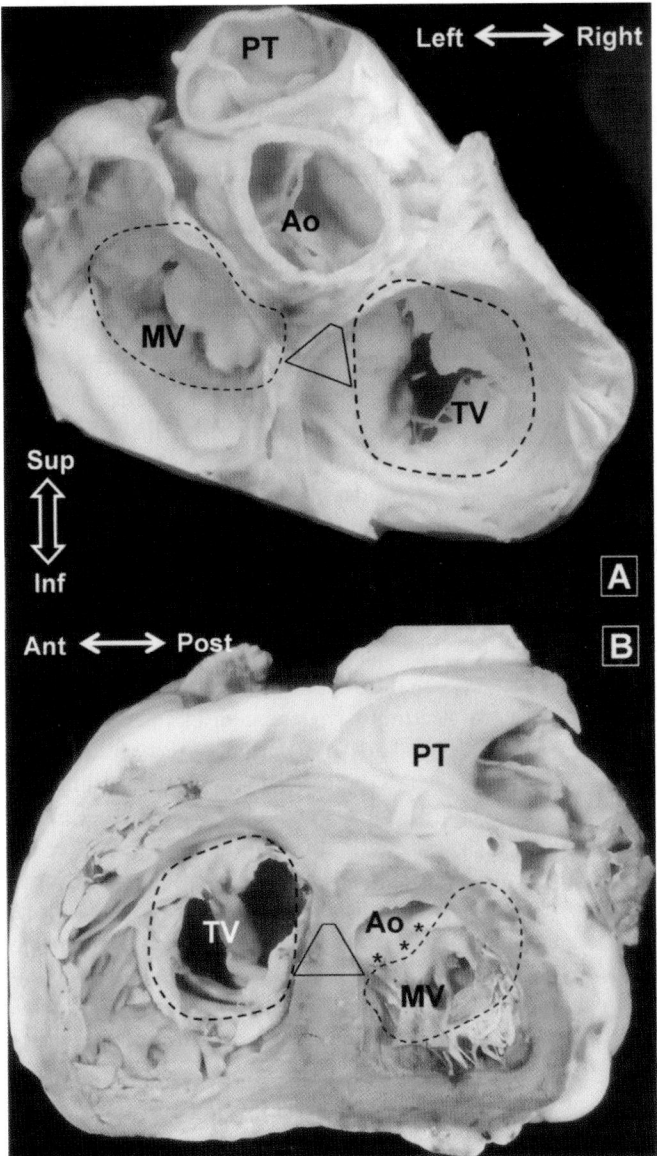

FIGURE 34-12. A. This view of the cardiac base with the *broken lines* representing the hinge lines (annulus) of the mitral and tricuspid valves and the *box* representing the extent of the septum at the atrioventricular junction illustrates how much of the junction is not septal. **B.** Viewed from the ventricular aspect and in attitudinal orientation, the atrioventricular junction is represented by the *broken lines*. Note the area of aortic-mitral valvar continuity indicated with *asterisks* and clearly not a septal area. Ao, aorta; MV, mitral valve; PT, pulmonary trunk; TV, tricuspid valve.

fibrofatty tissues together with the artery supplying the atrioventricular node (Fig. 34-13).[40,41]

THE VENTRICLES

Each ventricle has three components: the inlet containing the atrioventricular valve, the outlet leading to the arterial valve, and the apical trabecular component. The ventricular septum curves as it is traced from inlet toward the outlet portions allowing the right ventricle to lie anterosuperiorly over the left ventricle.

The curvature places the right ventricular outflow tract anteriorly and slightly leftward to that of the left ventricle's resulting in a

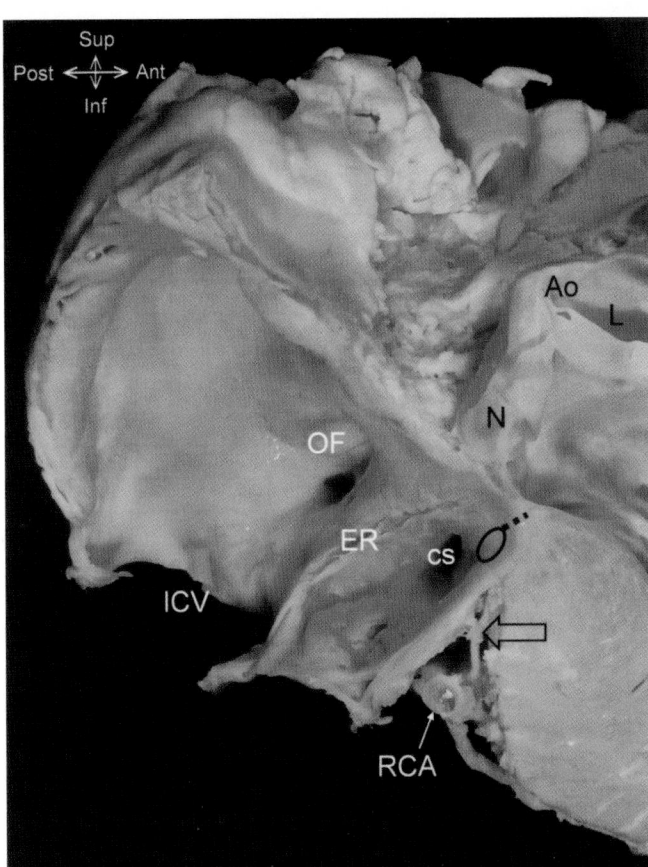

FIGURE 34-13. This longitudinal section through the inferior pyramidal space reveals the right atrial wall overlying the right coronary artery and the arterial branch (*open arrow*) supplying the atrioventricular node (*oval*). Note the proximity of the noncoronary aortic sinus to the right atrial wall and the His bundle (*dots*). Ao, aorta; CS, coronary sinus; ER, Eustachian ridge; ICV, inferior caval vein; N, noncoronary aortic sinus; OF, oval foramen; RCA, right coronary artery.

characteristic *crossover* relationship between right and left ventricular outflows (Fig. 34-14).

THE RIGHT VENTRICLE

The right ventricle in the normal heart is the most anteriorly situated cardiac chamber because it is located immediately behind the sternum. It is triangular in shape when viewed from the front. When seen from the apex, the right edge of the right ventricle is sharp forming the acute margin of the heart.

The right ventricular inlet extends from the hinge line (annulus) of the tricuspid valve to the papillary muscles. The leaflets of the tricuspid valve can be distinguished as septal, anterosuperior, and inferior or mural. The septal leaflet with its cords inserting directly to the ventricular septum is characteristic of the tricuspid valve. The medial papillary muscle, a small out-budding from the septum, supports the junction (commissure) between the septal and anterosuperior leaflets (Fig. 34-15). A larger papillary muscle, the anterior papillary muscle, supports the extensive anterosuperior leaflet and its junction with the inferior leaflet. The junction between anterosuperior and inferior leaflets is supported by a group of small papillary muscles, the inferior papillary muscles.

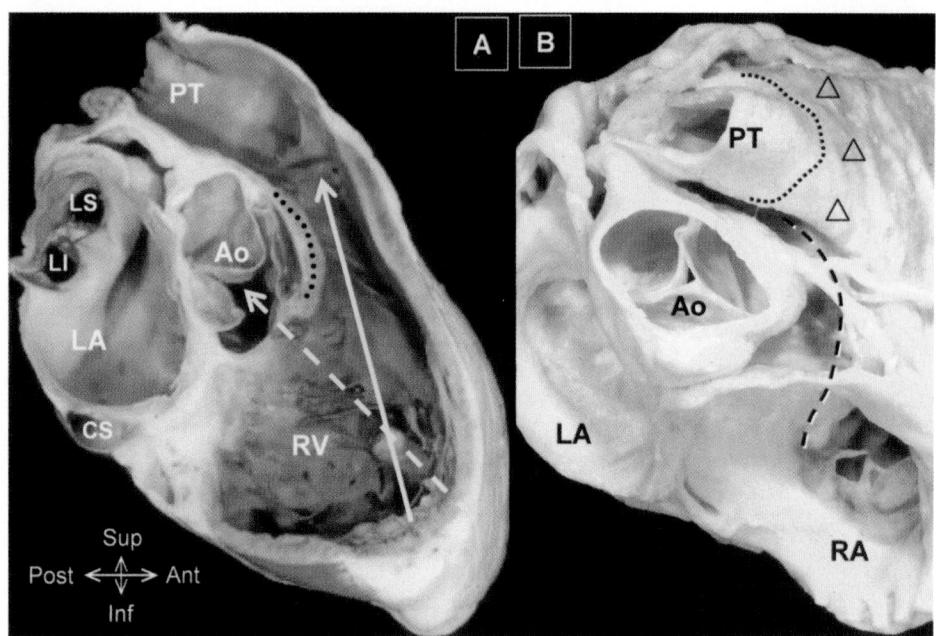

FIGURE 34–14. A. This sagittal section through a heart shows the aortic root in the middle. From the cardiac apex to the pulmonary valve, the right ventricular outflow tract (*solid arrow*) overlies the left ventricular outflow tract (*broken arrow*), which is behind the ventricular septum. The subpulmonary muscular infundibulum (*dots*) that lies anterior to the aortic valve is not septal. **B.** This dissection shows the relationship between the pulmonary and aortic valves. Note the musculature forming the freestanding subpulmonary infundibulum (*triangles*) that is proximal to the ventriculoarterial junction (*dotted line*). The deeper location of the ventricular septum is indicated by the *broken line*. Ao, aorta; CS, coronary sinus; LA, left atrium; LI, left inferior pulmonary vein; LS, left superior pulmonary vein; PT, pulmonary trunk; RA, right atrium; RV, right ventricle.

Coarse muscular trabeculations crisscross the apical portion. One of them, the moderator band, is characteristic of the right ventricle (see Fig. 34–15). This bridges the ventricular cavity between the body of the septomarginal trabeculation and the parietal wall, giving rise to the anterior papillary muscle along the way. Within its musculature runs a major fascicle of the right bundle branch. The septomarginal trabeculation itself is a Y-shaped muscular band that is adherent to the septal surface. In between its limbs lies the infolding of the heart wall forming the ventricular roof, an area also known as the supraventricular crest (see Fig. 34–15). This crest separates the two right heart valves and is an integral part of the outlet, continuous with the free-standing subpulmonary muscular infundibulum that is a tubelike structure supporting the pulmonary valve. Although ablationists refer to septal and free-wall portions of the right ventricular outflow tract, it should be noted that the infundibulum does not have a septal component (see Fig. 34–15) because the pulmonary valve can be resected surgically for the Ross procedure[42] without entering the left ventricle. The septal component of the right ventricular outlet is only in its most proximal part, where it continues into the supraventricular crest. Furthermore, the right ventricular outlet curves to pass anterior and cephalad to the left ventricular outlet (see Fig. 34–14). Any perforation in the *septal* part is more likely to go outside the heart than into the left ventricle (see Fig. 34–15). Two of the pulmonary sinuses are adjacent to two aortic sinuses, the right and left coronary sinuses, although the planes of the aortic and pulmonary valves are at and angle to one another (see Fig. 34–14). Thus, the main coronary arteries can also be at risk when ablating in the so-called *septal part* (see Figs. 34–14 and 34–15).

The infundibulum immediately beneath the pulmonary valve has a smooth wall. The crescentic hinge lines of the pulmonary leaflets cross the anatomic junction between ventricular musculature and arterial wall, enclosing within the sinuses small semilunar areas of myocardium (see Fig. 34–15).[43]

THE LEFT VENTRICLE

The left ventricle approximates to a conical shape. When the heart is viewed from the front, most of the left ventricle is behind the right ventricle. Its outlet overlaps its inlet. The hinge (annulus) of the mitral leaflets at the entrance to the inlet has a very limited attachment to septal structures (see Fig. 34–12). Compared to that of the tricuspid valve, the septal hinge line of the mitral valve is further away from the apex, and it does not have a septal leaflet (see Fig. 34–7). The larger portion of the valve is hinged to the parietal atrioventricular junction, whereas one-third is the span of fibrous continuity with the aortic valve (see Fig. 34–12). At the septal end of valvar fibrous continuity is the right fibrous trigone, and at the parietal end is the left fibrous trigone (Fig. 34–16A; see Fig. 34–12B). The right trigone in continuity with the membranous septum forms the central fibrous body. The two leaflets of the mitral valve are disproportionate in size. The *anterior* leaflet in continuity with the aortic valve is deep, whereas the mural (or *posterior*) leaflet is shallow. The mitral leaflets are attached by means of tendinous cords exclusively to two groups of papillary muscles.

The apical component of the left ventricle extends from the papillary muscles to the ventricular apex. At the apex, the muscular wall tapers to only 1 to 2 mm thick. The trabeculations are finer than those found in the right ventricle. Occasionally, fine muscular strands or so-called *false tendons* extend between the septum and the papillary muscles or the parietal wall.[44] Often, they carry the distal ramifications of the left bundle branch. In recent years they have been have been implicated in idiopathic left ventricular tachycardia.[45]

The left ventricular outlet is bordered by the muscular ventricular septum anterosuperiorly and the aortic (*anterior*) leaflet of the mitral valve posteroinferiorly (see Fig. 34–16). The upper part of the ventricular septum leading to the aortic valve is smooth. The common atrioventricular conduction bundle emerges from the central fibrous body to pass between the membranous septum and the crest of the muscular ventricular septum (see Fig. 34–16B). The landmark for the site of the atrioventricular conduction bundle is the fibrous body that adjoins the crescentic hinge lines of the right and noncoronary leaflets of the aortic valve. From here, the left bundle branch descends in the subendocardium and usually branches into three main fascicles that interconnect and further

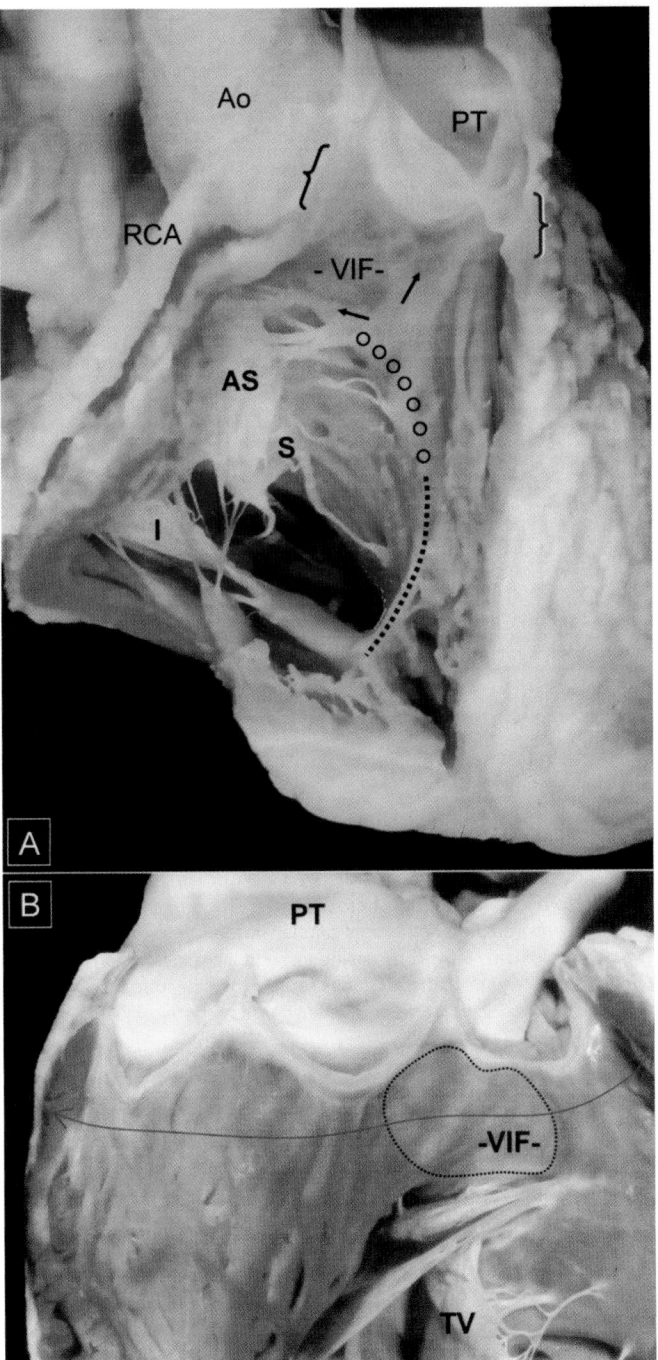

FIGURE 34–15. A. The inside of the right ventricle is displayed to show the supraventricular crest in between the pulmonary and tricuspid valves. The limbs (*arrows*) of the septomarginal trabeculation cradle the ventriculoinfundibular fold at the crest. The braces indicate the subpulmonary infundibulum. The course of the right bundle branch in the subendocardium of the septomarginal trabeculation is indicated by circles. One of its fascicles passes into the moderator band (*broken line*). **B.** The right ventricular outflow tract is displayed. The leaflets of the pulmonary valve have been removed to show the semilunar hinge lines crossing the ventriculoarterial junction. Each sinus thus includes a crescentic segment of ventricular wall (*dark areas*). *Double-headed arrow* indicates the free wall of the subpulmonary infundibulum. The area within the *dotted line* represents the so-called *septal* or *high septal* component but is actually free wall also. Ao, aorta; AS, anterosuperior; I, inferior; S, septal leaflet of tricuspid valve; PT, pulmonary trunk; RCA, right coronary artery; TV, tricuspid valve; VIF, ventriculoinfundibular fold.

divide into finer and finer branches as the *Purkinje* network (see below).

In the outlet, two leaflets of the aortic valve have muscular support, these being the ones adjacent to, or facing, the pulmonary valve. The third sinus, the noncoronary sinus, does not have muscular support. The facing aortic sinuses give rise to the right and left coronary arteries. Like the pulmonary valves, these two sinuses contain small segments of ventricular myocardium within (see Fig. 34–16A).[46] The musculature in the aortic sinuses can be a source of repetitive monomorphic ventricular tachycardia. Owing to the spatial relationship of the subpulmonary infundibulum and the left ventricular outlet (Fig. 34–17), the foci can be ablated from within the part of the right ventricular outlet that overlies the adjacent aortic sinuses.[47] Because the main coronary arteries arise from the arterial part of the sinuses, they are not in the immediate field. Ablations within the sinuses without trauma to the coronary arteries have also been reported.[48,49] The noncoronary aortic sinus, being immediately adjacent to the paraseptal region of the left and right atriums and close to the superior atrioventricular junction, can be used to map and ablate focal atrial tachycardia that have earliest activation in the vicinity of the His bundle area (see Fig. 34–13).[50]

THE CORONARY VEINS

The venous return from the myocardium is channelled either by means of small thebesian veins that open directly into the cardiac chambers or, more significantly, is collected by the greater coronary venous system that drains 85 percent of the venous flow.[51,52] The main coronary veins in the greater system are the great, middle, and small cardiac veins. The great and middle veins run alongside the anterior descending and posterior descending coronary arteries respectively and drain into the coronary sinus. As the great cardiac vein ascends into the left atrioventricular groove, it passes close to the first division of the left coronary artery and under the cover of the left atrial appendage. Approaching the coronary sinus, the great vein is joined by tributaries from the left ventricular obtuse margin and the inferior wall, as well as veins from the left atrium (Fig. 34–18). The distribution, courses, and calibres of the left ventricular veins vary from individual to individual. When using them for pacing lead implants it is worth noting that the left phrenic nerve running in the pericardium can pass across the obtuse marginal vein (see Fig. 34–2).[7] The left ventricular veins can be accessed for ablating ventricular tachycardia from a source close to the epicardium.[53] Although coronary veins are usually superficial to arteries, crossovers between arteries and veins are not uncommon.[54] Furthermore, when deploying catheters or wires in superficial veins, care should be taken because venous wall is thin and *unprotected* by muscle on the epicardial side.

The entrance of the vein of Marshall, or oblique left atrial vein, marks the venous end of the tube-shaped coronary sinus. The vein is a fibrous ligament in most individuals. Even when a lumen is present it is narrow, rarely exceeding 2 centimeters (cm) in length before tapering to a blind end (see Fig. 34–10). If adequately wide, this channel can be used for ablating the left atrial wall. In the absence of the vein of Marshall, or its remnant, the Vieussens valve is taken as the anatomic landmark for

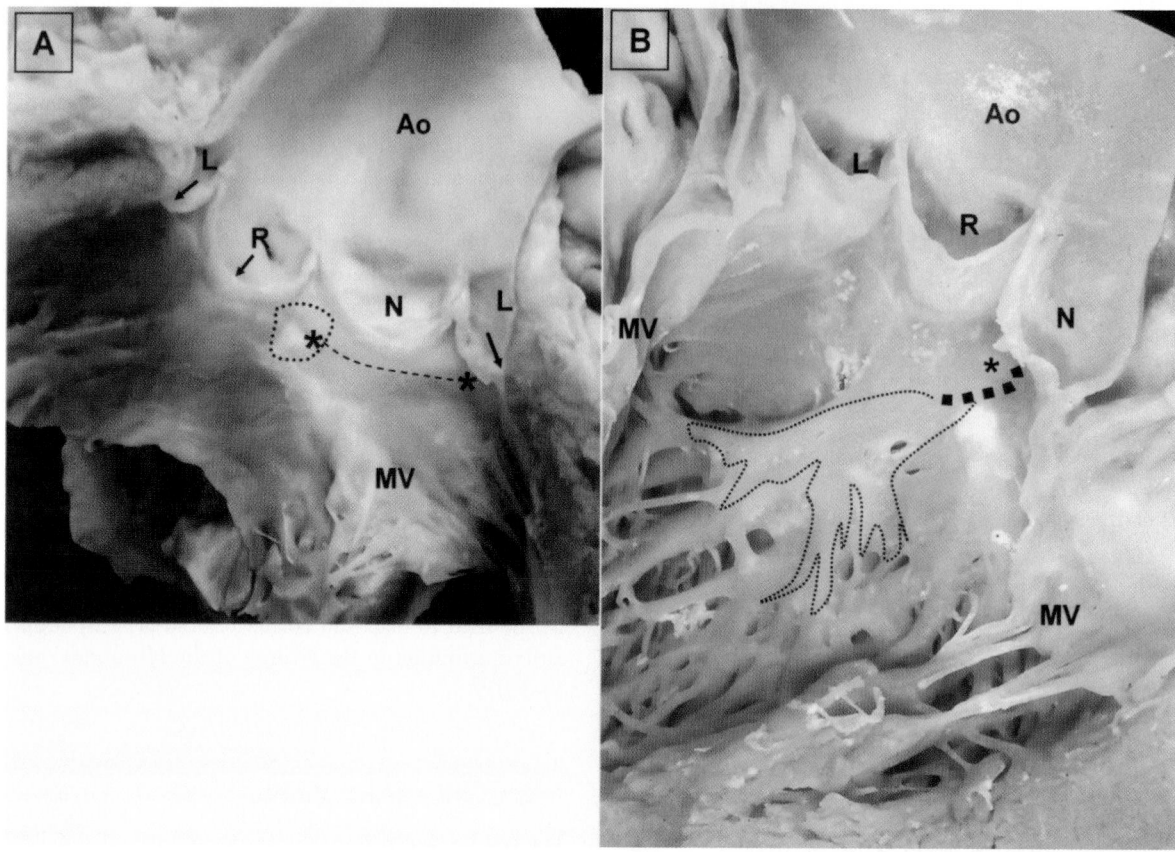

FIGURE 34–16. A. The left ventricular outflow tract incised through the left coronary aortic sinus is displayed to show the location of the membranous septum (*dotted shape*), and aortic-mitral fibrous continuity (*broken line*) with the fibrous trigones (*asterisks*) at each end. The aortic leaflets have been removed to show the muscular components (*arrows*) in the right and left coronary aortic sinuses that can be ablated for aortic sinus ventricular tachycardia. **B.** The aortic root is displayed by cutting through the *anterior* leaflet of the mitral valve. The atrioventricular conduction bundle (*broken line*) passes between the membranous septum (*asterisk*) and the muscular septum. The irregular shape represents the left bundle branch and its three fascicles. Ao, aorta; L, left coronary aortic sinus; MV, mitral valve; N, noncoronary aortic sinus; R, right coronary aortic sinus.

the junction between the coronary sinus and the great cardiac vein. Found in 80 to 90 percent of hearts, this very flimsy valve has one to three leaflets that can provide some resistance to the catheter.[19] Once past the Vieussens valve, a sharp bend in the great cardiac vein can cause further obstruction in 20 percent of cases.[20] Another marker for the junction between vein and coronary sinus is the end of the muscular sleeve around the sinus. But, in some cases, the sleeve can extend to 1 cm or more over the vein.[54] Bundles from the sleeve sometimes run into the left atrial wall and also cover the outer walls of adjacent coronary arteries.[55]

The middle cardiac vein drains into the coronary sinus just within the sinus os. Occasionally the middle vein enters the right atrium directly and opens adjacent to the os of the coronary sinus, providing the coronary sinus catheter with an alternative, but undesired, portal. The

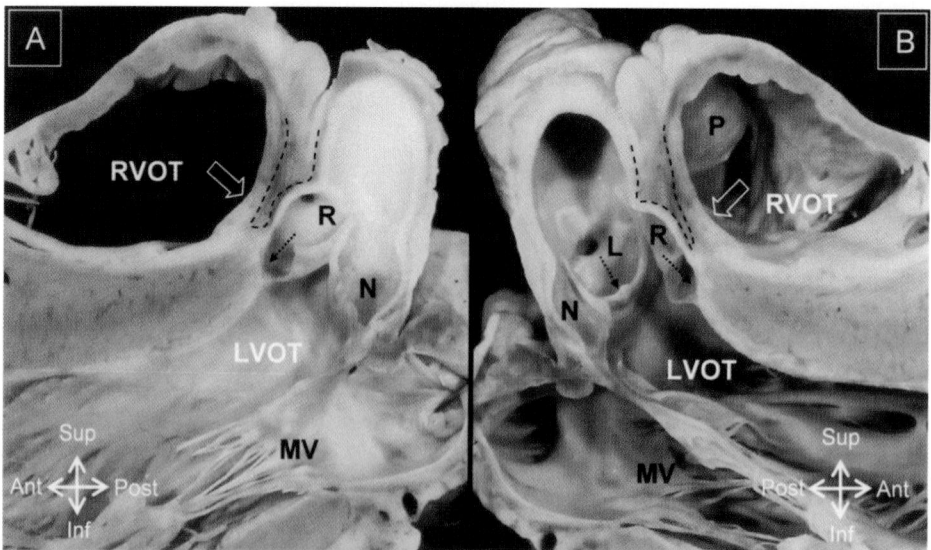

FIGURE 34–17. A and **B** are two halves of a heart cut longitudinally to show the relationship between left and right ventricular outflow tracts and why ablation of foci within the so-called *septal component* (*open arrows*) of the subpulmonary infundibulum can be approached from the adjacent aortic sinuses. Ablation of aortic sinus ventricular tachycardia target the muscle enclosed within the right and left coronary aortic sinuses (*arrows*). Note the epicardial fat (*within broken lines*) between the subpulmonary infundibulum and the aortic root. P, pulmonary valve; LVOT, left ventricular outflow tract; MV, mitral valve; N, noncoronary aortic sinus; R, right coronary aortic sinus; RVOT, right ventricular outflow tract.

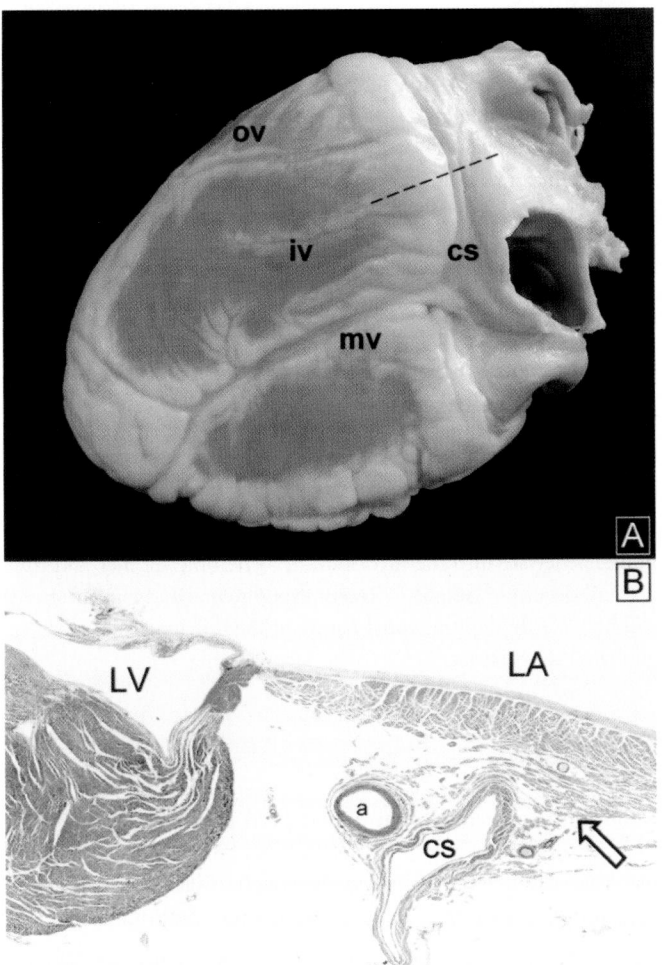

FIGURE 34–18. A. View of the diaphragmatic aspect showing cardiac veins draining into the coronary sinus. *Broken line* indicates plane of histologic section shown in (B). **B.** The coronary sinus has a muscular wall (*tissue stained pink*). This section shows muscular continuity (*arrow*) between the coronary sinus and the left atrial wall. The muscle has also surrounded the coronary artery. a, circumflex artery; CS, coronary sinus; iv, inferior left ventricular vein; LA, left atrium; LV, left ventricle; mv, middle cardiac vein; ov, left obtuse marginal vein.

middle vein passes just superficial to the right coronary artery at the cardiac crux. It is a useful portal for ablating accessory atrioventricular pathways located in the inferior pyramidal space.[56] Very rarely, the entrance of the middle vein is dilated and surrounded by a cuff of muscle giving the potential for accessory atrioventricular connections.[57,58]

The small cardiac vein receives tributaries from the right atrium and the inferior wall of the right ventricle before coursing in the right atrioventricular junction to open to the right margin of the coronary sinus orifice, or into the middle cardiac vein. When joined by the acute marginal vein, or vein of Galen, the small vein becomes larger. Several other veins, from the anterior surface of the right ventricle and from the acute margin, drain directly into the right atrium. In some hearts, the anterior veins merge into a venous lake in the right atrial wall. Again, these can be surrounded by a cuff of myocardium that gives the potential for accessory atrioventricular connection as the vein passes through the atrioventricular groove.[59]

THE CARDIAC CONDUCTION SYSTEM

Although much has been written about "specialized internodal tracts" connecting the sinus node to the atrioventricular node, their existence in the form as originally defined by early anatomists has never been demonstrated.[60–62] The myocardium between the nodes bears no histological characteristic of specialization or insulated bundles that in any way resemble the ventricular bundle branches.[63] Instead, the internodal myocardium is arranged in broad bands that surround the orifices of the large veins, the tricuspid valve, and the oval fossa. Bands such as the rim of the oval fossa and the terminal crest are raised ridges on the endocardial aspect and tend to have an orderly alignment of the myocardial fibers.[9] The Bachmann bundle and other interatrial bundles are not insulated by fibrous sheaths nor do they have well defined origins and terminations (see Fig. 34–9).

THE SINUS NODE

The sinus node is crescent like in shape with a mean length of 13.5 mm in the adult heart.[10,11] It is usually described as having a head, body, and tail, with the head portion situated cephalad and close to the superior margin of the terminal groove. In most cases the head is subepicardial, whereas the tail penetrates inferiorly into the myocardium of the terminal crest to lie closer to the subendocardium. The node is richly supplied with nerves from both the sympathetic chains and the vagus nerve. Nodal tissues are usually penetrated by a prominent nodal artery.[64] Although the specialized myocytes of the nodal cells are set in a fibrous matrix, the node is not encased in a fibrous sheath. The borders of the node are irregular with frequent interdigitations between nodal and ordinary atrial myocytes, facilitating communication between node and right atrial wall.[10,11]

THE ATRIOVENTRICULAR CONDUCTION SYSTEM

In the normal situation, the atrioventricular conduction system provides the only pathway of muscular continuity between atrial and ventricular myocardium. There is an interface of transitional cells between ordinary atrial myocardium and the histologically specialized cells that make up the atrioventricular node. These cells are arranged to provide anterior, inferior, and deep inputs to the compact atrioventricular node. The anterior input sweeps from the anterior margin of the oval fossa deep to the ordinary myocardium of the tricuspid vestibule. The inferior input approaches the compact node from the musculature in the floor of the coronary sinus and from the Eustachian ridge. The deep input bridges the compact node with the left atrial vestibule and inferior rim of the oval fossa.

The compact atrioventricular node described as the *Knoten* by Tawara[65] in his extensive 1906 monograph is located near the apex of the triangle of Koch (see Fig. 34–6). In the adult it is approximately 5 mm long and wide.[66] In the majority of hearts, inferior extensions from the node pass to the right and left sides of the artery that penetrates the compact node.[66,67] The right extension courses parallel and adjacent to the hinge of the tricuspid valve, whereas the left extension projects toward the mitral vestibule. The distance of the right inferior extension to the endocardial surface is approximately 1 to 5 mm. Put in the context of the right atrial landmarks of the triangle of Koch, the compact node is near the apex, but the right inferior extensions reach to the mid level of the triangle and can even extend to the vicinity of the coronary sinus in cases with small triangle.[68]

Superiorly, at the apex of the Koch triangle, the penetrating atrioventricular conduction bundle of His passes through the central fibrous body leftward. This short bundle of specialized myocardium encased in a fibrous sheath is a direct extension of the compact atrioventricular node, enabling atrial activity to be conveyed to the ventricles. As discussed previously, the emergence of the bundle in the ventricles is directly related to the membranous septum and the aortic outflow tract. The bundle is sandwiched between the membranous septum and the crest of the ventricular septum. After a short distance, on the left of the septal crest, the bundle bifurcates into the left and right bundle branches. The left bundle branch fans out as it descends in the subepicardium of the septal surface the left ventricle (see Fig. 34–16). In contrast, the right bundle branch is cordlike and descends through the musculature of the ventricular septum to emerge in the subendocardium at the base of the medial papillary muscle to run in the septomarginal trabeculation (see Fig. 34–15). Along its descent, a prominent branch crosses to the parietal wall within the moderator band. Both bundle branches are insulated as they descend toward the apical parts of the ventricles. The branches then ramify as the Purkinje fibers, these running in the subendocardium and into the myocardium like a network as shown in the diagrams in Tawara's monograph[65] and can be demonstrated in animal hearts by injections (Fig. 34–19). In the subendocardium of the ventricular walls, they can be traced crossing the ventricular cavities in *false tendons*. Recently, triggers of ventricular fibrillation have been mapped to the Purkinje system in the right ventricular outflow tract and successfully ablated.[69]

In some hearts, the atrioventricular bundle itself continues beyond the bifurcation as a third bundle. Termed the dead-end tract, this runs on the crest of the septum and, thus far, has not been ascribed any function.[70]

FAT PADS AND INNERVATION

Extracardiac nerves from the mediastinum reach the heart through the areas bounded by the serous pericardium. These sites around the great veins at the cardiac base and around the pulmonary trunk and aorta are referred to as the *hilum of the heart*.[71] Nerves from the venous part of the hilum extend mainly to the atria, whereas those from the arterial pole predominantly reach the ventricles, but there are also multiple connections. Several branches of mediastinal nerves between the aorta and the pulmonary trunk connect with the aortic root and the superior region of the left

atrium.[72] Six to ten collections of ganglia, ganglionated subplexuses of the epicardiac neural plexus, have been described in the human heart.[73,74] One-half of the subplexuses are located on the atria and the other half on the ventricles. Occasional ganglia are located in other atrial and ventricular regions of the epicardium.[72] The ganglionated subplexuses are generally associated with islands of adipose tissue referred to as fat pads that serve as visual landmarks to cardiac surgeons.[74] The atrial fat pads are located in the interatrial groove, at the cavo-atrial junctions and on the left atrial wall in the vicinity of the venoatrial junctions (Fig. 34–20). Pauza and colleagues[73] found up to 50 percent of all cardiac ganglia on the posterior and posterolateral surfaces of the left atrium, although Singh and colleagues[74] reported that the largest populations of ganglia are adjacent to the sinus and atrioventricular nodes reflecting different methodologies of studies. The ganglia within each subplexus are interconnected by thin nerves, although ganglia of adjacent subplexuses are also interconnected, forming the meshwork of epicardiac neural plexus. Further nerves penetrate into the myocardium to become thinner and thinner and devoid of ganglia.[71] Recent experimental and clinical studies will help clarify the functional nature of the different epicardial ganglionated subplexuses.[75–77]

CONCLUSIONS

Although the structure of the human heart remains unchanged over the ages, understanding of its anatomy has evolved over time as humankind develops imaging and therapeutic strategies, each calling for a revisit of anatomy. In recent decades, the development of electrophysiologic mapping and catheter-ablation techniques has out-

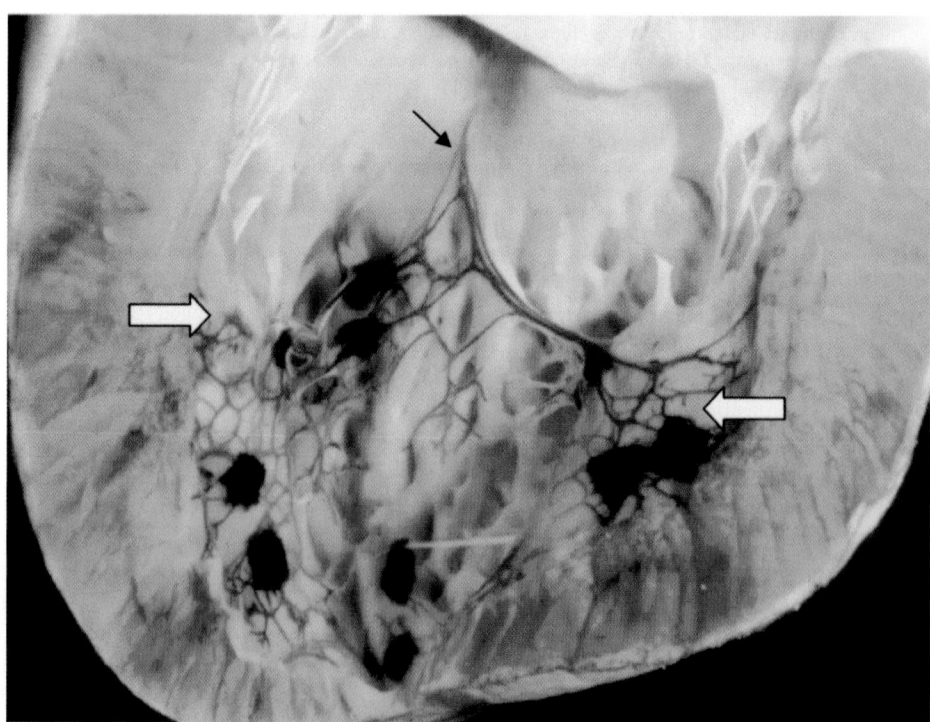

FIGURE 34–19. This preparation of a sheep heart shows the left bundle branch (*small arrow*) fanning out into interconnecting fascicles and *false tendons* carrying the distal ramifications across the cavity to the papillary muscles (*white arrows*).

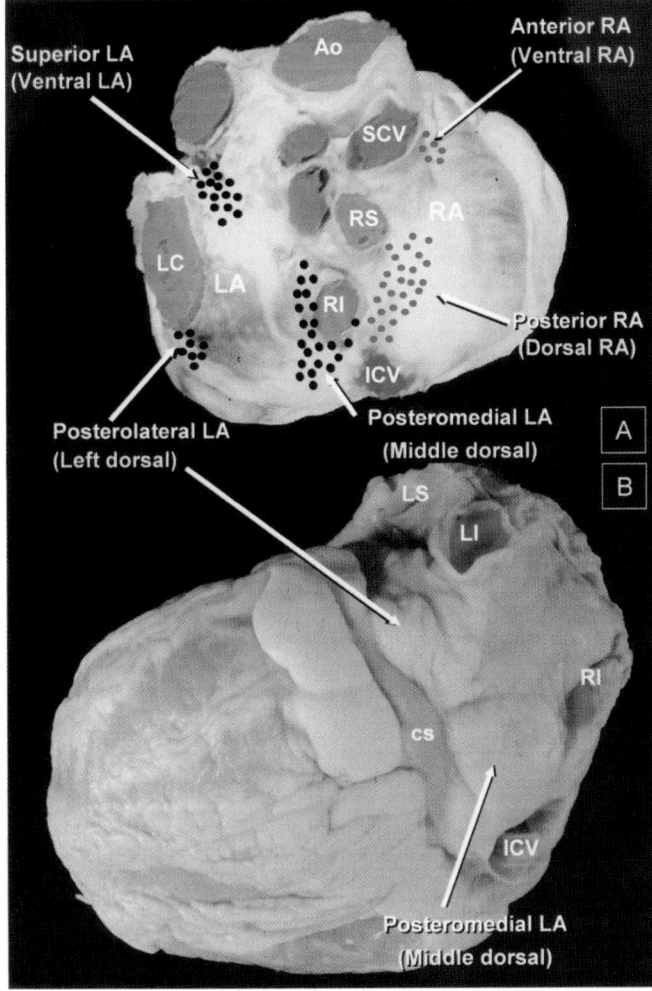

FIGURE 34–20. A and **B**. The atriums viewed from behind and left-inferior respectively to show the fat pads containing ganglionated plexuses (*represented by spots*). The naming of the plexuses is according to Armour et al[72] and Pauza et al[73] (*in brackets*). Ao, aorta; CS, coronary sinus; ICV, inferior caval vein; LA, left atrium; LC, left common pulmonary vein; LI, left inferior pulmonary vein; RA, right atrium; RI, right inferior pulmonary vein; RS, right superior pulmonary vein; SCV, superior caval vein.

paced the work of cardiac anatomists in many ways. Nevertheless, better understanding of detailed anatomy is relevant to clinical electrophysiologists not only to avoid or minimize complications during interventional procedures but also to provide the anatomical background for some of the substrates of certain arrhythmias. From the anatomical viewpoint, description of the heart in attitudinal orientation as originally promulgated by McAlpine[78] in his elegantly illustrated atlas is crucial in understanding living anatomy.

ACKNOWLEDGMENT

The Cardiac Morphology Unit at the Royal Brompton Hospital receives funding support from the Royal Brompton and Harefield Hospital Charitable Fund and the Royal Brompton and Harefield NHS Trust.

REFERENCES

1. Cosio FG, Anderson RH, Kuck K, et al. Living anatomy of the atrioventricular junctions. A guide to electrophysiological mapping. A consensus statement from the Cardiac Nomenclature Group of Arrhythmias, European Society of Cardiology, and the Task Force on Cardiac Nomenclature from NASPE. *Circulation.* 1999;100:e31-e37.

2. Walmsley T. *Quain's Elements of Anatomy. The Heart.* London: Longmans; 1929:28.

3. Doll N, Borger MA, Fabricius A, et al. Esophageal perforation during left atrial radiofrequency ablation: is the risk too high? *J Thorac Cardiovasc Surg.* 2003;125:836–842.

4. Lemola K, Sneider M, Desjardins B, et al. Computed tomographic analysis of the anatomy of the left atrium and the esophagus. Implications for left atrial catheter ablation. *Circulation.* 2004;110:3655–3660.

5. d'Avila A, Scanavacca M, Sosa E, et al. Pericardial anatomy for the interventional electrophysiologist. *J Cardiovasc Electrophysiol.* 2003;14:422–430.

6. Chaffanjon P, Brichon PY, Faure C, et al. Pericardial reflection around the venous aspect of the heart. *Surg Radiol Anat.* 1977;19:17–21.

7. Sanchez-Quintana, Cabrera JA, Climent V, et al. How close are the phrenic nerves to cardiac structures? Implications for cardiac interventionalists. *J Cardiovasc Electrophysiol.* 2005;16:309–313.

8. Ho SY, Sanchez-Quintana D, Cabrera JA, et al. Anatomy of the left atrium: Implications for radiofrequency ablation of atrial fibrillation. *J Cardiovasc Electrophysiol.* 1999;10:1525–33.

9. Ho SY, Anderson RH, Sanchez-Quintana D. Atrial structure and fibres: morphologic bases of atrial conduction. *Cardiovasc Res.* 2002;54:325–336.

10. Truex RC, Smythe MQ, Taylor MJ. Reconstruction of the human sinuatrial node. *Anat Rec.* 1967;159:371–378.

11. Sanchez-Quintana D, Cabrera C, Farre J, et al. Sinus node revisited in the era of electroanatomical mapping and catheter ablation. *Heart.* 2005;91:189–94.

12. Wu TJ, Yashima M, Xie F, et al. Role of pectinate muscle bundles in the generation and maintenance of intra-atrial reentry: potential implications for the mechanism of conversion between atrial fibrillation and atrial flutter. *Circ Res.* 1998;83;448–462.

13. Cabrera JA, Sanchez-Quintana D, Ho SY, et al. The architecture of the atrial musculature between the orifice of the inferior caval vein and the tricuspid valve: the anatomy of the isthmus. *J Cardiovasc Electrophysiol.* 1998;9:1186–1195.

14. Vobril ZB. Todaro's tendon in the heart. I. Todaro's tendon in the normal human heart. *Folia Morph Warsz.* 1967;15:187–192.

15. Ho SY, Anderson RH. How constant anatomically is the tendon of Todaro as a marker of the triangle of Koch? *J Cardiovasc Electrophysiol.* 2000;11:83–89.

16. McGuire MA. Koch's triangle: useful concept or dangerous mistake? *J Cardiovasc Electrophysiol.* 1999;10:1497–1500.

17. Janse MJ, Anderson RH, McGuire MA, et al. "AV nodal" reentry: Part I. "AV nodal reentry revisited. *J Cardiovasc Electrophysiol.* 1993;4:561–572.

18. Sanchez-Quintana D, Davies DW, Ho SY, et al. Architecture of the atrial musculature in and around the triangle of Koch: Its potential relevance to atrioventricular nodal reentry. *J Cardiovasc Electrophysiol.* 1997;8:1396–1407.

19. Ho SY, Sanchez-Quintana D, Becker AE. A review of the coronary venous system: a road less travelled. *Heart Rhythm.* 2004;1:107–112.

20. Corcoran SJ, Lawrence C, McGuire MA. The valve of Vieussens: an important cause of difficulty in advancing catheter into cardiac veins. *J Cardiovasc Electrophysiol.* 1999;10:804–808.

21. Cabrera JA, Sanchez-Quintana D, Ho SY, et al. Angiographic anatomy of the inferior right atrial isthmus in patients with and without history of common atrial flutter. *Circulation.* 1999;99:3017–3023.

22. Cabrera JA, Sanchez-Quintana D, Farre J, et al. The inferior right atrial isthmus: further architectural insights for current and coming ablation technologies. *J Cardiovasc Electrophysiol.* 2005;16:402–408.

23. Antz M, Otomo K, Arruda M, et al. Electrical conduction between the right atrium and the left atrium via the musculature of the coronary sinus. *Circulation.* 1998;98:1790–1795.

24. De Ponti R, Ho SY, Salerno-Uriarte JA, et al. Electroanatomic analysis of sinus impulse propagation in normal human atria. *J Cardiovasc Electrophysiol.* 2002;13:1–10.

25. Kim DT, Lai AC, Hwang C, et al. The ligament of Marshall: a structural analysis in human hearts with implications for atrial arrhythmias. *J Am Coll Cardiol.* 2000;36:1324–1327.

26. Veinot JP, Harrity PJ, Gentile F, et al. Anatomy of the normal left atrial appendage: a quantitative study of age-related changes in 500 autopsy hearts: implications for echocardiographic examination. *Circulation.* 1997;96:3112–3115.

27. Becker AE. Left atrial isthmus: anatomic aspects relevant for linear catheter ablation procedures in humans. *J Cardiovasc Electrophysiol.* 2004;15:809–812.

28. Wittkampf FHM, van Oosterhout MF, Loh P, et al. Where to draw the mitral isthmus line in catheter ablation of atrial fibrillation: histological analysis. *Eur Heart J.* 2005;26:689–695.

29. Papez JW. Heart musculature of the atria. *Am J Anat.* 1920–21;27:255–277.

30. Wang K, Ho SY, Gibson D, Anderson RH. Architecture of the atrial musculature in humans. *Br Heart J.* 1995;73:559–565.

31. Nathan H, Eliakin M. The junction between the left atrium and the pulmonary veins. *Circulation*. 1966;34:412–422.

32. Saito T, Waki K, Becker AE. Left atrial myocardial extension onto pulmonary veins in humans: anatomic observations relevant for atrial arrhythmias. *J Cardiovasc Electrophysiol*. 2000:11:888–894.

33. Ho SY, Cabrera JA, Tran VH, et al. Architecture of the pulmonary veins: relevance to radiofrequency ablation. *Heart*. 2001;86:265–270.

34. Tagawa M, Higuchi K, Chinushi M, et al. Myocardium extending from the left atrium onto the pulmonary veins: a comparison between subjects with and without atrial fibrillation. *Pacing Clin Electrophysiol*. 2001;24:1459–1463.

35. Burch GE, Romney RB. Functional anatomy and "throttle valve" action of the pulmonary veins. *Am Heart J*. 1954;47:58–66.

36. Brunton TL, Fayrer J. Note on independent pulsation of the pulmonary veins and vena cava. *Proc Royal Soc Lond*. 1876–1877;25:174–176.

37. Zipes DP, Knope RF. Electrical properties of the thoracic veins. *Am J Cardiol*. 1972;29:372–376.

38. Haissaguerre M, Jais P, Shah DC, et al. Spontaneous initiation of atrial fibrillation by ectopic beats originating in the pulmonary veins. *N Engl J Med*. 1998;339:659–665.

39. Wolff L, Parkinson J, White P. Bundle branch block with short P-R interval in healthy young people prone to paroxysmal tachycardia. *Am Heart J*. 1930;5:685–704.

40. Kozlowski D, Kozluk E, Adamowicz M, et al. Histological examination of the topography of the atrioventricular nodal artery within the triangle of Koch. *Pacing Clin Electrophysiol*. 1998;21:163–167.

41. Sanchez-Quintana D, Ho SY, Cabrera JA, et al. Topographic anatomy of the inferior pyramidal space: relevance to radiofrequency ablation. *J Cardiovasc Electrophysiol*. 2001;12:210–217.

42. Ross DN, Radley-Smith R, Somerville J. Pulmonary autograft replacement for severe aortic valve disease. *Br Heart J*. 1969;31:797–798.

43. Stamm C, Anderson R H, Ho S Y. Clinical anatomy of the normal pulmonary root compared with that in isolated pulmonary valvular stenosis. *J Am Coll Cardiol*. 1998;31:1420–1425.

44. Kervancioglu M, Ozbag D, Kervancioglu P, et al. Echocardiographic and morphologic examination of left ventricular false tendons in human and animal hearts. *Clin Anat*. 2003;16(5):389–395.

45. Thakur RK, Klein GJ, Sivaram CA, et al. Anatomic substrate for idiopathic left ventricular tachycardia. *Circulation*. 1996;93:497–501.

46. Sutton JPIII, Ho S Y, Anderson R H. The forgotten interleaflet triangles: a review of the surgical anatomy of the aortic valve. *Ann Thorac Surg*. 1995;59:419–427.

47. Ouyang F, Fotuhi P, Ho SY, et al. Repetitive monomorphic ventricular tachycardia originating from the aortic sinus cusp: electrocardiographic characterization for guiding catheter ablation. *J Am Coll Cardiol*. 2002;39:500–508.

48. Shimoike E, Ohnishi Y, Ueda N, et al. Radiofrequency catheter ablation of left ventricular outflow tract tachycardia from the coronary cusp: a new approach to the tachycardia focus. *J Cardiovasc Electrophysiol*. 1999;10:1005–1009.

49. Hachiya H, Aonuma K, Yamauchi Y, et al. How to diagnose, locate, and ablate coronary cusp ventricular tachycardia. *J Cardiovasc Electrophysiol*. 2002;13:551–556.

50. Ouyang F, Ma , Ho SY, Bansch D, et al. Focal atrial tachycardia originating from the non-coronary aortic sinus: electrophysiological characteristics and catheter ablation. *J Am Coll Cardiol*. 2006;48:122–131.

51. Lüdinghausen VM, Schott C. Microanatomy of the human coronary sinus and its major tributaries. In: *Myocardial Perfusion, Reperfusion, Coronary Venous Retroperfusion*. Meerbaum S, ed. Darmstadt: Steinkopff Verlag; 1990:93–122.

52. Gensini G, Giorgi SD, Coskun O, et al. Anatomy of the coronary circulation in living man. *Circulation*. 1965;31:778–784.

53. Stellbrink C, Dien B, Schauerte P, et al. Transcoronary venous radiofrequency catheter ablation of ventricular tachycardia. *J Cardiovasc Electrophysiol*. 1997;8:916–921.

54. Lüdinghausen VM, Ohmachi N, Boot C. Myocardial coverage of the coronary sinus and related veins. *Clin Anat*. 1992;5:1–15.

55. Chauvin M, Shah DC, Haissaguerre M, et al. The anatomic basis of connections between the coronary sinus musculature and the left atrium in humans. *Circulation*. 2000;101:647–652.

56. Kozlowski D, Kozluk E, Piatkowska A, et al. The middle cardiac vein as a key for "posteroseptal" space—a morphological point of view. *Folia Morph Warsz*. 2001;60:293–296.

57. Omran H, Pfeiffer D, Tebbenjohanns J, et al. Echocardiographic imaging of coronary sinus diverticula and middle cardiac veins in patients with preexcitation syndrome: impact on radiofrequency catheter ablation of posteroseptal accessory pathways. *Pacing Clin Electrophysiol*. 1995;18:1236–1243.

58. Ho SY, Russell G, Rowland E. Coronary venous aneurysms and accessory atrioventricular connections. *Br Heart J*. 1988;60:348–351.

59. Heaven DJ, Till JA, Ho SY. Sudden death in a child with an unusual accessory connection. *Europace*. 2000;2:224–227.

60. Mönckeberg JG. Beitrage zur normalen und pathologischen Anatomie des Herzens. *Verh Dtsch Pathol Ges*. 1910;14:64–71.

61. Aschoff L. Referat uber die Herzstorungen in ihren Beziehungen zu den Specifischen Muskelsyatem des Herzens. *Verh Dtsch Pathol Ges*. 1910;14:3–35.

62. Janse MJ, Anderson RH. Internodal atrial specialised pathways—fact or fiction? *Eur J Cardiol*. 1974;2:117–137.

63. Anderson RH, Ho SY, Smith A, Becker AE. The internodal atrial myocardium. *Anat Rec*. 1981;201:75–82.

64. Ryback R, Mizeres NJ. The sinus node artery in man. *Anat Rec*. 1965;153:23–30.

65. Tawara S. *Das Reizleitungssystem des Säugetierherzens. Eine Anatomisch-Histologische Studie Über das Atrioventrikularbündel ung die Purkinjeschen Fäden*. Jena: Gustav Fischer; 1906.

66. Ho SY, McCarthy KP, Ansari A, et al. Anatomy of the atrioventricular node and atrioventricular conduction system. *J Bifurcation & Chaos*. 2003;12:3665–3674.

67. Inoue S, Becker AE. Posterior extensions of the human compact atrioventricular node. A neglected anatomic feature of potential clinical significance. *Circulation*. 1998;87:188–193.

68. Ueng KC, Chen SA, Chiang CE, et al. Dimensions and related anatomical distance of Koch's triangle in patients with atrioventricular nodal reentrant tachycardia. *J Cardiovasc Electrophysiol*. 1996;7:1017–1023.

69. Haissaguerre M, Shah DC, Jais P, et al. Role of Purkinje conducting system in triggering of idiopathic ventricular fibrillation. *Lancet*. 2002;23;359:677–678.

70. Kurosawa H, Becker AE. Dead-end tract of the conduction axis. *Int J Cardiol*. 1985;7:13–20.

71. Pauza DH, Pauziene N, Tamasauskas KA, et al. Hilum of the heart. *Anat Rec*. 1997;248:322–324.

72. Armour JA, Murphy DA, Yuan B-X, et al. Gross and microscopic anatomy of the human intrinsic cardiac nervous system. *Anat Rec*. 1997;247:289–298.

73. Pauza DH, Skripka V, Pauzine N, et al. Morphology, distributions, and variability of the epicardial neural ganglionated subplexuses in the human heart. *Anat Rec*. 2000;259:353–382.

74. Singh S, Johnson PI, Lee RE, et al. Topography of cardiac ganglia in the adult human heart. *J Thorac Cardiovasc Surg*. 1996;112:943–953.

75. Nakajima K, Furukawa Y, Kurogouchi F, et al. Autonomic control of the location and rate of the cardiac pacemaker in the sinoatrial fat pad of parasympathetically denervated dog hearts. *J Cardiovasc Electrophysiol*. 2002;13:896–901.

76. Quan KJ, Lee JH, Van Hare GF, et al. Identification and characterization of atrioventricular parasympathetic innervation in humans. *J Cardiovasc Electrophysiol*. 2002;13:735–739.

77. Cummings JA, Gill I, Akhrass R, et al. Preservation of the anterior fat pad paradoxically decreases the incidence of postoperative atrial fibrillation in humans. *J Am Coll Cardiol*. 2004;43:994–1000.

78. McAlpine WA. *Heart and Coronary Arteries*. Berlin: Springer-Verlag; 1975:1.

CHAPTER 35

Mechanisms of Cardiac Arrhythmias and Conduction Disturbances

Charles Antzelevitch

Recent years have witnessed important advances in our understanding of the molecular and electrophysiologic mechanisms underlying the development of a variety of cardiac arrhythmias (Table 35–1) and conduction disturbances. Progress in our understanding of these phenomena has been fueled by innovative advances in our understanding of the genetic basis and predisposition for electrical dysfunction of the heart. These advances notwithstanding, our appreciation of the basis for many rhythm disturbances is incomplete. Chap. 35 examines our present understanding of cellular, ionic and molecular mechanisms responsible for cardiac arrhythmias, placing them in historical perspective whenever possible.

Arrhythmic activity can be categorized as passive (e.g., atrioventricular [AV] block) or active. The mechanisms responsible for active cardiac arrhythmias are generally divided into two major categories: (1) enhanced or abnormal impulse formation, and (2) reentry (Fig. 35–1). Reentry occurs when a propagating impulse fails to die out after normal activation of the heart and persists to reexcite the heart after expiration of the refractory period. Evidence implicating reentry as a mechanism of cardiac arrhythmias stems back to the turn of century.[1–3] *Phase 2 reentry*[4–7] and *fibrillatory conduction*[8,9] are interesting new concepts of reentrant activity advanced to explain the development of extrasystolic activity and atrial as well as ventricular fibrillation, respectively. Mechanisms responsible for abnormal impulse formation include enhanced automaticity and triggered activity. Automaticity can be further subdivided into normal and abnormal and triggered activity, consisting of: (1) early afterdepolarizations (EADs), and (2) delayed afterdepolarizations (DADs). Recent studies have identified a novel mechanism, termed *late phase 3 EAD*, representing a hybrid between those responsible for EAD and DAD activity.[10–12]

ABNORMAL IMPULSE FORMATION
【 】 NORMAL AUTOMATICITY

Automaticity is the property of cardiac cells to generate spontaneous action potentials. Spontaneous activity is the result of diastolic depolarization caused by a net inward current flowing during phase 4 of the action potential, which progressively brings the membrane potential to threshold. The sinoatrial (SA) node normally displays the highest intrinsic rate. All other pacemakers are referred to as subsidiary or latent pacemakers because they take over the function of initiating excitation of the heart only when the SA node is unable to generate impulses or when these impulses fail to propagate. There is a hierarchy of intrinsic rates of subsidiary pacemakers that have normal automaticity: atrial pacemakers have faster intrinsic rates than AV junctional pacemakers, and AV junctional pacemakers have faster rates than ventricular pacemakers.

The ionic mechanism underlying normal SA and AV nodes and Purkinje system automaticity include (1) a hyperpolarization-activated inward current (I_f),[13] and/or (2) decay of outward potassium current (I_K).[14] The contribution of I_f and I_K differs in SA/AV nodes and Purkinje fiber because of the different potential ranges of these two pacemaker types (i.e., –70 to –35 mV and –90 to –65 mV, respectively). The contribution of other voltage-dependent currents can also differ among the different cardiac

TABLE 35–1

Characteristics and Presumed Mechanisms of Cardiac Arrhythmia

TACHYCARDIA	MECHANISM	ORIGIN	RATE RANGE, BPM	AV OR VA CONDUCTION
Sinus tachycardia	Automatic (normal)	Sinus node	≥100	1:1
Sinus node reentry	Reentry	Sinus node and right atrium	110–180	1:1 or variable
Atrial fibrillation	Reentry, fibrillatory conduction, automatic	Atria, pulmonary veins, SVC	260–450	Variable
Atrial flutter	Reentry	Right atrium, left atrium (infrequent)	240–350, usually 300 ± 20	2:1 or variable
Atrial tachycardia	Reentry, automatic, triggered activity	Atria	150–240	1:1, 2:1, or variable
AV nodal reentry tachycardia	Reentry	AV node with an atrial component	120–250, usually 150–220	1:1
AV reentry (WPW or concealed accessory AV connection)	Reentry	Circuit includes accessory AV connection, atria, AV node, His-Purkinje system, ventricles	140–250, usually 150–220	1:1
Accelerated AV junctional tachycardia	Automatic	AV junction (AV node and His bundle)	61–200, usually 80–130	1:1 or variable
Accelerated idioventricular rhythm	Abnormal automaticity	Purkinje fibers	>60	Variable, 1:1, or AV dissociation
Ventricular tachycardia	Reentry, automatic, triggered	Ventricles	120–300, usually 140–240	AV dissociation, variable
Bundle branch reentrant tachycardia	Reentry	Bundle branches and ventricular septum	160–250, usually 195–240	AV dissociation, variable, or 1:1
Right ventricular outflow tract	Automatic, triggered activity	Right ventricular out-flow tract	120–200	AV dissociation, variable, or 1:1
Torsade de pointes tachycardia	Reentry	Ventricles	>200	AV dissociation

AV, atrioventricular; BPM, beats per minute; DAD, delayed afterdepolarization; EAD, early afterdepolarization; WPW, Wolff-Parkinson-White syndrome; SVC, superior vena cava.
Source: Modified from Waldo, Wit. Hurst's The Heart, 11th ed. With permission.

cell types. For example, L-type calcium current (I_{Ca}) participates in the late phase of diastolic depolarization in SA and AV nodes, but not in Purkinje fibers. In atrial pacemaker cells, low voltage-activated T-type I_{Ca}, has been shown to contribute by sarcoplasmic reticulum (SR) calcium release, which, in turn, stimulates the inward sodium-calcium (Na-Ca) exchange current (I_{Na-Ca}).[15] The action potential upstroke is provided largely by the fast sodium current in His-Purkinje system and predominantly by the slow calcium current in SA and AV nodes. A role for sustained inward current (I_{st}) as well as for Ca^{2+} release from the sarcoplasmic reticulum has been proposed as well.[16]

The rate at which pacemaking cells initiate impulses is determined by the interplay of three factors: (1) maximum dia-

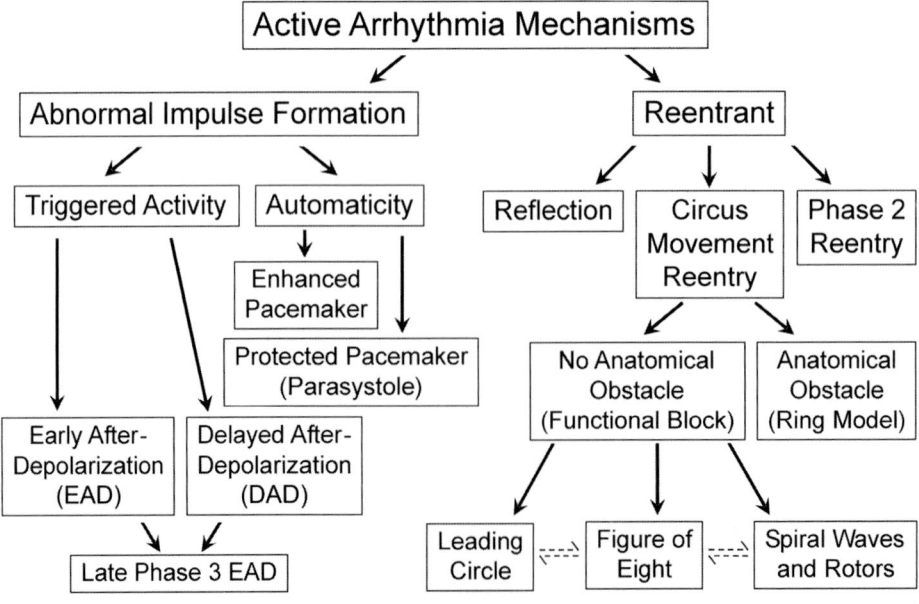

FIGURE 35–1. Classification of active cardiac arrhythmias.

stolic potential, (2) threshold potential, and (3) slope of phase 4 depolarization. A change in any one of these factors will alter the time required for phase 4 depolarization to carry the membrane potential from its maximum diastolic level to threshold and thus alter the rate of impulse initiation.

Parasympathetic and sympathetic influences as well as extracellular potassium levels can alter one or more of these three parameters and thus modulate the intrinsic rate of discharge of biological pacemakers. In general, β-adrenergic receptor stimulation increases, whereas muscarinic receptor stimulation reduces the rate of phase 4 depolarization. Parasympathetic agonists such as acetylcholine also hyperpolarize the cell leading to an increase in maximum diastolic potential. Acetylcholine (ACh) exerts these actions by activating a potassium (K) current, I_{K-ACh},[17] reducing inward Ca^{2+} current (I_{Ca}) as well as reducing the pacemaker current (I_f).[18] Vagal-induced hyperpolarization and slowing of phase 4 depolarization act in concert to reduce sinus rate and are the principal causes of sinus bradycardia.

Cells in the sinus node possess the fastest intrinsic rates. Thus the SA node is the primary pacemaker in the normal heart. When impulse generation or conduction within or out of the SA node is impaired, latent or subsidiary pacemakers within the atria or ventricle are capable of taking control of pacing the heart. The intrinsically slower rates of these latent pacemakers result in bradycardia.

Subsidiary atrial pacemakers with more negative diastolic potentials (–75 to –70 mV) than SA nodal cells are located at the junction of the inferior right atrium and the inferior vena cava, near or on the eustachian ridge.[19,20] Other atrial pacemakers have been identified in the crista terminalis[21] as well as at the orifice of the coronary sinus[22] and in the atrial muscle that extends into the tricuspid and mitral valves.[23,24] The cardiac muscle sleeves that extend into the cardiac veins (venae cavae and pulmonary veins) can also have the property of normal automaticity.[25] Latent pacemaking cells in the AV junction are responsible for AV junctional rhythms.[26] Both atrial and AV junctional subsidiary pacemakers are under autonomic control, with the sympathetic system increasing and parasympathetic system slowing the pacing rate.

The slowest subsidiary pacemakers are found in the His-Purkinje system in the ventricles of the heart. In the His-Purkinje system, parasympathetic effects are less apparent than those of the sympathetic system. Although acetylcholine produces little in the way of a direct effect, it can significantly reduce Purkinje automaticity by means of the inhibition of the sympathetic influence, a phenomenon termed *accentuated antagonism*.[27] As in the atria, sympathetic stimulation increases the rate of firing. In the His-Purkinje system, as in all pacemaker cells, an increase of extracellular potassium concentration increases inwardly rectifying K^+ current, (I_{K1}), thus reducing the rate of diastolic depolarization, whereas a decrease of extracellular potassium ($[K^+]_o$) has the opposite effect. A reduction in I_{K1} can also occur secondary to a mutation in *KCNJ2*, the gene that encodes for this channel, leading to increased automaticity and extrasystolic activity presumably arising from the Purkinje system.[28–30] Interestingly, because β-adrenergic stimulation is effective in augmenting I_{K1},[31] sympathetic stimulation can produce a paradoxical slowing of automaticity and ectopy in this setting.

【 】 ABNORMAL AUTOMATICITY

Abnormal automaticity or depolarization-induced automaticity is observed under conditions of reduced resting membrane potential,

such as ischemia, infarction, or other depolarizing influences (i.e., current injection). Abnormal automaticity is experimentally observed in tissues that normally develop diastolic depolarization (i.e., Purkinje fiber), as well as those that normally do not display this feature (e.g., ventricular or atrial myocardium). Compared to normal automaticity, abnormal automaticity in Purkinje fibers or ventricular and atrial myocardium is more readily suppressed by calcium channel blockers and shows little to no overdrive suppression.

Atrial and ventricular myocardial cells do not display spontaneous diastolic depolarization or automaticity under normal conditions, but can develop these characteristics when depolarized, resulting in the development of repetitive impulse initiation, a phenomenon termed *depolarization-induced automaticity*. The membrane potential at which abnormal automaticity develops ranges between –70 and –30 mV.

The rate of abnormal automaticity is substantially higher than that of normal automaticity and is a sensitive function of resting membrane potential (i.e., the more depolarized resting potential the faster the rate). Similar to normal automaticity, abnormal automaticity is enhanced by β-adrenergic agonists and by reduction of external potassium.

The ionic basis for diastolic depolarization in abnormal automaticity can be similar to that of normal automaticity, consisting of a time-dependent activation of sodium current[32] and pacemaker current I_f, as well as decay of I_K.[33,34] Experiments on depolarized human atrial myocardium from dilated atria indicate that Ca^{2+}-dependent processes also can contribute to abnormal pacemaker activity at low membrane potentials. It has been suggested that release of Ca^{2+} from the SR can activate sodium-calcium exchanger current, I_{Na-Ca}, leading to spontaneous diastolic depolarization and abnormal automaticity. This mechanism is similar to that that responsible for the generation of DADs (discussed below).

Action potential upstrokes associated with abnormal automaticity can be mediated either by sodium channel current (I_{Na}) or I_{Ca}, depending on the take-off potential. In the range of take-off potentials between approximately –70 and –50 mV, repetitive activity is dependent on I_{Na} and can be depressed or abolished by sodium channel blockers. In a take-off potential range of –50 to –30 mV, repetitive activity depends on I_{Ca} and can be abolished by calcium channel blockers.

Depolarization of membrane potential associated with disease states is most commonly a result of either: (1) an increase in extracellular potassium (K^+), which reduces the reversal potential for I_{K1}, the outward current that largely determines the resting membrane or maximum diastolic potential; (2) a reduced number of I_{K1} channels; (3) a reduced ability of the I_{K1} channel to conduct potassium ions; or (4) electrotonic influence of neighboring depolarized zone. An increase in $[K^+]_o$ reduces membrane potential, but does not induce abnormal automaticity. Indeed raising $[K^+]_o$ is effective in suppressing abnormal automaticity in atrial, ventricular, and Purkinje fibers.[35] This argues against abnormal automaticity being responsible for arrhythmias arising in acutely ischemic myocardium, where cells are partially depolarized by increased extracellular K^+.[36] As will be discussed later in the chapter, abnormal automaticity can occur in the border zone of an ischemic region, where electrotonic depolarization can occur in the absence of an increase in $[K^+]_o$.

Membrane depolarization can also occur as a result of a decrease in $[K]_i$, which has been shown to occur in Purkinje fibers surviving an infarct and to persist for at least 24 hours after coronary occlusion.[37] The reduction in $[K]_i$ contributes to the low membrane potential and the accompanying abnormal automaticity. Human tissues isolated from diseased atrial and ventricular myocardium show phase 4 depolarization and abnormal automaticity at membrane potentials in the range of –50 to –60 mV. It has been proposed that a decrease in membrane potassium conductance is an important cause of the low membrane potentials in the atrial fibers.[38]

Because the conductance of I_{K1} channels is a sensitive function of $[K^+]_o$, hypokalemia can lead to major reduction in inward rectifier current, leading to depolarization and the development of enhanced or abnormal automaticity, particularly in Purkinje pacemakers.

An example of an inherited disease involving a reduction in I_{K1} is Andersen-Tawil syndrome. A loss of function of I_{K1} occurs secondary to mutations in *KCNJ2*, the gene that encodes Kir2.1, the protein that forms the I_{K1} channel. Andersen-Tawil syndrome is associated with a very high level of ectopy thought to arise from enhanced pacemaker activity within the Purkinje system as a result of a reduced level of I_{K1}.[28–30,39,40]

AUTOMATICITY AS A MECHANISM OF CARDIAC ARRHYTHMIAS

Arrhythmias caused by abnormal automaticity can result from diverse mechanisms. Sinus bradycardia and tachycardia are caused by simple alteration of the rate of impulse initiation by the normal SA node pacemaker (see Table 35–1). Alterations in sinus rate can be accompanied by shifts of the origin of the dominant pacemaker within the sinus node or to subsidiary pacemaker sites elsewhere in the atria. Impulse conduction out of the SA mode can be impaired or blocked as a result of disease or increased vagal activity leading to development of bradycardia. AV junctional rhythms occur when AV junctional pacemakers located either in the AV node or in the His bundle take control of the heart, usually in the presence of AV block.[26]

Normal or subsidiary pacemaker activity also can be enhanced, leading to sinus tachycardia or a shift to ectopic sites within the atria, giving rise to atrial tachycardia. One cause can be enhanced sympathetic nerve activity. Another can be the flow of injury current between partially depolarized myocardium and normally polarized latent pacemaker cells.[41] This mechanism is thought to be responsible for ectopic beats that occur at the borders of ischemic zones.[42] Other causes of enhanced pacemaker activity include a decease in the extracellular potassium levels as well as acute stretch.[43] Stretch of the Purkinje system can occur in akinetic areas after acute ischemia or in ventricular aneurysms in hearts with healed infarcts. Accelerated idioventricular rhythms have been attributed to enhanced normal automaticity in the His-Purkinje system.[44] Although experimental and clinical three-dimensional mapping studies have shown that ventricular arrhythmias arising under conditions of acute ischemia, infarction, heart failure, and other cardiomyopathies can be ascribed to focal mechanisms,[45] it is often difficult to discern between automatic and focal reentrant (reflection, phase 2 reentry, and micro-reentry) mechanisms. It is noteworthy that myocytes isolated from failing and hypertrophied animal and human hearts have been shown to manifest diastolic depolarization[46,47] and to possess enhanced I_f pacemaker current[48] suggesting that these mechanisms contribute to extrasystolic and tachyarrhythmias arising with these pathologies.

Although automaticity is not responsible for most rapid tachyarrhythmias, it is can precipitate or trigger reentrant arrhythmias. Haissaguerre and coworkers have shown that atrial fibrillation (AF) can be triggered by rapid automaticity arising in the pulmonary veins.[49] It is noteworthy that atrial tissues isolated from patients with AF exhibit increased I_f-mRNA levels.[50]

The automaticity of all subsidiary pacemakers within the heart is inhibited when they are overdrive paced.[51] This inhibition is called *overdrive suppression*. Under normal condition all subsidiary pacemakers are overdrive-suppressed by SA nodal activity. Overdrive suppression is largely mediated by intracellular accumulation of Na^+ leading to enhanced activity of the sodium pump (sodium-potassium adenosine triphosphatase [Na^+-K^+ ATPase]), which generates a hyperpolarizing electrogenic current that opposes phase 4 depolarization.[52] The faster the overdrive rate or the longer the duration of overdrive, the greater the enhancement of sodium pump activity, so that the period of quiescence after cessation of overdrive is directly related to the rate and duration of overdrive.[53] The sinus node itself can be overdrive suppressed, although the degree of overdrive suppression is less than that of subsidiary pacemakers driven at comparable rates, likely because of the fact that the sinus node action potential upstroke is largely dependent on L-type Ca^{2+} channel current and less Na^+ accumulates intracellularly to stimulate the sodium pump.

PARASYSTOLE AND MODULATED PARASYSTOLE

Latent pacemakers throughout the heart are generally reset by the propagating wavefront initiated by the dominant pacemaker and are therefore unable to activate the heart. An exception to this rule occurs when the pacemaking tissue is protected from the impulse of sinus origin. A region of entrance block arises when cells exhibiting automaticity are surrounded by ischemic, infarcted, or otherwise compromised cardiac tissues that prevent the propagating wave from invading the focus, but which permit the spontaneous beat generated within the automatic focus to exit and activate the rest of the myocardium. A pacemaker region exhibiting entrance block and exit conduction defines a parasystolic focus.

The ectopic activity generated by a parasystolic focus is characterized by premature ventricular complexes with variable coupling intervals, fusion beats, and interectopic intervals that are multiples of a common denominator. This rhythm is fairly rare. Although it is usually considered benign, any premature ventricular activation can induce malignant ventricular rhythms in the ischemic myocardium or in the presence of a suitable myocardial substrate.

A variant of classical parasystole, termed modulated parasystole, was described by Moe and coworkers.[54,55] This variant of the arrhythmia was suggested to result from incomplete entrance block of the parasystolic focus. Electrotonic influences arriving early in the pacemaker cycle delayed and those arriving late in the cycle accelerated the firing of the parasystolic pacemaker, so that ventricular activity could entrain the partially protected pacemaker (Fig. 35–2). As a consequence, at select heart rate, extrasystolic activity generated by the entrained parasystolic pacemaker can mimic reentry, generating extrasystolic activity with fixed coupling (Figs. 35–3 and 35–4).[54–58] A recent study suggests that bidirectional modulated parasystole can also account for cyclic bursts of ventricular premature contractions.[59]

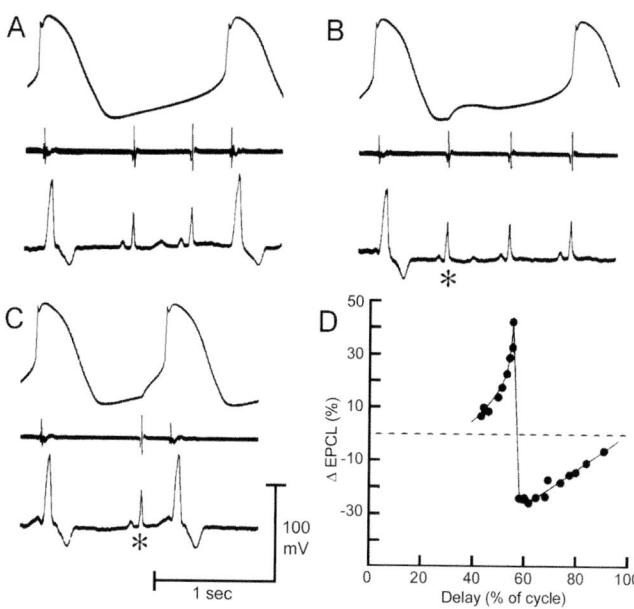

FIGURE 35–2. Electrotonic modulation of a parasystolic pacemaker. Traces were recorded from an experimental model consisting of a sucrose gap preparation in vitro coupled to the heart of an open chest dog. Traces (*top to bottom*): transmembrane potentials recorded from a distal segment of a Purkinje fiber-sucrose gap preparation, and a right ventricular electrogram and lead II ECG from the in vivo preparation. **A.** The Purkinje pacemaker was allowed to beat free of any influence from ventricular activation. **B** and **C.** Pacemaker activity of the Purkinje is electrotonically influenced by ventricular activation. An electrotonic influence arriving early in the pacemaker cycle delays the next discharge, whereas that arriving late, accelerates the next discharge. **D.** The electrotonic modulation of pacemaker discharge is described in the form of a phase-response curve. The percentage change in ectopic pacemaker cycle length is plotted as a function of the temporal position of the electrotonic influence in the pacemaker cycle. EPCL, ectopic pacemaker cycle length. *Source: From Antzelevitch, Bernstein, Feldman, et al.[57] Used with permission.*

[ ] AFTERDEPOLARIZATION AND TRIGGERED ACTIVITY

Oscillatory depolarizations that attend or follow the cardiac action potential and depend on preceding transmembrane activity for their manifestation are referred to as afterdepolarizations. Two subclasses traditionally recognized: (1) early, and (2) delayed. EADs interrupt or retard repolarization during phase 2 and/or phase 3 of the cardiac action potential, whereas DADs occur after full repolarization. When EAD or DAD amplitude suffices to bring the membrane to its threshold potential, a spontaneous action potential referred to as a triggered response is the result. These triggered events can be responsible for extrasystoles and tachyarrhythmias that develop under conditions predisposing to the development of afterdepolarizations.

Early Afterdepolarizations and Triggered Activity

Characteristics of Early Afterdepolarizations and Early Afterdepolarization-Induced Triggered Beats EADs are observed in isolated cardiac tissues exposed to injury, altered electrolytes, hypoxia, acidosis, catecholamines, and pharmacologic agents, including antiarrhythmic drugs. Ventricular hypertrophy and heart failure also predispose to the development of EADs.[60]

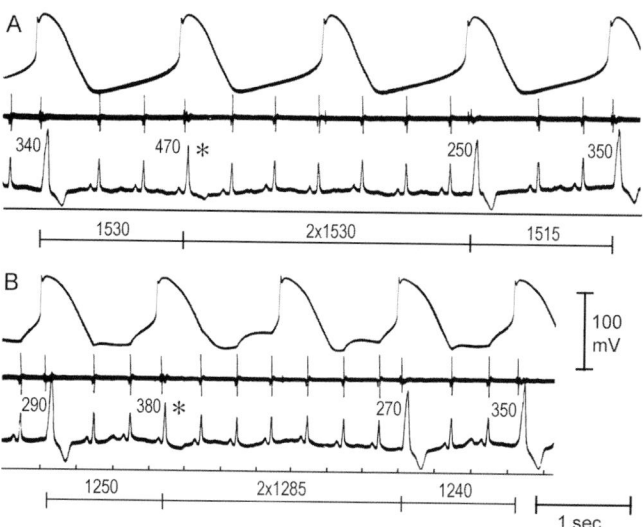

FIGURE 35–3. Patterns of classic parasystole generated by the experimental model described in Fig. 35–2 in the absence (**A**) and presence (**B**) of modulating influence from the ventricles. The lowest trace is a stimulus marker. Numbers denote the coupling intervals of the ectopic responses to the preceding normal beats (in milliseconds [msec]). *Asterisks* denote fusion beats. Classic parasystolic features are apparent in both cases. *Source: Antzelevitch, Bernstein, Feldman, et al.[57]*

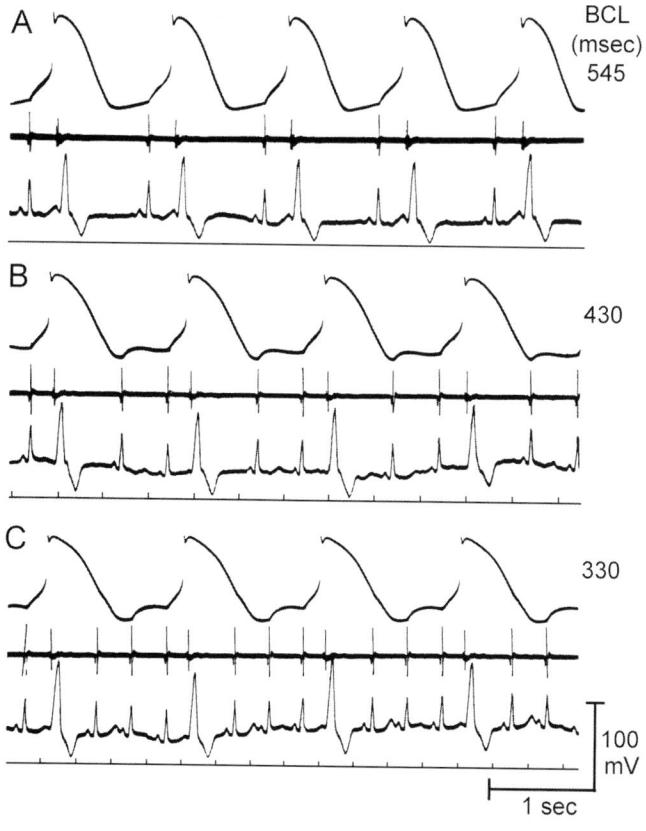

FIGURE 35–4. Records were obtained from the same preparation as in Fig. 35–2 but at different cycle lengths. At the basic cycle lengths shown, the activity generated was characteristic of reentry (fixed coupling of the premature beats to the basic beats). **A.** Bigeminy. **B.** Trigeminy. **C.** Quadrigeminy. BCL, basic cycle lengths. *Source: Antzelevitch, Bernstein, Feldman, et al.[57] Used with permission.*

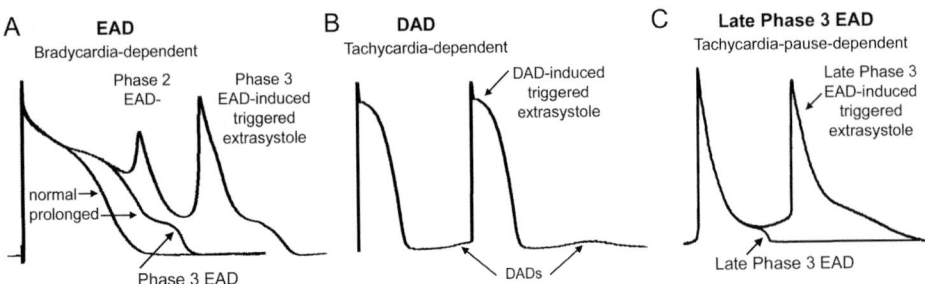

FIGURE 35–5. Afterdepolarizations. **A.** Phase 2 and 3 EADs and triggered extrasystole. **B.** DAD. **C.** Late phase 3 EAD. DAD, delayed afterdepolarization; EAD, early afterdepolarization.

EAD characteristics vary as a function of animal species, tissue or cell type, and the method by which the EAD is elicited. Although specific mechanisms of EAD induction can differ, a critical prolongation of repolarization accompanies most, but not all, EADs. Fig. 35–5 illustrates the two types of EAD generally encountered in Purkinje fiber. Oscillatory events appearing at potentials positive to –30 mV, are generally referred to as phase 2 EADs. Those occurring at more negative potentials are termed phase 3 EADs. Phase 2 and phase 3 EADs sometimes appear in the same preparation. The right panels show that triggered responses develop when the preparations are paced at slower rates.[61] In contrast to Purkinje fibers, EAD activity recorded in ventricular preparations are always phase 2 EADs.[62]

EAD-induced triggered activity is a sensitive function of stimulation rate. Agents with class III action generally induce EAD activity at slow stimulation rates and totally suppress EADs at rapid rates.[61,63] In contrast, β-adrenergic agonist–induced EADs are fast rate-dependent.[64,65] Recent studies have shown that in the presence of rapidly activating delayed rectifier current (rapid outward potassium current [I_{Kr}]) block, β-adrenergic agonists, and/or acceleration from an initially slow rate transiently facilitate the induction of EAD activity in ventricular M cells, but not in epicardium or endocardium and rarely in Purkinje fibers.[66] This biphasic effect is thought to be caused by an initial priming of sodium-calcium exchanger, which provides an electrogenic inward current (I_{Na-Ca}) that facilitates EAD development and prolongs action potential duration (APD). This early phase is followed by recruitment of slowly activating delayed rectifier current (slow outward potassium current [I_{Ks}]), which abbreviates APD and suppresses EAD activity.

Cellular Origin of Early Afterdepolarizations

EADs develop more in midmyocardial M cells and Purkinje fibers than in epicardial or endocardial cells when exposed to APD-prolonging agents[67] due to the presence of a weaker I_{Ks} in these cell types.[68] Block of I_{Ks} with chromanol 293B permits the induction of EADs in canine epicardial and endocardial tissues in response to I_{Kr} blockers such as E-4031 or sotalol.[69,70] The predisposition of cardiac cells to the development of EADs depends principally on the reduced availability of I_{Kr} and I_{Ks} as occurs in many forms of cardiomyopathy. Under these conditions, EADs can appear in any part of the ventricular myocardium.

Three-dimensional mapping of torsade de pointes (TdP) arrhythmias in canine experimental models suggest that the extrasystole that initiates TdP can originate from subendocardial, midmyocardium, or subepicardial regions of the left ventricle.[71,72] These data point to Purkinje fibers and M cells as the principal sources of

EAD-induced triggered activity in vivo. In the presence of combined I_{Kr} and I_{Ks} block, epicardium is often the first to develop an EAD. Although EAD-induced extrasystoles are capable of triggering TdP, the arrhythmia is considered by many, but not all, to be maintained by a reentrant mechanism.[73–75]

Ionic Mechanisms Responsible for the EAD

EADs are commonly associated with a prolongation of the repolarization phase caused by a reduction of net outward current secondary to an increase in inward currents and/or a decrease of outward currents. An EAD occurs when the balance of current active during phase 2 or 3 of the action potential shifts in the inward direction. If the change in current-voltage relation results in a region of net inward current during the plateau range of membrane potentials, it leads to a depolarization or EAD. Most pharmacological interventions or pathophysiological conditions associated with EADs can be categorized as acting predominantly through one of four different mechanisms: (1) A reduction of repolarizing potassium currents (I_{Kr}, class IA and III antiarrhythmic agents; I_{Ks}, chromanol 293B or I_{K1}); (2) an increase in the availability of calcium current (Bay K 8644, catecholamines); (3) an increase in the sodium-calcium exchange current caused by augmentation of intracellular calcium activity or upregulation of the exchanger; and (4) an increase in late sodium current (late I_{Na}) (aconitine, anthopleurin-A, and ATX-II). Combinations of these interventions (i.e., calcium loading and I_{Kr} reduction) or pathophysiological states can act synergistically to facilitate the development of EADs.[66,73,76–79]

The upstroke of the EAD is generally carried by calcium current. There is less agreement on the ionic basis for the critically important conditional phase of the EAD, defined as the period just before the EAD upstroke. Intracellular calcium levels and Na-Ca exchange current play pivotal roles in the conditional phase of isoproterenol-induced EADs.[64,65,80] Data from several investigator groups suggest that intracellular calcium levels do not influence the formation of this phase 2 EAD,[81–84] whereas others have presented strong evidence in support of the influence of intracellular calcium levels in the formation of at least the conditional phase of the EAD.[66,85] This discrepancy is in part caused by the type of tissues or cells studied.

There are important differences in the ionic mechanisms of EAD generation in canine Purkinje fibers and ventricular M cells. EADs induced in canine M cells are exquisitely sensitive to changes in intracellular calcium levels, whereas EADs elicited in Purkinje are largely insensitive.[66] Ryanodine, an agent known to block calcium release from the SR, abolishes EAD activity in canine M cells, but not in Purkinje fibers.[66] These distinctions can reflect differences in intracellular calcium handling in M cells, where the SR is well developed, as opposed to Purkinje fibers where the SR is poorly developed.

A sustained component of sodium channel current (I_{Na}) active during the action potential plateau, originating from channels that fail to inactivate and a nonequilibrium component arising from channels recovering from inactivation during phases 2 and 3, has been shown to contribute prominently the action potential duration and induction of EADs.[86–88] Calcium-calmodulin kinase II (CaMKII)has been linked to the development of EAD and TdP in cellular models where repolarization is prolonged.[89] Interestingly and somewhat unexpectedly, calmodulin binding to KCNQ1 was recently shown to be required for delivery of the channel protein to the cell surface; this chaperone effect is not dependent on calcium binding to calmodulin.[90–92] Failure of KvLQT1 (protein product of KCNQ1) to traffic to the membrane can prolong QT and facilitate the development of EADs.

Agents that inhibit I_{Ca}, CaMKII, and late I_{Na} have been shown to be effective in suppressing EAD activity.[93,94] The action of late I_{Na} blockers such as ranolazine and RSD1235 can be mediated by both a direct effect on the late inward current and indirectly by modulating calcium homeostasis.[95–99]

The Role of Early Afterdepolarizations in the Development of Cardiac Arrhythmias
As previously discussed, EAD-induced triggered activity is thought to be involved in precipitating TdP under conditions of congenital and acquired long QT syndromes.[100,101] EAD-like deflections have been observed in ventricular monophasic action potential (MAP) recordings immediately preceding TdP arrhythmias in the clinic as well as in experimental models of long QT syndrome (LQTS).[102–105]

EAD activity can also be involved in the genesis of cardiac arrhythmias in cases of hypertrophy and heart failure. These syndromes are commonly associated with prolongation of the ventricular action potential, which predisposes to the development of EADs.[43,47,106,107]

It is noteworthy that EADs developing in select transmural subtypes (such as M cells) can exaggerate transmural dispersion of repolarization (TDR), thus setting the stage for reentry. As will be discussed in more detail below, transmural dispersion of repolarization is thought to be the principal substrate permitting the development of TdP.

Delayed Afterdepolarization-Induced Triggered Activity
Oscillations of transmembrane activity that occur after full repolarization of the action potential and depend on previous activation of the cell for their manifestation are referred to as delayed afterdepolarizations (DADs). When DADs reach the threshold potential, they give rise to spontaneous action potentials generally referred to as triggered activity.

Causes and Origin of DAD-Induced Triggered Activity
DADs and DAD-induced triggered activity are observed under conditions that increase intracellular calcium, intracellular calcium $[Ca^{2+}]_i$, such as after exposure to toxic levels of cardiac glycosides (digitalis)[108,109] or catecholamines.[20,64,110] This activity is also apparent in hypertrophied and failing hearts[46] as well as in Purkinje fibers surviving myocardial infarction.[111] In contrast to EADs, DADs are always induced at relatively rapid rates.

Digitalis-induced DADs and triggered activity have been well characterized in isolated Purkinje fibers.[112] In the ventricular myocardium, they are less commonly observed in epicardial or endocardial tissues but readily induced in cells and tissues from the M region.[67] However, DADs are frequently observed in myocytes enzymatically dissociated from ventricular myocardium.[113] Digitalis, isoproterenol, high extracellular calcium ($[Ca^{2+}]_o$), or Bay K

8644, a calcium agonist, have been shown to cause DADs and triggered activity in tissues isolated from the M region but not in epicardial or endocardial tissues (see Fig. 35–5).[67,114–116] The failure of epicardial and endocardial cells to develop DADs has been ascribed to a high density of I_{Ks} in these tissues[68] as compared to M cells where I_{Ks} is small.[68] In support of this hypothesis, reduction of I_{Ks} can promote isoproterenol-induced DAD activity in canine and guinea pig endocardium and epicardium.[114]

Intervention capable of altering intracellular calcium, either by modifying transsarcolemmal calcium current or by inhibiting sarcoplasmic reticulum storage or release of calcium, can affect the manifestation of the DAD. DADs can also be modified by interventions capable of directly inhibiting or enhancing the transient inward current, I_{ti}. DADs are modified by extracellular K^+, Ca^{2+}, lysophosphoglycerides, and the metabolic factors such as adenosine triphosphate (ATP), hypoxia, and pH. Lowering extracellular K^+ (<4 millimolar [mM]) promote DADs, whereas increasing K^+ attenuates or totally suppresses DADs.[112] Lysophosphatidylcholine, in concentrations similar to those that accumulate in ischemic myocardium, have been shown to induce DAD activity.[117] Elevating extracellular Ca^{2+} promotes DADs,[112] and an increase of extracellular ATP potentiates isoproterenol-induced DAD.[118]

Agents that prolong action potential duration, such as quinidine and clofilium, facilitate the induction of DAD activity by augmenting calcium entry. Recent work indicates that calcium calmodulin (CaM) kinase can facilitate the induction of DADs by augmenting I_{Ca}.[93]

Under some pathophysiologic conditions, particularly those that predispose to the development of catecholaminergic ventricular tachycardia (VT), DAD activity can be observed to arise from epicardium.[119]

Delayed afterdepolarizations and triggered activity also can occur in the absence of pharmacologic agents, catecholamines, or an increase in extracellular Ca. DAD-induced triggered activity has been found in the upper pectinate muscles bordering the crista terminalis in the rabbit heart, branches of the sinoatrial ring bundle or transitional fibers between the ring bundle and ordinary pectinate muscle, rat ventricular muscle that is hypertrophic secondary to renovascular hypertension,[120] and ventricular myocardium from diabetic rats.[121] Abnormal SR function, in which the ability of the SR to sequester calcium during diastole is compromised, can lead to DADs. Such abnormal SR function can result from genetically based alterations in SR proteins and can be the cause of certain inherited ventricular tachyarrhythmias.[122]

Pharmacological agents that affect the release and reuptake of calcium by the SR, including caffeine and ryanodine, can also influence the manifestation of DADs and triggered activity. Low concentrations of caffeine facilitate Ca release from the SR and thus contribute to augmentation of DAD and triggered activity. High concentration of caffeine prevent Ca uptake by the SR and thus abolish I_{ti}, DADs, aftercontractions, and triggered activity. Doxorubicin, an anthracycline antibiotic, has been shown to be effective in suppressing digitalis-induced DADs, possibly through inhibition of the Na-Ca exchange mechanism.[123] Potassium channel activators, such as pinacidil, can also suppress DAD and triggered activity by activating ATP-regulated potassium current (I_{K-ATP}).[116,124] Flunarizine is another agent shown to suppress DAD and triggered activity, in part through inhibition of both L-type and T-type calcium current.[125,126] Ranolazine, an antianginal agent with potent late sodium channel blocking action, has also been shown to reduce the amplitude of delayed afterdepolarizations (DADs) induced by isoproterenol, forskolin or ouabain. [96,127,128]

Ionic Mechanisms Responsible for the Development of Delayed Afterdepolarizations

Delayed afterdepolarizations (DADs) and accompanying aftercontractions are caused by spontaneous release of calcium from the SR under calcium overload conditions. The afterdepolarization is believed to be induced by a transient inward current (I_{ti}) generated either by (1) a nonselective cationic current (I_{ns})[129,130]; (2) the activation of an electrogenic Na-Ca exchanger[129,131–133]; or (3) calcium-activated Cl^- current.[132,133] All are secondary to the release of Ca from the overloaded SR.

Role of Delayed Afterdepolarization-Induced Triggered Activity in the Development of Cardiac Arrhythmias

Although a wide variety of studies performed in isolated tissues and cells suggest an important role for DAD-induced triggered activity in the genesis of cardiac arrhythmias, especially bigeminal rhythms and tachyarrhythmias observed in the setting of digitalis toxicity,[112] little direct evidence of DAD-induced triggered activity is available in vivo. Consequently, even when triggered activity appears a likely mechanism, it is often impossible to completely rule out other mechanisms (e.g., reentry, enhanced automaticity, etc.).

Clinical arrhythmias suggested to be caused by DAD-induced triggered activity include: (1) *idiopathic right and left ventricular outflow tract ventricular tachyarrhythmias*[134–136]; and (2) *idioventricular rhythms*—accelerated atrioventricular (AV) junctional escape rhythms that occur as a result of digitalis toxicity or in a setting of myocardial infarction. Other possible *DAD-mediated* arrhythmias include exercise-induced adenosine-sensitive VT as described by Lerman and Belardinelli[137]; repetitive monomorphic VT caused presumably by cyclic adenosine monophosphate (cAMP)-mediated triggered activity[138]; supraventricular tachycardias, including arrhythmias originating in the coronary sinus[139]; and some heart failure-related arrhythmias.[45]

Pogwizd and coworkers demonstrated that ventricular arrhythmias associated with nonischemic cardiomyopathy are initiated by nonreentrant mechanisms, including DADs.[45] Ventricular arrhythmias associated with ischemic cardiomyopathy can also be initiated by DAD-induced triggered beats.[140] DADs have also been implicated in the reinitiation of ventricular fibrillation (VF) following failed defibrillation attempts. Flunarizine, a DAD inhibitor, significantly improved defibrillation efficacy.[126]

DADs are thought to play a prominent role in catecholaminergic or familial polymorphic VT, a rare, autosomal dominant inherited disorder, predominantly affecting children or adolescents with structurally normal hearts. It is characterized by bidirectional ventricular tachycardia (BVT), polymorphic VT (PVT), and a high risk of sudden cardiac death.[141] Recent molecular genetic studies have identified mutations in genes encoding for the cardiac ryanodine receptor 2 (RyR2) or calsequestrin 2 (CASQ2) in patients with this phenotype.[122,141–144] Several lines of evidence point to DAD-induced triggered activity (TA) as the mechanism underlying monomorphic or bidirectional VT in these patients. These include the identification of genetic mutations involving Ca^{2+} regu-

latory proteins, a similarity of the ECG features to those associated with digitalis toxicity, and the precipitation by adrenergic stimulation. A recent model of catecholaminergic polymorphic ventricular tachycardia (CPVT) developed using the left ventricular (LV) coronary-perfused wedge preparation was shown to recapitulate the electrocardiographic and arrhythmic manifestations of the disease, most of which were secondary to DAD-induced triggered activity.[119] DAD-induced extrasystolic activity arising from epicardium was also shown to provide the substrate for the development of reentrant tachyarrhythmias caused by reversal of the direction of activation of the ventricular wall.[119]

Late Phase 3 Early Afterdepolarizations and Their Role in Initiation of Atrial Fibrillation

Recent studies have uncovered a novel mechanism giving rise to triggered activity, termed *late phase 3 EAD*, which combines properties of both EAD and DAD, but has its own unique character. Late phase 3 EAD-induced triggered extrasystoles represent a new concept of arrhythmogenesis in which abbreviated repolarization permits *normal SR calcium release* to induce an EAD-mediated closely coupled triggered response, particularly under conditions permitting intracellular calcium loading.[10,11] These EADs are distinguished by the fact that they interrupt the final phase of repolarization of the action potential (late phase 3). In contrast to previously described DAD or intracellular calcium (Ca_i)-dependent EAD, it is *normal*, not spontaneous SR calcium release that is responsible for the generation of the EAD. Late phase 3 EADs are observed only when APD is markedly abbreviated as with acetylcholine (see Figs. 35–5 and 35–6).[10] Based on the time-course of contraction, levels of Ca_i would be expected to peak during the plateau of the action potential (membrane potential of approximately –5 mV) under control conditions but during the late phase of repolarization (membrane potential of approximately –70 mV)

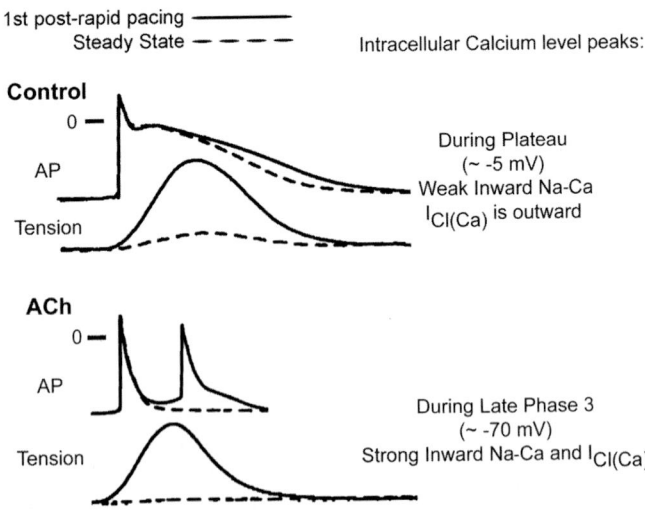

FIGURE 35–6. Proposed mechanism for the development of late phase 3 early afterdepolarizations (EADs). Shown are superimposed action potential (AP) and phasic tension recordings obtained under steady state conditions and during the first regular post–rapid pacing beat in control and in the presence of acetylcholine. See text for further discussion. ACh, acetylcholine; $I_{Cl(Ca)}$, calcium-activated chloride current; Na-Ca, sodium-calcium exchange. *Source: Reproduced with permission from Burashnikov, Antzelevitch.[10]*

in the presence of acetylcholine. As a consequence, the two principal calcium-mediated currents, I_{Na-Ca} and $I_{Cl(Ca)}$, would be expected to be weakly inward or even outward ($I_{Cl(Ca)}$) when APD is normal (control), but strongly inward when APD is very short (acetylcholine). Thus, abbreviation of the atrial APD, allows for a much stronger recruitment of both I_{Na-Ca} and $I_{Cl(Ca)}$ in the generation of a late phase 3 EADs. It is noteworthy that the proposed mechanism is similar to that thought to underlie the development of DADs and conventional Ca_i-dependent EAD.[133,145] The principal difference is that in the case of these DADs/EADs, I_{Na-Ca} and $I_{Cl(Ca)}$ are recruited secondary to a *spontaneous* release of calcium from the SR, whereas in the case of late phase 3 EADs, these currents are accentuated as a consequence of the *normal* SR release mechanisms.

In the isolated canine atria, late phase 3 EAD-induced extrasystoles have been shown to initiate AF, particularly following spontaneous termination of the arrhythmia (IRAF, immediate reinduction of AF).[10] The appearance of late phase 3 EAD immediately following termination of AF or rapid pacing has been recently reported by in the canine atria in vivo.[146] Patterson and colleagues[147] recently described "tachycardia-pause"-induced EAD in isolated superfused canine pulmonary vein muscular sleeve preparations in the presence of both simultaneous parasympathetic (to abbreviate APD) and sympathetic (to augment Ca_i) nerve stimulation. This EAD also appears during late phase 3 of the action potential, and a similar mechanism has been proposed.[147] A similar mechanism has recently been invoked to explain catecholamine-induced afterdepolarizations and VT in mice.[148]

REENTRANT ARRHYTHMIAS
[ ] CIRCUS MOVEMENT REENTRY

The circuitous propagation of an impulse around an anatomic or functional obstacle leading to reexcitation of the heart describes a circus movement reentry. Four distinct models of this form of reentry have been described: (1) the ring model, (2) the leading circle model, (3) the figure-of-eight model, and (4) the spiral wave model. The ring model of reentry differs from the other three in that an anatomic obstacle is required. The leading circle, figure-of-eight, and spiral wave models of reentry require only a functional obstacle.

Ring Model

The ring model is the simplest form of reentry. It first emerged as a concept shortly after the turn of the last century when A. G. Mayer reported the results of experiments involving the subumbrella tissue of a jellyfish (*Sychomedusa cassiopeia*).[1,149] The muscular disk did not contract until ringlike cuts were made and pressure and a stimulus applied. This caused the disc to "spring into rapid rhythmical pulsation so regular and sustained as to recall the movement of clockwork."[1] Mayer demonstrated similar circus movement excitation in rings cut from the ventricles of turtle hearts, but he did not consider this to be a plausible mechanism for the development of cardiac arrhythmias. His experiments proved valuable in identifying two fundamental conditions necessary for the initiation and maintenance of circus movement excita-

tion: (1) unidirectional block—the impulse initiating the circulating wave must travel in one direction only; and (2) for the circus movement to continue, the circuit must be long enough to allow each site in the circuit to recover before the return of the circulating wave.

G. R. Mines[150] was the first to develop the concept of circus movement reentry as a mechanism responsible for cardiac arrhythmias.[2] He confirmed Mayer's observations and suggested that the recirculating wave could be responsible for clinical cases of tachycardia.[150] This concept was reinforced with the discovery by Kent of an extra accessory pathway connecting the atrium and ventricle of a human heart.[151] The following three criteria developed by Mines for identification of circus movement reentry remains in use today:

1. An area of unidirectional block must exist.
2. The excitatory wave progresses along a distinct pathway, returning to its point of origin and then following the same path again.
3. Interruption of the reentrant circuit at any point along its path should terminate the circus movement.

Schmitt and Erlanger[152] in 1928 suggested that coupled ventricular extrasystoles in mammalian hearts could occur as a consequence of circus movement reentry within loops composed of terminal Purkinje fibers and ventricular muscle. Using a theoretical model consisting of a Purkinje bundle that divides into two branches that insert distally into ventricular muscle (Fig. 35–7), they suggested that a region of depression within one of the terminal Purkinje branches could provide for unidirectional block and conduction slow enough to permit successful reexcitation within a loop of limited size (i.e., 10 to 30 mm).

It was recognized that successful reentry could occur only when the impulse was sufficiently delayed in an alternate pathway to allow for expiration of the refractory period in the tissue proximal to the site of unidirectional block. Both conduction velocity and refractoriness determine the success or failure of reentry, and the general rule is that the length of the circuit (pathlength) must exceed or equal that of the wavelength, the wavelength being defined as the product of the conduction velocity and the refractory period or that part of the pathlength occupied by the impulse and refractory to reexcitation. The theoretical minimum path length required for development of reentry was initially thought to be quite long. In the early 1970s, micro-reentry within narrowly circumscribed loops was suggested to be within the realm of possibility. Cranefield, Hoffman, and coworkers[153] demonstrated that segments of canine Purkinje fibers that normally display impulse conduction velocities of 2 to 4 m/sec, can conduct impulses with apparent velocities of 0.01 to 0.1 m/sec when encased in high K^+ agar. This finding and the demonstration by Sasyniuk and Mendez in 1971[154] of a marked abbreviation of action potential duration and refractoriness in terminal Purkinje fibers just proximal to the site of block greatly reduced the theoretical limit of the pathlength required for the development of reentry. Single and repetitive reentry was reported by Wit and coworkers[155] in small loops of canine and bovine conducting tissues bathed in a high K^+ solution containing catecholamines, thus demonstrating reentry over a relatively small path. In some experiments, they used linear unbranched bundles of Purkinje tissue to demonstrate a phenome-

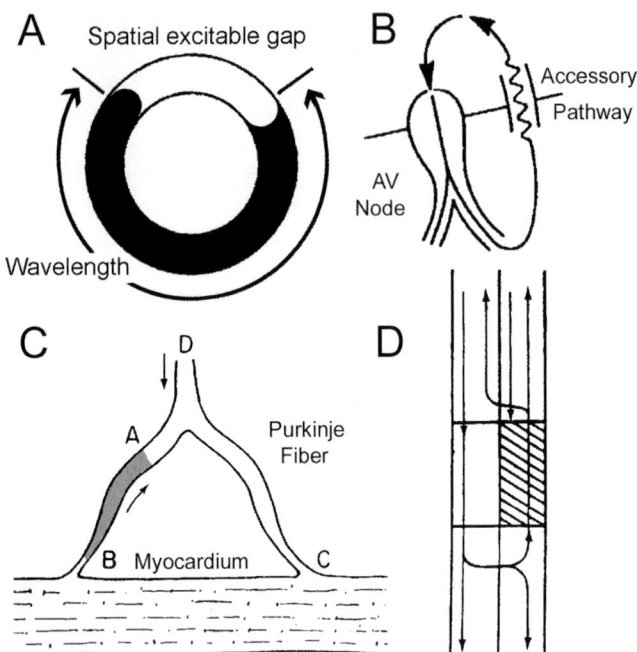

FIGURE 35-7. Ring models of reentry. **A.** Schematic of a ring model of reentry. **B.** Mechanism of reentry in the Wolff-Parkinson-White syndrome involving the atrioventricular (AV) node and an AV accessory pathway (AP). **C.** A mechanism for reentry in a Purkinje-muscle loop proposed by Schmitt and Erlanger. The diagram shows a Purkinje bundle (*D*) that divides into two branches, both connected distally to ventricular muscle. Circus movement was considered possible if the stippled segment, *A–B*, showed unidirectional block. An impulse advancing from *D* would be blocked at *A*, but would reach and stimulate the ventricular muscle at *C* by way of the other terminal branch. The wavefront would then reenter the Purkinje system at *B* traversing the depressed region slowly so as to arrive at *A* following expiration of refractoriness. **D.** Schematic representation of circus movement reentry in a linear bundle of tissue as proposed by Schmitt and Erlanger. The upper pathway contains a depressed zone (*shaded*) serves as a site of unidirectional block and slow conduction. Anterograde conduction of the impulse is blocked in the upper pathway but succeeds along the lower pathway. Once beyond the zone of depression, the impulse crosses over through lateral connections and reenters through the upper pathway. *Source: Panels C and D are from Schmitt FO, Erlanger J. Directional differences in the conduction of the impulse through heart muscle and their possible relation to extrasystolic and fibrillary contractions. Am J Physiol 1928;87:326–347, figures 5 and 6. Used with permission.*

non similar to that observed by Schmitt and Erlanger in which slow anterograde conduction of the impulse was at times followed by a retrograde wavefront that produced a "return extrasystole."[156] They proposed that the nonstimulated impulse was caused by a circus movement reentry made possible by longitudinal dissociation of the bundle, as in the Schmitt and Erlanger model (see Fig. 35-7). Noting that in many of their experiments "the rapid upstroke within the depressed segment occurs after the rapid upstroke of the normal fiber," Wit and coworkers also considered the possibility[156,157] that "the reflected impulse that travels slowly backward through the depressed segment is evoked by retrograde depolarization of the cells within the depressed segment by the rapid upstrokes of the cells beyond."[157] Thus arose the suggestion that reexcitation could occur in a single fiber through a mechanism other than circus movement, namely reflection. Although both explanations appeared plausible, proof for either was lacking

at the time. Direct evidence in support of reflection as a mechanism of reentrant activity did not emerge until the early 1980s, as discussed later.

These early pioneering studies led to our understanding of how anatomic obstacles such as the openings of the vena cava in the right atrium, an aneurysm in the ventricles, or the presence of bypass tracts between atria and ventricles (Kent bundle) can form a ringlike path for the development of extrasystoles, tachycardia, and flutter.

Leading Circle Model

That reentry could be initiated without the involvement of anatomic obstacles and that "natural rings are not essential for the maintenance of circus contractions" was first suggested by Garrey in 1924.[158] Nearly 50 years later, Allessie and coworkers[159–161] were the first to provide direct evidence in support of this hypothesis in experiments in which they induced a tachycardia in isolated preparations of rabbit left atria by applying properly timed premature extrastimuli. Using multiple intracellular electrodes, they showed that although the basic beats elicited by stimuli applied near the center of the tissue spread normally throughout the preparation, premature impulses propagate only in the direction of shorter refractory periods. An arc of block thus develops around which the impulse is able to circulate and reexcite the tissue. Recordings near the center of the circus movement showed only subthreshold responses. Thus arose the concept of the leading circle,[161] a form of circus movement reentry occurring in structurally uniform myocardium, requiring no anatomic obstacle. The functionally refractory region that develops at the vortex of the circulating wavefront prevents the centripetal waves from short circuiting the circus movement and thus serves to maintain the reentry. Because the head of the circulating wavefront usually travels on relatively refractory tissue, a fully excitable gap of tissue may not be present; unlike other forms of reentry the leading circle model may not be readily influenced by extraneous impulses initiated in areas outside the reentrant circuit and thus may not be easily entrained.

Subsequent studies later showed that the leading circle mechanism could mediate tachycardia induced in isolated ventricular tissues.[162] Allessie and coworkers[163] also described the development of circus movement reentry without the involvement of an anatomic obstacle in a two-dimensional model of ventricular epicardium created by freezing the endocardial layers of a Langendorf-perfused rabbit heart.

Functional arcs or lines of block attending the development of a circus movement reentry were shown to develop in in-vivo models of canine infarction in which a thin surviving epicardial rim overlay the infarcted ventricle.[164–166] The lines of block observed during tachycardia are usually oriented parallel to the direction of the myocardial fibers, suggesting that anisotropic conduction properties (faster conduction in the direction parallel to the long axis of the myocardial cells)[167] also play an important role in defining the functionally refractory zone. Dillon and coworkers[168] subsequently showed that the long lines of functional block that sustain reentry in the epicardial rim overlying canine infarction can represent zones of very slow conduction, implying that the dimensions of the area of functional block can in fact be relatively small and can even approach that of the vortex of functional block described by Allessie and coworkers.

Figure-of-Eight Model

The figure-of-eight model of reentry was first described by El-Sherif and coworkers in the surviving epicardial layer overlying infarction produced by occlusion of the left anterior descending artery in canine hearts in the late 1980s.[165,169,170] In the figure-of-eight model, the reentrant beat produces a wavefront that circulates in both directions around a long line of functional conduction block (Fig. 35–8) rejoining on the distal side of the block. The wavefront then breaks through the arc of block to reexcite the tissue proximal to the block. The single arc of block is thus divided into two, and the reentrant activation continues as two circulating wavefronts that travel in clockwise and counterclockwise directions around the two arcs in a pretzellike configuration. The diameter of the reentrant circuit in the ventricle can be as small as a few millimeters or as large as a several centimeters.

Spiral Waves and Rotors

First introduced by Rosenblueth and Weiner in 1946,[171] the concept of spiral waves has attracted a great deal of interest over the past decade. Originally used to describe reentry around an anatomic obstacle,[171] the term *spiral wave reentry* was later adopted to describe circulating waves in the absence of an anatomic obstacle,[172,173] similar to the circulating waves of the leading circle mechanism described by Allessie and colleagues.[159,161] Spiral wave theory has advanced our understanding of the mechanisms responsible for the functional form of reentry. Although leading circle and spiral wave reentry are considered by some to be similar, a number of distinctions have been suggested.[161,174–176] The curvature of the spiral wave is the key to the formation of the core.[176] The curvature of the wave forms a region of high impedance mismatch (sink-source mismatch), where the current provided by the reentering wavefront (source) is insufficient to charge the capacity and thus excite larger volume of tissue ahead (sink). A prominent curvature of the spiral wave is generally encountered following a wave break, a situation in which a planar wave encounters an obstacle and breaks up into two or more daughter waves. Because it has the greatest curvature, the broken end of the wave moves most slowly. As curvature decreases along the more distal parts of the spiral, propagation speed increases. Another difference between the leading circle and spiral wave is the state of the core; in former it is kept permanently refractory, whereas in the latter the core is excitable but not excited.

The term *spiral wave* is usually used to describe reentrant activity in two dimensions. The center of the spiral wave is called the *core* and the distribution of the core in three dimensions is referred to as the *filament* (Fig. 35–9). The three-dimensional form of the spiral wave forms a scroll wave.[177] In its simplest form, the scroll wave has a straight filament spanning the ventricular wall (i.e., from epicardium to endocardium). Theoretical studies have described three major scroll wave configurations with curved filaments (L-, U-, and O-shaped),[177] although numerous variations of these three-dimensional filaments in space and time are assumed to exist during cardiac arrhythmias.[177] Anisotropy and anatomic obstacles can substantially modify the characteristics and spatio-temporal behavior of the vortexlike reentries. As anatomic obstacles are introduced approaching a ring model of reentry, the curvature of the wave becomes less of a determinant of the characteristics of the arrhythmia.

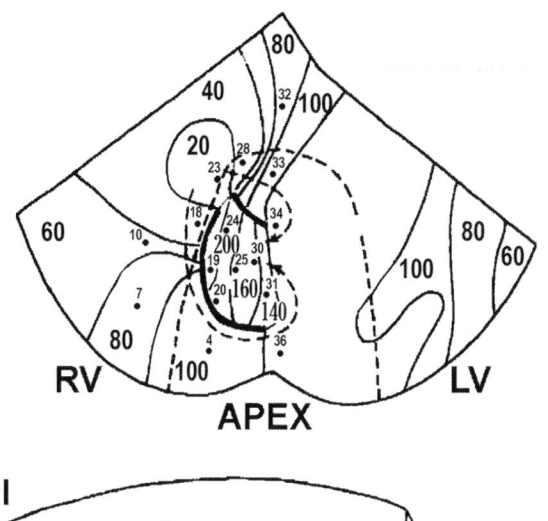

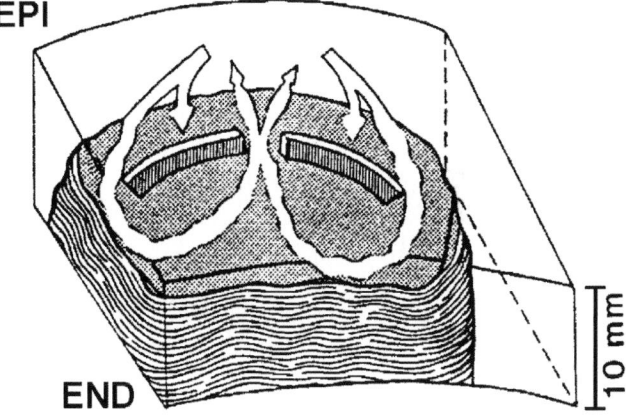

FIGURE 35–8. Figure-of-eight model of reentry. Isochronal activation map during monomorphic reentrant ventricular tachycardia occurring in the surviving epicardial layer overlying an infarction. Recordings were obtained from the epicardial surface of a canine heart 4 days after ligation of the left anterior descending coronary artery. Activation isochrones are drawn at 20 msec intervals. The reentrant circuit has a characteristic figure-of-eight activation pattern. Two circulating wavefronts advance in clockwise and counterclockwise directions, respectively, around two zones (*arcs*) of conduction block (*heavy solid lines*). The epicardial surface is depicted as if the ventricles were unfolded following a cut from the crux to the apex. A three-dimensional diagrammatic illustration of the ventricular activation pattern during the reentrant tachycardia is shown in the lower panel. END, endocardium; EPI, epicardium; LV, left ventricle; RV, right ventricle. *Source: El-Sherif N. Reentry revisited. PACE 1988;11:1358. Used with permission.*

Spiral wave activity has been used to explain the electrocardiographic patterns observed during monomorphic and polymorphic cardiac arrhythmias as well as during fibrillation.[173,178,179] Monomorphic VT results when the spiral wave is anchored and not able to drift within the ventricular myocardium. In contrast, a polymorphic VT such as that encountered with LQTS-induced TdP is caused by a meandering or drifting spiral wave. VF seems to be the most complex representation of rotating spiral waves in the heart. VF is often preceded by VT. One of the theories suggests that VF develops when a single spiral wave responsible for VT breaks up, leading to the development of multiple spirals that are continuously extinguished and re-created.

Reentrant mechanisms are thought to underlie the maintenance of most of rapid cardiac arrhythmias. The role of the reentrant models in the generation of these arrhythmias is discussed in this

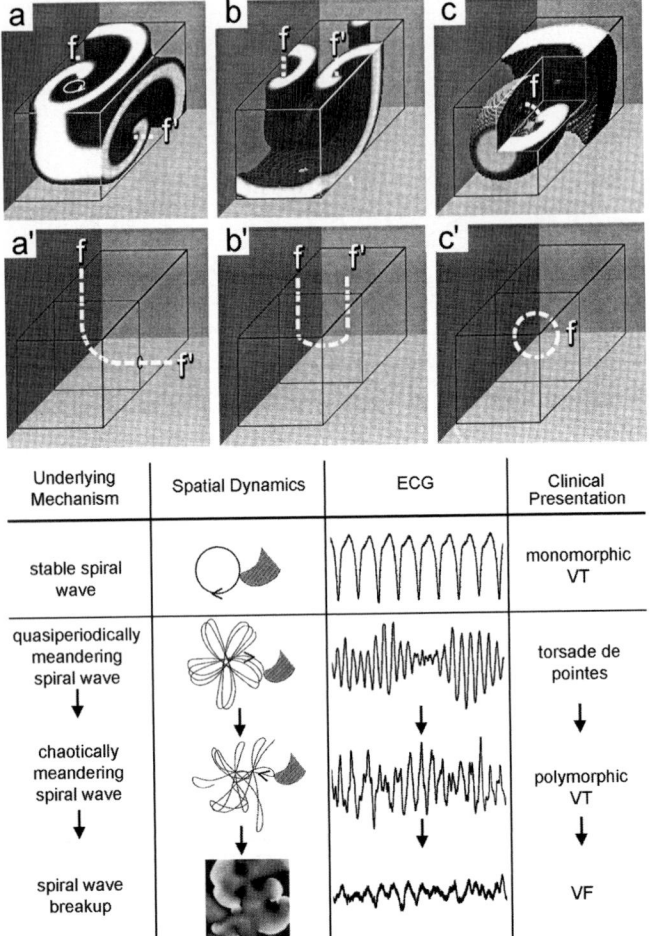

Underlying Mechanism	Spatial Dynamics	ECG	Clinical Presentation
stable spiral wave			monomorphic VT
quasiperiodically meandering spiral wave ↓			torsade de pointes ↓
chaotically meandering spiral wave ↓			polymorphic VT ↓
spiral wave breakup			VF

FIGURE 35–9. Schematic representation of basic scroll-type reentry in three-dimensional and spiral wave phenotypes with their possible clinical manifestations. **Top panel:** Basic configurations of vortexlike reentry in three dimensions: a and a, L-shaped scroll wave and filament, respectively. The scroll rotates in a clockwise direction (*on the top*) about the L-shaped filament (f,f') shown in a', b, and b', U-shaped scroll wave and filament, respectively. c and c, O-shaped wave and filament, respectively. **Bottom panel:** Four types of spiral wave phenotypes and associated clinical manifestations. A stable spiral wave mechanism gives rise to monomorphic ventricular tachycardia (VT) on the ECG. A quasi-periodic meandering spiral wave is responsible for torsade de pointes, whereas a chaotically meandering spiral wave is revealed as polymorphic VT. A ventricular fibrillation (VF) pattern is caused by spiral wave breakup. Second column, spiral waves are shown in *gray*; the path of their tip are shown as *solid lines. Source top panel: Pertsov AM, Jalife J.[177] Used with permission. Source bottom panel: Garfinkel A, Qu Z.[179] Used with permission.*

section. Some specific arrhythmogenic conditions where reentry plays a pivotal role (such as LQTS and Brugada syndrome as well as arrhythmias occurring during ischemia/infarct) are discussed in detail in the following sections. Some specific manifestations of the reentrant mechanism, such as reflection and phase 2 reentry, will be discussed separately as well.

Among the most representative clinical reentrant ring model equivalents are various forms of atrial flutter, involving superior or inferior venae cavae, tricuspid annulus, and so forth, as anatomic barriers to circulate around. Bundle-branch reentry and reentrant tachyarrhythmias in Wolff-Parkinson-White (WPW) preexcitation syndrome are also caused by the anatomically-determined pathway. Many forms of VT occurring under conditions of struc-

tural heart diseases are often maintained by anatomically-predetermined reentrant pathways.[180,181] Ventricular Purkinje fiber networks are thought to provide anatomic reentrant circuits as well.[182]

The figure-of-eight reentrant model can underlie ventricular arrhythmias originating from a thin surviving epicardial layer overlying infarction. It could be the result of either a functional or anatomic reentrant mechanism.

Although the leading circle and spiral wave models have some conceptual differences (discussed above), it is difficult to determine which of these is more likely to underlie a given functional reentrant arrhythmias in the heart. Comtois and colleagues[183] recently analyzed these two concepts of functional reentry and arrived at the conclusion that the spiral waves concept better explains functional reentrant cardiac arrhythmias and its pharmacological responses than the leading circuit concept, both in clinical and experimental settings.[183] The functional reentrant mechanisms can underlie many forms of tachyarrhythmias in ischemic or /infarcted hearts[184] and in structurally normal ventricles, as in the LQTS and Brugada syndrome.

A role for spiral waves in AF and VF is likely to be most common. Both AF and VF are considered to have similar spatio-temporal mechanisms. There are two major theories to explain AF/VF generation. The first, originally suggested by Gordon Moe and colleagues, proposes that cardiac fibrillation is maintained by the continuing development of multiple unstable reentrant wavelets.[185] This "multiple wavelet hypothesis" has been the dominating concept of AF and VF for more than three decades. Recent years have witnessed a revival of another theory for the maintenance of VF/AF known as the "single source hypothesis."[186,187] This theory proposes that AF/VF can be maintained by a single high frequency source, giving rise to impulse propagation with variable conduction block in the remainder of the ventricle (i.e., fibrillatory conduction), which accounts for the AF/VF pattern in the ECG.[186,188–191] It was first proved to occur in cardiac muscle in 1948.[186] A number of recent studies provide further proof for this concept.[188–191] A reentrant mechanism is believed to underlie a single source maintaining AV/VF in most cases (the so-called *mother rotor*).[187] However, a rapidly activating focal source (automatic or triggered activity) can cause some forms of AF/VF as well.[49,192,193] Fig. 35–10 illustrates an example of fibrillatory conduction in a patient with paroxysmal AF and shows its dependence on I_{K1} density in a mathematical model.

Whether AF/VF is caused by a single or multiple reentrant sources, wavebreak (i.e., conduction block) is an indispensable requirement for reentry to develop. Wavebreak occurs when a propagated activating waveform encounters an anatomic or functional (i.e, refractory state) obstacle. Anatomic heterogeneity is well recognized to promote wavebreak, reentry, and AF/VF in healthy and particularly in structurally abnormal ventricles.[194,195] Indeed, it has been shown that even in structurally normal ventricles, phase singularities during VF occur in a nonrandom spatial distribution, often colocalizing with normal anatomic heterogeneities.[196] It is well-appreciated that most cases of clinical VF take place in structurally-damaged ventricles. Many cases of clinical VF, however, occur in ostensibly normal hearts.

Experimental studies have shown that VF can develop spontaneously or can be readily induced in ischemic or infarcted ventricles.[184] In contrast, in healthy ventricles, VF rarely appears spontaneously and can be induced only with very aggressive electrical stimulation protocols, such as burst pacing and direct current of high intensity and long duration.

Interesting interactions have been described between anatomic obstacles and spiral waves.[195] It is noteworthy that the initial description of the spiral wave involved an anatomic obstacle.[171] Mathematical simulation and experimental studies have shown that an anatomic barrier can serve as a point/line of a wavebreak leading to the initiation of spiral wave, which subsequently can detach from the barrier and revolve independently of the barrier.[197] Another scenario is one in which the anatomic obstacle can serve as an anchor to stabilize a spiral wave.[195]

There are two fundamental hypotheses to explain wavebreak occurring in the absence of anatomic obstacles. The first involves spatial refractory period heterogeneity. Gordon Moe's multiple-wavelet concept is fundamentally based on spatial inhomogeneity of refractory periods, providing the substrate for conduction block and wavefront fragmentation (wavebreaks), leading to continuous appearance and disappearance of multiple wandering reentrant wavelets. The other concept of the spiral breakup, referred to as the *Restitution hypothesis*, was formulated less than a decade ago. It invokes temporal dynamic electrical heterogeneity (which is essentially determined by electrical restitution properties of the myocardium) to explain spiral wave instability and breakup during AF/VF. The original restitution hypothesis stipulates that the wavebreak occurs when the slope of the APD restitution curve (determined as the change in APD as a function the preceding diastolic interval) exceed a value of one. In its later versions, the restitution hypothesis includes the restitution of conduction velocity as well as other dynamic factors such as intracellular calcium cycling.[195] It has been shown that a steep relationship between conduction time and interstimulus interval might account for wavebreak and VF, particularly under conditions of depressed excitability.[198] Desynchronization of voltage and intracellular calcium cycling occurring during VF can affect wavebreak.[195,199] In addition to APD/conduction velocity restitution, a number of other factors have been shown to contribute to wave breakup during VF/AF, including cardiac memory, anatomic obstacles and anisotropy.[194,195]

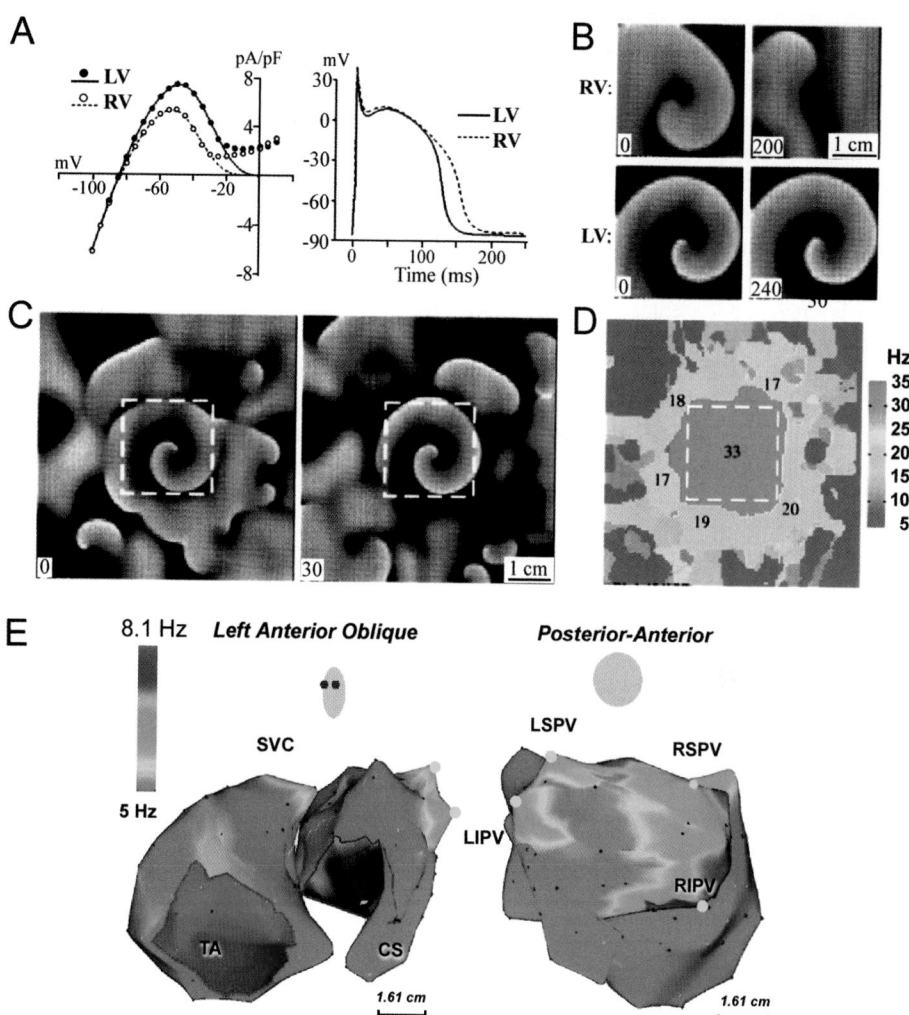

FIGURE 35–10. Computer simulations showing the role of inwardly rectifying K+ current (IK1) in maintaining a stable high-frequency rotor that results in fibrillatory conduction (**A–D**) and an example of fibrillatory conduction in a human patient with atrial fibrillation (AF) (**E**). **A.** Formulation of IK1 used in the model (*solid and broken lines*) with corresponding action potentials. **B.** Snapshots of numerical data; 3 × 3–cm² sheets simulating the right ventricle (*top*) and left ventricle (*bottom*). **C.** Snapshots of numerical data in the combined right ventricular (RV)-left ventricular (LV) model of 6 × 6 cm². **D.** Defibrillation (DF) map obtained from the model in panel C. Values in panels B and C are in milliseconds; in panel D, in hertz. *Broken lines* in panels C and D show the perimeter of the LV model (area, 2 × 2 cm²). **E.** Dominant frequency (DF) map obtained using spectral analysis (fast Fourier transform) of ~120 endocardial electrograms (CARTO) on the atrial surfaces in a patient with paroxysmal AF (6 hours). Note DF sites in each pulmonary vein. The rest of the atria activate at much slower frequencies as a result of fibrillatory conduction. CS, coronary sinus; Hz, hertz; LIPV, left inferior pulmonary vein; LSPV, left superior pulmonary vein; LV, left ventricle; ms, milliseconds; MA, mitral annulus; RIPV, right inferior pulmonary vein; RSPV, right superior pulmonary vein; RV, right ventricle; SVC, superior vena cava; TA, tricuspid annulus. *Source A, B, C, D: Samie, Berenfeld, Anumonwo, et al.[191] Used with permission. Source E: Sanders P, Berenfeld O, Hocini M, et al. Spectral analysis identifies sites of high-frequency activity maintaining atrial fibrillation in humans. Circulation. 2005;112:789. Used with permission.*

The role of spatial versus temporal electrical heterogeneity in wavebreak and the development of VF/AF is a topic of much debate.[194,195] The applicability of the restitution hypothesis is less obvious in the case of AF, than in the case of VF. Indeed, most of atria susceptible to AF, both in patients and experimental animal models, are associated with an abbreviation of refractoriness, loss of APD rate-adaptation, and flattening of the APD restitution curve.[200–202]

Many variation on these themes are possible. For example, it has been suggested that a single meandering spiral wave could underlie VF[203,204] as in the case of the Brugada syndrome.[205] All these concepts of VF/AF maintenance are not mutually exclusive. There are experimental and theoretical data supporting both the multiple-wavelet and single-source hypotheses.[191,206–211] It is possible that different mechanisms and manifestations of AF/VF can be operative depending on prevailing conditions (species, size of the heart, ischemia, time after the start of AF/VF, etc).[188,193,195,202,212] There are experimental data indicating that early stages of VF/AF are maintained by multiple wavelets and late stages of the arrhythmias by a single stable reentrant source.[188,212] It is thought that the functional spatial and temporal heterogeneities as well as anatomic structures interact synergistically to form wavebreak, thus contributing to the maintenance of AF/VF.[194,195] An increase of structural heterogeneity greatly promotes the probability of wavebreak and reentry, reducing the *amount* of functional spatial and temporal heterogeneities required for VF appearance.[195]

The ionic basis for the spatio-temporal behavior of reentrant rotor during VF is not completely understood. It was recently shown by Samie and colleagues[191] that the anterior LV region of the guinea pig heart displays earlier repolarization than right ventricular (RV) free wall during VF and that this region is the usual location of a stable rotor underlying VF in isolated guinea pig heart. Based on measurement of a higher density of background outward current, I_{K1}, in LV versus RV isolated myocytes, Samie and coworkers[191] proposed that the mechanism underlying the primary rotor and wavefront fragmentation can be related to gradients of refractoriness imposed by gradients in I_{K1} (see Fig. 35–10). Another recent paper suggests a dominant role for I_{Kr} in wavebreak dynamics during VF.[211] Higher levels of I_{Kr} and/or $I_{K(ACh)}$ in the left atrium, compared to right atrium, are thought to account for a shorter repolarization and left atrial location of rotor(s) during acute AF.[213,214]

【 】 REFLECTION

The concept of reflection was first suggested by studies of the propagation characteristics of slow action potential responses in K+-depolarized Purkinje fibers.[155] In strands of Purkinje fiber, Wit and coworkers demonstrated a phenomenon similar to that observed by Schmitt and Erlanger in which slow anterograde conduction of the impulse was at times followed by a retrograde wavefront that produced a "return extrasystole."[156] They proposed that the nonstimulated impulse was caused by circuitous reentry at the level of the syncytial interconnections, made possible by longitudinal dissociation of the bundle, as the most likely explanation for the phenomenon but also suggested the possibility of reflection. Direct evidence in support of reflection as a mechanism of arrhythmogenesis was provided by Antzelevitch and coworkers in the early 1980s.[215,216]

A number of models of reflection have been developed.[57,215–217] The first of these involves use of *ion-free* isotonic sucrose solution to create a narrow (1.5 to 2 mm) central inexcitable zone (gap) in unbranched Purkinje fibers mounted in a three-chamber tissue bath (Fig. 35–11).[215] In the sucrose-gap model, stimulation of the proximal (P) segment elicits an action potential that propagates to the proximal border of the sucrose gap. Active propagation across the sucrose gap is not possible because of the ion-depleted extracellular milieu, but local circuit current continues to flow through the intercellular low resistance pathways (a Ag/AgCl extracellular shunt pathway is provided). This local circuit or electrotonic current, very much reduced on emerging from the gap, gradually discharges the capacity of the distal (D) tissue thus giving rise to a depolarization that manifests as a either a subthreshold response (last distal response) or a foot-potential that brings the distal excitable tissue to its threshold potential (Fig. 35–12).[218] Active impulse propagation stops and then resumes after a delay that can be as long as several hundred milliseconds. When anterograde (P to D) transmission time is sufficiently delayed to permit recovery of refractoriness at the proximal end, electrotonic transmission of the impulse in the retrograde direction is able to reexcite the proximal tissue, thus generating a closely coupled reflected reentry. Reflection therefore results from the to-and-fro electrotonically-mediated transmission of the impulse across the same inexcitable segment; neither longitudinal dissociation nor circus movement need be invoked to explain the phenomenon.

A second model of reflection involved the creation of an inexcitable zone permitting delayed conduction by superfusion of a central segment of a Purkinje bundle with a solution designed to mimic the extracellular milieu at a site of ischemia.[216] The gap was shown to be largely comprised of an inexcitable cable across which conduction of impulses was electrotonically mediated.

Reflected reentry has been demonstrated in isolated atrial and ventricular myocardial tissues as well.[217,219,220] Reflection has also been demonstrated in Purkinje fibers in which a functionally inexcitable zone is created by focal depolarization of the preparation with long duration constant current pulses.[221] Reflection is also observed in isolated canine Purkinje fibers homogeneously de-

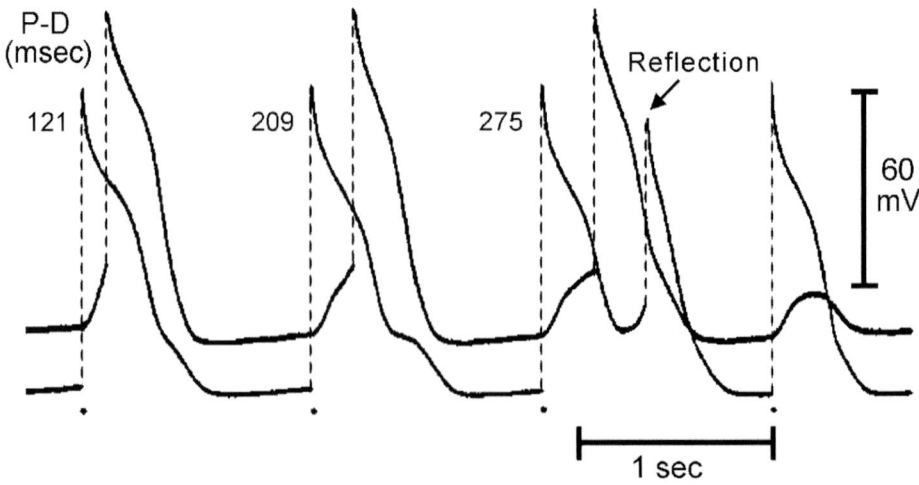

FIGURE 35–11. Delayed transmission and reflection across an inexcitable gap created by superfusion of the central segment of a Purkinje fiber with an *ion-free* isotonic sucrose solution. The two traces were recorded from proximal (P) and distal (D) active segments. P–D conduction time (indicated in the upper portion of the figure, in msec) increased progressively with a 4:3 Wenckebach periodicity. The third stimulated proximal response was followed by a reflection. *Source: Antzelevitch.[227] Used with permission.*

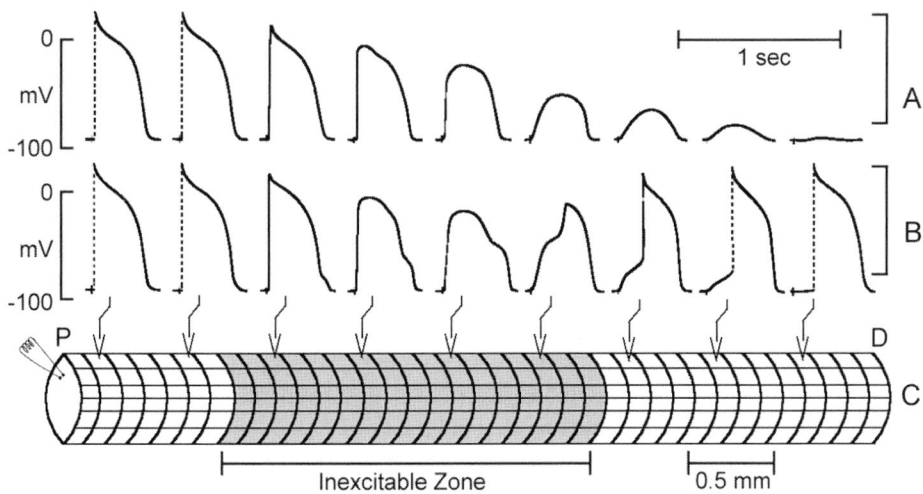

FIGURE 35–12. Discontinuous conduction (**B**) and conduction block (**A**) in a Purkinje strand with a central inexcitable zone (**C**). The schematic illustration is based on transmembrane recordings obtained from canine Purkinje fiber-sucrose gap preparations. An action potential elicited by stimulation of the proximal (P) side of the preparation conducts normally up to the border of the inexcitable zone. Active propagation of the impulse stops at this point, but local circuit current generated by the proximal segment continues to flow through the preparation encountering a cumulative resistance (successive gap junctions). Transmembrane recordings from the first few inexcitable cells show a response not very different from the action potentials recorded in the neighboring excitable cells, in spite of the fact that no ions may be moving across the membrane of these cells. The responses recorded in the inexcitable region are the electrotonic images of activity generated in the proximal excitable segment. The resistive-capacitive properties of the tissue lead to an exponential decline in the amplitude of the transmembrane potential recorded along the length of the inexcitable segment and to a slowing of the rate of change of voltage as a function of time. If, as in panel B, the electrotonic current is sufficient to bring the distal excitable tissue to its threshold potential, an action potential is generated after a step delay imposed by the slow discharge of the capacity of the distal (D) membrane by the electrotonic current (foot-potential). Active conduction of the impulse therefore stops at the proximal border of the inexcitable zone and resumes at the distal border after a step delay that can range from a few to tens or hundreds of milliseconds. *Source: Modified from Antzelevitch.[218] Used with permission.*

pressed with high K⁺ solution as well as in branched preparations of *normal* Purkinje fibers.[222]

Because the excitability of cardiac tissues continues to recover for hundreds of milliseconds after an action potential, impulse transmission across the inexcitable zone is a sensitive function of frequency.[215,223–226] As a consequence, the incidence and patterns of manifest ectopic activity encountered in models of reflection are highly rate-dependent.[57,220,224,227,228] Similar rate-dependent changes in extrasystolic activity are reported in patients with frequent extrasystoles evaluated with Holter recordings[229] and in patients evaluated by atrial pacing.[227,230] Reflection can occur within areas of limited size (as small as 1 to 2 mm²) and is expected to appear as focal in origin. Reflection has been suggested as the mechanism underlying reentrant extrasystolic activity in ventricular tissues excised from a 1-day-old infarcted canine heart[231] and in a clinical case of incessant ventricular bigeminy in a young patient with no evidence of organic heart disease.[232]

PHASE 2 REENTRY

Another reentrant mechanism that can appear to be of focal origin is Phase 2 reentry. Phase 2 reentry occurs when the dome of the action potential, most commonly epicardial, propagates from sites at which it is maintained to sites at which it is abolished, causing local reexcitation of the epicardium and the generation of a closely coupled extrasystole. A more detailed discussion of phase 2 reentry

and its role in the precipitation of VT/VF follows in the next section.

REENTRY CAUSED BY SPATIAL DISPERSION OF REPOLARIZATION

Studies conducted over the past 15 years have established that ventricular myocardium is not homogeneous, as previously thought but is comprised of at least three electrophysiologically and functionally distinct cell types: epicardial, M, and endocardial cells.[115,233] These three principal ventricular myocardial cell types differ with respect to phase 1 and phase 3 repolarization characteristics (Fig. 35–13). Ventricular epicardial and M, but not endocardial, cells generally display a prominent phase 1, because of a large 4-aminopyridine (4-AP) sensitive transient outward current (I_{to}), giving the action potential a spike and dome or notched configuration. These regional differences in I_{to}, first suggested on the basis of action potential data,[234] have now been directly demonstrated in a ventricular myocytes from a wide variety of species including canine,[235] feline,[236] and human.[237,238]

Differences in the magnitude of the action potential notch and corresponding differences in Ito have also been described between right and LV epicardium.[239] Similar interventricular differences in Ito have also been described for canine ventricular M cells.[240] This distinction is thought to form the basis for why the Brugada syndrome, a channelopathy-mediated form of sudden death, is a RV disease.

Myocytes isolated from the epicardial region of the LV wall of the rabbit show a higher density of cAMP-activated chloride current

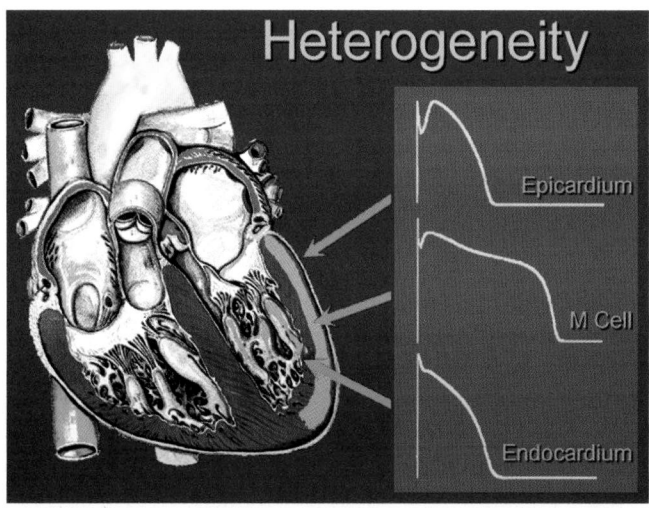

FIGURE 35–13. Action potential characteristics recorded from epicardial, M, and endocardial regions of the canine left ventricle.

when compared to endocardial myocytes.[241] I_{to2}, initially ascribed to a K^+ current, is now thought to be primarily because of the calcium-activated chloride current ($I_{Cl(Ca)}$) is also thought to contribute to the action potential notch, but it is not known whether this current, differs among the three ventricular myocardial cell types.[242]

Wang and coworkers reported two differences in Ca^{2+} channel properties between epicardial and endocardial canine ventricular cells. I_{Ca} was found to be larger in endocardial than in epicardial myocytes.[243] It is noteworthy that several other studies also conducted in canine ventricular myocytes failed to detect any difference in I_{Ca} among cells isolated from epicardium, M, and endocardial regions of the LV wall.[244,245]

Between the surface epicardial and endocardial layers are transitional and M cells. M cells are distinguished by the ability of their action potential to prolong disproportionately relative to the action potential of other ventricular myocardial cells in response to a slowing of rate and/or in response to action potential duration (APD)-prolonging agents (see Fig. 35–13).[115,246,247] In the dog, the ionic basis for these features of the M cell include the presence of a smaller slowly activating delayed rectifier current (I_{Ks}),[68] a larger late sodium current (late I_{Na})[86] and a larger Na-Ca exchange current (I_{Na-Ca}).[248] In the canine heart, the rapidly activating delayed rectifier (I_{Kr}) and inward rectifier (I_{K1}) currents are similar in the three transmural cell types. Transmural and apical-basal differences in the density of I_{Kr} channels have been described in the ferret heart.[249] I_{Kr} message and channel protein are much larger in the ferret epicardium. I_{Ks} is larger in M cells isolated from the right versus left ventricles of the dog.[240]

Histologically M cells are similar to epicardial and endocardial cells. Electrophysiologically and pharmacologically, they appear to be a hybrid between Purkinje and ventricular cells.[250] Like Purkinje fibers, M cells show a prominent APD prolongation and develop EADs in response to I_{Kr} blockers, whereas epicardium and endocardium do not. Like Purkinje fibers, M cells develop DADs in response to agents that calcium load or overload the cardiac cell; epicardium and endocardium do not. Unlike Purkinje fibers, M cells display an APD prolongation in response to I_{Ks} blockers; epicardium and endocardium also show an increase in APD in response to I_{Ks} blockers. Purkinje and M cells also respond differently to α-adrenergic agonists. α_1-Adrenoceptor stimulation produces APD prolongation in Purkinje fibers, but abbreviation in M cells, and little or no change in endocardium and epicardium.[251]

Distribution of M cells within the ventricular wall has been investigated in greatest detail in the left ventricle of the canine heart. Although transitional cells are found throughout the wall in the canine left ventricle, M cells displaying the longest action potentials (at basic cycle length [BCL] $\geq$ 2000 milliseconds [msec]) are often localized in the deep subendocardium to midmyocardium in the anterior wall,[252] deep subepicardium to midmyocardium in the lateral wall[246] and throughout the wall in the region of the RV outflow tracts.[233] M cells are also present in the deep cell layers of endocardial structures, including papillary muscles, trabeculae, and the interventricular septum.[253] Unlike Purkinje fibers, M cells are not found in discrete bundles or islets,[253,254] although there is evidence that they can be localized in discrete muscle layers. Cells with the characteristics of M cells have been described in the canine, guinea pig, rabbit, pig, and human ventricles (see Antzelevitch and coworkers).[250]

Amplification of transmural heterogeneities normally present in the early and late phases of the action potential can lead to the development of a variety of arrhythmias, including Brugada, long QT, and short QT syndromes as well as catecholaminergic VT (Table 35–2).

Brugada Syndrome

Brugada syndrome was introduced as a new clinical entity by Pedro and Josep Brugada in 1992.[255] The syndrome has attracted considerable interest because of its high incidence in many parts of the world and its association with high risk of sudden death, especially in males as they enter their third and fourth decade of life. A consensus report published in 2002 delineated diagnostic criteria for the syndrome.[256,257] A second consensus conference report published in 2005 focused on risk stratification schemes and approaches to therapy.[258,259]

Characterized by an ST-segment elevation in the right precordial ECG leads and a high incidence of sudden death in patients with structurally normal hearts, the Brugada syndrome generally manifests during adulthood. The average age at the time of initial diagnosis or sudden death is 40 ± 22 years of age. The youngest patient diagnosed with the syndrome is 2 days of age, and the oldest is 84 years of age. A recent report by Skinner and colleagues provides a direct link between sudden infant death syndrome (SIDS) and the Brugada syndrome.[260]

Sudden unexplained nocturnal death syndrome (SUNDS, also known as *sudden unexplained death syndrome* [SUDS]), a disorder most prevalent in Southeast Asia, and Brugada syndrome have recently been shown to be phenotypically, genetically, and functionally the same disorder.[261]

The majority of congenital Brugada syndrome patients are believed to possess a structurally normal heart, consistent with the notion that this is a primary electrical heart disease.[262] Although fibrosis and myocarditis can exacerbate or indeed trigger events in patients with the Brugada syndrome, it seems clear that in the vast majority of cases these structural changes are unrelated to arrhythmogenic right ventricular cardiomyopathy (ARVC) or arrhythmogenic right ventricular dysplasia (ARVD).

The first gene to be linked to the Brugada syndrome is *SCN5A*, the gene that encodes for the α subunit of the cardiac sodium channel.[263] More than 100 mutations in SCN5A have been linked to the syndrome in recent years (see Antzelevitch and coworkers[264] for references; also see www.fsm.it/cardmoc). Only a fraction of these mutations have been studied in expression systems and shown to result in loss of function due either to (1) failure of the sodium channel to express; (2) a shift in the voltage- and time-dependence of sodium channel current (I_{Na}) activation, inactivation, or reactivation; (3) entry of the sodium channel into an intermediate state of inactivation from which it recovers more slowly; or (4) accelerated inactivation of the sodium channel. Mutation in the *SCN5A* gene account for approximately 15 percent of Brugada syndrome probands. A higher incidence of *SCN5A* mutations has been reported in familial than in sporadic cases.[265] Of note, negative *SCN5A* results generally do not rule out causal gene mutations, because the promoter region, cryptic splicing mutations, or presence of gross rearrangements are generally not part of routine investigation. A recent report by Hong and coworkers[266]

TABLE 35–2

Genetic Disorders Caused by Ion Channelopathies

		RHYTHM	INHERITANCE	LOCUS	ION CHANNEL	GENE
Long QT syndrome (RW)	LQT1	TdP	AD	11p15	I_{Ks}	KCNQ1, KvLQT1
	LQT2	TdP	AD	7q35	I_{Kr}	KCNH2, HERG
	LQT3	TdP	AD	3p21	I_{Na}	SCN5A, Na$_v$1.5
	LQT4	TdP	AD	4q25		ANKB, ANK2
	LQT5	TdP	AD	21q22	I_{Ks}	KCNE1, minK
	LQT6	TdP	AD	21q22	I_{Kr}	KCNE2, MiRP1
	LQT7 (Andersen-Tawil syndrome)	TdP	AD	17q23	I_{K1}	KCNJ2, Kir 2.1
	LQT8 (Timothy syndrome)	TdP	AD	6q8A	I_{Ca-L}	CACNA1C, Ca$_v$1.2
	LQT9	TdP	AD	3p25	I_{Na}	CAV3, Caveolin-3
	LQT10	TdP	AD	11q23.3	I_{Na}	SCN4B. Na$_v$b4
LQT syndrome (JLN)		TdP	AR	11p15	I_{Ks}	KCNQ1, KvLQT1
		TdP	AR	21q22	I_{Ks}	KCNE1, minK
Brugada syndrome	BrS1	PVT	AD	3p21	I_{Na}	SCN5A, Na$_v$1.5
	BrS2	PVT	AD	3p24	I_{Na}	GPD1L
	BrS3	PVT	AD	12p13.3	I_{Ca}	CACNA1C, Ca$_V$1.2
	BrS4	PVT	AD	10p12.33	I_{Ca}	CACNB2b, Ca$_v$β$_{2b}$
Short QT syndrome	SQT1	VT/VF	AD	7q35	I_{Kr}	KCNH2, HERG
	SQT2	VT/VF	AD	11p15	I_{Ks}	KCNQ1, KvLQT1
	SQT3	VT/VF	AD	17q23.1–24.2	I_{K1}	KCNJ2, Kir2.1
	SQT4	VT/VF	AD	12p13.3	I_{Ca}	CACNA1C, Ca$_v$1.2
	SQT5	VT/VF	AD	10p12.33	I_{Ca}	CACNB2b, Ca$_v$β$_{2b}$
Catecholaminergic VT	CPVT1	VT	AD	1q42–43		RyR2
	CPVT2	VT	AR	1p13–21		CASQ2

AD, autosomal dominant; AR, autosomal recessive; JLN, Jervell and Lange–Nielsen; LQT, long QT; RW, Romano-Ward; TdP, torsade de pointes; VF, ventricular fibrillation; VT, ventricular tachycardia; PVT, polymorphic VT.

provided the first report of a dysfunctional sodium channel created by an intronic mutation giving rise to cryptic splice site activation in SCN5A in a family with the Brugada syndrome. The deletion of fragments of segments 2 and 3 of domain IV of SCN5A caused complete loss of function. Bezzina and coworkers recently provided interesting evidence in support of the hypothesis that an SCN5A promoter polymorphism common in Asians modulates variability in cardiac conduction and can contribute to the high prevalence of Brugada syndrome in the Asian population.[267] Sequencing of the SCN5A promoter identified a haplotype variant consisting of six polymorphisms in near-complete linkage disequilibrium that occurred at an allele frequency of 22 percent in Asian subjects and was absent in whites and blacks. The results of the study demonstrate that sodium channel transcription in the human heart can vary considerably among individuals and races and be associated with variable conduction velocity and arrhythmia susceptibility.

A second locus on chromosome 3, close to but distinct from SCN5A, has recently been linked to the syndrome[268] in a large pedigree in which the syndrome is associated with progressive conduction disease, a low sensitivity to procainamide, and a relatively good prognosis. The gene was recently identified as the glycerol-3-phosphate dehydrogenase 1-like gene (GPD1L). A mutation in GPD1L has been shown to result in a reduction of I_{Na}.[269]

The third and fourth genes associated with the Brugada syndrome encode the α1 (CACNA1C) and β (CACNB2b) subunits of the L-type cardiac calcium channel. Mutations in the α and β subunits of the calcium channel also lead to a shorter than normal QT interval, in some cases creating a combined Brugada/short-QT syndrome.[270]

Knowledge thus far gained through genetic analysis suggests that identification of specific mutations may not be very helpful in formulating a diagnosis or providing a prognosis. There are no clear hotspots, and mutations have been reported throughout the SCN5A gene. It is not clear whether some mutations are associated with a greater risk of arrhythmic events or sudden death. Genetic testing is recommended for support of the clinical diagnosis, for early detection of relatives at potential risk, and particularly for the purpose of advancing research and consequently our understanding of genotype-phenotype relations.

The cellular basis for the Brugada syndrome has come into focus in recent years. The concept of phase 2 reentry, which is a known trigger for the Brugada syndrome, was described in the early 1990s and evolved in parallel with the clinical discovery of the Brugada syndrome.[271–274] Studies conducted over the past decade suggest that rebalancing of the currents active at the end of phase 1, leading to an accentuation of the action potential notch in RV epicardium is responsible for the accentuated J wave or ST-segment elevation associated with the Brugada syndrome (see Antzelevitch[275] for references). Under normal conditions, the appearance of the epicardial action potential notch is caused principally by the interaction of two ion channel currents. The transient outward current (I_{to}), which activates during phase 0, contributes most prominently to phase 1 of the action potential, whereas the calcium inward current is largely responsible for the second upstroke, giving rise to the action potential dome.

Amplification of epicardial and transmural dispersion of repolarization secondary to the presence of genetic defects, pathophysiologic factors, and pharmacologic influences, leads to accentuation of the J wave and eventually to loss of the action potential dome, giving rise to extrasystolic activity in the form of phase 2 reentry. Activation of I_{to} leads to a paradoxical prolongation of APD in canine ventricular tissues[276] but to abbreviation of ventricular APD in species that normally exhibit brief action potentials (e.g., mouse and rat).[277] Pathophysiologic conditions (e.g., ischemia, metabolic inhibition) and some pharmacologic interventions (e.g., I_{Na} or I_{Ca} blockers or I_{K-ATP}, I_{to}, I_{Kr}, or I_{Ks} activators) can lead to marked abbreviation of the action potential in canine and feline[278] ventricular cells where I_{to} is prominent. Under these conditions, canine ventricular epicardium exhibits an all-or-none repolarization as a result of the shift in the balance of currents flowing at the end of phase 1 of the action potential. When phase 1 reaches approximately −30 mV, all-or-none repolarization of the action potential ensues leading to loss of the dome as the outward currents overwhelm the inward currents. Loss of the action potential dome generally occurs at some epicardial sites but not others, resulting in the development of a marked dispersion of repolarization within the epicardium as well as transmurally, between epicardium and endocardium. Propagation of the action potential dome from the epicardial site at which it is maintained to sites at which it is abolished can cause local reexcitation of the preparation. This mechanism, termed *phase 2 reentry*, produces extrasystolic beats capable of initiating circus movement reentry.[4] Phase 2 reentry occurs when RV epicardium is exposed to (1) K+-channel openers such as pinacidil[279]; (2) sodium channel blockers such as flecainide[280]; (3) increased $[Ca^{2+}]_o$[281]; (4) calcium channel blockers such as verapamil; (5) metabolic inhibition[282]; and (6) simulated ischemia.[4]

Prominent or otherwise abnormal J waves have long been linked to idiopathic VT and the Brugada syndrome.[255,283–286] The Brugada syndrome is characterized by exaggerated J waves that manifest as an ST-segment elevation in the right precordial leads.[255] A number of studies have highlighted the similarities between the conditions that predispose to phase 2 reentry and those that attend the appearance of the Brugada syndrome. Loss of the action potential dome in epicardium, but not endocardium generates a transmural current that manifests on the ECG as an ST-segment elevation, similar to that encountered in patients with the Brugada syndrome.[271,282,287] Evidence in support of a phase 2 reentrant mechanism in humans was recently provided by Thomsen and colleagues[5,6]

Autonomic neurotransmitters like acetylcholine facilitate loss of the action potential dome[288] by suppressing I_{Ca} and/or augment-

ing potassium current. β-adrenergic agonists restore the dome by augmenting I_{Ca}. Sodium channel blockers also facilitate loss of the canine RV action potential dome by means of a negative shift in the voltage at which phase 1 begins.[280,289] These findings are consistent with accentuation of ST-segment elevation in patients with the Brugada syndrome following vagal maneuvers or class I antiarrhythmic agents as well as normalization of the ST-segment elevation following β-adrenergic agents and phosphodiesterase III inhibitors.[271,290,291] Loss of the action potential dome is more readily induced in right versus left canine ventricular epicardium[239,282,287] because of the more prominent I_{to}-mediated phase 1 in action potentials in this region of the heart. This distinction is believed to be the basis for why the Brugada syndrome is a RV disease.

Thus accentuation of the RV epicardial action potential notch underlies the ST-segment elevation. Eventual loss of the dome of the RV epicardial action potential further exaggerates ST-segment elevation. The vulnerable window created within epicardium, as well as transmurally, serves as the substrate, and phase 2 reentry provides the extrasystole that serves as the trigger that precipitates episodes of VT and VF in the Brugada syndrome. Evidence in support of this hypothesis was recently provided in an arterially-perfused canine RV experimental model of the Brugada syndrome.[272] The VT and VF generated in these preparations is usually polymorphic, resembling a rapid form of TdP. This activity can be mechanistically related to the migrating spiral wave shown to generate a pattern resembling TdP associated with a normal or long QT interval.[105,173]

Although sodium channel block is capable in recapitulating the electrocardiographic and arrhythmic manifestations of the Brugada syndrome in experimental models,[272] a recent study reports that a combination of I_{Na} and I_{Ca} block is more effective than I_{Na} inhibition alone in precipitating the Brugada syndrome in the arterially-perfused wedge preparation (Fig. 35–14).[273] High concentrations of terfenadine (5 μM) produce a potent block of I_{Na} and I_{Ca}, leading to accentuation of the epicardial action potential notch following acceleration of the rate from a BCL of 800 msec to 400 msec. Accentuation of the notch is caused by the effect of the drug to depress phase 0, augment the magnitude of phase 1, and delay the appearance of the second upstroke. Because of use-dependent inhibition of I_{Na} and I_{Ca}, with continued rapid pacing, phase 1 becomes more accentuated, until all-or-none repolarization occurs at the end of phase 1 at some epicardial sites but not others, leading to the development of both epicardial (early diastolic relaxation [EDR]) and transmural dispersion of repolarization (Fig. 35–14C). Propagation of the dome from the region where it is maintained to the region at which it is lost then results in the development of local phase 2 reentry (Fig. 35–14D). Fig. 35–15 shows the ability of terfenadine-induced phase 2 reentry to generate an extrasystole, couplet and polymorphic VT/VF. An example of programmed electrical stimulation to initiate VT/VF under similar conditions is shown in Fig. 35–15D.

A high resolution optical mapping system that allows simultaneous recording of transmembrane action potentials from 256 sites along the transmural surface of the arterially-perfused canine RV wedge preparation has been used by Aiba and coworkers[292] to demonstrate that a steep repolarization gradient between the region at which the dome is lost and the region at which it is maintained is essential for the development of a closely coupled phase 2 reentrant extrasystole. This study also showed that reentry initially

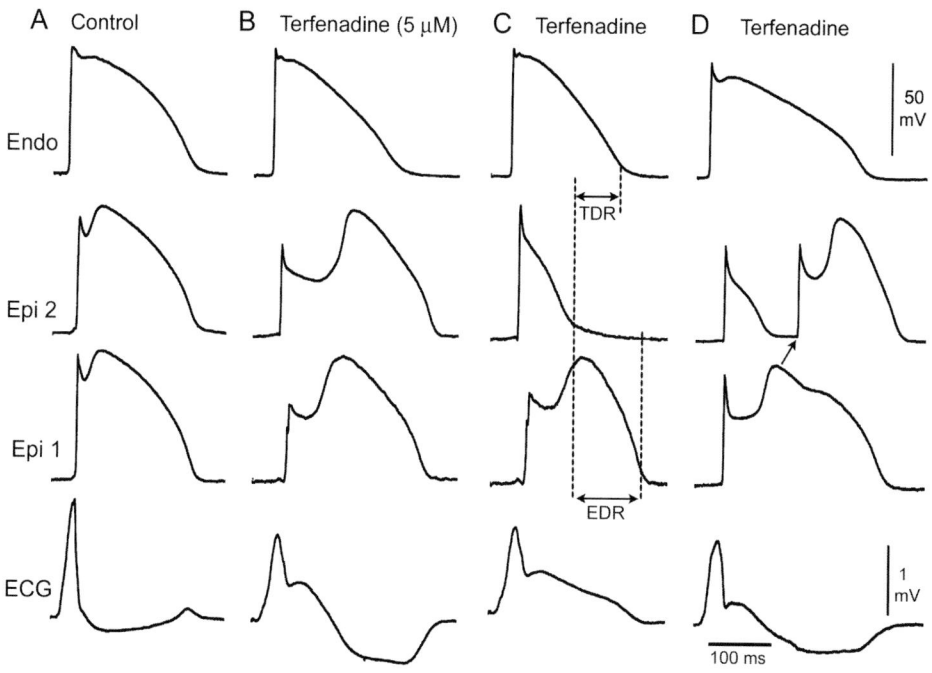

FIGURE 35–14. Experimental model of the Brugada syndrome. Terfenadine-induced ST-segment elevation, T-wave inversion, transmural and endocardial dispersion of repolarization, and phase 2 reentry. Each panel shows transmembrane action potentials from one endocardial (*top*) and two epicardial sites together with a transmural ECG recorded from a canine arterially-perfused right ventricular wedge preparation. **A.** Control (basic cycle length [BCL] 400 msec). **B.** Terfenadine (5 μM) accentuated the epicardial action potential notch creating a transmural voltage gradient that manifests as a ST-segment elevation or exaggerated J wave in the ECG. First beat recorded after changing from BCL 800 msec to BCL 400 msec. **C.** Continued pacing at BCL 400 msec results in all-or-none repolarization at the end of phase 1 at some epicardial sites but not others, creating a local epicardial dispersion of repolarization (EDR) as well as a transmural dispersion of repolarization. **D.** Phase 2 reentry occurs when the epicardial action potential dome propagates from a site where it is maintained to regions where it has been lost. *Source: Modified from Fish, Antzelevitch.[273] Used with permission.*

rotates in the epicardium and gradually shifts to a transmural orientation, responsible for nonsustained polymorphic VT or VF.

A recent report by Kurita and colleagues in which MAP electrodes where positioned on the epicardial and endocardial surfaces of the right ventricular outflow tract (RVOT) in patients with the Brugada syndrome provide further support.[293,294]

The marked accentuation of the epicardial action potential dome and the development of concealed phase 2 reentry suggest that activation forces can extend beyond the QRS in Brugada patients. Indeed, signal-averaged ECG (SAECG) recordings have demonstrated late potentials in patients with the Brugada syndrome, especially in the anterior wall of the RVOT.[295–298] The basis for these late potentials, which are commonly ascribed to delayed conduction within the ventricle, are largely unknown. Late potentials are often regarded as being representative of delayed activation of the myocardium, but in the case of the Brugada syndrome other possibilities exist. For example, the second upstroke of the epicardial action potential, thought to be greatly accentuated in Brugada syndrome[299] might be capable of generating late potentials when RVOT activation is otherwise normal. Moreover, the occurrence of phase 2 reentry, especially when concealed (i.e., when it fails to trigger transmural reentry), can contribute to the generation of delayed unipolar and late SAECG potentials.

The rate-dependence of the ECG sign can be helpful in discriminating between these two hypotheses (depolarization vs. re-

polarization defect). If the Brugada ECG sign is caused by delayed conduction in the RVOT, acceleration of the rate would be expected to further aggravate conduction and thus accentuate the ST-segment elevation and the right bundle-branch block (RBBB) morphology of the ECG. If, however, the Brugada ECG sign is secondary to accentuation of the epicardial action potential notch, at some point leading to loss of the action potential dome, acceleration of the rate would be expected to normalize the ECG, by restoring the action potential dome and reducing the notch. This occurs because the transient outward current, which is at the center of this mechanism, is less available at faster rates because of slow recovery from inactivation. Brugada patients usually display a normalization of their ECG or no change when heart rate is increased, thus favoring the second hypothesis.

Thus, the available data, both basic and clinical, point to transmural voltage gradients that develop secondary to accentuation of the epicardial notch and loss of the action potential dome as the predominant mechanism responsible for the Brugada ECG signature.

Although the genetic mutation responsible for the Brugada syndrome is equally distributed between the sexes, the clinical phenotype is 8 to 10 times more prevalent in males than in females. The basis for this sex-related distinction has been shown to be caused by a more prominent Ito-mediated action potential notch in the RV epicardium of males versus females.[300] The more prominent Ito causes the end of phase 1 of the RV epicardial action potential to repolarize to more negative potentials in tissue and arterially perfused wedge preparations from males, facilitating loss of the action potential dome and the development of phase 2 reentry and polymorphic VT.

The proposed cellular mechanism for the Brugada syndrome is summarized in Fig. 35–16. The available data support the hypothesis that the Brugada syndrome results from amplification of heterogeneities intrinsic to the early phases of the action potential among the different transmural cell types. The amplification is secondary to a rebalancing of currents active during phase 1, including a decrease in I_{Na} or I_{Ca} or augmentation of any one of a number of outward currents. ST-segment elevation similar to that observed in patients with the Brugada syndrome occurs as a consequence of the accentuation of the action potential notch, eventually leading to loss of the action potential dome in RV epicardium, where Ito is most prominent. Loss of the dome gives rise to both a transmural as well as epicardial dispersion of repolarization. The transmural dispersion is responsible for the development of ST-segment elevation and the creation of a vulnerable window across the ventricular wall, whereas the epicardial dispersion give to phase

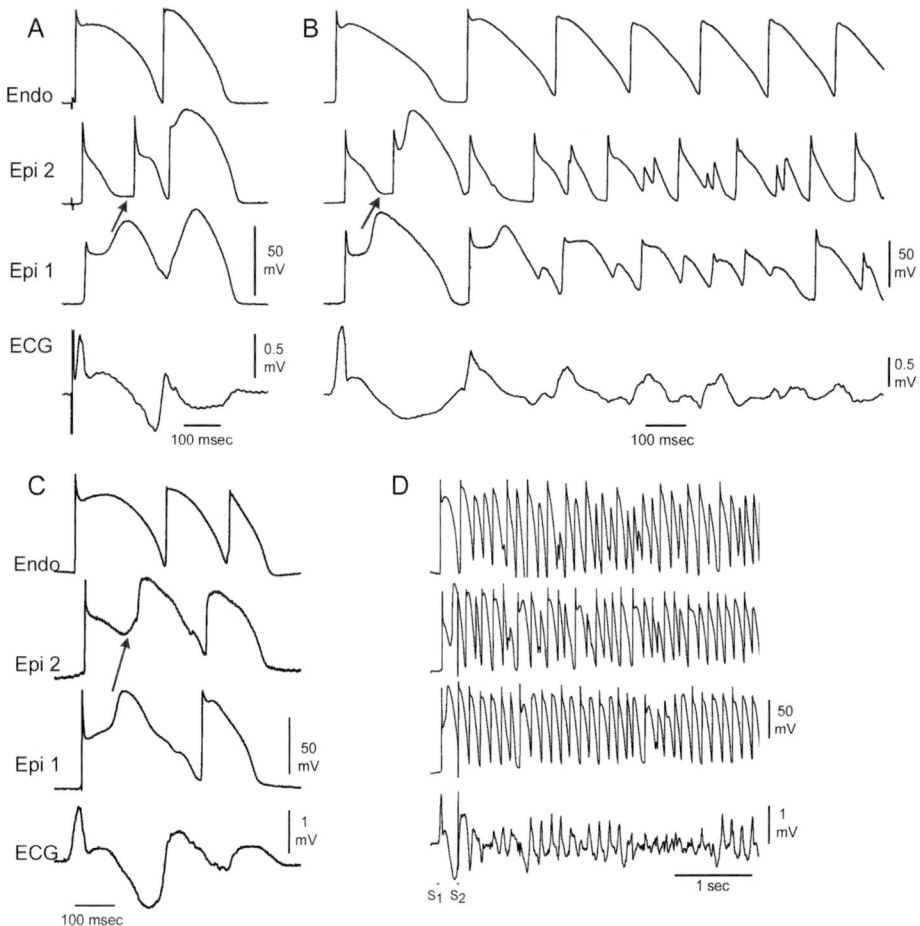

FIGURE 35–15. Spontaneous and programmed electrical stimulation-induced polymorphic ventricular tachycardia (VT) in right ventricular (RV) wedge preparations pretreated with terfenadine (5–10 µM). **A.** Phase 2 reentry in epicardium gives rise to a closely coupled extrasystole. **B.** Phase 2 reentrant extrasystole triggers a brief episode of polymorphic VT. **C.** Phase 2 reentry followed by a single circus movement reentry in epicardium gives rise to a couplet. **D.** Extrastimulus (S_1–S_2 = 250 msec) applied to epicardium triggers a polymorphic VT. S_1, first heart sound; S_2, second heart sound. *Source: Modified from Fish, Antzelevitch.[273] Used with permission.*

2 reentry, which provides the extrasystole that captures the vulnerable window, thus precipitating VT/VF. The VT generated is usually polymorphic, resembling a very rapid form of TdP.

The Long QT Syndrome

The long QT syndromes (LQTSs) are phenotypically and genotypically diverse but have in common the appearance of a long QT interval in the ECG, an atypical polymorphic VT known as TdP, and, in many but not all cases, a relatively high risk for sudden cardiac death.[301–303] Congenital LQTS is subdivided into ten genotypes distinguished by mutations in at least seven different ion genes and an structural anchoring protein located on chromosomes 3, 4, 6, 7, 11, 17, and 21 (see Table 35–2).[304–311] Timothy syndrome, also referred to as LQT8, is a rare congenital disorder characterized by multiorgan dysfunction including prolongation of the QT interval, lethal arrhythmias, webbing of fingers and toes, congenital heart disease, immune deficiency, intermittent hypoglycemia, cognitive abnormalities, and autism. Timothy syndrome has been linked to loss of voltage-dependent inactivation caused by mutations in $Ca_v 1.2$, the gene that encodes for an α

subunit of the calcium channel.[312] The most recent genes associated with LQTS are *CAV3,* which encodes caveolin-3 and *SCN4B,* which encodes $Na_v B4$, an auxiliary subunit of the cardiac sodium channel. Mutations in both genes produce a gain of function in late I_{Na}, causing an LQT3-like phenotype.[310,311]

Two patterns of inheritance have been identified: (1) a rare autosomal recessive disease associated with deafness (Jervell and Lange-Nielsen), caused by 2 genes that encode for the slowly activating delayed rectifier potassium channel (KCNQ1 and KCNE1); and (2) a much more common autosomal dominant form known a the Romano-Ward syndrome, caused by mutations in 10 different genes, including *KCNQ1* (KvLQT1; LQT1); *KCNH2* (HERG;LQT2); *SCN5A* ($Na_v 1.5$; LQT3); *ANKB* (LQT4); *KCNE1* (minK; LQT5); *KCNE2* (MiRP1; LQT6); *KCNJ2* (LQT7; Andersen syndrome), *CACNA1C* ($Ca_v 1.2$; LQT8; Timothy syndrome), *CAV3* (Caveolin-3; LQT9), and *SCN4B* ($Na_v B4$, LQT10). Six of the ten genes encode for cardiac potassium channels, one for the cardiac sodium channel (*SCN5A*), one for the β subunit of the sodium channel, one for caveolin-3 and one for a protein called ankyrin B (*ANKB*), which is involved in anchoring of ion channels to the cellular membrane.

The prevalence of this disorder is estimated at 1–2:10,000. The ECG diagnosis is based on the presence of prolonged repolarization (QT interval) and abnormal T-wave morphology.[313] In the different genotypes, cardiac events can be precipitated by physical or emotional stress (LQT1), a startle (LQT2), or can occur at rest or during sleep (LQT3). Anti-adrenergic intervention with β blockers is the mainstay of therapy. For patients unresponsive to this approach, implantable cardioverter-defibrillator (ICD) and/or cardiac sympathetic denervation can be therapeutic alternatives.[314,315]

Acquired LQTS refers to a syndrome similar to the congenital form but caused by exposure to drugs that prolong the duration of the ventricular action potential[316] or QT prolongation secondary to cardiomyopathies such as dilated or hypertrophic cardiomyopathy, as well as to abnormal QT prolongation associated with bradycardia or electrolyte imbalance.[87,317–320] The acquired form of the disease is far more prevalent than the congenital form, and in some cases can have a genetic predisposition.

Amplification of spatial dispersion of repolarization within the ventricular myocardium has been identified as the principal arrhythmogenic substrate in both acquired and congenital LQTS. The accentuation of spatial dispersion, typically secondary to an increase of transmural, trans-septal or apical-basal dispersion of re-

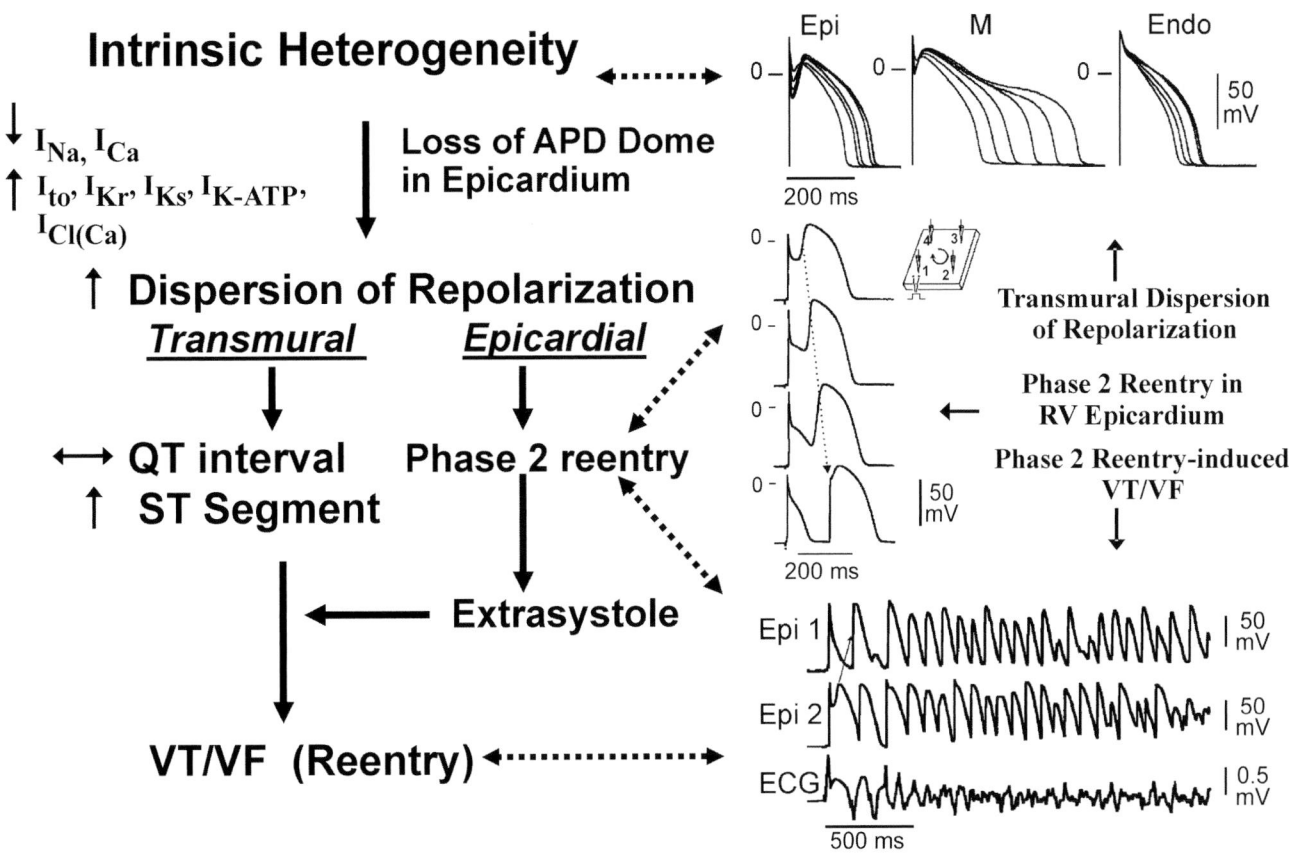

FIGURE 35–16. Cellular mechanisms proposed to underlie arrhythmogenesis in the Brugada syndrome. APD, action potential duration; Endo, endocardium; Epi, epicardium; I_{Ca}, calcium current; $I_{Cl(Ca)}$, calcium-activated chloride current; I_{K-ATP}, adenosine triphosphate-regulated potassium current; I_{Kr}, rapid outward potassium current; I_{Ks}, slow outward potassium current; I_{Na}, sodium channel current; I_{to}, transient outward current; VT/VF, ventricular tachycardia/ventricular fibrillation; RV, right ventricular. *Source: Modified from Antzelevitch C. The Brugada syndrome: diagnostic criteria and cellular mechanisms. Eur Heart J. 2001;22:356. Used with permission.*

polarization, and the development of early afterdepolarization (EAD)-induced triggered activity underlie the substrate and trigger for the development of TdP arrhythmias observed under LQTS conditions.[73,321] Models of the LQT1, LQT2, and LQT3, and LQT7 forms of LQTS have been developed using the canine arterially perfused LV wedge preparation (Fig. 35–17).[30,322,323] These models suggest that in the first three forms of LQTS, preferential prolongation of the M cell APD leads to an increase in the QT interval as well as an increase in transmural dispersion of repolarization , which contributes to the development of spontaneous as well as stimulation-induced TdP (Fig. 35–18).[80,324,325] The unique characteristics of the M cells are at the heart of the LQTS. The hallmark of the M cell is the ability of its action potential to prolong more than that of epicardium or endocardium in response to a slowing of rate. [233,246,326] This feature of the M cell is caused by weaker repolarizing current during phases 2 and 3 secondary to a smaller I_{Ks} and a larger late I_{Na} and I_{Na-Ca}[68,86,248] compared to epicardial and endocardial cells.

These ionic distinctions also sensitize the M cells to a variety of pharmacological agents. Agents that block I_{Kr}, I_{Ks}, or increase I_{Ca} or late I_{Na} generally produce a much greater prolongation of the APD of the M cell than of epicardial or endocardial cells (see Fig. 35–17). Differences in the time course of repolarization of the three predominant myocardial cell types have been shown to contribute prominently to the inscription of the T wave of the ECG.

Voltage gradients developing as a result of the different time course of repolarization of phases 2 and 3 in the three cell types give rise to opposing voltage gradients on either side of the M region, which are in large part responsible for the inscription of the T wave.[327] In the case of an upright T wave, the epicardial response is the earliest to repolarize, and the M cell action potential is the latest. Full repolarization of the epicardial action potential coincides with the peak of the T wave and repolarization of the M cells is coincident with the end of the T wave. The duration of the M cell action potential therefore determines the QT interval, whereas the duration of the epicardial action potential determines the QT_{peak} interval.

Experimental models that mimic the clinical congenital syndromes with respect to prolongation of the QT interval, T-wave morphology, and rate dependence of QT have been helpful in elucidation of the basis for sympathetic nervous system influences (see Fig. 35–17).[252,324,325,327,328]

The response to sympathetic activation displays a very different time-course in the case of LQT1 and LQT2, both in experimental models (see Fig. 35–17) and in the clinic.[321,329] In LQT1, β-adrenergic stimulation induces an increase in transmural dispersion of repolarization that is most prominent during the first 2 minutes, but which persists, although to a lesser extent, during steady-state. TdP incidence is enhanced during the initial period as well as during steady-state. In

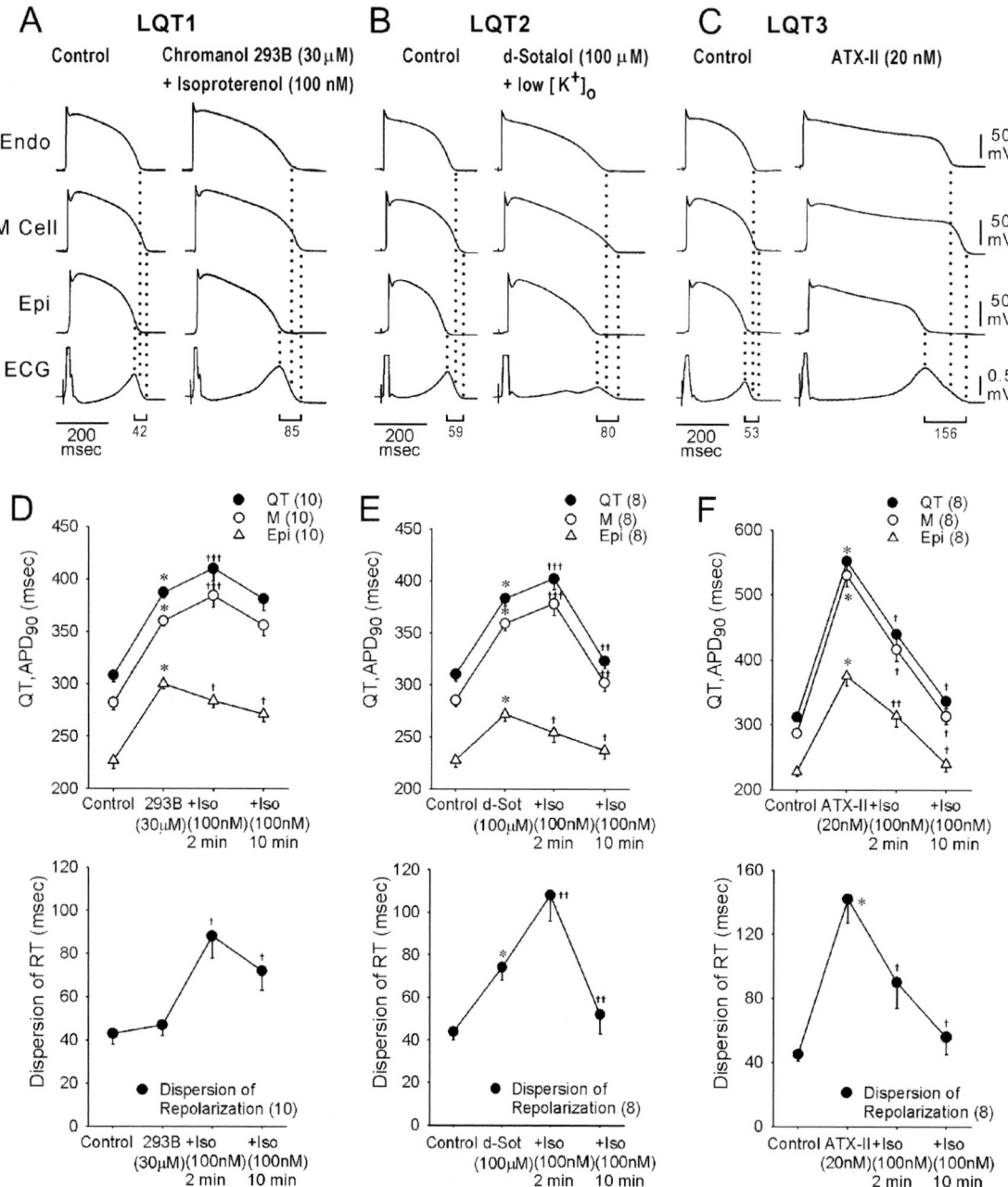

FIGURE 35–17. Transmembrane action potentials and transmural electrocardiograms in control and (**A**) LQT1, (**B**) LQT2, and (**C**) LQT3 models of long QT syndrome (LQTS) (arterially-perfused canine left ventricular wedge preparations). Isoproterenol + chromanol 293B (an I_{Ks} blocker), d-sotalol + low $[K^+]_o$, and ATX-II (an agent that slows inactivation of late I_{Na}) are used to mimic the LQT1, LQT2, and LQT3 syndromes, respectively. Panels **A, B,** and **C** depict action potentials simultaneously recorded from endocardial, M, and epicardial sites together with a transmural ECG. Basic cycle length (BCL) = 2000 msec. Transmural dispersion of repolarization across the ventricular wall, defined as the difference in the repolarization time between M and epicardial cells, is denoted below the ECG traces. Panels **D, E,** and **F** show the effect of isoproterenol in the LQT1, LQT2, and LQT3 models. In LQT1, isoproterenol produces a persistent prolongation of the APD_{90} of the M cell and of the QT interval (at both 2 and 10 min), whereas the APD_{90} of the epicardial cell is always abbreviated, resulting in a persistent increase in transmural dispersion of repolarization (**D**). In LQT2, isoproterenol initially prolongs (2 min) and then abbreviates the QT interval and the APD_{90} of the M cell to the control level (10 min), whereas the APD_{90} of epicardial cell is always abbreviated, resulting in a transient increase in transmural dispersion of repolarization (**E**). In LQT3, isoproterenol produced a persistent abbreviation of the QT interval and the APD_{90} of both M and epicardial cells (at both 2 and 10 min), resulting in a persistent decrease in transmural dispersion of repolarization (**F**). *, $p < .0005$ versus control; †, $p < .0005$; ††, $p < .005$; †††, $p < .05$ versus 293B, d-Sotalol, or ATX-II. 293B, chromanol 293B; d-Sot, d-Sotalol; Endo, endocardial; Epi, epicardial; Iso, isoproterenol. *Source: Modified from Shimizu, Antzelevitch[80]; Shimizu, Antzelevitch[324]; Shimizu, Antzelevitch.[325] Used with permission.*

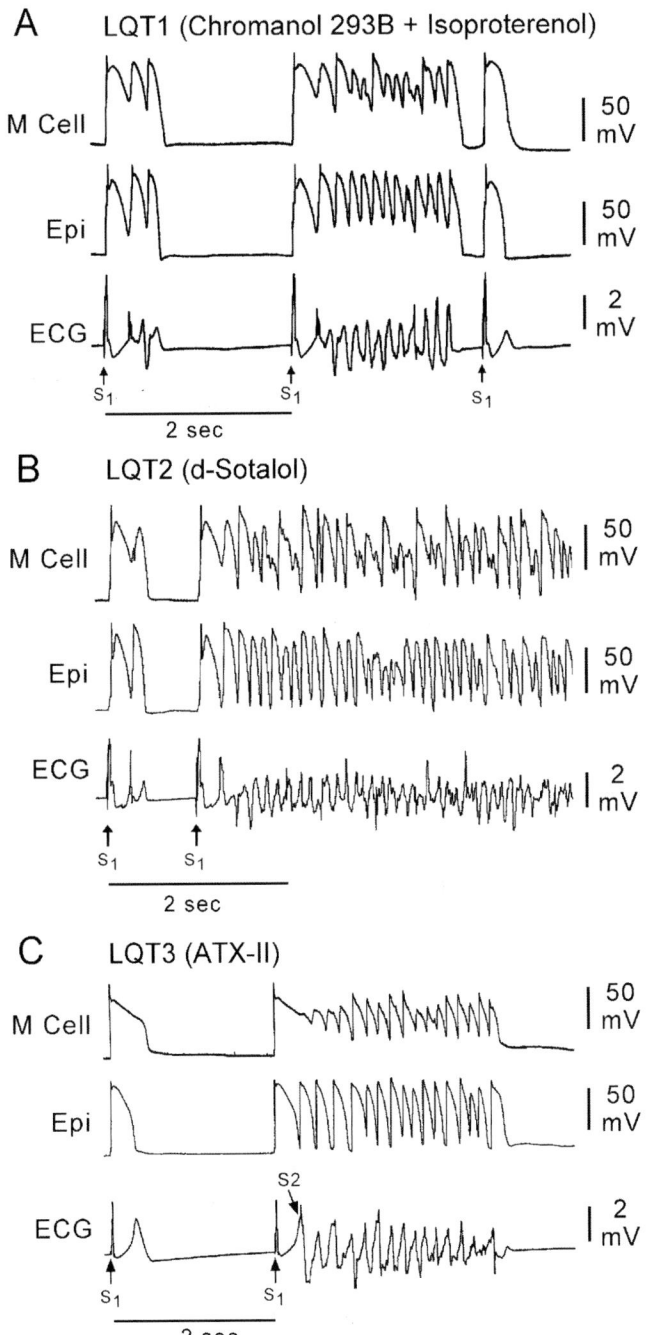

A LQT1 (Chromanol 293B + Isoproterenol)

M Cell

Epi

ECG

| 50 mV

| 50 mV

| 2 mV

S₁   S₁   S₁

2 sec

B LQT2 (d-Sotalol)

M Cell

Epi

ECG

| 50 mV

| 50 mV

| 2 mV

S₁   S₁

2 sec

C LQT3 (ATX-II)

M Cell

Epi

ECG

| 50 mV

| 50 mV

| 2 mV

S₂

S₁   S₁

2 sec

FIGURE 35-18. Polymorphic ventricular tachycardia displaying features of torsade de pointes (TdP) in the (**A**) LQT1, (**B**) LQT2, and (**C**) LQT3 models (arterially-perfused canine left ventricular wedge preparations). Isoproterenol + chromanol 293B, d-sotalol, and ATX-II are used to mimic the three LQTS syndromes, respectively. Each trace shows action potentials simultaneously recorded from M and epicardial cells together with a transmural ECG. The preparation was paced from the endocardial surface at a basic cycle length (BCL) of 2000 msec (S₁). **A** and **B**. Spontaneous TdP induced in the LQT1 and LQT2 models, respectively. In both models, the first groupings show spontaneous ventricular premature beat (or couplets) that fail to induce TdP, and a second grouping that show spontaneous premature beats that succeed. The premature response appears to originate in the deep subendocardium (M or Purkinje). **C.** Programmed electrical stimulation-induces TdP in the LQT3 model. ATX-II produced very significant dispersion of repolarization (first grouping). A single extrastimulus (S₂) applied to the epicardial surface at an S₁–S₂ interval of 320 msec initiates TdP (second grouping). Epi, epicardial; S₁, first heart sound; S₂, second heart sound. *Source: Modified from Shimizu, Antzelevitch*[80]*; Shimizu, Antzelevitch*[324]*; Shimizu, Antzelevitch.*[325] *Used with permission.*

LQT2, isoproterenol produces only a transient increase in transmural dispersion of repolarization that persists for less than 2 minutes. TdP incidence is therefore enhanced only for a brief period of time. These differences in time-course can explain the important differences in autonomic activity and other gene-specific triggers that contribute to events in patients with different LQTS genotypes.[321,330,331]

Although β blockers are considered the first line of therapy in patients with LQT1, they have not been shown to be beneficial in LQT3. Preliminary data suggest LQT3 patients might benefit from Na⁺ channel blockers, such as mexiletine and flecainide, but long-term data are not yet available.[332,333] Experimental data have shown that mexiletine reduces transmural dispersion and prevents TdP in LQT3 as well as LQT1 and LQT2, suggesting that agents that block the late sodium current can be effective in all forms of LQTS.[324,325] These observations suggest that a combination of β blockers and late sodium channel blockers can confer more protection in LQT1 and LQT2 than β blockade alone. Clinical data are not available as yet.

The T_{peak}–T_{end} interval has been shown to provide an index of transmural dispersion of repolarization.[233] The available data suggest that T_{peak}–T_{end} measurements are generally limited to precordial leads (V_1–V_6) because these leads more accurately reflect transmural dispersion of repolarization. Recent studies have also provided guidelines for the estimation of transmural dispersion of repolarization in the case of more complex T waves, including negative, biphasic, and triphasic T waves.[334] In these cases, the interval from the nadir of the first component of the T wave to the end of the T wave provides an accurate electrocardiographic approximation of transmural dispersion of repolarization.

The clinical applicability of these concepts remains to be carefully validated. Direct evidence in support of T_{peak}–T_{end} as an index to predict TdP in patients with LQTS was provided by Yamaguchi and coworkers.[335] These authors concluded that T_{peak}–T_{end} is more valuable than QTc and QT dispersion as a predictor of TdP in patients with acquired LQTS. Shimizu and colleagues demonstrated that T_{peak}–T_{end}, but not QTc, predicted sudden cardiac death in patients with hypertrophic cardiomyopathy.[336] Most recently, Watanabe and coworkers demonstrated that prolonged T_{peak}–T_{end} is associated with inducibility as well as spontaneous development of VT in high-risk patients with organic heart disease.[337]

Although further studies are needed to evaluate the usefulness of these noninvasive indices of electrical heterogeneity and their prognostic value in the assignment of arrhythmic risk, evidence is accumulating in support of the hypothesis that transmural dispersion of repolarization rather than QT prolongation underlies the substrate responsible for the development of TdP.[73,95,338–340]

Fig. 35–19 presents a working hypothesis for our understanding of the mechanisms underlying LQTS-related TdP based on available data. The hypothesis presumes the presence of electrical heterogeneity in the form of transmural dispersion of repolarization under baseline conditions and the amplification of transmural dispersion of repolarization by agents that reduce net repolarizing current by means of a reduction in I_{Kr}

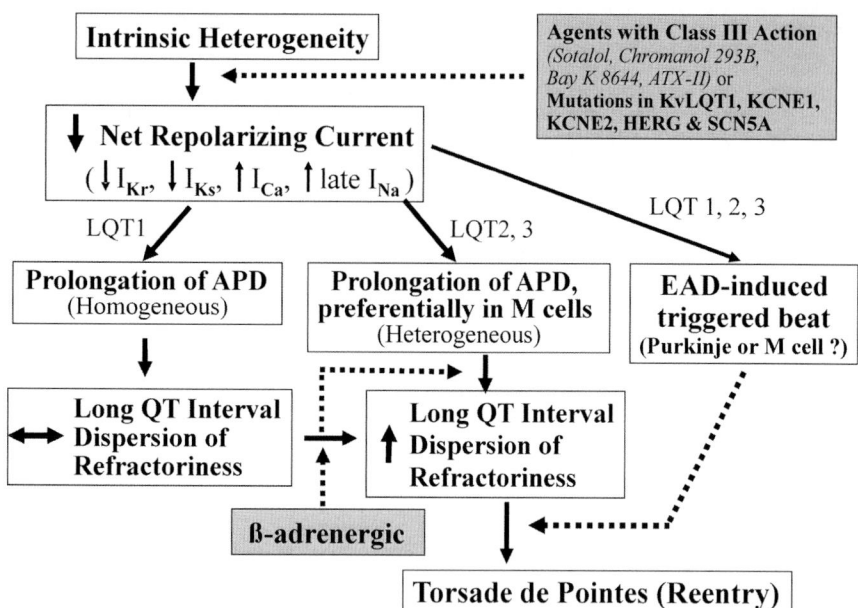

FIGURE 35–19. Proposed cellular and ionic mechanisms for the long-QT syndrome. APD, action potential duration; EAD, early afterdepolarization; I_{Ca}, calcium current; I_{Kr}, rapid outward potassium current; I_{Ks}, slow outward potassium current; I_{Na}, sodium channel current.

or I_{Ks} or augmentation of I_{Ca} or late I_{Na}. Conditions leading to a reduction in I_{Kr} or augmentation of late I_{Na} lead to a preferential prolongation of the M cell action potential. As a consequence, the QT interval prolongs and is accompanied by a dramatic increase in transmural dispersion of repolarization, thus creating a vulnerable window for the development of reentry. The reduction in net repolarizing current also predisposes to the development of EAD-induced triggered activity in M and Purkinje cells, which provide the extrasystole that triggers TdP when it falls within the vulnerable period. β-adrenergic agonists further amplify transmural heterogeneity (transiently) in the case of I_{Kr} block, but reduce it in the case of I_{Na} agonists.[80,341]

Not all agents that prolong the QT interval increase transmural dispersion of repolarization (TDR). Amiodarone, a potent antiarrhythmic agent used in the management of both atrial and ventricular arrhythmias, is rarely associated with TdP.[75] Chronic administration of amiodarone produces a greater prolongation of APD in epicardium and endocardium, but less of an increase, or even a decrease at slow rates, in the M region, thereby reducing TDR.[342] In a dog model of chronic complete atrioventricular block and acquired LQTS, 6 weeks of amiodarone was shown to produce a major QT prolongation without producing TdP. In contrast, after 6 weeks of dronedar-

one, TdP occurred in 4 of 8 dogs with the highest spatial dispersion of repolarization (105 ± 20 msec).[343] Sodium pentobarbital is another agent that prolongs the QT interval but reduces TDR. Pentobarbital has been shown to produce a dose-dependent prolongation of the QT interval, accompanied by a reduction in TDR from 51 to 27 msec.[344] TdP is never seen under these conditions, nor can it be induced with programmed stimulation. Amiodarone and pentobarbital have in common the ability to block I_{Ks}, I_{Kr}, and late I_{Na}. This combination produces a preferential prolongation of the APD of epicardium and endocardium so that the QT interval is prolonged, but TDR is actually reduced, and TdP does not occur.

Chromanol 293B, an I_{Ks} blocker, is another example of an agent that increases QT without augmenting TDR. Chromanol 293B prolongs APD of the three cell types homogeneously, neither increasing TDR nor widening the T wave. TdP is never observed under these conditions. This picture changes very quickly in the presence of β-adrenergic stimulation. Isoproterenol abbreviates the APD of epicardial and endocardial cells but not that of the M cell, resulting in a marked accentuation of TDR.[80] TdP develops under these conditions.

These findings have advanced our understanding of why long-QT patients, LQT1 in particular, are so sensitive to sympathetic influences, and provided further evidence in support of

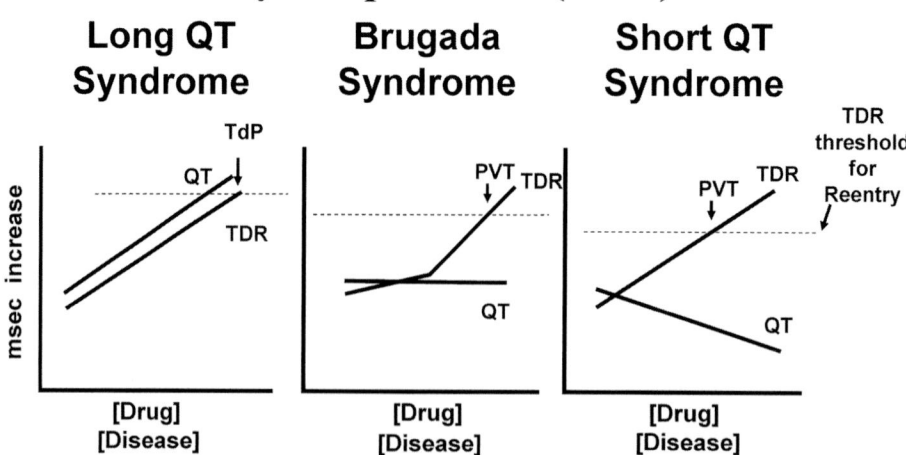

FIGURE 35–20. The role of transmural dispersion of repolarization in channelopathy-induced sudden death. In the long QT syndrome, QT increases as a function of disease or drug concentration. In the Brugada syndrome it remains largely unchanged, and in the short QT syndrome QT interval decreases as a function of disease or drug. The three syndromes have in common the ability to amplify transmural dispersion of repolarization, which results in the development of TdP when dispersion reaches the threshold for reentry. The threshold for reentry decreases as APD and refractoriness are reduced. PVT, polymorphic ventricular tachycardia; TDR, transmural dispersion of repolarization; TdP, torsade de pointes. *Source: Modified from Antzelevitch C, Oliva A. Amplification of spatial dispersion of repolarization underlies sudden cardiac death associated with catecholaminergic polymorphic VT, long QT, short QT and Brugada syndromes. J Intern Med. 2006;259:48. Used with permission.*

the hypothesis that the risks associated with LQTS are not caused by the prolongation of the QT interval but rather by the increase in spatial dispersion of repolarization that usually, but not always, accompanies the prolongation of the QT interval.

Short QT Syndrome

First proposed as a clinical entity by Gussak and colleagues in 2000,[345] the short QT syndrome (SQTS) is an inherited syndrome characterized by a QTc ≤300 to 340 msec and high incidence of VT/VF in infants, children, and young adults.[346] The familial nature of this sudden death syndrome was highlighted by Gaita and coworkers in 2003.[347] The first genetic defect responsible for the SQTS (SQTS1), reported by Brugada and colleagues in 2004, involved two different missense mutations (substitution of one amino acid for another) resulting in the same amino acid substitution in HERG (N588K), which caused a gain of function in the rapidly activating delayed rectifier channel, I_{Kr}.[348] A second gene reported by Bellocq and coworkers (SQTS2)[349] involved a missense mutation in KCNQ1 (KvLQT1), causing a gain of function in I_{Ks}. A third gene (SQT3), identified in 2005, involves *KCNJ2*, the gene that encodes for the inward rectifier channel. Mutations in *KCNJ2* caused a gain of function in I_{K1}, leading to an abbreviation of QT interval. SQT3 is associated with QTc intervals <330 msec, not quite as short as SQT1, and SQT2. Two additional genes recently linked to SQTS encode the α1 (CACNA1C) and β (CACNB2b) subunits of the L-type cardiac calcium channel. SQT4 caused by mutations in the α subunit of calcium channel have been shown to lead to QT interval <360 msec, whereas SQT5 caused by mutations in the β subunit of the calcium channel are characterized by QT intervals of 330 to 360 msec.[270] Mutations in the α and β subunits of the calcium channel can also lead to ST segment elevation, creating a combined Brugada/shortQT syndrome.[270]

In addition to an abbreviated QT interval, SQTS is characterized by the appearance of tall peaked often symmetrical T waves in the ECG. The augmented T_{peak}–T_{end} interval associated with this electrocardiographic feature of the syndrome suggests that TDR is significantly increased. Studies employing the left ventricular wedge model of the short QT syndrome have provided evidence in support of the hypothesis that an increase in outward repolarizing current can preferentially abbreviate endocardial/M cell thus increase TDR and create the substrate for reentry.[350] The potassium channel opener, pinacidil, used in this study caused a heterogeneous abbreviation of APD among the different cell types spanning the ventricular wall, thus creating the substrate for the genesis of VT under conditions associated with short QT intervals. Polymorphic VT could be readily induced with programmed electrical stimulation. The increase in TDR was further accentuated by isoproterenol, leading to easier induction and more persistent VT/VF. It is noteworthy that an increase of TDR to values greater than 55 msec was associated with inducibility of VT/VF. In LQTS models, a TDR of >90 msec is required to induce TdP. The easier inducibility in SQTS is caused by the reduction in the wavelength (product of refractory period and conduction velocity) of the reentrant circuit, which reduces

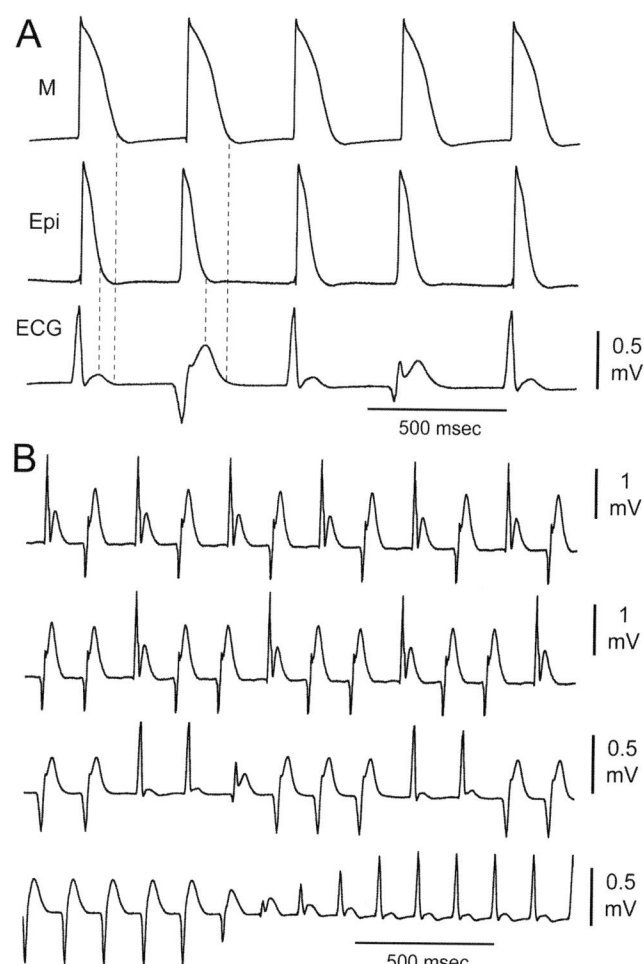

FIGURE 35–21. Experimental model of catecholaminergic ventricular tachycardia (VT). Bidirectional VT. **A.** Action potentials were simultaneously recorded from epicardial and M cells together with a transmural ECG in a left ventricular wedge preparation. Perfusion of isoproterenol (100 nM) in the presence of caffeine (300 mmol/L) produced a bidirectional ventricular rhythm as a consequence of alternation in the origin of ectopic activity between endocardium and epicardium. A marked change in T_{peak} to T_{end} interval (from 53 to 75 msec), and transmural dispersion of repolarization (from 51 to 73 msec) is observed. **B.** Bidirectional tachycardias displaying different patterns of alternations in the origin of the ectopic beat. This activity, presumably because of DAD-induced triggered beats, could be observed to generate a slow polymorphic VT. Because of their slow rates, these arrhythmias are unlikely to create hemodynamic compromise or to be responsible for sudden cardiac death. Epi, epicardial. *Source: Modified from Nam, Burashnikov, Antzelevitch.[119] Used with permission.*

the pathlength required for maintenance of reentry.[350] SQT4 and SQT5 have also been reported to exhibit abnormal rate-adaptation of the QT interval.[270]

The Role of TDR in Channelopathy-Induced Sudden Death
The three inherited and corresponding acquired sudden death syndromes discussed thus far differ with respect to the behavior of the QT interval (Fig. 35–20). In the LQTS, QT increases as a function of disease or drug concentration. In the Brugada syndrome it remains largely unchanged, and in the SQTS, QT interval decreases as a function of disease of drug. What these three syndromes have in common is an amplification of TDR, which results in the development of polymorphic VT when dispersion

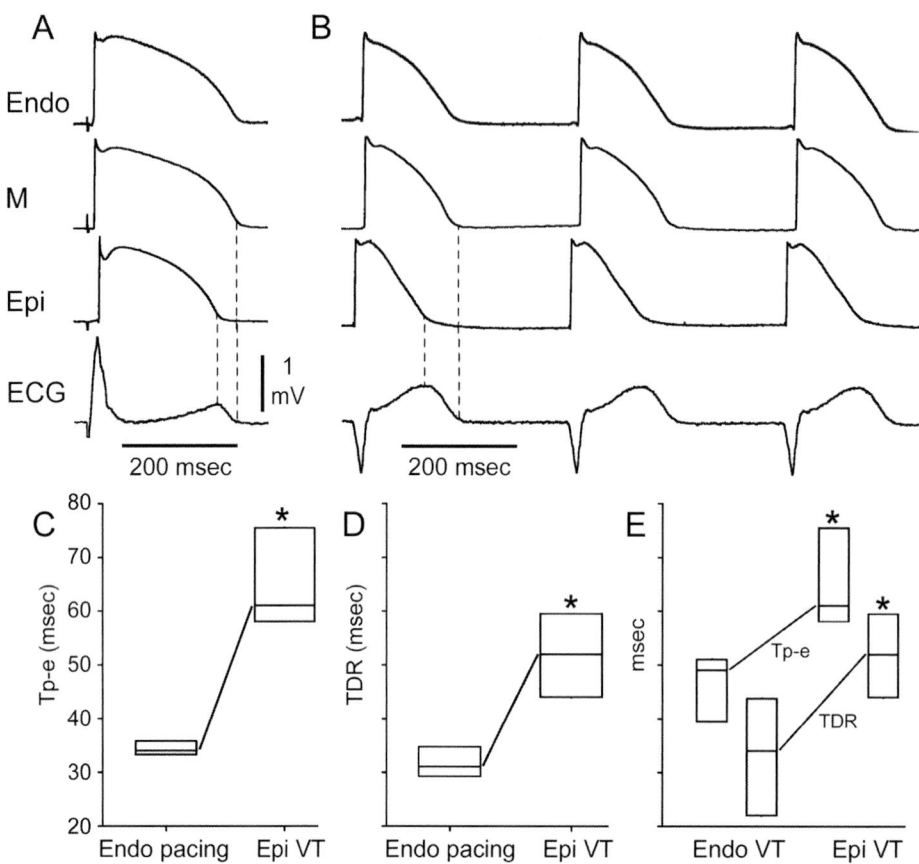

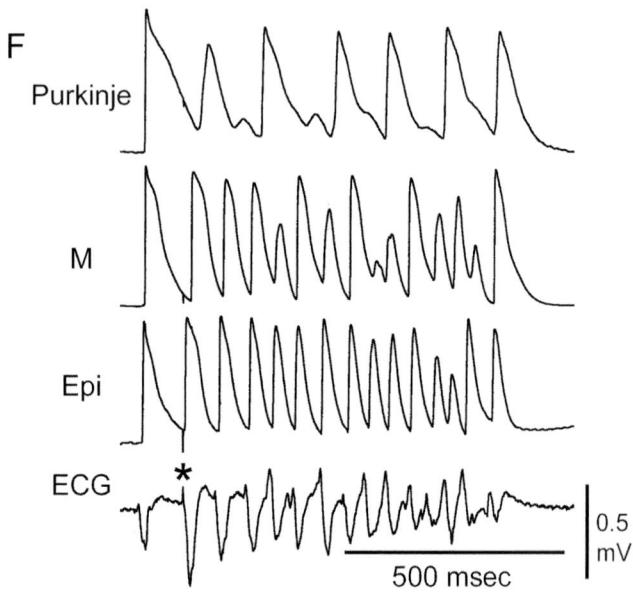

FIGURE 35–22. Experimental models of catecholaminergic ventricular tachycardia (VT). Development of epicardial VT is associated with an increase in transmural dispersion of repolarization **A.** T_{peak} to T_{end} interval (T_{p-e}) and transmural dispersion of repolarization in a left ventricular wedge preparation during endocardial pacing at a basic cycle length (BCL) of 2,000 msec are 36 and 34 msec, respectively. **B.** Reversal of the transmural sequence of activation as a consequence of the focal ventricular rhythm arising from epicardium, causes T_{p-e} and transmural dispersion of repolarization to increase to 57 and 52 msec, respectively. **C, D, E.** Comparison of T_{p-e} and transmural dispersion of repolarization values during endocardial pacing (caffeine only) and during VT (caffeine + isoproterenol). T_{p-e} and transmural dispersion of repolarization increased significantly during epicardial VT compared with those recorded during endocardial pacing at 2,000 msec (**C,D**) or during endocardial VT (**E**). Data are expressed as median (25, 75 percentile), (n = 7), *p < 0.05. **F.** Rapid polymorphic VT induced by single extrastimulus during a sustained episode of slow epicardial VT. Action potentials were recorded simultaneously from subendocardial Purkinje, M, and epicardial cells together with a transmural ECG. Perfusion of isoproterenol (100 nM) in the presence of caffeine (300 mmol/L) produced a slow monomorphic epicardial VT. A single extrastimulus (S$_2$, *) applied to the epicardial surface at an S$_1$–S$_2$ interval of 100 msec initiated a rapid polymorphic VT. Endo, endocardial; Epi, epicardial; S$_1$, first heart sound; S$_2$, second heart sound; TDR, transmural dispersion of repolarization. *Source: Modified from Nam, Burashnikov, Antzelevitch.*[119] *Used with permission.*

reaches the threshold for reentry. In the setting of a prolonged QT, we refer to it as Torsade de Pointes. It is noteworthy that the threshold for reentry decreases as APD and refractoriness are reduced, thus requiring a shorter pathlength for reentry, making it easier induce.

Catecholaminergic Polymorphic VT

CPVT is a rare, autosomal dominant or recessive inherited disorder, predominantly affecting children or adolescents with structurally normal hearts. It is characterized by bidirectional VT, polymorphic VT, and a high risk of sudden cardiac death (30 to 50 percent by 20 to 30 years of age).[351,141] Recent molecular genetic studies have identified mutations in genes encoding for the cardiac ryanodine receptor 2 (RyR2) or calsequestrin 2 (CASQ2) in patients with this phenotype.[122,142–144] Mutations in RyR2 cause autosomal dominant CPVT, whereas mutations in CASQ2 are responsible for either an autosomal recessive or dominant form of CPVT.

Numerous studies point to DAD-induced triggered activity (TA) as the mechanism underlying monomorphic or bidirectional

VT in patients with this syndrome. The cellular mechanisms underlying the various ECG phenotypes, and the transition of monomorphic VT to polymorphic VT or VF, were recently elucidated with the help of the coronary-perfused LV wedge preparation.[119] The wedge was exposed to low-dose caffeine to mimic the defective calcium homeostasis encountered under conditions that predispose to CPVT. The combination of isoproterenol and caffeine led to the development of DAD-induced triggered activity arising from the epicardium, endocardium, or M region (Fig. 35–21). Migration of the source of ectopic activity was responsible for the transition from monomorphic to slow polymorphic VT. Alternation of epicardial and endocardial source of ectopic activity gave rise to a bidirectional VT. The triggered activity-induced monomorphic, bidirectional, and slow polymorphic VT would be expected to be hemodynamically well tolerated because of the relatively slow rate of these rhythms and are unlikely to be the cause of sudden death in these syndromes.

Epicardial ectopy and VT were associated with an increased T_{peak}–T_{end} interval and transmural dispersion of repolarization caused by reversal of the normal transmural activation sequence (Fig. 35–22). The increase in TDR was sufficient to create the substrate for reentry and programmed electrical stimulation induced a rapid polymorphic VT that would be expected to lead hemodynamic compromise.[119] Thus, even in a syndrome in which arrhythmogenesis is traditionally ascribed to triggered activity, sudden death may be due to amplification of TDR, giving rise to reentrant VT/VF.

ACKNOWLEDGMENTS

Supported by grants from the National Institutes of Health (HL 47678), the American Heart Association, New York State Affiliate, and the Masons of New York State and Florida.

I am indebted to Dr. Alexander Burashnikov for his valuable assistance with discussion of spatio-temporal dynamics of reentrant waves.

REFERENCES

1. Mayer AG. *Rhythmical pulsations is scyphomedusae.* Carnegie Institute 1, publication 47; 1906.
2. Mines GR. On circulating excitations in heart muscles and their possible relation to tachycardia and fibrillation. *Trans R Soc Can.* 1914;8:43.
3. Lewis T. The broad features and time-relations of the normal electrocardiogram. Principles of interpretation. *The Mechanism and Graphic Registration of the Heart Beat.* 3rd ed. London: Shaw & Sons; 1925:44.
4. Lukas A, Antzelevitch C. Phase 2 reentry as a mechanism of initiation of circus movement reentry in canine epicardium exposed to simulated ischemia. *Cardiovasc Res.* 1996;32:593.
5. Antzelevitch C. In vivo human demonstration of phase 2 reentry. *Heart Rhythm.* 2005;2:804.
6. Thomsen PE, Joergensen RM, Kanters JK, et al. Phase 2 reentry in man. *Heart Rhythm.* 2005;2:797.
7. Yan GX, Joshi A, Guo D, et al. Phase 2 reentry as a trigger to initiate ventricular fibrillation during early acute myocardial ischemia. *Circulation.* 2004;110:1036.
8. Jalife J. Rotors and spiral waves in atrial fibrillation. *J Cardiovasc Electrophysiol.* 2003;14:776.
9. Cerrone M, Noujaim S, Jalife J. The short QT syndrome as a paradigm to understand the role of potassium channels in ventricular fibrillation. *J Intern Med.* 2006;259:24.
10. Burashnikov A, Antzelevitch C. Reinduction of atrial fibrillation immediately after termination of the arrhythmia is mediated by late phase 3 early afterdepolarization-induced triggered activity. *Circulation.* 2003;107:2355.
11. Burashnikov A, Antzelevitch C. Late-phase 3 EAD. A unique mechanism contributing to initiation of atrial fibrillation. *PACE.* 2006;29:290.
12. Patterson E, Lazzara R, Szabo B, et al. Sodium-calcium exchange initiated by the Ca2+ transient: an arrhythmia trigger within pulmonary veins. *J Am Coll Cardiol.* 2006;47:1196.
13. DiFrancesco D. The pacemaker current (I(f)) plays an important role in regulating SA node pacemaker activity. *Cardiovasc Res.* 1995;30:307.
14. Vassalle M. The pacemaker current (I(f)) does not play an important role in regulating SA node pacemaker activity. *Cardiovasc Res.* 1995;30:309.
15. Huser J, Blatter LA, Lipsius SL. Intracellular Ca²⁺ release contributes to automaticity in cat atrial pacemaker cells. *J Physiol.* 2000;524(pt 2):415.
16. Musa H, Lei M, Honjo H, et al. Heterogeneous expression of Ca(2+) handling proteins in rabbit sinoatrial node. *J Histochem Cytochem.* 2002;50:311.
17. Soejima M, Noma A. Mode of regulation of the ACh-sensitive K-channel by the muscarinic receptor in rabbit atrial cells. *Pflugers Arch.* 1984;400:424.
18. DiFrancesco D, Tromba C. Inhibition of the hyperpolarization-activated current (if) induced by acetylcholine in rabbit sino-atrial node myocytes. *J Physiol.* 1988;405:477.
19. Jones SB, Euler DE, Hardie E, et al. Comparison of SA nodal and subsidiary atrial pacemaker function and location in the dog. *Am J Physiol.* 1978;234:H471.
20. Rozanski GJ, Lipsius SL. Electrophysiology of functional subsidiary pacemakers in canine right atrium. *Am J Physiol.* 1985;249:H594.
21. Hogan PM, Davis LD. Evidence for specialized fibers in the canine right atrium. *Circ Res.* 1968;23:387.
22. Wit AL, Cranefield PF. Triggered and automatic activity in the canine coronary sinus. *Circ Res.* 1977;41:435.
23. Wit AL, Fenoglio JJ, Jr., Wagner BM, et al. Electrophysiological properties of cardiac muscle in the anterior mitral valve leaflet and the adjacent atrium in the dog. Possible implications for the genesis of atrial dysrhythmias. *Circ Res.* 1973;32:731.
24. Rozanski GJ. Electrophysiological properties of automatic fibers in rabbit atrioventricular valves. *Am J Physiol.* 1987;253:H720.
25. Chen YJ, Chen YC, Yeh HI, et al. Electrophysiology and arrhythmogenic activity of single cardiomyocytes from canine superior vena cava. *Circulation.* 2002;105:2679.
26. James TN, Isobe JH, Urthaler F. Correlative electrophysiological and anatomical studies concerning the site of origin of escape rhythm during complete atrioventricular block in the dog. *Circ Res.* 1979;45:108.
27. Levy MN. Sympathetic-parasympathetic interactions in the heart. *Circ Res.* 1971;29:437.
28. Donaldson MR, Yoon G, Fu YH, et al. Andersen-Tawil syndrome: a model of clinical variability, pleiotropy, and genetic heterogeneity 5. *Ann Med.* 2004;36(suppl 1):92.
29. Zhang L, Benson DW, Tristani-Firouzi M, et al. Electrocardiographic features in Andersen-Tawil syndrome patients with *KCNJ2* mutations: characteristic T-U-wave patterns predict the *KCNJ2* genotype. *Circulation.* 2005;111:2720.
30. Tsuboi M, Antzelevitch C. Cellular basis for electrocardiographic and arrhythmic manifestations of Andersen-Tawil syndrome (LQT7). *Heart Rhythm.* 2006;3:328.
31. Zitron E, Kiesecker C, Luck S, et al. Human cardiac inwardly rectifying current IKir2.2 is upregulated by activation of protein kinase A. *Cardiovasc Res.* 2004;63:520.
32. Rota M, Vassalle M. Patch-clamp analysis in canine cardiac Purkinje cells of a novel sodium component in the pacemaker range. *J Physiol.* 2003;548:147.
33. Katzung BG, Morgenstern JA. Effects of extracellular potassium on ventricular automaticity and evidence for a pacemaker current in mammalian ventricular myocardium. *Circ Res.* 1977;40:105.
34. Pappano AJ, Carmeliet EE. Epinephrine and the pacemaking mechanism at plateau potentials in sheep cardiac Purkinje fibers. *Pflugers Arch.* 1979;382:17.
35. Gadsby DC, Cranefield PF. Two levels of resting potential in cardiac Purkinje fibers. *J Gen Physiol.* 1977;70:725.
36. Kleber AG. Resting membrane potential, extracellular potassium activity, and intracellular sodium activity during acute global ischemia in isolated perfused guinea pig hearts. *Circ Res.* 1983;52:442.
37. Dresdner KP, Jr., Kline RP, Wit AL. Intracellular K⁺ activity, intracellular Na⁺ activity and maximum diastolic potential of canine subendocardial Purkinje cells from one-day-old infarcts. *Circ Res.* 1987;60:122.
38. Ten Eick RE, Singer DH. Electrophysiological properties of diseased human atrium. I. Low diastolic potential and altered cellular response to potassium. *Circ Res.* 1979;44:545.
39. Tristani-Firouzi M, Jensen JL, Donaldson MR, et al. Functional and clinical characterization of *KCNJ2* mutations associated with LQT7 (Andersen syndrome). *J Clin Invest.* 2002;110:381.
40. Tawil R, Ptacek LJ, Pavlakis SG, et al. Andersen's syndrome: potassium-sensitive periodic paralysis, ventricular ectopy, and dysmorphic features. *Ann Neurol.* 1994;35:326.

41. Katzung BG, Hondeghem LM, Grant AO. Letter: cardiac ventricular automaticity induced by current of injury. *Pflugers Arch.* 1975;360:193.

42. Janse MJ, Van Capelle FJL. Electrotonic interactions across an inexcitable region as a cause of ectopic activity in acute regional myocardial ischemia. A study in intact porcine and canine hearts and computer models. *Circ Res.* 1982;50:527.

43. Vermeulen JT. Mechanisms of arrhythmias in heart failure. *J Cardiovasc Electrophysiol.* 1998;9:208.

44. Katz LN, Pick A. *Clinical Electrocardiography. Part 1. The Arrhythmias.* Philadelphia, PA: Lea and Febiger; 1956:224, 225.

45. Pogwizd SM, McKenzie JP, Cain ME. Mechanisms underlying spontaneous and induced ventricular arrhythmias in patients with idiopathic dilated cardiomyopathy. *Circulation.* 1998;98:2404.

46. Vermeulen JT, McGuire MA, Opthof T, et al. Triggered activity and automaticity in ventricular trabeculae of failing human and rabbit hearts. *Cardiovasc Res.* 1994;28:1547.

47. Nuss HB, Kaab S, Kass DA, et al. Cellular basis of ventricular arrhythmias and abnormal automaticity in heart failure. *Am J Physiol.* 1999;277:H80.

48. Hoppe UC, Jansen E, Sudkamp M, et al. Hyperpolarization-activated inward current in ventricular myocytes from normal and failing human hearts. *Circulation.* 1998;97:55.

49. Haissaguerre M, Jais P, Shah DC, et al. Spontaneous initiation of atrial fibrillation by ectopic beats originating in the pulmonary veins. *N Engl J Med.* 1998;339:659.

50. Lai LP, Su MJ, Lin JL, et al. Measurement of funny current (I(f)) channel mRNA in human atrial tissue: correlation with left atrial filling pressure and atrial fibrillation. *J Cardiovasc Electrophysiol.* 1999;10:947.

51. Vassalle M. The relationship among cardiac pacemakers. Overdrive suppression. *Circ Res.* 1977;41:269.

52. Gadsby DC, Cranefield PF. Electrogenic sodium extrusion in cardiac Purkinje fibers. *J Gen Physiol.* 1979;73:819.

53. Vassalle M. Electrogenic suppression of automaticity in sheep and dog Purkinje fibers. *Circ Res.* 1970;27:361.

54. Jalife J, Moe GK. A biological model of parasystole. *Am J Cardiol.* 1979;43:761.

55. Jalife J, Antzelevitch C, Moe GK. The case for modulated parasystole. *PACE.* 1982;5:911.

56. Nau GJ, Aldariz AE, Acunzo RS, et al. Modulation of parasystolic activity by nonparasystolic beats. *Circulation.* 1982;66:462.

57. Antzelevitch C, Bernstein MJ, Feldman HN, et al. Parasystole, reentry, and tachycardia: a canine preparation of cardiac arrhythmias occurring across inexcitable segments of tissue. *Circulation.* 1983;68:1101.

58. Jalife J, Moe GK. Effect of electrotonic potentials on pacemaker activity of canine Purkinje fibers in relation to parasystole. *Circ Res.* 1976;39:801.

59. Ikeda N, Takeuchi A, Hamada A, et al. Model of bidirectional modulated parasystole as a mechanism for cyclic bursts of ventricular premature contractions. *Biol Cybern.* 2004;91:37.

60. Roden DM. Drug-induced prolongation of the QT interval. *N Engl J Med.* 2004;350:1013.

61. Davidenko JM, Cohen L, Goodrow RJ, et al. Quinidine-induced action potential prolongation, early afterdepolarizations, and triggered activity in canine Purkinje fibers. Effects of stimulation rate, potassium, and magnesium. *Circulation.* 1989;79:674.

62. Antzelevitch C, Sicouri S. Clinical relevance of cardiac arrhythmias generated by afterdepolarizations. Role of M cells in the generation of U waves, triggered activity and torsade de pointes. *J Am Coll Cardiol.* 1994;23:259.

63. Roden DM, Hoffman BF. Action potential prolongation and induction of abnormal automaticity by low quinidine concentrations in canine Purkinje fibers: relationship to potassium and cycle length. *Circ Res.* 1986;56:857.

64. Priori SG, Corr PB. Mechanisms underlying early and delayed afterdepolarizations induced by catecholamines. *Am J Physiol.* 1990;258:H1796.

65. Volders PGA, Kulcsar A, Vos MA, et al. Similarities between early and delayed afterdepolarizations induced by isoproterenol in canine ventricular myocytes. *Cardiovasc Res.* 1997;34:348.

66. Burashnikov A, Antzelevitch C. Acceleration-induced action potential prolongation and early afterdepolarizations. *J Cardiovasc Electrophysiol.* 1998;9:934.

67. Sicouri S, Antzelevitch C. Afterdepolarizations and triggered activity develop in a select population of cells (M cells) in canine ventricular myocardium: the effects of acetylstrophanthidin and Bay K 8644. *PACE.* 1991;14:1714.

68. Liu DW, Antzelevitch C. Characteristics of the delayed rectifier current (I_{Kr} and I_{Ks}) in canine ventricular epicardial, midmyocardial, and endocardial myocytes. *Circ Res.* 1995;76:351.

69. Burashnikov A, Antzelevitch C. Prominent IKs in epicardium and endocardium contributes to development of transmural dispersion of repolarization but protects against development of early afterdepolarizations. *J Cardiovasc Electrophysiol.* 2002;13:172.

70. Burashnikov A, Antzelevitch C. Failure of canine ventricular epicardial and endocardial cells to develop early afterdepolarization activity is due to the presence of a prominent IKs. *Circulation.* 1997;96:I-292.

71. El-Sherif N, Caref EB, Yin H, et al. The electrophysiological mechanism of ventricular arrhythmias in the long QT syndrome: tridimensional mapping of activation and recovery patterns. *Circ Res.* 1996;79:474.

72. Murakawa Y, Sezaki.K., Yamashita T, et al. Three-dimensional activation sequence of cesium-induced ventricular arrhythmias. *Am J Physiol.* 1997;273:H1377.

73. Belardinelli L, Antzelevitch C, Vos MA. Assessing Predictors of drug-induced torsade de pointes. *Trends Pharmacol Sci.* 2003;24:619.

74. Lankipalli RS, Zhu T, Guo D, et al. Mechanisms underlying arrhythmogenesis in long QT syndrome. *J Electrocardiol.* 2005;38(suppl):69.

75. Antzelevitch C. Role of transmural dispersion of repolarization in the genesis of drug-induced torsades de pointes. *Heart Rhythm.* 2005;2:S9.

76. Nattel S, Quantz MA. Pharmacological response of quinidine induced early afterdepolarizations in canine cardiac Purkinje fibers: insights into underlying ionic mechanisms. *Cardiovasc Res.* 1988;22:808.

77. Szabo B, Kovacs T, Lazzara R. Role of calcium loading in early afterdepolarizations generated by Cs in canine and guinea pig Purkinje fibers. *J Cardiovasc Electrophysiol.* 1995;6:796.

78. Patterson E, Scherlag BJ, Szabo B, et al. Facilitation of epinephrine-induced afterdepolarizations by class III antiarrhythmic drugs. *J Electrocardiol.* 1997;30:217.

79. Antzelevitch C. Cardiac repolarization. The long and short of it. *Europace.* 2005;7(suppl 2):3.

80. Shimizu W, Antzelevitch C. Differential effects of beta-adrenergic agonists and antagonists in LQT1 LQT2 and LQT3 models of the long QT syndrome. *J Am Coll Cardiol.* 2000;35:778.

81. Marban E, Robinson SW, Wier WG. Mechanism of arrhythmogenic delayed and early afterdepolarizations in ferret muscle. *J Clin Invest.* 1986;78:1185.

82. January CT, Riddle JM. Early afterdepolarizations: mechanism of induction and block: A role for L-type Ca^{2+} current. *Circ Res.* 1989;64:977.

83. Zeng J, Rudy Y. Early afterdepolarizations in cardiac myocytes: mechanism and rate dependence. *Biophys J.* 1995;68:949.

84. Ming Z, Nordin C, Aronson MD. Role of L-type calcium channel window current in generating current-induced early afterdepolarizations. *J Cardiovasc Electrophysiol.* 1994;5:323.

85. Patterson E, Scherlag BJ, Lazzara R. Early afterdepolarizations produced by d,l-sotalol and clofilium. *J Cardiovasc Electrophysiol.* 1997;8:667.

86. Zygmunt AC, Eddlestone GT, Thomas GP, et al. Larger late sodium conductance in M cells contributes to electrical heterogeneity in canine ventricle. *Am J Physiol.* 2001;281:H689.

87. Maltsev VA, Sabbah HN, Higgins RS, et al. Novel, ultraslow inactivating sodium current in human heart failure cardiomyocytes. *Circulation.* 1998;98:2545.

88. Clancy CE, Tateyama M, Liu H, et al. Non-equilibrium gating in cardiac Na+ channels: an original mechanism of arrhythmia. *Circulation.* 2003;107:2233.

89. Anderson ME. QT interval prolongation and arrhythmia: an unbreakable connection? *J Intern Med.* 2006;259:81.

90. Ghosh S, Nunziato DA, Pitt GS. KCNQ1 assembly and function is blocked by long-QT syndrome mutations that disrupt interaction with calmodulin. *Circ Res.* 2006;98:1048.

91. Shamgar L, Ma L, Schmitt N, et al. Calmodulin is essential for cardiac IKS channel gating and assembly: impaired function in long-QT mutations. *Circ Res.* 2006;98:1055.

92. Roden DM. A new role for calmodulin in ion channel biology. *Circ Res.* 2006;98:979.

93. Wu Y, Roden DM, Anderson ME. Calmodulin kinase inhibition prevents development of the arrhythmogenic transient inward current. *Circ Res.* 1999;84:906.

94. Anderson ME, Braun AP, Wu Y, et al. KN-93 an inhibitor of multifunctional Ca++/calmodulin-dependent protein kinase, decreases early afterdepolarizations in rabbit heart. *J Pharmacol Exp Ther.* 1998;287:996.

95. Antzelevitch C, Belardinelli L, Zygmunt AC, et al. Electrophysiologic effects of ranolazine: A novel anti-anginal agent with antiarrhythmic properties. *Circulation.* 2004;110:904.

96. Antzelevitch C, Belardinelli L, Wu L, et al. Electrophysiologic properties and antiarrhythmic actions of a novel anti-anginal agent. *J Cardiovasc Pharmacol Therapeut.* 2004;9(suppl 1):S65.

97. Undrovinas AI, Belardinelli L, Undrovinas NA, et al. Ranolazine improves abnormal repolarization and contraction in left ventricular myocytes of dogs with heart failure by inhibiting late sodium current. *J Cardiovasc Electrophysiol.* 2006;17:S161.

98. Wu L, Shryock JC, Song Y, et al. Antiarrhythmic effects of ranolazine in a guinea pig in vitro model of long-QT syndrome. *J Pharmacol Exp Ther.* 2004;310:599.

99. Orth PM, Hesketh JC, Mak CK, et al. RSD1235 blocks late I(Na) and suppresses early afterdepolarizations and torsades de pointes induced by class III agents. *Cardiovasc Res.* 2006;70:486.

100. Roden DM, Lazzara R, Rosen MR, et al. Multiple mechanisms in the long-QT syndrome: current knowledge, gaps, and future directions. *Circulation.* 1996;94:1996.

101. Antzelevitch C, Yan GX, Shimizu W, et al. Electrophysiologic characteristics of M cells and their role in arrhythmias. In Franz MR, ed. *Monophasic Action Potentials: Bridging Cell and Bedside.* Armonk, NY: Futura; 2000:583.

102. Ben-David J, Zipes DP. Differential response to right and left ansae subclaviae stimulation of early afterdepolarizations and ventricular tachycardia induced by cesium in dogs. *Circulation.* 1988;78:1241.

103. Shimizu W, Ohe T, Kurita T, et al. Early afterdepolarizations induced by isoproterenol in patients with congenital long QT syndrome. *Circulation.* 1991;84:1915.

104. Carlsson L, Abrahamsson C, Drews C, et al. Antiarrhythmic effects of potassium channel openers in rhythm abnormalities related to delayed repolarization in the rabbit. *Circulation.* 1992;85:1491.

105. Asano Y, Davidenko JM, Baxter WT, et al. Optical mapping of drug-induced polymorphic arrhythmias and torsade de pointes in the isolated rabbit heart. *J Am Coll Cardiol.* 1997;29:831.

106. Ben-David J, Zipes DP, Ayers GM, et al. Canine left ventricular hypertrophy predisposes to ventricular tachycardia induction by phase 2 early afterdepolarizations after administration of BAY K 8644. *J Am Coll Cardiol.* 1992;20(7):1576.

107. Volders PG, Sipido KR, Vos MA, et al. Cellular basis of biventricular hypertrophy and arrhythmogenesis in dogs with chronic complete atrioventricular block and acquired torsade de pointes. *Circulation.* 1998;98:1136.

108. Ferrier GR, Saunders JH, Mendez C. A cellular mechanism for the generation of ventricular arrhythmias by acetylstrophanthidin. *Circ Res.* 1973;32:600.

109. Rosen MR, Gelband H, Merker C, et al. Mechanisms of digitalis toxicity—effects of ouabain on phase four of canine Purkinje fiber transmembrane potentials. *Circulation.* 1973;47:681.

110. Marchi S, Szabo B, Lazzara R. Adrenergic induction of delayed afterdepolarizations in ventricular myocardial cells: beta-induction and alpha-Modulation. *J Cardiovasc Electrophysiol.* 1991;2:476.

111. Lazzara R, El-Sherif N, Scherlag BJ. Electrophysiological properties of canine Purkinje cells in one-day-old myocardial infarction. *Circ Res.* 1973;33:722.

112. Wit AL, Rosen MR. Afterdepolarizations and triggered activity: distinction from automaticity as an arrhythmogenic mechanism. In: Fozzard HA, et al, eds. *The Heart and Cardiovascular System.* New York: Raven Press; 1992: 2113.

113. Belardinelli LL, Isenberg G. Actions of adenosine and isoproterenol on isolated mammalian ventricular myocytes. *Circ Res.* 1983;53(3):287.

114. Burashnikov A, Antzelevitch C. Block of I(Ks) does not induce early afterpolarization activity but promotes beta-adrenergic agonist-induced delayed afterdepolarization activity. *J Cardiovasc Electrophysiol.* 2000;11:458.

115. Antzelevitch C, Sicouri S, Litovsky SH, et al. Heterogeneity within the ventricular wall. Electrophysiology and pharmacology of epicardial, endocardial, and M cells. *Circ Res.* 1991;69:1427.

116. Sicouri S, Antzelevitch C. Drug-induced afterdepolarizations and triggered activity occur in a discrete subpopulation of ventricular muscle cell (M cells) in the canine heart: quinidine and digitalis. *J Cardiovasc Electrophysiol.* 1993;4:48.

117. Pogwizd SM, Onufer JR, Kramer JB, et al. Induction of delayed afterdepolarizations and triggered activity in canine Purkinje fibers by lysophosphoglycerides. *Circ Res.* 1986;59:416.

118. Song Y, Belardinelli L. ATP promotes development of afterdepolarizations and triggered activity in cardiac myocytes. *Am J Physiol.* 1994;267:H2005.

119. Nam G-B, Burashnikov A, Antzelevitch C. Cellular mechanisms underlying the development of catecholaminergic ventricular tachycardia. *Circulation.* 2005;111:2727.

120. Aronson RS. Afterpotentials and triggered activity in hypertrophied myocardium from rats with renal-hypertension. *Circ Res.* 1981;48:720.

121. Nordin C, Gilat E, Aronson RS. Delayed afterdepolarizations and triggered activity in ventricular muscle from rats with streptozotocin-induced diabetes. *Circ Res.* 1985;57:28.

122. Priori SG, Napolitano C, Memmi M, et al. Clinical and molecular characterization of patients with catecholaminergic polymorphic ventricular tachycardia. *Circulation.* 2002;106:69.

123. Caroni P, Villani F, Carafoli E. The cardiotoxic antibiotic doxorubicin inhibits the Na+/Ca2+ exchange of dog heart sarcolemmal vesicles. *FEBS Lett.* 1981;130:184.

124. Spinelli W, Sorota S, Siegel MB, et al. Antiarrhythmic actions of the ATP-regulated K+ current activated by pinacidil. *Circ Res.* 1991;68:1127.

125. Vos MA, Gorgels APM, Leunissen JDM, et al. Flunarizine allows differentiation between mechanisms of arrhythmias in the intact heart. *Circulation.* 1990;81:343.

126. Chattipakorn N, Ideker RE. Delayed afterdepolarization inhibitor: a potential pharmacologic intervention to improve defibrillation efficacy. *J Cardiovasc Electrophysiol.* 2003;14:72.

127. Letienne R, Vie B, Puech A, et al. Evidence that ranolazine behaves as a weak beta1- and beta2-adrenoceptor antagonist in the cat cardiovascular system. *Naunyn Schmiedebergs Arch Pharmacol.* 2001;363:464.

128. Belardinelli L, Antzelevitch C, Fraser H. Inhibition of late (sustained/persistent) sodium current: a potential drug target to reduce intracellular sodium-dependent calcium overload and its detrimental effects on cardiomyocyte function. *Eur Heart J.* 2004;(suppl 6):i3.

129. Kass RS, Tsien RW, Weingart R. Ionic basis of transient inward current induced by strophanthidin in cardiac Purkinje fibres. *J Physiol (Lond).* 1978;281:209.

130. Cannell MB, Lederer WJ. The arrhythmogenic current I_{TI} in the absence of electrogenic sodium-calcium exchange in sheep cardiac Purkinje fibres. *J Physiol (Lond).* 1986;374:201.

131. Fedida D, Noble D, Rankin AC, et al. The arrhythmogenic transient inward current I_{ti} and related contraction in isolated guinea-pig ventricular myocytes. *J Physiol (Lond).* 1987;392:523.

132. Laflamme MA, Becker PL. Ca2+-induced current oscillations in rabbit ventricular myocytes. *Circ Res.* 1996;78:707.

133. Zygmunt AC, Goodrow RJ, Weigel CM. I_{NaCa} and $I_{Cl(Ca)}$ contribute to isoproterenol-induced delayed afterdepolarizations in midmyocardial cells. *Am J Physiol.* 1998;275:H1979.

134. Ritchie AH, Kerr CR, Qi A, et al. Nonsustained ventricular tachycardia arising from the right ventricular outflow tract. *Am J Cardiol.* 1989;64:594.

135. Wilber DJ, Blakeman BM, Pifarre R, et al. Catecholamine sensitive right ventricular outflow tract tachycardia: Intraoperative mapping and ablation of a free-wall focus. *PACE.* 1989;12:1851.

136. Cardinal R, Scherlag BJ, Vermeulen M, et al. Distinct activation patterns of idioventricular rhythms and sympathetically-induced ventricular tachycardias in dogs with atrioventricular block. *PACE.* 1992;15:1300.

137. Lerman BB, Belardinelli LL, West GA, et al. Adenosine-sensitive ventricular tachycardia: Evidence suggesting cyclic AMP-mediated triggered activity. *Circulation.* 1986;74:270.

138. Lerman BB, Stein K, Engelstein ED, et al. Mechanism of repetitive monomorphic ventricular tachycardia. *Circulation.* 1995;92:421.

139. Ter Keurs HE, Schouten VJA, Bucx JJ, et al. Excitation-contraction coupling in myocardium: implications of calcium release and Na+-Ca2+ exchange. *Can J Physiol Pharmacol.* 1987;65:619.

140. Rubart M, Zipes DP. Mechanisms of sudden cardiac death. *J Clin Invest.* 2005;115:2305.

141. Swan H, Piippo K, Viitasalo M, et al. Arrhythmic disorder mapped to chromosome 1q42-q43 causes malignant polymorphic ventricular tachycardia in structurally normal hearts. *J Am Coll Cardiol.* 1999;34:2035.

142. Priori SG, Napolitano C, Tiso N, et al. Mutations in the cardiac ryanodine receptor gene (hRyR2) underlie catecholaminergic polymorphic ventricular tachycardia. *Circulation.* 2001;103:196.

143. Laitinen PJ, Brown KM, Piippo K, et al. Mutations of the cardiac ryanodine receptor (RyR2) gene in familial polymorphic ventricular tachycardia. *Circulation.* 2001;103:485.

144. Postma AV, Denjoy I, Hoorntje TM, et al. Absence of calsequestrin 2 causes severe forms of catecholaminergic polymorphic ventricular tachycardia. *Circ Res.* 2002;91:e21.

145. Volders PG, Vos MA, Szabo B, et al. Progress in the understanding of cardiac early afterdepolarizations and torsades de pointes: time to revise current concepts. *Cardiovasc Res.* 2000;46:376.

146. Watanabe I, Okumura Y, Ohkubo K, et al. Steady-state and nonsteady-state action potentials in fibrillating canine atrium: alternans of action potential and late phase 3 early afterdepolarization as a precursor of atrial fibrillation. *Heart Rhythm.* 2005;2:S259.

147. Patterson E, Po SS, Scherlag BJ, et al. Triggered firing in pulmonary veins initiated by in vitro autonomic nerve stimulation 1. *Heart Rhythm.* 2005;2:624.

148. Kirchhof P, Klimas J, Fabritz L, et al. Mechanism of catecholamine-induced ventricular tachycardias in mice with heart-directed expression of junctin and triadin: shortening of action potentials and prolonging calcium transients. *Heart Rhythm.* 2005;2:S69.

149. Mayer AG. Rhythmical pulsations in Scyphomedusae. II. Carnegie Institute 115, publication 102; 1908.

150. Mines GR. On dynamic equilibrium in the heart. *J Physiol (Lond).* 1913;46:350.

151. Kent AFS. Observation on the auricula-ventricular junction of the mammalian heart. *Q J Exp Physiol.* 1913;7:193.

152. Schmitt FO, Erlanger J. Directional differences in the conduction of the impulse through heart muscle and their possible relation to extrasystolic and fibrillary contractions. *Am J Physiol.* 1928;87:326.

153. Cranefield PF, Klein HO, Hoffman BF. Conduction of the cardiac impulse. I. Delay, block and one-way block in depressed Purkinje fibers. *Circ Res.* 1971;28:199.

154. Sasyniuk BI, Mendez C. A mechanism for reentry in canine ventricular tissue. *Circ Res.* 1971;28:3.

155. Wit AL, Cranefield PF, Hoffman BF. Slow conduction and reentry in the ventricular conducting system. II. Single and sustained circus movement in networks of canine and bovine Purkinje fibers. *Circ Res.* 1972;30:11.

156. Wit AL, Hoffman BF, Cranefield PF. Slow conduction and reentry in the ventricular conducting system. I. Return extrasystoles in canine Purkinje fibers. *Circ Res.* 1972;30:1.

157. Cranefield P. *The Conduction of the Cardiac Impulse: The Slow Response and Cardiac Arrhythmias.* Mount Kisco, NY: Futura; 1975.

158. Garrey WE. Auricular fibrillation. *Physiol Rev.* 1924;4:215.

159. Allessie MA, Bonke FIM, Schopman JG. Circus movement in rabbit atrial muscle as a mechanism of tachycardia. *Circ Res.* 1973;33:54.

160. Allessie MA, Bonke FIM, Schopman JG. Circus movement in rabbit atrial muscle as a mechanism of tachycardia: II. The role of nonuniform recovery of excitability in the occurrence of unidirectional block as studied with multiple microelectrodes. *Circ Res.* 1976;39:168.

161. Allessie MA, Bonke FIM, Schopman JG. Circus movement in rabbit atrial muscle as a mechanism of tachycardia. III. The "leading circle" concept: a new model of circus movement in cardiac tissue without the involvement of an anatomical obstacle. *Circ Res.* 1977;41:9.

162. Kamiyama A, Eguchi K, Shibayama R. Circus movement tachycardia induced by a single premature stimulus on the ventricular sheet: evaluation of the leading circle hypothesis in the canine ventricular muscle. *Jpn Circ J.* 1986;50:65.

163. Allessie MA, Schalij MJ, Kirchhof CJ, et al. Experimental electrophysiology and arrhythmogenicity. Anisotropy and ventricular tachycardia. *Eur Heart J.* 1989;10(suppl E):2.

164. Wit AL, Allessie MA, Fenoglic JJ, Jr, et al. Significance of the endocardial and epicardial border zones in the genesis of myocardial infarction arrhythmias. In: Harrison D, ed. *Cardiac Arrhythmias: A Decade of Progress.* Boston: GK Hall; 1982:39.

165. El-Sherif N, Smith RA, Evans K. Canine ventricular arrhythmias in the late myocardial infarction period. 8. Epicardial mapping of reentrant circuits. *Circ Res.* 1981;49:255.

166. El-Sherif N, Mehra R, Gough WB, et al. Reentrant ventricular arrhythmias in the late myocardial infarction period. Interruption of reentrant circuits by cryothermal techniques. *Circulation.* 1983;68:644.

167. Spach MS, Kootsey JM, Sloan JD. Active modulation of electrical coupling between cardiac cells of the dog. A mechanism for transient and steady state variations in conduction velocity. *Circ Res.* 1982;51:347.

168. Dillon SM, Allessie MA, Ursell PC, et al. Influences of anisotropic tissue structure on reentrant circuits in the epicardial border zone of subacute canine infarcts. *Circ Res.* 1988;63:182.

169. El-Sherif N, Mehra R, Gough WB, et al. Ventricular activation pattern of spontaneous and induced ventricular rhythms in canine one-day-old myocardial infarction. Evidence for focal and reentrant mechanisms. *Circ Res.* 1982;51:152.

170. El-Sherif N. The figure 8 model of reentrant excitation in the canine postinfarction heart. In: Zipes DP, Jalife J, eds. *Cardiac Electrophysiology and Arrhythmias.* New York: Grune and Stratton; 1985:363.

171. Weiner N, Rosenblueth A. The mathematical formulation of the problem of conduction of impulses in a network of connected excitable elements, specifically in cardiac muscle. *Arch Inst Cardiol Mex.* 1946;16:205.

172. Davidenko JM, Kent PF, Chialvo DR, et al. Sustained vortex-like waves in normal isolated ventricular muscle. *Proc Natl Acad Sci U S A.* 1990;87:8785.

173. Pertsov AM, Davidenko JM, Salomonsz R, et al. Spiral waves of excitation underlie reentrant activity in isolated cardiac muscle. *Circ Res.* 1993;72:631.

174. Jalife J, Davidenko JM, Michaels DC. A new perspective on the mechanisms of arrhythmias and sudden cardiac death: spiral wave of excitation in heart muscle. *J Cardiovasc Electrophysiol.* 1991;2:S133.

175. Athill CA, Ikeda T, Kim YH, et al. Transmembrane potential properties at the core of functional reentrant wave fronts in isolated canine right atria. *Circulation.* 1998;98:1556.

176. Jalife J, Anumonwo JM, Delmar M, Davidenko JM. *Basic Cardiac Electrophysiology for the Clinician.* Armonk, NY: Futura Publishing; 1999.

177. Pertsov AM, Jalife J. Three-dimensional vortex-like reentry. In: Zipes DP, Jalife J, eds. *Cardiac Electrophysiology: From Cell to Bedside.* 2nd ed. Philadelphia, PA: W.B. Saunders; 1995:403.

178. Davidenko JM. Spiral wave activity: a possible common mechanism for polymorphic and monomorphic ventricular tachycardias. *J Cardiovasc Electrophysiol.* 1993;4:730.

179. Garfinkel A, Qu Z. Nonlinear dinamics of excitation and propagation in cardiac muscle. In: Zipes DP, Jalife J, eds. *Cardiac Electrophysiology: From Cell to Bedside.* 3rd ed. Philadelphia, PA: W.B. Saunders; 1999:315.

180. De Bakker JMT, Van Capelle FJL, Janse MJ, et al. Reentry as a cause of ventricular tachycardia in patients with chronic ischemic disease: electrophysiologic and anatomic correlation. *Circulation.* 1988;77:589.

181. Stevenson WG, Nademanee K, Weiss JN, et al. Programmed electrical stimulation at potential ventricular reentry circuit sites. Comparison of observations in humans with predictions from computer simulations. *Circulation.* 1989;80:793.

182. Berenfeld O, Jalife J. Purkinje-muscle reentry as a mechanism of polymorphic ventricular arrhythmias in a 3-dimensional model of the ventricles. *Circ Res.* 1998;82:1063.

183. Comtois P, Kneller J, Nattel S. Of circles and spirals: bridging the gap between the leading circle and spiral wave concepts of cardiac reentry. *Europace.* 2005;7(suppl 2):10.

184. Wit AL, Janse MJ. *The Ventricular Arrhythmias of Ischemia and Infarction. Electrophysiological Mechanisms.* Mount Kisco, NY: Futura; 1993.

185. Moe GK, Rheinboldt WC, Abildskov JA. A computer model of atrial fibrillation. *Am Heart J.* 1964;67:200.

186. Scherf D, Romano FJ, Terranova R. Experimental studies on auricular flutter and auricular fibrillation. *Am Heart J.* 1948;36:241.

187. Jalife J. Ventricular fibrillation: mechanisms of initiation and maintenance. *Annu Rev Physiol.* 2000;62:25.

188. Schuessler RB, Grayson TM, Bromberg BI, et al. Cholinergically mediated tachyarrhythmias induced by a single extrastimulus in the isolated canine right atrium. *Circ Res.* 1992;71:1254.

189. Chen J, Mandapati R, Berenfeld O, et al. High-frequency periodic sources underlie ventricular fibrillation in the isolated rabbit heart. *Circ Res.* 2000;86:86.

190. Zaitsev AV, Berenfeld O, Mironov SF, et al. Distribution of excitation frequencies on the epicardial and endocardial surfaces of fibrillating ventricular wall of the sheep heart. *Circ Res.* 2000;86:408.

191. Samie FH, Berenfeld O, Anumonwo J, et al. Rectification of the background potassium current: a determinant of rotor dynamics in ventricular fibrillation. *Circ Res.* 2001;89:1216.

192. Zhou S, Chang CM, Wu TJ, et al. Nonreentrant focal activations in pulmonary veins in canine model of sustained atrial fibrillation. *Am J Physiol Heart Circ Physiol.* 2002;283:H1244.

193. Everett TH, Wilson EE, Foreman S, et al. Mechanisms of ventricular fibrillation in canine models of congestive heart failure and ischemia assessed by in vivo noncontact mapping. *Circulation.* 2005;112:1532.

194. Ideker RE, Huang J. Our search for the porcine mother rotor. *Ann Noninvasive Electrocardiol.* 2005;10:7.

195. Weiss JN, Qu Z, Chen PS, et al. The dynamics of cardiac fibrillation. *Circulation.* 2005;112:1232.

196. Qin H, Huang J, Rogers JM, et al. Mechanisms for the maintenance of ventricular fibrillation: the nonuniform dispersion of refractoriness, restitution properties, or anatomic heterogeneities? *J Cardiovasc Electrophysiol.* 2005;16:888.

197. Cabo C, Pertsov AM, Davidenko JM, et al. Vortex shedding as a precursor of turbulent electrical activity in cardiac muscle. *Biophys J.* 1996;70:1105.

198. Wu TJ, Lin SF, Weiss JN, et al. Two types of ventricular fibrillation in isolated rabbit hearts: importance of excitability and action potential duration restitution. *Circulation.* 2002;106:1859.

199. Omichi C, Lamp ST, Lin SF, et al. Intracellular Ca dynamics in ventricular fibrillation. *Am J Physiol Heart Circ Physiol.* 2004;286:H1836.

200. Attuel P, Childers R, Cauchemez B, et al. Failure in the rate adaptation of the atrial refractory period: its relationship to vulnerability. *Int J Cardiol.* 1982;2:179.

201. Wijffels MC, Kirchhof CJ, Dorland R, et al. Atrial fibrillation begets atrial fibrillation. A study in awake chronically instrumented goats. *Circulation.* 1995;92:1954.

202. Burashnikov A, Antzelevitch C. Role of repolarization restitution in the development of coarse and fine atrial fibrillation in the isolated canine right atria. *J Cardiovasc Electrophysiol.* 2005;16:639.

203. Gray RA, Jalife J, Panfilov AV, et al. Mechanisms of cardiac fibrillation. *Science.* 1995;270:1222.

204. Janse MJ, Wilms-Schopman FJG, Coronel R. Ventricular fibrillation is not always due to multiple wavelet reentry. *J Cardiovasc Electrophysiol.* 1995;6:512.

205. Antzelevitch C. Ion channels and ventricular arrhythmias: cellular and ionic mechanisms underlying the Brugada syndrome. *Curr Opin Cardiol.* 1999;14:274.

206. Chen J, Mandapati R, Berenfeld O, et al. High-frequency periodic sources underlie ventricular fibrillation in the isolated rabbit heart. *Circ Res.* 2000;86:86.

207. Janse MJ, Van Capelle FJL, Morsink H, et al. Flow of "injury" current and patterns of excitation during early ventricular arrhythmias in acute regional myocardial ischemia in isolated porcine and canine hearts. Evidence for two different arrhythmogenic mechanisms. *Circ Res.* 1980;47:151.

208. Pogwizd SM, Corr PB. Mechanisms underlying the development of ventricular fibrillation during early myocardial ischemia. *Circ Res.* 1990;66:672.

209. Riccio ML, Koller ML, Gilmour RF Jr. Electrical restitution and spatiotemporal organization during ventricular fibrillation. *Circ Res.* 1999;84:955.

210. Weiss JN, Garfinkel A, Karagueuzian HS, et al. Chaos and the transition to ventricular fibrillation: a new approach to antiarrhythmic drug evaluation. *Circulation.* 1999;99:2819.

211. Choi BR, Liu T, Salama G. The distribution of refractory periods influences the dynamics of ventricular fibrillation. *Circ Res.* 2001;88:E49.

212. Chen PS, Wu TJ, Ting CT, et al. A tale of two fibrillations. *Circulation.* 2003;108:2298.

213. Li D, Zhang L, Kneller J, et al. Potential ionic mechanism for repolarization differences between canine right and left atrium. *Circ Res.* 2001;88:1168.

214. Sarmast F, Kolli A, Zaitsev A, et al. Cholinergic atrial fibrillation: I(K,ACh) gradients determine unequal left/right atrial frequencies and rotor dynamics. *Cardiovasc Res.* 2003;59:863.

215. Antzelevitch C, Jalife J, Moe GK. Characteristics of reflection as a mechanism of reentrant arrhythmias and its relationship to parasystole. *Circulation.* 1980;61:182.

216. Antzelevitch C, Moe GK. Electrotonically-mediated delayed conduction and reentry in relation to "slow responses" in mammalian ventricular conducting tissue. *Circ Res.* 1981;49:1129.

217. Rozanski GJ, Jalife J, Moe GK. Reflected reentry in nonhomogeneous ventricular muscle as a mechanism of cardiac arrhythmias. *Circulation.* 1984;69:163.

218. Antzelevitch C. Electrotonus and reflection. In: Rosen MR, Janse MJ, Wit AL, eds. *Cardiac Electrophysiology: A Textbook.* Mount Kisco, NY: Futura. 1990;491.

219. Lukas A, Antzelevitch C. Reflected reentry, delayed conduction, and electrotonic inhibition in segmentally depressed atrial tissues. *Can J Physiol Pharmacol.* 1989;67:757.

220. Davidenko JM, Antzelevitch C. The effects of milrinone on action potential characteristics, conduction, automaticity, and reflected reentry in isolated myocardial fibers. *J Cardiovasc Pharmacol.* 1985;7:341.

221. Rosenthal JE, Ferrier GR. Contribution of variable entrance and exit block in protected foci to arrhythmogenesis in isolated ventricular tissues. *Circulation.* 1983;67:1.

222. Antzelevitch C, Lukas A. Reflection and reentry in isolated ventricular tissue. In Dangman KH, Miura DS, eds. *Basic and Clinical Electrophysiology of the Heart.* New York: Marcel Dekker; 1991:251.

223. Antzelevitch C, Moe GK. Electrotonic inhibition and summation of impulse conduction in mammalian Purkinje fibers. *Am J Physiol.* 1983;245:H42.

224. Jalife J, Moe GK. Excitation, conduction, and reflection of impulses in isolated bovine and canine cardiac Purkinje fibers. *Circ Res.* 1981;49:233.

225. Davidenko JM, Antzelevitch C. Electrophysiological mechanisms underlying rate-dependent changes of refractoriness in normal and segmentally depressed canine Purkinje fibers. The characteristics of post-repolarization refractoriness. *Circ Res.* 1986;58:257.

226. Delmar M, Michaels DC, Jalife J. Slow recovery of excitability and the Wenckebach phenomenon in the single guinea pig ventricular myocyte. *Circ Res.* 1989;65:761.

227. Antzelevitch C. Clinical applications of new concepts of parasystole, reflection, and tachycardia. *Cardiol Clin.* 1983;1:39.

228. Davidenko JM, Antzelevitch C. The effects of milrinone on conduction, reflection, and automaticity in canine Purkinje fibers. *Circulation.* 69:1026, 984.

229. Winkle RA. The relationship between ventricular ectopic beat frequency and heart rate. *Circulation.* 1982;66:439.

230. Nau GJ, Aldariz AE, Acunzo RS, et al. Clinical studies on the mechanism of ventricular arrhythmias. In: Rosenbaum MB, Elizari MV, eds. *Frontier of Cardiac Electrophysiology.* Amsterdam: Martinus Nijhoff; 1983:239.

231. Rosenthal JE. Reflected reentry in depolarized foci with variable conduction impairment in 1 day old infarcted canine cardiac tissue. *J Am Coll Cardiol.* 1988;12:404.

232. Van Hemel NM, Swenne CA, De Bakker JMT, et al. Epicardial reflection as a cause of incessant ventricular bigeminy. *PACE.* 1988;11:1036.

233. Antzelevitch C, Shimizu W, Yan GX, et al. The M cell: its contribution to the ECG and to normal and abnormal electrical function of the heart. *J Cardiovasc Electrophysiol.* 1999;10:1124.

234. Litovsky SH, Antzelevitch C. Transient outward current prominent in canine ventricular epicardium but not endocardium. *Circ Res.* 1988;62:116.

235. Liu DW, Gintant GA, Antzelevitch C. Ionic bases for electrophysiological distinctions among epicardial, midmyocardial, and endocardial myocytes from the free wall of the canine left ventricle. *Circ Res.* 1993;72:671.

236. Furukawa T, Myerburg RJ, Furukawa N, et al. Differences in transient outward currents of feline endocardial and epicardial myocytes. *Circ Res.* 1990;67:1287.

237. Wettwer E, Amos GJ, Posival H, et al. Transient outward current in human ventricular myocytes of subepicardial and subendocardial origin. *Circ Res.* 1994;75:473.

238. Nabauer M, Beuckelmann DJ, Uberfuhr P, et al. Regional differences in current density and rate-dependent properties of the transient outward current in subepicardial and subendocardial myocytes of human left ventricle. *Circulation.* 1996;93:168.

239. Di Diego JM, Sun ZQ, Antzelevitch C. I_{to} and action potential notch are smaller in left vs. right canine ventricular epicardium. *Am J Physiol.* 1996;271:H548.

240. Volders PG, Sipido KR, Carmeliet E, et al. Repolarizing K+ currents ITO1 and IKs are larger in right than left canine ventricular midmyocardium. *Circulation.* 1999;99:206.

241. Takano M, Noma A. Distribution of the isoprenaline-induced chloride current in rabbit heart. *Pflugers Arch.* 1992;420:223.

242. Zygmunt AC. Intracellular calcium activates chloride current in canine ventricular myocytes. *Am J Physiol.* 1994;267:H1984.

243. Wang HS, Cohen IS. Calcium channel heterogeneity in canine left ventricular myocytes. *J Physiol.* 2003;547:825.

244. Cordeiro JM, Greene L, Heilmann C, et al. Transmural heterogeneity of calcium activity and mechanical function in the canine left ventricle. *Am J Physiol Heart Circ Physiol.* 2004;286:H1471.

245. Banyasz T, Fulop L, Magyar J, et al. Endocardial versus epicardial differences in L-type calcium current in canine ventricular myocytes studied by action potential voltage clamp. *Cardiovasc Res.* 2003;58:66.

246. Sicouri S, Antzelevitch C. A subpopulation of cells with unique electrophysiological properties in the deep subepicardium of the canine ventricle. The M cell. *Circ Res.* 1991;68:1729.

247. Anyukhovsky EP, Sosunov EA, Rosen MR. Regional differences in electrophysiologic properties of epicardium, midmyocardium and endocardium: In vitro and in vivo correlations. *Circulation.* 1996;94:1981.

248. Zygmunt AC, Goodrow RJ, Antzelevitch C. I(NaCa) contributes to electrical heterogeneity within the canine ventricle. *Am J Physiol Heart Circ Physiol.* 2000;278:H1671.

249. Brahmajothi MV, Morales MJ, Reimer KA, et al. Regional localization of ERG, the channel protein responsible for the rapid component of the delayed rectifier, K+ current in the ferret heart. *Circ Res.* 1997;81:128.

250. Antzelevitch C, Dumaine R. Electrical heterogeneity in the heart: Physiological, pharmacological and clinical implications. In: Page E, Fozzard HA, Solaro RJ, eds. *Handbook of Physiology. Section 2 The Cardiovascular System.* New York: Oxford University Press; 2001:654.

251. Burashnikov A, Antzelevitch C. Differences in the electrophysiologic response of four canine ventricular cell types to α_1-adrenergic agonists. *Cardiovasc Res.* 1999;43:901.

252. Yan GX, Shimizu W, Antzelevitch C. Characteristics and distribution of M cells in arterially-perfused canine left ventricular wedge preparations. *Circulation.* 1998;98:1921.

253. Sicouri S, Antzelevitch C. Electrophysiologic characteristics of M cells in the canine left ventricular free wall. *J Cardiovasc Electrophysiol.* 1995;6:591.

254. Sicouri S, Fish J, Antzelevitch C. Distribution of M cells in the canine ventricle. *J Cardiovasc Electrophysiol.* 1994;5:824.

255. Brugada P, Brugada J. Right bundle branch block, persistent ST segment elevation and sudden cardiac death: a distinct clinical and electrocardiographic syndrome: a multicenter report. *J Am Coll Cardiol.* 1992;20:1391.

256. Wilde AA, Antzelevitch C, Borggrefe M, et al. Proposed diagnostic criteria for the Brugada syndrome: consensus report. *Eur Heart J.* 2002;23:1648.

257. Wilde AA, Antzelevitch C, Borggrefe M, et al. Proposed diagnostic criteria for the Brugada syndrome: consensus report. *Circulation.* 2002;106:2514.

258. Antzelevitch C, Brugada P, Borggrefe M, et al. Brugada syndrome. Report of the Second Consensus Conference. Endorsed by the Heart Rhythm Society and the European Heart Rhythm Association. *Circulation.* 2005;111:659.

259. Antzelevitch C, Brugada P, Borggrefe M, et al. Brugada syndrome: report of the second consensus conference. *Heart Rhythm.* 2005;2:429.

260. Skinner JR, Chung SK, Montgomery D, et al. Near-miss SIDS due to Brugada syndrome. *Arch Dis Child.* 2005;90:528.

261. Vatta M, Dumaine R, Varghese G, et al. Genetic and biophysical basis of sudden unexplained nocturnal death syndrome (SUNDS), a disease allelic to Brugada syndrome. *Hum Mol Genet.* 2002;11:337.

262. Remme CA, Wever EFD, Wilde AAM, et al. Diagnosis and long-term follow-up of Brugada syndrome in patients with idiopathic ventricular fibrillation. *Eur Heart J.* 2001;22:400.

263. Chen Q, Kirsch GE, Zhang D, et al. Genetic basis and molecular mechanisms for idiopathic ventricular fibrillation. *Nature.* 1998;392:293.

264. Antzelevitch C, Brugada P, Brugada J, Brugada R. *The Brugada Syndrome: From Bench to Bedside.* Oxford: Blackwell Futura; 2005.

265. Schulze-Bahr E, Eckardt L, Breithardt G, et al. Sodium channel gene (SCN5A) mutations in 44 index patients with Brugada syndrome: different incidences in familial and sporadic disease. *Hum Mutat.* 2003;21:651.

266. Hong K, Guerchicoff A, Pollevick GD, et al. Cryptic 5 splice site activation in SCN5A associated with Brugada syndrome. *J Mol Cell Cardiol.* 2005;38:555.

267. Bezzina CR, Shimizu W, Yang P, et al. Common sodium channel promoter haplotype in Asian subjects underlies variability in cardiac conduction. *Circulation.* 2006;113:338.

268. Weiss R, Barmada MM, Nguyen T, et al. Clinical and molecular heterogeneity in the Brugada syndrome. A novel gene locus on chromosome 3. *Circulation.* 2002;105:707.

269. London B, Sanyal S, Michalec M, et al. AB16–1: A mutation in the glycerol-3-phosphate dehydrogenase 1-like gene (GPD1L) causes Brugada syndrome. *Heart Rhythm.* 2006;3:S32.

270. Antzelevitch C, Pollevick GD, Cordeiro JM, et al. Loss of function mutations in the cardiac calcium channel underlie a new clinical entity characterized by ST segment elevation, short QT intervals and sudden cardiac death. *Circulation.* 2007;115:442–449.

271. Yan GX, Antzelevitch C. Cellular basis for the electrocardiographic J wave. *Circulation.* 1996;93:372.

272. Yan GX, Antzelevitch C. Cellular basis for the Brugada syndrome and other mechanisms of arrhythmogenesis associated with ST segment elevation. *Circulation.* 1999;100:1660.

273. Fish JM, Antzelevitch C. Role of sodium and calcium channel block in unmasking the Brugada syndrome. *Heart Rhythm.* 2004;1:210.

274. Fish JM, Antzelevitch C. Cellular and ionic basis for the sex-related difference in the manifestation of the Brugada syndrome and progressive conduction disease phenotypes. *J Electrocardiol.* 2003;36:173.

275. Antzelevitch C. Brugada syndrome. *PACE.* 2006;29:1130.

276. Litovsky SH, Antzelevitch C. Rate dependence of action potential duration and refractoriness in canine ventricular endocardium differs from that of epicardium: role of the transient outward current. *J Am Coll Cardiol.* 1989;14:1053.

277. Kilborn MJ, Fedida D. A study of the developmental changes in outward currents of rat ventricular myocytes. *J Physiol (Lond).* 1990;430:37.

278. Furukawa Y, Akahane K, Ogiwara Y, et al. K⁺-Channel blocking and antimuscarinic effects of a novel piperazine derivative, INO 2628 on the isolated dog atrium. *Eur J Pharm.* 1991;193:217.

279. Di Diego JM, Antzelevitch C. Pinacidil-induced electrical heterogeneity and extrasystolic activity in canine ventricular tissues. Does activation of ATP-regulated potassium current promote phase 2 reentry? *Circulation.* 1993;88:1177.

280. Krishnan SC, Antzelevitch C. Flecainide-induced arrhythmia in canine ventricular epicardium. Phase 2 reentry? *Circulation.* 1993;87:562.

281. Di Diego JM, Antzelevitch C. High [Ca²⁺]-induced electrical heterogeneity and extrasystolic activity in isolated canine ventricular epicardium. Phase 2 reentry. *Circulation.* 1994;89:1839.

282. Antzelevitch C, Sicouri S, Lukas A, et al. Clinical implications of electrical heterogeneity in the heart: The electrophysiology and pharmacology of epicardial, M, and endocardial cells. In: Podrid PJ, Kowey PR, eds. *Cardiac Arrhythmia: Mechanism, Diagnosis and Management.* Baltimore, MD: William & Wilkins; 1995:88.

283. Kalla H, Yan GX, Marinchak R. Ventricular fibrillation in a patient with prominent J (Osborn) waves and ST segment elevation in the inferior electrocardiographic leads: a Brugada syndrome variant? *J Cardiovasc Electrophysiol.* 2000;11:95.

284. Yan GX, Lankipalli RS, Burke JF, et al. Ventricular repolarization components on the electrocardiogram: cellular basis and clinical significance. *J Am Coll Cardiol.* 2003;42:401.

285. Aizawa Y, Tamura M, Chinushi M, et al. Idiopathic ventricular fibrillation and bradycardia-dependent intraventricular block. *Am Heart J.* 1993;126:1473.

286. Bjerregaard P, Gussak I, Kotar Sl, et al. Recurrent syncope in a patient with prominent J-wave. *Am Heart J.* 1994;127:1426.

287. Lukas A, Antzelevitch C. Differences in the electrophysiological response of canine ventricular epicardium and endocardium to ischemia: role of the transient outward current. *Circulation.* 1993;88:2903.

288. Litovsky SH, Antzelevitch C. Differences in the electrophysiological response of canine ventricular subendocardium and subepicardium to acetylcholine and isoproterenol. A direct effect of acetylcholine in ventricular myocardium. *Circ Res.* 1990;67:615.

289. Krishnan SC, Antzelevitch C. Sodium channel block produces opposite electrophysiological effects in canine ventricular epicardium and endocardium. *Circ Res.* 1991;69:277.

290. Miyazaki T, Mitamura H, Miyoshi S, et al. Autonomic and antiarrhythmic drug modulation of ST segment elevation in patients with Brugada syndrome. *J Am Coll Cardiol.* 1996;27:1061.

291. Tsuchiya T, Ashikaga K, Honda T, et al. Prevention of ventricular fibrillation by cilostazol, an oral phosphodiesterase inhibitor, in a patient with Brugada syndrome. *J Cardiovasc Electrophysiol.* 2002;13:698.

292. Shimizu W, Aiba T, Kamakura S. Mechanisms of disease: current understanding and future challenges in Brugada syndrome. *Nat Clin Pract Cardiovasc Med.* 2005;2:408.

293. Antzelevitch C, Brugada P, Brugada J, et al. Brugada syndrome. A decade of progress. *Circ Res.* 2002;91:1114.

294. Kurita T, Shimizu W, Inagaki M, et al. The electrophysiologic mechanism of ST-segment elevation in Brugada syndrome. *J Am Coll Cardiol.* 2002;40:330.

295. Futterman LG, Lemberg L. Brugada. *Am J Crit Care.* 2001;10:360.

296. Nagase S, Kusano KF, Morita H, et al. Epicardial electrogram of the right ventricular outflow tract in patients with the Brugada syndrome: using the epicardial lead. *J Am Coll Cardiol.* 2002;39:1992.

297. Eckardt L, Bruns HJ, Paul M, et al. Body surface area of ST elevation and the presence of late potentials correlate to the inducibility of ventricular tachyarrhythmias in Brugada syndrome. *J Cardiovasc Electrophysiol.* 2002;13:742.

298. Ikeda T, Takami M, Sugi K, et al. Noninvasive risk stratification of subjects with a Brugada-type electrocardiogram and no history of cardiac arrest. *Ann Noninvasive Electrocardiol.* 2005;10:396.

299. Antzelevitch C. The Brugada syndrome: ionic basis and arrhythmia mechanisms. *J Cardiovasc Electrophysiol.* 2001;12:268.

300. Di Diego JM, Cordeiro JM, Goodrow RJ, et al. Ionic and cellular basis for the predominance of the Brugada syndrome phenotype in males. *Circulation.* 2002;106:2004.

301. Schwartz PJ. The idiopathic long QT syndrome: progress and questions. *Am Heart J.* 1985;109:399.

302. Moss AJ, Schwartz PJ, Crampton RS, et al. The long QT syndrome: prospective longitudinal study of 328 families. *Circulation.* 1991;84:1136.

303. Zipes DP. The long QT interval syndrome: a Rosetta stone for sympathetic related ventricular tachyarrhythmias. *Circulation.* 1991;84:1414.

304. Wang Q, Shen J, Splawski I, et al. *SCN5A* mutations associated with an inherited cardiac arrhythmia, long QT syndrome. *Cell.* 1995;80:805.

305. Mohler PJ, Schott JJ, Gramolini AO, et al. Ankyrin-B mutation causes type 4 long-QT cardiac arrhythmia and sudden cardiac death. *Nature.* 2003;421:634.

306. Plaster NM, Tawil R, Tristani-Firouzi M, et al. Mutations in Kir2.1 cause the developmental and episodic electrical phenotypes of Andersen's syndrome. *Cell.* 2001;105:511.

307. Curran ME, Splawski I, Timothy KW, et al. A molecular basis for cardiac arrhythmia: *HERG* mutations cause long QT syndrome. *Cell.* 1995;80:795.

308. Wang Q, Curran ME, Splawski I, et al. Positional cloning of a novel potassium channel gene: *KVLQT1* mutations cause cardiac arrhythmias. *Nat Genet.* 1996;12:17.

309. Splawski I, Tristani-Firouzi M, Lehmann MH, et al. Mutations in the hminK gene cause long QT syndrome and suppress I_Ks function. *Nat Genet.* 1997;17:338.

310. Ye B, Tester DJ, Vatta M, et al. AB1–1: Molecular and functional characterization of novel cav3-encoded caveolin-3 mutations in congenital long QT syndrome. *Heart Rhythm.* 2006;3:S1.

311. Domingo AM, Kaku T, Tester DJ, et al. AB16–6: sodium channel β4 subunit mutation causes congenital long QT syndrome. *Heart Rhythm.* 2006;3:S34.
312. Splawski I, Timothy KW, Sharpe LM, et al. Ca(V)1.2 calcium channel dysfunction causes a multisystem disorder including arrhythmia and autism. *Cell.* 2004;119:19.
313. Schwartz PJ, Priori SG, Napolitano C. The long QT syndrome. In: Zipes DP, Jalife J, eds. *Cardiac Electrophysiology: From Cell to Bedside.* 3rd ed. Philadelphia, PA: W.B. Saunders; 2000:597.
314. Moss AJ, Zareba W, Hall WJ, et al. Effectiveness and limitations of beta-blocker therapy in congenital long-QT syndrome. *Circulation.* 2000;101:616.
315. Schwartz PJ, Priori SG, Cerrone M, et al. Left cardiac sympathetic denervation in the management of high-risk patients affected by the long-QT syndrome. *Circulation.* 2004;109:1826–1833.
316. Bednar MM, Harrigan EP, Anziano RJ, et al. The QT interval. *Prog Cardiovasc Dis.* 2001;43:1.
317. Tomaselli GF, Marban E. Electrophysiological remodeling in hypertrophy and heart failure. *Cardiovasc Res.* 1999;42:270.
318. Sipido KR, Volders PG, De Groot SH, et al. Enhanced Ca(2+) release and Na/Ca exchange activity in hypertrophied canine ventricular myocytes: potential link between contractile adaptation and arrhythmogenesis. *Circulation.* 2000;102:2137.
319. Volders PG, Sipido KR, Vos MA, et al. Downregulation of delayed rectifier K(+) currents in dogs with chronic complete atrioventricular block and acquired torsades de pointes. *Circulation.* 1999;100:2455.
320. Undrovinas AI, Maltsev VA, Sabbah HN. Repolarization abnormalities in cardiomyocytes of dogs with chronic heart failure: role of sustained inward current. *Cell Mol Life Sci.* 1999;55:494.
321. Antzelevitch C, Shimizu W. Cellular mechanisms underlying the long QT syndrome. *Curr Opin Cardiol.* 2002;17:43.
322. Shimizu W, Antzelevitch C. Effects of a K(+) channel opener to reduce transmural dispersion of repolarization and prevent torsade de pointes in LQT1 LQT2 and LQT3 models of the long-QT syndrome. *Circulation.* 2000;102:706.
323. Antzelevitch C. Heterogeneity of cellular repolarization in LQTS. the role of M cells. *Eur Heart J.* 2001;(suppl)3:K-2.
324. Shimizu W, Antzelevitch C. Cellular basis for the ECG features of the LQT1 form of the long QT syndrome: effects of β-adrenergic agonists and antagonists and sodium channel blockers on transmural dispersion of repolarization and torsade de pointes. *Circulation.* 1998;98:2314.
325. Shimizu W, Antzelevitch C. Sodium channel block with mexiletine is effective in reducing dispersion of repolarization and preventing torsade de pointes in LQT2 and LQT3 models of the long-QT syndrome. *Circulation.* 1997;96:2038.
326. Anyukhovsky EP, Sosunov EA, Gainullin RZ, et al. The controversial M cell. *J Cardiovasc Electrophysiol.* 1999;10:244.
327. Yan GX, Antzelevitch C. Cellular basis for the normal T wave and the electrocardiographic manifestations of the long QT syndrome. *Circulation.* 1998;98:1928.
328. Shimizu W, Antzelevitch C. Cellular and ionic basis for T-wave alternans under long QT conditions. *Circulation.* 1999;99:1499.
329. Noda T, Takaki H, Kurita T, et al. Gene-specific response of dynamic ventricular repolarization to sympathetic stimulation in LQT1 LQT2 and LQT3 forms of congenital long QT syndrome. *Eur Heart J.* 2002;23:975.
330. Schwartz PJ, Priori SG, Spazzolini C, et al. Genotype-phenotype correlation in the long-QT syndrome: gene-specific triggers for life-threatening arrhythmias. *Circulation.* 2001;103:89.
331. Ali RH, Zareba W, Moss A, et al. Clinical and genetic variables associated with acute arousal and nonarousal-related cardiac events among subjects with long QT syndrome. *Am J Cardiol.* 2000;85:457.
332. Windle JR, Geletka RC, Moss AJ, et al. Normalization of ventricular repolarization with flecainide in long QT syndrome patients with SCN5A:DeltaKPQ mutation. *Ann Noninvasive Electrocardiol.* 2001;6:153.
333. Roden DM. Pharmacogenetics and drug-induced arrhythmias. *Cardiovasc Res.* 2001;50:224.
334. Emori T, Antzelevitch C. Cellular basis for complex T waves and arrhythmic activity following combined I(Kr) and I(Ks) block. *J Cardiovasc Electrophysiol.* 2001;12:1369.
335. Yamaguchi M, Shimizu M, Ino H, et al. T wave peak-to-end interval and QT dispersion in acquired long QT syndrome: a new index for arrhythmogenicity. *Clin Sci (Lond).* 2003;105:671.
336. Shimizu M, Ino H, Okeie K, et al. T-peak to T-end interval may be a better predictor of high-risk patients with hypertrophic cardiomyopathy associated with a cardiac troponin I mutation than QT dispersion. *Clin Cardiol.* 2002;25:335.
337. Watanabe N, Kobayashi Y, Tanno K, et al. Transmural dispersion of repolarization and ventricular tachyarrhythmias. *J Electrocardiol.* 2004;37:191.
338. Di Diego JM, Belardinelli L, Antzelevitch C. Cisapride-induced transmural dispersion of repolarization and torsade de pointes in the canine left ventricular wedge preparation during epicardial stimulation. *Circulation.* 2003;108:1027.
339. Antzelevitch C. Drug-induced Channelopathies. In: Zipes DP, Jalife J, eds. *Cardiac Electrophysiology. From Cell to Bedside.* 4th ed. New York: W.B. Saunders; 2004:151.
340. Fenichel RR, Malik M, Antzelevitch C, et al. Drug-induced torsade de pointes and implications for drug development. *J Cardiovasc Electrophysiol.* 2004;15:475.
341. Li GR, Feng J, Yue L, et al. Transmural heterogeneity of action potentials and Ito1 in myocytes isolated from the human right ventricle. *Am J Physiol.* 1998;275:H369.
342. Sicouri S, Moro S, Litovsky SH, et al. Chronic amiodarone reduces transmural dispersion of repolarization in the canine heart. *J Cardiovasc Electrophysiol.* 1997;8:1269.
343. van Opstal JM, Schoenmakers M, Verduyn SC, et al. Chronic amiodarone evokes no torsade de pointes arrhythmias despite QT lengthening in an animal model of acquired long-QT syndrome. *Circulation.* 2001;104:2722.
344. Shimizu W, McMahon B, Antzelevitch C. Sodium pentobarbital reduces transmural dispersion of repolarization and prevents torsade de pointes in models of acquired and congenital long QT syndrome. *J Cardiovasc Electrophysiol.* 1999;10:156.
345. Gussak I, Brugada P, Brugada J, et al. Idiopathic short QT interval: a new clinical syndrome? *Cardiology.* 2000;94:99.
346. Gussak I, Brugada P, Brugada J, et al. ECG phenomenon of idiopathic and paradoxical short QT intervals. *Cardiac Electrophysiol Rev.* 2002;6:49.
347. Gaita F, Giustetto C, Bianchi F, et al. Short QT syndrome: a familial cause of sudden death. *Circulation.* 2003;108:965.
348. Brugada R, Hong K, Dumaine R, et al. Sudden death associated with short QT-syndrome linked to mutations in HERG. *Circulation.* 2003;109:30.
349. Bellocq C, Van Ginneken AC, Bezzina CR, et al. Mutation in the KCNQ1 gene leading to the short QT-interval syndrome. *Circulation.* 2004;109:2394.
350. Extramiana F, Antzelevitch C. Amplified transmural dispersion of repolarization as the basis for arrhythmogenesis in a canine ventricular-wedge model of short-QT syndrome. *Circulation.* 2004;110:3661.
351. Leenhardt A, Lucet V, Denjoy I, et al. Catecholaminergic polymorphic ventricular tachycardia in children: a 7-year follow-up of 21 patients. *Circulation.* 1995;91:1512.

CHAPTER 36

Approach to the Patient with Cardiac Arrhythmias

Eric N. Prystowsky / Richard I. Fogel

The diagnosis and management of specific cardiac arrhythmias are detailed in other chapters in this textbook. This chapter provides the clinician with an approach to the overall evaluation of patients presumed to have a cardiac arrhythmia. Without a doubt, the two key elements in assessing patients are the history and, if available, the ECG rhythm strip obtained at the time of their symptom. Findings on the physical examination and judicious use of noninvasive and invasive tests can be quite helpful in certain circumstances.

HISTORY

It is imperative that a complete history of the patient's symptoms be obtained. Many elements must be sought for in this process, including (1) documentation of initial onset of symptoms; (2) complete characterization of symptoms; (3) identifying conditions that appear to initiate symptoms; (4) duration of episodes; (5) frequency of episodes; (6) pattern of symptoms over time, for example, better or worse; (7) effect of any treatment; and (8) family history of a similar problem. It is also important to ascertain any pertinent past medical history that might be helpful in the diagnosis. This might include history of myocardial infarction (MI), especially in a patient who presents with palpitations and syncope, or the recent initiation of an antihypertensive agent in a patient who now presents with dizzy spells. In our experience careful and thorough attention to obtaining the preceding information typically results in an efficient and focused approach to the patient's problem.

PHYSICAL EXAMINATION

Observations from the physical examination are helpful primarily to define whether cardiovascular disease is present. For example, in a patient who presents with dizzy spells or syncope, the presence of orthostatic hypotension, a carotid bruit, or decreased carotid pulses may be important findings that lead to a diagnosis of coronary artery disease. Most importantly, the presence of specific cardiac murmurs or an S_3 or S_4 gallop may direct the clinician toward a cardiac cause for the patient's symptoms. Also pay attention to the patient's gender, age, and physiognomy. Paroxysmal supraventricular tachycardia (PSVT) that occurs in a 12-year-old boy is more likely caused by atrioventricular reentry tachycardia, whereas PSVT presenting in a 45-year-old woman more commonly is caused by atrioventricular (AV) node reentry.

SYNCOPE, PRESYNCOPE, DIZZINESS

Patients with syncope, presyncope, or dizziness are often referred to the electrophysiologist for evaluation for fear that the symptoms are caused by an arrhythmia. Unless an ECG rhythm strip is recorded at the time of the patient's event, it is impossible to positively eliminate an arrhythmic cause. Regardless, a detailed history typically points in the correct direction (see Chap. 48). The ECG may disclose many clues to the cause of syncope, including MI, cardiac hypertrophy, sinus node dysfunction, conduction abnormality, Wolff-Parkinson-White syndrome, long or short QT interval, or Brugada syndrome. Evaluation of the echocardiogram may lead to a variety of cardiac diagnoses.

Neurally mediated syncope is very common. Typically the patient is in an upright position, either sitting or standing, and may recount a feeling of being hot or warm with or without concomitant nausea prior to loss of consciousness. Sweating is a common feature, but the patient may state that it occurred on regaining consciousness rather than prior to syncope. Normally the patient is alert on regaining consciousness but may feel fatigued. Although patients often state that their heart was *pounding* or faster than usual on awakening, they do not give a history of a rapid regular pulse that persists for minutes after the event. This latter feature should direct one to a possible arrhythmic cause for syncope. *Church* syncope, that is, patients who have presyncope or syncope during church services, is almost always vagally mediated in our experience.

Cardiac syncope is often sudden in onset and frequently unaccompanied by any prodrome. In some circumstances patients relate a feeling of rapid palpitations prior to loss of consciousness, and these individuals should be evaluated for a cardiac arrhythmia regardless of whether heart disease is present. One should remember that rapid PSVT as well as ventricular tachycardia can cause syncope. Unfortunately, a sudden loss of consciousness without prodrome is not specific for an arrhythmia, and patients with an arrhythmia can present with some features of a vasovagal syncope.

For patients who present with dizziness or presyncope, it is important to distinguish between vertigo and true light-headedness. Ask patients whether they feel like the room is spinning or they are spinning, compared with a sensation that *the lights are going out* or they are about to lose consciousness, especially if they are taking medication. Additional tests depend on the results of the initial workup as described earlier.

PALPITATIONS

Palpitations are described by patients in many ways including skipped beats, a sudden thump, hard beating, fluttering in the chest, a jittery sensation, a rapid pulse, or as merely a vague feeling that their heart is irregular. The authors have noted that many patients equate a *strong heartbeat* as palpitations, and it is important to distinguish this from irregular heartbeats. A premature atrial or ventricular complex often cannot be felt by the patient, and what they experience is the strong heartbeat that follows the pause. It may be useful to tap out various cadences for the patient. For example, to distinguish between atrial fibrillation (AF) and PSVT, tap out a rapid, irregular cadence compared with a rapid regular cadence—patients often recognize one over the other. Similarly, tap out a cadence of extra beats with a pause. Palpitations are often more prominent at night, especially when patients lie on their left side. Although these may be premature beats, often it is simply sinus rhythm.

Other historic features often tailor the initial workup. A rapid regular rhythm that occurs a few times per year and has been ongoing for many years is likely a form of PSVT. In the absence of a previous correlation with an ECG rhythm strip or 12-lead ECG, an electrophysiologic study typically is required

for diagnostic and/or therapeutic reasons. Noninvasive monitoring for such infrequent arrhythmias is usually futile, and an electrophysiologic study is preferred over prescription of an implantable loop recorder. In contrast, for patients with more frequent symptoms, noninvasive event recorder monitoring is often our choice, and a unique new form of technology using wireless outpatient continuous monitoring can even identify asymptomatic arrhythmic episodes (see Chap. 40). Even if sinus rhythm is identified as the cause of palpitations, the results are valuable to the patient. Most patients want a diagnosis and are reassured that their symptoms are not life-disturbing or life-threatening, often the reason that brought them to the physician.

Women might present with palpitations during the week prior to menstruation, and the diagnosis is often premature atrial or ventricular complexes that occur during a specific time of hormonal change. It is commonly believed that alcohol and caffeine are arrhythmogenic; and although this may be so in certain patients, it has been our experience that these agents typically play a minor role in patients who have arrhythmias. Obviously, patients with AF might have episodes during heavy alcohol intake, but such is usually not the case for PSVT and sustained ventricular tachycardia.

FATIGUE, CHEST PAIN, AND DYSPNEA

On occasion, patients present with symptoms such as fatigue, chest pain, or dyspnea that seem unrelated to an arrhythmia. This particularly is true for those who have AF. It is surprising how many patients with AF do not experience palpitations and present with either fatigue or shortness of breath. Thus, although these symptoms typically direct the clinician down another diagnostic road, remember that they might be caused by an arrhythmia. Of particular importance are patients who present with AF and symptoms of heart failure without palpitations. Often these individuals have tachycardia-mediated cardiomyopathy, and with appropriate control of the ventricular rate the ventricular function might even normalize. Because the patients do not experience palpitations, they typically present with symptoms of myocardial dysfunction secondary to the prolonged rapid ventricular rates experienced during AF.

ADJUNCTIVE TESTS

◖◗ ELECTROCARDIOGRAM

The ECG is covered elsewhere (Chap. 12), but two specific findings on the 12-lead ECG during PSVT (Fig. 36–1 and Fig. 36–2) should be emphasized. Fig. 36–1 demonstrates a pseudo r′ in ECG lead V$_1$ that is very typical for patients who present with AV node reentry. The pseudo r′ results from superimposition of the P wave on the end of the QRS complex and is noted best in ECG lead V$_1$. In contrast, the typical finding in patients with AV reentry caused by retrograde conduction over an accessory pathway (Wolff-Parkinson-White syndrome) is shown in Fig. 36–2. Note that the P wave is positioned in the early ST segment.

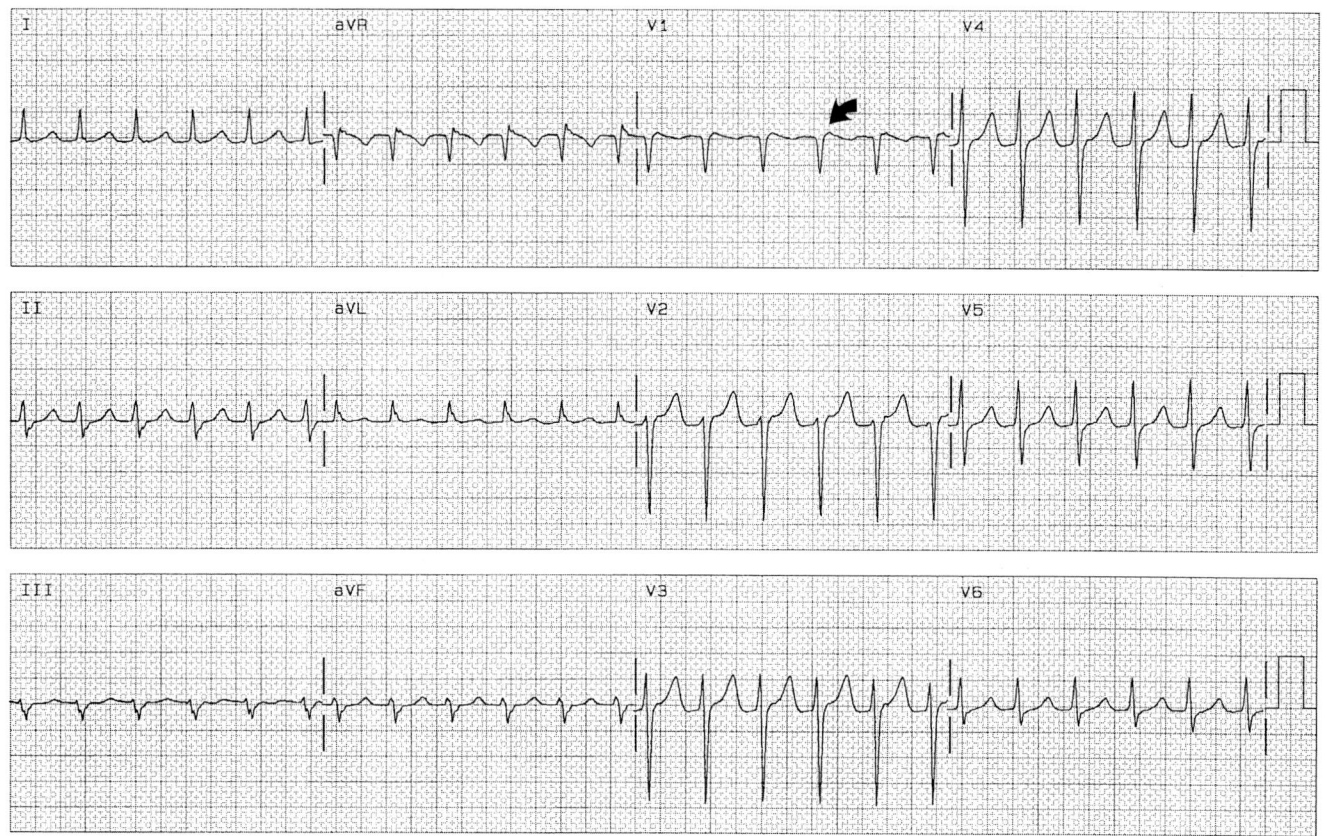

FIGURE 36–1. 12-lead electrocardiogram of atrioventricular node reentry. The *arrow* points to the retrograde P wave at the end of the QRS complex in V_1 and appears as a pseudo r′.

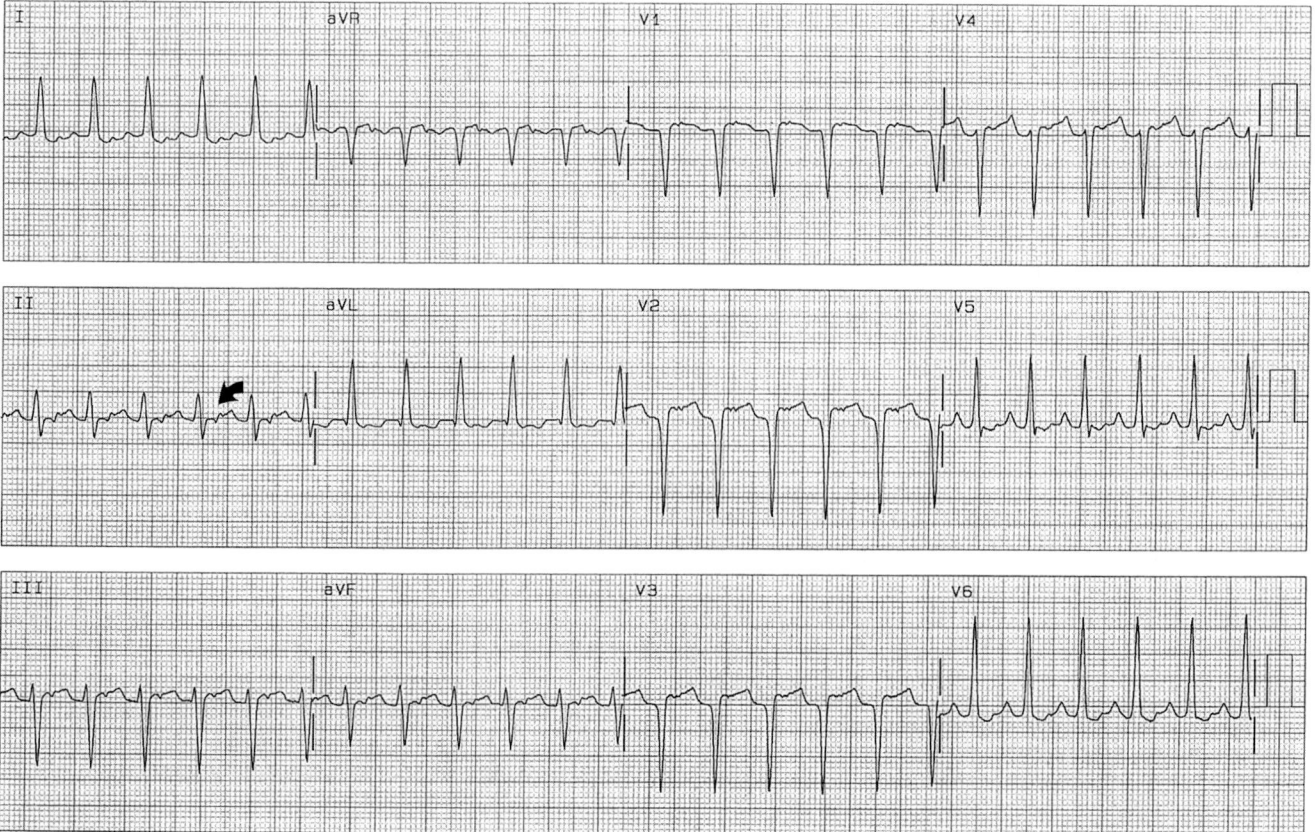

FIGURE 36–2. 12-lead electrocardiogram of atrioventricular reentry. The *arrow* points to the retrograde P wave in the early ST segment of lead II.

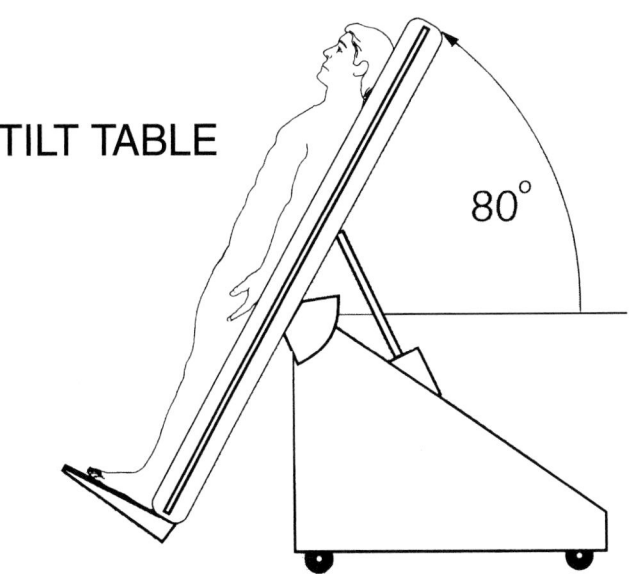

TILT TABLE

80°

FIGURE 36–3. Tilt table with footboard support. *Source: From Prystowsky EN, Klein GT. Cardiac Arrhythmias: An Integrated Approach for the Clinician. New York: McGraw-Hill; 1994:353. Reproduced with permission from McGraw-Hill.*

【 】 HEAD-UP TILT TABLE TESTING

Head-up tilt (HUT) table testing is a diagnostic technique to assess the susceptibility of an individual to neurally mediated syncope.[1] The protocol[1] for HUT generally involves footrest supported head-up tilting at 70 to 80 degrees for 30 to 45 minutes (Fig. 36–3). If HUT is negative, the test may be repeated following pharmacologic provocation. Several agents including sublingual nitroglycerin,[2] epinephrine,[3] and adenosine have been studied; however, most laboratories use isoproterenol at a dose of 1 to 3 μg/min. Repeat tilting is generally performed for 10 minutes after a steady state has been reached. Higher doses of isoproterenol, especially when coupled with longer durations of tilt, significantly decrease the specificity of the test.[3]

In control patients with no history of syncope, 70-degree head-up tilting has a specificity of approximately 90 percent.[4] In patients with unexplained syncope, HUT can yield a diagnosis in 40 to 64 percent,[5–8] particularly in the absence of other structural heart disease.

【 】 RISK-STRATIFICATION AFTER MYOCARDIAL INFARCTION

Risk stratification after MI may be divided into two categories. The first category includes signal-averaged electrocardiography (SAECG) to identify high-frequency potentials at the end of the QRS complex (late potentials) and microvolt changes in T-wave am-plitude. The second category assesses autonomic tone by analyzing spontaneous and induced changes in heart rate and blood pressure.

【 】 SIGNAL-AVERAGED ELECTROCARDIOGRAPHY

SAECG allows the identification of small potentials in the surface ECG that are not seen because their amplitude is less than the noise intrinsic to the ECG signal.[9] A more detailed description of the technique may be found elsewhere.[10] In brief, orthogonal surface XYZ ECG leads are acquired for approximately 200 beats and digitally stored. High-pass filtering minimizes the contribution of low-frequency content. The X, Y, and Z leads are then combined into a vector magnitude referred to as the *filtered QRS complex* (Fig. 36–4). Most commonly the SAECG has been used to identify late potentials appearing at the end of the QRS complex. These potentials correspond to fragmented electrical activity that is generated in areas of slow conduction either within or at the border zone of infarcts, which may be arrhythmogenic and prone to reentry.[11]

Three parameters have been identified to describe late potentials:

1. Filtered QRS duration (QRSd)
2. Root-mean-square voltage of the terminal 40 msec of the QRS complex (RMS40)
3. The duration of the low-amplitude signal (LAS) >40 mV

The latter two parameters represent the amplitude and duration of the late potential, respectively. With 40 Hz filtering, a QRSd >114 msec, RMS40 <20 mV, and LAS >38 msec are considered abnormal.[9] The interpretation of the SAECG is problematic in the presence of a significant baseline intraventricular conduction defect.

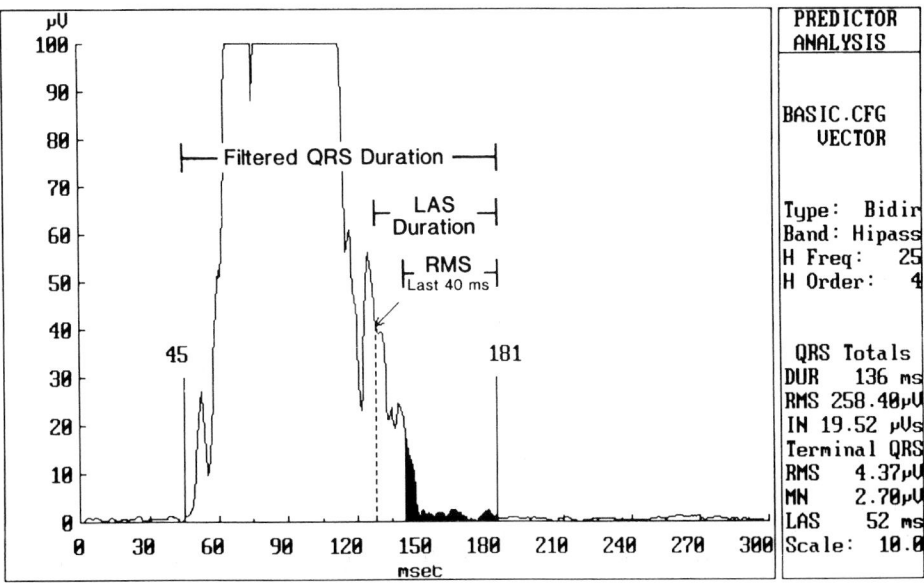

FIGURE 36–4. Positive signal-averaged electrocardiogram in a patient with sustained ventricular tachycardia. All three measured parameters are abnormal. Filtered QRS duration (DUR) is 136 msec; and the root-mean-square (RMS) voltage of the last 40 msec of the QS complex is 4.37 μV. LAS, low-amplitude signal. *Source: From Prystowsky EN, Klein GT. Cardiac Arrhythmias: An Integrated Approach for the Clinician. New York: McGraw-Hill; 1994:345. Reproduced with permission from McGraw-Hill.*

Late potentials are hypothesized to be associated with an increased incidence of ventricular arrhythmias and sudden death.[12–15] In some studies of patients after MI, the incidence of an arrhythmic event was 17 to 29 percent when late potentials were present.[13–19] When late potentials were absent, the incidence of sudden death was 3.5 to 5 percent. Late potentials were an independent risk factor when assessed along with left ventricular ejection fraction (EF).[14] The combination of an abnormal SAECG, reduced EF, and high-grade ectopy identified a population with a 50 percent risk in the same study.

MICROVOLT T-WAVE ALTERNANS

Microvolt T-wave alternans (MTWA) is a technique that measures small changes in T-wave amplitude that occur on an alternating beat-to-beat basis. These changes have been associated with an increased risk of malignant ventricular arrhythmias[16] and are thought to be caused by exaggerated repolarization heterogeneity.[17] Several techniques[18] have now been developed to detect and quantify these subtle variations in T-wave amplitude. The most common method involves the spectral analysis of a large number of beats. Using this technique, an *alternans power* and *alternans voltage* can be determined. The alternans voltage represents the magnitude of the variation of the alternans T-wave amplitude from the mean T-wave amplitude.

Rosenbaum and colleagues[19] reported the prospective assessment of MTWA in the prediction of sudden death and inducibility at electrophysiologic study in 83 patients. The presence of MTWA was an independent predictor of inducibility at the electrophysiology study (relative risk [RR] 5.2). Of 66 patients followed for up to 20 months, 13 had an arrhythmic event. The 20-month arrhythmic-free survival was 19 percent when MTWA was present, and 94 percent when MTWA was absent.

The most significant limitation of this technique is the requirement of atrial pacing to elevate heart rate. Because MTWA is heart rate dependent, other techniques that used exercise were developed.[20,21] Patients who developed MTWA at lower heart rates had a higher risk. Patients who developed MTWA only at high heart rates or did not develop MTWA were felt to be a lower risk.[22]

Subsequent clinical studies identified exercise-induced microvolt T-wave alternans as a predictor of arrhythmic risk.[22,23] The test is considered positive if the onset of sustained MTWA occurs at <110 beats/min, and negative if sustained MTWA does not occur at heart rates ≥105 beats/min. The most common causes of an indeterminate test are failure to attain an adequate heart rate, frequent ectopy, nonsustained alternans, and excessive background electrocardiographic noise. The predictive power of MTWA appears to be independent of other risk-stratifying techniques including heart rate variability, SAECG, baroreceptor sensitivity testing, ejection fraction, and electrophysiologic testing.[23]

Gehi and coworkers[24] performed a metaanalysis of 19 prospective studies involving 2608 patients with an average follow up of 21 months for a variety of cardiac problems and found the positive predictive value for arrhythmic events was 19.3 percent. The negative predictive value was 97.2 percent. The RR of a positive test for an arrhythmic event was 3.77. In patients with congestive heart failure and a nonischemic cardiomyopathy (seven studies), the predictive value of a positive test was 21.3 percent and of a nega-

tive test was 95.2 percent. In this population the RR was 3.67. In patients with congestive heart failure and an ischemic cardiomyopathy, the positive predictive value was 29.7 percent and the negative predictive value was 91.6 percent. However, this analysis included data from only 2 studies.

More recently, Chow and colleagues[25] reported the use of MTWA for risk stratification in 768 consecutive patients with an ischemic cardiomyopathy (EF <35 percent) and no history of ventricular arrhythmias. Of the 768 patients studied, 514 (67 percent) had a non-negative (positive or indeterminate) MTWA test. After multivariate analysis a non-negative MTWA test was associated with a higher risk of all cause mortality (hazard ratio 2.24) and arrhythmic mortality (hazard ratio 2.24).

Bloomfield and coworkers[26] studied 549 patients with an EF <40 percent, with no prior history of sustained ventricular arrhythmias, and 5 percent had an ischemic cardiomyopathy and 45 percent a prior MI. During a mean follow up of 20 months, there were 40 deaths and 11 nonfatal sustained ventricular arrhythmias treated by appropriate implantable cardioverter-defibrillator shocks. The 2-year event rate was 15 percent in patients with an abnormal MTWA and 2.5 percent in those with a normal test. The hazard ratio for an abnormal MTWA was 6.5.

HEART RATE VARIABILITY

Heart rate variability (HRV) analysis is based on subtle variations in sinus cycle length and has been used to assess cardiac autonomic status[27] by two methods. The time-domain methods identify the RR-interval sequences and then apply statistical techniques to express the variance. The most commonly employed measure is the standard deviation of normal-to-normal beats (SDNN), or of all RR intervals; however, multiple other measures have been used.

Frequency domain methods apply the fast Fourier transform to the RR-interval sequence to develop a power spectral density that describes how the variance of the signal (i.e., power) is distributed as a function of frequency. Three main spectral components have been identified: (1) very-low-frequency (<0.04 Hz), (2) low-frequency 0.04 to 0.15 Hz, and (3) high-frequency 0.15 to 0.40 Hz.[27]

HRV has been used for postmyocardial risk stratification. Several studies have shown that decreased heart rate variability is associated with an increased risk of sudden death.[28–31] An SDNN <50 to 70 msec appears to identify patients at highest risk. Kleiger and coworkers[29] demonstrated that the RR of mortality was 5.3 times higher for a group of patients following MI who had an SDNN <50 msec compared with a group with heart rate variability >100 msec. Results from the GISSI-2 trial demonstrated that the predictive ability of HRV was preserved following thrombolytic therapy.[32] Additionally, heart rate variability increases with β-blocker treatment[33] and is consistent with the protective effects of beta-adrenergic-blocking agents post-MI.

BAROREFLEX SENSITIVITY

Baroreflex sensitivity (BRS) testing is another technique to assess the cardiac autonomic nervous system. Typically, as carotid pressure rises, the RR interval is prolonged. The increase in carotid pressure is detected by the carotid sinus baroreceptors and results in vagal activation offsetting the rise in systemic blood pressure. Under normal circumstances there is resting vagal predominance and sympathetic inhibition. The theory underlying BRS sensitivity testing is that decreased BRS may be present post-MI and that a substantial reduction in BRS is a marker of increased risk for ventricular fibrillation.[34]

Most commonly, BRS is assessed by measuring the heart rate response following infusion of a vasoactive agent. Usually phenylephrine is given in doses to increase systolic blood pressure 20 to 40 mmHg. The changes in RR intervals are plotted against systolic blood pressure changes, and the slope is considered the BRS. In a group of normal controls, the average BRS was 14.8 ± 9 msec/mmHg.[35] Overall baroreceptor sensitivity decreases when the sympathetic nervous system is activated. An alternative technique employs neck collar suction to activate carotid baroreceptors.

In the Autonomic Tone and Reflexes After Myocardial Infarction (ATRAMI) study,[36] the investigators followed 1284 patients after MI and assessed BRS and HRV. Over an average of 21 months, there were 44 cardiac deaths and 5 nonfatal cardiac arrests. The multivariate risk of cardiac mortality was 2.8 when the BRS was <3 msec/mmHg, and 3.2 when the SDNN was <70 msec. In patients with BRS less than 3 msec/mmHg and SDNN <70 msec there was 17 percent mortality. In patients with BRS >3 and SDNN >70, the mortality was 2 percent. The ATRAMI investigators concluded that the analysis of vagal reflexes using BRS had prognostic value independent from left ventricular function and additive to the prognostic value of heart rate variability following MI.

CONCLUSION AND IMPLICATIONS

In the evaluation of patients with reduced left ventricular function to identify those at highest risk for arrhythmic death, the various noninvasive tests either alone or in combination have shown some value. They typically have relatively high-negative predictive value, but a weakness is their rather low-positive predictive value. The *optimum* risk stratification is yet to be found.

REFERENCES

1. Benditt DG, Ferguson DW, Grubb BP, et al. Tilt table testing for assessing syncope: an American College of Cardiology expert consensus document. *J Am Coll Cardiol* 1996;28:263–275.
2. Raviele A, Menozzi C, Brignole M, et al. Value of head-up tilt testing potentiated with sublingual nitroglycerin to assess the origin of unexplained syncope. *Am J Cardiol* 1995;76:267–272.
3. Calkins H, Kadish A, Sousa J, et al. Comparison of response to isoproterenol and epinephrine during head up tilt in suspected vasodepressor syncope. *Am J Cardiol* 1991;67:207–209.
4. Natale A, Akhtar M, Jazayeri M, et al. Provocation of hypotension during head-up tilt testing in subjects with no history of syncope or presyncope. *Circulation* 1995;92:54–58.
5. Raviele A, Gasparini G, DiPede F, et al. Usefulness of head-up tilt test in evaluating patients with syncope of unknown origin and negative electrophysiologic study. *Am J Cardiol* 1990;65:1322–1327.
6. Grubb BP, Temesy-Armos P, Hahn H, Elliot L. Utility of upright tilt table testing in the evaluation and management of syncope of unknown origin. *Am J Med* 1991;90:6–10.
7. Grubb BP, Wolfe D, Samoil D, et al. Recurrent unexplained syncope in the elderly: the use of head-upright tilt table testing in evaluation and management. *J Am Geriatr Soc* 1992;40:1123–1128.

8. Sra JS, Anderson AJ, Sheikh SH, et al. Unexplained syncope evaluated by electrophysiologic studies and head-up tilt testing. *Ann Intern Med* 1991;114:1013–1019.
9. Cain ME, Anderson JL, Arnsdorff MF, et al. American College of Cardiology expert consensus document: signal averaged electrocardiography. *J Am Coll Cardiol* 1996;27:238–249.
10. Simson MB. Use of signals in the terminal QRS complex to identify patients with ventricular tachycardia after myocardial infarction. *Circulation* 1981;64:235.
11. Simson MB, Untereker WJ, Speilman SR, et al. Relation between late potentials on the body surface and directly recorded fragmented electrograms in patients with ventricular tachycardia. *Am J Cardiol* 1983;51:105–112.
12. Gomes JA, Cain ME, Buxton AE, Josephson ME, Lee KL, Hafley GE. Prediction of long-term outcomes by signal-averaged electrocardiography in patients with unsustained ventricular tachycardia, coronary artery disease, and left ventricular dysfunction. *Circulation* 2001;104:436–441.
13. Denniss AR, Richards DA, Cody DV, et al. Prognostic significance of ventricular tachycardia and fibrillation induced at programmed stimulation and delayed potentials detected on the signal-averaged electrocardiograms of survivors of acute myocardial infarction. *Circulation* 1986;74:731–745.
14. Gomes JA, Winters SL, Stewart D, et al. A new noninvasive index to predict sustained ventricular tachycardia in the first year after myocardial infarction: bases on signal-averaged electrocardiogram, radionuclide ejection fraction and Holter monitoring. *J Am Coll Cardiol* 1987;10:349–357.
15. Kuchar DL, Thorburn CW, Sammel NL. Prediction of serious arrhythmic events after myocardial infarction: signal averaged electrocardiogram, Holter monitoring and radionuclide ejection fraction. *J Am Coll Cardiol* 1987;9:531–538.
16. Narayan SM. T-wave alternans and the susceptibility to ventricular arrhythmia. *J Am Coll Cardiol* 2006;47:269–281.
17. Armoundas AA, Tomaselli GF, Esperer HD. Pathophysiological basis and clinical application of T-wave alternans. *J Am Coll Cardiol* 2002;40:207–217.
18. Smith JM, Clancy EA, Valeri CR, et al. Electrical alternans and electrical instability. *Circulation* 1988;77:110–121.
19. Rosenbaum DS, Jackson LE, Smith JM, et al. Electrical alternans and vulnerability to ventricular arrhythmias. *N Engl J Med* 1994;330:235–241.
20. Rosenbaum DS, Albrecht O, Cohen RJ. Predicting sudden cardiac death from T wave alternans: promise and pitfalls. *J Cardiovasc Electrophysiol* 1996;7:1095–1111.
21. Hohnloser SH, Klinenheben T, Zabel M, et al. T wave alternans during exercise and atrial pacing in humans. *J Cardiovasc Electrophysiol* 1997;8:987–993.
22. Estes MNA, Michaud G, Zipes DP, et al. Electrical alternans during rest and exercise as predictors of vulnerability to ventricular arrhythmias. *Am J Cardiol* 1997;80:1314–1318.
23. Hohnloser SH, Klingenheben T, Yi-Gang L, et al. T wave alternans as a predictor of recurrent ventricular tachyarrhythmias in ICD recipients: prospective comparison with conventional risk markers. *J Cardiovasc Electrophysiol* 1989;9:1258–1268.
24. Gehi AK, Stein RH, Metz LD, Gomes JA. Microvolt T-wave alternans for the risk stratification of ventricular tachyarrhythmic events. *J Am Coll Cardiol* 2005;46:75–82.
25. Chow T, Kereiakes DJ, Bartone C, et al. Prognostic utility of microvolt T wave alternans in risk stratification of patients with ischemic cardiomyopathy. *J Am Coll Cardiol* 2006;47:1820–1827.
26. Bloomfield DM, Bigger JT, Steinman RC, et al. Microvolt T-wave alternans and the risk of death or sustained ventricular arrhythmias in patients with left ventricular dysfunction. *J Am Coll Cardiol* 2006;47:456–463.
27. Task force of the European Society of Cardiology and the North American Society of Pacing and Electrophysiology: heart rate variability—standards of measurement, physiologic interpretation and clinical use. *Circulation* 1996;93:1043–1065.
28. Farrell TG, Bashir Y, Gipps T, et al. Risk stratification for arrhythmic events in postinfarction patients based on heart rate variability, ambulatory electrocardiographic variables and signal averaged electrocardiogram. *J Am Coll Cardiol* 1991;18:687.
29. Kleiger RE, Miller JJP, Bigger JT, Moss AJ, and the Multicenter Post-Infarction Research Group. Decreased heart rate variability and its association with increased mortality after acute myocardial infarction. *Am J Cardiol* 1987;59:256–262.
30. Bigger JT, Fleiss JL, Steinmann RC, et al. Frequency domain measures of heart period variability and mortality after myocardial infarction. *Circulation* 1992;85:164–171.
31. Katz A, Liberty IF, Porath A, et al. A simple bedside test of 1-minute heart rate variability during deep breathing as a prognostic index after myocardial infarction. *Am Heart J* 1999;138:32–38.

32. Zuanetti G, Nelson JM; Lantini R, et al, on behalf of GISSI-2 Investigators. Prognostic significance of heart rate variability in postmyocardial infarction patients in the fibrinolytic era: the GISSI-2 results. *Circulation* 1996;94:432–436.

33. Sandrone G, Mortara A, Torzillo D, et al. Effects of beta blockers (atenolol or metoprolol) on heart rate variability after acute myocardial infarction. *Am J Cardiol* 1994;74:340–345.

34. Schwartz PJ, Vanoli W, Stramba-Basiele M, et al. Autonomic mechanisms and sudden death: new insights from the analysis of baroreceptor reflexes in conscious dogs with and without a myocardial infarction. *Circulation* 1988;78:969–979.

35. Bristow JD, Honour AJ, Pickering JW, et al. Cardiovascular and respiratory changes during sleep in normal and hypertensive subjects. *Cardiovasc Res* 1969;3:476–485.

36. LaRovere MT, Bigger JT, Marcus FL, et al, for the ATRAMI (Autonomic Tone and Reflexes After Myocardial Infarction) Investigators. Baroreflex sensitivity and heart-rate variability in prediction of total cardiac mortality after myocardial infarction. *Lancet* 1998;351:478–484.

Atrial Fibrillation, Atrial Flutter, and Atrial Tachycardia

Eric N. Prystowsky / Albert L. Waldo

Atrial fibrillation, atrial flutter, and atrial tachycardia are common arrhythmias associated with a variety of cardiac conditions. Indeed, atrial fibrillation is the most common sustained cardiac arrhythmia encountered in clinical practice and is increasing in prevalence.[1,2] These arrhythmias may be associated with deterioration of hemodynamics, a wide spectrum of symptoms, and significant morbidity, mortality, and medical costs. Perhaps because no single therapy has been shown to be ideal for all patients, there are a variety of treatment strategies that may be applied to these arrhythmias. These include no therapy at all, rhythm control and rate control, and these treatment strategies have both pharmacologic and nonpharmacologic options available.[3] This chapter describes the epidemiology, electrophysiologic mechanisms, and approach to management of patients with atrial fibrillation, atrial flutter, and atrial tachycardia.

ATRIAL FIBRILLATION

Atrial fibrillation (AF) is characterized by disorganized atrial electrical activation and uncoordinated atrial contraction. The surface electrocardiogram characteristically demonstrates rapid fibrillatory waves with changing morphology and rate and a ventricular rhythm that is irregularly irregular (Fig. 37–1). Most AF originates in one or more of the pulmonary veins (PVs), and because of disparate atrial refractory periods the rapid firing focus in the left atrium (LA) cannot be conducted in a 1:1 manner to the right atrium, which leads to fibrillatory conduction. Additionally, it is thought that a driver, perhaps a reentrant focus in the LA, acts in a similar manner.[4] Although the ECG has the characteristic appearance of disorganized atrial activation, further analysis may reveal what appears to be a regular rapid atrial rhythm, often seen best in lead V1 (see Fig. 37–1). Careful measurement will disclose variability in the P-P intervals, and this should not be misinterpreted as atrial flutter, or so-called *atrial fibrillation-flutter*. Atrial flutter, as discussed later, is a very regular rhythm with monotonous repetition of similar P waves with each cycle.

The ventricular rate during AF can be quite variable, and depends on autonomic tone, the electrophysiologic properties of the atrioventricular (AV) node, and the effects of medications that act on the AV conduction system. The ventricular rate may be very rapid (>300 beats/min) in patients with the Wolff-Parkinson-

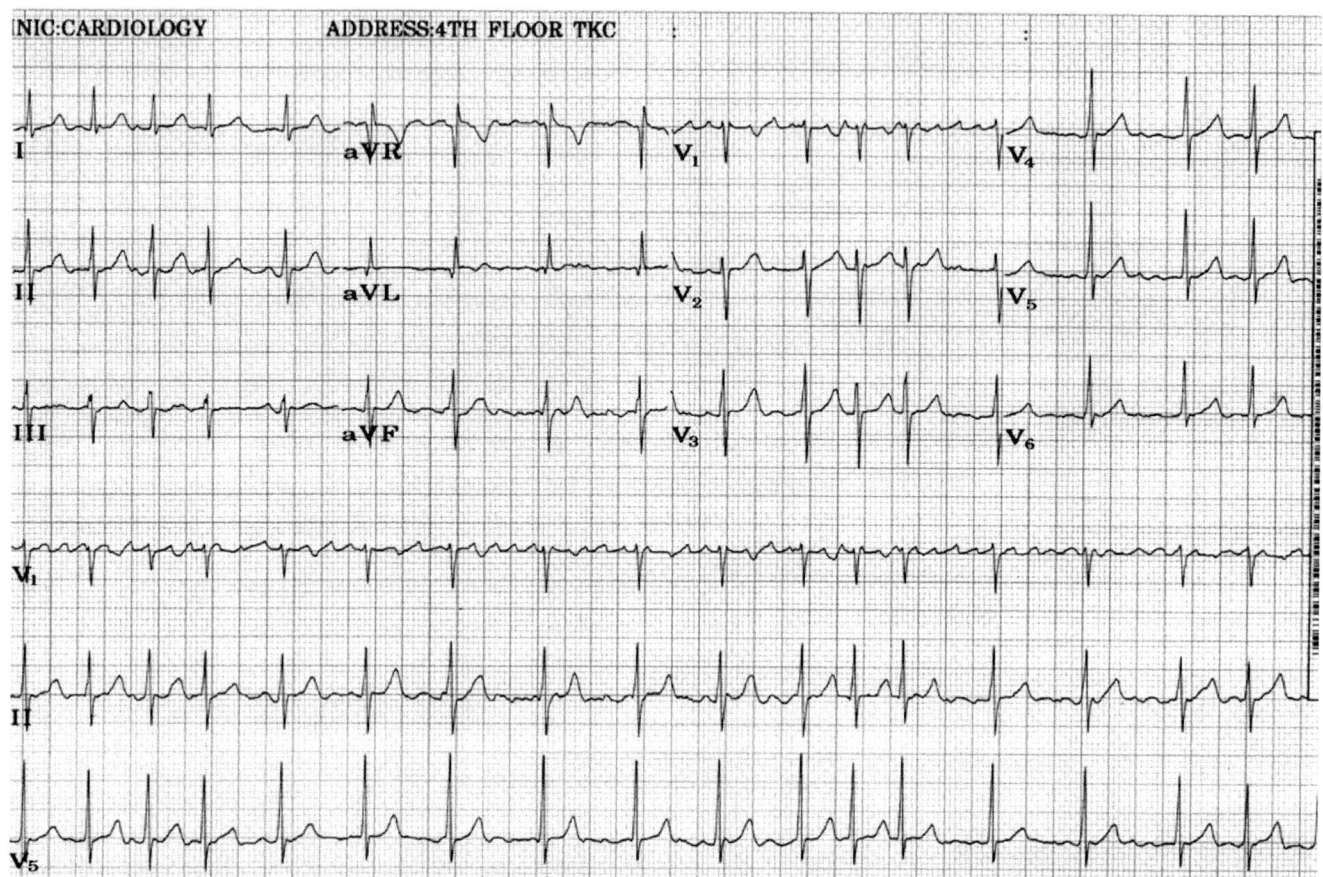

FIGURE 37–1. Twelve-lead electrocardiogram of atrial fibrillation. Note the rapid, irregular, changing, low-amplitude fibrillatory waves and an irregularly irregular ventricular response.

White (WPW) syndrome, with conduction over accessory pathways (wide preexcited QRS complexes) having short antegrade refractory periods (Fig. 37–2). A regular, slow ventricular rhythm during AF suggests a junctional rhythm, either as an escape mechanism with complete AV block or as an accelerated junctional pacemaker.

CLASSIFICATION

AF traditionally has been described as either paroxysmal or chronic. However, the definition of *chronic* varies greatly in the literature, often suggesting permanent AF. The American Heart Association (AHA), American College of Cardiology (ACC), and the European Society of Cardiology (ESC) have proposed a standardized classification scheme to describe AF, which we support.[3,5] At the initial detection of AF, it may be difficult to be certain of the subsequent pattern of duration and frequency of recurrences. Thus, a designation of *first detected* episode of AF is made on the initial diagnosis. When the patient has experienced two or more episodes, atrial AF is classified as *recurrent*. After the termination of an episode of AF, the rhythm can be classified as *paroxysmal* or *persistent*. Paroxysmal AF is characterized by self-terminating episodes that generally last <7 days (most <24 hours), whereas persistent AF generally lasts >7 days and often requires electrical or pharmacologic cardioversion. AF is classified as *permanent* when it has failed cardioversion or when further attempts to terminate the arrhythmia are deemed futile. It might be more appropriate to use

the term *established* rather than permanent, because these patients can undergo successful ablation to restore and maintain sinus rhythm precluding the concept of *permanent*. Although this classification scheme is generally useful, the pattern of AF may change in response to treatment. Thus, AF that has been persistent may become paroxysmal during pharmacologic therapy with antiarrhythmic medications.

EPIDEMIOLOGY

AF is the most common arrhythmia requiring treatment, with estimates of 2.2 to 5.0 million Americans and 4.5 million in the European Union experiencing paroxysmal or persistent AF.[1,3,6–10] This is likely an underestimate because many people with AF are asymptomatic. The overall prevalence in the general population is estimated to be 0.4 percent.[11] The incidence and prevalence of AF steadily increase with age, such that this arrhythmia occurs in <0.5 percent of the population <50 years of age and increases to approximately 2 percent at ages 60 to 69 years, 4.6 percent for ages 70 to 79 years, and 8.8 percent for ages 80 to 89 years.[7,12,13] The age-adjusted prevalence of AF is higher for men than women[7,8] and higher for whites than blacks.[9] Most cases of AF occur in patients with evidence of structural heart disease, but there may be no evidence of concomitant disease in >50 percent of patients with paroxysmal AF.[14–16] In contrast, >80 percent of patients with permanent AF have an identifiable underlying cause.[17]

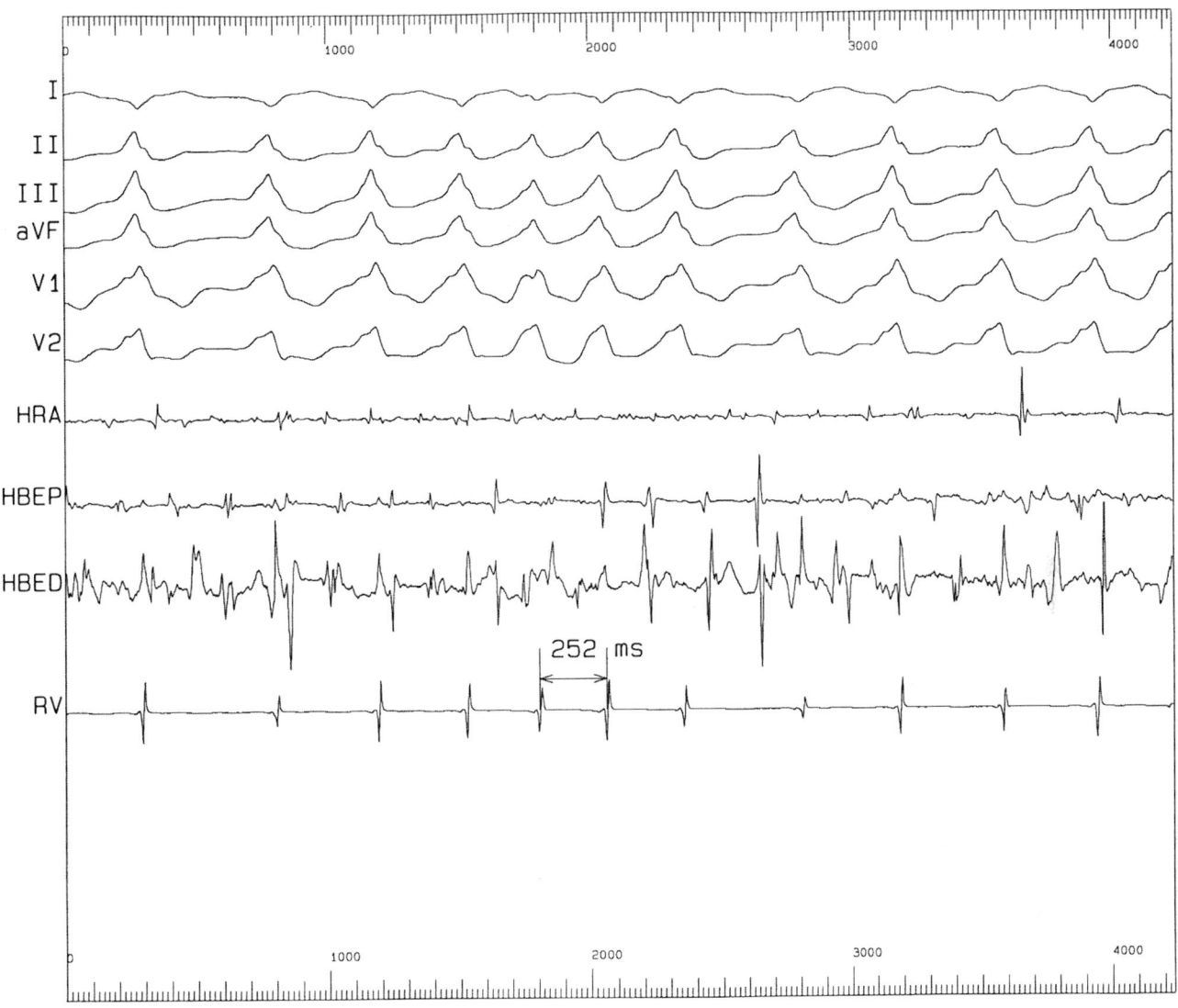

FIGURE 37–2. AF with rapid ventricular response over an accessory pathway. AF, atrial fibrillation; HBED, distal His bundle electrogram; HBEP, proximal His bundle electrogram; HRA, high right atrium; RV, right ventricle.

Familial AF can also occur.[3] In most circumstances the molecular abnormality is unknown. However, specific genetic defects have been identified in a few families.[18–21] In several Chinese families the defect has resulted in a gain in function and a short atrial refractoriness.[20,21]

AF confers an increased relative risk of overall mortality ranging from 1.4 times controls in the Manitoba Study[22] to 2.3 times controls in the Whitehall study[13] (average 1.7 times controls)[3] and is predominantly caused by stroke. The risk of stroke among patients with nonrheumatic AF is approximately 5 percent per year, with an average relative risk of stroke approximately 6 times that of age-matched controls.[12,13,16,23–26] In the absence of anticoagulation, the relative risk of stroke in patients with rheumatic AF is increased approximately 17-fold.[27] The Framingham Study demonstrated that the risk of stroke in AF is clearly related to age, with an annual risk of stroke of 1.5 percent in patients aged 50 to 59 years, which increased to 23.5 percent in patients aged 80 to 89 years.[12] The risk of stroke in nonvalvular AF has been estimated to be approximately 7 percent per year.[3,28–31] The development of AF is a strong predictor

of increased mortality in cardiac conditions such as hypertrophic or restrictive cardiomyopathy.[32–35]

PATHOPHYSIOLOGY

AF is associated with a wide variety of predisposing factors (Table 37–1). In the developed world, the most common clinical diagnoses associated with AF are hypertension and coronary artery disease.[9] The presence of congestive heart failure (CHF) markedly increases the risk of AF.[7–9] In developing countries hypertension, rheumatic valvular heart disease, and congenital heart disease are the most commonly related conditions.[36,37]

Two concepts of the underlying mechanism of AF have received considerable attention: factors that *trigger* the onset and factors that *perpetuate* this arrhythmia. Triggering foci of rapidly firing cells within the sleeve of atrial myocytes extending into the pulmonary veins have been clearly shown to be the underlying mechanism of most paroxysmal AF (Fig. 37–3).[38–40] In animal models these pulmonary vein foci manifest delayed afterpotentials and triggered activity in response to catecholamine stimulation, rapid

TABLE 37-1

Anatomic and Electrophysiologic Substrates Promoting the Initiation and/or Maintenance of Atrial Fibrillation

DISEASES	ANATOMIC	CELLULAR	ELECTROPHYSIOLOGIC
Part A. Substrate develops during sinus rhythm (remodeling related to stretch and dilatation). The main pathways involve the RAAS, TGF-β, and CTGF.			
Hypertension	Atrial dilatation	Myolysis	Conduction abnormalities
Heart failure	PV dilatation	Apoptosis, necrosis	ERP dispersion
Coronary disease	Fibrosis	Channel expression change	Ectopic activity
Valvular disease			
Part B. Substrate develops because of tachycardia (tachycardia-related remodeling, downregulation of calcium channel, and calcium handling).			
Focal AF	None or [b]	None or [b]	Ectopic activity
Atrial flutter	Atrial dilatation	Calcium channel downregulation	Microentry
	PV dilatation		Short ERP[c]
	Large PV sleeves	Myolysis	ERP dispersion[d]
	Reduced contractility[e]	Connexin downregulation	Slowed conduction
	Fibrosis	Adrenergic supersensitivity	
		Changed sympathetic innervation	

CTGF, connective tissue growth factor; ERP, effective refractory period; PV, pulmonary vein; RAAS, renin-angiotensin-aldosterone system; TGF-β, transforming growth factor β.

[a]Substrate develops either while in sinus rhythm, usually caused by ventricular remodeling, atrial pressure overload and subsequent atrial dilatation (Part A), or because of the rapid atrial rate during atrial fibrillation (AF), according to the principle that "AF begets AF" (Part B).
[b]The listed changes may only occur with prolonged episodes of AF at high atrial rate.
[c]Short ERP and slow conduction may produce short wavelength, thereby promoting further AF.
[d]ERP dispersion together with spontaneous or stretch-induced ectopic activity may initiate AF. Long ERPs occur in Bachmann bundle among other tissues.
[e]The reduction of atrial contractility during AF may enhance atrial dilatation, leading to persistent AF.
SOURCE: From Fuster V, Rydén LE, Cannon DS, et al.[3]

atrial pacing, or acute stretch.[37,41] The pulmonary veins of patients with paroxysmal AF demonstrate abnormal properties of conduction such that there is a markedly reduced effective refractory period within the pulmonary veins, progressive conduction delay within the pulmonary vein in response to rapid pacing or programmed stimulation, and often conduction block between the pulmonary vein and the LA (see Fig. 37-3).[42] Rapidly firing foci can often be recorded within the pulmonary veins with conduction block to the LA.[39,40] Discontinuous properties of conduction within the pulmonary vein may also provide a substrate for reentry within the pulmonary vein itself[43] (Fig. 37-4). Although most triggering foci that are mapped during electrophysiologic studies occur in the pulmonary veins in patients with paroxysmal AF, foci within the superior vena cava,[44] the ligament of Marshall,[45] and the musculature of the coronary sinus[46] have been identified (Fig. 37-5). Other sites of initiating foci may be recorded in the left atrial wall or along the crista terminalis in the right atrium.[47]

For patients with pulmonary vein foci, a primary increase in adrenergic tone followed by a marked vagal predominance has been reported just prior to the onset of paroxysmal AF.[48] A similar pattern of autonomic tone has been reported in an unselected group of patients with paroxysmal AF and a variety of cardiac conditions.[49] Vagal stimulation shortens the refractory period of atrial myocardium but with a nonuniform distribution of effect. These factors support the importance of vagal stimulation in the induction of paroxysmal AF.

A variety of electrophysiologic and structural factors promote the perpetuation of AF. Moe and colleagues[50,51] proposed the mul-

tiple wavelet hypothesis as the mechanism of AF. Fractionation of wavefronts traversing the atria into daughter wavelets has been proposed as the mechanism by which this nonrepeating arrhythmia perpetuate. The number of wavelets on the heart at any moment depends on the refractory period, conduction velocity, and anatomic obstacles in different portions of the atria. Li and colleagues demonstrated in a canine model of heart failure that interstitial fibrosis predisposed to intraatrial reentry and AF.[52] Fibrosis of the atria may produce inhomogeneity of conduction within the atria, leading to conduction block and intraatrial reentry.[53] A variety of clinical studies have demonstrated that patients with AF have delayed interatrial conduction and inhomogeneous dispersion of atrial refractory periods.[54] Long-standing AF results in loss of myofibrils, accumulation of glycogen granules, disruption in cell-to-cell coupling at gap junctions,[55] and organelle aggregates.[56,57] ADAMs (a disintegrin and metalloproteinase), a family of membrane-bound glycoproteins that regulate cell–cell and cell–matrix interactions, have been reported to double in concentration during AF in human biopsies of atrial myocardium. This increased disintegrin and metalloproteinase activity may be one mechanism contributing to atrial dilatation in AF. Thus, AF itself seems to produce a variety of alterations of atrial architecture that further contribute to atrial remodeling, mechanical dysfunction, and perpetuation of fibrillation.

In a population-based study of elderly patients without AF at baseline, Tsang and coworkers[23] demonstrated that AF developed in direct relations to the echocardiographic left atrial volume in-

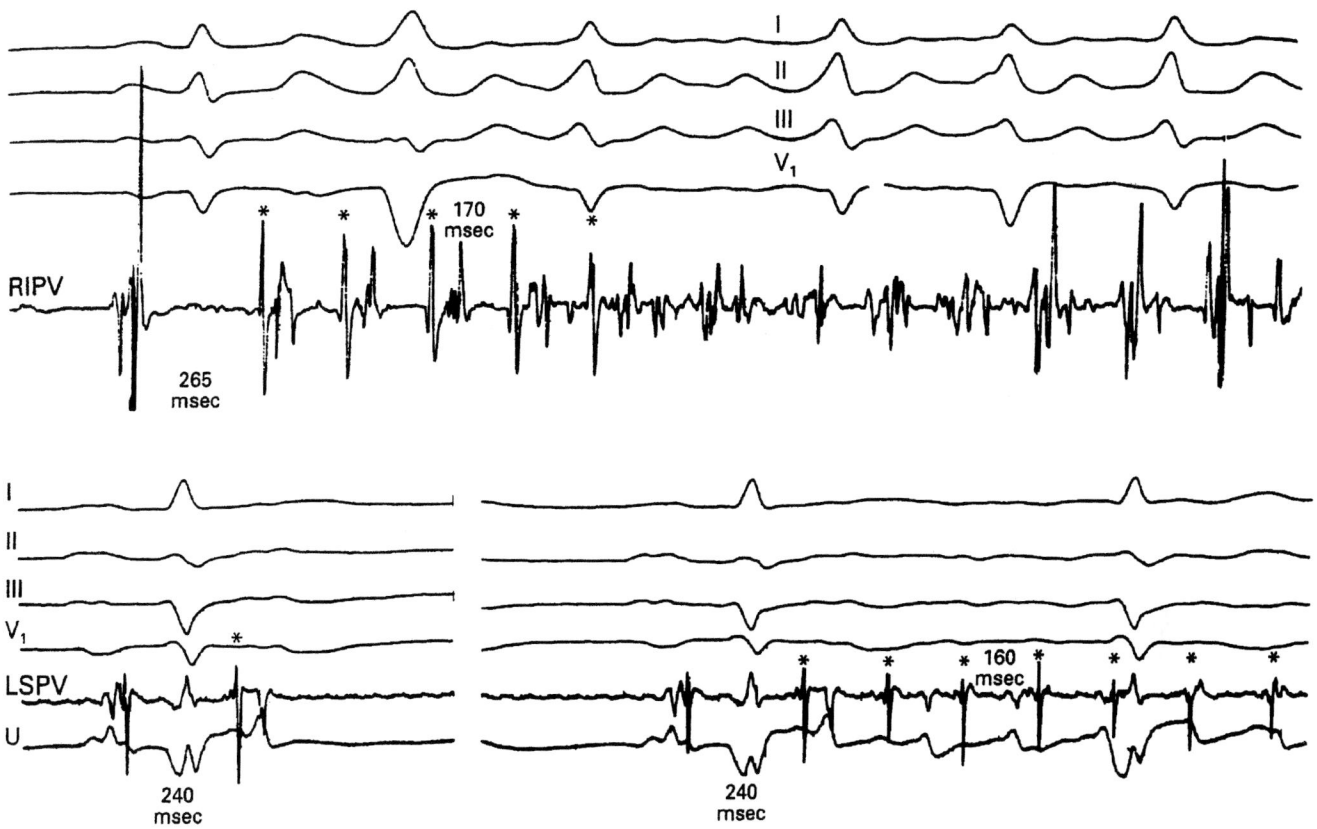

FIGURE 37–3. Top: Rapid firing in a pulmonary vein with the spontaneous onset of atrial fibrillation. **Bottom left:** Premature beats in a pulmonary vein (*asterisk*) with conduction block to the left atrium. **Bottom right:** Rapid firing at the same coupling interval conducts to the atrium with induction of atrial fibrillation. *Source: From Haisaguerre M, Jais P, Shah DC. Spontaneous initiation of atrial fibrillation by ectopic beats originating in the pulmonary veins. N Engl J Med 1998;339:659–666.*

dex. An even stronger predictor of the development of nonvalvular AF was a restrictive transmitral Doppler flow pattern. Thus, clinical evidence for diastolic dysfunction strongly supports the concept that myocardial stretch is an important mechanism of AF in the elderly. Altered stretch on atrial myocytes results in opening of stretch-activated channels.[37] Force transmitted to stretch-activated channels in the membrane or via cytoskeletal integrins produces opening of these channels as well as increasing local production of angiotensin II, which in turn increases L-type Ca^{2+} current and decreases the transient outward K^+ current. The antiarrhythmic effects of the angiotensin II receptor antagonist irbesartan have been demonstrated in patients undergoing electrical cardioversion.[58] Stretch-activated channels increase G protein–coupled pathways leading to increased protein kinase A and C activity and increased L-type Ca^{2+} current through the cell membrane and release of Ca^{2+} from the sarcoplasmic reticulum (promoting after depolarizations and triggered activity).[37]

AF also produces electrical remodeling that promotes further AF. The electrophysiologic changes typical of atrial myocytes during AF are a decrease in effective refractory period, decrease in action potential duration, reduction in the amplitude of the action potential plateau, and a loss of response of action potential duration to changes in rate (abnormal restitution).[59] Although the normal atrial action potential duration shortens in response to pacing at shorter cycle lengths, AF results in loss of this rate dependence of the action potential.[60–65] These changes can be attenuated by the sarcoplasmic reticulum's release of the calcium antagonist ry-

anodine, suggesting the importance of increased intracellular calcium to the maladaptation of atrial myocardium during AF. The reduction in the atrial effective refractory periods produced by AF are not uniform throughout the atria.[60] Most studies have demonstrated a reduction in atrial conduction velocity in response to prolonged rapid atrial rates.[61–63] The presence of underlying CHF may further interact with these electrophysiologic changes to promote AF. For example, Shinagawa and colleagues[60] reported that prolonged AF could be induced in 0 of 14 control dogs, 2 of 14 dogs with CHF, 4 of 12 dogs subjected to rapid atrial pacing at 400 beats/min for 1 week, and 8 of 13 dogs with both CHF and rapid atrial pacing. Similar data have been reported by Stambler and coworkers[64] in a canine, rapid ventricular pacing, heart failure model; however, importantly, in this model, the atrial effective refractory period increases, and the response of the action potential (restitution) is preserved.[64]

❲ ❳ HEMODYNAMIC EFFECTS

AF produces several adverse hemodynamic effects, including loss of atrial contraction, a rapid ventricular rate, and an irregular ventricular rhythm. The loss of mechanical AV synchrony may have a dramatic impact on ventricular filling and cardiac output when there is reduced ventricular compliance, as with left ventricular (LV) hypertrophy from hypertension, restrictive cardiomyopathy, hypertrophic cardiomyopathy, or the increased ventricular stiffness associated with aging. In addition, patients with mitral stenosis,

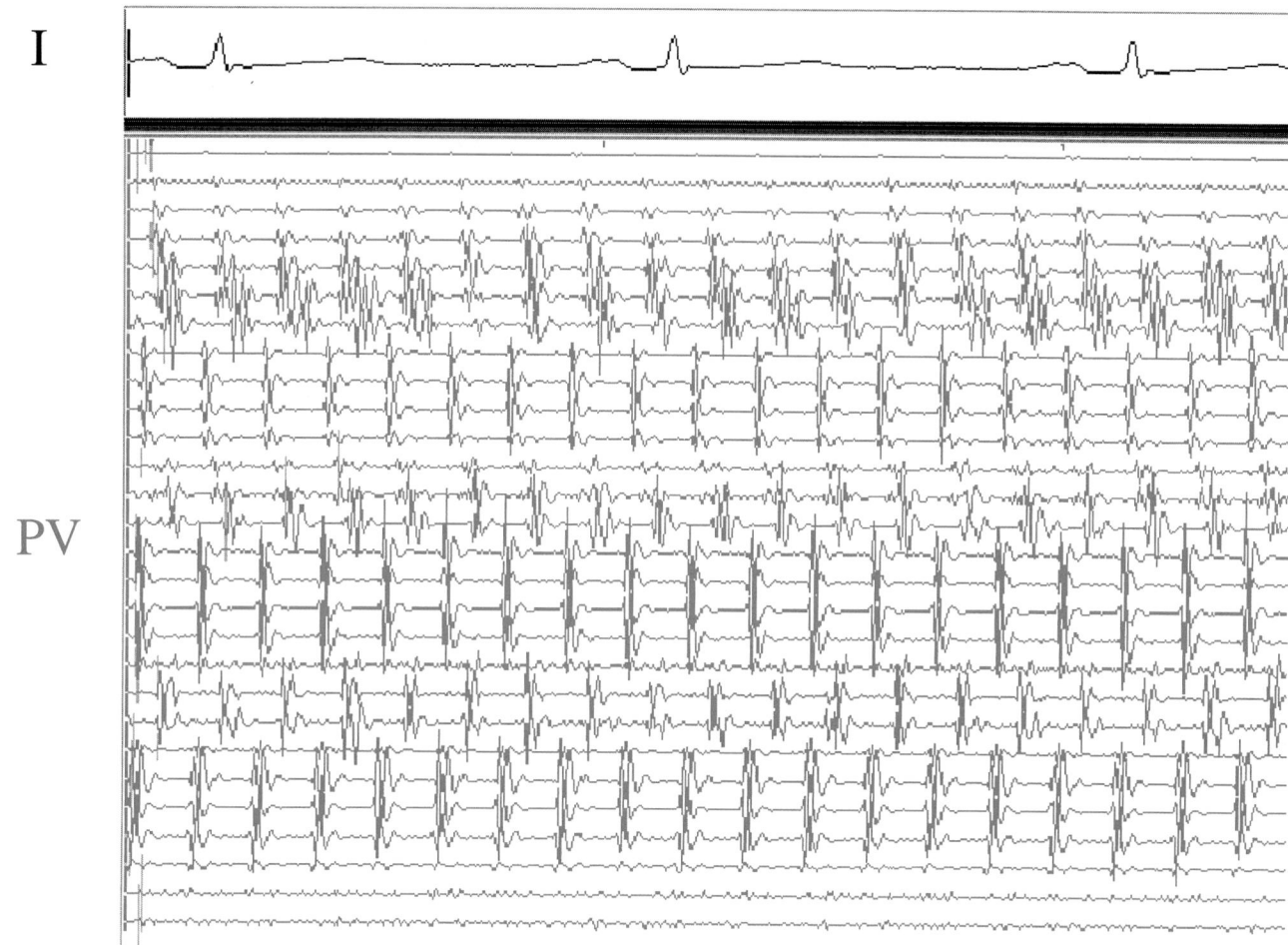

I

PV

FIGURE 37–4. Simultaneous recordings of surface electrocardiographic lead I and bipolar electrograms from the right superior pulmonary vein (PV) of a patient after catheter ablation at the ostium of the vein produced conduction block from the vein into the left atrium. Note the rapid, irregular electrical activity recorded with a 64-electrode basket catheter within the pulmonary vein, with sinus rhythm in the remainder of the atria as recorded on the surface electrocardiogram.

constrictive pericarditis, or right ventricular infarction typically experience marked hemodynamic deterioration at the onset of AF. The loss of AV synchrony results in a decrease in LV end-diastolic pressure (LVEDP) as the loading effect of atrial contraction is lost, thereby reducing stroke volume and LV contractility by the Frank-Starling mechanism. Although there is a reduction in the LVEDP, there is an increase in the left atrial mean diastolic pressure. Patients with significant restrictive physiology may experience pulmonary edema and/or hypotension with the onset of AF. In contrast, patients with dilated cardiomyopathy and high LV filling pressures may experience minimal hemodynamic compromise with AF if their LV compliance is not significantly impaired. The inappropriately rapid ventricular rate during AF also limits the duration of diastole and reduces ventricular filling. In occasional patients, the first clinical manifestation of AF may be CHF related to a tachycardia-induced cardiomyopathy.[65,66] This clinical syndrome is generally limited to patients who experience minimal or no palpitations during AF with a sustained ventricular rate >120 beats/min for sustained time periods. Because the patients do not experience symptoms, they do not seek medical care and thus often come to medical attention with signs and symptoms of heart failure. In these patients control of the ventricular rate by cardioversion, AV nodal–blocking medications, or catheter ablation typi-

cally reverses the impaired LV function within weeks. The irregular ventricular rhythm has adverse hemodynamic effects that are independent of the ventricular rate. Irregularity significantly reduces cardiac output[67] and coronary blood flow[68] compared with a regular ventricular rhythm at the same average heart rate. The effect of ventricular irregularity on coronary blood flow may explain in part why some patients with AF experience precordial pain in the presence of normal coronary arteriography.

Patients with heart failure often do worse when in AF, and it is difficult to know whether this is caused by loss of atrial contraction, too fast a ventricular rate, irregularity of rhythm, or a combination of factors. Recent ablation data demonstrate that successful maintenance of sinus rhythm in patients with previous persistent AF with good rate control can substantially improve LV function.[69,70]

Thromboembolism

Stroke is the most feared consequence of AF, and its prevention is a major focus of the management of patients with this condition. Most thrombi associated with AF arise within the left atrial appendage.[71] Flow velocity within the left atrial appendage is reduced during AF because of the loss of organized mechanical contrac-

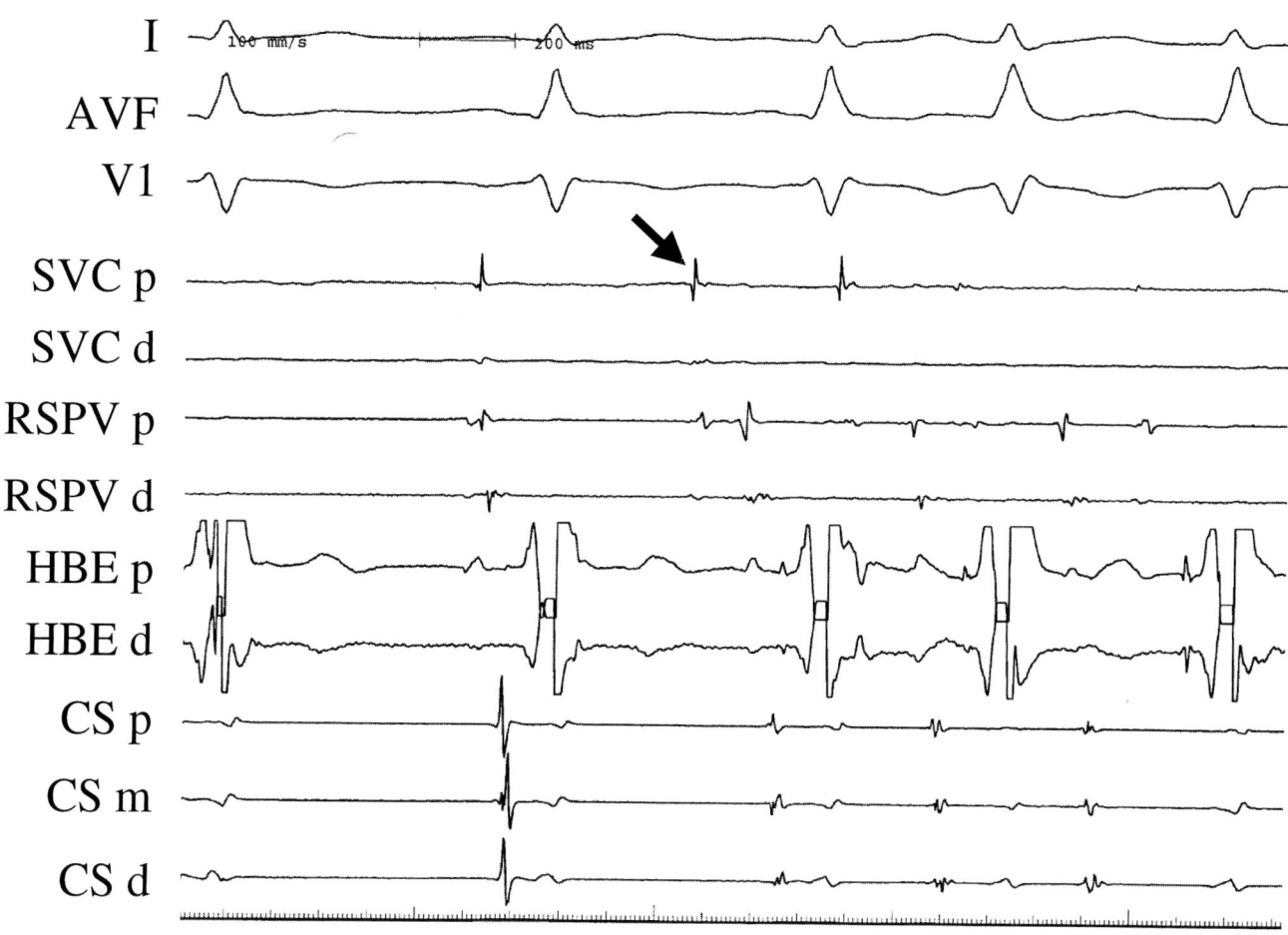

FIGURE 37–5. A rapidly firing focus in the superior vena cava (SVC) that induces atrial fibrillation. Surface leads I, aVF, and V₁ are recorded simultaneously with intracardiac bipolar electrograms from the SVC proximal (SVC p) and distal (SVC d) pairs, right superior pulmonary vein (RSPV p and RSPV d), His bundle (HBE p and HBE d), and coronary sinus (CS p, CS m, CS d). The *arrow* indicates early activation in the superior vena cava.

tion.[72] Compared with transthoracic echocardiogram, the transesophageal echocardiogram offers a much more sensitive and specific means of assessing left atrial thrombi and spontaneous echo contrast, an indicator of reduced flow.[73] Several factors contribute to the enhanced thrombogenicity of AF. Nitric oxide (NO) production in the left atrial endocardium is reduced in experimental AF, with an increase in levels of the prothrombotic protein plasminogen activator inhibitor 1 (PAI-1).[74] The lowest levels of NO and the highest levels of PAI-1 were recorded in the left atrial appendage during AF. Patients with AF have elevated levels of β-thromboglobulin and platelet factor 4[75,76]; elevated plasma levels of von Willebrand factor (vWF), soluble thrombomodulin, and fibrinogen have been reported in patients with permanent AF with no evidence of diurnal variation in thrombogenicity.[77,78] In the Stroke Prevention in Atrial Fibrillation (SPAF) III study,[79] increased plasma levels of vWF were strongly correlated with the clinical predictors of stroke in AF (age, prior cerebral ischemia, CHF, diabetes, and body mass index). There was a stepwise increase in vWF with increasing clinical risk of stroke in this population.

[ ] CLINICAL MANIFESTATIONS

Episodes of AF may be relatively short and self-terminating or persistent for weeks or months. Even in the same patient there is

substantial variability, making it difficult at times to label the patient as one with *paroxysmal* or *persistent* AF. However, most patients have a dominant pattern over time and are classified in that manner.

The clinical manifestations of AF range from no symptoms at all to profound hemodynamic deterioration with cardiogenic shock or even cardiac arrest in some patients with WPW syndrome. Cardiac arrest in WPW syndrome occurs when the very rapid ventricular response (e.g., 300 beats/min) over the accessory pathway degenerates into ventricular fibrillation (see Fig. 37–2).[80] Many patients experience minimal symptoms or may present with a vague sense of fatigue or effort intolerance. For others, the major symptom is palpitations, dyspnea, or dizziness; and many patients have multiple symptoms. Many patients with symptomatic AF also have asymptomatic episodes.[81,82] Several studies have reported a marked reduction in quality of life in patients with AF.[83–85] The Atrial Fibrillation Follow-up Investigation of Rhythm Management (AFFIRM) study[85] demonstrated that patients referred for randomization between rate-control and rhythm-control strategies have a reduced quality of life as compared with healthy controls. The ACC/AHA/ESC task force on practice guidelines has recommended that an evaluation for patients with AF should include at least certain elements[3] (Table 37–2). This evaluation

TABLE 37–2

Clinical Evaluation of Atrial Fibrillation

Minimum Evaluation	Additional Testing

1. To define history and physical examination
   Presence and nature of symptoms associated with AF
   Clinical type of AF (first episode, paroxysmal, persistent, or permanent)
   Onset of the first symptomatic attack or date of discover of AF
   Frequency, duration, precipitating factors, and modes of termination of AF
   Response to any pharmacologic agents that have been administered
   Presence of any underlying heart disease or other reversible conditions (e.g., hyperthyroidism or alcohol consumption)
2. To identify electrocardiogram
   Rhythm (verify AF)
   LV hypertrophy
   P-wave duration and morphology or fibrillatory waves
   Preexcitation
   Bundle-branch block
   Prior MI
   Other atrial arrhythmias
   To measure and follow the R-R, QRS, and QT intervals in conjunction with antiarrhythmic drug therapy
3. To identify transthoracic echocardiogram
   Valvular heart disease
   LA and RA size
   LV size and function
   Peak RV pressure (pulmonary hypertension)
   LV hypertrophy
   LA thrombus (low sensitivity)
   Pericardial disease
4. Blood tests of thyroid, renal, and hepatic function
   For a first episode of AF, when the ventricular rate is difficult to control
	One or several tests may be necessary
	1. Six-minute walk test
	   If the adequacy of rate control is in question
	2. Exercise testing
	   If the adequacy of rate control is in question (permanent AF)
	   To reproduce exercise-induced AF
	   To exclude ischemia before treatment of selected patients with a type 1C antiarrhythmic drug
	3. Holter monitoring or event recording
	   If diagnosis of the type of arrhythmia is in question
	   As a means of evaluating rate control
	4. Transesophageal echocardiography
	   To identify LA thrombus (in the LA appendage)
	   To guide cardioversion
	5. Electrophysiological study
	   To clarify the mechanism of wide-WRS-complex tachycardia
	   To identify a predisposing arrhythmia such as atrial flutter or paroxysmal supraventricular tachycardia
	   To seek sites for curative ablation or AV conduction block/modification
	6. To evaluate chest radiograph
	   Lung parenchyma, when clinical findings suggest an abnormality
	   Pulmonary vasculature, when clinical findings suggest an abnormality

AF, atrial fibrillation; AV, atrioventricular; LA, left atrial; LV, left ventricular; MI, myocardial infarction; RA, right atrial; RV, right ventricular. Type 1C refers to the Vaughn Williams classification of antiarrhythmic drugs.

includes a history and physical examination, electrocardiogram, chest radiograph, echocardiogram, and thyroid function studies.

[ ] TREATMENT

Anticoagulation

Stroke Risk and Stratification Schemes for Patients with Atrial Fibrillation The recognized risk factors for stroke are prior stroke or transient ischemic attack (TIA), hypertension, diabetes, heart failure, and age older than 75 years (Table 37–3).[3] Other stroke risk factors are mechanical prosthetic valve, mitral stenosis, coronary artery disease, thyrotoxicosis and female gender, LV dysfunction, and age older than 65 years.[3] Not all stroke risk factors have the same degree of association with

stroke in patients with AF, which is factored in when considering indications for oral anticoagulation therapy.

The CHADS$_2$ stroke risk stratification scheme, which is based on analysis of 1773 patients in the National Registry for Atrial Fibrillation, has gained considerable favor and is used in the ACC/AHA/ESC 2006 management guidelines to tailor therapy for stroke prevention.[3] The *C* in CHADS stands for recent CHF, *H* for hypertension, *A* for age older than 75 years, *D* for diabetes, and *S* for prior stroke or transient ischemic attack. Each category gets one point except stroke, which gets 2 because it is the most serious risk factor. The adjusted stroke rate per 100 patient years increases from 1.9 with a score of 1 to 18.2 with a score of 6 (see Table 37–3). Table 37–4 gives the new recommendations on antithrombotic therapy to prevent thromboembolism in patients with AF.[3] There is widespread consensus that all patients with rheumatic valvular heart dis-

TABLE 37–3

Stroke Risk in Patients with Nonvascular Atrial Fibrillation Not Treated with Anticoagulation According to the CHADS$_2$ Index

CHADS$_2$ RISK CRITERIA	SCORE
Prior stroke or TIA	2
Age >75 y	1
Hypertension	1
Diabetes mellitus	1
Heart failure	1

PATIENTS (N = 1733)	ADJUSTED STROKE RATE (%/Y)[a] (95% CI)	CHADS$_2$ SCORE
120	1.9 (1.2 to 3.0)	0
463	2.8 (2.0 to 3.8)	1
523	4.0 (3.1 to 5.1)	2
337	5.9 (4.6 to 7.3)	3
220	8.5 (6.3 to 11.1)	4
65	12.5 (8.2 to 17.5)	5
5	18.2 (10.5 to 27.4)	6

CHADS$_2$, Cardiac Failure, Hypertension, Age, Diabetes, and Stroke (Doubled); CI, confidence interval; TIA, transient ischemic attack.
[a]The adjusted stroke rate was derived from multivariate analysis assuming no aspirin usage.
Source: Data are from van Walraven WC, Hart RG, Wells GA, et al. A clinical prediction rule to identify patients with atrial fibrillation and a low risk for stroke while taking aspirin. Arch Intern Med 2003;163:936–943, and Gage BF, Waterman AD, Shannon W, et al. Validation of clinical classification schemes for predicting stroke: results from the National Registry of Atrial Fibrillation. JAMA 2001;285:2864–2870.

TABLE 37–4

Antithrombotic Therapy for Patients with Atrial Fibrillation

RISK CATEGORY	RECOMMENDED THERAPY
No risk factors	Aspirin, 81–325 mg daily
One moderate-risk factor	Aspirin, 81–325 mg daily, or warfarin (INR 2.0–3.0, target 2.5)
Any high-risk factor or >1 moderate-risk factor	Warfarin (INR 2.0–3.0, target 2.5)[a]

LESS VALIDATED OR WEAKER RISK FACTORS	MODERATE-RISK FACTORS	HIGH-RISK FACTORS
Female gender Age 65–74 y	Age ≥75 y Hypertension	Previous stroke, TIA, or embolism
Coronary artery disease	Heart failure LV ejection fraction 35% or less	Mitral stenosis Prosthetic heart valvae
Thyrotoxicosis	Diabetes mellitus	

INR, international normalized ratio; LV, left ventricular; TIA, transient ischemic attack.
[a]If mechanical valve, target international normalized ration (INR) greater than 2.5.

Meta-analysis of studies comparing aspirin with placebo suggest a relative risk reduction of approximately 22 percent with aspirin (Fig. 37–8). However, this is largely driven by the SPAF I data.[87] Comparisons of warfarin versus aspirin show superior-

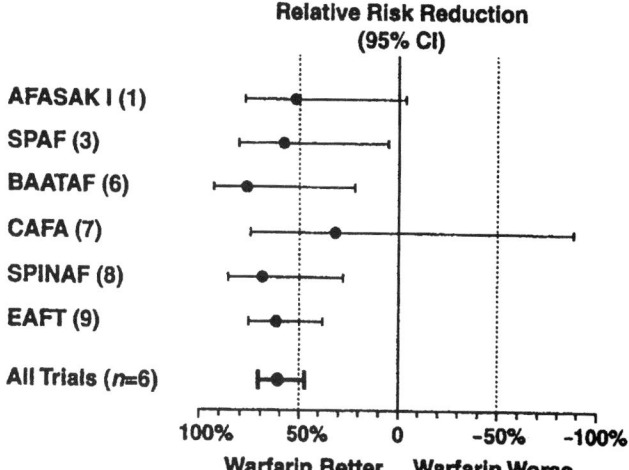

FIGURE 37-6. Effects of warfarin versus placebo on risk of stroke in six randomized, placebo-controlled clinical trials in nonvalvular atrial fibrillation. AFASAK I (1), The Copenhagen Atrial Fibrillation, Aspirin, and Anticoagulant Therapy Study; BAATAF (6), Boston Area Anticoagulation Trial for Atrial Fibrillation; CAFA (7), Canadian Atrial Fibrillation Anticoagulation; CI, confidence interval; EAFT (9), European Atrial Fibrillation Trial; SPAF (3), Stroke Prevention in Atrial Fibrillation; SPINAF (8), Stroke Prevention in Atrial Fibrillation. *Source: Adapted from Hart RG, Halperin JL.[26] With permission.*

ease and AF require anticoagulation with warfarin unless there is an absolute contraindication.

Warfarin is remarkably effective at reducing stroke risk in patients with AF. This was clearly demonstrated by a meta-analysis by the AF Investigators of five randomized, controlled clinical trials comparing warfarin versus placebo in patients with AF:

1. Copenhagen Atrial Fibrillation Aspirin and Anticoagulation (AFASAK) trial
2. SPAF trial
3. Boston Area Anticoagulation Trial for Atrial Fibrillation (BAATAF)
4. Canadian Atrial Fibrillation trial
5. Stroke Prevention in Nonrheumatic Atrial Fibrillation (SPINAF) trial (Fig. 37–6)

Using an intention-to-treat analysis that compared warfarin therapy with placebo, there was a 68 percent risk reduction in stroke for patients taking warfarin compared with patients taking placebo ($p < 0.001$).[25] Moreover, a subsequent on-treatment analysis demonstrated an 83 percent risk reduction in stroke when patients were taking warfarin compared with placebo.[86] Warfarin should be administered to achieve an international normalized ratio (INR) between 2 and 3, with a target INR of 2.5 to provide both efficacy and safety (Fig. 37–7).

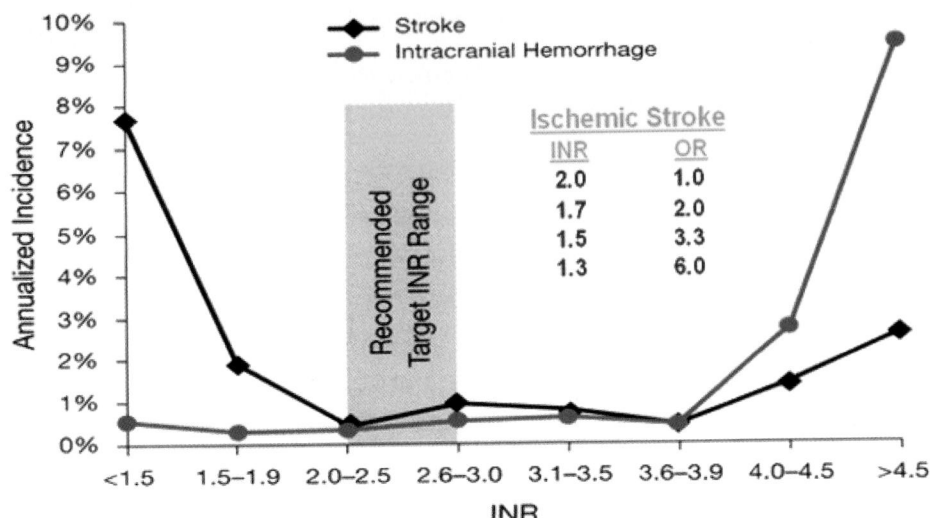

FIGURE 37-7. Annualized incidence of stroke or intracranial hemorrhage according to the international normalized ratio (INR). Note that when the INR decreases to <2.0, there is a steep rise in the odds ratio (OR) for stroke; but the incidence of intracranial hemorrhage remains low and flat (i.e., there is no associated decrease in intracranial hemorrhage). *Source: Modified after Hylek EM, Skates SJ, Sheehan MA, et al[90] and Hylek EM, Go AS, Chang Y, et al.[91]*

ity of warfarin (Fig. 37–9). In addition, the SPAF III trial[88] evaluated the benefit of an adjusted dose of warfarin (INR 2–3; target 2.5) versus low intensity, fixed-dose warfarin (INR 1.2–1.5) plus aspirin in patients with AF at high risk for stroke.[89] The trial was stopped early because the event rate in patients on the combination therapy was 7.9 percent per year versus an event rate on adjusted dose warfarin of 1.9 percent per year (*p* = 0.001).

Additional concerns using aspirin for stroke prevention in lieu of warfarin relate to severity of stroke.[90,91] Thus, these data found that warfarin with an INR ≥ 2 not only reduces the frequency of ischemic stroke, it also reduces the severity and risk of death from stroke compared to aspirin.

In summary, it is important that the risks of bleeding versus the benefits on stroke prevention always be weighed for each patient. However, the risk of stroke typically is greater than the risk of bleeding for most patients with AF at substantial risk for stroke. Thus, even though the ACC/AHA/ESC guidelines allow aspirin or warfarin therapy for patients who have one moderate-risk factor (see Table 37–4), we generally prefer warfarin for such patients. It is also important to remember that there is no difference in the indications for antithrombotic therapy between paroxysmal, persistent or permanent AF.

Cardioversion

Cardioversion can be accomplished using either antiarrhythmic drugs or the direct-current approach. In situations where urgent cardioversion is needed, such as marked hypotension, the direct-current approach is preferred. The need for anticoagulation prior to cardioversion must be considered. There is general consensus that AF that has been present for <48 hours can be

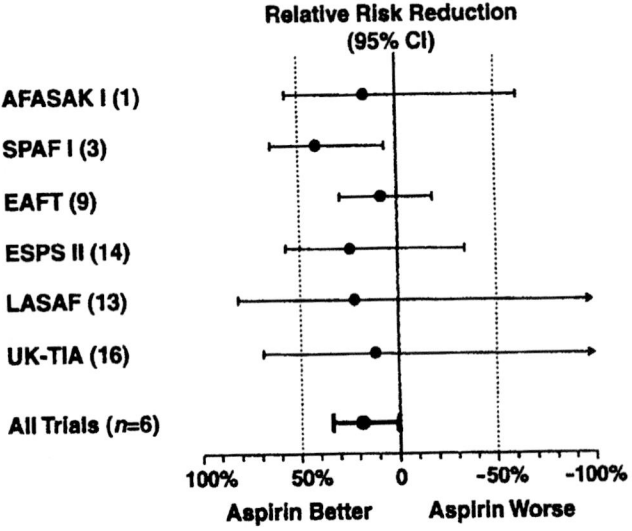

FIGURE 37-8. Effects of aspirin versus placebo on risk of stroke in five randomized, placebo-controlled trials in nonvalvular atrial fibrillation. AFASAK I (1), The Copenhagen Atrial Fibrillation, Aspirin, and Anticoagulant Therapy Study; CI, confidence interval; EAFT (9), European Atrial Fibrillation Trial; ESPS II (14), European Stroke Prevention Study; LASAF (13), Alternate-Day Dosing of Aspirin in Atrial Fibrillation Pilot Study Group; SPAF I (3), Stroke Prevention in Atrial Fibrillation; UK-TIA (16), United Kingdom Transient Ischaemic Attack Trial. *Source: Adapted from Hart RG, Halperin JL.[89] With permission.*

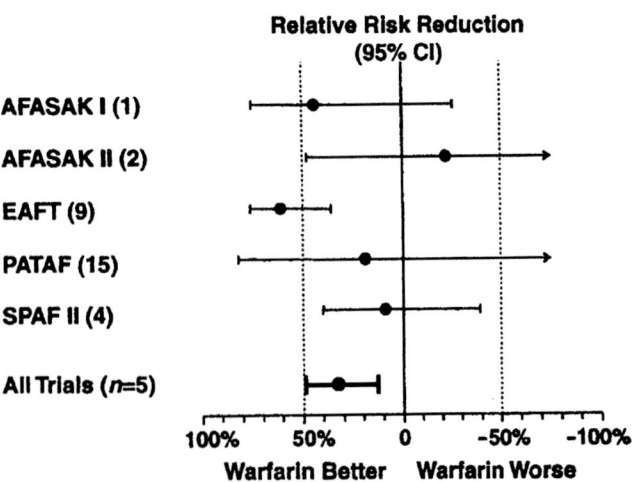

FIGURE 37-9. Effects of aspirin versus warfarin on risk of stroke in five randomized, controlled clinical trials in nonvalvular atrial fibrillation. AFASAK I (1) and AFASAK II (2), The Copenhagen Atrial Fibrillation, Aspirin, and Anticoagulant Therapy Study; EAFT (9), European Atrial Fibrillation Trial; PATAF (15), Primary Prevention of Arterial Thromboembolism in Nonrheumatic Atrial Fibrillation; SPAF II (3), Stroke Prevention in Atrial Fibrillation. *Source: Adapted from Hart RG, Halperin JL.[26] With permission.*

cardioverted without prior anticoagulation, but there are no randomized trial data to support this, and probable systemic emboli can occur in this situation.[92] Because often it is impossible to time accurately the onset of AF, anticoagulation therapy is recommended for AF of uncertain duration.

There are two basic strategies to deal with cardioversion: (1) oral warfarin with a therapeutic INR (2–3) for 3 to 4 weeks before cardioversion followed by continued warfarin thereafter or (2) transesophageal echocardiography (TEE) and heparin immediately before cardioversion followed by oral warfarin thereafter.[93] The Assessment of Cardioversion Using Transesophageal Echocardiography (ACUTE) study randomized 1222 patients with AF undergoing direct-current cardioversion between these strategies and found no difference in the rate of embolic events (0.5 percent TEE vs. 0.8 percent conventional) but a lower risk of bleeding complications (2.9 vs. 5.5 percent) and a shorter interval to cardioversion (3.0 vs. 31 days) in the TEE-guided group.[94] The important point is that left atrial mechanical function is significantly impaired for up to several weeks following cardioversion from AF to sinus rhythm. This *stunning* effect may occur after either electrical or pharmacologic cardioversion[95–97] and is more marked the longer the duration of AF. In patients without high-risk factors for stroke, anticoagulation can be discontinued approximately 4 weeks following cardioversion. If the patient has a standard indication for warfarin before cardioversion, anticoagulation should be continued indefinitely after cardioversion, with the exception of a clearly transient, reversible cause of AF.

Successful electrical cardioversion requires attention to details. Always be sure the patient is adequately anticoagulated. Rather than use handheld paddles, adhesive gel electrodes should be placed anteriorly over the sternum (with the upper edge at the sternal angle) and posteriorly (just to the left of the spine).[98] If cardioversion is not successful with this electrode position, try a different electrode placement such as right anterior-lateral configuration. The shock must be synchronized to the QRS complex, and it is important to select an ECG lead that has a prominent R-wave with no sensing of repolarization. Cardioversion shocks are painful and the patient requires adequate anesthesia. Biphasic waveforms clearly improve defibrillation efficacy at all energy settings as compared with monophasic shocks.[99,100] An initial shock energy of 200 J or more is recommended for both monophasic and biphasic wave forms.[3] However, in patients with smaller body habitus who have not had AF of long duration we typically start with approximately 120 J using biphasic waveform shocks. Another theoretical reason for using higher initial shock energies is to avoid initiating ventricular fibrillation if by accident the shock falls on the T-wave. A high-energy shock has a better chance of being above the lower limit of vulnerability to induce ventricular fibrillation. Consideration should be given to selected patients, for example, those with AF duration >3 months, to receive an antiarrhythmic drug prior to cardioversion to avoid immediate or early recurrence of AF.

The duration of AF is a major factor for cardioversion success using antiarrhythmic drugs, and AF lasting approximately 1 week has a substantial chance of cardioversion using oral flecainide, propafenone, dofetilide, and intravenous ibutilide.[3]

For longer duration AF, only dofetilide seems to have a reasonable chance of success, but amiodarone and ibutilide may be useful.[3] A single oral dose of propafenone (e.g., 600 mg) or flecainide (e.g., 300 mg) can be useful to convert recent-onset AF to sinus rhythm.[101–104] A recent study demonstrated the safety of the *pill-in-the-pocket* approach to outpatient conversion of AF in some patients.[105] Select patients were observed in hospital while being given a single oral loading dose of either propafenone or flecainide to convert AF. Those with success were allowed to self-administer the drug if they had a recurrence of AF, and few complications occurred during follow up. Because a type 1C drug may convert AF to atrial flutter, an AV nodal blocking agent should usually be administered concomitantly. Dofetilide is useful to convert AF of both short and long duration.[106,107] Intravenous ibutilide has also been demonstrated to provide effective cardioversion of recent-onset AF or flutter.[108–110] The risk of nonsustained or sustained torsade de pointes ventricular tachycardia was 3.6 percent. Thus, although effective, intravenous ibutilide requires monitoring for at least 4 hours after administration. Ibutilide is far more effective than intravenous procainamide (51 vs. 21 percent) for the acute termination of AF[110]; and intravenous amiodarone, because of its long interval from administration to electrophysiologic effect in the atria, has been demonstrated to be only marginally more effective than placebo.[111]

POSTOPERATIVE ATRIAL FIBRILLATION

AF may complicate the postoperative course of patients undergoing cardiac surgery, prolonging hospitalization and increasing costs. The mechanism may be related to pericarditis and high catecholamine concentrations in the myocardium. The most effective therapy to prevent AF is the routine use of β blockers throughout the perioperative period.[112] For patients without a preoperative history of AF, this arrhythmia is generally an acute, transient phenomenon that does not require long-term treatment.[113] Patients with postoperative AF are at risk for systemic emboli and anticoagulation should be considered.

RATE-CONTROL VERSUS RHYTHM-CONTROL STRATEGIES

Several prospective, randomized trials have been published comparing the strategies of rate control and rhythm control in patients with AF.[114–116] The AFFIRM trial enrolled 4060 patients aged older than 65 years or with risk factors for stroke, randomizing them to rate versus rhythm control.[114] Over a mean follow-up period of 3.5 years, there was no significant difference in overall mortality between the two groups (Fig. 37–10). The RACE trial[115] randomly assigned 522 patients with persistent AF after electrical cardioversion to either a rate-control or a rhythm-control treatment. There was no difference in the primary endpoint of the study (a composite of cardiovascular death, CHF, thromboemboli, bleeding, need for pacemaker, or serious drug side effects) between the two strategies. Thus, these studies indicate that both approaches have similar clinical outcomes provided that appropriate anticoagulation is maintained.

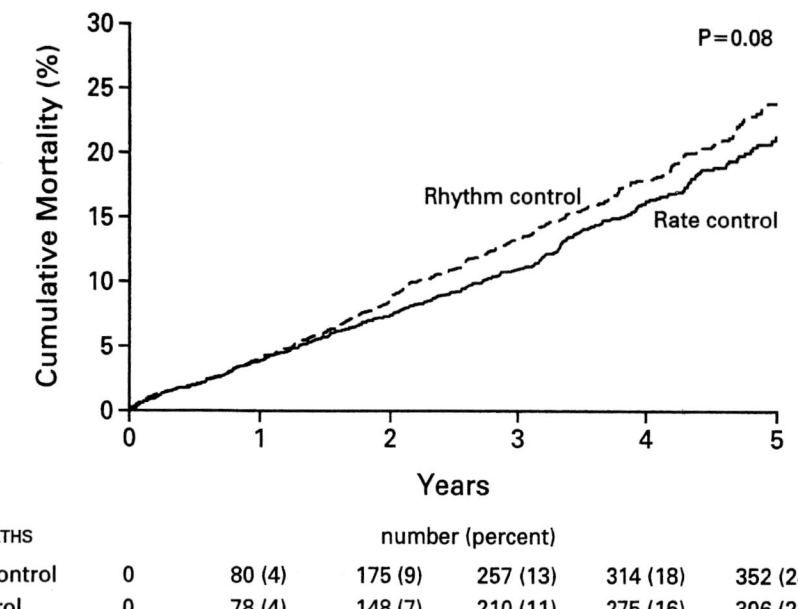

No. of Deaths			number (percent)			
Rhythm control	0	80 (4)	175 (9)	257 (13)	314 (18)	352 (24)
Rate control	0	78 (4)	148 (7)	210 (11)	275 (16)	306 (21)

FIGURE 37–10. Results of rate control versus rhythm control on overall survival in the AFFIRM trial. *Source: From Wyse DG, Waldo AL, DiMarco JP, et al. The Atrial Fibrillation Follow-Up Investigation of Rhythm Management (AFFIRM) investigators. A comparison of rate control and rhythm control in patients with atrial fibrillation. N Engl J Med 2002;347:1825–1833. With permission.*

In view of these randomized trials, how should an individual patient with AF be managed? First remember that patients enrolled in these and smaller such studies have been older and typically had one or more risk factors for stroke. The results concerning morbidity and mortality may not extend to other patient populations. In general the choice of strategy is determined by several factors such as paroxysmal versus persistent AF, severity and type of symptoms, associated cardiac and other medical diseases, age of patient, short- and long-term treatment goals, and choice of pharmacologic or nonpharmacologic therapy options. Our bias is to try and maintain sinus rhythm in younger patients with AF; but in the elderly, if symptoms can be controlled with a rate strategy, this would be our preference. Anticoagulation is needed in patients at high risk for stroke regardless of whether a rate or rhythm strategy is chosen.

[ ] CONTROL OF VENTRICULAR RATE

Control of the ventricular rate involves both acute and chronic phases. In the acute phase, intravenous diltiazem, metoprolol, esmolol, or verapamil have all been demonstrated to provide slowing of AV nodal conduction within 5 minutes; these drugs are indicated for patients with severe symptoms related to a rapid ventricular rate.[3] Intravenous digoxin requires a longer duration to achieve rate control and is less useful. For patients with only mild or moderate symptoms, oral medications that slow AV nodal conduction should be prescribed. After control of the resting ventricular rate has been achieved, attention is paid to the ambulatory heart rate. There is no overall agreement on what constitutes optimum rate control.[117] One set of criteria is 60 to 80 beats/min at rest and between 90 and 115 beats/min during moderate exercise.[3] It is also uncertain which

method is best to evaluate rate control, which has been done using a resting 12 ECG, 24-hour Holter monitor, exercise testing, and combinations of methods.[117] In essence, we want to achieve rate control for each patient during their usual daily activities, so we typically recommend titrating AV nodal blockers on an outpatient basis following the daily 24-hour heart rate plot as a guide.[117]

Digoxin may provide effective control of the resting heart rate but is often ineffective during exertion. β-Adrenergic blockers or calcium channel antagonists provide much better control of the ventricular rate during exercise and should be considered for most patients. Digoxin is most useful in the setting of impaired systolic function, and can be used in combination with β blockers or calcium antagonists if these agents do not provide adequate rate control. It may also be useful as a single agent in the elderly. Control of the ventricular rate can be especially challenging for patients with the tachycardia-bradycardia syndrome, who experience rapid ventricular rates during AF and sinus bradycardia or sinus pauses when AF terminates. Permanent pacemaker implantation is indicated for many of these patients.

[ ] ABLATION OF THE ATRIOVENTRICULAR NODE

Some patients may continue to experience significant symptoms from a rapid or irregular ventricular rhythm despite drug therapy. Chronically elevated ventricular rates (usually >120 beats/min) despite adequate trials of AV nodal blocking agents, can cause a tachycardia-induced cardiomyopathy.[65] Catheter ablation of the AV conduction system and permanent pacemaker implantation is a highly effective means of establishing permanent control of the ventricular rate during AF in selected patients.[118–120] Despite the many favorable effects of this procedure, there are several limitations. First, AV nodal ablation does not change the long-term need for anticoagulation. Second, although an adequate junctional escape rhythm is typically present after ablation, patients should be considered permanently pacemaker dependent. Third, because this procedure does not restore AV synchrony, patients who are highly dependent on mechanical atrial contraction often do not experience as much improvement as other patients. Fourth, right ventricular pacing produces an abnormal LV contraction sequence, and acute worsening of hemodynamics has been observed in some patients. In the Post AV Node Ablation Evaluation (PAVE) trial, patients who received biventricular versus RV apical pacing, especially those with abnormal LV ejection fractions before ablation, had longer 6-minute walking distances and higher LV ejection fractions after ablation.[121]

[ ] MAINTENANCE OF SINUS RHYTHM

When a rhythm control strategy is chosen for patients with paroxysmal or persistent AF, prophylactic treatment with antiarrhythmic drugs is usually needed to maintain sinus rhythm.[122] Although the ideal of pharmacologic therapy would be to prevent all recurrences of AF, this is unrealistic for many patients. Rather, marked reduction of the frequency, duration, and symptoms of AF may be a very acceptable clinical goal. In addition, the use of pharmacologic agents to prevent AF does not change the indication for anticoagulation.

As compared with drug therapy for life-threatening arrhythmias, the choice of pharmacologic agent is largely determined by the potential side effects of a given drug in an individual patient. The first drug chosen is usually associated with a low risk of serious side effects for that patient. For most patients a specific etiologic factor can not be identified for the initiation of AF. Conversely, if such an inciting factor is uncovered, therapeutic efforts should be targeted to eliminating it. Examples may be β blockers for exercise-induced AF, or avoidance of alcohol in selected individuals. Many agents have effectiveness to maintain sinus rhythm in patients with AF.[3,123–127] Because class IC drugs may suppress AF but promote atrial flutter, it is often prudent to combine them with a β blocker or calcium channel blocker to decrease the risk of atrial flutter with 1:1 ventricular response, a potentially life-threatening situation. Monitoring the QRS duration and PR interval helps during class IC therapy. If the QRS duration increases to 150 percent of the baseline value, reduce the dosage or discontinue the drug. Sotalol, dofetilide and amiodarone prolong ventricular refractoriness and the QT interval. Monitoring the QT interval during initiation of therapy is important. If possible avoid corrected QT intervals of >520 msec with sotalol and dofetilide, but longer QT intervals may occur without a risk of proarrhythmia in patients receiving amiodarone. Periodic ECGs should be obtained on an outpatient basis in patients receiving antiarrhythmic drugs, and efforts to avoid hypokalemia are important.

There are not much prospective data on the safety of initiating drugs in the outpatient setting, but some general rules are useful. Flecainide and sotalol can be initiated in patients without heart disease who are in sinus rhythm, and safety is maximized if AV nodal blockers are given first. Amiodarone can be used in patients with or without sinus rhythm, but frequent ECG monitoring, for example, by using event recorders is recommended to identify any potential bradycardia or tachycardia proarrhythmia. Sotalol may be administered to patients in sinus rhythm with minimal or no heart disease and normal QT interval and electrolyte status; the lowest dose should be used and an ECG should be obtained within days of starting sotalol to determine the QT interval. The same process should occur for any dose increase. Dofetilide must be started in hospital.

[ ] ANTIARRHYTHMIC DRUG SELECTION

Antiarrhythmic drugs are selected on a safety-first basis (Fig. 37–11). The ACC/AHA/ ESC guidelines[3] suggest for patients with no or minimal heart disease to start with flecainide, propafenone, or sotalol, agents with minimal noncardiac toxicity. The second-line therapy is either amiodarone/dofetilide or catheter ablation. Patients with hypertension who do not have substantial LV hypertrophy have a similar treatment algorithm; but those with substantial LV hypertrophy are considered at increased proarrhythmia risk with most drugs other than amiodarone, which becomes first-line therapy here. Catheter ablation is second-line treatment. Safety of drugs in coronary artery disease has been demonstrated for dofetilide/sotalol (first line) and amiodarone (second line), and catheter ablation is also second-line treatment. For patients with heart failure, first-line treatment can be either amiodarone or dofetilide,

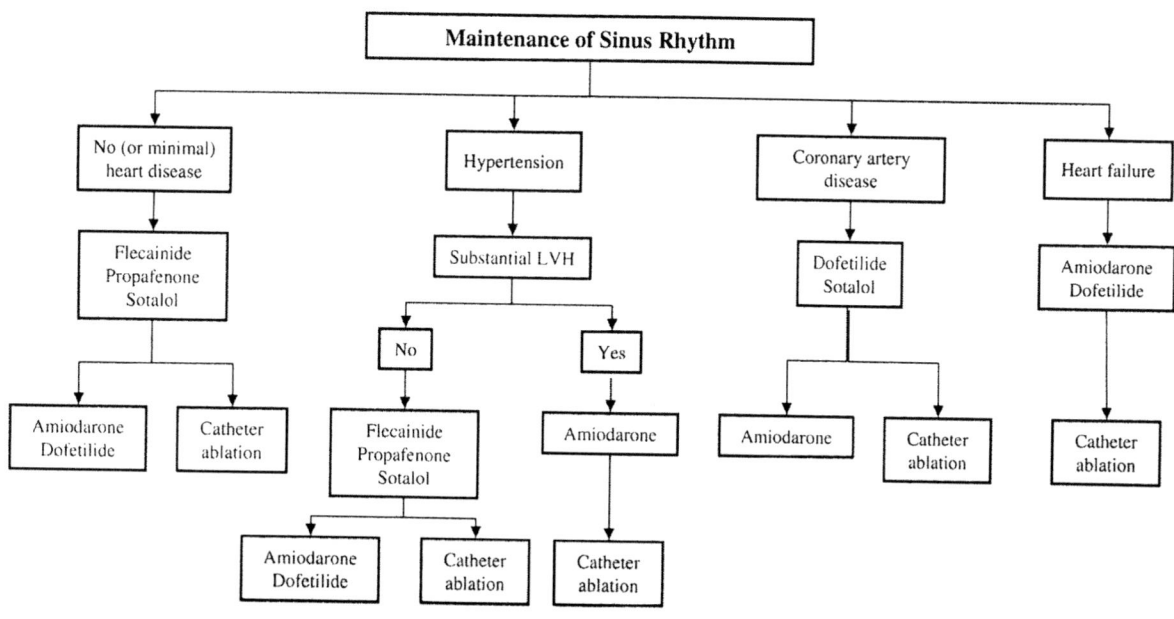

FIGURE 37–11. Proposed strategy for use of antiarrhythmic drugs to maintain sinus rhythm in patients with atrial fibrillation. LVH, left ventricular hypertrophy. *Source: Modified from Fuster V, Rydén LE, Cannom DS, et al.[3] With permission.*

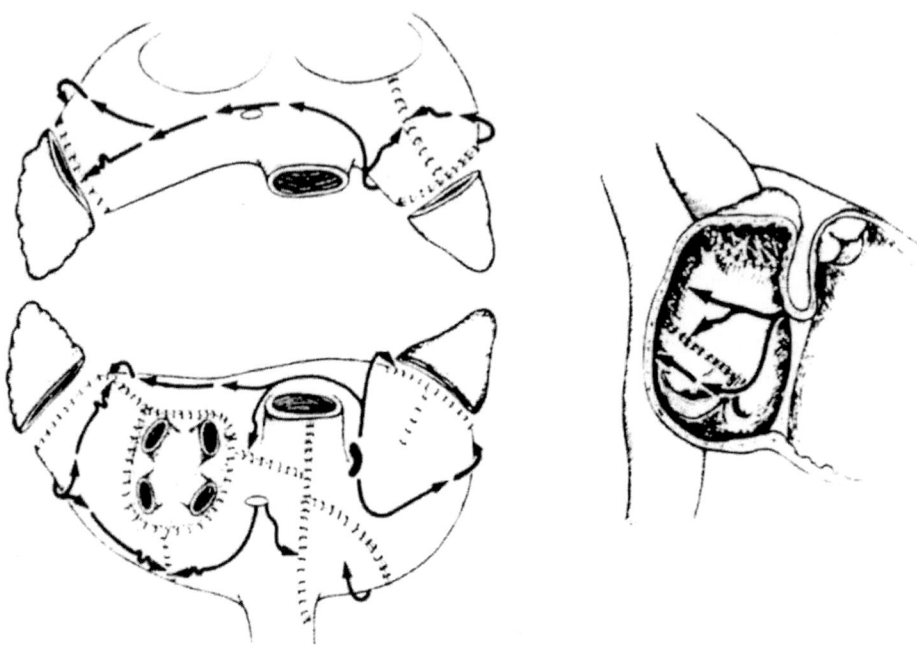

FIGURE 37–12. Diagram of surgical incisions and pathways for electrical propagation through the atria following the Cox-Maze III operation. *Source: From Cox JL, Boineau JP, Schuessler RB, et al. J Thorac Cardiovasc Surg 1995;110:473–484. With permission.*

but the authors prefer amiodarone in most circumstances, and ablation is second-line therapy. Recent data suggest that ablation to maintain sinus rhythm in patients with heart failure, even those with apparently good rate control, may confer beneficial effects on LV function.[69,70] The agents quinidine, procainamide, and disopyramide are currently considered as drugs of last resort.

Nontraditional Antiarrhythmic Agents

Several drugs used to treat other medical conditions have shown promise as adjuvant therapy in patients with AF. Drugs that modulate the rennin-angiotensin-aldosterone system, for example, angiotensin-converting enzyme inhibitors and angiotensin-receptor blockers, may decrease the incidence of AF.[58,128–133] These drugs can reduce atrial fibrosis and promote more favorable hemodynamics, but which of these actions is most important to reduce AF is not clear. Preliminary data also support the beneficial effect of statins to reduce AF.[134–136]

[ ] SURGICAL TREATMENT

Based on the pioneering research of Cox and coworkers, several surgical treatments (Fig. 37–12) for the prevention of AF have been developed.[137–141] Success rates have ranged from 70 to 95 percent.[139,140] For patients with AF who are undergoing cardiac surgery, consideration should be given to concomitant AF surgery. Otherwise, its role is typically for patients who require sinus rhythm for symptom relief and have failed to respond to antiarrhythmic drugs and catheter ablation.

[ ] CATHETER ABLATION

Recent approaches to catheter ablation of AF, especially paroxysmal AF, have been to eliminate triggering foci, primarily within

the pulmonary veins but also in the LA posterior wall, superior vena cava, crista terminalis, vein of Marshall, and coronary sinus.[3,39,40,44,47,69,142–151] Various techniques have been employed to isolate the pulmonary veins, including the use of intracardiac echocardiography[146] or an electroanatomical mapping system to guide delivery of radiofrequency energy circumferentially outside of the pulmonary veins.[148] Extensive areas of ablation targeting sites with complex fractionated electrograms has also been employed.[151] Success depends on operator experience,[150] but established laboratories generally report long-term success of approximately 70 to 85 percent in patients with paroxysmal AF, many of whom require more than one ablation to achieve success. Success rates for patients with persistent AF are lower.

In some patients, the site of initiation of atrial fibrillation is noted during the study (Fig. 37–13). Regardless, the goal is usually to isolate all of the pulmonary veins. Patients should have enough symptoms caused by AF to justify the risks of the procedure. The major risks of catheter ablation include pericardial tamponade, phrenic nerve injury, stroke, pulmonary vein stenosis, and atrioesophageal fistula.[152,153]

[ ] PACING

There is a higher risk of developing AF and stroke in patients receiving single-chamber, ventricular-based pacemakers (VVI or VVIR) compared with atrial-based pacing. However, it remains to be proven whether this is an adverse effect of VVI or VVIR pacing or an antiarrhythmic effect of atrial-based pacing. Although there has been much interest in atrial-based pacing from various site(s) and using a variety of pacing algorithms, pacing as primary therapy to prevent AF remains unproven.

ATRIAL FLUTTER

[ ] CLASSIFICATION AND MECHANISMS

There are several types of atrial flutter, all having rapid, regular atrial rates, generally 240 to 340 beats/min, because of a reentrant mechanism in the atria. Typical, also called *counterclockwise atrial flutter* is characterized by negative sawtooth flutter waves (Fig. 37–14), and reverse typical, also called *atypical* or *clockwise atrial flutter* by positive flutter waves in ECG leads II, III, and aVF (Fig. 37–15).[154] These two atrial flutter types share the same right atrial reentrant circuit. In typical atrial flutter, the reentrant wavefront travels up the interatrial septum and down the right atrial free wall, and vice versa in reverse atypical atrial flutter. Both types use the sub-Eustachian or cavotricuspid isthmus (i.e., the isthmus between the tricuspid annulus on one side and the inferior vena cava–

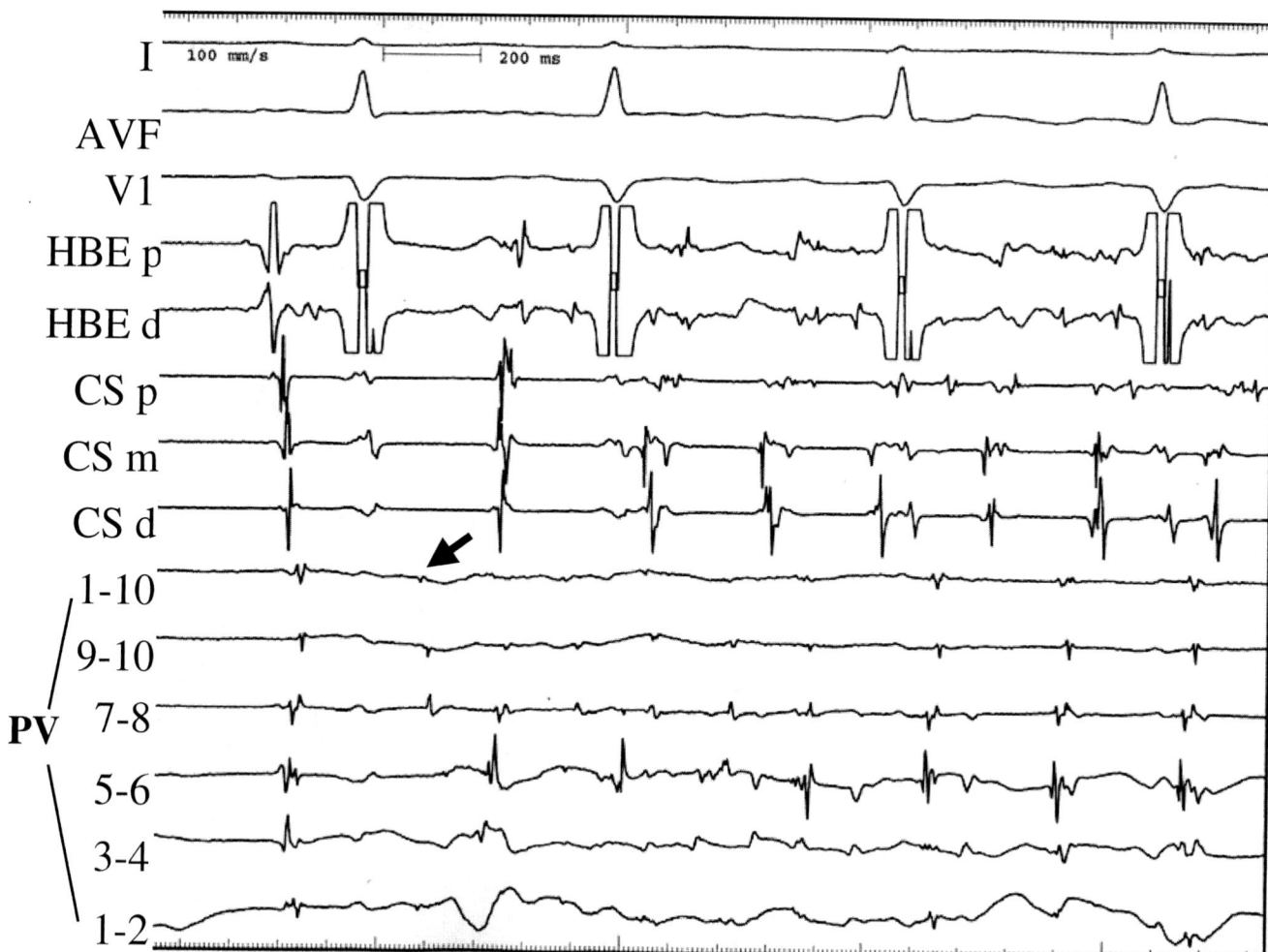

FIGURE 37–13. Spontaneous onset of AF by rapid firing from a pulmonary vein. The onset of AF (*arrow*) is produced by rapid firing from the pulmonary vein 1–10 electrode pair of a circular mapping catheter in the pulmonary vein (PV). Note that pulmonary vein activity occurs before the coronary sinus (CS) electrograms. AF, atrial fibrillation; HBE, His bundle electrogram; p, proximal; d, distal.

Eustachian ridge-coronary sinus on the other) as a part of the reentrant circuit.[155,156]

An important conceptual point is that the atrial flutter reentrant circuit usually is not simply present and waiting to be engaged. Almost always missing is the critical line of functional block between the venae cavae. In fact, it can be considered that the difference between the clinical development of AF and atrial flutter is whether or not this functional line of block between the venae cavae develops.[157] Moreover, this is an important part of the intricate relationship between AF and atrial flutter and may explain why, following successful ablation of the atrial flutter reentrant circuit, AF often becomes clinically manifest.

More recently, left atrial flutter, double wave reentry atrial flutter (two reentrant wave fronts simultaneously circulating in the same reentrant circuit),[158] lower loop and upper loop reentry atrial flutter (variants of typical atrial flutter),[159] and atrial flutter caused by reentry around a surgical incision (lesion reentry)[160] have also been described. Left atrial flutter may be caused by reentry around the mitral valve annulus, the pulmonary veins, or a region of block (usually anatomic) in the LA, such as secondary to the presence of a scar caused for any reason, including prior surgery or an ablation line.[161] Atrial flutter caused by a surgical lesion is common in patients after repair of congenital heart defects that involve one or more right atrial free wall incisions.[160] It has now been shown[162] that most (approximately two thirds) recurrent atrial flutter in patients following open heart surgical repair of congenital heart defects indeed uses the classical atrial flutter reentrant circuit.

【 】 EPIDEMIOLOGY

Atrial flutter often is a persistent rhythm, but more typically it is paroxysmal, lasting for variable periods. In most patients it is spontaneously induced by a premature atrial beat or beats that produce a transitional rhythm, resembling AF.[163–165] Atrial flutter commonly occurs in patients in the first week after open heart surgery.[166] Atrial flutter is also associated with chronic obstructive pulmonary disease, mitral or tricuspid valve disease, thyrotoxicosis, and postsurgical repair of certain congenital cardiac lesions (e.g., atrial septal defect, the Mustard procedure, the Senning procedure, or the Fontan procedure), as well as enlargement of the atria for any reason, especially the right atrium.[3,167] Atrial flutter occurs commonly in association with AF. Three out of every four patients with atrial flutter will, at some time, manifest clinical AF.[168] Furthermore, recent studies have indicated that atrial flutter per se may be associated with clot formation in the atria, with subsequent stroke or systemic embolism.[169–171]

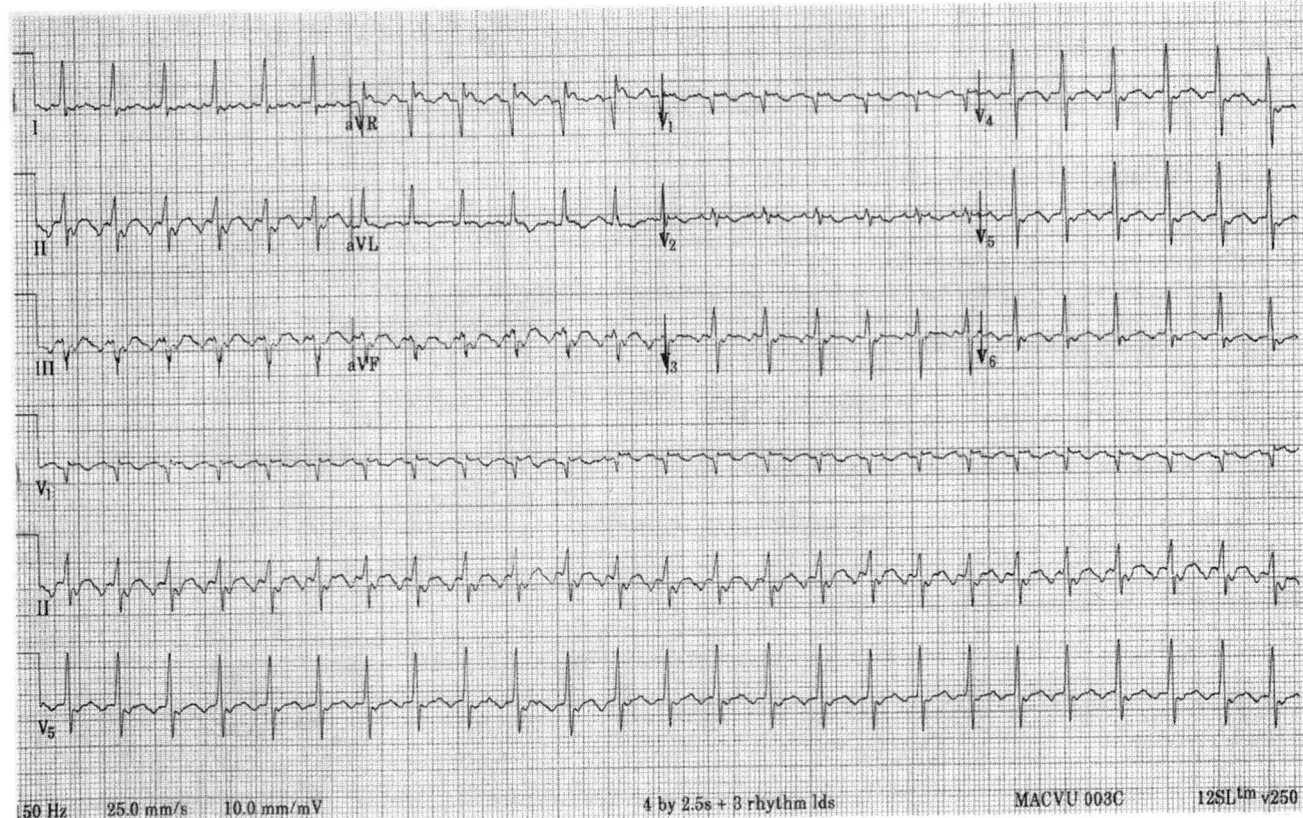

FIGURE 37–14. Twelve-lead electrocardiogram of typical atrial flutter. Note the negative flutter waves in leads II, III, and aVF and the upright flutter waves in lead V₁. This is characteristic of counterclockwise, isthmus-dependent atrial flutter.

【 】 DIAGNOSIS

Atrial flutter usually can be diagnosed from the ECG (see Fig. 37–14 and Fig. 37–15). The standard for the diagnosis of atrial flutter is the presence of atrial complexes of constant morphology, polarity, and cycle length. On occasion, the identification of atrial flutter complexes in the ECG may be difficult because of their temporal superimposition on other ECG deflections, such as the QRS complex or the T wave, or because of their very low amplitude. Use of vagal maneuvers or the intravenous administration of adenosine to prolong transiently AV conduction may result in AV nodal block and reveal atrial flutter complexes in the ECG if they are present.

【 】 MANAGEMENT

Acute Treatment of Atrial Flutter

Most often, atrial flutter should be treated acutely to restore sinus rhythm, or at the very least, to control the ventricular response rate as needed. Transthoracic direct current (DC) cardioversion of atrial flutter to sinus rhythm has a very high likelihood of success. Antiarrhythmic drug therapy to restore sinus rhythm is primarily intravenous ibutilide, which is associated with a 60 percent likelihood of converting recent atrial flutter to sinus rhythm.[108,172] Intravenous procainamide may also be useful in converting atrial flutter to normal sinus rhythm.[173]

Drug therapy may also be used to slow the ventricular response rate as needed. Useful agents include β blockers, vera-

pamil, diltiazem, and digitalis, alone or in combination. It is often difficult to achieve sufficient AV nodal block to slow adequately the ventricular response during atrial flutter, and 2:1 AV conduction frequently recurs. For this reason cardioversion to sinus rhythm is the best option, if possible. When using a class I antiarrhythmic drug, especially an Ic agent, to treat atrial flutter, care must be taken to provide adequate AV block. This is to avoid 1:1 AV conduction of a significantly slowed (e.g., to 170–200 beats/min) atrial flutter rate, which may also result in a very wide QRS complex tachycardia that can degenerate into ventricular tachycardia or fibrillation. Rapid atrial pacing can also be used to restore sinus rhythm.[166,174]

Long-Term Treatment of Atrial Flutter

Catheter Ablation Therapy Catheter ablation is highly successful, typically 90 percent or greater, to cure atrial flutter.[3] This coupled with the recognized difficulty in achieving adequate long-term suppression with antiarrhythmic drug therapy make catheter ablation a first-line treatment option for many patients.[175–177] Because classical atrial flutter is usually preceded by a variable period of AF, successful ablation of the atrial flutter reentrant circuit per se may not prevent either the new appearance or the recurrence of AF.

Antiarrhythmic Drug Therapy Selection of an antiarrhythmic drug to treat atrial flutter mirrors that to treat AF[3] (see Fig. 37–11). However, this form of therapy is no longer the treatment of choice for long-term therapy in most patients with atrial flutter, because catheter ablation to cure atrial flutter has superseded it.

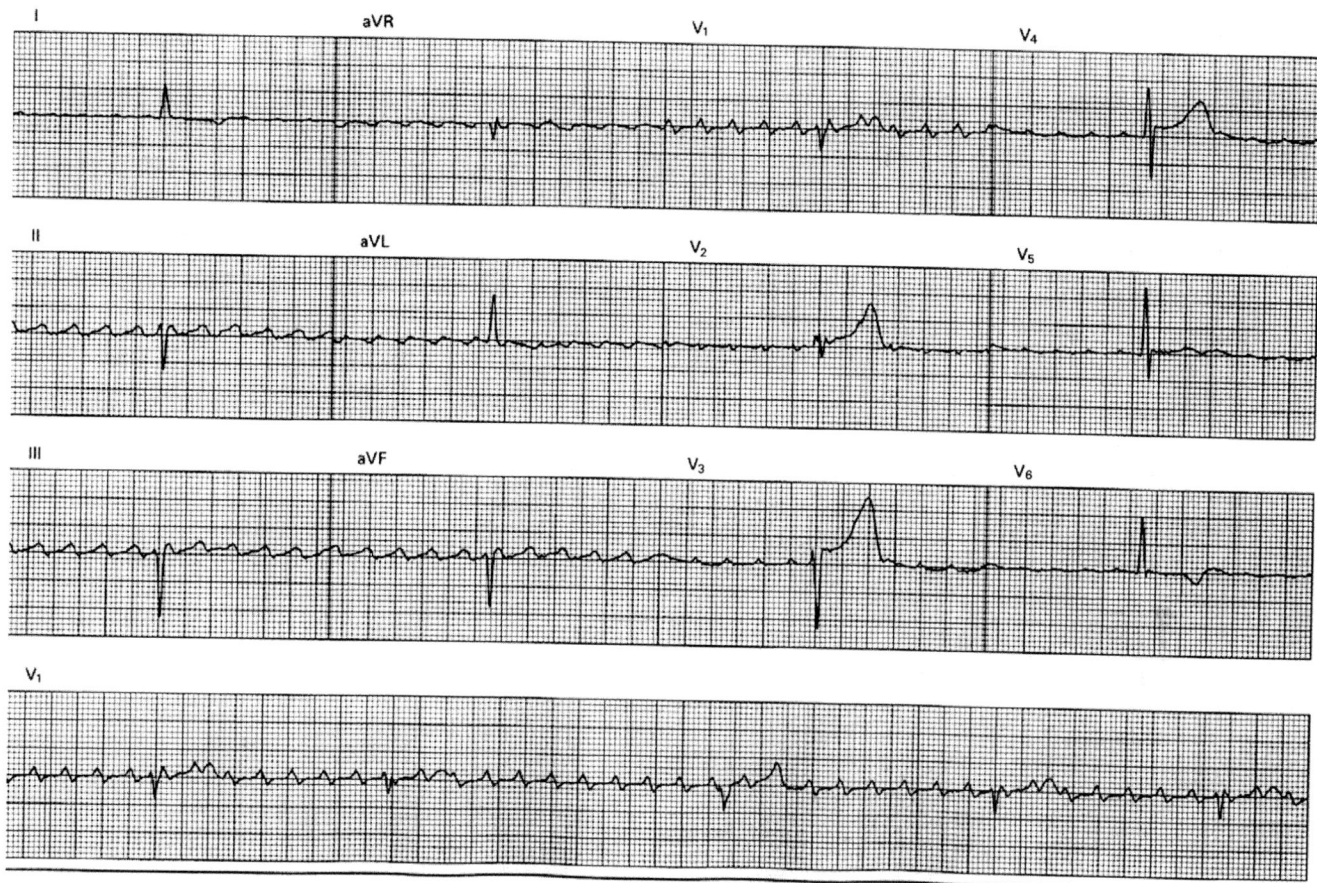

FIGURE 37–15. Twelve-lead electrocardiogram of a left atrial flutter that did not involve the usual cavotricuspid isthmus. Note the upright flutter waves in leads II, III, and aVF and the upright flutter waves in lead V₁.

Anticoagulant Therapy   In patients with atrial flutter, daily warfarin therapy to achieve an INR between 2 and 3 (target 2.5) is recommended using the same criteria as for AF.[3] In addition, several studies indicate that the incidence of stroke associated with atrial flutter approaches that of AF.[168–171]

Antitachycardia Pacemaker Therapy   Although available and effective,[178] little use has been made of implantation of an antitachycardia pacemaker to treat (interrupt) atrial flutter. Antitachycardia pacing can be used acutely in patients with atrial flutter who have an implanted pacemaker or defibrillator with the capability of temporary rapid atrial pacing therapies.

FOCAL ATRIAL TACHYCARDIA
【 】 CLASSIFICATION

The term atrial tachycardia refers to rapid (usually 130–250 beats/min), relatively regular rhythms that originate in the atria, do not require participation of either the sinus node or the AV node for maintenance, and are neither AF nor atrial flutter (Fig. 37–16).[154] Focal atrial tachycardia is characterized by atrial activation starting rhythmically at a small area (focus). Potential mechanisms include reentry, automaticity, and triggered activity. Foci are most frequently found in the pulmonary veins in the LA, and the crista terminalis in the right atrium[154,179] but can occur at various sites in both atria. When incessant, they may be associated with a dilated cardiomyopathy and CHF.[180,181]

【 】 MECHANISM

An automatic focus may demonstrate progressive rate increase at tachycardia onset (warm up) and/or progressive rate decrease before termination (cool down), does not respond to vagal maneuvers, and often displays an incessant nature. Focal atrial tachycardia caused by reentry generally can be induced by programmed electrical stimulation. During the arrhythmia the criteria for either manifest or concealed entrainment usually can be demonstrated, and the interval between the initiating beat and the first beat of the atrial tachycardia is usually inversely related.[154,180] Triggered activity is thought to be caused by delayed afterdepolarizations, and includes digitalis toxicity, but catecholamines can also precipitate focal atrial tachycardia due to this mechanism.[182–185]

【 】 EPIDEMIOLOGY

The incidence of focal atrial tachycardia increases with age, reportedly occurring in up to 13 percent of elderly subjects.[186,187] An increased incidence has been reported in patients with myocardial infarction,[188] nonischemic heart disease,[189] obstructive lung disease,[190] serum electrolyte disorders, and drug toxicity, especially caused by digitalis.[191] However, focal atrial tachycar-

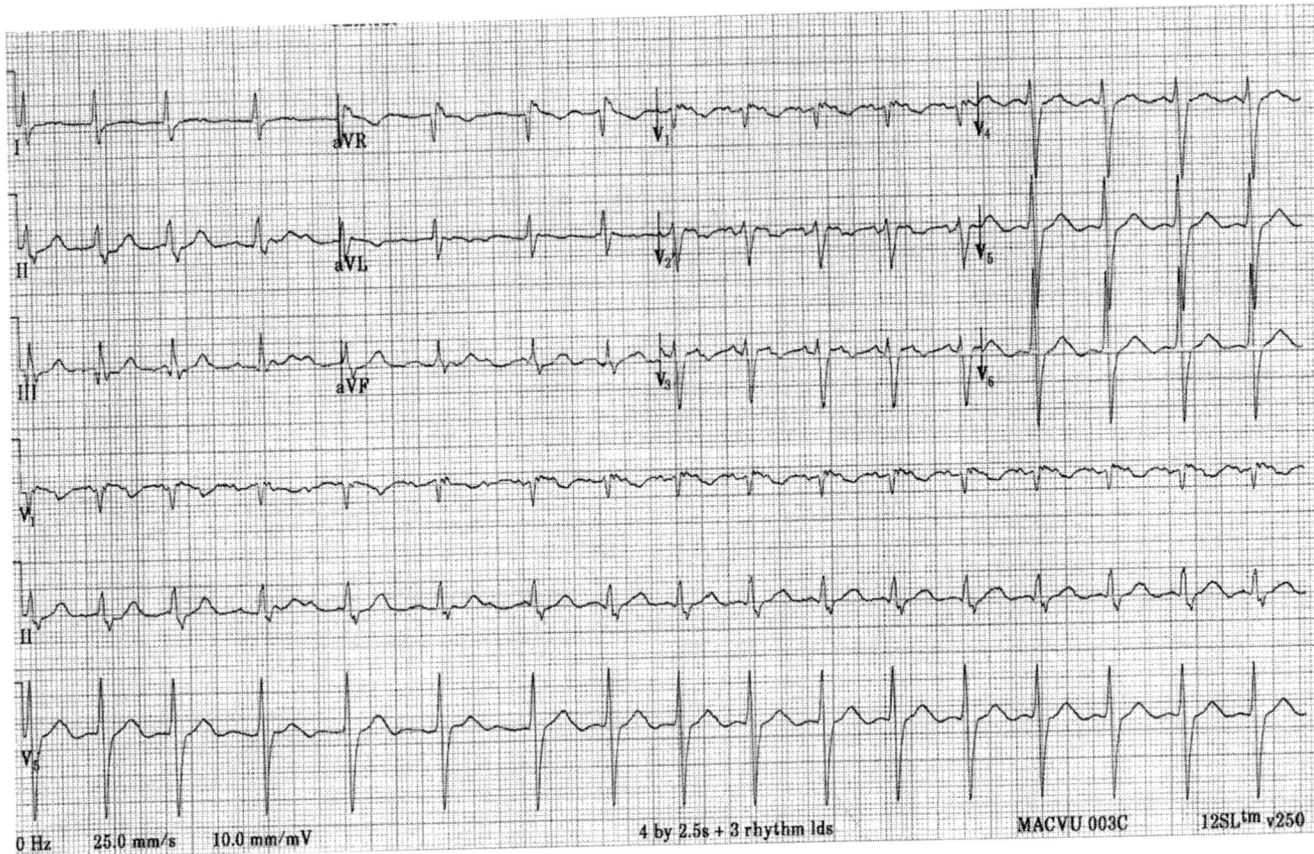

FIGURE 37–16. Surface electrocardiogram of an atrial tachycardia involving the right atrium. Note the discrete P waves with 2:1 AV conduction.

dia may occur in normal individuals,[192] and nonsustained episodes have been noted in 2 percent of healthy young adults.[179,193] Most episodes of focal atrial tachycardia are paroxysmal (deemed largely caused by reentry or triggered activity), but some episodes may be incessant (considered largely caused by automaticity).[194] Patients with atrial tachycardia secondary to an automatic mechanism are generally younger, with a mean age of 30 years.[180] In fact, automatic atrial tachycardias have been well described in children.[181]

[ ] DIAGNOSIS

A standard way to determine the presence or absence of an AV nodal independent atrial tachycardia is to demonstrate that despite the presence of conduction block at the AV node, the rhythm continues. Termination of a supraventricular tachycardia by a drug such as adenosine that causes transient AV node block generally supports the diagnosis of an underlying AV nodal dependent reentrant tachycardia, for example, AV node reentry. However, adenosine is known to terminate some atrial tachycardias,[180] so that termination of an atrial tachyarrhythmia after the administration of intravenous adenosine cannot be used per se to characterize the rhythm as AV nodal dependent. The same seems true for β blockers.[180] A useful sign of AV nodal dependence is consistent termination of tachycardia with a P wave without conduction to the ventricles. Unfortunately, termination with a conducted P-wave and no further arrhythmia can occur with AV nodal dependent and independent arrhythmias, and provides little diagnostic utility.

[ ] TREATMENT

For focal atrial tachycardia, especially in patients with clinically important (usually symptomatic, incessant, or both) atrial tachycardia, catheter ablation is usually the primary therapy regardless of the underlying mechanism. Reports of catheter ablation therapy for reentrant atrial tachycardia demonstrate a success rate >75 percent.[195]

Antiarrhythmic drug therapy of focal atrial tachycardia has not been predictably successful. For patients with infrequent episodes, treatment with either a β blocker or calcium channel blocker may be considered. Automatic atrial tachycardia appears more responsive to β blockers, whereas triggered arrhythmias appear to respond best to calcium channel blockers. For patients in whom the tachycardia is caused by digitalis toxicity, clearly the therapy is either to stop or reduce the dose of digitalis. Class IA or Class IC agents also have some reported success.

INAPPROPRIATE SINUS TACHYCARDIA

Sinus tachycardia is usually the result of an appropriate reflex controlled response. In recent years a syndrome originally called nonparoxysmal sinus tachycardia[196] but now called *inappropriate sinus tachycardia* (IST) has been described.[197] IST is an incessant and symptomatic tachycardia caused by inappropriately enhanced automaticity of sinus node pacemaker cells. It is characterized by an atrial rate ≥100 per minute at rest or with minimal activity; an inappropriate chronotropic response, with a rapid rise in heart rate with mild exertion; a normal P wave axis and morphology on the 12-lead ECG during tachycardia; and absence of an underlying cause.

MECHANISM

The mechanism of IST is not well understood. There is β-adrenergic hypersensitivity and depression of the efficient cardiovagal reflex, often superimposed on an abnormally high intrinsic heart rate.[196–198]

EPIDEMIOLOGY

Patients with this syndrome are usually relatively young and female.[197,198] They are frequently disabled by persistent palpitations, extreme dyspnea, chronic fatigue, and near syncope. To date, many patients described with this syndrome have been or were healthcare employees. There is no obvious reason to believe that such employment would render someone more prone to this arrhythmia, and it is more likely that these individuals are more savvy regarding health issues. The heart rate varies with activity but appears to be set 30 to 40 beats/min higher than normal. Surreptitious ingestion of drugs and Münchhausen syndrome must be excluded.

DIAGNOSIS

IST demonstrates a resting heart rate ≥100 per minute increasing rather rapidly with minimal exertion; P wave morphology consistent with a sinus focus; and secondary causes of sinus tachycardia (e.g., fever, anemia, etc.) have been excluded. A 24-hour ECG recording often provides important diagnostic information to differentiate IST from an atrial tachycardia arising near the sinus node. In IST the heart rate markedly slows during sleep, but only minimal changes in heart rate typically occur in atrial tachycardia throughout the day.

TREATMENT

Finding effective drug therapy for patients with this syndrome may be quite difficult. β Blockers, even in small doses, are often effective if tolerated. The problem is that many patients seem to require an increased level of adrenergic activity to function appropriately, and they often do not tolerate even minimal doses of β blockers. Occasionally, clonidine or even flecainide may be useful to slow the sinus rate and give patients some symptom relief. Catheter ablation of the sinus node may provide effective therapy.[198] However, even with sinus slowing, many patients still have troubling symptoms; ablation should be reserved only for patients who cannot tolerate or fail drug therapy and who are incapacitated by their symptoms.

SINUS NODE REENTRANT TACHYCARDIA

Sinus node reentrant tachycardia is thought to be caused by reentry within the tissue in or near the sinus node. This tachycardia is generally characterized by an atrial rate between 105 to150 beats/min, and a P wave morphology in the ECG similar to that of sinus rhythm. Marked cycle length variation during tachycardia is very common, and slowing prior to termination is frequent.

MECHANISM

As is evident from its name, this rhythm is caused by reentry involving the sinus node and perinodal tissue. It can usually be reproducibly induced during electrophysiological study using standard programmed pacing techniques in the atria.[182] Vagal maneuvers and administration of adenosine or verapamil result in termination of the arrhythmia.[199]

EPIDEMIOLOGY

Sinus node reentry is commonly induced during an electrophysiology study as a nonsustained and typically nonclinical arrhythmia in patients undergoing the study for other reasons. It rarely is severe enough to warrant therapy. However, sinus node reentry tachycardia can be associated with any of the classical symptoms associated with any tachycardia.

DIAGNOSIS

The rhythm is characterized by rapid rates (usual range 120–150) in which the P wave morphology in the 12-lead ECG is virtually identical to that during sinus rhythm. Its spontaneous onset and offset is abrupt, often with some slowing before termination. The tachycardia can be terminated with adenosine or with maneuvers that increase vagal tone.

TREATMENT

Intravenous adenosine, verapamil, and vagal maneuvers have been acutely used to terminate sustained episodes of sinus node reentry tachycardia. In several small series, radiofrequency ablation of the sinus node region has been shown to prevent recurrence of sinus node reentrant tachycardia.[200] Chronic therapy using pharmacologic agents has not been systematically studied. However, digitalis, a calcium channel blocker, or a β blocker alone or in combination may provide effective therapy.

MULTIFOCAL ATRIAL TACHYCARDIA

Multifocal atrial tachycardia (MAT) remains largely a descriptive entity with a need for better characterization.[201] MAT is usually diagnosed by ECG criteria that include an atrial rate greater that 100 beats/min with P waves of at least three distinct morphologies. The diagnosis of MAT can be difficult. The chaotic nature of the P wave morphology with varying AV intervals makes confusion with AF common.

MECHANISM

The mechanism underlying MAT is unknown. Several reports have noted that MAT cannot be induced or initiated by programmed stimulation. Thus, reentry seems an unlikely mechanism. Anecdotal reports of successful treatment of MAT with calcium channel or β blockers are consistent with both automatic and triggered mechanisms.

EPIDEMIOLOGY

MAT is often observed in patients with acute pulmonary disorders and associated hypoxia. Patients with MAT are usually acutely ill and often are receiving β agonists or theophylline preparations. As such, both β agonists and theophylline have been causally implicated. Data to support these observations as more than associations remain lacking. Regardless, efforts to discontinue these agents in affected patients seem reasonable. Anecdotal reports have also noted an association of MAT with pulmonary embolism, coronary artery disease, CHF, and electrolyte disturbances.

TREATMENT

The therapeutic issues revolve around the extent to which the rapid ventricular response rate during MAT affects the clinical condition of the patient. If the ventricular response is controlled (usually difficult), MAT per se probably shouldn't affect the patient's clinical course.

The basis for therapy should principally be correction of the underlying pulmonary problem. DC cardioversion has not provided successful therapy in patients with MAT. There is limited experience reported with the use of standard antiarrhythmic drugs. β Blockers have been used with success in selected patients. Precipitation of bronchospasm may be a potentially fatal complication when β blockers are used in acutely ill patients. Thus, short acting β_1 specific agents like esmolol seem most appropriate for initial use. Calcium channel blockers have been used with limited success. In selected patients, β blockers may have a role in the treatment of patients with MAT. It remains questionable whether or not antiarrhythmic drug therapy will affect outcome in this dramatically ill group of patients.[202]

REFERENCES

1. Chugh SS, Blackshear JL, Shen W-K, et al. Epidemiology and natural history of atrial fibrillation: clinical implications. *J Am Coll Cardiol* 2001;37:371–378.
2. Kopecky SL, Gersh BJ, McGoon MD, et al. The natural history of lone atrial fibrillation: a population-based study over three decades. *N Engl J Med* 1987;317:669–674.
3. Fuster V, Rydén LE, Cannom DS, et al. ACC/AHA/ESC 2006 guidelines for the management of patients with atrial fibrillation: a report of the American College of Cardiology/American Heart Association Task Force on Practice Guidelines and the European Society of Cardiology Committee for Practice Guidelines (Writing Committee to Revise the 2001 Guidelines for the Management of Patients With Atrial Fibrillation). *Eur Heart J* 2006;27(16):1979–2030.
4. Waldo AL. Mechanisms of atrial fibrillation. *J Cardiovasc Electrophysiol* 2003;14:5267–5274.
5. Levy S. Classification system of atrial fibrillation. *Curr Opin Cardiol* 2000;15:54–57.
6. Bialy D, Lehmann MH, Schumacher DN, et al. Hospitalization for arrhythmias in the United States: Importance of atrial fibrillation [abstract]. *J Am Coll Cardiol* 1992;19:41A.
7. Furberg CD, Psaty BM, Manolio TA, et al. Prevalence of atrial fibrillation in elderly subjects (the Cardiovascular Health Study). *Am J Cardiol* 1994;74:236–241.
8. Kannel WB, Abbott RD, Savage DD, McNamara PM. Coronary heart disease and atrial fibrillation: The Framingham Study. *Am Heart J* 1983;106:389–396.
9. Psaty BM, Manolio TA, Kuller LH, et al. Incidence of and risk factors for atrial fibrillation in older adults. *Circulation* 1997;96:2455–2461.
10. Miyasaka Y, Barnes ME, Gersh BJ, et al. Secular trends in incidence of atrial fibrillation in Olmsted County, Minnesota, 1980 to 2000 and implications on the projections for future prevalence. *Circulation* 2006;114:119–125.
11. Ostranderld JR, Brandt RL, Kjelsberg MO, Epstein FH. Electrocardiographic findings among the adult population of a total natural community, Tecumseh, Michigan. *Circulation* 1965;31:888–898.
12. Wolf PA, Abbott RD, Kannel WB. Atrial fibrillation as an independent risk factor for stroke. The Framingham Study. *Stroke* 1991;22:983–988.
13. Flegel KM, Shipley MJ, Rose G. Risk of stroke in nonrheumatic atrial fibrillation. *Lancet* 1987;1:526–529.
14. Levy S, Maarek M, Coumel P, et al. Characterization of different subsets of atrial fibrillation in general practice in France: the ALFA study. The College of French Cardiologists. *Circulation* 1999;99:3028–3035.
15. Murgatroyd FD, Gibson SM, Baiyan X, et al. Double-blind placebo-controlled trial of digoxin in symptomatic paroxysmal atrial fibrillation. *Circulation* 1999;99:2765–2770.
16. Evans W, Swann P. Lone auricular fibrillation. *Br Heart J* 1954;16:189–194.
17. Benjamin EJ, Levy D, Vaziri SM, et al. Independent risk factors for atrial fibrillation in a population-based cohort. The Framingham Heart Study. *JAMA* 1994;271:840–844.
18. Ellinor PT, Shin JT, Moore RK, et al. Locus for atrial fibrillation maps to chromosome 6q14–16. *Circulation* 2003;107:2880–2883.
19. Darbar D, Herron KJ, Ballew JD, et al. Familial atrial fibrillation is a genetically heterogeneous disorder. *J Am Coll Cardiol* 2003;41:2185–2192.
20. Chen YH, Xu SJ, Bendahhou S, et al. KCNQ1 gain-of-function mutation in familial atrial fibrillation. *Science* 2003;299:251–254.
21. Yang Y, Xia M, Jin Q, et al. Identification of a KCNE2 gain-of-function mutation in patients with familial atrial fibrillation. *Am J Hum Genet* 2004;75:899–905.
22. Krahn AD, Manfreda J, Tate RB, et al. The natural history of atrial fibrillation: Incidence, risk factors, and prognosis in the Manitoba followup study. *Am J Med* 1995;98:476–484.
23. Tsang TSM, Gersh BJ, Appleton CP, et al. Left ventricular diastolic dysfunction as a predictor of the first diagnosed nonvalvular atrial fibrillation in 840 elderly men and women. *J Am Coll Cardiol* 2002;40:1636–1644.
24. Wolf PA, Abbott RD, Kannel WB. Atrial fibrillation: a major contributor to stroke in the elderly. The Framingham Study. *Arch Intern Med* 1987;147:1561–1564.
25. Risk factors for stroke and efficacy of antithrombotic therapy in atrial fibrillation. Analysis of pooled data from five randomized controlled trials [published correction appears in *Arch Intern Med* 1994;154(19):2254]. *Arch Intern Med* 1994;154:1449–1457.
26. Hart RG, Halperin JL. Atrial fibrillation and thromboembolism: a decade of progress in stroke prevention. *Ann Intern Med* 1999;131:688–695.
27. Wolf PA, Dawber TR, Thomas HE Jr, Kannel WB. Epidemiologic assessment of chronic atrial fibrillation and risk of stroke. The Framingham study. *Neurology* 1978;28:973–977.
28. Feinberg WM, Seeger JF, Carmody RF, et al. Epidemiologic features of asymptomatic cerebral infarction in patients with nonvalvular atrial fibrillation. *Arch Intern Med* 1990;150:2340–2344.
29. Kempster PA, Gerraty RP, Gates PC. Asymptomatic cerebral infarction in patients with chronic atrial fibrillation. *Stroke* 1988;19:955–957.
30. Stroke Prevention in Atrial Fibrillation Study. Final results. *Circulation* 1991;84:527–539.
31. Petersen P, Madsen EB, Brun B, et al. Silent cerebral infarction in chronic atrial fibrillation. *Stroke* 1987;18:1098–1100.
32. Savage DD, Seides SF, Maron BJ, et al. Prevalence of arrhythmias during 24-hour electrocardiographic monitoring and exercise testing in patients with obstructive and nonobstructive hypertrophic cardiomyopathy. *Circulation* 1979;59:866–875.
33. Russell JW, Biller J, Hajduczok ZD, et al. Ischemic cerebrovascular complications and risk factors in idiopathic hypertrophic subaortic stenosis. *Stroke* 1991;22:1143–1147.
34. Robinson K, Frenneaux MP, Stockins B, et al. Atrial fibrillation in hypertrophic cardiomyopathy: a longitudinal study. *J Am Coll Cardiol* 1990;15:1279–1285.
35. Higashikawa M, Nakamura Y, Yoshida M, Kinoshita M. Incidence of ischemic strokes in hypertrophic cardiomyopathy is markedly increased if complicated by atrial fibrillation. *Jpn Circ J* 1997;61:673–681.
36. Lip GY, Beevers DG. ABCs of atrial fibrillation: history, epidemiology and importance of atrial fibrillation. *Br Med J* 1995;311:1361–1363.
37. Allessie MA, Boyden PA, Camm AJ, et al. Pathophysiology and prevention of atrial fibrillation. *Circulation* 2001;103:769–777.

38. Jais P, Haissaguerre M, Shah DC, et al. A focal source of atrial fibrillation treated by discrete radiofrequency ablation. *Circulation* 1997;95:572–576.

39. Haissaguerre M, Jais P, Shah DC, et al. Spontaneous initiation of atrial fibrillation by ectopic beats originating in the pulmonary veins. *N Engl J Med* 1998;339:659–666.

40. Chen SA, Hsieh MH, Tai CT, et al. Initiation of atrial fibrillation by ectopic beats originating from the pulmonary veins: electrophysiologic characteristics, pharmacologic responses and effects of radiofrequency ablation. *Circulation* 1999;100:1879–1886.

41. Cranefield P, Aronson R. *Cardiac Arrhythmias: The Role of Triggered Activity and Other Mechanisms.* New York: Futura; 1988.

42. Tse HF, Lau CP, Kou W, et al. Prevalence and significance of exit block during arrhythmias arising in pulmonary veins. *J Cardiovasc Electrophysiol* 2000;11:379–386.

43. Kumagai K, Ogawa M, Noguchi H, Yasuda T, Nakashima H, Saku K. Electrophysiologic properties of pulmonary veins assessed using a multielectrode basket catheter *J Am Coll Cardiol* 2004;43:2281–2289.

44. Tsai CF, Tai CT, Hsieh MH, et al. Initiation of atrial fibrillation by ectopic beats originating from the superior vena cava: electrophysiological characteristics and results of radiofrequency ablation. *Circulation* 2000;102:67–74.

45. Doshi RN, Wu TJ, Yashima M, et al. Relation between ligament of Marshall and adrenergic atrial tachyarrhythmia. *Circulation* 1999;100:876–883.

46. Chen PS, Chou CC. Coronary sinus as an arrhythmogenic structure. *J Cardiovasc Electrophysiol* 2002;13:863–864.

47. Chen SA, Tai CT, Yu WC, et al. Right atrial focal atrial fibrillation: electrophysiologic characteristics and radiofrequency catheter ablation. *J Cardiovasc Electrophysiol* 1999;10:328–335.

48. Zimmerman M, Kalusche D. Fluctuation in autonomic tone is a major determinant of sustained atrial arrhythmias in patients with focal ectopy originating from the pulmonary veins. *J Cardiovasc Electrophysiol* 2001;12:285–291.

49. Bettoni M, Zimmermann M. Autonomic tone variations before the onset of paroxysmal atrial fibrillation. *Circulation* 2002;105:2753–2759.

50. Moe GK, Abildskov JA. Atrial fibrillation as a self sustaining arrhythmia independent of focal discharge. *Am Heart J* 1959;58:59–70.

51. Moe GK, Abildskov JA. Observations on the ventricular dysrhythmia associated with atrial fibrillation in the dog heart. *Circ Res* 1964;4:447–460.

52. Li D, Fareh S, Leung TK, et al. Promotion of atrial fibrillation by heart failure in dogs: remodeling of a different sort. *Circulation* 1999;100:87–95.

53. Spach MS, Josephson ME. Initiating reentry: the role of nonuniform anisotropy in small circuits. *J Cardiovasc Electrophysiol* 1994;5:182–209.

54. Tai C-T, Chen S-A, Tzeng J-W, et al. Prolonged fractionation of paced right atrial electrograms in patients with atrial flutter and fibrillation. *J Am Coll Cardiol* 2001;37:1651–1657.

55. Polontchouk L, Haefliger J-A, Ebelt B, et al. Effects of chronic atrial fibrillation on gap junctions distribution in human and rat atria. *J Am Coll Cardiol* 2001;38:883–891.

56. Mary-Rabine L, Albert A, Pham TD, et al. The relationship of human atrial cellular electrophysiology to clinical function and ultrastructure. *Circ Res* 1983;52:188–199.

57. Ausma J, Wijffels M, Thoné F, et al. Structural changes of atrial myocardium due to sustained atrial fibrillation in the goat. *Circulation* 1997;96:3157–3163.

58. Madrid AH, Bueno MG, Rebollo JMG, et al. Use of irbesartan to maintain sinus rhythm in patients with long-lasting persistent atrial fibrillation: a prospective and randomized study. *Circulation* 2002;106:331–336.

59. Kim B-S, Kim Y-H, Hwang G-S, et al. Action potential duration restitution kinetics in human atrial fibrillation. *J Am Coll Cardiol* 2002;39:1329–1236.

60. Shinagawa K, Li D, Leung TK, Nattel S. Consequences of atrial tachycardia-induced remodeling depend on the preexisting atrial substrate. *Circulation* 2002;105:251–257.

61. Morillo CA, Klein GJ, Jones DL, et al. Chronic rapid atrial pacing: structural, functional, and electrophysiological characteristics of a new model of sustained atrial fibrillation. *Circulation* 1995;91:1588–1595.

62. Gaspo R, Bosch RF, Talajic M, et al. Functional mechanisms underlying tachycardia-induced sustained atrial fibrillation in a chronic dog model. *Circulation* 1997;96:4027–4035.

63. Elvan A, Wylie K, Zipes DP. Pacing-induced chronic atrial fibrillation impairs sinus node function in dogs: electrophysiological remodeling. *Circulation* 1996;94:2953–2960.

64. Stambler BS, Fenelon G, Shepard RK, Clemo HT, Guiraudon CM. Characterization of sustained atrial tachycardia in dogs with rapid ventricular pacing-induced heart failure. *J Cardiovasc Electrophysiol* 2003;14:499–507.

65. Grogan M, Smith HC, Gersh BJ, Wood DL. Left ventricular dysfunction due to atrial fibrillation in patients initially believed to have idiopathic dilated cardiomyopathy. *Am J Cardiol* 1992;69:1570–1573.

66. Kieny JR, Sacrez A, Facello A, et al. Increase in radionuclide left ventricular ejection fraction after cardioversion of chronic atrial fibrillation in idiopathic dilated cardiomyopathy. *Eur Heart J* 1992;13:1290–1295.

67. Clark DM, Plumb VJ, Epstein AE, Kay GN. Hemodynamic effects of an irregular sequence of ventricular cycle lengths during atrial fibrillation. *J Am Coll Cardiol* 1997;30:1039–1045.

68. Kochiadakis GE, Skalidis EI, Kalebubas D, et al. Effect of acute atrial fibrillation on phasic coronary blood flow pattern and flow reserve in humans. *Eur Heart J* 2002;23:734–741.

69. Hsu LF, Jais P, Sanders P, et al. Catheter ablation for atrial fibrillation in congestive heart failure. *N Engl J Med* 2004;351:2373–2383.

70. Gentlesk P, Sauer WH, Gerstenfeld EP, et al. Reversal of left ventricular dysfunction following ablation of atrial fibrillation. *J Cardiovasc Electrophysiol* January 2007;18(1)9–14.

71. Stoddard MF, Dawkins PR, Prince CR, Ammash NM. Left atrial appendage thrombus is not uncommon in patients with acute atrial fibrillation and a recent embolic event: a transesophageal echocardiographic study. *J Am Coll Cardiol* 1995;25:452–459.

72. Grimm RA, Stewart WJ, Maloney JD, et al. Impact of electrical cardioversion for atrial fibrillation on left atrial appendage function and spontaneous echo contrast: characterization by simultaneous transesophageal echocardiography. *J Am Coll Cardiol* 1993;22:1359–1366.

73. Mugge A, Kuhn H, Nikutta P, et al. Assessment of left atrial appendage function by biplane transesophageal echocardiography in patients with nonrheumatic atrial fibrillation: identification of a subgroup of patients at increased embolic risk. *J Am Coll Cardiol* 1994;23:599–607.

74. Cai H, Li Z, Goette A, et al. Downregulation of endocardial nitric oxide synthetase expression and nitric oxide production in atrial fibrillation: potential mechanisms for atrial thrombosis and stroke. *Circulation* 2002;1062854–1062858.

75. Heppel RM, Berkin KE, McLenachan JM, et al. Haemostatic and haemodynamic abnormalities associated with left atrial thrombosis in nonrheumatic atrial fibrillation. *Heart* 1977;77:407–411.

76. Sohara H, Amitani S, Kurose M, et al. Atrial fibrillation activates platelets and coagulation in a time-dependent manner: a study in patients with paroxysmal atrial fibrillation. *J Am Coll Cardiol* 1997;29:106–112.

77. Li-Saw-Hee FL, Blann AD, Lip GY. A cross-sectional and diurnal study of thrombogenesis among patients with chronic atrial fibrillation. *J Am Coll Cardiol* 2000;35:1926–1931.

78. Li-Saw-Hee FL, Blann AD, Lip GY. Effect of blood pressure on the hypercoagulable state in chronic atrial fibrillation. *Am J Cardiol* 2000;86:795–797.

79. Conway DSG, Pearce LA, Chin BSP, et al. Plasma von Willebrand factor and soluble P-selectin as indices of endothelial damage and platelet activation in 1321 patients with nonvalvular atrial fibrillation: relationship to stroke risk factors. *Circulation* 2002;106:1962–1967.

80. Klein GJ, Bashore TM, Seller TD, et al. Ventricular fibrillation in the Wolff-Parkinson-White syndrome. *N Engl J Med* 1979;301:1080–1085.

81. Israel CW, Gronefeld G, Ehrlich JR, et al. Long-term risk of recurrent atrial fibrillation as documented by an implantable monitoring device: implications for optimal patient care. *J Am Coll Cardiol* 2004;43:47–52.

82. Page RL, Tilsch TW, Connolly SJ, et al. Asymptomatic or "silent" atrial fibrillation: frequency in untreated patients and patients receiving azimilide. *Circulation* 2003;107:1141–1145.

83. Wood MA, Brown-Mahoney C, Kay GN, Ellenbogen KA. Clinical outcomes after ablation and pacing therapy for atrial fibrillation: a meta-analysis. *Circulation* 2000;101:1138–1144.

84. Dorian P, Jung W, Newman D, et al. The impairment of health-related quality of life in patients with intermittent atrial fibrillation: implications for the assessment of investigational therapy. *J Am Coll Cardiol* 2002;36:1303–1309.

85. Epstein AE, Vidaillet H, Greene HL, et al. Frequency of symptomatic atrial fibrillation in patients enrolled in the Atrial Fibrillation Follow-up Investigation of Rhythm Management (AFFIRM) study. *J Cardiovasc Electrophysiol* 2002;13:667–671.

86. Albers GW, Sherman DG, Gress DR, Paulseth JE, Petersen P. Stroke prevention in nonvalvular atrial fibrillation: a review of prospective randomized trials. *Ann Neurol* 1991;30:511–518.

87. Hart RG, Halperin JL. Atrial fibrillation and thromboembolism: a decade of progress in stroke prevention. *Ann Intern Med* 1999;131:492–501.

88. Adjusted-dose warfarin versus low-intensity, fixed-dose warfarin plus aspirin for high-risk patients with atrial fibrillation. Stroke Prevention in Atrial Fibrillation III Randomised Clinical Trial. *Lancet* 1996;348:633–638.

89. Stroke Prevention in Atrial Fibrillation III Study. Patients with nonvalvular atrial fibrillation at low risk of stroke during treatment with aspirin. The SPAF III Writing Committee for the Stroke Prevention in Atrial Fibrillation Investigators. *JAMA* 1998;279:1273–1277.

90. Hylek EM, Skates SJ, Sheehan MA, Singer DE. An analysis of the lowest effective intensity of prophylactic anticoagulation for patients with nonrheumatic atrial fibrillation. *N Engl J Med* 1996;335:540–546.

91. Hylek EM, Go AS, Chang Y, et al. Effect of intensity of oral anticoagulation on stroke severity and mortality in atrial fibrillation. *N Engl J Med* 2003;349:1019–1026.

92. Gallagher MM, Hennessy BJ, Edvardsson N, et al. Embolic complications of direct current cardioversion of atrial arrhythmias: association with low intensity of anticoagulation at the time of cardioversion. *J Am Coll Cardiol* 2002;40:926–933.

93. Klein EA. Assessment of Cardioversion Using Transesophageal Echocardiography (TEE) multicenter study (ACUTE I): clinical outcomes at eight weeks. *J Am Coll Cardiol* 2000;36:324.

94. Klein AL, Grimm RA, Murray RD, et al. Assessment of cardioversion using transesophageal echocardiography investigators: use of transesophageal echocardiography to guide cardioversion in patients with atrial fibrillation. *N Engl J Med* 2001;344:1411–1420.

95. Antonielli E, Pizzuti A, Bassignana A, et al. Transesophageal echocardiographic evidence of more pronounced left atrial stunning after chemical (propafenone) rather than electrical attempts at cardioversion from atrial fibrillation. *Am J Cardiol* 1999;84:1092–1010.

96. Bellotti P, Spirito P, Lupi G, Vecchio C. Left atrial appendage function assessed by transesophageal echocardiography before and on the day after elective cardioversion for nonvalvular atrial fibrillation. *Am J Cardiol* 1998;81:1199–1202.

97. Mitusch R, Garbe M, Schmucker G, et al. Relation of left atrial appendage function to the duration and reversibility of nonvalvular atrial fibrillation. *Am J Cardiol* 1995;75:944–947.

98. Botto GL, Politi A, Bonini W, et al. External cardioversion of atrial fibrillation: role of paddle position on technical efficacy and energy requirements. *Heart* 1999;82:726–730.

99. Mittal S, Ayati S, Stein KM, et al. Transthoracic cardioversion of atrial fibrillation: comparison of rectilinear biphasic versus damped sine wave monophasic shocks. *Circulation* 2000;101:1282–1287.

100. Page RL, Kerber RE, Russell JK, et al. Biphasic versus monophasic shock waveform for conversion of atrial fibrillation: the results of an international randomized, double-blind multicenter trial. *J Am Coll Cardiol* 2002;39:1956–1963.

101. Khan IA. Single oral loading dose of propafenone for pharmacological cardioversion of recent-onset atrial fibrillation. *J Am Coll Cardiol* 2001;37:542–547.

102. Boriani G, Martignani C, Biffi M, et al. Oral loading with propafenone for conversion of recent-onset atrial fibrillation: a review on in-hospital treatment. *Drugs* 2002;62:415–423.

103. Boriani G, Biffi M, Capucci A, et al. Oral propafenone to convert recent-onset atrial fibrillation in patients with and without underlying heart disease: a randomized, controlled trial. *Ann Intern Med* 1997;126:621–625.

104. Capucci A, Boriani G, Botto GL, et al. Conversion of recent-onset atrial fibrillation by a single oral loading dose of propafenone or flecainide. *Am J Cardiol* 1994;74:503–505.

105. Alboni P, Botto GL, Baldi N, et al. Outpatient treatment of recent-onset atrial fibrillation with the "pill-in-the-pocket" approach. *N Engl J Med* 2004;351:2384–2391.

106. Singh S, Zoble RG, Yellen L, et al. Efficacy and safety of oral dofetilide in converting to and maintaining sinus rhythm in patients with chronic atrial fibrillation or atrial flutter: the Symptomatic Atrial Fibrillation Investigative Research of Dofetilide (SAFIRE-D) Study. *Circulation* 2000;102:2385–2390.

107. Prystowsky EN, Freeland SA, Branyas NA, et al. Clinical experience with dofetilide in the treatment of patients with atrial fibrillation. *J Cardiovasc Electrophysiol* 2003;14:S287–S290.

108. Stambler BS, Wood MA, Ellenbogen KA, et al. Efficacy and safety of repeated intravenous doses of ibutilide for rapid conversion of atrial flutter or fibrillation: Ibutilide Repeat Dose Study Investigators. *Circulation* 1996;94:1613–1621.

109. Ellenbogen KA, Stambler BS, Wood MA, et al. Efficacy of intravenous ibutilide for rapid termination of atrial fibrillation and atrial flutter: a dose-response study. *J Am Coll Cardiol* 1996;28:130–136.

110. Volgman AS, Carberry PA, Stambler B, et al. Conversion efficacy and safety of intravenous ibutilide compared with intravenous procainamide in patients with atrial flutter or fibrillation. *J Am Coll Cardiol* 1998;31:1414–1419.

111. Galve E, Rius E, Ballester R, et al. Intravenous amiodarone in treatment of recent-onset atrial fibrillation: results of a randomized, controlled study. *J Am Coll Cardiol* 1996;27:1079–1082.

112. Crystal E, Connolly SJ, Sleik K, et al. Interventions on prevention of postoperative atrial fibrillation in patients undergoing heart surgery: a meta-analysis. *Circulation* 2002;106:75–80.

113. Lee JK, Klein GH, Krahn AD, et al. Rate-control versus conversion strategy in postoperative atrial fibrillation: a prospective, randomized pilot study. *Am Heart J* 2000;140:871–877.

114. Wyse DG, Waldo AL, DiMarco JP, et al. The Atrial Fibrillation Follow-up Investigation of Rhythm Management (AFFIRM) Investigators: a comparison of rate control and rhythm control in patients with atrial fibrillation. *N Engl J Med* 2002;347:1825–1833.

115. Van Gelder IC, Hagens VE, Bosker HA, et al. Rate Control versus Electrical Cardioversion for Persistent Atrial Fibrillation Study Group: a comparison of rate control and rhythm control in patients with recurrent persistent atrial fibrillation. *N Engl J Med* 2002;347:1834–1840.

116. Pelargonio G, Prystowsky EN. Rate versus rhythm control in the management of patients with atrial fibrillation. *Nat Clin Pract Cardiovasc Med* 2005;2:514–521.

117. Prystowsky, EN. Assessment of rhythm and rate control in patients with atrial fibrillation. *J Cardiovasc Electrophysiol* 2006;17(2):S7–S10.

118. Marshall HJ, Harris ZI, Griffith MJ, et al. Prospective randomized study of ablation and pacing versus medical therapy for paroxysmal atrial fibrillation: effects of pacing mode and mode-switch algorithm. *Circulation* 1999;99:1587–1592.

119. Kay GN, Ellenbogen KA, Giudici M, et al. The Ablate and Pace Trial: a prospective study of catheter ablation of the AV conduction system and permanent pacemaker implantation for treatment of atrial fibrillation: APT Investigators. *J Interv Card Electrophysiol* 1998;2:121–135.

120. Brignole M, Gianfranchi L, Menozzi C, et al. Assessment of atrioventricular junction ablation and DDDR mode-switching pacemaker versus pharmacological treatment in patients with severely symptomatic paroxysmal atrial fibrillation: a randomized controlled study. *Circulation* 1997;96:2617–2624.

121. Doshi RN, Daoud EG, Fellows C, et al. Left ventricular-based cardiac stimulation post AV nodal ablation evaluation (the PAVE study). *J Cardiovasc Electrophysiol* 2005;16:1160–1165.

122. Anderson JL, Gilbert EM, Alpert BL, et al. Prevention of symptomatic recurrences of paroxysmal atrial fibrillation in patients initially tolerating antiarrhythmic therapy: a multicenter, double-blind, crossover study of flecainide and placebo with transtelephonic monitoring. Flecainide Supraventricular Tachycardia Study Group. *Circulation* 1989;80:1557–1570.

123. Singh BN, Singh SN, Reda DJ, et al. Amiodarone versus sotalol for atrial fibrillation. *N Engl J Med* 2005;352:1861–1872.

124. Roy D, Talajic M, Dorian P, et al. Amiodarone to prevent recurrence of atrial fibrillation: Canadian Trial of Atrial Fibrillation Investigators. *N Engl J Med* 2000;342:913–920.

125. Van Gelder IC, Crijns HJ, van Gilst WH, et al. Efficacy and safety of flecainide acetate in the maintenance of sinus rhythm after electrical cardioversion of chronic atrial fibrillation or atrial flutter. *Am J Cardiol* 1989;64:1317–1321.

126. Pedersen OD, Bagger H, Keller N, et al. Efficacy of dofetilide in the treatment of atrial fibrillation-flutter in patients with reduced left ventricular function: a Danish investigation of arrhythmia and mortality on dofetilide (DIAMOND) substudy. *Circulation* 2001;104:292–296.

127. Torp-Pedersen C, Moller M, Bloch-Thomsen PE, et al. Dofetilide in patients with congestive heart failure and left ventricular dysfunction. Danish Investigations of Arrhythmia and Mortality on Dofetilide Study Group. *N Engl J Med* 1999;341:857–865.

128. Pedersen OD, Bagger H, Kober L, et al. Trandolapril reduces the incidence of atrial fibrillation after acute myocardial infarction in patients with left ventricular dysfunction. *Circulation* 1999;100:376–380.

129. Vermes E, Tardif JC, Bourassa MG, et al. Enalapril decreases the incidence of atrial fibrillation in patients with left ventricular dysfunction: insight from the Studies of Left Ventricular Dysfunction (SOLVD) trials. *Circulation* 2003;107:2926–2931.

130. Maggioni AP, Latini R, Carson PE, et al. Valsartan reduces the incidence of atrial fibrillation in patients with heart failure: results from the Valsartan Heart Failure Trial (Val-HeFT). *Am Heart J* 2005;149:548–557.

131. Wachtell K, Lehto M, Gerdts E, et al. Angiotensin II receptor blockade reduces new-onset atrial fibrillation and subsequent stroke compared to atenolol: the Losartan Intervention For End Point Reduction in Hypertension (LIFE) study. *J Am Coll Cardiol* 2005;45:712–719.

132. L'Allier PL, Ducharme A, Keller PF, et al. Angiotensin-converting enzyme inhibition in hypertensive patients is associated with a reduction in the occurrence of atrial fibrillation. *J Am Coll Cardiol* 2004;44:159–164.

133. Healey JS, Baranchuk A, Crystal E, et al. Prevention of atrial fibrillation with angiotensin-converting enzyme inhibitors and angiotensin receptor blockers: a meta-analysis. *J Am Coll Cardiol* 2005;45:1832–1839.
134. Siu CW, Lau CP, Tse HF. Prevention of atrial fibrillation recurrence by statin therapy in patients with lone atrial fibrillation after successful cardioversion. *Am J Cardiol* 2003;92:1343–1345.
135. Maron DJ, Fazio S, Linton MF. Current perspectives on statins. *Circulation* 2000;101:207–13.
136. Davignon J. Beneficial cardiovascular pleiotropic effects of statins. *Circulation* 2004;109:III39–III43.
137. Williams MR, Stewart JR, Bolling SF, et al. Surgical treatment of atrial fibrillation using radiofrequency energy. *Ann Thorac Surg* 2001;71:1939–1944.
138. Cox JL. Cardiac surgery for arrhythmias. *J Cardiovasc Electrophysiol* 2004;15:250–262.
139. Damiano RJ Jr, Gaynor SL, Bailey M, et al. The long-term outcome of patients with coronary disease and atrial fibrillation undergoing the Cox maze procedure. *J Thorac Cardiovasc Surg* 2003;126:2016–21.
140. Gillinov AM, McCarthy PM. Advances in the surgical treatment of atrial fibrillation. *Cardiol Clin* 2004;22:147–157.
141. Gaynor SL, Diodato MD, Prasad SM, et al. A prospective, single-center clinical trial of a modified Cox maze procedure with bipolar radiofrequency ablation. *J Thorac Cardiovasc Surg* 2004;128:535–542.
142. Oral H, Knight BP, Ozaydin M, et al. Segmental ostial ablation to isolate the pulmonary veins during atrial fibrillation: feasibility and mechanistic insights. *Circulation* 2002;106:1256–1262.
143. Haissaguerre M, Shah DC, Jais P, et al. Electrophysiological breakthroughs from the left atrium to the pulmonary veins. *Circulation* 2000;102:2463–2465.
144. Lin WS, Tai CT, Hsieh MH, et al. Catheter ablation of paroxysmal atrial fibrillation initiated by nonpulmonary vein ectopy. *Circulation* 2003;107:3176–3183.
145. Hocini M, Sanders P, Jais P, et al. Techniques for curative treatment of atrial fibrillation. *J Cardiovasc Electrophysiol* 1004;15:1467–1471.
146. Verma A, Marrouche NF, Natale A. Pulmonary vein antrum isolation: intracardiac echocardiography-guided technique. *J Cardiovasc Electrophysiol* 2004;15:1335–1340.
147. Wazni OM, Marouche NF, Martin DO, et al. Radiofrequency ablation vs antiarrhythmic drugs as first-line treatment of symptomatic atrial fibrillation; a randomized trial. *JAMA* 2005;293:2634–2640.
148. Pappone C, Santinelli V. The who, what, why and how-to guide for circumferential pulmonary vein ablation. *J Cardiovasc Electrophysiol* 2004;15:1226–1230.
149. Oral H, Scharf C, Chugh A, et al. Catheter ablation for paroxysmal atrial fibrillation: segmental pulmonary vein ostial ablation versus left atrial ablation. *Circulation* 2003;108:2355–2360.
150. Cappato R, Calkins H, Chen SA, et al. Worldwide survey on the methods, efficacy, and safety of catheter ablation for human atrial fibrillation. *Circulation* 2005;111:1100–1105.
151. Nademanee K, McKenzie J, Losar E, et al. A new approach for catheter ablation of atrial fibrillation: mapping of the electrophysiologic substrate. *J Am Coll Cardiol* 2004;43:2044–2053.
152. Pappone C, Oral H, Santinelli V, et al. Atrio-esophageal fistula as a complication of percutaneous transcatheter ablation of atrial fibrillation. *Circulation* 2004;109:2724–2726.
153. Scanavacca MI, D'avila A, Parga J, et al. Left atrial-esophageal fistula following radiofrequency catheter ablation of atrial fibrillation. *J Cardiovasc Electrophysiol* August 2004;15(8):960–962.
154. Saoudi N, Cosio F, Waldo A, et al. Classification of atrial flutter and regular atrial tachycardia according to electrophysiologic mechanism and anatomic bases. *J Cardiovasc Electrophysiol* 2001;12:852–866.
155. Cosío FG, Arribas F, Lopez-Gil M, Gonzalez D. Atrial flutter mapping and ablation. II. Radiofrequency ablation of atrial flutter circuits. *Pacing Clin Electrophysiol* 1996;19:965–975.
156. Cosío FG, Giocolea A, Lopez-Gil M, Arribas F, Barroso JL, Chicote R. Atrial endocardial mapping in the rare form of atrial flutter. *Am J Cardiol* 1990;66:715–720.
157. Waldo AL. The interrelationship between atrial fibrillation and atrial flutter. *Prog Cardiovasc Dis* 2005;48:41–56.
158. Cheng J, Scheinman MM. Acceleration of typical atrial flutter due to double wave reentry induced by programmed electrical stimulation. *Circulation* 1998;97:1589–1596.
159. Cheng J, Cabeen WR Jr, Scheinman MM. Right atrial flutter due to lower loop reentry: mechanism and anatomic substrates. *Circulation* 1999;99:1700–1705.
160. Triedman JK, Saul JP, Weindling SN, Walsh EP. Radiofrequency ablation of intra-atrial reentrant tachycardia after surgical palliation of congenital heart disease. *Circulation* 1995;91:707–714.
161. Jais P, Shah DC, Haissaguerre M, et al. Mapping and ablation of left atrial flutters. *Circulation* 2000;101:2928–2934.
162. Chan DP, Van Hare GF, Mackall JA, Carlson MD, Waldo AL. Importance of the atrial flutter isthmus in post-operative intra-atrial reentrant tachycardia. *Circulation*. 2000;102(11):1283–1289.
163. Waldo AL. Pathogenesis of atrial flutter. *J Cardiovasc Electrophysiol* 1998;9:518–525.
164. Shimizu A, Nozaki A, Rudy Y, Waldo AL. Onset of induced atrial flutter in the canine pericarditis model. *J Am Coll Cardiol* 1991;17:1223–1234.
165. Waldo AL, Cooper TB. Spontaneous onset of Type I atrial flutter in patients. *J Am Coll Cardiol* 1996;28:707–712.
166. Waldo AL, MacLean WAH. *Diagnosis and Treatment of Arrhythmias Following Open Heart Surgery: Emphasis on the Use of Epicardial Wire Electrodes.* New York: Futura, 1980.
167. Waldo AL. Clinical evaluation in therapy of patients with atrial fibrillation or flutter. In: Scheinman MM, ed. *Cardiology Clinics: Supraventricular Tachycardia.* 1990;8:479–490.
168. Biblo LA, Yuan Z, Quan KJ, Mackall JA, Rimm AA. Risk of stroke in patients with atrial flutter. *Am J Cardiol* 2001;87:17–20.
169. Black IW, Hopkins AT, Lee LC, Walsh WF. Evaluation of transesophageal echocardiography before cardioversion of atrial fibrillation and flutter in nonanticoagulated patients. *Am Heart J* 1993;126:375–381.
170. Wood KA, Eisenberg SJ, Kalman JM, et al. Risk of thromboembolism in chronic atrial flutter. *Am J Cardiol* 1997;79:1043–1047.
171. Seidl K, Haver B, Schwick NG, Zellner D, Zahn R, Senges J. Risk of thromboembolic events in patients with atrial flutter. *Am J Cardiol* 1998;82:580–584.
172. Stambler BS, Wood MA, Ellenbogen KA, Perry KT, Wakefield GK, Vander-Lust JT. Efficacy and safety of repeated intravenous doses of ibutilide for rapid conversion of atrial flutter or fibrillation. *Circulation* 1996;94:1613–1621.
173. Fenster PE, Comess KA, Marsh R, Katzenberg C, Hager WD. Conversion of atrial fibrillation to sinus rhythm by acute intravenous procainamide infusion. *Am Heart J* 1983;106:501–504.
174. Waldo AL, MacLean WAH, Karp RB, Kouchoukos NT, James TN. Entrainment and interruption of atrial flutter with atrial pacing: studies in man following open heart surgery. *Circulation* 1977;56:737–745.
175. Cosío FG, Arribas F, Lopez-Gil M, Gonzalez D. Atrial flutter mapping and ablation. II. Radiofrequency ablation of atrial flutter circuits. *Pacing Clin Electrophysiol* 1996;19:965–975.
176. Cauchemez B, Haissaguerre M, Fischer B, Thomas O, Clementy J, Coumel P. Electrophysiological effects of catheter ablation of inferior vena cava-tricuspid annulus isthmus in common atrial flutter. *Circulation* 1996;93:284–294.
177. Poty H, Saoudi N, Nair M, Anselme F, Letac B. Radiofrequency catheter ablation of atrial flutter: Further insights in to the various types of isthmus block: application to ablation during sinus rhythm. *Circulation* 1996;94:3204–3213.
178. Barold S, Wyndham CRC, Kappenberger LL, Abinader EG, Griffin JC, Falcoff MD. Implanted atrial pacemaker for paroxysmal atrial flutter: long term efficacy. *Ann Intern Med* 1987;107:144–149.
179. Callans DJ, Schwartzman D, Gottlieb CD, Marchlinski FE. Insights into the electrophysiology of atrial arrhythmias gained by the catheter ablation experience: "Learning while burning, Part II." *J Cardiovasc Electrophysiol* 1995;6:229–243.
180. Chen S-A, Chiang C-E, Yang C-J, et al. Sustained atrial tachycardia in adult patients; electrophysiological characteristics, pharmacological response, possible mechanisms, and effects of radiofrequency ablation. *Circulation* 1994;90:1262–1278.
181. Mehta AV, Sanchez GR, Sacks EJ, Casta A, Dunn JM, Donner RM. Ectopic automatic atrial tachycardia in children: clinical characteristics, management and follow up. *J Am Coll Cardiol* 1988;11:379–385.
182. Waldo AL, Wit AL. Mechanism of cardiac arrhythmias and conduction disturbances. In: Schlant RC, Alexander RW, eds. *Hurst's The Heart*. 8th ed. New York: McGraw-Hill; 1994:659–704.
183. Wit A, Cranefield PF. Triggered activity in cardiac muscle fibers of the simian mitral valve. *Circ Res* 1976;38:85–98.
184. Wit AL, Cranefield PF. Triggered and automatic activity in the canine coronary sinus. *Circ Res* 1977;41:435–445.
185. Rozanski GJ, Lipsius SL. Electrophysiology of functional subsidiary pacemakers in canine right atrium. *Am J Physiol* 1985;249:H594–H603.
186. Camm A, Evans K, Ward D, Martin A. The rhythm of the heart in active elderly subjects. *Am Heart J* 1980;99:598–603.
187. Fleig J, Kennedy H. Cardiac arrhythmias in a healthy elderly population. *Chest* 1982;81:302.

188. Cristal N, Szwarcberg J, Gueron M. Supraventricular arrhythmias in acute myocardial infarction. *Ann Intern Med* 1975;82:35–39.

189. Lazzeroni E, Domeniencci S, Finardi A, et al. Severity of arrhythmias and extent of hypertrophy in hypertrophic cardiomyopathy. *Am Heart J* 1989;118:734–738.

190. Holford F. Mithoefer J. Cardiac arrhythmias in hospitalized patients with chronic obstructive pulmonary disease. *Am Rev Respir Dis* 1973;108:879–885.

191. Storstein O, Hansteen V, Hatle L, Hillestad L, Storstein L. Studies on digitalis. XIII. A prospective study of 649 patients on maintenance treatment with digitoxin. *Am Heart J* 1977;93:434–443.

192. Brodsky M, Wu D, Denes P, Kanakis C, Rosen K. Arrhythmias documented by 24 hour continuous electrocardiographic monitoring in 50 male medical students without apparent heart disease. *Am J Cardiol* 1977;39:390–395.

193. Talan D, Bauernfeind R, Ashley W, Kanakis C, Rosen K. Twenty-four hour continuous ECG recordings in long-distance runners. *Chest* 1982;82(1):19–24.

194. Wellens H, Brugada P. Mechanisms of supraventricular tachycardia. *Am J Cardiol* 1988;62:10D–15D.

195. Poty H, Saoudi N, Haissaguerre M, Daou A, Clementy J, Letac B. Radiofrequency catheter ablation of atrial tachycardias. *Am Heart J* 1996;131:481–489.

196. Bauernfeind R, Amat-Y-Leon F, et al. Chronic nonparoxysmal sinus tachycardia in otherwise healthy persons. *Ann Intern Med* 1979;91:702–710.

197. Morillo C, Klein G, et al. Mechanism of "inappropriate" sinus tachycardia: role of sympathovagal balance. *Circulation* 1994;90:873–877.

198. Lee R, Kalman J, et al. Radiofrequency catheter modification of the sinus node for "inappropriate" sinus tachycardia. *Circulation* 1995;92:2929–2928.

199. Gomes J, Hariman R, Kang P, Chowdry I, et al. Sustained symptomatic sinus node reentrant tachycardia: incidence, clinical significance, electrophysiologic observations and the effects of antiarrhythmic agents. *J Am Coll Cardiol* 1985;5:45–57.

200. Narula OS. Sinus node re-entry: a mechanism for supraventricular tachycardia. *Circulation* 1974;50:1114–1128.

201. Scher D, Arsura E. Multifocal atrial tachycardia: mechanisms, clinical correlates, and treatment. *Am Heart J* 1989;118:574–580.

202. Arsura E, Lefkin A, Scher D, Solar M, Tessler S. A randomized, double-blind, placebo-controlled study of verapamil and metoprolol in treatment of multifocal atrial tachycardia. *Am J Med* 1988;85:519–524.

APPENDIX 37–1

Recommendations for Management of Patients with Atrial Fibrillation

1. *Pharmacologic Rate Control during Atrial Fibrillation*

   Class I

   1. Measurement of the heart rate at rest and control of the rate using pharmacological agents (either a β blocker or nondihydropyridine calcium channel antagonist, in most cases) are recommended for patients with persistent or permanent AF. *(Level of Evidence: B)*

   2. In the absence of preexcitation, intravenous administration of β blockers (esmolol, metoprolol, or propranolol) or nondihydropyridine calcium channel antagonists (verapamil, diltiazem, is recommended to slow the ventricular response to AF in the acute setting, exercising caution in patients with hypotension or heart failure (HF). *(Level of Evidence: B)*

   3. Intravenous administration of digoxin or amiodarone is recommended to control the heart rate in patients with AF and HF who do not have an accessory pathway. *(Level of Evidence: B)*

   4. In patients who experience symptoms related to AF during activity, the adequacy of heart rate control should be assessed during exercise, adjusting pharmacological treatment as necessary to keep the rate in the physiological range. *(Level of Evidence: C)*

   5. Digoxin is effective following oral administration to control the heart rate at rest in patients with AF and is indicated for patients with HF, left ventricular (LV) dysfunction, or for sedentary individuals. *(Level of Evidence: C)*

   Class IIa

   1. A combination of digoxin and either a β blocker or nondihydropyridine calcium channel antagonist is reasonable to control the heart rate both at rest and during exercise in patients with AF. The choice of medication should be individualized and the dose modulated to avoid bradycardia. *(Level of Evidence: B)*

   2. It is reasonable to use ablation of the AV node or accessory pathway to control heart rate when pharmacological therapy is insufficient or associated with side effects. *(Level of Evidence: B)*

   3. Intravenous amiodarone can be useful to control the heart rate in patients with AF when other measures are unsuccessful or contraindicated. *(Level of Evidence: C)*

   4. When electrical cardioversion is not necessary in patients with AF and an accessory pathway, intravenous procainamide or ibutilide is a reasonable alternative. *(Level of Evidence: C)*

   Class IIb

   1. When the ventricular rate cannot be adequately controlled both at rest and during exercise in patients with AF using a β blocker, nondihydropyridine calcium channel antagonist, or digoxin, alone or in combination, oral amiodarone may be administered to control the heart rate. *(Level of Evidence: C)*

   2. Intravenous procainamide, disopyramide, ibutilide, or amiodarone may be considered for hemodynamically stable patients with AF involving conduction over an accessory pathway. *(Level of Evidence: B)*

   3. When the rate cannot be controlled with pharmacological agents or tachycardia-mediated cardiomyopathy is suspected, catheter-directed ablation of the AV node may be considered in patients with AF to control the heart rate. *(Level of Evidence: C)*

   Class III

   1. Digitalis should not be used as the sole agent to control the rate of ventricular response in patients with paroxysmal AF. *(Level of Evidence: B)*

   2. Catheter ablation of the AV node should not be attempted without a prior trial of medication to control the ventricular rate in patients with AF. *(Level of Evidence: C)*

Recommendations for Management of Patients with Atrial Fibrillation *(continued)*

3. In patients with decompensated HF and AF, intravenous administration of a nondihydropyridine calcium channel antagonist may exacerbate hemodynamic compromise and is not recommended. *(Level of Evidence: C)*
4. Intravenous administration of digitalis glycosides or nondihydropyridine calcium channel antagonists to patients with AF and a preexcitation syndrome may paradoxically accelerate the ventricular response and is not recommended. *(Level of Evidence: C)*

2. *Preventing Thromboembolism*

(For recommendations regarding antithrombotic therapy in patients with AF undergoing cardioversion, see Section I.C.3.d.)

Class I

1. Antithrombotic therapy to prevent thromboembolism is recommended for all patients with AF, except those with lone AF or contraindications. *(Level of Evidence: A)*
2. The selection of the antithrombotic agent should be based upon the absolute risks of stroke and bleeding and the relative risk and benefit for a given patient. *(Level of Evidence: A)*
3. For patients without mechanical heart valves at high risk of stroke, chronic oral anticoagulant therapy with a vitamin K antagonist is recommended in a dose adjusted to achieve the target intensity international normalized ratio (INR) of 2.0 to 3.0, unless contraindicated. Factors associated with highest risk for stroke in patients with AF are prior thromboembolism (stroke, transient ischemic attack [TIA], or systemic embolism) and rheumatic mitral stenosis. *(Level of Evidence: A)*
4. Anticoagulation with a vitamin K antagonist is recommended for patients with more than 1 moderate risk factor. Such factors include age 75 y or greater, hypertension, HF, impaired LV systolic function (ejection fraction 35% or less or fractional shortening less than 25%), and diabetes mellitus. *(Level of Evidence: A)*
5. INR should be determined at least weekly during initiation of therapy and monthly when anticoagulation is stable. *(Level of Evidence: A)*
6. Aspirin, 81–325 mg daily, is recommended as an alternative to vitamin K antagonists in low risk patients or in those with contraindications to oral anticoagulation. *(Level of Evidence: A)*
7. For patients with AF who have mechanical heart valves, the target intensity of anticoagulation should be based on the type of prosthesis, maintaining an INR of at least 2.5. *(Level of Evidence: B)*
8. Antithrombotic therapy is recommended for patients with atrial flutter as for those with AF. *(Level of Evidence: C)*

Class IIa

1. For primary prevention of thromboembolism in patients with nonvalvular AF who have just 1 of the following validated risk factors, antithrombotic therapy with either aspirin or a vitamin K antagonist is reasonable, based upon an assessment of the risk of bleeding complications, ability to safely sustain adjusted chronic anticoagulation, and patient preferences: age greater than or equal to 75 y (especially in female patients), hypertension, HF, impaired LV function, or diabetes mellitus. *(Level of Evidence: A)*
2. For patients with nonvalvular AF who have 1 or more of the following less well-validated risk factors, antithrombotic therapy with either aspirin or a vitamin K antagonist is reasonable for prevention of thromboembolism: age 65 to 74 y, female gender, or CAD. The choice of agent should be based upon the risk of bleeding complications, ability to safely sustain adjusted chronic anticoagulation, and patient preferences. *(Level of Evidence: B)*
3. It is reasonable to select antithrombotic therapy using the same criteria irrespective of the pattern (i.e. paroxysmal, persistent, or permanent) of AF. *(Level of Evidence B)*
4. In patients with AF who do not have mechanical prosthetic heart valves, it is reasonable to interrupt anticoagulation for up to 1 wk without substituting heparin for surgical or diagnostic procedures that carry a risk of bleeding. *(Level of Evidence: C)*
5. It is reasonable to reevaluate the need for anticoagulation at regular intervals. *(Level of Evidence: C)*

Class IIb

1. In patients 75 y of age and older at increased risk of bleeding but without frank contraindications to oral anticoagulant therapy, and in other patients with moderate risk factors for thromboembolism who are unable to safely tolerate anticoagulation at the standard intensity of INR 2.0 to 3.0, a lower INR target of 2.0 (range 1.6 to 2.5) maybe be considered for primary prevention of ischemic stroke and systematic embolism. *(Level of Evidence: C)*
2. When surgical procedures require interruption of oral anticoagulant therapy for longer than 1 wk in high-risk patients, unfractionated heparin maybe be administered or low-molecular-weight heparin given by subcutaneous injection, although the efficacy of these alternatives in this situation is uncertain. *(Level of Evidence: C)*
3. Following percutaneous coronary intervention or revascularization surgery in patients with AF, low-dose aspirin (less than 100 mg per d) and/or clopidogrel (75 mg per d) may be given concurrently with anticoagulation to prevent myocardial ischemic events, but these strategies have not been thoroughly evaluated and are associated with an increased risk of bleeding. *(Level of Evidence: C)*

(continued)

APPENDIX 37–1

Recommendations for Management of Patients with Atrial Fibrillation *(continued)*

4. In patients undergoing percutaneous coronary intervention, anticoagulation may be interrupted to prevent bleeding at the site of peripheral arterial puncture, but the vitamin K antagonist should be resumed as soon as possible after the procedure and the dose adjusted to achieve an INR in the therapeutic range, Aspirin may be given temporarily during the hiatus, but the maintenance regimen should then consist of the combination of clopidogrel, 75 mg daily, plus warfarin (INR 2.0 to 3.0). Clopidogrel should be given for a minimum of 1 mo after implantation of the bare metal stent, at lease 3 mo for a sirolimus-eluting stent, at least 6 mo longer for a paclitaxel-eluting stent, and 12 mo or longer in selected patients, following which warfarin may be continued as monotherapy in the absence of a subsequent coronary event. When warfarin is given in combination with clopidogrel or low-dose aspirin, the dose intensity must be carefully regulated. *(Level of Evidence: C)*

5. In patients with AF younger than 60 y without heart disease or risk factors for thromboembolism (lone AF), the risk of thromboembolism is low without treatment and the effectiveness of aspirin for primary prevention of stroke relative to the risk of bleeding has not been established. *(Level of Evidence: C)*

6. In patients with AF who sustain ischemic stroke or systemic embolism during treatment with low-intensity anticoagulation (INR 2.0 to 3.0), rather than add an antiplatelet agent, it may be reasonable to raise the intensity of the anticoagulation to a maximum target INR of 3.0 to 3.5. *(Level of Evidence: C)*

Class III

Long-term anticoagulation with a vitamin K antagonist is not recommended for primary prevention of stroke in patients below the age of 60 y without heart disease (lone AF) or any risk factors for thromboembolism. *(Level of Evidence: C)*

3. *Cardioversion of Atrial Fibrillation*

a. *Pharmacological Cardioversion*

Class I

Administration of flecainide, dofetilide, propafenone, or ibutilide is recommended for pharmacological cardioversion of AF. *(Level of Evidence: A)*

Class IIa

1. Administration of amiodarone is a reasonable option for pharmacological cardioversion of AF. *(Level of Evidence: A)*

2. A single oral bolus dose of propafenone or flecainide ("pill-in-the-pocket") can be administered to terminate persistent AF outside the hospital once treatment has proved safe in hospital for selected patients without sinus or AV node dysfunction, bundle-branch block, QT interval prolongation, the Brugada syndrome, or structural heart disease. Before antiarrhythmic medication is initiated, a β blocker or nondihydropyridine calcium channel antagonist should be given to prevent rapid AV conduction in the event atrial flutter occurs. *(Level of Evidence: C)*

3. Administration of amiodarone can be beneficial on an outpatient basis in patients with paroxysmal or persistent AF when rapid restoration of sinus rhythm is not deemed necessary. *(Level of Evidence: C)*

Class IIb

Administration of quinidine or procainamide might be considered for pharmacological cardioversion of AF, but the usefulness of these agents is not well established. *(Level of Evidence: C)*

Class III

1. Digoxin and sotalol may be harmful when used for pharmacological cardioversion of AF and are not recommended. *(Level of Evidence: A)*

2. Quinidine, procainamide, disopyramide, and dofetilide should not be started out of hospital for conversion of AF to sinus rhythm. *(Level of Evidence: B)*

b. *Direct-Current Cardioversion*

Class I

1. When a rapid ventricular response does not respond promptly to pharmacological measures for patients with AF with ongoing myocardial ischemia, symptomatic hypotension, angina, or HF, immediate R-wave synchronized direct-current cardioversion is recommended. *(Level of Evidence: C)*

2. Immediate direct-current cardioversion is recommended for patients with AF involving preexcitation when very rapid tachycardia or hemodynamic instability occurs. *(Level of Evidence: B)*

3. Cardioversion is recommended in patients without hemodynamic instability when symptoms of AF are unacceptable to the patient. In case of early relapse of AF after cardioversion, repeated direct-current cardioversion attempts may be made following administration of antiarrhythmic medication. *(Level of Evidence: C)*

Class IIa

1. Direct-current cardioversion can be useful to restore sinus rhythm as part of a long-term management strategy for patients with AF. *(Level of Evidence: B)*

2. Patient preference is a reasonable consideration in the selection of infrequently repeated cardioversions for the management of symptomatic or recurrent AF. *(Level of Evidence: C)*

APPENDIX 37–1

Recommendations for Management of Patients with Atrial Fibrillation *(continued)*

Class III

1. Frequent repetition of direct-current cardioversion is not recommended for patients who have relatively short periods of sinus rhythm between relapses of AF after multiple cardioversion procedures despite prophylactic antiarrhythmic drug therapy. *(Level of Evidence: C)*

2. Electrical cardioversion is contraindicated in patients with digitalis toxicity or hypokalemia. *(Level of Evidence: C)*

c. *Pharmacological Enhancement of Direct-Current Cardioversion*

Class IIa

1. Pretreatment with amiodarone, flecainide, ibutilide, propafenone, or sotalol can be useful to enhance to the success of direct-current AF. *(Level of Evidence B)*

2. In patients who relapse to AF after successful cardioversion, it can be useful to repeat the procedure following prophylactic administration of antiarrhythmic medication. *(Level of Evidence: C)*

Class IIb

1. For patients with persistent AF administration of β blockers, disopyramide, diltiazem, dofetilide, procainamide, or verapamil maybe be considered, although the efficacy of these agents to enhance the success of direct-current cardioversion or to prevent early recurrence of AF is uncertain. *(Level of Evidence: C)*

2. Out-of-hospital initiation of antiarrhythmic medications may be considered in patients without heart disease to enhance the success of cardioversion of AF. *(Level of Evidence: C)*

3. Out-of-hospital administration of antiarrhythmic medications may be considered to enhance the success of cardioversion of AF in patients with certain forms of heart disease once the safety of the drug has been verified for the patient. *(Level of Evidence: C)*

d. *Prevention of Thromboembolism in Patients with Atrial Fibrillation Undergoing Cardioversion*

Class I

1. For patients with AF of 48-h duration of longer, or when the duration of AF is unknown, anticoagulation (INR 2.0 to 3.0) is recommended for at least 3 wk prior to and 4 wk after cardioversion , regardless of the method (electrical or pharmacological) used to restore sinus rhythm. *(Level of Evidence: B)*

2. For patients with AF or more than 48-h duration requiring immediate cardioversion because of hemodynamic instability, heparin should be administered concurrently (unless contraindicated) by an initial intravenous bolus injection followed by a continuous infusion in a dose adjusted to prolong the activated partial thromboplastin time to 1.5 to 2 times the reference control value. Thereafter, oral anticoagulation (INR 2.0 to 3.0) should be provided for at least 4 wk, as for patients undergoing elective cardioversion. Limited data support subcutaneous administration of low-molecular-weight heparin in this indication. *(Level of Evidence: C)*

3. For patients with AF of less than 48-h duration associated with hemodynamic instability (angina pectoris, myocardial infarction [MI], shock, or pulmonary edema), cardioversion should be performed immediately without delay for prior initiation of anticoagulation. *(Level of Evidence: C)*

Class IIa

1. During the 48 h after onset of AF, the need for anticoagulation before and after cardioversion maybe based on the patient's risk of thromboembolism.

2. As an alternative to anticoagulation prior to cardioversion of AF, it is reasonable to perform transesophageal echocardiography (TEE) in search of thrombus in the left atrium (LA) or left atrial appendage (LAA). *(Level of Evidence: B)*

2a. For patients with no identifiable thrombus, cardioversion is reasonable immediately after anticoagulation with unfractionated heparin (e.g., initiated by intravenous bolus injection and an infusion continued at a dose adjusted to prolong the activated partial thromboplastin time to 1.5 to 2 times the control value until oral anticoagulation has been established with an oral vitamin K antagonist (e.g., warfarin) as evidenced by an INR equal to or greater than 2.0). *(Level of Evidence: B)* Thereafter, continuation of oral anticoagulation (INR 2.0 to 3.0) is reasonable for a total anticoagulation period of at least 4 wk, as for patients undergoing elective cardioversion. *(Level of Evidence: B)* Limited data are available to support the subcutaneous administration of a low-molecular-weight heparin in this indication. *(Level of Evidence: C)*

2b. For patients in whom thrombus is identified by TEE, oral anticoagulation (INR 2.0 to 3.0) is reasonable for at least 3 wk prior to and 4 wk after restoration of sinus rhythm, and a longer period of anticoagulation may be appropriate even after apparently successful cardioversion, because the risk of thromboembolism often remains elevated in such cases. *(Level of Evidence: C)*

3. For patients with atrial flutter undergoing cardioversion, anticoagulation can be beneficial according to the recommendations as for patients with AF. *(Level of Evidence: C)*

(continued)

APPENDIX 37-1

Recommendations for Management of Patients with Atrial Fibrillation *(continued)*

4. *Maintenance of Sinus Rhythm*

Class I

Before initiating antiarrhythmic drug therapy, treatment of precipitating or reversible causes of AF is recommended. *(Level of Evidence: C)*

Class IIa

1. Pharmacological therapy can be useful in patients with AF to maintain sinus rhythm and prevent tachycardia-induced cardiomyopathy. *(Level of Evidence: C)*
2. Infrequent, well-tolerated recurrence of AF is reasonable as a successful outcome of antiarrhythmic drug therapy. *(Level of Evidence: C)*
3. Outpatient initiation of antiarrhythmic drug therapy is reasonable in patients with AF who have no associated heart disease when the agent is well-tolerated. *(Level of Evidence: C)*
4. In patients with lone AF without structural heart disease, initiation of propafenone or flecainide can be beneficial on an outpatient basis in patients with paroxysmal AF who are in sinus rhythm at the time of drug initiation. *(Level of Evidence: B)*
5. Sotalol can be beneficial to outpatients in sinus rhythm with little or no heart disease, prone to paroxysmal AF, if the baseline uncorrected QT interval is less than 460 ms, serum electrolytes are normal and risk factors associated with class III drug-related proarrhythmia are not present. *(Level of Evidence: C)*
6. Catheter ablation is a reasonable alternative to pharmacological therapy to prevent recurrent AF in symptomatic patients with little or no LA enlargement. *(Level of Evidence: C)*

Class III

1. Antiarrhythmic therapy with a particular drug is not recommended for maintenance of sinus rhythm in patients with AF who have well-defined risk factors for proarrhythmia with that agent. *(Level of Evidence: A)*
2. Pharmacological therapy is not recommended for maintenance of sinus rhythm in patients with advanced sinus node disease or atrioventricular (AV) node dysfunction unless they have a functioning electronic cardiac pacemaker. *(Level of Evidence: C)*

5. *Special Considerations*

a. *Postoperative Atrial Fibrillation*

Class I

1. Unless contraindicated, treatment with an oral β blocker to prevent postoperative AF is recommended for patients undergoing cardiac surgery. *(Level of Evidence: A)*.
2. Administration of AV nodal blocking agents is recommended to achieve rate control in patients who develop postoperative AF. *(Level of Evidence: B)*

Class IIa

1. Preoperative administration of amiodarone reduces the incidence of AF in patients undergoing cardiac surgery and represents appropriate prophylactic therapy for patients at high risk for postoperative AF. *(Level of Evidence: A)*
2. It is reasonable to restore sinus rhythm by pharmacological cardioversion in patients who develop postoperative AF as advised for nonsurgical patients. *(Level of Evidence: B)*
3. It is reasonable to administer antiarrhythmic medications in an attempt to maintain sinus rhythm in patients with recurrent or refractory postoperative AF, as recommended for other patients who develop AF. *(Level of Evidence: B)*
4. It is reasonable to administer antithrombotic medication in patients who develop postoperative AF, as recommended for nonsurgical patients. *(Level of Evidence: B)*

Class IIb

Prophylactic administration of sotalol may be considered for patients at risk of developing AF following cardiac surgery. *(Level of Evidence: B)*

b. *Acute Myocardial Infarction*

Class I

1. Direct-current cardioversion is recommended for patients with severe hemodynamic compromise or intractable ischemia, or when adequate rate control cannot be achieved with pharmacological agents in patients with acute MI and AF. *(Level of Evidence: C)*
2. Intravenous administration of amiodarone is recommended to slow a rapid ventricular response to AF and improve LV function in patients with acute MI. *(Level of Evidence: C)*
3. Intravenous β blockers and nondihydropyridine calcium antagonists are recommended to slow a rapid ventricular response to AF in patients with acute MI who do not display clinical LV dysfunction, bronchospasm, or AV block. *(Level of Evidence: C)*
4. For patients with AF and acute MI, administration of unfractionated heparin by either continuous intravenous infusion of intermittent subcutaneous injection is recommended in a dose sufficient to prolong the activated partial thromboplastin time to 1.5 to 2 times the control value, unless contraindications to anticoagulation exist. *(Level of Evidence: C)*

APPENDIX 37–1

Recommendations for Management of Patients with Atrial Fibrillation *(continued)*

Class IIa

Intravenous administration of digitalis is reasonable to slow a rapid ventricular response and improve LV function in patients with acute MI and AF associated with severe LV dysfunction and HF. *(Level of Evidence: C)*

Class III

The administration of class IC antiarrhythmic drugs is not recommended in patients with AF in the setting of acute MI. *(Level of Evidence: C)*

c. *Management of Atrial Fibrillation Associated With the Wolff-Parkinson-White (WPW) Preexcitation Syndrome*

Class I

1. Catheter ablation of the accessory pathway is recommended in symptomatic patients with AF who have WPW syndrome, particularly those with syncope due to rapid heart rate or those with a short bypass tract refractory period. *(Level of Evidence: B)*
2. Immediate direct-current cardioversion is recommended to prevent ventricular fibrillation in patients with a short anterograde bypass tract refractory period in whom AF occurs with a rapid ventricular response associated with hemodynamic instability. *(Level of Evidence: B)*
3. Intravenous procainamide or ibutilide is recommended to restore sinus rhythm in patients with WPW in whom AF occurs without hemodynamic instability in association with a wide QRS complex on the electrocardiogram (ECG) (greater than or equal to 120-ms duration) or with a rapid preexcited ventricular response. *(Level of Evidence: C)*

Class IIa

Intravenous flecainide or direct-current cardioversion is reasonable when very rapid ventricular rates occur in patients with AF involving conduction over an accessory pathway. *(Level of Evidence: B)*

Class IIb

It may be quite reasonable to administer intravenous quinidine, procainamide, disopyramide, ibutilide, or amiodarone to hemodynamically stable patients with AF involving conduction over an accessory pathway. *(Level of Evidence: B)*

Class III

Intravenous administration of digitalis glycosides or nondihydropyridine calcium channel antagonists is not recommended in patients with WPW syndrome who have preexcited ventricular activation during AF. *(Level of Evidence: B)*

d. *Hyperthyroidism*

Class I

1. Administration of a β blocker is recommended to control the rate of a ventricular response in patients with AF complicating thyrotoxicosis, unless contraindicated. *(Level of Evidence: B)*
2. In circumstances when a β blocker cannot be used, administration of a nondihydropyridine calcium channel antagonist (diltiazem or verapamil) is recommended to control the ventricular rate in patients with AF and thyrotoxicosis. *(Level of Evidence: B)*
3. In patients with AF associated with thyrotoxicosis, oral anticoagulation (INR 2.0 to 3.0) is recommended to prevent thromboembolism, as recommended for AF patients with other risk factors for stroke. *(Level of Evidence: C)*
4. Once a euthyroid state is restored, recommendations for antithrombotic prophylaxis are the same as for patients without hyperthyroidism. *(Level of Evidence: C)*

e. *Management of Atrial Fibrillation during Pregnancy*

Class I

1. Digoxin, a β blocker, or a nondihydropyridine calcium channel antagonist is recommended to control the rate of ventricular response in pregnant patients with AF. *(Level of Evidence: C)*
2. Direct-current cardioversion is recommended in pregnant patients who become hemodynamically unstable due to AF *(Level of Evidence: C)*
3. Protection against thromboembolism is recommended throughout pregnancy for all patients with AF (except for those with lone AF and/or low thromboembolic risk). Therapy (anticoagulant or aspirin) should be chose according to stage of pregnancy. *(Level of Evidence: C)*

Class IIb

1. Administration of heparin may be considered during the first trimester and last month of pregnancy for patients with AF and risk factors for thromboembolism. Unfractionated heparin may be administered either by continuous intravenous infusion in a dose sufficient to prolong the activated partial thromboplastin time to 1.5 to 2 times the control value or by intermittent subcutaneous injection in a dose of 10,000 to 20,000 units every 12 h adjusted to prolong the mid-interval (6 h after injection) activated partial thromboplastin time to 1.5 times control. *(Level of Evidence: B)*

(continued)

APPENDIX 37-1

Recommendations for Management of Patients with Atrial Fibrillation *(continued)*

2. Despite the limited data available, subcutaneous administration of low-molecular-weight heparin may be considered during the first trimester and last month of pregnancy for patients with AF and risk factors for thromboembolism. *(Level of Evidence: C)*

3. Administration of an oral anticoagulant may be considered during the second trimester for pregnant patients with AF at high thromboembolic risk. *(Level of Evidence: C)*

4. Administration of quinidine or procainamide may be considered to achieve pharmacological cardioversion in hemodynamically stable patients who develop AF during pregnancy. *(Level of Evidence: C)*

f. *Management of Atrial Fibrillation in Patients with Hypertrophic Cardiomyopathy (HCM)*

   Class I

   Oral anticoagulation (INR 2.0 to 3.0) is recommended in patients with HCM who develop AF, as for other patients at high risk of thromboembolism. *(Level of Evidence: B)*

   Class IIa

   Antiarrhythmic medications can be useful to prevent recurrent AF in patients with HCM. Available data are insufficient to recommend one agent over another in this situation, but (a) disopyramide combined with a β blocker or nondihydropyridine calcium channel antagonist or (b) amiodarone alone is generally preferred. *(Level of Evidence: C)*

g. *Management of Atrial Fibrillation in Patients with Pulmonary Disease*

   Class I

   1. Correction of hypoxemia and acidosis is the recommended primary therapeutic measure for patients who develop AF during an acute pulmonary illness or exacerbation of chronic pulmonary disease. *(Level of Evidence: C)*

   2. A nondihydropyridine calcium channel antagonist (diltiazem or verapamil) is recommended to control the ventricular rate in patients with obstructive pulmonary disease who develop AF. *(Level of Evidence: C)*

   3. Direct-current cardioversion should be attempted in patients with pulmonary disease who become hemodynamically unstable as a consequence of AF. *(Level of Evidence: C)*

   Class III

   1. Theophylline and β-adrenergic agonist agents are not recommended in patients with bronchospastic lung disease who develop AF. *(Level of Evidence: C)*

   2. β blockers, sotalol, propafenone, and adenosine are not recommended in patients with obstructive lung disease who develop AF *(Level of Evidence: C)*

SOURCE: From Fuster V, Rydén LE, Cannom DS, et al. ACC/AHA/ESC 2006 guidelines for the management of patients with atrial fibrillation: a report of the American College of Cardiology/American Heart Association Task Force on Practice Guidelines and the European Society of Cardiology Committee for Practice Guidelines (Writing Committee to Revise the 2001 Guidelines for the Management of Patients with Atrial Fibrillation). Circulation 2006;114:e257–354.

CHAPTER 38

Supraventricular Tachycardia: AV Nodal Reentry and Wolff-Parkinson-White Syndrome

Hugh Calkins

Supraventricular tachycardias (SVTs) include all tachyarrhythmias that either originate from or incorporate supraventricular tissue in a reentrant circuit. The ventricular rate may be the same or less than the atrial rate, depending on the atrioventricular (AV) nodal conduction. The term *paroxysmal supraventricular tachycardia* (PSVT) refers to a clinical syndrome characterized by a rapid, regular tachycardia with abrupt onset and termination. Approximately two-thirds of cases of PSVT result from AV nodal reentrant tachycardia (AVNRT). Orthodromic AV reciprocating tachycardia (AVRT), which involves an accessory pathway, is the second most common cause of PSVT, accounting for approximately one-third of cases. The term *Wolff-Parkinson-White syndrome* (WPW) designates a condition comprising both preexcitation and tachyarrhythmias. Atrial tachycardias, which arise exclusively from atrial tissue, account for approximately 5 percent of all cases of PSVT.[1-3] The purpose of this chapter is to review the mechanism, clinical features, and approach to diagnosis and treatment of AVNRT and accessory pathway–mediated tachycardias (including the WPW syndrome). Particular attention is focused on reviewing management guidelines developed by the American Heart Association, the American College of Cardiology (ACC), and also the Heart Rhythm Society (formerly known as the North American Society of Pacing and Electrophysiology).

ATRIOVENTRICULAR NODAL REENTRANT TACHYCARDIA

AVNRT is an important arrhythmia for several reasons. First, AVNRT is extremely common. Studies report that AVNRT occurs in approximately 10 percent of the general population and accounts for up to two-thirds of all cases of PSVT.[4] Although AVNRT can occur at any age, it is extremely uncommon prior to the age of 5 years. The usual age of onset is beyond the fourth decade and is later than the usual age of onset of accessory pathway-mediated tachycardias.[4-10] Women are affected twice as often as men.[6-10] A second reason for the importance of AVNRT is the fact that it can result in significant debility and decreased quality of life.[11]

⟦ ⟧ PATHOPHYSIOLOGIC BASIS OF ATRIOVENTRICULAR NODAL REENTRANT TACHYCARDIA

Anatomic Considerations of the Atrioventricular Node

Early descriptions of the AV nodal tissue came from Albert Kent more than a century ago.[12] The AV node is located epicardially, just underlying the right atrial epicardium, anterior to the nodal artery and between the coronary sinus and medial tricuspid valve leaflet. It comprises three different components: the transitional cell zone, the compact node, and the penetrating bundle of His (Fig. 38–1). The *compact* AV node refers to the most easily histologically distinguishable tissue located at the apex of the triangle of Koch (TOK). A zone of transitional cells is interposed between the compact node and the atrial myocardium. Transitional cells enter the triangle of Koch to join the compact node superiorly, inferiorly, posteriorly, and from the left. At its distal extent, the AV node is distinguished from the penetrating bundle, not so much by cellular characteristics as by the presence of a fibrous collar surrounding the specialized cells. Systematic anatomic investigation of the AV node in patients with AVNRT is lacking. No obvious histologic abnormalities have been identified among patients with AVNRT versus patients without AVNRT. Several recent autopsy studies have reported that the sites of successful slow pathway ablation were clearly away from the histologic compact AV node, approximately 1 or 2 cm inferior and posterior to it.[13–16]

Concept of Dual Pathways

The concept of dual AV nodal physiology was introduced by Moe and coworkers in the 1950s in an effort to explain AVNRT.[17] It was proposed that dual AV node physiology results from functional dissociation within the compact node into fast and slow pathways. Moe and colleagues went on to propose that AVNRT resulted from reentry within the AV node involving the fast and slow pathways. Subsequently, several investigators developed a catheter-based ablative technique that used direct current shocks[18,19] or radiofrequency energy[20–22] to eliminate the fast AV pathway and permanently eliminate AVNRT. Despite the excellent results of this procedure, it was complicated by a small but definite risk of AV block. A technique to interrupt slow pathway conduction without affecting normal AV conduction through the fast pathway by ablating small segments of myocardium in the posterior septum near the coronary sinus ostium was subsequently described.[5] This experience paved the way for the current approach using catheter ablation of this arrhythmia.[23–28]

Types of Atrioventricular Nodal Reentrant Tachycardia

Three types of AVNRT have been described (Table 38–1). Typical or slow/fast AVNRT is the most prevalent type, accounting for 85 to 90 percent of cases. Representing the other 10 to 15 percent of cases, atypical AVNRT can be further differentiated into fast/slow and slow/slow (or intermediate) AVNRT. Induction of typical and atypical AVNRT in the same patient is possible but unusual. The typical or slow/fast AVNRT is thought

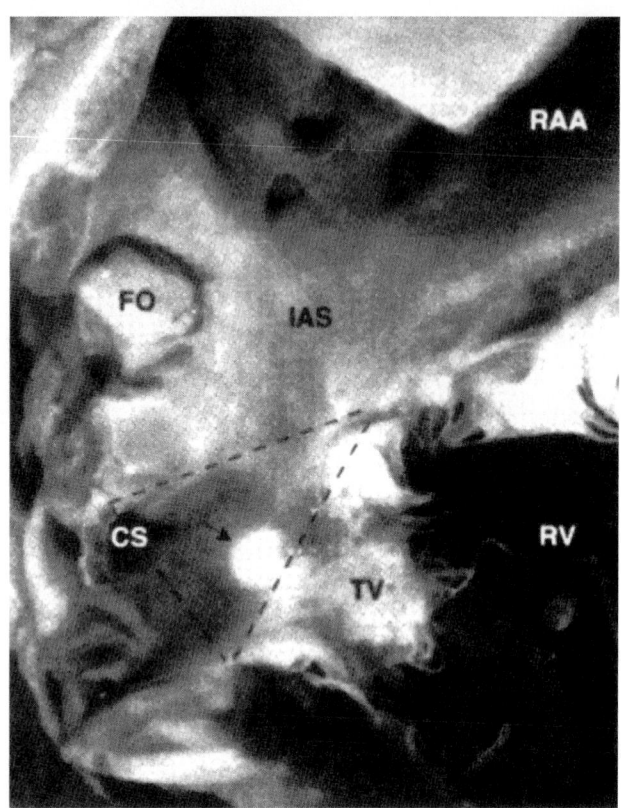

A

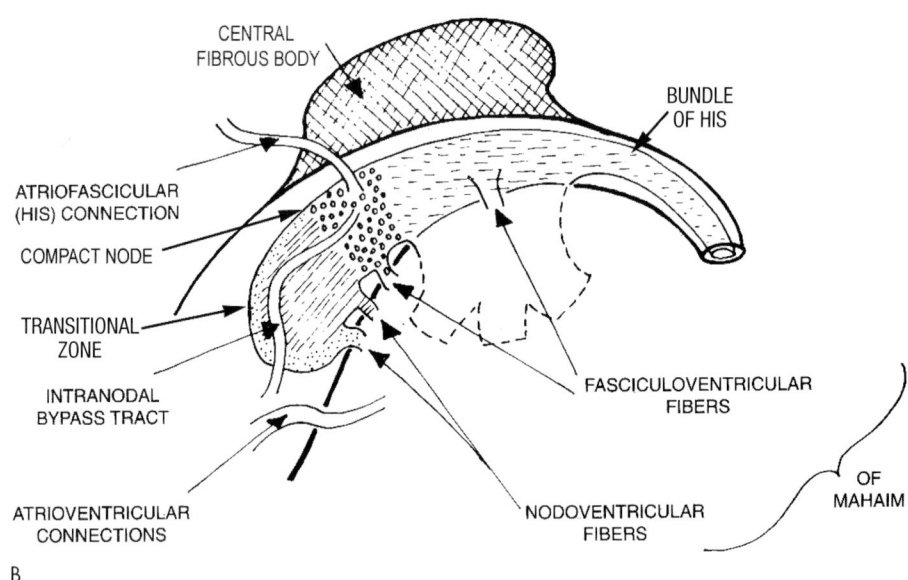

B

FIGURE 38–1. Structure of the atrioventricular (AV) node. **A.** Heart specimen from patient with AVNRT. Koch triangle is formed by tendon of Todaro, coronary sinus (CS), ostium, and septal attachment of tricuspid valve (TV). *Arrow* represents site of successful ablation. AVNRT, atrioventricular nodal reentrant tachycardia; IAS, interatrial septum; RV, right ventricle; FO, fossa ovalis; RAA, right atrial appendage. **B.** Schematic drawing depicting the three zones of the AV node and various types of perinodal and atrioventricular bypass tracts. *Sources: A, From Olgin JE, Ursell P, Kao AK, et al.[13] B, From McManus BM, Harji S, Wood SM. Morphologic features of normal and abnormal conductions systems. In: Singer I, ed. Interventional Electrophysiology. 2nd ed. New York: Lippincott Williams & Wilkins; 2001:23. With permission.*

to use the slow pathway for antegrade conduction and the fast pathway for retrograde conducion (Fig. 38–2). When an atrial premature complex blocks the fast pathway and proceeds slowly along the slow pathway, the fast pathway has enough time to re-

Differential Diagnosis for Types of Supraventricular Tachycardia Based on ECG Characteristics

I. Long–R-P tachycardia: R-P ≥ P-R
  i. Atypical AV nodal reentrant tachycardia
  ii. Atrial tachycardia
  iii. AVRT with a slowly conducting pathway (e.g., PJRT)
  iv. Sinus node reentry
  v. Sinus tachycardia
II. Short–R-P tachycardia R-P < P-R
  i. Typical AVNRT
  ii. AV reentry

AV, atrioventricular; AVNRT, atrioventricular nodal reentrant tachycardia; PJRT, permanent junctional reciprocating tachycardia.

cover from its refractoriness. This allows the impulse to activate the fast pathway retrogradely and return to the atrium, giving rise to an AV nodal reentrant echo beat. The impulse then travels down along the slow pathway again, continuation giving rise to AVNRT. It has been proposed that the fast/slow AVNRT uses the fast pathway for anterograde conduction and the slow pathway for retrograde conduction. The slow/slow AVNRT, conversely, requires presence of two or more slow pathways with different conduction properties and refractory periods; one slow pathway is used for antegrade conduction and the other slow pathway for retrograde conduction.

【 】 DIAGNOSIS

Clinical Features

Patients with AVNRT typically present with the clinical syndrome of paroxysmal supraventricular tachycardia.[20,29] Episodes may last from seconds to several hours. Patients often learn to use certain maneuvers such as carotid sinus massage or the Valsalva maneuver to terminate the arrhythmia, but many require pharmacologic treatment to achieve this. There is no significant association of AVNRT with other types of structural heart disease. The physical examination is usually remarkable only for a rapid, regular heart rate. At times, because of the simultaneous contraction of atria and ventricles, cannon A waves can be seen.

Electrocardiographic Characteristics

AVNRT is characterized by a tachycardia with a narrow QRS complex with sudden onset and termination generally at regular rates between 120 and 200 beats/min. Uncommonly, the rate can be as low as 110 beats/min; and occasionally, especially in children, it may exceed 200 beats/min. The rate of tachycardia may vary from episode to episode. In typical or slow/fast AVNRT, anterograde AV node conduction usually exceeds 200 msec. Because the retrograde conduction is through the fast pathway, the VA interval is short, resulting in superimposition of the P wave onto the QRS complex on the surface ECG. Usually, the P wave is obscured by the QRS or may be seen slightly before or after the QRS complex. The pres-

ence of a pseudo r wave in lead V$_1$ or pseudo S wave in leads II, III, and aVF suggests typical AVNRT (Fig. 38–3). Because of fast retrograde conduction, the R-P interval is shorter than the P-R interval.

In atypical fast/slow or slow/slow AVNRT, the AH interval is relatively short and the HA interval long. The P wave on surface ECG hence can be well delineated and is inverted in II, III, and aVF. The R-P interval is equal to or longer than the P-R interval (Fig. 38–4). This is one of the causes of *long R-P* tachycardia (see Table 38–1).

Functional bundle-branch block may develop, producing a wide QRS tachycardia. However, functional bundle-branch block should not affect the rate of tachycardia. Less commonly, dual pathways can be manifest on the ECG during sinus rhythm by sudden prolongation of the P-R interval, P-R alternans, and two QRS complexes in response to a single P wave[30] (Fig. 38–5).

Other ECG changes may be seen during or after the termination of AVNRT. Significant ST-segment depressions can be observed during tachycardia in nearly 25 to 50 percent of patients with AVNRT, and this is not predictive of ischemia.

Newly acquired T-wave inversions after termination of AVNRT, commonly in anterior or inferior leads, can be seen in nearly 40 percent of patients.[31] They may be seen immediately after termination of tachycardia or may develop within 6 hours,

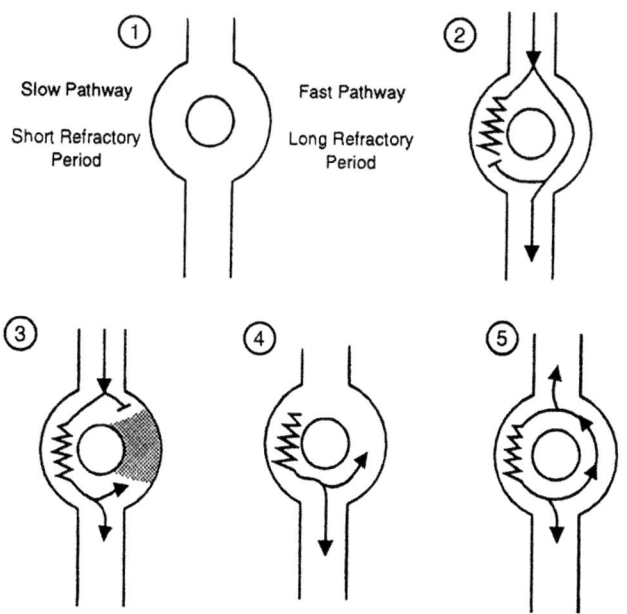

FIGURE 38–2. Schematic drawing showing dual atrioventricular (AV) nodal conduction. **1.** The two AV nodal pathways, one with fast conduction and a relatively long refractory period and a second with slower conduction and shorter refractory period. **2.** During sinus rhythm, impulses are conducted over both pathways but reach the bundle of His through the fast pathway. **3.** A premature atrial impulse finds the fast pathway still refractory and is conducted over the slow pathway. **4,5.** If the fast pathway has enough time to recover excitability, the impulse may reenter the fast pathway retrogradely and establish reentry. *Source: Modified from Fogel RI, Prystowsky EN. Atrioventricular nodal reentry. In: Podrid PJ, Kowey PR, eds. Cardiac Arrhythmia: Mechanisms, Diagnosis and Management. New York: Lippincott Williams & Wilkins; 2001:436. With permission.*

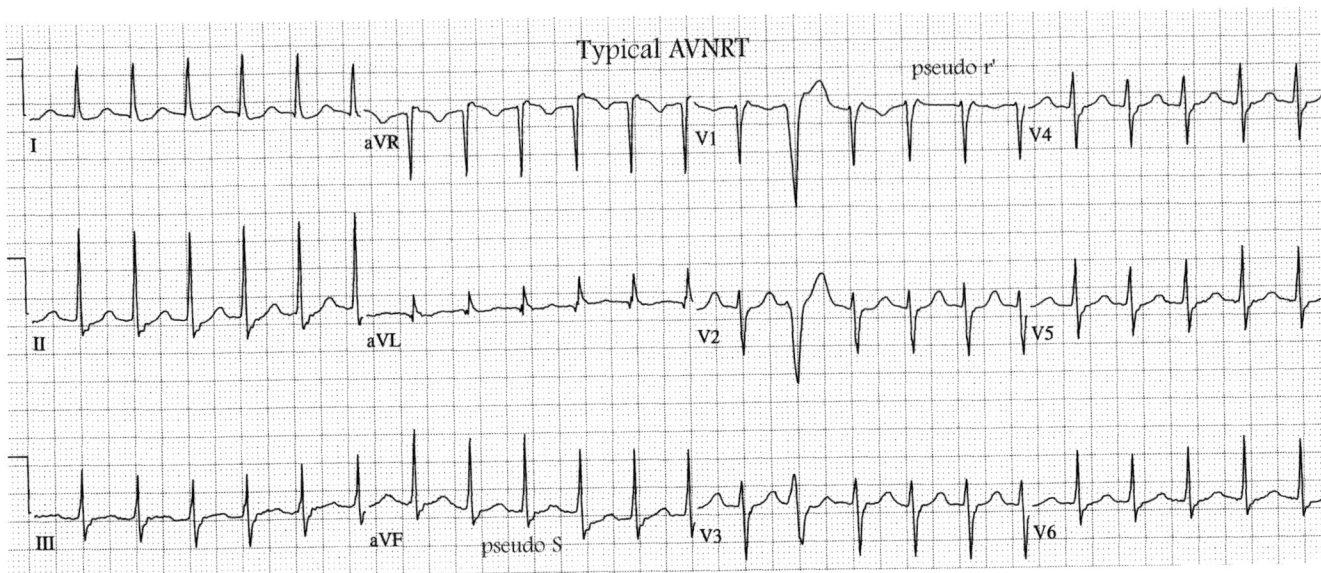

FIGURE 38–3. Twelve-lead ECG of a patient with typical AVNRT. Note the pseudo r and pseudo S waves, very typical of this arrhythmia.

and they can persist for a variable duration. This occurrence is also not related to rate or duration of tachycardia. This is also not the result of coronary artery disease but due to repolarization abnormalities, probably because of ionic current alterations resulting from the rapid rate.

A beat-to-beat oscillation in the QRS amplitude (i.e., QRS alternans) can be observed, although uncommonly, during episodes of AVNRT. Studies have reported that QRS alternans is observed more frequently in association with accessory pathway–mediated tachycardias than during AVNRT.[32,33]

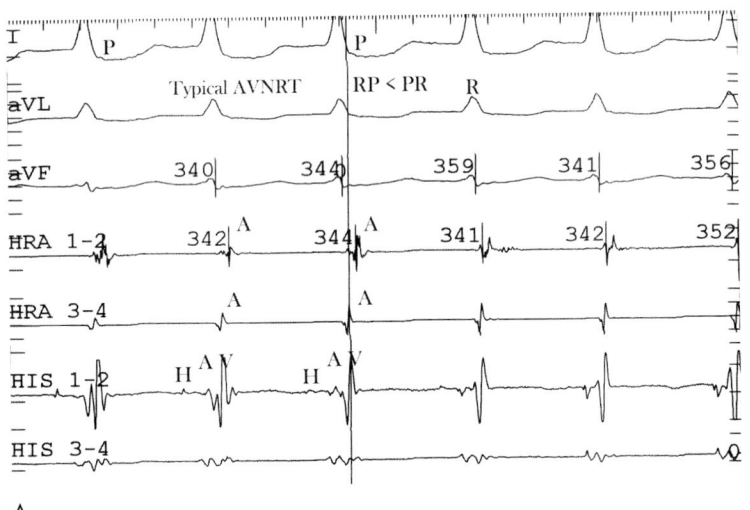

A

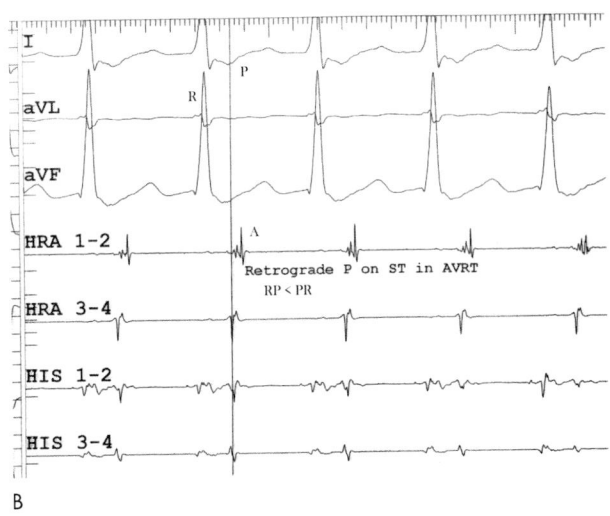

B

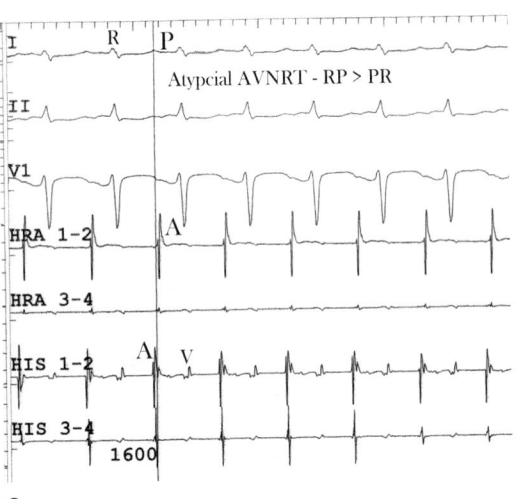

C

FIGURE 38–4. Surface ECG and intracardiac electrograms shown simultaneously in three different PSVTs. The vertical line in each of the panels shows the onset of atrial depolarization to indicate the timing of the P wave relative to the QRS. **A.** Typical AVNRT. **B.** AVRT involving an accessory pathway. **C.** Atypical AVNRT. R and P denote the corresponding waves on the surface ECG. A, atrial; AVNRT, atrioventricular nodal reentrant tachycardia; HRA, high right atrium; PSVT, paroxysmal supraventricular tachycardia; V, ventricular deflection.

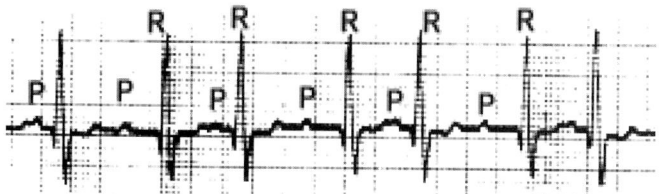

FIGURE 38–5. Rhythm strip of a patient during sinus rhythm. Note the sudden alternation of the P-R interval from beat to beat. P-R alternans is a manifestation of dual atrioventricular (AV) node physiology.

Electrophysiologic Testing

Dual AV nodal physiology can be demonstrated by two pacing techniques. Atrial pacing with introduction of PACs with increasing prematurity shows a gradual and progressive conduction delay in the AH interval. At a critical atrial coupling interval, a 10-msec decrement in the A_1A_2 results in a marked (>50-msec) prolongation of the A_2H_2 interval. It is a well-accepted convention that a 50-msec or greater increase in the AH interval in response to a 10-msec shortening of the A_1A_2 is considered evidence of dual AV node physiology. A plot of the A_1A_2 versus the A_2H_2 or the A_2H_2 versus the H_1H_2 shows a discontinuous curve (Fig. 38–6). The fast pathway has a shorter conduction time and longer refractory period and that the slow pathway has a longer conduction time and shorter refractory period. The abrupt increase in AV nodal conduction time is caused by block in the conduction of fast pathway with a selective conduction over the slow pathway (Fig. 38–7). Some patients with AVNRT may not have discontinuous refractory period curves and some patients without AVNRT can exhibit discontinuous refractory period curves. It has been estimated that *dual AV node physiology* is present in approximately 10 percent of the general population. Such existence in the latter patients is a benign finding. Multiple AV nodal pathways can be demonstrated in occasional patients. More than one pathway may be involved in clinical tachycardia. The development of a P-R interval that is greater than the atrial pacing cycle length during stable 1:1 AV conduction is a quite specific sign of slow AV nodal conduction.

Typical AVNRT is usually not inducible with ventricular pacing, whereas this is the rule with atypical AVNRT. Lack of reproducible arrhythmia induction is most often caused by block in retrograde fast pathway. Other causes include slow-pathway block and inability to achieve a critical delay in the AH interval.

During typical AVNRT the atrial and ventricular activation is nearly simultaneous, hence causing short AH intervals. An AH interval of <70 msec is virtually diagnostic of AVNRT[34] (see Fig. 38–7). Differentiation of AVNRT, particularly of the atypical type, from other forms of SVT can be challenging, requiring the use of several maneuvers at electrophysiologic study (EPS).[35]

[ ] MANAGEMENT

Because AVNRT is generally a benign arrhythmia that does not influence survival, the main reason for treating it is to alleviate symptoms. The threshold for initiation of therapy varies based on patient preference and also on the frequency and duration of the

episodes of tachycardia as well as the associated symptoms. The threshold for treatment also reflects whether the patient is a competitive athlete, a woman considering pregnancy, or someone with a high-risk occupation such as scuba diving. The North American Society for Pacing and Electrophysiology has recently developed a policy statement on catheter ablation. The recommendations made by this task force are reviewed at the end of this section.

Acute Management

The dependence of AVNRT on AV nodal conduction has important therapeutic implications. Because of the known influence of autonomic tone on AV nodal conduction, maneuvers that increase vagal tone, such as the Valsalva and Mueller maneuvers, gagging, carotid sinus massage, and occasionally exposing the face to ice water can been used to terminate the tachycardia. The effect of vagal maneuvers is most pronounced on the slow pathway.[34] Hence, in the slow/fast form of AVNRT, the tachycardia typically terminates in the anterograde direction; in the fast/slow type of AVNRT, the block is in the retrograde limb of the tachycardia circuit.

Adenosine, a purinergic blocking agent that causes acute and transient AV nodal blockade, is the drug of choice for acute termination of AVNRT. Multiple studies have shown that adenosine is nearly 100 percent effective in terminating AVNRT.[36,37] It has a rapid onset of action (seconds) and a short half life (<10 sec); moreover, it does not impair contractility. When used for termination of a narrow-complex tachycardia, an initial dose of 6 mg may be followed by 12 mg if the first dose is ineffective. Because of its short duration of action, it is essential that adenosine be administered as a rapid bolus. This is best achieved by having a syringe with adenosine and a 5-mL flush attached to the patient using a stopcock. In this fashion the dose of adenosine can be

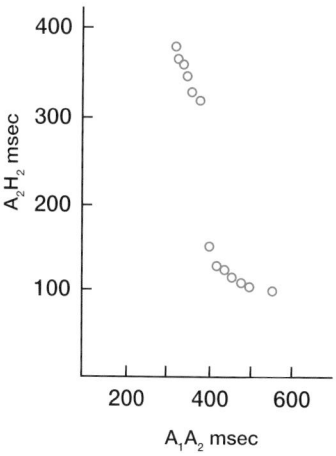

FIGURE 38–6. Atrioventricular (AV) nodal function curve in a patient with dual AV nodal physiology. As the coupling interval of A_1A_2 is progressively decreased, there is a progressive prolongation of A_2H_2 intervals. At a coupling interval of around 360 msec, there is a large jump in the A_2H_2 interval. This is caused by the fast pathway effectively reaching refractoriness at 360 msec and conduction proceeding over the slow pathway, which has a shorter refractory period but slower conduction. *Source: Modified with permission from Josephson M. Supraventricular tachycardias. In: Josephson M, ed. Clinical Cardiac Electrophysiology: Technique and Interpretation, 3rd ed. New York: Lippincott Williams & Wilkins, 2002:173.*

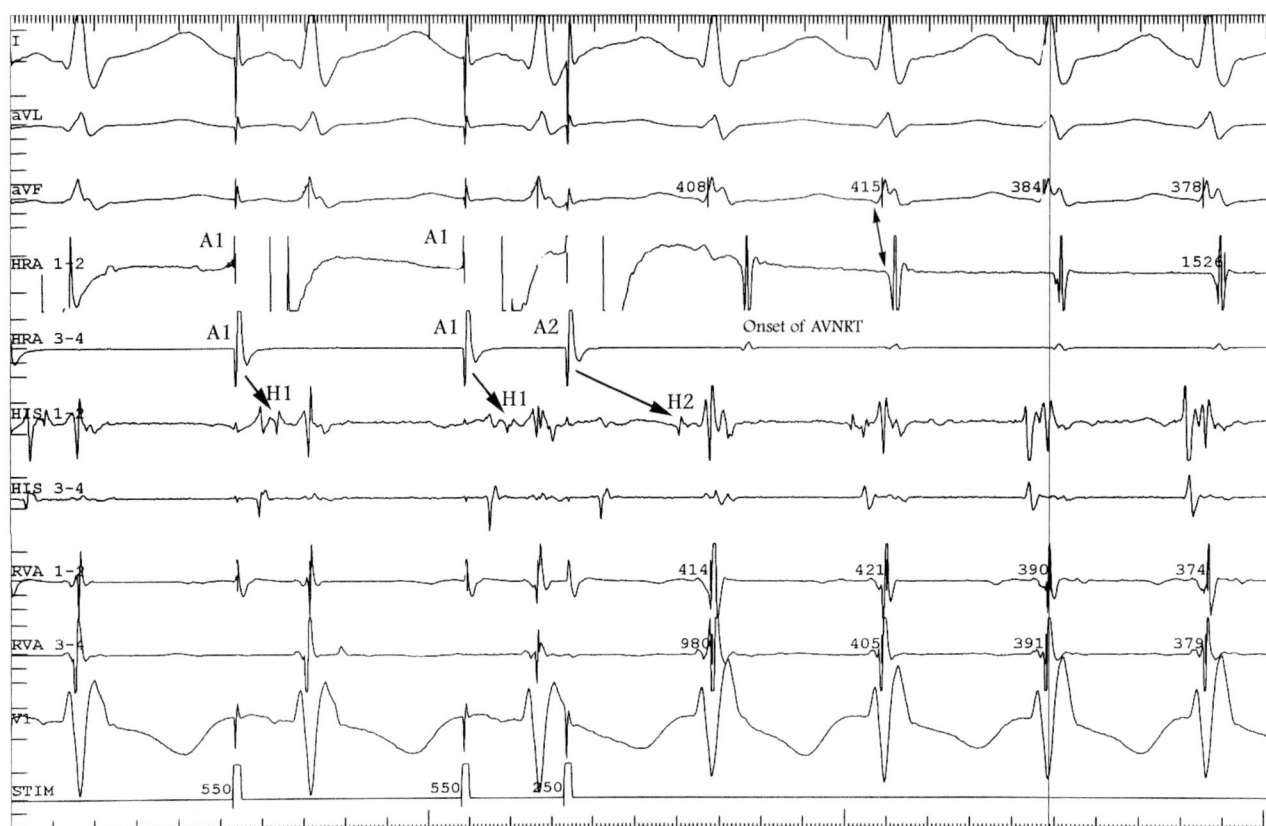

FIGURE 38–7. Electrophysiologic demonstration of dual atrioventricular nodal physiology and initiation of AVNRT. At an A_1A_2 coupling interval of 350 msec, there is a jump in the A_2H_2 interval (*arrows*). This is followed by initiation of tachycardia. Note the very short VA conduction time. A, atrial; AVNRT, atrioventricular nodal reentrant tachycardia; HRA, high right atrium.

followed immediately by a saline flush to ensure rapid delivery of the drug. Minor side effects, including transient dyspnea or chest pain, are common with adenosine. Sinus arrest or bradycardia may occur but resolve quickly if appropriate upward dosing is used. With termination of PSVT, atrial and ventricular premature beats are frequently seen; a few patients with adenosine-induced polymorphic ventricular tachycardia have been reported.[36] These patients had long baseline QT intervals and long pauses during adenosine-induced AV block. Adenosine shortens the atrial refractory period, and atrial ectopy may induce atrial fibrillation. This may be dangerous if the patient has an accessory pathway capable of rapid antegrade conduction. Because adenosine is cleared so rapidly, reinitiation of tachycardia after initial termination may occur. Either repeat administration of the same dose of adenosine or substitution of a calcium channel blocker will be effective. Adenosine mediates its effects via a specific cell surface receptor, the A_1 receptor. Theophylline and other methylxanthines block the A_1 receptor. Caffeine levels achieved after beverage ingestion may be overcome by the doses of adenosine used to treat PSVT.[38] Dipyridamole blocks adenosine elimination, thereby potentiating and prolonging its effects. Adenosine is also shown to produce faster termination of SVT in the presence of isoproterenol.[37] Cardiac transplant recipients are also unusually sensitive to adenosine. If adenosine is chosen in these latter situations, much lower starting doses (i.e., 1 mg) should be selected. Adenosine should also be used with great caution in patients with a history of asthma, as it may trigger bronchospasm.

Several other drugs that affect the AV node can also be used for acute termination of AVNRT. Verapamil, a calcium channel blocker, can terminate AVNRT and prevent induction. It slows conduction both in the slow and fast pathways, and termination is usually caused by anterograde block. A 5-mg bolus of verapamil may be followed by one or two additional 5-mg boluses 10 minutes apart if the initial dose does not terminate the tachycardia; this has been an effective regimen in up to 90 percent of patients.[37] Drugs that enhance vagal tone, such as digoxin, or that block the sympathetic effect, like β blockers, can also be used to terminate AVNRT.[39,40] Digoxin, which has a slower onset of action than the other AV nodal blockers, is not favored for the acute termination of AVNRT except if there are relative contraindications to the other agents. Class Ia and Class Ic sodium-channel blockers can also be employed in treating an acute event of AVNRT—a strategy that is rarely used when other regimens have failed. Unlike the other agents, the sodium-channel blocking agents depress retrograde fast-pathway conduction. If a patient's tachycardia cannot be terminated with intravenous drugs, direct-current shock cardioversion can always be used. Energies in the range of 10 to 50 J are usually adequate.

Long-Term Management

Catheter Ablation Catheter ablation of AVNRT is performed by ablating the slowly conducting portion of the AV node using the *posterior approach.* Once the diagnosis of AVNRT is established and the endpoint for ablation defined (either the presence of dual AV node physiology or reproducibly inducible AVNRT), the ablation catheter is positioned across the tricuspid valve at the level of the coronary sinus (CS) ostium (Fig. 38–8). The ablation catheter is then slowly withdrawn with clockwise catheter torque until a small multicomponent atrial electrogram is observed together with a large ventricular electrogram. The most common site of successful ablation is at the level of the superior aspect of the CS ostium[4,41] (see Fig. 38–8). In patients with unusual forms of AVNRT, the site of successful ablation is slightly inferior to the CS ostium or, at times, within the floor of the CS. Once an appropriate site is identified, radiofrequency (RF) energy is applied. The development of a junctional rhythm during RF application is a marker for a successful ablation site. If a junctional rhythm develops, VA conduction should be monitored carefully; if VA or AV conduction block is observed, RF energy should immediately be discontinued.

Successful ablation of AVNRT with the posterior approach is usually characterized by an increase in the AV block cycle length and in the AV nodal effective refractory period; a normal P-R interval on ECG and lack of inducibility of AVNRT both at baseline and during isoproterenol infusion are also seen. Retrograde conduction is generally not affected. The presence of >1 AV nodal echo beat or a P-R prolongation that exceeds the paced atrial cycle length during stable 1:1 AV conduction suggest that the AVNRT is likely to recur and will require further RF applications.

This technique was initially described by Jackman and coworkers[5] nearly a decade ago and has since been widely accepted as the standard approach. Calkins and colleagues[10] reported the largest multicenter experience with the posterior approach. In this trial of >1000 patients with AV tachycardias, 373 patients had AVNRT. The overall success rate of ablation was 97 percent. AV block is the most common complication, occurring in 0.5 to 1 percent of patients. The incidence of recurrence after successful ablation is approximately 3 percent. Because of the higher efficacy and lower incidence of AV block and arrhythmia recurrence and the greater likelihood of maintaining a normal P-R interval during sinus rhythm, the posterior approach is now considered the preferred approach to ablation of AVNRT.[23–27,42–45]

In the past several years cryoablation has become available as an alternative energy source for creation of myocardial lesions which can be used for treatment of AVNRT. The main advantage of cryoenergy, as compared to radiofrequency energy, is that the risk

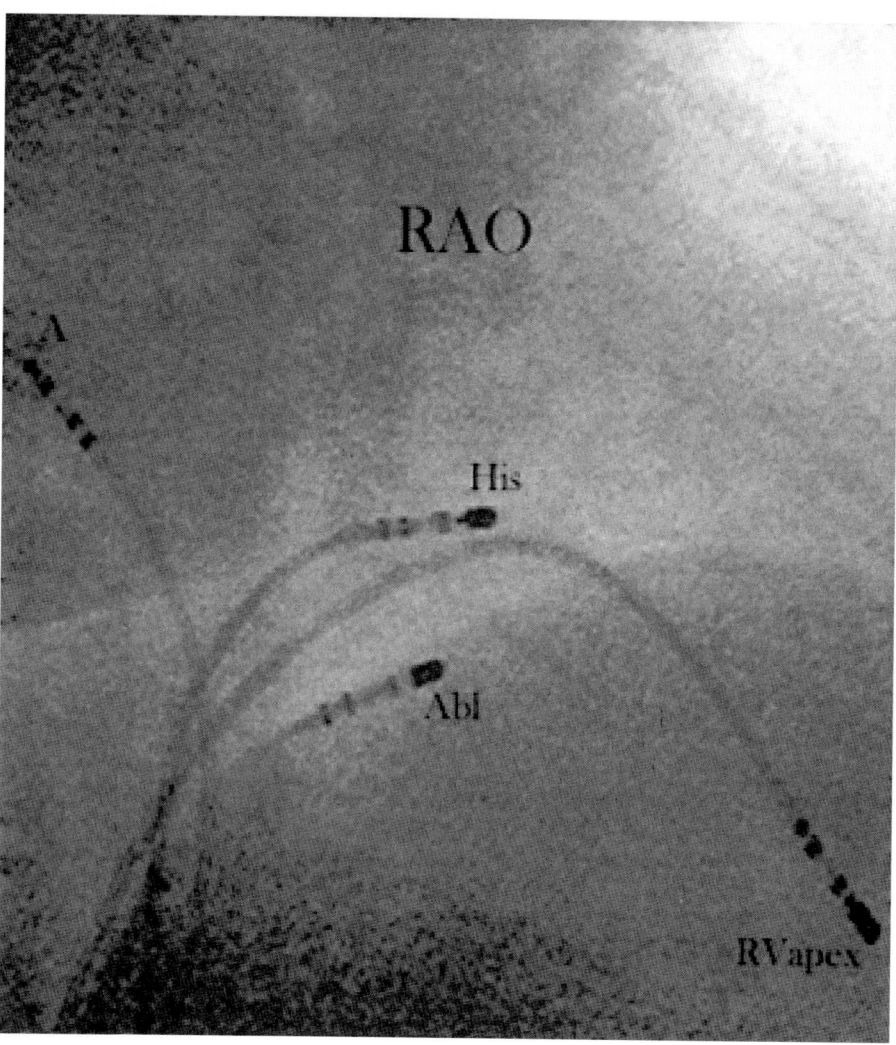

A

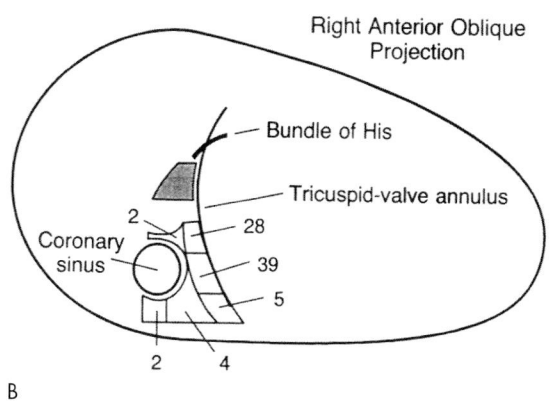

B

FIGURE 38–8. Site of slow-pathway ablation for AVNRT. **A.** Fluoroscopic images showing the alignment of the catheters during slow-pathway ablation. Note that the site of the slow pathway is a considerable distance from the site of the His bundle or compact atrioventricular node. **B.** Schematic showing the orientation of heart during corresponding fluoroscopic projection. The numbers represent the sites of successful slow-pathway ablation in corresponding patients. AVNRT, atrioventricular nodal reentrant tachycardia; RAO, right anterior oblique. *Source: Modified from Jackman WM, Beckman KJ, McClelland JH, et al.[5] With permission.*

of heart block appears to be lower.[46,47] This potential benefit must be balanced against longer procedure times and lower acute and long-term efficacy. Because of the implications of heart block in children, cryoablation has now become the preserved energy source for treatment of AVNRT in children.[46,47] In contrast, radiofrequency energy has remained the dominant ablation energy source for treatment of AVNRT in adults. This may change over time because data has emerged suggesting that higher acute and long-term success rates for catheter ablation of AVNRT with cryo-energy can be achieved by using larger ablation electrodes (6 mm vs. 4 mm).[48] Hopefully a randomized trial will be performed in the future to resolve this issue.

Medical Therapy Most pharmacologic agents that depress AV nodal conduction may be demonstrated to reduce the frequency of recurrences of AVNRT. These pharmacologic agents include β blockers, calcium channel blockers, class 1a antiarrhythmic agents such as procainamide and disopyramide, class 1c antiarrhythmic agents such as flecainide and propafenone, and class 3 antiarrhythmic agents such as sotalol (Betapace) and amiodarone. The best studied among these have been the class Ic antiarrhythmic agents.[49-55]

Henthorn and coworkers[49] studied 34 patients with PSVT, many of whom had documented or suspected AVNRT. Flecainide in doses up to 200 mg twice a day prevented recurrent tachycardia in 79 percent at 60 days, compared to 15 percent in the placebo arm ($p < 0.001$). The median time to the first recurrence of tachycardia increased from 11 days in the placebo arm to 55 days in the treated patients ($p < 0.001$). In dose-ranging studies, flecainide was effective in preventing SVT over a 1-month period in almost 60 percent of patients at a dose of 50 mg twice a day and 86 percent of patients at a dose of 150 mg twice a day.[50] The real advantage of flecainide is the minimal occurrence of extracardiac side effects, which are lower than with other antiarrhythmic drugs. In some cases of coexistent atrial tachycardia, flecainide can increase conduction through the AV node, resulting in rapid ventricular rates. Use of AV nodal blocking agents in such circumstances is highly advisable.

Pritchett and colleagues[53] reported similar efficacy with propafenone, the other currently available class Ic agent. They studied 33 patients with PSVT. The time to first recurrence of tachycardia was prolonged with propafenone ($p = 0.004$). Recurrence of tachycardia with treatment was decreased to one-fifth of the recurrence rate with placebo. The effective dose of propafenone is 150 to 300 mg three times a day for the long-term treatment of PSVT.

Sotalol, a class III agent, has been studied for long-term suppression of AVNRT. Huikuri and coworkers reported in a study that sotalol in a dose of 0.1 mg/kg prevented induction of AVNRT in 8 of 8 patients.[54] Sotalol in oral doses of 160 to 480 mg/d prevented long-term recurrence of SVT in all patients who took it chronically. Wanless and colleagues[55] observed, in a multicenter study, that the time to recurrence of PSVT was significantly less compared with placebo when patients were receiving sotalol 80 mg ($p = 0.018$) and sotalol 160 mg ($p = 0.0009$). Because of a higher incidence of side effects associated with amiodarone, it is rarely indicated for the treatment of AVNRT.

【 】 MANAGEMENT STRATEGY

Patients with AVNRT typically present with the clinical syndrome of PSVT. The diagnosis of PSVT can be made with a high degree of certainty based on the clinical history alone, even if the tachy-

cardia has never been documented by an ECG. Physicians may try to document the tachycardia with an ECG using either a 30-day event monitor or by instructing the patient to go to an emergency room or physician's office if another episode of tachycardia occurs. Because AVNRT is not a life-threatening arrhythmia, the primary indication for its treatment relates to its impact on a patient's quality of life. Patients who develop a highly symptomatic episode of PSVT, particularly if it requires an emergency room visit for termination, may elect to initiate therapy after a single episode. In contrast, a patient who presents with minimally symptomatic episodes of PSVT that terminate spontaneously or with a Valsalva maneuver may elect to be followed clinically without specific therapy.

Once it is decided to initiate treatment for AVNRT, the question arises of whether to initiate pharmacologic therapy or to use catheter ablation (see Appendix 38–1). Because of its greater than 95 percent efficacy and low incidence of complications, catheter ablation is now considered first-line therapy. The recently published National Association for Sport and Physical Education (NASPE) Policy Statement on Catheter Ablation includes catheter ablation of AVNRT using the posterior approach as a class 1 indication for catheter ablation. According to this statement, "for those patients in whom treatment of AVNRT is deemed necessary, ablation can be offered as an initial therapy option."[57] It is therefore reasonable to discuss catheter ablation with all patients suspected of having AVNRT. Depending on the frequency and severity of tachycardia episodes as well as the patient's lifestyle and preferences an individual may elect to be followed clinically without specific therapy, to begin a trial of pharmacologic therapy with a β blocker or calcium channel blocker, or to undergo electrophysiology (EP) testing and catheter ablation.

The recommendations for the long-term management of patients with recurrent AVNRT, which were developed by the ACC/AHA/ESC are shown on Table 38–2.[58] Catheter ablation is considered class 1 therapy for treatment of patients with poorly tolerated AVNRT with hemodynamic compromise, with recurrent

---

TABLE 38–2

Types of Accessory Pathway

I. Based on site of origin and insertion:
  a. Atrioventricular
    i. Right-sided: anteroseptal, RV free wall, posteroseptal
    ii. Left-sided: anteroseptal, LV free wall, posteroseptal
  b. Atriofascicular (Brechenmacher fibers)
  c. Nodofascicular (Mahaim fibers)
II. Based on direction of conduction:
  a. Antegrade
  b. Retrograde (concealed)
  c. Bidirectional
III. Based on conduction property:
  a. Slow, decremental
  b. Fast, nondecremental
IV. Based on number:
  a. Single
  b. Multiple

LV, left ventricle; RV, right ventricle.

symptomatic AVNRT, and who have experienced only a single episode of AVNRT who desire complete arrhythmia control. The indications for pharmacologic management are also provided.

ATRIOVENTRICULAR REENTRANT TACHYCARDIA AND WOLFF-PARKINSON-WHITE SYNDROME

Accessory pathways (APs) are important because they provide a substrate for antidromic and orthodromic AV reciprocating tachycardia, are associated with sudden cardiac death, and may be detected in asymptomatic patients on a routine screening ECG. The sections that follow cover the pathophysiology, diagnosis, and management of this fascinating clinical entity.

【 】 PATHOPHYSIOLOGY

The WPW syndrome was first described in 1930 in an article by Louis Wolff, Sir John Parkinson, and Paul Dudley White. The authors described 11 patients with recurrent tachycardia associated with an ECG pattern of "bundle-branch block with short P-R interval." Since publication of this initial report, our understanding of the anatomic and pathophysiologic features of preexcitation syndromes has improved enormously.[59]

Accessory pathways are anomalous, typically extranodal connections that connect the epicardial surfaces of the atrium and ventricle along the AV groove. Accessory bypass tracts, which conduct antegrade from the atrium to the ventricle and therefore are detectable on an ECG, are reportedly present in 0.15 to 0.25 percent of the general population. A higher prevalence of 0.55 percent has been reported in first-degree relatives of patients with WPW syndrome.

Classification

Accessory pathways can be classified based on their site of origin and insertion, location along the mitral or tricuspid annulus, type of conduction, and properties of conduction (decremental or nondecremental) (see Table 38–2). Accessory pathways usually exhibit rapid, nondecremental conduction, similar to that which is present in normal His-Purkinje tissue and atrial or ventricular myocardium. Approximately 8 percent of accessory pathways display decremental antegrade or retrograde conduction.[60] Accessory pathways, which are capable only of retrograde conduction, are referred to as *concealed*, whereas those capable of antegrade conduction are referred to as *manifest*, demonstrating preexcitation on a standard ECG (Fig. 38–9). Accessory pathways usually conduct both antegrade and retrograde. Antegrade-only accessory pathways are particularly uncommon. When present, they are usually right-sided and frequently demonstrate decremental conduction (Mahaim fiber). Concealed accessory pathways are less common, accounting for approximately 15 percent of all accessory pathways.[61] Patients with Ebstein anomaly who also have WPW syndrome frequently have more than one accessory pathway.

Variant accessory pathways include those that connect the atrium to the distal or compact AV node (James fibers), the atrium to the His bundle (the Brechenmacher fiber) and the AV node or

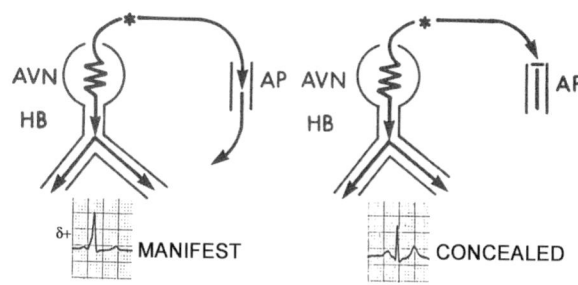

FIGURE 38–9. Atrioventricular conduction patterns and QRS morphologies during sinus rhythm for manifest and concealed accessory pathways. AP, accessory pathway; AVN, atrioventricular node; HB, His bundle. *Source: Modified from Cain ME, Luke RA, Lindsay BD.[83] With permission.*

His bundle to the distal Purkinje fibers or ventricular myocardium (the Mahaim fibers)[46] (see Fig. 38–1B).

Concept of Preexcitation

The hallmark of an accessory pathway function during sinus rhythm is depolarization of all or part of the ventricles earlier than expected if conduction has occurred only over the normal AV conduction system, resulting in preexcitation (Fig. 38–10).

The degree of shortening of the P-R interval and the extent of ventricular preexcitation depend on several factors, including location of the accessory pathway, the relationship between antegrade conduction times and refractory periods of the AV bypass tract, and the normal AV conduction system. A bypass tract that crosses the AV groove in the left lateral region may also result in inapparent preexcitation and minimal P-R–interval shortening during sinus rhythm due to greater interatrial distance for impulse propagation from the sinus node to this site of atrial input into the AP. Conversely, an AP on the right side is more likely to demonstrate marked preexcitation. Preexcitation may be less apparent during sinus tachycardia, when sympathetic tone is high and vagal tone low, resulting in faster AV node conduction time than that in the AP. On the other extreme, during conditions of slowed conduction through the AV node either by intrinsic nodal factors, withdrawal of sympathetic tone, or increased vagal tone, the amount of preexcitation apparent on the 12-lead ECG is maximized because of relatively greater conduction through the AP. Rapid intravenous administration of adenosine causing blocking or slowing of AV node conduction and exposing the anterograde AP conduction has been used as a diagnostic maneuver. The degree of preexcitation can also be enhanced with atrial pacing directly over the AP, eliminating the intraatrial conduction delay from the sinus node to the atrial insertion site of AP (Fig. 38–11).

Intermittent preexcitation is characterized by abrupt loss of delta wave, normalization of the QRS duration, and an increase in the P-R interval during a continuous ECG recording, often despite only minor variations in resting sinus rhythm heart rate. This should be distinguished from day-to-day variability in preexcitation or inapparent preexcitation caused by factors described above. The presence of intermittent preexcitation has been considered to suggest that the refractory period in the AP is long, making them very unlikely to mediate a rapid, preexcited ventricular response during atrial fibrillation.[47]

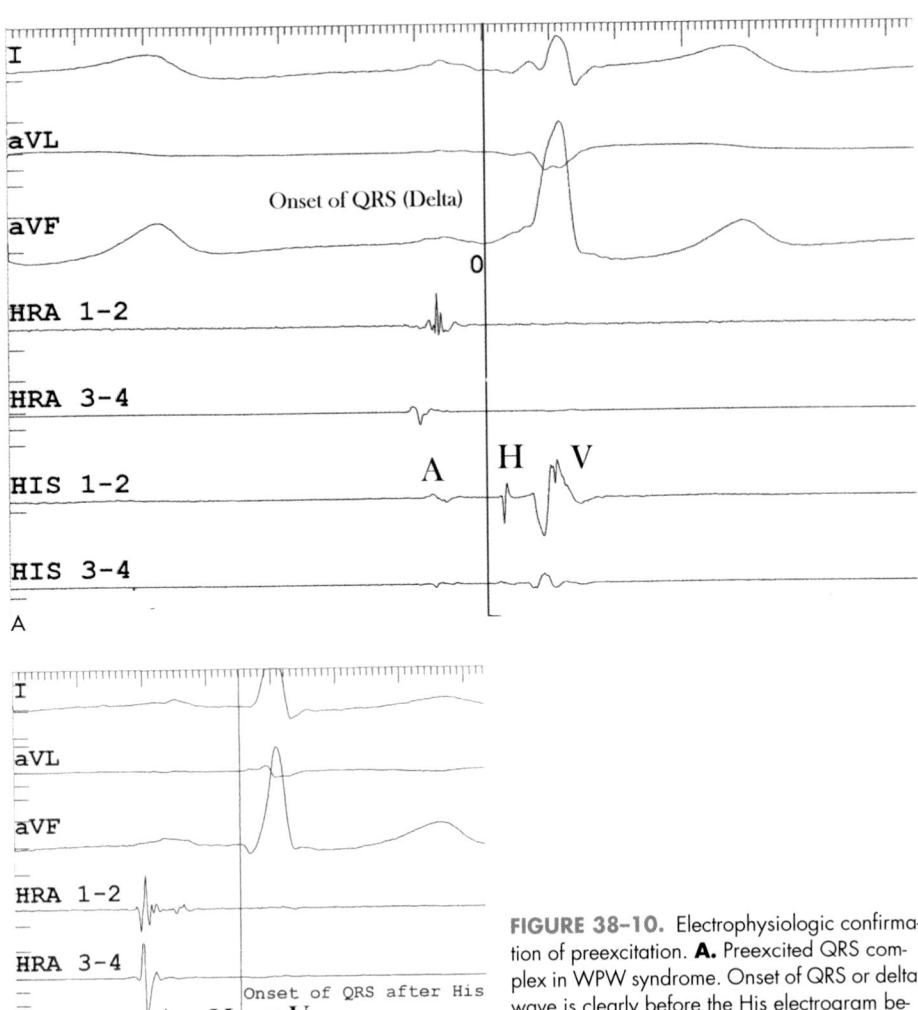

FIGURE 38–10. Electrophysiologic confirmation of preexcitation. **A.** Preexcited QRS complex in WPW syndrome. Onset of QRS or delta wave is clearly before the His electrogram before ablation. **B.** Loss of preexcitation and shift of onset of QRS to after His deflection postablation. A, atrial electrogram; H, His electrogram; HRA, high right atrium; HIS, His bundle electrogram; V, ventricular electrogram.

plex during orthodromic AVRT hence is not preexcited.

During antidromic AVRT, however, the reentrant impulse travels in the reverse direction, with conduction from the atrium to the ventricle occurring via the AP. Antidromic AV reciprocating tachycardia is rare, occurring in only 5 to 10 percent of patients with the WPW syndrome. APDs that occur at a coupling interval that is longer than the refractory period of the AP and shorter than the AV nodal refractory period can initiate the antidromic AVRT; the converse is true with a VPD. Susceptibility of antidromic AVRT appears to depend on the existence of adequate separation between the AP and the AV nodal tissue. Hence, most of the antidromic AVRTs seem to occur only with left-sided bypass tracts.[48]

Other forms of SVTs—like atrial tachycardia, junctional tachycardia, AVNRT, and even ventricular tachycardia—can occur in patients with bypass tracts. Dual AV nodal physiology has been noted in nearly 12 percent of patients with WPW syndrome.[62] Coexisting ventricular tachycardia is less likely because patients with WPW tend to present at a younger age and have less structural heart disease.

Atrial fibrillation is a less common but potentially more serious arrhythmia in patients with the WPW syndrome. If an AP has a short antegrade refractory period, atrial fibrillation can result in a rapid ventricular response with subsequent degeneration to ventricular fibrillation.[63–65] The risk of sudden death has been shown to be higher if the shortest RR interval is <250 msec during spontaneous or induced atrial fibrillation.[63] It has been estimated that one-third of patients with WPW syndrome also have atrial fibrillation.[66] APs appear to play a pathophysiologic role in the development of atrial fibrillation in these patients, as most are young and do not have structural heart disease. Furthermore, surgical or catheter ablation of APs usually results in elimination of atrial fibrillation as well.[67,68]

【 】 DIAGNOSIS
Clinical Features

Preexcitation occurs in the general population at a frequency of around 1.5 per 1000. Of these 50 to 60 percent of patients become symptomatic. Approximately one-third of all patients with PSVT are diagnosed as having an AP-mediated tachycardia. Patients with AP-mediated tachycardias most commonly present with the syndrome of PSVT. Population-based studies have demonstrated a bimodal distribution of symptoms for patients with preexcitation, with a peak in early childhood, followed by a second peak in young adulthood. Nearly 25 percent of patients will be-

Tachycardias Associated with Accessory Pathways

Tachycardias associated with APs can be subdivided into those in which the AP is necessary for initiation and maintenance of tachycardia and those in whom the AP acts as a bystander.

AV reentrant tachycardia (AVRT) is a macroreentrant tachycardia involving the atrium, the AP, the AV node, and the ventricle. AVRT is further subclassified into orthodromic and antidromic AVRT (Fig. 38–12). During orthodromic AVRT, the reentrant impulse utilizes the AV node and specialized conduction system for conduction from the atrium to the ventricle and utilizes the AP for conduction from the ventricle to the atrium. Orthodromic AVRT can be initiated by atrial or ventricular premature depolarizations (APDs or VPDs). APDs initiating the tachycardia block antegradely in the AP and conduct relatively slowly over the AV nodal tissue to the ventricles. The impulse then retrogradely conducts over the AP reentering the atria at the atrial insertion site of the pathway, thus completing the reentrant loop (Fig. 38–13). A VPD, conversely, blocks in the His-Purkinje system and retrogradely reaches the atria through retrogradely conducting AP. The impulse then antegradely conducts through the AV nodal tissue, completing the circuit. The QRS com-

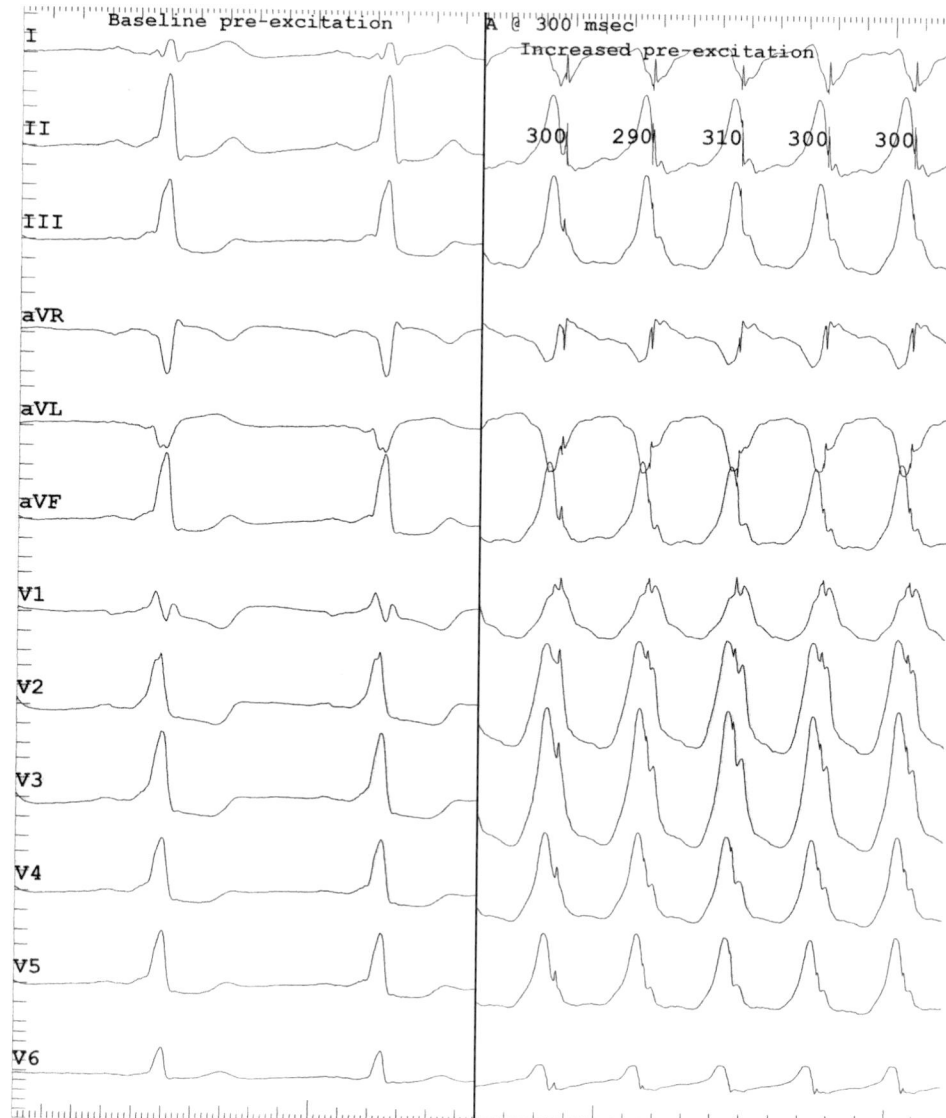

FIGURE 38–11. Increase in degree of preexcitation with atrial pacing. *Left panel* shows 12-lead ECG during sinus rhythm. Note the obvious increase in preexcitation in the *right panel* with atrial pacing at a cycle length of 300 msec (200 beats/min). Increase in atrial input causes decremental conduction in the atrioventricular node, resulting in increased conduction over the accessory pathway.

range from 0.15 to 0.39 percent.[69,72–74] It is distinctly unusual for cardiac arrest to be the first symptomatic manifestation of the WPW syndrome.[58,75] Given the high prevalence of atrial fibrillation among patients with WPW syndrome and the concern for sudden cardiac death resulting from rapid preexcited atrial fibrillation, the low annual incidence of sudden death among patients with the WPW syndrome is reassuring.

Patients with functioning AV bypass tracts tend to have certain congenital abnormalities, particularly Ebstein anomaly of the tricuspid valve. Nearly 10 percent of patients with Ebstein anomaly have preexcitation.[76,77] APs also commonly occur in patients with corrected transposition of great vessels. In this case, the Ebstein anomaly of the left (tricuspid) valve is associated with APs to the functioning systemic ventricle (anatomic right ventricle). In addition, multiple bypass tracts are frequently seen in Ebstein anomaly. Conversely, of patients with WPW syndrome presenting with SVT early in childhood, only 5 percent have Ebstein anomaly, despite the fact that it is the most common from of congenital heart disease associated with WPW syndrome. Interestingly, Deal and coworkers found that organic heart disease is less likely in patients with left-sided APs than in those with right-sided pathways (5 vs. 45 percent). In this study, organic heart disease was present in only 20 percent of the patients presenting with the WPW syndrome in the first 4 months of life.[76]

ECG Characteristics

The ECG hallmark of an antegradely conducting AP is the delta wave, along with a shorter than usual P-R interval. Conversely,

come asymptomatic over time. More than half the patients with an episode will suffer a recurrence.[69]

Symptoms range from palpitations to syncope.[69] As in AVNRT, episodes of tachycardia may be associated with dyspnea, chest pain, decreased exercise tolerance, anxiety, dizziness, or syncope. Although syncope is often considered a bad prognostic sign, the evidence is not clear. Auricchio and coworkers evaluated 101 consecutive patients with WPW syndrome, 36 of who had syncope. Although a higher percentage of patients who had syncope had a history of aborted sudden death (28 vs. 18 percent), the difference was not significant.[70] Leitch and colleagues investigated the mechanism of syncope in patients with PSVT and found that most had AVRT. Leitch and coworkers reported that syncope during SVT might, in fact, be caused by a vasodepressor mechanism and not to a rapid rate of tachycardia.[71] Physical examination demonstrates a fast, regular pulse with a constant-intensity first heart sound. The jugular venous pressure waveform is usually constant, but it can sometimes be elevated. The incidence of sudden cardiac death in patients with the WPW syndrome has been estimated to

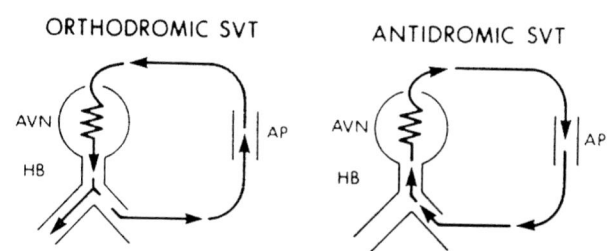

FIGURE 38–12. Schematic representation of the patterns of conduction through an accessory pathway (AP) and the normal conduction system (AVN-HB) during orthodromic AVRT and antidromic AVRT. AVN, atrioventricular node; AVRT, atrioventricular reciprocating tachycardia; HB, His bundle. *Source: Modified from Cain ME, Luke RA, Lindsay BD.[83] With permission.*

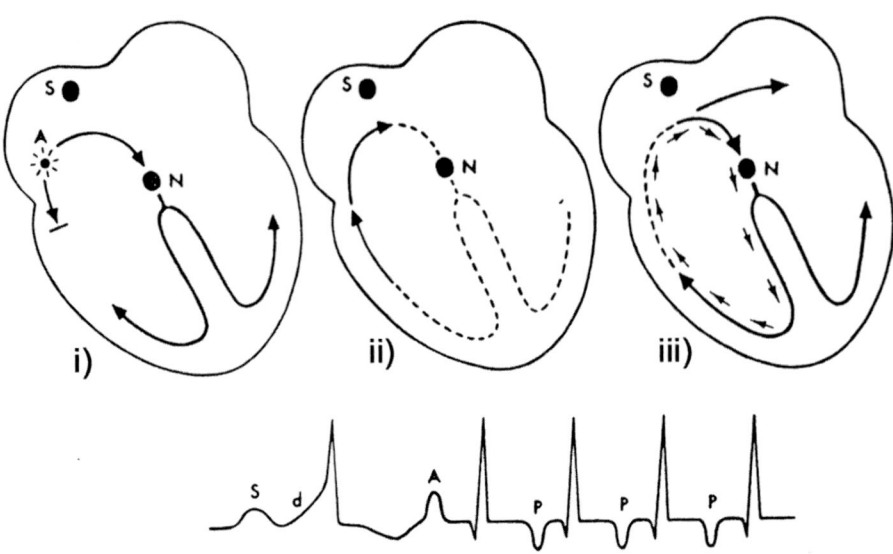

FIGURE 38-13. Schematic of initiation of orthodromic atrioventricular reentrant tachycardia. A diagrammatic ECG recording shows the first P wave of sinus-node (S) origin yielding a preexcited QRS complex with a delta wave (d) and short P-R interval (i). An ectopic atrial impulse (A) blocks antegradely in the bypass tract but still conducts over the atrioventricular node (N) and His-Purkinje system to the ventricles. This causes the second QRS complex to appear nonpreexcited (ii). The premature impulse continues to conduct retrogradely over the bypass tract, as the latter had time recover excitability while the impulse was conducting over the node (iii). The retrogradely conducted impulse has activated the atria from the bypass tracts' atrial insertion point and generated the first retrograde P wave (P) of AVRT. Reentrance of impulse through the node then occurs, causing AVRT to perpetuate. *Source: Modified from Chung EK. Wolff-Parkinson-White syndrome: current views. Am J Med 1977;62:261. With permission.*

the presence of retrograde conduction only in an AP will not be apparent on a surface ECG during sinus rhythm. ECG during orthodromic AVRT has a normal QRS complex with retrogradely conducting P wave after the completion of the QRS complex in the ST segment or early in the T wave (see Fig. 38-4), whereas the QRS during antidromic AVRT is fully preexcited.

Numerous algorithms have been described to localize the site of the AP using the axis of the delta wave and QRS morphology.[78-90] The location of the AP along the AV ring is classified variously into 5 or 10 regions, which can be broadly divided into those on the left and the right of the AV groove. Distribution along these lines is not homogenous. Some 46 to 60 percent of the pathways are found on the left free wall space. Nearly 25 percent are within the posteroseptal and midseptal spaces, 15 to 20 percent in the right free wall space, and 2 percent in the anteroseptal space.[78,79] The positive predictive value of these algorithms is better when the delta wave polarity is included and when algorithms involve less than six locations.[90] A simple algorithm that includes both the delta

wave axis and the QRS axis is shown in Fig. 38-14.

QRS alternans may be present in nearly 38 percent of patients with circus-movement tachycardia involving an AP.[91] Green and coworkers reported a series of 161 patients with SVT of who 36 had QRS alternans.[32] Of these 36 patients, 33 had AVRT (92 percent), 2 had AVNRT, and 1 had atrial tachycardia. The mechanism for this is unclear. Morady and colleagues proposed that it could be a rate-related phenomenon.[33] It could also be caused by oscillations in the relative refractory period of the His-Purkinje system.[92]

ST-segment depression may also occur during orthodromic AVRT. It may occur even in the young, who are unlikely to have coronary artery disease. The location of the ST-segment depression may vary with location of the AP. ST-segment depression in V_3 to V_6 is almost invariably seen with a left lateral pathway; a negative T wave in the inferior leads is associated with a posteroseptal or posterior pathway; and a negative or notched T wave in V_2 or V_3

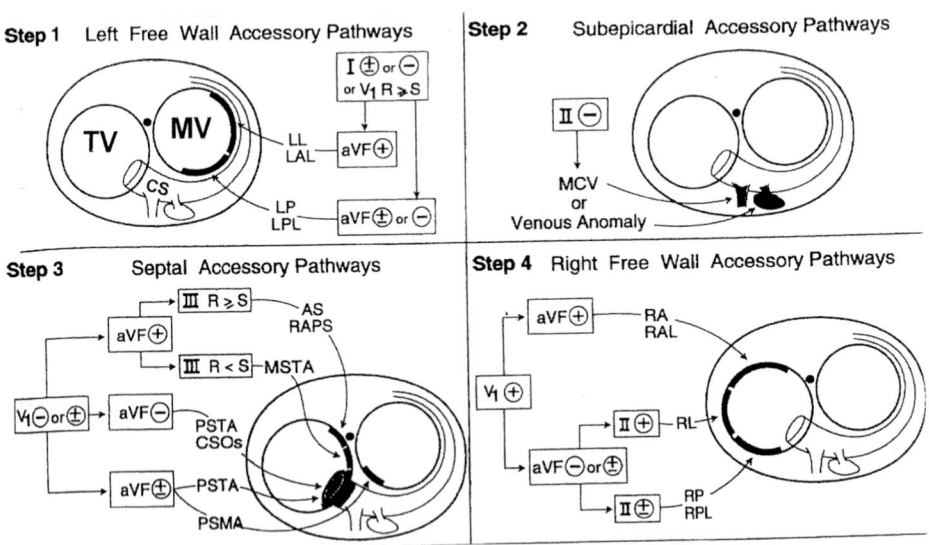

FIGURE 38-14. Localization of accessory pathways in patients with WPW syndrome. The line drawings illustrate the anatomic relationships between the tricuspid valve (TV), mitral valve (MV), coronary sinus (CS), atrioventricular conducting system, and accessory pathways. For each accessory pathway location indicated, the combination of QRS vectors most likely to result are shown, based on upright (+) or inverted (–) QRS waveforms. These vectorial guidelines are generally useful but not necessarily precise, because activation patterns from specific sites may vary in individual patients. AS, anteroseptal; CS, coronary sinus; CSOs, coronary sinus ostium; LAL, left anterolateral; LL, left lateral; LP, left posterior; LPL, left posterolateral; MCV, middle cardiac vein (coronary vein); MSTA, mid-septal tricuspid annulus; PSMA, posteroseptal mitral annulus; PSTA, posteroseptal tricuspid annulus; RA, right anterior; RAL, right anterolateral; RAPS, right anterior paraseptal; venous anomaly (coronary sinus diverticulum); RL, right lateral; RP, right posterior; RPL, right posterolateral; WPW, Wolff-Parkinson-White. *Source: From Arruda, McClelland, Wang, et al.[80] With permission.*

with a positive retrograde P wave in at least two inferior leads suggest an anteroseptal pathway. However, ST-segment depression occurring during orthodromic AVRT episodes in older patients or associated with symptoms of ischemia mandate the consideration of coexisting coronary artery disease.

Electrophysiologic Testing

EP study in patients with AVRT is done to not only confirm the presence of an AP and differentiate this condition from other forms of SVT but also to find the pathway participating in the tachycardia and aid in ablative therapy.

By definition, if an AP is present and conducting antegradely, some part of the ventricle begins activation earlier than expected, so that the H-V interval is less than normal at rest (see Fig. 38–10). Because the QRS complex is a fusion complex of conduction down both the AV node and the AP, slowing of conduction down the normal pathway results in an increasing degree of preexcitation.

Eccentric atrial activation with ventricular pacing makes it easy to identify the presence of an AP (Fig. 38–15). Retrograde conduction over most APs is nondecremental. Hence, in the absence of intraventricular conduction delay or presence of multiple bypass tracts, the VA conduction time is the same over a range of pace cycle lengths (see Fig. 38–15). The exception to this is the slowly conducting decremental posteroseptal pathway found in the permanent form of junctional reciprocating tachycardia, in which the VA conduction time increases with increasing ventricular pacing rate.

It is important and often challenging to differentiate retrograde conduction over septal pathway from conduction over the normal AV system. One maneuver that can make this differentiation is *differential pacing* (i.e., pacing both from the right ventricular apex and the RV base) and measuring the VA conduction time. Retrograde conduction over the normal AV conduction system is fastest when pacing from the apex, because conduction can occur rapidly over the His-Purkinje system. VA intervals are longer when the pacing site is moved from the apex to the base. The converse is true in the presence of an AP, with VA intervals shortest when pacing from the base, closer to the site of pathway insertion, than from the apex. The technique of *para-Hisian pacing* is useful in differentiating the anteroseptal pathway from AVNRT.

Development of bundle-branch block aberration during tachycardia can be useful in determining both presence of and participation of an AP in tachycardia (Fig. 38–16). An increase in tachycardia cycle length caused by an increase in VA conduction time with functional

bundle-branch block is consistent with the presence of an AP ipsilateral to the bundle-branch block.

【 】 MANAGEMENT

Catheter Ablation of APS

Catheter ablation of APs is performed in conjunction with a diagnostic EP test. Once the AP is localized to a region of the heart, precise mapping and ablation is performed using a steerable electrode catheter. No prospective randomized clinical trials have evaluated the safety and efficacy of catheter ablation of APs. However, the results of catheter ablation of APs have been reported in a large number of other trials.[93-98] The largest prospective, multicenter clinical trial to evaluate the safety and efficacy of radiofrequency ablation was reported by Calkins and colleagues.[10] This study involved analysis of 1050 patients, of whom 500 had APs. Overall success of catheter ablation in curing APs was 93 percent. The success rate for catheter ablation of left free-wall APs is slightly higher than for catheter ablation of right-sided APs (95 vs. 90 percent, *p* = 0.03). Following an initially successful procedure, recurrence of AP conduction is found in approximately 5 percent of patients. The recurrence-free interval postablation was also best with left-sided pathways (Fig. 38–17). APs that recur can usually be successfully ablated again. Complications associated with catheter ablation of APs may result from obtaining vascular access (hematomas, deep venous thrombosis, perforation of the aorta, arteriovenous fistula, pneumothorax), catheter manipulation (valvular damage, microemboli, perforation of the coronary sinus or myocardial

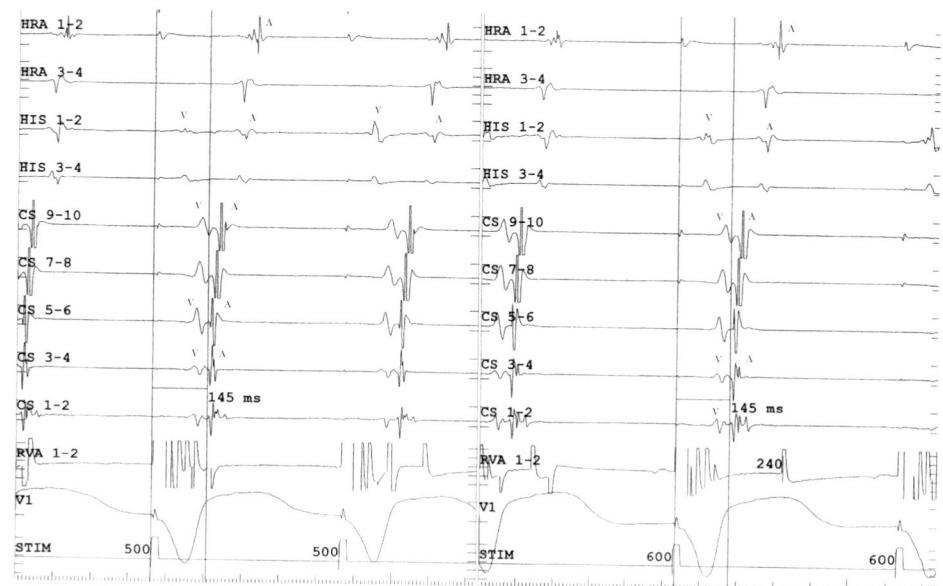

FIGURE 38–15. Nondecremental retrograde conduction in the accessory pathway. Note the eccentric activation of the atrium with pacing from the ventricle, with earliest atrial depolarization at the distal CS lead (CS 1–2). The *left panel* shows right ventricular pacing at a 120 beats/min (cycle length of 500 msec) and the *right panel* shows the same at 100 beats/min (cycle length of 600 msec). Note that the VA conduction time shown between the vertical lines remains the same with varying pacing rates. 1–2, distal electrodes; 3–4, proximal electrodes in each catheter; A, atrial electrogram; CS, coronary sinus; CS 9–20, the most proximal electrode in the CS catheter; HIS, His bundle electrogram; HRA, high right atrium; RVA, right ventricular apex; V, ventricular electrogram.

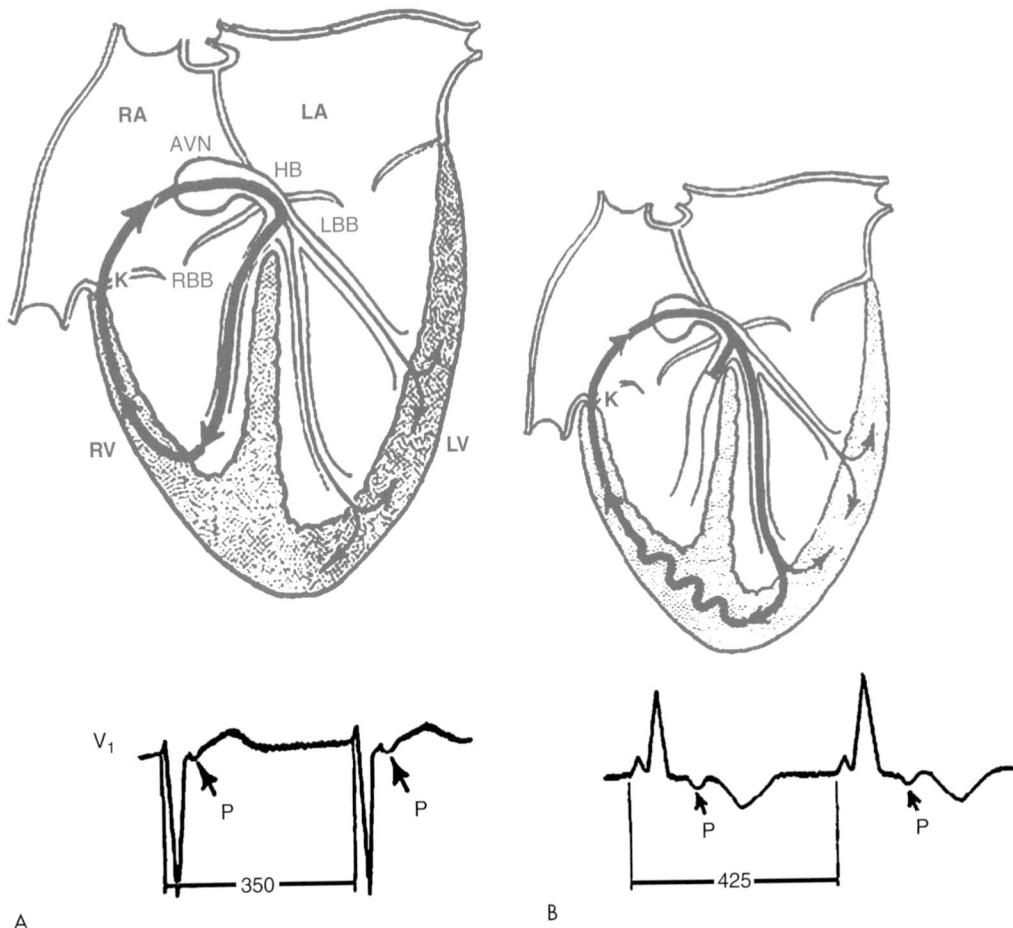

FIGURE 38–16. Effect of BBB on AVRT. **A.** AVRT involving a right-sided accessory pathway. Schematic at the bottom shows the ECG appearance of the tachycardia at a cycle length of 350 msec. **B.** Appearance of BBB on the same side leads to increase the cycle length of the tachycardia to 425 msec. See text for discussion. AVN, atrioventricular node; AVRT, atrioventricular reciprocating tachycardia; BBB, bundle-branch block; HB, His bundle; LA, left atrium; LBB, left bundle branch; LV, left ventricle; RA, right atrium; RBB, right bundle branch; RV, right ventricle. *Source: Modified from Josephson M. Preexcitation syndromes. In: Josephson M, ed. Clinical Cardiac Electrophysiology: Technique and Interpretation. 3rd ed. New York: Lippincott Williams & Wilkins; 2002:370. With permission.*

wall, coronary dissection and/or thrombosis), or delivery of RF energy (AV block, myocardial perforation, coronary artery spasm or occlusion, transient ischemic attacks, or cerebrovascular accidents).

Calkins and coworkers reported the incidence of major complications in their trial to be 3 percent and of minor complications around 8 percent.[10] The procedure-related mortality associated with catheter ablation of APs has ranged from 0 to 0.2 percent. The two most common types of major complications reported during catheter ablation of APs are inadvertent complete AV block and cardiac tamponade. The incidence of inadvertent complete AV block ranges from 0.17 to 1.0 percent. Most instances of complete AV block occur in the setting of the ablation of septal and posteroseptal APs. The frequency of cardiac tamponade as a result of the ablation of APs varies between 0.13 and 1.1 percent.

In the past several years, cryoablation has become available as an alternative energy source for creation of myocardial lesions which can be used for catheter ablation of accessory pathways. The main advantage of cryoenergy, compared to radiofrequency energy, is

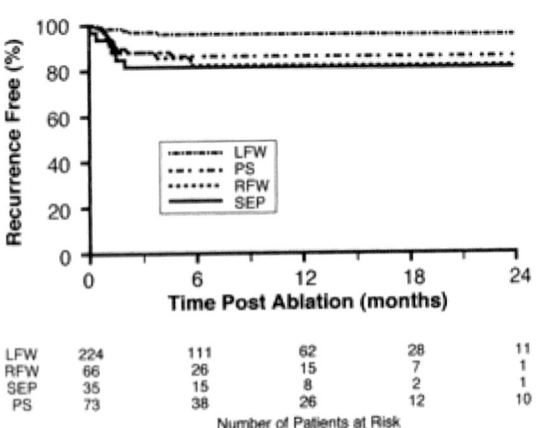

LFW	224	111	62	28	11
RFW	66	26	15	7	1
SEP	35	15	8	2	1
PS	73	38	26	12	10

Number of Patients at Risk

FIGURE 38–17. Kaplan-Meier curve showing freedom from arrhythmia recurrence among patients who underwent successful ablation of an AP subclassified by its location. This analysis was confined to patients in whom successful ablation was achieved with the investigational ablation system. AP, accessory pathway; LFW, left free wall; PS, posteroseptal; RFW, right free wall; SEP, septal. *Source: From Calkins H, Yong P, Miller JM, et al.[10] With permission.*

that the risk of heart block appears to be lower. This potential benefit must be balanced against longer procedure times and lower acute and long-term efficacy.[99] Because of the lower acute and long-term success rates of catheter ablation of accessory pathways using cryoenergy, this energy source is generally employed only for ablation of accessory pathways located in the anteroseptal and midseptal locations.

Medical Therapy

Antiarrhythmic drugs represent one therapeutic option for management of AP-mediated arrhythmias (Appendix 38–1). Antiarrhythmic drugs that primarily modify conduction through the AV node include verapamil, β blockers, and adenosine. In contrast, the antiarrhythmic drugs, which primarily modify conduction across the AP, consist of class 1 drugs such as procainamide, propafenone, and flecainide as well class 3 antiarrhythmic drugs such as sotalol and amiodarone. The approach to acute termination of these arrhythmias generally differs from that used for long-term suppression and prevention of further episodes of SVT. In general, the approach employed does not vary based on the specific tachycardia mechanism, which generally is unknown when the patient first presents to an emergency room. Pharmacologic agents are in general more effective in terminating an acute episode of tachycardia than in preventing future recurrences. Verapamil or diltiazem should not be administered intravenously to patients with atrial fibrillation and preexcitation, as they may accelerate conduction through the AP and precipitate a cardiac arrest.

There have been no controlled trials of drug prophylaxis involving patients with AV reentry. However, a number of small, nonrandomized trials have been performed. A subset of the patients in these studies had AV reentry as their underlying arrhythmia. Available data do not allow a comparison of the efficacy of these drugs.

Manolis and colleagues reported the largest published study evaluating the efficacy of propafenone in 11 adult patients, 9 of whom had a manifest AP. During 9 ± 6 months of followup, none of the 10 patients discharged on a combination of propafenone and a β blocker experienced a recurrence. No major side effects were reported.[100] Other small trials have evaluated the efficacy of propafenone in the treatment of AV reentry in children.[101–104] The largest of these involved 26 young children (younger than 10 years) with AV reentry.[101] Complete arrhythmia control was accomplished in 20 patients and partial control in one additional patient.

A number of studies have examined the acute and long-term efficacy of oral and intravenous flecainide in the treatment of patients with AV reentry. Helmy and coworkers reported the largest of these, involving 20 patients with AV reentry.[105] The oral administration of flecainide resulted in inability to induce sustained tachycardia in 17 of 20 patients. During 15 ± 7 months of followup on oral flecainide treatment, 3 patients developed a recurrence of tachycardia. The addition of a β blocker results in greater efficacy, with >90 percent of patients achieving abolition of symptomatic tachycardia. In addition to studies that specifically focused on patients with a known AV reentry, there have been several randomized trials evaluating the efficacy of flecainide in the treatment

of patients with paroxysmal SVT. The precise tachycardia mechanism in these patients was not determined.

Amiodarone has been evaluated in several trials for its efficacy in the treatment of patients with AP-mediated tachycardias.[106–109] However, these studies do not demonstrate that amiodarone is superior to class 1C antiarrhythmic agents or sotalol. Acute studies have also revealed that amiodarone does not consistently prolong the AP refractory period and, as a result, cannot be considered to be protective against sudden death in all patients with WPW syndrome.[109] As a result of these findings—combined with the well-recognized organ toxicity associated with amiodarone and the high rate of discontinuation of this drug because of noncardiac adverse effects—amiodarone generally does not play an important role in the treatment of patients with APs.

Verapamil, although less studied, can be moderately effective in the prevention of AVRT.[110] No studies have been performed to determine the short- or long-term efficacy of procainamide or quinidine in the treatment of AV reentry.

【 】 MANAGEMENT CONSIDERATIONS

Management of Asymptomatic Preexcitation

Most patients with asymptomatic preexcitation have a good prognosis. Because of the small but real risks associated with invasive procedures, EPS is not routinely recommended for risk stratification and/or ablative therapy. The NASPE Policy Statement on Catheter Ablation states that catheter ablation is not indicated (class 3) for patients with asymptomatic preexcitation unless they fall into a high-risk group, such as school bus drivers, pilots, and scuba divers.[110–113] The more recently published American College of Cardiology/American Heart Association/European Society of Cardiology (ACC/AHA/ESC) Guidelines for Management of Patients With Supraventricular Arrhythmias[58] gives catheter ablation a 2a classification for treatment of patients with asymptomatic preexcitation.

Several noninvasive and invasive tests have been proposed as useful in stratifying patients for the risk of sudden death. The detection of intermittent preexcitation—which is characterized by an abrupt loss of the delta wave, normalization of the QRS complex, and an increase in the P-R interval during a continuous ECG recording—is evidence that an AP has a relatively long refractory period and is unlikely to precipitate ventricular fibrillation.[48] The loss of preexcitation after administration of antiarrhythmic drugs like procainamide or ajmaline has also been used to indicate a low-risk subgroup.[114] These noninvasive tests are generally considered inferior to electrophysiologic testing in the assessment of risk of sudden cardiac death. Because of this, they play little role in patient management at present.

When screening studies are performed in patients with asymptomatic preexcitation, approximately 20 percent of those who are asymptomatic will demonstrate a rapid ventricular rate during atrial fibrillation induced at EPS.[110,111] Studies have identified markers that identify patients at increased risk.[47,66,114] These include (1) a short preexcited RR interval <250 msec during spontaneous or induced atrial fibrillation, (2) a history of symptomatic tachycardia, (3) multiple APs, and (4) Epstein anomaly. A short preexcited R-R interval during atrial fibrillation of >250 msec has been reported to have a negative predictive value of >95 percent.[70]

More recent evidence makes a stronger case for use of EPS in risk stratifying all asymptomatic patients with preexcitation.[115] Pappone and coworkers studied 212 consecutive asymptomatic WPW patients after a baseline EP test over 5 years.[116] After a mean follow up of 37.7 months, 33 patients became symptomatic. Of these, 29 had inducible SVT on EP test and only 4 were not inducible. More importantly, there were 3 sudden deaths in the entire population, and all those occurred in patients in whom AVRT and atrial fibrillation were inducible during EP test. In a more recent study, Pappone and colleagues examined the role of prophylactic catheter ablation in children with asymptomatic preexcitation.[117] Of the 165 eligible children, 60 were determined to be at high risk of an arrhythmia based on their results of EP testing. Of these 60 patients, 20 underwent prophylactic catheter ablation, 27 had no treatment, and 13 withdrew from the study. During a mean follow up of 34 months, 1 child in the ablation group (5 percent) and 12 in the control group (44 percent) had arrhythmic events. Among these 12 patients in the control group, two experienced ventricular fibrillation and one died suddenly. Based on the results of these studies, some members of the EP community have changed their clinical practice and are advocating screening EP studies and prophylactic catheter ablation when a high risk accessory pathway is uncovered. However, no consensus has been reached and many members of the EP community continue to manage patients with asymptomatic preexcitation in a more conservative fashion and only recommend EP testing in *high-risk* individuals.

Management of Symptomatic Wolff-Parkinson-White

The recently published NASPE Policy Statement on Catheter Ablation states that catheter ablation is considered first-line therapy (class 1) and the treatment of choice for patients with WPW syndrome—i.e., patients with manifest preexcitation along with symptoms.[117] It is curative in more than 95 percent of patients and has a low complication rate. It also obviates the unwanted side effects of antiarrhythmic agents. Catheter ablation is also considered first-line therapy (class 1) for patients with PSVT involving a concealed AP. However, because concealed APs are not associated with an increased risk of sudden cardiac death in these patients, catheter ablation can be presented as one of a number of potential therapeutic approaches including pharmacologic therapy and clinical followup alone (see discussion of management of AVNRT). When pharmacologic therapy is selected for patients with concealed APs, it is reasonable to consider a trial of β blocker therapy, calcium channel blocker therapy, or a class 1C antiarrhythmic agent. It is important to note that β blockers and calcium channel blockers generally are not recommended for the management of patients who have evidence of preexcitation.

The recommendations for the long term management of patients with accessory pathway mediated arrhythmias which were developed by the ACC/AHA/ESC are shown in Appendix 38–2.[58] Catheter ablation is considered class 1 therapy for treatment of patients with the WPW syndrome and also those with poorly tolerated AVRT in the absence of preexcitation. In contrast, catheter ablation received a 2a indication for treatment of patients who have had only a single episode of AVRT and also those with asymptomatic preexcitation.

REFERENCES

1. Wu D, Denes P, Amat-y-Leon F, Dhingra R, et al. Clinical, electrocardiographic and electrophysiologic observations in patients with paroxysmal supraventricular tachycardia. *Am J Cardiol* 1978;41:1045–1051.
2. Josephson ME, Wellens HJ. Differential diagnosis of supraventricular tachycardia. *Cardiol Clin* 1990;8(3):411–442.
3. Rostagno C, Paladini B, Taddei T, et al. Out-of-hospital symptomatic supraventricular arrhythmias: epidemiological aspects derived from 10 years experience of the Florence Mobile Coronary Care Unit. *G Ital Cardiol* 1993;23(6):549–562.
4. Denes P, Wu D, Dhingra RC, et al. Dual atrioventricular nodal pathways: a common electrophysiological response. *Br Heart J* 1975;37:1069–1076.
5. Jackman WM, Beckman KJ, McClelland JH, et al. Treatment of supraventricular tachycardia due to atrioventricular nodal reentry by radiofrequency catheter ablation of slow-pathway conduction. *N Engl J Med* 1992;327:313–318.
6. Haissaguerre M, Gaita F, Fischer B, et al. Elimination of atrioventricular nodal reentrant tachycardia using discrete slow potentials to guide application of radiofrequency energy. *Circulation* 1992;85:2162–2175.
7. Kay GN, Epstein AE, Dailey SM, et al. Selective radiofrequency ablation of the slow pathway for the treatment of atrioventricular reentrant tachycardia: evidence for involvement of perinodal myocardium within the reentrant circuit. *Circulation* 1992;85:1675–1688.
8. Goyal R, Zivin A, Souza J, et al. Comparison of the ages of tachycardia onset in patients with atrioventricular nodal reentrant tachycardia and accessory pathway–mediated tachycardia. *Am Heart J* 1996;132:765–767.
9. Clague JR, Dagres N, Kottkamp H, et al. Targeting the slow pathway for atrioventricular nodal reentrant tachycardia: Initial results and long-term follow-up in 379 consecutive patients. *Eur Heart J* 2001;22:82–88.
10. Calkins H, Yong P, Miller JM, Olshansky B, et al. Catheter ablation of accessory pathways, atrioventricular nodal reentrant tachycardia, and the atrioventricular junction: final results of a prospective, multicenter clinical trial. The Atakr Multicenter Investigators Group. *Circulation* 1999;99:262–270.
11. Bubien RS, Knotts-Dolson SM, Plumb VJ, Kay GN. Effect of radiofrequency catheter ablation on health-related quality of life and activities of daily living in patients with recurrent arrhythmias *Circulation* 1996;94:1585–1591.
12. Kent AFS. Researches on the structure and function of the mammalian heart. *J Physiol* 1893;14:233–254.
13. Olgin JE, Ursell P, Kao AK, et al. Pathological findings following slow pathway ablation for AV nodal reentrant tachycardia. *J Cardiovasc Electrophysiol* 1996;7:625–631.
14. Ho SW, McComb JH, Scott CD, et al. Morphology of the cardiac conduction system in patients with electrophysiologically proven dual atrioventricular nodal pathway. *J Cardiovasc Electrophysiol* 1993;4(5):504–512.
15. Sanchez-Quintana D, Davies DW, Ho SY, et al. Architecture of the atrial musculature in and around the triangle of Koch: its potential relevance to atrioventricular nodal reentry. *J Cardiovasc Electrophysiol* 1997;8:1396–1407.
16. Inoue S, Becker AE. Posterior extensions of the human compact atrioventricular node: a neglected anatomic feature of potential clinical significance. *Circulation* 1998;97:188–193.
17. Moe GK, Preston JB, Burlington H. Physiologic evidence for a dual AV transmission system. *Cir Res* 1956;4:357–375.
18. Haissaguerre M, Warin JF, Lemetayer P, et al. Closed chest ablation of retrograde conduction in patients with atrioventricular nodal reentrant tachycardia. *N Engl J Med* 1989;320:426–433.
19. Epstein LM, Scheinman MM, Langberg JJ, et al. Percutaneous catheter modification of the atrioventricular node. *Circulation* 1989;80:757–768.
20. Lee MA, Morady F, Kadish A, et al. Catheter modification of the atrioventricular junction with radiofrequency energy in patients with atrioventricular nodal reentry tachycardia. *Circulation* 1991;83:827–835.
21. Calkins H, Sousa J, El-Atassi R, et al. Diagnosis and cure of the Wolff-Parkinson-White syndrome or paroxysmal supraventricular tachycardia during a single electrophysiologic test. *N Engl J Med* 1991;324:1612–1618.

22. Goy JJ, Fromer M, Schlaepfer J, et al. Clinical efficacy of radiofrequency current in the treatment of patients with atrioventricular node reentrant tachycardia. *J Am Coll Cardiol* 1990;16:418–423.

23. Jazayeri MR, Hempe SL, Sra JS, et al. Selective transcatheter ablation of the fast and slow pathways using radiofrequency energy in patients with atrioventricular nodal reentrant tachycardia. *Circulation* 1992;85:1318–1328.

24. Kottkamp H, Hindricks G, Willems S, et al. An anatomically and electrogram-guided stepwise approach for effective and safe catheter ablation of the fast pathway for elimination of atrioventricular node reentrant tachycardia. *J Am Coll Cardiol* 1995;25:974–983.

25. Epstein LM, Lesh MD, Griffin JC, et al. A direct midseptal approach to slow atrioventricular nodal pathway ablation. *Pacing Clin Electrophysiol* 1995;18(pt 1):57–64.

26. Kalbfleisch SJ, Strickberger SA, Williamson B, et al. Randomized comparison of anatomic and electrogram mapping approaches to ablation of the slow pathway of atrioventricular node reentrant tachycardia. *J Am Coll Cardiol* 1994;23:716–723.

27. Janse MJ, Anderson RH, McGuire MA, Ho SY. "AV nodal" reentry: Part I. AV nodal reentry revisited. *J Cardiovasc Electrophysiol* 1993;4:561–572.

28. McGuire MA, Janse MJ, Ross DL. "AV nodal" reentry: Part II. AV nodal, AV junctional or atrionodal reentry? *J Cardiovasc Electrophysiol* 1993;4:573–586.

29. Josephson ME, Kastor JA. Paroxysmal supraventricular tachycardia: is atrium a necessary link? *Circulation* 1976;54:430.

30. Fisch C, Mandrola JM, Rardon DR. Electrocardiographic manifestations of dual atrioventricular node conduction during sinus rhythm. *J Am Coll Cardiol* 1997;29:1015–1022.

31. Paparella N, Ouyang F, Fuca G, et al. Significance of newly acquired negative T waves after interruption of paroxysmal reentrant supraventricular tachycardia with narrow QRS complex. *Am J Cardiol* 2000;85:261–263.

32. Green M, Heddle B, Dassen W, et al. Value of QRS alternation in determining the site of origin of narrow QRS supraventricular tachycardia. *Circulation* 1983;68:368–373.

33. Morady F, DiCarlo LA Jr, Baerman JM, et al. Determinants of QRS alternans during narrow QRS tachycardia. *J Am Coll Cardiol* 1987;9(3):489–499.

34. Chiou CW, Chen SA, Kung MH, et al. Effects of continuous enhanced vagal tone on dual atrioventricular node and accessory pathways. *Circulation* 2003;107(20):2583–2588.

35. Knight BP, Ebinger M, Oral H, Kim, et al. Diagnostic value of tachycardia features and pacing maneuvers during paroxysmal supraventricular tachycardia. *J Am Coll Cardiol* 2000;36:574–582.

36. DiMarco JP, Miles W, Akhtar M, et al. Adenosine for paroxysmal supraventricular tachycardia: dose ranging and comparison with verapamil: assessment in placebo-controlled, multicenter trials: the adenosine for PSVT study group. *Ann Intern Med* 1990;113:104–110.

37. Donahue KJ, Orias D, Berger RB, et al. Comparison of adenosine effects on atrioventricular node reentry and atrioventricular reciprocating tachycardias. *Clin Cardiol* 1998;21:743–745.

38. Ferguson JD, DiMarco JP. Contemporary management of paroxysmal supraventricular tachycardia. *Circulation* 2003;107:1096.

39. Wellens HJJ, Durer DR, Liem KL, et al. Effect of digitalis in patients with paroxysmal atrioventricular nodal tachycardia. *Circulation* 1975;52:779–788.

40. Wu D, Denes P, Dhingra RC, et al. The effects of propranolol on induction of AV nodal reentrant paroxysmal tachycardia. *Circulation* 1974;50:665–677.

41. Calkins H. Catheter ablation for cardiac arrhythmias. *Med Clin North Am* 2001;2:473–502.

42. Langberg JJ, Leon A, Borganelli M, et al. A randomized, prospective comparison of anterior and posterior approaches to radiofrequency catheter ablation of atrioventricular nodal reentry tachycardia. *Circulation* 1993;87(5):1551–1556.

43. Lickfett L, Pfeiffer D, Schimpf R, et al. Long-term follow-up of fast pathway radiofrequency ablation in atrioventricular nodal reentrant tachycardia. *Am J Cardiol* 2002;89(9):1124–1125.

44. Shieneman NM. NASPE survey on catheter ablation. *Pacing Clin Electrophysiol* 1995;18:1474.

45. Calkins H, Prystowsky E, Berger R, et al. Recurrences of conduction following radiofrequency catheter ablation procedures: relationship to ablation target and electrode temperature. *J Cardiovasc Electrophysiol* 1996;7:704.

46. Anderson RH, Becker AE, Brechenmacher C, et al. Ventricular pre-excitation: A proposed nomenclature for its substrates. *Eur J Cardiol* 1975;3(1):27–36.

47. Klein GJ, Gulamhusien SS. Intermittent preexcitation in the Wolff-Parkinson-White syndrome. *Am J Cardiol* 1983;52:292–296.

48. Cain ME, Luke RA, Lindsay BD. Diagnosis and localization of accessory pathways. *Pacing Clin Electrophysiol* 1992;15:801–824.

49. Henthorn RW, Waldo AL, Anderson JL, et al. Flecainide acetate prevents recurrence of symptomatic paroxysmal supraventricular tachycardia. The Flecainide Supraventricular Tachycardia Study Group. *Circulation* 1991;83:119–125.

50. Falk RH, Fogel RI. Flecainide. *J Cardiovasc Electrophysiol* 1994;5:964–981.

51. Anderson JL, Platt ML, Guarnieri T, et al. Flecainide acetate for paroxysmal supraventricular tachyarrhythmias: the flecainide supraventricular tachycardia study group. *Am J Cardiol* 1994;74:578–584.

52. Neuss H, Schlepper M. Long term efficacy and safety of flecainide of supraventricular tachycardia. *Am J Cardiol* 1988;62:56D–61D.

53. Pritchett ELO, McCarthy EA, Wilkinson WE, et al. Propafenone treatment of symptomatic paroxysmal supraventricular arrhythmias: A randomized, placebo-controlled cross-over trial in patients tolerating oral therapy. *Ann Intern Med* 1991;114:539-544.

54. Huikuri HV, Koistinen MJ, Takkunen JT. Efficacy of intravenous sotalol for suppressing inducibility of supraventricular tachycardias at rest and during isometric exercise. *Am J Cardiol* 1992;69(5):498–502.

55. Wanless RS, Anderson K, Joy M, et al. Multicenter comparative study of the efficacy and safety of sotalol in the prophylactic treatment of patients with paroxysmal supraventricular tachyarrhythmias. *Am Heart J* 1997;133(4):441–446.

56. Jensen-urstad M, Tabrizi F, Kenneback G, Wredlert C, Klang C. High success rate with cryomapping and cryoablation of atrioventricular nodal reentrytachycardia. *Pacing Clin Electrophysiol* 2006;29:487–489.

57. Scheinman M, Calkins H, Gillette P, et al. NASPE policy statement on catheter ablation: personnel, policy, procedures, and therapeutic recommendations. *Pacing Clin Electrophysiol* 2003;26:1–11.

58. Blomström-Lundqvist C, Scheinman MM, Aliot EM, et al. ACC/AHA/ESC Guidelines for the Management of Patients with Supraventricular Arrhythmias—Executive Summary: A Report of the American College of Cardiology/American Heart Association Task Force on Practice Guidelines and the European Society of Cardiology Committee for Practice Guidelines (Writing Committee to Develop Guidelines for the Management of Patients with Supraventricular Arrhythmias). *Circulation* 2003;108(15):1871–1909.

59. Wolff L, Parkinson J, White PD. Bundle-branch block with short PR interval in healthy young people prone to paroxysmal tachycardia. *Am Heart J* 1930;5:685–704.

60. Murdock CJ, Leitch JW, Teo WS, et al. Characteristics of accessory pathways exhibiting decremental conduction. *Am J Cardiol* 1991;67:506–510.

61. Ross DL, Uther JB. Diagnosis of concealed accessory pathways in supraventricular tachycardia. *Pacing Clin Electrophysiol* 1984;7:1069–1085.

62. Reyes W, Milstein S, Dunnigan A, et al. Indications for modification of coexisting dual atrioventricular node pathways in patients undergoing surgical ablation of accessory atrioventricular connections. *J Am Coll Cardiol* 1991;17:1561–1567.

63. Klein GJ, Bashore TM, Sellers TD, et al. Ventricular fibrillation in the Wolff-Parkinson-White syndrome. *N Engl J Med* 1979;301:1080–1085.

64. Dreifus LS, Haiat R, Watanabe Y, et al. Ventricular fibrillation: a possible mechanism of sudden death in patients with Wolff-Parkinson-White syndrome. *Circulation* 1971;43:520–527.

65. Wellens HJJ, Durrer D. Wolff-Parkinson-White syndrome and atrial fibrillation. *Am J Cardiol* 1974;34:777–782.

66. Campbell RWF, Smith R, Gallagher JJ, et al. Atrial fibrillation in the preexcitation syndrome. *Am J Cardiol* 1977;40:514–520.

67. Sharma AD, Klein GJ, Guiraudon GM, et al. Atrial fibrillation in patients with Wolff-Parkinson-White syndrome: incidence after surgical ablation of the accessory pathway. *Circulation* 1985;72:161–169.

68. Dagres N, Clague JR, Lottkamp H, et al. Impact of radiofrequency catheter ablation of accessory pathways on the frequency of atrial fibrillation during long-term follow-up: high recurrence rate of atrial fibrillation in patients older than 50 years of age. *Eur Heart J* 2001;22(5):423–427.

69. Munger TM, Packer DL, Hammill SC, et al. A population study of the natural history of Wolff-Parkinson-White syndrome in Olmsted Country, Minnesota, 1953–1989. *Circulation* 1993;87:866–873.

70. Auricchio A, Klein H, Trappe HJ, et al. Lack of prognostic value of syncope in patients with Wolff-Parkinson-White syndrome. *J Am Coll Cardiol* 1991;17:152–158.

71. Leitch JW, Klein GJ, Yee R, et al. Syncope associated with supraventricular tachycardia: an expression of tachycardia rate or vasomotor response? *Circulation* 1992;85(3):1064–1071.

72. Smith RF. The Wolff-Parkinson-White syndrome as an aviation risk. *Circulation* 1990;82:1718–1723.

73. Timmermans C, Smeets JL, Rodriguez LM, et al. Aborted sudden death in the Wolff-Parkinson-White syndrome. *Am J Cardiol* 1995;76:492–494.

74. Pappone C, Santinelli V, Rosanio S, et al. Usefulness of invasive electrophysiologic testing to stratify the risk of arrhythmic events in asymptomatic patients with Wolff-Parkinson-White pattern: results from a large prospective long-term follow-up study. *J Am Coll Cardiol* 2003;41(2):239–244.

75. Lundberg A. Paroxysmal atrial tachycardia in infancy: long term follow-up study of 49 subjects. *Pediatrics* 1982;70:638.

76. Deal BJ, Keana JF, Gillette PC, et al. Wolff-Parkinson-White syndrome and supraventricular tachycardia during infancy: management and follow-up. *J Am Coll Cardiol* 1985;5:130.

77. Lev M, Givson S, Miller RA. Ebsteins' disease with Wolff-Parkinson-White syndrome. *Am Heart J* 1955;49:724.

78. Gallager JJ, Pritchett ELC, Sealy WC, et al. The preexcitation syndromes. *Prog Cardiovasc Dis* 1978;20:285–327.

79. Ross DL, Uther JB. Diagnosis of concealed accessory pathways in supraventricular tachycardia. *Pacing Clin Electrophysiol* 1984;7:1069–1085.

80. Arruda MS, McClelland JH, Wang X, et al. Development and validation of an ECG algorithm for identifying accessory pathway ablation site in Wolff-Parkinson-White syndrome. *J Cardiovasc Electrophysiol* 1998;9(1):2–12.

81. Fitzpatrick AP, Gonzales RP, Lesh MD, et al. New algorithm for the localization of accessory atrioventricular connections using a baseline electrocardiogram. *J Am Coll Cardiol* 1994;23(1):107–116.

82. Lindsay BD, Crossen KJ, Cain ME. Concordance of distinguishing electrocardiographic features during sinus rhythm with the location of accessory pathways in the Wolff-Parkinson-White syndrome. *Am J Cardiol* 1987;59(12):1093–1102.

83. Cain ME, Luke RA, Lindsay BD. Diagnosis and localization of accessory pathway. *Pacing Clin Electrophysiol* 1992;15:801–824.

84. d'Avila A, Brugada J, Skeberis V, et al. A fast and reliable algorithm to localize accessory pathways based on the polarity of the QRS complex on the surface ECG during sinus rhythm. *Pacing Clin Electrophysiol* 1995;18(9 pt 1):1615–1627.

85. Milstein S, Sharma AD, Guiraudon GM, et al. An algorithm for the electrocardiographic localization of accessory pathways in the Wolff-Parkinson-White syndrome. *Pacing Clin Electrophysiol* 1987;10 (3 pt 1):555–563.

86. Xie B, Heald SC, Bashir Y, et al. Localization of accessory pathways from the 12-lead electrocardiogram using a new algorithm. *Am J Cardiol* 1994;74(2):161–165.

87. Haissaguerre M, Marcus F, Poquet F, et al. Electrocardiographic characteristics and catheter ablation of parahisian accessory pathways. *Circulation* 1994;90(3):1124–1128.

88. Diker E, Ozdemir M, Tezcan UK, et al. QRS polarity on 12-lead surface ECG: a criterion for the differentiation of right and left posteroseptal accessory atrioventricular pathways. *Cardiology* 1997;88(4):328–332.

89. Boersma L, Garcia-Moran E, Mont L, et al. Accessory pathway localization by QRS polarity in children with Wolff-Parkinson-White syndrome. *J Cardiovasc Electrophysiol* 2002;13(12):1222–1260.

90. Basiouny T, de Chillou C, Fareh S, et al. Accuracy and limitations of published algorithms using the twelve-lead electrocardiogram to localize overt atrioventricular accessory pathways. *J Cardiovasc Electrophysiol* 1999;10(10):1340–1349.

91. Kappenberger LJ, Fromer MA, Steinbrunn W, et al. Efficacy of amiodarone in the Wolff-Parkinson-White syndrome with rapid ventricular response via accessory pathway during atrial fibrillation. *Am J Cardiol* 1984;54(3):330–335.

92. Lai W, Voon W, Yen H, et al. Comparison of the electrophysiologic effects of oral sustained-release and intravenous verapamil in patients with paroxysmal supraventricular tachycardia. *Am J Cardiol* 1993;71:405–408.

93. Lesh MD, Van Hare G, Scheinman MM, et al. Comparison of the retrograde and transseptal methods for ablation of left free-wall accessory pathways. *J Am Coll Cardiol* 1993;22:542–549.

94. Jackman WM, Wang X, Friday KJ, et al. Catheter ablation of accessory atrioventricular pathways (Wolff-Parkinson-White syndrome) by radiofrequency current. *N Engl J Med* 1991;324:1605–1611.

95. Kuck KH, Schluter M, Geiger M, et al. Radiofrequency current catheter ablation of accessory atrioventricular pathways. *Lancet* 1991;337(8757):1557–1561.

96. Calkins H, Langberg J, Sousa J, et al. Radiofrequency catheter ablation of accessory atrioventricular connections in 250 patients: abbreviated therapeutic approach to Wolff-Parkinson-White syndrome. *Circulation* 1992;85:1337–1346.

97. Kay GN, Pressley JC, Packer DL, et al. Value of 12-lead electrocardiogram in discriminating atrioventricular nodal reciprocating tachycardia from circus movement atrioventricular utilizing a retrograde accessory pathway. *Am J Cardiol* 1987;59:296–300.

98. Tchou PJ, Lehmann MJ, Donga J, et al. Effect of sudden rate acceleration on the human His-Purkinje system: adaptation of refractoriness in a damped oscillatory pattern. *Circulation* 1986;73:920–929.

99. Drago F, DeSantis A, Grutter G, Silverti MS. Transvenous cryothermal catheter ablation of re-entry circuit located near the atrioventricular junction in pediatric patients. *J Am Coll Cardiol* 2005;45:1096–103.

100. Manolis AS, Katsaros C, Cokkinos DV. Electrophysiological and electropharmacological studies in pre-excitation syndromes: results with propafenone therapy and isoproterenol infusion testing. *Eur Heart J* 1992;13:1489–1495.

101. Janoušek J, Paul T, Reimer A, Kallfelz H. Usefulness of propafenone for supraventricular arrhythmias in infants and children. *Am J Cardiol* 1993;72:294–300.

102. Musto B, D'Onofrio A, Cavallaro C, Musto A. Electrophysiological effects and clinical efficacy of propafenone in children with recurrent paroxysmal supraventricular tachycardia. *Circulation* 1988;78:863–869.

103. Vignati G, Figini M, Figini A. The use of propafenone in the treatment of tachyarrhythmias in children. *Eur Heart J* 1993;14:546–550.

104. Vassiliadis, Papoutsakis P, Kallikazaros I, et al. Propafenone in the prevention of non-ventricular arrhythmias associated with the Wolff-Parkinson-White syndrome. *Int J Cardiol* 1990;27:63–70.

105. Helmy I, Scheinman MM, Herre JM, et al. Electrophysiologic effects of isoproterenol in patients with atrioventricular reentrant tachycardia treated with flecainide. *J Am Coll Cardiol* 1990;16:1649–1655.

106. Mason JW. Amiodarone. *N Engl J Med* 1987;316:455–466.

107. Rosenbaum MD, Chiale PA, Ryba D, et al. Control of tachyarrhythmias associated with Wolff-Parkinson-White syndrome by amiodarone hydrochloride. *Am J Cardiol* 1974;34:215–223.

108. Wellens HJJ, Lie KI, Bar FW, et al. Effect of amiodarone in the Wolff-Parkinson-White syndrome. *Am J Cardiol* 1976;38:189–194.

109. Hindricks G. The Multicenter European Radiofrequency Survey (MERFS): complications of radiofrequency catheter ablation of arrhythmias. The Multicenter European Radiofrequency Survey (MERFS) investigators of the Working Group on Arrhythmias of the European Society of Cardiology. *Eur Heart J* 1993;14:1644–1653.

110. Brembilla-Perrot B, Ghawi R. Electrophysiological characteristics of asymptomatic Wolff-Parkinson-White syndrome. *Eur Heart J* 1993;14:511–515.

111. Leitch JW, Klein GJ, Yee R, Murdock C. Prognostic value of electrophysiology testing in asymptomatic patients with Wolff-Parkinson-White pattern. *Circulation* 1990;82:1718–1723.

112. Priori SG, Aliot E, Blomström-Lundqvist C, et al. Task force on sudden cardiac death of the European society of cardiology. *Eur Heart J* 2001;22:1374–1450.

113. Zipes DP, DiMarco JP, Gillette PC, et al. Guidelines for clinical intracardiac electrophysiological and catheter ablation procedures: a report of the American College of Cardiology/American Heart Association Task Force on Practice Guidelines (Committee on Clinical Intracardiac Electrophysiologic and Catheter Ablation Procedures), developed in collaboration with the North American Society of Pacing and Electrophysiology. *J Am Coll Cardiol* 1995;26:555–573.

114. Wellens HJ, Bar FW, Gorgels AP, et al. Use of ajmaline in patients with the Wolff-Parkinson-White syndrome to disclose short refractory period of the accessory pathway. *Am J Cardiol* 1980;45:130–133.

115. Fitzsimmons PJ, McWhirter PD, Peterson DW, et al. The natural history of Wolff-Parkinson-White syndrome in 228 military aviators: a long-term follow-up of 22 years. *Am Heart J* 2001;142(3):530–536.

116. Pappone C, Santinelli V, Rosanio S. Usefulness of invasive electrophysiology testing to stratify the risk of arrhythmic events in asymptomatic patients with Wolff-Parkinson-White pattern: results from a large prospective long-term follow-up study. *J Am Coll Cardiol* 2003;41:239–244.

117. Pappone C, Manguso F, Santinelli R, et al. Radiofrequency ablation in children with asymptomatic Wolff-Parkinson-White syndrome. *N Engl J Med* 2004;351:1197–205.

APPENDIX 38–1

Recommendations for Long-Term Management of Patients with Recurrent AVNRT

CLINICAL PRESENTATION	RECOMMENDATION	CLASSIFICATION	LEVEL OF EVIDENCE
Poorly tolerated AVNRT with hemodynamic intolerance	Catheter ablation	1	B
	Verapamil, diltiazem, β blockers	2a	C
	Sotalol, amiodarone	2a	C
	Flecainide, propafenone	2a	C
Recurrent symptomatic AVNRT	Catheter ablation	1	B
	Verapamil	1	B
	Diltiazem, β blockers	1	C
	Digoxin	2b	C
	Verapamil, diltiazem, digoxin	3	C
Recurrent AVNRT unresponsive to β blockade or calcium channel blocker and patients not desiring RF ablation	Flecainide, propafenone, sotalol	2a	B
	Amiodarone	2b	C
AVNRT with infrequent or single episode in patient desiring complete control of arrhythmia	Catheter ablation	1	B
Documented PSVT with only dual AV-nodal pathways or single echo beats demonstrated during EP study and no identified cause of arrhythmia	Verapamil, diltiazem, β blockers	1	C
	Flecainide, propafenone	1	C
	Catheter ablation	1	B
Infrequent well tolerated AVNRT	No therapy	1	C
	Vagal maneuvers	1	B
	Pill in the pocket	1	B
	Verapamil, diltiazem, β blockers	1	B
	Catheter ablation	1	B

AV, atrioventricular; AVNRT, atrioventricular nodal reentrant tachycardia; CAD, coronary artery disease; EP, electrophysiology; LV, left ventricle; PSVT, paroxysmal supraventricular tachycardia; RF, radiofrequency.
aRelatively contraindicated for patients with CAD, LV dysfunction, or other significant heart disease.
SOURCE: Adapted from Blomström-Lundqvist, Scheinman, Aliot, et al.[58]

APPENDIX 38–2

Recommendations for Long-Term Management of Accessory Pathway-Mediated Arrhythmias

ARRHYTHMIA	RECOMMENDATION	CLASSIFICATION	LEVEL OF EVIDENCE
WPW syndrome, well tolerated	Catheter ablation	1	B
	Flecainide, propafenone	2a	C
	Sotalol, amiodarone, β blockers	2a	C
	Verapamil, diltiazem, digoxin	3	C
WPW syndrome (with AF with rapid conduction or poorly tolerated AVRT)	Catheter ablation	1	B
	Flecainide, propafenone	2a	C
	Sotalol, amiodarone	2a	C
	β blockers	2b	C
	Verapamil, diltiazem, digoxin	3	C
Single or infrequent AVRT (no preexcitation)	None	1	C
	Vagal maneuvers	1	B
	Pill in the pocket (verapamil, diltiazem, β blockers)	1	B
	Catheter ablation	2a	B
	Sotalol, amiodarone	2b	B
	Flecainide, propafenone	2b	C
	Digoxin	3	C
Preexcitation, asymptomatic	None	1	C
	Catheter ablation	2a	B

AF, atrial fibrillation; AVNRT, atrioventricular nodal reentrant tachycardia; WPW, Wolff-Parkinson-White.
SOURCE: *Adapted from Blomström-Lundqvist, Scheinman, Aliot, et al.*[58]

CHAPTER 39

Ventricular Arrhythmias

Robert W. Rho / Richard L. Page

INTRODUCTION

Ventricular arrhythmias occur commonly in clinical practice and range from benign asymptomatic premature ventricular complexes (PVCs) to ventricular fibrillation (VF) resulting in sudden death. The presence of structural heart disease plays a major role in risk stratification; however, it is important to recognize potentially lethal arrhythmias that may occur in structurally normal–appearing hearts. In general, management depends on the associated symptoms, hemodynamic consequences, and associated long-term prognosis. Initial management, risk stratification, and treatment of ventricular arrhythmias pose a significant challenge to clinicians. This chapter provides an overview of the clinical presentation, natural history, diagnosis, and therapeutic options for the ventricular arrhythmias encountered in clinical practice.

Care has been taken to incorporate the American College of Cardiology/American Heart Association/European Society of Cardiology (ACC/AHA/ESC) 2006 Guidelines for Management of Patients with Ventricular Arrhythmias and the Prevention of Sudden Cardiac Death.[1] As with all ACC/AHA guidelines, this document provides specific categories of recommendation, according to the level of evidence available (Table 39–1).

PREMATURE VENTRICULAR COMPLEXES

PVCs are commonly seen in clinical practice. The significance of PVCs depends on the frequency of PVCs, the presence and severity of structural heart disease, and the presence of associated symptoms.

PREMATURE VENTRICULAR COMPLEXES IN THE ABSENCE OF ORGANIC HEART DISEASE

PVCs occur frequently in the general population.[2] In general PVCs that occur in patients without structural heart disease are

TABLE 39-1

Classification of Recommendations and Levels of Evidence to Support Them[1]

Classification of Recommendations
- Class I: Conditions for which there is evidence and/or general agreement that a given procedure or treatment is beneficial, useful, and effective.
- Class II: Conditions for which there is conflicting evidence and/or divergence of opinion about the usefulness/efficacy of a procedure or treatment.
- Class IIa: Weight of evidence/opinion is in favor of usefulness/efficacy.
- Class IIb: Usefulness/efficacy is less established by evidence/opinion.
- Class III: Conditions for which there is evidence and/or general agreement that a procedure/treatment is not useful/effective and in some cases may be harmful.

Level of Evidence
- Level of Evidence A: Data derived from multiple randomized clinical trials or meta-analyses.
- Level of Evidence B: Data derived from a single randomized trial or nonrandomized studies.
- Level of Evidence C: Only consensus opinion of experts, case studies, or standard of care.

not associated with excess risk of sudden death. Kennedy and co-workers studied 73 patients with frequent ventricular ectopy and no structural heart disease on a 24-hour ambulatory (Holter) monitor. Patients were followed for an average of 6.5 years with no excess in mortality.[3] PVCs that occur in patients with a structurally normal heart warrant no therapy, unless significant symptoms are present.

[ ] PREMATURE VENTRICULAR COMPLEXES AFTER MYOCARDIAL INFARCTION

The relationship between PVCs following myocardial infarction (MI) and sudden death has been studied extensively. In general, the presence of PVCs after a MI is associated with an increased risk of sudden death when the frequency of PVCs exceeds >10 per hour. Patients with larger MIs and lower left ventricular ejection fractions (LVEFs) are at the greatest risk of sudden death.[4–8]

Data from trials of thrombolytic therapy have also shown an association between PVCs and sudden death. In an analysis of Gruppo Italiano per lo Studio della Sopravvivenza nell'Infarto Miocardico (GISSI)-2, Statters and colleagues[9] compared the prognostic value of PVCs among 680 patients who received or did not receive thrombolytics. They reported the greatest risk of sudden death among the patients who had greater than 10 PVCs per hour and did not receive thrombolytics. In contrast PVCs did not predict sudden death in patients who received thrombolytics until the frequency of PVCs were greater than 25 per hour. These observations reflect the contribution of infarct size and, by association, ejection fraction (EF) to the prognosis of patients who have experienced a MI.

[ ] TREATMENT OF PREMATURE VENTRICULAR COMPLEXES ASSOCIATED WITH AN ACUTE MYOCARDIAL INFARCTION

The association of PVCs with sudden death led to the routine use of intravenous lidocaine in patients suffering MIs.[10] Subsequent randomized controlled studies have demonstrated worse survival when PVCs or ventricular arrhythmias were treated with antiarrhythmic agents.[11,12] Based on these findings, the routine prophylactic use of antiarrhythmic agents for patients following a MI is not recommended. The treatment of PVCs and nonsustained ventricular tachycardia (VT) with antiarrhythmics is also not recommended unless they are associated with hemodynamic compromise (ACC/AHA/ESC practice guidelines[1]). In patients with frequent ventricular ectopy, electrolyte and acid-base imbalance should be vigilantly corrected. If frequent and persistent ventricular ectopy results in hemodynamic instability, a β-adrenergic blocking agent or amiodarone is the preferred pharmacologic intervention in this setting. Lidocaine may be considered temporarily when hemodynamically significant ventricular arrhythmias occur in the setting of acute MI.

The use of amiodarone in patients during and following an acute MI is debated. Amiodarone has unique pharmacologic properties beyond its effects on the cardiac sodium and potassium channels. It is also a β-adrenergic receptor blocker and a calcium channel blocker, and has anti-ischemic effects.[13] The European Myocardial Infarction Amiodarone Trial (EMIAT) was a study that randomized 1486 patients with an EF of <40 percent and prior MI to amiodarone or placebo. No difference in total mortality was observed in both groups after a mean follow up of 21 months.[14] In the Canadian Amiodarone Myocardial Infarction Arrhythmia Trial (CAMIAT), patients with prior MI and frequent ventricular ectopy (>10 PVCs per hour) were randomized to amiodarone or placebo. The primary endpoint (combined arrhythmic death and resuscitated VF) was observed in 0.6 percent of the amiodarone group and 3.3 percent of the placebo group (p = 0.016). Most of the benefit was in patients who were treated concomitantly with β-adrenergic blockers. Although a significant benefit in arrhythmic death was observed in the amiodarone group, no significant difference in total mortality was observed in this study.[15] A recent meta-analysis of 13 trials of amiodarone after MI or congestive heart failure reported a reduction in mortality and arrhythmic death in those patients treated with amiodarone.[16] However, based on the available information on amiodarone after MI, the prophylactic use of amiodarone in patients after a MI is not recommended for primary prevention. However, the use of amiodarone for the treatment of hemodynamically significant ventricular arrhythmias or other arrhythmias, such as atrial fibrillation, in the postinfarct setting appears to be safe.

Premature Ventricular Complexes and Nonsustained Ventricular Tachycardia in Nonischemic Cardiomyopathy

The association between PVCs in nonischemic cardiomyopathy and sudden death is less clear. Several large trials including Grupo de Estudio de la Sobrevida en la Insuficiencia Cardiaca en Argentina (GESICA) and the Vasodilator-Heart Failure Trial (VHeFT) have found that nonsustained VT is a risk factor for sudden death.[17,18] In

PVCs from the RV outflow tract

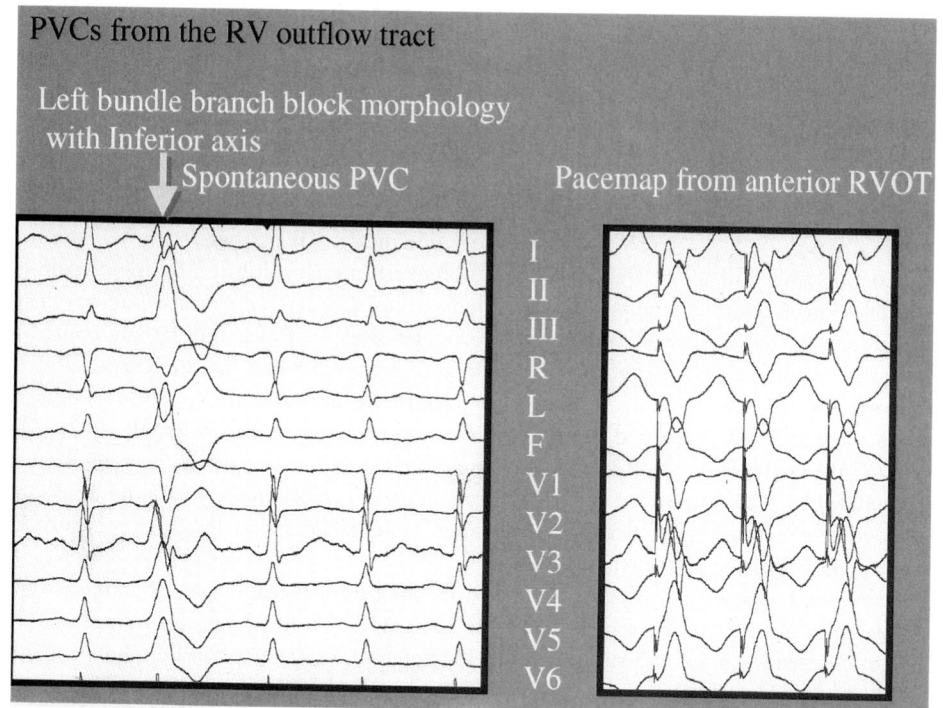

Left bundle branch block morphology with Inferior axis

Spontaneous PVC

Pacemap from anterior RVOT

I
II
III
R
L
F
V1
V2
V3
V4
V5
V6

FIGURE 39–1. Shown here is a typical PVC that originates from the RVOT. Characteristics of the QRS complex on a 12-lead electrocardiogram reveal a LBBB pattern in V1 and tall monophasic positive R-waves in leads II, III, and aVF. These PVCs were highly symptomatic in this 32-year old woman, despite aggressive pharmacologic treatment. She was brought to the electrophysiology laboratory for an electrophysiology study and radiofrequency ablation procedure. A mapping catheter is placed in the anterior RVOT at the site of origin of the PVC. Pacing from this site demonstrates a 12-lead QRS morphology that matches the spontaneously occurring PVC. A single radiofrequency ablation lesion successfully eliminates the PVC. LBBB, left bundle-branch block; PVC, premature ventricular complex; RV, right ventricular; RVOT, right ventricular outflow tract.

contrast Von Olshousen and coworkers[19] found only presence of a bundle-branch block and depressed EF predicted sudden death when they followed 73 patients with nonischemic cardiomyopathy and frequent PVCs for 3 years. In another study of ambulatory monitors performed in 674 patients with dilated cardiomyopathy, nonsustained VT was not associated with a lower survival rate.[20] Therefore, the clinical significance of asymptomatic nonsustained VT in patients with dilated cardiomyopathy remains unclear.

OUTFLOW TRACT PREMATURE VENTRICULAR COMPLEXES

PVCs originating from the right ventricular outflow tract (RVOT PVC) are characterized on the 12-lead electrocardiogram by a left bundle-block pattern in V1 and tall, monophasic R-waves in the inferior leads (Fig. 39–1). For most patients with structurally normal hearts who have RVOT PVCs, prognosis is good. This group of patients may manifest with frequent single PVCs or as repetitive salvos of monomorphic VT. The frequency of RVOT PVCs is often augmented by exercise; therefore, an exercise treadmill test is a useful diagnostic test. Symptomatic RVOT PVCs may respond to β-adrenergic blocking agents and calcium channel blockers. Radiofrequency catheter ablative therapy can be a curative treatment option for patients with symptomatic PVCs from the RVOT when drug therapy is proven ineffective (ACC/AHA/ESC practice guidelines [see Chapter 11][1]). In the workup of these patients, it is important

to rule out other causes of RVOT ectopy, such as arrhythmogenic right ventricular (RV) cardiomyopathy, a condition associated with sudden death and progressive RV failure.

EXERCISE-INDUCED PREMATURE VENTRICULAR COMPLEXES

The significance of PVCs in patients that occur during or in the recovery phase of exercise stress testing has been controversial, especially in patients with structurally normal hearts. A recent report of 6101 asymptomatic men who underwent exercise stress testing from the Paris Prospective Study reported that ventricular ectopy during exercise was associated with a relative risk of death from cardiovascular causes of 2.63 (95 percent confidence interval [CI] 1.93– 3.59) when followed for an average of 23 years.[21] In another study of 29,244 patients (70 percent men) without a history of heart failure or valve disease, the presence of frequent ventricular ectopy (defined by >7 PVCs/min) during recovery predicted an increased risk of death with an adjusted hazard ratio (HR) of 1.5 (95 percent CI 1.1–1.9; $p = 0.003$) but frequent ventricular ectopy during exercise did not predict increased risk of death. The mean follow up of this study was 5.3 years.[22] Specific treatment recommendations cannot be derived on the basis of these observational studies.

MANAGEMENT OF PATIENTS WITH PREMATURE VENTRICULAR COMPLEXES

Patients with PVCs should have an echocardiogram to assess left ventricular (LV) function. Patients with structurally normal hearts and asymptomatic PVCs do not require specific therapy. Patients with PVCs from the right ventricle, with RV dysfunction or enlargement, should undergo further workup to rule out arrhythmogenic right ventricular cardiomyopathy. This workup should include a cardiac MRI, a signal averaged electrocardiogram, and an electrophysiologic study.

In patients with symptomatic PVCs, therapy aimed at alleviating symptoms may be necessary. Initial treatment should include reassurance and the avoidance of exogenous stimulants or a trial of β-adrenergic blocking agents.

VENTRICULAR TACHYCARDIA IN PATIENTS WITH CORONARY ARTERY DISEASE

Ventricular tachycardia in patients with coronary disease ranges from nonsustained ventricular tachycardia (NSVT) to sustained

VT that leads to hemodynamic compromise and sudden death. The understanding of the pathophysiology of VT in patients with coronary artery disease has been greatly enhanced by animal studies, electrophysiologic studies in humans, and the results from recent multicenter randomized trials.

PATHOPHYSIOLOGY

The anatomic substrate from which sustained monomorphic VT originates usually involves an extensive healed scar following an acute MI. This substrate of healthy and damaged myocardium interlaced with fibrous scar is found primarily at the border zone of the scar (transition between scar and healthy tissue) and serves as a substrate for slowed conduction and reentry.[23,24] Evolution of the electrophysiologic substrate occurs over two weeks after a MI and then remains indefinitely.[25] The substrate may continue to be modified by subsequent ischemic insults as well as late ventricular remodeling and worsening pump function. These changes may lead to neurohormonal activation and progressive LV dilatation with regional and global elevations in wall tension, all of which may contribute to proarrhythmia. Patients with VT have a high risk of recurrence of VT even when heart failure and coronary ischemia are controlled.[26] Early data demonstrated that the risk of VT is highest during the first year (3–5 percent) after an MI but that new onset of VT may occur many years later.[6] However, recent evidence suggests that the risk of sudden death from ventricular arrhythmias remains high and may increase with time after an MI.[27,28] In general, patients with larger infarctions and lower EFs are at highest risk of fatal ventricular arrhythmias.

MECHANISM

The mechanism of VT in most cases is reentry. Ischemic VT usually is initiated, terminated, and reset with programmed electrical stimulation in the electrophysiology laboratory; this response to programmed electrical stimulation supports reentry as the mechanism for this form of VT.[29] The reentry circuit most frequently exists within the border zone of the scar.[23]

CLINICAL PRESENTATION AND MANAGEMENT

Symptoms associated with ischemic VT are variable. The main determinants of hemodynamic tolerance are the rate of the VT[30] and the degree of LV dysfunction.[31] The hemodynamic stability of sustained VT is not prognostic of mortality risk. In the AVID (Antiarrhythmics Versus Implantable Defibrillators) registry, patients with hemodynamically tolerated VT at presentation had similar mortality compared with patients with syncopal VT.[32]

Sustained Ventricular Tachycardia

Patients who present in clinically stable VT may be treated with antiarrhythmic drugs, antitachycardia pacing when available, or synchronized direct current (DC) cardioversion. Patients in VT with hemodynamic compromise, congestive heart failure, chest pain, or ischemia should be treated promptly with DC cardioversion (ACC/AHA/ESC practice guidelines[1]). In patients with stable sustained VT, intravenous procainamide is

a reasonable first choice (ACC/AHA/ESC practice guidelines[1]). However, intravenous procainamide may cause hemodynamic instability because of its negative inotropic effects. When antiarrhythmic drug therapy is chosen to prevent recurrence or when VT is accompanied by hemodynamic instability, amiodarone is the treatment of choice. The efficacy of amiodarone is superior to lidocaine or procainamide in this setting[33,34] (ACC/AHA/ESC practice guidelines[1]). All patients with VT should be treated with a β blocker unless prohibited by hypotension, bradycardia, or other clinical factors (i.e., reactive airway disease, vasospastic coronary disease). Reversible factors contributing to VT, such as congestive heart failure exacerbation, acute ischemia, or electrolyte abnormalities should be diagnosed rapidly and treated. In patients who have refractory VT despite aggressive treatment, a subset of patients may be treated successfully with an emergent radiofrequency catheter ablation procedure, mechanical ventricular assist devices, and cardiac transplantation.[35,36]

The primary goal for long-term management in patients who have presented with sustained VT is to prevent recurrence of VT and sudden death. LV function is a well-established independent risk factor for sudden cardiac death in patients with ventricular arrhythmias.[37–40] In a subanalysis of the Candesartan in Heart Failure Assessment of Reduction in Mortality and Morbidity (CHARM) study, evaluation of the impact of LVEF quartiles on long-term survival revealed a 39 percent relative risk of increased mortality for every 10 percent reduction in LVEF.[41]

Patients who present with sustained VT and an LVEF <35 percent should be considered for an implantable defibrillator. In patients with preserved LV function, the implantation of a defibrillator is controversial. A meta-analysis of the secondary prevention internal cardioverter-defibrillator (ICD) trials revealed that the patients who benefited from ICD therapy over amiodarone therapy were patients with EF <35 percent. Amiodarone was equivalent to ICD in patients with EF >35 percent.[42] Most patients with sustained VT should receive an implantable defibrillator (Table 39–2); but for some patients with preserved LV function, amiodarone is a reasonable alternative. Long-term toxicities (pulmonary, hepatic, thyroid, skin, etc.) and the high rate of drug cessation for intolerance to the medication remain practical limitations for chronic amiodarone therapy.

Before implantation of a cardiac defibrillator, it is important that VT is clinically well-controlled to prevent multiple shocks from the ICD. Reversible causes of VT should be corrected. Continued episodes of VT despite correcting reversible causes should be treated aggressively. Several studies have demonstrated the efficacy of antiarrhythmic agents in preventing ICD shocks. In a randomized controlled study of patients who had ICDs implanted for inducible or spontaneously occurring VT or VF, 412 patients were randomized to β-adrenergic blockers alone ($n = 140$), sotalol alone ($n = 134$), or amiodarone plus β blocker ($n = 140$). After a mean followup of 359 days, ICD shocks occurred in 38.5 percent of patients assigned to the β blocker group, 24.3 percent of patients in the sotalol group, and 10.3 percent in the amiodarone plus β blocker group. Amiodarone plus β blocker resulted in significantly fewer shocks compared to β blocker alone ($p = 0.006$).[43] The decision for empiric therapy with antiarrhythmic agents at the time of ICD implantation depends on whether VT or VF can be controlled clinically. A β-

TABLE 39-2

ACC/AHA/ESC 2006 Guidelines for Internal Cardioverter-Defibrillator Implantation[1]

Class I

1. ICD therapy is recommended for secondary prevention of SCD in patients who survived VF or hemodynamically unstable VT, or VT with syncope and who have an LVEF ≤40%, are receiving chronic optimal medical therapy, and have a reasonable expectation of survival with a good functional status for >1 year (Level of Evidence: A).
2. The ICD is effective therapy to reduce mortality by a reduction in SCD in patients with LV dysfunction caused by prior MI who present with hemodynamically unstable sustained VT, are receiving chronic optimal medical therapy, and have reasonable expectation of survival with a good functional status for >1 year (Level of Evidence: A).
3. An ICD should be implanted in patients with nonischemic DCM and significant LV dysfunction who have sustained VT or VF, are receiving chronic optimal medical therapy, and have reasonable expectation of survival with a good functional status for >1 year (Level of Evidence: A).
4. ICD therapy is recommended for primary prevention to reduce total mortality by a reduction in SCD in patients with LV dysfunction caused by prior MI who are at least 40 days post-MI, have an LVEF ≤30% to 40%, are NYHA functional class II or III, are receiving chronic optimal medical therapy, and have reasonable expectation of survival with a good functional status for >1 year (Level of Evidence: A).
5. ICD therapy is recommended for primary prevention to reduce total mortality by a reduction in SCD in patients with nonischemic heart disease who have an LVEF ≤30% to 35%, are NYHA functional class II or III receiving chronic optimal medical therapy, and who have reasonable expectation of survival with a good functional status for >1 year (Level of Evidence: B).

Class IIa

1. ICD implantation is reasonable for treatment of recurrent sustained VT in patients post-MI with normal or near normal ventricular function who are receiving chronic optimal medical therapy and have reasonable expectation of survival with a good functional status for >1 year (Level of Evidence: C).
2. Implantation of an ICD is reasonable in patients with LV dysfunction caused by prior MI who are at least 40 days post-MI, have an LVEF ≤30% to 35%, are NYHA functional class I on chronic optimal medical therapy, and who have reasonable expectation of survival with a good functional status for >1 year (Level of Evidence: B).
3. ICD implantation can be beneficial for patients with unexplained syncope, significant LV dysfunction, and nonischemic DCM who are receiving optimal medical therapy and who have a reasonable expectation of survival with a good functional status for >1 year (Level of Evidence: C).
4. ICD therapy is reasonable in patients who have recurrent stable VT, a normal or near normal LVEF, and optimally treated HF and who have a reasonable expectation of survival with a good functional status for >1 year (Level of Evidence: C).
5. ICD therapy combined with biventricular pacing can be effective for primary prevention to reduce total mortality by a reduction in SCD in patients with NYHA functional class III or IV receiving optimal medical therapy, in sinus rhythm with a QRS complex of at least 120 msec and who have reasonable expectation of survival with a good functional status for >1 year (Level of Evidence: B).
6. ICD therapy is reasonable for primary prevention to reduce total mortality by a reduction in SCD in patients with LV dysfunction caused by prior MI who are at least 40 days post-MI, have an LVEF ≤30% to 35%, are NYHA functional class I, are receiving chronic optimal medical therapy, and have reasonable expectation of survival with a good functional status for >1 year (Level of Evidence: B).

Class IIb

1. ICD therapy may be considered for primary prevention to reduce total mortality by a reduction in SCD in patients with nonischemic heart disease who have an LVEF ≤30% to 35%, are NYHA functional class I receiving chronic optimal medical therapy, and who have a reasonable expectation of survival with a good functional status for >1 year (Level of Evidence: B).

DCM, dilated cardiomyopathy; ICD, internal cardioverter-defibrillator; LV, left ventricular; LVEF, left ventricular ejection fraction; MI, myocardial infarction; NYHA, New York Heart Association; SCD, sudden cardiac death; VF, ventricular fibrillation; VT, ventricular tachycardia.

adrenergic blocking agent should be administered in all patients unless contraindicated.

When antiarrhythmic agents are initiated in patients with an implantable defibrillator, care must be taken in programming the implantable defibrillator because antiarrhythmic medications can have varying effects on defibrillation thresholds and may slow the rate of the VT.

Patients with ischemic cardiomyopathy and persistent VT refractory to medications may be successfully treated with radiofrequency catheter ablation techniques.[44,45] It should be emphasized that such ablation is adjuvant to ICD therapy and cannot be expected to obviate the need for an ICD (Table 39-3).

Nonsustained Ventricular Tachycardia

The evaluation and management of patients with asymptomatic nonsustained VT begins with the evaluation of the patient's LVEF. Patients with preserved LV function are generally at low risk and

TABLE 39-3

ACC/AHA/ESC 2006 Guidelines for the Role of Ablation in the Management of Ventricular Arrhythmias[1]

Class I

1. Ablation is indicated in patients who are otherwise at low risk for SCD and have sustained predominantly monomorphic VT that is drug resistant, are drug intolerant, or do not wish long-term drug therapy (Level of Evidence: C).
2. Ablation is indicated in patients with BBR VT (Level of Evidence: C).
3. Ablation is indicated as adjunctive therapy in patients with an ICD who are receiving multiple shocks as a result of sustained VT that is not manageable by reprogramming or changing drug therapy or do not wish long-term drug therapy (Level of Evidence: C).
4. Ablation is indicated in patients with Wolff-Parkinson-White syndrome resuscitated from sudden cardiac arrest caused by atrial fibrillation and rapid conduction over the accessory pathway causing VF (Level of Evidence: B).

Class IIa

1. Ablation can be useful therapy in patients who are otherwise at low risk for SCD and have symptomatic nonsustained monomorphic VT that is drug resistant, are drug intolerant, or do not wish long-term drug therapy (Level of Evidence: C).
2. Ablation can be useful therapy in patients who are otherwise at low risk for SCD and have frequent symptomatic predominantly monomorphic PVCs that are drug resistant, are drug intolerant, or do not wish long-term drug therapy (Level of Evidence: C).
3. Ablation can be useful in symptomatic patients with Wolff-Parkinson-White syndrome who have accessory pathways with refractory periods <240 msec in duration (Level of Evidence: B).

Class IIb

1. Ablation of asymptomatic PVCs may be considered when the PVCs are very frequent to avoid or treat tachycardia-induced cardiomyopathy (Level of Evidence: C).
2. Curative catheter ablation or amiodarone may be considered in lieu of ICD therapy to improve symptoms in patients with LV dysfunction caused by prior MI and recurrent hemodynamically stable VT whose LVEF is >40% (Level of Evidence: B).

Class III

1. Ablation of asymptomatic relatively infrequent PVCs is not indicated (Level of Evidence: C).

BBR, bundle branch reentrant; ICD, internal cardioverter-defibrillator; LV, left ventricular; LVEF, left ventricular ejection fraction; MI, myocardial infarction; PVC, premature ventricular complexes; SCD, sudden cardiac death; VT, ventricular tachycardia.

generally require no further treatment. Patients with low EF are at risk of sudden death. In patients with an LVEF of less than 40 percent, annual mortality of patients post-MI is estimated to be 8 to 10 percent.[46] The importance of treating these patients with an angiotensin-converting enzyme inhibitor (ACEI), aspirin, and a β-adrenergic receptor blocker cannot be over emphasized (ACC/AHA/ESC 2006 guidelines[1]).

Over the past several years, two important changes in the standard of care of patients with coronary artery disease at risk of malignant ventricular arrhythmias have occurred. First, programmed electrical stimulation at electrophysiologic study (EPS) has been demonstrated to be a poor risk stratification tool. Second, clinical documentation of NSVT is no longer necessary to identify patients that would benefit from primary prevention with an implantable cardiac defibrillator.

Previously, a diagnostic electrophysiologic study with programmed stimulation in the right ventricle was used to risk stratify asymptomatic postinfarct patients with NSVT.[47] However, an analysis of the Multicenter Unsustained Tachycardia Trial (MUSTT) registry data demonstrated patients with negative EPS who were followed in a registry had a high risk of arrhythmic death (12 percent over 12 months).[48] The high mortality rate in the patients that were noninducible at EPS in this study called into question the usefulness of programmed electrical stimulation as a risk stratification tool.

The need for NSVT to identify patients who would benefit from an ICD was invalidated by the Multicenter Automatic Defibrillator

Implantation Trial (MADIT) II study. This study randomized 1232 patients with ischemic cardiomyopathy on the basis of LV function alone (LVEF ≤30 percent) with no requirement for the documentation of NSVT. After an average follow up of 20 months, a significant reduction in all-cause mortality was observed in patients who received an ICD.[49] The Sudden Cardiac Death in Heart Failure Trial (SCD-HeFT) is the largest randomized primary prevention trial comparing ICD versus amiodarone versus optimal medical therapy in patients with LVEF <35 percent. This study did not require the presence of NSVT for enrollment. Patients enrolled in SCD-HeFT had New York Heart Association (NYHA) functional class II–III heart failure symptoms. After a 5-year follow-up period, this study demonstrated that (1) the annual mortality of patients on optimal medical therapy is 7 to 8 percent per year; (2) amiodarone, when used as a primary preventative agent, does not improve survival over good background medical therapy for heart failure; and (3) that an ICD decreases mortality by 23 percent compared with optimal medical therapy (HR = 0.77, CI 0.62–0.96, $p = 0.007$).[50]

Based on the recent literature guiding the primary prevention of sudden death in patients with coronary artery disease and depressed LV function, patients with ischemic cardiomyopathy with an EF of <35 percent should be treated according the ACC/AHA guidelines with appropriate pharmacological therapy for heart failure including ACEIs, angiotensin II receptor blocking agents, β-adrenergic receptor blockers, and aldosterone antagonists. Once they are adequately treated, an implantable cardiac defibrillator should be considered for primary prevention of sudden death regardless of whether they have NSVT clinically documented or not. The demonstration of spontaneously occurring nonsustained VT or sustained VT inducible on programmed electrical stimulation is no longer a necessary prerequisite to the implantation of an ICD (see Table 39–2).

VENTRICULAR TACHYCARDIA IN PATIENTS WITH NONISCHEMIC CARDIOMYOPATHY

Dilated cardiomyopathy is caused by a heterogeneous group of etiologies resulting in LV and/or RV failure. Causes of dilated cardiomyopathy include valvular heart disease, ethanol ingestion, viral infections, and cardiac sarcoidosis, among others. Sudden death in dilated cardiomyopathy is usually caused by a ventricular tachyarrhythmia. The contribution of bradyarrhythmias to the etiology of sudden death in patients with dilated cardiomyopathy may also be important. In a report of 157 cases of sudden death in idiopathic cardiomyopathy in which the rhythm preceding death was available from ambulatory monitoring, 62 percent of patients had organized VT that progressed to VF and 13 percent had primary VF but 17 percent had bradyarrhythmia.[51] In another report of 20 patients with severe dilated cardiomyopathy awaiting cardiac transplant, the cause of death was electromechanical dissociation/bradycardia in 13 out of 20 patients, and only 7 out of 20 died of a ventricular arrhythmia.[52] Although ventricular arrhythmias are the most frequent causes of sudden death, bradyarrhythmias may also play a role in some patients with severe dilated cardiomyopathy.[51–53]

【 】 PATHOPHYSIOLOGY

The pathogenesis of ventricular arrhythmias in dilated cardiomyopathy is not well understood and may reflect a variety of mechanisms. In a study of the autopsy findings in 152 patients with idiopathic dilated cardiomyopathy (IDCM), subendocardial scarring was present in 33 percent of patients. Histologic sectioning revealed multiple patchy areas of fibrosis in 57 percent of patients. These patchy areas of fibrosis, intermingled with viable myocardium, may serve as the substrate for reentry.[54] Changes in ventricular mechanics and geometry may alter regional refractoriness within the ventricle and also predispose to reentry, enhanced automaticity, or triggered activity.[55] Furthermore, the conduction system may also serve as a substrate for reentry in patients with dilated cardiomyopathy. Bundle-branch reentry (BBR) is a type of VT that uses the left and right bundle branches and a portion of the ventricular myocardium as its circuit. BBR is a common cause of sustained monomorphic VT in patients with dilated cardiomyopathy and may represent up to 41 percent of VTs present in this subgroup.[56] In another series of 26 patients with monomorphic VT and nonischemic cardiomyopathy, the etiology of VT was scar-related reentry in 62 percent, an ectopic focus in 27 percent, and BBR in 19 percent of patients.[57] The identification of BBR is important in patients with dilated cardiomyopathy because this arrhythmia may be treated with radiofrequency catheter ablation (see also ACC/AHA/ESC 2006 practice guidelines[1]).

Clinical Presentation and Management

Nonsustained VT is common in patients with dilated cardiomyopathy. NSVT is seen on 24-hour ambulatory and telemetry monitoring in 50 to 60 percent of these patients. Sustained VT or VF is thought to be the most common cause of death in dilated cardiomyopathy. The prevalence of NSVT increases with worsening heart failure symptoms. In patients with class I–II congestive heart failure, the prevalence of NSVT is 15 to 20 percent and in class IV heart failure the prevalence is 50 to 70 percent.[58–61] The significance of NSVT as an independent predictor of sudden death in this setting is unclear.

Patients with dilated cardiomyopathy should be treated with an ACEI and β blocker. The role of amiodarone in patients with nonischemic cardiomyopathy has evolved over recent years. The GESICA trial examined whether low-dose amiodarone (300 mg/d) would improve survival in patients with severe chronic heart failure (class II–IV and EF <35 percent). Although GESICA included patients with both ischemic and nonischemic VT, this South American trial had a high representation of patients with nonischemic cardiomyopathy (62 percent nonischemic, 10 percent with Chagas disease). In this trial 516 patients were randomized to amiodarone versus placebo and followed for a mean of 2 years. Amiodarone was associated with a 28 percent reduction in mortality in comparison to placebo (33.5 percent vs. 41.6 percent, $p = 0.024$).[62] Survival Trial of Antiarrhythmic Therapy in Congestive Heart Failure (CHF-STAT), a placebo-controlled, randomized trial of amiodarone that was conducted in North America, failed to show benefit to amiodarone; but the subgroup analysis of patients with nonischemic cardiomyopathy showed a trend toward lower mortality ($p = 0.07$).[13] The SCD-HeFT study was the largest study to date evaluating the efficacy of amiodarone versus placebo in ischemic and nonischemic cardiomyopathy. This study demonstrated no benefit of amiodarone over optimal medical treatment for the primary prevention of sudden death in patients with NYHA class II–III heart failure symptoms and an EF of <35 percent (HR = 1.06; 97.5 percent CI 0.86–1.30; $p = 0.53$). A subset analysis of this study demonstrated that amiodarone was associated with worse survival in patients with class III heart failure symptoms compared to optimal medical therapy alone.[50]

The role of an implantable cardiac defibrillator in the primary prevention of sudden death in patients with nonischemic cardiomyopathy has recently been established. Bansch and coworkers[63] randomized 104 patients with idiopathic dilated cardiomyopathy and LVEF ≤30 percent, with no prior history of VT or VF to two treatment arms: ICD or no ICD. After a mean followup of 5.5 years, no significant difference in survival was observed between patients with and without an ICD. Kadish and colleagues evaluated 458 patients with nonischemic cardiomyopathy and an EF <36 percent who were randomized to an ICD plus standard medical therapy versus standard medical therapy alone. After a mean follow-up period of 29 months, there were 28 deaths in the ICD group compared with 40 in the standard therapy group (HR 0.65, 95 percent CI 0.40 to 1.06, $p = 0.08$).[64] These two studies were underpowered to demonstrate benefit of the ICD in this group of patients with nonischemic cardiomyopathy. As previously mentioned, the SCD-HeFT trial enrolled 2521 patients with ischemic and nonischemic cardiomyopathy with NYHA class II–III heart failure symptoms and LVEF <35 percent. A 23 percent relative reduction in mortality was observed in the patients randomized to ICD compared with patients treated with optimal medical therapy only (HR = 0.77; 97.5 percent, CI 0.62–0.96; *p* = 0.007).[50]

Based on these findings, patients with nonischemic cardiomyopathy with an EF of <35 percent and NYHA class II–III heart failure symptoms should be considered for implantation of a cardiac defibrillator for primary prevention of sudden death (see Table 39–2). The importance of optimal medical therapy with an ACEI, β-adrenergic blocking agent, angiotensin II receptor blocker, and aldosterone antagonist cannot be overemphasized in this population of patients. Amiodarone provides no benefit in survival for the primary prevention of sudden death in this population.

Radiofrequency catheter ablation of VT in patients with drug refractory VT may serve as an adjunctive treatment option for patients with nonischemic cardiomyopathy suffering multiple recurrences of VT or frequent ICD therapies (see Table 39–3). In a series of 19 patients with nonischemic cardiomyopathy who had detailed mapping performed for VT, a modest-sized basal (perivalvular) area of endocardial electrogram abnormalities was observed. Most (88 percent) of the 57 VTs mapped in these patients had a site of origin near the base of the left ventricle within the region of abnormal electrograms.[65] Successful ablation of scar related VTs in patients with sarcoidosis, scleroderma, and Chagas disease have been reported; however, experience is limited.

[ ] VENTRICULAR TACHYCARDIA IN ARRHYTHMOGENIC RIGHT VENTRICULAR DYSPLASIA

Arrhythmogenic right ventricular dysplasia (ARVD) is characterized by fatty infiltration, fibrosis, and thinning of the right ventricle and is associated with ventricular arrhythmias and sudden death. It is the most common cause of exercise induced sudden death among young male athletes in Italy and may be responsible for up to 20 percent of sudden deaths in men younger than age 30 years old.[66] Although most cases appear to be sporadic, approximately 30 percent of patients have a family history of ARVD. Mutations in genes encoding for several cytoskeletal proteins such as plakoglobin, desmoplakin, and plakophilin-2 have been reported. The most frequently involved areas of the right ventricle are the posterior base, apex, and the infundibulum. These areas are collectively called the *triangle of dysplasia*. Diagnosis of ARVD can be difficult. Magnetic resonance imaging, echocardiography, electrocardiography, and signal averaged electrocardiogram may be helpful in the diagnosis.[67]

The electrocardiogram during sinus rhythm in ARVD has some distinctive features. T-wave inversion may be present in electrocardiographic leads V_1 to V_3. The prevalence of T-wave inversion increases over time. In patients with ARVD who present with VT, the prevalence of T-wave inversion in V_1 to V_3 increased from 50 to 98 percent during a follow-up period of 9.5 ± 3.2 years.[68] An increased QRS duration >110 msec in V_1 may be seen as a manifestation of delayed conduction in the Purkinje system in the free wall of the

[ ] BUNDLE-BRANCH REENTRY VENTRICULAR TACHYCARDIA

The clinical recognition of BBR VT is essential because this arrhythmia can potentially be cured by a radiofrequency ablation procedure.[56,57] The rate of BBR is usually rapid and may be associated with syncope. The sinus rhythm 12-lead electrocardiogram usually demonstrates an intraventricular conduction delay or a left bundle-branch block (LBBB). The 12-lead electrocardiogram during VT has a LBBB configuration (Fig. 39–2). The treatment of choice for this arrhythmia is radiofrequency ablation of the right bundle branch. Antiarrhythmic drugs for BBR are associated with a high recurrence rate. Patients with BBR with an EF <35 percent should receive an implantable defibrillator even after successful ablation of the right bundle, as they remain at risk for other lethal ventricular arrhythmias. The role of an ICD in patients with an EF >35 percent who have had a successful ablation for BBR is controversial.

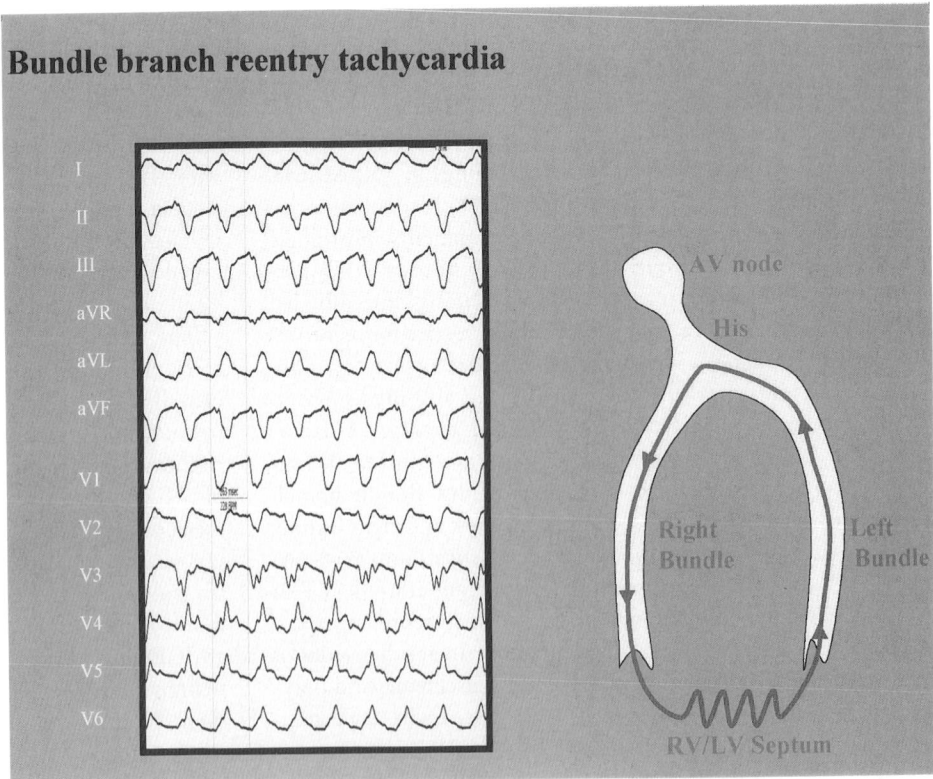

FIGURE 39–2. Bundle-branch reentry ventricular tachycardia. Note the left bundle-branch pattern and the left superior axis. The reentry circuit involves the right bundle branch as the anterograde limb and the left bundle branch as the retrograde limb, as depicted schematically on the right. AV, atrioventricular; LV, left ventricle; His, His bundle; RV, right ventricle.

right ventricle. Finally, epsilon waves, or small high frequency deflections found in the terminal portion of the QRS complex in leads V_1 to V_3 may be present, as shown in Fig. 39–3.[69]

The diagnosis of ARVD is challenging in some cases. A task force proposed several criteria for the diagnosis of ARVD. From this consensus of experts, several major and minor diagnostic criteria are described. The major criteria include the following:

- Severe dilatation and reduction in RVEF with normal LV function
- Localized RV aneurysms
- Severe segmental dilation of the RV
- Fibrofatty replacement of myocardium on endomyocardial biopsy
- An epsilon wave present on the 12-lead electrocardiogram
- A family history of ARVD confirmed at necropsy or surgery.

The minor criteria include the following:

- Mild global RV dilation or EF reduction with normal LV
- Mild segmental dilation of the RV
- Regional RV hypokinesia
- Inverted T-waves in the right precordial leads in the absence of a right bundle branch block (RBBB)
- Late potentials on a signal average electrocardiogram
- LBBB morphology ventricular arrhythmias (sustained or non-sustained)
- Frequent ventricular extrasystoles (>1000/24 hours)
- Family history of sudden death at age younger than age 35 years suspected to be caused by RV dysplasia

When secondary causes of RV enlargement or dysfunction are ruled out, the presence of two major criteria, one major and two minor criteria, or four minor criteria make the diagnosis of ARVD very likely.[69]

Patients with ARVD may present with stable monomorphic VT and sudden death. VT is characterized by a left LBBB pattern in V_1.

Multiple morphologies of VT are often present in a given individual. VT that originates from the infundibulum, or RVOT, may be difficult to distinguish from RVOT VT, which is a benign disease in patients with structurally normal hearts. Among these patients with VT that has a LBBB pattern in V_1, the presence of multiple morphologies of VT with a superior QRS axis (negative in leads II, III and aVF) should raise the suspicion for ARVD as the etiology.

Treatment of ventricular arrhythmias arising from ARVD is aimed at preventing sudden death and palliation of the clinical burden of VT. Clinical data on the efficacy of antiarrhythmic drugs and patient selection for implantable defibrillators is limited. Treatment of sustained VT may include amiodarone, β blockers, and sotalol as first line choices. Patients who have had sustained VT or a history of cardiac arrest from VF should receive an implantable defibrillator. Recurrent VT, not responsive to antiarrhythmic medications, can be successfully ablated by mapping guided by classic entrainment techniques (Table 39–4). An example of successful ablation of VT in patients with ARVD is provided in Fig. 39–4. Although ablation of one clinical VT may be successful, an ICD is often implanted due to the finding of multiple VT morphologies that occur with the progression of disease.

The Multidisciplinary Study of Right Ventricular Dysplasia is a multicenter collaborative study investigating the clinical findings and genetics of ARVD. A list of enrolling centers can be found at www.arvd.org or by calling the North American ARVD Registry (800-483-2662).[70]

【 】 VENTRICULAR TACHYCARDIA IN CARDIAC SARCOIDOSIS

Sarcoidosis is a granulomatous disease involving multiple organ systems. The incidence of cardiac symptoms in patients with sarcoidosis is relatively low.[71] However, 20 to 30 percent of patients with sarcoidosis are found to have evidence of cardiac involvement. Myocardial involvement may be diffuse but is frequently fo-

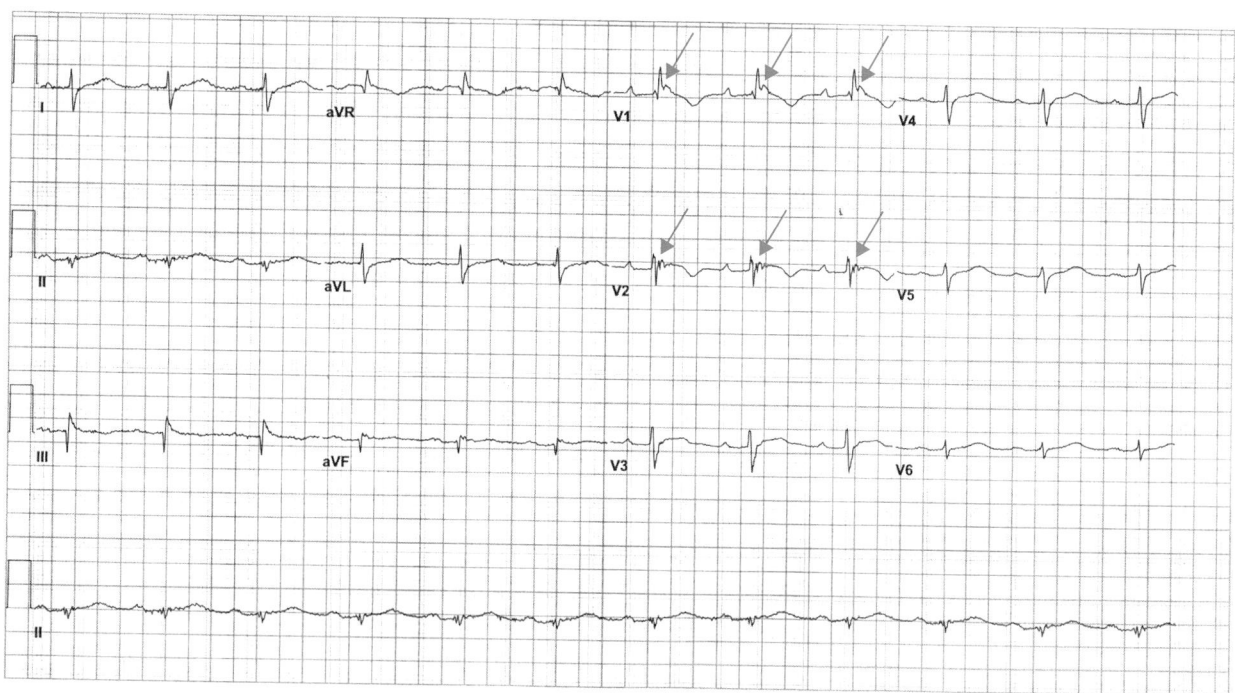

FIGURE 39–3. Epsilon waves (*arrows*) in a patient with arrhythmogenic right ventricular cardiomyopathy. This is an important diagnostic feature for this condition.

TABLE 39-4

ACC/AHA/ESC 2006 Guidelines for the Management of Ventricular Arrhythmias in Arrhythmogenic Right Ventricular Cardiomyopathy[1]

Class I

1. ICD implantation is recommended for prevention of SCD in patients with arrhythmogenic RV cardiomyopathy with documented sustained VT or VF who are receiving chronic optimal medical therapy and have reasonable expectation of survival with a good functional status for >1 year (*Level of Evidence: B*).

Class IIa

1. ICD implantation can be effective for prevention of SCD in patients with arrhythmogenic RV cardiomyopathy with extensive disease, including those with LV involvement, one or more family members affected with SCD, or undiagnosed syncope when VT or VF has not been excluded as the cause of syncope; are receiving chronic optimal medical therapy; and have reasonable expectation of survival with a good functional status for >1 year (*Level of Evidence: C*).
2. Amiodarone or sotalol can be effective for treatment of sustained VT or VF in patients with arrhythmogenic RV cardiomyopathy when ICD implantation is not feasible (*Level of Evidence: C*).
3. Ablation can be useful as adjunctive therapy in management of patients with arrhythmogenic RV cardiomyopathy with recurrent VT, despite optimal antiarrhythmic drug therapy (*Level of Evidence: C*).

Class IIb

1. EP testing might be useful for risk assessment of SCD in patients with arrhythmogenic RV cardiomyopathy (*Level of Evidence: C*).

EP, electrophysiologic; ICD, internal cardioverter-defibrillator; LV, left ventricular; RV, right ventricular; SCD, sudden cardiac death; VF, ventricular fibrillation; VT, ventricular tachycardia.

cal or patchy with a propensity for the basal free wall and the anteroapical septum.[71–73] The most common cardiac arrhythmias associated with cardiac sarcoidosis are VT and heart block (LBBB, RBBB, hemiblocks, complete heart block). The mechanism of VT is reentry within areas of patchy fibrosis, scarring, and granulomatous involvement of the myocardium.

Currently, there is insufficient data on the efficacy of specific treatment strategies in patients with ventricular arrhythmias caused by cardiac sarcoidosis. Until such data are available, patients with sustained VT may be treated initially with amiodarone and a β-adrenergic blocking agent. Implantation of a cardiac defibrillator should be considered, especially in patients with depressed LV function. Catheter ablation of VT is a reasonable option for those patients with VT refractory to antiarrhythmic medications.

VENTRICULAR ARRHYTHMIAS IN CHAGAS CARDIOMYOPATHY

Chagas disease is the major cause of VT in Central and South America. The protozoan, *Trypanosoma cruzi*, is transmitted to humans via the reduviid bug. The etiology of chronic Chagas cardiomyopathy is unknown but may be related to a cell mediated autoimmune reaction. Recurrent monomorphic VT is common in chronic Chagas cardiomyopathy. Most VTs can be induced with programmed stimulation and entrained during VT favoring reentry as the mechanism.

Histologic examination of patients with Chagas disease reveals focal and diffuse fibrosis of the myocardium, predominantly in the subepicardium and interspersed with surviving myocardial fibers. Regional wall-motion abnormalities are present often in the inferolateral wall of the LV. Apical septal and apical-inferior aneurysms have also been described.[74] Radiofrequency catheter ablation may be considered for the treatment of recurrent VT. This often requires epicardial mapping and ablation.[74–76]

IDIOPATHIC VENTRICULAR TACHYCARDIA

Idiopathic VT occurs in patients with structurally normal hearts, and represents approximately 10 percent of patients referred for evaluation of VT in one center.[77] The two main clinical entities of idiopathic VT include repetitive monomorphic VT (RVOT VT) and idiopathic left VT (fascicular VT or verapamil sensitive VT). The differentiation of these VTs from VTs associated with structural heart disease is important because they often respond well to drug therapies, are associated with an excellent prognosis, and can be cured with catheter ablation.

REPETITIVE MONOMORPHIC VENTRICULAR TACHYCARDIA

Repetitive monomorphic ventricular tachycardia (RMVT), also referred to as right ventricular outflow tract VT, was first described by Gallavardin in 1972 and is characterized by repetitive salvos of monomorphic nonsustained VT.[78] It occurs frequently in young middle-aged patients without structural heart disease. Men and women are affected equally.[79] This arrhythmia is usually provoked by exercise and emotional stress. Recurrence may be associated with exercise, stress, or caffeine, and in women it occurs more frequently during premenstrual, perimenopausal, and gestational periods.[80]

RMVT typically arises from the anterior septum of the RVOT immediately inferior to the pulmonary valve. Sites of origin of this VT have also been mapped to the free wall of the RVOT, LV outflow tract and aortic sinus of Valsalva, parahisian region, and in the pulmonary artery above the pulmonic valve.[81–85] The cellular mechanism of the tachycardia is thought to be caused by cyclic adenosine monophosphate–mediated triggered activity from delayed after depolarizations. This mechanism is supported by the sensitivity of the arrhythmia to adenosine infusion, which often terminates the arrhythmia.[86] The observation that this type of VT may originate from RVOT, the LV epicardium, LV outflow tract

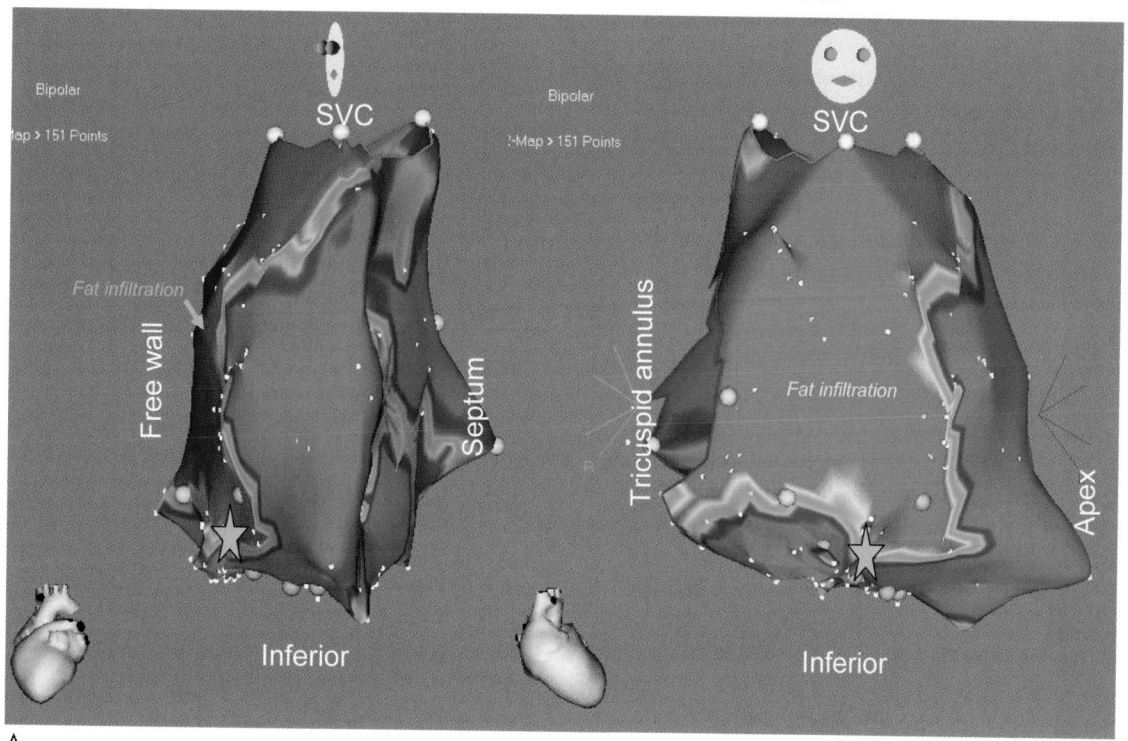

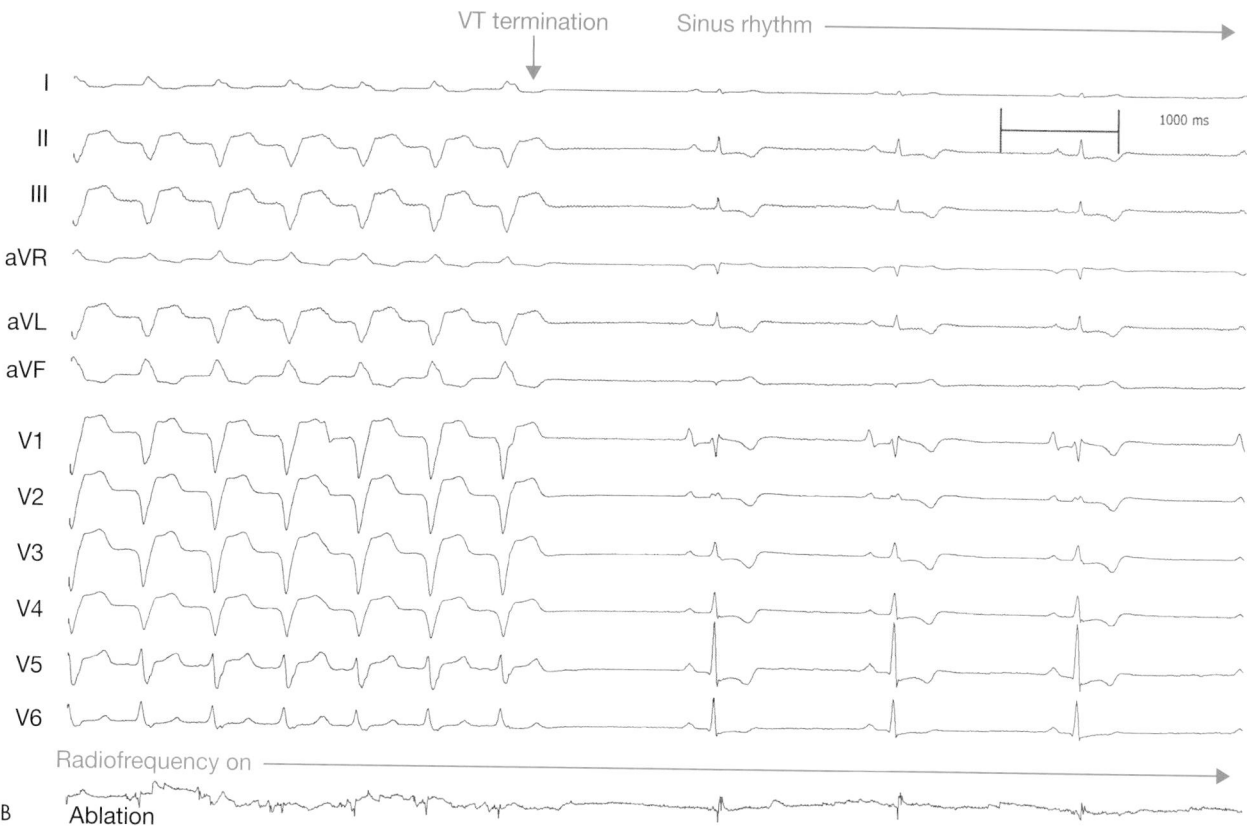

FIGURE 39-4. A. A voltage map of the right ventricle acquired using an electroanatomic mapping system (Biosense Webster). The red and grey areas indicate scar (low-amplitude signal <0.5 mV). The purple area represents healthy tissue (>1.5 mV signal amplitude). A right anterior oblique (RAO) and left anterior oblique (LAO) projection are shown. A large basal free wall scar is present, extending from the base to beyond the midcavity of the right ventricle. The blue star represents the site where the vulnerable isthmus of the ventricular tachycardia (VT) circuit is mapped. **B.** Application of a radiofrequency lesion to this site terminates VT.

and aortic sinus of Valsalva is interesting because myocardial cells of these regions of the heart share a common embryologic origin.[87]

RMVT has a characteristic pattern on the 12-lead electrocardiogram, with a LBBB morphology and inferior axis, consistent with a RVOT site of origin.[77] Most patients have a single VT morphology; the presence of multiple VT morphologies should alert the clinician to the possibility of arrhythmogenic RV dysplasia.[88]

Evaluation of patients with suspected RMVT includes an echocardiogram to confirm the absence of structural heart disease, ambulatory electrocardiogram monitoring, and exercise stress testing. In patients with RMVT an exercise stress test will induce the arrhythmia either during exercise or during recovery.

RMVT is associated with an excellent prognosis; therefore, treatment is aimed at the alleviation of symptoms. It is important to consider the diagnosis of ARVD in the workup of patients presenting with VT from the RVOT. β-Adrenergic receptor blockers and calcium channel antagonists are usually the first choice for the treatment of symptomatic VT, but their efficacy in preventing arrhythmia recurrence is modest. Verapamil was found to eliminate exercise-induced RMVT in 56 percent (*n* = 29) of patients who had RMVT induced during stress testing.[89] In general, β blockers are effective in approximately 25 to 50 percent of patients, whereas calcium channel blockers are effective in approximately 25 to 30 percent.[90] Catheter ablation is an attractive option for the treatment of RMVT, with success rates ranging from 80 to 100 percent[91,92] (Table 39–5).

IDIOPATHIC LEFT VENTRICULAR TACHYCARDIA

Idiopathic left VT (fascicular VT) is another ventricular arrhythmia found in patients with structurally normal hearts. A right bundle-branch pattern left superior axis VT characterizes the appearance of this VT on a 12-lead electrocardiogram. Belhassen was the first to describe the sensitivity of this tachycardia to verapamil.[93] Approximately 70 percent of patients with this form of VT are men. The resting electrocardiogram is usually normal. Patients usually have a structurally normal heart but may present with incessant fascicular VT. A reversible tachycardia mediated tachycardia has been described.[94] The site of origin of the tachycardia is usually in the region of the left posterior fascicle (inferior posterior LV septum). The ability to induce idiopathic left VT using programmed stimulation and the ability to entrain this tachycardia supports reentry as the mechanism for this arrhythmia.[95,96] The mechanism appears to be reentry around the distal Purkinje network of the left posterior fascicle, accounting for the relatively narrow QRS.[97]

The clinical features of this VT include (1) a structurally normal heart; (2) VT with a relatively narrow QRS (<140 msec), a RBBB pattern in V1, and superior limb lead axis (Fig. 39–5); (3) sensitivity to verapamil; (4) and induction with atrial pacing.[98] The arrhythmia usually presents in patients between ages 15 and 40 years of age. False tendons are found in a high percentage of patients with idiopathic left VT, but their anatomic and functional significance is unknown.[99,100] Patients with idiopathic left VT have a good prognosis.[90]

Idiopathic left VT responds well to verapamil for acute termination of VT as well as for long term arrhythmia control.[94,101–103] Membrane active antiarrhythmic medications are rarely indicated in the treatment of this arrhythmia and are usually ineffective.[103] In patients with poor control on verapamil, catheter ablation is an attractive option for treatment.[104–108]

TABLE 39–5

ACC/AHA/ESC 2006 Guidelines for the Management of Idiopathic Ventricular Tachycardia[1]

Class I
1. Catheter ablation is useful in patients with structurally normal hearts with symptomatic, drug-refractory VT arising from the RV or LV or in those who are drug intolerant or do not desire long-term drug therapy (Level of Evidence: C).

Class IIa
1. EP testing is reasonable for diagnostic evaluation in patients with structurally normal hearts with palpitations or suspected outflow tract VT (Level of Evidence: B).
2. Drug therapy with β blockers and/or calcium channel blockers (and/or IC agents in RVOT VT) can be useful in patients with structurally normal hearts with symptomatic VT arising from the right ventricle (Level of Evidence: C).
3. ICD implantation can be effective therapy for termination of sustained VT in patients with normal or near-normal ventricular function and no structural heart disease who are receiving chronic optimal medical therapy and have reasonable expectation of survival for >1 year (Level of Evidence: C).

EP, electrophysiologic; IC, intracardiac; ICD, internal cardioverter-defibrillator; LV, left ventricular; RV, right ventricular; RVOT, right ventricular outflow tract; VT, ventricular tachycardia.

ACCELERATED IDIOVENTRICULAR RHYTHM

Accelerated idioventricular rhythm (AIVR) is an automatic rhythm originating in the ventricle with rates between 40 to 120 beats/min. It is often seen gradually accelerating beyond the sinus rate, resulting in isorhythmic atrioventricular dissociation.[109] Fusion beats may be seen at the onset and termination of the arrhythmia. AIVR may be associated with ischemic cardiomyopathy, acute coronary syndromes, rheumatic heart disease, dilated cardiomyopathy, and in acute myocarditis.[110–113] Furthermore, AIVR has been described in patients with no apparent heart disease.[114] In the setting of acute coronary syndromes, AIVR is considered to be a noninvasive albeit nonspecific marker for successful reperfusion after thrombolytic therapy. The incidence of AIVR is not affected by the location of MI or the infarct size. Finally, the presence of AIVR after a MI is not associated with an increase in mortality.[115]

The mechanism of AIVR is thought to be increased automaticity in a region of the ventricle; however, in some instances, such as in myocardial ischemia and in digitalis toxicity, the mechanism may be caused by triggered activity.[116]

AIVR is a benign rhythm; no specific treatment is necessary. In the acute setting, when loss of atrioventricular synchrony results in hemodynamic compromise, atrial overdrive pacing or atropine may reestablish AV synchrony when the two rhythms are competing.

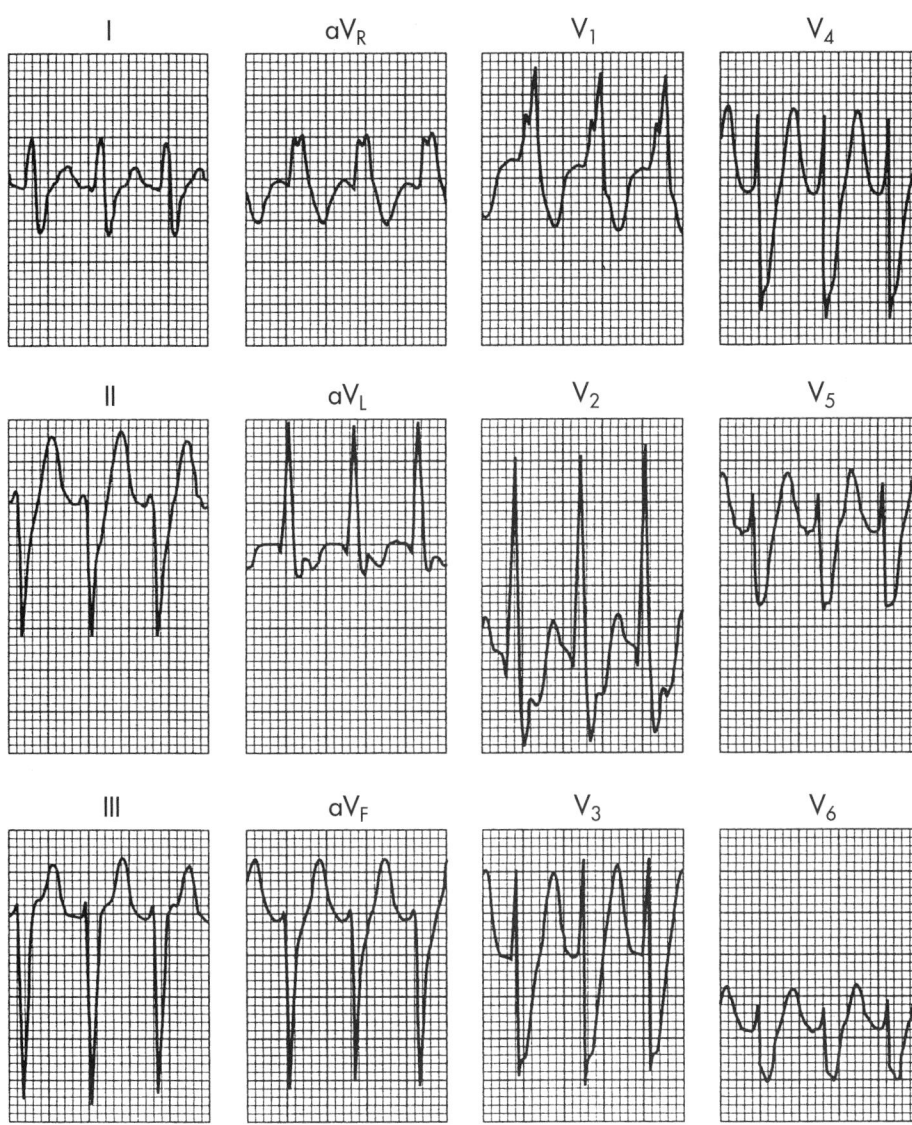

FIGURE 39–5. Idiopathic left ventricular tachycardia. The distinctive features are a right bundle branch morphology in V1 and a superior axis in the limb leads. *Source: From Marriott HJL, ed. Advanced Concepts in Arrhythmias, St. Louis: Mosby, 1998. Permission from Mosby, Inc.*

matical models, these functional reentry wavelets have the appearance of nonstationary rotating spiral waves.[119–121] The ever-changing pathways of these wavelets through the complex three-dimensional geometry of the ventricle accounts for the chaotic appearance of this rhythm on a rhythm strip or 12-lead electrocardiogram.

Coronary artery disease and resultant MI is the most common etiology of VF and cardiac arrest.[122] Other causes of VF include dilated cardiomyopathies,[123] hypertrophic cardiomyopathy,[124] myocarditis,[125] valvular heart disease,[126] congenital heart disease,[127] proarrhythmia from drugs,[128] acid-base and electrolyte abnormalities,[129,130] long QT syndrome,[131] short QT syndrome,[132] and atrial fibrillation in a patient with Wolff-Parkinson-White (WPW) syndrome with an anterogradely conducting bypass tract.[133]

Identification of the etiology of VF may be helpful in risk stratification and prevention of further bouts of VF. Revascularization of patients with myocardial ischemia caused by coronary disease, ablation of a bypass tract in a patient with VF because of WPW syndrome, or elimination of proarrhythmic drugs should minimize the risk of future VF episodes. However, patients with *reversible* causes of arrest may continue to be at risk for further bouts of VF. In an analysis of the AVID trial, Wyse and coworkers reported a similar mortality rate in patients with reversible cause of arrest compared with those considered to have a nonreversible cause of their VT or VF.[134]

VENTRICULAR FIBRILLATION

VF is characterized by rapid, chaotic, and asynchronous contraction of the left ventricle. The surface electrogram of VF reveals a rapid, irregular, dysmorphic pattern with no clearly defined QRS complex. VF is associated with rapid hemodynamic collapse and is the most common arrhythmia resulting in out-of-hospital cardiac arrest. Furthermore, patients who suffer a cardiac arrest have significant risk of subsequent arrest.[117]

【 】 MECHANISM

Our understanding of the mechanism of VF has been enhanced through animal and computer simulation models. Moe et al. stated that multiple wavelets of functional reentry can occur to sustain atrial fibrillation in the setting of significant dispersion of refractory periods.[118] Experimental studies in VF suggest functional reentry as the mechanism of propagation of VF. In mathe-

【 】 CLINICAL CHARACTERISTICS AND MANAGEMENT OF VENTRICULAR FIBRILLATION

Every year approximately 250,000 patients die from sudden cardiac death. In the early stages of cardiac arrest, VF is the most common arrhythmia encountered. Patients with VF require immediate defibrillation. Early defibrillation is an essential part of the AHA's *chain of survival*.[135] With every minute of delay in defibrillation for VF, the chance of survival decreases by 7 to 10 percent.[136] Determinants of successful defibrillation include time to defibrillation, energy delivered, defibrillation waveform, transthoracic impedance, shock electrode placement, surface area of the shock electrodes, and the patient's metabolic status (acid-base and electrolytes). Excessive energy and current may potentially cause irreversible myocardial necrosis and functional damage to the ventricular myocardium and conduction system,[137,138] but evidence of clinical importance of this postshock injury in humans has been difficult to demonstrate. For the traditional monophasic shock waveform, the recommended first shock energy is 200 J, followed by 300 and then 360 J. Biphasic waveforms appear to have an advantage over monophasic waveforms in that less energy is required for defibrillation and the lower-energy biphasic shocks result in less postshock ST segment abnormalities.[139] In a study comparing a nonescalating biphasic shock sequence (150J, 150J, 150J) to an escalating monophasic shock sequence (200J, 300J, 360J) in 115 victims of cardiac arrest, biphasic shocks were associated with higher rates of defibrillation and better cerebral function.[140]

Recognizing that early defibrillation is critical to survival in patients suffering VF arrest, significant technological advances have improved survival among patients suffering from VF arrest. One of these, the automated external defibrillator (AED), has the potential to significantly impact survival of out of hospital arrests. The AED has been proven to be safe, accurate, and effective even in the hands of nontraditional responders in a variety of public locations.[141,142]

The management of patients suffering VF arrest is aimed at determining its cause and treating potential recurrence. Because most cardiac arrests occur in patients with coronary artery disease, all patients should be evaluated for the presence of epicardial coronary disease (usually via coronary angiography). In addition, serial cardiac enzymes should be evaluated and an echocardiogram should be performed to assess LV function. In patients with structurally normal appearing hearts without evidence of ischemia or MI, other etiologies of VF should be considered, including WPW syndrome, proarrhythmia from medications, long QT syndrome, Brugada syndrome, short QT syndrome, and catecholaminergic VT.

When VF occurs during an acute MI, it usually occurs within the first four hours following onset of coronary occlusion. In GISSI-2 the incidence of early VF (occurring in the first 4 hours after presentation) was 3.1 percent, whereas the incidence of late VF (occurring in the subsequent 4–48 hours) was only 0.6 percent. Patients with early VF had a more complicated in-hospital course than matched controls. Both early (odds ratio [OR] 2.47, 95 percent CI 1.48 to 4.13) and late VF (OR 3.97, 95 percent CI 1.51 to 10.48) were independent predictors of in-hospital mortality. Postdischarge to 6-month death rates were similar for both early and late VF subgroups and controls.[143] Other studies have shown that VF associated with a Q-wave MI is associated with an increased in-hospital mortality but does not predict long-term survival among survivors of acute MI associated VF.[135,144] It is important to emphasize that all patients suffering an acute MI should undergo revascularization (if appropriate) and be treated with an aspirin, a β-adrenergic receptor blocker, a statin, and an ACEI.

In patients who present with VF arrest caused by chronic ischemic or nonischemic cardiomyopathy with a low LVEF, the recurrence rate of VF arrest is high. Aggressive therapy is indicated in this subgroup of patients. One-year survival of survivors of sudden death range between 70 and 84 percent.[145–147] Identification and treatment of reversible causes of VF, such as removal of proarrhythmic medications and correcting electrolyte abnormalities, should be performed without delay. Patients with long QT syndrome should be treated with a β-adrenergic receptor blocker, and temporary pacing should be considered if significant bradycardia is playing a role in arrhythmia recurrence (see below). When the

patient's workup is complete and all reversible causes or contributions to VF are corrected, most patients suffering VF arrest should undergo implantation of an ICD. Defibrillator implantation has become the mainstay of therapy for cardiac arrest survivors.

The implantable cardiac defibrillator has significantly affected outcomes from the primary and secondary treatment of patients suffering from ventricular arrhythmias. Currently, three general treatment options exist for patients with VT or VF: (1) antiarrhythmic drug therapy, (2) radiofrequency ablation procedures (VT), and (3) implantable cardiac defibrillators. Most patients with life-threatening ventricular arrhythmias receive an implantable defibrillator with antiarrhythmic drug therapy and radiofrequency catheter ablation as adjunctive treatment options (see Table 39–2).

POLYMORPHIC VENTRICULAR TACHYCARDIA

【 】 TORSADE DE POINTES AND LONG QT SYNDROME

The long QT syndromes are a heterogeneous group of disorders resulting from congenital or acquired defects in the ion currents underlying repolarization. Iatrogenic (drug-induced) causes are by far more common than congenital long QT. The prolongation of repolarization in long QT syndrome is associated with significant regional dispersion of refractory periods within the ventricular myocardium. Torsade de pointes (TdP) is the hallmark arrhythmia in the long QT syndrome. TdP is characterized by a rapid polymorphic VT that constantly changes (cycle length, axis, and morphology) in a pattern that appears to twist around a central axis. TdP may be repetitive, nonsustained, or sustained, and may degenerate into VF. Patients with long, repetitive salvos of TdP or sustained polymorphic VT/VF may manifest with presyncope or syncope. Although long QT syndrome is most commonly associated with TdP, other conditions such as hypokalemia, hypomagnesemia, severely altered nutritional states, and neurologic catastrophe have been associated with TdP.[148]

Other ventricular arrhythmias caused by genetic or acquired abnormalities of ion-channels include short QT syndrome, catecholaminergic VT, and Brugada syndrome. These are covered in greater detail in Chaps. 33, 81, and 82.

REFERENCES

1. ACC/AHA/ESC 2006 Guidelines for Management of Patients with Ventricular Arrhythmias and the Prevention of Sudden Cardiac Death. *J Am Coll Cardiol* 2006;48:e247–e346. Available at: www.content.onlinejacc.org/cgi/content. Accessed May 22, 2007.
2. Horan MJ, Kennedy HL. Ventricular ectopy: history, epidemiology, and clinical implications. *JAMA* 1984;251(3):380–386.
3. Kennedy HL, Whitlock JA, Sprague MK, et al. Long-term follow-up of asymptomatic healthy subjects with frequent and complex ventricular ectopy. *N Engl J Med* 1985;312:193–197.
4. Ruberman W, Weinblatt E, Frank CW, et al. Ventricular premature beats and mortality after myocardial infarction. *N Engl J Med* 1977;297:750–757.
5. Ruberman W, Weinblatt E, Goldberg JD, et al. Ventricular premature complexes and sudden death after myocardial infarction. *Circulation* 1981;64(2):297–305.
6. Andreson D, Bethge KP, Boissel JP, et al. Importance of quantitative analysis of ventricular arrhythmias for predicting the prognosis in low-risk postmyocardial infarction patients. European Infarction Study Group. *Eur Heart J* 1990;11(6):529–536.

7. Mukharji J, Rude RE, Poole WK, et al. Risk factors for sudden death after acute myocardial infarction: two-year follow-up. *Am J Cardiol* 1984;54(1):31–36.

8. Bigger JT Jr., Fleiss JL, Kleiger R, et al. The relationships among ventricular arrhythmias, left ventricular dysfunction, and mortality in the 2 years after myocardial infarction. *Circulation* 1984;69:250–258.

9. Statters DJ, Malik M, Redwood S, et al. Use of ventricular premature complexes for risk stratification after acute myocardial infarction in the thrombolytic era. *Am J Cardiol* 1996;77:133–138.

10. MacMahon S. Effects of prophylactic lidocaine in suspected acute myocardial infarction: an overview of results from the randomized, controlled trials. *JAMA* 1988;260:1910–1916.

11. Echt DS, Liebson PR, Mitchell LB, et al. Mortality and morbidity in patients receiving encainide, flecainide, or placebo. The Cardiac Arrhythmia Suppression Trial. *N Engl J Med* 1991;324:781–788.

12. Waldo A, Camm A, deRyuter H, et al. For the survival with oral d-sotalol (SWORD) investigators: effect of d-sotalol on mortality in patients with left ventricular dysfunction after recent and remote myocardial infarction. *Lancet* 1996;348:7–12.

13. Singh SN, Fletcher RD, Fisher SG, et al. Amiodarone in patients with congestive heart failure and asymptomatic ventricular arrhythmias. *N Engl J Med* 1995;333:77–82.

14. Julian D, Camm A, Frangin G, et al, for the European Myocardial Infarct Amiodarone Trial (EMIAT) investigators. Randomized trial of the effect of amiodarone on mortality in patients with left ventricular dysfunction after recent myocardial infarction: EMIAT. *Lancet* 1997;349:667–674.

15. Cairns J, Connolly S, Roberts R, Gent M. Randomised trial of outcome after myocardial infarction in patients with frequent or repetitive ventricular premature depolarisations: CAMIAT. Canadian Amiodarone Myocardial Infarction Arrhythmia Trial Investigators. *Lancet* 1997;349:675–682.

16. Connoly SJ. Meta-analysis of antiarrhythmic drug trials. *Am J Cardiol* 1999;84(9A);90R–93R.

17. Fletcher RD, Cintron GB, Johnson G, et al. Enalapril decreases prevalence of ventricular tachycardia in patients with chronic congestive heart failure. The V-HeFT II VA Cooperative Studies Group. *Circulation* 1993;87(6 suppl):VI49–VI55.

18. Doval HC, Nul DR, Grancelli HO, et al. Nonsustained ventricular tachycardia in severe heart failure. Independent marker of increased mortality due to sudden death. GESICA-GEMA Investigators. *Circulation* 1996;94:3198–3203.

19. Von Olshausen K, Stienen U, Schwarz F, et al. Long-term prognostic significance of ventricular arrhythmias in idiopathic dilated cardiomyopathy. *Am J Cardiol* 1988;61:146–151.

20. Singh SN, Fisher SG, Carson PE, et al. Prevalence and significance of nonsustained ventricular tachycardia in patients with premature ventricular contractions and heart failure treated with vasodilator therapy. *Am J Cardiol* 1998;32(4):942–947.

21. Jouven X, Zureikm J, Desnos M, et al. Long-term outcome in asymptomatic men with exercise-induced premature ventricular depolarizations. *N Engl J Med* 2000;343(12):826–833.

22. Frolkis JP, Pothier CE, Blackstone EH, et al. Frequent ventricular ectopy after exercise as a predictor of death. *N Engl J Med* 2003;348:781–790.

23. DeBakker JM, van Cappele F, Janse MJ, et al. Reentry as a cause of ventricular tachycardia in patients with chronic ischemic heart disease: electrophysiologic and anatomic correlation. *Circulation* 1988;77:589–606.

24. Josephson ME, Horowitz LN, Farshidi A, et al. Continuous local electrical activity: a mechanism of recurrent ventricular tachycardia. *Circulation* 1978;57:659–665.

25. McGuire M, Kuchar D, Ganis J, et al. Natural history of late potentials in the first ten days after acute myocardial infarction and relation to early ventricular arrhythmias. *Am J Cardiol* 1988;61:1187–1190.

26. A comparison of antiarrhythmic-drug therapy with implantable defibrillators in patients resuscitated from near-fatal ventricular arrhythmias. The Antiarrhythmics versus Implantable Defibrillators (AVID) Investigators. *N Engl J Med* 1997;337:1576–1584.

27. Pitt B, Remme W, Zannad F, et al. Eplerenone, a selective aldosterone blocker, in patients with left ventricular dysfunction after myocardial infarction. *N Engl J Med* 2003;348:1309–1322.

28. Wilber D, Wojciech Z, Hall WJ, et al. Time dependence of mortality risk and defibrillator benefit after myocardial infarction. *Circulation* 2004;109:1082–1084.

29. Josephson ME, Almendral JM, Buxton AE, et al. Mechanism of ventricular tachycardia. *Circulation* 1987;75:III41–III47.

30. Hamer AWF, Rubin SA, Peter CT, et al. Factors that predict syncope during ventricular tachycardia in patients. *Am Heart J* 1984;107:997–1005.

31. Lima JA, Weiss JL, Guzman PA, et al. Incomplete filling and incoordinate contraction as mechanisms of hypotension during ventricular tachycardia in man. *Circulation* 1983;68:928–938.

32. Anderson JL. Long term survival in the Antiarrhythmics Versus Implantable Defibrillators (AVID) Registry. *J Am Coll Cardiol* 1998;31:160A.

33. Levine JH, Scheinman MM, et al. Intravenous amiodarone for recurrent sustained hypotensive ventricular tachyarrhythmias. *J Am Coll Cardiol* 1996;27:67–75.

34. Gorgels AP, Van den Dool A, Hofs A, et al. Comparison of procainamide and lidocaine in terminating sustained monomorphic ventricular tachycardia. *Am J Cardiol* 1996;78:82–83.

35. Schwartzman D, Jadonath R, Callans DJ, et al. Radiofrequency catheter ablation for control of frequent ventricular tachycardia with healed myocardial infarction. *Am J Cardiol* 1995;75:297–299.

36. Iqbal I, Ventura HO, Smart FW, et al. Difficult cases in heart failure: left ventricular assist device implantation for the treatment of recurrent ventricular tachycardia in end stage heart failure. *Congest Heart Fail* 1999;5:129–130.

37. Wilber DJ, Garan H, Finkelstein D, et al. Out of hospital cardiac arrest: use of electrophysiologic testing in the prediction of long term outcome. *N Engl J Med* 1988;318:19–24.

38. Kim SG, Fischer J, Choue CW, et al. The influence of left ventricular function on the outcome of patients treated with implantable defibrillators. *Circulation* 1992. 85:1304–1310.

39. Curtis JP, Sokol SI, Wang Y, et al. The association of left ventricular ejection fraction, mortality, and cause of death in stable outpatients with heart failure. *J Am Coll Cardiol* 2003;42:736–742.

40. Caruso AC, Marcus FI, Hahn EA, Hartz VL, Mason JW. Predictors of arrhythmic death in the ESVEM trial. Electrophysiologic Study Versus Electromagnetic Monitoring. *Circulation* 1997;96:1888–1892.

41. Solomon SD, Anavekar N, Skali H, et al. Influence of ejection fraction on cardiovascular outcomes in a broad spectrum of heart failure patients. *Circulation* 2005;112:3738–3744.

42. Connolly SJ, Hallstrom AP, Cappato R, et al. Meta-analysis of the implantable cardioverter defibrillator secondary prevention trials. *Eur Heart J* 2000;21:2071–2078.

43. Connolly SJ, Dorian P, Roberts RS, et al. Comparison of beta-blockers, amiodarone plus beta-blockers, or sotalol for prevention of shocks from implantable cardioverter defibrillator: the OPTIC study: a randomized trial. *JAMA* 2006;295:211–213.

44. Soejima K, Suzuki M, Maisel WH, et al. Catheter ablation in patients with multiple and unstable ventricular tachycardias after myocardial infarction: short ablation lines guided by reentry circuit isthmuses and sinus rhythm mapping. *Circulation* 2001;104:664–669.

45. Marchlinski FE, Callans D, Gottlieb CD, et al. Linear ablation lesions for control of unmappable ventricular tachycardia in patients with ischemic and nonischemic cardiomyopathy. *Circulation* 2000;101:1288–1296.

46. Pfeffer MA, Braunwald E, Moye LA, et al. Effect of captopril on mortality and morbidity in patients with left ventricular dysfunction after myocardial infarction: results of the Survival and Ventricular Enlargement Trial. *N Engl J Med* 1992;327:669–677.

47. Wilber DJ, Olshansky B, Moran JF, et al. Electrophysiologic testing and nonsustained ventricular tachycardia: Use and limitation in patients with coronary artery disease and impaired ventricular function. *Circulation* 1990;82:350–358.

48. Buxton AE, Lee K, DiCarlo L, et al. Nonsustained ventricular tachycardia in coronary artery disease: relation to inducible sustained ventricular tachycardia. *Ann Intern Med* 1996;125:35–39.

49. Moss AJ, Zareba W, Hall WJ, et al. Prophylactic implantation of defibrillators in patients with myocardial infarction and reduced ejection fraction. *N Engl J Med* 2002;346:877–883.

50. Bardy GH, Lee KL, Mark DB, et al. Amiodarone or an implantable cardioverter-defibrillator for congestive heart failure *N Engl J Med* 2005;352:225–237.

51. Bayes de Luna A, Coumel P, Leclercq JF, et al. Ambulatory sudden cardiac death: mechanisms of production of fatal arrhythmia on the basis of data from 157 cases. *Am Heart J* 1989;117:115–159.

52. Luu M, Stevenson WG, Stevenson LW, et al. Diverse mechanisms of unexpected cardiac arrest in advanced heart failure. *Circulation* 1989;80:1675–1680.

53. Tamburro P, Wilber D. Sudden death in idiopathic dilated cardiomyopathy. *Am Heart J* 1992;124:1035–1045.

54. Franz MR, Burkoiff D, Yue DT, et al. Mechanically induced action potential changes and arrhythmia in isolated in situ canine hearts. *Cardiovasc Res* 1989;23:213–223.

55. Tchou P, Blanck Z, McKinnie J, et al. Mechanism of inducible ventricular tachycardia in patients with idiopathic dilated cardiomyopathy. *Circulation* 1983;67:674–680.

56. Chien WW, Scheinman M., Cohen TJ, et al. Importance of recording the right bundle branch deflection in the diagnosis of bundle branch reentrant ventricular tachycardia. *Pacing Clin Electrophysiol* 1992;15:1015–1024.

57. Delacretaz E, Stevenson W, Ellison K, et al. Mapping and radiofrequency catheter ablation of the three types of sustained monomorphic ventricular tachycardia in nonischemic cardiomyopathy. *Heart* 2000;11:11–17.

58. Stevenson LW, Fowler MB., Shroeder JS, et al. Poor survival in patients with idiopathic cardiomyopathy considered too well for transplantation. *Am J Med* 1987;83:871–876.

59. DeMaria R, Gavazzi A, Caroli A, et al. Ventricular arrhythmias in dilated cardiomyopathy as an independent prognostic hallmark. *Am J Cardiol* 1992;69:1451–1457.

60. Huang SK, Medsser JV, Denes P. Significance of ventricular tachycardia in idiopathic dilated cardiomyopathy: observations in 35 patients. *Am J Cardiol* 1983;51:507–512.

61. Kjekshus J. Arrhythmias and mortality in congestive heart failure. *Am J Cardiol* 1990;65:42I–48I.

62. Doval H, Nul DR, Grancelli H, Perrone SV, Bortman GR, Curiel R. Randomised trial of low-dose amiodarone in severe congestive heart failure. Grupo de Estudio de la Sobrevida en la Insuficiencia Cardiaca en Argentina (GESICA). *Lancet* 1994;344:493–498.

63. Bansch D, Antz M, Boczar M, et al. Primary prevention of sudden cardiac death in idiopathic dilated cardiomyopathy. The Cardiomyopathy Trial (CAT). *Circulation* 2002;105:1453–1458.

64. Kadish A, Dyer A, Daubert JP, et al: Prophylactic defibrillator implantation in patients with nonischemic dilated cardiomyopathy. *N Engl J Med* 2004;350:2151–2158.

65. Hsia HH, Callans DJ, Marchlinski FE. Characterization of endocardial electrophysiological substrate in patients with nonischemic cardiomyopathy and monomorphic ventricular tachycardia. *Circulation* 2003;108:704–710.

66. Corrado D, Basso C, Thiene G. Sudden cardiac death in young people with apparently normal heart. *Cardiovasc Res* 2001;50:339–408.

67. Marcus FI. Update of arrhythmogenic right ventricular dysplasia. *Card Electrophysiol Rev* 2002;6:54–56.

68. Jaoude SA, Leclercq JF, Coumel P. Progressive ECG changes in arrhythmogenic right ventricular disease. *Eur Heart J* 1996;17:1717–1722.

69. McKenna WJ, Thiene G, Nava, A, et al. Diagnosis of arrhythmogenic right ventricular dysplasia/cardiomyopathy: task force of the working group myocardial and pericardial disease of the European Society of Cardiology and of the Scientific Council on Cardiomyopathies of the International Society and Federation of Cardiology. *Br Heart J* 1994;71:215–219.

70. Marcus F, Calkins H. North American Arrhythmogenic Right Ventricular Dysplasia registry. Available at: http://www.arvd.org. Accessed June 15, 2006.

71. Silverman KJ, Hutchins GM, Bulkley BH, et al. Cardiac sarcoid: a clinicopathologic study of 84 unselected patients with systemic sarcoidosis. *Circulation* 1978;58:1204–1211.

72. Valantine H, McKenna WJ, Nihoyannopoulos P, et al. Sarcoidosis: a pattern of clinical and morphological presentation. *Br Heart J* 1987;57:256–263.

73. Roberts WC, McAllister, Jr. HA, Ferrans VJ. Sarcoidosis of the heart: a clinicopathologic study of 35 necropsy patients (group 1) and review of 78 previously described necropsy patients (group 11). *Am J Med* 1977;63:86–108.

74. Sosa E, Scanhavacca M, D'Avila A, et al. Endocardial and epicardial ablation guided by nonsurgical transthoracic epicardial mapping to treat recurrent ventricular tachycardia. *J Cardiovasc Electrophysiol* 1998;9:229–239.

75. Sosa E, Scanhavacca M, D'Avila A, et al. Radiofrequency catheter ablation of ventricular tachycardia guided by nonsurgical epicardial mapping in chronic Chagasic heart disease. *Pacing Clin Electrophysiol* 1999;22:128–130.

76. Sosa E, Scanavacca M, D'Avila A, et al. Transthoracic epicardial catheter ablation to treat recurrent ventricular tachycardia. *Curr Cardiol Rep* 2001;3:451–458.

77. Brooks R, Burgess JH. Idiopathic ventricular tachycardia: a review. *Medicine* 1988;67:271–294.

78. Gallavardin L. Extrasystolie ventriculaire a paroxysmes tachycardiques prolonges. *Arch Mal Coeur Vaiss* 1922;15:298–306.

79. Deal BJ, Miller SM, Scagliotti D, et al. Ventricular tachycardia in a young population without overt heart disease. *Circulation* 1986;73:1111–1118.

80. Marchlinski FE, Deely MP, Zado ES. Sex-specific triggers for right ventricular outflow tract tachycardia. *Am Heart J* 2000;139:1009–1013.

81. Calkins H, Kalbfleisch S, El-Atassi R. Relation between efficacy of radiofrequency catheter ablation and site of origin of idiopathic ventricular tachycardia. *Am J Cardiol* 1993;71:827–833.

82. Wilber D, Baerman J, Olshansky B. Adenosine-sensitive ventricular tachycardia: clinical characteristics and response to catheter ablation. *Circulation* 1993;87:126–134.

83. Hachiya H, Aonuma K, Yamauchi Y, et al. How to diagnose, locate, and ablate coronary cusp ventricular tachycardia. *J Cardiovasc Electrophysiol* 2002;13(6):551–556.

84. Yamauchi Y, Aonuma K, Takahashi A, et al. Electrocardiographic characteristics of repetitive monomorphic right ventricular tachycardia originating near the his-bundle. *J Cardiovasc Electrophysiol* 2005;16:1041–1048.

85. Sekiguchi Y, Aonuma K, Takahashi A, et al. Electrocardiographic and electrophysiologic characteristics of ventricular tachycardia originating within the pulmonary artery. *J Am Coll Cardiol* 2005;45:887–895.

86. Lerman BB, Stein K, Engelstein ED, et al. Mechanism of repetitive monomorphic ventricular tachycardia. *Circulation* 1995. 92(3):421–429.

87. Kochilas L, Merscher-Gomez S, Lu MM, et al. The role of neural crest during cardiac development in a mouse model of DiGeorge syndrome. *Dev Biol* 2002;251(1):157–166.

88. Marcus FI, Fontaine G, Guiraudon G. Right ventricular dysplasia: a report of 24 adult cases. *Circulation* 1982;65:384–390.

89. Gill JS, Blaszyk K, Ward DE, et al. Verapamil for the suppression of idiopathic ventricular tachycardia of left bundle branch block-like morphology. *Am Heart J* 1993;126(5):1126–1133.

90. Lerman B, Stein K, Markowitz S. Ventricular tachycardia in patients with structurally normal hearts. In: Zipes D, Jalife J, eds. *Cardiac Electrophysiology: From Cell to Bedside.* 3rd ed. Philadelphia: Saunders, 2000;640–656.

91. Callans D. Repetitive monomorphic idiopathic ventricular tachycardia. *J Am Coll Cardiol* 1997;29:1023–1027.

92. Globits S, Kreiner G, Frank H. Significance of morphological abnormalities detected by MRI in patients undergoing successful ablation of right ventricular outflow tract tachycardia. *Circulation* 1997;96:2633–2640.

93. Belhassen B, Laniado S. Response of recurrent sustained ventricular tachycardia to verapamil. *Br Heart J* 1981;46:679–682.

94. Ward D, Nathan A, Camm A. Fascular tachycardia sensitive to calcium antagonists. *Eur Heart J* 1984;5:896–905.

95. Okumura K, Yamahe H, Tsuchiya T, et al. Characteristics of slow conduction zone demonstrated during entrainment of idiopathic ventricular tachycardia of left ventricular origin. *Am J Cardiol* 1996;77(5):379–383.

96. Okumura K, Matsuyama K, Miyagi H, et al. Entrainment of idiopathic ventricular tachycardia of left ventricular origin with evidence for reentry with an area of slow conduction and effect of verapamil. *Am J Cardiol* 1988;62(10 pt 1):727–732.

97. Andrade F, Eslami M, Elias J. Diagnostic clues from the surface ECG to identify idiopathic (fascicular) ventricular tachycardia: correlation with electrophysiologic findings. *J Cardiovasc Electrophysiol* 1996;7:2–8.

98. Zipes D, Foster P. Atrial induction of ventricular tachycardia: reentry versus triggered activity. *Am J Cardiol* 1979;44:1–8.

99. Thakur RK, Klein GJ, Sivaram CA, et al. Anatomic substrate for idiopathic left ventricular tachycardia. *Circulation* 1996;93(3):497–501.

100. Ohe T. Idiopathic verapamil-sensitive sustained left ventricular tachycardia. *Clin Cardiol* 1993;16(2):139–141.

101. Ohe T, Shimomura K, Aihara N, et al. Idiopathic sustained left ventricular tachycardia: clinical and electrophysiologic characteristics. *Circulation* 1988;77(3):560–568.

102. Ohe T, Aihara N, Kamakura S, et al. Long-term outcome of verapamil-sensitive sustained left ventricular tachycardia in patients without structural heart disease. *J Am Coll Cardiol* 1995;25(1):54–58.

103. Mont L, Seixas T, Brugada P. The electrocardiographic, clinical and electrophysiologic spectrum of idiopathic monomorphic ventricular tachycardia. *Am Heart J* 1992;124:746–753.

104. Nakagawa H, Beckman KJ, McClelland JH, et al. Radiofrequency catheter ablation of idiopathic left ventricular tachycardia guided by a Purkinje potential. *Circulation* 1993;88(6):2607–2617.

105. Klein LS, Miles WM. Ablative therapy for ventricular arrhythmias. *Prog Cardiovasc Dis* 1995;37(4):225–242.

106. Coggins DL, Lee RJ, Swenney J, et al. Radiofrequency catheter ablation as a cure for idiopathic tachycardia of both left and right ventricular origin. *J Am Coll Cardiol* 1994;23(6):1333–1341.

107. Page RL, Shenasa H, Evans JJ, et al. Radiofrequency catheter ablation of idiopathic recurrent ventricular tachycardia with right bundle branch block, left axis morphology. *Pacing Clin Electrophysiol* 1993;16(2):327–336.

108. Lin D, Hsia HH, Gerstenfeld E, et al. Idiopathic fascicular left ventricular tachycardia: linear lesion strategy for noninducible or nonsustained tachycardia. *Heart Rhythm* 2005;9:934–939.

109. Gallagher JJ, Damato AN, Lau SH. Electrophysiologic studies during accelerated idioventricular rhythms. *Circulation* 1971;44(4):671–677.

110. Gressin V, Louvari D, Pezaano M, et al. Holter recording of ventricular arrhythmias during intravenous thrombolysis for acute myocardial infarction. *Am J Cardiol* 1992;69(3):152–159.

111. Rothfeld EL, Zucker IR, Leff NA, et al. Coexisting paroxysmal ventricular tachycardia and idioventricular rhythm in acute myocardial infarction. *J Electrocardiol* 1973;6(2):149–152.

112. Abreau P, Fernandes A, Ventosa A. Unsustained ventricular tachycardia and accelerated idioventricular rhythm-clinical and electrocardiographic features. *Rev Port Cardiol* 1992;11:641–648.

113. Nakagawa M, Hamaoka K, Okano S. Multiform accelerated idioventricular rhythm in a child with acute myocarditis. *Clin Cardiol* 1988;11:853–855.

114. Massumi RA, Ali N. Accelerated isorhythmic ventricular rhythms. *Am J Cardiol* 1970;26(2):170–185.

115. Norris R. Significance of idioventricular rhythms in acute myocardial infarction. *Am J Cardiol* 1974;34:667–670.

116. Sclarovsky S, Strasberg B, Fuchs J, et al. Multiform accelerated idioventricular rhythm in acute myocardial infarction: electrocardiographic characteristics and response to verapamil. *Am J Cardiol* 1983;52(1):43–47.

117. Eisenberg MS, Hallstrom A, Bergner L. Long-term survival after out-of-hospital cardiac arrest. *N Engl J Med* 1982;306(22):1340–1343.

118. Moe G, Rehinbolt W, Abildskov J. A computer model of atrial fibrillation. *Am Heart J* 1964;67:200–220.

119. Gray R, Jalife J, Panfilov A. Mechanisms of cardiac fibrillation. *Science* 1995;270:1222–1223.

120. Winfree A. Electrical turbulence in three-dimensional heart muscle. *Science* 1994;266:1003–1006.

121. Persov A, Davidenko R, Salomontsz J. Spiral waves of excitation underlie reentrant activity in isolated cardiac muscle. *Circ Res* 1993;72:631–650.

122. Davies M, Thomas A. Thrombosis and acute coronary artery lesions in sudden cardiac ischemic death. *N Engl J Med* 1984;310:1137–1140.

123. Packer M. Sudden unexpected death in patients with congestive heart failure: a second frontier. *Circulation* 1985;72:681–685.

124. Kowey P, Eisenberg R, Engel T. Sustained arrhythmias in hypertrophic obstructive cardiomyopathy. *N Engl J Med* 1984;310:1566–1567.

125. Strain J, Grose R, Factor S. Results of endomyocardial biopsy in patients with spontaneous ventricular tachycardia but without apparent structural heart disease. *Circulation* 1983;68:1171–1181.

126. Schwartz L, Goldfischer J, Sprague G. Syncope and sudden death in aortic stenosis. *Am J Cardiol* 1969;23:647–658.

127. Downar E, Harris L, Kimber S. Ventricular tachycardia after surgical repair of tetralogy of Fallot: results of intraoperative mapping studies. *J Am Coll Cardiol* 1992;20:648–655.

128. Roden D. Mechanisms and management of proarrhythmia. *Am J Cardiol* 1998;82:47I–57I.

129. Surawicz B. Ventricular fibrillation. *J Am Coll Cardiol* 1985;5:43B–54B.

130. Gerst P, Fleming W, Malm J. Increased susceptibility of the heart to ventricular fibrillation during metabolic acidosis. *Circ Res* 1966;19:63–70.

131. Jackman WM, Friday K, Anderson J. The long QT syndromes: a critical review, new clinical observations and a unifying hypothesis. *Prog Cardiovasc Dis* 1988;31:115–172.

132. Gaita F, Giustetto C, Bianchi F, et al. Short QT syndrome: a familial cause of sudden death. *Circulation* 2003;108:965–970.

133. Klein G, Bashore T, Sellers T. Ventricular fibrillation in the Wolff-Parkinson-White syndrome. *N Engl J Med* 1979;301:1080–1085.

134. Wyse DG, Friedman PL, Brodsky MA, et al. Life-threatening ventricular arrhythmias due to transient or correctable causes: high risk for death in follow-up. *J Am Coll Cardiol* 2001;38(6):1718–1724.

135. Cummins R, Ornato JP, Thies WH, et al. Improving survival from sudden cardiac arrest: the "chain of survival" concept. *Circulation* 1991;83:1832–1847.

136. Larsen MP, Eisenberg MS, Cummins RO, et al. Predicting survival from out-of-hospital cardiac arrest: a graphic model. *Ann Emerg Med* 1993;22:1652–1658.

137. Warner E, Dahl C, Ewy G. Myocardial injury from transthoracic defibrillator countershock. *Arch Path* 1975;99:55–59.

138. Weaver W, Copass M, Holstrom A. Ventricular defibrillation: comparative trial using 175 joule and 320 joule shocks. *N Engl J Med* 1982;307:1101–1106.

139. Bardy GH, Marchlinski FE, Sharma AD, et al. Multicenter comparison of truncated biphasic shocks and standard damped sine wave monophasic shocks for transthoracic ventricular defibrillation. Transthoracic Investigators. *Circulation* 1996;94(10):2507–2514.

140. Schneider T, Martens PR, Paschen H, et al. Multicenter, randomized, controlled trial of 150-J biphasic shocks compared with 200- 360-J monophasic shocks in the resuscitation of out-of-hospital cardiac arrest victims. Optimized Response to Cardiac Arrest (ORCA) Investigators. *Circulation* 2000;102(15):1780–1787.

141. Page RL, Joglar JA, Kowal RC, et al. Use of automated external defibrillators by a U.S. airline. *N Engl J Med* 2000;343(17):1210–1216.

142. Hallstrom A, Ornato JP, Weisfeldt M, et al, for the Public Access Defibrillation Trial Investigators. Public-access defibrillation and survival after out-of-hospital cardiac arrest. *N Engl J Med* 2004;351:637–646.

143. Volpi A, Cavalli A, Santaro L, et al. Incidence and prognosis of early primary ventricular fibrillation in acute myocardial infarction: results of the Gruppo Italiano per lo Studio della Sopravvivenza nell'Infarto Miocardico (GISSI-2) database. *Am J Cardiol* 1998;82(3):265–271.

144. Creed J, Packard JM, Lambrew CT, et al. Defibrillation and synchronized cardioversion. In: McIntyre K, Lewis A, eds. *Textbook of Advanced Cardiac Life Support.* Vol. 89. Dallas: American Heart Association, 1983.

145. Tofler GH, Stone PH, Muller JE, et al. Prognosis after cardiac arrest due to ventricular tachycardia or ventricular fibrillation associated with acute myocardial infarction (the MILIS Study). Multicenter Investigation of the Limitation of Infarct Size. *Am J Cardiol* 1987;60(10):755–761.

146. Nicod P, Gilpin E, Dittrich H, et al. Late clinical outcome in patients with early ventricular fibrillation after myocardial infarction. *J Am Coll Cardiol* 1988;11(3):464–470.

147. Cobbe S, Dalziel K, Ford I, et al. Survival of 1476 patients initially resuscitated from out of hospital cardiac arrest. *Br Med J* 1996;312:1633–1637.

148. Goldschlager N, Epstein AE, Grubb BP, et al. Etiologic considerations in the patient with syncope and an apparently normal heart. *Arch Intern Med* 2003;163:151–162.

CHAPTER 40

Bradyarrhythmias and Pacemakers

Pugazhendhi Vijayaraman / Kenneth A. Ellenbogen

BRADYARRHYTHMIAS

Bradyarrhythmias are most commonly caused by failure of impulse formation (sinus node dysfunction) or by failure of impulse conduction over the atrioventricular (AV) node/His-Purkinje system. Bradyarrhythmias may be caused by disease processes that directly alter the structural and functional integrity of the sinus node, atria, AV node, and His-Purkinje system or by extrinsic factors (autonomic disturbances, drugs, etc.) without causing structural abnormalities (Table 40–1).

【 】 ANATOMY OF THE SINUS NODE AND CONDUCTION SYSTEM

Sinoatrial Node

Normal electrical activation of the heart arises from the principal pacemaker cells that spontaneously depolarize, located laterally in the epicardial grove of the sulcus terminalis,[1] near the junction of the right atrium and the superior vena cava (Fig. 40–1). The sinus node in adults measures approximately 1 to 2 cm long and 0.5 mm wide. The central zone of the sinus node containing the principal pacemaker cells is small and located within a fibrous tissue matrix. In the periphery of the node along the crista terminalis, transitional cells with pacemaker function are also present. Experimental and clinical evidence now suggest that the sinus node region is less defined than previously appreciated. The principal pacemaker site within this region may migrate resulting in subtle alterations in P-wave morphology.[2] Once the impulse exits the sinus node and the perinodal tissues, it traverses the atrium to the AV node. The conduction of impulses from right to left atrium has been postulated to occur preferentially via Bachmann bundle, and secondarily across the musculature of the coronary sinus.

Atrioventricular Node

Once the sinus node impulse activates the atrium, electrical activation continues through the AV node with a conduction delay ensuring complete atrial contraction before initiation of ventricular conduction. The AV nodal complex is considered to have three related regions: (1) the transitional cell zone, (2) the compact AV node, and (3) the penetrating AV bundle.[3] The transitional zone consists of the main atrial approaches to the compact AV node. The compact AV node is shaped like a half oval and is located beneath the right atrial endocardium at the apex of the triangle of Koch. The triangle of Koch is formed by the base of the septal leaflet of the tricuspid valve and the tendon of Todaro (formed by the extension of the eustachian valve into the central fibrous body). The coronary sinus ostium is located at the base of this triangle. The distal end of the compact AV node enters the central fibrous body to become the penetrating bundle and continues in the membranous septum as the bundle of His. The speed of conduction through the AV nodal complex is at 0.03 m/sec, whereas the His-Purkinje fibers conduct at 2.4 m/sec.

TABLE 40–1

Classification of Bradyarrhythmias

Sinus Node Dysfunction
- Sinus bradycardia
- Sinus pauses, sinus arrest
- Sinoatrial exit block
- Tachycardia-bradycardia syndrome
- Chronotropic incompetence

AV Conduction Abnormalities
- First-degree heart block
- Second-degree heart block
  > Mobitz type I (Wenckebach)
  > Mobitz type II
  > 2:1 atrioventricular block
- High-grade atrioventricular block
- Third-degree (complete) heart block
- Atrioventricular dissociation

Bundle Branch Block
- Left bundle branch block
- Right bundle branch block
- Left anterior hemiblock
- Left posterior hemiblock
- Bifascicular block/trifascicular block
- Nonspecific intraventricular conduction defect

AV, atrioventricular.

His-Purkinje System

The penetrating part of the AV bundle continues through the annulus fibrosis into the membranous septum, along the crest of the left side of the interventricular septum for 1 to 2 cm and then divides into the right and left bundle branches. The right bundle branch continues intramyocardially along the right side of the interventricular septum and emerges subendocardially beneath the anterior papillary muscle of the right ventricle. The left bundle begins as a sheet of fascicles and runs along the left side of the interventricular septum, and soon separates into anterior and posterior

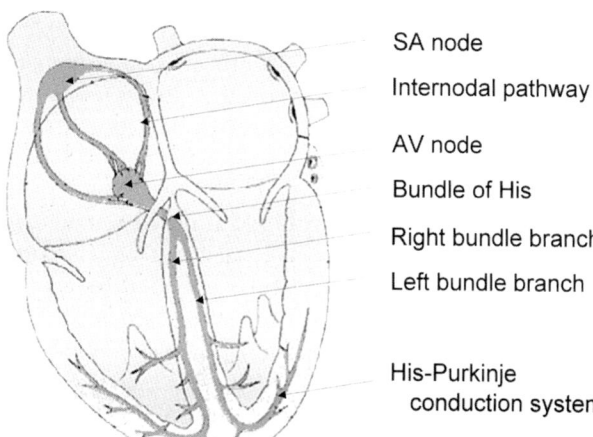

SA node

Internodal pathway

AV node

Bundle of His

Right bundle branch

Left bundle branch

His-Purkinje conduction system

FIGURE 40–1. Schematic representation of the cardiac conduction system. AV, atrioventricular; SA, sinoatrial.

sheets corresponding to the papillary muscles. In many hearts, the left bundle may appear more as a network rather than a well-defined bifascicular system. The terminal Purkinje fibers arising from the bundle branches form interweaving networks on the endocardial surface of both the right and left ventricles. The rapid conduction of electrical impulses across this network results in near simultaneous activation of both right and left ventricles.

Blood Supply

The sinus node receives its blood supply from the sinoatrial (SA) nodal artery arising from the right coronary artery in 59 percent of the patients, from the left circumflex artery in 38 percent, and from both arteries with a dual blood supply in 3 percent.[4] The AV node is supplied by the AV nodal artery arising from the right coronary artery in 90 percent of patients, whereas the left circumflex artery provides it in the remaining 10 percent of patients. The bundle of His is supplied by both the AV nodal artery and branches of the left anterior descending artery. The left bundle has a rich blood supply from the AV nodal artery, posterior descending artery, and branches of the left anterior descending artery.[5]

Innervation

The conduction system of the heart is significantly influenced by both the parasympathetic and sympathetic nervous system. The sinus node is richly innervated with postganglionic adrenergic and cholinergic nerve terminals. Vagal stimulation slows the sinus node discharge rate and increases the intranodal conduction time, occasionally to the point of sinus node exit block. Adrenergic stimulation increases the sinus node discharge rate. Parasympathetic tone predominates at rest in healthy individuals, and parasympathetic withdrawal occurs with increased sympathetic discharge during exercise and emotion. The effects of sympathetic and parasympathetic stimulation on the AV node are more pronounced than they are on the His-Purkinje system. Although sympathetic stimulation shortens AV-nodal conduction time and refractoriness, vagal stimulation prolongs AV-nodal conduction time and refractoriness. Both sympathetic and vagal stimulation have minimal effect on normal conduction in the His bundle.

SINUS NODE DYSFUNCTION

Sinus node dysfunction is a common clinical syndrome, comprising a wide range of electrophysiologic abnormalities from failure of impulse generation, failure of impulse transmission to the atria, inadequate subsidiary pacemaker activity, and increased susceptibility to atrial tachyarrhythmias.[6,7] This disorder has also been variably termed the *sick sinus syndrome, tachycardia-bradycardia syndrome, SA disease,* and *SA dysfunction.*

Pathophysiology

Disorders of sinus node dysfunction may be caused by intrinsic (processes that directly affect the anatomy and physiology of the sinus node and/or the surrounding atrial tissue) or extrinsic factors (processes that affect sinus node function in the absence of structural abnormalities) (Table 40–2). However, in some patients a combination of intrinsic and extrinsic factors may be responsible

TABLE 40–2

Etiology of Sinus Node Dysfunction

INTRINSIC	EXTRINSIC
Idiopathic degenerative disorder	Drugs
Ischemic heart disease	Antiarrhythmic agents
Chronic ischemia	Class IA—quinidine, procainamide
Acute myocardial infarction	Class IC—propafenone, flecainide
Hypertensive heart disease	Class II—β blockers
Cardiomyopathy	Class III—sotalol, amiodarone,
Trauma	dronedarone
Surgery for congenital heart disease	Class IV—diltiazem, verapamil
Heart transplant	Cardiac glycosides
Inflammation	Antihypertensive agents
Collagen vascular disease	Clonidine, reserpine, methyldopa
Rheumatic fever	Antipsychotic agents
Pericarditis	Lithium, phenothiazines, amitriptyline
Infection	Autonomically mediated
Viral myocarditis	Vasovagal syncope (cardioinhibitory)
Lyme disease (*Borrelia burgdorferi*)	Carotid sinus hypersensitivity
Neuromuscular disorder	Hypothyroidism
Friedreich ataxia	Intracranial hypertension
X-linked muscular dystrophy	Hypothermia
Familial disorder	Hyperkalemia
	Hypoxia

drugs used to maintain sinus rhythm in patients with atrial fibrillation may cause significant sinus node dysfunction especially in patients with underlying sinus node dysfunction. Other causes for sinus node dysfunction include electrolyte abnormalities such as hyperkalemia, hypothermia, intracranial hypertension, hypoxia, hypercapnia, and hypothyroidism.

Electrocardiographic Manifestations

A variety of electrocardiographic (ECG) abnormalities have been described in patients with sinus node dysfunction. Many of the ECG abnormalities that define sinus node dysfunction may be asymptomatic, and these abnormalities by themselves do not warrant therapy.

Sinus Bradycardia Sinus bradycardia is defined as a sinus rate <60 beats/min. In most instances sinus bradycardia is a benign arrhythmia. In healthy young adults and trained athletes, resting sinus bradycardia may be a normal phenomenon caused by increased vagal tone. Also sinus bradycardia during sleep in elderly individuals is common. Inability to increase sinus rates adequately during exercise is considered abnormal. Sinus bradycardia <40 beats/min (not associated with sleep or physical conditioning) is generally considered abnormal. Correlation of symptoms with sinus bradycardia is *critical* in the evaluation of these patients.

Sinus Pause and Sinus Arrest Sinus pause or arrest means failure of sinus node discharge with lack of atrial activation of sinus origin. This results in absence of P waves and periods of ventricular asystole if lower pacemakers (junctional or ventricular) do not initiate escape beats (Fig. 40-2). The resulting pause in sinus activity should not be in multiples of preceding sinus cycle length (P-P interval). Asymptomatic sinus pauses of up to 3 sec in duration are not uncommon in trained athletes.[15] Pauses longer than 3 sec need careful clinical correlation with symptoms and warrant further evaluation.

Sinoatrial Exit Block In SA exit block, as the name implies, the impulse is formed in the sinus node but fails to conduct to the atria, unlike sinus arrest. This particular arrhythmia is recognized on ECG by pauses resulting from the absence of normal P waves and the duration of the pause measuring an exact multiple of the preceding P-P interval (Fig. 40-3). SA block can also be described in the same way as AV block. In first-degree SA block, there is significant prolongation of the time for the sinus impulse to exit into the atria (SA conduction time). This cannot be identified clinically or electrocardiographically. Similar to AV block, second-degree SA block can be type I (Wenckebach) or type II. In type I there is pro-

for sinus node dysfunction. In patients with sinus node dysfunction, histopathologic evaluation has revealed the following patterns[8,9]: significant loss of nodal cells with replacement fibrosis, amyloid deposition in the nodal region, hypoplastic or atrophic sinus node, and no detectable morphologic abnormality.

While an idiopathic degenerative disorder of the sinus node is the most common cause for intrinsic sinus node dysfunction, ischemic heart disease is responsible in a significant number of patients. Chronic ischemia from sinus node artery disease[8] or acute myocardial infarction (MI),[10] especially inferior wall MI may result in sinus bradycardia, sinus arrest, and atrial tachyarrhythmias. Other potential causes include long-standing hypertension, cardiomyopathy (especially infiltrative disorders such as amyloidosis and sarcoidosis), inflammation, collagen vascular disease, and inherited neuromuscular disorders. In some cases the condition appears to be familial in origin.[11] Rare cases of sinus node dysfunction requiring pacemaker therapy have been reported with Lyme disease (*Borrelia burgdorferi* infection).[12] In children and young adults, damage to the sinus node during atrial surgery (closure of atrial septal defects of the sinus-venosus-type, mustard procedure for transposition of great arteries)[13] has been commonly associated with sinus node dysfunction. Sinus node dysfunction is also not uncommon in the donor hearts of patients with orthotopic cardiac transplantation.[14]

The most important causes of sinus node dysfunction in patients without structural abnormalities are drugs and autonomic nervous system influences (see Table 40–2). Drugs may alter sinus node function by direct pharmacologic effects on nodal tissue or indirectly by neurally mediated effects.[15] Antiarrhythmic

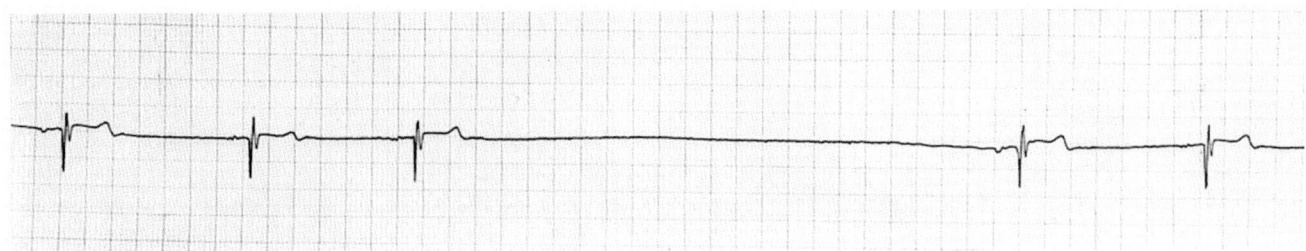

FIGURE 40-2. Telemetry strip demonstrating sinus bradycardia followed by 4.6-sec sinus pause.

gressive prolongation of SA conduction, manifested on surface ECG as progressive shortening of P-P interval, prior to the pause created by loss of a P wave. In type II SA exit block, the P-P intervals remain constant before the pause. Third-degree or complete SA block will manifest as absence of P waves, with long pauses resulting in lower pacemaker escape rhythm; it is impossible to diagnose with certainty without invasive sinus node recordings.

Tachycardia-Bradycardia Syndrome Sinus bradycardia interspersed with periods of atrial tachyarrhythmias is a common manifestation of sinus node dysfunction. The atrial tachyarrhythmias usually range from paroxysmal atrial tachycardia to atrial flutter and atrial fibrillation. Apart from underlying sinus bradycardia of varying severity, these patients often experience prolonged sinus arrest and asystole upon termination of the atrial tachyarrhythmias, resulting from suppression of sinus node and secondary pacemakers (Fig. 40–4). Long sinus pauses that occur following electrical cardioversion of atrial fibrillation are another manifestation of sinus node dysfunction. Therapeutic strategies to control tachyarrhythmias often result in the need for pacemaker therapy. These patients are at increased risk for thromboembolism,[16] and the issue of long-term anticoagulation should be addressed to prevent strokes.

Chronic atrial fibrillation with a slow ventricular response in the absence of AV nodal blocking drugs may also be a manifestation of sinus node dysfunction. These patients may demonstrate very slow ventricular rates at rest or during sleep and occasionally have long pauses. They may also conduct rapidly and develop symptoms caused by tachycardia during exercise. Occasionally they may develop complete AV block with a junctional or ventricular escape rhythm.

Persistent Atrial Standstill Atrial standstill is a rare clinical syndrome in which there is no spontaneous atrial activity and the atria cannot be electrically stimulated.[17] The surface ECG usu-

ally reveals junctional bradycardia without atrial activity. This must be differentiated from fine atrial fibrillation with complete heart block. Intracardiac electrograms fail to show any atrial activity. Atria are generally fibrotic and without any functional myocardium. Myocarditis, amyloidosis, and familial etiology have been recognized as causes in some cases. Lack of mechanical atrial contraction poses a high risk for thromboembolism in these patients.

Chronotropic Incompetence Chronotropic incompetence is the inability of the sinus node to achieve at least 80 percent of the age predicted heart rate. It is present in approximately 20 to 60 percent of patients with sinus node dysfunction.[18] Although the resting heart rates may be normal, these patients may have either the inability to increase their heart rate during exercise or have unpredictable fluctuations in heart rate during activity. Some patients may initially experience a normal increase in heart rate with exercise, which then plateaus or decreases inappropriately. Chronotropic incompetence may be secondary to intrinsic sinus node dysfunction or secondary to drugs with negative chronotropic effects.

Clinical Presentation

Even though sinus node dysfunction can occur in any age group, more than half the patients affected are older than 50 years of age at the time of diagnosis. The incidence of sinus node dysfunction is equal in both men and women. Patients with sinus node dysfunction commonly present with symptoms of syncope, near syncope, or dizzy spells, predominantly related to prolonged sinus pauses. Patients with sinus bradycardia or chronotropic incompetence, however, may present with decreased exercise capacity or fatigue. Patients with atrial fibrilla-

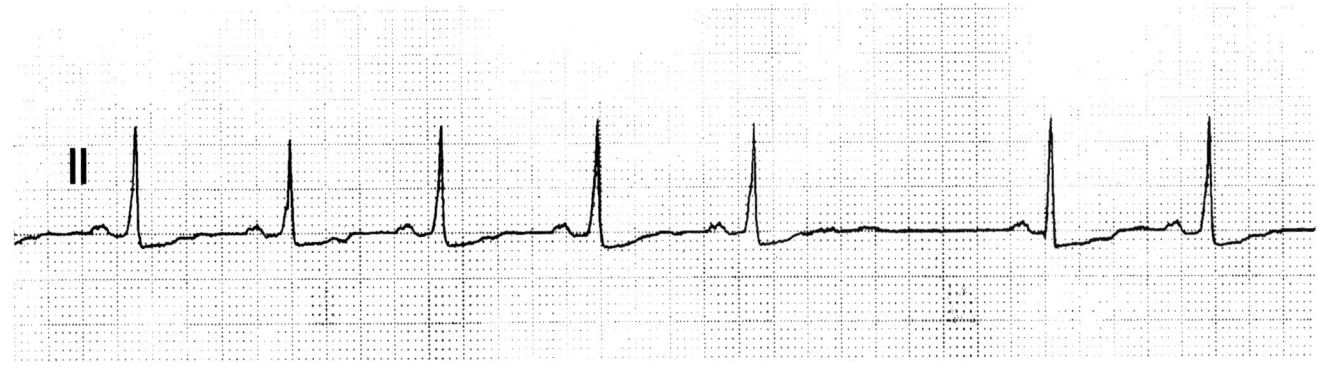

FIGURE 40-3. Telemetry strip demonstrating a sinus pause twice the length of the preceding P-P interval suggesting sinoatrial exit block.

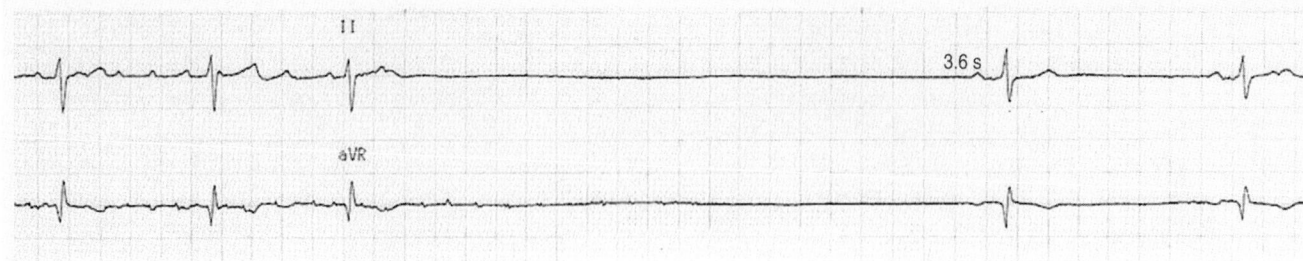

FIGURE 40-4. An example of atrial tachyarrhythmia terminating with 3.6-sec sinus pause.

tion may also present with palpitations or congestive heart failure. Elderly individuals may have unexplained confusion or memory loss. Occasionally, stroke may be the first manifestation of sinus node dysfunction in patients presenting with paroxysmal atrial fibrillation and thromboembolism.

Diagnostic Evaluation

The diagnosis of sinus node dysfunction in patients who present with typical symptoms and ECG findings is straightforward. However, because of the intermittent nature of the symptoms and rhythm manifestations, the diagnosis can be time consuming and frustrating. A number of noninvasive and invasive tests are available to assist in the evaluation.

Electrocardiographic Recordings Documentation of the various arrhythmias associated with sinus node dysfunction can be obtained with routine telemetric monitoring during hospitalization or with outpatient ambulatory 24- to 48-hour Holter recordings. If the symptoms are infrequent in nature, event recorders capable of intermittent or continuous monitoring can be used. If other noninvasive and invasive tests are inconclusive, patients may benefit from an implantable loop recorder, which has the ability to record both patient-triggered and automatic device-triggered events over a period of 18 to 24 months. Exercise testing to assess chronotropic incompetence can be valuable in select patients. Many patients with sinus node dysfunction may achieve peak heart rates similar to matched controls during specific exercise protocols; however, the time course of heart rate acceleration during activity and deceleration after activity may be markedly abnormal.[19]

Autonomic Testing Abnormalities of autonomic control of sinus node alone or in association with intrinsic sinus node disease can result in clinical symptoms and electrocardiographic findings of sinus node dysfunction. This can be assessed by observing the response of heart rate and rhythm with carotid sinus massage, head-up tilt testing, and Valsalva maneuver. Pharmacologic evaluation of the sinus node can be performed with atropine, isoproterenol, and propranolol. Following injection of atropine 0.04 mg/kg intravenously, the heart rate increases by 15 percent and to more than 90 beats/min. Isoproterenol infusion at 1 to 3 μg/min increases heart rate by 25 percent. Patients with sinus node dysfunction show blunted heart rate responses to the preceding infusions. Another method to assess sinus node function is to measure the intrinsic heart rate (IHR) of the sinus node when the autonomic influence is negated by both atropine (0.04 mg/kg) and propranolol (0.2 mg/kg), using the following equation[20]:

$$IHR = 117.2 - (0.53 \times age) \text{ beats/min}$$

Patients with sinus node dysfunction demonstrate a decreased intrinsic heart rate.

Electrophysiology Study Invasive electrophysiology study, in addition to assessing sinus node function, offers insight into other potential etiologies for symptoms of syncope and palpitations (AV block, supraventricular tachycardia, ventricular tachycardia [VT]). The sinus node recovery time (SNRT) is a measure of sinus node automaticity and is measured as the longest pause after atrial overdrive pacing.[21] SA conduction time (SACT) is a measure of the interval from sinus node depolarization to activation of atrial muscle.

Management

Pharmacologic Treatment Theophylline and β-adrenergic agonists have been used to treat symptomatic bradycardia. Although they have been shown to increase the heart rate and reduce the duration of sinus pauses, they do not prevent recurrent syncope.[21,22] In patients with extrinsic causes for sinus node dysfunction, treatment should be directed toward the underlying etiology. Drugs known to depress sinus node function can be switched to other agents that lack effects on the cardiac conduction system. This is not possible, however, in many patients. Patients with paroxysmal atrial tachyarrhythmias either require drugs to maintain sinus rhythm or agents to control ventricular rate, both of which may have significant depressant effects on sinus node function. In many of these patients pacemaker therapy becomes essential. At the time of diagnosis of sinus node dysfunction, the incidence of atrial fibrillation is reported to be approximately 8 percent and the likelihood of developing new atrial fibrillation in this group of patients is approximately 5 percent per year.[23] The prevalence of thromboembolism was reported to be 15.2 percent in this group. This underscores the importance of monitoring for atrial fibrillation and the need for oral anticoagulation in intermediate to high-risk patients.

Pacing Therapy in Sinus Node Dysfunction The current indications for pacing in the setting of sinus node dysfunction are shown in Table 40-3. In this and subsequent tables, the format used for American Heart Association (AHA)/American College of Cardiology (ACC) guidelines is used, with class I to III indications denoting the degree of agreement for a given procedure or treatment that is useful and effective.

TABLE 40–3

Indications for Pacing in Sinus Node Dysfunction (ACC/AHA/NASPE 2002 Revised Guidelines)

Class I
1. Sinus node dysfunction with documented symptomatic bradycardia or sinus pauses. Sinus node dysfunction as a result of essential long-term drug therapy of a type and dose, for which there are no acceptable alternatives *(Level of evidence: C).*
2. Symptomatic chronotropic incompetence *(Level of evidence: C).*

Class IIa
1. Sinus node dysfunction occurring spontaneously or as a result of necessary drug therapy, with heart rates <40 beats/min when a clear association between significant symptoms consistent with bradycardia and the actual presence of bradycardia has not been documented *(Level of evidence: C).*
2. Syncope of unexplained origin when major abnormalities of sinus node function are discovered or provoked in electrophysiologic studies *(Level of evidence: C).*

Class IIb
1. In minimally symptomatic patients, chronic heart rates <40 bpm while awake *(Level of evidence: C).*

Class III
1. Sinus node dysfunction in asymptomatic patients, including those in whom substantial sinus bradycardia (heart rate <40 bpm) is a consequence of long-term drug treatment.
2. Sinus node dysfunction in patients with symptoms suggestive of bradycardia that are clearly documented as not associated with a slow heart rate.
3. Sinus node dysfunction with symptomatic bradycardia caused by nonessential drug therapy.

ACC, American College of Cardiology; AHA, American Heart Association; NASPE, National Association for Sports and Physical Education.

Sinus node dysfunction is the most common indication for permanent pacemaker implantation in North America, accounting for over 40 to 60 percent of new pacemaker implants.[24] The optimal pacemaker choice is influenced by a number of factors. At the time of diagnosis of sinus node dysfunction, 17 percent of patients have been reported to have AV conduction abnormalities in the form of a P-R interval >240 msec, bundle-branch block, H-V interval prolongation, AV Wenckebach rates <120 beats/min, and second- or third-degree AV block. The incidence of new AV block developing over time was reported to be <2.7 percent per year.[23] Generally, if the patient has persistent atrial fibrillation, a single-chamber ventricular pacemaker (VVIR) is recommended. In all other situations a rate-responsive dual-chamber pacemaker (DDDR) is used, whereas a single-chamber atrial pacemaker (AAIR) can be implanted if no evidence of AV conduction disease is present.

Clinical Trials and Pacing Mode Many nonprospective, nonrandomized studies have suggested significant survival benefits with physiologic pacing compared to ventricular demand pacing (VVI mode) in patients with sinus node dysfunction. This led to randomized, large-scale prospective trials, the results of which are summarized in Table 40–4. The first randomized trial comparing atrial to ventricular pacing in 225 patients with sick sinus syndrome demonstrated significant reduction in the incidence of atrial fibrillation, thromboembolism, and cardiovascular mortality in the atrial pacing group.[25] Subsequent large-scale trials have not confirmed these mortality or stroke prevention benefits. The Canadian Trial of Physiologic Pacing (CTOPP)[27] randomized patients with symptomatic bradycardia without chronic atrial fibrillation to receive either a physiologic (atrial or dual-chamber) pacemaker or a ventricular pacemaker and showed no difference in stroke or cardiovascular mortality, but a decreased annual rate of atrial fibrillation in the physiologic pacing group (5.3 percent) compared to the ventricular pacing group (6.6 percent). Another large randomized trial of dual-chamber pacing versus ventricular pacing was MOST (Mode Selection Trial in sinus node dysfunction),[28] which also confirmed the benefit of dual-chamber pacing to reduce the risk for atrial fibrillation. The United Kingdom Pacing and Cardiovascular Events (UKPACE) trial compared dual chamber pacing to single-chamber ventricular pacing in patients older than 70 years of age with high grade atrioventricular block.[29] Over a mean follow-up period of 4.6 years there was no difference in annual mortality, atrial fibrillation or heart failure between the groups. In a recent meta-analysis of randomized pacing modes, atrial based pacing was associated with a significant reduction in atrial fibrillation of approximately 20 percent (95 percent confidence interval [CI]: 0.77–0.89, $p = 0.00003$) and a borderline significant reduction in the risk of stroke of 19 percent (95 percent CI: 0.67–0.99, $p = 0.035$). The use of atrial based pacing did not reduce mortality or the incidence of congestive heart failure.[30]

The failure to easily demonstrate clinical benefits of dual-chamber pacing has forced a rethinking of *physiologic pacing.* It is now well accepted that long-term right ventricular (RV) pacing causes a deterioration of left ventricular (LV) function through complex effects on regional ventricular wall strain and loading conditions. This deterioration is thought to result from intraventricular dyssynchrony between different regions of the left ventricle induced by RV apical pacing. Sweeney and coworkers demonstrated, by careful review of data from MOST, that an increase in the frequency of ventricular pacing in patients with sick sinus syndrome who had a narrow native QRS complex was associated with an increased incidence of atrial fibrillation and congestive heart failure.[31] These observations were confirmed by Wilkoff and colleagues in the Dual Chamber and VVI Implantable Defibrillator (DAVID) study, in which backup ventricular pacing and dual-chamber pacing were prospectively compared in patients with dual-chamber defibrillators.[32] The primary end point was a composite of congestive heart failure, hospitalization, and death, which was increased by a factor of 1.6 in patients with an increased frequency of ventricular pacing. Thus, RV pacing is a double-edged sword, conferring atrioventricular synchrony but at the same time possibly negating its benefit by inducing ventricular dysfunction.

【 】 CAROTID SINUS HYPERSENSITIVITY AND VASOVAGAL SYNCOPE

The pathophysiology, diagnosis, and specific management of these disorders are discussed separately in Chap. 48. A hypersensitive re-

TABLE 40-4

Randomized Trials of Pacing Modes in Patients with Sinus Node Dysfunction and/or Atrioventricular Block

TRIAL	INDICATION	MODE COMPARISON	NO. OF PATIENTS	FOLLOW-UP	ENDPOINTS	RESULTS
Danish[25]	SSS	AAI vs. VVI	225	8 y	Total mortality, AF, thrombo-embolism	Atrial pacing significantly reduced mortality (RR 0.66), AF (RR 0.54), and stroke (RR 0.47)
PASE[49]	SSS and AVB	DDDR vs. VVIR	407	30 mo	Primary: QOL Secondary: Total mortality, stroke, AF, HF	No change in QOL, mortality, stroke or AF, improved QOL in SSS patients with physiologic pacing
CTOPP[27]	SSS and AVB	DDDR/AAIR vs VVIR	2568	3 y	Primary: Stroke, CV mortality Secondary: Total mortality, AF, hospitalization for HF	No reduction in mortality or stroke; relative risk reduction of 18% for AF with physiologic pacing
MOST[28]	SSS	DDDR vs VVIR	2010	33 mo	Primary: Total mortality, stroke Secondary: Composite of death, stroke, or hospital for HF, AF, QOL, HF score	No difference in primary or secondary endpoint except for AF; lower incidence of AF with DDD pacing (hazard ratio of 0.79)
UKPACE[29]	AVB	DDDR vs. VVIR	2021	4.6 y	Primary: Total mortality Secondary: HF, AF, composite of stroke, TIA or thromboembolic events	No difference in primary (mortality 7.4% vs. 7.2%) or secondary endpoints

AF, atrial fibrillation; AVB, atrioventricular block; CTOPP, Canadian trial of physiologic pacing; CV, cardiovascular; HF, heart failure; MOST, mode selection trial; PASE, pacemaker selection in the elderly; QOL, quality of life; RR, relative risk; SSS, sick sinus syndrome; TIA, transient ischemic attack; UKPACE, United Kingdom Pacing and Cardiovascular Events.

sponse to carotid sinus stimulation of 5 to 10 sec is defined as asystole caused by sinus arrest or AV block of more than 3 sec (cardioinhibitory), a substantial symptomatic decrease in systolic blood pressure of 50 mmHg or more, (vasodepressor) or both (mixed). The pathophysiology of carotid sinus syncope is complex and poorly understood and is hypothesized to result from abnormalities of neuromuscular structures surrounding the carotid sinus mechanoreceptors, a central defect of the autonomic nervous system and association with atherosclerotic disease. Carotid sinus syncope predominantly occurs in elderly males with associated coronary artery disease. Although carotid sinus hypersensitivity is common, carotid sinus syncope is relatively rare accounting for 11 to 19 percent of patients with syncope of undetermined cause.[33] For patients with recurrent or severe carotid sinus syncope of the cardioinhibitory type, permanent pacemaker implantation is the accepted and proven modality of treatment as evidenced by many small randomized trials.[34] DDI or DDD pacemakers are generally

the accepted mode of pacing for patients with carotid sinus syncope, whereas AAI pacing is contraindicated because many patients may demonstrate associated AV block. The current indications for pacing in hypersensitive carotid sinus syndrome and neurocardiogenic syncope are shown in Table 40-5.

Vasovagal syncope is a common condition caused by inappropriate reflex vasodilation and bradycardia, and occasionally even asystole. Dual-chamber pacemakers with *rate-drop response* or *rate hysteresis* feature are currently a treatment option in a select group of patients with recurrent syncope and refractory to conventional medical therapy. Three randomized but nonplacebo-controlled trials have assessed the role of permanent pacemakers in patients with vasovagal syncope and cardioinhibitory response during tilt-table testing (Table 40-6).[35-37] The results of these trials are somewhat contradictory, and as a result most clinicians refer pacing therapy to patients who are severely symptomatic and refractory to medical therapy.

TABLE 40–5

Recommendations for Permanent Pacing in Hypersensitive Carotid Sinus Syndrome and Neurocardiogenic Syncope

Class I

1. Recurrent syncope caused by carotid sinus stimulation; minimal carotid sinus pressure induces ventricular asystole of >3-sec duration in the absence of any medication that depresses the sinus node or AV conduction (Level of evidence: C).

Class IIa

1. Recurrent syncope without clear, provocative events and with a hypersensitive cardioinhibitory response (Level of evidence: C).
2. Significantly symptomatic and recurrent neurocardiogenic syncope associated with bradycardia documented spontaneously or at the time of tilt-table testing (Level of evidence: C).

Class III

1. A hyperactive cardioinhibitory response to carotid sinus stimulation in the absence of symptoms or in the presence of vague symptoms such as dizziness, light-headedness, or both.
2. Recurrent syncope, light-headedness, or dizziness in the absence of a hyperactive cardioinhibitory response.
3. Situational vasovagal syncope in which avoidance behavior is effective.

AV, atrioventricular.

DISORDERS OF ATRIOVENTRICULAR CONDUCTION

AV block occurs when atrial conduction to the ventricle is blocked at a time when the AV junction is not physiologically refractory. This can be caused by conduction block in the atrium, AV node, and/or His-Purkinje system. Using His-bundle electrogram recordings, three anatomic sites of AV block can be identified: AV nodal, intra-Hisian, or infra-Hisian. Block at the AV nodal level implies a favorable prognosis while block at or below the His-bundle level implies an unfavorable prognosis. Surface ECGs often provide adequate information to make a diagnosis regarding the site of the block, whereas occasionally intracardiac recordings are necessary to confirm the level of the block.

Pathophysiology of Atrioventricular Block

Transient or persistent AV block of varying degrees can occur in a variety of clinical situations (Table 40–7). Heightened vagal tone in athletes or during sleep may be associated with first-degree or type I second-degree AV block and occasionally even complete heart block. The AV block in these situations is usually preceded by slowing of the heart rate. Vagally mediated AV block may occur in response to various stimuli such as carotid sinus hypersensitivity, coughing, swallowing, or micturition.[35] Varying degrees of heart block have been described in a large variety of infectious diseases. Heart block associated with endocarditis may be transient or permanent. In patients with endocarditis and ring abscess, heart block may not resolve and pacing may be required. With Lyme disease cardiac involvement may occur in 8 to 10 percent of patients. More than 50 percent of patients with cardiac involvement may develop advanced heart block requiring temporary pacing.[36] Even complete AV block generally re-

TABLE 40–6

Randomized Trials of Permanent Pacing in Patients with Recurrent Vasovagal Syncope

TRIAL	INCLUSION CRITERIA	TREATMENT GROUPS	NO. OF PATIENTS	FOLLOW-UP	ENDPOINTS	RESULTS
VPS	Syncope × 6, positive tilt-table test with relative bradycardia	DDD pacer with RDR vs. no pacer	54	15 mo	First recurrence of syncope	85% relative risk reduction for recurrent syncope (22% in pacemaker vs. 70% in no pacemaker arm)
VASIS	>3 syncope in last 2 y, positive tilt-table test with HR <40 or asystole <3 sec, age >40 y	DDI pacer with rate hysteresis vs. no pacer	42	3.7 y (mean)	First recurrence of syncope	Significant reduction in recurrent syncope (5% in pacemaker arm vs. 61% in no pacer arm)
SYDIT	>3 syncope in last 2 y, positive tilt-table test with relative bradycardia, age >35 y	DDD pacer with RDR vs. atenolol	93	17 mo (mean)	First recurrence of syncope	Significant reduction in recurrent syncope, 4.3% in pacer group vs. 25.5% in atenolol group
VPS II	>5 syncope/lifetime or >2 syncope/2 y, positive tilt-table test with relative bradycardia, age >19 y	DDD pacer with RDR vs. pacer in ODO mode	100	6 mo	First recurrence of syncope	Nonsignificant reduction in recurrent syncope (DDD paced patients 30 vs. 40% in ODO)

HR, heart rate; RDR, rate drop response; SYDIT, Syncope Diagnosis and Treatment study; VASIS, Vasovagal Syncope International Study; VPS, Vasovagal Pacemaker Study.

TABLE 40–7

Etiology of Atrioventricular Block

REVERSIBLE	PERMANENT
Physiologic	Idiopathic fibrosis
Heightened vagal tone (athletes, sleep apnea)	Lev disease
	Lenegre disease
Autonomic mediated	Congenital
Carotid sinus hypersensitivity	Congenital heart disease
Neurocardiogenic syncope	Maternal systemic lupus erythematosus
Coronary artery disease	Coronary artery disease
Acute myocardial infarction	Acute myocardial infarction
Angina (Prinzmetal)	Ischemic cardiomyopathy
Infectious disease	Cardiomyopathy
Infective endocarditis	Infiltrative disease
Myocarditis	Amyloidosis
Viral, rickettsial, Lyme disease,	Sarcoidosis
Rheumatic fever	Hemochromatosis
Metabolic	Infectious disease
Hyperkalemia	Endocarditis
Hypermagnesemia	Syphilis
Addison disease	Tuberculosis
Traumatic	Chagas disease
Catheter induced	Collagen vascular disease
Radiofrequency energy	Systemic lupus erythematosus
Surgery	Rheumatoid arthritis
Drug induced	Scleroderma
Digitalis	Traumatic
β Blockers	Surgery
Calcium channel blockers	Radiofrequency ablation
Class III antiarrhythmic agents	Radiation
Class I antiarrhythmic agents	Tumors
Adenosine	Mesothelioma
Lithium	Rhabdomyoma
	Hodgkin lymphoma
	Melanoma
	Neuromuscular disease
	Myotonic dystrophy
	Kearns-Sayre Syndrome
	Erb dystrophy
	X-linked muscular dystrophy
	Peroneal muscular atrophy

AV block occurs in 12 to 25 percent of all patients with acute MI; first-degree AV block occurs in 2 to 12 percent, second-degree AV block in 3 to 10 percent; and third-degree AV block in 3 to 7 percent.[40] Ischemic injury can produce conduction block at any level of the AV or intraventricular conduction system. Second-degree type I AV block occurs more commonly in inferior than anterior MIs. Inferior infarctions are often associated early on with increased vagal tone causing sinus bradycardia and AV block. Most patients are asymptomatic, and rarely type I AV block may progress to complete AV block. Second-degree type II AV block occurs in 1 percent of patients with acute MI and predominantly occurs in patients with anterior infarctions. The risk of progression to complete AV block is high in these patients. Complete AV block can occur in both inferior and anterior infarctions. In inferior MIs, the block is at the level of the AV node and the escape rhythm typically arises from the AV junction, with a narrow QRS and an escape rate of 40 to 60 beats/min. The prognosis in these patients is generally good as the AV block resolves in most patients within a few days. Complete AV block resulting from anterior infarction is usually at the His or infra-Hisian level, and the escape rhythm is from the distal Purkinje fibers or the ventricle, with a wide QRS interval and a rate of 20 to 40 beats/min. Because of the coexisting extensive infarction and pump failure, AV block resulting from anterior infarctions are associated with high mortality. In patients with acute MI, temporary pacing is generally indicated in patients with complete AV block at any level, type II second-degree AV block, and in patients with type I second-degree AV block if associated with symptomatic bradycardia. Although the incidence of complete AV block in acute MIs has decreased following thrombolytic therapy, the mortality still remains high.[41] The indications for permanent pacing in patients with acute MI are listed in Table 40–8. Patients with coronary artery disease and ischemic cardiomyopathy may develop persistent AV block. AV nodal block can occur transiently during episodes of ischemia especially with Prinzmetal's angina.

A variety of uncommon autoimmune, oncologic, infectious, and iatrogenic disorders can also lead to heart block and are listed in Table 40–7. Certain neuromuscular disorders (myotonic dystrophy, Kearns-Sayre syndrome, peroneal muscular atrophy, Erb limb-girdle dystrophy, and X-linked muscular dystrophies) may give rise to progressive and insidiously developing conduction disorders of the His-Purkinje system. Myotonic dystrophy and Kearns-Sayre syndrome are associ-

solves in 1 to 2 weeks, and permanent pacing is seldom necessary. Chagas cardiomyopathy may be associated with persistent AV block.

Idiopathic progressive fibrosis of the conduction system is a common cause of acquired AV block. Also known as idiopathic bilateral bundle-branch fibrosis, Lev disease is characterized by progressive replacement of the proximal bundle branches by fibrosis as a result of the aging process exaggerated by hypertension and arteriosclerosis.[37] Lenègre disease is a variant of idiopathic conduction disorder involving young patients and the peripheral parts of the bundle branches.[38] Some cases of Lenègre disease may be caused by mutations in the sodium channel gene SCN5a, causing a hereditary form of AV conduction disease.[39]

TABLE 40-8

Indications for Pacing in Atrioventricular Block Associated with Acute Myocardial Infarction

Class I

1. Persistent second-degree atrioventricular (AV) block in the His-Purkinje system with bilateral bundle-branch block or third-degree AV block within or below the His-Purkinje system after AMI (Level of evidence: B).
2. Transient advanced (second- or third-degree) infranodal AV block and associated bundle-branch block. If the site of block is uncertain, an electrophysiology study may be necessary (Level of evidence: B).
3. Persistent and symptomatic second- or third-degree AV block (Level of evidence: C).

Class IIb

1. Persistent second- or third-degree AV block at the AV node level (Level of evidence: B).

Class III

1. Transient AV block in the absence of intraventricular conduction defects (Level of evidence: B).
2. Transient AV block in the presence of isolated left anterior fascicular block (Level of evidence: B).
3. Acquired left anterior fascicular block in the absence of AV block (Level of evidence: B).
4. Persistent first-degree AV block in the presence of bundle-branch block that is old or age indeterminate (Level of evidence: B).

ated with high incidence of unpredictable and rapidly progressive conduction system disease.[42] Complete heart block may occur after aortic or mitral valve replacement surgery, and rarely after coronary artery bypass surgery. Preoperative right bundle-branch block and multivalve surgery involving the tricuspid valve were shown to be strong independent predictors of postoperative heart block requiring permanent pacemaker implantation.[43] Complete AV block is more common after surgical procedures to correct ventricular septal defects, tetralogy of Fallot, AV canal defects, or myectomy for hypertrophic obstructive cardiomyopathy. Congenital heart diseases such as corrected transposition of great arteries, ostium primum atrial septal defects, and ventricular septal defects may be associated with complete heart block. Congenital complete AV block is a rare anomaly that results from abnormal embryonic development of the AV node and is not associated with structural heart disease in 50 percent of cases. Congenital complete heart block is also associated with maternal lupus erythematosus. Most children with isolated congenital complete AV block have a stable escape rhythm with a narrow complex. Pacing is generally indicated in children with complete heart block if the heart rate in the awake child is <50 beats/min or if associated with LV systolic dysfunction or ventricular arrhythmias. The indications for pacing in children, adolescents, and patients with congenital heart disease are outlined in Table 40-9.

Electrocardiographic Manifestations

First-Degree Atrioventricular Block Prolongation of the P-R interval to >200 msec constitutes first-degree AV block. It is most commonly caused by conduction delay within the AV node and occasionally caused by intraatrial or infra-Hisian conduction delay. If the QRS duration is normal, the site of conduction delay is almost always within the AV node. If first-degree AV block occurs in the presence of bundle-branch block, the conduction delay can be in the AV node (60 percent of cases), His-Purkinje system, or both. Patients with first-degree AV block have an excellent prognosis even when associated with chronic bifascicular block as the rate of progression to third-degree AV block is low, and no specific therapy is indicated.[44]

Second-Degree Atrioventricular Block Second-degree AV block is characterized by intermittent failure of conduction from the atria to the ventricles. If the AV block occurs with the atrial rate in the physiologic range, it is considered a primary arrhythmia. AV block in the setting of atrial tachyarrhythmias is generally a normal response. Based on the electrocardiographic patterns, second-degree AV block is classified into Mobitz types I and II.

Second-degree AV Block of the Wenckebach Type (Mobitz Type I) Second-degree AV block of the Wenckebach type (Mobitz type I) is characterized by the following features: (1) progressive prolongation of the P-R interval prior to a nonconducted P wave, (2) P-R interval prolongation at progressively decreasing increments, (3) progressive shortening of R-R intervals, (4) pause encompassing the blocked P wave shorter than the sum of two P-P cycles, and (5) the last conducted P-R interval prior to the blocked P wave longer than the next conducted P-R interval (Fig. 40-5). Type I second-degree AV block often occurs with regularity leading to patterns of *group beating*. When type I second-degree AV block occurs in association with a normal QRS interval, block is almost always in the AV node. In the presence of a prolonged QRS interval, block may be in the AV node, His-Purkinje (rare), or both. Very long P-R intervals are usually caused by a block in the AV node. Type I second-degree AV block occurs in a small percentage of normal people and not uncommonly in well-trained athletes. Most patients are asymptomatic, whereas some develop symptomatic bradycardia, near syncope, or occasionally syncope caused by progression to complete AV block.

Mobitz Type II Second-Degree AV block is characterized by (1) constant P-P intervals and R-R intervals; (2) constant P-R intervals prior to a nonconducted P wave; and (3) pause encompassing the nonconducted P wave equal to two P-P cycles. Type II AV block usually occurs in the presence of bundle-branch block and is almost always caused by a block in the His-Purkinje system (Fig. 40-6). Type II AV block rarely occurs in patients with normal QRS duration. Type II AV block frequently progresses to a complete AV block and may result in syncopal attacks.

2:1 Atrioventricular Block In this form of second-degree AV block, every other P wave is not conducted, making it difficult to diagnose the level of AV block (Fig. 40-7). A 2:1 AV block pattern with normal QRS duration or with a very long P-R interval generally suggests block in the AV node. A 2:1 AV block pattern in the presence of bundle-branch block favors block below the AV node but is not diagnostic. A prolonged electrocardiographic recording may sometimes reveal a transition to varying degrees of AV block (3:2 or 4:3), with type I

TABLE 40–9

Indications for Pacing in Children, Adolescents, and Patients with Congenital Heart Disease

Class I

1. Advanced second- or third-degree atrioventricular (AV) block associated with symptomatic bradycardia, ventricular dysfunction, or low cardiac output (*Level of evidence: C*).
2. Sinus node dysfunction with correlation of symptoms during age-inappropriate bradycardia. The definition of bradycardia varies with the patient's age and expected heart rate (*Level of evidence: B*).
3. Postoperative advanced second- or third-degree AV block that is not expected to resolve or persists at least 7 days after cardiac surgery (*Level of evidence: B,C*).
4. Congenital third-degree AV block with a wide QRS escape rhythm, complex ventricular ectopy, or ventricular dysfunction (*Level of evidence: B*).
5. Congenital third-degree AV block in the infant with the ventricular rate less than 50 to 55 bpm or with congenital heart disease and a ventricular rate <70 beats/min (*Level of evidence: B,C*).
6. Sustained pause-dependent VT, with or without prolonged QT, in which the efficacy of pacing is thoroughly documented (*Level of evidence: B*).

Class IIa

1. Bradycardia-tachycardia syndrome with the need for long-term antiarrhythmic treatment other than digitalis (*Level of evidence: C*).
2. Congenital third-degree AV block beyond the first year of life with an average heart rate <50 beats/min caused by abrupt pauses in ventricular rate that are two or three times the basic cycle length, or associated with symptoms due to chronotropic incompetence (*Level of evidence: B*).
3. Long-QT syndrome with 2:1 AV or third-degree AV block (*Level of evidence: B*).
4. Asymptomatic sinus bradycardia in the child with complex congenital heart disease with resting heart rate <40 beats/min or pauses in ventricular rate more than 3 sec (*Level of evidence: C*).
5. Patients with congenital heart disease and impaired hemodynamics due to sinus bradycardia or loss of AV synchrony (*Level of evidence: C*).

Class IIb

1. Transient postoperative third-degree AV block that reverts to sinus rhythm with residual bifascicular block (*Level of evidence: C*).
2. Congenital third-degree AV block in the asymptomatic infant, child, adolescent, or young adult with an acceptable rate, narrow QRS complex, and normal ventricular function (*Level of evidence: B*).
3. Asymptomatic sinus bradycardia in the adolescent with congenital heart disease with resting heart rate <40 beats/min or pauses in ventricular rate > 3 sec (*Level of evidence: C*).
4. Neuromuscular diseases with any degree of AV block (including first-degree AV block), with or without symptoms, because there may be unpredictable progression of AV conduction disease.

Class III

1. Transient postoperative AV block with return of normal AV conduction (*Level of evidence: B*).
2. Asymptomatic postoperative bifascicular block with or without first-degree AV block (*Level of evidence: C*).
3. Asymptomatic type I second-degree AV block (*Level of evidence: C*).
4. Asymptomatic sinus bradycardia in the adolescent with longest R-R interval <3 sec and minimum heart rate >40 bpm (*Level of evidence: C*).

or type II features that aids in the diagnosis. Intracardiac recordings with a His-bundle catheter is sometimes necessary to determine the site of the block. In patients with a 2:1 AV block, vagal maneuvers are helpful in diagnosing the level of AV block. Carotid sinus stimulation may worsen the degree of block if it is in the AV node, whereas slowing of the sinus rate may paradoxically improve the ratio of AV conduction and increase ventricular rate if the block is located in the His-Purkinje system. Similarly, atropine improves AV nodal conduction, but the increased sinus rate may worsen the ratio of AV conduction in patients with His-Purkinje block, resulting in worsened bradycardia. Hence, atropine should be used with caution in patients with a 2:1 AV block and bundle-branch block where His-Purkinje disease is strongly suspected.

High-Grade Atrioventricular Block

When two or more consecutive atrial impulses do not conduct to the ventricle, it is defined as high-grade AV block. It may be associated with a junctional or ventricular escape rhythm. Occasionally, runs of consecutive atrial impulses may fail to conduct to the ventricles for up to 10 to 20 sec with or without an escape rhythm resulting in ventricular asystole and syncope. The block is usually initiated by a conducted or blocked atrial or ventricular premature beat. The block persists until terminated by an escape beat. Unless a clearly defined reversible etiology is identified, permanent pacing is indicated.

Third-Degree Atrioventricular Block

Complete or third-degree AV block is characterized by failure of all P waves to conduct to the ventricle. This results in complete dissociation of P waves and QRS complexes. Complete AV block may occur as a result of block in the AV node or at the His-Purkinje level. In patients with block at the AV node level, the escape rhythm is usually junctional, with a narrow QRS complex (unless associated with preexisting bundle-branch block), at rates of 40 to 60 beats/min (Fig. 40–8). In complete heart block resulting from His-Purkinje disease, the escape rhythm is ventricular in origin, with a wide QRS interval and at rates of 20 to 40 beats/min.

Atrioventricular Dissociation

This rhythm is characterized by atrial and ventricular activity independent of each other. AV dissociation may be secondary to AV block (complete heart block) or physiologic refractoriness. AV dissociation can occur when the sinus rate is slower than the secondary junctional or ventricular pacemaker as in patients with sinus bradycardia. In contrast, AV dissociation can also occur in the presence of normal sinus rhythm and accelerated junctional (junctional tachycardia) or ventricular (VT) rhythm with retrograde conduction block. In patients with complete heart block, the atrial rate is

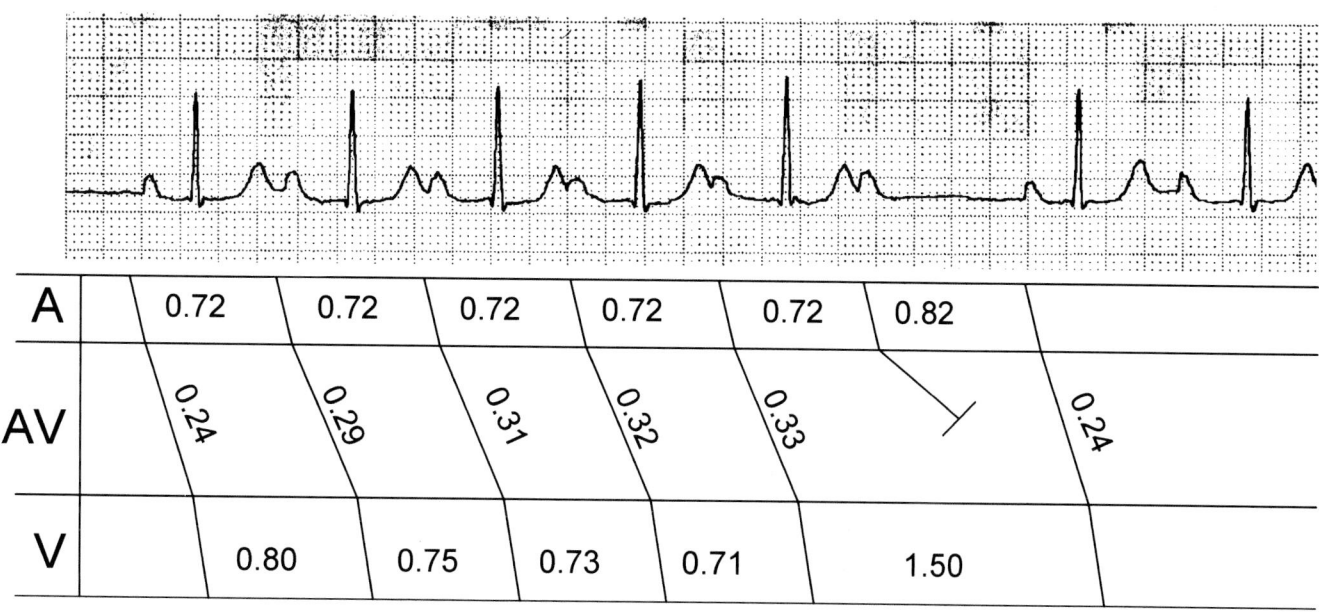

A	0.72	0.72	0.72	0.72	0.72	0.82	
AV	0.24	0.29	0.31	0.32	0.33		0.24
V		0.80	0.75	0.73	0.71	1.50	

FIGURE 40-5. Type I second-degree atrioventricular (AV) block. A 6:5 AV Wenckebach periodicity is shown. Note that the P-R interval progressively lengthens with a decreasing increment. This results in shortening of R-R intervals. The last conducted P-R interval (0.33 sec) is significantly longer than the next conducted P-R interval (0.24 sec).

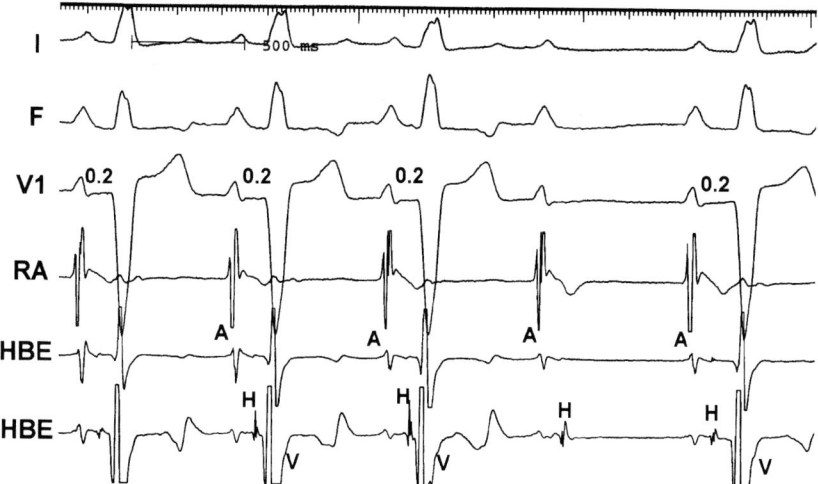

FIGURE 40-6. Type II second-degree atrioventricular block. Surface electrocardiogram (ECG); leads I, aVF, and V_1 and intracardiac electrograms from the right atrial (RA), proximal, and distal His bundle electrogram (HBE) catheters are shown. Surface ECGs show that the P-R intervals are constant at 0.2 sec with a left bundle-branch block morphology of the QRS complex, and the fourth P wave is not followed by a QRS complex. The HBEs reveal that the site of block of the fourth P wave is below the His bundle.

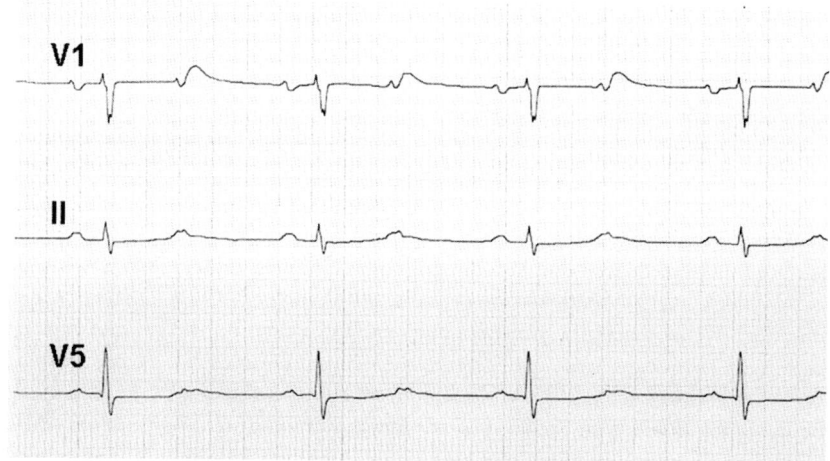

FIGURE 40-7. Surface electrocardiogram from leads V_1, II, and V_5 demonstrating 2:1 atrioventricular (AV) block with narrow QRS complexes. Although a definite diagnosis of type I or type II AV block cannot be made, longer rhythm strip recordings might reveal Wenckebach periodicity. Vagal maneuvers or exercise might assist further in the final diagnosis.

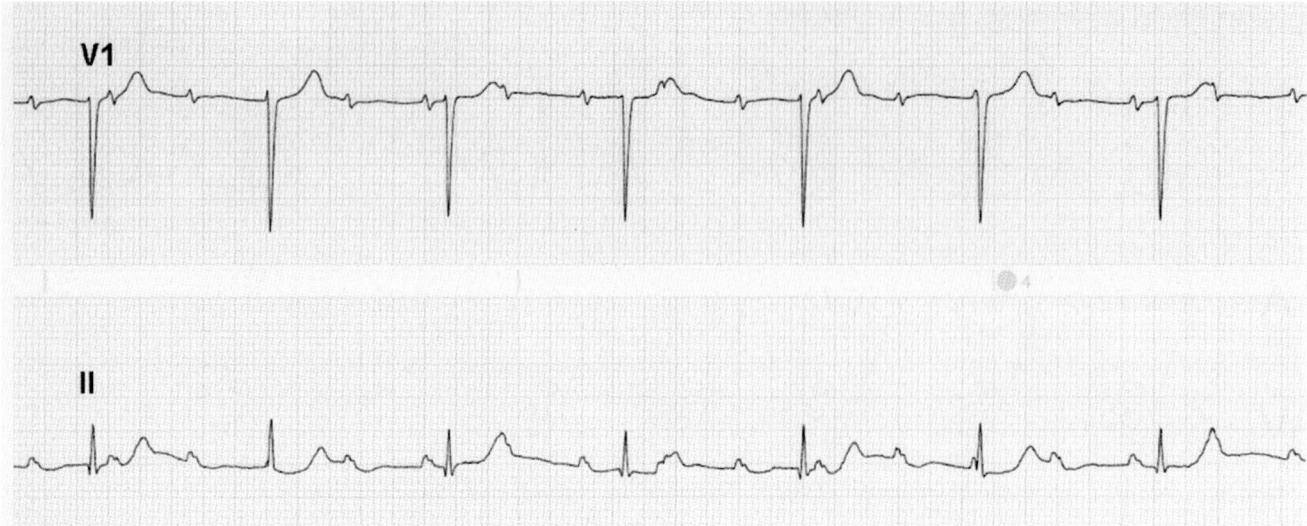

FIGURE 40–8. Complete heart block. Surface leads V₁ and II shows sinus tachycardia at 120 beats/min and is completely dissociated from a regular junctional (narrow QRS complexes) escape rhythm at 54 beats/min. The site of atrioventricular (AV) block is most likely within the AV node.

faster than is the ventricular rate, whereas in AV dissociation the ventricular rate is faster than is the atrial rate. Although AV dissociation is present in complete heart block, it is not synonymous. AV dissociation is usually a manifestation of another rhythm abnormality such as complete heart block, sinus bradycardia, or VT. Treatment is usually directed toward the underlying cause.

Clinical Presentation

Symptoms in patients with AV conduction abnormalities are generally caused by bradycardia and loss of AV synchrony. Patients with significantly prolonged P-R intervals may behave in a similar fashion to patients with pacemaker syndrome because of loss of AV synchrony. In patients with structural heart disease and LV dysfunction, this may result in worsening of heart failure. Symptoms caused by more advanced AV block may range from exercise intolerance, easy fatigability, dyspnea on exertion, dizzy spells, and near syncope to frank syncope. In patients with paroxysmal or intermittent complete heart block, these symptoms are episodic, and routine ECGs may not be diagnostic. Children and adolescents with isolated complete heart block may be generally asymptomatic, whereas some may develop symptoms later as adults because of chronotropic incompetence. Other late signs and symptoms include the development of congestive heart failure and nonsustained VT. Children with complete heart block associated with structural heart disease are symptomatic very early on and have an increased risk for sudden death.[45]

Diagnostic Evaluation

The prognosis and treatment of AV block depends on its association with symptoms and the level of AV block. Routine 12-lead surface ECGs adequately establish the diagnosis of varying degrees of AV block in many patients. Analyzing the P-R interval, QRS duration, Wenckebach phenomenon, and ventricular rates on the surface ECG provides important clues to the level of AV block. In certain situations such as 2:1 AV block, additional maneuvers may be necessary to establish the level of AV block. Responses to carotid sinus massage, atropine, and exercise are often very helpful.

In patients with complete heart block at the level of the AV node, the resultant junctional escape rhythm usually accelerates with exercise in contrast to the ventricular escape rhythm with infranodal block, which usually remains unchanged.

In patients with paroxysmal symptoms of near syncope or syncope and no significant conduction abnormalities on the surface ECG, prolonged electrocardiographic monitoring with 24- to 48-hour Holter recordings or 30-day event monitors may be helpful. An implantable loop recorder may be necessary to establish the diagnosis, particularly in patients with infrequent symptoms. Electrophysiology study is indicated in patients with syncope or near syncope in whom high-grade AV block is suspected as the cause. In patients with structural heart disease, in addition to AV conduction disease, VT can also be a major etiology for syncope; and electrophysiology study can be very useful in establishing the diagnosis.

Management

Identifying transient or reversible causes for AV conduction disturbances is the first step in management. Withdrawal of any offending drugs, correction of any electrolyte abnormalities, or treatment of any infectious processes should be considered prior to permanent pacing therapy. If the drugs causing AV block are essential for treatment of other medical conditions, permanent pacing may be considered. In patients with advanced AV block and hemodynamic decompensation unresponsive to drug therapy such as atropine or isoprenaline, as in digitalis toxicity, hyperkalemia, acute anterior MI, or Lyme myocarditis, temporary pacing should be instituted until AV block resolves or permanent pacing can be initiated. Temporary pacing can be accomplished by transcutaneous pacing systems in those patients at low to moderate risk for developing complete heart block or in patients with complete heart block and hemodynamically stable escape rhythms. Transcutaneous pacing for prolonged periods is very uncomfortable and transvenous pacing should be performed in patients with need for continuous active pacing.

Permanent pacemaker implantation is indicated in most patients with advanced heart block associated with symptoms. Permanent pacemakers are also indicated in asymptomatic patients with complete heart block and infra-Hisian second-degree AV block. Permanent pacing has clearly been shown to decrease mortality in patients with advanced heart block and syncope.[46] The indications for pacing in children with AV block and in adults with acquired heart block are described in Table 40–9 and Table 40–10, respectively (see also Chap. 11).

Most patients with AV block require dual-chamber pacemakers, because this mode of pacing maintains AV synchrony and prevents development of pacemaker syndrome. In patients with associated sinus node dysfunction, dual-chamber pacemakers with rate-responsive function (DDDR) are the preferred mode of choice. In patients with normal sinus node function and AV block, VDD pacing using a single lead with a series of electrodes for atrial sensing and ventricular pacing and sensing is an ideal mode of pacing, because it provides AV synchrony and rate-responsiveness and is superior to single-chamber VVI pacing. In patients with chronic atrial fibrillation and bradycardia, rate-responsive single-chamber ventricular pacing (VVIR) is adequate. Early studies of comparison of pacing modes in a small number of patients with AV block had shown that physiologic pacing (DDD or VDD) enhanced survival compared to VVI pacing.[47,48] However, prospective, randomized, large-scale trials showed that dual-chamber pacing provided little benefit over ventricular pacing for the prevention of death (see Table 40–4).[27] The incidence of pacemaker syndrome was as high as 26 percent in patients with ventricular pacing necessitating crossover to dual-chamber pacing in the Pacemaker Selection in the Elderly trial.[49]

Bundle-Branch Block

Conduction disturbances that occur at various levels of the branches of the His-Purkinje system are described as bundle-branch block or intraventricular conduction defects (IVCDs). In patients with isolated chronic right or left bundle-branch block, the progression to advanced AV block is rare. Patients with bifascicular block (right bundle-branch block and left anterior or posterior fascicular block) or left bundle-branch block and left axis deviation have a 6 percent annual incidence of progression to complete heart block.[50,51] In patients with acute MI, the development of new

bifascicular block and first-degree AV block is associated with a very high risk (40 percent) for progression to high-grade AV block. These patients are generally recommended to undergo prophylactic temporary pacing.[40] Alternating bundle-branch block, even in asymptomatic patients, is a sign of advanced conduction distur-

---

TABLE 40–10

Indications for Pacing in Acquired Atrioventricular Block in Adults

Class I

1. Third-degree and advanced second-degree atrioventricular (AV) block at any anatomic level, associated with any one of the following conditions:
   a. Bradycardia with symptoms (including heart failure) presumed to be caused by AV block *(Level of evidence: C)*.
   b. Arrhythmias and other medical conditions requiring drugs that result in symptomatic bradycardia *(Level of evidence: C)*.
   c. Documented periods of asystole ≥3.0 sec or any escape rate <40 beats/min in awake, symptom free patients *(Levels of evidence: B,C)*.
   d. After catheter ablation of the AV junction *(Levels of evidence: B,C)*. There are no trials to assess outcome without pacing, and pacing is virtually always planned in this situation unless the operative procedure is AV junction modification.
   e. Postoperative AV block that is not expected to resolve after cardiac surgery *(Level of evidence: C)*.
   f. Neuromuscular diseases with AV block, such as myotonic muscular dystrophy, Kearns-Sayre syndrome, Erb dystrophy, and peroneal muscular atrophy, with or without symptoms, because there may be unpredictable progression of AV conduction disease *(Level of evidence: B)*.
2. Second-degree AV block regardless of type or site of block, with associated symptomatic bradycardia *(Level of evidence: B)*.

Class IIa

1. Asymptomatic third-degree AV block at any anatomic site with average awake ventricular rates of 40 beats/min or faster especially if cardiomegaly or left ventricular dysfunction is present *(Levels of evidence: B,C)*.
2. Asymptomatic type II second-degree AV block with a narrow QRS. When type II second-degree AV block occurs with a wide QRS, pacing becomes a class I recommendation *(Level of evidence: B)*.
3. Asymptomatic type I second-degree AV block at intra- or infra-His levels found at electrophysiology study performed for other indications *(Level of evidence: B)*.
4. First- or second-degree AV block with symptoms similar to those of pacemaker syndrome *(Level of evidence: B)*.

Class IIb

1. Marked first-degree AV block (>0.30 sec) in patients with LV dysfunction and symptoms of congestive heart failure in whom a shorter AV interval results in hemodynamic improvement, presumably by decreasing left atrial filling pressure *(Level of evidence: C)*.
2. Neuromuscular diseases such as myotonic muscular dystrophy, Kearns-Sayre syndrome, Erb dystrophy, and peroneal muscular atrophy with any degree of AV block (including first-degree AV block) with or without symptoms, because there may be unpredictable progression of AV conduction disease *(Level of evidence: B)*.

Class III

1. Asymptomatic first-degree AV block *(Level of evidence: B)*.
2. Asymptomatic type I second-degree AV block at the AV nodal level or not known to be intra- or infra-Hisian *(Levels of evidence: B,C)*.
3. AV block expected to resolve and/or unlikely to recur (e.g., drug toxicity, Lyme disease, or during hypoxia in sleep apnea syndrome in absence of symptoms) *(Level of evidence: B)*.

bance in the His-Purkinje system and is considered a class I indication for permanent pacing. In patients with bundle-branch block, His-bundle recordings can occasionally be helpful in identifying patients at high risk for progression to high-grade AV block. The incidental findings of markedly prolonged H-V interval ($\geq$100 msec) or atrial-pacing-induced infra-Hisian block[52] that is not physiologic during an electrophysiology study are considered to indicate high risk for progression to advanced AV block, and prophylactic permanent pacing is recommended (Table 40–11). Intraventricular conduction disturbances are usually associated with significant structural heart disease, especially dilated (ischemic or idiopathic) cardiomyopathies, and are a marker of poor prognosis both in terms of advanced heart failure and increased mortality in these patients (discussed later in this chapter).

PACEMAKERS

The science of cardiac pacing is only approximately 50 years old and has seen tremendous growth and evolution. Since the introduction of transvenous pacing in 1958,[26] the field of cardiac pacing has benefited greatly from advances made in electronics, computer technology, power sources, and miniaturization. The rapid growth in pacemaker design and functions has made the understanding of these devices more complex and difficult. As the po-

TABLE 40–11

Indications for Pacing in Chronic Bifascicular and Trifascicular Block

Class I
1. Intermittent third-degree atrioventricular (AV) block *(Level of evidence: B)*.
2. Type II second-degree AV block *(Level of evidence: B)*.
3. Alternating bundle-branch block *(Level of evidence: C)*.

Class IIa
1. Syncope not demonstrated to be caused by to AV block when other likely causes have been excluded, specifically ventricular tachycardia *(Level of evidence: B)*.
2. Incidental finding at electrophysiology study of markedly prolonged HV interval (greater than or equal to 100 ms) in asymptomatic patients *(Level of evidence: B)*.
3. Incidental finding at electrophysiology study of pacing induced infra-His block that is not physiologic *(Level of evidence: B)*.

Class IIb
1. Neuromuscular diseases such as myotonic muscular dystrophy, Kearns-Sayre syndrome, Erb dystrophy, and peroneal muscular atrophy with any degree of fascicular block with or without symptoms, because there may be unpredictable progression of AV conduction disease *(Level of evidence: C)*.

Class III
1. Fascicular block without AV block or symptoms *(Level of evidence: B)*.
2. Fascicular block with first-degree AV block without symptoms.

tential indications for pacing had expanded, prospective, randomized trials to assess the efficacy of these devices have become an integral part of the discipline.

PACEMAKER SYSTEM

A permanent pacemaker system consists of an implanted pulse generator and the leads through which it delivers electrical stimuli in the various chambers of the heart. The pacemaker is composed of the pulse generator, housing the complex electronic circuitry and the battery, the power source. The pulse generator contains an output circuit, sensing circuit, timing circuit, and telemetry coil that sends and receives programing instructions and diagnostic information. Most current devices also have another circuit for the rate-adaptive sensor. Modern pacemakers almost exclusively use lithium-iodine batteries as their power source. The advantages of the lithium-iodine battery is that it has a high-energy density, long shelf life, low battery life loss caused by internal self-discharge, and predictable characteristics that allow early warning of battery depletion. Most single-chamber pacemakers have an expected battery longevity of 7 to 12 years, whereas dual-chamber pacemakers have an expected longevity of 6 to 10 years. Most pacemakers generate 2.8 V at the beginning of life. When the voltage nears the end of life (2.1 to 2.4 V), several elective replacement indicators in the pacemaker are activated. The common indicators of elective replacement of the pacemaker are as follows:

- Percent or fixed decrease in pacing rate on magnet application or free running rate
- Increase in pulse-width duration
- Change to a simpler pacing mode (DDDR to VVI; VVIR to VOO)
- Reduced battery voltage
- Elevated battery impedance
- Restricted programmability

Once the elective replacement indicators are activated, the pacemaker is generally replaced within weeks to months, earlier if the patient is pacemaker dependent. When the battery reaches the end of life (EOL, <2.1 V), the pacemaker changes to the simplest mode (VOO), fails to communicate or reprogram, fails to pace or sense, and may function erratically. If the pacemaker reaches end of life, it should be replaced immediately.

Pacemaker Leads

Permanent pacing leads have five major components: (1) electrodes, (2) conductors, (3) insulation, (4) connector pin, and (5) fixation mechanism. The pacing leads may be unipolar or bipolar. Although most of the leads used are bipolar in configuration, it is essential to understand both lead systems. In unipolar leads, only a single electrode is present at the lead tip (cathode) in contact with the myocardial tissue and the surface of the pacemaker-can acts as the anodal terminal. Bipolar lead systems have a cathodal tip electrode and an anodal ring electrode, 10 to 20 mm proximal to the tip electrode. Unipolar leads have a simple structural design and excellent durability but may infrequently exhibit skeletal myopotential oversensing, far-field sensing, crosstalk (atrial stimulus sensed by ventricular channel), and skeletal muscle stimulation. Many newer pacemakers with bipolar leads allow a change in configuration of the pacing/sensing function to unipolar or bipolar, as the situation warrants. Contemporary electrodes have a small tip surface area with a porous or roughened surface and steroid-eluting capability that reduces stimulation thresholds, decreases current drain, and improves sensing. The electrodes are connected to the connecter pin at the proximal end of the leads by the conductor wires that are usually made of Elgiloy (alloy of nickel). The materials used for insulation of the pacing leads are of silicone rubber and polyurethane varieties. Polyurethane insulation has the advantage of having high tear strength, low friction, and smaller diameter and is relatively nonthrombogenic compared to silicone-insulated leads.

The most commonly used transvenous endocardial leads have either a passive or an active fixation mechanism to avoid early dislodgement. The passive fixation mechanisms include tines, fins, or wings that are entrapped within the trabeculae of the right sided heart chambers and are subsequently covered by fibrous tissue. Most contemporary active fixation leads use an extendable/retractable or exposed screw mechanism. The active fixation leads allow precise positioning of the pacing lead in locations other than the right atrial appendage or RV apex. They reduce the acute dislodgement rates of the right atrial leads and are also easier to extract compared to the passive fixation leads.

Pacemaker Implantation

Almost all pacemaker implantations are performed transvenously under local anesthesia and conscious sedation using the cephalic, subclavian, or axillary veins. Axillary vein access avoids the potential complication of compression damage to the leads inserted via medial subclavian puncture in the tight costoclavicular angle. The pulse generator is usually placed in the upper pectoral region subcutaneously, and occasionally the pacemaker is implanted behind the pectoral muscle or behind the breast via an inframammary approach, especially in young women.

Pacing Site The atrial lead is generally placed in the right atrial appendage; however, in patients with prior cardiac surgery, the atrial septum or the lateral wall is preferred. It is preferable to avoid the atrial free-wall with active fixation leads, because this has the potential to cause delayed, serious pericardial effusion and/or cardiac tamponade.[53] Atrial septal pacing and Bachmann bundle pacing[54] have been tested in an attempt to reduce the frequency of episodes of atrial fibrillation. Similarly, dual-site atrial pacing with one atrial lead placed in the atrial appendage and a second atrial lead placed around the coronary sinus ostium has been shown to have a variable effect on the frequency of episodes of paroxysmal atrial fibrillation.[55] The ventricular lead is typically placed in the RV apex. However, attempts to maintain the normal sequence of ventricular activation by high septal pacing near the His-bundle and the RV outflow tract, especially in patients with cardiomyopathies, have suggested hemodynamic benefits by improving cardiac output compared to RV apical pacing.[56] A randomized crossover trial of patients with congestive heart failure, LV dysfunction (ejection fraction [EF] <40 percent), and chronic atrial fibrillation pacing from right ventricular outflow tract (RVOT) or dual-site RV pacing (RVOT + RV apex) did not consistently improve quality of life or other clinical outcomes compared with RV apical pac-

ing.[57] Deshmukh and colleagues[58] as well as Occhetta and coworkers[59] have demonstrated that direct His-bundle pacing is a viable approach for permanent cardiac pacing in patients with dilated cardiomyopathy and atrial fibrillation and preserves LV function compared to RV apical pacing.

With the advent of biventricular pacing for hemodynamic improvement in patients with advanced heart failure and intraventricular conduction disturbances, more patients will receive biventricular pacing systems. The LV lead is placed in the posterior or lateral vein of the left ventricle through the coronary sinus. Epicardial pacing via thoracotomy must be considered in occasional patients with inadequate venous access, phrenic nerve stimulation, or mechanical prosthetic tricuspid valve; undergoing cardiac surgery; with right to left shunting; and who have failed transvenous LV lead placement.

Pacing Threshold and Sensing Atrial and ventricular leads are placed into the appropriate chambers and sutured in place after ensuring adequate pacing and sensing thresholds. The basic premise in obtaining acute pacing and sensing thresholds during implant is that these thresholds may degenerate over time, and adequate safety margins must be maintained to ensure safe long-term pacing and sensing. It is essential to understand the strength-duration curve (Fig. 40–9). The strength-duration curve for stimulation is the quantity of voltage required to stimulate the heart at a series of pulse widths. As shown in the figure, increasing the pulse width beyond 0.6 msec usually does not decrease the voltage threshold. At implant, an atrial pacing threshold of <1.5 V and ventricular threshold of <1 V should be obtained. The threshold commonly increases over the next 2 to 4 weeks, reaches a peak, and then decreases to a chronic threshold level after 6 to 8 weeks. With steroid-eluting leads, the acute rise in threshold is ameliorated and the chronic threshold is significantly lower than in nonsteroid-eluting leads.[60] During initial programing, the pacing output is programed at 3 to 5 times the threshold voltage with a pulse width of 0.4 to 0.5 msec. At the 2- to 3-month follow-up visit, the output is decreased to no less than twice the threshold to maintain an adequate safety margin and prevent battery drain. Some newer pacemakers have algorithms that enable the device to confirm capture.[61] These algorithms may determine pacing threshold at programed time intervals or on a beat-by-beat basis. Using algorithms to automatically check pacing-capture thresholds, these pacers adjust pacing voltages to just above the pacing threshold to reduce current drain and prolong battery longevity.

Sensing is usually measured as the peak-to-peak or base-to-peak amplitude of the intracardiac electrogram in millivolts. The ventricular electrograms should measure at least 5 mV and frequently measure in excess of 10 to 20 mV. Ventricular sensitivity (the level in millivolts that the intracardiac electrogram must exceed to be sensed by the device) is generally programed between 2 to 3 mV so that an adequate safety margin exists for sensing intrinsic ventricular depolarization without the risk of oversensing T waves or other artifacts. Atrial electrograms are smaller in amplitude than ventricular electrograms; however, a minimum atrial electrogram of 1 to 2 mV should be obtained. In patients with paroxysmal atrial fibrillation or flutter, the atrial electrogram during tachycardia might be smaller than during sinus rhythm. The atrial sensitivity is usually programed at 0.5 mV; however, the sensitivity may have to be adjusted depending on the size of the far-field ventricular electro-

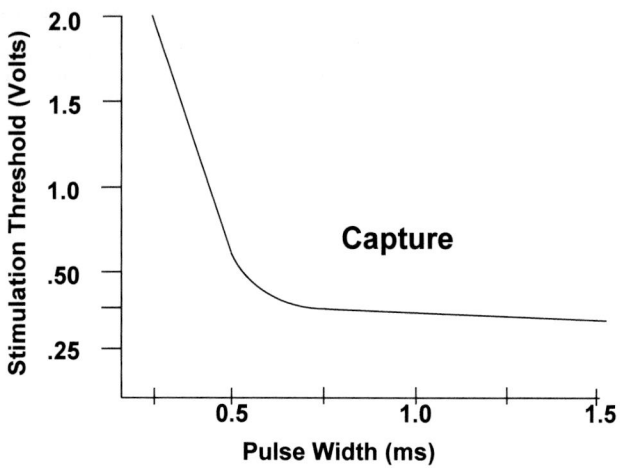

FIGURE 40–9. Strength-duration curve. This curve is obtained by plotting the voltage threshold obtained at various pulse widths. When programing the pacemaker output, this curve should be considered to ensure at least two times the safety margin. Increasing the pulse width beyond 0.6 msec generally does not decrease the voltage threshold.

gram and associated atrial arrhythmias. Newer pacemakers also incorporate algorithms that automatically adjust sensitivity to the size of the atrial or ventricular signal.

Impedance Lead impedance is the resistance to the flow of current from the generator to the myocardial tissue through the lead. Although there is a wide variability of normal lead impedances (250–1200 Ω), chronic lead impedances should not vary widely between outpatient follow-up visits. A fractured lead exhibits markedly elevated lead impedance. Insulation breaks manifest by reduced lead impedances. Lead fractures or insulation breaks often are intermittent problems. Therefore, normal lead impedances and pacing and sensing thresholds do not rule out these problems. The leads can be stressed by having the patient change position and do various provocative arm movements (e.g., isometric exercise) to facilitate diagnosis of lead-related problems that are not otherwise observed. Many pacemakers intermittently monitor lead impedance and alert the physician to measured impedances that are out of the typical range.

Pacemaker Nomenclature

The North American Society of Pacing and Electrophysiology (NASPE) and the British Pacing and Electrophysiology Group

(BPEG) have established a five-letter pacemaker code to describe the basic pacemaker mode and function (Table 40–12).[62] The first letter represents the chamber being paced: *A* for atrium, *V* for ventricle, and *D* for both atrium and ventricle. The second letter refers to the chamber in which sensing occurs: Codes are similar to those for the first position. The third position describes the response of the pacemaker to a sensed event: *I* for inhibition, *T* for triggered, and *D* for both inhibition and triggering. The pacemaker can either inhibit (I) pacing output from one or both of its leads, or it can trigger (T) pacing after the sensed event. In a DDD pacemaker, a sensed atrial event inhibits the atrial pacing channel and triggers ventricular pacing after a programmable AV delay. The fourth position refers to the programmability of the device: *R* for rate-responsive pacing; the letters *C* (communicating), *P* (simple programmable), and *M* (multiprogrammable) are obsolete because all current devices are fully programmable. The fifth position refers to antitachycardia function; with the evolution of implantable defibrillators, this position is rarely used. With the evolution of biventricular pacemakers, the pacemaker code currently in practice needs to be revised.

【 】 PACING MODES
VVI Mode

As the pacemaker code indicates, the ventricle is the chamber sensed and paced, with inhibition of ventricular pacing in response to a sensed ventricular event. A sensed or paced ventricular event initiates two timing cycles:

1. A refractory period that is programmable (ventricular refractory period) during which period no ventricular sensing occurs to prevent inappropriate sensing of T waves. Any ventricular event occurring during this interval will also not reset the timing cycle.
2. A lower-rate interval (LRI), which corresponds to the programed pacing rate. If there is no sensed ventricular event following the end of the ventricular refractory period and this interval expires, the pacemaker initiates a paced ventricular event. If a ventricular event is sensed following the ventricular refractory period (VRP), the pacemaker resets the timing cycle to begin a new LRI and VRP (Fig. 40–10).

VVI pacing is the most commonly used pacing mode. Although it is a simple pacing mode and offers protection against brad-

TABLE 40–12

The Pacemaker Code

I	II	III	IV	V
CHAMBER-PACED	CHAMBER-SENSED	RESPONSE TO SENSING	PROGRAMMABILITY/ RATE RESPONSE	ANTITACHYCARDIA FUNCTION(S)
O (None)	O (None)	O (None)	O (None)	O (None)
A (Atrium)	A (Atrium)	I (Inhibit)	R (Rate responsive)	P (Antitachycardia pacing)
V (Ventricle)	V (Ventricle)	T (Triggered)	P (Simple programmable)	S (Shock)
D (Dual)	D (Dual)	D (I + T)	M (Multiprogrammable)	D (P + S)
S (Single chamber)	S (Single chamber)		C (Communicating)	

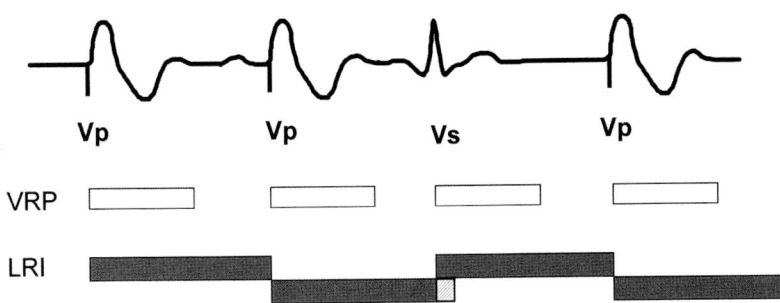

FIGURE 40–10. Single-chamber ventricular inhibited pacing mode. The first two beats are ventricular-paced (Vp) events. The third beat is a ventricular-sensed (Vs) event. A Vs or Vp event starts a lower-rate interval (LRI) at the end of which ventricular pacing is initiated. A sensed- or paced event also initiates a ventricular refractory period (VRP) during which no sensing will occur. The LRI following a sensed event can be separately programed at a longer interval to allow for native rhythm. This is called *hysteresis*.

yarrhythmias, loss of AV synchrony is not well tolerated in many patients and may lead to pacemaker syndrome (discussed later in the chapter). In patients with chronic atrial fibrillation, this is an ideal pacing mode, especially if rate-responsiveness is available.

AAI Mode

Similar to VVI mode, sensing and pacing occurs in the atrium, with the atrial pacing channel inhibited in response to a sensed atrial activity. An atrial refractory period (ARP) and a lower-rate interval (LRI) are initiated in response to a sensed or paced atrial event. AAIR pacing with rate-responsiveness is an excellent pacing mode in patients with sinus node dysfunction and normal AV conduction. Patients with sinus node dysfunction may develop AV block, which may be a source of concern when using AAI pacing. However, with careful selection of patients, including normal P-R intervals, absence of bundle-branch block, and AV Wenckebach phenomenon occurring at atrial pacing rates of more than 120 beats/min, the risk of development of second- or third-degree AV block is <0.6 percent per year.[63]

VOO/AOO Modes

In these asynchronous pacing modes, there is no sensing. The chamber is paced asynchronously at the lower-rate limit. The timing cycle consists of only an LRI and will not be reset by any intrinsic activity. Because there is no sensing, there are no refractory periods. This mode is rarely used except during procedures using constant electrocautery to avoid inhibition of pacing caused by sensing of the high-frequency impulses of electrocautery. When a magnet is applied over the pulse generator, the pacemaker switches to an asynchronous mode (VVI to VOO, DDD to DOO). The obvious disadvantage of this pacing mode is the possibility of asynchronous pacing during the vulnerable period and initiation of either atrial or ventricular fibrillation (extremely rare).

VDD Mode

In this mode the pacemaker paces only the ventricle, senses in both the atrium and the ventricle, and responds to atrial sensing with ventricular pacing. The ventricular channel is also inhibited by spontaneous ventricular activity. A sensed atrial event will start an atrioventricular interval (AVI) followed by ventricular pacing. If spontaneous AV conduction occurs before the termination of

the AVI, ventricular pacing is inhibited. If there is no spontaneous atrial activity, ventricular pacing occurs at the lower-rate limit as in a VVI pacemaker. However, because there is no atrial pacing, this mode should not be used in patients with sinus node dysfunction. In patients with normal sinus node function and AV block, this is an excellent mode choice.

DDD Mode

A DDD pacemaker senses and paces in both the atrium and the ventricle, and the response to sensing involves both inhibition and triggered output. The DDD pacemaker uses numerous timing cycles, and it is essential to understand the following intervals. Most modern pacemaker timing cycles are ventricular based (with some modifications) and are explained as such.

The LRI starts with a sensed or paced ventricular event and ends with a paced ventricular event, and consists of two portions. The ventricular event initiates an atrial escape interval (AEI) or VA interval at the end of which atrial pacing is initiated. The atrial paced or sensed event initiates the AVI at the end of which ventricular pacing is initiated. So, LRI = VA interval + AVI. A sensed atrial event occurring before the completion of the VA interval terminates this interval and starts the AVI. A sensed ventricular event occurring before the completion of the AVI will terminate this interval and the LRI and reinitiate the LRI. A sensed or paced ventricular event will also initiate the ventricular refractory period (VRP) to avoid T-wave oversensing and simultaneously initiates the postventricular atrial refractory period (PVARP). The PVARP helps prevent the sensing and tracking of any retrograde P waves. This refractory period is programmable and is essential to the prevention of pacemaker mediated, endless-loop tachycardia, which is an arrhythmia where the dual chamber pacemaker serves as the antegrade limb and the patient's retrograde conduction as the retrograde limb. The AV interval and the PVARP together constitute the total atrial refractory period (TARP) during which period the atrial channel remains refractory and will not be tracked. This in essence determines the upper rate interval (URI) or the maximal tracking rate interval (MTRI) in a DDD pacemaker.

In patients with DDD pacemakers, four different rhythm scenarios are possible, and many patients exhibit more than one scenario:

1. Normal sinus rhythm with no atrial or ventricular pacing: Here the patient's rate is faster than the programed lower rate of the pacemaker, and the native P-R interval is shorter than the programed AV interval as a result of which both the atrial and ventricular channels are inhibited (Fig. 40–11A).
2. Atrial sensed, ventricular pacing: The patient's atrial rate is faster than the lower-rate limit; and the AV conduction interval is longer than the programed AV interval, or there is no AV conduction resulting in sensing of P waves and triggering of the ventricular channel after the programed AV interval. In this situation the patient is ventricularly paced at the patient's sinus rate until the upper rate limit (Fig. 40–11B).
3. Atrial paced and ventricular sensed: In this situation the patient's atrial rate is slower than the programed lower rate and the patient's AV conduction interval shorter than the programed AV interval. Here the patient is atrially paced at the lower-rate limit (Fig. 40–11C).

4. Atrial and ventricular pacing: Here the sinus rate is slower than the lower-rate limit, and AV conduction is longer or absent resulting in atrial and ventricular pacing at the lower-rate limit (Fig. 40–11D).

ATRIOVENTRICULAR INTERVAL

The AV interval following a sensed atrial event is usually programed to a shorter value than the AV interval following a paced atrial event and is termed *differential AV interval.* Some DDD pacemakers also have the added capability of shortening the AV interval with increase in heart rates and is called *dynamic,* or *rate-adaptive, AV interval.* Another available feature increasingly incorporated into modern pacemakers is AV hysteresis or Search AV+ in which the device periodically increases the AV interval to allow native AV conduction and intrinsic ventricular activation.

The paced AV interval is considered as a single interval with two subportions. The initial interval is the blanking period (12 to 50 msec, programmable) during which the ventricular channel is blanked to avoid ventricular sensing of the atrial pacing artifact. If a spontaneous ventricular event occurs in this period it will not be sensed. The second portion of the AV interval is the crosstalk-sensing window during which a ventricular event is sensed if it occurs and leads to ventricular safety pacing with a shorter AV interval of 100 to 110 msec. This is to avoid *cross talk* or inhibition of the ventricular channel by sensing of the atrial pacing artifact (Fig. 40–12).

UPPER RATE BEHAVIOR

In VDD and DDD modes, in addition to the programed lower-rate limit, there is an upper rate limit beyond which ventricular tracking of atrial events will not occur. When the atrial rate exceeds the programed upper rate limit the pacemaker will exhibit either Wenckebach or 2:1 AV block behavior. When the patient with complete heart block exercises to a sinus rate beyond the upper rate limit of the pacemaker, the P wave that is sensed is followed by ventricular pacing with prolongation of the AV interval beyond the programed value, to avoid violating the upper rate limit for pacing. When one subsequent P wave falls in the postventricular atrial refractory period, it will not be tracked re-

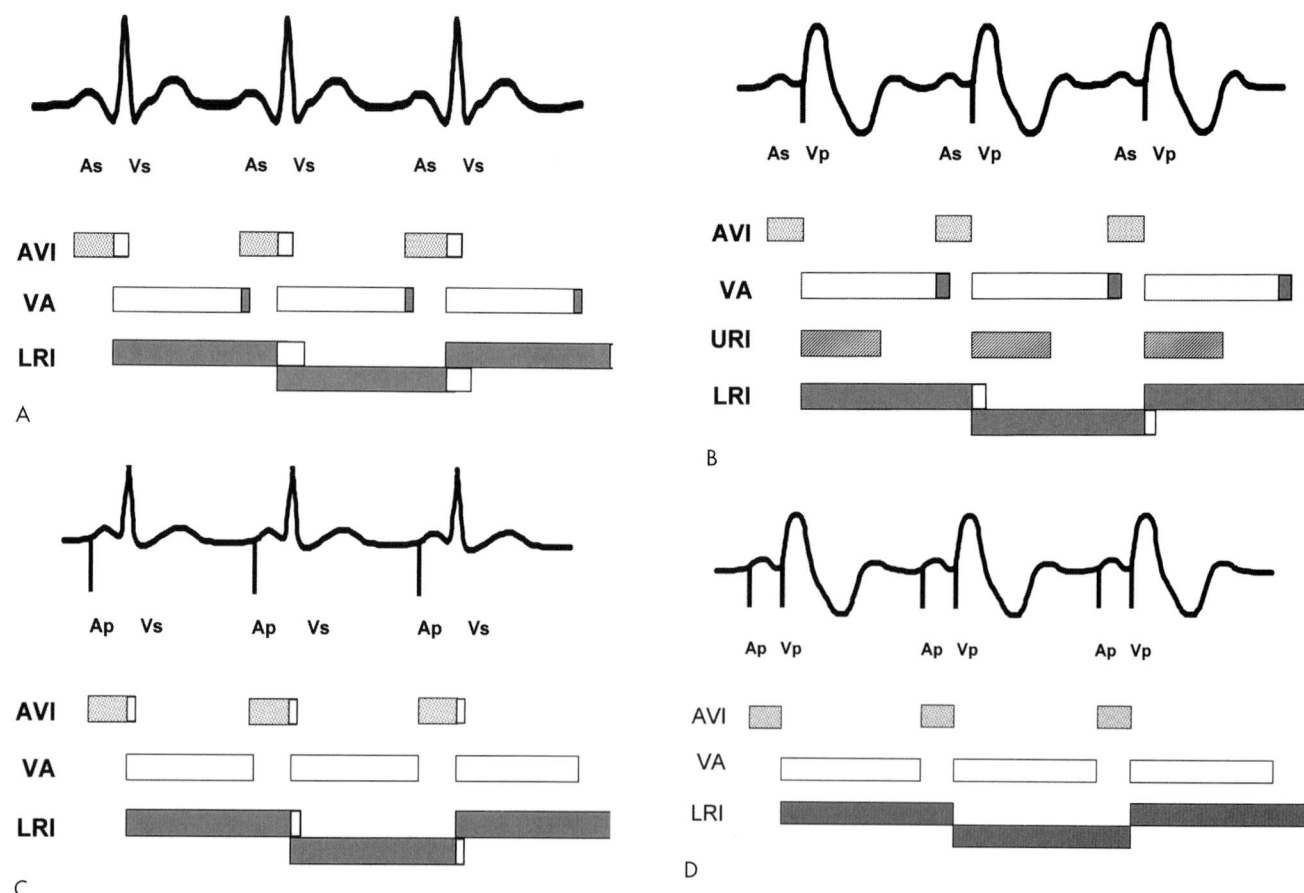

FIGURE 40–11. A. DDD pacing mode: atrial- and ventricular-sensed. In this example, atrial-sensed activity (As) initiates an atrioventricular interval (AVI) and normal conduction results in a ventricular-sensed (Vs) event that terminates the AV interval and the lower-rate interval (LRI) and initiates an LRI and the atrial escape interval (VA). Spontaneous atrial activity (As) again terminates the VA interval and starts a new AV interval. **B.** DDD pacing mode: As ventricular pacing. In this example the As event leads to Vp at the completion of the programed AVI, because there is no native AV conduction to the ventricle. The Vp event starts the VA interval, the LRI, and the upper-rate interval (URI). The VA and the LRIs are terminated by the spontaneous atrial activity that starts a new AV interval. **C.** DDD pacing mode: atrial-paced–ventricular-sensed. In this example Ap starts the AVI but is terminated by the ventricular event that occurs prior to the completion of the AV interval. The Vs event initiates the VA and the LRI. If there is no spontaneous atrial activity, the VA interval times out and Ap occurs. **D.** DDD pacing mode: atrial- and ventricular-paced. The Ap event starts the AVI, at the completion of which the ventricle is paced because there is no spontaneous ventricular activity. The Vp event initiates the VA interval and results in atrial pacing as there is no spontaneous atrial activity. Both Ap and Vp occur at the LRI.

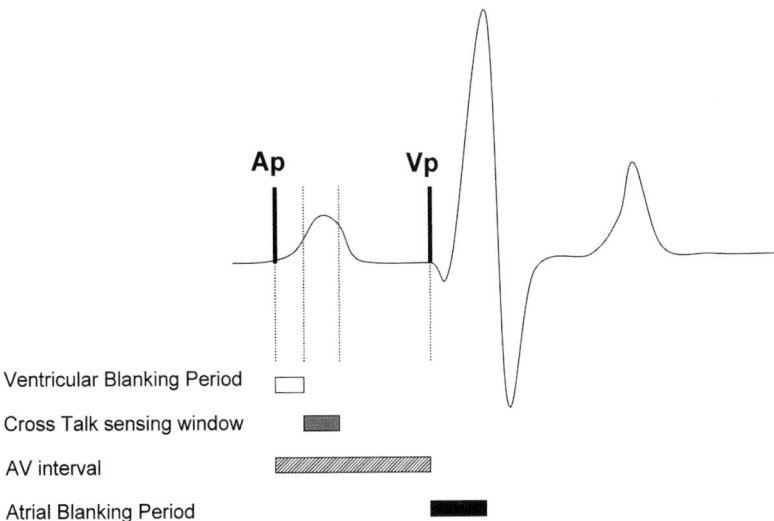

FIGURE 40–12. Atrioventricular (AV) interval and blanking periods. The AV interval following atrial pacing has two subportions. During the initial ventricular blanking period, sensing is suspended to avoid ventricular sensing of the leading edge of the atrial pacing artifact. During the second portion (crosstalk sensing window), if ventricular activity is sensed, ventricular pacing occurs with a shorter AV delay. The purpose of this safety feature (ventricular safety pacing) is to avoid inhibition of the ventricular channel by sensing of the atrial pacing artifact during this time window. Similar to the ventricular blanking period, there is an atrial blanking period following ventricular pacing, during which sensing is suspended in the atrial channel to avoid atrial oversensing of the far-field ventricular pacing artifact. Ap, atrial paced; Vp, ventricular paced.

sulting in *pacemaker* Wenckebach behavior (Fig. 40–13). When the atrial rate increases further such that every other P wave falls in the total atrial refractory period (TARP), 2:1 pacemaker AV block pattern occurs. The TARP should be programed shorter than the upper rate interval to prevent sudden development of 2:1 pacemaker AV block.

In young patients with complete heart block, the upper rate of the pacemaker should be programed to faster rates corrected for the patient's age to prevent Wenckebach behavior of the pacemaker during exercise. Programing dynamic AV interval and dynamic PVARP allows the TARP to be shorter at higher pacing rates and avoid sudden slowing of ventricular pacing rates. Another option is rate-responsive features where a separately programmable sensor rate allows the pacemaker to continue to pace at the sensor-driven rate during exercise.

【 】 MODE SWITCH

When pacemaker patients with AV block (in DDD or VDD mode) develop atrial tachyarrhythmias (atrial tachycardia, flutter, or fibrillation), many atrial events are sensed and ventricular tracking occurs up to the programed upper rate of the device. The surface ECG typically shows an irregular ventricular paced rhythm at rates close to the upper rate limit of the device. Occasionally in patients with slower atrial flutter, every other atrial electrogram may fall in the PVARP resulting in 2:1 AV block. In patients with intact conduction, the ventricular rates are determined by the patient's intrinsic AV conduction.

In patients with persistent atrial tachyarrhythmias, reprograming the pacemaker to DDI(R) or VVI(R) mode avoids rapid ventricular tracking of the atrial arrhythmias. Automatic mode switching is a programmable option in all current generation pacemakers for patients with paroxysmal atrial tachyarrhythmias (Fig. 40–14). When the atrial rate exceeds the programed mode switch rate, the device automatically changes its mode to either the VVI or DDI, in which ventricular tracking of atrial-sensed events do not occur. Current devices can also provide a complete history of mode-switch episodes with regard to the duration and frequency of these episodes and may also provide electrograms to confirm their nature. During followup of these devices, it is important to monitor for these mode-switch episodes and confirm by reviewing the electrograms that they truly represent atrial tachyarrhythmias. Arrhythmia logs from the device provide a very efficient way of assessing the effects of various drug therapies in patients with atrial fibrillation.

Managed Ventricular Pacing

It is now well accepted that long-term RV pacing causes a deterioration of LV function through complex effects on regional ventricular wall strain and loading conditions. Newer pacemakers employ different AV interval algorithms to search for intrinsic conduction and avoid unnecessary ventricular pacing. Electrocardiograms obtained during such pacemaker behavior may cause concern for the interpreting physicians unaware of these pacemaker functions. Unlike traditional mode switch from DDD to VVI or DDI mode during atrial tachyarrhythmias, newer pacemakers can switch pacing mode from AAI(R) to DDD(R) in the Managed Ventricular Pacing (MVP) mode or the AAIsafeR2 mode. The MVP mode provides functional AAI(R) pacing with the safety of dual chamber ventricular support

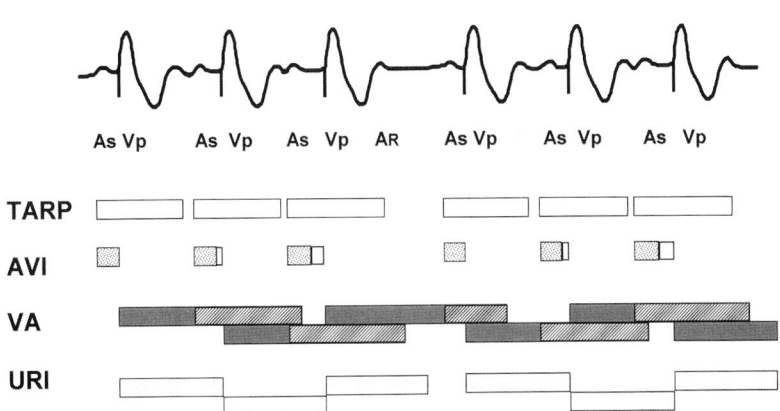

FIGURE 40–13. DDD pacemaker: Wenckebach behavior at upper rate limit. The first beat shows the ventricular paced (Vp) event synchronized to the atrial-sensed (As) event at the programed AV interval (AVI). The next atrial event initiates an AVI; but when the AVI times out, the upper rate limit has not been satisfied so the AVI is prolonged. When the upper rate limit is satisfied, ventricular pacing occurs. Because of the delayed ventricular pacing, the next P wave falls even earlier into the next cardiac cycle and the AVI extension is even greater. The next P wave falls within the total atrial refractory period (TARP) and is not sensed. This atrial event (AR) is not followed by ventricular pacing. The following P wave occurs before the VA interval expires and tracking occurs at the programed AV delay since the upper rate limit cannot be exceeded. URI, upper rate interval.

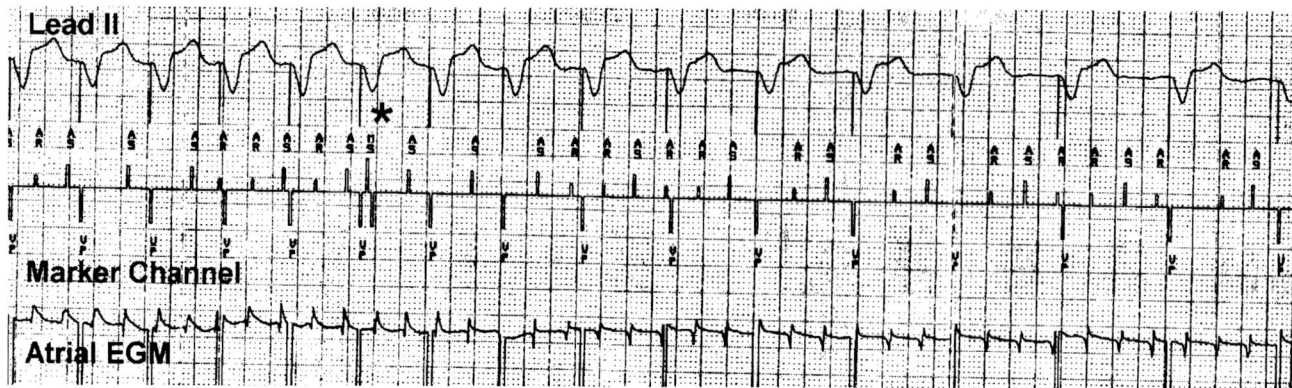

FIGURE 40–14. Mode switch behavior of DDD pacemaker during atrial flutter. Surface lead II, marker channel, and atrial electrograms (EGMs) are shown. In the beginning of the tracing, atrial flutter is sensed and the ventricle is paced at, but does not exceed, the upper rate limit of 110 beats/min. Once atrial tachyarrhythmia detection criteria are met, mode switch occurs (*). Pacemaker switches mode to DDI (no atrial tracking) at 70 beats/min with rate-smoothing function to avoid an abrupt change in pacing rate.

in the presence of transient or persistent loss of conduction (Fig. 40–15A and Fig. 40–15B). The criterion to switch to backup ventricular pacing is loss of AV conduction for two out of the last four pacing cycles (the four most recent A-A intervals). This allows fast switch to DDD(R) mode but does not cause false switching on a single nonconducted atrial event.

RATE-RESPONSIVE PACING

Rate-responsive pacing refers to the ability of the pacemaker to increase its lower rate in response to physiologic stimuli. Simple VVI and AAI pacemakers do not have the ability to increase their pacing rates in response to exercise. In patients with normal sinus node function and DDD pacemakers, the ventricular pacing rate increases in response to an increase in sinus rate and is physiologic. However, in the presence of sinus node dysfunction, the pacing rate does not increase commensurate with the increase in physiologic need. Rate-responsive pacemakers provide the ability to increase pacing rates through special sensors incorporated in the pacing system that monitor various physiologic processes. Based on information from the sensors, the lower rate of the pacemakers constantly varies up to the upper sensor rate. At any point in time, the sensor rate overrides the programed lower rate of the pacemaker. Rate-responsive pacing is available in most current pacemakers in VVIR, AAIR, DDIR, and DDDR modes. In patients with sinus node dysfunction, rate-responsive pacing in AAIR, DDIR, or DDDR mode is preferable to nonsensor-driven pacing. Also, in patients with chronic atrial fibrillation and heart block, VVIR pacing is preferable to VVI pacing. In patients with severe coronary artery disease, it may be necessary to limit the programed upper rate limit. The ideal mode for pacing is decided based on information regarding sinus node function, AV nodal function, atrial arrhythmias, and heart rate response to exercise (Fig. 40–16).

Rate-Responsive Sensors

An ideal rate-responsive pacing system should provide rate response appropriate for the metabolic demand during a wide range of activities. The optimal sensor should provide the following:

• Proportionate increase in heart rate to match increase in metabolic demand
• Appropriate rapid change in heart rate with exercise onset

• High sensitivity and specificity
• Appropriate slowing of heart rate following exercise

Sensors available or under development can be classified using a physiologic or technical classification system. In physiologic classification[64] the sensors are classified according to the physiologic level at which they sense (Table 40–13).

Activity Sensors Activity-based sensors using piezoelectric crystals or accelerometers to detect vibration are the most widely used sensors. While the piezoelectric crystal senses vibration associated with up-and-down motion, the accelerometer detects anteroposterior motion of the body. Accelerometer-based sensors provide adequate and quick increases in heart rate during treadmill exercise as compared to that of piezoelectric crystals. Although both sensors have been shown to provide excellent rate-responsiveness, direct manual pressure, walking down stairs, horseback riding, or riding on a bumpy street can cause an inappropriate increase in heart rate with the piezoelectric crystal-based sensor. These activity-based sensors do not provide adequate heart rate response with emotional stress or isometric exercises.

Minute-Ventilation Sensor The specificity and sensitivity of minute-ventilation sensing pacemakers for changes in metabolic workload are excellent. Current pulses are emitted from the pacemaker can, and the proximal ring electrode of the RV lead (or right atrial lead) and transthoracic impedances are measured. Measurement of phasic impedance changes provides respiratory rate and tidal volume information, thus determining the minute ventilation. The minute ventilation changes are used to calculate the pacing rate and have excellent correlation with exercise. Minute-ventilation sensing pacemakers can inappropriately increase pacing rates with hyperventilation, coughing, and mechanical ventilation and in patients with chronic obstructive pulmonary disease exacerbations.

Dual Sensors Most of the currently available sensors have an excellent track record, but they may occasionally respond to nonphysiologic stimuli. A multisensor rate-responsive pacemaker can improve specificity by having one sensor verify the other sensor (e.g., sensor crosschecking). A combination of two sensors can

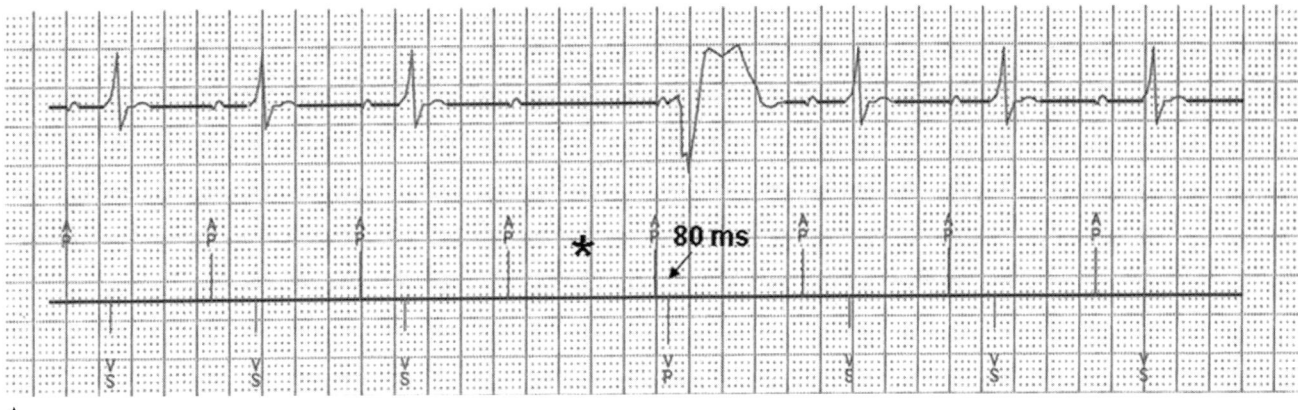

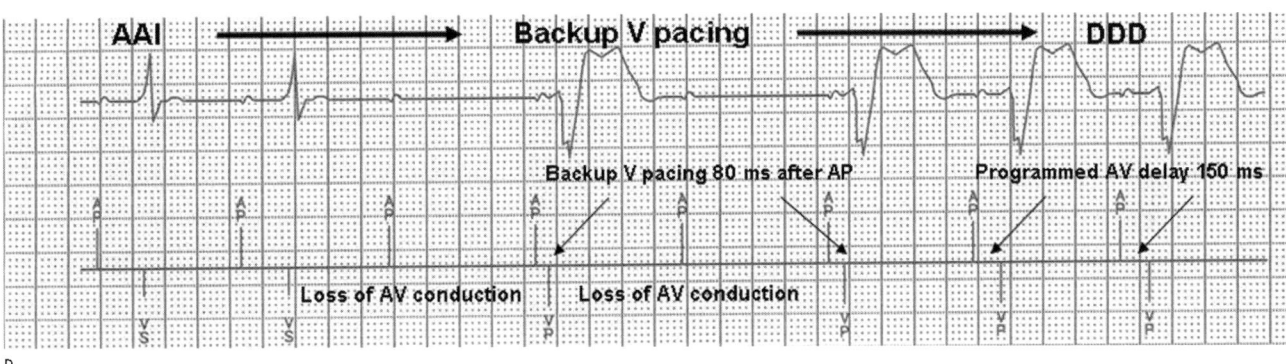

FIGURE 40-15. Managed Ventricular Pacing (MVP). **A.** Primarily, MVP mode looks like AAI(R) mode, *except* that it allows for prolonged AV interval. It is an atrial-based pacing (Ap) mode that looks for any consecutive A-A intervals without associated ventricular events. For occasional, single, nonconducted normal atrial contractions, the device provides backup ventricular pacing to ensure ventricular support. The backup ventricular pace (Vp) is scheduled to occur after any A-A interval in which there is no Vp event (*). The Vp occurs 80 msec after the scheduled Ap (if pacing is occurring in the chamber), *or* after the inhibited atrial pace (i.e., 80 msec after the escape A-A interval). **B.** MVP switches from AAI(R) operation to DDD(R) operation when there is evidence of persistent loss of AV conduction. The criterion to switch is loss of AV conduction for 2 out of the last 4 pacing cycles (the four most recent A-A intervals). The strip illustration shows that immediately after the first A-A interval with no conducted ventricular sensed event (Vs), a backup Vp is delivered 80 msec after the scheduled Ap. Then a second A-A interval occurs with no conducted Vs event. Again, the backup Vp is delivered followed by a permanent switch to DDD(R) operation where in the AV delay is the programed paced (or sensed) AV delay of 150 msec. AV, atrioventricular.

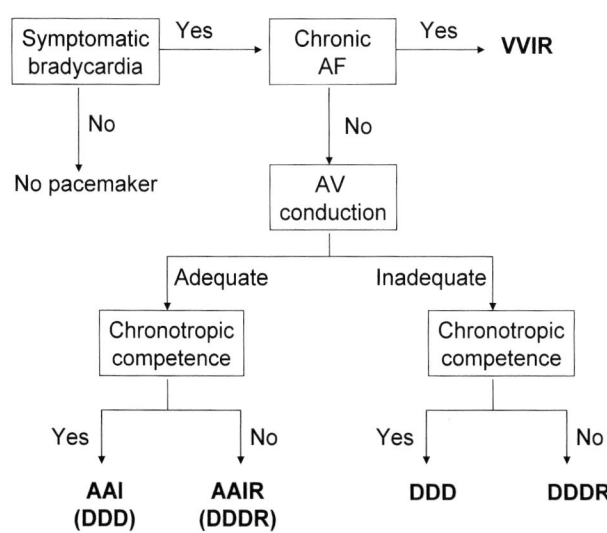

FIGURE 40-16. Pacemaker mode selection. AF, atrial fibrillation; AV, atrioventricular.

TABLE 40-13

Physiologic Classification of Sensors

TYPE	DESCRIPTION	PHYSIOLOGIC PARAMETERS
Primary	Physiologic factors that modulate sinus function	Catecholamine level Autonomic nervous system activity
Secondary	Physiologic parameters that are the consequence of exercise	QT,[a] respiratory rate[a] Minute ventilation,[a] temperature[a] pH, stroke volume Preejection interval, Sv_{O_2} Peak endocardial acceleration
Tertiary	External changes that result from exercise	Vibration[a] Acceleration[a]

[a]Available clinically.

better simulate the normal sinus node response. Both sensors must indicate a need for rate response to allow an increase in sensor-driven heart rate. Some sensor systems provide the advantage of more physiologic pacing during steady state but have a slow response time during initiation of exercise. Other sensors, particularly activity sensors, have faster response times at initiation of activity but may not produce physiologic responses during peak or steady-state activity. Pacemakers with dual sensors can provide patients with rapid responses during the start of exercise and then use a more physiologic sensor (minute ventilation) to provide more proportional heart rate responses during steady state (e.g., sensor blending).[65]

[ ] INDICATIONS FOR PACING

The guidelines of the ACC and the AHA and the North American Society of Pacing and Electrophysiology for the implantation of pacemakers were revised and updated in 2002. The indications for permanent pacing can be considered in categories of bradyarrhythmia and nonbradyarrhythmia. The bradyarrhythmic indications were discussed in the earlier part of this chapter.

Pacing to Prevent or Terminate Tachyarrhythmias

Pacing can help prevent and terminate tachyarrhythmias. The long QT syndrome is characterized by abnormally prolonged ventricular repolarization with the tendency to develop pause-dependent ventricular arrhythmias (torsade de pointes), syncope, and sudden death. In patients with long QT syndrome, recurrent pause-dependent VT may be prevented by continuous pacing; and pacing, in addition to β blockade, has been shown to shorten QT interval and prevent sudden death in high-risk patients.[66]

Reentrant supraventricular arrhythmias such as AV node reentrant tachycardia, AV reentrant tachycardia, and atrial flutter may be terminated by a variety of pacing methods that include programed stimulation and short bursts of rapid overdrive pacing.[67] These antitachycardia pacemakers must detect a tachyarrhythmia and then spontaneously initiate an antitachycardia pacing algorithm, or they can be programed to respond to external magnet application. With significant advances with catheter ablation, the need for pacemakers to treat supraventricular arrhythmias has virtually vanished.

Further trials are ongoing to determine the best pacing algorithms and atrial lead locations to prevent or terminate atrial fibrillation.[68] The indications for pacemaker therapy to prevent or treat tachyarrhythmias are shown in Table 40–14.

Pacing in Dilated Cardiomyopathy

Permanent dual-chamber pacing with a short AV delay and a conventional pacemaker (ventricular lead in the RV apex) was initially proposed a decade ago as adjuvant treatment of advanced heart failure.[69] However, initially encouraging results were not confirmed in several subsequent, small randomized, prospective studies.[70–72] Bakker and colleagues first suggested a clinical benefit from biventricular pacing in heart failure patients with intraventricular conduction disorder.[73] Thereafter, biventricular pacing has been studied in a number of acute and short-term studies followed by many prospective, randomized trials,[74–76] the results of which

---

(**TABLE 40–14**

Indications for Pacing to Prevent or Terminate Tachycardias

Class I
1. Sustained pause-dependent ventricular tachycardia, with or without prolonged QT, in which the efficacy of pacing is thoroughly documented (Level of evidence: C).

Class IIa
1. High-risk patients with congenital long-QT syndrome (Level of evidence: C).
2. Symptomatic recurrent supraventricular tachycardia that is reproducibly terminated by pacing in the unlikely event that catheter ablation and/or drugs fail to control the arrhythmia or produce intolerable side effects (Level of evidence: C).

Class IIb
1. Recurrent SVT or atrial flutter that is reproducibly terminated by pacing as an alternative to drug therapy or ablation (Level of evidence: C).
2. AV reentrant or AV node-reentrant supraventricular tachycardia not responsive to medical or ablative therapy (Level of evidence: C).
3. Prevention of symptomatic, drug refractory recurrent atrial fibrillation in patients with coexisting sinus node dysfunction (Level of evidence: B).

Class III
1. Tachycardias frequently accelerated or converted to fibrillation by pacing.
2. The presence of accessory pathways with the capacity for rapid anterograde conduction whether or not the pathways participate in the mechanism of the tachycardia.
3. Frequent or complex ventricular ectopic activity without sustained VT in the absence of the long QT syndrome.
4. Torsade de pointes VT due to reversible causes.

AV, atrioventricular; SVT, supraventricular tachycardia; VT, ventricular tachycardia.

---

are summarized in Table 40–15. Approximately 30 percent of the patients with chronic heart failure manifest intraventricular conduction disorder with QRS intervals longer than 130 msec.[87] Intraventricular conduction disturbances of the left bundle-branch block–type lead to delay in the activation of LV free wall as compared to the septum and right ventricle resulting in intra- and interventricular mechanical dyssynchrony. Ventricular dyssynchrony is associated with paradoxical septal motion, decreased diastolic filling times, prolonged mitral regurgitation, and reduced LV stroke volume. Biventricular pacing by simultaneous pacing of the right and left ventricle has been shown to coordinate the septal and the LV free-wall contraction and decrease right and left atrial filling pressures and mitral regurgitation, as well as improve diastolic filling, cardiac output, and left ventricular ejection fraction (LVEF) in patients with severe LV systolic dysfunction and prolonged IVCD.[88] Biventricular pacing also has been shown to reduce myocardial oxygen consumption with improvement in ventricular contraction.[89–91]

TABLE 40–15

Trials of Biventricular Pacing for Heart Failure

STUDY	INCLUSION CRITERIA	DESIGN	ENDPOINTS	RESULTS
PATH–CHF[74]	NYHA class II–IV QRS >120 ms Sinus rate >55 beats/min	Longitudinal study with second placebo control phase. First and third periods are crossovers between BiV and LV pacing ($n = 42$)	Primary: Peak VO$_2$, Peak VO$_2$ at anaerobic threshold, 6-min walk; secondary: QOL, hospitalization, NYHA class	CRT improved functional capacity, QOL and functional status
InSync[75]	NYHA class III–IV, LVEF <35% QRS >150 ms, LVEDD >60 mm pacing indication allowed	Prospective longitudinal trial ($n = 103$)	Primary: 6-min walk, ORS width; secondary: QOL, NYHA class	CRT improved functional class, QOL and 6-min walk
MUSTIC SR[92]	NYHA class III, LVEF <35% LVEDD >60 mm, QRS >150 ms 6-min walk <450 m, NSR	Prospective, randomized, single-blind crossover study ($n = 67$)	Primary: 6-min walk, QOL, NYHA class; secondary: hospitalization, peak VO$_2$	Improved 6-min walk, QOL, peak VO$_2$ and reduced hospitalizations. patients preferred biventricular pacing
MUSTIC AF[76]	NYHA class III, LVEF <35% LVEDD >60 mm, QRS >150 ms 6-min walk <450 m, AF	Prospective, randomized, single-blind crossover study ($n = 64$)	Primary: 6-min walk, QOL, NYHA class; secondary: hospitalization, peak VO$_2$	Improved 6-min walk, QOL, peak VO$_2$ and reduced hospitalizations; patients preferred biventricular pacing
MIRACLE[94]	NYHA class III, LVEF <35% LVEDD >55 mm, QRS >130 ms Stable 3-mo regimen of BB and ACEI	Prospective, randomized, double-blind, parallel, controlled trial for 6 months ($n = 300$)	Primary: 6-min walk, QOL, NYHA class, device and lead safety; secondary: Neurohormone levels, echo indices, peak VO$_2$	Improved NYHA class, 6-min walk, QOL, LVEF, ventricular volumes and mitral regurgitation
InSync III[90]	NYHA class IIIIV, LVEDD >55 mm, LVEF <35%, QRS >130 ms	Prospective, nonrandomized trial to evaluate safety and efficacy of InSync III device, OTW lead, and programmable RV-LV timing	Safety and efficacy of InSync III device and OTW lead performance QOL, functional capacity	Device and lead safety confirmed. QOL, functional capacity and 6-min walk improved compared to historic control from MIRACLE
VENTAK CHF/ CONTAK CD[96]	NYHA class II–IV, LVEF <35% QRS >120 ms, ICD indication Normal sinus node	6-month parallel, double-blind trial between CRT and no CRT, beginning 1 mo after implant ($n = 581$)	Primary: Effectiveness and safety of ICD + CRT Secondary: NYHA class, QOL, 6-min walk, peak VO$_2$	Device safety confirmed; peak VO$_2$ improved; Class III and IV patients without RBBB showed QOL improvement
InSync ICD[95]	NYHA class II–IV, LVEF <35% LVEDD >55 mm, QRS >130 ms ICD indication	Prospective, longitudinal trial to evaluate safety and efficacy of CRT in CHF patients with ICD indication ($n = 84$)	Primary: 6-min walk, effectiveness and safety of ICD + CRT; Secondary: NYHA class, QOL	CRT – ICD safe to use; Improvement in endpoints for NYHA class III and IV only

(continued)

TABLE 40–15

Trials of Biventricular Pacing for Heart Failure *(continued)*

STUDY	INCLUSION CRITERIA	DESIGN	ENDPOINTS	RESULTS
COMPANION[78]	NYHA class III–IV, EF <35% QRS >120 ms, P-R >150 ms, no indication for pacer or ICD	Randomized, open-label, 3-arm study of optimal drug therapy, CRT and CRT-ICD (n = 2200)	Combined all cause mortality and hospitalization, QOL, functional capacity, peak exercise performance	Terminated early after 1520 patients, with 40% reduction in mortality with CRT-ICD; significant reduction in hospitalization in CRT and CRT-ICD groups
CARE–HF[80]	NYHA class III–IV, EF <35%, QRS >120 ms, no conventional indications for pacer or ICD, no AF	Randomized, open-label, study of optimal drug therapy vs. CRT	Primary: Composite of death from any cause and unplanned hospitalization for major cardiac event Secondary: Death from any cause, QOL, NYHA class	Primary: 55% vs. 39% (HR 0.63) Secondary: Mortality 30% vs. 20%; Improved NYHA class and QOL

ACEI, angiotensin-converting enzyme inhibitor; AF, atrial fibrillation; BB, β blocker; BiV, biventricular; CARE-HF, Cardiac Resynchronization Heart Failure; CHF, congestive heart failure; COMPANION, Comparison of Medical Therapy Pacing and Defibrillation in Heart Failure; CRT, cardiac resynchronization therapy; EF, ejection fraction; HF, heart failure; ICD, implantable cardioverter defibrillator; LV, left ventricle; LVEDD, left ventricle end diastolic diameter; MIRACLE, Muticenter InSync Randomized Clinical Evaluation; MUSTIC AF, Mutisite Stimulation in Cardiomyopathy Atrial Fibrillation; MUSTIC SR, Multisite Stimulation in Cardiomyopathy Sinus Rhythm; NYHA, New York Heart Association; NSR, normal sinus rhythm; OTW, over the wire; PATH-CHF, Pacing Therapies in Congestive Heart Failure; QOL, quality of life; RV, right ventricular; RBBB, right bundle-branch block; VO_2, oxygen uptake.

Clinical Trials The Multisite Stimulation in Cardiomyopathy (MUSTIC) trial was the first randomized, prospective study of biventricular pacing (see Table 40–15).[92] There was a significant improvement in the 6-minute walk distance, quality of life, and reduction in hospitalizations in the pacing group as compared to the non-pacing group. Biventricular pacing was the preferred pacing mode in >80 percent of patients. In a long-term open-label follow up of these patients, significant clinical benefits were maintained at 24 months.[93] The Multicenter InSync Randomized Clinical Evaluation (MIRACLE) study was a prospective, randomized, placebo-controlled, double-blind trial of patients with class III to IV heart failure, LVEF of 35 percent or less, and QRS duration of 130 msec or longer.[94] Patients who received biventricular pacing experienced significant improvement in the 6-minute distance walked (+39 min vs. +10 min, $p = 0.005$), functional class, quality of life, and EF (+4.6 vs. 0.2 percent, $p < 0.001$). Both trials showed significant clinical improvement in patients with biventricular pacing despite maximal medical therapy for congestive heart failure with β blockers, diuretics, digoxin, and angiotensin-converting enzyme inhibitors.

Meta-analysis pooling data from 4 studies showed that cardiac resynchronization therapy (CRT) reduced death from progressive heart failure by 51 percent compared to control (odds ratio, 0.49; 95 percent CI, 0.25 to 0.93), and reduced heart failure hospitalization by 29 percent (odds ratio, 0.71; CI, 0.53 to 0.96). CRT was not associated with a statistically significant effect on nonheart failure mortality or a reduction in the number of patients experiencing VT or ventricular fibrillation.[95] Preliminary experience with a biventricular pacemaker in combination with an implantable cardioverter defibrillator (ICD) has been published.[77,96] The early termination of the COMPANION (Comparison of Medical, Resynchronization, and Defibrillation Therapies in Heart Failure) trial has answered the question regarding the mortality benefit of ICD therapy combined with biventricular pacing in this patient group.[78] The trial was terminated prematurely after enrolling almost 1600 patients, because initial results demonstrated that combined biventricular pacemaker–ICDs reduced mortality by 40 percent (19–11 percent) compared to optimal medical therapy, whereas biventricular pacemakers alone showed only a 15-percent reduction in mortality. CARE-HF (Cardiac Resynchronization Heart Failure) trial[80] enrolled 813 patients with severe New York Heart Association (NYHA) class III to IV heart failure, reduced LVEF of <35 percent, cardiac dyssynchrony with QRS duration >120 msec, and randomized to optimal medical therapy versus biventricular pacing and followed for a mean of 29.4 months. The primary endpoint of composite of death from any cause and unplanned hospitalization for a major cardiac event was reached in 55 percent of medical therapy group compared to 39 percent in the biventricular pacing group. All-cause mortality was 30 percent in the medical therapy group compared to 20 percent in the biventricular pacing group. This is the first study to demonstrate a mortality benefit from the biventricular pacemaker alone.

Biventricular Pacemaker System In addition to the usual right atrial and RV lead, the biventricular pacing system uses an additional lead to pace the left ventricle. Most leads have been specifically designed with a lumen to allow for passage of the lead over a guidewire into the coronary venous system and further manipulated through the vein branches until an adequate site with acceptable pacing and sensing thresholds is located on the LV epicardium. Acute data indicate that optimal hemodynamic response in most patients is obtained if the LV lead is placed in a posterolateral, lateral, or anterolateral vein to provide resynchronization therapy.[74] Fig. 40–17 demonstrates an occlusive venogram of the

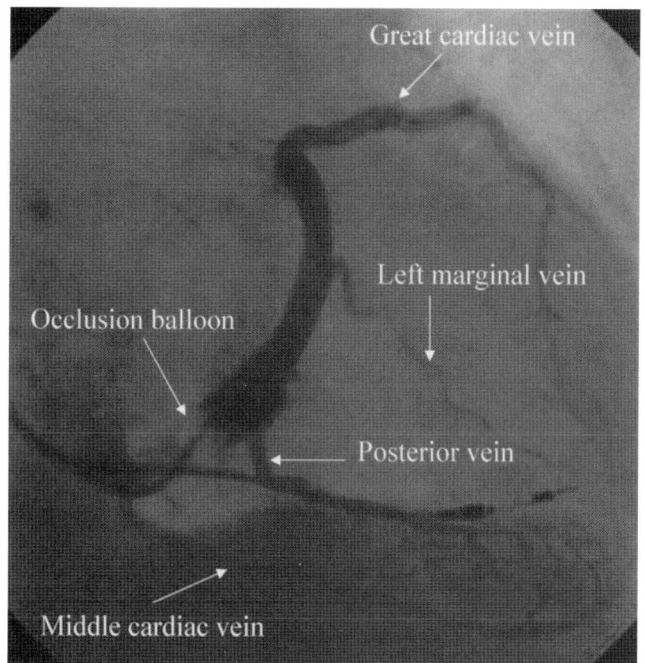

FIGURE 40–17. Right anterior oblique view of an occlusive venogram of the great cardiac vein and the other branch veins of the coronary sinus (left marginal vein, left posterior vein, and the middle cardiac vein).

coronary sinus, showing great cardiac vein and branch vein anatomy. Chest radiographs in posteroanterior and lateral views of a patient with a biventricular pacemaker is shown in Fig. 40–18. Fig. 40–19 demonstrates the ECGs of this patient in sinus rhythm with left bundle-branch block and with biventricular stimulation, respectively. The hallmark of LV capture is a R/S ratio ≥1 in lead V1 or R/S ratio ≤1 in lead I. The sensitivity of these findings to correctly identify loss of LV capture is 94 percent.[97] The preferred pacing mode is VDD, in which both ventricles are paced simultaneously following sensed atrial activity with a short AV interval. The InSync III trial suggested a possible increased hemodynamic benefit with sequential biventricular pacing by varying the interventricular activation sequence compared to simultaneous biventricular pacing.[90] For this therapy to be effective, the patients must maintain ventricular pacing (>90 percent ventricular pacing). Biventricular pacing has also been shown to improve functional status and heart failure symptoms in patients with chronic atrial fibrillation and AV-node ablation.[76,91] The current indications for pacing in patients with dilated cardiomyopathy are shown in Table 40–16.

Pacing in Hypertrophic Cardiomyopathy

Dynamic LV outflow tract obstruction is present in approximately 25 percent of patients with hypertrophic cardiomyopathy. Symptoms such as dyspnea, angina, palpitations, and syncope may coexist in patients with LV outflow obstruction. Although the severity of symptoms does not correlate well with the severity of obstruction, reduction or elimination of the outflow gradient seems to correlate with clinical improvement. RV apical pacing results in preexcitation of the interventricular septum and reverses the ventricular activation sequence leading to an increase in the outflow tract diameter and reduction of the outflow gradient. Although gradient reduction may reduce effective cardiac workload, abnormal ventricular activation from pacing may cause impaired relaxation and may be more detrimental in patients with preexisting diastolic abnormalities.

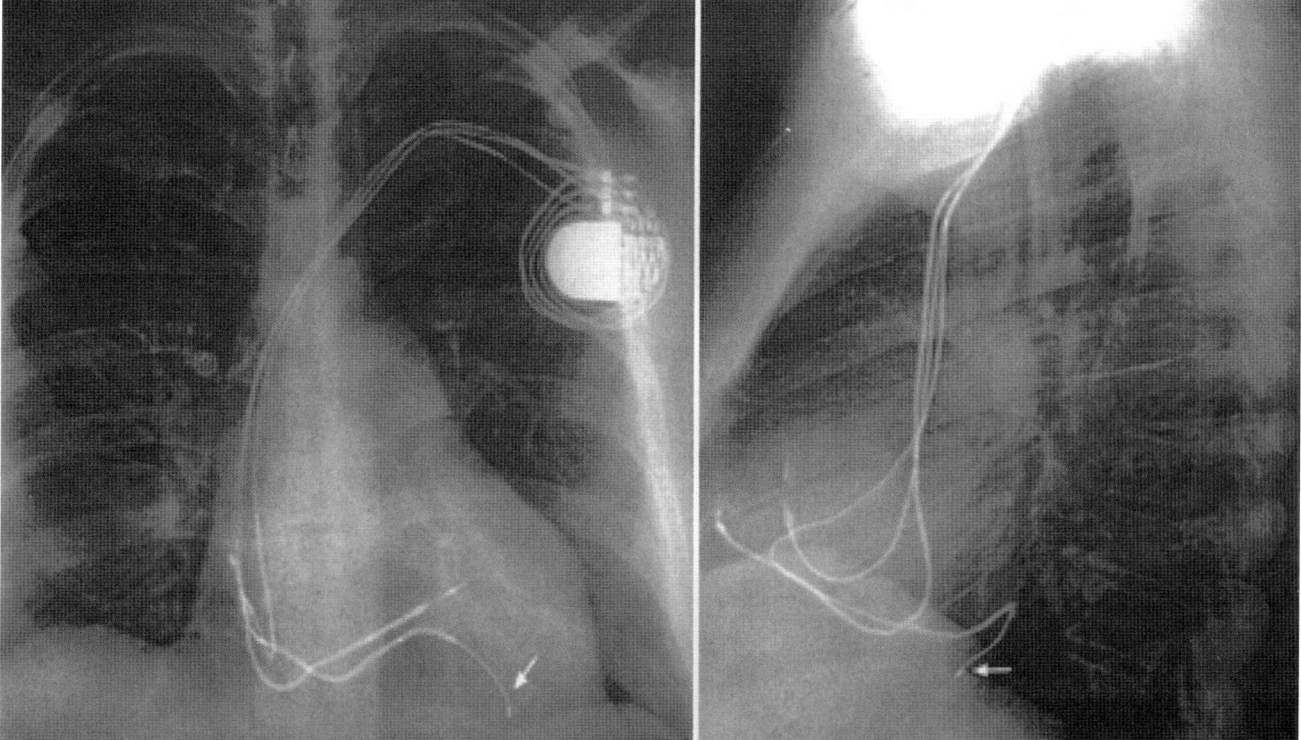

FIGURE 40–18. Posteroanterior and lateral chest radiographs demonstrating the right atrial, right ventricular, and the left ventricular (LV) leads in a patient with a biventricular pacemaker. The LV lead (*arrow*) is placed in the posterolateral vein branch of the coronary sinus allowing for simultaneous activation of the septum and the LV free wall.

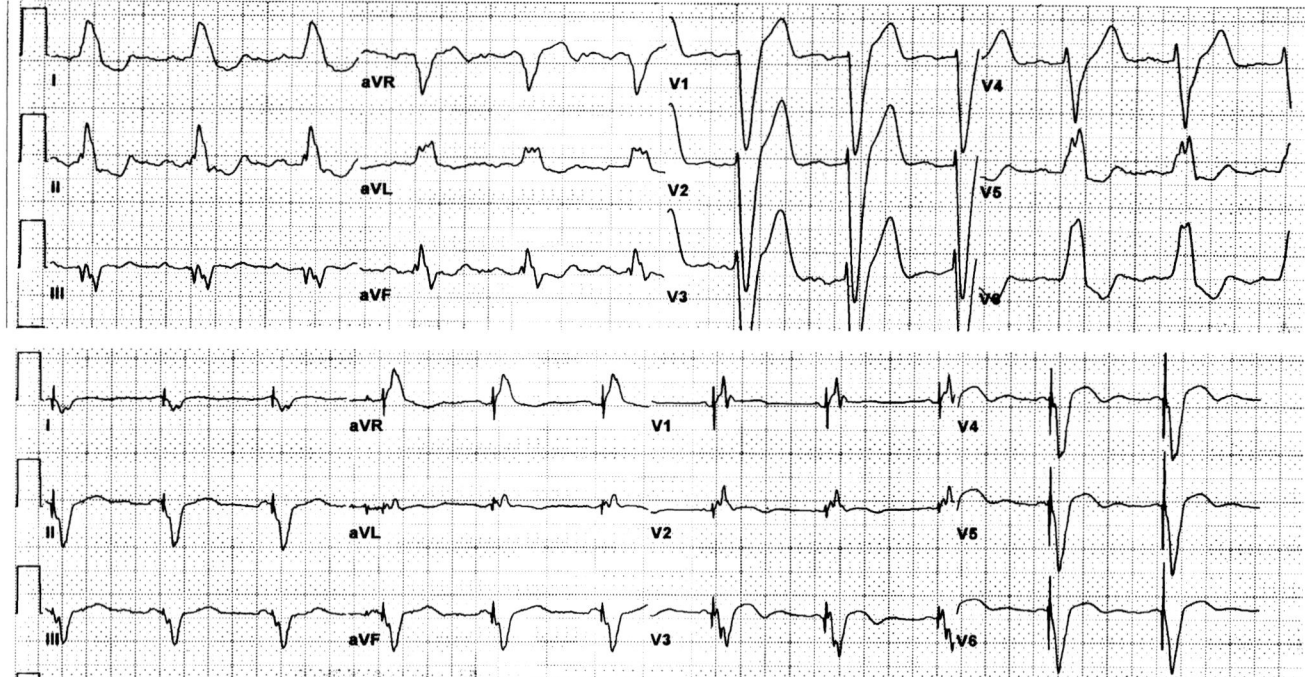

FIGURE 40–19. Electrocardiogram of biventricular pacing. Normal sinus rhythm with left bundle-branch block and QRS width of 200 msec (*top*). Atrial-sensed biventricular stimulation; note how the paced QRS complex has narrowed significantly from the baseline (*bottom*).

Hassenstein and Wolter reported in 1967 that RV pacing resulted in significant reduction of the LV outflow gradient in patients with hypertrophic cardiomyopathy.[98] Subsequent to this and a few other reports, many small and large observational studies suggested reduction of the outflow tract gradient, modest improvement in exercise tolerance, and favorable changes in the degree of angina, syncope, and functional class following dual-chamber pacemaker implantation.[99] Subsequent placebo-controlled, blinded, randomized studies have shown only modest benefit with pacemaker therapy. For example, the Pacing in Hy-

pertrophic Cardiomyopathy (PIC) trial examined 83 patients with hypertrophic cardiomyopathy and randomized to DDD pacing or AAI pacing for 12 weeks and then crossed over. DDD pacing was associated with 51-percent reduction in the LV outflow gradient and 63 percent improvement in functional class. DDD pacing, however, did not improve exercise tolerance. At the end of 6 months, 76 patients preferred the active DDD pacing mode.[100] Dual-chamber pacing is considered only for patients who are not surgical candidates or who cannot tolerate or fail medical therapy (Table 40–17).

PACEMAKER COMPLICATIONS

Patients undergoing a new pacemaker system implantation are generally monitored in the hospital for a day in anticipation of any

TABLE 40–16

Indications for Pacing in Dilated Cardiomyopathy

Class I
1. Class I indications for sinus node dysfunction or atrioventricular (AV) block as previously described *(Level of evidence: C)*.

Class IIa
1. Biventricular pacing in medically refractory, symptomatic New York Heart Association class III or IV patients with idiopathic dilated or ischemic cardiomyopathy, prolonged QRS interval (≥130 ms), LV end-diastolic diameter ≥55 mm and ejection fraction ≥35% *(Level of evidence: A)*.

Class III
1. Asymptomatic dilated cardiomyopathy.
2. Symptomatic dilated cardiomyopathy when patients are rendered asymptomatic by drug therapy.
3. Symptomatic ischemic cardiomyopathy when the ischemia is amenable to intervention.

LV, left ventricular.

TABLE 40–17

Indications for Pacing in Hypertrophic Obstructive Cardiomyopathy

Class I
1. Class I indications for sinus node dysfunction or AV block as previously described *(Level of evidence: C)*.

Class IIb
1. Medically refractory, symptomatic hypertrophic cardiomyopathy with significant resting or provoked left ventricular outflow tract obstruction *(Level of evidence: A)*.

Class III
1. Patients who are asymptomatic or medically controlled.
2. Symptomatic patients without evidence of left ventricular outflow tract obstruction (see Chap. 11).

AV, atrioventricular.

untoward complications. The various complications associated with pacemakers are outlined in Table 40–18.

Pneumothorax

At the time of implantation, subclavian or axillary venous access can rarely result in pneumothorax, hemothorax, or hemopneumothorax. This can occur from inadvertent puncture and laceration of the subclavian vein or the subclavian artery or the lung. The use of venograms to locate the venous system in difficult cases and the routine use of axillary venous access have reduced these complications significantly. Occasionally, air embolism may occur during cephalic vein or subclavian vein cannulation. The use of *safe sheaths* with one-way valve mechanism minimizes this risk.

Cardiac Perforation

Cardiac perforation resulting in pericardial effusion and occasionally cardiac tamponade is a rare but potentially life-threatening complication of pacemaker lead insertion. This may be recognized at the time of lead insertion by fluoroscopic position of the lead, right bundle-branch block morphology of the paced QRS complex, diaphragmatic stimulation, or hypotension resulting from cardiac tamponade. If identified at the time of implantation, lead withdrawal and repositioning is usually not associated with tamponade. In patients with chest pain, friction rub, and a small pericardial effusion, serial echocardiograms may be performed to assess for hemodynamic deterioration. Cardiac perforation and pericarditis may also develop as a late complication and occasionally lead to tamponade weeks to months after the pacemaker implantation, especially with active fixation leads.[79]

Hematomas

Hematomas occurring at the pacemaker pocket site can vary from a small ecchymosis to large and tense swelling. Most small hematomas can be managed conservatively with cold compresses and

TABLE 40–18
Pacemaker Complications

ACUTE	SUBACUTE OR CHRONIC
Pneumothorax	Venous occlusion
Hemothorax	Infection
Air embolism	Pacemaker allergy
Cardiac perforation and tamponade	Twiddler syndrome
	Pacemaker syndrome
Coronary sinus dissection	Pacemaker-mediated arrhythmias
Coronary vein perforation	
Pocket hematoma	Pacemaker-mediated tachycardia
Venous thrombosis	
Lead dislodgement	Runaway pacemaker
Infection (pocket, sepsis)	Lead Failure
Loose setscrews	Pacemaker malfunction
Diaphragmatic stimulation	Electromagnetic interference

withdrawal of antiplatelet or antithrombotic agents. Occasionally, large hematomas that compromise the suture line or skin integrity may have to be surgically evacuated. In patients who require therapeutic anticoagulation, heparin should be delayed for at least 24 to 48 hours after implantation to avoid bleeding complications.

Venous Occlusion

Venous occlusion may result from acute subclavian or axillary vein thrombosis and lead to ipsilateral arm edema and thrombosis. Venous thrombosis is generally treated with heparin and 3 to 6 months of warfarin. Rarely invasive surgical interventions may be required. Up to 30 to 40 percent of patients undergoing pacemaker implantation may develop partial to complete venous occlusion over time and may remain asymptomatic because of the development of venous collaterals.[101] Occasionally, superior vena caval occlusion leading to superior vena cava syndrome may result from pacemaker lead implantation.[81]

Infection

The use of prophylactic antibiotics and pocket irrigation with antibiotic solutions has decreased the rate of acute infections following pacemaker implantations to <1 to 2 percent in most series. Although early infections are generally caused by *Staphylococcus aureus* and may be aggressive, late infections associated with pacemakers are usually caused by *Staphylococcus epidermidis* and their course tends to be indolent. The signs of infection include local inflammation and abscess formation, erosion of the pacer, and fever with positive blood cultures without an identifiable focus of infection. Occasionally the infected pacemaker tends to erode through the skin. Transesophageal echocardiography helps determine whether vegetations are present on the pacemaker leads. Removal of the pacemaker leads and generator is usually required to completely eliminate pacemaker infections.[102]

Lead Dislodgement

Leads may dislodge from the initial implant site in the first few days to few weeks following the implantation. Active and passive fixation mechanisms of leads help prevent this complication. Atrial lead dislodgement is slightly more common than it is for ventricular leads. Although passive fixation leads are stable in the atrial appendage, active fixation leads are necessary to prevent dislodgment in patients with prior cardiac surgery. Lead dislodgment may result in an increase in pacing thresholds, failure to capture, or failure to sense. Lead dislodgment may be radiographically visible or it may be a *microdislodgment*, where there is no radiographic change in position, but there is significant increase in pacing threshold and/or decline in the electrogram amplitude.

Diaphragmatic/Phrenic Nerve Stimulation

Diaphragmatic/phrenic nerve stimulation may lead to significant discomfort. This phenomenon is most commonly in patients with LV coronary vein branch lead placement for biventricular stimulation. During implant, high-output pacing at maximal voltage and pulse width should be tested routinely to avoid diaphragmatic stimulation.

Twiddler Syndrome

Twiddler syndrome is a term applied to patients who intentionally or unintentionally manipulate their pulse generator, causing twisting of the entire pacemaker system. This leads to lead dislodgment or fracture.

Pacemaker Syndrome

The constellation of neurologic and cardiovascular signs and symptoms resulting from deleterious hemodynamics induced by ventricular pacing has been termed *pacemaker syndrome.* The variety of symptoms and signs associated with pacemaker syndrome are listed in Table 40–19. They are attributable to a decrease in cardiac output and arterial pressure caused by loss of AV synchrony or to cardiovascular or humoral reflexes elicited by increases in pulmonary venous or right atrial pressures. The basis for pacemaker syndrome is not only loss of AV synchrony but also the presence of ventriculoatrial (VA) conduction. Atrial contraction against closed AV valves leads to increases in jugular and pulmonary venous pressure causing cough and malaise in patients with intact cardiac function and congestive heart failure in other patients with structural heart disease. The symptoms may vary from mild to severe and the onset of symptoms range from acute to chronic.

The exact incidence of pacemaker syndrome is unknown, but severe manifestations are expected to occur in 5 to 7 percent of ventricularly paced patients. Milder symptoms or significant drops in systolic blood pressure and cardiac output during ventricular pacing occur in >20 percent of patients.[84] In the Pacemaker Selection in the Elderly trial, 26 percent of the patients in the ventricular pacing arm crossed over to the DDD pacing mode because of symptoms caused by pacemaker syndrome.[51]

The management of pacemaker syndrome usually requires restoration of AV synchrony. In many patients, an upgrade to a dual-chamber pacer is indicated. In some patients with intact sinus and AV conduction, lowering the pacing rate in VVI mode and using the hysteresis mode may promote sinus rhythm, lessening the symptoms associated with pacemaker syndrome.

TABLE 40–19

Symptoms and Signs of Pacemaker Syndrome

SYMPTOMS	SIGNS
Neck pulsations	Cannon A waves
Fatigue	Elevated jugular venous
Palpitations	pressure
Cough	Palpable liver pulsations
Apprehension	Peripheral edema
Chest fullness	S_3 gallop
Choking sensation	Pulmonary rales
Orthopnea	Drop in systolic blood pres-
Exertional dyspnea	sure >20 mmHg during
Dizziness, near syncope, or	ventricular pacing
syncope	
Confusion, altered mental	
state	

Pacemaker-Mediated Arrhythmias

Pacemaker-Mediated Tachycardia Pacemaker-mediated tachycardia (PMT), or *endless-loop tachycardia,* is a well-recognized arrhythmia mediated by the pacemaker in patients with atrial-sensed ventricular pacing systems. In patients with intact VA conduction, a premature ventricular contraction may result in retrograde conduction to the atria, which, if outside the PVARP, is sensed and followed by ventricular pacing after the programed AV interval. The paced ventricular event will again be followed by VA conduction resulting in endless-loop tachycardia. PMT can be prevented by programing the PVARP to be longer than the native VA conduction time. However, if the VA interval is very long, the PVARP cannot be lengthened as this will limit the upper rate. Modern pacemakers have several options to prevent or terminate PMT. One such feature is automatic extension of PVARP following a sensed premature ventricular beat to prevent tracking of retrogradely conducted P waves. If PMT is established (atrial-sensed ventricular pacing close to the upper rate limit with stable VA intervals), the PVARP is automatically extended to a longer interval of 500 msec for one cycle, usually terminating the tachycardia (Fig. 40–20).

Lead Failure

The pacemaker leads are subject to long-term complications. The insulation of the leads may break, leading to problems with oversensing (caused by electrical noise), undersensing, and failure to capture (caused by current leak). This problem often manifests intermittently and may be difficult to detect during a routine pacer check. The patient may complain of pectoral muscle stimulation caused by current leakage around an insulation break. An abnormally low impedance with demonstrable lead malfunction is diagnostic for insulation break. Leads may also fracture over time. Early lead fractures lead to increased impedances associated with failure to capture, oversensing, and undersensing. Lead damage can occur at the site of venous access (subclavian vein) in the costoclavicular space causing the crush syndrome.

【 】 PACEMAKER SYSTEM MALFUNCTION: TROUBLESHOOTING

Pacemaker system malfunction can be secondary to pacemaker circuitry failure or to lead dysfunction. Not uncommonly what appears to be pacemaker malfunction may actually represent normal functioning of the pacemaker: A pacing artifact may be delivered in the middle of the normal QRS and may represent pseudofusion (caused by late sensing) and not undersensing. Unexplained longer pauses after sensed, but not paced, complexes might suggest oversensing; but it may represent normal function caused by hysteresis. Major electrocardiographic abnormalities of pacemaker system malfunction is broadly categorized into the following: failure to capture, failure to output, undersensing, and oversensing.

Failure to Capture

The loss of pacemaker capture occurs when there is a visible pacing stimulus and no atrial or ventricular depolarization. The differential diagnosis of failure to capture is outlined in Table 40–20. Failure to capture may be intermittent or persistent. Lead dislodgment can

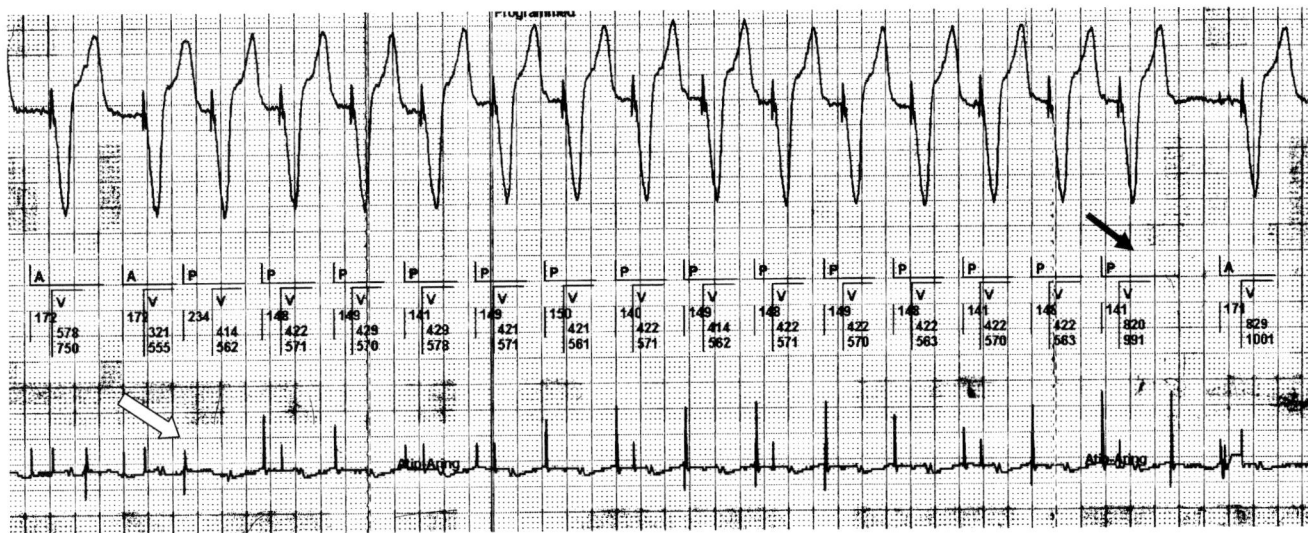

FIGURE 40–20. Pacemaker-mediated tachycardia. Surface electrocardiogram; marker channel with AV, VA, and VV intervals; and intracardiac atrial electrograms are displayed. The atrium is paced (A) at subthreshold output leading to noncapture resulting in atrioventricular dissociation. The second-paced ventricular event is followed by a native P wave with a VA interval of 320 msec (PVARP 275 msec) and is sensed leading to ventricular pacing. This is followed by a retrogradely conducted P wave (*open arrow*), with a VA interval of 420 msec, and sets up the endless-loop tachycardia. Because the ventricular pacing rate is above the programed pacemaker-mediated tachycardia rate of 100 beats/min, the device automatically extends the PVARP on the second-to-last ventricular paced beat to 500 msec (*arrow*), resulting in nonsensing of the retrograde P wave terminating the tachycardia. PVARP, postventricular atrial refractory period.

cause obvious failure to capture. An increase in the pacing threshold above the programed pacing output can occur as a result of the rise of the threshold within a few weeks following lead placement because of drug therapy, electrolytes, MI, or ischemia. Fracture of the lead, insulation breaks, and loose setscrews are mechanical problems that can cause failure to capture (Fig. 40–21). Last, battery depletion may cause the pacing output to decline sufficiently such that pacing failure occurs. Loss of capture requires a check of the pacing threshold and of pacing lead impedance and a chest radiograph. For instance, if the problem is an elevated pacing threshold, pacing outputs must be increased. Abnormal lead impedances may confirm a lead failure and the need for lead replacement. Functional noncapture occurs when a stimulus falls during the physiologic refractory period of a native depolarization. It may be secondary to undersensing or as a function of the pacing mode (AOO, VOO).

Failure to Output

Another pacing system malfunction is the absence of pacing stimuli and hence no capture. In bipolar systems the pacing artifact is

diminutive especially if isoelectric in some surface leads. It is important to record multiple leads simultaneously. Failure to output is often caused by oversensing and inhibition of pacing output and less commonly caused by circuitry failure (Table 40–21). Oversensing may be caused by T waves, P waves, or far-field R waves and may cause inhibition of pacing output. In unipolar systems, oversensing of myopotentials is common. A loose setscrew may cause noise and oversensing leading to inhibition of pacing output (Fig. 40–22). Electromagnetic signals from arc welding and electrocautery may be sensed by the pacemaker. Occasionally, the ventricular channel may be inhibited by oversensing the atrial channel output (crosstalk). If the absence of pacing output is caused by oversensing, a magnet application changes the pacemaker to an asynchronous mode to eliminate the pauses. In generator component malfunction, there is no delivery of pacing output by the device and magnet application does not restore pacing output. Systematic analysis of the pacing parameters, evaluation of lead impedances at rest, and provocative isometric exercises and chest radiograph may help identify the cause.

Oversensing

In a single-chamber pacemaker oversensing leads to inhibition of the pacing channel and causes inappropriate pauses. However, in dual-chamber pacemakers oversensing elicits either inappropriate inhibition or triggering, depending on the channel in which oversensing occurs and the programed pacing mode. Oversensing in the ventricular channel in the DDD or DDI mode results in inhibition of both atrial and ventricular outputs and resetting of timing cycles. In patients with complete heart block, this may result in ventricular asystole (Fig. 40–23). Oversensing in the atrial channel can lead to inappropriate triggering of ventricular output. The various etiologies of oversensing were discussed in the previous section. One example of oversensing peculiar to dual-chamber pacemakers is crosstalk. The atrial channel output can

TABLE 40–20

Differential Diagnosis of Failure to Capture

ETIOLOGY	PACING THRESHOLD	IMPEDANCE
Lead dislodgement	Elevated	Normal
Lead insulator failure	Elevated	Decreased
Lead conductor fracture	Elevated	Increased
Loose setscrew	Elevated	Increased
Battery depletion	Normal	Normal
Functional noncapture	Normal	Normal

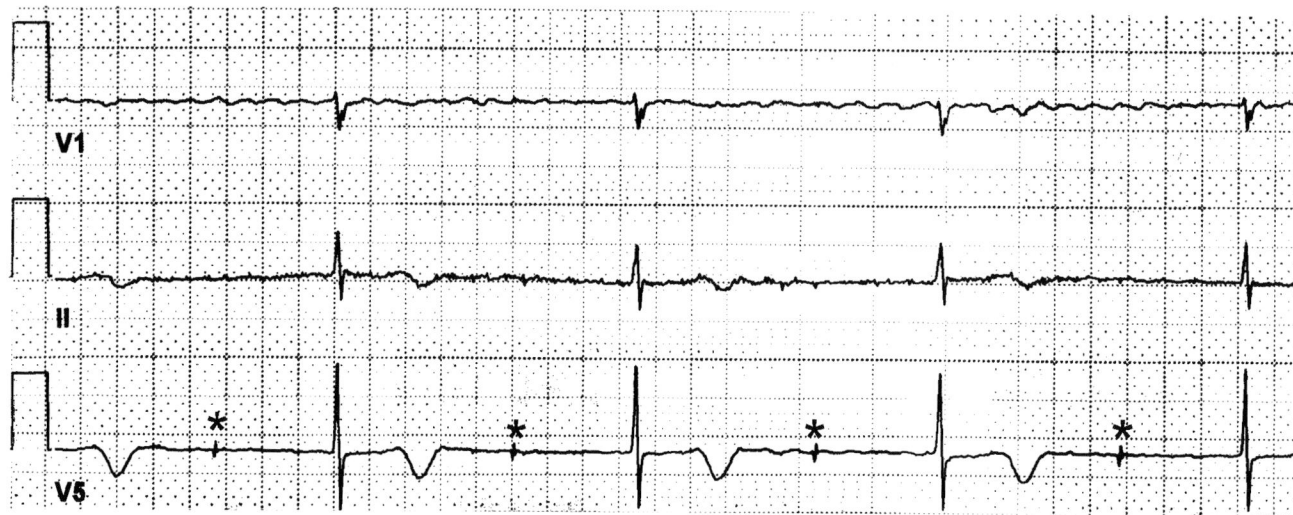

FIGURE 40–21. Failure to capture. Surface electrocardiogram of a patient with VVI pacemaker at a lower-rate limit of 60 ppm is shown at the bottom. The pacemaker spikes (*) are not followed by ventricular depolarization (no capture). Patient has spontaneous ventricular activity at 35 beats/min. The device clearly senses the ventricular event because the pacemaker spike appears 1000 msec (60 ppm) after the sensed event. On interrogation of the device, His lead impedance was significantly lower (300 Ω) than the implant values; and His pacing threshold had increased significantly. These findings are consistent with lead failure secondary to insulation break. Chest radiograph revealed evidence of insulation break at the subclavian venous access site. VVI, ventricular demand pacing.

be sensed in the ventricular channel as a far-field signal and inhibit the ventricular pacing output. In patients with complete heart block, this can result in ventricular asystole. Although far more common with unipolar systems, crosstalk can also occur in bipolar pacing systems. To prevent this phenomenon, there is a programmable ventricular blanking period (51–150 msec) following atrial pacing during which the ventricular channel is refractory. Additionally, there is a crosstalk sensing window following the blanking period during which a ventricular event, if sensed, will lead to ventricular pacing with a shorter AV interval. Oversensing due to lead fracture, insulation break, or other electrode problems will usually be random and erratic. With early lead problems, the malfunction is typically intermittent and may be exacerbated by certain body positions or motions. In later stages, the combination of oversensing, undersensing, and failure to capture is almost always diagnostic of a lead-related problem. Programing to an asynchronous mode may temporarily control this problem while awaiting lead replacement, which should be carried out as promptly as possible.

Undersensing

An inadequate intracardiac signal can lead to undersensing. The intracardiac electrograms can deteriorate because of inflammation or scar formation at the tissue lead interface. Additionally, some drugs, electrolyte abnormalities, infarction, ischemia, lead fracture, or insulation breaks can all lead to undersensing. Cardioversion or defibrillation can also cause attenuation of intracardiac electro-

grams. Usually, undersensing is a greater problem in the atrium than the ventricle. The atrial electrograms are typically significantly lower in amplitude during atrial fibrillation than they are during sinus rhythm. The optimal solution is to program an enhanced sensitivity (decreased sensing level, e.g., from 1.5 mV–0.55 mV). With bipolar systems, the programed sensitivity can usually be reduced to as low as 0.18 mV in the atrium in some devices, without oversensing of myopotentials or other extraneous

TABLE 40–21

Differential Diagnosis of Failure to Output

ETIOLOGY	DIAGNOSIS/MANAGEMENT
Oversensing T wave, P wave, R wave Myopotential/diaphragmatic Electromagnetic interference Crosstalk Make–break potential	Application of magnet eliminates pauses Reduce sensitivity Change unipolar to bipolar sensing
Insulation failure	Pauses persist despite magnet application Impedance low; replace lead
Open circuit Conductor fracture Loose setscrew	Pauses persist despite magnet application Impedance high Chest x-ray may show conductor deformity Loosely seated lead pin
Component malfunction	Pauses persist despite magnet application Replace pulse generator
Pseudomalfunction Hysteresis Mode switching Pacemaker-mediated tachycardia intervention	Pauses follow only sensed beats Reassurance

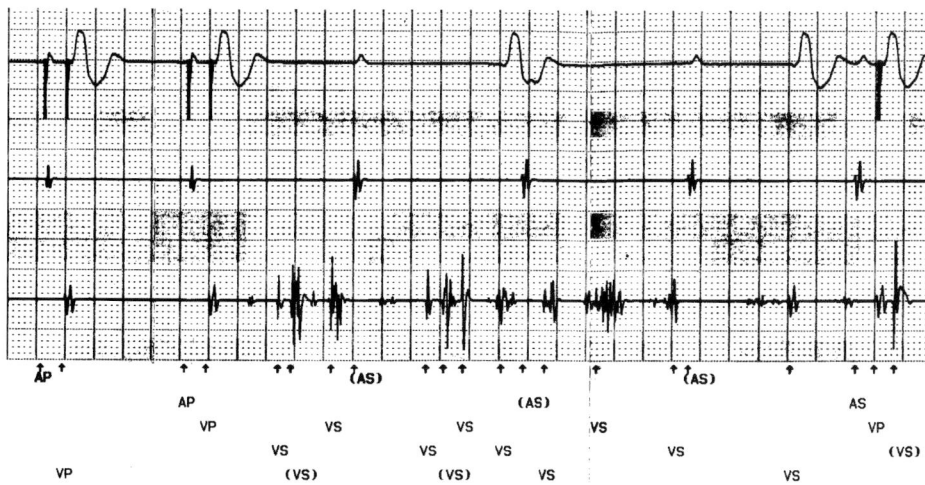

FIGURE 40–22. Failure to output. Surface electrocardiogram and atrial and ventricular electrograms with pacemaker event markers are shown. In this patient with dual-chamber pacemaker, loose setscrew resulted in noise on the ventricular channel leading to oversensing and inhibition of the ventricular output. Ap, atrial paced; As, atrial sensed; Vp, ventricular paced; Vs, ventricular sensed.

signals. Other etiologies for undersensing occur when intrinsic atrial or ventricular complexes fall within one of the programed refractory periods. Undersensing can also result when a pacemaker is inadvertently programed to an asynchronous mode (occasionally occurring with battery depletion or pacemaker generator reset).

【 】 ELECTROMAGNETIC INTERFERENCE

Electromagnetic interference (EMI) is defined as any nonphysiologic electrical signal that interferes with pacemaker function. EMI can originate from a variety of sources both within the hospital environment and outside. EMI can result in the inhibition of the pacemaker, inappropriate triggering, noise reversion, resetting of the pacemaker parameters, and occasionally damage to the circuitry or electrode–myocardial interface[85]; unipolar pacemakers are more susceptible to EMI than bipolar pacemakers. EMI has become an increasingly important problem because sources of interference are ubiquitous in the hospital and workplace.

In the hospital environment, the most common sources of EMI include electrocautery and defibrillation. Electrocautery can cause inhibition of the pacemaker; and in a pacemaker-dependent patient, this may result in severe bradycardia or asystole. Specific perioperative management of a device includes the following[103]:

- Identify the type of the device and its manufacturer; identifying the manufacturer is essential.
- Identify if the patient is dependent on the device for antibradycardia pacing; this may be obtained from the history of syncope, complete heart block, or AV node ablation requiring pacemaker placement. Interrogating the device may help identify if the patient has a stable underlying escape rhythm.
- Determine if EMI is likely to occur during the procedure. The device should be reprogramed to asynchronous mode (VOO or DOO) or triggered mode (VVT), especially if the patient is dependent. Rate adaptive pacing function should be turned off. Antitachyarrhythmia functions should be suspended (if an ICD). The surgeon should be advised to use a bipolar electrocautery (if possible) to minimize EMI.

- Place a magnet over the pacemaker to convert this device to function in an asynchronous mode (VVI to VOO or DDD to DOO) for as long as the magnet remains over the device. Removing the magnet returns the device to its original mode. In patients with ICDs, placing a magnet disables its antitachycardia therapies. However, this will not alter its pacemaker function. Magnets should be used when reprograming options are not immediately available. All operating room personnel including the surgeon, anesthesiologist, and nursing staff must be aware of the presence of the device, the potential for electromagnetic interference encountered in the operating room, and corrective techniques. An external defibrillator with transcutaneous pacing capabilities should be readily available.

- Intraoperatively, electrocardiographically monitor all patients to assess for device inhibition and with peripheral pulse evaluation (plethysmography or arterial pressure, etc.) in case of electrocautery-induced artifact on telemetry. Individuals performing the procedure should be advised to avoid electrocautery in the immediate field of the device generator and leads. Electrocautery should be used in short, intermittent, and irregular bursts.

- If the patient requires electrical cardioversion, deliver the shock as far as possible from the pulse generator and place the defibrillation pads on an axis perpendicular to that of the leads and pulse generator (to avoid transient undersensing or pacing inhibition).

- Interrogate devices postprocedure to assess for threshold changes and to reprogram the device to its original function if necessary.

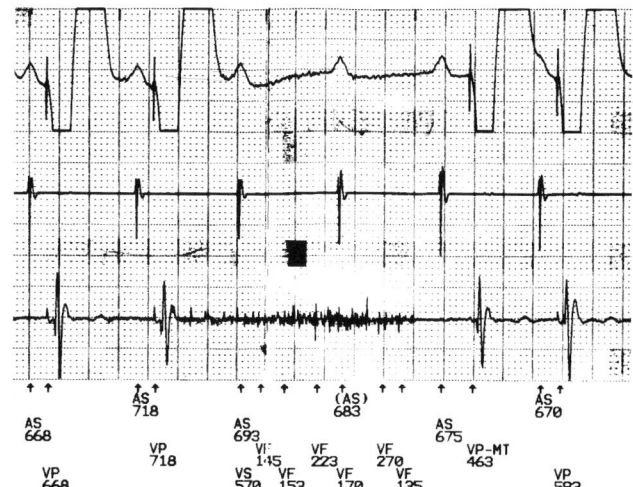

FIGURE 40–23. Oversensing of diaphragmatic myopotentials. Surface electrocardiogram and atrial and ventricular electrograms with event markers are shown. In this patient with a dual-chamber defibrillator, deep respiration reproduced the diaphragmatic myopotentials resulting in inhibition of ventricular output. The patient developed dizzy spells caused by underlying complete heart block. The ventricular lead was repositioned in the RV outflow tract eliminating the diaphragmatic oversensing. As, atrial sensed; VF, ventricular fibrillation; Vp, ventricular paced; Vs, ventricular sensed.

Other potential sources of EMI in the hospital include extracorporeal lithotripsy, radiation therapy, and MRI. Generally, MRI should be avoided in patients with pacemakers because it is potentially hazardous, most commonly when it causes rapid pacing triggered by the pulsing of the magnetic field. Other potential complications related to MRI include device reprograming, reed switch closure, heating at the myocardial-lead interface, and mechanical movement of the device. Approaches to minimize the risk of MRI to patients consist of programing the device to asynchronous mode, reducing the pacemaker output, limiting the MRI to areas remote from the device, and monitoring blood pressure and ECG during the MRI scanning. However, at present MRI should be considered strongly contraindicated in patients with implantable devices. Lithotripsy can also result in inappropriate inhibition or oversensing, especially in rate-responsive pacemakers with piezoelectric crystals. The pacemaker should generally be programed to VVI or VOO mode with the rate-responsive feature turned off prior to lithotripsy. Radiation therapy should be avoided directly over the field of the pacemaker. If shielding the pacemaker and limiting the field of radiation cannot be performed with safety, repositioning of the pacemaker prior to radiotherapy should be considered. Other possible EMI sources in the hospital include therapeutic diathermy, radiofrequency catheter ablation, transcutaneous electric nerve stimulation (TENS) units, and spinal cord stimulators.

Daily sources of EMI include digital cellular phones, electronic article surveillance devices, metal detectors, and electric razors; and work or industrial environment sources include high-voltage power lines, transformers, welding, and electric motors. Activated digital cell phones should not be placed in the breast pocket ipsilateral to the pacemaker, and the phone should be held to the ear contralateral to the pacemaker. Electronic surveillance devices or antitheft devices present in most stores and libraries can cause transient asynchronous pacing, atrial oversensing with tracking, and ventricular oversensing and inhibition. Patients with pacemakers should quickly walk through these devices and avoid lingering near them. Common household appliances such as electric can openers, stereos, televisions, video recorders, power tools, electric blankets, electric shavers, microwave ovens, and electric lawnmowers do not cause any pacemaker interference.

❘ ❘ DEVICE RECALL, ADVISORY, AND ALERTS

Currently, there are approximately 2 million patients with implantable pacemakers or defibrillators worldwide. In the year 2005, >400,000 patients received a new pacemaker or defibrillator implant in the United States alone. As the number of implantable cardiac devices has increased, device alerts and advisories have become a part of routine clinical practice. When a physician is faced with the management of a patient with an implanted device that has been the subject of a recall or advisory, the major concern facing the clinician is how to manage the patient and whether the device must be replaced. Compared to other medical devices, these devices are unique because they are often implanted for life-threatening problems for which device failure may be causally linked to death or poor outcome. A recent review by Maisel and colleagues of device manufacturer performance reports issued between 1990 and 2002 found that >17,000 devices were explanted during this timeframe for confirmed malfunction.[85,86] The explanted devices were evenly split among pacemakers and ICDs; but when comparing the number of implants in each category, ICDs ap-

peared to be four times more likely to malfunction and require explantation. A meta-analysis of device registries found that pacemaker reliability has improved markedly and consistently over the past 20 years.[86]

There are a wide variety of malfunctions that have been reported with pacemakers and ICDs. These include both hardware component malfunction and software problems. In general, hardware malfunction tends to be far more common than software malfunction and are also more problematic for physicians and patients. Among hardware problems, battery/capacitor and electrical issues account for more than half of the reported malfunctions. Gould and Krahn[104] reported the results from a multicenter Canadian study of the consequences of various ICD advisories. From approximately 18 percent (533 of 2915 patients) of devices electively replaced because of advisories, complications were observed in 8.1 percent of cases within 2.7 months following ICD generator replacement (5.8 percent were major complications requiring re-operation, including two deaths). In contrast, there were *only* three (0.1 percent) device malfunctions from the devices that were included in advisories but no clinical complications from these malfunctions.

Currently, several groups have recently provided specific recommendations or guidelines for managing patients with devices affected by recalls or advisories.[82,105–107] The Heart Rhythm Society has proposed a series of recommendations for physicians and industry. Device manufacturers and the Food and Drug Administration (FDA) notify physicians and patients after determining a device problem by an advisory; however, decisions about management are left to physicians. All patients with devices affected by recall, advisories, or alerts should be seen in the office for immediate device interrogation and discussion of the implications of the notification to the patient and their immediate and long-term device management and clinical status.[107] The patient's indication for device implantation and relative device dependence should be discussed, and well as potential consequences of device failure. The decision regarding which patients affected by the advisory/recall should undergo device replacement may be difficult for both the patient and the physician. Pacemaker dependence, ICDs implanted for secondary prevention, and high likelihood of device failure are some of the factors that lead to consideration for device replacement. Alternately, patients may be scheduled for more frequent in-clinic followup or by transtelephonic or computer-based remote monitoring based on a careful review of the company, FDA, and any outside physician panel recommendations. Patients should be instructed to present to device clinic or use remote followup whenever any symptoms (i.e., syncope, presyncope, palpitations, angina, etc.) or other symptoms that suggest possible device malfunction are experienced. Device self-monitoring capabilities and the ability to do intensive remote followup allows for more reliable device followup in the future. Remote automatic checks with wireless or internet-based physician notification schemes may improve monitoring of device performance, but currently office interrogations remain the most commonly used modality for followup. Diagnostic tools are being developed to help detect potential hardware problems which could lead to malfunction.

REFERENCES

1. Katz LN, Pick A. *Clinical Electrocardiography. Part I. The Arrhythmias.* Philadelphia: Lea & Febiger; 1956:20.
2. Benditt DG, Sakaguchi S, Goldstein MA, et al. Sinus node dysfunction, pathophysiology, clinical features, evaluation, and treatment. In: Zipes DP, Jaliffe J, eds.

Cardiac Electrophysiology: From Cell to Bedside. 2nd ed. Philadelphia: Saunders; 1995:1215–1247.

3. Hecht HH, Kossmann CE, Childers RW, et al. Atrioventricular and intraventricular conduction: revised nomenclature and concepts. *Am J Cardiol* 1973;31:232–244.

4. Kyrialikdis MK, Kouraouklis CB, Papaioannou JT, et al. Sinus node coronary arteries studied with angiography. *Am J Cardiol* 1983;51:749–750.

5. Frink RJ, James TN. Normal blood supply to the human His bundle and proximal bundle branches. *Circulation* 1973;43:491–502.

6. Ferrer MI. The sick sinus syndrome. *Circulation* 1973;47:635.

7. Moss AJ, Davis RJ. Brady-tachy syndrome. *Prog Cardiovasc Dis* 1974;16:439–454.

8. Evans R, Shaw D. Pathological studies in sinoatrial disorder (sick sinus syndrome). *Br Heart J* 1977;39:778.

9. Thery C, Gosselin B, Lekieffre J, et al. Pathology of the sinoatrial node: correlation with electrophysiological findings in 111 patients. *Am Heart J* 1977;93:735.

10. Adgey AAJ, Geddes JS, Mulho JF. Incidence, significance and management of early bradyarrhythmia complicating acute myocardial infarction. *Lancet* 1968;2:1097–1101.

11. Barak M, Herschkowitz S, Shapiro I, et al. Familial combined sinus node and atrioventricular conduction dysfunctions. *Int J Cardiol* 1987;15:231–239.

12. Bartunek P, Nemec J, Mrazek V, et al. Borrelia burgdorferi as a cause of sick sinus syndrome. *Cas Lek Cesk* 1996;135:729–731.

13. Greenwood RD, Rosenthal A, Sloss LJ, et al. Sick sinus syndrome after surgery for congenital heart disease. *Circulation* 1975;52:208–213.

14. Bexton RS, Nathan AW, Hellerstrand KJ, et al. Sinoatrial function after cardiac transplantation. *J Am Coll Cardiol* 1984;3:712–723.

15. Talan DA, Bauernfeind RA, Ashley WW, et al. Twenty-four hour continuous ECG recordings in long distance runners. *Chest* 1982;82:19–24.

16. Fairfax AJ, Lambert CD, Leatham A. Systemic embolism in chronic sinoatrial disorder. *N Engl J Med* 1976;295:190–192.

17. Talwar KK, Dev V, Chopra P, et al. Persistent atrial standstill: clinical, electrophysiological and morphological study. *Pacing Clin Electrophysiol* 1991;14:1274–1280.

18. Gwynn N, Leman R, Kratz, et al. Chronotropic incompetence: a common and progressive finding in pacemaker patients. *Am Heart J* 1992;123:1216.

19. Forbath P, Darling DS, Quimet S. Adapting the rate modulation to the type of chronotropic incompetence. *PACE* 1991;14:685.

20. Jose AD, Collison D. The normal range and determinants of intrinsic heart rate in man. *Cardiovasc Res* 1970;4:160.

21. Avery P, Small J, Shaw DB. Xamoterol in sinus node disease. *Int J Cardiol* 1993;40:45.

22. Alboni P, Menozzi C, Brignole M, et al. Effect of permanent pacemaker and oral theophylline in sick sinus syndrome, the THEOPACE study: A randomized controlled trial. *Circulation* 1997;96(1):260–266.

23. Sutton R, Kenny RA. The natural history of sick sinus syndrome. *Pacing Clin Electrophysiol* 1986;9:1110.

24. Bernstein AD, Parsonnet V. Survey of cardiac pacing and implanted defibrillator practice patterns in the United States in 1997. *Pacing Clin Electrophysiol* 2001;24(5):842–855.

25. Andersen HR, Nielsen JC, Thomsen PEB, et al. Long-term follow up of patients from a randomized trial of atrial versus ventricular pacing for sick sinus syndrome. *Lancet* 1997;350:1210–1216.

26. Furman S, Schwedel JB. An intracardiac pacemaker for Stokes-Adams seizures. *N Engl J Med* 1959;261:943–948.

27. Connolly SJ, Kerr CR, Gent M, et al. Effects of physiologic pacing versus ventricular pacing on the risk of stroke and death due to cardiovascular causes. *N Engl J Med* 2000;342:1385–1391.

28. Lamas GA, Lee KL, Sweeney M, et al. Ventricular pacing or dual chamber pacing for sinus node dysfunction. *N Engl J Med* 2002;346:1854–1862.

29. Toff WD, Camm JA, Skehn JD, et al. Single chamber versus dual chamber pacing for high-grade atrioventricular block. *N Engl J Med* 2005;353:145–155.

30. Healey JS, Toff WD, Lamas GA, et al. Cardiovascular outcomes with atrial-based pacing compared with ventricular pacing: meta-analysis of randomized trials, using individual patient data. *Circulation* 2006;114:11–17.

31. Sweeney MO, Helkamp AS, Ellenbogen KA, et al. Adverse effect of ventricular pacing on heart failure and atrial fibrillation among patients with a normal QRS duration in a clinical trial of pacemaker therapy for sinus node dysfunction. *Circulation* 2003;107:2932–2937.

32. Wilkoff BL, Cook JR, Epstein AE, et al. Dual chamber pacing or ventricular backup pacing in patients with an implantable defibrillator: the Dual chamber and VVI implantable defibrillator (DAVID) trial. *JAMA* 2002;288:3115–3123.

33. Teichman SL, Felder SD, Matos JA. The value of electrophysiologic studies in syncope of undetermined origin: report of 150 cases. *Am Heart J* 1985;110:469.

34. Katritsis D, Ward DE, Camm AJ. Can we treat carotid sinus syndrome? *PACE* 1991;14:1367.

35. Strasberg B, Lam W, Swiryn S, et al. Symptomatic spontaneous paroxysmal AV nodal block due to localized hyperresponsiveness of the AV node to vagotonic reflexes. *Am Heart J* 1982;103:79.

36. Steere AC, Batsford WP, Weinberg M, et al. Lyme carditis: cardiac abnormalities of Lyme disease. *Ann Intern Med* 1980;93(1):8.

37. Lev M. The pathology of complete AV block. *Prog Cardiovasc Dis* 1964;6:317.

38. Lenègre J. Etiology and pathology of bilateral bundle branch fibrosis in relation to complete heart block. *Prog Cardiovasc Dis* 1964;6:409.

39. Probst V, Kyndt F, Potet F, et al. Haploinsufficiency in combination with aging causes SCN5A-linked hereditary Lenègre disease. *J Am Coll Cardiol* 2003;41:643–652.

40. Ellenbogen KA, de Guzman M, Kawanishi DT, et al. Pacing for acute and chronic AV conduction system disease. In: Ellenbogen KA, Kay GN, Wilkoff BL, eds. *Clinical Cardiac Pacing and Defibrillation.* Philadelphia: Saunders; 2000:426–454.

41. Harpaz, D, Behar S, Gottileb S, et al. Complete atrioventricular block complicating acute myocardial infarction in the thrombolytic era. *J Am Coll Cardiol* 1999;34:1721–1728.

42. Perloff JK. The heart in neuromuscular disease. In: O'Rourke RA, ed. *Current Problems in Cardiology.* Chicago: Year Book; 1986:513–517.

43. Koplan BA, Stevenson WG, Epstein LM, et al. Development and validation of a simple risk score to predict the need for permanent pacing after cardiac valve surgery. *J Am Coll Cardiol* 2003;41:795–801.

44. McAnulty JH, Rahimtoola SH, Murphy E, et al. Natural history of "high risk" bundle-branch block: final report of a prospective study. *N Engl J Med* 1982;307:137–143.

45. Camm AJ, Bexton RS. Congenital complete heart block. *Eur Heart J* 1984;5:115–117.

46. Donmoyer TL, DeSanctis RW, Austen WG. Experience with implantable pacemakers using myocardial electrodes in the management of heart block. *Ann Thorac Surg* 1967;3:218–227.

47. Alpert MA, Curtiss JJ, Sanfelippo JF, et al. Comparative survival after permanent ventricular and dual chamber pacing for patients with chronic high-degree atrioventricular block with and without preexistent congestive heart failure. *J Am Coll Cardiol* 1986;7:925.

48. Linde-Edelstam C, Gulberg B, Norlander R, et al. Longevity in patients with high degree atrioventricular block paced in the atrial synchronous mode or the fixed rate ventricular inhibited mode. *Pacing Clin Electrophysiol* 1992;15:304.

49. Lamas GA, Orav EJ, Stambler BS, et al. Quality of life and clinical outcomes in elderly patients treated with ventricular pacing as compared with dual chamber pacing. *N Engl J Med* 1998;338:1097–1104.

50. Dhingra RC, Amat-Y-Leon F, Wyndham C, et al. Significance of left axis deviation in patients with left bundle branch block. *Am J Cardiol* 1978;42:551–556.

51. Smith RF, Jackson DH, Harthorne JW, et al. Acquired bundle branch block in a healthy population. *Am Heart J* 1970;80:746–751.

52. Scheinman MM, Peters RW, Suave MJ, et al. Value of the H-Q interval in patients with bundle branch block and the role of prophylactic permanent pacing. *Am J Cardiol* 1982;50:1316–1322.

53. Ellenbogen KA, Wood MA, Shepahrd RK. Delayed complications following pacemaker implantation. *Pacing Clin Electrophysiol* 2002;8:1155–1158.

54. Bailin SJ, Johnson WB, Hoyt R. A prospective randomized trial of Bachmann's bundle pacing for the prevention of atrial fibrillation (abstract). *J Am Coll Cardiol* 1997;29:74A.

55. Saksena S, Prakash A, Ziegler P, et al. Improved suppression of recurrent atrial fibrillation with dual-site right atrial pacing and antiarrhythmic drug therapy. *J Am Coll Cardiol* 2002;40(6):1140–1150.

56. de Cock CC, Meyer A, Kamp O, et al. Hemodynamic benefits of right ventricular outflow tract pacing: comparison with right ventricular apex pacing. *Pacing Clin Electrophysiol* 1998;21(3):536–541.

57. Stambler BS, Ellenbogen KA, Zhang X, et al. Right ventricular outflow versus apex pacing in pacemaker patients with congestive heart failure an atrial fibrillation. *J Cardiovasc Electrophysiol* 2003;14:1180–1186.

58. Deshmukh PM, Casavant DA, Romanyshyn M, et al. Permanent, direct His-bundle pacing: a novel approach to cardiac pacing in patients with normal His-Purkinje activation. *Circulation* 2000;101:869–877.

59. Occhetta E, Bortnik M, Magnani A, et al. Prevention of ventricular desynchronization by permanent para-Hisian pacing after atrioventricular node ablation in chronic atrial fibrillation: a crossover, blinded, randomized study versus apical right ventricular pacing. *J Am Coll Cardiol* 2006;47:1938–1945.

60. Ellenbogen KA, Wood MA, Gilligan DM, et al. Steroid eluting high impedance pacing leads decrease short and long-term current drain: results from a multicenter clinical trial of CapSure Z investigators. *PACE* 1999;22:39–48.

61. Clarke M, Liu B, Schuller H, et al. Automatic adjustment of pacemaker stimulation output correlated with continuously monitored capture thresholds: a multicenter study. *PACE* 1998;21:1567–1575.

62. Bernstein AD, Camm AJ, Fletcher R, et al. The NASPE/BPEG generic pacemaker code for antibradyarrhythmia and adaptive rate pacing and antitachyarrhythmia devices. *PACE* 1987;10:794–799.

63. Andersen HR, Nielsen JC, Thomsen PEB, et al. Atrioventricular conduction during long-term follow-up of patients with sick sinus syndrome. *Circulation* 1998;98:1315–1321.

64. Rickards AF, Donaldson RM. Rate-responsive pacing. *Clin Prog Pacing Electrophysiol* 1983;1:12–19.

65. Leung SK, Lau CP, Tng MO. Cardiac output is a sensitive indicator of difference in exercise performance between single and dual sensor pacemakers. *PACE* 1998;21:35–41.

66. Eldar M, Griffin JC, Van Hare GF, et al. Combined use of beta-adrenergic blocking agents and long-term cardiac pacing for patients with the long-QT syndrome. *J Am Coll Cardiol* 1992;20:830–837.

67. Ward DE, Camm AJ, Spurrell RA. The response of regular supraventricular tachycardia to right heart stimulation. *PACE* 1979;2:586–595.

68. Knight BP, Gersh BJ, Carlson MD, et al. Role of permanent pacing to prevent atrial fibrillation: Science Advisory from the American Heart Association Council on Clinical Cardiology and the Quality of Care and Outcomes Research Interdisciplinary Working Group, in Collaboration with the Heart Rhythm Society. *Circulation* 20055;111:240–243.

69. Hochleitner H, Hortnagl H, Ng CK, et al. Usefulness of physiologic dual chamber pacing in drug resistant idiopathic dilated cardiomyopathy. *Am J Cardiol* 1990;66:198–202.

70. Linde C, Gadler F, Edner M, et al. Results of atrioventricular synchronous pacing with optimized delay in patients with severe congestive heart failure. *Am J Cardiol* 1995;75:919–923.

71. Gold MR, Feliciano Z, Gottlieb SS, et al. Dual chamber pacing with a short atrioventricular delay in congestive heart failure: a randomized study. *J Am Coll Cardiol* 1995;26:967–973.

72. Innes D, Leitch JW, Fletcher PJ. VDD pacing at short atrioventricular intervals does not improve cardiac output in patients with dilated heart failure. *PACE* 1994;17:959–965.

73. Bakker P, Chin K, Sen A, et al. Biventricular pacing improves functional capacity in patients with end stage heart failure (abstract). *PACE* 1995;18:825.

74. Auricchio A, Stellbrink C, Block M, et al. Effect of pacing chamber and atrioventricular delay on acute systolic function of paced patients with congestive heart failure. The Pacing Therapies for Congestive Heart Failure Study Group. The Guidant Congestive Heart Failure Research Group. *Circulation* 1999;99:2993–3001.

75. Gras D, Mabo P, Tang T, et al. Multisite pacing as a supplemental treatment of congestive heart failure: preliminary results of the Medtronic Inc. InSync Study. *Pacing Clin Electrophysiol* 1998;2:2249–2255.

76. Daubert JC, Linde C, Cazeau S, et al. Clinical effects of biventricular pacing in patients with severe heart failure and chronic atrial fibrillation: results from the Multisite Stimulation in Cardiomyopathy-MUSTIC-study group II [abstract]. *Circulation* 2000;102(suppl II):693.

77. Kuhlkamp V. Initial experience with an implantable cardioverter-defibrillator incorporating cardiac resynchronization therapy. *J Am Coll Cardiol* 2002;39:790–797.

78. Bristow MR, Saxon LA, Boehmer J, et al. Cardiac-resynchronization therapy with or without an implantable defibrillator in advanced chronic heart failure. *N Engl J Med* 2004;350:2140–2150. .

79. Ellenbogen KA, Wood MA, Shepard RK. Delayed complications following pacemaker implantation. *Pacing Clin Electrophysiol* 2002;25:1155–1158.

80. Cleland JGF, Daubert J-C, Erdmann E, et al. The effect of cardiac resynchronization on morbidity and mortality in heart failure. *N Engl J Med* 2005;352:1539–1549.

81. Mazzetti H, Dussaut A, Tentori C, et al. Superior vena cava occlusion and/or syndrome related to pacemaker leads. *Am Heart J* 1993;125:831–837.

82. Amin MS, Matchar DB, Wood MA, Ellenbogen KA. Management of recalled pacemakers and implantable cardioverter-defibrillators: a decision analysis model. *JAMA* 2006 July 26;296(4):414–420.

83. Pinski Sl, Trohman RG. Interference in implanted cardiac devices. *Pacing Clin Electrophysiol* 2002;25:1367–1381.

84. Travill CM, Sutton R, Pacemaker syndrome: an iatrogenic condition. *Br Heart J* 1992;68:163.

85. Maisel WH. Safety issues involving medical devices: implications of recent implantable cardioverter-defibrillator malfunctions. *JAMA* 2005;294:955–958.

86. Maisel WH, Moynahan M, Zuckerman BD, et al. Pacemaker and ICD generator malfunctions: analysis of Food and Drug Administration annual reports. *JAMA* 2006;295(16):1901–1906.

87. Farwell D, Patel NR, Hall A, et al. How many people with heart failure are appropriate for biventricular resynchronization? *Eur Heart J* 2000;21:1246–1250.

88. Auricchio A, Stellbrink C, Block M, et al. Effect of pacing chamber and atrioventricular delay on acute systolic function of paced patients with congestive heart failure. *Circulation* 1999;99:2993–3001.

89. Nelson G, Berger RD, Feltics BJ, et al. Left or biventricular pacing improves cardiac function at diminished energy cost in patients with dilated cardiomyopathy and left bundle branch block. *Circulation* 2000;102:3053–3059.

90. Leon A, Brozena S, Liang CS, et al. Effect of cardiac resynchronization therapy with sequential biventricular pacing in Doppler derived left ventricular stroke volume, functional status and exercise capacity in patients with ventricular dysfunction and conduction delay. The US InSync III trial [abstract]. *PACE* 2002;24:141.

91. Leon AR, Greenberg JM, Kanuru N, et al. Cardiac resynchronization in patients with congestive heart failure and chronic atrial fibrillation. *J Am Coll Cardiol* 2002;39:1258–1263.

92. Cazeau S, LeClercq C, Lavergne T, et al. Effects of multisite biventricular pacing in patients with heart failure and intraventricular conduction delay. *N Engl J Med* 2001;344:873–880.

93. Linde C, Leclercq C, Rex S, et al. Long-Term benefits of biventricular pacing in congestive heart failure: results from the Multisite Stimulation In Cardiomyopathy (MUSTIC) Study. *J Am Coll Cardiol* 2002;40:111–118.

94. Abraham WT, Fisher WG, Smith AL, et al. Cardiac resynchronization in chronic heart failure. *N Engl J Med* 2002;346:1845–1853.

95. Bradley DJ, Bradley EA, Baughman KL, et al. Cardiac resynchronization and death from progressive heart failure: a meta-analysis of randomized controlled trials. *JAMA* 2003;289:730–740.

96. Higgins SL, Young P, Scheck D, et al. Biventricular pacing diminishes the need for implantable cardioverter defibrillator therapy. *J Am Coll Cardiol* 2000;36:824–827.

97. Ammann P, Sticherling C, Kalusche D, et al. *Ann Intern Med* 2005;142:968–973.

98. Hassenstein VP, Wolter HH. Therapeutische beherrschung einer bedrohmichen situation bei der idiopathischen hypertrophischen subaortenstenose. *Verh Dtsch Ges Kreislaufforsch* 1967;33:242–246.

99. Sorajja P, Elliott PM, McKenna WJ. Pacing in hypertrophic cardiomyopathy. *Cardiol Clin* 2000;18:67–79.

100. Appenberger L, Linde C, Daubert C, et al. Pacing in hypertrophic cardiomyopathy: a randomized crossover study. PIC study group. *Eur Heart J* 1997;18:1249–1256.

101. Oginosawa Y, Abe H, Nakashima Y. The incidence and risk factors for venous obstruction after implantation of transvenous pacing leads. *Pacing Clin Electrophysiol* 2002;25:1605–1611.

102. Smith HJ, Fernot NE, Byrd CL, et al. Five-years experience with intravascular lead extraction. *Pacing Clin Electrophysiol* 1994;17:2016.

103. American Society of Anesthesiologists Task Force on Perioperative Management of Patients with Cardiac Rhythm Management Devices. Practice advisory for the perioperative management of patients with cardiac rhythm management devices: pacemakers and implantable cardioverter defibrillators. A report by the American Society of Anesthesiologists Task Force on Perioperative Management of Patients with Cardiac Rhythm Management Devices. *Anesthesiology* 2005;103:186–198.

104. Gould PA, Krahn AD; Canadian Heart Rhythm Society Working Group on Device Advisories. Complications associated with implantable cardioverter-defibrillator replacement in response to device advisories. *JAMA* 2006;295(16):1907–1911.

105. Santini M, Brachmann J, Cappato R, et al. Recommendations of the European Cardiac Arrhythmia Society Committee on Device Failures and Complications. *PACE* 2006;29:653–669.

106. Auricchio A, Gropp M, Ludgate S, et al. European Heart Rhythm Association Guidance Document on cardiac rhythm management product performance. *Europace* 2006;8:313–332.

107. Carlson MD, Wilkoff BL, Maisel WH, et al. Recommendations from the Heart Rhythm Society Task Force on Device Performance Policies and Guidelines. *Heart Rhythm* 2006;10:1250–1273.

CHAPTER 41

Long-Term Continuous Electrocardiographic Recording

Eric N. Prystowsky / Benzy J. Padanilam

Long-term electrocardiographic recording is a method of recording the ECG over an extended time period.[1] Technological advances in the past few years have provided a diversity of recording, transmitting, and analysis systems.

INDICATIONS

Ambulatory ECG recording may be helpful in diagnosing and, less frequently, quantitating cardiac arrhythmias. The recording of an arrhythmia during a patient's symptoms may be the only means of diagnosis, particularly when the two are relatively infrequent (Fig. 41–1). The recording of a normal rhythm during symptoms may prove equally valuable in excluding an arrhythmia as the cause for the symptoms.[2]

Detection of asymptomatic arrhythmias using ambulatory ECG recordings (e.g., nonsustained ventricular tachycardia) may be indicated in certain patients for assessing risk for future cardiac events. These may include patients with hypertrophic cardiomyopathy and those postmyocardial infarction with left ventricular (LV) dysfunction. Patients who are treated for arrhythmias, such as atrial fibrillation or ventricular tachycardia, may benefit from ambulatory ECG recordings for assessing the efficacy of therapy. An example is determining the ventricular rate control over 24 hours in patients with persistent atrial fibrillation. Other potential uses of ambulatory ECG are detection of myocardial ischemia from ST segment or T-wave changes, measurement of heart rate variability and QT dispersion. However, technical limitations, including nonstandard lead positioning and low-fidelity recordings, lead to uncertainty of the significance of ST segment and T-wave changes. Even more important than these technical considerations are certain physiologic limitations. For instance, standing, hy-

perventilation, eating, anxiety, use of drugs, and changes in autonomic tone are all daily events that may result in depression of the ST segment or inversion of the T wave to simulate ischemic changes. The American College of Cardiologists/American Heart Association (ACC/AHA) clinical practice *Guidelines for Ambulatory Electrocardiography,* provide a more complete consideration of clinical indications for ambulatory ECG recordings[3] (see Appendix 41–1).

RECORDING TECHNIQUES

Four general types of devices are currently available: continuous recorders, intermittent or event recorders, instruments for real-time recording and transmission of ECGs, and implantable recorders (Table 41–1).

【 】 CONTINUOUS RECORDERS

The ECG can be recorded continuously on cassette tape or digitally in solid-state memory. The tape recorder is a battery-powered, miniature device with a very slow tape speed that is small enough to be suspended by a strap over the shoulder or around the waist. The leads are usually attached to the patient's precordial skin using adhesive patches.

All digital recording systems amplify, digitize, and store the ECG in solid-state memory. Two types of digital recorders are available. In the first, each QRS complex is recorded, similar in this sense to the continuous tape recording. "Full disclosure" of the ECG is provided by enhanced storage capacity on a memory card the size of a credit card. With the second, microcomputers and microelectronic circuits sample the cardiac rhythm in real time as it is being recorded, convert the ana-

Rapid Heartbeat Symptom

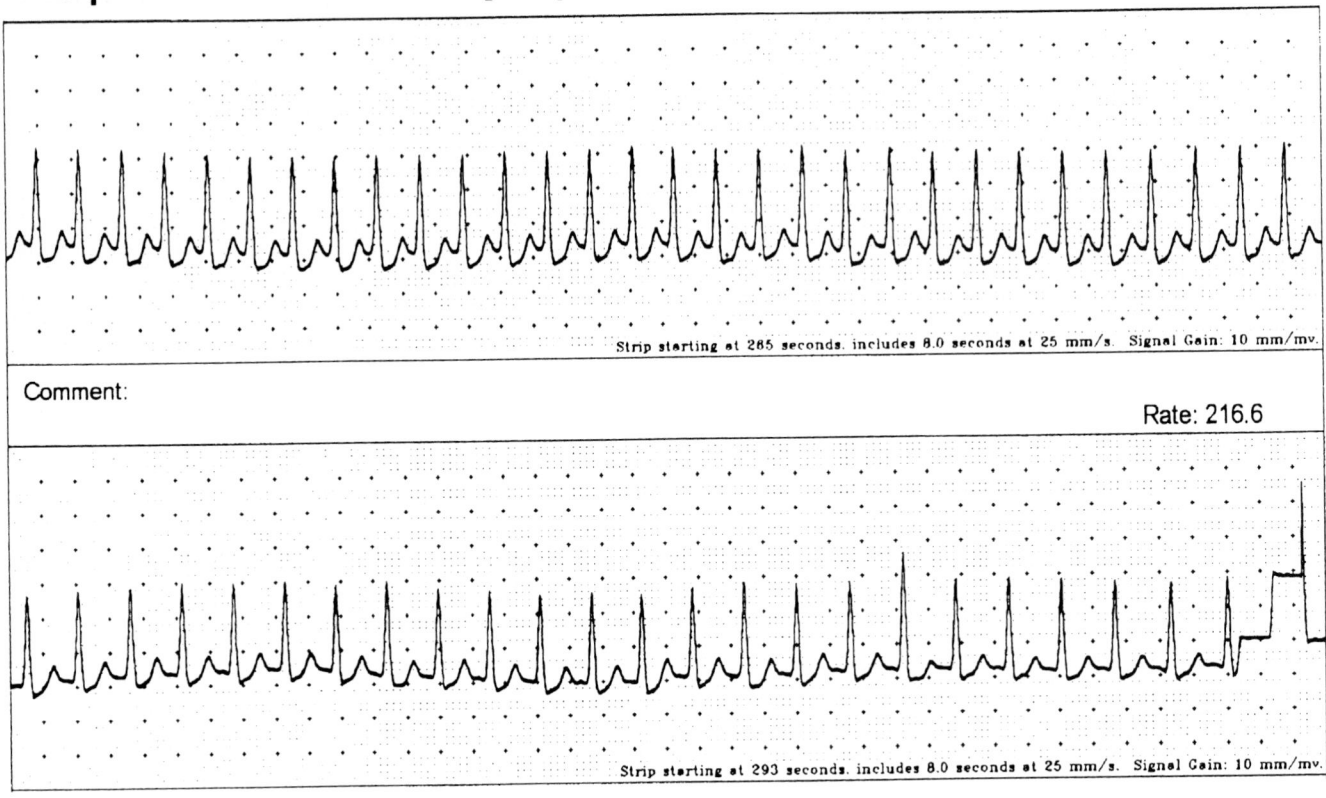

Strip starting at 285 seconds. includes 8.0 seconds at 25 mm/s.   Signal Gain: 10 mm/mv.

Comment:

Rate: 216.6

Strip starting at 293 seconds. includes 8.0 seconds at 25 mm/s.   Signal Gain: 10 mm/mv.

FIGURE 41-1. An episode of rapid paroxysmal supraventricular tachycardia captured with a handheld event recorder during a typical period of symptoms.

logue signal into a digital signal, and analyze the data in terms of maximal and minimal rates, RR intervals, and changes in RR intervals. This instrument differs in that the actual ECG has not been recorded on tape; only the histogram has been stored. Selected brief segments of the patient's ECG can also be stored, however. Microcomputers are available that can analyze electronic data over periods of up to several days.

【 】 EVENT RECORDERS

This alternative method records not continuously, but only when the patient activates the device. There are two basic types of event recorders, which differ on the basis of their memory—postevent recorders and preevent recorders. In the postevent recorder, without memory, the patient usually wears the recorder continuously, activating it when symptoms appear. The device does not record the ECG until it is activated. Alternatively, the patient may carry a miniature solid-state recorder with which the symptomatic rhythm can be recorded simply by placing the unit on the precordium or, in some cases, on the wrist. The recorded data are stored in memory until the patient submits the information either directly or transtelephonically to an ECG recorder. With a preevent recorder, employing a memory loop, the rhythm is monitored continuously. Patients activate the unit when they experience symptoms and the loop recorder is capable of recording ECG several seconds or minutes before and after a recognized event; the number of events that can be recorded and the allotment of recording time prior to and after activation of the unit are programmable.

The limitations of traditional event recorders include their inability to record asymptomatic arrhythmias, inability for the patient to transmit specific symptoms with each event, and missed events be-

cause of patient error in activating the device.[2] A newer mobile cardiac outpatient telemetry system consists of a three-electrode, two-channel sensor transmitting wirelessly to a portable monitor, which analyzes and stores ECG data.[4] Significant arrhythmias, whether symptomatic or asymptomatic, are transmitted automatically by the wireless network to a central monitoring station and analyzed by trained personnel. In a study of 100 patients using this system, a clinically defined significant arrhythmia was found in 51 patients, in 25 of whom (49 percent) the arrhythmia was asymptomatic.[4]

【 】 IMPLANTABLE RECORDERS

A miniaturized event recorder can be implanted subcutaneously on the precordium. It can be manually activated by the patient to record an ECG when symptoms occur, and high and low heart rate limit parameters can be programmed for the device to record events automatically. These devices are particularly useful to capture events that occur relatively infrequently—for example, a few times per year.[5] Event recording is also provided by some newer-generation pacemakers and implantable cardioverter/defibrillators that automatically recognize and record abnormal rhythms.

【 】 REAL-TIME MONITORING

These devices acquire data and transmit the ECG information directly and transtelephonically, in real time, without recording the data in the unit. The patient's ECG can be transmitted daily, or even multiple times each day, to a recording station. Routine transtelephonic pacemaker evaluations use such systems.

TABLE 41–1

Types of Electrocardiographic Recording Instruments

TYPE	RECORDING	SCANNING	TRANSMITTING
Continuous			
Analogue	All ECG complexes, "full disclosure"	Technician with computer assistance, templating, area determination, and superimposition	None
Digital—continuous recording	All ECG complexes, "full disclosure"	Technician with computer assistance, templating, area determination, and superimposition	Transtelephonic
Digital—real-time analysis	Computer analysis of ECG and selected ECG printouts	Real time by microprocessor with retrospective technician editing	None
Event Recorder			
"Postevent," nonlooping, without memory Handheld or worn	ECG, selected by patient activation	Direct visualization	Transtelephonic
"Preevent," looping, with memory, monitor worn with attached electrodes	ECG, selected by patient activation, with memory of preevent	Direct visualization	Transtelephonic
Continuous mobile outpatient telemetry system	ECG, selected by patient or automatic	Direct visualization; technician with computer assistance	Transtelephonic
Implantable Devices			
Subcutaneous, implanted digital recorder	ECG, selected by patient activation with memory of preevent or automatic	Direct visualization	Direct telemetry
Automatic electronic sensor in ICD or pacemaker	ECG, when activated by ICD discharge or recognized by sensor in pacemaker, with memory	Direct visualization of analysis or ECG	Direct telemetry
Real Time			
Real-time transtelephonic monitoring	ECG at central monitoring station—no recording at device	Direct visualization	Transtelephonic

SCANNING AND ANALYSIS TECHNIQUES

The recording can be analyzed by scanning the tape or digital record at high speed, by printing it out directly, or—as in the case of microcomputers—by processing during the recording and printing out the analysis at the end of sampling. Scanning techniques include technician-dependent analysis, in which a technician interprets the cardiac rhythm as it is played back at high speed on an oscilloscope at 30 to 240 times the speed of the actual event. One technique superimposes each QRS complex on the immediately preceding complex so that identical QRS contours present as a stationary image. Variations in QRS contour then become readily apparent. A computer can be interfaced with the scanner to quantitate the data even more accurately. The playback analysis can occur at up to 240 times the normal rate. Electronic analyzers and scanners, can be programmed to recognize the patient's own QRS complex template and then to recognize any deviation from normal. The computer program can provide summaries of heart rates, heart rate variability, frequency of premature atrial or ventricular extrasystoles, coupling intervals, arrhythmias, and variations in QRS, ST, QT, or T-wave pattern during any time period. When arrhythmias or pattern changes are detected, an automatic ECG printout can be triggered.

SELECTION OF DEVICE AND DURATION OF RECORDING

The selection of a long-term ECG recording system depends on the individual patient's needs.[2-5] If a precise count of ectopy is required, a continuous recorder with computer-based analysis is essential. If the purpose of the recording is to detect episodic arrhythmic events such as ventricular tachycardia or atrial fibrillation, an event recorder would be an excellent choice. An event recorder provides an opportunity to monitor over prolonged periods of time and is of benefit to the patient whose symptoms do not occur on a daily basis. When the goal is to correlate the patient's ECG pattern with symptoms that are very infrequent (e.g., every few months) an implantable loop recorder may be the best choice. A preevent loop recorder is needed for evaluation of symptoms of brief duration (such as syncope without warning) and allows the patient to activate the recorder after the event. The monitoring period must be extended sufficiently to incorporate a symptomatic period, which may be hours to months. For assessment of ventricular rate control for a patient with atrial fibrillation, a 24-hour ECG monitoring period is usually sufficient. However, continuous outpatient telemetry monitoring,[4,6] performed for 1–2 weeks, may be advantageous in the titration of oral medications (e.g., β blockers, calcium channel

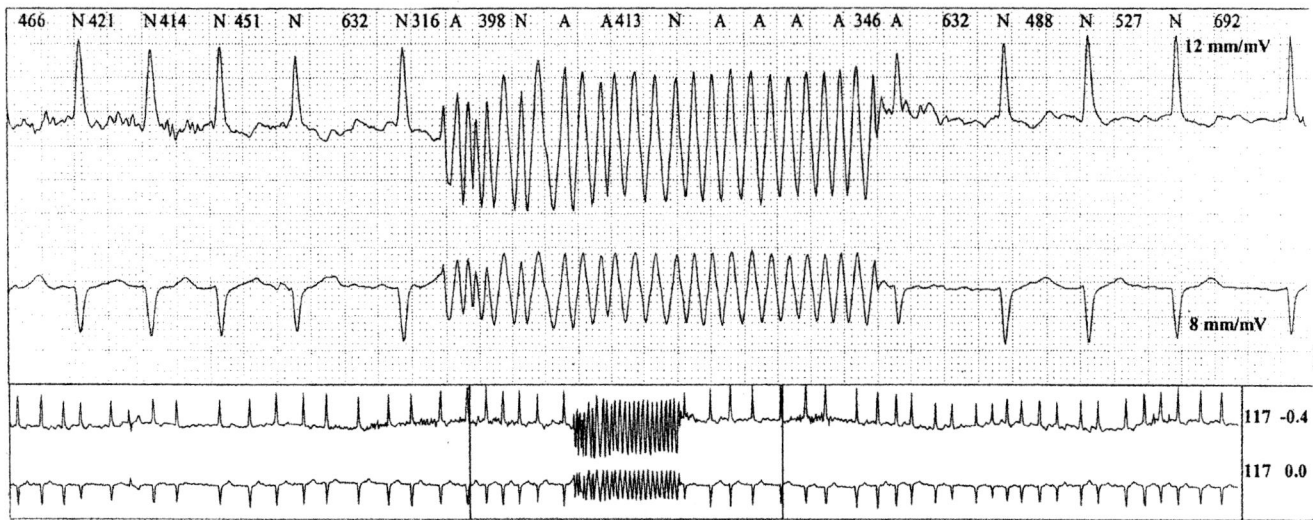

FIGURE 41–2. Artifact recorded from a Holter monitor mimicking ventricular tachycardia most likely caused by a loose electrode. The artifacts are distinguished from true ventricular tachycardia by their appearance (spike-like features), non-physiologic short coupling intervals with normal QRS complexes, and presence of normal QRS complexes that can be measured "marching through" the artifacts.

blockers, digoxin) in patients with atrial fibrillation and uncontrolled ventricular rates.

ARTIFACTS AND ERRORS

Artifacts registered during prolonged ECG recording have mimicked virtually every variety of cardiac arrhythmias and have led to misdiagnosis and inappropriate treatment.[7,8] Artifacts can occur at different levels of the recording process. *Patient-related* artifacts may result from involuntary muscle contractions (e.g., tremors, rigors, hiccoughs) and body movements (e.g., changing body position, brushing teeth, combing hair). The Parkinson disease tremor often has a frequency of 4 to 5 per second and when captured on an ECG, can be mistaken for atrial flutter or ventricular tachycardia.

A second type of artifact may occur during *data recording and processing*. Recording system artifacts can occur for a variety of reasons, including loose skin–electrode contact, lead fractures, processing errors, altered tape speed in the recorder and incomplete erasure of a previous recording. The most common artifact

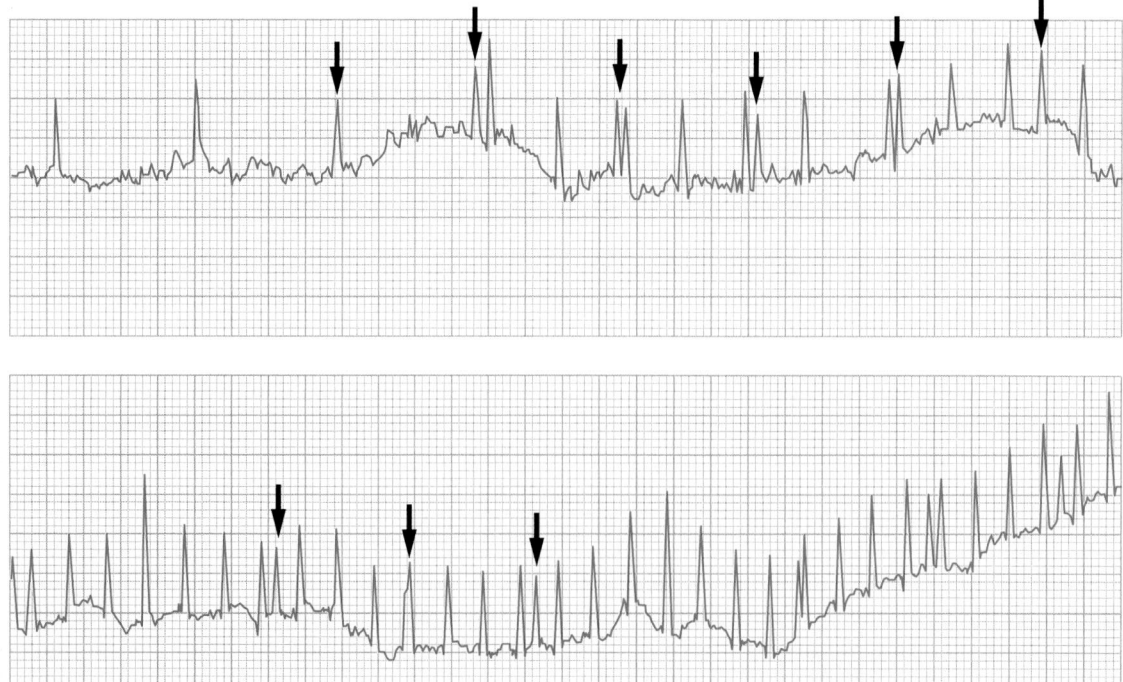

FIGURE 41–3. Artifacts mimicking supraventricular tachycardia. Nonphysiologic short coupling intervals are apparent between artifacts and the native QRS complexes. Note the undulating ECG baseline. The first three QRS complexes on the top panel have a cycle length of 760 ms. The *arrows* point to native QRS complexes "marching through" the artifacts at similar cycle lengths.

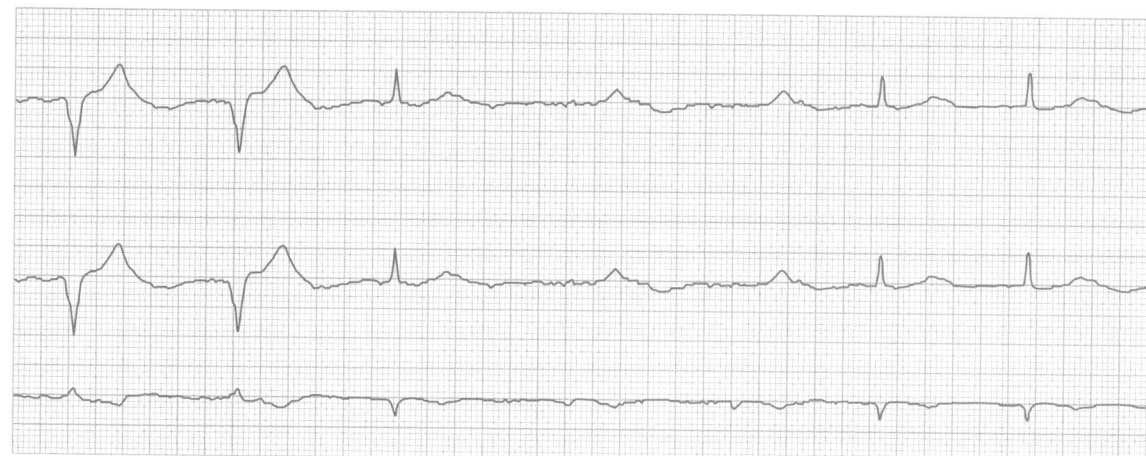

FIGURE 41–4. High frequency dropout. QRS complexes are "dropped out" from the fourth and fifth beats. Presence of T-wave recordings for these beats indicates the mechanism of the "pause" in the rhythm to be a recording artifact caused by high-frequency signal dropout. The similar T-wave morphology of the beats without an obvious preceding QRS complex compared with the narrow QRS complexes, and more than one ECG lead showing the same findings make this unlikely to be caused by QRS axis changes resulting in isoelectric recordings.

probably is that resulting from a loose electrode (Figs. 41–2 and 41–3) or mechanical "stimulation" of the electrode. High-frequency signal dropout (Fig. 41–4) or generation of a high-frequency signal mimicking pacing artifacts can occur from processing errors, especially in digital systems. Failure of either the battery or the motor of the recorder generally results in a slowing of the tape speed as the ECG is recorded. When played back, the heart rate appears fast, mimicking a tachycardia (Fig. 41–5). The interpreter may be alerted to the artifact by the concomitant shortening of all ECG intervals (PR, QRS, QT, and RR). Conversely, transient slowing or sticking of the tape during playback may mimic bradycardia, atrioventricular (AV) block and intraventricular conduction delays (Fig. 41–6). Recording an ECG on a previously used tape that is incompletely erased can result in the simultaneous registration of two ECGs and possible misinterpretation of a "parasystolic" ectopic rhythm (Fig. 41–7). The artifact can be identified by "looking through" longer rhythm strips where nonphysiologic QRS coupling intervals may become apparent. Rare clinical scenarios where this can occur without being an artifact are Siamese twins and "piggyback heart transplantations" where two independent cardiac rhythms are simultaneously recorded.

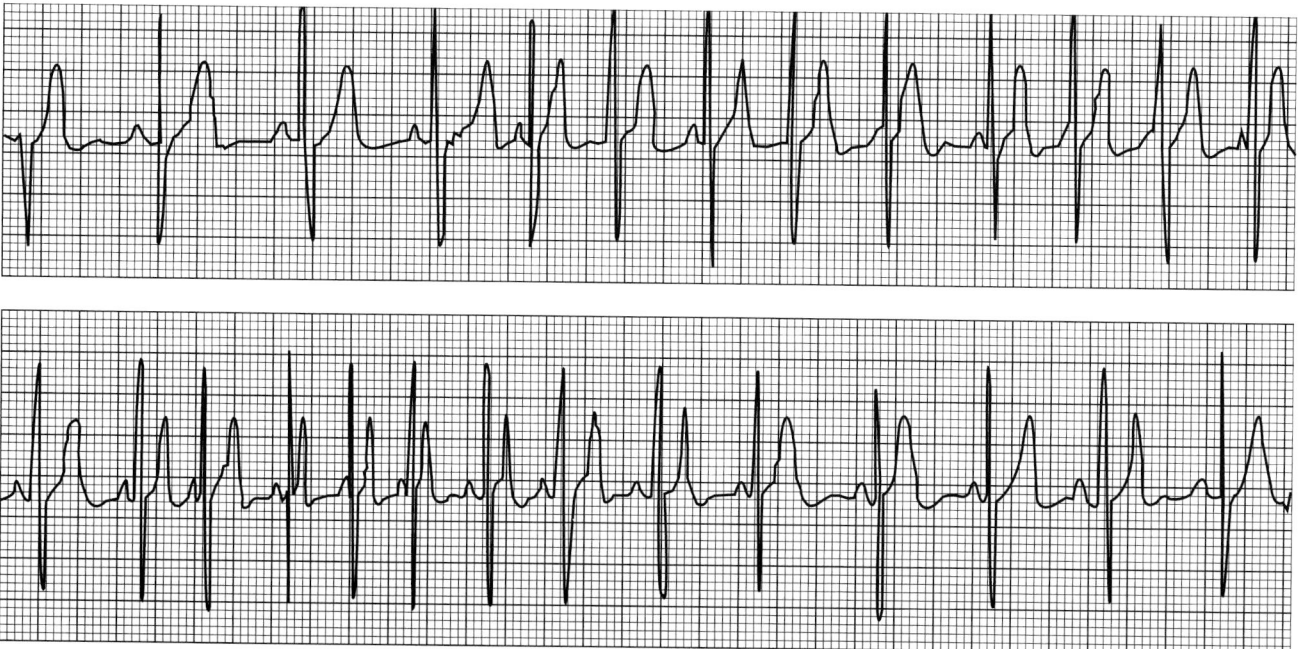

FIGURE 41–5. Deceleration of tape during recording. Supraventricular tachycardia is simulated toward the end of the top and beginning of the second trace as the tape, which transiently slowed as a result of battery failure during recording, was played back on recording paper at proper speed. Note the foreshortening of the duration of the P wave, PR interval, QRS complex, and QT interval.

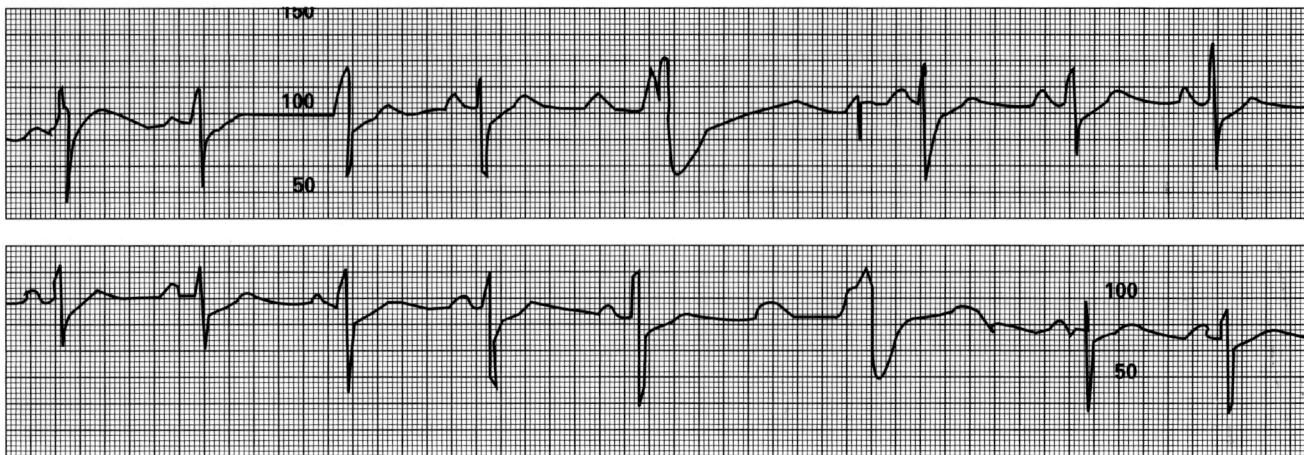

FIGURE 41-6. Deceleration of tape during playback. Slowing or sticking of the tape during playback spreads out the P wave, PR interval, and QRS complex to resemble sinus deceleration or transient atrioventricular or intraventricular conduction delay (fifth complex in top trace; sixth complex in bottom trace).

External interferences also offer a very common cause for ECG artifacts. "Noise" can occur in the recordings because of external sources such as 60 Hz from alternating current or electromagnetic interference from mechanical devices. Simultaneous use of a variety of medical equipment (e.g., infusion pumps, transcutaneous or implanted nerve stimulators) may result in ECG artifacts mimicking atrial or ventricular arrhythmias. Implanted or external nerve stimulators in some patients can result in an atrial flutter like appearance, but can be distinguished by its rate, "spike-like" nature of the artifacts, and appearance of sinus P waves in some recording leads.

Most of these artifacts are readily identifiable from their characteristic appearances. One should "look through" the artifacts for normal background ECG appearance. Quite often QRS complexes can be identified and "marched out" at cycle lengths similar to the sinus rhythm cycle lengths before the beginning of the artifacts. Look for high-frequency (spike-like activity) or low-frequency signals inconsistent with the normal PQRST waves. Nonphysiologic (e.g., <140 milliseconds) coupling intervals between QRS complexes and unstable ECG baselines are sometimes more apparent at the beginning or the ending of the recorded artifacts. Lack of clinical correlation to an

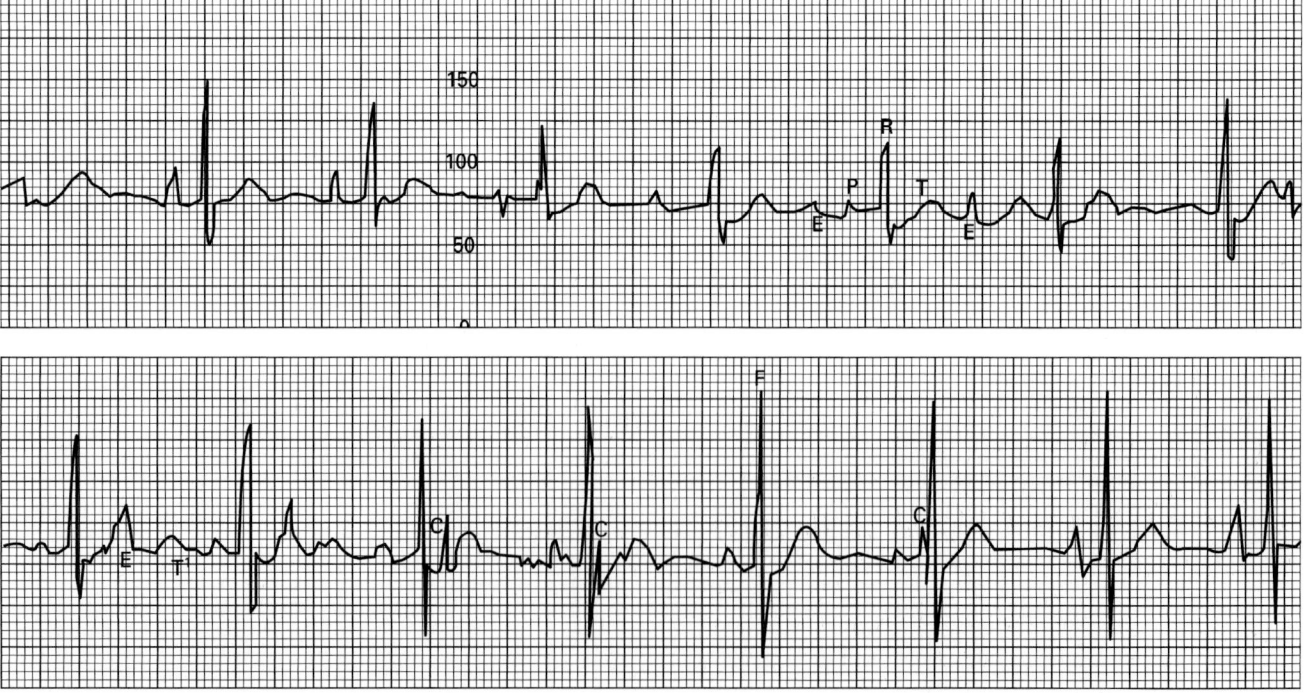

FIGURE 41-7. Incomplete erasure of tape. Two independent ventricular rhythms are identified: a larger QRS, labeled *R*, whose P wave and T wave are also labeled, and a smaller QRS, considered "ectopic" and labeled *E*; its T wave is labeled *T*. Alternatively, ectopic complex E may be misinterpreted to represent a parasystolic rhythm even fusing with complex R at F. The very short coupling intervals (*C*) preclude this possibility and indicate that the ECG record of one patient is superimposed on that of another.

identified "arrhythmia" may be a useful feature, but beware that some serious cardiac arrhythmias can be asymptomatic. Ultimately, the keys to identifying artifacts are the clinician's familiarity with the various types of artifacts and the careful analysis of the ECG.

REFERENCES

1. Holter NJ. New method for heart studies: Continuous electrocardiography of active subjects over long periods is now practical. *Science* 1961;134:1214–1220.
2. Fogel R, Evans J, Prystowsky E. Utility and cost of event recorders in the diagnosis of palpitations, presyncope and syncope. *Am J Cardiol* 1997;79:207–208.
3. ACC/AHA. Guidelines for ambulatory electrocardiography: a report of the American College of Cardiology/American Heart Association Task Force on Practice Guidelines. *J Am Coll Cardiol* 1999;34:(3)917–948.
4. Joshi AK, Kowey PR, Prystowsky EN, et al. First experience with a mobile cardiac outpatient telemetry (MCOT) system for the diagnosis and management of cardiac arrhythmias. *Am J Cardiol* 2005;95:878–881.
5. Krahn A, Klein G, Yee R, Takle-Newhouse T. Use of an extended monitoring strategy in patients with problematic syncope. *Circulation* 1999;99(3):406–410.
6. Prystowsky EN. Assessment of rhythm and rate control in patients with atrial fibrillation. *J Cardiovasc Electrophysiol* 2006;17:S7–S10.
7. Krasnow AZ, Bloomfield DK. Artifacts in portable electrocardiographic monitoring. *Am Heart J* 1976;91:349–357.
8. Knight BP, Pelosi F, Michaud GF, et al. Clinical consequences of electrocardiographic artifact mimicking ventricular tachycardia. *N Engl J Med* 1999;341:1270–1274.

APPENDIX 41–1

ACC/AHA Guidelines for Ambulatory Electrocardiography

A. INDICATIONS FOR AMBULATORY ECG (AECG) TO ASSESS SYMPTOMS POSSIBLY RELATED TO RHYTHM DISTURBANCES

Class I
1. Patients with unexplained syncope, near syncope, or episodic dizziness in whom the cause is not obvious
2. Patients with unexplained recurrent palpitation

Class IIb
3. Patients with episodic shortness of breath, chest pain, or fatigue that is not otherwise explained
4. Patients with neurologic events when transient atrial fibrillation or flutter is suspected
5. Patients with symptoms such as syncope, near syncope, episodic dizziness, or palpitation in whom a probable cause other than an arrhythmia has been identified but in whom symptoms persist despite treatment of this other cause

Class III
6. Patients with symptoms such as syncope, near syncope, episodic dizziness, or palpitation in whom other causes have been identified by history, physical examination, or laboratory tests
7. Patients with cerebrovascular accidents, without other evidence of arrhythmia

B. INDICATIONS FOR AECG ARRHYTHMIA DETECTION TO ASSESS RISK FOR FUTURE CARDIAC EVENTS IN PATIENTS WITHOUT SYMPTOMS FROM ARRHYTHMIA

Class IIb
1. Postmyocardial infarction (MI) patients with LV dysfunction (ejection fraction ≥40%)
2. Patients with congestive heart failure (CHF)
3. Patients with idiopathic hypertrophic cardiomyopathy

Class III
4. Patients who have sustained myocardial contusion
5. Systemic hypertensive patients with LV hypertrophy
6. Post-MI patients with normal LV function
7. Preoperative arrhythmia evaluation of patients for noncardiac surgery
8. Patients with sleep apnea
9. Patients with valvular heart disease

C. INDICATIONS FOR MEASUREMENT OF HEART RATE VARIABILITY (HRV) TO ACCESS RISK FOR FUTURE CARDIAC EVENTS IN PATIENTS WITHOUT SYMPTOMS FROM ARRHYTHMIA

Class IIb
1. Post-MI patients with LV dysfunction
2. Patients with CHF
3. Patients with idiopathic hypertrophic cardiomyopathy

Class III
4. Post-MI patients with normal LV function
5. Diabetic subjects to evaluate for diabetic neuropathy
6. Patients with rhythm disturbances that preclude HRV analysis (i.e., atrial fibrillation)

(continued)

APPENDIX 41–1

ACC/AHA Guidelines for Ambulatory Electrocardiography (*continued*)

D. INDICATIONS FOR AECG TO ASSESS ANTIARRHYTHMIC THERAPY

Class I

1. To assess antiarrhythmic drug response in individuals in whom baseline frequency of arrhythmia has been characterized as reproducible and of sufficient frequency to permit analysis

Class IIa

2. To detect proarrhythmic responses to antiarrhythmic therapy in patients at high risk

Class IIb

3. To assess rate control during atrial fibrillation
4. To document recurrent or asymptomatic nonsustained arrhythmias during therapy in the outpatient setting

E. INDICATIONS FOR AECG TO ASSESS PACEMAKER AND INTRACARDIAC CARDIOVERTER-DEFIBRILLATOR (ICD) FUNCTION

Class I

1. Evaluation of frequent symptoms of palpitation, syncope, or near syncope to assess device function to exclude myopotential inhibition and pacemaker-mediated tachycardia and to assist in the programming of enhanced features such as rate responsivity and automatic mode switching
2. Evaluation of suspected component failure or malfunction when device interrogation is not definitive in establishing a diagnosis
3. To assess the response to adjunctive pharmacological therapy in patients receiving frequent ICD therapy

Class IIb

4. Evaluation of immediate postoperative pacemaker function after pacemaker or ICD implantation as an alternative or adjunct to continuous telemetric monitoring
5. Evaluation of the rate of supraventricular arrhythmias in patients with implanted defibrillators

Class III

6. Assessment of ICD/pacemaker malfunction when device interrogation, ECG, or other available data (chest radiograph and so forth) are sufficient to establish an underlying cause/diagnosis
7. Routine followup in asymptomatic patients

F. INDICATIONS FOR AECG FOR ISCHEMIA MONITORING

Class IIa

1. Patients with suspected variant angina

Class IIb

2. Evaluation of patients with chest pain who cannot exercise
3. Preoperative evaluation for vascular surgery of patient who cannot exercise
4. Patients with known coronary artery disease (CAD) and atypical chest pain syndrome

Class III

5. Initial evaluation of patients with chest pain who are able to exercise
6. Routine screening of asymptomatic subjects

G. INDICATIONS FOR AECG MONITORING IN PEDIATRIC PATIENTS

Class I

1. Syncope, near syncope, or dizziness in patients with recognized cardiac disease, previously documented arrhythmia, or pacemaker dependency
2. Syncope or near syncope associated with exertion when the cause is not established by other methods
3. Evaluation of patients with hypertrophic or dilated cardiomyopathies
4. Evaluation of possible or documented long QT syndromes
5. Palpitations in the patient with prior surgery for congenital heart disease and significant residual hemodynamic abnormalities
6. Evaluation of antiarrhythmic drug efficacy during rapid somatic growth
7. Asymptomatic congenital complete AV block, nonpaced

APPENDIX 41-1

ACC/AHA Guidelines for Ambulatory Electrocardiography *(continued)*

Class IIa

8. Syncope, near syncope, or sustained palpitation in the absence of a reasonable explanation and where there is not overt clinical evidence of heart disease
9. Evaluation of cardiac rhythm after initiation of an antiarrhythmic therapy, particularly when associated with a significant proarrhythmic potential
10. Evaluation of cardiac rhythm after transient AV block associated with heart surgery or catheter ablation
11. Evaluation of rate-responsive or physiologic pacing function in symptomatic patients

Class IIb

12. Evaluation of asymptomatic patients with prior surgery for congenital heart disease, particularly when there are either significant or residual hemodynamic abnormalities, or a significant incidence of late postoperative arrhythmias
13. Evaluation of the young patient (<3 years old) with a prior tachyarrhythmia to determine if unrecognized episodes of the arrhythmia recur
14. Evaluation of the patient with a suspected incessant atrial tachycardia
15. Complex ventricular ectopy on ECG or exercise test

Class III

16. Syncope, near syncope, or dizziness when a noncardiac cause is present
17. Chest pain without clinical evidence of heart disease
18. Routine evaluation of asymptomatic individuals for athletic clearance
19. Brief palpitation in the absence of heart disease
20. Asymptomatic Wolff-Parkinson-White syndrome

SOURCE: ACC/AHA Guidelines for ambulatory electrocardiography.[3]

CHAPTER (42)

Techniques of Electrophysiologic Evaluation

Masood Akhtar

The recording of intracavitary electrocardiographic signals and various forms of pacing programs have experienced enormous growth during the past three decades. Recordings of intracardiac signals from the region of the His bundle, initially made by Scherlag et al,[1] were rapidly applied to clinical problems including atrioventricular (AV) blocks and supraventricular and ventricular tachyarrhythmias.[1–10] Such recordings were then complemented by pacing to unmask sinus node dysfunction and AV conduction abnormalities, as well as to initiate supraventricular tachycardias (SVTs).[3–8] Intracardiac electrophysiologic studies (EPSs) have since been found to be useful for a variety of cardiac arrhythmias, including sinus node dysfunction, intraventricular and AV conduction disturbances, SVTs, ventricular tachycardias (VTs), preexcitation syndromes, and atrial and ventricular fibrillation (VF). Such studies are now also employed as a prelude to correction of various arrhythmias and conduction defects. This chapter addresses recording and pacing techniques and their clinical usefulness.[9–12]

TECHNIQUES OF INTRACARDIAC ELECTROPHYSIOLOGIC STUDIES

The exact type of electrical signal recordings, specific equipment used, and pacing protocol depend on the nature of the clinical problem, the type of electrophysiologic assessment, and the anticipated course of action. Routine cardiac EPSs are performed while patients are in a nonsedated postabsorptive state.[13] Although some degree of sedation is advisable in apprehensive patients, the use of drugs that may alter the properties of the cardiac conduction sys-

tem should be avoided. Antiarrhythmic drugs are usually—but not always—stopped prior to these studies. In selected cases, antiarrhythmic drugs may be continued if a clinical event occurred while the patient was on a specific agent.

The typical electrode catheters used for both recording and cardiac stimulation are multipolar (sizes varying from 4 to 8 French [Fr]). Catheters can be inserted via peripheral veins such as the antecubital, femoral, subclavian, or internal jugular veins. For most electrophysiologic testing, the catheter is placed in the high right atrium, at the His bundle (Fig. 42–1), or at the right bundle-branch region across the tricuspid valve and right ventricular apex, septum, or outflow. For accessory pathways or AV junctional tachycardias, a catheter is placed in the region of the coronary sinus. Heparin may be given as needed. For a routine study, left-sided heart catheterization is seldom necessary. In patients with VT and/or left-sided accessory pathways and atrial fibrillation, however, this is performed for diagnostic or therapeutic purposes. More recently, transseptal catheterization via the right atrium to get access to pulmonary veins in atrial fibrillation ablation is invaluable. As the knowledge regarding the origins of arrhythmias has grown, catheters with special designs (e.g., lasso, baskets) have emerged and newer locations are being increasingly used. Continuous heparinization is desirable for left-heart catheterization to avoid thromboembolic complications.

▌❩ ELECTROPHYSIOLOGIC RECORDINGS

Once the electrode catheters are placed appropriately, the connections are made via a junction box and isolation units to prevent excess current in the event of random electrical surges. Electrograms are displayed simultaneously on a multichannel oscilloscopic recorder. In addition to the intracardiac signals, several unfiltered surface electrocardiographic leads (i.e., X, Y, and Z, or leads I and II, or aVF and V_1) are recorded. Although appropriately placed electrode catheters will record desired signals at any filtering frequency, filter settings between 30 to 40 and 500 Hz are best suited for sharp intracardiac signals such as those from the His bundle and accessory pathways (Fig. 42–2). Undesirable low-frequency signals can be reduced by a high-pass filter setting of more than 50 to 100 Hz. On the other hand, 60-cycle interference can be eliminated with a low-pass filter setting at 50 Hz. All equipment is reliably grounded.

The main value of intracardiac/electrocardiographic tracings is the timing of electrical events and determining the direction of impulse propagation. To acquire true local electrical activity, a bipolar electrogram with an interelectrode distance of less than 1 cm is desirable. When unipolar electrograms are obtained, a rapid intrinsic deflection will identify a point of local activation. For routine intracardiac electrocardiographic studies, unipolar electrograms provide a relatively limited advantage over bipolar signals, thus the latter are more often used. For patients with atrial fibrillation, which seems primarily a left atrial arrhythmia originating in the pulmonary veins, left atrial catheterization is necessary.

The foregoing description relates to the standard diagnostic invasive EPS. In other clinical situations, different types of diagnostic methods are employed. For instance, during intraoperative mapping, direct placement of electrodes over the epicardium or endocardium is necessary to get appropriate signals for identifying the precise origin and route of impulse propagation.[14] These electrodes can be in the form of either handheld probes or plaques that can be placed or sutured over the myocardium. Socks and balloons incorporating several electrodes can also be used for epicardial and endocardial mapping techniques, respectively.[15,16] All electrical signals can be recorded on either a disk or frequency-modulated tape for permanent storage. Catheterization into the pericardial space using an epicardial approach has also been used to ablate certain types of tachycardias more easily accessed in this manner.[17]

More recently, several other types of mapping and recording equipment have emerged to locate the origin of cardiac arrhythmias more accurately. Two of the systems likely to find clinical utility in the mapping of arrhythmic origins are (1) nonfluoroscopic electromagnetic endocardial mapping (CARTO, Biosense [Cordis Webster], Marlton, NJ) and (2) noncontact mapping (EnSite, Endocardial Solutions, Saint Paul, MN).

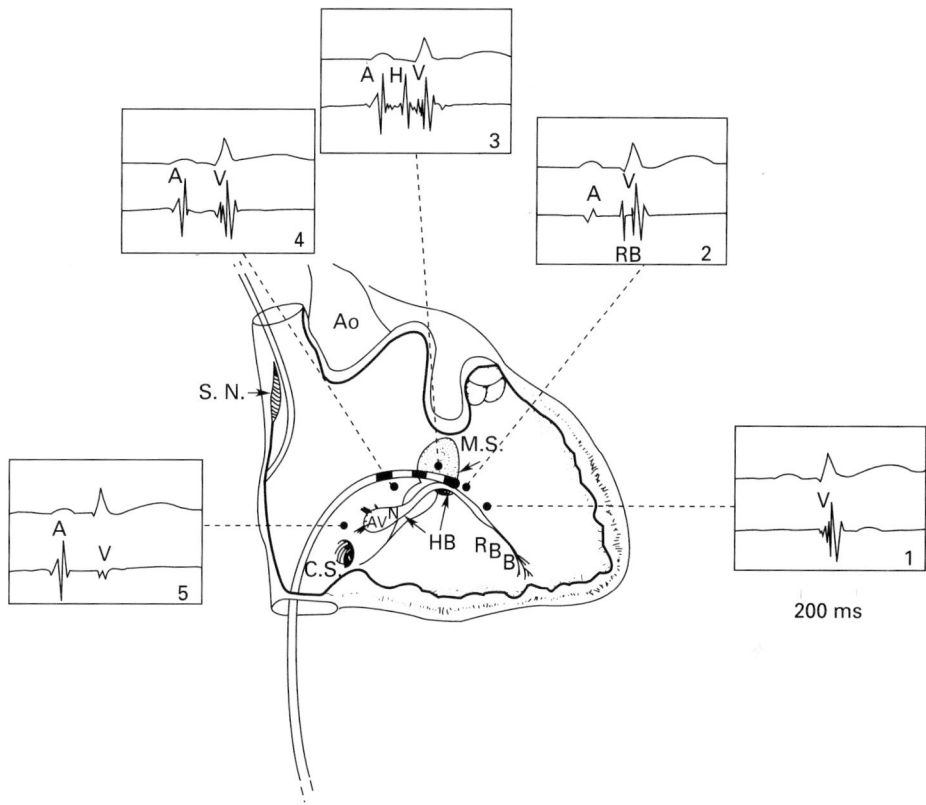

FIGURE 42–1. Intracardiac recordings from the specialized conduction system in the atrioventricular (AV) junction. The recording of various electrograms along the right side of the interventricular septum with gradual withdrawal of the catheter across the tricuspid valve is shown. The intracardiac recordings are labeled. Numbers 1 through 5 refer to intracardiac location of catheters along with corresponding electrogram. A, atrial deflection; Ao, aorta; AVN, atrioventricular node; CS, coronary sinus; H and RB, His and right bundle potentials; HB, His bundle; MS, membranous septum; RBB, right bundle branch; SN, sinus node; V, ventricular deflection. *Source: From Gallagher JJ, Damato AN. Technique of recording His bundle activity in man. In: Grossman W, ed. Cardiac Catheterization and Angiography. Philadelphia: Lea & Febiger, 1980:283. Reproduced with permission from the publisher and authors.*

The Biosense CARTO System

The CARTO system consists of a magnetic field generator locator pad placed under the patient table, a sensor-mounted catheter and a reference catheter placed intracardially, a mapping system, and a graphic computer.[18] The catheter tip allows orientation in relation to the reference signal. The accuracy of catheter tip position is within a millimeter of arrhythmia location in this low magnetic field. By moving the sensor sequentially, one can generate a three-dimensional (3D) activation map. By color coding, both the earliest and the latest directions of electrical activation can be recorded. Once the initial fluoroscopy-guided placement of reference catheter and other catheters is satisfactory, several points are acquired. A 3D map is generated, and sensor-mounted catheters are manipulated further without the help of fluoroscopy. Figure 42–3 shows a typical map generated during this technique.

The EnSite 3000 System

Noncontact mapping can be done using the Endocardial Solutions EnSite 3000 system.[19] This is a relatively new endocardial 3D mapping system that takes a different approach to such mapping (Fig. 42–4). Like the CARTO system, the EnSite 3000 system also makes use of an amplifier and computer system with custom software. The EnSite catheter uses a balloon design with a 64-elec-

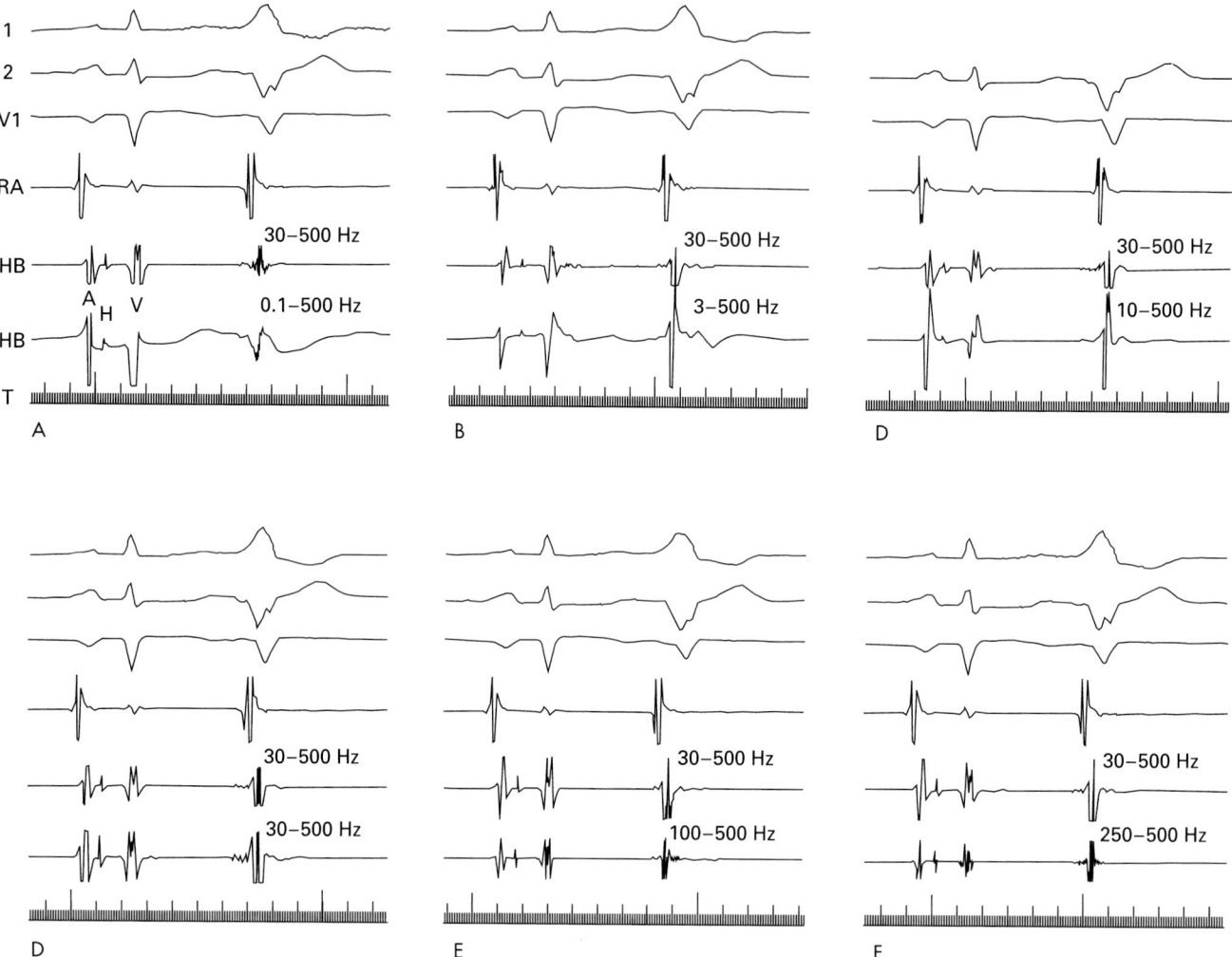

FIGURE 42–2. Effects of various filtering frequencies on the morphologic appearance of intracardiac electrograms **A** through **F**. The tracings from top to bottom are electrocardiographic leads I, II, V₁, right atrial (RA), two His bundle (HB) electrograms, and time (T) line. Similar abbreviations are used in subsequent figures and tracings. In each panel, the first beat is of sinus origin and is followed by a spontaneous ventricular premature beat. The top HB, RA, and RV are filtered at 30 to 500 Hz (i.e., the usual filtering frequencies). The bottom HB tracing shows the effect of various filtering frequencies on the appearance. The low-frequency signals are mostly eliminated at high-bandpass filter frequency settings above 10 Hz (**C**). The low-bandpass filter settings above 500 Hz generally do not have a significant effect on the intracardiac electrogram appearance. It should be pointed out that the high-bandpass setting reduces the overall magnitude of the electrogram, necessitating an increase in amplification. It should also be noted that the HB deflection can be clearly identified at all frequencies depicted. *Source: From Akhtar M.*[13] *Reproduced with permission from the publisher and authors.*

trode array arranged over the outside of the balloon. This balloon is positioned in the center of the chamber and does not come in contact with the walls of the chamber being mapped. Employing data from the 64-electrode-array catheter, the computer uses sophisticated algorithms to compute an *inverse solution* to determine the activation sequence on the endocardial surface. Data from all points in the chamber are acquired simultaneously.

Because data from the entire chamber are collected simultaneously with the EnSite 3000 system, it can be used to map nonsustained rhythms such as premature atrial complexes, irregular rhythms such as atrial fibrillation or polymorphic VT, and rhythms that are not hemodynamically stable. The system is highly useful for identifying focal arrhythmias (Fig. 42–4) and atrial flutter.

The Navex System

Further improvements in technology will enable the operator an anatomic view of the cardiac chambers noninvasively. Navex is a

step in the right direction. Navex (Endocardial Solutions, St. Paul, MN) is a method for catheter tracking and location, recording ablation lesion location, and cardiac chamber anatomy reconstruction.[20–22] Based on the LocaLisa (Medtronic Inc., Minneapolis, MN) technology, this system combines catheter location and tracking features of LocaLisa with the ability to create an anatomic model of the cardiac chamber using only a single, conventional electrophysiology catheter and skin patches (Fig. 42–5). This approach may be useful in treating certain types of arrhythmias where the ablation strategy is primarily anatomically based; it could possibly be combined with other technologies for treating complex arrhythmias.

Current Improvements in the New Mapping System

One of the areas producers of cardiac mapping systems have targeted for improvement is in the reproduction of the patient-specific cardiac chamber anatomy. This includes importing scan data from an imaging modality such as computed tomography or magnetic resonance imaging into the mapping application. Segmented 3D models of the cardiac chamber, can then be imported directly into the mapping application and synchronized, or registered. The end goal of registration is to provide the operator with real-time catheter location and tracking along with a highly accurate, patient specific anatomic model of the cardiac chamber undergoing mapping. Importing image data from CT or MRI is now possible using a process known as digital image fusion.[23,24]

【 】 PROGRAMMED ELECTRICAL STIMULATION

After satisfactory placement of the electrode catheters, patches, or other forms of recording equipment, baseline recordings are made and programmed stimulation is initiated from various cardiac chambers. For ventricular stimulation, the pacing sites are typically the right ventricular apex and outflow tract. Endocardial left ventricular (LV) pacing is seldom used, but when it is done, it is used for tachycardia induction. A variety of pacing programs can be used, depending on the nature of the underlying arrhythmic problem under investigation. At least two formats of pacing protocol are common. The first is in-

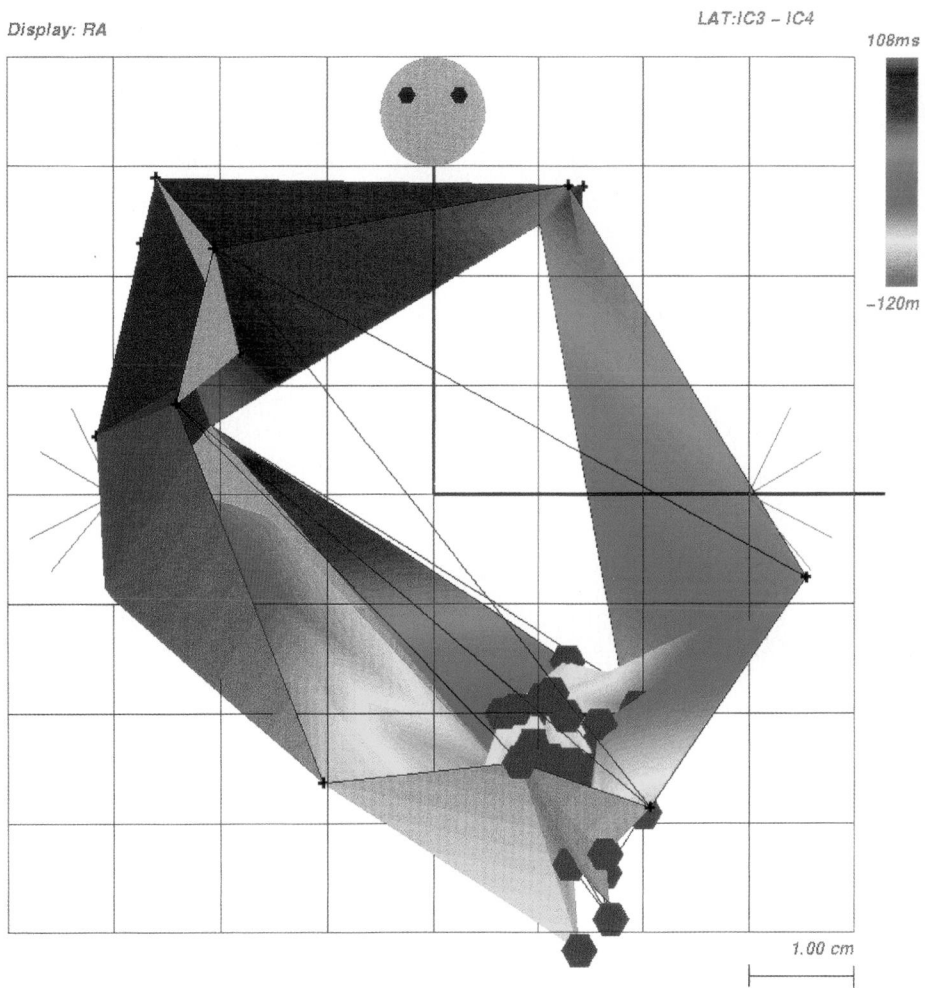

Display: RA

LAT: IC3 – IC4

108ms

–120m

1.00 cm

FIGURE 42–3. Anterior–posterior view of the right atrium during typical, inferior vena cava (IVC)–tricuspid valve annulus isthmus-dependent atrial flutter using the Biosense CARTO system. The red shows the earliest activation with respect to the timing reference (typically the proximal coronary sinus recording), and the blue and the violet represent areas of late activation. The gray areas are where early activation meets late activation, a characteristic of reentrant tachycardias. The brown hexagons mark the location of radiofrequency lesions positioned on the isthmus to ablate the atrial flutter. RA, right atrium.

cremental atrial or ventricular pacing, which is pacing at a constant cycle length with gradual shortening until the occurrence of a desirable event, such as induction of a tachycardia or production of AV or ventriculoatrial (VA) block. Bursts of pacing at a constant cycle length are also used to induce SVT, VT, or VF or for study of sinus node function and integrity of subsidiary pacemakers. Ramp and auto decremental are pacing variations of burst pacing wherein the pacing cycle length interval is progressively decreased to improve consecutive capture of paced area.

The second pacing format is premature (or extra) stimulation from atrial or ventricular sites. For the study of a physiologic phenomenon, refractory periods, and conduction characteristics, a single extra stimulus is usually applied after a series of beats with a constant cycle length (Fig. 42–6). The scanning is initiated late during electrical diastole, and the coupling interval is progressively decreased until the atrial and/or ventricular muscle is refractory. For induction of SVTs, single, double, or more extra stimuli may be delivered (Fig. 42–7). For the induction of VT, up to three ventricular extra stimuli are employed. The sen-

sitivity of pacing protocols seems to be directly related to the number of extra stimuli used.[25] This occurs, however, at the expense of specificity when polymorphic VT/VF can be induced at very short coupling intervals by using multiple extra stimuli. Regardless of the pacing protocol, the induction of sustained monomorphic VT constitutes a specific response and is seldom induced in patients not prone to such arrhythmias clinically. In contrast, the induction of polymorphic VT/VF with three extra stimuli at short coupling intervals can be nonspecific and does not provide a reliable guide for serial drug testing. Both polymorphic VT and VF can be avoided to a great extent at short coupling intervals (<200 milliseconds) if the induction of latency between the stimulus artifact and the local ventricular electrograms is avoided.[25-27]

During routine EPSs, a variety of electrophysiologic parameters are measured, including sinus node function and intraatrial, AV nodal, and His-Purkinje system conduction. Initiation of SVT and VT is attempted to determine the mechanisms, the site of origin (by pacing and mapping techniques), prognostication and the potential of overdrive termination as a therapy option. After base-

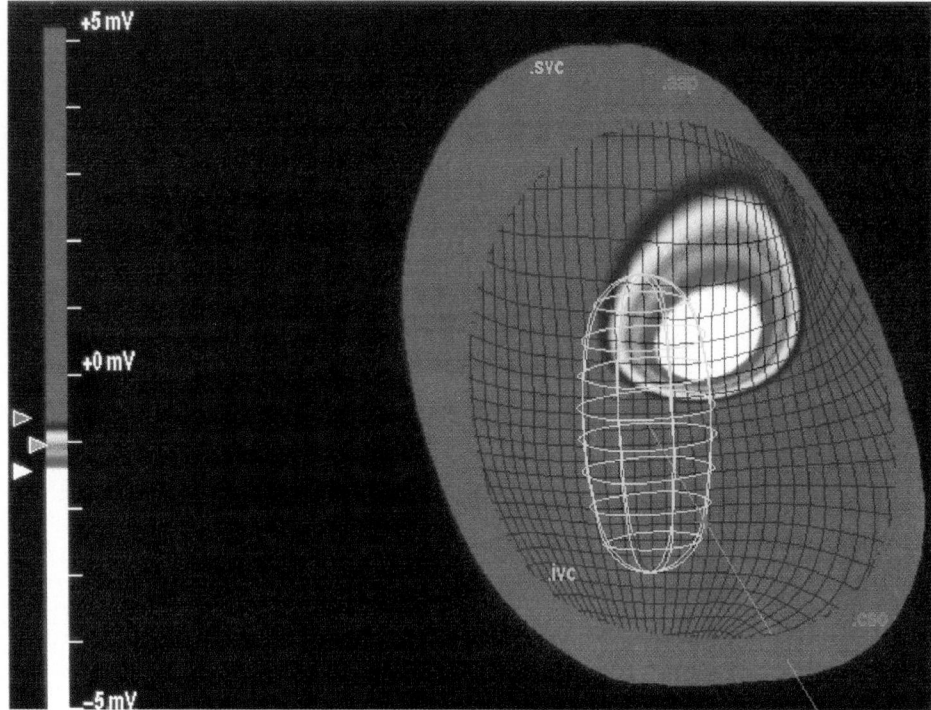

FIGURE 42–4. Activation of the right atrium during focal atrial tachycardia, mapped with the Endocardial Solutions EnSite 3000 system. The white represents tissue that is fully activated, and purple is tissue that is not yet activated. IVC, inferior vena cava; SVC, superior vena cava.

line studies, intravenous drugs may be administered to facilitate either induction of tachycardias, aggravation of sinus node function, or production of AV block (Fig. 42–8), or to determine drug efficacy.[25–27] The role of EPSs in patient management has evolved over the past decades from a purely diagnostic method to a frequently applied therapeutic tool. A brief outline of the value of clinical EPSs in various arrhythmia settings is outlined separately under diagnostic and therapeutic categories, below.

INVASIVE ELECTROPHYSIOLOGIC STUDIES FOR DIAGNOSIS

[ ] SINUS NODE DYSFUNCTION[3,4,28,29]

EPSs are performed to detect suspected sinus node dysfunction in patients with dizziness, presyncope, syncope, and the like, in whom the diagnosis cannot be made noninvasively. The most frequently performed test is that of sinus node suppression by using overdrive atrial pacing. After pacing at several basic cycle lengths for a period of approximately 30 seconds or longer, the pacing is interrupted. The resultant escape interval, which is called *sinus node recovery time*, is measured. By deducting the predominant sinus cycle length from this interval, one can obtain the so-called *corrected sinus node recovery time*. In one study,[3] sinus node recovery time in patients with sinus node disease averaged 3087 milliseconds; it averaged 1073 milliseconds in normal individuals. In another series,[6] the value for corrected sinus node recovery time was less than 525 milliseconds in normal individuals and exceeded those values in patients with overt sinus node dysfunction.

In the vast majority of patients with true sinus node disease, sinoatrial conduction abnormalities are the predominant reason for sinus node dysfunction. The sinoatrial conduction time in the absence of obvious sinus node disease is less than 100 milliseconds. The sensitivity of sinus node recovery time for the detection of sinus node dysfunction is 54 percent, whereas that of sinoatrial conduction time is 51 percent, with a combined sensitivity of the two tests of around 64 percent. Poor sensitivity of such testing relates in part to the fact that, in previous studies, documented episodes of sinus bradycardia or sinus arrest because of neurocardiogenic mechanisms may have been included as examples of sinus node dysfunction.[30] The specificity of the two tests combined is approximately 88 percent. It is important to test the AV conduction in patients with sinus node dysfunction, as the former is also frequently abnormal. In patients with bradycardia/tachycardia syndrome, tachycardias are frequent, particularly those arising in the atrium, and testing may also be necessary for the proper diagnosis and therapy of the concomitant tachyarrhythmia.

[ ] ATRIOVENTRICULAR BLOCK

In asymptomatic patients with first-degree AV block (prolonged PR interval), electrophysiologic assessment is unnecessary, regardless of the QRS morphology of the conducted beats. In asymptomatic individuals with second-degree AV block, electrophysiologic assessment is used to find the site of the block (Fig. 42–9). Patients with intra- or infra-Hisian block tend to have a more unpredictable course, and permanent

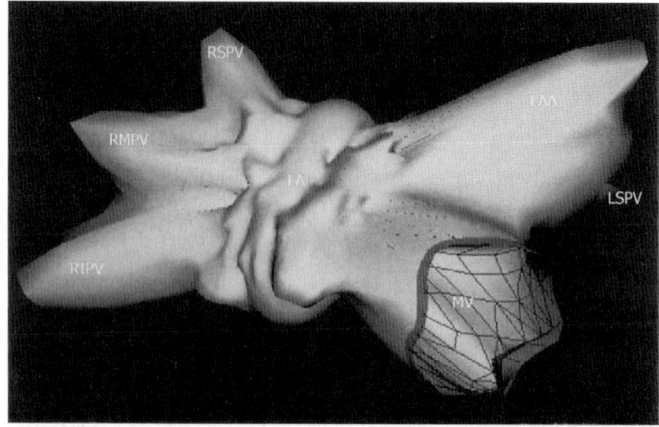

FIGURE 42–5. Anatomic reconstruction of the left atrium in a patient using Navex, anterior–posterior projection. A cutout is shown at the location of the mitral valve. LA, left atrium; LAA, left atrial appendage; LSPV, left superior pulmonary vein; MV, mitral valve; RIPV, right inferior pulmonary vein; RMPV, right middle pulmonary vein emptying directly into the left atrium; RSPV, right superior pulmonary vein.

pacing is desirable.³¹ Even though the intranodal block usually presents as Wenckebach phenomenon or Mobitz type I, it is not uncommon to see Wenckebach phenomena within the His-Purkinje system or within the His bundle. There is no difference in prognosis regardless of how the infra- or intra-Hisian second-degree block manifests itself; that is, type I versus type II (Fig. 42–9). On occasion, intranodal blocks are preceded by no discernible change in PR interval and, from a surface electrocardiogram, may appear as forms of Mobitz type II. The absolute length of the PR interval is usually quite diagnostic in that it is markedly prolonged (i.e., >300 milliseconds), and there is a PR shortening exceeding 100 milliseconds following the block beat (Fig. 42–9). In symptomatic patients with second-degree AV block, the role of EPS is limited because permanent pacing is the appropriate intervention. On the other hand, if the patient's symptoms cannot be explained on the basis of AV block and may be related to another arrhythmia, such as VT, EPS should be considered. In patients with third-degree or complete AV block, EPSs are seldom required; permanent pacing is the obvious option in symptomatic patients.

A discernible His bundle recording enables one to determine the exact site of AV conduction abnormality—that is, proximal to, within, or distal to the His bundle region. This, in combination with surface electrocardiographic morphology of conducted beats, enables one to identify precisely the location of conduction abnormality.

If 1:1 AV conduction is noted during EPS in patients suspected of intermittent AV block, incremental atrial pacing should be done to see whether AV block can be reproduced. AV block in the His-Purkinje system is abnormal during incremental atrial pacing but may be a physiologic response during atrial extrastimulation (see Fig. 42–6A). First- and second-degree blocks in the AV node are considered physiologic responses during incremental atrial pacing or atrial extrastimulation (see Fig. 42–6B).

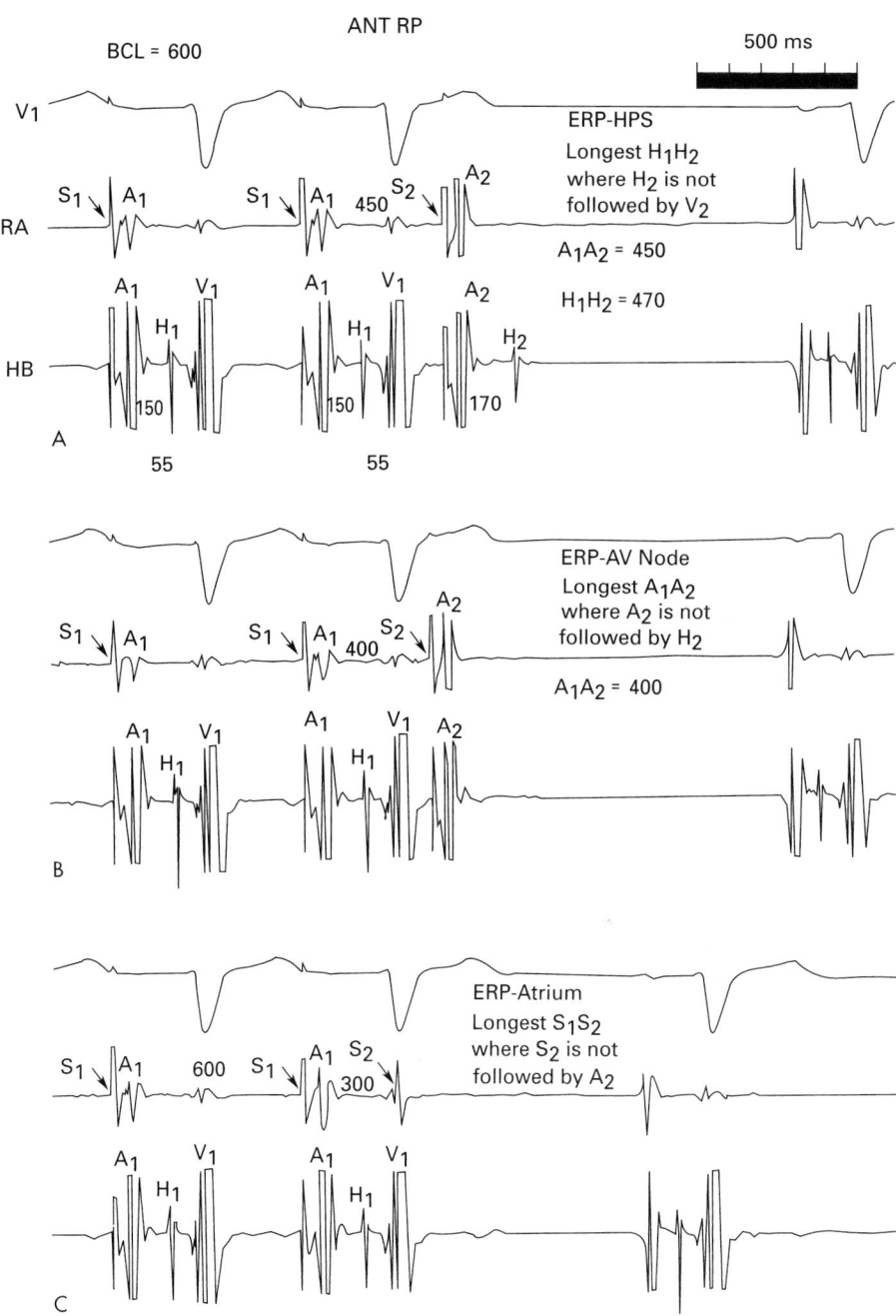

FIGURE 42–6. Determination of cardiac refractory periods during atrial pacing (**A** through **C**). During a basic cycle-length pacing at 600 milliseconds (S₁S₁ or A₁A₁), atrial premature stimulation (S₂ or A₂) at progressively shorter coupling intervals (S₁S₂ or A₁A₂) is depicted. The definition of the effective refractory period (ERP) of the His-Purkinje system (HPS), atrioventricular node, and atrium are labeled. ANT RP, antegrade refractory period. *Source: From Akhtar M.¹³ Reproduced with permission from the publisher and authors.*

WIDE QRS TACHYCARDIA

Wide QRS tachycardia occurs as a consequence of a variety of electrophysiologic mechanisms, both from supraventricular and ventricular origins in the presence or absence of accessory pathways (Fig. 42–10).³² The underlying nature of the wide QRS tachycardia is critical for both prognosis and therapy. EPSs have proven invaluable for distin-guishing the various etiologies (Fig. 42–11). With few exceptions, when the nature of the arrhythmic problem is not known and the direction of therapy is not clear, patients with wide QRS tachycardia should undergo EPS. This is particularly true in situations where nonpharmacologic therapy is the desired goal.

UNEXPLAINED SYNCOPE

Unexplained syncope³²⁻³⁸ may be caused by cardiovascular mechanisms. Electrophysiologic evaluation constitutes an integral part of the evaluation of patients with unexplained syncope, especially those with

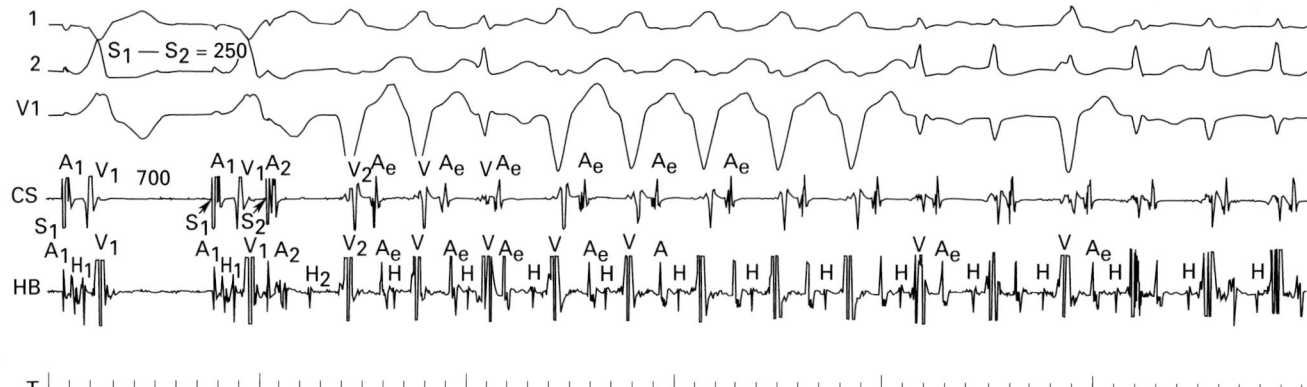

FIGURE 42–7. Induction of supraventricular tachycardia (SVT) in Wolff-Parkinson-White syndrome. The tracings are labeled. Atrial pacing from coronary sinus (CS) is done at a 700-millisecond basic cycle. During the basic drive pacing, left free wall accessory pathway conduction to the ventricle produces ventricular preexcitation. A single premature beat (S_2) blocks in the accessory pathway (AP) and conducts over the normal pathway with a left bundle-branch block morphology, and the SVT is initiated. Note the intermittent normalization of the QRS complex during this SVT. *Source: From Jazayeri M, Caceres J, Tchou P, et al. Electrophysiologic characteristics of sudden QRS axis deviation during orthodromic tachycardia. J Clin Invest 1989;83:952–959. Reproduced with permission from the publisher and authors.*

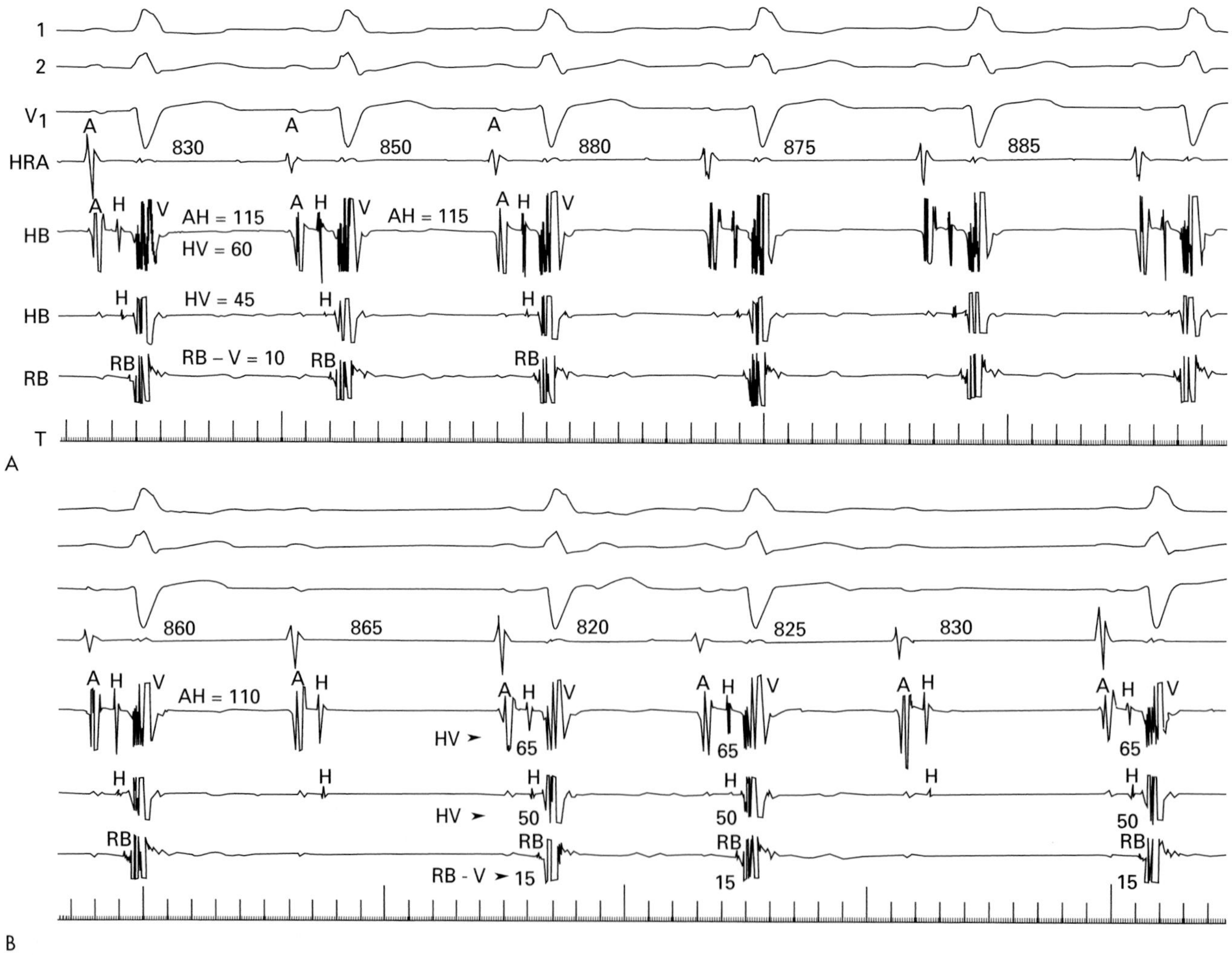

FIGURE 42–8. Atrioventricular (AV) block in the His-Purkinje system (HPS). **A.** Control. A 1:1 AV conduction is depicted in a patient with unexplained syncope. Following 150 mg of intravenous procainamide (**B**), a second-degree AV block in the HPS is noted (i.e., His bundle potential is not followed by a QRS complex), an abnormal response to a small dose of procainamide suggesting AV block in the HPS as a potential cause of syncope.

heart disease. During such studies, all arrhythmic possibilities—such as sinus node dysfunction, AV conduction abnormalities, SVT, and VT—should be excluded. Neurocardiogenic mechanisms constitute the most common causes of syncope in patients without structural heart disease, and incomplete assessment of these patients may lead to inappropriate therapy (Fig. 42–12).[30–33] The possibility of neurocardiogenic dysfunction should always be considered in younger patients (<50 years of age) with syncope and documented bradycardia (sinus arrest or AV block) and can be unmasked on a tilt table. The triage of patients toward one or the other, that is, electrophysiologic testing versus head-up tilt, is fairly simple and predicted by clinical history and the presence or absence of structural heart disease.[30–38] Patients with underlying structural heart disease—such as old myocardial infarction, primary myocardial disease, or poor LV function—generally have underlying VT to explain the symptoms of syncope (Fig. 42–13). When arrhythmias occur in patients without overt structural heart disease, sinus node dysfunction, AV block (particularly intra-Hisian block), or SVTs are likely. Less frequently, VT can occur in the absence of an overt structural heart disease.

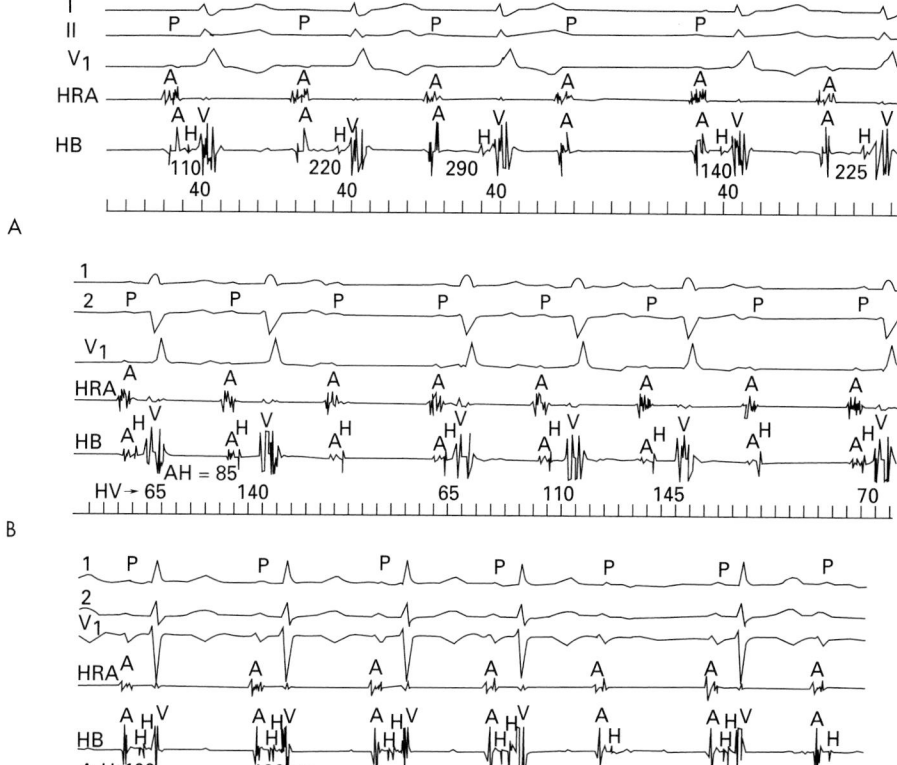

FIGURE 42–9. His bundle (HB) electrograms in atrioventricular (AV) block. The tracings are from three different patients with second-degree AV block. In **A** and **B**, the conducted QRS complexes are wide and associated with bundle branch block. In **A**, the block is within the AV node (i.e., the A wave on the HB is not followed by an HB deflection). In **B**, it can be appreciated that the block is distal to the HB even though the surface electrocardiogram (ECG) demonstrates a Wenckebach phenomenon. The latter can obviously occur in the His-Purkinje system as well, as depicted in this figure. **C.** The site of the block is within the HB. This is suggested by split HB potentials (labeled H and H+), and the block is distal to the H but proximal to the H+. Intra-His block is difficult to diagnose from the surface ECG but can be suspected when a Mobitz type II occurs in association with a normal PR interval and a narrow QRS complex. *Source: From Akhtar M.[13] Reproduced with permission from the publisher and authors.*

❨ ❩ SURVIVORS OF SUDDEN CARDIAC ARREST

In many patients with documented episodes of cardiac arrest from the onset, VF can be documented as the initial cause. Patients dying suddenly often have underlying structural heart disease (usually coronary artery disease or primary myocardial disease) and are prone to VT/VF because of electrical instability. It seems prudent to investigate both the nature and extent of organic heart disease and also to assess vulnerability to recurrent VT/VF. At present, EPS is considered a routine part of the overall patient assessment in this group of individuals.[10,39,40]

EPSs in survivors of VT/VF are desirable for a variety of reasons; four are listed here:

1. Occasionally the underlying VT leading to cardiac arrest is bundle-branch reentry (Fig. 42–14). In our group's experience almost 40 percent of patients with monomorphic VT in association with idiopathic dilated cardiomyopathy and valvular heart disease have bundle-branch reentry as the underlying mechanism. We feel this arrhythmia is preferably managed with bundle-branch ablation, which is curative, rather than with an implantable cardioverter defibrillator (ICD) alone.

2. Several VT morphologies or other types of tachycardia may be induced in addition to VT. Lack of awareness of such arrhythmias may complicate patient management. For example, the coexistence of rapid SVT may require separate attention to prevent unnecessary ICD shocks.

3. In some cases, supraventricular arrhythmia may trigger VT/VF. This may happen in patients with, for example, severe coronary artery disease, congestive heart failure, or Wolff-Parkinson-White syndrome. Elimination of the underlying causes is a more rational therapeutic approach in such cases.

4. Patients with VT/VF often have underlying sick sinus syndrome or AV block, which can be further aggravated with antiarrhythmic drugs and may require permanent pacing. Assessment for this eventuality can be done during the conduct of an EPS and may help selection of a particular device. Because of the increasing flexibility of these devices, this need for EPS may be less relevant in the future.

INVASIVE CARDIAC ELECTROPHYSIOLOGIC STUDIES FOR THERAPEUTIC INTERVENTION

Because of the episodic nature of most cardiac arrhythmias, the efficacy of any therapeutic intervention is difficult to assess unless the ar-

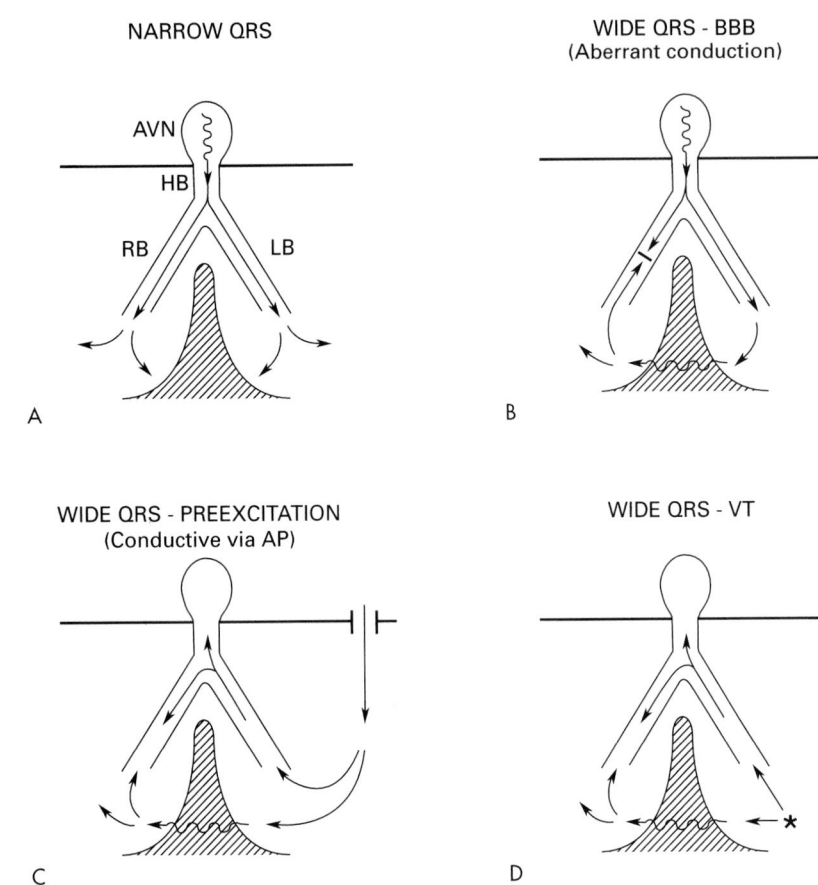

NARROW QRS

A

WIDE QRS - BBB
(Aberrant conduction)

B

WIDE QRS - PREEXCITATION
(Conductive via AP)

C

WIDE QRS - VT

D

FIGURE 42–10. Wide QRS tachycardia. Routes of impulse propagation during a wide QRS tachycardia in various settings are depicted. It should be noted that only in **A** and **B** is His bundle activation expected to precede ventricular activation. This helps the delineation from other causes of wide QRS tachycardia shown in **C** and **D**.

rhythmia in question can be replicated. Diagnostic EPS provides that opportunity, and it seems logical to use the same tool to assess therapeutic interventions.[40–46] This method to assess efficacy can be applied for both pharmacologic and nonpharmacologic therapy.

PHARMACOLOGIC THERAPY

It is arguable whether the assessment of pharmacologic intervention is essential in patients with relatively benign cardiac arrhythmias. The clinical course can be observed to determine whether control has been achieved. With life-threatening tachycardias, such as VT/VF, or with severe manifestations of cardiac arrhythmias, such as syncope or presyncope, it is desirable to assess efficacy of pharmacologic intervention (Fig. 42–15).[43,44] A technique of drug testing has been developed whereby the elimination of inducibility of a given tachycardia is assessed following a drug administration. Both the drug's efficacy or inefficacy can be evaluated by this method. When drug therapy does eliminate induction of a previously inducible tachycardia, the addition of isoproterenol will frequently demonstrate reversal of therapeutic drug effect.[45,46] This is helpful in considering additional β blocker therapy, which can be accomplished with ease in patients with good LV function, whereas the addition of β blockers may pose a problem in patients with VT and poor LV function. Failure of serial drug testing is associated with a significant recurrence rate and is a strong indication for nonpharmacologic intervention.

Some controversy has arisen regarding the value of EPS for predictive drug efficacy in comparison to ambulatory monitoring.[41] However, because of the infrequency of spontaneous VT/VF in most patients with life-threatening ventricular arrhythmias, ambulatory monitoring is an impractical approach. At present, serial drug studies with multiple oral antiarrhythmic agents are seldom carried out for SVT or VT.[42–46]

NONPHARMACOLOGIC THERAPY

Nonpharmacologic intervention has become an integral part of patient management in cardiac arrhythmias. With documented cardiac arrest from VF, implantation of an automatic ICD is fairly common and electrophysiologic assessment before such therapy is routine.[10,47] Both preimplant and postimplant electrophysiologic evaluation can be done through permanent leads of an ICD through a wand and programmer. Pacing, antitachycardia function, low-energy cardioversion, and cardiac defibrillation can all be programmed with newer devices. When problems are encountered following discharge of a patient with an ICD, electrophysiologic reassessment via ICD is frequently necessary, both for reprogramming and for troubleshooting. For assessment of certain other electrophysiologic parameters (e.g., AV conduction and mechanism of SVTs), however, transvenous catheterization may be necessary.

Patients with coronary artery disease and mappable VT are also candidates for VT surgery when it cannot be managed with an ICD, antiarrhythmic drugs, and/or catheter ablation.[48–50] Preoperative EPS assessment for this possibility is important. Surgery for VT in the form of endocardial resection or cryoablation can be performed very effectively and relatively safely in patients with an LV ejection fraction greater than 20 percent. This curative procedure provides effective control in approximately 75 percent of the patients who have monomorphic VT that can be appropriately mapped; it may be considered when other forms of therapies are ineffective.

Surgery for SVT has gone through a significant evolution. The introduction of catheter ablative techniques has made it rare for patients to undergo surgery for Wolff-Parkinson-White syndrome and/or AV nodal reentrant tachycardia. Some individuals with resistant atrial fibrillation and flutter and those who fail catheter ablative therapy may still be considered candidates for such a procedure, but this is now becoming less frequent.

CATHETER ABLATION TECHNIQUES[51–55]

The realization that the origin of VT and SVT can be effectively mapped has made the catheter ablative technique a rational approach. The radiofrequency form of energy delivered through a catheter has permitted controlled trauma to cardiac tissue to abolish or modify reentrant circuits. This is true for both SVT and VT. Unifocal atrial tachycardia, AV nodal reentry of all varieties, and ac-

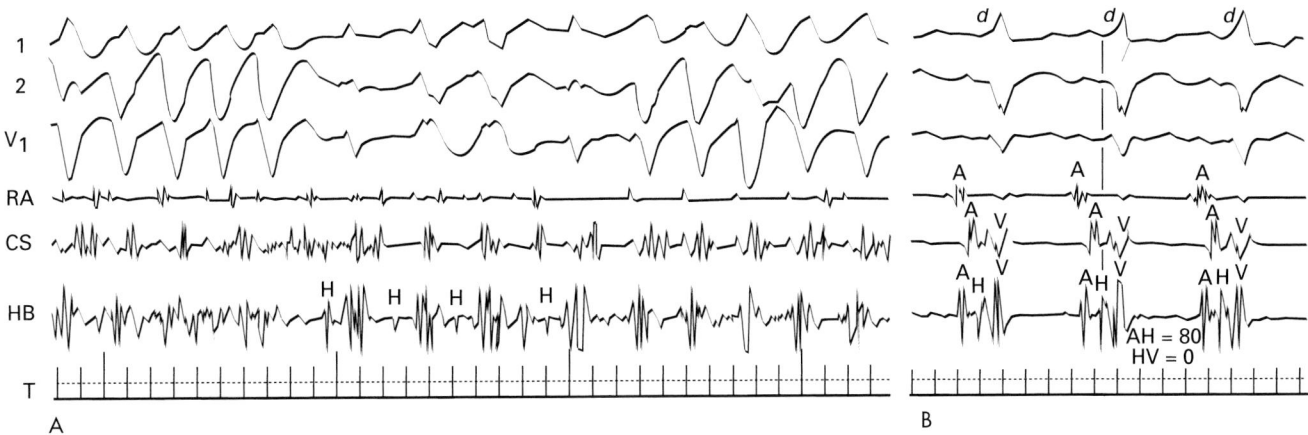

FIGURE 42–11. Wide QRS tachycardia. **A.** Wide QRS complexes of at least two varieties are seen. Those showing a left bundle-branch block pattern are a result of conduction over an accessory pathway, whereas those with a right bundle-branch pattern are aberrant in nature. Note the His bundle activation prior to both narrow and aberrant complexes but not before preexcited complexes. A right posteroseptal preexcitation can be appreciated in **B**, with a short PR, a delta wave (*d*), a His to ventricle (HV) of zero, Q wave in lead 2 and a complex in lead V₁.

cessory pathways including atriofascicular fibers can be cured in over 90 percent of patients with radiofrequency catheter ablation. Among the VTs, bundle-branch reentry tachycardia seen in association with dilated cardiomyopathy (both ischemic and nonischemic) and valvular disease is an ideal substrate for catheter ablation. Patients with monomorphic VT associated with myocardial scarring or other substrates can also be considered candidates, particularly when they are not suitable for VT surgery and have failed drug therapy. Additionally, in patients with incessant VT or frequency VT with inadequate control despite ICD therapy, VT ablation should be considered. By using electromagnetic mapping, the scarred area is mapped during sinus rhythm and ablation of this substrate can effectively eliminate VT. The noncontact mapping techniques outlined above are likely to further help improve the ablation success rate with unifocal or possibly multifocal tachycardias.

IATROGENIC PROBLEMS ENCOUNTERED DURING ELECTROPHYSIOLOGIC STUDIES

Mechanical irritation from catheters during placement, even when they are not being manipulated, can cause a variety of arrhythmias and conduction disturbances.[56] These include induction of atrial, junctional, and ventricular ectopic beats and right bundle-branch block and

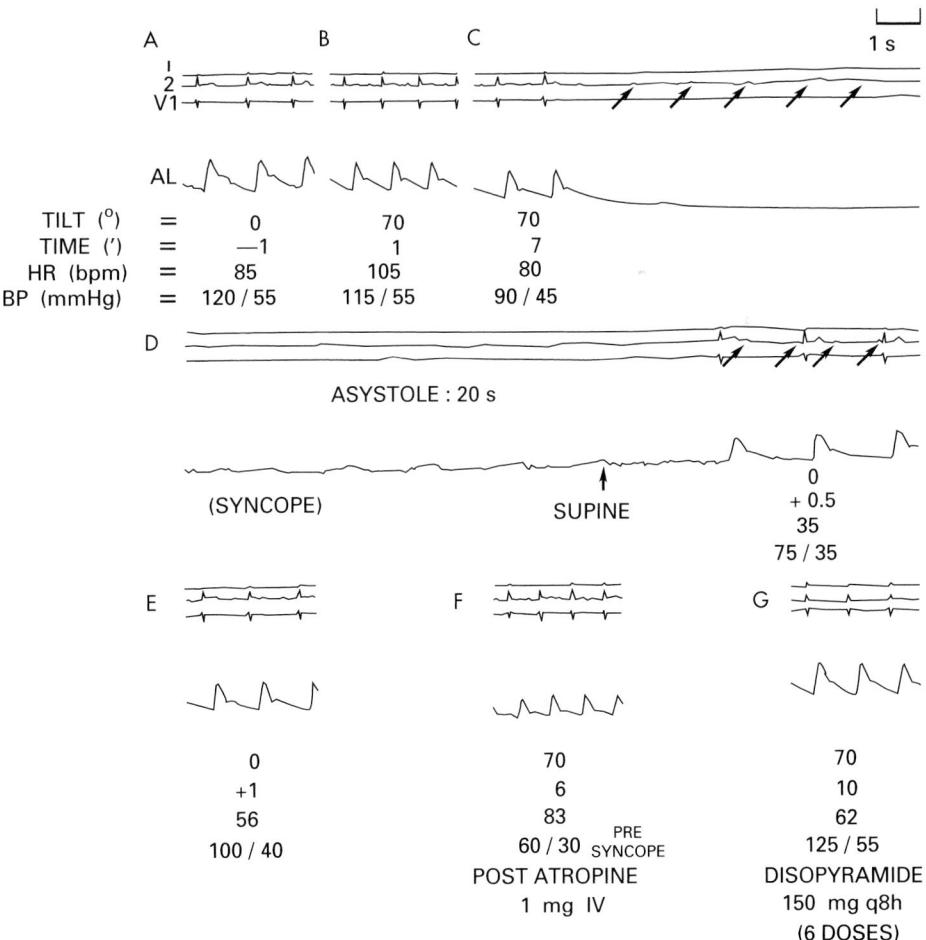

FIGURE 42–12. Asystole in neurocardiogenic syncope. Note the normal heart rate (HR) and blood pressure (BP) in supine position. At the beginning of head-up tilt at 70 degrees (**B**), some degree of tachycardia is noted. Seven minutes after the onset of tilt (**C**), an episode of atrioventricular block occurs and is followed by sinus arrest and a total asystole of 20 seconds. Syncopal episodes follow. Presyncope is still present when asystole is prevented by atropine (**F**). Findings in **C** might tempt one to prescribe permanent pacing, an inappropriate choice of therapy. In this patient with neurocardiogenic syncope, disopyramide (**G**) prevented hypotension and syncope without the need for a permanent pacemaker. This patient has remained asymptomatic on this therapy for more than 10 years now. *Source: From Akhtar M.[27] Reproduced with permission from the publisher and authors.*

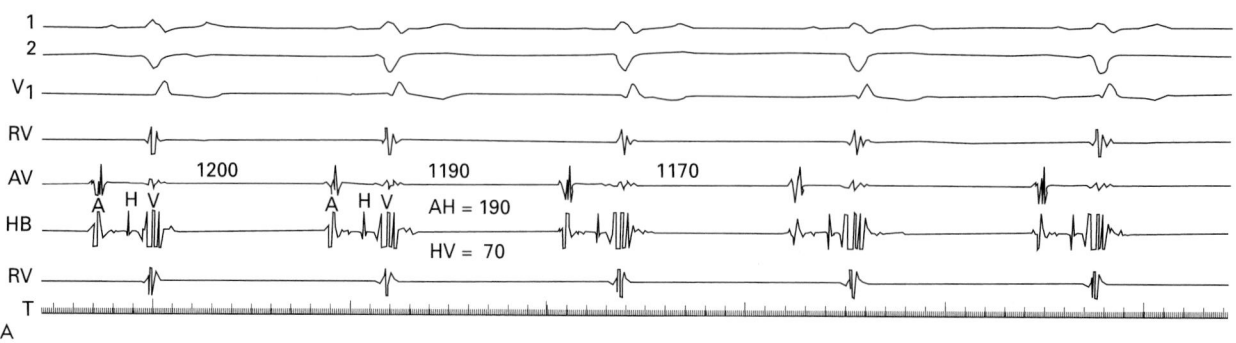

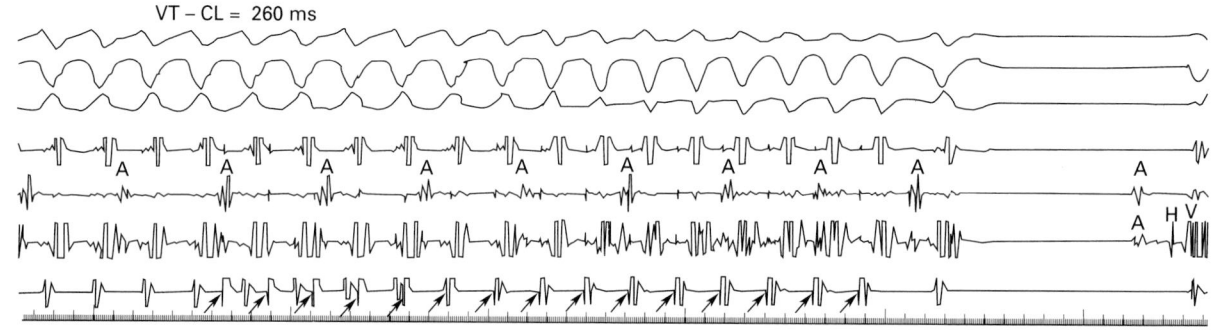

FIGURE 42–13. Arrhythmic causes of syncope. **A.** Sinus rhythm in a patient with unexplained syncope. Sinus bradycardia, bifascicular block, and a long PR interval from surface electrocardiogram suggest possible bradycardia etiology. In this patient, however, ventricular tachycardia (**B**) was inducible with ventricular extrastimulation and was the actual cause of syncope. Control of ventricular tachycardia (VT) without a pacemaker was sufficient to prevent syncope in this patient. Termination of tachycardia and restoration of sinus rhythm are shown in **B**.

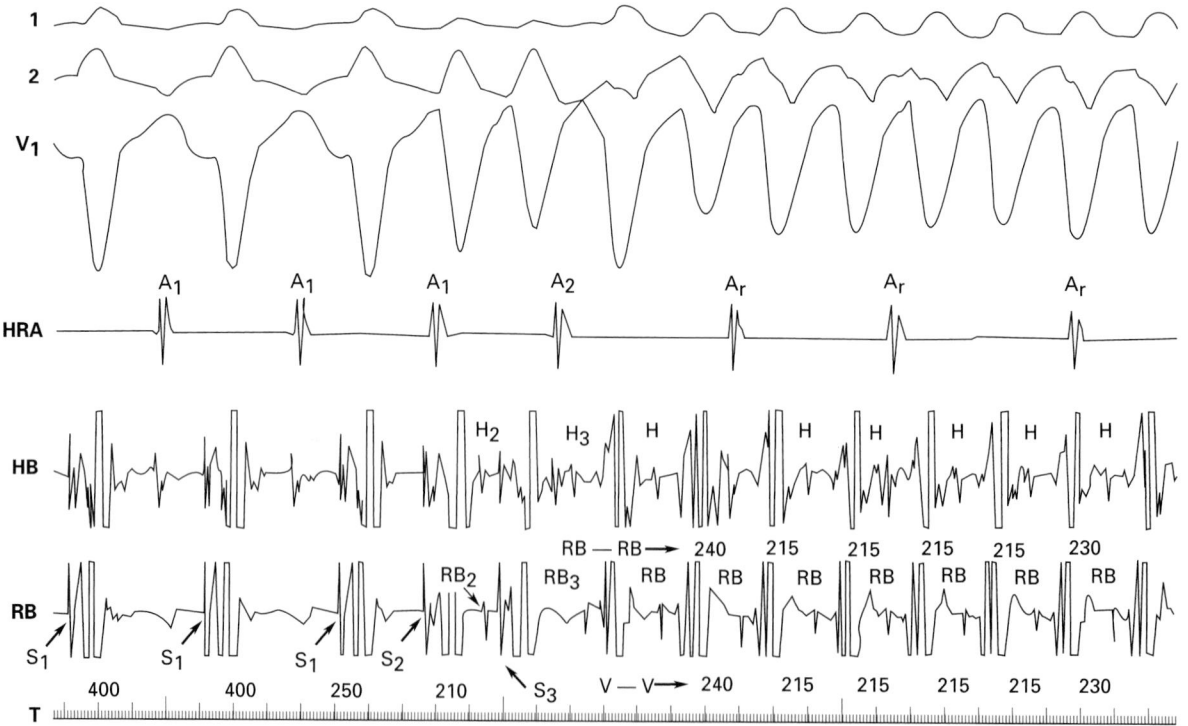

FIGURE 42–14. Induction of sustained ventricular tachycardia a result of bundle-branch reentry. The surface electrocardiogram and intracardiac tracings are labeled. Basic cycle length (S_1S_1) is 400 milliseconds during ventricular pacing. Sustained bundle-branch reentry is induced with two extra stimuli (S_2S_3). Note that the His bundle and right bundle (RB) deflections precede the QRS, suggesting supraventricular tachycardia with aberrant conduction. However, there is 2:1 ventricular atrial (VA) block, indicating the ventricular nature of this tachycardia. Without His bundle/ right bundle (HB/RB) recordings, the diagnosis can be difficult and, consequently, the likelihood of inappropriate therapy will be high. RB-RB and V-V (ventricular) intervals are labeled. *Source: From Jazayeri M, Sra J, Akhtar M. Wide QRS complexes: electrophysiologic basis of a common electrocardiographic diagnosis. J Cardiovasc Electrophysiol 1992;3:36–39. Reproduced with permission from the publisher and authors.*

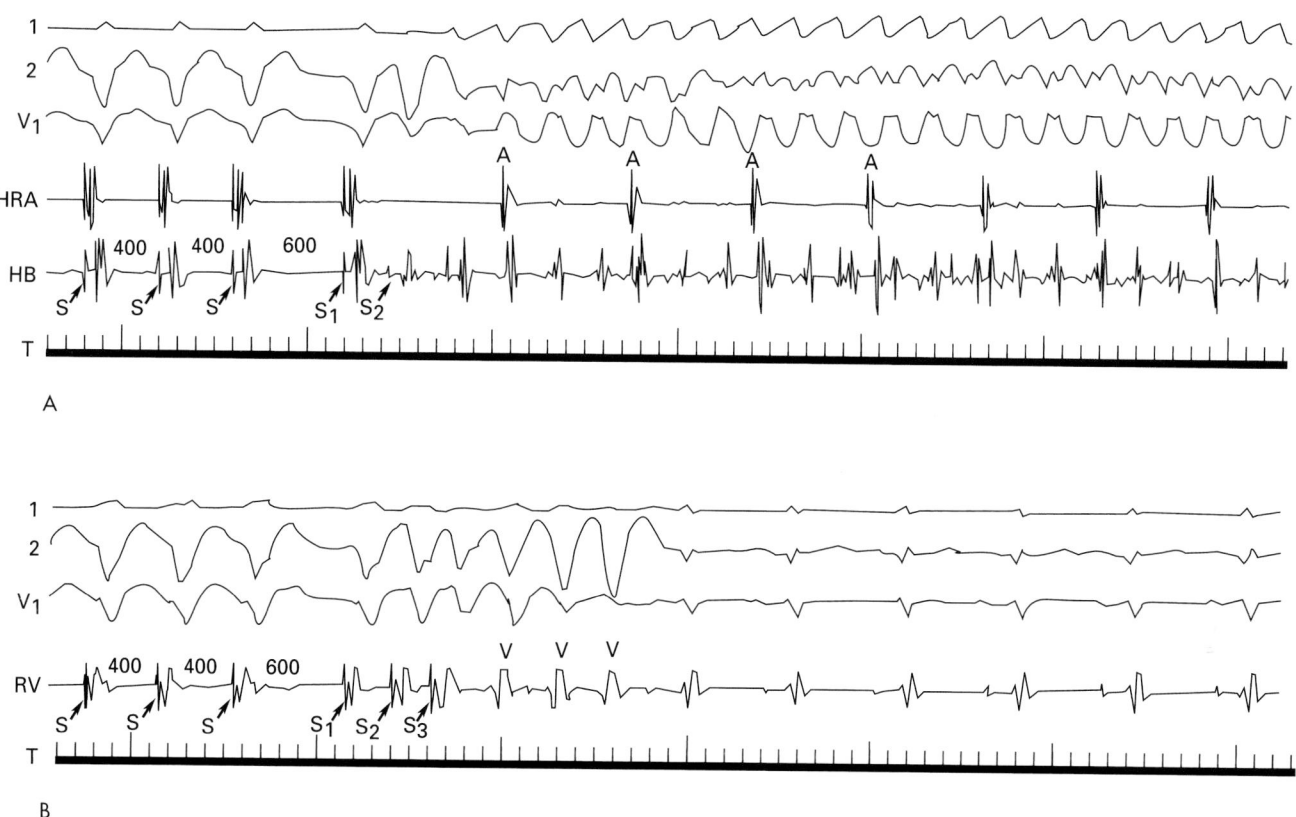

FIGURE 42–15. A. Control. **B.** Postprocainamide (PA) + mexiletine. Initiation of sustained monomorphic ventricular tachycardia (VT) of myocardial origin is shown in A. After oral procainamide and mexiletine, the sustained VT could not be induced despite using a more aggressive pacing protocol.

thus AV block in the His-Purkinje system in patients with preexisting left bundle branch block during right ventricular catheterization.[56] Obviously, AV block in the His-Purkinje system can occur in patients with preexisting right bundle-branch block during LV catheterization. Ventricular stimulation can also occur from physical movement of the ventricular catheter coincident with atrial contraction, producing electrocardiographic patterns of ventricular preexcitation. Recognition of all these iatrogenic patterns is important for avoiding misinterpretation of electrophysiologic phenomena and the significance of findings in the laboratory.

Certain types of arrhythmias must be avoided at all costs, such as atrial fibrillation and VF. Atrial fibrillation will obviously not permit study of any other form of SVT, and VF will require prompt sedation and cardioversion, making it difficult to continue the EPS. If atrial fibrillation must be initiated for diagnostic purposes (i.e., to assess ventricular response over the accessory pathway in Wolff-Parkinson-White syndrome), it should be done at the end of the study. Patients with a prior history of atrial fibrillation are more prone to the occurrence of sustained atrial fibrillation in the laboratory. Frequently, this will occur during initial placement of catheters; excessive manipulation of catheters in the atria should therefore be avoided. Catheter trauma resulting in abolition of accessory pathway conduction or the reentrant pathway may make the curative ablation difficult or impossible.

【 】 RISKS AND COMPLICATIONS

The complication rate is relatively low when only right-heart catheterization is done; additionally, there is almost negligible mortality.[57,58] Other complications include deep venous thrombosis, int-

racavitary thrombosis, pulmonary or systemic embolism, infection at catheter sites, systemic infection, pneumothorax, hemothorax perforation of a cardiac chamber or coronary sinus, pericardial effusion, or tamponade. Potentially lethal arrhythmias such as rapid VT or VF are common in the laboratory. These are not necessarily counted as complications, however, but are often expected and anticipated. Nonetheless, their common occurrence makes the electrophysiology laboratory a place for only highly trained personnel equipped to handle such problems.

REFERENCES

1. Scherlag BJ, Lau SH, Helfant RH, et al. Catheter technique for recording His bundle activity in man. *Circulation* 1969;39:13–18.
2. Goldreyer BN, Bigger JT. Spontaneous and induced reentrant tachycardia. *Ann Intern Med* 1969;70:87–98.
3. Mandel WJ, Hayakawa H, Danzig R, Marcus HS. Evaluation of sinoatrial node function in man by overdrive suppression. *Circulation* 1971;44:59–66.
4. Narula OS, Samet P, Javier RP. Significance of the sinus node recovery time. *Circulation* 1972;45:140–158.
5. Damato AN, Lau SH, Helfant RH, et al. A study of heart block in man using His bundle recordings. *Circulation* 1969;39:297–305.
6. Narula OS, Scherlag BJ, Samet P, Javier RP. Atrioventricular block: localization and classification by His bundle recordings. *Am J Med* 1971;50:146–165.
7. Goldreyer BN, Damato AN. The essential role of atrioventricular conduction delay in the initiation of paroxysmal supraventricular tachycardia. *Circulation* 1971;43:679–687.
8. Wellens HJJ, Schuilenberg RM, Durrer D. Electrical stimulation of the heart in patients with the Wolff-Parkinson-White syndrome type A. *Circulation* 1971;43:99–114.
9. Mason JW, Winkel RA. Electrode catheter arrhythmia induction in the selection and assessment of antiarrhythmic drug therapy for recurrent ventricular tachycardia. *Circulation* 1978;58:971–985.

10. Ruskin JN, DiMarco JP, Garan H. Out of hospital cardiac arrest: electrophysiologic observations in selection of long-term antiarrhythmic therapy. *N Engl J Med* 1980;303:607–613.

11. Nelson GS, Berger RD, Fetics BJ, et al. Left ventricular or biventricular pacing improves cardiac function at diminished energy cost in patients with dilated cardiomyopathy and left bundle-branch block. *Circulation* 2000;102:3053–3059.

12. Auricchio A, Kloss M, Trautmann SI, et al. Exercise performance following cardiac resynchronization therapy in patients with heart failure and ventricular conduction delay. *Am J Cardiol* 2002;89:198–203.

13. Akhtar M. Invasive cardiac electrophysiologic studies: an introduction. In: Parmley WW, Chatterjee K, eds. *Cardiology*, vol 1: *Physiology, Pharmacology, Diagnosis.* Philadelphia: Lippincott, 1991:6.54–6.67.

14. Josephson ME, Harken PH, Horowitz LN. Endocardial excision: a new surgical technique for the treatment of recurrent ventricular tachycardia. *Circulation* 1979;60:1430–1439.

15. Fann JI, Loeb JM, LoCicero J III, et al. Endocardial activation mapping and endocardial pace-mapping using a balloon apparatus. *Am J Cardiol* 1985;55:1076.

16. Mickleborough LL, Harris L, Downar E, et al. A new intraoperative approach for endocardial mapping of ventricular tachycardia. *J Thorac Cardiovasc Surg* 1988;95:271.

17. Sosa E, Scanavacca M, d'Avila A, et al. Endocardial and epicardial ablation guided by nonsurgical transthoracic epicardial mapping to treat recurrent ventricular tachycardia. *J Cardiovasc Electrophysiol* 1998;9:229–239.

18. Gepstein L, Hayam G, Ben-Haim SA. A novel method for nonfluoroscopic catheter-based electroanatomical mapping of the heart. *Circulation* 1997;95:1611–1622.

19. Schilling RJ, Peters NS, Davies DW. A non-contact catheter for simultaneous endocardial mapping in the human left ventricle: comparison of contact and reconstructed electrograms during sinus rhythm. *Circulation* 1998;98:887–898.

20. Wittkampf F, Wever E, Derksen R, et al. LocaLisa new technique for real-time 3-dimensional localization of regular intracardiac electrodes. *Circulation* 1999;99:1312–1317.

21. Wittkampf F, Wever E, Derksen R, et al. Accuracy of the LocaLisa system in catheter ablation procedures. *J Electrocardiol* 1999;32(Suppl):7–12.

22. Wittkampf F, Loh P, Derksen R, et al. Real-time, three-dimensional, nonfluoroscopic localization of the lasso catheter. *J Cardiovasc Electrophysiol* 2002;13:630.

23. Sra J, Krum D, Malloy A, et al. Registration of three-dimensional left atrial computed tomographic images with projection images obtained using fluoroscopy. *Circulation* 2005;112:3763–3768.

24. Ector J, De Buck S, Adams J, et al. Cardiac three-dimensional magnetic resonance imaging and fluoroscopy merging: a new approach for electroanatomic mapping to assist catheter ablation. *Circulation* 2005;112:3769–3776.

25. Brugada P, Green M, Abdollah H, Wellens HJ. Significance of ventricular arrhythmias initiated by programmed ventricular stimulation: the importance of the type of ventricular arrhythmia induced and the number of premature stimuli required. *Circulation* 1984;69:87–92.

26. Avitall B, McKinnie J, Jazayeri M, et al. Induction of ventricular fibrillation versus monomorphic ventricular tachycardia during programmed stimulation: role of premature beat conduction delay. *Circulation* 1992;85:1271–1278.

27. Akhtar M. Clinical application of electrophysiologic studies in the management of patients requiring pacemaker therapy. In: Barold S, ed. *Modern Cardiac Pacing.* Mount Kisco, NY: Futura, 1985:3.

28. Hariman RJ, Krongrad E, Boxer RA, et al. Method for recording electrical activity of the sinoatrial node and automatic atrial foci during cardiac catheterization in human subjects. *Am J Cardiol* 1980;45:775–781.

29. Gomes JA. The sick sinus syndrome and evaluation of the patient with sinus node disorders. In: Parmley WW, Chatterjee K, eds. *Cardiology*, vol 1: *Physiology, Pharmacology, Diagnosis.* Philadelphia: Lippincott, 1991:6.100–6.111.

30. Sra JS, Jazayeri MR, Avitall B, et al. Comparison of cardiac pacing with drug therapy in the treatment of neurocardiogenic (vasovagal) syncope with bradycardia or asystole. *N Engl J Med* 1993;328:1085–1090.

31. Dhingra RC, Wyndham CRC, Bauernfiend R, et al. Significance of block distal to the His bundle induced by atrial pacing in patients with chronic bifascicular block. *Circulation* 1979;60:1455–1464.

32. Akhtar M, Jazayeri M, Avitall B, et al. Electrophysiologic spectrum of wide QRS complex tachycardia. In: Zipes DP, Jalife J, eds. *Cardiac Electrophysiology: From Cell to Bedside.* Orlando, FL: WB Saunders, 1990:635.

33. Sra J, Anderson A, Sheikh S, et al. Unexplained syncope evaluated by electrophysiologic studies and head-up tilt testing. *Ann Intern Med* 1991;114:1013–1019.

34. DiMarco JP, Garan H, Ruskin JN. Cardiac electrophysiologic techniques in recurrent syncope of unknown cause. *Ann Intern Med* 1981;95:542–548.

35. Akhtar M, Shenasa M, Denker S, et al. Role of cardiac electrophysiologic studies in patients with unexplained recurrent syncope. *Pacing Clin Electrophysiol* 1983;6:192–201.

36. Morady F, Scheinman MM. The role and limitations of electrophysiologic testing in patients with unexplained syncope. *Int J Cardiol* 1983;4:229–234.

37. Teichman SL, Felder DS, Matos JA, et al. The value of electrophysiologic studies in syncope of undetermined origin: Report of 150, cases. *Am Heart J* 1985;110:469–479.

38. Moazez F, Peter T, Simonson J, et al. Syncope of unknown origin: Clinical noninvasive and electrophysiologic determinants of arrhythmia induction and symptom recurrence during long-term follow-up. *Am Heart J* 1991;121:81–88.

39. Akhtar M, Garan H, Lehmann MH, Troup PJ. Sudden cardiac death: Management of high-risk patients. *Ann Intern Med* 1991;114:499–512.

40. Morady F, Scheinman MM, Hess DS, et al. Electrophysiologic testing in the management of survivors of out-of-hospital arrest. *Am J Cardiol* 1983;51:85–89.

41. Mason JW. A comparison of electrophysiologic testing with Holter monitoring to predict antiarrhythmic-drug efficacy for ventricular tachyarrhythmias. *N Engl J Med* 1993;329:445–451.

42. Wu D, Wyndham CR, Denes P, et al. Chronic electrophysiological study in patients with recurrent paroxysmal tachycardia: a new method for developing successful oral antiarrhythmic therapy. In: Kulbertus HE, ed. *Reentrant Arrhythmias.* Baltimore: University Park Press, 1976:294.

43. Horowitz LN, Josephson ME, Farshidi A, et al. Recurrent sustained ventricular tachycardia: role of the electrophysiologic study in selection of antiarrhythmic regimens. *Circulation* 1978;58:986–997.

44. Mason JW, Winkle RA. Accuracy of ventricular tachycardia induction study for predicting long-term efficacy and inefficacy of antiarrhythmic drugs. *N Engl J Med* 1980;303:1073–1077.

45. Niazi I, Naccarelli G, Dougherty A, et al. Treatment of atrioventricular node reentrant tachycardia with encainide: reversal of drug effect with isoproterenol. *J Am Coll Cardiol* 1989;13:904–910.

46. Jazayeri M, Van Wyhe G, Avitall B, et al. Isoproterenol reversal of antiarrhythmic effects in patients with inducible sustained ventricular tachyarrhythmias. *J Am Coll Cardiol* 1989;14:705–711.

47. Akhtar M, Avitall B, Jazayeri M, et al. Role of implantable cardioverter defibrillator therapy in the management of high risk patients. *Circulation* 1992;85(Suppl I):I131–I139.

48. Josephson ME, Harken AH, Horowitz LN. Long-term results of endocardial resection from sustained ventricular tachycardia in coronary disease patients. *Am Heart J* 1982;104:51–57.

49. Caceres J, Werner P, Jazayeri M, et al. Efficacy of cryosurgery alone for refractory monomorphic sustained ventricular tachycardia due to inferior wall infarct. *J Am Coll Cardiol* 1988;11:1254–1259.

50. Caceres J, Akhtar M, Werner P, et al. Cryoablation of refractory sustained ventricular tachycardia due to coronary artery disease. *Am J Cardiol* 1989;63:296–300.

51. Jackman WM, Wang X, Friday KJ, et al. Catheter ablation of accessory atrioventricular pathways (Wolff-Parkinson-White syndrome) by radiofrequency current. *N Engl J Med* 1991;324:1605–1611.

52. Calkins H, Sousa J, El-Atassi R, et al. Diagnosis and cure of the Wolff-Parkinson-White syndrome or paroxysmal supraventricular tachycardias during a single electrophysiologic test. *N Engl J Med* 1991;324:1612–1618.

53. Jazayeri M, Hempe SL, Sra JS, et al. Selective transcatheter ablation of the fast and slow pathways using radiofrequency energy in patients with atrioventricular nodal reentrant tachycardia. *Circulation* 1992;85:1318–1328.

54. Saoudi N, Atallah G, Kirkorian G, Touboul P. Catheter ablation of the atrial myocardium in human type I atrial flutter. *Circulation* 1990;81:762–771.

55. Klein LS, Shih HT, Hackett FK, et al. Radiofrequency catheter ablation of ventricular tachycardia in patients without structural heart disease. *Circulation* 1992;85:1666–1674.

56. Akhtar M, Damato AN, Gilbert-Leeds CJ, et al. Induction of iatrogenic electrocardiographic patterns during electrophysiologic studies. *Circulation* 1977;56:60–65.

57. Di Marco JP, Garan H, Ruskin JN. Complications in patients undergoing cardiac electrophysiologic procedures. *Ann Intern Med* 1982;97:490–493.

58. Horowitz L. Risks and complications of clinical cardiac electrophysiologic studies: a prospective analysis of 1000 consecutive patients. *J Am Coll Cardiol* 1987;9:1261–1268.

CHAPTER 43

Antiarrhythmic Drugs

Peter R. Kowey / Gan-Xin Yan / Harry Crijns

INTRODUCTION

Antiarrhythmic drug therapy is the mainstay of treatment of patients with nearly every form of cardiac arrhythmia. An in-depth knowledge of the pharmacology of antiarrhythmic drugs, including their pharmacokinetics and pharmacodynamics, is essential to their successful and safe implementation.

PHARMACOKINETICS OF ANTIARRHYTHMIC DRUGS

Pharmacokinetic describes the relationship between drug administration and plasma concentration. It is assumed that the plasma concentration reflects, in a general sense, myocardial concentrations, and thus the availability of the drug at its site of action. The pharmacokinetics of antiarrhythmic drugs are variable and not predictable by drug classification or by knowledge of the drug's chemical structure.

【 】 ABSORPTION/BIOAVAILABILITY

Absorption describes the movement of orally administered drug from the gut lumen to the systemic circulation and the efficiency of this absorption is defined as bioavailability. Those factors that influence passage of the drug through the gut wall into the portal circulation and through the liver will have an effect on drug bioavailability. Thus, diseases that affect bowel motility, bowel wall blood flow, gastric and bowel pH, and presystemic or "first-pass" hepatic clearance will to some extent influence the amount of drug that is available to the systemic circulation.

A common way to extend interdosing intervals during treatment with drugs that have a relatively short plasma half-life is to formulate them into a sustained-release preparation. Changes in bowel pH and other conditions within the gut influence the amount of drug that is released from sustained-release preparations, which, in turn, has an effect on the amount of drug that is absorbed from the gastrointestinal tract. Drugs can also have altered absorption because of intraluminal binding by other substances, such as milk and antacids. Finally, the physiochemical properties of the drug itself can have an effect on absorption.

Varying the salt of the drug can change solubility and thus its rate of absorption. Drug solubility is also determined by the pH of its medium. Weak bases are rapidly dissolved in acid medium. Antacids, by increasing gut pH, can slow the absorption of a weakly basic drug. In clinical situations, high intestinal pH, caused by such factors as bacterial overgrowth syndrome, can reduce the bioavailability of antiarrhythmic drugs. Thus, for patients with serious arrhythmias, especially those that are controlled by drugs that have a relatively narrow toxic-to-therapeutic ratio,

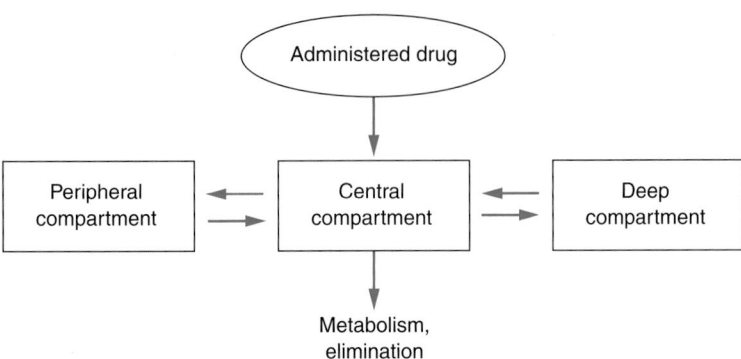

FIGURE 43-1. Pharmacokinetic compartments. Administered drug enters a highly perfused central compartment and then is redistributed to peripheral compartments and more slowly equilibrating deep compartments. *Source: Reproduced from Siddoway L.[10] With permission.*

reassessing plasma concentration or clinical efficacy during conditions of altered bowel physiology or pathology is relevant.

Finally, many antiarrhythmic drugs have a *food-fast effect*; that is, the bioavailability of a drug may be changed several fold in the presence of food or during fasting. A notable example is oral amiodarone, which is three times more bioavailable after a high-fat meal.[1] For such drugs, providing the patient with specific information as to the timing of drug ingestion with relationship to meals is important to maintain a predictable and reproducible plasma concentration over the course of therapy.

Generic antiarrhythmic drugs are approved by demonstration of *bioequivalence*. Thus, variations in formulation that can occur with generic drugs are permissible as long as there is a clear demonstration that the same amount of the generic drug is absorbed and available to the systemic circulation as the proprietary compound. Regulatory agencies have specified limits in the difference in bioavailability that may be allowed for the approval of new formulations.[2]

DISTRIBUTION

Following absorption, drug is distributed to various parts of the body and the pattern of distribution is determined by the amount of blood flow to different tissues (Fig. 43–1). Organs with high blood flow, such as the heart, liver, brain, and kidney, are generally exposed to the drug early and these organs are generally referred to as the *central compartment*. However, drugs nearly always redistribute from the central compartment to other tissues or sites of metabolism and elimination. They may distribute to muscle, skin, and adipose tissue, generally in a second phase. These less-perfused organs are considered to be the *peripheral compartment*. Finally, some drugs may distribute very slowly to tissues and organs that have low blood flow and may be referred to as the *deep compartment*. When the relative concentrations of drugs in all compartments reach equilibrium, *steady state* has been reached.

Volume of distribution is the term used to describe the virtual pool into which a drug is administered. The magnitude of the volume of distribution is dependent on the perfusion of tissues, the concentration of plasma and tissue proteins that bind drug, and the physiochemical properties of the drug as it relates to its binding to tissue and plasma proteins. The volume of distribution is changed in many pathologic conditions, including congestive heart failure. Because organ perfusion is reduced, the volume of distribution of the central compartment is smaller in heart failure, making more of the drug available to active binding sites in the heart. Consequently, patients with congestive heart failure have increased sensitivity to the electrophysiologic properties of commonly used agents.[3]

Critically important among the factors that modulate volume of distribution is protein binding. Most antiarrhythmic drugs are bound to varying extents in plasma to α_1-acid glycoprotein. A variation in protein binding changes the amount of unbound drug that is available to exert a pharmacologic effect. Protein binding is modulated by changes in the concentration of binding proteins, fluctuations in drug concentration, and interactions with drugs competing for binding by the same proteins. The latter is the explanation for drug interactions that occur during simultaneous dosing with drugs such as digoxin and quinidine.[4] Changes in plasma and tissue pH can also change protein binding by altering the ionized state of the antiarrhythmic drug. Such alterations are probably only important during marked alterations in pH as may occur during severe acidosis.

DRUG METABOLISM

The metabolism of drugs in general, as well as in antiarrhythmic drugs, can be divided into two phases: the first phase changes the drug into more polar metabolites via oxidation–reduction reactions. During the second phase, drugs are conjugated to endogenous ligands, such as glucuronide or sulfate. The majority of drug metabolism occurs in the liver with oxidative metabolism usually occurring via the cytochrome P450 enzyme system. However, the metabolism of rapidly cleared drugs may occur in lung, plasma, vascular endothelium, or even red blood cells.

Knowledge of the relative concentration of active metabolites and their electrophysiologic action is critical to understanding the net pharmacologic effect of an antiarrhythmic drug. An example of an active metabolite is 5-hydroxypropafenone, a metabolite that has similar electrophysiologic effects to those of the parent compound but with slightly less potency.[5] The 5-hydroxy metabolite of propafenone possesses little β-adrenergic blocking activity. Thus, the presence of higher concentrations of the metabolite would be associated with less rate slowing in extensive metabolizers compared with a small percentage of individuals who are poor metabolizers of propafenone who manifest a greater β-blocking effect. Similarly, N-acetylprocainamide, the principal metabolite of procainamide, has a greater repolarization effect than the parent drug procainamide. N-acetylprocainamide (NAPA) is renally eliminated and so in a rapid acetylator with renal impairment, a greater effect on QT interval might be expected compared with an individual who has lesser amounts of the metabolite in the circulation.[6]

The relative concentration of parent and metabolite in any individual is genetically determined.[7] Differences in drug metabolism have been demonstrated for several antiarrhythmic drugs, including propafenone and procainamide. Genetic polymorphisms have been most extensively described for the oxidative P450 enzyme system. Population studies demonstrate that this enzyme system is expressed in a bimodal pattern, with subjects having either "extensive" or "poor" metabolic capability. The poor metabolizer phenotype is expressed in approximately 10 percent of the population in whom parent drug plasma concentration is increased, clearance is reduced, and elimination half-life prolonged. P450 enzyme isoforms have been identified that are responsible for the metabolism of specific agents and now can be identified by genotyping. Careful monitoring of patients during drug initiation to detect differences in response that may be caused by relative concentration of parent and metabolite is critically important for patient safety.

CYP2D6 is the enzyme responsible for the metabolism of propafenone, flecainide, acebutolol, metoprolol, and propranolol. Most patients are *extensive metabolizers*, which means that a large percentage of the parent compound is transformed into a metabolite with activity that is identical to, similar to, or dissimilar from the parent. CYP3A4 is the most prevalent enzyme in the liver and metabolizes many antiarrhythmic drugs, including quinidine, lidocaine, mexiletine, and many calcium channel blockers. This enzyme is inhibited by cimetidine, erythromycin, and grapefruit juice. Use of these agents causes accumulation of higher concentrations of the parent compound and thus an exaggerated electrophysiologic affect.

Metabolism issues are important in predicting the interaction of antiarrhythmic drugs with other agents, including other cardiac and noncardiac drugs that may be metabolized by the same pathways. These drugs may interfere with metabolism either by occupying the enzyme site or by having a direct effect on the activity of the enzyme. The relative affinity of the drug for the enzyme system is predictive, in many cases, of the potency of the drug interaction that might occur with commonly used agents such as digoxin and warfarin.[7]

ELIMINATION

Drug elimination occurs via a number of routes in addition to hepatic metabolism. *Clearance* is the term that describes removal of

drug from plasma and is defined as the volume of plasma cleared of drug per unit of time. The sum of all individual clearances is called total-body clearance and is the most reliable indicator of the rate of metabolism and elimination of drug. Other methods of quantifying elimination are less satisfactory. Terms such as *half-life* can be altered both by changes in clearance and by volume of distribution.

Clearance generally begins with *presystemic clearance*, which is the metabolism of the drug during its passage through the liver before reaching the systemic circulation, as previously described. A number of drugs, such as lidocaine,[8] undergo extensive first-pass clearance, which obviates their oral use. Other drugs with less-extensive first-pass clearance may be given at high doses so as to make some of the drug available to the systemic circulation. Examples include propafenone, propranolol, and verapamil. Although most drugs have a linear relationship between oral dose and plasma concentration during first-pass metabolism, others such as propafenone exhibit *saturable kinetics*, resulting in a nonlinear rise in plasma concentration during increases in oral dosing. This also results in a change in the ratio of parent drug to metabolite when the oxidative enzyme in the liver becomes saturated.

Despite its limitations, the concept of half-life can be used to describe the time required for drug elimination. Half-life is defined as the time required for the plasma concentration to drop by 50% (Fig. 43–2). For drugs that have more than one pharmacologic compartment, more than one half-life may be defined. For example, the drop in plasma concentration after administration of an intravenous bolus of a drug can be divided into its "distribution period" when the drug is distributed from the central to the peripheral compartments, and an "elimination period" during which time the drug is cleared from the central compartment by metabolism and elimination. Conversely when a drug is administered by mouth, it is usually absorbed at a rate slower than the rate of distribution of the drug. Therefore, the distribution phase may be masked by the slow absorption of the drug.

As can be seen from Fig. 43–2, the time required to achieve a steady-state plasma concentration during chronic therapy can be estimated from the elimination half-life. After approximately 3.3 half-lives, 90 percent of the steady-state plasma concentration has been reached during loading or removed during washout. Thus for a drug with a half-life of 8 hours, 24 hours is sufficient to reach near steady-state levels.

For those drugs that have a longer half-life and therefore a longer time to achieve steady state, a *loading period* may be used to bring plasma concentrations into a desired range more rapidly. Lidocaine is an excellent example of this principle. Using fixed infusion rates without loading would require more than 6 hours for lidocaine to achieve a steady-state plasma concentration. In the setting of treatment of patients with severe arrhythmias, this time period is unacceptably long. Therefore, bolus doses are given to fill the central compartment and to replace the amount of drug leaving the plasma through distribution to peripheral compartments.[8] Once steady state has been achieved—that is, when there is no more movement of drug from central to peripheral compartments—the drug can be administered as a maintenance infusion that is given at the same rate at which the drug is eliminated.

Amiodarone represents the most complicated example of drug loading to balance distribution and elimination.[9] Amiodarone is

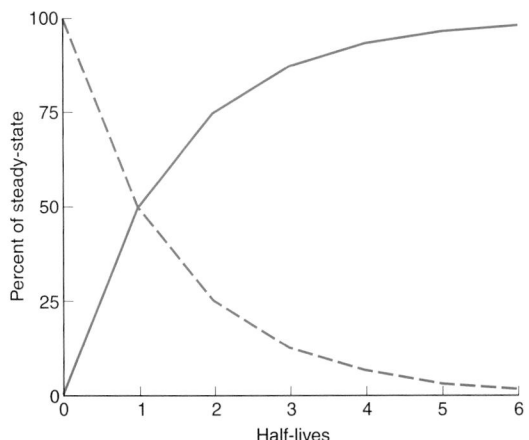

FIGURE 43–2. Time required for accumulation and elimination of drug. After initiation of drug therapy (*solid line*), 50 percent of steady-state drug concentrations are achieved in 1 half-life and 90 percent in 3.3 half-lives. Similarly, after drug is stopped (*broken line*), concentration drops by 90 percent after 3.3 half-lives. *Source: Reproduced from Siddoway L.[10] With permission.*

generally considered to have three compartments, all of which need to be saturated to achieve steady state. Large doses of oral drug are given over several weeks to achieve saturation of the peripheral and deep compartments. However, because the myocardial half-life of the drug is significantly shorter than the half-life of deeper compartments, the drug is given daily to maintain equilibrium in the myocardium.

Knowledge of the elimination half-life is critical for designing proper interdosing intervals for most oral antiarrhythmic drugs. The main considerations in determining how frequently a drug has to be administered are half-life and *therapeutic range*, defined as the minimum and maximum plasma concentrations that will achieve clinical benefit without exposing patients to toxicity.[10] The larger the ratio of maximum to minimum therapeutic effect, the longer may be the intradosing interval, during which time high peak and low trough concentrations will be achieved. Reducing peaks and valleys requires shorter interdosing intervals. For most drugs, knowledge of renal elimination kinetics is critical in formulating an effective interdosing interval and finding an adequate dose to achieve a therapeutic effect. A notable example of this principle is sotalol. Sotalol is entirely eliminated through the kidney. An estimate of creatinine clearance is necessary to select an appropriate dose and dosing interval.

One caveat in designing dosing schedules is the problem of active metabolites. Metabolites may have pharmacokinetics that are distinct from the parent.[5,6] For drugs that have metabolites that are active and have longer half-lives than the parent, interdosing intervals might need to be extended to account for the metabolite's effect. Accumulation of a metabolite with higher than necessary dosing frequency can produce toxicity that may be life-threatening.

Finally, drug half-life may be determined not only by the rate but also by the route of elimination. A prime example is adenosine, which is rapidly taken up and metabolized by erythrocytes and vascular endothelium, and thus eliminated in prompt fashion.[11] Drugs with rapid offset of effect frequently are eliminated by routes other than the kidney, or they may be distributed quickly from the central compartment as in the case of ibutilide.[12]

SPECIAL POPULATIONS
【 】 THE ELDERLY

The elderly are particularly prone to overdosing with antiarrhythmic drugs. There are several physiologic changes associated with aging that make drug accumulation more likely. These include reduction in lean body mass, fall in renal function, alterations in hepatic metabolism, and changes in receptor affinity.[13] The elderly also have increases in glycoprotein concentrations and reduction in serum albumin concentrations that may alter the ability of drugs to bind to plasma proteins, in effect raising free concentrations. Reduced receptor affinity and stimulation of adenylate cyclase attenuate the effects of catecholamines, and may make these patients more susceptible to the depressant effects of β-adrenergic blocking agents. Reduction in the activity of the renin–aldosterone system and arterial wall elasticity make elderly patients more susceptible to the develop-

ment of orthostatic hypotension. Although it is clear that aging also affects the density of ion channels, no age-related changes in the physiology of the ion channel per se has been documented. Because of these physiologic changes, elderly patients in general should be started on a smaller dose of an antiarrhythmic drug with slow upward dose titration to clinical effect or to tolerance.

【 】 OBESE PATIENTS

In general, patients with larger body size require higher doses of drugs to achieve a therapeutic plasma concentration. However, drugs may distribute differently in adipose tissue compared with muscle and other tissue. Thus, if adjustment in dose is made only on the basis of the patient's weight, some drugs will be overdosed.

【 】 CONGESTIVE HEART FAILURE

The central volume of distribution of an antiarrhythmic drug is generally reduced in congestive heart failure, necessitating reduction in initial dose.[14] Congestive heart failure also gives rise to derangements of liver and renal blood flow with reduction in clearance of the drug and high extraction ratios. For all of these reasons, as well as altered sensitivity to drug and altered plasma protein binding, drugs should be administered in low dose to patients with congestive heart failure with slow upward dose titration, as in the elderly.

【 】 RENAL FAILURE

Drug and metabolites can accumulate in patients with renal failure, depending on the proportion of the drug that is eliminated by the kidney. Drugs such as sotalol, which are exclusively renally eliminated, are particularly important in this regard.[15] Fortunately, most drugs have other routes of elimination, which can at least partly compensate for reduced elimination because of renal failure. Amiodarone is an example of a drug that is not at all eliminated by the kidney and which can be safely administered to patients on renal dialysis and to patients who are functionally anephric.

【 】 HEPATIC DISEASE

Fortunately, until hepatic disease is far advanced, hepatic metabolism and elimination of most drugs is not significantly compromised. Short of liver cirrhosis, it can be assumed the drugs will be metabolized and eliminated normally, even in patients who have elevated transaminase and bilirubin concentrations.[10]

【 】 DRUG INTERACTIONS

Antiarrhythmic drug interactions are ubiquitous and, unfortunately, underappreciated by practicing physicians. This is a complex issue as drug interactions may occur for a number of reasons, including inhibition or enhancement of drug metabolism and elimination, displacement of drug from plasma or tissue-binding sites, competition for receptor sites, and additive pharmacodynamic effects.[10] Table 43–1 outlines common drug interactions. Interaction of drugs at the level of the P450 enzyme system is responsible for an appreciable number of drug interactions in clinical practice. Other important drug interactions occur because of interference with elimination, such as when digoxin clearance is reduced by agents such as propafenone, flecainide, and amiodarone. The mechanism of this interaction has been described best for quinidine, which also dislodges digoxin from tissue-binding sites, leading to potentially toxic digoxin levels. Among the assorted other mechanisms for kinetic interactions is reduced hepatic blood flow by β-adrenergic blockers, which can result in reduction of the clearance of high extraction drugs such as lidocaine.

MECHANISMS UNDERLYING ANTIARRHYTHMIC AND PROARRHYTHMIC EFFECTS

The development of cardiac arrhythmias and drug-induced proarrhythmias can be a result of abnormal impulse formation (i.e., enhanced automaticity and triggered activities) and/or reentry (see Chap. 35). This section provides a brief overview of ionic and cellular mechanisms underlying antiarrhythmic and proarrhythmic effects of the drugs.

ION CHANNEL PHYSIOLOGY

Antiarrhythmic drugs exert their effects on cardiac electrical impulse formation and propagation via their interaction with ionic channels, or with membrane receptors and cellular pumps that subsequently influence ionic currents across the cell membrane. Cardiac ionic currents commonly targeted by antiarrhythmic drugs include inward sodium current (I_{Na}), L-type calcium current ($I_{Ca,L}$) and delayed rectifier outward potassium current (I_K).

Antiarrhythmic drugs that block the sodium channel appear to bind selectively to the channel during only one or two of the states and dissociate from the channel during the other states (Fig. 43–3). Therefore, a sodium channel blocker will block the sodium channel differently depending on pathologic conditions. Because the maximal velocity of change in membrane potential during phase 0 (V_{max}) is correlated with I_{Na} and the major driving force for electrical conduction in atrial, His-Purkinje and ventricular tissues, sodium channel blockers that bind to the

TABLE 43-1

Drug Interactions

	DIGOXIN	β BLOCKERS	WARFARIN
Quinidine	↑		
Flecainide	↑		
Propafenone	↑	↑	↑
Sotalol			
Dofetilide			
Amiodarone	↑	↑	↑
Verapamil	↑	↑	

↑ Indicates increased serum concentration of one of the three reference drugs.

Channel state	State of the m gate	State of the h gate
Resting (R)	Closed	Open
Open (O)	Open	Open
Inactivated (I)	Open	Closed

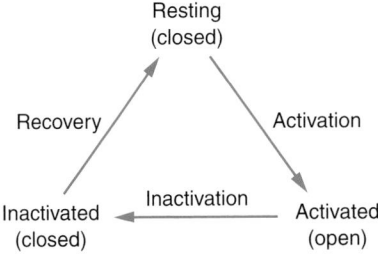

FIGURE 43–3. Schematic of sodium channel gating. Depolarization of the cell membrane opens the m gate (activation) and initiates the process (i.e., inactivation) for closing the h gate in the same time, so that the sodium channel remains open only transiently (1 to 2 milliseconds) before cycling into the inactivated state. Recovery of the sodium channel from the inactivated state for reopening is voltage and time dependent.

channel during the open state, like class Ia and Ic drugs, cause conduction slowing that manifests as QRS widening on the body surface ECG. On the other hand, sodium channel blockers that predominantly bind to the channel in the inactivated state, like class Ib drugs, have only a modest effect on action potential phase 0. In ischemic myocardium with reduced membrane potential, voltage- and time-dependent recovery of sodium channel from inactivation is delayed, so that binding of class Ib drugs to the channel is significantly increased. This explains the greater activity of class Ib antiarrhythmic drugs under conditions of myocardial ischemia. In contrast, atrial repolarization is faster compared with the ventricles, and is associated with rapid transition of the atrial sodium channel from the inactivated to the resting state. Therefore, class Ib drugs play little role in atrial arrhythmias. A few channels may remain open through sustained depolarization, the so-called *late* (or *slow*) I_{Na},[16] and contribute to the action potential duration. Compared with the epicardium and endocardium, the submyocardium of the left ventricle (M cells) has a larger late I_{Na}.[17,18] Blockade of the late I_{Na} causes action potential shortening, whereas an increase in this current by drugs like ibutilide leads to action potential lengthening.

$I_{Ca,L}$ is responsible for the prolonged plateau phase (phase 2) of the action potentials of atrial, His-Purkinje, and ventricular cells, and is the major inward current responsible for phase 0 depolarization in sinus and atrioventricular (AV) nodal cells. Consequently, calcium channel blockade causes slight action potential shortening in the atria, His-Purkinje system, and the ventricles, depresses the slope of diastolic depolarization and action potential amplitude, and prolongs the effective refractory period in sinus and AV nodal cells. L-type calcium channels may reactivate during the action potential plateau under conditions of delayed ventricular repolarization (i.e., long QT syndrome). This may lead to phase 2 early afterdepolarization (EAD) capable of initiating a specific form of polymorphic ventricular tachycardia termed *torsade de pointes*.[19] In addition, larger calcium influx via L-type calcium channel increases the likelihood of calcium overloading in the sarcoplasmic reticulum (SR) under certain pathologic conditions. Oscillatory release of calcium from SR increases Na/Ca exchange, resulting in the genesis of delayed afterdepolarization (DAD) and triggered activity.[20]

The delayed rectifier outward potassium current is responsible for phase 3 repolarization and blockade of this current leads to an increase in action potential duration and effective refractory period in the atria, AV node, His-Purkinje fibers, the ventricles, and accessory pathways. The delayed rectifier outward potassium current consists of two components: one activates rapidly (I_{Kr}) and another that activates slowly (I_{Ks}).

Use Dependence

The class Ic drugs dissociate from the sodium channel in the resting state very slowly, exhibiting strong use dependence, manifest as an increase in sodium channel blockade during tachycardia. This is thought to be responsible for the increased efficacy of the class antiarrhythmic Ic drugs in slowing and converting tachycardia with minimal effects at normal sinus rates.

Reverse Use Dependence

As opposed to the use dependence observed for drugs that block the sodium and calcium channels, inhibition of I_{Kr} is enhanced during bradycardia when the channel is "not frequently used," leading to more significant action potential prolongation at slow heart rates. The mechanism is probably related to the dependence of I_{Kr} blockade on extracellular potassium concentration.[21] Reverse use-dependent properties of antiarrhythmic drugs may reduce their efficacy in tachycardias, and predispose to bradycardia-dependent proarrhythmias.

【 】 REENTRY

Development of reentry using an anatomical circuit is determined by the wavelength of the reentrant wavefront and the size of the circuit. The wavelength of the reentrant wavefront is equal to the product of the conduction velocity times the effective refractory period of myocardial tissue in the pathway, and should be significantly less than the length of the reentrant circuit for the maintenance of circus movement. Conduction velocity of the electrical impulse in the atria, His-Purkinje, and the ventricles is largely determined by the intensity of the fast inward sodium current that contributes to the rapid upstroke (V_{max}) of the action potential. For example, class Ic antiarrhythmic drugs may predispose to the development of monomorphic ventricular tachycardia in patients with coronary artery disease because of reduction of the V_{max} of the action potential and slowing of conduction.[22] On the other hand, antiarrhythmic drugs that prolong the refractory period and therefore the wavelength of a reentrant wavefront are useful in suppressing reentrant arrhythmias.

【 】 ABNORMAL IMPULSE FORMATION

Abnormal Automaticity

Normal automaticity of cardiac cells is the consequence of spontaneous diastolic depolarization caused by a net inward current during phase 4 of action potential. Abnormal automaticity, which is caused by either enhanced normal automaticity or spontaneous activity in ventricular and atrial myocardium, may occur with heightened β-adrenergic tone, or reduced resting membrane potentials, such as ischemia or infarction.[23]

Afterdepolarization and Triggered Activity

Afterdepolarization can be divided into two subclasses: EADs and DADs. EADs often occur in M cells or endocardium because these action potentials prolong disproportionally with drugs that block I_{Kr}, an ionic current targeted by most QT-prolonging drugs.[19,24] Antiarrhythmic drugs like mexiletine that inhibit $I_{Ca,L}$ or shorten action potential duration by blocking sodium current suppress EADs. Calcium channel and β-adrenergic blockers suppress DADs and, therefore, DAD-mediated arrhythmias by reducing intracellular calcium overload.

【 】 PROARRHYTHMIA

Proarrhythmic and antiarrhythmic effects of a drug are two sides of the same coin. Antiarrhythmic drugs that are intended to suppress arrhythmias may potentially worsen a preexisting arrhythmia or cause a new arrhythmia. The mechanisms responsible for cardiac arrhythmias are complicated, and any intervention may be antiarrhythmic in some circumstances and proarrhythmic in others.

Atrial Proarrhythmias

When class I antiarrhythmic drugs are used for the treatment of supraventricular tachycardia, they can cause atrial flutter, often with slower rates (approximately 150 to 200 beats/min). This is seen in patients with atrial fibrillation treated with the class Ic drugs flecainide and propafenone. The slowed atrial flutter may be associated with 1:1 AV conduction with markedly high ventricular rates. Therefore, dosing with an AV nodal blocking agent should be considered with a sodium channel blocker in patients with atrial fibrillation and intact AV nodes.

Adenosine and digitalis occasionally promote the development of atrial fibrillation by shortening atrial effective refractory period. Shortening of the refractory period reduces the wavelength of reentrant wavefront, so that reentry can occur in smaller reentrant substrates.

Ventricular Proarrhythmias

Ventricular proarrhythmias can generally be divided into two categories based on mechanisms and ECG features: monomorphic ventricular tachycardia and a specific form of polymorphic ventricular tachycardia termed *torsade de pointes* (TdP).

A key factor in the genesis of monomorphic ventricular tachycardia is the availability of an anatomical reentrant pathway. Any drug that causes conduction slowing more than effective refractory period prolongation has the potential to facilitate the development of reentrant arrhythmias. Class Ic drugs have the highest risk to cause this type of proarrhythmia and to increase mortality in patients with coronary artery disease and left ventricular systolic dysfunction.[25–27] Myocardial ischemia seems to play a pivotal role in the genesis of proarrhythmia with class Ic drugs. Conversely, proarrhythmia rates are nearly zero when class Ic drugs are used for atrial arrhythmias in patients with a structurally normal heart.[28]

TdP requires QT prolongation.[29] An example is "quinidine syncope" in patients who have taken quinidine for the treatment of atrial fibrillation and experienced recurrent syncope or cardiac arrest as the result of QT prolongation and TdP. It is widely accepted that TdP is initiated by EAD-dependent triggered activity and maintains itself via functional reentry.[19] Class Ia and class III antiarrhythmic drugs that block I_{Kr} and/or increase late I_{Na} may facilitate the development of TdP. Interestingly, amiodarone, a commonly used class III antiarrhythmic drug, significantly prolongs the QT interval but rarely causes TdP. Amiodarone prolongs the action potential duration without producing EADs and reduces transmural dispersion of repolarization, probably as a consequence of its effects on multiple ionic channels and receptors.[30]

Marked QT prolongation and resultant TdP are more likely to occur in patients with reduced repolarization reserve. Clinical diseases or conditions that are associated with reduced repolarization reserve include congenital long QT syndrome, bradycardia, female gender, ventricular hypertrophy, electrolyte disturbances such as hypokalemia and hypomagnesemia, and coadministration of other QT-prolonging agents or drugs that delay clearance of the drugs from the body.

HEMODYNAMIC EFFECTS

A number of antiarrhythmic drugs have significant hemodynamic effects that may limit their usefulness under certain clinical situations. It is well known that class I drugs reduce myocardial contractility and may exacerbate congestive heart failure.[31] Among the sodium channel blockers, class Ic drugs and disopyramide exert the most potent negative inotropic effect; β-adrenergic and calcium channel blockers also are negative inotropic agents, because of their inhibitory effect on inward L-type calcium current. Although β-adrenergic blockers, when used in patients with compensated heart failure, reduce symptoms of heart failure and improve survival, their use in patients with decompensated heart failure who need inotropic support of intravenous agents should be avoided.

The majority of class III antiarrhythmic drugs are well tolerated hemodynamically in patients with heart failure. Data from clinical trials show that dofetilide and amiodarone do not significantly affect the hemodynamic state of patients with severe left ventricular dysfunction and heart failure.[32,33] However, d,l-sotalol should be used cautiously in patients with significant heart failure because its β-adrenergic blocking effect may exacerbate heart failure.

ANTIARRHYTHMIC DRUG CLASSIFICATION

The antiarrhythmic drug classification system most often employed was originally put forth by Vaughn-Williams and modified by Harrison. This classification is relatively simple and useful. It assumes that each antiarrhythmic drug has a predominant electrophysiologic mechanism of action and has a primary therapeutic application (Table 43–2).

Class I Antiarrhythmic Drugs

According to the original schema, drugs that have an effect on sodium channels were placed in class I. It was later recognized that the relative potency of all of these drugs varied, and that some had additional electrophysiologic effects differentiating them from others (see Table 43–2). For that reason, subclasses a, b, and c were used to designate these differences. The class Ia agents, including quinidine, procainamide, and disopyramide, exert an intermediate effect to block the fast sodium current and prolong the action potential duration by blocking outward potassium current. The class Ib agents, including lidocaine, mexiletine, and tocainide, are the weakest sodium blockers that produce little change in the QRS duration in normal cardiac tissues and have a negligible effect on repolarization. The class Ic drugs, including flecainide and propafenone, have a more potent effect on the sodium current, leading to depression of phase 0 of the action potential and exhibiting more use dependence, that is, inhibiting the sodium current and slowing conduction during tachycardia.

Class II Antiarrhythmic Drugs

These agents act indirectly on ionic currents primarily by inhibiting sympathetic activity through β-adrenergic blockade, leading to

TABLE 43–2

Vaughan-Williams Classification of Antiarrhythmic Drugs

CLASS		ACTION	DRUGS
I		Sodium channel blockade	
	Ia	Moderate phase 0 depression and conduction slowing, prolonging of action potential duration	Quinidine, procainamide, disopyramide
	Ib	Minimal effect on phase 0 upstroke No change or shortening of action potential duration	Lidocaine, mexiletine, tocainide
	Ic	Marked phase 0 depression and conduction slowing, little effect on repolarization	Flecainide, propafenone, moricizine
II		β-Adrenergic blockade	Propranolol, metoprolol, atenolol, esmolol, acebutolol
III		Potassium channel blockade	d,l-Sotalol, dofetilide, amiodarone, bretylium, ibutilide
IV		Calcium channel blockade	Verapamil, diltiazem

TABLE 43–3

Threshold Effects of Some Antiarrhythmic Drugs

DRUG	PACING THRESHOLD	DEFIBRILLATION THRESHOLD
Quinidine	Increase	Increase
Procainamide	Increase	No change
Lidocaine	No change	Increase
Mexiletine	Slight increase	Increase
Flecainide	Increase	Increase
Propafenone	Increase	No change
β Blockers	Variable	No change
Sotalol	No change	Decrease
Dofetilide	No change	Decrease
Azimilide	No change	Decrease
Ibutilide	No change	Decrease
Amiodarone	Variable	Increase
Verapamil	Increase	No change
Digitalis	Decrease	No change or decrease

SOURCE: Modified with permission from Reiffel JA, Coromilas J, Zimmerman JM, Spotnitz HM. Drug-device interactions: clinical considerations. PACE 1985;8:369–373.

sinus rhythm slowing and PR interval prolongation under physiologic conditions.

Class III Antiarrhythmic Drugs

Class III antiarrhythmic drugs are those that extend the action potential duration, thereby increasing the effective refractory period. There is a great deal of heterogeneity within this class as the drugs may act on any of several different ion channels to reduce the net repolarizing current and prolong refractoriness Most of the class III drugs demonstrate reverse use dependence, with their maximal effect on repolarization at slower heart rates, which may be counterproductive for effective arrhythmia termination. Amiodarone, ibutilide, and azimilide have a fairly homogeneous effect on refractoriness across a range of cycle lengths.

Class IV Antiarrhythmic Drugs

Class IV antiarrhythmic drugs are L-type calcium channel blockers. Here, again, there is substantial heterogeneity within the class. This may be particularly important as the calcium antagonists have a variable effect on slow channels in the heart versus the peripheral circulation.

This Vaughn-Williams classification schema has been used as a conversational shorthand to facilitate exchange of information about the electrophysiologic properties of antiarrhythmic drugs. But it has a number of important drawbacks: First, many of the currently available drugs have multiple actions. Second, the metabolites of some of the drugs may be primarily responsible for at least some of the antiarrhythmic actions, such as procainamide and its metabolite N-acetylprocainamide. Third, the scheme does not account for important differences

seen when the drugs are used in diverse patients populations; for example, the incidence and nature of proarrhythmia as it relates to presence, type, and severity of underlying structural heart diseases.

Because of the limitations of the Vaughan-Williams classification of antiarrhythmic drugs, an alternative approach has been proposed, termed the *Sicilian gambit,* in which antiarrhythmic drugs are classed based on their differential effects on (1) channels, (2) receptors, and (3) transmembrane pumps.[34] The Sicilian gambit has not had a major impact on clinical practice.

DRUG–DEVICE INTERACTIONS[35]

Patients with devices may require concomitant drug therapy for a variety of reasons, the most common being to reduce arrhythmia frequency. An antiarrhythmic drug can cause excessive rate slowing that mandates placement of a bradycardia pacing device. Drugs can also have an impact on the pacing threshold and the thresholds for arrhythmia termination (Table 43–3). In general, drugs that reduce the sodium current should be expected to raise pacing and defibrillation thresholds, while potassium channel blockers reduce the defibrillation threshold and exert little effect on capture threshold. Drugs can change ventricular tachycardia rate and thus the efficiency of detection and termination algorithms.

ANTIARRHYTHMIC DRUGS AND PREGNANCY

Antiarrhythmic drugs have played a central role in the treatment of arrhythmias in the mother as well as the fetus. Table 43–4 summarizes the use of antiarrhythmic drugs and their potential side effects in pregnancy.

Quinidine and procainamide have been safely used for the treatment of maternal and fetal arrhythmias. Quinidine can cause thrombocytopenia and eighth nerve damage in the fetus; chronic administration of procainamide may be associated with autoimmune responses such as lupus-like syndrome. There is limited experience with the use of disopyramide but it can cause uterine contraction and premature labor. Lidocaine is well tolerated and widely used in pregnancy. Intravenous lidocaine is administered primarily for the acute management of life-threatening ventricular arrhythmias. Experience with mexiletine, flecainide, and propafenone in pregnancy is relatively limited.[36,37] Because propafenone and flecainide have good transplacental passage, both have been used as the second-line of therapy for sustained fetal supraventricular arrhythmias, particularly in the presence of hydrops fetalis, which are refractory to digoxin.[37]

β-Adrenergic blockers are primarily used to treat hypertension and thyrotoxicosis in pregnancy. These agents are generally safe for the mother and the fetus. β-Adrenergic blockers are useful in the treatment of supraventricular tachycardia, atrial fibrillation or atrial flutter, idiopathic ventricular tachycardia, and long QT syndrome. Prophylactic treatment with β-adrenergic blockers significantly reduces the risk of cardiac events in patients with the congenital long QT syndrome, particularly in the postpartum period when patients are at the highest risk.[38]

The adverse effects of β-adrenergic blockers include bradycardia, hypoglycemia, fetal apnea, premature labor and metabolic abnormalities, but these effects occur more frequently in high-risk patients.[39] Because β-adrenergic blockers may cause intrauterine growth retardation,[40] the use of β-adrenergic blockers in the first trimester of pregnancy should be avoided. Although some β-adrenergic blockers, such as propranolol, atenolol, labetalol, nadolol, and metoprolol, are excreted in breast milk, significant bradycardia in infants may be seen, although rarely.

There is relatively limited experience with the use of class III antiarrhythmic drugs in pregnancy. Sotalol has been used in the treatment of refractory maternal and fetal supraventricular and ventricular arrhythmias. Amiodarone should be totally avoided or used with extreme caution for arrhythmias that are refractory to other drugs and are life-threatening. Amiodarone causes hypothyroidism or hyperthyroidism, congenital abnormalities, bradycardia, premature labor, low birth weight, and prematurity.[41,42] Amiodarone is excreted in breast milk and can cause hypothyroidism or hyperthyroidism, but not significant bradycardia, in breast-fed infants.

Calcium channel blockers, like verapamil and diltiazem, have been used for supraventricular tachycardia and control of the ventricular response to atrial fibrillation or flutter in pregnancy. These agents are also useful in the treatment of selected idiopathic ventricular tachycardias. Calcium channel blockers are considered to be relatively safe, although they have the potential to cause hypotension, heart block, bradycardia, and exacerbation of heart failure in mother and fetus.

Digoxin has a long record of safety for the treatment of supraventricular tachycardia including AV nodal reentrant tachycardia and atrial fibrillation or flutter in pregnancy.[43] Because digoxin can cross the placenta, it has been used to treat fetal supraventricular tachycardia. It is often administered in a relatively large dose to the mother to obtain a therapeutic plasma concentration in the fe-

TABLE 43–4

Antiarrhythmic Drugs and Pregnancy

DRUG	FDA CLASS[a]	INDICATIONS	POSSIBLE ADVERSE EFFECTS	COMMENTS
Quinidine	C	SVT/CBT and VT	Maternal and fetal thrombocytopenia, eighth nerve toxicity, and TdP	Long record of safety
Procainamide	C	SVT/CBT, VT, or undiagnosed WCT	Lupus-like syndrome with long-term use and TdP	Long record of safety
Disopyramide	C	Limited experience Induction of labor	Premature labor and TdP	Limited experience
Lidocaine	B	VT	CNS adverse effects and bradycardia	Long record of safety
Mexiletine	C	VT	CNS adverse effects and fetal bradycardia	Limited usage
Flecainide	C	SVT/CBT and selected VT	?	Used in fetal SVT with hydrops fetalis
Propafenone	C	SVT/CBT and selected VT	?	Used in fetal SVT with hydrops fetalis
β Blockers	B-D	SVT, AF/AFL, selected VT, and LQTS	Intrauterine growth retardation, fetal bradycardia, hypoglycemia, and apnea	Generally safe Avoid during first trimester
Sotalol	B	SVT and VT	Bradycardia and TdP	Limited experience
Amiodarone	D	Life-threatening VT	Fetal hyper- or hypothyroidism, growth retardation, prematurity, bradycardia, and malformation	Avoid during first trimester
Ibutilide	C	Acute termination of AF/AFL	TdP	No experience
Verapamil	C	SVT, AF/AFL, and selected VT	Maternal hypotension, fetal bradycardia, and AV block	Relatively safe
Diltiazem	C	SVT and AF/AFL	Maternal hypotension, fetal bradycardia, and AV block	Verapamil preferred
Digoxin	C	SVT and AF/AFL	Low birth weight and premature labor	Long record of safety
Adenosine	C	Acute termination of the mother's SVT	Transient dyspnea and fetal bradycardia	Short duration of effect

AF/AFL, atrial fibrillation/flutter; AV, atrioventricular; CNS, central nervous system; LQTS, long QT syndrome; SVT, supraventricular tachycardia; SVT/CBT, supraventricular tachycardia utilizing concealed bypass tract; TdP, torsade de pointes; VT, ventricular tachycardia; WCT, wide complex tachycardia; ?, unknown.
[a]FDA pregnancy categories: A, no risk demonstrated in well-controlled studies in humans; B, no evidence of risk in humans; C, risk can't be ruled out; D, positive evidence of risk in pregnancy; X, contraindicated in pregnancy.
SOURCE: Modified with permission from Joglar JA, Page RL. Antiarrhythmic drugs in pregnancy. Curr Opin Cardiol 2001;16: 40–45.

tus because transplacental passage of digoxin may be impaired by some pathologic conditions, such as hydrops fetalis.[37,43] Digoxin is associated with premature labor and low birth weight. Adenosine is used for the acute termination of supraventricular tachycardia and is not associated with adverse effects in the mother or fetus. Fetal bradycardia may occur occasionally, but is usually very brief because of the drug's short half-life.

ANTIARRHYTHMIC DRUGS

❚❩ CLASS I ANTIARRHYTHMIC DRUGS

Class Ia: Quinidine

Electrophysiology The main actions of quinidine include conduction slowing and action potential prolongation. Action potential duration prolongation relates to block of the delayed rectifier potassium current (I_{Kr}). Quinidine also inhibits the transient-outward current (Ito) and may thereby prevent ventricular fibrillation in the Brugada syndrome.[44,45] Apart from these effects on cardiac sodium and potassium channels, quinidine has vagolytic effects leading to increased sinus rate and enhanced AV nodal conduction. Dose-related changes in the electrocardiogram include increases in the PR, QRS, and QT intervals.

Pharmacokinetics and Dosing Quinidine sulfate is usually administered every 6 hours, but it must be kept in mind that interindividual differences in its elimination half-life may vary from 3 to 19 hours. Quinidine is eliminated by both hepatic metabolism (50 to 90 percent) and renal elimination (10 to 30 percent). Therapeutic plasma concentrations range between 2 and 7 μg/mL. Because the quinidine content in the different forms of quinidine (sulfate, gluconate, and polygalacturonate) differs, one needs to adjust dose when one form is substituted for another. The usual effective dosage of quinidine sulfate ranges from 800 to 2400 mg/d. In patients with heart failure or structural heart disease, and in those with the congenital long QT syndrome, hypokalemia, or a history of torsade de pointes, quinidine should be withheld.[46] In combination with digitalis, dosages of both drugs should be kept lower than usual.

Indication Quinidine is used in supraventricular and ventricular arrhythmias.[47,48] However, at present there is no large role for quinidine in the management of cardiac arrhythmias.

Adverse Effects Quinidine can cause diarrhea that can be very troublesome. Rare adverse reactions include fever, rash, tinnitus, thrombocytopenia, and granulomatous hepatitis. Atrial and ventricular proarrhythmia may occur. Torsade de pointes usually occurs in patients (more often in women than in men) with low serum concentrations of quinidine, hypokalemia, poor ventricular function, and bradycardia.[49]

Class Ia: Disopyramide

Electrophysiology Disopyramide's effects on automaticity, conduction, and refractoriness in atrial and ventricular tissue are similar to those of quinidine and procainamide. It has more marked

anticholinergic effects than quinidine. In addition, it is more negatively inotropic.

Pharmacokinetics Ninety percent of an oral dose of disopyramide is absorbed and its bioavailability is approximately 80 percent. It is excreted in the urine, 55 percent unchanged and partially as the active N-monodealkylated metabolite. The half-life varies from 4 to 10 hours, but may lengthen to as much as 15 hours in cardiac patients. In patients with renal failure and congestive heart failure, its elimination half-life is significantly increased. Therapeutic levels vary between 2 and 5 mg/L.

Dosing Dosage ranges from 100 to 400 mg three to four times per day with the short-acting form, or twice daily when a sustained preparation is used. The maximum dose should not exceed 800 mg/d. The therapeutic plasma concentration may not always be reliable because of variable protein binding. The initial dosage of disopyramide should be reduced to 50 to 100 mg every 12 hours in patients with renal insufficiency or decreased hepatic function.

Indication Disopyramide may be used for treatment of ventricular or atrial arrhythmias.

Adverse Effects Disopyramide's subjective toxicity is primarily a result of its anticholinergic activity and includes dry mouth, blurred vision, urinary retention (also in women), constipation, and worsening of glaucoma. If needed, a long-acting cholinesterase inhibitor pyridostigmine (or physostigmine and neostigmine) can be given with disopyramide to minimize anticholinergic adverse effects. Disopyramide is contraindicated in patients with uncompensated heart failure because it can worsen left ventricular function. It may cause atrial and ventricular proarrhythmias.

Class Ia: Procainamide

Electrophysiology Procainamide slows conduction and decreases the automaticity and excitability of atrial and ventricular myocardium and Purkinje fibers. It also prolongs action potential duration and refractoriness but this is mainly caused by the active metabolite of procainamide, NAPA, which lacks class I activity. Compared with quinidine, procainamide has very little vagolytic activity and prolongs the QT interval less.

Pharmacokinetics Procainamide is 95 percent absorbed in the small intestine, with bioavailability of approximately 85 percent. Procainamide is acetylated in the liver to an active metabolite, NAPA. The rate of acetylation depends on a genetically determined acetylation phenotype. In rapid acetylators (slightly more than half of the population), NAPA levels usually exceed that of the parent compound. The usual effective plasma concentration for procainamide is 4 to 8 mg/L. From 30 to 60 percent of the drug is excreted unchanged in the urine and the remainder is excreted as NAPA. The short half-life of elimination after oral administration (2 to 4 hours in patients with normal renal function), necessitates dosing every 3 to 6 hours. Dosing every 6, 8, or 12 hours is possible with sustained-release preparations. NAPA has a half-life of 6 hours.

Dosing Procainamide can be administered intravenously or taken orally in a shorter-acting or sustained-release formulation. The procainamide dose usually is 50 mg/kg per day, if cardiac and renal function is normal; the average dosage is thus 1500 to 4000 mg/d, administered in two to four doses, depending on the formulation. Intravenous procainamide requires loading doses of 10 to 15 mg/kg given at 100 mg/min, depending on blood pressure. This can be followed by a 1 to 4 mg/min intravenous infusion.

During chronic therapy, levels of NAPA may accumulate to effective or toxic levels in some individuals, resulting in achievement of maximum pharmacologic effect long after procainamide has reached steady state. Thus, dosage should be initiated at conservative levels, and the patient should be monitored carefully until both procainamide and its metabolite have reached steady state.

Indication Both intravenous and oral procainamide may be used to convert and treat patients with supraventricular and ventricular tachycardia. Intravenous procainamide is one of the parenteral treatments of choice for termination of ventricular tachyarrhythmias and is more likely to terminate ventricular tachycardia (VT) than lidocaine.[50]

Adverse Effects Procainamide may cause nausea, anorexia, vomiting, and rash. End-organ toxicity of concern is rare granulocytosis that usually occurs during the first 3 months of treatment. The major limiting adverse reaction with procainamide is the development of a systemic lupus-like reaction in 10 to 20 percent of patients. This is more likely to occur in slow acetylators, in whom procainamide levels are high and NAPA levels are low. Procainamide has a mild negative inotropic effect.[51] Procainamide can cause high-degree AV block and ventricular proarrhythmia, including new-onset, sustained, monomorphic VT or torsade de pointes, the latter likely related to NAPA.

Class Ib: Lidocaine

Electrophysiology Lidocaine may suppress abnormal automaticity as may occur in myocardial ischemia. Apart from this, lidocaine also shows significant conduction-slowing effects in ischemic tissue. Lidocaine has little to no effect on normal atrial, AV nodal, or accessory pathway tissue; thus it is ineffective in treating supraventricular arrhythmias.

Pharmacokinetics Lidocaine administered as an intravenous bolus is distributed rapidly into the intravascular compartment and then diffuses quickly into the peripheral compartment (biphasic disposition). Lidocaine has a half-life of 1.5 to 2 hours in the second pass of redistribution, with extensive metabolism occurring hepatically. Because of this, a bolus load must be given before continuous infusion. The time required to reach steady-state conditions is approximately 8 to 10 hours in normal individuals and up to 24 hours in patients with heart failure and/or liver disease.

Dosing Recommended dosing includes a loading bolus infusion of 75 to 200 mg intravenously followed by a 1- to 4-mg/min maintenance infusion. Within 15 minutes of the first bolus, a second bolus of 100 mg can be given to maintain levels. Initial loading regimens do not require adjustment in patients with renal or liver disease. However, maintenance doses must be decreased in liver disease and heart failure to compensate for decreased clearance.

Indication Lidocaine is useful in the acute treatment of ischemic ventricular arrhythmias. A meta-analysis, however, suggests that lidocaine should not be routinely used in these patients.

Adverse Effects Lidocaine has dose-related neurologic and gastrointestinal adverse effects. A rapid bolus can induce tinnitus or seizures. High plasma levels are associated with drowsiness, dysarthria, confusion, hallucinations, and even coma. Gastrointestinal side effects include nausea and vomiting. Lidocaine is well tolerated hemodynamically. Lower dosages are needed in patients with heart failure and in the elderly.

Other Class Ib Drugs

Mexiletine and tocainide are orally active drugs with effects like lidocaine. Tocainide is rarely used at present. Mexiletine may be used in patients with long QT_3 syndrome because it blocks late sodium current, which is responsible for the lengthening of repolarization and torsade de pointes.[52] Because congestive heart failure significantly affects mexiletine clearance, dose adjustments and careful monitoring are required in congestive heart failure patients who are receiving mexiletine. Class Ib drugs have little, if any, effect on hemodynamics and myocardial contractility, and may be safely used in heart failure patients.

Class Ic: Flecainide

Electrophysiology Flecainide slows conduction in the atria, AV node, His-Purkinje system, ventricles, and accessory pathways. It also prolongs refractoriness, especially in the atria.

Pharmacokinetics Flecainide's bioavailability is 90 to 95 percent. Because its half-life is approximately 20 hours, a twice-daily dosing scheme must be followed when using the normal formulation. Although flecainide is mostly metabolized in the liver, kidney excretion is quite important. The dose of flecainide should be reduced in renal failure patients.

Dosing Therapy is usually initiated at 100 mg twice daily, but one should start lower dosages in elderly and low-body-weight patients, as well as in patients with decreased renal function. The maximum dose is three times 100 mg or two times 150 mg. Therapeutic levels vary between 0.2 and 1.0 μg/mL. Prolongation of the PR and QRS intervals occur when therapeutic plasma levels are achieved. QRS duration should not exceed 125 to 140 percent of baseline provided that the drug is avoided in patients with wide drug-free QRS duration (>120 milliseconds). In appropriate patients, exercise testing should be done before starting treatment to check for ventricular ischemia. Also, after reaching steady-state plasma concentration, exercise testing may be done to exclude excessive QRS widening, which is associated with ventricular proarrhythmia.

Indication Flecainide is a class Ic antiarrhythmic agent used in ventricular and supraventricular arrhythmias.[53–57] However, it should be avoided in patients with ischemia and ventricular scar, such as coronary artery disease patients, especially after myocardial infarction.[26]

Adverse Effects Flecainide is usually well tolerated. Noncardiac side effects, which are dose-related, include dizziness, uncertain gait, difficulty in focusing vision, and sometimes headache. In patients with structural heart disease, flecainide may cause sudden death, new-onset, sustained ventricular tachycardia, and aggravation of heart failure.[58] In patients without significant heart disease and supraventricular tachycardia or atrial fibrillation, there is no such risk.[59] Obviously, it must be avoided in patients with Brugada syndrome. Flecainide may worsen sinus node dysfunction, and because of its slowing effects on the His-Purkinje conduction, it may cause atrioventricular block.

Class Ic: Propafenone

Electrophysiology Propafenone differs from flecainide because of its β-blocking activity and it blocks sodium channels in both the activated and the inactivated state. The clinical electrophysiologic effects are the same as with flecainide.

Pharmacokinetics Propafenone is completely absorbed. Thereafter, it undergoes first-pass hepatic elimination. Metabolism of propafenone occurs by the CYP2D6 enzyme system. Ten percent of patients are poor metabolizers with a prolonged half-life of the parent compound. The half-life of the parent compound is around 6 hours. Poor metabolizers may have half-lives between 10 and 12 hours. The major metabolites of propafenone are 5-hydroxypropafenone (active) and *N*-debutyl propafenone. Although the half-life of propafenone is only 6 hours, steady state is not usually reached for 72 hours because of the active metabolite's half-life.

Dosing The recommended starting dosage of propafenone is 150 mg three times a day. The dosage may be increased to 225 to 300 mg three times per day. A sustained-release form of this drug is available.

Indications Its indications are similar to those of flecainide.[60,61]

Adverse Effects Subjective and cardiac adverse effects are similar to flecainide. A rash is seen in approximately 3 percent of patients. Rarely propafenone causes neutropenia or lupus syndrome. Propafenone can raise digoxin levels by 40 to 60 percent. Propafenone may also increase warfarin levels.

【 】 CLASS II AGENTS (β BLOCKERS)
Electrophysiology

β Blockers may prevent shortening of refractoriness at all levels in the heart. They also block adrenergic activation of calcium chan-

nels. β Blockers decrease resting and maximum exercise heart rate, prolong sinus node recovery time, and increase PR and AH intervals. In addition, they prolong the refractoriness of the atrioventricular node. In addition, β_2 receptors are implicated in ischemia-dependent ventricular fibrillation, which may be prevented by nonselective β blockade.[62]

Pharmacokinetics

Pharmacokinetics may differ significantly among β blockers. As a general pattern, β blockers may be eliminated through hepatic metabolism or excreted by the kidney. Bioavailability of these drugs is quite variable and their plasma half-life is short.

Indications

β Blockers affect AV nodal conduction and slow the ventricular response over the AV node during atrial fibrillation and may be effective in terminating AV and AV nodal reentry, or preventing such arrhythmias. β Blockers are contraindicated in patients with a preexcited ventricular response during atrial fibrillation. β Blockers may suppress nonsustained ventricular arrhythmias, especially in patients with an underlying adrenergic mechanism. Consequently, they are the drugs of choice in exercise-induced arrhythmias and in patients with long QT syndrome, especially LQT1.

Dosing

β Blockers are usually titrated to resting heart rate and, if needed, to heart rate during exercise. Dosing schemes and actual dosages vary.

Adverse Effects

Abrupt withdrawal of β blockers in coronary artery disease patients may lead to worsening angina, myocardial infarction, and even sudden death. Blockade of the β receptor may mask signs of hypoglycemia in diabetics. Adverse effects caused by exaggerated therapeutic effects include bradycardias in patients with sick sinus syndrome or atrioventricular nodal conduction disturbances. Heart failure in patients with significant left ventricular systolic disease is another important adverse effect of all β blockers. Nonselective β blockers may cause bronchial constriction. Nonselective β blockers may also worsen claudication or Raynaud phenomenon. Other frequently observed complaints during β-blocker therapy are fatigue (through lowering of contractility and cardiac output, or through central nervous system effects), impotence, depression, hallucinations, nightmares, and insomnia.[63]

【 】 CLASS III DRUGS
Ibutilide

Electrophysiology Ibutilide prolongs repolarization both in atrial and ventricular myocardium.[64,65] It increases atrial and ventricular refractoriness, as well as refractoriness of the atrioventricular node, His-Purkinje system, and accessory pathways.[66] Electrocardiographic changes with ibutilide include mild slowing of the sinus rate and prolongation of the QT interval. The QT interval returns to baseline within 2 to 4 hours after stopping infusion. After drug conversion of atrial flutter or fibrillation, patients need to stay on a monitor until the QT interval has normalized.

Pharmacokinetics Ibutilide has a half-life of 2 to 12 hours. It is extensively metabolized by the liver to eight metabolites. Only one metabolite exhibits antiarrhythmic activity, but its level does not exceed 10 percent of the parent drug. This metabolite does not determine efficacy of ibutilide, but may play a role in its late proarrhythmic effects.

Dosing Ibutilide should be administered under continuous ECG monitoring. The recommended dose varies with patient size: for patients weighing less than 60 kg, 0.01 mg/kg is infused over 10 minutes. If flutter or fibrillation does not terminate 10 minutes after the end of the infusion, a second bolus (same dose over 10 minutes) can be given. For patients weighing more than 60 kg, a fixed dose of 1 mg is given over 10 minutes, which—if unsuccessful—may be followed by a similar second infusion.[67] Arrhythmia termination is usually seen within 40 to 60 minutes after start of infusion. Then the infusion may be stopped and the patient is monitored for at least 4 hours. During and after infusion, aberrant conduction masquerading as monomorphic ventricular tachycardia may occur similar to dofetilide.[57] Before discharging the patient, the QT should have normalized. With excessive QT prolongation or with development of torsade de pointes, drug administration must be stopped immediately. Intravenous magnesium may help suppress further torsade de pointes and may be given beforehand.

Indication Ibutilide is approved for intravenous termination of recent onset atrial flutter and fibrillation. Its efficacy is higher in flutter, as well as in patients with shorter arrhythmia duration.[68] It may also safely convert atrial fibrillation to sinus rhythm in patients after cardiac surgery and in those with the Wolff-Parkinson-White syndrome.

Adverse Effects Because of the short-term application, noncardiac side effects are infrequent and include nausea, headache, and renal failure. Transient hypotension, sinus bradycardia, and atrioventricular block may also occur sporadically. Ibutilide does not exhibit negative inotropic effects but may cause vasodilation leading to hypotension. Polymorphic VT occurs in 4 to 8 percent of patients and torsade de pointes requiring cardioversion in approximately 2 percent. Women, patients with heart failure, low potassium or magnesium, or a low ventricular rate, and patients who are receiving the higher dosage are at increased risk of torsade de pointes. Considering the above, ibutilide is contraindicated in patients with severe structural heart disease and heart failure, prolonged QT interval, or underlying sinus node disease.

Sotalol

Sotalol may be effective in atrial and ventricular arrhythmias.[57,69]

Electrophysiology d,l-Sotalol is a racemic mixture of d and l isomers that both contribute to its antiarrhythmic actions.[70] The d isomer blocks I_{Kr} and the l isomer prolongs repolarization and exhibits β-blocking activity. The latter effect is dose dependent, is not cardioselective, and is not associated with intrinsic sympathomimetic activity. Sotalol prolongs the atrial and ventricular action potential and refractory period. It also slows atrioventricular nodal conduction (as reflected by the AH interval) and may prolong the refractory period of accessory atrioventricular connections.[71,72] There is a risk of torsade de pointes, especially at a low ventricular rate. On the electrocardiogram one may see sinus bradycardia and prolonged PR and QT (by 80–90 milliseconds) intervals, all in a dose-dependent manner.

Pharmacokinetics and Dosing Sotalol should not be used in patients who have contraindications for β blockade or in patients with acquired or congenital long QT syndrome. To observe for proarrhythmic effects, sotalol should preferably be initiated in-hospital. The same holds for increases of the dosage. The initial dose of sotalol in adults is 80 mg twice daily. However, doses as low as twice 40 mg daily may be effective. Depending on the patient's response, the dose may be increased to 240 or 320 mg/d. Dose adjustments should be made at 3-day intervals while monitoring the QT interval. A therapeutic response is usually obtained at a total daily dose of 160 to 320 mg/d given in two or three divided doses. The proarrhythmia risk increases dose dependently.[73] Concomitant administration with other QT-prolonging drugs should be avoided. Dosing intervals depend on creatinine clearance.

Indication and Efficacy Sotalol can prevent recurrence of ventricular tachycardia and fibrillation and supraventricular tachycardias, especially atrial fibrillation.[74]

Adverse Effects The main side effects are fatigue, bradycardia, and proarrhythmia. Sometimes the β-blocking activity precipitates heart failure. Excessive QT prolongation (>500 milliseconds) should prompt discontinuation of sotalol. Sotalol must be avoided in patients with asthma, substantial sinus bradycardia, second- and third-degree atrioventricular block, cardiogenic shock, or uncontrolled heart failure. For its class III action, it must be avoided in congenital and acquired long QT syndrome.

Amiodarone

Electrophysiology The electrophysiologic effects of intravenous amiodarone differ from oral amiodarone. Oral amiodarone has a delayed onset of action that usually takes at least 2 to 3 days or longer, whereas intravenous amiodarone is effective within 1–12 hours. Although oral amiodarone is classified as a class III antiarrhythmic agent, it also has classes I, II, and IV activity. It prolongs repolarization both in the atria and the ventricles as a consequence of blockade of I_{Kr}. The electrocardiogram shows QT prolongation, often marked; sinus bradycardia, PR lengthening, and an increase in QRS duration may occur. Amiodarone rarely causes torsade de pointes.[73,75] Short-term intravenous amiodarone produces only little conduction slowing or action potential prolongation in the atria and ventricles. Conversely, quite quickly after the start of infusion, amiodarone prolongs atrioventricular nodal conduction time and refractoriness. Supposedly, the acute effects of intravenous amiodarone depend in part on its sympatholytic and calcium channel-blocking activity.

Pharmacokinetics Amiodarone has a large volume of distribution, and a long half-life of more than 50 days on average. Consequently, it takes months before blood levels reach equilibrium and vice versa, and it takes 9 months before amiodarone is expelled completely from the body, reaching clinically insignificant levels only after 3 months. The bioavailability of amiodarone varies between 30 and 50 percent. It is not dialyzable and is extensively metabolized to desethylamiodarone. Intravenous amiodarone has complex pharmacokinetics. Peak serum concentrations range from 5 to 41 mg/L after a 15-minute infusion. Because of the rapid distribution, serum levels decrease rapidly within 30 to 45 minutes after stopping the infusion.

Dosing The delayed effect with oral therapy largely relates to the fact that amiodarone is highly lipophilic, resulting in a very large volume of distribution. Therapeutic blood levels are in the 1 to 2.5 mg/L range for both the parent compound and the metabolite. Applying the lowest possible dose may help to reduce side effects. Amiodarone may raise the plasma concentration of digoxin, potentially leading to digoxin toxicity. It may also interfere with the metabolism of vitamin K antagonists, often requiring a reduction in the dose of oral anticoagulant.

The recommended loading dose for ventricular arrhythmias is 800 to 1600 mg/d (in divided doses) for up to 2 to 3 weeks.[75] Thereafter, the dose can be reduced to a maintenance level of 400 to 600 mg/d with the goal to reduce it to the lowest dose possible, for example, 200–300 mg/d. Treatment for atrial fibrillation can be started on an outpatient basis especially if there is no underlying heart disease, a normal QT, and no marked bradycardia or signs of sinus node disease. Loading and maintenance doses in atrial fibrillation are 600 to 800 mg/d in two divided doses for 2 to 4 weeks, followed by maintenance dose of 200 to 400 mg/d and lowered at 3 to 6 months to 100 to 300 mg/d.[75] In patients with ventricular fibrillation who do not respond to electrical countershocks, 5 mg/kg to a maximum of 300 mg is given rapidly into a peripheral vein. For acute rate control or acute conversion of atrial fibrillation, an initial intravenous loading dose of 150 mg is given over 10 minutes. Alternatively, 300 mg in 30 minutes may be given. More rapid infusion increases the risk of hypotension. The loading dose may be followed by a continuous infusion as needed up to a dose of 1200 mg/d. Repeated 150-mg boluses can be given over 10 to 30 minutes for recurrent arrhythmias.[75]

Indications Amiodarone is used in ventricular and supraventricular arrhythmias.[74–77] Intravenous amiodarone is primarily given for the short-term treatment and prophylaxis of recurrent ventricular fibrillation and for hemodynamically unstable ventricular tachycardia that is refractory to other therapies.[75] Because intravenous amiodarone prolongs AV nodal conduction and refractoriness it is very effective in slowing the ventricular rate in critically ill patients with acute atrial fibrillation.[76] It is also used to prevent atrial fibrillation after cardiac surgery.

Adverse Effects Adverse effects leading to discontinuation of amiodarone occurs in 3 to 4 percent of patients. Minor side effects that seldom require drug discontinuation include corneal microdeposits, asymptomatic transient elevation of hepatic enzymes, photosensitivity of the skin, blue-gray skin discoloration, and subjective gastrointestinal side effects. Very few cases of optic neuritis causing blindness have been reported. Amiodarone-induced hypothyroidism occurs in approximately 8 percent of patients and requires the addition of thyroid replacement. Drug-induced hyperthyroidism (2 percent) may require discontinuation of therapy. Liver and thyroid function tests should be done on a regular basis.[75] The most serious adverse effect is interstitial pneumonitis or bronchiolitis obliterans. Patients with baseline abnormal chest radiographs or pulmonary function tests have a higher incidence of pulmonary fibrosis. This adverse effect is dose related and occurs rarely if less than 400 mg/d is used. However, acute pneumonitis may occur even after a few weeks of amiodarone therapy. Neurologic side effects, including a peripheral neuropathy and myopathy, usually resolve on lowering the dose, but may produce unstable gait in the elderly. Drug-induced bradycardia may require permanent pacing in up to 2 percent of patients. Torsade de pointes and incessant ventricular tachycardias are rare.

Dofetilide

Electrophysiology Dofetilide is one of several methane sulfonamides that selectively block IKr. As a consequence, dofetilide prolongs the QT interval without changing PR or QRS interval. It also lengthens the refractory period of atrial, ventricular, and accessory pathway tissue.

Pharmacokinetics Dofetilide is almost completely absorbed with bioavailability exceeding 90 percent. The elimination half-life averages 8 to 9 hours. Excretion is half unchanged via the kidney, the other half is metabolized in the liver. Dose adjustment is needed in case of decreased renal function. Dofetilide is metabolized mainly by the CYP 3A4 family. This means that it may interact with drugs like erythromycin, ketoconazole, verapamil, cimetidine, and certain antibiotics. There is a good correlation between plasma levels and the QT interval.

Dosing In patients with normal renal function, the dosage is 500 μg twice daily; if the renal function is abnormal, the dosage is 250 μg twice daily. Dose reduction is also mandatory if the QT interval increases to above 500 milliseconds.

Indications Dofetilide is used for conversion of atrial fibrillation and atrial flutter to normal sinus rhythm, and for maintenance of normal sinus rhythm thereafter.[57,78] It may also be used to prevent recurrences of paroxysmal atrial fibrillation.

Adverse Effects Torsade de pointes may occur in up to 4 percent of cases and dofetilide should not be used in patients with the long QT syndrome and in patients with severe renal dysfunction. It does not affect contractility or hemodynamics. With precautions, it is safe to use in postinfarct and heart-failure patients, with neutral effects on overall survival.[79,80]

CLASS IV DRUGS
Nondihydropyridine Calcium Channel Blockers

Electrophysiology The nondihydropyridine calcium channel blockers (class IV antiarrhythmic drugs) verapamil and diltiazem affect calcium-dependent slow action potentials in the sinus and atrioventricular nodes. They do not have an effect on sodium-dependent fast action potentials in the myocardium and His-Purkinje tissues. These effects result in slowing the ventricular rate during atrial fibrillation or flutter and termination of AV nodal-dependent arrhythmias, for example, AV node reentry, and their prevention.

Pharmacokinetics Most of ingested verapamil is absorbed, but because of extensive first-pass metabolism, only 20 percent is bioavailable. Renal excretion is limited. After oral administration, peak levels occur in 2 hours. The plasma half-life is 3 to 7 hours.

Dosing Intravenous verapamil—usually 5 to 10 mg—acts within minutes. Infusion should be given slowly—over minutes—to avoid the hypotension that is caused by vasodilatation. The infusion may be repeated if arrhythmia persists. The dose for continuous infusions is 0.005 mg/kg per minute. The total daily oral dose ranges from 120 to 320 mg but sometimes also to 720 mg/d.

The oral diltiazem dose ranges between 90 and 360 mg. The short-term intravenous dose is 0.25 mg/kg. Like verapamil, diltiazem may be repeated in a dose of 25 mg if necessary. Continuous infusions are set at a rate of 10 to 15 mg/h.

Indications Verapamil and diltiazem are mainly used in paroxysmal supraventricular tachycardias and for rate control in atrial fibrillation. Verapamil is also used to treat multifocal atrial tachycardia mainly aiming at slowing heart rate; conversion is infrequent. Some idiopathic ventricular tachycardias, particularly in the left ventricle, are verapamil sensitive and may be successfully treated with this.

Adverse Effects Verapamil should be avoided in patients with hypotension, systolic dysfunction, and heart failure, especially in postinfarct patients.[81,82] Combination with β blockers may exacerbate heart failure in susceptible patients.[83] Diltiazem may be less negatively inotropic. Verapamil and diltiazem should be avoided in the Wolff-Parkinson-White syndrome complicated by atrial fibrillation because they may facilitate conduction over the accessory pathway.

OTHER ANTIARRHYTHMIC DRUGS
Adenosine

Electrophysiology Rapid injection of adenosine yields a biphasic heart rate effect. Early after injection, sinus bradycardia occurs followed by sinus tachycardia. Adenosine has negative chronotropic and dromotropic effects on the sinoatrial and AV nodes, but it has no effect on the His-Purkinje system or ventricular refractoriness. The negative dromotropic effects may lead to transient complete atrioventricular block. Adenosine has no effect on accessory atrioventricular connections although slowing of conduction may be seen in pathways with decremental conduction.

Pharmacokinetics Adenosine is quickly cleared by cellular metabolism. Adenosine enters the circulation and metabolizes to inosine and adenosine monophosphate with an elimination half-life of 10 seconds or less. Onset of action is within 1 minute. Aminophylline counteracts adenosine, whereas dipyridamole, a strong adenosine uptake inhibitor, may potentiate adenosine.

Dosing The dose of adenosine is 6 to 12 mg by bolus. Additional rapid injections may be given up to 36 mg. Most patients will respond to lower dosages.

Indications Adenosine effectively converts reentrant paroxysmal supraventricular tachycardia requiring the atrioventricular node as part of the tachycardia circuit with more than half of patients responding to 6 mg and an additional third responding when given an injection of 12 mg.[84,85] Conversion usually occurs within 1 minute. Adenosine may convert uncommon ventricular tachycardias that depend on catecholamine sensitive calcium entry. It is ineffective in terminating most atrial tachycardias, as well as atrial flutter and fibrillation. Adenosine is contraindicated in patients with preexcited atrial fibrillation because it may produce ventricular fibrillation by facilitation of conduction over the accessory pathway. It is also contraindicated in patients with sick sinus syndrome or second-degree atrioventricular block, unless an artificial pacemaker has been implanted. Bronchospasm has been reported in asthmatic patients when adenosine is used intravenously. Theophylline has been recommended to reverse the effects of adenosine and should be kept ready in susceptible patients. Caffeine and theophylline antagonize the actions of adenosine.[86]

Adverse Effects Most commonly encountered acute but transient adverse effects include dyspnea and unpleasant feeling in the chest. Serious adverse events are prolonged ventricular asystole, ventricular tachycardia, or polymorphic ventricular tachycardia, or even ventricular fibrillation; torsade de pointes may also be seen in patients at risk for bradycardia-dependent arrhythmias, particularly those with a prolonged QT interval. Atrial fibrillation is another proarrhythmic event which may be seen after injection of adenosine.

Digitalis

Electrophysiology Digitalis enhances vagal activity and thus slows sinus node automaticity and prolongs atrioventricular nodal conduction and refractoriness.[87] By enhancing intracellular calcium via inhibition of the sarcolemmal Na^+-K^+-ATPase and thereby a decrease in Ca^{2+} extrusion by the Na^+-Ca^{2+} exchanger, digitalis may produce proarrhythmias.

Pharmacokinetics The bioavailability of digoxin tablets is between 65 and 85 percent. Up to 80 percent is excreted unchanged in the urine. Renal failure prolongs the half life of digoxin and decreases its extravascular volume of distribution. Digitoxin has a longer elimination half-life (>7 days) and undergoes primarily hepatic metabolization rather than renal excretion.

Dosing Digoxin may be given orally, intravenously, or intramuscularly. For convenience, the *rule of 70* can be used. Digoxin dose should be reduced to 0.125 mg if one of the following is present: age >70 years, body weight below 70 kg, or creatinine level above 70 µmol/L. If more than one of these factors is present, the dose should not exceed 0.0625 mg/d.

The total intravenous loading dose digoxin lies between 0.75 and 1.5 mg, whereas the oral loading dose varies between 1 and 2 mg. The loading dose need not be modified in patients with renal dysfunction. When the normal maintenance dose of 0.125 to 0.25 mg daily is started without a load, steady-state plasma concentrations are only reached after approximately 7 to 10 days. Quinidine, verapamil, and amiodarone may increase serum digoxin concentrations, and when used concomitantly, one should consider lowering the dose of digoxin. Absorption of digoxin may be reduced with antacids. By causing hypokalemia, diuretics may enhance digitalis toxicity.

Indications Digitalis may be used to control the ventricular rate in atrial fibrillation or to prevent reentrant arrhythmias involving the atrioventricular node. Digoxin may be used during pregnancy and lactation.

Adverse Effects Noncardiac adverse effects include nausea, headache, visual scotomas, and changes in color perception. Ventricular bigeminy, nonparoxysmal junctional tachycardia, paroxysmal atrial tachycardia with atrioventricular nodal block, and bidirectional ventricular tachycardia are manifestations of digitalis toxicity.

REFERENCES

1. Meng X, Mojaverian P, Doedee M, et al. Bioavailability of amiodarone tablets administered with and without food in healthy subjects. *Am J Cardiol* 2001;87:432–435.
2. Reiffel JA, Kowey PR. Generic antiarrhythmics are not therapeutically equivalent for the treatment of tachyarrhythmias. *Am J Cardiol* 2000;85:1151–1153.
3. Flaker GC, Blackshear JL, McBride R, Kronmal RA, Halperin JL, Hart RG. Antiarrhythmic drug therapy and cardiac mortality in atrial fibrillation. The Stroke Prevention in Atrial Fibrillation Investigators. *J Am Coll Cardiol* 1992;20:527–532.
4. Doering W. Quinidine-digoxin interaction: pharmacokinetics, underlying mechanism and clinical implications. *N Engl J Med* 1979;301:400–404.
5. Siddoway LA, Thompson KA, McAllister CB, et al. Polymorphism of propafenone metabolism and disposition in man: clinical and pharmacokinetic consequences. *Circulation* 1987;75:785–791.
6. Winkle RA, Jaillon P, Kates RE, Peters F. Clinical pharmacology and antiarrhythmic efficacy of *N*-acetylprocainamide. *Am J Cardiol* 1981;47:123–130.
7. Roden DM, Kim RB. Pharmacokinetics, pharmacodynamics, pharmacogenetics, and drug interactions. In: Zipes DP, Jalife J, eds. *Cardiac Electrophysiology: From Cell to Bedside*. Philadelphia: WB Saunders, 2000:882–889.
8. Collinsworth KA, Kalman SM, Harrison DC. The clinical pharmacology of lidocaine as an antiarrhythmic drug. *Circulation* 1974;50:1217–1230.
9. Mason JW. Amiodarone. *N Engl J Med* 1987;316:455–466.
10. Siddoway L. Pharmacologic principles of antiarrhythmic drugs. In: Podrid PJ, Kowey PR, eds. Cardiac Arrhythmias. Baltimore: Williams & Wilkins, 1995:355–368–889.
11. DiMarco JP, Sellers TD, Lerman BB, Greenberg ML, Berne RM, Belardinelli L. Diagnostic and therapeutic use of adenosine in patients with supraventricular tachyarrhythmias. *J Am Coll Cardiol* 1985;6:417–425.
12. Naccarelli GV, Lee KS, Gibson JK, VanderLugt J. Electrophysiology and pharmacology of ibutilide. *Am J Cardiol* 1996;78:12–16.
13. Vestal RE, Wood AJ, Shand DG. Reduced beta-adrenoceptor sensitivity in the elderly. *Clin Pharmacol Ther* 1979;26:181–186.
14. Naccarelli GV, Sager PT, Singh BN. Antiarrhythmic agents. In: Podrid PJ, Kowey PR, eds. Cardiac Arrhythmias. Philadelphia: Lippincott Williams & Wilkins, 2001:265–301.
15. Hanyok JJ. Clinical pharmacokinetics of sotalol. *Am J Cardiol* 1993;72:19A–26A.
16. Patlak JB, Ortiz M. Two modes of gating during late Na⁺ channel currents in frog sartorius muscle. *J Gen Physiol* 1986;87:305–326.
17. Antzelevitch C, Yan GX, Shimizu W, et al. Electrical heterogeneity, the ECG, and cardiac arrhythmias. In: Zipes DP, Jalife J, eds. Cardiac Electrophysiology: From Cell to Bedside. Philadelphia: WB Saunders, 1999:222–238.
18. Zygmunt AC, Eddlestone GT, Thomas GP, Nesterenko VV, Antzelevitch C. Larger late sodium conductance in M cells contributes to electrical heterogeneity in canine ventricle. *Am J Physiol Heart Circ Physiol* 2001;281:H689–H697.
19. Yan GX, Wu Y, Liu T, Wang J, Marinchak RA, Kowey PR. Phase 2 early afterdepolarization as a trigger of polymorphic ventricular tachycardia in acquired long-QT syndrome: direct evidence from intracellular recordings in the intact left ventricular wall. *Circulation* 2001;103:2851–2856.
20. Nam GB, Burashnikov A, Antzelevitch C. Cellular mechanisms underlying the development of catecholaminergic ventricular tachycardia. *Circulation* 2005;111:2727–2733.
21. Yang T, Roden DM. Extracellular potassium modulation of drug block of I_{Kr}. Implications for torsade de pointes and reverse use-dependence. *Circulation* 1996;93:407–411.
22. Levine JH, Morganroth J, Kadish AH. Mechanisms and risk factors for proarrhythmia with type Ia compared with Ic antiarrhythmic drug therapy. *Circulation* 1989;80:1063–1069.
23. Carmeliet E. Cardiac ionic currents and acute ischemia: from channels to arrhythmias. *Physiol Rev* 1999;79:917–1017.
24. Yan GX, Rials SJ, Wu Y, et al. Ventricular hypertrophy amplifies transmural repolarization dispersion and induces early afterdepolarization. *Am J Physiol* 2001;281:H1968–H1975.
25. Herre JM, Titus C, Oeff M, et al. Inefficacy and proarrhythmic effects of flecainide and encainide for sustained ventricular tachycardia and ventricular fibrillation. *Ann Intern Med* 1990;113:671–676.
26. CAST Investigators. Preliminary report: effect of encainide and flecainide on mortality in a randomized trial of arrhythmia suppression after myocardial infarction. *N Engl J Med* 1989;321:406–412.
27. Greene HL, Roden DM, Katz RJ, Woosley RL, Salerno DM, Henthorn RW. The Cardiac Arrhythmia Suppression Trial: first CAST…then CAST-II. *J Am Coll Cardiol* 1992;19:894–898.
28. Pritchett EL, Wilkinson WE. Mortality in patients treated with flecainide and encainide for supraventricular arrhythmias. *Am J Cardiol* 1991;67:976–980.
29. Yan GX, Lankipalli RS, Burke JF, Musco S, Kowey PR. Ventricular repolarization components on the electrocardiogram: cellular basis and clinical significance. *J Am Coll Cardiol* 2003;42:401–409.
30. van Opstal JM, Schoenmakers M, Verduyn SC, et al. Chronic amiodarone evokes no torsade de pointes arrhythmias despite QT lengthening in an animal model of acquired long-QT syndrome. *Circulation* 2001;104:2722–2727.
31. Ravid S, Podrid PJ, Lampert S, Lown B. Congestive heart failure induced by six of the newer antiarrhythmic drugs. *J Am Coll Cardiol* 1989;14:1326–1330.
32. Torp-Pedersen C, Moller M, Bloch-Thomsen PE, et al. Dofetilide in patients with congestive heart failure and left ventricular dysfunction. Danish Investigations of Arrhythmia and Mortality on Dofetilide Study Group. *N Engl J Med* 1999;341:857–865.
33. Singh SN, Fletcher RD, Fisher SG, et al. Amiodarone in patients with congestive heart failure and asymptomatic ventricular arrhythmia. Survival Trial of Antiarrhythmic Therapy in Congestive Heart Failure. *N Engl J Med* 1995;333:77–82.
34. Breithardt G, Cain ME, El-Sherif N, et al. Standards for analysis of ventricular late potentials using high-resolution or signal-averaged electrocardiography. A statement by a task force committee of the European Society of

Cardiology, the American Heart Association, and the American College of Cardiology. *Circulation* 1991;83:1481–1488.

35. Bollmann A, Husser D, Cannom DS. Antiarrhythmic drugs in patients with implantable cardioverter-defibrillators. *Am J Cardiovasc Drugs* 2005;5:371–378.

36. Gregg AR, Tomich PG. Mexiletine use in pregnancy. *J Perinatol* 1988;8:33–35.

37. Vergani P, Mariani E, Ciriello E, et al. Fetal arrhythmias: natural history and management. *Ultrasound Med Biol* 2005;31:1–6.

38. Rashba EJ, Zareba W, Moss AJ, et al. Influence of pregnancy on the risk for cardiac events in patients with hereditary long QT syndrome. LQTS Investigators. *Circulation* 1998;97:451–456.

39. Joglar JA, Page RL. Treatment of cardiac arrhythmias during pregnancy: safety considerations. *Drug Saf* 1999;20:85–94.

40. Joglar JA, Page RL. Antiarrhythmic drugs in pregnancy. *Curr Opin Cardiol* 2001;16:40–45.

41. Magee LA, Downar E, Sermer M, Boulton BC, Allen LC, Koren G. Pregnancy outcome after gestational exposure to amiodarone in Canada. *Am J Obstet Gynecol* 1995;172:1307–1311.

42. Bartalena L, Bogazzi F, Braverman LE, Martino E. Effects of amiodarone administration during pregnancy on neonatal thyroid function and subsequent neurodevelopment. *J Endocrinol Invest* 2001;24:116–130.

43. Fouron JC. Fetal arrhythmias: the Saint-Justine hospital experience. *Prenat Diagn* 2004;24:1068–1080.

44. Yan GX, Antzelevitch C. Cellular basis for the Brugada syndrome and other mechanisms of arrhythmogenesis associated with ST-segment elevation. *Circulation* 1999;100:1660–1666.

45. Mizusawa Y, Sakurada H, Nishizaki M, Hiraoka M. Effects of low-dose quinidine on ventricular tachyarrhythmias in patients with Brugada syndrome: low-dose quinidine therapy as an adjunctive treatment. *J Cardiovasc Pharmacol* 2006;47:359–364.

46. Kay GN, Plumb VJ, Arciniegas JG, Henthorn RW, Waldo AL. Torsade de pointes: the long-short initiating sequence and other clinical features: observations in 32 patients. *J Am Coll Cardiol* 1983;2:806–817.

47. Juul-Moller S, Edvardsson N, Rehnqvist-Ahlberg N. Sotalol versus quinidine for the maintenance of sinus rhythm after direct current conversion of atrial fibrillation. *Circulation* 1990;82:1932–1939.

48. Belhassen B, Viskin S, Fish R, Glick A, Setbon I, Eldar M. Effects of electrophysiologic-guided therapy with Class IA antiarrhythmic drugs on the long-term outcome of patients with idiopathic ventricular fibrillation with or without the Brugada syndrome. *J Cardiovasc Electrophysiol* 1999;10:1301–1312.

49. Roden DM, Woosley RL, Primm RK. Incidence and clinical features of the quinidine-associated long QT syndrome: implications for patient care. *Am Heart J* 1986;111:1088–1093.

50. Gorgels AP, van den DA, Hofs A, et al. Comparison of procainamide and lidocaine in terminating sustained monomorphic ventricular tachycardia. *Am J Cardiol* 1996;78:43–46.

51. Gottlieb SS, Weinberg M. Comparative hemodynamic effects of mexiletine and quinidine in patients with severe left ventricular dysfunction. *Am Heart J* 1991;122:1368–1374.

52. Napolitano C, Bloise R, Priori SG. Gene-specific therapy for inherited arrhythmogenic diseases. *Pharmacol Ther* 2006;110:1–13.

53. Crijns HJ, den Heijer P, van Wijk LM, Lie KI. Successful use of flecainide in atrial fibrillation with rapid ventricular rate in the Wolff-Parkinson-White syndrome. *Am Heart J* 1988;115:1317–1321.

54. Benhorin J, Taub R, Goldmit M, Kerem B, Kass RS, Windman I, Medina A. Effects of flecainide in patients with new SCN5A mutation: mutation-specific therapy for long-QT syndrome? *Circulation* 2000;101:1698–1706.

55. Naccarelli GV, Dorian P, Hohnloser SH, Coumel P. Prospective comparison of flecainide versus quinidine for the treatment of paroxysmal atrial fibrillation/flutter. The Flecainide Multicenter Atrial Fibrillation Study Group. *Am J Cardiol* 1996;77:53A–59A.

56. Crijns HJ, van Wijk LM, Van Gilst WH, Kingma JH, van Gelder IC, Lie KI. Acute conversion of atrial fibrillation to sinus rhythm: clinical efficacy of flecainide acetate. Comparison of two regimens. *Eur Heart J* 1988;9:634–638.

57. Crijns HJ, van Gelder IC, Kingma JH, Dunselman PH, Gosselink AT, Lie KI. Atrial flutter can be terminated by a class III antiarrhythmic drug but not by a class IC drug. *Eur Heart J* 1994;15:1403–1408.

58. Tarin N, Farre J, Rubio JM, Tunon J, Castro-Dorticos J. Brugada-like electrocardiographic pattern in a patient with a mediastinal tumor. *PACE* 1999;22:1264–1266.

59. Pritchett EL, Wilkinson WE, Clair WK, McCarthy EA. Comparison of mortality in patients treated with propafenone to those treated with a variety of antiarrhythmic drugs for supraventricular arrhythmias. *Am J Cardiol* 1993;72:108–110.

60. Meinertz T, Lip GY, Lombardi F, et al. Efficacy and safety of propafenone sustained release in the prophylaxis of symptomatic paroxysmal atrial fibrillation (The European Rythmol/Rhythmonorm Atrial Fibrillation Trial [ERAFT] Study). *Am J Cardiol* 2002;90:1300–1306.

61. Capucci A, Boriani G, Botto GL, et al. Conversion of recent-onset atrial fibrillation by a single oral loading dose of propafenone or flecainide. *Am J Cardiol* 1994;74:503–505.

62. Billman GE, Castillo LC, Hensley J, Hohl CM, Altschuld RA. Beta$_2$-adrenergic receptor antagonists protect against ventricular fibrillation: in vivo and in vitro evidence for enhanced sensitivity to beta$_2$-adrenergic stimulation in animals susceptible to sudden death. *Circulation* 1997;96:1914–1922.

63. Ko DT, Hebert PR, Coffey CS, Sedrakyan A, Curtis JP, Krumholz HM. Beta-blocker therapy and symptoms of depression, fatigue, and sexual dysfunction. *JAMA* 2002;288:351–357.

64. Murray KT. Ibutilide. *Circulation* 1998;97:493–497.

65. Lee KS. Ibutilide, a new compound with potent class III antiarrhythmic activity, activates a slow inward Na$^+$ current in guinea pig ventricular cells. *J Pharmacol Exp Ther* 1992;262:99–108.

66. Glatter KA, Dorostkar PC, Yang Y, et al. Electrophysiological effects of ibutilide in patients with accessory pathways. *Circulation* 2001;104:1933–1939.

67. Ellenbogen KA, Clemo HF, Stambler BS, Wood MA, VanderLugt JT. Efficacy of ibutilide for termination of atrial fibrillation and flutter. *Am J Cardiol* 1996;78:42–45.

68. Vos MA, Golitsyn SR, Stangl K, et al. Superiority of ibutilide (a new class III agent) over DL-sotalol in converting atrial flutter and atrial fibrillation. The Ibutilide/Sotalol Comparator Study Group. *Heart* 1998;79:568–575.

69. Singh BN, Singh SN, Reda DJ, et al. Amiodarone versus sotalol for atrial fibrillation. *N Engl J Med* 2005;352:1861–1872.

70. Hohnloser SH, Woosley RL. Sotalol. *N Engl J Med* 1994;331:31–38.

71. Nademanee K, Feld G, Hendrickson J, Singh PN, Singh BN. Electrophysiologic and antiarrhythmic effects of sotalol in patients with life-threatening ventricular tachyarrhythmias. *Circulation* 1985;72:555–564.

72. Mitchell LB, Wyse DG, Duff HJ. Electropharmacology of sotalol in patients with Wolff-Parkinson-White syndrome. *Circulation* 1987;76:810–818.

73. Hohnloser SH, Klingenheben T, Singh BN. Amiodarone-associated proarrhythmic effects. A review with special reference to torsade de pointes tachycardia. *Ann Intern Med* 1994;121:529–535.

74. Fuster V, Ryden LE, Cannom DS, et al. ACC/AHA/ESC 2006 guidelines for the management of patients with atrial fibrillation-executive summary: a report of the American College of Cardiology/American Heart Association Task Force on practice guidelines and the European Society of Cardiology Committee for Practice Guidelines (Writing Committee to Revise the 2001 Guidelines for the Management of Patients with Atrial Fibrillation). *Eur Heart J* 2006;27:1979–2030.

75. Goldschlager N, Epstein AE, Naccarelli G, Olshansky B, Singh B. Practical guidelines for clinicians who treat patients with amiodarone. Practice Guidelines Subcommittee, North American Society of Pacing and Electrophysiology. *Arch Intern Med* 2000;160:1741–1748.

76. Clemo HF, Wood MA, Gilligan DM, Ellenbogen KA. Intravenous amiodarone for acute heart rate control in the critically ill patient with atrial tachyarrhythmias. *Am J Cardiol* 1998;81:594–598.

77. Roy D, Talajic M, Dorian P, et al. Amiodarone to prevent recurrence of atrial fibrillation. Canadian Trial of Atrial Fibrillation Investigators. *N Engl J Med* 2000;342:913–920.

78. Singh S, Zoble RG, Yellen L, et al. Efficacy and safety of oral dofetilide in converting to and maintaining sinus rhythm in patients with chronic atrial fibrillation or atrial flutter: the Symptomatic Atrial Fibrillation Investigative Research on Dofetilide (SAFIRE-D) study. *Circulation* 2000;102:2385–2390.

79. Torp-Pedersen C, Moller M, Bloch-Thomsen PE, et al. Dofetilide in patients with congestive heart failure and left ventricular dysfunction. Danish Investigations of Arrhythmia and Mortality on Dofetilide Study Group. *N Engl J Med* 1999;341:857–865.

80. Singh SN, Lazin A, Cohen AJ, Johnson MC, Fletcher RD. Sotalol-Induced torsades de pointes successfully treated with hemodialysis after failure of conventional therapy. *Am Heart J* 1991;121:601–602.

81. Effect of verapamil on mortality and major events after acute myocardial infarction (the Danish Verapamil Infarction Trial II—DAVIT II). *Am J Cardiol* 1990;66:779–785.

82. The effect of diltiazem on mortality and reinfarction after myocardial infarction. The Multicenter Diltiazem Postinfarction Trial Research Group. *N Engl J Med* 1988;319:385–392.

83. Singh BN, Nademanee K, Baky SH. Calcium antagonists. Clinical use in the treatment of arrhythmias. *Drugs* 1983;25:125–153.

84. DiMarco JP, Sellers TD, Lerman BB, Greenberg ML, Berne RM, Belardinelli L. Diagnostic and therapeutic use of adenosine in patients with supraventricular tachyarrhythmias. *J Am Coll Cardiol* 1985;6:417–425.

85. DiMarco JP, Sellers TD, Berne RM, West GA, Belardinelli L. Adenosine: electrophysiologic effects and therapeutic use for terminating paroxysmal supraventricular tachycardia. *Circulation* 1983;68:1254–1263.

86. Waxman HL, Myerburg RJ, Appel R, Sung RJ. Verapamil for control of ventricular rate in paroxysmal supraventricular tachycardia and atrial fibrillation or flutter: a double-blind randomized cross-over study. *Ann Intern Med* 1981;94:1–6.

87. Hauptman PJ, Kelly RA. Digitalis. *Circulation* 1999;99:1265–1270.

CHAPTER (44)

Treatment of Cardiac Arrhythmias with Catheter-Ablative Techniques

Usha B. Tedrow / William G. Stevenson

INTRODUCTION

Successful catheter ablation requires precise localization of the source of the arrhythmia, accurate placement of the ablation catheter, and achievement of an adequate ablation lesion. Catheter positioning is assisted by fluoroscopy. Sophisticated mapping systems can also display catheter position and create a three-dimensional depiction of the anatomy, reducing radiation exposure. MRI and CT data can also be integrated with these systems, facilitating complex ablation procedures. Ablation is most commonly performed by application of radiofrequency (RF) current applied through a large-tip electrode on a steerable catheter to heat the tissue. Freezing with cryoablation catheters is also now available. Serious complications of catheter ablation are infrequent and most often related to the catheterization procedure, usually including vascular injury, and cardiac perforation with tamponade.

REENTRANT SUPRAVENTRICULAR TACHYCARDIA

【 】 ATRIOVENTRICULAR NODAL REENTRANT TACHYCARDIA

Catheter ablation for atrioventricular nodal reentrant tachycardia (AVNRT) is recommended when episodes are poorly tolerated or re-

sistant to medical therapy, or if the patient desires control of the arrhythmia without medications.[1] The atrioventricular (AV) node consists of a compact portion and adjoining lobes. In patients with AVNRT, the lobe that extends along the tricuspid annulus toward the coronary sinus likely forms a functional pathway for slow conduction between the os of the coronary sinus and the septal leaflet of the tricuspid valve (Fig. 44–1) that can be ablated without damaging conduction through the compact portion of the AV node.[2] Success is achieved in more than 95 percent of patients. Heart block is the major risk, requiring permanent pacemaker implantation occurs in approximately 0.8 percent of patients. Cryoablation may be associated with a lower risk of heart block, but lower long-term success rates.[3]

【 】 ATRIOVENTRICULAR RECIPROCATING TACHYCARDIA

Patients with atrioventricular reciprocating tachycardia (AVRT) have an accessory pathway connecting atrium and ventricle and bypassing the His-Purkinje system. If the pathway has manifest antegrade conduction, the ECG shows preexcitation, a hallmark of the Wolff-Parkinson-White syndrome. Accessory pathways conducting only from ventricle to atrium are termed *concealed* because during sinus rhythm preexcitation is absent, but AVRT still can occur. Catheter ablation is the standard of care for symptomatic Wolff-Parkinson-White syndrome, or for concealed accessory

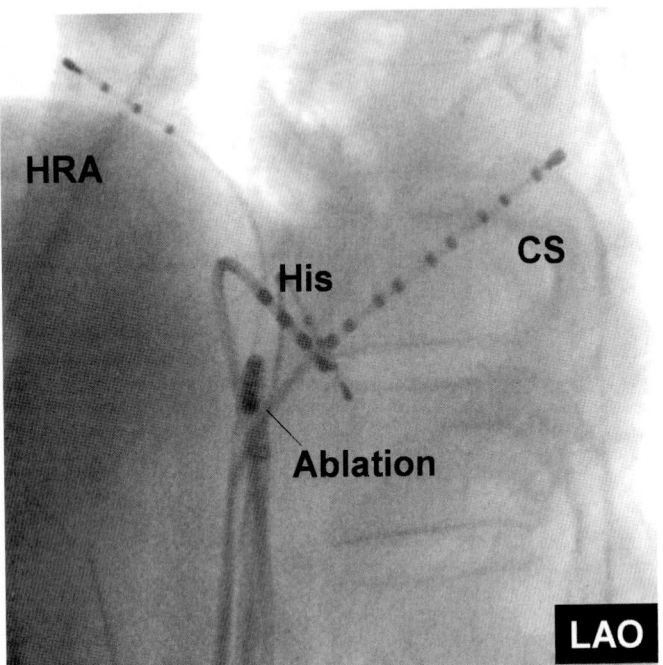

FIGURE 44–1. AV nodal reentry tachycardia. Shown is a left anterior oblique fluoroscopic image indicating the ablation catheter position for ablation of the slow AV nodal pathway. Quadripolar catheters are located in the high right atrium (HRA) and His bundle (His) positions. A decapolar catheter is seen in the coronary sinus (CS). The ablation catheter is seen just lateral to the CS os on the tricuspid valve annulus.

pathways causing symptomatic tachycardias when pharmacologic therapy is ineffective or not desirable.[1]

Accessory pathways can be located along the mitral (Fig. 44–2A) or tricuspid annulus, or in the septum. Location determines whether an arterial, venous, or transseptal approach is required. Success rates are 95 percent (Fig. 44–2B), slightly lower with septal pathways and greater with free wall pathways, with a risk of recurrent pathway conduction after healing of 3 to 10 percent.[1] Serious complications related to left- or right-heart catheterization can occur, but are uncommon. Heart block can occur with ablation of septal pathways located close to the AV node.

REGULAR ATRIAL ARRHYTHMIAS
[ ] FOCAL ATRIAL TACHYCARDIA

Focal atrial tachycardias (ATs) tend to occur in specific anatomic locations: along the crista terminalis, tricuspid or mitral annulus, coronary sinus musculature, atrial appendages, and in the pulmonary veins. The tachycardia must be present or provocable to be localized for ablation (Fig. 44–3).[4,5] Inability to induce the arrhythmia can thwart successful ablation. Ablation is successful in more than 80% of patients with a recurrence rate after successful ablation of approximately 8 percent.[1] Significant complications occur in 1 to 2 percent of patients.

[ ] MODIFICATION OF SINUS NODE FUNCTION FOR INAPPROPRIATE SINUS TACHYCARDIA

Patients with inappropriate sinus tachycardia have sinus tachycardia without a discernible cause. Catheter ablation is a last resort

when severe symptoms do not respond to pharmacologic therapy. Ablation of the rapidly firing regions, typically located in the superior medial portion of the crista terminalis near the septum often slows the sinus rate.[6,7] Ablation of the entire sinus node, with permanent pacemaker implantation is recommended by some centers and can require epicardial ablation.[7,8] Long-term success is limited; more than 20 to 50 percent of patients have recurrent symptoms, some despite improvement in heart rate. Potential complications include narrowing of the superior vena cava, right phrenic nerve paralysis, and the need for chronic pacing.

[ ] ATRIAL FLUTTER AND OTHER MACROREENTRANT ATRIAL TACHYCARDIAS

Common atrial flutter is caused by a large macroreentrant circuit with a wavefront revolving around the tricuspid annulus. In typical counterclockwise atrial flutter, the wavefront proceeds up the atrial septum and down the right atrial free wall. P waves are negative in the inferior leads, positive in V_1 and negative in V_6. The circuit can also revolve in the clockwise direction, giving rise to positive P waves in the inferior leads and a negative deflection in V_1. Reentry is dependent on conduction through the cavotricuspid isthmus bounded by the tricuspid valve annulus, inferior vena cava, eustachian ridge, and coronary sinus os. Other atrial tachycardias can mimic atrial flutter, and in patients with prior atrial surgery or ablation, common atrial flutter may have an atypical ECG appearance. Once the diagnosis is confirmed by entrainment and activation mapping, a series of ablation lesions is placed across the cavotricuspid isthmus, creating a line of conduction block (Fig. 44–4).

Success is achieved in more than 95 percent of patients and recurrences are less frequent than in those managed with antiarrhythmic drug therapy.[9] Approximately 20 to 30 percent of patients also have atrial disease that leads to atrial fibrillation in the next 20 months. A history of atrial fibrillation and depressed ventricular function increase the risk of subsequent atrial fibrillation.[10]

Other macroreentrant circuits can occur in the left or right atrium that do not involve the cavotricuspid isthmus. Arrhythmias from reentry occurring around atrial scars from prior heart surgery, such as atrial septal defect repair, Fontan repair, mitral valve surgery, and atrial maze surgery, or after catheter ablation for atrial fibrillation are referred to as "lesion-related" or "scar-related" macroreentrant ATs.[1] Catheter ablation is more difficult, with success rates of 80 to 85 percent, and more frequent late recurrences than are observed for common flutter.[11]

ATRIAL FIBRILLATION
[ ] ATRIOVENTRICULAR JUNCTION ABLATION FOR RATE CONTROL

In patients with atrial fibrillation (AF), catheter ablation of the AV junction to produce complete heart block with implantation of a permanent pacemaker can be used to control the ventricular rate. The procedure is generally reserved for older patients who may already have an implanted pacemaker or defibrillator, who cannot tolerate rate-control medications, and who are not candidates for

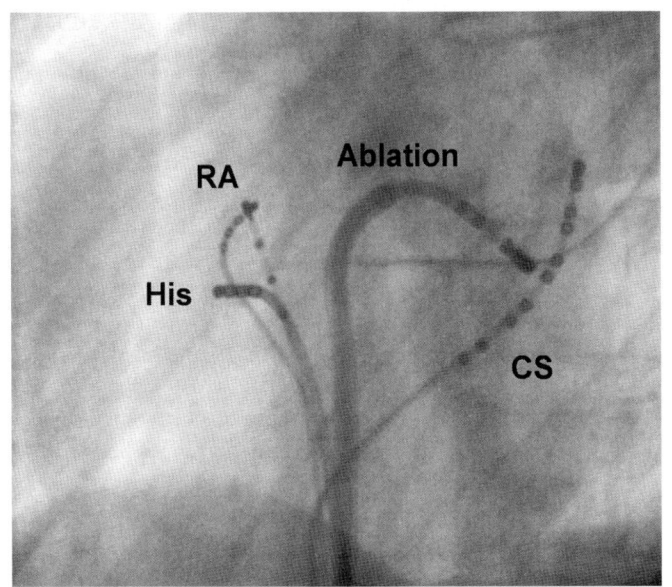

A

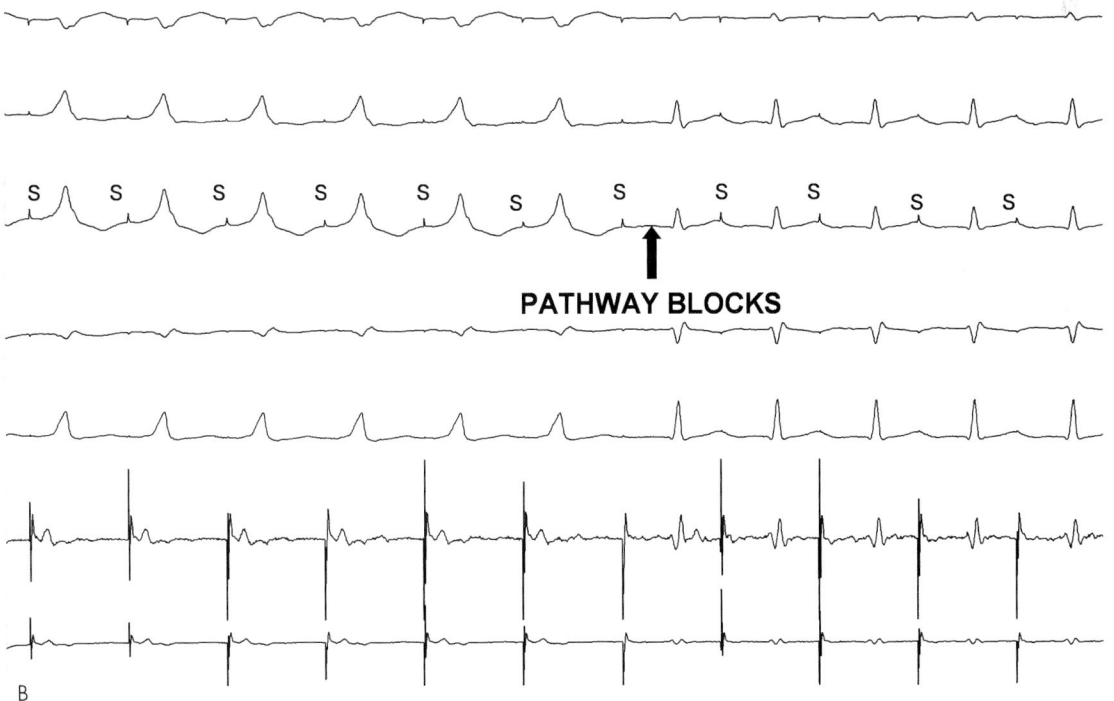

B

FIGURE 44–2. A. Ablation of a left-sided accessory pathway in a patient with Wolff-Parkinson-White syndrome. Shown is a left anterior oblique fluoroscopic image depicting catheter position for transablation of a left-sided accessory pathway by a transeptal approach. A decapolar catheter is seen in the coronary sinus (CS). The ablation catheter (Ablation) is passed through a sheath that crosses the fossa ovalis into the left atrium for mapping along the tricuspid valve annulus. **B.** Five surface ECG leads and 2 intracardiac leads depict ablation of a left lateral accessory pathway during atrial pacing. The right atrium is being paced (pacing stimuli indicated by S). Pacing stimuli initially conduct from the atrium to the ventricles over the AV node and an accessory pathway producing a pattern of ventricular preexcitation with a wide QRS with a slurred initial delta wave. The pathway blocks within seconds of the application of radiofrequency energy with sudden narrowing of the QRS complex indicating that conduction to the ventricles is occurring only over the normal conduction system of AV node and His bundle.

other rhythm-control strategies. After ablation, rate-control medications are not required and the ventricular rate is regularized, which may confer some hemodynamic advantage. Anticoagulation for thromboembolic risk is still required. For patients with previously uncontrolled ventricular rates, quality of life, exercise tolerance, and ejection fraction can improve.[12]

Benefits must be weighed against potential disadvantages. Following the abrupt decrease in heart rate, cases of sudden death have occurred, likely as a result of polymorphic ventricular tachycardia. Pacing the ventricle at 90 beats per minute for the first several weeks and then gradually reducing the rate over time reduces the risk.[13] Right ventricular (RV) pacing can have adverse hemodynamic consequences in some patients with poor left ventricular (LV) function. Biventricular pacing likely reduces this risk.[12] In patients with biventricular pacing for heart failure, AV junction abla-

tion is occasionally needed to ensure continuous biventricular capture without competition from conducted supraventricular beats.

ATRIAL FIBRILLATION ABLATION FOR MAINTAINING SINUS RHYTHM

Sleeves of myocardium extending along the pulmonary veins are often important sites for the initiation and maintenance of AF. The majority of focal triggers that initiate paroxysmal AF are in these regions.[14] Although ablation strategies vary, most target areas within the atrium that encircle the broader, antral regions of the pulmonary veins, often with the goal of electrically isolating these regions with additional lesions to address other atrial regions that promote AF in some patients.[15–17] Extensive series of lesions are usually placed in the left atrium. Intracardiac echocardiography

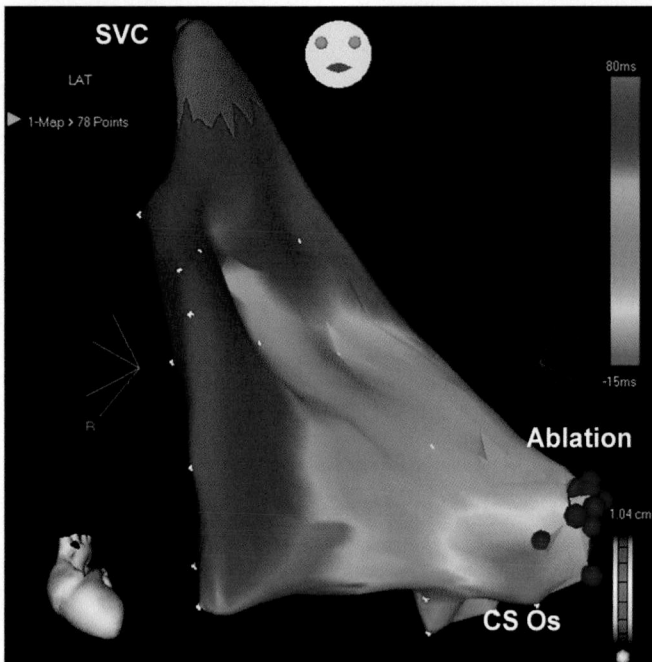

FIGURE 44–3. Activation map of focal atrial tachycardia originating from the coronary sinus os. Shown is an electroanatomic map of the right atrium created by moving a catheter point by point throughout the atrium. Sensing of a low-energy electromagnetic field is used to calculate the position of the catheter in three-dimensional space without the need for fluoroscopy. The superior vena cava (SVC) is marked in gray. Colors indicate activation times during tachycardia. The earliest area of activation appears red, whereas progressively later activation is indicated by orange, yellow, green, blue, and purple, respectively. In this case, activation originated at the os of the coronary sinus and spread rightward across the atrium from that site. Ablation lesions placed at the early region, indicated by the small red spheres, abolished the tachycardia.

and three-dimensional mapping systems that incorporate anatomy from MRI or CT images are helpful (Fig. 44–5) adjuncts to facilitate ablation strategies.[18]

Success varies with the type of AF and severity of underlying heart disease. Young patients with paroxysmal AF without structural heart disease have the best outcome. More than 80 percent have sinus rhythm after the initial healing phase following ablation. Reported followup periods are still relatively short, with few studies reporting data beyond 1 year. Success rates are lower for patients with persistent or permanent AF.[15]

Following ablation recurrent ATs and AF can occur and often dissipate spontaneously over a period of several weeks as ablation lesions heal and the atrium remodels. A second procedure is required in 20 to 50 percent of patients. Antiarrhythmic medications are often continued for 1 to 3 months after ablation. Anticoagulation with warfarin is required as well.

Major procedural complications include myocardial perforation with tamponade (1 to 2 percent) and stroke (0.5 to 1 percent). Severe pulmonary vein stenosis has been reported in (2 to 6 percent) of patients and can present months after the procedure with dyspnea, pneumonia, or pulmonary infiltrate, but can also be asymptomatic.[19] Death from atrioesophageal fistulae, presenting days to a few weeks after the procedure with endocarditis, septic emboli, or gastrointestinal bleeding, has been reported (<0.5 percent estimated).[20] Appropriate patient selection requires adequate assessment of risks and benefits

for each individual patient. The risks and benefits can be expected to improve as this relatively new procedure continues to evolve.

VENTRICULAR TACHYCARDIA

【 】 IDIOPATHIC VENTRICULAR TACHYCARDIA

Idiopathic ventricular tachycardia (VT) occurs in the absence of structural heart disease and is often amenable to catheter ablation. The most common form originates from a focus in the right ventricular outflow tract, beneath the pulmonary valve and may cause exercise-induced VT, repetitive bursts of monomorphic VT, or symptomatic premature ventricular contractions.[21] The VT has a pattern of left bundle-branch block in V_1 with an inferiorly directed axis. Ablation is performed at the area of earliest activation in the outflow tract, with successful elimination of tachycardia in more than 80 percent of patients. Occasionally outflow tract VT originates from sites adjacent to the aortic annulus, the left ventricular outflow tract, or in the epicardium. Catheter ablation can be thwarted because of lack of inducibility of the VT for mapping and occasionally because of an atypical location.

The most common form of left-sided idiopathic VT originates from the left ventricular apical septum.[22] This arrhythmia is characterized on surface ECG by a pattern of right bundle-branch block in lead V_1, usually with a superiorly directed axis. It often responds to verapamil and can be mistaken for supraventricular tachycardia (SVT) with aberrancy. It appears to be caused by reentry involving ramifications of the Purkinje system. Ablation targeting characteristic electrograms in the reentry region is successful in more than 80 percent of patients. Significant complications are infrequent, although femoral arterial and retrograde aortic left ventricular catheterization are usually required.

【 】 VT AFTER MYOCARDIAL INFARCTION AND SCAR-RELATED REENTRY

Sustained VT associated with structural heart disease is associated with a risk of sudden death. Most patients receive an implanted cardioverter defibrillator (ICD) that can terminate VT when it occurs, either with shocks or by antitachycardia pacing. Catheter ablation is an important alternative to antiarrhythmic drug therapy for reducing the frequency of symptomatic VT and can be lifesaving if VT becomes incessant.

Any ventricular scar can cause VT. Myocardial infarction is the most common cause, but fibrosis from idiopathic dilated cardiomyopathy, sarcoidosis, arrhythmogenic right ventricular dysplasia, and Chagas disease can also result in VT substrate. Prior cardiac surgery such as repair of tetralogy of Fallot also causes scar-related VT. Areas of conduction block with intervening regions of slow conduction in the scar region support reentry. The resulting VT is typically monomorphic with each QRS complex resembling the preceding and following QRS. The ECG morphology of the VT suggests the location of the scar and region where the reentry wavefront propagates away from the scar to produce the QRS complex. VTs with a left bundle-branch block configuration in V_1 often originate from the RV or the interventricular septum. Those with right bundle-branch block usually originate from the LV.

During mapping, areas of scar are identified as regions with abnormal, low-voltage electrograms that can be highlighted on three-dimensional anatomic maps (Fig. 44–6).[23–25] Pacing from the map-

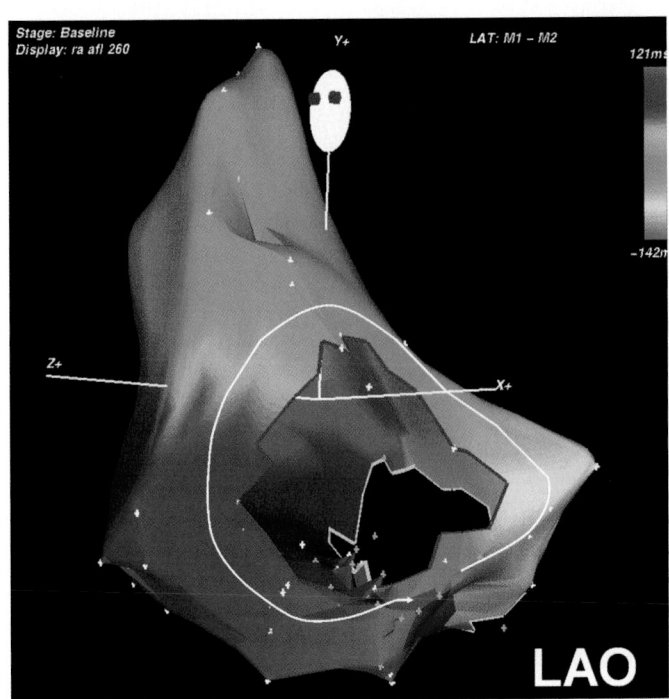

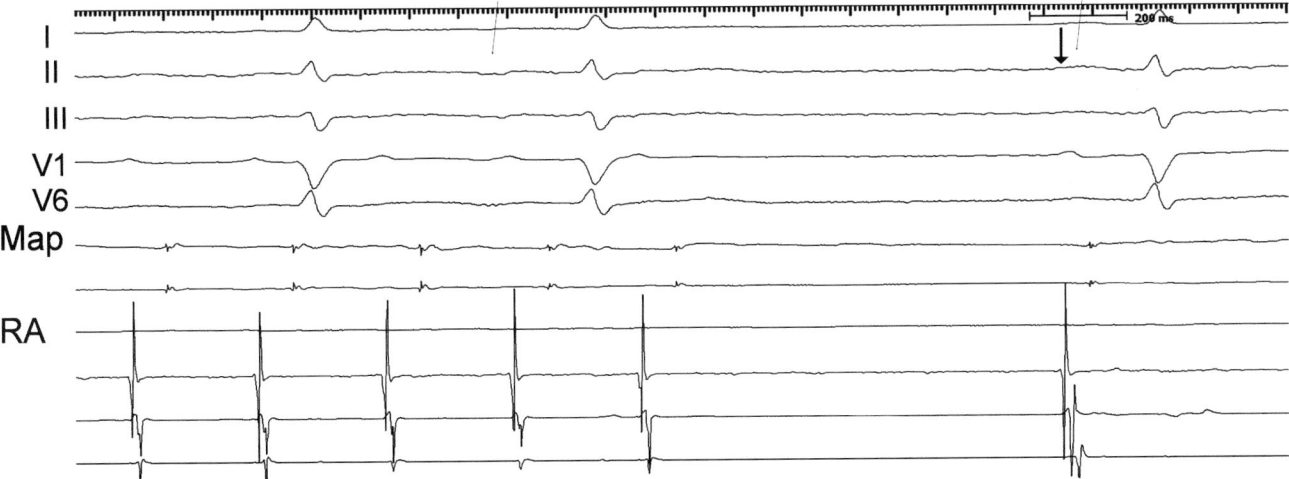

FIGURE 44-4. Mapping and ablation of typical counterclockwise atrial flutter. At the top is an activation map of the right atrium during counterclockwise atrial flutter as viewed in an left anterior oblique projection. Activation circulates up the interatrial septum, across the roof, down the free wall, and through the cavotricuspid isthmus. A line of RF lesions was placed across this isthmus, which blocked conduction in the isthmus terminating atrial flutter. The tracing at the bottom shows surface ECG leads and intracardiac recordings from the mapping catheter (Map) and lateral right atrium (RA) during RF ablation. Atrial flutter terminates and is followed by sinus rhythm (*arrow*).

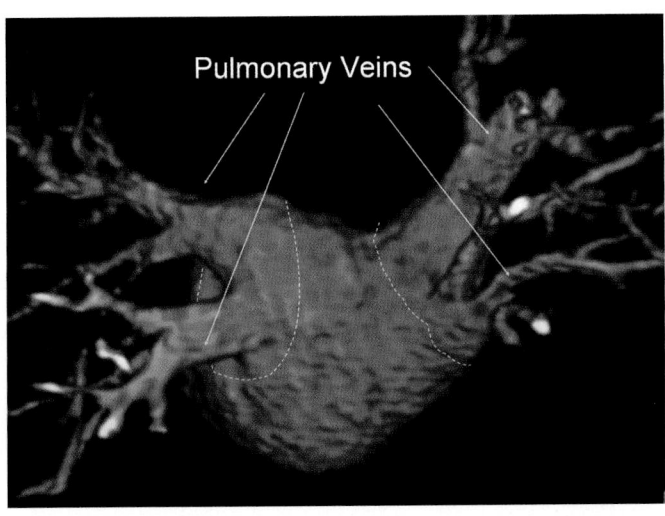

FIGURE 44-5. Left atrial ablation for atrial fibrillation. A magnetic resonance image of the left atrium and pulmonary veins from a patient with atrial fibrillation viewed from a posterior projection. The four pulmonary veins are indicated by *arrows*. The *dashed lines* indicate the typical location desired for antral ablation for atrial fibrillation, avoiding ablation within the veins themselves.

ping catheter during sinus rhythm (*pace mapping*) also helps identify the exit region. Identification of the scar region during stable sinus rhythm, referred to as *substrate mapping*, allows some VTs that are hemodynamically unstable to be targeted. Ablation then targets conducting channels through the scar region, or the border of the scar region that contains the exit. Ablation of scar-related VTs is more difficult than ablation for SVTs and has lower success rates. The scar region is typically large, usually contains multiple potential reentry circuits that cause different morphologies of VT inducible by electrical stimulation, and parts of the VT circuit can be deep within the myocardium or in the epicardium.[26–28] Some epicardial VTs can be approached by a subxiphoid percutaneous puncture into the pericardial space for mapping and ablation when pericardial scarring from prior surgery or proximity of the VT circuit to an epicardial coronary artery is not present.

In two recent multicenter ablation trials, acute success, abolishing one or more VTs, was achieved in more than 70 percent of patients.[29,30] Approximately half of the patients experienced at least one episode of VT during followup, although the frequency of episodes were reduced in the majority. The procedure can be lifesaving when VT is incessant. Procedure-related mortality was approximately 3 percent, some from uncontrollable VT when the procedure fails. Stroke, perforation with tamponade, femoral hematomas, and heart block from septal ablation also can occur.[31]

Bundle-branch reentry VT is a type of VT that is particularly susceptible to ablation, and is found in approximately 6 percent of patients with VT and structural heart disease. A diseased Purkinje system supports a reentry circuit revolving up one bundle branch and down the contralateral bundle branch. These patients often have intraventricular conduction delay or a pattern of left bundle-branch block during sinus rhythm and advanced ventricular dysfunction.[32] Catheter ablation of the right bundle branch is curative. Dual-chamber ICD implantation or even biventricular pacing is often warranted because of residual impaired AV conduction and the presence of other VTs in the setting of impaired ventricular function.

[ ] ABLATION FOR ELECTRICAL STORM AND VENTRICULAR FIBRILLATION

Repetitive episodes of ventricular fibrillation causing *electrical storm* are sometimes initiated by ectopic foci in the Purkinje system or RV outflow tract. Idiopathic ventricular fibrillation, acute and chronic myocardial infarction, long QT syndrome, and Brugada syndrome are commonly associated with electrical storm.[33] Such cases are rare, but ablation targeting the initiating foci during periods of electrical storm with a strategy similar to that used for idiopathic VT can be lifesaving.

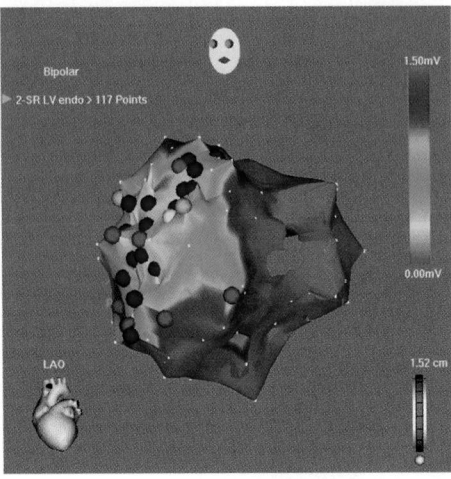 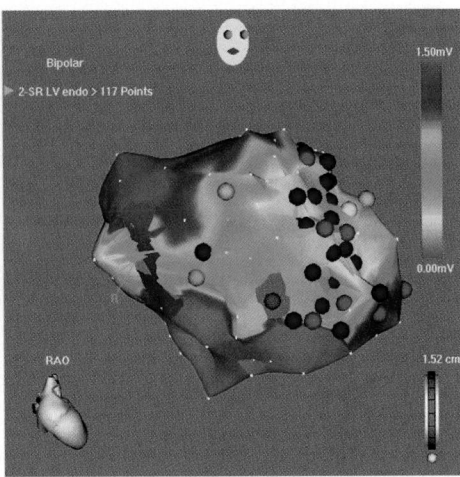

LAO   **RAO**

FIGURE 44–6. Electroanatomic voltage map of the left ventricle in a patient with sustained monomorphic VT caused by an old anterior wall myocardial infarction. A right anterior oblique (RAO) and left anterior oblique (LAO) projection are shown. In contrast to the maps shown in Figures 44–3 and 44–4, the color coding indicates the bipolar voltage acquired at each point in the map during sinus rhythm. Normal voltage is that above 1.5 mV, and is purple. Voltage progressively decreases as colors proceed to blue, green, yellow, orange, and red. The large low-voltage region is consistent with a prior anteroseptal infarction. Additional pacing at sites in the infarct region (red and yellow spheres) suggested a broad channel for conduction with exits at the superior and inferior margins of the infarct region. A series of RF lesions placed through the presumptive channel region (maroon spheres) abolished inducible ventricular tachycardia.

CONCLUSION

Catheter ablation offers an alternative to antiarrhythmic drug therapy for most tachyarrhythmias. Appropriate patient selection depends on an individualized assessment of risks and benefits. Ablation is a reasonable first-line therapy for most symptomatic supraventricular tachycardias caused by accessory pathways, atrial flutter, AV node reentrant tachycardia, and idiopathic VT. Its use for atrial fibrillation is increasing and further studies will continue to define the risks and benefits. Catheter ablation is an important adjunctive therapy to an implanted defibrillator for patients with recurrent VT associated with structural heart disease and can be lifesaving for patients with incessant VT or electrical storms.

REFERENCES

1. Blomstrom-Lundqvist C, Scheinman MM, Aliot EM, et al. ACC/AHA/ESC guidelines for the management of patients with supraventricular arrhythmias—executive summary: a report of the American College of Cardiology/American Heart Association Task Force on Practice Guidelines and the European Society of Cardiology Committee for Practice Guidelines (Writing Committee to Develop Guidelines for the Management of Patients With Supraventricular Arrhythmias). *Circulation* 2003;108:1871–1909.
2. Wu J, Olgin J, Miller JM, et al. Mechanisms underlying the reentrant circuit of atrioventricular nodal reentrant tachycardia in isolated canine atrioventricular nodal preparation using optical mapping. *Circ Res* 2001;88:1189–1195.
3. Friedman PL, Dubuc M, Green MS, et al. Catheter cryoablation of supraventricular tachycardia: results of the multicenter prospective "frosty" trial. *Heart Rhythm* 2004;1:129–138.
4. Dong J, Zrenner B, Schreieck J, et al. Catheter ablation of left atrial focal tachycardia guided by electroanatomic mapping and new insights into interatrial electrical conduction. *Heart Rhythm* 2005;2:578–591.
5. Badhwar N, Kalman JM, Sparks PB, et al. Atrial tachycardia arising from the coronary sinus musculature: electrophysiological characteristics and long-term outcomes of radiofrequency ablation. *J Am Coll Cardiol* 2005;46:1921–1930.

6. Lee RJ, Kalman JM, Fitzpatrick AP, et al. Radiofrequency catheter modification of the sinus node for "inappropriate" sinus tachycardia. *Circulation* 1995;92:2919–2928.

7. Marrouche NF, Beheiry S, Tomassoni G, et al. Three-dimensional nonfluoroscopic mapping and ablation of inappropriate sinus tachycardia. Procedural strategies and long-term outcome. *J Am Coll Cardiol* 2002;39:1046–1054.

8. Callans DJ, Ren JF, Schwartzman D, et al. Narrowing of the superior vena cava-right atrium junction during radiofrequency catheter ablation for inappropriate sinus tachycardia: analysis with intracardiac echocardiography. *J Am Coll Cardiol* 1999;33:1667–1670.

9. Natale A, Newby KH, Pisano E, et al. Prospective randomized comparison of antiarrhythmic therapy versus first-line radiofrequency ablation in patients with atrial flutter. *J Am Coll Cardiol* 2000;35:1898–1904.

10. Paydak H, Kall JG, Burke MC, et al. Atrial fibrillation after radiofrequency ablation of type I atrial flutter: time to onset, determinants, and clinical course. *Circulation* 1998;98:315–322.

11. Delacretaz E, Ganz LI, Soejima K, et al. Multi atrial macro-re-entry circuits in adults with repaired congenital heart disease: entrainment mapping combined with three-dimensional electroanatomic mapping. *J Am Coll Cardiol* 2001;37:1665–1676.

12. Doshi RN, Daoud EG, Fellows C, et al. Left ventricular-based cardiac stimulation post AV nodal ablation evaluation (the PAVE study). *J Cardiovasc Electrophysiol* 2005;16:1160–1165.

13. Ozcan C, Jahangir A, Friedman PA, et al. Sudden death after radiofrequency ablation of the atrioventricular node in patients with atrial fibrillation. *J Am Coll Cardiol* 2002;40:105–110.

14. Haissaguerre M, Jais P, Shah DC, et al. Spontaneous initiation of atrial fibrillation by ectopic beats originating in the pulmonary veins. *N Engl J Med* 1998;339:659–666.

15. Verma A, Natale A. Should atrial fibrillation ablation be considered first-line therapy for some patients? Why atrial fibrillation ablation should be considered first-line therapy for some patients. *Circulation* 2005;112:1214–1222; discussion 1231.

16. Oral H, Pappone C, Chugh A, et al. Circumferential pulmonary-vein ablation for chronic atrial fibrillation. *N Engl J Med* 2006;354:934–941.

17. Pappone C, Santinelli V. Segmental pulmonary vein isolation versus the circumferential approach: is the tide turning? *Heart Rhythm* 2004;1:326–328.

18. Dong J, Dickfeld T, Lamiy SZ, et al. Catheter ablation of atrial fibrillation guided by registered computed tomographic image of the atrium. *Heart Rhythm* 2005;2:1021–1022.

19. Cappato R, Calkins H, Chen SA, et al. Worldwide survey on the methods, efficacy, and safety of catheter ablation for human atrial fibrillation. *Circulation* 2005;111:1100–1105.

20. Pappone C, Oral H, Santinelli V, et al. Atrio-esophageal fistula as a complication of percutaneous transcatheter ablation of atrial fibrillation. *Circulation* 2004;109:2724–2726.

21. Joshi S, Wilber DJ. Ablation of idiopathic right ventricular outflow tract tachycardia: current perspectives. *J Cardiovasc Electrophysiol* 2005;16 Suppl 1:S52–S58.

22. Ouyang F, Cappato R, Ernst S, et al. Electroanatomic substrate of idiopathic left ventricular tachycardia: unidirectional block and macroreentry within the Purkinje network. *Circulation* 2002;105:462–469.

23. Marchlinski FE, Callans DJ, Gottlieb CD, et al. Linear ablation lesions for control of unmappable ventricular tachycardia in patients with ischemic and nonischemic cardiomyopathy. *Circulation* 2000;101:1288–1296.

24. Soejima K, Stevenson WG, Maisel WH, et al. Electrically unexcitable scar mapping based on pacing threshold for identification of the reentry circuit isthmus: feasibility for guiding ventricular tachycardia ablation. *Circulation* 2002;106:1678–1683.

25. Brunckhorst CB, Stevenson WG, Soejima K, et al. Relationship of slow conduction detected by pace-mapping to ventricular tachycardia re-entry circuit sites after infarction. *J Am Coll Cardiol* 2003;41:802–809.

26. Soejima K, Stevenson WG, Sapp JL, et al. Endocardial and epicardial radiofrequency ablation of ventricular tachycardia associated with dilated cardiomyopathy: the importance of low-voltage scars. *J Am Coll Cardiol* 2004;43:1834–1842.

27. Berruezo A, Mont L, Nava S, et al. Electrocardiographic recognition of the epicardial origin of ventricular tachycardias. *Circulation* 2004;109:1842–1847.

28. Sosa E, Scanavacca M, d'Avila A, et al. Nonsurgical transthoracic epicardial catheter ablation to treat recurrent ventricular tachycardia occurring late after myocardial infarction. *J Am Coll Cardiol* 2000;35:1442–1449.

29. Calkins H, Epstein A, Packer D, et al. Catheter ablation of ventricular tachycardia in patients with structural heart disease using cooled radiofrequency energy: results of a prospective multicenter study. Cooled RF Multi Center Investigators Group. *J Am Coll Cardiol* 2000;35:1905–1914.

30. Stevenson W, Wilber D, Natale A, et al. Multicenter trial of irrigated RF ablation with electroanatomic mapping for ventricular tachycardia after myocardial infarction. *Circulation* 2004;110 Suppl:1869.

31. Scheinman MM, Huang S. The 1998 NASPE prospective catheter ablation registry. *Pacing Clin Electrophysiol* 2000;23:1020–1028.

32. Tchou P, Jazayeri M, Denker S, et al. Transcatheter electrical ablation of right bundle branch. A method of treating macroreentrant ventricular tachycardia attributed to bundle branch reentry. *Circulation* 1988;78:246–257.

33. Haissaguerre M, Extramiana F, Hocini M, et al. Mapping and ablation of ventricular fibrillation associated with long-QT and Brugada syndromes. *Circulation* 2003;108:925–928.

CHAPTER 45

Indications and Techniques of Electrical Defibrillation and Cardioversion

Richard E. Kerber

HISTORY OF DEFIBRILLATION AND CARDIOVERSION

The deleterious effects of uncontrolled electrical current on cardiac rhythm were first recognized early in the 20th century. Concerned by accidental electrocutions of its line workers, the Consolidated Edison Company of New York supported research on the mechanisms and treatment of electrical accidents. Investigators at Johns Hopkins Hospital developed techniques of defibrillation—the termination of ventricular fibrillation—by an electrical shock in the 1930s.[1] The first human defibrillation, in the operating room, was performed by Claude Beck in 1947.[2] Transchest defibrillation using alternating current became a clinical reality when introduced by Paul Zoll in 1956,[3] and direct current defibrillation was pioneered by Bernard Lown in 1962.[4] The work of Zoll and Lown in combination with the description of closed-chest cardiac massage by Jude and colleagues in 1960[5] have formed the foundation of cardiopulmonary resuscitation from cardiac arrest for more than 40 years.

Lown used a damped sinusoidal waveform, which—at the usually encountered human transthoracic impedance (70 to 80 ohms)—was effectively monophasic. In the Soviet Union, Gurvich described an underdamped sinusoidal waveform that was effectively biphasic[6]; this waveform was not used in the West.

More recently, truncated exponential biphasic waveforms have now become the standard for transchest defibrillation; this is discussed in the section on New Waveforms.

In this chapter, the term *defibrillation* refers to the electrical termination of ventricular fibrillation (VF); *cardioversion* refers to the electrical termination of atrial fibrillation, atrial flutter, and supraventricular and ventricular tachycardias.

MECHANISMS OF DEFIBRILLATION AND CARDIOVERSION

How does an electric shock terminate a cardiac arrhythmia? There are three principal hypotheses. The critical mass hypothesis suggests that some proportion of the myocardium (not necessarily all) must be depolarized, so that the remaining muscle is inadequate to maintain the arrhythmia.[7] The upper limit of vulnerability hypothesis argues that a sufficient current density throughout the ventricle must be achieved lest fibrillation be reinitiated by a subthreshold current density.[8] Jones' group[9] states that defibrillating shocks must prolong refractoriness in sufficient myocardium to terminate VF. These concepts are not mutually exclusive; all may be applicable. Whether they also apply to the atrial myocardium for the termination of atrial fibrillation by electrical shock is not known. More organized arrhythmias, such as ventricular tachycardia and atrial flutter, terminate with lower energy than VF and atrial fibrillation,[10] likely because only regional depolarization in the path of an advancing wavefront is required.

SHOULD DEFIBRILLATION BE PERFORMED IMMEDIATELY UPON DISCOVERY OF VF, OR SHOULD IT BE PRECEDED BY A PERIOD OF CARDIOPULMONARY RESUSCITATION?

VF, a lethal arrhythmia, demands prompt termination as a lifesaving maneuver. The American Heart Association has encouraged immediate defibrillation of a victim of VF on the arrival of personnel equipped with a defibrillator. However, two recent investigations, by Cobb et al.[11] and Wik et al.,[12] show that if the initial application of shock is delayed (usually as a consequence of late arrival of rescuers at the scene of the cardiac arrest), a brief period of cardiopulmonary resuscitation (CPR) (ventilation, closed-chest compression) *prior* to the first shock will favorably enhance outcome. (A third clinical trial, by Jacobs et al.,[13] did not find that a period of CPR before defibrillation facilitates resuscitation.) These observations led Weisfeldt and Becker to propose a three-phase model of VF-induced cardiac arrest[14]: (1) The *electrical* phase consists of the first 4 minutes of VF. Shocks administered during this period have a high likelihood of achieving VF termination and resumption of spontaneous circulation. (2) The *circulatory* phase lasts from 4 to 10 minutes of VF. Shocks should be delayed in favor of a period of 1 to 3 minutes of CPR, including epinephrine or vasopressin, to restore a more favorable milieu for defibrillation. (3) The *metabolic* phase begins after 10 minutes of VF. In this phase, changes in myocardial metabolism after prolonged VF require aggressive and invasive measures for reversal, such as cardiopulmonary bypass and/or hypothermia. Shocks given during this period without such preparatory measures are likely to result in pulseless electrical activity or asystole—conditions associated with a very low likelihood of survival.

The phases of VF/cardiac arrest outlined above are time-based. Could we achieve a more sophisticated insight into the myocardial milieu and thereby determine whether immediate electrical shock or preshock pharmacologic or other resuscitative maneuvers should be employed in each particular case? Such insight might be afforded by a detailed analysis of the electrocardiographic VF signal itself. Experimental and clinical studies have shown that changes in VF frequency and amplitude occur over time. Such changes can be modulated pharmacologically, may correlate with coronary perfusion pressure (the difference between aortic and right atrial pressure during cardiac arrest), and may predict the response to a defibrillating shock.[15–18] With better understanding of the VF signal and its rela-

tionship to the state of the myocardium, the optimal timing of the electrical shock could be guided by a microprocessor-based analysis of the VF signal integrated into the defibrillator, which would instantly instruct the operator whether to deliver a shock or employ other supportive measures such as continuing CPR and administering vasopressors. Defibrillators employing such sophisticated techniques of VF analysis are now commercially available.

WHO SHOULD BE CARDIOVERTED FROM ATRIAL FIBRILLATION/ATRIAL FLUTTER, AND WHEN SHOULD THIS BE PERFORMED?

Sinus rhythm improves cardiac performance, especially in patients with mitral stenosis, left ventricular hypertrophy (aortic stenosis, hypertension, idiopathic hypertrophic subaortic stenosis), and/or diminished myocardial reserve (congestive heart failure, myocardial ischemia, and infarction). The coordinated atrial contraction of sinus rhythm improves ventricular filling, and cardiac rate is usually slower. Patients with these conditions are thus candidates for *elective* cardioversion. *Urgent* cardioversion may be required for patients with atrial or ventricular arrhythmias who are hypotensive and/or in pulmonary edema.

In some cases, treatment of an underlying or causative condition may restore sinus rhythm without the necessity of electrical cardioversion. Common causes of atrial arrhythmias include hyperthyroidism, pulmonary embolism, congestive heart failure, and mitral stenosis. Postoperative cardiac patients frequently experience transient rhythm disturbances that may spontaneously revert to sinus rhythm.

Important factors that determine the immediate and long-term success of cardioversion of atrial arrhythmias include the duration of the arrhythmia, the extent of atrial fibrosis, and the size of the left atrium. High success rates have been reported for cardioversion of atrial fibrillation and atrial flutter, especially when the new biphasic waveforms are used. High transthoracic impedance (TTI)—the resistance of the chest to the flow of electrical current—degrades current flow. Because current across the heart is what accomplishes the termination of the arrhythmia, high TTI may reduce the success of defibrillation or cardioversion, especially if the operator has selected a low shock energy.[19]

THROMBOEMBOLISM

There is a significant risk of thromboembolism after cardioversion. Three factors contribute to this risk: (1) If there is a preexisting thrombus in the fibrillating atrium (especially likely in the left atrial appendage), the electrical shock and/or the resumption of atrial contraction may dislodge the thrombus. (2) The shock itself may have thrombogenic effects. (3) With prolonged atrial fibrillation an atrial myopathy develops, which results in a slow return to normal atrial contraction following cardioversion. To prevent thromboembolism, therapeutic anticoagulation (international normalized ratio [INR] 2.0 to 3.0) for 3 weeks prior to cardioversion and 4 weeks afterward is traditionally recommended.[20]

The risk of thromboembolism associated with atrial fibrillation and cardioversion is higher in patients with mitral stenosis, a large left atrium from any cause, chronic atrial fibrillation of long duration, previous thromboembolic events, diabetes, or hypertension. Although transthoracic echocardiography is able to image the left atrial cavity well, it is usually unsatisfactory for visualization of the left atrial appendage, the site of most atrial thrombi. However, the newer technique of transesophageal echocardiography (TEE) images the left atrial appendage well and is highly sensitive to the presence of thrombi. Manning et al.[21] reported no embolic events during the cardioversion of atrial fibrillation when transesophageal echocardiography showed no thrombi were present in the atrial appendage and the patient received intravenous heparin for 2 days before cardioversion. This approach is known as *TEE-guided cardioversion.*[22] If a thrombus in the left atrial appendage is seen by TEE, cardioversion should be delayed, anticoagulation for 3 weeks should be undertaken. Some clinicians repeat the TEE to ensure that the thrombus has lysed. Although thromboembolism after cardioversion of atrial flutter is less common, it has been reported, as have conditions associated with thromboembolism, such as left atrial "smoke" (spontaneous ultrasound contrast) on transesophageal echocardiography.[23,24] Thus, anticoagulation before cardioversion of atrial flutter of more than short duration should be undertaken, similar to atrial fibrillation.[25]

At present TEE and cardioversion are generally carried out as two separate procedures, both requiring conscious sedation or anesthesia. Recently the two procedures have been combined by adding an electrode to the external surface of the transesophageal echo probe. Another electrode is placed on the anterior chest wall using a self-adhesive electrode pad. This allows a cardioverting DC shock to be delivered, using the esophageal–chest pathway. Because the esophageal electrode is close to the heart and the pathway is shortened, less energy—typically 20 to 50 J—is required to terminate atrial fibrillation using this esophageal cardioversion technique. Initial clinical experience with this combined TEE–cardioversion approach has been reported.[26]

Whether the traditional or TEE-guided anticoagulation scheme is used, it is considered mandatory to maintain anticoagulation for at least 4 weeks after cardioversion, because in the absence of anticoagulation thrombi may form postcardioversion and embolism may occur despite a negative TEE precardioversion.[21–25] Patients with paroxysmal atrial fibrillation, or those considered at high risk of recurrence of atrial fibrillation after cardioversion may require permanent anticoagulation. Antiarrhythmic drugs such as amiodarone may facilitate cardioversion and maintenance of sinus

rhythm after cardioversion. It is customary to withhold digitalis on the day of cardioversion (although this practice is not consistent with the long half-life of this drug). Digitalis-toxic rhythms should not be cardioverted, as the enhanced automaticity of such arrhythmias, combined with the shock could result in ventricular fibrillation or ventricular tachycardia.[27]

TECHNIQUES OF CARDIOVERSION AND DEFIBRILLATION

[ ] ANESTHESIA

Because the electrical current passing across the thorax causes a painful tetanic contraction, elective cardioversion, in this author's opinion, should be performed under general anesthesia; conscious sedation is often inadequate, with the patient experiencing and remembering severe discomfort. Bag-valve ventilation without endotracheal intubation is usually sufficient, but the presence of an anesthesiologist assures the ability to perform rapid endotracheal intubation if necessary.

[ ] SYNCHRONIZATION

It is essential to synchronize the electrical discharge on the R wave of the QRS complex; if the shock falls in the vulnerable period of the cardiac cycle, VF may be induced (Fig. 45–1). This is the most frequent serious complication of elective cardioversion of atrial arrhythmias and usually results from the operator's failure to enable properly the synchronizing device or to verify that the R wave of the ECG lead chosen is sufficiently tall to be recognized by the synchronizer. Recognition of the R wave of ventricular tachycardia is sometimes difficult owing to the morphology of the arrhythmia. If the patient is hemodynamically unstable owing to rapid ventricular tachycardia, unsynchronized shocks may be necessary.

[ ] ELECTRODES

Electrode placement on the chest is important to maximize current flow through the heart, which is what actually terminates the arrhythmia. Only a small proportion—as low as 4 percent—of the total transchest current flow actually traverses the heart.[28] Numer-

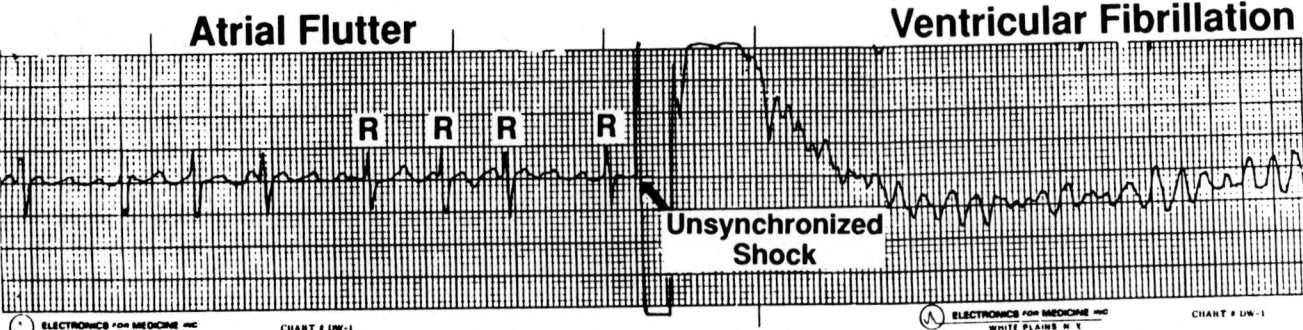

FIGURE 45–1. A complication of cardioversion: induction of ventricular fibrillation. The ventricular arrhythmia occurred because the operator failed to enable the synchronizer, resulting in inadvertent delivery of the shock on the vulnerable T wave instead of the intended delivery on the R wave. This complication is preventable by enabling the synchronizer and checking that it is properly functioning before shock delivery. *Source: From Kerber RE. Transchest cardioversion: optimal techniques. In: Tacker WA, ed. Defibrillation of the Heart: ICDs, AEDs and Manual. St. Louis: Mosby-Year Book, 1994:164. With permission.*

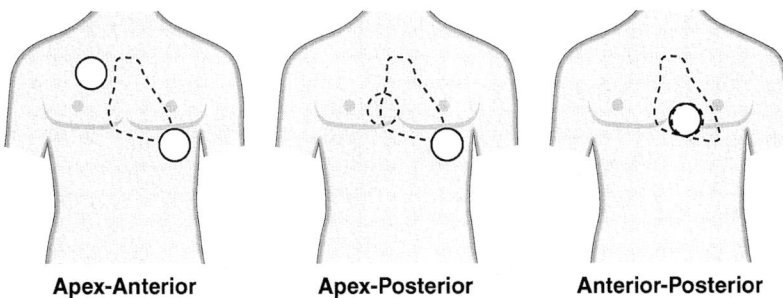

Apex-Anterior   **Apex-Posterior**   **Anterior-Posterior**

FIGURE 45–2. Electrode positions commonly used for transthoracic defibrillation and cardioversion. The apex-anterior position is most commonly used, but all are effective. If shocks given from one electrode pair position fail to terminate the arrhythmia, it is the author's practice to quickly change to another position and repeat the shocks. *Source: From Kerber RE. Transchest cardioversion: optimal techniques. In: Tacker WA, ed. Defibrillation of the Heart: ICDs, AEDs and Manual. St. Louis: Mosby-Year Book, 1994:163. With permission.*

ous pathways have been used successfully, including apex–high right parasternal, anteroposterior, and apex–right infrascapular (Fig. 45–2). The apex–high right parasternal is most frequently used. Although it has been difficult to demonstrate the superiority of any one pathway over others in clinical studies, one pathway might prove superior in the individual patient. Thus, it is the author's practice to move the electrodes to an alternate pathway when a patient whose atrial arrhythmia is expected to respond to elective cardioversion fails to convert with the initial shocks.

Electrodes should not be placed directly over the site of implanted pacemaker or defibrillator generators.[29] Although manufacturers commonly mark electrodes to indicate the location of chest placement, electrode polarity does not seem to influence shock success for either monophasic or biphasic waveforms.[30]

Electrode size influences the impedance of the chest; larger electrodes yield lower impedance, thereby improving current flow and increasing the likelihood of arrhythmia termination. For adult humans, the optimal paddle size appears to be 8 to 12 cm in diameter.[31,32] The Association for the Advancement of Medical Instrumentation recommends a minimum electrode contact area of 50 cm² for each electrode. The total area of both electrodes should be at least 150 cm².[33] Smaller pediatric paddles have been manufactured for children, but adult-size paddles should be used for children who weigh more than 10 kg (approximately 1 year old). This minimizes transthoracic impedance.[34]

Gels or pastes should not be smeared across the chest between paddle electrodes; the electrical current may follow the low-impedance pathway created by the paste, deflecting current away from the heart.[35] In women, the apex electrode should be placed adjacent to or under the breast; placement on the breast results in a high transthoracic impedance and degrades current flow.[36]

Cutaneous erythema after shocks is often noted at the location of the electrode placement. Skin biopsies show that these are first-degree burns.[37] Because there is preferential current flow at the edges of these electrodes, the erythema typically is most intense at the edges of the electrode location, outlining the electrode shape. Self-adhesive electrode pads constructed to have increased impedance at the pad edges allow more homogeneous current flow and may minimize these burns.[38]

Self-adhesive electrode pads for defibrillation have other advantages. They allow continuous monitoring of cardiac rhythm before

and after the shock as well as more physical separation of the generator from the patient (thus reducing the chance of the operator inadvertently receiving a shock); they also facilitate arrhythmia documentation. These pads are universally used in the new automated external defibrillators (AEDs), which are discussed in the section on Automated External Defibrillators.

NEW WAVEFORMS FOR DEFIBRILLATION AND CARDIOVERSION

For many years truncated exponential biphasic waveforms have been used instead of damped sinusoidal monophasic waveforms for implantable cardioverter defibrillators. Their superiority for *transthoracic* defibrillation and cardioversion has been demonstrated, initially in the operating room and electrophysiology laboratory, where VF is deliberately induced,[39] and subsequently during out-of-hospital cardiac arrest.[40] They are also superior for the electrical cardioversion of atrial arrhythmia.[41,42] At any energy level, these biphasic waveforms yield higher rates of arrhythmia termination than damped sinusoidal monophasic waveforms. This has resulted in lower energy recommendations for biphasic defibrillation and cardioversion; however, clinical considerations (left atrial size, duration of arrhythmia) may suggest higher or lower energies. The American Heart Association has stated that biphasic waveform shocks of ≥200 J are safe and effective for defibrillation,[43] and similar biphasic shock energies are highly effective for cardioversion.[41,42] Whether biphasic shocks of >200 J for defibrillation will be necessary for a significant number of VF patients is not known at present.

"Smart" biphasic waveform defibrillators incorporate technology to measure transthoracic impedance during the shock and instantaneously alter the waveform duration and/or voltage to compensate for impedance. Still other available defibrillators use a rectilinear near-rectangular fixed-pulse-duration waveform.[41] Any of these biphasic waveform variants will be superior to the traditional damped sinusoidal monophasic waveform; whether any one biphasic waveform is superior to another for human defibrillation and cardioversion has yet to be established.

New waveforms for defibrillation have been investigated in animal models. These include sawtooth-shaped biphasic waveforms[44] and multipulse multipathway shocks.[45] These have not yet been used for transthoracic defibrillation in humans. Triphasic and quadriphasic waveforms do not require additional capacitors or elaborate circuitry; these show superiority in animal studies.[46–48]

MYOCARDIAL DAMAGE FROM DEFIBRILLATION AND CARDIOVERSION

Although a lifesaving technique, direct current shocks may cause myocardial damage, especially when repeated high-energy discharges are administered.[49] Shocks cause mitochondrial dysfunction and free radical generation in the myocardium proportional to the energy used.[50,51] Antioxidant strategies to minimize shock-induced cardiac damage have been investigated in experimental animals.[51,52] Reducing shock energy/current, as well as minimizing the number of shocks delivered, will limit shock-induced myocardial damage. Some clinicians delay repeating a failed shock (for atrial fibrillation) for 1 or 2 minutes in the hope of preventing damage, but there is no convincing evidence for this approach; the author's practice is to repeat shocks as necessary without delay. Biphasic waveforms seem to be less toxic, perhaps simply by requiring less energy to achieve defibrillation.[53]

AUTOMATED EXTERNAL DEFIBRILLATORS AND PUBLIC ACCESS DEFIBRILLATION

In the 1980s, efforts to reduce the mortality associated with out-of-hospital cardiac arrest emphasized training of emergency medical technicians to recognize VF and to defibrillate using traditional manual defibrillators. Subsequently, AEDs were introduced. These small, light, and relatively inexpensive devices acquire an ECG via self-adhesive monitor-defibrillator pads applied to the cardiac arrest victim's thorax. A microprocessor in the defibrillator analyzes the ECG thus acquired; if the algorithm for VF is satisfied, the device sounds a warning and then delivers a shock. The ease of application and use of these devices make training requirements minimal, and biphasic waveforms in presently available units enhance the effectiveness of these AEDs. Requirements for AED algorithm performance and safety have been published.[54] Initial experience with AEDs has been reported from aircraft, airports, and gambling casinos[55-57]; all reports are highly favorable. Many communities are now equipping "first responders," such as police officers, firefighters, and security guards, with AEDs.[58] Placement of AEDs in areas known to have a high rate of cardiac arrest—airports, prisons, gyms—is an appropriate and cost-effective strategy.[55-59] Controlled trials of this strategy show its effectiveness.[60] The American Heart Association strongly supports these efforts under the rubric of *Public Access Defibrillation*.[61,62]

HOME DEFIBRILLATORS

Although widespread placement of AEDs in public spaces will improve survival after cardiac arrest, it is known that more than two-thirds of cardiac arrests occur at home.[59,63] Should AEDs be placed in homes of patients with known heart disease who have an increased risk of cardiac arrest? (Patients who are at the highest risk, e.g., those with ischemic heart disease with ejection fractions less than 30 percent, should receive an implanted cardioverter defibrillator.) For an AED to be effective when used to treat a cardiac arrest at home, the following must happen: (1) a spouse (or family member/friend) previously trained in AED use, must be at home; (2) the spouse must witness the arrest; (3) the spouse must retrieve the AED; (4) the spouse must correctly apply and turn on the AED; and (5) the AED must be in proper operating condition. These requirements are not trivial, and initial experience with AED use at home suggested that in an emergency, spouses, often elderly, may forget to retrieve their AED and/or be unable to apply and use it correctly.[63]

One potential solution to this problem is the recent development of a wearable defibrillator.[64,65] The patient wears a vest in which electrodes are incorporated and an ECG is fed to a defibrillator that is worn in a holster-like device (Fig. 45–3). The ECG is continuously analyzed; if the VF algorithm is satisfied the device initially delivers an audible and tactile alarm. If VF is not actually present (for example, if one of the ECG leads in the vest loses skin contact and the resultant artifact simulates VF), the patient has about 30 seconds to disable the device; if it is not disabled during the alert period, the defibrillator charges and then automatically delivers a biphasic shock. Initial clinical experience has been favorable.[64,65]

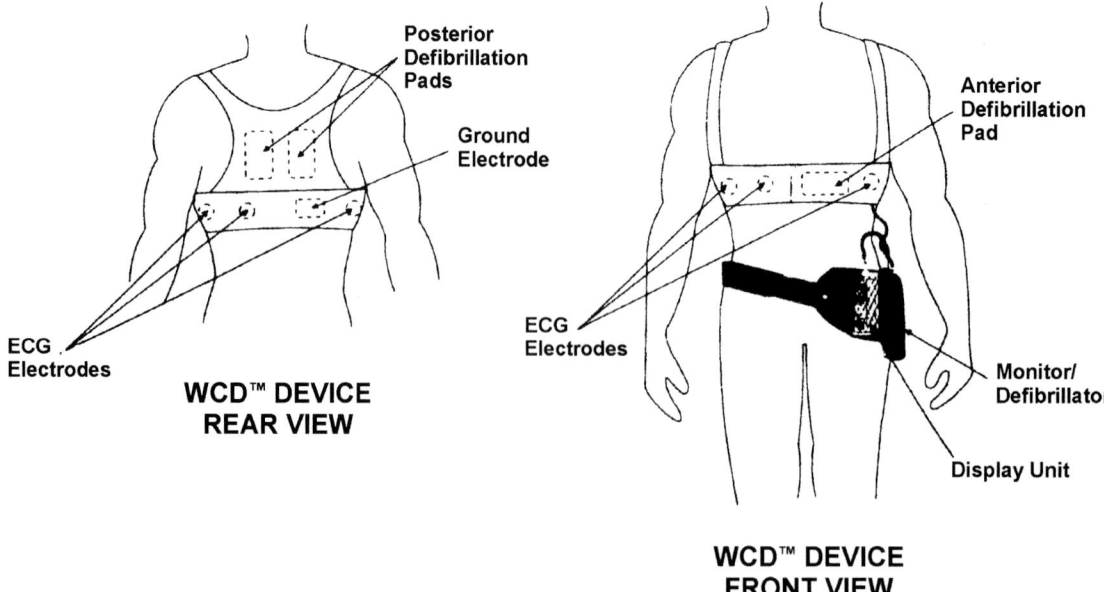

FIGURE 45–3. A wearable, fully automatic defibrillator. The patient wears electrodes in a vest; the ECG is continuously analyzed. If the algorithm for VF is satisfied, the device initiates an audible and tactile alarm; this allows the device to be disabled by the patient if the "arrhythmia" was artifactual (e.g., a loose or faulty lead). If the device is not disabled within 20 to 30 seconds, a shock is delivered automatically. *Source: Reprinted from Aurrichio A, Klein H, Geller C, et al.[64] with permission from Excerpta Medica, Inc.*

HYPOTHERMIA

Two recent multicenter trials have shown that the deliberate induction of hypothermia by application of external cooling devices affords protection to the brains of patients who have been defibrillated and resuscitated from VF/VT (ventricular tachycardia) but who remain comatose after resuscitation (i.e., anoxic encephalopathy).[66,67] By cooling such patients to about 91.4°F (33°C) for 24 to 36 hours, neurologic outcome improved. This strategy has been endorsed by the American Heart Association.[43] Could hypothermia applied before or during VF/VT (i.e., intraarrest hypothermia) facilitate defibrillation and resuscitation? Recent animal studies in mice and pigs suggest this is so.[68–72] A major challenge is to develop methods to lower core temperature in patients to about 91.4°F (33°C) rapidly—within a few minutes—in order to render this a feasible strategy for intraarrest application, because external cooling in patients requires several hours to reach 91.4°F (33°C). Experimental methods currently being evaluated include intravenous iced saline, chemical slurries, and intrapulmonary cold perfluorocarbons. This is a fertile field for future research.

CONCLUSION

As the professional baseball player and folk philosopher Yogi Berra may have said, "Predictions are difficult—especially about the future." Nevertheless, I offer some predictions about the state of the art of defibrillation and cardioversion in the next decade. The ECG signal of VF will be analyzed quickly and automatically and shock timing will be guided by information extracted from the ECG. Defibrillators in public places will become as common and accepted as fire extinguishers, and brief training in their use will be widespread, thanks largely to the Public Access Defibrillation program of the American Heart Association. Finally, defibrillators in the homes of patients with ischemic heart disease and/or a known propensity to arrhythmia (perhaps revealed by genetic analysis) will be an accepted part of cardiovascular therapy. These strategies hold great promise for combating the international epidemic of sudden cardiac death.

REFERENCES

1. Hooker DR, Kowenhoven WB, Langworth CR. The effect of alternating electrical currents on the heart. *Am J Physiol* 1933;103:444–454.
2. Beck C, Prichard WH, Feil HS. Ventricular fibrillation of long duration abolished by electrical shock. *JAMA* 1947;135:985–986.
3. Zoll PM, Linenthal AJ, Gibson W. Termination of ventricular fibrillation in man by externally applied electric countershock. *N Engl J Med* 1956;254:727–732.
4. Lown BR, Amarasingham R, Newman J. New method for terminating cardiac arrhythmias: use of synchronized capacity discharge. *JAMA* 1962;182:548–555.
5. Kowenhoven WB, Jude JR, Knickerbocker CG. Closed-chest cardiac massage. *JAMA* 1960;173:94–97.
6. Gurvich NL, Yuniev GS. Restoration of regular rhythm in the mammalian fibrillating heart. *Am Rev Soviet Med* 1945;3:236–239.
7. Zipes DP, Fisher J, King RM, et al. Termination of ventricular fibrillation in dogs by depolarizing a critical amount of myocardium. *Am J Cardiol* 1975;36:37–44.
8. Shibata N, Chen PS, Dixon EG, et al. Epicardial activation after unsuccessful defibrillation shocks in dogs. *Am J Physiol* 1988;255:H902–H909.
9. Jones JL. Waveforms for implantable cardioverter defibrillators (ICDs) and transchest defibrillation. In: Tacker WA, ed. *Defibrillation of the Heart: ICDs, AEDs and Manual.* St. Louis: Mosby-Year Book, 1994:46–81.
10. Kerber RE, Kienzle MG, Olshansky B, et al. Ventricular tachycardia rate and morphology determine energy and current requirements for transthoracic cardioversion. *Circulation* 1992;85:158–163.
11. Cobb L. Fahrenbruch CE, Walsh JR, et al. Influence of cardiopulmonary resuscitation prior to defibrillation in patients with out-of-hospital ventricular fibrillation. *JAMA* 1999;281:1182–1188.
12. Wik L, Hansen TB, Fylling F, et al. Delaying defibrillation to give basic cardiopulmonary resuscitation to patients with out-of-hospital ventricular fibrillation. *JAMA* 2003;289:1389–1395.
13. Jacobs IG, Finn JC, Oxer HF, Jelinek GA. CPR before defibrillation in out-of-hospital cardiac arrest: A randomized trial. *Emerg Med Australas* 2005;17:39–45.
14. Weisfeldt M, Becker L. Resuscitation after cardiac arrest: a three-phase time-sensitive model. *JAMA* 2002;288:3035–3038.
15. Strohmenger HU, Lindner KH, Brown CG. Analysis of the ventricular fibrillation amplitude and frequency parameters as predictors of countershock success in humans. *Chest* 1997;111:584–589.
16. Eftesol T, Sunde K, Aase SO, et al. Predicting outcome of defibrillation by spectral characterization and nonparameter classification of VF in patients with out-of-hospital cardiac arrest. *Circulation* 2000;102:1523–1529.
17. Watson JN, Uchaipichet N, Addison PS, et al. Improved prediction of defibrillation success for out-of-hospital VF cardiac arrest using wavelet transform methods. *Resuscitation* 2004;63:269–275.
18. Callaway CW, Menegazzi JJ. Waveform analysis of ventricular fibrillation to predict defibrillation. *Curr Opin Crit Care* 2005;11:192–199.
19. Kerber RE, Martins JB, Kienzle MG, et al. Energy, current and success in defibrillation and cardioversion: clinical studies using an automated impedance-based energy adjustment method. *Circulation* 1988;77:1038–1046.
20. Albers GW, Dalen JE, Laupacis A, et al. Antithrombotic therapy in atrial fibrillation. *Chest* 2001;119:194S–206S.
21. Manning W, Silverman DI, Gordon SPF, et al. Cardioversion from atrial fibrillation without prolonged anticoagulation with use of transesophageal echocardiography to exclude the presence of atrial thrombi. *N Engl J Med* 1993;328:750–755.
22. Klein A, Grimm RA, Black IW, et al. Cardioversion guided by transesophageal echocardiography: The ACUTE pilot study. *Ann Intern Med* 1997;126:200–209.
23. Black I, Hopkins AP, Lee CLL, et al. Evaluation of transesophageal echocardiography before cardioversion of atrial fibrillation and atrial flutter in nonanticoagulated patients. *Am Heart J* 1993;126:375–381.
24. Arnold AZ, Mick MJ, Mazurek RP, et al. Role of prophylactic anticoagulation for direct current cardioversion in patients with atrial fibrillation or atrial flutter. *J Am Coll Cardiol* 1992;19:851–855.
25. Olshansky B, Kerber RE. Cardioversion of atrial flutter. In: Waldo AL, Touboul P, eds. *Atrial Flutter: Advances in Mechanism and Management.* Armonk, NY: Futura, 1996;387–409.
26. Scholten MF, Thornton AF, Jordaens LJ, et al. Usefulness of transesophageal echocardiography using a combined probe when converting atrial fibrillation to sinus rhythm. *Am J Cardiol* 2005;94:470–473.
27. Lown B, Krieger R, Williams J. Cardioversion and digitalis drugs: changed threshold to electric shock in digitized animals. *Circ Res* 1965;17:519–531.
28. Lerman BB, Deale OS. Relation between transcardiac and transthoracic current during defibrillation in humans. *Circ Res* 1990;67:1420–1426.
29. Aylward P, Blood R, Tonkin A. Complications with defibrillation with permanent pacemakers in situ (abstr). *Pacing Clin Electrophysiol* 1988;2:462.
30. Karlsson G, Zhang Y, Davies LR, et al. Does electrode polarity alter the energy requirements for transthoracic biphasic waveform defibrillation? Experimental studies. *Resuscitation* 2001;51:77–81.
31. Sirna SJ, Ferguson DW, Charbonnier F, et al. Electrical cardioversion in humans: factors affecting transthoracic impedance. *Am J Cardiol* 1988;62:1048–1058.
32. Kerber RE, Martins JB, Kelly K, et al. Self-adhesive pre-applied electrode pads for defibrillation and cardioversion. *J Am Coll Cardiol* 1984;3:815–820.
33. Association for the Advancement of Medical Instrumentation. *American National Standard: Medical Electrical Equipment. Part 2–4: Particular Requirements for the Safety of Cardiac Defibrillators (Including Automated External Defibrillators).* ANSI/AAMI DF80–2003. Arlington, VA: AAMI 2003.
34. Atkins D, Kerber RE. Pediatric defibrillation: Importance of paddle size in determining transthoracic impedance. *Pediatrics* 1988;82:914–918.
35. Caterine MR, Yoerger DM, Spencer KT, et al. Effect of electrode position and gel-application technique on predicted transcardiac current during transthoracic defibrillation. *Ann Emerg Med* 1997;29:588–595.

36. Pagan-Carlo LA, Spencer KT, Robertson CE, et al. Transthoracic defibrillation: importance of avoiding electrode placement directly on the female breast. *J Am Coll Cardiol* 1996;27:449–452.

37. Pagan-Carlo LA, Stone MS, Kerber RE. Nature and determinants of skin burns after transthoracic cardioversion. *Am J Cardiol* 1997;79:689–691.

38. Garcia L, Pagan-Carlo LA, Stone MS, et al. High perimeter impedance defibrillation electrodes reduce skin burns in transthoracic cardioversion. *Am J Cardiol* 1998;82:1125–1127.

39. Bardy GH, Marchlinski FE, Sharma AD, et al. Multicenter comparison of truncated biphasic shocks and standard damped sine waveform modified shocks for transthoracic ventricular defibrillation. *Circulation* 1996;94:2507–2514.

40. Schneider T, Martens PR, Paschen H, et al. Multicenter randomized controlled trial of 150 J biphasic shocks compared with 200–360 J monophasic shocks in the resuscitation of out-of-hospital cardiac arrest victims. *Circulation* 2000;102:1780–1787.

41. Mittal S, Ayati S, Stein KM, et al. Transthoracic cardioversion of atrial fibrillation: comparison of rectilinear biphasic vs. damped sine monophasic shocks. *Circulation* 2000;101:1282–1287.

42. Page RL, Kerber RE, Russell JK, et al. Biphasic versus monophasic shock waveform for conversion of atrial fibrillation. *J Am Coll Cardiol* 2002;39:1956–1963.

43. American Heart Association guidelines 2005 for cardiopulmonary resuscitation and emergency cardiac care. *Circulation* 2005;112:IV-1–IV-41.

44. Yamanouchi Y, Brewer JE, Mowrey KA. Sawtooth first phase biphasic defibrillation waveforms: a comparison with standard waveform in clinical devices. *J Cardiovasc Electrophysiol* 1997;8:517–528.

45. Pagan-Carlo LA, Allan JJ, Spencer KT, et al. Encircling overlapping multi-pulse shock waveforms for transthoracic defibrillation. *J Am Coll Cardiol* 1998;32:2065–2071.

46. Jones JL, Jones RE. Improved safety factor for triphasic defibrillator waveforms. *Circ Res* 1989;64:1172–1177.

47. Zhang Y, Ramabadran R, Boddicker K, et al. Triphasic shocks are superior to biphasic shocks for transthoracic defibrillation: experimental studies. *J Am Coll Cardiol* 2003;42:568–575.

48. Zhang Y, Rhee B, Davis L, et al. Quadriphasic waveforms are superior to triphasic waveforms for transthoracic defibrillation in a cardiac arrest swine model with high impedance. *Resuscitation* 2006;68:251–258.

49. Warner ED, Dahl C, Ewy GA. Myocardial injury from transthoracic defibrillator countershock. *Arch Pathol* 1975;99:55–59.

50. Trouton PG, Allen JD, Yong LK, et al. Metabolic changes in mitochondrial dysfunction early following transthoracic countershocks in dogs. *Pacing Clin Electrophysiol* 1989;12:1827–1834.

51. Caterine MR, Spencer KT, Pagan Carlo LA, et al. Direct current shocks to the heart generate free radicals: An electron paramagnetic resonance study. *J Am Coll Cardiol* 1996;28:1598–1609.

52. Clark CB, Zhang Y, Martin SM, et al. The nitric oxide synthase inhibitor N^G-nitro-L-arginine decreases defibrillation-induced free radical generation. *Resuscitation* 2003;57:101–108.

53. Tang W, Weil MH, Sun S, et al. The effects of biphasic and conventional monophasic defibrillation post-resuscitation myocardial function. *J Am Coll Cardiol* 1999;34:815–822.

54. Kerber RE, Becker LB, Bourland JD, et al. Automatic external defibrillators for public access defibrillation: recommendations for specifying and reporting arrhythmia analysis algorithm performance, incorporating new waveforms, and enhancing safety. *Circulation* 1997;95:1677–1682.

55. Page RL, Joglar J, Kowal RC, et al. Use of automated defibrillators by a U.S. airline. *N Engl J Med* 2000;343:1210–1216.

56. Valenzuela T, Roe DJ, Nichol G, et al. Outcomes of rapid defibrillation by security officers after cardiac arrest in casinos. *N Engl J Med* 2000;343:1206–1209.

57. Caffrey SL, Willoughby P, Pepe PE, et al. Public use of automated external defibrillators. *N Engl J Med* 2002;347:1242–1247.

58. White RD, Asplin BR, Bugliosi TF, et al. High discharge survival rate after out-of-hospital ventricular fibrillation with rapid defibrillation by police and paramedics. *Ann Emerg Med* 1996;28:480–485.

59. Weaver DL, Peberdy MA. Defibrillation in public places—one step closer to home. *N Engl J Med* 2002;347:1223–1224.

60. PAD Trial Investigators. Public access defibrillation and survival after out-of-hospital cardiac arrest. *N Engl J Med* 2004;351:637–646.

61. Weisfeldt ML, Kerber RE, McGoldrick RP, et al. American Heart Association report on public access defibrillation conference, December 8–10, 1994: Automatic External Defibrillation Task Force. *Circulation* 1995;92:684–692.

62. Hazinski MF, Idris A, Kerber RE, et al. Lay rescuer automatic external defibrillator ("public access defibrillator") programs. Lessons learned from an international multicenter trial. *Circulation* 2005;111:3336–3340.

63. Eisenberg MS, Moore J, Cummins RO, et al. Use of the automatic external defibrillator in homes of survivors of out-of-hospital ventricular fibrillation. *Am J Cardiol* 1989;63:443–446.

64. Aurrichio A, Klein H, Geller C, et al. Clinical efficacy of the wearable cardioverter defibrillator in acutely terminating episodes of ventricular fibrillation. *Am J Cardiol* 1998;81:1253–1257.

65. Feldman A, Klein H, Tchou P, et al. Use of a wearable defibrillator in terminating tachyarrhythmias in patients at high risk for sudden death. *Pacing Clin Electrophysiol* 2004;27:4–9.

66. Hypothermia After Cardiac Arrest Study Group. Mild therapeutic hypothermia to improve the neurologic outcome after cardiac arrest. *N Engl J Med* 2002;346:549–556.

67. Barnard SA, Gray TW, Brist MD, et al. Treatment of comatose survivors of out-of-hospital cardiac arrest with induced hypothermia. *N Engl J Med* 2002;346:557–563.

68. Rhee BJ, Zhang Y, Boddicker K, et al. Effect of hypothermia on transthoracic defibrillation in a swine model. *Resuscitation* 2005;65:79–85.

69. Boddicker K, Zhang Y, Zimmerman MB, et al. Hypothermia improves defibrillation success and resuscitation outcomes from ventricular fibrillation. *Circulation* 2005;111:3195–3201.

70. Abela BS, Zhao D, Alvarado T, et al. Intra-arrest cooling improves outcomes in a murine cardiac arrest model. *Circulation* 2004;109:2786–2791.

71. Dendi R, Zhang Y, Brooks L, et al. Rapid cardiopulmonary intra-arrest hypothermia improves resuscitation outcomes from ventricular fibrillation cardiac arrest [abstract]. *Circulation* 2005;112:II-323.

72. Nordmark J, Rubertsson R. Induction of mild hypothermia with infusion of cold (4°C) fluid during CPR. *Resuscitation* 2005;66:357–365.

CHAPTER 46

The Implantable Cardioverter Defibrillator

Christian Wolpert / Martin Borggrefe

INTRODUCTION

After Zacouto and Bouvrain developed the concept of an automatic device that monitors the heart rhythm, paces, and defibrillates, Mirowski implanted the first implantable defibrillator in humans in 1980.[1,2] Since these early days of this revolutionary therapy, great progress has been made in defibrillation waveforms, transvenous implantation and increasing miniaturization. After Luderitz and coworkers implanted an antitachycardia pacemaker together with a separate intracardiac cardioverter-defibrillator (ICD) and tested the efficacy of antitachycardia pacing by an implantable device, these features were soon implemented in one device.[3] Not much later biphasic shock waveforms were developed, which dramatically reduced the defibrillation thresholds and made fully transvenous implantation feasible.[4] The main diagnostic pitfalls of ICD therapy—the inability to analyze the underlying rhythms leading to ICD therapy and inappropriate therapies—have been in part overcome by the introduction of stored electrograms and enhanced detection criteria. With the addition of biventricular pacing and its integration into defibrillator devices, ICD therapy has become a combined electrical treatment for patients with malignant ventricular tachyarrhythmias and those with severe heart failure.[5] Prospective trials in high-risk patients have extended indications in primary prevention of sudden death.[6,7]

DEVICE FUNCTIONALITY

The implantable defibrillator system consists of a pulse generator and a right ventricular lead, (additive atrial lead in dual-chamber ICDs, additive coronary sinus lead in biventricular ICDs) which serves for heart rate detection, pacing and defibrillation therapy. The generator contains the lithium battery, the capacitors and the pace-sense circuits as well as the other electronic components. The housing of the defibrillator can serve further as one defibrillation electrode (*active can*). The leads are connected to the generator through plugs in the connector, which is attached to the can.

There are different leads available for transvenous implant. Some have one ventricular defibrillation coil electrode; others have two defibrillation electrodes—one distally in the right ventricle and the other on the proximal portion of the lead at the junction of the superior vena cava and the right atrium. In the setting of high defibrillation threshold for patients in whom ventricular fibrillation cannot be terminated by a shock within the required safety margin using the conventional leads, further subcutaneous finger or patch electrodes can be added.

For rate sensing and pacing, true bipolar and integrated bipolar leads are available.

SENSING

The rate signal is derived from either between the distal tip and the distal coil of the right ventricular lead (integrated bipolar sensing) or from the distal tip to distal ring electrode (true bipolar sensing). The intracardiac signal is amplified, filtered, and rectified. The sensing varies depending on the underlying rhythm and the amplitude of the signal and therefore modern ICDs use automatic gain control, which ensures adjustment of the signal. Autoadjustment decreases the sensitivity exponentially to a preprogrammed value following a sensed event (i.e., R wave). This is mainly aimed at avoidance of T-wave sensing.

Beside the automatic gain control, the sensitivity threshold can be programmed in all defibrillators to different levels depending on the individual intracardiac R-wave and T-wave amplitude. After sensing and pacing blanking periods are either fixed or freely programmable, depending on the manufacturer.

PACING

All defibrillators use bipolar pacing for stimulation. In addition to baseline pacing there is a separately programmable postshock pacing output to pace in postshock asystole or postshock atrioventricular (AV)-block.

Pacing is delivered from the right ventricular lead or from the coronary sinus or epicardial left ventricular lead in biventricular ICDs.

DETECTION

All modern devices provide different detection zones for ventricular tachycardia and ventricular fibrillation. The detection zones are programmable to different heart rates (cycle lengths). Most devices have two zones programmable for VT. In whichever zone a rhythm is detected, the programmed mode of therapy for that zone is delivered.

The detection criterion is fulfilled if the programmed number of intervals to detect (NID) is reached. The NID is programmable and varies among the manufacturers. Commonly, the criterion for ventricular fibrillation is a duration of a prespecified number of seconds of consecutive R waves within the ventricular fibrillation (VF), or a given number of intervals with a rate higher than the cut-off rate.

Once this criterion is met, the therapy is delivered. However, between the arrhythmia detection and the shock delivery, the capacitors are charged. At the end of charging, a second look to the rate is applied to avoid delivering a shock in nonsustained or self-terminating ventricular tachycardia (VT). If the heart rate exceeds the detection rate during this second look, the therapy is delivered. If the rhythm has returned to normal rate during the charging period, the therapy is withheld (*noncommitted shock*).

Following the therapy delivery a period of redetection starts and, if the criterion for VT/VF redetection is fulfilled, a second therapy is delivered, this time without a second look (*committed shock*).[8]

The detection for ventricular tachycardia is different from the detection of ventricular fibrillation. For VT detection a consecutive number of intervals above the programmed cut-off rate have to occur in order to meet the criterion. When detection is met, immediate therapy is delivered. In most of the cases an antitachycardia pacing attempt is programmed as first therapy. After this therapy a redetection window starts, which, if fulfilled, will prompt additional therapies.

When one interval within a detection period is longer than the programmed detection cycle length, then the counter is reset. This is designed to avoid inappropriate therapy during atrial tachyarrhythmias with rapid conduction to the ventricle. It is based on the observation that VT is less likely than rapid atrial fibrillation to be interrupted by a long cycle.

Further criteria to avoid inappropriate ICD therapies for supraventricular tachycardias are based on cycle-length stability, tachycardia onset characteristics, and QRS width or morphology. The rate stability criterion measures the RR interval stability during a rhythm inside the VT detection zone and compares the difference of cycle lengths in a given number of cycles. When the variability of the cycle lengths is higher than the programmed value, the rhythm will be rejected as being of supraventricular origin. In case of regular cycle lengths the tachycardia is classified as VT. The onset criterion compares the cycle length immediately preceding the arrhythmia onset to the cycle length of the initial beats of the arrhythmia and requires a certain percentage of difference for classification as VT. If the difference is smaller than the programmed value, the rhythm is classified as supraventricular tachycardia.

Finally, devices can compare the morphology of the QRS complex during tachycardia to a QRS template of a normal sinus beat. If a preprogrammed degree of congruency is not fulfilled, the tachycardia is classified as being of ventricular origin. If the congruency of the sinus template and the tachycardia complex is high, it is detected as supraventricular tachycardia.

DUAL-CHAMBER DETECTION

In dual-chamber defibrillators, the atrial sensing is incorporated into the detection algorithm. The algorithms differ among manufacturers. The underlying principle is that the atrial rate, AV-association, and stability form the basis of all algorithms. Dual-chamber detection reduces the likelihood of inappropriate ICD therapies compared to single-chamber ICD detection.

Prospective studies demonstrate that by using dual-chamber detection, sensitivity is not reduced and therapy is not delayed compared with single-chamber detection.[9,10]

INTRACARDIAC CARDIOVERSION AND DEFIBRILLATION

The defibrillator provides both synchronous cardioversion and defibrillation. The shock strength can be programmed to different energies. The number of therapies for one episode is limited to a maximum number of shocks. Most defibrillators are programmed to the maximum available energy for treatment of VF. Inside the VT zone, low-energy cardioversion can be programmed. The delay between the arrhythmia onset and therapy delivery depends on the capacitor charging time, which itself depends on the energy programmed. The higher the energy, the longer the capacitor charge requires, with maximum energy usually taking between 5 and 10 seconds.

ANTITACHYCARDIA PACING

Antitachycardia pacing can be delivered as fixed burst pacing or auto-decremental burst pacing (ramp pacing). The number of stimuli and the coupling interval of the pacing stimuli can be programmed and depends on the tachycardia cycle length. Within one detection zone different pacing modes can be programmed in sequence.

Antitachycardia pacing is effective in terminating monomorphic ventricular tachycardia 85 percent to more than 90 percent of the time.[11–14] This feature helps avoid unnecessary shocks in regular VT. A high success rate is also seen for tachycardias faster than 200 beats per minute (Fig. 46–1).[15,16]

STORED ENDOCARDIAL ELECTROGRAMS AND DEVICE DATA STORAGE

Devices can provide endocardial electrograms with the date, time, and duration of the episodes, and with the tachycardia rate and morphology characteristics. Morphology interpretation is often difficult. In dual-chamber defibrillators, an additional atrial electrogram is recorded.[17]

AUTOMATIC DEVICE INTEGRITY MEASUREMENTS

In recent device generations, automatic measurements of battery status and lead impedance, or noise signal detection, are provided. These features help to detect lead integrity problems and changes in battery voltage at an early stage. Some devices have a so-called *patient alert feature*, which provides an audible signal to the patient when an alarm condition has occurred.[18]

FOLLOWUP PROCEDURES

Patients are typically seen for routine followup interrogation every 3–6 months. Before device interrogation and testing, patients should undergo a physical examination and be interviewed for any symptoms of heart failure or palpitations during the previous fol-

lowup interval. The current medication should be checked for any potential changes in drugs or dosage.

During the visits the battery status, pace/sense, and impedance characteristics are assessed. Further data storage and stored electrograms are retrieved and reviewed. Radiographs are performed annually to ensure lead and device location. In patients in whom amiodarone therapy is initiated, a retesting of the defibrillation safety margin under conscious sedation may be indicated, because amiodarone can increase the defibrillation thresholds.[19]

If a spontaneous arrhythmia or a shock has occurred, review of the endocardial electrograms and device data will help to classify the arrhythmia, assess the appropriateness of therapy, and guide reprogramming. The site of implant should be inspected to identify potential infection of the pocket, skin erosion or device dislodgement/migration. Superficial venous collaterals are sometimes a clinical sign of subclavian vein stenosis or chronic occlusion.

Some clinics now use transtelephonic device interrogation, and studies are evaluating the effectiveness of this approach.

ICD IMPLANTATION

Most ICD implantations are performed under conscious sedation by cardiologists.[20] The implantation technique is similar to the implantation of normal antibradycardia pacemakers. After an incision in the left pectoral region, the lead is inserted by puncture of the subclavian vein or the left cephalic vein or another side branches. The right ventricular screw-in, or tine lead, is then advanced to the right ventricular apex under fluoroscopic guidance, with the ventricular coil electrode parallel and close to the interventricular septum. This position achieves the best possible defibrillation performance.[21] If necessary, a dual-coil electrode or additional subcutaneous leads can be implanted to improve the electrical field for defibrillation.

Prophylactic antibiotics are generally administered (Fig. 46–2).

DEFIBRILLATION THRESHOLD TESTING

Intraoperative defibrillation testing is performed after connection of the device to the lead, with the device in the pocket. The patient should be connected to a surface ECG and to an external defibrillator, which is necessary to provide external rescue shocks if internal defibrillation fails. Commonly, ventricular fibrillation is

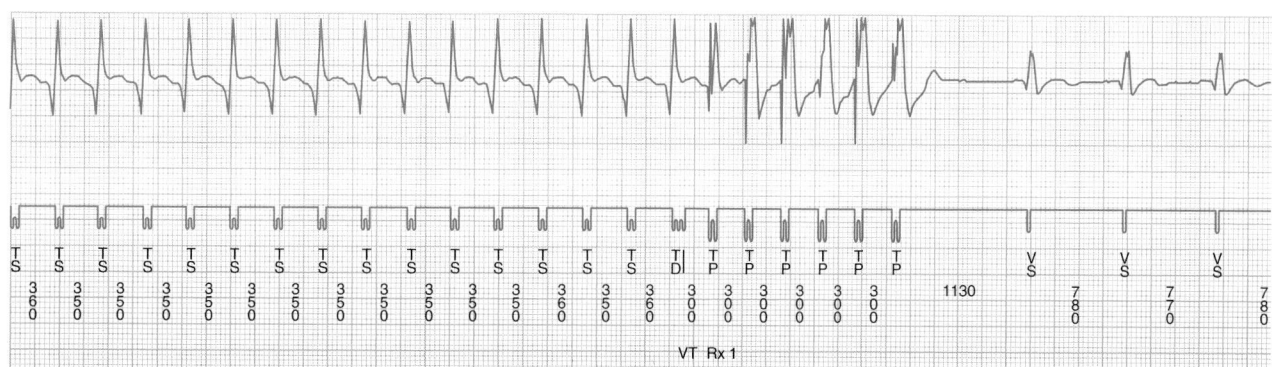

FIGURE 46–1. The stored electrogram depicts a ventricular tachycardia with a cycle length of 350 milliseconds, which is terminated by antitachycardia pacing with a burst of 6 stimuli and a coupling interval of 81 percent. After the programmed number of intervals to detect (NID) has occurred, the detection criterion for ventricular tachycardia is met (TD) and the therapy is immediately delivered. Following the last pacing stimulus, the rhythm returns to a normal heart rate. RX, therapy; TD, tachycardia detection; TS, tachycardia sense; TP, tachycardia pace; VS, ventricular sense; VT, ventricular tachycardia.

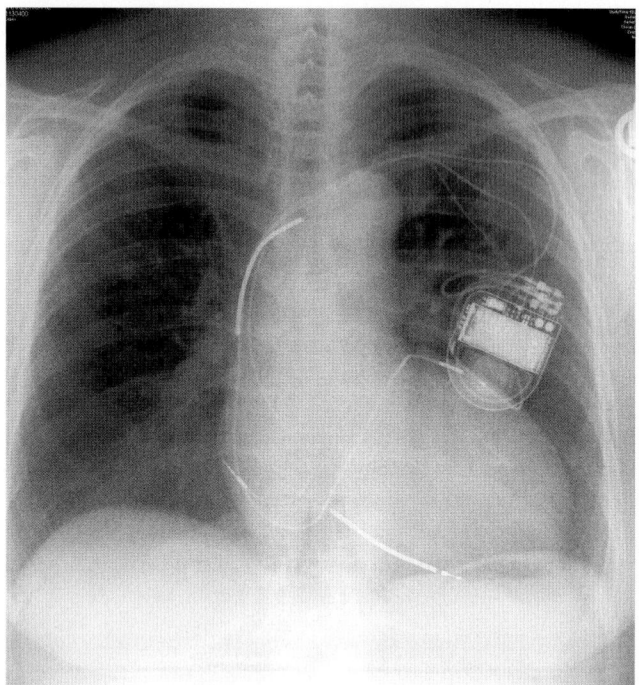

FIGURE 46–2. Posterior–anterior chest radiograph of a biventricular ICD. The leads are placed in the right atrium, in the right ventricular apex, and in a posterolateral venous branch of the coronary sinus. The device is placed subpectorally on the left side.

induced by the ICD programmer through T-wave shocks, programmed stimulation, or burst pacing. The first shock should be programmed for at least 10 joules below the maximum shock output, and the second shock (that follows an unsuccessful defibrillation) to the maximum output. If the second shock fails, an external rescue shock is delivered. Allow 3 to 5 minutes for the patient to recover from ischemia and/or hemodynamic compromise between two inductions of ventricular fibrillation.

During implantation, termination of ventricular fibrillation has to be demonstrated at an energy level that is at least 10 joules below the maximum energy available, which is achievable in nearly all patients. Successful termination of VF should be reproduced. The average defibrillation threshold (DFT) for active can devices is 10 to 15 joules.[22] Many physicians use two tests at 10 or 15 joules below the maximum capacity of the device as successful implant criterion.

When defibrillation fails at the 10-joule margin, several options are available, including reversing shock polarity, changing the pulse duration for phase 1 and phase 2 of the biphasic shock, and implanting a dual-coil electrode or adding a subcutaneous array, finger, or patch electrode. Epicardial implantation of ICD leads has become a rare last resort. Intraoperative testing is always performed at the minimal sensitivity level to ensure proper detection of small intracardiac signals during VF. Careful evaluation of the intracardiac signals and continuous detection of fibrillation cycles are necessary.

DEVICE PROGRAMMING

In most patients, it is useful to program a two-zone detection—one for ventricular tachycardia and one for ventricular fibrillation. In some patients with both slow and fast VT, as well as VF, a three-zone program may be critical to tier therapy for the different tachyarrhythmias.[16]

Because the probability of experiencing VT, which can to a great extent be terminated by painless antitachycardia pacing, is much higher than suffering primary ventricular fibrillation both in primary and secondary prevention,[16] programming should allow for antitachycardia pacing for most VT rhythms. The VT detection is commonly set to a cycle length of more than 40 milliseconds longer than the documented VT or, when programmed empirically, to a cycle length of 350 to 400 milliseconds. In progressive heart failure, some patients develop slow VT over time and may experience a VT below the programmed cut-off rate.[23,24] After the addition of rate-slowing drugs, such as class III antiarrhythmic drugs, the VT detection boundary should be adjusted, because spontaneous VT may be significantly slower.

Enhanced detection criteria should be activated to avoid inappropriate shocks for supraventricular rhythms. In general, programming of enhanced detection criteria and detection boundaries have to balance maximum specificity and utmost sensitivity (Figs. 46–3 and 46–4).

INDICATIONS

ICD FOR SECONDARY PREVENTION

Therapy with the implantable defibrillator is most effective in the treatment of sudden cardiac death and is superior to antiarrhythmic drug treatment. However, the benefit of ICD therapy is not equal for different subpopulations and may vary among patients with different degrees of heart failure and comorbidities.

Three prospective randomized trials were carried out to assess the effect of ICD therapy on total mortality in patients who had experienced aborted sudden cardiac death or hemodynamically non-tolerated ventricular tachycardia: the CASH (Cardiac Arrest Study Hamburg) trial, the CIDS (Canadian Implantable Defibrillator Study) trial, and the AVID (Antiarrhythmics Versus Implantable Defibrillator) trial.[25–27]

In the CIDS trial, 659 patients who had suffered from ventricular fibrillation, symptomatic VT, or syncope with inducible ventricular tachyarrhythmias were randomized to either receive an ICD or amiodarone treatment.[26] There was a 20 percent reduction in total mortality and 33 percent reduction in sudden arrhythmic death after 5 years of followup in the ICD treatment group, but these results were not statistically significant ($p = 0.14$ and $p = 0.09$).

The AVID trial was the largest randomized trial to compare the effect of an ICD or conventional treatment on mortality in patients who survived sudden death or hemodynamically nontolerated VT.[27] In more than 1000 patients, mortality was reduced in the ICD arm by 29 percent at 3 years. However, the effect was stronger in patients with a left ventricular ejection fraction of less than 35 percent than in patients with a better ejection fraction.

In the CASH trial,[25] 346 cardiac arrest survivors were randomized to an ICD or drug treatment. The trial resulted in a reduction of mortality by 37 percent in patients with an ICD versus conventionally treated patients ($p = 0.047$).

Although there are no trials that prospectively compared ICD to conventional treatment separately for patients with a severely reduced ejection fraction and an ejection fraction greater than 35 percent, ICD treatment has become accepted therapy for second-

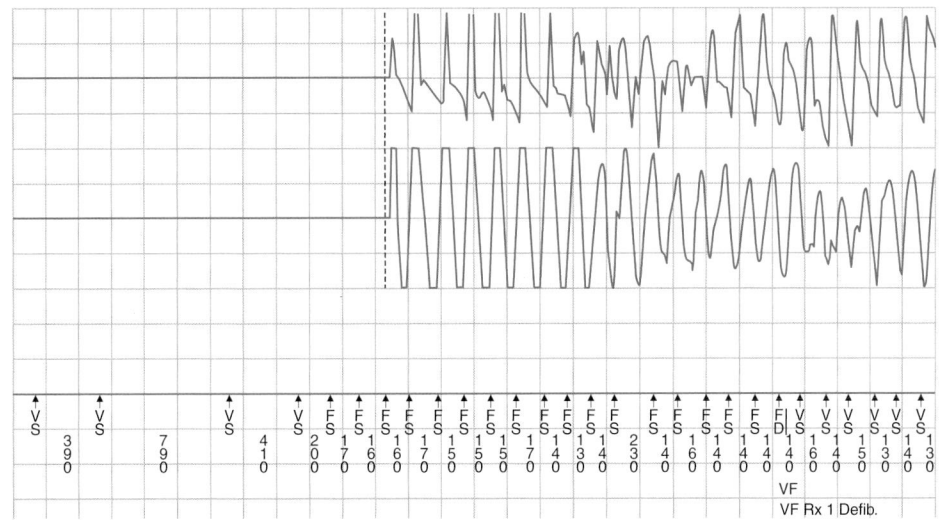

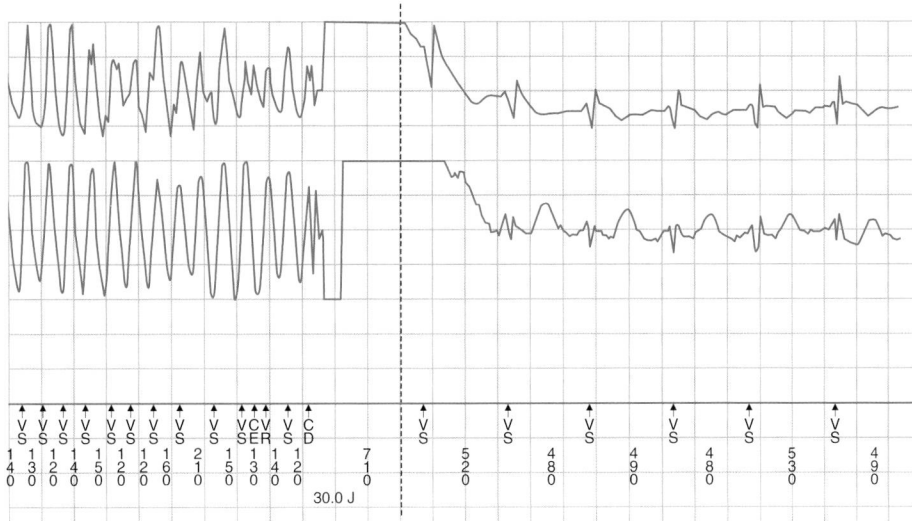

FIGURE 46-3. Stored electrogram of an episode of ventricular fibrillation. After the arrhythmia is initiated and the number of intervals to detect for ventricular fibrillation detection is met, the capacitor starts charging. At the end of charging, a second look at the rhythms is performed to see if the high ventricular rate is still present, and then the shock is delivered and restores normal sinus rhythm. CD, capacitor discharge; CE, charging end; FD, fibrillation detect; FS, fibrillation sense; VS, ventricular sense.

ary prevention of sudden cardiac death irrespective of left ventricular ejection fraction.

The indication for an ICD for secondary prevention is accepted not only for patients with coronary artery disease and idiopathic dilated cardiomyopathy, the two leading underlying structural diseases leading to sudden cardiac death, but also for less-common diseases, such as hypertrophic cardiomyopathy, idiopathic ventricular fibrillation, and arrhythmogenic right ventricular disease.

[ ] ICD FOR PRIMARY PREVENTION

Following the trials on secondary prevention, other trials evaluated the effect of ICD therapy on mortality in patients at a high risk for future sudden cardiac death. The first trials were the MADIT I (Multicenter Automatic Defibrillator Implantation Trial) and the MUSTT (Multicenter Unsustained Tachycardia Trial).[28–31] The MUSTT included patients with an ejection fraction of less than 40 percent, nonsustained VT, and inducible VT or VF by programmed

stimulation. Patients were randomized to receive either an ICD, electrophysiologically guided antiarrhythmic drugs, or no antiarrhythmic treatment.[29] Mortality was reduced significantly in the arm that received either an ICD or an electrophysiologically guided antiarrhythmic drug, but the beneficial effect was limited only to those who received an ICD. Of note, the antiarrhythmic drugs that were used were mainly class I agents.

The MADIT investigated patients with a coronary artery disease, prior myocardial infarction more than 3 weeks prior, nonsustained VT on Holter-ECG and inducible VT, which was not suppressed by procainamide.[28] In this trial, patients were randomized to either an ICD-implantation or conventional treatment. The trial resulted in a significant reduction of mortality in the ICD arm. Furthermore, a high rate of appropriate shocks was documented in this patient population. The main criticism of this trial was the difference in β-blocker treatment between the two groups and the small population size. The MADIT II was designed to assess the effect of ICD treatment in patients with an ejection fraction of less than 30 percent and previous myocardial infarction.[32] A total of 1232 patients were enrolled in a 3:2 ratio to receive an ICD or best medical therapy. The trial was prematurely stopped because of superiority of ICD treatment with a 31 percent risk reduction. The absolute mortality rate in the ICD arm was 14.2 percent versus 19.8 percent in the control group.

The conclusion was that ICD significantly improves survival in coronary artery disease with prior myocardial infarction and severely reduced left ventricular function. Finally, in a post-hoc analysis, it was shown that patients benefit most if they have a QRS duration of greater than 150 milliseconds.

In contrast to the results of trials that included patients with a prior "old" myocardial infarction (MI), the first trial on ICD use in patients with severely reduced left ventricular (LV) function and recent MI (within 1 month) demonstrated that ICD does not improve overall outcome when implanted early after acute MI. The DINAMIT (Defibrillator in Acute Myocardial Infarction Trial) randomized 676 patients with an acute MI, ejection fraction <35 percent and elevated heart rate with a mean RR interval of <750 milliseconds or reduced heart rate variability with a SDANN of <70 milliseconds to receive either an ICD or best medical therapy.[33] Patients received an ICD within 6 to 40 days after acute MI. After 2 years, a higher mortality of nonarrhythmic cause was observed in the ICD group compared to the control arm, although mortality from sudden arrhythmic death was significantly reduced (p =

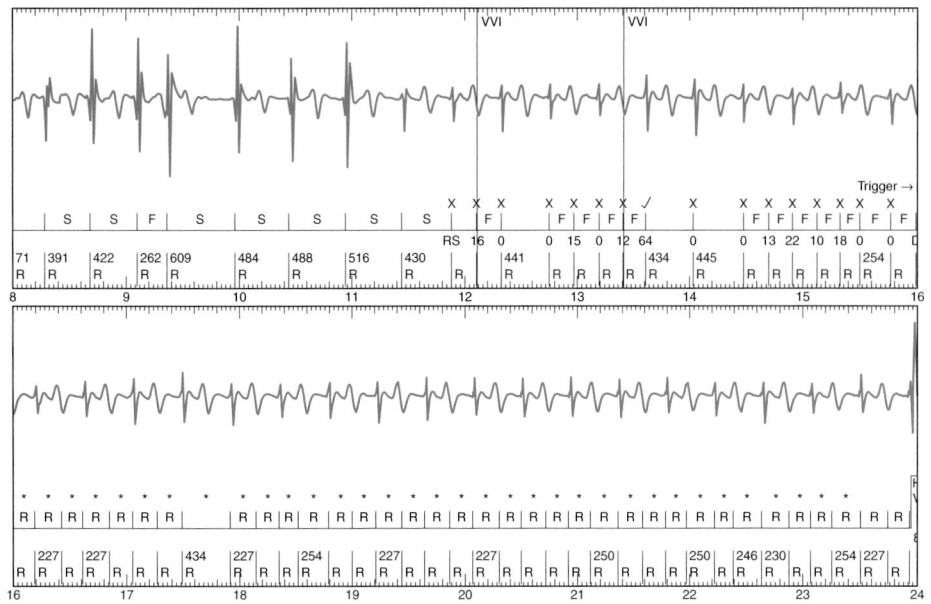

FIGURE 46–4. Stored endocardial electrogram of an episode with intermittent oversensing of T waves in a patient with Brugada syndrome. The additionally sensed T wave results in the false initiation of VT/VF detection. During this period, the cycle length intervals range between 227 and 254 milliseconds, thus imitating a fast ventricular tachycardia. F, fibrillation interval; R, ventricular event; S, sinus interval.

0.009). Consequently, ICD therapy in this clinical setting seems to be of no benefit early after MI.

The second largest group of patients at risk for cardiac arrest suffers from idiopathic nonischemic dilated cardiomyopathy (DCM).

Based on data from the 1980s the first trial designed to assess the effect of ICD therapy on survival in patients with DCM was the Cardiomyopathy Trial (CAT).[34] It was based on the assumption that 1-year mortality in patients with DCM and an ejection fraction of less than 30 percent is approximately 12 percent. Patients with an ejection fraction of less than 30 percent, a recent diagnosis of DCM (<9 months) were randomized to ICD or conventional treatment. Of note, at that time β-blocker treatment was considered contraindicated in severe heart failure. The trial was stopped for futility, because the event rate in both groups was so low that the trial was not powered for the main study hypothesis. Even after 5 years no significant difference in mortality could be found for treatment with an ICD or conventional drug therapy.

Subsequently, two major trials on primary prevention were carried out in patients with nonischemic dilated cardiomyopathy, the AMIOVIRT (Amiodarone Versus Implantable Cardioverter-Defibrillator Trial) and the DEFINITE (Defibrillators in Non-Ischemic Cardiomyopathy Treatment Evaluation) trial.[35,36]

AMIOVIRT randomized patients with an ejection fraction of less than 35 percent and asymptomatic nonsustained VT to ICD therapy or amiodarone treatment.[35] The trial also failed to demonstrate a superiority of the ICD and had a low mortality rate.

The largest trial in patients with idiopathic dilated cardiomyopathy is the DEFINITE trial.[37] In this trial, 458 patients with an idiopathic dilated cardiomyopathy, a left ventricular ejection fraction of less than 35 percent, and premature ventricular contractions or nonsustained VT, were enrolled and randomized to ICD treatment or conventional treatment. There was a strong trend toward a better outcome in patients with an ICD with reduction in total mortality (*p* = 0.08), and a significant reduction

of mortality from arrhythmic death (*p* = 0.006). The mortality rate at 2 years was 14.1 and 7.9 percent in the conventional and the ICD arms, respectively.

Although these trials were not conclusive with regard to the role of ICD in idiopathic cardiomyopathy, the recently published SCD-HeFT (Sudden Cardiac Death in Heart Failure Trial) revealed that in patients with a left ventricular ejection fraction (LVEF) <35 percent and heart failure with New York Heart Association (NYHA) class II or III symptoms, the ICD significantly reduced overall mortality.[38] Interestingly, in this trial the percentage of patients with nonischemic cardiomyopathy was 48 percent. Post-hoc analysis pointed to a better hazard risk ratio in patients with a nonischemic etiology than in patients with an ischemic etiology of heart failure.

[ ] ICD IN PATIENTS WITH SEVERE LEFT VENTRICULAR DYSFUNCTION

In previous trials in secondary prevention, patients with severely reduced left ventricular function benefited most from ICD therapy. Consequently, two major trials investigated the impact of ICD therapy on mortality in patients with severe left ventricular dysfunction and clinical signs of heart failure and in patients with heart failure and increased QRS duration. The SCD-HeFT trial enrolled 2521 patients with an ejection fraction of less than 35 percent and NYHA class II or III congestive heart failure.[38] Patients were randomized to either ICD therapy, best medical therapy, or best medical therapy plus amiodarone. The trial resulted in a significant risk reduction for overall mortality in the ICD arm versus both other treatment modalities. Of note, there was an even higher mortality in the amiodarone arm. In this trial, a shock-only device was implanted, which was programmed to a VF cut-off rate at 187 beats/min and ventricular-inhibited (VVI) pacing at 34 beats/min. ICD therapy was associated with a decreased risk of death of 23 percent (*p* = 0.007). The absolute decrease in mortality was 7.2 percent after 5 years. The COMPANION (Comparison of Medical Therapy, Pacing and Defibrillation in Chronic Heart Failure) trial enrolled patients with NYHA class III or IV congestive heart failure and a QRS duration >120 milliseconds.[39] Patients were randomized to either conventional treatment, a resynchronization pacemaker device, or treatment with an ICD and biventricular pacing. There was a significant difference in risk of the combined end point death or hospitalization for heart failure when comparing patients with conventional therapy to patients who received a biventricular ICD (*p* < 0.001). Risk reduction was 40 percent comparing the pacemaker-ICD arm to conventional therapy.

The results are in line with the observation of the MADIT II, where post-hoc analysis revealed a greater benefit for patients with a severely reduced LV function and a QRS duration longer than 150 milliseconds (Tables 46–1 and 46–2).[32]

TABLE 46–1

Trials on Primary and Secondary Prevention of Sudden Death

STUDY	INCLUSION CRITERIA	MAIN END POINTS	CONTROL TREATMENT	NO. OF PATIENTS	MAIN RESULTS
Secondary prevention					
AVID[24]	Cardiac arrest survivors	Total mortality	Amiodarone or sotalol	1016	Significant improvement in overall survival in the ICD treatment arm
	Syncopal VT	Mode of death			
	Symptomatic sustained VT and LVEF ≤40%				
CIDS[23]	Cardiac arrest survivors	Total mortality	Amiodarone	659	No significant improvement of survival in the ICD treatment arm
	Syncope with symptomatic sustained VT, LVEF ≤35% or inducible VT and syncope				
CASH[40]	Cardiac arrest survivors	Total mortality	Amiodarone or metoprolol, propafenone	288	Significant improvement in overall survival in the ICD treatment arm
Primary prevention in CAD					
MADIT I[25]	Q-wave MI, asymptomatic NSVT	Total mortality	Conventional	196	Significant improvement in overall survival in the ICD treatment arm
	LVEF ≤35% Inducible and nonsuppressible VT with procainamide				
MADIT II[27]	Prior myocardial infarction, LVEF ≤30%	Total mortality	Conventional	1232	Significant improvement in overall survival in the ICD treatment arm
CABG-Patch[41]	CABG surgery	Total mortality	No ICD	900	No significant improvement of survival in the ICD treatment arm
	LVEF ≤35% Abnormal SAECG				
MUSTT[26]	Coronary artery disease	Sudden arrhythmic death or spontaneous sustained VT	Conventional	2202	>70% reduction of risk of arrhythmic death or cardiac arrest
	LVEF ≤40%				>50% reduction in overall mortality
	Nonsustained VT Inducible VT/VF				
DINAMIT[28]	Acute MI (6–40 days)	Total mortality	Conventional	674	No significant difference in overall survival between ICD and control arm
	LVEF ≤35% Heart rate >80 beats/min				

(continued)

TABLE 46–1

Trials on Primary and Secondary Prevention of Sudden Death *(continued)*

STUDY	INCLUSION CRITERIA	MAIN END POINTS	CONTROL TREATMENT	NO. OF PATIENTS	MAIN RESULTS
Primary prevention in IDC					
CAT[29]	Nonischemic dilated cardiomyopathy	Total mortality	Conventional	104	No significant difference in mortality between ICD and control arm
	NYHA class II or III	Sudden death			
	LVEF ≤30%				
AMIOVIRT[30]	Nonischemic dilated cardiomyopathy	Total mortality	Amiodarone	103	No significant difference in mortality between ICD and control arm
	Nonsustained VT LVEF ≤35%				
DEFINITE[31]	Nonischemic cardiomyopathy	Total mortality	Conventional	450	No significant difference in overall mortality (*p* = 0.08) Significant risk reduction of arrhythmic death in the ICD arm
	Nonsustained VT				
	LVEF ≤35%				
Primary prevention in severe left ventricular dysfunction					
SCD-HeFT[33]	Ischemic or nonischemic cardiomyopathy	Total mortality	Conventional	2521	Significant risk reduction in overall mortality in ICD treatment arm
	NYHA class II or III LVEF ≤35%		Amiodarone		
COMPANION[34]	NYHA classes II–IV LVEF ≤35%	Total mortality Hospitalization	Conventional Biventricular pacemaker	1520	Significant risk reduction in mortality and hospitalization for heart failure in patients treated with biventricular ICD vs. conventional treatment
	QRS >120 msec PR >150 msec No conventional indication for pacemaker or ICD				

AMIOVIRT, Amiodarone Versus Implantable Cardioverter defibrillator Trial; AVID, The Antiarrhythmics versus Implantable Defibrillators; CABG, coronary artery bypass grafting; CABG-Patch, coronary artery bypass grafting-patch; CAD, coronary artery disease; CASH, Cardiac Arrest Study Hamburg; CAT, Cardiomyopathy Trial; CIDS, Canadian Implantable Defibrillator Study; COMPANION, Comparison of Medical Therapy, Pacing and Defibrillation in Chronic Heart Failure Trial; DEFINITE, Defibrillators in Non-Ischemic Cardiomyopathy Treatment Evaluation; DINAMIT, Defibrillator in Acute Myocardial Infarction Trial; IDC, idiopathic dilated cardiomyopathy; LVEF, left ventricular ejection fraction; MADIT, Multicenter Automatic Defibrillator Implantation Trial; MI, myocardial infarction; MUSTT, Multicenter Unsustained Tachycardia Trial; NYHA, New York Heart Association; SCD-HeFT, Sudden Cardiac Death in Heart Failure Trial; VF, ventricular fibrillation; VT, ventricular tachycardia.

ICD IN OTHER CLINICAL SETTINGS

❬ ❭ HYPERTROPHIC CARDIOMYOPATHY

The annual risk of sudden death in hypertrophic cardiomyopathy is approximately 1 to 3 percent in the overall population and approximately 6 percent in younger patients.[42–44] There is no clear role for implantable cardioverter-defibrillator therapy for primary prevention, because risk stratification in this patient population is difficult. The risk of future sudden death seems to be elevated for patients with syncope, nonsustained VT, or a wall thickness of >30 mm. Programmed ventricular stimulation for risk assessment does not play a role in hypertrophic cardiomyopathy.

TABLE 46–2

ACC/AHA/ESC Guidelines for Management of Patients with Ventricular Arrhythmias and the Prevention of Sudden Cardiac Death 2006

UPDATED INDICATIONS FOR ICD IMPLANTATION

Chronic Ischemic Heart Disease
Class I
- Ischemic heart disease, ≥40 days post MI, LVEF ≤30% to 40%, NYHA functional class II or III, life expectancy >1 year
- Hemodynamically unstable sustained VT

Class IIa
- Ischemic cardiomyopathy, ≥40 days post-MI, LVEF ≤30% to 40%, NYHA functional class I, life expectancy >1 year

Nonischemic Dilated Cardiomyopathy
Class I
- Patients with sustained VT or VF
- Nonischemic dilated cardiomyopathy, LVEF ≤30% to 35%, NYHA functional class II or III, life expectancy >1 year

Class IIa
- Nonischemic dilated cardiomyopathy, significant LV dysfunction, and unexplained syncope

Class IIb
- Nonischemic dilated cardiomyopathy, LVEF ≤30% to 35%, NYHA functional class I, life expectancy >1 year

LVEF, left ventricular ejection fraction; MI, myocardial infarction; NYHA, New York Heart Association; VF, ventricular fibrillation; VT, ventricular tachycardia.
Source: Adapted from the ACC/AHA/ESC Guidelines for management of patients with ventricular arrhythmias and the prevention of sudden cardiac death 2006.[66]

ICD implantation is indicated in patients with sustained monomorphic VT or aborted sudden death. The annual rate of appropriate ICD therapy in patients who received an ICD for secondary prevention is high enough to accept ICD therapy for these patients. Regarding primary prevention, there are only sparse data on ICD therapy rates after implantation. Because inappropriate therapy for atrial fibrillation is of general concern in ICD patients, it is very important to program devices in hypertrophic cardiomyopathy specifically to avoid inappropriate discharge, because the risk of atrial fibrillation in these patients is high. Furthermore, T-wave oversensing may be an issue in these patients. In patients where right ventricular pacing is able to reduce the intraventricular gradient, selection of a dual-chamber device may be considered in individual cases.

ARRHYTHMOGENIC RIGHT VENTRICULAR CARDIOMYOPATHY

A subgroup of patients with a right ventricular cardiomyopathy is at an increased risk of sustained monomorphic VT and sudden death. These patients may need an implantable defibrillator to treat VT and VF and thereby reduce the risk from sudden death.[45] To date, there is no clear role for ICD in primary prevention in arrhythmogenic right ventricular cardiomyopathy and the treatment is mainly used in patients with sustained hemodynamically nontoler-

ated VT and/or syncope and inducible VT/VF. In advanced stages of arrhythmogenic right ventricular cardiomyopathy with a severely enlarged right ventricle, problems with placement of the right ventricular leads are frequently encountered, because local fibrofatty displacement of myocardial tissue results in deterioration of intracardiac signal quality and high stimulation thresholds. This may also occur during later followup as a consequence of disease progression. Special care should be taken when implanting the lead in aneurysmal-altered regions of the heart to avoid lead perforation.

CHANNELOPATHIES AND CONGENITAL ARRHYTHMIC DISORDERS

With increasing knowledge in the field of genetics and molecular mechanisms in patients with malignant ventricular tachyarrhythmias, an increasing number of patients with so-called *idiopathic ventricular tachycardia* or fibrillation are being diagnosed with specific entities such as new forms of long QT syndrome, Brugada syndrome, the short QT syndrome and catecholaminergic polymorphic ventricular tachycardia (CPVT).[46–49]

In these patients ICDs are inserted when patients survive an episode of aborted sudden cardiac death or sustained monomorphic or polymorphic VT, which cannot be controlled by antiarrhythmic drugs, as in CPVT or long QT syndrome.

ICD therapy is effective in reducing mortality in high risk patients with a long QT syndrome.[50–52] An ICD is generally indicated for patients with aborted sudden death, recurrent torsade de pointes tachycardia despite β-blocker therapy or pacemaker therapy in long QT syndrome, or aborted sudden death or recurrent polymorphic VT despite β-blocker treatment in CPVT. The current guidelines also provide a class II indication for ICD treatment in these diseases, when familial sudden death is present in younger relatives with the disease.[6]

The role of ICD therapy in secondary prevention of sudden death in Brugada syndrome is established, but there is debate on its role in primary prevention. The Second Brugada Consensus Conference gives some recommendations on the use of ICDs based on the restricted current knowledge on the event rates and risk factors.[49,53]

Because ICD implantation in these rare diseases is performed in younger patients and sometimes in children, special emphasis on detection algorithms is warranted to avoid inappropriate ICD discharge. Further psychological support should be provided in these patients to improve quality of life and address age-related psychological issues.

In short QT syndrome, a recently discovered new form of channelopathy, ICD therapy may be recommended in patients with previous syncope and/or familial sudden death. However, there have been only relatively few cases identified, so that there are no conclusive data. When ICD therapy is used, special attention should be given to the problem of T-wave oversensing, which can be suppressed by reprogramming the sensing parameters in most of the cases.[54]

COMPLICATIONS OF ICD THERAPY

LEAD DYSFUNCTION, INFECTION, IMPLANTATION

Implantation has an intra- and perioperative risk of approximately 1 to 3 percent, including a death rate of ≤1 percent, perforation and cardiac tamponade of ≤1 percent, and acute lead dysfunction.[55-57] During followup, the most feared complication is lead or pocket infection, which generally requires the removal of the complete system. It is reported to occur in 1 to 2 percent of patients. The most frequently found organism is *Staphylococcus aureus*. Infection risk seems to be a little higher at time of battery or lead replacement than at the initial implantation.[54]

Lead dislodgment can occur shortly after implantation or at any time during followup. In patients in whom the lead is completely dislodged, monitoring and timely removal of the lead is mandatory to avoid mechanically induced arrhythmias.

Lead dysfunction from insulation breakage or insulation erosion is most frequently preceded by inappropriate ICD therapy caused by electrical noise on the rate electrogram. It usually displays high, frequent, irregular signals with pseudo-RR intervals at the resolution boundary of the device. Some newer devices provide a counter for these specific signals to detect the problems early and avoid inappropriate discharges.[58] Sometimes, the electrical noise is not found during real-time recording at rest and can only be provoked by specific maneuvers. Breakage or partial disruption of the lead are most commonly detected by a change in the signal amplitude, a rise in pacing thresholds, and an increase in lead impedance. Other potential reasons for lead dysfunction may be a loose connection of the lead at the header or the so-called *subclavian crush syndrome*, where there is a breakage as a result of compression of the lead at the first rib.

INAPPROPRIATE ICD THERAPIES AND ELECTRICAL STORM

The most frequent complication of ICD therapy is inappropriate ICD therapy. The vast majority of inappropriate shocks or antitachycardia pacing attempts are caused by atrial tachyarrhythmias with rapid ventricular response and sinus tachycardia. They occur in up to 30 percent of patients with single-chamber ICDs.[59] Apart from adding antiarrhythmic drugs, many of the inappropriate therapies can be avoided by reprogramming the device by changing detection boundaries or activating enhanced detection criteria. Although sinus tachycardia can be better distinguished from VT by activating the sudden-onset criterion, discrimination of ventricular tachycardia from atrial fibrillation may require using QRS width or morphology criteria. In dual-chamber devices, additional criteria can be programmed to include the rate information from the atrial lead.

Another potential cause for inappropriate ICD therapy is T-wave oversensing. In most devices, this problem can be eliminated by decreasing the ventricular sensitivity level. In this case, proper reliable detection of ventricular fibrillation should be tested at the altered sensitivity level.

In dual-chamber devices with integrated atrial antitachycardia therapies, R-wave oversensing in the atrial channel may lead to false detection of atrial flutter during sinus tachycardia. In this case, the atrial sensitivity level may be decreased and continuous atrial sensing be ensured thereafter.

A serious clinical problem is the occurrence of electrical storm, which is defined as repetitive ventricular tachycardia or fibrillation with recurrent ICD therapies within 24 hours or a few days (Fig. 46–5). It has been reported to occur in up to 25 percent of all ICD recipients.[41,60,61] When acute ischemia is excluded as a trigger for these frequent VT/VF, the use of β blockers, class III drugs, sedation and/or narcosis, and catheter ablation for treatment of VT are effective.

Electrical proarrhythmia induced by the ICD can be caused by inappropriate antitachycardia pacing, low-energy cardioversion or shocks into supraventricular rhythms. Another cause is asynchronous pacing caused by sensing failure.

PSYCHOSOCIAL ISSUES

In the early days of implantable defibrillator therapy, the device was considered lifesaving. With the increasing ease of implantation and the growing number of patients who receive the device for primary prevention, and who, therefore, have no history of recurrent syncope or resuscitation, perception of the device may be altered and it is sometimes perceived as an intrusive therapy.

Although prospective data on quality of life demonstrate a good quality of life for the majority of patients, appropriate or inappropriate shocks have a significant impact on the quality of life. Psychological support groups may be helpful for patients with either uncontrolled fears or a history of repetitive shocks that have caused anxiety or depression.[62,63]

DRIVING AND THE ICD

There are no generally applicable driving guidelines and legislation varies widely internationally. Physicians often ask their patients not to drive for at last 6 months after ICD implantation secondary prevention. During this period, spontaneous ventricular tachyarrhythmias and their response to ICD therapy, as well as the symptoms associated with the VT/VF episodes, can be assessed. For primary prevention, there currently is no overall recommendation. How-

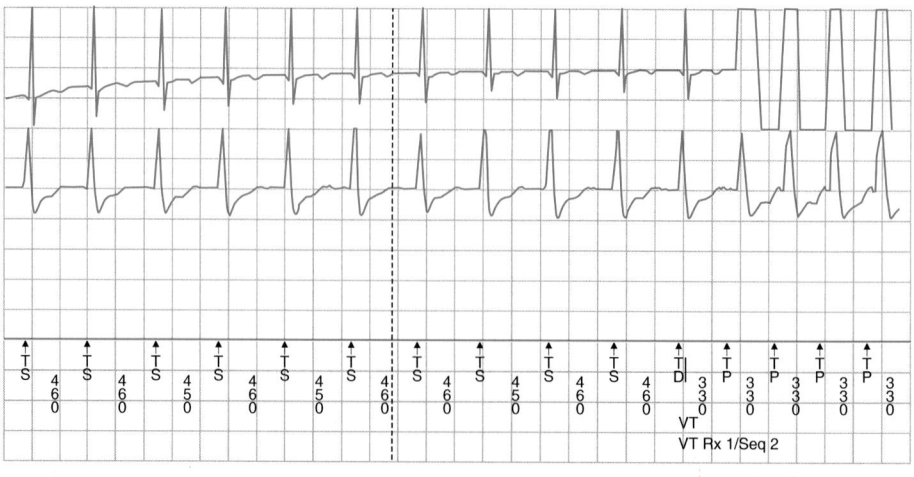

FIGURE 46–5. This stored endocardial electrogram strip displays in the *upper tracing* a near-field, and in the *lower tracing* a far-field, electrogram during a ventricular tachycardia.

ever, because the number of patients with an ICD for primary pro-phylaxis is growing, this issue must be addressed in the future. In the existing literature, there are no data available that shows an in-creased risk of car accidents in ICD recipients compared with the general population.[64,65]

REFERENCES

1. Hoffmann T, Zacouto F. On the mechanism of heart arrest and its elimina-tion by controlled electrical stimulation.. *Langenbecks Arch Klin Chir Ver Dtsch Z Chir* 1961;298:762–765.

2. Mirowski M, Reid PR, Mower MM, et al. Termination of malignant ventric-ular arrhythmias with an implanted automatic defibrillator in human beings. *N Engl J Med.* 1980;303:322–324.

3. Luderitz B, Gerckens U, Manz M. Automatic implantable cardioverter/defibrilla-tor (AICD) and antitachycardia pacemaker (Tachylog): combined use in ventric-ular tachyarrhythmias. *Pacing Clin Electrophysiol* 1986;9:1356–1360.

4. Block M, Hammel D, Borggrefe M, et al. Initial clinical experiences with a transvenous-subcutaneous defibrillation system. *Z Kardiol* 1991;80:657–664.

5. Le Franc P, Klug D, Lacroix D, et al. Triple chamber pacemaker for end-stage heart failure in a patient with a previously implanted automatic defibrillator. *Pacing Clin Electrophysiol* 1998;21:1672–1675.

6. Gregoratos G, Abrams J, Epstein AE, et al. ACC/AHA/NASPE 2002 guideline update for implantation of cardiac pacemakers and antiarrhythmia devices: sum-mary article: a report of the American College of Cardiology/American Heart Association Task Force on Practice Guidelines (ACC/AHA/NASPE Committee to Update the 1998 Pacemaker Guidelines). *Circulation* 2002;106:2145–2161.

7. Priori SG, Aliot E, Blomstrom-Lundqvist C, et al. [Task Force on Sudden Cardiac Death, European Society of Cardiology. Summary of recommenda-tions.] *Ital Heart J Suppl* 2002;3:1051–1065.

8. Hurwitz JL, Hook BG, Flores BT, et al. Importance of abortive shock capa-bility with electrogram storage in cardioverter-defibrillator devices. *J Am Coll Cardiol* 1993;21:895–900.

9. Bansch D, Steffgen F, Gronefeld G, et al. The 1+1 trial: a prospective trial of a dual- versus a single-chamber implantable defibrillator in patients with slow ventricular tachycardias. *Circulation* 2004;110:1022–1029.

10. Friedman PA, McClelland RL, Bamlet WR, et al. Dual-chamber versus sin-gle-chamber detection enhancements for implantable defibrillator rhythm diagnosis: the detect supraventricular tachycardia study. *Circulation* 2006;113:2871–2879.

11. Fromer M, Brachmann J, Block M, et al. Efficacy of automatic multimodal device therapy for ventricular tachyarrhythmias as delivered by a new implantable pacing cardioverter-defibrillator. Results of a European multi-center study of 102 implants. *Circulation* 1992;86:363–374.

12. Almendral J, Arenal A, Villacastin JP, et al. The importance of antitachycar-dia pacing for patients presenting with ventricular tachycardia. *Pacing Clin Electrophysiol* 1993;16:535–539.

13. Jimenez-Candil J, Arenal A, Garcia-Alberola A, et al. Fast ventricular tachy-cardias in patients with implantable cardioverter-defibrillators: efficacy and safety of antitachycardia pacing. A prospective and randomized study. *J Am Coll Cardiol* 2005;45:460–461.

14. Schaumann A, von zur Muhlen F, Herse B, et al. Empirical versus tested anti-tachycardia pacing in implantable cardioverter defibrillators: a prospective study including 200 patients. *Circulation* 1998;97:66–74.

15. Wathen MS, Sweeney MO, DeGroot PJ, et al. Shock reduction using anti-tachycardia pacing for spontaneous rapid ventricular tachycardia in patients with coronary artery disease. *Circulation* 2001;104:796–801.

16. Wathen MS, DeGroot PJ, Sweeney MO, et al. Prospective randomized mul-ticenter trial of empirical antitachycardia pacing versus shocks for spontane-ous rapid ventricular tachycardia in patients with implantable cardioverter-defibrillators: Pacing Fast Ventricular Tachycardia Reduces Shock Therapies (PainFREE Rx II) trial results. *Circulation* 2004;110:2591–2596.

17. Grimm W, Flores BF, Marchlinski FE. Symptoms and electrocardiographi-cally documented rhythm preceding spontaneous shocks in patients with implantable cardioverter-defibrillator. *Am J Cardiol* 1993;71:1415–1418.

18. Duru F, Luechinger R, Scharf C, et al. Automatic impedance monitoring and patient alert feature in implantable cardioverter defibrillators: being alert for the unexpected! *J Cardiovasc Electrophysiol* 2005;16:444–448.

19. Brunn J, Bocker D, Weber M, et al. Is there a need for routine testing of ICD defibrillation capacity? Results from more than 1000 studies. *Eur Heart J* 2000;21:162–169.

20. Pacifico A, Wheelan KR, Nasir N, Jr, et al. Long-term follow-up of cardio-verter-defibrillator implanted under conscious sedation in prepectoral subfas-cial position. *Circulation* 1997;95:946–950.

21. Winter J, Zimmermann N, Lidolt H, et al. Optimal method to achieve con-sistently low defibrillation energy requirements. *Am J Cardiol* 2000;86:71K–75K.

22. Bardy GH, Dolack GL, Kudenchuk PJ, et al. Prospective, randomized com-parison in humans of a unipolar defibrillation system with that using an additional superior vena cava electrode. *Circulation* 1994;89:1090–1093.

23. Bansch D, Castrucci M, Bocker D, et al. Ventricular tachycardias above the initially programmed tachycardia detection interval in patients with implant-able cardioverter-defibrillators: incidence, prediction and significance. *J Am Coll Cardiol* 2000;36:557–565.

24. Sadoul N, Mletzko R, Anselme F, et al. Incidence and clinical relevance of slow ventricular tachycardia in implantable cardioverter-defibrillator recipi-ents: an international multicenter prospective study. *Circulation* 2005;112:946–953.

25. Kuck KH, Cappato R, Siebels J, et al. Randomized comparison of antiar-rhythmic drug therapy with implantable defibrillators in patients resuscitated from cardiac arrest: the Cardiac Arrest Study Hamburg (CASH). *Circulation* 2000;102:748–754.

26. Connolly SJ, Gent M, Roberts RS, et al. Canadian implantable defibrillator study (CIDS): a randomized trial of the implantable cardioverter defibrillator against amiodarone. *Circulation* 2000;101:1297–1302.

27. A comparison of antiarrhythmic-drug therapy with implantable defibrillators in patients resuscitated from near-fatal ventricular arrhythmias. The Antiar-rhythmics versus Implantable Defibrillators (AVID) Investigators. *N Engl J Med* 1997;337:1576–1583.

28. Moss AJ, Hall WJ, Cannom DS, et al. Improved survival with an implanted defibrillator in patients with coronary disease at high risk for ventricular arrhythmia. Multicenter Automatic Defibrillator Implantation Trial Investi-gators. *N Engl J Med* 1996;335:1933–1940.

29. Buxton AE, Fisher JD, Josephson ME, et al. Prevention of sudden death in patients with coronary artery disease: the Multicenter Unsustained Tachycar-dia Trial (MUSTT). *Prog Cardiovasc Dis* 1993;36:215–226.

30. The CABG Patch Trial Investigators and Coordinators. The Coronary Artery Bypass Graft (CABG) Patch Trial. *Prog Cardiovasc Dis* 1993;36:97–114.

31. Bigger JT Jr. Prophylactic use of implanted cardiac defibrillators in patients at high risk for ventricular arrhythmias after coronary-artery bypass graft sur-gery. Coronary Artery Bypass Graft (CABG) Patch Trial Investigators. *N Engl J Med* 1997;337:1569–1575.

32. Moss AJ, Zareba W, Hall WJ, et al. Prophylactic implantation of a defibrilla-tor in patients with myocardial infarction and reduced ejection fraction. *N Engl J Med* 2002;346:877–883.

33. Hohnloser SH, Kuck KH, Dorian P, et al. Prophylactic use of an implantable cardioverter-defibrillator after acute myocardial infarction. *N Engl J Med* 2004;351:2481–2488.

34. Bansch D, Antz M, Boczor S, et al. Primary prevention of sudden cardiac death in idiopathic dilated cardiomyopathy: the Cardiomyopathy Trial (CAT). *Circulation* 2002;105:1453–1458.

35. Strickberger SA, Hummel JD, Bartlett TG, et al. Amiodarone versus implantable cardioverter-defibrillator: randomized trial in patients with nonischemic dilated cardiomyopathy and asymptomatic nonsustained ven-tricular tachycardia—AMIOVIRT. *J Am Coll Cardiol* 2003;41:1707–1712.

36. Kadish A, Dyer A, Daubert JP, et al. Prophylactic defibrillator implantation in patients with nonischemic dilated cardiomyopathy. *N Engl J Med* 2004;350:2151–2158.

37. Kadish A, Quigg R, Schaechter A, Anderson KP, Estes M, Levine J. Defibril-lators in nonischemic cardiomyopathy treatment evaluation. *Pacing Clin Electrophysiol*, 2000;23:338–343.

38. Bardy GH, Lee KL, Mark DB, et al. Amiodarone or an implantable cardio-verter-defibrillator for congestive heart failure. *N Engl J Med* 2005;352:225–237.

39. Bristow MR, Saxon LA, Boehmer J, et al. Cardiac-resynchronization therapy with or without an implantable defibrillator in advanced chronic heart fail-ure. *N Engl J Med* 2004;350:2140–2150.

40. Knuefermann P, Wolpert C, Spehl S, et al. [Implantable cardioverter/defibril-lator: long-term stability of the defibrillation threshold with a unipolar elec-trode configuration ("active-can").] *Z Kardiol* 2000;89:774–780.

41. Credner SC, Klingenheben T, Mauss O, et al. Electrical storm in patients with transvenous implantable cardioverter-defibrillators: incidence, man-agement and prognostic implications. *J Am Coll Cardiol* 1998;32:1909–1915.

42. Maron BJ, Shen WK, Link MS, et al. Efficacy of implantable cardioverter-defibrillators for the prevention of sudden death in patients with hypertrophic cardiomyopathy. *N Engl J Med* 2000;342:365–373.

43. Maron BJ. Hypertrophic cardiomyopathy: a systematic review. *JAMA* 2002;287:1308–1320.

44. Maron BJ, McKenna WJ, Elliott P, et al. Hypertrophic cardiomyopathy. *JAMA* 1999;282:2302–2303.

45. Corrado D, Leoni L, Link MS, et al. Implantable cardioverter-defibrillator therapy for prevention of sudden death in patients with arrhythmogenic right ventricular cardiomyopathy/dysplasia. *Circulation* 2003;108:3084–3091.

46. Priori SG, Napolitano C, Memmi M, et al. Clinical and molecular characterization of patients with catecholaminergic polymorphic ventricular tachycardia. *Circulation* 2002;106:69–74.

47. Gaita F, Giustetto C, Bianchi F, et al. Short QT syndrome: pharmacological treatment. *J Am Coll Cardiol* 2004;43:1494–1499.

48. Wolpert C, Schimpf R, Veltmann C, et al. Clinical characteristics and treatment of short QT syndrome. *Expert Rev Cardiovasc Ther* 2005;3:611–617.

49. Antzelevitch C, Brugada P, Borggrefe M, et al. Brugada syndrome: report of the second consensus conference. *Heart Rhythm* 2005;2:429–440.

50. Zareba W, Moss AJ, Daubert JP, et al. Implantable cardioverter defibrillator in high-risk long QT syndrome patients. *J Cardiovasc Electrophysiol* 2003;14:337–341.

51. Priori SG, Aliot E, Blomstrom-Lundqvist C, et al. Task Force on Sudden Cardiac Death of the European Society of Cardiology. *Eur Heart J* 2001;22:1374–1450.

52. Priori SG, Schwartz PJ, Napolitano C, et al. Risk stratification in the long-QT syndrome. *N Engl J Med* 2003;348:1866–1874.

53. Brugada J, Brugada R, Brugada P. Determinants of sudden cardiac death in individuals with the electrocardiographic pattern of Brugada syndrome and no previous cardiac arrest. *Circulation* 2003;108:3092–3096.

54. Chambers ST. Diagnosis and management of staphylococcal infections of pacemakers and cardiac defibrillators. *Intern Med J* 2005;35(Suppl 2):S63–S71.

55. Alter P, Waldhans S, Plachta E, et al. Complications of implantable cardioverter defibrillator therapy in 440 consecutive patients. *Pacing Clin Electrophysiol* 2005;28:926–932.

56. Hauser RG, Cannom D, Hayes DL, et al. Long-term structural failure of coaxial polyurethane implantable cardioverter defibrillator leads. *Pacing Clin Electrophysiol* 2002;25:879–882.

57. Hauser RG, Hayes DL, Epstein AE, et al. Multicenter experience with failed and recalled implantable cardioverter-defibrillator pulse generators. *Heart Rhythm* 2006;3:640–644.

58. Auer J, Berent R, Eber B. Patient alert and cardiac defibrillators. *J Am Coll Cardiol* 2005;45:966; author reply 966.

59. Dorian P, Philippon F, Thibault B, et al. Randomized controlled study of detection enhancements versus rate-only detection to prevent inappropriate therapy in a dual-chamber implantable cardioverter-defibrillator. *Heart Rhythm* 2004;1:540–547.

60. Arya A, Haghjoo M, Dehghani MR, et al. Prevalence and predictors of electrical storm in patients with implantable cardioverter-defibrillator. *Am J Cardiol* 2006;97:389–392.

61. Exner DV, Pinski SL, Wyse DG, et al. Electrical storm presages nonsudden death: the antiarrhythmics versus implantable defibrillators (AVID) trial. *Circulation* 2001;103:2066–2071.

62. Luderitz B, Jung W, Deister A, et al. Patient acceptance of the implantable cardioverter defibrillator in ventricular tachyarrhythmias. *Pacing Clin Electrophysiol* 1993;16:1815–1821.

63. Sweeney MO, Wathen MS, Volosin K, et al. Appropriate and inappropriate ventricular therapies, quality of life, and mortality among primary and secondary prevention implantable cardioverter defibrillator patients: results from the Pacing Fast VT REduces Shock ThErapies (PainFREE Rx II) trial. *Circulation* 2006;111:2898–2905.

64. Jung W, Luderitz B. European policy on driving for patients with implantable cardioverter defibrillators. *Pacing Clin Electrophysiol* 1996;19:981–984.

65. Trappe HJ, Wenzlaff P, Grellman G. Should patients with implantable cardioverter-defibrillators be allowed to drive? Observations in 291 patients from a single center over an 11-year period. *J Interv Card Electrophysiol* 1998;2:193–201.

66. Zipes DP, Camm AJ, Borggrefe M, et al. ACC/AHA/ESC 2006 guidelines for management of patients with ventricular arrhythmias and the prevention of sudden cardiac death: a report of the American College of Cardiology/American Heart Association Task Force and the European Society of Cardiology Committee for Practice Guidelines (Writing Committee to Develop Guidelines for Management of Patients With Ventricular Arrhythmias and the Prevention of Sudden Cardiac Death). *Circulation* 2006;114:e385–e484.

CHAPTER 47

Pediatric Arrhythmias

Ronald J. Kanter / Timothy Knilans

The physiology, natural history, and treatment options of arrhythmias in the fetus, infant, child, and teenager are influenced by developmental changes in cardiac dimensions and hemodynamics, pharmacokinetics and pharmacodynamics of antiarrhythmic drugs, and specific electrophysiologic features of the maturing heart. Furthermore, a growing understanding of the developmental changes in myocyte ion channels, intercellular connections, and autonomic nervous system influences is helping to unravel our knowledge of the gross changes that occur during maturation. Finally, cardiac arrhythmias in the young are relatively more likely to be related to structural congenital heart disease, compared with arrhythmias in adults.

This chapter focuses on arrhythmia substrates in patients having congenital heart disease, arrhythmias exclusive to the pediatric age range, and pharmacologic and nonpharmacologic treatment of these arrhythmias in children.

clearly is derived from specialized tissue in the intersegmental zones of the primitive heart tube. Currently, the favored concept involves a single ring of tissue that arises in the primary junction between the primitive ventricle and the bulbus cordis, and that stains with antibodies to chicken ganglion nodosum (Fig. 47–1). As the rightward portion of the primitive atrium forms a connection with the bulbus cordis, and the outflow tracts form and septate, a portion of this encircling ring of specialized conduction tissue is carried rightward and superiorly to create relationships with the right atrioventricular (AV) ring and the aortic valve annulus. Normally, the majority of this tissue involutes, leaving only those portions associated with the lower interatrial septum, the central fibrous body, and the crest of the muscular septum to become the compact AV node and the penetrating bundle. Reports of dissections of the specialized conduction systems from malformed hearts have proved complementary and have resulted in the accurate prediction of the anatomy of the conduction system in many forms of complex congenital heart disease.

CONGENITAL ABNORMALITIES OF THE SPECIALIZED CONDUCTION SYSTEM

Although there is not yet consensus regarding the precise embryogenesis of the specialized conduction system in the human heart, it

LEVOTRANSPOSITION OF THE GREAT ARTERIES

In levotransposition of the great arteries (l-TGA), also known as *congenitally corrected transposition*, there are both AV and ven-

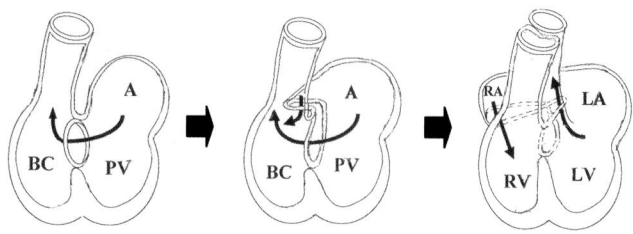

FIGURE 47–1. The prevailing model of development of the specialized cardiac condition system in the human supports the concept that the specialized AV conduction system develops only from a ring of tissue encircling the primary interventricular junction. This tissue persists into the rightward expansion of the atrioventricular junction (*middle* and *right*) and accounts for the entire AV node and penetrating bundle. A, atrial mass; BC, bulbus cordis; LA, left atrium; LV, left ventricle; PV, primitive ventricle; RA, right atrium.

triculoarterial discordance. Therefore, systemic venous return enters the pulmonary arteries, and pulmonary venous return is directed to the aorta, as they should. The majority have associated structural defects, most commonly ventricular septal defect (VSD) and/or pulmonic stenosis. The specialized AV conduction system is also structurally different, usually giving a QS or qR pattern in V_1 and an rS or RS pattern in V_6 on a standard electrocardiogram (ECG; Fig. 47–2). In most patients having situs solitus and l-TGA, the AV node is located anteriorly in the right atrium near the mitral–pulmonary junction. The His bundle is relatively elongated as it crosses anterior to the pulmonary valve annulus before bifurcating on the anterior ventricular septum. When a VSD is also present, the His bundle borders the anterosuperior quadrant of the defect. A second, hypoplastic posterior AV node may also be present just anterior to the coronary sinus. Rarely, it also connects with the ventricular mass via a separate posterior penetrating bundle, or to the anterior AV node via a sling of conduction tissue (so-called *Mönckeberg sling*). Congenitally corrected transposition may also exist in the presence of situs inversus. In such cases, the AV node is usually located in a normal location at the apex of the triangle of Koch, especially if there is accompanying pulmonic stenosis or atresia.[1] As in most complex congenital heart defects, the location of the specialized AV conduction system appears to be dictated by the alignment of the inlet portion of the ventricular septum with the annulus fibrosus.

Pathologic series of heart specimens having l-TGA demonstrate that the elongated penetrating bundle is either infiltrated with fibrous tissue or is completely disrupted. Data analysis shows an approximately 2 percent per year risk of developing AV block after diagnosis. It is generally recommended that prophylactic pacemaker placement is not necessary in children, if their heart rates were greater than 50 beats/min. In patients also having a VSD requiring surgical closure, the risk of intraoperative AV block is higher than it is in patients not having l-TGA. Special surgical handling of the superior portion of the defect is required to avoid this complication. In such cases, if AV block is avoided, the risk of late AV block is not increased. Atrioventricular block is congenital in 3.7 to 18.2 percent of infants having l-TGA,[2-4] and seems to be more prevalent in those having intact ventricular septum than in those also having a VSD.[4]

Patients having l-TGA have a higher-than-expected incidence of paroxysmal supraventricular tachycardia (PSVT), usually, atrioventricular reciprocating tachycardia (AVRT), using one or more accessory AV connections associated with the left-sided tricuspid valve. As a separate concern, because patients with l-TGA have a high incidence of structural tricuspid valve (systemic AV valve) abnormalities, atrial fibrillation also occurs commonly later in life. Tricuspid regurgitation is associated with increased mortality at 20 years' followup. Finally, symptomatic ventricular tachycardia (VT) may also occur, generally in patients >30 years old and having l-TGA.

【 】 TRICUSPID ATRESIA

Tricuspid atresia is a congenital abnormality of alignment in which there is no connection between the atrial mass and the morphologically right ventricle. The right atrium ends in a muscular floor, and its only outlet is an atrial septal communication. The atrial and ventricular septa form normally (usually with a VSD). This causes the AV node to be located posterolateral to the blind-ending dimple in the muscular floor of the right atrium, maintaining a normal relationship with the tendon of Todaro and coronary sinus.

The surface ECG reflects hemodynamic and anatomic influences, with right atrial enlargement in almost all, left axis deviation in approximately 75 percent, and a short PR interval (<0.10 seconds) in up to 12 percent (see Fig. 47–2). Preexcitation occurs in between 0.29 percent and 0.51 percent. However, electrophysiologic evaluation of these patients demonstrates that only approximately 10 percent have a true accessory pathway, prompting the use of the term *pseudopreexcitation* in the others. Hence clinical arrhythmias secondary to structural conduction system abnormalities are uncommon in patients having tricuspid atresia. When accessory pathways are present, they are right-sided, including septal. An interesting form of Wolff-Parkinson-White pattern may occur following an older form of the Fontan operation, in which the right atrial appendage is anastomosed to the right ventricular infundibulum. Acquired conduction across suture lines may give the appearance of a right anteroseptal accessory pathway and may even predispose to AVRT.[5] It may also be treated by standard catheter ablation techniques.[5]

【 】 EBSTEIN ANOMALY OF THE TRICUSPID VALVE

In this disease, the tricuspid valve does not differentiate properly from the right ventricle, resulting in distal displacement of the tricuspid valve leaflets into the right ventricle. There may be significant tricuspid regurgitation into that thin-walled, hypocontractile portion of the right ventricle between the tricuspid valve leaflet coaptation plane and the normally positioned annulus. In moderate or severe cases, there may be chronic cyanosis, severe volume overload of both atria, and sometimes right ventricular outflow tract obstruction. Abnormalities of the right bundle branch and accessory AV connections are intrinsic malformations that are variably present. This combination of physiologic and anatomic abnormalities results in a patient group with a high incidence of arrhythmias. Even from early childhood, the ECG

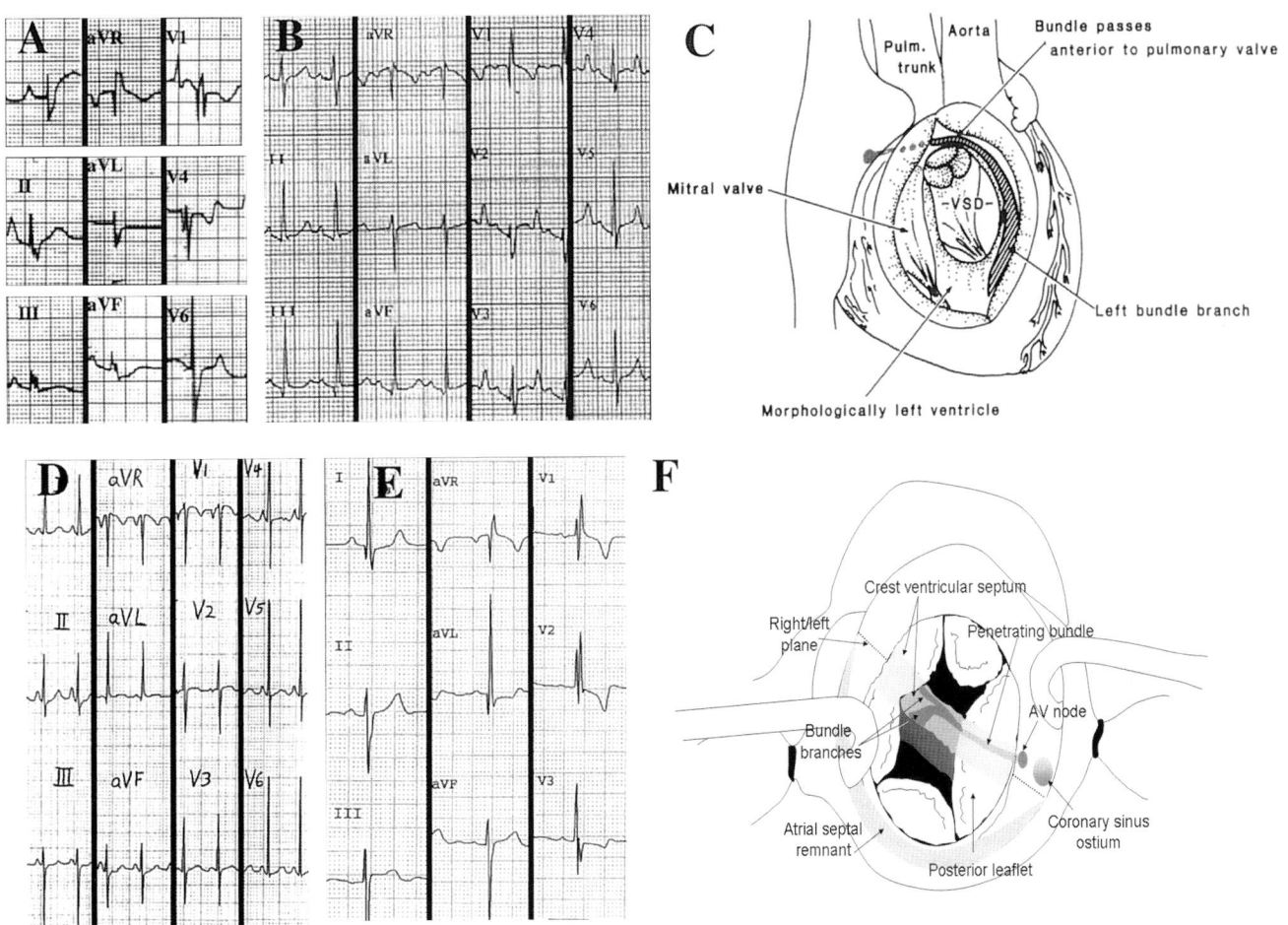

FIGURE 47–2. Examples of electrocardiograms from patients with congenital heart disease, who have both structural abnormalities of the specialized conduction system and abnormalities of cardiac chamber size due to the hemodynamic alterations. **A.** An 8-year-old with severe Ebstein anomaly of the tricuspid valve, showing marked right atrial enlargement and incomplete right bundle-branch block. **B.** A 3-year-old with l-TGA and pulmonic stenosis, showing a septal q in V$_1$ and RS in V$_6$, as well as right ventricular hypertrophy. **C.** The cardiac anatomy of l-TGA, showing the specialized conduction system and its relationships to a VSD. **D.** A 6-month-old with tricuspid atresia, illustrating left axis deviation, right atrial enlargement, and paucity of right-sided forces (abnormal R:S ratio in V$_1$). **E.** A 3-year-old with AV septal defect, demonstrating left axis deviation and right ventricular hypertrophy (RSR' in V$_1$). **F.** Anatomic location of the AV conduction system in hearts with AV septal defect, from the surgeon's perspective.

from moderately or severely affected patients shows marked right atrial enlargement and—if Wolff-Parkinson-White (WPW) syndrome is not present—right ventricular conduction delay (see Fig. 47–2).

WPW syndrome occurs in 10 to 21 percent of patients having the Ebstein anomaly. Paroxysmal supraventricular tachycardia contributes to morbidity but not to risk of sudden death, and its incidence increases with age at presentation. In an older large series of 220 cases of Ebstein anomaly, arrhythmia was the most common presenting symptom (42 percent) in the adolescent and adult age group, but not in children. Actuarial survival was 59 percent at 10 years, but sudden death accounted for only 14 percent of deaths. In retrospective analysis of predictors of long-term survival in 48 patients, 14 percent died by 5 months, none of whom had WPW syndrome. Of surviving patients, 24 percent had WPW syndrome, and there was 68 percent long-term survival (11 years mean followup). Although atrial fibrillation was associated with nonsurvival (p = 0.03), WPW syndrome did not appear to play a role in any deaths. Of eight older patients having experienced sudden cardiac death, ventricular fibrillation related to severe cardiomegaly was thought to be the cause. Most tachycardias associated with accessory pathways can now be treated nonpharmacologically.

❚ ❭ ATRIOVENTRICULAR SEPTAL DEFECT

In all forms of atrioventricular septal defect (AVSD), there are predictable abnormalities of the specialized AV conduction system. Embryologically, the AV node always forms at the insertion of the inlet ventricular septum and the atrial septum. Because of the location of the AV septal deficiency in this disease, there is posteroinferior displacement of the AV node toward the ostium of the coronary sinus (see Fig. 47–2). There is also a longer-than-normal penetrating bundle and relative hypoplasia of the anterior portion of the left bundle branch, resulting in the characteristic ECG findings: left axis deviation of the QRS complex with a superior counterclockwise vector loop in the frontal plane (see Fig. 47–2). Accessory AV connections may also exist in patients with AVSD, and they tend to be posteroseptal in location.

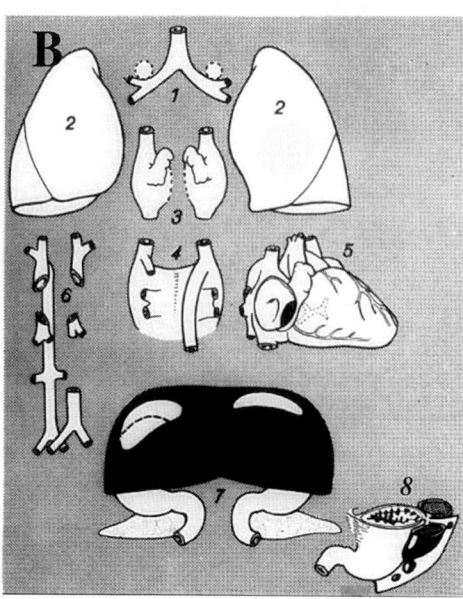

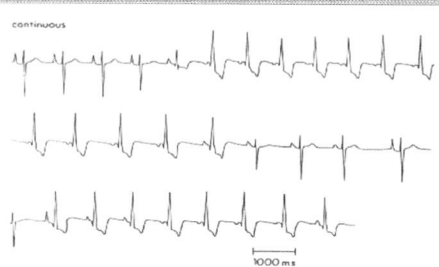

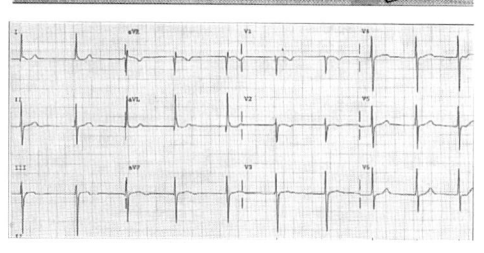

FIGURE 47–3. The heterotaxies. Characteristic gross organ abnormalities (*top*) and typical ECG findings (*bottom*) in **A.** Right atrial isomerism ("asplenia"). **B.** Left atrial isomerism ("polysplenia"). **A** depicts eparterial bronchi (*1*), trilobed lungs (*2*), mirror-image right atrial appendages (*3*), and total anomalous pulmonary venous return (*4*). The rhythm strip shows evidence of duplicated conduction systems, with QRS axis changes following P-wave morphology and PR-segment changes. **B** shows hyparterial bronchi (*1*), bilobed lungs (*2*), mirror-image left atrial appendages (*3*), ipsilateral pulmonary venous return and azygos continuation of lower body venous return because of interrupted inferior vena cave (*4*), and multiple small spleens (*8*). The 12-lead electrocardiogram shows junctional rhythm. Common to both entities are common atrium, AV septal defect, and outflow tract obstructions (*5*); abnormalities in systemic venous return (*6*); and midline liver with gut malrotation (*7*). *Source: The anatomic figures are adapted with permission from the March of Dimes. In: Van Mierop LHS, Gessner IH, Schiebler GL. Asplenia and polysplenia syndromes. Birth Defects 1972;8:36–43.*

[ ] HETEROTAXIES

The heterotaxy syndromes are patterns of malformation involving multiple organs and thought to occur as a result of failure of lateralization of thoracic and abdominal viscera into either a normal pattern (situs solitus) or inverted pattern (situs inversus). They usually involve the cardiovascular system, often with severe congenital malformations. They are categorized as either right atrial isomerism or left atrial isomerism, although there is great variability within each group (Fig. 47–3). The cardiac conduction system may be structurally abnormal, and congenital or acquired AV block is the most important clinical conduction defect.

ARRHYTHMIAS ASSOCIATED WITH COMMON CONGENITAL HEART DEFECTS

Among the most prevalent congenital heart defects are the VSD, the atrial septal defect (ASD), pulmonary valve stenosis, and aortic valve stenosis.

[ ] ATRIAL SEPTAL DEFECT

A nonsinus atrial rhythm may coexist in up to 10 percent of children and young adults with sinus venosus ASDs[6] but much less commonly in those having isolated ostium secundum ASDs. Since chronic left-to-right shunting results in dilatation of the right atrium and right ventricle in both lesions, the relatively proximate location of sinus venosus defects with respect to the sinoatrial node may play a role in this observation. When considering older adults having ASDs, however, the incidence of sinoatrial node dysfunction has been reported to be 22 to 65 percent. Starting in early childhood, and probably as a consequence of right ventricular stretch, right ventricular conduction delay is ubiquitous.

After childhood repair of ASD, the late-term (mean: 26 years) incidence of symptomatic atrial tachyarrhythmia is only approximately 4 percent.[7] Atrial flutter and/or fibrillation are increasingly prevalent with increasing age at ASD presentation, increasing pulmonary-to-systemic flow ratio, and increasing pulmonary artery pressure. This prevalence approaches 50 percent in patients >50 years old and 80 percent in octogenarians. Surgical repair later in life may not protect these patients from atrial tachyarrhythmias. In an old series of 123 patients who had undergone repair of ostium secundum or sinus venosus ASDs at the Mayo Clinic, late followup (27 to 32 years) revealed that the incidence of atrial flutter or fibrillation increased directly with age at repair: 4 percent if operated on at ≤11 years old, 17 percent if operated on at 12 to 24 years old, 41 percent if operated on at 25 to 41 years old, and 59 percent if operated on at >41 years old. More recent reports show additional risk factors for late postoperative atrial flutter or fibrillation: the presence of preoperative atrial flutter or fibrillation and the occurrence of immediate postoperative atrial flutter or fibrillation or junctional rhythm, as well as older age at surgery (>40 years).[8] Pacemaker requirement for new onset sinus node dysfunction or AV block is low in all groups, ranging from 0 to 3.7 percent.[6,8]

When postoperation atrial flutter does occur, it seems to be potentiated by slow conduction within either the low lateral right atrium (between the atriotomy scar and the orifice of the inferior vena cava) or the subtricuspid isthmus. Catheter ablation within these zones is highly effective in long-term relief of tachycardia.[9]

Starting in the late 1990s, techniques using catheter-delivered devices to permanently close many secundum ASDs began to supplant surgery. Transient AV block has been reported in up to 6 percent of these procedures[10] but with permanent AV block in only 0.1 percent at medium-term followup.[11] The incidence of symptomatic atrial tachyarrhythmias following device closure is negligible in children and only approximately 1 percent per year in adults, unless present prior to the procedure.[12]

[ ] VENTRICULAR SEPTAL DEFECT

Patients having a VSD develop chronic volume overload in the right ventricle, left atrium, and left ventricle proportionate to the size of the left-to-right shunt. In patients with large defects, pulmonary and right ventricular hypertension may also occur. The long-term effects of having a VSD were investigated as part of the Second Natural History Study, published in 1993. Among 2408 patients entered into this study between 1958 and 1969, 93 percent were younger than 18 years old at entry. At the time of followup, ambulatory ECG (Holter) data from 419 patients having a VSD demonstrated that 15.3 percent had supraventricular arrhythmias versus 5 percent of controls (p <0.0001). Compared with age-appropriate controls, premature ventricular beats were more frequent in 11 to 17 percent of patients younger than 40 years old (>4 per hour) and in 22 to 39 percent of those greater than 40 years old (>8 per hour). These incidences related to disease severity, occurring in 12 percent of those medically managed, in 20 percent of those surgically managed, and in 80 percent of those having Eisenmenger physiology. The presence of *serious ventricular arrhythmias* (defined as the presence of ventricular couplets, multiform premature ventricular beats, or ventricular tachycardia) was determined from some combination of ECG, Holter, and exercise testing in all 1252 patients having a VSD. Table 47–1 shows the incidences of and independent risk factors for having serious ventricular arrhythmias. Although this work demonstrated

that arrhythmia risk is related to severity of hemodynamic alterations, even small VSDs may be associated with symptomatic arrhythmias in adulthood, especially ventricular tachycardia and atrial fibrillation.

Catheter-delivered devices have been used to close muscular VSDs since about 1998. This technique is not associated with long-term arrhythmias or conduction defects,[13] except perhaps when performed in young infants.[14] Newer devices for perimembranous defects do seem to carry risk of AV block,[15] although sufficient experience is not yet available.

[ ] PULMONIC STENOSIS

Pulmonic stenosis results in right ventricular hypertension and hypertrophy proportionate to the degree of outflow tract obstruction. Treatment with surgical or balloon valvotomy can cause right ventricular volume overload from valve insufficiency. In the Second Natural History Study, among 182 patients having Holter data, 18.9 percent had supraventricular arrhythmias versus 5 percent of controls (p <0.001), although this incidence was not influenced by prior valvotomy. However, only those having prior valvotomy had more premature ventricular beats than controls (p <0.0001), suggesting a role for volume loading from pulmonary valve insufficiency. Table 47–1 shows the incidence of "serious" ventricular arrhythmia. The incidence did not increase with lesion severity, and the overall incidence of ventricular tachycardia (2 percent) was not greater than that of control patients. However, the severity of hemodynamic abnormality as represented by New York Heart Association (NYHA) class and by the presence of cardiomegaly was related to the likelihood of serious ventricular arrhythmia.

TABLE 47–1

Serious Ventricular Arrhythmias in Patients Having Ventricular Septal Defect, Pulmonic Stenosis, or Aortic Stenosis

| CONGENITAL HEART DEFECT | SERIOUS VENTRICULAR ARRHYTHMIAS[a] | | | SUDDEN UNEXPLAINED DEATH |
	INCIDENCE (%)	INDEPENDENT RISK FACTORS	ODDS RATIO	INCIDENCE (%)
Ventricular septal defect	31.4	Main pulmonary artery pressure[b]	1.49	4.0
		Age[c]	1.51	
		NYHA class[c]	8.53	
		Cardiomegaly[c]	2.79	
Pulmonic stenosis	29.7	Age[b]	1.05	0.5
		Age[c]	1.04	
		NYHA Class[c]	7.93	
		Cardiomegaly[c]	3.21	
Aortic stenosis	44.8	Left ventricular end-diastolic pressure[b]	2.02	5.4
		Aortic regurgitation[c]	11.70	
		Gender[c]	4.10	
		Prior aortic valve replacement[c]	4.80	

NYHA, New York Heart Association.
[a]Defined as ventricular couplets, multiform ventricular premature beats, or ventricular tachycardia.
[b]Upon entry into First Natural History Study.
[c]Upon entry into Second Natural History Study.

【 】 AORTIC STENOSIS

Aortic stenosis results in left ventricular hypertension and hypertrophy proportionate to the severity of obstruction. Aortic valve insufficiency may be associated naturally or occur following surgical or balloon valvotomy. As ventricular compliance worsens, subendocardial ischemia eventually results from a decreasing diastolic transmural coronary perfusion gradient. In the Second Natural History Study, among 134 patients having Holter data, 24.8 percent had supraventricular arrhythmias versus 5 percent of controls (p <0.001), unrelated to prior valvotomy. As in the case of pulmonic stenosis, 13 percent of patients having undergone prior valvotomy had premature ventricular beats at a rate exceeding normal for age (p <0.0001 vs. controls). The incidences of serious ventricular arrhythmias were high in these patients, as depicted in Table 47–1, with an overall incidence of VT (13 percent) much greater than in controls. This incidence increased with increasing lesion severity, unlike that in patients with pulmonic stenosis. Independent predictors of risk of serious ventricular arrhythmias were identified only in patients having undergone valvotomy or valve surgery (see Table 47–1) and included hemodynamic, demographic, and surgical procedure characteristics.

Among patients having all types of congenital heart diseases, the relationship of serious ventricular arrhythmia (from noninvasive monitoring) to symptoms or to sudden cardiac death is tenuous, at best. As Table 47–1 illustrates, this relationship is also unclear in patients having VSD, pulmonic stenosis, or aortic stenosis. Although the incidence of serious ventricular arrhythmia is similar among the three groups, the risk of unexpected sudden death is significantly higher among VSD (4 percent) and aortic stenosis (5.4 percent) patients, as compared with controls. Patients with aortic stenosis or VSD and severe hemodynamic alterations do require close surveillance.

ARRHYTHMIAS LONG-TERM FOLLOWING CONGENITAL HEART SURGERY

This section considers four categories of arrhythmias that are of clinical concern long-term following congenital heart surgery: (1) SAND and (2) intraatrial reentry tachycardia following complex atrial surgery, especially atrial redirection procedures (Mustard and Senning operations) and atriopulmonary connections in patients with a single functional ventricle (Fontan operation); (3) AV block following VSD closure; and (4) ventricular tachyarrhythmias following ventricular outflow tract surgeries, such as tetralogy of Fallot.

【 】 SINOATRIAL NODE DYSFUNCTION AND INTRAATRIAL REENTRY TACHYCARDIA

The longest experience with arrhythmias following atrial surgery is with the Mustard and Senning operations for dextrotransposition of the great arteries (d-TGA). These operations are intended to direct the systemic venous return to the mitral valve and pulmonary venous return to the tricuspid valve and involve creation of an intraatrial baffle with prosthetic material or pericardium (Mustard operation) or atrial wall itself (Senning). These suture lines may damage the sinus node, perinodal structures, and their blood supplies. Symptomatic bradycardia presents as exercise intolerance, fatigue, or presyncope and syn-

cope. intraatrial reentry tachycardia (IART; referred to as *atrial flutter* in older literature) may rarely predispose to sudden death. (*IART* and *atrial flutter* are used interchangeably in this chapter.)

Incidence and "Natural History"

When evaluated by ambulatory ECG monitoring 5 to 10 years postoperatively, between 20 and 40 percent of patients having Mustard procedures are still in sinus rhythm; between 7 and 35 percent are in junctional rhythm, up to 40 percent are in slow ectopic atrial rhythm, and 10 percent have atrial flutter. In an older series of 249 patients, there was a 2.4 percent per year loss of sinus rhythm, and the presence of junctional rhythm carried a 2.1-fold increased risk of developing atrial flutter (p <0.05). At 23 years median followup of 86 adults who had undergone the Mustard operation, up to 48 percent had a history of supraventricular tachycardia (mostly IART) and up to 22 percent had pacemakers. Risk factors for supraventricular tachycardia include pulmonary hypertension, right ventricular dysfunction, and junctional rhythm. Sinoatrial node dysfunction appears to be more common following the Mustard procedure than following the Senning operation.

Sudden death occurs late after these operations in between 3 and 15 percent of patients, and the presence of atrial flutter increases this risk up to 4.7-fold (p <0.01). The mechanism of sudden death has been thought to be 1:1 AV conduction during atrial flutter, either directly causing ventricular fibrillation or followed by marked overdrive suppression of all subsidiary pacemakers with resultant asystole. However, primary ventricular tachycardia in those having depressed right ventricular function may also contribute to this risk.

Because the Fontan-style operations have gone through several iterations, the incidences and prevalences of atrial tachyarrhythmias must be interpreted cautiously. Among >2600 patients having undergone any kind of Fontan operation over two decades of publications, atrial tachycardia occurs in 0 to 57 percent of patients, at followup ranging from 3 months to 14 years.[16–20] The prevalences vary according to Fontan type: 12 to 57 percent for atriopulmonary/Bjork type Fontans; 3 to 26 percent for lateral tunnel/total cavopulmonary connections[18–20]; and 0 to 9 percent for extracardiac conduits.[18,20] Risk factors for the development of atrial tachycardias include duration of followup, right atrial enlargement, AV valve surgery, early postoperative arrhythmias, atriopulmonary connection (vs. lateral tunnel), and lateral tunnel (vs. extracardiac conduit). Moreover, animal studies and clinical reports show a lower incidence of immediate and medium-term (2 to 8 years) postoperative atrial tachycardias in TCPC (total cavopulmonary connection) patients when the crista terminalis is not violated by suture lines. Most centers have evolved to extracardiac conduits whenever possible to prevent hypertension in any portion of the atrial mass.

The incidence of pacemaker requirement in patients following the modified Fontan operation ranges from 5 to 16 percent. The indications include tachycardia–bradycardia syndrome, congenital AV block, or postoperative AV block. The reported incidence of late arrhythmic death overall is 2 to 3 percent. These data will also be influenced by newer surgical techniques.

Noninvasive Evaluation

Even if there are no symptoms, electrocardiographic signs of sinus node dysfunction following atrial surgery requires regular surveillance. Otherwise, 24-hour ambulatory ECGs are sufficient every 2 to 5 years. In patients having chronic fatigue and in those having syncope or dizziness at rest or with exercise, a 24-hour ECG and exercise test should be performed. It should be recognized that the maximum attained heart rate in these patients is usually below predicted, often with an abnormally pronounced reduction in heart rate during the immediate postexercise recovery phase. This relatively sudden drop in heart rate immediately following exercise may correlate with the frequently observed fatigue and dizziness that many patients experience immediately following exercise.

For patients having less frequent paroxysmal episodes of syncope, dizziness, or palpitations, ambulatory electrocardiographic monitoring systems or insertable loop recorders having memory are useful.

Electrophysiologic Testing

Prolongation of the sinus node or pacemaker recovery times has been reported in greater than 50 percent, prolongation of the sinoatrial conduction time in greater than 33 to 50 percent, intraatrial conduction delay in 76 to 90 percent, and increased atrial effective refractory period in 40 to 45 percent of patients following Mustard or Fontan operations. In one report of Mustard patients, sustained atrial reentry tachycardia was inducible in 51 percent of patients, half of whom later developed spontaneous atrial flutter. AV conduction is usually normal.

Following atrial surgery, electrophysiologic study is indicated for any patient who has experienced syncope, presyncope, or palpitations suggestive of a tachyarrhythmia; or who has documented nonsinus tachycardia. (If atrial flutter is the cause of symptoms, it can be argued that electrophysiologic study can be deferred unless catheter ablation is to be performed.) Even if noninvasive monitoring shows bradycardia as the source for syncope, cardiac catheterization and electrophysiologic study may be useful prior to pacemaker implantation for several reasons: (1) evaluation of AV nodal function; (2) identification and possible ablation of coexisting tachyarrhythmias; and (3) demonstration of venous and atrial anatomy pertinent to permanent lead implantation.

Management

The recommendations of the American Heart Association (AHA)/ American College of Cardiology (ACC)/North American Society of Pacing and Electrophysiology Joint Committee on Pacing as they relate to patients who have undergone atrial surgery[21] are to insert a pacemaker in any patient with (1) "symptomatic" bradycardia (dizziness, light-headedness, and near or frank syncope) correlated with sudden severe bradycardia; marked exercise intolerance and chronotropic incompetence; or congestive heart failure and chronic bradycardia (class I indication); (2) tachycardia–bradycardia syndrome requiring treatment with an antiarrhythmic drug (other than digitalis) that could suppress the sinus node (class IIa indication); or (3) a resting heart rate <30 beats/min or pauses exceeding 3 seconds (class IIa indication in a child, class IIb in a teenager). These recommendations are only guidelines; we have offered permanent pacing in children having less-defined symptoms of fatigue, morning headaches, or daytime somnolence and only moderate bradycardia while awake. The interplay with hemodynamic function is not well defined by these recommendations. A small series has described the value of atrial pacing in Fontan patients having protein-losing enteropathy.[22]

Because sudden death in patients having the Mustard or Senning operation is most likely linked to *tachy*arrhythmias, complete arrhythmia suppression is often the goal of therapy. Occasionally, patients having impaired AV conduction remain asymptomatic with atrial flutter, as a consequence of 2–4:1 AV conduction, and may not require aggressive treatment. Patients who present with atrial flutter (with or without symptoms) should undergo transvenous or transesophageal overdrive pacing termination or direct current cardioversion. Chronic treatment with an AV node-blocking agent alone following a first episode is reasonable until a timeline of recurrences is established, especially if that event is not associated with syncope or other evidence for severe cardiovascular decompensation. Following recurrences, three options are available: antitachycardia pacing (with an AV node blocking drug); class I (with an AV node blocking drug and bradycardia pacing) or class III agents (with bradycardia pacing); or radiofrequency catheter ablation. Implantation of an antitachycardia pacemaker may obviate the need for potentially proarrhythmic drugs, but safety and efficacy of this modality must be demonstrated by electrophysiologic testing in the drug-free state. Radiofrequency ablation of IART can now be performed with success rates at long-term followup of 70 to 80 percent. This is now our preferred approach in patients with recurrent IART (Fig. 47–4).

Pharmacologic suppression of atrial tachycardias is more difficult following Fontan-type operations. The importance of AV synchrony and adequate diastolic filling time makes arrhythmia control especially crucial. Combinations of antiarrhythmic drugs, often including amiodarone, is often necessary. However, there is an unusually high incidence of amiodarone-induced thyrotoxicosis in Fontan patients. Antitachycardia pacing is occasionally helpful but may result in dangerous rhythm acceleration.

Because of an unpredictable imbalance in natural anticoagulant and procoagulant factors, Fontan patients with atrial tachyarrhythmias may be at unusually high risk for atrial and pulmonary thrombosis, sometimes with catastrophic results. Transesophageal echocardiography should be performed prior to conversion of IART in these patients, because transthoracic echocardiography has been shown to underestimate the prevalence of thrombus. Warfarin should be used for at least 3 weeks following cardioversion, although its efficacy is somewhat controversial in this patient group.[23]

Radiofrequency catheter ablation of IART is more difficult in these patients, because of the frequent presence of multiple tachycardia circuits and the increased atrial wall thickness, compared with atria after other heart operations. In the large series of patients undergoing catheter ablation for IART after surgery for congenital heart disease by Triedman et al.,[24] 63 patients had undergone the Fontan operation. Multivariate factors relating to acute success included use of an irrigated ablation catheter (odds ratio: 3.8) and, inversely, a history of atrial fibrillation (odds ratio: 0.43). Favorable outcome at medium-term followup was related to complete procedural success (odds ratio: 3.9), the use of an electroanatomic mapping technique (odds ratio: 2.4), and, inversely, the number of IART circuits (odds ratio: 0.58).[25] Following the atriopulmonary connection-type of Fontan procedure, corridors of conduction critical to IART circuits and amenable to ablation seem to be clustered in the posterolateral right atrium associated with the atriotomy scar, in the subtricuspid isthmus (when present), and related to the atriopulmonary connection itself (Fig.

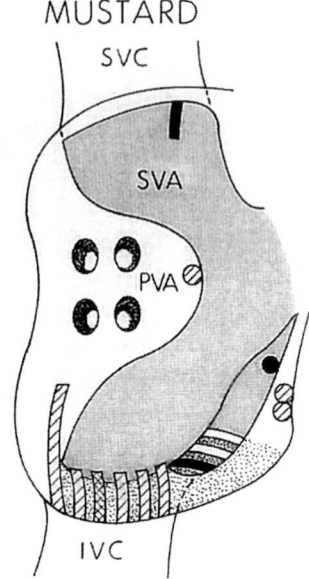

MUSTARD   SENNING

● ■ SUCCESSFUL SYSTEMIC VENOUS
(focal, linear)

⌀, ▨ SUCCESSFUL PULM. VENOUS
(focal, linear)

▭ UNSUCCESSFUL SYSTEMIC
VENOUS LINEAR

▩ UNSUCCESSFUL PULM.
VENOUS LINEAR

FIGURE 47–4. Successful and unsuccessful radiofrequency catheter ablation sites from patients having undergone the Mustard or Senning operations for d-TGA. Rectangular sites represent linear lesions for intraatrial reentry tachycardia, and circular sites represent focal lesions for "focal atrial tachycardia." In the figure depicting the Mustard operation, the *gray region* represents the systemic venous atrium, and the *stippled zone* represents the subtricuspid isthmus. In the figure showing the Senning operation, the *lightly shaded* area is a part of the systemic venous atrium, whose roof (atrial freewall flap to the viewer's left) has been removed from its attachment to the atrial septal remnant (*vertical dashed line*); and a portion of the pulmonary venous atrium adjacent to the tricuspid valve is visible to the viewer's right of the vertical dashed line. IVC, inferior vena cava; MV, mitral valve; PVA, pulmonary venous atrium; SVA, systemic venous atrium; SVC, superior vena cava; TV, tricuspid valve. *Source: Reproduced with permission from Kanter RJ, Papagiannis J, Carboni MP, et al. Radiofrequency catheter ablation of supraventricular tachycardia substrates after Mustard and Senning operations for d-transposition of the great arteries. J Am Coll Cardiol 2000;35:428–441.*

47–5). Standard techniques for identifying ideal targets for ablation in macroreentry atrial tachycardias, such as demonstration of diastolic potentials and concealed entrainment mapping, may not be effective in these patients.[26,27] Successful ablation of >70 percent of these circuits is now being achieved, although the recurrence rate is approximately 50 percent at 2 to 3 years' followup.[24,28] Among patients having IART following newer Fontan-type operations, catheter access to the tachycardia circuits may require novel approaches, including transthoracic puncture.[29]

【 】 ARRHYTHMIAS FOLLOWING VENTRICULAR SURGERY

Postoperative AV block and ventricular tachyarrhythmias are the major clinical concerns in patients having undergone ventricular surgery. Based on patients having undergone repair of tetralogy of Fallot, it was once believed that the occurrence of sudden death was related to sudden AV block; but it is now understood that the main etiologies are ventricular tachycardia and fibrillation. In general, complexity of the congenital lesion relates to the potential for residual hemodynamic abnormalities and risk of sudden death. This section considers con-

duction disturbances and ventricular tachyarrhythmias separately. Most data are based on patients having tetralogy of Fallot because of the high natural incidence of this defect.

Conduction Disturbance

Incidence and Clinical Significance Repair of tetralogy of Fallot requires closure of a perimembranous VSD and enlargement of the right ventricular outflow tract ("infundibulectomy"). Using this repair as a model for conduction system damage, approximately 80 percent of patients have complete fight bundle-branch block (RBBB), an additional 11 percent have the combination of RBBB with left axis deviation, and 3 percent have the combination of RBBB, left axis deviation, and first-degree AV block. Accordingly, the presence of a prolonged H-V interval or AV block at a slow atrial paced rate in any such patient having syncope may help guide clinical decision making. Permanent complete AV block occurs in <1 percent of operated patients in the modern surgical era.[30] However, in Hokanson's series, even transient complete AV block may be associated with late risk of sudden death.[25] Isolated RBBB has specific clinical implications: (1) It will never be possible to identify progressive ventricular dilatation or hypertrophy from the ECG. (2) We are now learning that the dyssynchronous ventricular activation, which results from bundle-branch block, may be deleterious to overall myocardial performance. Modern echographic techniques, including tissue Doppler strain imaging and the Tei index, can identify patients with decreased regional and global left ventricular dysfunction,[31] decreased exercise capability,[32] and increased risk of ventricular arrhythmias.[32] And (3) in the presence of proximal RBBB, the development of left bundle-branch block, which occasionally occurs later in life, places these patients at risk for complete AV block.

Among other congenital defects known to be associated with surgical complete AV block, AV septal defect is associated with 3 to 4 percent incidence; VSD with congenitally corrected transposition, 10 percent; and isolated perimembranous VSD, <1 percent.

Evaluation Based on old data, the ECG findings of RBBB and left axis deviation is usually associated with normal Q-wave-to-right-ventricular-apex activation times; and RBBB, left axis deviation, and first-degree AV block is usually associated with normal H-V intervals in these patients. Hence, the terms *bifascicular* and *trifascicular* block may not be appropriate, unless there are intracardiac conduction interval abnormalities. In the absence of symptoms, even "true" bifascicular or trifascicular block requires intervention in only certain circumstances: type II second-degree AV block during sinus rhythm; complete AV block; or marked H-V interval prolongation (>100 milliseconds). In the presence of syncope (and no inducible tachyarrhythmias), there is concern with any H-V interval prolongation or block below the His

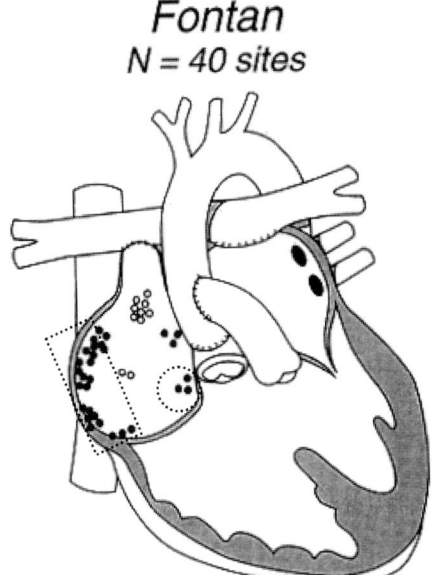

Fontan
N = 40 sites

FIGURE 47–5. Successful radiofrequency catheter ablation sites in patients having had a Fontan operation (predominantly atriopulmonary connection) and intraatrial reentry tachycardia. *Open circles* are anterior, mostly associated with the right atrial appendage-to-pulmonary artery anastomosis; *closed circles within the dotted rectangle* are in the region of the right atriotomy; and *closed circles within the dotted circle* are in the region of the subtricuspid isthmus (when present). *Source: Adapted with permission from Collins KK, Love BA, Walsh EP, et al. Location of acutely successful radiofrequency catheter ablation of intraatrial reentrant tachycardia in patients with congenital heart disease. Am J Cardiol 2000;86:969–974.*

bundle at atrial paced rates below 120 per minute. In the presence of transient postoperative second-degree AV block or complete AV block (lasting less than 10 days postoperatively), 24-hour ECG monitoring should be performed prior to discharge and then regularly.

In the patient who has had an operation on the ventricles and who has had syncope or presyncope, documentation of that patient's rhythm during symptoms is mandatory. Following repair of tetralogy of Fallot, for example, syncope secondary to AV block, ventricular arrhythmias, atrial flutter with rapid AV conduction, and supraventricular tachycardia are known to occur. Although diagnostic techniques such as attached ambulatory event recorders ("loop recorders") or insertable loop recorders are reasonable first approaches, there is a tendency toward invasive electrophysiologic testing very early in that patient's course.

Management Based on the AHA/ACC/North American Society of Pacing and Electrophysiology (now the Heart Rhythm Society) Joint Committee on Pacing, a pacemaker should be implanted in any child with type II second-degree or complete AV block lasting more than 10 days postoperatively following heart surgery (class I indication).[21] In our opinion, similar consideration should be given to the patient with syncope and either a prolonged H-V interval or AV block below the His at atrial paced rates below the 120 per minute. Asymptomatic patients with prolonged H-V interval or AV block below the His at atrial paced rates below 120 per minute should be followed closely with 24-hour ambulatory ECG monitoring and exercise testing.

Occasional patients undergo pacemaker insertion in the postoperative period but later regain AV conduction. In Batra's series, among 72 patients having complete postoperative AV block during surgery

for congenital heart disease (1.3 percent), 7 (9.6%) regained AV conduction at 18 to 113 days postoperation.[33] None redeveloped AV block at 4.4 ± 2.6 years of followup. Whether this is an endorsement for relaxing long-term followup of the conduction system of these patients is unknown. We know of one patient who redeveloped AV block 16 years following transient block during aortic valve replacement at 7 years of age.

Ventricular Tachyarrhythmias and Sudden Death

Incidence and Risk Factors Following surgical correction of common congenital heart defects, the long-term incidence of sudden cardiac death is 25 to 100 times greater than age-matched controls. This risk is greatest among patients having had cyanotic heart disease or left ventricular outflow tract obstructive lesions, ranging from 1.5/1000 patient-years for tetralogy of Fallot to 4.9 and 5.4/1000 patient-years for aortic stenosis and atrial switch operation for d-TGA, respectively. Furthermore, this risk increases incrementally, 20 years after surgery.

Evaluation A main goal of routine evaluation of patients following ventricular surgery is to identify individuals who are at risk for symptoms or death from ventricular arrhythmias. At least in patients having undergone tetralogy of Fallot repair, the 12-lead ECG may be an especially valuable screen for patients at risk of having dangerous ventricular arrhythmias. An increased QRS duration appears to be sensitive and perhaps specific for such risk, with a cutoff value of ≥180 ms providing the greatest accuracy. The coexistence of increased JT-interval dispersion may enhance the positive and negative predictive value, suggesting that both repolarization and depolarization abnormalities are important. A rapid increase of these measurements is especially ominous. The chest radiograph, 24-hour ECG, exercise tests, and echocardiogram also have roles in routine patient surveillance. Application of magnetic resonance imaging to quantify pulmonary valve regurgitant and ventricular ejection fractions and tissue Doppler imaging to identify ventricular dyssynchrony are newer modalities being investigated. In patients with poor hemodynamics, followup is stricter than it is in those with excellent hemodynamics. Equivocal or minor symptoms may be evaluated with event recorders, but paroxysmal palpitations or syncope merit invasive electrophysiologic testing.

We recommend invasive electrophysiologic testing following ventricular surgery in patients having sustained palpitations or syncope. The demonstration of symptomatic sustained monomorphic VT by noninvasive means is an indication for electrophysiologic testing if catheter ablation is anticipated. In the era of implantable cardioverter-defibrillators, electrophysiologic testing as a guide for antiarrhythmic drug selection is becoming antiquated. In the absence of symptoms, ventricular programmed stimulation could also be considered if a patient has impaired hemodynamics or markedly prolonged QRS duration, *plus* high-grade ventricular ectopy. The indication to proceed to programmed stimulation is enhanced by a history of older age at repair and/or prior palliative surgery.[34]

Management Symptomatic VT requires treatment. In the current era of device and ablation therapy, antiarrhythmic drug therapy has become less popular. Nevertheless, medium-term efficacy of phenytoin and propranolol has been reported, using serial electrophysiology studies and clinical followup. Amiodarone and sotalol are also potentially efficacious drugs. Class Ia drugs are not very useful for sustained VT in these patients, and class Ic agents may be especially proarrhythmic. Because of potential drug side effects, suboptimal efficacy, and difficulty in proving efficacy, non-pharmacologic therapies are now favored. Following complete tachycardia circuit mapping in the electrophysiology laboratory, surgical resection, cryoablation, and microwave ablation have all met with variable success. Radiofrequency catheter ablation has been used to successfully interrupt macroreentry VT circuits in several patients, even when there are multiple VT circuits and when VT is poorly hemodynamically tolerated. Newer electroanatomic mapping systems are very helpful in these patients. Programmed ventricular stimulation prior to hospital discharge and again at several months postablation is recommended to ensure successful elimination of VT substrate, unless an implantable cardioverter-defibrillator is also used. The implantable cardioverter-defibrillator is an excellent primary treatment modality for infrequent sustained monomorphic VT and is mandatory for patients having resuscitated sudden death. They provide antitachycardia pacing as well as the safety net of cardioversion or defibrillation, if necessary.

Less clear are the indications for treating asymptomatic patients with high-grade ventricular ectopy by ambulatory monitoring. If their hemodynamics are acceptable, we would only follow these patients closely. In those with poor hemodynamics, options include ventricular programmed stimulation to help identify patients with inducible sustained tachycardia; surgical correction of hemodynamic abnormality when possible; or empiric implantation of implantable cardioverter-defibrillators. Until there are randomized clinical trials involving treatment and nontreatment of such patients, the best approach remains unclear.

In summary, in patients who have undergone ventricular surgery, we recommend consideration of treatment for those who fall into the following categories: asymptomatic patients with poor hemodynamics and high-grade ventricular ectopy; asymptomatic patients with poor hemodynamics and inducible sustained VT during electrophysiologic testing; and any patient with clinical sustained VT.

SPECIFIC ARRHYTHMIAS IN THE YOUNG

This section discusses arrhythmias specific to or requiring special considerations in children and teenagers.

【 】 CONGENITAL HEART BLOCK

Once the diagnosis of congenital heart block has been made by fetal ultrasonography, frequent followup is required. Close observation for findings of fetal heart failure are critical to avoid fetal demise. Reversal of the destructive process occurring in the fetal conduction system with maternally administered dexamethasone has been shown in small studies without control subjects[35–37] where findings of endocardial fibroelastosis and second-degree AV block were reversed. Another study showed reversal of signs of myocarditis in fetuses in a triplet pregnancy, but no reversal of complete AV bock in one fetus and, indeed, progression to second-

degree AV block in another fetus in the same pregnancy despite treatment with dexamethasone.[38] In another study, dexamethasone was shown to improve some cases of intrauterine antibody-mediated second-degree AV block, only to have it progress later to complete AV block.[39] Yet another study showed the delivery of a healthy child at 31 weeks gestation after treatment with dexamethasone, azathioprine, and plasmapheresis in a mother with two previous fetal losses to complete AV block from SSA antibodies.[40] Maternally administered steroids carry significant potential adverse effects[41] and reversal or prevention of progression of AV block with maternally administered steroids has not been proven by controlled studies. Such studies are currently ongoing.

Table 47–2 lists specific indications for permanently pacing children with congenital complete AV block. In addition, it is becoming increasingly apparent that virtually all patients with congenital heart block should receive a pacemaker by early adulthood. This notion is supported by a longitudinal study from Sweden, which showed a disturbing incidence of sudden death among previously asymptomatic individuals with congenital heart block who had not been paced. We recommend permanent pacing for all patients with complete AV block who are older than 15 years of age.

【 】 SUPRAVENTRICULAR TACHYCARDIA AND WOLFF-PARKINSON-WHITE SYNDROME

The age distribution of different types of supraventricular tachycardia in the pediatric age range has been estimated by esophageal electrophysiology studies, by measuring the ventricular-atrial (V-A) interval from the atrial electrogram recorded from an esophageal catheter. AV reentrant tachycardia (in which the V-A interval is >70 milliseconds) is thought to represent approximately 80 percent of supraventricular tachycardia in infancy. This may underestimate the frequency of AV nodal reentrant tachycardia in this age group which, in our experience, may be atypical in form and thus have a longer V-A interval. Ventricular stimulation, which is rarely performed in infants is required to differentiate these diagnoses. AV nodal reentry tachycardia is at least as frequent as AV reentry in older teenagers. Evidence for dual AV nodal physiology by established criteria in adults is seen in 50 percent or fewer of pediatric patients with AV nodal reentrant tachycardia[42] and is only slightly more commonly than in control patients.[43]

Among neonates having the Wolff-Parkinson-White syndrome, approximately 25 to 35 percent will experience disappearance of the delta wave, often by 1 year of age. The recurrence rate of supraventricular tachycardia following neonatal presentation has been reported to occur late in approximately one-third of cases. However, older children experiencing their first episode of supraventricular tachycardia are far less likely to experience spontaneous resolution of their arrhythmia substrate. After the neonatal period, the peak age for the initial episode of supraventricular tachycardia is about 8 years of age. This may be related to cardiac dimensional changes, functional changes of the conduction system, and the accessory connection, maturation of the autonomic nervous system, and/or the influences of increased physical activity and caffeine use. In some cases, accessory AV connections and their associated tachycardias may be acquired by surgical intervention for congenital heart disease with electrical connection of the right atrial appendage to the right ventricular outflow tract.[5]

TABLE 47-2

Recommendations for Permanent Pacing in Children, Adolescents, and Patients with Congenital Heart Disease

Class I: Conditions for which there is evidence and/or general agreement that cardiac pacing is beneficial, useful, and effective.

1. Advanced second- or third-degree atrioventricular (AV) block associated with symptomatic bradycardia, ventricular dysfunction or low cardiac output. *(Level of evidence: C)*
2. Sinus node dysfunction with correlation of symptoms during age-inappropriate bradycardia. The definition of bradycardia varies with the patient's age and expected heart rate. *(Level of evidence: B)*
3. Postoperative advanced second- or third-degree AV block that is not expected to resolve or persists at least 7 days after cardiac surgery. *(Level of evidence: B, C)*
4. Congenital third-degree AV block with a wide QRS escape rhythm, complex ventricular ectopy, or ventricular dysfunction. *(Level of evidence: B)*
5. Congenital third-degree AV block in the infant with a ventricular rate less than 50 to 55 beats/min or with congenital heart disease and a ventricular rate less than 70 beats/min. *(Level of evidence: B, C)*
6. Sustained pause-dependent ventricular tachycardia (VT), with or without prolonged QT, in which the efficacy of pacing is thoroughly documented. *(Level of evidence: B)*

Class IIa: Conditions for which there is conflicting evidence and/or a divergence of opinion about the usefulness/efficacy of cardiac pacing. Weight of evidence/opinion is in favor of usefulness/efficacy.

1. Bradycardia–tachycardia syndrome with the need for long-term antiarrhythmic treatment other than digitalis. *(Level of evidence: C)*
2. Congenital third-degree AV block beyond the first year of life with an average heart rate less than 50 beats/min, abrupt pauses in ventricular rate that are two or three times the basic cycle length, or associated with symptoms caused by chronotropic incompetence. *(Level of evidence: B)*
3. Long–QT syndrome with 2:1 AV or third-degree AV block. *(Level of evidence: B)*
4. Asymptomatic sinus bradycardia in the child with complex congenital heart disease with resting heart rate less than 40 beats/min or pauses in ventricular rate more than 3 s. *(Level of evidence: C)*
5. Patients with congenital heart disease and impaired hemodynamics caused by sinus bradycardia or loss of AV synchrony. *(Level of evidence: C)*

Class IIb: Usefulness/efficacy is less well established by evidence/opinion.

1. Transient postoperative third-degree AV block that reverts to sinus rhythm with residual bifascicular block. *(Level of evidence: C)*
2. Congenital third-degree AV block in the asymptomatic infant, child, adolescent, or young adult with an acceptable rate, narrow QRS complex, and normal ventricular function. *(Level of evidence: B)*
3. Asymptomatic sinus bradycardia in the adolescent with congenital heart disease with resting heart rate less than 40 beats/min or pauses in ventricular rate more than 3 seconds. *(Level of evidence: C)*
4. Neuromuscular diseases with any degree of AV block (including first-degree AV block), with or without symptoms, because there may be unpredictable progression of AV conduction disease.

Class III: Conditions for which there is evidence and/or general agreement that cardiac pacing is not useful/effective and in some cases may be harmful.

1. Transient postoperative AV block with return of normal AV conduction. *(Level of evidence: B)*
2. Asymptomatic postoperative bifascicular block with or without first-degree AV block. *(Level of evidence: C)*
3. Asymptomatic type I second-degree AV block. *(Level of evidence: C)*
4. Asymptomatic sinus bradycardia in the adolescent with longest RR interval less than 3 seconds and minimum heart rate more than 40 beats/min. *(Level of evidence: C)*

Level of evidence:

A: If the data were derived from multiple randomized clinical trials involving a large number of individuals.
B: If the data were derived from a limited number of trials involving a comparatively small number of patients or from well-designed data analyses of nonrandomized studies or observational data registries.
C: If the consensus of experts was the primary source of the recommendation.

Natural history studies in children with asymptomatic ventricular preexcitation are very limited in number and duration of followup. A prospective study in children and adults reported that 3 of 212 patients having asymptomatic ventricular preexcitation went on to have cardiac arrest at 5-year followup.[44] The 3 patients were 21 to 25 years of age, and all had multiple accessory AV connections and a short preexcited R-R interval during induced atrial

fibrillation of 230 milliseconds or less. This risk for catastrophic events in patients with ventricular preexcitation may increase in the presence of digoxin and seems to be related to heightened adrenergic state. This combination of facts and impressions has directed most experts to recommend that no child having the Wolff-Parkinson-White syndrome and supraventricular tachycardia receive digoxin, and that nonpharmacologic therapy be considered first-line treatment for the combination of the Wolff-Parkinson-White syndrome and supraventricular tachycardia when β-blocker therapy is contraindicated beyond 2 to 5 years of age. It is further recommended that children older than the age of 5 years who have asymptomatic ventricular preexcitation and who wish to participate in sports or require stimulant therapy undergo risk assessment for sudden death. This can be accomplished noninvasively with the demonstration of intermittent ventricular preexcitation on routine ECGs, Holter monitors, or exercise tests because of "phase 3" accessory pathway block. Care must be taken to evaluate the specific cause of intermittency of ventricular preexcitation.[45] If ventricular preexcitation is persistent by noninvasive studies, the majority of practicing electrophysiologists will use invasive (esophageal) studies for risk stratification of asymptomatic pediatric patients to select appropriate patients for catheter ablation.[46,47]

Approximately 10 percent of supraventricular tachycardia in children of all ages is primary atrial; either incessant automatic atrial tachycardia or a paroxysmal form, using a nonspecified but usually reentrant mechanism. When incessant atrial tachycardia occurs in infancy and early childhood, pharmacologic control (usually sotalol or amiodarone) may be advisable, because there is a possibility that the tachycardia will spontaneously resolve.[48] In children who are older than 3 years of age, spontaneous resolution is less likely and antiarrhythmic drugs are frequently less successful.[48] By contrast, adult patients with incessant atrial tachycardia have documented spontaneous resolution without surgical or catheter ablation intervention in one third of patients. The anatomic distribution of atrial tachycardia foci in children is similar to that reported in adults: the ostia of the pulmonary veins, along the crista terminalis from the sinus node to the coronary sinus ostium, and, less commonly, along the AV valve annuli. Atrial tachycardia foci from the pulmonary vein ostia and chaotic atrial tachycardia of infancy may involve similar substrates to that causing focal atrial fibrillation in adults.

Tachycardia-induced cardiomyopathy in childhood most commonly results from incessant atrial tachycardia[49] or the permanent form of junctional reciprocating tachycardia (a type of orthodromic AV reentrant tachycardia). Much less commonly, incessant ventricular tachycardia or automatic junctional tachycardia may be the etiology. Because children who are younger than 3 years of age are preverbal, they are more likely to present with advanced signs of congestive heart failure than are older children. Management consists of aggressive pharmacologic treatment of congestive heart failure (including digoxin) and either antiarrhythmic drug therapy or radiofrequency ablation. When multiple foci of atrial tachycardia are suspected, radiofrequency ablation is less likely to be successful, and drug management may be preferable until ventricular function improves, and the child is better able to tolerate a prolonged procedure. The permanent form of junctional reciprocating tachycardia is very amenable to radiofrequency ablation,[50] although risk of damage to the AV node may be a concern in young infants, depending on the location of accessory pathway and cryothermal ablation may be preferable.[51]

[ ] CHAOTIC ATRIAL TACHYCARDIA

This uncommon tachycardia seems to occur mostly in infants who are younger than 1 year of age.[52] Unlike adults, in whom it is mostly associated with chronic obstructive pulmonary disease and theophylline use (and is usually referred to as *multifocal atrial tachycardia*), it is usually an isolated phenomenon in the child. Coexisting respiratory infections are present in about one-third of these infants, and structural heart defects are seen in a similar number.[52] The diagnosis is based on the ECG and requires (1) ≥3 ectopic P-wave morphologies; (2) irregular P-P intervals; (3) isoelectric baseline between P waves; and (4) rapid rate.[52] Absence of a dominant atrial pacemaker has also been considered a diagnostic criteria. The atrial rate is typically between 250 and 600 beats/min. The ventricular response rate varies from 110–250 beats/min and results in echocardiographic evidence of tachycardia-induced cardiomyopathy in one-fourth of patients.[52] Less commonly, overt congestive heart failure may occur. The mechanism of chaotic atrial tachycardia is not primary reentry, because it is unresponsive to adenosine, direct current cardioversion, and overdrive pacing. It has been theorized to use a triggered mechanism, although calcium channel blockers are also not efficacious. A rapid automatic mechanism with variable exit points seems to be the most plausible mechanism. Thus chaotic atrial tachycardia in infancy could be analogous to focal atrial fibrillation in adults (i.e., multiple reentry wavelets generated by a single non-reentry generator). This is supported by a single case report describing successful treatment of chaotic atrial tachycardia by ablating a single atrial focus.

Infants who are having chaotic atrial tachycardia generally have an excellent outcome, typically with complete resolution by 1 year of age.[52] Sudden death has been reported in older series and may have been related to digitalis toxicity and factors not directly related to the arrhythmia. If the ventricular response rate cannot be reliably controlled with digoxin, an oral β blocker or calcium channel blocker may be added; or pharmacologic cardioversion to sinus rhythm may be accomplished with oral amiodarone, flecainide, or propafenone. Once sinus rhythm is established and ventricular function returns to normal, the antiarrhythmic drug is generally empirically discontinued after 6 months of treatment or 1 year of age. Close followup including ambulatory ECGs is then required.

[ ] CONGENITAL AUTOMATIC JUNCTIONAL TACHYCARDIA

Automatic junctional tachycardia that presents in the first year of life is usually considered "congenital." It is defined as a regular narrow QRS tachycardia with AV dissociation and a ventricular rate faster than the atrial rate. It is not terminable with overdrive atrial pacing, adenosine, or cardioversion, proving the mechanism to be enhanced automaticity of a portion of the AV junction, below the atrial myocardium, and above the bundle branches—most likely the His bundle.

Most cases present in the first months of life and are sporadic, although a familial predisposition is well known.[53] As a result of its incessant nature, affected infants usually present with signs of congestive heart failure secondary to tachycardia-induced cardiomyopathy. The ventricular rate ranges from 140 to 370 beats/min (mean: 230 beats/min).

The primary goal of therapy is to reduce the ventricular rate to <150 beats/min in young infants in order to allow recovery of ventricular function. Amiodarone has been shown to be most efficacious, although sotalol, flecainide, propranolol, and propafenone may also be used. Digoxin alone is ineffective. If pharmacologic treatment fails, catheter ablation of the junctional focus with preservation of normal AV conduction may be successful[54,55]—even in neonates. Reports of the technical aspects of radiofrequency catheter ablation suggest the use of low-energy "test" applications to regions of the proximal His bundle until acceleration occurs, followed by slightly higher energy until the arrhythmia disappears. Atrial overdrive pacing will allow monitoring of AV conduction during energy delivery.[54] Cryothermal catheter ablation of this arrhythmia has been undertaken in a few as yet unpublished cases.

POSTOPERATIVE AUTOMATIC JUNCTIONAL TACHYCARDIA

Postoperative automatic junctional tachycardia generally occurs within 24 hours after congenital heart operations. It reportedly occurs in up to 8 percent of open heart operations, most commonly following tetralogy of Fallot repair, Mustard operation for d-TGA, VSD closure, arterial switch procedure, AVSD repair, repair of total anomalous pulmonary venous return, and the Fontan operation.[56] These operations have in common the placement of suture lines near the penetrating bundle of His, which may result in a transient period of injury, and edema of the bundle; or, when it occurs following procedures remote from this structure, there may be pressure on the bundle, as may occur with postoperative pulmonary artery hypertension or from cardiopulmonary bypass cannulae or retrograde cardioplegia delivered into the coronary sinus. Longer bypass and cross-clamp times also are risk factors for this arrhythmia.[57] Postoperative automatic junctional tachycardia has previously had a reported mortality rate of up to 50 percent caused by the adverse effect of both rate-related reduction in ventricular filling and loss of AV asynchrony. Less-severe forms of postoperative automatic junctional rhythm are seen. A review of pediatric patients (ages 1 day to 10.5 years) monitored following cardiac surgery at the Children's Hospital of Philadelphia showed a 5.6 percent incidence rate of this rhythm in all patients operated on during the study period. Of the patients with postoperative automatic junctional tachycardia, only 39 percent received therapeutic intervention.[58] This rhythm, however, may be underdiagnosed.[59]

If the patient's hemodynamic status can be improved, given time, postoperative automatic junctional tachycardia generally resolves. The goals of therapy are to reduce the ventricular rate to less than 180 per minute in infants and less than 150 per minute in older children. Successful reduction in rate has been reported in a small series of patients using a variety of antiarrhythmic agents. Moderate hypothermia (89.6° to 93.2°F [32° to 34°C]) has been used in the past to control this arrhythmia, but usually requires pharmacologic paralysis and may result in metabolic acidosis. Intravenous amiodarone is a widely used agent for treatment of this arrhythmia.[60] Hypotension, especially during the intravenous administration of amiodarone, is a definite risk, but is usually successfully treated with administration of intravenous fluid and calcium. Atrial pacing at a rate faster than that of the junctional tachycardia, or AV sequential pacing if AV block is present at rates which are required, should be employed to achieve AV association. Success seems to be related to early intervention.

Patients refractory to all measures may be considered for transcatheter or surgical His bundle ablation and dual-chamber pacemaker implantation. With early intervention, the use of atrial pacing and antiarrhythmic agents such as intravenous amiodarone, and, occasionally, with aggressive hemodynamic support using extracorporeal circulation[61] or ventricular assist, this irreversible and unappealing therapy can nearly always be avoided.

THERAPIES FOR PEDIATRIC ARRHYTHMIAS

This section addresses treatment concepts in children with special attention to those differences from treating adults with arrhythmias.

ANTIARRHYTHMIC DRUGS

With increasing use of catheter ablation as first-line treatment in older children with tachyarrhythmia, acute and chronic pharmacologic intervention is significantly less frequently used.[62] Nevertheless, drug therapy remains a necessary part of the armamentarium for treating arrhythmias in children for several reasons: fetal tachycardia does not currently have alternate therapies; control of tachycardia in the infant with medications likely carries less risk than ablative therapies; and, in this population, the natural history of the disease may favor spontaneous resolution. In older children, drugs are useful in acute treatment of tachycardias and in chronic treatment of tachycardias that are not amenable to curative treatments. Table 47–3 and this section present basic concepts of antiarrhythmic drug pharmacology, classification, and specific applications.

Bioavailability of antiarrhythmic drugs after oral administration is reduced in young infants as a consequence of relative achlorhydria (until about 3 years of age; e.g., this reduces phenytoin absorption), delayed gastric emptying (until 6 to 8 months of age), and immature gut motility (until about 4 years of age). "First-pass" elimination of propranolol, lidocaine, and verapamil is similar in children and adults. Likewise, the effects of coexisting congestive heart failure, intestinal mucosal edema, and other drugs on bioavailability of these agents are similar to those in adults.

Drugs are eliminated by some combination of hepatic or red blood cell biotransformation, renal excretion, pulmonary exhalation, and fecal excretion. The volume of blood totally "cleared" of a drug (so-called *clearance*) is reduced in the presence of renal or hepatic dysfunction, reduced blood flow to that organ, elevated plasma protein binding, and in the presence of immature organ function. Hepatic biotransformation of most drugs is markedly reduced in young infants until enzyme maturation occurs by about 6 months. Hence, drug half-lives are longer until that age. Most antiarrhythmic drug excretion occurs in the kidneys as a result of a combination of glomerular filtration, tubular secretion, and tubular reabsorption. At birth, these three processes are 20 to 30 percent that of an adult, reaching maturity by 1 year (filtration), 1 year (secretion), and 6 months (reabsorption). Renal parenchymal disease and decreased renal perfusion, as in cases of congestive heart failure, obviously prolong the elimination half-life.

The clinical importance of drug metabolites (e.g., procainamide and propafenone), drug–drug interactions (e.g., amiodarone), pharmacokinetic interactions with non-antiarrhythmic drugs (e.g., alteration of gastric pH with antacids; enhancement of biotransformation with phenobarbital; inhibition of transformation with cimetidine; urinary acidification or alkalinization), and pharmacodynamic interactions (e.g., increased myocardial sensitivity to digoxin from di-

TABLE 47–3

Use of Antiarrhythmic Drugs in Children

DRUG	HALF-LIFE	INTRAVENOUS DOSING	ORAL DOSING	TRANS-PLACENTAL PASSAGE (%)	PREGNANCY CATEGORY/ SAFETY FOR FETUS	PASSAGE IN BREAST MILK	INDICATIONS
CLASS Ia							
Disopyramide	4.5–7.8 h	Not available	10–30 mg/kg/d (infants); 10–20 mg/kg/d (children); 6–15 mg/kg/d (adolescents); 400–800 mg/d (adults) q6h (regular), q12h (sustained release); maximum: 1600 mg/d)	39	C	50–90% maternal blood level; safe for infant	PSVT; AFl; AF; VT in CHD with good ventricular function
Quinidine	30–90 min (sulfate); 3.4–4.0 h (gluconate)	Not recommended	30–60 mg/kg/d (450–900 mg/m2); q4–6h; 10 mg/kg/d (adult); 20% higher if gluconate	24–94	C	Reported to occur; safe for infant	Rarely used because of "quinidine syncope"; PSVT; AFl; AF; VT in CHD
Procain-amide	1.7 h (children); 2.5–4.7 h (adults) (short acting), 6–7 h (slow release); shorter in children; longer in neonates	10–15 mg/kg over 20 min; maintenance: 30–80 µg/kg/min	50–100 mg/kg/d	25–100	C	Reported to occur; safe for infant	PSVT; AFl; AF; AET; VT in CHD; postoperative JET
CLASS Ib							
Moricizine	1.5–3.5 h; biologic $T_{1/2}$ 48 h	Not available	200 mg/m2/d (initial) increase to 600 mg/m2/d; q8h	Not known	B	Not known	AET; VT; PSVT
Lidocaine	3.2 h (neonate); 1.5–2 h (children and adults)	1 mg/kg, may repeat twice; maintenance: 20–50 µg/kg/min	Not effective	50	B (fetal bradycardia reported; generally safe for fetus)	40% maternal blood level; safe for infant	VT, especially ischemic
Mexiletine	6.3–11.8 h	Not available	Infants: 8–25 mg/kg/d; children: 4.5–15 mg/kg/d; max: 600–1200 mg/d; q8h	100 (equivalent to maternal blood level)	C	100% maternal blood level; safe for infant	VT
Phenytoin	75 ± 64 h (premature); 21 ± 12 h (term); 8 ± 4 h (1 mo); 22 ± 7 h (child–adult)	10–15 mg/kg over 1 h	Load: 15 mg/kg ÷ q 6 h (day 1), 7.5 mg/kg ÷ q6h (day 2); maintenance: 0–2 wk: 4–8 mg/kg/d q12h; 2 wks–2 y: 8–12 mg/kg/d q8h; 3–12 y: 5–6 mg/kg/d q12h; >12 y: 4.5 mg/kg/d q12h	Excellent	D (11% have "fetal hydantoin syndrome", 31% have lesser manifestations)	Safe for infant	VT
Tocainide	15 h (adult)	Not available	Children: 350–700 mg/m²/d	Not known	C	Not known	VT

	Half-life	IV dose	Oral dose	Transplacental passage	Pregnancy category	Breast milk	Indications
CLASS Ic Flecainide	29 h (newborn); 11–12 h (infant); 8 h (children) 12–27 h (adult)	1–2 mg/kg over 5–10 min	1–6 mg/kg/d or 50–150 mg/m²/d q8h (children) & q12h (newborn, infant and adult); maximum: 400 mg/d; avoid administration with milk-based formulas in infants	100 (equivalent to maternal blood level)	C	Concentrated (2.3–3.7:1); safe for infant	PSVT; AF1; AF; PJRT; VT; fetal tachycardias; JET
Propafenone	4.7 ± 1.3 h (extensive metabolizer); 16.8 ± 10.6 h (slow, 10% population); ↑ with time in both groups	0.2 mg/kg q10min to effect (max, 2 mg/kg); maint: 4–7 µg/kg/min	200–600 mg/m²/d q6–8h; maximum: 900 mg/d	Not known	C	Not known	PSVT; AF1; AF; PJRT; VT; infantile CAT; JET
CLASS II Atenolol	16–35 h (newborn); 3.5–7 h (children); 6–9 h (adults)	No pediatric data	0.8–1.5 mg/kg/d q12–24h; when used for potentially life-threatening arrhythmia (LQTS), q12h recommended	100 maternal blood level	D	Concentrated (1.5–6.8:1); fetal bradycardia	PSVT; rate control in AF1 and AF; VT in normal heart; LQTS
Esmolol	4.5 ± 2.1 min (children); 9 min (adults)	Load: 500 µg/kg over 1 min; maint: 50–600 µg/kg/min	Not applicable	Not known	C	Not known	PSVT; rate control in AF1 and AF
Nadolol	20–24 h (adults); shorter in infants and children	Not available	1–2 mg/kg/d q day	Some passage occurs	C (hypoglycemia; symptomatic bradycardia)	Concentrated (3:1); fetal bradycardia	PSVT; rate control in AF1 and AF; VT in normal heart; LQTS
Propranolol	3.9–6.4 h (children); 4–6 h (adults)	0.01–0.15 mg/kg over 5 min	1–5 mg/kg/d q6–8h (short acting); q12–24h (time release); when used for potentially life-threatening arrhythmia (LQTS), q12h recommended	100 maternal blood level	C (IUGR; hypoglycemia; respiratory depression)	64% maternal plasma level; safe for infant	PSVT; rate control in AF1 and AF; VT in normal heart; LQTS
CLASS III Amiodarone	8–107 d; biphasic elimination (plasma level 50% after 10 d; rebounds days 12–21; falls again)	Load: 2–5 mg/kg over 5–30 min (repeat as needed: then 0.4–1.0 mg/kg/h)	Load: 10 mg/kg/d q8–12h (up to 60 mg/kg/d × ≤ 3 d, if necessary); then, 5 mg/kg/d × 2 mos; then, wean to 2.5 mg/kg/d	10–25 maternal blood level	D (prematurity 12%; IUGR 21%; hypothyroidism 9%)	Exceeds maternal plasma level; safe for infant	PSVT; AF1; AF; VT; JET; AET
Sotalol	9.5 h (children); 7–18 h (adult); β-blocking effect longer	Not available	2–8 mg/kg/d (2–4 mg/kg/d) for neonates, 3–6 mg/kg/d for children <6 y and 2–4 mg/kg/d for children >6 y or 40–250 mg/m2/d q8–12h; maximum dose 640 mg/d; usual adult starting dose: 160 mg/d	5–100 maternal blood level	B (asymptomatic bradycardia)	Concentrated (5.4:1); may not be important	PSVT; AF1; AF; VT

(continued)

TABLE 47-3

Use of Antiarrhythmic Drugs in Children *(continued)*

DRUG	HALF-LIFE	INTRAVENOUS DOSING	ORAL DOSING	TRANS-PLACENTAL PASSAGE (%)	PREGNANCY CATEGORY/ SAFETY FOR FETUS	PASSAGE IN BREAST MILK	INDICATIONS
CLASS IV Verapamil	2.5–7 h (infancy); 5–12 h with chronic use	0.1 mg/kg over 2 min (max: 10 mg); infusion: 5 μ/kg/min; not <1 y of age	3–10 mg/kg/d q8h (short-acting); q day (time release)	15–50 maternal level	C	23–100% maternal blood level; safe for infant	PSVT; rate control in AFl and AF; fetal PSVT; occasional forms of VT in normal heart
DIGOXIN Digoxin	61–170 h (premature); 35–45 h (term); 18–25 h (infant); 35 h (child); 38–48 h (adult)	Oral load (3 doses/16–24 h): 30 µg/kg (premature), 35 (term), 40–50 (<2 y), 30–40 (>2 y); maintenance: 1/4 load ÷ q12h; intravenous dose: 75–80% oral		Similar to maternal level	C	Similar to maternal blood level; safe for infant	PSVT; fetal PSVT

AET, atrial ectopic tachycardia; AF, atrial fibrillation; AFl, atrial flutter; CAT, chaotic atrial tachycardia; CHD, congenital heart disease; IUGR, intrauterine growth rate; JET, junctional ectopic tachycardia; LQTS, long QT syndrome; PJRT, permanent form of junctional reciprocating tachycardia; PSVT, paroxysmal supraventricular tachycardia; VT, ventricular tachycardia. United States FDA Pregnancy Categories: A, Controlled studies in women fail to demonstrate a risk to the fetus in the first trimester, and the possibility of fetal harm appears remote. B, Animal studies do not indicate a risk to the fetus and there are no controlled human studies, or animal studies do show an adverse effect on the fetus but well-controlled studies in pregnant women have failed to demonstrate a risk to the fetus. C, Studies have shown that the drug exerts animal teratogenic or embryocidal effects, but there are no controlled studies in women, or no studies are available in either animals or women. D, Positive evidence of human fetal risk exists, but benefits in certain situations (e.g., life-threatening situations or serious diseases for which safer drugs cannot be used or are ineffective) may make use of the drug acceptable despite its risks. X, Studies in animals or humans demonstrate fetal abnormalities or there is evidence of fetal risk based on human experience, or both, and the risk clearly outweighs any possible benefit.

uretic-induced hypokalemia) is similar to that in adults and is not further discussed.

Table 47–3 presents commonly available antiarrhythmic drugs (including digoxin); they are organized according to the Vaughan-Williams classification. Important considerations regarding drug use in the pediatric age range that are different from adults (half-life, intravenous dosing, oral dosing), or that are specific to infants (transplacental passage, safety to the fetus, and passage in breast milk), are also included.

【 】 CATHETER ABLATION

Transcatheter delivery of radiofrequency energy to arrhythmia substrates was shown to be efficacious in children initially through small series in the early 1990s. The Pediatric Radiofrequency Registry of North America subsequently provided the first large experience with this treatment. In the late 1990s, Van Hare organized the Prospective Assessment of Pediatric Catheter Ablation project (so-called *PAPCA*) to further define efficacy and safety.[63] Cryothermal catheter ablation was first reported in 1999 and has been used for ablation of tachyarrhythmia substrates in pediatric patients.[51,64] This section focuses on catheter ablation in children, radiofrequency and cryothermal, and how its application is different from that in adults.

Patient Size and Physiology

Catheter design and the electronics of radiofrequency energy delivery have heretofore limited the size of the catheter tip to no smaller than 3 mm in length of the distal electrode and no smaller than 5 French in circumference. Hence, lesion size cannot be focused any smaller than about 3 mm in diameter and depth. Studies in a maturing lamb model demonstrated substantial growth of scar depth and width at the ventricular level; increase of scar width only at the atrial level; and only minimal scar growth when lesions were delivered at the annulus fibrosis. Similar studies have not yet been reported with cryothermal ablation. The potential for "collateral damage" is of greatest concern regarding the AV node and coronary arteries. In children who are younger than 3 years of age, the base of the Koch triangle is only 3 to 5 mm and the length is only 3 to 6 mm. Given that the minimal lesion size with radiofrequency ablation is comparable to these dimensions, septal accessory pathways and AV nodal reentrant tachycardia present particular risk for infants and young children. Cryothermal catheter ablation probably offers greater safety, but still may pose risk in smaller patients. Endocardial to coronary artery distances in children who are younger than 7 years of age are less than or equal to 4 mm in 76 percent and less than or equal to 5 mm in 96 percent. The shortest distance from endocardial surface to coronary artery appears to be in the region of the coronary sinus os and greatest in the right anteroseptal area.[65] Although reports of obvious clinical damage to coronary arteries from catheter ablation are few,[66,67] concern for longer-term coronary problems in children following ablation remain. Cryothermal ablation may offer more safety in this regard.[68]

The physics of radiofrequency energy delivery from an internal catheter to an external dispersion pad is also different from that in adults. Unlike adults, among patients with <1.5 m² body surface area, there is no correlation between patient size and impedance load. Therefore, applied power is similar to that for adults. It appears that thermistor- and thermocouple-linked closed-loop systems are as safe in children as they are in adults. Experience with irrigated tipped catheters in children is limited, but it is a promising modality in patients having complex atrial arrhythmias following Fontan operation in whom increased atrial wall thickness is a limiting factor for standard ablation catheters.[69]

Complete electrophysiologic testing and catheter ablation[70] can, if necessary, be performed in even the smallest patients, despite limited venous capacity by using creative catheter combinations. For example, atrial electrogram recording and pacing can be performed from an esophageal electrode catheter; three 2-French quadripolar electrode catheters can be placed through a single 7-French triple-lumen sheath or through a 5-French single lumen sheath; and a single catheter may be used for both right ventricular apical pacing and sensing and His bundle recording. The normal femoral vein can easily accommodate up to 5-mm net circumference (5 French) in children weighing >2.0 kg, 6 French if >3.0 kg, 7 French if >5 kg, 9 French if >10 kg, 11 French if >25 kg, and 14 French for larger patients. Venous obstruction has been reported when a total of 18 French (5 + 6 + 7) catheters were placed in children 8 to 21 years of age. Arterial damage is of greater concern and is largely preventable with the widespread use of the transseptal approach to the left side of the heart.

The coexistence of congenital heart defects presents additional concerns. Femoral venous access may be obviated by iliofemoral vein thrombosis as a result of prior catheterizations, or there may be congenital interruption of the suprarenal inferior vena cava. In these instances, inferior access to the atria by cannulation of a hepatic vein[71] or advancing catheters via the azygous vein[72] has allowed for successful catheter ablation.

In patients who are having complex congenital heart disease, complete knowledge of the cardiac anatomy is mandatory. This requires availability of prior echocardiograms, MRI or CT scans and surgical reports, use of biplane fluoroscopy, and capacity to perform venography, atriography, and ventriculography during electrophysiologic testing. The location of accessory pathways and AV nodes/His bundles may be predicted by knowledge of the anatomy, but the operator should be prepared to perform meticulous mapping. Intracardiac ultrasound and electroanatomic mapping techniques are emerging technologies whose usefulness in congenital heart disease is just being realized.[73,74]

Although radiation exposure during pediatric catheter ablation has decreased over time,[75] it is still a matter of concern.[76] The use of three-dimensional electroanatomic mapping has further reduced, and in some cases eliminated, radiation exposure.[77]

Other Considerations for Pediatric Catheter Ablation

Technical considerations aside, developmentally, children have varying degrees of comprehension of the procedure that they are about to undergo. Age-appropriate reading material (including coloring books), play therapy, and opportunities to speak with same-age patients who have undergone ablations are useful techniques to help children have an atraumatic experience. General anesthesia or deep sedation is usually used for the procedure. Sedation is preferred in cases of highly sensitive arrhythmias, such as atrial tachycardia. When general anesthesia is used, propofol and isoflurane are equally useful, and neither suppresses arrhythmia inducibility.[78] Propofol may slow AV node conduction velocity, and isoflurane increases the corrected QT interval.[78] An advantage of general anesthesia is that it permits muscle relaxation during the period of radiofrequency energy delivery, thus helping to prevent catheter dislodgement as may occur during spontaneous respiration. The phenomenon of "cryoadhesion" or fixation of the catheter to its point of endocardial contact once the catheter tip temperature is less than 32°F (0°C) plus the relative absence of pain during cryoenergy delivery compared with radiofrequency energy delivery make such strict immobilization less critical. The selection of sedation versus anesthesia should be individualized, but, in general, patients who are younger, or who have structural heart disease, coexisting medical problems, or potential airway obstruction, are at higher risk for sedation and are better candidates for anesthesia.

Indications for Catheter Ablation in Children

In May 2000, an Expert Consensus Conference was held by the North American Society for Pacing and Electrophysiology. The report from this conference was published in 2002 and established consensus recommendations for the performance of radiofrequency catheter ablation in pediatric patients;[79] Table 47–4 summarizes the recommendations. With continued refinement of radiofrequency catheter ablation and expanded use of cryothermal ablation, indications for these procedures continue to be debated in pediatric patients.[80] Radiofrequency ablation is more cost-effective than medical treatment for supraventricular tachycardia in children, with ablation cost equaling medical care cost after 5.1 years and being 3.4 times less after 20 years.[81] It is useful in pediatric patients with ventricular tachycardia.[82]

Results of Catheter Ablation in the Young

To date, the only large prospective analysis of pediatric patients undergoing radiofrequency catheter ablation for AV reciprocating or AV nodal reentrant tachycardias has been the PAPCA project.[83] There were 481 patients ranging in age from 0 to 21 years enrolled in this cohort, and patients with congenital heart disease were excluded. The overall acute success rate was 95.7 percent, ranging

---

TABLE 47–4

Indications for Radiofrequency Catheter Ablation in Pediatric Patients

Class I: There is consistent agreement and/or supportive data that catheter ablation is likely to be medically beneficial or helpful for the patient.
1. Wolff-Parkinson-White (WPW) syndrome following an episode of aborted sudden cardiac death.
2. The presence of WPW syndrome associated with syncope when there is a short preexcited R-R interval during atrial fibrillation (preexcited R-R interval, 250 milliseconds) or the antegrade effective refractory period of the accessory pathway measured during programmed electrical stimulation is <250 ms.
3. Chronic or recurrent supraventricular tachycardia (SVT) associated with ventricular dysfunction.
4. Recurrent ventricular tachycardia (VT) that is associated with hemodynamic compromise and is amenable to catheter ablation.

Class IIa: There is a divergence of opinion regarding the benefit or medical necessity of catheter ablation, the majority of opinions/data are in favor of the procedure.
1. Recurrent and/or symptomatic SVT refractory to conventional medical therapy and age >4 years.
2. Impending congenital heart surgery when vascular or chamber access may be restricted following surgery.
3. Chronic (occurring for >6 to 12 months following an initial event) or incessant SVT in the presence of normal ventricular function.
4. Chronic or frequent recurrences of intraatrial reentrant tachycardia (IART).
5. Palpitations with inducible sustained SVT during electrophysiological testing.

Class IIb: There is clear divergence of opinion regarding the need for the procedure.
1. Asymptomatic preexcitation (WPW pattern on an electrocardiograph), age >5 years, with no recognized tachycardia, when the risks and benefits of the procedure and arrhythmia have been clearly explained.
2. SVT, age >5 years, as an alternative to chronic antiarrhythmic therapy which has been effective in control of the arrhythmia.
3. SVT, age <5 years (including infants), when antiarrhythmic medications, including sotalol and amiodarone, are not effective or associated with intolerable side effects.
4. IART, one to three episodes per year, requiring medical intervention.
5. Atrioventricular node (AVN) ablation and pacemaker insertion as an alternative therapy for recurrent or intractable IART.
6. One episode of VT associated with hemodynamic compromise and which is amenable to catheter ablation.

Class III: There is agreement that catheter ablation is not medically indicated and/or the risk of the procedure may be greater than the benefit for the patient.
1. Asymptomatic WPW syndrome, age <5 years.
2. SVT controlled with conventional antiarrhythmic medications, age <5 years.
3. Nonsustained, paroxysmal VT, which is not considered incessant (i.e., present on monitoring for hours at a time or on nearly all strips recorded during any 1-hour period) and where no concomitant ventricular dysfunction exists.
4. Episodes of nonsustained SVT that do not require other therapy and/or are minimally symptomatic.

from 97.8 percent for left free-wall pathways to 90.8 percent for right free-wall pathways. Complications from the electrophysiology study itself occurred in 4.2 percent of patients and from catheter ablation, in 4 percent. Recurrence was seen in 7 percent, 9.2 percent, and 10.7 percent of the patients at 2, 6, and 12 months after ablation, respectively. Recurrence rate varied by arrhythmia substrate with 24.6 percent recurrence for right septal pathways, 15.8 percent for right free-wall, 9.3 percent for left free-wall, 4.8 percent for left septal, and 4.8 percent for AV nodal reentry.[84] Other reports have confirmed similar results of radiofrequency catheter ablation in children.[85,86] Cryothermal catheter ablation in pediatric patients has been applied to treatment of all tachyarrhythmia substrates, but has been most widely used in situations where radiofrequency ablation is particularly problematic like AV nodal reentry and septal accessory pathways. Several case series from single institutions and one multicenter study have been reported. Acute success from ablation of AV nodal reentry has ranged from 83 to 96 percent and of AV reentry from 60 to 92 percent. Recurrence of tachycardia substrate after successful cryoablation has been reported to range from 8 to 45 percent in relatively short-term followup.[87–93]

【 】 PACEMAKERS AND IMPLANTABLE CARDIOVERTER-DEFIBRILLATORS IN CHILDREN

Technologic advances in implanted cardiac rhythm management devices and lead hardware have benefited children greatly, especially as a result of significant downsizing of pulse generators and lead bodies.[94] Consequently, pediatric electrophysiologists have shifted investigative efforts to other areas: cellular, tissue, and whole-organ responses to artificial pacing of the immature heart; optimization of pacing modes in children with congenital heart disease; and development of low-threshold, high-impedance epicardial leads for infants and for children with intracardiac shunts or single-ventricle physiology. This section considers pediatric pacing and how it differs from that in adults.

Indications for Pacing in Children

Indications for permanent pacing in children, adolescents, and patients with congenital heart disease appear in the ACC/AHA/North American Society for Pacing and Electrophysiology *2002 Guideline Update for Implantation of Cardiac Pacemakers and Antiarrhythmia Devices*.[21] These indications are categorized according to consensus of opinion, and each recommendation is annotated to indicate degree of support in the scientific literature. These recommendations appear as Table 47–2.

Psychologic and Social Aspects of Pacing in the Young

The need for a permanent pacemaker may be viewed as a chronic disease by a child or teenager. When compared to a group of children having undergone congenital heart surgery but not requiring pacemaker implantation, and to a group of healthy controls, children with pacemakers demonstrated healthy psychosocial adaptation, using denial and intellectualization to deal with stresses. Although they largely maintained a healthy self-image, they were

sensitive to very real negative peer responses. In pediatric patients with cardiac pacemakers, an increased requirement for psychiatric treatment related to disturbed family dynamics as well as abnormal body images, compared with controls, has been demonstrated. Furthermore, compared with adults, children and teenagers have greater difficulty incorporating their pacemaker into their body image. These studies underscore the importance of normalization of the other aspects of the lifestyle of a child with a pacemaker, at least within the constraints of safety considerations. Interest in sports participation among school-age children has increased dramatically since the 1960s. There is general agreement that contact sports, such as wrestling, American football, and rugby, are forbidden in children with pacemakers. We view high-endurance activities, such as basketball, soccer, track, and swimming, as permissible in children who are not "pacemaker dependent." This may be defined by the clinical demonstration that a stable escape rate compatible with life will not occur following interruption of pacing. (We expect a 1- to 5-second pause following abrupt loss of capture as a consequence of overdrive suppression, and do not consider that observation, alone, as life-threatening.) Placement of a second pacing system may be indicated in some patients with extreme pacemaker dependence.[95] All families must be informed of the increased risk of transvenous lead damage by activities that require excessive movement about the shoulders, such as swimming, basketball, and gymnastics.

Implantable Cardioverter/Defibrillators in Children

The treatment of conditions predisposing to sudden cardiac death is discussed in Chapter 49, according to disease type. Treatment algorithms for conditions in which life-threatening ventricular tachyarrhythmias exist have changed because of the advances in implantable cardioverter-defibrillator technology. It has been clearly shown that these devices permit greater longevity among affected adults who have acceptable cardiac function.[96] Alexander et al. reported the use of implanted defibrillators in 76 children and young adults with congenital heart disease.[97] Device therapy was shown to effectively manage malignant arrhythmias, but the complications of inappropriate shocks[98] and arrhythmia storm emphasize the need for concomitant medical and ablative therapy. As with cardiac pacing in pediatric patients, implantable cardioverter-defibrillator lead failure was relatively frequent.[97] Because of these advances, implantable cardioverter-defibrillators are now considered first- or second-line therapy for children and teenagers who are clearly at risk for sudden cardiac death based on the occurrence of resuscitated events in the presence of certain chronic cardiac conditions[99] such as dilated or hypertrophic cardiomyopathy, primary ventricular fibrillation, unstable ventricular tachycardia and congenital heart disease, and the long QT syndrome. Implantable cardioverter-defibrillator placement in pediatric and congenital heart disease patients who are awaiting heart transplantation is particularly beneficial.[100] The role of the implantable cardioverter-defibrillator in combination with antiarrhythmic drugs is an area of ongoing investigation.

Technically, active can devices may be placed in a subpectoral position in children as small as 25-kg body weight. In smaller children, adequate defibrillation thresholds have been demonstrated when the defibrillator is placed subcutaneously in the left upper quadrant of the abdomen, and the lead is tunneled to the left subclavian vein. For infants and toddlers, creative patch placement subcutaneously and/or superficial to the pericardium is efficacious and avoids complications associated with epicardial patch placement.[101,102] Leads having coils designed for transvenous use may also be used in an epicardial or extracardiac thoracic position and may provide adequate defibrillation thresholds.[103]

Children with implantable cardioverter-defibrillators not only have the emotional burden of knowing that they have an implanted artificial device, but must also deal with the underlying and presumably life-threatening cardiovascular condition. Not surprisingly, nearly half of all adolescents having implantable cardioverter-defibrillators show signs of depression and/or anxiety.[104]

REFERENCES

1. Anderson RH. The conduction tissues in congenitally corrected transposition. *Ann Thorac Surg* 2004;77:2163–2166.
2. Sharland G, Tingay R, Jones A, Simpson J. Atrioventricular and ventriculoarterial discordance (congenitally corrected transposition of the great arteries): echographic features, associations, and outcomes in 34 fetuses. *Heart* 2005;91:1453–1458.
3. Chiappa E, Micheletti A, Sciaronne A, Botta G, Abbruzzese P. The prenatal diagnosis of short-term outcome for patients with congenitally corrected transposition. *Cardiol Young* 2004;14:265–276.
4. Kofali G, Elsharshari H, Ozer S, Celiker A, Ozme S, Demiricin M. Incidence of dysrhythmias in congenitally corrected transposition of the great arteries. *Turk J Pediatr* 2002;44:219–223.
5. Hager A, Zrenner B, Brodherr-Heberlein S, Steinbauer-Rosenthal I, Schreieck J, Hess J. Congenital and surgically acquired Wolff-Parkinson-White syndrome in patients with tricuspid atresia. *J Thorac Cardiovasc Surg* 2005;130:48–53.
6. Walker RE, Mayer JE, Alexander ME, Walsh EP, Berul CI. Paucity of sinus node dysfunction following repair of sinus venosus defects in children. *Am J Cardiol* 2001;15:1223–1226.
7. Roos-Hesselink JW, Meijboom FJ, Spitaels SEC, et al. Excellent survival and low incidence of arrhythmias, stroke and heart failure after surgical ASD closure at young age. *Eur Heart J* 2003;24:190–197.
8. Oliver JM, Gallego P, Gonzalez A, Benito F, Mesa JM, Sobrino JA. Predisposing conditions for atrial fibrillation in atrial septal defect with and without operative closure. *Am J Cardiol* 2002;89:39–43.
9. Magnin-Poull I, De Chillou C, Miljoen H, Andronache M, Aliot F. Mechanism of right atrial tachycardia occurring late after closure of atrial septal defects. *J Cardiovasc Electrophysiol* 2005;16:681–687.
10. Suda K, Raboisson MJ, Piette E, Dahdah NS, Miro J. Reversible AV block associated with closure of atrial septal defects using the Amplatzer device. *J Am Coll Cardiol* 2004;43:1677–1682.
11. Chessa M, Carminati M, Butera G, et al. Early and late complications associated with transcatheter occlusion of secundum atrial septal defect. *J Am Coll Cardiol* 2002;39:1061–1065.
12. Silversides CK, Siu SC, McLaughlin PR, et al. Symptomatic atrial arrhythmias and transcatheter closure of atrial septal defects in adult patients. *Heart* 2004;90:1194–1198.
13. Arora R, Trehan V, Thakur AK, Mehta V, Sengupta PP, Nigam M. Transcatheter closure of congenital muscular ventricular septal defect. *J Interv Cardiol* 2004;17:109–115.
14. Thanopoulos BD, Rigby ML. Outcome of transcatheter closure of muscular ventricular septal defects with the Amplatzer ventricular septal defect occluder. *Heart* 2005;91:513–516.
15. Yip WC, Zimmerman F, Hijazi ZM. Heart block and empirical therapy after transcatheter closure of perimembranous ventricular septal defect. *Catheter Cardiovasc Interv* 2005;66:436–441.
16. Sugimoto S, Takagi N, Hachiro Y, Abe T. High frequency of arrhythmias after Fontan operation indicates earlier anticoagulant therapy. *Intern J Cardiol* 2001;78:33–39.
17. Ghai A, Harris L, Harrison DA, Webb GD, Siu SC. Outcomes of late atrial tachyarrhythmias in adults after the Fontan operation. *J Am Coll Cardiol* 2001;37:585–592.
18. Azackie A, McCrindle BW, Van Arsdell G, et al. Extracardiac conduit versus lateral tunnel cavopulmonary connections at a single institution: Impact on outcomes. *J Thorac Cardiovasc Surg* 2001;122:1219–1228.

19. Stamm C, Friehs I, Mayer JE Jr, et al. Long-term results of the lateral tunnel Fontan operation. *J Thorac Cardiovasc Surg* 2001;121:28–41.
20. Ovroutski S, Dahnert I, Alexi-Meskishvili V, Numberg JH, Hetzer R, Lange PE. Preliminary analysis of arrhythmias after the Fontan operation with extracardiac conduit compared with intra-atrial lateral tunnel. *Thorac Cardiovasc Surg* 2001;49:334–337.
21. Gregoratos G, Abrams J, Epstein AE, et al. ACC/AHA/NASPE 2002 guideline update for implantation of cardiac pacemakers and antiarrhythmia devices—summary article: a report of the American College of Cardiology/American Heart Association Task Force on Practice Guidelines (ACC/AHA/NASPE Committee to Update the 1998, Pacemaker Guidelines). *J Am Coll Cardiol* 2002;40:1703–1719.
22. Cohen MI, Rhodes LA, Wernovsky G, et al. Atrial pacing: an alternative treatment for protein-losing enteropathy after the Fontan operation. *J Thorac Cardiovasc Surg* 2001;121:582–583.
23. Varma C, Warr MR, Hendles AL, Paul NS, Webb GD, Therrien J. Prevalence of "silent" pulmonary emboli in adults after the Fontan operation. *J Am Coll Cardiol* 2003;41:2252–2258.
24. Triedman JK, Alexander ME, Love BA. Influence of patient factors and ablative technologies on outcomes of radiofrequency catheter ablation of intra-atrial reentrant tachycardia in patients with congenital heart disease. *J Am Coll Cardiol* 2002;39:1827–1835.
25. Hokanson JS, Moller JH. Significance of early transient complete heart block as a predictor of sudden death late after operative correction of tetralogy of Fallot. *Am J Cardiol* 2001;87:1271–1277.
26. Triedman JK, Alexander ME, Berul CI, Bevilacqua LM, Walsh EP. Electroanatomic mapping of entrainment and exit zones in patients with repaired congenital heart disease and intraatrial reentry tachycardia. *Circulation* 2001;103:2060–2065.
27. Nakagawa H, Shah N, Matsudaira K, et al. Characterization of reentrant circuit in macroreentrant right atrial tachycardia after surgical repair of congenital heart disease: isolated channels between scars allow "focal" ablation. *Circulation* 2001;103:699–709.
28. Kannankeril PJ, Anderson ME, Rottman JN, Wathen MS, Fish FA. Frequency of late recurrence of intra-atrial reentry tachycardia after radiofrequency ablation in patients with congenital heart disease. *Am J Cardiol* 2003;92:879–881.
29. Nehgme RA, Carboni MP, Care J, Murphy JD. Transthoracic percutaneous access for electroanatomic mapping and catheter ablation of atrial tachycardias in patients with a lateral tunnel Fontan. *Heart Rhythm* 2006;3:37–43.
30. Anderson HO, deLeval MR, Tsang VT, Elliott MJ, Anderson RH, Cook AC. Is complete heart block after surgical closure of ventricular septum still an issue? *Ann Thorac Surg* 2006;82:948–956.
31. Abd El Rahman MY, Hui W, Yigitbasi M, et al. Detection of left ventricular asynchrony in patients with right bundle branch block after repair of tetralogy of Fallot using tissue Doppler imaging-derived strain. *J Am Coll Cardiol* 2005;45:915–921.
32. D'Andrea A, Caso P, Sarubbi B, et al. Right ventricular myocardial activation delay in adult patients with right bundle-branch block late after repair of tetralogy of Fallot. *Eur J Echocardiogr* 2004;5:123–131.
33. Batra AS, Wells WJ, Hinoki KW, Stanton RA, Silka MJ. Late recovery of atrioventricular conduction after pacemaker implantation for complete heart block associated with surgery for congenital heart disease. *J Thorac Cardiovasc Surg* 2003;125:1291–1293.
34. Khairy P, Landzberg MJ, Gatzoulis MA, et al. Value of programmed ventricular stimulation after tetralogy of Fallot repair: a multicenter study. *Circulation* 2004;109:1994–2000.
35. Kleinman CS, Nehgme RA. Cardiac arrhythmias in the human fetus. *Pediatr Cardiol* 2004;25(3):234–251.
36. Raboisson MJ, Fouron JC, Sonesson SE, Nyman M, Proulx F, Gamache S. Fetal Doppler echocardiographic diagnosis and successful steroid therapy of Luciani-Wenckebach phenomenon and endocardial fibroelastosis related to maternal anti-Ro and anti-La antibodies. *J Am Soc Echocardiogr* 2005;18(4):375–380.
37. Jaeggi ET, Silverman ED, Yoo SJ, Kingdom J. Is immune-mediated complete fetal atrioventricular block reversible by transplacental dexamethasone therapy? *Ultrasound Obstet Gynecol* 2004;23(6):602–605.
38. Fesslova V, Mannarino S, Salice P, et al. Neonatal lupus: fetal myocarditis progressing to atrioventricular block in triplets. *Lupus* 2003;12(10):775–778.
39. Askanase AD, Friedman DM, Copel J, Dische MR, Dubin A, Starc TJ, et al. Spectrum and progression of conduction abnormalities in infants born to mothers with anti-SSA/Ro-SSB/La antibodies. *Lupus* 2002;11(3):145–151.
40. Yang CH, Chen JY, Lee SC, Luo SF. Successful preventive treatment of congenital heart block during pregnancy in a woman with systemic lupus erythe-

matosus and anti-Sjögren's syndrome A/Ro antibody. *J Microbiol Immunol Infect* 2005;38(5):365–369.

41. Breur JM, Visser GH, Kruize AA, Stoutenbeek P, Meijboom EJ. Treatment of fetal heart block with maternal steroid therapy: case report and review of the literature. *Ultrasound Obstet Gynecol* 2004;24(4):467–472.

42. Lee PC, Chen SA, Chiang CE, Tai CT, Yu WC, Hwang B. Clinical and electrophysiological characteristics in children with atrioventricular nodal reentrant tachycardia. *Pediatr Cardiol* 2003;24(1):6–9.

43. Blurton DJ, Dubin AM, Chiesa NA, Van Hare GF, Collins KK. Characterizing dual atrioventricular nodal physiology in pediatric patients with atrioventricular nodal reentrant tachycardia. *J Cardiovasc Electrophysiol* 2006;17(6):638–644.

44. Pappone C, Santinelli V, Rosanio S, et al. Usefulness of invasive electrophysiologic testing to stratify the risk of arrhythmic events in asymptomatic patients with Wolff-Parkinson-White pattern: results from a large prospective long-term follow-up study. *J Am Coll Cardiol* 2003;41(2):239–244.

45. Cnota JF, Ross JE, Knilans TK, Epstein MR. Does intermittent accessory pathway block during slow sinus atrial rhythm always imply a low risk for rapid AV conduction of preexcited atrial fibrillation? *Cardiology* 2002;98(1–2):106–108.

46. Campbell RM, Strieper MJ, Frias PA, Collins KK, Van Hare GF, Dubin AM. Survey of current practice of pediatric electrophysiologists for asymptomatic Wolff-Parkinson-White syndrome. *Pediatrics* 2003;111(3):e245–e247.

47. Niksch AL, Dubin AM. Risk stratification in the asymptomatic child with Wolff-Parkinson-White syndrome. *Curr Opin Cardiol* 2006;21(3):205–207.

48. Salerno JC, Kertesz NJ, Friedman RA, Fenrich AL Jr. Clinical course of atrial ectopic tachycardia is age-dependent: results and treatment in children <3 or > or = 3 years of age. *J Am Coll Cardiol* 2004;43(3):438–444.

49. Horenstein MS, Saarel E, Dick M, Karpawich PP. Reversible symptomatic dilated cardiomyopathy in older children and young adolescents due to primary non-sinus supraventricular tachyarrhythmias. *Pediatr Cardiol* 2003;24(3):274–279.

50. Drago F, Silvetti MS, Mazza A, et al. Permanent junctional reciprocating tachycardia in infants and children: effectiveness of medical and non-medical treatment. *Ital Heart J* 2001;2(6):456–461.

51. Gaita F, Montefusco A, Riccardi R, et al. Cryoenergy catheter ablation: a new technique for treatment of permanent junctional reciprocating tachycardia in children. *J Cardiovasc Electrophysiol* 2004;15(3):263–268.

52. Bradley DJ, Fischbach PS, Law IH, Serwer GA, Dick M 2nd. The clinical course of multifocal atrial tachycardia in infants and children. *J Am Coll Cardiol* 2001;38(2):401–408.

53. Sarubbi B, Musto B, Ducceschi V, et al. Congenital junctional ectopic tachycardia in children and adolescents: a 20, year experience based study. *Heart* 2002;88(2):188–190.

54. Fukuhara H, Nakamura Y, Ohnishi T. Atrial pacing during radiofrequency ablation of junctional ectopic tachycardia—a useful technique for avoiding atrioventricular bloc. *Jpn Circ J* 2001;65(3):242–244.

55. Bae EJ, Kang SJ, Noh CI, Choi JY, Yun YS. A case of congenital junctional ectopic tachycardia: diagnosis and successful radiofrequency catheter ablation in infancy. *Pacing Clin Electrophysiol* 2005;28(3):254–257.

56. Batra AS, Chun DS, Johnson TR, et al. A prospective analysis of the incidence and risk factors associated with junctional ectopic tachycardia following surgery for congenital heart disease. *Pediatr Cardiol* 2006;27(1):51–55.

57. Delaney JW, Moltedo JM, Dziura JD, Kopf GS, Snyder CS. Early postoperative arrhythmias after pediatric cardiac surgery. *J Thorac Cardiovasc Surg* 2006;131(6):1296–1300.

58. Hoffman TM, Bush DM, Wernovsky G, et al. Postoperative junctional ectopic tachycardia in children: incidence, risk factors, and treatment. *Ann Thorac Surg* 2002;74(5):1607–1611.

59. Gengsakul A, Potts JE, Sandhu A, et al. Documenting junctional ectopic tachycardia following pediatric open heart surgery. *J Med Assoc Thai* 2005;88 Suppl 3:S214–S222.

60. Laird WP, Snyder CS, Kertesz NJ, Friedman RA, Miller D, Fenrich AL. Use of intravenous amiodarone for postoperative junctional ectopic tachycardia in children. *Pediatr Cardiol* 2003;24(2):133–137.

61. Walker GM, McLeod K, Brown KL, Franklin O, Goldman AP, Davis C. Extracorporeal life support as a treatment of supraventricular tachycardia in infants. *Pediatr Crit Care Med* 2003;4(1):52–54.

62. Pfammatter JP, Pavlovic M, Bauersfeld U. Impact of curative ablation on pharmacologic management in children with reentrant supraventricular tachycardias. *Int J Cardiol* 2004;94(2–3):279–282.

63. Van Hare GF, Carmelli D, Smith WM, et al. Prospective assessment after pediatric cardiac ablation: design and implementation of the multicenter study. *Pacing Clin Electrophysiol* 2002;25(3):332–341.

64. Perry JC. State-of-the-art pediatric interventional electrophysiology: transvenous cryoablation establishes its niche. *Heart Rhythm* 2006;3(3):259–260.

65. Al-Ammouri I, Perry JC. Proximity of coronary arteries to the atrioventricular valve annulus in young patients and implications for ablation procedures. *Am J Cardiol* 2006;97(12):1752–1755.

66. Weiss C, Becker J, Hoffmann M, Willems S. Can radiofrequency current isthmus ablation damage the right coronary artery? Histopathological findings following the use of a long (8 mm) tip electrode. *Pacing Clin Electrophysiol* 2002;25(5):860–862.

67. Sassone B, Leone O, Martinelli GN, Di Pasquale G. Acute myocardial infarction after radiofrequency catheter ablation of typical atrial flutter: histopathological findings and etiopathogenetic hypothesis. *Ital Heart J* 2004;5(5):403–407.

68. Lustgarten DL, Bell S, Hardin N, Calame J, Spector PS. Safety and efficacy of epicardial cryoablation in a canine model. *Heart Rhythm* 2005;2(1):82–90.

69. Blaufox AD, Numan MT, Laohakunakorn P, Knick B, Paul T, Saul JP. Catheter tip cooling during radiofrequency ablation of intra-atrial reentry: effects on power, temperature, and impedance. *J Cardiovasc Electrophysiol* 2002;13(8):783–787.

70. Kolditz DP, Blom NA, Bokenkamp R, Schalij MJ. Low-energy radiofrequency catheter ablation as therapy for supraventricular tachycardia in a premature neonate. *Eur J Pediatr* 2005;164(9):559–562.

71. Sreeram N. Transhepatic approach for catheter interventions in infants and children with congenital heart disease. *Clin Res Cardiol* 2006;95(6):329–333.

72. Kilic A, Amasyali B, Kose S, Aytemir K, Kursaklioglu H, Lenk MK. Successful catheter ablation of a right-sided accessory pathway in a child with interruption of the inferior vena cava and azygos continuation. *Int Heart J* 2005;46(3):537–541.

73. Samii SM, Cohen MH. Ablation of tachyarrhythmias in pediatric patients. *Curr Opin Cardiol* 2004;19(1):64–67.

74. Van Hare GF, Dubin AM, Collins KK. Invasive electrophysiology in children: state of the art. *J Electrocardiol* 2002;35 Suppl:165–174.

75. Kugler JD, Danford DA, Houston KA, Felix G. Pediatric radiofrequency catheter ablation registry success, fluoroscopy time, and complication rate for supraventricular tachycardia: comparison of early and recent eras. *J Cardiovasc Electrophysiol* 2002;13(4):336–341.

76. Campbell RM, Strieper MJ, Frias PA, et al. Quantifying and minimizing radiation exposure during pediatric cardiac catheterization. *Pediatr Cardiol* 2005;26(1):29–33.

77. Drago F, Silvetti MS, Di Pino A, Grutter G, Bevilacqua M, Leibovich S. Exclusion of fluoroscopy during ablation treatment of right accessory pathway in children. *J Cardiovasc Electrophysiol* 2002;13(8):778–782.

78. Erb TO, Kanter RJ, Hall JM, Gan TJ, Kern FH, Schulman SR. Comparison of electrophysiologic effects of propofol and isoflurane-based anesthetics in children undergoing radiofrequency catheter ablation for supraventricular tachycardia. *Anesthesiology* 2002;96(6):1386–1394.

79. Friedman RA, Walsh EP, Silka MJ, et al. NASPE Expert Consensus Conference: radiofrequency catheter ablation in children with and without congenital heart disease. Report of the writing committee. North American Society of Pacing and Electrophysiology. *Pacing Clin Electrophysiol* 2002;25(6):1000–1017.

80. Campbell RM, Strieper MJ, Frias PA. The role of radiofrequency ablation for pediatric supraventricular tachycardia. *Minerva Pediatr* 2004;56(1):63–72.

81. Vida VL, Calvimontes GS, Macs MO, Aparicio P, Barnoya J, Castaneda AR. Radiofrequency catheter ablation of supraventricular tachycardia in children and adolescents : feasibility and cost-effectiveness in a low-income country. *Pediatr Cardiol* 2006;27(4):434–439.

82. Laohakunakorn P, Paul T, Knick B, Blaufox AD, Long B, Saul JP. Ventricular tachycardia in nonpostoperative pediatric patients: role of radiofrequency catheter ablation. *Pediatr Cardiol* 2003;24(2):154–160.

83. Van Hare GF, Javitz H, Carmelli D, et al. Prospective assessment after pediatric cardiac ablation: demographics, medical profiles, and initial outcomes. *J Cardiovasc Electrophysiol* 2004;15(7):759–770.

84. Van Hare GF, Javitz H, Carmelli D, et al. Prospective assessment after pediatric cardiac ablation: recurrence at 1 year after initially successful ablation of supraventricular tachycardia. *Heart Rhythm* 2004;1(2):188–196.

85. Bae EJ, Ban JE, Lee JA, et al. Pediatric radiofrequency catheter ablation: results of initial 100 consecutive cases including congenital heart anomalies. *J Korean Med Sci* 2005;20(5):740–746.

86. Celiker A, Kafali G, Karagoz T, Ceviz N, Ozer S. The results of electrophysiological study and radio-frequency catheter ablation in pediatric patients with tachyarrhythmia. *Turk J Pediatr* 2003;45(3):209–216.

87. Papez AL, Al-Ahdab M, Dick M 2nd, Fischbach PS. Transcatheter cryotherapy for the treatment of supraventricular tachyarrhythmias in children: a single center experience. *J Interv Card Electrophysiol* 2006.

88. Collins KK, Dubin AM, Chiesa NA, Avasarala K, Van Hare GF. Cryoablation versus radiofrequency ablation for treatment of pediatric atrioventricular nodal reentrant tachycardia: initial experience with 4-mm cryocatheter. *Heart Rhythm* 2006;3(5):564–570.

89. Miyazaki A, Blaufox AD, Fairbrother DL, Saul JP. Cryo-ablation for septal tachycardia substrates in pediatric patients: mid-term results. *J Am Coll Cardiol* 2005;45(4):581–588.

90. Kirsh JA, Gross GJ, O'Connor S, Hamilton RM. Transcatheter cryoablation of tachyarrhythmias in children: initial experience from an international registry. *J Am Coll Cardiol* 2005;45(1):133–136.

91. Kriebel T, Broistedt C, Kroll M, Sigler M, Paul T. Efficacy and safety of cryo-energy in the ablation of atrioventricular reentrant tachycardia substrates in children and adolescents. *J Cardiovasc Electrophysiol* 2005;16(9):960–966.

92. Drago F, De Santis A, Grutter G, Silvetti MS. Transvenous cryothermal catheter ablation of re-entry circuit located near the atrioventricular junction in pediatric patients: efficacy, safety, and midterm follow-up. *J Am Coll Cardiol* 2005;45(7):1096–1103.

93. Bar-Cohen Y, Cecchin F, Alexander ME, Berul CI, Triedman JK, Walsh EP. Cryoablation for accessory pathways located near normal conduction tissues or within the coronary venous system in children and young adults. *Heart Rhythm* 2006;3(3):253–258.

94. Walsh EP, Cecchin F. Recent advances in pacemaker and implantable defibrillator therapy for young patients. *Curr Opin Cardiol* 2004;19(2):91–96.

95. Villain E, Eliasson H, Sidi D. Redundant pacing in a child. *Pacing Clin Electrophysiol* 2004;27(8):1161–1163.

96. Chatrath R, Porter CB, Ackerman MJ. Role of transvenous implantable cardioverter-defibrillators in preventing sudden cardiac death in children, adolescents, and young adults. *Mayo Clin Proc* 2002;77(3):226–231.

97. Alexander ME, Cecchin F, Walsh EP, Triedman JK, Bevilacqua LM, Berul CI. Implications of implantable cardioverter defibrillator therapy in congenital heart disease and pediatrics. *J Cardiovasc Electrophysiol* 2004;15(1):72–76.

98. Korte T, Koditz H, Niehaus M, Paul T, Tebbenjohanns J. High incidence of appropriate and inappropriate ICD therapies in children and adolescents with implantable cardioverter defibrillator. *Pacing Clin Electrophysiol* 2004;27(7):924–932.

99. Stefanelli CB, Bradley DJ, Leroy S, Dick M 2nd, Serwer GA, Fischbach PS. Implantable cardioverter defibrillator therapy for life-threatening arrhythmias in young patients. *J Interv Card Electrophysiol* 2002;6(3):235–244.

100. Dubin AM, Berul CI, Bevilacqua LM, et al. The use of implantable cardioverter-defibrillators in pediatric patients awaiting heart transplantation. *J Card Fail* 2003;9(5):375–379.

101. Ten Harkel AD, Witsenburg M, de Jong PL, Jordaens L, Wijman M, Wilde AA. Efficacy of an implantable cardioverter-defibrillator in a neonate with LQT3 associated arrhythmias. *Europace* 2005;7(1):77–84.

102. Kriebel T, Ruschewski W, Paul T. Implantation of an "extracardiac" internal cardioverter defibrillator in a 6-month-old infant. *Z Kardiol* 2005;94(6):415–418.

103. Stephenson EA, Batra AS, Knilans TK, et al. A multicenter experience with novel implantable cardioverter defibrillator configurations in the pediatric and congenital heart disease population. *J Cardiovasc Electrophysiol* 2006;17(1):41–46.

104. Eicken A, Kolb C, Lange S, et al. Implantable cardioverter defibrillator (ICD) in children. *Int J Cardiol* 2006;107(1):30–35.

PART 7

Syncope, Sudden Death, and Cardiopulmonary Resuscitation

CHAPTER 48

Diagnosis and Management of Syncope

Mark D. Carlson / Blair P. Grubb

INTRODUCTION

Syncope is a sudden loss of consciousness and postural tone caused by transient decreased cerebral blood flow; it is associated with spontaneous recovery. The occurrence of syncope in the general population, as reflected in the Framingham Study, is 3.0 percent in men and 3.5 percent in women in the general population.[1] As a general rule, the incidence of syncope increases with age. In the United States, 1 to 2 million patients are evaluated for syncope annually, 3 to 5 percent of emergency department visits, and 1 to 6 percent of urgent hospital admissions are for syncope.[2–5] As a result, management of syncope is associated with significant resource use and expense.[6–8]

Syncope can occur suddenly, without warning, or may be preceded by a prodrome of presyncope, including lightheadedness, dizziness but not true vertigo, nausea, a feeling of warmth, diaphoresis, and blurred or tunnel vision. Self-limited episodes of presyncope can occur in the absence of loss of consciousness.

CAUSES OF SYNCOPE

The causes of syncope include *cardiovascular disorders, disorders of vascular tone or blood volume,* and *cerebrovascular disorders.* The relative incidence of these categories varies with the clinical site from which the patients are selected; in hospitalized patients, syncope is most often a result of a cardiovascular disorder, whereas in the emergency room, other causes of syncope predominate.[4] In many cases, the cause of syncope may be multifactorial. Furthermore, in up to 50 percent of cases the cause of syncope cannot be determined with certainty even after a rigorous evaluation.

Recent studies document the widely divergent mortality risks associated with an episode of syncope, ranging from those that are benign to cardiac arrhythmias that are potentially lethal.[9] Syncope caused by cardiovascular disorders is associated with the highest risk for mortality, approaching 50 percent over 5 years and 30 percent in the first year after diagnosis.[4] Furthermore, among patients with certain cardiac diseases, including hypertrophic cardiomyopathy, the long QT syndrome, and others, those with syncope are at greater risk for mortality.[10] The mortality rate is lower among patients with syncope from other causes (30 percent over 5 years and <10 percent in the first year) but still substantial. Syncope that is not associated with cardiac disease and is of undetermined cause is usually associated with the lowest mortality risk (6 to 10 percent over 3 years and 24 percent over 5 years).[2,4,7] Syncope can impact quality of life for patients and their families, particularly when it occurs abruptly without warning and is recurrent or when it is likely to occur in relationship to certain activities. In such cases, patients may need to adjust their lifestyle or change occupation.

For prognostic and therapeutic reasons, it is important to distinguish syncope from other causes of transient loss of consciousness, including seizures, psychogenic seizures, hypoglycemia, pharmacologic agents and trauma. In some cases, this may prove difficult because reduced cerebral blood flow associated with syncope can cause tonic-clonic movements similar to those that occur with certain seizures. In one study, syncope had been misdiagnosed as seizures in 38 percent of patients who continued to have episodes despite adequate anticonvulsant therapy.[11]

CARDIOVASCULAR DISORDERS

Syncope can occur from either severe obstruction of cardiac output or disturbances of cardiac rhythm.[4,12–24] Obstructive lesions and arrhythmias frequently coexist; indeed, one abnormality may accentuate the effects of the other. Table 48–1 lists the cardiovascular disorders that may be associated with syncope.

Syncope Related to Obstruction of Cardiac Output

Obstruction to cardiac output in the left or right side of the heart may cause syncope. The relationship of syncope to exertion may provide clues to the etiology. Loss of consciousness during or immediately after exertion can occur with any of the cardiac causes of syncope but is particularly common and may be the presenting symptom in patients with certain obstructive lesions, including aortic stenosis and hypertrophic cardiomyopathy. Studies suggest that in such patients, failure of cardiac output to increase adequately during exercise together with a reflex decrease in peripheral vascular resistance may play a role.[25] Nonexertional syncope related to acute decreases in preload or afterload or to inotropic stimulation may also occur in either aortic stenosis or hypertrophic cardiomyopathy (see also Chap. 30). Transient arrhythmias can also induce syncope in patients with obstructive lesions. Syncope is an ominous sign in patients with hypertrophic cardiomyopathy, portending a significant risk for sudden cardiac death.[10,25–27] Syncope in patients with aortic stenosis suggests that the obstruction is severe.

Malfunction of a left-sided prosthetic heart valve can produce transient and profound obstruction to blood flow resulting in syncope (see Chap. 79). Mitral stenosis can produce cardiac syncope but usually does so only when tachycardia or other arrhythmias occur (see also Chap. 77). A left atrial myxoma may cause syncope by obstructing left ventricular filling. In some cases, the obstruction of left ventricular inflow is posturally induced.

Obstruction in the pulmonary vasculature as a result of pulmonary artery hypertension, pulmonary stenosis, or pulmonary embolism can cause syncope. Pulmonary embolism as a cause of syncope should be suspected in paraplegic patients and in those who have been at prolonged bedrest.[28,29] In tetralogy of Fallot, because the right ventricular outflow obstruction is often fixed, the magnitude of flow through the right-to-left shunt increases when systemic resistance falls during exertion. This shunting can result in marked arterial hypoxia, which may precipitate syncope. Cardiac tamponade, which affects both the right and the left sides of the heart, rarely causes syncope. The likelihood of syncope is increased by concomitant arrhythmias.

Syncope Related to Cardiac Arrhythmia

Arrhythmias are a common cause of syncope and must be considered in any patient, particularly when cardiac disease is present. Either extreme of ventricular rate (bradycardia or tachycardia) can depress cardiac output to the point of critical hypotension with cerebral hypoperfusion and syncope. The arrhythmias that produce syncope most often are caused by sinoatrial disease (bradycardia, exit block or pauses), high-grade atrioventricular (AV) block, and ventricular tachycardia. Although arrhythmias are usually secondary to disorders such as ischemic heart disease, cardiomyopathy, valvular heart disease, and primary conduction system disease, they can, on occasion occur in the absence of apparent heart disease.

Primary degenerative disease of the sinus node and the specialized conduction tissue is the most common cause of sinoatrial disease (*sick sinus syndrome;* see Chap. 40). The sick sinus syndrome may be manifested by persistent or episodic sinus bradycardia or sinoatrial exit block, often with impaired junctional escape rhythm. The presence of alternating sinus bradycardia or sinoatrial block with atrial tachyarrhythmias is referred to as the *bradycardia–tachycardia syndrome.* Syncope often occurs with asystole or bradycardia at the termination of tachycardia because of overdrive suppression of the sinoatrial and junctional pacemakers.[30] AV and intraventricular conduction defects are more prevalent in the sick sinus syndrome and, along with ventricular tachyarrhythmias, may be responsible for syncope in these patients.[21]

High-grade AV block may be a result of disease of either the AV node or the His-Purkinje system. Conduction block in the AV node is usually associated with a junctional pacemaker, a normal QRS complex, and a heart rate that can sustain blood pressure adequate to maintain consciousness, whereas AV block as a result of His-Purkinje system disease is usually associated with a wide complex idioventricular escape rhythm that may be too slow to maintain adequate blood pressure. Bifascicular block in the presence of a prolonged PR interval suggests that His-Purkinje system disease is present and is associated with a substantial risk of developing high-grade AV block and syncope. Progression to high-grade AV block in patients with bifascicular block and a normal PR interval is less common.

Sinus bradycardia, AV block, or cardiac asystole may be mediated by reflex vagal mechanisms and have been observed in a variety of disease states or during diagnostic procedures. Transient sinus bradycardia or AV block also can occur in apparently healthy young individuals, certain of whom may have mitral valve prolapse.[22]

Supraventricular tachyarrhythmias rarely cause syncope unless they occur in the presence of other abnormalities that decrease cerebral perfusion (decreased cardiac output because of structural heart disease, a neurocardiogenic reaction, disorders of vascular

TABLE 48–1

Cardiac Disorders Associated with Syncope

Obstructive
  Aortic stenosis
  Hypertrophic cardiomyopathy
  Mitral stenosis
  Prosthetic mitral or aortic valve malfunction
  Atrial myxoma
  Pulmonary embolism
  Pulmonary hypertension
  Tetralogy of Fallot
  Cardiac tamponade
Arrhythmic
  Sinoatrial disease
  Atrioventricular block
  Supraventricular tachyarrhythmias
  Ventricular tachycardia
  Pacemaker disorders

control, or reduced blood volume). As is the case for other causes of syncope, a neurocardiogenic reaction may be precipitated by the hemodynamic effects of arrhythmias.[31] In such cases, syncope may be related to vasomotor factors and not be solely a result of heart rate.[30,31] Syncope can occur in patients with the Wolff-Parkinson-White (WPW) syndrome who experience atrial fibrillation and a very rapid ventricular rate as a consequence of conduction across an accessory atrioventricular connection.

Ventricular tachycardia is the most common arrhythmic cause of syncope and often occurs in the setting of structural heart disease. In the United States, ventricular tachycardia is usually associated with previous myocardial infarction and depressed left ventricular ejection fraction, but it can occur also in nonischemic cardiomyopathy.

Ventricular tachycardia may also cause syncope in patients with normal left ventricular (LV) function (i.e., long QT syndrome, Brugada syndrome, right ventricular outflow tract ventricular tachycardia, arrhythmogenic right ventricular cardiomyopathy [ARVC], and idiopathic left ventricular tachycardia).[32–35] Syncope is considered to be an ominous sign, portending a high risk for sudden cardiac arrest in patients with long QT syndrome, Brugada syndrome, and ARVC.

Torsade de pointes can cause syncope in patients with either congenital or acquired long QT syndrome (see Chaps. 39 and 47). A normal QT interval does not preclude the diagnosis of long QT syndrome because prolongation of repolarization can be intermittent. In some heritable forms of the syndrome, QT prolongation and ventricular tachycardia can be triggered by exercise or a startle response.[36,37] Although a number of drugs can prolong ventricular repolarization, the most frequent causes of acquired long QT syndrome are antiarrhythmic drugs (types Ia and III) and electrolyte disorders (hypokalemia and hypomagnesemia). A pause preceding the onset of tachycardia is common, because the early afterdepolarizations thought to be responsible for torsade de pointes in some long QT syndrome patients are bradycardia dependent.[23,37,38]

A variety of other drugs may produce or aggravate arrhythmias, resulting in syncope or presyncope. Type Ic antiarrhythmic drugs may cause ventricular arrhythmias in patients with structural heart disease. β-Adrenoceptor antagonists, calcium-channel blockers, digoxin, sotalol, and amiodarone are some of the agents that most commonly cause significant sinus bradycardia or AV block. Theophylline and β agonists, used for therapy of chronic obstructive pulmonary disease, may precipitate ventricular or supraventricular arrhythmias. Therapy with diuretics can cause hypokalemia and hypomagnesemia. Both caffeine and alcohol may precipitate either atrial or ventricular tachyarrhythmias.

In the patient who has an artificial ventricular pacemaker, near syncope or syncope may be secondary to pacemaker malfunction or to the pacemaker syndrome (see Chap. 40). Dual-chamber pacemakers can produce pacemaker-mediated tachycardias when there is retrograde conduction of the ventricular impulse to the atria. Improvements in technology have reduced the incidence of this complication.[39,40]

【 】 DISORDERS OF VASCULAR CONTROL OR BLOOD VOLUME

Disorders of vascular control or blood volume that can cause syncope include the reflex syncopes and a number of causes for orthostatic intolerance (Table 48–2).[41,42] Under normal circumstances, systemic blood pressure is regulated by a complex process that includes the musculature, the venous valves, the autonomic nervous system, and the rennin–aldosterone–angiotensin system. Knowledge of these processes is a prerequisite to understanding the disorders of vascular control or blood volume that can cause syncope.

Maintenance of Postural Blood Pressure

A principal stress imposed while standing is produced by gravity displacing venous blood downward to a level below the heart. Although the renin–aldosterone–angiotensin system regulates long-

---

TABLE 48–2

Disorders of Vascular Control and Blood Volume

Reflex syncope
  Neurocardiogenic
  Situational
  Carotid sinus hypersensitivity
Orthostatic intolerance
  Autonomic nervous system disorders
    Primary autonomic failure
      Pure autonomic failure
      Multiple system atrophy
      Postural orthostatic tachycardia syndrome
        Peripheral or partial dysautonomic
        Hyperadrenergic
      Acute autonomic failure
    Secondary autonomic failure
      Amyloidosis
      Diabetes
      Sarcoidosis
      Renal failure
      Cancer
      Nerve growth factor deficiency
      β-Hydroxylase deficiency
    Pharmacologic agents
    Certain heavy metals
      Mercury
      Lead
      Arsenic
      Iron
Intravascular volume depletion
  Anemia
  Blood loss
  Dehydration
  Diuretics
Venous pooling/vasodilation
  Prolonged bed rest
  Prolonged weightlessness
  Pregnancy
  Venous varicosities
  Pharmacologic agents
  Hyperbradykininism
  Mastocytosis
  Carcinoid syndrome

term blood pressure responses to upright posture, the autonomic nervous system provides the majority of the short- and medium-term responses to postural change.[43]

In the normal supine individual, approximately one quarter of the blood volume is in the thorax. On standing, there is a gravity-mediated displacement of between 300 and 800 mL of blood to both the dependent extremities and the inferior mesenteric area.[44] Approximately 50 percent of this displacement occurs within the first few seconds of standing, resulting in a drop in venous return to the heart and a mean fall in stroke volume of approximately 40 percent.[44] In the normal subject, accommodation to this change in posture occurs in less than 1 minute.

Immediately on standing, muscle contractions in the legs, abdomen, and arms, in concert with the venous valvular system, support blood pressure by facilitating venous return.[44,45] However, this alone is insufficient to maintain venous return and systemic blood pressure. The reduction in venous return with upright posture is followed by a slow progressive fall in arterial pressure and cardiac filling that produces less stretch and reduces the discharge rate of aortic arch and carotid sinus baroreceptors. Fibers from these mechanoreceptors travel with unmyelinated vagal fibers from the atria and the ventricles to the nucleus tractus solitarii and other areas of the medulla that modulate vascular tone. In the resting supine position, impulses from these fibers increase efferent parasympathetic activity and have an inhibitory effect on efferent sympathetic activity to the heart. After standing, the drop in arterial pressure receptor firing in the carotid sinuses decreases efferent vagal activity and increases efferent sympathetic activity producing a reflex increase in heart rate and peripheral vasoconstriction. As a result, assumption of upright posture results in a 10 to 15 beats/min increase in heart rate, minimal change in systolic blood pressure, and an approximately 10 mmHg increase in diastolic blood pressure.[46]

Any inability of this complex process to respond adequately or in a coordinated manner may result in varying degrees of postural hypotension and ultimately loss of consciousness. Failure of one component may be compensated for by increased action of another component. For example, a failure of the peripheral vasculature to constrict during upright posture may be compensated for by increased heart rate and myocardial contractility sufficient to maintain blood pressure. Nonetheless, compensatory mechanisms may not be sufficient, or may not be sustainable over long periods of time. Furthermore, compensatory mechanisms, if not modulated, may result in orthostatic hypertension and inappropriate sinus tachycardia.

Reflex Syncope

In each of the reflex syncopes there is a sudden failure of the autonomic nervous system to maintain sufficient vascular tone during periods of gravitational stress resulting in hypotension (and sometimes bradycardia). The two types most commonly encountered are neurocardiogenic (vasodepressor or vasovagal) syncope and the carotid sinus syndrome.[47] The other forms of reflex syncope are frequently grouped together under the term *situational* because they occur in association with specific activities or conditions (such as micturition, defecation, swallowing, coughing, postprandial). It is important to realize that the reflexes responsible for neurocardiogenic syncope are normal; healthy individuals will experience neurocardiogenic syncope in the setting of a stimulus that is sufficiently strong and prolonged. However, some individuals develop

neurocardiogenic syncope frequently and with relatively little provocation, suggesting that disorders of autonomic control exist.

Neurocardiogenic syncope can be quite diverse in presentation and tends to occur more often in young people.[48] The episodes often include three stages: a prodrome (nausea, sweating, lightheadedness, or visual alterations), abrupt loss of consciousness, and rapid recovery without a postictal state. However, close to one-third of patients (often elderly) experience little if any prodrome and report a sudden loss of consciousness (drop attack).

The etiology of neurocardiogenic syncope is poorly understood. It can be provoked by prolonged standing, warm environments, emotional distress, and pain, although episodes can occur also without an identifiable trigger.[48] Many episodes of neurocardiogenic syncope are provoked by prolonged orthostatic stress.[49–51] Gravity-mediated displacement of blood and venous pooling in dependent areas decreases venous return to the heart, resulting in a reflex-mediated increase in myocardial contractility that activates ventricular mechanoreceptors that would normally fire only during stretch.[50] This sudden increase in neural traffic to the medulla appears to mimic the conditions seen in hypertension, resulting in a "paradoxic" decrease in sympathetic activity that results in hypotension (vasodepressor response), and in some cases, an increase in vagal efferent activity that results in bradycardia.[51] Other nonorthostatic stimuli (such as fear, fright or epileptic discharges) can provoke virtually identical responses, suggesting that these patients may have an inherent predisposition to these events.[48] During head upright tilt-table testing individuals susceptible to neurocardiogenic syncope demonstrate a precipitous fall in blood pressure that is frequently (but not always) followed by a fall in heart rate (on occasion to the point of asystole).[47]

Carotid Sinus Hypersensitivity

Syncope caused by carotid sinus hypersensitivity is most common in men ≥50 years old and is precipitated by pressure on the carotid sinus baroreceptors, typically in the setting of shaving, a tight collar, or turning the head to one side. Activation of carotid sinus baroreceptors gives rise to impulses to the medulla oblongata that, in turn, activate efferent sympathetic nerve fibers to the heart and blood vessels, cardiac vagal efferent nerve fibers, or both. In patients with carotid sinus hypersensitivity, these responses may cause sinus arrest or AV block (a cardioinhibitory response), vasodilatation (a vasodepressor response), or both (a mixed response). The underlying mechanisms responsible for the syndrome are not clear, and validated diagnostic criteria do not exist.

Some investigators have noted that the hemodynamic responses observed in neurocardiogenic syncope and carotid sinus hypersensitivity are similar, suggesting that the two syndromes may represent different aspects of the same condition.[52] Others have proposed that each of the reflex syncopes may occur in predisposed individuals when rapid activation of neuroreceptors from multiple sites (esophagus, bladder, rectum, or cough) activates a similar response.[51] Recent observations concerning defecation syncope support this.[47] What seems to distinguish the reflex syncopes from the other autonomic syndromes is that between episodes of syncope these patients rarely complain of symptoms referable to the autonomic nervous system. Consequently, in the reflex syncopes the autonomic nervous system functions normally, despite being at times "hypersensitive," in contrast to other conditions wherein the autonomic system appears to "fail," operating at a level insufficient for the body's needs, thereby resulting in drawing levels of orthostatic intolerance.[47]

Syndromes of Orthostatic Intolerance

Orthostatic hypotension may occur as a result of hypovolemia or disturbances in vascular control (see Table 48–2). The latter may occur because of agents that affect the vasculature directly or to primary or secondary abnormalities of autonomic control. During the last two decades, several autonomic disorders have been identified that can impact vascular control and cause syncope.[47] The system presented here corresponds with that developed by the American Autonomic Society and attempts to present these disorders in a clinically useful framework.[41,42] Primary autonomic disorders that affect vascular control are often idiopathic, occur in the absence of other disease states that affect the autonomic nervous system, and may follow either an acute or chronic course. In contrast, the secondary forms occur in conjunction with another illness (such as amyloidosis or diabetes), in the setting of a known biochemical or structural alteration, or following exposure to various drugs or toxins (heavy metals, alcohol or some chemotherapeutic agents) (Tables 48–2 and 48–3).[41,42]

Primary Causes of Autonomic Failure

Pure Autonomic Failure
Bradbury and Eggleston first reported an autonomic failure syndrome in 1925, coining the term *idiopathic orthostatic hypotension* to describe the disorder.[53] In the interim, it has become apparent that this term insufficiently describes the diffuse state of autonomic failure present in these patients, as evidence by impaired bladder, bowel, thermoregulatory, motor, and sexual function (all in the absence of somatic nerve involvement). Currently the condition is referred to as *pure autonomic failure* (PAF).[54] Onset of symptoms in PAF is usually between ages 50 and 75 years and affects twice as many men as women.[55] PAF is manifested by orthostatic hypotension, syncope, and near syncope, neurocardiogenic bladder, constipation, heat intolerance, inability to sweat, and erectile dysfunction.

TABLE 48–3

Pharmacologic Agents That May Cause or Worsen Orthostatic Intolerance

Angiotensin-converting enzyme inhibitors
α Receptor blockers
Calcium channel blockers
β Blockers
Phenothiazines
Tricyclic antidepressants
Bromocriptine
Opiates
Diuretics
Hydralazine
Ganglionic-blocking agents
Nitrates
Sildenafil citrate
Monoamine oxidase inhibitors
Chemotherapeutic agents
   Vincristine
   Vinblastine

Typically, the onset of symptoms is gradual and insidious, often with sensations of positional weakness, lightheadedness, and dizziness.[56] Male patients often report that the earliest signs of PAF were erectile dysfunction and diminished libido; women often report that their earliest symptoms were urinary retention and incontinence.[57] Although not the initial symptom, syncope may be the event that prompts the patient to seek medical attention. Whereas PAF may result in severe functional impairment, it infrequently leads to death.[57]

Multiple System Atrophy
Multiple system atrophy (MSA) is a more severe form of autonomic failure, first reported by Shy and Drager in 1960.[58] In contrast to PAF, these patients display not only significant orthostatic hypotension, but also urinary and rectal incontinence, anhidrosis, iris atrophy, external ocular palsy, erectile dysfunction, rigidity, and tremor. As with PAF, the condition is twice as common in men as women and usually starts in the fifth and sixth decades of life.[55] Although MSA may initially be indistinguishable from PAF, patients with MSA eventually experience somatic nervous system involvement.[59]

MSA is subclassified into three groups according to the somatic system involvement.[55,56] Group I patients exhibit a muscle tremor similar to that seen in Parkinson disease, (also referred to by some as suffering from striatonigral degeneration).[60] As opposed to patients with true Parkinson disease, MSA patients display more rigidity than tremor and the tremor usually lacks the "lead pipe" or "cogwheel" rigidity observed in Parkinson disease.[61,62] Patients with the parkinsonism form of MSA often show a loss of facial expression as well as limb akinesia.

Group II (olivopontocerebellar degenerative atrophy) patients demonstrate pronounced cerebellar and/or pyramidal signs and symptoms.[63] These patients display both gait disturbance and a truncal ataxia severe enough to prevent standing without assistance. They may have a mild intention tremor and severe slurring of speech with impaired diction. Group III (mixed) patients display features of both the parkinsonian and cerebellar groups.[59]

The frequency of MSA may be underappreciated, as an autopsy study found that between 7 and 22 percent of patients thought to have Parkinson disease during life had neuropathologic changes consistent with the disorder.[61] MSA is relentlessly progressive, with the vast majority of patients dying within 5 to 8 years after onset of the illness, (although occasional patients have been reported to have lived up to 20 years).[56] Aspiration, apnea, and respiratory failure are the most frequent terminal events.

Postural Orthostatic Tachycardia Syndrome
Postural orthostatic tachycardia syndrome (POTS) is a somewhat less severe autonomic insufficiency in which heart rate increases excessively in response to upright posture.[64] There are two primary forms of the disorder. The more common type is referred to as the peripheral (or partial) dysautonomic form.[65] These individuals appear to suffer from an inability to increase adequately peripheral vascular resistance in the face of continuing orthostatic stress. This leads to a greater than normal amount of blood pooling in the dependent areas of the body (including the mesenteric vasculature) which is then compensated for by an excessive increase in both heart rate and myocardial contractility.

Patients with dysautonomic POTS experience constant tachycardia (up to 160 beats/min) while standing, and often complain of palpitation, exercise intolerance, fatigue, lightheadedness, cognitive impairment, visual disturbances, dizziness, near syncope, and syncope. Patients may complain of heat intolerance and that they constantly feel cold. Heart rate increases greater than 30 beats/min or to a rate greater than 120 beats/min, usually with minimal drop in blood pressure during the first 10 minutes of upright tilt.[66] Approximately 10 percent of dysautonomic POTS patients progress to PAF. Dysautonomic POTS often occurs following a viral infection, surgery, or trauma. Recent studies suggest a link between dysautonomic POTS and the joint hypermobility syndrome.[47,67]

A second primary form of POTS is referred to as the *hyperadrenergic*, β *hypersensitivity*, or *central* form. This form is thought to be associated with a failure of normal feedback mechanisms above the level of the baroreflex. Whereas the initial heart rate response to postural changes is adequate, the brain appears to be unable to discontinue the response, allowing heart rate to continue to rise. These patients may also be noted to have significant orthostatic *hypertension*. Although supine serum catecholamine levels are normal, upright levels are often quite elevated (over 600 mg/dL) and these patients often display an excessive response to an infusion of isoproterenol (a greater then 30 beats/min increase in response to 1 μg/min). In contrast to patients with the peripheral dysautonomic form, patients with hyperadrenergic POTS complain more often of tremor, hyperhidrosis, diarrhea, panic attacks, and severe migraines headaches. Recent studies in a family with several affected members identified genes that appear to be responsible for hyperadrenergic POTS.[68] A defect was found in the genetic code for a protein that functions to recycle norepinephrine in the intrasynaptic cleft, allowing for excessively high serum levels of norepinephrine. Additional studies suggest that there may be several different genetic forms of the disorder.[69]

Acute Autonomic Failure Although less common than the other autonomic disorders, acute autonomic failure is dramatic in presentation.[70] The onset is surprisingly rapid and is characterized by severe widespread failure of both parasympathetic and sympathetic components of the autonomic nervous system, while the somatic system is unaffected. Patients may have such profound orthostatic hypotension that merely attempting to sit up in bed causes syncope.[71] Many suffer from complete anhidrosis and disturbances in bowel and bladder function that result in abdominal pain, cramping, bloating, nausea and vomiting. Cardiac denervation is common, resulting in a fixed heart rate of 45 to 50 beats/min and chronotropic incompetence.[72] Most of these patients have high circulating levels of antibodies to acetylcholine receptors within the ganglia of the autonomic nervous system, supporting the idea that the disorder is autoimmune in nature.[73]

Secondary Causes of Autonomic Dysfunction

A wide variety of conditions may cause orthostatic hypotension by disturbing normal autonomic function (see Table 48–2).[41,42] Almost any systemic illness that affects multiple organ systems (such as diabetes mellitus, amyloidosis, sarcoidosis, renal failure, and certain cancers) may disrupt autonomic function sufficiently so as to result in orthostatic hypotension and syncope. A subgroup of patients with autonomic failure syndrome (especially diabetic patients) have a combination of supine hypertension and orthostatic

hypertension, thought to be caused by a failure to properly vasoconstrict when upright or properly vasodilate when supine.[74] It is not uncommon for these patients to exhibit a 100-point fall in systolic blood pressure on standing. In some hypertensive patients, a rapid fall in blood pressure may exceed the brain's autoregulatory ability to maintain perfusion, causing syncope even though the systemic blood pressure may at the time be in a relatively normal range.[75] Some investigators suggest that there may be an association between Alzheimer disease and orthostatic hypotension as a consequence of effects on autonomic control.[76] Isolated enzyme abnormalities may also cause orthostatic hypotension, examples of which are nerve growth factor deficiency and β-hydroxylase deficiency.[74] In addition, certain pharmacologic agents may either produce or contribute to orthostatic hypotension by interfering with autonomic control (see Table 48–3).

Additional Causes of Orthostatic Intolerance

Intravascular volume depletion, venous pooling, certain pharmacologic agents, and a number of endogenous vasodilators may cause orthostatic hypotension and syncope. Anemia, acute blood loss, dehydration may cause intravascular volume depletion. Venous pooling is more common in older individuals who have incompetent venous valves in the lower extremities. Individuals subjected to prolonged periods of bedrest or weightlessness often experience orthostatic hypotension. In addition to those pharmacologic agents that interfere with autonomic vascular control, a number of pharmacologic agents can cause orthostatic hypotension by reducing intravascular volume or causing vasodilatation. Certain endogenous vasodilators may cause syncope when they are present in high concentrations.

Clinical Presentation

The principal feature shared by the syndromes of orthostatic intolerance is a disturbance in cardiovascular regulation sufficiently profound so as to result in orthostatic hypotension. Symptoms, the response to tilt testing (see Diagnostic Tests below), and the company they keep may assist in differentiating among the disorders. Symptoms are related to both the rate and magnitude of change in blood pressure.

On occasion it may be difficult to fully distinguish between the various autonomic nervous system disorders as there is a considerable degree of overlap between them and because our understanding of mechanisms remains incomplete. In addition, these disorders should be distinguished from neurocardiogenic syncope. Patients with neurocardiogenic syncope tend to experience an abrupt fall in blood pressure that is commonly associated with definitive prodrome. In dysautonomic syncope the drop in blood pressure tends to be slow and may not be perceived, resulting in a "drop attack" with little or no warning, particularly in older patients.[74] Those who experience a prodrome report feeling lightheaded, dizzy, and blurred or tunnel vision. In contrast to reflex syncope, dysautonomic syncope is seldom associated with either bradycardia or diaphoresis.[56] Patients with the dysautonomic forms of syncope find that symptoms are more common in the morning after awaking from sleep and are made worse by situations that enhance peripheral venous pooling (extreme heat, fatigue, dehydration, and alcohol). Patients suffering from PAF and MSA may display severe chronotropic incompetence with a relatively fixed heart rate (usually around 50 to 70 beats/min).[57]

CEREBROVASCULAR DISORDERS

A number of cerebrovascular disorders can cause syncope. Syncope can occur in patients with extensive occlusive disease of the origins of the brachiocephalic vessels, such as pulseless disease (e.g., aortic arch syndrome and Takayasu arteritis).[4,77] With lesser degrees of cerebral occlusive disease, as with atherosclerotic narrowing, transient lowering of arterial pressure such as that immediately following assumption of the upright posture may be followed by vague symptoms suggesting impaired cerebral blood flow. In patients with cerebrovascular occlusive disease, a transient decrease in cardiac output and arterial pressure may provoke syncope at levels of arterial pressure that would otherwise be tolerated (see Multifactorial Syncope below).

Impairment in or loss of consciousness in relation to changing positions of the head, particularly hyperextension and lateral rotation, has been attributed to mechanical narrowing of the vertebral arteries by skeletal deformities of the cervical spine. Such symptoms have been observed in patients with Klippel-Feil deformity, cervical spondylosis, and severe cervical osteoarthritis. Altered consciousness is often preceded by vestibular symptoms. However, when vertigo is a predominant symptom, the syndrome of benign postural vertigo must be considered.

Syncope in the *subclavian steal syndrome* is caused by major occlusive disease of the subclavian artery proximal to the origin of the vertebral artery. During upper extremity exercise, blood flow is shunted retrograde, by the circle of Willis, to the distal subclavian artery. The consequent decrease in cerebral circulation induces cerebral ischemia.[77] This syndrome is suggested by the findings of diminished brachial arterial pressure on the affected side, a bruit that is maximal over the supraclavicular area adjacent to the origin of the vertebral artery, and the induction of symptoms by exercise of the involved extremity.

Although focal neurologic symptoms and signs are the usual neurologic manifestations of cerebral emboli, transient loss of consciousness can be a primary presenting symptom. Syncopal episodes are more likely to occur when atherosclerotic occlusive disease involves the vertebrobasilar system, with compromised perfusion to the medullary arousal center. In vertebrobasilar vascular insufficiency, syncope or presyncope is nearly always preceded by symptoms of vertigo, diplopia, dysarthria, and ataxia. The episodes are generally attributed to microemboli arising from an atherosclerotic plaque, although vasospasm or postural hypotension may contribute.

SYNCOPE OF UNDETERMINED CAUSE

Despite careful diagnostic evaluation, the cause of syncope cannot be defined in as many as 50 percent of patients.[4] Unexplained syncope has a broad spectrum of etiologies. The varying mortality rate among patients with syncope of undetermined cause likely reflects the varying incidence of undetected cardiac syncope. A certain number of these patients may have experienced syncope from multiple causes.[78,79]

MULTIFACTORIAL SYNCOPE

The cause of syncope is often multifactorial. Patients with structural heart disease or cerebrovascular disease may be predisposed to lose consciousness when blood pressure is compromised because of other causes, such as orthostatic hypotension, a neurocardiogenic reaction, cerebrovascular disease, or an arrhythmia. In addition, patients may have more than one abnormality that alone can cause syncope. In these patients the history may provide clues that enable the clinician to identify the cause of a particular event.

APPROACH TO THE PATIENT

The diagnosis of syncope can be challenging, in part because the cause, like the event, may be only transiently apparent. One of the most important goals is to determine if the patient has a cause for syncope that is potentially life-threatening. This is particularly important because many of the life-threatening causes for syncope can be treated effectively to prolong and improve the quality of life. However, exclusion of a life-threatening cause is not the only goal. The efficacy of therapy depends to a great extent on an accurate diagnosis.

HISTORY AND PHYSICAL EXAMINATION

The history and physical examination remain of paramount importance and may alone diagnose the etiology or distinguish syncope from other causes of loss of consciousness.[80–92] The history should include questions about when the first event occurred, how often and in what settings syncope has occurred, and external factors that can contribute to syncope including medications, diet pills, dietary supplements, and illicit drugs. Symptoms, the patient's posture, and activities preceding the event may provide clues to the cause. Elderly patients who experience lightheadedness or syncope immediately after assuming upright posture may have orthostatic hypotension. Bradycardia, caused by sinus node dysfunction or atrioventricular block, should be suspected in the elderly who experience abrupt loss of consciousness without warning. Neurocardiogenic syncope should be suspected in young patients without apparent structural heart disease who lose consciousness after standing for a prolonged period or after venipuncture. Neurocardiogenic syncope rarely occurs in individuals when they are supine. Syncope while shaving or after turning one's head to the side suggests that carotid sinus hypersensitivity may be the cause.

Whenever possible, the history should include observations of the patient during an episode. Tonic-clonic movements may accompany loss of postural tone if cerebral anoxia is prolonged. Although trauma can occur with syncope, tongue biting and incontinence are more commonly associated with seizures.[92] The time course of the event may suggest an etiology of syncope. Most episodes of syncope are brief, seconds to minutes, though episodes in patients with dysautonomias may be more prolonged. Typically, neurocardiogenic syncope is associated with spontaneous recovery of consciousness within seconds when the patient becomes supine. Unlike seizure disorders, patients rarely experience prolonged confusion or disorientation after an episode of syncope. Patients should be asked whether a family history exists for cardiovascular

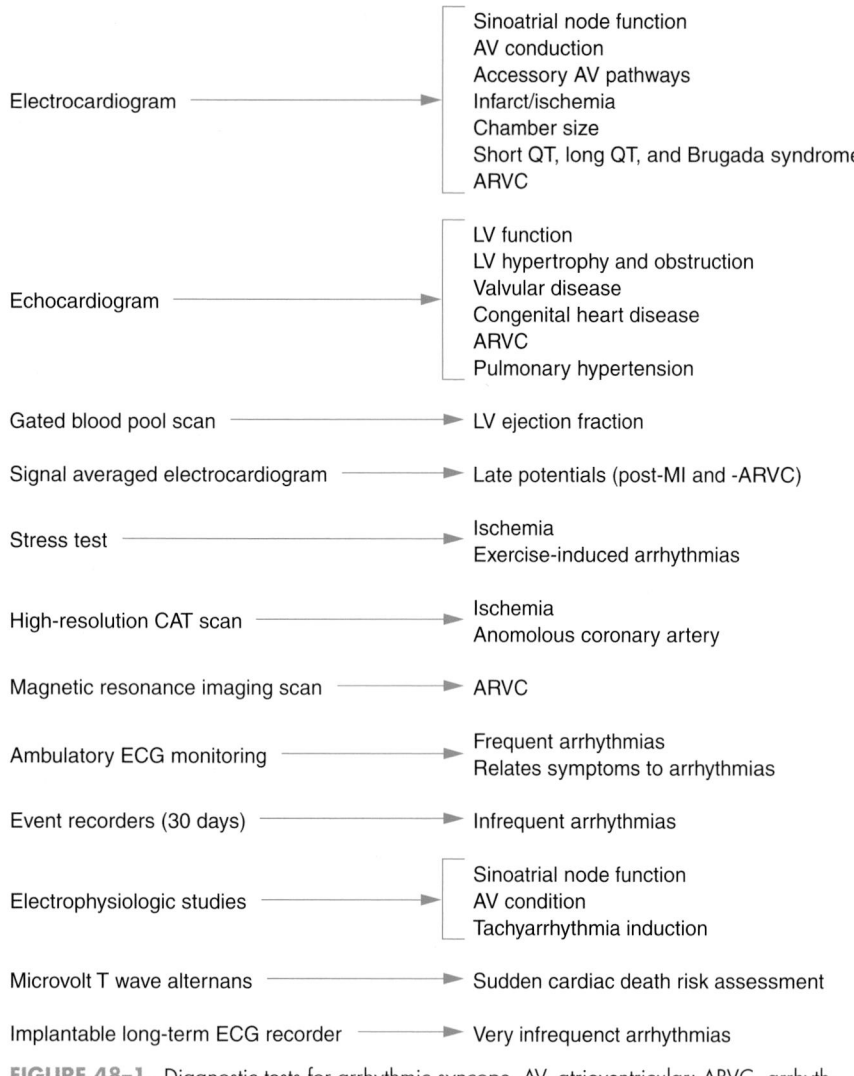

Electrocardiogram	→	Sinoatrial node function AV conduction Accessory AV pathways Infarct/ischemia Chamber size Short QT, long QT, and Brugada syndromes ARVC
Echocardiogram	→	LV function LV hypertrophy and obstruction Valvular disease Congenital heart disease ARVC Pulmonary hypertension
Gated blood pool scan	→	LV ejection fraction
Signal averaged electrocardiogram	→	Late potentials (post-MI and -ARVC)
Stress test	→	Ischemia Exercise-induced arrhythmias
High-resolution CAT scan	→	Ischemia Anomolous coronary artery
Magnetic resonance imaging scan	→	ARVC
Ambulatory ECG monitoring	→	Frequent arrhythmias Relates symptoms to arrhythmias
Event recorders (30 days)	→	Infrequent arrhythmias
Electrophysiologic studies	→	Sinoatrial node function AV condition Tachyarrhythmia induction
Microvolt T wave alternans	→	Sudden cardiac death risk assessment
Implantable long-term ECG recorder	→	Very infrequenct arrhythmias

FIGURE 48–1. Diagnostic tests for arrhythmic syncope. AV, atrioventricular; ARVC, arrhythmogenic right ventricular cardiomyopathy; LV, left ventricular.

disease, neurologic disorders, and early sudden death. A thorough list of prescription and nonprescription medications, supplements, and herbal remedies should be obtained.

Physical Examination

The physical examination should include evaluation of blood pressure and heart rate in the supine, sitting, and upright positions, and again in the upright position 3 to 5 minutes after standing to determine if abnormal changes in orthostatic control are present. Blood pressure should be determined with the arm extended horizontally so as to diminish the hydrostatic effect that occurs when the arm is in a dependant position.[55] Traditionally, orthostatic hypotension has been defined as a fall in systolic blood pressure of at least 20 mmHg or at least 10 mmHg fall in diastolic blood pressure during the first 2 minutes of standing. It should be kept in mind, however, that in some patients, a less dramatic fall in blood pressure may be associated with symptoms.[47]

Cardiac auscultation, especially when combined with appropriate physical maneuvers, may reveal evidence for structural heart disease. When the cause of syncope is unknown, an attempt to reproduce the event may assist in determining the cause. A Valsalva maneuver may reproduce cough syncope; hyperventilation for 2 to 3 minutes may reproduce episodes that are related to anxiety. Although carotid sinus massage may induce significant bradycardia in susceptible individual, it is not recommended for those who may have carotid atherosclerotic disease because the procedure may cause plaque to embolize. The absence of a carotid bruit does not exclude the presence of an atheroma that could be dislodged during carotid sinus massage. In a patient with syncope, a pause of longer than 3 seconds during carotid sinus massage suggests that carotid sinus hypersensitivity may be the cause.

【 】 DIAGNOSTIC TESTS

The history and physical examination guide the choice of diagnostic tests. Blood tests that may contribute to diagnosis include a complete blood count to evaluate for anemia, serum electrolytes, including potassium and magnesium, to evaluate for abnormalities that might cause or aggravate arrhythmias, supine and upright serum catecholamine levels when hyperadrenergic postural orthostatic tachycardia is suspected, and drug levels when the patient's medication or an illicit drug has the potential to precipitate an arrhythmia.

Although it is unlikely alone to provide a diagnosis, almost all patients should undergo a 12-lead surface electrocardiogram because it may identify abnormalities that can predispose to syncope, including prior infarction, ventricular preexcitation (WPW syndrome), AV or bundle-branch block, short or long QT interval, incomplete right bundle-branch block with right precordial ST-segment elevation (Brugada syndrome), epsilon waves, or right precordial T-wave inversion suggestive of ARVC. A transthoracic echocardiogram should be performed whenever heart disease is considered to be in the differential diagnosis.

Transthoracic echocardiography can identify a number of structural abnormalities that are associated with obstructive and arrhythmic causes for syncope. An echocardiogram should be performed whenever the diagnosis of structural heart disease is considered to be significantly likely. Gated blood pool scanning measures left ventricular ejection fraction, but does not provide as much information about cardiac valvular abnormalities.

Patients who are at risk for coronary artery disease should undergo a stress test. In patients who are at high risk for or who are known to have coronary artery disease, cardiac catheterization may be indicated. The use of new high-fidelity computed axial tomography scans to identify coronary artery disease and anomalous coronary arteries is evolving.

Because of their transient nature, arrhythmic causes of syncope may be very difficult to diagnose. Testing for structural heart disease is important to identify patients at risk for arrhythmia and to determine prognosis when an arrhythmia is diagnosed. Figure 48–1 lists the various diagnostic tests used for the evaluation of arrhythmic syncope. The 12-lead surface electrocardiogram is usually of limited use other than to reveal cardiac abnormalities that predispose to arrhythmia. The signal-averaged ECG, which was developed to detect late potentials following myocardial infarction, is rarely used for that purpose in light of the several clinical trials that demonstrated that patients with a left ventricular ejection fraction ≥ 35 percent and the presence of heart failure predict benefit from an implantable cardioverter defibrillator.[93–96] Patients with arrhythmogenic right ventricular cardiomyopathy may also have an abnormal signal-averaged ECG.[97] Cardiac MRI may also be useful in establishing the diagnosis of arrhythmogenic right ventricular cardiomyopathy.

In addition to its use to detect myocardial ischemia, an exercise stress test should be performed when exertional arrhythmias are suspected and ambulatory monitoring has failed to document arrhythmia.[98,99] Continuous ECG monitoring (Holter monitor) is a widely used screening test for suspected arrhythmic syncope but it has a low yield in unselected patients. One 24-hour monitoring period may not be sufficient for detecting transient rhythm disturbances. However, the diagnostic yield increases only slightly with more prolonged monitoring.[98–100] When a Holter monitor does not document an arrhythmia, a patient-activated ECG device (event recorder) may prove efficacious, particularly if the episodes are infrequent (days to weeks). In patients without implantable defibrillators, event recorders should not be used when life-threatening arrhythmias are thought to be the likely cause of symptoms.[101–103]

Patients in whom syncope is very infrequent (weeks to months between episodes) may benefit from an implantable loop recorder, a small device that is surgically placed subcutaneously in the chest, can store up to 45 minutes of retrospective electrocardiographic data, and can record automatically or be activated by the patient. Implantable loop recorders provide diagnostic information in up to two-thirds of patients with syncope of undetermined cause.[104,105] A diagnostic strategy beginning with the implantable loop recorder may be more cost-effective than the traditional approach (external event recorder, tilt-table and electrophysiologic testing) in some patients.[106]

When noninvasive testing does not diagnose arrhythmic causes, an electrophysiologic study may be useful in high-risk patients (i.e., those with structural heart disease, suspicious arrhythmia by ECG monitoring, or recurrent syncope) to assess sinus and AV node function and susceptibility to supraventricular and ventricular tachyarrhythmias. The yield of electrophysiologic testing in patients with an otherwise normal evaluation for syncope is approximately 3 percent.[106] Furthermore, the sensitivity of electrophysiologic testing for bradyarrhythmias is low.[107] However, electrophysiologic testing can be useful in stratifying risk among symptomatic patients with bundle-branch block and in those with bifascicular block. Patients who receive a permanent pacemaker on the basis of electrophysiologic testing also have a favorable prognosis, with a low rate of symptom recurrence.[108–113]

Patients without identifiable heart disease are less likely to have the cause of syncope identified by electrophysiologic study. In patients with coronary artery disease, particularly those with previous myocardial infarction, the cause of syncope most commonly identified by electrophysiologic study is ventricular tachycardia.[107]

The use of the microvolt T-wave alternans test to stratify risk for ventricular arrhythmias is evolving. The test is most useful when performed during exercise and appears to have a strong negative predictive value.[114–117]

Tilt-table testing is the only method employed for the diagnosis of neurocardiogenic syncope that has undergone extensive evaluation.[118–121] Tilt-table testing is based on the principle that orthostatic stress, such as that provided by a period of prolonged upright posture, can produce venous pooling and thus provoke the aforementioned responses in susceptible individuals. As opposed to standing, the patient is placed on a table that can incline up to an angle of 60 to 70°. In this position, the skeletal muscle pump is inhibited and the autonomic nervous system must function alone to maintain blood pressure. The absence of compensatory mechanisms in the presence of a stimulus (prolonged upright posture) may provide the opportunity to observe heart rate and blood pressure patterns that provoke syncope.

Table 48–4 lists the indications for tilt-table testing. A positive test is one that provokes a hypotensive episode (or in the case of POTS, a tachycardic episode) that reproduces the patient's symptoms.[121] A young, otherwise healthy individual with a history that strongly suggests neurocardiogenic syncope and no evidence of life-threatening condition, may not require tilt-table testing after an initial episode of syncope.[122] The specificity of tilt-table testing is reported to be near 90 percent, but lower when pharmacologic provocation is employed. The sensitivity of the test is reported to be between 20 and 74 percent, the variability a result of differences in study populations, protocols, and the absence of a true "gold standard" to which the results of the test can be compared.[118,120,123–132] The reproducibility of the test (in a time frame ranging from several hours to weeks) is 80 to 90 percent for an initially positive response, but less for an initially negative response (ranging from 30 to 90 percent).

It is important to remember that the type of autonomic stress provided by tilt-table testing is different from that which the pa-

---

TABLE 48–4

Head-Up Tilt-Table Testing

Indications for head-up title-table testing

1. Unexplained recurrent syncope or single syncopal episode associated with injury (or significant risk of injury) in absence of organic heart disease.
2. Unexplained recurrent syncopal episodes or single syncopal episode associated with injury (or significant risk of injury) in setting of organic heart disease after exclusion of potential cardiac cause of syncope
3. After identification of a cause of recurrent syncope in situations in which determination of an increased predisposition to neurocardiogenic syncope could alter treatment

Conditions in which tilt-table testing may be useful

1. Differentiating conclusive syncope from epilepsy
2. Evaluation of recurrent near syncope or dizziness
3. Evaluation of syncope in autonomic failure syndromes
4. Exercise- or postexercise-induced syncope in absence of organic heart disease in whom exercise stress testing cannot reproduce an episode
5. Evaluation of recurrent unexplained falls

tient encounters clinically. The International Study of Syncope of Unknown Etiology (ISSUE) compared heart rates during syncopal episodes induced during tilt-table testing with those that occurred spontaneously (as documented by an implantable loop recorder) and showed that spontaneous events were more likely to be associated with significant bradycardia.[119]

Abnormal tilt-table responses can be classified into five groups.[118] The first is referred to as a *classic neurocardiogenic response*, which is characterized by an abrupt drop in blood pressure. When accompanied by a significant drop in heart rate, this is referred to as a *vasovagal response*; in the absence of a decrease in heart rate, a *vasodepressor response*. A second pattern referred to as a *dysautonomic (or delayed orthostatic)*, is characterized by a gradual progressive fall in blood pressure with relatively little change in heart rate. This pattern is often noted in the autonomic failure syndromes. The third pattern, termed a *postural tachycardic response*, is associated with a >30 beats/min increase in heart rate (or a heart rate of >120 beats/min) during the first 10 minutes of the baseline tilt. The fourth pattern is called *cerebral syncope*. These patients experience syncope in the absence of systematic hypotension concomitant with intense cerebral vasoconstriction (as determined by transcranial Doppler), as well as cerebral hypoxia (as determined by electroencephalogram). The fifth response pattern is *psychogenic*. These patients are noted to experience loss of consciousness in the absence of systemic hypotension or any observable change in electroencephalogram or transcranial Doppler recording.[132] These patients are often found to suffer from psychiatric disorders that range from conversion reactions to severe depression.[133] Patients suffering from conversion reactions are not consciously aware of these events.[134] Many patients with psychogenic syncope are young women who have been victims of sexual abuse.[133]

【 】 TREATMENT

Treatment of syncope depends to a great extent on the cause. However, regardless of the etiology, patients should be counseled to minimize exposure to factors that have or are likely to provoke a syncopal episode. This is particularly important for individuals with neurocardiogenic syncope in whom prolonged standing or specific environmental factors have played a role in initiating syncope. Patients should be counseled to avoid situations in which they or others could be injured were they to lose consciousness, particularly when syncope occurs frequently, abruptly, and without warning. Finally, patients should be counseled to take measures (i.e., lie down) to minimize or avoid syncope should they experience prodromal symptoms.

A patient who has lost consciousness should be placed in a position that maximizes cerebral blood flow, offers protection from trauma, and secures the airway. Whenever possible, the patient should be placed supine with the head turned to the side to prevent aspiration and the tongue from blocking the airway. Assessment of the pulse and direct cardiac auscultation may assist in determining if the episode is associated with a bradyarrhythmia or tachyarrhythmia. Clothing that fits tightly around the neck or waist should be loosened.

Syndromes of Orthostatic Intolerance

Therapies for the syndromes of orthostatic intolerance target the various components of the complex mechanisms responsible for control of systemic blood pressure including blood volume, the skeletal muscle pump, heart rate, and central and peripheral components of the autonomic nervous system. Table 48–5 lists therapies and the syndromes for which they are used. Moderate aerobic and isometric exercises are of paramount importance as these therapies enhance skeletal muscle pump function and, thereby, venous return to the heart. Patients with orthostatic hypotension should be instructed to move their legs prior to rising in order to facilitate venous return and to rise slowly and systematically (supine to seated, seated to standing) from the bed or a chair. Whenever possible, medications that aggravate the problem (e.g., vasodilators, diuretics) should be discontinued.

A variety of physical maneuvers have been employed to treat the syndromes of orthostatic intolerance. Tilt training has been advocated; for neurocardiogenic syncope, however, long-term compliance is often poor.[135–137] Isometric countermaneuvers, such as tensing of the arm and leg muscle, can sometimes prevent neurocardiogenic syncope if used at the first onset of symptoms.[138,139] Sleeping with the head of the bed elevated 6 inches above the feet is reported to be useful in neurocardiogenic syncope and the autonomic failure syndromes. Elastic support stockings can be helpful in some patients; to be truly effective, however, they must be waist high and provide a minimum of 30 mmHg of ankle counterpressure.

In some patients, salt and water loading increase intravascular volume and are effective in controlling syncope. However, many patients require pharmacologic therapy. β-Adrenoceptor antagonists were one of the first agents used to prevent neurocardiogenic syncope.[140] Theoretically, the negative inotropic effect of these drugs reduces the degree of cardiac mechanoreceptor activation provoked by a sudden drop in venous return. However, randomized trials of β blockers have yielded mixed results. In the Prevention of Syncope Trial (POST), metoprolol was ineffective in patients who were younger than 42 years of age, but decreased the incidence of syncope in patients who were older than 42 years of age, raising the possibility that there may be important age-related differences in response to pharmacotherapy.[141]

The mineralocorticoid, fludrocortisone, in addition to promoting sodium and fluid retention, appears to enhance peripheral α-receptor sensitivity (promoting vasoconstriction).[142] Its role in treating neurocardiogenic syncope is not well defined.

Several vasoconstrictive agents have been employed as treatments. The first of these were ephedra alkaloids such as Dexedrine and methylphenidate, both of which are α-receptor stimulants.[143] Midodrine, another α-agonist, has been approved by the U.S. Food and Drug Administration for the treatment of symptomatic orthostatic hypotension and was shown to be effective in preventing neurocardiogenic syncope in two randomized trials.[144,145] Bupropion is a norepinephrine and dopamine reuptake inhibitor that has been useful in certain patients. It tends to have fewer sexual side effects but may aggravate hypertension. Other vasoconstrictive substances, such as theophylline, ephedrine, and yohimbine, also are reported to be effective; however, tolerance of these agents is often poor.

The α_2-receptor agonist clonidine causes a paradoxic increase in blood pressure in patients with autonomic failure and a high degree of postganglionic sympathetic impairment. These individuals appear to have reduced peripheral sympathetic stimulation but increased density of postjunctional α_2 receptors throughout the vasculature. Whereas clonidine causes a reduction in central sympa-

TABLE 48–5

Orthostatic Intolerance Syndrome Therapies

TREATMENT	APPLICATION	FORM EFFECTIVE IN				PROBLEMS
		NCS	PD	HA	OH	
Reconditioning	Aerobic exercise 20 min 3 times/wk	X	X	X	X	If done too vigorously may worsen symptoms
Physical maneuvers (tilt training, etc.)	30 min 3 times/d	X				Noncompliance is common
Sleeping with head tilted upright	During sleep	X		X	X	
Hydration	2 L PO/d	X	X		X	Edema
Salt	2–4 g/d	X	X		X	Edema
Fludrocortisone	0.1–0.2 mg PO qd	X	X		X	Hypokalemia, hypomagnesemia, edema
Metoprolol	25–100 mg bid	X				Fatigue
Labetalol	100–200 mg PO bid			X		Fatigue
Midodrine	5–10 mg PO tid	X	X		X	Nausea, scalp itching, supine hypertension
Methylphenidate	5–10 mg PO tid	X	X	X		Anorexia, insomnia, dependency
Bupropion	150–300 mg XL/qd		X	X	X	Tremor, agitation, insomnia
Clonidine	0.1–0.3 mg PO bid 0.1–0.3 mg patch qwk			X		Dry mouth, blurred vision
Pyridostigmine	30–60 mg PO/d		X		X	Nausea, diarrhea
SSRI-escitalopram	10 mg PO/d	X	X		X	Tremor, agitation, sexual problems
Erythropoietin	10,000–20,000 μg sq q/week	X	X		X	Pain at injection site, expensive
Octreotide	50–200 micrograms SC tid		X	X	X	Nausea, diarrhea, gallstone
Permanent pacing		X				

HA, hyperadrenic postural orthostatic tachycardia syndrome; NCS, neurocardiogenic syncope; OH, orthostatic hypotension; PD, partial dysautonomia postural orthostatic tachycardia syndrome; SSRI, selective serotonin reuptake inhibitor.

thetic output with subsequent blood pressure reduction in normal subjects, in patients with autonomic failure, the vasoconstrictive effects of the drug seem to predominate.[74] Clonidine may be most useful in patients with both hyper- and hypotensive episodes.

Recent investigations suggest that the acetylcholinesterase inhibitor pyridostigmine may be an effective agent for both orthostatic hypotension and postural tachycardia syndrome. Randomized, double-blind, placebo-controlled trials show that the agent is safe and effective and seems to be able to prevent falls in blood pressure without exacerbating supine hypertension.[146–148]

Evidence that serotonin plays a vital role in regulation of heart rate and blood pressure and the postulated role of serotonin in neurocardiogenic syncope has led to the investigation of selective serotonin reuptake inhibitors as a treatment for the disorder. Several open-label trials and one double-blind, randomized, placebo-controlled trial have demonstrated that the serotonin reuptake inhibitors prevent recurrent neurocardiogenic syncope.[149–152]

It has been observed that many patients suffering from the autonomic failure syndromes have some degree of anemia. In 1993, Hoeldtke and Streeten published a landmark study demonstrating that erythropoietin given by subcutaneous injection would not only raise red cell counts but would also prevent orthostatic hypotension.[153] Other studies have confirmed these findings, dem-

onstrating that erythropoietin is an effective treatment for orthostatic hypotension.[154–156] Erythropoietin has vasoconstrictive effects (related to its effects on peripheral metric oxide) that are independent of its effect on red cell production.[155]

Octreotide, a synthetic somatostatin analogue, causes splanchnic mesenteric vasoconstriction, thus enhancing venous return to the heart. Biofeedback therapy also has been useful in preventing neurocardiogenic syncope provoked by a variety of psychogenic stimuli.[48]

Despite several trials evaluating its efficacy, the role of permanent cardiac pacing for neurocardiogenic syncope remains somewhat controversial. Initial randomized trials reported that pacing was effective in preventing syncope.[157–159] However, because all patients who received a pacemaker were paced and patients in the control group did not receive a pacemaker, there were concerns that the observed benefit could be a result of placebo effect. In two ensuing studies pacemakers were implanted in all patients who were then randomized to having the pacemaker programmed to an "on" or "off" mode. The Vasovagal Pacemaker Study II (VPS 2) reported no significant reduction in the time to a first recurrence of syncope during dual chamber pacing over 6 months of follow up.[160] The Vasovagal Syncope and Pacing Trial (SYNPACE) also reported that there was no significant difference between the "on" and "off" groups.[161] However, they did observe that the subgroup of patients who had demonstrated asystole during tilt-table testing had a significant increase in time to first syncope recurrence compared to those with bradycardia alone (91 vs. 11 days). The recent ISSUE II trial reported that permanent pacing in patients with periods of asystole had a significant reduction in the frequency of syncope.[162] Patients with the cardioinhibitory or mixed forms of carotid sinus hypersensitivity may benefit also from permanent pacing. In SAFE PACE, permanent pacing reduced falls, recurrent syncope, and injuries in elderly patients with frequent nonaccidental falls and cardioinhibitory carotid sinus hypersensitivity.[163]

For patients who suffer from syncope with little or no prodrome, in whom other forms of therapy have failed, permanent pacing can potentially reduce the frequency of syncope or prolong the time from onset of symptoms to loss of consciousness. This may allow the patient sufficient time to take evasive action (i.e., lie down) and prevent injury if not loss of consciousness.

In contrast to reflex syncope, the autonomic failure syndromes can be associated with symptoms in addition to hypotension some of which are easier to control then others. In addition, some of the autonomic disorders are chronic and progressive necessitating treatment alterations to meet the patient's changing needs. The patient with a severe form of autonomic neuropathy may encounter a wide range of both personal and social difficulties that may include psychosocial problems that necessitate a multidisciplinary approach, including social work, psychological therapy, and physical therapy.

Cerebrovascular Disorders

The treatment of recurrent syncope in cerebrovascular disease is predicated on an accurate diagnosis. In this regard, it is essential to segregate the potential contribution of cardiac and vascular factors and their interplay. Anticoagulants and/or platelet antiaggregant agents are recommended for the prevention of embolic disease from the heart or central vessels. Endarterectomy or percutaneous dilatation should be considered in carotid arterial occlusive disease.

Cardiovascular Disorders

Obstructive Heart Disease Cardiac surgery is often the treatment of choice for patients with syncope caused by obstructive heart disease. Patients with hypertrophic cardiomyopathy and syncope may respond well to pharmacologic therapy but certain patients may respond to A-V sequential pacing.[164–172] However, in patients with severe obstruction and persistent symptoms, surgery should be considered. High-risk patients with hypertrophic cardiomyopathy benefit from placement of an implantable cardioverter defibrillator.[173–175] Among all patients with obstructive heart disease and recurrent syncope, the diagnosis of fixed pulmonary hypertension is most difficult to treat because effective therapeutic options are limited (see Chap. 71).

Arrhythmic Syncope Detailed discussions of therapy for cardiac arrhythmias are presented in Chaps. 33 to 47 of this book. General principles of arrhythmia management as they apply to patients with syncope are summarized here. Treatment of arrhythmic syncope requires accurate definition of the arrhythmia associated with syncope or presyncope.

The bradycardic rhythm disturbances responsible for syncope, primarily AV and sinoatrial pauses or exit block, usually require the implantation of a permanent pacemaker.[166] However, patients who are receiving drugs that cause or contribute to the bradyarrhythmia may benefit from withdrawal or substitution of the offending agent. Patients with bradycardia–tachycardia syndrome usually require pacemaker therapy, because the antiarrhythmic agents required for control of the tachycardia often further suppress sinoatrial function. A select group of patients with symptomatic sick sinus syndrome may benefit from oral theophylline.[176]

Implicit in the approach to the tachycardias causing syncope is the accurate diagnosis of a specific tachycardia. The definition of the tachycardia and the response to antiarrhythmic therapy are often achieved best in the electrophysiologic laboratory. Patients with syncope caused by supraventricular tachycardia associated with an atrioventricular accessory pathway are most often treated with catheter ablation.[176,177] Catheter ablation is also a successful mode of therapy in patients with AV nodal reentry supraventricular tachycardia, atrial flutter, and some atrial tachycardias (see Chap. 44).

Implantable cardioverter-defibrillators (ICDs) are the first-line therapy for ventricular tachycardia in the setting of structural heart disease. It is important to recognize that some patients may continue to experience presyncope or even syncope if cerebral hypoperfusion occurs before the ICD terminates the arrhythmia. Some patients may require additional antiarrhythmic drugs to reduce the frequency of shocks from the ICD. Ventricular tachycardia ablation may be palliative for slower ventricular tachycardia, which requires frequent ICD shocks. Catheter ablation may be effective also for right ventricular outflow tract tachycardia, bundle-branch reentrant tachycardia, fascicular tachycardias, and idiopathic left ventricular tachycardia.

In patients with polymorphic ventricular tachycardia in the setting of a long QT interval (torsade de pointes), the potential offending drug(s) (usually an antiarrhythmic drug) should be stopped. Acute therapy includes intravenous magnesium and measures to increase the heart rate and shorten electrical diastole (i.e., cardiac pacing). Long-term therapy for congenital long QT syndrome may include β blockers, permanent pacing, an implantable defibrillator, and lifestyle changes.

Pacemaker-induced hypotension and syncope are rectified by changing from ventricular pacing to AV sequential pacing when hypotension is a result of loss of atrial transport or neurocardiogenic response is responsible for symptoms. Pacemaker-mediated tachycardia can usually be corrected by reprogramming the pacemaker. Pacemaker malfunction or myopotential inhibition requires a change in programming or replacing the defective system component.

Patients who are known to have a normal heart and for whom the history strongly suggests vasovagal or situational syncope may be treated as outpatients if the episodes are neither frequent nor severe. Patients with syncope should be hospitalized with continuous electrocardiographic monitoring if there is a reasonable likelihood that the episode resulted from a life-threatening abnormality or if recurrence with significant injury seems likely. In the Syncope Evaluation in the Emergency Department Study (SEEDS), a syncope unit in the emergency room reduced hospital admission and total length of hospital stay without affecting recurrent syncope or mortality.[178]

Syncope of Unknown Cause

Treatment of syncope can be particularly challenging when the cause is unknown. Often, treatment must be targeted to the most likely cause and to prolong life. This is particularly true for patients in whom an arrhythmia is the likely (but undocumented) cause of syncope. Certain patients who are at high risk for sudden cardiac arrest may benefit from an implantable cardioverter defibrillator even when it is not clear that a ventricular arrhythmia caused syncope. Patients with certain cardiac conduction abnormalities may benefit from a permanent pacemaker.

CONCLUSION

Syncope, transient loss of consciousness and postural tone as a result of decreased cerebral blood flow with spontaneous recovery, is common and can occur because of a number of underlying mechanisms and disorders, some of which may be normal or benign and do not require therapy (a single episode of neurocardiogenic syncope), and others that are life-threatening and require intervention (e.g., ventricular arrhythmias, aortic stenosis). Identifying the cause for syncope is important for establishing a prognosis and to guide therapy. In addition, syncope must be distinguished from other causes of loss of consciousness (e.g., seizures, trauma, metabolic abnormalities, certain drugs). Syncope can be classified as cardiac, noncardiac, unknown origin, or multifactorial. The history, physical examination, and certain tests can be used to identify the likely cause and guide therapy in many cases. Yet in many cases, the cause may remain obscure, more than one explanation may exist, or syncope may have occurred as a result of more than one process. In these cases, clinical judgement and assessment of the risks and benefits of therapies are required for effective management.

REFERENCES

1. Savage DD, Corwin L, McGee DL, et al. Epidemiologic features of isolated syncope: the Framingham Study. *Stroke* 1985;16:626–629.
2. Kapoor WN. Evaluation and outcome of patients with syncope. *Medicine (Baltimore)* 1990;69:160–175.
3. Day SC, Cook EF, Funkenstein H, Goldman L. Evaluation and outcome of emergency. room patients with transient loss of consciousness. *Am J Med* 1982;73:15–23.
4. Kapoor WN, Karpf M, Wieand S, Peterson JR, Levey GS. A prospective evaluation. and follow-up of patients with syncope. *N Engl J Med* 1983;309:197–204.
5. Manolis AS, Linzer M, Salem D, Estes NA III. Syncope: current diagnostic evaluation and management. *Ann Intern Med* 1990;112:850–863.
6. Calkins H, Byrne M, el-Atassi R, Kalbfleisch S, Langberg JJ, Morady F. The economic burden of unrecognized vasodepressor syncope. *Am J Med* 1993;95:473–479.
7. Olshansky B. Syncope: overview and approach to management. In: Grubb BP, Olshansky B, eds. *Syncope: Mechanisms and Management.* Armonk, NY: Futura, 1998:15–71.
8. Krahn AD, Klein GJ, Yee R, Manda V. The high cost of syncope: cost implications of new insertable loop recorder in the investigation of recurrent syncope. *Am Heart J* 1999;137:870–877.
9. Soteriades ES, Evans JC, Larson MG, et al. Incidence and prognosis of syncope. *N Engl J Med* 2002;347:878.
10. Kofflard MJ, Ten Cate FJ, van der Lee C, van Domburg RT. Hypertrophic cardiomyopathy in a large community-based population: clinical outcome and identification of risk factors for sudden cardiac death and clinical deterioration. *J Am Coll Cardiol* 2003;19(6):987–983.
11. Zaidi A, Clough P, Cooper P, Scheepers B, Fitzpatrick AP. Misdiagnosis of epilepsy: many seizure-like attacks have a cardiovascular cause. *J Am Coll Cardiol* 2000;36(1):181–184.
12. Aminoff MJ, Scheimman MM, Griffin JC, et al. Electrocerebral accompaniments of syncope associated with malignant ventricular arrhythmias. *Ann Intern Med* 1988;108:791–796.
13. Constantin L, Martins JB, Fincham RW, et al. Bradycardia and syncope as manifestations of partial epilepsy. *J Am Coll Cardiol* 1990;15:900–905.
14. Grech ED, Ramsdale DR. Exertional syncope in aortic stenosis: evidence to support inappropriate left ventricular baroreceptor response. *Am Heart J* 1991;121:603–606.
15. Schwartz LS, Goldfisher J, Sprague GJ, et al. Syncope and sudden death in aortic stenosis. *Am J Cardiol* 1969;23:647–658.
16. Nienaber CA, Hiller S, Speilmann RP, et al. Syncope in hypertrophic cardiomyopathy: multivariate analysis of prognostic determinants. *J Am Coll Cardiol* 1990;15:948–955.
17. Dressler W. Effort syncope as an early manifestation of primary pulmonary hypertension. *Am J Med Sci* 1952;223:131–143.
18. Scarpa WJ. The sick sinus syndrome. *Am Heart J* 1983;92:648–651.
19. Talwar KK, Edvardsson N, Varnauskas E. Paroxysmal vagally mediated AV block with recurrent syncope. *Clin Cardiol* 1985;8:337–340.
20. Beder SD, Cohen MH, Riemenschneider TA. Occult arrhythmias as the etiology of unexplained syncope in children with structurally normal hearts. *Am Heart J* 1985;109:309–313.
21. Brignole M, Menozzi C, Moya A, et al. Mechanism of syncope in patients with bundle branch block and negative electrophysiological test. *Circulation* 2001;104:2045–2050.
22. Boudoulas H, Wooley CF. *Mitral Valve: Floppy Mitral Valve, Mitral Valve Prolapse, Mitral Valvular Regurgitation,* 2d ed. Armonk, NY: Futura, 2000.
23. Moss AJ, Schwartz PJ, Crampton RS, et al. The long QT syndrome: prospective longitudinal study of 328 families. *Circulation* 1991;84:1136–1144.
24. Menozzi C, Brignole M, Alboni P, et al. The natural course of untreated sick sinus syndrome and identification of the variables predictive of unfavorable outcome. *Am J Cardiol* 1998;82:1205–1209.
25. Spirito P, Seidman C, McKenna WJ, Maron BJ. The management of hypertrophic cardiomyopathy. *N Engl J Med* 19997;336:775–785.
26. Maron BJ. Hypertrophic cardiomyopathy: a systematic review. *JAMA* 2002;287:1308–1320.
27. Elliott PM, Poloniecki J, Dickie S, et al. Sudden death in hypertrophic cardiomyopathy: identification of high risk patients. *J Am Coll Cardiol* 2000;36:2212–2218.
28. Mikhail GW, Gibbs JSR, Yacoub MH. Pulmonary and systemic arterial pressure changes during syncope in primary pulmonary hypertension. *Circulation* 2001;104:1326–1327.
29. Chen SY, Wang YH, Hwang JJ, et al. Pulmonary embolism presenting as syncope in paraplegia: a case report. *Arch Phys Med Rehabil* 1995;76:387–390.
30. Brignole M, Gianfranchi L, Menozzi C, et al. Role of autonomic reflexes in syncope associated with paroxysmal atrial fibrillation. *J Am Coll Cardiol* 1993;22:1123–1129.
31. Leitch JW, Klein GJ, Yee R, et al. Syncope associated with supraventricular tachycardia. *Circulation* 1992;85:1064–1071.
32. Antzelevitch C, Brugada P, Brugada J, et al. Brugada syndrome: a decade of progress. *Circ Res* 2002;91:1114–1118.
33. Wilde AA, Antzelevitch C, Borggrefe M, et al. Proposed diagnostic criteria for the Brugada syndrome: consensus report. *Circulation* 2002;106:2514–2519.
34. Priori SG, Napolitano C, Gasparini M, et al. Natural history of Brugada syndrome: insights for risk stratification and management. *Circulation* 2002;105:1342–1347.
35. Gemayel C, Pelliccia A, Thompson P. Arrhythmogenic right ventricular cardiomyopathy. *J Am Coll Cardiol* 2001;38:1773–1781.
36. Splawski I, Shen J, Timothy KW, Lehmann MH, et al. Spectrum of mutations in long-QT syndrome genes. *KVLQT1, HERG, SCN5A, KCNE1,* and *KCNE2. Circulation* 2000;102:1178–1185.
37. Zareba W, Moss AJ, Schwartz PJ, et al. Influence of the genotype on the clinical course of the long-QT syndrome. *N Engl J Med* 1998;339:960–965.
38. Menozzi C, Brignole M, Garcia-Civera R, et al. Mechanism of syncope in patients with heart disease and negative electrophysiologic test. *Circulation* 2002;105:2741–2745.
39. Ausubel K, Boal BH, Furmen S. Pacemaker syndrome: definition and evaluation. *Cardiol Clin* 1985;3:587–589.
40. Lamas GA, Orav EJ, Stambler BS, et al. Quality of life and clinical outcomes in elderly patients treated with ventricular pacing as compared with dual-chamber pacing. *N Engl J Med* 1998;338:1097–1104.
41. Consensus Committee of the American Autonomic Society and the American Academy of Neurology on the definition of orthostatic hypotension, pure autonomic failure and multiple system atrophy. *Neurology* 1996;46:1470–1471.

42. Mathias C. The classification and nomenclature of autonomic disorders: ending chaos, restoring conflict and hopefully achieving clarity. *Clin Auton Res* 1995;5:307–310.

43. Joyner M, Shepard T. Autonomic regulation of the circulation. In: Low P, ed. *Clinical Autonomic Disorders,* 2d ed. Philadelphia: Lippincott-Raven, 1997:61–71.

44. Streeten D. Physiology of the microcirculation. In: Streeten D, ed. *Orthostatic Disorders of the circulation.* New York: Plenum, 1987:1–12.

45. Thompson WO, Thompson PK, Daily ME. The effect of upright posture on the composition and volume of the blood in man. *J Clin Invest* 1988;5:573–609.

46. Wieling W, van Lieshout JJ. Maintenance of postural normotension in humans. In: Low P, ed. *Clinical Autonomic Disorders,* 2d ed. Philadelphia: Lippincott-Raven, 1997:73–82.

47. Grubb BP. Neurocardiogenic syncope and related disorders of orthostatic intolerance. *Circulation* 2005;111:2997–3006.

48. Grubb BP. Neurocardiogenic syncope. In: Grubb BP, Olshanski B. *Syncope: Mechanisms and Management.* Malden, MA: Blackwell-Futura, 2005:47–71.

49. Mosqueda-Garcia R, Farlan R, Tank J, Fernandez-Violante R. The elusive pathophysiology of neurally-mediated syncope. *Circulation* 2000;102:2898–2906.

50. Kosinski D, Grubb BP, Temesy-Armos P. Pathophysiology aspects of neurocardiogenic syncope. *Pacing Clin Electrophysiol* 1995;18:716–721.

51. Morillo CA, Ellenbogen A, Pava LF. Pathophysiologic basic for vasodepressor syncope. In: Klein G, ed. *Syncope: Cardiology Clinics of North America.* Philadelphia: WB Saunders, 1997:15:233–250.

52. Sutton R, Peterson M. The clinical spectrum of neurocardiogenic syncope. *J Cardiovasc Electrophysiol* 1995;6:569–576.

53. Bradbury S, Eggleston C. Postural hypotension: a report of three cases. *Am Heart J* 1925;I:73–86.

54. Freeman R. Pure autonomic failure. In: Robertson D, Biaggiona I, eds. *Disorders of the Autonomic Nervous System.* Luxembourg: Harwood Academic, 1995:83–106.

55. Low PA, Banister R. Multiple system atrophy and pure autonomic failure. In: Low P, ed. *Clinical Autonomic Disorders,* 2d ed. Philadelphia: Lippincott-Raven, 1997:555–575.

56. Mathias C, Bannister R. Clinical features and evaluation of the primary chromic autonomic failure syndromes. In: Mathias C, Bannister R eds. *Autonomic Failure: A Textbook of Clinical Disorders of the Autonomic Nervous System,* 45th ed. Oxford, UK: Oxford University Press, 1999:307–320.

57. Schatz IT. Pure autonomic failure. In: Robertson D, Low RA, Polinsky RJ, eds. *Primer on the Autonomic Nervous System.* San Diego, CA: Academic Press, 1996:239–242.

58. Shy GM, Drager GA. A neurologic syndrome associated with orthostatic hypotension. *Arch Neurol* 1960;3:511–527.

59. Polinsky RT. Multiple system atrophy and Shy-Drager syndrome. In: Robertson D, Low RA, Polinsky RT, eds. *Primary on the Autonomic Nervous System.* San Diego, CA: Academic Press, 1996:222–226.

60. Fearnley TM, Less AT. Striatonigral degeneration: a clinicopathologic study. *Brain* 1990;113:1823–1842.

61. Hughes AJ, Daniel DE, Kilford L, Less AJ. Accuracy of clinical diagnosis of idiopathic Parkinson's disease: a clinico-pathologic study of 100 cases. *J Neurol Neurosurg Pyschiatry* 1992;55:181–184.

62. Jellinger KA. Pathology of Parkinson's disease: changes other than the nigro-striatal pathway. *Mol Chem Neuropathol* 1991;14:153–197.

63. Gilman S, Quinn NP. The relationship of multiple system atrophy and other forms of late onset cerebellar atrophy. *Neurology* 1996;46:1197–1199.

64. Kanjwal Y, Kosinski D, Grubb BP. The postural tachycardia syndrome: definitions, diagnosis, and management. *Pacing Clin Electrophysiol* 2003;26:1747–1757.

65. Grubb BP, Kosinski D, Boehm K, Kip K. The postural tachycardia syndrome: a neurocardiogenic variant identified during head upright tilt table testing. *Pacing Clin Electrophysiol* 1997;20:2205–2212.

66. Low P, Novak Y, Novak P, Sandroni P, Schondorf R, Opfer-Gehrking L. Postural tachycardia syndrome. In: Low P, ed. *Clinical Autonomic Disorders,* 2d ed. Philadelphia: Lippincott-Raven, 1997:681–698.

67. Grubb BP, Kosinski D, Grubb BP. Postural tachycardia, orthostatic intolerance and chronic fatigue syndrome. In: Grubb B, Olshansky B. *Syncope: Mechanisms and Management.* Malden, MA: Blackwell-Futura, 2005:225–244.

68. Shannon J, Flatten NL, Jordan T, et al. Orthostatic intolerance and tachycardia associated with norepinephrine-transporter deficiency. *N Engl J Med* 2000;342:541–549.

69. Garland EM, Winker R, Williams SM, et al. Endothelial NO synthase polymorphisms and postural tachycardia syndrome. *Hypertension* 2005;46(5):1103–1110.

70. Grubb BP, Kosinski DJ. Acute pandysautonomic syncope. *Eur J Cardiac Pacing Electrophysiol* 1997;7:10–14.

71. Low P, McLeed T. Autonomic neuropathies. In: Low P, ed. *Clinical Autonomic Disorders,* 2d ed. Philadelphia: Lippincott-Raven, 1997:464–486.

72. Yaki MD, Fronera AT. Acute autonomic neuropathy. *Arch Neurol* 1975;32:132–133.

73. Verino S, Low P, Fearly R, Stewart J, Farrujia G, Lennon V. Autoantibodies to ganglionic acetylcholine receptors in autoimmune autonomic neuropathies. *N Engl J Med* 2000;343:347–355.

74. Grubb BP, Kosinski D. Orthostatic hypotension: causes, classification and treatment. *Pacing Clin Electrophysiol* 2003;26:892–901.

75. Grubb BP, Kanjwal Y, Kosinski D. Hypertensive syncope: loss of consciousness in hypertensive patients in the absence of systemic hypotension. *Heart Rhythm* 2004;1:S259.

76. Passant V, Warkentine S, Karlson, Nisson K, Edvinsson L, Gustafson L. Orthostatic hypotension in organic dementia: relationship between blood pressure, cortical blood flow, and syncope. *Clin Auton Res* 1996;6:29–36.

77. Bousser MG, Dubois B, Castaigne P. Transient loss of consciousness in ischemic cerebral events: a study of 557 ischemic strokes and transient ischemic attacks. *Ann Intern Med* 1980;132:300–307.

78. Krahn AD, Klein GJ, Fitzpatrick A, et al. Predicting the outcome of patients with unexplained syncope undergoing prolonged monitoring. *Pacing Clin Electrophysiol* 2002;25:37–41.

79. Menozzi C, Brignole M, Garcia-Civera R, et al. International study on syncope of uncertain etiology investigators. Mechanism of syncope in patients with heart disease and negative electrophysiologic test. *Circulation* 2002;105:2741–2745.

80. Boudoulas H, Lewis RP. Cardiac syncope: diagnosis, mechanism, and management. In: Hurst JW, ed. *The Heart,* 6th ed. New York: McGraw-Hill, 1986:321.

81. Calkins H, Shyr Y, Frumin H, et al. The value of the clinical history in the differentiation of syncope due to ventricular tachycardia, atrioventricular block, and neurocardiogenic syncope. *Am J Med* 1995;98:365–373.

82. Kapoor WN. Current evaluation and management of syncope. *Circulation* 2002;106:1606–1609.

83. Gilman JK. Syncope in the emergency department. *Emerg Med Clin North Am* 1995;13:955–971.

84. Kroenke K, Lucas CA, Rosenberg ML, et al. Causes of persistent dizziness: a prospective study of 100 patients in ambulatory care. *Ann Intern Med* 1992;117:898–904.

85. Krahn AD, Klein GJ, Norris C, et al. The etiology of syncope in patients with negative tilt table and electrophysiological testing. *Circulation* 1995;92:1819–1824.

86. Schaal SF, Nelson SD, Boudoulas H, Lewis RP. Syncope. *Curr Probl Cardiol* 1992;14:211–264.

87. Alboni P, Brignole M, Menozzi C, et al. Diagnostic value of history in patients with syncope with or without heart disease. *J Am Coll Cardiol* 2001;37:1921–1928.

88. Brignole M, Alboni P, Benditt D, et al. Guidelines on management (diagnosis and treatment) of syncope. European Task Force on Syncope. European Society of Cardiology. *Eur Heart J* 2001;22:1256–1306.

89. Linzer M, Yang EH, Estes NA, Wang P, Vorperian VR, Kapoor WN. Diagnosing syncope, part 1: value of history, physical examination, and electrocardiography; Clinical Efficacy Assessment Project for the American College of Physicians. *Ann Intern Med* 1997;126:989–996.

90. Kapoor WN. Syncope. *N Engl J Med* 2000;343:1856–1862.

91. Delanty N, Vaughan CJ, French JA. Medical causes of seizures. *Lancet* 1998;352:383–390.

92. Sheldon R, Rose S, Ritchie D, et al. Historical criteria that distinguish syncope from seizures. *J Am Coll Cardiol* 2002;40:142–148.

93. Winters SL, Stewart D, Gomes JA. Signal averaging of the surface QRS complex predicts inducibility of ventricular tachycardia in patients with syncope of unknown origin: a prospective study. *J Am Coll Cardiol* 1987;10:775–781.

94. Nalos PC, Gang ES, Mandel WJ, et al. The signal-averaged electrocardiogram as a screening test for inducibility of sustained ventricular tachycardia in high-risk patients: a prospective study. *J Am Coll Cardiol* 1987;9:539–548.

95. Cain ME, Anderson JL, Arnsdorf MF, et al. ACC Expert Consensus Document: signal-averaged electrocardiography. *J Am Coll Cardiol* 1996;27:238–249.

96. Steinberg JS, Prystowsky E, Freedman RA, et al. Use of the signal-averaged electrocardiogram for predicting inducible ventricular tachycardia in patients with unexplained syncope: relation to clinical variables in a multivariate analysis. *J Am Coll Cardiol* 1994;23:99–106.

97. Corrado D, Basso C, Thiene G, et al. Spectrum of clinicopathologic manifestations of arrhythmogenic right ventricular cardiomyopathy dysplasia: a multicenter study. *J Am Coll Cardiol* 1997;30:1512–1520.

98. Boudoulas H, Schaal SF, Lewis RP, et al. Superiority of 24-hour outpatient monitoring over multi-stage exercise testing for the evaluation of syncope. *J Electrocardiol* 1979;12:103–108.

99. Boudoulas H, Geleris P, Schaal SF, et al. Comparison between electrophysiologic studies and ambulatory monitoring in patients with syncope. *J Electrocardiol* 1983;16:91–96.

100. Dewey RC, Capeless MA, Levy AM. Use of ambulatory electrocardiographic monitoring to identify high-risk patients with congenital complete heart block. *N Engl J Med* 1987;316:835–839.

101. Linzer M, Prystowsky EN, Brunetti LL, et al. Recurrent syncope of unknown origin diagnosed by ambulatory continuous loop ECG recording. *Am Heart J* 1988;116:1632–1634.

102. Fetter JG, Stanton MS, Benditt DG, et al. Transtelephonic monitoring and transmission of stored arrhythmia detection and therapy data from an implantable cardioverter defibrillator. *Pacing Clin Electrophysiol* 1995;18:1531–1539.

103. Kinlay S, Leitch JW, Neil A, et al. Cardiac event recorders yield more diagnoses and are more cost-effective than 48-hour Holter monitoring in patients with palpitations. *Ann Intern Med* 1996;24:16–20.

104. Krahn AD, Klein GJ, Yee R, et al. Use of an extended monitoring strategy in patients with problematic syncope. *Circulation* 1999;99:406–410.

105. Zimetbaum PJ, Kim KY, Josephson ME, et al. Diagnostic yield and optimal duration of continuous-loop event monitoring for the diagnosis of palpitations. *Ann Intern Med* 1998;128:890–895.

106. Krahn AD, Klein GJ, Yee R, Hoch JS, Skanes AC. Cost implications of testing strategy in patients with syncope: randomized assessment of syncope trial. *J Am Coll Cardiol* 2003;42(3):502–504.

107. Brembilla-Perrot B, Suty-Selton C, Beurrier D, et al. Differences in mechanisms and outcomes of syncope in patients with coronary disease or idiopathic left ventricular dysfunction as assessed by electrophysiologic testing. *J Am Coll Cardiol* 2004;44(3):594–601.

108. Kushner JA, Kou WH, Kadish AM, et al. Natural history of patients with unexplained syncope and a nondiagnostic electrophysiologic study. *J Am Coll Cardiol* 1989;74:391–396.

109. Boudoulas H, Schaal SF, Lewis RP. Electrophysiologic risk factors in syncope. *J Electrocardiol* 1978;11:339–342.

110. Englund A, Bergfeldt L, Rehnqvist N, et al. Diagnostic value of programmed ventricular stimulation in patients with bifascicular block: a prospective study of patients with and without syncope. *J Am Coll Cardiol* 1995;26:1508–1515.

111. Bellinder G, Nordlander R, Pehrsson SK, et al. Atrial pacing in the management of sick sinus syndrome: long-term observation for conduction disturbances and supraventricular tachyarrhythmias. *Eur Heart J* 1986;7:105–109.

112. Moss AJ, Liu JE, Gottlieb S, et al. Efficacy of permanent pacing in the management of high-risk patients with long QT syndrome. *Circulation* 1991;84:1524–1529.

113. Link MS, Kim KMS, Homoud MK, et al. Long-term outcome of patients with syncope associated with coronary artery disease and a nondiagnostic electrophysiologic evaluation. *Am J Cardiol* 1999;83:1334–1337.

114. Chow T, Kereiakes DJ, Bartone C, et al. Prognostic utility of microvolt T-wave alternans in risk stratification of patients with ischemic cardiomyopathy. *J Am Coll Cardiol* 2006;47(9):1820–1827.

115. Bloomfield DM, Bigger JT, Steinman RC, et al. Microvolt T-wave alternans and the risk of death or sustained ventricular arrhythmias in patients with left ventricular dysfunction. *J Am Coll Cardiol* 2006;47(2):456–463.

116. Gehi AK, Stein RH, Metz LD, Gomes JA. Microvolt T-wave alternans for the risk stratification of ventricular tachyarrhythmic events: a meta-analysis. *J Am Coll Cardiol* 2005;46(1):75–82.

117. Bloomfield DM, Steinman RC, Namerow PB, et al. Microvolt T-wave alternans distinguishes between patients likely and patients not likely to benefit from implanted cardiac defibrillator therapy: a solution to the Multicenter Automatic Defibrillator Implantation Trial (MADIT) II conundrum. Circulation 2004;110(14):1885–1889.

118. Grubb BP, Kosinski D. Tilt table testing: concepts and limitations. *Pacing Clin Electrophysiol* 1997;20:781–787.

119. Krahn A, Klein GJ, Yee R, Skanes AC. Randomized assessment of syncope trial: conventional diagnosis testing versus a prolonged monitoring strategy. *Circulation* 2001;104:46–51.

120. Benditt D, Ferguson D, Grubb BP, Kapoor WN, Kugler L, Lerman BB. Tilt table testing for accessing syncope and its treatment: an American College of Cardiology Consensus document. *J. Am Coll Cardiol* 1996;28:263–267.

121. Brignole M, Alboni P, Benditt L, et al. Guidelines on the management, diagnosis and treatment of syncope. *Eur Heart J* 2001;22:1256–1306.

122. Strickberger SA, Benson DW, Biaggioni I, et al. AHA/ACCF Scientific Statement on the evaluation of syncope: from the American Heart Association Councils on Clinical Cardiology, Cardiovascular Nursing, Cardiovascular Disease in the Young, and Stroke, and the Quality of Care and Outcomes Research Interdisciplinary Working Group; and the American College of Cardiology Foundation: in collaboration with the Heart Rhythm Society: endorsed by the American Autonomic Society. *Circulation* 2006;113(2):316–327.

123. Almquist A, Goldenberg IF, Milstein S, et al. Provocation of bradycardia and hypotension by isoproterenol and upright posture in patients with unexplained syncope. *N Engl J Med* 1989;320:346–351.

124. Fitzpatrick AP, Theodorakis G, Vardas P, et al. Methodology of head-up tilt testing in patients with unexplained syncope. *J Am Coll Cardiol* 1991;17:125–130.

125. Bloomfield D, Maurer M, Bigger JT. Effects of age on outcome of tilt-table testing. *Am J Cardiol* 1999;83:1055–1058.

126. Moya A, Brignole M, Menozzi C, et al. Mechanism of syncope in patients with isolated syncope and in patients with tilt-positive syncope. *Circulation* 2001;104:1261–1267.

127. Sneddon JF, Slade A, Seo H, et al. Assessment of the diagnostic value of head-up tilt testing in the evaluation of syncope in hypertrophic cardiomyopathy. *Am J Cardiol* 1994;73:601–604.

128. Kenny RA, Bayliss J, Ingram A, et al. Head-up tilt: a useful test for investigating unexplained syncope. *Lancet* 1986;1:1352–1355.

129. Morello CA, Klein GJ, Zandri S, et al. Diagnostic accuracy of a low-dose isoproterenol head-up tilt protocol. *Am Heart J* 1995;129:901–906.

130. Natale A, Akhtar M, Jazayeri M, et al. Provocation of hypotension during head-up tilt testing in subjects with no history of syncope or presyncope. *Circulation* 1995;92:54–58.

131. Sheldon R, Rose S, Flanagan P, et al. Risk factors for syncope recurrence after a positive tilt-table test in patients with syncope. *Circulation* 1996;93:973–981.

132. Grubb BP, Samoil D, Kosinski D, et al. Cerebral syncope: loss of consciousness associated with cerebral vasoconstriction in the absence of systematic hypotension. *Pacing Clin Electrophysiol* 1988;21:652–658.

133. Grubb BP, Gerald G, Wolfe DA, Samoil D, Davenport CW, Homan RW. Syncope and seizure of psychogenic origin: identification with head upright tilt table testing. *Clin Cardiol* 1992;15:839–842.

134. Kouakam C, Lacriox D, Klug D, Baux P, Marquie C, Kacet S. Prevalence and significance of psychiatric disorders in patients evaluated for recurrent neurocardiogenic syncope. *Am J Cardiol* 2002;89:530–535.

135. Ector H, Reybrouck T, Heidbuchel H, Gewillig M, Van de Weif F. Tilt training: a new treatment for recurrent neurocardiogenic syncope or severe orthostatic intolerance. *Pacing Clin Electrophysiol* 1998;21:193–196.

136. Di Girolamo E, Di Iorio C, Leonzio L, Sabatini P, Barsotti A. usefulness of tilt training program for the prevention of refractory neurocardiogenic syncope in adolescents: a controlled study. *Circulation* 1999;100:1798–1801.

137. Abe H, Kondo S, Kohshi K, Nakashima Y. Usefulness of orthostatic self training for the prevention of neurocardiogenic syncope. *Pacing Clin Electrophysiol* 2002;25:1454–1458.

138. Brignole M, Croci F, Menozzi C, et al. Isometric arm counter-pressure maneuvers to abort impending vasovagal syncope. *J Am Coll Cardiol* 2002;40:2054–2060.

139. Krediet P, van Dijk N, Linzer M, Liehout J, Wieling W. Management of vasovagal syncope: controlling or aborting faints by leg crossing and muscle tensing. *Circulation* 2002;106:1684–1689.

140. Brignole M. Randomized trials of neurally mediated syncope. *J Cardiovasc Electrophysiol* 2003;14:564–569.

141. Sheldon R, Connolly S, Rose S, et al. Prevention of Syncope Trial (POST). A randomized placebo controlled trial of metoprolol in the prevention of vasovagal syncope. *Circulation* 2006;113:1164–1170.

142. Hickler RB, Thompson GR, Fox LM, Hamlin JT. Successful treatment of orthostatic hypotension with 9-X-fluohydrocortisone. *N Engl J Med* 1959;263:788–791.

143. Grubb BP, Kosinski D, Mouhaffel A, Pathoulakis A. Utility of methylphenidate in the therapy of refractory neurocardiogenic syncope. *Pacing Clin Electrophysiol* 1996;19:836–840.

144. McTavish D, Goa KL. Misodren: a review of its pharmacologic properties and therapeutic use in orthostatic hypotension and secondary hypotensive disorders. *Drugs* 1989;38:757–777.

145. Jankovic J, Gilden JL, Hiner BC, et al. Neurocardiogenic orthostatic hypotension a double blind placebo controlled study with midodren. *Am J Med* 1993;95:38–48.

146. Singer W, Opfen-Gehrking, McPhee BR, Hiltz MJ, Bharucha AE, Low P. Acetylcholinesterase inhibition: a novel approach in the treatment of orthostatic hypotension. *J Neurol Neurosurg Psychiatry* 2003;74:1294–1298.

147. Raj S, Black B, Biaggioni I, Harris P, Robertson D. Acetylcholinesterase inhibition improves tachycardia in postural tachycardia syndrome. *Circulation* 2005;111:2734–2740.

148. Singer W, Sandroni O, Opfer-Gehrking TL, et al. Pyridostigmine treatment trial in neurogenic orthostatic hypotension. *Arch Neurol* 2006;63:513–518.

149. Grubb BP, Kara BJ. The postural role of serotonin in the pathogenesis of neurocardiogenic syncope and related autonomic disturbances. *J Interv Card Electrophysiol* 1998;2:325–332.

150. Grubb BP, Samoil D, Kosinski D, Wolfe D, Lorton M, Madu E. Fluoxetine hydrochloride for the treatment of severe refractory orthostatic hypotension. *Am J Med* 1994;97:366–368.

151. Di Gerolamo E, Di Iorio C, Leonzio L, Barbone C, Barsotti A. Effects of paroxetine hydrochloride, a selective serotonin reuptake inhibitor, on refractory vasovagal syncope: a randomized, double blind, placebo-controlled study. *J Am Coll Cardiol* 1999;33:1227–1230.

152. Grubb BP, Kosinski D. Preliminary observations on the use of venlafaxine hydrochloride in refractory orthostatic hypotension. *J Serotonin Res* 1996;6:89–94.

153. Hoeldkte RD, Streeten DH. Treatment of orthostatic hypotension with erythropoietin. *N Engl J Med* 1993;329:611–615.

154. Biaggioni S, Robertson D, Krantz S, Jones M, Hale V. The anemia of primary autonomic failure and its reversal with recombinant erythropoietin. *Ann Intern Med* 1994;121:181–186.

155. Grubb BP, Lachant N, Kosinski D. Erythropoietin as a therapy for severe refractory orthostatic hypotension. *Clin Auton Res* 1994;4:212.

156. Kawakami K, Abe H, Harayama N. Successful treatment of severe orthostatic hypotension with erythropoietin. *Pacing Clin Electrophysiol* 2003;26:105–107.

157. Conolly SJ, Sheldon R, Roberts RS, Gent M. The North American Vasovagal Pacemaker study (VPS): a randomized trial of permanent cardiac pacing for the prevention of vasovagal syncope. *J Am Coll Cardiol* 1999;33:16–20.

158. Sutton R, Brignole M, Menozzi C, et al. Dual-chamber pacing in the treatment of neurally mediated tilt-positive cardioinhibitory syncope: pacemaker versus no therapy: a multicenter randomized study. *Circulation* 2000;102:294–299.

159. Ammirati F, Colivicchi F, Santini M. Permanent cardiac pacing vs. medical treatment for the prevention of recurrent vasovagal syncope: a multicenter, randomized, controlled trial. *Circulation* 2001;104:52–57.

160. Connolly SJ, Sheldon R, Thorpe KE, et al. Pacemaker therapy for prevention of syncope in patients with recurrent severe vasovagal syncope: second Vasovagal Pacemaker Study (VPSII). *JAMA* 2003;289:2224–2229.

161. Giada F, Raviele A, Menozzi C, et al. The vasovagal syncope and pacing trial (Synpace): a randomized placebo-controlled study of permanent pacing for treatment of recurrent vasovagal syncope. *Pacing Clin Electrophysiol* 2003;26:1016.

162. Brignole M, Sutton R, Menozzi C, et al. Early application of an implantable loop recorder allows effective specific therapy in patients with recurrent suspected neurally mediated syncope. *Eur Heart J* 2006;27:1085–1092.

163. Kenny RA, Richardson DA, Steen N, Bexton RS, Shaw FE, Bond J. Carotid sinus syndrome: a modifiable risk factor for nonaccidental falls in older adults (SAFE PACE). *J Am Coll Cardiol* 2001;38(5):1491–1496.

164. Nishimura RA, Giuliani ER, Brandenburg RO, et al. Hypertrophic cardiomyopathy. In: Giuliani ER, Gersh BJ, McGoon MD, eds. *Mayo Clinic Practice of Cardiology*, 3d ed. St. Louis: Mosby, 1996:689.

165. Henein MY, O'Sullivan CA, Ramzy IS, et al. Electromechanical left ventricular behavior after nonsurgical septal reduction in patients with hypertrophic obstructive cardiomyopathy. *J Am Coll Cardiol* 1999;34:1117–1122.

166. Ommen SR, Nishimura RA, Squires RW, et al. Comparison of dual-chamber pacing versus septal myectomy for the treatment of patients with hypertrophic obstructive cardiomyopathy. *J Am Coll Cardiol* 1999;34:191–196.

167. Fananapazir L. Advances in molecular genetics and management of hypertrophic cardiomyopathy. *JAMA* 1999;281:1746–1747.

168. Henein MY, O'Sullivan C, Sutton GC, et al. Stress-induced left ventricular outflow tract obstruction: a potential cause of dyspnea in the elderly. *J Am Coll Cardiol* 1997;30:1301–1307.

169. Spirito P, Maton BJ. Perspectives on the role of new treatment strategies in hypertrophic obstructive cardiomyopathy. *J Am Coll Cardiol* 1999;33:1071–1075.

170. Kappenberger L, Linde C, McKenna DW, et al. Pacing in hypertrophic obstructive cardiomyopathy: a randomized crossover study. *Eur Heart J* 1997;18:1249–1256.

171. Suda K, Kohl T, Kovalchin JP, et al. Echocardiographic predictors of poor outcome in infants with hypertrophic cardiomyopathy. *Am J Cardiol* 1997;80:595–600.

172. Knight C, Kurbaan AS, Seggewiss H, et al. Nonsurgical septal reduction for hypertrophic obstructive cardiomyopathy: outcome in the first series of patients. *Circulation* 1997;95:2075–2081.

173. Maron BJ, Shen WK, Link MS, et al. Efficacy of implantable cardioverter-defibrillators for the prevention of sudden cardiac death in patient with hypertrophic cardiomyopathy. *N Engl J Med* 2000;342:365–373.

174. Gregoratos G, Abrams J, Epstein AE, et al. ACC/AHA/NASPE 2002 Guideline update for implantation of cardiac pacemakers and antiarrhythmia devices—summary article: a report of the American College of Cardiology/American Heart Association Task Force on Practice Guidelines (ACC/AHA/NASPE Committee to Update the 1998 Pacemaker Guidelines). *J Am Coll Cardiol* 2002;40:1703–1719.

175. Alboni P, Menozzi C, Brignole M, et al. Effects of permanent pacemaker and oral theophylline in sick sinus syndrome the THEOPACE study: a randomized controlled trial. *Circulation* 1997;96:260–266.

176. Jackman WM, Xunzhang W, Friday K, et al. Catheter ablation of accessory atrioventricular pathways (Wolff-Parkinson-White syndrome) by radiofrequency current. *N Engl J Med* 1991;324:1605–1611.

177. Calkins H, Sousa J, El-Atassi R, et al. Diagnosis and cure of the Wolff-White-Parkinson syndrome or paroxysmal supraventricular tachycardia during a single electrophysiologic test. *N Engl J Med* 1991;324:1612–1618.

178. Shen WK, Decker WW, Smars PA, et al. Syncope Evaluation in the Emergency Department Study (SEEDS): a multidisciplinary approach to syncope management. *Circulation* 2004;110:3636–3645.

CHAPTER (49)

Sudden Cardiac Death

Matthew R. Reynolds / Duane S. Pinto /
Mark E. Josephson

DEFINITION OF SUDDEN CARDIAC DEATH

Sudden cardiac death (SCD) describes the unexpected natural death from a cardiac cause within a short time period from the onset of symptoms in a person without any prior condition that would appear fatal. It is most often caused by a sustained ventricular tachyarrhythmia. Although many cardiovascular disorders increase the risk of SCD, the presence or absence of preexisting cardiovascular disease is unnecessary.[1] Prodromal symptoms such as palpitations, chest pain, and dyspnea may suggest a cardiovascular etiology such as arrhythmia, ischemia, or congestive heart failure, but are not specific. The definition of SCD includes the time interval from onset of the symptoms leading to collapse and then to death, the unexpected nature of the event, and the specific cause of death. More recent definitions have focused on time intervals of 1 hour or less, which normally identify SCD populations having a 90 percent or more proportion of arrhythmic death.[2,3] Because 80 percent of SCDs occur in the home environment, and up to 40 percent of sudden deaths are not witnessed, the information necessary to establish a diagnosis of SCD is frequently lacking.[4,5]

EPIDEMIOLOGY

【 】 INCIDENCE

SCD accounts for more than 400,000 deaths yearly in the United States, with exact totals depending on the definition used.[1,6] When the definition of SCD is restricted to death less than 2 hours from onset of symptoms, 12 percent of all natural deaths are sudden and 88 percent of these are a result of cardiac disease. In autopsy-based studies, a cardiac etiology of sudden death has been reported in 60 to 70 percent of sudden death victims.[5]

The U.S. Centers for Disease Control and Prevention estimated the SCD incidence per 1000 persons in 1999 to be 2.1 in men and 1.4 in women, resulting in 462,340 deaths of a total of 728,743 deaths from cardiac disease.[6] The average age of cardiac arrest victims is around 65 years, and 70 to 80 percent are men.[7] In the United

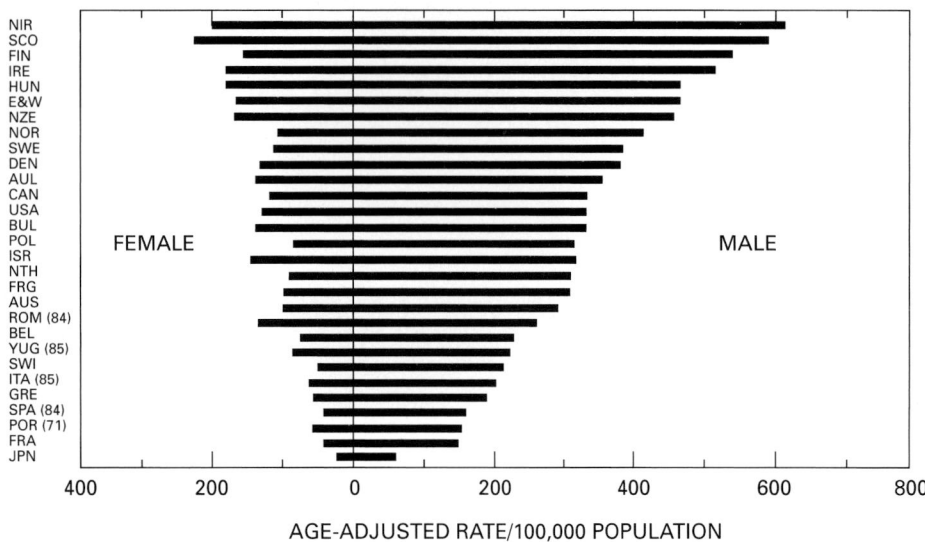

FIGURE 49–1. SCD rates by gender and country, ages 35 to 74 years, compiled by the World Health Organization, Geneva (1986) from death certificates. *Source: From Manolio TA, Furberg CD. Epidemiology of SCD. In: Akhtar M, Myerburg RJ, Ruskin JN, eds. SCD. Baltimore: Williams & Wilkins; 1994:3. Reproduced with permission from the publisher and authors.*

States, several population-based studies have documented an age-adjusted decline in SCD rates of more than 8 percent over the last 15 years.[1] SCD rates in other developed countries are comparable to those in the United States: the World Health Organization reported an annual incidence of SCD of 1.9 per 1000 persons in men and 0.6 per 1000 persons in women.[8] SCD rates in developing countries are considerably lower, paralleling the rates of ischemic heart disease, the most common substrate for SCD in developed nations (Fig. 49–1).

[ ] INFLUENCE OF AGE, RACE, AND GENDER

Age

The incidence of SCD increases with the higher prevalence of ischemic heart disease at older ages (Fig. 49–2).[9] Among sudden natural deaths, the proportion with cardiac causes also increases with advancing age. Among patients with coronary heart disease (CHD), however, the proportion of coronary deaths that are sudden decreases from more than 74 percent of deaths in those ages 35 to 44 years to <60 percent of those ages 75 to 84 years.[1,9]

SCD accounts for approximately 20 percent of all sudden deaths in patients younger than age 20 years.[10] Although structural cardiac abnormalities can be identified in the majority of young victims of SCD,[11] recent autopsy-based studies suggest that 20 to 35 percent of sudden deaths in young adults occur in the absence of identifiable structural abnormalities.[12,13] Many of these are likely a result of genetically based arrhythmogenic disorders. These topics are discussed in further detail below (see also Chaps. 33 and 47).

Racial Differences

Numerous studies show that the annual incidence of SCD is higher in African Americans than in whites.[1,14] An analysis of cardiac death rates in the United States between 1989 and 1998 showed that the age-adjusted rates of SCD per 1000 persons were 5.0 for black men, 4.1 for white men, and 2.1 for Asian men. Likewise, in a recent analysis of sudden deaths in young female military recruits, African American

women were found to have a risk ratio of 10.2 compared with women of other races.[15] The reasons for these findings are unclear. Postmortem analyses show that differences in rates of sudden death may be a result of an increased prevalence of hypertension, left ventricular hypertrophy, diabetes, and tobacco use.[16] Other factors that must be considered include limitations in access to preventive care,[17] prehospital delays in patient activation of emergency medical services, and denial or self-treatment of prodromal symptoms. These issues warrant further investigation.

Gender

SCD has a much higher incidence in men than in women, reflecting gender differences in the incidence of CHD.[1,9] Between 70 and 89 percent of SCDs occur in men, and the annual incidence of SCD in men is overall three to four times higher than in women. As is the case with coronary disease, however, this disparity decreases with advancing age, with a male-to-female ratio for SCD of 7:1 in 45- to 64-year-olds but only 2:1 in 65- to 74-year-olds.

Women are more likely than men (64 vs. 50 percent) to suffer SCD without prior evidence of coronary heart disease.[9] Among survivors of cardiac arrest, women are more likely than men to have other forms of structural heart disease (valvular heart disease,

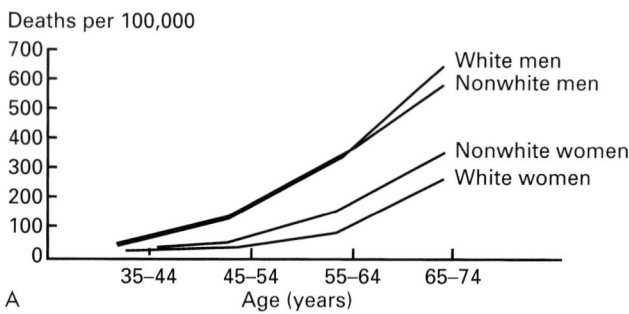

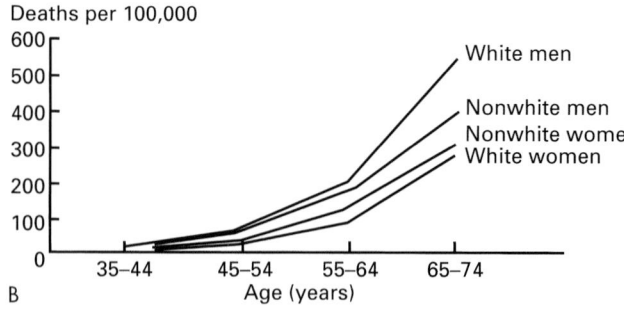

FIGURE 49–2. Plots of mortality rates (deaths per 100,000 persons) for ischemic heart disease occurring (**A**) out of hospital or in the emergency room (an estimate for SCD rate) and (**B**) occurring in the hospital, by age, gender, and race in 40 states during 1985. *Source: From the National Center for Health Statistics. Reproduced from Gillum RF. Sudden coronary death in the United States: 1980–1985. Circulation 1989;79(4):756–765, with permission.*

dilated cardiomyopathy) or a structurally normal heart.[18] A greater percentage of sudden deaths occur outside of the hospital in women, and the aforementioned decline in sudden death rates has been noted to be smaller in women (6 percent) than in men (12 percent). In fact, the rate of sudden death has increased by 21 percent in women ages 35 to 44 years. The reasons for these findings are myriad and may include less-aggressive treatment[17,19] or patients' lack of awareness of the importance of cardiovascular signs and symptoms. For example, less than 10 percent of women consider heart disease their greatest health concern.[20] Continued efforts are needed to raise awareness regarding the risks of SCD—and heart disease in general—in women.

[ ] RISK FACTORS FOR SCD

Only a fraction of patients survive a cardiac arrest, and there has been considerable interest in identifying populations at risk for sustained ventricular arrhythmias. Because more than 80 percent of SCDs occur in patients with underlying coronary disease, the risk factors for SCD largely reflect those for CHD. Left ventricular dysfunction and CHD confer the highest risk for SCD.[21] In the Framingham study, a multivariate model based on various risk factors found that 53 percent of men and 42 percent of women who were at risk for sudden death were in the upper decile of this analysis (Fig. 49–3).[9]

Despite the fact that numerous population-based studies have shown a strong relationship between risk factors for CHD and SCD, no study has identified a single set of risk factors that are specific for SCD (Table 49–1).[21,22] The inability to determine risk factors that are specific for SCD reflects the fact that these factors are linked to chronic disease processes that create the structural basis for sustained arrhythmia. These structural abnormalities may be

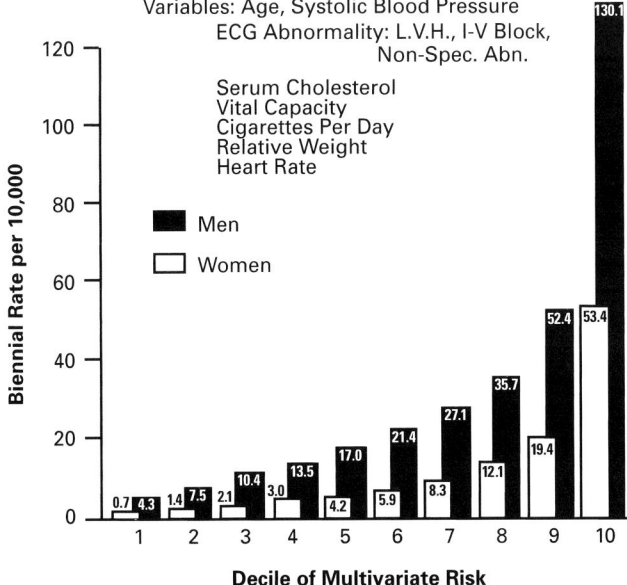

FIGURE 49–3. Risk of SCD by decile of multivariate risk: 26-year follow-up, the Framingham Study. ECG, electrocardiographic; I-V, intraventricular; LVH, left ventricular hypertrophy; Non-Spec. Abn., nonspecific abnormality. Source: Reproduced from Kannel WB, Schatzkin A. Sudden death: lessons from subsets in population studies. *J Am Coll Cardiol* 1985;5(6 Suppl):141B–149B, with permission.

TABLE 49–1

Age-Adjusted Risk Factors for Sudden Cardiac Death in Population-Based Studies

STUDY	STUDY POPULATION	RISK FACTORS FOR SCD
Kannel et al.[9,22] (Framingham Study)	5128 men and women, age 30–62, no CHD at entry: 546 CHD deaths over 26 years, 46% (men) and 35% (women) SCD	Men LVH (by ECG) Cholesterol Systolic blood pressure Relative body weight Cigarette smoking Women Vital capacity Cholesterol Serum glucose
Hinkle et al.[21]	269,755 men, age 20–65: 1839 CHD deaths over 5 years, 60% SCD	Hypertension Cigarette smoking Alcohol History of CHD LVH (by ECG) Enlarged heart (CXR) CHF PVCs
Wannamethee et al.[255]	7735 British men, age 40–59: 488 CHD events, 117 SCD over 8 years	History of CHD Physical inactivity Systolic blood pressure Cholesterol Cigarette smoking Physical inactivity Arrhythmia Resting heart rate >90 beats/min Alcohol
Albert et al.[256]	121,701 women age 30–55: 1110 CV deaths, 244 SCD over 12 years	Diabetes mellitus Hypertension Cigarette smoking Family history CHD Obesity

CHD, coronary heart disease; CHF, congestive heart failure; CXR, chest x-ray; HDL, high-density lipoproteins; LVH, left ventricular hypertrophy; PVC, premature ventricular contraction; SCD, sudden cardiac death.
Source: Data from Wannamethee G, Shaper AG, MacFarlane PW, et al.[255] and Albert CM, Chae, CU, Grodstein F, et al.[256]

necessary but are insufficient to cause an episode of SCD. To date, primary prevention of sudden death has mainly focused on modifying atherosclerotic risk factors and heart failure, but individuals with these disorders signify only a small fraction of those who will experience sudden arrhythmic death. In the future, genotypic analysis may improve the stratification of risk for sudden death. Novel markers to assess risk of sudden death are currently under investigation. Hemostatic factors,[23] inflammatory markers such as C-reactive protein,[24] and polymorphisms in cardiac β receptors[25,26] show promise. A challenge for the future will be to use knowledge of these indicators to further understand the mechanisms of sudden death as well as the interplay of environmental and genetic predispositions so that patients at high-risk for malignant arrhythmias can be targeted for intervention.

Lifestyle Factors

Observations suggest that changes in lifestyle factors, such as alcohol consumption, cigarette smoking, exercise and stress, are potentially important in modifying the risk of dying suddenly.[22,27,28] Individuals who consume large amounts of alcohol (more than 5 drinks per day) have increased risks of ventricular arrhythmia and SCD.[29] However, a prospective analysis of 21,537 subjects in the Physicians Health Study demonstrated a decreased risk of SCD in men who consumed light-to-moderate amounts of alcohol (2 to 6 drinks per week) compared with those who rarely or never consumed alcohol.[27]

Cigarette smoking is one of the few coronary risk factors that is associated with a disproportionate number of sudden deaths. In the Framingham Study, the annual incidence of SCD increased from 13 per 1000 in nonsmokers to 31 per 1000 in those smoking more than 20 cigarettes per day.[30] Smoking induces physiologic changes that predispose to SCD, such as increased platelet adhesiveness and catecholamine release, decreased ventricular fibrillation threshold, acceleration of heart rate, increased blood pressure, coronary spasm, reduced oxygen-carrying capacity by accumulation of carboxyhemoglobin, and impairment of myoglobin use.[30] A postmortem study linked smoking and the presence of acute coronary thrombus. Fresh thrombus was found in more than 50 percent of men who died suddenly, and cigarette smoking was a risk factor in 75 percent of these men, compared with 41 percent of the men with stable plaques.[31] Those who stop smoking have a prompt reduction in CHD mortality rate irrespective of the duration of previous smoking.[32]

There are many reports linking stress, particularly emotional stress, to SCD. Patients experiencing intense anger tend to have higher rates of implantable cardioverter-defibrillator (ICD) discharge[28] and an estimated seven times greater relative risk of appropriate discharge occurs during mental and physical stress.[33] In the hours following the Northridge, California earthquake of 1994, there was a more than fourfold increase in SCD, illustrating the role of emotional stress as trigger for SCD.[34]

Although there is increasing evidence that regular physical activity may help prevent CHD and its complications, the benefits of vigorous exercise in patients with known CHD is controversial. Several clinical and autopsy-based studies report exercise as a trigger for SCD.[35,36] Emergency medical records show that 11 to 17 percent of adults with CHD and SCD collapse during or immediately after exertion, but the amount of exertion is rarely quantified.[37] The increased risk of cardiac arrest caused by ventricular fibrillation during or after exercise is also evident from cardiac rehabilitation programs and from exercise stress testing of patients with heart disease. Cardiac arrest rates of 1 in 12,000 to 15,000 (rehabilitation) and 1 per 2000 (stress testing) are reported. These rates are at least six times higher than those for patients not known to have heart disease.[37]

Although the absolute risk of sudden death during any particular episode of vigorous exertion is low (1 sudden death per 1.51 million episodes of exertion), the Physicians Health Study esti-

mated that the risk of sudden death increases more than 16-fold in the first 30 minutes of vigorous activity. Nevertheless, there is ample experimental evidence that regular exercise may prevent ischemia-induced ventricular fibrillation and death,[38] and habitual vigorous exercise attenuates the relative risk of sudden death associated with vigorous exertion.[36] It appears that regular participation in moderate-intensity activities is associated with reduced rates of cardiovascular morbidity and mortality; the risks of SCD and myocardial infarction are transiently increased during acute bouts of high-intensity activity.

SCD in competitive athletes is rare (see Chap. 100). Collapse usually occurs during or shortly after exercise. Unfortunately, SCD is often the first manifestation of the underlying cardiac disease that is present in the majority of these patients.[39] Age is the most useful variable in predicting the type of underlying cardiac disease (Fig. 49-4). In athletes younger than 35 years of age, the majority of SCDs arise from a variety of congenital cardiovascular diseases, most commonly hypertrophic cardiomyopathy and congenital coronary artery anomalies.[40] Less common structural conditions include myocarditis, aortic dissection (e.g., related to Marfan syndrome), aortic stenosis, dilated cardiomyopathy, and arrhythmias associated with mitral valve prolapse. Other disorders such as arrhythmogenic right ventricular cardiomyopathy (ARVC) may be more frequent in endemic areas.[41] SCD among young athletes without structurally identifiable cardiac abnormalities is reportedly rare,[39] but was recently found to be much more common among young active-duty military members.[13] These cases are likely to be related to inherited arrhythmia disorders such as long QT syndrome, Wolff-Parkinson-White syndrome, and others (see Chap. 33 and below). Coronary artery disease is an uncommon cause of SCD in athletes younger than age 35 years.[42]

Screening programs for identifying relatively rare cardiac abnormalities in large populations of asymptomatic athletes are costly and inefficient, but are still pursued because of the dramatic and often public nature of SCD in athletes, and the medical-legal climate. Consequently, guidelines for such screening have been published, and focus on detailed personal and family history, physical examination, and ECG, with echocardiography and other noninvasive tests reserved for those with positive findings during the initial evaluation.[43] Guidelines have also been published outlining which athletes with cardiac arrhythmias can participate in competitive athletics (see Chap. 100).[44]

Blunt, nonpenetrating, and usually innocent-appearing chest blows leading to ventricular arrhythmia and sudden death have also been reported as causes of SCD in young persons.[45] Termed *commotio cordis,* these events often occur during organized sports, but also occur in other settings. Most deaths occur as a result of low-energy and -velocity projectiles striking the chest.

MECHANISM OF SCD

【 】 RELATIONSHIP BETWEEN STRUCTURE AND FUNCTION IN SCD

The vast majority of patients who have experienced SCD have cardiac structural abnormalities. In the adult population, these consist predominantly of CHD, cardiomyopathies, valvular heart disease,

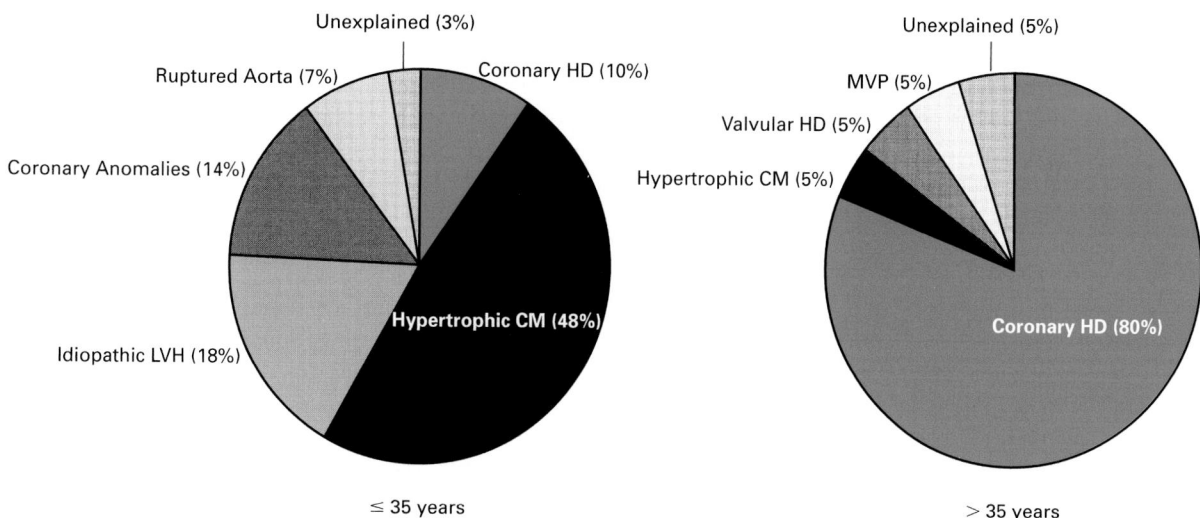

FIGURE 49–4. Causes of SCD in competitive athletes by age group. There is evidence for structural heart disease in nearly all athletes who die suddenly of cardiac causes. In athletes younger than age 35 years, hypertrophic cardiomyopathy is more prevalent, whereas in those older than age 35 years, coronary heart disease is the most frequent cause. CM, cardiomyopathy; HD, heart disease; LVH, left ventricular hypertrophy; MVP, mitral valve prolapse. *Source: Reproduced from Maron BJ, Epstein SE, Roberts WC. Causes of sudden death in competitive athletes. J Am Coll Cardiol 1986;7:204–214, with permission.*

and abnormalities of the conduction system. These structural changes provide the substrate for ventricular tachyarrhythmias, which represent the cause of SCD in most cases. It is important to recognize the role of triggering factors, such as ischemia, hemodynamic changes, fluctuations in the autonomic nervous system, electrolyte abnormalities, and proarrhythmic effects of drugs in the initiation of ventricular arrhythmias resulting in SCD (Fig. 49–5).[46,47] Strategies aimed at eliminating or reducing the triggers of arrhyth-

mias may prove to be effective short- and midterm solutions as most structural abnormalities, once present, cannot be cured.

【 】 TACHYARRHYTHMIAS VERSUS BRADYARRHYTHMIAS IN SCD

Ventricular fibrillation is the first recorded rhythm in approximately 75 percent of patients who have cardiac arrest.[48] Sustained

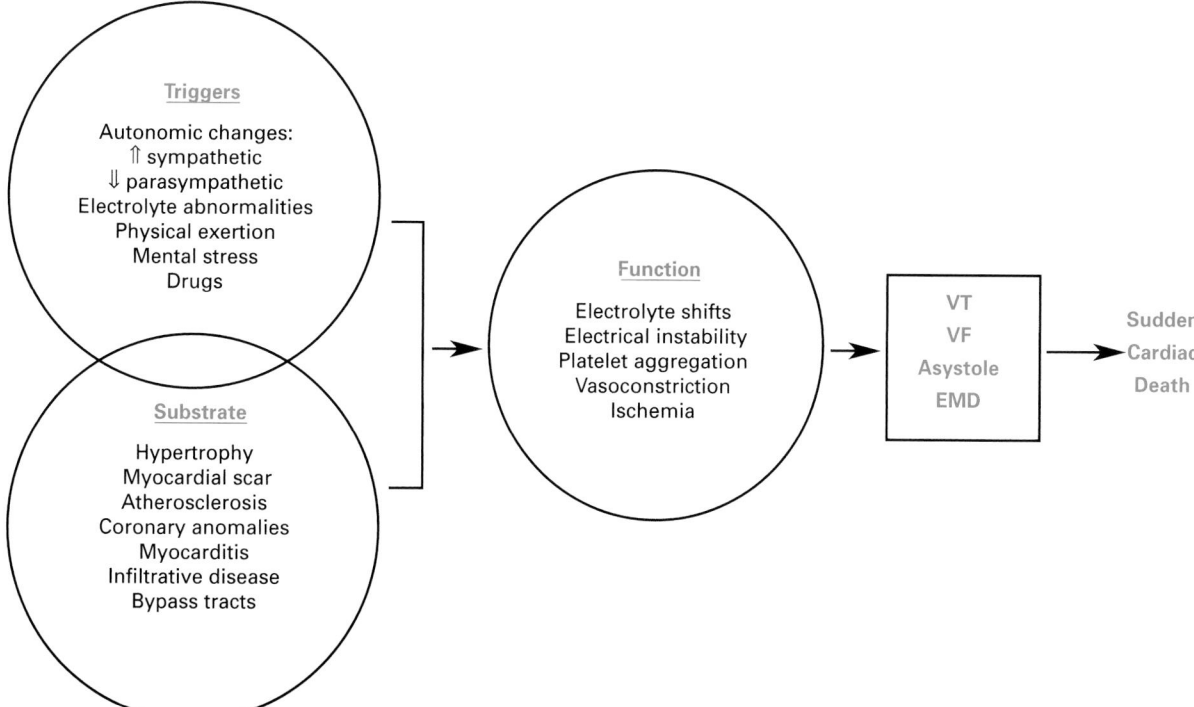

FIGURE 49–5. Interaction between structural cardiac abnormalities, functional changes, and triggering factors in the pathophysiology of SCD. The role of triggering factors, such as changes in autonomic tone or reflexes, is increasingly being recognized. EMD, electromechanical dissociation; VF, ventricular fibrillation; VT, ventricular tachycardia.

ventricular tachycardia is only rarely (less than 2 percent) documented as the initial rhythm, but it is unknown how often it precedes and precipitates ventricular fibrillation. In a series of 157 ambulatory patients who were wearing an ECG monitor at the time of their cardiac arrest, primary ventricular fibrillation was documented in 8 percent, ventricular tachycardia degenerating into ventricular fibrillation in 62 percent, and torsade de pointes in 13 percent.[49] Likewise, in patients with implantable cardioverter defibrillators, 90 percent of appropriate arrhythmia detections are for VT rather than VF.[50]

Electromechanical dissociation and asystole are found in approximately 30 percent of patients experiencing cardiac arrest, and this finding is usually related to the time interval from collapse to first monitoring of the rhythm, suggesting that it is often a later manifestation of cardiac arrest.[48] The incidence of bradycardia as the first documented rhythm varies according to the population studied. In patients who have died suddenly while wearing an ambulatory ECG monitor, bradyarrhythmias as the initial rhythm were documented infrequently, and ventricular tachyarrhythmias were most often the mode of cardiac arrest, even in patients with preexisting atrioventricular or intraventricular conduction defects.[49] In a small group of patients with severe congestive heart failure who were awaiting cardiac transplantation, bradycardia or electromechanical dissociation at the time of death was more frequent than ventricular arrhythmia.[51] We believe that in this population, bradycardia reflects the unrelenting failure of the severely impaired heart and is not a primary cause of sudden death unless the bradyarrhythmia allows for the development of a tachyarrhythmia. An understanding of the mechanisms responsible for ventricular arrhythmia is essential in its prevention and treatment, but a complete discussion is beyond the scope of this chapter (see Chaps. 35 and 39).

ELECTROPHYSIOLOGIC EFFECTS OF ISCHEMIA

Acute myocardial ischemia leads to intracellular and extracellular acidosis and loss of myocellular membrane integrity with efflux of potassium and influx of calcium. These biochemical abnormalities have electrophysiologic consequences, including a decrease in the amplitude and upstroke velocity of the cardiac action potential, inhomogeneous depolarization of the resting membrane potential, and shortening of action potential duration.[52] Fast sodium and slow calcium channels in partially depolarized fibers may remain inactive, thereby prolonging refractoriness even after completion of repolarization. This may further contribute to electrical inhomogeneities within and around the ischemic zone, causing conduction delays, unidirectional block, and reentrant arrhythmias.[53]

Ventricular arrhythmias during experimental coronary occlusion occur in two peaks, one between 2 and 8 minutes (phase IA) and a second at 15 to 45 minutes (phase IB). Rapid polymorphic ventricular tachycardia and fibrillation are the characteristic arrhythmias during the early stages of ischemia.[54] Activation mapping during ventricular fibrillation has demonstrated that the initial arrhythmias are caused by reentry, which is facilitated by the inhomogeneous conduction velocities and refractory periods in and around the ischemic zone. The second peak

of ventricular arrhythmias coincides with a peak in catecholamine release. Automatic and triggered rhythms are implicated in these arrhythmias. Reentrant rhythms may also occur, attributed to cellular uncoupling related to impaired function of gap junctions.[55]

Within the first 3 days of myocardial infarction, SCD may occur as a result of ventricular fibrillation initiated by early, frequent premature ventricular complexes (PVCs). Such PVCs have been shown in experimental models to be predominantly caused by impulse formation consistent with abnormal automaticity. Other manifestations of abnormal automaticity are the accelerated idioventricular rhythms signifying reperfusion. These arrhythmias appear to arise, for the most part, from surviving Purkinje fibers in the subendocardial border zone of a transmural infarction. They have no prognostic significance for development of late arrhythmias and usually subside after 2 to 3 days at about the same time that the resting membrane potential and action potential duration of Purkinje fibers normalize.[52]

In the late phases following myocardial infarction, when the infarction is healed, reentrant excitation is the principal mechanism of ventricular arrhythmias. Critical areas of the reentrant circuit are formed by surviving myocardial cells in the epicardial and endocardial border zone of a healed infarction as well as surviving intramural fibers within the infarct zone.[56] It appears that the rate, time, and degree of myocardial reperfusion influence the incidence, rate, and duration of these arrhythmias. More work is needed to further define these relationships (see Chap. 35).

MECHANOELECTRICAL FEEDBACK

Left ventricular dysfunction has been identified as the strongest independent predictor of SCD.[57] Despite the clinical recognition that acute heart failure can precipitate ventricular tachyarrhythmias, the mechanism by which this occurs is incompletely understood. Besides mechanisms related to acute and chronic ischemia, it has been shown that acute changes in the mechanical state of the heart related to altered preload and contractility can have direct electrophysiologic effects that may precipitate arrhythmias; this relationship is referred to as *mechanoelectrical feedback*. An increase in right ventricular pressure shortens action potential duration in humans.[58] An increase in both left ventricular preload and contractility shortens action potential duration and refractoriness in the canine ventricle as well.[59] There is some evidence that these changes may be mediated through the β-adrenergic receptor. Downstream effects leading to fluctuation of intracellular calcium levels or to an increase in a cyclic adenosine monophosphate-mediated potassium current may serve as the cellular mechanism by which this phenomenon occurs.[59] Recent mechanistic evidence has also pointed to calcium handling in the sarcoplasmic reticulum, mediated by defective regulation of the cardiac ryanodine receptor.[60]

CARDIAC DISEASES ASSOCIATED WITH SCD

Table 49–2 summarizes cardiac abnormalities associated with sudden death.

ISCHEMIC HEART DISEASE

Coronary Atherosclerosis

In survivors of cardiac arrest, CHD is present in 40 to 86 percent of patients, depending on age and gender of the population.[61] Patients with known coronary heart disease accounted for 20 to 34 percent of SCDs in the Framingham cohort.[9] SCD was the first symptom of CHD in approximately 10 percent of all coronary events.

Although the majority of patients who suffer SCD have severe multivessel coronary disease, fewer than half of the patients resuscitated from ventricular fibrillation evolve evidence of myocardial infarction by elevated cardiac enzymes, and less than 20 percent have Q-wave myocardial infarction.[48] Holter monitoring at the time of arrest infrequently shows evidence of ischemic ECG changes before the event.[46,62] In postmortem examinations and in catheterization studies, there was a significant (75 to 85 percent) stenosis in at least two major coronary arteries in as many as 76 percent of patients. Detailed pathologic studies confirm the presence of acute coronary arterial lesions (plaque fissure, plaque hemorrhage, and thrombosis) in up to 95 percent of patients who die suddenly, but only a fraction have total occlusion.[31,63]

Coronary collateralization may play an important role in the presentation of coronary artery disease as SCD. It is hypothesized

---

TABLE 49–2

Cardiac Abnormalities Associated with Sudden Cardiac Death

ISCHEMIC HEART DISEASE

Coronary atherosclerosis
  Acute myocardial infarction
  Chronic ischemic cardiomyopathy
Anomalous origin of coronary arteries
Hypoplastic coronary artery

Coronary artery spasm
Coronary artery dissection
Coronary arteritis
Small vessel disease

NONISCHEMIC HEART DISEASE

Cardiomyopathies
  Idiopathic dilated cardiomyopathy
  Hypertrophic cardiomyopathy
  Hypertensive cardiomyopathy
  Arrhythmogenic right ventricular cardiomyopathy
Infiltrative and inflammatory heart disease
  Sarcoidosis
  Amyloidosis
  Hemochromatosis
  Myocarditis
Valvular heart disease
Aortic stenosis
  Aortic regurgitation
  Mitral valve prolapse
  Infective endocarditis
  Congenital heart disease
Tetralogy of Fallot
  Transposition of the great vessels (post–Mustard-Senning)
  Ebstein anomaly
  Pulmonary vascular obstructive disease
  Congenital aortic stenosis
  Primary electrical abnormalities
Long QT syndrome
Short QT syndrome
Wolff-Parkinson-White syndrome
Congenital atrioventricular block
Idiopathic ventricular tachycardia
Idiopathic ventricular fibrillation
  Syndrome of right bundle-branch block, ST elevation, and sudden death (Brugada syndrome)
  Catecholaminergic polymorphic ventricular tachycardia
Nocturnal death in Southeast Asian men

Drug-induced and other toxic agents
  Antiarrhythmic drugs (class Ia, Ic, and III)
  Erythromycin
  Clarithromycin
  Astemizole
  Terfenadine
  Pentamidine
  Ketoconazole
  Trimethoprim-sulfamethoxazole
  Psychotropic drugs (tricyclic antidepressants, haloperidol, phenothiazines, chloral hydrate)
  Probucol
  Cisapride
  Cocaine
  Chloroquine
  Alcohol
  Phosphodiesterase inhibitors
  Organophosphates
Electrolyte abnormalities
  Hypokalemia
  Hypomagnesemia
  Hypocalcemia
  Anorexia nervosa and bulimia
  Liquid protein dieting
  Diuretics

that chronic ischemia may be a stimulus for development of coronary collaterals, which, in turn, could have a protective effect during acute coronary occlusion. The mitigating effect of coronary collateralization is supported by a study of exercise testing in 894 healthy men followed for a mean of 12.7 years. In this study, the initial coronary event was acute myocardial infarction or SCD in 73 percent of those with a normal stress test result, as opposed to 20 percent of those with an abnormal stress test result.[64] These findings might also be related to ischemic preconditioning, which is associated with reductions in ventricular fibrillation (VF) in animal models.[65]

Nonatherosclerotic Disease of the Coronary Arteries

Several nonatherosclerotic diseases of the coronary arteries are associated with increased risk of SCD precipitated by cardiac ischemia. Congenital coronary artery anomalies, found in approximately 1 percent of all patients undergoing angiography and in 0.3 percent of patients undergoing autopsy, have been complicated by SCD, often exercise-related, in up to approximately 30 percent of patients.[66] Origin of the left main coronary artery from the right aortic sinus or origin of the right coronary artery from the left coronary sinus are the variants most frequently associated with SCD.

Life-threatening ventricular arrhythmias and SCD have been described in patients with coronary artery spasm (Prinzmetal or variant angina). Significant arrhythmias during attacks of variant angina have been documented in these patients.[67] Calcium channel blockers are effective in many patients in preventing coronary spasm and appear also to protect from malignant ventricular arrhythmias if the attacks can be completely abolished. The major predictors of major coronary events in this population include systemic hypertension, luminal irregularities on coronary arteriography, and QT dispersion.[67]

SCD has been described as a rare complication of coronary artery dissection in Marfan syndrome, during the puerperium, secondary to trauma or coronary catheterization, as a consequence of syphilitic aortitis, or as an extension of aortic dissection. Myocardial bridges have been reported in association with SCD during exercise, but they are also an incidental finding at autopsy in up to 25 percent of patients dying of other causes.[68] Coronary arteritis and subsequent infarction have been reported in Kawasaki disease, giant cell arteritis, Behçet disease, systemic lupus erythematosus, and Churg-Strauss syndrome. Coronary occlusion can also occur as a complication of infective endocarditis, particularly involving the aortic valve (see Chap. 55).

[ ] CARDIOMYOPATHIES
Idiopathic Dilated Cardiomyopathy

Idiopathic dilated cardiomyopathy is the substrate for approximately 10 percent of SCDs in the adult population. The mortality rate for idiopathic dilated cardiomyopathy is high, reaching 10 to 50 percent annually, and is most closely tied to the severity of pump dysfunction.[69] Mortality rates are higher among patients with advanced heart failure, but the proportion of SCDs is not increased.[70] In an overview of 14 studies including 1432 patients

with idiopathic dilated cardiomyopathy, the mean mortality rate after a followup of 4 years was 42 percent, with 28 percent of deaths classified as sudden.[69] SCD in idiopathic dilated cardiomyopathy is usually attributed to both polymorphic and monomorphic ventricular tachyarrhythmias occurring in the setting of a high frequency of complex ventricular ectopy.[71] The terminal event may, however, also be a result of pump failure with asystole or electromechanical dissociation, especially in patients with advanced left ventricular dysfunction.[51]

Risk stratification of patients with idiopathic dilated cardiomyopathy is difficult because there are few clinical predictors specific for SCD. The only clinical variable that identifies patients with a higher risk of SCD is unexplained syncope, and these patients should undergo further evaluation. The prognostic value of simple and complex PVCs as well as nonsustained ventricular tachycardia (NSVT) is limited by the extremely high prevalence of these arrhythmias in patients with idiopathic dilated cardiomyopathy.[71] The induction of polymorphic ventricular tachycardia or fibrillation during electrophysiologic testing is nonspecific, and the probability of inducing sustained monomorphic ventricular tachycardia (VT) in this population is less than 10 percent.[72] Consequently, an electrophysiology study is not considered a useful screening tool in patients with nonischemic cardiomyopathy. However, when sustained monomorphic VT occurs in patients with dilated cardiomyopathy, the mechanism is usually reentrant and potentially amenable to catheter ablation (see Chaps. 29 and 44).[73]

Hypertrophic Cardiomyopathy

Hypertrophic cardiomyopathy (HCM), caused by a variety of mutations in genes encoding cardiac sarcomere proteins, is classically associated with asymmetric septal hypertrophy and myofibrillar disarray, but has diverse clinical presentations. The incidence of SCD in selected families with hypertrophic cardiomyopathy treated at large referral centers has been reported as high as 2 to 4 percent per year in adults and 4 to 6 percent per year in children and adolescents,[74] but is probably closer to 1 percent per year in unselected populations.[75,76]

A number of factors have been studied to aid in distinguishing the minority of HCM patients who are at high risk for SCD from the majority of patients who are at a much lower risk. The highest-risk features include a clinical history of spontaneous ventricular arrhythmias, sudden death in family members, onset of symptoms in childhood, and syncope or near-syncope, especially when exertional or recurrent and unrelated to neurocardiogenic mechanisms.[76] Other risk factors with a lower predictive value include extreme left ventricular wall thickness (e.g., greater than 3.0 cm),[77] hypotensive response to exercise,[78] unsustained ventricular tachycardia during ambulatory monitoring (particularly repetitive or prolonged bursts), and significant (greater than 30 to 50 mmHg) resting left ventricular outflow tract gradient. Although none of these factors alone have a high positive predictive value, they do have high negative predictive value, particularly in combination.[76] The decision to implant an ICD in a patient who has only one risk factor is uncertain and should be based on clinician and patient tolerance for risk.

Because of the clinical heterogeneity of HCM, there is hope that genotypic analysis will provide further guidance on SCD risk. For example, some mutations of the β-myosin heavy chain appear to be associated with a benign prognosis, whereas mutations in cardiac troponin T are associated with a mild degree of hypertrophy but a high incidence of SCD in selected kindreds.[79,80] As with most genetic disorders, however, the phenotypic expression of the same genetic abnormality is highly variable in HCM, and clinical decisions cannot be reliably made at this time based solely on genotype (see Chaps. 30 and 81).

Hypertensive Cardiomyopathy

Left ventricular hypertrophy (LVH) is one of the strongest independent risk factors for acute myocardial infarction, congestive heart failure, and sudden death.[81,82] In the Framingham Study, ECG evidence of LVH doubled the risk of SCD. Echocardiographic studies showed an incremental risk for cardiovascular deaths of 1.73 in men and 2.12 in women for each 50-g increment in the left ventricular mass index.[83] Decreased coronary blood flow, decreased flow reserve, and endothelial dysfunction may all be factors favoring the development of transient ischemia in the setting of LVH, and long-term, repeated transient ischemic episodes can lead to interstitial fibrosis, which may underlie the arrhythmias in this population.[84] Another potential contributing factor to the increased risk of SCD in hypertensive cardiomyopathy are electrolyte disturbances associated with diuretic therapy.[85]

Arrhythmogenic Right Ventricular Cardiomyopathy

ARVC is characterized by fatty or fibrofatty replacement of myocardium, primarily in the right ventricle, and ventricular tachyarrhythmias, usually of right ventricular (RV) origin. It is a rare cause of SCD, except in a few endemic regions, and is a familial disorder in approximately 30 percent of cases. The diagnosis is most easily made by magnetic resonance imaging; consensus diagnostic criteria were published in 1994.[86]

Multiple genetic mutations have now been reported as causing ARVC. The first reported mutation involves the cardiac ryanodine receptor (*RyR2*), the major calcium release channel on the sarcoplasmic reticulum in cardiomyocytes.[87] More recently, mutations have been reported from genes encoding four related proteins (plakoglobin,[88] desmoplakin,[89] plakophilin-2,[90] and desmoglein-2[91]) that are associated with desmosomes, which anchor intermediate filaments to the cell membrane in adjoining cells. An autosomal recessive mutations of the plakoglobin gene causes Naxos disease, characterized by ARVC and skin and hair abnormalities.[88] Desmosomal proteins are now thought to be involved in at least 40 percent of ARVC cases, but mutations of unrelated proteins, including transforming growth factor β_3,[92] also have been reported.

Recurrent ventricular tachycardia with multiple left bundle-branch block morphologies typifies ARVC. Patchy myocarditis, programmed cell death, and/or congenital abnormalities of development appear to lead to myocardial atrophy and repair by fibrofatty replacement, which forms the basis for ventricular reentry. The left ventricle and ventricular septum can be involved, especially later in the course of the disease, and such involvement confers a poor prognosis.[93]

The electrocardiographic manifestations of ARVC in sinus rhythm include T-wave inversion in V_1-V_3 or complete or incomplete right bundle-branch block. Intraventricular conduction delay may produce a terminal notch on the QRS complex, called an epsilon wave, in approximately 50 percent of patients. Ventricular ectopy is usually of a left bundle-branch pattern with a QRS axis between 90 degrees and +110 degrees and generally arises from one of three sites of fatty degeneration. Called the *triangle of dysplasia*, these sites are the right ventricular outflow and inflow tract and apex. Any patient with frequent premature beats of a left bundle-branch morphology and left-axis deviation should be evaluated for this disorder, which must be differentiated from the usually benign right ventricular outflow-tract tachycardia.

The course and prognosis of ARVC are highly variable and difficult to predict even in patients with overt disease and significant ventricular arrhythmias. ICDs are the primary therapy in those patients with sustained ventricular tachycardia with hemodynamic compromise or ventricular fibrillation, and nonrandomized studies suggest improved survival in patients with serious symptoms and high-risk mutations.[94,95] Sustained, tolerated VT can be treated successfully with catheter ablation,[96] but because ARVC tends to be a progressive condition, these patients are usually treated with ICDs as well. More data are required to define which asymptomatic patients with ARVC benefit from this therapy (see Chaps. 32 and 81).

【 】 VALVULAR HEART DISEASE

Aortic Valve Disease

The risk of SCD in asymptomatic patients with aortic stenosis or regurgitation appears to be low.[97,98] In contrast, there appears to be an increased risk of SCD following aortic valve replacement for aortic stenosis or regurgitation. In 831 patients receiving a Bjork-Shiley prosthesis in the aortic (341 patients), mitral (345 patients), or double-valve (145 patients) position, the incidence of SCD in the subgroups was 1.8 percent, 3.5 percent, and 4 percent, respectively, over a follow-up period of 7 years.[99] Malignant tachyarrhythmias have been suggested as the cause of SCD in such patients. Transient complete heart block is relatively common following both aortic (17.6 percent) and mitral (13 percent) valve replacement, pointing to bradyarrhythmias as another potential precipitating factor for SCD[100] (see Chap. 75).

Mitral Valve Prolapse

Whether or not mitral valve prolapse (MVP) is a cause of SCD is controversial. The prevalence of MVP is sufficiently high that its presence may just be a coincidental finding in victims of SCD. In a prospective 8-year study of 237 asymptomatic or minimally symptomatic patients with echocardiographically documented MVP, survival was not significantly different from that for a matched control population.[101] On the other hand, MVP may not always be benign. Patients with MVP associated with mitral regurgitation and left ventricular dysfunction clearly carry a risk for such complications as infective endocarditis, cerebroembolic events, and SCD.[102] In a significant number of victims of SCD, especially young women, MVP is the only structural cardiac disease identified.[103] Several echocardiographic risk factors for SCD have been identified in asymptomatic or mildly symptomatic MVP patients without significant mitral regurgitation, including increased mitral valve annular circumference, thickness of the anterior and posterior mitral valve leaflets, presence and extent of endocardial plaque, and presence or absence of redundant mitral valve leaflets on M-mode echocardiography.[101,104] The most important prognostic indicators for sudden death in MVP are probably a history of syncope and a family history of sudden death at a young age, as well as significant mitral regurgitation, abnormal left ventricular function and a long QT interval (see Chap. 76).[104]

[ ] INFLAMMATORY AND INFILTRATIVE MYOCARDIAL DISEASE

Any inflammatory disease can cause SCD as a consequence of either ventricular tachyarrhythmias or complete heart block. Histologic findings suggestive of myocarditis have been reported in 10 to 44 percent of young victims of SCD.[105] In adults, the diagnosis of myocarditis is made much less frequently, perhaps because of concurrent structural heart disease or because the late manifestations of the disease are indistinguishable from idiopathic dilated cardiomyopathy (see Chap. 32). In South America, however, myocarditis as a consequence of specific pathogens such as Chagas disease, is the most frequent cause of cardiomyopathy and related SCD.[106] Patients with infective endocarditis may also be at risk for SCD caused by acute coronary emboli from valvular vegetations. More often, SCD is caused by acute hemodynamic deterioration caused by valvular failure. Intramyocardial abscesses can also precipitate ventricular tachycardia and lead to SCD.

Infiltrative cardiomyopathies, such as primary or secondary amyloidosis, hemochromatosis, or sarcoidosis, are associated with predominantly cardiac conduction defects, as well as ventricular tachyarrhythmias and SCD. Ventricular tachycardia is sometimes the mode of presentation of sarcoidosis, can usually be reproduced by programmed electrical stimulation, and is associated with a high rate of recurrent arrhythmia and SCD (see Chap. 31).[107]

[ ] CONGENITAL HEART DISEASE

A 25- to 100-fold increased risk of SCD as a consequence of arrhythmia, increasing primarily in the second postoperative decade, has been found predominantly in four congenital conditions: tetralogy of Fallot, transposition of the great arteries, aortic stenosis, and pulmonary vascular obstruction.[108] In patients who have undergone reparative surgery for tetralogy of Fallot, a QRS duration of 180 milliseconds or more was found to be the most sensitive predictor of SCD and ventricular tachyarrhythmias in 793 adults and correlated with other parameters of right ventricular volume overload. Older age at repair also increased the risk of arrhythmia.[109] Electrophysiology testing is useful in evaluating the risk of ventricular arrhythmias in patients late after surgical repair of tetralogy of Fallot,[110] as these patients can be uniquely susceptible to reentrant VT.

Transposition of the great arteries (after Mustard and Senning procedures) is associated with at least a 6 percent risk of late SCD, which is, in some cases, caused by sinus node dysfunction, and in other cases, by ventricular tachyarrhythmias (see Chaps. 82 and 83).[111] Arterial-switch surgery for transposition may result in fewer late-term arrhythmias.

SCD is often (45 to 60 percent) the mode of death in patients with primary or secondary pulmonary hypertension (see Chap. 71). Death can be precipitated by general anesthesia, dehydration, exertion, or pregnancy. Any process that decreases systemic vascular resistance increases right-to-left shunting and decreases pulmonary flow. The resultant peripheral desaturation may trigger lethal arrhythmias and SCD.[112]

The SCD risk in congenital aortic stenosis is estimated to be 1 percent and occurs predominantly in symptomatic patients with severe left ventricular hypertrophy. The Ebstein anomaly is frequently (up to 25 percent) associated with the presence of accessory pathways and the Wolff-Parkinson-White syndrome, which carries a small risk of SCD (see below). Congenital heart block without associated structural heart disease occurs in 1 of 20,000 infants, and a moderate decrease in heart rate is usually well tolerated. A maternal risk factor is systemic lupus erythematosus. As previously noted, patients with severe bradycardia, however, have a tendency to develop ventricular arrhythmias. Pacemaker therapy has virtually eliminated the risk of SCD in this population.[112]

[ ] PRIMARY ELECTRICAL ABNORMALITIES
Long QT Syndrome

Sudden cardiac death is one of the hallmarks of the idiopathic long QT syndrome (LQTS), a group of genetically distinct disorders resulting from mutations in one of seven genes encoding cardiac ion channels or auxiliary ion-channel subunits (see also Chap. 33).[113,114] The long QT interval reflects abnormal prolongation of repolarization caused by defects in outward currents (potassium) or impaired inactivation of inward currents (sodium). Prolonged repolarization enhances the propensity to develop early afterdepolarizations leading to triggered activity that is the initiating mechanism for torsade de pointes (see Chap. 35). Other characteristics of this disorder, in addition to the prolonged QT interval (>440 milliseconds for males or >460 milliseconds for females, corrected for heart rate), include abnormal T-wave contours, relative sinus bradycardia, a family history of early sudden death, and a propensity for recurrent syncope and sudden cardiac death because of polymorphic ventricular tachycardia (torsade de pointes) and ventricular fibrillation. The rare autosomal recessive Jervell-Lange-Nielsen syndrome is also associated with congenital deafness.

More than 90 percent of the congenital forms of LQTS have been linked to specific chromosomal defects, resulting in a genetically based classification (LQT1 through LQT7) with important functional and prognostic implications.[114] Multiple mutations have been identified in each gene, and this locus heterogeneity appears to be important prognostically. The risk of sudden death in LQTS is influenced by the duration of the QT interval, corrected for heart rate (QTc), the specific genetic defect, gender, family history, and possibly other factors.[115]

Torsade de pointes can be triggered by different stimuli, typically involving high adrenergic states such as exercise or sudden arousal (startle). Cardiac events associated with exercise, especially with swimming, dominate the clinical picture of LQTS1 patients, and auditory stimuli tend to be a trigger for arrhythmic events in LQTS2 patients.[116] The frequency with which sudden deaths attributed to electrolyte or drug effects actually occur in unrecognized or subclinical carriers of LQTS genetic mutations is unknown, but these factors can precipitate torsade de pointes in known LQTS patients. Registry data suggest a >50 percent risk by age 40 years of syncope, cardiac arrest, or sudden death for LQT1,

LQT2, and male LQT3 gene carriers with QT intervals >500 milliseconds.[115] Lower levels of risk have been reported for other mutations and for patients with shorter QT intervals.

β Blockers are a mainstay of treatment for LQTS patients, and nonrandomized data suggest these drugs reduce mortality. In the past, pacemakers were used in some patients to avoid bradycardia and pauses, which exacerbate QT prolongation and torsade de pointes, and left-sided sympathectomy has also been used in selected cases. Implantable defibrillators are clearly indicated for sudden death survivors, and may also be appropriate for LQTS patients with syncope and other high-risk features.

Short QT Syndrome

Different mutations in a few of the same genes previously shown to cause long QT syndrome have recently been identified as causing a distinct syndrome characterized by shorter than normal corrected QT intervals (less than 300 to 320 milliseconds) and a propensity for both atrial fibrillation and sudden cardiac death at potentially very young ages.[117,118] The first familial analysis identified gain-of-function mutations in the KCNH2 (or hERG) gene, which codes for the potassium channel responsible the rapidly activating delayed rectifier (I_{Kr}) current.[117] Although loss-of-function mutations in this gene cause LQT2, the mutations in these families were associated with short QT intervals and unusually short atrial and ventricular refractory periods at electrophysiologic study.[119] Since this first description, two additional genetic mutations have been reported: a de novo gain of function mutation in the KCNQ1 gene (responsible for the subunit of the KvLQT1 protein [I_{Ks}]),[120] and a mutation in the KCNJ2 gene (coding the inwardly rectifying Kir2.1 [I_{K1}] channel), associated with a unique T-wave morphology.[121] Based on these preliminary data, short QT syndrome appears to be another uncommon genetically based condition responsible for some sudden deaths in infancy, childhood, and early adulthood.[118] The frequency, full range of genotypes and phenotypes, and optimal therapy of this condition require further study to define (see Chap. 33).

Idiopathic Polymorphic Ventricular Tachycardias and Idiopathic Ventricular Fibrillation

Several additional types of idiopathic polymorphic ventricular tachycardias have been described and are associated with an unfavorable prognosis. These arrhythmias include idiopathic ventricular fibrillation, torsade de pointes with normal QT and a short coupling interval,[122] and catecholaminergic polymorphic ventricular tachycardia. They can occur in sporadic or familial forms and are frequently, though not uniformly, associated with catecholamine release during physical or emotional stress.

Catecholaminergic polymorphic VT, characterized initially by a pattern of bidirectional VT first described in children, has been linked to mutations in the cardiac ryanodine receptor (*RyR2*)[123] and calsequestrin (*CASQ2*)[124] genes, both of which encode proteins involved in the handling of calcium by the sarcoplasmic reticulum. Patients with *RyR2* mutations have also presented with polymorphic ventricular tachycardia and ventricular fibrillation in adulthood. These arrhythmias are at least partly responsive to β blockers.[123] The pathophysiologic mechanisms underlying short-coupled torsade de pointes and other forms of idiopathic VF have not yet been characterized.

Although the list of potential causes of SCD continues to grow, a definite cause cannot be established in a minority of patients who suffer cardiac arrest. These instances of SCD without evident cause are sometimes attributed to idiopathic ventricular fibrillation. The incidence of idiopathic ventricular fibrillation is higher in selected populations such as younger patients (up to 14 percent in patients younger than 40 years of age[125]) or female survivors of SCD unrelated to myocardial infarction (10 percent[18]). The risk of recurrent ventricular fibrillation in this young and otherwise healthy patient population ranges between 22 and 37 percent at 2 to 4 years.[126] In survivors of cardiac arrest caused by idiopathic ventricular fibrillation, the diagnosis is made by exclusion if extensive cardiac workup reveals no diagnostic abnormality.

Brugada Syndrome

The syndrome of SCD associated with complete or incomplete right bundle-branch block and ST-segment elevation in V_1-V_3 in patients without demonstrable structural heart disease is known as the Brugada syndrome.[127] Three ST-segment morphologies have been described. The type 1 electrocardiographic pattern is characterized by upward convex, "coved" ST-segment elevation of 2 mm or greater followed by a negative T wave. By consensus guidelines,[128] the diagnosis of Brugada syndrome is made by the presence of the type I pattern in at least two leads (V_1-V_3) in the absence of other factor(s) that could account for the ECG abnormality (Table 49–3) when one of the following clinical criteria is present: documented ventricular fibrillation; polymorphic ventricular tachycardia; a family history of sudden death (age <45

TABLE 49–3

Abnormalities That Can Lead to ST-Segment Elevation in the Right Precordial Leads[a]

Right or left bundle-branch block, left ventricular hypertrophy
Acute myocardial ischemia or infarction
Acute myocarditis
Right ventricular ischemia or infarction
Dissecting aortic aneurysm
Acute pulmonary thromboemboli
Various central and autonomic nervous system abnormalities
Heterocyclic antidepressant overdose
Duchenne muscular dystrophy
Friedreich ataxia
Thiamine deficiency
Hypercalcemia
Hyperkalemia
Cocaine intoxication
Mediastinal tumor compressing the right ventricular outflow tract
Arrhythmogenic right ventricular dysplasia/cardiomyopathy
Long QT syndrome type 3
Early repolarization syndrome
Other normal variants (particularly in men)

[a]The final two conditions that can lead to ST-segment elevation are more likely to give rise to type 2 and type 3 ECGs. Most conditions mentioned in this table can give rise to type 1 ECG.
SOURCE: From Wilde AAM, Antzelevitch C, Borggrefe M, et al. Proposed diagnostic criteria for the Brugada syndrome: consensus report. Circulation 2002;106:2514–2519, with permission.

years); coved-type ECGs in family members; electrophysiologic inducibility; syncope; or nocturnal agonal respiration. The type 2 ECG pattern has J-wave elevation of ≥2 mm, a downsloping ST segment that remains ≥1 mm above the baseline, and then a positive or biphasic T wave, resulting in a "saddleback" appearance, whereas the type 3 pattern has a coved or saddleback shape with less than 1 mm of ST elevation. The diagnosis is also confirmed in patients with clinical predictors and type 2 or 3 electrocardiographic patterns that convert to type 1 after administration of a sodium channel blocking drug. The ECG manifestations of Brugada syndrome can by dynamic, even in clearly affected patients.

Mutations in the sodium channel gene *SCN5A* have been implicated as the cause of Brugada syndrome in many families.[129] Different mutations of the same gene are also responsible for LQTS type 3. Other ion channels and proteins are suspected to be causative as well because only approximately 20 percent of Brugada syndrome cases have been linked to *SC5NA*.[130]

Brugada syndrome has a particular high prevalence—and striking male predominance[131]—in southeast Asia. Brugada syndrome is now thought to be the explanation behind sudden, unexpected nocturnal death syndromes described prior to Brugada's work in young, apparently healthy males from Southeast Asia,[132] and variably known as *laitai* (Laos: "death during sleep"), *bangungut* (Philippines: "to rise and moan in sleep followed by death"), and *pokkuri* (Japan: "unexpected sudden death at night").[131,133,134]

The mutations in the Brugada syndrome are not associated with structural heart disease and seem to lead to an acceleration of recovery of the sodium channel or nonfunctional sodium channels. There is a transmural dispersion of repolarization and refractoriness. Local reexcitation via a phase 2 reentry mechanism can occur leading to the development of very closely coupled premature ventricular contractions that trigger ventricular tachycardia and fibrillation.[135,136]

Symptomatic patients have a high incidence of SCD; those who have syncope, ventricular tachycardia, or a prior history of cardiac arrest should be treated with ICD implantation. High rates of inducible polymorphic VT/VF have been reported during electrophysiologic studies of such subjects. Thus it has been proposed that family members of symptomatic patients who also have spontaneously abnormal ECGs undergo electrophysiologic studies for risk stratification and consider ICD implantation if VF is induced.[128] However, the clinical benefit of this strategy is unproven, and at least one group has found the electrophysiologic study to be poorly predictive in this setting.[130] Studies have shown a lower risk of sudden death in asymptomatic patients who are not inducible at electrophysiologic study and most agree that ICD placement is not beneficial in this setting.[137] There is also data suggesting that the incidence of sudden death in asymptomatic patients with a diagnostic ECG only after provocative testing also is also low.[130] Preliminary data suggest that quinidine, because of its inhibitory effects on the transient outward (I_{to}) current, may be beneficial in Brugada syndrome. Two groups have reported large reductions in electrophysiologic inducibility and clinical events in patients treated with this agent (see Chaps. 33 and 81).[138,139]

Wolff-Parkinson-White Syndrome

The risk of SCD in patients with Wolff-Parkinson-White syndrome is less than 1 per 1000 patient-years of followup.[140] Al-

though a rare event, it is an important one to consider, as it usually occurs in otherwise healthy individuals and, in the era of catheter ablation of accessory pathways, is a curable cause of SCD. The mechanism of SCD in most patients with Wolff-Parkinson-White is most likely the development of atrial fibrillation with rapid ventricular rates as a result of antegrade conduction over an accessory pathway and subsequent degeneration into ventricular fibrillation. The best predictor for development of ventricular fibrillation during atrial fibrillation is the spontaneous occurrence of a rapid ventricular response over the accessory pathway, with the shortest interval between preexcited ventricular beats (i.e., those conducted over the accessory pathway) being less than 220 milliseconds, but the specificity of this finding specificity is low.[141,142] Spontaneous or exercise-induced intermittent loss of preexcitation is helpful in identifying patients that will have a slower ventricular response in atrial fibrillation, and may be at lower risk for sudden death.

In symptomatic patients, an electrophysiologic study offers the opportunity to assess conduction properties of the accessory pathways, the propensity to develop tachyarrhythmias, and the possibility of cure with minimal risk with catheter ablation. A diagnostic electrophysiologic study can also be helpful in identifying patients with asymptomatic preexcitation who are at high risk for arrhythmic complications. One randomized study[143] in adults found a reduction in symptomatic arrhythmias—mainly atrioventricular reentrant tachycardia—over time with this approach, with no difference in mortality. Consequently, an electrophysiologic study for asymptomatic patients with preexcitation on ECG, with selective prophylactic ablation for patients with high-risk findings, is considered a class IIa intervention by consensus guidelines[144] and may be especially appropriate in patients with high-risk occupations (e.g., pilots). Alternatively, careful observation of such patients is considered a class I intervention.

[ ] DRUGS AND OTHER TOXIC AGENTS

Proarrhythmia

The paradox that antiarrhythmic agents can cause arrhythmias has been recognized since quinidine's introduction in 1918.[145] The most common form of proarrhythmia, seen with Vaughan-Williams class Ia and class III antiarrhythmics, stems from QT interval prolongation resulting from blockade of repolarizing potassium currents (primarily I_{Kr}) and is, accordingly, sometimes referred to as the *acquired* long QT syndrome. In these cases, the initiation of the arrhythmia is often triggered by bradycardia or a characteristic "long-short" coupling interval that initiates a pause-dependent prolongation of the QT interval. The ventricular tachycardia in this setting is usually of the typical torsade de pointes morphology. This form of proarrhythmia, seen in a dose-dependent manner in 2 to 5 percent of patients treated with quinidine, sotalol, or dofetilide, may be facilitated by electrolyte abnormalities such as hypokalemia or hypomagnesemia. It usually occurs within 3 days of drug initiation, has greater prevalence in women than men,[146] and concomitant therapy with digitalis and diuretic agents may predispose patients to this complication (see Chaps. 35 and 43).[147]

Besides antiarrhythmic drugs, many other commonly used medications with diverse actions have been implicated in ventricular proarrhythmia. Common examples include erythromycin, terfenadine, astemizole, pentamidine, and certain psychotropic drugs, such as tricyclic antidepressants and antipsychotics. Most of these drugs produce toxicity by prolonging repolarization and QTc, leading to torsade de pointes; some do so by interacting with the metabolism of other QT-prolonging agents. A few drugs (cisapride, terfenadine, astemizole) were withdrawn from the U.S. market because of such concerns. The list of medications reported to cause this complication is constantly growing (see Table 49–2), and a registry of drugs associated with this complication exists. An updated list of these drugs can be found online at www.torsades.org.

Proarrhythmia with different underlying mechanisms has been seen with other drugs that do not prolong the QT interval. For example, the Cardiac Arrhythmia Suppression Trial (CAST) showed an increased mortality rate in postinfarction patients treated with class Ic antiarrhythmic drugs encainide or flecainide compared with placebo, despite antiarrhythmic efficacy as documented by the suppression of PVCs.[148] It is believed that these potent sodium channel blockers exacerbate ischemia-induced myocardial conduction delays and promote reentrant ventricular tachycardias.[149] Class Ic antiarrhythmic agents can also lead to by proarrhythmia by converting atrial fibrillation to atrial flutter at slower-than-usual atrial rates, allowing one-to-one conduction of the flutter waves (referred to as *enhanced atrioventricular nodal conduction*). For this reason, nodal-blocking agents should be administered concomitantly with these medications. Phosphodiesterase inhibitors and other positive inotropic agents may promote arrhythmias via another mechanism. Possibly by increasing the intracellular calcium level, these medications have been shown to be proarrhythmic and to increase the risk of SCD, despite their beneficial effects on hemodynamic parameters.[150]

Cocaine and Alcohol

Widespread use of cocaine in the United States led to the realization that this drug can precipitate life-threatening cardiac events, including SCD. The combination of alcohol and cocaine is especially dangerous because of the generation of a unique metabolite, cocaethylene, that has enhanced cardiotoxicity.[151] Cocaine causes coronary vasoconstriction, increases cardiac sympathetic effects, increases action potential duration, and precipitates cardiac arrhythmias irrespective of the amount ingested, prior use, or whether there is an underlying cardiac abnormality. The combination of increased oxygen demand because of sympathetic stimulation and diminished coronary flow as a result of vasoconstriction may precipitate ischemia-induced arrhythmias and SCD (see Chap. 93).

Electrolyte Abnormalities

Hypokalemia is often found in patients during and following resuscitation from a cardiac arrest. Although it can be a secondary phenomenon caused by catecholamine-induced potassium shift into the cells, primary hypokalemia is clearly arrhythmogenic. There is an almost linear inverse relationship between serum potassium concentration and the probability of ventricular tachycardia in patients with acute myocardial infarction.[152] Electrolyte abnormalities are thought to play a role in the sudden death of patients treated with non–potassium-sparing diuretics[153] and in

those with severe eating disorders or who abuse diuretics or are on liquid-protein diets.

A decrease in the extracellular potassium level hypopolarizes the resting membrane potential, shortens the plateau duration, prolongs the phase of rapid repolarization in ventricular fibers, and causes an increase in pacemaker activity in Purkinje cells, triggering ventricular arrhythmias.[154] These changes in repolarization may increase the dispersion of the recovery of excitability and facilitate reentrant ventricular arrhythmias.[154] Many of the electrophysiologic effects of hypokalemia are similar to those caused by digitalis and catecholamine stimulation, explaining the high risk of ventricular arrhythmias when a combination of these factors is present.

Magnesium deficiency and changes in intracellular concentration of calcium can also be arrhythmogenic.[154] Increased intracellular calcium is believed to play a significant role in arrhythmias associated with digitalis glycosides, catecholamine-induced ventricular tachycardia, reperfusion arrhythmias, and the proarrhythmic effect seen with phosphodiesterase inhibitors and other positive inotropic agents (see Chap. 35).

CLINICAL PRESENTATION AND MANAGEMENT OF THE PATIENT WITH CARDIAC ARREST

OUT-OF-HOSPITAL CARDIAC ARREST

Approximately 80 percent of cardiac arrests occur at home, and about 60 percent are witnessed.[4] Because most patients are found in ventricular fibrillation, the time to successful defibrillation is a key element in the acute management of the cardiac arrest victim (see Chap. 50). The importance of early intervention is reflected in the *chain of survival* concept of emergency cardiac care systems: early access, early cardiopulmonary resuscitation (CPR), early defibrillation, and early advanced cardiac life support.[155] This concept has led to the development of tiered medical emergency systems in most urban areas. Following activation of the emergency call (911) system, the first response consists of the nearest emergency medical technicians or fire department that is trained to provide basic CPR and defibrillation. The second response is by paramedics who are trained in advanced cardiac life support, including endotracheal intubation, intravenous medications, and additional defibrillation if necessary.

Initiation of bystander CPR is another important element of early intervention and improves the chances of successful resuscitation. Retrospective studies show that bystander CPR more than doubles the odds of survival following cardiac arrest.[156] The earlier CPR is performed, the greater the proportion of patients who are found in ventricular fibrillation as opposed to bradycardia or asystole, and there is an increased rate of successful defibrillation in these patients. Data from two studies suggests that a period of effective CPR prior to defibrillation when emergency response times are greater than 4 to 5 minutes may improve survival.[157,158] Community-based CPR training programs result in a higher likelihood of bystander CPR being administered in out-of-hospital cardiac arrest.

To improve the time to initial defibrillation, early defibrillation by nonmedical personnel has been advocated. The widespread use of automated external defibrillators (AEDs) has the potential to improve significantly the availability of early defibrillation. AEDs are relatively simple and inexpensive devices that have an automatic detection and treatment algorithm for ventricular tachyarrhythmias. One study evaluating the use of these devices in casinos demonstrated a remarkable 74 percent survival rate for those who received their first defibrillation no later than 3 minutes after a witnessed collapse and 49 percent for those who received their first defibrillation after more than 3 minutes.[159] Improvements in other settings have also been noted.[160] For example, in the Piacenza region of Italy, 173,114 persons were instructed in the use of AEDs and survival to hospital discharge following cardiac arrest improved from 3.3 percent to 10.5 percent.[161] Likewise, a large North American multi-center study involving lay volunteers in 993 community units found an improvement in survival to hospital discharge after cardiac arrest from 14 percent to 23 percent when training in the use of AEDs was added to traditional CPR education.[162] It is hoped that ongoing efforts to improve the science behind resuscitation guidelines and the availability of early defibrillation will continue to improve the outcomes of cardiac arrest in all settings.

SURVIVAL AND PROGNOSIS AFTER CARDIAC ARREST

Marked differences in survival rates following out-of-hospital cardiac arrest have been reported in different communities. Survival rates are lowest in large cities such as New York (1.4 percent) and Chicago (4 percent)[122] and highest (29 percent) in Seattle, a mid-sized urban community where many of the early intervention concepts have been pioneered.[163] The in-hospital mortality rate following successful resuscitation outside the hospital remains as high as 90 percent in some populations (Fig. 49–6).[163,164] Important factors associated with increased in-hospital mortality rates after out-of-hospital resuscitation are cardiogenic shock after defibrillation, age 60 years or greater, requirement of four or more shocks for defibrillation, absence of an acute myocardial infarction, and coma on admission to the hospital.[48,165]

Survival depends largely on the initial recorded rhythm. Some 40 to 60 percent of patients who are found in ventricular fibrillation are successfully resuscitated, but only a fraction will survive to

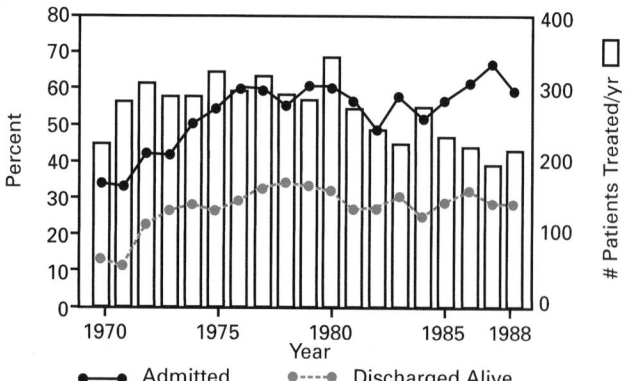

FIGURE 49–6. Percentage of out-of-hospital cardiac arrest victims admitted to the hospital by emergency medical service personnel and subsequently discharged alive during the period from 1970 to 1988. *Source: Reproduced from Cobb LA, et al. Community-based interventions for SCD: Impact, limitations, and changes. Circulation 1992;85:I98–I102 with permission.*

be discharged from the hospital. The outcome is much better in the smaller (less than 7 percent) group of patients where ventricular tachycardia is the initial documented rhythm, for whom the survival rate is more than 85 percent to hospital admission and over 75 percent to discharge. Bradycardias and electromechanical dissociation as the presenting rhythms are associated with the worst prognosis, and very few (less than 5 percent) of these patients survive to discharge from the hospital.[166] A higher burden of comorbid conditions such as heart failure, diabetes, chronic pulmonary disease, hypertension, and prior myocardial infarction, as well as recent symptoms prior to the event, are associated with worse outcomes.[167]

MANAGEMENT OF CARDIAC ARREST SURVIVORS AND RISK STRATIFICATION FOR SCD

ESTABLISHING THE UNDERLYING CARDIAC PATHOLOGY

The initial management following successful resuscitation from cardiac arrest consists of establishing cardiopulmonary stabilization, after which every effort should be made to determine the cause of cardiac arrest and likelihood of recurrence. For this, the underlying cardiac disease should first be determined. History and physical examination may provide the first clues. Myocardial infarction must be excluded by serum biomarker measurements and electrocardiography. Echocardiographic studies can determine left ventricular function, regional wall motion abnormalities, valvular heart disease, or cardiomyopathies. Stress-imaging studies can demonstrate inducible ischemia. Cardiac catheterization is often recommended to evaluate the coronary anatomy and hemodynamic parameters. Other tests, such as radionuclide studies, magnetic resonance imaging, or cardiac biopsy, may be necessary in selected patients. As discussed above, an underlying cardiac disease can be found in most patients.

Primary versus Secondary Cardiac Arrest

An important question following cardiac arrest is whether it was primarily caused by acute circulatory, or respiratory failure, or an arrhythmia. Although all these events are usually present during the arrest, it is important to distinguish whether the arrhythmia preceded or followed the hemodynamic collapse. Although several clinical and historical clues help to answer this question (Table 49–4), the distinction sometimes cannot be made with certainty. Separating primary from secondary cardiac arrest has important prognostic and therapeutic consequences. In 142 survivors of cardiac arrest with coronary artery disease, the 1-year survival rate was 89 percent, 80 percent, and 71 percent in the patients classified as having had cardiac arrest secondary to acute myocardial infarction (44 percent of patients), secondary to an ischemic event (34 percent), or because of a primary arrhythmic event (22 percent), respectively.[168] Patients who present with cardiac arrest secondary (and within 48 hours) to an acute transmural myocardial infarction have a prognosis similar to patients who have an acute myocardial infarction without an arrhythmia.[48] Specific antiarrhythmic therapy is therefore usually not recommended if cardiac

TABLE 49-4

Differences in Clinical Status Immediately before Death in Patients Dying Primarily of Arrhythmia versus Circulatory Failure

CLINICAL STATUS IMMEDIATELY BEFORE DEATH	ARRHYTHMIC DEATHS (N = 82)	CIRCULATORY FAILURE DEATHS (N = 59)
Comatose	0/82 (0%)	56/59 (95%)
Standing or actively moving	39/82 (48%)	0/59 (0%)
Terminal arrhythmia		
Ventricular fibrillation	15/18 (83%)	3/9 (33%)
Asystole	3/18 (17%)	6/9 (67%)
Duration of terminal illness		
<1 h	53/82 (65%)	4/59 (7%)
>24 h	17/82 (21%)	48/59 (81%)
Nature of terminal illness		
Acute cardiac events	80/82 (98%)	8/59 (14%)
Noncardiac events	1/82 (1%)	51/59 (86%)

SOURCE: *Modified from Hinkle LE Jr, Thaler HT. Clinical classification of cardiac deaths. Circulation 1982;65(3):457–464,with permission.*

arrest occurs during or within 2 days of an acute ST-elevation myocardial infarction. In contrast, if the arrhythmia is the primary event and only low-level biomarker evidence of myocardial infarction develops secondary to the acute hemodynamic deterioration during the arrhythmia, then antiarrhythmic therapy is recommended unless a transient or reversible cause is identified.

Every effort should be made to exclude potentially reversible causes of SCD, including transient ischemic episodes in patients who are candidates for revascularization and in whom the onset of the arrhythmia is clearly preceded by ischemic ECG changes or symptoms. Other reversible etiologies for cardiac arrest include transient severe electrolyte disturbances and proarrhythmic effects of antiarrhythmic drugs and other pharmacologic agents (see Drugs and Other Toxic Agents above). It can be difficult to establish a causal relationship between the proarrhythmic agent and the malignant ventricular arrhythmia in come cases. Pathologic prolongation of the QTc interval preceding initiation of the arrhythmia and return of the QTc interval to normal following discontinuation of the presumed proarrhythmic agent are strongly suggestive.

Another setting in which a reversible etiology for cardiac arrest is often present is in the hemodynamically unstable patient in the early postoperative period following cardiac surgery. Infusion of positive inotropic and pressor agents, electrolyte imbalances, acidosis, and hypoxia are often precipitating factors. Nevertheless, one should be cautious in assigning, as the primary cause of arrest, a functional trigger such as ischemia or electrolyte imbalance. In the patient with structural heart disease, especially myocardial infarction, the underlying anatomic substrate should be considered the primary disorder, and eliminating transient perturbations such as drug effects, hypoxia, and ischemia may not be sufficient in eliminating the risk for recurrent arrest. In fact, patients from the Antiarrhythmics Versus Implantable Defibrillator (AVID) registry who were thought to have arrested from a transient or correctable cause (and were therefore excluded from the trial) had a mortality rate that was similar to the general population of patients with ventricular fibrillatory arrest.[169]

[ ] RISK STRATIFICATION FOR SCD

A variety of means have been evaluated to assist in prospectively identifying individuals at high risk for sudden cardiac death in order to target them for preventative therapies. Such methods have most often been applied to patients with dilated cardiomyopathy and/or prior myocardial infarction, as these are the most common conditions associated with sudden cardiac death. At present there is no universal agreement on the optimal approach to sudden death risk stratification, in part because each of these methods possess, at best, moderate sensitivity and specificity for predicting future events, and in part because only a few of the techniques have been used in prospective clinical trials of effective interventions. The use of different risk stratification methods in the selection of candidates for prophylactic ICD implantation remains a point of controversy.

Clinical History

Several prognostic variables for SCD are related to clinical history. In the AVID registry, these included age >65 years, reduced ejection fraction, history of congestive heart failure, atrial fibrillation, prior pacemaker, diabetes, and smoking.[170] Interestingly, the hemodynamic impact of the qualifying arrhythmia was not a predictor of outcome in this study. Syncope in patients with a left ventricular ejection fraction below 30 percent is associated with increased risk of SCD (approximately 50 percent at 3 years) irrespective of finding an arrhythmic cause.[171] Patients with a history of unexplained, impaired consciousness, especially if associated with congestive heart failure or other structural heart disease, should also be considered at high risk for sudden death and warrant further therapy or risk stratification. In patients with unexplained syncope and structural heart disease, the induction of sustained VT or VF at electrophysiology study is considered a class I indication of ICD implantation.[172]

Left Ventricular Function

Left ventricular dysfunction is a major independent predictor of total and sudden cardiac mortality rates in patients with ischemic as well as nonischemic cardiomyopathy and has become a singular criterion in the selection of patients for prophylactic ICDs.[173] Assessment of left ventricular function by clinical history (e.g., a history of congestive heart failure) and by either noninvasive (echocardiography, nuclear imaging, MRI) or invasive means (angiography) is essential in the evaluation of a patient who is at risk for SCD.[57] Unfortunately, detection of severe left ventricular dysfunction serves to predict the total cardiac mortality rate but does not distinguish patients who will die suddenly from those who will die of progressive congestive heart failure.[174,175]

Electrocardiographic Abnormalities

In survivors of out-of-hospital cardiac arrest, the presence of atrioventricular block or intraventricular conduction defects on ambulatory ECG (72 hours) is associated with a higher recurrence rate of cardiac arrest.[166] Other ECG parameters reported to be associated independently with an increased risk of SCD are prolongation of the QT interval,[176] increased dispersion of the QT interval,[177] atrial fibrillation, left bundle-branch block, left ventricular hypertrophy,[82] and an increase in resting heart rate above 90 beats/min, particularly in men without a history of coronary artery disease.[178]

Detection of NSVT by ambulatory ECG monitoring has been reported to be of value in the risk stratification of patients for SCD, particularly following myocardial infarction.[57,179] The incidence of SCD in the 2 years following myocardial infarction in 766 patients enrolled in a prospective multicenter study increased with the frequency of PVCs detected during 24-hour ECG monitoring from 3 percent for less than 1 per hour to 14 percent for greater than 30 per hour; similarly, patients with NSVT had a higher (17 percent) incidence of SCD than did those with single PVCs (6 percent).[179] The prognostic value of ambulatory ECG monitoring in patients with congestive heart failure is limited by the high incidence of these arrhythmias (up to 88 percent) in this population, resulting in a low specificity of this parameter.[180]

Autonomic Markers

There is increasing evidence that cardiac abnormalities associated with a high risk of SCD are accompanied by changes in autonomic function. Myocardial infarction, for instance, causes regional cardiac sympathetic and parasympathetic denervation.[181] This autonomic heterogeneity may predispose to arrhythmia development by creating dispersion of refractoriness and/or conduction. Mathematical analyses of ambulatory ECG recordings have generated several measurements related to autonomic function associated with an increased risk of sudden and total cardiac death in postmyocardial infarction (MI) and heart-failure populations. Reported measures include depressed heart rate variability, baroreceptor sensitivity, and heart rate turbulence.

Reduced baroreflex sensitivity and heart rate variability reflect impairment in the vagal efferent component of the autonomic nervous system, and may help to predict cardiovascular mortality rates and arrhythmic events, particularly in patients following myocardial infarction. In one prospective study of 6693 unselected patients who underwent 24-hour ECG monitoring, those with reduced heart rate variability had a fourfold higher risk of SCD than did patients with higher variability.[182] Another study compared the relative usefulness of these measures alone and in combination by measuring baroreflex sensitivity, heart rate variability, 24-hour ECG recording, and left ventricular ejection fraction in more than 1000 patients after myocardial infarction.[183] In that study, NSVT, abnormal heart rate variability, and baroreflex sensitivity each were independently predictive of worse outcomes. The combination of all three risk factors signified a 22-fold increased risk of death, but the positive predictive value was only approximately 20 percent. A recent analysis from the DEFINITE trial showed very low mortality rates in nonischemic cardiomyopathy patients with preserved heart rate variability, suggesting that these patients may not benefit from ICD implantation.[184]

These findings underscore the usefulness of identifying patients who are at low risk for adverse events with negative test findings, as well as the limitations of predicting events based on positive results.

Signal-Averaged Electrocardiography

Late potentials, microvolt waveforms extending the duration of a filtered QRS complex detected by signal-averaged electrocardiography (SAECG), are helpful in the risk stratification of patients following myocardial infarction. The prognostic significance of late potentials has been demonstrated in several studies, which reported a 17 to 29 percent incidence of SCD, ventricular fibrillation, or sustained ventricular tachycardia in patients with an abnormal SAECG, in contrast to 0.8 to 3.5 percent in those without.[185] Although the negative predictive value of a normal SAECG is good, the application of SAECG in risk stratification for SCD is limited by a low positive predictive value in patients following myocardial infarction, as well as by its poor sensitivity in patients with nonischemic cardiomyopathies (see Chap. 42).[186]

T-Wave Alternans

Macroscopic T-wave changes with an alternating-beat pattern have been observed in patients with long QT syndrome prior to onset of ventricular fibrillation as well as in the setting of mechanical alternans, as is sometimes present during cardiac tamponade. Recent studies indicate that T-wave alternans that is discernible only by computer-averaging techniques may be a more ubiquitous phenomenon that can identify patients who are at risk for ventricular arrhythmias.[187]

Techniques for computer-assisted detection of microvolt-level T-wave alternans have been developed and may provide a useful method for assessing susceptibility to SCD. The presence of sustained microvolt-level T-wave alternans, typically measured noninvasively during exercise treadmill testing, correlates well with the result of electrophysiologic testing and has been shown in multiple series to be associated with a two- to fourfold increased risk for SCD and/or total mortality, after adjusting for other factors.[188–190] In these series, abnormal test results had a roughly 80 percent sensitivity for serious arrhythmic events over 1 to 2 years of followup, with negative predictive values consistently greater than 95 percent. A strategy incorporating T-wave alternans testing into clinical decision making could improve the cost-effectiveness of ICDs for primary prevention candidates.[191]

Electrophysiologic Studies

Electrophysiologic studies have advanced our understanding of life-threatening ventricular arrhythmias and facilitated the development of new therapies for their prevention and treatment. Induction of sustained monomorphic ventricular tachycardia is the generally accepted end point for programmed ventricular stimulation, whereas induction of nonsustained ventricular arrhythmias, polymorphic VT, or ventricular fibrillation may be nonspecific findings depending on the aggressiveness of the stimulation protocol.[192,193] Information obtained during electrophysiologic studies—such as VT rate, morphology, origin, mechanism, and hemodynamic stability—is valuable in planning appropriate therapy.

In patients who present with sustained monomorphic VT, the clinical rhythm is reproducibly inducible in the majority, especially in those with prior myocardial infarction.[193] Electrophysiologic testing is also useful in patients with structural heart disease who present with unexplained syncope. VT is the most common abnormal finding in these patients, but demonstration of His-Purkinje conduction disease or hemodynamically unstable supraventricular tachycardia can also be important. In survivors of cardiac arrest caused by ventricular fibrillation, the value of electrophysiologic testing is less clear, but may be of diagnostic usefulness in selected circumstances.

In the past, serial electrophysiologic testing was performed to assess the efficacy of antiarrhythmic drugs in suppressing inducible arrhythmias. Given the observed superiority of ICDs over antiarrhythmic drugs in clinical trials for both primary and secondary sudden death prevention, this practice essentially has been abandoned. The electrophysiologic laboratory continues, however, to offer the therapeutic option of VT ablation for recurrent VT in patients with both ischemic and nonischemic heart disease, particularly those who experience frequent ICD shocks.

The role of electrophysiologic testing in selection of patients for primary prevention with ICDs remains somewhat unsettled. Early studies suggested relatively low rates of VT inducibility in patients with nonischemic cardiomyopathy and no history of sustained arrhythmia. Thus electrophysiologic testing has never been widely advocated as a tool for selecting nonischemic patients for ICDs because of low sensitivity in this population (see Device Therapy below). Although electrophysiologic testing does predict future arrhythmic events independent of ejection fraction in the presence of prior MI, concern has been raised regarding the poor negative predictive value of electrophysiologic studies in patients with severely compromised ejection fraction (<30 percent).[194] Electrophysiologic inducibility (as well as nonsustained VT on ambulatory monitoring) was an entry criterion for MUSTT (Multicenter Unsustained Tachycardia Trial) and MADIT (Multicenter Automatic Defibrillator Implantation Trial), the first major clinical trials to demonstrate a survival benefit for ICDs over drug therapy in the primary prevention of sudden cardiac death (Table 49–5).[195,196] MUSTT and MADIT included post-MI patients with ejection fractions below 40 percent and 35 percent, respectively. More recent ICD trials, which enrolled post-MI patients with ejection fractions less than 30 to 35 percent, did not require electrophysiologic inducibility for enrollment.[197,198] Although these trials did show survival benefit for ICD implantation compared with control therapy, the magnitude of this benefit was significantly smaller than in the earlier trials that used in electrophysiologic studies for risk stratification (see Chap. 42).

TREATMENT OPTIONS FOR PATIENTS AT RISK FOR SCD

[ ] PHARMACOLOGIC THERAPY

Several medications reduce the risk of SCD in patients known to have cardiac disease. Some, such as the statins and aspirin, reduce sudden death by reducing the incidence of coronary plaque rupture or platelet aggregation and thrombosis (see Chaps. 26 and 52). β Blockers stabilize autonomic balance, improve pump func-

tion, and help reduce ischemia, while angiotensin-converting enzyme (ACE) inhibitors reduce the incidence of sudden death through similar and probably other mechanisms (see Chaps. 26 and 52).

β Blockers

Of all the therapies currently available for the prevention of SCD, none are better established or more universally applicable in patients with coronary heart disease than β blockers.[199] In a review of 19,000 postmyocardial infarction patients who were randomized to β blockers or placebo, active treatment was associated with a decrease in total mortality of 20 percent, of SCD 30 percent, and of reinfarction 35 to 40 percent.[200] The Metoprolol CR/XL Randomized Intervention Trial in Congestive Heart Failure (MERIT-HF) demonstrated a 34 percent decrease in the all-cause mortality rate, 38 percent decrease in the cardiovascular mortality rate, and a 41 percent decrease in the sudden death rates in 3991 patients who were randomized to β blockers or placebo while being treated with standard medical therapy, including ACE inhibition, digitalis, and diuretics.[201]

β Blockers are effective in the setting of ventricular arrhythmias provoked by a high sympathetic tone, as in patients with congenital long QT syndrome, arrhythmogenic right ventricular dysplasia, or congestive heart failure (CHF). Importantly, the beneficial effects of β blockers on cardiac mortality are most pronounced in patients who are at higher risk for sudden cardiac death, such as those with CHF, atrial and ventricular arrhythmias, post-MI, and diabetes (see Chap. 36).[199]

Angiotensin-Converting Enzyme Inhibitors

Reduced total mortality rates have been proven with the use of ACE inhibitors in patients with impaired ejection fraction with or without mild heart failure symptoms after myocardial infarction[202] and with established heart failure.[203–205] Although the mortality benefit from ACE inhibitors is thought to stem primarily from a reduction in pump failure, a specific reduction in the incidence of sudden death may be present as well. Although data from individual trials has conflicted on this issue, a meta-analysis including over 15,000 post-MI patients reported a 20 percent reduction in sudden cardiac death in ACE inhibitor-treated subjects (odds ratio [OR] 0.80; 95 percent confidence interval [CI] 0.70 to 0.92).[206] Whether these results also pertain to angiotensin-receptor blockers is not known.

The protection afforded by ACE inhibitors may extend to patients with vascular disease in general. A recent trial of patients with preserved ventricular function who were 55 years or older and had vascular disease or diabetes and one other coronary risk factor found significantly fewer patients treated with ramipril had a cardiac arrest (relative risk: 0.62; $p = 0.02$).[207]

Beta-Hydroxy-Beta-Methylglutaryl-Coenzyme A (HMG-CoA) Reductase Inhibitors

The beneficial effects of statins for patients with atherosclerotic heart disease, and vascular disease in general, continue to mount. Recent reports suggest that, in addition to preventing vascular events, statins reduce SCD and appropriate shocks in patients with ICDs.[208] A report from the MADIT II trial found that time-dependent exposure to statins was associated with a nearly 30 per-

Trials for Primary Prevention of Sudden Cardiac Death

	N	CAD	LOW EF	PVCS	NSVT	THERAPY	FOLLOW-UP (MONTHS)	FINDINGS	COMMENTS
CORONARY ARTERY DISEASE									
Class IC									
CAST, 1989	1498	+	+	+	−	Encainide or flecainide vs. placebo	10	7.7% mortality (treatment) vs. 3.0% (placebo)	Terminated prematurely because of excess mortality in treatment group
CAST II, 1992	1325	+	+	+	−	Moricizine vs. placebo	14 days	2.6% death or cardiac arrest (treatment) vs. 0.5% (placebo)	Terminated prematurely because of excess mortality in treatment group
Amiodarone									
BASIS, 1990	312	+	−	+	−	Amiodarone vs. mexiletine or quinidine vs. placebo	72	5% mortality (amiodarone) vs. 10% (class I) vs. 13% (placebo)	Amiodarone improved survival, non-significant trend with Holter-guided PVC suppression
EMIAT, 1997	1486	+	+	−	−	Amiodarone vs. placebo	21	7.2% mortality (both groups), 35% RR in arrhythmic death	Amiodarone reduced arrhythmic death rate without affecting total survival
CAMIAT, 1997	1202	+	−	+	−	Amiodarone vs. placebo	21	3.3% VF/SCD (amiodarone) vs. 6.0% (placebo), RR 21.2%	Prophylactic amiodarone improved survival for frequent/repetitive PVCs
ICD									
MADIT, 1996	196	+	+	+	+	ICD vs. conventional therapy	27	15.7% mortality (ICD) vs. 38.6% (no ICD), RR 46%	Terminated prematurely because of significant ICD benefit
CABG-Patch, 1997	900	+	+	−	−	ICD vs. no ICD at time of CABG	36	No difference in all-cause mortality	All patients had abnormal SAECG; no benefit of prophylactic ICD
MUSTT, 1999	704	+	+	+	+	EP-guided or ICD vs. no antiarrhythmic therapy	60	25% mortality (EP-guided or ICD) vs. 32% (no therapy)	EP-guided therapy with ICDs, but not with antiarrhythmic drugs, reduces the risk of SCD
MADIT-2, 2002	1232	+	+	−	−	ICD vs. conventional therapy	20	15.7% mortality (ICD) vs. 19.8% (no ICD), RR 31%	Patients on average were 3 years post-infarction
DINAMIT, 2004	674	+	+	−	−	ICD vs. conventional therapy	30	18.7% mortality (ICD) vs. 17.0% (no ICD); HR 1.08	ICDs reduced arrhythmic death, but increased nonarrhythmic death
Sotalol									
Julian et al., 1982	1456	+	−	−	−	d,l-Sotalol vs. placebo	12	7.3% mortality (sotalol) vs. 8.9% (placebo), RR 18%	d,l-Sotalol may reduce mortality by up to 25%
SWORD, 1996	3121	+	+	−	−	d-Sotalol vs. placebo	5	5.0% mortality (sotalol) vs. 3.1% (placebo)	Trial terminated because of excess mortality in the treatment group

CHF TRIALS (NON-ISCHEMIC OR MIXED POPULATION)

Trial, Year	N					Design	EF	Results	Comment
GESICA, 1994	516	~1/3	+	−	−	Amiodarone vs. standard therapy	24	33.5% mortality (amiodarone) vs. 41.4% (control)	Amiodarone improved survival in symptomatic heart failure
CHF-STAT, 1995	674	~2/3	+	−	−	Amiodarone vs. placebo	45	30.6% mortality (amiodarone) vs. 29.2% (placebo)	No survival benefit with amiodarone; trend to improved survival in DCM
DEFINITE, 2004	458	−	+	+	+	ICD vs. standard therapy	29	7.9% mortality (ICD) vs. 14.1% (no ICD) at 2 years: HR 0.65 (0.40–1.06), $p = 0.08$	Statistically significant reduction in SCD from arrhythmia
COMPANION, 2004	1520	~1/2	+	−	−	Med Rx vs. CRT-P vs. CRT-D	16	1-yr mortality 19% (med Rx) vs. 15% (CRT-P) vs. 12% CRT-D	Mortality a secondary end point; CRT-D vs. med Rx $p = 0.003$
SCD-HeFT, 2005	2521	~1/2	+	−	−	ICD vs. amiodarone vs. placebo	45	22% mortality (ICD) vs. 28% (amiodarone) and 29% (placebo); HR (ICD vs. placebo) 0.77	Amiodarone of no benefit vs. placebo; single-lead, shock-only ICDs used

+, Inclusion criterion; −, not inclusion criterion; amio, amiodarone; CAD, coronary artery disease; CHF, congestive heart failure; DCM, dilated cardiomyopathy; EF, ejection fraction; ICD, implantable cardioverter/defibrillator; NSVT, nonsustained ventricular tachycardia; PVCs, premature ventricular contractions; RR, risk reduction; SCD, sudden cardiac death; VF, ventricular fibrillation; HR, hazard ratio; CRT-P, cardiac resynchronization therapy pacemaker; CRT-D, cardiac resynchronization therapy defibrillator. See text for clinical trial abbreviations.

SOURCE: Modified with permission from Welch PJ, Page RL, Hamdan MH. Management of ventricular arrhythmias: a trial-based approach. J Am Coll Cardiol 1999;34:621–630.

cent reduction in appropriate ICD therapy for VT/VF or cardiac death, after adjustment for other factors.[209] Whether this effect of statins is mediated through prevention of coronary ischemic events, or through some other mechanism, is unknown.

Class I Antiarrhythmic Agents

The efficacy and safety of antiarrhythmic drugs in preventing sudden death has been disappointing (see Table 49–5). In fact, for patients with advanced heart failure and/or prior MI, only two antiarrhythmic drugs—amiodarone and dofetilide—lack evidence of *increased* mortality compared with placebo. The landmark CAST I and CAST II trials revealed increased mortality in post-MI patients with frequent ventricular ectopy treated for primary prevention with Vaughn-Williams Class Ic agents encainide, flecainide, and moricizine.[148,210,211] Likewise, the propafenone arm of the secondary prevention CASH (Cardiac Arrest Study Hamburg) trial was terminated early because of excess mortality compared with the other groups.[212]

A meta-analysis of lidocaine in acute myocardial infarction suggested an increase in in-hospital mortality rate despite a reduction in the prevalence of ventricular fibrillation.[213] Empiric use of class Ia drugs for long-term management in cardiac arrest survivors was also shown to increase mortality in a nonrandomized series.[214] No other class I antiarrhythmic drug has been shown to prolong survival in any patient group studied (see Chap. 43).

Sotalol

The effect of the class III agent sotalol on sudden death in high-risk patients is somewhat uncertain, in part because the commercially available preparation of the drug is a racemic mixture of *d* and *l* stereoisomers. The *d* isomer is a potent class III antiarrhythmic agent while the *l* isomer has nonselective β-blocking effects. Consequently, separating out potentially detrimental and beneficial effects of sotalol is difficult. In the Electrophysiologic Study Versus Electrocardiographic Monitoring (ESVEM) study, which enrolled patients with sustained ventricular tachycardia (75 percent), syncope, or cardiac arrest, sotalol appeared to be both safer and more effective than a variety of class I agents.[215]

However, when the class III effects of *d*-sotalol are separated from the β-blocking properties of *l*-sotalol, the drug appears less safe. *d*-Sotalol was compared with placebo in more than 3000 patients in the Survival with Oral *d*-Sotalol (SWORD) trial of post-MI patients with ejection fractions ≤40 percent, and was associated with a statistically significant increase in total mortality.[216] Sotalol prolongs the QT interval and can cause torsade de pointes, which has been reported to occur in up to 8 percent of treated patients.

Dofetilide

Unlike sotalol and the Vaughn-Williams class I agents, dofetilide, a newer class III antiarrhythmic drug devoid of β-blocking properties, has established safety with careful use in heart failure and post-MI patients. Dofetilide was studied in heart failure (DIAMOND-CHF; N = 1518)[217] and post-MI populations (DIAMOND-MI; N = 1510)[218] and showed a neutral effect on mortality in both. The drug was effective in converting atrial fibrillation and maintaining sinus rhythm—its only FDA-approved

indication—as well as in decreasing hospitalizations for heart failure.

Amiodarone

Amiodarone is widely considered the most effective antiarrhythmic agent for therapy of supraventricular and ventricular arrhythmias (see Chap. 43).[219,220] It is a class III antiarrhythmic agent with additional class I, II, and IV properties and has unusual pharmacokinetics, with a delayed onset of action and long elimination half-life after chronic therapy. Both oral and intravenous versions are available.

Several placebo-controlled randomized studies showed that amiodarone significantly reduced SCD rates following myocardial infarction, but its effects on total mortality are questionable.[221] The Basel Antiarrhythmic Study of Infarct Survival (BASIS) showed that amiodarone significantly reduced total mortality at 1 year from 13 percent to 5 percent (see Table 49–5).[222] On the other hand, amiodarone therapy did not reduce the total mortality rate but was shown to be safe compared with placebo in nearly 2700 postmyocardial infarction patients enrolled in the Canadian Amiodarone Myocardial Infarction Arrhythmia Trial (CAMIAT)[223] and the European Myocardial Infarction Amiodarone Trial (EMIAT)[224] despite a 50 percent risk reduction in the arrhythmic mortality rate (see Table 49–5). Post-hoc analysis of the pooled CAMIAT and EMIAT trial data showed a significant reduction in total mortality for amiodarone when combined with β blockers.[225]

In patients with congestive heart failure, prophylactic therapy with amiodarone decreased the mortality rate (by 28 percent) in the Argentine Grupo de Estudio de la Sobrevida en la Insuficiencia Cardiaca en Argentina (GESICA) trial,[226] but not in the Survival Trial of Antiarrhythmic Therapy in Congestive Heart Failure (CHF-STAT).[227] Comparison of the two patient populations suggested that prophylactic amiodarone may be more beneficial in patients with nonischemic cardiomyopathy, found in greater number in the GESICA study (see Table 49–5).

Thus individual trials comparing amiodarone with placebo suggest a consistent reduction in sudden death, but an inconsistent effect on total mortality. Two meta-analyses of all placebo-controlled amiodarone trials prior to SCD-HeFT (Sudden Cardiac Death in Heart Failure Trial) were published; both concluded that amiodarone reduces the total mortality of post-MI and heart failure populations by approximately 10 percent.[228,229] Therefore, in our opinion, amiodarone is the drug of choice when antiarrhythmic drug treatment is required for patients with left ventricular dysfunction and congestive heart failure. Sotalol may be considered in those patients with left ventricular systolic dysfunction without congestive symptoms.

Given its status as the most effective drug for the prevention and treatment of ventricular arrhythmias, amiodarone served as an active control against ICDs in the AVID, CASH, and CIDS (Canadian Implantable Defibrillator Study) studies,[230–232] as well as the recently completed SCD-HeFT trial.[197] Most of the control group patients in the MADIT I trial were also treated with amiodarone. In all cases, amiodarone was inferior to ICD therapy on the end point of total mortality (see Device Therapy section), although β blocker use was not balanced between groups in several of these trials. Perhaps most disappointing was the complete lack of efficacy for amiodarone compared with placebo on the end point of total mortality in SCD-HeFT.[197]

In contrast to the oral version, relatively strong evidence supports the use of intravenous amiodarone for out-of-hospital cardiac arrest and recurrent unstable ventricular arrhythmias. The efficacy of intravenous amiodarone in patients with recurrent, hemodynamically unstable ventricular tachycardia refractory to lidocaine, procainamide, and bretylium was approximately 40 percent in one prospective study, with suppression of about 80 percent of the arrhythmias within 48 hours.[233] The use of intravenous amiodarone in out-of-hospital cardiac arrest was recently studied in two important randomized trials. In the first, community patients receiving a 300-mg bolus of intravenous amiodarone for VT/VF refractory to three external shocks had an improved rate of survival to hospital admission compared with placebo-treated patients. [164] In the second trial, intravenous amiodarone proved superior to intravenous lidocaine for the same indication.[234] Neither trial was sufficiently powered to detect a difference in survival to hospital discharge.

【 】 DEVICE THERAPY

The ICD was initially developed to recognize ventricular fibrillation or rapid VT and terminate it automatically by delivering one or more high-energy shocks (see Chap. 46).[235] The first generation of defibrillators required a thoracotomy to place the sensing and defibrillator leads epicardially and the generator size mandated implantation of the device in an abdominal pocket. The reduced size of defibrillators now allows for transvenous, endocardial lead systems that integrate pacing, sensing and high-voltage defibrillation abilities. Current generation defibrillators have the additional ability to deliver low-energy cardioversion, antitachycardia pacing for VT, and antibradycardia pacing, and have all the features of the most sophisticated pacemakers, including the capacity to provide resynchronization therapy through simultaneous pacing of both right and left (through the coronary venous system) ventricles.[236] Given the excellent safety of current ICD implantation techniques and performance of ICD systems, a major challenge has been the identification of patient populations most appropriate for this potentially lifesaving therapy. Criteria for patient selection continue to evolve.

Three major trials of ICDs for secondary prevention were conducted (see Chap. 46). Each enrolled patient was successfully resuscitated from VF arrest or hemodynamically nontolerated VT without a transient reversible cause, and all three trials compared ICDs with amiodarone (the CASH trial had additional propafenone[212] and metoprolol arms). The CIDS[230] randomized 659 patients to ICD or amiodarone. After 3 years of followup, ICDs were associated with a 33 percent reduction in arrhythmic death and a 20 percent reduction in mortality that did not reach statistical significance. CASH reported a nonsignificant 23 percent reduction of all-cause mortality at 2 years in the ICD arm compared with the drug arm (metoprolol or amiodarone).[231] The AVID trial, the largest and most recent secondary prevention ICD trial,[232] randomized 1016 patients to ICD or amiodarone, and found a significant improvement in survival at 3 years for ICD patients (75 percent vs. 64 percent, $p = 0.02$). Thus, while the CIDS and CASH trials did not reach statistical significance, the treatment effect was in the same direction, and the three trials were generally regarded as consistent. Consequently, ICDs are considered by consensus guidelines[172] as a class I indication for patients with cardiac arrest from VF or VT not caused by a transient or reversible cause, and for patients with spontaneous sustained VT in association with structural heart disease.[173]

A number of randomized studies looking at the *primary prevention* or prophylactic use of defibrillators in high-risk populations have been published (see Table 49–5; see also Chap. 46). These studies varied considerably in patient population, entry criteria, and nature of control group therapy, but in aggregate support an expansion in the use of ICDs for primary prevention.

The Coronary Artery Bypass Graft (CABG) Patch Trial found no significant difference in the primary end point of total mortality in patients with ejection fractions of <30 percent and an abnormal SAECG randomized to ICD or no ICD at the time of coronary artery bypass grafting.[237] The findings were attributed to the benefit of complete revascularization in preventing sudden cardiac death and possibly to the poor positive predictive value of the SAECG. Two studies—MADIT and MUSTT—enrolled patients with ejection fractions less than 35 or 40 percent because of prior infarctions who also had nonsustained VT on ambulatory monitoring and inducible VT at the time of invasive electrophysiologic studies.[195,196] In both MADIT and MUSTT, ICD therapy was associated with significant (relative risk: 51 to 59 percent) reductions in total mortality over 3 to 5 years of followup, compared with no antiarrhythmic therapy (MUSTT; Fig. 49–7) or "standard" therapy consisting of primarily amiodarone (MADIT).

The MUSTT/MADIT entry criteria remained the standard of care for selecting post-MI patients for ICDs until the publication of the MADIT II trial, which included patients with ejection fractions less than 30 percent caused by prior MI, without further risk stratification.[198] MADIT II patients were randomized to ICD implantation or standard medical therapy without antiarrhythmic drugs. MADIT II reported a decrease in total mortality from 20 to 14 percent over 20 months in favor of the ICD group.[198] SCD-HeFT, which comprised a roughly even split between ischemic and nonischemic cardiomyopathy patients, similarly found a 7 percent absolute mortality difference (22 vs. 29 percent) between ICD and standard medical therapy over 45 months for patients with ejection fractions below 35 percent and New York Heart Association (NYHA) class II or III heart failure.[197]

ICDs do not appear to be of benefit immediately following large myocardial infarctions. The Defibrillator in Acute Myocardial Infarction Trial (DINAMIT) randomized 674 patients with recent (6 to 40 days) MI, an ejection fraction less than 35 percent, and a depressed heart rate variability on 24-hour monitoring to ICD or no ICD.[238] In contrast to other trials that excluded patients with very recent infarcts, DINAMIT found no benefit from prophylactic ICD implantation.

Based on the above trials, consensus guidelines have classified ICDs as a class I intervention in patients with prior MI, left ventricular dysfunction, nonsustained VT, and inducible VT at electrophysiologic study.[172] In earlier guidelines, ICD implantation was listed as a class IIa intervention for patients with prior MI and an ejection fraction below 30 percent with no further testing, provided the patient was more than 1 month post-MI and 3 months postrevascularization.[172] This was upgraded to a class I recommen-

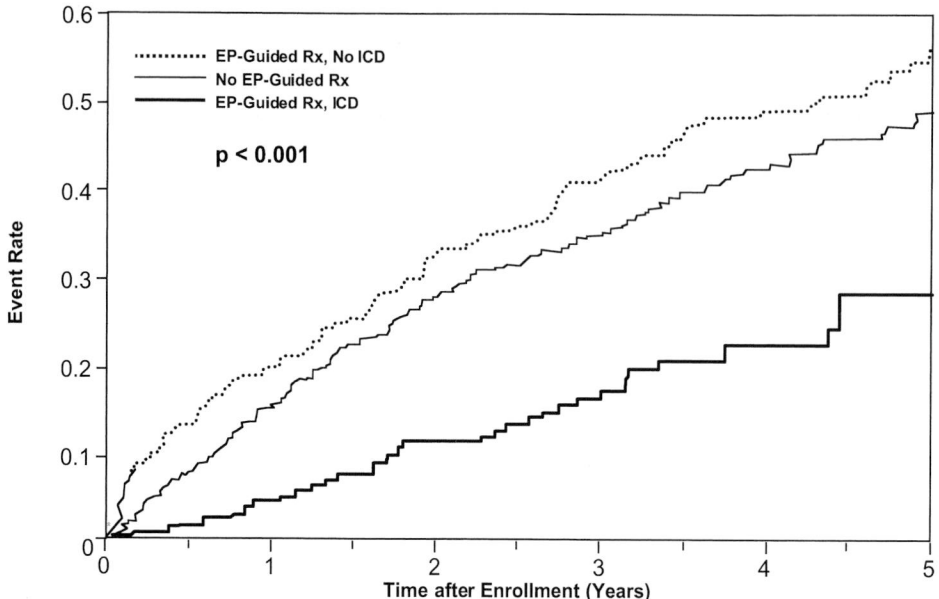

FIGURE 49–7. Kaplan-Meier estimates of the rates of overall mortality in a randomized trial between electrophysiologically guided therapy versus no antiarrhythmic therapy. (Multicenter Unsustained Tachycardia Trial [MUSTT]). The *p* value refers to two comparisons: between the patients in the group assigned to electrophysiologically guided therapy who received treatment with a defibrillator and those who did not receive such treatment, and between the patients assigned to electrophysiologically guided therapy who received treatment with a defibrillator and those assigned to no antiarrhythmic therapy. *Source: Reproduced from the MUSTT Investigators with permission. Buxton AE, Lee KL, Fisher JD, Josephson ME, Prystowsky EN, Hafley G. A randomized study of the prevention of sudden death in patients with coronary artery disease. Multicenter Unsustained Tachycardia Trial Investigators. N Engl J Med 1999;341(25):1882–1890.*

ter a median of 45 months, all-cause mortality in the ICD, amiodarone, and placebo arms was 22, 28, and 29 percent, respectively. The benefit of ICDs in the trial was highly statistically significant and appeared similar between ischemic and nonischemic subgroups, but was greater for patients with class II, compared with class III, heart failure—an observation not seen in other ICD trials. Recent consensus guidelines on heart failure management recommend ICDs for patients with left ventricular ejection fractions less than or equal to 30 percent, NYHA class II or III heart failure symptoms on optimal medical therapy and expected survival of more than 1 year with good functional status (class I recommendation, level of evidence: B).[173]

ICDs have also been used in less-common conditions associated with a high risk of sudden cardiac death, including hypertrophic cardiomyopathy, congenital long QT syndrome, and the Brugada syndrome. Nonrandomized series suggest a salutary effect on survival in carefully selected patients with these disorders. Because of a lack of evidence from randomized trials, ICD implantation in these cases is presently a class IIb recommendation.[172]

Finally, the feasibility and safety of combining defibrillation with cardiac resynchronization therapy (CRT) pacing in a single device have been established.[244] Although both CRT-pacemakers and CRT-defibrillators reduce mortality in patients with left ventricular systolic dysfunction, severe heart failure symptoms, and wide QRS duration on ECG, the incremental benefit of CRT-defibrillators over CRT-pacemakers remains uncertain.[236,245]

dation, when class II or III heart failure is present, in more recent heart failure guidelines following the publication of the SCD-HeFT trial results.[173] However, because of the smaller relative benefit from ICDs seen in less-selected trial populations, the high cost, and the potential morbidity of ICD therapy,[239] debate continues regarding the optimal methods of risk stratification and patient selection.[240]

Several ICD primary prevention trials in patients with nonischemic cardiomyopathy and heart failure have also been conducted, but the results have not been as consistently positive as in the post-MI population. Two early trials (the Cardiomyopathy Trial [CAT][241] and Amiodarone Versus Implantable Cardioverter-Defibrillator Trial [AMIOVIRT][242]) compared ICDs versus either standard medical therapy or amiodarone, respectively, in nonischemic cardiomyopathy patients but were too small to find differences between groups. The Defibrillators in Nonischemic Cardiomyopathy Treatment Evaluation (DEFINITE) trial enrolled 458 nonischemic cardiomyopathy patients with an ejection fraction under 35 percent, symptomatic heart failure, and either nonsustained VT or frequent PVCs on Holter monitoring and randomized them to standard medical therapy with or without ICDs.[243] All-cause mortality at 2 years was 13.8% with standard medical therapy versus 8.1% for medical therapy plus ICD, a result which fell just short of statistical significance (*p* = 0.06).

Finally, the aforementioned SCD-HeFT enrolled more than 2500 patients with class II (70 percent) and III heart failure and ejection fractions less than 35 percent because of either ischemic or nonischemic cardiomyopathy, and randomized them to ICD, amiodarone, or placebo, in addition to standard medical therapy.[197] Af-

⟦ ⟧ ROLE OF SURGERY

Revascularization

There is a reduced prevalence of SCD after coronary artery bypass grafting,[246] and attempts should be made to identify and revascularize ischemic myocardium so as to mitigate arrhythmic risk. While it is accepted that coronary artery bypass grafting reduces ventricular arrhythmias, the effect is unpredictable. Among the 13,476 patients in the Coronary Artery Surgical Study (CASS) registry, all of whom had significant coronary artery disease, operable vessels, and no significant valvular disease, the mean incidence of SCD during the 4.6-year average followup was 5.2 percent in patients who were treated medically and 1.8 percent in those who were treated surgically.[246] The beneficial effect of coronary artery bypass grafting was even more pronounced in the subgroup of patients with reduced left ventricular ejection fraction and multivessel disease, where the survival rate free from SCD at 5 years was 91 percent for the surgical group versus 69 percent for the medical group.

The failure of ICDs to save lives in the CABG-Patch trial suggests that revascularization reduced the risk of sudden death to such a degree that no incremental advantage of ICD therapy could be detected.[237,247] Importantly, patients with a preexisting history of ventricular fibrillation or ventricular tachycardia were excluded in this trial. Analysis of data from the AVID registry shows that patients with VT or VF who underwent revascularization after the index arrhythmia had improved survival compared to those who did not undergo revascularization.[248] Nevertheless, ICD implantation offered a similar survival advantage to AVID registry patients with coronary artery disease, whether or not they were revascularized, pointing out that coronary artery bypass grafting is not necessarily sufficient for removing the arrhythmic substrate.

The protective effect of coronary artery bypass grafting against recurrent cardiac arrest appears to be best in patients who have reversible ischemia as the major pathophysiologic factor in SCD. These patients are characterized by critical coronary artery disease, significant regions of myocardium at risk for ischemia, and no inducible monomorphic ventricular arrhythmias at electrophysiologic study.[249,250] Despite the encouraging results of coronary artery bypass grafting in survivors of cardiac arrest, it should be noted that only a minority of these patients are candidates for operative revascularization and that scar-mediated, monomorphic ventricular tachycardia is often uncontrolled by myocardial revascularization alone.[251] The relative benefits of partial or complete percutaneous revascularization compared to coronary artery bypass grafting in this setting are also unclear.

Antiarrhythmia Surgery

Electrophysiologically guided subendocardial resection and cryoablation are potentially curative surgical options in patients with recurrent monomorphic VT in whom areas of slow conduction around myocardial scars are critical for sustaining VT. Long-term followup of this operative technique has yielded a clinical success rate of nearly 90 percent in eliminating the presenting rhythm in patients who survive surgery. This approach was limited by the high surgical mortality rate of 10 to 15 percent in early series[252]; however, these data, gathered in the 1980s, may exaggerate the operative risk, given improvements in surgical technique over time. The best candidates for electrophysiologically guided subendocardial resection are patients who require coronary revascularization and who have a well-defined left ventricular aneurysm.

Catheter Ablation Therapy

Catheter ablation of arrhythmias has emerged as a curative approach for many supraventricular arrhythmias and a few specific forms of VT.[142] The role of catheter ablation in the prevention of SCD is less-well established, but this therapy form has been successfully employed in selected cases. Rarely, supraventricular tachycardias with a rapid ventricular response may degenerate into fatal ventricular tachyarrhythmias and cardiac arrest.[253] Radiofrequency catheter ablation can eliminate the risk of a rapid ventricular response by abolishing conduction over an accessory pathway in patients with Wolff-Parkinson-White syndrome, or it can slow or completely block conduction over the atrioventricular node in patients with atrial arrhythmias and rapid, medically uncontrolled atrioventricular conduction. Radiofrequency catheter ablation can potentially prevent SCD in patients

with documented and inducible bundle-branch reentrant VT as the only mechanism of cardiac arrest.[254] Improved mapping techniques of VT circuits, better catheters, and perhaps other energy sources may help improve the efficacy of catheter ablation for VT and potentially expand its role in the prevention of SCD (see Chap. 44).

REFERENCES

1. Zheng ZJ, Croft JB, Giles WH, Mensah GA. Sudden cardiac death in the United States, 1989 to 1998. *Circulation* 2001;104(18):2158–2163.
2. Goldstein S. The necessity of a uniform definition of sudden coronary death: witnessed death within 1 hour of the onset of acute symptoms. *Am Heart J* 1982;103(1):156–159.
3. Hinkle LE Jr, Thaler HT. Clinical classification of cardiac deaths. *Circulation* 1982;65(3):457–464.
4. de Vreede-Swagemakers JJ, Gorgels AP, Dubois-Arbouw WI, et al. Out-of-hospital cardiac arrest in the 1990s: a population-based study in the Maastricht area on incidence, characteristics and survival. *J Am Coll Cardiol* 1997;30(6):1500–1505.
5. Leach IH, Blundell JW, Rowley JM, Turner DR. Acute ischaemic lesions in death due to ischaemic heart disease. An autopsy study of 333 cases of out-of-hospital death. *Eur Heart J* 1995;16(9):1181–1185.
6. Centers for Disease Control and Prevention. State-specific mortality from sudden cardiac death—United States, 1999. *MMWR Morb Mortal Wkly Rep* 2002;51(6):123–126.
7. Eisenberg MS, Horwood BT, Cummins RO, Reynolds-Haertle R, Hearne TR. Cardiac arrest and resuscitation: a tale of 29 cities. *Ann Emerg Med* 1990;19(2):179–186.
8. Registers MIC. *Public Health in Europe 5.* Copenhagen: Regional Office for Europe, World Health Organization, 1976.
9. Kannel WB, Cupples LA, D'Agostino RB. Sudden death risk in overt coronary heart disease: the Framingham Study. *Am Heart J* 1987;113(3):799–804.
10. Wren C, O'Sullivan JJ, Wright C. Sudden death in children and adolescents. *Heart* 2000;83(4):410–413.
11. Maron BJ, Gohman TE, Aeppli D. Prevalence of sudden cardiac death during competitive sports activities in Minnesota high school athletes. *J Am Coll Cardiol* 1998;32(7):1881–1884.
12. Tiziana CR, Autore C, Romeo D, et al. Sudden cardiac death in younger adults: autopsy diagnosis as a tool for preventive medicine. *Hum Pathol* 2006;37(7):794–801.
13. Eckart RE, Scoville SL, Campbell CL, et al. Sudden death in young adults: a 25-year review of autopsies in military recruits. *Ann Intern Med* 2004;141(11):829–834.
14. Becker LB, Han BH, Meyer PM, et al. Racial differences in the incidence of cardiac arrest and subsequent survival. The CPR Chicago Project. *N Engl J Med* 1993;329(9):600–606.
15. Eckart RE, Scoville SL, Shry EA, Potter RN, Tedrow U. Causes of sudden death in young female military recruits. *Am J Cardiol* 2006;97:1756–1758.
16. Asher CR, Topol EJ, Moliterno DJ. Insights into the pathophysiology of atherosclerosis and prognosis of black Americans with acute coronary syndromes. *Am Heart J* 1999;138(6 Pt 1):1073–1081.
17. Gauri AJ, Davis A, Hong T, Burke MC, Knight BP. Disparities in the use of primary prevention and defibrillator therapy among blacks and women. *Am J Med* 2006;119(2):167e17–167e21.
18. Albert CM, McGovern BA, Newell JB, Ruskin JN. Sex differences in cardiac arrest survivors. *Circulation* 1996;93(6):1170–1176.
19. Schulman KA, Berlin JA, Harless W, et al. The effect of race and sex on physicians' recommendations for cardiac catheterization. *N Engl J Med* 1999;340(8):618–626.
20. Mosca L, Jones WK, King KB, Ouyang P, Redberg RF, Hill MN. Awareness, perception, and knowledge of heart disease risk and prevention among women in the United States. American Heart Association Women's Heart Disease and Stroke Campaign Task Force. *Arch Fam Med* 2000;9(6):506–515.
21. Hinkle LE Jr. Short-term risk factors for sudden death. *Ann N Y Acad Sci* 1982;382:22–38.
22. Kannel WB, Thomas HE Jr. Sudden coronary death: the Framingham Study. *Ann N Y Acad Sci* 1982;382:3–21.
23. Soeki T, Tamura Y, Shinohara H, Sakabe K, Onose Y, Fukuda N. Plasma concentrations of fibrinolytic factors in the subacute phase of myocardial infarction predict recurrent myocardial infarction or sudden cardiac death. *Int J Cardiol* 2002;85(2–3):277–283.
24. Albert CM, Campos H, Stampfer MJ, et al. Blood levels of long-chain n-3 fatty acids and the risk of sudden death. *N Engl J Med* 2002;346(15):1113–1118.
25. Sotoodehnia N, Siscovick DS, Vatta M, et al. Beta₂-adrenergic receptor genetic variants and risk of sudden cardiac death. *Circulation* 2006;113(15):1842–1848.
26. Lanfear DE, Jones PG, Marsh S, Cresci S, McLeod HL, Spertus JA. Beta₂-adrenergic receptor genotype and survival among patients receiving beta-blocker therapy after an acute coronary syndrome. *JAMA* 2005;294(12):1526–1533.
27. Albert CM, Manson JE, Cook NR, Ajani UA, Gaziano JM, Hennekens CH. Moderate alcohol consumption and the risk of sudden cardiac death among US male physicians. *Circulation* 1999;100(9):944–950.
28. Lampert R, Joska T, Burg MM, Batsford WP, McPherson CA, Jain D. Emotional and physical precipitants of ventricular arrhythmia. *Circulation* 2002;106(14):1800–1805.
29. McElduff P, Dobson AJ. Case fatality after an acute cardiac event: the effect of smoking and alcohol consumption. *J Clin Epidemiol* 2001;54(1):58–67.
30. Kannel WB. Update on the role of cigarette smoking in coronary artery disease. *Am Heart J* 1981;101(3):319–328.
31. Burke AP, Farb A, Malcom GT, Liang YH, Smialek J, Virmani R. Coronary risk factors and plaque morphology in men with coronary disease who died suddenly. *N Engl J Med* 1997;336(18):1276–1282.
32. Hallstrom AP, Cobb LA, Ray R. Smoking as a risk factor for recurrence of sudden cardiac arrest. *N Engl J Med* 1986;314(5):271–275.
33. Fries R, Konig J, Schafers HJ, Bohm M. Triggering effect of physical and mental stress on spontaneous ventricular tachyarrhythmias in patients with implantable cardioverter-defibrillators. *Clin Cardiol* 2002;25(10):474–478.
34. Leor J, Poole WK, Kloner RA. Sudden cardiac death triggered by an earthquake. *N Engl J Med* 1996;334(7):413–419.
35. Burke AP, Farb A, Malcom GT, Liang Y, Smialek JE, Virmani R. Plaque rupture and sudden death related to exertion in men with coronary artery disease. *JAMA* 1999;281(10):921–926.
36. Albert CM, Mittleman MA, Chae CU, Lee IM, Hennekens CH, Manson JE. Triggering of sudden death from cardiac causes by vigorous exertion. *N Engl J Med* 2000;343(19):1355–1361.

37. Cobb LA, Weaver WD. Exercise: a risk for sudden death in patients with coronary heart disease. *J Am Coll Cardiol* 1986;7(1):215–219.
38. Lemaitre RN, Siscovick DS, Raghunathan TE, Weinmann S, Arbogast P, Lin DY. Leisure-time physical activity and the risk of primary cardiac arrest. *Arch Intern Med* 1999;159(7):686–690.
39. Maron BJ. Sudden Death in Young Athletes. *N Engl J Med* 2003;349(11):1064–1075.
40. Maron BJ, Roberts WC, McAllister HA, Rosing DR, Epstein SE. Sudden death in young athletes. *Circulation* 1980;62(2):218–229.
41. Corrado D, Thiene G, Nava A, Rossi L, Pennelli N. Sudden death in young competitive athletes: clinicopathologic correlations in 22 cases. *Am J Med* 1990;89(5):588–596.
42. Maron BJ, Shirani J, Poliac LC, Mathenge R, Roberts WC, Mueller FO. Sudden death in young competitive athletes. Clinical, demographic, and pathological profiles. *JAMA* 1996;276(3):199–204.
43. Maron BJ, Zipes DP, et al. 36th Bethesda Conference: eligibility recommendations for competitive athletes with cardiovascular abnormalities. *J Am Coll Cardiol* 2005;45(8):1312–1375.
44. Zipes DP, Ackerman MJ, Estes NA 3rd, Grant AO, Myerburg RJ, Van Hare G. 36th Bethesda Conference. Task force 7: arrhythmias. *J Am Coll Cardiol* 2005;45(8):1354–1363.
45. Maron BJ, Poliac LC, Kaplan JA, Mueller FO. Blunt impact to the chest leading to sudden death from cardiac arrest during sports activities. *N Engl J Med* 1995;333:337–342.
46. Myerburg RJ, Kessler KM, Bassett AL, Castellanos A. A biological approach to sudden cardiac death: structure, function and cause. *Am J Cardiol* 1989;63(20):1512–1516.
47. Willich SN, Maclure M, Mittleman M, Arntz HR, Muller JE. Sudden cardiac death. Support for a role of triggering in causation. *Circulation* 1993;87(5):1442–1450.
48. Greene HL. Sudden arrhythmic cardiac death—mechanisms, resuscitation and classification: the Seattle perspective. *Am J Cardiol* 1990;65(4):4B–12B.
49. Bayes de Luna A, Coumel P, Leclercq JF. Ambulatory sudden cardiac death: mechanisms of production of fatal arrhythmia on the basis of data from 157 cases. *Am Heart J* 1989;117(1):151–159.
50. Wathen MS, DeGroot PJ, Sweeney MO, et al. Prospective randomized multicenter trial of empirical antitachycardia pacing versus shocks for spontaneous rapid ventricular tachycardia in patients with implantable cardioverter-defibrillators: Pacing Fast Ventricular Tachycardia Reduces Shock Therapies (PainFREE Rx II) trial results. *Circulation* 2004;110(17):2591–2596.
51. Luu M, Stevenson WG, Stevenson LW, Baron K, Walden J. Diverse mechanisms of unexpected cardiac arrest in advanced heart failure. *Circulation* 1989;80(6):1675–1680.
52. Janse MJ, Wit AL. Electrophysiological mechanisms of ventricular arrhythmias resulting from myocardial ischemia and infarction. *Physiol Rev* 1989;69(4):1049–1169.
53. Dillon SM, Allessie MA, Ursell PC, Wit AL. Influences of anisotropic tissue structure on reentrant circuits in the epicardial border zone of subacute canine infarcts. *Circ Res* 1988;63(1):182–206.
54. Pogwizd SM, Corr PB. Mechanisms underlying the development of ventricular fibrillation during early myocardial ischemia. *Circ Res* 1990;66(3):672–695.
55. De Groot JR, Coronel R. Acute ischemia-induced gap junctional uncoupling and arrhythmogenesis. *Cardiovasc Res* 2004;62(2):323–334.
56. Josephson ME, Horowitz LN, Farshidi AK. Recurrent sustained ventricular tachycardia. 1. Mechanisms. *Circulation* 1978;57:431–440.
57. The Multicenter Postinfarction Research Group. Risk stratification and survival after myocardial infarction. *N Engl J Med* 1983;309(6):331–336.
58. Levine JH, Guarnieri T, Kadish AH, White RI, Calkins H, Kan JS. Changes in myocardial repolarization in patients undergoing balloon valvuloplasty for congenital pulmonary stenosis: evidence for contraction–excitation feedback in humans. *Circulation* 1988;77(1):70–77.
59. Lerman BB, Engelstein ED, Burkhoff D. Mechanoelectrical feedback: role of beta-adrenergic receptor activation in mediating load-dependent shortening of ventricular action potential and refractoriness. *Circulation* 2001;104(4):486–490.
60. Wehrens XH, Lehnart SE, Marks AR. Ryanodine receptor-targeted anti-arrhythmic therapy. *Ann N Y Acad Sci* 2005;1047:366–375.
61. Goldstein S, Landis JR, Leighton R, et al. Characteristics of the resuscitated out-of-hospital cardiac arrest victim with coronary heart disease. *Circulation* 1981;64(5):977–984.
62. Bigger JT Jr. Patients with malignant or potentially malignant ventricular arrhythmias: opportunities and limitations of drug therapy in prevention of sudden death. *J Am Coll Cardiol* 1985;5(6 Suppl):23B–26B.
63. Davies MJ. Anatomic features in victims of sudden coronary death. Coronary artery pathology. *Circulation* 1992;85(1 Suppl):I19–I24.
64. McHenry PL, J OD, Morris SN, Jordan JJ. The abnormal exercise electrocardiogram in apparently healthy men: a predictor of angina pectoris as an initial coronary event during long-term follow-up. *Circulation* 1984;70(4):547–551.
65. Cinca J, Warren M, Carreno A, et al. Changes in myocardial electrical impedance induced by coronary artery occlusion in pigs with and without preconditioning: correlation with local ST-segment potential and ventricular arrhythmias. *Circulation* 1997;96(9):3079–3086.
66. Taylor AJ, Rogan KM, Virmani R. Sudden cardiac death associated with isolated congenital coronary artery anomalies. *J Am Coll Cardiol* 1992;20(3):640–647.
67. Parchure N, Batchvarov V, Malik M, Camm AJ, Kaski JC. Increased QT dispersion in patients with Prinzmetal's variant angina and cardiac arrest. *Cardiovasc Res* 2001;50(2):379–385.
68. Roberts WC, Dicicco BS, Waller BF, et al. Origin of the left main from the right coronary artery or from the right aortic sinus with intramyocardial tunneling to the left side of the heart via the ventricular septum. The case against clinical significance of myocardial bridge or coronary tunnel. *Am Heart J* 1982;104(2 Pt 1):303–305.
69. Tamburro P, Wilber D. Sudden death in idiopathic dilated cardiomyopathy. *Am Heart J* 1992;124(4):1035–1045.
70. Packer M. Lack of relation between ventricular arrhythmias and sudden death in patients with chronic heart failure. *Circulation* 1992;85(1 Suppl):I50–I56.
71. Larsen L, Markham J, Haffajee CI. Sudden death in idiopathic dilated cardiomyopathy: role of ventricular arrhythmias. *Pacing Clin Electrophysiol* 1993;16(5 Pt 1):1051–1059.
72. Grimm W, Hoffmann J, Menz V, Luck K, Maisch B. Programmed ventricular stimulation for arrhythmia risk prediction in patients with idiopathic dilated cardiomyopathy and nonsustained ventricular tachycardia. *J Am Coll Cardiol* 1998;32:739–745.
73. Soejima K, Stevenson WG, Sapp JL, Selwyn AP, Couper G, Epstein LM. Endocardial and epicardial radiofrequency ablation of ventricular tachycardia associated with dilated cardiomyopathy: the importance of low-voltage scars. *J Am Coll Cardiol* 2004;43(10):1834–1842.
74. McKenna WJ, Camm AJ. Sudden death in hypertrophic cardiomyopathy. Assessment of patients at high risk. *Circulation* 1989;80(5):1489–1492.
75. Spirito P, Rapezzi C, Autore C, et al. Prognosis of asymptomatic patients with hypertrophic cardiomyopathy and nonsustained ventricular tachycardia. *Circulation* 1994;90(6):2743–2747.
76. Maron BJ. Hypertrophic cardiomyopathy: a systematic review. *JAMA* 2002;287(10):1308–1320.
77. Spirito P, Bellone P, Harris KM, Bernabo P, Bruzzi P, Maron BJ. Magnitude of left ventricular hypertrophy and risk of sudden death in hypertrophic cardiomyopathy. *N Engl J Med* 2000;342(24):1778–1785.
78. Sadoul N, Prasad K, Elliott PM, Bannerjee S, Frenneaux MP, McKenna WJ. Prospective prognostic assessment of blood pressure response during exercise in patients with hypertrophic cardiomyopathy. *Circulation* 1997;96(9):2987–2991.
79. Marian AJ, Roberts R. Molecular genetic basis of hypertrophic cardiomyopathy: genetic markers for sudden cardiac death. *J Cardiovasc Electrophysiol* 1998;9(1):88–99.
80. Moolman JC, Corfield VA, Posen B, et al. Sudden death due to troponin T mutations. *J Am Coll Cardiol* 1997;29(3):549–555.
81. Zehender M, Faber T, Koscheck U, Meinertz T, Just H. Ventricular tachyarrhythmias, myocardial ischemia, and sudden cardiac death in patients with hypertensive heart disease. *Clin Cardiol* 1995;18(7):377–383.
82. Zimetbaum PJ, Buxton AE, Batsford W, et al. Electrocardiographic predictors of arrhythmic death and total mortality in the multicenter unsustained tachycardia trial. *Circulation* 2004;110(7):766–769.
83. Levy D, Garrison RJ, Savage DD, Kannel WB, Castelli WP. Prognostic implications of echocardiographically determined left ventricular mass in the Framingham Heart Study. *N Engl J Med* 1990;322(22):1561–1566.
84. Tanaka M, Fujiwara H, Onodera T, Wu DJ, Hamashima Y, Kawai C. Quantitative analysis of myocardial fibrosis in normals, hypertensive hearts, and hypertrophic cardiomyopathy. *Br Heart J* 1986;55(6):575–581.
85. Siscovick DS, Raghunathan TE, Psaty BM, et al. Diuretic therapy for hypertension and the risk of primary cardiac arrest. *N Engl J Med* 1994;330(26):1852–1857.
86. McKenna WJ, Thiene G, Nava A, et al. Diagnosis of arrhythmogenic right ventricular dysplasia/cardiomyopathy. Task Force of the Working Group Myocardial and Pericardial Disease of the European Society of Cardiology and of the Scientific Council on Cardiomyopathies of the International Society and Federation of Cardiology. *Br Heart J* 1994;71(3):215–218.
87. Tiso N, Stephan DA, Nava A, et al. Identification of mutations in the cardiac ryanodine receptor gene in families affected with arrhythmogenic right ventricular cardiomyopathy type 2 (ARVD2). *Hum Mol Genet* 2001;10(3):189–194.
88. Protonotarios N, Tsatsopoulou A, Anastasakis A, et al. Genotype-phenotype assessment in autosomal recessive arrhythmogenic right ventricular cardiomyopathy (Naxos disease) caused by a deletion in plakoglobin. *J Am Coll Cardiol* 2001;38(5):1477–1484.
89. Norman M, Simpson M, Mogensen J, et al. Novel mutation in desmoplakin causes arrhythmogenic left ventricular cardiomyopathy. *Circulation* 2005;112(5):636–642.
90. Syrris P, Ward D, Asimaki A, et al. Clinical expression of plakophilin-2 mutations in familial arrhythmogenic right ventricular cardiomyopathy. *Circulation* 2006;113(3):356–364.
91. Pilichou K, Nava A, Basso C, et al. Mutations in desmoglein-2 gene are associated with arrhythmogenic right ventricular cardiomyopathy. *Circulation* 2006;113(9):1171–1179.
92. Beffagna G, Occhi G, Nava A, et al. Regulatory mutations in transforming growth factor-beta3 gene cause arrhythmogenic right ventricular cardiomyopathy type 1. *Cardiovasc Res* 2005;65(2):366–373.
93. Corrado D, Basso C, Thiene G, et al. Spectrum of clinicopathologic manifestations of arrhythmogenic right ventricular cardiomyopathy/dysplasia: a multicenter study. *J Am Coll Cardiol* 1997;30(6):1512–1520.
94. Hodgkinson KA, Parfrey PS, Bassett AS, et al. The impact of implantable cardioverter-defibrillator therapy on survival in autosomal-dominant arrhythmogenic right ventricular cardiomyopathy (ARVD5). *J Am Coll Cardiol* 2005;45(3):400–408.
95. Corrado D, Leoni L, Link MS, et al. Implantable cardioverter-defibrillator therapy for prevention of sudden death in patients with arrhythmogenic right ventricular cardiomyopathy/dysplasia. *Circulation* 2003;108(25):3084–3091.
96. Kottkamp H, Hindricks G. Catheter ablation of ventricular tachycardia in ARVC. Is curative treatment at the horizon? *J Cardiovasc Electrophysiol* 2006;17(5):477–479.
97. Pellikka PA, Nishimura RA, Bailey KR, Tajik AJ. The natural history of adults with asymptomatic, hemodynamically significant aortic stenosis. *J Am Coll Cardiol* 1990;15(5):1012–1017.
98. Bonow RO, Lakatos E, Maron BJ, Epstein SE. Serial long-term assessment of the natural history of asymptomatic patients with chronic aortic regurgitation and normal left ventricular systolic function. *Circulation* 1991;84(4):1625–1635.
99. Alvarez L, Escudero C, Figuera D, Castillo-Olivares JL. Late sudden cardiac death in the follow-up of patients having a heart valve prosthesis. *J Thorac Cardiovasc Surg* 1992;104(2):502–510.
100. Keefe DL, Griffin JC, Harrison DC, Stinson EB. Atrioventricular conduction abnormalities in patients undergoing isolated aortic or mitral valve replacement. *Pacing Clin Electrophysiol* 1985;8(3 Pt 1):393–398.
101. Nishimura RA, McGoon MD, Shub C, Miller FA Jr, Ilstrup DM, Tajik AJ. Echocardiographically documented mitral-valve prolapse. Long-term follow-up of 237 patients. *N Engl J Med* 1985;313(21):1305–1309.
102. Marks AR, Choong CY, Sanfilippo AJ, Ferre M, Weyman AE. Identification of high-risk and low-risk subgroups of patients with mitral-valve prolapse. *N Engl J Med* 1989;320(16):1031–1036.
103. Vohra J, Sathe S, Warren R, Tatoulis J, Hunt D. Malignant ventricular arrhythmias in patients with mitral valve prolapse and mild mitral regurgitation. *Pacing Clin Electrophysiol* 1993;16(3 Pt 1):387–393.
104. Puddu PE, Pasternac A, Tubau JF, Krol R, Farley L, de Champlain J. QT interval prolongation and increased plasma catecholamine levels in patients with mitral valve prolapse. *Am Heart J* 1983;105(3):422–428.
105. Liberthson RR. Sudden death from cardiac causes in children and young adults. *N Engl J Med* 1996;334(16):1039–1044.
106. Ramos SG, Matturri L, Rossi L, Rossi MA. Lesions of mediastinal paraganglia in chronic chagasic cardiomyopathy: cause of sudden death? *Am Heart J* 1996;131(2):417–420.
107. Winters SL, Cohen M, Greenberg S, et al. Sustained ventricular tachycardia associated with sarcoidosis: assessment of the underlying cardiac anatomy and the prospective utility of programmed ventricular stimulation, drug therapy and an implantable antitachycardia device. *J Am Coll Cardiol* 1991;18(4):937–943.
108. Silka MJ, Hardy BG, Menashe VD, Morris CD. A population-based prospective evaluation of risk of sudden cardiac death after operation for common congenital heart defects. *J Am Coll Cardiol* 1998;32(1):245–251.
109. Gatzoulis MA, Balaji S, Webber SA, et al. Risk factors for arrhythmia and sudden cardiac death late after repair of tetralogy of Fallot: a multicentre study. *Lancet* 2000;356(9234):975–981.
110. Khairy P, Landzberg MJ, Gatzoulis MA, et al. Value of programmed ventricular stimulation after tetralogy of Fallot repair: a multicenter study. *Circulation* 2004;109(16):1994–2000.
111. Gelatt M, Hamilton RM, McCrindle BW, et al. Arrhythmia and mortality after the Mustard procedure: a 30-year single-center experience. *J Am Coll Cardiol* 1997;29(1):194–201.
112. Moss AJ, Adams FH. *Heart Disease in Infants, Children and Adolescents Including the Fetus and Young Adult*, 5th ed. Baltimore: Williams & Wilkins, 1995.
113. Vincent GM, Timothy KW, Leppert M, Keating M. The spectrum of symptoms and QT intervals in carriers of the gene for the long-QT syndrome. *N Engl J Med* 1992;327(12):846–852.

114. Shah M, Akar FG, Tomaselli GF. Molecular basis of arrhythmias. *Circulation* 2005;112(16):2517–2529.
115. Priori SG, Schwartz PJ, Napolitano C, et al. Risk stratification in the long-QT syndrome. *N Engl J Med* 2003;348(19):1866–1874.
116. Wilde AA, Jongbloed RJ, Doevendans PA, et al. Auditory stimuli as a trigger for arrhythmic events differentiate HERG-related (LQTS2) patients from KVLQT1-related patients (LQTS1). *J Am Coll Cardiol* 1999;33(2):327–332.
117. Brugada R, Hong K, Dumaine R, et al. Sudden death associated with short-QT syndrome linked to mutations in HERG. *Circulation* 2004;109(1):30–35.
118. Schimpf R, Wolpert C, Gaita F, Giustetto C, Borggrefe M. Short QT syndrome. *Cardiovasc Res* 2005;67(3):357–366.
119. Hong K, Bjerregaard P, Gussak I, Brugada R. Short QT syndrome and atrial fibrillation caused by mutation in KCNH2. *J Cardiovasc Electrophysiol* 2005;16(4):394–396.
120. Bellocq C, van Ginneken ACG, Bezzina CR, et al. Mutation in the KCNQ1 gene leading to the short QT-interval syndrome. *Circulation* 2004;109:2394–2397.
121. Priori SG, Pandit SV, Rivolta I, et al. A novel form of short QT syndrome (SQT3) is caused by a mutation in the KCNJ2 gene. Circ Res 2005;96(7):800–807.
122. Leenhardt A, Glaser E, Burguera M, Nurnberg M, Maison-Blanche P, Coumel P. Short-coupled variant of torsade de pointes. A new electrocardiographic entity in the spectrum of idiopathic ventricular tachyarrhythmias. *Circulation* 1994;89(1):206–215.
123. Priori SG, Napolitano C, Memmi M, et al. Clinical and molecular characterization of patients with catecholaminergic polymorphic ventricular tachycardia. *Circulation* 2002;106(1):69–74.
124. Lahat H, Pras E, Olender T, et al. A missense mutation in a highly conserved region of CASQ2 is associated with autosomal recessive catecholamine-induced polymorphic ventricular tachycardia in Bedouin families from Israel. *Am J Hum Genet* 2001;69(6):1378–1384.
125. Morady F, Scheinman MM, Hess DS, Chen R, Stanger P. Clinical characteristics and results of electrophysiologic testing in young adults with ventricular tachycardia or ventricular fibrillation. *Am Heart J* 1983;106(6):1306–1314.
126. Wever EF, Hauer RN, Oomen A, Peters RH, Bakker PF, Robles de Medina EO. Unfavorable outcome in patients with primary electrical disease who survived an episode of ventricular fibrillation. *Circulation* 1993;88(3):1021–1029.
127. Brugada P, Brugada J. Right bundle branch block, persistent ST segment elevation and sudden cardiac death: a distinct clinical and electrocardiographic syndrome. A multicenter report. *J Am Coll Cardiol* 1992;20(6):1391–1396.
128. Antzelevitch C, Brugada P, Borggrefe M, et al. Brugada syndrome: report of the second consensus conference (endorsed by the Heart Rhythm Society and the European Heart Rhythm Association). *Circulation* 2005;111:659–670.
129. Chen Q, Kirsch GE, Zhang D, et al. Genetic basis and molecular mechanism for idiopathic ventricular fibrillation. *Nature* 1998;392(6673):293–296.
130. Priori SG, Napolitano C, Gasparini M, et al. Natural History of Brugada syndrome: Insights for Risk Stratification and Management. *Circulation* 2002;105(11):1342–1347.
131. Nademanee K, Veerakul G, Nimmannit S, et al. Arrhythmogenic marker for the sudden unexplained death syndrome in Thai men. *Circulation* 1997;96(8):2595–2600.
132. Kirschner RH, Eckner FA, Baron RC. The cardiac pathology of sudden, unexplained nocturnal death in Southeast Asian refugees. *JAMA* 1986;256(19):2700–2705.
133. Gotoh K. A histopathological study on the conduction system of the so-called "Pokkuri disease" (sudden unexpected cardiac death of unknown origin in Japan). *Jpn Circ J* 1976;40(7):753–768.
134. Corrado D, Nava A, Buja G, et al. Familial cardiomyopathy underlies syndrome of right bundle branch block, ST segment elevation and sudden death. *J Am Coll Cardiol* 1996;27(2):443–448.
135. Antzelevitch C, Brugada P, Brugada J, et al. Brugada syndrome: a decade of progress. *Circ Res* 2002;91(12):1114–1118.
136. Lukas A, Antzelevitch C. Phase 2 reentry as a mechanism of initiation of circus movement reentry in canine epicardium exposed to simulated ischemia. *Cardiovasc Res* 1996;32(3):593–603.
137. Priori SG, Aliot E, Blomstrom-Lundqvist C, et al. Task Force on Sudden Cardiac Death of the European Society of Cardiology. *Eur Heart J* 2001;22(16):1374–1450.
138. Belhassen B, Glick A, Viskin S. Efficacy of quinidine in high-risk patients with Brugada syndrome. *Circulation* 2004;110:1731–1737.
139. Hermida JS, Denjoy I, Clerc J, et al. Hydroquinidine therapy in Brugada syndrome. *J Am Coll Cardiol* 2004;43:1853–1860.
140. Munger TM, Packer DL, Hammill SC, et al. A population study of the natural history of Wolff-Parkinson-White syndrome in Olmsted County, Minnesota, 1953–1989. *Circulation* 1993;87(3):866–873.
141. Klein GJ, Bashore TM, Sellers TD, Pritchett EL, Smith WM, Gallagher JJ. Ventricular fibrillation in the Wolff-Parkinson-White syndrome. *N Engl J Med* 1979;301(20):1080–1085.
142. Jackman WM, Wang XZ, Friday KJ, et al. Catheter ablation of accessory atrioventricular pathways (Wolff-Parkinson-White syndrome) by radiofrequency current. *N Engl J Med* 1991;324(23):1605–1611.
143. Pappone C, Santinelli V, Manguso F, et al. A randomized study of prophylactic catheter ablation in asymptomatic patients with the Wolff-Parkinson-White syndrome. *N Engl J Med* 2003;349:1803–1811.
144. Blomstrom-Lundqvist C, Scheinman MM, Aliot EM, et al. ACC/AHA/ESC guidelines for the management of patients with supraventricular arrhythmias—executive summary: a report of the American College of Cardiology/American *Heart* Association Task Force on Practice Guidelines and the European Society of Cardiology Committee for Practice Guidelines (Writing Committee to Develop Guidelines for the Management of Patients With Supraventricular Arrhythmias). *Circulation* 2003;108(15):1871–1909.
145. Frey W. Weitere Erfahrungen mit Chinidin bei absoluter Herzunregelma bigkeit. *Wein Klin Wochenschr* 1918;55:849–853.
146. Lehmann MH, Hardy S, Archibald D, Quart B, MacNeil DJ. Sex difference in risk of torsade de pointes with *d,l*-sotalol. *Circulation* 1996;94(10):2535–2541.
147. Minardo JD, Heger JJ, Miles WM, Zipes DP, Prystowsky EN. Clinical characteristics of patients with ventricular fibrillation during antiarrhythmic drug therapy. *N Engl J Med* 1988;319(5):257–262.
148. Echt DS, Liebson PR, Mitchell LB, et al. Mortality and morbidity in patients receiving encainide, flecainide, or placebo. The Cardiac Arrhythmia Suppression Trial. *N Engl J Med* 1991;324(12):781–788.
149. Nattel S, Pedersen DH, Zipes DP. Alterations in regional myocardial distribution and arrhythmogenic effects of aprindine produced by coronary artery occlusion in the dog. *Cardiovasc Res* 1981;15(2):80–85.
150. Packer M, Medina N, Yushak M. Hemodynamic and clinical limitations of long-term inotropic therapy with amrinone in patients with severe chronic heart failure. *Circulation* 1984;70(6):1038–1047.
151. Hearn WL, Flynn DD, Hime GW, et al. Cocaethylene: a unique cocaine metabolite displays high affinity for the dopamine transporter. *J Neurochem* 1991;56(2):698–701.
152. Nordrehaug JE, Johannessen KA, von der Lippe G. Serum potassium concentration as a risk factor of ventricular arrhythmias early in acute myocardial infarction. *Circulation* 1985;71(4):645–649.
153. Hoes AW, Grobbee DE, Peet TM, Lubsen J. Do non-potassium-sparing diuretics increase the risk of sudden cardiac death in hypertensive patients? Recent evidence. *Drugs* 1994;47(5):711–733.
154. Gettes LS. Electrolyte abnormalities underlying lethal and ventricular arrhythmias. *Circulation* 1992;85(1 Suppl):I70–6.
155. Cummins RO, Ornato JP, Thies WH, Pepe PE. Improving survival from sudden cardiac arrest: the "chain of survival" concept. A statement for health professionals from the Advanced Cardiac Life Support Subcommittee and the Emergency Cardiac Care Committee, American Heart Association. *Circulation* 1991;83(5):1832–1847.
156. Valenzuela TD, Roe DJ, Cretin S, Spaite DW, Larsen MP. Estimating effectiveness of cardiac arrest interventions: a logistic regression survival model. *Circulation* 1997;96(10):3308–3313.
157. Cobb LA, Fahrenbruch CE, Walsh TR, et al. Influence of cardiopulmonary resuscitation prior to defibrillation in patients with out-of-hospital ventricular fibrillation. *JAMA* 1999;281(13):1182–1188.
158. Wik L, Hansen TB, Fylling F, et al. Delaying defibrillation to give basic cardiopulmonary resuscitation to patients with out-of-hospital ventricular fibrillation: a randomized trial. *JAMA* 2003;289(11):1389–1395.
159. Valenzuela TD, Roe DJ, Nichol G, Clark LL, Spaite DW, Hardman RG. Outcomes of rapid defibrillation by security officers after cardiac arrest in casinos. *N Engl J Med* 2000;343(17):1206–1209.
160. Page RL, Joglar JA, Kowal RC, et al. Use of automated external defibrillators by a U.S. airline. *N Engl J Med* 2000;343(17):1210–1216.
161. Capucci A, Aschieri D, Piepoli MF, Bardy GH, Iconomu E, Arvedi M. Tripling survival from sudden cardiac arrest via early defibrillation without traditional education in cardiopulmonary resuscitation. *Circulation* 2002;106(9):1065–1070.
162. The Public Access Defibrillation Trial Investigators. Public access defibrillation and survival after out-of-hospital cardiac arrest. *N Engl J Med* 2004;351(7):637–646.
163. Cobb LA, Weaver WD, Fahrenbruch CE, Hallstrom AP, Copass MK. Community-based interventions for sudden cardiac death. Impact, limitations, and changes. *Circulation* 1992;85(1 Suppl):I98–I102.
164. Kudenchuk PJ, Cobb LA, Copass MK, et al. Amiodarone for resuscitation after out-of-hospital cardiac arrest due to ventricular fibrillation. *N Engl J Med* 1999;341(12):871–878.
165. Dickey W, Adgey AA. Mortality within hospital after resuscitation from ventricular fibrillation outside hospital. *Br Heart J* 1992;67(4):334–338.
166. Myerburg RJ, Conde CA, Sung RJ, et al. Clinical, electrophysiologic and hemodynamic profile of patients resuscitated from prehospital cardiac arrest. *Am J Med* 1980;68(4):568–576.
167. Hallstrom AP, Cobb LA, Yu BH. Influence of comorbidity on the outcome of patients treated for out-of-hospital ventricular fibrillation. *Circulation* 1996;93(11):2019–2022.
168. Kempf FC Jr, Josephson ME. Cardiac arrest recorded on ambulatory electrocardiograms. *Am J Cardiol* 1984;53(11):1577–1582.
169. Wyse DG, Friedman PL, Brodsky MA, et al. Life-threatening ventricular arrhythmias due to transient or correctable causes: high risk for death in follow-up. *J Am Coll Cardiol* 2001;38(6):1718–1724.
170. Pinski SL, Yao Q, Epstein AE, et al. Determinants of outcome in patients with sustained ventricular tachyarrhythmias: the antiarrhythmics versus implantable defibrillators (AVID) study registry. *Am Heart J* 2000;139(5):804–813.
171. Middlekauff HR, Stevenson WG, Saxon LA. Prognosis after syncope: impact of left ventricular function. *Am Heart J* 1993;125(1):121–127.
172. Gregoratos G, Abrams J, Epstein AE, et al. ACC/AHA/NASPE 2002 guideline update for implantation of cardiac pacemakers and antiarrhythmia devices: summary article: a report of the American College of Cardiology/American Heart Association Task Force on Practice Guidelines (ACC/AHA/NASPE Committee to Update the 1998 Pacemaker Guidelines). *Circulation* 2002;106(16):2145–2161.
173. Hunt SA, Abraham WT, Chin MH, et al. ACC/AHA 2005 guideline update for the diagnosis and management of chronic heart failure in the adult: a report of the American College of Cardiology/American Heart Association Task Force on Practice Guidelines (Writing Committee to Update the 2001 Guidelines for the Evaluation and Management of Heart Failure): developed in collaboration with the American College of Chest Physicians and the International Society for Heart and Lung Transplantation: endorsed by the Heart Rhythm Society. *Circulation* 2005;112(12):e154–235.
174. Tomaselli GF, Beuckelmann DJ, Calkins HG, et al. Sudden cardiac death in heart failure. The role of abnormal repolarization. *Circulation* 1994;90(5):2534–2539.
175. Wilson JR, Schwartz JS, Sutton MS, et al. Prognosis in severe heart failure: relation to hemodynamic measurements and ventricular ectopic activity. *J Am Coll Cardiol* 1983;2(3):403–410.
176. Algra A, Tijssen JG, Roelandt JR, Pool J, Lubsen J. QTc prolongation measured by standard 12-lead electrocardiography is an independent risk factor for sudden death due to cardiac arrest. *Circulation* 1991;83(6):1888–1894.
177. Barr CS, Naas A, Freeman M, Lang CC, Struthers AD. QT dispersion and sudden unexpected death in chronic heart failure. *Lancet* 1994;343(8893):327–329.
178. Shaper AG, Wannamethee G, Macfarlane PW, Walker M. Heart rate, ischaemic heart disease, and sudden cardiac death in middle-aged British men. *Br Heart J* 1993;70(1):49–55.
179. Bigger JT Jr, Fleiss JL, Kleiger R, Miller JP, Rolnitzky LM. The relationships among ventricular arrhythmias, left ventricular dysfunction, and mortality in the 2 years after myocardial infarction. *Circulation* 1984;69(2):250–258.
180. Chakko CS, Gheorghiade M. Ventricular arrhythmias in severe heart failure: incidence, significance, and effectiveness of antiarrhythmic therapy. *Am Heart J* 1985;109(3 Pt 1):497–504.
181. Barber MJ, Mueller TM, Henry DP, Felten SY, Zipes DP. Transmural myocardial infarction in the dog produces sympathectomy in noninfarcted myocardium. *Circulation* 1983;67(4):787–796.
182. Algra A, Tijssen JG, Roelandt JR, Pool J, Lubsen J. Heart rate variability from 24-hour electrocardiography and the 2-year risk for sudden death. *Circulation* 1993;88(1):180–185.
183. La Rovere MT, Pinna GD, Hohnloser SH, et al. Baroreflex sensitivity and heart rate variability in the identification of patients at risk for life-threatening arrhythmias: implications for clinical trials. *Circulation* 2001;103(16):2072–2077.
184. Rashba EJ, Estes NA, Wang P, et al. Preserved heart rate variability identifies low-risk patients with nonischemic dilated cardiomyopathy: results from the DEFINITE trial. *Heart Rhythm* 2006;3(3):281–286.
185. Simson MB. Noninvasive identification of patients at high risk for sudden cardiac death. Signal-averaged electrocardiography. *Circulation* 1992;85(1 Suppl):I145–I151.
186. Mancini DM, Wong KL, Simson MB. Prognostic value of an abnormal signal-averaged electrocardiogram in patients with nonischemic congestive cardiomyopathy. *Circulation* 1993;87(4):1083–1092.

187. Rosenbaum DS, Jackson LE, Smith JM, Garan H, Ruskin JN, Cohen RJ. Electrical alternans and vulnerability to ventricular arrhythmias. *N Engl J Med* 1994;330(4):235–241.
188. Ikeda T, Saito H, Tanno K, et al. T-wave alternans as a predictor for sudden cardiac death after myocardial infarction. *Am J Cardiol* 2002;89(1):79–82.
189. Chow T, Kereiakes DJ, Bartone C, et al. Prognostic utility of microvolt T-wave alternans in risk stratification of patients with ischemic cardiomyopathy. *J Am Coll Cardiol* 2006;47(9):1820–1827.
190. Bloomfield DM, Bigger JT, Steinman RC, et al. Microvolt T-wave alternans and the risk of death or sustained ventricular arrhythmias in patients with left ventricular dysfunction. *J Am Coll Cardiol* 2006;47(2):456–463.
191. Chan PS, Stein K, Chow T, Fendrick M, Bigger JT, Vijan S. Cost-Effectiveness of a microvolt T-wave alternans screening strategy for implantable cardioverter-defibrillator placement in the MADIT-II-eligible population. *J Am Coll Cardiol* 2006;48(1):112–121.
192. DiCarlo LA Jr, Morady F, Schwartz AB, et al. Clinical significance of ventricular fibrillation-flutter induced by ventricular programmed stimulation. *Am Heart J* 1985;109(5 Pt 1):959–963.
193. Ruskin JN. Role of invasive electrophysiological testing in the evaluation and treatment of patients at high risk for sudden cardiac death. *Circulation* 1992;85(1 Suppl):I152–I159.
194. Buxton AE, Lee KL, DiCarlo L, et al. Electrophysiologic testing to identify patients with coronary artery disease who are at risk for sudden death. Multicenter Unsustained Tachycardia Trial Investigators. *N Engl J Med* 2000;342(26):1937–1945.
195. Buxton AE, Lee KL, Fisher JD, Josephson ME, Prystowsky EN, Hafley G. A randomized study of the prevention of sudden death in patients with coronary artery disease. Multicenter Unsustained Tachycardia Trial Investigators. *N Engl J Med* 1999;341(25):1882–1890.
196. Moss AJ, Hall WJ, Cannom DS, et al. Improved survival with an implanted defibrillator in patients with coronary disease at high risk for ventricular arrhythmia. Multicenter Automatic Defibrillator Implantation Trial Investigators. *N Engl J Med* 1996;335(26):1933–1940.
197. Bardy GH, Lee KL, Mark DB, et al. Amiodarone or an implantable cardioverter-defibrillator for congestive heart failure. *N Engl J Med* 2005;352(3):225–237.
198. Moss AJ, Zareba W, Hall WJ, et al. Prophylactic implantation of a defibrillator in patients with myocardial infarction and reduced ejection fraction. *N Engl J Med* 2002;346(12):877–883.
199. Kendall MJ, Lynch KP, Hjalmarson A, Kjekshus J. Beta-blockers and sudden cardiac death. *Ann Intern Med* 1995;123(5):358–367.
200. Singh BN. Advantages of beta blockers versus antiarrhythmic agents and calcium antagonists in secondary prevention after myocardial infarction. *Am J Cardiol* 1990;66(9):9C-20C.
201. Goldstein S, Hjalmarson A. The mortality effect of metoprolol CR/XL in patients with heart failure: results of the MERIT-HF Trial. *Clin Cardiol* 1999;22 Suppl 5:V30–V35.
202. Pfeffer MA, Braunwald E, Moye LA, et al. Effect of captopril on mortality and morbidity in patients with left ventricular dysfunction after myocardial infarction. Results of the survival and ventricular enlargement trial. The SAVE Investigators. *N Engl J Med* 1992;327(10):669–677.
203. The CONSENSUS Trial Study Group. Effects of enalapril on mortality in severe congestive heart failure. Results of the Cooperative North Scandinavian Enalapril Survival Study (CONSENSUS). *N Engl J Med* 1987;316(23):1429–1435.
204. The SOLVD Investigators. Effect of enalapril on survival in patients with reduced left ventricular ejection fractions and congestive heart failure. *N Engl J Med* 1991;325(5):293–302.
205. The SOLVD Investigators. Effect of enalapril on mortality and the development of heart failure in asymptomatic patients with reduced left ventricular ejection fractions. *N Engl J Med* 1992;327(10):685–691.
206. Domanski MJ, Exner DV, Borkowf CB, Geller NL, Rosenberg Y, Pfeffer MA. Effect of angiotensin converting enzyme inhibition on sudden cardiac death in patients following acute myocardial infarction. A meta-analysis of randomized clinical trials. *J Am Coll Cardiol* 1999;33(3):598–604.
207. The Heart Outcomes Prevention Evaluation Study Investigators. Effects of an angiotensin-converting-enzyme inhibitor, ramipril, on cardiovascular events in high-risk patients. *N Engl J Med* 2000;342(3):145–153.
208. Chiu JH, Abdelhadi RH, Chung MK, et al. Effect of statin therapy on risk of ventricular arrhythmia among patients with coronary artery disease and an implantable cardioverter-defibrillator. *Am J Cardiol* 2005;95(4):490–491.
209. Vyas AK, Guo H, Moss AJ, et al. Reduction in ventricular tachyarrhythmias with statins in the Multicenter Automatic Defibrillator Implantation Trial (MADIT)-II. *J Am Coll Cardiol* 2006;47(4):769–773.
210. The Cardiac Arrhythmia Suppression Trial (CAST) Investigators. Preliminary report: effect of encainide and flecainide on mortality in a randomized trial of arrhythmia suppression after myocardial infarction. *N Engl J Med* 1989;321(6):406–412.
211. The Cardiac Arrhythmia Suppression Trial II Investigators. Effect of the antiarrhythmic agent moricizine on survival after myocardial infarction. *N Engl J Med* 1992;327(4):227–233.
212. Siebels J, Cappato R, Ruppel R, Schneider MA, Kuck KH. Preliminary results of the Cardiac Arrest Study Hamburg (CASH). CASH Investigators. *Am J Cardiol* 1993;72(16):109F-13F.
213. Hine LK, Laird N, Hewitt P, Chalmers TC. Meta-analytic evidence against prophylactic use of lidocaine in acute myocardial infarction. *Arch Intern Med* 1989;149(12):2694–2698.
214. Moosvi AR, Goldstein S, VanderBrug Medendorp S, et al. Effect of empiric antiarrhythmic therapy in resuscitated out-of-hospital cardiac arrest victims with coronary artery disease. *Am J Cardiol* 1990;65(18):1192–1197.
215. Mason JW. A comparison of electrophysiologic testing with Holter monitoring to predict antiarrhythmic-drug efficacy for ventricular tachyarrhythmias. Electrophysiologic Study Versus Electrocardiographic Monitoring Investigators. *N Engl J Med* 1993;329(7):445–451.
216. Waldo AL, Camm AJ, deRuyter H, et al. Effect of *d*-sotalol on mortality in patients with left ventricular dysfunction after recent and remote myocardial infarction. The SWORD Investigators. Survival With Oral *d*-Sotalol. *Lancet* 1996;348(9019):7–12.
217. Torp-Pedersen C, Moller M, Bloch-Thomsen PE, et al. Dofetilide in patients with congestive heart failure and left ventricular dysfunction. Danish Investigations of Arrhythmia and Mortality on Dofetilide Study Group. *N Engl J Med* 1999;341(12):857–865.
218. Kober L, Bloch Thomsen PE, Moller M, et al. Effect of dofetilide in patients with recent myocardial infarction and left-ventricular dysfunction: a randomised trial. *Lancet* 2000;356(9247):2052–2058.
219. Connolly SJ, Dorian P, Roberts RS, et al. Comparison of beta-blockers, amiodarone plus beta-blockers, or sotalol for prevention of shocks from implantable cardioverter defibrillators: the OPTIC Study: a randomized trial. *JAMA* 2006;295(2):165–171.
220. Singh BN, Singh SN, Reda DJ, et al. Amiodarone versus sotalol for atrial fibrillation. *N Engl J Med* 2005;352(18):1861–1872.
221. Nademanee K, Singh BN, Stevenson WG, Weiss JN. Amiodarone and post-MI patients. *Circulation* 1993;88(2):764–774.
222. Burkart F, Pfisterer M, Kiowski W, Follath F, Burckhardt D. Effect of antiarrhythmic therapy on mortality in survivors of myocardial infarction with asymptomatic complex ventricular arrhythmias: Basel Antiarrhythmic Study of Infarct Survival (BASIS). *J Am Coll Cardiol* 1990;16(7):1711–1718.
223. Cairns JA, Connolly SJ, Roberts R, Gent M. Randomised trial of outcome after myocardial infarction in patients with frequent or repetitive ventricular premature depolarisations: CAMIAT. Canadian Amiodarone Myocardial Infarction Arrhythmia Trial Investigators. *Lancet* 1997;349(9053):675–682.
224. Julian DG, Camm AJ, Frangin G, et al. Randomised trial of effect of amiodarone on mortality in patients with left-ventricular dysfunction after recent myocardial infarction: EMIAT. European Myocardial Infarct Amiodarone Trial Investigators. *Lancet* 1997;349(9053):667–674.
225. Boutitie F, Boissel JP, Connolly S, et al. Amiodarone interaction with beta-blockers: analysis of the merged EMIAT and CAMIAT databases. *Circulation* 1999;99:2268–2275.
226. Doval HC, Nul DR, Grancelli HO, Perrone SV, Bortman GR, Curiel R. Randomised trial of low-dose amiodarone in severe congestive heart failure. Grupo de Estudio de la Sobrevida en la Insuficiencia Cardiaca en Argentina (GESICA). *Lancet* 1994;344(8921):493–498.
227. Singh SN, Fletcher RD, Fisher SG, et al. Amiodarone in patients with congestive heart failure and asymptomatic ventricular arrhythmia. Survival Trial of Antiarrhythmic Therapy in Congestive Heart Failure. *N Engl J Med* 1995;333(2):77–82.
228. Sim I, McDonald KM, Lavori PW, Norbutas CM, Hlatky MA. Quantitative overview of randomized trials of amiodarone to prevent sudden cardiac death. *Circulation* 1997;96(9):2823–2829.
229. Connolly S. Evidence-based analysis of amiodarone efficacy and safety. *Circulation* 1999;100:2025–2034.
230. Connolly SJ, Gent M, Roberts RS, et al. Canadian implantable defibrillator study (CIDS): a randomized trial of the implantable cardioverter defibrillator against amiodarone. *Circulation* 2000;101(11):1297–1302.
231. Kuck KH, Cappato R, Siebels J, Ruppel R. Randomized comparison of antiarrhythmic drug therapy with implantable defibrillators in patients resuscitated from cardiac arrest: the Cardiac Arrest Study Hamburg (CASH). *Circulation* 2000 Aug 15;102(7):748–754.
232. The Antiarrhythmics versus Implantable Defibrillators (AVID) Investigators. A comparison of antiarrhythmic-drug therapy with implantable defibrillators in patients resuscitated from near-fatal ventricular arrhythmias. *N Engl J Med* 1997;337(22):1576–1583.
233. Levine JH, Massumi A, Scheinman MM, et al. Intravenous amiodarone for recurrent sustained hypotensive ventricular tachyarrhythmias. Intravenous Amiodarone Multicenter Trial Group. *J Am Coll Cardiol* 1996;27(1):67–75.
234. Dorian P, Cass D, Schwartz B, Cooper R, Gelaznikas R, Barr A. Amiodarone as compared with lidocaine for shock-resistant ventricular fibrillation. *N Engl J Med* 2002;346(12):884–890.
235. Mirowski M, Reid PR, Mower MM, et al. Termination of malignant ventricular arrhythmias with an implanted automatic defibrillator in human beings. *N Engl J Med* 1980;303(6):322–324.
236. Bristow MR, Saxon LA, Boehmer J, et al. Cardiac-resynchronization therapy with or without an implantable defibrillator in advanced chronic heart failure. *N Engl J Med* 2004;350(21):2140–2150.
237. Bigger JT Jr. Prophylactic use of implanted cardiac defibrillators in patients at high risk for ventricular arrhythmias after coronary-artery bypass graft surgery. Coronary Artery Bypass Graft (CABG) Patch Trial Investigators [see comments]. *N Engl J Med* 1997;337(22):1569–1575.
238. Hohnloser SH, Kuck KH, Dorian P, et al. Prophylactic use of an implantable cardioverter-defibrillator after acute myocardial infarction. *N Engl J Med* 2004;351(24):2481–2488.
239. Reynolds MR, Cohen DJ, Kugelmass AD, et al. The frequency and incremental cost of major complications among medicare beneficiaries receiving implantable cardioverter-defibrillators. *J Am Coll Cardiol* 2006;47(12):2493–2497.
240. Gehi A, Haas D, Fuster V. Primary prophylaxis with the implantable cardioverter-defibrillator: the need for improved risk stratification. *JAMA* 2005;294(8):958–960.
241. The Cardiomyopathy Trial Investigators. Cardiomyopathy trial. *Pacing Clin Electrophysiol* 1993;16(3 Pt 2):576–581.
242. Strickberger SA, Hummel JD, Bartlett TG, et al. Amiodarone versus implantable cardioverter-defibrillator: randomized trial in patients with nonischemic dilated cardiomyopathy and asymptomatic nonsustained ventricular tachycardia—AMIOVIRT. *J Am Coll Cardiol* 2003;41(10):1707–1712.
243. Kadish A, Dyer A, Daubert JP, et al. Prophylactic defibrillator implantation in patients with nonischemic dilated cardiomyopathy. *N Engl J Med* 2004;350(21):2151–2158.
244. Young JB, Abraham WT, Smith AL, et al. Combined cardiac resynchronization and implantable cardioversion defibrillation in advanced chronic heart failure: the MIRACLE ICD Trial. *JAMA* 2003;289(20):2685–2694.
245. Cleland JG, Daubert JC, Erdmann E, et al. The effect of cardiac resynchronization on morbidity and mortality in heart failure. *N Engl J Med* 2005;352(15):1539–1549.
246. Holmes DR Jr, Davis KB, Mock MB, et al. The effect of medical and surgical treatment on subsequent sudden cardiac death in patients with coronary artery disease: a report from the Coronary Artery Surgery Study. *Circulation* 1986;73(6):1254–1263.
247. Veenhuyzen GD, Singh SN, McAreavey D, Shelton BJ, Exner DV. Prior coronary artery bypass surgery and risk of death among patients with ischemic left ventricular dysfunction. *Circulation* 2001;104(13):1489–1493.
248. Cook JR, Rizo-Patron C, Curtis AB, et al. Effect of surgical revascularization in patients with coronary artery disease and ventricular tachycardia or fibrillation in the Antiarrhythmics Versus Implantable Defibrillators (AVID) Registry. *Am Heart J* 2002;143(5):821–826.
249. Wilber DJ, Garan H, Finkelstein D, et al. Out-of-hospital cardiac arrest. Use of electrophysiologic testing in the prediction of long-term outcome. *N Engl J Med* 1988;318(1):19–24.
250. Every NR, Fahrenbruch CE, Hallstrom AP, Weaver WD, Cobb LA. Influence of coronary bypass surgery on subsequent outcome of patients resuscitated from out of hospital cardiac arrest. *J Am Coll Cardiol* 1992;19(7):1435–1439.
251. Kelly P, Ruskin JN, Vlahakes GJ, Buckley MJ, Jr., Freeman CS, Garan H. Surgical coronary revascularization in survivors of prehospital cardiac arrest: its effect on inducible ventricular arrhythmias and long-term survival. *J Am Coll Cardiol* 1990;15(2):267–273.
252. Hargrove WCd, Josephson ME, Marchlinski FE, Miller JM. Surgical decisions in the management of sudden cardiac death and malignant ventricular arrhythmias. Subendocardial resection, the automatic internal defibrillator, or both. *J Thorac Cardiovasc Surg* 1989;97(6):923–928.
253. Wang YS, Scheinman MM, Chien WW, Cohen TJ, Lesh MD, Griffin JC. Patients with supraventricular tachycardia presenting with aborted sudden death: incidence, mechanism and long-term follow-up [see comments]. *J Am Coll Cardiol* 1991;18(7):1711–1719.
254. Langberg JJ, Desai J, Dullet N, Scheinman MM. Treatment of macroreentrant ventricular tachycardia with radiofrequency ablation of the right bundle branch. *Am J Cardiol* 1989;63(13):1010–1013.
255. Wannamethee G, Shaper AG, MacFarlane PW, et al. Risk factors for sudden cardiac death in middle-aged British men. *Circulation* 1995;91:1749–56.
256. Albert CM, Chae, CU, Grodstein F, et al. Prospective study of sudden cardiac death among women in the United States. *Circulation* 2003;107:2096–2101.

CHAPTER (50)

Cardiopulmonary and Cardiocerebral Resuscitation

Gordon A. Ewy

INTRODUCTION

Sudden death is a leading cause of mortality in the United States, Canada, and Europe.[1] The major cause of unexpected sudden death is out-of-hospital cardiac arrest. Over the past few centuries, resuscitation techniques have been diverse and initially were focused on victims of drowning. Although cardiopulmonary resuscitation (CPR) has been in existence for almost a half century, the survival rates have remained essentially unchanged.[1-9] Survival rates are dismal in the absence of early defibrillation with only a few percent of out-of-hospital cardiac arrest victims resuscitated and returned to normal or near-normal function.

This chapter addresses the latest recommendations for CPR—*2005 American Heart Association Guidelines for Cardiopulmonary Resuscitation and Emergency Cardiovascular Care*, here after referred to as *2005 Guidelines*, by summarizing the major changes from the better known *2000 Guidelines*.[8] This chapter also highlights the shortcomings of these recommenda-

tions for cardiac arrest, and emphasizes a different approach called *cardiocerebral resuscitation*.

Cardiocerebral resuscitation emphasizes the importance of near continuous, uninterrupted chest compressions, and deemphasizes positive-pressure ventilations, but otherwise employs many components of standard CPR but often in different sequences.

BACKGROUND

The technique of closed-chest "cardiac massage" for cardiac arrest was first published in 1960, and since the survival rate in this initial report was 70 percent (14/20) it quickly became the preferred technique for both in-hospital and prehospital treatment of cardiac arrest.[10] Closed-chest cardiac massage extends the period of time from the onset of ventricular fibrillation (VF) to possible successful closed chest defibrillation.[1,10]

The discoverers of closed-chest cardiac massage, Kouwenhoven, Jude, and Knickerbocker, stated that "assisted ventilation was not necessary as the victim gasped" during continuous closed-chest compressions.[11] Several of their initial patients received chest compression without positive-pressure ventilation.[10]

Others advocated ventilation for both cardiac and respiratory arrests and this view has persisted.[12] The possible reasons and justifications for this view are: (1) the emphasis of therapy for out-of-hospital arrests was historically based on the resuscitation of drowning victims; (2) it was thought that lay individuals could not reliably differentiate between respiratory and cardiac arrest; (3) gasping did not always occur in patients with cardiac arrest; and (4) studies in volunteer medical students given drugs to produce temporary paralysis showed that blood gases rapidly deteriorated without assisted ventilations.[12] This latter study was of little relevance, as the normal cardiac output in these students created significant ventilation-to-perfusion mismatch. Nevertheless, closed-chest cardiac massage was merged with mouth-to-mouth or assisted ventilation to form what became known as CPR.[1,2,5–8]

By 1966, standardized methods for performing and teaching CPR had been published. A few years later, the American Heart Association (AHA) adopted CPR as one of its main focus areas, developed standards for CPR and emergency cardiac care (ECC), and spearheaded a campaign to disseminate the techniques of CPR and ECC to both professionals and the public. As new information became available, "Standards" became "Standards and Guidelines" and finally just "Guidelines."[2,5–7,13,14] In 2000, the *Guidelines for CPR and Emergency Cardiac Care (ECC)* were published in collaboration with the International Liaison Committee on Resuscitation (ILCOR).[13] ILCOR joined for the consensus conference in 2005, but published separate guidelines.[1,9]

Unfortunately, in spite of the international efforts in the development, promulgation and periodic updates of the guidelines for CPR, as noted above, survival rates for out-of-hospital victims of cardiac arrest in the absence of early defibrillation remain dismal.[15] In New York, Chicago, and Los Angeles, the reported overall survival from out-of-hospital cardiac arrest is approximately 1 percent—near that defined as medically futile.

One of the many reasons the *Guidelines*-advocated approach to out-of-hospital cardiac arrest in adults are suboptimal is that the same technique is advocated for two entirely different pathophysiologic conditions: sudden collapse cardiac arrests as a result of VF or pulseless ventricular tachycardia (arrhythmogenic arrests), and cardiac arrest precipitated by primary respiratory failure (asphyxial arrests). The *Guidelines'* emphasis on mouth-to-mouth "rescue breathing" as an integral part of CPR contributes to the fact that only approximately 20 percent of individuals with out-of-hospital cardiac arrest have CPR initiated by a lay bystander.[16–18] Other *1992 Guidelines* and *2000 Guidelines* recommendations for emergency medical services (EMS) resuscitation, such as early intubation, defibrillation first, escalating energy of up to three consecutive shocks for VF, prolonged periods without chest compressions required by automated external defibrillators (AEDs), and frequent pulse and rhythm checks resulted in chest compressions being performed by EMS personnel only half of the time—further contributing to the poor survival rates.[19,20] Fortunately, some of these latter EMS issues were addressed in the *2005 Guidelines*.[1]

2005 GUIDELINES RECOMMENDATIONS FOR CPR

【 】 CARDIOPULMONARY RESUSCITATION

Cardiopulmonary resuscitation has been defined as chest compression and assisted ventilations. Ventilations, or "rescue breathing," is considered important for children in cardiac arrest because a respiratory problem often initiates the event and VF or asystole is a relatively late event.[7,21–23] Consequently, CPR is indicated for respiratory arrest and appears to be critical in subjects after the complete loss of arterial pressure secondary to asphyxial cardiac arrest.[24]

Unlike primary cardiac arrest caused by sudden onset of VF or pulseless ventricular tachycardia (VT), cardiac arrest secondary to hypoxia is associated with severely abnormal arterial blood gases. The typical sequence for untreated respiratory arrest is hypoxia followed in several minutes by pulseless hypotension, leading to hypoxic ischemia and, finally, cardiac arrest.

Treated early in this sequence, before hypotension ensues, the only intervention that is usually necessary is relieving the cause of the hypoxia. An example of asphyxial arrest is the so-called *café coronary* where aspiration of a large piece of food obstructs the trachea. The Heimlich maneuver (Henry J. Heimlich MD, Xavier University, Cincinnati, Ohio), or similar maneuver, abruptly increases the intrathoracic pressure, causing a forceful expulsion of air from the lungs, which may be all that is needed to relieve an obstruction. Assisted ventilation may be all that is necessary in a patient with respiratory depression or respiratory arrest secondary to drug overdose or other causes of severe hypoxia before cardiac arrest has ensued.

Once hypotension ensues, however, both chest compression and assisted ventilation are needed. In a realistic swine model of pediatric asphyxia, Berg et al. produced hypoxic arrest by clamping the endotracheal tube until the loss of arterial pressure—a process that took a variable period of time averaging 9 minutes.[24] In this study, the swine with hypoxic arrest were randomized to one of four different interventions, each of 8 minutes duration: (1) chest compressions plus ventilations, (2) chest compressions only, (3) assisted ventilations only, or (4) no CPR.[24] Arterial blood gas oxygen saturation after 1 minute of intervention was 87 ± 6 percent in the chest compressions plus assisted ventilations group, compared to only 17 ± 5 percent in the chest compression only group. The Pco_2 was 45 ± 8 mmHg in the chest compressions plus assisted ventilations group, compared to 97 ± 5 mmHg for the chest compressions only group, and associated pH values were 7.20 versus 7.10, respectively.[24] The 24-hour neurologically normal survival was 7 of 10 for the group receiving both chest compressions and ventilations, but only 1 of 14 for those treated with chest compressions only ($p < 0.05$).[24]

Nevertheless, studies suggest that early chest-compression-only by a bystander is helpful in some of these cases. In an experiment where interventions were begun earlier in the hypoxic arrest, that is, when the peak systolic aortic pressures had decreased to 50 mmHg, survival was similar with chest compression plus ventilation, chest compression only, or assisted ventilation only, but each was significantly better than no CPR.[25] These types of experiments have led to the advice in respiratory arrest, "do something, as something is better than nothing."[1] This philosophy is supported by the findings of Sirbaugh et al.[23] Forty-one pediatric respiratory arrest patients who received bystander CPR survived and were neurologically normal, whereas only 6 of 300 (2 percent) of patients who did not receive bystander CPR prior to EMS arrival survived and 5 of the 6 (83 percent) had bad neurologic outcomes.[23]

【 】 MAJOR CHANGES FOR LAY RESCUER

The major changes of *2005 American Heart Association Guidelines for Cardiopulmonary Resuscitation* for the lay rescuer might be summarized as follows[1]: start CPR as soon as collapse occurs, activate the EMS system by calling 911, and use an AED if available.[1] Push hard, push fast, allow full chest recoil, and minimize interruptions of chest compressions.[1]

Specific *2005 Guidelines* changes included the recommendation of "a single (universal) chest compression:ventilation ratio of 30:2 for single rescuers of victims of all ages (except newborn infants)."[1] "This recommendation is designed to simplify teaching and provide longer periods of uninterrupted chest compressions."[1] The *2005 Guidelines* recommendation is for each breath to be administered within 1 second,[1] and delivered with enough volume to cause a visible rise in the anterior chest wall. In certification sessions it is stressed that administration of the two rescue breaths should be completed quickly, interrupting chest compression for only 10 seconds.[1] While this recommendation is well intended to minimize interruptions of chest compression, providing two respirations without interrupting chest compressions for more than 10 seconds is nearly impossible for a single lay rescuer.[26,27]

Minor changes in the *2005 Guidelines* include the elimination of the recommendations that lay individuals assess the pulse or check for other for "signs of circulation" before initiating CPR. The recommended hand position for chest compressions is also simplified and is "the center of the chest at the nipple line."[1]

【 】 THREE TIME-SENSITIVE PHASES OF VENTRICULAR FIBRILLATION BASIS FOR CHANGES

Some of the changes made in the *2005 Guidelines*, as well as some of the recommendations of cardiocerebral resuscitation, are based on Weisfeldt and Becker's three-phase, time-sensitive model of cardiac arrest as a consequence of untreated VF.[28] This model explains why several of the past recommendations for resuscitation of patients with cardiac arrest as a consequence of VF were ineffective.

The first, or electrical, phase of VF, lasts for about 4 to 5 minutes. During this time, the most important therapeutic intervention is prompt defibrillation. Although the heart is fibrillating, the myocardium has not yet used up its energy stores or undergone serious cellular damage and is able to respond to the defibrillation shock and generate a perfusing rhythm. This is why implantable cardioverter defibrillators work so well and why AEDs have been employed so successfully in patients with out-of-hospital cardiac arrest in selected settings, including airplanes, airports, casinos, and in communities where prompt defibrillation was possible.[29–32]

The second, or circulatory, phase of untreated VF lasts for a variable period of time, but typically from about 5 to 15 minutes after the onset of VF. During this time, the continued lack of myo-

cardial perfusion during the uncoordinated myocyte contractions results in declining myocardial energy stores and the accumulation of toxic metabolites. Defibrillation first during this "circulatory" phase rarely results in a perfusing rhythm, but rather in pulseless electrical activity (PEA) or asystole. The most crucial intervention during this second or circulatory phase of VF cardiac arrest is restoring myocardial blood flow by the generation of adequate coronary perfusion pressure with chest compressions prior to and immediately after defibrillation attempts.[33] Chest compressions during the circulatory phase of VF increase the amplitude and the frequency spectrum of the fibrillation waveforms and improve the chances of restoring a perfusing rhythm following defibrillation.[34]

The third or metabolic phase of VF follows the circulatory phase. Immediate defibrillation during this phase is almost universally unsuccessful. Survival rates of individuals found in this state, in the absence of youth and/or hypothermia, are uniformly poor.

【 】 *2005 GUIDELINES* CHANGES FOR EMERGENCY MEDICAL SERVICES

Several important changes were made in the *2005 Guidelines* for advanced cardiac life support.[1] Chest compression prior to defibrillation results in improved survival during the circulatory phase of ventricular fibrillation. Therefore, the *2005 Guidelines* recommend that "Emergency Medical Services (EMS) providers may consider the provision of about 5 cycles (or about 2 minutes) of CPR before defibrillation for unwitnessed arrest, particularly when the interval from the call to the EMS dispatcher response at the scene is more than 4 to 5 minutes."[1]

A single defibrillation shock (rather than the three stacked shocks previously recommended) is to be followed immediately by about 2 minutes of chest compressions prior to rhythm checks. Specifically, rescuers "should not check the rhythm or a pulse immediately after shock delivery—they should immediately resume CPR, beginning with chest compressions, and should check the rhythm after 5 cycles (or about 2 minutes) of CPR."[1]

The recommendation to administer only one shock followed immediately by CPR (beginning with chest compressions) instead of three stacked shocks for the treatment of ventricular fibrillation/pulseless ventricular tachycardia "...is based on the high first-shock success rate of new defibrillators and the knowledge that if the first shock fails, intervening chest compressions may improve oxygen and substrate delivery to the myocardium, making the subsequent shock more likely to result in defibrillation."[1]

These changes were made because research had shown that excessive no-flow time can be consumed while AEDs analyzed the cardiac rhythm before and after shock delivery.[35] Research also showed that a period of chest compressions to produce blood flow preceding and following defibrillation could improve defibrillation success and patient outcome.[36,37]

SHORTCOMINGS OF PREVIOUS GUIDELINES
【 】 POOR SURVIVAL RATES

Return of spontaneous circulation (ROSC), being alive at hospital admission, or being alive at some later designated time were all used previously as criteria for survival for out-of-hospital cardiac arrest. Most such "survivors" ultimately died before being discharged from the hospital, making these definitions inappropriate. In addition, different definitions of survival made comparisons of different approaches to CPR difficult.

A more clinically relevant definition of "survival" has been introduced: neurologically normal survival at hospital discharge or at a specified time after discharge for humans, or neurologically intact survival at 24 or 48 hours for experimental animals.[38–40] When definitions of survival such as neurologically normal or near normal are used, it is clear that survival rates for out-of-hospital cardiac arrest with cardiopulmonary resuscitation have been very low and, with the exceptions of early application of an AED have remained stagnant over the last few decades.[15]

Most survivors of out-of-hospital cardiac arrest are found in the subset of patients with a bystander-witnessed arrest and a shockable rhythm on arrival of EMS with a defibrillator.[29–32] In this subset of patients, survival in 2002 in Los Angeles was 6 percent, survival from 1992 to 2002 in Tucson, Arizona averaged 10 percent, whereas in Rock and Walworth Counties, Wisconsin during 2000 to 2003 it was 20 percent.[41,42] These survival differences probably reflect differences in EMS response times.

[ ] CHEST COMPRESSION RATES CORRELATE WITH SURVIVAL

Abella et al. reported that suboptimal compression rates during in-hospital cardiac arrest correlated with poor ROSC.[43] Although survival rates were not reported, there would be no survival in those without ROSC. In this study, ROSC was significantly higher for patients receiving more than 87 compressions per minute than those receiving fewer than 72 compressions per minute.[43] In this in-hospital study, ventilations were given quickly by a second rescuer. In the out-of-hospital situation, where a single bystander is performing CPR, if every set of 15 compressions is interrupted for 14 to 16 seconds to deliver the recommended two ventilations, the individual will not receive enough chest compressions for ROSC. In fact, if every set of 30 compressions is interrupted 14 to 16 seconds for single bystander CPR, the delivered chest compressions would still fall short of the near 90 compressions needed for ROSC in this in-hospital population. Several studies have suggested improved survival with greater compressions-to-ventilation ratios.[44,45]

[ ] DELETERIOUS EFFECTS OF POSITIVE-PRESSURE VENTILATIONS

From their inception, the standards and guidelines[1,2,5–9] for a bystander's response to out-of-hospital cardiac arrest have emphasized the imperative of mouth-to-mouth ventilation, paradoxically called "rescue breathing." While mouth-to-mouth ventilation may "rescue" an individual with respiratory arrest, this approach actually decreases the likelihood of a "rescue" in a much larger group of patients—those with a primary cardiac arrest.[46]

Mouth-to-mouth positive ventilations for primary cardiac arrest are detrimental for several reasons: (1) Bystander reluctance to perform mouth-to-mouth breathing dramatically decreases the frequency with which resuscitative efforts are initiated. (2) Both ob-

servational and experimental studies have long reported that survival is better in patients with cardiac arrest who receive chest-compression-only CPR than in those in whom no bystander rescue efforts were initiated until the actual or simulated arrival of EMS personnel.[47,48] (3) Mouth-to-mouth ventilations by single bystanders requires inordinately long interruptions of essential chest compressions.[26] (4) During cardiac arrest, mouth-to-mouth or positive-pressure ventilation increases intrathoracic pressures, thereby reducing the return of venous blood to the chest. Decreased venous return to the chest further compromises the already marginal coronary and cerebral blood flow extant during cardiac arrest and resuscitation.[49,50] This phenomenon is made worse when a forceful ventilation is given while the chest is being compressed.[50] (5) With sudden unexpected cardiac collapse from VF, the pulmonary veins, the left heart and the entire arterial system are filled with oxygenated blood and the recommended two ventilations do not increase arterial saturation.[1,46,51] (6) Mouth-to-mouth ventilation is not necessary in a significant number of victims of cardiac arrest because they initially gasp, and if chest compressions are initiated early and continued, many of these patients will continue to gasp, thereby providing physiologic ventilation that facilitates both oxygenation and venous return to the chest.[52–54] (7) It is known that survival from experimentally induced cardiac arrest is best correlated with the coronary and cerebral perfusion produced by chest compressions.[33,55] And, finally, (8) it has been shown in nonparalyzed swine studies of cardiac arrest that survival is dramatically better with chest-compression-only resuscitation than with *2000 Guidelines*-recommended ventilations plus chest compressions during prolonged arrests, when chest compressions were interrupted for a realistic 16 seconds to provide the two mouth-to-mouth breaths between each set of 15 chest compressions.[56]

CARDIOCEREBRAL RESUSCITATION FOR CARDIAC ARREST

CPR should be reserved for respiratory arrest. Cardiocerebral resuscitation (CCR), a new approach to cardiac arrest, improves survival of these patients by increasing the prevalence of bystander initiated resuscitation, by limiting interruptions of chest compressions throughout the process of resuscitation thereby enhancing cardiac and cerebral perfusion, by assuring coronary perfusion prior to defibrillation in the circulatory phase of ventricular fibrillation arrest, by the immediate resumption of chest compressions during the post defibrillation pulseless electrical activity, and by eliminating the negative effects of positive pressure ventilation during early resuscitation phases of cardiac arrest.[41,42,46,57]

During cardiac arrest and resuscitation efforts, the perfusion pressures generated by chest compressions are very much less than those developed by the beating heart. Accordingly, any interruption of chest compressions has a negative effect on cerebral and myocardial perfusion and decreases the chance of neurologically intact survival.[46,56] Consequently, the delivery of near-continuous, appropriate chest compressions is a fundamental tenet of CCR.

The emphasis on limiting interruptions of chest compressions is based on research that showed that the major determinant of neurologically intact survival from prolonged cardiac arrest because of VF is the perfusion pressures generated by chest compressions rather

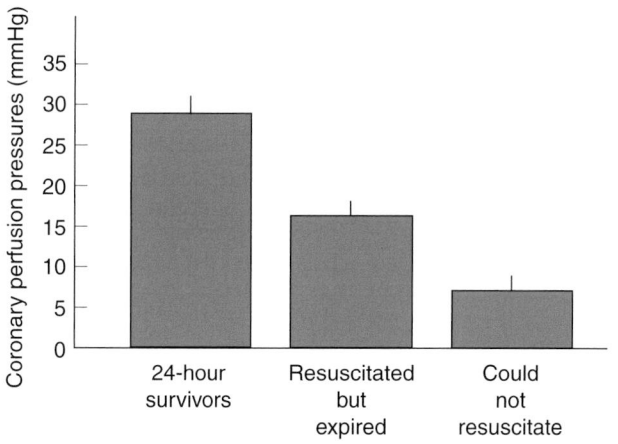

FIGURE 50–1. Relation of coronary perfusion pressures generated during prolonged cardiac arrest secondary ventricular fibrillation to survival. *Source: Modified from Kern KB, Ewy GA, Vorhees WD, Babbs CF, Tacker WA.[33]*

than the blood gas composition, acid–base balance, or the frequency or strength of defibrillation shocks (Fig. 50–1).[33,38,46,55,58,59]

Interruptions of chest compressions immediately curtail blood flow (Fig. 50–2), and resumption takes several compressions to restore good perfusion pressures (Fig. 50–3). There should be no interruptions of chest compressions for anything but rhythm analysis and defibrillation until the return of spontaneous circulation or the termination of the resuscitation effort. Pulse checks are to be done only during pauses in chest compressions for rhythm analysis.[41]

There are now survival observations in man that indicate that chest-compression-only CPR is better than doing nothing[60] and that chest compression only is better than compression plus rescue breathing.[61] The survey of survivors of the SOS-KANTO study showed that the overall survival of out-of-hospital cardiac arrest was 2.2 percent for those who were not receiving bystander CPR when the EMS arrived, 4.2 percent for those who were receiving chest compressions plus mouth-to-mouth breathing, and 6.2 per-

cent for those receiving chest-compression-only bystander CPR.[61] More importantly, they found that in the subset of patients with the greatest chance of survival—those with witnessed arrest and a shockable ventricular arrhythmia on arrival of the EMS personnel, the survival was twice as great in those who had received bystander chest compression alone than in those who received chest compression plus mouth-to-mouth ventilation.[62]

WILL CHANGES MAKE A DIFFERENCE?

Although the *2005 Guidelines* have incorporated many of the same changes for EMS system as cardiocerebral resuscitation, the *2005 Guidelines* still recommend positive-pressure ventilation and have not been compared to the approach advocated in the *2000 Guidelines*. In contrast the Wisconsin experience of using CCR found that this approach dramatically improved survival compared with CPR.[41] Patients with witnessed cardiac arrest, who had a shockable rhythm on survival of the EMS, had a dramatically improved survival.[41] During the 3 years before the initiation of CCR, the neurologically normal survival of this group was 15 percent.[41] During the year CCR was instituted, the survival of this group was 45 percent.[41] This approach was initiated in several municipal fire departments in Arizona in 2004 and 2005 and has tripled survival.

COMPONENTS OF CARDIOCEREBRAL RESUSCITATION

Cardiocerebral resuscitation has three components: the "lay component" for the public, the EMS component, and the postresuscitation component.[42,46,63] The first or lay component is directed toward the public to emphasize the importance of activating the EMS system, beginning chest-compression-only bystander CCR, and using an AED if available.

Bystanders are taught to call 911 to activate the EMS as soon as possible and then to begin continuous chest compressions.[46,64] They are instructed to place the heel of one hand in the center of the patient's chest, with the heel of the other on top of the first, lock the elbows so the arms are straight, and with the shoulders above the center of the patient's chest, to fall so the weight of their upper body compresses the patient's chest. The compression rate should be 100 per minute. Lifting the hands completely off the chest after each compression to allow full chest recoil is specifically emphasized.[65] If more than one rescuer is present, they are to trade off doing chest compressions after each 100 or 200 compressions, as properly done continuous chest compressions at 100 per minute is very tiring, especially for older individuals. If an AED is readily available, they are to instruct someone to get it, or if they are alone, to get it themself and follow the directions and voice prompts.[46,63]

The second component of CCR consists of new recommendations for EMS personnel.[41,42,46,57,63,66] "Chest-compression-only" dispatch-directed bystander resuscitation

180 mm Hg

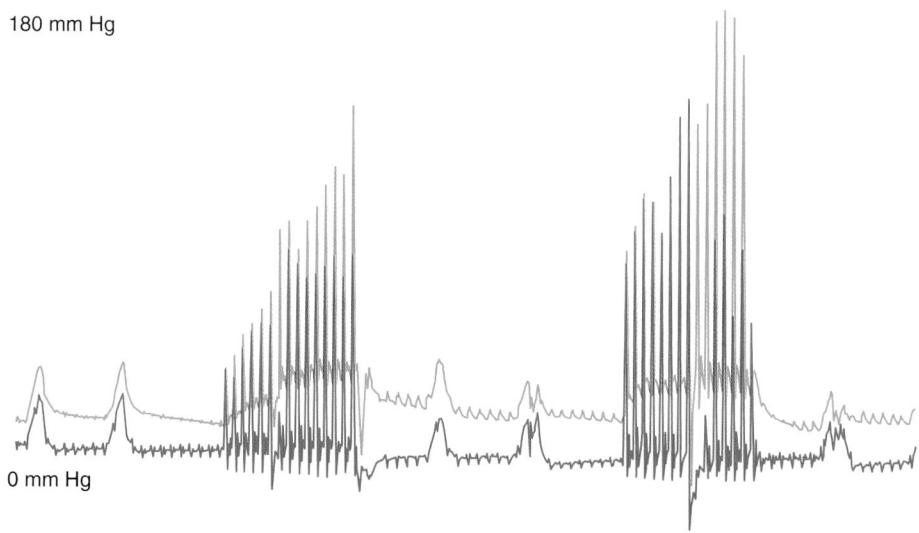

0 mm Hg

FIGURE 50–2. Simultaneous aortic (red) and right atrial (blue) pressure tracings from a swine undergoing CPR during prolonged VF arrest. Two ventilations are provided for every 15 chest compressions. There is a realistic 16-second interruption of chest compression to simulate a single bystander delivering "rescue breathing." The chest compression rate is 100 per minute.

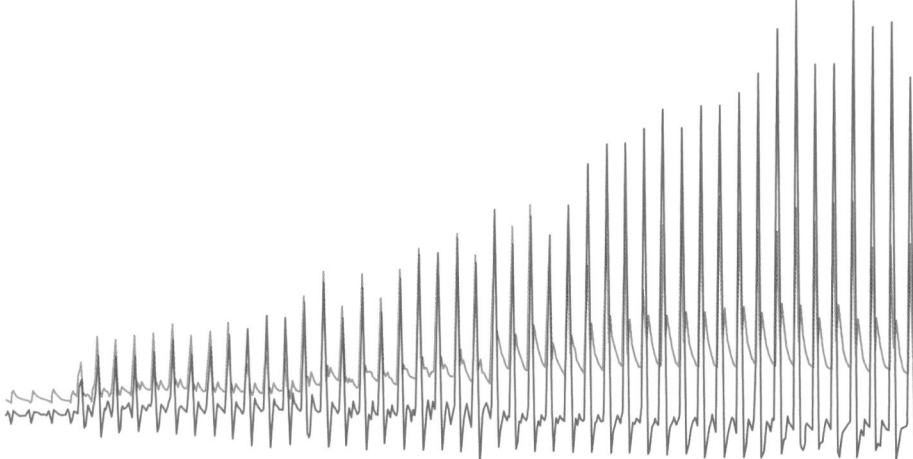

FIGURE 50–3. Simultaneous aortic (red) and right atrial (blue) pressure tracings from a swine undergoing the initiation of continuous chest compressions for cardiac arrest as a consequence of VF. Note that with the initiation of chest compressions it takes some time for the coronary perfusion pressures (aortic diastolic minus the right atrial diastolic pressure) to increase. The chest compression rate is 100 per minute.

which time immediate defibrillation should be attempted.

Emphasis is also placed on minimizing the time between cessation of chest compressions and delivery of shocks and resumption of chest compressions.

Three sequential shocks of increasing energy were not and are not recommended for cardiocerebral resuscitation and are no longer recommended in the *2005 Guidelines*.[41,42,66] Stacked shocks were recommended in previous CPR guidelines because high-energy (360-J) shocks from monophasic wave defibrillators resulted in a higher incidence of postdefibrillation heart block.[67] This complication (heart block) is rare when biphasic defibrillators are used.

Why 200 chest compressions immediately after the defibrillator shock? Following prolonged VF arrest in animal models, a direct current shock frequently defibrillated the subject into a nonperfusing rhythm—PEA.[42,46,68] Resuming chest compressions to restore coronary perfusion pressures was highly successful in converting PEA to a perfusing rhythm.

instructions are given. Once the EMS personnel arrive, they are to follow the algorithm for cardiocerebral resuscitation (Fig. 50–4).

Law officers and other EMS rescuers who are equipped with AEDs are to defibrillate immediately only if they personally witness the collapse or if good continuous chest compressions are being provided by a bystander when they arrive. Otherwise, they are to perform uninterrupted chest compressions for 2 minutes (200 compressions) before defibrillation. To assure prompt defibrillation when only one rescuer is on the scene, the AED pads are to be quickly attached before chest compressions are initiated. If two rescuers are available, one begins chest compressions while the other attaches the defibrillator pads. If a shockable rhythm is present, a single defibrillation shock (preferably biphasic) is delivered, followed immediately by an additional 200 chest compressions prior to rhythm and pulse analysis. Note that the latter approach has also been recommended in the *2005 Guidelines*.[1]

Cardiocerebral resuscitation simplifies the EMS decision-making process. It is very often difficult to ascertain an accurate downtime in emergency circumstances and place the victim in the electrical or the circulatory phase of VF arrest. Because previous reports in humans did not demonstrate a detrimental effect of performing chest compressions prior to defibrillation during the electrical phase,[36,37] CCR advocates 2 minutes (200 compressions) of continuous chest compressions prior to defibrillation in all cases except those where the AED-equipped rescuer witnesses the collapse, at

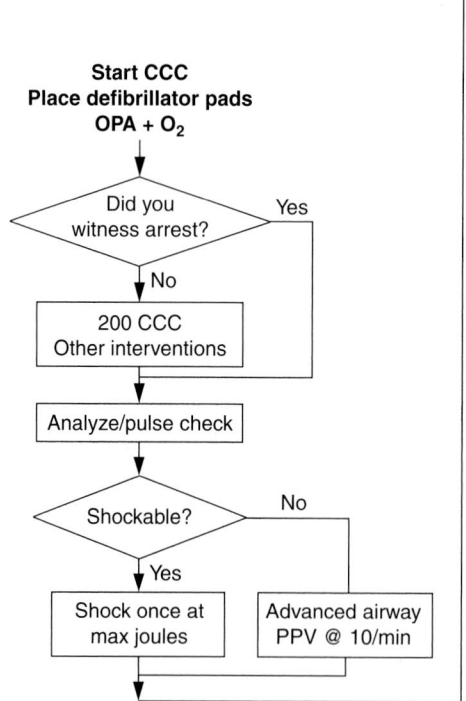
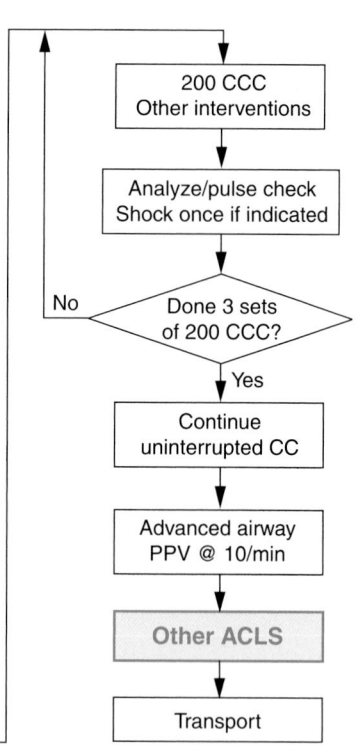

FIGURE 50–4. Cardiocerebral resuscitation algorithm for cardiac arrest. "Other interventions" include switch pumper (individual doing chest compressions) every 2 minutes, start intravenous or intraosseous access for drug injections (epinephrine every 3 minutes), and amiodarone 300-mg bolus (for recurrent VT). If no return of spontaneous circulation after one set of 200 chest compressions, analysis, shock and 200 chest compressions, and two additional sets of shock and 200 chest compressions, place an advance airway and ventilate with positive-pressure ventilations (limit to 10 per minute), and consider other advanced cardiac life support interventions, including mechanical chest compression and transfer. ACLS, advanced cardiac life support; CC, chest compression; CCC, continuous chest compressions at 100 per minute; O$_2$, high-flow oxygen; OPA, oral pharyngeal airway; PPV, positive-pressure ventilation.

Observational studies by paramedic units found that a pulse was rarely, if ever, present after the initial defibrillation, and therefore immediate chest compressions are now also recommended by the *2005 Guidelines*.[1]

TECHNIQUE OF CHEST COMPRESSIONS

Full chest recoil during the release phase of each chest compression is extremely important.[1,65,69] During the decompression or release phase of chest compression, a small negative pressure is created within the chest as the chest wall recoils back to its resting position.[70] This draws venous blood back into the right heart from the systemic veins and may draw air into the airways.[70] Incomplete chest recoil compromises perfusion because it interferes with the generation of this negative pressure in the chest, and thus decreases venous blood return to the heart. As a consequence, cardiac output and perfusion pressures are reduced and self-ventilation is curtailed. Incomplete chest recoil has been reported in 46 percent of simulated resuscitations performed by paramedics.[69] Furthermore, when incomplete chest recoil was combined with excessive ventilations, perfusion was severely compromised.[69]

ROLE OF GASPING OR AGONAL RESPIRATIONS

Gasping is not uncommon following the onset of VF or VT. When it occurs with out-of-hospital cardiac arrest, it is both fortunate and unfortunate. It is fortunate because if chest compressions are promptly initiated, the subject is likely to continue to gasp and provide self-respirations. However, gasping may be unfortunate as most lay individuals interpret this as an indication that the individual is still breathing. Accordingly, they are likely to neither initiate bystander CPR nor activate the EMS as soon as they should. Public education on this issue is essential for improving prompt initiation of bystander chest compressions.

Clark et al. reported that gasping or agonal breathing was observed in 56 percent of out-of-hospital VF cardiac arrests and was highly correlated with survival.[71] Others have shown similar results in the animal laboratory.[72,73] Animal research laboratories that use paralysis as part of the protocol when studying CPR eliminate this physiologically important reflex. This is one reason that some investigators have not found improved survival with chest-compression-only approaches to cardiac resuscitation.

CARDIOCEREBRAL RESUSCITATION DELAYS POSITIVE PRESSURE VENTILATIONS BY EMS

Another major difference between CCR and CPR is in the recommendations for ventilation. The three cardiocerebral resuscitation recommendations concerning airway management and ventilations in cardiac arrest can be summarized as follows: (1) Bystander or first responders are to perform continuous chest compressions without ventilations or so-called *rescue breathing*. (2) Initial EMS airway management is limited to assuring an open airway and administration of high-flow supplemental oxygen via a nonrebreather mask. (3) Advanced airway management and assisted ventilations for patients with cardiac arrest is initiated only after ROSC in those who need it, or in those without ROSC after three sequences of defibrillation and 200 chest compressions. Ventilations should be performed in a manner that minimizes their negative impact upon perfusion pressures.[41]

Each of these three recommendations represents a deviation from the CPR guidelines and each is counterintuitive to the ABCs (airway, breathing, circulation) that has been taught for decades. Cardiocerebral resuscitation does not advocate the elimination of ventilations; instead, it emphasizes the beneficial effects of negative intrathoracic pressure respiration, for example, gasping or agonal breathing, and the possible beneficial effects of chest wall recoil and deemphasizes the use of positive-pressure ventilation early in the course of a cardiac arrest.[41,42,46]

EXCESSIVE VENTILATIONS BY EMS PERSONNEL CAN BE DEADLY

There are several problems with positive-pressure ventilation. Because it often takes considerable time to establish an airway by intubation, the result is prolonged interruption of chest compressions during the critical circulatory phase of VF arrest. For this reason, intubation is initially not allowed in cardiocerebral resuscitation.[41,46] But even bag-mask ventilation can be detrimental as excessive positive-pressure and/or rapid ventilation is common with intubation and there is no reason to believe that it will be less common with bag-mask ventilation.[49] Excessive pressure ventilation during cardiac arrest increases mean intrathoracic pressure impedes venous return to the chest, reducing cerebral and myocardial perfusion in spite of continued chest compressions.[49,50,72]

Aufderheide et al. found that "there is an inversely proportional relationship between mean intrathoracic pressure, coronary perfusion pressure and survival from cardiac arrest."[49,74] Observations of hospital-based responders to cardiac arrest, as well as those made on paramedics, found that both professionals almost always performed assisted ventilation at excessively high rates.[75] They both delivered an average of 37 ventilations per minute, rather than the 10–12 per minute recommended by the *Guidelines*. Even after retraining they ventilated at 22 per minute.[49]

Cardiocerebral resuscitations protocols minimize these adverse effects of excessive positive pressure ventilations by advocating the placement of an oropharyngeal device.[41] Oxygenation is provided by high-flow oxygen via a nonrebreather mask in the initial phases of treatment.[41] Positive pressure ventilation is delayed until after ROSC, or if the patient is not awake, after three shocks, each followed by 200 chest compressions.[41]

The first person with an AED to arrive applies the defibrillator pads and begins chest compressions; the second person places an oropharyngeal airway and a nonrebreather mask with high-flow oxygen (passive oxygen insufflation).[41] Gasping and/or chest wall recoil provides respiration. This approach has another major benefit; freeing another professional for other critically important duties during the cardiac arrest, such as spelling the person doing chest compressions and/or obtaining vascular access for intravenous therapies.[41]

HEMODYNAMICS OF CARDIAC ARREST

Ventricular fibrillation results in totally uncoordinated contractile activity of the ventricular myocytes, resulting in almost immediate cessation of effective ventricular pump function. However, antegrade blood flow continues after cardiac arrest until the pressure gradient between the arterial and venous pressures is completely dissipated, and the pressures in the arterial and venous systems equalize[76] at the "mean circulatory filling pressure" of Guyton.[77] Because of a variety of compensatory mechanisms, including increased sympathetic activity and the fact that some microvascular beds close, the equilibrium between the arterial and venous systems does not occur until about 5 minutes of VF in animal models.[76] One result of the shift of blood from the arterial to the venous circuits is prompt distension of the right ventricle (Fig. 50–5). It had been postulated that the shift in blood from the arterial to the venous vascular beds significantly decreases left ventricular volume, perhaps explaining why chest compressions prior to defibrillation are necessary for the left ventricle to fill and generate a more effective arterial pressure.[78] However, magnetic resonance imaging of the closed chest animal models of VF did not show a dramatic decrease in left ventricular volume until the development of "stone heart" (extreme myocardial contraction) (Fig. 50–6) several minutes later.[79]

The changes in coronary blood flow and carotid blood flow in response to ventricular fibrillation are different.[76] Carotid blood flow declines exponentially to zero over approximately 4 minutes, but coronary blood flow rapidly declines to zero by 1 minute. For the next 2 minutes coronary blood flow is retrograde before again becoming zero.[76]

【 】 MECHANISM OF BLOOD FLOW DURING CARDIAC ARREST AND CLOSED-CHEST COMPRESSION

Closed-chest compressions during cardiac arrest result in phasic forward blood flow. The mechanisms responsible for forward

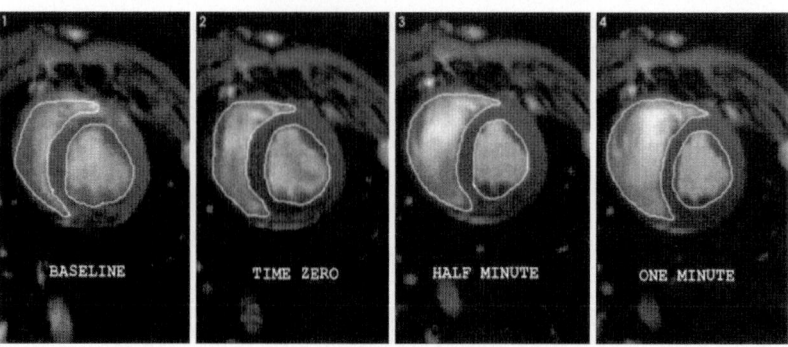

FIGURE 50–5. Magnetic resonance images of swine chest at baseline and during the first minute of ventricular fibrillation. Note that the right ventricular (RV) volume increases by approximately 50 percent within 1 minute of the onset of ventricular fibrillation. *Source: Courtesy of Dr. Vincent Sorrell.*

blood flow during closed-chest compressions are variable and depend on several factors. Of the factors identified, perhaps the most important is the duration between the onset of ventricular fibrillation arrest and initiation of chest compressions.[80] Another important determinant is the technique used for chest compressions[81] and the patient's chest wall configuration.

According to the cardiac compression theory, direct compression of the left and right ventricles between the sternum and the vertebral column creates a pressure gradient between the ventricles and the great vessels. This pressure gradient closes the mitral and tricuspid valves and ejects blood forward out of the ventricles. The ventricles then refill during the decompression phase.

When closed-chest cardiac massage was introduced in the 1960s, it was assumed that the mechanism of blood flow was much the same as with open-chest cardiac massage, wherein the heart was grasped in the hand and the flow was produced by squeezing the fibrillating left ventricle. This was the presumed operative mechanism of forward blood flow during CPR until a study was done in hu-

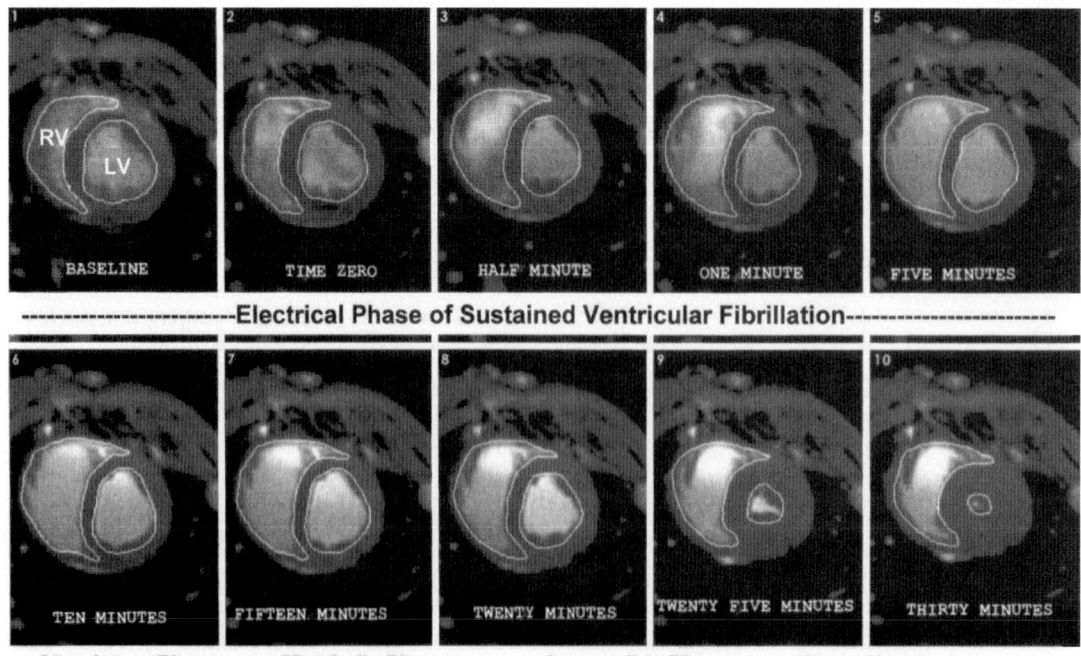

FIGURE 50–6. Magnetic resonance images of swine chest at baseline and periodically until 30 minutes of cardiac arrest as a consequence of ventricular fibrillation. Note the development of "stone heart."

mans by researchers at Johns Hopkins, which was published in 1980.[82] Their data suggested that the mechanism of blood flow during chest compression was the "thoracic pump" mechanism[82]: external chest compression increases intrathoracic pressure, forcing blood to flow from the thorax (Fig. 50–7). Retrograde flow from the right heart to the systemic veins is prevented by the jugular venous valves at the thoracic outlet. According to this paradigm, the heart acts merely as a passive conduit without having a pump function. The assumption that thoracic pump mechanism was of major importance was supported by the then popular theory of "cough resuscitation," which had been popularized by Criley et al.[83,84]

However, the Johns Hopkins study, while performed in humans, was performed late in cardiac arrest, after the house staff had decided that resuscitation was unlikely.[82] Thus these hemodynamic measurements were made after prolonged cardiac arrest when one would expect the onset of myocardial stiffness and swelling that progress to stone heart.[85,86] With these developments, the thoracic pump is the mechanism of blood flow during chest compressions, but resuscitation and survival are unlikely.[81,85,87]

Transesophageal echocardiography evaluations in humans during cardiac arrest and CPR have shown both mechanisms—cardiac compression in some and the thoracic pump in others. However, cardiac compression mechanism was more likely to be seen in patients studied early after arrest and the thoracic pump mechanism when cardiac arrest patients were studied later.[87] And in one such study, survival only occurred among those studied early; there were no survivors among those who demonstrated the thoracic pump mechanism.[87]

It is probable that in younger individuals with compliant chest walls and/or narrow anterior posterior chest dimensions, the cardiac pump is the predominant mechanism and that they are more likely to be resuscitated. In patients with severe emphysema and a "barrel chest," the mechanism of blood flow is likely because of the thoracic pump mechanism, but these patients are also unlikely to be revived by closed-chest compressions.

The actual mechanism of forward blood flow during resuscitation is of great import, as guidelines for CPR have been altered dramatically, depending on the alleged or accepted operative mechanism. Based on the "thoracic pump" theory, the 1980 AHA guidelines recommended a chest compression rate of 60 per minute, and stated that "compression should be sustained for 0.5 second, with relaxation given for equal period."[5] In hindsight this was a disaster, as this resulted in too few compression per minute for single rescuers. Resuscitation is rare with so few chest compressions.[43]

This recommendation of 60 compressions per minute was not accepted by many clinicians who had years of experience with successful resuscitations using much faster chest compression rates. Accordingly investigators from The University of Arizona and Duke Medical Schools performed studies in animals and found that the optimal chest compression rates for survival from VF arrest were 80 to 120 per minute.[88] Because a chest compression rate of 120 per minute was thought to be too fatiguing for the general public, the 1992 AHA guidelines compromised and recommended rates of 80 to 100 per minute.[7] The group supporting the thoracic pump theory accepted this change only because it is easier to obtain a 50 percent compression–to-relaxation ratio at faster rates. The *2005 Guidelines* recommend a compression rate of 100 per minute.

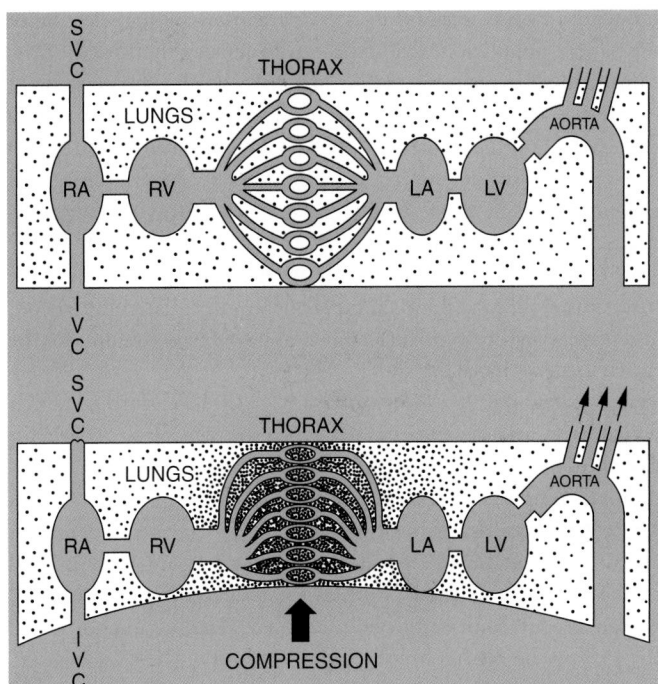

FIGURE 50–7. Schematic representation of the "thoracic pump" mechanism of blood flow during external chest compression. In this model, the heart is a passive conduit. The *top* drawing shows the thorax during hands off, whereas the *bottom* drawing shows it during chest compression, the secondary increase in intrathoracic pressures. IVC, inferior vena cava; LA, left atrium; LV, left ventricle; RA, right atrium; RV, right ventricle; SVC, superior vena cava. *Source: Modified from Ewy GA. Cardiopulmonary resuscitation. Med Times 1983;3:60–69.*

MECHANICAL DEVICES FOR RESUSCITATION

A mechanical piston device that depresses the sternum via a compressed gas-powered plunger mounted on a backboard has been available for years. This device (Thumper, Michigan Instruments Inc., Grand Rapids, Michigan) "may be considered," according to the AHA *2005 Guidelines*, "for patients in cardiac arrest in circumstances that make manual resuscitation difficult (Level of Evidence Class IIb)."[1]

More recently the AutoPulse, a device composed of a pneumatically or electrically actuated constricting band and backboard, became available. This type of device is referred to as a load-distributing band. It was designed on the principle of the "thoracic pump" mechanism for blood flow during cardiac arrest and chest compression. Different results were found in two different studies published in 2006.[89] The first was a prospective cluster-randomized multicenter clinical trial involving five communities that included 1071 patients who experienced out-of-hospital nontraumatic cardiac arrest.[89] This study was terminated early by the data safety and monitoring board.[90] Survival to hospital discharge was lower with the AutoPulse than with manual CPR (6 percent vs. 10 percent).[89] The other study was a prospective, pre- and postobservational study of a single EMS system.[91] Resuscitation outcomes were compared before and after an urban EMS system switched from manual CPR to the AutoPulse device.[91] Survival to hospital discharge was higher in the AutoPulse phase than in the manual CPR phase (10 percent vs. 3 percent).[91] The results are no doubt influenced by the details of its use—perhaps including selection of the patient population with respect to presenting rhythm, the time from cardiac arrest to initiation of CPR, time to deployment of the device, duration of chest compressions interruptions to apply the device, and the influence of it deployment on time to defibrillation.[90] A post-hoc analysis suggests that shorter response times appear to benefit from manual CPR and those with longer response times may benefit from the load-distributing band CPR.[90] This would make sense as it appears that early in an arrest the mechanism of blood flow is more likely to be cardiac compression, and later in an arrest the mechanism of blood flow is more like the thoracic pump mechanism.

Active compression–decompression CPR is performed either with a hand-held device equipped with a suction cup to actively lift the anterior chest during decompression[92] or a mechanical gas-powered piston that not only depresses the sternum via a compressed gas but also actively retracts with a suction cup on the chest,[93] such as the LUCAS (Lund University Cardiac Assist System).[93] Such devices show promise in the experimental laboratory[93] and are used in some countries in Europe.[94] The suction portion of the LUCAS device has been modified, and the LUCAS is now approved for sale in the United States.

In some cases of optimal CPR, either manual or with mechanical devices, the forward blood flow is so good that the patient awakes and sedation is necessary. This needs emphasis, as all too often when the patient begins moving, manual chest compressions are stopped until the patient becomes unresponsive—a procedure that should be deplored.

Mechanical devices should not be used early in resuscitation efforts. Like endotracheal intubation for assisted ventilation, with or without devices that decrease intrathoracic pressures with positive pressure ventilations, they may be indicated in patients who do not respond to the initial resuscitation attempts, but in whom there is a reasonable chance of survival with more aggressive therapy.

DRUG THERAPY

The guidelines for drug therapy in patients with cardiac arrest were little changed. Epinephrine remains the drug of choice, although vasopressin is an option if the arrest persists after the first dose of epinephrine.[1] One dose of vasopressin is considered an option to epinephrine.[1] With persistent ventricular fibrillation, amiodarone has surfaced as the antiarrhythmic drug of choice. However, the aqueous formation may cause vasodilation, and therefore amiodarone, if used, should always be preceded by at least one dose of epinephrine.[1]

The most important intravenous (IV) or intraosseous (IO) medication during prolonged cardiac arrest is epinephrine, which increases systemic vascular resistance, thereby increasing coronary and cerebral perfusion.[1] It is the α-, not the β-adrenergic effects of epinephrine that are important.[95–97] Epinephrine plus β blockers was effective for use in resuscitation, whereas epinephrine plus α blockers was not.[95,97] Studies from several laboratories showed that α agonists were as effective as epinephrine.[98] Nevertheless, because epinephrine is equally effective and has a long history of use, it is the recommended drug of choice during prolonged arrest.

The *2005 Guidelines* states, "It is appropriate to administer a 1-mg dose of epinephrine IV/IO every 3 to 5 minutes during adult cardiac arrest (Class IIb). Higher doses may be indicated to treat specific problems, such as β-blocker or calcium channel blocker overdose."[1] Because of epinephrine's β-adrenergic effects, repeated doses may result in recurrent ventricular arrhythmias so it may be desirable to give intravenous β blockers as an antiarrhythmic during resuscitation if several doses of epinephrine have been administered. High-dose epinephrine is not recommended.[1]

Vasopressin is a nonadrenergic peripheral vasoconstrictor whose use during cardiac arrest has been recommended. However, in two large randomized trials in humans, the administration of 40 IU of vasopressin (with the dose repeated in one study) there was no increase in ROSC when compared to the injection of 1 mg of epinephrine.[1] The *2005 Guidelines*, in its Advanced Cardiac Life Support (ACLS) pulseless arrest algorithm, indicates that a single dose of vasopressin may be substituted for the first 1 of 2 epinephrine doses.[1] However, the International Consensus Conference concluded that there is insufficient evidence to support or refute the use of vasopressin as an alternative to, or in combination with, epinephrine in any cardiac arrest rhythm.[9]

The major problem with drug therapy during out-of-hospital cardiac arrest is that it usually takes too long to obtain intravenous access, often because the EMS team is busy with chest compression, defibrillation, and ventilation. Delay reduces the effectiveness of all drugs, including epinephrine. On the other hand, if the patient responds to early defibrillation, epinephrine is neither necessary nor indicated.

Amiodarone is an antiarrhythmic drug that was shown to be beneficial in two blinded studies in adults with out-of-hospital cardiac arrest.[99,100] The administration of amiodarone (300 mg or 5 mg/kg) by paramedics to patients with refractory VF in out-of-hospital settings improved survival to hospital admission when compared with administration of placebo[99] or lidocaine (1.5 mg/kg).[100]

POSTRESUSCITATION DYSFUNCTION

The major concern of aggressive management of patient with cardiac arrest has always been that the patient will survive in a vegetative state with severe neurologic impairment from the global ischemia. In one early study, only one-fourth of patients who were resuscitated from cardiac arrest subsequently had good neurologic function.[101] Clinical experience suggests that survival with normal neurologic function may be even worse in patients who are comatose following cardiac arrest.

The best prognostic sign in cardiac arrest patients after ROSC is regaining consciousness, a gradual process that may take days to evolve. There are, at present, no clinically relevant, reliable predictive tools that can be used in recently resuscitated, comatose patients to distinguish who will or who will not wake up.[102]

Although neurologic function after prolonged cardiac arrest is of major concern, there is almost always other organ dysfunction as well, a syndrome referred to as *postresuscitation disease*. This is a multiorgan pathophysiologic state that affects almost all body systems, but especially the cardiovascular, nervous, pulmonary, renal, and metabolic systems.[103] Postresuscitation disease is postulated to consist of four different pathophysiologic mechanisms: (1) perfusion failure consisting of multifocal no-reflow phenomenon; (2) reperfusion injuries from oxygen free radicals, invasion of inflammatory cells, defects in injured mitochondria, and triggered programmed cell death; (3) postanoxic viscera damage and dysfunction; and (4) blood derangement from stasis during the arrest.[104]

Myocardial dysfunction after resuscitation from cardiac arrest has been described in clinical studies as well as animal models. In a study of 165 patients who had ROSC after out-of-hospital cardiac arrest, 55 percent had hemodynamic instability requiring vasoactive drugs during the first 72 hours following resuscitation.[105] The left ventricular ejection fraction was depressed in all patients. Of clinical import is the observation that hemodynamic instability was not predictive of neurologic outcome and myocardial dysfunction appeared to be reversed by 72 hours.[105]

In animal models, the myocardial dysfunction has been shown to be related to the duration of arrest and resuscitation. Kern et al. noted progressive systolic and diastolic progressive dysfunction, but if the animals survived, these abnormalities spontaneously recovered.[106] In these animals, myocardial function could be improved with dobutamine but not with intraaortic balloon counterpulsation.[106]

POSTRESUSCITATION CARE
[ ] HYPOTHERMIA THERAPY

One of the most promising approaches to resuscitated cardiac arrest patients with coma is hypothermia.[102,107] It has long been known that survival after cardiac arrest was more likely in cold water drowning or hypothermic states, suggesting a protective effect of hypothermia. However, hypothermia activates shivering, and in postcardiac arrest comatose patients, shivering-produced thermogenesis is potentially deleterious. Uncontrolled hypothermia results in catecholamine release, and vasoconstriction. Many of the early studies using moderate (82.4 to 89.6°F [28 to 32°C]) or severe (<82.4°F [28°C]) hypothermia for cerebral protection had worse survival than normothermic controls.[102] In contrast, therapeutic, controlled mild hypothermia (89.6 to 93.2°F [32 to 34°C]) appears to be beneficial for preserving cerebral function.

One of the earlier reports of beneficial effects of hypothermia for comatose survivors of cardiac arrest was that by Benson et al.[108] Only 1 of 7 patients survived without cooling compared with 6 of 12 who survived after being cooled to 87.8 to 89.6°F (31 to 32°C).[108]

The Hypothermia after Cardiac Arrest (HACA) study group performed the largest randomized clinical trial of hypothermia to date.[109] In this multicenter trial, adult patients who remained comatose after resuscitation from cardiac arrest were randomized to therapeutic mild hypothermia or normothermia.[109] Inclusion criteria were an arrest of presumed cardiac etiology, an estimated downtime no longer than 15 minutes, and a time to ROSC of no more than 60 minutes from collapse.[109] Only 8 percent of all patients in cardiac arrest met these criteria. Patients in the hypothermic group had an external cooling device applied that was set to a target temperature of 89.6 to 93.2°F (32 to 34°C). The temperature was continuously monitored by a bladder catheter. It took an average of 8 hours to reach the target temperature, but once achieved, it was maintained for 24 hours, followed by passive rewarming over 8 hours.[109] All patients were intubated, sedated, and paralyzed. Standard critical care was delivered to both groups. Neurologic outcome was assessed at 6 months postresus-

citation. Fifty-five percent of patients in the hypothermic group had a favorable neurologic outcome, compared to 39 percent in the normothermic group ($p = 0.009$).[109] Sepsis was more common in the hypothermic group, although the difference between groups was not significant.[109]

Barnard et al. also studied adult patients with out-of-hospital cardiac arrest from VF.[110] Patients with ROSC were randomized to hypothermic and normothermic groups. Patients in the hypothermic group were cooled with ice packs as soon as possible with the goal of reaching a core temperature of 91.4°F (33°C).[110] This temperature was maintained for 12 hours after which patients were actively warmed over 8 hours. At discharge, 49 percent of the patients in the hypothermic group had a good neurologic outcome compared to 26 percent in the normothermic group ($p = 0.011$).[110] The mortality was 51 percent in the hypothermic group and 68 percent in the normothermic group, but this difference was not statistically significant.[110]

Hachimi-Idrissi et al. evaluated a helmet cooling device containing a solution of aqueous glycerol that was placed around the head and neck of the patient.[111] Patients were successfully cooled to a target bladder temperature of 93.2°F (34°C) for a maximum of 24 hours without incurring hypothermia-related complications.[111]

The ILCOR issued an advisory statement in 2003 recommending "[u]nconscious adult patients with spontaneous circulation after out-of-hospital cardiac arrest should be cooled to [89.6 to 93.2°F] 32 to 34°C for 12 to 24 hours when the initial rhythm was ventricular fibrillation (VF). Such cooling may be beneficial for other rhythms or in-hospital cardiac arrest."[112] Similar recommendations were echoed in the 2005 Guidelines and by ILCOR.[1,9]

The mechanism of action of hypothermia is unknown, but is thought to be related to its inhibitory effect on adverse enzymatic and chemical reactions that are initiated by the global ischemia. It is well known that cooling slows chemical reactions. Thus it is logical to assume that the sooner therapeutic cooling is begun, the better. Laboratory experiments support this assumption.[113]

Seizures, myoclonus, or shivering may occur, necessitating sedation and intermittent or continuous neuromuscular blockade. However, the use of continuous neuromuscular blockage could mask seizure activity.[102] Accordingly, seizure control is an important part of hypothermia therapy postcardiac arrest and requires neurology consultation and continuous electroencephalographic monitoring.

Therapeutic hypothermia may be associated with hyperglycemia.[114] Although control of blood glucose in the range of 80 to 110 mg/dL has not been specifically studied in postcardiac arrest patients, studies of patients with stroke or other serious cardiovascular conditions suggest that control of blood glucose is another important therapeutic goal.

[ ] MYOCARDIAL INFARCTION CAUSING CARDIAC ARREST

Many cardiac arrests are caused by myocardial ischemia or infarction. Many postcardiac arrest patients require urgent cardiac catheterization to determine the etiology and if a reversible cause is present. This is especially true if the patient's electrocardiogram is consistent with an acute myocardial infarction. Some may have acute coronary occlusion that is amenable to percutaneous coronary intervention.

ENDING RESUSCITATIVE EFFORTS

The cost of providing emergency medical service to victims of out-of-hospital cardiac arrest is considerable. At one end of the spectrum of patients with out-of-hospital cardiac arrest are those in whom the arrest was not witnessed, or in whom the arrest was witnessed but no bystander resuscitation efforts were made, or for whom the arrival of those delivering emergency medical services was prolonged. This subset of patients has little chance of survival. Studies have found that, if in addition, a defibrillator shock is not delivered or advised and there is no ROSC, almost no one lives.[115] Transportation of these moribund patients to the hospital emergency department consumes resources, puts the public and the providers at risk during transportation, increases costs, and may decrease the availability of emergency medical services and emergency department resources for other patients. It has therefore been acknowledged by expert groups that there are some patients with little or no chance of survival for whom continued efforts at resuscitation in the field are perhaps not merited.

For services delivering advanced cardiac life support in England, the *Recognition of Life Extinct* (ROLE) guidelines state that "resuscitation attempts should be terminated when the patient remains in asystole despite full advanced life support procedures for more than 20 minutes."[116] The AHA *2005 Guidelines* state that "resuscitation efforts should be continued until "reliable criteria indicating irreversible death are present."[1] This position leaves more latitude for the judgment of the medical personnel involved, but is more difficult to apply uniformly in practice.

In many areas of the world, victims of out-of-hospital cardiac arrest are not attended by paramedics capable of delivering the full spectrum of advanced cardiac life support, but by emergency medical technicians equipped with first-aid measures and an automated external defibrillator. These responders are in need of guidelines for termination of resuscitation. Morrison et al. (Termination of Resuscitation investigators)[115] prospectively validated their previously published "termination of resuscitation prediction rule" for automated external defibrillator-equipped emergency medical services personnel responding to out-of-hospital cardiac arrest. They found that only 0.5 percent of arrest victims survived if (1) there was no ROSC, (2) no shocks were administered, and (3) the arrest was not witnessed by EMS personnel. When (4) "response time greater than 8 minutes" was retrospectively added to the prediction rule, the survival rate was 0.3 percent, and when (5) "not bystander witnessed" was added, no patient survived. These findings suggest that it is possible to objectively select a group of cardiac arrest patients in whom resuscitation efforts can be discontinued and the patient pronounced in the field. This approach would result in the transportation of far fewer patients.

There is a caveat to the study by Morrison et al.[117] The study was conducted during a time when emergency medical personnel followed the *2000 Guidelines*, which are no longer considered optimal. The Morrison study was also done during a time when bystander-initiated CPR used a ventilation-to-compression ratio that is no longer recommended in adults.[1] Since the completion of the study, the *2005 Guidelines*, which differ in a number of ways from the *2000 Guidelines*, were published. Furthermore, newer approaches to out-of-hospital cardiac arrest, such as cardiocerebral resuscitation, may result in a paradigm shift in the entire approach to out-of-hospital cardiac arrest.[41,42,46,66]

REFERENCES

1. American Heart Association. 2005 American Heart Association guidelines for cardiopulmonary resuscitation and emergency cardiovascular care. *Circulation* 2005;112(Suppl IV):IV-1–IV-211.
2. Standards for cardiopulmonary resuscitation (CPR) and emergency cardiac care (ECC). II. Basic life support. *JAMA* 1974;227(Suppl 7):833–868.
3. Engdahl J, Bang A, Lindqvist J, Herlitz J. Time trends in long-term mortality after out-of-hospital cardiac arrest, 1980 to 1998, and predictors for death. *Am Heart J* 2003;145:826–833.
4. Rea T, Eisenberg M, Becker L, Murray J, Hearne T. Temporal trends in sudden cardiac arrest: a 25-year emergency medical services perspective. *Circulation* 2003;107:2780–2785.
5. Standards and guidelines for cardiopulmonary resuscitation (CPR) and emergency cardiac care (ECC). *JAMA* 1980;244(5):453–509.
6. Standards and guidelines for cardiopulmonary resuscitation (CPR) and emergency cardiac care (ECC). *JAMA* 1986;255(21):2905–2989.
7. American Heart Association. Guidelines for cardiopulmonary resuscitation and emergency cardiac care. Emergency Cardiac Care Committee and Subcommittees, American Heart Association. *JAMA* 1992;268(16):2171–2302.
8. American Heart Association in collaboration with the International Liaison Committee on Resuscitation. Guidelines for cardiopulmonary resuscitation and emergency cardiac care: international consensus on science. *Circulation* 2000;102(Suppl I):I-1–I-403.
9. International Liaison Committee on Resuscitation. 2005 International consensus on cardiopulmonary resuscitation and emergency cardiovascular care science with treatment recommendations. *Resuscitation* 2005;67:181–341.
10. Kouwenhoven WB, Jude JR, Knickerbocker GG. Closed-chest cardiac massage. *JAMA* 1060;173:1064–1067.
11. Kouwenhoven WB, Jude JR, Knickerbocker GB. Demonstration of the technique of CPR for New York Society of Anesthesiologist 1960. (Copy of demonstration provided on CD by J.R. Jude).
12. Safar P, Brown T, Holtey W, Wilder R. Ventilation and circulation with closed-chest cardiac massage in man. *JAMA* 1961;176:574–576.
13. American Heart Association in collaboration with International Liaison Committee on Resuscitation. Guidelines 2000 for cardiopulmonary resuscitation and emergency cardiovascular care: international consensus on science. *Circulation* 2000;102(Suppl I (8)):I-1–I-348.
14. American Heart Association. International liaison committee on resuscitation 2005 international consensus on cardiopulmonary resuscitation and emergency cardiovascular care science with treatment recommendations. Part 2 adult basic life support. *Circulation* 2005:112:5–16.
15. Eckstein M, Stratton S, Chan L. Cardiac arrest resuscitation evaluation in Los Angeles: CARE-LA. *Ann Emerg Med* 2005;45:504–509.
16. Herlitz J, Ekstrom I, Wennerblom B, Axelsson A, Bang A, Holmberg S. Effects of bystander initiated cardiopulmonary resuscitation on ventricular fibrillation and survival after witnessed cardiac arrest outside hospital. *Br Heart J* 1994;72:408–412.
17. Wenzel V, Kern KB, Hilwig RW, et al. Effects of intravenous arginine vasopressin on epicardial coronary artery cross sectional area in a swine resuscitation model. *Resuscitation* 2005;64(2):219–226.
18. Stiell IG, Wells GA, Field B, et al. Advanced cardiac life support in out-of-hospital cardiac arrest. *N Engl J Med* 2004;351(7):647–656.
19. Wik L, Kramer-Johansen J, Myklebust H, et al. Quality of cardiopulmonary resuscitation during out-of-hospital cardiac arrest. *JAMA* 2005;293:299–304.
20. Valenzuela TD, Kern KB, Clark LL, et al. Interruptions of chest compressions during emergency medical systems resuscitation. *Circulation* 2005;112(9):1259–1265.
21. Berg RA. Role of mouth-to-mouth rescue breathing in bystander cardiopulmonary resuscitation for asphyxial cardiac arrest. *Crit Care Med* 2000;28(11 Suppl):N193–N195.
22. Mogayzel C, Quan L, Graves JR, Tiedeman D, Fahrenbruch C, Herndon P. Out-of-hospital ventricular fibrillation in children and adolescents: causes and outcomes. *Ann Emerg Med* 1995;25(4):484–491.
23. Sirbaugh PE, Pepe PE, Shook JE, et al. A prospective, population-based study of the demographics, epidemiology, management, and outcome of out-

of-hospital pediatric cardiopulmonary arrest. *Ann Emerg Med* 1999;33:174–184.

24. Berg RA, Hilwig RW, Kern KB, Babar I, Ewy GA. Simulated mouth-to-mouth ventilation and chest compressions (bystander cardiopulmonary resuscitation) improves outcome in a swine model of prehospital pediatric asphyxial cardiac arrest. *Crit Care Med* 1999;27(9):1893–1899.

25. Berg RA, Hilwig RW, Kern KB, Ewy GA. "Bystander" chest compressions and assisted ventilation independently improve outcome from piglet asphyxial pulseless "cardiac arrest." *Circulation* 2000;101:1743–1748.

26. Assar D, Chamberlain D, Colquhoun M, et al. Randomised controlled trials of staged teaching for basic life support. 1. Skill acquisition at bronze stage. *Resuscitation* 2000;45:7–15.

27. Heidenreich J, Higdon T, Kern K, et al. Single rescuer cardiopulmonary resuscitation: "two quick breaths"—an oxymoron. *Resuscitation* 2004;62:283–289.

28. Weisfeldt M, Becker L. Resuscitation after cardiac arrest: a 3-phase time-sensitive model. *JAMA* 2002;288:3035–3038.

29. Page R, Joglar J, Kowal R, et al. Use of automated external defibrillators by a U.S. airline. *N Engl J Med* 2000;343(17):1210–1216.

30. Caffrey S, Willoughby P, Pepe P, Becker L. Public use of automated external defibrillators. *New England J Medicine* 2002;347(16):1242–1247.

31. Valenzuela T, Roe D, Nichol G, Clark L, Spaite D, Hardman R. Outcomes of rapid defibrillation by security officers after cardiac arrest in casinos. *N Engl J Med* 2000;343(17):1206–1209.

32. The Public Access Defibrillation Trial Investigators. Public-access defibrillation and survival after out-of-hospital cardiac arrest. *N Engl J Med* 2004;351(7):637–646.

33. Kern KB, Ewy GA, Voorhees WD, Babbs CF, Tacker WA. Myocardial perfusion pressure: a predictor of 24-hour survival during prolonged cardiac arrest in dogs. *Resuscitation* 1988;16:241–250.

34. Berg RA, Hilwig RW, Kern KB, Ewy GA. Precountershock cardiopulmonary resuscitation improves ventricular fibrillation median frequency and myocardial readiness for successful defibrillation from prolonged ventricular fibrillation: a randomized controlled swine study. *Ann Emerg Med* 2002;40:563–570.

35. Yu T, Weil M, Tang W, et al. Adverse outcomes of interrupted precordial compression during automated defibrillation. *Circulation* 2002;106:368–372.

36. Cobb L, Fahrenbruch C, Walsh T, Compass M, Olsufka M. Influence of cardiopulmonary resuscitation prior to defibrillation in patients with out-of-hospital ventricular fibrillation. *JAMA* 1999;281:1182–1188.

37. Wik L, Hansen TB, Fylling F, et al. Delaying defibrillation to give basic cardiopulmonary resuscitation to patients with out-of-hospital ventricular fibrillation: a randomized trial. *JAMA* 2003;289:1389–1395.

38. Sanders A, Ewy G, Taft T. Prognostic and therapeutic importance of the aortic diastolic pressure in resuscitation from cardiac arrest. *Crit Care Med* 1984;12:871–873.

39. Sanders AB, Kern KB, Bragg S, Ewy GA. Neurologic benefits from the use of early cardiopulmonary resuscitation. *Ann Emerg Med* 1987;16(2):142–146.

40. Sanders AB, Kern KB, Berg RA, Hilwig RW, Heidenrich J, Ewy GA. Survival and neurologic outcome after cardiopulmonary resuscitation with four different chest compression-ventilation ratios. *Ann Emerg Med* 2002;40(6):553–562.

41. Kellum MJ, Kennedy KW, Ewy GA. Cardiocerebral resuscitation improves survival of patients with out-of-hospital cardiac arrest. *Am J Med* 2006;119:335–340.

42. Kern K, Valenzuela T, Clark L, et al. An alternative approach to advancing resuscitation science. *Resuscitation* 2005;64:261–268.

43. Abella BS, Sandbo N, Vassilatos P, et al. Chest compression rates during cardiopulmonary resuscitation are suboptimal. A prospective study during in-hospital cardiac arrest. *Circulation* 2005;111:428–434.

44. Sanders A, Kern K, Berg R, Hilwig R, Heidenrich J, Ewy G. Survival and neurologic outcome after cardiopulmonary resuscitation with four different chest compression-ventilations ratios. *Ann Emerg Med* 2002;40:553–562.

45. Dorph E, Wik L, Stromme TA, Eriksen M, Steen PA. Quality of CPR with three different ventilation:compression ratios. *Resuscitation* 2003;58:193–201.

46. Ewy G. Cardiocerebral resuscitation: the new cardiopulmonary resuscitation. *Circulation* 2005;111:2134–2142.

47. Van Hoeyweghen RJ, Bossaert LL, Mullie A, et al. Quality and efficiency of bystander CPR. Belgian Cerebral Resuscitation Study Group. *Resuscitation* 1993;26(1):47–52.

48. Berg RA, Kern KB, Sanders AB, Otto CW, Hilwid RW, Ewy GA. Cardiopulmonary resuscitation: Bystander cardiopulmonary resuscitation: is ventilation necessary? *Circulation* 1993;88:1907–1915.

49. Aufderheide T, Sigurdsson G, Pirrallo R, et al. Hyperventilation-induced hypotension during cardiopulmonary resuscitation. *Circulation* 2004;109:1960–1965.

50. Aufderheide TP, Lurie KG. Death by hyperventilation: a common and life-threatening problem during cardiopulmonary resuscitation. *Crit Care Med* 2004;32(9 Suppl):S345–S351.

51. Meursing B, Wulterkens D, Kesteren RV. The ABC of resuscitation and the Dutch (re)treat. *Resuscitation* 2005;64:279–286.

52. Chandra NC, Gruben KG, Tsitlik JE, et al. Observations of ventilation during resuscitation in a canine model. *Circulation* 1994;90(6):3070–3075.

53. Noc M, Weil M, Tang W, al. e. Mechanical ventilation may not be essential for initial cardiopulmonary resuscitation. *Chest* 1995;108(821–827).

54. Yang L, Weil MH, Noc M, Tang W, Turner T, Gazmuri RJ. Spontaneous gasping increases the ability to resuscitate during experimental cardiopulmonary resuscitation. *Crit Care Med* 1994;22(5):879–883.

55. Sanders A, Ogle M, Ewy G. Coronary perfusion pressure during cardiopulmonary resuscitation. *Am J Emerg Med* 1985;3:11–14.

56. Kern KB, Hilwig RW, Berg RA, Berg MD, Sanders AB, Ewy GA. Importance of continuous chest compressions during cardiopulmonary resuscitation: improved outcome during a simulated single lay-rescuer scenario. *Circulation* 2002;105:645–649.

57. Ewy G. A new approach for out-of-hospital CPR. A bold step forward. *Resuscitation* 2003;58:271–272.

58. Kern KB, Hilwig RW, Berg RA, Sanders AB, Ewy GA. Importance of continuous chest compressions during cardiopulmonary resuscitation: improved outcome during a simulated single lay-rescuer scenario. *Circulation* 2002;105(5):645–649.

59. Sanders A, Kern K, Atlas M, Bragg S, Ewy G. Importance of the duration of inadequate coronary perfusion pressure on resuscitation from cardiac arrest. *J Am Coll Cardiol* 1985;6:113–118.

60. Becker L, Berg R, Pepe P, et al. A reappraisal of mouth-to-mouth ventilation during bystander- initiated cardiopulmonary resuscitation. A statement for healthcare professionals from the Ventilation Working Group of the Basic Life Support and Pediatric Life Support Subcommittees, American Heart Association. *Circulation* 1997;96:2102–2112.

61. SOS-KANTO Study Group. Cardiopulmonary resuscitation by bystanders with chest compression only: an observational study. *Lancet* 2007;369:920–926.

62. Ewy GA. Cardiac arrest: guidelines changes urgently needed. *Lancet* 2007;369:882–884.

63. Ewy GA, Kern KB, Sanders AB, et al. Cardiocerebral resuscitation for cardiac arrest. *Am J Med* 2006;119(1):6–9.

64. Ewy GA. Cardiopulmonary resuscitation—strengthening the links in the chain of survival. *N Engl J Med* 2000;342(21):1599–1601.

65. Aufderheide T, Pirrallo R, Yannopoulos D, et al. Incomplete chest wall decompression: a clinical evaluation of CPR performance by EMS personnel and assessment of alternative manual chest compression–decompression techniques *Resuscitation* 2005;64(3):353–362.

66. Ewy GA. Cardiocerebral resuscitation should replace cardiopulmonary resuscitation for out-of-hospital cardiac arrest. *Curr Opin Crit Care* 2006;12:189–192.

67. Weaver WD, Cobb LA, Copass MK, Hallstrom AP. Ventricular defibrillation—a comparative trial using 175-J and 320-J shocks. *N Engl J Med* 1982;307:1101–1106.

68. Berg MD, Clark LL, Valenzuela TD, Kern KB, Berg RA. Post-shock chest compression delays with automated external defibrillator use. *Resuscitation* 2005;64:287–291.

69. Aufderheide TP. The problem with the benefit of ventilations: should our approach be the same in cardiac and respiratory arrest? *Curr Opin Crit Care* 2006;12:207–212.

70. Lurie K, Voelckel W, Plaisance P, et al. Use of an inspiratory impedance threshold valve during cardiopulmonary resuscitation: a progress report. *Resuscitation* 2000;44:219–230.

71. Clark J, Larsen M, Culley L, Graves J, Eisenberg M. Incidence of agonal respiration in sudden cardiac arrest. *Ann Emerg Med* 1991;21:1464–1467.

72. Noc M, Weil MH, Sun S, Tang W, Bisera J. Spontaneous gasping during cardiopulmonary resuscitation without mechanical ventilation. *Am J Respir Crit Care Med* 1994;150(3):861–864.

73. Srinivasan V, Nadkarni VM, Yannopoulos D, et al. Spontaneous gasping decreases intracranial pressure and improves cerebral perfusion in a pig model of ventricular fibrillation. *Resuscitation* 2006;69(2):329–334.

74. Aufderheide TP. The problem with and benefit of ventilations: should our approach be the same in cardiac and respiratory arrest? *Curr Opin Crit Care* 2006;12:207–212.

75. Milander MM, Hiscok PS, Sanders AB, Kern KB, Berg RA, Ewy GA. Chest compression and ventilation rates during cardiopulmonary resuscitation: the effects of audible tone guidance. *Acad Emerg Med* 1995;2:708–713.

76. Andreka P, Frenneaux MP. Haemodynamics of cardiac arrest and resuscitation. *Curr Opin Crit Care* 2006;12:198–203.

77. Guyton AC, Polizio D, Armstrong GG. Mean circulatory filling pressure measured immediately after cessation of heart pumping. *Am J Physiol* 1954;179:261–267.

78. Steen S, Liao Q, Pierre L, Paskevicius A, Sjoberg T. The critical importance of minimal delay between chest compressions and subsequent defibrillation: a haemodynamic explanation. *Resuscitation* 2003;58:249–258.

79. Berg RA, Sorrell VL, Kern KB, et al. Magnetic resonance imaging during untreated ventricular fibrillation reveals prompt right ventricular overdistention without left ventricular volume loss. *Circulation* 2005;111:1136–1140.

80. Higano ST, Oh JK, Ewy GA, Seward JB. The mechanism of blood flow during closed chest cardiac massage in humans: transesophageal echocardiographic observations. *Mayo Clin Proc* 1990;65:1432–1440.

81. Raessler KL, Kern KB, Sanders AB, Tacker WA Jr, Ewy GA. Aortic and right atrial systolic pressures during cardiopulmonary resuscitation: a potential indicator of the mechanism of blood flow. *Am Heart J* 1988;115:1021–1029.

82. Rudikoff MT, Maughan WL, Effron M, Freund P, Weisfeldt ML. Mechanisms of blood flow during cardiopulmonary resuscitation. *Circulation* 1980;61:345–352.

83. Criley JM, Blaufuss AH, Kissel GL. Cough-induced cardiac compression. Self-administered from of cardiopulmonary resuscitation. *JAMA* 1976;236:1246–1250.

84. Niemann JT, Rosborough J, Hausknecht M, Brown D, Criley JM. Cough-CPR: documentation of systemic perfusion in man and in an experimental model: a "window" to the mechanism of blood flow in external CPR. *Crit Care Med* 1980;8:141–146.

85. Klouche K, Weil MH, Sun S, et al. Evolution of the stone heart after prolonged cardiac arrest. *Chest* 2002;122:1006–1011.

86. Berg RA, Sorrell VL, Kern KB, et al. Magnetic resonance imaging during untreated ventricular fibrillation reveals prompt right ventricular overdistention without left ventricular volume loss. *Circulation* 2005;111:1136–1140.

87. Ma MH-M, Hwang J-J, L-P. L, et al. Transesophageal echocardiography assessment of mitral valve position and pulmonary venous flow during cardiopulmonary resuscitations in humans. *Circulation* 1995;92:854–861.

88. Feneley MP, Maier GW, Kern KB, et al. Influence of compression rate on initial success of resuscitation and 24-hour survival after prolonged manual cardiopulmonary resuscitation in dogs. *Circulation* 1988;77:240–250.

89. Hallstrom A, Rea TD, Sayre MR, et al. Manual chest compression vs use of an automated chest compression device during resuscitation following out-of-hospital cardiac arrest: a randomized trial. *JAMA* 2006;295:2620–2628.

90. Lewis RJ, Niemann JT. Manual vs device-assisted CPR. reconciling apparently contradictory results. *JAMA* 2006;295:2661–2664.

91. Ong ME, Ornato JP, Edwards DP, et al. Use of an automated, load-distributing band chest compression device for out-of-hospital cardiac arrest resuscitation. *JAMA* 2006;295:2629–2637.

92. Plaisance P, Lurie KG, Vicaut E, et al. A comparison of standard cardiopulmonary resuscitation and active compression-decompression resuscitation for out-of-hospital cardiac arrest. French Active Compression–Decompression Cardiopulmonary Resuscitation Study Group. *N Engl J Med* 1999;341:569–575.

93. Steen S, Liao Q, Pierre L, Paskevicius A, Sjoberg T. Evaluation of LUCAS, a new device for automatic mechanical compression and active decompression resuscitation. *Resuscitation* 2002;55:285–299.

94. Steen S, Sjoberg T, Olsson P, Young M. Treatment of out-of-hospital cardiac arrest with LUCAS, a new device for automatic mechanical compression and active decompression resuscitation. *Resuscitation* 2005;67:25–30.

95. Otto CW, Yakaitis RW, Blitt CD. Mechanism of action of epinephrine in resuscitation from asphyxial arrest. *Crit Care Med* 1981;9:321–324.

96. Otto CW, Yakaitis RW, Ewy GA. Effect of epinephrine on defibrillation in ischemic ventricular fibrillation. *Am J Emerg Med* 1985;3:285–291.

97. Yakaitis RW, Otto CW, Blitt CD. Relative importance of alpha and beta adrenergic receptors during resuscitation. *Crit Care Med* 1979;7:293–296.

98. Otto CW, Yakaitis RW, Redding JS, Blitt CD. Comparison of dopamine, dobutamine, and epinephrine in CPR. *Crit Care Med* 1981;9(9):640–643.

99. Kudenchuk PJ, Cobb LA, Copass MK, et al. Amiodarone for resuscitation after out-of-hospital cardiac arrest due to ventricular fibrillation. *N Engl J Med* 1999;341:871–878.

100. Dorian P, Cass D, Schwartz B, Cooper R, Gelaznikas R, Barr A. Amiodarone as compared with lidocaine for shock-resistant ventricular fibrillation. *N Engl J Med* 2002;346:884–890.

101. Brain Resuscitation Clinical Trial II Study Group. A randomized clinical study of a calcium-entry blocker (lidoflazine) in the treatment of comatose survivors of cardiac arrest. *N Engl J Med* 1991;324:1225–12231.

102. Sanders AB. Therapeutic hypothermia after cardiac arrest. *Curr Opin Crit Care* 2006;12:213–217.

103. Negovsky VA. Postresuscitation disease. *Crit Care Med* 1988;16:942–946.

104. Holzer M BS, Hachimi-Idrissi S, Roine RO, Sterz F, Mullner M. Hypothermia for neuroprotection after cardiac arrest: Systematic review and individual patient data meta-analysis. *Crit Care Med* 2005;33:414–418.

105. Laurent I, Monchi M, Chiche JD, et al. Reversible myocardial dysfunction in survivors of out-of-hospital cardiac arrest. *J Am Coll Cardiol* 2002;40:2110–2116.

106. Kern KB, Hilwig RW, Berg RA, et al. Postresuscitation left ventricular systolic and diastolic dysfunction. Treatment with dobutamine. *Circulation* 1997;95:2610–2613.

107. Holzer M, Bernard S, Hachimi-Idrissi S, et al. Hypothermia for neuroprotection after cardiac arrest: systematic review and individual patient data meta-analysis. *Crit Care Med* 2005;33:414–418.

108. Benson DW, Williams GR, Spencer FC, Yates AJ. The use of hypothermia after cardiac arrest. *Anesth Analg* 1959;38:423–428.

109. Hypothermia After Cardiac Arrest Group. Mild hypothermia to improve neurologic outcome after cardiac arrest. *N Engl J Med* 2002;346:549–556.

110. Bernard SA, Gray TW, Buist MD, et al. Treatment of comatose survivors of out-of-hospital cardiac arrest with induced hypothermia. *N Engl J Med* 2002;346:557–563.

111. Hachimi-Idrissi S, Come L, Ebinger G, Others M. Mild hypothermia induces by a helmet device: a clinical feasibility study. *Resuscitation* 2001;51:275–281.

112. Nolan JP, Morley PT, Vanden Hoek TL, Hickey RW. Therapeutic hypothermia after cardiac arrest: ILCOR advisory statement. *Resuscitation* 2003;57:231–237.

113. Nozari A, Safar P, Stezoski SW, et al. Critical time window for intra-arrest cooling with cold saline flush in a dog model of cardiopulmonary resuscitation. *Circulation* 2006;113:2690–2696.

114. Bernard S, Buist M. Induced hypothermia in critical care medicine: a review. *Crit Care Med* 2003;31(7):2041–2051.

115. Morrison LJ, Visentin LM, Kiss A, et al. Validation of a termination of resuscitation prediction rules in out-of-hospital cardiac arrests. *N Engl J Med* 2006;355(5):478–487.

116. ROLE. Available at: http://www.asancep.org.uk/JRCALC/publications/doc/ROLE_Most_Final_March2003.pdf.

117. Ewy GA. Cardiopulmonary resuscitation: when is enough enough? *N Engl J Med* 2006;355(5):510–512.

PART 8 — Coronary Heart Disease

CHAPTER (51)

Preventive Strategies
for Coronary Heart Disease

David J. Maron / Paul M. Ridker / Scott M. Grundy /
Thomas A. Pearson

Primary prevention refers to strategies to prevent clinical manifestations of disease in asymptomatic individuals. Secondary prevention refers to efforts to prevent recurrent clinical events in patients with established disease. Prevention of coronary heart disease (CHD) requires identification and treatment of risk factors and the judicious use of medications that have demonstrated efficacy in clinical trials. *Risk factor management prevents and treats coronary atherosclerosis, and should be included as an integral part of any management plan for the many acute and chronic manifestations of this disease.* The intensity of preventive intervention should correspond to the patient's level of absolute risk. This chapter reviews risk assessment for primary prevention, provides an overview of CHD

risk factors, discusses the efficacy of risk factor interventions and drug therapy, and provides practical recommendations for implementing preventive cardiology practice. (Certain risk factors, such as diabetes and hypertension, are reviewed more comprehensively in other chapters.) The approach to risk assessment and management presented in this chapter is based on the American Heart Association guidelines for primary prevention of cardiovascular disease,[1] the American Heart Association/American College of Cardiology (AHA/ACC) guidelines for secondary prevention,[2] and the recommendations of the National Cholesterol Education Program (NCEP) Adult Treatment Panel III (ATP III)[3] and the American Diabetes Association.[4] Where appropriate, this chapter also provides updated information that was not available at the time each of these guidelines was created.

RISK ASSESSMENT BASED ON CLINICAL CONDITIONS AND RISK FACTOR EVALUATION

[ ] CATEGORIES OF ABSOLUTE RISK

In most current risk algorithms, absolute risk is divided into three categories: high, intermediate, and low. Patients at high risk deserve intensive risk-reduction therapy. Those at intermediate risk are also candidates for clinical intervention to the extent that therapy is effective, safe, and cost-effective. Finally, most lower-risk persons should be encouraged by their physicians to follow public health recommendations for primary prevention of CHD, but some may benefit from risk-reducing drug therapy. Each category of absolute risk can be expressed in quantitative terms such that those with less than a 10 percent 10-year risk are considered "low risk," those with a 10 to 20 percent 10-year risk are considered "intermediate risk," and those with a greater than 20 percent 10-year risk are considered "high risk" (Table 51–1). Patients without CHD whose absolute 10-year risk for CHD equals that of patients who already manifest clinical CHD are said to have a *CHD risk equivalent*. It is recognized that there are limitations to this approach as these risk estimates are highly dependent on age, and that lifetime risk may be more appropriate than 10-year risk in several prevention settings.[5,6]

[ ] IDENTIFICATION OF VERY-HIGH-RISK PATIENTS

An update to the NCEP ATP III guidelines proposed a new classification of patients as very high risk who deserve especially aggressive low-density lipoprotein cholesterol (LDL-C) lowering.[7] These individuals are those with the presence of established cardiovascular disease plus (1) multiple major risk factors (especially diabetes), (2) severe and poorly controlled risk factors (especially continued cigarette smoking), (3) the metabolic syndrome (especially triglycerides ≥200 mg/dL plus non–high-density lipoprotein cholesterol [HDL-C] ≥130 mg/dL with HDL-C <40 mg/dL), and (4) patients with acute coronary syndromes. Clinical trial data also indicate that those with established coronary disease and elevated levels of C-reactive protein (CRP) represent a very high risk group.[8] A national survey of outpatients with CHD found that 75 percent meet the criteria for very high risk.[9]

[ ] IDENTIFICATION OF HIGH-RISK PATIENTS

Clinical Coronary Heart Disease

Included in the category of clinical CHD are a history of acute coronary syndromes, stable angina, and coronary revascularization procedures. Evidence from clinical trials of cholesterol-lowering therapy indicates that patients with a prior history of myocardial infarction (MI) have a 10-year risk for recurrent nonfatal or fatal MI of about 26 percent.[10,11] Patients with stable angina pectoris have a 10-year risk for acute MI of approximately 20 percent.[12,13]

Noncoronary Atherosclerosis

Patients in this group include those with peripheral arterial disease, abdominal aortic aneurysm, and symptomatic carotid artery disease or asymptomatic disease with greater than 50 percent stenosis.[3] The absolute risk for MI in patients with noncoronary atherosclerosis equals that for recurrent MI in patients with established CHD.

Diabetes

Patients with diabetes, particularly middle-age and older patients with type 2 diabetes, who do not manifest CHD commonly carry a risk for major coronary events equivalent to that of nondiabetic patients with established CHD.[14] Moreover, many patients with type 2 diabetes have had a silent MI, and many others have silent ischemia. Thus most patients with diabetes are at high risk, and ATP III has designated diabetes as a CHD equivalent.

Multiple Risk Factors without Clinical Coronary Heart Disease

Persons without known atherosclerosis who have multiple risk factors (other than diabetes) often have risk that is equivalent to CHD. The absolute risk for the development of CHD over the next decade can be estimated by Framingham risk tables (Tables 51–2 and 51–3). These tables show absolute risk for *hard CHD* (nonfatal and fatal MI) and exclude *soft CHD* (stable and unstable angina). *A CHD risk equivalent is defined when the absolute 10-year risk for hard CHD events exceeds 20 percent.*

Selection of Patients for Advanced Risk Assessment Using Emerging Risk Factors When patients without known atherosclerotic disease have a 10-year risk for hard CHD between 5 and 20 percent (i.e., intermediate risk), they are potential candidates for advanced risk assessment. There has been intensive research to identify new risk factors that will improve the accuracy of prognosis. These so-called *emerging risk factors* are divided into three categories: nontraditional lipid risk factors, nonlipid risk factors, and subclinical atherosclerotic disease (Table 51–4). ATP III does not recommend routine measurement of any of these factors. However, evidence is accumulating to justify the measurement of certain factors to (1) elevate persons with multiple risk factors and intermediate risk to the category of CHD risk equivalent, and (2) guide the decision about use and intensity of drug therapy to lower LDL-C.[15] In particular, recent prospective data demonstrate that the addition of CRP for risk prediction among those with 5 to <10 and 10 to <20 percent

TABLE 51-1

Risk Categories

RISK CATEGORY	10-YEAR ABSOLUTE RISK FOR MYOCARDIAL INFARCTION (NONFATAL + FATAL)
High	>20%
Intermediate	10–20%
Low	<10%

TABLE 51–2

Estimate of 10-Year Risk for Men (Framingham Point Scores)

AGE	POINTS
20–34	–9
35–39	–4
40–44	0
45–49	3
50–54	6
55–59	8
60–64	10
65–69	11
70–74	12
75–79	13

TOTAL CHOLESTEROL	POINTS AT AGES 20–39	POINTS AT AGES 40–49	POINTS AT AGES 50–59	POINTS AT AGES 60–69	POINTS AT AGES 70–79
<160	0	0	0	0	0
160–199	4	3	2	1	0
200–239	7	5	3	1	0
240–279	9	6	4	2	1
≥280	11	8	5	3	1

	POINTS AT AGES 20–39	POINTS AT AGES 40–49	POINTS AT AGES 50–59	POINTS AT AGES 60–69	POINTS AT AGES 70–79
Nonsmoker	0	0	0	0	0
Smoker	8	5	3	1	1

HDL	POINTS
≥60	–1
50–59	0
40–49	1
>40	2

SYSTOLIC BLOOD PRESSURE	IF UNTREATED	IF TREATED
<120	0	0
120–129	0	1
130–139	1	2
140–159	1	2
≥160	2	3

POINT TOTAL	10-YEAR RISK	POINT TOTAL	10-YEAR RISK
<0	<1%	9	5%
0	1%	10	6%
1	1%	11	8%
2	1%	12	10%
3	1%	13	12%
4	1%	14	16%
5	2%	15	20%
6	2%	16	25%
7	3%	≥17	≥30%
8	4%		

SOURCE: From Third Report of the National Cholesterol Education Program (NCEP) Expert Panel on Detection, Evaluation, and Treatment of High Blood Cholesterol in Adults (Adult Treatment Panel III) final report. Circulation 2002;106:3143–3421, with permission.

TABLE 51-3

10-Year Risk Estimates for Women (Framingham Point Scores)

AGE	POINTS
20–34	–7
35–39	–3
40–44	0
45–49	3
50–54	6
55–59	8
60–64	10
65–69	12
70–74	14
75–79	16

TOTAL CHOLESTEROL	POINTS AT AGES 20–39	POINTS AT AGES 40–49	POINTS AT AGES 50–59	POINTS AT AGES 60–69	POINTS AT AGES 70–79
<160	0	0	0	0	0
160–199	4	3	2	1	1
200–239	8	6	4	2	1
240–279	11	8	5	3	2
≥280	13	10	7	4	2

	POINTS AT AGES 20–39	POINTS AT AGES 40–49	POINTS AT AGES 50–59	POINTS AT AGES 60–69	POINTS AT AGES 70–79
Nonsmoker	0	0	0	0	0
Smoker	9	7	4	2	1

HDL	POINTS
≥60	–1
50–59	0
40–49	1
<40	2

SYSTOLIC BLOOD PRESSURE	IF UNTREATED	IF TREATED
<120	0	0
120–129	1	3
130–139	2	4
140–159	3	5
≥160	4	6

POINT TOTAL	10-YEAR RISK	POINT TOTAL	10-YEAR RISK
<9	<1%	17	5%
9	1%	18	6%
10	1%	19	8%
11	1%	20	11%
12	1%	21	14%
13	2%	22	17%
14	2%	23	22%
15	3%	24	27%
16	4%	≥25	≥30%

SOURCE: From Third Report of the National Cholesterol Education Program (NCEP) Expert Panel on Detection, Evaluation, and Treatment of High Blood Cholesterol in Adults (Adult Treatment Panel III) final report. Circulation 2002;106:3143–3421, with permission.

TABLE 51-4

Emerging Risk Factors

Lipid
- Triglycerides
- Lipoprotein remnant particles
- Lipoprotein(a)
- Small LDL particles
- HDL subspecies
- Apolipoprotein B
- Apolipoprotein AI
- Total cholesterol/HDL cholesterol ratio

Nonlipid
- Homocysteine
- Thrombogenic/hemostatic factors
- Inflammatory markers
- Impaired fasting glucose

Detection of subclinical atherosclerosis
- Ankle brachial index
- Tests for myocardial ischemia
- Tests for atherosclerotic plaque burden (e.g., coronary calcium scanning, carotid sonography)

HDL, high-density lipoprotein; LDL, low density lipoprotein.

10-year risks correctly reclassifies between 20 and 30 percent of all patients.[16] However, unlike CRP, several of these emerging tests are not commercially available, not well standardized, and are expensive. The NCEP recommends that they be considered optional modifiers of therapy, used only as an adjunct to adjust the estimate of absolute risk status obtained using major risk factors.[17] If such testing is done, it should always be preceded by determination of Framingham risk scoring, which will provide greater perspective on a person's absolute risk than will advanced measures.

High-Risk Patients Identified by Major Risk Factors Plus Subclinical Atherosclerosis

Many patients will have multiple CHD risk factors but have an absolute 10-year risk <20 percent by the Framingham risk score. Some of these patients are undoubtedly at higher risk because of advanced subclinical coronary atherosclerosis. If the latter can be identified noninvasively, the projected risk level can be raised to that of a CHD risk equivalent.[18] Noninvasive testing in asymptomatic patients has been controversial.[19] Many have expressed concern that asymptomatic patients with advanced subclinical atherosclerosis will be labeled as having CHD and referred inappropriately for invasive procedures. *Noninvasive testing in asymptomatic patients should be used for risk assessment (prognosis) and not for diagnosis of "coronary artery disease."* (An important exception is for patients with diabetes who may have atypical or no symptoms associated with myocardial ischemia.) The goal of such testing is to add to the accuracy of risk prediction from conventional risk factors, and thus to identify persons who will benefit most from intensive medical therapy for risk reduction. The goal is not case finding for invasive coronary interventions.

Some authorities question whether the scientific evidence supporting noninvasive testing in asymptomatic patients is adequate to justify its recommendation and believe that Framing-

ham risk scoring is sufficient for risk stratification. It is also important to recognize that imaging tests do not detect *risk factors* for atherosclerosis but rather the disease itself, and thus that screening can only succeed after the disease is well-established and not in the earliest phases when lifestyle preventive efforts need initiation. Nonetheless, noninvasive imaging tests that have been suggested to improve risk prediction beyond the Framingham risk score are exercise treadmill testing (see Chap. 14), coronary calcium scanning,[20] and carotid ultrasonography.[21,22] In addition to risk stratification, patients who visualize their atherosclerotic disease may improve use of and adherence to statin therapy.[23] Simple evaluation of the ankle-brachial index (ABI) has also been shown to be an effective method for detecting subclinical atherosclerosis. Given that the ABI can be performed easily in the primary care office at exceptionally low cost, this technique should be widely considered, especially as it will also detect clinically important peripheral disease. An additional advantage of the ABI is that it focuses responsibility for prevention appropriately in the primary care physician's office.

High-Risk Patients Identified by Major Risk Factors Plus Inflammatory Markers

Substantial evidence indicates that high-sensitivity C-reactive protein independently predicts coronary events and improves risk stratification in intermediate-risk patients.[15,24] The AHA and Centers for Disease Control and Prevention recommend the optional use of CRP in the evaluation of patients at intermediate risk to help direct further evaluation and therapy (see C-Reactive Protein below).[24] As described above, CRP levels are effective for the correct reclassification of many patients at intermediate risk and thus may provide a simple and inexpensive method to improve the targeting of statin therapy to those in greatest need.[16]

IDENTIFICATION OF INTERMEDIATE-RISK PATIENTS

Patients at intermediate risk are those without known atherosclerosis but with two or more conventional risk factors whose 10-year risk for CHD is 10 to 20 percent. These patients are candidates for treatment of major risk factors and evidence-based pharmacologic interventions. For example, low-dose aspirin is recommended by the AHA[1]; hypertension should be treated with antihypertensive agents to normalize blood pressure[25]; and cholesterol-lowering drugs are indicated if the goals of therapy are not achieved by lifestyle changes.[3]

RISK ASSESSMENT IN ELDERLY PATIENTS

The predictive power of conventional risk factors declines in older patients, and age becomes the predominant risk factor. For these reasons, noninvasive measures of myocardial ischemia, coronary or carotid plaque burden, or markers of inflammation may be especially useful in differentiating between intermediate- and high-risk elderly patients. Mounting evidence that aggressive medical therapy significantly reduces risk for CHD in the older population increases the need to define absolute risk in this population more accurately.[7]

LOWER-RISK PATIENTS

People in this category usually have one or no conventional risk factors. Less-intensive therapies are indicated for patients with a single risk factor. An important question is how to manage patients with a single categorical risk factor but who are otherwise at low risk. A fundamental principle of primary prevention is that *all categorical risk factors must be treated, regardless of absolute risk.*[26] For example, cigarette smoking can cause cancer and cardiovascular disease even in the absence of other risk factors, and hypertension alone can cause stroke or heart failure. Although a person with only one risk factor—such as hypertension, smoking, or hypercholesterolemia—has less than a 10 percent 10-year risk of CHD, the presence of a single major risk factor at 50 years of age is associated with substantially increased lifetime risk for CHD and markedly shorter survival.[27] Therefore, some individuals with only one major risk factor may be candidates for pharmacologic therapy to decrease the risk for CHD and increase survival.

RISK FACTORS FOR WHICH INTERVENTIONS HAVE PROVED TO LOWER RISK OF CORONARY HEART DISEASE

LIPID DISORDERS

Low-Density Lipoprotein Cholesterol

LDL-C is a major cause of CHD, and controlled clinical trials show that lowering LDL-C reduces risk for CHD. Accordingly, the NCEP has identified LDL-C as the primary target of lipid-lowering therapy. Five decades of research on the role of LDL-C in the pathogenesis of CHD represents one of the major advances in modern medicine and public health. This evidence is summarized briefly.

Low-Density Lipoprotein Cholesterol as the Primary Atherogenic Agent Studies in laboratory animals indicate that raising serum levels of LDL-C initiates and sustains atherogenesis (see Chap. 52). Moreover, humans with genetic forms of severely elevated LDL-C exhibit premature atherosclerotic disease.[26] These examples demonstrate that elevated LDL-C alone, without the presence of another risk factor, is independently atherogenic. For many years, it was believed that the major action of low-density lipoprotein (LDL) was merely to deposit its cholesterol within the arterial wall. More recently, LDL has been found to be proinflammatory, setting into motion the chronic inflammatory response that is the hallmark of the atherosclerotic lesion. Elevated LDL appears to be involved with all stages of atherogenesis: endothelial dysfunction, plaque formation and growth, plaque instability and disruption, and thrombosis. Elevated levels of LDL-C in the plasma lead to increased retention of LDL particles in the arterial wall, their oxidation, and secretion of various inflammatory mediators and chemoattractants (see Chap. 52). Treatment of elevated LDL-C levels has been shown to reestablish normal coronary endothelial function.[28,29]

The primacy of LDL as a pathogenic agent is supported by epidemiologic data of several types. In different populations, the risk for CHD is positively correlated with serum total cholesterol concentration, which in turn is highly correlated with LDL-C. The association between LDL-C levels and CHD risk is almost linear on a log scale.[7,30] These observations strongly suggests that elevated LDL-C is the *primary* risk factor.

Primary and Secondary Prevention Numerous cholesterol-lowering trials have used dietary and drug interventions. One trial also induced cholesterol lowering by intestinal surgery.[31] Primary and secondary prevention trials with older cholesterol-lowering drugs demonstrated reduced risk for CHD but failed to reduce total mortality. This left many clinicians skeptical of the benefits of cholesterol-lowering therapy. The introduction of beta-hydroxy-beta-methylglutaryl-coenzyme A (HMG-CoA) reductase inhibitors (statins), more powerful LDL-lowering drugs, made possible a more effective test of the cholesterol hypothesis. Since 1993, several large primary and secondary prevention trials with statins using clinical end points have been completed, as summarized in Table 51–5.[10,11,32–49] As a whole, these trials document convincingly that cholesterol-lowering therapy with statins is both safe and effective for reducing CHD risk. The mechanism by which LDL-C lowering reduces clinical end points is suggested by angiographic studies and, more recently, by studies using intravascular ultrasound. Most statin trials with imaging end points demonstrated that marked reductions of LDL-C slow progression, and in some cases induce regression, of coronary lesions.[50,51] Although measurable changes in lesion size were small in angiographic studies, the incidence of major coronary events was reduced strikingly in those studies sufficiently powered. This observation engendered the concept that LDL-C reduction *stabilizes* coronary lesions by changing their composition rather than causing them to substantially enlarge the coronary lumen (see Chap. 52). In fact, intravascular ultrasound studies have demonstrated that for lesions causing <50 percent stenosis, progression of coronary atherosclerosis can be associated with a paradoxical *increase* in lumen cross-sectional area (so-called *positive remodeling*), whereas regression is not associated with any change in lumen area. The greatest regression in atherosclerosis among statin-treated patients appears to be among those who not only reduce LDL-C, but who also reduce CRP levels.[52] When a patient treated with a statin develops CHD, the initial presentation is more likely to be stable angina and less likely to be an acute MI.[53]

Practice Recommendations for Lowering Low-Density Lipoprotein Cholesterol LDL-C lowering can be accomplished with dietary and drug therapies (Tables 51–6 and 51–7). With the availability of powerful statins, there is an unfortunate tendency of physicians to minimize the importance of dietary therapy when treating patients. The benefit of the Mediterranean diet, as demonstrated persuasively in the Lyon Diet Heart Study,[54] is often overlooked. Patients should be advised to reduce intake of cholesterol-raising fatty acids (saturated and *trans*-fatty acids) and dietary cholesterol. The major sources of dietary saturated fatty acids are dairy fats (e.g., milk, butter, cream, cheese, and ice cream) and animal fats (e.g., fatty cuts of meat [especially hamburger], fatty processed meats, lard, and tallow). *Trans*-fatty acids are present in shortening, hard margarine, and processed foods containing these forms of fat, such as french fries. *Trans*-fatty acids have markedly adverse effects on serum lipids, causing a rise in LDL-C, a reduction in

TABLE 51–5

Large Clinical Outcome Studies Using Statins

STUDY NAME	SAMPLE SIZE N (% WOMEN)	PATIENT CHARACTERISTICS	STUDY DESIGN	PRIMARY END POINT	MAIN RESULTS RRR	ARR	NNT
				SECONDARY PREVENTION IN STABLE CHD PATIENTS			
4S[32]	4444 (19%)	CHD, high LDL-C	Simvastatin 20–40 mg/d vs. placebo	Total mortality	30% (p = 0.0003)	3.3%	30
CARE[10]	4159 (14%)	MI 3 to 20 months prior	Pravastatin 40 mg/d vs. placebo	CHD death or nonfatal MI	24% (p = 0.003)	3.0%	33
LIPID[11]	9014 (17%)	CHD	Pravastatin 40 mg/d vs. placebo	CHD death	24% (p <0.001)	1.9%	53
LIPS[33]	1677 (16%)	Post-PCI	Fluvastatin 80 mg/d vs. placebo	Cardiac death, nonfatal MI, or repeat intervention	22% (p = 0.01)	5.3%	19
GREACE[34]	1600 (22%)	CHD	Atorvastatin titrated from 10 mg/d to 80 mg/d to achieve LDL-C <100 mg/dL vs. usual care	Death, nonfatal MI, unstable angina, heart failure, coronary revascularization, or stroke	51% (p <0.0001)	12.5%	8
ALLIANCE[35]	2442 (18%)	CHD, high LDL-C	LDL-C goals of <80 mg/dL or atorvastatin dose of 80 mg/d vs. usual care	Cardiac death, nonfatal MI, resuscitated cardiac arrest, coronary revascularization, or unstable angina	17% (p = 0.02)	4.0%	25
TNT[36]	10,001 (19%)	CHD, LDL-C <130 mg/dL on atorvastatin 10 mg/d	Atorvastatin 10 mg/d (LDL-C goal 100 mg/dL) vs. 80 mg/d (LDL-C goal 75 mg/dL)	CHD death, nonfatal MI, resuscitated cardiac arrest, or stroke	22% (p <0.001)	2.2%	45
IDEAL[37]	8888 (19%)	CHD	Atorvastatin 80 mg/d vs. simvastatin 20 mg/d	CHD death, nonfatal MI, or resuscitated cardiac arrest	11% in favor of atorvastatin (p = 0.07)	1.1%	91
				SECONDARY PREVENTION AFTER ACUTE CORONARY SYNDROME			
MIRACL[38]	3086 (35%)	Acute coronary syndrome	Atrovastatin 80 mg/d vs. placebo	Total mortality, nonfatal MI, resuscitated cardiac arrest, or recurrent acute coronary syndrome	16% (p = 0.048)	2.6%	38
PROVE IT[39]	4162 (22%)	Acute coronary syndrome	Atrovastatin 80 mg/d vs. pravastatin 40 mg/d	Total mortality, nonfatal MI, unstable angina, coronary revascularization, or stroke	16% in favor of atorvastatin (p = 0.005)	3.9%	26
A to Z[40]	4497 (25%)	Acute coronary syndrome	Simvastatin 40 mg/d for 1 month followed by 80 mg/d vs. placebo for 4 months followed by simvastatin 20 mg/d	Cardiovascular death, nonfatal MI, acute coronary syndrome, or stroke	11% in favor of high-dose simvastatin (p = 0.14)	2.3%	43

(continued)

TABLE 51-5

Large Clinical Outcome Studies Using Statins (continued)

STUDY NAME	SAMPLE SIZE N (% WOMEN)	PATIENT CHARACTERISTICS	STUDY DESIGN	PRIMARY END POINT	MAIN RESULTS RRR	ARR	NNT
MIXED PRIMARY AND SECONDARY PREVENTION STUDIES							
HPS[41]	20,536 (25%)	CHD, noncoronary atherosclerosis, or diabetes	Simvastatin 40 mg/d vs. placebo	Total mortality	13% (p <0.0003)	1.8%	56
ALLHAT-LLT[42]	10,335 (49%)	Hypertensive with ≥1 other risk factors; 14% had CHD at baseline	Pravastatin 40 mg/d vs. usual care	Total mortality	1% (p = 0.88)	0.4%	250
PROSPER[43]	5804 (52%)	70–82 years old with history (44%) or risk factors for coronary, cerebral, or peripheral vascular disease	Pravastatin 40 mg/d vs. placebo	CHD death, nonfatal MI, or stroke	15% (p = 0.014)	2.1%	48
ALERT[44]	2102 (34%)	Renal transplant patients	Fluvastatin 40 mg/d vs. placebo	Cardiac death, nonfatal MI, or coronary revascularization	17% (p = 0.139)	2%	50
PRIMARY PREVENTION							
WOSCOPS[45] AFCAPS/TexCAPS[46]	6595 (0%) 6605 (15%)	High LDL-C Low HDL-C	Pravastatin 40 mg/d vs. placebo Lovastatin 20–40 mg/d vs. placebo	CHD death or nonfatal MI Fatal or nonfatal MI, unstable angina, or sudden cardiac death	31% (p <0.001) 37% (p <0.001)	2.4% 2.8%	42 36
ASCOT-LLA[47]	10,305 (19%)	Hypertensive with ≥3 other CHD risk factors	Atorvastatin 10 mg/d vs. placebo	CHD death and nonfatal MI	36% (p <0.0005)	1.1%	91
CARDS[48]	2838 (32%)	Type 2 diabetes and ≥1 of the following: retinopathy, albuminuria, current smoking, or hypertension	Atorvastatin 10 mg/d vs. placebo	Acute coronary syndrome, coronary revascularization, or stroke	37% (p = 0.001)	3.2%	31
4D[49]	1255 (46%)	Type 2 diabetes on dialysis	Atorvastatin 20 mg/d vs. placebo	Cardiovascular death, nonfatal MI, or stroke	8% (p = 0.37)	1.0%	100

4D, Deutsche Diabetes Dialyse Studie; 4S, Scandinavian Simvastatin Survival Study; A to Z, Aggrastat to Zocor; AFCAPS/TexCAPS, Air Force/Texas Coronary Atherosclerosis Prevention Study; ALERT, Assessment of LEscol in Renal Transplantation; ALLHAT-LLT, Antihypertensive and Lipid-Lowering Treatment to Prevent Heart Attack Trial; ALLIANCE, Aggressive Lipid-Lowering Initiation Abates New Cardiac Events; ASCOT-LLA, Anglo-Scandinavian Cardiac Outcomes Trial–Lipid Lowering Arm; CARDS, Collaborative Atorvastatin Diabetes Study; HPS, Heart Protection Study; IDEAL, Incremental Decrease in Endpoints through Aggressive Lipid Lowering; CARE, Cholesterol and Recurrent Events; GREACE, GREek Atorvastatin and Coronary-heart-disease Evaluation; LIPID, Long-Term Intervention with Pravastatin in Ischaemic Disease; LIPS, Lescol Intervention Prevention Study; MIRACL, Myocardial Ischemia Reduction with Aggressive Cholesterol Lowering; PROSPER, Prospective Study of Pravastatin in the Elderly at Risk; PROVE IT, Pravastatin or Atorvastatin Evaluation and Infection Therapy; TNT, Treating to New Targets; WOSCOPS, West of Scotland Coronary Prevention Study.

ARR, absolute risk reduction; CHD, coronary heart disease; HDL-C, high-density lipoprotein cholesterol; LDL-C, low-density lipoprotein cholesterol; MI, myocardial infarction; n, number of subjects; NNT, number needed to treat to prevent 1 primary end point (100/ARR); RRR, relative risk reduction.

1210

TABLE 51–6

American Heart Association Guide to Primary Prevention of Cardiovascular Disease: Risk Intervention

RISK INTERVENTION AND GOALS	RECOMMENDATIONS
SMOKING Goal: Complete cessation; no exposure to environmental tobacco smoke.	Ask about tobacco use status at every visit. Advise every tobacco user to quit. Assess the tobacco user's willingness to quit. Assist by counseling and developing a plan for quitting. Arrange followup, referral to special programs, or pharmacotherapy. Urge avoidance of exposure to secondhand smoke at work or home.
BP CONTROL Goal: <140/90 mmHg; <130/85 mmHg if renal insufficiency or heart failure is present or <130/80 mmHg if diabetes is present.	Promote healthy lifestyle modification. Advocate weight reduction; reduction of sodium intake; consumption of fruits, vegetables, and low-fat dairy products; moderation of alcohol intake; and physical activity in persons with BP of ≥130 mmHg systolic or 80 mmHg diastolic. For persons with renal insufficiency or heart failure, initiate drug therapy if BP is ≥130 mmHg systolic or 85 mmHg diastolic (≥80 mmHg diastolic for patients with diabetes). Initiate drug therapy for those with BP ≥140/90 mmHg if 6 to 12 months of lifestyle modification is not effective, depending on the number of risk factors present.
DIETARY INTAKE Goal: An overall healthy eating pattern.	Advocate consumption of a variety of fruits, vegetables, grains, low-fat or nonfat dairy products, fish, legumes, poultry, and lean meats. Match energy intake with energy needs. Reduce saturated fats (<10% of calories), cholesterol (<300 mg/d), and *trans*-fatty acids by substituting grains and unsaturated fatty acids from fish, vegetables, legumes, and nuts. Limit salt intake to <6 g/d. Limit alcohol intake (≤2 drinks per day in men, ≤1 drink per day in women) among those who drink.
ASPIRIN Goal: Low-dose aspirin in persons at higher CHD risk (especially those with 10-year risk of CHD ≥10%).	Do not recommend for patients with aspirin intolerance. Do not use in persons at increased risk for gastrointestinal bleeding and hemorrhagic stroke. Consider 75–160 mg aspirin per day for persons at higher risk (especially those with 10-year risk of CHD of ≥10%).
BLOOD LIPID MANAGEMENT Primary goal: LDL-C <160 mg/dL if ≤1 risk factor is present; LDL-C <130 mg/dL if ≥2 risk factors are present and 10-year CHD risk is <20%; or LDL-C <100 mg/dL if ≥2 risk factors are present and 10-year CHD risk is ≥20% or if patient has diabetes. Secondary goals (if LDL-C is at goal range): If triglycerides are <200 mg/dL, then use non–HDL-C as a secondary goal: non–HDL-C <190 mg/dL for ≤1 risk factor; non–HDL-C <160 mg/dL for ≥2 risk factors and 10-year CHD risk ≤20%; non–HDL-C <130 mg/dL for diabetics or for ≥2 risk factors and 10-year CHD risk >20%. Other targets for therapy: triglycerides <150 mg/dL; HDL-C <40 mg/dL in men and <50 mg/dL in women.	If LDL-C is above goal range, initiate additional therapeutic lifestyle changes consisting of dietary modifications to lower LDL-C: <7% of calories from saturated fat, cholesterol <200 mg/d, and, if further LDL-C lowering is required, dietary options (plant stanols/sterols not to exceed 2 g/d and/or increased viscous [soluble] fiber [10–25 g/d]), and additional emphasis on weight reduction and physical activity. If LDL-C is above goal range, rule out secondary causes (liver function test, thyroid-stimulating hormone level, urinalysis). After 12 weeks of therapeutic lifestyle change, consider LDL-lowering drug therapy if ≥2 risk factors are present, 10-year risk is >10%, and LDL-C is ≥130 mg/dL; ≥2 risk factors are present, 10-year risk is <10%, and LDL-C is ≥160 mg/dL; or ≤1 risk factor is present and LDL-C is ≥190 mg/dL. Start drugs and advance dose to bring LDL-C to goal range, usually a statin but also consider bile acid-binding resin or niacin. If LDL-C goal not achieved, consider combination therapy (statin + resin, statin + niacin). After LDL-C goal has been reached, consider triglyceride level: If 150–199 mg/dL, treat with therapeutic lifestyle changes. If 200–499 mg/dL, treat elevated non–HDL-C with therapeutic lifestyle changes and, if necessary, consider higher doses of statin or adding niacin or fibrate. If >500 mg/dL, treat with fibrate or niacin to reduce risk of pancreatitis. If HDL-C is <40 mg/dL in men and <50 mg/dL in women, initiate or intensify therapeutic lifestyle changes. For higher-risk patients, consider drugs that raise HDL-C (e.g., niacin, fibrates, statins).
PHYSICAL ACTIVITY Goal: At least 30 minutes of moderate-intensity physical activity on most (and preferably all) days of the week.	If cardiovascular, respiratory, metabolic, orthopedic, or neurologic disorders are suspected, or if patient is middle-aged or older and is sedentary, consult physician before initiating vigorous exercise program. Moderate-intensity activities (40 to 60% of maximum capacity) are equivalent to a brisk walk (15–20 minutes per mile). Additional benefits are gained from vigorous-intensity activity (>60% of maximum capacity) for 20–40 minutes on 3–5 days per week. Recommend resistance training with 8–10 different exercises, 1–2 sets per exercise, and 10–15 repetitions at moderate intensity ≥2 days per week. Flexibility training and an increase in daily lifestyle activities should complement this regimen.

(continued)

TABLE 51–6

American Heart Association Guide to Primary Prevention of Cardiovascular Disease: Risk Intervention *(continued)*

RISK INTERVENTION AND GOALS	RECOMMENDATIONS
WEIGHT MANAGEMENT Goal: Achieve and maintain desirable weight (body mass index 18.5–24.9 kg/m²). When body mass index is ≥25 kg/m², waist circumference at iliac crest level ≤40 inches in men, ≤35 inches in women.	Initiate weight-management program through caloric restriction and increased caloric expenditure as appropriate. For overweight/obese persons, reduce body weight by 10% in first year of therapy.
DIABETES MANAGEMENT Goals: Normal fasting plasma glucose (<110 mg/dL) and near normal HbA1c (<7%).	Initiate appropriate hypoglycemic therapy to achieve near-normal fasting plasma glucose or as indicated by near-normal HbA1c. First step is diet and exercise. Second-step therapy is usually oral hypoglycemic drugs: sulfonylureas and/or metformin with ancillary use of acarbose and thiazolidinediones. Third-step therapy is insulin. Treat other risk factors more aggressively (e.g., change BP goal to <130/80 mmHg and LDL-C goal to <100 mg/dL).

BP, blood pressure; CHD, coronary heart disease; LDL-C, low-density lipoprotein cholesterol; HDL-C, high-density lipoprotein cholesterol.

SOURCE: From Pearson TA, Blair SN, Daniels SR, et al. AHA guidelines for primary prevention of cardiovascular disease and stroke: 2002 update: consensus panel guide to comprehensive risk reduction for adult patients without coronary or other atherosclerotic vascular diseases. Circulation 2002;106:388–391, with permission.

HDL-C, a rise in triglycerides, a reduction in LDL diameter, and a rise in lipoprotein(a).[55] Per calorie consumed, *trans*-fats appear to increase the risk of CHD more than any other dietary variable. Dietary cholesterol is found in egg yolks, dairy fats, and other animal products. Current intake of cholesterol-raising fatty acids in the United States is approximately 11 percent of total calories.[27] For patients on cholesterol-lowering therapy, this should be reduced to less than 7 percent. Dietary cholesterol should be low-

TABLE 51–7

American Heart Association/American College of Cardiology Secondary Prevention for Patients with Coronary and Other Vascular Disease

	INTERVENTION RECOMMENDATIONS WITH CLASS OF RECOMMENDATION
SMOKING Goal: Complete cessation; no exposure to environmental tobacco smoke	Ask about tobacco use status at every visit. Advise every tobacco user to quit. Assess the tobacco user's willingness to quit. Assist by counseling and developing plan for quitting. Arrange followup, referral to special programs, or pharmacotherapy (including nicotine replacement and bupropion) Urge avoidance of exposure to environmental tobacco smoke at work and home.
BLOOD PRESSURE CONTROL Goal: <140/90 mmHg or <130/80 mmHg if patient has diabetes or chronic kidney disease	For all patients: Initiate or maintain lifestyle modification—weight control; increased physical activity; alcohol moderation; sodium reduction; and emphasis on increased consumption of fresh fruits, vegetables, and low-fat dairy products. For patients with blood pressure ≥140/90 mmHg (or ≥130/80 mmHg for individuals with chronic kidney disease or diabetes): As tolerated, add blood pressure medication, treating initially with β-blockers and/or ACE inhibitors, with addition of other drugs such as thiazides as needed to achieve goal blood pressure. (A) [For compelling indications for individual drug classes in specific vascular diseases, see Seventh Report of the Joint National Committee on Prevention, Detection, Evaluation, and Treatment of High Blood Pressure.[25]]

TABLE 51-7

American Heart Association/American College of Cardiology Secondary Prevention for Patients with Coronary and Other Vascular Disease *(continued)*

	INTERVENTION RECOMMENDATIONS WITH CLASS OF RECOMMENDATION
LIPID MANAGEMENT	**For all patients:**
Goal: LDL-C <100 mg/dL; if triglycerides are ≥200 mg/dL, non–HDL-should be <130 mg/dL (non–HDL-C = total cholesterol minus HDL-C)	Start dietary therapy. Reduce intake of saturated fats (to <7% of total calories), *trans*-fatty acids, and cholesterol (to <200 mg/d)
	Adding plant stanol/sterols (2 g/d) and viscous fiber (>10 g/d) will further lower LDL-C. Promote daily physical activity and weight management.
	Encourage increased consumption of omega-3 fatty acids in the form of fish or in capsule form (1 g/d) for risk reduction. For treatment of elevated triglycerides, higher doses are usually necessary for risk reduction.
	For lipid management:
	Assess fasting lipid profile in all patients, and within 24 hours of hospitalization for those with an acute cardiovascular or coronary event. For hospitalized patients, initiate lipid-lowering medication as recommended below before discharge according to the following schedule:
	LDL-C should be <100 mg/dL, and
	Further reduction of LDL-C to <70 mg/dL is reasonable.
	If baseline LDL-C is ≥100 mg/dL, initiate LDL-lowering drug therapy.
	If on-treatment LDL-C is ≥100 mg/dL, intensify LDL-lowering drug therapy (may require LDL-lowering drug combination).
	If baseline LDL-C is 70 to 100 mg/dL, it is reasonable to treat to LDL-C <70 mg/dL.
	If triglycerides are 200 to 499 mg/dL, non-HDL-should be <130 mg/dL and
	Further reduction of non-HDL-C to <100 mg/dL is reasonable.
PHYSICAL ACTIVITY	For all patients, assess risk with physical activity history and/or an exercise test, to guide prescription.
Goal: 30 minutes, 7 days per week (minimum 5 days per week)	For all patients, encourage 30 to 60 minutes of moderate-intensity aerobic activity, such as brisk walking, on most, preferably all, days of the week, supplemented by an increase in daily lifestyle activities (e.g., walking breaks at work, gardening, household work).
	Encourage resistance training 2 days per week.
	Advise medically supervised programs for high-risk patients (e.g., recent acute coronary syndrome or revascularization, heart failure).
WEIGHT MANAGEMENT	Assess body mass index and/or waist circumference on each visit and consistently encourage weight maintenance/reduction through an appropriate balance of physical activity, caloric intake, and formal behavioral programs when indicated to maintain/achieve body mass index between 18.5 and 24.9 kg/m²
Goal: Body mass index: 18.5 to 24.9 kg/m² Waist circumference: men <40 inches, women <35 inches	If waist circumference (measured horizontally at the iliac crest) is ≥35 inches in women and ≥40 inches in men, initiate lifestyle changes and consider treatment strategies for metabolic syndrome as indicated.
	The initial goal of weight loss therapy should be to reduce body weight by approximately 10% from baseline.
	With success, further weight loss can be attempted if indicated through further assessment.

ACE, angiotensin-converting enzyme; HDL-C, high-density lipoprotein cholesterol; LDL-C, low density lipoprotein cholesterol
SOURCE: *Reprinted with permission from Smith SC Jr, Allen J, Blair SN, et al.[2]*

TABLE 51–8

Comparative Efficacy of the Six Currently Available Statins on Lipids and Lipoproteins in Patients without Hypertriglyceridemia Changes in Lipid and Lipoprotein Levels[a]

ROSUVA-STATIN	ATORVA-STATIN	SIMVA-STATIN	LOVA-STATIN	PRAVA-STATIN	FLUVA-STATIN	TOTAL	LDL-C	HDL-C	TRIGLYCER-IDES
—	—	10	20	20	40	−22%	−27%	+4–8%	−10–15%
5	10	20	40	40	80	−27%	−34%	+4–8%	−10–20%
10	20	40	80	80	—	−32%	−41%	+4–8%	−15–25%
20	40	80	—	—	—	−37%	−48%	+4–8%	−20–30%
40	80	—	—	—	—	−42%	−55%	[b]	−25–35%

[a]For the purpose of illustration, the lipid and lipoprotein responses are based on short-term clinical trials and are approximations of what might be observed in clinical practice.
[b]The increase in HDL-C for atorvastatin is in the range of 4–8%; the rise for rosuvastatin is 8–14%.

ered to less than 200 mg/d. There is growing interest in obtaining further risk reduction by use of dietary adjuncts. A daily intake of 2 to 3 g/d of plant stanols or sterol esters will reduce LDL-C concentrations from 6 to 15 percent beyond that which can be achieved by reducing cholesterol-raising fatty acids and cholesterol in the diet.[3] Consuming 5 to 10 g of viscous fiber per day reduces LDL-C levels by approximately 5 percent. Unsaturated fatty acids (monounsaturated, n-6 polyunsaturated, and n-3 polyunsaturated fatty acids) will lower LDL and may reduce global risk for CHD via several other mechanisms.[56–58] When combined with a low-saturated-fat, low-trans-fat diet, the addition of plant sterols, viscous fibers, and nuts can reduce LDL-C comparable to the effect of a low-dose statin.[59]

Statin Efficacy Statins are the most effective cholesterol-lowering drugs available. Table 51–8 compares the efficacy of the currently available statins.

Statin Safety No increase in noncardiovascular mortality has been observed in subjects randomized to active treatment in any of the large statin trials. Furthermore, none of these trials suggests a lower boundary below which LDL-C lowering is ineffective or dangerous. In the Pravastatin or Atorvastatin Evaluation and Infection Therapy (PROVE IT) trial, the subgroups that achieved LDL-C <40 mg/dL and 40 to 60 mg/dL had fewer major cardiac events with no significant difference in safety outcomes.[60] Most patients tolerate statins with few side effects. Occasional patients will have a mild rise in liver transaminases, but this change is not believed to be an indication of hepatotoxicity. Statin-induced myopathy, defined as a serum creatine kinase level of more than 10 times the upper limit of normal, has been observed in 0.1 to 0.5 percent of patients treated with statins during randomized controlled trials.[61] In a series of 45 cases of statin-induced myopathy, the average duration of statin therapy prior to symptom onset was 6 months, and muscle pain resolved after an average of 2 months.[62] In that series, 4 of 10 patients tolerated another statin without recurrent symptoms. Some patients receiving statins develop muscle symptoms but have normal serum creatine kinase levels. Biopsy-confirmed myopathy has been documented in such patients;[63] consequently, normal creatine kinase levels do not rule out statin-induced myopathy in patients with muscle symptoms. The frequency of this condition is unknown.

Rhabdomyolysis, characterized by muscle weakness, myoglobinuria, and renal failure, is a rare complication of statin therapy. In a series of patients with statin-associated myopathy, 13 percent developed rhabdomyolysis requiring hospitalization.[62] Table 51–9 lists risk factors for myopathy and rhabdomyolysis.[64] Analysis from a database of more than 250,000 patients from managed care health plans found the average incidence of rhabdomyolysis for monotherapy with atorvastatin, pravastatin, or simvastatin was 0.44 per 10,000 person-years.[61] The average incidence rose to nearly 6 per

TABLE 51–9

Risk Factors for Severe Myopathy from Statin Therapy

- Age >80 years
- Small body frame and frailty
- Multisystem disease (e.g., chronic renal insufficiency, especially as a result of diabetes)
- Multiple medications
- Specific concomitant medications or consumptions (with various statins, check package insert for warnings)
  - Fibrates (especially gemfibrozil, but other fibrates too)
  - Nicotinic acid (rarely)
  - Cyclosporine
  - Azole antifungals
  - Itraconazole and ketoconazole
  - Macrolide antibiotics
  - Erythromycin and clarithromycin
  - HIV protease inhibitors
  - Nefazodone (antidepressant)
  - Verapamil
  - Large quantities of grapefruit juice (>1 quart per day)
  - Alcohol abuse (independently predisposes to myopathy)
- Perioperative periods[a]
- Acute illnesses[a]

[a]In most patients admitted to the hospital for acute illnesses or surgery, statin therapy should be temporarily discontinued.
SOURCE: Adapted from Pasternak RC, Smith SC Jr, Bairey-Merz CN, et al. ACC/AHA/NHLBI clinical advisory on the use and safety of statins. Circulation 2002;106;1024–1028, with permission.

TABLE 51–10

Drug Therapy Consideration and Goals of Therapy for Primary Prevention

		LDL CHOLESTEROL	
RISK CATEGORY	10-YEAR RISK FOR CHD	LEVEL AT WHICH TO CONSIDER DRUG THERAPY	PRIMARY GOAL OF THERAPY
Multiple (2+) risk factors	>20% (includes all CHD risk equivalents[a])	>100 mg/dL[b]	<100 mg/dL
	10–20%	≥130 mg/dL[c]	<130 mg/dL
	<10%	≥160 mg/dL	<130 mg/dL
0–1 risk factor	<10%	≥190 mg/dL[d]	<160 mg/dL

[a]Most patients with CHD risk equivalents have multiple risk factors and a 10-year risk >20 percent. They include patients with noncoronary forms of clinical atherosclerosis, diabetes, and multiple (2+) risk factors with a 10-year risk >20 percent by Framingham scoring.
[b]When LDL cholesterol is >130 mg/dL, a cholesterol-lowering drug can be started concomitantly with therapeutic lifestyle change (TLC). If baseline LDL cholesterol is 100–129 mg/dL, TLC should be started immediately. Concomitant use of drugs is optional; several options for drug therapy are available (e.g., statins, bile acid sequestrants, fibrates, nicotinic acid).
[c]When LDL cholesterol is in the range of 130–159 mg/dL, drug therapy can be used if necessary to reach the LDL-cholesterol goal of <130 mg/dL, after an adequate trial of TLC.
[d]When LDL cholesterol is in the range of 160–189 mg/dL, use of cholesterol-lowering drugs is optional, depending on response to TLC diet.

10,000 person-years when these statins were combined with a fibrate. The rate for monotherapy with cerivastatin, which has been withdrawn from the market, was greater than 5 per 10,000 person-years, and the risk rose to approximately 1 in every 10 patients per year who were treated with cerivastatin plus a fibrate.

Pleiotropic Effects Statins may confer benefits that go beyond LDL-C lowering. These potential benefits, known as *pleiotropic effects*, include antiinflammatory, vascular, and immune-altering properties. The existence of cardiovascular pleiotropic effects has been questioned, because in patients with stable coronary disease there is a linear relationship between LDL-C reduction and event reduction, regardless of the method by which LDL-C is reduced (i.e., diet, bile acid-binding resins, ileal bypass, and different statins).[65–67] Proposed noncardiovascular benefits of statins include a reduced risk of breast cancer,[68,69] colon cancer,[70] osteoporosis,[71] and severe sepsis,[72] and attenuation of multiple sclerosis.[73] Of these proposed pleiotropic effects, data are strongest for antiinflammatory effects and all statins lower CRP in a manner only partially related to LDL reduction.[74] Furthermore, in clinical trials of both primary and secondary prevention, the magnitude of benefit attributable to statin therapy is greater among those with elevated CRP levels.[75,76]

Goals of Therapy for LDL Cholesterol Tables 51–10 and 51–11 summarize the NCEP ATP III LDL-C goals and recommendations for initiation of drug therapy.

Combination Therapy for LDL-C Lowering For every doubling of the dose of a statin, LDL-C will fall by only approximately 6 percent. Another strategy to achieve NCEP LDL-C goals is to add another agent to a statin, namely ezetimibe, niacin, or a bile acid sequestrant. Another rationale for combining other lipid medications with statins is that statin monotherapy reduces the relative risk of coronary events by approximately 30 percent, meaning that 70 percent of events are *not* prevented. Improving *other* elements of disordered lipid metabolism beyond LDL-C, such as remnant lipoproteins or low HDL-C, may improve clinical outcomes, and

this hypothesis is being tested in large scale clinical trials. Table 51–12 summarizes the efficacy of different classes of lipid-altering medications. Ezetimibe is primarily effective in lowering LDL-C. It is well-tolerated and has an excellent safety profile when combined with statins.[77] When patients are already taking a statin, the addition of ezetimibe will result in an approximately 25 percent additional LDL-C lowering.[78] The addition of ezetimibe to statin therapy also leads to a further reduction in CRP even though ezetimibe on its own has no effect on this inflammatory biomarker. It is important to recognize, however, that no clinical end point trials using ezetimibe as monotherapy or in combination with statins have been completed. Niacin should be considered in combination with a statin when triglycerides are elevated and/or HDL-C is reduced in combination with high LDL-C. Only about three-fourths of patients can remain on niacin in the long-term because of flushing, itching, skin rash, a rise in plasma glucose,

TABLE 51–11

Drug Therapy Consideration and Goals of Therapy for Secondary Prevention

	LDL CHOLESTEROL	
RISK CATEGORY	LEVEL AT WHICH TO CONSIDER DRUG THERAPY[c]	PRIMARY GOAL OF THERAPY
Very High[a]	≥70 mg/dL	<70 mg/dL
High[b]	≥100 mg/dL	<100 mg/dL

[a]Defined as patients with established cardiovascular disease plus (1) multiple major risk factors (especially diabetes), (2) severe and poorly controlled risk factors (especially continued cigarette smoking), (3) multiple risk factors of the metabolic syndrome (especially triglycerides ≥200 mg/dL plus non–HDL-C ≥130 mg/dL with HDL-C <40 mg/dL), and (4) patients with acute coronary syndromes.
[b]Defined as patients with CHD without high-risk characteristics as indicated above, or patients with CHD risk equivalents.
[c]The authors recommend statin therapy in all high- and very-high-risk patients regardless of baseline LDL-C.

TABLE 51–12

Efficacy of Different Classes of Lipid-Altering Medications

DRUG	RANGE OF LIPID AND LIPOPROTEIN EFFECTS (% CHANGE)		
	LDL CHOLESTEROL	HDL CHOLESTEROL	TRIGLYCERIDES
Statins	−20–55	+5–15	−10–20
Niacin	−10–25	+10–35	−25–50
Resins	−15–30	+3–5	a
Fibrates	−10–15a	+10–20	−35–50
Ezetimibe	−15–25	+2–3	−5–10
Omega-3 fatty acids	+5–10	+1–3	−20–30

aMay increase in patients with preexisting hypertriglyceridemia.

uric acid, and liver transaminases, and, rarely, frank hepatotoxicity. Extended-release and slow-release niacin is better tolerated than immediate-release niacin, but the dose should not exceed 2000 mg/d. In the long-term followup of the Coronary Drug Project, niacin reduced total mortality.[79] Niacin is attractive for combined drug therapy with statins because the combination has a very low risk of severe myopathy, and statin–niacin therapy produces marked clinical and angiographic benefits in patients with low HDL-C and CHD.[80] Bile acid sequestrants are safe to use in combination with statins, but their use is limited because of inconvenience, gastrointestinal side effects, and interference with the absorption of other drugs.

Atherogenic Dyslipidemia: Hypertriglyceridemia, Low High-Density Lipoprotein, and Small, Dense Low-Density Lipoprotein

Although high LDL-C is the primary lipid risk factor, other lipid parameters increase the risk of CHD in persons with or without an elevated LDL-C. Specifically, the combination of elevated concentrations of triglycerides, small, dense LDL-C, and low levels of HDL-C is referred to as *atherogenic dyslipidemia*. This is a complex dyslipidemia that usually results from a generalized metabolic disorder related to *insulin resistance*. Patients with insulin resistance often have the metabolic syndrome (see Metabolic Syndrome below). Although an elevated LDL-C deserves primary emphasis for management, atherogenic dyslipidemia is assuming increasing importance as a contributor to CHD because of the growing prevalence of obesity, diabetes, and the metabolic syndrome. Patients with atherogenic dyslipidemia often have concomitant abnormalities of inflammation (elevated CRP) and hypofibrinolysis (elevated plasminogen activator inhibitor 1 [PAI-1]).

Relation of Atherogenic Dyslipidemia to CHD It has been difficult to establish whether the individual components of atherogenic dyslipidemia are independent risk factors because each of the three lipid components is highly correlated with the other two. Nevertheless, there is growing evidence for independent atherogenicity of each component. For triglycerides, meta-analyses of multiple prospective studies strongly suggest that elevated serum triglycerides are an independent risk factor for CHD.[81] Other prospective studies show that a low level of HDL-C is an independent risk factor.[82] Two important mechanisms by which high-density lipoprotein (HDL) is thought to play a protec-

tive role against atherosclerosis are reverse cholesterol transport and inhibition of LDL oxidation.[83] A lesser body of data also suggests that small, dense LDL particles are more atherogenic than normal-size LDL.[84]

Prevention of CHD among Subjects with Atherogenic Dyslipidemia Clinical trials to support therapy of atherogenic dyslipidemia are less robust than those supporting therapy to lower LDL-C. Nonetheless, there is a growing body of evidence to support a moderate efficacy of drugs that target atherogenic dyslipidemia to reduce major coronary events. The drugs that most effectively modify atherogenic dyslipidemia are fibrates and niacin. Several trials with fibrates have shown a significant reduction of major coronary events. The largest of these include the World Health Organization clofibrate trial,[85] the Helsinki Heart Study gemfibrozil trial,[86] and the Veterans Affairs HDL Intervention Trial (VA-HIT) with gemfibrozil.[87,88] Another trial, the Bezafibrate Infarction Prevention Study,[89] was negative overall but showed risk reduction in the subgroup with hypertriglyceridemia. In the Diabetes Atherosclerosis Intervention Study (DAIS) of approximately 400 patients with diabetes and baseline coronary angiograms, those assigned fenofibrate had less angiographic progression than those randomized to placebo.[90] There were fewer clinical events in the fenofibrate group, but this was not statistically significant and the study was not powered to evaluate clinical outcomes. The Fenofibrate Intervention and Event Lowering in Diabetes (FIELD) study found no significant difference in CHD death and nonfatal MI among type 2 diabetics who were randomly treated with fenofibrate versus placebo.[91] Patients randomized to placebo had a higher rate of starting statin therapy, which might have masked a treatment benefit from fenofibrate. Fibrates are not recommended as first-line drugs to reduce LDL-cholesterol levels.

The role of fibrates as add-on therapy to statins is being evaluated in ongoing clinical trials. As noted above, the risk for severe myopathy is increased in patients treated with statins and fibrates. Fenofibrate and bezafibrate are less likely to cause myopathy when used in combination with statins than is gemfibrozil.[92–94] At the present time, it is prudent to limit the use of statin and fibrate combination to higher-risk patients. Fenofibrate can be combined safely with ezetimibe in patients with atherogenic dyslipidemia.[95]

Niacin lowers triglycerides, lowers the concentration of small, dense LDL particles, and raises HDL-C concentration. Niacin has more side effects than fibrates. (See discussion about niacin under Combination Therapy for LDL-C Lowering above.)

Novel therapies for raising HDL-C are under development. A recombinant apolipoprotein A (apoA)-1 Milano/phospholipid complex administered intravenously produced significant regression of coronary atherosclerosis as measured in a small study using intravascular ultrasound.[96] Pharmacologic inhibition of cholesteryl ester transfer protein is capable of raising HDL-C by 50 to 100 percent, and studies are underway to evaluate the impact of cholesteryl ester transfer protein inhibitors on atherosclerosis.[97]

ATHEROGENIC DIET

An atherogenic diet and a lack of physical activity are considered leading preventable causes of death, second only to tobacco use.[98] Considerable epidemiologic data indicate that populations with diets high in saturated and *trans*-fatty acids have higher rates of CHD.[57,99] Conversely, those populations that consume large amounts of calories as vegetables, cereals, and fish have lower rates of CHD.[99] Populations that consume larger amounts of sodium in their diet have higher average blood pressures.[100] Caloric imbalance, in part a result of excess calorie consumption, is related to the rising prevalence of obesity and diabetes. On an individual basis, clinical trials of modified diets have demonstrated reductions in angiographic progression[101] and significant reductions in recurrence of clinical events.[54]

It has been assumed that the harmful effects of the Western diet have been mediated by saturated fats, *trans*-fatty acids, dietary cholesterol, and sodium via their effects on traditional risk factors such as LDL-C, body weight, hyperglycemia, and blood pressure. Part of the effect of a Western diet appears to be attributable to these factors. However, there is evidence for other mechanisms. The Western Electric Study adjusted for traditional factors and continued to find an independent risk associated with dietary cholesterol.[102] The Lyon Diet Heart Study compared a Mediterranean-type diet high in α-linolenic acid with the AHA diet and showed a 65 percent reduction in recurrent coronary events despite no demonstrable change in any of the traditional risk factors.[54] Potential mechanisms responsible for these benefits include antioxidant, antiinflammatory, and antiplatelet effects. Fish consumption and supplementation with omega-3 fatty acids appear to promote cardiovascular health and specifically to protect against sudden death through many possible mechanisms, including antiarrhythmic, antithrombotic, hypolipidemic, and antiinflammatory effects.[56,103,104]

Primary Prevention

Two primary prevention dietary trials with interventions lasting more than 1 year and using clinical end points have been conducted, and these demonstrated significant reductions in clinical events associated with reduced saturated fat and increased polyunsaturated fat intake.[105,106]

Secondary Prevention

Angiographic studies of low-fat diets, such as the STARS trial[107] and the Lifestyle Heart Study,[101] produced a marked reduction in LDL-C and slowed progression of coronary atherosclerosis. However, these studies were too small to test for clinical end-point reduction. The Oslo Diet-Heart Study demonstrated a significant reduction in reinfarction rates with an intervention consisting of a low-saturated-fat diet and smoking cessation.[108] The Lyon Diet Heart Study, with a Mediterranean-type diet enriched in α-linolenic acid, demonstrated a 65 percent reduction in recurrent cardiac events and death over a 4-year period of followup.[54] *The magnitude of benefit in the* Lyon Diet Heart Study *was greater than that shown in any trial of lipid-lowering drugs.*

Practice Recommendations

The current dietary recommendations emphasize a well-balanced diet low in saturated fat, cholesterol, and sodium, while rich in fruits and vegetables.[3,99] Very-low-fat diets are poorly complied with and have few long-term safety and efficacy data to support them.[109] A diet with less than 30 percent of calories from fat is generally recommended, but with caloric content compatible with the maintenance of ideal body weight. For patients with vascular disease or hyperlipidemia, less than 7 percent of calories from saturated fat and less than 200 mg of dietary cholesterol per day are suggested. Monounsaturated fats and omega-3 fatty acids from fish may be a beneficial source of calories, as compared with carbohydrates.[56,110] Consultation with a registered dietitian or other nutrition specialist can be valuable as part of a risk-modification program in high-risk patients.

CIGARETTE SMOKING

A strong dose–response relationship between cigarette smoking and CHD has been observed in both sexes, in the young, in the elderly, and in all racial groups.[111] Cigarette smoking increases risk two- to threefold and interacts with other risk factors to multiply risk. There is no evidence that filters or other modifications of the cigarette reduce risk. Pipe smoking and cigar smoking increase the risk of CHD. More than 1 in every 10 cardiovascular deaths in the world in the year 2000 were attributable to smoking.[112]

Exposure to environmental tobacco smoke, or passive smoking, is now recognized as a modifiable risk factor.[111] In a meta-analysis of 18 epidemiologic studies, exposure to tobacco smoke by nonsmokers was consistently associated with a 20 to 30 percent increase in risk.[113] This is in addition to an increased risk for respiratory tract cancers and other smoking-related diseases.

Pathophysiologic studies have identified multiple mechanisms through which cigarette smoking may cause CHD.[111] Oxidative stress plays a central role in smoking-mediated dysfunction of nitric oxide biosynthesis in endothelial cells. Cigarette smoking also lowers HDL-C. These effects, along with direct effects of carbon monoxide and nicotine, produce endothelial damage. Smokers have increased vascular reactivity, reduced oxygen-carrying capacity, a lower threshold for myocardial ischemia, and increased risk of coronary spasm. Cigarette smoking is also associated with increased levels of fibrinogen and increased platelet aggregability.

Primary Prevention

Cessation of smoking is associated with a precipitous fall in CHD events. *In a previous smoker, the relative risk declines nearly to that of a nonsmoker in a year or less.*[114] It is estimated that a 35-year-old who quits smoking extends his or her survival by 3 to 5 years,[115] with much of the improved life expectancy caused by a reduction in risk for CHD death.

Secondary Prevention

Compared with a post-MI patient who continues to smoke, one who quits smoking reduces the risk of a second MI by 50 percent.[116,117] *The benefits of achieving complete abstinence from smoking for a patient with CHD compare favorably with the health benefits of any intervention in modern cardiology.*

Practice Recommendations

Nothing less than complete cessation of smoking and other tobacco use should be acceptable in patients with cardiovascular disease. Moreover, the home and work environments to which patients return should be smoke free, both to encourage cessation and to reduce the risk from passive smoking. Cardiovascular specialists often have unique and time-limited opportunities to influence the behaviors of patients. After an acute event, the patient and his or her family members may be especially receptive to a smoking cessation intervention.

Smoking cessation guidelines emphasize that tobacco use status be documented in every patient and that every smoker should be offered one or more of three effective treatment interventions.[118] Even a brief intervention may be effective and should, at a minimum, be provided to every patient who uses tobacco (see Table 51–7). The elements of a treatment program found to be effective include social support, skills training, problem solving, and nicotine replacement or other pharmacologic intervention. More intense efforts by the care provider to achieve complete cessation will generally result in a greater success rate. The huge reduction in risk resulting from smoking cessation in the patient with cardiovascular disease provides a strong rationale for sustained and intense efforts to be expended.

Addiction to tobacco is a major barrier to cessation, and a number of pharmacologic agents can be recommended as an adjunct to a concurrent behavioral intervention on the basis of clinical trials demonstrating significantly increased rates of smoking cessation.[119] Sustained-release bupropion, nicotine gum, nicotine inhaler, nicotine nasal spray, and nicotine patch are all first-line drugs to prevent nicotine withdrawal. The safety of using nicotine replacement in patients with coronary disease was initially a concern. Clinical trials of nicotine replacement therapy in patients with stable CHD suggest that nicotine does not increase cardiovascular risk. At worst, the risks of nicotine replacement therapy are no greater than those of cigarette smoking. The risks of nicotine replacement for smokers, even for those with underlying cardiovascular disease, are small and are overwhelmed by the benefits of smoking cessation.[120] Lastly, in addition to bupropion, there is now a second nonnicotine smoking cessation drug, varenicline, approved by the Food and Drug Administration.[121]

Smoking cessation is associated with weight gain, on average 4.4 kg for men and 5.0 kg for women.[122] Because the health hazards of smoking greatly exceed the risks of moderate weight gain, cigarette smokers should be given the clear message that smoking cessation is of the highest priority even if it results in weight gain.

【 】 HYPERTENSION

Several major prospective epidemiologic studies have found that both systolic and diastolic hypertension have a strong, positive, continuous, and graded relationship to CHD without evidence of a threshold risk level of blood pressure (see also Chap. 70).[25] A widened pulse pressure, an indicator of arterial stiffness, is another blood pressure parameter that predicts CHD.[123] *Hypertension clusters with insulin resistance, hyperinsulinemia, glucose intolerance, dyslipidemia, left ventricular hypertrophy, and obesity and occurs in isolation in less than 20 percent of individuals.*[124] The potential mechanisms by which hypertension may cause coronary events include impaired endothelial function, increased endothelial permeability to lipoproteins, increased adherence of leukocytes, increased oxidative stress, hemodynamic stress triggering acute

plaque rupture, and increased myocardial wall stress and oxygen demand.

Primary Prevention

The benefits of reducing blood pressure on the risks of major cardiovascular disease are well established. A meta-analysis of 17 randomized controlled trials of antihypertensive drugs (vs. placebo or usual care) in more than 47,000 men and women with mild to moderate hypertension found that stroke was reduced by 38 percent and CHD was reduced by 16 percent.[125] The mean difference in diastolic blood pressure over 5 years between treatment and control groups was only 5 to 6 mmHg. An important subset in whom events were reduced was composed of elderly subjects with isolated systolic hypertension (systolic blood pressure ≥160 mmHg; diastolic blood pressure ≤90 mmHg).

The comparative effect of different blood pressure-lowering regimens is less well established. The Blood Pressure Lowering Treatment Trialists' Collaboration analyzed data from 29 randomized trials (n = 162,341) to compare the efficacy of angiotensin-converting enzyme (ACE) inhibitors, calcium channel blockers, angiotensin receptor blockers (ARBs), and diuretics or β blockers on the risks of major cardiovascular events and death.[126] In placebo-controlled trials, the relative risks of total major cardiovascular events were reduced by regimens based on ACE inhibitors (relative risk reduction [RRR] 22 percent; 95 percent confidence interval [CI] 17–27) or calcium channel blockers (RRR 18 percent; 95 percent CI 5–29). Greater risk reductions were produced by regimens that targeted lower blood pressure goals (RRR 15 percent; 95 percent CI 5–24). ARB-based regimens reduced the risks of major cardiovascular events (RRR 10 percent; 95 percent CI 4–17) compared with control regimens. There were no significant differences in total major cardiovascular events between regimens based on ACE inhibitors, calcium antagonists, or diuretics or β blockers, although ACE-inhibitor-based regimens reduced blood pressure less. Treatment with any commonly used regimen reduces the risk of total major cardiovascular events, and larger reductions in blood pressure produce larger reductions in risk. Thiazide diuretics and β blockers are independently associated with a higher risk of new-onset type 2 diabetes.[127]

Blood pressure can be lowered by weight loss, exercise, salt restriction, and avoidance of alcohol,[25] but the long-term usefulness of these measures to prevent CHD in hypertensives has not been tested in randomized controlled studies.

Secondary Prevention

Clinical trials to test the effect of blood pressure lowering per se in CHD patients have not been performed.

Practice Recommendations

The Joint National Committee (JNC) on Detection, Evaluation, and Treatment of High Blood Pressure recommends a treatment goal of <140/90 mmHg.[25] A goal of <130/85 mmHg is appropriate for patients with renal insufficiency or congestive heart failure. A goal of <130/80 mmHg is recommended for patients with diabetes.[1] See Chap. 70 for a complete discussion of the treatment of hypertension.

RISK FACTORS FOR WHICH INTERVENTIONS ARE LIKELY TO LOWER RISK OF CORONARY HEART DISEASE

LEFT VENTRICULAR HYPERTROPHY

Left ventricular hypertrophy (LVH), defined either by electrocardiography or echocardiography, is a potent independent risk factor for CHD, roughly doubling the risk of cardiovascular death in both men and women.[128] LVH is the adaptive response of the heart to chronic pressure or volume overload. In addition to hypertension, LVH is associated with obesity, excessive salt intake, advanced age, and heredity.[129] Progressive LVH may lead to decreased left ventricular compliance, decreased coronary reserve, ventricular ectopy, and impaired systolic function. The Framingham Heart Study observed that electrocardiographic (ECG) evidence of LVH regression was associated with a reduction in cardiovascular disease morbidity and mortality.[130] Another observational, prospective evaluation of LVH using echocardiography indicated an improved prognosis among patients with a reduction of left ventricular mass on antihypertensive therapy.[131] Most antihypertensive drugs can reduce LVH, although not all drugs are equally effective in this regard despite their equipotent blood pressure-lowering capabilities. An analysis of double-blind, randomized, controlled studies with parallel group design indicates that ACE inhibitors reduced left ventricular mass by 12 percent, calcium channel blockers by 11 percent, β blockers by 5 percent, and diuretics by 8 percent.[132]

Two large trials provide insight into the clinical relevance of LVH regression. In the Heart Outcomes Prevention Evaluation (HOPE) trial, ramipril resulted in more frequent prevention or regression of LVH compared with placebo. This effect of ramipril on LVH was independent of blood pressure changes and was associated with reduced risk of death, MI, stroke, and heart failure.[133] In the LIFE trial, losartan-based antihypertensive therapy resulted in fewer cardiovascular events and greater LVH regression than atenolol-based treatment.[134] Both the HOPE and the LIFE trials used ECG definitions of LVH.

THE METABOLIC SYNDROME

See Chap. 91 for a complete discussion of the metabolic syndrome.

The NCEP published diagnostic criteria for the metabolic syndrome, a condition characterized by multiple metabolic risk factors and increased risk for CHD,[3] and those criteria have subsequently been revised.[135] Approximately one-fourth of U.S. adults, or 47 million U.S. residents, have the metabolic syndrome.[136] The prevalence increases with age, rising from roughly 7 percent in young adults to more than 40 percent in people age ≥60 years. After adjusting for conventional risk factors, men with the metabolic syndrome are three to four times more likely to die from CHD over an 11-year followup period than are men without the metabolic syndrome.[137]

Patients with the metabolic syndrome should be counseled to make intensive lifestyle changes, especially weight reduction and increased physical activity. Furthermore, in higher-risk patients with the metabolic syndrome, drug therapies directed toward the metabolic risk factors are indicated.

DIABETES MELLITUS

See Chap. 90 for a complete discussion of diabetes and CHD.

Diabetes mellitus is an independent risk factor for CHD, increasing risk for type 1 as well as type 2 patients by two to four times.[14,138] At least 65 percent of people with diabetes die from cardiovascular disease.[4,27] Approximately 25 percent of MI survivors have diabetes. *Diabetic patients without a history of MI have as high a risk of coronary mortality as do nondiabetic patients with a history of MI.*[14] Once patients with type 2 diabetes suffer a myocardial infarction, their prognosis for recurrent MI and survival is much worse than that for CHD patients without diabetes.[14]

Diabetes abolishes the usual protection from CHD afforded a premenopausal woman. Diabetic women have twice the risk of recurrent MI compared with diabetic men.[139] The greater risk of CHD in type 2 diabetic women compared to diabetic men may be explained in part by the greater adverse effect of diabetes on lipoproteins in women.[140]

Potential mechanisms by which diabetes may cause atherosclerosis include low HDL-C, high triglycerides, increased lipoprotein remnant particles, increased small, dense LDL-C, elevated lipoprotein(a) concentration, enhanced lipoprotein oxidation, glycation of LDL-C, increased fibrinogen, increased platelet aggregability, increased CRP and PAI-1, impaired fibrinolysis, increased von Willebrand factor, hyperinsulinemia, and impaired endothelial function.

Primary and Secondary Prevention

Tight glycemic control in patients with type 1 and type 2 diabetes prevents microvascular complications.[141,142] Intensive glycemic control in patients with type 1 diabetes is associated with a dramatic reduction in major cardiovascular events,[143] but the impact of glycemic control on macrovascular complications in patients with type 2 remains uncertain, and awaiting the outcome of large-scale, randomized, controlled trials currently in progress. Pharmacologic interventions to control dyslipidemia and hypertension have been shown to have a clearly favorable effect on CHD in type 2 diabetics.[144]

Practice Recommendations

Weight loss and exercise are key therapeutic interventions because they improve the constellation of metabolic abnormalities that accompany type 2 diabetes. Although the optimal proportion of dietary fat and carbohydrate is controversial, calorie restriction for obesity and avoidance of sugar and saturated fat are recommended. *β Blockers should not be withheld from diabetic patients following MI unless strong contraindications exist, because diabetic MI survivors have fewer deaths if treated with a β blocker.*[145] Although there is no consistent evidence to support chronic intensive glycemic control as a strategy to reduce macrovascular end points, fasting glucose and glycosylated hemoglobin (HbA1c) should be reduced to near normal (HbA1c <7 percent) to prevent microvascular complications.[4] The AHA, NCEP, and American Diabetes Association guidelines recommend a more aggressive LDL-C goal (<100 mg/dL) in primary prevention of CHD in diabetics.[1,3,4] The LDL-C goal for patients with diabetes who have CHD is <70 mg/dL.[7] The blood pressure goal for patients with diabetes is <130/80 mmHg.

【 】 PHYSICAL INACTIVITY

Physical inactivity is an independent risk factor for CHD and roughly doubles the risk.[146] There is a dose–response relation between the amount of exercise performed weekly, from 700 to 2000 kcal of energy, and death from cardiovascular disease and all causes. Data linking sedentary lifestyle with CHD derive from numerous lines of evidence, including animal studies, observational studies, and clinical trials. Moderate-intensity exercise reduces coronary atherosclerosis and widens coronary arteries in monkeys fed an atherogenic diet compared with monkeys fed the same diet but forced to be sedentary. Physical activity slows the progression of angiographically defined coronary atherosclerosis in humans.[146] More than 50 observational studies, primarily of men, have established that physical fitness, on-the-job physical activity, and leisure-time physical activity reduce the risk of CHD.[147] These studies of physical activity are subject to important potential biases, including self-selection and unmeasured confounding variables. An observational study of 73,743 postmenopausal women indicated that both walking and vigorous exercise are associated with substantial reductions in cardiovascular events, and that prolonged sitting predicts increased risk.[148] The risk of MI and sudden cardiac death is greatest during exercise, but the overall risk of sudden cardiac death is reduced among those who exercise regularly.[149] The greatest potential for reduced mortality is in sedentary individuals who become moderately active.[146] Moderate-intensity activity, as opposed to high-intensity activity, produces most of the beneficial effects of physical activity on cardiovascular mortality. A prospective study of more than 72,000 apparently healthy female nurses indicated that brisk walking and vigorous exercise are associated with substantial and similar reductions in coronary events.[150] Shorter exercise sessions can reduce CHD risk as effectively as longer sessions, provided that the total energy expended is similar.[151] In addition to decreasing myocardial oxygen demand and increasing myocardial efficiency and electrical stability, other potential mechanisms of benefit include increasing HDL-C, lowering triglycerides, reducing blood pressure, reducing obesity, improving insulin sensitivity, decreasing platelet aggregation, and increasing fibrinolysis.[147]

Primary Prevention

A randomized, controlled trial of physical activity for primary prevention of CHD is not likely to be conducted because of cost and compliance issues.

Secondary Prevention

Meta-analyses of randomized trials of cardiac rehabilitation with exercise in more than 4000 MI survivors demonstrated a 20 to 25 percent reduction in cardiovascular mortality, although there were no significant differences in nonfatal reinfarction (see Chap. 67 on cardiac rehabilitation).[152,153] Most of the studies combined exercise training with other risk-factor modification.

Practice Recommendations

Every adult with or without CHD should accumulate 30 minutes or more of moderate-intensity physical activity on most, preferably all, days.[1,2] Only 30 percent of U.S. adults report regular leisure-time physical activity defined as light-to-moderate activity for ≥30 minutes, ≥5 times per week or vigorous activity for ≥20 minutes, ≥3 times per week.[27] Twenty-four percent of U.S. adults report no leisure-time physical activity. Large-scale studies indicate that high-intensity physical activity is *not* required to achieve a mortality benefit, and that 200 calories expended daily in moderate-intensity physical activity will confer the majority of CHD risk reduction that exercise can provide. To accomplish this requires about 30 minutes of brisk walking; however, intermittent activity also provides substantial benefit. Therefore, the minimal goal of 30 minutes can be accumulated in short bouts of typical daily activities like walking, climbing stairs, housework, and gardening. Exercise testing should be recommended to apparently healthy men older than age 45 years and women older than age 55 years who are sedentary, as well as to younger adults with coronary risk factors, particularly if they have diabetes, if the individual plans to start a *vigorous* physical activity program (intensity >60 percent individual maximum oxygen consumption).[154] For secondary prevention, exercise testing is recommended to guide exercise prescription, and high-risk patients should exercise in a medically supervised setting.[2] Structured exercise programs, whether on site or at home, help compliance with an exercise prescription.

【 】 OBESITY

See Chap. 91 for a more complete discussion on obesity.

Obesity is defined by the AHA as a major risk factor for CHD.[155] Obesity is associated with insulin resistance, hyperinsulinemia, type 2 diabetes, hypertension, low HDL-C, hypertriglyceridemia, small dense LDL, inflammation and elevated CRP, thrombosis, diastolic dysfunction, and LVH.[155] In women, obesity contributes independently from physical inactivity to the development of CHD.[156] Obesity accelerates the progression of coronary atherosclerosis in adolescent and young adult men,[157] and it is associated with an increase in cardiovascular and all-cause mortality.[155] Body mass index (BMI) has been adopted widely as a measure of adiposity. BMI is calculated as weight (kg)/height squared (m^2) and is estimated as [weight (pounds)/height (inches)^2] × 704.5. *Normal* weight is defined as a BMI of 18.5 to 24.9, *overweight* is defined as a BMI of 25 to 29.9, and *obesity* is defined as a BMI ≥ 30. The number of overweight and obese adults in the United States has increased dramatically over the past few decades. The latest U.S. survey data indicate that 34 percent of adults in the United States were overweight and an additional 32 percent were obese.[158] BMI correlates with total body fat content. Abdominal obesity adds to the health risks of obesity, and waist circumference correlates positively with abdominal fat content. In some recent analyses, the waist-to-hip ratio has been suggested as a better measure of obesity than the BMI.

In univariate analysis, many observational studies have found obesity strongly and positively correlated with the risk of CHD. In multivariate analysis—when controlling statistically for risk factors such as hypertension, diabetes, and dyslipidemia—obesity is not usually found to be an independent risk factor. This reflects the fact that many of the adverse consequences of obesity are mediated through resultant metabolic risk factors acting as pathogenetic links in the causal pathway. Nevertheless, some large prospective observational studies of long duration indicate that obesity is independently related to coronary and cardiovascular mortality in men and women.[159–161] Weight loss improves insulin sensitivity and glucose disposal, reduces HbA1c in patients with type 2 diabetes, reduces blood pressure and triglycerides, produces a modest reduction in LDL-C, and increases HDL-C.[155]

Primary and Secondary Prevention

Although weight loss leads to a number of favorable short-term changes in metabolism, it is unknown whether long-term weight loss results in reduced CHD events. No primary or secondary prevention trials of weight loss have been conducted.

Practice Recommendations

BMI should be calculated and listed as a vital sign. Waist circumference should be measured in patients with a BMI ≥25.[1,2] Overweight and obese patients should be treated with diet and exercise and waist circumference should be monitored. The initial goal of weight-loss therapy is to reduce body weight by 10 percent from baseline in 12 months. The waist circumference goal is ≤40 inches in men and ≤35 inches in women. Lost weight is usually regained unless a program consisting of dietary therapy, physical activity, and behavior therapy is continued indefinitely.

Currently approved prescription medications for weight loss can help carefully selected obese patients lose weight and reduce the rate at which weight is regained.[162] Rimonabant is a cannabinoid receptor type 1 blocker being developed for the treatment of multiple cardiometabolic risk factors, including abdominal obesity.[163] Fenfluramine and dexfenfluramine were withdrawn from the market because of associated valvular heart disease. CHD end point trials with weight-loss drugs have not been conducted.

RISK FACTORS FOR WHICH INTERVENTIONS HAVE NOT BEEN SHOWN TO LOWER RISK OF CORONARY HEART DISEASE

LIPOPROTEIN(a)

Lipoprotein(a) [Lp(a)] consists of an LDL particle linked via a disulfide bond to an apoA polypeptide chain. Because of homology between apoA and plasminogen, Lp(a) has been hypothesized to serve as a competitive inhibitor for plasminogen binding and thus may inhibit endogenous fibrinolysis.[164] Lp(a) is largely genetically determined, and distributions differ between men and women, as well as between races.

Several retrospective case-control studies support the view that Lp(a) is an independent risk factor for thromboembolic disease. However, results of the major prospective studies evaluating baseline Lp(a) concentration and future risks of MI and stroke are inconsistent.[165] A possible explanation of these divergent results may be that Lp(a) adds to risk only among patients who are at high risk from other factors, such as high LDL-C, low HDL-C, or high fi-

brinogen.[166,167] Nevertheless, a meta-analysis of prospective studies with at least 1 year of followup demonstrated a clear association between Lp(a) and CHD, but causality remains uncertain.[165]

Primary and Secondary Prevention

Although niacin and estrogen reduce Lp(a) levels in some patients, no clinical trials have been conducted to test whether reducing plasma levels reduces clinical events.

Practice Recommendations

It is not yet clear whether Lp(a) provides information incremental to the conventional lipid profile, and no recommendation for screening can be made. If elevated levels prove to increase risk among hypercholesterolemic individuals, it may be prudent to lower levels of LDL-C even more aggressively in such individuals than current guidelines dictate. Knowledge of Lp(a) levels may also be useful in the selection of agents to lower LDL-C (e.g., niacin) and may identify a possible treatable cause in the occasional patient with CHD and none of the major risk factors.

HYPERHOMOCYSTEINEMIA

Homocysteine is a highly reactive sulfur-containing amino acid that is an intermediary product of methionine metabolism. B vitamins have a primary role as cofactors and substrates in homocysteine metabolism such that there is an inverse relationship between plasma homocysteine concentration and levels of folic acid, vitamin B_6, and vitamin B_{12}. Hyperhomocysteinemia is an independent risk marker for cardiovascular disease in several groups of high-risk subjects.[168] Homocysteine and its derivatives cause endothelial dysfunction, arterial intimal-medial thickening, oxidation of LDL-C, and a procoagulant state. The normal fasting levels of homocysteine are between 5 and 15 μmol/L. Hyperhomocysteinemia may be classified as moderate (16 to 30 μmol/L), intermediate (31 to 100 μmol/L), or severe (>100 μmol/L).[168] The most important factor affecting plasma concentration is dietary intake of folate and vitamins B_6 and B_{12}. Other causes of hyperhomocysteinemia include increased age, male sex, menopause, smoking, heavy coffee intake, alcohol, and certain drugs (e.g., bile acid-binding resins, niacin, estrogen-containing oral contraceptives, cyclosporine, and metformin).

A series of cross-sectional and case-control studies and a meta-analysis of 27 observational studies strongly support an independent association between total plasma homocysteine level and increased risk of CHD, cerebrovascular disease, and peripheral vascular disease.[168] Prospective cohort studies have been somewhat conflicting. A large cohort study from Norway reported a relative risk of CHD of 1.4 for every 4 μmol/L increase in plasma homocysteine.[169]

Primary and Secondary Prevention

Notwithstanding the observational data, two large clinical randomized placebo controlled trials in high-risk subjects found no reduction in cardiovascular events from supplementation with folate and vitamins B_6 and B_{12},[170,171] and a *harmful* effect from vitamin B_6 was suggested in one of these studies.[171] These large, negative trials corroborate earlier studies that failed to show a reduction in stroke risk with folate supplementation.[172]

Practice Recommendations

Measurement and treatment of homocysteine are not recommended.

【 】 OXIDATIVE STRESS

Oxidative modification of LDL-C has been hypothesized to play a major role in the initiation and progression of atherosclerosis. Naturally occurring antioxidants such as vitamins E, C, and beta-carotene have been studied as agents for both primary and secondary prevention. Observational epidemiologic studies support the hypothesis that increased dietary intake of antioxidants is associated with reduced cardiovascular risk, with the strongest evidence for vitamin E.[173,174]

Primary Prevention

In the Alpha-Tocopherol, Beta-Carotene Cancer Prevention Study, which enrolled 29,133 male smokers, there was no evidence that vitamin E (given as 50 mg of α-tocopherol daily) reduced the subsequent risk of CHD or stroke, and a small increase in rates of cerebral hemorrhage was reported.[175] In the same trial, beta-carotene was associated with a small increase in lung cancer and deaths caused by CHD. In the Carotene and Efficacy Trial—conducted among 18,314 smokers, former smokers, and asbestos-exposed workers—the combined use of 30 mg/d of beta-carotene plus 25,000 IU of retinol was associated with a small but statistically significant increase in lung cancer and all-cause mortality, as well as a nonsignificant increase in cardiovascular mortality.[176] In contrast, among 22,071 men participating in the Physicians' Health Study who were randomly allocated to 50 mg of beta-carotene on alternate days for a period of 12 years, supplementation resulted in no evidence of benefit or harm in terms of the incidence of cardiovascular disease or cancer.[177] Similarly, among 39,876 apparently healthy U.S. women participating in the Women's Health Study who were randomly assigned to receive vitamin E or placebo and were followed for an average of 10 years, supplementation resulted in no significant effects on the incidences of myocardial infarction or stroke.[178] There was a significant 24 percent reduction in cardiovascular death, but there was no significant effect of vitamin E on total mortality.

Secondary Prevention

Three large, randomized, placebo-controlled trials have tested the hypothesis that vitamin E supplementation might reduce cardiovascular events. The HOPE trial found no overall benefit among 2545 women and 6996 men with cardiovascular disease or diabetes plus at least one additional risk factor randomly allocated to vitamin E 400 IU versus placebo.[179] Similarly, the Heart Protection Study of 20,536 high-risk individuals found no cardiovascular benefit over 5 years from antioxidant vitamin supplementation with 600 mg of vitamin E, 250 mg of vitamin C, and 20 mg of beta-carotene daily.[180] Lastly, the GISSI-Prevenzione trial found no reduction in cardiovascular events from 300 mg daily vitamin E supplementation compared with placebo among 11,324 MI survivors.[181]

Practice Recommendations

Supplementation with beta-carotene, vitamin C, and vitamin E appears to offer no benefit for CHD prevention. Observational evidence supports the consumption of diets rich in fruits and vegetables.

ALCOHOL AND CORONARY HEART DISEASE

Heavy alcohol intake is associated with increased risk of death from several causes and is a major public health concern. However, cross-sectional, case-control, and prospective cohort studies indicate that mild to moderate alcohol consumption is associated with reduced rates of CHD compared with no alcohol consumption.[182,183] These studies suggest a J-shaped relationship between the level of alcohol consumption and total mortality, such that a protective effect is apparent at low levels of consumption (one to two beverages daily), whereas there is substantial hazard among heavy consumers. In large part, this dose-dependent balance reflects summation of three effects: (1) a positive association between alcohol use and cancer; (2) a U-shaped relationship between alcohol use and total cardiovascular disease because of increased risks of cardiomyopathy, sudden death, and hemorrhagic stroke among heavy drinkers; and (3) a well-established L-shaped protective effect for coronary disease.[184] In a large Danish population-based cohort, women who drank at least once a week had a lower risk of CHD than women who drank less frequently, although more frequent alcohol consumption did not result in additional risk reduction.[185] Among men in the same cohort, an inverse association was found between drinking frequency and CHD risk across the entire range of drinking frequencies.

Several mechanisms have been proposed for the cardioprotective effect of moderate alcohol use. Alcohol intake increases total HDL-cholesterol levels as well as HDL2 and HDL3 subfractions.[186–189] Alcohol consumption also has potentially beneficial effects on fibrinolytic function,[190,191] platelet aggregation,[192,193] inflammation, oxidation, and endothelial function.[194]

Primary and Secondary Prevention

There have been no randomized trials of alcohol use for primary or secondary prevention.

Practice Recommendations

How best to advise patients concerning the potential use of alcohol for cardiovascular protection is a complex process because of the potential for abuse.[194,195] Abstinence is advised for patients who are pregnant or who have hepatic disorders, pancreatic disease, congestive heart failure, idiopathic cardiomyopathy, or degenerative neurologic conditions. On the other hand, the recommendation to drink moderately (one drink per day for women and two drinks per day for men) may be safe when made on a case-by-case basis in the absence of a history of abuse or medical contraindication.[195] Whether specific beverage type matters in terms of cardiovascular protection is uncertain. Evidence indicating benefits for white wine, red wine, beer, and liquor suggest that alcohol content rather than type is the more important predictor of cardiovascular risk reduction.[182,183]

UNMODIFIABLE RISK FACTORS

【 】 AGE AND SEX AS RISK FACTORS FOR ATHEROSCLEROTIC DISEASE

The incidence and prevalence of CHD increase sharply with age, so that age might be considered one of the most potent cardiovascular risk factors.[27] Atherosclerotic involvement of the coronary arteries is well established in men by young adulthood, as shown in Korean War and Vietnam War casualties.[196,197] CHD incidence rates in men are similar to those in women who are 10 years older than the men.[198] Approximately 52 percent of women and 46 percent of men will eventually die of atherosclerotic disease.[27] The increased risk for men and older persons provides the rationale for more intense management of modifiable risk factors in these subgroups. Persons at very advanced age should have the risks and benefits of preventive cardiology interventions weighed on an individual basis.

POSTMENOPAUSAL STATUS

CHD is relatively uncommon in premenopausal women. There is a dramatic rise in CHD incidence in women after age 55 years, coinciding with increasing age and a decline in endogenous estrogen levels. Early menopause (natural or surgical) is associated with increased CHD risk. These observations are consistent with the hypothesis that estrogen deficiency permits or promotes CHD and that estrogen reduces risk. Numerous observational studies show that postmenopausal users of estrogen replacement therapy have a 40 to 50 percent lower risk of initial CHD events compared with nonusers.[199,200] Because of their observational design, these studies were subject to selection bias and uncontrolled or unknown confounding variables. In most of these studies, estrogen replacement therapy was unopposed by concomitant progestin therapy. Estrogen raises HDL-C and lowers LDL-C, small, dense LDL-C, and Lp(a). Additional proposed mechanisms by which estrogen may confer benefit include favorable effects on fibrinogen, plasma viscosity, plasminogen activator inhibitor-1, tissue-type plasminogen activator, insulin sensitivity, homocysteine, and markers of platelet aggregation and endothelial cell activation. Furthermore, estrogen enhances endothelium-dependent and endothelium-independent coronary vasodilation and inhibits intimal hyperplasia and smooth muscle migration, promotes angiogenesis, and has antioxidant properties. On the other hand, hormone replacement therapy increases triglycerides, CRP levels, coagulation factor VII, and prothrombin fragments 1 and 2.[200,201] In contrast to oral estrogen, transdermal estrogen decreases plasma triglyceride concentration and produces larger LDL particles resistant to oxidation.[201]

Primary Prevention

The Women's Health Initiative (WHI) conducted the first randomized, controlled, primary prevention trial of postmenopausal hormones in which 16,608 postmenopausal women ages 50 to 79 years with an intact uterus at baseline were randomized to conjugated equine estrogens 0.625 mg/d plus medroxyprogesterone acetate 2.5 mg/d or placebo.[199] The planned duration of the trial was 8.5 years. The primary outcome was nonfatal MI and CHD death. The primary adverse outcome was invasive breast cancer. The study was terminated prematurely because women in the active hormone group had an excess incidence of invasive breast cancer. Estimated hazard ratios (nominal 95 percent CIs) for other outcomes were as follows: CHD, 1.29 (1.02 to 1.63); stroke, 1.41 (1.07 to 1.85); pulmonary embolism, 2.13 (1.39 to 3.25); colorectal cancer, 0.63 (0.43 to 0.92); endometrial cancer, 0.83 (0.47 to

1.47); hip fracture, 0.66 (0.45 to 0.98); and death as a result of other causes, 0.92 (0.74 to 1.14). Absolute excess risks per 10,000 person-years attributable to estrogen plus progestin were 7 more CHD events, 8 more strokes, 8 more pulmonary emboli, and 8 more invasive breast cancers, while absolute risk reductions per 10,000 person-years were 6 fewer colorectal cancers and 5 fewer hip fractures. The absolute excess risk of events included in the global index was 19 per 10,000 person-years. All-cause mortality was not affected. The investigators concluded that the risk of estrogen plus progestin exceeded the benefit for the primary prevention of CHD and recommended that this regimen should not be initiated or continued for primary prevention of CHD.

Secondary Prevention

The Heart and Estrogen Progestin Replacement Study (HERS) investigated the impact of estrogen plus progestin on the risk of CHD in 2763 postmenopausal women with established coronary disease and an intact uterus.[202] Subjects were randomly assigned 0.625 mg of conjugated equine estrogens plus 2.5 mg of medroxyprogesterone daily or a placebo, with a mean followup of 4 years. There was no difference in the primary end point of nonfatal MI or CHD death. The lack of an overall effect occurred despite a net 11 percent lower LDL level and 10 percent higher HDL level in the hormone treatment group. Although there was no difference overall between groups, there was a statistically significant time trend, with more CHD events in the hormone group in year 1 and fewer events in years 4 and 5. More women in the hormone group suffered venous thromboembolic events and gallbladder disease. A report of the unblinded followup after an additional 2.7 years (HERS II) was completed in 2321 subjects.[203] There were no significant decreases in rates of any cardiovascular events among women assigned to hormone therapy compared with placebo in HERS, HERS II, or overall. The investigators concluded that postmenopausal hormone therapy should not be used to reduce risk for CHD in women with established CHD.

Practice Recommendations

On the basis of WHI and HERS, women with and without CHD who have not been on hormone replacement therapy should not be started on hormone therapy for primary or secondary prevention.[199,200,203,204] The decision to continue or discontinue hormone therapy should be based on established noncardiovascular benefits and risks, and patient preference. In chronic users of hormone therapy, medication should be discontinued, at least temporarily, if a woman develops an acute coronary syndrome or is immobilized. Oral estrogen therapy is contraindicated in women with hypertriglyceridemia (e.g., serum triglycerides >400 mg/dL), but transdermal estrogen might be an appropriate substitute in such women for noncardiovascular indications.[201]

SOCIOECONOMIC STATUS: AN UNMODIFIABLE CORONARY RISK FACTOR?

At any one point in time, markedly different CHD rates may be observed between socioeconomic subgroups of the population, as defined by occupation, education, income, and other measures. As a group becomes affluent, its members use their new wealth to purchase high-fat and high-salt foods, tobacco products, and auto-mobiles. Less-affluent groups lag behind this development, achieving access to these potentially deleterious products later. Affluent groups then learn about and adopt healthful lifestyles, reducing deleterious behaviors. Again, less-affluent and less-educated groups lag behind, eventually exceeding the rates of CHD in those educated groups whose CHD rates have begun to fall.

Currently, persons with low socioeconomic status are at high risk for CHD. A number of mechanisms may explain this.[205] First, risk factors for atherosclerosis—such as smoking, hypertension, obesity, and sedentary lifestyle—are higher in persons with low socioeconomic status. Second, some of these risk factors, as well as psychosocial responses to stressors, may increase exposure to CHD triggers in these groups. Finally, these groups have less access to care.

[ ] FAMILY HISTORY OF EARLY ONSET CORONARY HEART DISEASE

More than 35 case-control and prospective studies have consistently identified an association between CHD and a history of first-degree relatives with early onset CHD.[206] This risk generally persists even after adjustment for other risk factors. The family history most predictive of coronary disease is that of a first-degree relative developing CHD at an early age. Although CHD in a male relative with onset at age 55 years or younger or a female relative with onset at age 65 years or younger is defined as a positive family history, the larger the number of relatives with early onset CHD or the younger the age of CHD onset in the relative, the stronger is the predictive value.[207,208]

Although considered a nonmodifiable risk factor, a positive family history should result in the careful screening of individual risk factors known to aggregate in families.156 Such familial aggregations may represent monogenic factors with known phenotypic expressions and inheritance patterns, polygenic factors with less-clear modes of expression and inheritance, or shared environments. In early CHD families, Williams et al. estimate that only 10 percent of families will not have a concordant risk factor,[208] most of which are amenable to intervention. Thus, family members of patients with CHD at a young age represent fruitful targets for risk factor assessment. However, risk factor screening often does not extend beyond the coronary patient. A strong recommendation that siblings and children of early CHD patients be screened for CHD risk factors should be delivered to each patient and their family members.

ADDITIONAL EMERGING RISK FACTORS
[ ] INFLAMMATORY MARKERS
Fibrinogen

Inflammation is involved in the initiation, growth, and complication of the atherosclerotic plaque.[24,209] This provides the rationale for the use of inflammatory markers as indicators of atherosclerosis and predictors of atherosclerotic complications. *Several studies have shown that plasma fibrinogen level predicts the future risk of MI and stroke.*[166,210] When pooled, these studies indicate that individuals with fibrinogen concentrations in the upper third of the control distribution have a relative risk of future cardiovascular disease 2.0 to 2.5 times that of individuals with lower levels.[210] High fibrinogen

levels result in increased whole-blood viscosity and may play a direct role in atherogenesis and platelet aggregation. Fibrinogen levels increase with smoking, age, oral contraceptive use, and diabetes, and decrease with physical activity.[211] This risk variable is poorly correlated with dyslipidemia and therefore may provide additional prognostic information beyond lipid and lipoprotein measurement. Unfortunately, clinical assays for fibrinogen remain poorly standardized as several methods of measurement are used. Newer mass based immunoassays for fibrinogen may improve this current limitation.

C-Reactive Protein

The desirable characteristics of a laboratory test to assess inflammation are stability of the analyte, the commercial availability of the assay, standardization of the assay to allow comparison of the results, and the precision of the assay as measured by the coefficient of variation.[24] Given these considerations, high-sensitivity CRP is currently the best candidate assay to identify and monitor the inflammatory process. CRP is an acute-phase reactant derived from the liver. *CRP is increased with hypertension, obesity, cigarette smoking, metabolic syndrome, diabetes, low HDL-C/high triglycerides, postmenopausal hormone use, chronic infections, and chronic inflammation. CRP is decreased with moderate alcohol consumption, physical activity, weight loss, and treatment with statins, fibrates, niacin, thiazolidinediones, and angiotensin receptor blockade.*[24,212,213]

Several nested case-control studies, as well as large-scale prospective studies, have shown a single, nonfasting measure of CRP to be a potent predictor of first cardiovascular events among men, women, the elderly, those with metabolic syndrome or diabetes, and smokers.[24,212] Exercise frequency and body mass both correlate with CRP levels,[214,215] but CRP levels correlate minimally with lipid levels. CRP has an independent association with incident coronary events after adjusting for conventional risk factors using the Framingham Risk Score, including LDL cholesterol.[24,212] CRP is a stronger predictor of risk than LDL cholesterol or nuclear magnetic resonance-based evaluation of LDL-C particle size and concentration.[212] CRP can differentiate patients with the metabolic syndrome into relatively low-, moderate-, and high-risk groups. *Consequently, CRP is an independent predictor of incident cardiovascular events that adds prognostic information to lipid screening,* to the metabolic syndrome, and to the Framingham Risk Score. Moreover, the addition of CRP to traditional Framingham Risk Factors correctly reclassifies a large proportion of individuals otherwise considered at "intermediate risk" and thus may provide an improved method for risk stratification.[16]

Weight loss, diet, exercise, and smoking cessation all reduce CRP levels.[212] Statins lower CRP levels by 15 to 25 percent as early as 6 weeks after initiation of therapy.[212] Statin therapy results in a greater clinical benefit when levels of CRP are elevated,[76,216] and statins lower CRP levels in a manner largely independent of LDL cholesterol levels.[216,217]

Survival data from the Women's Health Study demonstrate event-free survival was worse for those with elevated CRP and low LDL than for those with elevated LDL and low CRP.[24] The magnitude of relative risk reduction attributable to low-dose aspirin in reducing risk of first MI appears to be greatest among those with elevated CRP and declines proportionately in direct relation to CRP levels.[212]

Primary Prevention A randomized, placebo-controlled trial is in progress to determine whether long-term treatment with rosuvastatin will reduce cardiovascular end points among apparently healthy individuals with low LDL-C and elevated CRP.[218]

Secondary Prevention Prespecified analysis of the PROVE IT trial found that achieving a lower CRP level with statin therapy is associated with a lower risk of recurrent events in patients with acute coronary syndromes. In that trial of acute coronary syndrome patients, those who achieved the "dual goals" of LDL-C <70 mg/dL and CRP levels <2 mg/L on statin therapy had markedly improved event-free survival compared with those who achieved only one or neither of these poststatin targets.[8]

Practice Recommendations The AHA and Centers for Disease Control *endorse the optional use of CRP in primary prevention of patients at intermediate risk to help direct further evaluation and therapy (class IIa, level of evidence B).* For the purpose of cardiovascular risk prediction, a "high-sensitivity" CRP (hsCRP) test is required. *In patients with stable coronary disease or acute coronary syndromes, hsCRP measurement may be useful as an independent marker for assessing probability of recurrent events. Measurement of hsCRP for widespread global screening of the adult population is not recommended.*[24] *hsCRP measurement may be useful to monitor therapy in patients with established CHD.*[8] Low risk is defined as <1.0 mg/L, average risk is 1.0 to 3.0 mg/L, and high risk is >3.0 mg/L. These risk categories correspond to approximate tertiles of hsCRP in the adult population. The high risk tertile carries a twofold increase in relative risk compared with the low-risk tertile.[24] However, the relationship between hsCRP and vascular risk is linear across a wide range of levels such that those with hsCRP <0.5 mg/L are at very low risk, whereas those with persistently elevated levels of 10 mg/L are at markedly elevated risk.[219]

ENDOGENOUS FIBRINOLYSIS: TISSUE-TYPE PLASMINOGEN ACTIVATOR, PAI-1, AND D-DIMER

The activity of the endogenous fibrinolytic system reflects a balance between plasma concentration of tissue-type plasminogen activator (tPA) and its primary inhibitor, PAI-1. Prospective studies of initially healthy individuals,[220,221] as well as of patients with known CHD,[222] indicate that elevated antigen levels of both enzymes are associated with increased risk of future MI. D-Dimer and tPA concentrations are elevated in relatives of patients with premature CHD compared with healthy controls.[223]

Because both tPA and PAI-1 contribute to the net fibrinolytic balance, it has been hypothesized that individuals at risk for future vascular occlusive events suffer from a net inhibition of fibrinolytic function, a finding supported in at least one prospective study.[224] Other data, however, indicate that elevations of D-dimer are also associated with increased risk of future MI.[225] Because plasma D-dimer levels increase with fibrinogen turnover, these data raise the possibility that the endogenous fibrinolytic system is activated among individuals at risk.

Evidence is not available to support fibrinogen reduction as a measure to prevent CHD. Many factors affect endogenous fibrinolytic activity, including obesity, estrogen status, and exercise. In addition, pharmacologic interventions may soon be available that can favorably shift fibrinolytic function in an attempt to reduce

vascular risk. To date, aspirin therapy, alcohol use, and ACE inhibitors have all shown promise in this regard.[226]

OTHER PHARMACOLOGIC THERAPY

ANTIPLATELET AND ANTICOAGULANT THERAPY

Primary Prevention

Several prevention trials of aspirin have been completed in healthy men. The largest of these, the Physicians' Health Study, enrolled 22,071 apparently healthy male physicians 40 to 84 years of age and randomized them to 325 mg of aspirin on alternate days or to placebo.[227] Aspirin resulted in a highly statistically significant 44 percent reduction in nonfatal MI with no benefit or significant hazard for stroke.

By contrast, the results of the Women's Health Study, a large randomized trial of low-dose aspirin in the primary prevention of cardiovascular disease in women were not fully consistent with the findings in men. The study randomized 39,876 initially healthy women 45 years of age or older to receive 100 mg of aspirin on alternate days or placebo and then monitored the women for 10 years for a first major cardiovascular event (i.e., nonfatal myocardial infarction, nonfatal stroke, or death from cardiovascular causes).[228] In this trial, aspirin use was associated with a nonsignificant 9 percent reduction in risk for a first cardiovascular event that was almost entirely attributable to a statistically significant 17 percent reduction in stroke. This stroke reduction was the result of a 24 percent reduction in ischemic stroke and a nonsignificant increase in the risk of hemorrhagic stroke. In contrast with prior studies in men, aspirin had no significant effect on the risk of fatal or nonfatal MI. Subgroup analyses showed that aspirin significantly reduced the risk of major cardiovascular events, ischemic stroke, and MI among women 65 years of age or older. Thus, although the dose of aspirin used in the Women's Health Study (100 mg every other day) was less than that used in the Physicians' Health Study (325 mg every other day), this lower dose appeared adequate for prevention of heart disease in women older than the age of 65 years.

A sex-specific meta-analysis was performed of randomized controlled trials of aspirin for the primary prevention of cardiovascular events in women and men has confirmed the findings of the individual trials cited above.[229] Among 51,342 women, aspirin therapy was associated with a significant 12 percent reduction in cardiovascular events (nonfatal MI, nonfatal stroke, and cardiovascular death) and a 17 percent reduction in stroke, primarily as a consequence of reduced rates of ischemic stroke. *There was no significant effect on MI or cardiovascular mortality in women.* Among 44,114 men, aspirin therapy was associated with a significant 14 percent reduction in cardiovascular events and a 32 percent reduction in MI. *There was no significant effect on stroke or cardiovascular mortality in men.* Hence, for women and men, aspirin therapy reduces the risk of a composite of cardiovascular events because of its effect on reducing the risk of ischemic stroke in women and MI in men. For clinical purposes, it is important to recognize that when compared to men, women suffer a proportionately higher percentage of strokes as compared to myocardial infarction.

The CHARISMA trial compared the combination of clopidogrel (75 mg/d) plus aspirin (75 to 162 mg/d) versus placebo plus aspirin in more than 15,000 patients with established cardiovascular disease or multiple risk factors.[230] The primary end point was a composite of MI, stroke, or cardiovascular death. There was no significant difference in the primary end point between groups. In the asymptomatic cohort, there was a suggestion of harm from clopidogrel with more primary end points and a higher rate of death. Although use of clopidogrel remains important for patients with recent stent placement, its use in primary prevention cannot be recommended.

Secondary Prevention

The Antiplatelet Trialists' collaborative meta-analysis of randomized trials of antiplatelet therapy among high-risk patients with preexisting vascular disease reviewed 287 studies involving 135,000 patients in comparisons of antiplatelet therapy versus control and 77,000 in comparisons of different antiplatelet regimens.[231] Overall, allocation to antiplatelet therapy reduced serious vascular events by approximately 25 percent. Aspirin was the most widely studied drug, with doses of 75 to 150 mg daily at least as effective as higher doses. Large-scale randomized comparisons of the effects of other antiplatelet drugs versus aspirin was available only for clopidogrel. Clopidogrel reduced serious vascular events by 10 percent compared with aspirin ($p = 0.03$), making that drug an appropriate alternative for patients with a contraindication to aspirin. Addition of dipyridamole to aspirin produced no additional benefit to that derived from aspirin alone.

A meta-analysis of 31 trials evaluated the role of chronic oral anticoagulant therapy in the secondary prevention of coronary disease.[232] Moderate-intensity (international normalized ratio [INR] 2 to 3) and high-intensity (INR 2.8 to 4.8) anticoagulation are effective in reducing MI and stroke, but increase the risk of bleeding. In the presence of aspirin, low-intensity anticoagulation does not appear to be superior to aspirin alone, whereas moderate- to high-intensity anticoagulation and aspirin versus aspirin alone appears promising and the bleeding risk is modest.[232,233]

Practice Recommendations

Low-dose aspirin, 75–160 mg/d, is recommended for primary prevention among individuals with a 10-year risk of CHD greater than or equal to 10 percent.[1] For secondary prevention, 75 to 160 mg of aspirin daily is recommended, with treatment continued indefinitely.[2] See Chaps. 61, 62, and 65 for recommendations regarding antiplatelet therapy following acute coronary syndromes, or percutaneous coronary intervention with stent placement, coronary artery bypass grafting.

【 】 β-ADRENERGIC BLOCKING AGENTS

β-Adrenergic blocking agents reduce heart rate, systemic blood pressure, and ventricular contractility—all factors that decrease myocardial oxygen consumption. β Blockers further have antiarrhythmic properties and appear to increase thresholds for ventricular fibrillation.[234]

Primary Prevention

Few clinical trial data are available that directly test β-blocking agents in the primary prevention of MI. The use of this class of agents in the treatment of hypertension, however, has been shown to be efficacious for CHD prevention,[235] and β blockers have few long-term side effects. When a patient treated with a β blocker develops CHD, the initial presentation is more likely to be stable angina and less likely to be an acute MI.[53]

Secondary Prevention

The usefulness of β-blocking agents in the acute, subacute, and chronic phases following MI has been demonstrated in many clinical trials. Overview analyses indicate that therapy with β blockers reduces mortality approximately 20 percent compared with placebo.[236,237] The mortality effect of long-term β blockade results primarily from prevention of sudden death (pooled relative risk = 0.68), presumably as a consequence of a reduction in the incidence and complexity of ventricular arrhythmias. β Blockers have also proven effective in reducing rates of nonfatal reinfarction (pooled relative risk = 0.74), an effect more likely to result from chronic reductions in heart rate, contractility, and vascular stress.

Practice Recommendations

For primary prevention, β blockers are recommended as first-line therapy for hypertension.[25] For secondary prevention, β blockers are recommended for all patients who have had MI, an acute coronary syndrome, or left ventricular dysfunction with or without heart failure symptoms, and continued indefinitely unless contraindicated.[2] β Blockers should be considered as chronic therapy for all other patients with coronary or other vascular disease or diabetes unless contraindicated.

【 】 RENIN–ANGIOTENSIN SYSTEM BLOCKERS
Angiotensin-Converting Enzyme Inhibitors

Primary Prevention There are no large, primary prevention, placebo-controlled trials using ACE inhibitors. Meta-analysis of trials comparing ACE inhibitors with other drug classes found no significant differences in total major cardiovascular events between regimens based on ACE inhibitors, calcium antagonists, diuretics, or β blockers, although ACE inhibitor-based regimens reduced blood pressure less.[126]

Secondary Prevention ACE inhibitors were first recognized to reduce mortality in patients with heart failure and reduced left ventricular ejection fraction.[238] Subsequently, this class of agents was recognized as important adjunctive therapy following acute MI. The primary rationale for using these agents in this setting is based on the experimental observation that ACE inhibition slows the process of ventricular remodeling. This effect appears time-dependent in that the use of ACE inhibition after MI requires a sufficient length of therapy to result in detectable changes in ventricular volumes and size. The observation in several trials that rates of recurrent MI may also be reduced with ACE inhibition raises the possibility that these agents also result in enhanced endogenous fibrinolysis.

A meta-analysis of placebo-controlled trials testing ACE inhibitors in patients with coronary disease and preserved left ventricular systolic function found a significant modest beneficial effect on cardiovascular outcomes.[239] There were 16,772 patients randomized to ACE inhibitors and 16,728 randomized to placebo. ACE inhibitors were associated with a 17 percent relative risk reduction in cardiovascular mortality (95 percent CI 0.72–0.96, $p = 0.01$), 16 percent reduction in nonfatal MI (95 percent CI 0.75 to 0.94, $p = 0.003$), and 13 percent reduction in all-cause mortality (95 percent CI 0.81 to 0.94, $p = 0.0003$).

Angiotensin-Receptor Blockers

In the LIFE study, the ARB losartan significantly reduced cardiovascular death, MI, and stroke compared with atenolol in patients with hypertension and left ventricular hypertrophy.[134] In meta-analysis, ARB-based regimens reduced the risks of major cardiovascular events by 10 percent compared with control regimens.[126] For a complete discussion about ARBs in the treatment of heart failure, see Chap. 26.

Practice Recommendation Based on recent, large, randomized, controlled clinical trials, it appears that ACE inhibitors are at least as effective as diuretics in the primary prevention of CHD death or nonfatal MI,[240,241] although national guidelines continue to recommend diuretics or β blockers as first-line agents for the treatment of hypertension.[25] ACE inhibitors and ARBs are appropriate first-line antihypertensive therapy in patients with diabetes and hypertension, and they are an excellent second step after diuretic therapy in hypertensive patients.[25] For secondary prevention, ACE inhibitors should be prescribed indefinitely to all patients following MI and to patients with a left ventricular ejection fraction ≤40 percent, and in those with hypertension, diabetes, or chronic kidney disease, unless contraindicated.[2] ACE inhibitors should be considered as chronic therapy for all other patients with coronary or other atherosclerotic vascular disease. Among lower-risk patients with normal left ventricular ejection fraction in whom cardiovascular risk factors are well controlled and revascularization has been performed, use of ACE inhibitors may be considered optional. ARBs should be prescribed for patients who are intolerant of ACE inhibitors and have heart failure or have had an MI with left ventricular ejection fraction ≤40 percent. ARBs should be considered in other patients with CHD or other atherosclerotic disease who are ACE inhibitor intolerant.

THE PRACTICE OF PREVENTIVE CARDIOLOGY

The evidence for a causal role of risk factors in the etiology of CHD and the feasibility and efficacy of risk factor modification in lowering CHD risk is among the most convincing in all of medicine. Despite this, there are inexcusable gaps in our identification and treatment of coronary risk factors and the application of evidence-based guidelines, even in patients at highest risk.[242–245] An analysis of 138,001 patients from 1470 U.S. hospitals in the National Registry of Myocardial Infarction 3 revealed that only 32 percent of patients hospitalized with acute MI were discharged on lipid-lowering medication.[244] In another study, only 18 percent of 20,809 patients hospitalized with an acute coronary syndrome were discharged on lipid-lowering therapy.[246] Quality improvement initiatives, such as the AHA's hospital-based *Get With the Guidelines* and the ACC's hospital- and office-based *Guidelines Applied in*

Practice, may be making inroads. Data from 3377 U.S. hospitals in 1994 show that upon discharge from acute MI admission, 95 percent of patients were prescribed aspirin, 80 percent of patients with systolic dysfunction were prescribed ACE inhibitors, 93 percent were prescribed β blockers, and 84 percent of smokers were provided smoking-cessation counseling.[27] Data for the year 2004 from 336 hospitals participating in the AHA *Get With the Guidelines* program, including 74,848 patients who were admitted for acute cardiovascular events, showed that upon discharge 92 percent of patients were prescribed aspirin, 67 percent were prescribed ACE inhibitors, 86 percent were prescribed β blockers, 79 percent of patients with LDL-C >100 mg/dL were prescribed lipid medication, 82 percent of smokers were provided smoking-cessation counseling, and 64 percent were referred for cardiac rehabilitation.[27]

The implementation of evidence-based therapies in the outpatient setting has proved more challenging. Among 48,586 outpatients with CHD from 140 medical practices (80 percent cardiology), only 39 percent were treated with lipid-lowering medications and only 11 percent were documented to have LDL-C levels <100 mg/dL.[247] In a national survey of 4885 outpatients, overall 67 percent achieved their LDL cholesterol treatment goal, including 89 percent, 76 percent, and 57 percent, respectively, in the 0 or 1 risk factor, >2 risk factors or CHD, and CHD risk equivalent categories.[9] Patients with diabetes (55 percent) and other CHD risk equivalents (40 percent) were less likely to have achieved their LDL cholesterol targets than were patients with CHD (62 percent). Of the 1447 patients with cardiovascular disease, 75 percent could be classified as very high risk according to ATP III, of whom only 18 percent had an LDL cholesterol level of <70 mg/dL. These results show improved lipid management compared with previous national surveys, but large gaps remain. Once prescribed, long-term adherence to secondary prevention therapies is suboptimal. Data from the Duke Databank for Cardiovascular Disease indicate that although use of evidence-based therapies among CHD patients is increasing, consistent use is poor: 71 percent for aspirin, 20 percent for ACE inhibitors, 46 percent for β blockers, and 44 percent for lipid medication.[248] Thus preventive cardiology strategies backed by strong evidence for efficacy and cost-effectiveness are simply not being applied uniformly or widely, constituting a missed opportunity to reduce the burden of disease.

【 】 BARRIERS TO IMPLEMENTATION OF PREVENTIVE CARDIOLOGY SERVICES

A number of barriers to the implementation of preventive services can be identified at the patient, physician, healthcare setting, and community society levels (Table 51–13).[249,250] The improved implementation of proven interventions therefore requires a variety of strategies targeted at patients, healthcare providers, inpatient care settings, ambulatory care settings, and health systems.

【 】 STRATEGIES TO IMPROVE PREVENTIVE CARDIOLOGY SERVICES

Improving Patient Compliance

Although there is a pervasive tendency to blame the patient, healthcare providers can take a number of actions to improve their

TABLE 51–13

Barriers to Implementation of Preventive Services

Patient
  Lack of knowledge and motivation
  Lack of access to care
  Cultural factors
  Social factors
Physician
  Problem-based focus
  Feedback on prevention is negative or neutral
  Time constraints
  Lack of incentives, including reimbursement
  Lack of training
  Poor knowledge of benefits
  Perceived ineffectiveness
  Lack of skills
  Lack of specialist–generalist communication
  Lack of perceived legitimacy
  Healthcare settings (hospitals, practices, etc.)
  Acute care priority
  Lack of resources and facilities
  Lack of systems for preventive services
  Time and economic constraints
  Poor communication between specialty and primary care
    providers
  Lack of policies and standards
Community/society
  Lack of policies and standards
  Lack of reimbursement

SOURCE: *From Pearson TA, McBride PE, Miller NH, et al. 27th Bethesda Conference: matching the intensity of risk factor management with the hazard for coronary disease events. Task Force 8. Organization of preventive cardiology service. J Am Coll Cardiol 1996;27:1039–1047, with permission.*

patients' compliance with the treatment regimen.[251] These include (1) encouragement to engage in prevention and treatment behaviors essential to adherence with a regimen, such as acceptance and understanding of the need to control risk factors; (2) establishment of specific behavioral or physiological goals; (3) skills training of patients for adopting and maintaining the recommended behaviors; (4) recommending self-monitoring of progress toward the goals; and (5) helping patients anticipate and resolve problems that keep the goals from being realized. This will require regular communication between providers and patients about the goals and actions agreed on.

Improving Performance by Healthcare Providers

Providers must foster effective communication both with their patients and with other health professionals on the preventive cardiology team. Strategies to improve this communication include verbal and written instructions, negotiation of goals and a plan with the patient, and anticipation of barriers to successful attainment of goals. There also must be documentation and monitoring of progress toward goals, with assessment of patient compliance at each visit and reminder systems (e.g., listing smoking status as a vital

sign) to assure that risk factors are identified and attended to. One barrier to physician action in this area is a perceived lack of legitimacy by cardiovascular specialists for involvement in risk-factor management. *Professional societies counter this problem by strongly recommending that risk-factor management should be part of the optimal care of patients who are at high risk for cardiovascular disease and therefore should be considered the responsibility of all healthcare providers.*

Improving the Inpatient Care Setting

Admission to an inpatient unit provides an enormous opportunity for risk-factor modification and behavior change that should not be missed for several reasons. First, the opportunity to reduce short-term risk in patients following infarction or revascularization has not been extensively studied, but several interventions such as antiplatelet therapy, ACE inhibitors, β blockers, and even lipid management appear to provide benefit within days or weeks. Second, the patient and family are aroused to the risk of disability and death, and their receptivity to behavior-change messages is likely highest at this time. Finally, the message communicated to the patient and their primary care provider is that, along with revascularization and pharmacotherapy, behavior change is an important, integral part of their care.

The inpatient setting can be reorganized to provide efficient risk-factor assessment and management. The joint ACC/AHA guidelines for preventing MI and death in patients with atherosclerosis provide a convenient list of risk-factor goals and modification strategies (see Table 51–7).[2] These can be transcribed onto a simple checklist or integrated into more elaborate, perhaps computerized, care protocols. The cardiovascular specialist should confirm the diagnosis of prevalent risk factors, set goals for treatment, and integrate a treatment plan into the overall regimen of care. However, the physician is often not the best person to carry out the plan, partly because of time constraints and acute care focus. A better model is the multidisciplinary team approach, with nurses, nutritionists, pharmacists, and exercise physiologists assigned specific tasks for the patient's care. Factors associated with improved inpatient post-MI β-blocker prescription are shared goals among clinical and administrative staff, substantial administrative support, strong physician leadership advocating β-blocker use, and use of credible data feedback.[252] In one study, routine implementation of secondary prevention guidelines in all hospitalized CHD patients resulted in increased use of aspirin (68 to 92 percent), β blockers (12 to 62 percent), ACE inhibitors (6 to 58 percent), and statins (6 to 86 percent), which were associated with a reduction in recurrent MI and 1-year mortality.[245] The AHA *Get With the Guidelines* is based on the foregoing principles.

Improving the Ambulatory Care Setting

The AHA guidelines for primary prevention of cardiovascular diseases (see Table 51–6) and for comprehensive risk reduction for patients with coronary and other vascular disease (see Table 51–7) provide clear risk-factor goals and risk-reduction strategies.[1,2] The office or clinic should strive to develop an environment supportive of risk factor management, including staff trained in behavior-modification skills, followup protocols, and tracking systems and reminders. A clear assignment of tasks and responsibilities is important, with defined roles for the physician, nurse, nutritionist, and even receptionist.

A number of specialty units might be convenient platforms for risk-factor management. Cardiac rehabilitation has been documented, in meta-analyses of randomized clinical trials, to reduce coronary disease recurrence and death significantly, especially when the service includes risk-factor modification. The patient's extended exposure (after 12 weeks or longer) to a supportive environment provides the opportunity for behavior change, monitoring, and reinforcement. When compared with a contemporary cardiac rehabilitation program, a cardiovascular risk-reduction program supervised by a physician and case managed by a nurse, and a similar program administered by exercise physiologists and guided by a computerized participant management system, produce similarly effective risk-factor change.[253]

Improving the Health System

Supportive of this are a large number of guidelines from professional societies, expert bodies, and governmental agencies that promote preventive cardiology practices. The joint ACC/AHA guidelines in risk reduction are coordinated with more extensive guidelines for individual risk factors, including dyslipidemia,[3] hypertension,[25] smoking,[254] cardiac rehabilitation,[255] and obesity.[31,55] These provide clear recommendations for healthcare providers as to the goals and scenarios required for optimal risk reduction. Increasingly, these guidelines are being used in quality assurance programs that use provision of preventive services and attainment of risk factor goals as quality-of-care indicators. The use of preventive cardiology services as quality indicators has motivated healthcare systems to implement reorganization and reallocation of resources that are effective in improving preventive cardiology care. In addition, the AHA has created a guide for community leaders to reduce the burden of cardiovascular disease at the community level.[256]

REFERENCES

1. Pearson TA, Blair SN, Daniels SR, et al. AHA guidelines for primary prevention of cardiovascular disease and stroke: 2002 update: consensus panel guide to comprehensive risk reduction for adult patients without coronary or other atherosclerotic vascular diseases. *Circulation* 2002;106:388–391.
2. Smith SC Jr, Allen J, Blair SN, et al. AHA/ACC guidelines for secondary prevention for patients with coronary and other atherosclerotic vascular disease: 2006 update: endorsed by the National Heart, Lung, and Blood Institute. *Circulation* 2006;113:2363–2372.
3. Third Report of the National Cholesterol Education Program (NCEP) Expert Panel on Detection, Evaluation, and Treatment of High Blood Cholesterol in Adults (Adult Treatment Panel III) final report. *Circulation* 2002;106:3143–3421.
4. Standards of medical care in diabetes—2006. *Diabetes Care* 2006;29(Suppl 1):S4–S42.
5. Ridker PM, Cook N. Should age and time be eliminated from cardiovascular risk prediction models? Rationale for the creation of a new national risk detection program. *Circulation* 2005;111:657–658.
6. Lloyd-Jones DM, Leip EP, Larson MG, et al. Prediction of lifetime risk for cardiovascular disease by risk factor burden at 50 years of age. *Circulation* 2006;113:791–798.
7. Grundy SM, Cleeman JI, Merz CN, et al. Implications of recent clinical trials for the National Cholesterol Education Program Adult Treatment Panel III guidelines. *Circulation* 2004;110:227–239.
8. Ridker PM, Cannon CP, Morrow D, et al. C-reactive protein levels and outcomes after statin therapy. *N Engl J Med* 2005;352:20–28.
9. Davidson MH, Maki KC, Pearson TA, et al. Results of the National Cholesterol Education (NCEP) program evaluation project utilizing novel e-technology (NEPTUNE) II survey and implications for treatment under the recent NCEP Writing Group recommendations. *Am J Cardiol* 2005;96:556–563.
10. Sacks FM, Pfeffer MA, Moye LA, et al. The effect of pravastatin on coronary events after myocardial infarction in patients with average cholesterol levels. Cholesterol and Recurrent Events Trial investigators. *N Engl J Med* 1996;335:1001–1009.
11. Prevention of cardiovascular events and death with pravastatin in patients with coronary heart disease and a broad range of initial cholesterol levels. The Long-Term Intervention with Pravastatin in Ischaemic Disease (LIPID) Study Group. *N Engl J Med* 1998;339:1349–1357.
12. Cleland JG. Can improved quality of care reduce the costs of managing angina pectoris? *Eur Heart J* 1996;17 Suppl A:29–40.
13. Juul-Moller S, Edvardsson N, Jahnmatz B, et al. Double-blind trial of aspirin in primary prevention of myocardial infarction in patients with stable chronic angina pectoris. The Swedish Angina Pectoris Aspirin Trial (SAPAT) Group. *Lancet* 1992;340:1421–1425.
14. Haffner SM, Lehto S, Ronnemaa T, et al. Mortality from coronary heart disease in subjects with type 2 diabetes and in nondiabetic subjects with and without prior myocardial infarction. *N Engl J Med* 1998;339:229–234.
15. Tsimikas S, Willerson JT, Ridker PM. C-reactive protein and other emerging blood biomarkers to optimize risk stratification of vulnerable patients. *J Am Coll Cardiol* 2006;47:C19–C31.
16. Cook NR, Buring JE, Ridker PM. The effect of including C-reactive protein in cardiovascular risk prediction models for women. *Ann Intern Med* 2006;145:21–29.
17. Executive summary of the third report of the National Cholesterol Education Program (NCEP) Expert Panel on Detection, Evaluation, and Treatment of High Blood Cholesterol in Adults (Adult Treatment Panel III). *JAMA* 2001;285:2486–2497.
18. Smith SC Jr, Amsterdam E, Balady GJ, et al. Prevention Conference V. Beyond secondary prevention: identifying the high-risk patient for primary prevention: tests for silent and inducible ischemia: Writing Group II. *Circulation* 2000;101:E12–E16.
19. O'Rourke RA, Brundage BH, Froelicher VF, et al. American College of Cardiology/American Heart Association Expert consensus document on electron-beam computed tomography for the diagnosis and prognosis of coronary artery disease: committee members. *Circulation* 2000;102:126–140.
20. Greenland P, Smith SC Jr, Grundy SM. Improving coronary heart disease risk assessment in asymptomatic people: role of traditional risk factors and noninvasive cardiovascular tests. *Circulation* 2001;104:1863–1867.
21. Hodis HN, Mack WJ, LaBree L, et al. The role of carotid arterial intima-media thickness in predicting clinical coronary events. *Ann Intern Med* 1998;128:262–269.
22. van der Meer IM, Bots ML, Hofman A, et al. Predictive value of noninvasive measures of atherosclerosis for incident myocardial infarction: the Rotterdam Study. *Circulation* 2004;109:1089–1094.
23. Kalia NK, Miller LG, Nasir K, et al. Visualizing coronary calcium is associated with improvements in adherence to statin therapy. *Atherosclerosis* 2006;185:394–399.
24. Pearson TA, Mensah GA, Alexander RW, et al. Markers of inflammation and cardiovascular disease: application to clinical and public health practice: a statement for healthcare professionals from the Centers for Disease Control and Prevention and the American Heart Association. *Circulation* 2003;107:499–511.
25. Chobanian AV, Bakris GL, Black HR, et al. The seventh report of the Joint National Committee on Prevention, Detection, Evaluation, and Treatment of High Blood Pressure: the JNC 7 report. *JAMA* 2003;289:2560–2572.
26. Goldstein JL, Kita T, Brown MS. Defective lipoprotein receptors and atherosclerosis. Lessons from an animal counterpart of familial hypercholesterolemia. *N Engl J Med* 1983;309:288–296.
27. Thom T, Haase N, Rosamond W, et al. Heart disease and stroke statistics—2006 update: a report from the American Heart Association Statistics Committee and Stroke Statistics Subcommittee. *Circulation* 2006;113:e85–e151.
28. Treasure CB, Klein JL, Weintraub WS, et al. Beneficial effects of cholesterol-lowering therapy on the coronary endothelium in patients with coronary artery disease. *N Engl J Med* 1995;332:481–487.
29. Klocke FJ, Baird MG, Lorell BH, et al. ACC/AHA/ASNC guidelines for the clinical use of cardiac radionuclide imaging—executive summary: a report of the American College of Cardiology/American Heart Association Task Force on Practice Guidelines (ACC/AHA/ASNC Committee to Revise the 1995 Guidelines for the Clinical Use of Cardiac Radionuclide Imaging). *Circulation* 2003;108:1404–1418.
30. Stamler J, Wentworth D, Neaton JD. Is relationship between serum cholesterol and risk of premature death from coronary heart disease continuous and

graded? Findings in 356,222 primary screenees of the Multiple Risk Factor Intervention Trial (MRFIT). *JAMA* 1986;256:2823–2828.

31. Buchwald H, Varco RL, Matts JP, et al. Effect of partial ileal bypass surgery on mortality and morbidity from coronary heart disease in patients with hypercholesterolemia. Report of the Program on the Surgical Control of the Hyperlipidemias (POSCH). *N Engl J Med* 1990;323:946–955.

32. Randomised trial of cholesterol lowering in 4444 patients with coronary heart disease: the Scandinavian Simvastatin Survival Study (4S). *Lancet* 1994;344:1383–1389.

33. Serruys PW, de Feyter P, Macaya C, et al. Fluvastatin for prevention of cardiac events following successful first percutaneous coronary intervention: a randomized controlled trial. *JAMA* 2002;287:3215–3222.

34. Athyros VG, Papageorgiou AA, Mercouris BR, et al. Treatment with atorvastatin to the National Cholesterol Educational Program goal versus "usual" care in secondary coronary heart disease prevention. The Greek atorvastatin and coronary-heart-disease evaluation (GREACE) study. *Curr Med Res Opin* 2002;18:220–228.

35. Koren MJ, Hunninghake DB. Clinical outcomes in managed-care patients with coronary heart disease treated aggressively in lipid-lowering disease management clinics: the alliance study. *J Am Coll Cardiol* 2004;44:1772–1779.

36. LaRosa JC, Grundy SM, Waters DD, et al. Intensive lipid lowering with atorvastatin in patients with stable coronary disease. *N Engl J Med* 2005;352:1425–1435.

37. Pedersen TR, Faergeman O, Kastelein JJ, et al. High-dose atorvastatin vs usual-dose simvastatin for secondary prevention after myocardial infarction: the IDEAL study: a randomized controlled trial. *JAMA* 2005;294:2437–2445.

38. Schwartz GG, Olsson AG, Ezekowitz MD, et al. Effects of atorvastatin on early recurrent ischemic events in acute coronary syndromes: the MIRACL study: a randomized controlled trial. *JAMA* 2001;285:1711–1718.

39. Cannon CP, Braunwald E, McCabe CH, et al. Intensive versus moderate lipid lowering with statins after acute coronary syndromes. *N Engl J Med* 2004;350:1495–1504.

40. de Lemos JA, Blazing MA, Wiviott SD, et al. Early intensive vs a delayed conservative simvastatin strategy in patients with acute coronary syndromes: phase Z of the A to Z trial. *JAMA* 2004;292:1307–1316.

41. MRC/BHF Heart Protection Study of cholesterol lowering with simvastatin in 20,536 high-risk individuals: a randomised placebo-controlled trial. *Lancet* 2002;360:7–22.

42. Major outcomes in moderately hypercholesterolemic, hypertensive patients randomized to pravastatin vs usual care: the Antihypertensive and Lipid-Lowering Treatment to Prevent Heart Attack Trial (ALLHAT-LLT). *JAMA* 2002;288:2998–3007.

43. Shepherd J, Blauw GJ, Murphy MB, et al. Pravastatin in elderly individuals at risk of vascular disease (PROSPER): a randomised controlled trial. *Lancet* 2002;360:1623–1630.

44. Holdaas H, Fellstrom B, Jardine AG, et al. Effect of fluvastatin on cardiac outcomes in renal transplant recipients: a multicentre, randomised, placebo-controlled trial. *Lancet* 2003;361:2024–2031.

45. Shepherd J, Cobbe SM, Ford I, et al. Prevention of coronary heart disease with pravastatin in men with hypercholesterolemia. West of Scotland Coronary Prevention Study Group. *N Engl J Med* 1995;333:1301–1307.

46. Downs JR, Clearfield M, Weis S, et al. Primary prevention of acute coronary events with lovastatin in men and women with average cholesterol levels: results of AFCAPS/TexCAPS. Air Force/Texas Coronary Atherosclerosis Prevention Study. *JAMA* 1998;279:1615–1622.

47. Sever PS, Dahlof B, Poulter NR, et al. Prevention of coronary and stroke events with atorvastatin in hypertensive patients who have average or lower-than-average cholesterol concentrations, in the Anglo-Scandinavian Cardiac Outcomes Trial—Lipid Lowering Arm (ASCOT-LLA): a multicentre randomised controlled trial. *Lancet* 2003;361:1149–1158.

48. Colhoun HM, Betteridge DJ, Durrington PN, et al. Primary prevention of cardiovascular disease with atorvastatin in type 2 diabetes in the Collaborative Atorvastatin Diabetes Study (CARDS): multicentre randomised placebo-controlled trial. *Lancet* 2004;364:685–696.

49. Wanner C, Krane V, Marz W, et al. Atorvastatin in patients with type 2 diabetes mellitus undergoing hemodialysis. *N Engl J Med* 2005;353:238–248.

50. Nissen SE, Tuzcu EM, Schoenhagen P, et al. Effect of intensive compared with moderate lipid-lowering therapy on progression of coronary atherosclerosis: a randomized controlled trial. *JAMA* 2004;291:1071–1080.

51. Sipahi I, Tuzcu EM, Schoenhagen P, et al. Paradoxical increase in lumen size during progression of coronary atherosclerosis: observations from the REVERSAL trial. *Atherosclerosis* 2006;189:229–235.

52. Nissen SE, Tuzcu EM, Schoenhagen P, et al. Statin therapy, LDL cholesterol, C-reactive protein, and coronary artery disease. *N Engl J Med* 2005;352:29–38.

53. Go AS, Iribarren C, Chandra M, et al. Statin and beta-blocker therapy and the initial presentation of coronary heart disease. *Ann Intern Med* 2006;144:229–238.

54. de Lorgeril M, Salen P, Martin JL, et al. Mediterranean diet, traditional risk factors, and the rate of cardiovascular complications after myocardial infarction: final report of the Lyon Diet Heart Study. *Circulation* 1999;99:779–785.

55. Mozaffarian D, Katan MB, Ascherio A, et al. Trans fatty acids and cardiovascular disease. *N Engl J Med* 2006;354:1601–1613.

56. Kris-Etherton PM, Harris WS, Appel LJ. Fish consumption, fish oil, omega-3 fatty acids, and cardiovascular disease. *Circulation* 2002;106:2747–2757.

57. Kris-Etherton P, Daniels SR, Eckel RH, et al. Summary of the Scientific Conference on Dietary Fatty Acids and Cardiovascular Health : Conference Summary From the Nutrition Committee of the American Heart Association. *Circulation* 2001;103:1034–1039.

58. Kris-Etherton P, Eckel RH, Howard BV, et al. AHA Science Advisory: Lyon Diet Heart Study. Benefits of a Mediterranean-style, National Cholesterol Education Program/American Heart Association Step I Dietary Pattern on Cardiovascular Disease. *Circulation* 2001;103:1823–1825.

59. Jenkins DJ, Kendall CW, Marchie A, et al. Effects of a dietary portfolio of cholesterol-lowering foods vs lovastatin on serum lipids and C-reactive protein. *JAMA* 2003;290:502–510.

60. Wiviott SD, Cannon CP, Morrow DA, et al. Can low-density lipoprotein be too low? The safety and efficacy of achieving very low low-density lipoprotein with intensive statin therapy: a PROVE IT-TIMI 22 substudy. *J Am Coll Cardiol* 2005;46:1411–1416.

61. Graham DJ, Staffa JA, Shatin D, et al. Incidence of hospitalized rhabdomyolysis in patients treated with lipid-lowering drugs. *JAMA* 2004;292:2585–2590.

62. Hansen KE, Hildebrand JP, Ferguson EE, et al. Outcomes in 45 patients with statin-associated myopathy. *Arch Intern Med* 2005;165:2671–2676.

63. Phillips PS, Haas RH, Bannykh S, et al. Statin-associated myopathy with normal creatine kinase levels. *Ann Intern Med* 2002;137:581–585.

64. Pasternak RC, Smith SC Jr, Bairey-Merz CN, et al. ACC/AHA/NHLBI clinical advisory on the use and safety of statins. *Circulation* 2002;106:1024–1028.

65. Davidson MH. Clinical significance of statin pleiotropic effects: hypotheses versus evidence. *Circulation* 2005;111:2280–2281.

66. Robinson JG, Smith B, Maheshwari N, et al. Pleiotropic effects of statins: benefit beyond cholesterol reduction? A meta-regression analysis. *J Am Coll Cardiol* 2005;46:1855–1862.

67. LaRosa JC. At the heart of the statin benefit. *J Am Coll Cardiol* 2005;46:1863.

68. Cauley JA, Zmuda JM, Lui LY, et al. Lipid-lowering drug use and breast cancer in older women: a prospective study. *J Womens Health (Larchmt)* 2003;12:749–756.

69. Cauley JA, McTiernan A, Rodabough RJ, et al. Statin use and breast cancer: prospective results from the Women's Health Initiative. *J Natl Cancer Inst* 2006;98:700–707.

70. Poynter JN, Gruber SB, Higgins PD, et al. Statins and the risk of colorectal cancer. *N Engl J Med* 2005;352:2184–2192.

71. Hatzigeorgiou C, Jackson JL. Hydroxymethylglutaryl-coenzyme A reductase inhibitors and osteoporosis: a meta-analysis. *Osteoporos Int* 2005;16:990–998.

72. Almog Y, Shefer A, Novack V, et al. Prior statin therapy is associated with a decreased rate of severe sepsis. *Circulation* 2004;110:880–885.

73. Vollmer T, Key L, Durkalski V, et al. Oral simvastatin treatment in relapsing-remitting multiple sclerosis. *Lancet* 2004;363:1607–1608.

74. Jain MK, Ridker PM. Anti-inflammatory effects of statins: clinical evidence and basic mechanisms. *Nat Rev Drug Discov* 2005;4:977–987.

75. Ridker PM, Rifai N, Clearfield M, et al. Measurement of C-reactive protein for the targeting of statin therapy in the primary prevention of acute coronary events. *N Engl J Med* 2001;344:1959–1965.

76. Ridker PM, Rifai N, Pfeffer MA, et al. Inflammation, pravastatin, and the risk of coronary events after myocardial infarction in patients with average cholesterol levels. Cholesterol and Recurrent Events (CARE) Investigators. *Circulation* 1998;98:839–844.

77. Bruckert E, Giral P, Tellier P. Perspectives in cholesterol-lowering therapy: the role of ezetimibe, a new selective inhibitor of intestinal cholesterol absorption. *Circulation* 2003;107:3124–3128.

78. Meyers CD, Moon YS, Ghanem H, et al. Type of preexisting lipid therapy predicts LDL-C response to ezetimibe. *Ann Pharmacother* 2006;40:818–823.

79. Canner PL, Berge KG, Wenger NK, et al. Fifteen year mortality in Coronary Drug Project patients: long-term benefit with niacin. *J Am Coll Cardiol* 1986;8:1245–1255.

80. Brown BG, Zhao XQ, Chait A, et al. Simvastatin and niacin, antioxidant vitamins, or the combination for the prevention of coronary disease. *N Engl J Med* 2001;345:1583–1592.

81. Austin MA. Plasma triglyceride as a risk factor for cardiovascular disease. *Can J Cardiol* 1998;14 Suppl B:14B–17B.

82. Vega GL, Grundy SM. Hypoalphalipoproteinemia (low high density lipoprotein) as a risk factor for coronary heart disease. *Curr Opin Lipidol* 1996;7:209–216.

83. Brewer HB Jr. Increasing HDL cholesterol levels. *N Engl J Med* 2004;350:1491–1494.

84. Austin MA. Triglyceride, small, dense low-density lipoprotein, and the atherogenic lipoprotein phenotype. *Curr Atheroscler Rep* 2000;2:200–207.

85. A co-operative trial in the primary prevention of ischaemic heart disease using clofibrate. Report from the Committee of Principal Investigators. *Br Heart J* 1978;40:1069–1118.

86. Frick MH, Elo O, Haapa K, et al. Helsinki Heart Study: primary-prevention trial with gemfibrozil in middle-aged men with dyslipidemia. Safety of treatment, changes in risk factors, and incidence of coronary heart disease. *N Engl J Med* 1987;317:1237–1245.

87. Rubins HB, Robins SJ, Collins D, et al. Gemfibrozil for the secondary prevention of coronary heart disease in men with low levels of high-density lipoprotein cholesterol. Veterans Affairs High-Density Lipoprotein Cholesterol Intervention Trial Study Group. *N Engl J Med* 1999;341:410–418.

88. Otvos JD, Collins D, Freedman DS, et al. Low-density lipoprotein and high-density lipoprotein particle subclasses predict coronary events and are favorably changed by gemfibrozil therapy in the Veterans Affairs High-Density Lipoprotein Intervention Trial. *Circulation* 2006;113:1556–1563.

89. Secondary prevention by raising HDL cholesterol and reducing triglycerides in patients with coronary artery disease: the Bezafibrate Infarction Prevention (BIP) study. *Circulation* 2000;102:21–27.

90. Effect of fenofibrate on progression of coronary-artery disease in type 2 diabetes: the Diabetes Atherosclerosis Intervention Study, a randomised study. *Lancet* 2001;357:905–910.

91. Keech A, Simes RJ, Barter P, et al. Effects of long-term fenofibrate therapy on cardiovascular events in 9795 people with type 2 diabetes mellitus (the FIELD study): randomised controlled trial. *Lancet* 2005;366:1849–1861.

92. Kyrklund C, Backman JT, Kivisto KT, et al. Plasma concentrations of active lovastatin acid are markedly increased by gemfibrozil but not by bezafibrate. *Clin Pharmacol Ther* 2001;69:340–345.

93. Prueksaritanont T, Zhao JJ, Ma B, et al. Mechanistic studies on metabolic interactions between gemfibrozil and statins. *J Pharmacol Exp Ther* 2002;301:1042–1051.

94. Pan WJ, Gustavson LE, Achari R, et al. Lack of a clinically significant pharmacokinetic interaction between fenofibrate and pravastatin in healthy volunteers. *J Clin Pharmacol* 2000;40:316–323.

95. McKenney JM, Farnier M, Lo KW, et al. Safety and efficacy of long-term co-administration of fenofibrate and ezetimibe in patients with mixed hyperlipidemia. *J Am Coll Cardiol* 2006;47:1584–1587.

96. Nissen SE, Tsunoda T, Tuzcu EM, et al. Effect of recombinant apoA-I Milano on coronary atherosclerosis in patients with acute coronary syndromes: a randomized controlled trial. *JAMA* 2003;290:2292–2300.

97. Forrester JS, Makkar R, Shah PK. Increasing high-density lipoprotein cholesterol in dyslipidemia by cholesteryl ester transfer protein inhibition: an update for clinicians. *Circulation* 2005;111:1847–1854.

98. Mokdad AH, Marks JS, Stroup DF, et al. Actual causes of death in the United States, 2000. *JAMA* 2004;291:1238–1245.

99. Hu FB, Willett WC. Optimal diets for prevention of coronary heart disease. *JAMA* 2002;288:2569–2578.

100. Intersalt: an international study of electrolyte excretion and blood pressure. Results for 24 hour urinary sodium and potassium excretion. Intersalt Cooperative Research Group. *BMJ* 1988;297:319–328.

101. Ornish D, Brown SE, Scherwitz LW, et al. Can lifestyle changes reverse coronary heart disease? The Lifestyle Heart Trial. *Lancet* 1990;336:129–133.

102. Shekelle RB, Stamler J. Dietary cholesterol and ischaemic heart disease. *Lancet* 1989;1:1177–1179.

103. Hu FB, Bronner L, Willett WC, et al. Fish and omega-3 fatty acid intake and risk of coronary heart disease in women. *JAMA* 2002;287:1815–1821.

104. Marchioli R, Barzi F, Bomba E, et al. Early protection against sudden death by n-3 polyunsaturated fatty acids after myocardial infarction: time-course analysis of the results of the Gruppo Italiano per lo Studio della Sopravvivenza nell'Infarto Miocardico (GISSI)-Prevenzione. *Circulation* 2002;105:1897–1903.

105. Turpeinen O, Karvonen MJ, Pekkarinen M, et al. Dietary prevention of coronary heart disease: the Finnish Mental Hospital Study. *Int J Epidemiol* 1979;8:99–118.

106. Dayton S, Hashimoto S, Pearce ML. Influence of a diet high in unsaturated fat upon composition of arterial tissue and atheromata in man. *Circulation* 1965;32:911–924.

107. Watts GF, Lewis B, Brunt JN, et al. Effects on coronary artery disease of lipid-lowering diet, or diet plus cholestyramine in the St Thomas' Atherosclerosis Regression Study (STARS). *Lancet* 1992;339:563–569.

108. Leren P. The Oslo diet-heart study. Eleven-year report. *Circulation* 1970;42:935–942.

109. Lichtenstein AH, Van Horn L. Very low fat diets. *Circulation* 1998;98:935–939.

110. Kris-Etherton PM. Monounsaturated fatty acids and risk of cardiovascular disease. *Circulation* 1999;100:1253–1258.

111. U.S. Department of Health and Human Services. The health consequences of smoking: a report of the surgeon general. Public Health Service Centers for Disease Control and Prevention, National Center for Chronic Disease Prevention and Health Promotion, Office on Smoking and Health. Atlanta, GA: USDHHS, 2004.

112. Ezzati M, Henley SJ, Thun MJ, et al. Role of smoking in global and regional cardiovascular mortality. *Circulation* 2005;112:489–497.

113. He J, Vupputuri S, Allen K, et al. Passive smoking and the risk of coronary heart disease—a meta-analysis of epidemiologic studies. *N Engl J Med* 1999;340:920–926.

114. Gordon T, Kannel WB, McGee D, et al. Death and coronary attacks in men after giving up cigarette smoking. A report from the Framingham study. *Lancet* 1974;2:1345–1348.

115. Tsevat J, Weinstein MC, Williams LW, et al. Expected gains in life expectancy from various coronary heart disease risk factor modifications. *Circulation* 1991;83:1194–1201.

116. Wilhelmsson C, Vedin JA, Elmfeldt D, et al. Smoking and myocardial infarction. *Lancet* 1975;1:415–420.

117. Hermanson B, Omenn GS, Kronmal RA, et al. Beneficial six-year outcome of smoking cessation in older men and women with coronary artery disease. Results from the CASS registry. *N Engl J Med* 1988;319:1365–1369.

118. Fiore M BW, Cohen S, et al. Smoking cessation: clinical practice guidelines no. 18. Washington , DC: Public Health Service, U.S. Department of Health and Human Services, 1996.

119. Hughes JR, Goldstein MG, Hurt RD, et al. Recent advances in the pharmacotherapy of smoking. *JAMA* 1999;281:72–76.

120. Benowitz NL, Gourlay SG. Cardiovascular toxicity of nicotine: implications for nicotine replacement therapy. *J Am Coll Cardiol* 1997;29:1422–1431.

121. Coe JW, Brooks PR, Vetelino MG, et al. Varenicline: an $alpha_4beta_2$ nicotinic receptor partial agonist for smoking cessation. *J Med Chem* 2005;48:3474–3477.

122. Flegal KM, Troiano RP, Pamuk ER, et al. The influence of smoking cessation on the prevalence of overweight in the United States. *N Engl J Med* 1995;333:1165–1170.

123. Vaccarino V, Holford TR, Krumholz HM. Pulse pressure and risk for myocardial infarction and heart failure in the elderly. *J Am Coll Cardiol* 2000;36:130–138.

124. Kannel WB. Blood pressure as a cardiovascular risk factor: prevention and treatment. *JAMA* 1996;275:1571–1576.

125. Collins R, MacMahon S. Blood pressure, antihypertensive drug treatment and the risks of stroke and of coronary heart disease. *Br Med Bull* 1994;50:272–298.

126. Turnbull F. Effects of different blood-pressure-lowering regimens on major cardiovascular events: results of prospectively-designed overviews of randomised trials. *Lancet* 2003;362:1527–1535.

127. Taylor EN, Hu FB, Curhan GC. Antihypertensive medications and the risk of incident type 2 diabetes. *Diabetes Care* 2006;29:1065–1070.

128. Levy D, Garrison RJ, Savage DD, et al. Prognostic implications of echocardiographically determined left ventricular mass in the Framingham Heart Study. *N Engl J Med* 1990;322:1561–1566.

129. Harjai KJ. Potential new cardiovascular risk factors: left ventricular hypertrophy, homocysteine, lipoprotein(a), triglycerides, oxidative stress, and fibrinogen. *Ann Intern Med* 1999;131:376–386.

130. Levy D, Salomon M, D'Agostino RB, et al. Prognostic implications of baseline electrocardiographic features and their serial changes in subjects with left ventricular hypertrophy. *Circulation* 1994;90:1786–1793.

131. Verdecchia P, Schillaci G, Borgioni C, et al. Prognostic significance of serial changes in left ventricular mass in essential hypertension. *Circulation* 1998;97:48–54.

132. Schlaich MP, Schmieder RE. Left ventricular hypertrophy and its regression: pathophysiology and therapeutic approach: focus on treatment by antihypertensive agents. *Am J Hypertens* 1998;11:1394–1404.

133. Mathew J, Sleight P, Lonn E, et al. Reduction of cardiovascular risk by regression of electrocardiographic markers of left ventricular hypertrophy by the angiotensin-converting enzyme inhibitor ramipril. *Circulation* 2001;104:1615–1621.

134. Devereux RB, Dahlof B, Gerdts E, et al. Regression of hypertensive left ventricular hypertrophy by losartan compared with atenolol: the Losartan Intervention for Endpoint Reduction in Hypertension (LIFE) trial. *Circulation* 2004;110:1456.

135. Grundy SM, Brewer HB Jr, Cleeman JI, et al. Definition of metabolic syndrome: report of the National Heart, Lung, and Blood Institute/American Heart Association conference on scientific issues related to definition. *Circulation* 2004;109:433–438.

136. Ford ES, Giles WH, Dietz WH. Prevalence of the metabolic syndrome among U.S. adults: findings from the third National Health and Nutrition Examination Survey. *JAMA* 2002;287:356–359.

137. Lakka HM, Laaksonen DE, Lakka TA, et al. The metabolic syndrome and total and cardiovascular disease mortality in middle-aged men. *JAMA* 2002;288:2709–2716.

138. Krolewski AS, Kosinski EJ, Warram JH, et al. Magnitude and determinants of coronary artery disease in juvenile-onset, insulin-dependent diabetes mellitus. *Am J Cardiol* 1987;59:750–755.

139. Abbott RD, Donahue RP, Kannel WB, et al. The impact of diabetes on survival following myocardial infarction in men vs women. The Framingham Study. *JAMA* 1988;260:3456–3460.

140. Walden CE, Knopp RH, Wahl PW, et al. Sex differences in the effect of diabetes mellitus on lipoprotein triglyceride and cholesterol concentrations. *N Engl J Med* 1984;311:953–959.

141. The effect of intensive treatment of diabetes on the development and progression of long-term complications in insulin-dependent diabetes mellitus. The Diabetes Control and Complications Trial Research Group. *N Engl J Med* 1993;329:977–986.

142. Intensive blood-glucose control with sulphonylureas or insulin compared with conventional treatment and risk of complications in patients with type 2 diabetes (UKPDS 33). UK Prospective Diabetes Study (UKPDS) Group. *Lancet* 1998;352:837–853.

143. Nathan DM, Cleary PA, Backlund JY, et al. Intensive diabetes treatment and cardiovascular disease in patients with type 1 diabetes. *N Engl J Med* 2005;353:2643–2653.

144. Libby P, Plutzky J. Diabetic macrovascular disease: the glucose paradox? *Circulation* 2002;106:2760–2763.

145. Gundersen T, Kjekshus J. Timolol treatment after myocardial infarction in diabetic patients. *Diabetes Care* 1983;6:285–290.

146. Fletcher GF, Balady G, Blair SN, et al. Statement on exercise: benefits and recommendations for physical activity programs for all Americans. A statement for health professionals by the Committee on Exercise and Cardiac Rehabilitation of the Council on Clinical Cardiology, American Heart Association. *Circulation* 1996;94:857–862.

147. Haskell W. Sedentary lifestyle as a risk factor for coronary heart disease. In: Pearson T, ed. *Primer in Preventive Cardiology.* Dallas, TX: American Heart Association, 1994:173–187.

148. Manson JE, Greenland P, LaCroix AZ, et al. Walking compared with vigorous exercise for the prevention of cardiovascular events in women. *N Engl J Med* 2002;347:716–725.

149. Albert CM, Mittleman MA, Chae CU, et al. Triggering of sudden death from cardiac causes by vigorous exertion. *N Engl J Med* 2000;343:1355–1361.

150. Manson JE, Hu FB, Rich-Edwards JW, et al. A prospective study of walking as compared with vigorous exercise in the prevention of coronary heart disease in women. *N Engl J Med* 1999;341:650–658.

151. Lee IM, Sesso HD, Paffenbarger RS Jr. Physical activity and coronary heart disease risk in men: does the duration of exercise episodes predict risk? *Circulation* 2000;102:981–986.

152. Oldridge NB, Guyatt GH, Fischer ME, et al. Cardiac rehabilitation after myocardial infarction. Combined experience of randomized clinical trials. *JAMA* 1988;260:945–950.

153. O'Connor GT, Buring JE, Yusuf S, et al. An overview of randomized trials of rehabilitation with exercise after myocardial infarction. *Circulation* 1989;80:234–244.

154. Lauer M, Froelicher ES, Williams M, et al. Exercise testing in asymptomatic adults: a statement for professionals from the American Heart Association Council on Clinical Cardiology, Subcommittee on Exercise, Cardiac Rehabilitation, and Prevention. *Circulation* 2005;112:771–776.

155. Poirier P, Giles TD, Bray GA, et al. Obesity and cardiovascular disease: pathophysiology, evaluation, and effect of weight loss: an update of the 1997 American Heart Association Scientific Statement on Obesity and Heart Disease from the Obesity Committee of the Council on Nutrition, Physical Activity, and Metabolism. *Circulation* 2006;113:898–918.

156. Wada K, Tamakoshi K, Yatsuya H, et al. Association between parental histories of hypertension, diabetes and dyslipidemia and the clustering of these disorders in offspring. *Prev Med* 2006;42:358–363.

157. McGill HC Jr, McMahan CA, Herderick EE, et al. Obesity accelerates the progression of coronary atherosclerosis in young men. *Circulation* 2002;105:2712–2718.

158. Ogden CL, Carroll MD, Curtin LR, et al. Prevalence of overweight and obesity in the United States, 1999–2004. *JAMA* 2006;295:1549–1555.

159. Hubert HB, Feinleib M, McNamara PM, et al. Obesity as an independent risk factor for cardiovascular disease: a 26-year follow-up of participants in the Framingham Heart Study. *Circulation* 1983;67:968–977.

160. Manson JE, Willett WC, Stampfer MJ, et al. Body weight and mortality among women. *N Engl J Med* 1995;333:677–685.

161. Jousilahti P, Tuomilehto J, Vartiainen E, et al. Body weight, cardiovascular risk factors, and coronary mortality. 15-year follow-up of middle-aged men and women in eastern Finland. *Circulation* 1996;93:1372–1379.

162. Yanovski SZ, Yanovski JA. Obesity. *N Engl J Med* 2002;346:591–602.

163. Gelfand EV, Cannon CP. Rimonabant: a cannabinoid receptor type 1 blocker for management of multiple cardiometabolic risk factors. *J Am Coll Cardiol* 2006;47:1919–1926.

164. Scanu AM. Lipoprotein(a). A genetic risk factor for premature coronary heart disease. *JAMA* 1992;267:3326–3329.

165. Danesh J, Collins R, Peto R. Lipoprotein(a) and coronary heart disease. Meta-analysis of prospective studies. *Circulation* 2000;102:1082–1085.

166. Cantin B, Despres JP, Lamarche B, et al. Association of fibrinogen and lipoprotein(a) as a coronary heart disease risk factor in men (The Quebec Cardiovascular Study). *Am J Cardiol* 2002;89:662–666.

167. von Eckardstein A, Schulte H, Cullen P, et al. Lipoprotein(a) further increases the risk of coronary events in men with high global cardiovascular risk. *J Am Coll Cardiol* 2001;37:434–439.

168. Mangoni AA, Jackson SH. Homocysteine and cardiovascular disease: current evidence and future prospects. *Am J Med* 2002;112:556–565.

169. Nygard O, Nordrehaug JE, Refsum H, et al. Plasma homocysteine levels and mortality in patients with coronary artery disease. *N Engl J Med* 1997;337:230–236.

170. Lonn E, Yusuf S, Arnold MJ, et al. Homocysteine lowering with folic acid and B vitamins in vascular disease. *N Engl J Med* 2006;354:1567–1577.

171. Bonaa KH, Njolstad I, Ueland PM, et al. Homocysteine lowering and cardiovascular events after acute myocardial infarction. *N Engl J Med* 2006;354:1578–1588.

172. Toole JF, Malinow MR, Chambless LE, et al. Lowering homocysteine in patients with ischemic stroke to prevent recurrent stroke, myocardial infarction, and death: the Vitamin Intervention for Stroke Prevention (VISP) randomized controlled trial. *JAMA* 2004;291:565–575.

173. Rimm EB, Stampfer MJ, Ascherio A, et al. Vitamin E consumption and the risk of coronary heart disease in men. *N Engl J Med* 1993;328:1450–1456.

174. Stampfer MJ, Hennekens CH, Manson JE, et al. Vitamin E consumption and the risk of coronary disease in women. *N Engl J Med* 1993;328:1444–1449.

175. The effect of vitamin E and beta carotene on the incidence of lung cancer and other cancers in male smokers. The Alpha-Tocopherol, Beta Carotene Cancer Prevention Study Group. *N Engl J Med* 1994;330:1029–1035.

176. Omenn GS, Goodman GE, Thornquist MD, et al. Effects of a combination of beta carotene and vitamin A on lung cancer and cardiovascular disease. *N Engl J Med* 1996;334:1150–1155.

177. Hennekens CH, Buring JE, Manson JE, et al. Lack of effect of long-term supplementation with beta carotene on the incidence of malignant neoplasms and cardiovascular disease. *N Engl J Med* 1996;334:1145–1149.

178. Lee IM, Cook NR, Gaziano JM, et al. Vitamin E in the primary prevention of cardiovascular disease and cancer: the Women's Health Study: a randomized controlled trial. *JAMA* 2005;294:56–65.

179. Yusuf S, Dagenais G, Pogue J, et al. Vitamin E supplementation and cardiovascular events in high-risk patients. The Heart Outcomes Prevention Evaluation Study Investigators. *N Engl J Med* 2000;342:154–160.

180. MRC/BHF Heart Protection Study of antioxidant vitamin supplementation in 20,536 high-risk individuals: a randomised placebo-controlled trial. *Lancet* 2002;360:23–33.

181. Dietary supplementation with n-3 polyunsaturated fatty acids and vitamin E after myocardial infarction: results of the GISSI-Prevenzione trial. Gruppo Italiano per lo Studio della Sopravvivenza nell'Infarto miocardico. *Lancet* 1999;354:447–455.

182. Rimm EB, Giovannucci EL, Willett WC, et al. Prospective study of alcohol consumption and risk of coronary disease in men. *Lancet* 1991;338:464–468.

183. Mukamal KJ, Conigrave KM, Mittleman MA, et al. Roles of drinking pattern and type of alcohol consumed in coronary heart disease in men. *N Engl J Med* 2003;348:109–118.

184. Maclure M. Demonstration of deductive meta-analysis: ethanol intake and risk of myocardial infarction. *Epidemiol Rev* 1993;15:328–351.

185. Tolstrup J, Jensen MK, Tjonneland A, et al. Prospective study of alcohol drinking patterns and coronary heart disease in women and men. *BMJ* 2006;332:1244–1248.

186. Haskell WL, Camargo C Jr, Williams PT, et al. The effect of cessation and resumption of moderate alcohol intake on serum high-density-lipoprotein subfractions. A controlled study. *N Engl J Med* 1984;310:805–810.

187. Suh I, Shaten BJ, Cutler JA, et al. Alcohol use and mortality from coronary heart disease: the role of high-density lipoprotein cholesterol. The Multiple Risk Factor Intervention Trial Research Group. *Ann Intern Med* 1992;116:881–887.

188. Gaziano JM, Buring JE, Breslow JL, et al. Moderate alcohol intake, increased levels of high-density lipoprotein and its subfractions, and decreased risk of myocardial infarction. *N Engl J Med* 1993;329:1829–1834.

189. Langer RD, Criqui MH, Reed DM. Lipoproteins and blood pressure as biological pathways for effect of moderate alcohol consumption on coronary heart disease. *Circulation* 1992;85:910–915.

190. Ridker PM, Vaughan DE, Stampfer MJ, et al. Association of moderate alcohol consumption and plasma concentration of endogenous tissue-type plasminogen activator. *JAMA* 1994;272:929–933.

191. Hendriks HF, Veenstra J, Velthuis-te Wierik EJ, et al. Effect of moderate dose of alcohol with evening meal on fibrinolytic factors. *BMJ* 1994;308:1003–1006.

192. Deykin D, Janson P, McMahon L. Ethanol potentiation of aspirin-induced prolongation of the bleeding time. *N Engl J Med* 1982;306:852–854.

193. Elmer O, Goransson G, Zoucas E. Impairment of primary hemostasis and platelet function after alcohol ingestion in man. *Haemostasis* 1984;14:223–228.

194. Goldberg IJ. To drink or not to drink? *N Engl J Med* 2003;348:163–164.

195. Pearson TA, Terry P. What to advise patients about drinking alcohol. The clinician's conundrum. *JAMA* 1994;272:967–968.

196. Enos WFJ, Beyer JC, Holmes RH. Pathogenesis of coronary disease in American soldiers killed in Korea. *JAMA* 1955;58:912.

197. McNamara JJ, Molot MA, Stremple JF, et al. Coronary artery disease in combat casualties in Vietnam. *JAMA* 1971;216:1185–1187.

198. Castelli WP. Epidemiology of coronary heart disease: the Framingham study. *Am J Med* 1984;76:4–12.

199. Rossouw JE, Anderson GL, Prentice RL, et al. Risks and benefits of estrogen plus progestin in healthy postmenopausal women: principal results from the Women's Health Initiative randomized controlled trial. *JAMA* 2002;288:321–333.

200. Mosca L, Collins P, Herrington DM, et al. Hormone replacement therapy and cardiovascular disease: a statement for healthcare professionals from the American Heart Association. *Circulation* 2001;104:499–503.

201. Wakatsuki A, Okatani Y, Ikenoue N, et al. Different effects of oral conjugated equine estrogen and transdermal estrogen replacement therapy on size and oxidative susceptibility of low-density lipoprotein particles in postmenopausal women. *Circulation* 2002;106:1771–1776.

202. Hulley S, Grady D, Bush T, et al. Randomized trial of estrogen plus progestin for secondary prevention of coronary heart disease in postmenopausal women. Heart and Estrogen/progestin Replacement Study (HERS) Research Group. *JAMA* 1998;280:605–613.

203. Grady D, Herrington D, Bittner V, et al. Cardiovascular disease outcomes during 6.8 years of hormone therapy: Heart and Estrogen/progestin Replacement Study follow-up (HERS II). *JAMA* 2002;288:49–57.

204. Mosca L, Appel LJ, Benjamin EJ, et al. Evidence-based guidelines for cardiovascular disease prevention in women. American Heart Association scientific statement. *Arterioscler Thromb Vasc Biol* 2004;24:e29–e50.

205. Kaplan GA, Keil JE. Socioeconomic factors and cardiovascular disease: a review of the literature. *Circulation* 1993;88:1973–1998.

206. Hopkins PN, Williams RR. Human genetics and coronary heart disease: a public health perspective. *Annu Rev Nutr* 1989;9:303–345.

207. Rissanen AM. Familial aggregation of coronary heart disease in a high incidence area (North Karelia, Finland). *Br Heart J* 1979;42:294–303.

208. Williams RR, Hopkins PN, Wu LL, et al. Evaluating family history to prevent early coronary heart disease. In: Pearson TA, ed. *Primer in Preventive Cardiology.* Dallas, TX: American Heart Association, 1994:93–106.

209. Libby P, Ridker PM, Maseri A. Inflammation and Atherosclerosis. *Circulation* 2002;105:1135–1143.

210. Ernst E, Resch KL. Fibrinogen as a cardiovascular risk factor: a meta-analysis and review of the literature. *Ann Intern Med* 1993;118:956–963.

211. Abramson JL, Vaccarino V. Relationship between physical activity and inflammation among apparently healthy middle-aged and older U.S. adults. *Arch Intern Med* 2002;162:1286–1292.

212. Ridker PM. Clinical application of C-reactive protein for cardiovascular disease detection and prevention. *Circulation* 2003;107:363–369.

213. Ridker PM, Danielson E, Rifai N, et al. Valsartan, blood pressure reduction, and C-reactive protein. Primary report of the Val-MARC trial. *Hypertension* 2006;48:73–79.

214. Smith JK, Dykes R, Douglas JE, et al. Long-term exercise and atherogenic activity of blood mononuclear cells in persons at risk of developing ischemic heart disease. *JAMA* 1999;281:1722–1727.

215. Visser M, Bouter LM, McQuillan GM, et al. Elevated C-reactive protein levels in overweight and obese adults. *JAMA* 1999;282:2131–2135.

216. Albert MA, Danielson E, Rifai N, et al. Effect of statin therapy on C-reactive protein levels: the pravastatin inflammation/CRP evaluation (PRINCE): a randomized trial and cohort study. *JAMA* 2001;286:64–70.

217. Ridker PM, Rifai N, Pfeffer MA, et al. Long-term effects of pravastatin on plasma concentration of C-reactive protein. The Cholesterol and Recurrent Events (CARE) Investigators. *Circulation* 1999;100:230–235.

218. Ridker PM, on behalf of the JSG. Rosuvastatin in the primary prevention of cardiovascular disease among patients with low levels of low-density lipoprotein cholesterol and elevated high-sensitivity c-reactive protein: rationale and design of the JUPITER trial. *Circulation* 2003;108:2292–2297.

219. Ridker PM, Cook N. Clinical usefulness of very high and very low levels of C-reactive protein across the full range of Framingham risk scores. *Circulation* 2004;109:1955–1959.

220. Ridker PM, Vaughan DE, Stampfer MJ, et al. Endogenous tissue-type plasminogen activator and risk of myocardial infarction. *Lancet* 1993;341:1165–1168.

221. Thogersen AM, Jansson JH, Boman K, et al. High plasminogen activator inhibitor and tissue plasminogen activator levels in plasma precede a first acute myocardial infarction in both men and women: evidence for the fibrinolytic system as an independent primary risk factor. *Circulation* 1998;98:2241–2247.

222. Thompson SG, Kienast J, Pyke SD, et al. Hemostatic factors and the risk of myocardial infarction or sudden death in patients with angina pectoris. European Concerted Action on Thrombosis and Disabilities Angina Pectoris Study Group. *N Engl J Med* 1995;332:635–641.

223. Mills JD, Mansfield MW, Grant PJ. Tissue plasminogen activator, fibrin D-dimer, and insulin resistance in the relatives of patients with premature coronary artery disease. *Arterioscler Thromb Vasc Biol* 2002;22:704–709.

224. Meade TW, Ruddock V, Stirling Y, et al. Fibrinolytic activity, clotting factors, and long-term incidence of ischaemic heart disease in the Northwick Park Heart Study. *Lancet* 1993;342:1076–1079.

225. Ridker PM, Hennekens CH, Cerskus A, et al. Plasma concentration of cross-linked fibrin degradation product (D-dimer) and the risk of future myocardial infarction among apparently healthy men. *Circulation* 1994;90:2236–2240.

226. Vaughan DE, Rouleau JL, Ridker PM, et al. Effects of ramipril on plasma fibrinolytic balance in patients with acute anterior myocardial infarction. HEART Study Investigators. *Circulation* 1997;96:442–447.

227. Final report on the aspirin component of the ongoing Physicians' Health Study. Steering Committee of the Physicians' Health Study Research Group. *N Engl J Med* 1989;321:129–135.

228. Ridker PM, Cook NR, Lee IM, et al. A randomized trial of low-dose aspirin in the primary prevention of cardiovascular disease in women. *N Engl J Med* 2005;352:1293–1304.

229. Berger JS, Roncaglioni MC, Avanzini F, et al. Aspirin for the primary prevention of cardiovascular events in women and men: a sex-specific meta-analysis of randomized controlled trials. *JAMA* 2006;295:306–313.

230. Bhatt DL, Fox KA, Hacke W, et al. Clopidogrel and aspirin versus aspirin alone for the prevention of atherothrombotic events. *N Engl J Med* 2006;354:1706–1717.

231. Collaborative meta-analysis of randomised trials of antiplatelet therapy for prevention of death, myocardial infarction, and stroke in high risk patients. *BMJ* 2002;324:71–86.

232. Anand SS, Yusuf S. Oral anticoagulant therapy in patients with coronary artery disease: a meta-analysis. *JAMA* 1999;282:2058–2067.

233. Hurlen M, Abdelnoor M, Smith P, et al. Warfarin, aspirin, or both after myocardial infarction. *N Engl J Med* 2002;347:969–974.

234. Stone PH SF. *Strategies for secondary prevention.* London: Oxford University Press, 1996.

235. Wikstrand J, Warnold I, Olsson G, et al. Primary prevention with metoprolol in patients with hypertension. Mortality results from the MAPHY study. *JAMA* 1988;259:1976–1982.

236. Yusuf S, Peto R, Lewis J, et al. Beta blockade during and after myocardial infarction: an overview of the randomized trials. *Prog Cardiovasc Dis* 1985;27:335–371.

237. Lau J, Antman EM, Jimenez-Silva J, et al. Cumulative meta-analysis of therapeutic trials for myocardial infarction. *N Engl J Med* 1992;327:248–254.

238. Khalil ME, Basher AW, Brown EJ Jr, et al. A remarkable medical story: benefits of angiotensin-converting enzyme inhibitors in cardiac patients. *J Am Coll Cardiol* 2001;37:1757–1764.

239. Al-Mallah MH, Tleyjeh IM, Abdel-Latif AA, et al. Angiotensin-converting enzyme inhibitors in coronary artery disease and preserved left ventricular systolic function: a systematic review and meta-analysis of randomized controlled trials. *J Am Coll Cardiol* 2006;47:1576–1583.

240. Major outcomes in high-risk hypertensive patients randomized to angiotensin-converting enzyme inhibitor or calcium channel blocker vs diuretic: the Antihypertensive and Lipid-Lowering Treatment to Prevent Heart Attack Trial (ALLHAT). *JAMA* 2002;288:2981–2997.

241. Wing LM, Reid CM, Ryan P, et al. A comparison of outcomes with angiotensin-converting enzyme inhibitors and diuretics for hypertension in the elderly. *N Engl J Med* 2003;348:583–592.

242. Rogers WJ, Canto JG, Lambrew CT, et al. Temporal trends in the treatment of over 1.5 million patients with myocardial infarction in the U.S. from 1990 through 1999: the National Registry of Myocardial Infarction 1, 2 and 3. *J Am Coll Cardiol* 2000;36:2056–2063.

243. Krumholz HM, Radford MJ, Wang Y, et al. National use and effectiveness of beta-blockers for the treatment of elderly patients after acute myocardial infarction: National Cooperative Cardiovascular Project. *JAMA* 1998;280:623–629.

244. Fonarow GC, French WJ, Parsons LS, et al. Use of lipid-lowering medications at discharge in patients with acute myocardial infarction: data from the National Registry of Myocardial Infarction 3. *Circulation* 2001;103:38–44.

245. Fonarow GC, Gawlinski A, Moughrabi S, et al. Improved treatment of coronary heart disease by implementation of a Cardiac Hospitalization Atherosclerosis Management Program (CHAMP). *Am J Cardiol* 2001;87:819–822.

246. Aronow HD, Topol EJ, Roe MT, et al. Effect of lipid-lowering therapy on early mortality after acute coronary syndromes: an observational study. *Lancet* 2001;357:1063–1068.

247. Sueta CA, Chowdhury M, Boccuzzi SJ, et al. Analysis of the degree of undertreatment of hyperlipidemia and congestive heart failure secondary to coronary artery disease. *Am J Cardiol* 1999;83:1303–1307.

248. Newby LK, LaPointe NM, Chen AY, et al. Long-term adherence to evidence-based secondary prevention therapies in coronary artery disease. *Circulation* 2006;113:203–212.

249. Kottke TE, Blackburn H, Brekke ML, et al. The systematic practice of preventive cardiology. *Am J Cardiol* 1987;59:690–694.

250. Pearson TA, McBride PE, Miller NH, et al. 27th Bethesda Conference: matching the intensity of risk factor management with the hazard for coronary disease events. Task Force 8. Organization of preventive cardiology service. *J Am Coll Cardiol* 1996;27:1039–1047.

251. Miller NH, Hill M, Kottke T, et al. The multilevel compliance challenge: recommendations for a call to action. A statement for healthcare professionals. *Circulation* 1997;95:1085–1090.

252. Bradley EH, Holmboe ES, Mattera JA, et al. A qualitative study of increasing beta-blocker use after myocardial infarction: why do some hospitals succeed? *JAMA* 2001;285:2604–2611.

253. Gordon NF, English CD, Contractor AS, et al. Effectiveness of three models for comprehensive cardiovascular disease risk reduction. *Am J Cardiol* 2002;89:1263–1268.

254. *Treating Tobacco Use and Dependence: A Clinical Practice Guideline.* Washington, DC: U.S. Department of Health and Human Services, 2000.

255. Wenger NK, Froelicher ES, Smith LK. *Cardiac Rehabilitation as Secondary Prevention.* Bethesda, MD: National Heart, Lung, and Blood Institute, 1995.

256. Pearson TA, Bazzarre TL, Daniels SR, et al. American Heart Association guide for improving cardiovascular health at the community level: a statement for public health practitioners, healthcare providers, and health policy makers from the American Heart Association Expert Panel on Population and Prevention Science. *Circulation* 2003;107:645–651.

CHAPTER (52)

Atherothrombosis: Role of Inflammation

Prediman K. Shah / Erling Falk / Valentin Fuster

INTRODUCTION

Occlusive arterial disease resulting from atherosclerosis is a leading cause of death and disability throughout industrialized nations and is soon expected to rival other diseases in developing nations as well.[1,2] This global burden of cardiovascular disease carries with it a heavy financial burden.[3] Arterial occlusive disorders include atherosclerosis of native arteries, an accelerated variant of atherosclerosis involving vein grafts, allograft vasculopathy of transplanted organs, and restenosis resulting from neointima formation following angioplasty and stenting. An improved understanding of the pathophysiology of atherosclerosis and thrombosis is likely to lead to improved prevention, diagnosis, and treatment of this common disorder.

Atherosclerosis involves the buildup of a plaque composed of variable amounts of lipoproteins, extracellular matrix (collagen, proteoglycans, glycosaminoglycans), calcium, vascular smooth muscle cells, inflammatory cells (chiefly monocyte-derived macrophages, T lymphocytes, mast cells, dendritic cells), and new blood vessels (angiogenesis). A body of evidence now suggests that atherosclerosis represents a chronic inflammatory response to vascular injury caused by a variety of agents that activate or injure endothelium and promote lipoprotein infiltration, retention, and modification, combined with inflammatory cell entry, retention and activation (Table 52–1).[4–6]

INFLAMMATORY SIGNALING AND SITES OF PREDILECTION FOR ATHEROSCLEROSIS DEVELOPMENT

The sites of predilection for atherosclerosis are characterized by low and/or oscillatory shear stress, evidence of endothelial activation with expression of leukocyte adhesion molecules, and increased influx and/or prolonged retention of lipoproteins.[7–9] Specific arterial sites, such as branches, bifurcations, and curvatures, cause characteristic alterations in the flow of blood, including decreased shear stress and increased turbulence. Changes in flow alter the expression of genes that have elements in their promoter regions that respond to shear stress. For example, the genes for intracellular adhesion molecule-1, platelet-derived growth factor B chain, and tissue factor in endothelial cells have these elements, and their expression is increased by reduced shear stress.[10–18] Recent studies demonstrate that in vitro application of flow patterns observed at sites of predilection for atherosclerosis to endothelial cells activates a broad-based proinflammatory gene program, whereas application of flow patterns observed at atherosclerosis-resistant sites inhibits proinflammatory signaling, in part through activation of Kruppel-like factor (KLF-2), a novel transcription factor.[19]

Rolling and adherence of inflammatory cells (monocytes and T cells) occur at these sites as a result of the upregulation of proin-

TABLE 52–1

Key Steps in Atherogenesis Highlighting Role of Inflammation at Various Steps

1. Endothelial activation with increased infiltration of atherogenic lipoproteins at sites of low or oscillating shear stress (branch points and flow dividers)
2. Subendothelial retention and modification of atherogenic lipoproteins (LDL/VLDL)
3. Endothelial activation with increased mononuclear leukocyte (inflammatory cell) adhesion, chemotaxis, and subendothelial recruitment
4. Subendothelial inflammatory cell activation with lipid ingestion through monocyte scavenger receptor expression resulting in foam cell formation
5. Intimal migration and proliferation of medial/adventitial smooth muscle cells/myofibroblasts in response to growth factors released by activated monocytes with matrix production and formation of fibrous cap and fibrous plaque
6. Abluminal plaque growth with positive (outward) arterial adventitial remodeling preserving lumen size in early stages; later plaque growth or negative remodeling results in luminal narrowing
7. Angiogenesis because of angiogenic stimuli produced by inflammatory cells (macrophages) and other arterial wall cells (VEGF, IL-8)
8. Death of foam cells by necrosis/apoptosis leading to necrotic lipid-core formation
9. Plaque disruption (rupture of fibrous cap or endothelial erosion) because of inflammatory cell-mediated matrix degradation and death of matrix-synthesizing smooth muscle cells
10. Exposure of thrombogenic substrate (lipid-core containing tissue factor derived from inflammatory cells) following plaque disruption with arterial thrombosis

IL, interleukin; LDL, low-density lipoprotein; VEGF, vascular endothelial growth factor; VLDL, very-low-density lipoprotein.

flammatory adhesion molecules on both the endothelium and the leukocytes. At these sites, specific molecules form on the endothelium that are responsible for the adherence, migration, and accumulation of monocytes and T cells. Such adhesion molecules, which act as receptors for glycoconjugates and integrins present on monocytes and T cells, include several selectins, intercellular adhesion molecules, and vascular cell adhesion molecules.[10–18] Molecules associated with the migration of leukocytes across the endothelium, such as platelet-endothelial cell adhesion molecules act in conjunction with chemoattractant molecules generated by the endothelium, smooth muscle, and monocytes—such as monocyte chemotactic protein-1 (MCP-1), osteopontin, and modified low-density lipoprotein (LDL)—to attract monocytes and T cells into the artery.[7–18] Chemokines may be involved in the chemotaxis and accumulation of macrophages in fatty streaks.[20,21] Activation of monocytes and T cells leads to upregulation of receptors on their surfaces, such as the mucin-like molecules that bind selectins, inte-

grins that bind adhesion molecules of the immunoglobulin superfamily, and receptors that bind chemoattractant molecules. These ligand-receptor interactions further activate mononuclear cells, induce cell proliferation, and help define and localize the inflammatory response at the site of lesions.

In genetically modified mice that are deficient in apolipoprotein E (and have hypercholesterolemia), intercellular adhesion molecule-1 (ICAM-1) is constitutively increased at lesion-prone sites long before the lesions develop.[8] In contrast, vascular cell adhesion molecule-1 (VCAM-1) is absent in normal mice but is present at the same sites as ICAM-1 in mice with apolipoprotein E deficiency.[8] Mice that are completely deficient in ICAM-1, P-selectin, CD18, or combinations of these molecules, have reduced atherosclerosis in response to lipid feeding. Proteolytic enzymes may cleave adhesion molecules such that in situations of chronic inflammation it may be possible to measure the "shed" molecules in plasma as markers of a sustained inflammatory response to help identify patients at risk for atherosclerosis or other inflammatory diseases.[22–27]

ENDOTHELIAL ACTIVATION AND INFLAMMATION IN INITIATION AND PROGRESSION OF ATHEROSCLEROSIS

Several studies suggest that one of the earliest steps in atherogenesis is endothelial activation or injury/dysfunction with infiltration and retention and modification of atherogenic lipoproteins (predominantly the apoB-containing lipoproteins) in the subendothelial space of the vessel wall (Table 52–2).[28–39]

Various factors that may contribute to endothelial activation or the development of endothelial injury/dysfunction predisposing to atherosclerosis, including risk factors such as elevated and modified LDL/very-low-density lipoprotein (VLDL) cholesterol; reduced high-density lipoprotein (HDL) cholesterol; oxidant stress caused by cigarette smoking, hypertension, and diabetic mellitus; genetic alterations; infectious microorganisms; estrogen deficiency; and advancing age.[31,32,37] Endothelial activation and injury/dysfunction may manifest in (1) increased adhesiveness of the endothelium to inflammatory cells (leukocytes) or platelets, (2) increased vascular permeability, (3) change from an anticoagulant to a procoagulant phenotype, (4) change from a vasodilator to a vasoconstrictor phenotype or, (5) change from a growth-inhibiting to a growth-promoting phenotype through elaboration of cytokines. Abnormal vasomotor function has been one of the most well-studied manifestations of endothelial dysfunction in subjects with either established atherosclerosis or in those with risk factors for atherosclerosis. Normal healthy endothelium produces nitric oxide from arginine through the action of a family of enzymes known as nitric oxide synthases.[31,32,37] Nitric oxide acts as a local vasodilator by increasing smooth muscle cell cyclic guanosine monophosphate levels, while at the same time inhibiting platelet aggregation and smooth muscle cell proliferation.[31,32,37] In the presence of risk factors, a reduced vasodilator response to endothelium-dependent vasodilator stimuli or even paradoxical vasoconstrictor response to such stimuli have been observed in large vessels as well as in the microcirculation, even in absence of structural abnormalities in the vessel wall.[31,32,37] These abnormal vasomotor responses have been attributed to reduced bioavailability of endothelium-derived

TABLE 52–2

Endothelial Activation/Dysfunction in Atherosclerosis

Phenotypic features
1. Reduced vasodilator and increased vasoconstrictor capacity
   Enhanced oxidant stress with increased inactivation of nitric oxide
   Increased expression of endothelin
2. Enhanced leukocyte (inflammatory cell) adhesion and recruitment
   Increased adhesion molecule expression (ICAM, VCAM)
   Increased chemotactic molecule expression (MCP-1, IL-8)
3. Increased prothrombotic and reduced fibrinolytic phenotype
4. Increased growth-promoting phenotype

Factors contributing to endothelial activation/dysfunction
1. Dyslipidemia and atherogenic lipoprotein modification
   Elevated LDL, VLDL, LP(a)
   LDL modification (oxidation, glycation)
   Reduced HDL
2. Increased angiotensin II and hypertension
3. Insulin resistance and diabetes
4. Estrogen deficiency
5. Smoking
6. Hyperhomocysteinemia?
7. Advancing age
8. Infection?

HDL, high-density lipoprotein; ICAM, intercellular adhesion molecule; IL, interleukin; LDL, low-density lypoprotein; LP(a), lipoprotein (a); MCP-1, monocyte chemotactic protein-1; VCAM, vascular cell adhesion; VLDL, very-low-density lipoprotein.

relaxing factor(s), specifically nitric oxide, as a result of rapid inactivation of nitric oxide by oxidant stress or excess generation of asymmetric dimethylarginine and/or increased production of vasoconstrictors such as endothelin.[31,32,37]

A major contributor to endothelial injury is LDL-cholesterol modified by processes such as oxidation, glycation (in diabetes), aggregation, association with proteoglycans, or incorporation into immune complexes.[31–33,36,38–40] Oxidized LDL is present in the atherosclerotic lesions of both experimental animals and humans.[41] Subendothelial retention of LDL particles results in progressive oxidation and its subsequent internalization by macrophages through the scavenger receptors.[36,38,39] The internalization leads to the formation of lipid peroxides and facilitates the accumulation of cholesterol esters, even finally resulting in the formation of foam cells. Once modified and taken up by macrophages, LDL activates the foam cells. In addition to its ability to injure these cells, modified LDL is chemotactic for other monocytes and can upregulate the expression of genes for macrophage colony-stimulating factor (M-CSF) and monocyte chemotactic protein derived from endothelial cells.[42–45] Thus, it may help expand the inflammatory response by stimulating the replication of monocyte-derived macrophages and the entry of new monocytes into lesions. Continued inflammatory response stimulates migration and proliferation of smooth muscle cells that accumulate within the ar-

eas of inflammation to form an intermediate fibroproliferative lesion resulting in thickening of the artery wall.

The inflammatory and immune response in atherosclerosis consists of accumulation of monocyte-derived macrophages and specific subtypes of T lymphocytes at every stage of the disease.[5,46–52] The fatty streak, the earliest type lesion, common in infants and young children, consists of monocyte-derived macrophages, macrophage-derived foam cells, and T lymphocytes. The critical role of the macrophage in atherogenesis is supported by the virtual absence (or drastic reduction) of atherosclerosis when M-CSF null genotype is introduced in murine models of severe dyslipidemia induced by a diet or genetic manipulation.[53,54]

Continued inflammation results in increased numbers of macrophages and lymphocytes, which both emigrate from the blood and multiply within the lesion. Activation of these cells leads to the release of proteolytic enzymes, cytokines, chemokines, and growth factors, which can induce further damage and eventually lead to focal necrosis. Necrosis and/or apoptosis of foam cells results in the formation of the necrotic lipid core in the plaque.[55] Thus, cycles of accumulation of mononuclear cells, migration and proliferation of smooth muscle cells, and formation of fibrous tissue lead to further enlargement and restructuring of the lesion, so that it becomes covered by a fibrous cap that overlies a core of lipid and necrotic tissue resulting in the formation of an advanced and complicated atherosclerotic plaque.

The inflammatory response itself can influence lipoprotein transfer within the vessel wall. Proinflammatory cytokines, such as tumor necrosis factor-α (TNF-α), interleukin (IL)-1, and M-CSF increase binding of LDL to endothelium and smooth muscle and increase the transcription of the LDL-receptor gene.[56] After binding to scavenger receptors in vitro, modified LDL initiates a series of intracellular events that include the induction of proteases and inflammatory cytokines.[56] Thus, a vicious circle of inflammation, modification of lipoproteins, and further inflammation can be maintained in the artery by the presence of these modified lipoproteins.

Monocyte-derived macrophages are present in various stages of atherosclerosis and act as scavenging and antigen-presenting cells. They produce cytokines, chemokines, growth-regulating molecules, tissue factor, metalloproteinases, and other hydrolytic enzymes. The continuing entry, survival, and replication of monocytes/macrophages in lesions depend in part on growth factors, such as M-CSF and granulocyte-macrophage colony-stimulating factor (GM-CSF), whereas IL-2 is involved in a similar manner for T lymphocytes. Recent experimental observations suggest that in and out trafficking of macrophages within the atherosclerotic vascular wall may be regulated by the microenvironment within the lesion with ingress and retention being promoted by a proinflammatory milieu related to oxidized lipids whereas egress via the lumen or via transformation into migratory dendritic cells and subsequent immigration to regional lymph nodes is associated with reduced proinflammatory lipids in the lesion; an environment promoted by high HDL levels favoring lesion regression.[57] Dendritic cells have been identified within the subendothelium and the adventitia of normal blood vessels. An increase in the number and activity of subendothelial dendritic cells has been observed in the atherosclerotic lesion raising the possibility that dendritic cells may be involved in the pathophysiology of atherosclerosis.[58,59]

Activated macrophages as well as lesional smooth muscle cells express class II histocompatibility antigens, such as HLA-DR, that allow them to present antigens to T lymphocytes.[5,46–52,56] Atherosclerotic lesions contain both CD4 and CD8 T cells, implicating the immune system in atherogenesis.[5,46–52] T-cell activation, following antigen processing, results in production of various cytokines, such as interferon-γ (INF-γ) and TNF-α and -β, which can further enhance the inflammatory response. Antigens presented include oxidized LDL and heat shock protein 60, which may participate in the immune response in atherosclerosis.[5,46–52]

Macrophages, T cells, endothelial cells, and smooth muscle cells in the atherosclerotic lesions express CD40 ligand and its receptor, which may play a role in atherogenesis by regulating the function of inflammatory cells.[60–63] The antiatherogenic effects of CD40-blocking antibodies in the murine model of atherosclerosis suggests that CD40-mediated signaling may play an important role in atherogenesis.[64]

Platelet adhesion and mural thrombosis are ubiquitous in the generation of advanced atherosclerotic lesions in humans and some animals.[56] Platelets can adhere to dysfunctional endothelium, exposed collagen, and macrophages. When activated, platelets release their granules, which contain cytokines and growth factors that, together with thrombin, may contribute to the migration and proliferation of smooth muscle cells and monocytes. Activation of platelets leads to the formation of free arachidonic acid, which can be transformed into prostaglandins such as thromboxane A_2, one of the most potent vasoconstricting and platelet-aggregating substances known, or into leukotrienes, which can amplify the inflammatory response.

Angiotensin II, a potent vasoconstrictor, may also contribute to atherogenesis by stimulating the growth of smooth muscle, increasing oxidant stress, inducing LDL oxidation, and promoting an inflammatory response.[56,65–68]

Elevated plasma homocysteine concentrations, resulting from enzymatic defects or vitamin deficiency, may facilitate atherothrombosis by inducing endothelial dysfunction with reduction in vasodilator capacity and enhanced prothrombotic phenotype and smooth muscle replication.[69–73] However, although numerous observational studies have found a positive association between hyperhomocysteinemia and increased risk of atherosclerotic cardiovascular disease,[69–73] recent clinical trials failed to reduce the risk of recurrent vascular events in high-risk patients by lowering the homocysteine level with folic acid and B vitamins.[74,75]

TRIGGERS OF INFLAMMATION IN ATHEROSCLEROSIS

It is likely that a number of stimuli are responsible for provoking and sustaining a chronic inflammatory response in the vessel wall in atherosclerosis. Among the key potential culprits are the modified lipoproteins and infectious agents (Table 52–3). Oxidatively modified lipoproteins can induce a variety of proinflammatory genes in the vessel wall that are responsible for recruiting and activating inflammatory cells such as ICAM- and VCAM-type adhesion molecules, chemotactic cytokines such as MCP-1, IL-8, and colony-stimulating factors such as M-CSF. In addition to modified lipoproteins, there is now a body of indirect evidence suggesting that arterial wall infec-

TABLE 52–3

Potential Role of Infection in Atherothrombosis

Infectious organisms implicated
1. Viruses
   Herpes virus
   Cytomegalovirus
2. Bacteria
   Chlamydia pneumoniae
   Helicobacter pylori
   Porphyromonas gingivalis?

Mechanism(s) by which infections may contribute to atherothrombosis
1. Direct infection of the vascular wall with endothelial injury, inflammatory cell recruitment, and activation (*C. pneumoniae*, herpes virus, cytomegalovirus)
2. Immune-mediated vascular injury through molecular mimicry (*C. pneumoniae*)
3. Remote infections with systemic activation of the inflammatory response (*H. pylori*, *P. gingivalis*)

tions with organisms such as *Chlamydia pneumoniae*, cytomegalovirus (CMV)/herpes virus, as well as remote infections such as chronic bronchitis, gingivitis, and *Helicobacter pylori* infection may affect inflammation, thereby contributing to atherogenesis and/or plaque disruption and thrombosis in the presence of preexisting atherosclerosis.[76–88] Increased titers of antibodies to these organisms have been used as a predictor of further adverse events in patients who have had a myocardial infarction. Organisms, particularly *C. pneumoniae*, have been identified in atheromatous lesions in coronary arteries and in other organs obtained at autopsy. The case for *C. pneumoniae* is of particular interest because acceleration of atherosclerosis with *C. pneumoniae* infection has been demonstrated in both the hypercholesterolemic rabbit and in genetically hyperlipidemic mice.[84,85] In addition, pilot clinical trials of antichlamydial macrolide antibiotics have raised the possibility that such therapy may reduce the risk of recurrent coronary events.[86,87] In vitro studies suggest that *C. pneumoniae* can trigger proatherogenic events, such as foam cell formation, procoagulant activity, and metalloproteinase activity in monocytes, probably mediated by its heat shock protein 60.[76] Molecular antigenic mimicry between certain chlamydia antigens and myosin have also raised the additional possibility that such antigenic mimicry could be involved in an immune-mediated vascular and myocardial injury.[88] However, recent large-scale clinical trials have failed to demonstrate any clinical benefit of using antibiotics targeting *C. pneumoniae*, raising questions about a link between this infection and atherothrombosis.[89–92]

INNATE IMMUNITY, TOLL-LIKE RECEPTORS AND ATHEROSCLEROSIS

Toll-like receptors are a family of transmembrane receptors that serve as signaling receptors in the innate immune system; their ligation by exogenous and possibly endogenous ligands triggers a proinflammatory signaling cascade in various cells linking innate immunity to inflammation.[93,94] Recent studies show that Toll-like receptors are expressed in murine and human atherosclerotic lesions and that hyperlipidemia induces proinflammatory signaling, in part through these receptors and their downstream adaptor molecules, such as MyD88 (myeloid differentiation factor) contributing to vascular inflammation, neointimal hyperplasia, and atherosclerosis in murine models.[94–96]

INFLAMMATION, ANGIOGENESIS, AND ATHEROSCLEROSIS

Angiogenesis or neovascularization is an essential process that supports chronic inflammation and fibroproliferation, processes that are involved in atherogenesis. Several studies demonstrate increased angiogenesis in atherosclerotic lesions, and hypercholesterolemia increases adventitial neovascularity in porcine arteries before the development of an atherosclerotic lesion.[97–100] Concomitant development of vasa vasorum with advanced lesion formation in aortas of hypercholesterolemic mice was recently demonstrated after scanning with microcomputed tomography.[101] Proinflammatory chemokines, such as IL-8, and other angiogenic growth factors, such as vascular endothelial growth factor, have been demonstrated in atherosclerotic lesions where they could contribute to angiogenesis.[102] Angiogenesis may contribute to plaque progression by providing a source of intraplaque hemorrhage, which, in turn, may provide red cell membrane-derived cholesterol, contributing to the expansion of the necrotic lipid core.[103] In addition, neovascular channels may also provide a source of inflammatory cells into the vessel wall; thus angiogenesis and inflammation appear to be linked pathophysiologic processes.[103–105] Recently, the ability of macrophages to undergo transdifferentiation into functional endothelial cells was demonstrated, suggesting yet another potential direct link between inflammation and angiogenesis.[106] Recent preliminary data demonstrating an inhibitory effect of angiostatin in murine models of atherosclerosis suggests the potential proatherogenic role for angiogenesis.[107]

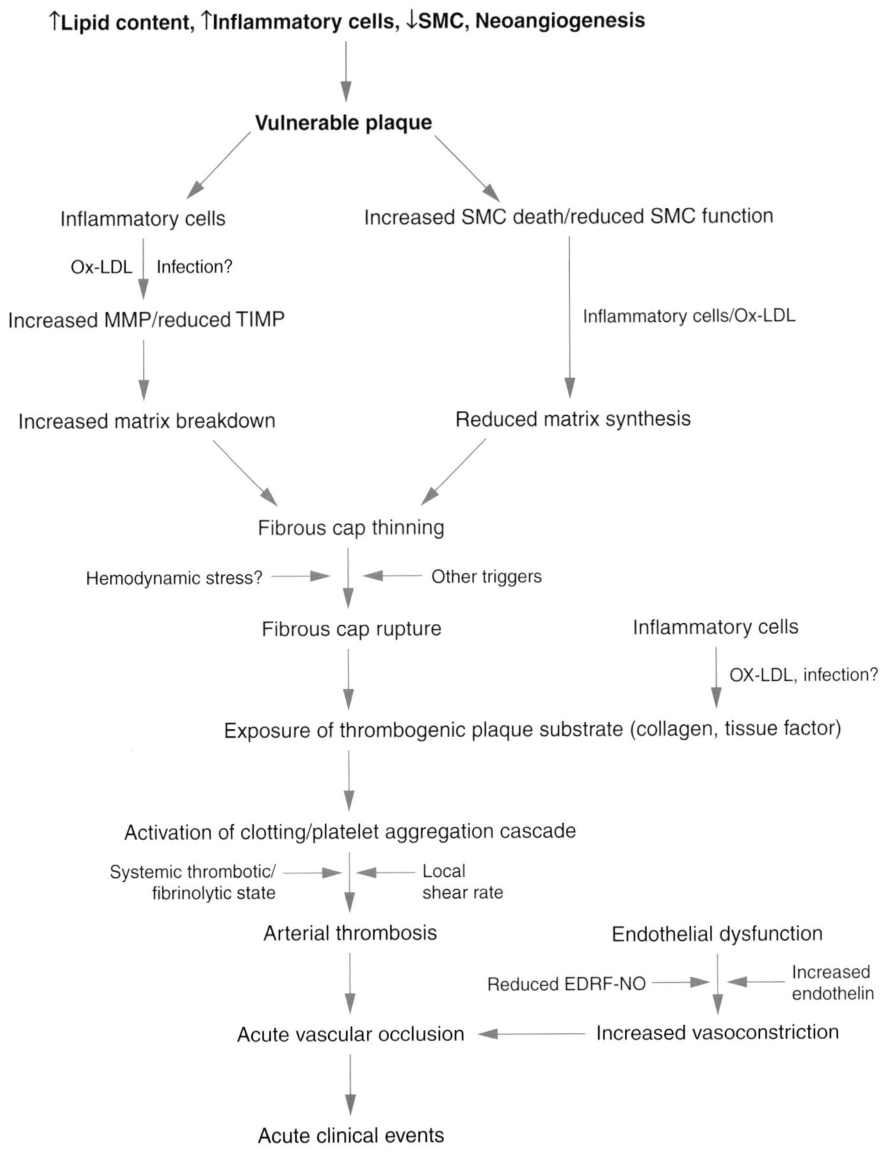

INFLAMMATION, PLAQUE RUPTURE, AND THROMBOSIS

Thrombosis-complicating atherosclerosis is the mechanism by which atherosclerosis leads to acute ischemic syndromes of unstable angina, non–ST-elevation, and ST-elevation myocardial infarction and many cases of sudden cardiac death.[108–113] In most cases, coronary thrombosis occurs as a result of uneven thinning and rupture of the fibrous cap, often at the shoulders of a lipid-rich lesion where macrophages and T cells enter, accumulate, and are activated, and where apoptosis may occur (Fig. 52–1).[108–111] Thinning of the fibrous cap may result from elaboration of matrix-degrading metalloproteinases (MMPs) such as collagenases (MMP-1, MMP-13), gelatinases (MMP-2, MMP-9), elastases (MMP-12), stromelysins (MMP-3), and/or other proteases, such as cathepsins, by inflammatory cells, chiefly macrophages.[110,111,114,115] These proteases may be induced or activated by oxidized LDL, cell-to-cell interaction between macrophages and activated T cells, CD40 ligation, mast cell-derived proteases, oxidant radicals, matrix proteins such as tenascin-C, and infectious agents.[110,111,114–116] Thinning may also result from increased smooth muscle cell death by apoptosis/necrosis and consequent reduced matrix production.[117,118] Death of vascular smooth muscle cells in the atherosclerotic lesion may be triggered by

↑Lipid content, ↑Inflammatory cells, ↓SMC, Neoangiogenesis

Vulnerable plaque

Inflammatory cells

Ox-LDL | Infection?

Increased MMP/reduced TIMP

Increased matrix breakdown

Increased SMC death/reduced SMC function

Inflammatory cells/Ox-LDL

Reduced matrix synthesis

Fibrous cap thinning

Hemodynamic stress? → ← Other triggers

Fibrous cap rupture

Inflammatory cells

OX-LDL, infection?

Exposure of thrombogenic plaque substrate (collagen, tissue factor)

Activation of clotting/platelet aggregation cascade

Systemic thrombotic/ fibrinolytic state → ← Local shear rate

Arterial thrombosis

Endothelial dysfunction

Reduced EDRF-NO → ← Increased endothelin

Acute vascular occlusion ← Increased vasoconstriction

Acute clinical events

FIGURE 52–1. Schematic describing the pathways and steps involved in disruption of atherosclerotic plaques with consequent thrombosis. EDRF-NO, endothelium-derived relaxing factor-nitric oxide; MMP, matrix metalloproteinase; Ox-LDL, oxidized low-density lipoprotein; SMC, smooth muscle cell; TIMP, tissue inhibitor of metalloproteinase.

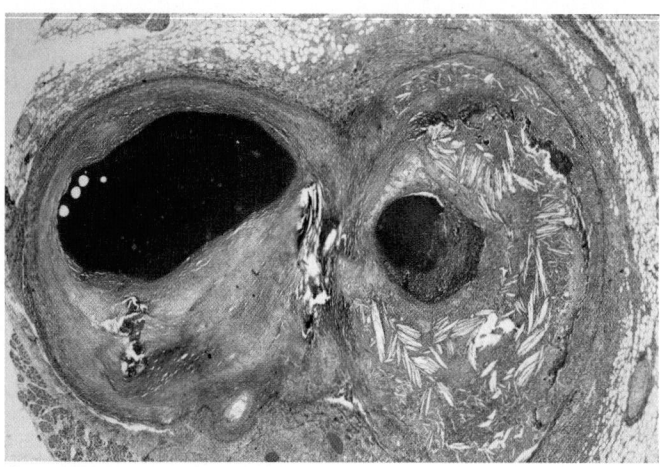
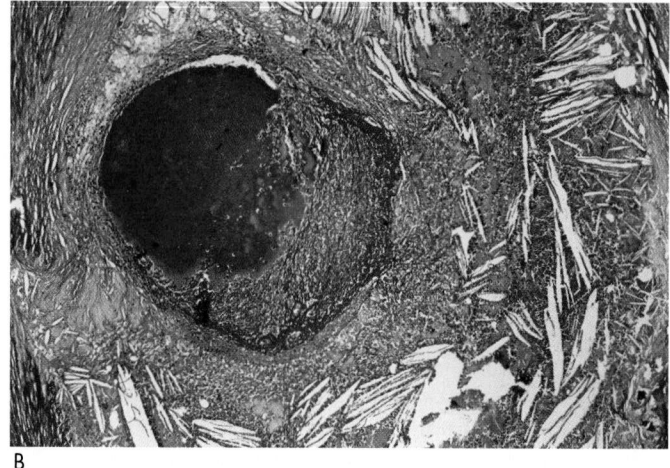

A B

FIGURE 52–2. Plaque rupture. **A.** Cross-section of a coronary artery cut just distal to a bifurcation. The atherosclerotic plaque to the left (circumflex branch) is fibrotic and partly calcified, whereas the plaque to the right (marginal branch) is lipid-rich with a nonoccluding thrombus superimposed. **B.** Higher magnification of the plaque-thrombus interface reveals that the fibrous cap overlying the lipid-rich necrotic core is extremely thin, inflamed, and ruptured with a real defect—a gap—in the cap. Both arteries contain contrast medium injected postmortem. Trichrome stain, staining collagen blue and thrombus red.

macrophages, as well as by subsets of T cells that are present in atherosclerotic plaques and in the circulating blood of patients with acute coronary syndromes. [119,120]

Inflammatory cells, specifically the macrophages, are also the main source of tissue factor in the atherosclerotic plaque. [121–123] Tissue factor, when exposed to circulating blood, interacts with activated factor VII to generate activated factor X; activated factor X, in turn, cleaves thrombin from prothrombin. Thrombin is involved in recruiting and activating platelets as well as the clotting cascade, thereby initiating thrombus formation. Tissue factor expression is increased in atherosclerotic plaques, particularly in unstable coronary syndromes. [122,123] The lipid core of the atheromatous lesion is heavily impregnated with tissue factor derived from dead (possibly apoptotic) macrophages and foam cells, accounting for its high thrombogenicity. [124] Macrophage tissue factor expression may be induced by a variety of signals in the atherosclerotic plaque, including various cytokines, infectious agents, and oxidized lipoproteins. Fur-

thermore, elevated levels of blood-borne tissue factor may also be detected in patients with acute coronary syndromes. [125] Thrombosis may also occur on a proteoglycan-rich matrix without a large lipid core, and in such cases, evidence of superficial endothelial erosion is found. [126] This plaque erosion may account for thrombosis in a relatively higher proportion of young victims of sudden death, particularly in premenopausal women who smoke. [126] The precise molecular basis for these plaque erosions is not clear, although endothelial desquamation through activation of basement membrane-degrading MMP may be involved. [115]

Plaques with a large necrotic core, activated inflammatory cell infiltration, and a thinned fibrous cap are considered vulnerable or thrombosis-prone plaques (Fig. 52–2). [127] Their identification may be particularly difficult because they may not produce symptoms because of lack of flow-limiting stenoses and may thus escape detection by stress testing and even angiography (Fig. 52–3). [113,128] Plaque rupture is responsible for approximately 75 percent of fatal coronary thrombi (80 percent in men and 60 percent in women; Table 52–4). [108] Furthermore, multiple ruptured and inflamed plaques often coexist in the coronary arteries of patients with acute coronary syndromes, indicating that a local-culprit lesion-based approach is not enough to eliminated the risk of recurrent events, but systemic treatment is (also) necessary. [129–131] Inflammation in atherosclerosis may be accompanied by elevation of circulating proinflammatory markers such as C-reactive protein, IL-6, serum amyloid A, and a variety of soluble leukocyte adhesion molecules. [132–137] Elevated C-reactive protein levels are associated with an increased risk of adverse cardiac events in patients with symptomatic vascular disease, as well as in asymptomatic patients who are at risk for vascular disease. [132–135,137] However, the predictive value of C-reactive protein beyond that provided by conventional risk factors seems to be limited. [138–140]

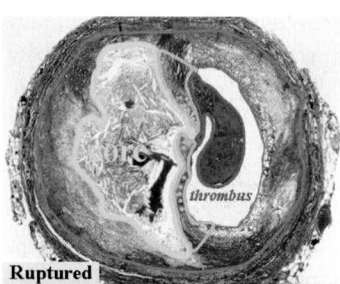
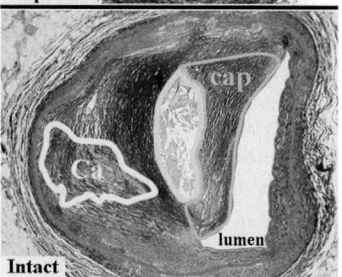

- Plaque size ↑
- Necrotic core ↑
  - ~34% of plaque area*
  - ~38 mm² & ~9 mm long*
- Fibrous cap
  - thickness ↓, ~23 μm (95% <65 μm)*
  - macrophages ↑, ~26% of cap*
  - smooth muscle cells ↓ (apoptosis)
  - thrombus ↑
- Expansive remodeling ↑
- Angiogenesis ↑
  - intraplaque hemorrhage
- Perivascular inflammation
- Calcification ↓ & spotty

FIGURE 52–3. Vulnerable coronary plaque: potential targets for imaging. *Source: Reprinted from Kolodgie FD, Virmani R. Heart 2004;90:1385–91.*

CONCLUSIONS

Atherosclerosis is a complex disease process that involves lipoprotein influx, lipoprotein modification, increased prooxidant stress, and inflammatory, angiogenic, and fibroproliferative responses in-

TABLE 52–4

Worldwide, 1114 (76%) of 1460 Fatal Coronary Thrombi Were Precipitated by Plaque Rupture

PATIENTS	AGE (Y)[a]	N	RUPTURE	STUDY[b]
Hospital, —	—	19	19 = 100%	Chapman, 1965
Hospital, —	—	17	17 = 100%	Constantinides, 1966
Hospital, AMI + SCD	58	40	39 = 98%	Friedman et al., 1966
Hospital, AMI	62	88	71 = 81%	Bouch et al., 1970
Hospital, AMI	53	20	68 = 75%	Sinapius, 1972
Coroner, SCD	53	20	19 = 95%	Friedman et al., 1973
Hospital, AMI	67	76	69 = 91%	Horie et al., 1978
Coroner, SCD	<65	32	26 = 81%	Tracy et al., 1985
Medical Exam, SCD	<70	61	39 = 64%	El Fawal et al., 1987
Hospital, AMI	—	83	52 = 63%	Yutani at al., 1987
Coroner, —	—	85	71 = 84%	Richardson et., 1989
Hospital, AMI	63	20	12 = 60%	van der Wal et al., 1994
Coroner, SCD	—	202	143 = 71%	Davies, 1997
Hospital, AMI	69	291	218 = 75%	Arbustini et al., 1999
Hospital, AMI	61	61	56 = 92%	Shi et al., 1999
Hospital, AMI	69	100	82 = 81%	Kojima et al., 2000
Medical Exam, SCD	48	125	74 = 59%	Virmani et al., 2000
Total AMI + SCD		1460	1114 = 76%	Wordwide

—, Not reported; AMI, acute myocardial infarction; SCD, sudden coronary death.
[a]Mean.
[b]For details, see Falk and Shah.[108]

termingled with extracellular matrix and lipid accumulation, resulting in the formation of an atherosclerotic plaque. Endothelial activation/dysfunction is common in atherosclerosis and often manifests as a reduced vasodilator or enhanced vasoconstrictor phenotype that contributes to luminal compromise. Thrombosis resulting from plaque rupture or superficial erosion complicates atherosclerosis, often resulting in abrupt luminal occlusion with resultant acute ischemic syndromes. Infectious agents may contribute to the inflammatory response and thus to destabilization of lesions. An improved understanding of the pathophysiology of atherosclerosis is providing novel directions for its prevention and treatment. In particular, the recognition of the important role of inflammation could lead to novel therapeutic interventions directed at selective inhibition of inflammatory cascade in the vessel wall. Targeting inflammatory triggers such as lipoproteins, angiotensin II, possible infectious agents, and others is likely to lead to improved outcomes in patients with atherosclerosis.

REFERENCES

1. Mackay J, Mensah G. *The Atlas of Heart Disease and Stroke*. World Health Organization and U.S. Centers for Disease Control and Prevention 2004. Available at http://www.who.int/cardiovascular_diseases/resources/atlas/en/.
2. *A Race Against Time. The Challenge of Cardiovascular Disease in Developing Economies*. New York, Columbia University, 2004. Available at http://www.earth.columbia.edu/news/2004/images/raceagainsttime_FINAL_0410404.pdf.
3. Fuster V. Cardiovascular disease and the UN Millennium Development Goals: a serious concern. *Nat Clin Pract Cardiovasc Med* 2006;3:401.
4. Libby P. Inflammation in atherosclerosis [review]. *Nature* 2002;420:868–874.
5. Hansson GK. Inflammation, atherosclerosis, and coronary artery disease. *N Engl J Med* 2005;352:1685–1695.
6. Nilsson J, Hansson GK, Shah PK. Immunomodulation of atherosclerosis: implications for vaccine development. *Arterioscler Thromb Vasc Biol* 2005;25:18–28.
7. McMillian DE. Blood flow and the localization of atherosclerotic plaques. *Stroke* 1985;16:582–587.
8. Langille BL, Dajnowiec D, Gotlieb AI. The role of rheology in atherothrombotic coronary artery disease. In: Fuster V, Topol EJ, Nabel EG, eds. *Atherothrombosis and Coronary Artery Disease*, 2d ed. Philadelphia: Lippincott Williams & Wilkins, 2005;561–568.
9. Cheng C, Tempel D, van Haperen R, et al. Atherosclerotic lesion size and vulnerability are determined by patterns of fluid shear stress. *Circulation* 2006;113:2744–2753.
10. Nagel T, Resnick N, Atkinson WJ, Dewey CF Jr, Gimbrone MA Jr. Shear stress selectively upregulates intercellular adhesion molecule-1, expression in cultured human vascular endothelial cells. *J Clin Invest* 1994;94:885–891.
11. Resnick N, Collins T, Atkinson W, Bonthron DT, Dewey CF Jr, Gimbrone MA Jr. Platelet-derived growth factor B chain promoter contains a cis-acting fluid shear-stress-responsive element. *Proc Natl Acad Sci U S A* 1993;90:4591–4595.
12. Lin MC, Almus-Jacobs F, Chen HH, et al. Shear stress induction of the tissue factor gene. *J Clin Invest* 1997;99:737–744.
13. Mondy JS, Lindner V, Miyashiro JK, Berk BC, Dean RH, Geary RL. Platelet-derived growth factor ligand and receptor expression in response to altered blood flow in vivo. *Circ Res* 1997;81:320.
14. Nakashima Y, Raines EW, Plump AS, Breslow JL, Ross R. Upregulation of VCAM-1, and ICAM-1, at atherosclerosis-prone sites on the endothelium in the ApoE-deficient mouse. *Arterioscler Thromb Vasc Biol* 1998;18:842–851.
15. Cybulsky MI, Charo IF. Leukocytes, adhesion molecules, and chemokines in atherothrombosis. In: Fuster V, Topol EJ, Nabel EG, eds. *Atherothrombosis and Coronary Artery Disease*, 2d ed. Philadelphia: Lippincott Williams & Wilkins, 2005;489–503.
16. Muller WA, Weigl SA, Deng X, Phillips DM. PECAM-1, is required for transendothelial migration of leukocytes. *J Exp Med* 1993;178:449–460.

17. Giachelli CM, Lombardi D, Johnson RJ, Murry CE, Almeida M. Evidence for a role of osteopontin in macrophage infiltration in response to pathological stimuli in vivo. *Am J Pathol* 1998;152:353–358.

18. Nagel T, Resnick N, Dewey CF Jr, Gimbrone MA Jr. Vascular endothelial cells respond to spatial gradients in fluid shear stress by enhanced activation of transcription factors. *Arterioscler Thromb Vasc Biol* 1999;19:1825–1834.

19. Parmar KM, Larman HB, Dai G, et al. Integration of flow-dependent endothelial phenotypes by Kruppel-like factor 2. *J Clin Invest* 2006;116:49–58.

20. Boisvert WA, Santiago R, Curtiss LK, Tekeltaub RA. A leukocyte homologue of the IL-8, receptor CXCR-2, mediates the accumulation of macrophages in atherosclerotic lesions of LDL receptor- deficient mice. *J Clin Invest* 1998;101:353–363.

21. Tedgui A, Mallat Z. Cytokines in atherosclerosis: pathogenic and regulatory pathways. *Physiol Rev* 2006;86:515–581.

22. Herren B, Raines EW, Ross R. Expression of a disintegrin-like protein in cultured human vascular cells and in vivo. *FASEB J* 1997;11:173–180.

23. Black RA, Rauch CT, Kozlosky CJ, et al. A metalloproteinase disintegrin that releases tumor-necrosis factor-(alpha) from cells. *Nature* 1997;385:729–733.

24. Moss ML, Jin S-LC, Milla ME, et al. Cloning of a disintegrin metalloproteinase that processes precursor tumour necrosis factor-(alpha). *Nature* 1997;385:733–736.

25. De Caterina R, Basta G, Lazzerini G, et al. Soluble vascular cell adhesion molecule-1, as a biohumoral correlate of atherosclerosis. *Arterioscler Thromb Vasc Biol* 1997;17:2646–2654.

26. Hwang S-J, Ballantyne CM, Sharrett AR, et al. Circulating adhesion molecules VCAM-1, ICAM-1, and E-selectin in carotid atherosclerosis and incident coronary heart disease cases: the Atherosclerosis Risk in Communities (ARIC) study. *Circulation* 1997;96:4219–4225.

27. Lind L. Circulating markers of inflammation and atherosclerosis. *Atherosclerosis* 2003;169:203–214.

28. Napoli C, D'Armiento FP, Mancini FP, et al. Fatty streak formation occurs in human fetal aortas and is greatly enhanced by maternal hypercholesterolemia: intimal accumulation of low density lipoprotein and its oxidation precede monocyte recruitment into early atherosclerotic lesions. *J Clin Invest* 1997;100:2680–2690.

29. Stary HC, Chandler AB, Glagov S, et al. A definition of initial, fatty streak, and intermediate lesions of atherosclerosis: a report from the Committee on Vascular Lesions of the Council on Atherosclerosis, American Heart Association. *Circulation* 1994;89:2462–2478.

30. Simionescu N, Vasile E, Lupu F, Popescu G, Simionescu M. Prelesional events in atherogenesis: accumulation of extracellular cholesterol-rich liposomes in the arterial intima and cardiac valves of the hyperlipidemic rabbit. *Am J Pathol* 1986;123:109–125.

31. Kinlay S, Ganz P. Role of endothelial dysfunction in coronary artery disease and implications for therapy. *Am J Cardiol* 1997;80:111–161.

32. Lerman A, Edwards BS, Hallett JW, Heublein DM, Sandberg SM, Burnett JC Jr. Circulating and tissue endothelin immunoreactivity in advanced atherosclerosis. *N Engl J Med* 1991;325:997–1001.

33. Steinberg D. Low-density lipoprotein oxidation and its pathobiological significance. *J Biol Chem* 1997;272:20963–20966.

34. Khoo JC, Miller E, McLoughlin P, Steinberg D. Enhanced macrophage uptake of low density lipoprotein after self-aggregation. *Arteriosclerosis* 1988;8:348–358.

35. Khoo JC, Miller E, Pio F, Steinberg D, Witztum JL. Monoclonal antibodies against LDL further enhance macrophage uptake of LDL aggregates. *Arterioscler Thromb* 1992;12:1258–1266.

36. Navab M, Berliner JA, Watson AD, et al. The Yin and Yang of oxidation in the development of the fatty streak: a review based on the 1994 George Lyman Duff Memorial Lecture. *Arterioscler Thromb Vasc Biol* 1996;16:831–834.

37. Bonetti PO, Lerman LO, Lerman A. Endothelial dysfunction: a marker of atherosclerotic risk. *Arterioscler Thromb Vasc Biol* 2003;23:168–175.

38. Skalen K, Gustafsson M, Rydberg EK, et al. Subendothelial retention of atherogenic lipoproteins in early atherosclerosis. *Nature* 2002;417:750–754.

39. Williams KJ, Tabas I. Lipoprotein retention—and clues for atheroma regression. *Arterioscler Thromb Vasc Biol* 2005;25:1536–1540.

40. Griendling KK, Alexander RW. Oxidative stress and cardiovascular disease. *Circulation* 1997;96:3264–3265.

41. Yla-Herttuala S, Palinski W, Rosenfeld ME, et al. Evidence for the presence of oxidatively modified low density lipoprotein in atherosclerotic lesions of rabbit and man. *J Clin Invest* 1989;84:1086–1095.

42. Han J, Hajjar DP, Febbraio M, Nicholson AC. Native and modified low-density lipoproteins increase functional expression of the macrophage class B scavenger receptor, CD36. *J Biol Chem* 1997;272:1654–1659.

43. Rajavashisth TB, Andalibi A, Territo MC, et al. Induction of endothelial cell expression of granulocyte and macrophage colony-stimulating factors by modified low-density lipoproteins. *Nature* 1990;344:254–257.

44. Quinn MT, Parthasarathy S, Fong LG, Steinberg D. Oxidatively modified low density lipoproteins: A potential role in recruitment and retention of monocyte/ macrophages during atherogenesis. *Proc Natl Acad Sci U S A* 1987;84:2995–2998.

45. Leonard EJ, Yoshimura T. Human monocyte chemoattractant protein-1, (MCP-1). *Immunol Today* 1990;11:97–101.

46. Jonasson L, Holm J, Skalli O, Bondjers G, Hansson GK. Regional accumulations of T cells, macrophages, and smooth muscle cells in the human atherosclerotic plaque. *Arteriosclerosis* 1986;6:131–138.

47. Van der Wal AC, Das PK, Bentz van de Berg D, van der Loos CM, Becker AE. Atherosclerotic lesions in humans: In situ immunophenotypic analysis suggesting an immune mediated response. *Lab Invest* 1989;166–170.

48. Schönbeck U, Libby P. Cytokines and growth regulatory molecules. In: Fuster V, Topol EJ, Nabel EG, eds. *Atherothrombosis and Coronary Artery Disease*, 2d ed. Philadelphia: Lippincott Williams & Wilkins, 2005:547–559.

49. Raines EW, Libby P, Rosenfeld ME. The role of macrophages. In: Fuster V, Topol EJ, Nabel EG, eds. *Atherothrombosis and Coronary Artery Disease*. Philadelphia: Lippincott Williams & Wilkins 2005:505–520.

50. Hansson GK, Libby P. The role of lymphocyte. In: Fuster V, Topol EJ, Nabel EG, eds. *Atherothrombosis and Coronary Artery Disease*, 2d ed. Philadelphia: Lippincott Williams & Wilkins, 2005:521–528.

51. Hansson GK, Jonasson L, Siefert PS, Stemme S. Immune mechanisms in atherosclerosis. *Arteriosclerosis* 1989;9:567–578.

52. Stemme S, Faber B, Holm J, Wiklund O, Witztum JL, Hansson GK. T lymphocytes from human atherosclerotic plaques recognize oxidized low density lipoprotein. *Proc Natl Acad Sci U S A* 1995;92:3893–3897.

53. Qiao J-H, Tripathi J, Mishra NK, et al. Role of macrophage colony-stimulating factor in atherosclerosis: studies of osteopetrotic mice. *Am J Pathol* 1997;150:1687–1699.

54. Rajavashisth T, Qiao JH, Tripathi S, et al. Heterozygous osteopetrotic (op) mutation reduces atherosclerosis in LDL receptor-deficient mice. *J Clin Invest* 1998;101:2702–2710.

55. Tabas I. Consequences and therapeutic implications of macrophage apoptosis in atherosclerosis: the importance of lesion stage and phagocytic efficiency. *Arterioscler Thromb Vasc Biol* 2005;25:2255- 64.

56. Ross R. Atherosclerosis: an inflammatory disease. *N Engl J Med* 1999;340:115–126.

57. Llodra J, Angeli V, Liu J, Trogan E, Fisher EA, Randolph GJ. Emigration of monocyte-derived cells from atherosclerotic lesions characterizes regressive, but not progressive, plaques. *Proc Natl Acad Sci U S A* 2004;101(32):11779–11784.

58. R.S. Lord and Y.V. Bobryshev, Clustering of dendritic cells in athero-prone areas of the aorta, *Atherosclerosis* 146, (1999), pp 197–198.

59. Yilmaz, Lochno M, Traeg F, et al. Emergence of dendritic cells in rupture-prone regions of vulnerable carotid plaques, *Atherosclerosis* 2004;176:101–110.

60. Hollenbaugh D, Mischel-Petty N, Edwards CP, et al. Expression of functional CD40, by vascular endothelial cells. *J Exp Med* 1995;182:33–40.

61. Mach F, Schonbeck U, Bonnefoy J-Y, Pober JS, Libby P. Activation of monocyte/macrophage functions related to acute atheroma complication by ligation of CD40: induction of collagenase, stromelysin, and tissue factor. *Circulation* 1997;96:396–399.

62. Schonbeck U, Mach F, Sukhova GK, et al. Regulation of matrix metalloproteinase expression in human vascular smooth muscle cells by T lymphocytes: a role for CD40, signaling in plaque rupture? *Circ Res* 1997;81:448–454.

63. Schonbeck U, Mach F, Bonnefoy J-Y, Loppnow H, Flad H-D, Libby P. Ligation of CD40, activates interleukin 1(beta)-converting enzyme (caspase-1) activity in vascular smooth muscle and endothelial cells and promotes elaboration of active interleukin 1(beta). *J Biol Chem* 1997;272:19569–19574.

64. Mach F, Schonbeck U, Sukhova GK, Atkinson E, Libby P. Reduction of atherosclerosis in mice by inhibition of CD40 signaling. *Nature* 1998;394:200–203.

65. Dzau VJ, Chobanian AV. Role of angiotensin in the pathobiology of cardiovascular disease. In: Fuster V, Topol EJ, Nabel EG, eds. *Atherothrombosis and Coronary Artery Disease*, 2d ed. Philadelphia: Williams & Wilkins, 2005:191–197.

66. Gibbons GH, Pratt RE, Dzau VJ. Vascular smooth muscle cell hypertrophy vs. hyperplasia: Autocrine transforming growth factor-beta 1, expression determines growth response to angiotensin II. *J Clin Invest* 1992;90:456–461.

67. Lacy F, O'Connor DT, Schmid-Schonbein GW. Plasma hydrogen peroxide production in hypertensive and normotensive subjects as genetic risk of hypertension. *J Hypertens* 1998;16:291–303.

68. Swei A, Lacy F, DeLano FA, Schmid-Schoenbein GW. Oxidative stress in the Dahl hypertensive rat. *Hypertension* 1997;30:1628–1633.

69. Nehler MR, Taylor LM Jr, Porter JM. Homocysteinemia as a risk factor for atherosclerosis: a review. *Cardiovasc Surg* 1997;6:559–567.

70. Nygard O, Nordrehaug JE, Refsum H, Ueland PM, Farstad M, Vollset SE. Plasma homocysteine levels and mortality in patients with coronary artery disease. *N Engl J Med* 1997;337:230–236.

71. Malinow MR. Plasma homocyst(e)ine and arterial occlusive disease diseases: a mini-review. *Clin Chem* 1995;41:173–176.

72. Verhoef P, Stampfer MJ. Prospective studies of homocysteine and cardiovascular disease. *Nutr Rev* 1995;53:283–288.

73. Omenn GS, Beresford SSA, Motulsky AG. Preventing coronary heart disease: B vitamins and homocysteine. *Circulation* 1998;97:421–424.

74. Lonn E, Yusuf S, Arnold MJ, et al. Homocysteine lowering with folic acid and B vitamins in vascular disease. *N Engl J Med* 2006;354:1567–1577.

75. Bonaa KH, Njolstad I, Ueland PM, et al. Homocysteine lowering and cardiovascular events after acute myocardial infarction. *N Engl J Med* 2006;354:1578–1588.

76. Libby P, Egan D, Skarlatos S. Roles of infectious agents in atherosclerosis and restenosis: an assessment of the evidence and need for future research. *Circulation* 1997;96:4095–4103.

77. Hendrix MG, Salimans MM, van Boven CP, Bruggeman CA. High prevalence of latently present cytomegalovirus in arterial walls of patients suffering from grade III atherosclerosis. *Am J Pathol* 1990;136:23–28.

78. Jackson LA, Campbell LA, Schmidt RA, et al. Specificity of detection of *Chlamydia pneumoniae* in cardiovascular atheroma: evaluation of the innocent bystander hypothesis. *Am J Pathol* 1997;150:1785–1790.

79. Thom DH, Wang SP, Grayston JT, et al. *Chlamydia pneumoniae* strain TWAR antibody and angiographically demonstrated coronary artery disease. *Arterioscler Thromb* 1991;11:547–551.

80. Melnick JL, Adam E, Debakey ME. Cytomegalovirus and atherosclerosis. *Eur Heart J* 1993;14(Suppl K):30–38.

81. Hajjar DP, Fabricant CG, Minick CR, Fabricant J. Virus-induced atherosclerosis: herpesvirus infection alters aortic cholesterol metabolism and accumulation. *Am J Pathol* 1986;122:62–70.

82. Nicholson AC, Hajjar DP. Herpesviruses in atherosclerosis and thrombosis: etiologic agents or ubiquitous bystanders? *Arterioscler Thromb Vasc Biol* 1998;18:339–348.

83. Shah PK. Plaque disruption and coronary thrombosis: new insight into pathogenesis and prevention. *Clin Cardiol* 1997;20(II):38–44.

84. Muhlestein JB, Anderson JL, Hammond EH, et al. Infection with *Chlamydia pneumoniae* accelerates the development of atherosclerosis and treatment with azithromycin prevents it in a rabbit model. *Circulation* 1998;97:633–636.

85. Hu H, Pierce GN, Zhong G. The atherogenic effects of chlamydia are dependent on serum cholesterol and specific to *Chlamydia pneumoniae*. *J Clin Invest* 1999;103:747–753.

86. Gurfinkel E, Bozovich G, Daroca A, Beck E, Mautner B. Randomized trial of roxithromycin in non- Q-wave coronary syndromes: ROXIS Pilot Study. ROXIS Study Group [see comments]. *Lancet* 1997;350:404–407.

87. Gupta S, Leatham EW, Carrington D, Mendall MA, Kaski JC, Camm AJ. Elevated *Chlamydia pneumoniae* antibodies, cardiovascular events, and azithromycin in male survivors of myocardial infarction. *Circulation* 1997;96:404–407.

88. Bachmaier K, Neu N, de la Maza LM, Pal S, Hessel A, Penninger JM. *Chlamydia* infections and heart disease linked through antigenic mimicry. *Science* 1999;283:1335–1339.

89. Cercek B, Shah PK, Noc M, et al. Effect of short-term treatment with azithromycin on recurrent ischemic events in patients with acute coronary syndrome in the Azithromycin in Acute Coronary Syndrome (AZACS) trial: a randomised controlled trial. *Lancet* 2003;361(9360):809–813.

90. O'Connor CM, Dunne MW, Pfeffer MA, et al. Azithromycin for the secondary prevention of coronary heart disease events: the WIZARD study: a randomized controlled trial. *JAMA* 2003;290(11):1459–1466.

91. Cannon CP, Braunwald E, McCabe CH, et al. Antibiotic treatment of *Chlamydia pneumoniae* after acute coronary syndrome. *N Engl J Med* 2005;352(16):1646–1654.

92. Grayston JT, Kronmal RA, Jackson LA, et al. Azithromycin for the secondary prevention of coronary events. *N Engl J Med* 2005;352(16):1637–1645.

93. Xu XH, Shah PK, Faure E, et al. Toll-like receptor-4, is expressed by macrophages in murine and human lipid-rich atherosclerotic plaques and upregulated by oxidized LDL. *Circulation* 2001;104:3103–3108.

94. Michelsen KS, Doherty TM, Shah PK, Arditi M. TLR signaling: an emerging bridge from innate immunity to atherogenesis. *J Immunol* 2004;173:5901–5907.

95. Michelsen KS, Wong MH, Shah PK, et al. Lack of Toll-like receptor 4, or myeloid differentiation factor 88, reduces atherosclerosis and alters plaque phenotype in mice deficient in apolipoprotein E. *Proc Natl Acad Sci U S A* 2004;101:10679–10684.

96. Bjorkbacka H, Kunjathoor VV, Moore KJ, et al. Reduced atherosclerosis in MyD88-null mice links elevated serum cholesterol levels to activation of innate immunity signaling pathways. *Nat Med* 2004;10:416–421.

97. Folkman J. Angiogenesis in cancer, vascular, rheumatoid and other diseases. *Nat Med* 1995;1:27–31.

98. Barger AC, Beeuwkes R, Iainey LL, Silverman KJ. Hypothesis: vasa vasorum and neovascularization of human coronary arteries. *N Engl J Med* 1984;310:175–177.

99. O'Brien ER, Garvin MR, Dev R, et al. Angiogenesis in human atherosclerotic plaques. *Am J Pathol* 1994;145:883–894.

100. Kwon HM, Sangiorgi G, Ritman EL, et al. Enhanced coronary vasa vasorum neovascularization in experimental hypercholesterolemia. *J Clin Invest* 1998;101:1551–1556.

101. Langheinrich AC, Michniewicz A, Sedding DG, et al. Correlation of vasa vasorum neovascularization and plaque progression in aortas of apolipoprotein E(/)/low-density lipoprotein(/) double knockout mice. *Arterioscler Thromb Vasc Biol* 2006;26:347–352.

102. Wang N, Tabas I, Winchester R, Ravalli S, Rabbani L, Tall A. Interleukin-8 is induced by cholesterol loading of macrophages and expressed by macrophage foam-cells in human atheroma. *J Biol Chem* 1996;271:8837–8842.

103. Virmani R, Kolodgie FD, Burke AP, et al. Atherosclerotic plaque progression and vulnerability to rupture: angiogenesis as a source of intraplaque hemorrhage. *Arterioscler Thromb Vasc Biol* 2005;25(10):2054.

104. Moreno PR, Purushothaman KR, Sirol M, Levy AP, Fuster V. Neovascularization in human atherosclerosis. *Circulation* 2006;113:2245–2252.

105. Herrmann J, Lerman LO, Mukhopadhyay D, Napoli C, Lerman A. Angiogenesis in atherogenesis. *Arterioscler Thromb Vasc Biol* 2006;26(9):1948–1957.

106. Sharifi BG, Zeng Z, Wang L, et al. Pleiotrophin induces transdifferentiation of monocytes into functional endothelial cells. *Arterioscler Thromb Vasc Biol* 2006;26(6):1273–1280.

107. Moulton KS, Heller E, Konerding MA, Flynn E, Palinski W, Folkman J. Angiogenesis inhibitor endostatin or TNP-470, reduces intimal neovascularization and plaque growth in apolipoprotein E deficient mice. *Circulation* 1999;99:1726–1732.

108. Falk E, Shah PK. Pathogenesis of atherothrombosis—role of vulnerable, ruptured, and eroded plaques. In: Fuster V, Topol EJ, Nabel EG, eds. *Atherothrombosis and Coronary Artery Disease*, 2d ed. Philadelphia: Lippincott Williams & Wilkins, 2005:451–465.

109. Lee RT, Libby P. The unstable atheroma. *Arterioscler Thromb Vasc Biol* 1997;17:1859–1867.

110. Shah PK. Role of inflammation and metalloproteinases in plaque disruption and thrombosis. *Vasc Med* 1998;3:199–206.

111. Shah PK. Plaque disruption and thrombosis. Potential role of inflammation and infection. *Cardiol Clin* 1999;17:271–281.

112. Fuster V, Moreno PR, Fayad ZA, Corti R, Badimon JJ. Atherothrombosis and high-risk plaque: part I. evolving concepts. *J Am Coll Cardiol* 2005;46:937–954.

113. Falk E. Pathogenesis of atherosclerosis. *J Am Coll Cardiol* 2006;47(Suppl):C7–C12.

114. Xu XP, Meisel SR, Ong JM, et al. Oxidized low-density lipoprotein regulates matrix metalloproteinase-9 and its tissue inhibitor in human monocyte-derived macrophages. *Circulation* 1999;99:993–998.

115. Rajavashisth TB, Xu XP, Jovinge S, et al. Membrane type 1 matrix metalloproteinase expression in human atherosclerosis plaques: evidence for activation by proinflammatory mediators. *Circulation* 1999;99:3103–3109.

116. Wallner K, Shah PK, Fishbein MC, Forrester JS, Kaul S, Sharifi BG. Tenascin-C is expressed in macrophage-rich human coronary atherosclerotic plaque. *Circulation* 1999;16:1284–1289.

117. Geng Y-J, Libby P. Evidence for apoptosis in advanced human atheroma: colocalization with interleukin-1 beta-converting enzyme. *Am J Pathol* 1995;147:251–266.

118. Wallner K, Li Chen, Shah PK, Wu KJ, Schwartz S, Sharifi BG. The EGF-L domain of tenascin-C is pro-apoptotic for cultured smooth muscle cells. *Arterioscler Thromb Vasc Biol* 2004;24:1416–1421.

119. Pryshchep S, Sato K, Goronzy JJ, Weyand C. T cell recognition and killing of vascular smooth muscle cells in acute coronary syndrome. *Circ Res* 2006;98:1168–1176.

120. Flavahan NA. A farewell kiss triggers a broken heart. *Circ Res* 2006;98:1117–1119.

121. Wilcox JN, Smith KM, Schwartz SM, Gordon D. Localization of tissue factor in the normal vessel wall and in the atherosclerotic plaque. *Proc Natl Acad Sci U S A* 1989;86:2839–2843.

122. Moreno PR, Bernardi VH, López-Cuéllar J, et al. Macrophages, smooth muscle cells, and tissue factor in unstable angina. Implications for cell-mediated thrombogenicity in acute coronary syndromes. *Circulation* 1996;94:3090–3097.

123. Toschi V, Gallo R, Lettino M, et al. Tissue factor modulates the thrombogenicity of human atherosclerotic plaque. *Circulation* 1997;95:594–599.

124. Fernandez-Ortiz A, Badimon JJ, Falk E, et al. Characterization of the relative thrombogenicity of atherosclerotic plaque components: Implications for consequences of plaque rupture. *J Am Coll Cardiol* 1994;23:1562–1569.

125. Steffel J, Luscher TF, Tanner FC. Tissue factor in cardiovascular diseases: molecular mechanisms and clinical implications. *Circulation* 2006;113:722–731.

126. Burke AP, Farb A, Malcom GT, Liang Y, Smialek J, Virmani R. Effect of risk factors on the mechanism of acute thrombosis and sudden coronary death in women. *Circulation* 1998;97(21):2110–2116.

127. Schaar JA, Muller JE, Falk E, et al. Terminology for high-risk and vulnerable coronary artery plaques. *Eur Heart J* 2004;25:1077–1082.

128. Fuster V, Fayad ZA, Moreno PR, Poon M, Corti R, Badimon JJ. Atherothrombosis and high-risk plaque: part II. Approaches by non-invasive computed tomographic/magnetic resonance imaging. *J Am Coll Cardiol* 2005;46:1209–1218.

129. Tanaka A, Shimada K, Sano T, et al. Multiple plaque rupture and C-reactive protein in acute myocardial infarction. *J Am Coll Cardiol* 2005;45:1594–1599.

130. Mauriello A, Sangiorgi G, Fratoni S, et al. Diffuse and active inflammation occurs in both vulnerable and stable plaques of the entire coronary tree: a histopathologic study of patients dying of acute myocardial infarction. *J Am Coll Cardiol* 2005;45:1585–1593.

131. Libby P. Act local, act global: inflammation and the multiplicity of "vulnerable" coronary plaques. *J Am Coll Cardiol* 2005;45:1600–1602.

132. Ridker PM, Cushman M, Stampfer MJ, Tracy RP, Hennekens CH. Inflammation, aspirin, and the risk of cardiovascular disease in apparently healthy men. *N Engl J Med* 1997;336:973–979.

133. Haverkate F, Thompson SG, Pyke SD, Gallimore JR, Pepys MB. Production of C-reactive protein and risk of coronary events in stable and unstable angina: European Concerted Action on Thrombosis and Disabilities Angina Pectoris Study Group. *Lancet* 1997;349:462–466.

134. Toss H, Lindahl B, Siegbahn A, Wallentin L. Prognostic influence of increased fibrinogen and C-reactive protein levels in unstable coronary artery disease. *Circulation* 1997;96:4204–4210.

135. Berk BC, Weintraub WS, Alexander RW. Elevation of C-reactive protein in "active" coronary artery disease. *Am J Cardiol* 1990;65:168–172.

136. Levenson J, Giral P, Razavian M, Gariepy J, Simon A. Fibrinogen and silent atherosclerosis in subjects with cardiovascular risk factors. *Arterioscler Thromb Vasc Biol* 1995;15:1263–1268.

137. Libby P, Ridker PM, Maseri A. Inflammation and atherosclerosis. *Circulation* 2002;105:1135–1143.

138. Danesh J, Wheeler JG, Hirschfield GM, et al. C-reactive protein and other circulating markers of inflammation in the prediction of coronary heart disease. *N Engl J Med* 2004;350:1387–1397.

139. Tracy RP, Kuller LH. C-reactive protein, heart disease risk, and the popular media. *Arch Intern Med* 2005;165:2058–2060.

140. Blankenberg S, McQueen MJ, Smieja M, et al. Comparative impact of multiple biomarkers and N-terminal pro-brain natriuretic peptide in the context of conventional risk factors for the prediction of recurrent cardiovascular events in the Heart Outcomes Prevention Evaluation (HOPE) study. *Circulation* 2006;114:201–208.

CHAPTER (53)

Coronary Thrombosis:
Local and Systemic Factors

Juan Jose Badimon / Borja Ibanez /
Valentin Fuster / Lina Badimon

The formation of an acute thrombus on a ruptured coronary atherosclerotic lesion, obstructing coronary blood flow and reducing the oxygen supply to the myocardium, leads to the onset of acute coronary syndromes (ACSs). These thrombotic episodes largely occur in response to atherosclerotic lesions that have progressed to a high-risk inflammatory/prothrombotic stage. Although they are distinct from one another, the atherosclerotic and thrombotic processes appear to be closely interrelated, causing ACSs through a complex, multifactorial process called atherothrombosis. ACSs represent a spectrum of ischemic myocardial events that share similar pathophysiology; they include unstable angina/non–ST-segment elevation myocardial infarction, ST-segment elevation myocardial infarction, and sudden cardiac death.

Atherosclerosis is a systemic disease involving the intima of large and medium-sized arteries, including the aorta, carotids, coronaries, and peripheral arteries, that is characterized by intimal thickening as a consequence of the accumulation of cells and lipids (Fig. 53–1).[1] Lipid accumulation results from an imbalance between the mechanisms responsible for the influx and efflux of lipids into the arterial wall.[2] Secondary changes may occur in the underlying media and adventitia, particularly in advanced disease stages. The early atherosclerotic lesions might progress without compromising the lumen because of compensatory vascular enlargement (Glagovian remodeling).[3] Importantly, the culprit lesions leading to ACS are usually mildly stenotic and thus barely detected by angiography (Fig. 53–2).[4] These high-risk rupture-prone lesions usually have a large lipid core, a thin fibrous cap, and a high density of inflammatory cells (particularly at the shoulder region, where disruptions most often occur).

Recent evidences have highlighted the importance of lesion neovascularization and blood extravasation in plaque destabilization and plaque growth.[5-7] Leaky vasa vasorum with the subsequent red blood cell extravasation has been postulated as a major source for intraplaque cholesterol deposition. This change in composition, characterized by increased extracellular cholesterol within the lipid core and excessive macrophage infiltration, increases the vulnerability of the atherosclerotic lesions. In fact, postmortem studies show a strong correlation between macrophage infiltration and increased vasa vasorum in human atherosclerotic lesions. Preexisting vasa vasorum in the adventitia are thought to spread into the intima, prompting intimal neovascularization.[6]

Inflammation is another important process affecting plaque progression, vulnerability, and subsequent thrombus formation. Inflammation could be considered as the link between atherosclerosis and thrombosis. In fact, the relation of inflammation and atherothrombosis could represent different faces of the same disease. Under "healthy" circumstances, the normally functional endothelial monolayer creates an antiatherogenic environment protecting against atherogenesis. This protection is achieved by releasing a series of antithrombotic and vasoactive substances (e.g., nitrous oxide

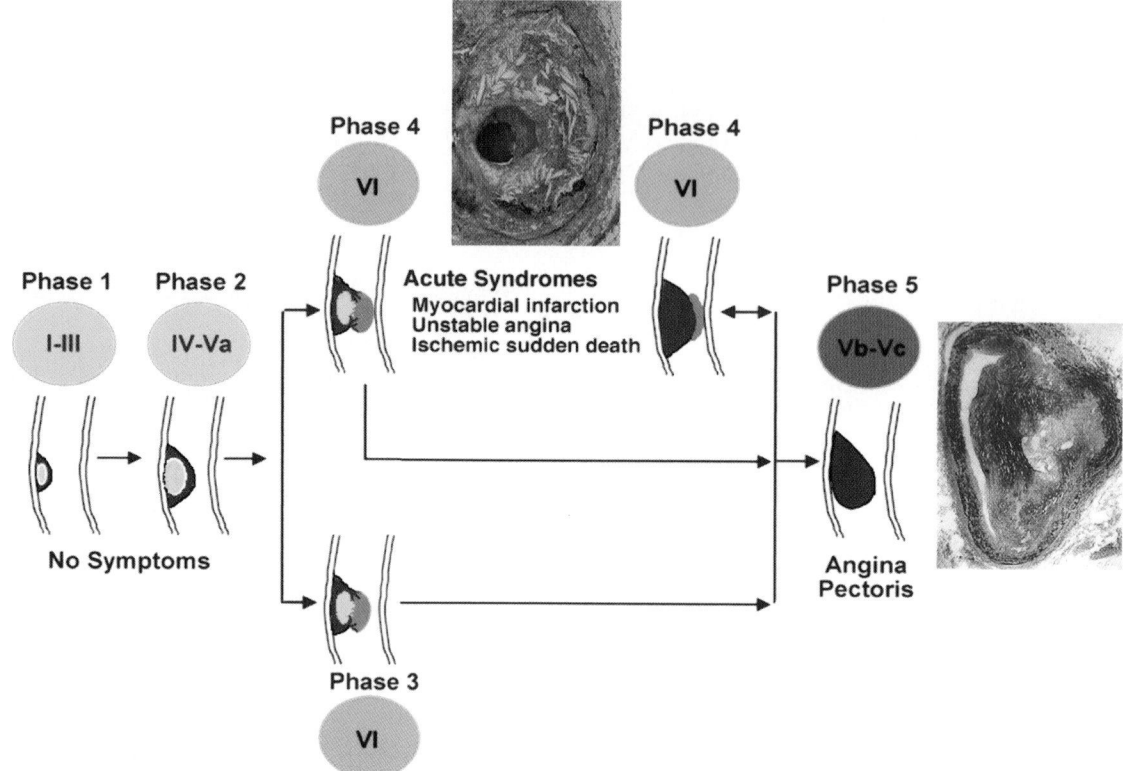

FIGURE 53-1. Simplified diagram of the evolution of coronary atherosclerosis. Phases and morphology of lesion progression.

[NO], prostaglandin I_2 [PGI$_2$], tissue plasminogen activator [tPA]). The initial pathologic manifestation of arthrosclerosis is a dysfunctional endothelium. The dysfunctional endothelium, characterized by a reduced NO and PGI$_2$ synthesis, facilitates the permeability of circulating lipids into the subendothelial space and, by exposing adhesive proteins of the selectin family, it facilitates the "homing" of the circulating monocytes on the endothelium. Vascular cell adhesion molecule-1 (VCAM-1) is implicated in early adhesion of mononuclear leukocytes to arterial endothelium at sites of atheroma initiation.[8] In addition to VCAM-1, P- and E-selectin also seem to contribute to leukocyte recruitment to the nascent atheroma plaque.[9,10] There are many other "inflammatory" molecules implicated in atherogenesis (e.g., monocyte chemotactic protein-1 [MCP-1], T lymphocytes, interleukin [IL]-1, IL-6).

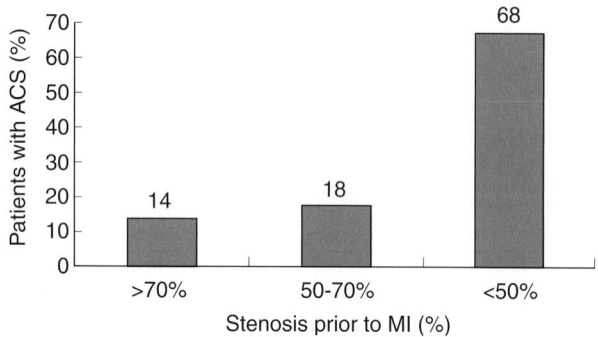

FIGURE 53-2. Relation of coronary stenosis severity (angiography) and presentation of acute coronary events from four studies with a total of 200 patients. ACS, acute coronary syndrome; MI, myocardial infarction. *Source: Modified with permission from Falk E, Shah PK, Fuster V. Coronary plaque disruption. Circulation 1995;92:657–671.*

Platelets also play an important role in the inflammatory environment. Although formerly platelets were suggested to be passive players, as they are organelles lacking a nucleus, currently we know that they are very active, being important not only in thrombosis itself, but in perpetuating the inflammatory environment. Platelets secrete various vasoactive chemokines and cytokines (e.g., CD40L, thrombospondin, platelet activating factor, RANTES [regulated on activation, normal T-cell expressed and secreted], extractable nuclear antigen [ENA]-78, macrophage inflammatory protein [MIP], CXCL4 [chemokine (C-X-C motif) ligand 4]) with autocrine and paracrine effects. Also very important is the notion that free cholesterol, major component of atherosclerotic plaques, is one the most inflammatory substances triggering the recruitment of more macrophages. Therefore, inflammation plays a dual role on atherothrombosis, at both the vascular and circulating level.

A reliable, noninvasive imaging tool able to detect early atherosclerotic disease and characterize lesion composition would be clinically advantageous. Although MRI has been widely tested for plaque composition analysis,[11] other imaging techniques, like computed tomography[12] and radionuclide imaging (positron emission tomography),[13] also have been used for this enterprise (see Chaps. 21 to 23). The reliable noninvasive plaque characterization, and eventually the vulnerable plaque identification, would improve our understanding of the pathophysiologic mechanisms of atherothrombosis and help in the risk stratification of the patients in order to select the appropriate approach.[14]

Growing thrombi on atherosclerotic vessels may occlude the lumen locally or embolize and be washed away by the blood flow to occlude distal vessels. However, thrombi may be physiologically and/or spontaneously lysed by mechanisms that block thrombus propagation. Thrombus size, location, and composition are regulated by local fluid dynamic conditions (mechanical effects), thrombogenicity of exposed substrate (local molecular effects), relative concentration of fluid phase and cellular blood components (local cellular effects), and the efficiency of the physiologic mechanisms of control of the system, mainly fibrinolysis.[15] Similarly, the size and stability of the thrombus, are major modulators for the severity of the ACS.

CELLULAR AND MOLECULAR MECHANISMS IN THROMBUS FORMATION

Although several decades ago the endothelium was viewed as a simple barrier separating the fluid phase of the blood from the highly thrombogenic smooth muscle vascular wall, today we know that the endothelium is a critical player in the maintenance of the normal function of the arterial bed.[16] The endothelium (endothelial cells) constantly secretes substances (e.g., hormones, growth factors) into the vascular lumen to maintain vascular tone and to avoid abnormal platelet adhesion/activation and clot formation. When the endothelium is damaged and cannot perform this crucial task, it is dysfunctional. Endothelial dysfunction, as well as a discontinuity of the endothelial integrity, triggers a series of biochemical and molecular reactions aimed at preventing excessive blood loss and repairing the vessel wall. Vasoconstriction and platelet adhesion at the site of injury combine to form a hemostatic aggregate as the first step in vessel wall repair and the hemostasis. A few platelets may interact with injured and dysfunctional endothelium and release growth factors which stimulate intimal hyperplasia.[8] Several layers of platelets may be deposited on the lesion with mild injury, and may or may not evolve to become a mural thrombus. The release of platelet growth factors may contribute significantly to accelerated intimal hyperplasia, as occurs in the coronary vein grafts within the first postoperative year. With severe injury and exposure of components of deeper layers of the vessel, as in spontaneous plaque rupture or in angioplasty, marked platelet aggregation with mural thrombus formation follows. Vascular injury of this magnitude also stimulates thrombin formation through both the intrinsic (surface-activated) and extrinsic (tissue factor-dependent) coagulation pathways (Fig. 53–3).

【 】 PLATELETS

Plaque rupture facilitates the interaction of inner plaque components with the circulating blood. Among these components, tissue factor (TF) exhibits a potent activating effect on platelets and coagulation. There is now an understanding of the biochemical events involved in platelet activation.[17–20] At the site of vascular lesions, circulating von Willebrand factor (vWF) binds to the exposed collagen which subsequently binds to the glycoprotein (GP) Ib/IX receptor on the platelet membrane.[21–23] Under pathologic

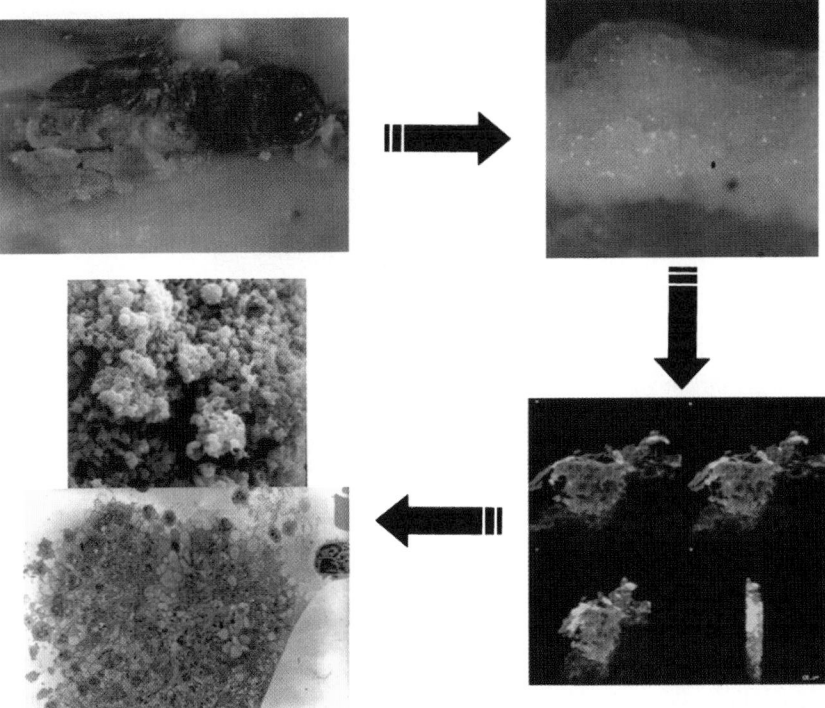

FIGURE 53–3. Images of thrombosis. From naked eye observation to immunohistochemistry (*green*, platelets; *red*, fibrinogen) and electronic microscopy (*top*, scanning; *bottom*, transmission).

conditions and in response to changes in shear stress, vWF can be secreted from the storage organelles in platelets or endothelial cells, reinforcing the activation process. Although GPIb/IX–vWF interaction is enough to promote binding of platelets to subendothelium, it is highly transient, resulting in rapid dislocation of platelet to the site of injury. GPVI binding to matrix collagen has slower binding kinetics, but once initiated promotes a firm adhesion of platelet to the vessel surface[24] (Fig. 53–4 shows mechanisms and agonists involved in platelet adhesion, activation and aggregation).[25] Finally, both GPIb/IX and GPVI also regulate platelet–leukocyte adhesion and thereby are implicated in other vascular process, such as inflammation and atherosclerosis.[26–28] Exposed matrix from the vessel wall and thrombin generated by activation of the coagulation cascade, as well as epinephrine and adenosine diphosphate (ADP), are powerful platelet agonists. Each agonist stimulates the discharge of calcium and promotes the subsequent release of its granular content. Platelet-related ADP and 5-hydroxytryptamine (5HT) stimulate adjacent platelets, further enhancing the process of platelet aggregation. Arachidonate, which is released from the platelet membrane by the stimulatory effect of collagen, thrombin, ADP, and 5HT, promotes the synthesis of thromboxane A_2 by the sequential effects of cyclooxygenase (COX) and thromboxane synthetase. Thromboxane A_2 not only promotes further platelet aggregation but is also a potent vasoconstrictor (Figs. 53–4 and 53–5).[29] The initial recognition of damaged vessel wall by platelets involves (1) adhesion, activation, and adherence to recognition sites on the thromboactive substrate (extracellular matrix proteins such as vWF, collagen, fibronectin, vitronectin, laminin); (2) spreading of the platelet on the surface; and (3) aggregation of platelets to form a platelet plug or white

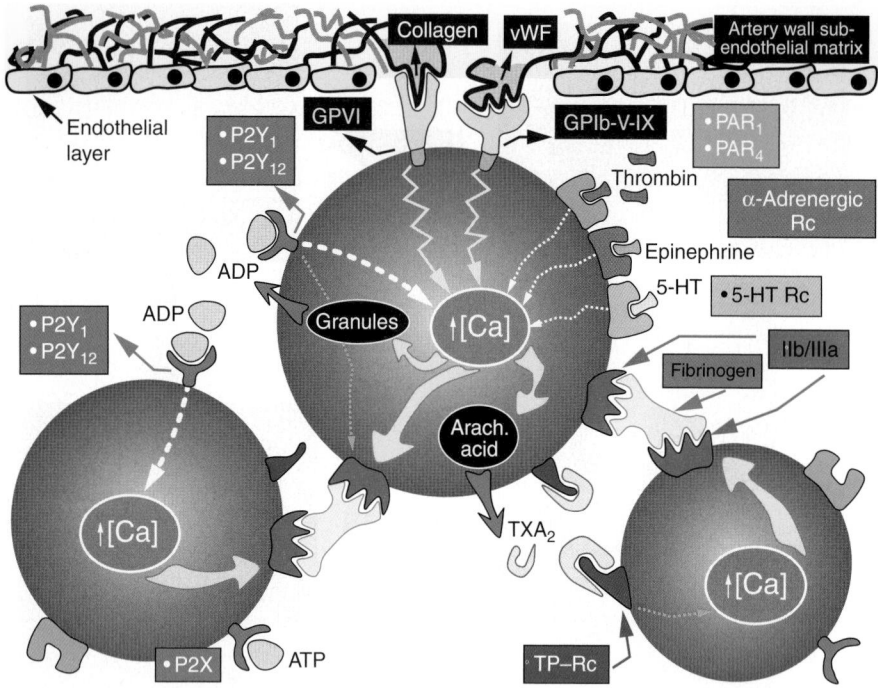

FIGURE 53-4. Mechanisms and agonists involved in platelet adhesion, activation, and aggregation. GP, glycoprotein; 5HT, 5-hydroxytryptamine (serotonin); PAR, protease-activated receptor; TP, thromboxane receptor, TXA, thromboxane; vWF, von Willebrand factor. *Source: Reprinted from Ibanez B, Vilahur G, Badimon JJ. Eur Heart J Suppl 2006. Under permission of the copyright holder, Oxford University Press.*

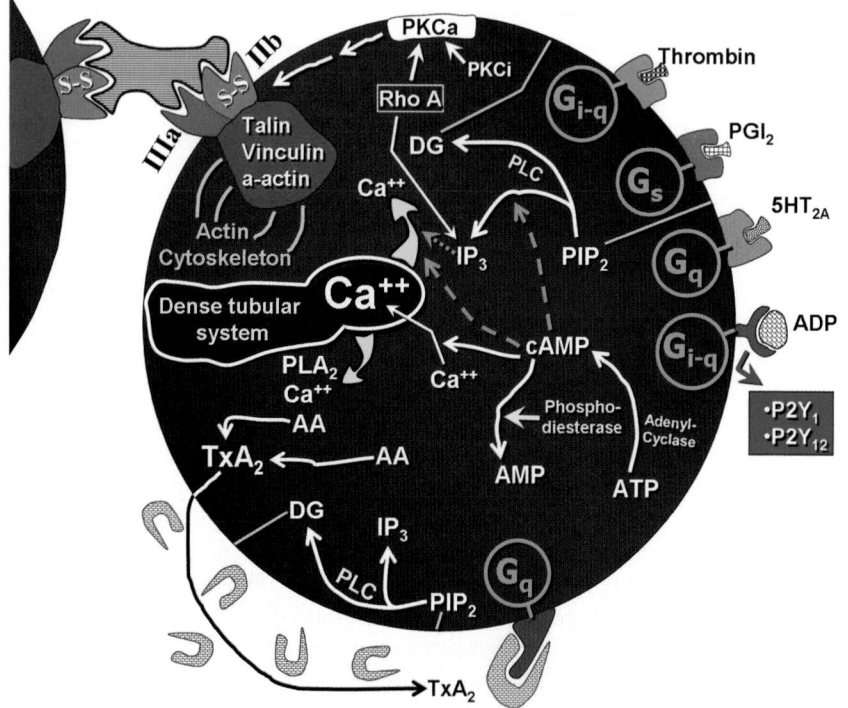

FIGURE 53-5. Signal transduction mechanisms of platelet activation and aggregation. AA, arachidonic acid; DG, diacylglycerol; Gs, Gi, Gp, Gq, guanine nucleotide-binding regulatory proteins; IIb/IIIa, receptor glycoprotein for adhesive protein ligands (mainly fibrinogen and vWF); IP_3, inositol 1,4,5-triphosphate; PLA_2, phospholipase A_2; PGI_2, prostacyclin; PIP_2, phosphoinositol diphosphate; PKCi and PKCa, protein kinase C, inactivated and activated; PLC, phospholipase C; TxA_2, thromboxane A_2.

thrombus (Fig. 53–6 shows the processes implicated in the formation of a thrombus after a plaque disruption).[25] The efficiency of platelet recruitment depends on the underlying substrate and local geometry (local factors). A final step involving the recruitment of other blood cells also occurs; erythrocytes, neutrophils, and occasionally monocytes are found on evolving mixed thrombus.

Platelet function depends on the adhesive interaction of several compounds. Most of the glycoproteins on the platelet membrane surface are receptors for adhesive proteins. Many of these receptors have been identified, cloned, sequenced, and classified within large gene families that mediate a variety of cellular interactions (Table 53–1).[30–32] The most abundant is the integrin family, which includes, GPIIb/IIIa, GPIc/IIa, the fibronectin receptor, and the vitronectin receptor, in decreasing order of magnitude. Another gene family present in the platelet membrane glycocalyx is the leucine-rich glycoprotein family represented by the GPIb/IX complex, receptor for vWF, on unstimulated platelets that mediates adhesion to subendothelium and GPV. Other genes include the selectins (such as GMP-140) and the immunoglobulin domain protein (human leukocyte antigen [HLA] class I antigen and platelet endothelial cell adhesion molecule-1 [PECAM-1]). Unrelated to any other gene family is the GPIV(IIIa) (see Table 53–1).[30]

Randomly distributed on the surface of resting platelets are about 50,000 molecules of GPIIb/IIIa. The complex is composed of one molecule of GPIIb (disulfide-linked large and light chains) and one of GPIIIa (single polypeptide chain). It is a Ca^{2+}-dependent heterodimer, noncovalently associated on the platelet membrane.[33] Calcium is required for maintenance of the complex and for binding of adhesive proteins.[34,35] On activated platelets, the GPIIb/IIIa is a receptor for fibrinogen, fibronectin, vWF, vitronectin, and thrombospondin.[36]

The GPIb/IX complex consists of two disulfide-linked subunits (GPIbα and GPIbβ) tightly (not covalently) complexed with GPIX in a 1:1 heterodimer. GPIbβ and GPIX are transmembrane glycoproteins and form the larger globular domain. The elongated, protruding part of the receptor corresponds to GPIbα. The major role of GPIb/IX is to bind immobilized vWF on the exposed vascular subendothelium and initiate adhesion of platelets. GPIb does not bind soluble vWF in plasma; apparently it undergoes a conforma-

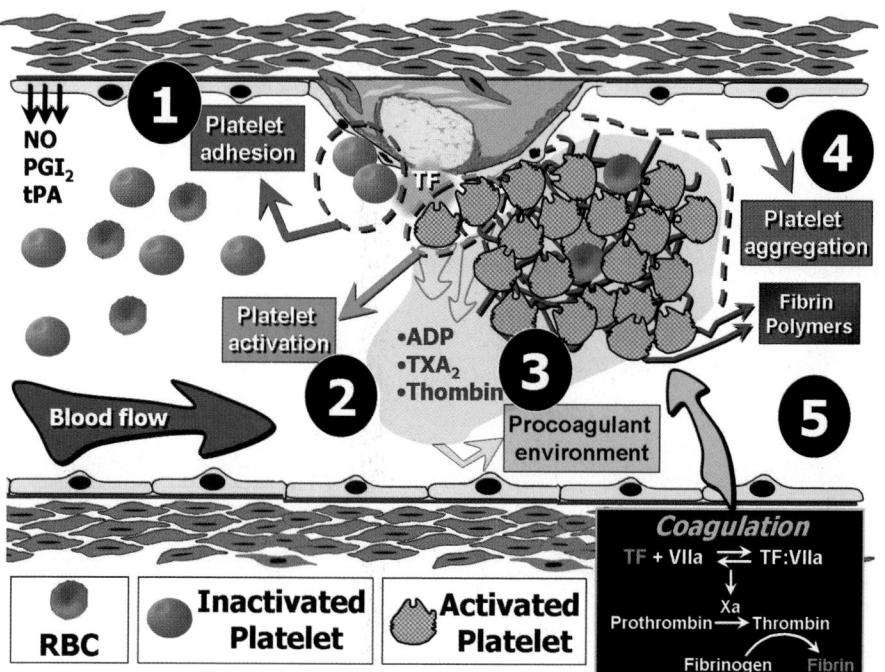

FIGURE 53–6. Mechanism involved in thrombus formation. Healthy endothelium (*left*) presents antithrombotic properties since it is able to release vascular protective substances such as nitric oxide (NO), prostacyclin (PGI$_2$), tissue plasminogen activator (tPA) and tissue factor pathway inhibitor (TFPi). On the contrary, dysfunctional endothelium (*right*) not only favors platelet adhesion, activation and aggregation, but also promotes vascular lipid deposition, macrophage migration and tissue factor (TF) expression (activation of the coagulation cascade). Following platelet adhesion, activation is characterized by platelet shape change. Activated platelets secrete different agonists prompting activation of circulating platelets, and a procoagulant environment. This prothrombotic milieu will favor thrombus formation and the subsequent clinical manifestations. Source: Reprinted from Ibanez B, Vilahur G, Badimon JJ. *Eur Heart J* Suppl 2006. Under permission of the copyright holder, Oxford University Press.

tional change upon binding to the extracellular matrix and then exposes a recognition sequence for GPIb/IX. The cytoplasmic domain of GPIb/IX has a major function in linking the plasma membrane to the intracellular actin filaments of the cytoskeleton and functions to stabilize the membrane and to maintain the platelet shape.[37,38]

Thrombin plays an important role in the pathogenesis of arterial thrombosis. It is one of the most potent known agonists for platelet activation and recruitment. In addition, thrombin is critical in the maintenance of the fibrin mesh. The thrombin receptor has 425 amino acids with seven transmembrane domains and a large NH$_2$-terminal extracellular extension that is cleaved by thrombin to produce a "tethered" ligand that activates the receptor to initiate signal transduction.[39,40] Thrombin is a critical enzyme in early thrombus formation, cleaving fibrinopeptides A and B from fibrinogen to yield insoluble fibrin, which effectively anchors the evolving thrombus. Both free and fibrin-bound thrombin are able to convert fibrinogen to fibrin, allowing propagation of thrombus at the site of injury.

Platelet activation triggers intracellular signaling and expression of platelet membrane receptors for adhesion and initiation of cell contractile processes that induce shape change and secretion of the granular contents. The expression of the integrin IIb/IIIa (αIIbβ_3) receptors for adhesive glycoprotein ligands (mainly fibrinogen and vWF) in the circulation initiates platelet-to-platelet interaction. The process is perpetuated by the arrival of platelets from the circulation. Most of the glycoproteins in the platelet membrane surface are receptors for adhesive proteins or mediate cellular interactions. von Willebrand factor binds to platelet membrane glycoproteins in both adhesion (platelet–substrate interaction) and aggregation (platelet–platelet interaction), leading to thrombus formation, as seen in perfusion studies conducted at high shear rates.[41–45] Ligand binding to the different membrane receptors triggers platelet activation with different relative potencies. There is great interest in the platelet ADP receptors (P2Y, P2X) because of available pharmacologic inhibitors. The P2Y1 receptor is responsible for inositol trisphosphate formation through activation of phospholipase C, leading to transient increase in the concentration of intracellular calcium, platelet shape change, and weak transient platelet aggregation.[46–48] Pharmacologic data reveal an essential role for the P2Y1 receptor in the initiation of platelet ADP-induced activation, thromboxane A$_2$ generation and platelet activation in response to other agonists.[49] The P2Y12 receptor is responsible for completion of the

TABLE 53–1

Platelet Membrane Glycoprotein Receptors

GLYCOPROTEIN RECEPTOR	FUNCTION	LIGAND
GP IIb/IIIa	Aggregation, adhesion at high shear rate	Fg, vWF, Fn, Ts, Vn
Receptor Vn	Adhesion	Vn, vWF, Fn, Fg, Ts
GP Ia/IIa	Adhesion	C
GP Ic/IIa	Adhesion	Fn
GP IcN/IIa	Adhesion	Ln
GP Ib/IX	Adhesion	vWF, T
GP V	Unknown	Substrate T
GP IV (GP IIIb)	Adhesion	Ts, C
GMP-140 (PADGEM)	Interaction with leukocytes	Unknown
PECAM-1 (GP IIa)	Unknown	Unknown

C, collagen; Fg, fibrinogen; Fn, fibronectin; Ln, laminin; PECAM-1, platelet endothelial cell adhesion molecule 1; Ts, thrombospondin; Vn, vitronectin; vW, von Willebrand factor.

platelet aggregation response to ADP.[50] There are several signalling molecules downstream of P2Y12 activation like cyclic adenosine monophosphate (cAMP), vasodilator-stimulated phosphoprotein (VASP) dephosphorylation, phosphoinositide 3-kinase, and Rap1B.[51-55] Pharmacologic approaches show a role for the P2Y12 receptor in dense granule secretion, fibrinogen-receptor activation, P-selectin expression, and thrombus formation, identifying it as a central mediator of the hemostatic response.[56-60] Both P2Y12 and P2Y1 are indirectly involved in platelet P-selectin exposure and formation of platelet-leukocyte conjugates, which leads to leukocyte-tissue factor exposure.[61-63] Although not activated by ADP, platelets possess a third purinergic receptor (P2X1), which is a fast adenosine triphosphate (ATP)-gated calcium channel receptor mainly involved in platelet shape change. Figure 53–7 shows in detail the platelet purinergic receptors. The most recent advances in antiplatelet therapy related to the inhibition of the P2Y12 receptors are focused on the availability of faster acting and reversible inhibitors.[64,64-66]

[ ] COAGULATION SYSTEM

During plaque rupture, in addition to platelet deposition in the injured area, the clotting mechanism is activated by the exposure of the plaque contents. The activation of coagulation leads to the generation of thrombin, which is a powerful platelet agonist in addition to being an enzyme that catalyzes the formation and polymerization of fibrin. Fibrin is essential in the stabilization of the platelet thrombus and its ability to withstand removal forces by flow, shear, and high intravascular pressure. The efficacy of fibrinolytic agents demonstrates the importance of fibrin in thrombosis associated with myocardial infarction.

The blood coagulation system involves a sequence of reactions integrating zymogens (proteins susceptible to activation into enzymes via limited proteolysis) and cofactors (nonproteolytic enzyme activators) in three groups: (1) the contact activation (generation of factor XIa via the Hageman factor), (2) the conversion of factor X to factor Xa in a complex reaction requiring the participation of factors IX and VIII, and (3) the conversion of prothrombin to thrombin and fibrin formation (Fig. 53–8, *left panel*).[67]

It has been suggested that glycosaminoglycans and sulfatides are the triggering surfaces for in vivo initiation of contact activation; however, the physiologic role of coagulation contact activation is unclear, because the absence of Hageman factor, prekallikrein, or high-molecular-weight kininogen does not induce a clinically apparent pathology. On the contrary, factor XI deficiency is associated with abnormal bleeding. Activated factor XI induces the acti-

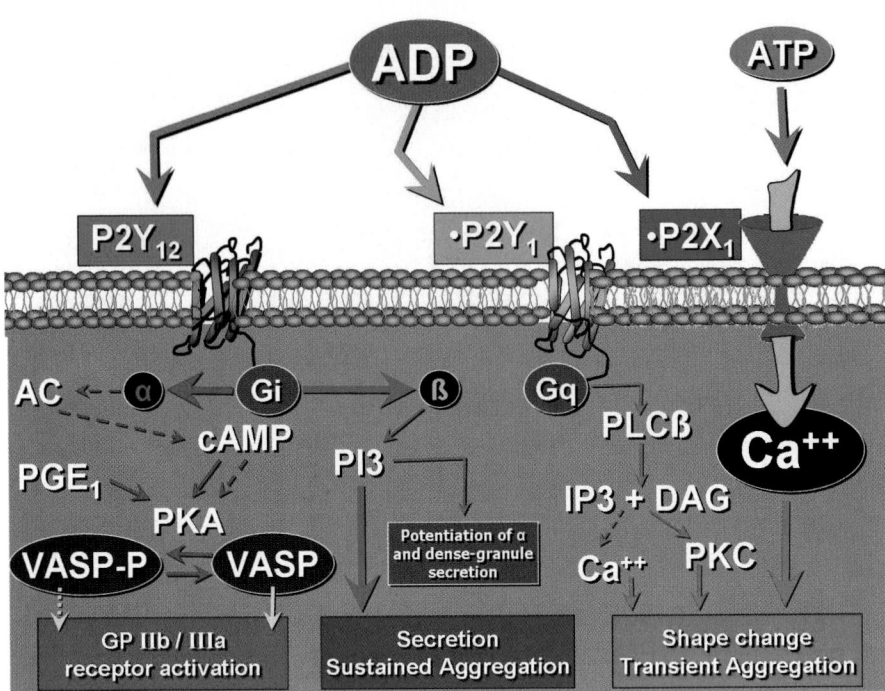

FIGURE 53–7. P2Y platelet receptors. P2Y receptors can be clearly divided into two subgroups: the Gq-coupled subtypes P2Y1 and the Gi-coupled P2Y12. P2Y1 that is responsible for platelet shape change and calcium mobilization is coupled to Gq and activates phospholipase Cβ (PLCβ) that is responsible for the formation of inositol (1,4,5)-trisphosphate (IP$_3$) and diacylglycerol (DAG), an activator of protein kinase C (PKC). IP$_3$ causes calcium mobilization from internal stores. The P2Y12 receptor couples primarily to Gαi$_2$ inhibition of adenylyl cyclase (AC). The subsequent decrease in cyclic adenosine monophosphate (cAMP) production leads, in turn, to a reduction in the activation of specific protein kinases (PKA), which can no longer phosphorylate the vasodilator-stimulated phosphoprotein (VASP); VASP phosphorylation is crucial for GPIIb/IIIa receptor inhibition. The subunit β activates the phosphatidylinositol-3-kinase, which is an important signaling molecule for P2Y12-mediated platelet-dense granule secretion and GPIIb/IIIa receptor activation. Finally, P2X1 is a gated cation channel protein activated by adenosine triphosphate (ATP). This activation leads to increase intraplatelet calcium, platelet shape change, and transient and weak platelet aggregation response. *Source: Reprinted from Ibanez B, Vilahur G, Badimon JJ. Eur Heart J Suppl 2006. Under permission of the copyright holder, Oxford University Press.*

vation of factor IX in the presence of Ca^{2+}. Factor IXa forms a catalytic complex with factor VIII on a membrane surface and efficiently activates factor X in the presence of Ca^{2+}. Factor IX is a vitamin K-dependent enzyme, as are factors II, VII and X, prothrombin, and proteins C and S.

Citrate is calcium chelant frequently used in studies of platelet–vessel wall interaction. Its anticoagulant properties are based on its action over calcium. It blocks not only the coagulation cascade, because the coagulation reactions do not proceed further than the activation of factor XI because of their dependence on Ca^{2+}, but also inhibits platelet activation because of the central role of calcium in platelet activation (see Fig. 53–4). Platelets may provide the membrane requirements for the activation of factor X, although the participation of cells of the vessel wall (in exposed injured vessels) has not been excluded.[68] As such, endothelial cells in culture have been shown to support the activation of factor X.[45] Factor VIII forms a noncovalent complex with vWF in plasma, and its function in coagulation is the acceleration of the effects of IXa on the activation of X to Xa. Absence of factor VIII or IX produces the hemophilic syndromes (see Fig. 53–8, *left panel*).[69]

The TF pathway, previously known as the extrinsic coagulation pathway, through the TF–factor VIIa complex in the presence of

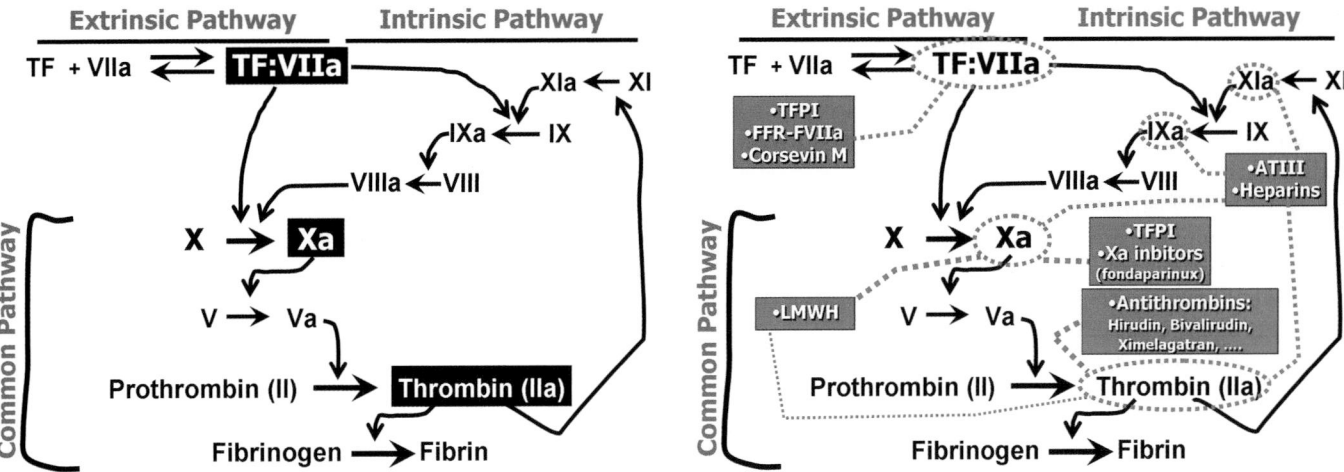

FIGURE 53-8. Simplified diagram of the coagulation cascade, with specific therapeutic targets for inhibitor drugs.

Ca^{2+}, induces the formation of Xa. A second TF-dependent reaction catalyzes the transformation of IX into IXa. Tissue factor is an integral membrane protein that serves to initiate the activation of factors IX and X and to localize the reaction to cells on which TF is expressed. Other cofactors include factor VIIIa, which binds to platelets and forms the binding site for IXa, thereby forming the machinery for the activation of X; and factor Va, which binds to platelets and provides a binding site for Xa. The human genes for these cofactors have been cloned and sequenced. In physiologic conditions, no cells in contact with blood contain active TF, although cells such as monocytes and polymorphonuclear leukocytes can be induced to synthesize and express TF.[68]

Activated Xa converts prothrombin into thrombin. The complex that catalyzes the formation of thrombin consists of factors Xa and Va in a 1:1 complex. This activation results in the cleavage of fragment 1.2 and formation of thrombin from fragment 2. The interaction of the four components of the "prothrombinase complex" (Xa, Va, phospholipid, and Ca^{2+}) enhances the efficiency of the reaction.[70]

Activated platelets provide a procoagulant surface for the assembly and expression of both intrinsic Xase and prothrombinase enzymatic complexes.[71-73] These complexes respectively catalyze the activation of factor X to factor Xa and prothrombin to thrombin. The expression of activity is associated with the binding of both of the proteases, factor IXa and factor Xa, and the cofactors, VIIIa and Va, to procoagulant surfaces. The binding of IXa and Xa is promoted by VIIIa and Va, respectively, such that Va and likely VIIIa provide the equivalent of receptors for the proteolytic enzymes.[73,74] The surface of the platelet expresses the procoagulant phospholipids that bind coagulation factors and contribute to the procoagulant activity of the cell.[74]

Thrombin acts on multiple substrates, including fibrinogen, factors XIII, V, and VIII, and protein C, in addition to its effects on platelets. It plays a central role in hemostasis and thrombosis. The catalytic transformation of fibrinogen into fibrin is essential in the formation of the hemostatic plug and in the formation of arterial thrombi. Thrombin binds to the fibrinogen central domain and cleaves fibrin-

opeptides A and B, resulting in the formation of fibrin monomer and polymer formation.[75] The fibrin mesh holds the platelets together and contributes to the attachment of the thrombus to the vessel wall.

SPONTANEOUS FIBRINOLYSIS

The control of the coagulation reactions occurs by diverse mechanisms, such as hemodilution and flow effects, proteolytic feedback by thrombin, inhibition by plasma proteins (such as antithrombin III) and endothelial cell–localized activation of an inhibitory enzyme (protein C), and fibrinolysis (Fig. 53-9). Although antithrombin III readily inactivates thrombin in solution, its catalytic site is inaccessible while bound to fibrin; however, it may still cleave fibrinopeptides, even in the presence of heparin. Thrombin has a specific receptor in endothelial cell surfaces, thrombomodulin, which triggers a physiologic anticoagulation system.[76] The thrombin–thrombomodulin complex serves as a receptor for the vitamin K-dependent protein C, which is activated and released from the endothelial cell surface. Thrombin generated at the site of injury binds to thrombomodulin, an endothelial surface-membrane

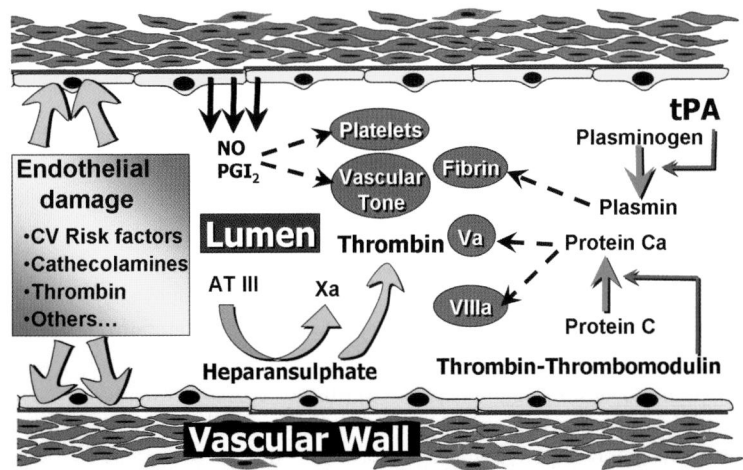

FIGURE 53-9. Simplified diagram of the physiologic anticoagulation system.

protein, initiating activation of protein C, which, in turn (in the presence of protein S), inactivates factors Va and VIIIa and limits thrombin effects. Loss of Va decreases the role of thrombin formation to negligible levels.[77] Thrombin stimulates successive release of both tPA and plasminogen activator inhibitor type 1 from endothelial cells, thus initiating endogenous lysis through plasmin generation from plasminogen by tPA with subsequent modulation through plasminogen activator inhibitor type 1. Consequently, thrombin plays a pivotal role in maintaining the complex balance of initial prothrombotic reparative events and subsequent endogenous anticoagulant and fibrinolytic pathways. Figure 53–10 illustrates the pivotal role of thrombin in the different mechanisms exposed here.

Endogenous fibrinolysis, a repair mechanism, involves catalytic activation of zymogens, positive and negative feedback control, and inhibitor blockade (see Fig. 53–9).[78,79] Blood clotting is blocked at the level of the prothrombinase complex by the physiologic anticoagulant-activated protein C and oral anticoagulants. Oral anticoagulants prevent posttranslational synthesis of γ-carboxyglutamic acid groups on the vitamin K-dependent clotting factors, preventing binding of prothrombin and Xa to the membrane surface. Activated protein C cleaves factor Va, rendering it functionally inactive.

ROLE OF LOCAL FACTORS IN THE REGULATION OF CORONARY THROMBOSIS

The cellular and molecular mechanisms of platelet deposition and thrombus formation following vascular damage are modulated by the type of injury, the local geometry at the site damage (degree of stenosis) and local hemodynamic conditions.[80–83] Similarly, three major factors also determine the vulnerability of the fibrous: (1) circumferential wall stress, or cap "fatigue"; (2) lesion characteristics (location, size, and consistency); and (3) blood-flow characteristics.[84]

[ ] EFFECTS DERIVED FROM THE SEVERITY OF VESSEL WALL DAMAGE

Exposure of deendothelialized vessel wall, native fibrillar collagen type I bundles with a rough surface, or atherosclerotic plaque components at similar blood shear rate conditions leads to increasing degrees of platelet deposition.[80] Thromboplastin or tissue factor,[85] readily available in the atherosclerotic intimal space exposed by endothelial loss, contributes to the high thrombogenicity of atherosclerotic plaques. Overall, it is likely that when injury to the vessel wall is mild, the thrombogenic stimulus is relatively limited and the resulting thrombotic occlusion is transient, as occurs in unstable angina. On the other hand, deep vessel injury secondary to plaque rupture or ulceration results in exposure of collagen, tissue factor, and other elements of the vessel matrix, leading to relatively persistent thrombotic occlusion and myocardial infarction.

It is likely that the nature of the substrate exposed after spontaneous or angioplasty-induced plaque rupture determines whether an unstable plaque proceeds rapidly to an occlusive thrombus or persists as nonocclusive mural thrombus. The analysis of the relative contribution of different components of human atherosclerotic plaques (fatty streaks, sclerotic plaques, fibrolipid plaques,

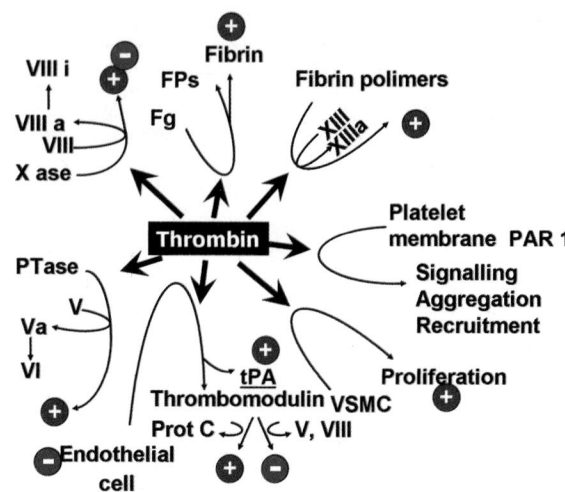

FIGURE 53–10. Role of thrombin in different pathways of coagulation. Thrombin plays a critical role in the maintenance of physiologic fibrinolysis system, but also in thrombosis.

atheromatous plaques, hyperplastic cellular plaque, and normal intima) to acute thrombus formation has shown that the atheromatous core is up to sixfold more active than the other substrates in triggering thrombosis.[86] The atheromatous core remained the most thrombogenic substrate when the various components were normalized by the degree of irregularity, as defined by the roughness index. Therefore ruptured plaques with a large atheromatous core are at high risk of leading to ACS.[86] The plaque TF content is directly related to its thrombogenicity.[87] As proof of concept, we showed that local tissue blockade of TF, by treatment with tissue factor pathway inhibitor, significantly reduces thrombosis.[88] Recently, the use of active site-inhibited recombinant FVIIa (FFr-FVIIa) was shown to significantly reduce thrombus growth on severely damaged vessels.

Monocytes/macrophages are key to the development of vulnerable plaques.[89] The vulnerable plaques (American Heart Association [AHA] types IV and Va), commonly composed of an abundant lipid core separated from the lumen by a thin fibrotic cap, are particularly soft and prone to disruption.[90] A high density of activated inflammatory cells has been detected in the disrupted areas of atherectomy specimens from patients with ACS.[91] These cells are capable of degrading extracellular matrix by secreting proteolytic enzymes, such as matrix metalloproteinases.[92] In addition, T cells isolated from rupture-prone sites can stimulate macrophages to produce metalloproteinases and may predispose to the disruption of lesions by weakening their fibrous caps.[93] Leukocytes, their enzymes, and their activation, play a critical role in the plaque vulnerability and its ruspture.[94–96] Recently, links between the activity of the leukocyte enzyme myeloperoxidase (MPO) and features of vulnerable plaque have been reported.[97] MPO has been implicated in endothelial cell loss/denudation, and development of a prothrombotic environment. Low-density lipoprotein (LDL) has been shown to downregulate the expression of lysil-oxidase (LOX) in vascular wall cells.[98] LOX is an enzyme that contributes to the maturation of the elastin and collagen fibrils of the extracellular matrix. Its decrease is associated with increased permeability of the vascular wall and hence may contribute to plaque destabilization. Cell apoptosis and microparticles with procoagulant activity and postulated apoptotic origin have also been linked to inflammation and thrombosis.[99,100]

Macrophages are suggested to play a key role in inducing plaque rupture by secreting proteases that destroy the extracellular matrix that provides physical strength to the fibrous cap. Recently, it was demonstrated that macrophage-mediated matrix degradation by matrix metalloproteinases (MMP) can induce plaque rupture. MMP-9 enhances elastin degradation and induces significant plaque disruption when overexpressed by macrophages in advanced atherosclerotic lesions of apoE/ mice.[101] Other MMP also has been implicated in different stages of atherosclerotic plaque progression.[102–105]

【 】 EFFECTS DERIVED FROM GEOMETRY

Platelet deposition is directly related to the degree of stenosis in the presence of the same degree of injury, indicating a shear-induced platelet activation.[82,83] In addition, analysis of the axial distribution of platelet deposition indicates that the apex, and not the flow recirculation zone distal to the apex, is the segment of greatest platelet accumulation. These data suggest that the severity of the acute platelet response to plaque disruption depends in part on the sudden changes in geometry following rupture.[15] Interestingly, hemodynamic effects play a role in the regulation of the thrombotic response in different arteries. In the absence of atherosclerotic changes in the porcine normolipemic model, the dilation of carotid and coronary arteries in the same animal produced significantly different levels of platelet deposition in the arterial beds, with the coronaries triggering a significantly greater deposition than the carotids.[106] Also it has been shown in apolipoprotein E-deficient (apoE/) mice that lowered shear stress induces larger lesions with a vulnerable plaque phenotype, whereas vortices with oscillatory shear stress induce stable lesions.[107]

Spontaneous lysis of thrombus does occur, not only in unstable angina, but also in acute myocardial infarction.[108] In these patients, as well as in those undergoing thrombolysis for acute infarction, the presence of a residual mural thrombus predisposes to recurrent thrombotic vessel occlusion.[2,109–111] Two main contributing factors for the development of rethrombosis have been identified. First, because platelet deposition increases with increasing degrees of vessel stenosis, residual mural thrombus encroaching into the vessel lumen may result in an increased shear rate, which facilitates the activation and deposition of platelets on the lesion.[82,83] Second, a fragmented thrombus appears to present one of the most powerful thrombogenic surfaces. A gradual increase in platelet deposition in the area of maximal stenosis may be followed by an abrupt decrease in platelet deposition, probably as a result of spontaneous embolization of the thrombus or platelet deaggregation.[112] Such an episode can be immediately followed by a rapid increase in platelet deposition, suggesting that the remaining thrombus is markedly thrombogenic. In fact, platelet deposition is increased two to four times on residual thrombus compared with deeply injured arterial wall, and thrombus continues to grow during heparin therapy. However, it is inhibited by specific antithrombin treatment.[113]

A specific antithrombin such as r-hirudin (a recombinant molecule that blocks both the catalytic site and the anion-exosite of the thrombin molecule) is capable of significantly inhibiting the secondary growth.[113] Thus, following lysis, thrombin becomes exposed to the circulating blood, leading to activation of the platelets, coagula-

tion, and further thrombosis. The antithrombin activity of heparin is limited for three main reasons. First, a residual thrombus contains active thrombin bound to fibrin, which is thus poorly accessible to the large heparin–antithrombin III complexes; second, a platelet-rich arterial thrombus releases large amounts of platelet factor 4, which may inhibit heparin; third, fibrin II monomer, formed by the action of thrombin on fibrinogen, may also inhibit heparin. Conversely, molecules of hirudin and other specific antithrombins are at least 10 times smaller than the heparin–antithrombin III complex, have no natural inhibitors, and thus have greater access to thrombin bound to fibrin. These findings clarify the clinical observations in patients with acute myocardial infarction undergoing thrombolysis, which have shown that residual stenosis is in part related to residual nonlysed thrombus.[114] The effects of different antithrombotic treatment regimens on thrombus formation triggered by a residual mural thrombus have been evaluated, and specific thrombin inhibition has been shown to be the most effective method of slowing the progression of thrombus growth when compared to aspirin, heparin, or both.[112,115]

The fact that a clear predilection exists for lesion formation at arterial branch points strongly indicates the important influence of local hemodynamics and rheologic conditions on atherosclerosis. Furthermore, vascular-cell gene-expression profiles are also modulated by acute changes in flow profiles.[116]

ROLE OF SYSTEMIC FACTORS IN THE REGULATION OF CORONARY THROMBOSIS

The severity of coronary thrombosis and associated ACS is modulated by the magnitude and/or stability of the formed thrombus.[84] In addition, successive events of plaque disruption and asymptomatic thrombus formation have been postulated to be responsible for the rapid progression of disease in certain patients.[84,117] Once a plaque ruptures, in addition to the local factors mentioned above, there are systemic factors that modulate, predispose, or lead to ACS. In fact, current knowledge supports the concept that rupture of atherosclerotic plaques happens more frequently than initially thought. This disruption occurs in an asymptomatic fashion and thus, remains clinically unnoticed. Postmortem evidence has demonstrated the existence of repeated and healed thrombotic episodes within the same lesion.[118] This plaque rupture without a superimposed thrombus suggest that, in addition to local factors implicated in coronary thrombosis, there are other circulating systemic factors modulating coronary thrombosis (Table 53–2). This knowledge led to the concept of vulnerable patient as a composite of vulnerable plaque plus vulnerable blood.[119,120]

One-third of ACS cases, particularly those involving ischemic sudden cardiac death, develop without plaque disruption but just superficial erosion of a markedly stenotic and fibrotic plaque.[121] Under such conditions, thrombus formation (TF) seems to depend on the hyperthrombogenic state triggered by systemic factors (Table 53–3). Indeed, systemic factors—including elevated LDL, decreased high-density lipoprotein, cigarette smoking, diabetes, and dysregulated hemostasis—are associated with increased thrombotic complications.[122–125] Our group has reported an increased blood thrombogenicity associated with both hyperlipemia and diabetes; more importantly, the effective management of these risk factors normalized this increased blood thrombogenicity.[126–128]

TABLE 53–2

Factors Implicated in Thrombus Formation

	PLAQUE DISRUPTION	RHEOLOGY	BLOOD THROMBOGENICITY
Coronaries	+++	++	+
Carotids	++	+	++
Peripherals	+	++	+++

As was stated above, TF is a major local player in the vulnerability and thrombogenicity of atherosclerotic plaques. TF is highly expressed in atherosclerotic plaques, and its content has been related to plaque thrombogenicity.[88] More recent is the knowledge of the existence of a blood-borne pool of TF that may play a critical role in the propagation of thrombosis.[129,130] Moreover, it has been reported that polymorphonuclear leukocytes might be involved in the transport of circulating TF to platelets.[131] High plasma levels of TF antigen,[132] and TF-positive microparticles with procoagulant activity[133,134] have been reported in patients with ACS. It seems that blood-borne TF plays an important role in the blood thrombogenicity, and in the thrombotic complications of plaque disruption/erosion. Our group found that increased levels of circulating TF activity are associated with cardiovascular risk factors,[135] epidemiologically linked to a high incidence of atherothrombotic complications. In addition, we found that patients with improvement in glycemic control show a reduction in circulating TF,[135] suggesting that circulating TF may be the mechanism of action responsible for the increased thrombotic complications associated with the presence of these cardiovascular risk factors. Figure 53–11 shows the possible cellular sources of circulating blood borne TF.

Thrombogenic systemic factors can be modulated by controlling the cardiovascular risk factors and by dietary and pharmacologic strategies. The development of additional novel therapeutic approaches depends on the increasing knowledge of the pathogenesis of ACS.

Atherosclerosis and inflammation could represent different faces from the same disease. Currently, it is well known that inflammatory circulating markers correlate with cardiovascular events and severity of the disease. Several inflammatory markers are being postulated as having a significant prognostic value for recurrent cardiovascular events.[136] Given the role of inflammation on atherosclerosis, it is plausible to think that drugs directed against inflammation (like COX-2 inhibitors and nonsteroidal antiinflammatory drugs [NSAIDs]) could render a positive impact in the prevention of cardiovascular events. However, several studies associ-

ated a significant increased in cardiovascular events with the use of COX-2 inhibitors. At the time it was thought that NSAIDs did not have the same association with cardiovascular events and could even be protective; however, it has been demonstrated that NSAIDs also seem to have a negative impact in cardiovascular disease patients.[137,138] Consequently, it is clear that the best weapon to treat inflammation in cardiovascular disease is an aggressive management of all the cardiovascular risk factors (e.g., by use of statins, angiotensin-converting enzyme inhibitors, hypoglycemic agents, antiplatelets). Interestingly the use of these therapeutic interventions not only offers significant benefits, but also reduces the systemic levels of proinflammatory markers.[136] This emphasizes the idea that atherothrombotic disease and inflammation could be two faces of the same disease rather than two different entities.

The antithrombotic agents presently used in clinical practice can be subdivided into three categories, according to their mechanism of action: fibrinolytics, inhibitors of the intrinsic coagulation cascade, and antiplatelet agents. Among the novel antithrombotic strategies that are reaching clinical research are the inhibitors of the TF:FVIIa pathway, direct factor Xa inhibitors, and direct thrombin inhibitors (DTIs). The newly generated understanding of the role of TF in atherothrombosis has suggested the inhibition of its pathway as a new antithrombotic approach. The biochemistry of TF and the clotting cascade has identified TF:VIIa, factor Xa, and thrombin as potential targets (see Fig. 53–8, *left panel*).

Several direct and specific antagonists to each of these targets have been developed and are being investigated in the clinical arena. Specific anti-TF antibodies, recombinant forms of endogenous tissue factor pathway inhibitors, inhibitors of factor VIIa,[139] and factor Xa in-

TABLE 53–3

Factors Modulating Thrombus Formation

LOCAL FLUID DYNAMICS	NATURE OF THE EXPOSED SUBSTRATE	SYSTEMIC THROMBOGENIC FACTORS
Shear stress	Degree of injury (mild vs. severe arterial injury)	Hypercholesterolemia
Tensile stress	Composition of atherosclerotic plaque	Catecholamines (smoking, cocaine, stress, etc.)
	Residual mural thrombus	Smoking
		Diabetes
		Homocysteine
		Lipoprotein(a)
		Infections (*Chlamydia pneumoniae, Helicobacter,* cytomegalovirus)
		Hypercoagulable state (Fg, vWF, TF, FVII)
		Defective fibrinolytic state, etc.

Fg, fibrinogen; FVII, factor VII; TF, tissue factor; VWF, von Willebrand factor.

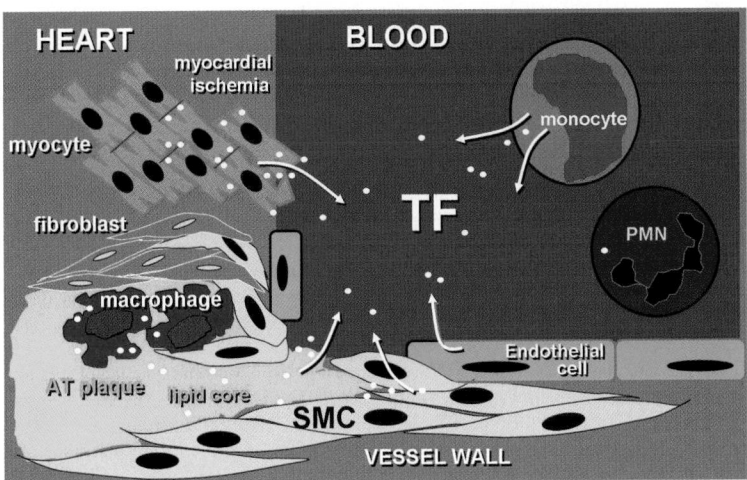

FIGURE 53–11. Suggested sources of circulating tissue factor (TF).

hibitors may afford at least a theoretical advantage over therapies that target more "downstream" components of the coagulation cascade.

DTIs inhibit thrombin by directly binding to exosite 1 and/or the active site of thrombin. DTIs produce a predictable anticoagulant response because they exhibit minimal binding to plasma proteins or cellular elements and inhibit fibrin-bound thrombin as well as fluid-phase thrombin.[140] The intravenous DTIs approved in the United States by the Food and Drug Administration (FDA) for anticoagulation in patients with heparin-induced thrombocytopenia are the recombinant hirudin, lepirudin, and Argatroban. Ximelagatran is an oral DTI that acts by direct and reversible inhibition of thrombin and was expected to replace warfarin. After analyzing 5 phase III pivotal trials involving 30,698 subjects, using ximelagatran,[141–145] in 2004 the FDA Cardiovascular and Renal Drug Advisory Committee concluded that the benefit-to-risk ratio of ximelagatran was unfavorable. Ximelagatran hepatic toxicity was a key feature leading the Cardiovascular and Renal Drug Advisory Committee to that decision.

Direct factor Xa inhibitors are also under investigation at the clinical level. Selective factor Xa inhibitors would effectively block coagulation because factor Xa is positioned at the start of the common pathway of the extrinsic and intrinsic coagulation systems (see Fig. 53–8). The indirect factor Xa inhibitor fondaparinux is the first of the selective factor Xa inhibitors to receive FDA approval for the prevention and treatment of venous thromboembolism, although various direct factor Xa inhibitors, including the oral agents LY517717 and BAY 59-7939, are under clinical development. Fondaparinux inhibits thrombin generation, formation, and growth. Its action is exerted selectively toward factor Xa, contrary to the action of unfractionated heparin and low-molecular-weight heparin, which act on a number of coagulation factors. Unfractionated heparin has equipotent activity against factors IIa and Xa, but also acts on factors IXa, XIa, and XIIa in an antithrombin-dependent manner. Low-molecular-weight heparins, which are prepared by chemical or enzymatic depolymerization of unfractionated heparin, have relatively more antifactor Xa than antifactor IIa activity (Fig. 53–8, *right panel*, shows the site of action of the different drugs targeting the coagulation cascade).

The superiority of fondaparinux versus low-molecular-weight heparin was shown in the prevention of deep venous thrombosis af-

ter major orthopedic surgery.[146,147] In acute myocardial infarction, the PENTALYSE study found that the pentasaccharide was as safe and effective as unfractionated-heparin; it also showed a trend toward fewer complications.[148] The thromboprophylactic efficacy and safety of fondaparinux were analyzed in a meta-analysis involving 7344 patients who were undergoing major orthopedic surgery.[149] Overall, fondaparinux reduced the incidence of venous thromboembolism from 14 percent in the enoxaparin-treated group to 7 percent.[150] The OASIS-5 trial reported similar short-term efficacy of fondaparinux compared with enoxaparin in preventing ischemic events in patients with unstable angina/non–ST-segment elevation myocardial infarction, with a large reduction in bleeding.[151] This resulted in significant reductions in mortality, myocardial infarction, and strokes at 3 to 6 months. The OASIS-6 trial[152] demonstrates a moderate reduction in mortality and reinfarction with the use of fondaparinux compared with usual care in ST-segment elevation myocardial infarction patients who are not treated with percutaneous coronary intervention.

Other approaches, still in early preclinical phase, are inhibitors of GPIb receptor (anti-vWF),[153] inhibitors of vWF-collagen binding (Saratin), and inhibitors of the adenosine diphosphate receptor P2T,[154] among others.

SUMMARY

The formation of a thrombus within a coronary artery with obstruction of coronary blood flow and reduction in oxygen supply to the myocardium produce the several types of ACS. These thrombotic episodes largely occur in response to atherosclerotic lesions that have progressed to a high-risk inflammatory/prothrombotic stage by a process modulated by local and systemic factors. Although distinct from one another, these atherosclerotic and thrombotic processes appear to be closely interrelated as the cause of ACS through a complex multifactorial process called *atherothrombosis*. The cellular and molecular mechanisms at play in the formation, growth, and stabilization of a coronary thrombus are being thoroughly investigated, and many of the activation pathways and receptor–ligand interactions have been identified. Inflammation has been revealed as a great player in the systemic and diffuse pattern of atherothrombotic disease. Strategies combining dietary, pharmacologic-medical, and interventional-surgical therapies have enjoyed considerable success in the prevention and treatment of major cardiovascular events. These regimens focus on inhibiting the various pathways involved in thrombus generation. Novel strategies based on the knowledge of the biochemistry of platelet aggregation and the coagulation process as well as the geometric conditions encountered in the circulation are presently in different stages of development and clinical trials. Advances in noninvasive imaging techniques will help to identify plaques at risk and reduce the clinical impact of atherothrombosis.

ACKNOWLEDGMENTS

The work reported in this review has been partially supported by grants from PNS SAF2006/0991 (Spain), FIS Ciber03–2006 (Spain) (LB), Fundación "La Caixa," and Fundación Conchita Rábago de Jiménez Díaz.

REFERENCES

1. Corti R, Badimon JJ. Biologic aspects of vulnerable plaque. *Curr Opin Cardiol* 2002;17(6):616–625.
2. Moreno PR, Fuster V. New aspects in the pathogenesis of diabetic atherothrombosis. *J Am Coll Cardiol* 2004;44(12):2293–2300.
3. Glagov S, Weisenberg E, Zarins CK, Stankunavicius R, Kolettis GJ. Compensatory enlargement of human atherosclerotic coronary arteries. *N Engl J Med* 1987;316(22):1371–1375.
4. Tousoulis D, Davies G, Stefanadis C, Toutouzas P, Ambrose JA. Inflammatory and thrombotic mechanisms in coronary atherosclerosis. *Heart* 2003;89(9):993–997.
5. Moreno PR, Purushothaman KR, Fuster V, et al. Plaque neovascularization is increased in ruptured atherosclerotic lesions of human aorta: implications for plaque vulnerability. *Circulation* 2004;110(14):2032–2038.
6. Virmani R, Kolodgie FD, Burke AP, et al. Atherosclerotic plaque progression and vulnerability to rupture: angiogenesis as a source of intraplaque hemorrhage. *Arterioscler Thromb Vasc Biol* 2005;25(10):2054–2061.
7. Fuster V, Moreno PR, Fayad ZA, Corti R, Badimon JJ. Atherothrombosis and high-risk plaque: part I. evolving concepts. *J Am Coll Cardiol* 2005;46(6):937–954.
8. Libby P. Inflammation in atherosclerosis. *Nature* 2002;420(6917):868–874.
9. Johnson RC, Chapman SM, Dong ZM, et al. Absence of P-selectin delays fatty streak formation in mice. *J Clin Invest* 1997;99(5):1037–1043.
10. Dong ZM, Chapman SM, Brown AA, Frenette PS, Hynes RO, Wagner DD. The combined role of P- and E-selectins in atherosclerosis. *J Clin Invest* 1998;102(1):145–152.
11. Wilensky RL, Song HK, Ferrari VA. Role of magnetic resonance and intravascular magnetic resonance in the detection of vulnerable plaques. *J Am Coll Cardiol* 2006;47(8 Suppl):C48–C56.
12. Viles-Gonzalez JF, Poon M, Sanz J, et al. In vivo 16-slice, multidetector-row computed tomography for the assessment of experimental atherosclerosis: comparison with magnetic resonance imaging and histopathology. *Circulation* 2004;110(11):1467–1472.
13. Davies JR, Rudd JH, Weissberg PL, Narula J. Radionuclide imaging for the detection of inflammation in vulnerable plaques. *J Am Coll Cardiol* 2006;47(8 Suppl):C57–C68.
14. Corti R, Fuster V, Badimon JJ, Hutter R, Fayad ZA. New understanding of atherosclerosis (clinically and experimentally) with evolving MRI technology in vivo. *Ann N Y Acad Sci* 2001;947:181–195.
15. Badimon L, Chesebro JH, Badimon JJ. Thrombus formation on ruptured atherosclerotic plaques and rethrombosis on evolving thrombi. *Circulation* 1992;86(6 Suppl):III74–III85.
16. Viles-Gonzalez JF, Fuster V, Badimon JJ. Atherothrombosis: a widespread disease with unpredictable and life-threatening consequences. *Eur Heart J* 2004;25(14):1197–1207.
17. Badimon JJ, Fuster V, Chesebro JH, Badimon L. Coronary atherosclerosis. A multifactorial disease. *Circulation* 1993;87(3 Suppl):II3–II16.
18. Savage B, Cattaneo M, Ruggeri ZM. Mechanisms of platelet aggregation. *Curr Opin Hematol* 2001;8(5):270–276.
19. Brass LF. The biochemistry of platelet activation. In: Hoffman R, Benz EJ Jr, Shattil SJ, eds. *Hematology: Basic Principles and Practice*. New York: Churchill Livingstone, 1991:1176–1197.
20. Colman RW, Walsh PN. Mechanisms of platelet aggregation. In: Colman RW, Hirsh J, Marder VJ, Salzman E, eds. *Hemostasis and Thrombosis: Basic Principles and Clinical Practice*. Philadelphia: Lippincott, 1987:594–605.
21. Ruggeri ZM. Mechanisms initiating platelet thrombus formation. *Thromb Haemost* 1997;78(1):611–616.
22. Ruggeri ZM. Platelets in atherothrombosis. *Nat Med* 2002;8(11):1227–1234.
23. Alevriadou BR, Moake JL, Turner NA, et al. Real-time analysis of shear-dependent thrombus formation and its blockade by inhibitors of von Willebrand factor binding to platelets. *Blood* 1993;81(5):1263–1276.
24. Nieswandt B, Watson SP. Platelet-collagen interaction: is GPVI the central receptor? *Blood* 2003;102(2):449–461.
25. Ibanez B, Vilahur G, Badimon JJ. Pharmacology of thienopyridines. Rationale for dual pathway inhibition. Eur Heart J Suppl 2006;8:G3–G9.
26. Gawaz M. Role of platelets in coronary thrombosis and reperfusion of ischemic myocardium. *Cardiovasc Res* 2004;61(3):498–511.
27. Andrews RK, Gardiner EE, Shen Y, Berndt MC. Platelet interactions in thrombosis. *IUBMB Life* 2004;56(1):13–18.
28. Weyrich AS, Lindemann S, Zimmerman GA. The evolving role of platelets in inflammation. *J Thromb Haemost* 2003;1(9):1897–1905.
29. Badimon L, Badimon JJ, Fuster V. Pathogenesis of thrombosis. In: Verstraete M, Fuster V, Topol E, eds. *Cardiovascular Thrombosis: Thrombocardiology*. Philadelphia: Lippincott-Raven, 1998:23–44.
30. Kieffer N, Phillips DR. Platelet membrane glycoproteins: functions in cellular interactions. *Annu Rev Cell Biol* 1990;6:329–357.
31. Kunicki TJ. Organization of glycoproteins within the platelet plasma membrane. In: George JN, Nurden AT, Philips DR, eds. *Platelet Membrane Glycoproteins*. New York: Plenum Press, 1985:87–101.
32. Watson SP, Auger JM, McCarty OJ, Pearce AC. GPVI and integrin alphaIIb beta3 signaling in platelets. *J Thromb Haemost* 2005;3(8):1752–1762.
33. Fox JE. Transmembrane signaling across the platelet integrin glycoprotein IIb-IIIa. *Ann N Y Acad Sci* 1994;714:75–87.
34. Calvete JJ. On the structure and function of platelet integrin alpha IIb beta 3 the fibrinogen receptor. *Proc Soc Exp Biol Med* 1995;208(4):346–360.
35. Beer J, Coller BS. Evidence that platelet glycoprotein IIIa has a large disulfide-bonded loop that is susceptible to proteolytic cleavage. *J Biol Chem* 1989;264(29):17564–17573.
36. Plow EF, Ginsberg MH, Marguerie GA. Expression and function of adhesive proteins on the platelet surface. In: Phillips DR, Shuman MA, eds. *Biochemistry of Platelets*. New York: Academic Press, 1986:225–256.
37. Fox JE, Boyles JK, Berndt MC, Steffen PK, Anderson LK. Identification of a membrane skeleton in platelets. *J Cell Biol* 1988;106(5):1525–1538.
38. Meyer D, Girma JP. von Willebrand factor: structure and function. *Thromb Haemost* 1993;70(1):99–104.
39. Vu TK, Hung DT, Wheaton VI, Coughlin SR. Molecular cloning of a functional thrombin receptor reveals a novel proteolytic mechanism of receptor activation. *Cell* 1991;64(6):1057–1068.
40. Bode W. The structure of thrombin: a janus-headed proteinase. *Semin Thromb Hemost* 2006;32 Suppl 1:16–31.
41. Coughlin SR. Thrombin receptor structure and function. *Thromb Haemost* 1993;70(1):184–187.
42. Sakariassen KS, Bolhuis PA, Sixma JJ. Human blood platelet adhesion to artery subendothelium is mediated by factor VIII–Von Willebrand factor bound to the subendothelium. *Nature* 1979;279(5714):636–638.
43. Badimon L, Badimon JJ, Turitto VT, Fuster V. Role of von Willebrand factor in mediating platelet-vessel wall interaction at low shear rate; the importance of perfusion conditions. *Blood* 1989;73(4):961–967.
44. Nemerson Y. Overview of hemostasis. In: Spaet TH, ed. *Hemostasis and Thrombosis: Basic Principles and Clinical Practice*. Philadelphia: Lippincott, 1987:3–17.
45. Rimon S, Melamed R, Savion N, Scott T, Nawroth PP, Stern DM. Identification of a factor IX/IXa binding protein on the endothelial cell surface. *J Biol Chem* 1987;262(13):6023–6031.
46. Hechler B, Leon C, Vial C, et al. The P2Y1 receptor is necessary for adenosine 5-diphosphate-induced platelet aggregation. *Blood* 1998;92(1):152–159.
47. Savi P, Beauverger P, Labouret C, et al. Role of P2Y1 purinoceptor in ADP-induced platelet activation. *FEBS Lett* 1998;422(3):291–295.
48. Jin J, Daniel JL, Kunapuli SP. Molecular basis for ADP-induced platelet activation. II. The P2Y1 receptor mediates ADP-induced intracellular calcium mobilization and shape change in platelets. *J Biol Chem* 1998;273(4):2030–2034.
49. Leon C, Vial C, Gachet C, et al. The P2Y1 receptor is normal in a patient presenting a severe deficiency of ADP-induced platelet aggregation. *Thromb Haemost* 1999;81(5):775–781.
50. Nurden P, Savi P, Heilmann E, et al. An inherited bleeding disorder linked to a defective interaction between ADP and its receptor on platelets. Its influence on glycoprotein IIb-IIIa complex function. *J Clin Invest* 1995;95(4):1612–1622.
51. Geiger J, Brich J, Honig-Liedl P, et al. Specific impairment of human platelet P2Y(AC) ADP receptor-mediated signaling by the antiplatelet drug clopidogrel. *Arterioscler Thromb Vasc Biol* 1999;19(8):2007–2011.
52. Trumel C, Payrastre B, Plantavid M, et al. A key role of adenosine diphosphate in the irreversible platelet aggregation induced by the PAR1-activating peptide through the late activation of phosphoinositide 3-kinase. *Blood* 1999;94(12):4156–4165.
53. Jackson SP, Schoenwaelder SM, Goncalves I, et al. PI 3-kinase p110beta: a new target for antithrombotic therapy. *Nat Med* 2005;11(5):507–514.
54. Lova P, Paganini S, Sinigaglia F, Balduini C, Torti M. A Gi-dependent pathway is required for activation of the small GTPase Rap1B in human platelets. *J Biol Chem* 2002;277(14):12009–12015.
55. Woulfe D, Jiang H, Mortensen R, Yang J, Brass LF. Activation of Rap1B by G(i) family members in platelets. *J Biol Chem* 2002;277(26):23382–23390.
56. Dangelmaier C, Jin J, Smith JB, Kunapuli SP. Potentiation of thromboxane A_2-induced platelet secretion by Gi signaling through the phosphoinositide-3 kinase pathway. *Thromb Haemost* 2001;85(2):341–348.
57. Quinton TM, Kim S, Dangelmaier C, et al. Protein kinase C- and calcium-regulated pathways independently synergize with Gi pathways in agonist-induced fibrinogen receptor activation. *Biochem J* 2002;368(Pt 2):535–543.

58. Nieswandt B, Schulte V, Zywietz A, Gratacap MP, Offermanns S. Costimulation of Gi- and G12/G13-mediated signaling pathways induces integrin alpha IIbbeta 3 activation in platelets. *J Biol Chem* 2002;277(42):39493–39498.

59. Storey RF, Judge HM, Wilcox RG, Heptinstall S. Inhibition of ADP-induced P-selectin expression and platelet-leukocyte conjugate formation by clopidogrel and the P2Y12 receptor antagonist AR-C69931MX but not aspirin. *Thromb Haemost* 2002;88(3):488–494.

60. Andre P, Delaney SM, LaRocca T, et al. P2Y12 regulates platelet adhesion/activation, thrombus growth, and thrombus stability in injured arteries. *J Clin Invest* 2003;112(3):398–406.

61. Leon C, Ravanat C, Freund M, Cazenave JP, Gachet C. Differential involvement of the P2Y1 and P2Y12 receptors in platelet procoagulant activity. *Arterioscler Thromb Vasc Biol* 2003;23(10):1941–1947.

62. Leon C, Freund M, Ravanat C, Baurand A, Cazenave JP, Gachet C. Key role of the P2Y(1) receptor in tissue factor-induced thrombin-dependent acute thromboembolism: studies in P2Y(1)-knockout mice and mice treated with a P2Y(1) antagonist. *Circulation* 2001;103(5):718–723.

63. Leon C, Alex M, Klocke A, et al. Platelet ADP receptors contribute to the initiation of intravascular coagulation. *Blood* 2004;103(2):594–600.

64. Husted S, Emanuelsson H, Heptinstall S, Sandset PM, Wickens M, Peters G. Pharmacodynamics, pharmacokinetics, and safety of the oral reversible P2Y12 antagonist AZD6140 with aspirin in patients with atherosclerosis: a double-blind comparison to clopidogrel with aspirin. *Eur Heart J* 2006;27(9):1038–1047.

65. Greenbaum AB, Grines CL, Bittl JA, et al. Initial experience with an intravenous P2Y12 platelet receptor antagonist in patients undergoing percutaneous coronary intervention: results from a 2-part, phase II, multicenter, randomized, placebo- and active-controlled trial. *Am Heart J* 2006;151(3):689.

66. Wiviott SD, Antman EM, Winters KJ, et al. Randomized comparison of prasugrel (CS-747 LY640315), a novel thienopyridine P2Y12 antagonist, with clopidogrel in percutaneous coronary intervention: results of the Joint Utilization of Medications to Block Platelets Optimally (JUMBO)-TIMI 26 trial. *Circulation* 2005;111(25):3366–3373.

67. Viles-Gonzalez JF, Badimon JJ. Atherothrombosis: the role of tissue factor. *Int J Biochem Cell Biol* 2004;36(1):25–30.

68. Nemerson Y. Mechanisms of coagulation. In: Williams WJ, Beutler E, Erslev AJ, Lichtman MA, eds. *Hematology*. New York: McGraw-Hill, 1990:1295–1304.

69. Colman RW, Marder VJ, Salzman EW. Overview of hemostasis. In: Colman RW, Hirsh J, Marder VJ, Salzman EW, eds. *Hemostasis and Thrombosis: Basic Principles and Clinical Practice*. Philadelphia: Lippincott, 1993:3–18.

70. Mann KG. Membrane-bound enzyme complexes in blood coagulation. In: Spaet TH, ed. *Progress in Hemostasis and Thrombosis*. New York: Grune & Stratton, 1984:1–23.

71. Mann KG, Nesheim ME, Church WR, Haley P, Krishnaswamy S. Surface-dependent reactions of the vitamin K-dependent enzyme complexes. *Blood* 1990;76(1):1–16.

72. Rawala-Sheikh R, Ahmad SS, Ashby B, Walsh PN. Kinetics of coagulation factor X activation by platelet-bound factor IXa. *Biochemistry* 1990;29(10):2606–2611.

73. Ahmad SS, London FS, Walsh PN. The assembly of the factor X-activating complex on activated human platelets. *J Thromb Haemost* 2003;1(1):48–59.

74. Nesheim ME, Furmaniak-Kazmierczak E, Henin C, Cote G. On the existence of platelet receptors for factor V(a) and factor VIII(a). *Thromb Haemost* 1993;70(1):80–86.

75. Comp PC. Kinetics of plasma coagulation factors. In: Williams WJ, Beutler E, Erslev AJ, Lichtman MA, eds. *Hematology*. New York: McGraw-Hill, 1990:1285–1290.

76. Esmon NL, Owen WG, Esmon CT. Isolation of a membrane-bound cofactor for thrombin-catalyzed activation of protein C. *J Biol Chem* 1982;257(2):859–864.

77. Nemerson Y, Williams WJ. Biochemistry of plasma coagulation factors. In: Williams WJ, Beutler E, Erslev AJ, Lichtman MA, eds. *Hematology*. New York: McGraw-Hill, 1990:1267–1284.

78. Francis CW, Marder VJ. Physiologic regulation and pathologic disorders of fibrinolysis. In: Colman RW, Hirsh J, Marder VJ, Salzman EW, eds. *Hemostasis and Thrombosis: Basic Principles and Clinical Practice*. Philadelphia: Lippincott, 1987:358–379.

79. Collen D, Lijnen HR. Molecular and cellular basis of fibrinolysis. In: Hoffman R, Benz EJ Jr, Shattil SJ, eds. *Hematology: Basic Principles and Practice*. New York: Churchill-Livingstone, 1991:1232–1242.

80. Badimon L, Badimon JJ, Turitto VT, Vallabhajosula S, Fuster V. Platelet thrombus formation on collagen type I. A model of deep vessel injury. Influence of blood rheology, von Willebrand factor, and blood coagulation. *Circulation* 1988;78(6):1431–1442.

81. Badimon L, Badimon JJ, Galvez A, Chesebro JH, Fuster V. Influence of arterial damage and wall shear rate on platelet deposition. Ex vivo study in a swine model. *Arteriosclerosis* 1986;6(3):312–320.

82. Badimon L, Badimon JJ. Mechanisms of arterial thrombosis in nonparallel streamlines: platelet thrombi grow on the apex of stenotic severely injured vessel wall. Experimental study in the pig model. *J Clin Invest* 1989;84(4):1134–1144.

83. Lassila R, Badimon JJ, Vallabhajosula S, Badimon L. Dynamic monitoring of platelet deposition on severely damaged vessel wall in flowing blood. Effects of different stenoses on thrombus growth. *Arteriosclerosis* 1990;10(2):306–315.

84. Fuster V, Badimon L, Badimon JJ, Chesebro JH. The pathogenesis of coronary artery disease and the acute coronary syndromes (1). *N Engl J Med* 1992;326(4):242–250.

85. Mackman N. Role of tissue factor in hemostasis, thrombosis, and vascular development. *Arterioscler Thromb Vasc Biol* 2004;24(6):1015–1022.

86. Fernandez-Ortiz A, Badimon JJ, Falk E, et al. Characterization of the relative thrombogenicity of atherosclerotic plaque components: implications for consequences of plaque rupture. *J Am Coll Cardiol* 1994;23(7):1562–1569.

87. Toschi V, Gallo R, Lettino M, et al. Tissue factor modulates the thrombogenicity of human atherosclerotic plaques. *Circulation* 1997;95(3):594–599.

88. Badimon JJ, Lettino M, Toschi V, et al. Local inhibition of tissue factor reduces the thrombogenicity of disrupted human atherosclerotic plaques: effects of tissue factor pathway inhibitor on plaque thrombogenicity under flow conditions. *Circulation* 1999;99(14):1780–1787.

89. Libby P, Simon DI. Inflammation and thrombosis: the clot thickens. *Circulation* 2001;103(13):1718–1720.

90. Davies MJ. Stability and instability: two faces of coronary atherosclerosis. The Paul Dudley White Lecture 1995. *Circulation* 1996;94(8):2013–2020.

91. Moreno PR, Falk E, Palacios IF, Newell JB, Fuster V, Fallon JT. Macrophage infiltration in acute coronary syndromes. Implications for plaque rupture. *Circulation* 1994;90(2):775–778.

92. Galis ZS, Khatri JJ. Matrix metalloproteinases in vascular remodeling and atherogenesis: the good, the bad, and the ugly. *Circ Res* 2002;90(3):251–262.

93. Libby P. Current concepts of the pathogenesis of the acute coronary syndromes. *Circulation* 2001;104(3):365–372.

94. Buffon A, Biasucci LM, Liuzzo G, D'Onofrio G, Crea F, Maseri A. Widespread coronary inflammation in unstable angina. *N Engl J Med* 2002;347(1):5–12.

95. Gurm HS, Lincoff AM, Lee D, et al. Outcome of acute ST-segment elevation myocardial infarction in diabetics treated with fibrinolytic or combination reduced fibrinolytic therapy and platelet glycoprotein IIb/IIIa inhibition: lessons from the GUSTO V trial. *J Am Coll Cardiol* 2004;43(4):542–548.

96. Brennan ML, Penn MS, Van LF, et al. Prognostic value of myeloperoxidase in patients with chest pain. *N Engl J Med* 2003;349(17):1595–1604.

97. Sugiyama S, Kugiyama K, Aikawa M, Nakamura S, Ogawa H, Libby P. Hypochlorous acid, a macrophage product, induces endothelial apoptosis and tissue factor expression: involvement of myeloperoxidase-mediated oxidant in plaque erosion and thrombogenesis. *Arterioscler Thromb Vasc Biol* 2004;24(7):1309–1314.

98. Rodriguez C, Raposo B, Martinez-Gonzalez J, Casani L, Badimon L. Low density lipoproteins downregulate lysyl oxidase in vascular endothelial cells and the arterial wall. *Arterioscler Thromb Vasc Biol* 2002;22(9):1409–1414.

99. Mallat Z, Tedgui A. Current perspective on the role of apoptosis in atherothrombotic disease. *Circ Res* 2001;88(10):998–1003.

100. Mallat Z, Hugel B, Ohan J, Leseche G, Freyssinet JM, Tedgui A. Shed membrane microparticles with procoagulant potential in human atherosclerotic plaques: a role for apoptosis in plaque thrombogenicity. *Circulation* 1999;99(3):348–353.

101. Gough PJ, Gomez IG, Wille PT, Raines EW. Macrophage expression of active MMP-9 induces acute plaque disruption in apoE-deficient mice. *J Clin Invest* 2006;116(1):59–69.

102. Turu MM, Krupinski J, Catena E, et al. Intraplaque MMP-8 levels are increased in asymptomatic patients with carotid plaque progression on ultrasound. *Atherosclerosis* 2006;187(1):161–169.

103. Kuzuya M, Nakamura K, Sasaki T, Cheng XW, Itohara S, Iguchi A. Effect of MMP-2 deficiency on atherosclerotic lesion formation in apoE-deficient mice. *Arterioscler Thromb Vasc Biol* 2006;26(5):1120–1125.

104. de NR, Verkleij CJ, von der Thusen JH, et al. Lesional overexpression of matrix metalloproteinase-9 promotes intraplaque hemorrhage in advanced lesions but not at earlier stages of atherogenesis. *Arterioscler Thromb Vasc Biol* 2006;26(2):340–346.

105. Sluijter JP, Pulskens WP, Schoneveld AH, et al. Matrix metalloproteinase 2 is associated with stable and matrix metalloproteinases 8 and 9 with vulnerable carotid atherosclerotic lesions: a study in human endarterectomy specimen pointing to a role for different extracellular matrix metalloproteinase inducer glycosylation forms. *Stroke* 2006;37(1):235–239.

106. Badimon JJ, Ortiz AF, Meyer B, et al. Different response to balloon angioplasty of carotid and coronary arteries: effects on acute platelet deposition and intimal thickening. *Atherosclerosis* 1998;140(2):307–314.

107. Cheng C, Tempel D, van HR, et al. Atherosclerotic lesion size and vulnerability are determined by patterns of fluid shear stress. *Circulation* 2006;113(23):2744–2753.

108. Fuster V, Chesebro JH. Mechanisms of unstable angina. *N Engl J Med* 1986;315(16):1023–1025.

109. Van LJ, De GH, Verstraete M, Van de WF. Angiographic assessment of the infarct-related residual coronary stenosis after spontaneous or therapeutic thrombolysis. *J Am Coll Cardiol* 1990;16(7):1545–1549.

110. Corti R, Fuster V, Badimon JJ. Pathogenetic concepts of acute coronary syndromes. *J Am Coll Cardiol* 2003;41(4 Suppl S):7S–14S.

111. Davies SW, Marchant B, Lyons JP, et al. Coronary lesion morphology in acute myocardial infarction: demonstration of early remodeling after streptokinase treatment. *J Am Coll Cardiol* 1990;16(5):1079–1086.

112. Meyer BJ, Badimon JJ, Mailhac A, et al. Inhibition of growth of thrombus on fresh mural thrombus. Targeting optimal therapy. *Circulation* 1994;90(5):2432–2438.

113. Badimon L, Badimon JJ, Lassila R. Thrombin inhibition by hirudin decreases platelet thrombus growth on areas of severe vessel wall injury [abstract]. *J Am Coll Cardiol* 1989;13:145.

114. Waller BF, Rothbaum DA, Pinkerton CA, et al. Status of the myocardium and infarct-related coronary artery in 19 necropsy patients with acute recanalization using pharmacologic (streptokinase, r-tissue plasminogen activator), mechanical (percutaneous transluminal coronary angioplasty) or combined types of reperfusion therapy. *J Am Coll Cardiol* 1987;9(4):785–801.

115. Meyer BJ, Badimon JJ, Chesebro JH, Fallon JT, Fuster V, Badimon L. Dissolution of mural thrombus by specific thrombin inhibition with r-hirudin: comparison with heparin and aspirin. *Circulation* 1998;97(7):681–685.

116. Gosgnach W, Challah M, Coulet F, Michel JB, Battle T. Shear stress induces angiotensin converting enzyme expression in cultured smooth muscle cells: possible involvement of bFGF. *Cardiovasc Res* 2000;45(2):486–492.

117. Burke AP, Kolodgie FD, Farb A, et al. Healed plaque ruptures and sudden coronary death: evidence that subclinical rupture has a role in plaque progression. *Circulation* 2001;103(7):934–940.

118. Kolodgie FD, Gold HK, Burke AP, et al. Intraplaque hemorrhage and progression of coronary atheroma. *N Engl J Med* 2003;349(24):2316–2325.

119. Naghavi M, Libby P, Falk E, et al. From vulnerable plaque to vulnerable patient: a call for new definitions and risk assessment strategies: Part I. *Circulation* 2003;108(14):1664–1672.

120. Naghavi M, Libby P, Falk E, et al. From vulnerable plaque to vulnerable patient: a call for new definitions and risk assessment strategies: Part II. *Circulation* 2003;108(15):1772–1778.

121. Virmani R, Kolodgie FD, Burke AP, Farb A, Schwartz SM. Lessons from sudden coronary death: a comprehensive morphological classification scheme for atherosclerotic lesions. *Arterioscler Thromb Vasc Biol* 2000;20(5):1262–1275.

122. Burke AP, Farb A, Pestaner J, et al. Traditional risk factors and the incidence of sudden coronary death with and without coronary thrombosis in blacks. *Circulation* 2002;105(4):419–424.

123. Shah PK. Thrombogenic risk factors for atherothrombosis. *Rev Cardiovasc Med* 2006;7(1):10–16.

124. Markovitz JH, Tolbert L, Winders SE. Increased serotonin receptor density and platelet GPIIb/IIIa activation among smokers. *Arterioscler Thromb Vasc Biol* 1999;19(3):762–766.

125. Badimon JJ, Badimon L, Turitto VT, Fuster V. Platelet deposition at high shear rates is enhanced by high plasma cholesterol levels. In vivo study in the rabbit model. *Arterioscler Thromb* 1991;11(2):395–402.

126. Osende JI, Badimon JJ, Fuster V, et al. Blood thrombogenicity in type 2 diabetes mellitus patients is associated with glycemic control. *J Am Coll Cardiol* 2001;38(5):1307–1312.

127. Rauch U, Crandall J, Osende JI, et al. Increased thrombus formation relates to ambient blood glucose and leukocyte count in diabetes mellitus type 2. *Am J Cardiol* 2000;86(2):246–249.

128. Corti R, Badimon JJ. Value or desirability of hemorheological-hemostatic parameter changes as endpoints in blood lipid-regulating trials. *Curr Opin Lipidol* 2001;12(6):629–637.

129. Giesen PL, Rauch U, Bohrmann B, et al. Blood-borne tissue factor: another view of thrombosis. *Proc Natl Acad Sci U S A* 1999;96(5):2311–2315.

130. Giesen PL, Fyfe BS, Fallon JT, et al. Intimal tissue factor activity is released from the arterial wall after injury. *Thromb Haemost* 2000;83(4):622–628.

131. Rauch U, Bonderman D, Bohrmann B, et al. Transfer of tissue factor from leukocytes to platelets is mediated by CD15 and tissue factor. *Blood* 2000;96(1):170–175.

132. Soejima H, Ogawa H, Yasue H, et al. Heightened tissue factor associated with tissue factor pathway inhibitor and prognosis in patients with unstable angina. *Circulation* 1999;99(22):2908–2913.

133. Mallat Z, Benamer H, Hugel B, et al. Elevated levels of shed membrane microparticles with procoagulant potential in the peripheral circulating blood of patients with acute coronary syndromes. *Circulation* 2000;101(8):841–843.

134. Tedgui A, Mallat Z. Apoptosis as a determinant of atherothrombosis. *Thromb Haemost* 2001;86(1):420–426.

135. Sambola A, Osende J, Hathcock J, et al. Role of risk factors in the modulation of tissue factor activity and blood thrombogenicity. *Circulation* 2003;107(7):973–977.

136. Jaffe AS, Babuin L, Apple FS. Biomarkers in acute cardiac disease. The present and the future. *J Am Coll Cardiol* 2006;48(1):1–11.

137. Bresalier RS, Sandler RS, Quan H, et al. Cardiovascular events associated with rofecoxib in a colorectal adenoma chemoprevention trial. *N Engl J Med* 2005;352(11):1092–1102.

138. Chan AT, Manson JE, Albert CM, et al. Nonsteroidal antiinflammatory drugs, acetaminophen, and the risk of cardiovascular events. *Circulation* 2006;113(12):1578–1587.

139. Erhardtsen E, Nilsson P, Johannessen M, Thomsen MS. Pharmacokinetics and safety of FFR-rFVIIa after single doses in healthy subjects. *J Clin Pharmacol* 2001;41(8):880–885.

140. Bauer KA. New anticoagulants: anti IIa vs anti Xa—is one better? *J Thromb Thrombolysis* 2006;21(1):67–72.

141. Albers GW, Diener HC, Frison L, et al. Ximelagatran vs warfarin for stroke prevention in patients with nonvalvular atrial fibrillation: a randomized trial. *JAMA* 2005;293(6):690–698.

142. Fiessinger JN, Huisman MV, Davidson BL, et al. Ximelagatran vs low-molecular-weight heparin and warfarin for the treatment of deep vein thrombosis: a randomized trial. *JAMA* 2005;293(6):681–689.

143. Francis CW, Davidson BL, Berkowitz SD, et al. Ximelagatran versus warfarin for the prevention of venous thromboembolism after total knee arthroplasty. A randomized, double-blind trial. *Ann Intern Med* 2002;137(8):648–655.

144. Olsson SB. Stroke prevention with the oral direct thrombin inhibitor ximelagatran compared with warfarin in patients with non-valvular atrial fibrillation (SPORTIF III): randomised controlled trial. *Lancet* 2003;362(9397):1691–1698.

145. Wahlander K, Eriksson-Lepkowska M, Nystrom P, et al. Antithrombotic effects of ximelagatran plus acetylsalicylic acid (ASA) and clopidogrel plus ASA in a human ex vivo arterial thrombosis model. *Thromb Haemost* 2006;95(3):447–453.

146. Eriksson BI, Bauer KA, Lassen MR, Turpie AG. Fondaparinux compared with enoxaparin for the prevention of venous thromboembolism after hip-fracture surgery. *N Engl J Med* 2001;345(18):1298–1304.

147. Turpie AG, Bauer KA, Eriksson BI, Lassen MR. Postoperative fondaparinux versus postoperative enoxaparin for prevention of venous thromboembolism after elective hip-replacement surgery: a randomised double-blind trial. *Lancet* 2002;359(9319):1721–1726.

148. Coussement PK, Bassand JP, Convens C, et al. A synthetic factor-Xa inhibitor (ORG31540/SR9017A) as an adjunct to fibrinolysis in acute myocardial infarction. The PENTALYSE study. *Eur Heart J* 2001;22(18):1716–1724.

149. Turpie AG, Bauer KA, Eriksson BI, Lassen MR. Fondaparinux vs enoxaparin for the prevention of venous thromboembolism in major orthopedic surgery: a meta-analysis of 4 randomized double-blind studies. *Arch Intern Med* 2002;162(16):1833–1840.

150. Simoons ML, Bobbink IW, Boland J, et al. A dose-finding study of fondaparinux in patients with non-ST-segment elevation acute coronary syndromes: the Pentasaccharide in Unstable Angina (PENTUA) Study. *J Am Coll Cardiol* 2004;43(12):2183–2190.

151. Yusuf S, Mehta SR, Chrolavicius S, et al. Comparison of fondaparinux and enoxaparin in acute coronary syndromes. *N Engl J Med* 2006;354(14):1464–1476.

152. Yusuf S, Mehta SR, Chrolavicius S, et al. Effects of fondaparinux on mortality and reinfarction in patients with acute ST-segment elevation myocardial infarction: the OASIS-6 randomized trial. *JAMA* 2006;295(13):1519–1530.

153. Cauwenberghs N, Meiring M, Vauterin S, et al. Antithrombotic effect of platelet glycoprotein Ib-blocking monoclonal antibody Fab fragments in nonhuman primates. *Arterioscler Thromb Vasc Biol* 2000;20(5):1347–1353.

154. Ingall AH, Dixon J, Bailey A, et al. Antagonists of the platelet P2T receptor: a novel approach to antithrombotic therapy. *J Med Chem* 1999;42(2):213–220.

CHAPTER (54)

Coronary Blood Flow and Myocardial Ischemia

Christophe Depre / Stephen F. Vatner / Garrett J. Gross

There are two major components to this chapter: (1) regulation of coronary blood flow, mainly under physiologic conditions, and (2) mechanisms of myocardial ischemia, both reversible and irreversible, where coronary blood flow is compromised.

REGULATION OF CORONARY BLOOD FLOW

The defining characteristic of the coronary circulation is the direct relationship existing between coronary blood flow and myocardial oxygen consumption. The physiologic rationale is based on the requirement for coronary blood flow to meet the energy requirements of the heart. The main parameters dictating cardiac oxygen consumption are heart rate (chronotropy), cardiac contractility (inotropy) and left ventricular (LV) wall stress. Whereas coronary perfusion at rest in humans represents about 200 mL/min, it can increase up to 1000 mL/min on maximal exercise. The difference between values at rest and maximal levels of coronary flow represents the coronary flow reserve. The mechanisms by which the coronary bed adapts blood flow to the cardiac workload represent one component of coronary autoregulation, that is, the recruitment of the coronary flow reserve to match coronary blood flow (O_2 supply) to energy needs (O_2 demand). This is accomplished via metabolic byproducts and adenosine, but it can also be modu-

lated through an integrated regulation of substance release from the endothelium or from the myocardium itself, neural control, myocardial compressive forces and aortic perfusion pressure. First, the myogenic tone of the small-caliber coronary resistance vessels is controlled by endothelial factors (such as nitric oxide), metabolic products (such as adenosine), and by the autonomic nervous system (both cholinergic and α- and β-adrenergic receptors). Second, this chemical control of coronary flow is additional to the control exerted by physical forces (aortic perfusion pressure and intramyocardial compression forces). All of these components are discussed in the first part of this chapter.

【 】 UNIQUE CHARACTERISTICS OF CORONARY BLOOD FLOW

Phasic Flow

In contrast to most other vascular beds, the myocardium is perfused mainly during diastole and shows a sharp decrease in perfusion during systole, which can be attributed to myocardial compression (Fig. 54–1). The myocardial compressive forces are largely responsible for this phasic nature of coronary perfusion throughout the cardiac cycle. Because of this, a measurement of mean coronary vascular resistance is less meaningful than a calculation of vascular resistance at end-diastole prior to atrial contraction when compressive forces are

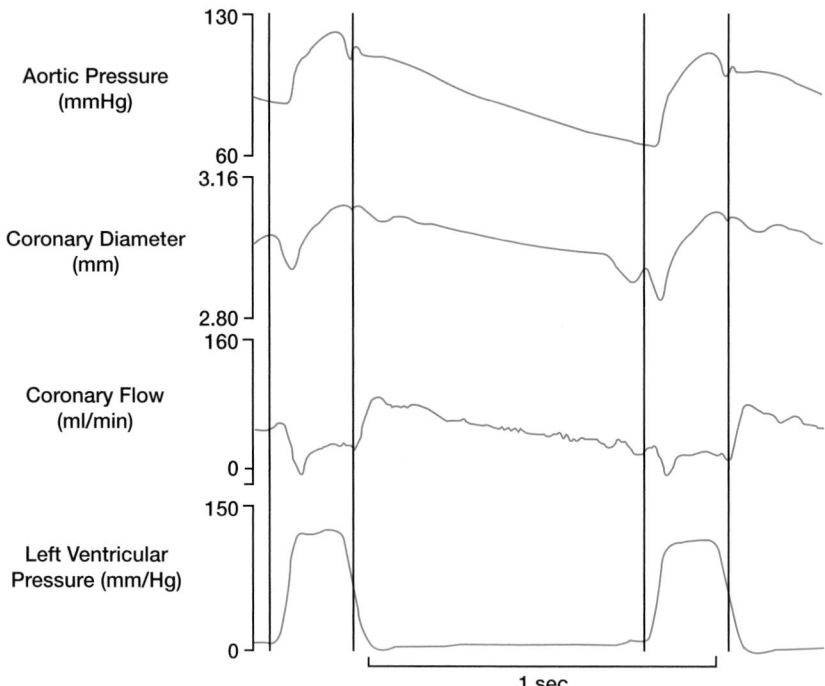

FIGURE 54–1. Phasic nature of coronary flow during the cardiac cycle. This Figure illustrates the profile of aortic pressure, coronary diameter, coronary blood flow, and left ventricular pressure, during the cardiac cycle in the conscious dog. Vertical lines indicate the duration of systole, and indicate that the large coronary arteries follow arterial pressure and are at a maximum, whereas the coronary blood flow is minimal during systole due to extravascular compression. *Source: Reprinted with permission from Vatner SF, Pagani M, Manders WT, Pasipoularides AD. Alpha adrenergic vasoconstriction and nitroglycerin vasodilation of large coronary arteries in the conscious dog. J Clin Invest 1980;65:5–14.*

minimal. A fall of coronary perfusion at the onset of ventricular systole is caused by the squeezing forces of the contracting myocardium, when the intraventricular pressure that opposes coronary flow is roughly equal to the aortic perfusion pressure. Blood flow through large coronary arteries can even be transiently reversed during early systole. Reciprocally, ventricular relaxation during diastole is accompanied by a drop in intraventricular pressure that is far greater than the decrease in aortic pressure, which allows optimal coronary perfusion early in diastole. In addition, the position of the coronary ostia just above the aortic valve leaflets favors the perfusion of the coronary bed during diastole by a retrograde blood flow from the ascending aorta. As a consequence, systole contributes for less than 20 percent of the total coronary flow during a cardiac cycle at rest. However, the fraction of coronary blood flow during systole can rise, particularly when tachycardia compromises diastole, as during electrical pacing or exercise (Fig. 54–2).

Transmural Flow

In a normal heart, the blood flow to the subendocardium is approximately 125 percent of that in the subepicardium,[1] that is, the subendocardial-to-subepicardial (endo-epi) ratio, one index of myocardial ischemia, is above unity in the normally perfused heart. However, this ratio drops dramati-

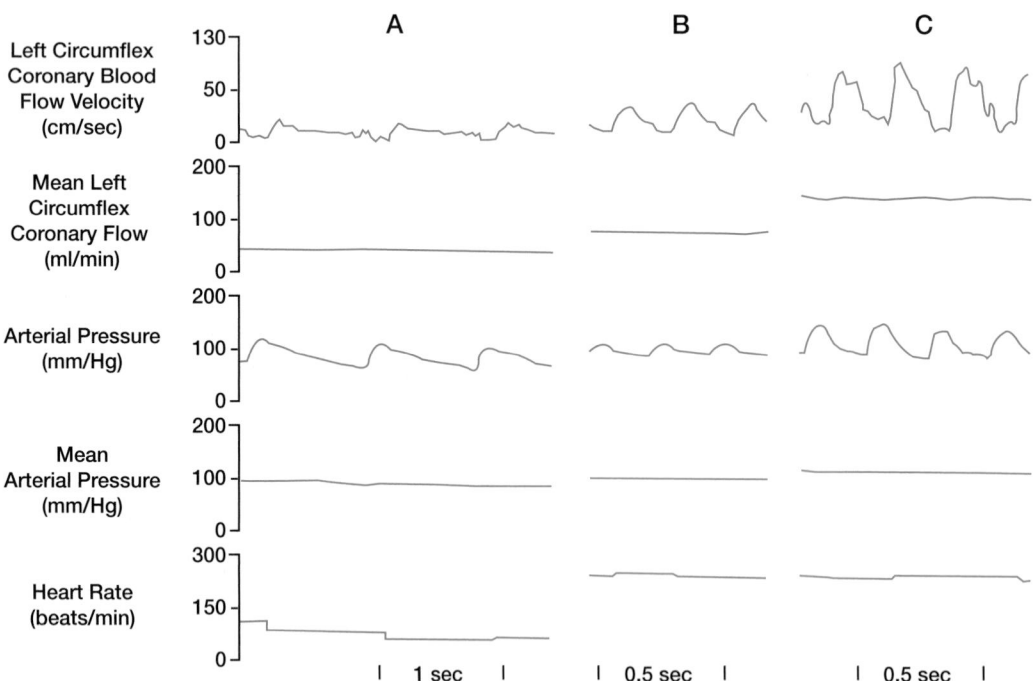

FIGURE 54–2. Regulation of coronary flow and heart rate by exercise. Comparison of coronary flow, aortic pressure, and heart rate in a dog at rest, during an atrial stimulation at a frequency of 248 beats/min, and during exercise at the same atrial frequency. Note that roughly one-third of the coronary hyperemia of exercise can be ascribed simply to the increase in heart rate. *Source: Reprinted with permission from Vatner SF, Higgins CB, Franklin D, Braunwald E. Role of tachycardia in mediating the coronary hemodynamic response to severe exercise. J App Physiol 1972;32:380–385.*

cally in conditions of reduced perfusion pressure or during coronary artery constriction or occlusion, particularly in situations with well-developed coronary collaterals, which favor the subepicardium. In that condition, the maintained subepicardial perfusion is at the expense of the subendocardium, and represents the basis of subendocardial ischemia. A reversed subendocardial-to-subepicardial flow ratio is the hallmark of myocardial ischemia. Furthermore, a vasodilator, for example, isoproterenol, can increase blood flow to the subepicardium at the expense of the subendocardium, a condition referred to as *coronary steal*. Another condition in which the subendocardial coronary flow will decrease, but not to the same extent as in ischemia, is cardiac hypertrophy. Not only the coronary arteries use their mechanism of autoregulation because of the higher energy demand of the hypertrophied heart, but also the compressive forces become much larger, especially in the subendocardium.[2]

Extravascular Compression

As mentioned above, the compressive forces are largely responsible for the phasic nature of coronary flow. The subendocardium is the region most vulnerable to changes in physical forces. Not only the subendocardium is submitted to the highest compressive force during systole, but the subendocardial flow also can be impaired during diastole in conditions of increased LV wall stress, such as during the advanced stage of cardiac hypertrophy or during heart failure. An important distinction must be made for coronary blood flow to the left ventricle and right ventricle because of compressive forces, which are lower in the right ventricle. Correspondingly, the fraction of systolic coronary blood flow is slightly higher to the right ventricle than to the left, whereas the total flow is less in the right ventricle as a consequence of the lower level of wall stress.[3]

Oxygen Extraction

Coronary oxygen extraction is almost maximal at rest. Myocardial oxygen extraction at rest averages 75 to 80 percent, and therefore it may increase only by a slight margin, up to a maximum of 90 percent, upon maximal demand, such as heavy exercise. As a consequence, the main mechanism to bring more oxygen to the myocardium upon increased demand is to increase coronary blood flow.

【 】 CONTROL OF CORONARY BLOOD FLOW BY MYOCARDIAL METABOLIC DEMAND

The primary determinant of coronary blood flow is myocardial oxygen consumption ($M\dot{V}O_2$),[4] which is calculated as the product of coronary blood flow and the arteriovenous (A-V) O_2 difference. As noted above, because A-V O_2 difference cannot increase greatly, an increase in $M\dot{V}O_2$ must be accompanied by an increase in coronary blood flow. Because cardiac work is tightly coupled to $M\dot{V}O_2$, the fact that heart rate increases threefold and contractility fivefold, along with increases in LV wall motion during maximal exercise, results in a requirement for a fivefold increase in coronary blood flow observed in that condition. Consequently, the main determinants of $M\dot{V}O_2$ are those factors primarily involved in regulating myocardial metabolic demand (heart rate and contractility) and LV wall stress.

Heart Rate

Heart rate is the principal mechanism by which cardiac output can be increased. In humans, heart rate increases by about threefold during intense exercise as a result of an adrenergic stimulation from both neural and circulating catecholamines.[5] Heart rate is probably the factor that affects $M\dot{V}O_2$ the most. Increasing the heart rate to the same level as reached during exercise in an experimental preparation will increase coronary blood flow by 50 percent.[6] During intense exercise, heart rate accounts for approximately 30 percent of the increase in coronary flow (see Fig. 54–2). In the case of tachycardia, the oxygen demand increases not only strictly because of a higher heart rate, but also because it decreases the diastolic time of coronary perfusion. Clinically, the Framingham study has shown that individuals with higher heart rates at rest have a higher probability of cardiovascular mortality.

Myocardial Contractility

The increase in contractile state of the myocardium is critical for adjustments to exercise and response to sympathetic stimulation. For example, during intense exercise, LV dP/dt (rate of change of LV systolic pressure), an index of contractility, can also increase four- to fivefold, which permits stroke volume to increase despite increases in heart rate. This increase in myocardial contractility also increases $M\dot{V}O_2$, which requires a commensurate increase in coronary blood flow.

LV Wall Stress

LV systolic wall stress correlates directly with $M\dot{V}O_2$. The formula for LV wall stress demonstrates that this critical determinant of $M\dot{V}O_2$ is directly proportional to LV pressure and LV diameter or volume, and inversely proportional to LV wall thickness. Accordingly, with LV hypertrophy caused by pressure overload, which increases LV systolic pressure, the wall stress is normalized by the LV hypertrophy, that is, increased wall thickness. For that reason, baseline myocardial blood flow per gram of tissue remains essentially at normal levels, 1.0 mL/min per g, in LV hypertrophy. For the same level of ventricular hypertrophy, that is, where wall thickness is reduced by LV dilation, $M\dot{V}O_2$ will increase much more than in a condition of normalized wall stress.[7] In patients with systemic hypertension, for example, $M\dot{V}O_2$ increases, compared to normotensive subjects, before wall stress is normalized. This increased oxygen requirement implies a recruitment of the coronary flow reserve already at rest.

The Adenosine Hypothesis

As developed by Berne et al., the most potent stimulus that suppresses the myogenic tone and therefore dilates the coronary vasculature is adenosine.[8] The ratio between the coronary blood flow after administration of adenosine and the flow at rest represents the coronary blood flow reserve. In normal individuals, this ratio is between 4 and 5, the flow ranging from 200 mL/min at rest to 1000 mL/min at maximal exercise in well-trained athletes. In cardiac myocytes in vivo, adenosine is formed when the rate of adenosine triphosphate (ATP) degradation exceeds the rate of ATP regeneration. This biochemical mechanism is extremely sensitive because the concentration of adenosine in cardiac tissue is about

1000-fold lower than the concentration of ATP. Therefore, even a minute imbalance between ATP degradation and synthesis will result in an increase of adenosine that will be qualitatively, if not quantitatively, very significant. Adenosine production is triggered by hypoxia, either in conditions of ischemia or when oxygen demand increases, such as during exercise. The "adenosine hypothesis" stipulates that the adenosine released from the myocytes binds to A_2 receptors on the smooth muscle cells of the coronary bed, which stimulates vasodilation through production of cyclic adenosine monophosphate.[9] The resulting decrease in vascular resistance increases the coronary flow, which restores the balance between oxygen demand and supply. The same adenosine that is formed under these conditions will bind A_1 receptors on the cardiac myocytes to decrease inotropy, and will trigger the mechanisms of preconditioning.[10] Inhibition of adenosine receptors does not abolish the coronary autoregulation in absence of ischemia, suggesting that, in physiologic conditions, the endothelial control of coronary flow predominates, whereas in ischemic conditions, the metabolic control takes over through the production of adenosine. However, nitric oxide production increases in conditions of ischemia[11] and may therefore be complementary to the effects of adenosine.

Coronary Autoregulation

Coronary autoregulation represents a mechanism by which the coronary artery can maintain a constant flow that matches the metabolic demand independently of the perfusion pressure. The coronary flow can increase up to fivefold between the basal state and the maximal perfusion, which represents the coronary flow reserve. Therefore, coronary autoregulation represents a mechanism by which the coronary flow reserve can be recruited to maintain the desired perfusion level. It is important to note that there are two distinct definitions of coronary autoregulation: the one controlled by the perfusion pressure and the one that is an adaptation of coronary resistance to the metabolic demand. These two components, or definitions of coronary autoregulation, are discussed next.

Autoregulation by Pressure
Coronary autoregulation is a mechanism intrinsic to myogenic tone in the coronary vessels by which the coronary artery maintains a constant blood flow in the face of variations in perfusion pressure.[12] The vascular smooth muscle cells making the tunica media of the coronary arteriole are rich in stretch-operated ion channels activated by shear stress and which stimulate cell contraction. The high myogenic tone that results from the contractile activity of the smooth muscle cells translates in a high resistance to flow. This process allows keeping the flow constant when the perfusion pressure varies between 40 and 140 mmHg.[12] These values were first established in experimental models, and subsequently confirmed in humans. The result is that, in cases of severe coronary artery stenosis or in shock, when the vascular resistance has fallen to its maximal capacity, the flow becomes directly proportional to the perfusion pressure.

Coronary Autoregulation by Metabolic Demand
The main cause of coronary stenosis and obstruction of a coronary artery is atherosclerosis. The single most important parameter of a coronary stenosis is the extent of reduction of the internal luminal diameter because, according to the laws of hydrodynamics, the drop in perfusion pressure across the stenosis is inversely proportional to the fourth power of the minimal luminal diameter. In other words, even a slight decrease in diameter will result in a major loss of pressure. As an example, it has been calculated that an atherosclerotic plaque progressing from an 80 percent to a 90 percent obstruction of the vessel diameter would result in a threefold increase in coronary resistance. The effect of coronary obstruction on blood flow therefore depends largely on the extent of the stenosis. For example, although minor obstructions do not have hemodynamic repercussions, a coronary stenosis obstructing at least 40 percent of the vessel diameter results in a drop of perfusion pressure, which requires a matching decrease of coronary resistance to maintain the normal flow at rest.[13] The decreased resistance is mediated mainly by adenosine release from the myocardium supplied by the obstructed artery. This process requires recruiting the coronary blood flow reserve already at rest, and therefore limits the capacity to exercise. If the obstruction progresses, the coronary blood flow reserve will progressively decrease. When the coronary stenosis becomes so severe that it occludes at least 80 percent of the vessel diameter, the coronary reserve will be totally recruited at rest, and, at that point, any further obstruction will result in a limitation of blood flow already at rest. This concept is further developed below in the section on Coronary Blood Flow Reserve.

【 】 CONTROL OF CORONARY BLOOD FLOW BY NON-METABOLIC FACTORS
Control of Flow by the Endothelium

The endothelium both produces vasoactive substances (nitric oxide, prostacyclin, endothelin-1) and responds to circulating factors (e.g., epinephrine, serotonin). The overall function of the endothelium is to increase the flow through the arteries, if we exclude the tonic vasoconstriction induced by endothelin-1. Consequently, endothelial dysfunction resulting from endothelial damage that accompanies most risk factors (in particular atherosclerosis) will result in increased vascular resistance and impaired flow. The most potent vasodilator released by the endothelium is nitric oxide (NO), which is produced by the stimulation of the cholinergic cascade, and which immediately diffuses as a gas from the endothelium to the surrounding vascular smooth muscle cells where it induces a cyclic guanosine monophosphate-dependent muscular relaxation.[14] Paradoxically, acetylcholine provokes vasoconstriction in isolated coronary arteries in vitro. These apparently contradictory results can be reconciled in light of the seminal observation by Furchgott and Zawadzki[15] that acetylcholine induces vasoconstriction, rather than vasodilation, in isolated aortic rings denuded of endothelial cells, but in vessels with endothelium intact, acetylcholine induces prominent vasodilation. NO is the main mediator of the vasodilatory effect of acetylcholine (which is released physiologically through the parasympathetic neural stimulation) but its production is also increased by stimulation of the α-adrenergic receptors. In addition to NO, another potent vasodilator released by the endothelium is prostacyclin, which is involved in the normal vasodilation at rest and in the adaptation to increased shear stress.

Blocking prostacyclin synthesis with cyclooxygenase inhibitors (e.g., aspirin, indomethacin) can reduce the coronary blood flow at rest in patients.

Control by the Autonomic Nervous System

Parasympathetic (Muscarinic) Receptor Control

The release of NO by stimulation of endothelial cells by acetylcholine (the parasympathetic neurotransmitter) remains one of the most important mechanisms of vasodilation throughout the vasculature, which is reflected by the use of nitrates to decrease the preload in patients with coronary artery disease. Vagal stimulation has a vasodilatory effect in the coronary bed, thereby increasing coronary blood flow. In addition to a direct effect on the coronary bed, the parasympathetic tone reduces heart rate, arterial pressure and inotropy, which altogether reduce the oxygen demand of the myocardium.[16] However, when these parameters are kept constant in experimental preparations where both heart rate and perfusion pressure can be controlled, vagal stimulation still increases coronary flow. This effect is reproduced by administration of acetylcholine and is blocked by atropine. It is now well established that endothelial dysfunction and reduced NO production, which often accompanies atherosclerosis, increases the frequency of coronary vasospasm. Even if the coronary obstruction resulting from the atherosclerotic plaque is minor, the risk of vasospasm in that condition may be sufficient to induce ischemia and even myocardial infarction.

α-Adrenergic Receptor Control

The stimulation of cardiac sympathetic nerves markedly increases coronary blood flow, as a consequence of the increased metabolic demand induced by the increase in workload (heart rate, contractility, LV wall stress) resulting from catecholamine release. This increased metabolic demand is blocked by pretreatment with a β-adrenergic antagonist, which unmasks a vasoconstrictive effect.[17] This vasoconstriction, in turn, can be blocked by an α-adrenergic antagonist.[18] These results indicate that sympathetic stimulation in vivo increases heart rate and inotropy mainly through the β-adrenergic receptors, whereas stimulation of the α receptors induces a vasoconstrictive response. Similarly, direct stimulation of α_1-adrenergic receptors with pharmacologic agonists can provoke vasoconstriction in coronary vessels. An important consequence of the α-adrenergic–mediated vasoconstriction in a context of increased workload is an increase in oxygen extraction,[19] which might be particularly relevant during exercise. The vasoconstriction resulting from α-adrenergic receptor stimulation is increased in patients with coronary artery disease,[20] probably reflecting the partial use of the coronary flow reserve in that situation. The α-adrenergic tone of the coronary arteries can be activated by stimulation of reflex pathways, such as carotid baroreceptors upon carotid sinus hypotension, as well as by direct sympathomimetic stimulation. Similarly, stimulation of the carotid chemoreceptor, pulmonary infla-

tion reflex, and arterial baroreceptor hypertension induce coronary vasodilation that results from a withdrawal of the α-adrenergic tone, potentially with a smaller vagal component contributing to the vasodilation (Fig. 54–3).

β-Adrenergic Receptor Control

Stimulation of the β-adrenergic receptors achieves coronary vasodilation through two complementary mechanisms. Binding of the receptors in the coronary vessel itself will stimulate a Gs protein-mediated relaxation of the vascular smooth muscle cells.[21] In addition, binding of the receptors on the cardiac cells will stimulate a Gs protein-mediated increase in contractility, which, together with the increase in heart rate, will increase the metabolic demand and activate the recruitment of the coronary flow reserve through adenosine release. Whereas the β_2 receptors are mainly responsible for the direct vasodilatory mechanism, the contribution of the β_1 receptor predominates for the metabolic effect resulting from increased workload.[22] As a consequence, treatment of patients with β blockers will reduce coronary flow and may exacerbate coronary vasospasm. However, the negative inotropy and reduction of heart rate following administration of β blockers markedly reduce the risk of exercise-induced angina,

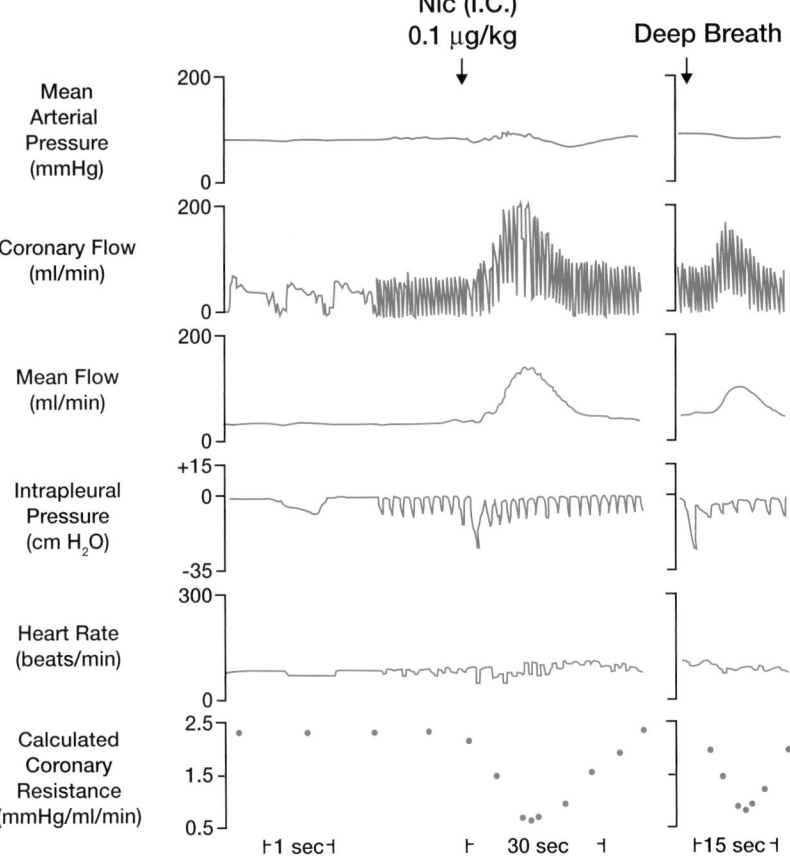

FIGURE 54–3. Reflex adaptation of coronary flow. Effects of intracarotid (I.C.) administration of nicotine (Nic), at a dose that has no systemic effect, but which stimulates the carotid chemoreflex, resulting in increases in respiration depth, as reflected by the change in intrapleural pressure, and marked increase in coronary blood flow and decreases in collateral coronary vascular resistance. The reflex coronary vasodilation can be mimicked by a spontaneous deep breath (*right panel*), which stimulates the pulmonary inflation reflex. The effect of nicotine can be reproduced by an episode of spontaneous deep breath. *Source: Reprinted with permission from Vatner SF, McRitchie RJ. Interaction of the chemoreflex and the pulmonary inflation reflex in the regulation of coronary circulation in conscious dogs. Circ Res 1975;37:664–673.*

do provide protection following myocardial infarction, and, accordingly, are used widely in patients with ischemic heart disease as well as in hypertension.

CONTROL OF CORONARY BLOOD FLOW IN LARGE ARTERIES

Under normal circumstances, large coronary arteries participate very little in the regulation of coronary resistance because the chemical control of coronary blood flow is mainly performed at the level of small-caliber resistance vessels. However, the large coronary arteries play a major role in the regulation of coronary flow in pathologic settings, especially in conditions of coronary vasospasm and obstruction by an atherosclerotic plaque when blood flow becomes largely dependent on perfusion pressure, and by shear stress (flow-dependent regulation of flow). The physical components of coronary flow include the coronary perfusion pressure, flow-dependent regulation, as well as control by neurohumoral mechanisms. In contrast to the phasic measurement of coronary blood flow, the phasic measurement of large coronary artery diameter parallels that of aortic pressure (see Fig. 54–1).

Flow-Dependent Dilation

Because NO production is also increased by shear stress, it represents an excellent mediator of autoregulation in conditions of increased cardiac output, such as during exercise.[23] This mechanism represents the molecular basis of flow-dependent coronary vasodilation. The increased shear stress in conditions of increased flow, which is mainly determined by the viscosity of the blood and its velocity, represents a stimulus for NO production that is followed by vasodilation and subsequent decrease in shear stress. One of the first investigations was by Hintze and Vatner, who observed that following a temporary coronary artery occlusion during the reactive hyperemia phase, the large coronary arteries dilated (termed "reactive dilation"), which was entirely dependent upon the increase in coronary blood flow.[24]

Reactive Hyperemia

The best experimental method to gauge the coronary flow reserve is a transient occlusion of a large coronary artery. Upon reperfusion, the coronary flow reserve is fully recruited, inducing transiently a maximal flow called *reactive hyperemia*,[25] which is accompanied by an increased diameter of the coronary artery (*reactive dilation*),[24] discussed earlier. Whereas the reactive hyperemia results mainly from adenosine release, the reactive dilation is caused by the NO-mediated response to increased shear stress following the increase in flow a result of the hyperemia. This experiment shows that an obstacle to coronary flow is the most potent mechanism to challenge the system of autoregulation. When this system reaches its limits in the resistance vessels, the flow becomes mainly dependent on the perfusion pressure in the large coronary arteries.

Regulation by Aortic Pressure

Coronary perfusion pressure is directly proportional to the aortic pressure. It has been known for more than a century that increas-

ing the perfusion pressure in an isolated preparation has a positive inotropic effect on cardiac contractility, a phenomenon known as the *Anrep effect*.[26] However, changes in aortic pressure are not necessarily accompanied by parallel changes in coronary flow because the coronary circulation adapts its resistance primarily to the oxygen needs. This is because the aortic perfusion pressure also represents the cardiac afterload, an important determinant of LV wall stress and of $M\dot{V}O_2$. Because any increase in aortic pressure increases the metabolic demand of the myocardium, variations in vascular resistance, rather than changes in perfusion pressure, are the main mediators of flow autoregulation. For example, coronary flow can increase up to fivefold in conditions of maximal exercise despite a limited increase in aortic pressure because of the combined vasodilatory effects of metabolic and endothelial effectors. Reciprocally, a drop in aortic pressure provokes an increase in heart rate, which may also activate the mechanisms of metabolic autoregulation, as well as the myogenic component through the change in pressure and myogenic tone.

Autonomic Control

Large coronary arteries react to both cholinergic and adrenergic stimulation. Similarly to the resistance vessels, nitroglycerin induces a marked vasodilation of large arteries, whereas α-adrenergic stimulation results in vasoconstriction and a β-adrenergic stimulation in vasodilation. However, the large coronary arteries are relatively more sensitive to the α-adrenergic–mediated vasoconstriction than the resistance vessels. Interestingly, α-adrenergic stimulation induces vasoconstriction despite an increase in both preload and afterload that should theoretically result in a pressure-induced dilation of the coronary artery. The β-adrenergic vasodilation of the large arteries is also specific (i.e., mediated by vascular receptors), as it can be dissociated from changes in other cardiac parameters, such as heart rate.[21] The cholinergic effect is reversed in conditions of endothelial dysfunction, according to the Furchgott paradigm.[15]

CORONARY BLOOD FLOW RESERVE

The coronary flow reserve represents the difference between coronary flow at rest and maximal perfusion. The main condition recruiting the coronary flow reserve in the normal heart is exercise. However, this reserve is already recruited at rest in the diseased heart, in conditions such as ischemic heart disease.

Effects of Exercise

The massive increase in myocardial metabolic demands during exercise requires a matching increase in coronary blood flow because, as mentioned earlier, coronary oxygen extraction is almost maximal already at rest, and the maximal increases in heart rate, LV wall stress and myocardial contractility during exercise increase $M\dot{V}O_2$ and secondarily coronary blood flow. As a consequence, the only mechanism to bring more oxygen to the myocardium upon increased demand is to increase the flow (see Fig. 54–2). All the mechanisms of coronary flow regulation participate in this adaptation. The increased oxygen demand results from an increase in heart rate, cardiac contractility and ventricular wall stress from the adrenergic stimulation. Variations of pressure in large coronary arteries during exercise are intertwined with variations of resistance in smaller vessels. For instance, an increase in heart rate will shorten the time of ventricular relaxation during which the perfusion pressure is optimal, but a metabolic effect usually accompanies this situation to maintain or increase the coronary flow.[27] It results that, during exercise, the contribution of systole to the coronary blood flow increases to about 40 percent, whereas it represents only 15 to 20 percent at rest. During exercise, coronary resistance decreases through the three mechanisms described above; that is, flow-mediated dilation and NO release, metabolic dilation by adenosine, and β-adrenergic vasodilation. It has been demonstrated experimentally that exercise is also accompanied by a vasoconstrictive α-adrenergic stimulation.[18] Although counterintuitive, this mechanism could balance an excessive decrease in coronary resistance, and could also improve myocardial oxygen extraction. In addition, the aortic perfusion pressure also increases, thereby improving the flow through large coronary arteries.

Flow Reserve in the Diseased Heart

The considerations detailed above apply only to the normal heart. For example, limited coronary reserve in the hypertrophied heart severely impairs its capacity to exercise. It was demonstrated in the canine model of both right and left ventricular hypertrophy that the animals present a massive postexercise coronary hyperemia, suggesting a perfusion deficit of the hypertrophied ventricle during exercise.

Ischemic heart disease is another pathologic condition that limits the coronary flow reserve. The purpose of the coronary flow reserve in that condition is to maintain a normal flow at rest as long as possible. As mentioned above, a coronary obstruction that occludes at least 40 percent of the vessel diameter will recruit the coronary flow reserve in order to maintain a normal flow in rest conditions. Above that threshold of 40 percent, the coronary flow reserve is recruited to an extent that is proportional to the severity of the stenosis. When patients with coronary obstruction start exercising, the increased energy demand will not be matched properly by an increased oxygen supply because the coronary flow cannot increase further proportionally to the metabolic needs, which will trigger an episode of exercise- or stress-induced angina. If the atherosclerotic plaque obstructs at least 80 percent of the vessel diameter (which corresponds to approximately 95 percent of the cross-sectional area), the coronary flow reserve will be compromised at rest. Coronary flow will be directly related to perfusion pressure.[28] If the obstruction becomes any worse than 80 percent (typically, if a thrombus forms on an ulcerated plaque), the coronary blood flow will become insufficient even at rest, which results in episodes of unstable angina (pain in absence of increased workload). This situation is "unstable" because a thrombotic plaque can rapidly evolve into total coronary occlusion and subsequent myocardial infarction.

Beside the mechanical obstacle created by the plaque, other factors limit the blood flow in an atherosclerotic artery. An additional reason for the lack of increased flow in response to increased shear stress in the diseased artery is that endothelial dysfunction frequently is superimposed on atherosclerosis, which limits the recruitment of NO-mediated vasodilation. In all cases, the coronary flow reserve in the subendocardium is recruited faster than in the

subepicardium. There is a point at which the subendocardial arterioles are fully dilated (and therefore, the subendocardial flow becomes directly proportional to the perfusion pressure), whereas the subepicardial arteries retain some autoregulation.[29] At that point, any further dilation in the subepicardium redistributes the flow from the subendocardium to the subepicardium (*coronary steal*) and exacerbate subendocardial ischemia. In addition, in case of thrombus formation, the serotonin released by activated platelets also promotes vasospasm in a context of endothelial dysfunction. Thus, limitations of coronary flow reserve become an integral component of coronary artery disease, and of the mechanisms of myocardial ischemia that are described below.

MECHANISMS OF REVERSIBLE MYOCARDIAL ISCHEMIA

Myocardial ischemia is the result of an imbalance between myocardial oxygen supply and myocardial oxygen demand and has a variety of consequences (Fig. 54–4) depending on the severity of the reduction in coronary blood flow, the length of the ischemic insult, the area of myocardium subserved by the occluded artery and the presence of collateral vessels from other adjacent vascular beds within the heart. These consequences of ischemia include angina pectoris, myocardial stunning, myocardial hibernation, pre- or postconditioning, or under the most severe instances, a myocardial infarction with subsequent heart failure. Of course, the hemodynamic determinants of oxygen demand will also influence the outcome and include heart rate, wall stress, and myocardial contractility. Although a reduction or abolition in coronary blood flow is thought to usually be detrimental to the myocardium, there are instances where brief periods of coronary artery occlusion followed by intermittent periods of reperfusion prior to a more prolonged coronary occlusion is beneficial to the heart and makes it resistant to stunning or infarction, a phenomenon termed *myocardial* or *ischemic preconditioning* (IPC).[30] There is also recent evidence to suggest that an IPC protocol administered immediately on reperfusion can also result in a reduction in infarct size as compared to a control group, a phenomenon termed *postconditioning* (POC).[31] Both of these potentially clinically applicable phenomena are discussed in more detail in the Myocardial Preconditioning and Myocardial Postconditioning sections.

ANGINA PECTORIS

Secondary or Effort-Induced Angina

Myocardial ischemia does not generally occur via a total coronary artery occlusion but usually results from one of two sequelae of events that result in the clinical syndrome of angina pectoris. In the majority of cases, a single stenosis or multiple flow-limiting coronary artery stenoses are present in one or more of the major epicardial coronary arteries and no symptoms of ischemia occur at rest, but often occur when the patient exercises or is under other potentially stressful conditions, that is, oxygen demand exceeds oxygen supply. This situation is often termed *secondary angina* because the ischemia is secondary to an increase in oxygen requirements and is relieved when the patient stops exercising or removes him- or her-

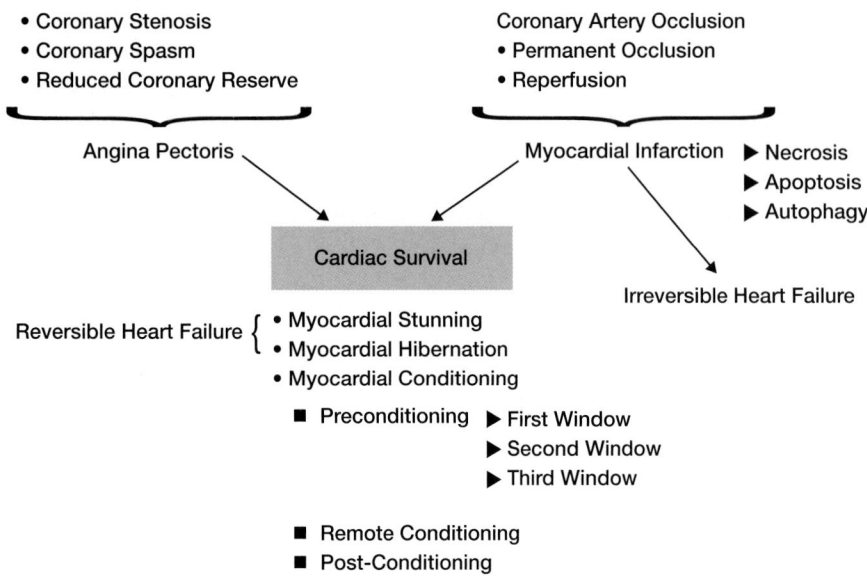

FIGURE 54-4. Paradigms of myocardial ischemia. Coronary stenosis leads to the different forms of angina and is reversible on reperfusion by angioplasty or coronary bypass surgery. Repetitive bouts of ischemia on coronary stenosis can lead to the formation of survival syndromes (stunning, hibernation, and conditioning). Coronary occlusion also leads to myocardial infarction, which evolves into heart failure in absence of early reperfusion, or leads to survival mechanisms if reperfused.

self from a stressful situation, or when a rapidly acting antianginal drug is administered, such as sublingual nitroglycerin. These patients usually present with a decrease in the ST segment on the electrocardiogram, which is indicative of severe subendocardial ischemia. Subendocardial ischemia normally occurs in secondary angina because of the worsening of a *trans*-stenotic pressure gradient, which does not generally produce ischemia at rest as normal flow is maintained by a compensatory dilation distal to the stenosis. As described in the first part of the chapter, it generally requires a reduction in the resting epicardial diameter of 85 to 90 percent of a major coronary artery to produce regional ischemia at rest. Usually, the acute increase in blood flow that occurs across a flow-limiting stenosis during stress or exercise markedly reduces the poststenotic pressure that is the major determinant of blood flow to the subendocardium. Along with the increase in the *trans*-stenotic pressure gradient and reduction in subendocardial perfusion, an acute increase in left ventricular filling or end-diastolic pressure may also occur because of regional ischemia, and this may result in a further reduction in the poststenotic diastolic perfusion pressure and subendocardial perfusion, a condition termed *diastolic crunch*. In the presence of a prolonged flow-limiting stenosis and intermittent episodes of ischemia, coronary artery collaterals from other vascular beds may be stimulated to grow and the distal coronary pressure may increase, thereby increasing the coronary flow reserve to the affected area and reducing the significance of the flow-limiting stenosis and increasing the anginal or ischemic threshold.

Another mechanism shown to be responsible for ischemia distal to a flow-limiting coronary artery stenosis is the coronary steal described in the first part of this chapter. This situation is present when vasodilation occurs in a coronary bed with a much greater coronary flow reserve than an adjacent coronary bed. This may occur during exercise or in the presence of certain arteriolar vasodilators and may result in steal from the subendocardium to the sub-

epicardium, which is termed transmural steal, or from areas perfused by collaterals where dilation of an artery feeding the collaterals may have a stenosis, and poststenotic dilation will decrease the collateral perfusion pressure and collateral flow. This scenario is termed *lateral coronary steal*. Generally, steal does not occur in the presence of currently used antianginal drugs, such as the nitrates or calcium channel blockers, as these drugs selectively dilate large coronary conductance vessels as opposed to the more distal arterioles.

Collateral blood vessels are stimulated to grow as a result of the poststenotic pressure gradient that develops as a result of atherosclerosis in the large epicardial coronary arteries and/or as a result of the intermittent episodes of ischemia that develop as a result of single or multiple flow-limiting coronary artery stenoses present in the vascular bed. Generally, these collaterals develop from small preexisting anastomoses that are preformed and connect the vascular beds, although in some cases these vessels appear to be newly formed. The collateral circulation is very species dependent, with numerous collaterals being found in guinea pig hearts, fewer in dogs and humans, and essentially none in other animal species such as rabbits, pigs, rats, sheep, mice, and nonhuman primates. In young humans, before coronary artery disease has progressed, collaterals are also sparse. However, in older patients, coronary artery disease has largely induced collateral formation. These preexisting anastomoses progressively form over several months to years by increasing in width and developing a smooth muscle coat and endothelial cells, and may reach diameters of 200 to 400 μm. These vessels may proliferate to the point where they may prevent ischemia in vascular beds distal to a total coronary artery occlusion at rest or during mild stress.

Primary Angina or Vasospasm

The second major type of angina is the result of spasm of a major coronary artery, which is termed *primary* or *variant angina* because the ischemia occurs as the result of a primary decrease in oxygen supply, that is, coronary blood flow, without a change in myocardial oxygen demand. This syndrome was originally noted by Prinzmetal et al., and is often referred to as *Prinzmetal angina*. Some patients show evidence of microvascular spasm or thrombosis, which is responsible for the ischemia and symptoms, but these are more difficult to diagnose by commonly used angiographic techniques. Coronary spasm can occur in an area of the artery with or without the presence of a stenotic lesion detectable by angiography.[32,33] Coronary spasm is often associated with ST segment elevation on the electrocardiogram, which is indicative of severe transmural myocardial ischemia. In some cases, subendocardial ischemia and ST-segment depression is observed if the occlusion is incomplete. Coronary spasm can be reproduced by the intracoronary administration of ergonovine into the affected segment of the vascular tree, which is relieved by intracoronary nitroglycerin. Similar to secondary angina, this syndrome can be quickly relieved in outpatients by the sublingual administration of nitroglycerin or isosorbide dinitrate, which are effective vasodilators for large coronary arteries. Although the precise mechanism responsible for coronary spasm has not been identified, a number of vasoconstrictor substances have been proposed to be responsible, including sympathomimetic amines such as norepinephrine or epinephrine, serotonin, histamine, endothelin, thromboxane A_2, and acetylcholine, which all act on G protein-coupled receptors. Increases in extracellular K^+ or Ca^{2+}, which would be expected to result in membrane depolarization and vasoconstriction, also have been implicated in being causative in spasm. That Ca^{2+} channel blockers are the mainstays in therapy in preventing coronary spasm supports the possibility that these latter two mechanisms are key components of spasm.

Unstable Angina Pectoris

Unstable angina is characterized by a sudden worsening of chronic angina in which angina may appear at rest with an increased frequency and severity. These patients are often prone to develop an acute myocardial infarction as a result of plaque rupture, thrombosis and coronary vasoconstriction or spasm. Another feature of unstable angina is a reduction in the ischemic threshold during exercise, which is suggestive of an increased severity of a flow-limiting stenosis. Usually, these patients cannot be controlled by pharmacologic therapy alone and require coronary angioplasty with a stent placement, or in extreme cases, coronary artery bypass surgery.

Angina Resulting from Microvascular Dysfunction (Syndrome X)

A number of patients with angiographically normal coronary arteries have a positive exercise stress test with ST segment depression on the ECG and perfusion defects indicative of myocardial ischemia and classic angina pectoris. This condition is often termed *cardiac syndrome X* and most often occurs in postmenopausal women. Although the exact etiology of this syndrome is uncertain, there is strong evidence that this may be the result of microvascular dysfunction, particularly of endothelial cells. Evidence for microvascular dysfunction has been suggested by exercise-induced perfusion abnormalities by radionuclide imaging, a reduced left ventricular ejection fraction during exercise compared with control patients, by the presence of ST-segment changes indicative of subendocardial ischemia during exercise, and the perception of classic anginal pain during exercise that may persist for up to 30 minutes following exercise. These patients often respond poorly to sublingual nitrates and demonstrate a variable response to β-receptor blockers and calcium antagonists. Women with syndrome X had impaired vasodilator responses to acetylcholine, an endothelium-dependent vasodilator, and to sodium nitroprusside, an endothelium-independent vasodilator, which clearly suggested a generalized impaired vasodilator function in these patients.[34] However, other investigators have failed to show microvascular dysfunction uniformly in patients with syndrome X, and have suggested other possibilities exist to explain the pain that these patients feel, including an abnormality in pain perception, estrogen-related hormonal irregularities, insulin resistance, and a psychological basis. Thus, although microvascular dysfunction appears to be involved in many of these patients, this syndrome may be multifactorial, and a comprehensive treatment regimen may be necessary in treating this disorder.

There are a number of other consequences that occur when the myocardium is subjected to brief periods of myocardial ischemia and reperfusion, or to prolonged low flow. These syndromes are termed *myocardial stunning* and *hibernating myocardium*, respectively. The consequences and potential mechanisms of these two syndromes on myocardial cell injury are described later in this chapter.

Symptoms of Angina Pectoris

The primary manifestation of myocardial ischemia is angina pectoris, irrespective of the type of angina and the causal factors involved. Unfortunately, myocardial ischemia appears to occur in approximately 70 percent of cases without the symptoms of chest pain, a syndrome known as *silent ischemia* and anginal pain may occur in the absence of myocardial ischemia, most notably as a result of esophageal spasm or some other form of gastrointestinal disorder. Typically, the pain of angina occurs retrosternally and may manifest as a crushing, burning, or squeezing-type of discomfort. The pain may spread to the lower part of the neck and radiate down the left arm or either arm in some cases. The pain may be mild or intense and persists for approximately 5 to 10 minutes and is usually relieved rapidly by the administration of nitroglycerin sublingually. If three sequential tablets of nitroglycerin do not relieve the pain, it is likely the result of an ongoing myocardial infarction or the pain is from an extracardiac source. Chemical mediators such as adenosine, which is known to be released in large quantities during ischemia, are most likely responsible for the pain of angina or a myocardial infarction via activation of sensory nerves surrounding the coronary arteries. These nerves project to the dorsal roots of the spinal cord, where they converge on thalamic centers, and finally to the cortex. Unfortunately, nerves from other visceral organs have a similar distribution, which is responsible for nonspecific cardiac pain that often is mistaken for angina.

【 】 REVERSIBLE MYOCARDIAL ISCHEMIA: SURVIVAL MECHANISMS

Until the mid 1960s, myocardial ischemia was thought to result in irreversible myocyte damage. However, this concept was challenged with the discovery that early reperfusion may lead to contractile recovery of the ischemic territory. This proof of principle that ischemia does not necessarily mean death led the path to the unraveling of physiologic conditions in which ischemia–reperfusion boosts the survival capacity of the myocardium. The three most common conditions of cardiac cell survival in a context of ischemia–reperfusion are described as myocardial stunning, ischemic preconditioning, and hibernating myocardium.

Myocardial Stunning

Heyndrickx et al.[35] were the first to demonstrate that reversibly injured myocardium following a 5- or 15-minute episode of ischemia and reperfusion resulted in a deficit in regional contractile function in dogs following reperfusion that lasted for 6 hours following 5 minutes of ischemia and greater than 24 hours following 15 minutes of ischemia (Fig. 54–5). This phenomenon was termed *myocar-*

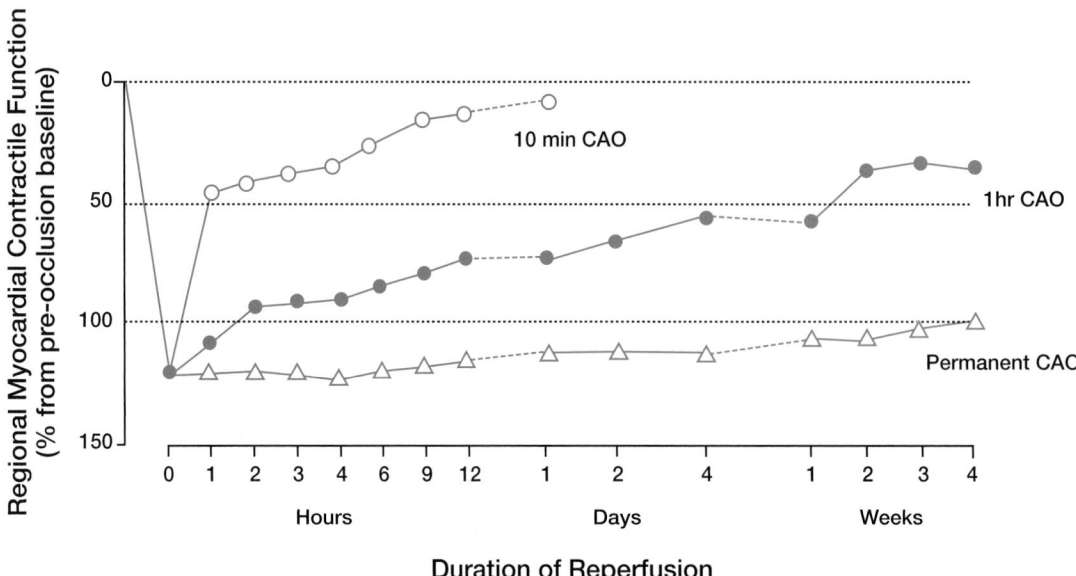

FIGURE 54–5. Importance of early reperfusion on postischemic function recovery. This figure compares the extent of recovery of cardiac contraction after a coronary occlusion (CAO) of 10 minutes or 1 hour, with reperfusion, compared to a permanent occlusion. The delayed recovery of function that occurs with reperfusion is a result of myocardial stunning. *Source: Reprinted with permission from Depre C, Vatner SF. Mechanisms of reversible ischemic dysfunction. In: Walsh RA, ed. Molecular Mechanisms of Cardiac Hypertrophy and Failure. London: Taylor & Francis, 2005:221–246; adapted with permission from Lavallee M, Cox D, Patrick T, et al. Salvage of myocardial function by coronary artery reperfusion 1, 2 and 3 hours after occlusion in conscious dogs. Circ Res 1983;53:235–47.*

dial stunning, which can be defined as a prolonged and fully reversible dysfunction of the ischemic heart that persists after reperfusion despite the normalization of blood flow. Another characteristic of myocardial stunning is that the affected area is responsive to inotropic stimulation by catecholamines such as dobutamine, or by noncatecholamine-positive inotropes such as milrinone, without any deleterious consequences following inotropic support. In other words the time course of stunning is not altered by the increase in contractile function produced by the positive inotropes.

Clinical Relevance Initially described in animal models, myocardial stunning also occurs in the clinical setting. Stunning can occur in a number of conditions, including following exercise in the presence of a flow-limiting stenosis, following a brief period of total coronary occlusion such as might occur in patients with primary angina caused by spasm, or following global ischemia after cardiopulmonary bypass. Stunning may even occur in combination with a myocardial infarction where the subendocardium is infarcted and the overlying reversibly injured subepicardium may be stunned for a prolonged period of time, perhaps days to weeks. Characteristically, stunned myocardium does not result in electrocardiographic abnormalities and coronary blood flow to the stunned area is usually normal, which suggests that there is a flow–function mismatch. Myocardial stunning can occur because of the ischemic bout that is induced by angioplasty. The occlusion caused by the balloon inflation, followed by the reperfusion when the balloon deflates, triggers an ischemic attack that, in turn, stuns the myocardium. However, the ischemic attack induced by this procedure is not long enough to cause any long-term damage, and the myocardium resumes normal function soon after. Angina is also believed to induce stunning. Jeroudi et al.[36] found that patients with angina experienced wall motion abnormalities that per-

sisted for close to 24 hours, even after flow had been normalized and chest pain subsided. The findings of this study are rather vague, as the delay of improvement can be linked to other factors, such as short-lived ischemic episodes that occur persistently, but sporadically, or myocardial hibernation.[37] Also, the systolic function of patients who have been treated for acute myocardial infarction with thrombolytic therapy does not normalize until several days afterwards. This delay in the improvement of myocardial function is strongly suggestive of myocardial stunning. Stress-induced ischemia is also believed to result in stunning. Ambrosio et al.[38] demonstrated that after an exercise-induced ischemic episode, myocardial function remains depressed even after termination of exercise and normalization of perfusion levels. Stunning is also a very dire consequence of cardiac surgery, because the stunning would involve the entire left and right ventricles. This type of postoperative stunning, which may occur after cardiopulmonary bypass, may be alleviated by the use of inotropes.

Mechanisms of Stunning Although there is no unified view of the pathogenesis of myocardial stunning, mainly because of species differences, the two main trigger mechanisms seem to be Ca^{2+} and oxygen radicals.

Although the seminal description of stunning was made in a large mammalian model,[35] the Ca^{2+} hypothesis was largely developed in rodent models. During stunning in rodents, transient Ca^{2+} overload activates the Ca^{2+}-dependent protease calpain I, which degrades, affects the phosphorylation state, and induce covalent modifications of myofilaments, such as troponin I.[39] As a result, there is a decreased responsiveness to $Ca,^{2+}$ manifested by a decrease in the maximal force and a relative insensitivity to extracellular Ca^{2+} concentration. However, these data obtained in rodents differ radically from what is observed in larger mammals. As shown by Kim et al.[40] in a pig model of myocardial stunning where intracellular Ca^{2+} handling in myocytes from stunned and nonischemic regions can be compared in the same heart, the impaired contractile function observed in vivo was also present in isolated myocytes in vitro in this model. In this study, both Ca^{2+} transients and L-type Ca^{2+} current density were decreased in stunned myocytes, which indicates that the mechanisms of contractile dysfunction in the pig involve impaired Ca^{2+} handling. Importantly, there is no degradation of troponin I in the pig model of stunning.[41] Reciprocally, the mechanisms of stunning most described in large mammals appear to be primarily the result of the effect of reactive oxygen species (ROS) released during the first few minutes of reperfusion and the subsequent impairment in calcium handling by the myocyte. The oxyradical hypothesis was pioneered by Bolli's laboratory via a series of elegant experiments using pharmacologic tools and free radical spin-trap agents in anesthetized and conscious animals. Initially, evidence for the role of ROS in stunning was published by three laboratories nearly simultaneously.[42–44] All three laboratories showed that the combination of two free radical scavengers, superoxide dismutase (SOD) and catalase, a superoxide scavenger and hydrogen peroxide scavenger, respectively, attenuated stunning in anesthetized animals.

Myocardial Hibernation

Myocardial hibernation represents a condition of chronic ventricular dysfunction in patients with coronary artery disease, which is progressively reversible after revascularization.[45] The time to restoration of regional contractile function usually occurs within days, months, or up to a year in patients, depending on the length and severity of the previous flow reduction and the underlying ultrastructural damage of the affected area of myocardium. The term *hibernation* referring to this condition was first used by Diamond et al. in 1978,[46] but was not widely recognized until Rahimtoola demonstrated the importance of this paradigm.[45]

Myocardial hibernation was first proposed to represent a condition in which a prolonged subacute or chronic state of myocardial ischemia results in a new equilibrium in which myocardial necrosis is not present because myocardial metabolism and function are both reduced to match a concomitant reduction in coronary blood flow as a result of the presence of a moderate to severe flow-limiting stenosis (*smart heart* hypothesis).[45] Initially, this phenomenon was based totally on clinical observations because of the difficulty in producing a stable animal model of hibernation that could be distinguished from that of myocardial stunning, which has some characteristics in common with myocardial hibernation. An alternative mechanism was subsequently proposed in which the myocardium is subject to repetitive episodes of ischemia–reperfusion resulting from an imbalance between myocardial metabolic demand, which can increase during exertion, and myocardial oxygen supply, which cannot increase appropriately because of the coronary artery disease and limited coronary reserve. This imbalance results in repetitive episodes of ischemic dysfunction followed by stunning that eventually create a sustained depression of contractile function (*repetitive stunning* hypothesis).[47]

The pathophysiology of myocardial hibernation depends to a large extent on the mechanisms of coronary blood flow reserve. As described in the first part of this chapter, the coronary blood flow reserve represents the difference between maximal coronary blood flow on complete vasodilation and coronary flow at rest. In patients with ischemic heart disease, the coronary flow reserve decreases in response to the coronary stenosis, when the only possible mechanism to maintain normal coronary flow at rest is to decrease the downstream vascular resistance by vasodilation.[28] When the stenosis becomes critical, the coronary flow reserve is totally recruited to maintain resting blood flow, and therefore any stimulus of increased oxygen demand (such as exercise) will automatically induce ischemia. These small, repetitive episodes of ischemia, which are not necessarily symptomatic, are followed by transient regional dysfunction upon restoration of the balance between energy demand and supply at reperfusion. Although a single episode of ischemia–reperfusion induces only a short-term myocardial dysfunction (which represents myocardial stunning, as detailed above), the repetition of such episodes can lead to prolonged and maintained regional dysfunction. Consequently, hibernating myocardium is submitted to repetitive bouts of ischemia because of normally occurring increases in myocardial metabolic demand in the face of significant coronary stenosis and limited coronary reserve, yet it does not develop irreversible damage. Revascularization (either by bypass surgery or by percutaneous angioplasty) represents the only avenue to restore normal contractile function by restoring the coronary flow reserve, unless collaterals form naturally to bypass the diseased vessel. Figure 54–6 summarizes the mechanisms of these two hypotheses to explain myocardial hibernation.

Clinical Relevance Whereas stunning and preconditioning were described initially in animal models, myocardial hibernation is primarily a clinical observation. The diagnosis of myocardial hibernation is of importance in patients with chronic coronary artery disease because the restoration of coronary flow reserve in hibernating myocardium by coronary revascularization is followed by an improvement of contractile performance, whereas the untreated condition leads to heart failure. The diagnosis of this condition is facilitated by the observation that human hibernating myocardium has a glucose uptake that is higher than the uptake in normal myocardium,[48] which confirms the maintained viability and, therefore, the potential recovery of this territory. Based on the pathophysiologic mechanisms described above, it is easy to understand that revascularization (either by bypass surgery or by percutaneous angioplasty) represents the only avenue to restore normal contractile function by restoring the coronary flow reserve, unless collaterals form naturally to bypass the diseased vessel.

Mechanisms of Hibernation There is no animal model that fully reproduces the long-term condition of myocardial hibernation found in patients, in whom the condition can take years to develop. However, several models reproduce the hallmarks of human hibernating myocardium,[49] including chronic dysfunction, loss of myofibrils, accumulation of glycogen, alteration of Ca^{2+} metabolism, gene response and some extent of cell degeneration.

Models of Coronary Stenosis Induction of 1 to 5 hours of coronary stenosis was used as a model of "short-term hibernation" in the pig,[50–52] which demonstrated the possibility of a short-term perfusion–contraction matching. The effects of 24-hour partial stenosis were also examined,[53,54] but this model induces suben-

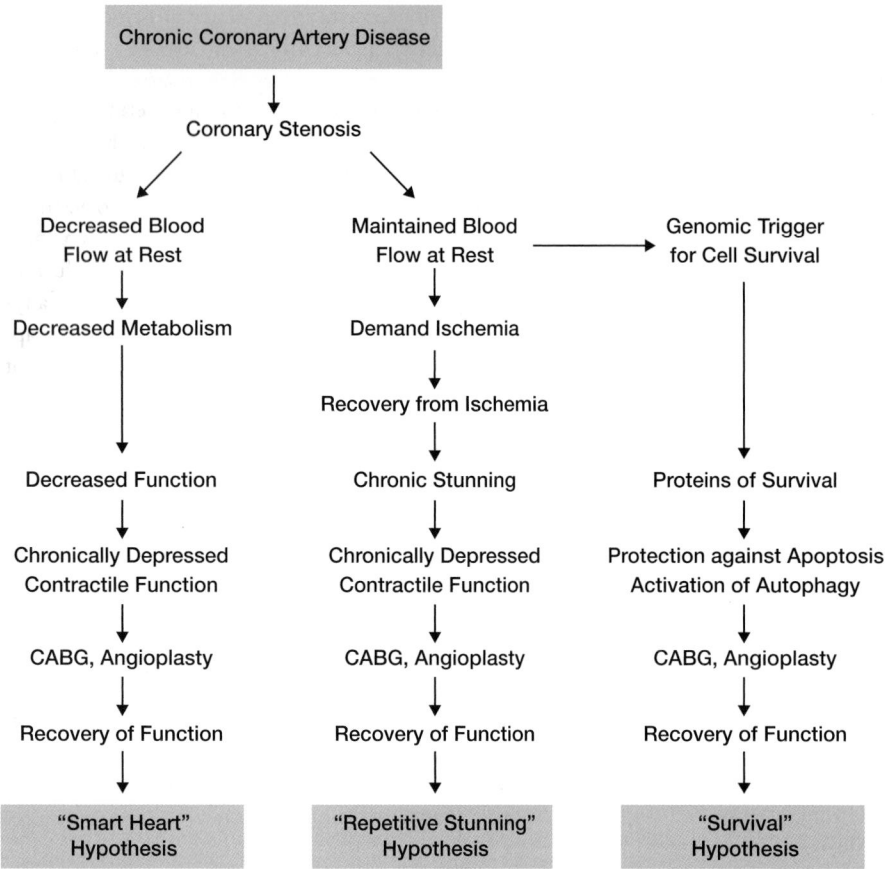

FIGURE 54–6. Pathophysiology of myocardial hibernation. The figure illustrates the "smart heart" hypothesis compared to the "repetitive stunning" hypothesis, and shows how an adaptation of gene expression and intracellular processes (such as autophagy) may underlie the maintained viability of the hibernating tissue. CABG, coronary artery bypass grafting. *Source: Reprinted with permission from Depre C, Vatner SF. Mechanisms of reversible ischemic dysfunction. In: Walsh RA, ed. Molecular Mechanisms of Cardiac Hypertrophy and Failure. London: Taylor & Francis, 2005:221–246.*

docardial necrosis, which is contradictory with the concept of hibernating myocardium. Two models simulate the chronic contractile dysfunction by hypoperfusion[55,56] but with divergent results because of differences in perfusion.

Models of Repetitive Stunning The induction of multiple episodes of myocardial stunning by excitement in conscious pigs leads to a stable chronic contractile dysfunction and the pathognomonic histologic features of hibernating myocardium.[56] More recently, it was demonstrated in the pig that persistent stunning can lead to hibernation.[57] In that model, swine hearts were submitted to repetitive episodes of 90-minute coronary stenosis followed by 12 hours reperfusion, and this cycle was repeated up to six times. After the first ischemic episode, the regional function was depressed despite a normalization of blood flow, reflecting persistent stunning, but there was no further decrease in ventricular function after the following episodes of coronary stenosis, reflecting the mismatch between blood flow and contractile function that characterizes myocardial hibernation.[57] This model also showed the metabolic characteristics of hibernating myocardium, such as a higher dependence on glucose and glycogen accumulation.[57]

Genomics of Survival The maintained viability of the hibernating heart in a context of prolonged ischemia strongly suggests the

possibility of a genomic adaptation in this condition. Recently, the concept of a genomic survival program was tested in the swine model of repetitive stunning described above, in which repetitive episodes of coronary stenosis and reperfusion lead to a chronic reduction in contractility and the morphologic hallmarks of hibernation.[57] Major survival genes progressively increased as ischemia was repeated,[58] including anti-apoptotic, cytoprotective, and growth-promoting genes. Genes of cell survival were tested in human hibernating myocardium as well, by comparing the tissue samples obtained from the hibernating territory and from the normal remote area of the heart of patients scheduled for surgical revascularization of the dysfunctional myocardium. In this setting, all the genes described above in animal models, and their corresponding proteins, were significantly upregulated in hibernating compared to remote myocardium.[58] Therefore, human hibernating myocardium develops an endogenous genomic mechanism of cytoprotection that sustains cell survival in prolonged conditions of ischemia. These results provide a molecular mechanism for maintained cardiac cell viability in ischemic territory, and they underlie the potential for functional recovery of hibernating myocytes.

Myocardial Preconditioning

IPC was first described by Murry et al.[30] in 1986 in a landmark study in dogs in which they showed that four 5-minute periods of coronary artery occlusion interspersed with 10-minute periods of reperfusion prior to the longer index ischemic period of 40 minutes followed by 72 hours of reperfusion resulted in a marked 70 percent reduction in infarct size as compared to a nonpreconditioned group. This finding stimulated a tremendous amount of interest by both basic scientists and clinicians to uncover the possible mechanisms responsible for this marked protective effect as an important therapeutic target for treating patients with ischemic heart disease. IPC occurs in two phases termed *acute IPC* and the *second window of protection* (SWOP) or *delayed preconditioning* and has a duration of 1 to 2 hours following reperfusion in the acute phase, which disappears for up to 12 to 24 hours later, at which time the second window appears and has a duration from 24 to 96 hours, depending on species and preconditioning stimulus.[10] The protective effect of acute IPC to reduce infarct size is generally more robust (50 to 80 percent decrease in infarct size) than the delayed phase where the infarct size reduction is generally 30 to 40 percent of the risk zone. The ceiling of protection is limited to a 30- to 45-minute index ischemic period in smaller animals such as rabbits, rats, and mice, whereas the index ischemic period can be increased to 60 to 90 minutes in larger animal species such as the dog heart. Furthermore, IPC occurs in other organs besides the heart, including skeletal muscle, intestine, liver, kidneys, and brain. Additionally, ischemia in one organ can produce a protective response in another distal organ, a phenomenon termed *remote preconditioning*. Remote preconditioning has not been as well characterized as classical preconditioning but a role for adenosine, opioids, and K_{ATP} channels have been observed so there are obvious similarities between these different modes of preconditioning, which requires further investigation.

Clinical Relevance Because IPC is a very reproducible and powerful cardioprotective mechanism in all animal models studied, the question becomes whether this phenomenon occurs in humans and can it be harnessed for use in clinical medicine. Although acute IPC occurs in human myocardium, the characteristic parameters, such as the window and ceiling of protection, are not as well-defined as in animal models where experimental conditions can be more rigorously controlled. The demonstration of IPC in isolated human ventricular myocytes was published in 1994 by Ikonomidis et al.[59] These investigators also showed that adenosine and protein kinase C (PKC) were both involved in the protection observed. Delayed IPC in human heart was first demonstrated in 1993.[60] Yellon et al., using an atrial trabeculae preparation obtained from human hearts, demonstrated the possible signaling pathways involved in patients,[60] including the adenosine receptors and the δ-opioid receptors as triggers of the preconditioning response, and PKC and the mitochondrial K_{ATP} channel as an end effector in the protection observed. A number of investigations have demonstrated that patients who warmup with brief periods of exercise can exercise longer when exposed to another bout of exercise approximately 1 to 2 hours later. Although this may be a form of preconditioning, it is still uncertain that the same signaling pathways are involved in IPC and warmup angina. Results from a TIMI-9B study[61] showed a protective effect 24 to 72 hours after the onset of a myocardial infarction, which suggest that the protection observed was similar to the phenomenon of delayed IPC. However, no mechanistic studies have been performed in tissue obtained from these patients, so it remains to be seen if this phenomenon is really the result of delayed IPC. Another clinical situation where IPC can be studied in humans more easily is that of coronary angioplasty. A series of balloon inflations results in a preconditioning-like response as indicated by smaller changes in the ST segment of the electrocardiogram following the initial balloon inflation.[62] Several other studies suggested a role for opioids, bradykinin, and the antianginal drug nitroglycerin in a similar model of IPC in man.

Mechanisms of Preconditioning The mechanisms of IPC vary widely depending on the window of protection that is considered. We describe separately the first and second windows, then allude to a possible third window of cardioprotection conferred by repetitive stunning.

First Window Generally, the ischemic stimulus releases several mediators from myocardial tissues or blood vessels such as adenosine, opioids, and bradykinin that act on G_i protein-coupled receptors to trigger the preconditioning response. There is also accumulating evidence that activation of these receptors produces a small release of ROS, which may serve as signaling molecules to further activate a number of kinases within the cell. Transactivation of a tyrosine kinase receptor, the epidermal growth factor receptor, appears to occur in opioid and bradykinin-induced signaling, but not following adenosine receptor signaling.[10] The phosphatidylinositol 3-kinase (PI3K)/Akt pathway also appears to signal via opioid and bradykinin receptors, and eventually PKCε is activated by all the triggers of IPC. Activation of PKCε is a central convergence point in acute IPC and further activates the mitochondrial K_{ATP} channel, which prevents the opening of the mitochondrial permeability transition pore (MPTP) at reperfusion, and thereby prevents both necrosis and apoptosis. There is also recent evidence for an important role for the inhibition of glycogen synthase kinase-3β (GSK3β), which appears to be upstream from the mitochondrial K_{ATP} channel, as a major determinant as to whether the preconditioning stimulus has a memory phase or not.[63] Other kinases, such as ERK (extracellular regulated kinase) 1/2, S6K-1, p38 MAPK (mitogen-activated protein kinase), and mTOR (mammalian target of rapamycin), also are involved in preconditioning produced by various stimuli; Fig. 54–7 summarizes the major signaling pathways involved in acute or classic IPC.

Second Window Delayed IPC or SWOP has more potential clinical relevance than classic preconditioning as it has a much

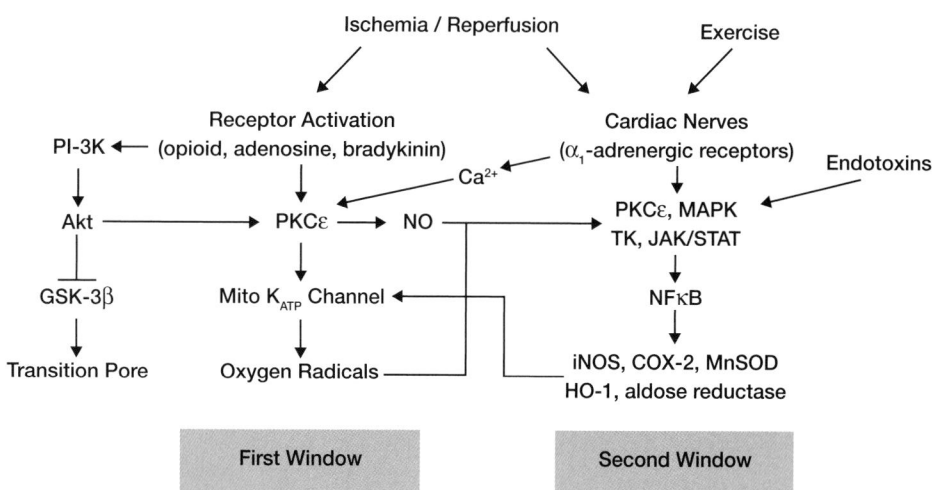

FIGURE 54–7. Mechanisms of the first and second windows of preconditioning. The figure illustrates the triggering by ischemia–reperfusion or by exercise through bradykinin, opioid, or adenosine receptors, or by Ca^{2+}, and the resulting signaling cascade from PKC to the mitochondrial K_{ATP} channel. The mechanisms of the first window in turn activate the second window through NFκB (nuclear factor kappa B) and the subsequent gene response. COX-2, cyclooxygenase-2; GSK, glycogen synthase kinase; HO-1, heme oxygenase 1; iNOS, induced nitric oxide synthase; JAK/STAT, Janus kinase/signal transducer and activator of transcription; K_{ATP}, potassium adenosine triphosphate; MAPK, mitogen-activated protein kinase; MnSOD, manganese superoxide dismutase; PI3K, phosphoinositide 3 kinase; PKC, protein kinase C; TK, thymidine kinase.

more persistent effect and may last up to 4 days.[10] Some of the same triggers that mediate the early window of IPC are involved in the initiation of delayed IPC. These include adenosine acting via its A_1 receptor, opioids acting via δ or κ receptors, bradykinin, and NO. The sarcolemmal and mitochondrial K_{ATP} channels both appear to trigger and/or mediate delayed IPC. These stimuli appear to initiate delayed preconditioning by triggering the release of ROS, which activates a number of intracellular kinases and transcription factors, resulting in the upregulation of several key enzymes responsible for the cardioprotection observed. The kinases involved upstream of transcription include PKCε or PKCδ, tyrosine kinases, mitogen-activated protein (MAP) kinases such as p38 MAPK and ERK 1/2 and the Janus kinase/signal transducer and activator of transcription (JAK/STAT) pathway. Nuclear factor kappa B (NFκB) appears to be a key transcription factor that is activated and translocates to the nucleus to produce gene transcription to upregulate distal mediators such as the manganese-dependent superoxide dismutase (MnSOD), the inducible isoform of NO synthase (iNOS), heat shock proteins (HSPs), cyclooxygenase-2 (COX-2) and heme oxygenase-1 (HO-1) to name a few.[64] These key enzymes translate signals to produce cardioprotective end products such as NO, prostaglandins, HSPs, and other yet-to-be-discovered cardioprotective substances.[64] The end effector for protection appears to be similar to early IPC and is most likely the mitochondrial K_{ATP} channel and the prevention of the MPTP opening.[65] Two mediators of the second window, upregulation of iNOS and COX-2, are not required for the first window of preconditioning. Very recent data indicate that cardiac sympathetic nerves and α_1-adrenergic receptors also are required for the second window of preconditioning,[66] because the second window, including iNOS and COX-2 upregulation, cannot be demonstrated in the denervated heart. Exercise is also a physiologic stimulus of both first and second windows of preconditioning, which activates the PKC pathway through an increase in Ca^{2+} flux mediated by the adrenergic receptors. Figure 54–7 schematically summarizes the factors involved in SWOP or delayed IPC.

A Third Window of Protection Patients with myocardial hibernation are submitted to repetitive stunning, which, as described above, activates a cardiac genomic program of cell survival (see Fig. 54–6). This survival adaptation could theoretically elicit a cardioprotection comparable to IPC. This hypothesis was recently tested in the swine model of repetitive stunning described above, and these animals were compared to pigs submitted to a classic protocol of IPC. In that model, upon induction of lethal ischemia, the cardioprotection conferred by repetitive stunning is quantitatively equivalent to that resulting from IPC. However, the pigs submitted to repetitive stunning and which have a genomic activation of survival mechanisms, do not show the molecular characteristics of the second window, such as an increase in iNOS or in COX-2. Also, pretreatment with an NO synthase inhibitor prevents the cardioprotection by IPC but fails to prevent the protection by repetitive stunning. Consequently, repetitive stunning induces powerful protection against lethal myocardial ischemia that lasts longer than the classic IPC and that proceeds through radically different mechanisms, which we coin a *third window* of cardioprotection. This protection may be very relevant clinically because the regulation of survival genes observed in the model of

repetitive stunning reproduces the pattern found in patients with coronary artery disease.[58]

Myocardial Postconditioning

Although the recently named phenomenon of myocardial POC primarily deals with reducing reperfusion injury, we devote a section of this chapter to this phenomenon because it is related to the use of multiple episodes of ischemia for therapeutic benefit in patients subjected to a previous bout of prolonged ischemia. POC is defined as the decrease in infarct size that results from brief periods of ischemia alternating with brief periods of reperfusion applied immediately after reperfusion following lethal ischemia. In this sense, POC is closely related to IPC but it may have more clinical usefulness as it is administered at reperfusion, which has much more clinical relevance, as opposed to IPC, which is only effective as a pretreatment intervention.

Clinical Relevance POC has a broad array of protective mechanisms and although much work still remains in this field, POC appears to possibly have great clinical potential, particularly in situations where an angioplasty catheter and balloon is in place at the time of reperfusion to control the reflow periods early in reperfusion. Two clinical studies suggesting that POC has clinical benefit in patients already have been published.[67,68] The first study showed that the patients postconditioned by angioplasty had a reduction in the magnitude of ST-segment elevation and produced a faster recovery of the ST segment on reperfusion.[67] In the second study, patients had a total coronary artery occlusion and were subjected to a stent placement in the occluded artery, followed by POC with angioplasty. The patients who had been subjected to POC had a smaller infarct size and an improvement in overall coronary blood flow.[68] These results are quite promising and suggest that more extensive clinical trials are necessary to confirm the efficacy of POC in the treatment of patients subjected to angioplasty/stent placement during an ongoing myocardial infarction.

Mechanism of Postconditioning POC was first identified by Vinten-Johansen et al.[31] and has been shown to reduce a number of indices of reperfusion injury, such as infarct size, apoptosis, myocardial stunning, micro- and macrovascular dysfunction, metabolic dysfunction, and impaired blood flow. Many of the triggers of IPC are also involved in POC, such as adenosine, opioids, and bradykinin. POC also appears to protect cardiac myocytes and endothelial cells against injury caused by cytokines, neutrophils, ROS, and other inflammatory mediators.

IRREVERSIBLE MYOCARDIAL ISCHEMIA AND MYOCARDIAL INFARCTION

Tennant and Wiggers performed the seminal observation that the regional dysfunction which accompanies coronary artery occlusion remains reversible if the ischemic period is brief.[69] Jennings and Sommers demonstrated that this occlusion in the dog consisted of 8 minutes.[70] Subsequently, it became clear from the pathologic studies that reversibility of ischemic damage could be promoted by limiting the time of hypoperfusion. These experimental works still represent the foundation of early reperfusion in patients with coronary artery occlusion. In four decades, the belief that coronary artery occlusion results in myocardial infarction and irreversible damage evolved into the understanding that viability can be maintained by early reperfusion and through a spectrum of survival and cardioprotective mechanisms described above.

MECHANISMS RESPONSIBLE FOR MYOCARDIAL INFARCTION

An acute myocardial infarction usually results from a marked impairment in blood flow produced by a coronary occlusion resulting from a severe atherosclerotic plaque or from a thrombosis caused by platelet aggregation at the site of an unstable plaque that ruptured. Less frequently, embolic phenomena or vasospasm can result in coronary artery occlusion and myocardial infarction. There are a series of biochemical and functional consequences that occur as a result of a severe, prolonged ischemic insult, including a loss of mitochondrial ATP production, a compensatory increase in anaerobic glycolysis with the accumulation of hydrogen ions and lactate production, which leads to tissue acidosis and an impairment in glycolysis and fatty acid metabolism. Functionally, these changes are accompanied by a rapid loss of contractile function in the affected region and electrical abnormalities that may result in severe arrhythmias. Increases in cytosolic and mitochondria calcium also occurs, which leads to the activation of proteases, disruption of myocyte ultrastructure, cell swelling, and, eventually, to the physical disruption of the sarcolemmal membrane and cell death. The patterns of cell death are discussed in the next sections, but it is first necessary to emphasize the importance of early reperfusion as the most powerful mechanism to prevent cell death.

IMPORTANCE OF EARLY REPERFUSION IN ISCHEMIC REVERSIBILITY

Ross et al. extensively demonstrated the importance of early reperfusion in the limitation of contractile dysfunction and irreversible ischemic damage.[71] Dogs submitted to reperfusion, even up to 6 hours of coronary occlusion, resulted in a smaller infarct size, especially in the subepicardium,[72] than dogs submitted to chronic coronary occlusion.[70] Time-course experiments in conscious animals defined the window during which myocardial salvage is possible.[73] Although earlier reperfusion exposes to a higher risk of tachyarrhythmias, it is accompanied, in the acute phase, by an improved cardiac contractile function[71] and, at a later time point, by decreased infarct size.[74] Interestingly, ischemic preconditioning also enhances the rate of tachyarrhythmias, while resulting in reduced necrosis. Figure 54–5 is an example of this principle. Whereas short-term (10-minute) coronary occlusion is followed by myocardial stunning, 1-hour occlusion leads to irreversible damage, which is, however, significantly less than the damage caused by a permanent coronary occlusion (see Fig. 54–5). These seminal investigations paved the way for early revascularization of occluded arteries by thrombolysis or by angioplasty. The TIMI trial was the first multicenter demonstration in a large series of patients that early reperfusion is the optimal method to salvage myocardial tissue, to preserve ventricular function and to improve sur-

vival. These studies also illustrated that cardiac function in an ischemic territory may recover only weeks to months after reperfusion. This finding is of the greatest importance in the assessment of functional recovery after bypass surgery in patients with chronic ventricular dysfunction (hibernating myocardium).

NECROSIS (ONCOSIS)

Morphologically, a myocardial infarction starts in the most ischemic area of the heart, the subendocardium, and proceeds in a wavefront from the subendocardium to subepicardium. Cell death starts 20 to 30 minutes after occlusion in the subendocardium, and is usually complete within 3 to 6 hours unless timely reperfusion occurs to halt this process. A number of stages occur during the progression to necrotic cell death. Initially, there are alterations in ionic movements into and out of the cell, including K^+ and ATP efflux and an influx of Na^+ and Ca^{2+}, resulting in cell swelling. Mitochondrial ATP production ceases and glycolysis becomes the major source of ATP synthesis, with the deleterious consequences of increases in cytosolic H^+ ions and lactate, resulting in intracellular acidosis and decreased myofilament Ca^{2+} sensitivity. The lack of oxygen also leads to an increase in ROS production by the mitochondrial electron transport chain and other sources, such as xanthine oxidase, arachidonic acid metabolism, catecholamine metabolism, and activation of neutrophils and macrophages. All these changes lead to lipid peroxidation and damage to the cellular cytoskeleton and loss of sarcolemmal integrity, and, finally, to cell death. Ischemic necrosis typically involves a region of myocardium in which myocytes, blood vessels, and fibroblasts are all affected. Histologically, the myocytes show increased eosinophilia, loss of striations, and nuclear lysis (karyolysis). The release of cell contents incites an acute inflammatory response with subsequent replacement of the necrotic region with fibrous connective tissue. In the area of infarction, the structural remodeling may lead to congestive heart failure.[75]

APOPTOSIS OR PROGRAMMED CELL DEATH

Apoptosis, first described in 1972 as a mode of cell death separate from cellular necrosis,[76] has become a subject of intense investigation over the past years. In contrast to necrosis, apoptosis occurs on a cell-by-cell basis but may affect both nonmyocytes and myocytes. Rather than undergoing lysis, the nucleus of the apoptotic cell condenses and fragments. The DNA of the apoptotic cell is broken down into multimers of nucleosomes, contrasting with the random fragments created during necrosis. In the terminal stage of apoptosis, the affected cell is ingested locally by phagocytosis or else breaks up into membrane-bound apoptotic bodies. Typically, the apoptotic demise of a cell does not induce inflammation. The otherwise sharp distinction between necrosis and apoptosis can be blurred in ischemia when apoptosis is initiated early and later necrosis ensues.

There are two major pathways responsible for apoptosis: the death receptor pathway and the mitochondrial pathway. The death receptor pathway is stimulated by ligands, particularly the Fas-ligand which binds to its receptor on the cell membrane, the Fas-associating protein with death domain (FADD), activating pro-caspase-8, and, eventually, caspase-3, resulting in cell death several hours after activation, possibly continuing for days to even months in some cases. The more commonly activated mitochondrial proapoptotic pathway is primarily activated via the caspase cascade initiated by the release of cytochrome c from the intermembrane space, which, in conjunction with the apoptosis activating factor (Apaf-1), activates procaspase-9 and, eventually, caspase-3, the protease responsible for cell death in both pathways. There are a number of pro- and antiapoptotic proteins and ligands acting through death receptors that also regulate the mitochondria, including Bcl-2, an antiapoptotic protein, and bax, a proapoptotic protein. It is thought that the ratio of these two proteins determines whether the cell will live or die. Although some promising data has been obtained with caspase inhibitors in reducing infarct size and preventing cellular remodeling, the use of caspase inhibitors in humans remains to be addressed in future studies.

Whereas both necrosis (oncosis) and apoptosis result in the death of myocytes, the distinction between the two is important in evaluating damage to the myocardium. To recapitulate, cells undergoing necrotic death lose sarcolemmal integrity, swell, exhibit increased permeability, lyse their nuclei, induce an acute inflammatory reaction, and result in a dense, collagenous scar. In early stages, regions of necrosis can be identified by examining slices of myocardium for the loss of NADH using the absence of reduction of a tetrazolium salt. Cells dying by apoptosis maintain membrane integrity early, shrink, undergo nuclear condensation and fragmentation, form apoptotic vesicles and are removed by macrophages with little trace. The presence of specific DNA cleavage sites provides a convenient means of identifying apoptotic cells early in the sequence of events. At the cellular level terminal deoxynucleotidyl transferase-mediated deoxyuridine triphosphate nick-end labeling (TUNEL) or another probe (hairpin 1, hairpin oligonucleotide with single-base 3 overhangs) for the specific site of DNA cleavage can identify presumptive apoptotic nuclei. Chromatographic ladders of DNA extracted from damaged tissue also identify apoptosis, as does the binding of annexin V to phosphatidylserine abnormally present on the external surface of the still impermeable sarcolemma. Immunohistochemical identification of activated caspase 3 is yet another method for the identification of apoptotic myocytes.

AUTOPHAGY

Autophagy is a degradation process of endogenous proteins and organelles by the lysosomes, which is typically activated in conditions of energy deprivation. Through autophagy, the cell can recycle denatured proteins or dysfunctional organelles, which represents an important mechanism to maintain homeostasis. Although autophagy is also observed in conditions of cell death, its mechanisms are very different from necrosis or apoptosis, because the recycling of proteins by autophagy might rather be a survival mechanism to generate energy and new peptides. This hypothesis was demonstrated in the swine model of repetitive stunning described above, a model in which apoptosis is activated rapidly but transiently by ischemia, whereas a sustained activation of mechanisms of autophagy is observed at a later time point as ischemia is repeated.[77] This observation, which was also made in human hibernating myocardium,[78] suggests that autophagy may be a long-term survival mechanism[79] additional to the genomic mechanisms described above to sustain the viability of chronically ischemic myocardium (see Fig. 54–6). A cardioprotective role for autophagy during ischemia–reperfusion was recently demonstrated in vitro.[80]

CARDIAC REMODELING AFTER PERMANENT OCCLUSION

Cardiac remodeling initially is an attempt to compensate for the loss of cardiac muscle, but eventually represents one of the most common etiologies of heart failure. At the physiologic level, cardiac remodeling can be defined as the process of modifying ventricular size, shape, and function as a consequence of increased load, decreased contractility, and neurohormonal regulation. At the molecular level, ventricular remodeling is defined as an association of cellular hypertrophy, apoptosis, and extracellular fibrosis. Irreversible ischemic damage and the fibrotic scar that ensues impair the homogeneity of contraction in the ventricle, which results in a change of its geometry to a spherical shape. This anatomic modification increases both end-diastolic ventricular pressure and volume, which results in a right shift of the Starling curve and a decreased output. This raise in ventricular pressure and dimension automatically results in an increased wall stress that further impairs the external work of the ventricle. The only mechanism to counteract this increased wall stress is an adjustment in wall thickness. This cannot be achieved in the peri-infarct territory (adjacent zone), which is subject to stretching and volume overload, resulting in an increased rate of apoptosis and wall thinning. At the remote noninfarcted territory, which is submitted to both volume and pressure overload, a pattern of cellular hypertrophy develops to increase the wall thickness. The neurohormonal trigger of this hypertrophic response consists essentially in a hyperactivation of both the renin–angiotensin and the sympathetic systems, which results from the decreased cardiac output that inevitably accompanies the formation of scar tissue and ventricular remodeling. This process continues until the heart reaches a new equilibrium in wall stress, that is, a new balance between ventricular pressure and wall thickness. However, if untreated, this equilibrium is fragile in the chronic setting by exposing the cardiac cells to higher energetic and contractile demand, which will inevitably lead to more cell death, wall stress, and neurohormonal response, resulting in a spiraling progression into clinical heart failure.

The best way to limit the damage of ventricular remodeling in patients consists of reducing the infarct size and reducing the wall stress that increases following the changes in shape and loading conditions of the ventricular chamber. A reduction in infarct size is best achieved, as described above, by early reperfusion after coronary artery occlusion. The medical approach to decreasing wall stress mainly involves the inhibitors of the angiotensin-converting enzyme (ACE) and β blockers. The mechanisms of ACE inhibition involve a decrease in afterload, a decrease in the extent of scar tissue, an inhibition of apoptosis, and a decrease in the hypertrophic response of the ventricle. β Blockers are a classic category of drugs for patients with ischemic heart disease and previous myocardial infarction, which prevent the sympathetic overdrive resulting from the decreased inotropic performance of the remodeled ventricle. As with ACE inhibitors, β blockers improve both the contractile performance and survival of patients with ischemic heart disease.

REFERENCES

1. Feigl EO. Coronary physiology. *Physiol Rev* 1983;63(1):1–205.
2. Hittinger L, Mirsky I, Shen YT, Patrick TA, Bishop SP, Vatner SF. Hemodynamic mechanisms responsible for reduced subendocardial coronary reserve in dogs with severe left ventricular hypertrophy. *Circulation* 1995;92(4):978–986.
3. Murray PA, Vatner SF. Fractional contributions of the right and left coronary arteries to perfusion of normal and hypertrophied right ventricles of conscious dogs. *Circ Res* 1980;47(2):190–200.
4. Braunwald E. Control of myocardial oxygen consumption: physiologic and clinical considerations. *Am J Cardiol* 1971;27(4):416–432.
5. Saltin B, Astrand PO. Maximal oxygen uptake in athletes. *J Appl Physiol* 1967;23(3):353–358.
6. Vatner SF, Pagani M. Cardiovascular adjustments to exercise: hemodynamics and mechanisms. *Prog Cardiovasc Dis* 1976;19(2):91–108.
7. Rooke GA, Feigl EO. Work as a correlate of canine left ventricular oxygen consumption, and the problem of catecholamine oxygen wasting. *Circ Res* 1982;50(2):273–286.
8. Berne RM. Cardiac nucleotides in hypoxia: possible role in regulation of coronary blood flow. *Am J Physiol* 1963;204:317–322.
9. Berne RM. The role of adenosine in the regulation of coronary blood flow. *Circ Res* 1980;47(6):807–813.
10. Yellon D, Downey J. Preconditioning the Myocardium: From Cellular Physiology to Clinical Cardiology. *Physiol Rev* 2003;83(4):1113–1151.
11. Depre C, Fierain L, Hue L. Activation of nitric oxide synthase by ischaemia in the perfused heart. *Cardiovascular Research* 1997;33(1):82–87.
12. Shaw RF, Mosher P, Ross J Jr, Joseph JI, Lee AS. Physiologic principles of coronary perfusion. *J Thorac Cardiovasc Surg* 1962;44:608–616.
13. Gould KL, Lipscomb K. Effects of coronary stenoses on coronary flow reserve and resistance. *Am J Cardiol* 1974;34(1):48–55.
14. Ignarro LJ, Cirino G, Casini A, Napoli C. Nitric oxide as a signaling molecule in the vascular system: an overview. *J Cardiovasc Pharmacol* 1999;34(6):879–886.
15. Furchgott RF, Zawadzki JV. The obligatory role of endothelial cells in the relaxation of arterial smooth muscle by acetylcholine. *Nature* 1980;288(5789):373–376.
16. Daggett WM, Nugent GC, Carr PW, Powers PC, Harada Y. Influence of vagal stimulation on ventricular contractility, O2 consumption, and coronary flow. *Am J Physiol* 1967;212(1):8–18.
17. Feigl EO. Sympathetic control of coronary circulation. *Circ Res* 1967;20(2):262–271.
18. Murray PA, Vatner SF. alpha-Adrenoceptor attenuation of the coronary vascular response to severe exercise in the conscious dog. *Circ Res* 1979;45(5):654–660.
19. Eckstein RW, Stroud M, III, Eckel R, Dowling CV, Pritchard WH. Effects of control of cardiac work upon coronary flow and O2 consumption after sympathetic nerve stimulation. *Am J Physiol* 1950;163(3):539–544.
20. Mudge GH Jr, Grossman W, Mills RM Jr, Lesch M, Braunwald E. Reflex increase in coronary vascular resistance in patients with ischemic heart disease. *N Engl J Med* 1976;295(24):1333–1337.
21. Vatner SF, Hintze TH, Macho P. Regulation of large coronary arteries by beta-adrenergic mechanisms in the conscious dog. *Circ Res* 1982;51(1):56–66.
22. Ross G, Jorgensen CR. Effects of a cardio-selective beta-adrenergic blocking agent on the heart and coronary circulation. *Cardiovasc Res* 1970;4(2):148–153.
23. Niebauer J, Cooke JP. Cardiovascular effects of exercise: role of endothelial shear stress. *J Am Coll Cardiol* 1996;28(7):1652–1660.
24. Hintze TH, Vatner SF. Reactive dilation of large coronary arteries in conscious dogs. *Circ Res* 1984;54(1):50–57.
25. Olsson RA. Myocardial reactive hyperemia. *Circ Res* 1975;37(3):263–270.
26. Anrep G. On the part played by the suprarenals in the normal vascular reactions of the body. *J Physiol* 1912;45:307–317.
27. Raff WK, Kosche F, Lochner W. [Heart rate and extravascular component of coronary resistance]. *Pflugers Arch* 1971;323(3):241–249.
28. Uren NG, Melin JA, De Bruyne B, Wijns W, Baudhuin T, Camici PG. Relation between myocardial blood flow and the severity of coronary-artery stenosis. *N Engl J Med* 1994;330(25):1782–1788.
29. Harrison DG, Florentine MS, Brooks LA, Cooper SM, Marcus ML. The effect of hypertension and left ventricular hypertrophy on the lower range of coronary autoregulation. *Circulation* 1988;77(5):1108–1115.
30. Murry CE, Jennings RB, Reimer KA. Preconditioning with ischemia: a delay of lethal cell injury in ischemic myocardium. *Circulation* 1986;74:1124–1136.
31. Zhao Z-Q, Corvera JS, Halkos ME, et al. Inhibition of myocardial injury by ischemic postconditioning during reperfusion: comparison with ischemic preconditioning. *Am J Physiol Heart Circ Physiol* 2003;285(2):H579–H588.
32. Maseri A. Abnormal coronary vasomotion in ischemic heart disease. *J Cardiovasc Pharmacol* 1992;20:S30–S31.
33. Maseri A, Davies G, Hackett D, Kaski JC. Coronary artery spasm and vasoconstriction. The case for a distinction. *Circulation* 1990;81(6):1983–1991.
34. Jadhav ST, Ferrell WR, Petrie JR, et al. Microvascular function, metabolic syndrome, and novel risk factor status in women with cardiac syndrome X. *Am J Cardiol* 2006;97(12):1727–1731.
35. Heyndrickx GR, Millard RW, McRitchie RJ, Maroko PR, Vatner SF. Regional myocardial functional and electrophysiological alterations after brief coronary artery occlusion in conscious dogs. *J Clin Invest* 1975;56:978–985.
36. Jeroudi MO, Cheirif J, Habib G, Bolli R. Prolonged wall motion abnormalities after chest pain at rest in patients with unstable angina: a possible manifestation of myocardial stunning. *Am Heart J* 1994;127(5):1241–1250.
37. Bolli R. Myocardial "stunning" 20 years later: a summary of current concepts regarding its pathophysiology, pathogenesis, and clinical significance. *Dialogues Cardiovasc Med* 1996;1(1):5–12.
38. Ambrosio G, Betocchi S, Pace L, et al. Prolonged impairment of regional contractile function after resolution of exercise-induced angina. Evidence of myocardial stunning in patients with coronary artery disease. *Circulation* 1996;94(10):2455–2464.
39. Gao WD, Liu Y, Mellgren R, Marban E. Intrinsic myofilament alterations underlying the decreased contractility of stunned myocardium. A consequence of Ca2+-dependent proteolysis? *Circ Res* 1996;78:455–465.
40. Kim S-J, Kudej RK, Yatani A, et al. A novel mechanism for myocardial stunning involving impaired Ca2+ handling. *Circ Res* 2001;89(9):831–837.
41. Thomas SA, Fallavollita JA, Lee TC, Feng J, Canty JM Jr. Absence of troponin I degradation or altered sarcoplasmic reticulum uptake protein expression after reversible ischemia in swine. *Circ Res* 1999;85(5):446–456.
42. Gross GJ, Farber NE, Hardman HF, Warltier DC. Beneficial actions of superoxide dismutase and catalase in stunned myocardium of dogs. *Am J Physiol* 1986;250(3 Pt 2):H372–H377.
43. Myers ML, Bolli R, Lekich RF, Hartley CJ, Roberts R. Enhancement of recovery of myocardial function by oxygen free-radical scavengers after reversible regional ischemia. *Circulation* 1985;72(4):915–921.
44. Przyklenk K, Kloner RA. Superoxide dismutase plus catalase improve contractile function in the canine model of the "stunned myocardium." *Circ Res* 1986;58(1):148–156.
45. Rahimtoola SH. A perspective on the three large multicenter randomized clinical trials of coronary bypass surgery for chronic stable angina. *Circulation* 1985;72:V123–V135.
46. Diamond GA, Forrester JS, deLuz PL, Wyatt HL, Swan HJ. Post-extrasystolic potentiation of ischemic myocardium by atrial stimulation. *Am Heart J* 1978;95(2):204–209.
47. Vanoverschelde JL, Wijns W, Depre C, et al. Mechanisms of chronic regional postischemic dysfunction in humans. New insights from the study of noninfarcted collateral-dependent myocardium. *Circulation* 1993;87(5):1513–1523.
48. Tamaki N, Yonekura Y, Yamashita K, et al. Positron emission tomography using fluorine-18, deoxyglucose in evaluation of coronary artery bypass grafting. *Am J Cardiol* 1989;64(14):860–865.
49. Borgers M, Ausma J. Structural aspects of the chronic hibernating myocardium in man. *Basic Res Cardiol* 1995;90:44–46.
50. Arai AE, Pantely GA, Anselone CG, Bristow J, Bristow JD. Active downregulation of myocardial energy requirements during prolonged moderate ischemia in swine. *Circ Res* 1991;69(6):1458–1469.
51. Schulz R, Guth BD, Pieper K, Martin C, Heusch G. Recruitment of an inotropic reserve in moderately ischemic myocardium at the expense of metabolic recovery. A model of short-term hibernation. *Circ Res* 1992;70(6):1282–1295.
52. Schulz R, Rose J, Martin C, Brodde OE, Heusch G. Development of short-term myocardial hibernation. Its limitation by the severity of ischemia and inotropic stimulation. *Circulation* 1993;88(2):684–695.
53. Kudej RK, Ghaleh B, Sato N, Shen YT, Bishop SP, Vatner SF. Ineffective perfusion-contraction matching in conscious, chronically instrumented pigs with an extended period of coronary stenosis. *Circ Res* 1998;82(11):1199–1205.
54. Chen C, Chen L, Fallon JT, et al. Functional and structural alterations with 24-hour myocardial hibernation and recovery after reperfusion: a pig model of myocardial hibernation. *Circulation* 1996;94(3):507–516.
55. Fallavollita JA, Perry BJ, Canty JM Jr. 18F-2-deoxyglucose deposition and regional flow in pigs with chronically dysfunctional myocardium. Evidence

for transmural variations in chronic hibernating myocardium. *Circulation* 1997;95(7):1900–1909.

56. Shen YT, Vatner SF. Mechanism of impaired myocardial function during progressive coronary stenosis in conscious pigs: hibernation versus stunning? *Circ Res* 1995;76:479–488.

57. Kim SJ, Peppas A, Hong SK, et al. Persistent stunning induces myocardial hibernation and protection: flow/function and metabolic mechanisms. *Circ Res* 2003;92(11):1233–1239.

58. Depre C, Kim SJ, John AS, et al. Program of cell survival underlying human and experimental hibernating myocardium. *Circ Res* 2004;95(4):433–440.

59. Ikonomidis JS, Tumiati LC, Weisel RD, Mickle DA, Li RK. Preconditioning human ventricular cardiomyocytes with brief periods of simulated ischaemia. *Cardiovasc Res* 1994;28(8):1285–1291.

60. Yellon DM, Alkhulaifi AM, Pugsley WB. Preconditioning the human myocardium. *Lancet* 1993;342(8866):276–277.

61. Kloner RA, Shook T, Antman EM, et al. Prospective temporal analysis of the onset of preinfarction angina versus outcome: an ancillary study in TIMI-9B. *Circulation* 1998;97(11):1042–1045.

62. Tomai F, Crea F, Chiariello L, Gioffre PA. Ischemic preconditioning in humans: models, mediators, and clinical relevance. *Circulation* 1999;100(5):559–563.

63. Juhaszova M, Zorov DB, Kim S-H, et al. Glycogen synthase kinase-3 beta mediates convergence of protection signaling to inhibit the mitochondrial permeability transition pore. *J Clin Invest* 2004;113(11):1535–1549.

64. Bolli R. The late phase of preconditioning. *Circ Res* 2000;87(11):972–983.

65. Gross GJ, Peart JN. KATP channels and myocardial preconditioning: an update. *Am J Physiol Heart Circ Physiol* 2003;285(3):H921–H930.

66. Kudej RK, Shen YT, Peppas AP, et al. Obligatory role of cardiac nerves and alpha$_1$-adrenergic receptors for the second window of ischemic preconditioning in conscious pigs. *Circ Res* 2006;99(11):1270–1276.

67. Laskey WK. Brief repetitive balloon occlusions enhance reperfusion during percutaneous coronary intervention for acute myocardial infarction: a pilot study. *Catheter Cardiovasc Interv* 2005;65(3):361–367.

68. Staat P, Rioufol G, Piot C, et al. Postconditioning the human heart. *Circulation* 2005;112(14):2143–2148.

69. Tennant T, Wiggers CJ. Effect of coronary occlusion on myocardial contraction. *Am J Physiol* 1935;112:351–361.

70. Sommers HM, Jennings RB. Experimental acute myocardial infarction; histologic and histochemical studies of early myocardial infarcts induced by temporary or permanent occlusion of a coronary artery. *Lab Invest* 1964;13:1491–1503.

71. Maroko PR, Libby P, Ginks WR, et al. Coronary artery reperfusion. I. Early effects on local myocardial function and the extent of myocardial necrosis. *J Clin Invest* 1972;51(10):2710–2716.

72. Kloner RA, Ganote CE, Whalen DA Jr, Jennings RB. Effect of a transient period of ischemia on myocardial cells. II. Fine structure during the first few minutes of reflow. *Am J Pathol* 1974;74(3):399–422.

73. Lavallee M, Cox D, Patrick T, Vatner S. Salvage of myocardial function by coronary artery reperfusion 1, 2, and 3 hours after occlusion in conscious dogs. *Circ Res* 1983;53:235–247.

74. Ginks WR, Sybers HD, Maroko PR, Covell JW, Sobel BE, Ross J Jr. Coronary artery reperfusion. II. Reduction of myocardial infarct size at 1 week after the coronary occlusion. *J Clin Invest* 1972;51(10):2717–2723.

75. Buja LM. Myocardial ischemia and reperfusion injury. *Cardiovasc Pathol* 2005;14(4):170–175.

76. Kerr JF, Wyllie AH, Currie AR. Apoptosis: a basic biological phenomenon with wide-ranging implications in tissue kinetics. *Br J Cancer* 1972;26(4):239–257.

77. Yan L, Vatner DE, Kim S-J, et al. Autophagy in chronically ischemic myocardium. *Proc Nat Acad Sci U S A* 2005;102(39):13807–13812.

78. Elsasser A, Vogt AM, Nef H, et al. Human hibernating myocardium is jeopardized by apoptotic and autophagic cell death. *J Am Coll Cardiol* 2004;43(12):2191–2199.

79. Yan L, Sadoshima J, Vatner DE, Vatner SF. Autophagy: a novel protective mechanism in chronic ischemia. *Cell Cycle* 2006;5(11):1175–1177.

80. Hamacher-Brady A, Brady NR, Gottlieb RA. Enhancing macroautophagy protects against ischemia/reperfusion injury in cardiac myocytes. *J Biol Chem* 2006;281(40):29776-29787.

CHAPTER (55)

Nonatherosclerotic Coronary Heart Disease

Bruce F. Waller

Although atherosclerotic disease of the coronary arteries is the most common cause of luminal narrowing and coronary heart disease, there are multiple nonatherosclerotic (congenital and acquired) causes of severe luminal narrowing and subsequent clinical coronary events (angina pectoris, acute myocardial infarction, and sudden death) (Table 55–1).

Various nonatherosclerotic coronary artery diseases can reduce or interrupt coronary blood flow by three mechanisms: (1) fixed luminal obstructions (internal narrowing), (2) encroachment of the lumen by disease of the arterial wall or adjacent tissues (external narrowing), or (3) both.[1] Reduction in coronary arterial blood flow may also result from dynamic changes in the walls of an otherwise normal artery (spasm) or from a disproportion of myocardial oxygen supply and demand. In view of current trends toward rapid coronary artery reperfusion to salvage jeopardized myocardium during

TABLE 55–1

Nonatherosclerotic Causes of Coronary Artery Disease (Coronary Heart Disease)

Congenital anomalies	Buerger disease
Anomalous origin from the aorta	Giant cell arteritis
Right-from-left sinus of Valsalva	Metabolic disorders
Left-from-right sinus of Valsalva	Mucopolysaccharidoses (Hurler, Hunter)
Single coronary artery	Homocystinuria
Atresia of coronary ostium	Fabry disease
High-takeoff coronary ostium	Amyloid
Ostial ridges	Intimal proliferation
Anomalous origin from the pulmonary trunk	Irradiation therapy
Fistula	Cardiac transplantation
Myocardial bridges (tunneled epicardial artery)	Fibromuscular hyperplasia (methysergide therapy)
Embolus	Ostial cannulation
Natural	Transluminal balloon angioplasty
Thrombus	Idiopathic infantile arterial calcification (juvenile internal sclerosis)
Tumor	Cocaine
Calcium	External compression
Vegetation (infective, noninfective)	Aortic aneurysm
Iatrogenic	Tumor metastases
Cardiac surgery	Muscle bridges
Cardiac catheterization	Thrombosis without underlying atherosclerotic plaque
Coronary angioplasty	Polycythemia
Prosthetic valves	Thrombocytosis
Paradoxical	Hypercoagulability
Dissection	Substance abuse
Coronary artery	Cocaine
Aortic	Amphetamines
Spasm	Myocardial oxygen demand–supply disproportion
Trauma	Aortic stenosis
Nonpenetrating	Systemic hypotension
Penetrating	Carbon monoxide poisoning
Surgery	Increased myocardial function (thyrotoxicosis)
Catheterization	Intramural coronary artery disease (small vessel disease)
Arteritis	Hypertrophic cardiomyopathy
Takayasu disease	Amyloid
Polyarteritis nodosa	Cardiac transplantation
Systemic lupus erythematosus	Neuromuscular
Kawasaki syndrome (mucocutaneous lymph node syndrome)	Diabetes mellitus
Syphilis	Normal coronary arteries
Other infections (infective endocarditis, *Salmonella*, parasites)	

SOURCES: Adapted from Waller,[1] Alpert, Braunwald,[2] Cheitlin et al.,[3] and Baim and Harrison.[3a]

evolving acute myocardial infarction, the various nonatherosclerotic etiologies of coronary artery disease must be considered.

FREQUENCY OF NONATHEROSCLEROTIC CORONARY NARROWING PRODUCING FATAL MYOCARDIAL INFARCTION

Approximately 4 to 7 percent of all patients with acute myocardial infarction and nearly four times this percentage for patients younger than age 35 years do not have atherosclerotic coronary artery disease as demonstrated by coronary arteriography, at necropsy, or both.[1–5]

Because coronary angiography simply represents an image of one lumen, the specificity for etiology of the coronary luminal narrowing is extremely low. Review of necropsy studies[1–3] suggests that approximately 95 percent of patients with fatal acute myocardial infarction have at least one major epicardial coronary artery with severe luminal narrowing or total occlusion (Fig. 55–1). The remaining 5 percent of patients apparently have normal major epicardial coronary arteries. Of the 95 percent of patients with severe coronary luminal narrowing, 95 percent have typical atherosclerotic plaque with a superimposed thrombus in 85 percent.

The remaining 5 percent of the patients with severe coronary luminal narrowing have a host of etiologies (see Table 55–1), in-

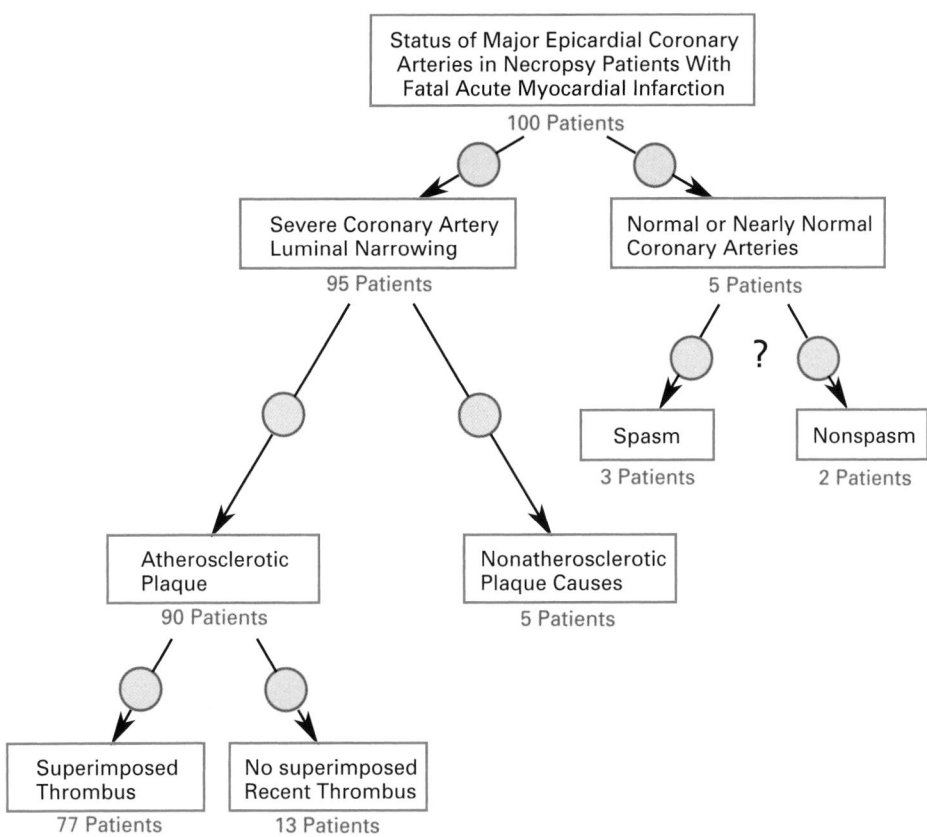

Status of Major Epicardial Coronary
Arteries in Necropsy Patients With
Fatal Acute Myocardial Infarction

100 Patients

Severe Coronary Artery
Luminal Narrowing

95 Patients

Normal or Nearly Normal
Coronary Arteries

5 Patients

?

Spasm

3 Patients

Nonspasm

2 Patients

Atherosclerotic
Plaque

90 Patients

Nonatherosclerotic
Plaque Causes

5 Patients

Superimposed
Thrombus

77 Patients

No superimposed
Recent Thrombus

13 Patients

FIGURE 55–1. Diagram displaying the approximate breakdown of status of major epicardial coronary arteries in necropsy patients with fatal acute myocardial infarction. *Source: From Waller BF. Exercise related sudden death in young (age <30 years) and old (age >30 years) conditioned athletes. In: Wenger NK, ed. Exercise and the Heart, 2d ed. Cardiovascular Clinics. Philadelphia: FA Davis, 1985:9–73. Reproduced with permission from the publisher, editor, and author.*

cluding coronary arteritis, trauma, systemic metabolic disorders, intimal fibrous proliferation, and coronary emboli. In medical centers with large populations of cardiac transplant patients, the incidence of nonatherosclerotic coronary disease will exceed 5 percent because of the frequency of intimal fibrous proliferation in the coronary arteries late after transplantation. Of the 5 percent of patients seen at necropsy after fatal acute myocardial infarction with normal or nearly normal epicardial coronary arteries, 50 to 60 percent likely represent clinical coronary spasm, but the remaining 40 to 50 percent represent a combination of congenital coronary artery anomalies, spontaneous recanalization, and mismatches of coronary supply and myocardial demand.

In the presence of acute myocardial infarction, there is a greater than 90 percent chance that the underlying etiology in the Western world is coronary atherosclerosis. Many other diseases have been associated with myocardial infarction.[4] The epicardial coronary arteries, intramural coronary arteries or both are affected (see Table 55–1).[5]

CONGENITAL CORONARY ARTERY ANOMALIES

Variation in the origin, course, or distribution of the epicardial coronary arteries are found in 1 to 2 percent of the population (Table 55–2; Fig. 55–2).[1,6–12]

Certain types of these anomalies—including ostial lesions, passage of a major artery between the walls of the pulmonary trunk, a major coronary artery originating from the pulmonary trunk, or perhaps myocardial "bridges"—may produce ischemia with subsequent myocardial infarction.

The incidence of coronary anomalies at routine autopsy varies from 0.3 to 0.6 percent.[11] The incidence of major coronary anomalies, causing acute myocardial infarction at autopsy (<35 years of age) was 4 percent (5/120). Angiographically, the incidence of coronary arterial anomalies ranges from 0.6 to 1.55 percent. Virmani et al. reported 232 necropsy patients at the Armed Forces Institute of Pathology with isolated coronary anomalies associated with sudden death (see Table 55–2).[4]

ORIGIN OF BOTH RIGHT AND LEFT CORONARY ARTERIES FROM THE SAME SINUS OF VALSALVA

When either the right or left coronary artery arises from the left or right sinus of Valsalva, respectively, the anomalous vessel transverses the base of the heart in a course anterior to the pulmonary trunk, posterior to the aorta, or between the aorta and pulmonary trunk (Figs. 55–3 and 55–4). At least 43 cases have been reported with necropsy where the origin of the left main coronary artery is from the right sinus with passage between the aorta and pulmonary trunk.[6] In 79 percent of these patients, death was related to the anomaly with sudden death or an acute myocardial infarction. At necropsy, 5 of 26 patients younger than age 20 years had myocardial infarcts.[6] When the right coronary artery originates from the left sinus of Valsalva and passes between the aorta and pulmonary trunk, symptoms of myocardial ischemia, infarction, or sudden death may occur.[6] Of 12 patients with this anomaly, 3 died suddenly and 2 had angina or syncope. At necropsy, transmural ventricular scars (healed infarction) were seen in two patients.

The mechanism of ischemia, infarction, and/or sudden death in this coronary anomaly appears related to the shape of the coronary ostium of the anomalous vessel (see Fig. 55–4). Normally, the coronary ostia are round to oval in shape, but in this anomaly, the coronary artery has an acute angle of takeoff that makes the ostium slit-like in shape. With increased cardiac output, the aorta dilates with stretching of the aortic wall, so that this slit-like ostium may become severely narrowed (Figs. 55–3 to 55–6). It is unlikely that there is "compression" of the anomalous coronary artery by the aorta and pulmonary trunk, in view of the marked differences in diastolic pressures. There

TABLE 55-2

Certain Coronary Arterial Anomalies Associated with Clinical Coronary Events or Coronary Artery Narrowing

Anomalous origin of one or more coronary arteries from the aorta
  Origin of both right (R) and left (L) from same sinus of Valsalva
    R + LM (left main) from right sinus
    R + LM (left main) from left sinus
  Single coronary artery
    Arising from right sinus
    Arising from left sinus
    Arising from posterior sinus
Anomalous origin of one or more coronary arteries from pulmonary trunk (PT)
  Origin of R from PT
  Origin of LM from PT
  Origin of left anterior descending from PT
  Origin of left circumflex from PT
Coronary artery atresia
  Atresia of R
  Atresia of LM
High-takeoff coronary ostia
Ostial narrowing
  Syphilis
  Takayasu disease (pulseless disease)
  Fibromuscular hyperplasia (drug induced)
  Aortic valve surgery
  Fibrous ridges
  Protruding masses
    Calcific nodules
    Supravalvular aortic stenosis
    Aortic dissection
    Adhesion of aortic cusp to sinus wall
    Embolism
    Fibroelastosis
Coronary artery fistula
Myocardial bridges

is likely an anterior shift of the anomalous vessel rather than a vise-like compression.

SINGLE CORONARY ARTERY

Origin of the entire coronary circulation from a single aortic ostium is termed *single coronary*. This anomaly is rare in the absence of other associated anomalies of the heart (see Fig. 55–1). One or more branches of the single artery may cross the base of the heart in a fashion described above and thus may be exposed to the risks of ischemia owing to acute angulation. Angina pectoris and myocardial lactate production have been demonstrated in patients with single coronary arteries where coronary atherosclerosis or an anomalous coronary artery passage was absent.

CORONARY ARTERY ATRESIA

Atresia of one of the two main coronary ostia may be associated with myocardial ischemia and infarction in infancy or childhood. The involved vessel becomes dependent on collateral coronary blood flow from the contralateral coronary artery.

HIGH-TAKEOFF CORONARY OSTIA

Normally, the coronary ostia are located within the sinuses of Valsalva, which optimizes coronary artery blood flow in diastole. Location of the ostia in the tubular portion of the aorta (i.e., "high-takeoff" position) may be associated with decreased coronary perfusion (Figs. 55–7 and 55–8). Morphologic evidence of chronic ischemia has been reported in a patient with a high-takeoff right coronary artery who had right and left ventricular (LV) wall scarring.[10–12] High-takeoff position of the coronary ostium also has been postulated as a cause of sudden coronary death. In a series of 54 major and minor coronary artery anomalies, coronary artery ostia arose above the sinotubular junction in 2, the right coronary artery ostium arose high in 5, and the left coronary artery ostium was in a high-takeoff position in 3.[13] In two cases of high origin of the right coronary artery ostium, ischemia and death were attributed to the ostial lesion in one.

OSTIAL FIBROUS RIDGES

Nonatherosclerotic causes of coronary ostial narrowing include syphilis,[14] Takayasu disease (pulseless disease),[15] fibromuscular hyperplasia associated with methysergide therapy,[16] aortic valve surgery with or without coronary artery cannulation,[17] and ostial valve-like ridges (see Fig. 55–7). A nonatherosclerotic fibrous shelf-like ridge can project from the wall of aorta into the left main ostium.[12] It may have been responsible for chronic ischemia and myocardial necrosis. Baroldi summarized the other rare diseases that may narrow or occlude the coronary ostia as follows[14]: (1) a nonatheromatous, calcific protrusion from the sinotubular junction into the right or left ostium; (2) saccular aneurysm of the aorta; (3) aortic dissection extending into the coronary ostium—the right ostium being involved more commonly than the left; (4) supravalvular aortic stenosis with severe intimal thickening; (5) obliteration of the ostium as a result of adhesion of the free edge of an aortic cusp to the aortic wall above the coronary ostium; (6) occlusion by embolus (see Coronary Artery Emboli section); and (7) occlusive fibroelastosis.

ANOMALOUS ORIGIN OF ONE OR TWO CORONARY ARTERIES FROM THE PULMONARY TRUNK

Anomalous origin of a coronary artery from the pulmonary trunk (Figs. 55–9 and 55–10) may be responsible for myocardial ischemia and infarction in infants and children. In more than 90 percent of cases,[5,6] the left main is the anomalous artery; thus the anteroseptal and anterolateral left ventricular myocardium may be at jeopardy for injury. Asymptomatic older patients with this coro-

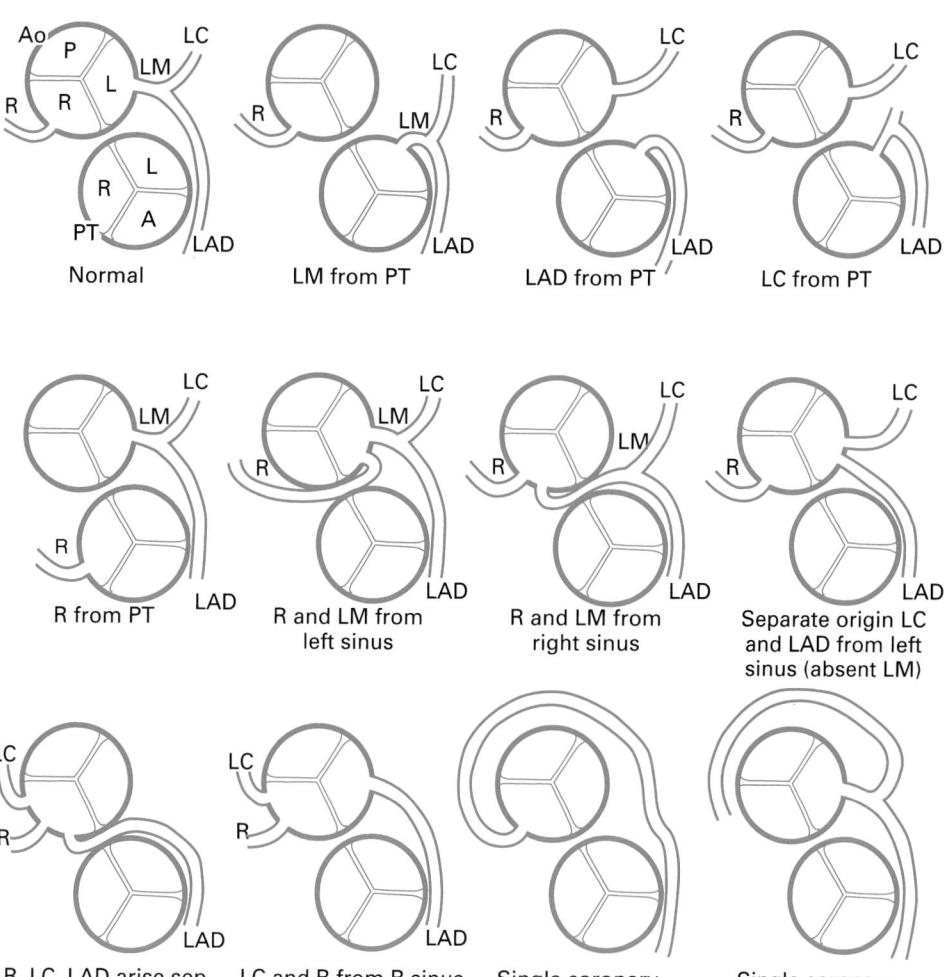

FIGURE 55-2. Diagram showing various congenital coronary artery anomalies that are associated with clinical symptomatic heart disease. A, anterior cusp; Ao, aorta; L, left cusp; LAD, left anterior descending; LC, left circumflex; LM, left main; P, posterior cusp; PT, pulmonary trunk; R, right cusp or right coronary artery.

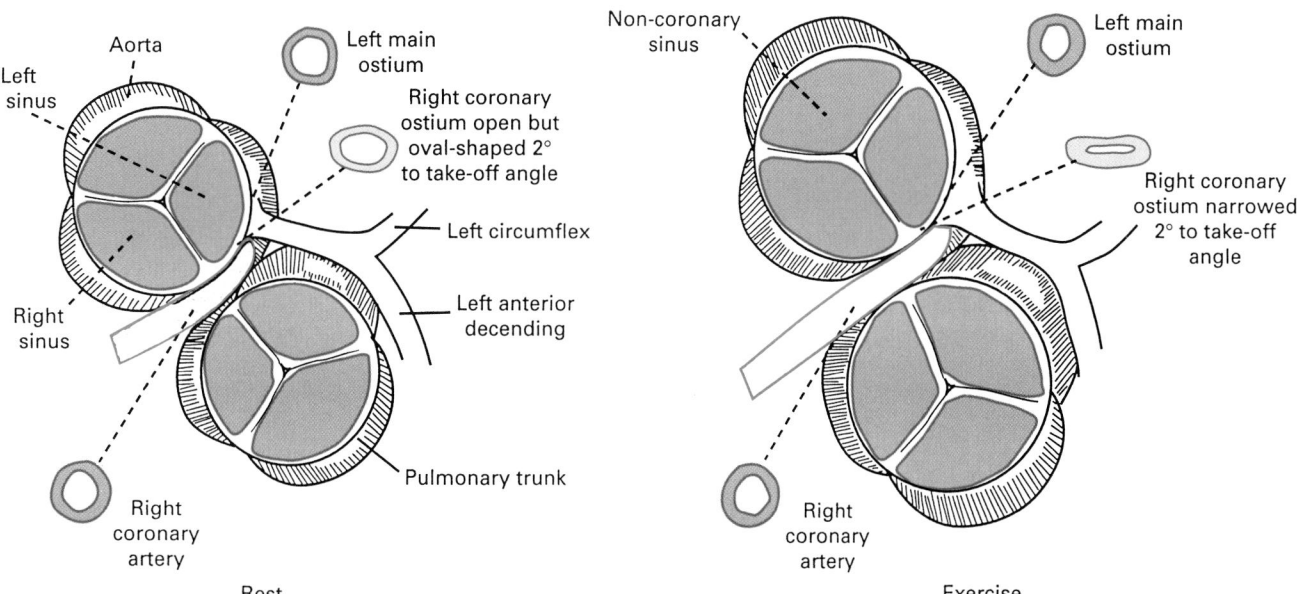

FIGURE 55-3. Diagram showing the proposed mechanism of myocardial ischemia produced by anomalous origin of the right coronary artery from the left sinus of Valsalva. With exercise, the aorta and pulmonary trunk dilate, thereby reducing the already narrowed coronary ostium of the anomalous right coronary. *Source: From Waller BF. Exercise related sudden death in young (age <30 years) and old (age >30 years) conditioned athletes. In: Wenger NK, ed. Exercise and the Heart, 2d ed. Cardiovascular Clinics. Philadelphia: FA Davis, 1985:9–73. Reproduced with permission from the publisher, editor, and author.*

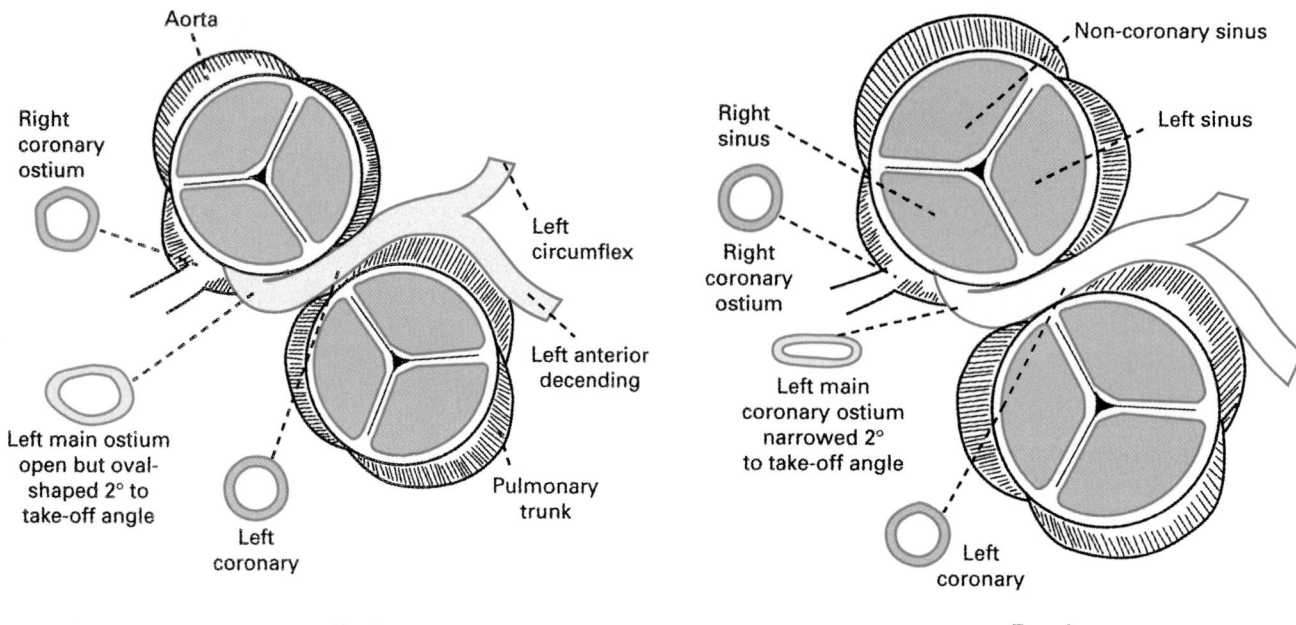

FIGURE 55–4. Diagram showing the proposed mechanism of myocardial ischemia produced by anomalous origin of the left coronary artery from the right sinus of Valsalva. With exercise, the aorta and pulmonary trunk dilate, thereby reducing the already narrowed coronary ostium of the anomalous left coronary. *Source: From Waller BF. Exercise related sudden death in young (age <30 years) and old (age >30 years) conditioned athletes. In: Wenger NK, ed. Exercise and the Heart, 2d ed. Cardiovascular Clinics. Philadelphia: FA Davis, 1985:9–73. Reproduced with permission from the publisher, editor, and author.*

nary anomaly are usually found when they present with an abnormal electrocardiogram (ECG), a systolic murmur, or sudden death.[6] The murmur and abnormal ECG are the result of papillary muscle and/or anteroseptal myocardial wall damage.

MYOCARDIAL BRIDGES ("TUNNELED" EPICARDIAL CORONARY ARTERY)

The coronary arteries may dip into the myocardium for varying lengths and then reappear on the heart's surface (Figs. 55–11 to

55–18). The muscle overlying the intramyocardial segment of the epicardial coronary artery is termed a *myocardial bridge*, and the artery coursing within the myocardium is called a *tunneled artery* (see Figs. 55–11 to 55–13).[15–24] Tunneled coronary arteries have long been recognized anatomically,[15] but suggested associations between myocardial ischemia and myocardial bridges have heightened their clinical relevance.[16]

Also, tunneled coronary arteries are presumed to be congenital in origin. At least three factors are postulated to account for differences between the high frequency of tunneled major coronary arteries observed at necropsy and the lower frequency of tunneled coronary arteries observed angiographically[17,23] or associated with symptoms of myocardial ischemia (18 percent): (1) length of the tunneled coronary segment, (2) degree of systolic compression, and (3) heart rate. Longer tunneled segments of coronary arteries, more severe systolic

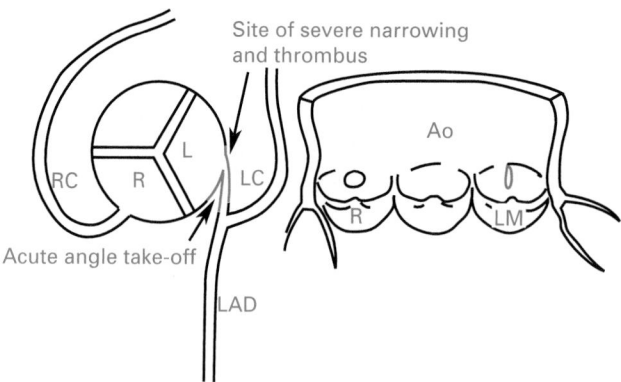

FIGURE 55–5. Diagram showing acute angle takeoff of the left main coronary artery with ostial ridge and slit-like orifice. The proximal left main is occluded by atherosclerotic plaque and thrombus, but the remaining vessels are normal. Accelerated coronary atherosclerosis may result from the acute angle takeoff malformation. Ao, aorta; L, left cusp; LAD, left anterior descending; LC, left circumflex; LM, left main; R, right cusp; RC, right coronary. *Source: From Menke DM, Jordan MD, Sut CH, Aust CH, Waller BF. Isolated and severe left main coronary atherosclerosis and thrombosis: a complication of acute angle takeoff of the left main coronary artery. Am Heart J 1986;112:1319–1320. Reproduced with permission from the publisher and author.*

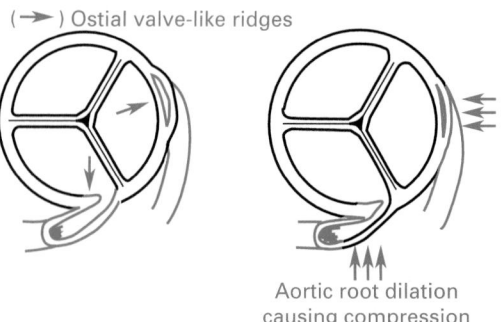

FIGURE 55–6. Diagram illustrating ostial valve-like ridges and the proposed mechanism of ostial compression with aortic root dilation. *Source: From Virmani R, Chun PKC, Goldstein RE, Rabinowitz M, McAllister HA. Acute takeoffs of the coronary arteries along the aortic wall and congenital coronary ostial valve-like ridges: association with sudden death. J Am Coll Cardiol 1984;3:766–771. Reproduced with permission from the publisher and author.*

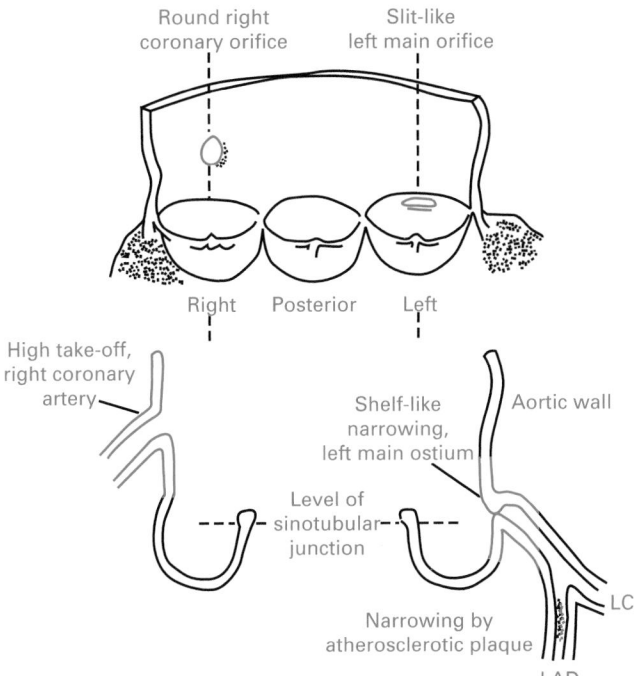

FIGURE 55–7. Diagram showing high takeoff position of the right coronary artery and the nonatherosclerotic fibrous ridge occluding the left main coronary ostium. LAD, left anterior descending; LC, left circumflex. *Source: From Foster L, Waller BF, Pless JE. Hypoplastic coronary arteries and high takeoff position of the right coronary artery. Chest 1985;88:299–301. Reproduced with permission from the publisher and author.*

diameter narrowing of the tunneled segment,[16] and tachycardia may contribute to the production of myocardial ischemia with myocardial bridging (see Figs. 55–17 and 55–18). The length of coronary tunneling may not always be an important factor in causing myocardial ischemia, as three cases with left main intramyocardial tunneling of greater than 40 mm have been described without evidence of myocardial ischemia[16] (Fig. 55–19).

CORONARY ARTERY FISTULA

A coronary artery fistula is an abnormal communication between an epicardial coronary artery and a cardiac chamber, major vessel (vena cava, subpulmonary veins, pulmonary artery), or other vascular structure (mediastinal vessels, coronary sinus) (Fig. 55–20).[5,25–32] This infrequent abnormality can affect any age and is the most important hemodynamically significant coronary artery anomaly.[5,25–32] Many are small and found incidentally during coronary arteriography, whereas others are identified as the cause of a continuous murmur, myocardial ischemia angina, acute myocardial infarction, sudden death coronary steal, congestive heart failure, endocarditis, stroke, arrhythmias, coronary aneurysm formation (rupture, emboli), or superior vena cava syndrome.[25–29] Of more than 33,000 patients undergoing coronary arteriography, coronary artery fistula occurred in 0.1 percent, whether as a result of congenital or ac-

quired causes (Table 55–3). Fistulas from the right coronary artery are more common than from the left coronary artery and more than 90 percent of the fistulas drain into the venous circulation. Most fistulas are single communications, but multiple fistulas have been identified. The natural history of coronary artery fistulas is variable, with long periods of stability in some and sudden onset or gradual progression of symptoms in others. Spontaneous closure is uncommon. Surgical repair of the fistula is recommended for symptomatic patients and for those asymptomatic patients at risk for future complications (coronary steals, aneurysms, large shunts). Transcatheter embolization of fistulas has been reported. Direct connection between a major epicardial coronary artery and a cardiac chamber or major vessel is the most common hemodynamically significant coronary artery anomaly (see Fig. 55–19). Myocardial ischemia has been documented in some patients with coronary artery fistulas who have no evidence of coronary atherosclerosis.[5]

Treatment of symptomatic, clinically recognized myocardial bridges has involved and calcium channel blockers (control of tachycardia and antispasmodic effects) and surgery. Several cases have now been reported[24] in which *supraarterial myotomy* (release of myocardial bridge, excision of myocardial bridge) has resulted in relief of symptoms and improvement in previously abnormal nuclear imaging tests. High-frequency intraoperative echocardiography has been used to image the intramyocardial coronary artery before and after surgical release.[24]

CORONARY ANEURYSMS

Congenital coronary artery aneurysms are found most commonly in the right coronary artery.[32] Abnormal flow patterns within the aneurysm may lead to thrombus formation, with subsequent ves-

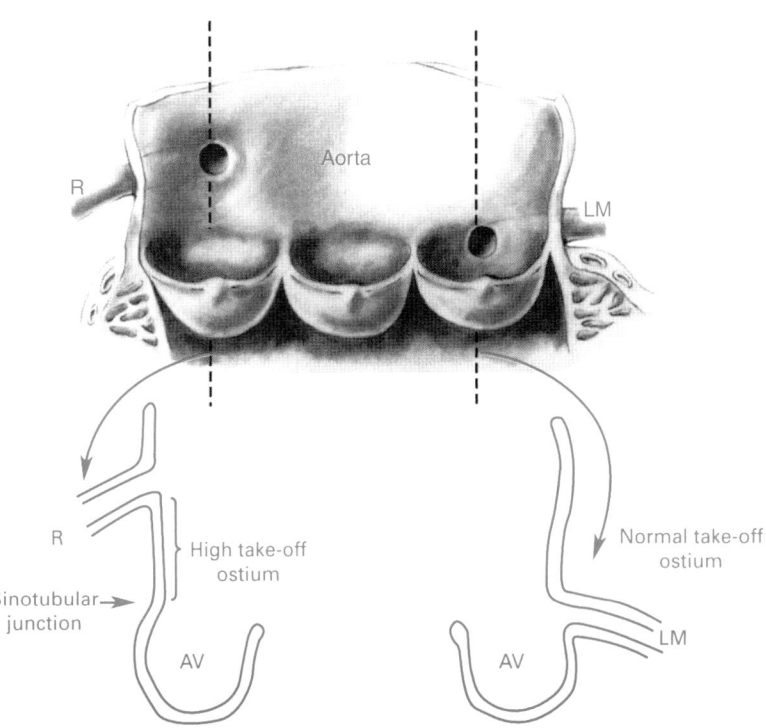

FIGURE 55–8. Diagram showing origin of right coronary ostium above the sinotubular junction—"high-takeoff position." AV, aortic valve; L, left cusp; LM, left main; R, right cusp or right coronary artery.

CORONARY ARTERIES ARISING FROM PULMONARY TRUNK
ASSOCIATED WITH MYOCARDIAL INFARCTION

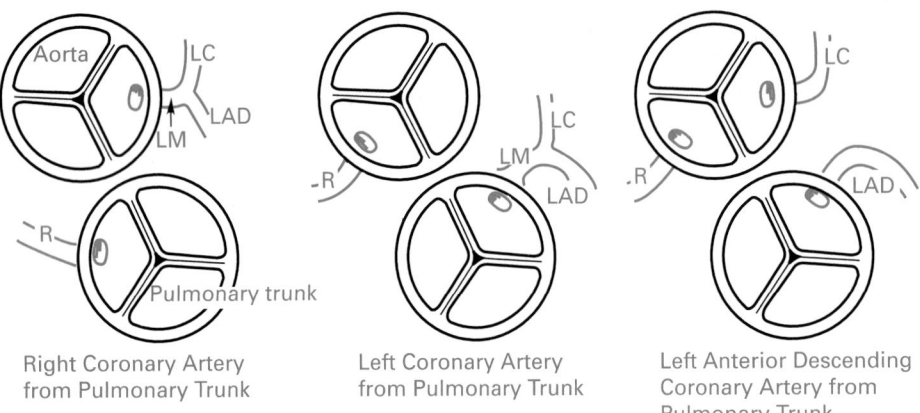

Right Coronary Artery
from Pulmonary Trunk

Left Coronary Artery
from Pulmonary Trunk

Left Anterior Descending
Coronary Artery from
Pulmonary Trunk

FIGURE 55–9. Anomalous origin of one or two major epicardial coronary arteries from the pulmonary trunk. LAD, left anterior descending; LC, left circumflex; LM, left main; R, right cusp. *Source: From Waller BF. Atherosclerotic and nonatherosclerotic coronary artery factors in acute myocardial infarction. In: Pepine CJ, ed. Acute Myocardial Infarction. Philadelphia: FA Davis, 1989:29–104. Reproduced with permission from the publisher, editor, and author.*

sel occlusion, distal thromboembolization, and myocardial infarction.[33] In general, angina pectoris or acute myocardial infarction present in patients who are younger than 20 years of age should prompt suspicion of a congenital coronary artery anomaly or a congenital coronary artery aneurysm.[32] Coronary artery aneurysms are found in approximately 1.5 percent of patients studied at necropsy or by coronary arteriography.

Coronary artery aneurysms, which may be multiple, can be congenital or the result of atherosclerosis, trauma, angioplasty, atherectomy, laser procedures, arteritis (including syphilis), mycotic emboli, mucocutaneous lymph node syndrome (Kawasaki disease), systemic lupus erythematosus, or dissection (spontaneous or secondary) (see Table 55–3). Atherosclerosis-induced aneurysms are thought to result from primary thinning and/or destruction of the media and may represent up to 50 percent of the causes (Table 55–4). Angioplasty, atherectomy, vasculitis, and arteritis may also damage the arterial wall (media) and lead to coronary aneurysms.

CORONARY ARTERY EMBOLI

Coronary arterial emboli (Figs. 55–21 to 55–25) are clinically suspected in patients who develop severe chest pain with acute myocardial infarction in the presence of a prosthetic left-sided valve,

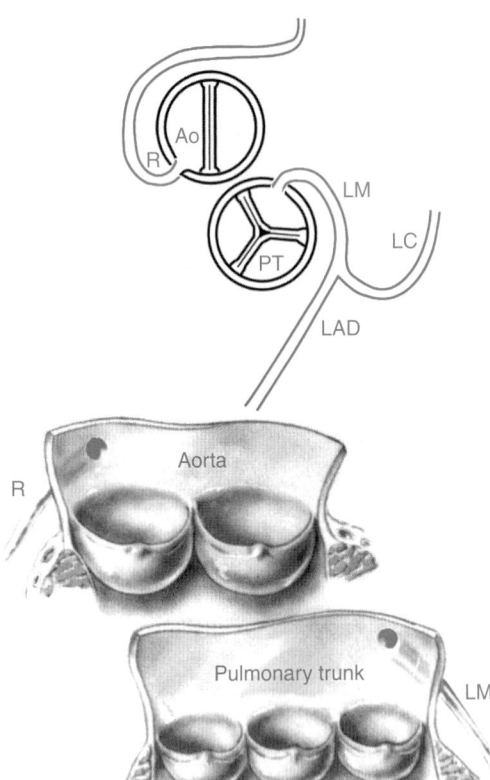

FIGURE 55–10. Anomalous origin of the main (LM) coronary artery from the pulmonary trunk causing acute myocardial infarction in an infant. Of interest is both the anomalous LM and normal right coronary arteries arise in high-takeoff positions from the pulmonary trunk and aorta (Ao) respectively. LAD, left anterior descending; LC, left circumflex; PT, pulmonary trunk; R, right cusp or right coronary artery.

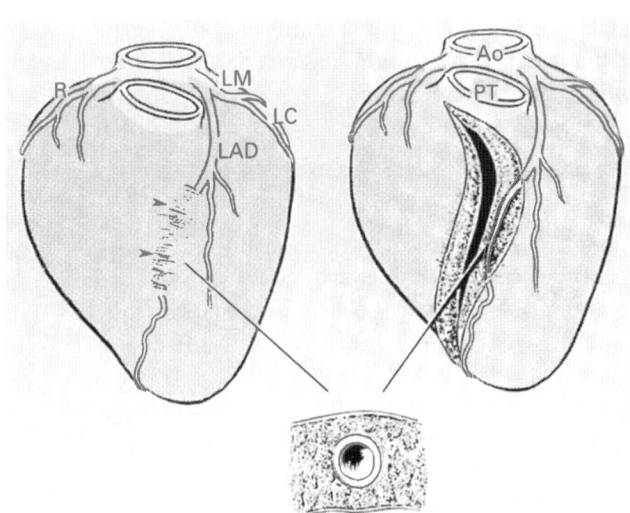

FIGURE 55–11. *Left:* Diagram showing tunneled left anterior descending coronary artery (LAD) (*arrowheads*). *Right:* Opened left ventricle showing intramyocardial segment. *Below:* Transverse section of left ventricular wall showing tunneled coronary artery surrounded by myocardium. Ao, aorta; LC, left circumflex; LM, left main; PT, pulmonary trunk. *Source: From Waller BF. Atherosclerotic and nonatherosclerotic coronary artery factors in acute myocardial infarction. In: Pepine CJ, ed. Acute Myocardial Infarction. Philadelphia: FA Davis, 1989:29–104. Reproduced with permission from the publisher, editor, and author.*

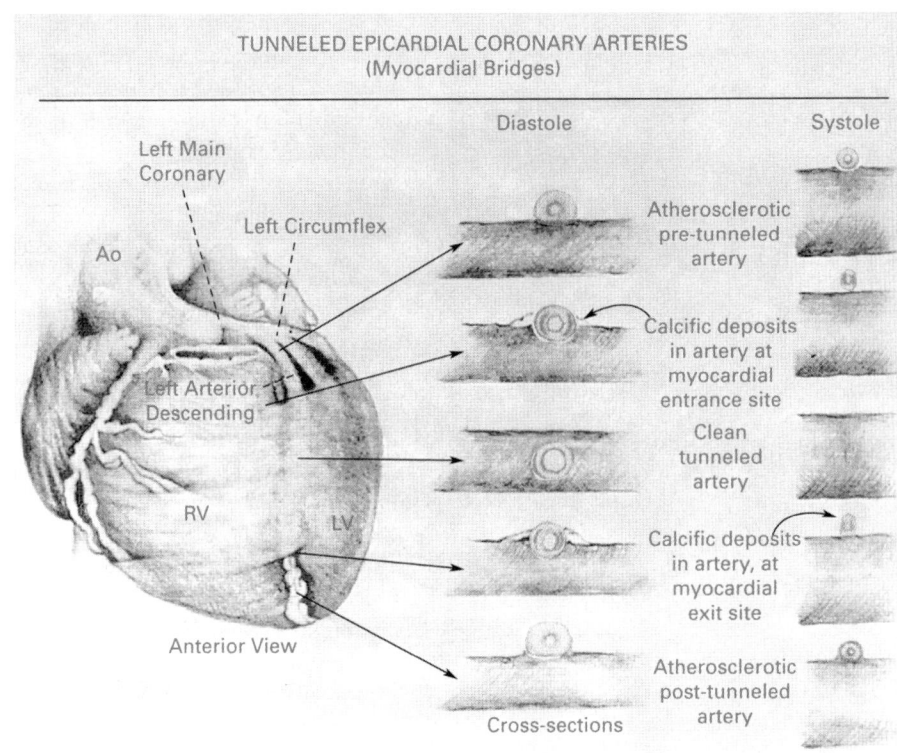

TUNNELED EPICARDIAL CORONARY ARTERIES
(Myocardial Bridges)

FIGURE 55-12. Diagram showing segments of tunneled and nontunneled epicardial coronary artery with changes during ventricular systole and diastole. Ao, aorta; LV, left ventricle; RV, right ventricle. *Source: From Waller BF. Exercise related sudden death in young (age <30 years) and old (age >30 years) conditioned athletes. In: Wenger NK, ed. Exercise and the Heart, 2d ed. Cardiovascular Clinics. Philadelphia: FA Davis, 1985:9–73. Reproduced with permission from the publisher, editor, and author.*

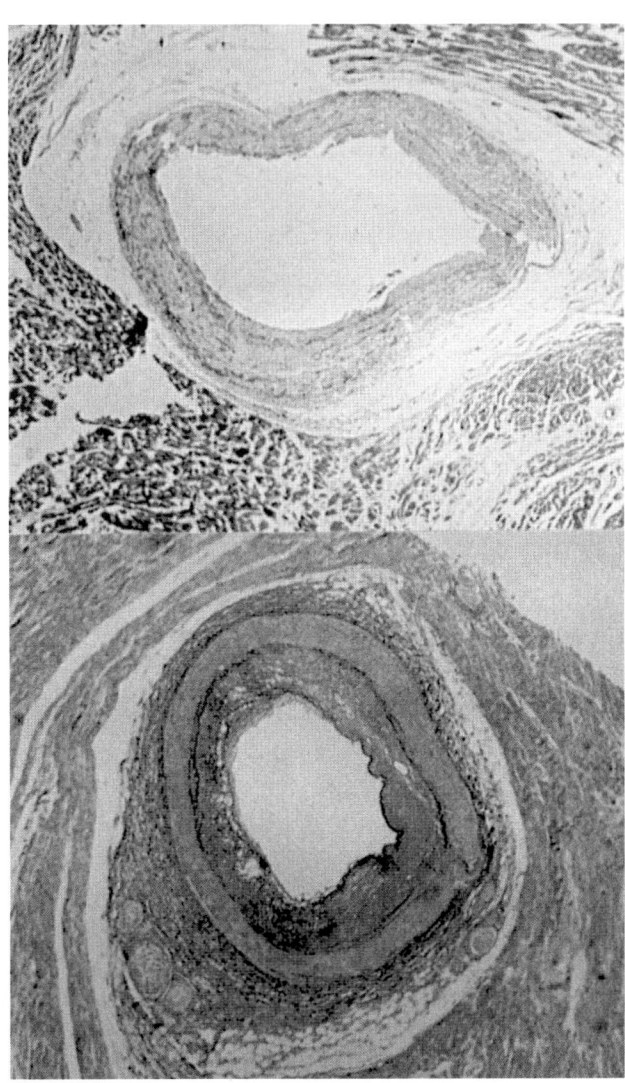

FIGURE 55-13. Tunneled epicardial coronary arteries. Two examples of tunneled left anterior descending coronary arteries. Each artery is surrounded by myocardium. *Source: From Waller BF. Atherosclerotic and nonatherosclerotic coronary artery factors in acute myocardial infarction. In: Pepine CJ, ed. Acute Myocardial Infarction. Philadelphia: FA Davis, 1989:29–104. Reproduced with permission from the publisher, editor, and author.*

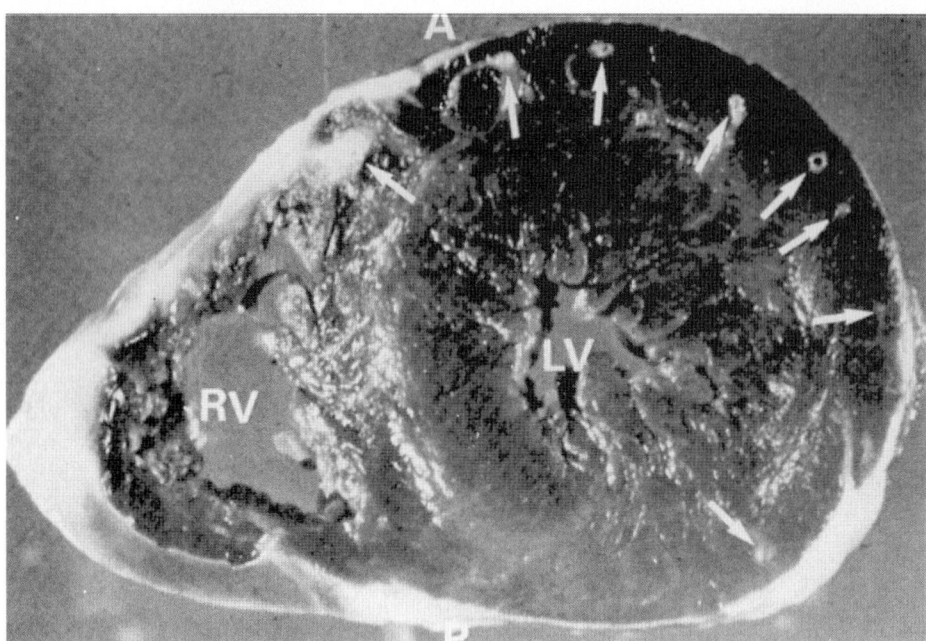

FIGURE 55–14. Transverse section of ventricular myocardium showing the "arcade" of tunneled epicardial coronary arteries (*arrows*). A, anterior; LV, left ventricle; P, posterior; RV, right ventricle. *Source: From Waller BF. Atherosclerotic and nonatherosclerotic coronary artery factors in acute myocardial infarction. In: Pepine CJ, ed. Acute Myocardial Infarction. Philadelphia: FA Davis, 1989:29–104. Reproduced with permission from the publisher, editor, and author.*

Coronary emboli can be caused by natural, iatrogenic, or "paradoxical" causes (see Figs. 55–21 to 55–25). Coronary embolism most often involves the left anterior descending coronary artery. Coronary artery embolism of tumor fragments or thrombus from the surface of tumors is an unusual cause of acute myocardial infarction. Left-sided primary cardiac tumors (myxoma, angiosarcomas, rhabdomyosarcoma, rhabdomyoma, fibrosarcoma, lipoma papillary fibrosarcoma) or metastatic cardiac tumors (primary or metastatic pulmonary tumors, osteogenic sarcoma, renal cell carcinoma) can cause coronary emboli traveling from left atrium or left ventricle to the coronary circulation. Right-sided cardiac primary or metastatic tumors can only produce coronary emboli in the presence of an intracardiac shunt.

Coronary embolism is suspected as the cause of acute myocardial infarction when, at necropsy, the zone of necrosis is large but discrete (insufficient time to develop effective collaterals). Embolic coronary artery lesions can resolve completely and spontaneously and provide an explanation for angiographically normal coronary arteries several months following an acute myocardial infarction.

active infective endocarditis, native left-sided valve stenosis, atrial fibrillation, left ventricular aneurysm, dilated cardiomyopathy (see Fig. 55–22), known cardiac tumor, or during cardiac catheterization or cardiac surgery.

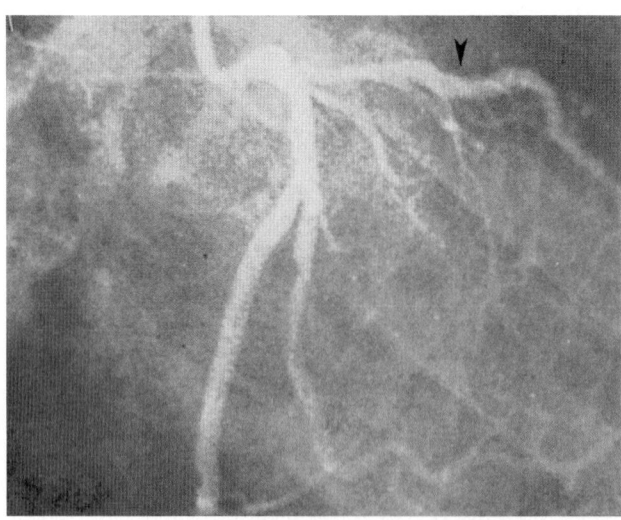
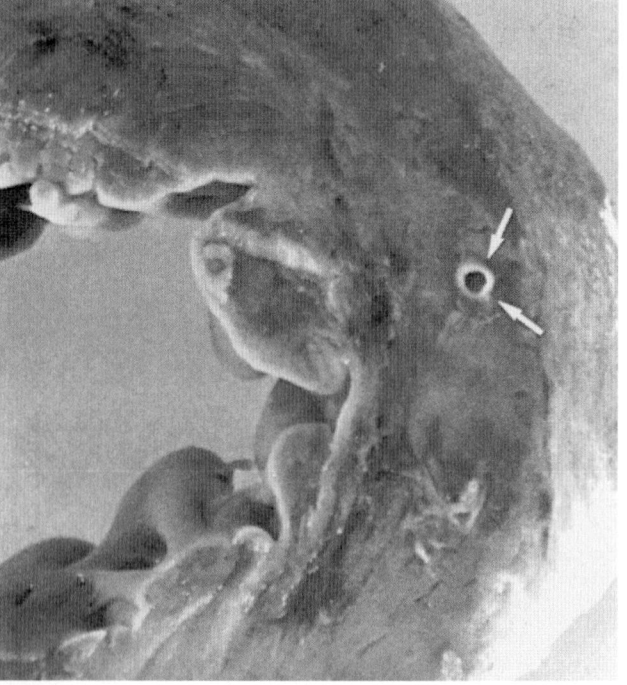

FIGURE 55–15. Tunneled epicardial coronary artery. **A.** Coronary angiogram showing tunneled segment of epicardial coronary artery. **B.** Corresponding segment of tunneled left circumflex coronary artery (*arrow*). *Source: From Waller BF. Atherosclerotic and nonatherosclerotic coronary artery factors in acute myocardial infarction. In: Pepine CJ, ed. Acute Myocardial Infarction. Philadelphia: FA Davis, 1989:29–104. Reproduced with permission from the publisher, editor, and author.*

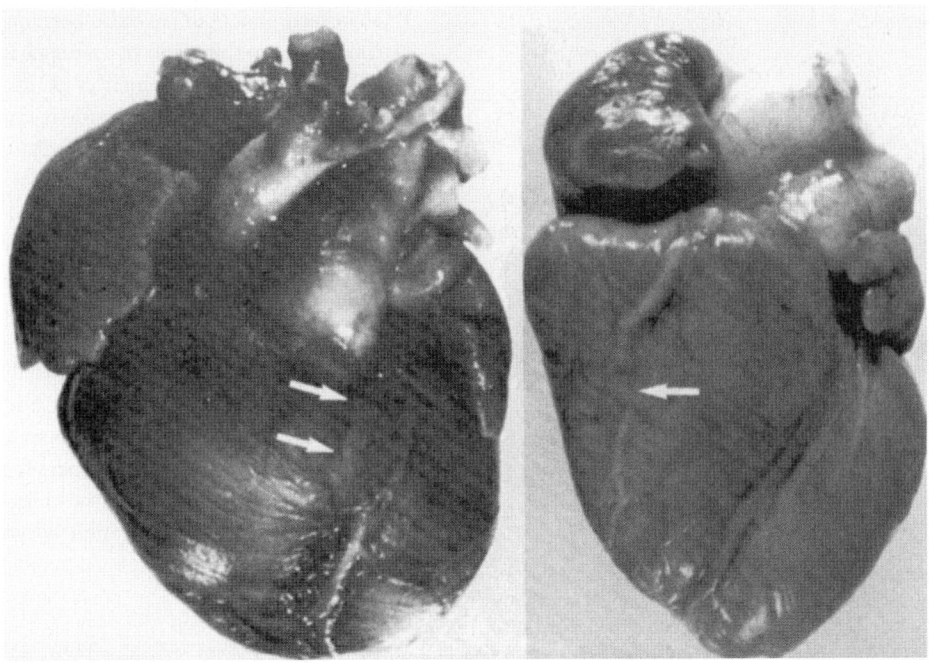

FIGURE 55–16. Tunneled left anterior epicardial coronary arteries from two newborn infants. *Left:* Tunneled left anterior descending. *Right:* Tunneled marginal branch of right coronary artery. *Source: From Waller BF. Atherosclerotic and nonatherosclerotic coronary artery factors in acute myocardial infarction. In: Pepine CJ, ed. Acute Myocardial Infarction. Philadelphia: FA Davis, 1989:29–104. Reproduced with permission from the publisher, editor, and author.*

eased coronary artery is more likely to impact proximally. Emboli to the left main coronary arteries are rare but usually fatal (see Fig. 55–24).

CORONARY ARTERY DISSECTION

Separation of the media by hemorrhage with or without an associated intimal tear is termed *coronary artery dissection.* The medial separation forces the intimal-medial layer (wall of true channel) toward the true coronary lumen and produces distal myocardial ischemia/infarction (Figs. 55–26 and 55–27). Coronary artery dissections may be primary or secondary.[34] Secondary coronary artery dissections are more frequent, especially those associated as an extension from aortic root dissection (8 percent).[5] Primary coronary artery dissections may occur spontaneously or as a consequence of coronary angioplasty or angiography, cardiac surgery, or chest trauma (0.3 percent).[34] Most spontaneous coronary artery dissections occur in women who are most commonly postpartum; they may be associated with coronary artery wall eosinophils.[35–39] The left anterior descending artery is the one most frequently involved. Systemic hypertension does not appear to provide a significant factor of risk.[32]

Spontaneous coronary artery dissection may result in sudden death or acute myocardial infarction and subsequent death. Spontaneous coronary artery dissection that becomes chronic (chronic dissection) may result in congestive heart failure. This

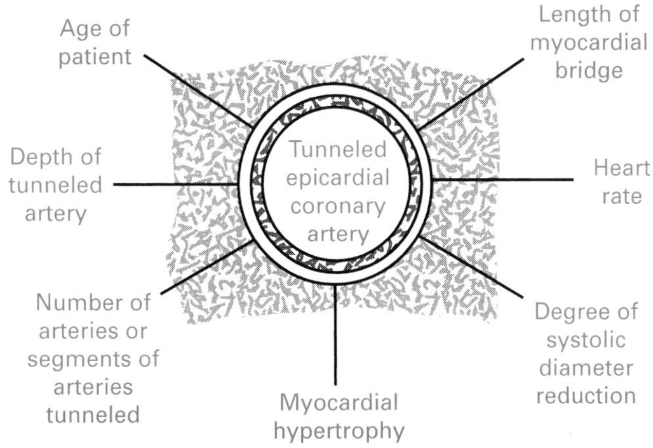

The consequences of coronary embolism depend on two major factors (see Fig. 55–25): the size of the embolus and the size of the lumen of the artery in which it becomes impacted. The smaller the embolus, the greater the chance that it will travel distally to a small coronary arterial segment and the less the likelihood of myocardial infarction or fatal arrhythmia.[32] An embolus so small that it travels distally and impacts in a single intramural vessel is probably clinically silent and observed only at necropsy.[32,33] An embolus to a previously normal coronary artery is likely to migrate distally and result in localized myocardial infarction because of absence of collaterals. An embolus traveling to a previously dis-

FIGURE 55–17. Diagram showing some of the clinical and anatomic factors in a tunneled epicardial coronary artery. *Source: From Waller BF. Atherosclerotic and nonatherosclerotic coronary artery factors in acute myocardial infarction. In: Pepine CJ, ed. Acute Myocardial Infarction. Philadelphia: FA Davis, 1989:29–104. Reproduced with permission from the publisher, editor, and author.*

Age of patient / Length of myocardial bridge / Depth of tunneled artery / Tunneled epicardial coronary artery / Heart rate / Number of arteries or segments of arteries tunneled / Myocardial hypertrophy / Degree of systolic diameter reduction

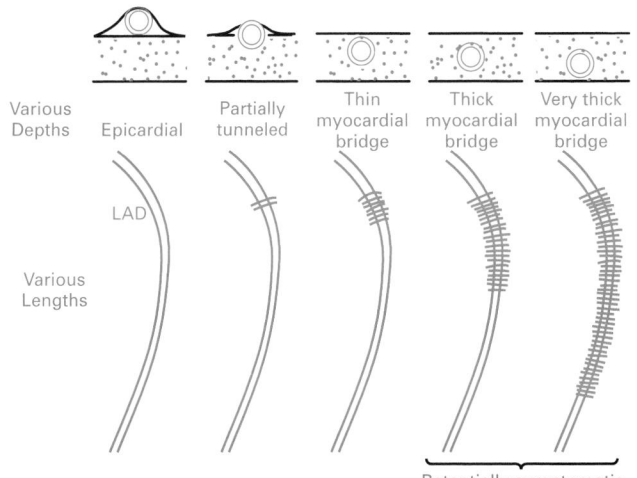

FIGURE 55–18. Diagram showing morphologic variations in tunneling (length of tunneled segment, depth of tunneled segment). LAD, left anterior descending *Source: From Waller BF. Atherosclerotic and nonatherosclerotic coronary artery factors in acute myocardial infarction. In: Pepine CJ, ed. Acute Myocardial Infarction. Philadelphia: FA Davis, 1989:29–104. Reproduced with permission from the publisher, editor, and author.*

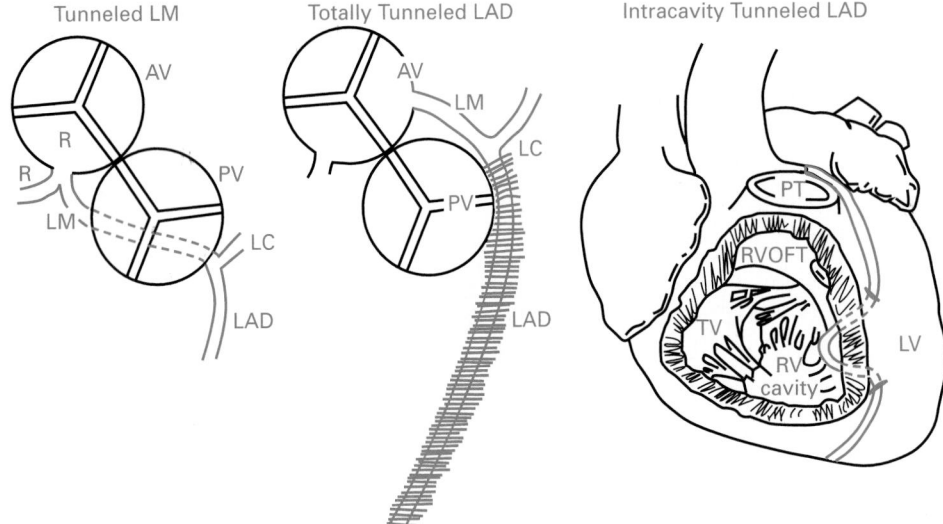

FIGURE 55-19. Diagram showing extremes of tunneled coronary arteries: left main (LM) tunneled through the ventricular septum, total length of the left anterior descending (LAD) located within the myocardium, tunneled segment of LAD becoming intracavitary. AV, aortic valve; LC, left circumflex; LV, left ventricular; PT, pulmonary trunk; PV, pulmonary valve; R, right cusp or right coronary artery; RV, right ventricle; RVOFT, right ventricular outflow tract; TV, tricuspid valve. *Source: From Waller BF. Atherosclerotic and nonatherosclerotic coronary artery factors in acute myocardial infarction. In: Pepine CJ, ed. Acute Myocardial Infarction. Philadelphia: FA Davis, 1989:29–104. Reproduced with permission from the publisher, editor, and author.*

circumstance is found primarily in postpartum women.[39] In a series reported by DeMaio[40] and Nishikawa et al.,[39] 75 percent of cases were diagnosed only at autopsy and 75 percent of these patients were women (half of women were postpartum).[39] In a few patients with multivessel coronary artery dissection, systemic hypertension was the only association identified. Acute spontaneous coronary artery dissection thrombolytic therapy may extend the dissection process or promotion rupture of the false channel because of "engorgement" tearing a thin medial-adventitial wall of the false channel. Recognition of the associated causes and conditions of spontaneous coronary artery dissection (including absence of classic coronary atherosclerotic disease risk factors) should alert clinicians to the possibility of coronary dissection producing acute myocardial infarction and use of urgent coronary arteriography instead of automatic infusion of thrombolytic agents.

Localized and limited coronary artery dissection (i.e., intimal-medial tear) appears necessary for a clinically successful coronary artery balloon angioplasty procedure. Coronary angioplasty dissections viewed in short- or long-axis tomographic images help distinguish dissections that are *therapeutic* (mechanism) from those that are *complications of angioplasty* (complications). In the short-axis image, dissection involving more than 50 percent of the coronary media circumference has been considered a complication. Similarly, in the long-axis image, dissections (antegrade, retrograde, or both) longer

than 1 cm in length have also been defined as a complication of angioplasty (Fig. 55–28). A combination of dissection >50 percent of short-axis circumference and >1-cm antegrade or retrograde of long-axis length may result in "intussusception" of intimal-medial tissue. Spiral dissections ("the ugly") are among the most serious dissection injuries after balloon angioplasty (Fig. 55–29). The spiral dissection as reviewed angiographically appears to alternate from side to side, extending antegrade and retrograde (Fig. 55–29A), or it has an unaltered dissection course but appears alternating from limited angiographic views (Fig. 55–29B).

CORONARY ARTERY SPASM

Coronary artery luminal narrowing produced by spasm has been associated with angina pectoris, acute myocardial infarction, and sudden death[41–52] (see Chap. 56). Despite the extensive clinical information about coronary artery spasm, relatively few necropsy data are available.[41–46] Smooth muscle cells in the coronary artery wall may contract in response to various neurologic and pharmacologic stimuli and temporarily reduce the vessel lumen. Specific pathogenesis of this disorder is unknown.[43] Enhanced α-adrenergic tone[49] and various vasoactive substances—such as histamine, catecholamines, prostaglandins, thromboxane[47–49] are presently thought to be relevant factors. Necropsy findings have been reviewed in 13 previously reported cases and in 3 new cases (Figs. 55–30 and 55–31).[43–52]

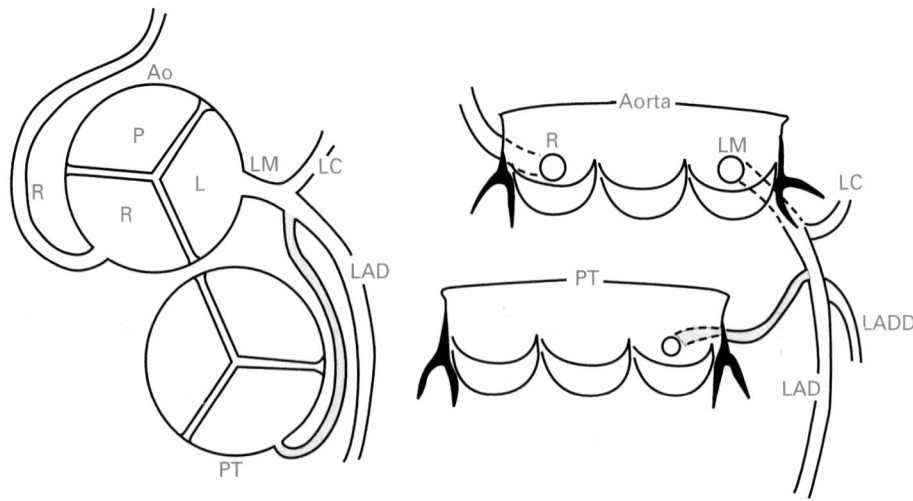

FIGURE 55-20. Diagram showing coronary artery fistula connecting pulmonary trunk and left anterior descending (LAD) artery. It originally was misdiagnosed as an anomalous coronary artery. Ao, aorta; L, left; LC, left circumflex; LADD, diagonal branch of LAD; LM, left main; PT, pulmonary trunk; R, right.

TABLE 55-3

Causes and Associations of Coronary Artery Fistula

Congenital
  Embryonic
  Multiple; systemic hemangioma
Acquired
  Closed-chest ablation of accessory pathway
  Percutaneous coronary balloon angioplasty
  Hypertrophic cardiomyopathy
  Right/left ventricular septal myectomy
  Penetrating and nonpenetrating trauma
  Acute myocardial infarction
  Dilated cardiomyopathy
  Mitral valve surgery
  "Sign" of mural thrombus
  Tumor
  Permanent pacemaker placement
  Cardiac transplant
  Endomyocardial biopsy
  Coronary artery bypass grafting

TABLE 55-4

Causes of Coronary Arterial Aneurysms

Atherosclerosis (destruction of coronary media)
Trauma
Angioplasty
Atherectomy
Laser
Arteritis (including syphilis, lupus erythematosus)
Mycotic emboli
Mucocutaneous lymph node syndrome (Kawasaki disease)
Congenital
Dissection
Neoplasm
Connective tissue disorders (Ehlers-Danlos, Marfan)

Most of the 13 previous patients with clinical evidence of spasm had significant fixed coronary luminal narrowing caused by atherosclerotic plaque, although coronary angiograms during life did not recognize these lesions found at necropsy.[35,52] In one of the original patients described by Prinzmetal et al.,[44] both major epicardial coronary arteries were "markedly sclerotic," and the "posterior coronary artery" was 80 percent narrowed. Of the subsequent 12 necropsy patients, 10 had at least one major artery severely narrowed by atherosclerotic plaque at necropsy.[41-44] The three necropsy patients with clinical spasm[35,43] all had severe luminal coronary narrowing by atherosclerotic plaque at least in the artery in which spasm had been demonstrated during life (see Figs. 55-30 and 55-31). In general, histologic sections of the left anterior descending artery at the site of spasm disclosed luminal concentric plaque that had a predominance of smooth muscle cells, suggesting that the lesion may have been responsive to pharmacologic and neurologic stimuli compared with "garden-variety" fibrotic and calcified atherosclerotic plaque (see Fig. 55-31). In a patient with normal angiograms and documented myocardial infarction, "intimal ridges" were observed on postmortem angiography; these were interpreted as evidence of spasm.[51]

Similar ridges have been noted at necropsy in a patient with coronary artery spasm.[52] Histology of the ridges disclosed typical atherosclerotic plaque,[53] suggesting that varying degrees of dynamic muscular contraction may be superimposed upon fixed atherosclerotic lesions, presumably related to the amount of smooth muscle present. Coronary artery smooth muscle depletion ("medial attenuation"), which accompanies advanced degrees of luminal narrowing by atherosclerotic plaque, suggests diminished potential for coronary wall spasm.[53] It was recently suggested that medial "contraction" bands may represent a morphologic–histologic marker for arteries that have spasm during life (see Chap. 56).[54]

Eccentric atherosclerotic plaques have a segment of disease-free wall with preserved media which presumably has the potential for spasm (see Chap. 56).[55] In patients with clinical coronary spasm, unstable and stable angina pectoris, and episodes of silent myocardial ischemia, where 448 segments were narrowed by more than 75 percent in cross-sectional area by plaques, 15 percent of these segments had a variable arc of disease-free wall with normal media. Other studies have found a similar 15 to 20 percent of the coronary wall normal in 70 percent of cases studied.[56-59] This disease-free coronary segment represents a site of "vasospastic potential" and could convert a hemodynamically insignificant lesion of less than 50 percent cross-sectional area into a hemodynamically significant one of more than 75 percent narrowing.

Three newly recognized associations and/or causes of coronary spasm include general anesthesia, "allergic angina" (histamine-induced),[45] and postpartum bromocriptine usage. Acute ST-segment elevation has been noted following induction of general an-

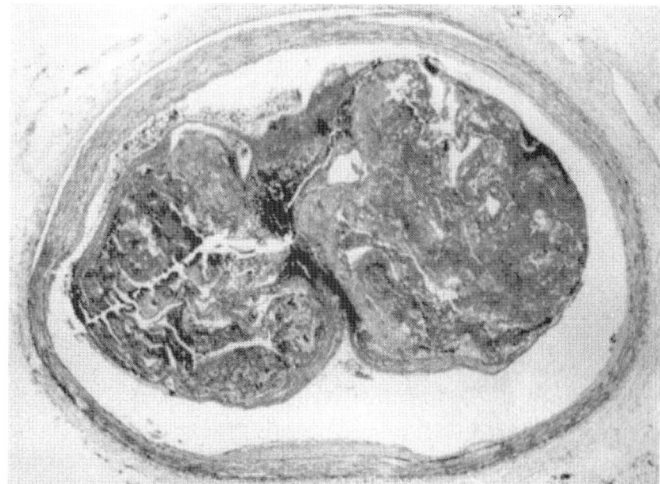

FIGURE 55-21. Coronary artery embolus. Fibrin-platelet thrombus occluding the left anterior descending coronary artery. The source of the embolus was not established, but the patient had recently undergone cardiac surgery. *Source: From Waller BF. Atherosclerotic and nonatherosclerotic coronary artery factors in acute myocardial infarction. In: Pepine CJ, ed. Acute Myocardial Infarction. Philadelphia: FA Davis, 1989:29–104. Reproduced with permission from the publisher, editor, and author.*

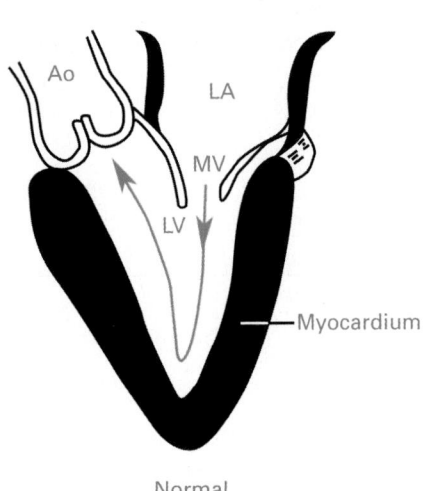

Normal

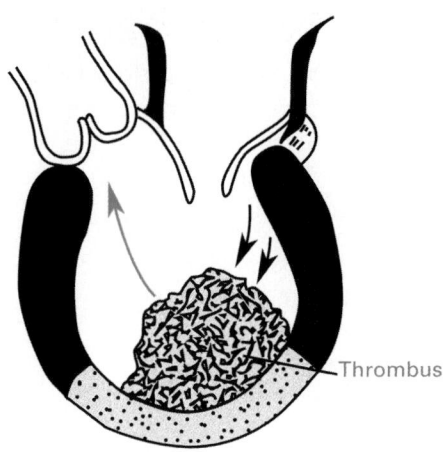

Idiopathic Dilated
Cardiomyopathy

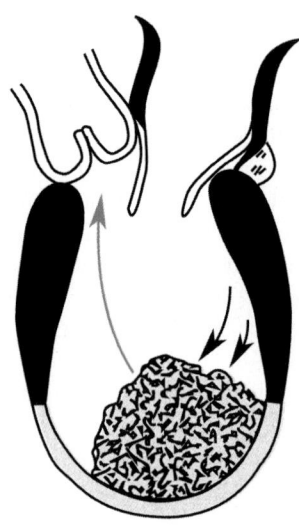

Coronary Dilated
Cardiomyopathy

("Ischemic Cardiomyopathy")

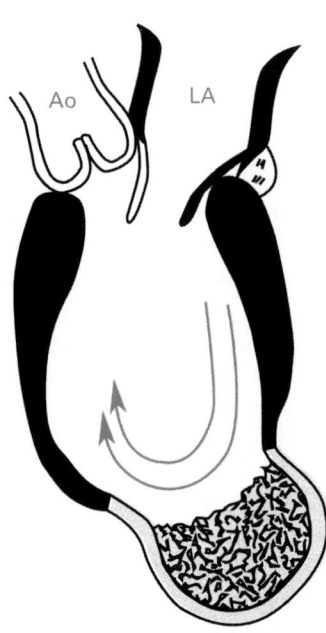

Left Ventricular Aneurysm

FIGURE 55–22. Diagram showing factors associated with emboli from left ventricular (LV) thrombus in three conditions: (1) idiopathic dilated cardiomyopathy (IDC); (2) coronary dilated cardiomyopathy (CDC); and (3) left ventricular aneurysm. Thrombus protruding into the left ventricular (LV) cavity (IDC, CDC) is more likely to embolize than thrombus protected within the sac of a LV aneurysm. Underlying myocardial contraction is more likely to propel thrombus out the LV outflow tract than paradoxical motion of LV aneurysm. Ao, aorta; LA, left atrium; MV, mitral valve. *Source: From Cabin HS, Roberts WC. Left ventricular aneurysm, intraaneurysmal thrombus and systemic embolus in coronary heart disease. Chest 1980;77:586–590. Reproduced with permission from the publisher, editor, and author.*

esthesia in some patients with angiographically normal coronary arteries. In postpartum women receiving bromocriptine in the presence of pregnancy-induced hypertension, acute myocardial infarction has occurred. Coronary spasm also occurs with balloon angioplasty and coronary interventional procedures,[46] catheter-related angiography, and neurofibromatosis.[47]

Endothelial cell dysfunction has been proposed to explain coronary vasospasm.[48] In response to increases in shear stress, platelet products and other agonists, normal endothelial cells release endothelium-derived relaxing factor (nitric oxide), resulting in vaso-

dilation.[48] When endothelium is damaged, as occurs with hypertension, elevated cholesterol, smoking, or use of cocaine, endothelial nitric oxide is reduced or lost. Thus when platelets aggregate at such sites with release of vasospastic substances such as serotonin and thromboxane A_2, arterial smooth muscle cells contract, causing spasm.

Pheochromocytomas result in excess catecholamine production coronary artery vasoconstriction has been reported with the excess catecholamine production resulting in decreased myocardial perfusion, myocardial inflammation, cell deaths, and fibrosis.

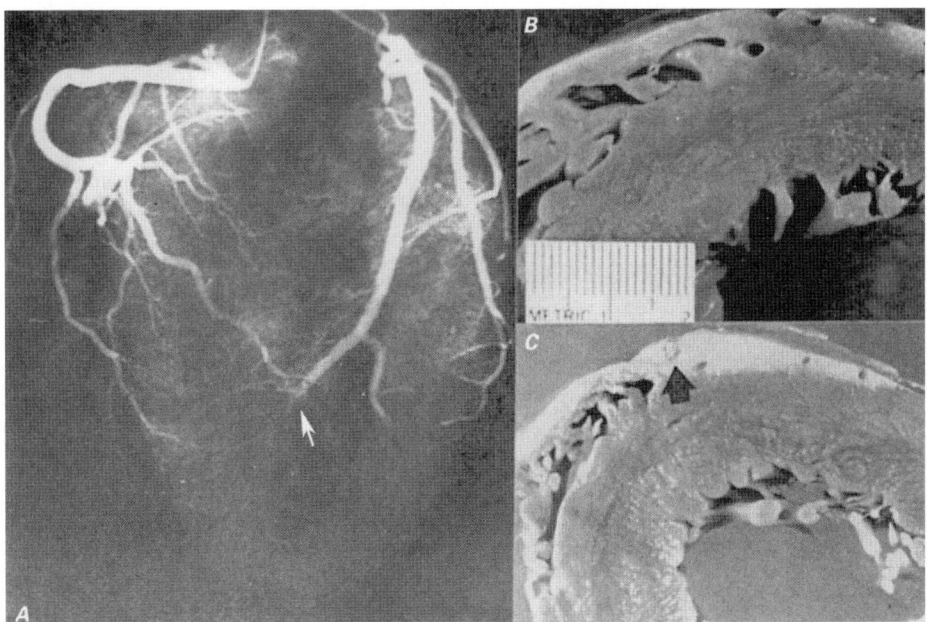

FIGURE 55–23. Coronary artery embolus **A.** Postmortem coronary angiogram showing normal epicardial coronary arteries except for sudden cutoff of the distal third of the left anterior coronary artery (*arrow*). **B.** Portion of anterior left ventricle and proximal left anterior descending coronary artery showing normal artery. **C.** Site (*arrow*) of embolic occlusion of the left anterior descending coronary artery. The remaining distal left anterior descending, right, left circumflex, and left main coronary arteries were normal. *Source: From Waller BF. Atherosclerotic and nonatherosclerotic coronary artery factors in acute myocardial infarction. In: Pepine CJ, ed. Acute Myocardial Infarction. Philadelphia: FA Davis, 1989:29–104. Reproduced with permission from the publisher, editor, and author.*

CORONARY ARTERY TRAUMA

Coronary artery trauma may produce myocardial ischemia and/or acute myocardial infarction. Traumatic injury may result from a nonpenetrating blunt chest wall injury such as a steering-wheel injury, penetration trauma such as a laceration from a stab wound or bullet, coronary bypass surgery as from inadvertent ligation, laceration, or intimal dissection, or after coronary angiography or angioplasty resulting in dissection, rupture, or embolus.

Nonpenetrating trauma may produce coronary injury and subsequent myocardial infarction as a consequence of coronary dissection, contusion and thrombosis, fistula formation, and/or coronary artery aneurysm formation.[5] Extensive coronary artery dissections occur more commonly as the result of catheter or cannula injury in normal or nearly normal arteries as opposed to coronary arteries with severe atherosclerotic plaque.

CORONARY ARTERY ARTERITIS (VASCULITIS)

Epicardial coronary arteritis (vasculitis) is a rare event but has been reported in several conditions (Table 55–5). The resulting coronary injury may lead to myocardial ischemia/infarction with or without associated coronary artery thrombosis. This type of coronary artery damage has been classified by route(s) of entry: *direct extension* from adja-

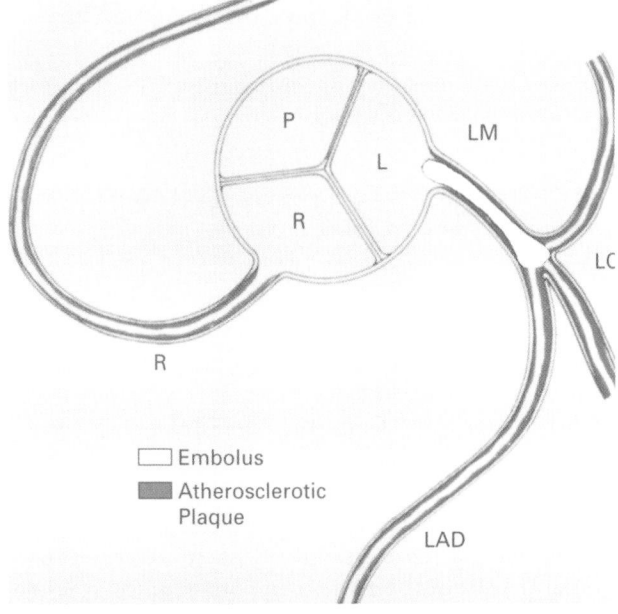

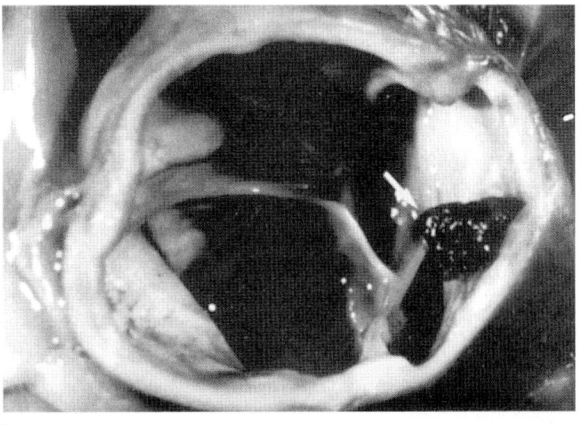

FIGURE 55–24. Coronary artery embolism. **A.** Diagram showing location and extent of occlusion of the left main (LM) coronary artery by an embolus. **B.** Photograph of aortic root showing embolus protruding from the LM coronary ostium (*arrow*). L, left; LAD, left anterior descending; LC, left circumflex; P, pulmonary; R, right. *Source: From Waller BF, Dixon DS, Kem RW, Roberts WC. Embolus to the left main coronary artery. Am J Cardiol 1982;50:658–660. Reproduced with permission from the publisher, editor, and author.*

CORONARY ARTERIAL EMBOLI

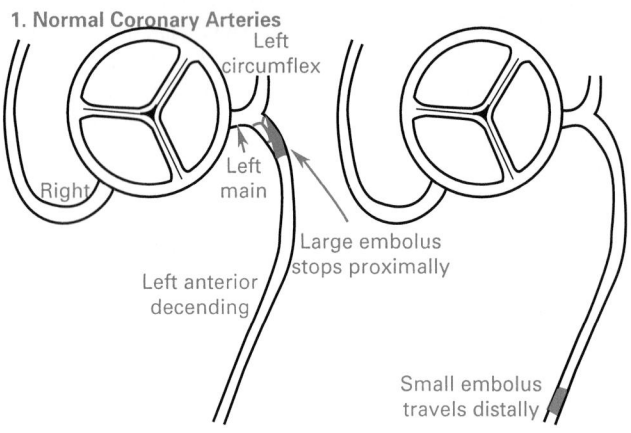

1. Normal Coronary Arteries

Left
circumflex

Right

Left
main

Left anterior
decending

Large embolus
stops proximally

Small embolus
travels distally

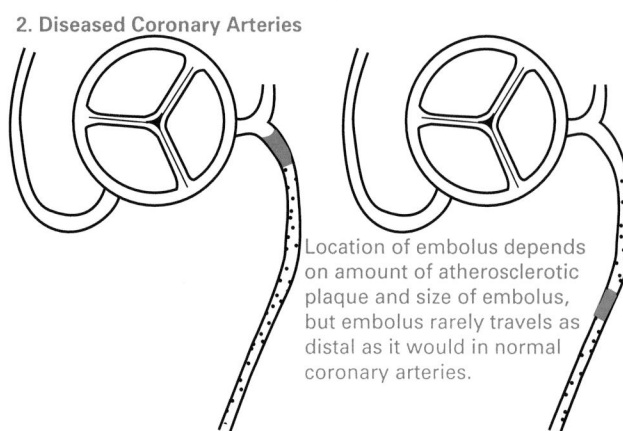

2. Diseased Coronary Arteries

Location of embolus depends
on amount of atherosclerotic
plaque and size of embolus,
but embolus rarely travels as
distal as it would in normal
coronary arteries.

FIGURE 55–25. Coronary emboli in normal and diseased arteries. Source: From Waller BF. Atherosclerotic and nonatherosclerotic coronary artery factors in acute myocardial infarction. In: Pepine CJ, ed. Acute Myocardial Infarction. Philadelphia: FA Davis, 1989:29–104. Reproduced with permission from the publisher, editor, and author.

cent organ or tissue infections, for example, epicardial or myocardial abscess from aortic valve endocarditis, pericardial infections such as tuberculosis; *hematogenous spread* through the coronary lumen or vasa vasorum; and *unknown* route of entry. In the direct extension route of entry, the adventitial layer of the artery is initially involved, whereas in the hematogenous route, the coronary intimal layer is initially involved.

Evidence of coronary arteritis has included the following: (1) focal artery necrosis with or without calcification; (2) acute coronary artery thrombosis or recanalized thrombus associated with underlying atherosclerotic plaque; (3) rupture of the vessel wall unassociated with trauma or an interventional procedure; (4) coronary artery wall thickening with secondary luminal narrowing; and (5) wall thickening with aneurysm formation.[58] Specific coronary lesions may also be seen with systemic diseases such as tuberculosis or polyarteritis periarteritis.

A more recent classification of coronary vasculitides has been based upon known and unknown causes and involvement of size of vessel (medium-size, small-size; Table 55–6).[59] With the exception of infectious angiitis resulting from syphilitic, mycobacterial or rickettsial infection, the causes and pathogenesis of most coronary vasculitides are either unknown or incompletely understood.

Vasculitic syndromes may be caused by deposition of immune complex in the vessel walls.[59–64] The specific antigen has been identified in only a few cases, such as hepatitis B. Circulating immune complexes associated with hepatitis B infection may cause more than one type of vasculitic syndrome,[59] producing periarteritis nodosa in arteries of muscles and hypersensitivity angiitis in venules while eliciting the production of antiimmunoglobulin antibodies, leading to cryoglobulinemia. Thus, a classification of vasculitides *based solely* on immunologic studies is incomplete.[59]

GENERAL CONCEPTS

The earliest vasculitic syndrome was named *periarteritis nodosa*[64] because of the nodules along the course of small arteries.[59] Because the inflammatory changes are not only periarterial, *polyarteritis* may be a better term. Periarteritis nodosa has become a "wastebasket designation" of any vasculitis whose cause is unknown.[59] The term *necrotizing angiitis*[65] is used to designate arterial and venous lesions; there are five types of necrotizing angiitis[65]: (1) hypersensitivity angiitis, (2) allergic granulomatous angiitis, (3) rheumatoid arteritis, (4) periarteritis nodosa, and (5) temporal arteritis. The term *hypersensitivity angiitis* has been considered synonymous with small-vessel vasculitis and is used to imply that the angiitis is caused by an allergic response to proteins, drugs, vaccines, or infections.[59] Allergic *granulomatous angiitis* (Churg-Strauss syndrome) is a variant of polyarteritis characterized by necrotizing vasculitis with extravascular granulomas and eosinophilia associated with asthma or allergic rhinitis.[59,66–68] *Rheumatic arteritis* describes vascular lesions in rheumatic diseases with both rheumatic and necrotizing vascular lesions. *Temporal arteritis* (giant cell arteritis) involves large and small extracranial arteries, including the coronary arteries, and blindness may be a serious complication.[59,69–72] Despite its limitations, this classification[65] remains a basis for the diagnosis of vasculitides. The classification of coronary vasculitis is closely tied to that of vasculitides in general[65] and relates to the predominant type and size of vessels affected (see Table 55–6).[73]

INFECTIOUS ANGIITIS

Various microorganisms may cause vasculitis in vessels of any size and involve the vessel by extension of the acute or chronic infective process from an adjacent tissue or organ or from the lumen by hematogenous spread. The inflammatory response produces variable reactions including suppurative inflammation bacteria, proliferative response (typhoid[74]), hemorrhagic (anthrax), and histiocytic and granulomatous response (leprosy, syphilis, tuberculosis).[4,59] The most important angiitic infections affecting the coronary arteries are syphilis, tuberculosis, and syphilitic arteritis. All three stages of syphilis show arteritic features. The most important vascular lesion of tertiary syphilis, coronary ostial stenosis, seen in up to 4 percent of patients with tertiary syphilis,[5,75–77] can occur independent of aortic involvement.[59]

Syphilitic arteritis is characterized by a chronic inflammation with adventitial fibrosis and patchy destruction of media with a

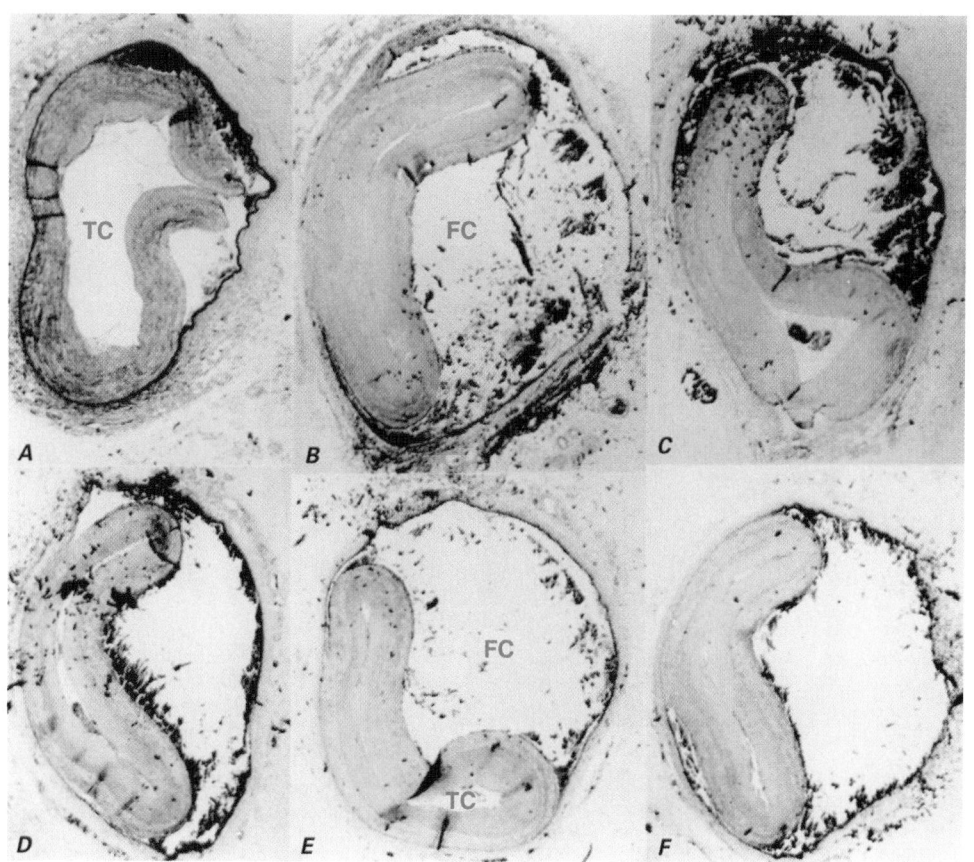

FIGURE 55–26. Coronary artery dissection. Serial cross-section (**A** to **F**) showing dissection of the left anterior descending coronary artery. The true channel (TC) is severely compromised by external compression from the false channel (FC) ("dissection channel"). *Source: From Waller BF. Atherosclerotic and nonatherosclerotic coronary artery factors in acute myocardial infarction. In: Pepine CJ, ed. Acute Myocardial Infarction. Philadelphia: FA Davis, 1989:29–104. Reproduced with permission from the publisher, editor, and author.*

these infections consist of a lymphomononuclear infiltrate with or without thrombosis. A direct toxic effect from rickettsiae may produce angiitis.[83] Viruses also have been implicated in vasculitis by direct invasion of immunologic mechanisms.[59] Virus-induced vasculitides in humans are represented by polyarteritis associated with hepatitis B antigenemia[59] and herpes zoster.[59]

NONINFECTIOUS ANGIITIS

Various noninfectious causes of angiitis involve large- to medium-size (predominately medium- and small-size) blood vessels (see Table 55–6).[59]

TAKAYASU ARTERITIS

Takayasu disease (pulseless disease) is one of the coronary vasculitides associated with aortitis; others are temporal arteritides and rheumatic disease. Takayasu disease is a chronic, occlusive inflammatory disease of unknown etiology[59,84–87] with a worldwide distribution and greater incidence in young to middle-aged female Asians.[86,87] Involvement of the coronary arteries occurs in 15 to 25 percent of cases and may be the lethal complication (Fig. 55–33),[85–87] commonly involving the coronary ostium[85] with segmental involvement of distal coronary arteries.[88–91] Rarely, diffuse coronary arteritis is produced by Takayasu disease.[92]

Takayasu arteritis[93,94] should be considered in a patient without classic atherosclerotic risk factors who is younger than age 40 years and who presents with acute myocardial infarction. The average age at onset of symptoms is about 24 years and another coronary event occurs in 40 percent in the next 10 years.[93,94]

GRANULOMATOUS GIANT CELL ARTERITIS (TEMPORAL ARTERITIS)

Granulomatous giant cell arteritis may occur independently or, more commonly, may be associated with temporal arteritis in 10 to 15 percent of patients.[59,95–97] Histologically proven giant cell coronary arteritis is rare, and cases leading to fatal myocardial infarction are even rarer (Fig. 55–34).[59,95–97]

The arterial wall lesion is a granulomatous inflammation with giant cells found along degenerative internal elastic membrane.[98] The intima becomes greatly thickened and, ultimately, the vessel is converted into a fibrous cord. Luminal thrombosis may also be present in the 16 cases of temporal arteritis reported by Harrison[99]: only 1 case involved the epicardial coronary arteries. Giant cell arteritis of the intramural (intramyocardial) coronary

lymphoplasmacytic infiltrate. Gummas can be found in 20 percent of cases,[78] but spirochetes are rarely detected.[59] The first 3 to 4 mm of the left and right coronary arteries may be involved with an obliterative arteritis; angina and acute myocardial infarction may result from syphilitic involvement.

TUBERCULOUS ARTERITIS

Tuberculous coronary arteritis occurs mainly in patients with pericardial and myocardial tuberculosis.[79,80] Granuloma may involve the adventitia, intima, or the entire wall and result from several infectious angiitic agents. Endocarditis and septicemia are the most common underlying causes of infectious angiitis and mycotic aneurysm formation.[59] Any type of gram-positive or gram-negative organism may be involved. Myocarditis with abscesses and pericarditis frequently accompany infectious coronary angiitis. Mucormycosis, aspergillosis, and *Candida* (Fig. 55–32) are examples of fungi and systemic yeast infections associated with coronary angiitis. Malarial parasites and parasitized red blood cells also may plug larger coronary arteries.[81] *Schistosoma haematobium* has been found in a major epicardial coronary artery associated with myocardial infarction.[82] Rickettsial infections may produce angiitis in small vessels of the heart[59];

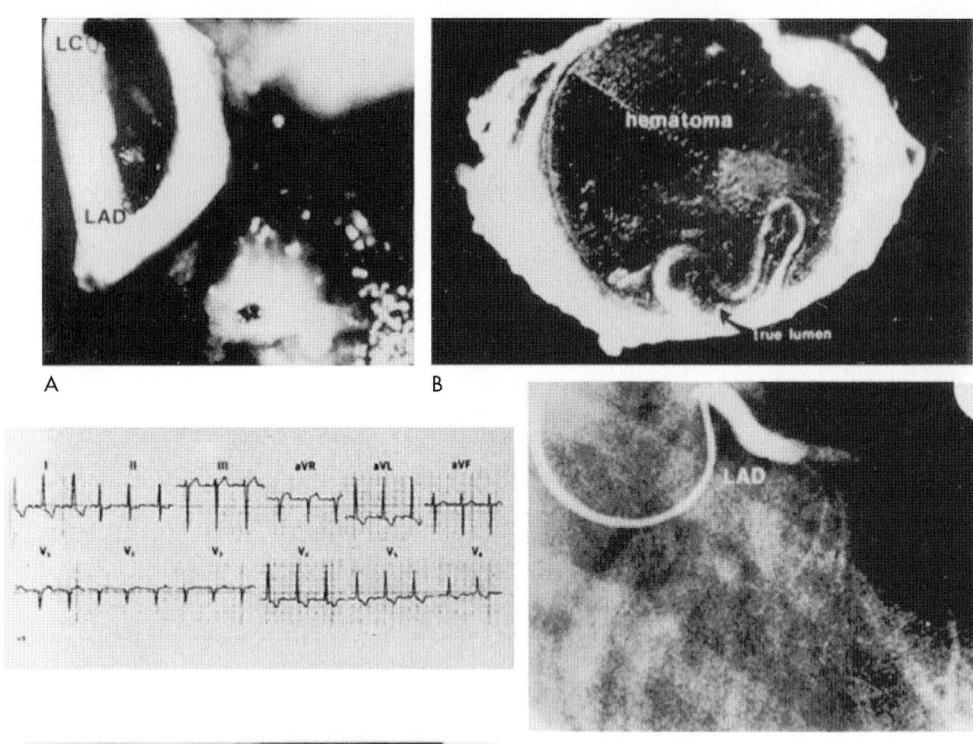

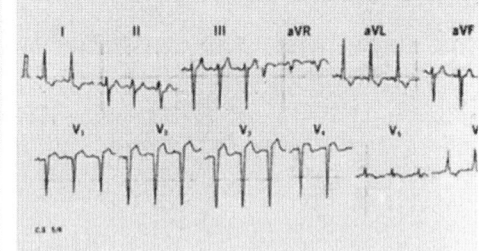

FIGURE 55-27. Coronary artery dissection. Occlusion of the left anterior descending (LAD) artery due to dissection. **A.** The LAD and left circumflex (LC) are seen through the left main artery. **B.** Cross section shows hematoma in false channel severely narrows native (true channel) unobstructed lumen. **C.** Sequential electrocardiographic and angiographic findings. *Source: From Isner JM, Donaldson RF. Coronary angiographic and morphologic correlation. In: Waller BF, ed. Cardiac Morphology. Cardiology Clinics. Philadelphia: WB Saunders, 1984:571–592. Reproduced with permission from the publisher, editor, and author.*

FIGURE 55-28. Diagram showing morphologic definition of coronary artery dissections in balloon angioplasty (long-axis plane): localized (mechanism) (1 cm in total dissection length) and extensive (complications) (>1 cm in total length). *Source: From Waller BF, Orr CM, Pinkerton CA, Van Tassel J, Peters T, Slack JD. Coronary balloon angioplasty dissections: The good, the bad, and the ugly. J Am Coll Cardiol 1992;20:701–706. Reproduced with permission from the author, editor, and publisher.*

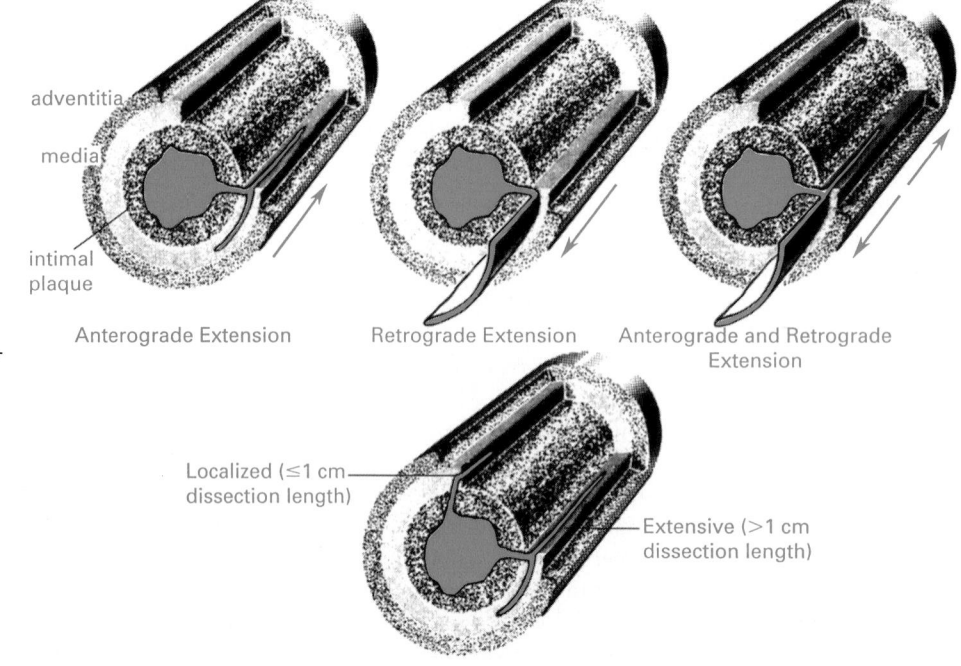

arteries may also occur in association with temporal arteritis and giant cell arteritis.

ARTERITIS OF RHEUMATIC DISEASE

Rheumatic diseases commonly affect the aorta and are morphologically indistinguishable from granulomatous aortitis.[59,100–102] Coronary arteritis at necropsy has been detected in up to 20 percent of patients with rheumatoid arthritis, usually involving small intramural vessels.[100–103] The small-vessel arteritis may also involve conduction system vessels leading to various forms of heart block (see Chap. 88). Rheumatoid coronary vasculitis producing myocardial infarction is rare.[104,105] Histologically, extraaortic rheumatoid vasculitis (coronary artery vasculitis) is usually a polyarteritis type of necrotizing angiitis[59,106,107] and not a giant cell arteritis (Fig. 55–35). Small myocardial vessels may also be severely narrowed in ankylosing spondylosis. Occlusion of the left main ostium has been described.[108]

THROMBOANGIITIS OBLITERANS (BUERGER DISEASE)

Thromboangiitis obliterans (Buerger disease), which is very rare (Fig. 55–36),[59,109] is a nonatherosclerotic, occlusive, inflammatory vascular disease of unknown cause occurring mainly in young males who are heavy smokers of cigarettes.[59] In a few patients, the coronary arteries have shown focal polymorphonuclear infiltrates, histiocytes, and giant cells with or without coronary artery thrombosis.[110] Coronary involvement is rare,[110] although coronary thrombosis may be seen. Buerger disease involving a saphenous vein bypass graft has also been documented.[111]

POLYARTERITIS GROUP OF NECROTIZING ANGIITIS

CLASSIC POLYARTERITIS NODOSA

Classic polyarteritis nodosa is a chronic systemic disease manifest by infarction or hemorrhage in various target organs as the result of necrotizing vasculitis. Male patients are affected twice as often as female, with a mean age of 45 years.[59,112,113] It is probably the most common cause of coronary angiitis with both epicardial and intramural coronary arteries being affected (Fig. 55–37).[112,113] In a review of 66 necropsy cases, 41 (62 percent) had involvement of the epicardial coronary arteries, including 25 cases (61 percent) with involvement of both the epicardial and intramural coronary arteries, while 16 cases (39 percent) had only involvement of the intramural arteries. Frequently, various stages of acute disease and healing are seen in the same arterial segment. The acute phase has an acute cellular reaction with destruction of the media and internal elastic membrane.[114,115] The healing stage results in fibrous internal proliferation. Coronary arteries may dilate to form small berry-like aneurysms (becoming occluded by thrombus), rupture, or produce fatal myocardial infarction,[116–118] pericardial tamponade, or sudden death.

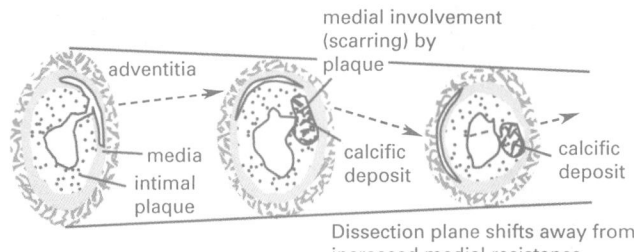

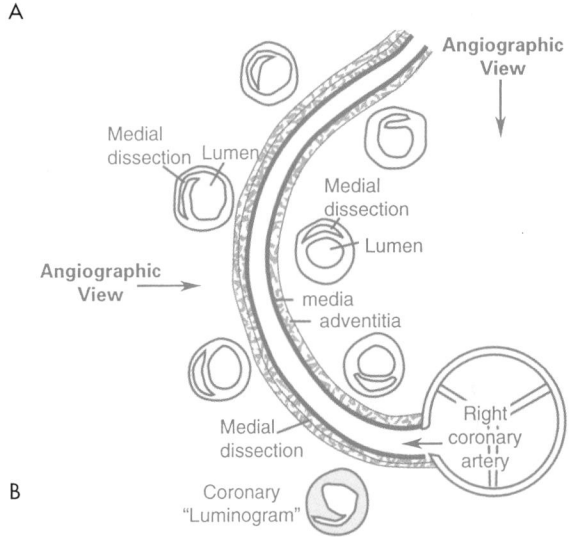

FIGURE 55–29. Diagram showing pathologic change accounting for angiographic appearance of coronary artery "spiral" dissection. **A.** Alteration in course of dissection. **B.** Angiographic appearance of unaltered course of dissection. *Source: From Waller BF, Orr CM, Pinkerton CA, Van Tassel J, Peters T, Slack JD. Coronary balloon angioplasty dissections: The good, the bad, and the ugly. J Am Coll Cardiol 1992;20:701–706. Reproduced with permission from the author, editor, and publisher.*

INFANTILE POLYARTERITIS

Polyarteritis nodosa occurring in infants younger than 2 years of age (infantile polyarteritis) differs from the clinical pathologic features of classical polyarteritis nodosa.[59,119–121] Infantile disease involves a higher frequency (79 percent) of coronary vasculitis and aneurysmal disease of the coronary arteries with sparing of vessels in other locations.[59,119–121] Kawasaki disease may involve children up to 8 or 10 years of age[59] rather than being confined to patients younger than 2 years as in infantile polyarteritis.[122]

KAWASAKI DISEASE (MUCOCUTANEOUS LYMPH NODE SYNDROME)

Kawasaki disease, or mucocutaneous lymph node syndrome, is an acute febrile exanthematous illness of children that was first described in the Japanese literature in 1967 and reported in the English literature in 1974.[123] It was subsequently reported in children worldwide and in all racial groups.[124] In approximately 20 percent of children with the acute illness, a vasculitis of the coronary vasa vasorum leads to coronary arterial aneurysm formation, thrombosis, acute myocardial infarction, and sudden

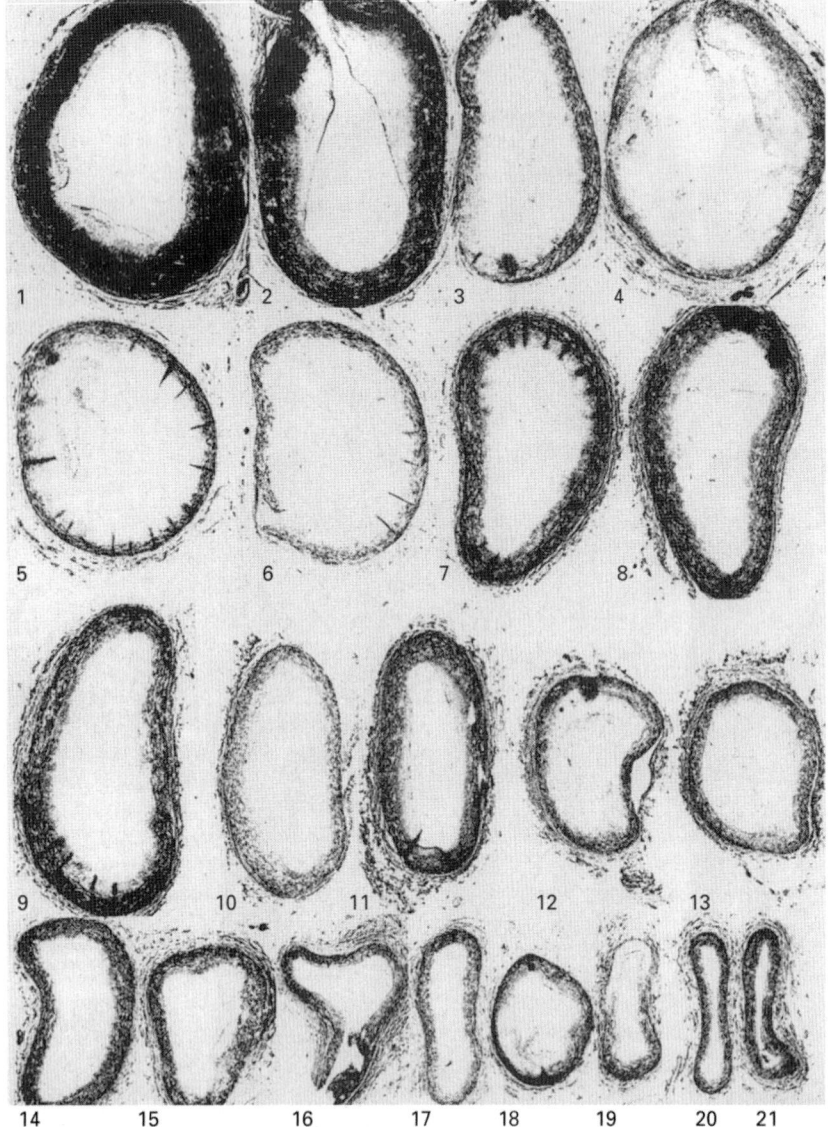

FIGURE 55–30. Coronary artery spasm. Composite of coronary artery cross sections of a patient with coronary spasm during life. Clinical spasm involved segments 3 to 7. Severe atherosclerotic plaque is seen in 8 of the 21 segments. *Source: From Roberts WC, Curry RC, Isner JM, et al. Sudden death in Prinzmetal's angina with coronary spasm documented by angiography: analysis of 3 necropsy patients. Am J Cardiol 1982;50:203–210. Reproduced with permission from the author, editor, and publisher.*

two-thirds of vessels. The likelihood of resolution of coronary artery aneurysms in Kawasaki disease is determined largely by the initial size of the aneurysm. Takahashi et al. reported regression of coronary aneurysms associated with *age* of the patient (regression more likely in children younger than age 1 year), aneurysm *morphology* (saccular more common than fusiform type), and *vessel location* of the aneurysm (regression more likely with distal coronary artery location). Angiographic regression of aneurysms occurs by intimal proliferation within the aneurysm or recanalization of a previously thrombotically occluded aneurysm. Necropsy "regressed coronary artery aneurysms" are historically abnormal and show reduced vascular reactivity.

Pathologically, the acute phase shows a necrotizing angiitis involving media and adventitial layers. Some children have survived into adulthood, with coronary artery aneurysms identified later in life (see Figs. 55–38 and 55–39).[129] The differential diagnosis of coronary artery aneurysms in adults includes previously undiagnosed Kawasaki disease, presumably occurring during childhood. Coronary arteriography results in 1100 children ages 4 months to 13 years identified 262 (24 percent) patients with the disease. In these, coronary occlusion was present in 76 percent; segmental stenosis in 5.7 percent; localized stenosis in 23.7 percent; aneurysms in 35.5 percent; and dilatation in 27.5 percent. The incidence of both occlusion and segmental stenosis was lowest in the group studied shortly after the onset of the illness, whereas the prevalence of coronary aneurysm was highest in this early group.

[ ] ALLERGIC GRANULOMATOSIS AND ANGIITIS: WEGENER GRANULOMATOSIS AND CHURG-STRAUSS SYNDROME

Wegener granulomatosis is a necrotizing vasculitis of unknown cause, classically involving the upper and lower respiratory tracts and the kidneys.[38,130,131] Cardiovascular involvement in Wegener granulomatosis was described in one of three cases reported in 1936. About 30 additional necropsy cases were described subsequently, 14 of which (48 percent) showed small-vessel necrotizing coronary vasculitis (Fig. 55–40).[38] Fibrinoid necrosis of the small- and medium-size coronary arteries and occlusion of larger epicardial coronary arteries with myocardial infarction have been reported. In a large clinical series of patients with Wegener granulomatosis, 12 percent had cardiac involvement, largely manifested by pericarditis and coronary arteritis.[131] Some patients with this disease develop unusual cardiac complications, such as pericardial tamponade and later constrictive pericarditis, high-grade atrioventricular block, and atrial tachycardia resistant to usual treat-

death.[123,124] Estimates of death from acute infarction or ventricular analytic range from 1 to 2 percent.[125] Late presentation with myocardial infarction secondary to dislodged aneurysmal thrombosis may also occur (Figs. 55–38 and 55–39).[125,126]

Coronary artery ectasia or coronary artery aneurysms occur in 15 to 25 percent of children with Kawasaki disease who do *not* receive treatment with gamma globulin in the acute phase.[127,128] Coronary artery dilation (detectable echocardiographically) can be seen as early as 4 days after the first appearance of fever, with maximal dilation peaking at 4 weeks after illness onset.[129] Coronary aneurysms in early Kawasaki disease occur mainly in the proximal segments of the major coronary arteries. The presence of distal coronary aneurysms is nearly always associated with proximal coronary aneurysms. Coronary aneurysms resolve angiographically 1 to 2 years after disease onset in about half to

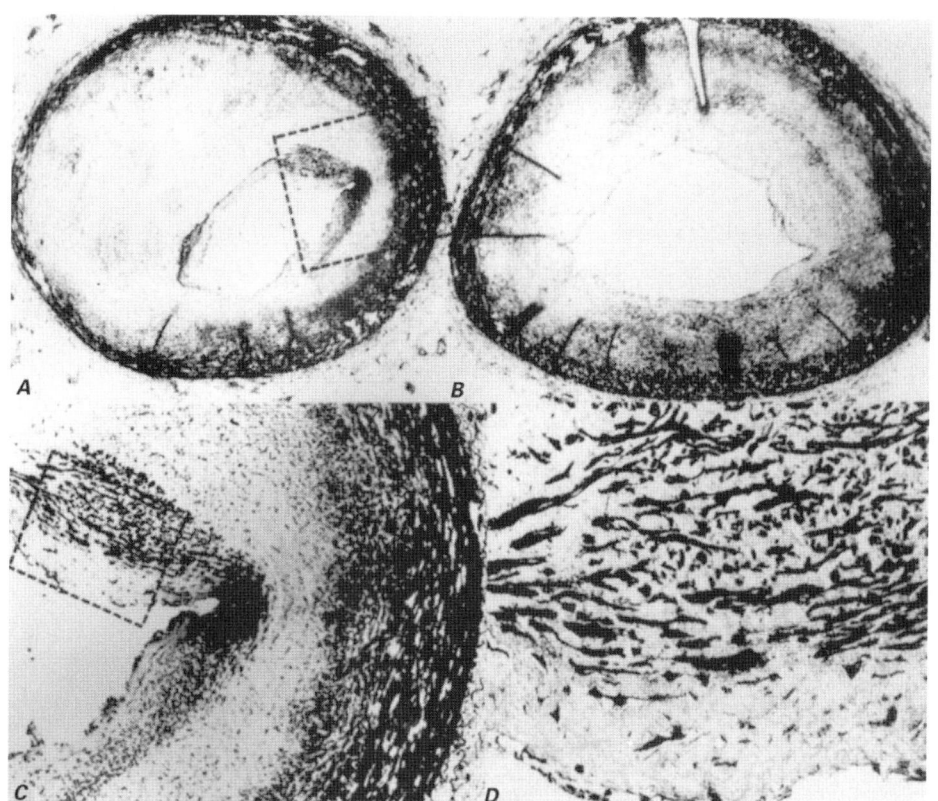

FIGURE 55–31. Coronary artery spasm. **A** and **B.** Histology sections of the left anterior descending coronary artery at the approximate site of spasm showing severe luminal narrowing. **C** and **D.** Higher magnifications of the internal plaque showing the predominance of smooth muscle cells. *Source: From Roberts WC, Curry RC, Isner JM, et al. Sudden death in Prinzmetal's angina with coronary spasm documented by angiography: analysis of 3 necropsy patients. Am J Cardiol 1982;50:203–210. Reproduced with permission from the author, editor, and publisher.*

leads to fatal coronary thrombosis and myocardial infarction,[59,135] rarely associated with thrombotic occlusion of all three major arteries.[135] Smaller intramural coronary arteries are also involved frequently with fibrinoid necrosis and subsequent fibrosis. Recently myocardial infarction has been seen with a proximal right coronary artery aneurysm at necropsy. It was postulated that the coronary aneurysm represented a sequela of systemic lupus erythematosus arteritis similar to Kawasaki disease.[136] Necrotizing vasculitis occurs less commonly in other entities of collagen vascular disease such as dermatopolymyositis, systemic sclerosis, Behçet syndrome, and Cogan syndrome.[59] The antiphospholipid syndrome is characterized by arterial and venous thrombus in the *absence* of underlying coronary atherosclerosis in patients with lupus. The antiphospholipid antibiotics are associated with unstable angina and acute myocardial infarction.

ment measures. In this series,[131] all patients improved with cyclophosphamide therapy.

Churg-Strauss syndrome (allergic granulomatosis and angiitis) is a variant of polyarteritis nodosa[59] occurring in patients with asthma or an allergy history.[132] It is characterized by necrotizing angiitis with extravascular granulomas and eosinophilia. The heart is commonly involved with this disease, with granulomatous vasculitis of the coronary arteries (see Fig. 55–40; Chap. 88). Granulomatous myocarditis may occur with or without the coronary angiitis.[133]

HYPERSENSITIVITY ANGIITIS (ALLERGIC VASCULITIS)

Hypersensitivity angiitis describes a miscellaneous group of necrotizing vasculitides that involve both epicardial and intramural coronary arteries.[59] This includes drug-induced vasculitis,[137] which, when generalized, may involve the heart. Histologically, drug-induced vasculitis cannot be separated from primary vasculitis or from hypersensitivity angiitis associated with a known underlying disease or malignancy such as serum sickness, mixed cryoglobulinemia, or Schönlein-Henoch purpura (see Table 55–6).[59] Correct diagnosis cannot be made without clinical information about drug usage. Organ-transplantation arteritis[59,138] is also in this category, representing a form of immune-mediated vascular injury.

COLLAGEN VASCULAR DISEASE VASCULITIS

Collagen vascular diseases generally involve arthritis, myositis, carditis, dermatitis, and inflammatory vascular changes to varying degrees.[134] They include systemic lupus erythematosus, rheumatoid vasculitis, systemic sclerosis, and polymyositis. Rheumatoid vasculitis is discussed in Chapter 88. A common condition with coronary vasculitis is systemic lupus erythematosus. Several young patients with this disease and absent coronary atherosclerosis have suffered acute myocardial infarction. Giant coronary artery aneurysms also are associated with systemic lupus erythematosus and acute myocardial infarction. At necropsy, the coronary arteries have shown internal fibrous proliferation, possibly representing healed arteritis. Necrotizing vasculitis frequently

METABOLIC DISORDERS NARROWING CORONARY ARTERIES

Specific metabolic substances may accumulate in the walls of large and small coronary arteries as a result of inborn errors of metabolism. The deposition of this material may severely narrow the coronary artery lumen and produce acute myocardial infarction.[5] Inherited inborn errors of metabolism that are known to affect major epicardial coronary arteries include Hunter and Hurler diseases (mucopolysaccharidoses).[139] The involvement of the coronary arteries in these disorders may be so severe as to occlude totally the vessel and to produce myocardial ischemia/infarction. Other disorders of metabolism, such as primary oxalosis, Fabry disease, Sandhoff disease (gan-

TABLE 55–5

Some Conditions Associated with Coronary Artery Arteritis (Vasculitis)

Tuberculosis
Polyarteritis nodosa
Giant cell arteritis
Systemic lupus erythematosus
Buerger disease (thromboangiitis obliterans)
Wegener granulomatosis
Salmonella
Leprosy
Mucocutaneous lymph node syndrome
Takayasu disease
Typhus
Infective endocarditis
Rheumatic diseases
Ankylosing spondylitis
Syphilis
Malaria
Schistosoma haematobium
Rickettsial infections
Viruses

SOURCE: *Waller BF. Atherosclerotic and nonatherosclerotic coronary artery factors in acute myocardial infarction. In: Pepine CJ, ed. Acute Myocardial Infarction. Philadelphia: FA Davis, 1989:29–104. Reproduced with permission from the author, editor, and publisher.*

INTIMAL PROLIFERATION

Fibrous hyperplasia and smooth muscle proliferation in the coronary arteries may severely narrow the lumen and produce myocardial ischemia/infarction. The process may be associated with mediastinal irradiation,[141] fibromuscular hyperplasia of the renal arteries,[5] the use of methysergide,[142] ostial cannulation during cardiac surgery, aortic valve replacement, and unknown causes.[143] Up to 50 percent of patients who undergo cardiac transplantation develop significant narrowing of epicardial coronary arteries or total occlusion by intimal fibrous proliferation within 3 to 5 years after transplantation. Myocardial infarction and sudden death may result from this "chronic rejection" process.

Fibrosis of the intramural vessels may also occur. Intimal damage from immunologic rejection is believed to be the basis for the accelerated intimal fibrous hyperplasia involving the coronary arteries. A morphologic assessment of 61 human cardiac allografts of short- and long-term survival has been provided.[144] Allographs were divided into two groups: fibrous lesions confined to the proximal regional of epicardial arteries and those with diffuse necrotizing vasculitis of the entire system. Disease in the proximal region begins as concentric fibrous thickening. Diffuse disease (necrotizing vasculitis) is invariably associated with acute myocardial rejection with severe intimal lesions of large and small epicardial and

TABLE 55–6

Classification of Vasculitides

1. **Infectious angiitis**
   Syphilitic
   Mycobacterial
   Pyogenic bacteria or fungal
   Rickettsial
   Viral
   Whipple bacillus
2. **Noninfectious angiitis**
   A. Involving large, medium-sized, and small blood vessels
      Takayasu arteritis
      Granulomatous (giant cell) arteritis
      Cranial (temporal) arteritis and extracranial giant cell arteritis
      Disseminated visceral granulomatous angiitis
      Granulomatous angiitis of the central nervous system
      Arteritis of rheumatic–rheumatoid disease and spondyloarthropathies
   B. Involving predominantly medium-size and small blood vessels
      Thromboangiitis obliterans (Buerger disease)
      Polyarteritis (periarteritis)
      Polyarteritis nodosa
      Infantile polyarteritis
      Microscopic polyarteritis
      Kawasaki disease
      Pathergic–allergic granulomatosis and angiitis
      Wegener granulomatosis
      Churg-Strauss syndrome
      Necrotizing sarcoid granulomatosis
      Vasculitis of collagen vascular disease
      Rheumatic fever
      Relapsing polychondritis
      Rheumatoid arthritis
      Systemic sclerosis
      Seronegative arthropathies
      Sjögren syndrome
      Systemic lupus erythematosus
      Behçet syndrome
      Cogan syndrome
      Dermatomyositis/polymyositis
   C. Involving predominantly small blood vessels
      Hypersensitivity angiitis (*synonym:* leukocytoclastic or allergic vasculitis)
      Serum sickness
      Mixed cryoglobulinemia
      Schönlein-Henoch purpura
      Drug-induced angiitis
      Hypocomplementemia
      Inflammatory bowel disease
      Malignancy-associated vasculitis
      Primary biliary cirrhosis
      Retroperitoneal fibrosis
      Goodpasture syndrome

SOURCE: *Lie JT. Coronary vasculitis: a review in the current scheme of classification of vasculitis. Arch Pathol Lab Med 1987;111:224–233. Reproduced with permission from the author, editor, and publisher.*

gliosidoses),[140] and homocystinuria, may affect smaller coronary vessels by severe intimal proliferation.

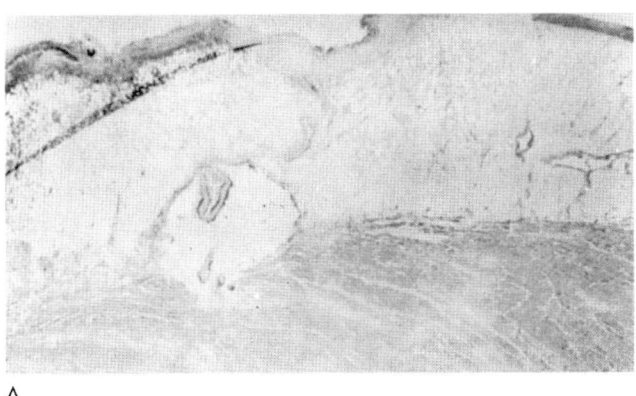
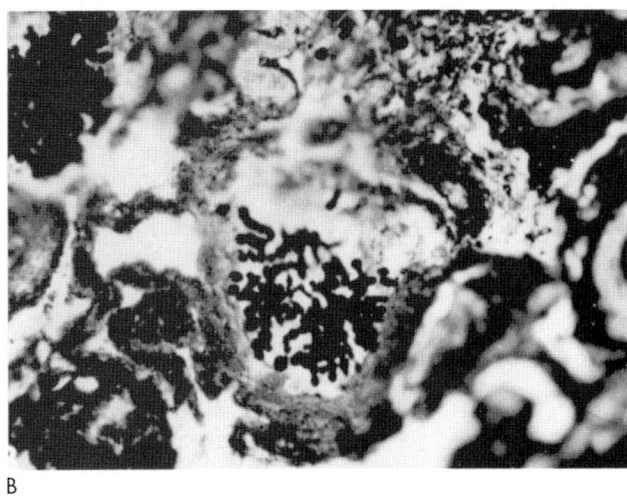

FIGURE 55–32. Coronary arteritis. **A.** Extensive yeast (*Candida*) pericarditis, which involves the adventitial layer of a branch of a major subepicardial coronary artery. **B.** Close-up shows the budding yeast organisms (GMS [Gomori methenamine-silver] stain). *Source: From Waller BF. Atherosclerotic and nonatherosclerotic coronary artery factors in acute myocardial infarction. In: Pepine CJ, ed. Acute Myocardial Infarction. Philadelphia: FA Davis, 1989:29–104. Reproduced with permission from the author, editor, and publisher.*

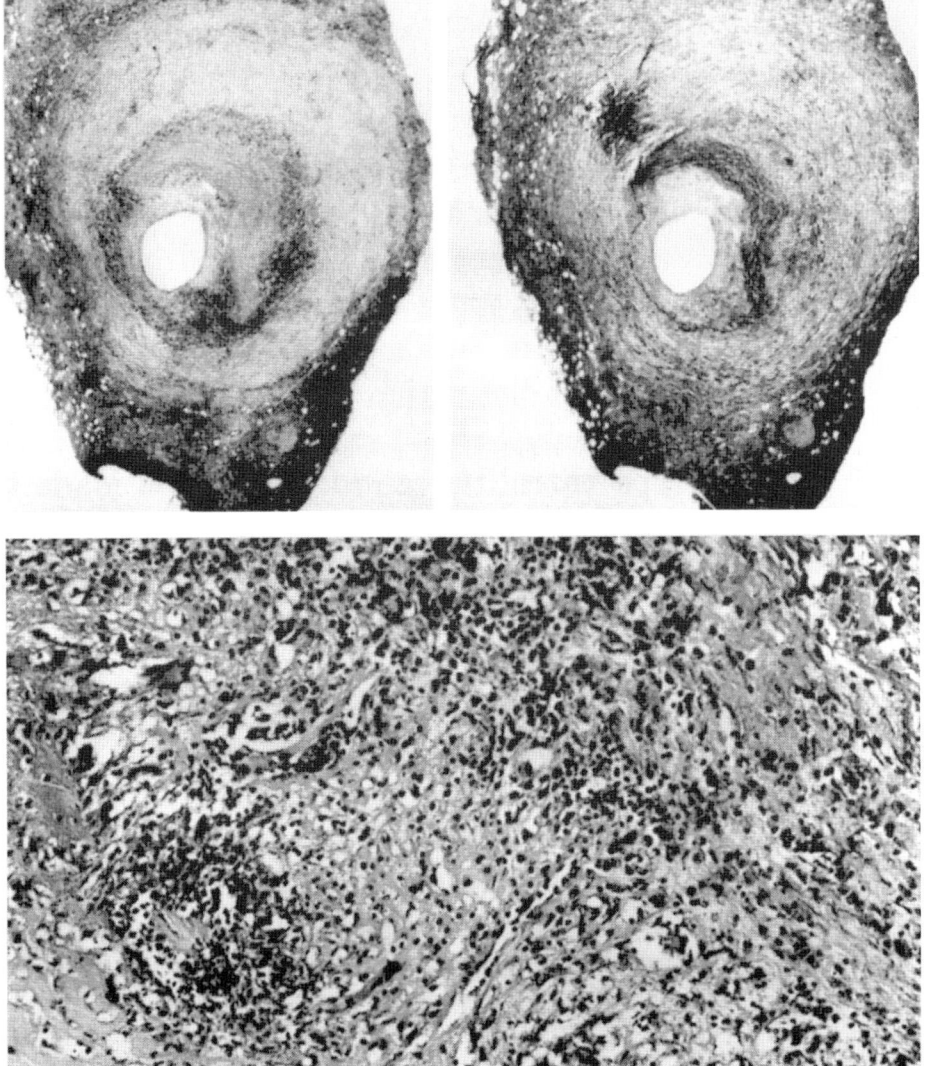

FIGURE 55–33. *Top:* Matching hematoxylin-eosin (*left*) and elastic stain (*right*) sections of coronary artery in Takayasu arteritis. Note transmural fibrosis and inflammatory infiltrate in media of artery (× 16). *Bottom:* Close-up view of lymphoplasmacytic infiltrate with giant cells in media of coronary artery (× 160). *Source: From Lie JT. Coronary vasculitis: a review in the current scheme of classification of vasculitis. Arch Pathol Lab Med 1987;111:224–233. Reproduced with permission from the author, editor, and publisher.*

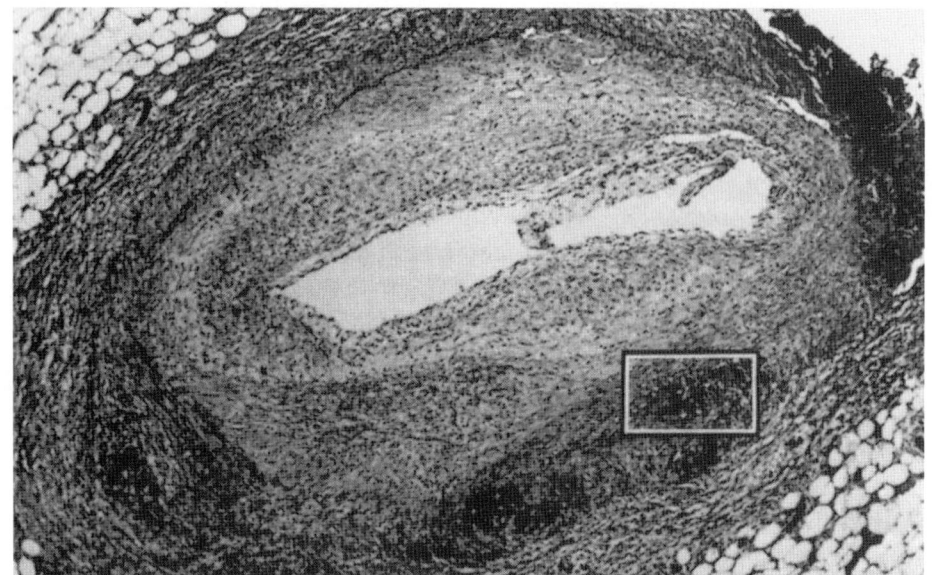

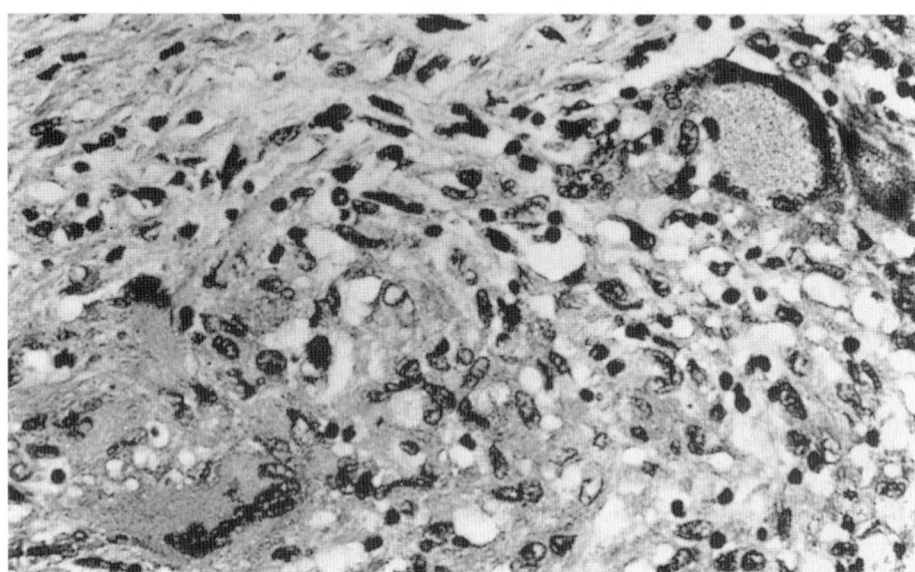

FIGURE 55–34. *Top:* Low-power view of granulomatous coronary arteritis associated with giant cell aortitis (hematoxylin-eosin, × 40). *Bottom:* Close-up view of boxed area (hematoxylin-eosin × 400). *Source: From Lie JT. Coronary vasculitis: a review in the current scheme of classification of vasculitis. Arch Pathol Lab Med 1987;111:224–233. Reproduced with permission from the author, editor, and publisher.*

intramural arteries.[144] These authors and others postulate that disease results from healing of a necrotizing vasculitis.

Intravascular ultrasound has shown intimal hyperplasia; its severity predicted the development of cardiac events, including myocardial infarction, unstable angina, and sudden death, despite the presence of a normal coronary arteriogram.

A similar histologic picture of intimal fibrous proliferation is seen in epicardial coronary arteries late after undergoing percutaneous balloon angioplasty (Fig. 55–41). Intimal fibrous proliferation of the left main coronary artery has been reported late after balloon angioplasty of a lesion in the proximal left anterior descending coronary artery.[145] This may be a result of intimal reaction from balloon rubbing of the intimal surface and/or extension of the fibrous process from the angioplasty dilation site.

EXTERNAL COMPRESSION

External compression of the epicardial coronary arteries may result in severe luminal narrowing and progressive myocardial ischemia. External compression of a major epicardial coronary artery has been reported in patients with sinus of Valsalva aneurysms, chronic aortic dissection,[146] and epicardial tumor metastases.[147] Myocardial bridging (external muscle compression during ventricular systole) was reviewed in the Myocardial Bridges section.

METASTATIC IMPLANTS

Myocardial metastatic lesions from various tumors—including carcinomas, sarcomas, and lymphomas—may mimic a healed

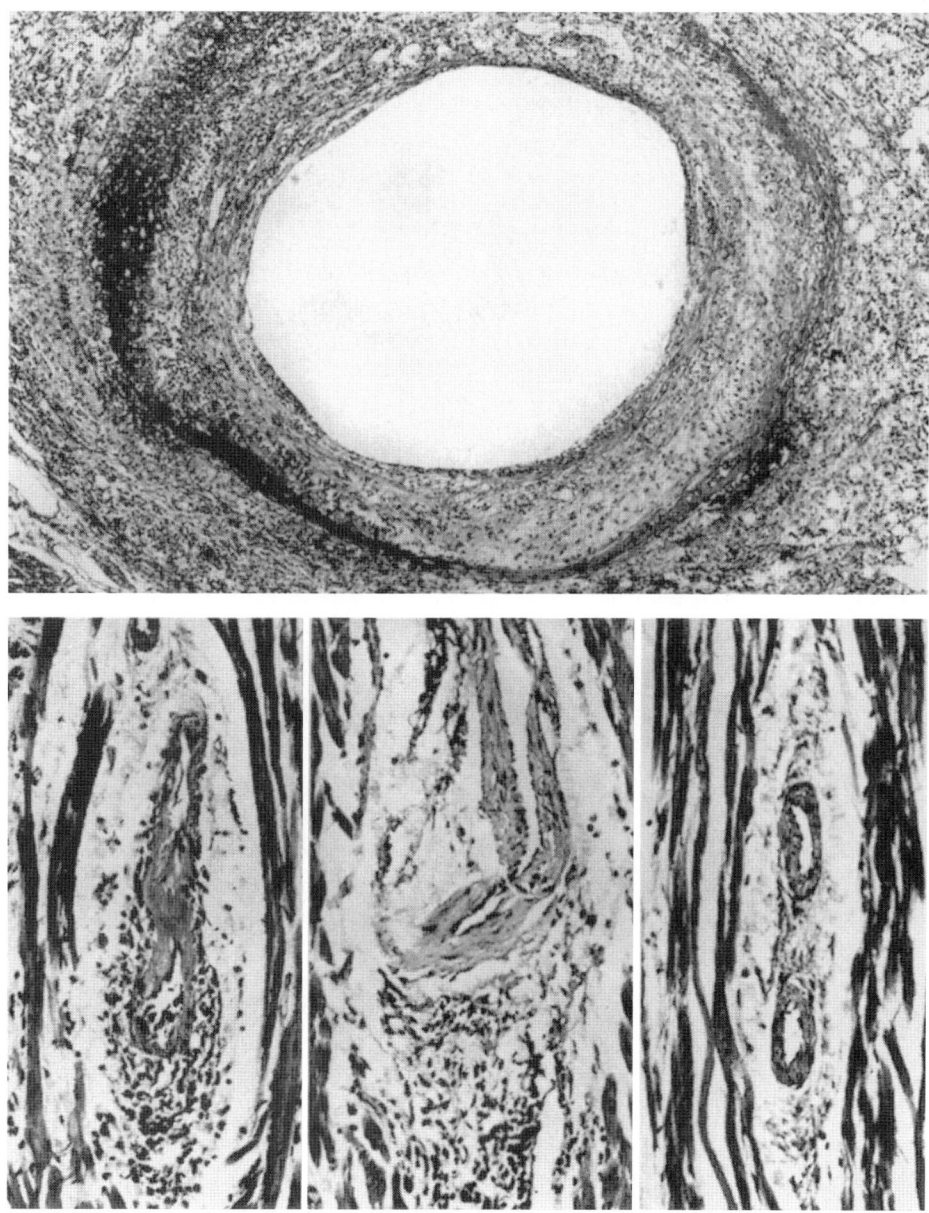

FIGURE 55–35. *Top:* Polyarteritis type necrotizing angiitis of epicardial coronary artery in rheumatoid arthritis (hematoxylin-eosin, × 160). *Bottom:* Variations of small-vessel coronary arteritis in rheumatic fever (hematoxylin-eosin, × 160). *Source: From Lie JT. Coronary vasculitis: a review in the current scheme of classification of vasculitis. Arch Pathol Lab Med 1987;111:224–233. Reproduced with permission from the author, editor, and publisher.*

myocardial infarct at necropsy (Fig. 55–42). The discrete location or locations of these metastatic deposits generally are unrelated to specific coronary arterial supply zones, and the lesions are usually surrounded by normal myocardium. These two gross observations suggest the lesions are metastatic tumor implants rather than healed myocardial infarcts.

RADIATION-INDUCED CORONARY DISEASE

Intimal proliferation of epicardial coronary arteries involving the ostium, main segment, or both is well known and increasingly reported.[148] "Accelerated" or "premature" coronary atherosclerosis

has been noted in young individuals who had previously undergone mediastinal irradiation for various types of malignancies.[149–151] Internal proliferation following mediastinal radiation 5 to 10 years earlier is described as "intimal thickening *without* medial abnormalities." The intimal lesions (ostial or main segment of artery) consists of fibrous tissue *without* extra cellular lipid deposits.[149] Coronary ostial stenosis has an incidence of 0.13 to 2.7 percent of patients undergoing mediastinal irradiation treatment.[149] A few patients have developed acute myocardial infarction or unstable angina as a result of the radiation-induced lesions treated by myocardial revascularization or angioplasty.

Because of their fibrous nature, many radiation-induced lesions do not provide the best substrate for dilation techniques. Chemo-

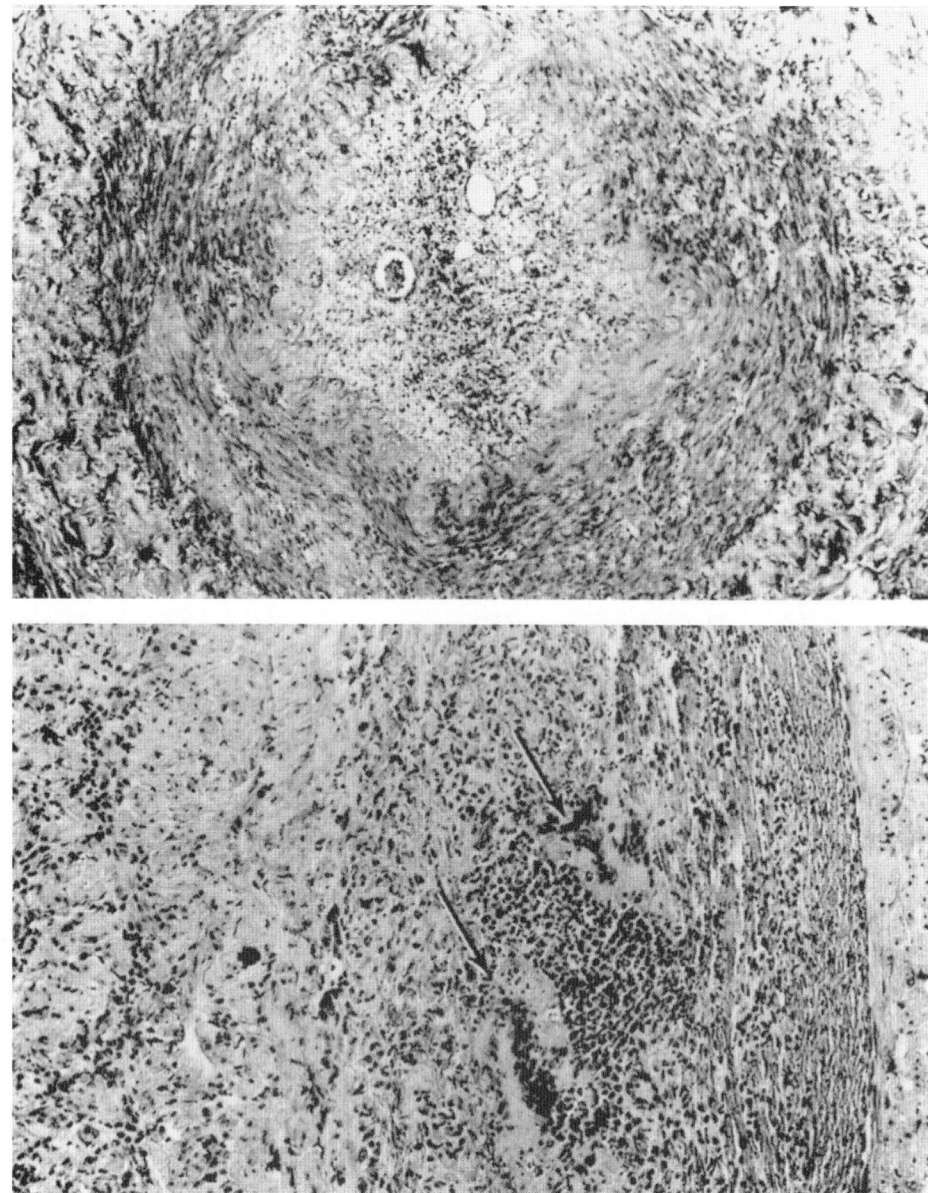

FIGURE 55-36. *Top:* Subacute stage of Buerger disease of coronary artery with organizing thrombus (hematoxylin-eosin, × 160). *Bottom:* Involvement of coronary vein in Buerger disease with typical intraluminal microabscesses and giant cells (*arrows*) (hematoxylin-eosin, × 160). Source: From Lie JT. Coronary vasculitis: a review in the current scheme of classification of vasculitis. Arch Pathol Lab Med 1987;111:224–233. Reproduced with permission from the author, editor, and publisher.

therapy-induced myocardial infarction in a young man without coronary disease has been reported.[152] Cardiac invasion by tumor, hypercoagulable states, and coronary artery spasm are possible etiologies.[152] Vascular toxicity, including myocardial infarction has been reported following antineoplastic regimens containing *Vinca* alkaloids.[152]

CORONARY ARTERY THROMBOSIS WITHOUT UNDERLYING ATHEROSCLEROTIC PLAQUE (THROMBOSIS IN SITU)

Thrombotic occlusion of the coronary system unassociated with underlying atherosclerotic plaque may be seen with several hematologic diseases: thrombocytopenic purpura, leukemia,[153] polycy-

themia vera, sickle cell anemia, and primary thrombocytosis.[154] Occasionally, acute myocardial infarction may be the initial manifestation of these hematologic disorders. A main factor responsible for the myocardial ischemia in these conditions is blockage of small intramural coronary vessels by platelet aggregates. These platelet aggregates initially may form in the major coronary arteries, then embolize distally.

SUBSTANCE ABUSE (COCAINE)

Cocaine abuse is now a major health hazard; more than 22 million Americans have tried cocaine at least once, and 5 million Americans are current users.[155] Recent reports document that cocaine abuse can result in myocardial ischemia and infarction in the ab-

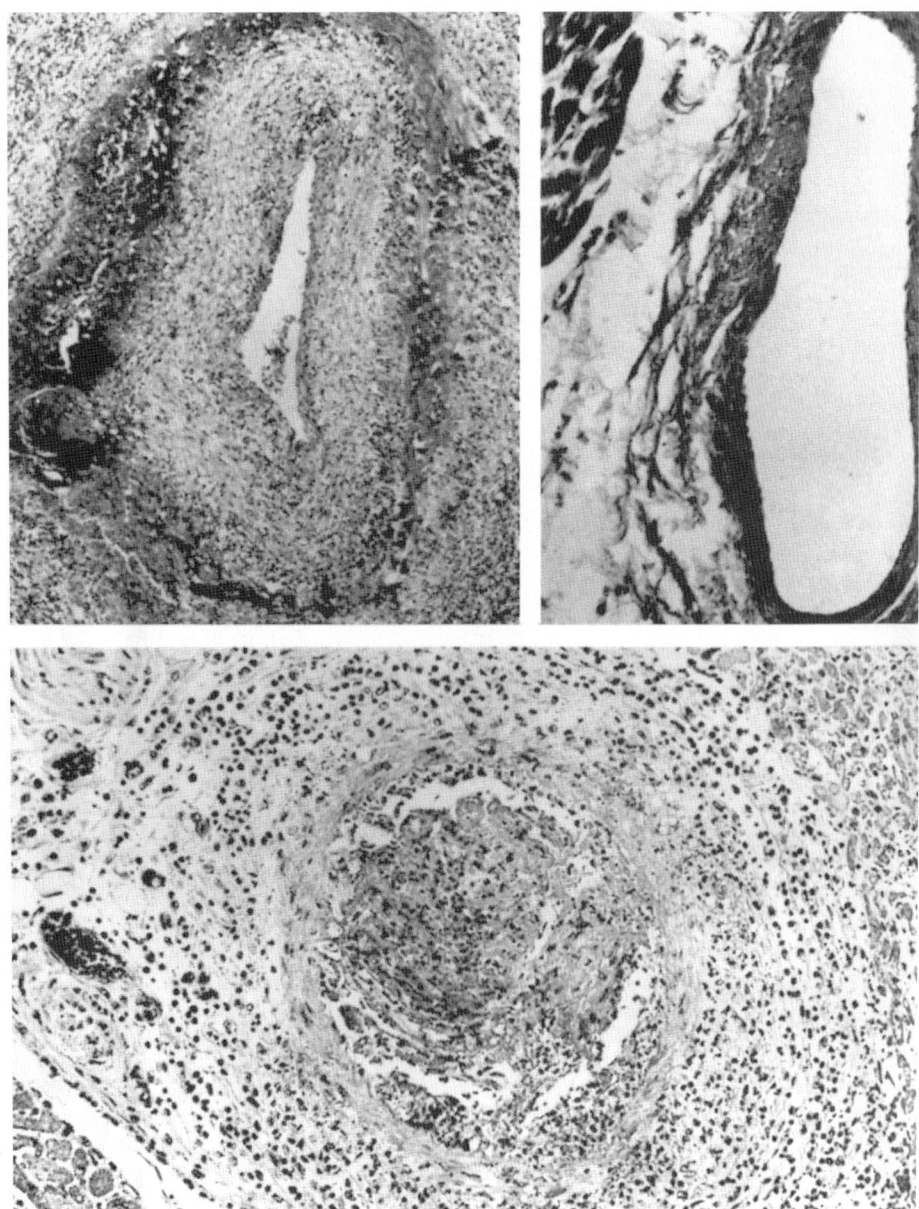

FIGURE 55–37. *Top:* Necrotizing angiitis (*left*) and histologically normal (*right*) segments of epicardial coronary arteries in classic polyarteritis nodosa (hematoxylin-eosin, × 16). *Bottom:* Necrotizing angiitis with fibrinoid necrosis of intramural coronary artery (hematoxylin-eosin, × 160). *Source: From Lie JT. Coronary vasculitis: a review in the current scheme of classification of vasculitis. Arch Pathol Lab Med 1987;111:224–233. Reproduced with permission from the author, editor, and publisher.*

sence of coronary artery disease,[155–157] and cocaine-induced coronary artery vasoconstriction has been reported in patients following the intranasal administration of cocaine.

Several instances of coronary artery thrombosis and spasm have been reported in patients who abuse cocaine. Acute coronary thrombosis in association with cardiac events—including angina, acute myocardial infarction, and sudden death—has been reported.[158] In some instances, there is underlying atherosclerotic plaque; in others, the coronary arteries are normal. Coronary thrombosis occurring in coronary arteries free of atherosclerotic plaque suggests the role of cocaine-induced spasm, massive norepinephrine release in the heart, or possible primary thrombogenicity of cocaine or its metabolites. Coronary spasm is associated with cocaine use and is postulated as a mechanism

of myocardial infarction in cocaine users with clean coronary arteries.[159] In such cases, fibrointimal proliferation with coronary narrowing was attributed to underlying coronary artery spasm that caused focal vessel endothelial injury, platelet adherence, and aggregation. Platelets liberate platelet-derived growth factor, which can induce intimal proliferative lesions. In patients with underlying coronary plaque, cocaine-induced spasm also may produce endothelial disruption at the surface of the plaque and promote platelet aggregation and further vasoconstriction from the release of platelet prostaglandins.

Two drugs are the center of debate over their potential for abuse versus use as psychotherapeutic agents and their complication in induction of arrhythmias.[160] Use of MDMA ("Ecstasy"; 3,4-methylenedioxymethamphetamine) and MDEA ("Eve"; 3,4-methy

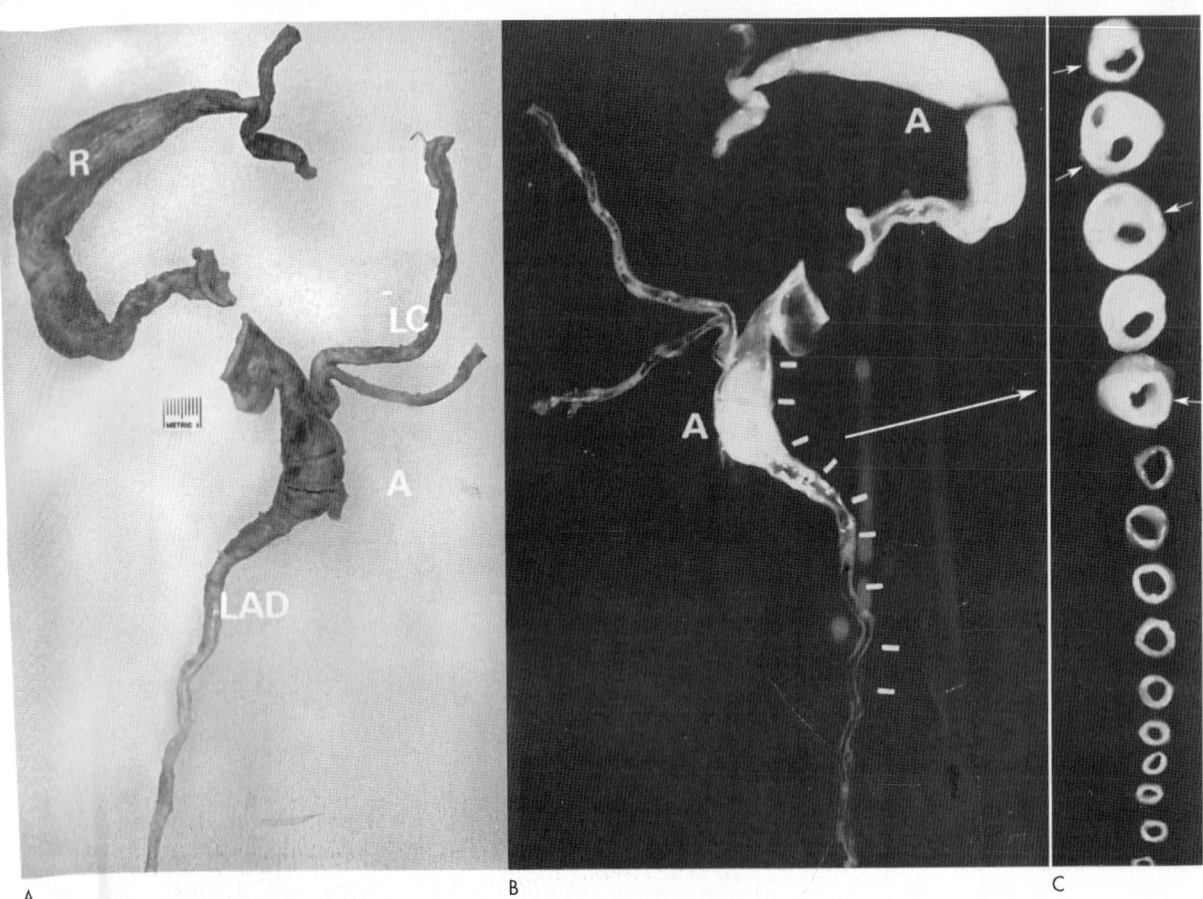

A   B   C

FIGURE 55-38. A. Epicardial coronary artery aneurysm involving the proximal left anterior descending (LAD) and right coronary artery (A) from an adult with probable Kawasaki disease as a child. **B.** Radiograph of coronary arterial tree in **A** showing calcific deposits. **C.** Cross section of the aneurysm shown in **A**. *Arrows* indicate calcific deposits. LC, left circumflex.

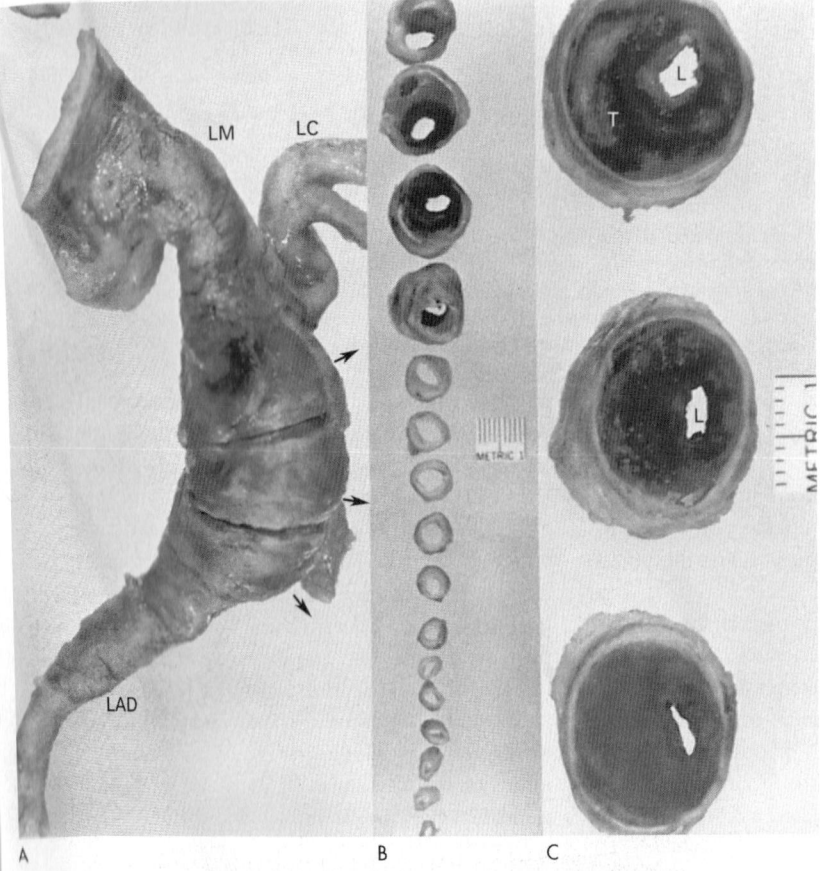

A   B   C

FIGURE 55-39. A. Close-up of left anterior descending (LAD) coronary aneurysm from Fig. 55-38 with cross-sections displayed in **B.** Note the intraaneurysmal thrombus. **C.** Close-up of three transverse sections of coronary aneurysm shown in **A** and **B**. LC, left circumflex; LM, left main.

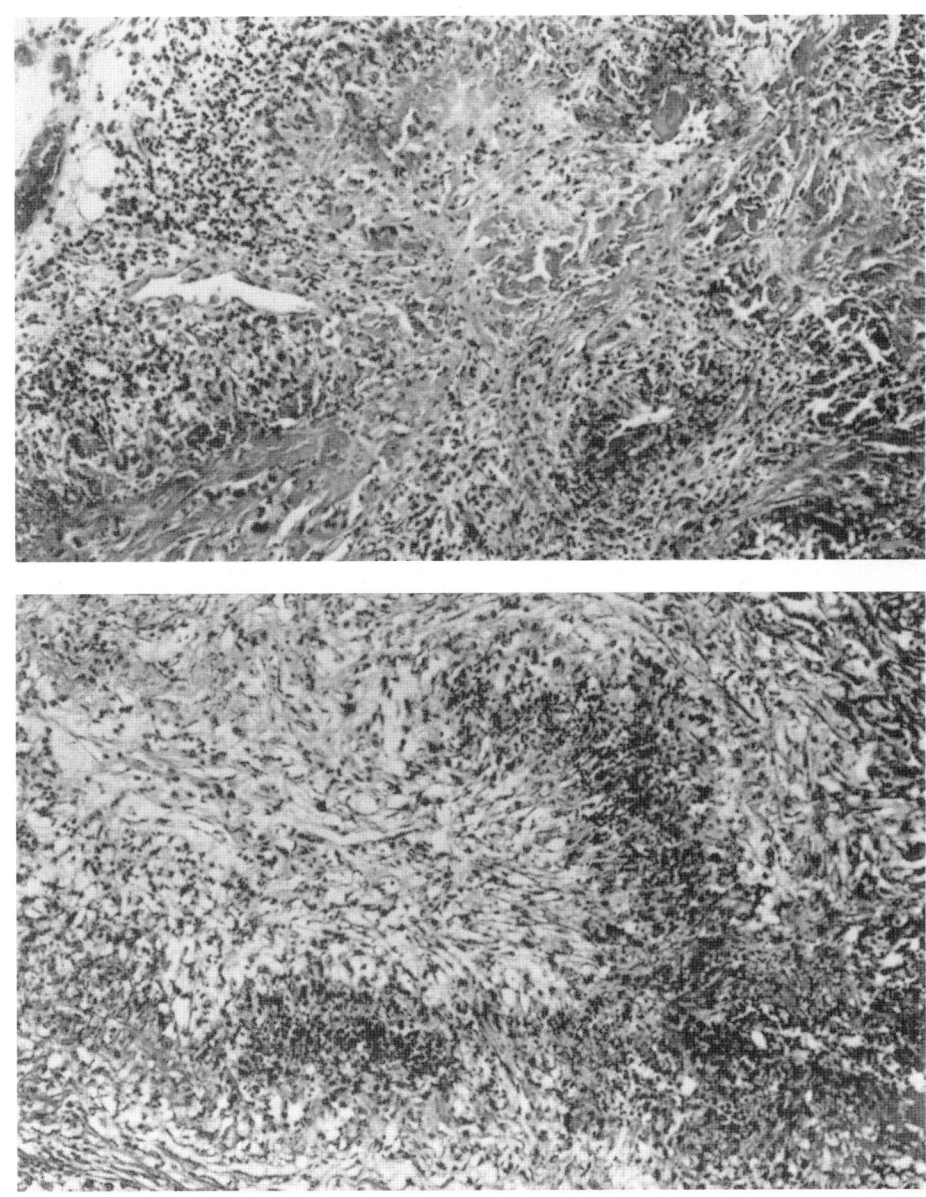

FIGURE 55–40. Granulomatous necrotizing angiitis of coronary arteries in Wegener granulomatosis (*top*) and Churg-Strauss syndrome (*bottom*) (hematoxylin-eosin, × 160). *Source: From Lie JT. Coronary vasculitis: a review in the current scheme of classification of vasculitis. Arch Pathol Lab Med 1987;111:224–233. Reproduced with permission from the author, editor, and publisher.*

enedioxymethamphetamine) is associated with five sudden deaths.[160] In three of these deaths, Eve and Ecstasy may have induced fatal arrhythmias.

MYOCARDIAL OXYGEN DEMAND–SUPPLY DISPROPORTION

In this category are disease states in which there is failure to deliver adequate oxygen to the myocardium over a prolonged period, or increased myocardial wall tension requiring increased oxygen supply. The classic example of the first situation is carbon monoxide poisoning,[4] which is associated with extensive nontransmural infarction in the presence of normal epicardial coronary arteries. Prolonged shock from any cause can also result in extensive non-transmural necrosis and is frequently associated with transmural necrosis of the papillary muscles. One example of increased myocardial wall tension requiring increased coronary oxygen supply is aortic valve stenosis[4] (see Chap. 56). In the face of increased oxygen demand with increased muscle mass, coronary blood supply may be limited by poor perfusion resulting from the lower coronary arterial pressure. In addition, poor perfusion results from the high coronary resistance caused by increased wall pressure on the intramural coronary arteries and the high left ventricular end-diastolic pressure from a stiff ventricle, with further limitation of the time in diastole for coronary blood flow occasioned by tachycardia.[4] Excessive myocardial oxygen demand exceeding supply and resulting in myocardial ischemia/infarction may also be seen in thyrotoxicosis,[161] which reflects increased metabolic rates and the adverse affects of tachycardia.

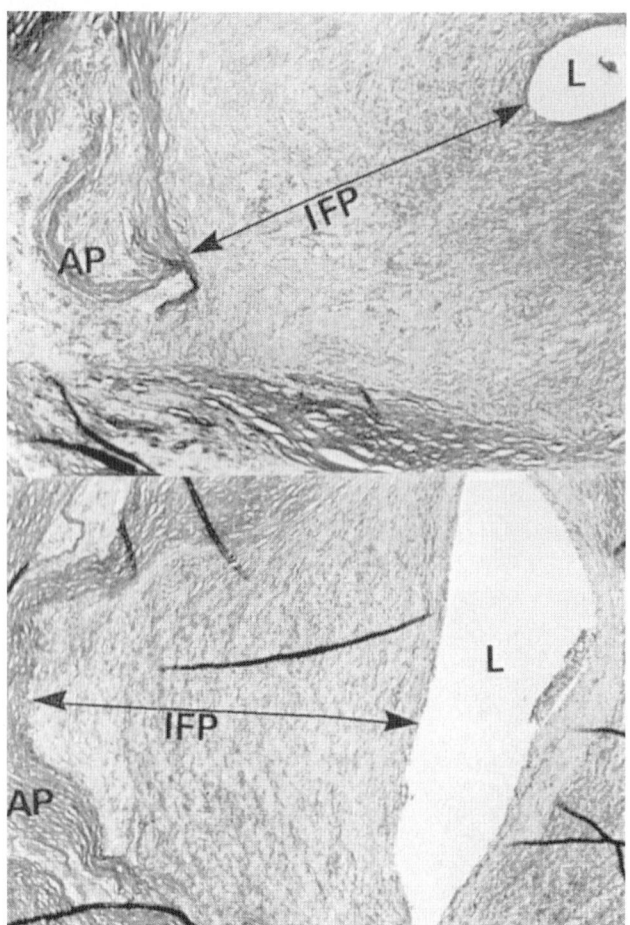

FIGURE 55–41. Intimal fibrous proliferation. Severe luminal narrowing of the left anterior descending coronary artery by intimal fibrous proliferation (IFP) several months after percutaneous balloon angioplasty. The IFP superimposes underlying atherosclerotic plaque (AP). L, lumen. *Source: From Waller BF. Atherosclerotic and nonatherosclerotic coronary artery factors in acute myocardial infarction. In: Pepine CJ, ed. Acute Myocardial Infarction. Philadelphia: FA Davis, 1989:29–104. Reproduced with permission from the author, editor, and publisher.*

Left ventricular hypertrophy is an independent risk factor of cardiac mortality in renal failure patients. Arrhythmias, LV dysfunction and myocardial ischemia may result from the left ventricular hypertrophy from multiple factors, such as small-vessel smooth-muscle hypertrophy vascular endothelial abnormalities microvascular calcification and alterations in oxygen demand and supply.

INTRAMURAL CORONARY ARTERY DISEASE (SMALL-VESSEL DISEASE)

Acute myocardial infarction may result from abnormally thickened or totally occluded intramural coronary arteries in the presence of normal extramural (epicardial) coronary arteries. A few of the conditions in this category include hypertrophic cardiomyopathy, diabetes mellitus, amyloid heart disease,[161] neuromuscular disorders (Friedreich ataxia, progressive muscular dystrophy), cardiac transplantation, rheumatoid arthritis, collagen–vascular disorders (scleroderma, systemic lupus erythematosus), metabolism

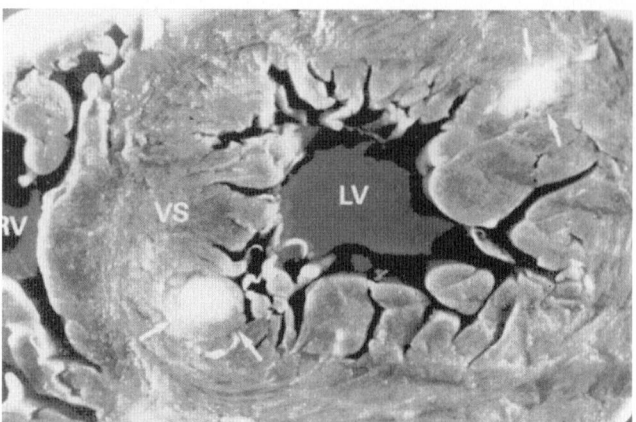

FIGURE 55–42. Metastatic deposits mimicking myocardial infarction. Transverse section of cardiac ventricle showing two discrete myocardial metastatic deposits of lymphoma. These whitish deposits may be mistakenly interpreted as healed myocardial infarctions in a patient with clean epicardial coronary arteries. LV, left ventricle; RV, right ventricle; VS, ventricular septum. *Source: From Waller BF. Atherosclerotic and nonatherosclerotic coronary artery factors in acute myocardial infarction. In: Pepine CJ, ed. Acute Myocardial Infarction. Philadelphia: FA Davis, 1989:29–104. Reproduced with permission from the author, editor, and publisher.*

abnormalities (mucopolysaccharidoses, gangliosidoses), and polyarteritis nodosa.[162]

Histologic abnormalities of small vessel coronary arteries are reported in individuals who have died from toxic oil syndrome involving rapeseed oil adulterated with aniline.[163] Many of those who later died had scleroderma-like illnesses. Dense fibrosis of the sinus node, resembling scleroderma, was found with cystic degeneration of the sinus node (resembling lupus erythematosus) and fibromuscular dysplasia of small coronary vessels.

NORMAL EPICARDIAL CORONARY ARTERIES

There are relatively few necropsy reports of patients with acute myocardial infarction who had angiographically normal coronary arteries and normal coronary arteries at necropsy.[3,4,164,165] Of 100 consecutive necropsy cases of acute myocardial infarction (AMI),[3] 7 percent had infarcts without evidence of coronary luminal narrowing. In 10 patients with a typical picture of AMI who died within 25 days of onset of symptoms, the coronary arterial systems showed minimal or no luminal narrowing by atherosclerosis. No thrombotic material was observed in the coronary arteries despite the fact that the AMI was 2 days old in five patients and 3 to 4 days old in three patients. Possible explanations for this include coronary artery spasm, coronary artery disease in vessels too small to be visualized angiographically, and coronary artery thrombosis or embolus with subsequent clot lysis. Myocardial infarction in postpartum women with normal epicardial coronary arteries has included two additional causes for possible spasm in these patients: bromocriptine used for suppression of lactation[166] and antiphospholipid syndrome with elevated anticardiolipin antibody levels, false-positive syphilis serology, and a history of deep venous thrombosis.[165]

SYNDROME X

The syndrome of angina or angina-like pain with angiographically normal coronary arteries is referred to as *syndrome X*.[167] The cause of symptoms in this syndrome is unclear, but true myocardial ischemia (lactate production during exercise) likely results from microvascular dysfunction or spasm (microvascular angina) or abnormal pain perception or sensitivity (sympathovagal imbalance with sympathic predominance).[167] In patients with evidence of myocardial ischemia, the incidence of coronary calcific deposits on CT-scanning is higher than normal controls (63 percent vs. 22 percent) but lower than patients with coronary artery atherosclerosis (63 percent vs. 96 percent) (see Chap. 64).

REFERENCES

1. Waller BF. Atherosclerotic and nonatherosclerotic coronary artery factors in acute myocardial infarction. In: Pepine CJ, ed. *Acute Myocardial Infarction.* Philadelphia: FA Davis, 1989:29–104.
2. Eliot RS, Baroldi G. Necropsy studies in myocardial infarction with minimal or no coronary luminal reduction due to atherosclerosis. *Circulation* 1974;49:1127–1131.
3. Cheitlin MD, McAllister HA, deCastro CM. Myocardial infarction without atherosclerosis. *JAMA* 1975;231:951–959.
3a. Baim DS, Harrison DC. Nonatherosclerotic coronary heart disease (including coronary artery spasm). In: Husrt JW, et al (eds). *The Heart,* 5th ed. New York: McGraw-Hill, 1982:1158–1170.
4. Virmani R, Forman MB, eds. *Nonatherosclerotic Ischemic Heart Disease.* New York: Raven Press, 1989:1–428.
5. Cheitlin MD, Virmani R. Myocardial infarction in the absence of coronary atherosclerotic disease. In: Virmani R, Forman MB, eds. *Nonatherosclerotic Ischemic Heart Disease.* New York: Raven Press, 1989:1–30.
6. Roberts WC. Major anomalies of coronary arterial origin seen in adulthood. *Am Heart J* 1986;111:941–963.
7. Roberts WC, Siegel RJ, Zipes DP. Origin of the right coronary artery from the left sinus of Valsalva and its functional consequences: analysis of 10 necropsy patients. *Am J Cardiol* 1982;49:863–868.
8. Waller BF. Exercise related sudden death in young (age <30 years) and old (age >30 years) conditioned athletes. In: Wenger NK, ed. *Exercise and the Heart,* 2d ed. *Cardiovascular Clinics.* Philadelphia: FA Davis, 1985:9–73.
9. Virmani R, Chun PKC, Goldstein RE, Rabinowitz M, McAllister HA. Acute takeoffs of the coronary arteries along the aortic wall and congenital coronary ostial valve-like ridges: association with sudden death. *J Am Coll Cardiol* 1984;3:766–771.
10. Foster L, Waller BF, Pless JE. Hypoplastic coronary arteries and high takeoff position of the right coronary artery. *Chest* 1985;88:299–301.
11. Chetlin MD. Coronary arterial anomalies: clinical and angiographic aspects. In: Virmani R, Forman MB, eds. *Nonatherosclerotic Ischemic Heart Disease.* New York: Raven Press, 1989:125–152.
12. Foster L, Waller BF. Nonatherosclerotic fibrous ridges: A previously unrecognized cause of ostial left main stenosis. *J Indiana State Med Assoc* 1983;76:682–683.
13. Alexander RW, Griffith GC. Anomalies of the coronary arteries and their clinical significance. *Circulation* 1956;14:800–805.
14. Baroldi G. Diseases of the coronary arteries. In: Silver MD, ed. *Cardiovascular Pathology.* New York: Churchill Livingstone, 1983:341.
15. Young JA, Sengupta A, Khaja FU. Coronary arterial stenosis, angina pectoris and atypical coarctation of the aorta due to nonspecific arteritis: Treatment, with aortocoronary bypass graft. *Am J Cardiol* 1973;32:356–361.
16. Faruqui AM, Maloy WC, Felner JM, Schlant RC, Logan WD, Symbas P. Symptomatic myocardial bridging of the coronary artery. *Am J Cardiol* 1978;41:1305–1310.
17. Kramer JR, Kitazume H, Proudin WI, Sones IM. Clinical significance of isolated coronary bridges: benign and frequent condition involving the left anterior descending artery. *Am Heart J* 1982;103:283–288.
18. Roberts WC, Dicicco BS, Waller BF, Kishel JC, McManus BM, Dawson SL. Origin of the left main from the right coronary artery or from the right aortic sinus with intramyocardial tunneling to the left side of the heart via the ventricular septum: the case against clinical significance of myocardial bridge or coronary tunnel. *Am Heart J* 1982;104:303–305.
19. Angelini P, Trivellato M, Donis J, Leachman RD. Myocardial bridges: a review. *Prog Cardiovasc Dis* 1983;26:75–88.
20. Carvalho VB, Macruz R, Decort LV, et al. Hemodynamic determinants of coronary constriction in human myocardial bridges. *Am Heart J* 1984;108:73–80.
21. Greenspan M, Iskandrian AS, Catherwood E, Kimbiris D, Bemis CE, Segal BL. Myocardial bridging of the left anterior descending artery: evaluation using exercise thallium-201 myocardial scintigraphy. *Catheter Cardiovasc Diagn* 1980;6:173–180.
22. Ferreira AG Jr, Trotter SE, Konig B Jr, Decourt LV, Fox K, Olsen EG. Myocardial bridges: morphological and functional aspects. *Br Heart J* 1991;66:364–367.
23. Wymore P, Yedlicka JW, Garcia-Medina V, et al. The incidence of myocardial bridges in heart transplants. *Cardiovasc Int Radiol* 1989;12:202–206.
24. Watanabe G, Ohhira M, Takemura H, Tanaka N, Iwa T. Surgical treatment for myocardial bridge using intraoperative echocardiography. *J Cardiovasc Surg* 1989;30:1009–1012.
25. Gupta NC, Beauvais J. Physiologic assessment of coronary artery fistula. *Clin Nucl Med* 1991;16:40–42.
26. Sethia B, Pollock JC. Coronary artery fistula following rupture of aneurysm of the sinus node artery into the right atrium. *Thorac Cardiovasc Surg* 1985;33:191–192.
27. Bata IR, MacDonald RG, O'Neill BJ. Coronary artery fistula as a complication of percutaneous transluminal coronary angioplasty. *Can J Cardiol* 1993;9:331–335.
28. Fyfe DA, Edwards WD, Driscoll DJ. Myocardial ischemia in patients with pulmonary atresia and intact ventricular septum. *J Am Coll Cardiol* 1986;8:402–406.
29. Uchida N, Baudet E, Roques X, Laborde N, Billes MA. Surgical experience of coronary artery–right ventricular fistula in a heart transplant patient. *Eur J Cardiothorac Surg* 1995;9:106–108.
30. Lee RT, Mudge GH, Colucci WS. Coronary artery fistula after mitral valve surgery. *Am Heart J* 1988;115:1128–1130.
31. Henzlova MJ, Nath H, Bucy RP, Bourge RC, Kirklin JK, Rogers WJ. Coronary artery to right ventricle fistula in heart transplant recipients: a complication of endomyocardial biopsy. *J Am Coll Cardiol* 1989;14:258–261.
32. Sapin P, Frantz E, Jain A, Nichols TC, Dehmer GJ. Coronary artery fistula: an abnormality affecting all age groups. *Medicine* 1990;69:101–113.
33. Glickel SZ, Maggs PR, Ellis FH. Coronary artery aneurysm. *Ann Thorac Surg* 1978;25:372–376.
34. Waller BF, Dixon DS, Kem RW, Roberts WC. Embolus to the left main coronary artery. *Am J Cardiol* 1982;50:658–660.
35. Isner JM, Donaldson RF. Coronary angiographic and morphologic correlation. In: Waller BF, ed. *Cardiac Morphology. Cardiology Clinics.* Philadelphia: WB Saunders, 1984:571–592.
36. Mather PJ, Hansen CL, Goldman B, et al. Postpartum multivessel coronary dissection. *J Heart Lung Transplant* 1994;13:533–537.
37. Wasserman L, Wolf P, Podolin R, Bloor CM. Dissecting aneurysm of a coronary artery due to percutaneous transluminal balloon angioplasty. *Am J Cardiovasc Pathol* 1990;3:271–274.
38. Ehya H, Weitzner S. Postpartum dissecting aneurysm of coronary arteries in a patient with sarcoidosis. *South Med J* 1980;73:87–88.
39. Nishikawa H, Nakanishi S, Nishiyama S, et al. Primary coronary artery dissection: its incidence, mode of the onset and prognostic evaluation. *J Cardiol* 1988;18:307–317.
40. DeMaio SJ Jr, Kinsella SH, Silverman ME. Clinical course and long-term prognosis of spontaneous coronary artery dissection. *Am J Cardiol* 1989;64:471–475.
41. Prinzmetal M, Kennamer R, Merliss R, Wada T. Angina pectoris: I. A variant form of angina pectoris. Preliminary report. *Am J Med* 1959;27:375–388.
42. Maseri A, L'Abbate A, Baroldi G, et al. Coronary vasospasm as a possible cause of myocardial infarction: a conclusion derived from the study of ""preinfarction"" angina. *N Engl J Med* 1978;299:1271–1277.
43. Roberts WC, Curry RC, Isner JM, et al. Sudden death in Prinzmetal's angina with coronary spasm documented by angiography: analysis of 3 necropsy patients. *Am J Cardiol* 1982;50:203–210.
44. Brown BF. Coronary vasospasm: observations linking the clinical spectrum of ischemic heart disease to the dynamic pathology of coronary, atherosclerosis. *Arch Intern Med* 1981;141:716–722.
45. Kounis NG, Zavras GM. Histamin induced coronary artery spasm: the concept of allergic angina. *Br J Clin Pract* 1991;45:121–128.
46. Fischell TA. Coronary artery spasm after percutaneous transluminal coronary angioplasty: pathophysiology and clinical consequences. *Cathet Cardiovasc Diagn* 1990;19:1–3.

47. Halper J, Factor SM. Coronary lesions in neurofibromatosis associated with vasospasm and myocardial infarction. *Am Heart J* 1984;108:420–422.

48. Shepherd JT, Katusic ZS, Vedernikov Y, Vanhoutte PM. Mechanisms of coronary vasospasm: Role of endothelium. *J Mol Cell Cardiol* 1991;23(Suppl 1):125–131.

49. Hillis LD, Braunwald E. Coronary artery spasm. *N Engl J Med* 1978;299:695–702.

50. Maseri A, Severi S, De Nes M, et al. ""Variant"" angina: one aspect of a continuous spectrum of vasospastic myocardial ischemia. *Am J Cardiol* 1978;42:1019–1035.

51. El-Maraghi NRH, Sealey BJ. Recurrent myocardial infarction in a young man with coronary arterial spasm, demonstrated at autopsy. *Circulation* 1980;61:199–207.

52. Isner JM, Donaldson RF, Katsas GC. Spasm at autopsy: a prospective study [abstract]. *Circulation* 1983;68:III-1028.

53. Isner JM, Fortin AH, Fortin RV. Depletion of smooth muscle from the media of atherosclerotic coronary arteries: a potential factor in the pathogenesis of myocardial ischemia and the variable response to anti-anginal therapy [abstract]. *Clin Res* 1983;31:193A.

54. Factor SM, Cho S. Smooth muscle contraction bands in the media of coronary arteries: a postmortem marker of antemortem coronary spasm? *J Am Coll Cardiol* 1985;6:1329–1337.

55. Waller BF. The eccentric coronary atherosclerotic plaque: morphologic observations and clinical relevance. *Clin Cardiol* 1988;12:14–20.

56. Quyyumi AA, Al-Rufaii HK, Olsen EGJ, Fox KM. Coronary anatomy in patients with various manifestations of three vessel coronary artery disease. *Br Heart J* 1985;54:362–366.

57. Saner HE, Gobel FL, Salomonowitz E, Erlich DA, Edwards JE. The disease-free wall in coronary atherosclerosis: its relation to degree of obstruction. *J Am Coll Cardiol* 1985;6:1096–1099.

58. Manion WC. Infectious angiitis. In: Orbison JL, Smith DE, eds. *The Peripheral Blood Vessels.* Baltimore: Williams & Wilkins, 1963:221.

59. Lie JT. Coronary vasculitis: a review in the current scheme of classification of vasculitis. *Arch Pathol Lab Med* 1987;111:224–233.

60. Christian CL, Sergent JS. Vasculitis syndromes: clinical and experimental models. *Am J Med* 1976;61:385–392.

61. Conn DL, McDuffie FC, Holley KE, Schroeter AL. Immunologic mechanisms in systemic vasculitis. *Mayo Clin Proc* 1976;51:511–518.

62. Fauci AS, Hayne BF, Katz P. The spectrum of vasculitis: clinical, pathogenic, immunologic, and therapeutic considerations. *Ann Intern Med* 1978;89:660–676.

63. Soter NA, Austen KF. Pathogenetic mechanisms in necrotizing vasculitides. *Clin Rheum Dis* 1980;6:233–253.

64. Kussmaul A, Maier R. Uber eine bisher nicht beschriebene eigenthumliche Arterienerkrankung (periarteritis nodosa), die mit Morbus Brightii und rapid fortschreitender allgemeiner Muskellahmung einhergeht. *Disch Arch Klin Med* 1866;1:484–518.

65. Zeek PM. Periarteritis nodosa: a critical review. *Am J Clin Pathol* 1952;22:777–790.

66. Churg J, Strauss L. Allergic granulomatosis, allergic angiitis, and periarteritis nodosa. *Am J Pathol* 1951;27:277–294.

67. Churg J. Allergic granulomatosis and granulomatous vascular syndromes. *Ann Allergy* 1963;21:619–628.

68. Lanham JG, Elkon KB, Pusey CD, Hughes GF. Systemic vasculitis with asthma and eosinophilia: a clinical approach to the Churg-Strauss syndrome. *Medicine* 1984;63:65–81.

69. Huthinson J. Diseases of the arteries: On a peculiar form of thrombotic arteritis of the aged which is sometimes productive of gangrene. *Arch Surg Lond* 1890;1:323–329.

70. Horton BT, Magath TB, Brown GE. An undescribed form of arteritis of the temporal vessels. *Mayo Clin Proc* 1932;7:700–701.

71. Horton BT, Magath TB, Brown GE. Arteritis of the temporal vessels. *Arch Intern Med* 1934;53:400–410.

72. Ostberg G. On arteritis: with special reference to polymyalgia arteritica. *Acta Pathol Microbiol Immunol Scand A* 1973;237:1–59.

73. Somer T. Thrombo-embolic and vascular complications in vasculitis syndromes. *Eur Heart J* 1993;14(Suppl K):24–29.

74. Allen AC, Spitz S. A comparative study of the pathology of scrub typhus (Tsutsugamushi disease) and other rickettsial diseases. *Am J Pathol* 1945;21:603–682.

75. Moritz AR. Syphilitic coronary arteritis. *Arch Pathol Lab Med* 1931;11:44–59.

76. Bruenn HG. Syphilitic disease of the coronary arteries. *Am Heart J* 1934;9:421–436.

77. Holt S. Syphilitic ostial occlusion. *Br Heart J* 1977;39:469–470.

78. Heggtveit HA. Syphilitic aortitis: a clinicopathologic study of 100 cases, 1950 to 1960. *Circulation* 1964;29:346–355.

79. Rose AG. Cardiac tuberculosis. A study of 19 patients. *Arch Pathol Lab Med* 1987;111:422–426.

80. Gouley BA, Bellet S, McMillan TM. Tuberculosis of the myocardium: report of six cases with observations on involvement of coronary arteries. *Arch Intern Med* 1933;51:244–263.

81. Merkel WC. Plasmodium falciparum malaria: the coronary and myocardial lesions observed in autopsy in two cases of acute fulminating *P. falciparum* infection. *Arch Pathol* 1946;41:290–298.

82. Gazayerli M. Unusual site of a schistosome worm in the circumflex branch of the left coronary artery. *J Egypt Med Assoc* 1939;22:34–39.

83. Moe JB, Mosher DF, Kenyon RH, White JD, Stookey JL, Bagley LR. Functional and morphological changes during experimental Rocky Mountain spotted fever in guinea pigs. *Lab Invest* 1976;35:235–245.

84. Heibel RH, O'Toole JD, Curtiss EI, Medsger TA, Reddy SP, Shaver JA. Coronary arteritis in systemic lupus erythematosus. *Chest* 1976;69:700–703.

85. Cipriano PR, Silverman JF, Perlroth MG, Grupp RB, Wexler L. Coronary arterial narrowing in Takayasu's aortitis. *Am J Cardiol* 1977;39:744–750.

86. Judge RD, Currier RD, Gracie WA, Figley MM. Takayasu's arteritis and the aortic arch syndrome. *Am J Med* 1962;32:379–392.

87. Strachan RW. The natural history of Takayasu's arteriopathy. *Q J Med* 1964;33:57–69.

88. Hachiya J. Current concepts of Takayasu's arteritis. *Semin Roentgenol* 1970;5:245–259.

89. Lupi-Herrera E, Sanchez-Torres G, Marcus-Hamer J, Mispireta J, Horowitz S, Vela JE. Takayasu's arteritis: clinical study of 107 cases. *Am Heart J* 1977;93:94–103.

90. Ischikawa K. Natural history and classification of occlusive thromboarteriopathy (Takayasu's disease). *Circulation* 1978;57:27–35.

91. Rose AG, Sinclair-Smith CC. Takayasu's arteritis: a study of 16 cases. *Arch Pathol Lab Med* 1980;104:231–237.

92. Case 46–1967. Case records of the Massachusetts General Hospital: weekly clinicopathological exercise. *N Engl J Med* 1967;277:1025–1033.

93. Sibramanyan R, Joy J, Balakrishnan KG. Natural history of aortoarteritis (Takayasu's disease) *Circulation* 1989;80:429–435.

94. Kihara M, Kimura K, Yakuwa H. Isolated left coronary ostial stenosis as the sole arterial involvement in Takayasu's disease. *J Intern Med* 1992;232:353–356.

95. Lie JT, Failoni DD, Davis DC. Temporal arteritis with giant cell aortitis, coronary arteritis, and myocardial infarction. *Arch Pathol Lab Med* 1986;110:857–860.

96. Klein RG, Hunder GG, Stanson AW, Sheps SG. Large vessel involvement in giant cell (temporal) arteritis. *Ann Intern Med* 1975;83:806–812.

97. Harris M. Dissecting aneurysm of the aorta due to giant cell arteritis. *Br Heart J* 1968;30:840–844.

98. Ainsworth RW, Gresham GA, Balmforth GV. Pathologic changes in temporal arteries removed from unselected cadavers. *J Clin Pathol* 1961;14:115–119.

99. Harrison CV. Giant-cell or temporal arteritis: a review. *J Clin Pathol* 1948;1:197–211.

100. Paulley JW. Coronary ischemia and occlusion in giant cell (temporal) arteritis. *Acta Med Scand* 1980;208:257–263.

101. Zvaifler NJ, Weintraub AM. Aortitis and aortic insufficiency in chronic rheumatic disorders: a reappraisal. *Arthritis Rheum* 1963;6:241–245.

102. Heggtveit HA, Hennigar GR, Morrione TG. Pan aortitis. *Am J Pathol* 1963;42:151–172.

103. Reimer KA, Rodgers RF, Oyasu R. Rheumatoid arthritis with rheumatoid heart disease and granulomatous aortitis. *JAMA* 1976;235:2510–2512.

104. Swezey RL. Myocardial infarction due to rheumatoid arthritis. *JAMA* 1967;199:855–857.

105. Voyles WF, Searles RP, Bankhurst AD. Myocardial infarction caused by rheumatoid vasculitis. *Arthritis Rheum* 1980;23:860–883.

106. Glass D, Soter NA, Schur PH. Rheumatoid vasculitis. *Arthritis Rheum* 1976;19:950–952.

107. Scott DG, Bacon PA, Tribe CR. Systemic rheumatoid vasculitis: a clinical and laboratory study of 50 cases. *Medicine* 1981;60:288–297.

108. Grismer JT, Anderson WR, Weiss L. Chronic occlusive rheumatic coronary vasculitis and myocardial dysfunction. *Am J Cardiol* 1976;20:739–745.

109. Gilkes R, Dow J. Aortic involvement in Buerger's disease. *Br J Med* 1973;46:110–114.
110. Saphir O. Thromboangiitis obliterans of the coronary arteries and its relation to arteriosclerosis. *Am Heart J* 1936;12:521–535.
111. Lie JT. Thromboangiitis obliterans (Buerger's disease) in a saphenous vein arterial graft. *Hum Pathol* 1987;18:402–404.
112. Fronert PP, Sheps SG. Long-term follow-up study of polyarteritis nodosa. *Am J Med* 1967;43:8–14.
113. Leib ES, Restivo C, Paulus HE. Immunosuppressive and corticosteroid therapy of polyarteritis nodosa. *Am J Med* 1979;67:941–947.
114. Arkin A. A clinical and pathological study of periarteritis nodosa. *Am J Pathol* 1930;6:401–426.
115. Sinclair W, Nitsch E. Polyarteritis nodosa of the coronary arteries: report of a case with rupture of an aneurysm and intrapericardial hemorrhage. A*m Heart J* 1949;38:898–904.
116. Przybojewski JZ. Polyarteritis nodosa in the adult: report of a case with repeated myocardial infarction and a review of cardiac involvement. *S Afr Med J* 1981;60:512–518.
117. Swalwell CI, Reddy SK, Rao VJ. Sudden death due to unsuspected coronary vasculitis. *Am J Forens Med Pathol* 1991;12:306–312.
118. Sugihara N, Genda A, Shimizu M, et al. Intramural coronary angiitis of periarteritis nodosa proved by endomyocardial biopsy. *Am Heart J* 1990;119:1414–1416.
119. Ettinger RE, Nelson AM, Buske EC, Lie JT. Polyarteritis nodosa in childhood: a clinical pathologic study. *Arthritis Rheum* 1979;22:820–825.
120. Petty RE, Maligilavy DB, Cassidy JT, Sullivan DB. Polyarteritis in childhood: a clinical description of eight cases. *Arthritis Rheum* 1977;20:392–394.
121. Roberts FB, Fetterman GH. Polyarteritis nodosa in infancy. *J Pediatr* 1963;63:519–529.
122. Tanaka N, Naoe S, Masuda H, Ueno T. Pathological study of sequelae of Kawasaki disease (MCLS): with special reference to the heart and coronary arterial lesions. *Acta Pathol Japon* 1986;36:1513–1527.
123. Kawasaki T, Kosaki F, Okawa S, Shigematsu I, Yanagawa H. A new infantile acute febrile mucocutaneous lymph node syndrome (MLNS) prevailing in Japan. *Pediatrics* 1974;54:271–276.
124. Melish ME. Kawasaki syndrome (the mucocutaneous lymph node syndrome). *Annu Rev Med* 1982;33:569–585.
125. Fukushige J, Nihill MR, McNamara DG. Spectrum of cardiovascular lesions in mucocutaneous lymph node syndrome. *Am J Cardiol* 1980;45:98–107.
126. Kitamura S, Kawashima Y, Fujita T, Mori T, Oyama C, Fujino M. Aortocoronary bypass grafting in a child with coronary artery obstruction due to mucocutaneous lymph node syndrome: report of a case. *Circulation* 1976;53:1035–1040.
127. Sakai Y, Takayanagi K, Inoue T, et al. Coronary artery aneurysms and congestive heart failure: possible long term course of Kawasaki disease in an adult. A case report. *Angiology* 1988;39:625–630.
128. Kato H, Ichinose E, Kawasaki T. Myocardial infarction in Kawasaki disease: clinical analyses in 195 cases. *J Pediatr* 1986;108:923–928.
129. Fuiwara T, Fujiwara H, Hamashima Y. Frequency and size of coronary arterial aneurysm at necropsy in Kawasaki disease. *Am J Cardiol* 1987;59:808–811.
130. Parrillo JE, Fauci AS. Necrotizing vasculitis, coronary angiitis and the cardiologist. *Am Heart J* 1980;99:547–554.
131. Schiavone WA, Ahmad M, Ockner SA. Unusual cardiac complications of Wegener's granulomatosis. *Chest* 1985;88:745–748.
132. Lie JT. Classification of vasculitis and a reappraisal of allergic granulomatosis and angiitis. *Mt Sinai J Med* 1986;53:429–439.
133. Cupps TR, Fauci AS. *The Vasculitides.* Philadelphia: WB Saunders, 1981:211.
134. Rich AR. Hypersensitivity in disease, with special reference to periarteritis nodosa, rheumatic fever, disseminated lupus erythematosus, and rheumatoid arthritis. *Harvey Lect* 1947;42:106–147.
135. Bonfiglio TA, Botti RE, Hagstrom JWC. Coronary arteritis, occlusion and myocardial infarction due to lupus erythematosus. *Am Heart J* 1972;83:153–158.
136. Sumino H, Kanda T, Sasaki T, Kanazawa N, Takeuch H. Myocardial infarction secondary to coronary aneurysm in systemic lupus erythematosus: an autopsy case. *Angiology* 1995;46:527–530.
137. Mullick FG, McAllister HA, Wagner BM, Fenoglio JJ Jr. Drug related vasculitis: Clinicopathologic correlation in 30 patients. *Hum Pathol* 1979;10:313–325.
138. Uys CJ, Rose AG. Pathologic findings in long-term cardiac transplants. *Arch Pathol Lab Med* 1984;108:112–116.
139. Renteria VG, Ferrans VJ, Roberts WC. The heart in the Hurler syndrome: gross histologic and ultrastructural observations in five necropsy cases. *Am J Cardiol* 1976;38:487–501.
140. Blieden LC, Desnick RJ, Carter JB, Krivit W, Moller JH, Sharp HL. Cardiac involvement in Sandhoff's disease: an inborn error of glycosphingolipid metabolism. *Am J Cardiol* 1974;34:83–88.
141. Brosius FC III, Waller BF, Roberts WC. Radiation heart disease: analysis of 16 young (aged 15 to 33 years) necropsy patients who received over 3500 rads to the heart. *Am J Med* 1981;70:519–530.
142. Brill IC, Brodeur MTH, Oyama AA. Myocardial infarction in two sisters less than 20 years old. *JAMA* 1971;217:1345–1348.
143. Dominguez FE, Tate LG, Robinson MJ. Familial fibromuscular dysplasia presenting as sudden death. *Am J Cardiovasc Pathol* 1988;2:269–272.
144. Johnson DE, Gao SZ, Schroeder JS, DeCampl WM, Billingham ME. The spectrum of coronary artery pathologic findings in human cardiac allografts. *J Heart Transplant* 1989;8:349–359.
145. Waller BF, Pinkerton CA, Foster LN. Morphologic evidence of accelerated left main coronary artery stenosis: a late complication of percutaneous transluminal angioplasty of the proximal left anterior descending coronary artery. *J Am Coll Cardiol* 1987;9:1019–1023.
146. Giritsky AS, Ricci MT, Reitz BA, Shumway NE. Extrinsic coronary artery obstruction by chronic aortic dissection. *Ann Thorac Surg* 1981;32:289–293.
147. Gardia-Rinaldi R, Von Koch L, Howell JP. Aneurysm of the sinus of Valsalva producing obstruction of the left main coronary artery. *J Thorac Cardiovascular Surg* 1976;72:123–126.
148. Applefeld MM, Wiernik PH. Cardiac disease after radiation therapy for Hodgkin's disease: analysis of 48 patients. *Am J Cardiol* 1983;51:1679–1681.
149. Grollier G, Commeau P, Mercier V, et al. Post radiotherapeutic left main coronary ostial stenosis: clinical and histological study. *Eur Heart J* 1988;9:567–570.
150. Mittal B, Deutsch M, Thompson M, Dameshek HL. Radiation induced accelerated coronary arteriosclerosis. *Am J Med* 1986;81:183–184.
151. Om A, Ellahham S, Vetrovec GW. Radiation induced coronary artery disease. *Am Heart J* 1992;124:1598–1602.
152. House KW, Simon SR, Pugh RP. Chemotherapy induced myocardial infarction in a young man with Hodgkin's disease. *Clin Cardiol* 1992;15:122–125.
153. Fomina LG. A case of myocardial infarct in acute leukemia. *Sov Med* 1960;24:141–143.
154. Spach MS, Howell DA, Harris JS. Myocardial infarction and multiple thrombosis in a child with primary thrombocytosis. *Pediatrics* 1963;31:268–276.
155. Simpson RW, Edwards WD. Pathogenesis of cocaine-induced ischemic heart disease. *Arch Pathol Lab Med* 1986;110:479–484.
156. Zimmerman FH, Gustafson GM, Kemp HG. Recurrent myocardial infarction associated with cocaine abuse in a young man with normal coronary arteries: evidence for coronary artery spasm culminating in thrombosis. *J Am Coll Cardiol* 1987;9:964–968.
157. Perreault CL, Hauge NL, Morgan KG, Allen PD, Morgan JP. Negative inotropic and relaxant effects of cocaine on myopathic human ventricular myocardium and epicardial coronary arteries in vitro. *Cardiovasc Res* 1993;27:262–268.
158. Hollander JE, Hoffman RS. Cocaine-induced myocardial infarction: an analysis and review of the literature. *J Emerg Med* 1992;10:169–177.
159. Wetli CV, Wright RK. Death caused by recreational cocaine use. *JAMA* 1979;241:2519–2522.
160. Dowling GP, McDonough ET, Bost RO. Eve and ecstasy: a report of five deaths associated with the use of MDEA and MDMA. *J Am Coll Cardiol* 1987;257:1615–1617.
161. Masani ND, Northbridge DB, Hall RJ. Severe coronary vasospasm associated with hyperthyroidism causing myocardial infarction. *Br Heart J* 1995;74:700–701.
162. Mosseri M, Yarom R, Gotsman MS, Hasin Y. Histologic evidence for small vessel coronary artery disease in patients with angina pectoris and patent large coronary arteries. *Circulation* 1986;74:964–972.
163. James TN, Posada de la Paz M, Abaitua Borda I, Gomez-Sanchez MA, Martinez-Tello FJ, Soldevilla LB. Histologic abnormalities of large and small coronary arteries, neural structures, and the conduction system of the heart found in postmortem studies of individuals dying from the toxic oil syndrome. *Am Heart J* 1991;121:803–815.
164. Friedberg CK, Horn H. Acute myocardial infarction not due to coronary artery occlusion. *JAMA* 1939;112:1675–1679.

165. Baroldi G, Scomazzoni X. *Coronary Circulation in the Normal and Pathologic Heart.* Washington, DC: American Registry of Pathology, Armed Forces Institute of Washington DC, U.S. Government Printing Office 1967:1–80.

166. Department of Health and Human Services, Food and Drug Administration Docket No. 94N-0304. Notice of hearing on proposal to withdraw approval of the indication for prevention of physiological lactation: bromocriptine. Center for Drug Evaluation and Research, 7500 Standish Pl, Rockville MD, pp 1–12.

167. Cannon RO III, The sensitive heart. A syndrome of abnormal cardiac pain perception. *JAMA* 1995;273:883–886.

CHAPTER 56

Definitions of Acute Coronary Syndromes

Michael C. Kim / Annapoorna S. Kini / Valentin Fuster

INTRODUCTION

Coronary heart disease (CHD) is a worldwide health epidemic. In the United States, for example, it is estimated that 13.7 million Americans have CHD, including more than 7.2 million individuals who already have had a myocardial infarction.[1] In the group of persons older than 30 years of age, 213 per 100,000 individuals have CHD.[1] Although age-specific events related to CHD have fallen dramatically in the last few decades, the overall prevalence has risen as populations age and patients survive the initial coronary or cardiovascular event. The Centers for Disease Control and Prevention estimates that life expectancy in America might be increased by 7 years if CHD and its complications were eradicated.[2] Worldwide 30 percent of all deaths can be attributed to cardiovascular disease, of which more than half are caused by CHD, and the forecasts for the future estimate a growing number as a consequence of lifestyle changes in developing countries.[2] Globally, of those dying from cardiovascular diseases, 80 percent are in developing countries and not in the Western world.[2]

CHD represents a continuum of disease pathologies and its subsequent risks. CHD has been classified as chronic CHD, acute coronary syndromes, and sudden death. CHD may present clinically in many ways, extending from an asymptomatic finding to unexpected cardiac collapse. Chronic CHD is always secondary to coronary atherosclerosis, leading to mismatch of coronary blood flow and adenosine triphosphate homeostasis (imbalance of supply and demand) and a stable pattern of coronary ischemia. The clinical pattern includes stable angina pectoris and myocardial hibernation.[3] This chapter, however, focuses on a more high-risk population, those with acute coronary syndromes.

ACUTE CORONARY SYNDROMES

Acute coronary syndrome (ACS) is a unifying term representing a common end result, acute myocardial ischemia. Acute ischemia is usually, but not always, caused by atherosclerotic plaque rupture, fissuring, erosion, or a combination with superimposed intracoronary thrombosis, and is associated with an increased risk of cardiac death and myonecrosis.[4] It encompasses acute myocardial infarction (resulting in ST elevation or non-ST elevation) and unstable angina. Recognizing a patient with ACS is important because the diagnosis triggers both triage and management. Those deemed to have an acute coronary syndrome in the emergency department should be triaged immediately to an area with continuous electrocardiographic monitoring and defibrillation capability. An ECG should be obtained and accurately interpreted within 10 minutes. Those patients with suspected ACS should be managed immediately with antiplatelet and anticoagulant therapies and considered for immediate revascularization mechanically or pharmacologically if new ST-elevation is noted.[5]

Because of the life-threatening nature of an ACS, it is prudent to have a low threshold in suspecting a patient with acute chest pain as potentially having an ACS. Because the efficient diagnosis and optimal management of these patients are derived from information mostly only readily available from initial clinical presentation, there is overlap of those with true ACS and those that ultimately do not have CHD as a cause of their cardiac symptoms. In addition, it may not be possible to differentiate patients with myocardial infarction (either ST-elevation or non–ST-elevation) from those with unstable angina in the initial hours as the biomarkers of myonecrosis can be normal initially.

Nonetheless, proper initial triage of patients suspected to have acute coronary ischemia should eventually identify patients as having (1) ACS; (2) a non-ACS cardiovascular condition such as myocarditis/myopericarditis, stress-related cardiomyopathy, aortic dissection, or pulmonary embolism; (3) a noncardiac cause of chest pain such as gastroesophageal reflux; and (4) a noncardiac condition that is yet undefined, such as sepsis.[6] ACS patients with new evidence of ST-segment elevation on the presenting ECG are labeled as having an ST-segment elevation myocardial infarction (STEMI) and should be considered for immediate reperfusion therapy by thrombolytics or percutaneous coronary intervention (PCI); those without ST-segment elevation but with evidence of myonecrosis are deemed to have a non–ST-segment elevation myocardial infarction (NSTEMI); and those without any evidence of myonecrosis are diagnosed with unstable angina (Fig. 56–1).

DEFINITION OF UNSTABLE ANGINA

Unstable angina is usually secondary to reduced myocardial perfusion resulting from coronary artery atherothrombosis. In this event, however, the nonocclusive thrombus that developed on a disrupted atherosclerotic plaque does not result in any biochemical evidence of myocardial necrosis. Unstable angina and NSTEMI can be viewed as very closely related clinical conditions with similar presentations and pathogenesis but of differing severity.

Because of the lack of objective data associated with the condition, unstable angina (also known as *preinfarction angina, intermediate coronary syndrome,* and *acute coronary insufficiency*) must be diagnosed from careful history taking and is thus the most subjective of the

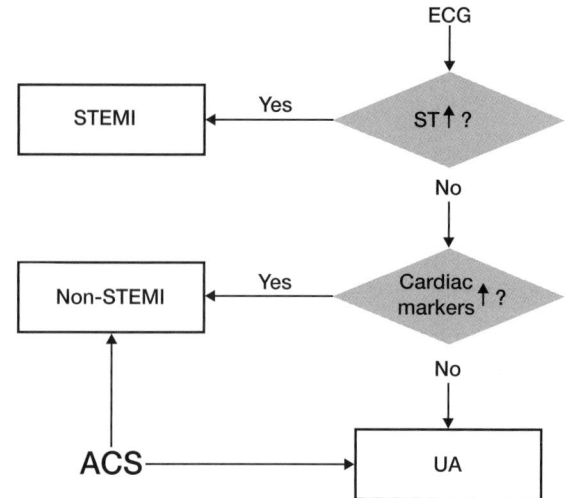

FIGURE 56–1. Acute chest pain syndromes: classification. ACS, acute coronary syndrome; NSTEMI, non–ST-segment elevation myocardial infarction; STEMI, ST-segment elevation myocardial infarction; UA, unstable angina.

ACS diagnoses. The Agency for Health Care Policy and Research has published guidelines listing features that signify the likelihood of signs and symptoms suggestive of an ACS likely caused by CHD (Table 56–1).[7] There are three principal presentations of unstable angina: (1) rest angina or angina with minimal exertion usually lasting at least 20 minutes; (2) new-onset severe angina, usually defined as occurring within the last month; and (3) crescendo angina, defined as previously diagnosed angina that has become distinctly more frequent, longer in duration, or more severe in nature.[8]

TABLE 56–1

Likelihood That Signs and Symptoms Represent an Acute Coronary Syndrome Secondary to Coronary Artery Disease

FEATURE	HIGH LIKELIHOOD: ANY OF THE FOLLOWING	INTERMEDIATE LIKELIHOOD: ABSENCE OF HIGH-LIKELIHOOD FEATURES AND PRESENCE OF ANY OF THE FOLLOWING	LOW LIKELIHOOD: ABSENCE OF HIGH- OR INTERMEDIATE-LIKELIHOOD FEATURES BUT MAY HAVE
History	Chest or left arm pain or discomfort as chief symptom reproducing documented angina; known history of CAD, including MI	Chest or left arm pain or discomfort as chief symptom; age >70 years; male sex; diabetes mellitus	Probable ischemic symptoms in absence of any of the intermediate likelihood characteristics; recent cocaine use
Examination	Transient MR, hypotension, diaphoresis, pulmonary edema or rales	Extracardiac vascular disease	Chest discomfort reproduced by palpation
ECG	New, or presumably new, transient, ST-segment deviation (≥ 0.05 mV) or T-wave inversion (≥ 0.2 mV) with symptoms	Fixed Q waves; abnormal ST segments or T waves not documented to be new	T-wave flattening or inversion in leads with dominant R waves; normal ECG
Cardiac markers	Elevated cardiac TnI, TnT, or CK-MB	Normal	Normal

CAD, coronary artery disease; CK-MB, creatine kinase myocardial band; MI, myocardial infarction; MR, mitral regurgitation; TnI, troponin I; TnT, troponin T.

TABLE 56-2

Grading of Angina Pectoris According to Canadian Cardiovascular Society Classification

CLASS	DESCRIPTION OF STAGE
I	"Ordinary physical activity does not cause...angina," such as walking or climbing stairs. Angina occurs with strenuous, rapid or prolonged exertion at work or recreation.
II	"Slight limitation of ordinary activity." Angina occurs on walking or climbing stairs rapidly; walking uphill; walking or stair climbing after meals; in cold, in wind, or under emotional stress; or only during the few hours after awakening. Angina occurs on walking >2 level blocks and climbing >1 flight of ordinary stairs at normal pace and under normal conditions.
III	"Marked limitation of ordinary physical activity." Angina occurs on walking 1 to 2 level blocks and climbing 1 flight of ordinary stairs under normal conditions and at normal pace.
IV	"Inability to carry on any physical activity" without discomfort—anginal symptoms may be present at rest.

Because of the heterogenous nature of the patients who fall under these loose definitions, many classification schemes have been proposed for unstable angina. Although not devised precisely to help define unstable angina, the Canadian Cardiovascular Society (CCS) has developed an easy classification system to grade anginal symptoms (Table 56–2).[9] Class I angina is the least symptomatic and denotes that ordinary physical activity does not illicit anginal symptoms. Class II angina implies anginal symptoms that slightly impair ordinary activity such as walking >2 blocks or climbing >1 flight of stairs. Class III angina is defined as symptoms that limit markedly ordinary physical activity such as walking <1 block or climbing <1 flight of stairs. Finally, Class IV angina is symptoms at rest or that cause an inability to carry on any physical activity without discomfort. Using this classification, crescendo angina can be defined as symptoms that result in at least 1 CCS class increase or to at least CCS class III severity.[10]

Braunwald developed a useful classification of unstable angina by assessing risk.[11] By differentiating the severity and clinical circumstances surrounding the presentation of unstable angina and considering also the presence or absence of ECG changes and the intensity of medical therapy, Braunwald has estimated the risk of death or myocardial infarction (MI) at 1 year. In terms of severity, class I unstable angina is new onset or accelerated angina but with no rest pain. Class II presents with rest angina within the last month but not within the previous 48 hours. Class III angina presents at rest and within the last 48 hours of initial evaluation. In terms of clinical circumstances, class A represents unstable angina in the setting of a secondary noncoronary cause of demand ischemia such as anemia, hypotension, or prolonged tachycardia. Class B is worsening primary CHD in the absence of extracardiac conditions. Class C is postinfarction unstable angina within 2 weeks of a documented MI (Table 56–3). Furthermore, patients fared worse over the following 12 months if they presented with transient ST-T–wave changes during pain and if they had angina despite maximal antiischemic therapy. In summary, patients with a 48-hour pain-free interval and the absence of ECG changes were at decreased risk, whereas those with postinfarction angina and the need for maximal medical therapy have the highest risk of death or MI over the next 1 year after presentation with unstable angina.

The Agency for Health Care Policy and Research (AHCPR) also has published guidelines assessing the short-term risk of death or nonfatal MI in patients with unstable angina using similar clinical features (Table 56–4). It should be noted that an elevated level of a cardiac marker such as a troponin places the patient at high risk. These patients would now be considered to have a NSTEMI instead of high risk unstable angina. The risk of death at 6 months with unstable angina is approximately 3 percent versus 9 percent with NSTEMI, illustrating the importance of an accurate diagnosis.[11]

Although nonocclusive thrombus on a preexisting atherosclerotic plaque is the most common cause of unstable angina/NSTEMI, other causes may lead to acute coronary ischemia (Table 56–5).[6] A less-common cause is dynamic obstruction of an

TABLE 56-3

Braunwald Classification of Unstable Angina

SEVERITY	CLINICAL CIRCUMSTANCES		
	A. DEVELOPS IN PRESENCE OF EXTRACARDIAC CONDITION THAT INTENSIFIES MYOCARDIAL ISCHEMIA (SECONDARY UA)	B. DEVELOPS IN ABSENCE OF EXTRACARDIAC CONDITION (PRIMARY UA)	C. DEVELOPS WITHIN 2 WEEKS AFTER ACUTE MI (POSTINFARCT UA)
I.	IA	IB	IC
II.	IIA	IIB	IIC
III.	IIIA	IIIB	IIIC

MI, myocardial infarction; UA, unstable angina.

TABLE 56–4

Short-Term Risk of Death or Nonfatal Myocardial Infarction in Patients with Unstable Angina

FEATURE	HIGH RISK: AT LEAST 1 OF THE FOLLOWING FEATURES MUST BE PRESENT	INTERMEDIATE RISK: NO HIGH-RISK FEATURE BUT MUST HAVE 1 OF THE FOLLOWING	LOW RISK: NO HIGH- OR INTERMEDIATE-RISK FEATURE BUT MAY HAVE ANY OF THE FOLLOWING
History	Accelerating tempo of ischemic symptoms in preceding 48 h	Prior MI, peripheral or cerebrovascular disease or CABG, prior aspirin use	
Character of pain	Prolonged ongoing (>20 min) rest pain	Prolonged (>20 min) rest angina, now resolved, with moderate or high likelihood of CAD; rest angina (<20 min) or relieved with rest or sublingual NTG	New-onset or progressive CCS class III or IV angina within the past 2 weeks without prolonged (>20 min) rest pain but with moderate or high likelihood of CAD (see Table 56–1).
Clinical findings	Pulmonary edema, most likely caused by ischemia; new or worsening MR murmur; S_3 or new/worsening rales; hypotension, bradycardia, tachycardia; age >75 years	Age >70 years	
ECG	Angina at rest with transient ST-segment changes >0.05 mV; bundle-branch block, new or presumed new; sustained ventricular tachycardia	T-wave inversions >0.2 mV; Pathologic Q waves	Normal or unchanged ECG during an episode of chest discomfort
Cardiac markers	Elevated (e.g., TnT or TnI >0.1 ng/mL)	Slightly elevated (e.g., TnT >0.01 bnut <0.1 ng/mL)	Normal

CABG, coronary artery bypass graft; CAD, coronary artery disease; CCS, Canadian Cardiovascular Society; MI, myocardial infarction; MR, mitral regurgitation; NTG, nitroglycerin; Tn, troponin.

epicardial artery leading to intense focal spasm (Prinzmetal angina). It is thought that this spasm is caused by hypercontractility of vascular smooth muscle and/or endothelial dysfunction. Abnormal constriction of small intramural resistance vessels can also lead to dynamic obstruction and acute ischemia. A third cause of unstable angina is severe mechanical obstruction without spasm or thrombus. An example would be restenosis after PCI or some patients with progressive atherosclerosis. A fourth cause is arterial inflammation and/or infection. It is thought that chronic inflammation perhaps related to infection lead to activation of macrophages and T-lymphocytes at the shoulder of a vulnerable plaque and increased expression of metalloproteinase resulting in disruption and rupture of the plaque. Finally, a fifth cause of unstable angina is alluded to in Braunwald's classification, namely unstable angina from a secondary cause. These patients generally have chronic stable CHD that worsens as a result of a noncoronary condition that increases myocardial oxygen demand, such as fever, tachycardia, reduced coronary blood flow caused by hypotension, and reduced blood myocardial oxygen content such as with hypoxemia or anemia. These causes are not mutually exclusive.

NON–ST-SEGMENT ELEVATION MYOCARDIAL INFARCTION

For many years, the diagnosis of an acute myocardial infarction was defined by the World Health Organization as having two of the following three criteria: (1) typical ischemic chest pain; (2) typical ECG pattern including the development of Q waves; (3) typical rise and fall in serum markers of myocardial injury, usually creatine kinase myocardial band (CK-MB).[12] If the patient did not have evidence of ST elevation or Q waves, and the CK-MB was elevated, the patient was diagnosed with a NSTEMI. Those patients with acute ischemic chest pain without evidence of ST elevation or Q waves and who had negative CK-MB levels were thought to have unstable angina.

With the introduction of serum troponin levels, which were much more sensitive and specific for myonecrosis than CK-MB levels, a joint European Society of Cardiology (ESC) and American College of Cardiology (ACC) committee convened and in 2000 proposed the following definition of an acute, evolving, or recent MI: Typical rise and gradual fall of serum troponin levels or

TABLE 56–5

Secondary Precipitants of Myocardial Ischemia

INCREASED MYOCARDIAL OXYGEN DEMAND

Fever
Thyrotoxicosis
Tachycardia
Malignant hypertension
Pheochromocytoma
Aortic stenosis
High output state
Pregnancy
Drugs, cocaine, amphetamine

DECREASED OXYGEN SUPPLY

Anemia
Hypoxemia
Carbon monoxide poisoning
Polycythemia vera
Hyperviscosity syndromes

a more rapid rise and fall of serum CK-MB levels in addition to presenting with either ischemic symptoms, development of pathologic Q waves on ECG, ST-segment changes indicative of ischemia, or coronary artery intervention (e.g., PCI).[13]

Patients presenting with NSTEMI have an intermediate risk of acute complications when compared to unstable angina (lower risk) and STEMI (higher risk) with a 30-day mortality rate of approximately 5 percent.[11] Interestingly, at 6 months, patients who present with NSTEMI actually have a higher mortality rate than do those with STEMI.[11] Because evidence of myonecrosis is required, the diagnosis of NSTEMI is less subject to error versus unstable angina, and requires more careful monitoring and aggressive therapy. In fact, the most important reason to differentiate true unstable angina from NSTEMI is in the management strategy during the early hospitalization period. It is becoming increasingly evident from recent large, randomized, multicenter clinical trials that early aggressive management with enhanced antiplatelet (clopidogrel and glycoprotein IIb/IIIa inhibitors) and earlier angiography/mechanical revascularization is superior to conservative traditional medical therapy and ischemia-guided revascularization (see Fig. 56–1).[14–16]

BIOMARKERS OF MYONECROSIS

Because the diagnosis of NSTEMI implies ischemia severe enough to cause sufficient myocardial damage to release detectable quantities of a marker of myocardial injury, it is important to discuss the different cardiac markers of injury. Biochemical markers such as troponins, creatinine kinase, and myoglobin are useful both prognostically and for the diagnosis of myonecrosis.[17] An ideal cardiac marker would be very specific to cardiac muscle and absent from nonmyocardial tissue. It would be released quickly into the peripheral blood after onset of injury and reflect quantitatively the magnitude of necrosis. Finally, the

marker should be easy to use, quick to measure, cheap to measure, and stable in vitro. Each laboratory should know the 99th percentile limits of the measurement.

Until recently creatine kinase (CK) activity has been the most widely used serum cardiac marker for the evaluation of ACS. Although this marker is very sensitive for detecting myocardial damage (average time to peak is 24 hours and becomes initially elevated in 4 to 8 hours after insult) and can accurately predict the magnitude of necrosis, several limitations do exist with this marker. CK levels are elevated in patients with muscle disease, alcohol intoxication, skeletal muscle trauma, seizures, vigorous exercise, thoracic outlet syndrome, and pulmonary embolism. Even the more cardiac muscle specific myocardial band (MB) isoform may be present in the tongue, small intestine, uterus, and prostate.

Recent methods to improve specificity include measurement of CK-MB levels by specific enzyme immunoassays that use monoclonal antibodies directed against CK-MB (mass method) and by measuring CK-MB isoforms. The mass method of CK-MB levels has proved to be more accurate than traditional radioimmunoassay or agarose gel electrophoresis methods, especially in patients presenting within 4 hours of injury. CK-MB isoforms exist in only one form in cardiac muscle (CK-MB2) but exists in different isoforms in the plasma (CK-MB1). An absolute value of CK-MB2 of greater than 1 U/L and a ratio of CK-MB2:CK-MB1 of greater than 2.5 has significantly improved the sensitivity of diagnosing myonecrosis at 6 hours.[18] However, these isoform assays are not readily available and are still limited by specificity issues concerning CK-MB levels in the heart versus other tissues.

Cardiac troponins represent a major clinical shift in the diagnosis of NSTEMI. The troponin complex consists of three subunits that regulate contraction of cardiac muscle: Troponin I (TnI), TnT, and TnC. Troponin C binds to calcium; TnI binds to actin and inhibits the actin-myosin interaction; TnT binds to tropomyosin, which attaches the troponin complex to the thin filament. Monoclonal antibody-based immunoassays have been developed to detect the cardiac-specific TnT and TnI. Because cardiac and smooth muscle share isoforms for TnC, no immunoassays of TnC have been developed to date. Because of the increased sensitivity and specificity of cardiac troponins relative to CK, it is estimated that up to 30 percent of patients who present with rest pain and normal CK-MB levels and who were previously diagnosed with unstable angina, should be reclassified as having NSTEMI when assessed with troponins.[19] There is some controversy as to whether the subgroup of patients with negative CK-MB levels and minor elevations in troponins should be labeled as having high-risk unstable angina or NSTEMI. Some investigators have used the term *microinfarction* or *minor myocardial damage* to describe this situation.[20] Similarly, there is controversy regarding the labeling of a patient with no significant ECG changes and a minor troponin elevation as having unstable angina or NSTEMI.

Regardless of the etiology of troponin release, an elevated level implies a worse prognosis.[21,22] An elevated troponin level indicates a higher risk subgroup independent of ECG presentation and predischarge exercise testing.[23] There is an incremental risk of death or MI in patients with elevated troponins that can be seen in a quantitative fashion, even in patients with chronic renal insufficiency.[24] Even patients in whom CK-MB levels are within normal limits, troponin elevation signifies an increased risk of death when compared with those without elevation.[25]

It should be emphasized that cardiac troponins should be used only as one tool in the initial evaluation along with the history, physical examination (heart failure, hypotension, tachycardia, mitral regurgitation all portend a poor prognosis), and baseline ECG in making a diagnosis of ACS. Most patients with high-risk clinical and ECG features will have elevated troponin levels. Still, it has been documented that decompensated heart failure can elevate troponin levels, indicating that myocardial damage from any etiology may lead to elevated levels.[26]

An elevated troponin level is an easy and objective method for identifying high-risk ACS patients. For example, glycoprotein IIb/IIIa inhibitor in the acute medical management of coronary ischemia is mostly beneficial in patients with elevated troponin levels.[27,28] Furthermore, there is convincing data that early angiography and mechanical revascularization is superior to medical therapy in patients with NSTEMI and troponin elevation.[12–14]

Myoglobin is a low-molecular-weight heme protein found in both cardiac and skeletal muscle. Although not specific for cardiac muscle, it is released very rapidly from necrotic myocardium, usually within 2 hours after onset of injury. Levels are only elevated for 24 hours, limiting the time period of use. Confirmation of myonecrosis should be made with a more specific marker such as cardiac troponins or CK-MB levels. Because of its high sensitivity, however, myoglobin measurements made within 4 to 8 hours of symptom onset can be used to rule out a myocardial infarction if normal levels are documented.[29]

The Diagnostic Marker Cooperative Study evaluated the role of these biochemical markers in the evaluation of ACS patients.[30] This large, multicenter, randomized, double-blind study of patients suspected of a MI in the emergency department compared the sensitivity and specificity of both cardiac troponin assays, CK-MB mass levels, CK-MB isoforms, and myoglobin for the diagnosis of myonecrosis. Within the first 6 hours of symptom onset, CK-MB isoforms and myoglobin were the most efficient for diagnosis, whereas both cardiac troponins proved to be the most cardiac specific and were very useful for the late diagnosis of MI as their levels usually remain elevated for 7–14 days (Table 56–6).

In summary, cardiac troponins have become the biochemical marker of choice in the evaluation of myonecrosis and the diagnosis of NSTEMI. Its greater sensitivity and specificity for cardiac muscle damage, in addition to its proven prognostic value, has established its current clinical position. CK-MB levels by mass method remains a reliable method to diagnose more than minor myocardial damage. CK-MB isoforms are particularly useful in detecting early myocardial damage. Because of its high sensitivity to detect myonecrosis, myoglobin levels can be used in the early hours after symptom onset to rule out myocardial infarction. Table 56–7 summarizes the strengths and weaknesses of each cardiac marker.

Research continues on new biochemical cardiac markers for injury. For example, there has been much interest in documenting levels of inflammatory markers such as C-reactive protein, serum amyloid A, and interleukin-6 in patients with unstable angina.[31–33] Although there is hard evidence now that these inflammatory markers can help to risk-stratify patients with unstable angina/NSTEMI on presentation, they are not valid for diagnosing myonecrosis at this time. Levels of circulating soluble adhesion molecules, such as E-selectin and intercellular adhesion molecule-1, are under investigation.[34] Finally, markers of the coagulation cascade, such as fibrinopeptide and fibrinogen levels, appear to signify an increased risk of death in ACS patients.[35,36] Clinically, none of these markers are currently accepted as a biochemical means of demonstrating myocardial infarction.

ST-SEGMENT ELEVATION MYOCARDIAL INFARCTION

STEMI represents the most lethal form of acute coronary syndrome, one in which a completely occlusive thrombus results in total cessation of coronary blood flow in the territory of the occluded artery and the resultant ST-segment elevation on the ECG. Typically, new Q waves evolve because of full- or nearly full-thickness necrosis of the ventricular wall supplied by the occluded artery. As this may only occur in up to 70 percent of patients and because a minority of patients without ST-segment elevation can eventually develop new Q waves, the nomenclature has changed from Q-wave myocardial infarction to STEMI.[37,38]

The actual diagnosis of an STEMI does not completely rely on the ECG itself, as the name might imply. As mentioned earlier, the classic World Health Organization criteria for an acute myocardial infarction requires that two of the following three elements be

---

TABLE 56–6

European Society of Cardiologists/American College of Cardiology Definition of Myocardial Infarction

The diagnosis of acute myocardial infarction (MI) requires the following criteria for acute, evolving, or recent MI—a typical rise and gradual fall (troponin) or more rapid rise and fall (creatine kinase myocardial band) of biochemical markers of myocardial necrosis with at least one of the following:

- Ischemic symptoms;
- Development of pathologic Q waves on the electrocardiogram;
- Electrocardiogram changes indicative of ischemia (ST segment elevation or depression);
- Coronary artery intervention (e.g., coronary angioplasty); or
- Pathologic findings of an acute MI.

Criteria for established MI includes:

- Development of new pathologic Q waves on serial electrocardiograms. The patient may or may not remember previous symptoms. Biochemical markers of myocardial necrosis may have normalized, depending on the length of time that has passed since the infarct developed; or
- Pathologic findings of a healed or healing MI.

TABLE 56–7

Biochemical Cardiac Markers for the Evaluation and Management of Patients with Suspected Acute Coronary Syndrome but without ST-Segment Elevation of 12-Lead Echocardiogram

MARKER	ADVANTAGES	DISADVANTAGES	POINT OF CARE TEST AVAILABLE?	COMMENT	CLINICAL RECOMMENDATION
CK-MB	1. Rapid, cost-efficient, accurate assay 2. Ability to detect early reinfarction	1. Loss of specificity in setting of skeletal muscle disease of injury, including surgery 2. Low sensitivity during very early MI (<6 h after symptom onset) or later after symptom onset (>36 h) and for minor myocardial damage (detectable with troponins)	Yes	Familiar to majority of clinicians	Prior standard and still acceptable diagnostic test in most clinical circumstances
CK-MB isoforms	1. Early detection of MI	1. Specificity profile similar to that of CK-MB 2. Current assays require special expertise	No	Experience to date predominantly in dedicated research centers	Used for extremely early (3–6 h after symptom onset) detection of MI in centers with demonstrated familiarity with assay technique
Myoglobin	1. High sensitivity 2. Useful in early detection of MI 3. Detection of reperfusion 4. Most useful in ruling out MI	1. Very low specificity in setting of skeletal muscle injury or disease 2. Rapid return to normal range limits sensitivity for later presentations	Yes	More convenient early marker than CK-MB isoforms because of greater availability of assays for myoglobin; rapid-release kinetics make myoglobin useful for non-invasive monitoring of reperfusion in patients with established MI	
Cardiac troponins	1. Powerful tool for risk stratification 2. Greater sensitivity and specificity than CK-MB 3. Detection of recent MI up to 2 weeks after onset 4. Useful for selection therapy 5. Detection of reperfusion	1. Low sensitivity in very early phase of MI (<6 h after symptom onset) and requires repeat measurement at 8–12 h, if negative 2. Limited ability to detect late minor reinfarction	Yes	Data on diagnostic performance and potential therapeutic implications increasingly available from clinical trials	Useful as a single test to efficiently diagnose NSTEMI (including minor myocardial damage), with serial measurements; clinicians should familiarize themselves with diagnostic "cutoffs" used in their local hospital laboratory

CK-MB, creatine kinase myocardial band; MI, myocardial infarction; NSTEMI, non–ST-segment elevation myocardial infarction.

present: (1) a history suggestive of coronary ischemia for a prolonged period of time (>30 minutes), (2) evolutionary changes on serial ECGs suggestive of myocardial infarction, and (3) a rise and fall in serum cardiac markers consistent with myonecrosis. Only two of the three criteria are needed because of the wide variability in the pattern of patient presentation with acute myocardial infarction. It has been estimated that up to one-third of patients with STEMI do not describe classic chest pain.[39] On the other hand, because of the multitude of etiologies producing chest pain, objective evidence of myocardial necrosis is needed in order to confirm a MI. ST-segment elevation from noncoronary causes such as pericarditis, left ventricular hypertrophy, or J-point elevation must be differentiated from true myocardial ischemia.

The accurate diagnosis of STEMI is of paramount importance for two reasons. First, the diagnosis mandates immediate consideration for reperfusion therapy, either by thrombolytic agents or by mechanical revascularization, most probably PCI. Mortality has been significantly decreased by reperfusion within 12 hours of onset of symptoms in patients with STEMI.[40] However, both pharmacologic and mechanical means of reperfusion have potentially fatal side effects or complications and should not be employed unless diagnosis is relatively certain. To prevent unnecessary dangers, thrombolytic agents are only recommended for at least a 2-mm ST-segment elevation in at least two contiguous leads in the precordium or at least a 1-mm ST-segment elevation in two contiguous limb leads in addition to biochemical marker data and clinical history.[41] It should be noted that a new left bundle-branch block in the clinical setting of an acute myocardial infarction also meets criteria for aggressive revascularization therapy with thrombolytic agents or by mechanical means.

PERIPROCEDURAL MYOCARDIAL INFARCTION

Periprocedural CK-MB or troponin release can be seen in up to 50 percent of patients who undergo PCI. The etiology of this may be obvious and apparent on angiography such as no reflow, thrombus formation, side-branch closure, or coronary dissection. However, up to 30 percent of CK-MB or troponin release cannot be predicted during the procedure. These instances are usually caused by distal embolization of plaque during the procedure itself, for example, during atherectomy, ballooning, or stent placement. It is important to recognize periprocedural NSTEMI because the release of detectable biomarkers do not indicate the usual high-risk state seen in patients with spontaneous NSTEMI. In fact, only patients with CK-MB levels greater than five or eight times normal after a PCI may have long-term deleterious outcomes. Furthermore, elevated troponin levels near the time of the procedure do not add any prognostic information on top of CK-MB in this setting.

CONCLUSIONS

The definitions of acute coronary syndromes have become more important as new therapies have been developed. Unstable angina, NSTEMI, and STEMI all share similar pathophysiologic characteristics but the severity of their clinical presentations differs. By

accurately diagnosing each patient as having unstable angina, NSTEMI, or STEMI, the medical team can treat each appropriately. Medical therapy alone might be sufficient for the majority of patients with unstable angina. Those patients with NSTEMI may require more urgent mechanical revascularization and more intensive antiplatelet/antithrombotic therapy. Patients with STEMI require emergent revascularization therapy if possible in addition to aggressive secondary treatment of CHD such as statins, blockers, and angiotensin-converting enzyme inhibitors.

Finally, it is important to diagnose accurately and define the grades of ACS for physicians to assess the benefits and risks of the ever-evolving and available therapies for each individual patient. Bleeding may occur in low-risk patients who are too aggressively treated, whereas reinfarction may occur in higher-risk patients who do not receive adequate medical and/or mechanical therapies. To this end, cardiac troponins, a more accurate biochemical marker of myonecrosis, is especially useful in diagnosing the higher-risk NSTEMI patients who previously may have been erroneously diagnosed and treated as unstable angina.

REFERENCES

1. The American Heart Association. *2004 Heart and Stroke Statistical Update.* Dallas, TX: American Heart Association, 2004.
2. Anderson RN. *U.S. Decennial Life* Tables for 1989–91. *Vol. 1 No. 4. United States Life Tables. Eliminating Certain Causes of Death.* Hyattsville, MD: National Center for Health Statistics, 1999.
3. Fuster V, Badimon L, Badimon JJ, Chesebro JH. The pathogenesis of coronary artery disease and the acute coronary syndromes. Part 1. *N Engl J Med* 1992:326;242–250.
4. Fuster, V, Moreno PR, Fayad ZA, Corti R, Badimon JS. Atherothrombosis and high-risk plaque: part 1: evolving concepts. *J Am Coll Cardiol* 2005;46:937–954.
5. Braunwald, E, Mark DB, Jones RH, et al. *Unstable Angina: Diagnosis and Management.* AHCPR Publication 94–0602.Rockville, MD: Agency for Health Care Policy and Research and the National Heart, Lung, and Blood Institute, U.S. Public Health Service, U.S. Department of Health and Human Services; 1994:1.
6. Braunwald E, Antman EM, Beasley, et al. ACC/AHA guideline for the management of patients with unstable angina and non-ST-segment elevation myocardial infarction: a report of the American College of Cardiology/American Heart Association Task Force on Practice Guidelines (Committee on the Management of Patients with Unstable Angina). *J Am Coll Cardiol* 2002;40:1366–1374.
7. Braunwald E. Unstable angina: an etiologic approach to management [editorial]. *Circulation* 1998;98:2219–2222.
8. Betriu A, Heras M, Cohen M, Fuster V. Unstable angina: outcome according to clinical presentation. *J Am Coll Cardiol* 1992;19:1659–1663.
9. Campeau L. Grading of angina pectoris [letter]. *Circulation* 1976;54:522.
10. Braunwald E. Unstable angina: a classification. *Circulation* 1989;80:410–414.
11. Fuster V, Badimon L, Badimon JJ, Chesebro JH. The pathogenesis of coronary artery disease and the acute coronary syndromes. Part 2. *N Engl J Med* 1992;326:310–318.
12. Cannon CP, Weintraub WS, Demopolous LA, et al. Comparison of early invasive and conservative strategies in patients with unstable coronary syndromes treated with the glycoprotein IIb/IIIa inhibitor tirofiban. *N Engl J Med* 2001;344:1879–1887.
13. The Fragmin and Fast Revascularization During Instability in Coronary Artery Disease Investigators: Invasive compared with non-invasive treatment in unstable coronary artery disease: FRISC II prospective randomized multicentre study. *Lancet* 1999;354:708–715.
14. Fox KAA, Poole-Wilson PA, Henderson RA, et al.. Interventional versus conservative treatment for patients with unstable angina or non-ST-elevation myocardial infarction: the British Heart Foundation RITA 3 randomised trial. *Lancet* 2002;360:743–751.
15. Roberts R, Fromm RE. Management of acute coronary syndromes based on risk stratification by biochemical markers: an idea whose time has come. *Circulation* 1998;98:1831–1833.

16. Mair J, Morandell D, Genser N, Lechleitner P, Dienstl F, Puschendorf B. Equivalent early sensitivities of myoglobin, creatinine kinase MB mass, creatinine kinase isoform ratios, and cardiac troponins I and T for acute myocardial infarction. *Clin Chem* 1995;41:1266–1272.

17. Puleo PR, Meyer D, Wathen C, et al. Use of a rapid assay of subforms of creatinine kinase-MB to diagnose or rule out acute myocardial infarction. *N Engl J Med* 1994;331:561–566.

18. Apple FS, Falahati A, Paulsen PR, Miller EA, Sharkey SW. Improved detection of minor ischemic myocardial injury with measurement of serum cardiac troponin I. *Clin Chem* 1997;43:2047–2051.

19. Bertrand ME, Simoons ML, Fox KA, et al. Management of acute coronary syndromes: acute coronary syndromes without ST-elevation: recommendations of the Task Force of the European Society of Cardiology. *Eur Heart J* 2000;21:1406–1432.

20. Hamm CW, Goldmann BU, Heesschen C, Kreymann G, Berger J, Meinertz T. Emergency room triage of patients with acute chest pain by means of rapid testing for cardiac troponin T or troponin I. *N Engl J Med* 1997;337:1648–1653.

21. Ohman EM, Armstrong PW, Christenson RH, et al. Cardiac troponin T levels for risk stratification in acute myocardial ischemia. *N Engl J Med* 1996;335:1333–1341.

22. Antman EM, Tanasijevic MJ, Thompson B, et al. Cardiac-specific troponin I levels to predict the risk of mortality in patients with acute coronary syndromes. *N Engl J Med* 1996;335:1342–1349.

23. Galvani M, Ottani F, Ferrini D, et al. Prognostic influence of elevated troponin I in patients with unstable angina. *Circulation* 1997;95:2053–2059.

24. Aviles RJ, Askari AT, Lindahl B, et al. Troponin T levels in patients with acute coronary syndromes, with or without renal dysfunction. *N Engl J Med* 2002;346:2047–2052.

25. Stubbs P, Collinson P, Moseley D, Greenwood T, Noble M. Prospective study of the role of cardiac troponin T in patients admitted with unstable angina. *BMJ* 1996;313:262–264.

26. Del Carlo CH, O'Connor CM. Cardiac troponins in congestive heart failure. *Am Heart J* 1999;138:646–653.

27. Hamm CW, Heeschen C, Goldmann B, et al. Benefit of abciximab in patients with refractory unstable angina in relation to serum troponin T levels. *N Engl J Med* 1999;340:1623–1629.

28. Heeschen C, Hamm CW, Goldmann B, et al. Platelet receptor inhibition in ischemic syndrome management. Troponin concentrations for stratification of patients with acute coronary syndromes in relation to therapeutic efficacy of tirofiban. *Lancet* 1999;354:1757–1762.

29. Zaninotto M, Altinier S, Lachin M, Celegon L, Plebani M. Strategies for the early diagnosis of acute myocardial infarction using biochemical markers. *Am J Clin Pathol* 1999;111:399–405.

30. Zimmerman J, Fromm R, Meyer D, et al. Diagnostic Marker Cooperative Study for the diagnosis of myocardial infarction. *Circulation* 1999;99:1671–1677.

31. Morrow DA, Rifai N, Antman EM, et al. C-reactive protein is a potent predictor of mortality independently of and in combination with troponin T in acute coronary syndromes: a TIMI 11A substudy. Thrombolysis in Myocardial Infarction. *J Am Coll Cardiol* 1998;31:1460–1465.

32. Morrow DA, Rifai N, Antman EM, et al. Serum amyloid A predicts early mortality in acute coronary syndromes. A TIMI 11A substudy. *J Am Coll Cardiol* 2000;35:358–362.

33. Biasucci LM, Vitelli A, Liuzzo G, et al. Elevated levels of interleukin-6 in unstable angina. *Circulation* 1996;94:874–877.

34. Ghasias NK, Shahi CN, Foley B, et al. Elevated levels of circulating soluble adhesion molecules in peripheral blood of patients with unstable angina. *Am J Cardiol* 1997;80:617–619.

35. Ardissino D, Merlini PA, Gamba G, et al. Thrombin activity and early outcome in unstable angina pectoris. *Circulation* 1996;93:1634–1639.

36. Becker RC, Cannon CP, Bovill EG, et al. Prognostic value of plasma fibrinogen concentration in patients with unstable angina and non–Q-wave myocardial infarction (TIMI IIIB Trial). *Am J Cardiol* 1996;78:142–147.

37. Myocardial infarction redefined—a consensus document of the Joint European Society of Cardiology/American College of Cardiology Committee for the redefinition of myocardial infarction. *J Am Coll Cardiol* 2000;36:959–969.

38. Pedoe-Tunstall H, Kuulasmaa K, Amouyel P, et al. Myocardial infarction and coronary deaths in the World Health Organization MONICA Project. *Circulation* 1994;90:583–612.

39. Canto JG, Every NR, Magid DJ, et al. The volume of primary angioplasty procedures and survival after acute myocardial infarction. National Registry of Myocardial Infarction 2 Investigators. *N Engl J Med* 2000;342:1573–1580.

40. Califf RM. Ten years of benefit from a one-hour intervention. *Circulation* 1998;98:2649–2651.

41. Ryan TJ, Antman EM, Brooks NH, et al. 1999 Update: ACC/AHA guidelines for the management of patients with acute myocardial infarction: executive summary and recommendations: a report of the American College of Cardiology/American Heart Association Task Force on Practice Guidelines (Committee on Management of Acute Myocardial Infarction). *Circulation* 1999;100:1016–1030.

CHAPTER 57

Pathology of Myocardial Ischemia, Infarction, Reperfusion, and Sudden Death

Allen P. Burke / Renu Virmani

PATHOPHYSIOLOGY OF MYOCARDIAL ISCHEMIA

The major cause of acute myocardial infarction is coronary atherosclerosis with superimposed luminal thrombus, which accounts for more than 80 percent of all infarcts. Myocardial infarctions resulting from nonatherosclerotic diseases of the coronary arteries are rare. In past decades, there have been several trends regarding the epidemiology and outcome of patients hospitalized with acute myocardial infarction. Over the time span from 1975 to 2001, patients became significantly older, were more likely to be women, and were more likely to receive effective cardiac medications. Despite a greater prevalence of comorbidities, hospital survival rates have improved over time.[1]

【 】 MECHANISMS OF MYOCARDIAL INJURY

The normal function of the heart muscle is supported by high rates of myocardial blood flow, oxygen consumption, and combustion of fat and carbohydrates (glucose and lactate). Under normal aerobic conditions, cardiac energy is derived from fatty acids, supplying 60 to 90 percent of the energy for adenosine triphosphate (ATP) synthesis (Fig. 57–1). The rest of the energy (10 to 40 percent) comes from oxidation of pyruvate formed from glycolysis and lactate oxidation. Almost all of the ATP formed comes from oxidative phosphorylation in the mitochondria; only a small amount of ATP (<2 percent) is synthesized by glycolysis. Approximately two-thirds of the ATP used by the heart goes to contractile shortening, and the remaining one-third is used by sarcoplasmic reticulum Ca^{2+} ATPase and other ion pumps.

Sudden occlusion of a major branch of a coronary artery shifts aerobic or mitochondrial metabolism to anaerobic glycolysis within seconds of reduced arterial flow. Myocardial ischemia primarily affects mitochondrial metabolism resulting in decrease in ATP formation by shutting off oxidative phosphorylation. The reduced aerobic ATP formation stimulates glycolysis and an increase in myocardial glucose uptake and glycogen breakdown (Fig. 57–2). Decreased

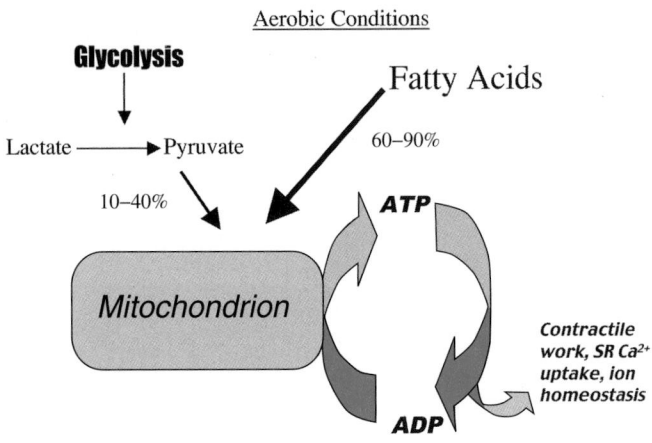

FIGURE 57–1. Cardiac energy metabolism under normal aerobic conditions. Fatty acids are the primary source of energy for the heart, supplying 60 to 90 percent of the energy for adenosine triphosphate (ATP) synthesis. The balance (10 to 40 percent) comes from the oxidation of pyruvate formed from glycolysis and lactate oxidation. Almost all of the ATP formation comes from oxidative phosphorylation in the mitochondria; only a trivial amount of ATP (<2 percent of the total) is synthesized by glycolysis. ADP, adenosine diphosphate; SR, sarcoplasmic reticulum. *Source: Reproduced with permission from Stanley WC. Changes in cardiac metabolism: a critical step from stable angina to ischemic cardiomyopathy. Eur Heart J Suppl 2001;3 Suppl O:O3, Fig. 1.*

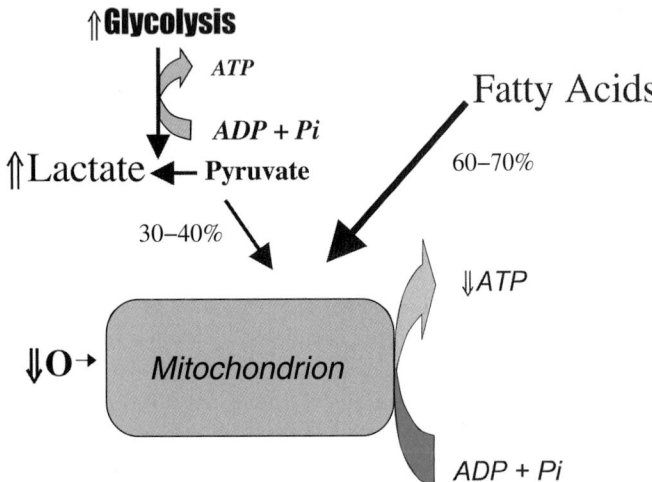

FIGURE 57–2. Cardiac energy metabolism during ischemia of moderate severity (approximately 40 percent of normal blood flow). The *up* and *down* arrows indicate the changes compared with normal conditions. Relative to aerobic conditions, ischemia results in an increase in glycolysis without an increase in the rate of pyruvate oxidation, thus causing lactate to accumulate in the cell. Despite accelerated glycolysis and lactate production, the relatively high rate of residual oxygen consumption is fueled primarily by the oxidation of fatty acids. ADP, adenosine diphosphate; ATP, adenosine triphosphate; Pi, inorganic phosphate. *Source: Reproduced with permission from Stanley WC. Changes in cardiac metabolism: a critical step from stable angina to ischemic cardiomyopathy. Eur Heart J Suppl 2001;3 Suppl O:O5, Fig. 4.*

ATP inhibits Na$^+$, K$^+$-ATPase, increasing intracellular Na$^+$ and Cl, leading to cell swelling. Derangements in transport systems in the sarcolemma and sarcoplasmic reticulum increase cytosolic Ca^{2+}, inducing activation of proteases and alterations in contractile proteins. Pyruvate is not readily oxidized in the mitochondria leading to the production of lactate, a fall in intracellular pH, and a reduction in contractile function. The fall in pH also leads to greater ATP requirement in order to maintain Ca^{2+} homeostasis.[2]

Electron microscopic alterations result from reversible and irreversible myocardial ischemic injury, and are similar across animal species, with some variation in time course. Reversibly injured myocytes are edematous and swollen from the osmotic overload. The cell size is increased with a decrease in the glycogen content.[3–5] The myocyte fibrils are relaxed and thinned; I-bands are prominent secondary to noncontracting ischemic myocytes.[6] The nuclei show mild condensation of chromatin at the nucleoplasm. The cell membrane (sarcolemma) is intact and no breaks can be identified. The mitochondria are swollen, with loss of normal dense mitochondrial granules and incomplete clearing of the mitochondrial matrix, but without amorphous or granular flocculent densities (Fig. 57–3A and B). Irreversibly injured myocytes contain shrunken nuclei with marked chromatin margination. The two hallmarks of irreversible injury are cell membrane breaks and mitochondrial presence of small osmiophilic amorphous densities.[7] The densities are composed of lipid, denatured proteins, and calcium.[8] The cell membrane breaks are small and are associated with subsarcolemmal blebs of edema fluid. (Fig. 57–3B).

Irreversible ischemic injury is characterized by a variety of processes involving the sarcolemmal membrane eventuating in its disruption and cell death. Increased cytosolic Ca^{2+} and mitochondrial impairment cause phospholipase activation, and release of lysophospholipids and free fatty acids, which are incorporated within the cell and damaged by peroxidative damage from free radicals and toxic oxygen species. Cleavage of anchoring cytoskeletal proteins and progressive increases in cell membrane permeability result in physical disruption and cell death.[8]

[ ] APOPTOSIS VERSUS ONCOSIS: MECHANISMS OF MYOCYTE CELL DEATH, INCLUDING AUTOPHAGIC CELL DEATH

There are two basic types of cell death: oncosis, which results in cell swelling and is associated with ischemic damage, and apoptosis, which results from cell shrinkage. In general, oncosis results from events exogenous to the cell, whereas apoptosis is programmed, and is ATP dependent. Oncosis is independent of energy supply and caspase activity. Because apoptosis is energy dependent, it has not been classically implicated in ischemic myocyte death; however, experiments have suggested that apoptosis is involved in the first hours of ischemic injury, especially during reperfusion. The detection of apoptosis depends on identifying the final outcome of the apoptotic pathway (double-stranded DNA fragmentation), but there are issues of specificity associated with detection of these fragments by the most commonly used technique, terminal deoxynucleotidyl transferase-mediated biotinylated deoxyuridine triphosphate nick-end labeling (TUNEL). Other features of apoptosis that can be assayed include activation of cytosolic aspartate-specific cysteine proteases, or caspases; cytochrome

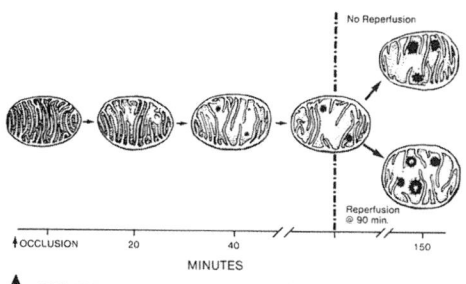

A SEQUENTIAL CHANGES IN MITOCHONDRIA

B

FIGURE 57–3. A. Sequential changes within mitochondria with varying time intervals of myocardial ischemia. At 20 minutes of ischemia, there is mild mitochondrial swelling. Matrix space between cristae show disorganization. At 40 minutes of ischemia, there is greater mitochondrial swelling, and prominent amorphous matrix densities are present, which indicate irreversible injury. With longer duration of coronary occlusion, mitochondria show larger amorphous matrix densities, and they also become more numerous. On reperfusion, both amorphous and granular densities are seen. Granular densities, however, seem larger and more fully developed. *Source: Adapted with permission of American Heart Association from Jennings RB, Ganote CE.*[7] **B.** Electron micrographs showing progressive changes in mitochondria as a result of ischemia in the canine model. *Panel a:* Mitochondria showing reversible changes of ischemia after 10 minutes of coronary occlusion and reperfusion: mitochondria are swollen, there is clearing of mitochondrial matrix, and some cristae show disorganization. *Panel b:* Similar changes as in *panel a* with only one of the mitochondria showing amorphous matrix densities (*arrowhead*) after 90 minutes of ischemia. *Panel c:* Note the presence of large amorphous matrix densities (*arrowheads*) in two of the three mitochondria, in a dog with 120 minutes of coronary occlusion. *Panel d:* Ischemic myocyte with mitochondria containing multiple large amorphous matrix densities (*arrowheads*) after 3 days of permanent coronary occlusion. Note the break in the plasma lemma (*arrow*). *Source: Reproduced with permission from the American Heart Association from Virmani R, Forman MB, Kolodgie FD.*[5]

C release in mitochondria; and selective alteration of cell membranes with an increased expression of phosphatidylserine in the outer membrane, with preservation of selective membrane permeability (generally accomplished by annexin-V labeling). Various of these alterations have been described in ischemic myocardium, but the current consensus is that apoptosis and oncosis proceed together in ischemic myocytes, with oncosis dominating, especially in end stages.[8]

Autophagic, or ubiquitin-related, cell death is characterized ultrastructurally by autophagic vacuoles, cellular degeneration, and nuclear disassembly.[9] Autophagic cell death is energy dependent like apoptosis but, in contrast to apoptosis, is caspase independent. The formation of autophagic vacuoles involves posttranslational modification of proteins by linkage to numerous ubiquitin molecules, making them susceptible to proteasomal digestion. A variety of proteins, including cathepsin D, cathepsin B, heat shock

cognate protein Hsc73, beclin 1, and the processed form of microtubule-associated protein 1 light chain 3 are known to mediate autophagy. Autophagic cell death has been described in hypertrophied and failing myocardium, and has been identified as increasing in hibernating myocardium.[10] The initiation of autophagy does not always result in death of the cell, as autophagy may be responsible for the turnover of unnecessary or dysfunctional organelles and cytoplasmic proteins. In a model of repetitive ischemia in the pig, autophagic cell death has been demonstrated to occur later than apoptosis, and, inversely, suggested a protective effect against ischemia-induced apoptosis.[11]

【 】 EVOLUTION OF MYOCARDIAL INFARCTION, DETERMINANTS OF INFARCT SIZE, AND VENTRICULAR REMODELING

Myocardial ischemia occurs when oxygen supply does not meet myocardial demand, and necrosis or infarction occurs when ischemia is severe and prolonged. Although biochemical and functional abnormalities begin almost immediately at onset of ischemia, severe loss of myocardial contractility occurs within 60 seconds, while other changes take a more protracted course; for example, the loss of viability (irreversible injury) takes at least 20 to 40 minutes following total occlusion of blood flow.

Two zones of myocardial damage occur: a central zone with no flow or very low flow, and a zone of collateral vessels in a surrounding marginal zone. The survival of the marginal zone is dependent on the level of ischemia and the duration of ischemia. In autopsy hearts, the size of the ischemic zone surrounding an acute myocardial infarction is associated with increased apoptosis and degree of occlusion of the infarct-related artery.[12] The extent of coronary collateral flow is one of the principal determinants of infarct size. Indeed, at autopsy it is not uncommon to see chronic total coronary occlusion and an absence of myocardial infarction in the distribution of that artery. Absence of myocardial ischemia (revealed by electrocardiographic changes or angina during transient coronary balloon occlusion) is associated with presence of well-developed collateral vessels, suggesting that the patients with well-developed collateral vessels have a low risk of developing acute myocardial infarction upon abrupt closure of the culprit coronary artery.[13] Collaterals are better developed in patients with angina and in younger individuals as compared to older patients with acute infarcts.[14] Because infarct size is an important determinant of survival as well as development of congestive heart failure, efforts have been directed to limit infarct size by early reperfusion, reduction of myocardial oxygen demand, and prevention of reperfusion injury. In 1971, Page et al. showed that infarcts ≤40 percent of left ventricle are predictors of cardiogenic shock and death.[15]

Reimer and Jennings, initially in 1979, showed that if a canine coronary artery was occluded for 15 minutes, 40 minutes, 3 hours, or permanently for 4 days, myocardial necrosis progressed as a "wave front phenomenon" (Fig. 57–4A).[16,17] The extent of myocardial necrosis therefore depended on the duration of coronary occlusion. After only 15 minutes of occlusion, no infarct occurred. At 40 minutes, the infarct was subendocardial, involving only the papillary muscle, resulting in 28 percent of the myocardium at risk. At 3 hours following coronary artery occlusion and reper-

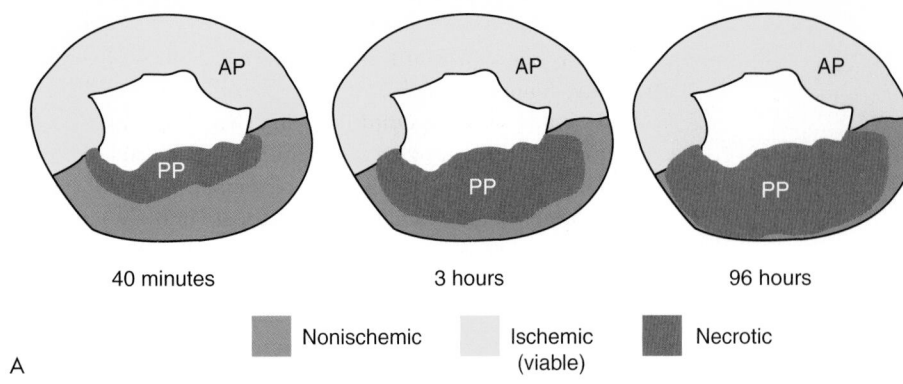

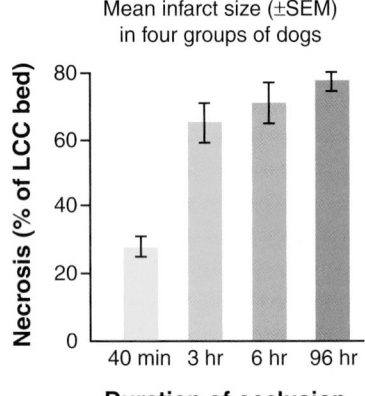

FIGURE 57–4. **A.** Progression of cell death versus time after experimental occlusion of the left circumflex coronary artery in the dog. Necrosis occurs first in the subendocardial region of the myocardium. With extension of the occlusion time, a wavefront of cell death moves from the subendocardial zone across the wall to involve progressively more of the transmural thickness of the ischemic zone. AP, anterior; PP, posterior. **B.** Infarct size variation with increasing duration of coronary occlusion. Infarct size dramatically increases from 40 minutes to 3 hours; however, there is very little increase between 3 and 6 hours and between 6 and 96 hours of coronary artery occlusion. LCC, left circumflex coronary bed. *Source: Reproduced by permission from Reimer KA, Jennings RB. The "wavefront phenomenon" of myocardial ischemic cell death. II. Transmural progression of necrosis with the framework of ischemic bed size (myocardium at risk) and collateral flow. Lab Invest 1979;40:633–644.*

processes involved in postinfarction ventricular dilatation are known as *ventricular remodeling*. In general, transmural extent of necrosis is a major determinant of infarct expansion (remodeling), based on large infarct size and the persistence of the occlusion. The preservation of islands of viable myocardium in the subepicardial regions is associated with decreased remodeling or infarct expansion. Other factors that are implicated in reduced ventricular remodeling include microvascular integrity[19] and initial ventricular compliance, as measured by mitral deceleration time.[20] The effect of reperfusion on ventricular remodeling is clear as far as early reperfusion is concerned, as there are definite benefits in reducing infarct size and expansion. The benefits of late reperfusion, beyond myocardial salvage, are unclear. It has been demonstrated that remodeling is affected by the presence of viable zones after successful late percutaneous coronary intervention.[21] In general, the mechanisms of ventricular remodeling are poorly understood, because different techniques have been used to assess myocardial viability in human subjects, in animal studies, and in postmortem specimens. The release of matrix metalloproteinases are now being linked to remodeling.

[ ] THE NO-REFLOW PHENOMENON AND REPERFUSION INJURY

The no-reflow phenomenon was originally described by Kloner and Jennings in 1974 in an experimental canine model of myocardial infarction.[22] They demonstrated homogenous distribution of thioflavin S dye after 40 minutes of ischemia and reperfusion. However, after 90 minutes of ischemia, areas of no-reflow were identified mainly in the subendocardial regions as zones not staining with thioflavin S. By electron microscopy they showed swollen endothelial protrusions and membrane-bound intraluminal bodies, which obstructed the capillary lumen and resulted in plugging of the capillaries by red cells, neutrophils, platelets, and fibrin thrombi. The areas not stained by thioflavin S were characterized by low regional myocardial blood flow. The term *reperfusion injury* was coined to describe reperfusion-related expansion or worsening of the ischemic cardiac injury as assessed by contractile performance, the arrhythmogenic threshold, conversion of reversible to irreversible myocyte injury and microvessel dysfunction. Recent studies show that angiographic no-reflow is a strong predictor of major cardiac events, like congestive heart failure, malignant arrhythmias, and cardiac death, after acute myocardial infarction. The major mediators of reperfusion injury are oxygen radicals, calcium loading, and neutrophils.[23]

fusion the infarct was significantly smaller compared with non-reperfused permanently occluded infarct (62 percent of area at risk). The infarct size was the greatest in permanent occlusion, becoming transmural involving 75 percent of the area at risk (Fig. 57–4B).[6] In the dog model, it is impossible to achieve 100 percent infarction of the area at risk because of species-related native collaterals. In humans, it has been shown that approximately 40 percent of patients with acute myocardial infarction have well-developed collateral circulation.[14]

Other than the presence of collateral circulation, factors that influence infarct size include preconditioning, which may greatly reduce infarct size, and reperfusion. However, there is a balance between benefits of reperfusion in reducing infarct size, and reperfusion injury, which is dependent on time of onset. In general, if reperfusion is instituted within 2 to 3 hours of the onset of ischemia, the degree of myocardial salvage greatly exceeds damage from free radicals and calcium loading caused by reperfusion.

It was documented in the late 1970s that transmural infarcts may increase in size for weeks after the initial event, and the degree of this expansion is associated with a decrease in survival rate.[18] The

MICROEMBOLIZATION

Acute coronary thrombosis with or without percutaneous intervention results in the embolization of microparticles, including fragments of fibrin-platelet thrombus and necrotic core. Coronary microembolization is associated with arrhythmias, contractile dysfunction, microinfarcts, and reduced coronary reserve.[24] Autopsy studies show a 13 percent rate of microembolization in cardiac disease, often associated with focal myocyte necrosis.[25] The rate of coronary microembolization is highest in documented epicardial coronary thrombosis, reaching 30 to 54 percent[26,27] and even higher in acute infarcts (79 percent) in acute myocardial infarcts.[28] Little data is available that compares acute plaque rupture with acute plaque erosion and the rate of embolization, but we have noted a higher rate of thrombotic microembolization with plaque erosion. In hearts with acute coronary thrombi, evidence of distal embolization was more frequent in erosions than ruptures (74 percent vs. 40 percent, $p = .03$).

ISCHEMIC PRECONDITIONING

Ischemic preconditioning was first described by Murry et al., in 1986, when they observed that canine myocardial infarct size was markedly reduced if it follows four brief episodes of 5 minutes of occlusion followed by 5 minutes of reperfusion.[29] Preconditioning has also been observed with only one episode of brief occlusion followed by reperfusion. If the duration between ischemic preconditioning and the long duration of occlusion is extended to 24 to 96 hours, the protective effect is markedly reduced.[30] The original description of preconditioning was applied only to infarct size reduction; this definition is now extended to cardiac function and arrhythmias, although the latter are not as consistent.[31]

The mechanisms of preconditioning are unclear, but it has been shown that preconditioning reduces the energy demand of the myocardium, both in animals and man. Two phases of preconditioning have been described: the classical initial phase, operative for 1 to 2 hours prior to sustained coronary occlusion; and the delayed phase, operative 24 hours after the precondition, known as the *second window of protection* (SWOP).[8] Classical preconditioning is associated with activation of adenosine receptors, activation of protein kinase C coupled to G proteins, and opening of ATP-dependent potassium channels. The mechanism of SWOP is less clear, and is believed to involve a kinase cascade, including mitogen-activated protein kinases and nuclear factor kappa B, which increase levels of superoxide dismutase, nitric oxide synthase, cyclooxygenase-2, and heat shock proteins, thereby creating a protective milieu for the cardiomyocyte.

Clinically, Yellon et al. showed that intermittent aortic cross-clamping could precondition the human left ventricle during coronary artery bypass surgery, resulting in preservation of ATP levels.[32] Other observations that confirm the existence of preconditioning in patients have been observed in patients undergoing percutaneous transluminal coronary angioplasty (PTCA). Repeated balloon inflations of 60 to 90 seconds are associated with decreasing chest pain, a reduction in ST-segment elevation, and a decrease in lactate production with subsequent inflations; the foregoing phenomenon are observed irrespective of the presence or absence of collaterals.[33] In the Thrombolysis in Myocardial Infarction (TIMI)-9 study, the timing of angina in relationship to myocardial infarction was studied, only patients with angina within 24 hours of infarction showed smaller infarct size and better clinical outcome.[34]

The mediators of preconditioning are believed to involve the K_{ATP} channel and specific isoforms of protein kinase C (PKC). The protective effect of temporary ischemia can be blocked by pretreatment of the myocardium with inhibitors of K_{ATP} channel, such as glibenclamide and 5-hydrocydeconate (5HD).[35,36] Similarly, inhibitors of PKC and tyrosine kinase, but not PKC alone, will prevent ischemic preconditioning. Also similarly, agonists of adenosine (A_1 receptor) will pharmacologically precondition the heart against ischemia.[37]

HIBERNATING MYOCARDIUM

Left ventricular systolic dysfunction caused by ischemia may arise in dead myocardium or from hypocontractile areas of viable myocardium. In the early 1980s, Rahimtoola found significant improvement in left ventricular function after coronary revascularization in a subset of patients with depressed ventricular performance. He postulated that the mechanism of poor myocardial contractility was chronic ischemia,[38] which could be improved by revascularization. The premise behind this rationale was dependent on the surviving myocardium being in a functional, albeit depressed, state, suggesting that the myocardium may adapt to chronic ischemia by decreasing its contractility but preserving viability.[39] Reversibly dysfunctional tissue is commonly referred to as *hibernating myocardium*.[40] Sheiban et al.[41] demonstrated that 5 to 7 minutes of angioplasty balloon inflations in the coronary arteries of patients undergoing interventional procedures, followed by tracking of the resolution of the regional wall-motion abnormalities over the next 5 days, showed persistence of regional wall-motion abnormalities for up to 36 hours. Similarly, return of left ventricular function has been studied following acute myocardial infarction. Delayed recovery of wall motion was observed in the infarct region, with a positive change in wall motion from 0.2 at 3 days to 1.0 at 6 months in patients with reperfusion but not in those without reperfusion, as measured by the centerline method.[42]

Clinical functional techniques such as stress echocardiography and cardiac magnetic resonance are more specific, but less sensitive, than nuclear modalities, which assess perfusion and metabolic activity, in the detection of hibernating myocardium.[40,43] The concept of myocardial hibernation was initially based on clinical observation. Subsequently, there have been a number of experimental studies to support the concept that ischemia is not the result of simple inadequacy of blood flow for myocardial contraction, but that there is a stepwise decrease in function based on incremental decrease in oxygen-supplying perfusion (so-called *perfusion–contraction matching*). There is evidence that repeated episodes of ischemia–reperfusion may result in a state of chronic hibernation, with alterations in the flow–function relationship and decreased oxygen demand. Chronically hibernating myocardium demonstrates alterations in adrenergic control and calcium responsiveness. Substances that are upregulated in chronic hibernating myocardium include heat shock protein, hypoxia-inducible factor, inducible nitric oxide synthase, cyclooxygenase-2, and monocyte chemotactic protein. Because some of these pathways are involved in preconditioning, a relationship between cardiac hibernation and preconditioning is postulated.

Morphologically, hibernating myocytes show loss of contractile elements, especially in the perinuclear region, and occasionally throughout the cytoplasm. The space left by the dissolution of the myofibrils is occupied by glycogen, as evidenced by the strong positivity for the periodic acid-Schiff reagent. Ultrastructurally, there is depletion of sarcomeres, most pronounced in the perinuclear region, with increased glycogen. The nuclei are enlarged, with a tortuous nuclear membrane and evenly distributed heterochromatin. The mitochondria are elongated, shrunken, and osmiophilic.[44] The interstitium shows an increase in connective tissue. Increased numbers of apoptotic myocytes, using the technique of DNA nick-end labeling, have been demonstrated,[45] as well as an increase in autophagic and oncotic cell death.[10,46]

The composition and distribution of sarcomeric, cytoskeletal, and membrane-associated proteins is significantly altered in chronic myocardial hibernation.[47,48] There is a disorderly increase in cytoskeletal desmin, tubulin and vinculin, with a decrease in contractile proteins myosin, titin, and -actinin. More recently, decreased connexin 43, a membrane transport protein, has been associated with reduced gap junction size and a proposed propensity for arrhythmias in the hibernating state.[49]

PLAQUE MORPHOLOGY AND SITE OF THROMBUS IN ACUTE MYOCARDIAL INFARCTION

The vast majority of myocardial infarctions occur in patients with coronary atherosclerosis, and of these myocardial infarctions, more than 90 percent are associated with superimposed luminal thrombus. Arbustini et al. found coronary thrombi in 98 percent of patients dying with clinically documented acute myocardial infarction, and of these thrombi, 75 percent were caused from plaque rupture and 25 percent from plaque erosion. There are gender differences in the causation of coronary thrombi leading to acute myocardial infarcts, as Arbustini showed that 37 percent of thrombi in women were erosion, as compared to only 18 percent in men.[50] Although an individual severe stenosis is more likely to become occluded by a thrombus than a lesion with less-severe stenosis, the less-severely narrowed plaques give rise to more occlusions, as there are many more sites that are mild to moderately narrowed.[51] We have observed that the mean percent stenosis underlying coronary plaque erosion is 70 percent versus 80 percent at the site of plaque rupture; however, 82 percent of fatal plaque erosions result in total occlusions, compared to only 57 percent of plaque ruptures.[52] The culprit coronary artery of infarction at autopsy most frequent is the left anterior descending artery (approximately 50 percent), followed by the right coronary artery (30 to 45 percent) and then the left circumflex (15 to 20 percent). No thrombi are found in fewer than 5 percent of acute myocardial infarctions.

PATHOLOGY OF ACUTE MYOCARDIAL INFARCTION

[ ] GROSS PATHOLOGIC FINDINGS

The earliest change that can be grossly discerned in the evolution of acute myocardial infarction—pallor of the myocardium—occurs 12 hours or later after the onset of irreversible ischemia. The gross detection of infarction can be enhanced by the use of tetrazolium salt solutions, which form a colored precipitate on gross section of fresh heart tissue in the presence of dehydrogenase-mediated activity. The tetrazolium salts (nitroblue tetrazolium [NBT] and 2,3,5-triphenyltetrazolium chloride [TTC]) are dyes that are sensitive to the presence of tissue dehydrogenase enzyme activity, which is depleted in the infarcted myocardium. It has been shown that myocardial infarct can be detected by NBT as early as 2 to 3 hours in the dog and in a little less time in the pig because of poor collaterals.[53] Red color (TTC) or blue color (NBT) will only form in the normal noninfarcted myocardium, thus revealing the pale, nonstained, infarcted region (Fig.

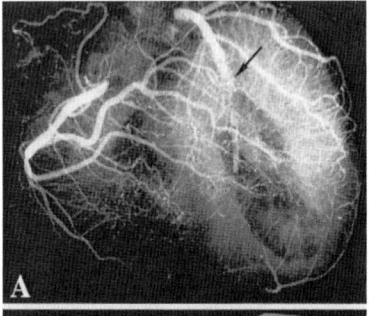
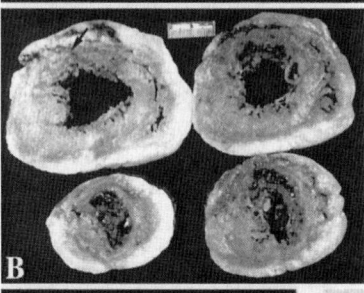
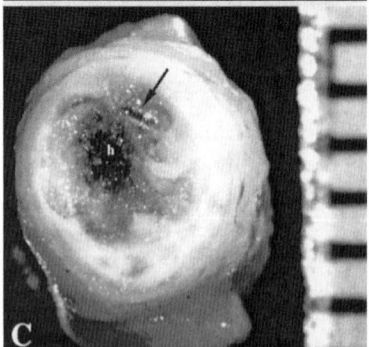
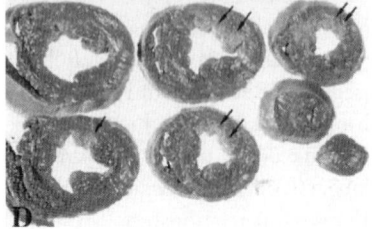

FIGURE 57–5. Regional distribution of vascular supply to the ventricles with right coronary artery dominance. **A.** Postmortem angiogram of the heart in a patient with acute myocardial infarction with total occlusion (*arrow*) of the proximal left anterior descending coronary artery in a 65-year-old female who presented with persistent chest pain of 6 hours duration. **B.** At autopsy she had a hemopericardium with rupture site (*arrow*) identified on the anterior wall of the left ventricle. Note extensive hemorrhagic (h) transmural infarction involving the anterior wall of the left ventricle near the base of the heart (*upper slices*) and extending into the septum in the mid and apical slices (*lower slices*). **C.** Gross photography of the left anterior descending coronary artery showing hemorrhage into the necrotic core and a >90 percent luminal narrowing; barium is seen within the lumen (*arrow*). **D.** Dog heart slices following 15 minutes incubation in 2% triphenyltetrazolium chloride (TTC) at 98.6°F (37°C). The animal had undergone 60 minutes of left anterior descending (LAD) coronary artery occlusion distal to the first diagonal branch followed by reperfusion and sacrificed at 24 hours. Injecting monastery dye following reocclusion of the LAD and just prior to sacrifice identified the myocardium at risk of infarction. The heart was sliced and then immersed in TTC. The viable myocardium at risk stains red and area not at risk is blue-red, where as the infarcted region is creamy white (*arrows*).
Source: Reproduced with permission from Virmani R, Burke AP, Farb A, Atkinson J, eds. Cardiovascular Pathology, 2nd ed. Philadelphia: WB Saunders, 2001: Vol 40, Fig. 5–4.

57–5). In humans, the necrotic myocardium can be detected within 2 to 3 hours after infarct by immersion of the fresh heart slices in a solution of TTC or NBT. TTC staining has a diagnostic sensitivity of 77 percent and a specificity of 93 percent compared with routine histology with predictive values of positive and negative test of 81 and 91 percent, respectively.[54]

At approximately 24 hours after the onset of irreversible ischemia, the pallor is enhanced (Fig. 57–6). However, in this era of thrombolytic therapy with percutaneous intervention, most in-hospital patients will have received tissue plasminogen activator, streptokinase, or glycoprotein IIb/IIIa inhibitors with balloon angioplasty and stenting, which lyse the thrombus and restore blood flow into the area of infarction. Consequently, in a reperfused infarct, the infarcted region will appear red from trapping of the red cells and hemorrhage from the rupture of the necrotic capillaries (Fig. 57–7). However, if there has been no reperfusion, the area of the infarct is better defined at 2 to 3 days with a central area of yellow discoloration that is surrounded by a thin rim of highly vascularized hyperemia (Fig. 57–6). At 5 to 7 days, the regions are much more distinct, with a central soft area and a depressed hyperemic border. At 1 to 2 weeks, the infarct begins to heal with infiltration by macrophages as well as early fibroblasts at the margins. At the same time, the infarct begins to be more depressed, especially at the margins where organization takes place, and there is a white hue to the borders (Table 57–1 and Fig. 57–6). Healing may be complete as early as 4 to 6 weeks in small infarcts, or may take as long as 2 to 3 months when the area of infarction is large. Healed infarcts are white from the scarring and the ventricular wall may or may not be thinned (aneurysmal). In general, infarcts that are transmural and confluent are likely to result in thinning, whereas subendocardial and nonconfluent infarcts are not.

[ ] LIGHT MICROSCOPIC FINDINGS IN NONREPERFUSED INFARCTION

The earliest morphologic characteristic of myocardial infarction that can be discerned, between 12 and 24 hours after onset of chest pain, is the hypereosinophilic myocyte (Fig. 57–8). Despite the hypereosinophilia of the cytoplasm, which is seen best on routine hematoxylin-eosin staining, the myocyte striations appear normal and some chromatin condensation may be seen in the nucleus. The area of infarction may show interstitial edema; however, this change is difficult to appreciate in human autopsy hearts and better appreciated in animal experiments. It has been suggested in experimentally induced infarction that the appearance of "wavy fibers" may be the earliest change and is thought to be the result of stretching of the ischemic noncontractile fibers by the adjoining viable contracting myocytes. Wavy fiber change is, however, nonspecific and occurs in the absence of ischemia, especially in the right ventricle. Neutrophil infiltration is present by 24 hours at the border areas. As the infarct progresses between 24 and 48 hours, coagulation necrosis is established with various degrees of nuclear pyknosis, early karyorrhexis, and karyolysis. The myocyte striations are preserved and the sarcomeres elongate. The border areas show prominent neutrophil infiltration by 48 hours (Fig. 57–8).

At 3 to 5 days the central portion of the infarct shows loss of myocyte nuclei and striations; in smaller infarcts neutrophils invade within the infarct and fragment, resulting in more severe karyorrhexis (nuclear dust). Loss of myocyte striations is best appreciated by using the Mallory trichrome stain. Markers of ischemia include hypoxia-inducible factor-1 and cyclooxygenase-2, which can be demonstrated immunohistochemically.[12] The influx of inflammatory cells, including mast cells, induces a cascade of chemokines which suppress further inflammation and result in scar tissue.[55,56] Macrophages and fibroblasts begin to appear in the border areas. By 1 week, neutrophils decline and granulation tissue is established with neocapillary invasion and lymphocytic and plasma cell infiltration. Although lymphocytes may be seen as early as 2 to 3 days, they are not prominent in any stage of infarct evolution. Eosinophils may be seen within the inflammatory infiltrate but are only present in 24 percent of infarcts.[57] There is phagocytic removal of the necrotic myocytes by macrophages, and pigment is seen within macrophages.

By the second week, fibroblasts are prominent but their appearance may be seen as early as day 4 at the periphery of the infarct. There is continued removal of the necrotic myocytes as the fibroblasts are actively producing collagen and angiogenesis occurs in the area of healing. The healing continues, and depending on the extent of necrosis, the healing may be complete as early as 4 weeks, or require 8 weeks or longer to complete (see Fig. 57–8). The central area of infarction may remain unhealed, showing mummified myocytes for extended periods, despite the fact that the infarct borders are completely healed. For this reason, it is important to evaluate the age of the infarct by examining the border with noninfarcted muscle.

The magnitude of repair and healing is dependent not only on infarct size, but also on local and systemic factors. If there is good collateral blood flow locally, healing will be relatively rapid, especially at the lateral borders where viable myocardium interdigitates with necrotic myocardium. There may be various levels of healing within an infarct, because of differences in blood flow in adjoining vascular beds caused by variable extent of coronary narrowing. The border areas may show hemorrhage and contraction band necrosis, depending upon regional variations in blood flow. Systemic factors that influence repair of myocardium are the systemic blood pressure and cardiac output, which are severely decreased in heart of patients with multisystem failure.

[ ] LIGHT MICROSCOPIC APPEARANCE OF REPERFUSED ACUTE MYOCARDIAL INFARCTION

In dogs, the amount of myocardium that can be salvaged depends on the duration of total occlusion of the artery supplying the area of infarction. The maximal salvage is possible, both in dogs and humans, if the artery is opened within 6 hours. The myocardium in the dog following 90 minutes of occlusion followed by reperfusion and sacrifice at 24 hours shows a hemorrhagic infarct limited to the area of occlusion, which is subendocardial in extent. Hemorrhage occurs when the myocardial blood flow during the occlusion period is less than one-fifth of normal. The myocytes are thin, hypereosinophilic, devoid of nuclei or showing karyorrhexis, with

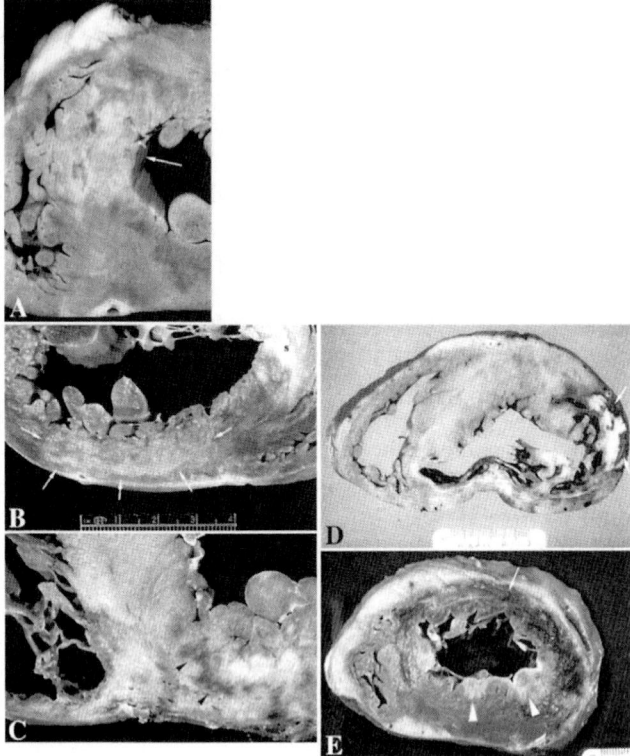

FIGURE 57–6. Gross photographs of the hearts with varying ages of acute myocardial infarction. **A.** A 50-year-old hyperlipidemic and hypertensive male presented with unstable angina, underwent emergency percutaneous transluminal coronary angioplasty (PTCA) of the left anterior descending coronary artery (LAD), died 20 hours following onset of chest pain. At autopsy he had a pale, ill-defined, slightly raised region in the anterior ventricular septum suggestive of an acute transmural infarct (*arrow*), which was confirmed by the presence of hypereosinophilic myocytes localized to the septum with sparing of the subendocardial myocytes. The LAD at the PTCA site was totally occluded by a luminal thrombus and an underlying 60 percent atherosclerotic lesion. **B.** Another high power view of a different acute transmural myocardial infarct involving the posterior wall of the heart, well-defined, pale, creamy tan, slightly raised infarct. Note the absence of hyperemia in the border region—the infarct is 24 to 36 hours old. An older infarct can be seen in the septum. **C.** An older infarct dated 36 to 72 hours showing hyperemic areas (*arrow heads*) surrounding the subendocardial infarct (age 3 days), with paler area in the outer half of the posterior wall of the left ventricle (infarct extension). The more recent infarct involves the posterior portion of the ventricular septum and the posterior wall of the right ventricle (36 to 48 hours). **D.** Gross photograph of a heart slice, close to the base of the heart shows 1-week-old acute transmural myocardial infarct involving the posterolateral wall of the heart. Note the marked pale region in the inner two-thirds of the infarct, with surrounding prominent hyperemic zone (*arrows*). Also present is a healed transmural myocardial infarct involving the posterior wall and posteroseptal region of the heart. The patient died in severe congestive heart failure. **E.** Gross photograph of a transmural healing myocardial infarct involving the septum, anterior, and lateral wall of the left ventricle in an apical slice of the heart. Note the depressed, gelatinous appearance (*arrow*) of the infarct, which is 3 weeks old. Focal areas of scarring can be seen (*arrowheads*). *Source: Reproduced with permission from Virmani R, Burke AP, Farb A, Atkinson J, eds. Cardiovascular Pathology, 2nd ed. Philadelphia: WB Saunders, 2001: Vol 40, Fig. 5–5.*

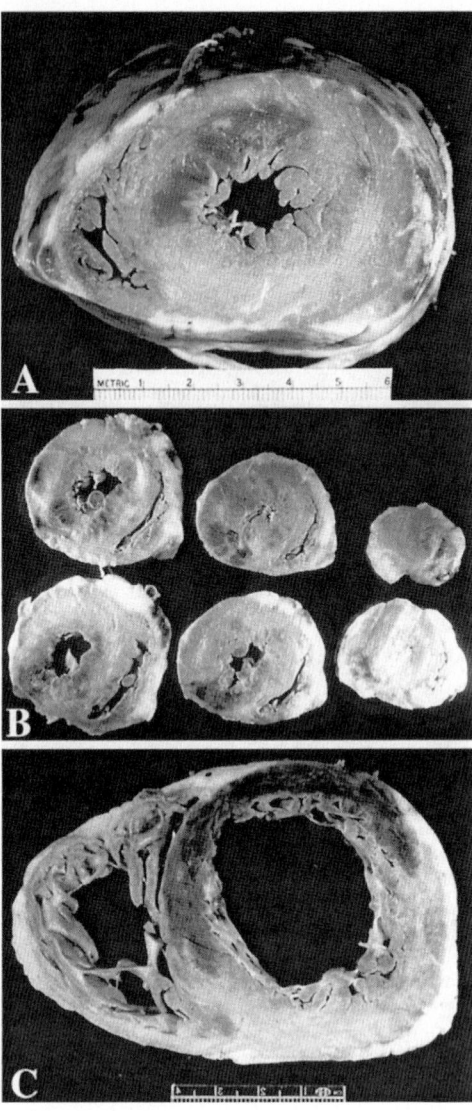

FIGURE 57–7. A. A 47-year-old black male presented with unstable angina that evolved into a Q-wave infarct. On catheterization, he had a total occlusion of the left anterior descending coronary artery and severe stenosis of the right and left circumflex coronary arteries. The patient underwent emergency bypass graft to all three vessels. He died secondary to refractory arrhythmias on the third hospital day. Note subendocardial hyperemic region in the anteroseptal wall of the left ventricle. **B.** Patient presented with acute myocardial infarction of 6 hours duration, received streptokinase in the emergency room, and died 2 days after successful reperfusion of a cerebral bleed. Note a hemorrhagic transmural infarct involves the posteroseptal wall of the left ventricle, extending from the base to the apex of the heart with approximately 20 to 25 percent of the myocardium infarcted. **C.** A 60-year-old male admitted with onset of chest pain while mowing the lawn. He did not seek medical treatment until 8 hours after onset of chest pain. The patient received streptokinase, developed arrhythmias, was treated with lidocaine, went into cardiogenic shock, and died 3 days after infarction. Note the transmural confluent hemorrhagic infarct of the anteroseptal wall of the left ventricle involving at least 40 percent of the left ventricle. *Source: Reproduced with permission from Virmani R, Burke AP, Farb A, Atkinson J, eds. Cardiovascular Pathology, 2nd ed. Philadelphia: WB Saunders, 2001: Vol 40, Fig. 5–6.*

TABLE 57–1

Gross and Microscopic Evolution of Reperfused and Non-Reperfused Acute Myocardial Infarct

TIME OF OCCLUSION	PERMANENT OCCLUSION/ NO REPERFUSION		REPERFUSION FOLLOWING OCCLUSION	
	GROSS	HISTOLOGIC	GROSS	HISTOLOGIC
12 hours	No change/pallor	Wavy fibers	Mottled, prominent hemorrhage	CBN
24–48 hours	Pallor-yellow, soft	Hypereosinophilic fibers, PMNs at borders	Prominent hemorrhage	Hypereosinophilic fibers + CBN + PMNs + hemorrhage throughout
3–5 days	Yellow center, hyperemic borders	Large number of PMNs at border, coagulation necrosis, loss of nuclei	Prominent hemorrhage	Aggressive phagocytosis profuse fibroblast infiltration + collagen
6–10 days	Yellow, depressed central infarct, tan-red margins	Mummified fibers in center, macrophage phagocytosis + granulation tissue at borders	Depressed red-brown infarct with gray-white intermingled	Aggressive healing with greater collagen
10–14 days	Gray red borders, infiltrating central tan-yellow infarct if large	Marked granulation tissue, collagen deposition, subendocardial myocyte sparing	Gray-white intermingled with brown	Aggressive healing with greater collagen
2–8 weeks	Gelatinous to gray-white scar, greater healing at border zone	Collagen deposition with prominent large capillaries	White intermingled with groups of myocytes with red myocardium	Collagen intermingled with groups of myocytes

CBN, contraction band necrosis; PMN, polymorphonuclear cell.
SOURCE: Reprinted with permission from Virmani R, Burke AP, Farb A, Atkinson J, eds. Cardiovascular Pathology, 2nd ed. Philadelphia: WB Saunders; 2001: Vol 40, Table 57–1.

ill-defined borders and interspersed areas of interstitial hemorrhage. There is a diffuse but mild neutrophil infiltration. Within 2 to 3 days, macrophage infiltration is obvious and there is phagocytosis of necrotic myocytes and early stages of granulation tissue. The infarct healing in the dog is more rapid than that in man, most likely a result of nondiseased adjoining coronary arteries (collaterals) and a lack of underlying myocardial disease. In humans with acute myocardial infarction, there is often chronic ischemia secondary to extensive atherosclerotic disease.

In humans, if reperfusion occurs within 4 to 6 hours following onset of chest pain or ECG changes, there is myocardial salvage and the infarct is likely to be subendocardial without transmural extension. There will be a nearly confluent area of hemorrhage within the infarcted myocardium, with extensive contraction band necrosis. The extent of hemorrhage is dependent on the extent of reperfusion of the infarct, as well as the extent of capillary necrosis. The larger the infarct, and the longer the duration of the infarct, the more the hemorrhage. The degree of hemorrhage may be variable and nonuniform, as blood flow is dependent upon the residual area of coronary narrowing and the amount of thrombolysis. Within a few hours of reperfusion, neutrophils are evident within the area of necrosis, but they are usually sparse (Fig. 57–9). In contrast to nonreperfused infarcts, neutrophils do not show concentration at the margins. However, reperfused infarcts often demonstrate areas of necrosis at the periphery with interdigitation with noninfarcted myocar-

dium. Macrophages begin to appear by day 2 or 3 and stromal cells show enlarged nuclei and nucleoli by days 3 and 4 (Fig. 57–9). Neutrophil debris, which may be concentrated at the border areas in cases of incomplete reperfusion, is seen by 3 to 5 days. Fibroblasts appear by days 3 to 5, with an accelerated rate of healing as compared to nonreperfused infarcts. By 1 week there is collagen deposition with disappearance of neutrophils and prominence of macrophages containing pigment derived from ingested myocytes (Fig. 57–9). Angiogenesis is prominent and lymphocytes are often seen. Infarcts at 5 to 10 days are more cellular and there is prominent myocytolysis (loss of myofibrils). As early as 2 to 3 weeks subendocardial infarcts may be fully healed (Fig. 57–9). Five to 10 layers of subendocardial myocytes are spared without necrosis. However, myofibrillar loss, which is a result of ischemia not severe enough to cause cell death, is prominent in this subendocardial zone. Larger infarcts, and those reperfused after 6 hours, take longer to heal. Infarcts reperfused after 6 hours show larger areas of hemorrhage as compared to occlusions with more immediate reperfusion (see Fig. 57–7). However, myocytes maintain their striations, become stretched and elongated, and as they do not respond to calcium influx, do not show significant contraction band necrosis. Despite the fact that reperfusion should occur within 6 hours of occlusion for maximal myocyte salvage, there appears to be some benefit in opening an artery regardless of the duration of coronary occlusion.

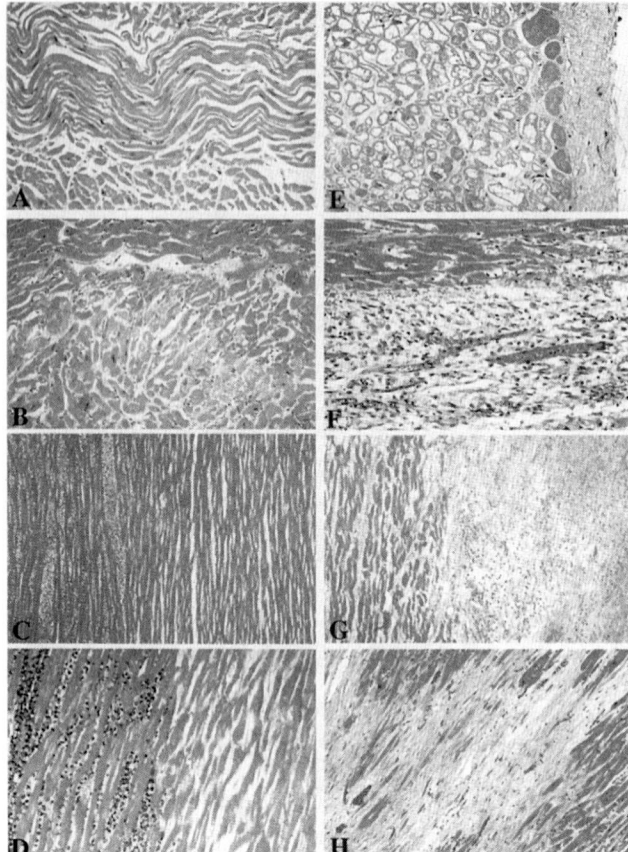

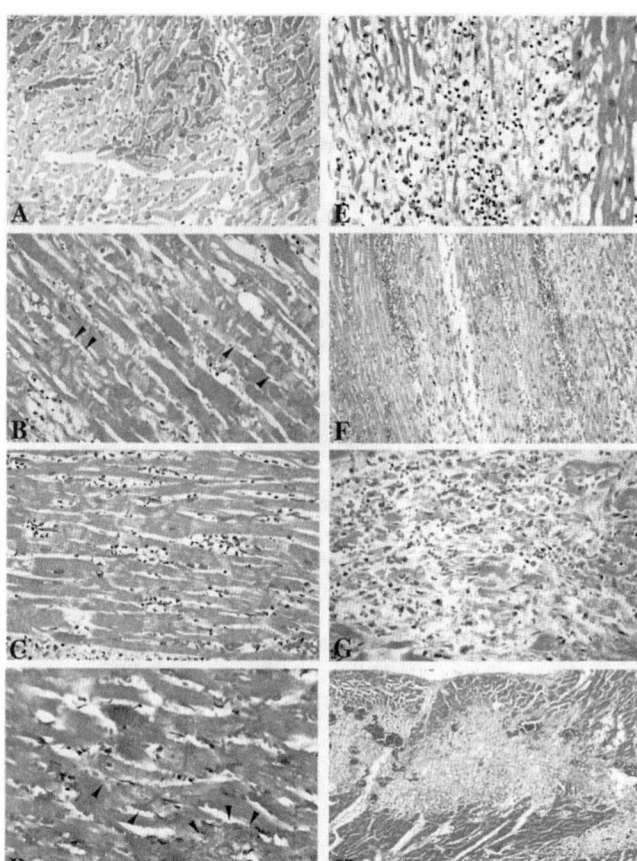

FIGURE 57–8. Histologic characteristics of myocardial infarction following total occlusion of a coronary artery. **A.** The earliest change seen is within 12 hours after the onset of chest pain and has been described as wavy fibers with elongation of myocytes, and narrowing of the myocyte diameter. **B.** Hypereosinophilic myocyte fibers representing early features of coagulation necrosis can be seen between 12 and 24 hours after onset of chest pain, the nucleus is intact, and the cross-striations are well seen. **C.** By 48 to 72 hours the neutrophils are now concentrated at the border of the infarcted and viable myocardium, the extent of neutrophil infiltration depends upon the collateral flow as well as the extent of coronary perfusion of the adjacent bed. The central zone of infarction now shows all the features of coagulation necrosis with karyolysis and loss of cross striations. **D.** Photomicrograph showing high-power view of the border zone of a 5-day-old infarct with marked neutrophil infiltration that have undergone karyopyknosis and karyorrhexis and the adjoining infarcted myocardium shows coagulation necrosis with loss of nuclei and cross-striations. **E.** A high-power view of the subendocardial region, which is usually ischemic but viable, showing myocyte vacuolization and loss of myofibrils. **F.** Almost complete removal of the necrotic myocardium, note presence of neovascular channels and surrounding macrophages and few lymphocytes (granulation tissue) at 7 to 10 days following acute myocardial infarction. **G.** The infarct is heavily infiltrated with fibroblasts with early collagen deposition and interspersed neocapillaries and few lymphocytes, infarct age 3 to 4 weeks. **H.** A fully healed infarct with dense collagen and few interspersed myocytes at the border region of the healed infarct. Infarct age may be 6 weeks or older. *Source: Reproduced with permission from Virmani R, Burke AP, Farb A, Atkinson J, eds. Cardiovascular Pathology, 2nd ed. Philadelphia: WB Saunders, 2001: Vol 40, Fig. 5–7.*

FIGURE 57–9. Histologic characteristics of a reperfused infarct following occlusion and reperfusion either with thrombolysis (tissue plasminogen activator [tPA], streptokinase, or glycoprotein IIb/IIIa) or balloon angioplasty with or without stenting or surgical revascularization. **A.** A cross section of myocytes shows necrosis with interstitial hemorrhage. Note pale myocyte nuclei and very early neutrophil infiltration. **B.** Myocytes cut longitudinally in a patient who was admitted with chest pain of 2 hours duration followed by infusion of streptokinase. The patient died within 6 hours. Note the extensive contraction band necrosis (dark bands alternating with lighter bands, *arrowheads*), a hallmark of reperfusion injury. There are interstitial red cells and a few neutrophils, which were scattered throughout the infarct. **C.** Note the number of neutrophils is greater than the previous example. There is mild red cell extravasation and contraction band necrosis. The duration of chest pain was 3 hours prior to reperfusion and the patient died 24 hours later. **D.** It is not uncommon to see single or a few necrotic myocytes with calcification (*arrowheads*) in patients with reperfused infarcts. **E.** Note the presence of macrophages and lymphocytes with early dissolution of the necrotic myocytes. These areas of necrosis are interdigitating with viable noninfarcted myocardium (4- to 5-day-old reperfused infarct). **F.** Note interstitial hemorrhage and infiltrating macrophages seen in the lower fifth and the right third of photomicrograph. **G.** High-power view of another infarct showing dissolution of the infarct and replacement with macrophages and early angiogenesis. Hemorrhage is still present, but no neutrophils are seen (5- to 7-day-old infarct). **H.** Low-power view of a healing infarct at 7 to 10 days; note angiogenesis and early replacement fibrosis. *Source: Reproduced with permission from Virmani R, Burke AP, Farb A, Atkinson J, eds. Cardiovascular Pathology, 2nd ed. Philadelphia: WB Saunders, 2001: Vol 40, Fig. 5–8.*

COMPLICATIONS OF MYOCARDIAL INFARCTION

The in-hospital and late survival rates of patients with acute myocardial infarction improved remarkably from the 1970s to early 1980s, from 16 percent in the 1970s to 8 to 10 percent in the early 1990s. The reasons are multifactorial and include myocardial salvage from reperfusion, small infarction, and remodeling.[58] However, the incidence of cardiogenic shock in community studies has not declined.[59] The complications of myocardial infarction may manifest immediately or may appear late, and are dependent on the location and extent of infarction. The acute complications consist of arrhythmias and sudden death, cardiogenic shock, infarct extension, fibrinous pericarditis, cardiac rupture including papillary muscle rupture, and mural thrombus and embolization.

ARRHYTHMIAS AND SUDDEN DEATH

Arrhythmias after myocardial infarction are varied, and include ventricular arrhythmias (the major source of sudden death), conduction system disturbances, and atrial arrhythmias. Almost 90 percent of patients develop a cardiac rhythm abnormality after acute infarction.

Tachyarrhythmias that occur during acute myocardial infarction (MI) often result from reperfusion, altered automatic tone or hemodynamic instability. In all patients, ventricular tachyarrhythmias are seen in 67 percent of cases within the first 12 hours of acute myocardial infarction.[60] Ventricular fibrillation occurs in approximately 4.5 percent of cases, with the greatest incidence in the first hour.[61] Sudden death occurs in 25 percent of patients after myocardial infarction, often before patients reach the hospital. The proportion of deaths from ischemic heart disease that are sudden is almost 60 percent.

Ventricular arrhythmias are important markers of electrical instability and are helpful in predicting patients who will die suddenly after myocardial infarction. Several types of tachyarrhythmias are associated with decreased survival, including subacute and late premature ventricular complexes, nonsustained ventricular tachycardia of late onset, and sustained monomorphic ventricular tachycardia in the acute post-MI phase. Early mortality is higher when ventricular fibrillation occurs in the acute phase after infarction, but if the patient survives, long-term prognosis is unaffected.[62]

The mechanism of postinfarct arrhythmias involve the adjoining ischemic but noninfarcted myocardium. In this acidotic arrhythmogenic zone, there is the release of metabolites such as potassium, calcium, and catecholamines, with low levels ATP and hypoxemia.[63] Later in the course of myocardial infarction, arrhythmias may occur as a result of scar tissue surrounding viable myocytes.[64] Experimental data suggest an association between sodium (Na^+) channel loss-of-function and sudden cardiac death. An effect of oxidative stress on Na^+ channel function has been postulated to play a role in postinfarct arrhythmias. Na^+ channel dysfunction may involve lipid peroxidation.[65]

Arrhythmias in the remodeled ischemic myocardium evolve from sites of slow conduction near the border zone, which is characterized by rate-dependent slowing and reentry. It is believed that blockade of the Na^+ channel is responsible for this slowing as cells of the epicardial border zone show postrepolarization refractoriness, a key requirement for the initiation of ischemia-related ventricular tachycardia.

There are emerging clinical imaging techniques to measure areas at risk for arrhythmias. Infarct surface area and mass, as measured by cardiac magnetic resonance imaging, are better identifiers of patients who have a substrate for inducible ventricular tachycardia than left ventricular ejection fraction.[66] The extent of the peri-infarct zone measured by magnetic resonance imaging is correlated with the risk of arrhythmias.[67] The role of adrenergic imbalance in the generation of arrhythmias associated with acute coronary syndromes has been emphasized.[68]

After acute infarction, 25 percent of patients experience a cardiac conduction disturbance within 24 hours. Bradyarrhythmias during the first few hours of acute MI are triggered from inferior myocardial infarction and are usually benign, with conduction disease beyond the first 24 hours requiring the most attention. Conduction disturbances (right bundle-branch block and left anterior fascicular block) resulting from anterior MI are associated with higher mortality because of necrosis of the conduction system.

Atrial fibrillation occurs in approximately 5 to 10 percent of patients postinfarction, especially in older patients with heart failure.[69]

CARDIOGENIC SHOCK

Heart failure after myocardial infarction ranges from pulmonary congestion to profound organ hypoperfusion, or cardiogenic shock. Cardiogenic shock is caused by decreased systemic cardiac output in the presence of adequate intravascular volume. Cardiogenic shock after myocardial infarction usually occurs if there is loss of at least 40 percent of the left ventricular mass, either acutely or in combination with scarred myocardium from old healed infarcts.[15,70] In approximately 10 percent of patients who develop cardiogenic shock, shock occurs before hospitalization immediately upon presentation. Much more commonly, shock develops while the patient is in the hospital, presumably from infarct extension (Fig. 57–10A).[71] As a proportion of short-term deaths after myocardial infarction, cardiogenic shock accounts for 44 percent. The remainder of deaths are the result of cardiac rupture (26 percent) and arrhythmias (16 percent).[64] Patients with extension of infarction (reinfarction) into subendocardial zones remote from the larger infarct may develop cardiogenic shock (Fig. 57–10B). In turn, cardiogenic shock renders the remaining viable myocardium prone to ischemic necrosis because of poor perfusion.

Two related but distinct complications of myocardial infarction are infarct extension and infarct expansion, or remodeling (see the Evolution of Myocardial Infarction section). Infarct extension results from an incremental increase in absolute necrotic myocardium, and may be the result of infarction remote from the original infarct in either the right or left ventricle (see Fig. 57–10). It has been suggested that the more general term *recurrent infarction* be used for infarct extension.[72] Infarct extension usually occurs between 2 and 10 days following infarction, at a time when ECG changes are evolving and the troponin I or T is still high. However, the rapidly falling serum creatine kinase myocardial band (CK-MB) after the first 24 hours may be useful for the detection of infarct extension along with new Q wave on ECG. The risk factors associated with infarct expansion are cardiogenic shock, subendocardial infarct, female gender, and previous infarcts.

RUPTURE OF THE MYOCARDIAL FREE WALL

Left ventricular rupture results in cardiac tamponade, and if there is prolonged survival, pseudoaneurysm formation. The incidence of rupture of the left ventricular free wall is between 10 and 20 percent; patients with first infarct have a rate of approximately 18 percent.[73] In contrast, rupture of the ventricular septum is only 2 percent.[73] Left ventricular wall rupture is seven times more common than right ventricle rupture.[74] Although reperfusion therapy

FIGURE 57–10. **A.** A 54-year-old male with history of acute myocardial infarction had an anteroseptal transmural myocardial infarction. On day 3, the patient went into severe congestive heart failure and died on day 10. Note the markedly thinned transmural anteroseptal infarct (*arrowheads*) involving 60 percent of the basal slice of the heart. The anteroseptal region shows infarct expansion. **B.** A 47-year-old man presented with chest pain, elevated creatine kinase (CK) and creatine kinase myocardial band (CK-MB), and a non–Q-wave myocardial infarction involving the posterior wall of the left ventricle on ECG. Patient had an uneventful hospital course with cardiac enzymes (CK-MB) falling close to baseline. On hospital day 3 he developed another episode of chest pain with a rise in cardiac enzymes and new ECG changes of ST-segment elevation in precordial leads. The patient was diagnosed with infarct extension and right ventricular infarction. The ventricular slice shows an older subendocardial infarct with hyperemic border (*arrowheads*) and a more recent infarction involving full thickness of the posterior wall and portion of the ventricular septum of the left ventricle with extension into the posterior wall of the right ventricle (*arrows*). **C.** A 51-year-old male presented with chest pain of longer than 24 hours' duration. A diagnosis of acute myocardial infarction involving the inferior wall of the left ventricle and a right atrial infarction was made. Note the hemorrhagic right atrial border and that the tip is pale and dusky; the surface shows fibrin deposits on the pericardial surface. *Source: Reproduced with permission from Virmani R, Burke AP, Farb A, Atkinson J, eds. Cardiovascular Pathology, 2nd ed. Philadelphia: WB Saunders, 2001: Vol 40, Fig. 5–9.*

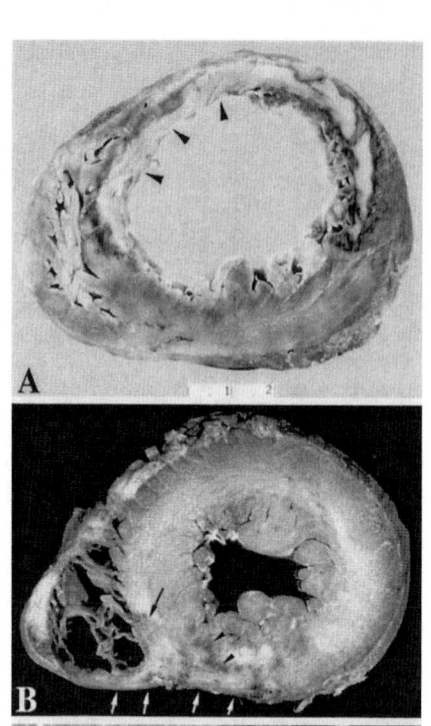
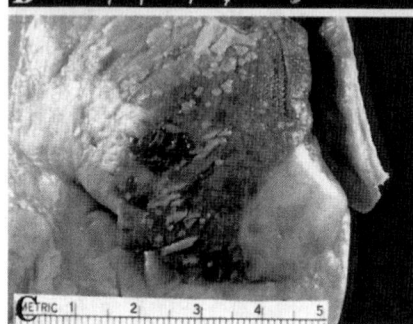

has reduced the incidence of cardiac rupture, late thrombolytic therapy may increase the risk of cardiac rupture (Fig. 57–11).

Factors associated with cardiac rupture include female gender, age older than 60 years, hypertension, and first MI. Additional risk factors include multivessel atherosclerotic disease, absence of ventricular hypertrophy, poor collateral flow, transmural infarct involving at least 20 percent of the wall, and location of the infarct in the mid anterior or lateral wall of the left ventricle.[75] Transthoracic echocardiography is a fast and sensitive test for the diagnosis; contrast echocardiography also has been suggested.[76]

Defective cardiac remodeling, involving matrix metalloproteinases and the extracellular matrix, may predispose the heart for rupture. In addition to surgery, management includes hemodynamic monitoring, blockers, and angiotensin-converting enzyme inhibitors in select cases.[77]

Cardiac rupture usually occurs within 1 to 4 days following the infarct, which is when coagulation necrosis and neutrophilic infiltration are at their peak and have weakened the left ventricular wall. However, at least 13 to 28 percent of ruptures occur within 24 hours of onset of infarction when inflammation and necrosis are not prominent.[74] Infarcts with rupture contain more extensive inflammation and are more likely to demonstrate eosinophils as compared to nonruptured infarcts.[78] Rupture most frequently occurs at the border of the infarcted region with the

viable myocardium. Ruptures usually are not seen beyond 10 days after healing occurs. However, ruptures in infarcts with healing generally occur in the center of the infarct, unlike earlier ruptures (see Fig. 57–11). Nearly half the deaths from cardiac rupture occur as out-of-hospital sudden deaths, and therefore are never seen by the clinician.[74] The mortality rate in the prethrombolytic era was extremely high, with 50 percent mortality in surgically treated patients and 90 percent mortality in medically treated patients. Surgical options include both open procedures and percutaneous seals.[79]

Myocardial rupture, in addition to the free wall, may involve solely the papillary muscle or the ventricular septum. Ruptures of the ventricular septum are classified into simple or complex. Simple ruptures have a discreet defect and a direct through-and-through communication across the septum, are usually associated with anterior myocardial infarction, and are located in the apex. Complex ruptures are characterized by extensive hemorrhage with irregular serpiginous borders of the necrotic muscle, usually occur in inferior infarcts, and involve the basal inferoposterior septum.[80]

Rupture of papillary muscle is less common than septal or free wall rupture, and may occur as a complication of small subendocardial or larger transmural myocardial infarctions. More than 80 percent of infarcts underlying papillary muscle rupture involve the posteromedial muscle, which has a single blood supply from the right coronary artery (see Fig. 57–11). Because the anterolateral papillary muscle has a dual blood supply from the left anterior descending and the left circumflex coronary artery, it rarely undergoes isolated ischemic rupture. However, it may rarely rupture if there is a single supply via one diagonal branch.[81] The patient with papillary muscle rupture presents with sudden mitral regurgitation with variable severity. Diagnosis is made by transesophageal echocardiography, including transgastric imaging.[82] Operative mortality is high, but there is good long-term survival after operative repair.[83,84]

⟦ ⟧ RIGHT-SIDED AND ATRIAL INFARCTION

Right ventricular infarction is a common complication of inferior transmural myocardial infarction (see Fig. 57–10B). Its pathophysiology and clinical manifestations are distinctly different from those of left ventricular infarction. Necropsy studies demonstrate right ventricular infarction in 14 to 60 percent of patients who die with inferior left ventricular myocardial infarction, and is usually seen as a triad of findings consisting of inferior–posterior wall, posterior septum, and posterior right ventricular wall necrosis, which is contiguous and, rarely, with anterolateral right ventricular wall extension.[85] We reported that 78 percent of right ventricular infarctions occurring in patients with inferior left ventricular infarcts had concomitant right ventricular hypertrophy.[86] Isolated right ventricular infarction may occur infrequently in the absence of coronary disease in patients with chronic lung disease and right ventricular hypertrophy.[87] Atrial infarction occurs in 10 percent of all left ventricular inferior wall infarcts, and typically involves the right atrium.[88]

Right ventricular cardiogenic shock after acute infarction is associated with younger age, lower prevalence of previous infarctions, fewer anterior infarct locations, and less multivessel disease.[89]

〖 〗 PERICARDIAL EFFUSION AND PERICARDITIS

Pericardial effusion is reported in 25 percent of patients with acute myocardial infarcts and is more common in patients with anterior myocardial infarction, large infarcts, and congestive heart failure.[90] Pericardial effusion secondary to acute myocardial infarction may occur as a transudative effusion, or as an exudate, in association with acute pericarditis.

Myocardial infarction-associated pericarditis is a common cause of chest pain following MI, its frequency depending on how it is defined. Pericarditis occurs less often than pericardial effusion, and is seen only in transmural acute myocardial infarction. Pericarditis, in contrast to postinfarction effusions, may be localized to the area of necrosis, and is accompanied by chest pain. The incidence appears to have decreased in the era of thrombolytic therapy, the incidence of pleuropericardial chest pain has remained constant.[91] Pericardial involvement is related to infarct size and is associated with poor prognosis. Postinfarction syndrome (Dressler syndrome) consists of pleuropericardial chest pain, friction rub, fever, leukocytosis, and pulmonary infiltrates, occurs weeks to months after myocardial infarction, and is often recurrent. Previously reported to occur in 3 to 4 percent of all cases of myocardial infarction, its incidence had been greatly reduced because of the extensive use of thrombolysis and treatments that dramatically decrease the size of myocardial necrosis and modulated the immune system.[92]

Pericarditis consists of fibrin deposition in addition to inflammation, and may be present from day 1 postinfarction to as late as 6 weeks postinfarction. Pericardial effusion after myocardial infarction usually takes several months to reabsorb. In Dressler syn-

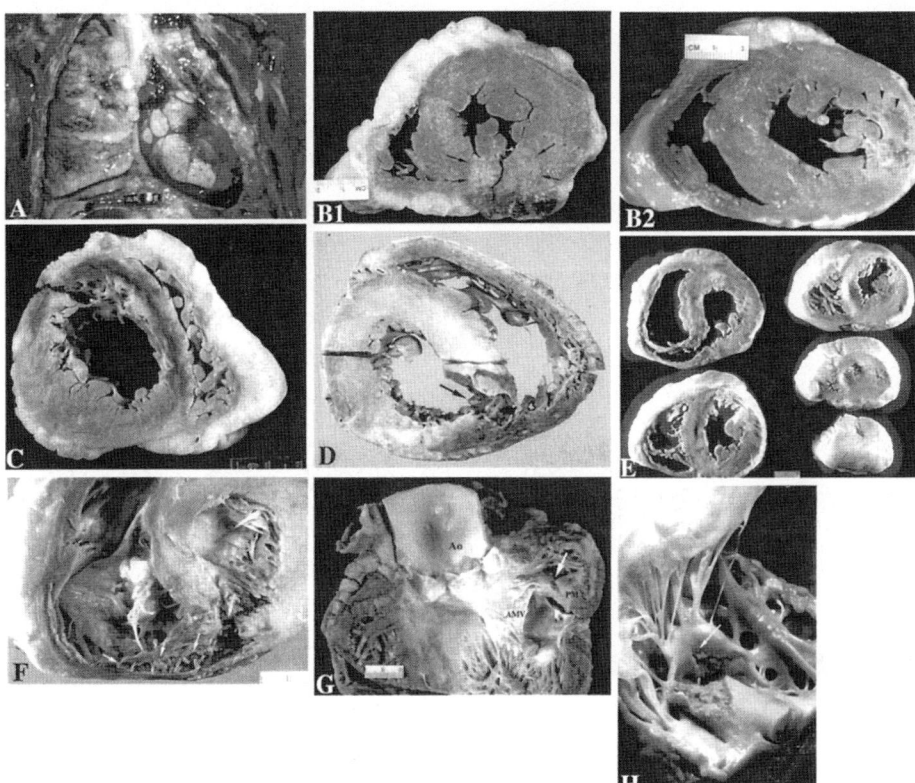

FIGURE 57-11. Ruptured acute myocardial infarction. **A.** Hemopericardium in a 70-year-old male with history of chest pain and diagnosis of acute transmural infarction who died suddenly while walking to the bathroom 24 hours after admission. The pericardium contained 300 mL of blood and a rupture site was identified on the posterior wall of the left ventricle (**B1**). Note the early transmural infarct (pale area on the posterior wall [*arrows*]) with the rupture site close to the viable myocardium but within the infarct zone. **B2** shows a lateral wall rupture. Note that the rupture site is close to the viable and infarcted myocardium (*arrowheads*). **C.** A 50-year-old man presented with chest pain of 7 hours' duration. He received streptokinase and underwent balloon angioplasty of the proximal left anterior descending coronary artery. At autopsy, the patient had hemopericardium and a transmural hemorrhagic reperfused infarct that involved the anteroseptal wall of left ventricle. The rupture occurred close to the viable myocardium on the anterior wall. **D.** Rupture of the posterior ventricular septum (*arrow*) 2 weeks following an acute myocardial infarction. The patient died with severe congestive heart failure, and the diagnosis of ventricular septal rupture was clinically missed. (A four-chamber cut had been made prior to short-axis slicing.) **E.** Ventricular septal rupture involving the inferobasal portion of the heart, which extends through the posterior septum and into the right ventricular, causing a dissection of the posterior wall of the right ventricle. **F.** A high-power view of the inferobasal portion of the heart showing the rupture through the septum extending into the right ventricle and piercing the right ventricular wall (*arrow* along the rupture tract). **G.** A patient with transmural myocardial infarction of the posterior wall of the left ventricle with rupture of one of the two heads of posteromedial (PM) papillary muscle (*arrow*). The base of the heart has been opened along the left ventricular outflow tract (Ao, aorta; AMV, anterior mitral leaflet). **H.** High-power view showing total severance of one of the papillary heads (*arrow*) of the posteromedial papillary muscle. *Source: Reproduced with permission from Virmani R, Burke AP, Farb A, Atkinson J, eds. Cardiovascular Pathology, 2nd ed. Philadelphia: WB Saunders, 2001: Vol 40, Fig. 5–10.*

drome, there is localized fibrinous pericarditis along with neutrophil infiltration.

〖 〗 CHRONIC CONGESTIVE HEART FAILURE

Patients with large acute myocardial infarction and persistent ischemia are the most likely to develop heart failure. The occurrence of heart failure has long been recognized as a strong predictor of increased morbidity and mortality after myocardial infarction. The therapeutic impact of renin–angiotensin system inhibition, early -blockade, and aggressive reperfusion strategies have been investigated in a number of clinical trials.[93] Newer approaches, in-

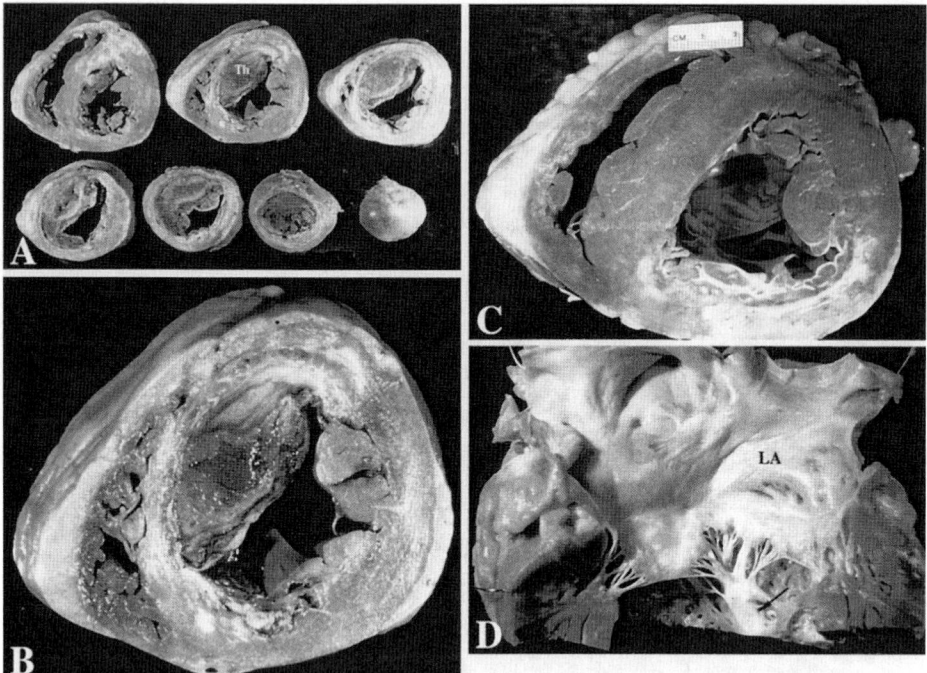

FIGURE 57–12. Thrombus left ventricle with healed myocardial infarct. **A.** Ventricular slices of a heart with healed myocardial infarction involving the anteroseptal wall of the left ventricle with extension from the base to the apex, note dilatation of the left ventricular cavity and presence of an organizing thrombus (Th). **B.** Closeup of the basal ventricular slice (middle slice from top row in **A**). Note the large transmural healed infarct with overlying organizing infarct. At autopsy, patient had multiple infarcts in the kidneys and one in the spleen. **C.** A 60-year-old man with congestive heart failure and mitral regurgitation who had a healed myocardial infarction of the posterolateral wall of the left ventricle at autopsy. **D.** Note scarred and thinned posteromedial papillary muscle (*arrow*), whereas the anterolateral papillary muscle is hypertrophied. Note the dilated left atrium (LA). *Source: Reproduced with permission from Virmani R, Burke AP, Farb A, Atkinson J, eds. Cardiovascular Pathology, 2nd ed. Philadelphia: WB Saunders, 2001: Vol 40, Fig. 5–11.*

cluding inhibition of nitric oxide synthase and new mechanical support devices, may further decrease mortality rates, which nevertheless remain high.[94]

At autopsy, congestive heart failure is characterized by dilatation of both atria and the ventricles, which show either a large healed infarct (Fig. 57–12) or multiple smaller infarcts with or without a transmural scar.[95] Scarring of the inferior wall of the left ventricle often involves the posteromedial papillary muscle, which gives rise to mitral regurgitation, contributing to congestive heart failure (Fig. 57–12).[95] Microscopically, the subendocardial regions of ischemia will show myocytes with myofibrillar loss and which are rich in glycogen, suggesting a state of hibernation (see Hibernating Myocardium section).[96] It is sometimes difficult to differentiate ischemic cardiomyopathy from idiopathic dilated cardiomyopathy when infarcts are few and small and only one vessel disease is present; in such situations we tend to call these idiopathic dilated cardiomyopathy with incidental coronary artery disease.[97]

[ ] TRUE AND FALSE ANEURYSM

The overall incidence of left ventricular aneurysm is currently nearly 12 percent.[98] Angiographically, single-vessel disease, proximal left anterior descending artery stenosis, total left anterior descending coronary artery (LAD) occlusion, end-diastolic pressure, and left ventricular score are higher in patients who develop aneurysms after infarction, as compared to nonaneurysmal infarcts. By

multivariate analysis, single-vessel disease, absence of previous angina, total LAD occlusion, and female gender are independent determinants of left ventricular aneurysm formation after anterior infarct.[99] Patients receiving thrombolytic therapy and exhibiting a patent infarct-related artery have a lower incidence of aneurysm formation.[98]

A large acute transmural myocardial infarct that has undergone expansion is the most likely infarct that will result in a true aneurysm. The pulsatile force from the blood in the cavity stretches and thins the necrotic muscle, which heals forming the wall of a true aneurysm.[100] An aneurysm is defined clinically as a discrete thinned segment of the left ventricle that protrudes during both systole and diastole and has a broad neck (Fig. 57–13). Morphologically the wall of a true aneurysm develops after myocardial infarction and consists of fibrous tissue with or without interspersed myocytes. In contrast, a false aneurysm has a small neck (from a prior rupture of the free wall of the left ventricle caused by infarct and is contained by the adherent pericardium) and a wall of the aneurysm is formed by fibrous pericardium (not from the left ventricular myocardial infarction and healing), and the aneurysm is usually filled by a thrombus that is organizing (Fig. 57–13). False aneurysms often require urgent surgical repair because of their propensity to rupture; false aneurysms may also give rise to congestive heart failure. The cavity of the false aneurysm is usually filled with large blood clots, both old and new. The presence of hypertension and the use of steroids and nonsteroidal antiinflammatory drug may promote aneurysm formation.[101]

Aneurysms are usually associated with two-or-more-vessel coronary disease with poorly developed collaterals.[102] Four of five aneurysms involve the anteroapical wall of the left ventricle and are four times more frequent in this wall than in the inferior or posterior wall. The pericardium is usually adherent to the aneurysm and may calcify. True aneurysm rarely rupture, whereas rupture is more common of a false aneurysm (see Fig. 57–13).[103] The cavity of the aneurysm usually contains an organizing thrombus and the patient may present with embolic complications. The mortality is significantly higher in patients with aneurysm than without.

Mills et al. suggested that aneurysmectomy should be performed in patients having true aneurysms because of poor prognosis. They reported a 27 percent 3-year survival in an autopsy series and a 70 percent survival in the Coronary Artery Surgery Study.[104] Percutaneous closure has also been successfully reported.[105] The survival of patients with pseudoaneurysm is also better following surgery. It has been said that more than half of pseudoaneurysms are located in the posterior or inferior walls whereas true aneurysms mostly involve the anterior wall. There is speculation regarding the reasons for these differences because large inferoposterior infarcts that could lead to aneurysms are more often fatal and posterior rupture is more often contained by the pericardium, allowing pseudoaneurysm to develop.[106]

[ ] MURAL THROMBUS AND EMBOLIZATION

Mural thrombus forming on the endocardial surface over the area of the acute infarction occurs in 20 percent of all patients. However, the incidence is 40 percent for anterior infarcts and 60 percent for apical infarcts.[107] Patients with left ventricular thrombi have poorer global left ventricular function and poorer prognosis than those patients without thrombi.[108] The poor prognosis is secondary to complications of a large infarct and not from emboli.[107] It is reported that those that form thrombi have endocardial inflammation during the phase of acute infarction. The thrombi tend to organize, but the superficial portions may embolize in approximately 10 percent of cases (Fig. 57–14).[108] The usual sites of symptomatic embolization are the brain, eyes, kidney, spleen, bowel, legs, and coronary arteries. Symptomatic emboli are usually caused by larger fragments, whereas small particles of thrombus that embolize generally do not cause symptoms.[109] The risk of embolization is greatest in the first few weeks of acute myocardial infarction.[110]

PATHOLOGY OF SUDDEN CORONARY DEATH

[ ] INCIDENCE OF CORONARY THROMBOSIS

The frequency of coronary thrombosis in sudden coronary death varies from 20 to 70 percent.[111–113] The time interval between onset of symptoms and death, the presence of concurrent conditions that may cause arrhythmias (scars, ventricular hypertrophy), and the type of prodromal symptom (stable angina, unstable angina, no apparent symptoms) all affect the incidence of thrombi in coronary sudden cardiac death. Coronary thrombosis may occur over two major substrates: rupture of thin-cap fibroatheroma, and plaque erosion. The latter

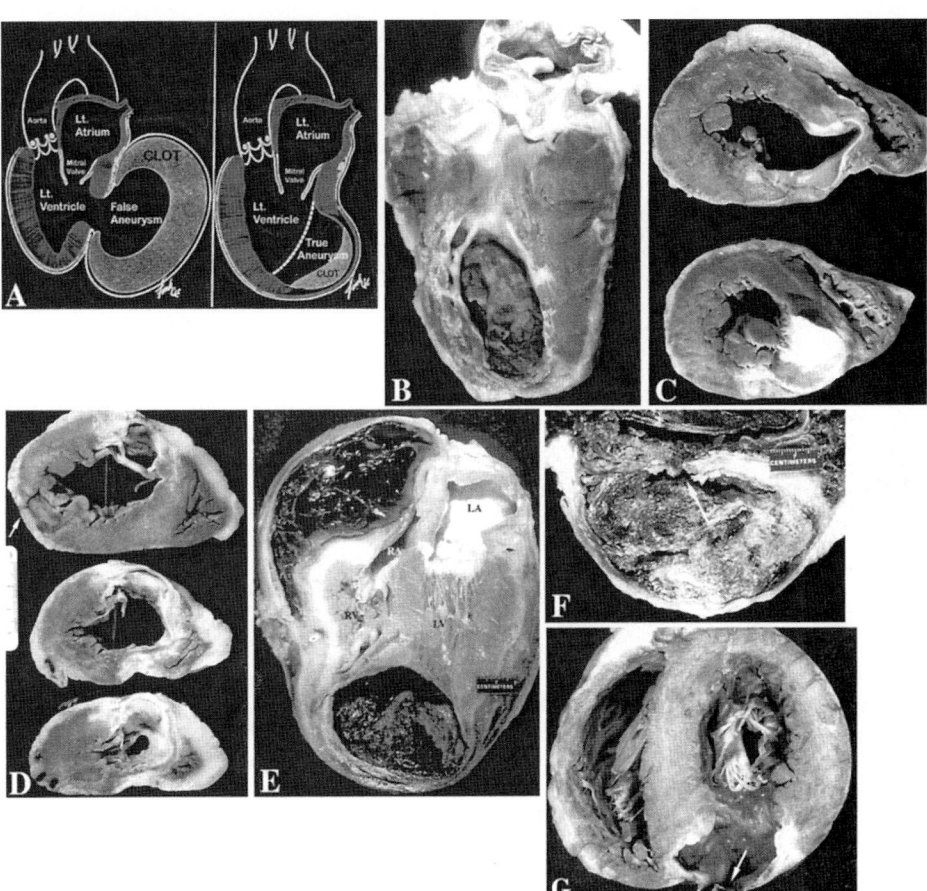

FIGURE 57–13. A. Diagram of a false (*left*) and a true (*right*) aneurysm. Note a rupture of the left ventricular wall with the blood contained by the pericardial wall. The left ventricle does not form the wall of the aneurysm and the neck of the aneurysm is narrow. The wall of the true aneurysm is formed by the wall of the infarcted myocardium and the neck of the aneurysm is wide. *Source: Courtesy of Dr. William C. Roberts.* **B.** A true aneurysm is seen at the apex of the heart involving the anteroseptal apical two-thirds of the left ventricle. The aneurysm is filled with a thrombus and there is endocardial thickening around the edges of the infarct. **C.** Healed transmural infarction of the posteroseptal wall of the left ventricle. Note the thinned and bulging aneurysm of the posterior and septal wall with marked endocardial thickening. No thrombus was identified within the cavity of the aneurysm. **D.** A 54-year–old man died suddenly without any significant medical history. At autopsy there was cardiac tamponade with ventricular rupture of the posterolateral wall (*arrow*) secondary to a transmural acute infarction. Ventricular slices of the heart showing presence of a localized small anterior aneurysm from a healed myocardial infarction involving the anterior and septal wall of the left ventricle. Note organizing thrombus in the aneurysmal cavity. **E.** False aneurysm. A 47-year-old male presented with sudden onset shortness of breath and died in the emergency room. At autopsy there was a loculated hemopericardium and a left ventricular anteroapical aneurysm secondary to a healed myocardial infarction with overlying thrombus. Four-chamber cut of the heart showed extensive adhesions between the visceral and the parietal pericardium, and loculated fresh blood was present in the pericardial space above the right atrium (RA) and right ventricle (RV), as well as organizing hemorrhage around the heart. (LA, left atrium, LV, left ventricle) **F.** A deeper posterior cut revealed the rupture site in the aneurysmal wall (*arrow*). Note the narrow communicating neck of the true aneurysm with the false aneurysm. A diagnosis of rupture of a true aneurysm with a secondary false aneurysm was made. **G.** Rupture of a healed inferior wall aneurysm (*arrow*) in a 56-year-old male who developed chest pain and died while undergoing a stress test. At autopsy, there was hemopericardium (500 mL). *Source: Reproduced with permission from Virmani R, Burke AP, Farb A, Atkinson J, eds.* Cardiovascular Pathology, *2nd ed. Philadelphia: WB Saunders, 2001: Vol 40, Fig. 5–12.*

occur in men and women younger than age 50 years and are less common, whereas plaque rupture is more common, occurs at all ages in adults, and is associated with hypercholesterolemia. We have shown in sudden coronary death that coronary thrombosis is most frequently the result of plaque rupture (65 percent) and less frequently from plaque erosion (30 to 35 percent), and uncommonly from calcified nodule (2 to 5 percent).[52,114]

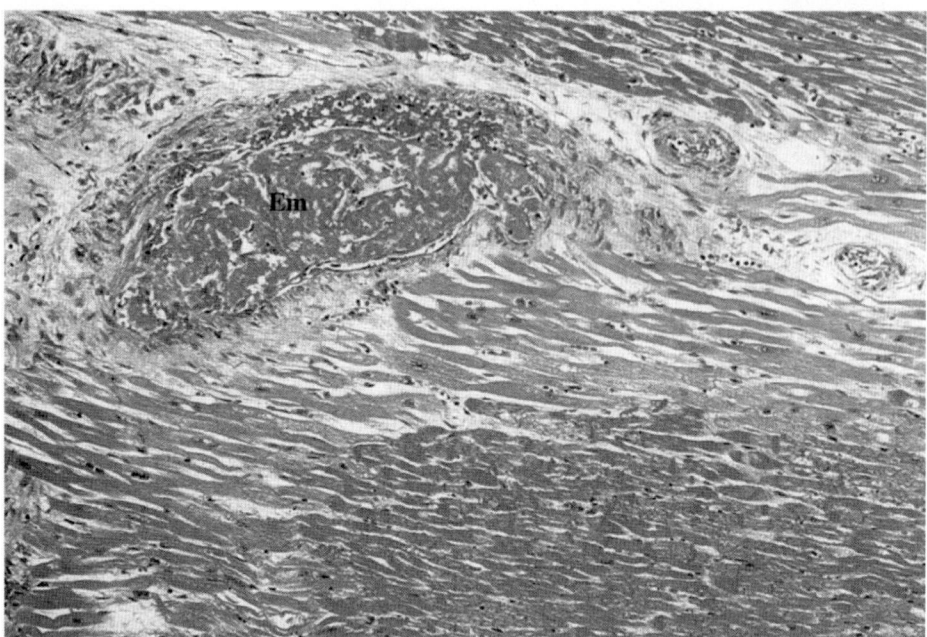

FIGURE 57-14. Intramyocardial thrombus with surrounding acute myocardial infarction in a patient with history of myocardial infarction 6 months prior to current presentation with chest pain. On echocardiography he had a thrombus in the left ventricular cavity overlying the healed infarct. No acute thrombus was seen in any of the epicardial coronary arteries at autopsy. However, the anterolateral wall of the left ventricle showed intramyocardial coronary emboli (Em) and surrounding infarction of less than 24 hours' duration. *Source: Reproduced with permission from Virmani R, Burke AP, Farb A, Atkinson J, eds. Cardiovascular Pathology, 2nd ed. Philadelphia: WB Saunders, 2001: Vol 40, Fig. 5–13.*

❚ ❩ MYOCARDIAL FINDINGS

In our series of sudden coronary death with epicardial thrombosis, there is an approximate 10 percent incidence of acute myocardial infarction, 40 percent incidence of healed myocardial infarction, and in 40 percent no myocardial ischemia is identified.[115] In these cases, it is presumed that ischemia has not been manifest because of the short time interval between thrombosis and death. In sudden coronary death victims without epicardial thrombi, there is a low incidence of acute myocardial infarction (4 percent), with a 60 percent rate of healed infarct, and 35 percent without evidence of acute or healed infarct. Consequently, given that approximately 50 percent of cases of sudden coronary death occur in the absence of coronary thrombosis, 15 to 40 percent of hearts will demonstrate stable coronary atherosclerotic plaque in the absence of acute or healed infarction in the ventricles. The role of cardiac hypertrophy and other arrhythmogenic factors in these deaths has not been studied in detail.

REFERENCES

1. Goldberg RJ, Spencer FA, Yarzebski J, et al. A 25-year perspective into the changing landscape of patients hospitalized with acute myocardial infarction (the Worcester Heart Attack Study). *Am J Cardiol* 2004;94(11):1373–1378.
2. Stanley WC. Cardiac energetics during ischaemia and the rationale for metabolic interventions. *Coron Artery Dis* 2001;12(Suppl 1):S3–S7.
3. Jennings RB, Ganote CE. Mitochondrial structure and function in acute myocardial ischemic injury. *Circ Res* 1976;38(5 Suppl 1):I80–I91.
4. Jennings RB, Ganote CE, Reimer KA. Ischemic tissue injury. *Am J Pathol* 1975;81(1):179–198.
5. Virmani R, Forman MB, Kolodgie FD. Myocardial reperfusion injury. Histopathological effects of perfluorochemical. *Circulation* 1990;81(3 Suppl):IV57–IV68.
6. Jennings RB, Steenbergen C Jr, Reimer KA. Myocardial ischemia and reperfusion. *Monogr Pathol* 1995;37:47–80.
7. Jennings RB, Ganote CE. Structural changes in myocardium during acute ischemia. *Circ Res* 1974;35 Suppl 3:156–172.
8. Buja LM. Myocardial ischemia and reperfusion injury. *Cardiovasc Pathol* 2005;14(4):170–175.
9. Knaapen MW, Davies MJ, De Bie M, Haven AJ, Martinet W, Kockx MM. Apoptotic versus autophagic cell death in heart failure. *Cardiovasc Res* 2001;51(2):304–312.
10. Elsasser A, Vogt AM, Nef H, et al. Human hibernating myocardium is jeopardized by apoptotic and autophagic cell death. *J Am Coll Cardiol* 2004;43(12):2191–2199.
11. Yan L, Vatner DE, Kim SJ, et al. Autophagy in chronically ischemic myocardium. *Proc Natl Acad Sci U S A* 2005;102(39):13807–13812.
12. Abbate A, Bussani R, Biondi-Zoccai GG, et al. Infarct-related artery occlusion, tissue markers of ischaemia, and increased apoptosis in the peri-infarct viable myocardium. *Eur Heart J* 2005;26(19):2039–2045.
13. Miwa K, Fujita M, Kameyama T, Nakagawa K, Hirai T, Inoue H. Absence of myocardial ischemia during sudden controlled occlusion of coronary arteries in patients with well-developed collateral vessels. *Coron Artery Dis* 1999;10(7):459–463.
14. Fujita M, Nakae I, Kihara Y, et al. Determinants of collateral development in patients with acute myocardial infarction. *Clin Cardiol* 1999;22(9):595–599.
15. Page DL, Caulfield JB, Kastor JA, DeSanctis RW, Sanders CA. Myocardial changes associated with cardiogenic shock. *N Engl J Med* 1971;285(3):133–137.
16. Reimer KA, Jennings RB. The "wavefront phenomenon" of myocardial ischemic cell death. II. Transmural progression of necrosis within the framework of ischemic bed size (myocardium at risk) and collateral flow. *Lab Invest* 1979;40(6):633–644.
17. Reimer KA, Jennings RB, Tatum AH. Pathobiology of acute myocardial ischemia: metabolic, functional and ultrastructural studies. *Am J Cardiol* 1983;52(2):72A–81A.
18. Eaton LW, Weiss JL, Bulkley BH, Garrison JB, Weisfeldt ML. Regional cardiac dilatation after acute myocardial infarction: recognition by two-dimensional echocardiography. *N Engl J Med* 1979;300(2):57–62.
19. Bolognese L, Carrabba N, Parodi G, et al. Impact of microvascular dysfunction on left ventricular remodeling and long-term clinical outcome after primary coronary angioplasty for acute myocardial infarction. *Circulation* 2004;109(9):1121–1126.
20. Cerisano G, Bolognese L, Carrabba N, et al. Doppler-derived mitral deceleration time: an early strong predictor of left ventricular remodeling after reperfused anterior acute myocardial infarction. *Circulation* 1999;99(2):230–236.
21. Bellenger NG, Yousef Z, Rajappan K, Marber MS, Pennell DJ. Infarct zone viability influences ventricular remodelling after late recanalisation of an occluded infarct related artery. *Heart* 2005;91(4):478–483.
22. Kloner RA, Ganote CE, Jennings RB. The "no-reflow" phenomenon after temporary coronary occlusion in the dog. *J Clin Invest* 1974;54(6):1496–1508.
23. Moens AL, Claeys MJ, Timmermans JP, Vrints CJ. Myocardial ischemia/reperfusion-injury, a clinical view on a complex pathophysiological process. *Int J Cardiol* 2005;100(2):179–190.
24. Heusch G, Schulz R, Haude M, Erbel R. Coronary microembolization. *J Mol Cell Cardiol* 2004;37(1):23–31.
25. El-Maraghi N, Genton E. The relevance of platelet and fibrin thromboembolism of the coronary microcirculation, with special reference to sudden cardiac death. *Circulation* 1980;62(5):936–944.
26. Davies MJ, Thomas AC, Knapman PA, Hangartner JR. Intramyocardial platelet aggregation in patients with unstable angina suffering sudden ischemic cardiac death. *Circulation* 1986;73(3):418–427.
27. Falk E. Unstable angina with fatal outcome: dynamic coronary thrombosis leading to infarction and/or sudden death. Autopsy evidence of recurrent

mural thrombosis with peripheral embolization culminating in total vascular occlusion. *Circulation* 1985;71(4):699–708.

28. Frink RJ, Rooney PA Jr, Trowbridge JO, Rose JP. Coronary thrombosis and platelet/fibrin microemboli in death associated with acute myocardial infarction. *Br Heart J* 1988;59(2):196–200.

29. Murry CE, Jennings RB, Reimer KA. Preconditioning with ischemia: a delay of lethal cell injury in ischemic myocardium. *Circulation* 1986;74(5):1124–1136.

30. Kuzuya T, Hoshida S, Yamashita N, et al. Delayed effects of sublethal ischemia on the acquisition of tolerance to ischemia. *Circ Res* 1993;72(6):1293–1299.

31. Hagar JM, Hale SL, Kloner RA. Effect of preconditioning ischemia on reperfusion arrhythmias after coronary artery occlusion and reperfusion in the rat. *Circ Res* 1991;68(1):61–68.

32. Yellon DM, Alkhulaifi AM, Pugsley WB. Preconditioning the human myocardium. *Lancet* 1993;342(8866):276–277.

33. Kloner RA, Yellon D. Does ischemic preconditioning occur in patients? *J Am Coll Cardiol* 1994;24(4):1133–1142.

34. Kloner RA, Shook T, Antman EM, et al. Prospective temporal analysis of the onset of preinfarction angina versus outcome: an ancillary study in TIMI-9B. *Circulation* 1998;97(11):1042–1045.

35. Critz SD, Liu GS, Chujo M, Downey JM. Pinacidil but not nicorandil opens ATP-sensitive K$^+$ channels and protects against simulated ischemia in rabbit myocytes. *J Mol Cell Cardiol* 1997;29(4):1123–1130.

36. Kloner RA, Jennings RB. Consequences of brief ischemia: stunning, preconditioning, and their clinical implications: part 2. *Circulation* 2001;104(25):3158–3167.

37. Takano H, Bolli R, Black RG Jr, et al. A(1) or A(3) adenosine receptors induce late preconditioning against infarction in conscious rabbits by different mechanisms. *Circ Res* 2001;88(5):520–528.

38. Rahimtoola SH, Grunkemeier GL, Teply JF, et al. Changes in coronary bypass surgery leading to improved survival. *JAMA* 1981;246(17):1912–1916.

39. Heusch G, Schulz R, Rahimtoola SH. Myocardial hibernation: a delicate balance. *Am J Physiol Heart Circ Physiol* 2005;288(3):H984–H999.

40. Bhatia G, Sosin M, Leahy JF, Connolly DL, Davis RC, Lip GY. Hibernating myocardium in heart failure. *Expert Rev Cardiovasc Ther* 2005;3(1):111–122.

41. Sheiban I, Tonni S, Marini A, Trevi G. Clinical and therapeutic implications of chronic left ventricular dysfunction in coronary artery disease. *Am J Cardiol* 1995;75(13):23E–30E.

42. Schmidt WG, Sheehan FH, von Essen R, Uebis R, Effert S. Evolution of left ventricular function after intracoronary thrombolysis for acute myocardial infarction. *Am J Cardiol* 1989;63(9):497–502.

43. Gerber BL, Belge B, Legros GJ, et al. Characterization of acute and chronic myocardial infarcts by multidetector computed tomography: comparison with contrast-enhanced magnetic resonance. *Circulation* 2006;113(6):823–833.

44. Vanoverschelde JL, Wijns W, Depre C, et al. Mechanisms of chronic regional postischemic dysfunction in humans. New insights from the study of noninfarcted collateral-dependent myocardium. *Circulation* 1993;87(5):1513–1523.

45. Lim H, Fallavollita JA, Hard R, Kerr CW, Canty JM Jr. Profound apoptosis-mediated regional myocyte loss and compensatory hypertrophy in pigs with hibernating myocardium. *Circulation* 1999;100(23):2380–2386.

46. Schwarz ER, Schaper J, vom Dahl J, et al. Myocyte degeneration and cell death in hibernating human myocardium. *J Am Coll Cardiol* 1996;27(7):1577–1585.

47. Elsasser A, Schaper J. Hibernating myocardium: adaptation or degeneration? *Basic Res Cardiol* 1995;90(1):47–48.

48. Elsasser A, Schlepper M, Klovekorn WP, et al. Hibernating myocardium: an incomplete adaptation to ischemia. *Circulation* 1997;96(9):2920–2931.

49. Kaprielian RR, Gunning M, Dupont E, et al. Downregulation of immunodetectable connexin43, and decreased gap junction size in the pathogenesis of chronic hibernation in the human left ventricle. *Circulation* 1998;97(7):651–660.

50. Arbustini E, Dal Bello B, Morbini P, et al. Plaque erosion is a major substrate for coronary thrombosis in acute myocardial infarction. *Heart* 1999;82(3):269–272.

51. Falk E, Shah PK, Fuster V. Coronary plaque disruption. *Circulation* 1995;92(3):657–671.

52. Farb A, Burke AP, Tang AL, et al. Coronary plaque erosion without rupture into a lipid core. A frequent cause of coronary thrombosis in sudden coronary death. *Circulation* 1996;93(7):1354–1363.

53. Vargas SO, Sampson BA, Schoen FJ. Pathologic detection of early myocardial infarction: a critical review of the evolution and usefulness of modern techniques. *Mod Pathol* 1999;12(6):635–645.

54. Adegboyega PA, Adesokan A, Haque AK, Boor PJ. Sensitivity and specificity of triphenyl tetrazolium chloride in the gross diagnosis of acute myocardial infarcts. *Arch Pathol Lab Med* 1997;121(10):1063–1068.

55. Frangogiannis NG. Chemokines in the ischemic myocardium: from inflammation to fibrosis. *Inflamm Res* 2004;53(11):585–595.

56. Frangogiannis NG, Entman ML. Identification of mast cells in the cellular response to myocardial infarction. *Methods Mol Biol* 2006;315:91–101.

57. Cowan MJ, Reichenbach D, Turner P, Thostenson C. Cellular response of the evolving myocardial infarction after therapeutic coronary artery reperfusion. *Hum Pathol* 1991;22(2):154–163.

58. Hohnloser SH, Gersh BJ. Changing late prognosis of acute myocardial infarction: impact on management of ventricular arrhythmias in the era of reperfusion and the implantable cardioverter-defibrillator. *Circulation* 2003;107(7):941–946.

59. Menon V, Hochman JS. Management of cardiogenic shock complicating acute myocardial infarction. *Heart* 2002;88(5):531–537.

60. Campbell RW, Murray A, Julian DG. Ventricular arrhythmias in first 12 hours of acute myocardial infarction. Natural history study. *Br Heart J* 1981;46(4):351–357.

61. Perron AD, Sweeney T. Arrhythmic complications of acute coronary syndromes. *Emerg Med Clin North Am* 2005;23(4):1065–1082.

62. Khairy P, Thibault B, Talajic M, et al. Prognostic significance of ventricular arrhythmias post-myocardial infarction. *Can J Cardiol* 2003;19(12):1393–1404.

63. Corr PB, Sobel BE. Mechanisms contributing to dysrhythmias induced by ischemia and their therapeutic implications. *Adv Cardiol* 1978;22:110–129.

64. Stevenson WG, Linssen GC, Havenith MG, Brugada P, Wellens HJ. The spectrum of death after myocardial infarction: a necropsy study. *Am Heart J* 1989;118(6):1182–1188.

65. Fukuda K, Davies SS, Nakajima T, et al. Oxidative mediated lipid peroxidation recapitulates proarrhythmic effects on cardiac sodium channels. *Circ Res* 2005;97(12):1262–1269.

66. Bello D, Fieno DS, Kim RJ, et al. Infarct morphology identifies patients with substrate for sustained ventricular tachycardia. *J Am Coll Cardiol* 2005;45(7):1104–1108.

67. Yan AT, Shayne AJ, Brown KA, et al. Characterization of the peri-infarct zone by contrast-enhanced cardiac magnetic resonance imaging is a powerful predictor of post-myocardial infarction mortality. *Circulation* 2006;114(1):32–39.

68. Bacaner M, Brietenbucher J, LaBree J. Prevention of ventricular fibrillation, acute myocardial infarction (myocardial necrosis), heart failure, and mortality by bretylium: is ischemic heart disease primarily adrenergic cardiovascular disease? *Am J Ther* 2004;11(5):366–411.

69. Bhatia GS, Lip GY. Atrial fibrillation post-myocardial infarction: frequency, consequences, and management. *Curr Heart Fail Rep* 2004;1(4):149–155.

70. Califf RM, Bengtson JR. Cardiogenic shock. *N Engl J Med* 1994;330(24):1724–1730.

71. Holmes DR Jr, Bates ER, Kleiman NS, et al. Contemporary reperfusion therapy for cardiogenic shock: the GUSTO-I trial experience. The GUSTO-I Investigators. Global Utilization of Streptokinase and Tissue Plasminogen Activator for Occluded Coronary Arteries. *J Am Coll Cardiol* 1995;26(3):668–674.

72. Califf RM. Myocardial reperfusion: is it ever too late? *J Am Coll Cardiol* 1989;13(5):1130–1132.

73. Figueras J, Cortadellas J, Soler-Soler J. Left ventricular free wall rupture: clinical presentation and management. *Heart* 2000;83(5):499–504.

74. Batts KP, Ackermann DM, Edwards WD. Postinfarction rupture of the left ventricular free wall: clinicopathologic correlates in 100 consecutive autopsy cases. *Hum Pathol* 1990;21(5):530–535.

75. Pohjola-Sintonen S, Muller JE, Stone PH, et al. Ventricular septal and free wall rupture complicating acute myocardial infarction: experience in the Multicenter Investigation of Limitation of Infarct Size. *Am Heart J* 1989;117(4):809–818.

76. Naik H, Sherev D, Hui PY. The rapid diagnosis of pseudoaneurysm formation in left ventricular free wall rupture. *J Invasive Cardiol* 2004;16(7):390–392.

77. Wehrens XH, Doevendans PA. Cardiac rupture complicating myocardial infarction. *Int J Cardiol* 2004;95(2–3):285–292.

78. Atkinson JB, Robinowitz M, McAllister HA, Virmani R. Association of eosinophils with cardiac rupture. *Hum Pathol* 1985;16(6):562–568.

79. Birnbaum Y, Chamoun AJ, Anzuini A, Lick SD, Ahmad M, Uretsky BF. Ventricular free wall rupture following acute myocardial infarction. *Coron Artery Dis* 2003;14(6):463–470.

80. Birnbaum Y, Fishbein MC, Blanche C, Siegel RJ. Ventricular septal rupture after acute myocardial infarction. *N Engl J Med* 2002;347(18):1426–1432.

81. Wada H, Yasu T, Murata S, et al. Rupture of the anterolateral papillary muscle caused by a single diagonal branch obstruction. *Circ J* 2002;66(9):872–873.

82. Kim MY, Park CH, Lee JA, Song JH, Park SH. Papillary muscle rupture after acute myocardial infarction--the importance of transgastric view of TEE. *Korean J Intern Med* 2002;17(4):274–277.

83. Minami H, Mukohara N, Obo H, et al. Papillary muscle rupture following acute myocardial infarction. *Jpn J Thorac Cardiovasc Surg* 2004;52(8):367–371.

84. Chen Q, Darlymple-Hay MJ, Alexiou C, et al. Mitral valve surgery for acute papillary muscle rupture following myocardial infarction. *J Heart Valve Dis* 2002;11(1):27–31.

85. Isner JM, Roberts WC. Right ventricular infarction complicating left ventricular infarction secondary to coronary heart disease. Frequency, location, associated findings and significance from analysis of 236 necropsy patients with acute or healed myocardial infarction. *Am J Cardiol* 1978;42(6):885–894.

86. Forman MB, Wilson BH, Sheller JR, et al. Right ventricular hypertrophy is an important determinant of right ventricular infarction complicating acute inferior left ventricular infarction. *J Am Coll Cardiol* 1987;10(6):1180–1187.

87. Kopelman HA, Forman MB, Wilson BH, et al. Right ventricular myocardial infarction in patients with chronic lung disease: possible role of right ventricular hypertrophy. *J Am Coll Cardiol* 1985;5(6):1302–1307.

88. Lazar EJ, Goldberger J, Peled H, Sherman M, Frishman WH. Atrial infarction: diagnosis and management. *Am Heart J* 1988;116(4):1058–1063.

89. Pfisterer M. Right ventricular involvement in myocardial infarction and cardiogenic shock. *Lancet* 2003;362(9381):392–394.

90. Sugiura T, Iwasaka T, Takayama Y, et al. Factors associated with pericardial effusion in acute Q wave myocardial infarction. *Circulation* 1990;81(2):477–481.

91. Aydinalp A, Wishniak A, van den Akker-Berman L, Or T, Roguin N. Pericarditis and pericardial effusion in acute ST-elevation myocardial infarction in the thrombolytic era. *Isr Med Assoc J* 2002;4(3):181–183.

92. Bendjelid K, Pugin J. Is Dressler syndrome dead? *Chest* 2004;126(5):1680–1682.

93. Spencer FA, Meyer T. Heart failure and shock complicating acute coronary syndromes. *Curr Cardiol Rep* 2005;7(4):276–282.

94. Duvernoy CS, Bates ER. Management of cardiogenic shock attributable to acute myocardial infarction in the reperfusion era. *J Intensive Care Med* 2005;20(4):188–198.

95. Virmani R, Roberts WC. Quantification of coronary arterial narrowing and of left ventricular myocardial scarring in healed myocardial infarction with chronic, eventually fatal, congestive cardiac failure. *Am J Med* 1980;68(6):831–838.

96. Kloner RA, Bolli R, Marban E, Reinlib L, Braunwald E. Medical and cellular implications of stunning, hibernation, and preconditioning: an NHLBI workshop. *Circulation* 1998;97(18):1848–1867.

97. Atkinson JB, Virmani R. Congestive heart failure due to coronary artery disease without myocardial infarction: clinicopathologic description of an unusual cardiomyopathy. *Hum Pathol* 1989;20(12):1155–1162.

98. Tikiz H, Balbay Y, Atak R, Terzi T, Genc Y, Kutuk E. The effect of thrombolytic therapy on left ventricular aneurysm formation in acute myocardial infarction: relationship to successful reperfusion and vessel patency. *Clin Cardiol* 2001;24(10):656–662.

99. Tikiz H, Atak R, Balbay Y, Genc Y, Kutuk E. Left ventricular aneurysm formation after anterior myocardial infarction: clinical and angiographic determinants in 809 patients. *Int J Cardiol* 2002;82(1):7–14; discussion 14–16.

100. Hamer DH, Lindsay J Jr. Redefining true ventricular aneurysm. *Am J Cardiol* 1989;64(18):1192–1194.

101. Friedman BM, Dunn MI. Postinfarction ventricular aneurysms. *Clin Cardiol* 1995;18(9):505–511.

102. Forman MB, Collins HW, Kopelman HA, et al. Determinants of left ventricular aneurysm formation after anterior myocardial infarction: a clinical and angiographic study. *J Am Coll Cardiol* 1986;8(6):1256–1262.

103. MacDonald ST, Mitchell AR, Timperley J, Forfar JC. Left ventricular pseudoaneurysm and rupture after limited myocardial infarction. *J Am Soc Echocardiogr* 2005;18(9):980.

104. Mills NL, Everson CT, Hockmuth DR. Technical advances in the treatment of left ventricular aneurysm. *Ann Thorac Surg* 1993;55(3):792–800.

105. Gladding PA, Ruygrok PN, Greaves SC, Gerber IL, Hamer AW. Images in cardiovascular medicine. Percutaneous closure of a left ventricular free-wall rupture site. *Circulation* 2006;113(18):e748–e749.

106. Brown SL, Gropler RJ, Harris KM. Distinguishing left ventricular aneurysm from pseudoaneurysm. A review of the literature. *Chest* 1997;111(5):1403–1409.

107. Fuster V, Halperin JL. Left ventricular thrombi and cerebral embolism. *N Engl J Med* 1989;320(6):392–394.

108. Keeley EC, Hillis LD. Left ventricular mural thrombus after acute myocardial infarction. *Clin Cardiol* 1996;19(2):83–86.

109. Meltzer RS, Visser CA, Fuster V. Intracardiac thrombi and systemic embolization. *Ann Intern Med* 1986;104(5):689–698.

110. Kupper AJ, Verheugt FW, Peels CH, Galema TW, Roos JP. Left ventricular thrombus incidence and behavior studied by serial two-dimensional echocardiography in acute anterior myocardial infarction: left ventricular wall motion, systemic embolism and oral anticoagulation. *J Am Coll Cardiol* 1989;13(7):1514–1520.

111. Davies MJ, Bland JM, Hangartner JR, Angelini A, Thomas AC. Factors influencing the presence or absence of acute coronary artery thrombi in sudden ischemic death. *Eur Heart J* 1989;10:203–208.

112. Farb A, Tang AL, Burke AP, Sessums L, Liang Y, Virmani R. Sudden coronary death. Frequency of active coronary lesions, inactive coronary lesions, and myocardial infarction. *Circulation* 1995;92(7):1701–1709.

113. Scott RF, Briggs TS. Pathologic findings in pre-hospital deaths due to coronary atherosclerosis. *Am J Cardiol* 1971;29:782–787.

114. Virmani R, Kolodgie FD, Burke AP, Farb A, Schwartz SM. Lessons from sudden coronary death: A comprehensive morphological classification scheme for atherosclerotic lesions. *Arterioscler Thromb Vasc Biol* 2000;20(5):1262–1275.

115. Virmani R, Kolodgie FD, Burke AP, Farb A, Schwartz SM. Lessons from sudden coronary death: a comprehensive morphological classification scheme for atherosclerotic lesions. *Arterioscler Thromb Vasc Biol* 2000;20(5):1262–1275.

CHAPTER (58)

Molecular and Cellular Mechanisms of Myocardial Ischemia–Reperfusion Injury

Cyril Ruwende / Scott Visovatti / David J. Pinsky

INTRODUCTION

Normal cardiac function is predicated on a continuous supply of oxygen and nutritive substances. When coronary perfusion is interrupted, profound myocardial damage can occur at both microscopic and macroscopic levels. Clinically, this scenario gives rise to acute coronary syndromes manifesting as angina, or in the most severe form, acute myocardial infarction. The onset of ischemia triggers homeostatic processes geared at limiting damage, but which may act in concert with processes associated with reperfusion, to actually exacerbate injury. These potentially deleterious effects of reperfusion have been described as *reperfusion injury*, or, more aptly, as *ischemia–reperfusion injury*, because the pathology associated with reperfusion occurs only in the setting of antecedent ischemia. Ischemia–reperfusion injury is a complex process that is brought about by the interaction of a number of endothelial cells and different inflammatory cells with components of the coagulation and complement cascades. This interplay promotes the formation of harmful substances which may further amplify myocardial cell death after an ischemic insult.

PATHOPHYSIOLOGY OF MYOCARDIAL ISCHEMIA

Myocardial ischemia occurs when there is a demand–supply mismatch between the myocardium's energy requirement and the oxygen supply from myocardial perfusion.[1] With compromise of coronary arterial flow, a number of electrical, mechanical, and chemical changes take place in the ischemic area of myocardium. The myocardium becomes cyanotic with consumption of freely diffusible oxygen and oxymyoglobin oxygen stores causing decreased tissue oxygen tension.[2] With increasing tissue hypoxia, intracellular respiration shifts from its aerobic to its anaerobic form. Adenosine triphosphate (ATP) stores are rapidly depleted,[3] causing adenosine diphosphate (ADP), adenosine monophosphate (AMP), and adenosine to accumulate in the tissue. At this time point, the ischemic region of myocardium loses its ability to maintain the negative resting membrane potential.[4] Diminished ATP stores and or alteration in availability of Ca^{2+} leads to cessation of cardiac contraction.[5] This is followed by a distension of the ischemic myocardium, which perhaps occurs as the result of stretch caused by tugging by adjacent nonischemic (and still contracting) muscle.[6] Characteristic metabolic changes occur in the ischemic tissue, including an accumulation of tissue lactate,[3,7] H[+] ions,[8] phosphate[7] and potassium.[9,10] There is also a rise in tissue tension of carbon dioxide (P_{CO_2}),[11] as an accumulating byproduct of cellular metabolism in the absence of an egress mechanism during the stasis that characterizes ischemia. In addition, mitochondrial calcium increases,[12] a process that may further contribute to ischemic contracture, and perhaps even the ultimate death of the vulnerable myocyte. Arterioles exhibit a profound vasodilator response,[11] which under nonobstructive conditions might result in a restoration of nutritive flow, but under severe ischemic conditions is often futile. If complete obstruction to blood flow persists for as little as 20 minutes, myocardial necrosis may be observed.[13] Under circumstances in which myocardial reperfusion is reestablished with great rapidity, mechanical function can return to near baseline levels.[14]

When ischemic myocardial tissue is subjected to detailed histopathologic examination, there are characteristic structural changes, one of the earliest of which includes a decrease in the size and number of glycogen granules within the myocytes. The amount of glycogen decreases significantly following 30 minutes of ischemia, and almost disappears during the subsequent 2.5 hours.[15–17] Myofibrils then appear to arrest in a relaxed state.[18] Ischemic tissue shows marked enlargement of interfibrillar and subsarcolemmal spaces with swelling of transverse tubules (T-tubules). Mitochondria also appear swollen and demonstrate decreased matrix density.[15–17] This swelling reflects changes in intracellular fluid distribution and increases in myocardial water content, which can represent nearly a 50 percent increase following an extended period of interrupted blood flow.[19,20] In addition to the contribution of intracellular shifts of fluid, there is an expansion of the extracellular water content, presumably brought about by increases in vascular permeability in vessels in the ischemic zone.[21–23]

There remains considerable controversy in the field as to the precise point in this complex process at which the death of cardiac myocytes becomes irreversible. There are many pathologic mechanisms that are triggered, which, if they remain unchecked, certainly lead to the inevitable death of the myocyte. However, other death-sparing pathways may be simultaneously activated and counterbalance the prodeath signals. Consequently, the ultimate fate of the cardiac myocyte is determined by the prevailing balance of forces promoting or inhibiting its death. Clinically, it is often difficult to know where this balance lies, or whether a given therapy will hasten or salvage myocyte death. An ischemic insult can be considered to cause irreversible myocyte death if it is of sufficient magnitude and duration so that cells continue their march toward death even after restoration of blood supply.[24] Dead myocytes exhibit a characteristic histologic appearance, including the presence of contraction bands[25–27] and amorphous densities within swollen mitochondria.[27] Irreversible damage to mitochondria and cell membranes causes the release into blood of numerous plasma markers, which can be used to diagnostically quantify the degree of myocardial necrosis in patients. Markers of cardiac myocyte death appear in the plasma, as plasma membrane integrity is compromised; these include enzymes such as lactate dehydrogenase (LDH), creatinine phosphokinase (CK), serum glutamic oxaloacetic transaminase (sGOT), and other intracellular proteins, such as myoglobin,

troponins T and I, and cardiac-specific myosin light chains.[28] The other factor that contributes to rapid washout of these markers into blood is reperfusion of myocardium following the period of ischemia. Integration of the area under the time–activity curves provides a rough estimate of extent and degree of infarction,[29] although the presence of reperfusion causes early washout peaks, which can somewhat confound quantitative interpretation of this information. There is now greater appreciation of the role of inflammation, vascular remodeling, and plaque vulnerability in modulating ischemic injury in acute coronary syndromes, and an emerging literature points to other potential markers of adverse outcomes that include C-reactive protein,[30] N-terminal probrain natriuretic peptide (NT pro-BNP),[31] soluble CD40 ligand,[32,33] myeloperoxidase,[34] metalloproteinases,[35] tissue inhibitors of metalloproteinases (TIMP),[36] and adiponectin.[37]

PATHOPHYSIOLOGY OF MYOCARDIAL ISCHEMIA–REPERFUSION INJURY

CELLULAR FACTORS

Neutrophil Activation

Neutrophils (polymorphonuclear leukocytes) are key cellular effectors in the pathogenesis of myocardial ischemic–reperfusion damage. There are compelling data from animal studies showing the protective effects of therapies that either interfere with neutrophil adhesion mechanisms or compromise neutrophil function prior to ischemia and reperfusion.[38–40] A number of events must occur for recruitment of the requisite quantity of the neutrophils to elicit myocardial damage in the setting of ischemia/reperfusion. Neutrophils are activated and recruited by pro-inflammatory signals such as tumor necrosis factor (TNF)-α, complement fragments, and cytokines which are released by the ischemic–reperfused myocardium itself,[41–45] or other resident or vascular cells in the vicinity. Intravascular neutrophils decelerate[46] and begin to adhere to endothelium primarily through an interaction via P-selectin glycoprotein-1 (PSGL-1) and L-selectin on the neutrophil, and P-selectin on the endothelium. PSGL-1 is the most well-characterized ligand for all selectins and its dual roles include mediation attachment of leukocytes to the activated endothelium,[47–49] as well as signal transduction for leukocyte activation.[50–53] Whereas L-selectin is constitutively expressed on the neutrophil cell surface, P-selectin is stored in α granules of platelets and Weibel-Palade bodies of endothelial cells, and is rapidly translocated to the cell surface of these cells within minutes of cardiac reperfusion.[54] Hypoxia itself is sufficient to induce endothelial surface expression of P-selectin.[55] This interaction brings the neutrophils into close approximation with the vascular wall, thereby facilitating the engagement of other cognate receptors, such as L-selectin, platelet activating factor, intercellular adhesion molecule-1 (ICAM-1) on the endothelial cells, and leukocyte β$_2$-integrins (CD11/CD18 complex) on the neutrophils.[42] Migration across cell junctions requires interaction between neutrophils and endothelial platelet endothelial cell adhesion molecule (PECAM), another immunoglobulin adhesion molecule. Blockage of PECAM using antibody fragments decreases neutrophil accumulation and infarct size in rat myocardium during ischemic reperfusion.[56]

Infiltration of neutrophils into the ischemic zone begins within 60 minutes after the onset of ischemia, and increases significantly for up to 90 minutes after reperfusion. A canine model comparing permanent occlusion with reperfusion following temporary occlusion showed that accumulation of neutrophils in myocardium was augmented by 80 percent in reperfused infarcts, likely because of reperfusion-facilitated neutrophil entry into necrotic regions.[57] Stimulation of neutrophils by chemotactic factors and cytokines elicits the respiratory burst characterized by sudden release of oxygen-derived free radicals including superoxide anion, hypochlorous acid, hydroxyl radical, chloramine and hydrogen peroxide.[42] This cytotoxic milieu damages endothelial cells and impairs physiologic vasodilatory and anticoagulant mechanisms. These events promote increases in vascular permeability, leukocyte infiltration, and neutrophil and platelet activation and adhesion, thereby further amplifying reactive oxygen species release and exacerbating reperfusion injury.

Thromboresistance: Endothelial Cells and Platelets

The intact endothelium that lines blood vessels maintains an anticoagulant phenotype to maintain blood fluidity. Normally the luminal surface of vascular endothelium repels platelets and coagulant events, and prevents contact of the coagulation system with the subjacent and highly procoagulant endothelial matrix (which is rich in collagen and tissue factor).[58] The endothelial surface is rich in heparin-like proteoglycans that can function to accelerate the inactivation of coagulation proteases by antithrombin III. The other mechanism by which prevention of clot formation is achieved involves the membrane-spanning thrombin-binding protein thrombomodulin, which converts thrombin into a potent protein C activator.[59] In addition, local production of nitric oxide potently inhibits platelet aggregation.

Under conditions associated with tissue hypoxia, such as in myocardial ischemia, the endothelium develops a procoagulant phenotype. Macrophages, monocyte and endothelial cell expression of tissue factor increases, while endothelial cell expression of thrombomodulin is significantly reduced.[60–63] Moreover, retraction of endothelial cell margins exposes the procoagulant subendothelial matrix to circulating elements of the coagulation cascade. Additionally, hypoxia triggers the calcium-dependent exocytosis of Weibel-Palade bodies, leading to increased secretion of von Willebrand factor.[64] In addition, platelet adhesion and aggregation are aided by the superoxide-mediated decline in nitric oxide (NO) levels that occurs with reperfusion,[65–67] which contributes to a local prothrombotic diathesis. Platelets activated by ischemia–reperfusion not only aggregate and cause microvascular plugging, but they also release products such as thromboxane and serotonin that give rise to microvascular inflammation and spasm.[68]

[ ] SUBCELLULAR FACTORS
Mitochondrial Permeability Transition

Because of their key roles as metabolic energy producers and regulators of apoptosis, mitochondria play a central role in cell survival.[69] Mitochondrial injury is believed to be an important component in the pathobiology of ischemia–reperfusion injury. Arguably the most critical factor in determining mitochondrial injury is opening of the permeability transition pores (PTPs), large proteins that form nonselective pores in the inner mitochondrial membrane. The PTP opening leads to immediate depolarization of the mitochondrial membrane and transforms the mitochondria from net ATP producers to net ATP consumers by reversing ATP synthesis in an attempt to maintain the membrane potential. PTPs are believed to be sensitive to calcium, reduction–oxidation, voltage, and pH states.[70] Ischemia serves to prime the mitochondrial permeability transition, whereas reperfusion triggers the process. Under ischemic conditions, activated fatty acids accumulate in the myocardium and not only decrease the rate of ATP synthesis, but also increase both inner mitochondrial membrane leakiness and cytochrome c mobilization and release.[71] During ischemia, acidosis, elevated magnesium levels, and diminished electron transport generally keep PTPs closed; however, with reperfusion, mitochondria are placed at high risk of PTP opening because of the associated reactive oxygen species burst and clearing of acidosis, as well as the elevated calcium and inorganic phosphorous levels.[70]

Intracellular Calcium Overload and the Development of Hypercontracture

Cytosolic calcium overload is believed to be an important mechanism underlying development of ischemic contracture and cardiomyocyte death.[72,73] Whereas ischemia disrupts the capacity of myocytes to regulate calcium, it is reperfusion that dramatically leads to intracellular accumulation of toxic levels of calcium.[74,75] There are several potential mechanisms for this phenomenon.[76] One is related to increased sarcolemmal calcium entry via L-type calcium channels that occurs as a consequence of sodium overload.[77,78] Another possibility links increased myocyte entry of calcium to a perturbation in calcium handling by the sarcoplasmic reticulum secondary to ATP depletion-related disruption of the sarcolemmal membrane.[76] Additionally, there is evidence to suggest that reperfusion injury causes significant myofilament desensitization to calcium. Moreover, in the minutes following reperfusion, intracellular calcium overload and depletion of ATP levels give rise to hypercontracture or sustained shortening and stiffening that causes myocardial stiffness and leads to tissue necrosis.

[ ] HUMORAL FACTORS
Oxygen-Derived Free Radical Release

With reperfusion of previously ischemic myocardium, the reintroduction of abundant oxygen immediately evokes a burst of potent oxygen-derived free radicals, such as superoxide anion, hydroxyl radical, hydrogen peroxide, and peroxynitrite.[79–81] These reactive oxygen species are generated by endothelial cells, recruited/activated leukocytes, and even the myocytes themselves. They are in most instances the byproduct of mitochondrial respiration, catecholamine oxidation, the Haber-Weiss pathway, and the enzyme activities of xanthine oxidase, cytochrome oxidase, and cyclooxygenase.[82–87] The overwhelming increase in oxygen-derived free radicals can peak within minutes but may persist for many hours following restoration of blood flow. This overwhelms the tissues' antioxidant capacity, which leads to protein denaturation, inactivation of key homeostatic enzymes and peroxidation of lipid membranes.[88–90] These processes cause loss of membrane integrity, ultimately giving rise to necrosis and cell death. There are several lines of evidence confirming the in vivo formation of reactive oxygen species in the human heart.

Nitric Oxide

The specific role of NO in myocardial damage and ischemic–reperfusion injury remains controversial. To the extent that endothelial injury and dysregulation of microvascular tone are features of myocardial ischemia–reperfusion injury, it is hardly surprising that NO is implicated in this phenomenon.[91] NO causes relaxation of vascular smooth muscle by activating intracellular guanylate cyclase, causing an increase in cyclic guanosine monophosphate levels.[92] In addition to its vasodilatory function, NO has other important vascular functions as well, such as inhibition of platelet adhesion and aggregation, inhibition of neutrophil adhesion, and maintenance of endothelial restricted diffusion.[93–96] NO may have dual roles in determining cell survival in myocardial ischemia–reperfusion injury. On the one hand, NO can inhibit apoptotic death of myocytes via nitrosylation of active sites of caspases.[97] On the other hand, high NO levels may directly contribute to myocyte apoptosis. Although the synthesis of NO is ongoing during the ischemic phase, reoxygenation triggers a precipitous drop in NO, and this decline is precipitated by the quenching effect of reactive oxygen species generated during reperfusion.[91,98] Several studies demonstrate that administration of NO donors, or induction/overexpression of the enzyme responsible for synthesis of NO, may potentially prevent myocardial ischemia–reperfusion injury.[94,99–102] Curiously, there is equally compelling evidence that pharmacologic inhibition of nitric oxide production may also reduce infarct size, probably by preventing peroxynitrite formation from NO and superoxide during reperfusion.[103–106]

Complement Activation

Activation of complement system has been implicated in ischemia reperfusion injury.[107] Activation of complement by either the classic, alternate, or mannose-binding pathways causes cleavage of the C3 component, which causes formation of the anaphylotoxins (C3a and C5a) and the membrane attack complex (C5b-9; MAC). The MAC is the final effector that punctures the target cell, causing rapid dissipation of ionic gradients and extrusion of cytoplasmic contents. Complement activation elicits myocardial damage in ischemia reperfusion injury via two mechanisms. First, the anaphylotoxins (C3a and C5a) and chemotactic factor C4a augment superoxide production and cellular release of histamine and platelet activating factor, thereby increasing vascular permeability, as well as attracting neutrophils to the ischemic area.[107] Even small amounts of C5b-9, below the threshold levels required for cell lysis, may trigger translocation of P-selectin to the endothelial surface, further contributing to neutrophil adhesion. Second, activation of the complement system also causes direct myocardial damage through the formation of the MAC. MAC has been detected using immunohistochemical techniques in areas of myocardial infarction with relatively little deposition in adjacent nonischemic regions.[108] In experimental models, there is a plethora of evidence indicating that local activation of the complement system is harmful to the heart. In one model, depletion of complement by the administration of cobra venom toxin significantly reduced ischemic injury,[109,110] while in other models, soluble complement inhibitors (sCR-1) or a C1 esterase inhibitor eliminated the deleterious effect of complement cascade activation on myocardium.[107,111,112]

Renin–Angiotensin System

Apoptosis has been noted to increase during the reperfusion of myocardial ischemic injury.[113] Given the multiple, complex mechanisms at work in the ischemic milieu, it is helpful to think of the process of accelerated apoptosis as an increase in the ratio of proapoptotic to antiapoptotic mechanisms. Two such opposing processes are triggered by the proteins bcl-2 (antiapoptotic) and Bax (proapoptotic).[114] In the setting of ischemia–reperfusion, p53 is a transcriptional regulator that helps shift the ratio in favor of apoptosis through direct activation of the Bax gene,[115] activation of caspases, and upregulation of the renin–angiotensin system. The renin–angiotensin system produces angiotensin II, which induces apoptosis directly through increased cytosolic Ca^{2+} release.[116] Furthermore, blockade of the angiotensin II receptor AT1 with quinaprilat decreases p53 and Bax, indicating that the renin–angiotensin system may have an important potentiating effect on p53.[113] Binding of angiotensin II to vascular AT1 receptors contributes further to ischemia–reperfusion injury by limiting forward flow, despite removal of the obstruction. Angiotensin II also may directly exacerbate microvascular vasoconstriction and promote diastolic dysfunction by boosting intracellular myocyte calcium levels.

MECHANISMS OF CARDIAC MYOCYTE DEATH

Myocardial ischemic injury results from a mismatch between myocyte oxygen demand and arterial oxygen delivery. ATP production by mitochondrial oxidative phosphorylation is profoundly dependent upon an adequate supply of oxygen, and hypoxemia leads to a rapid decrease in ATP production. Compensatory anaerobic glycolysis produces ATP less efficiently and leads to the accumulation of hydrogen ions and lactate. The resulting acidosis eventually inhibits glycolysis. Without ATP, ion transport mechanisms such as the Na^+, K^+-ATPase are inhibited, leading to an efflux of K^+ and an influx of Na^+, Ca^{2+}, Cl, and H_2O. The increase in intracellular Ca^{2+} augmented by dysregulation of transport systems in the sarcolemma and sarcoplasmic reticulum activates proteases which alter contractile proteins. Thus, myocyte contractility is impaired despite elevated cytosolic Ca^{2+}.[78] Activation of phospholipase also occurs, and results in the release of free fatty acids and lysophospholipids, which incorporate into membranes and further impair function. Free fatty acids such as these are targets of reactive oxygen species, which are present in the ischemic milieu. This ATP-independent process of dysregulated cell membrane permeability, accumulation of electrolytes and other prooncotic molecules within the myocyte and resultant cell swelling is termed *oncosis*, and ultimately results in irreversible injury and cell lysis (Fig. 58–1).

Not all myocytes die as the result of cell swelling caused by oncosis. *Apoptosis* is a complex process of programmed cell death that is the result of endogenous or exogenous stimuli, which results in death following cell shrinkage (Fig. 58–2). First described

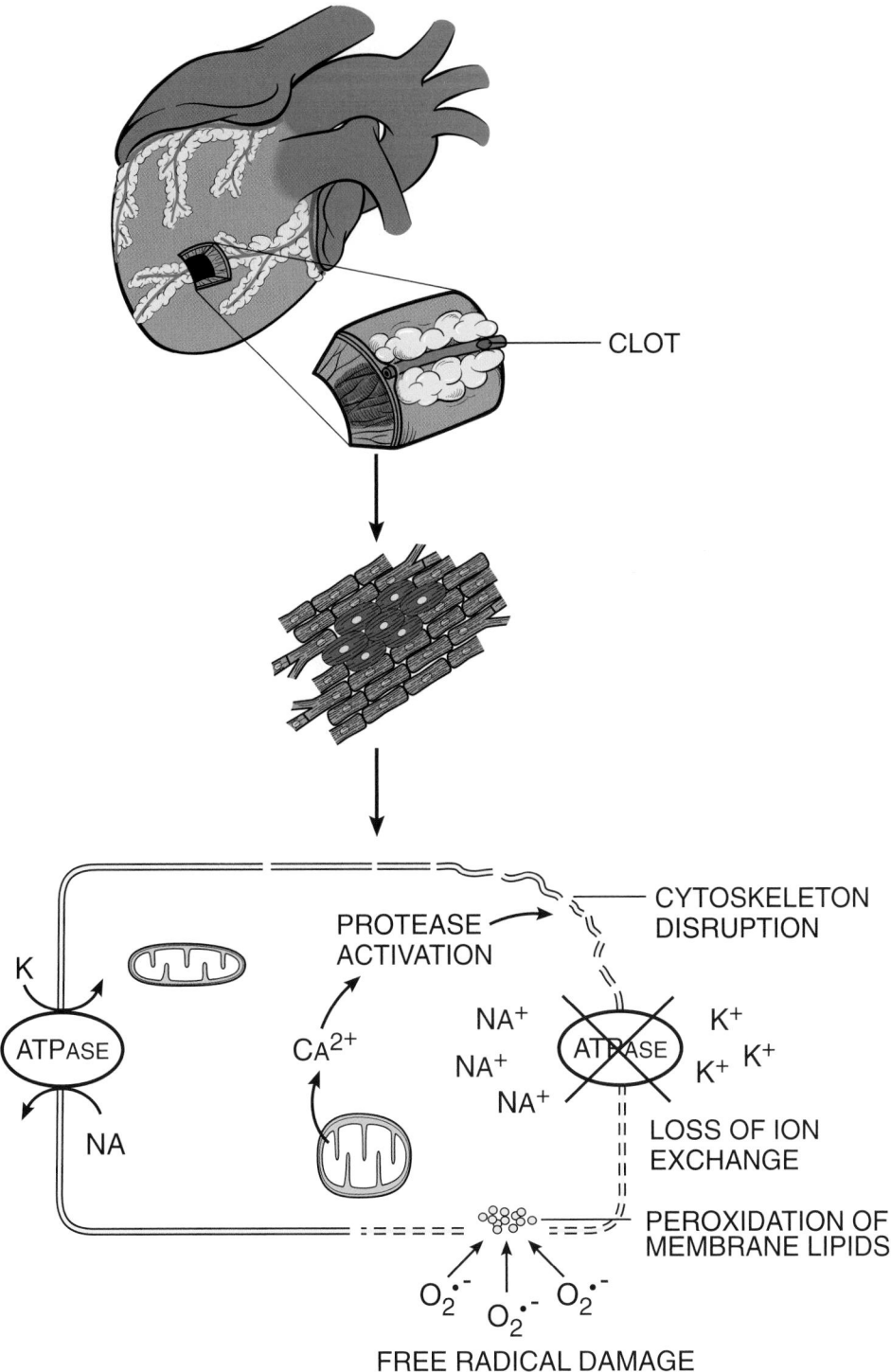

FIGURE 58–1. Ischemia-induced myocyte death. Obstruction of the arterial lumen by clot leads to gross anatomic and intracellular ischemic changes. The left side of the cell represented in the lower portion of the image shows normal cell function and morphology. The right side of the same cell portrays the major cellular effects of ischemia: free radicals damage the cell wall, mitochondrial dysfunction leads to mitochondrial swelling and release of stored calcium, calcium activates proteases that destroy the cytoskeleton, and dysfunction of ion exchange pumps eliminates vital ion concentration gradients.

the TNF receptor gene superfamily) or by activators such as cytochrome c[122] or apoptosis-inducing factor[123] released by mitochondria. The cytochrome c is released along with other proapoptotic factors and Ca^{2+} on opening of mitochondrial PTPs.[124] The tumor-suppressor gene p53 also activates the caspase cascade through gene induction, although this process has not been elucidated fully.[124] After activation by proteolytic processing of their zymogen precursors, caspases affect cell disintegration by cleaving substrates such as structural proteins, DNA repair enzymes, and protein kinases.[125–127] The caspase cascade results in a sequence of morphologic changes that begin with mitochondrial and cytosolic swelling (Fig. 58–2). Shortly thereafter, the cell membrane begins to bleb and then disintegrates. Pyknosis (chromatin condensation) and *karyohexis* (fragmentation of the nucleus) ensue. These processes result in cell shrinkage into what has been described as an apoptotic body, which is eliminated by phagocytes[123] (Fig. 58–3). The translocation of phosphatidylserine from the inner to the outer leaflet of the cell membrane allows phagocytes with specific phosphatidylserine receptors to identify and remove the apoptotic cell.[128] It has been postulated that this complex cascade, replete with redundant systems, confers the survival advantage of facilitating cell death without an inflammatory response.[129] Regulation of caspase activity occurs through a family of proteins known as *inhibitors of apoptosis*.[130] Historically, the process of apoptosis in the setting of myocardial ischemia has been studied using both terminal deoxynucleotidyl transferase-mediated deoxyuridine triphosphate biotin nick-end labeling by light microscopy[131] and genomic deoxyribonucleic acid (DNA) ladder detection. However, it has been shown that some dying myocytes identified by these processes are actually undergoing concomitant oncosis and apop-

by Kerr et al.[117] in rat breast carcinomas in 1972, and later by Gottlieb et al. in rabbit myocytes,[118] apoptosis is an ATP-dependent[119] process that culminates in chromosomal DNA fragmentation. The process most commonly begins with activation of a family of cysteine aspartyl proteases known as *caspases*.[120] Caspases are activated by cell surface death receptors[121] (part of

tosis, necessitating the use of additional techniques, such as the assessment of cell membrane integrity using electron microscopy[132] or molecular probes[133] to identify apoptotic myocytes with greater specificity.

Studies specific to myocyte apoptosis implicate various apoptotic pathways in multiple clinical cardiac diseases. For example,

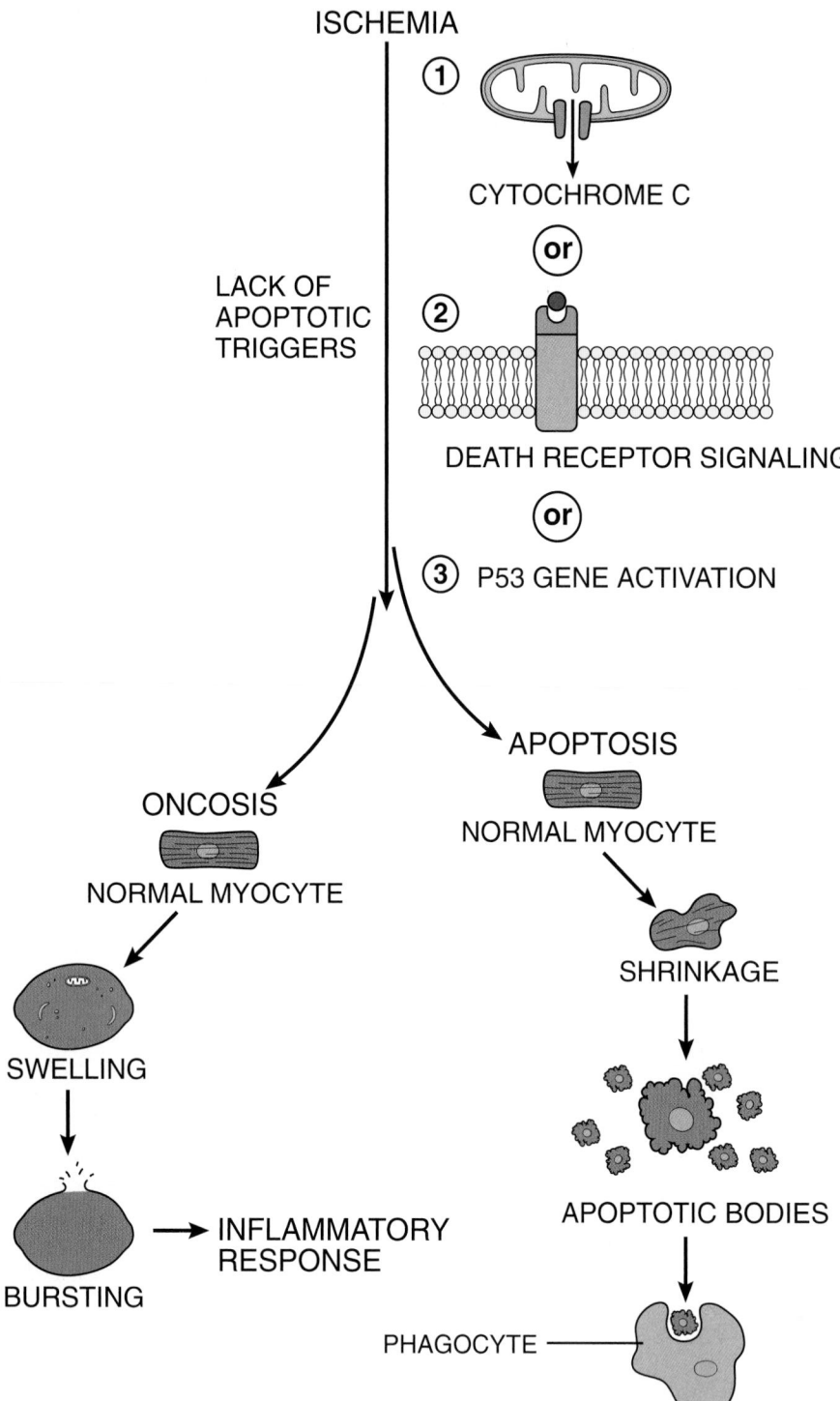

FIGURE 58–2. Oncosis and apoptosis. Ischemic injury can send a cell down one of two pathways: a lack of a specific proapoptotic trigger results in oncosis, a process that ultimately leads to swelling of the cell, lysis, and an inflammatory response that may further impair cardiac function. Specific triggers result in cell death by the programmed, energy-dependent process of apoptosis. Instead of swelling, the apoptotic cell shrinks and breaks into apoptotic bodies that are engulfed by macrophages. Apoptosis does not generally result in an inflammatory response.

optosis has also been found in the myocardium of patients with essential hypertension without coronary artery disease or heart failure.[136]

The elucidation of apoptosis has identified multiple targets for therapeutic strategies. Caspase inhibition by Asp-Glu-Val-aspartic acid aldehyde (DEVD-CHO)[137] or minocycline,[138] inhibition of mitochondrial PTP opening using cyclosporine A,[139] inhibition of STAT1 (an inducer of proapoptotic genes for caspase-1, Fas, and FasL, and inhibitor of antiapoptotic genes Bcl-2 and Bcl-x),[140] and downregulation of proapoptotic GSK3β using a beta-hydroxy-beta-methylglutaryl-coenzyme A (HMG-CoA) reductase inhibitor[141] are some of the more promising investigations into limiting apoptosis following myocardial ischemia.

PATHOLOGIC AND CLINICAL CONSEQUENCES OF MYOCARDIAL ISCHEMIA–REPERFUSION

There are several scenarios in which myocardial ischemia–reperfusion occurs. The first scenario involves reperfusion (spontaneous, pharmacologic, or percutaneous) following acute coronary syndromes, or exercise-induced ischemia.[142–144] The second setting involves reperfusion of a globally ischemic myocardium as occurs during the cardiac arrest of open heart surgery or cardiac transplantation.

【 】 MYOCARDIAL STUNNING

See discussion in Chap. 54 on coronary blood flow.

【 】 MICROVASCULAR ENDOTHELIAL DYSFUNCTION AND NO-REFLOW

Impaired loss of coronary vasodilatory reserve, vasospasm, tissue edema and microvascular obstruction secondary to downstream microembolization of platelets, neutrophils, thrombus, and atheroma particles all act in concert to cause microvascular dysfunction that may lead to electrical instability and cell death (Fig. 58–4).[66,91] In its most severe form, this microvascular dysfunction manifests as the *no-reflow phenomenon*.[145] This syndrome is associated with tissue hypoperfusion in the absence of a significant obstruction in the epicardial coronary vessel, and is detectable with nuclear scintigraphy,

caspase-3 activation by cytochrome c has been shown to induce apoptosis in the myocardium of end-stage heart failure patients.[134] The clinical significance of this observation, however, remains uncertain. Myocyte apoptosis in the infarct zone is a major determinant of adverse left ventricular remodeling 10 to 60 days following acute myocardial infarction.[135] Increased ap-

Nonapoptotic

Apoptotic

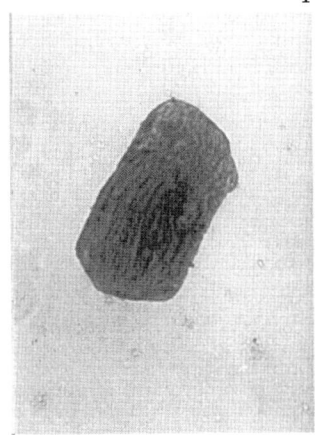
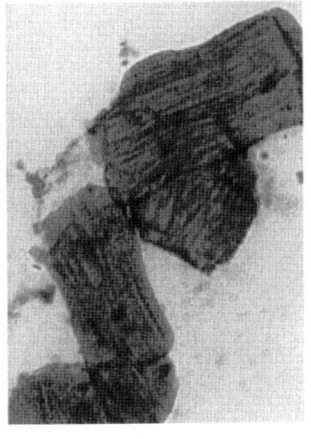
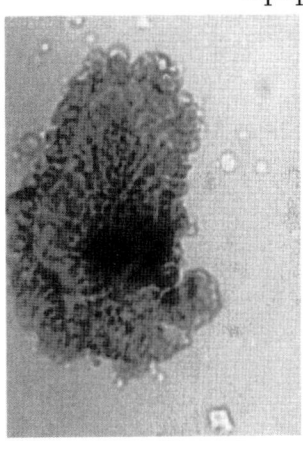
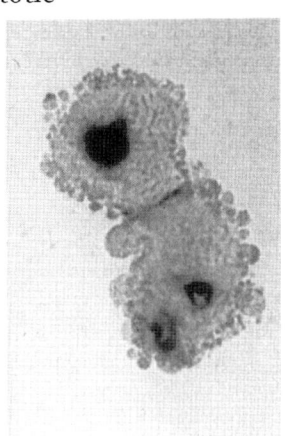

FIGURE 58–3. Examples of isolated nonapoptotic and apoptotic adult rat ventricular myocytes in culture. Note the condensation of nuclear chromatin (pyknosis), nuclear fragmentation (karyohexis), and membrane blebbing in the apoptotic cells. Image prepared using TUNNEL staining. *Source: Reprinted with permission from Pinsky DJ, Aji W, Szabolcs M, et al. Nitric oxide triggers programmed cell death (apoptosis) of adult rat ventricular myocytes in culture. Am J Physiol 1999;277(3 Pt 2):H1189–H1199.*

contrast echocardiography, positron emission tomography, and magnetic resonance angiography.[146–148] In acute coronary syndromes, no-reflow is associated with incomplete ST-segment recovery[149] and with increased infarct sizes, as well as a greater incidence of major adverse cardiac outcomes, such as arrhythmias, myocardial rupture, adverse left ventricular remodeling, and death.[150–153]

MYOCYTE DEATH AND NECROSIS

Contraction-band necrosis occurs within minutes of reperfusion following myocardial ischemia and results in infarct extension.[87] Reperfusion induces contraction necrosis in myocytes irreversibly injured by the preceding ischemic insult. Reperfusion often gives rise to local hemorrhage caused by leakage from damaged vessels, as well as accelerated release of cardiac biomarkers of myocardial infarction. Although all these changes take place in irreversibly damaged myocardium, there is evidence that reperfusion can lead to the conversion from reversible to irreversible injury of a population of myocytes that have been compromised during the preceding ischemia.[154]

REPERFUSION ARRHYTHMIA

Reperfusion following myocardial ischemia may lead to life-threatening arrhythmias.[155] The most common reperfusion arrhythmia in humans is accelerated idioventricular rhythm. While accelerated idioventricular rhythm is usually a benign rhythm, ventricular tachycardia and ventricular fibrillation are important causes of sudden death following restoration of antegrade flow.[156]

DIASTOLIC DYSFUNCTION

To the extent that the pathophysiologic changes of ischemia–reperfusion interfere with both the active and passive phases of diastole, it is likely that this phenomenon also causes diastolic dysfunction. Intracellular calcium loading and ATP depletion within cardiac myocytes during ischemia–reperfusion injury gives rise to hypercontracture and myocardial stiffening, both of which inter-

fere with diastolic function. Moreover, ATP depletion with attendant derangements in myocardial energy metabolism likely interferes with the active phase of diastole.

THERAPEUTIC APPROACHES TO ISCHEMIA–REPERFUSION INJURY IN CLINICAL PRACTICE

Although the phenomenon of ischemia–reperfusion is well established in research settings, its clinical relevance in humans remains controversial. Understanding of these basic pathophysiologic mechanisms that ultimately trigger myocyte death has led to new therapies designed to reduce the tissue injury that accompanies myocardial ischemia and reperfusion. Research on the cellular and molecular mechanisms of preconditioning in particular has facilitated clinical trials of therapeutic agents that mimic the cardioprotective effects of this phenomenon. Unfortunately, other than early reperfusion, few of the multiple therapies for ischemia–reperfusion have yielded consistent clinical benefit.

Numerous treatment agents have been considered, with most based on an understanding of either the triggers or mediators of ischemia. The myriad of therapies include but are not restricted to adenosine; opioids; bradykinin B_2 receptor antagonists; ATP-sensitive potassium channel openers; nucleoside transport inhibitors; angiotensin-converting enzyme and angiotensin II antagonists; statins; volatile anesthetics; NO donors; adenosine receptor agonists; sodium–calcium exchange inhibitors; sodium–hydrogen exchange inhibitors; complement inhibitors; xanthine oxidase inhibitors; antioxidant vitamins; specific inhibitors of fatty acid oxidation; hypothermia; hyperbaric oxygen; and distal protection devices. By and large, studies of these agents have either been negative or associated with worrisome safety issues.

Arguably, the most encouraging clinical trials have involved the use of intravenous adenosine infusions as in the Acute Myocardial Infarction Study of Adenosine (AMISTAD) trials.[157–159] AMISTAD I used a 70 μg/kg/min infusion versus placebo control in 236 individuals who had received thrombolytic therapy for an acute ST-elevation myocardial infarction. Although there was

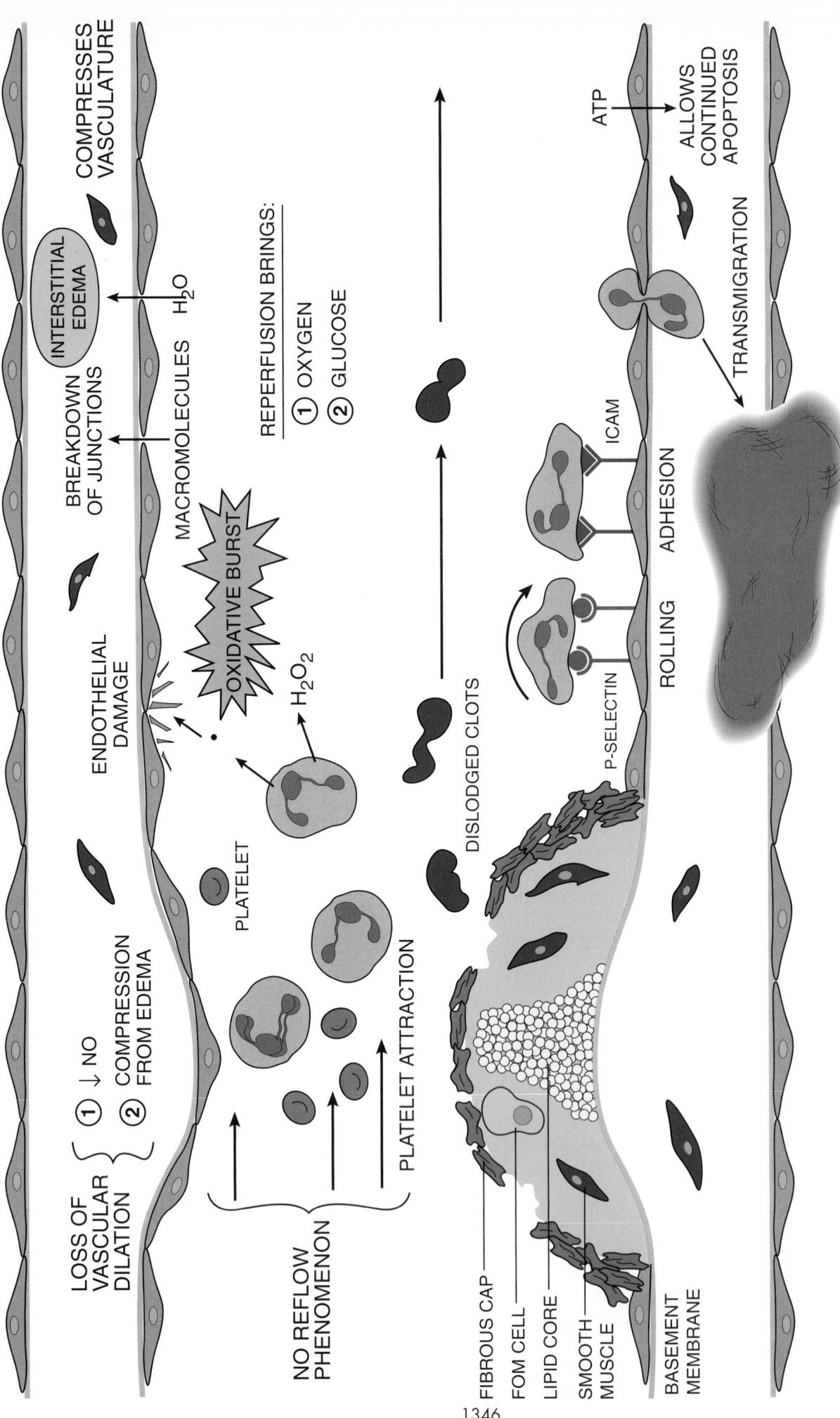

FIGURE 58–4. Ischemia–reperfusion injury. Occlusion of the arterial lumen by clot leads to tissue ischemia and a downstream accumulation of the products of anaerobic metabolism. Once blood flow is reestablished, a series of detrimental processes are initiated. The *no-reflow phenomenon* occurs when blood flow through the vessel continues to be impeded by a combination of residual plaque and clot, impaired vascular dilation, and activated platelets and leukocytes. In addition to inhibiting blood flow, the leukocytes adhere to endothelium and transmigrate into the damaged myocardium where they cause inflammation. Leukocytes also use newly delivered oxygen to create radicals that cause an oxidative burst that injures endothelium. Endothelial damage impairs the production of nitric oxide, leading to a loss of dilation. The vessel lumen is further narrowed by extraluminal edema caused by fluid loss through the damaged vessel walls.

no significant difference in infarct size in the two groups, subgroup analysis indicated a significant reduction in infarct size in individuals with anterior myocardial infarctions. The followup study (AMISTAD II) enrolled 2118 acute myocardial infarction individuals who had been reperfused with either thrombolytic or percutaneous therapy and randomized them to placebo versus two doses of adenosine infusions of 50 and 70 µg/kg/min. There were no significant differences in infarct sizes between control and pooled adenosine groups (27 percent vs. 17 percent), but the high-dose adenosine group (70 µg/kg/min) exhibited a significantly lower infarct size (11 percent vs. control 27 percent, $p = 0.023$).

Several angioplasty studies also have demonstrated that ischemic preconditioning via repetitive brief inflation–deflation maneuvers reduces chest pain, ST-segment elevation, CK release, and lactate levels. A 2005 study by Staat et al. provided solid clinical evidence supporting the clinical relevance of ischemia–reperfusion, as well as encouraging data regarding the therapeutic use of postconditioning to limit ischemia–reperfusion.[159] After direct stenting, subjects randomized to postconditioning had four repeated episodes of 1 minute inflation and 1 minute deflation of the angioplasty balloon. Compared to control, the postconditioning group had greater myocardial perfusion and smaller infarct sizes as measured by creatine kinase release.

Post-hoc analysis of the GUARDIAN trial demonstrated that pretreatment with the Na^+/H^+ exchange inhibitor cariporide yielded a significant reduction in the primary end point of death and/or myocardial infarction at 36 days postcoronary artery bypass graft.[160] A subsequent study, the EXPEDITION trial, also showed a reduction in perioperative myocardial infarction with cariporide treatment, although this advantage was offset by an increase in stroke incidence in the drug group.[161] Acadesine, an adenosine-regulating agent substance that increases adenosine levels in ischemic tissue, amplifies adenosine-mediated cardioprotective effects. A recent study by Mangano et al. demonstrated improved 2-year mortality rates in postcoronary artery bypass graft patients with reperfusion myocardial infarction who had received acadesine treatment (6.5 percent) versus control (28.7 percent; $p = 0.006$).[162]

CONCLUSION

Over the last decade there have been significant strides made in determining the molecular and cellular underpinnings of ischemic preconditioning and the pathophysiology of myocardial ischemia–reperfusion. There is now greater, albeit incomplete, understanding of the complex interplay of recruited cellular (neutrophils, platelets) and subcellular (calcium homeostasis, mitochondrial) effector mechanisms, with humoral factors (reactive oxygen species, cytokines, coagulation, and complement cascades). Better characterization of the factors that govern the extent of reperfusion-associated myocardial injury following ischemia remains an important research imperative. With growing acceptance that myocardial ischemia–reperfusion is a clinically relevant entity, a major challenge for researchers in this field is to continue to harness the vast molecular knowledge on myocardial ischemia–reperfusion to identify novel therapeutic strategies for well-designed clinical trials of reperfusion in acute coronary syndromes, as well as perioperative reperfusion in open heart surgery.

REFERENCES

1. Jennings RB. Myocardial ischemia observations, definitions and speculations. *J Mol Cell Cardiol* 1970;1:345–349.
2. Sayen JJ, Sheldon WF, Peirce G, Kuo PT. Polarographic oxygen, the epicardial electrocardiogram and muscle contraction in experimental acute regional ischemia of the left ventricle. *Circ Res* 1958;6:779–798.
3. Braasch W, Gudbjarnason S, Puri PS, Ravens KG, Bing RJ. Early changes in energy metabolism in the myocardium following acute coronary artery occlusion in anesthetized dogs. *Circ Res* 1968;23:429–438.
4. Jennings RB. Early phase of myocardial ischemic injury and infarction. *Am J Cardiol* 1969;24:753–765.
5. Katz AM, Hecht HH. The early "pump" failure of the ischemic heart [editorial]. *Am J Med* 1969;47:497–502.
6. Kloner RA, Ellis SG, Lange R, Braunwald E. Studies of experimental coronary artery reperfusion. Effects on infarct size, myocardial function, biochemistry, ultrastructure and microvascular damage. *Circulation* 1983;68:I8–I15.
7. Herdson PB, Kaltenbach JP, Jennings RB. Fine structural and biochemical changes in dog myocardium during autolysis. *Am J Pathol* 1969;57:539–557.
8. Krug A. Der Fruhnachweis des Herzinfarktes durch Bestimmung der Wasserstoffionenkonzentration im Hermuskel mit Idicatorpapier. *Virchows Arch* 1965;338:330–341.
9. Berne RM, Rubio R. Acute coronary occlusion: early changes that induce coronary dilatation and the development of collateral circulation. *Am J Cardiol* 1969;24:776–781.
10. Harris AS, Bisteni A, Russell RA, Brigham JC, Firestone JE. Excitatory factors in ventricular tachycardia resulting from myocardial ischemia; potassium a major excitant. *Science* 1954;119:200–203.
11. Corr PB, Gross RW, Sobel BE. Arrhythmogenic amphiphilic lipids and the myocardial cell membrane. *J Mol Cell Cardiol* 1982;14:619–626.
12. Ferrari R, Ceconi C, Curello S, Alfieri O, Visioli O. Myocardial damage during ischaemia and reperfusion. *Eur Heart J* 1993;14 Suppl G:25–30.
13. Jennings RB, Sommers HM, Smyth GA, Flack HA, Linn H. Myocardial necrosis induced by temporary occlusion of a coronary artery in the dog. *Arch Pathol* 1960;70:68–78.
14. Tennant R, Wiggers, CJ. The effect of coronary occlusion on myocardial contraction. *Am J Physiol* 1935;112:351–361.
15. Kloner RA, DeBoer LW, Carlson N, Braunwald E. The effect of verapamil on myocardial ultrastructure during and following release of coronary artery occlusion. *Exp Mol Pathol* 1982;36:277–286.
16. Kloner RA, Rude RE, Carlson N, Maroko PR, DeBoer LW, Braunwald E. Ultrastructural evidence of microvascular damage and myocardial cell injury after coronary artery occlusion: which comes first? *Circulation* 1980;62:945–952.
17. Sobel RE, ed. *Acute Myocardial Infarction*. Philadelphia: WB Saunders, 1992.
18. Jennings RB, Reimer KA. Salvage of ischemic myocardium. *Mod Concepts Cardiovasc Dis* 1974;43:125–130.
19. Garcia-Dorado D, Oliveras J. Myocardial oedema: a preventable cause of reperfusion injury? *Cardiovasc Res* 1993;27:1555–1563.
20. Garcia-Dorado D, Theroux P, Munoz R, et al. Favorable effects of hyperosmotic reperfusion on myocardial edema and infarct size. *Am J Physiol* 1992;262:H17–H22.
21. Dauber IM, VanBenthuysen KM, McMurtry IF, et al. Functional coronary microvascular injury evident as increased permeability due to brief ischemia and reperfusion. *Circ Res* 1990;66:986–998.
22. Pilati CF. Macromolecular transport in canine coronary microvasculature. *Am J Physiol* 1990;258:H748–H753.
23. Steenbergen C, Hill ML, Jennings RB. Volume regulation and plasma membrane injury in aerobic, anaerobic, and ischemic myocardium in vitro. Effects of osmotic cell swelling on plasma membrane integrity. *Circ Res* 1985;57:864–875.
24. Jennings RB, Ganote CE, Reimer KA. Ischemic tissue injury. *Am J Pathol* 1975;81:179–198.
25. Baroldi G. Different types of myocardial necrosis in coronary heart disease: a pathophysiologic review of their functional significance. *Am Heart J* 1975;89:742–752.
26. Hutchins GM, Bulkley BH. Correlation of myocardial contraction band necrosis and vascular patency. A study of coronary artery bypass graft anastomoses at branch points. *Lab Invest* 1977;36:642–648.
27. Jennings RB, Schaper J, Hill ML, Steenbergen C Jr, Reimer KA. Effect of reperfusion late in the phase of reversible ischemic injury. Changes in cell volume, electrolytes, metabolites, and ultrastructure. *Circ Res* 1985;56:262–278.
28. Adams JE 3rd, Abendschein DR, Jaffe AS. Biochemical markers of myocardial injury. Is MB creatine kinase the choice for the 1990s? *Circulation* 1993;88:750–763.

29. Devries SR, Jaffe AS, Geltman EM, Sobel BE, Abendschein DR. Enzymatic estimation of the extent of irreversible myocardial injury early after reperfusion. *Am Heart J* 1989;117:31–36.

30. Arroyo-Espliguero R, Avanzas P, Cosin-Sales J, Aldama G, Pizzi C, Kaski JC. C-reactive protein elevation and disease activity in patients with coronary artery disease. *Eur Heart J* 2004;25:401–408.

31. Heeschen C, Hamm CW, Mitrovic V, Lantelme NH, White HD. N-terminal pro-B-type natriuretic peptide levels for dynamic risk stratification of patients with acute coronary syndromes. *Circulation* 2004;110:3206–3212.

32. Heeschen C, Dimmeler S, Hamm CW, et al. Soluble CD40 ligand in acute coronary syndromes. *N Engl J Med* 2003;348:1104–1111.

33. Varo N, de Lemos JA, Libby P, et al. Soluble CD40L: risk prediction after acute coronary syndromes. *Circulation* 2003;108:1049–1052.

34. Baldus S, Heeschen C, Meinertz T, et al. Myeloperoxidase serum levels predict risk in patients with acute coronary syndromes. *Circulation* 2003;108:1440–1445.

35. Zeng B, Prasan A, Fung KC, et al. Elevated circulating levels of matrix metalloproteinase-9, and -2, in patients with symptomatic coronary artery disease. *Intern Med J* 2005;35:331–335.

36. Cavusoglu E, Ruwende C, Chopra V, et al. Tissue inhibitor of metalloproteinase-1 (TIMP-1) is an independent predictor of all-cause mortality, cardiac mortality, and myocardial infarction. *Am Heart J* 2006;151:1101.e1–1101.e8.

37. Cavusoglu E, Ruwende C, Chopra V, et al. Adiponectin is an independent predictor of all-cause, cardiac mortality, and myocardial infarction in patients presenting with chest pain. *Eur Heart J* 2006;27(19):2300–2309.

38. Hoffmann G, Gobel BO, Harbrecht U, Vetter H, Dusing R. Platelet cAMP and cGMP in essential hypertension. *Am J Hypertens* 1992;5:847–850.

39. Ma XL, Lefer DJ, Lefer AM, Rothlein R. Coronary endothelial and cardiac protective effects of a monoclonal antibody to intercellular adhesion molecule-1, in myocardial ischemia and reperfusion. *Circulation* 1992;86:937–946.

40. Ma XL, Tsao PS, Lefer AM. Antibody to CD-18, exerts endothelial and cardiac protective effects in myocardial ischemia and reperfusion. *J Clin Invest* 1991;88:1237–1243.

41. Detmers PA, Lo SK, Olsen-Egbert E, Walz A, Baggiolini M, Cohn ZA. Neutrophil-activating protein 1/interleukin 8, stimulates the binding activity of the leukocyte adhesion receptor CD11b/CD18, on human neutrophils. *J Exp Med* 1990;171:1155–1162.

42. Kilgore KS, Lucchesi BR. Reperfusion injury after myocardial infarction: the role of free radicals and the inflammatory response. *Clin Biochem* 1993;26:359–370.

43. Peveri P, Walz A, Dewald B, Baggiolini M. A novel neutrophil-activating factor produced by human mononuclear phagocytes. *J Exp Med* 1988;167:1547–1559.

44. Rot A. Endothelial cell binding of NAP-1/IL-8: role in neutrophil emigration. *Immunol Today* 1992;13:291–294.

45. Vinten-Johansen J. Involvement of neutrophils in the pathogenesis of lethal myocardial reperfusion injury. *Cardiovasc Res* 2004;61:481–497.

46. Mayadas TN, Johnson RC, Rayburn H, Hynes RO, Wagner DD. Leukocyte rolling and extravasation are severely compromised in P selectin-deficient mice. *Cell* 1993;74:541–554.

47. Hicks AE, Nolan SL, Ridger VC, Hellewell PG, Norman KE. Recombinant P-selectin glycoprotein ligand-1, directly inhibits leukocyte rolling by all 3 selectins in vivo: complete inhibition of rolling is not required for antiinflammatory effect. *Blood* 2003;101:3249–3256.

48. Hirata T, Merrill-Skoloff G, Aab M, Yang J, Furie BC, Furie B. P-selectin glycoprotein ligand 1 (PSGL-1) is a physiological ligand for E-selectin in mediating T helper 1 lymphocyte migration. *J Exp Med* 2000;192:1669–1676.

49. Norman KE, Katopodis AG, Thoma G, et al. P-selectin glycoprotein ligand-1 supports rolling on E- and P-selectin in vivo. *Blood* 2000;96:3585–3591.

50. Evangelista V, Manarini S, Sideri R, et al. Platelet/polymorphonuclear leukocyte interaction: P-selectin triggers protein-tyrosine phosphorylation-dependent CD11b/CD18 adhesion: role of PSGL-1 as a signaling molecule. *Blood* 1999;93:876–885.

51. Simon SI, Hu Y, Vestweber D, Smith CW. Neutrophil tethering on E-selectin activates beta 2 integrin binding to ICAM-1 through a mitogen-activated protein kinase signal transduction pathway. *J Immunol* 2000;164:4348–4358.

52. Hidari KI, Weyrich AS, Zimmerman GA, McEver RP. Engagement of P-selectin glycoprotein ligand-1 enhances tyrosine phosphorylation and activates mitogen-activated protein kinases in human neutrophils. *J Biol Chem* 1997;272:28750–28756.

53. Haller H, Kunzendorf U, Sacherer K, et al. T cell adhesion to P-selectin induces tyrosine phosphorylation of pp125 focal adhesion kinase and other substrates. *J Immunol* 1997;158:1061–1067.

54. Weyrich AS, Buerke M, Albertine KH, Lefer AM. Time course of coronary vascular endothelial adhesion molecule expression during reperfusion of the ischemic feline myocardium. *J Leukoc Biol* 1995;57:45–55.

55. Pinsky D, Naka Y, Liao H, et al. Hypoxia-induced exocytosis of endothelial cell Weibel-Palade bodies: a mechanism for rapid neutrophil recruitment following cardiac preservation. *J Clin Invest* 1996;97:493–500.

56. Gumina RJ, el Schultz J, Yao Z, et al. Antibody to platelet/endothelial cell adhesion molecule-1 reduces myocardial infarct size in a rat model of ischemia-reperfusion injury. *Circulation* 1996;94:3327–3333.

57. Chatelain P, Latour JG, Tran D, de Lorgeril M, Dupras G, Bourassa M. Neutrophil accumulation in experimental myocardial infarcts: relation with extent of injury and effect of reperfusion. *Circulation* 1987;75:1083–1090.

58. Gerlach MC, S Ogawa, D Stern. Perturbation of endothelial barrier and coagulant properties by environmental factors. In: Simionescu M. *Endothelial Cell Dysfunction*. New York: Plenum Press, 1991:525–545.

59. Esmon CT. The regulation of natural anticoagulant pathways. *Science* 1987;235:1348–1352.

60. Koga S, Ogawa S, Kuwabara K, et al. Synthesis and release of interleukin 1, by reoxygenated human mononuclear phagocytes. *J Clin Invest* 1992;90:1007–1015.

61. Shreeniwas R, Koga S, Karakurum M, et al. Hypoxia-mediated induction of endothelial cell interleukin-1 alpha. An autocrine mechanism promoting expression of leukocyte adhesion molecules on the vessel surface. *J Clin Invest* 1992;90:2333–2339.

62. Ogawa S, Clauss M, Kuwabara K, et al. Hypoxia induces endothelial cell synthesis of membrane-associated proteins. *Proc Natl Acad Sci U S A* 1991;88:9897–9901.

63. Pober JS. Warner-Lambert/Parke-Davis award lecture. Cytokine-mediated activation of vascular endothelium. Physiology and pathology. *Am J Pathol* 1988;133:426–433.

64. Pinsky DJ, Naka Y, Liao H, et al. Hypoxia-induced exocytosis of endothelial cell Weibel-Palade bodies. A mechanism for rapid neutrophil recruitment after cardiac preservation. *J Clin Invest* 1996;97:493–500.

65. Lefer AM. Role of selectins in myocardial ischemia-reperfusion injury. *Ann Thorac Surg* 1995;60:773–777.

66. Lefer AM, Lefer DJ. The role of nitric oxide and cell adhesion molecules on the microcirculation in ischaemia-reperfusion. *Cardiovasc Res* 1996;32:743–751.

67. Weyrich AS, Ma XL, Lefer AM. The role of L-arginine in ameliorating reperfusion injury after myocardial ischemia in the cat. *Circulation* 1992;86:279–288.

68. Xiao CY, Hara A, Yuhki K, et al. Roles of prostaglandin I(2) and thromboxane A(2) in cardiac ischemia-reperfusion injury: a study using mice lacking their respective receptors. *Circulation* 2001;104:2210–2215.

69. Newmeyer DD, Ferguson-Miller S. Mitochondria: releasing power for life and unleashing the machineries of death. *Cell* 2003;112:481–490.

70. Honda HM, Korge P, Weiss JN. Mitochondria and ischemia/reperfusion injury. *Ann N Y Acad Sci* 2005;1047:248–258.

71. Korge P, Honda HM, Weiss JN. Effects of fatty acids in isolated mitochondria: implications for ischemic injury and cardioprotection. *Am J Physiol Heart Circ Physiol* 2003;285:H259–H269.

72. Owen P, Dennis S, Opie LH. Glucose flux rate regulates onset of ischemic contracture in globally underperfused rat hearts. *Circ Res* 1990;66:344–354.

73. Opie LH. The mechanism of myocyte death in ischaemia. *Eur Heart J* 1993;14 Suppl G:31–33.

74. Shen AC, Jennings RB. Kinetics of calcium accumulation in acute myocardial ischemic injury. *Am J Pathol* 1972;67:441–452.

75. Shen AC, Jennings RB. Myocardial calcium and magnesium in acute ischemic injury. *Am J Pathol* 1972;67:417–440.

76. Bolli R, Marban E. Molecular and cellular mechanisms of myocardial stunning. *Physiol Rev* 1999;79:609–634.

77. Kusuoka H, Camilion de Hurtado MC, Marban E. Role of sodium/calcium exchange in the mechanism of myocardial stunning: protective effect of reperfusion with high sodium solution. *J Am Coll Cardiol* 1993;21:240–248.

78. Buja LM. Myocardial ischemia and reperfusion injury. *Cardiovasc Pathol* 2005;14:170–175.

79. Beard T, Carrie D, Boyer MJ, et al. [Production of oxygen free radicals in myocardial infarction treated by thrombolysis. Analysis of glutathione peroxidase, superoxide dismutase and malondialdehyde]. *Arch Mal Coeur Vaiss* 1994;87:1289–1296.

80. Roberts MJ, Young IS, Trouton TG, et al. Transient release of lipid peroxides after coronary artery balloon angioplasty. *Lancet* 1990;336:143–145.

81. Kim KB, Chung HH, Kim MS, Rho JR. Changes in the antioxidative defensive system during open heart operations in humans. *Ann Thorac Surg* 1994;58:170–175.

82. Ide T, Tsutsui H, Kinugawa S, et al. Mitochondrial electron transport complex I is a potential source of oxygen free radicals in the failing myocardium. *Circ Res* 1999;85:357–363.

83. Boveris A, Chance B. The mitochondrial generation of hydrogen peroxide. General properties and effect of hyperbaric oxygen. *Biochem J* 1973;134:707–716.

84. Lucchesi BR, Werns SW, Fantone JC. The role of the neutrophil and free radicals in ischemic myocardial injury. *J Mol Cell Cardiol* 1989;21:1241–1251.

85. Zweier JL, Kuppusamy P, Lutty GA. Measurement of endothelial cell free radical generation: evidence for a central mechanism of free radical injury in postischemic tissues. *Proc Natl Acad Sci U S A* 1988;85:4046–4050.

86. Babbs CF, Cregor MD, Turek JJ, Badylak SF. Endothelial superoxide production in the isolated rat heart during early reperfusion after ischemia. A histochemical study. *Am J Pathol* 1991;139:1069–1080.

87. Moens AL, Claeys MJ, Timmermans JP, Vrints CJ. Myocardial ischemia/reperfusion-injury, a clinical view on a complex pathophysiological process. *Int J Cardiol* 2005;100:179–190.

88. McCord JM. Oxygen-derived free radicals in postischemic tissue injury. *N Engl J Med* 1985;312:159–163.

89. Lefer DJ, Scalia R, Campbell B, et al. Peroxynitrite inhibits leukocyte-endothelial cell interactions and protects against ischemia-reperfusion injury in rats. *J Clin Invest* 1997;99:684–691.

90. Mehta JL, Nichols WW, Donnelly WH, et al. Protection by superoxide dismutase from myocardial dysfunction and attenuation of vasodilator reserve after coronary occlusion and reperfusion in dog. *Circ Res* 1989;65:1283–1295.

91. Lefer AM, Tsao PS, Lefer DJ, Ma XL. Role of endothelial dysfunction in the pathogenesis of reperfusion injury after myocardial ischemia. *FASEB J* 1991;5:2029–2034.

92. Moncada S, Palmer RM, Higgs EA. Nitric oxide: physiology, pathophysiology, and pharmacology. *Pharmacol Rev* 1991;43:109–142.

93. Kubes P, Granger DN. Nitric oxide modulates microvascular permeability. *Am J Physiol* 1992;262:H611–H615.

94. Lefer AM. Attenuation of myocardial ischemia-reperfusion injury with nitric oxide replacement therapy. *Ann Thorac Surg* 1995;60:847–851.

95. Lefer DJ, Nakanishi K, Johnston WE, Vinten-Johansen J. Antineutrophil and myocardial protecting actions of a novel nitric oxide donor after acute myocardial ischemia and reperfusion of dogs. *Circulation* 1993;88:2337–2350.

96. Sneddon JM, Vane JR. Endothelium-derived relaxing factor reduces platelet adhesion to bovine endothelial cells. *Proc Natl Acad Sci U S A* 1988;85:2800–2804.

97. Leist M, Single B, Naumann H, et al. Inhibition of mitochondrial ATP generation by nitric oxide switches apoptosis to necrosis. *Exp Cell Res* 1999;249:396–403.

98. Pinsky D, Patton S, Mesaros S, et al. Mechanical transduction of nitric oxide synthesis in the beating heart. *Circ Res* 1997;81:372–379.

99. Mizuno T, Watanabe M, Sakamoto T, Sunamori M. L-Arginine, a nitric oxide precursor, attenuates ischemia-reperfusion injury by inhibiting inositol-1,4,5-triphosphate. *J Thorac Cardiovasc Surg* 1998;115:931–936.

100. Beresewicz A, Karwatowska-Prokopczuk E, Lewartowski B, Cedro-Ceremuazynska K. A protective role of nitric oxide in isolated ischaemic/reperfused rat heart. *Cardiovasc Res* 1995;30:1001–1008.

101. Kanno S, Lee PC, Zhang Y, et al. Attenuation of myocardial ischemia/reperfusion injury by superinduction of inducible nitric oxide synthase. *Circulation* 2000;101:2742–2748.

102. Brunner F, Maier R, Andrew P, Wolkart G, Zechner R, Mayer B. Attenuation of myocardial ischemia/reperfusion injury in mice with myocyte-specific overexpression of endothelial nitric oxide synthase. *Cardiovasc Res* 2003;57:55–62.

103. Parrino PE, Laubach VE, Gaughen JR Jr, et al. Inhibition of inducible nitric oxide synthase after myocardial ischemia increases coronary flow. *Ann Thorac Surg* 1998;66:733–739.

104. Flogel U, Decking UK, Godecke A, Schrader J. Contribution of NO to ischemia-reperfusion injury in the saline-perfused heart: a study in endothelial NO synthase knockout mice. *J Mol Cell Cardiol* 1999;31:827–836.

105. Igarashi J, Nishida M, Hoshida S, et al. Inducible nitric oxide synthase augments injury elicited by oxidative stress in rat cardiac myocytes. *Am J Physiol* 1998;274:C245–C252.

106. Woolfson RG, Patel VC, Neild GH, Yellon DM. Inhibition of nitric oxide synthesis reduces infarct size by an adenosine-dependent mechanism. *Circulation* 1995;91:1545–1551.

107. Homeister JW, Lucchesi BR. Complement activation and inhibition in myocardial ischemia and reperfusion injury. *Annu Rev Pharmacol Toxicol* 1994;34:17–40.

108. Homeister JW, Satoh P, Lucchesi BR. Effects of complement activation in the isolated heart. Role of the terminal complement components. *Circ Res* 1992;71:303–319.

109. Crawford MH, Grover FL, Kolb WP, et al. Complement and neutrophil activation in the pathogenesis of ischemic myocardial injury. *Circulation* 1988;78:1449–1458.

110. Maroko PR, Carpenter CB, Chiariello M, et al. Reduction by cobra venom factor of myocardial necrosis after coronary artery occlusion. *J Clin Invest* 1978;61:661–670.

111. Weisman HF, Bartow T, Leppo MK, et al. Soluble human complement receptor type 1: in vivo inhibitor of complement suppressing post-ischemic myocardial inflammation and necrosis. *Science* 1990;249:146–151.

112. Pugsley MK, Abramova M, Cole T, Yang X, Ammons WS. Inhibitors of the complement system currently in development for cardiovascular disease. *Cardiovasc Toxicol* 2003;3:43–70.

113. Kossmehl P, Kurth E, Faramarzi S, et al. Mechanisms of apoptosis after ischemia and reperfusion: role of the renin-angiotensin system. *Apoptosis* 2006;11:347–358.

114. Misao J, Hayakawa Y, Ohno M, Kato S, Fujiwara T, Fujiwara H. Expression of bcl-2 protein, an inhibitor of apoptosis, and Bax, an accelerator of apoptosis, in ventricular myocytes of human hearts with myocardial infarction. *Circulation* 1996;94:1506–1512.

115. Miyashita T, Reed JC. Tumor suppressor p53 is a direct transcriptional activator of the human bax gene. *Cell* 1995;80:293–299.

116. Pierzchalski P, Reiss K, Cheng W, et al. p53 Induces myocyte apoptosis via the activation of the renin-angiotensin system. *Exp Cell Res* 1997;234:57–65.

117. Kerr JF, Wyllie AH, Currie AR. Apoptosis: a basic biological phenomenon with wide-ranging implications in tissue kinetics. *Br J Cancer* 1972;26:239–257.

118. Gottlieb RA, Burleson KO, Kloner RA, Babior BM, Engler RL. Reperfusion injury induces apoptosis in rabbit cardiomyocytes. *J Clin Invest* 1994;94:1621–1628.

119. Li P, Nijhawan D, Budihardjo I, et al. Cytochrome c and dATP-dependent formation of Apaf-1/caspase-9 complex initiates an apoptotic protease cascade. *Cell* 1997;91:479–489.

120. Alnemri ES, Livingston DJ, Nicholson DW, et al. Human ICE/CED-3 protease nomenclature. *Cell* 1996;87:171.

121. Ashkenazi A, Dixit VM. Death receptors: signaling and modulation. *Science* 1998;281:1305–1308.

122. Atlante A, Calissano P, Bobba A, Azzariti A, Marra E, Passarella S. Cytochrome c is released from mitochondria in a reactive oxygen species (ROS)-dependent fashion and can operate as a ROS scavenger and as a respiratory substrate in cerebellar neurons undergoing excitotoxic death. *J Biol Chem* 2000;275:37159–37166.

123. Yaoita H, Ogawa K, Maehara K, Maruyama Y. Apoptosis in relevant clinical situations: contribution of apoptosis in myocardial infarction. *Cardiovasc Res* 2000;45:630–641.

124. Gustafsson AB, Gottlieb RA. Mechanisms of apoptosis in the heart. *J Clin Immunol* 2003;23:447–459.

125. Logue SE, Gustafsson AB, Samali A, Gottlieb RA. Ischemia/reperfusion injury at the intersection with cell death. *J Mol Cell Cardiol* 2005;38:21–33.

126. Thornberry NA, Lazebnik Y. Caspases: enemies within. *Science* 1998;281:1312–1316.

127. Salvesen GS, Dixit VM. Caspases: intracellular signaling by proteolysis. *Cell* 1997;91:443–446.

128. Fadok VA, Voelker DR, Campbell PA, Cohen JJ, Bratton DL, Henson PM. Exposure of phosphatidylserine on the surface of apoptotic lymphocytes triggers specific recognition and removal by macrophages. *J Immunol* 1992;148:2207–2216.

129. Scarabelli TM, Gottlieb RA. Functional and clinical repercussions of myocyte apoptosis in the multifaceted damage by ischemia/reperfusion injury: old and new concepts after 10 years of contributions. *Cell Death Differ* 2004;11 Suppl 2:S144–S152.

130. Goyal L. Cell death inhibition: keeping caspases in check. *Cell* 2001;104:805–808.

131. Gavrieli Y, Sherman Y, Ben-Sasson SA. Identification of programmed cell death in situ via specific labeling of nuclear DNA fragmentation. *J Cell Biol* 1992;119:493–501.

132. Ohno M, Takemura G, Ohno A, et al. "Apoptotic" myocytes in infarct area in rabbit hearts may be oncotic myocytes with DNA fragmentation: analysis by immunogold electron microscopy combined with in situ nick-end labeling. *Circulation* 1998;98:1422–1430.

133. Buja LM, Entman ML. Modes of myocardial cell injury and cell death in ischemic heart disease. *Circulation* 1998;98:1355–1357.

134. Narula J, Pandey P, Arbustini E, et al. Apoptosis in heart failure: release of cytochrome c from mitochondria and activation of caspase-3 in human cardiomyopathy. *Proc Natl Acad Sci U S A* 1999;96:8144–8149.

135. Abbate A, Biondi-Zoccai GG, Bussani R, et al. Increased myocardial apoptosis in patients with unfavorable left ventricular remodeling and early symptomatic post-infarction heart failure. *J Am Coll Cardiol* 2003;41:753–760.

136. Gonzalez A, Lopez B, Ravassa S, et al. Stimulation of cardiac apoptosis in essential hypertension: potential role of angiotensin II. *Hypertension* 2002;39:75–80.

137. Balsam LB, Kofidis T, Robbins RC. Caspase-3 inhibition preserves myocardial geometry and long-term function after infarction. *J Surg Res* 2005;124:194–200.

138. Scarabelli TM, Stephanou A, Pasini E, et al. Minocycline inhibits caspase activation and reactivation, increases the ratio of XIAP to smac/DIABLO, and reduces the mitochondrial leakage of cytochrome C and smac/DIABLO. *J Am Coll Cardiol* 2004;43:865–874.

139. Nazareth W, Yafei N, Crompton M. Inhibition of anoxia-induced injury in heart myocytes by cyclosporin A. *J Mol Cell Cardiol* 1991;23:1351–1354.

140. Townsend PA, Scarabelli TM, Pasini E, et al. Epigallocatechin-3-gallate inhibits STAT-1 activation and protects cardiac myocytes from ischemia/reperfusion-induced apoptosis. *FASEB J* 2004;18:1621–1623.

141. Bergmann MW, Rechner C, Freund C, Baurand A, El Jamali A, Dietz R. Statins inhibit reoxygenation-induced cardiomyocyte apoptosis: role for glycogen synthase kinase 3beta and transcription factor beta-catenin. *J Mol Cell Cardiol* 2004;37:681–690.

142. Kloner RA, Arimie RB, Kay GL, et al. Evidence for stunned myocardium in humans: a 2001 update. *Coron Artery Dis* 2001;12:349–356.

143. Kloner RA, Jennings RB. Consequences of brief ischemia: stunning, preconditioning, and their clinical implications: part 1. *Circulation* 2001;104:2981–2989.

144. Kloner RA, Jennings RB. Consequences of brief ischemia: stunning, preconditioning, and their clinical implications: part 2. *Circulation* 2001;104:3158–3167.

145. Kloner RA, Ganote CE, Jennings RB. The "no-reflow" phenomenon after temporary coronary occlusion in the dog. *J Clin Invest* 1974;54:1496–1508.

146. Schofer J, Montz R, Mathey DG. Scintigraphic evidence of the "no reflow" phenomenon in human beings after coronary thrombolysis. *J Am Coll Cardiol* 1985;5:593–598.

147. Maes A, Van de Werf F, Nuyts J, Bormans G, Desmet W, Mortelmans L. Impaired myocardial tissue perfusion early after successful thrombolysis. Impact on myocardial flow, metabolism, and function at late follow-up. *Circulation* 1995;92:2072–2078.

148. Wu KC, Zerhouni EA, Judd RM, et al. Prognostic significance of microvascular obstruction by magnetic resonance imaging in patients with acute myocardial infarction. *Circulation* 1998;97:765–772.

149. Claeys MJ, Bosmans J, Veenstra L, Jorens P, De Raedt H, Vrints CJ. Determinants and prognostic implications of persistent ST-segment elevation after primary angioplasty for acute myocardial infarction: importance of microvascular reperfusion injury on clinical outcome. *Circulation* 1999;99:1972–1977.

150. Abbo KM, Dooris M, Glazier S, O'Neill WW, Byrd D, Grines CL, Safian RD. Features and outcome of no-reflow after percutaneous coronary intervention. *Am J Cardiol* 1995;75:778–782.

151. Morishima I, Sone T, Mokuno S, et al. Clinical significance of no-reflow phenomenon observed on angiography after successful treatment of acute myocardial infarction with percutaneous transluminal coronary angioplasty. *Am Heart J* 1995;130:239–243.

152. Erlebacher JA, Weiss JL, Weisfeldt ML, Bulkley BH. Early dilation of the infarcted segment in acute transmural myocardial infarction: role of infarct expansion in acute left ventricular enlargement. *J Am Coll Cardiol* 1984;4:201–208.

153. Ito H, Maruyama A, Iwakura K, et al. Clinical implications of the "no reflow" phenomenon. A predictor of complications and left ventricular remodeling in reperfused anterior wall myocardial infarction. *Circulation* 1996;93:223–228.

154. Piper HM, Meuter K, Schafer C. Cellular mechanisms of ischemia–reperfusion injury. *Ann Thorac Surg* 2003;75:S644–S648.

155. Manning AS, Hearse DJ. Reperfusion-induced arrhythmias: mechanisms and prevention. *J Mol Cell Cardiol* 1984;16:497–518.

156. Goldberg S, Greenspon AJ, Urban PL, et al. Reperfusion arrhythmia: a marker of restoration of antegrade flow during intracoronary thrombolysis for acute myocardial infarction. *Am Heart J* 1983;105:26–32.

157. Mahaffey KW, Puma JA, Barbagelata NA, et al. Adenosine as an adjunct to thrombolytic therapy for acute myocardial infarction: results of a multicenter, randomized, placebo-controlled trial: the Acute Myocardial Infarction Study of Adenosine (AMISTAD) trial. *J Am Coll Cardiol* 1999;34:1711–1720.

158. Ross AM, Gibbons RJ, Stone GW, Kloner RA, Alexander RW. A randomized, double-blinded, placebo-controlled multicenter trial of adenosine as an adjunct to reperfusion in the treatment of acute myocardial infarction (AMISTAD-II). *J Am Coll Cardiol* 2005;45:1775–1780.

159. Staat P, Rioufol G, Piot C, et al. Postconditioning the human heart. *Circulation* 2005;112:2143–2148.

160. Boyce SW, Bartels C, Bolli R, et al. Impact of sodium-hydrogen exchange inhibition by cariporide on death or myocardial infarction in high-risk CABG surgery patients: results of the CABG surgery cohort of the GUARDIAN study. *J Thorac Cardiovasc Surg* 2003;126:420–427.

161. Menzter. Effects of Na+H+ exchange inhibition by cariporide on death and nonfatal myocardial infarction in patients undergoing coronary artery bypass graft surgery: the EXPEDITION study. *Circ J* 2003;108.

162. Mangano DT, Miao Y, Tudor IC, Dietzel C. Post-reperfusion myocardial infarction: long-term survival improvement using adenosine regulation with acadesine. *J Am Coll Cardiol* 2006;48:206–214.

CHAPTER (59)

Unstable Angina and Non–ST-Segment Elevation Myocardial Infarction

James A. de Lemos / Robert A. O'Rourke

INTRODUCTION

As discussed in detail in Chap. 56, *acute coronary syndrome* (ACS) is a useful operative term for referring to any pattern of clinical symptoms that is consistent with acute myocardial ischemia (Fig. 59–1).[1] This chapter is confined to two closely related forms of ACS, namely unstable angina (UA) and non–ST-segment elevation myocardial infarction (NSTEMI). The latter (Fig. 59–1) usually does not progress to a Q-wave myocardial infarction (QWMI) but rather to a non–Q-wave myocardial infarction (NQMI). Early revascularization therapy—thrombolysis or percutaneous coronary intervention (PCI)—may "convert" a potential ST-segment elevation myocardial infarction (STEMI) to a NQMI. Infrequently, an NSTEMI evolves to become a QWMI by electrocardiography (ECG).

UA and the closely related condition, NSTEMI are very common manifestations of coronary artery disease (CAD).[2]

Previously, these two forms of ACS had been classified separately as unstable angina and NQMI. However, the usual underlying pathophysiologic mechanism for both involves the rupture (most commonly) or erosion of an atherosclerotic plaque with thrombus formation that severely obstructs the coronary artery lumen. There is a complex overlap between the two syndromes. Accordingly, patients with either of these syndromes are frequently treated identically, with individual variations in management depending on the classification of high, intermediate, or low risk.[1] They differ primarily in whether the ischemia is severe enough to cause sufficient myocardial damage to release detectable quantities of a marker of myocardial injury (troponin I, troponin T, or creatine kinase myocardial band [CK-MB]). In recent years, considerable new information has come to light concerning the diagnosis and subsequent management of patients with either of these two types of ACS.[1]

1351

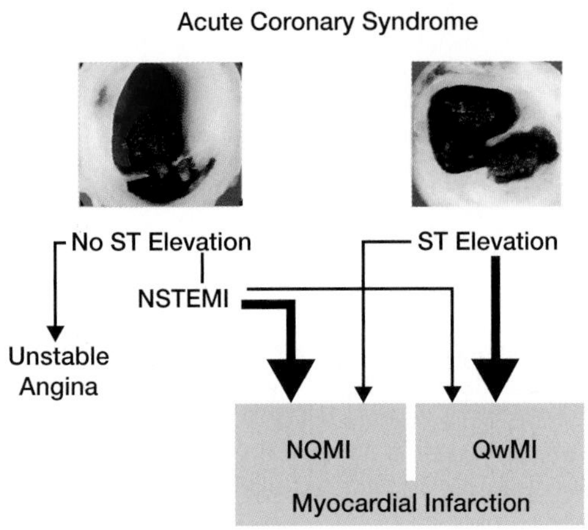

Acute Coronary Syndrome

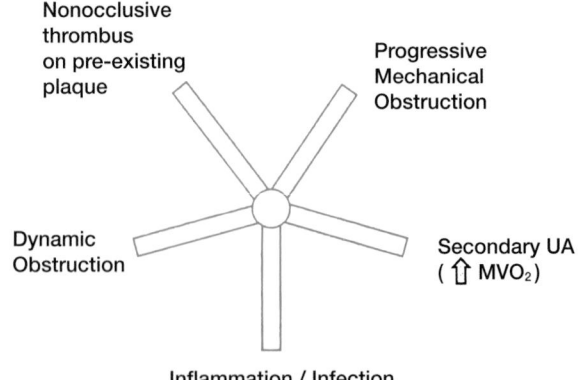

FIGURE 59–1. Nomenclature and pathophysiology of ACS. Patients with ischemic discomfort may present with or without ST-segment elevation on the ECG. The majority of patients with ST-segment elevation (*large arrows*) have complete thrombotic occlusion of an epicardial coronary artery and ultimately develop a Q-wave myocardial infarction (QWMI), whereas a minority (*small arrow*) develop a non–Q-wave myocardial infarction (NQMI). Patients who present without ST-segment elevation tend to have nonocclusive thrombus and experience either unstable angina or a non–ST-segment elevation myocardial infarction (NSTEMI). *Source: Adapted from Davies MJ. Pathophysiology of Acute Coronary Syndromes. Heart 2003;83:361.*

A practical approach to the patient with UA/NSTEMI in the emergency department was published recently as an American Heart Association (AHA) Scientific Statement.[3]

Serum biochemical markers such as troponins I and T, B-type natriuretic peptide (BNP) and N-terminal pro-BNP (NT pro-BNP) and C-reactive protein (CRP) enable more accurate risk stratification. Newer therapies, specifically low-molecular-weight heparin, platelet glycoprotein (GP) IIb/IIIa receptor antagonists and clopidogrel, have improved outcomes in high-risk patients, specifically when combined with the use of PCI and drug-eluting coronary artery stents.[1]

This chapter discusses the current management of patients with UA/NSTEMI and also discusses another angina syndrome that is not "stable"—namely, *variant angina*.

DEFINITION AND CLASSIFICATION

UA/NSTEMI is also termed *non–ST-elevation ACS*. Angiographic, intravascular ultrasound and angioscopic studies indicate that UA/NSTEMI usually results from the disruption of an atherosclerotic plaque with a subsequent cascade of pathologic processes that decrease coronary blood flow. Most patients who die during UA/NSTEMI do so because of sudden death or the development of a new or recurrent myocardial infarction (MI). Effective diagnosis and optimal management of these patients is initiated based on information readily available at the time of presentation, and updated using new information accumulated over time.[1] Initial diagnosis may be challenging as NSTEMI often cannot be differentiated from UA at the time of initial presentation. Initial management of patients with UA/NSTEMI differs from those with STEMI, who are treated with early reperfusion therapy (see Chap. 60).

The patient with symptoms consistent with ACS should be placed in an environment with the capability for continuous electrocardiographic recording and defibrillation and where a 12-lead ECG can be obtained expeditiously and interpreted accurately within 10 minutes. The most urgent priority is to identify patients with STEMI who should be considered for immediate reperfusion therapy. Each patient should have a provisional diagnosis, ruled in or ruled out, of (1) ACS, which, in turn, is classified as STEMI, NSTEMI, or UA; (2) a non-ACS cardiovascular condition; (3) another specific noncardiac disease (e.g., esophageal spasm); or (4) a noncardiac condition that is undefined. Also, the initial assessment should include risk determination and treatment of life-threatening events.[1]

CAUSES

UA and NSTEMI are characterized by an imbalance between myocardial oxygen supply and demand. The most common cause of UA/NSTEMI is reduced myocardial perfusion because of coronary artery luminal narrowing caused by a nonocclusive thrombus that developed following rupture or erosion of an atherothrombotic plaque (Fig. 59–2). The thrombus is usually not occlusive and microembolization of platelet aggregates and components of the disruptive plaque are likely responsible for the release of biochemical markers of myocardial injury in many patients. A second, but much less common, cause (Fig. 59–2) is dynamic obstruction, which may be a result of intense focal spasm of a segment of an epicardial coronary artery (Prinzmetal or variant angina, as discussed specifically in the section Variant [Prinzmetal] Angina below). A third cause of UA/NSTEMI is severe narrowing without spasm or thrombosis. This occurs in some patients with progressive atherosclerosis or with restenosis after PCI. Arterial inflammation is operative in each of the above causes of UA/STEMI, but plays a particularly important role in plaque rupture.[4] Secondary UA/NSTEMI occurs when the precipitating condition is extrinsic to the coronary arterial bed (Fig. 59–2). Such patients have underlying coronary atherosclerotic narrowing that limits

FIGURE 59–2. Framework for considering the pathophysiologic components that contribute to unstable angina in a specific patient. Varying contributions are possible from each of the five arms. Some patients will have predominantly one cause, whereas in others, two or more mechanisms will contribute significantly. MVO_2, myocardial oxygen consumption; UA, unstable angina. *Source: From Braunwald E. Unstable angina: an etiologic approach to management. Circulation 1998;98: 2219–2222, with permission.*

myocardial perfusion; they also often have prior chronic stable angina. UA/NSTEMI occurs with sudden increases in myocardial oxygen demands (e.g., fever, tachycardia), reductions in coronary blood flow, (e.g., hypotension), or diminution in myocardial oxygen delivery (e.g., severe anemia).

INITIAL PRESENTATION

There are three principal manifestations of UA/NSTEMI: (1) rest angina; (2) new-onset severe angina; and (3) increasing angina.[1] Criteria for diagnosis of UA/NSTEMI are based on duration and intensity of angina as graded according to the Canadian Cardiovascular Society Classifications (see Chaps. 11 and 12).

The designation of three specific forms of UA/NSTEMI is useful because the pathophysiology, prognosis, and management of these forms are different. The de novo form resulting from the development of an unstable coronary plaque was described above. Other settings include UA/NSTEMI within 6 months after PCI, which is most often caused by restenosis. Intravenous nitroglycerin provides effective therapy and repeat PCI is usually performed. UA/NSTEMI in a patient with previous coronary bypass surgery often involves advanced atherothrombosis of venous bypass grafts and a lower likelihood of long-term symptomatic relief compared with other patients with UA.

ACS may present with "atypical" symptoms, which include acute dyspnea, indigestion, unusual locations of pain, agitation, altered mental status, profound weakness, and syncope. Such presentations are more common in women, the elderly, and patients with long-standing diabetes mellitus, and are associated with higher risk for death and major complications.[5]

PATHOPHYSIOLOGY

Table 59–1 lists the factors that modulate the development and complications of ACS.

PLAQUE DISRUPTION OR EROSION

Many of the mechanical, cellular, and molecular factors contributing to plaque disruption have been elucidated in recent years (see Chaps. 52 and 56).[4,6,7] *Plaque rupture* most commonly occurs at the shoulder region of the plaque, where the plaque joins the adjacent vessel wall: this area of the plaque is commonly infiltrated with inflammatory cells and is subjected to high shear forces.[6,7] Plaques prone to rupture ("high risk" or "vulnerable" plaques) tend to have a thin fibrous cap and a large lipid pool, which influence the biomechanical properties of the plaque and increases the likelihood of rupture (Fig. 59–3). Conversely, fibrosis and calcification appear to decrease the risk of rupture.[4,7,8]

Erosion is a less-common precipitant of ACS and usually occurs centrally through a thinning cap rather than at the plaque shoulders.[4,8] Erosion appears to be more common among women who smoke, whereas plaque rupture occurs more frequently in hyperlipidemic men.[7,8]

INFLAMMATION

Inflammation plays a central role in plaque disruption and ACS (Fig. 59–4). Macrophages and T lymphocytes accumulate in atherothrombotic plaques because of the expression of adhesion molecules on monocytes, endothelial cells, and leukocytes, and the release of proinflammatory cytokines and chemokines (such as monocyte chemoattractant protein-1) that recruit additional inflammatory cells into the region.[9]

The matrix metalloproteinases—which include collagenases and gelatinases—are released from macrophages and degrade the collagen that provides strength to the fibrous cap.[6] Tissue inhibi-

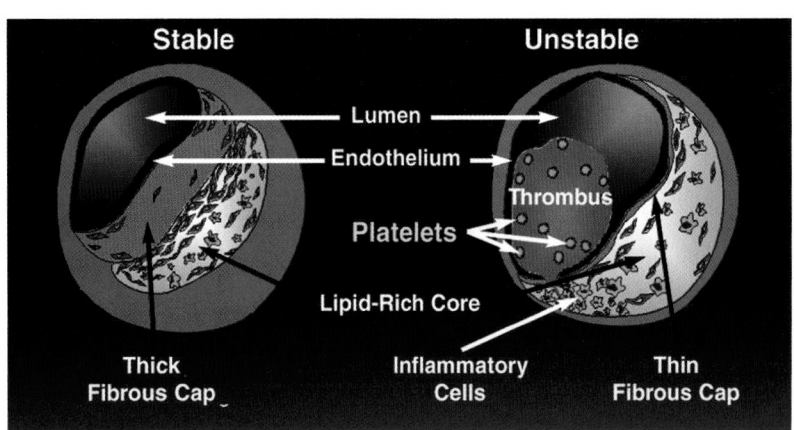

FIGURE 59–3. Characteristics of the unstable and stable plaque. Although the stable plaque may be associated with significant luminal narrowing, it tends to have a thick fibrous cap, a small lipid core, and a paucity of inflammatory cells. In contrast, the unstable plaque tends to have a large lipid core and a thin fibrous cap. Inflammatory cells accumulate at the shoulder region and contribute to plaque rupture with subsequent thrombus formation.

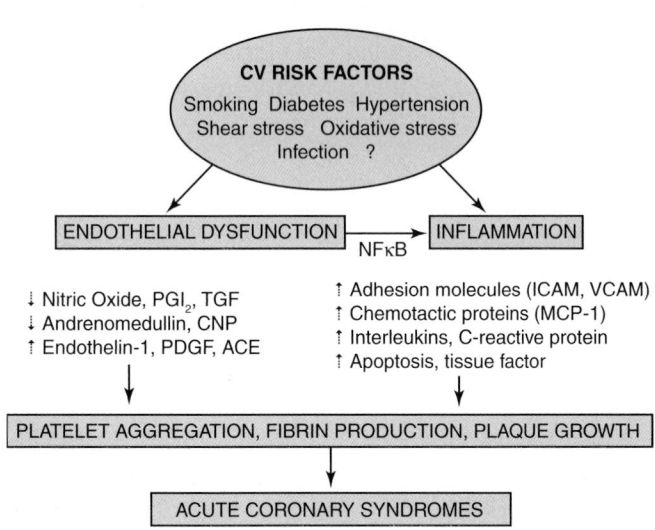

FIGURE 59–4. Link between cardiovascular risk factors, endothelial dysfunction, inflammation, and acute coronary syndromes. Endothelial dysfunction can be caused by many proinflammatory atherogenic factors. Endothelial cells thereafter increase expression of adhesion molecules. ACE, angiotensin converting enzyme; CNP, c-type natriuretic peptide; ICAM, intercellular adhesion molecule; MCP-1, monocyte chemoattractant protein-1; NF, nuclear factor kappa; PDGF, platelet-derived growth factor; PGI$_2$, prostaglandin; TGF, transforming growth factor; VCAM, vascular cell adhesion molecule.

tors of matrix metalloproteinases are normally expressed by vascular smooth muscle cells. In the vulnerable areas of the fibrous cap, however, macrophages predominate and smooth muscle cells are sparse, creating an imbalance between matrix degrading enzymes and their inhibitors.[6] Together, these findings indicate that an inflammatory stimulus causes a "biochemical storm" within the high-risk plaque, leading to rupture of its fibrous cap.

It is now believed that in at least in some individuals with UA/NSTEMI, inflammation may be a much more widespread process. Patients with unstable angina have been demonstrated to have neutrophil activation throughout the coronary tree, including sites remote from the culprit stenosis.[10] The clinical manifestations of this phenomenon are now recognized to include the occurrence of multiple, simultaneous complex coronary plaques at the time of presentation in some patients with UA/NSTEMI.[11]

【 】 INFECTION

The stimulus initiating the acute inflammatory process in UA has not been clearly delineated. Atherothrombosis, as defined by the "response to injury" hypothesis, is a chronic, low-grade inflammatory condition. Controversy persists as to whether infectious agents play a primary role either in atherothrombosis or in the transformation of stable to unstable CAD.

Chlamydia pneumoniae, cytomegalovirus, and *Helicobacter pylori* have been identified within human atherosclerotic lesions. Furthermore, antibodies against *Chlamydia* heat shock proteins can cross-react against heat shock proteins produced by endothelium, resulting in endothelial damage and accelerated atherosclerosis.[12]

Although antibodies to *Chlamydia*, cytomegalovirus, and *H. pylori* are found more often in patients with atherothrombosis than in controls, these associations do not indicate causality. Antibodies to

these agents because of prior infection are found in a high proportion of the population. Moreover, a series of large, randomized, controlled trials has failed to show benefit from prolonged treatment with antibiotic regimens that have activity against *Chlamydia*.[13,14]

【 】 PLATELETS AND LEUKOCYTES

Platelet activation and deposition onto the exposed thrombogenic surface of a ruptured plaque is important in the pathogenesis of UA/NSTEMI. Indeed, a distinguishing feature of thrombosis in the arterial as compared with the venous circulation is the critical role of activated platelets. When stimulated by factors such as collagen, epinephrine, adenosine diphosphate (ADP), and thrombin, platelets become activated, undergo a conformational change, and secrete the contents of their α granules, which contain vasoconstrictive substances such as thromboxane A$_2$ and serotonin, as well as procoagulant substances such as fibrinogen and von Willebrand factor. In addition, activation of the platelet causes an increase in surface expression and binding affinity of GPIIb/IIIa receptors, which bind fibrinogen and von Willebrand factor to cause platelet aggregation.[15] Activated platelets also release soluble CD40 ligand, which is now recognized as an important immunoregulatory and proinflammatory molecule that may link platelet activation and inflammation.[16] Activated platelets and leukocytes interact in the acute phase of UA/NSTEMI to facilitate platelet-thrombus deposition.[17]

【 】 THROMBOSIS AND FIBRINOLYSIS

The interplay of activated platelets and leukocytes stimulates the coagulation system. Monocytes release tissue factor, a small glycoprotein that initiates the extrinsic clotting cascade, resulting in an augmentation in thrombin generation.[4] Tissue factor is also present in the lipid-rich core of atherothrombotic plaques and is likely one of the major determinants of the thrombogenicity of ruptured plaques.[4] Tissue factor initiates the extrinsic coagulation cascade, resulting in activation of factor X to factor Xa, which can then convert prothrombin to thrombin. Using phospholipid from the membrane of the activated platelet, thrombin catalyzes the conversion of fibrinogen to fibrin, forming the platelet-fibrin clot that obstructs coronary blood flow in ACS.

【 】 EMBOLIZATION AND THE CORONARY MICROCIRCULATION

Embolization of platelet-thrombus and plaque material from the site of the ruptured plaque can lead to microvascular obstruction and initiate a cascade of events including local inflammation and tissue injury, vasoconstriction, and in situ propagation of platelet-leukocyte aggregates. This is an important contributing factor to adverse outcomes in UA/NSTEMI and a target for pharmacotherapy. Troponin elevation appears to identify patients with UA/NSTEMI who are more likely to have microvascular obstruction.[18]

【 】 VASOCONSTRICTION

Culprit lesions in UA/NSTEMI demonstrate an increased response to vasoconstrictor stimuli compared to other coronary artery segments or culprit lesions of patients with stable angina.

Vasoconstriction or the lack of appropriate vasodilation probably contributes significantly to the development of ischemic episodes in patients with UA and is a potential target for therapy.

[ ] ANGIOGRAPHIC CHARACTERISTICS OF THE CULPRIT LESION

The angiographic characteristics of the culprit lesion have been defined before, during, and after an episode of UA. If a patient with UA has had a prior coronary angiogram, the culprit lesion has usually progressed markedly since the time of the prior angiogram. At the time of UA/NSTEMI, the culprit lesion is likely to be asymmetric or eccentric, with a narrow base or neck. Lesions with irregular borders, overhanging edges, or obvious thrombus at angiography are more likely to initiate another cardiac event in the ensuing months.[19]

DIAGNOSIS

Patients with suspected ACS must be evaluated expeditiously. Decisions based on the early evaluation have important clinical and economic consequences. A prompt and accurate diagnosis permits the timely initiation of appropriate therapy which is paramount.

Patients with chest pain lasting for longer than 20 minutes, stuttering chest pain, hemodynamic instability, recent syncope or presyncope should be referred to a hospital emergency department.[1]

[ ] INITIAL EVALUATION

In a patient with known CAD, typical symptoms are highly likely to be caused by myocardial ischemia, especially if the current symptoms are identical to previous episodes when CAD was objectively documented as the cause. The evaluation of a patient with UA/NSTEMI requires not only the establishment of the diagnosis but also an assessment of the short-term risk, which determines the intensity of initial and often subsequent treatment.

[ ] HISTORY

When unstable angina is suspected in a patient younger than age 50 years, it is particularly important to consider cocaine use. Cocaine can cause coronary vasospasm and thrombosis in addition to its direct effect on heart rate and blood pressure; it has been implicated as a cause of ACS.[1]

Patients with ACS often experience discomfort typical of angina but the episodes are more severe and prolonged; they often occur at rest and commonly are precipitated by less exertion than previously. Also, chest discomfort because of UA/NSTEMI is less likely to be relieved by nitroglycerin than is stable angina. Some patients may have no chest discomfort but present solely with jaw, neck, ear, arm, and epigastric discomfort, or with dyspnea in the absence of pain. These should be considered as "angina equivalents."

Evaluation of patients with suspected UA/NSTEMI should include the physician's opinion of whether the chest discomfort's *likelihood* of being caused by myocardial ischemia is in one of three categories: high, intermediate, or low (Table 59–2).

Nausea, sweating, or shortness of breath may accompany episodes of chest discomfort. In elderly or diabetic patients, these symptoms may be the only indication that myocardial ischemia is present. Both groups of patients have an increased incidence of multivessel disease. Women also present certain challenges with regard to diagnosis. On the one hand, they have a lower probability of underlying significant coronary heart disease than men. On the other hand, women are also more likely than men to have ACS with an "atypical" presentation.[5]

[ ] THE ELECTROCARDIOGRAM

The diagnostic yield of the 12-lead ECG is enhanced greatly if it can be recorded during an episode of chest discomfort. Although a normal ECG during chest pain does not rule out ACS, it is a favorable prognostic sign. Transient ST-segment depression of at least 0.5 mm (Fig. 59–5) that appears during chest discomfort and disappears after relief provides objective evidence of transient myocardial ischemia. When it is a constant finding with or without chest pain, it is less specific. A common ECG pattern in patients with unstable angina is a persistent negative T wave over the involved area (Fig. 59–6). Deeply negative T waves across all the precordial leads suggest a proximal, severe, left anterior descending coronary artery stenosis as the culprit lesion.

TABLE 59–2

Likelihood That Unstable Angina Symptoms Are Caused by Myocardial Ischemia

HIGH LIKELIHOOD

Known coronary disease (particularly recent percutaneous coronary intervention)
Typical angina reproducing prior documented angina
Hemodynamic or ECG changes during pain
Variant angina
ST-segment elevation or depression of at least 0.5 mm
Marked symmetric T-wave inversion in multiple precordial leads
Elevated cardiac enzymes

INTERMEDIATE LIKELIHOOD

Absence of high-likelihood features and any of the following:
Typical angina in a patient without prior documented angina
Atypical anginal symptoms in diabetics or in nondiabetics with two or more other risk factors
Male gender
Age >70
Extracardiac vascular disease
T-wave inversion of at least 1 mm in leads with dominant R waves

LOW LIKELIHOOD

Absence of high- or intermediate-likelihood features but may have:
Chest pain, probably not angina
One risk factor but not diabetes
T waves flat or inverted <1 mm in leads with dominant R waves
Normal ECG

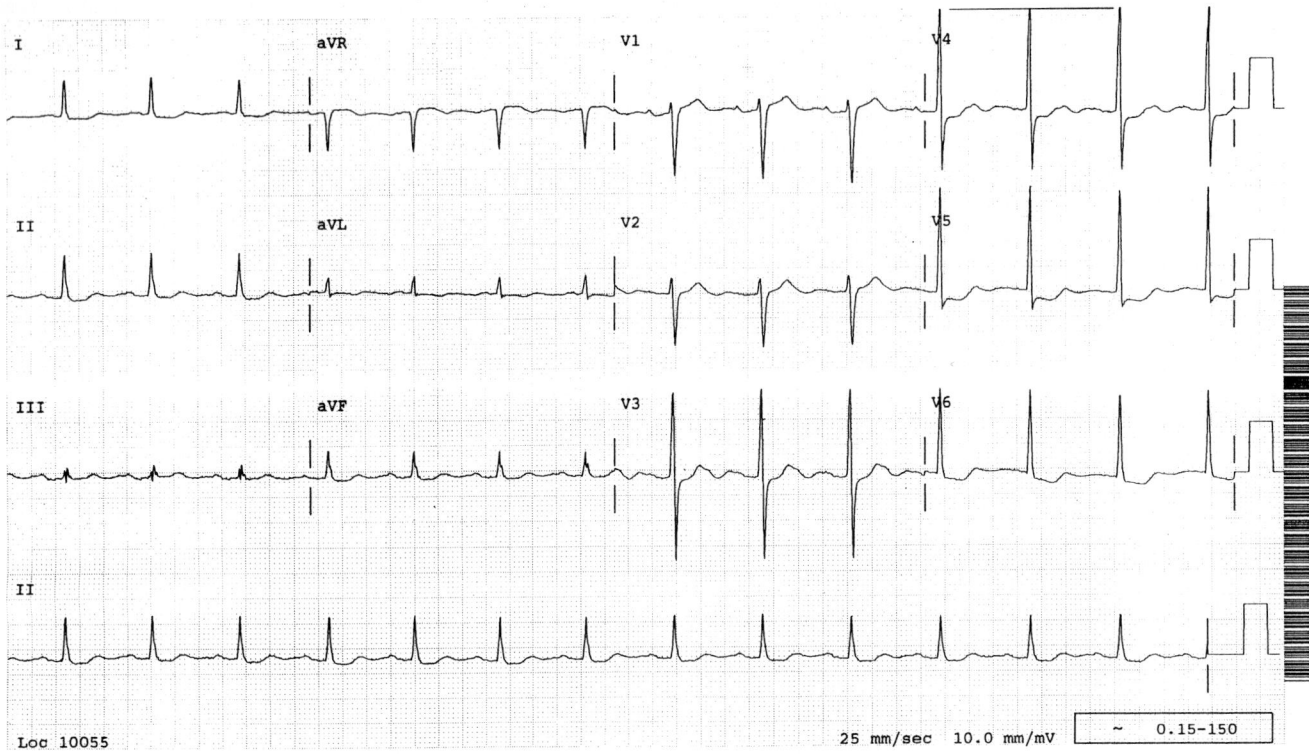

FIGURE 59–5. Electrocardiogram recorded during an episode of chest pain at rest in a patient with unstable angina. ST-segment depression >1 mm is present in leads V_4 to V_6. This abnormality was not present on the baseline tracing. The chest pain and ST-segment depression disappeared promptly after the administration of sublingual nitroglycerin.

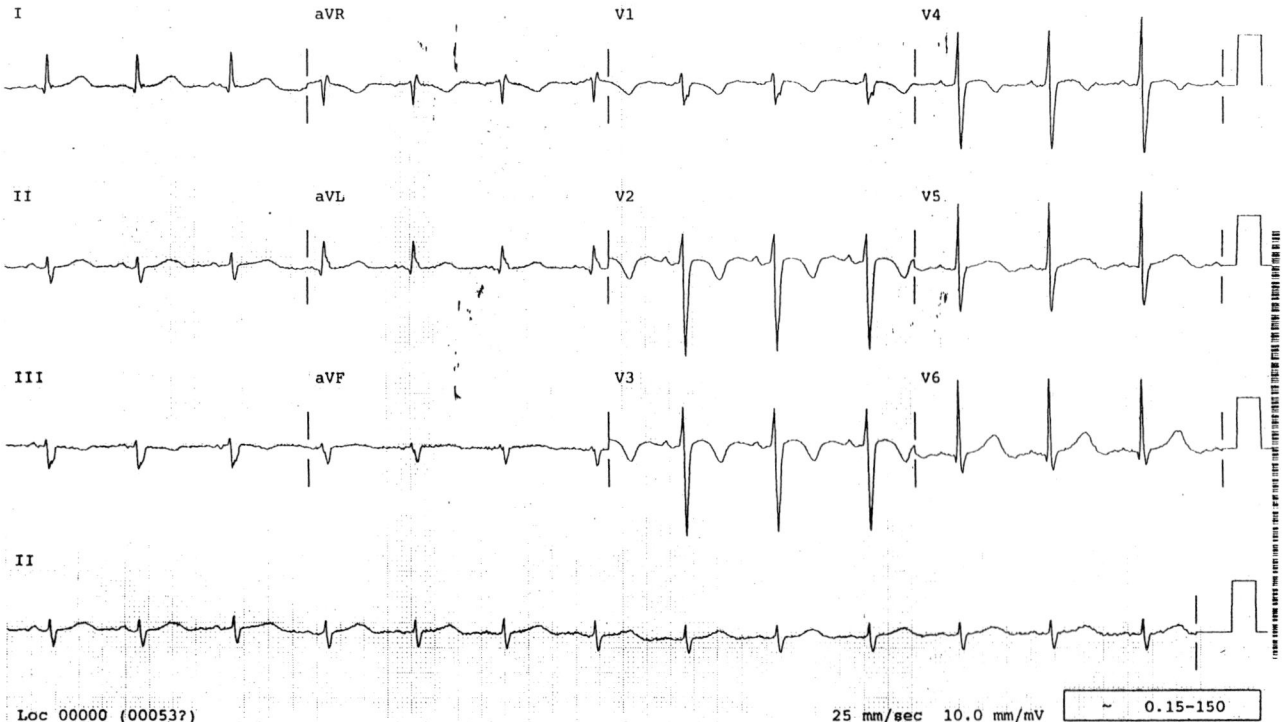

FIGURE 59–6. Electrocardiogram recorded during a pain-free interval from a patient hospitalized with unstable angina. The negative T waves in leads V_1 to V_4 had been upright on a previous tracing. The culprit lesion was located in the left anterior descending coronary artery.

In UA/NSTEMI patients, the ECG may show Q waves from an old infarction or a left bundle-branch block resulting from extensive prior left ventricular (LV) damage. Patients with such findings are at increased risk.[20]

ECG abnormalities may appear or progress in the absence of new symptoms or signs in patients with ACS. Accordingly, it is appropriate to obtain serial ECGs during the first 48 hours, as well as during recurrent episodes of chest pain.

[ ] BIOCHEMICAL CARDIAC MARKERS

Biochemical cardiac markers are useful for both the diagnosis of myocardial necrosis and the estimation of prognosis. Traditionally, elevated serum levels of creatine kinase or its myocardial band (MB) isoenzyme were used to distinguish between UA and acute MI. The widespread availability of assays for cardiac troponins has improved the ability to diagnose lesser degrees of myocardial necrosis. The absence of cardiac troponins T (cTnT) and I (cTnI) from adult skeletal muscle confers very high cardiac specificity and has allowed the diagnostic threshold for troponin assays to approach zero, resulting in high sensitivity of cTnT and cTnI to detect cardiac injury. As many as one-third of patients with a clinical syndrome consistent with UA will have elevated levels of troponin T or I on admission or soon thereafter.[1] Many of these will have normal levels of CK-MB. Numerous studies have demonstrated that even minor troponin elevations are independent predictors of adverse events in populations with non-ST elevation ACS.[21] It is now clear that patients who have isolated elevation in troponin levels should be classified as having a NSTEMI, *provided the clinical syndrome is consistent with ACS.*

Troponins are not specific for the *etiology* of cardiac injury. Multiple acute illnesses besides ACS may cause cardiac injury and lead to troponin elevation (Table 59–3). Moreover, in the general population, diabetes, LV hypertrophy, LV dysfunction or heart failure, and moderate renal insufficiency may be associated with chronic cTnT elevation, even in the absence of signs and symptoms of ischemia (Fig. 59–7).[22] It is important to interpret troponin values in the context of the clinical presentation and available clinical information. In most non-ACS conditions associated with cardiac injury, patients with detectable troponin are at increased risk for adverse cardiac outcomes.[23–25] However, it should be recognized that in patients with atypical presentations, particularly if they have underlying LV hypertrophy, heart failure, chronic kidney disease, or diabetes, the elevation in troponin may be the result of a cause other than ACS. Particular consideration should be given to the diagnosis of pulmonary embolism.

Interpreting troponins in patients with renal failure presents unique problems. While persistent troponin elevation occurs in patients on hemodialysis in the absence of signs of ACS, detectable

TABLE 59–3

Causes of Troponin Elevation Other Than Acute Coronary Syndromes

Pulmonary embolus
Myocarditis
Cardiac contusion
Congestive heart failure
Chemotherapy (Adriamycin, 5-fluorouracil)
Cardioversion or radiofrequency ablation
Septic shock
Extreme endurance athletics
Renal failure

cTnT or cTnI is still associated with very high cardiac event rates.[24–27] Knowledge of prior troponin values may help to assess whether a current troponin elevation is new (i.e., potentially caused by ACS) or chronic. Demonstration of a transient rise and fall in troponin values may not improve specificity for ACS. If ACS is suspected, troponin elevation should be interpreted similarly in patients with and without renal failure.

[ ] ACUTE MYOCARDIAL PERFUSION IMAGING

Intermittent reductions in coronary blood flow distal to the culprit coronary stenosis can occur in UA without either ECG changes or elevation in cardiac enzymes. Acute rest myocardial perfusion imaging with sestamibi is a relatively sensitive and specific diagnostic test for ACS. Sestamibi is more useful than thallium for this purpose because imaging can be delayed for up to several hours after injection as a result of minimal redistribution of this imaging agent. ECG-gated images provide an assessment of wall motion in addition to perfusion (see Chap. 19).

The sensitivity and negative predictive value of acute rest perfusion imaging is extremely high if sestamibi is injected during an episode of chest pain, but sensitivity decreases if the injection is done within the ensuing hours. However, acute rest imaging will be normal in a few (<5 percent) patients with ACS.

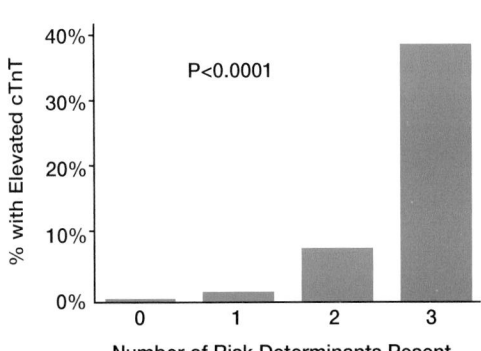

Risk Determinant	Odds Ratio
Diabetes	4.6
Hypertrophy	5.4
Congestive Heart Failure	5.3
Chronic Kidney Disease	20.4

FIGURE 59–7. Troponin T elevation in the general population. Among 3557 participants from the general population enrolled in the Dallas Heart Study, 0.7 percent had detectable troponin T levels in the absence of signs of cardiac ischemia. Variables associated with troponin elevation included diabetes, left ventricular (LV) hypertrophy, evidence of heart failure, and moderate or severe renal insufficiency (*left panel*). In the absence of one of these criteria, troponin elevation was extremely rare, but the probability of elevated cardiac troponin T (cTnT) increased markedly in proportion to the number of these factors present (*right panel*). *Source: Adapted from Wallace TW, Abdullah SM, Drazner MH, et al.*[22]

❪ ❫ CHEST PAIN UNITS

The evaluation of patients with chest pain who may have UA or MI is often difficult and uncertain. Hospitalizing all such patients for an extensive workup is unwise and results in unnecessary tests with patient risk and expense. However, missing the diagnosis of MI is the leading cause of malpractice claims for emergency room physicians. The chest pain unit was developed as a solution to these problems.[1]

Most chest pain units are in or near the emergency department and use a set of criteria to select *low-risk* patients. Criteria usually include chest pain or related symptoms that may indicate myocardial ischemia but with a normal or unchanged ECG and a normal initial set of cardiac enzymes. In most units, cTnT or cTnI is measured every 3 to 4 hours for 6 to 12 hours' duration, sometimes with other serum markers. Some chest pain units measure myoglobin serially over 90 to 180 minutes in a rapid "rule out MI" protocol,[28] but this strategy has not been widely adopted. Myeloperoxidase and ischemia-modified albumin are under active investigation as tools to further risk-stratify troponin-negative patients.

Patients receive an aspirin, an intravenous line, ECG monitoring, and a 12-lead ECG at specific intervals. If no evidence of active CAD is detected, a stress test may be performed for diagnostic and prognostic purposes or the patient may be discharged and sent home.[1]

Chest pain units are reported to reduce the rate of missed MIs from approximately 5 percent to 0.5 percent, as estimated from return visits within 72 hours.[29,30]

RISK STRATIFICATION

Initial risk assessment of UA/NSTEMI requires both establishing the diagnosis and determining the short-term risk. This risk assessment dictates the appropriate intensity of initial therapy. At the low end of the risk scale, a patient may be discharged home with aspirin and β blockers, often with an early outpatient stress test. By contrast, high-risk patients may be hospitalized in a coronary care unit, treated with multiple drugs, and undergo coronary angiography urgently as a prelude to revascularization.

❪ ❫ CLINICAL FEATURES

The American College of Cardiology (ACC)/AHA *2002 Guideline Update for the Management of Patients with UA and Non–ST-Segment Elevation Myocardial Infarction* categorizes patients with UA into low-, intermediate-, and high-risk groups (Table 59–4).[1] High-risk patients have ongoing chest pain that lasts longer than 20 minutes, reversible ST-segment changes of at least 0.5 mm, elevated markers of myonecrosis, or signs of significant LV dysfunction. Low-risk patients have worsening angina without rest pain, are age 65 years or younger, have a normal or unchanged ECG without evidence of previous infarction, and have normal cardiac enzymes.

The risk assessment should be updated during hospitalization. Continuing angina with ST changes despite medical therapy is an ominous sign that should prompt urgent coronary arteriography with probable revascularization. Episodes of silent ST depression detected by ambulatory ECG recordings predict an unfavorable course.

❪ ❫ THE ELECTROCARDIOGRAM

The ECG is too often overlooked as a powerful risk stratification tool in patients with UA/NSTEMI. Even minor ST depression (>0.5 mV) is associated is associated with a markedly increased mortality rate. Among 9461 patients enrolled in the PURSUIT (Platelet Glycoprotein IIb/IIIa in Unstable Angina: Receptor Suppression Using Integrilin Therapy) study, mortality at 30 days was 5.1 percent in patients with ST depression versus 2.1 percent among those without ST depression.[31] Patients with isolated T-wave inversion have a more favorable prognosis than do those with ST depression.[32]

❪ ❫ BIOCHEMICAL MARKERS

Troponin measurements should be used in the risk stratification of patients with UA/NSTEMI to supplement the assessment from clinical and ECG data. Elevated troponin levels strongly predict coronary events over the short-term. The combination of troponin elevation and ST-segment depression identifies a group at particularly high risk.[33,34] Measuring troponin not just at baseline but also at 8 to 16 hours after admission adds useful prognostic information.[33]

Coronary angiographic trials have demonstrated that in patients with ACS, troponin elevation is associated with multivessel coronary disease, complex lesion morphology, and visible thrombus, as well as with impairment in microvascular function, which is indicative of distal embolization of plaque material and platelet thrombus to the coronary microcirculation.[18] These findings have been confirmed using intravascular ultrasound[35] and explain the consistent association between troponin elevation, even at low levels, and recurrent ischemic events in patients with ACS. The association of troponin elevation with high-risk coronary lesion morphology provides mechanistic insight into studies demonstrating that patients with even minor elevations in cTnT or cTnI derive substantial benefit from an aggressive approach with respect to GPIIb/IIIa inhibitors, low-molecular-weight heparin and an early invasive management strategy.[36–38]

The clinical significance of minor (borderline) elevation in cardiac troponins has generated controversy, because most immunoassays have high variability near the lower limits of detection. An ACC/European Society of Cardiology committee has argued that the diagnostic threshold for MI should be set at the lowest level at which the coefficient of variation (CV) is <10 percent.[39] However, several studies show that patients with "borderline" troponin values (between the lower limit of detection and the level of 10 percent CV) have similar ischemic event rates and derive similar benefit from aggressive therapy as do patients with more markedly elevated troponin values.[37,40] In the Dallas Heart Study, Wallace et al. observed similar cardiac structural and functional abnormalities among patients with borderline versus higher cTnT values.[22] These data argue strongly that *any* detectable level of troponin with a valid assay should be considered indicative of myocardial injury.

Plasma levels of BNP and the N-terminal fragment of its prohormone (NT pro-BNP) may rise in response to cardiac ischemia in proportion to the size and severity of the ischemic insult.[41] In patients with UA/NSTEMI, higher levels of BNP or NT pro-BNP measured at presentation or during hospitalization are asso-

TABLE 59-4

Short-Term Risk of Death or Nonfatal Myocardial Infarction in Patients with Unstable Angina[a]

FEATURE	HIGH RISK: AT LEAST ONE OF THE FOLLOWING FEATURES MUST BE PRESENT	INTERMEDIATE RISK: NO HIGH-RISK FEATURE BUT MUST HAVE ONE OF THE FOLLOWING FEATURES	LOW RISK: NO HIGH- OR INTERMEDIATE-RISK FEATURE BUT MAY HAVE ANY OF THE FOLLOWING FEATURES
History	Accelerating tempo of ischemic symptoms in preceding 48 h	Prior MI, peripheral or disease, or CABG, prior aspirin use	New-onset or progressive CCS class III or IV angina the past 2 weeks without prolonged (>20 min) rest pain but with moderate or high likelihood of CAD
Character of pain	Prolonged ongoing (>20 min) rest pain	Prolonged (>20 min) rest angina, now resolved, with moderate or high likelihood of CAD Rest angina (<20 min) or relieved with rest or sublingual NTG	
Clinical findings	Pulmonary edema, most likely caused by ischemia New or worsening MR murmur S_3 or new/worsening rales Hypotension, bradycardia, tachycardia Age >75 years	Age >70 years	
ECG	Angina at rest with transient ST-segment changes >0.05 mV Bundle-branch block, new or presumed new Sustained ventricular tachycardia	T-wave inversions >0.2 mV Pathologic Q waves	Normal or unchanged ECG during an episode of chest discomfort
Cardiac markers	Elevated (e.g., cTnT ≥0.01 ng/mL or cTnI >0.1 ng/mL)	Normal	Normal

CABG, coronary artery bypass graft; CAD, coronary artery disease; CCC, Canadian cardiovascular class; CCS, Canadian Cardiovascular Society; ECG, electrocardiogram; MI, myocardial infarction; MR, mitral regurgitation; NTG, nitroglycerin; TnI, troponin I; TnT, troponin T.
[a]Estimation of the short-term risk of death and nonfatal cardiac ischemic events in unstable angina is a complex multivariable problem that cannot be fully specified in a table such as this; thus, this table is meant to offer general guidance and illustration rather than rigid algorithms.
SOURCE: Adapted from Braunwald E, Antman EM, Beasly JW, et al.[1]

ciated with a markedly increased risk for subsequent death or heart failure, even among patients with normal troponin levels and no evidence of heart failure[42–44] (Fig. 59–8). In a recent substudy of the Aggrastat to Zocor (A to Z) trial involving 2901 patients with ACS, those with persistent BNP elevation >80 pg/mL at 4 or 12 months after ACS had a three- to fourfold increased risk for death at 2 years, compared to patients with persistently low BNP levels.[45] These findings suggest that serial BNP or NT pro-BNP measurements may provide incremental prognostic value in patients following ACS. Despite robust and reproducible prognostic data, the therapeutic implications of isolated BNP or NT pro-BNP elevation in patients with UA/NSTEMI have not been delineated. Thus, currently, we recommend only selective measurement of BNP and NT pro-BNP in patients with ACS.

Several studies have also evaluated CRP measurement early after ACS, where levels typically rise markedly in response to cardiac injury. In a FRISC (Fragmin During Instability in Coronary Artery Disease) II substudy, CRP levels >10 mg/L were associated with increased risk of cardiovascular death at all troponin levels.[46] In a large substudy involving more than 6900 patients from the GUSTO (Global Utilization of Streptokinase and Tissue Plasminogen Activator for Occluded Arteries) IV trial, a CRP >10 mg/L was associated with a higher rate of death at 1 year in multivariate analyses.[47] However, CRP appears to provide less prognostic information than troponins and BNP/NT pro-BNP. Moreover, the therapeutic implications of early CRP elevation have not been well studied. CRP measurements in the chronic phase of coronary disease and for population screening are discussed in Chap. 51.

Newer Biomarkers

Myeloperoxidase (MPO) is a neutrophil enzyme that has been postulated to play a role in low-density lipoprotein (LDL) oxidation. Among 604 patients presenting to an emergency room with chest pain, initial plasma MPO levels predicted the risk of MI and of major adverse cardiac events at 30 days and 6 months, even among those with negative cTnT levels.[48] The prognostic value of MPO appeared to be particularly robust when measured early after symptom onset, when troponin elevation may not have yet occurred. However, MPO is a *nonspecific marker* of inflammation

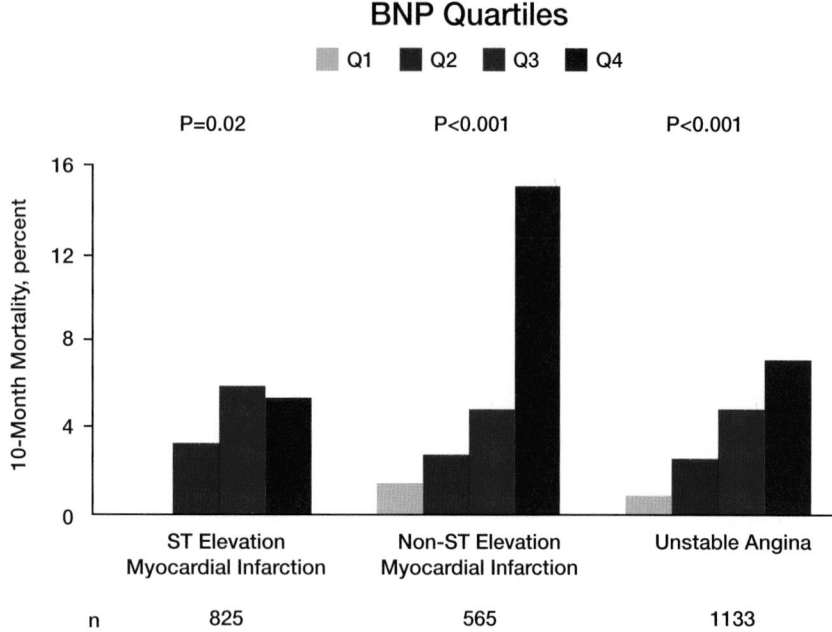

BNP Quartiles

■ Q1 ■ Q2 ■ Q3 ■ Q4

FIGURE 59–8. Association between levels of B-type natriuretic peptide (BNP) and mortality across the spectrum of acute coronary syndrome in the OPUS-TIMI 16 study. A robust association between BNP (measured within the first few days after presentation) and 10-month mortality was observed for patients with ST-segment elevation myocardial infarction, non–ST-segment elevation myocardial infarction, and unstable angina. This difference persisted after adjustment for known risk predictors and variables associated with heart failure. Source: Adapted with permission from de Lemos JA, Morrow DA, Bentley JH, et al.[42]

and oxidative stress, and elevated levels do not alter therapy in ACS at this time.

The ability of albumin to bind transitional metals such as copper and cobalt is altered in the setting of ischemia. The albumin cobalt binding test measures ischemia-modified albumin (IMA). In one study of 208 patients presenting to the emergency room with chest pain consistent with ACS, sensitivity of IMA to diagnose ACS was 82 percent; and the combined sensitivity of the ECG, cTnT, and IMA was 95 percent, significantly higher than the 53 percent sensitivity of the ECG and cTnT alone.[49] A recent meta-analysis has validated the high sensitivity and negative predictive value of IMA for detecting ACS, especially in combination with troponin and ECG measurements;[50] specificity, however, is very poor.[49] Increased IMA values are found with infection, cancer, renal or liver disease, and ischemia in organs other than the heart. Thus, most patients with an elevated IMA value will have "false-positive" evaluations for ischemia.

Despite the promise of newer biomarkers for risk stratification in ACS, in practice the only markers that should be measured routinely for risk stratification are troponin I or T.[1]

TABLE 59–5

American College of Cardiology/American Heart Association Recommendations for Noninvasive Risk Stratification

HIGH RISK (>3% ANNUAL MORTALITY RATE)

1. Severe resting LV dysfunction (LVEF <0.35)
2. High-risk treadmill (score ≤−11)
3. Severe exercise LV dysfunction (exercise LVEF <0.35)
4. Stress-induced large perfusion defect (particularly if anterior)
5. Stress-induced multiple perfusion defects of moderate size
6. Large, fixed perfusion defect with LV dilation or increased lung uptake
7. Stress-induced moderate perfusion defect with LV dilation or increased lung uptake (thallium 201)
8. Echocardiographic wall motion abnormality (involving more than two segments) developing at a low dose of dobutamine (≤10 mg/kg/min) or at a low heart rate (≤120 beats/min)
9. Stress echocardiographic evidence of extensive ischemia

INTERMEDIATE RISK (1 TO 3 % ANNUAL MORTALITY RATE)

1. Mild/moderate resting LV dysfunction (LVEF 0.35–0.49)
2. Intermediate-risk treadmill score (score −11 to +5)
3. Stress-induced moderate perfusion defect without LV dilation or increased lung intake
4. Limited stress echocardiographic ischemia with a wall motion abnormality only at higher doses or dobutamine involving ≤2 segments

LOW RISK (<1% ANNUAL MORTALITY RATE)

1. Low-risk treadmill (score ≥+5)
2. Normal or small myocardial perfusion defect at rest or with stress
3. Normal stress echocardiographic wall motion or no change of limited resting wall motion abnormalities during stress

LV, left ventricular; LVEF, left ventricular ejection fraction.

STRESS TESTING

Stress testing (Table 59–5) is often used for risk assessment in patients with UA/NSTEMI. Low-risk and some intermediate-risk patients who stabilize with medical therapy undergo stress testing for advanced risk stratification. Those with high-risk findings, such as large, reversible perfusion defects or ST-segment depression at low exercise levels, should undergo coronary arteriography; those with negative or low-risk results can be treated medically (see Chap. 19). This approach has been validated in patients with UA/NSTEMI, demonstrating that high-risk abnormalities correlate with a higher event rate during followup.

Patients who complete a stay in a chest pain unit without objective evidence of myocardial ischemia can safely undergo stress testing for diagnosis and prognostic purposes either immediately or as an outpatient within the next 24 to 48 hours.

In patients who are unable to exercise, pharmacologic testing with dipyridamole, adenosine, or dobutamine can be used as the stress and sestamibi imaging or echocardiography can be used as a method of assessment (see Chaps. 14, 16, and 19). Stress testing is not needed in patients whose clinical features already put them at high risk; and should proceed directly to coronary arteriography.

CORONARY ANGIOGRAPHY

Risk in coronary patients traditionally has been assessed according to the number of vessels with >50 percent diameter stenosis and the presence and severity of LV dysfunction. However, the relative prognostic impact is probably less with ACS, as the risk of short-term events is dominated by features of the *culprit lesion,* such as whether it induces ST-segment depression or troponin release.

Among patients with UA/NSTEMI who undergo arteriography, approximately 25 percent will have one-vessel disease, 25 percent will have two-vessel disease, and 25 percent will have three-vessel disease. Ten percent will have significant main stenosis, and the other 15 percent will have coronary luminal narrowing of <50 percent or normal vessels on arteriography.[51] Patients with left main stenosis of at least 50 percent, or three-vessel disease with LV dysfunction, derive a survival benefit from coronary artery bypass surgery. Importantly, patients with *no* significant lesions at angiography benefit from a reorientation of their management. Noncardiac causes of chest pain should be considered (including pulmonary embolism), as well as "syndrome X" and variant angina. If the coronaries are completely normal, antithrombotic and antiplatelet drugs can often be discontinued, and the need for antianginal medication reassessed. Patients who are most likely to have no significant lesions at angiography tend to be women with no ECG changes. Nevertheless, the finding of no significant lesions at angiography is usually unanticipated. Importantly, symptomatic patients with "normal" coronary artery contrast laminography may have severe coronary atherosclerosis on intravascular ultrasound, with coronary artery remodeling (see Chap. 18).

RISK MODELS AND RISK SCORES

Risk models and scores predict a probability for adverse outcomes based on combinations of clinical, ECG, and laboratory data available at presentation. The TIMI and PURSUIT scores were derived from clinical trial databases, whereas the GRACE (Global Registry of Acute Coronary Events) score was derived from a large international registry.[31,52,53] Although all three methods discriminate patients at high versus low risk for short- and intermediate-term adverse outcomes, the GRACE model provides better calibration between predicted and observed rates of death.[54,55] The TIMI score does not include any measurement of heart failure. The GRACE model was developed in a less-selected patient population and includes renal insufficiency as a variable, which are two potential advantages over the other methods. The major advantage of the TIMI score is that it is a simple integer sum that can be calculated at the bedside without a calculator (Fig. 59–9), whereas PURSUIT and GRACE use weighted averages of multiple risk factors and may require a computer to calculate. None of the models incorporates information from newer biomarkers such as troponin, BNP, or CRP.

In summary, the short-term outcome of UA/NSTEMI can be predicted by a variety of methods (see Table 59–4).[1] The most important of these are the clinical presentation, ECG findings, elevated troponin levels, and continuing episodes of pain despite medical therapy.

PROGNOSIS

Prognosis in patients with UA or UA/NSTEMI depends on the combination of the morbidity or mortality expected from the extent of coronary stenosis and LV dysfunction and the short-term risk associated with the culprit lesion and the unstable state of ACS. Risk is highest early after the onset of symptoms.

Published reports concerning UA are influenced by patient selection and treatment and can be quite misleading. The inclusion and exclusion criteria for clinical trials introduce bias by often eliminating low- or high-risk patients. Comparisons of incidence and outcome of UA/NSTEMI since the adoption of routine troponin testing are problematic, as the proportion of patients classified as NSTEMI has increased and overall mortality risk of NSTEMI may have fallen as a consequence.[56]

Recent data from the GRACE study show a 6-month mortality rate of 6.2 percent in patients with NSTEMI and 3.6 percent in those with unstable angina. Rehospitalization rates over the 6

Variables

1. Age ≥65 y
2. ≥3 CAD risk factors
   (high cholesterol,
   family history,
   hypertension
   diabetes, smoking)
3. Prior coronary stenosis >50%
4. Aspirin in last 7 days
5. ≥2 anginal events in ≤24 h
6. ST-segment deviation
7. Elevated cardiac markers
   (CK-MB or troponin)

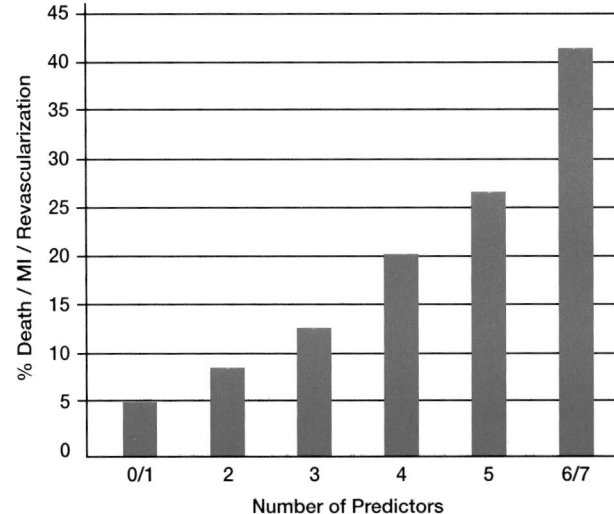

FIGURE 59–9. The TIMI risk score for unstable angina/non–ST-segment elevation myocardial infarction. This simple integer score incorporates variables that can be measured at the bedside and provides both prognostic information as well as a tool to select patients for more or less aggressive treatment algorithms. CAD, coronary artery disease; CK-MB, creatinine kinase myocardial band; MI, myocardial infarction. *Source: Adapted from Antman EM, Cohen M, Bernink PJ, et al.*[52]

month period were approximately 20 percent and revascularization rates approximately 15 percent.[57]

TREATMENT OVERVIEW

The aims of therapy for UA/NSTEMI patients are to control symptoms and prevent further episodes of myocardial ischemia and/or necrosis. β Blockers, nitrates, and, to a lesser extent, calcium channel blockers reduce the risk of recurrent ischemia. Revascularization eliminates ischemia in many patients. The risk of MI is diminished by antiplatelet and antithrombotic drugs. Aggressive statin therapy plays an increasingly important role following ACS.

Hospitalized moderate- to high-risk ACS patients should be treated with aspirin (ASA), clopidogrel, antithrombin therapy, a β blocker, statin, and, in selected individuals, a GPIIb/IIIa inhibitor.[1] Furthermore, critical decisions are required regarding the angiographic strategy. One option, commonly termed the *early invasive strategy*, incorporates an angiographic approach in which coronary angiography and revascularization are performed unless a contraindication exists. Previously, the most common approach included an initial period of medical stabilization. More recently, many physicians are taking an earlier aggressive approach, with coronary angiography and revascularization performed within 24 hours of admission when possible. The rationale for earlier intervention includes the demonstrated protective effects of adjunctive antiplatelet and antithrombin therapy on procedural outcome; recent data demonstrating no advantage for the "cooling off" period before catheterization[58]; and the desire to shorten hospital stays as much as possible. The alternative approach, the *early conservative strategy*, is guided by myocardial ischemia, with angiography reserved for patients with recurrent ischemia at rest or a high-risk noninvasive evaluation for ischemia. This strategy is better described as *selective invasive* as it requires aggressive medical intervention and risk stratification. Regardless of the angiographic strategy, an assessment of LV function should be strongly considered because it is imperative to treat patients who have impaired LV systolic function with both angiotensin-converting enzyme (ACE) inhibitors and β blockers unless contraindicated, and when appropriate, coronary artery bypass graft (CABG) surgery. When the coronary angiogram is performed, a left ventriculogram usually should be obtained at the same time. When coronary angiography is not scheduled, the patient is evaluated at rest and/or with stress for inducible myocardial ischemia or LV systolic dysfunction.

[ ] USE OF ANTIISCHEMIC DRUGS

Also see Chaps. 60 and 64.

Table 59–6 lists the class I recommendations of the ACC/AHA guidelines for antiischemic therapy in the presence or absence of continuing ischemia or high-risk features.[1]

Nitrates

Nitroglycerin (NTG), an endothelium-independent vasodilator, has both peripheral and coronary vascular effects; it reduces myocardial oxygen demand while enhancing myocardial oxygen delivery. By dilating the capacitance vessels, it diminishes myocardial preload, thereby reducing LV wall tension, a determinant of myo-

TABLE 59–6

American College of Cardiology/American Heart Association Class I Recommendations for Antiischemic Therapy in the Presence or Absence of Continuing Ischemia or High-Risk Features[a]

PRESENT	ABSENT
Bedrest with continuous ECG monitoring	
Supplemental O₂ to maintain SaO₂ >90 percent	
NTG IV	
β Blockers, oral or IV	β Blockers, oral
Morphine IV for pain, anxiety, pulmonary congestion	
IABP if ischemia or hemodynamic instability persists	
ACE inhibitor for control of hypertension or LV dysfunction after MI	ACE inhibitor for control of hypertension or LV dysfunction after MI

ACE, angiotensin-converting enzyme; ECG, electrocardiogram; EF, ejection fraction; IABP, intraaortic balloon pump; LV, left ventricular; MI, myocardial infarction; NTG, nitroglycerin.
[a]Recurrent angina and/or ischemia-related ECG changes (greater than or equal to 0.05-mV ST-segment depression or bundle-branch block) at rest or low-level activities; or ischemia associated with CHF symptoms, S₃ gallop, or new or worsening mitral regurgitation; or hemodynamic instability or depressed LV function (EF <0.40 on noninvasive study); or malignant ventricular arrhythmia.

cardial oxygen consumption (MVO_2). NTG promotes the dilation of large coronary arteries as well as collateral vessels and redistributes coronary blood flow to ischemic regions.

Patients whose symptoms are not relieved with three 0.4-mg sublingual NTG tablets or spray taken 5 minutes apart may benefit from intravenous NTG, and such therapy is recommended in the absence of contraindications for patients with ongoing ischemia or heart failure. The use of sildenafil (Viagra) within the previous 24 hours or one of the longer-acting phosphodiesterase-5 inhibitors (tadalafil or vardenafil) within 48 to 72 hours, or the presence of hypotension are important contraindications. Nitrates should not be administered routinely in the absence of ongoing chest pain or heart failure symptoms.

Morphine Sulfate

Morphine sulfate (1 to 5 mg IV) is recommended for patients whose symptoms are not relieved after three serial sublingual NTG tablets or whose symptoms recur despite adequate antiischemic therapy. Unless contraindicated by hypotension or intolerance, morphine may be administered along with intravenous NTG, with careful blood pressure monitoring, and may be repeated every 5 to 30 minutes as needed to relieve symptoms.

β-Adrenergic Blockers

β Blockers competitively block the effects of catecholamines on cell membrane β receptors, reducing heart rate, contractility, and blood pressure. All of these effects reduce MVO_2. In UA/NSTEMI, the primary benefits of β blockers are a result of effects on β_1-adrenergic receptors that decrease cardiac work and myocardial oxygen demand. Slowing of the heart rate has several desirable effects, reducing MVO_2 and also increasing the duration of diastole and diastolic pressure time, a determinant of coronary and collateral flow (see Chap. 61).

β Blockers should be started early in the absence of contraindications. In low-risk patients without active ischemia, oral administration is appropriate. In high-risk patients, as well as in patients with ongoing rest pain, these agents should be initiated *intravenously* and transitioned to an oral regimen.[1] Intravenous administration should be avoided in patients with evidence of heart failure or borderline hemodynamic status.[59]

The choice of β blocker for an individual patient is based primarily on pharmacokinetic and side-effect criteria. Esmolol can be used if an ultrashort-acting agent is required.[1]

The contraindications to β blocker use on an acute basis include significant sinus bradycardia (heart rate <50 beats/min), hypotension (systolic blood pressure <90 mmHg), or evidence of significant heart failure (rales > lung bases). If there are concerns about possible intolerance to β-blockers, initial selection should favor a short-acting β_1-specific drug such as metoprolol. Mild wheezing or a history of chronic obstructive pulmonary disease does not preclude use of a β blocker, but selecting a short-acting cardioselective agent at a reduced dose is prudent.[1]

Support for the beneficial effects of β blockers in patients with UA/NSTEMI is based on limited randomized clinical trials, pathophysiologic considerations, and extrapolation from experience with patients who have other types of ischemic syndromes (see Chap. 60).

Calcium Antagonists

These agents reduce cell transmembrane inward calcium flux, which inhibits both myocardial and vascular smooth muscle contraction; some also slow atrioventricular (AV) conduction and depress sinus node function. Agents in this class vary in the degree to which they produce vasodilation, decrease myocardial contractility, cause AV block, and sinus node slowing (see Chap. 61). Nifedipine and amlodipine have the greatest vasodilatory effect but little or no AV or sinus node effects, whereas verapamil and diltiazem have prominent AV and sinus node effects, as well as some peripheral arterial dilatory effects.[1]

Calcium antagonists may be used to control ongoing or recurring ischemia-related symptoms in patients who are already receiving adequate doses of nitrates and β blockers, in patients who are unable to tolerate adequate doses these agents, and in those patients with variant angina. Several randomized trials assessing the use of rate-limiting calcium antagonists such as diltiazem or verapamil suggest that these agents relieve or prevent symptoms and ischemia but that these agents should be avoided in patients with heart failure or known LV dysfunction, as they have been shown to increase mortality in this setting.[1] Rapid-release short-acting dihydropyridines (e.g., nifedipine) *must be avoided* in ACS because they cause adverse outcomes.

Angiotensin-Converting Enzyme Inhibitors and Angiotensin Receptor Antagonists

ACE inhibitors reduce mortality rates in patients with acute MI or those who recently had an MI and have LV systolic dysfunction.[60]

They are also effective in patients with high-risk chronic CAD, including those with normal LV function.[61] Accordingly, ACE inhibitors should be used in such patients as well as in those with hypertension that is not controlled with β blockers (see Chap. 61). Angiotensin receptor blockers are effective alternatives to ACE inhibitors in patients with LV dysfunction or heart failure following acute MI. However, angiotensin receptor blockers should only be used in place of ACE inhibitors in patients with ACE inhibitor intolerance.

[ ] ANTIPLATELET THERAPY

Antiplatelet and antithrombotic agents are cornerstone therapies to passivate the active disease process and prevent complications, including death and recurrent ischemic events.[1] Currently, a combination of ASA, clopidogrel, antithrombin therapy (unfractionated heparin, low-molecular-weight heparin [LMWH], fondaparinux, or bivalirudin) and in certain instances a platelet GPIIb/IIIa receptor antagonist, represents the most effective therapy. The intensity of treatment is tailored to individual risk.[1]

Aspirin

By irreversibly inhibiting cyclooxygenase-1 within platelets, ASA prevents the formation of thromboxane A_2, thereby diminishing platelet activation and aggregation promoted by this pathway but not by others. Clinical trials in patients with UA/NSTEMI have consistently documented a marked benefit from ASA independent of differences in study design.[62,63]

It appears reasonable to initiate ASA treatment in patients with UA/NSTEMI at a dose of 160 or 325 mg.[1] Patients who present with suspected ACS who are not already receiving ASA may chew the first dose to rapidly establish a high blood level. Subsequent doses may be swallowed. Thereafter, daily doses of 75 to 325 mg are prescribed and continued indefinitely. Because bleeding risk is higher with increasing aspirin dosages, an 81-mg dose is recommended for long-term therapy in most patients.

Adenosine Diphosphate Receptor Antagonists

Ticlopidine and clopidogrel are thienopyridine derivatives that block the binding of ADP to the P_2Y_{12} receptor on the platelet surface, inhibiting ADP-mediated platelet activation and aggregation by approximately 50 to 60 percent. Clopidogrel has replaced ticlopidine for essentially all indications. Early clinical experience with clopidogrel was derived from the Clopidogrel versus Aspirin in Patients at Risk of Ischaemic Events (CAPRIE) trial.[64] A total of 19,185 patients with recent ischemic stroke, MI, or symptomatic peripheral arterial disease were randomized to receive 325 mg/d of ASA or 75 mg/d of clopidogrel, and followed for 1 to 3 years. The *composite outcome* of ischemic stroke, MI, or vascular death was reduced slightly in the clopidogrel arm, from 5.83 to 5.32 percent (relative risk [RR] reduction 8.7 percent; $p = 0.043$). The benefit of clopidogrel was modest, and the drug is expensive. Thus, aspirin has remained the agent of choice when only a single agent is used. Clopidogrel monotherapy is indicated for patients with frank allergy or serious intolerance to aspirin.[1]

Because aspirin and clopidogrel antagonize platelet function via nonredundant pathways, combined use of the two agents represents an attractive antiplatelet strategy. The Clopidogrel in Unstable Angina to Prevent Recurrent Ischemic Events (CURE) trial randomized 12,562 patients with UA/NSTEMI to aspirin alone or to the combination of aspirin and clopidogrel for 3 to 12 months (average 9 months).[65] The *composite end point* of CV death, MI, or stroke occurred in 11.5 percent of patients assigned to placebo versus 9.3 percent assigned to clopidogrel (RR 0.80; *p* <0.001). Importantly, this benefit was similar whether patients were managed with medical therapy or with coronary revascularization (Fig. 59–10).[66] Major bleeding was increased in the clopidogrel arm (3.7 percent vs. 2.7 percent; *p* = 0.003). Bleeding was notably increased in patients who underwent CABG surgery within the first 5 days of stopping clopidogrel.[65]

In the PCI-CURE study, which was a subgroup analysis of CURE consisting of the 2658 patients who underwent PCI after UA/NSTEMI, cardiovascular death or MI was reduced by 31 percent in the clopidogrel-plus-aspirin group versus the aspirin-alone group (*p* = 0.002).[67] In the Clopidogrel for the Reduction of Events During Observation (CREDO) trial,[68] 2116 patients scheduled to undergo PCI were randomized to clopidogrel or to placebo in addition to aspirin. A 27 percent reduction in the *composite outcome* of CV death, MI, or stroke was reported in patients treated with combination clopidogrel and ASA for 1 year (8.5 vs. 11.5 percent; *p* = 0.02).[68] As with CURE, there was an increased risk of major bleeding in the combination-therapy group (8.8 vs. 6.7 percent; *p* = 0.07), but this was almost entirely in the group that underwent CABG. Thus, it may be difficult to modify this bleeding risk without delaying a patient's surgery for at least 5 days after having received a dose of clopidogrel.

It is important to recognize that the PCI-CURE and CREDO trials were performed before newer drug-eluting stents (DESs) were available. DESs inhibit vascular smooth muscle cell proliferation and prevent in-stent restenosis; however, they also delay regrowth of the protective vascular endothelium, which results in a longer time period during which patients are at risk for stent thrombosis.[69] As a result, *the absolute minimum requirement* is for 3 months of clopidogrel following placement of a sirolimus-eluting stent and 6 months following placement of a paclitaxel-eluting stent.[70] Because stent thrombosis has been observed up to and even beyond 1 year following placement of a DES, the most recent

update to the ACC/AHA PCI guidelines recommends 1 year of clopidogrel following DES placement if the patient is not at high risk for bleeding.[70] Patients who, for any reason, are poor candidates for long-term clopidogrel should not receive a DES.

Loading clopidogrel prior to catheterization presents logistical challenges, mostly related to the possibility that the patient will require CABG and thus might be at risk for delayed surgery or excess bleeding. There does appear to be a modest benefit associated with the clopidogrel loading dose administered at least 12 to 24 hours prior to PCI.[71] Clopidogrel often is not started until it is clear that CABG will not be needed within the next several days. If patients are not pretreated with clopidogrel, a loading dose (often 600 mg) can be given on the catheterization table if a PCI is to be carried out immediately.

GPIIb/IIIa Inhibitors

When the platelet is activated, the number of GPIIb/IIIa receptors on the platelet surface increase in number, and demonstrate improved binding affinity for fibrinogen. The binding of fibrinogen to receptors on different platelets results in aggregation. The platelet GPIIb/IIIa receptor antagonists act by occupying the receptors sites, thus opposing fibrinogen and von Willebrand binding. The occupancy of ≥ 80 percent of the receptor sites and inhibition of platelet aggregation to ADP by ≥ 80 percent results in potent antithrombotic effects. The various GPIIb/IIIa antagonists, however, possess significantly different pharmacokinetic and pharmacodynamic properties (see Chap. 61).

The role of GPIIb/IIIa inhibitors in the contemporary treatment of patients with ACS continues to evolve. Two broad strategies characterize current use of these agents in ACS. The first is an "upstream" strategy in which either eptifibatide or tirofiban is administered in the emergency department or hospital for medical stabilization, usually in anticipation of an early invasive approach to PCI. The second strategy defers upstream use of these agents, and uses either eptifibatide or abciximab as adjunctive therapy immediately prior to PCI.

Upstream GPIIb/IIIa Treatment

In the Platelet Receptor Inhibition in Ischemic Syndrome Management in Patients Limited by Unstable Signs and Symptoms

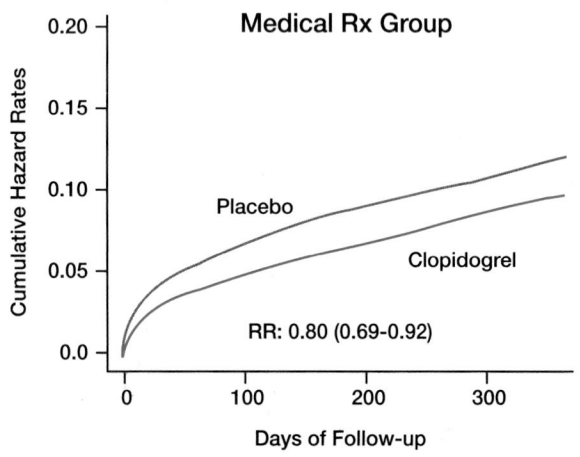
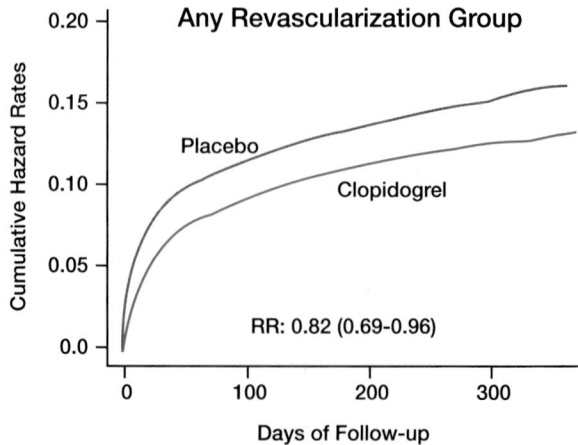

FIGURE 59–10. Comparison of clopidogrel with placebo in the CURE trial, in subgroups defined by revascularization strategy. A similar benefit was observed for clopidogrel whether patients were managed with medical therapy or revascularization (PCI or CABG). *Source: Adapted from Fox K, Mehta SR, Peters R, et al.[66]*

(PRISM-PLUS) trial, the composite outcome of death, MI, or refractory ischemia at the end of a 48-hour infusion period was reduced from 5.6 percent with unfractionated heparin (UFH) and aspirin to 3.8 percent with *tirofiban*, UFH, and aspirin (RR 0.67; $p = 0.01$). Eptifibatide was studied in the PURSUIT trial,[72] which randomized 10,948 patients with UA/NSTEMI to eptifibatide or placebo. The incidence of death or MI at 30 days was reduced from 15.7 percent in the placebo arm to 14.2 percent in the eptifibatide arm ($p = 0.03$).[72] Upstream abciximab was studied in the GUSTO IV-ACS trial,[73] which enrolled 7800 patients with UA/NSTEMI who were not intended to undergo revascularization. No benefit for upstream abciximab was observed. Accordingly, abciximab is not indicated for management of patients with UA/ NSTEMI in whom an early invasive management strategy is *not planned*.[1]

In a meta-analysis of upstream therapy, Boersma et al. reported a very modest reduction in death or MI during 72 hours of medical stabilization, followed by a robust benefit following PCI (Fig. 59–11).[74] In a subsequent meta-analysis, a gradient of benefit was observed based on the approach to revascularization. Among patients undergoing PCI, death and MI were significantly reduced (odds ratio [OR] 0.82; $p = 0.02$) whereas no benefit was observed for patients managed medically (OR 0.95; $p = 0.27$).[75] Finally, a significant 15 percent risk reduction was found among troponin-positive patients but no benefit was seen among troponin-negative patients.[76]

Adjunctive GPIIb/IIIa Use during PCI

Despite support from the ACC/AHA guidelines,[1] upstream GPIIb/IIIa inhibitor use has not increased in the United States for several reasons. First, catheterization and PCI occur earlier than in previous eras. Second, only 40 to 50 percent of patients managed with an early invasive treatment strategy actually undergo PCI during the index hospitalization.[77] It may be more cost-efficient in many patients to defer GPIIb/IIIa until the cardiac catheterization has been performed and PCI is imminent.

The efficacy of GPIIb/IIIa antagonists during PCI has been documented in numerous trials, including UA patients.[1] Abciximab has been studied primarily in PCI trials, and its adjunctive administration prior to PCI consistently showed a significant reduction in the rate of periprocedural MI and the need for urgent revascularization.[1] In the CAPTURE trial among troponin-positive patients, abciximab was associated with a 68 percent relative risk reduction in death or MI, whereas no benefit was observed for troponin-negative patients.[78] More recently, the Intracoronary Stenting and Antithrombotic Regimen: Rapid Early Action for Coronary Treatment (ISAR-REACT)-2 study compared abciximab versus placebo immediately prior to PCI in 2022 patients

with UA/NSTEMI who were treated with aspirin and clopidogrel. Abciximab reduced the primary end point of death or MI by 25 percent ($p = 0.03$). This benefit was restricted to patients with elevated troponin values.[79]

In general, aspirin and UFH or LMWH are administered to all patients with UA/NSTEMI. Clopidogrel is usually given (300- to 600-mg loading dose) prior to or at the time of PCI. In many centers, it is not given until the patient has been ruled out for coronary bypass surgery. The GPIIb/IIIa inhibitors are usually reserved for high-risk patients who are likely to undergo early PCI and may be administered either upstream or at the time of PCI.

【 】 ANTICOAGULANT THERAPY

Anticoagulants available for parenteral use include UFH, various LMWHs, synthetic pentasaccharides, and the direct-acting anti-thrombins hirudin and bivalirudin; for oral use, warfarin remains available (see Chap. 53).[1]

UFH is a heterogenous mixture of polysaccharides of various molecular weights, which accelerate the action of circulating anti-thrombin, a proteolytic enzyme that inactivates factor IIa (thrombin), factor IXa, and factor Xa. UFH prevents thrombus generation but is not active against clot-bound thrombin. LMWHs are relatively more potent inhibitors of factor Xa than of thrombin. Relative to UFH, LMWH has decreased nonspecific binding, a longer half-life, and predictable anticoagulation, permitting once- or twice-daily subcutaneous administration. Use of LMWHs does not usually require laboratory monitoring, except during pregnancy. Direct thrombin inhibitors act by binding directly to the anion binding and catalytic sites of thrombin to produce potent, predictable anticoagulation. Unlike UFH and LMWH, these agents also are active against clot-bound thrombin (see Chap. 53).[80]

Most of the benefits of the various anticoagulants are short-term and not maintained on a long-term basis once therapy is discontinued (see Chap. 53). Continuation of ASA after discontinua-

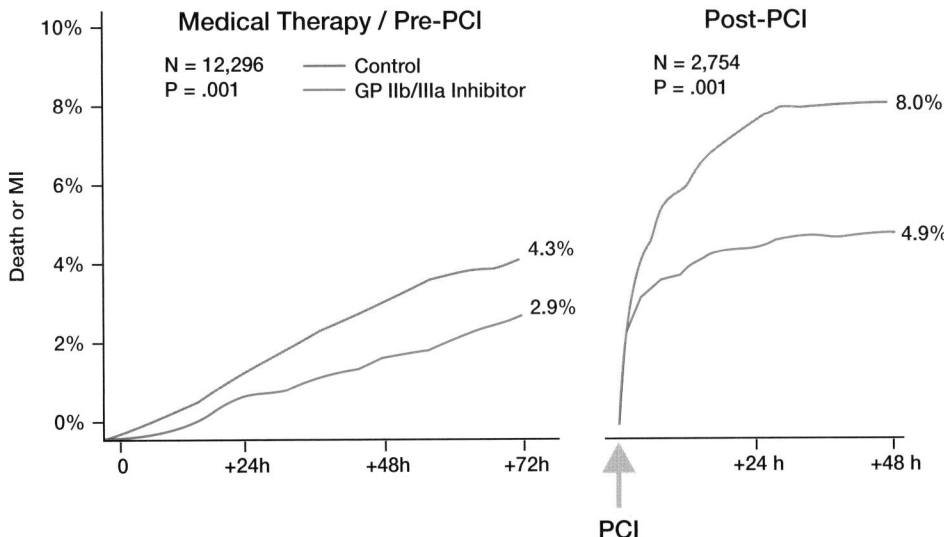

FIGURE 59–11. Glycoprotein (GP) IIb/IIIa inhibitor benefits during medical stabilization and following percutaneous coronary intervention (PCI). In this meta-analysis of patients treated with "upstream" GPIIb/IIIa inhibitors, the benefit of GPIIb/IIIa inhibitor therapy was quantitatively greater post-PCI compared to the period of medical stabilization prior to PCI. MI, myocardial infarction. *Source: Adapted with permission from Boersma E, Akkerhuis KM, Theroux P, et al.*[74]

tion of antithrombin therapy appears to partially mitigate this reactivation process.

Unfractionated Heparin

Several trials have compared UFH with placebo and form the basis of the class I recommendation for use of UFH with ASA for patients with UA/NSTEMI.[1] In a meta-analysis of six trials with end point assessment varying from 2 to 12 weeks, death or MI was reduced by 33 percent in UFH-treated patients ($p = 0.06$).[81]

Pharmacokinetic limitations of UFH translate into poor bioavailability and marked variability in anticoagulant response. UFH requires monitoring with the activated partial thromboplastin time (aPTT; see Chap. 53). A weight-adjusted regimen is recommended, with an initial bolus of 60 to 70 U/kg (maximum: 5000 U) and an initial infusion of 12 to 15 U•kg[1]•h[1] (maximum: 1000 U/h). Guideline committees recommend dosage adjustments of the nomograms to correspond to a therapeutic range equivalent to heparin levels of 0.3 to 0.7 U/mL by antifactor Xa determinations, which correlates with aPTT values between 60 and 80 seconds.[1]

Serial platelet counts are necessary to monitor for heparin-induced thrombocytopenia. Thrombocytopenia from heparin takes two forms: a mild decrease in platelet counts (rarely <100,000/μL) that occurs early (1 to 4 days) after initiation of therapy, reverses quickly after discontinuation of heparin, and is of little clinical consequence. The more severe form of thrombocytopenia is an immune-mediated thrombocytopenia that typically occurs >5 days from therapy, although it may occur earlier in patients who have received heparin within the previous 3 to 4 months. Heparin immune thrombocytopenia is caused by a heparin-dependent, antiplatelet antibody that can activate normal platelets. This syndrome often causes thrombosis that can produce severe morbidity and mortality.

Low-Molecular-Weight Heparin

Several large, randomized trials have directly compared LMWH with UFH (Fig. 59–12; see Chap. 53). Important differences have emerged depending on the approach (early or later) to revascularization employed.

Among the earlier trials, Fragmin in Unstable Coronary Artery Disease (FRIC),[82] which randomized 1482 patients with UA/NSTEMI to dalteparin or to UFH, and Fraxiparine in Ischaemic Syndrome (FRAXIS)[83] which randomized 3468 patients with UA/NSTEMI to nadroparin or to UFH, did not demonstrate benefit of the LMWH over UFH (see Chap. 53). In contrast, the ESSENCE[84] and TIMI 11B[85] trials found benefit from enoxaparin compared with UFH in patients with non–ST-elevation ACS. In ESSENCE, the composite outcome of death, MI, or recurrent angina at 14 days was reduced by 16.2 percent with enoxaparin ($p = 0.02$), and in TIMI 11B, the composite end point of death, MI, or urgent revascularization at 8 days was reduced by 17 percent ($p = 0.048$). Both trials reported a small excess in bleeding in the enoxaparin arms.

More recently, enoxaparin and UFH have been compared among patients treated with contemporary therapies that include GPIIb/IIIa inhibitors and early coronary intervention. In the Integrilin and Enoxaparin Randomized Assessment of Acute Coronary Syndromes

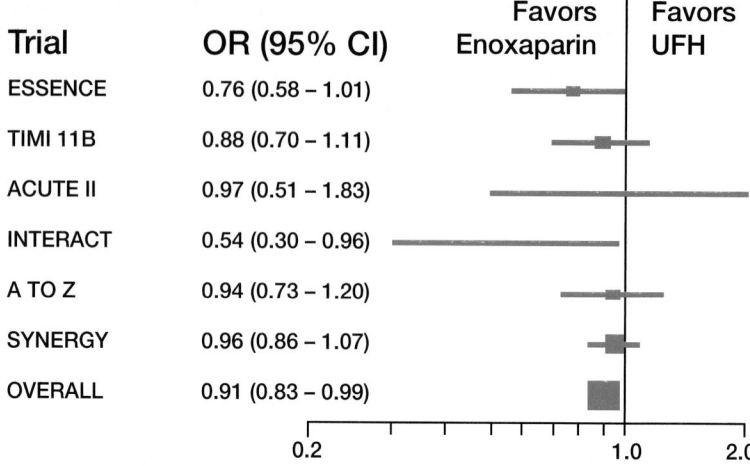

Trial	OR (95% CI)	
ESSENCE	0.76 (0.58 – 1.01)	
TIMI 11B	0.88 (0.70 – 1.11)	
ACUTE II	0.97 (0.51 – 1.83)	
INTERACT	0.54 (0.30 – 0.96)	
A TO Z	0.94 (0.73 – 1.20)	
SYNERGY	0.96 (0.86 – 1.07)	
OVERALL	0.91 (0.83 – 0.99)	

FIGURE 59–12. Comparison of enoxaparin and unfractionated heparin (UFH) in unstable angina/non–ST-segment elevation myocardial infarction. A systematic overview of death/myocardial infarction (MI) at 30 days including 21,946 patients enrolled in 6 trials. Overall, a significant reduction in death/MI was observed (10.1 percent vs. 11.0 percent; OR, 0.91; 95 percent confidence interval [CI], 0.83 to 0.99). *Source: Adapted with permission from Peterson JL, Mahaffey KW, Hasselblad V, et al.[122]*

Treatment (INTERACT) trial, enoxaparin and UFH were compared in patients treated with eptifibatide and aspirin.[86] The group treated with enoxaparin had lower rates of ischemic ECG changes, as well as lower rates of death or MI at 30 days (5 percent vs. 9 percent; $p = 0.03$). Bleeding risk was not increased.

The Aggrastat (A phase) of the A to Z trial was an open label non-inferiority trial comparing enoxaparin with UFH in 3987 patients with UA/NSTEMI who were treated with tirofiban and aspirin.[87] The primary outcome of death, recurrent MI, or refractory ischemia at 7 days occurred in 8.4 percent of patients in the enoxaparin arm versus 9.4 percent in the UFH arm (hazard ratio [HR] 0.88; 95 percent confidence interval [CI] 0.71 to 1.08). This result met the definition for noninferiority. Bleeding trended slightly higher in the enoxaparin arm but was not statistically different. Importantly, among patients managed with an initial conservative strategy, enoxaparin was associated with a statistically significant 28 percent reduction in the primary composite end point.[88]

The Superior Yield of the New Strategy of Enoxaparin, Revascularization, and Glycoprotein IIb/IIIa Inhibitors (SYNERGY) trial was a recent large (n = 10,027) open-label superiority trial comparing enoxaparin with UFH among patients with a planned early invasive treatment strategy.[89] GPIIb/IIIa inhibitors were used in >50 percent of patients. The primary end point of death or nonfatal MI occurred in 14.0 percent of patients randomized to enoxaparin versus in 14.5 percent of patients randomized to UFH (HR 0.96; 95 percent CI 0.86 to 1.06). Rates of thrombolysis in myocardial infarction major bleeding events defined by the TIMI criteria were increased among patients receiving enoxaparin (9.1 percent vs. 7.6 percent). "Pretreatment" with antithrombin drugs prior to randomization may have diluted the ability to detect true differences between the two treatment arms in this trial. Alternatively, early PCI and enoxaparin "compete" to prevent recurrent ischemic events caused by the culprit lesion. In trials where conservative approaches to catheterization and PCI were used, such as ESSENCE, TIMI 11B, INTERACT, and the early conservative subgroup of A to Z, enoxaparin demonstrated significant advantages over UFH. In contrast, among invasively managed patients in the A to Z and SYNERGY trials, results were very similar between enoxaparin and UFH.

Practical Issues Regarding LMWHs

Because the level of anticoagulant activity cannot easily be measured in patients who are receiving LMWH, interventional cardiologists have expressed concern about the substitution of LMWH for UFH in patients who are scheduled for catheterization with possible PCI. One common approach is to use LMWH during the period of initial stabilization, but to hold the dose on the morning of the procedure.[1] If an intervention is required and more than 12 hours has elapsed since the last dose of LMWH, UFH can be used for PCI according to usual practice patterns. If 8–12 hours have elapsed since the last dose of enoxaparin, either 3000 U of UFH or 0.3 mg/kg of enoxaparin can be given during PCI. An alternative approach is to continue enoxaparin through the procedure. This strategy does not appear to cause excess procedural thrombotic complications but is associated with a modest increase in vascular access site bleeding.[89] Because the anticoagulant effect of UFH can be more readily reversed, it is preferred in patients who are likely to undergo CABG within 24 hours.

It is important to recognize that LMWH agents are cleared predominantly via renal mechanisms, and that dose adjustment is needed with severe (glomerular filtration rate <30 mL/min) and possibly also with moderate renal insufficiency. Additionally, few data are available in the morbidly obese and it is not known whether dosing should be based on actual or lean body mass. We recommend using LMWH with caution in patients with significant renal insufficiency and in patients with morbid obesity. In such patients, UFH, which can be titrated to an easily measured aPTT goal, represents an excellent alternative. Alternatively, when LMWH is used in high-risk groups (e.g., pregnancy), factor Xa levels can be measured.

Fondaparinux

Fondaparinux is a synthetic pentasaccharide that can bind antithrombin and inactivate factor Xa. It has no effect on thrombin and thus is a pure factor Xa inhibitor. It offers predictable pharmacokinetics and a half-life of 15 hours, allowing once-daily subcutaneous dosing without a need for routine laboratory monitoring. In the Organization for the Assessment of Strategies for Ischemic Syndromes (OASIS)-5 trial,[90] which enrolled >20,000 patients with UA/NSTEMI, fondaparinux 2.5 mg/d and enoxaparin 1 mg/kg bid yielded similar rates of the primary end point of death, MI, or refractory ischemia at 9 days (5.8 percent vs. 5.7 percent). Major bleeding events were significantly reduced by 48 percent with fondaparinux. Mortality trended lower in the fondaparinux group at 30 days (2.9 percent vs. 3.5 percent; $p = 0.02$) and at 180 days (5.8 percent vs. 6.5 percent; $p = 0.05$); all but 3 of the 64 excess deaths with enoxaparin were associated with major or minor bleeding.[90]

However, several caveats to the OASIS trial merit mention. First, patients were allowed entry with a creatinine up to 3.0 mg/dL. Major bleeding risk was particularly high among those patients treated with weight-adjusted enoxaparin who had a creatinine clearance <30 mL/min (9.9 percent rate of major bleeding). Second, UFH was administered after randomization in a larger proportion of enoxaparin-treated patients, a practice that is thought to increase bleeding risks.[89] Finally, the long half-life of fondaparinux may create logistical problems in centers that perform early cardiac catheterization.

Direct Thrombin Inhibitors

Hirudin is the prototype of the direct thrombin inhibitors. This agent has been extensively studied in patients with ACS where it has shown only small reductions in MI at a cost of excess bleeding.[80] Recombinant hirudin (lepirudin) is presently only indicated in patients with heparin-induced thrombocytopenia.

Bivalirudin (Hirulog) is a semisynthetic direct-acting antithrombin that differs from hirudin by having a shorter half-life, only providing transient reversible inhibition of the active site of thrombin, and undergoing only modest renal clearance. In the Randomized Evaluation in PCI Linking Angiomax to Reduced Clinical Events (REPLACE) II trial,[91] bivalirudin alone was "noninferior" to the combination of UFH plus GPIIb/IIIa inhibitor with regard to death, MI, or urgent revascularization at 30 days (OR 1.09; 95 percent CI 0.90 to 1.32). Major bleeding was significantly lower in the bivalirudin arm (2.4 percent vs. 4.1 percent; p<0.001). The Acute Catheterization and Urgent Intervention Triage Strategy (ACUITY) trial was a complex trial performed in 13,819 patients with UA/NSTEMI, all of whom underwent cardiac catheterization within 72 hours. Patients were randomized to one of three arms: UFH or enoxaparin plus routine GPIIb/IIIa inhibition; bivalirudin plus routine GPIIb/IIIa inhibition; or bivalirudin alone (with provisional GPIIb/IIIa use only). Preliminary results from this trial largely support the findings from REPLACE II, demonstrating lower bleeding rates without a significant increase in ischemic complications in patients treated with bivalirudin alone compared with UFH (or enoxaparin) plus a GPIIb/IIIa inhibitor.[92] Importantly, however, in the GPIIb/IIIa arms, no safety or efficacy benefits of bivalirudin were noted over UFH or enoxaparin. While this study confirms bivalirudin as a safe and lower-cost alternative to UFH plus GPIIb/IIIa inhibitors during PCI, the role of this agent outside the cardiac catheterization laboratory requires further study. In patients receiving GPIIb/IIIa inhibitors, bivalirudin offers no benefit over UFH.

Long-Term Anticoagulation

Several studies have evaluated the combination of warfarin and aspirin after ACS. In initial trials, low-fixed-dose warfarin was not superior to aspirin monotherapy, and the combination was associated with excess bleeding risk. More recently, several studies have shown that the combination of aspirin and warfarin may be effective in preventing ischemic events post-ACS when the international normalized ratio (INR) is maintained at a higher level consistently and carefully monitored.[93,94] However, these findings are of questionable significance in light of the results of the CURE trial, which demonstrated similar benefit with a simpler (and safer) regimen of aspirin and clopidogrel.[65] Warfarin should be prescribed for UA/NSTEMI patients who also have other well-proven indications for warfarin, such as atrial fibrillation and mechanical prosthetic heart valves. In such patients, combination with low-dose aspirin is reasonable if the bleeding risk is not markedly increased.

❙❘ THROMBOLYSIS

Thrombolytic agents in UA/NSTEMI have had no significant beneficial effect and actually increased the risk of MI in TIMI IIIB.[95]

EARLY CONSERVATIVE VERSUS INVASIVE STRATEGIES

Two broad strategies may be employed with regard to the early use of coronary angiography and revascularization following non–ST-elevation ACS. In the *early invasive* strategy, patients are referred for coronary angiography, typically within 48 hours of presentation, with coronary revascularization (either PCI or CABG) performed based on anatomic findings identified during angiography. In the *early conservative* strategy, which is more appropriately termed a *selective invasive* strategy, angiography is deferred, and reserved for patients with spontaneous recurrent ischemia or significant ischemia detected on a predischarge noninvasive evaluation. Both strategies should incorporate aggressive antiplatelet and antithrombotic strategies as described above. Proponents of the early invasive strategy argue that it allows earlier and more definitive risk stratification. It identifies the 10 to 15 percent of patients with no significant coronary stenoses and the approximately 20 percent of patients with three-vessel or left main CAD. Proponents of the early conservative strategy argue that the high- and low-risk patients also can be identified with appropriate noninvasive imaging.

Several large, randomized, controlled trials performed over the past decade have compared routine early invasive with selective invasive strategies in patients with non–ST-elevation ACS, with conflicting results (Fig. 59–13).[77,95–99] Comparisons are difficult because the studies included heterogeneous patient populations and the comparisons cannot account for the rapid advances in PCI technology and medical therapies over time.

Trials performed prior to coronary stenting, including TIMI 3B and VANQUISH, failed to demonstrate an advantage for the routine early invasive approach compared to the selective invasive approach.[95,96] Subsequently, the FRISC II study compared a routine invasive strategy in which catheterization was performed after an average of 6 days of aggressive medical therapy with a conservative strategy in which catheterization was only performed for markedly

positive findings on a predischarge stress test (0.3-mV ST depression).[97] In this study, the primary composite outcome of death or MI at 6 months was reduced by 22 percent in the invasive therapy group ($p = 0.03$),[97] and by 1 year mortality was significantly lower in the invasive arm.[100] Importantly, this is the only study to report a mortality advantage in favor of the routine invasive approach. Benefit from the invasive strategy was greatest in higher-risk patients, defined based on ST depression at entry, elevated troponin values, and age >65 years. Benefit from the invasive strategy was particularly marked among those patients with both elevated cTnT and ST depression.[101]

In the TACTICS-TIMI 18 trial, 2220 patients with UA or NSTEMI were treated with ASA, UFH, and tirofiban, and randomized to early invasive or early conservative strategies.[77] Death, MI, or rehospitalization for ACS at 6 months occurred in 15.9 percent of patients assigned to the invasive strategy versus in 19.4 percent of patients assigned to the conservative strategy ($p = 0.025$). The benefit of the early invasive approach was confined to patients at intermediate or high risk, as defined using troponin elevation or the TIMI Risk Score (Fig. 59–14).[77]

The Randomized Intervention Trial of Unstable Angina (RITA)-3 trial demonstrated a significant reduction in the primary composite outcome of death, MI, or refractory ischemia at 4 months in favor of an early invasive strategy (RR 0.66; $p = 0.001$) but no significant difference in the coprimary end point of death or MI at 1 year (RR 0.91; $p = 0.58$).[98] Five-year outcomes from this trial were recently reported.[102] Death or MI was reduced from 20 percent in the invasive arm to 16.6 percent in the conservative arm (OR 0.78, $p = 0.04$), with similar proportional reductions in death and MI individually. Benefits from the invasive approach were mainly seen in higher-risk patients.[102]

The most recent trial, Invasive versus Conservative Treatment in Unstable Coronary Syndromes (ICUTUS), challenges the positive findings of FRISC-II, TACTICS-TIMI 18, and RITA-3. In this trial, performed in 1200 patients with NSTEMI (cTnT >0.03 µg/L), the primary outcome of death, MI, or rehospitalization for angina at 1 year occurred in 22.7 percent of patients in the early invasive group versus 21.2 percent in the selective invasive group (RR 1.07; $p = 0.33$). Mortality rates were identical between the two groups, but MI occurred significantly more often in the invasive arm (15 percent vs. 10 percent; $p = 0.005$).[99] Importantly, a conservative MI definition was used in which any elevation in CK-MB above the upper limit of normal was classified as an MI. This differs considerably from procedural MI definitions used in most other trials.

Integrating the results of these trials presents a clearer but inconsistent picture. First, mortality rates appear to be similar between routine and selective invasive strategies, when a low threshold for crossover to angiography is used in patients who fail conservative management. On the other hand, nonfatal recurrent ischemic events are significantly reduced by an early invasive strategy, particularly among patients at high risk, including those with elevated troponin levels, new ST-segment depression, or clinical or hemodynamic instability. Moreover, this strategy appears to be cost-effective.[103] Thus, in high-risk patients, a routine invasive strategy is generally preferred if there are no contraindications to coronary angiography and if the patient is a good candidate for prolonged clopidogrel ther-

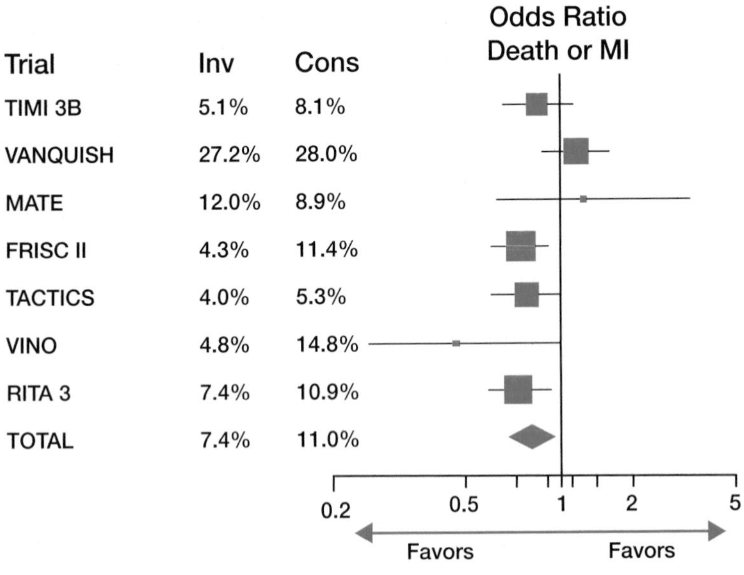

Trial	Inv	Cons	Odds Ratio Death or MI
TIMI 3B	5.1%	8.1%	
VANQUISH	27.2%	28.0%	
MATE	12.0%	8.9%	
FRISC II	4.3%	11.4%	
TACTICS	4.0%	5.3%	
VINO	4.8%	14.8%	
RITA 3	7.4%	10.9%	
TOTAL	7.4%	11.0%	

FIGURE 59–13. Meta-analysis comparing invasive (INV) and conservative (Cons) approaches to revascularization in unstable angina/non–ST-segment elevation myocardial infarction (MI). *Source: Adapted with permission from Mehta S, Cannon CP, Fox KA, et al.*[123]

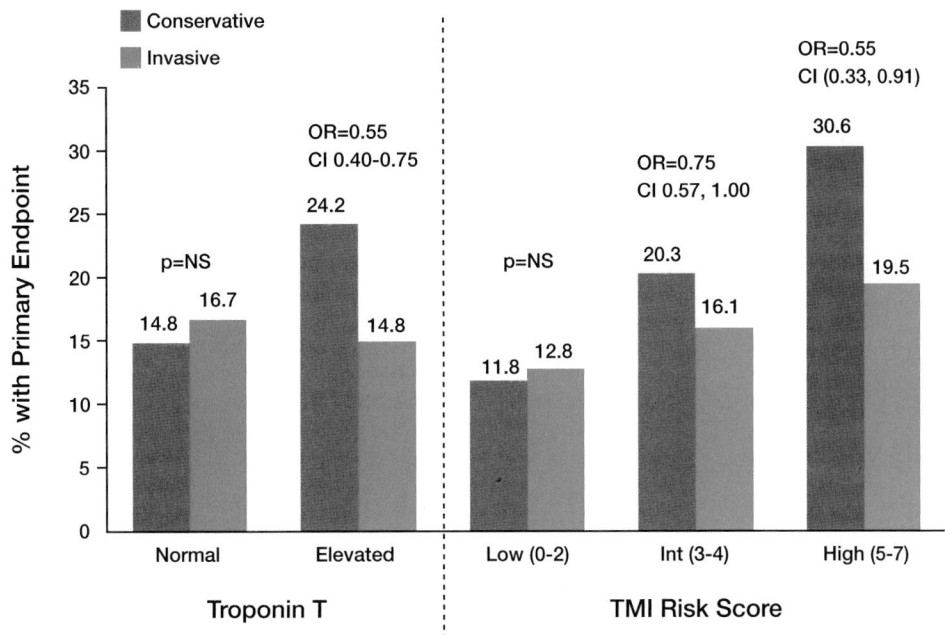

FIGURE 59–14. Comparison of routine invasive and selective invasive (conservative) strategies according to risk stratification results. In the TACTICS-TIMI 18 study, among patients with elevated troponin T levels, or intermediate or high TIMI risk scores, the routine invasive strategy significantly reduced the primary end point of death, MI, or rehospitalization for acute coronary syndrome at 6 months. In contrast, among low-risk patients with normal troponin values or low TIMI risk scores, no advantage was present for the invasive strategy. *Source: Adapted from Cannon CP, Weintraub WS, Demopoulos LA, et al.[77]*

apy.[1] Among intermediate-risk patients, the benefits of an invasive approach are attenuated but still present, whereas among low risk patients, no benefit exists for the routine invasive approach (see Fig. 59–14). Thus careful integration of risk-stratification data with patient preference is needed to achieve appropriate use of coronary revascularization.[104] Table 59–7 presents the ACC/AHA guidelines for selecting between conservative versus invasive approaches in ACS.

【 】 NONINVASIVE TEST SELECTION

A detailed discussion of noninvasive stress testing in CAD is presented in the ACC/AHA *Guidelines for Exercise Testing*, ACC/AHA *Guidelines for the Clinical Use of Cardiac Radionuclide Imaging*, and ACC/AHA *Guidelines for the Clinical Application of Echocardiography*. Coronary angiography is usually indicated in patients with UA/NSTEMI who either have recurrent symptoms of ischemia despite adequate medical therapy or who are at high risk as categorized by clinical signs (congestive heart failure, malignant ventricular arrhythmias) or noninvasive test findings (significant LV dysfunction: ejection fraction less than 0.35, large anterior or multiple perfusion defects) (see Table 59–5).

CORONARY REVASCULARIZATION

Coronary revascularization (PCI or CABG) is done to improve prognosis, relieve symptoms, prevent ischemic complications, and improve functional capacity. The decision to proceed from diagnostic angiography to revascularization is influenced not only by the coronary anatomy but also by a number of additional factors, including anticipated life expectancy, LV function, comorbidity, functional capacity, severity

of symptoms, and quantity of viable myocardium at risk. Careful clinical judgement is required when deciding which lesions identified at coronary angiography merit revascularization.

Data from both retrospective observations and randomized clinical trials indicate that PCI can lead to angiographic success in most patients with UA/NSTEMI. Procedural safety in these patients is enhanced by the addition of GPIIb/IIIa receptor inhibitors to the standard regimen of ASA, clopidogrel, antithrombin agents, and antiischemic medications. Patients with multivessel CAD can now often undergo complete revascularization with use of multidrug-eluting stents. Indeed, the rapid advances in PCI technology *appear* to have outpaced clinical trial data. As a result, few adequate data are available to guide selection between PCI and CABG in patients with ACS and multivessel CAD. An exception may be in patients with diabetes, in whom CABG is preferred for most patients with diffuse multivessel disease.[1]

TABLE 59–7

American College of Cardiology/American Heart Association Class I Recommendations for Early Conservative versus Invasive Strategies

An early invasive strategy in patients with unstable angina/non–ST-segment elevation myocardial infarction and any of the following high-risk indicators:

Recurrent angina/ischemia at rest or with low-level activities despite intensive antiischemic therapy

Elevated TnT or TnI

New or presumably new ST-segment depression

Recurrent angina/ischemia with CHF symptoms, an S_3 gallop, pulmonary edema, worsening rales, or new or worsening MR

High-risk findings on noninvasive stress testing

Depressed LV systolic function (e.g., EF <0.40 on noninvasive study)

Hemodynamic instability

Sustained ventricular tachycardia

PCI within 6 months

Prior CABG

In the absence of these findings, either an early conservative or an early invasive strategy in hospitalized patients without contraindications for revascularization.

CABG, coronary artery bypass graft; CHF, congestive heart failure; EF, ejection fraction; LV, left ventricular; MR, mitral regurgitation; PCI, percutaneous coronary intervention; TnI, troponin I; TnT, troponin T.

In general, the indications for CABG in UA/NSTEMI are similar to those for stable angina.[1] High-risk patients with LV dysfunction, patients with diabetes mellitus and multivessel CAD, and those with two-vessel disease with severe proximal involvement of the left anterior descending artery or severe three-vessel or left main disease should be considered for CABG. However, some of these patients may be candidates for multivessel PCI.[105] Thus, selection between PCI and CABG in patients with multivessel CAD without diabetes is based on patient preference, lesion morphology, and the likelihood of a complete revascularization result with PCI.[105]

POSTHOSPITAL DISCHARGE AND CARE

The risk of progression to MI or the development of recurrent MI or death is highest during the first few months after the index ACS event. At 1 to 3 months after the acute phase, most patients resume a clinical course similar to that in patients with chronic stable CAD (see Chap. 64).

The broad goals during the hospital discharge phase are twofold: (1) to prepare the patient for normal activities to the extent possible and (2) to use the acute event as an opportunity to reevaluate long-term care, particularly lifestyle and risk-factor modification. *Aggressive risk-factor modification* is the mainstay of the long-term management of stable CAD (see Chap. 64). Patients who have undergone successful PCI with an uncomplicated course are usually discharged the next day, and patients who undergo uncomplicated CABG are generally discharged 4 to 7 days after CABG. Medical management of low-risk patients after noninvasive stress testing and coronary arteriography can typically be accomplished rapidly with discharge on the day of testing or the day after. Medical management of high-risk patients who are unsuitable for or unwilling to undergo revascularization may require prolonged hospitalization.

The goals for continued medical therapy after discharge relate to potential prognostic benefits (primarily shown for ASA, clopidogrel, β blockers, statins, and ACE inhibitors, especially for left ventricular ejection fraction less than 0.40), control of ischemic symptoms (nitrates, β blockers, and calcium antagonists), and treatment of major risk factors such as hypertension, smoking, hyperlipidemia, and diabetes mellitus (see Chap. 90). Thus, the selection of a medical regimen is individualized to the specific needs of each patient based on the in-hospital findings and events, the risk factors for CAD, drug tolerability, or the type of recent procedure.

[ ] TIMING AND INTENSITY OF LIPID LOWERING

A recent series of large randomized controlled trials has evaluated the role of statin therapy in patients with ACS. In the Myocardial Ischemia Reduction with Aggressive Cholesterol Lowering (MIRACL) study, 3086 patients were randomized to treatment with atorvastatin 80 mg/d or placebo 24 to 96 hours after an ACS.[106] After 16 weeks, the primary end point of death, MI, resuscitated cardiac arrest, or recurrent myocardial ischemia was reduced from 17.4 percent in the placebo group to 14.8 percent in the atorvastatin group (p = 0.048).

The Zocor (Z) phase of the A to Z trial compared an early intensive statin regimen (40 mg followed by 80 mg simvastatin) with a

delayed and less-intensive regimen (placebo for 4 months followed by 20 mg simvastatin) for up to 24 months in 4497 patients with ACS.[107] The primary end point of cardiovascular death, MI, readmission for ACS, or stroke occurred in 14.4 percent of patients in the early intensive statin arm versus in 16.7 percent of patients in the delayed, less-intensive arm (HR 0.89; 95 percent CI 0.76 to 1.04). CV death was reduced by 25 percent in the early intensive statin arm (p = 0.05). During the first 4 months, no difference was evident between treatment groups, but from 4 to 24 months the primary end point was reduced in the intensive statin group. The findings are generally consistent with a "lower is better" approach to LDL cholesterol management after ACS.

In the Pravastatin or Atorvastatin Evaluation and Infection Therapy (PROVE IT)-TIMI 22 trial an intensive statin regimen of atorvastatin 80 mg was compared with a standard statin regimen of pravastatin 40 mg/d among 4162 patients with ACS. The atorvastatin arm achieved an average LDL cholesterol of 62 mg/dL versus an average of 95 mg/dL in the pravastatin arm. The primary end point of death, MI, unstable angina, or revascularization after 30 days was reduced by 16 percent in the atorvastatin arm (p <0.0001). The National Cholesterol Education Panel now endorses an optional LDL target of 70 mg/dL in patients following ACS.[108]

VARIANT (PRINZMETAL) ANGINA

In 1959, Prinzmetal described a syndrome characterized by angina at rest with transient marked ST-segment elevation.[109] Exercise tolerance usually was well preserved, and the attacks were cyclic in nature, often occurring in the early morning hours (see Chap. 64). The episodes lasted no longer than ordinary anginal episodes, and the ST-segment elevation disappeared rapidly as the chest pain receded. Ventricular arrhythmias and AV block sometimes occurred at the peak of an attack, and both MI and sudden death were common consequences (see Chap. 49).

With the use of coronary angiography, it soon became evident that the syndrome was caused by coronary spasm, usually focal and often at the site of a coronary artery stenosis. The underlying coronary lesion varies from subtotal occlusion to a very mild stenosis; in some cases the coronary arteries are angiographically normal. Coronary spasm occurs in more than one artery in some patients, and the site of spasm can fluctuate from one coronary artery to another.

[ ] PATHOPHYSIOLOGY

Many etiologic explanations for variant angina have been proposed and rejected. Current thought focuses on abnormalities in nitric oxide activity at sites of coronary spasm.[110] A mutation of the endothelial nitric oxide synthetase (eNOS) gene is reportedly more common in patients with coronary spasm than in controls.[111]

Coronary spasm usually is localized to the site of an atherosclerotic lesion. Even variant angina patients with no angiographic evidence of luminal narrowing invariably will have atherosclerosis demonstrable by intracoronary vascular ultrasound (IVUS) at the site of focal spasm. Asian patients with variant angina more commonly have generalized coronary artery inflammation and hyperactivity, whereas in white patients, the abnormality is more focal.

Severe spasm rapidly induces transmural ischemia, resulting in segmental myocardial dyskinesis and ST-segment elevation. If the ischemic zone is large, cardiac output and systemic arterial pressure decrease. The risks of serious ventricular arrhythmias and conduction abnormalities (including compete heart block) increase in proportion to the severity and extent of ischemia. Prolonged spasm can lead to MI, which is sometimes associated with coronary thrombus.

CLINICAL FEATURES

Variant angina is uncommon, and the presenting symptoms are usually not distinguishable from UA. Angina at rest occurs with a cyclic pattern, and episodes are more common in the early morning hours. Exertional angina coexists in more than half of these patients, but with a greater variability in ischemic threshold. Variant angina can occur during the recovery phase of MI or in the early hours after coronary bypass surgery or PCI.

Variant angina is more common in heavy cigarette smokers, but their age, sex, and risk-factor profiles are otherwise similar to those of other coronary patients.[112] Of patients with variant angina, 25 percent have a history of migraine headaches, and approximately 25 percent have symptoms of Raynaud's phenomenon. Thus in some cases, variant angina may be part of a more generalized vasospastic diathesis. Syncope, likely caused by ischemia-induced ventricular arrhythmia or AV block, during rest angina is a clue to the diagnosis. Rare cases of life-threatening ventricular arrhythmias caused by silent myocardial ischemia during coronary spasm have been reported.

Cocaine causes coronary vasoconstriction and can precipitate coronary spasm, sometimes with myocardial infarction. This topic is discussed in Chaps. 52, 60, and 61.

Physical examination of variant angina patients between attacks usually reveals no abnormalities. Routine laboratory tests, including cardiac enzymes, are normal.

DIAGNOSTIC PROCEDURES

Variant angina can be diagnosed most easily by an ECG recording during an episode of rest angina. The ST-segment elevation that occurs during an attack disappears promptly after the administration of nitroglycerin. Coronary spasm can induce ST elevation, ST depression, or pseudonormalization of abnormally negative T waves. When variant angina is a consideration, ambulatory ECG monitoring or an event monitor sometimes can be useful to confirm the diagnosis. Exercise testing will provoke angina with ST-segment elevation in approximately one-third of patients with variant angina during an active phase of the disease. Provocative testing has been used to confirm the diagnosis of variant angina when a spontaneous attack cannot be documented. The cold pressor response, exercise, and hyperventilation are physiologic stimuli for coronary spasm, but each is too insensitive to be reliable clinically. Ergonovine and acetylcholine provoke coronary spasm with a sensitivity of approximately 90 percent in patients with variant angina. Intracoronary acetylcholine is probably the preferred method, but a temporary pacemaker should be placed before right coronary (or dominant left coronary) injections are done because of the high incidence of bradyarrhythmias and conduction disturbances. All attempts to induce coronary spasm should be performed in the catheterization laboratory.

All patients with variant angina should undergo coronary angiography unless an absolute contraindication is present. Coronary angiography is the only certain method to distinguish between patients who have severe organic multivessel disease and those who have only mild luminal narrowings or angiographically normal arteries. An IVUS study (see Chap. 18) may reveal more disease than is indicated by angiography.

TREATMENT

Variant angina is often difficult to treat because attacks are unpredictable and often occur without an obvious precipitating factor. The aim of therapy is the elimination of all attacks. Spontaneous remission is a common outcome, but MI is a frequent consequence within the first 3 months after diagnosis, particularly in those patients with underlying multivessel disease. Nitroglycerin relieves variant angina attacks within minutes and should be used promptly. Long-acting nitrates initially are effective in preventing variant angina attacks, but the development of nitrate tolerance may limit their usefulness. A 12-hour nitrate-free period should be provided every day.

Calcium channel blockers are very effective in preventing attacks of variant angina. More than 50 percent of patients treated with one of these drugs become completely asymptomatic, but higher doses are frequently required. For example, long-acting nifedipine 80 mg/d, diltiazem 360 mg/d, verapamil 480 mg/d, or amlodipine 20 mg/d are commonly used doses. The efficacy of these drugs in preventing variant angina is about equal. Patients with an incomplete response to one drug often become angina-free on a combination of nifedipine (or amlodipine) and either diltiazem or verapamil. Treatment with calcium channel blockers likely reduces the risk of MI.[113,114]

Approximately 20 percent of variant angina patients will not respond to treatment with two calcium channel blockers plus a long-acting nitrate. Although not approved by the U.S. Food and Drug Administration for this indication, amiodarone,[115] guanethidine,[116] and clonidine[117] are reportedly effective in some of these refractory patients. Patients with variant angina should also be treated with low-dose aspirin to reduce the risk of MI, even though very high doses of aspirin have been reported to aggravate coronary spasm.[118]

CABG surgery should be considered in patients with multivessel CAD, even though operative mortality and perioperative MI rates are higher than in comparable patients without variant angina.[119,120] Nevertheless, surgery almost invariably eliminates variant angina, and the long-term outcome is excellent. Bypass surgery will be successful when the anastomosis can be placed distal to the site of focal spasm but not when diffuse spasm involves the entire artery. Bypass surgery is *not* indicated when there are no significant stenoses present.

Many patients with variant angina have coronary lesions that are ideal for PCI. When such patients are pretreated with calcium channel blockers and are given intracoronary nitroglycerin during the procedure, the primary success rate is high. With angioplasty alone, restenosis occurs more often than usual. Coronary stenting appears to be more effective, abolishing spasm at the stented site in most patients. However, spasm may recur in other arterial segments.[121] PCI, like CABG, is not indicated for patients with coronary spasm who have normal or nearly normal arteries on coronary angiography.

[ ] PROGNOSIS

The long-term prognosis of variant angina is typically favorable. The extent and severity of the underlying coronary disease appear to be the most important factors influencing the outcome. One-year survival without infarction in a consecutive series of 217 patients was 93 percent for those without significant CAD, 86 percent for patients with single-vessel disease, and 65 percent for patients with multivessel disease. At 5 years, the corresponding figures were 83 percent, 74 percent, and 44 percent, respectively. Other factors correlating with a poor outcome include the presence of LV dysfunction, ventricular arrhythmias during attacks, multivessel spasm, and the absence of treatment with calcium channel blockers. Fortunately, the majority of patients will become angina-free within months or years. Variant angina will occasionally recur after a long asymptomatic interval. More commonly, patients will develop further manifestations of coronary atherothrombosis.

REFERENCES

1. Braunwald E, Antman EM, Beasley JW, et al. ACC/AHA 2002 guideline update for the management of patients with unstable angina and non–ST-segment elevation myocardial infarction—summary article: a report of the American College of Cardiology/American Heart Association task force on practice guidelines (Committee on the Management of Patients with Unstable Angina). *J Am Coll Cardiol* 2002;40:1366–1374.
2. National Center of Health Statistics. *Detailed Diagnoses and Procedures: National Hospital Discharge Survey 1996*. Hyattsville, MD: National Center for Health Statistics, 1998.
3. Gibler WB, Cannon CP, Blomkains AL, et al. Practical implementation of the Guidelines for Unstable Angina/Non–ST-Segment Elevation Myocardial Infarction in the emergency department. An AHA scientific statement. *Circulation* 2005;111:2699–2710.
4. Fuster V, Moreno PR, Fayad ZA, Corti R, Badimon JJ. Atherothrombosis and high-risk plaque: part I. evolving concepts. *J Am Coll Cardiol* 2005;46:937–954.
5. Canto JG, Shlipak MG, Rogers WJ, et al. Prevalence, clinical characteristics, and mortality among patients with myocardial infarction presenting without chest pain. *JAMA* 2000;283:3223–3229.
6. Libby P. Molecular bases of the acute coronary syndromes. *Circulation* 1995;91:2844–2850.
7. Kolodgie FD, Virmani R, Burke AP, et al. Pathologic assessment of the vulnerable human coronary plaque. *Heart* 2004;90:1385–1391.
8. Virmani R, Burke AP, Farb A, Kolodgie FD. Pathology of the unstable plaque. *Prog Cardiovasc Dis* 2002;44:349–356.
9. Libby P, Ridker PM, Maseri A. Inflammation and atherosclerosis. *Circulation* 2002;105:1135–1143.
10. Buffon A, Biasucci LM, Liuzzo G, D'Onofrio G, Crea F, Maseri A. Widespread coronary inflammation in unstable angina. *N Engl J Med* 2002;347:5–12.
11. Goldstein JA, Demetriou D, Grines CL, Pica M, Shoukfeh M, O'Neill WW. Multiple complex coronary plaques in patients with acute myocardial infarction. *N Engl J Med* 2000;343:915–922.
12. Mayr M, Metzler B, Kiechl S, et al. Endothelial cytotoxicity mediated by serum antibodies to heat shock proteins of *Escherichia coli* and *Chlamydia pneumoniae*: immune reactions to heat shock proteins as a possible link between infection and atherosclerosis. *Circulation* 1999;99:1560–1566.
13. Andraws R, Berger JS, Brown DL. Effects of antibiotic therapy on outcomes of patients with coronary artery disease: a meta-analysis of randomized controlled trials. *JAMA* 2005;293:2641–2647.
14. Grayston JT, Kronmal RA, Jackson LA, et al. Azithromycin for the secondary prevention of coronary events. *N Engl J Med* 2005;352:1637–1645.
15. Ruggeri ZM. Platelets in atherothrombosis. *Nat Med* 2002;8:1227–1234.
16. Libby P, Simon DI. Inflammation and thrombosis: the clot thickens. *Circulation* 2001;103:1718–1720.
17. Michelson AD, Barnard MR, Krueger LA, Valeri CR, Furman MI. Circulating monocyte-platelet aggregates are a more sensitive marker of in vivo platelet activation than platelet surface P-selectin: studies in baboons, human coronary intervention, and human acute myocardial infarction. *Circulation* 2001;104:1533–1537.
18. Wong GC, Morrow DA, Murphy S, et al. Elevations in troponin T and I are associated with abnormal tissue level perfusion: a TACTICS-TIMI 18 substudy. Treat Angina with Aggrastat and Determine Cost of Therapy with an Invasive or Conservative Strategy-Thrombolysis in Myocardial Infarction. *Circulation* 2002;106:202–207.
19. Ambrose JA, Winters SL, Stern A, et al. Angiographic morphology and the pathogenesis of unstable angina pectoris. *J Am Coll Cardiol* 1985;5:609–616.
20. Petrina M, Goodman SG, Eagle KA. The 12-lead electrocardiogram as a predictive tool of mortality after acute myocardial infarction: current status in an era of revascularization and reperfusion. *Am Heart J* 2006;152:11–18.
21. Heidenreich PA, Alloggiamento T, Melsop K, McDonald KM, Go AS, Hlatky MA. The prognostic value of troponin in patients with non-ST elevation acute coronary syndromes: a meta-analysis. *J Am Coll Cardiol* 2001;38:478–485.
22. Wallace TW, Abdullah SM, Drazner MH, et al. Prevalence and determinants of troponin T elevation in the general population. *Circulation* 2006;113:1958–1965.
23. Yalamanchili K, Sukhija R, Aronow WS, Sinha N, Fleisher AG, Lehrman SG. Prevalence of increased cardiac troponin I levels in patients with and without acute pulmonary embolism and relation of increased cardiac troponin I levels with in-hospital mortality in patients with acute pulmonary embolism. *Am J Cardiol* 2004;93:263–264.
24. deFilippi C, Wasserman S, Rosanio S, et al. Cardiac troponin T and C-reactive protein for predicting prognosis, coronary atherosclerosis, and cardiomyopathy in patients undergoing long-term hemodialysis. *JAMA* 2003;290:353–359.
25. Ammann P, Maggiorini M, Bertel O, et al. Troponin as a risk factor for mortality in critically ill patients without acute coronary syndromes. *J Am Coll Cardiol* 2003;41:2004–2009.
26. Apple FS, Murakami MM, Pearce LA, Herzog CA. Predictive value of cardiac troponin I and T for subsequent death in end-stage renal disease. *Circulation* 2002;106:2941–2945.
27. Aviles RJ, Askari AT, Lindahl B, et al. Troponin T levels in patients with acute coronary syndromes, with or without renal dysfunction. *N Engl J Med* 2002;346:2047–2052.
28. McCord J, Nowak RM, McCullough PA, et al. Ninety-minute exclusion of acute myocardial infarction by use of quantitative point-of-care testing of myoglobin and troponin I. *Circulation* 2001;104:1483–1488.
29. Goldman L, Cook EF, Johnson PA, Brand DA, Rouan GW, Lee TH. Prediction of the need for intensive care in patients who come to the emergency departments with acute chest pain. *N Engl J Med* 1996;334:1498–1504.
30. Farkouh ME, Smars PA, Reeder GS, et al. A clinical trial of a chest-pain observation unit for patients with unstable angina. Chest Pain Evaluation in the Emergency Room (CHEER) Investigators. *N Engl J Med* 1998;339:1882–1888.
31. Boersma E, Pieper KS, Steyerberg EW, et al. Predictors of outcome in patients with acute coronary syndromes without persistent ST-segment elevation. Results from an international trial of 9461 patients. The PURSUIT Investigators. *Circulation* 2000;101:2557–2567.
32. Mueller C, Neumann FJ, Perach W, Perruchoud AP, Buettner HJ. Prognostic value of the admission electrocardiogram in patients with unstable angina/non–ST-segment elevation myocardial infarction treated with very early revascularization. *Am J Med* 2004;117:145–150.
33. Newby LK, Christenson RH, Ohman EM, et al. Value of serial troponin T measures for early and late risk stratification in patients with acute coronary syndromes. The GUSTO-IIa Investigators. *Circulation* 1998;98:1853–1859.
34. Lindahl B, Venge P, Wallentin L, and the FRISC study group. Troponin T identifies patients with unstable coronary artery disease who benefit from long-term antithrombotic protection. *J Am Coll Cardiol* 1997;29:43–48.
35. Fuchs S, Stabile E, Mintz GS, et al. Intravascular ultrasound findings in patients with acute coronary syndromes with and without elevated troponin I level. *Am J Cardiol* 2002;89:1111–1113.
36. Morrow DA, Antman EM, Tanasijevic M, et al. Cardiac troponin I for stratification of early outcomes and the efficacy of enoxaparin in unstable angina: a TIMI-11B substudy. *J Am Coll Cardiol* 2000;36:1812–1817.
37. Morrow DA, Cannon CP, Rifai N, et al. Ability of minor elevations of troponins I and T to predict benefit from an early invasive strategy in patients with unstable angina and non-ST elevation myocardial infarction: results from a randomized trial. *JAMA* 2001;286:2405–2412.
38. Heeschen C, Hamm CW, Goldmann B, Deu A, Langenbrink L, White HD. Troponin concentrations for stratification of patients with acute coronary

syndromes in relation to therapeutic efficacy of tirofiban. PRISM Study Investigators. Platelet Receptor Inhibition in Ischemic Syndrome Management. *Lancet* 1999;354:1757–1762.

39. Alpert JS, Thygesen K, Antman E, Bassand JP. Myocardial infarction redefined—a consensus document of the Joint European Society of Cardiology/American College of Cardiology Committee for the redefinition of myocardial infarction. *J Am Coll Cardiol* 2000;36:959–969.

40. Pham MX, Whooley MA, Evans GT Jr, et al. Prognostic value of low-level cardiac troponin-I elevations in patients without definite acute coronary syndromes. *Am Heart J* 2004;148:776–782.

41. Sabatine MS, Morrow DA, de Lemos JA, et al. Acute changes in circulating natriuretic peptide levels in relation to myocardial ischemia. *J Am Coll Cardiol* 2004;44:1988–1995.

42. de Lemos JA, Morrow DA, Bentley JH, et al. The prognostic value of B-type natriuretic peptide in patients with acute coronary syndromes. *N Engl J Med* 2001;345:1014–1021.

43. Morrow DA, de Lemos JA, Sabatine MS, et al. Evaluation of B-type natriuretic peptide for risk assessment in unstable angina/non–ST-elevation myocardial infarction: B-type natriuretic peptide and prognosis in TACTICS-TIMI 18. *J Am Coll Cardiol* 2003;41:1264–1272.

44. James SK, Lindahl B, Siegbahn A, et al. N-terminal pro-brain natriuretic peptide and other risk markers for the separate prediction of mortality and subsequent myocardial infarction in patients with unstable coronary artery disease: a Global Utilization of Strategies To Open occluded arteries (GUSTO)-IV substudy. *Circulation* 2003;108:275–281.

45. Morrow DA, de Lemos JA, Blazing MA, et al. Prognostic value of serial B-type natriuretic peptide testing during follow-up of patients with unstable coronary artery disease. *JAMA* 2005;294:2866–2871.

46. Lindahl B, Toss H, Siegbahn A, Venge P, Wallentin L. Markers of myocardial damage and inflammation in relation to long-term mortality in unstable coronary artery disease. FRISC Study Group. Fragmin During Instability in Coronary Artery Disease. *N Engl J Med* 2000;343:1139–1147.

47. James SK, Armstrong P, Barnathan E, et al. Troponin and C-reactive protein have different relations to subsequent mortality and myocardial infarction after acute coronary syndrome: a GUSTO-IV substudy. *J Am Coll Cardiol* 2003;41:916–924.

48. Brennan ML, Penn MS, Van Lente F, et al. Prognostic value of myeloperoxidase in patients with chest pain. *N Engl J Med* 2003;349:1595–1604.

49. Sinha MK, Roy D, Gaze DC, Collinson PO, Kaski JC. Role of "ischemia modified albumin," a new biochemical marker of myocardial ischaemia, in the early diagnosis of acute coronary syndromes. *Emerg Med J* 2004;21:29–34.

50. Peacock F, Morris DL, Anwaruddin S, et al. Meta-analysis of ischemia-modified albumin to rule out acute coronary syndromes in the emergency department. *Am Heart J* 2006;152:253–262.

51. Luchi RJ, Scott SM, Dupree RH, and the Principal Investigators and their Associates of Veterans Administration Cooperative Study No 28. Comparison of medical and surgical treatment for unstable angina pectoris. *N Engl J Med* 1987;316:977–984.

52. Antman EM, Cohen M, Bernink PJ, et al. The TIMI risk score for unstable angina/non-ST elevation MI. A method for prognostication and therapeutic decision making. *JAMA* 2000;284:835–842.

53. Eagle KA, Lim MJ, Dabbous OH, et al. A validated prediction model for all forms of acute coronary syndrome: estimating the risk of 6-month postdischarge death in an international registry. *JAMA* 2004;291:2727–2733.

54. Yan AT, Jong P, Yan RT, et al. Clinical trial--derived risk model may not generalize to real-world patients with acute coronary syndrome. *Am Heart J* 2004;148:1020–1027.

55. de Araujo Goncalves P, Ferreira J, Aguiar C, Seabra-Gomes R. TIMI, PURSUIT, and GRACE risk scores: sustained prognostic value and interaction with revascularization in NSTE-ACS. *Eur Heart J* 2005;26:865–872.

56. Watkins S, Thiemann D, Coresh J, Powe N, Folsom AR, Rosamond W. Fourteen-year (1987 to 2000) trends in the attack rates of, therapy for, and mortality from non-ST-elevation acute coronary syndromes in four United States communities. *Am J Cardiol* 2005;96:1349–1355.

57. Goldberg RJ, Currie K, White K, et al. Six-month outcomes in a multinational registry of patients hospitalized with an acute coronary syndrome (the Global Registry of Acute Coronary Events [GRACE]). *Am J Cardiol* 2004;93:288–293.

58. Neumann FJ, Kastrati A, Pogatsa-Murray G, et al. Evaluation of prolonged antithrombotic pretreatment ("cooling-off" strategy) before intervention in patients with unstable coronary syndromes: a randomized controlled trial. *JAMA* 2003;290:1593–1599.

59. Chen ZM, Pan HC, Chen YP, et al. Early intravenous then oral metoprolol in 45,852 patients with acute myocardial infarction: randomised placebo-controlled trial. *Lancet* 2005;366:1622–1632.

60. ACE Inhibitor Myocardial Infarction Collaborative Group. Indications for ACE inhibitors in the early treatment of acute myocardial infarction: systematic overview of individual data from 100,000 patients in randomized trials. *Circulation* 1998;97:2202–2212.

61. Yusuf S, Sleight P, Pogue J, Bosch J, Davies R, Dagenais G. Effects of an angiotensin-converting-enzyme inhibitor, ramipril, on cardiovascular events in high-risk patients. The Heart Outcomes Prevention Evaluation Study Investigators. *N Engl J Med* 2000;342:145–153.

62. Antiplatelet Trialists' Collaboration. Collaborative overview of randomised trials of antiplatelet therapy—I: prevention of death myocardial infarction and stroke by prolonged antiplatelet therapy in various categories of patients. *BMJ* 1994;308:81–106.

63. Antithrombotic Trialists' Collaboration. Collaborative meta-analysis of randomised trials of antiplatelet therapy for prevention of death, myocardial infarction, and stroke in high risk patients. *BMJ* 2002;324:71–86.

64. CAPRIE Steering Committee. A randomised, blinded, trial of clopidogrel versus aspirin in patients at risk of ischaemic events (CAPRIE). *Lancet* 1996;348:1329–1339.

65. Yusuf S, Zhao F, Mehta SR, Chrolavicius S, Tognoni G, Fox KK. Effects of clopidogrel in addition to aspirin in patients with acute coronary syndromes without ST-segment elevation. *N Engl J Med* 2001;345:494–502.

66. Fox KA, Mehta SR, Peters R, et al. Benefits and risks of the combination of clopidogrel and aspirin in patients undergoing surgical revascularization for non-ST-elevation acute coronary syndrome: the Clopidogrel in Unstable angina to prevent Recurrent ischemic Events (CURE) Trial. *Circulation* 2004;110:1202–1208.

67. Mehta SR, Yusuf S, Peters RJ, et al. Effects of pretreatment with clopidogrel and aspirin followed by long-term therapy in patients undergoing percutaneous coronary intervention: the PCI-CURE study. *Lancet* 2001;358:527–533.

68. Steinhubl SR, Berger PB, Mann JT 3rd, et al. Early and sustained dual oral antiplatelet therapy following percutaneous coronary intervention: a randomized controlled trial. *JAMA* 2002;288:2411–2420.

69. Iakovou I, Schmidt T, Bonizzoni E, et al. Incidence, predictors, and outcome of thrombosis after successful implantation of drug-eluting stents. *JAMA* 2005;293:2126–2130.

70. Smith SC Jr, Feldman TE, Hirshfeld JW Jr, et al. ACC/AHA/SCAI 2005, Guideline Update for Percutaneous Coronary Intervention—summary article: a report of the American College of Cardiology/American Heart Association Task Force on Practice Guidelines (ACC/AHA/SCAI Writing Committee to Update the 2001, Guidelines for Percutaneous Coronary Intervention). *Circulation* 2006;113:156–175.

71. Steinhubl SR, Berger PB, Brennan DM, Topol EJ. Optimal timing for the initiation of pre-treatment with 300 mg clopidogrel before percutaneous coronary intervention. *J Am Coll Cardiol* 2006;47:939–943.

72. The PURSUIT Trial Investigators. Inhibition of platelet glycoprotein IIb/IIIa with eptifibatide in patients with acute coronary syndromes. The PURSUIT Trial Investigators. Platelet Glycoprotein IIb/IIIa in Unstable Angina: Receptor Suppression Using Integrilin Therapy. *N Engl J Med* 1998;339:436–443.

73. The GUSTO IV Investigators. Effect of glycoprotein IIb/IIIa receptor blocker abciximab on outcome in patients with acute coronary syndromes without early coronary revascularisation: the GUSTO IV-ACS randomised trial. *Lancet* 2001;357:1915–1924.

74. Boersma E, Akkerhuis KM, Theroux P, Califf RM, Topol EJ, Simoons ML. Platelet glycoprotein IIb/IIIa receptor inhibition in non-ST-elevation acute coronary syndromes: early benefit during medical treatment only, with additional protection during percutaneous coronary intervention. *Circulation* 1999;100:2045–2048.

75. Roffi M, Chew DP, Mukherjee D, et al. Platelet glycoprotein IIb/IIIa inhibition in acute coronary syndromes. Gradient of benefit related to the revascularization strategy. *Eur Heart J* 2002;23:1441–1448.

76. Boersma E, Harrington RA, Moliterno DJ, et al. Platelet glycoprotein IIb/IIIa inhibitors in acute coronary syndromes: a meta-analysis of all major randomised clinical trials. *Lancet* 2002;359:189–198.

77. Cannon CP, Weintraub WS, Demopoulos LA, et al. Comparison of early invasive and conservative strategies in patients with unstable coronary syndromes treated with the glycoprotein IIb/IIIa inhibitor tirofiban. *N Engl J Med* 2001;344:1879–1887.

78. Hamm CW, Heeschen C, Goldmann B, et al. Benefit of abciximab in patients with refractory unstable angina in relation to serum troponin T levels. *N Engl J Med* 1999;340:1623–1629.

79. Kastrati A, Mehilli J, Neumann FJ, et al. Abciximab in patients with acute coronary syndromes undergoing percutaneous coronary intervention after clopidogrel pretreatment: the ISAR-REACT 2 randomized trial. *JAMA* 2006;295:1531–1538.

80. Di Nisio M, Middeldorp S, Buller HR. Direct thrombin inhibitors. *N Engl J Med* 2005;353:1028–1040.

81. Oler A, Whooley MA, Oler J, Grady D. Adding heparin to aspirin reduces the incidence of myocardial infarction and death in patients with unstable angina. A meta-analysis. *JAMA* 1996;276:811–815.

82. Klein W, Buchwald A, Hillis SE, et al. Comparison of low-molecular-weight heparin with unfractionated heparin acutely and with placebo for 6 weeks in the management of unstable coronary artery disease. Fragmin in unstable coronary artery disease study (FRIC). *Circulation* 1997;96:61–68.

83. Group FS. Comparison of two treatment durations (6 days and 14 days) of a low molecular weight heparin with a 6-day treatment of unfractionated heparin in the initial management of unstable angina or non–Q-wave myocardial infarction: FRAXIS. *Eur Heart J* 1999:1553–1562.

84. Cohen M, Demers C, Gurfinkel EP, et al. A comparison of low-molecular-weight heparin with unfractionated heparin for unstable coronary artery disease. *N Engl J Med* 1997;337:447–452.

85. Antman EM, McCabe CH, Gurfinkel EP, et al. Enoxaparin prevents death and cardiac ischemic events in unstable angina/non–Q-wave myocardial infarction. Results of the thrombolysis in myocardial infarction (TIMI) 11B trial. *Circulation* 1999;100:1593–1601.

86. Goodman SG, Fitchett D, Armstrong PW, Tan M, Langer A. Randomized evaluation of the safety and efficacy of enoxaparin versus unfractionated heparin in high-risk patients with non–ST-segment elevation acute coronary syndromes receiving the glycoprotein IIb/IIIa inhibitor eptifibatide. *Circulation* 2003;107:238–244.

87. Blazing MA, de Lemos JA, White HD, et al. Safety and efficacy of enoxaparin vs unfractionated heparin in patients with non-ST-segment elevation acute coronary syndromes who receive tirofiban and aspirin: a randomized controlled trial. *JAMA* 2004;292:55–64.

88. de Lemos JA, Blazing MA, Wiviott SD, et al. Enoxaparin versus unfractionated heparin in patients treated with tirofiban, aspirin and an early conservative initial management strategy: results from the A phase of the A-to-Z trial. *Eur Heart J* 2004;25:1688–1694.

89. Ferguson JJ, Califf RM, Antman EM, et al. Enoxaparin vs unfractionated heparin in high-risk patients with non–ST-segment elevation acute coronary syndromes managed with an intended early invasive strategy: primary results of the SYNERGY randomized trial. *JAMA* 2004;292:45–54.

90. Yusuf S, Mehta SR, Chrolavicius S, et al. Comparison of fondaparinux and enoxaparin in acute coronary syndromes. *N Engl J Med* 2006;354:1464–1476.

91. Lincoff AM, Bittl JA, Harrington RA, et al. Bivalirudin and provisional glycoprotein IIb/IIIa blockade compared with heparin and planned glycoprotein IIb/IIIa blockade during percutaneous coronary intervention: REPLACE-2 randomized trial. *JAMA* 2003;289:853–863.

92. Stone GW. *The Acuity Trial.* Oral presentation at the American College of Cardiology Meeting, Atlanta, GA, 2006.

93. van Es RF, Jonker JJ, Verheugt FW, Deckers JW, Grobbee DE. Aspirin and Coumadin after acute coronary syndromes (the ASPECT-2 study): a randomised controlled trial. *Lancet* 2002;360:109–113.

94. Hurlen M, Abdelnoor M, Smith P, Eriksssen J, Arnesen H. Warfarin, aspirin, or both after myocardial infarction. *N Engl J Med* 2002;347:969–974.

95. The TIMI IIIB Investigators. Effects of tissue plasminogen activator and a comparison of early invasive and conservative strategies in unstable angina and non–Q-wave myocardial infarction: Results of the TIMI IIIB Trial. *Circulation* 1994;89:1545–1556.

96. Boden WE, O'Rourke RA, Crawford MH, et al. Outcomes in patients with acute non–Q-wave myocardial infarction randomly assigned to an invasive as compared with a conservative strategy. *N Engl J Med* 1998;338:1785–1792.

97. Fragmin and Fast Revascularisation During Instability in Coronary Artery Disease (FRISC II) Investigators. Invasive compared with non-invasive treatment in unstable coronary-artery disease: FRISC II prospective randomised multicentre study. *Lancet* 1999;354:708–715.

98. Fox KA, Poole-Wilson PA, Henderson RA, et al. Interventional versus conservative treatment for patients with unstable angina or non-ST-elevation myocardial infarction: the British Heart Foundation RITA 3 randomised trial. Randomized Intervention Trial of Unstable Angina. *Lancet* 2002;360:743–751.

99. de Winter RJ, Windhausen F, Cornel JH, et al. Early invasive versus selectively invasive management for acute coronary syndromes. *N Engl J Med* 2005;353:1095–1104.

100. Wallentin L, Lagerqvist B, Husted S, Kontny F, Stahle E, Swahn E. Outcome at 1 year after an invasive compared with a non-invasive strategy in unstable

101. coronary-artery disease: the FRISC II invasive randomised trial. FRISC II Investigators. Fast Revascularisation During Instability in Coronary Artery Disease. *Lancet* 2000;356:9–16.

101. Diderholm E, Andren B, Frostfeldt G, et al. The prognostic and therapeutic implications of increased troponin T levels and ST depression in unstable coronary artery disease: the FRISC II invasive troponin T electrocardiogram substudy. *Am Heart J* 2002;143:760–767.

102. Fox KA, Poole-Wilson P, Clayton TC, et al. 5-Year outcome of an interventional strategy in non–ST-elevation acute coronary syndrome: the British Heart Foundation RITA 3 randomised trial. *Lancet* 2005;366:914–920.

103. Mahoney EM, Jurkovitz CT, Chu H, et al. Cost and cost-effectiveness of an early invasive vs conservative strategy for the treatment of unstable angina and non–ST-segment elevation myocardial infarction. *JAMA* 2002;288:1851–1858.

104. Bhatt DL, Roe MT, Peterson ED, et al. Utilization of early invasive management strategies for high-risk patients with non–ST-segment elevation acute coronary syndromes: results from the CRUSADE Quality Improvement Initiative. *JAMA* 2004;292:2096–2104.

105. Ong AT, Serruys PW. Complete revascularization: coronary artery bypass graft surgery versus percutaneous coronary intervention. *Circulation* 2006;114:249–255.

106. Schwartz GG, Olsson AG, Ezekowitz MD, et al. Effects of atorvastatin on early recurrent ischemic events in acute coronary syndromes: the MIRACL study: a randomized controlled trial. *JAMA* 2001;285:1711–1718.

107. de Lemos JA, Blazing MA, Wiviott SD, et al. Early intensive vs a delayed conservative simvastatin strategy in patients with acute coronary syndromes: phase Z of the A to Z trial. *JAMA* 2004;292:1307–1316.

108. Grundy SM, Cleeman JI, Merz CN, et al. Implications of recent clinical trials for the National Cholesterol Education Program Adult Treatment Panel III guidelines. *Circulation* 2004;110:227–239.

109. Prinzmetal M, Kennamer R, Merliss R, Wada T, Bor N. Angina pectoris. I. A variant form of angina pectoris; preliminary report. *Am J Med* 1959;27:375–388.

110. Kugiyama K, Yasue H, Okumura K, et al. Nitric oxide activity is deficient in spasm arteries of patients with coronary spastic angina. *Circulation* 1996;94:266–271.

111. Egashira K, Katsuda Y, Mohri M, et al. Basal release of endothelium-derived nitric oxide at site of spasm in patients with variant angina. *J Am Coll Cardiol* 1996;27:1444–1449.

112. David PR, Waters DD, Scholl JM, et al. Percutaneous transluminal coronary angioplasty in patients with variant angina. *Circulation* 1982;66:695–702.

113. Chahine RA, Feldman RL, Giles TD, et al. Randomized placebo-controlled trial of amlodipine in vasospastic angina. Amlodipine Study 160 Group. *J Am Coll Cardiol* 1993;21:1365–1370.

114. Yasue H, Takizawa A, Nagao M, et al. Long-term prognosis for patients with variant angina and influential factors. *Circulation* 1988;78:1–9.

115. Rutitzky B, Girotti AL, Rosenbaum MB. Efficacy of chronic amiodarone therapy in patients with variant angina pectoris and inhibition of ergonovine coronary constriction. *Am Heart J* 1982;103:38–43.

116. Frenneaux M, Kaski JC, Brown M, Maseri A. Refractory variant angina relieved by guanethidine and clonidine. *Am J Cardiol* 1988;62:832–833.

117. Miwa K, Kambara H, Kawai C. Exercise-induced angina provoked by aspirin administration in patients with variant angina. *Am J Cardiol* 1981;47:1210–1214.

118. Shubrooks SJ Jr, Bete JM, Hutter AM Jr, et al. Variant angina pectoris: Clinical and anatomic spectrum and results of coronary bypass surgery. *Am J Cardiol* 1975;36:142–147.

119. Bertrand ME, LaBlanche JM, Thieuleux FA, Fourrier JL, Traisnel G, Asseman P. Comparative results of percutaneous transluminal coronary angioplasty in patients with dynamic versus fixed coronary stenosis. *J Am Coll Cardiol* 1986;8:504–508.

120. Freemantle N, Calvert M, Wood J, Eastaugh J, Griffin C. Composite outcomes in randomized trials: greater precision but with greater uncertainty? *JAMA* 2003;289:2554–2559.

121. Tanabe Y, Itoh E, Suzuki K, et al. Limited role of coronary angioplasty and stenting in coronary spastic angina with organic stenosis. *J Am Coll Cardiol* 2002;39:1120–1126.

122. Petersen, JL, Mahaffey KW, Hasselblad, V, et al. Efficacy and bleeding complications among patients randomized to enoxaparin or unfractionated heparin for antithrombin therapy in non–ST-segment elevation acute coronary syndromes: a systematic overview. *JAMA* 2004;292:89–96.

123. Mehta, SR, Cannon CP, Fox, KA, et al. Routine vs selective invasive strategies in patients with acute coronary syndromes: a collaborative meta-analysis of randomized trials. *JAMA* 2005;293:2908–2971.

CHAPTER (60)

ST-Segment Elevation Myocardial Infarction

Eric H. Yang / Bernard J. Gersh / Robert A. O'Rourke

EPIDEMIOLOGY

Coronary artery disease is the leading cause of morbidity and mortality in Western society and is a worldwide epidemic. In 2001, it was estimated that worldwide, ischemic heart disease was responsible for 11.8 percent of all deaths (5.7 million) in low-income countries and 17.3 percent (1.36 million) of all deaths in high-income countries.[1] Approximately 865,000 Americans suffer from an acute myocardial infarction (AMI) per year, one-third of which are caused by an acute ST-segment elevation myocardial infarction (STEMI).[2] The incidence of AMI has declined over the past two decades from 244 per 100,000 population in 1975 to 184 per 100,000 population in 1995.[3] The in-hospital mortality rate also has declined from 18 percent in 1975 to 12 percent in 1995. Despite these improvements, AMI continues to be a serious public health problem and it has been estimated that the number of years of life lost because of an AMI is 14.2 years and the cost to American society (both direct and indirect) is $142.5 billion per year.[2]

The management of STEMI patients is complex, multidisciplinary, and involves the following three different stages of care: (1) emergency department, (2) cardiac catheterization laboratory, and (3) coronary care unit. This chapter discusses the diagnosis and management of STEMI patients in each of these three settings. The pathophysiology of disease is discussed in Chap. 57 and the acute coronary syndromes of unstable angina and non ST-elevation myocardial infarction are discussed in Chap. 59.

DIAGNOSIS

【 】 SYMPTOMS

The classic symptom of AMI is precordial or retrosternal discomfort that is commonly described as a pressure, crushing, aching, or burning sensation. Radiation of the discomfort to the neck, back, or arms frequently occurs, and the pain is usually persistent. The discomfort typically achieves maximum intensity over several minutes and can be associated with nausea, diaphoresis, generalized weakness, and a fear of impending death. Some patients, particular the elderly, may also present with syncope, unexplained nausea and vomiting, acute confusion, agitation, or palpitations.

Approximately 20 percent of AMI patients are asymptomatic or have atypical symptoms that are not initially recognized. Painless myocardial infarction occurs more frequently in the elderly, women, diabetics, and postoperative patients. These patients tend to present with dyspnea or frank congestive heart failure as their initial symptom.[4]

PHYSICAL EXAMINATION

Patients can appear anxious and uncomfortable. Those with substantial left ventricular (LV) dysfunction at presentation may have tachycardia, pulmonary rales, tachypnea, and a third heart sound. The presence of a mitral regurgitant murmur suggests ischemic dysfunction of the mitral valve apparatus, rupture, or ventricular remodeling.

In patients with right ventricular infarction, increased jugular venous pressure, Kussmaul sign (rise in jugular venous pressure with inspiration), and a right ventricular third sound may be present. Such patients virtually always have inferior infarctions, usually without evidence of left-heart failure, and may have exquisite blood pressure sensitivity to nitrates or hypovolemia. In patients with extensive left ventricular dysfunction, shock is indicated by hypotension, diaphoresis, cool skin and extremities, pallor, oliguria, and possible confusion.

ELECTROCARDIOGRAM

The classic initial electrocardiographic (ECG) manifestation of STEMI are discussed in Chap. 13 and involve an increase in the amplitude of the T wave (peaking), followed within minutes by ST-segment elevation. The R wave may initially increase in height but soon decreases, and often Q waves form. If the jeopardized myocardium is reperfused, the ST segment may promptly revert to normal, although T waves can remain inverted, and Q waves may or may not regress. Persistent ST-segment elevation after restoration of flow in the epicardial coronary artery is a marker of failed myocardial perfusion and associated with an adverse prognosis. In the absence of reperfusion, the ST segment gradually returns to baseline in several hours to days, and T waves become symmetrically inverted. Failure of the T wave to invert in 24 to 48 hours suggest regional pericarditis.

The specific leads with ST-elevation can help localize the infarct (see Chap. 13): ST-segment elevation in the inferior, anterior, or high lateral leads is seen with infarction of the corresponding areas of myocardium. ST-segment elevation in lead aVR is more frequent in patients with left main artery occlusion than in patients with left anterior descending coronary artery or right coronary artery occlusion.[5] In a study of STEMI patients, ST-segment elevation in lead aVR that was greater than or equal to the extent of ST-segment elevation in lead V_1 had 81 percent accuracy for diagnosing left main occlusion.[5] ST elevation in lead V_1, in the setting of inferior myocardial infarction (MI) suggests right ventricular (RV) involvement.

New onset left bundle-branch block (LBBB) in the setting of chest pain is considered as a STEMI. The diagnosis of STEMI in the setting of old LBBB can be difficult. Findings suggesting STEMI include (1) a pathologic Q wave in leads I, aVL, V_5, or V_6 (two leads); (2) precordial R-wave regression; (3) late notching of the S wave in V_1 to V_4; and (4) deviation of the ST segment in the same direction as that of the major QRS deflection.[6] Similar findings may be expected in right ventricular pacing with left bundle-

branch block structure of the QRS. In a recent study, patients with paced rhythm had higher in-hospital and 1-year mortality, in part because of undertreatment, which illustrates the difficulty of AMI diagnosis in this setting.[7]

Analysis of ECG data from the Global Use of Strategies to Open Occluded Coronary Arteries (GUSTO) I study identified three criteria for diagnosing myocardial infarction in the presence of the LBBB: (1) ST-segment elevation ≥ 1 mm concordant with the QRS complex; (2) ST-segment depression ≥ 1 mm in leads V_1, V_2, or V_3; and (3) ST-segment elevation ≥ 5 mm discordant with the QRS.[8]

The ECG, however, has several limitations: (1) even though ST-segment elevation usually signifies acute coronary occlusion, acute coronary occlusion may not cause ST-segment elevation in certain circumstances such as a circumflex artery occlusion; (2) in addition, not all ST-segment elevation is caused by AMI; and (3) finally, an old LBBB limits the usefulness of the ECG for AMI diagnosis.

LABORATORY STUDIES

Damaged cardiomyocytes release several proteins in the circulation including myoglobin, creatine kinase (CK) and its myocardial band isoenzyme (CK-MB), troponins (I and T), myoglobin, aspartate aminotransferase, and lactate dehydrogenase (see Chap. 59). Figure 60–1 shows the timing of release.[9] Cardiac troponins are currently the preferred biomarkers for myocardial damage because of their high sensitivity and specificity.[10] CK-MB is the best alternative, if cardiac troponin assays are not available. CK-MB because of its more rapid appearance and disappearance from the blood can be used (1) in patients presenting early after symptom onset; (2) to time the onset of injury if the troponin is increased; and (3) to detect reinfarction later in the hospital course. Determinations of total CK, aspartate aminotransferase, and lactate dehy-

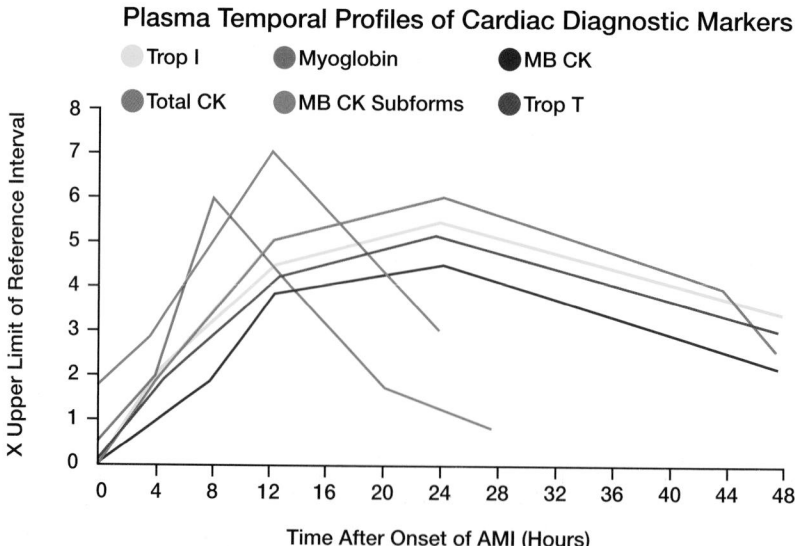

FIGURE 60–1. Shown here is the temporal profile of the diagnostic biomarkers used for detecting acute myocardial infarction (AMI). The plasma temporal profile for early detection is illustrated for myoglobin and myocardial band (MB) creatinine kinase (CK) subforms. The markers MB CK, total CK, and cardiac troponins (Trop) I and T are all released with a similar initial time profile. However, troponins I and T remain elevated for 10 to 14 days and thus are better markers for late diagnosis than that of MB CK.

drogenase are no longer recommended. Blood sampling for biomarker determination is recommended at hospital admission, at 6 to 9 hours, and at 12 to 24 hours if the earlier samples were negative and the clinical index of suspicion is high (see Chap. 59).[10]

Myoglobin

Myoglobin is a 17.8-kDa protein that is released from injured myocardial cells. As shown in Fig. 60–1, myoglobin release occurs within hours after the onset on infarction, reaches peak levels at 1 to 4 hours, and remains elevated for about 24 hours. Although the rapid rise allows for its use as an early marker for STEMI, myoglobin is not specific to myocardial cells and should not be used in isolation as a method for diagnosing myocardial infarction.

CK-MB

The MB isoenzyme of creatine kinase is present in largest concentration in myocardium, although small amounts (1 to 2 percent) can be found in skeletal muscle, tongue, small intestine, and diaphragm. CK-MB appears in serum within about 3 hours after the onset of infarction, reaches peak levels at 12 to 24 hours, and has a mean duration of activity of 1 to 3 days.[9] Other cardiac, but non-AMI etiologies of increased CK-MB levels can occur after cardioversion, cardiac surgery, myopericarditis, percutaneous coronary intervention (PCI), and occasionally after rapid tachycardia. Noncardiac causes of increased CK-MB levels may occur with hypothyroidism, extensive skeletal muscle trauma, rhabdomyolysis, the muscular dystrophies, and some other neuromuscular disorders.

Occasionally, the concentration of CK-MB isoenzyme may be increased in the presence of normal total levels of CK enzyme. This finding usually indicates a small amount of myocardial necrosis in a patient whose baseline total CK enzyme level is at the low-normal end of the range (see Chap. 59).

Troponins

The cardiac troponins regulate the interaction of actin and myosin and are more cardiac specific than CK-MB. There are two isoforms of cardiac troponin: T and I. Their levels start to rise 3 to 12 hours after the onset of ischemia, peak at 12 to 24 hours, and may remain elevated for 8 to 21 days (troponin T) or 7 to 14 days (troponin I). Elevated troponin levels correlate with pathologically proven myocardial necrosis and indicate poor prognosis in patients with suspected acute coronary syndromes (see Chap. 59).[11-15]

MANAGEMENT IN THE EMERGENCY DEPARTMENT

【 】 PREHOSPITAL DIAGNOSIS

Rapid diagnosis is a pivotal component of the management of STEMI patients. Early diagnosis can be achieved with a prehospital ECG that is obtained in the field by emergency medical personnel and transmitted to an emergency department physician or cardiologist on-call. This allows for early administration of thrombolytic therapy or activation of the cardiac catheterization team prior to arrival of the patient and has been demonstrated in several studies to reduce both the door-to-needle and door-to-

balloon time.[16-18] Although the American College of Cardiology (ACC)/American Heart Association (AHA) guidelines for STEMI considers the prehospital electrocardiogram as a class IIa indication,[19] analysis of data from the National Registry of Myocardial Infarction revealed that only 4.5 percent (1599/35,370) of patients receiving thrombolytic therapy and 8 percent (1696/21,277) of patients undergoing primary PCI had a prehospital electrocardiogram.[16] The analysis also showed that a prehospital electrocardiogram resulted in a significantly shorter door-to-needle time (24.6 vs. 34.7 minutes, p <0.0001) for those receiving thrombolytic therapy and a shorter door-to-balloon time (94 vs. 110 minutes, p <0.0001) for primary PCI patients.[16]

【 】 TRIAGE AND EVALUATION IN THE EMERGENCY DEPARTMENT

The cornerstone of STEMI therapy is a rapid and accurate evaluation in the emergency department. All patients presenting with complaints of chest discomfort should be rapidly triaged and allowed to bypass the emergency department waiting room. An ECG should be obtained within the first 10 minutes of arrival at the emergency department and a focused history and physical examination assessing the symptoms and signs described in the diagnosis section of this chapter should be quickly performed.

The physical examination also provides a method for the risk stratification of STEMI patients. As shown in Table 60–1, the Killip classification can be used as method to stratify patients and predict clinical outcomes.[20] With modern therapy, the mortality of those in cardiogenic shock has improved from 83 percent to approximately 60 percent.

The Clinical Practice Guidelines recommend the following (see Chap. 11)[19]:

Class I

1. *The targeted history of STEMI patients taken in the emergency department should ascertain whether the patient has had prior episodes of myocardial ischemia, such as stable or unstable angina, MI, coronary bypass surgery, or PCI. Evaluation of the patient's complaints should focus on chest discomfort, associated symptoms, sex- and age-related differences in presentation, hypertension, diabetes mellitus, possibility of aortic dissection, risk of bleeding, and clinical cerebrovascular disease (amaurosis fugax, face/limb weak-*

TABLE 60–1

Killip Classification for Patients with ST-Segment Elevation Myocardial Infarction

KILLIP CLASS		HOSPITAL MORTALITY (%)
I	No congestive heart failure	6
II	Mild congestive heart failure, rales, S_3, congestion on chest radiograph	17
III	Pulmonary edema	38
IV	Cardiogenic shock	81[a]

[a]Has improved to approximately 60 percent with current therapy.

ness or clumsiness, face/limb numbness or sensory loss, ataxia, or vertigo). (Level of Evidence: C)

2. A physical examination should be performed to aid in the diagnosis and assessment of the extent, location, and presence of complications of STEMI. (Level of Evidence: C)

3. A brief, focused, and limited neurologic examination to look for evidence of prior stroke or cognitive deficits should be performed on STEMI patients before administration of fibrinolytic therapy. (Level of Evidence: C)

4. A 12-lead ECG should be performed and shown to an experienced emergency physician within 10 minutes of emergency department arrival on all patients with chest discomfort (or anginal equivalent) or other symptoms suggestive of STEMI. (Level of Evidence: C)

5. If the initial ECG is not diagnostic of STEMI but the patient remains symptomatic, and there is a high clinical suspicion for STEMI, serial ECGs at 5- to 10-minute intervals or continuous 12-lead ST-segment monitoring should be performed to detect the potential development of ST elevation. (Level of Evidence: C)

6. In patients with inferior STEMI, right-sided ECG leads should be obtained to screen for ST elevation suggestive of RV infarction. (Level of Evidence: B)

【 】 INITIAL THERAPY IN THE EMERGENCY DEPARTMENT

The initial management of patients in the emergency department includes the use of oxygen, aspirin, β blockers, analgesia, nitroglycerin, and anticoagulation with heparin.

Oxygen

Low-flow oxygen therapy delivered by nasal cannula should be routinely given during the first 24 to 48 hours and perhaps several days after acute myocardial infarction in most patients. Although routine use of supplemental oxygen is common practice, hard evidence supporting its use is lacking. Mild hypoxemia is not uncommon, even in the absence of apparent pulmonary congestion. Additionally, some patients may have dyspnea related to acute changes in left ventricular compliance and secondarily increased pulmonary interstitial fluid. The *Clinical Practice Guidelines* recommend the following (see Chap. 11)[19]:

Class I

1. Supplemental oxygen should be administered to patients with arterial oxygen desaturation (SaO$_2$ less than 90 percent). (Level of Evidence: B)

Class IIa

1. It is reasonable to administer supplemental oxygen to all patients with uncomplicated STEMI during the first 6 hours. (Level of Evidence: C)

Aspirin

Aspirin decreases mortality in myocardial infarction and should be administered as early as possible and continued indefinitely in pa-

tients with acute coronary syndromes. In cases of aspirin allergy or major intolerance, clopidogrel should be substituted. In the International Study of Infarct Survival 2 (ISIS-2), 77,187 STEMI patients were randomized to treatment with aspirin, streptokinase, or placebo. The 5-week incidence of vascular death decreased by 23 percent with aspirin and heparin, by 25 percent with streptokinase and heparin, and by 41 percent with the combination of all three agents.[21] Thus, the effect of aspirin was surprisingly nearly as great as that of streptokinase alone in that study, and the benefits of each were partially additive. Thus 160 to 325 mg of chewable aspirin should be given to patients at presentation, with a subsequent dose of 75 to 325 mg daily. For those with a history of a documented significant adverse reaction to aspirin, 300 mg of clopidogrel can be used as an alternative. The *Clinical Practice Guidelines* recommend the following (see Chap. 11)[19]:

Class I

1. Aspirin should be chewed by patients who have not taken aspirin before presentation with STEMI. The initial dose should be 162 mg (Level of Evidence: A) to 325 mg (Level of Evidence: C). Although some trials have used enteric-coated aspirin for initial dosing, more rapid buccal absorption occurs with non–enteric-coated aspirin formulations.

β Blockers

The results of clinical trials investigating the use of β blockers in acute coronary syndromes have documented a decrease in early and late mortality. In pooled data from 28 trials of β blockers, the average mortality decrease was 28 percent at 1 week, with the majority of benefit occurring in the first 48 hours.[22] Specifically, reinfarction was reduced by 18 percent and cardiac arrest by 15 percent.[22] The long-term effects of β blockade for the secondary prevention of death after MI were established by large-scale randomized trials. In a recent meta-analysis of 82 randomized trials of β blockers, there was a significant reduction in long-term, but not short-term, mortality.[23] The number of patients needed to treat with a β blocker to prevent 1 death over 2 years was 42, compared to 24 for thrombolytics, 94 for standard-dose statins, and 153 for antiplatelet agents.

Traditionally, metoprolol has been the agent of choice and was initially administered intravenously followed by an oral dose. The Thrombolysis in Myocardial Infarction (TIMI) 2B study of early (immediate intravenous load followed by oral dosing) versus delayed (no intravenous load) therapy in STEMI patients who were undergoing reperfusion therapy with thrombolytic therapy showed no difference between the two groups in mortality or ejection fraction at the time of discharge.[24] Data from COMMIT (Clopidogrel and Metoprolol in Myocardial Infarction Trial), which involved 45,852 patients, demonstrated that β blockade resulted in a 15 to 20 percent relative risk reduction in recurrent infarction, but in a 30 percent relative increase in the risk of cardiogenic shock.[25] Therefore, the use of β blockade in patients with evidence of hemodynamic instability should be delayed until the patients become stable. Also, the routine initial intravenous dose should be reconsidered as standard therapy. Finally, the benefits of β blockade in patients undergoing primary PCI remains unclear and there have been no randomized prospective studies. The *Clinical Practice Guidelines* recommend the following (see Chap. 11)[19]:

Class I

1. Oral β-blocker therapy should be administered promptly to those patients without a contraindication, irrespective of concomitant fibrinolytic therapy or performance of primary PCI. (Level of Evidence: A)

Class IIa

1. It is reasonable to administer IV β blockers promptly to STEMI patients without contraindications, especially if a tachyarrhythmia or hypertension is present. (Level of Evidence: B)

Analgesia

Morphine is frequently used for pain relief and is best administered intravenously in boluses of 1 to 2 mg, to a maximum of 10 to 15 mg for a normal adult. Respiratory depression can occur and care must be taken not to over sedate patients. Morphine should be used with caution in patients with hemodynamic instability because of its effects on reducing cardiac preload. The *Clinical Practice Guidelines* recommend the following (see Chap. 11)[19]:

Class I

1. Morphine sulfate (2 to 4 mg IV with increments of 2 to 8 mg IV repeated at 5- to 15-minute intervals) is the analgesic of choice for management of pain associated with STEMI. (Level of Evidence: C)

Nitrates

Nitrates cause non–endothelium-dependent coronary vasodilatation, systemic venodilatation, reduced cardiac preload, and enhanced perfusion of ischemic myocardial zones (see Chap. 64). Animal and human data demonstrate that nitrate use may result in a reduction of infarct size.[26,27] For patients with *symptomatic* ischemia, however, intravenous nitroglycerin may be very effective, although nitroglycerin tolerance has been observed as early as 12 hours after institution of intravenous therapy. Often, hemodynamic intolerance to nitroglycerin may be a problem, especially in patients with inferior infarction, hemodynamically significant right ventricular infarction, or concomitant aortic valve stenosis, or among the elderly, particularly in the setting of preexisting volume depletion. Often the hypotension is accompanied by a bradycardia as a manifestation of the von Bezold-Jarisch reflex.

Intravenous nitroglycerin should be initiated at 5 to 10 μg/min and gradually increased with a goal of a 10 to 30 percent reduction in systolic blood pressure and symptomatic pain relief. In most patients, use of this agent will be tapered within 24 to 36 hours. Nitrates should not be administered to patients with recent sildenafil use. In addition, approximately 40 percent of patients with an inferior STEMI will have involvement of the right ventricle and nitrates should be used with caution in these patients in order to avoid profound hypotension, which usually responds promptly to intravenous volume replacement. The *Clinical Practice Guidelines* recommend the following (see Chap. 11)[19]:

Class I

1. Patients with ongoing ischemic discomfort should receive sublingual nitroglycerin (0.4 mg) every 5 minutes for a total of 3 doses, after which an assessment should be made about the need for intravenous nitroglycerin. (Level of Evidence: C)

2. Intravenous nitroglycerin is indicated for relief of ongoing ischemic discomfort, control of hypertension, or management of pulmonary congestion. (Level of Evidence: C)

Class III

1. Nitrates should not be administered to patients with systolic blood pressure less than 90 mmHg or greater than or equal to 30 mmHg below baseline, severe bradycardia (less than 50 beats/min), tachycardia (more than 100 beats/min), or suspected RV infarction. (Level of Evidence: C)

2. Nitrates should not be administered to patients who have received a phosphodiesterase inhibitor for erectile dysfunction within the last 24 hours (48 hours for tadalafil). (Level of Evidence: B)

Heparin

Anticoagulation with heparin is essential in the management of STEMI. Currently two forms of heparin are used: unfractionated heparin and low-molecular-weight heparin (LMWH). The use and pharmacology of these agents is explained in detail in Chap. 59.

When bound to antithrombin III, unfractionated heparin inactivates factor Xa and thrombin. Its use has been widely studied and unfractionated heparin is considered a class I indication for patients with STEMI undergoing primary PCI or receiving fibrin specific thrombolytic agents.[19] An initial bolus of 60 U/kg (4000 U maximum) followed by a 12 U/kg/h (1000 U/h maximum) infusion should be administered promptly. A goal activated partial thromboplastin time (aPTT) of 1.5 to 2.0 times normal should be achieved. The anticoagulation effects of unfractionated heparin, however, can be variable as a consequence of unpredictable protein binding.

The LMWHs are glycosaminoglycans consisting of chains of alternating residues of D-glucosamine and uronic acid. When compared to unfractionated heparin, they have a more predictable anticoagulation effect as a result of a longer half-life, better bioavailability, and dose-independent clearance. Unlike unfractionated heparin, the LMWHs have a great activity against factor Xa than thrombin and their anticoagulation effect cannot be measured with standard laboratory tests.[28]

The use of the LMWH enoxaparin in conjunction with thrombolysis has been studied in the ASSENT 3 (Assessment of the Safety and Efficacy of a New Thrombolytic Regimen) and TIMI-25 EXTRACT (Enoxaparin and Thrombolysis Reperfusion for Acute Myocardial Infarction Treatment) trials.[29,30] In the ASSENT 3 trial, patients treated with enoxaparin plus tenecteplase had a lower combined end point of 30-day mortality, in-hospital rein-farction, and in-hospital refractory ischemia than did those treated with unfractionated heparin plus tenecteplase (11.4 vs. 15.4 percent; $p = 0.0002$). The TIMI-25 EXTRACT trial randomized 20,506 patients undergoing thrombolytic therapy for STEMI to anticoagulation with enoxaparin through the entire index hospitalization or unfractionated heparin for the initial 48 hours. The combined primary end point of death or recurrent MI at 30 days occurred in 9.9 percent of patients in the enoxaparin group and in 12 percent of those in the heparin group (p <0.001).

Because of the delay in the onset of action of subcutaneous administration, an initial intravenous loading dose of 30 mg of enoxaparin followed by the traditional 1 mg/kg subcutaneous dose every 12 hours was used in both trials for patients younger than 75 years of age. Use of enoxaparin, however, was associated with a higher risk of minor and major bleeding when compared to unfractionated heparin (UFH) in the TIMI-25 EXTRACT trial.[30] The *Clinical Practice Guidelines* recommend the following (see Chap. 11)[19]:

Class I

1. *Patients undergoing percutaneous or surgical revascularization should receive UFH. (Level of Evidence: C)*

2. *UFH should be given intravenously to patients undergoing reperfusion therapy with alteplase, reteplase, or tenecteplase with dosing as follows: bolus of 60 U/kg (maximum 4000 U) followed by an infusion of 12 U/kg/h (maximum 1000 U) initially adjusted to maintain aPTT at 1.5 to 2.0 times control (approximately 50 to 70 seconds). (Level of Evidence: C)*

3. *UFH should be given intravenously to patients treated with nonselective fibrinolytic agents (streptokinase, anistreplase, urokinase) who are at high risk for systemic emboli (large or anterior MI, atrial fibrillation, previous embolus, or known left ventricular thrombus). (Level of Evidence: B)*

4. *Platelet counts should be monitored daily in patients taking UFH. (Level of Evidence: C)*

Class IIb

1. *It may be reasonable to administer UFH intravenously to patients undergoing reperfusion therapy with streptokinase. (Level of Evidence: B)*

2. *LMWH might be considered an acceptable alternative to UFH as ancillary therapy for patients younger than 75 years of age who are receiving fibrinolytic therapy, provided that significant renal dysfunction (serum creatinine greater than 2.5 mg/dL in men or 2.0 mg/dL in women) is not present. Enoxaparin (30-mg IV bolus followed by 1.0 mg/kg SC every 12 hours until hospital discharge) used in combination with full-dose tenecteplase is the most comprehensively studied regimen in patients younger than 75 years of age. (Level of Evidence: B)*

Class III

1. *LMWH should not be used as an alternative to UFH as ancillary therapy in patients older than 75 years of age who are receiving fibrinolytic therapy. (Level of Evidence: B)*

2. *LMWH should not be used as an alternative to UFH as ancillary therapy in patients younger than 75 years of age who are receiving fibrinolytic therapy but have significant renal dysfunction (serum creatinine greater than 2.5 mg/dL in men or 2.0 mg/dL in women). (Level of Evidence: B)*

Direct Thrombin Inhibitors

Direct thrombin inhibitors bind directly to thrombin and have been used as an alternative to heparin in patients with heparin-induced thrombocytopenia. Several studies have compared direct thrombin inhibitors to heparin for the management of STEMI patients.[31,32] The Hirulog and Early Reperfusion or Occlusion (HERO)-2 trial randomized 17,073 STEMI patients to the direct thrombin inhibitor bivalirudin or heparin. Thirty-day mortality was similar in both groups; the incidence of reinfarction was decreased at the cost of an increased risk of mild and moderate bleeding.[31] A recent meta-analysis of 11 randomized trials demonstrated that compared with heparin, direct thrombin inhibitors were associated with a lower risk of death or myocardial infarction both at the end of treatment (4.3 percent vs. 5.1 percent, $p = 0.001$) and at 30 days (7.4 percent vs. 8.2 percent, $p = 0.02$).[33] This difference was primarily a result of a reduction in the incidence of reinfarction (2.8 percent vs. 3.5 percent, p <0.001) with no difference in mortality (1.9 percent vs. 2.0 percent, $p = 0.69$). There was no excess in intracranial hemorrhage with any direct thrombin inhibitor.[33] The *Clinical Practice Guidelines* recommend the following (see Chap. 11)[19]:

Class IIa

1. *In patients with known heparin-induced thrombocytopenia, it is reasonable to consider bivalirudin as a useful alternative to heparin to be used in conjunction with streptokinase. Dosing according to the HERO-2 regimen (a bolus of 0.25 mg/kg followed by an intravenous infusion of 0.5 mg/kg/h for the first 12 hours and 0.25 mg/kg/h for the subsequent 36 hours)[33] is recommended, but with a reduction in the infusion rate if the partial thromboplastin time is above 75 seconds within the first 12 hours. (Level of Evidence: B)*

Factor Xa Inhibitors

The factor Xa inhibitor fondaparinux was investigated in the OASIS-6 (Organization for the Assessment of Strategies for Ischemic Syndromes) trial. In this study, 12,092 STEMI patients were randomized to fondaparinux for 8 days or placebo with standard heparin therapy.[34] The primary end point of death or reinfarction at 30 days occurred in 9.7 percent of patients in the fondaparinux group and 11.2 percent of those in the placebo group ($p = 0.008$). Patients treated with thrombolytic therapy had the most benefit and there was no significant increase in the rate of bleeding.

【 】 REPERFUSION STRATEGIES

The main goal of STEMI management is rapid reperfusion to establish coronary blood flow to ischemic myocardium. Currently, there are three main reperfusion strategies: thrombolytic therapy, primary PCI, and thrombolytic-facilitated primary PCI.

Thrombolytic Therapy

Thrombolytic therapy for STEMI has been shown to be effective in numerous randomized trials involving more than 100,000 patients.[35] It is widely available, easily administered, and is relatively inexpensive. However, only approximately 50 percent of STEMI patients are eligible for thrombolytic therapy (Table 60–2), and only 50 to 60 percent of patients treated with thrombolytics will achieve complete reperfusion (TIMI grade III flow). In addition, 10 to 20 percent of patients will experience reocclusion and 1 percent will suffer from a stroke caused by intracranial hemorrhage. Thrombolytic therapy is most effective when given within 3 hours from onset of chest pain.[36]

Although streptokinase is still widely used around the world, fibrin-specific agents are almost exclusively used in the United States. These therapies are summarized in Table 60–3 and are molecular modifications of the tissue plasminogen activator (tPA) molecule. The impetus for their development was the hope that increasing fibrin specificity (TNK), or prolonging the plasma half-life (reteplase [rPA], tenecteplase [TNK], lanoteplase [nPA]) would increase TIMI-3 flow rates in the infarct-related artery beyond the approximately 50 percent found at 90-minute angiography for tPA. Phase 1 and 2 trials of these agents have shown TIMI-3 flow rates in excess of 60 percent; however, there was no significant reduction in mortality or in the incidence of stroke.[37,38] The *Clinical Practice Guidelines* recommend the following (see Chap. 11)[19]:

Class I

1. In the absence of contraindications, fibrinolytic therapy should be administered to STEMI patients with symptom onset within the prior 12 hours and ST elevation greater than 0.1 mV in at least two contiguous precordial leads or at least two adjacent limb leads. (Level of Evidence: A)

2. In the absence of contraindications, fibrinolytic therapy should be administered to STEMI patients with symptom onset within the prior 12 hours and new or presumably new LBBB. (Level of Evidence: A)

Class IIa

1. In the absence of contraindications, it is reasonable to administer fibrinolytic therapy to STEMI patients with symptom onset within the prior 12 hours and 12-lead ECG findings consistent with a true posterior MI. (Level of Evidence: C)

2. In the absence of contraindications, it is reasonable to administer fibrinolytic therapy to patients with symptoms of STEMI beginning within the prior 12 to 24 hours who have continuing ischemic symptoms and ST elevation greater than 0.1 mV in at least two contiguous precordial leads or at least two adjacent limb leads. (Level of Evidence: B)

Class III

1. Fibrinolytic therapy should not be administered to asymptomatic patients whose initial symptoms of STEMI began more than 24 hours earlier. (Level of Evidence: C)

2. Fibrinolytic therapy should not be administered to patients whose 12-lead ECG shows only ST-segment depression except if a true posterior MI is suspected. (Level of Evidence: A)

Primary PCI

Approximately 95 percent of patients who are treated with primary PCI obtain complete reperfusion versus 50 to 60 percent of patients who are treated with thrombolytics. Primary PCI is also associated with a lower risk of stroke and diagnostic angiography quickly defines coronary anatomy, left ventricular (LV) function, and mechanical complications. However, invasive cardiovascular services are only available at <10 percent of hospitals in the United States and require a significant investment in infrastructure, personnel, and training, as well as maintenance in case volume and expertise.

A meta-analysis by Keeley et al. of 23 trials that included 3872 patients treated with primary PCI and 3867 patients treated with thrombolytics showed that PCI was superior to thrombolytic therapy.[39] Primary PCI was associated with a lower mortality rate (7 percent vs. 9 percent; $p = 0.0002$), less reinfarction (3 percent vs. 7 percent; $p = 0.0001$), and fewer strokes (1 percent vs. 2 percent; $p = 0.0004$) at 30 days when compared to thrombolysis. PCI capability, however, is only available at <50 percent of hospitals in the United States and each 30-minute delay from symptom onset to balloon inflation

---

TABLE 60–2

Absolute and Relative Contraindications for Thrombolytic Therapy in Patients with ST-Segment Elevation Myocardial Infarction

ABSOLUTE CONTRAINDICATIONS

Any prior intracranial hemorrhage
Known structural cerebral vascular lesion
Known intracranial neoplasm
Ischemic stroke within the past 3 months (except for acute stroke within 3 hours)
Suspected aortic dissection
Active bleeding or bleeding diathesis (excluding menses)
Significant closed-head or facial trauma within 3 months

RELATIVE CONTRAINDICATIONS

History of chronic, severe, poorly controlled hypertension
Systolic pressure >180 mmHg or diastolic 110 mmHg
History of prior ischemic stroke >3 months previously, dementia, or known intracranial pathology not covered in absolute contraindications
Recent (within 2 to 4 weeks) internal bleeding
Noncompressible vascular punctures
Pregnancy
Active peptic ulcer
Current use of anticoagulants: the higher the international normalized ratio, the higher the risk of bleeding
For streptokinase/anistreplase: prior exposure (more than 5 days previously) or prior allergic reaction to these agents

TABLE 60–3

Fibrin-Specific Thrombolytic Agents

CHARACTERISTIC	ALTEPLASE (tPA)	RETEPLASE (rPA)	TENECTEPLASE (tPA)	LANOTEPLASE (nPA)
Immunogenicity	No	No	No	?
Plasminogen activation	Direct	Direct	Direct	Direct
Fibrin specificity	++	+	+++	+
Plasma half-life	4 to 6 min	18 min	20 min	37 min
Dose	15-mg bolus plus 90-min infusion up to 85 mg	10+10-MU double bolus 30 min apart	± 0.5 mg/kg single bolus	120 KU/kg single bolus
PAI-1 resistance	No	?	Yes	?
Genetic alteration to native tPA	No	Yes	Yes	Yes
	Recombinant version	Finger, EGF, and kringle-1 regions deleted	2 single amino acid substitutions in kringle-1 and substitution of 4 amino acids in catalytic domain	Finger, EGF regions deleted and glycosylation sites in kringle-1 domain modified

EGF, epidermal growth factor; PAI, plasminogen activator inhibitor; nPA, lanoteplase; rPA, reteplase; tPA, tissue plasminogen activator.

TABLE 60–4

Trials Comparing In-hospital Thrombolysis with Transfer for Percutaneous Coronary Intervention (PCI) in Patients Presenting <12 Hours from the Onset of Chest Pain

		DEATH, REINFARCTION, DISABLING STROKE AT 30 DAYS		
	N	THROMBOLYSIS	TRANSFER FOR PCI	P VALUE
PRAGUE-2[133]	850	15.2%	8.4%	<0.003
AIR PAMI[134]	138	13.6%	8.4%	0.33
DANAMI-2[135]	1572	13.7%	8.0%	<0.001

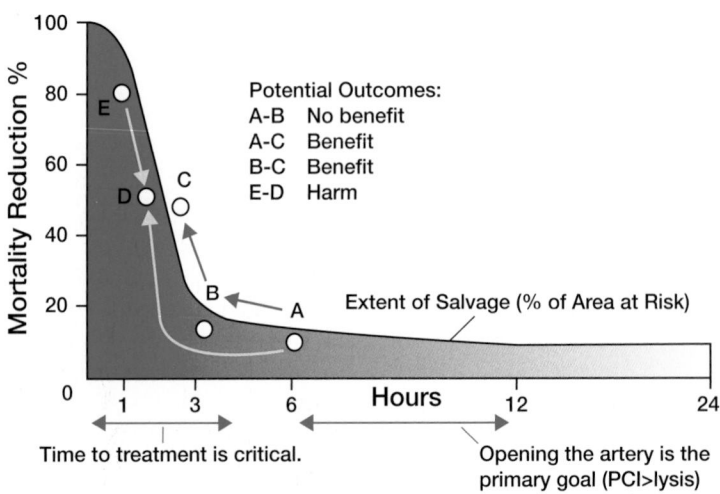

FIGURE 60–2. Relationship between mortality reduction and extent of myocardial salvage. *Source: Adapted with permission from Gersh, Stone, White, et al.[36]*

during primary PCI is associated with a 7.5 percent relative increase in mortality at 1 year.[40] In addition, a meta-analysis of data from 23 trials that included 7739 patients, which compared thrombolytic therapy to primary PCI by Nallamothu and Bates, demonstrated that the mortality advantage of primary PCI is lost if the door-to-balloon time is 60 minutes greater than the door-to-needle time for thrombolytic therapy.[41]

Three large-scale, randomized trials have compared thrombolysis to transfer for primary PCI in STEMI patients (Table 60–4). The combined end point of death, reinfarction, and disabling stroke at 30 days was significantly lower in the patients treated with primary PCI. Although transfer for primary PCI appears to be the treatment of choice, two important points need to be made. First, the transport time in these trials was extremely short (median time in the DANAMI-2 trial was 32 minutes) and these times may not be achievable outside of a clinical trial and in areas in which longer distances and weather may play a substantial role in hindering rapid transport. Second, thrombolytic therapy still has a critically important role during the "golden hour" (Fig. 60–2) of myocardial infarction or when there is a delay in transfer.[36] The mortality rates and infarct size in patients treated with thrombolytic therapy within the first 60 to 90 minutes of symptoms are extremely low, suggesting that thrombolytic therapy still plays a vital role in the management of patients presenting to hospitals without primary PCI capability. Also, the benefit of primary PCI appears to be mainly in high-risk patients, which were a minority of the patients in the trial (Fig. 60–3).[42] The *Clinical Practice Guidelines* recommend the following (see Chap. 11)[19]:

Class I

1. *General considerations: If immediately available, primary PCI should be performed in patients with STEMI (including true posterior MI) or MI with new or presumably new LBBB who can undergo PCI of the infarct artery within 12 hours of symptom onset, if performed in a timely fashion (balloon inflation within 90 minutes of presentation) by persons skilled in the procedure (individuals who perform more than 75 PCI procedures per year). The procedure should be supported by experienced personnel in an appropriate laboratory environment (a laboratory that performs more than 200 PCI procedures per year, of which at least 36 are primary PCI for STEMI, and has cardiac surgery capability). (Level of Evidence: A)*

2. *Specific considerations:*

   a. *Primary PCI should be performed as quickly as possible with a goal of a medical contact-to-balloon or door-to-balloon interval of within 90 minutes. (Level of Evidence: B)*

   b. *If the symptom duration is within 3 hours and the expected door-to-balloon time minus the expected door-to-needle time is:*

      i. *within 1 hour, primary PCI is generally preferred. (Level of Evidence: B)*

      ii. *greater than 1 hour, fibrinolytic therapy (fibrin-specific agents) is generally preferred. (Level of Evidence: B)*

   c. *If symptom duration is greater than 3 hours, primary PCI is generally preferred and should be performed with a medical contact-to-balloon or door-to-balloon interval as short as possible and a goal of within 90 minutes. (Level of Evidence: B)*

   d. *Primary PCI should be performed for patients younger than 75 years old with ST elevation or LBBB who develop shock within 36 hours of MI and are suitable for revascularization that can be performed within 18 hours of shock unless further support is futile because of the patient's wishes or contraindications/unsuitability for further invasive care. (Level of Evidence: A)*

   e. *Primary PCI should be performed in patients with severe congestive heart failure and/or pulmonary edema (Killip class 3) and onset of symptoms within 12 hours. The medical contact-to-balloon or door-to-balloon time*

should be as short as possible (i.e., goal within 90 minutes). (Level of Evidence: B)

Class IIa

1. *Primary PCI is reasonable for selected patients age 75 years or older with ST elevation or LBBB or who develop shock within 36 hours of MI and are suitable for revascularization that can be performed within 18 hours of shock. Patients with good prior functional status who are suitable for revascularization and agree to invasive care may be selected for such an invasive strategy. (Level of Evidence: B)*

2. *It is reasonable to perform primary PCI for patients with onset of symptoms within the prior 12 to 24 hours and one or more of the following:*

   a. *Severe congestive heart failure (Level of Evidence C)*

   b. *Hemodynamic or electrical instability (Level of Evidence: C)*

   c. *Persistent ischemic symptoms. (Level of Evidence: C)*

Class IIb

1. *The benefit of primary PCI for STEMI patients eligible for fibrinolysis is not well established when performed by an operator who performs fewer than 75 PCI procedures per year. (Level of Evidence: C)*

Class III

1. *PCI should not be performed in a noninfarct artery at the time of primary PCI in patients without hemodynamic compromise. (Level of Evidence: C)*

2. *Primary PCI should not be performed in asymptomatic patients more than 12 hours after onset of STEMI if they are hemodynamically and electrically stable. (Level of Evidence: C)*

- DANAMI-2
- 1,527 patients
- Stratified by TIMI risk score

  ■ Fibrinolysis
  ■ PPCI

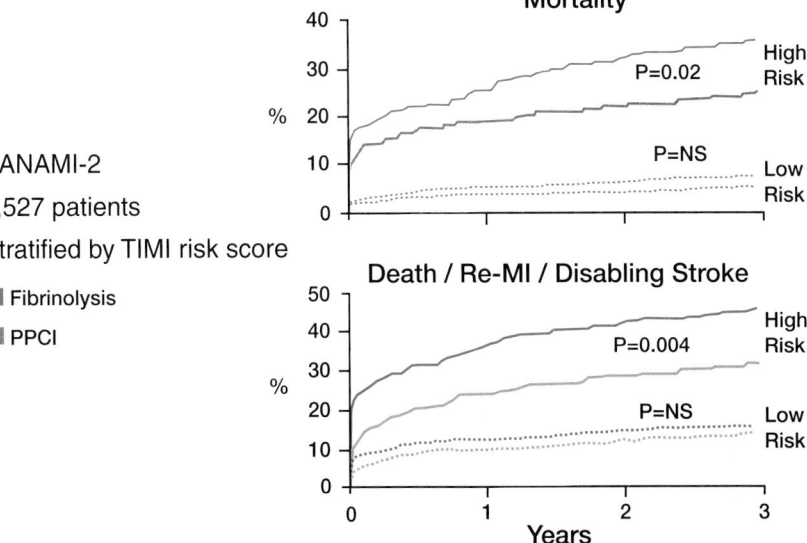

FIGURE 60–3. Risk stratification and the results of primary PCI in patients from the DANAMI 2 trial. MI, myocardial infarction; PPCI, primary percutaneous coronary intervention; TIMI, Thrombolysis in Myocardial Infarction. *Source: Modified from Thune, Hoefsten, Lindholm, et al.[42]*

Thrombolytic-Facilitated PCI

Thrombolytic-facilitated PCI refers to the pretreatment with thrombolytics in STEMI patients as a bridge to immediate PCI. This pretreatment has been proposed as a method to initiate earlier reperfusion and reduce ischemic time and infarct size in patients who experience a delay before the onset of PCI. Thrombolytic facility therapy, however, can also expose patients to a higher risk of bleeding. Currently, three trials have investigated the use of thrombolytic-facilitated PCI in STEMI. In the BRAVE (Bavarian Reperfusion Alternatives Evaluation) study, 253 STEMI patients undergoing primary PCI were randomized to pretreatment with a glycoprotein IIb/IIIa inhibitor (abciximab) alone, or half-dose thrombolytic (reteplase) plus abciximab.[43] The primary end point of total infarct size was similar between the two groups (11.5 percent abciximab only vs. 13 percent in the combination group; $p = 0.81$). In addition, there was no difference in the combined secondary end point of death, recurrent MI, or stroke (4.7 percent abciximab only vs. 6.4 percent in the combination group; $p = 0.56$). Major bleeding complications were more frequent in the combination group, although this was not statistically significant (1.6 percent abciximab only vs. 5.6 percent in the combination group; $p = 0.16$).

The ASSENT 4 trial randomized 1666 STEMI patients undergoing immediate PCI to pretreatment with a thrombolytic (tenecteplase) or placebo. The Data Safety Monitoring Board halted the trial prior to the enrollment of the 4000 anticipated patients because of an increased 30-day mortality rate in the facilitated PCI group (6.0 percent vs. 3.8 percent; $p = 0.004$).[44] Patients in the thrombolytic plus PCI group also had a greater incidence of stroke (1.81 percent vs. 0 percent; $p <0.001$), bleeding (31.3 percent vs. 23.4 percent; $p <0.001$), and reinfarction (4.1 percent vs. 1.9 percent; $p = 0.01$).

The CAPITAL-AMI (Combined Angioplasty and Pharmacological Intervention versus Thrombolysis Alone in Acute Myocardial Infarction) study randomized 170 STEMI patients to treatment with TNK alone, or TNK followed by immediate PCI.[45] The composite primary end point of death, reinfarction, recurrent unstable ischemia, or stroke at 6 months occurred in 24.4 percent of the patients in the TNK group and in 11.6 percent of patients in the TNK plus PCI group ($p = 0.04$). This difference was mainly driven by a reduction in the rate of recurrent unstable ischemia (20.7 percent vs. 8.1 percent; $p = 0.03$). However, it is important to note that the trial did not include a group that was treated with primary PCI alone.

The WEST (Which Early ST-elevation Myocardial Infarction Therapy) trial randomized 304 STEMI patients presenting within 6 hours from the onset of symptoms to one of three treatment strategies: TNK alone, TNK followed by mandatory angiography within 24 hours, or primary PCI.[46] The combined 30-day end point of death, reinfarction, refractory ischemia, congestive heart failure, cardiogenic shock, and major ventricular arrhythmias was similar in all three groups. There was, however, a significant lower rate of death and reinfarction in the primary PCI group compared with the two TNK-treated groups (4 percent vs. 13 percent; $p = 0.021$).

In the ongoing FINESSE (Facilitated Intervention with Enhanced Reperfusion Speed to Stop Events) trial, STEMI patients undergoing immediate PCI are randomized to receive one of the following three strategies: half-dose thrombolytic (reteplase) plus a glycoprotein IIb/IIIa inhibitor (abciximab), early administration of abciximab, or late administration of abciximab.

Until the results of the FINESSE trial become available, the current data clearly do not support the use of thrombolytic-facilitated PCI. The preferred reperfusion strategies for STEMI patients should continue to be thrombolytic therapy or primary PCI.

[ ] SELECTION OF THE OPTIMAL REPERFUSION STRATEGY

Figures 60–4, 60–5, and 60–6 show a systematic, evidence-based framework for selecting reperfusion strategies in STEMI patients. STEMI patients presenting to PCI-capable hospitals should undergo primary PCI with a target door-to-balloon time of <90 minutes. If the hospital does not have PCI capability, the clinician must first determine if the patient is eligible for thrombolytic therapy (see Table 60–2). Patients ineligible for thrombolytic therapy should be transferred for primary PCI. For those who are eligible for thrombolytic therapy, the clinician must then consider two important factors: duration from onset of symptoms ("fixed" ischemia time) and transport time to the nearest PCI facility ("incurred" ischemia time). These two factors can be incorporated into a 2 × 3 table to select a reperfusion strategy (Fig. 60–6).

Patients facing a transport time <30 minutes should be transferred for primary PCI. Thrombolytic-eligible patients who present <2 to 3 hours from onset of symptoms and have >30 minutes transport time should receive thrombolytic therapy. Patients presenting >2 to 3 hours after the onset of chest pain and have a transport time of 60 minutes or less should be promptly transported for primary PCI. If the anticipated transport time is >60 minutes, patients can be treated with either thrombolytic therapy or primary PCI. The choice of using thrombolytic therapy should always be considered along with the risk of bleeding in each individual patient.

All patients receiving thrombolytic therapy should also be transferred to a PCI facility for potential failure to reperfuse

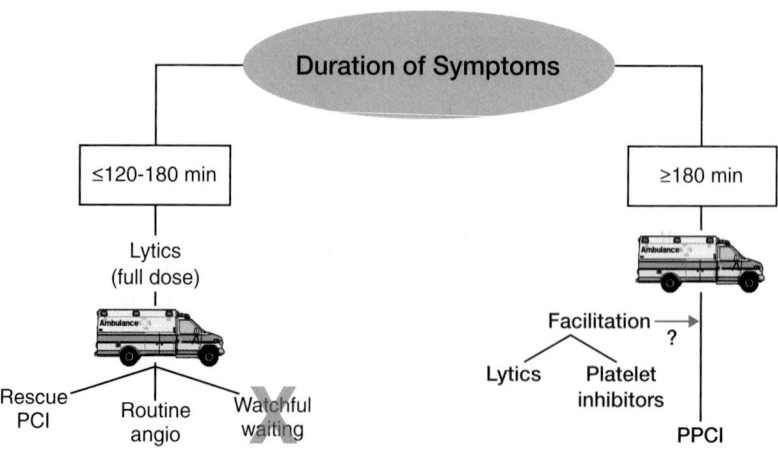

FIGURE 60–4. Reperfusion strategies in community hospitals. angio, Angiogram; PPCI, primary percutaneous coronary intervention.

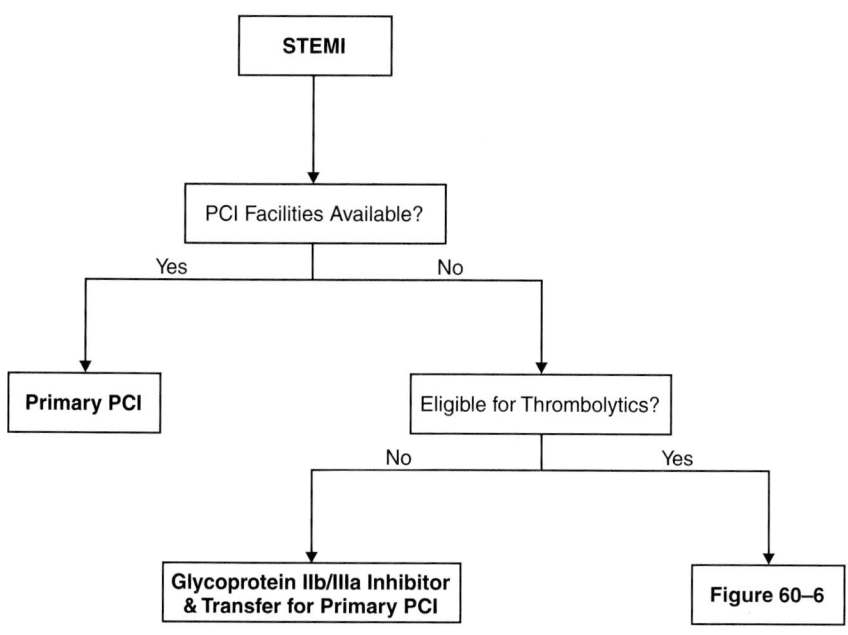

FIGURE 60–5. Algorithm for deciding a reperfusion strategy in ST-segment elevation myocardial infarction (STEMI) patients. PCI, percutaneous coronary intervention.

(ongoing chest pain or <50 percent resolution of ST-segment elevation at 90 minutes) and rescue PCI. Recent randomized data suggest that all STEMI patients who are treated with thrombolytic therapy benefit from routine coronary angiography during the index hospitalization.[47]

[ ] ADJUVANT ANTIPLATELET THERAPY

Clopidogrel

Clopidogrel is an oral thienopyridine prodrug whose active metabolite inhibits the activation of platelets by adenosine diphosphate. Its antiplatelet effects are more potent than aspirin and less potent than the glycoprotein IIb/IIIa inhibitors.

Use with Thrombolytic Therapy Clopidogrel in combination with thrombolytic therapy has been studied in the CLARITY-TIMI 28 (Clopidogrel as Adjunctive Reperfusion Therapy–Thrombolysis in Myocardial Infarction 28) trial.[48] In this trial, 3491 STEMI patients 75 years of age or younger who were treated with thrombolytics were randomized to therapy with aspirin plus placebo or aspirin plus clopidogrel. Clopidogrel was given as a 300-mg loading dose within minutes of thrombolysis and 75 mg daily thereafter. The composite primary end point of death, reinfarction prior to angiography, or occluded infarct-related artery at angiography occurred in 15 percent of patients in the clopidogrel group and in 22 percent of patients in the placebo group (*p* <0.001).[48] The use of clopidogrel was not associated with a higher rate of major or minor bleeding.

Although a loading dose of 300 mg of clopidogrel was not associated with a greater risk of bleeding, patients older than 75 years of age were excluded from the study. Patients older than 75 years of age were included in the COMMIT[25] (a randomized, placebo-controlled trial of adding clopidogrel to aspirin in 46,000 acute myocardial infarction patients), which randomized 45,849 STEMI patients treated with thrombolysis to therapy with aspirin plus placebo or aspirin plus clopidogrel. Unlike the CLARITY trial, a 300-mg loading dose was not given. Instead, patients randomized to the clopidogrel arm received 75 mg of clopidogrel at the time of thrombolysis and then 75 mg daily for the duration of hospitalization. Patients in the clopidogrel arm had a lower rate of the composite end point of death, reinfarction, or stroke (9.3 percent versus 10.1 percent; *p* = 0.002) and no increase in major or minor bleeding.

The data from these two trials suggest that patients treated with thrombolytics should receive clopidogrel. For patients older than 75 years of age, 75 mg of clopidogrel without a loading dose should be used. In patients 75 years of age or younger, the current data suggest a 300-mg loading-dose followed by 75 mg daily of clopidogrel is beneficial and safe.

Use with Primary PCI Although data from the PCI-CURE (Clopidogrel in Unstable Angina to Prevent Recurrent Ischemic Events) trial (effects of pretreatment with clopidogrel and aspirin followed by long-term therapy in patients undergoing percutaneous coronary intervention)[49] demonstrated that the early use of clopidogrel in non ST-elevation acute coronary syndrome patients who eventually undergo PCI is of benefit (see Chap. 59), their use in the setting of primary PCI for STEMI is unknown. No studies have compared early administration of clopidogrel to the early use

Transport Time ("Incurred Ischemic Time")	Duration from Onset of Symptoms ("Fixed Ischemic Time")	
	0–3 Hours	>3 Hours
0–30 Minutes	PCI + GP IIb/IIIa	PCI + GP IIb/IIIa
30–60 Minutes	Thrombolytic + Clopidogrel	PCI + GP IIb/IIIa
>60 Minutes	Thrombolytic + Clopidogrel	Thrombolytic + Clopidogrel or PCI + GP IIb/IIIa

FIGURE 60–6. Table organizing the treatment strategies for thrombolytic eligible ST-segment elevation myocardial infarction patients who present to hospitals without facilities for percutaneous coronary intervention. GPIIb/IIIa, glycoprotein IIb/IIIa inhibitor; lytics, thrombolysis (patients should be immediately transferred to a PCI facility after thrombolysis); PCI, transfer for percutaneous coronary intervention.

of glycoprotein IIb/IIIa inhibitors in STEMI patients. *Therefore, clopidogrel should not be used in STEMI patients prior to visualization of the coronary anatomy at the time of coronary angiography.*

Glycoprotein IIb/IIIa Inhibitors

Glycoprotein IIb/IIIa inhibitors are potent agents that inhibit the final common pathway for platelet aggregation. There are currently three intravenous agents available in the United States: abciximab, tirofiban, and eptifibatide.

Use with Thrombolytic Therapy

Thrombolysis has been shown to be a potent activator of platelets[50] and the concomitant use of aspirin along with thrombolysis has been shown to be beneficial.[51] Two dose-finding studies[52,53] have shown that the glycoprotein IIb/IIIa inhibitor abciximab, when used in combination with half-dose thrombolytics, improves coronary artery blood flow in STEMI patients. Three subsequent randomized trials (Table 60–5) have investigated combination therapy with a glycoprotein IIb/IIIa inhibitor and half-dose thrombolytic therapy.[29,54,55] The largest of the trials was the GUSTO-V trial, which included 16,588 patients with STEMI who presented within 6 hours from the onset of chest pain. The primary end point, 30-day mortality, occurred in 5.6 percent of patients treated with abciximab plus half-dose reteplase and in 5.9 percent of patients treated with full-dose reteplase ($p = 0.43$).[54] Patients treated with the combination therapy had a higher rate of major (1.1 percent vs. 0.5 percent; $p < 0.0001$) and minor bleeding (20 percent vs. 11.4 percent; $p < 0.0001$).[54] This increased risk of bleeding and lack of survival benefit with combination therapy was also seen in the ASSENT-3[29] and INTEGRITI (Integrilin and Tenecteplase in Acute Myocardial Infarction)[55] trials (Table 60–5). Based on the results of these three trials, glycoprotein IIb/IIIa inhibitors should not be used in combination with thrombolytic therapy.

Use with Primary PCI

The early (prior to arrival in the catheterization laboratory) versus delayed (at the time of catheterization) use of glycoprotein IIb/IIIa inhibitors in STEMI patients was investigated in eight randomized trials (Table 60–6) involving abciximab,[56–58] tirofiban,[59–61] and eptifibatide.[62,63] A meta-analysis of six of these trials by Montalescot et al. showed that early administration of glycoprotein IIb/IIIa inhibitors in STEMI patients was associated with a greater prevalence of TIMI 2 or 3 flow (41.7 percent vs. 29.8 percent; $p < 0.001$) in the infarct-related artery prior to PCI.[64] Because prior studies have shown that better coronary artery flow after PCI is associated with less in-hospital and 1-year adverse outcomes,[65–67] early administration of glycoprotein IIb/IIIa inhibitors should probably be encouraged. The *Clinical Practice Guidelines* recommend the following (see Chap. 11)[19]:

Class IIa

1. It is reasonable to start treatment with abciximab as early as possible before primary PCI (with or without stenting) in patients with STEMI. (Level of Evidence: B)

Class IIb

1. Treatment with tirofiban or eptifibatide may be considered before primary PCI (with or without stenting) in patients with STEMI. (Level of Evidence: C)

MANAGEMENT IN THE CARDIAC CATHETERIZATION LABORATORY

【 】 RAPID TRANSPORT PROTOCOL

For STEMI patients who present to hospitals without PCI capabilities, a well-developed plan for transfer to a PCI hospital is essential. This plan should be evidence based, easy to activate, and time efficient. It requires a multidisciplinary approach and coordination of personnel at the PCI facility, community hospital, and emergency transport service.

The Mayo Clinic developed a "Fast Track" protocol to facilitate the management and transport of STEMI patients from surrounding community hospitals. The protocol has 23 activated regional hospitals and 3 helicopters covering a service area extending 100 nautical miles. This rapid transport protocol involves four key concepts:

1. The identification and elimination of inefficient practices involved in the management of STEMI patients from referring hospitals.
2. Developing an evidence-based protocol to standardize the care of STEMI patients.
3. Implicating a communication network to ensure easy activation of the rapid transport protocol system by community hospitals.
4. Reducing the time for activation of the cardiac cath lab team.

The implication of these processes has resulted in a significant reduction in the median door-to-balloon times from 202 to 107 minutes in all STEMI patients transferred to the Mayo Clinic.[68]

Primary PCI should be performed by operators who perform at least 75 PCIs per year, 36 of which are primary PCI for STEMI patients in a catheterization laboratory that performs at least 200 PCIs per year. The *Clinical Practice Guidelines* recommend the following (see Chap. 11)[19]:

Class I

1. Every community should have a written protocol that guides emergency medical services system personnel in determining where to take patients with suspected or confirmed STEMI. (Level of Evidence: C)

2. Hospitals should establish multidisciplinary teams (including primary care physicians, emergency medicine physicians, cardiologists, nurses, and laboratorians) to develop guideline-based, institution-specific written protocols for triaging and managing patients who are seen in the prehospital setting or present to the emergency department with symptoms suggestive of STEMI. (Level of Evidence: B)

【 】 PRIMARY PCI WITHOUT ONSITE SURGICAL BACKUP

Primary PCI at centers without surgical backup has been proposed as a possible method of increasing the availability of PCI to STEMI patients. Aversano et al. conducted the multicenter, prospective, randomized C-PORT (Atlantic Cardiovascular Patient Outcomes Research Team) trial to investigate the feasibility of off-

TABLE 60-5

Randomized Trials Comparing Combination Therapy with a Glycoprotein IIb/IIIa Inhibitor Plus Half-Dose Thrombolytic Therapy to Full Dose Thrombolytics in Patients with ST-Segment Elevation Myocardial Infarction

	N	GLYCOPROTEIN IIB/IIIA INHIBITOR	THROMBOLYTIC AGENT	MORTALITY RATE (%)		MAJOR BLEEDING RATE (%)	
				COMBINATION THERAPY	THROMBOLYTIC-ONLY THERAPY	COMBINATION THERAPY	THROMBOLYTIC-ONLY THERAPY
GUSTO-V[46]	16588	Abciximab	Reteplase	5.6	5.9	1.1	0.5
ASSENT-3[25]	6095	Abciximab	Tenecteplase	6.6	6.0	4.3	2.2
INTEGRITI[47]	438	Eptifibatide	Tenecteplase	3.0	5.0	7.6	2.5

ASSENT, Assessment of the Safety and Efficacy of a New Thrombolytic; GUSTO, Global Utilization of Streptokinase and Tissue Plasminogen Activator for Occluded Arteries; INTEGRITI, Integrilin and Tenecteplase in Acute Myocardial Infarction.

TABLE 60-6

Early Administration of Glycoprotein IIb/IIIa Inhibitors in ST-Segment Elevation Myocardial Infarction Patients Undergoing Primary Percutaneous Coronary Intervention

	N	AGENT	TIMI 2 OR 3 FLOW (PERCENT OF PATIENTS)		P VALUE
			EARLY ADMINISTRATION	LATE ADMINISTRATION	
Zorman et al.[48]	112	Abciximab	32	13	0.04
REOMOBILE[49]	100	Abciximab	52	48	NS
ERAMI[50]	74	Abciximab	31	26	NS
On-TIME[53]	307	Tirofiban	43	34	0.04
TIGER-PA[51]	100	Tirofiban	46	18	0.007
Cullip et al.[52]	58	Tirofiban	39	27	NS
Cullip et al.[54]	60	Eptifibatide	57	13	<0.01
INTAMI[55]	102	Eptifibatide	42	33	0.01

site primary PCI. In this study, 11 centers with cardiac catheterization facilities, but no surgical backup, randomized 451 thrombolytic therapy-eligible STEMI patients to thrombolytic therapy or primary PCI at the community hospital. The composite primary end point of death, recurrent MI, and stroke at 6 months occurred in 19.9 percent of those in the thrombolytic group and 12.4 percent of those in the PCI group ($p = 0.03$).[69]

Our own experience with offsite primary PCI was been positive. Of the 1007 PCIs performed at a Mayo Clinic affiliate hospital between 1999 and 2005, 285 were primary PCIs for STEMI patients.[70] There was a 93 percent success rate without any major complications and no patients required emergency bypass surgery. The survival of primary PCI patients treated at the offsite catheterization laboratory was identical to those treated at the Mayo Clinic.

Although these results suggest that primary PCI at sites without surgical backup is feasible, many cardiologists believe that offsite PCI may not be as successful outside of a clinical trial, or where the quality control may not be as rigorous and the intervention cardiologists not as experienced. Data from our center, however, suggest that good clinical outcomes can occur if a program emphasizing quality control and experienced interventionalists is developed. The ACC/AHA guidelines for PCI recommend[71]:

Class IIb

1. *Primary PCI for patients with STEMI might be considered in hospitals without onsite cardiac surgery, provided that appropriate planning for program development has been accomplished, including appropriately experienced physician-operators (more than 75 total PCIs and, ideally, at least 11 primary PCIs per year for STEMI), an experienced catheterization team on a 24 hours per day, 7 days per week call schedule, and a well-equipped catheterization laboratory with digital imaging equipment, a full array of interventional equipment, and intraaortic balloon pump capability, and provided that there is a proven plan for rapid transport to a cardiac surgery operating room in a nearby hospital with appropriate hemodynamic support capability for transfer. The procedure should be limited to patients with STEMI or MI with new or presumably new left bundle-branch block on ECG, and should be performed in a timely fashion (goal of balloon inflation within 90 minutes of presentation) by persons skilled in the procedure (at least 75 PCIs per year) and at hospitals performing a minimum of 36 primary PCI procedures per year. (Level of Evidence: B)*

Class III

1. *Primary PCI should not be performed in hospitals without onsite cardiac surgery and without a proven plan for rapid transport to a cardiac surgery operating room in a nearby hospital, or without appropriate hemodynamic support capability for transfer. (Level of Evidence: C)*

[ ] DISTAL PROTECTION AND THROMBECTOMY DEVICES

Distal embolization of the intracoronary thrombus at the time of PCI and subsequent no-reflow is a concern. To prevent embolization, distal protection devices have been used in STEMI patients. The

EMERALD (Enhanced Myocardial Efficacy and Recovery by Aspiration of Liberated Debris) trial investigated the use of the Guidewire Plus distal occlusion device in 501 STEMI patients. Participants were randomized to conventional primary PCI or PCI with the Guidewire Plus device. The primary end point of ST-segment resolution measured 30 minutes after PCI by continuous Holter monitoring and infarct size measured by technetium (Tc)-99m sestamibi imaging between days 5 and 14 was similar between both groups.[72] Another distal protection device, the Filter Wire-EX, was investigated in the PROMISE (Protection Devices in PCI Treatment of Myocardial Infarction for Salvage of Endangered Myocardium) trial. Two hundred AMI patients undergoing PCI were randomized to conventional therapy or PCI with the Filter Wire-EX distal protection device.[73] The primary end point of maximal adenosine-induced Doppler flow velocity in the recanalized infarct artery was similar in both groups. The secondary end point of infarct size as determined by MRI was also similar between the two groups.

Mechanical debulking of intracoronary thrombus has also been proposed as a method to reduce distal embolization. The AIMI (AngioJet Rheolytic Thrombectomy In Patients Undergoing Primary Angioplasty for Acute Myocardial Infarction) trial randomized 480 STEMI patients to conventional PCI or PCI plus rheolytic thrombectomy with the AngioJet thrombectomy device. Patients in the thrombectomy group had a larger infract size (12.5 percent vs. 9.8 percent; $p = 0.03$) and a lower rate of postprocedure TIMI 3 flow (92 percent vs. 96 percent; $p < 0.02$). Thus the routine use of distal protection devices or thrombectomy is not supported by the current data.

[ ] ANGIOPLASTY VERSUS STENT PLACEMENT

Two large, randomized studies have investigated whether STEMI patients undergoing primary PCI should be managed with angioplasty alone or undergo stent placement. The Stent-PAMI (Primary Angioplasty in Myocardial Infarction Study Group) trial randomized 900 STEMI patients who were to undergo primary PCI to either angioplasty alone or stent placement.[74] The combined primary end point of death, nonfatal reinfarction, disabling stroke, or target-vessel revascularization at 6 months occurred in 12.6 percent of those in the stent group and in 20.1 percent in the angioplasty group ($p < 0.01$). Because there was no significant difference between the two groups in mortality (4.2 percent vs. 2.7 percent; $p = 0.27$), the results were mainly driven by the decrease need for revascularization in the stent group (20.3 percent vs. 33.5 percent; $p = 0.001$).

In the CADILLAC (Controlled Abciximab and Device Investigation to Lower Late Angioplasty Complications) trial, 2082 STEMI patients who were to undergo primary PCI were randomized in a 2×2 manner to angioplasty or stenting followed by heparin alone or heparin plus the glycoprotein IIb/IIIa inhibitor abciximab.[75] The combined primary end point of death, reinfarction, disabling stroke, and target-vessel revascularization at 6 months occurred in 20 percent of patients in the angioplasty-alone group, 16.5 percent of those in the angioplasty-plus-abciximab group, 11.5 percent in the stenting-alone group, and in 10.2 percent of those in the stent-plus-abciximab group ($p = 0.001$ for trend). As in the Stent-PAMI trial, the primary end point was driven by the decrease need for revascularization in those treated with coronary stenting.

Based on these two trials, STEMI patients who are to undergo primary PCI should be treated with coronary stenting so as to reduce restenosis and the need for repeat revascularization. Because there is no significant difference in mortality or reinfarction, angioplasty alone is a reasonable treatment for patients in whom stenting is not technically possible or not desired. The latter scenario is often encountered in STEMI patients who require coronary artery bypass surgery in the near future for noninfarct-related arteries, and in those patients with comorbid conditions that prevent them from taking dual antiplatelet therapy.

[ ] DRUG-ELUTING STENTS

Several studies have demonstrated that drug-eluting stents significantly reduce the occurrence of restenosis in patients undergoing PCI.[76–79] These studies, however, were in patients who were undergoing elective PCI and did not include STEMI patients. The preliminary results of two randomized studies investigating the use of drug-eluting stents for primary PCI in STEMI patients were recently presented. In the TYPHOON (Trial to Assess the Use of the Cypher Stent in Acute Myocardial Infarction Treated with Balloon Angioplasty) trial, 712 STEMI patients who were to undergo primary PCI were randomized to receive either a Cypher drug-eluting stent or a bare metal stent.[80] The combined primary end point of death, reinfarction, or target-vessel revascularization at 1 year occurred in 7.3 percent of the patients in the Cypher group and in 14.3 percent of patients in the bare metal stent group (p = 0.0036). The end point, however, was mainly driven by a reduction in target-vessel revascularization (3.7 percent vs. 12.6 percent; p <0.0001). Rates of stent thrombosis were similar in both groups (3.4 percent Cypher vs. 3.6 percent bare metal).

The PASSION (Paclitaxel Eluting Stent versus Conventional Stent in ST-segment Elevation Myocardial Infarction) trial randomized 619 STEMI patients who were to undergo primary PCI to the Taxus drug-eluting stent or to an Express bare metal stent.[81] Unlike the TYPHOON trial, use of the Taxus drug-eluting stent *was not* associated with a significant difference in the 1 year combined primary end point of death, reinfarction, or target-vessel revascularization (8.7 percent Taxus vs. 12.6 percent bare metal; p = 0.12). The rate of target vessel revascularization was 6.2 percent in the Taxus group and 7.4 percent in the bare metal group (p = 0.23).

Consequently, the use of drug-eluting stents in the setting of STEMI is unclear at this time. For those patients who do receive a drug-eluting stent, the importance of dual antiplatelet therapy must be emphasized. A registry of acute myocardial infarction patients who received drug-eluting stents revealed that 13.6 percent of patients stop taking clopidogrel after the first month of therapy. These patients had a 1-year mortality rate of 7.5 percent, which was significantly greater than the death rate of .7 percent in those who were compliant with dual antiplatelet therapy.[82]

MANAGEMENT IN THE CORONARY CARE UNIT
[ ] THROMBOLYTIC-TREATED PATIENTS

On arrival in the coronary care unit (CCU), the first objective in the evaluation of thrombolytic-treated patients is to determine if reperfusion has been achieved. Successful thrombolysis is defined as complete resolution of chest pain and at least 50 percent ST-segment resolution 60 to 90 minutes after the initiation of thrombolytic therapy.[83] For those patients who fail to reperfuse or who develop recurrent ischemia or infarction, three treatment options are available: conservative management, repeat lysis, or rescue PCI (Fig. 60–7). In the REACT (Rescue Angioplasty after Failed Thrombolytic Therapy for Acute Myocardial Infarction) trial, 427 STEMI patients who failed initial thrombolytic therapy were randomized to one of these three treatment options.[84] The combined primary end point of death, reinfarction, or severe heart failure within 6 months occurred in 29.8 percent of patients in the conservative group, in 31 percent of those receiving repeat thrombolysis, and in 15.3 percent of patients in the rescue PCI group (p = 0.004). There was no significant difference in mortality and the results were mainly driven by a decrease in the reinfarction rate (8.5 percent conservative group, 10.6 percent repeat thrombolysis group, 2.1 percent rescue PCI group; p <0.01). Because rescue PCI appears to be the treatment of choice for patients who fail thrombolytic therapy, all patients who are given thrombolytics should be immediately transported to a PCI center in case of the need for rescue PCI.

If initial thrombolysis is successful, further risk stratification is needed. All patients with an ejection fraction less than 0.40 should undergo coronary angiography. Patients with an interpretable ECG and who are able to exercise can undergo a submaximal exercise treadmill test prior to discharge. For those who are unable to exercise, a pharmacologic stress test with imaging can be performed. If the initial ECG is uninterpretable, stress testing (either with exercise, if the patient is able, or pharmacologic) with imaging must be performed. Patients with abnormal stress testing should undergo coronary angiography prior to discharge.

As an increasingly used alternative to stress testing, STEMI patients successfully treated with thrombolysis undergo routine coronary angiography prior to discharge. In the GRACIA 1 (Grupo de Análisis de la Cardiopatía Isquémica Aguda) trial, 500 STEMI patients who were successfully treated with thrombolytic therapy were randomized to immediate coronary angiography within 24 hours of presentation or ischemic-driven (positive stress test prior to discharge) coronary angiography.[47] Of those who underwent immediate angiography, 80 percent underwent PCI of the infarct-

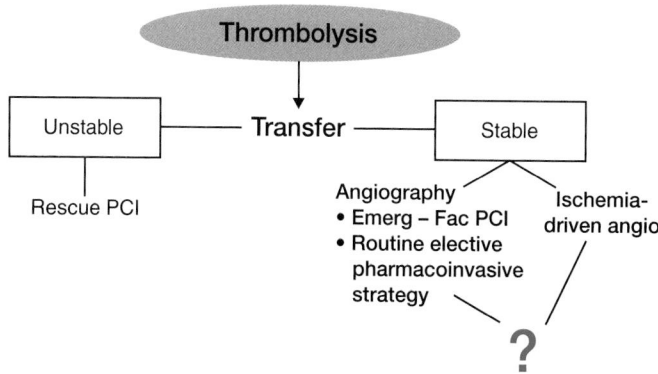

FIGURE 60–7. Potential postthrombolytic treatment strategies. Fac, facilitated; PCI, percutaneous coronary intervention.

related artery, 2 percent had bypass surgery, 1 percent had PCI of a noninfarct-related artery, and 16 percent had no intervention. The 1-year combined primary end point of death, reinfarction, and revascularization occurred in 9 percent of the immediate-angiography group and in 21 percent in the ischemic-driven group (*p* = 0.0008). The end point was driven by a decrease in revascularization (4 percent vs. 12 percent; *p* = 0.001) with only a trend for a reduction in death or reinfarction (7 percent vs. 12 percent; *p* = 0.07) in the immediate-angiography group. The *Clinical Practice Guidelines* recommend the following (see Chap. 11)[19]:

Class I

1. Exercise testing should be performed either in the hospital or early after discharge in STEMI patients who are not selected for cardiac catheterization and without high-risk features to assess the presence and extent of inducible ischemia. (Level of Evidence: B)

2. In patients with baseline abnormalities that compromise ECG interpretation, echocardiography or myocardial perfusion imaging should be added to standard exercise testing. (Level of Evidence: B)

Class IIa

1. It is reasonable to perform routine PCI in patients with LV ejection fraction less than or equal to 0.40, congestive heart failure, or serious ventricular arrhythmias. (Level of Evidence: C)

2. It is reasonable to perform PCI when there is documented clinical heart failure during the acute episode, even though subsequent evaluation shows preserved LV function (LV ejection fraction greater than 0.40). (Level of Evidence: C)

3. It is reasonable to monitor the pattern of ST elevation, cardiac rhythm, and clinical symptoms over the 60 to 180 minutes after initiation of fibrinolytic therapy. Noninvasive findings suggestive of reperfusion include relief of symptoms, maintenance or restoration of hemodynamic and or electrical stability, and a reduction of at least 50 percent of the initial ST-segment elevation injury pattern on a followup ECG 60 to 90 minutes after initiation of therapy. (Level of Evidence: B)

Class IIb

1. Routine PCI might be considered as part of an invasive strategy after fibrinolytic therapy. (Level of Evidence: B)

2. Exercise testing might be considered before discharge of patients recovering from STEMI to guide the postdischarge exercise prescription or to evaluate the functional significance of a coronary lesion previously identified at angiography. (Level of Evidence: C)

Class III

1. Exercise testing should not be performed within 2 to 3 days of STEMI in patients who have not undergone successful reperfusion. (Level of Evidence: C)

2. Exercise testing should not be performed to evaluate patients with STEMI who have unstable postinfarction angina, decompensated congestive heart failure, life-threatening cardiac arrhythmias, noncardiac conditions that severely limit their ability to exercise, or other absolute contraindications to exercise testing.[10,75] (Level of Evidence: C)

3. Exercise testing should not be used for risk stratification in patients with STEMI who have already been selected for cardiac catheterization. (Level of Evidence: C)

[ ] PHARMACOTHERAPY

Inhibition of the Renin–Angiotensin–Aldosterone System

Angiotensin-Converting Enzyme Inhibitors Nine trials, with cumulative enrollment of more than 100,000 patients, have documented the effects of angiotensin-converting enzyme (ACE) inhibitors on mortality in a prospective randomized fashion. These trials can be conveniently divided into those in which all patients were given the drug and those in which drug administration was limited to only patients who were at higher risk. The four nonselective trials include the Cooperative New Scandinavian Enalapril Survival Study-2 (CONSENSUS-2),[85] the Gruppo Italiano per lo Studio della Sopravvivenza nell'Infarto Miocardico-3 (GISSI-3),[86] the ISIS-4,[87] and the Chinese Cardiac Study (CCS-1).[88] In CONSENSUS-2, intravenous enalaprilat was administered within 24 hours of presentation followed by oral enalapril.[85] In the remaining studies, patients did not receive an initial IV load and in three of these four trials, the drug was initiated within 24 hours of presentation. In CONSENSUS-2, mortality was nonsignificantly increased in the treatment group, but in the remaining three trials, a statistically significant reduction in mortality was observed in the treatment group with about 5 lives saved per 1000 patients receiving ACE-inhibitor therapy.

Five trials studied the selective use of ACE inhibitors after acute myocardial infarction. These included the Survival And Ventricular Enlargement (SAVE) study,[89] the Trandolapril Cardiac Evaluation (TRACE) study,[90] the Acute Infarction Ramipril Efficacy (AIRE) study,[91] the Survival of Myocardial Infarction Long-Term Evaluation (SMILE) study,[92] and the Captopril and Thrombolysis Study (CATS).[93] In SAVE and TRACE, patients were selected by laboratory evidence of a left ventricular ejection fraction of less than 40 percent or wall-motion abnormality. In AIRE, transient heart failure was the entrance criterion. Clinically and statistically significant mortality reduction of 40 to 70 lives saved per 1000 patients treated was documented in 4 of these 5 trials.

Based on the results of these trials, it is reasonable to initiate therapy with ACE inhibitors within the first 24 hours as long as no contraindications exist and the patient is hemodynamically stable. Patients with an ejection fraction greater than 45 percent and no clinical evidence of heart failure, significant mitral regurgitation, or hypertension, can have therapy discontinued after determination of risk status while still hospitalized. Because captopril has the shortest half-life, overdosing and inadvertent hypotension may be most easily correctable with the use of this agent. In addition, the short half-life allows for more rapid titration. Intravenous administration is unnecessary unless the patient is unable to take oral medication. Duration of treatment is uncertain; however, many patients will be treated indefinitely.

Angiotensin Receptor Blockers Additional blockade of the renin–angiotensin system with the angiotensin receptor blocker valsartan was investigated in VALIANT (Valsartan in Acute Myocardial Infarction Trial).[94] This was a prospective, randomized, double-blinded trial involving 14,808 AMI patients complicated by impaired LV function (ejection fraction ≤0.35 on echocardiography or contrast angiography and ≤0.40 on radionuclide ventriculography) who were randomized to one of three groups: captopril only, valsartan only, or both captopril and valsartan. After a median followup of 25 months, the primary end point of cardiovascular death was 16.9 percent in the captopril group, 16.8 percent in the valsartan group, and 16.9 percent in the combination group (p = NS). The combination group, however, experienced a statistically significant greater amount of hypotension and renal dysfunction. The results of VALIANT suggest that valsartan is as effective as captopril in the management of AMI patients with LV dysfunction, but the combination of an ACE inhibitor and an angiotensin receptor blocker should be avoided.

In the OPTIMAAL (Optimal Trial in Myocardial Infarction with the Angiotensin II Antagonist Losartan), 5477 acute myocardial infarction patients were randomized to therapy with losartan or captopril.[95] The 3-year primary end point of all-cause mortality occurred in 18 percent of patients in the losartan groups and in 16 percent of those in the captopril group (p = 0.07). These studies suggest that ACE inhibitors should be used as primary therapy and angiotensin receptor blockers in those who cannot tolerate ACE inhibitors.

Aldosterone Antagonist The use of an aldosterone antagonist in patients with AMI complicated by LV dysfunction was studied in the EPHESUS (Eplerenone Post-Acute Myocardial Infarction Heart Failure Efficacy and Survival Study) trial.[96] The 6642 patients with AMI and a resulting ejection fraction <0.40 were randomized to the aldosterone antagonist eplerenone or placebo 3 to 14 days after admission. After a median followup of 16 months, the primary end point of death from any cause occurred in 14.4 percent of patients in the eplerenone group and 16.7 percent of patients in the placebo group (p = 0.008). As expected, eplerenone use was associated with a greater amount of hyperkalemia and less hypokalemia. Based on the results of the EPHESUS trial, it is reasonable to use an aldosterone antagonist in conjunction with β blockade and ACE inhibition in patients with AMI and subsequent LV dysfunction (ejection fraction <0.40). Diligent monitoring of the serum potassium must occur with patients who are treated with an aldosterone antagonist.

The *Clinical Practice Guidelines* recommend the following (see Chap. 11)[19]:

Class I

1. An ACE inhibitor should be administered orally during convalescence from STEMI in patients who tolerate this class of medication, and it should be continued over the long-term. (Level of Evidence: A)

2. An angiotensin receptor blocker should be administered to STEMI patients who are intolerant of ACE inhibitors and have either clinical or radiologic signs of heart failure or a LV ejection fraction less than 0.40. Valsartan and candesartan have demonstrated efficacy for this recommendation. (Level of Evidence: B)

3. Long-term aldosterone blockade should be prescribed for post-STEMI patients without significant renal dysfunction (creatinine should be less than or equal to 2.5 mg/dL in men and less than or equal to 2.0 mg/dL in women) or hyperkalemia (potassium should be less than or equal to 5.0 mEq/L) who are already receiving therapeutic doses of an ACE inhibitor, have a LV ejection fraction of less than or equal to 0.40, and have either symptomatic heart failure or diabetes. (Level of Evidence: A)

Class IIa

1. In STEMI patients who tolerate ACE inhibitors, an angiotensin receptor blocker can be useful as an alternative provided there are either clinical or radiologic signs of heart failure or the LV ejection fraction is less than 0.40. Valsartan and candesartan have established efficacy for this recommendation. (Level of Evidence: B)

β Blockade Initiation of β-blockade therapy in the CCU is essential in the management of STEMI patients. β Blockers have both acute and long-term benefits in STEMI patients treated with either lysis or primary PCI. A meta-analysis of 24,000 AMI patients demonstrated a significant 14 percent reduction in acute mortality and a 23 percent reduction in long-term mortality. Short-acting β blockade with metoprolol should be initiated as early as possible and rapidly titrated to the maximally tolerated dose. In patients who present with shock or heart failure, the initiation of β blockers should be delayed until patients become hemodynamically stable. The *Clinical Practice Guidelines* recommend the following (see Chap. 11)[19]:

Class I

1. Patients receiving β blockers within the first 24 hours of STEMI without adverse effects should continue to receive them during the early convalescent phase of STEMI. (Level of Evidence: A)

2. Patients without contraindications to β blockers who did not receive them within the first 24 hours after STEMI should have them started in the early convalescent phase. (Level of Evidence: A)

3. Patients with early contraindications within the first 24 hours of STEMI should be reevaluated for candidacy for β-blocker therapy. (Level of Evidence: C)

Aspirin The use of aspirin in the initial management of STEMI patients was previously discussed. Once initiated, patients should remain on aspirin indefinitely. A dose between 75 and 162 mg/d is recommended, and no specific study has been performed to determine if one dose is superior. Patients who are allergic to aspirin should be given 75 mg of clopidogrel daily. The *Clinical Practice Guidelines* recommend the following (see Chap. 11)[19]:

Class I

1. Aspirin 162 to 325 mg should be given on day 1 of STEMI and in the absence of contraindications should be continued indefinitely on a daily basis thereafter at a dose of 75 to 162 mg. (Level of Evidence: A)

2. A thienopyridine (preferably clopidogrel) should be administered to patients who are unable to take aspirin because of hypersensitivity or major gastrointestinal intolerance. (Level of Evidence: C)

Thienopyridines A thienopyridine—ticlopidine or clopidogrel—should be given in addition to aspirin to patients who are receiving coronary artery stenting. The minimal duration of therapy depends on the type of stent implanted. Patients with bare metal stents should be treated for a minimum of 30 days, whereas those with a Cypher drug-eluting stent need a minimum of 3 months. Patients with Taxus drug-eluting stents should be on dual antiplatelet therapy for at least 6 months. Long-term use of dual antiplatelet therapy was investigated in the CREDO (Clopidogrel for the Reduction of Events During Observation) trial. In this study, use of aspirin plus clopidogrel for 1 year resulted in a 27 percent relative risk reduction in the combined primary end point of death, MI, or stroke (*p* = 0.02). The CREDO trial, however, did not include STEMI patients.

STEMI patients who receive clopidogrel and require bypass surgery should be off the medication for 5 to 7 days prior to surgery because of the risk of bleeding and the long half-life of clopidogrel.[97] The *Clinical Practice Guidelines* recommend the following (see Chap. 11)[19]:

Class I

1. For patients taking clopidogrel for whom coronary artery bypass graft is planned, the drug should be withheld for at least 5 days if possible, and preferably for 7, unless the urgency for revascularization outweighs the risks of bleeding. (Level of Evidence: B)

2. For patients who have undergone diagnostic cardiac catheterization and for whom PCI is planned, clopidogrel should be started and continued for at least 1 month after bare metal stent implantation and for infarction, several months after drug-eluting stent implantation (3 months for sirolimus, 6 months for paclitaxel) and for up to 12 months in patients who are not at high risk for bleeding. (Level of Evidence: B)

Statins Several trials have demonstrated that statins should be used in the secondary prevention of patients with coronary artery disease.[98] In addition to lowering low-density lipoprotein (LDL) cholesterol, statins also improve endothelial function, have antiplatelet effects, and reduce inflammation.[99] The benefits of initiating statin therapy during the acute setting in STEMI patients was investigated in the PROVE-IT (Pravastatin or Atorvastatin Evaluation and Infection Therapy) TIMI 22 trial.[100] In this study, 4162 acute coronary syndrome patients (33 percent with STEMI) were randomized to standard therapy with 40 mg of pravastatin or to intense lipid-lowering therapy with atorvastatin 80 mg daily within the first 10 days of hospitalization for acute coronary syndrome. The combined primary end point of death from any cause, myocardial infarction, documented unstable angina requiring rehospitalization, revascularization (performed at least 30 days after randomization), and stroke occurred in 26.3 percent of the patients in the pravastatin group and 22.4 percent

of patients in the atorvastatin group (*p* = 0.005). The final LDL was 95 mg/dL in the pravastatin group and 62 mg/dL in the atorvastatin group (*p* <0.001).

It is therefore reasonable to initiate statin therapy during the acute setting of STEMI. Although the data are not clear regarding the benefits of early statin use, STEMI patients are more likely to be on statin therapy in the post MI period if treatment is initiated during the index hospitalization. An LDL goal of less than 70 mg/dL should be achieved.

Several studies have investigated the long-term benefits of statin therapy as secondary prevention in patients with coronary artery disease. These studies are discussed in detail in Chap. 51.

❴ ❵ HEMODYNAMIC COMPLICATIONS

The most common major complications include: cardiogenic shock, right ventricular infarction, acute mitral regurgitation, ventricular septum rupture, and free wall rupture.

Cardiogenic Shock

Cardiogenic shock as a result of severe LV dysfunction occurs in approximately 7 percent of patients with myocardial infarction and has a historic mortality of approximately 80 percent.[101] A recent population-based study analyzed temporal trends in cardiogenic shock complicating acute myocardial infarction in 9076 patients between the years 1975 and 1997. The frequency of cardiogenic shock remained relatively stable at 7.1 percent, and the mortality rate was approximately 72 percent. There was a trend toward increased in-hospital survival in the mid to late 1990s, which correlated with the increased application of reperfusion technologies.[101]

The goals for treatment are twofold: first, hemodynamic stabilization to ensure adequate oxygenation, acid–base balance, and tissue perfusion; and second, rapid investigation of any potentially reversible causes for the patient's condition. Hypovolemia, which is more common in older patients, those receiving chronic diuretic therapy, and those receiving narcotics or preload-reducing agents, must be corrected. Hemodynamic monitoring by using a balloon-tipped pulmonary artery catheter allows immediate access to valuable hemodynamic information. Forrester and others[102,103] described the treatment of patients on the basis of hemodynamic subsets related to pulmonary artery wedge pressure and cardiac output (Table 60–7). The basic goals of this approach include adjustment of the intravascular volume status to bring the pulmonary artery capillary wedge pressure to 18 to 20 mmHg and optimization of

TABLE 60–7

Forrester Classification of Myocardial Infarction

	CARDIAC INDEX (L/MIN/M²)	WEDGE (mmHG)
Class I	>2.2	<18
Class II	>2.2	>18
Class III	<2.2	<18
Class IV	<2.2	>18

cardiac output with inotropic and/or vasodilating agents. Severely hypotensive patients can be temporarily aided by intraaortic balloon pumping or possibly by a ventricular-assist device. However, the benefits from these mechanical treatments are often temporary, and there may be a significant risk of complications.

Many observational studies suggest that reperfusion therapy, especially with primary PCI, can reduce the incidence of cardiogenic shock. In one of the largest observational series, 1321 patients with shock in the GUSTO-1 trial were analyzed with respect to revascularization within 30 days versus no revascularization therapy. After multivariable logistic regression analysis, revascularization was independently associated with reduced 1-year mortality (odds ratio [OR] 0.6; 95 percent confidence interval [CI] 0.4 to 0.9; $p = 0.007$). In-hospital mortality; however, remained high at 56 percent.[104]

The "Should We Emergently Revascularize Occluded Coronaries for Cardiogenic Shock" (SHOCK) trial evaluated the effect of early revascularization in acute myocardial infarction complicated by cardiogenic shock.[105,106] The 302 patients with shock caused by left ventricular dysfunction complicating myocardial infarction were randomly assigned to either emergency revascularization ($n = 152$), or initial medical stabilization ($n = 150$). Eighty-six percent of patients in both groups had intraaortic balloon counterpulsation placement, and revascularization was accomplished by either coronary artery bypass grafting or angioplasty. The median time from symptom onset to revascularization was approximately 12 hours. The revascularization group had lower all-cause mortality at 30 days (46.7 percent vs. 56 percent; $p = 0.11$), 6 months (50.3 percent vs. 63.1 percent; $p = 0.027$), and 1 year (53.3 percent vs. 64.4 percent; $p <0.03$). There was an interaction between the effect of therapy and age, in that only patients younger than age 75 years benefited from revascularization. Although the 20 percent relative mortality reduction was more modest than expected on the basis of observational studies, only eight patients would have to receive early revascularization to prevent one death at 6 months. This result compares very favorably with benefits achieved by fibrinolytic therapy or primary PCI in patients without shock.

Although vasoconstriction has traditionally been associated with cardiogenic shock, vasodilatation can also be present. The mechanism of vasodilatation occurs from an increase in inducible nitric oxide synthase and subsequent increased production of nitric oxide. Use of the nitric oxide synthase inhibitor N^G-monomethyl-L-arginine (L-NMMA), has been proposed as a potential therapy for these patients with vasodialtion.[107] The *Clinical Practice Guidelines* recommend the following (see Chap. 11)[19]:

Class I

1. Intraaortic balloon counterpulsation is recommended for STEMI patients when cardiogenic shock is not quickly reversed with pharmacologic therapy. The intraaortic balloon pump is a stabilizing measure for angiography and prompt revascularization. (Level of Evidence: B)

2. Intraarterial monitoring is recommended for the management of STEMI patients with cardiogenic shock. (Level of Evidence: C)

3. Early revascularization, either PCI or coronary artery bypass graft, is recommended for patients younger than 75 years old with ST elevation or LBBB who develop shock

within 36 hours of MI and who are suitable for revascularization that can be performed within 18 hours of shock unless further support is futile because of the patient's wishes or contraindications/unsuitability for further invasive care. (Level of Evidence: A)

4. Fibrinolytic therapy should be administered to STEMI patients with cardiogenic shock who are unsuitable for further invasive care and do not have contraindications to fibrinolysis. (Level of Evidence: B)

5. Echocardiography should be used to evaluate mechanical complications unless these are assessed by invasive measures. (Level of Evidence: C)

Class IIa

1. Pulmonary artery catheter monitoring can be useful for the management of STEMI patients with cardiogenic shock. (Level of Evidence: C)

2. Early revascularization, either PCI or coronary artery bypass graft, is reasonable for selected patients age 75 years or older with ST elevation or LBBB who develop shock within 36 hours of MI and who are suitable for revascularization that can be performed within 18 hours of shock. Patients with good prior functional status who agree to invasive care may be selected for such an invasive strategy. (Level of Evidence: B)

Right Ventricular Infarction

Involvement of the right ventricle is a common sequela of acute inferior myocardial infarction,[108] especially after proximal right coronary artery occlusion.[109] However, hemodynamically significant dominant RV dysfunction is much less common, occurring in relatively few patients with right ventricular infarction (RVI).

The diagnosis of hemodynamically significant RVI rests on the clinical triad of hypotension, increased jugular venous pressure, and clear lung fields in a patient with acute inferior MI. Additional diagnostic techniques that can document RV involvement include ST-segment elevation in right–sided chest leads (V_3R or V_4R), visualization of RV wall-motion abnormalities, and RV dilatation on radionuclide angiography or echocardiography.

Hemodynamic measurements in patients with significant RVI demonstrate elevation of the right atrial pressure, usually more than 10 mmHg, and often show a right atrial pressure/pulmonary artery wedge pressure ratio of 0.8 or more. However, in cases with significant LV dysfunction and increased wedge pressure, this ratio may be lower and does not exclude the presence of significant RV involvement. Rarely, substantial arterial desaturation may be observed because of opening of a patent foramen ovale as a result of increased right atrial pressure and right-to-left atrial shunting. The incidence of bradyarrhythmias is increased in patients with RVI and can be detrimental because an increased heart rate may be necessary to compensate for the decrease in RV (and as a result LV) stroke volume caused by the RVI. Similarly, high–grade atrioventricular block may lead to loss of the atrioventricular synchrony with RV underfilling and further decrease in the RV and LV stroke volume.[110]

Treatment of RVI initially involves volume loading with normal saline to achieve a pulmonary artery wedge pressure of 18 to 20 mmHg. In some patients, this alone is sufficient to improve cardiac output and systemic pressure. However, some patients will not respond to fluid-loading alone. This may be a result of marked right ventricular enlargement within a relatively noncompliant pericardium, which may result in functional LV compression because of ventricular interaction. In addition to volume loading, use of dobutamine improves cardiac index.[111] Patients requiring temporary pacing for heart block may also benefit from arteriovenous sequential pacing rather than lone ventricular pacing. Reperfusion by thrombolysis,[112] and especially with primary PCI,[113] improves both RV function and clinical outcomes.

The natural history of dominant RVI may be favorable because the right ventricle is very resistant to ischemia and usually recovers.[108] Most patients, even those with substantial RV dysfunction, spontaneously improve in 48 to 72 hours after the acute event. Patients in shock may benefit from angioplasty of the occluded right coronary artery or from temporary use of a right ventricular assist device; however, many of these patients have associated significant LV dysfunction, which complicates the picture.[114] The overall balance between the extent of RV and LV dysfunction is a major determinant of long-term outcome and the majority of patients with RVI and significant hemodynamic compromise usually have evidence of extensive biventricular infarction and cardiogenic shock. The *Clinical Practice Guidelines* recommend the following (see Chap. 11)[19]:

Class I

1. *Patients with inferior STEMI and hemodynamic compromise should be assessed with a right precordial V_4R lead to detect ST-segment elevation and an echocardiogram to screen for RV infarction. (See the ACC/AHA/ASE [American Society of Echocardiography] 2003 Guideline Update for the Clinical Application of Echocardiography.[226]) (Level of Evidence: B)*

2. *The following principles apply to therapy for patients with STEMI and RV infarction and ischemic dysfunction:*

   a. *Early reperfusion should be achieved if possible. (Level of Evidence: C)*

   b. *Atrioventricular synchrony should be achieved, and bradycardia should be corrected. (Level of Evidence: C)*

   c. *Right ventricular preload should be optimized, which usually requires initial volume challenge in patients with hemodynamic instability provided the jugular venous pressure is normal or low. (Level of Evidence: C)*

   d. *Right ventricular afterload should be optimized, which usually requires therapy for concomitant LV dysfunction. (Level of Evidence: C)*

   e. *Inotropic support should be used for hemodynamic instability not responsive to volume challenge. (Level of Evidence: C)*

Class IIa

1. *After infarction that leads to clinically significant RV dysfunction, it is reasonable to delay coronary artery bypass graft surgery for 4 weeks to allow recovery of contractile performance. (Level of Evidence: C)*

Acute Mitral Regurgitation

Severe mitral regurgitation caused by papillary muscle rupture is responsible for approximately 5 percent of deaths in AMI patients. Rupture may be complete or partial, and it usually involves the posteromedial papillary muscle because its blood supply is derived only from the posterior descending artery, whereas the anterolateral papillary muscle has a dual blood supply from both the left anterior descending and the circumflex coronary arteries. Most patients have relatively small areas of infarction with poor collaterals, and up to half of the patients may have single–vessel disease.

The clinical presentation of papillary muscle rupture is the acute onset of pulmonary edema, usually within 2 to 7 days after inferior MI. The characteristics of the murmur vary; as a result of a rapid increase of pressure in the left atrium, no murmur may be audible. Thus a high degree of suspicion, especially in patients with inferior wall infarction is necessary for diagnosis. Two-dimensional echocardiographic examination demonstrates the partially or completely severed papillary muscle head and a flail segment of the mitral valve. LV function is hyperdynamic as a result of the severe regurgitation into the low-impedance left atrium; this finding alone, in a patient with severe congestive heart failure, should suggest the diagnosis.

The cornerstones of successful therapy are prompt diagnosis and emergency surgery. Emergent placement of an intraaortic balloon pump and blood pressure control is also beneficial. The current approach of emergency surgery accrues an overall operative mortality of 0 to 21 percent, but this appears to be decreasing, and the late results of this approach can be excellent.[115,116] The *Clinical Practice Guidelines* recommend the following (see Chap. 11)[19]:

Class I

1. *Patients with acute papillary muscle rupture should be considered for urgent cardiac surgical repair, unless further support is considered futile because of the patient's wishes or contraindications/unsuitability for further invasive care. (Level of Evidence: B)*

2. *Coronary artery bypass graft surgery should be undertaken at the same time as mitral valve surgery. (Level of Evidence: B)*

Ventricular Septal Rupture

Rupture of the ventricular septum occurs in 1 percent to 3 percent of acute infarctions and causes approximately 5 percent of peri-infarction deaths. The substrate is quite similar to that of free-wall rupture in terms of number of vessels diseased and infarct size. Typically, ventricular septal rupture (VSR) associated with anterior infarction is located in the apical septum, and those associated with inferior infarction is located in the basal inferior septum. The prevalences of anterior and inferior infarctions are approximately equal, unlike papillary muscle rupture.[117]

The diagnosis should be suspected clinically when a new pansystolic murmur is present. As with other cardiac ruptures, surgical management is advocated, although the outcome is not as gratifying as in acute mitral regurgitation, because the extent of myocardial necrosis is generally larger.[118,119] Percutaneous closure using occluding devices has been done in nonsurgical candidates with variable results: three of seven patients survived to hospital discharge in one report.[120]

The outcome of 91 patients seen in a single institution with VSR after acute myocardial infarction was reviewed by Lemery et al.[118] Advanced age, cardiogenic shock, and long delay between septal rupture and surgery correlated with adverse outcome. In patients with cardiogenic shock and ventricular septal defect, only those operated on within 48 hours survived; thus the proportion surviving in this group was only 38 percent. For patients not in shock, mortality was similar for surgery either within 2 to 14 days or after 14 days; however, the clinical course was unpredictable, with rapid deterioration and death in approximately 50 percent of these patients.

The incidence and outcome of periinfarction ventricular septal defect in the fibrinolytic era was reported in a study from the GUSTO-1 database.[119] In 84 patients (0.2 percent), ventricular septal defect developed after fibrinolysis, and the median time from symptom onset to the diagnosis of ventricular septal defect was 1 day. Mortality at 30 days in this group was 73.8 percent, and in patients selected for surgical repair versus those managed medically, 30-day mortality was 47 percent versus 94 percent, respectively. All patients presenting in Killip class III or IV died regardless of therapy; however, 1-year survival was excellent in patients surviving the initial 30 days after infarction. The *Clinical Practice Guidelines* recommend the following (see Chap. 11)[19]:

Class I

1. Patients with STEMI complicated by the development of a VSR should be considered for urgent cardiac surgical repair, unless further support is considered futile because of the patient's wishes or contraindications/unsuitability for further invasive care. (Level of Evidence: B)

2. Coronary artery bypass grafting should be undertaken at the same time as repair of the VSR. (Level of Evidence: B)

Free Wall Rupture

Rupture of the free wall of the left ventricle occurs in 1 percent to 4.5 percent of AMI patients and accounts for 10 to 15 percent of early AMI deaths.[121–126] Rupture is more common in women, the elderly, and persons with delayed admission to hospital.[121,123,126] Although any wall may be involved, rupture of the lateral wall is probably most common. Rupture occurs within the first 5 days of infarction in 50 percent of cases, and within 14 days in 87 percent of cases. The area of rupture always occurs within the area of infarction but usually is eccentrically located near the junction with normal myocardium. The incidence of rupture has decreased in the fibrinolytic era, but the timing is earlier (24 to 48 hours).[123] Further decrease in the rate of rupture can be achieved by primary PCI.[122,126] Survival to discharge in patients with cardiogenic shock included in the SHOCK trial[105] was 39.3 percent, similar to the survival of the other patients.[127]

The clinical presentation is usually sudden electromechanical dissociation. Most patients die even when rapid resuscitative measures, including pericardiocentesis, intraaortic balloon pump insertion, and emergent cardiac surgery, are attempted.[128] Surgical correction of acute free-wall rupture is the treatment of choice, even though surgical mortality can be high.[129] Surgical correction can be challenging because of the friability of the tissue that surrounds the rupture. A sutureless patch technique has shown encouraging initial results.[130] Early diagnosis is critical and can be achieved by a high degree of suspicion in any patient with sudden hemodynamic deterioration, particularly in the absence of evidence for recurrent ischemia or infarct extension.

Alternatively, rupture may be subacute, with periodic small amounts of blood leaking into the pericardial space.[128,131] ECG evidence of regional pericarditis may be a warning of impending rupture. Persistent and severe pericardial pain also may be a manifestation of this phenomenon, and the subsequent inflammatory process may serve to wall off the area of pericardial leakage from the remaining pericardial space forming a false or pseudoaneurysm of the left ventricle. The entity is easily and reliably detected by two-dimensional echocardiography and, when acute, mandates early surgical intervention because of the risk of further expansion of the false aneurysm or rupture producing tamponade and death. Chronic LV false aneurysm has a relatively low risk of rupture. Survival is reduced from multiple causes. In one observational series of 21 patients followed for a mean of 3.6 years, mortality was 64 percent, although no patient died of rupture.[132] The *Clinical Practice Guidelines* recommend the following (see Chap. 11)[19]:

Class I

1. Patients with free-wall rupture should be considered for urgent cardiac surgical repair, unless further support is considered futile because of the patient's wishes or contraindications/unsuitability for further invasive care. (Level of Evidence: B)

2. Coronary artery bypass grafting should be undertaken at the same time as repair of free wall rupture. (Level of Evidence: C)

【 】 ELECTRICAL COMPLICATIONS

Bradyarrhythmias

Bradyarrhythmias usually result from ischemic injury to the sinus node/conduction system or abnormal reflexes that are vagally mediated or both. The blood supply to the sinus node arises from the proximal right coronary artery in 55 percent of patients and from the proximal left circumflex in the remainder. The blood supply to the atrioventricular node arises from the distal branches of the right coronary artery in 90 percent of patients and from the distal portions of the left circumflex artery in the remaining 10 percent of patients. The right bundle branch is supplied primarily by the septal perforator vessels originating from the left anterior descending artery, as is the distal portion of the anterior left bundle branch. The main left bundle branch has a dual supply from both distal branches of the right coronary and proximal circumflex vessels, and the posterior division of the left bundle branch is supplied from branches of the circumflex coronary artery.

In general, conduction disturbances associated with inferoposterior infarction are related to enhanced vagal activity, tend to be more transient, are often responsive to atropine, and imply a somewhat more benign outcome than those involved in anterior infarction. Conversely, major conduction disturbances associated with anterior infarction usually imply extensive septal necrosis and more significant reduction in LV function.

Sinus Bradycardia Sinus bradycardia and sinus pauses are usually benign. First-degree atrioventricular block occurs in 4 percent to 13 percent of myocardial infarctions. Observation and avoidance of any medications that might prolong atrioventricular conduction are required.

Second–Degree Atrioventricular Block This usually develops within the first 24 hours of myocardial infarction in 3 percent to 10 percent of individuals. With type I second–degree atrioventricular block, progressive prolongation of the PR interval is observed. This is usually seen in inferoposterior infarction and may often respond to atropine. A narrow QRS complex is usually present, and temporary pacing is not needed unless the ventricular rate decreases to less than 45 beats/min or symptoms of impaired perfusion develop. Type II second-degree atrioventricular block is identified by intermittent dropped beats in the absence of progressive PR prolongation and implies extensive infranodal conduction system injury. Often the QRS complex is wide, indicating associated bundle–branch block, and progression to complete heart block occurs in approximately one-third of these patients. Most patients with anterior infarction and type II second-degree atrioventricular block need temporary transvenous pacing because of the unpredictable risk of complete heart block.

Complete Heart Block This occurs in 3 percent to 12 percent of acute myocardial infarctions.[133,134] In general, patients with inferoposterior infarction progress to third-degree heart block after a period of second–degree heart block and again may demonstrate some responsiveness to atropine or aminophylline.[135] A stable junctional escape rhythm is often present, and recovery tends to occur within 3 to 7 days. The occurrence of complete heart block in a patient with inferior infarction confers a 1.5- to 4-fold increase in risk of in-hospital mortality.[133,134] Consequently, these patients should be carefully observed, often with standby temporary transcutaneous pacing patches in place. Complete heart block in the presence of anterior infarction usually indicates an extensive area of myocardial necrosis and has a poor prognosis. Most patients require temporary transvenous pacing, and some physicians advocate permanent transvenous pacing. Late mortality in these patients is usually the result of contractile failure or ventricular fibrillation rather than persistent, high-grade atrioventricular block.

Bundle-Branch Block The occurrence of any new bundle-branch block with acute myocardial infarction also identifies patients with extensive infarction who are at higher risk for complications. Unifascicular block, especially left anterior hemiblock, occurs in approximately 5 percent of patients and has a relatively benign prognosis. Complete right or left bundle-branch block occurs in 10 to 15 percent of patients and most commonly (two-thirds of cases) involves the right bundle branch. Both LBBB and right bundle-branch block are associated with higher in-hospital and long-term mortality[136] In the past, the new occurrence of left or right bundle-branch block has been a generally accepted indication for temporary transvenous pacing.

Permanent transvenous pacing is indicated in patients with persistent complete or high-grade atrioventricular block or persistent type II second-degree atrioventricular block after myocardial infarction and in patients with a new bundle-branch block and transient but resolved complete heart block during the acute course of infarction. Occasionally, patients may require an electrophysio-logic study to determine the site of atrioventricular block and to aid in the decision about whether permanent pacing is indicated. Permanent pacing also may be indicated in the rare patient with profound sinus node dysfunction. However, this complication is rarely related to myocardial infarction. The *Clinical Practice Guidelines* recommend the following (see Chap. 11)[19]:

Class I

1. Permanent ventricular pacing is indicated for persistent second-degree atrioventricular block in the His-Purkinje system with bilateral bundle-branch block or third degree atrioventricular block within or below the His-Purkinje system after STEMI. (Level of Evidence: B)

2. Permanent ventricular pacing is indicated for transient advanced second- or third-degree infranodal atrioventricular block and associated bundle-branch block. If the site of block is uncertain, an electrophysiology study may be necessary. (Level of Evidence: B)

3. Permanent ventricular pacing is indicated for persistent and symptomatic second- or third-degree atrioventricular block. (Level of Evidence: C)

Class IIb

1. Permanent ventricular pacing may be considered for persistent second- or third-degree atrioventricular block at the atrioventricular node level. (Level of Evidence: B)

Class III

1. Permanent ventricular pacing is not recommended for transient atrioventricular block in the absence of intraventricular conduction defects. (Level of Evidence: B)

2. Permanent ventricular pacing is not recommended for transient atrioventricular block in the presence of isolated left anterior fascicular block. (Level of Evidence: B)

3. Permanent ventricular pacing is not recommended for acquired left anterior fascicular block in the absence of atrioventricular block. (Level of Evidence: B)

4. Permanent ventricular pacing is not recommended for persistent first-degree atrioventricular block in the presence of bundle-branch block that is old or of indeterminate age. (Level of Evidence: B)

Tachyarrhythmias

Multiple factors play a role in the genesis of tachyarrhythmias in patients with myocardial infarction. Decreased blood flow leads to anaerobic metabolism, and decreased venous outflow allows accumulation of by-products of this process, resulting in acidosis, increase in extracellular potassium concentration, and an increase in intracellular calcium concentration. In addition to these ionic changes, there may be alterations in sympathetic and vagal tone and increased concentrations of circulating catecholamines. The electrophysiologic correlates of these cellular abnormalities include slowing of conduction and prolongation of refractoriness, which coupled with the inhomogeneous nature of the infarction process, produces an ideal situation for the occurrence of reentrant arrhythmias. The presence of injury currents may directly enhance phase IV depolarization of Purkinje cells, resulting in increased automaticity. Fiber stretch, resulting from increased atrial and ventricular end-diastolic pressures, is also arrhythmogenic. Finally, reperfusion, possibly caused by intracellular calcium overload or production of free oxygen radicals, may generate reperfusion arrhythmias that may be either automatic or reentrant.

Supraventricular Arrhythmias

Sinus tachycardia may occur in up to 25 percent of patients with acute infarction and often results from pain, anxiety, and sometimes hypovolemia. Persistent sinus tachycardia may be a marker of severe LV dysfunction and is a poor prognostic sign. After relief of pain and assessment for the presence of pulmonary congestion, it is desirable to decrease the heart rate to less than 70 beats/min by intravenous administration of β-adrenergic–receptor blockers. A short-acting β-adrenergic–receptor blocker, such as esmolol, may be appropriate for patients in whom the extent of left ventricular dysfunction is of particular concern.

Atrial fibrillation occurs in 10 to 15 percent of patients with acute infarction.[137,138] Its early presence signifies atrial ischemia; later it may also represent atrial stretch caused by increasing filling pressures, which is why it is associated with such an adverse prognosis. Immediate cardioversion is the best treatment for patients with symptomatic rapid atrial fibrillation or in whom the rapid ventricular response produces ischemia. If the ventricular response is only moderate and the patient is asymptomatic, diltiazem or esmolol (in patients with a normal ejection fraction) given intravenously is useful for control of heart rate, along with digoxin given orally; the latter may take 4 to 8 hours for full effect. Recurrent episodes of atrial fibrillation should be suppressed with an antiarrhythmic agent such as procainamide, or intravenous amiodarone. The treatment of atrial flutter is similar to that of atrial fibrillation, except that drug treatment is less effective in controlling the ventricular response. Occasionally atrial overdrive pacing may be used to terminate atrial flutter without resorting to cardioversion. Atrial fibrillation in the setting of AMI, especially if it occurs after admission, is associated with higher mortality and incidence of stroke.[137,138] The *Clinical Practice Guidelines* recommend the following (see Chap. 11)[19]:

Class I

1. *Sustained atrial fibrillation and atrial flutter in patients with hemodynamic compromise should be treated with one or more of the following:*

    a. *Synchronized cardioversion with an initial monophasic shock of 200 J for atrial fibrillation and 50 J for flutter, preceded by brief general anesthesia or conscious sedation whenever possible. (Level of Evidence: C)*

    b. *For episodes of atrial fibrillation that do not respond to electrical cardioversion or recur after a brief period of sinus rhythm, the use of antiarrhythmic therapy aimed at slowing the ventricular response is indicated. One or more of these pharmacologic agents may be used:*

        i. *Intravenous amiodarone. (Level of Evidence: C)*

        ii. *Intravenous digoxin for rate control, principally for patients with severe LV dysfunction and heart failure. (Level of Evidence: C)*

2. *Sustained atrial fibrillation and atrial flutter in patients with ongoing ischemia but without hemodynamic compromise should be treated with one or more of the following:*

    a. *β-Adrenergic blockade is preferred, unless contraindicated. (Level of Evidence: C)*

    b. *Intravenous diltiazem or verapamil. (Level of Evidence: C)*

    c. *Synchronized cardioversion with an initial monophasic shock of 200 J for atrial fibrillation and 50 J for flutter, preceded by brief general anesthesia or conscious sedation whenever possible. (Level of Evidence: C)*

3. *For episodes of sustained atrial fibrillation or flutter without hemodynamic compromise or ischemia, rate control is indicated. In addition, patients with sustained atrial fibrillation or flutter should be given therapy with anticoagulants. Consideration should be given to conversion of sinus rhythm in patients without a history of atrial fibrillation or flutter prior to STEMI. (Level of Evidence: C)*

4. *Reentrant paroxysmal supraventricular tachycardia, because of its rapid rate, should be treated with the following in the sequence shown:*

    a. *Carotid sinus massage. (Level of Evidence: C)*

    b. *Intravenous adenosine (6 mg IV over 1 to 2 seconds; if no response, 12 mg IV after 1 to 2 minutes may be given; repeat 12 mg dose if needed. (Level of Evidence: C)*

    c. *Intravenous β-adrenergic blockade with metoprolol (2.5 to 5.0 mg every 2 to 5 minutes to a total of 15 mg over 10 to 15 minutes) or atenolol (2.5 to 5.0 mg over 2 minutes to a total of 10 mg in 10 to 15 minutes). (Level of Evidence: C)*

    d. *Intravenous diltiazem (20 mg [0.25 mg/kg]) over 2 minutes followed by an infusion of 10 mg/h. (Level of Evidence: C)*

    e. *Intravenous digoxin, recognizing that there may be a delay of at least 1 hour before pharmacologic effects appear (8 to 15 μg/kg [0.6 to 1.0 mg in a person weighing 70 kg]). (Level of Evidence: C)*

Class III

1. *Treatment of atrial premature beats is not indicated. (Level of Evidence: C)*

Ventricular Tachyarrhythmias

Accelerated idioventricular rhythm may occur in up to 40 percent of continuously monitored patients and may be a marker of reperfusion in some. This rhythm disturbance is generally considered benign and is usually untreated. (see Chap. 12). The *Clinical Practice Guidelines* recommend the following (see Chap. 11)[19]:

Class III

1. *Antiarrhythmic therapy is not indicated for accelerated idioventricular rhythm. (Level of Evidence: C)*

2. *Antiarrhythmic therapy is not indicated for accelerated junctional rhythm. (Level of Evidence: C)*

Ventricular tachycardia occurs in up to 15 percent of patients during acute myocardial infarction. The ventricular rate is usually between 140 and 200 beats/min, and this rhythm disturbance may degenerate to ventricular fibrillation. The rhythm disturbance usually responds to lidocaine given intravenously. However, procainamide, bretylium, cardioversion, ventricular overdrive pacing, or amiodarone may all be required in the acute stages for resistant cases. The use of lidocaine prophylactically for prevention of ventricular tachycardia is not currently recommended. Pooled results of studies showed that the incidence of ventricular tachycardia was decreased, but fatal asystole was more common and no survival advantage was proved.

Ventricular fibrillation is seen in approximately 8 percent of patients surviving to hospitalization for acute infarction. It is more frequent in large ST–elevation infarcts and may occur with or without warning arrhythmias. The occurrence of ventricular fibrillation within the first 24 hours of hospitalization was previously thought not to confer any long-term risk to patients successfully resuscitated; however, some studies indicate a poorer outcome for patients with ventricular fibrillation at any time during their hospital course. Ventricular fibrillation or tachycardia occurring late in the hospital course may be the result of pump failure, severe electrolyte imbalance, effects of antiarrhythmic medications, or other metabolic derangements; it is usually associated with decreased left ventricular systolic function and portends a poor prognosis. Sustained monomorphic ventricular tachycardia (VT), occurring early or late during the hospital course, is not common but implies a fixed arrhythmogenic substrate and a propensity for recurrence after dismissal. An invasive electrophysiologic study can be justified in these patients before discharge from the hospital. The *Clinical Practice Guidelines* recommend the following (see Chap. 11)[19]:

Class I

1. Sustained (more than 30 seconds or causing hemodynamic collapse) polymorphic VT should be treated with an unsynchronized electric shock with an initial monophasic shock energy of 200 J; if unsuccessful, a second shock of 200 to 300 J should be given, and, if necessary, a third shock of 360 J. (Level of Evidence: B)

2. Episodes of sustained monomorphic VT associated with angina, pulmonary edema, or hypotension (blood pressure less than 90 mmHg) should be treated with a synchronized electric shock of 100 J of initial monophasic shock energy. Increasing energies may be used if not initially successful. Brief anesthesia is desirable if hemodynamically tolerable. (Level of Evidence: B)

3. Sustained monomorphic VT not associated with angina, pulmonary edema, or hypotension (blood pressure less than 90 mmHg) should be treated with:

a. Amiodarone: 150 mg infused over 10 minutes (alternative dose 5 mg/kg); repeat 150 mg every 10 to 15 minutes as needed. Alternative infusion: 360 mg over 6 hours (1 mg/min), then 540 mg over the next 18 hours (0.5 mg/min). The total cumulative dose, including additional doses given during cardiac arrest, must not exceed 2.2 g over 24 hours. (Level of Evidence: B)

b. Synchronized electrical cardioversion starting at monophasic energies of 50 J (brief anesthesia is necessary). (Level of Evidence: B)

Class IIa

1. It is reasonable to manage refractory polymorphic VT by:

a. Aggressive attempts to reduce myocardial ischemia, and adrenergic stimulation, including therapies such as β-adrenoceptor blockade, intraaortic balloon pump use, and consideration of emergency PCI/coronary artery bypass graft surgery. (Level of Evidence: B)

b. Aggressive normalization of serum potassium to greater than 4.0 mEq/L and of magnesium to greater than 2.0 mg/dL. (Level of Evidence: C)

c. If the patient has bradycardia to a rate less than 60 beats/min or long QTc, temporary pacing at a higher rate may be instituted. (Level of Evidence: C)

Class IIb

1. It may be useful to treat sustained monomorphic VT not associated with angina, pulmonary edema, or hypotension (blood pressure less than 90 mmHg) with a procainamide bolus and infusion. (Level of Evidence: C)

Class III

1. The routine use of prophylactic antiarrhythmic drugs (i.e., lidocaine) is not indicated for suppression of isolated ventricular premature beats, couplets, runs of accelerated idioventricular rhythm, and nonsustained VT. (Level of Evidence: B)

2. The routine use of prophylactic antiarrhythmic therapy is not indicated when fibrinolytic agents are administered. (Level of Evidence: B)

3. Treatment of isolated ventricular premature beats, couplets, and nonsustained VT is not recommended unless they lead to hemodynamic compromise. (Level of Evidence: A)

Implantable Cardiac Defibrillator Several trials have demonstrated a mortality benefit with the use of implantable cardiac defibrillators (ICDs) as primary prevention for sudden cardiac death in patients with chronic ischemic cardiomyopathy. The DINAMIT (Defibrillator in Acute Myocardial Infarction Trial) investigated the used of ICD therapy early after AMI. In this study, 674 patients within 6 to 40 days after an AMI with subsequent left ventricular dysfunction (ejection fraction <35 percent) were randomized to ICD therapy or placebo. After a median followup period of 30 months there was no significant difference in the mortality rate between the two groups. These results were somewhat surprising given that the highest incidence of sudden cardiac death in the VALIANT trial occurred during the first 3 months postmyocardial infarction.[139]

AMI patients with left ventricular dysfunction should not receive an ICD during the early period for prophylactic indications. ICD therapy is recommended in those who have recurrent sustained episodes of ventricular tachycardia during the post-MI period. A repeat assessment of left ventricular dysfunction 30 to 40 days after the acute event should be performed and those with an ejection fraction less than 35 percent should receive and ICD. Antiarrhythmic therapy has not been demonstrated to prevent sudden cardiac death in the post-MI setting in patients without sustained ventricular arrhythmias. The *Clinical Practice Guidelines* recommend the following (see Chap. 11)[19]:

Class I

1. *An implantable cardioverter defibrillator (ICD) is indicated for patients with ventricular fibrillation or hemodynamically significant sustained VT more than 2 days after STEMI, provided the arrhythmia is not judged to be caused by transient or reversible ischemia or reinfarction. (Level of Evidence: A)*

2. *An ICD is indicated for patients without spontaneous ventricular fibrillation or sustained VT more than 48 hours after STEMI whose STEMI occurred at least 1 month previously, who have an LV ejection fraction between 0.31 and 0.40, demonstrate additional evidence of electrical instability (e.g., nonsustained VT), and have inducible ventricular fibrillation or sustained VT on electrophysiology testing. (Level of Evidence: B)*

Class IIa

1. *If there is reduced LV ejection fraction (0.30 or less) at least 1 month post-STEMI and 3 months after coronary artery revascularization, it is reasonable to implant an ICD in post-STEMI patients without spontaneous ventricular fibrillation or sustained VT more than 48 hours after STEMI. (Level of Evidence: B)*

Class IIb

1. *The usefulness of an ICD is not well established in STEMI patients without spontaneous ventricular fibrillation or sustained VT more than 48 hours after STEMI who have a reduced LV ejection fraction (0.31 to 0.40) at least 1 month after STEMI but who have no additional evidence of electrical instability (e.g., nonsustained VT). (Level of Evidence: B)*

2. *The usefulness of an ICD is not well established in STEMI patients without spontaneous ventricular fibrillation or sustained VT more than 48 hours after STEMI who have a reduced LV ejection fraction (0.31 to 0.40) at least 1 month after STEMI and additional evidence of electrical instability (e.g., nonsustained VT) but who do not have inducible ventricular fibrillation or sustained VT on electrophysiology testing. (Level of Evidence: B)*

Class III

1. *An ICD is not indicated in STEMI patients who do not experience spontaneous ventricular fibrillation or sustained VT more than 48 hours after STEMI and in whom the LV ejection fraction is greater than 0.40 at least 1 month after STEMI. (Level of Evidence: C)*

SECONDARY PREVENTION

See also Chap. 51.

Cholesterol Management

In accordance with the National Cholesterol Education Program (NCEP) Expert Panel on Detection, Evaluation, and Treatment of High Blood Cholesterol in Adults (Adult Treatment Panel III) guidelines, patients with coronary artery disease should meet the following lipid goals: LDL <100 mg/dL, high-density lipoprotein (HDL) >40 mg/dL in men and >50 mg/dL in women, and a serum triglyceride level <150 mg/dL.[140] New data from the PROVE-IT and the TNT (Treating to New Targets) trials suggest that a goal LDL of <70 mg/dL may further reduce future events.[100,141]

The benefits of statins for secondary prevention were described in Chapter 51. The use of niacin and fibrates has also been studied. In the coronary drug project, the use of niacin reduced nonfatal myocardial infarction and total mortality at 15 years of followup.[142] The Veterans Affairs High-Density Lipoprotein Cholesterol Intervention Trial (VA-HIT) randomized 2531 men with coronary artery disease (CAD), HDL level ≤40 mg/dL, LDL level ≤140 mg/dL, and triglyceride level ≤300 mg/dL to gemfibrozil (1200 mg/d) or placebo.[143] After a median followup of 5.1 years the gemfibrozil group had a lower incidence of nonfatal myocardial infarction (11.6 percent vs. 14.5 percent; $p = 0.02$) and CAD death (7.4 percent vs. 9.3 percent; $p = 0.07$). Therefore, gemfibrozil should be considered for CAD patients with a low HDL who do not have a high LDL. The *Clinical Practice Guidelines* recommend the following (see Chap. 11)[19]:

Class I

1. *Dietary therapy that is low in saturated fat and cholesterol (less than 7 percent of total calories as saturated fat and less than 200 mg/d cholesterol) should be started on discharge after recovery from STEMI. Increased consumption of the following should be encouraged: omega-3 fatty acids, fruits, vegetables, soluble (viscous) fiber, and whole grains. Calorie intake should be balanced with energy output to achieve and maintain a healthy weight. (Level of Evidence: A)*

2. *A lipid profile should be performed, or obtained from recent past records, for all STEMI patients, preferably after they have fasted and within 24 hours of symptom onset. (Level of Evidence: C)*

3. *The target LDL cholesterol level after STEMI should be substantially less than 100 mg/dL. (Level of Evidence: A)*

   a. *Patients with LDL cholesterol 100 mg/dL or above should be prescribed drug therapy on hospital discharge, with preference given to statins. (Level of Evidence: A)*

   b. *Patients with LDL cholesterol less than 100 mg/dL or unknown LDL cholesterol levels should be prescribed statin therapy on hospital discharge. (Level of Evidence: B)*

4. *Patients with non–high-density lipoprotein cholesterol levels less than 130 mg/dL who have an HDL cholesterol level less than 40 mg/dL should receive special emphasis on*

nonpharmacologic therapy (e.g., exercise, weight loss, and smoking cessation) to increase HDL. (Level of Evidence: B)

Class IIa

1. It is reasonable to prescribe drug therapy at hospital discharge to patients with non-HDL cholesterol greater than or equal to 130 mg/dL, with a goal of reducing non-HDL cholesterol to substantially less than 130 mg/dL. (Level of Evidence: B)

2. It is reasonable to prescribe drugs such as niacin or fibrate therapy to raise HDL cholesterol levels in patients with LDL cholesterol less than 100 mg/dL and non-HDL cholesterol less than 130 mg/dL but HDL cholesterol less than 40 mg/dL despite dietary and other nonpharmacologic therapy. Dietary-supplement niacin must not be used as a substitute for prescription niacin, and over-the-counter niacin should be used only if approved and monitored by a physician. (Level of Evidence: B)

3. It is reasonable to add drug therapy with either niacin or a fibrate to diet regardless of LDL and HDL levels when triglyceride levels are greater than 500 mg/dL. In this setting, non-HDL cholesterol (goal substantially less than 130 mg/dL) should be the cholesterol target rather than LDL cholesterol. Dietary-supplement niacin must not be used as a substitute for prescription niacin, and over-the-counter niacin should be used only if approved and monitored by a physician. (Level of Evidence: B)

Weight Loss

Obesity is a risk factor for coronary artery disease. It is estimated that 65 percent of the population in the United States is overweight or obese and the number appears to be increasing especially among children and adolescents.[144] Weight loss via diet and exercise is an important aspect of secondary prevention among STEMI patients. A goal reduction of 10 percent in body weight over a period of 6 months should be obtained. The *Clinical Practice Guidelines* recommend the following (see Chap. 11)[19]:

Class I

1. Measurement of waist circumference and calculation of body mass index are recommended. Desirable body mass index range is 18.5 to 24.9 kg/m². A waist circumference greater than 40 inches in men and 35 inches in women would result in evaluation for metabolic syndrome and implementation of weight-reduction strategies. (Level of Evidence: B)

2. Patients should be advised about appropriate strategies for weight management and physical activity (usually accomplished in conjunction with cardiac rehabilitation). (Level of Evidence: B)

3. A plan should be established to monitor the response of body mass index and waist circumference to therapy (usually accomplished in conjunction with cardiac rehabilitation). (Level of Evidence: B)

Smoking Cessation

Tobacco abuse is one of the leading modifiable risk factors for coronary artery disease. Smoking cessation counseling during the initial

hospital stay for STEMI patients with tobacco abuse should be routinely offered. Strategies to help patients with smoking cessation include nicotine replacement and bupropion therapy. The *Clinical Practice Guidelines* recommend the following (see Chap. 11)[19]:

Class I

Patients recovering from STEMI who have a history of cigarette smoking should be strongly encouraged to stop smoking and to avoid secondhand smoke. Counseling should be provided to the patient and family, along with pharmacologic therapy (including nicotine replacement and bupropion) and formal smoking cessation programs as appropriate. (Level of Evidence: B)

All STEMI patients should be assessed for a history of cigarette smoking. (Level of Evidence: A)

Glucose Control

Hyperglycemia is a risk factor for coronary artery disease. Tight glucose control, defined as a hemoglobin A1c of less than 7 percent, results in a 2.7 percent absolute reduction in myocardial infarction.[145] Therefore, all STEMI patients should be screened for diabetes and those with elevated blood glucose levels should receive aggressive management. The *Clinical Practice Guidelines* recommend the following (see Chap. 11)[19]:

Class I

Hypoglycemic therapy should be initiated to achieve hemoglobin A1c of less than 7 percent. (Level of Evidence: B)

Class III

Thiazolidinediones should not be used in patients recovering from STEMI who have New York Heart Association class III or IV heart failure. (Level of Evidence: B)

Depression

Many patients suffer from depression after myocardial infraction. It has been estimated that 45 percent of patients treated for an acute myocardial infraction suffer from a depressive episode within 4 months of an acute myocardial infarction.[146] Depression after myocardial infraction is associated with a decrease in compliance with medications use, exercise, and diet.[147] In addition to poor compliance, depression also results in a four- to fivefold increase in mortality after myocardial infarction.[148–150] Consequently, it is important to diagnose and treat depression in postinfraction patients.

Cardiac Rehabilitation

Rehabilitation after myocardial infraction is an important aspect of secondary prevention and is described in Chap. 67.

CONCLUSION

Despite the numerous improvements in the management of STEMI, it remains one of the leading causes of morbidity and mortality worldwide. The key steps in the management of these patients include rapid diagnosis, prompt delivery of initial therapeutic agents, immediate reperfusion, and diligent in-hospital management, which includes the aggressive implementation of secondary prevention strategies. Future improvements in each of these categories, some of which are logistical, need to be made if any significant reductions in the morbidity and mortality are to be obtained. The persistently high mortality of myocardial infarction in the elderly provides a formidable, but highly important challenge for the future.

REFERENCES

1. Lopez AD, Mathers CD, Ezzati M, Jamison DT, Murray CJ. Global and regional burden of disease and risk factors, 2001: systematic analysis of population health data. *Lancet* 2006;367:1747–1757.

2. *Heart Disease and Stroke Statistics—2006 Update*. Dallas, TX: American Heart Association, 2006.

3. Goldberg RJ, Yarzebski J, Lessard D, Gore JM. A two-decades (1975 to 1995) long experience in the incidence, in-hospital and long-term case-fatality rates of acute myocardial infarction: a community-wide perspective. *J Am Coll Cardiol* 1999;33:1533–1539.

4. Madias JE CG, Choudry M, Chalavarya G, Kegan M. Correlates and in-hospital outcome of painless presentation of acute myocardial infarction: a prospective study of a consecutive series of patients admitted to the coronary care unit. *J Investig Med* 1195;43:567–574.

5. Yamaji H, Iwasaki K, Kusachi S, et al. Prediction of acute left main coronary artery obstruction by 12-lead electrocardiography. ST segment elevation in lead aVR with less ST segment elevation in lead V(1). *J Am Coll Cardiol* 2001;38:1348–1354.

6. Hands ME, Cook EF, Stone PH, et al. Electrocardiographic diagnosis of myocardial infarction in the presence of complete left bundle-branch block. *Am Heart J* 1988;116:23–31.

7. Rathore SS, Weinfurt KP, Gersh BJ, Oetgen WJ, Schulman KA, Solomon AJ. Treatment of patients with myocardial infarction who present with a paced rhythm. *Ann Intern Med* 2001;134:644–651.

8. Sgarbossa EB, Pinski SL, Barbagelata A, et al. Electrocardiographic diagnosis of evolving acute myocardial infarction in the presence of left bundle-branch block. GUSTO-1 (Global Utilization of Streptokinase and Tissue Plasminogen Activator for Occluded Coronary Arteries) Investigators. *N Engl J Med* 1996;334:481–487.

9. Wu AH, Apple FS, Gibler WB, Jesse RL, Warshaw MM, Valdes R Jr. National Academy of Clinical Biochemistry Standards of Laboratory Practice: recommendations for the use of cardiac markers in coronary artery diseases. *Clin Chem* 1999;45:1104–1121.

10. Alpert JS, Thygesen K, Antman E, Bassand JP. Myocardial infarction redefined—a consensus document of The Joint European Society of Cardiology/American College of Cardiology Committee for the redefinition of myocardial infarction. *J Am Coll Cardiol* 2000;36:959–969.

11. Galvani M, Ottani F, Ferrini D, et al. Prognostic influence of elevated values of cardiac troponin I in patients with unstable angina. *Circulation* 1997;95:2053–2059.

12. Newby LK, Christenson RH, Ohman EM, et al. Value of serial troponin T measures for early and late risk stratification in patients with acute coronary syndromes. The GUSTO-IIa Investigators. *Circulation* 1998;98:1853–1859.

13. Ohman EM, Armstrong PW, Christenson RH, et al. Cardiac troponin T levels for risk stratification in acute myocardial ischemia. GUSTO IIA Investigators. *N Engl J Med* 1996;335:1333–1341.

14. Hamm CW, Ravkilde J, Gerhardt W, et al. The prognostic value of serum troponin T in unstable angina. *N Engl J Med* 1992;327:146–150.

15. Wallentin L, Lagerqvist B, Husted S, Kontny F, Stahle E, Swahn E. Outcome at 1 year after an invasive compared with a non-invasive strategy in unstable coronary-artery disease: the FRISC II invasive randomised trial. FRISC II Investigators. Fast Revascularisation During Instability in Coronary artery disease. *Lancet* 2000;356:9–16.

16. Curtis JP, Portnay EL, Wang Y, et al. The pre-hospital electrocardiogram and time to reperfusion in patients with acute myocardial infarction, 2000–2002: findings from the National Registry of Myocardial Infarction-4. *J Am Coll Cardiol* 2006;47:1544–1552.

17. Kereiakes DJ, Brian Gibler W, Martin LH, Pieper KS, Anderson LC. Relative importance of emergency medical system transport and the prehospital electrocardiogram on reducing hospital time delay to therapy for acute myocardial infarction: a preliminary report from the Cincinnati Heart Project. *Am Heart J* 1992;123:835–840.

18. Canto M, John G, Rogers M, William J, Bowlby R, Laura J. The prehospital electrocardiogram in acute myocardial infarction: is its full potential being realized? *J Am Coll Cardiol* 1997;29:498–505.

19. Antman EM, Anbe DT, Armstrong PW, et al. ACC/AHA guidelines for the management of patients with ST-elevation myocardial infarction: a report of the American College of Cardiology/American Heart Association Task Force on Practice Guidelines (Committee to Revise the 1999 Guidelines for the Management of patients with acute myocardial infarction). *J Am Coll Cardiol* 2004;44:e1–e211.

20. Killip T 3rd, Kimball JT. Treatment of myocardial infarction in a coronary care unit. A two-year experience with 250 patients. *Am J Cardiol* 1967;20:457–464.

21. Randomised trial of intravenous streptokinase, oral aspirin, both, or neither among 17,187 cases of suspected acute myocardial infarction: ISIS-2. ISIS-2 (Second International Study of Infarct Survival) Collaborative Group. *Lancet* 1988;2:349–360.

22. Lau J, Antman EM, Jimenez-Silva J, Kupelnick B, Mosteller F, Chalmers TC. Cumulative meta-analysis of therapeutic trials for myocardial infarction. *N Engl J Med* 1992;327:248–254.

23. Freemantle N, Cleland J, Young P, Mason J, Harrison J. Beta blockade after myocardial infarction: systematic review and meta regression analysis. *BMJ* 1999;318:1730–1737.

24. Roberts R, Rogers W, Mueller H, et al. Immediate versus deferred beta-blockade following thrombolytic therapy in patients with acute myocardial infarction. Results of the Thrombolysis in Myocardial Infarction (TIMI) II-B Study. *Circulation* 1991;83:422–437.

25. COMMIT (ClOpidogrel and Metoprolol in Myocardial Infarction Trial) collaborative group. Early intravenous then oral metoprolol in 45,852 patients with acute myocardial infarction: randomised placebo-controlled trial. *Lancet* 2005;366:1622–1632.

26. Jugdutt BI, Warnica JW. Intravenous nitroglycerin therapy to limit myocardial infarct size, expansion, and complications. Effect of timing, dosage, and infarct location. *Circulation* 1988;78:906–919.

27. Jugdutt BI, Becker LC, Hutchins GM, Bulkley BH, Reid PR, Kallman CH. Effect of intravenous nitroglycerin on collateral blood flow and infarct size in the conscious dog. *Circulation* 1981;63:17–28.

28. Weitz JI. Low-molecular-weight heparins. *N Engl J Med* 1997;337:688–699.

29. Van de Werf FJ, Armstrong PW, Granger C, Wallentin L. Efficacy and safety of tenecteplase in combination with enoxaparin, abciximab, or unfractionated heparin: The ASSENT-3 randomised trial in acute myocardial infarction. *Lancet* 2001;358:605–613.

30. Antman EM, Morrow DA, McCabe CH, et al. Enoxaparin versus unfractionated heparin with fibrinolysis for st-elevation myocardial infarction. *N Engl J Med* 2006;354:1477–1488.

31. White H. Thrombin-specific anticoagulation with bivalirudin versus heparin in patients receiving fibrinolytic therapy for acute myocardial infarction: the HERO-2 randomised trial. *Lancet* 2001;358:1855–1863.

32. A comparison of recombinant hirudin with heparin for the treatment of acute coronary syndromes. The Global Use of Strategies to Open Occluded Coronary Arteries (GUSTO) IIb investigators. *N Engl J Med* 1996;335:775–782.

33. Direct thrombin inhibitors in acute coronary syndromes: principal results of a meta-analysis based on individual patients' data. *Lancet* 2002;359:294–302.

34. The OASIS-6 Trial Group. Effects of fondaparinux on mortality and reinfarction in patients with acute ST-segment elevation myocardial infarction: the OASIS-6 randomized trial. *JAMA* 2006;295:1519–1530.

35. Van de Werf F, Baim DS. Reperfusion for ST-segment elevation myocardial infarction: an overview of current treatment options. *Circulation* 2002;105:2813–2816.

36. Gersh BJ, Stone GW, White HD, Holmes DR, Jr. Pharmacological facilitation of primary percutaneous coronary intervention for acute myocardial infarction: is the slope of the curve the shape of the future? *JAMA* 2005;293:979–986.

37. A comparison of reteplase with alteplase for acute myocardial infarction. The Global Use of Strategies to Open Occluded Coronary Arteries (GUSTO III) Investigators. *N Engl J Med* 1997;337:1118–1123.

38. Single-bolus tenecteplase compared with front-loaded alteplase in acute myocardial infarction: the ASSENT-2 double-blind randomised trial. Assessment of the Safety and Efficacy of a New Thrombolytic Investigators. *Lancet* 1999;354:716–722.

39. Keeley EC, Boura JA, Grines CL. Primary angioplasty versus intravenous thrombolytic therapy for acute myocardial infarction: a quantitative review of 23 randomised trials. *Lancet* 2003;361:13–20.

40. De Luca G, Suryapranata H, Ottervanger JP, Antman EM. Time delay to treatment and mortality in primary angioplasty for acute myocardial infarction: every minute of delay counts. *Circulation* 2004;109:1223–1225.

41. Nallamothu BK, Bates ER. Percutaneous coronary intervention versus fibrinolytic therapy in acute myocardial infarction: is timing (almost) everything? *Am J Cardiol* 2003;92:824–826.

42. Thune JJ, Hoefsten DE, Lindholm MG, et al. Simple risk stratification at admission to identify patients with reduced mortality from primary angioplasty. *Circulation* 2005;112:2017–2021.

43. Kastrati A, Mehilli J, Schlotterbeck K, et al. Early administration of reteplase plus abciximab vs abciximab alone in patients with acute myocardial infarction referred for percutaneous coronary intervention: a randomized controlled trial. *JAMA* 2004;291:947–954.

44. Van de Werf F. *ASSENT 4*. European Society of Cardiology Congress. Stockholm, Sweden, 2005.

45. Le May MR, Wells GA, Labinaz M, et al. Combined Angioplasty and Pharmacological Intervention Versus Thrombolysis Alone in Acute Myocardial Infarction (CAPITAL AMI Study). *J Am Coll Cardiol* 2005;46:417–424.

46. Armstrong PW, WEST Steering Committee. A comparison of pharmacologic therapy with/without timely coronary intervention vs. primary percutaneous intervention early after ST-elevation myocardial infarction: the WEST (Which Early ST-elevation myocardial infarction Therapy). *Eur Heart J* 2006;27:1530–1538.

47. Fernandez-Aviles PF, Alonso PJJ, Castro-Beiras PA, et al. Routine invasive strategy within 24 hours of thrombolysis versus ischaemia-guided conservative approach for acute myocardial infarction with ST-segment elevation (GRACIA-1): a randomised controlled trial. *Lancet* 2004;364:1045–1053.

48. Sabatine MS, Cannon CP, Gibson CM, et al. Addition of clopidogrel to aspirin and fibrinolytic therapy for myocardial infarction with ST-segment elevation. *N Engl J Med* 2005;352:1179–1189.

49. Mehta SR, Yusuf S, Peters RJ, et al. Effects of pretreatment with clopidogrel and aspirin followed by long-term therapy in patients undergoing percutaneous coronary intervention: the PCI-CURE study. *Lancet* 2001;358:527–533.

50. Weitz J, Califf R, Ginsberg J, Hirsh J, Theroux P. New antithrombotics. *Chest* 1995;108:471S–485.

51. Randomised trial of intravenous streptokinase, oral aspirin, both, or neither among 17,187 cases of suspected acute myocardial infarction. ISIS-2. *Lancet* 1988;332:349–360.

52. Antman EM, Giugliano RP, Gibson CM, et al. Abciximab facilitates the rate and extent of thrombolysis: results of the thrombolysis in myocardial infarction (TIMI) 14 trial. *Circulation* 1999;99:2720–2732.

53. Trial of abciximab with and without low-dose reteplase for acute myocardial infarction. *Circulation* 2000;101:2788–2794.

54. Topol EJ. Reperfusion therapy for acute myocardial infarction with fibrinolytic therapy or combination reduced fibrinolytic therapy and platelet glycoprotein IIb/IIIa inhibition: The GUSTO V randomised trial. *Lancet* 2001;357:1905–1914.

55. Giugliano RP, Roe MT, Harrington RA, et al. Combination reperfusion therapy with eptifibatide and reduced-dose tenecteplase for ST-elevation myocardial infarction: results of the Integrilin and tenecteplase in acute myocardial infarction (INTEGRITI) Phase II Angiographic trial. *J Am Coll Cardiol* 2003;41:1251–1260.

56. Zorman S, Zorman D, Noc M. Effects of abciximab pretreatment in patients with acute myocardial infarction undergoing primary angioplasty. *Am J Cardiol* 2002;90:533–536.

57. Arntz H-R, Schroder J, Pels K. Prehospital versus periprocedural administration of abciximab in STEMI. early and late results from the randomised REOMOBILE study. *Eur Heart J* 2003;24:268.

58. Mesquita Gabriel H, Oliveira J, et al. Early administration of abciximab bolus in the emergency room improves microperfusion after primary percutaneous coronary intervention, as assessed by TIMI frame count: results of the ERAMI trial. *Eur Heart J* 2003;24:543.

59. Lee DP, Herity NA, Hiatt BL, et al. Adjunctive platelet glycoprotein IIb/IIIa receptor inhibition with tirofiban before primary angioplasty improves angiographic outcomes: results of the TIrofiban Given in the Emergency Room before Primary Angioplasty (TIGER-PA) pilot trial. *Circulation* 2003;107:1497–1501.

60. Cutlip DE, Ricciardi MJ, Ling FS, et al. Effect of tirofiban before primary angioplasty on initial coronary flow and early ST-segment resolution in patients with acute myocardial infarction. *Am J Cardiol* 2003;92:977–980.

61. van't Hof AWJ, Ernst N, de Boer M-J, et al. Facilitation of primary coronary angioplasty by early start of a glycoprotein 2b/3a inhibitor: results of the ongoing tirofiban in myocardial infarction evaluation (On-TIME) trial. *Eur Heart J* 2004;25:837–846.

62. Cutlip DE, Cove CJ, Irons D, et al. Emergency room administration of eptifibatide before primary angioplasty for ST elevation acute myocardial infarction and its effect on baseline coronary flow and procedure outcomes. *Am J Cardiol* 2001;88:62–64.

63. Zeymer U, Zahn R, Schiele R, et al. Early eptifibatide improves TIMI 3 patency before primary percutaneous coronary intervention for acute ST elevation myocardial infarction: results of the randomized Integrilin in acute myocardial infarction (INTAMI) pilot trial. *Eur Heart J* 2005:ehi293.

64. Montalescot G, Borentain M, Payot L, Collet JP, Thomas D. Early vs late administration of glycoprotein IIb/IIIa inhibitors in primary percutaneous coronary intervention of acute ST-segment elevation myocardial infarction: a meta-analysis. *JAMA* 2004;292:362–366.

65. Mehta RH, Harjai KJ, Cox D, et al. Clinical and angiographic correlates and outcomes of suboptimal coronary flow inpatients with acute myocardial infarction undergoing primary percutaneous coronary intervention. *J Am Coll Cardiol* 2003;42:1739–1746.

66. Kenner MD, Zajac EJ, Kondos GT, et al. Ability of the no-reflow phenomenon during an acute myocardial infarction to predict left ventricular dysfunction at one-month follow-up. *Am J Cardiol* 1995;76:861–868.

67. Ito H, Maruyama A, Iwakura K, et al. Clinical implications of the "no reflow" phenomenon: a predictor of complications and left ventricular remodeling in reperfused anterior wall myocardial infarction. *Circulation* 1996;93:223–228.

68. Ting H, Bell M, Bresnahan J, et al. *Mayo Fast Track Protocol for STEMI*. Chicago, SCAI: 2006.

69. Aversano T, Aversano LT, Passamani E, et al. Thrombolytic therapy vs primary percutaneous coronary intervention for myocardial infarction in patients presenting to hospitals without on-site cardiac surgery: a randomized controlled trial. *JAMA* 2002;287:1943–1951.

70. Ting HH, Raveendran G, Lennon RJ, et al. A total of 1,007 percutaneous coronary interventions without onsite cardiac surgery: acute and long-term outcomes. *J Am Coll Cardiol* 2006;47:1713–1721.

71. Smith J, Sidney C, Feldman TE, et al. ACC/AHA/SCAI 2005 Guideline Update for Percutaneous Coronary Intervention—summary article: a report of the American College of Cardiology/American Heart Association Task Force on Practice Guidelines (ACC/AHA/SCAI Writing Committee to Update the 2001 Guidelines for Percutaneous Coronary Intervention). *J Am Coll Cardiol* 2006;47:216–235.

72. Stone GW, Webb J, Cox DA, et al. Distal microcirculatory protection during percutaneous coronary intervention in acute ST-segment elevation myocardial infarction: a randomized controlled trial. *JAMA* 2005;293:1063–1072.

73. Gick M, Jander N, Bestehorn H-P, et al. Randomized evaluation of the effects of filter-based distal protection on myocardial perfusion and infarct size after primary percutaneous catheter intervention in myocardial infarction with and without ST-segment elevation. *Circulation* 2005;112:1462–1469.

74. Grines CL, Cox DA, Stone GW, et al. Coronary angioplasty with or without stent implantation for acute myocardial infarction. *N Engl J Med* 1999;341:1949–1956.

75. Stone GW, Grines CL, Cox DA, et al. Comparison of angioplasty with stenting, with or without abciximab, in acute myocardial infarction. *N Engl J Med* 2002;346:957–966.

76. Morice M-C, Serruys PW, Sousa JE, et al. A randomized comparison of a sirolimus-eluting stent with a standard stent for coronary revascularization. *N Engl J Med* 2002;346:1773–1780.

77. Moses JW, Leon MB, Popma JJ, et al. Sirolimus-eluting stents versus standard stents in patients with stenosis in a native coronary artery. *N Engl J Med* 2003;349:1315–1323.

78. Stone GW, Ellis SG, Cox DA, et al. A polymer-based, paclitaxel-eluting stent in patients with coronary artery disease. *N Engl J Med* 2004;350:221–231.

79. Dibra A, Kastrati A, Mehilli J, et al. Paclitaxel-eluting or sirolimus-eluting stents to prevent restenosis in diabetic patients. *N Engl J Med* 2005;353:663–670.

80. American College of Cardiology. *Trial to Assess the Use of the Cypher Stent in Acute Myocardial Infarction Treated with Balloon Angioplasty (TYPHOON)*. Atlanta, GA: 2006.

81. American College of Cardiology. *Paclitaxel-Eluting Stent Versus Conventional Stent in ST-segment Elevation Myocardial Infarction (PASSION Trial)*. Atlanta, GA: 2006.

82. Spertus JA, Kettelkamp R, Vance C, et al. Prevalence, predictors, and outcomes of premature discontinuation of thienopyridine therapy after drug-eluting stent placement: results from the PREMIER registry. *Circulation* 2006;113:2803–2809.

83. de Lemos JA, Braunwald E. ST segment resolution as a tool for assessing the efficacy of reperfusion therapy. *J Am Coll Cardiol* 2001;38:1283–1294.

84. Gershlick AH, Stephens-Lloyd A, Hughes S, et al. Rescue angioplasty after failed thrombolytic therapy for acute myocardial infarction. *N Engl J Med* 2005;353:2758–2768.

85. Swedberg K, Held P, Kjekshus J, Rasmussen K, Ryden L, Wedel H. Effects of the early administration of enalapril on mortality in patients with acute myo-

cardial infarction. Results of the Cooperative New Scandinavian Enalapril Survival Study II (CONSENSUS II). *N Engl J Med* 1992;327:678–684.

86. GISSI-3: effects of lisinopril and transdermal glyceryl trinitrate singly and together on 6-week mortality and ventricular function after acute myocardial infarction. Gruppo Italiano per lo Studio della Sopravvivenza nell'infarto Miocardico. *Lancet* 1994;343:1115–1122.

87. ISIS-4: a randomised factorial trial assessing early oral captopril, oral mononitrate, and intravenous magnesium sulphate in 58,050 patients with suspected acute myocardial infarction. ISIS-4 (Fourth International Study of Infarct Survival) Collaborative Group. *Lancet* 1995;345:669–685.

88. Oral captopril versus placebo among 13,634 patients with suspected acute myocardial infarction: interim report from the Chinese Cardiac Study (CCS-1). *Lancet* 1995;345:686–687.

89. Pfeffer MA, Braunwald E, Moye LA, et al. Effect of captopril on mortality and morbidity in patients with left ventricular dysfunction after myocardial infarction. Results of the survival and ventricular enlargement trial. The SAVE Investigators. *N Engl J Med* 1992;327:669–677.

90. Kober L, Torp-Pedersen C, Carlsen JE, et al. A clinical trial of the angiotensin-converting-enzyme inhibitor trandolapril in patients with left ventricular dysfunction after myocardial infarction. Trandolapril Cardiac Evaluation (TRACE) Study Group. *N Engl J Med* 1995;333:1670–1676.

91. Effect of ramipril on mortality and morbidity of survivors of acute myocardial infarction with clinical evidence of heart failure. The Acute Infarction Ramipril Efficacy (AIRE) study investigators. *Lancet* 1993;342:821–828.

92. Ambrosioni E, Borghi C, Magnani B. The effect of the angiotensin-converting-enzyme inhibitor zofenopril on mortality and morbidity after anterior myocardial infarction. The Survival of Myocardial Infarction Long-Term Evaluation (SMILE) study investigators. *N Engl J Med* 1995;332:80–85.

93. Kingma JH, van Gilst WH, Peels CH, Dambrink JH, Verheugt FW, Wielenga RP. Acute intervention with captopril during thrombolysis in patients with first anterior myocardial infarction. Results from the Captopril and Thrombolysis Study (CATS). *Eur Heart J* 1994;15:898–907.

94. Pfeffer MA, McMurray JJV, Velazquez EJ, et al. Valsartan, captopril, or both in myocardial infarction complicated by heart failure, left ventricular dysfunction, or both. *N Engl J Med* 2003;349:1893–1906.

95. Dickstein K, Kjekshus J. Effects of losartan and captopril on mortality and morbidity in high-risk patients after acute myocardial infarction: the OPTIMAAL randomised trial. *Lancet* 2002;360:752–760.

96. Pitt B, Remme W, Zannad F, et al. Eplerenone, a selective aldosterone blocker, in patients with left ventricular dysfunction after myocardial infarction. *N Engl J Med* 2003;348:1309–1321.

97. Mehta RH, Roe MT, Mulgund J, et al. Acute clopidogrel use and outcomes in patients with non-st-segment elevation acute coronary syndromes undergoing coronary artery bypass surgery. *J Am Coll Cardiol* 2006;48:281–286.

98. LaRosa JC, He J, Vupputuri S. Effect of statins on risk of coronary disease: a meta-analysis of randomized controlled trials. *JAMA* 1999;282:2340–2346.

99. Ray KK, Cannon CP. The potential relevance of the multiple lipid-independent (pleiotropic) effects of statins in the management of acute coronary syndromes. *J Am Coll Cardiol* 2005;46:1425–1433.

100. Cannon CP, Braunwald E, McCabe CH, et al. Intensive versus moderate lipid lowering with statins after acute coronary syndromes. *N Engl J Med* 2004;350:1495–1504.

101. Goldberg RJ, Gore JM, Alpert JS, et al. Cardiogenic shock after acute myocardial infarction. Incidence and mortality from a community-wide perspective, 1975 to 1988. *N Engl J Med* 1991;325:1117–1122.

102. Forrester JS, Diamond G, Chatterjee K, Swan HJ. Medical therapy of acute myocardial infarction by application of hemodynamic subsets (second of two parts). *N Engl J Med* 1976;295:1404–1413.

103. Forrester JS, Diamond G, Chatterjee K, Swan HJ. Medical therapy of acute myocardial infarction by application of hemodynamic subsets (first of two parts). *N Engl J Med* 1976;295:1356–1362.

104. Berger PB, Tuttle RH, Holmes DR Jr, et al. One-year survival among patients with acute myocardial infarction complicated by cardiogenic shock, and its relation to early revascularization: results from the GUSTO-I trial. *Circulation* 1999;99:873–878.

105. Hochman JS, Sleeper LA, White HD, et al. One-year survival following early revascularization for cardiogenic shock. *JAMA* 2001;285:190–192.

106. Hochman JS, Sleeper LA, Webb JG, et al. Early revascularization in acute myocardial infarction complicated by cardiogenic shock. SHOCK Investigators. Should we emergently revascularize occluded coronaries for cardiogenic shock? *N Engl J Med* 1999;341:625–634.

107. Cotter G, Kaluski E, Blatt A, et al. L-NMMA (a nitric oxide synthase inhibitor) is effective in the treatment of cardiogenic shock. *Circulation* 2000;101:1358–1361.

108. Goldstein JA. Pathophysiology and management of right heart ischemia. *J Am Coll Cardiol* 2002;40:841–853.

109. Bowers TR, O'Neill WW, Pica M, Goldstein JA. Patterns of coronary compromise resulting in acute right ventricular ischemic dysfunction. *Circulation* 2002;106:1104–1109.

110. Goldstein JA, Barzilai B, Rosamond TL, Eisenberg PR, Jaffe AS. Determinants of hemodynamic compromise with severe right ventricular infarction. *Circulation* 1990;82:359–368.

111. Dell'Italia L, Starling M, Blumhardt R, Lasher J, O'Rourke R. Comparative effects of volume loading, dobutamine, and nitroprusside in patients with predominant right ventricular infarction. *Circulation* 1985;72:1327–1335.

112. Zehender M, Kasper W, Kauder E, et al. Eligibility for and benefit of thrombolytic therapy in inferior myocardial infarction: focus on the prognostic importance of right ventricular infarction. *J Am Coll Cardiol* 1994;24:362–369.

113. Bowers TR, O'Neill WW, Grines C, Pica MC, Safian RD, Goldstein JA. Effect of reperfusion on biventricular function and survival after right ventricular infarction. *N Engl J Med* 1998;338:933–940.

114. Zeymer U, Neuhaus KL, Wegscheider K, Tebbe U, Molhoek P, Schroder R. Effects of thrombolytic therapy in acute inferior myocardial infarction with or without right ventricular involvement. HIT-4 Trial Group. Hirudin for Improvement of Thrombolysis. *J Am Coll Cardiol* 1998;32:876–881.

115. Nishimura RA, Schaff HV, Gersh BJ, Holmes DR Jr, Tajik AJ. Early repair of mechanical complications after acute myocardial infarction. *JAMA* 1986;256:47–50.

116. Nishimura RA, Schaff HV, Shub C, Gersh BJ, Edwards WD, Tajik AJ. Papillary muscle rupture complicating acute myocardial infarction: analysis of 17 patients. *Am J Cardiol* 1983;51:373–377.

117. Birnbaum Y, Wagner GS, Gates KB, et al. Clinical and electrocardiographic variables associated with increased risk of ventricular septal defect in acute anterior myocardial infarction. *Am J Cardiol* 2000;86:830–834.

118. Lemery R, Smith HC, Giuliani ER, Gersh BJ. Prognosis in rupture of the ventricular septum after acute myocardial infarction and role of early surgical intervention. *Am J Cardiol* 1992;70:147–151.

119. Crenshaw BS, Granger CB, Birnbaum Y, et al. Risk factors, angiographic patterns, and outcomes in patients with ventricular septal defect complicating acute myocardial infarction. *Circulation* 2000;101:27–32.

120. Landzberg MJ, Lock JE. Transcatheter management of ventricular septal rupture after myocardial infarction. *Semin Thorac Cardiovasc Surg* 1998;10:128–132.

121. Honan MB, Harrell FE Jr, Reimer KA, et al. Cardiac rupture, mortality and the timing of thrombolytic therapy: a meta-analysis. *J Am Coll Cardiol* 1990;16:359–367.

122. Kinn JW, O'Neill WW, Benzuly KH, Jones DE, Grines CL. Primary angioplasty reduces risk of myocardial rupture compared to thrombolysis for acute myocardial infarction. *Cathet Cardiovasc Diagn* 1997;42:151–157.

123. Becker RC, Gore JM, Lambrew C, et al. A composite view of cardiac rupture in the United States National Registry of Myocardial Infarction. *J Am Coll Cardiol* 1996;27:1321–1326.

124. Purcaro A, Costantini C, Ciampani N, et al. Diagnostic criteria and management of subacute ventricular free wall rupture complicating acute myocardial infarction. *Am J Cardiol* 1997;80:397–405.

125. Becker RC, Hochman JS, Cannon CP, et al. Fatal cardiac rupture among patients treated with thrombolytic agents and adjunctive thrombin antagonists—observations from the thrombolysis and thrombin inhibition in myocardial infarction 9 study. *J Am Coll Cardiol* 1999;33:479–487.

126. Solodky A, Behar S, Herz I, et al. Comparison of incidence of cardiac rupture among patients with acute myocardial infarction treated by thrombolysis versus percutaneous transluminal coronary angioplasty. *Am J Cardiol* 2001;87:1105–1108.

127. Slater J, Brown RJ, Antonelli TA, et al. Cardiogenic shock due to cardiac free-wall rupture or tamponade after acute myocardial infarction: A report from the SHOCK Trial Registry. *J Am Coll Cardiol* 2000;36:1117–1122.

128. Lopez-Sendon J, Gonzalez A, Lopez de Sa E, et al. Diagnosis of subacute ventricular wall rupture after acute myocardial infarction: sensitivity and specificity of clinical, hemodynamic and echocardiographic criteria. *J Am Coll Cardiol* 1992;19:1145–1153.

129. Montoya A, McKeever L, Scanlon P, Sullivan HJ, Gunnar RM, Pifarre R. Early repair of ventricular septal rupture after infarction. *Am J Cardiol* 1980;45:345–348.

130. Padro JM, Caralps JM, Montoya JD, Camara ML, Garcia Picart J, Aris A. Sutureless repair of postinfarction cardiac rupture. *J Card Surg* 1988;3:491–493.

131. Frances C, Romero A, Grady D. Left ventricular pseudoaneurysm. *J Am Coll Cardiol* 1998;32:557–561.

132. Yeo TC, Malouf JF, Reeder GS, Oh JK. Clinical characteristics and outcome in postinfarction pseudoaneurysm. *Am J Cardiol* 1999;84:592–5 A8.

133. Archbold RA, Sayer JW, Ray S, Wilkinson P, Ranjadayalan K, Timmis AD. Frequency and prognostic implications of conduction defects in acute myocardial infarction since the introduction of thrombolytic therapy. *Eur Heart J* 1998;19:893–898.

134. Rathore SS, Gersh BJ, Berger PB, et al. Acute myocardial infarction complicated by heart block in the elderly: Prevalence and outcomes. *Am Heart J* 2001;141:47–54.

135. Goodfellow J, Walker PR. Reversal of atropine-resistant atrioventricular block with intravenous aminophylline in the early phase of inferior wall acute myocardial infarction following treatment with streptokinase. *Eur Heart J* 1995;16:862–865.

136. Brilakis ES, Wright RS, Kopecky SL, Reeder GS, Williams BA, Miller WL. Bundle-branch block as a predictor of long-term survival after acute myocardial infarction. *Am J Cardiol* 2001;88:205–209.

137. Crenshaw BS, Ward SR, Granger CB, Stebbins AL, Topol EJ, Califf RM. Atrial fibrillation in the setting of acute myocardial infarction: the GUSTO-I experience. *J Am Coll Cardiol* 1997;30:406–413.

138. Pedersen OD, Bagger H, Kober L, Torp-Pedersen C. The occurrence and prognostic significance of atrial fibrillation/-flutter following acute myocardial infarction. *Eur Heart J* 1999;20:748–754.

139. Solomon SD, Zelenkofske S, McMurray JJV, et al. Sudden death in patients with myocardial infarction and left ventricular dysfunction, heart failure, or both. *N Engl J Med* 2005;352:2581–2588.

140. Executive summary of the third report of the National Cholesterol Education Program (NCEP) Expert Panel on Detection, Evaluation, and Treatment of High Blood Cholesterol in Adults (Adult Treatment Panel III). *JAMA* 2001;285:2486–2497.

141. LaRosa JC, Grundy SM, Waters DD, et al. Intensive lipid lowering with atorvastatin in patients with stable coronary disease. *N Engl J Med* 2005;352:1425–1435.

142. Canner PL, Berge KG, Wenger NK, et al. Fifteen-year mortality in Coronary Drug Project patients: long-term benefit with niacin. *J Am Coll Cardiol* 1986;8:1245–1255.

143. Rubins HB, Robins SJ, Collins D, et al. Gemfibrozil for the secondary prevention of coronary heart disease in men with low levels of high-density lipoprotein cholesterol. Veterans Affairs High-Density Lipoprotein Cholesterol Intervention Trial Study Group. *N Engl J Med* 1999;341:410–418.

144. Weiss R, Dziura J, Burgert TS, et al. Obesity and the metabolic syndrome in children and adolescents. *N Engl J Med* 2004;350:2362–2374.

145. UK Prospective Diabetes Study (UKPDS) G. Intensive blood-glucose control with sulphonylureas or insulin compared with conventional treatment and risk of complications in patients with type 2 diabetes (UKPDS 33). *Lancet* 1998;352:837–853.

146. Schleifer SJ, Macari-Hinson MM, Coyle DA, et al. The nature and course of depression following myocardial infarction. *Arch Intern Med* 1989;149:1785–1789.

147. Ziegelstein RC, Fauerbach JA, Stevens SS, Romanelli J, Richter DP, Bush DE. Patients with depression are less likely to follow recommendations to reduce cardiac risk during recovery from a myocardial infarction. *Arch Intern Med* 2000;160:1818–1823.

148. Frasure-Smith N, Lesperance F, Talajic M. Depression and 18-month prognosis after myocardial infarction. *Circulation* 1995;91:999–1005.

149. Frasure-Smith N, Lesperance F, Talajic M. Depression following myocardial infarction. Impact on 6-month survival. *JAMA* 1993;270:1819–1825.

150. Bush DE, Ziegelstein RC, Tayback M, et al. Even minimal symptoms of depression increase mortality risk after acute myocardial infarction. *Am J Cardiol* 2001;88:337–341.

CHAPTER (61)

Pharmacologic Therapy for Acute Coronary Syndromes

Santo Dellegrottaglie / Antony H. Gershlick / Massimo Chiariello / Bernard J. Gersh

INTRODUCTION

During the last three decades, improvements in pharmacologic therapy have significantly contributed to a better prognosis in patients with acute coronary syndrome (ACS). The term *acute coronary syndrome* encompasses different clinical entities associated with acute myocardial ischemia, including ST-segment elevation myocardial infarction (STEMI; see Chap. 60), and non–ST-segment elevation myocardial infarction (NSTEMI) and unstable angina (UA; see Chap. 59). The two clinical types of ACS are discussed in their entirety in Chaps. 59 and 60. This chapter further elucidates the pharmacotherapy of these two common syndromes.

Although a common underlying pathophysiologic mechanism (i.e., atherosclerotic plaque rupture/erosion) explains the majority of ACS cases, some key differences in the characteristics of the triggered process are responsible for the varied clinical presentations (see Chaps. 59 and 60). These result in important differences in the therapeutic approach for different forms of ACS.

UA and NSTEMI represent two closely related conditions whose pathogenesis and clinical presentation are similar but of differing severity. In patients with NSTEMI, ischemia is severe enough to cause sufficient myocardial damage to release detectable quantities of markers of myocardial injury. However, biomarkers of necrosis may become detectable in the bloodstream hours after the onset of symptoms (see Chap. 59). Thus, at the time of presentation, patients with UA or NSTEMI may be indistinguishable, resulting in UA and NSTEMI frequently being considered a single clinical entity.

UNSTABLE ANGINA/NON–ST-SEGMENT ELEVATION MYOCARDIAL INFARCTION

Patients with UA/NSTEMI present a substantial but heterogeneous risk of death (between 2.5 and 5 percent) and of subsequent reinfarction (between 3 and 12 percent).[1,2] To select the most appropriate treatment for each patient with UA/NSTEMI, the risk for subsequent events should be assessed at admission and, then, repeatedly during hospitalization. Several risk stratification tools (e.g., TIMI [Thrombolysis in Myocardial Infarction] risk score, GRACE [Global Registry of Acute Coronary Events] risk score), based on the consideration of some baseline variables that are part of routine medical evaluation, have been developed.[3] Apart from age and a previous history of coronary artery disease, clinical examination, ECG, and cardiac biomarkers (see Chap. 59) provide the key elements for risk assessment in UA/NSTEMI patients (Table 61–1).

TABLE 61–1

Elements for Risk Stratification in Patients with Unstable Angina/Non–ST-Segment Elevation Myocardial Infarction

FEATURE	HIGH RISK	INTERMEDIATE RISK	LOW RISK
History	Accelerating tempo of ischemic symptoms in preceding 48 h	Previous MI, peripheral or cerebrovascular disease, or CABG; previous aspirin use	
Character of pain	Prolonged ongoing (>20 min) rest pain	Prolonged (>20 min) rest angina, now resolved, with moderate or high likelihood of CAD; rest angina (>20 min) or relieved with rest or sublingual NTG	New-onset or progressive CCS class III or IV angina within previous 2 weeks without prolonged rest pain but with moderate-high likelihood for CAD
Clinical findings	Pulmonary edema most likely result of ischemia; new or worsening MR murmur, S_3 or new/worsening rales; hypotension, bradycardia, tachycardia; age >75 y	Age >70 y	
ECG	Angina at rest with transient ST-segment changes >0.05 mV; bundle-branch block, new or presumed new; sustained ventricular tachycardia	T-wave inversions >0.2 mV; pathologic Q waves	Normal or unchanged ECG during episode of chest discomfort
Cardiac markers	Elevated (eg, troponin T >0.1 ng/mL)	Slightly elevated (e.g., troponin T >0.01 but <0.1 ng/mL)	Normal

CABG, coronary artery bypass graft; CCS, Canadian Cardiovascular Society; MR, mitral regurgitation; NTG: nitroglycerin.
SOURCE: Braunwald E, Antman EM, Beasley JW, et al. ACC/AHA guideline update for the management of patients with unstable angina and non–ST-segment elevation myocardial infarction—2002: summary article: a report of the American College of Cardiology/American Heart Association Task Force on Practice Guidelines (Committee on the Management of Patients With Unstable Angina). Circulation 2002;106:1893–1900.

Based on the measured level of risk, patients may be managed through an early invasive or an early conservative strategy (Fig. 61–1).[4] The early routine invasive strategy generally consists of diagnostic coronary angiography and angiographically directed revascularization within 48 hours of symptom onset and is indicated in patients with high-risk features.[5,6] In contrast, the conservative strategy is recommended in patients who are at lower risk and relies on noninvasive evaluation of ischemia after a period of observation, with catheterization only if ischemia recurs or is unresolved. Patients with an intermediate level of risk may be managed either with an early conservative or an early invasive strategy.

Regardless of treatment strategy, a combined antiischemic and antithrombotic therapy is recommended for all patients with UA/NSTEMI (Table 61–2).[7,8]

ANTIISCHEMIC TREATMENT

Bedrest needs to be strictly observed at admission, but cautious mobilization may be allowed in patients without ongoing chest pain or ischemic ECG changes for at least 24 hours. Subsequent activity should not be inappropriately restricted, especially in older patients.[7]

Patients with respiratory distress or other high-risk features should receive supplemental oxygen to maintain an arterial oxygen saturation >90 percent.

Recommended antiischemic medications include sublingually or intravenously administered nitrates for relief of recurrent ischemia and associated symptoms and, in the absence of contrain-

dications, an intravenously administered β blocker for management of ongoing ischemia (followed by an orally administered β blocker). As an alternative, heart-rate-limiting calcium antagonists may be used in stable patients with contraindications to β blockers. Morphine sulfate is indicated to control symptoms in patients who are nonresponsive to full antiischemic therapy.

NITRATES

The rationale for using nitrates in UA/NSTEMI is derived from pathophysiologic principles and extensive, although uncontrolled, clinical observations.[9] The major therapeutic benefit of nitrates is related to the marked vasodilator effects, which lead to a reduction in myocardial preload and left ventricular (LV) end-diastolic volume, resulting in decreased myocardial oxygen demand. In addition, nitrates enhance myocardial oxygen delivery by inducing a dilation of normal and atherosclerotic coronary arteries.

Sublingual or buccal spray nitrates (0.3 to 0.6 mg) are indicated in patients with ischemic chest pain. In cases with persistence of symptoms after three doses administered 5 minutes apart, intravenous nitroglycerin (5 to 10 μg/min) is recommended. The rate of infusion may be increased by 10 μg/min every 5 minutes (to a maximum of 200 μg/min) until a satisfactory symptom response is noted or significant side effects occur (notably headache or hypotension).[7]

A marked fall in blood pressure with nitrates should always raise the suspicion of underlying hypovolemia, particularly in the elderly. Also, the use of sildenafil (or other drugs of the same class)

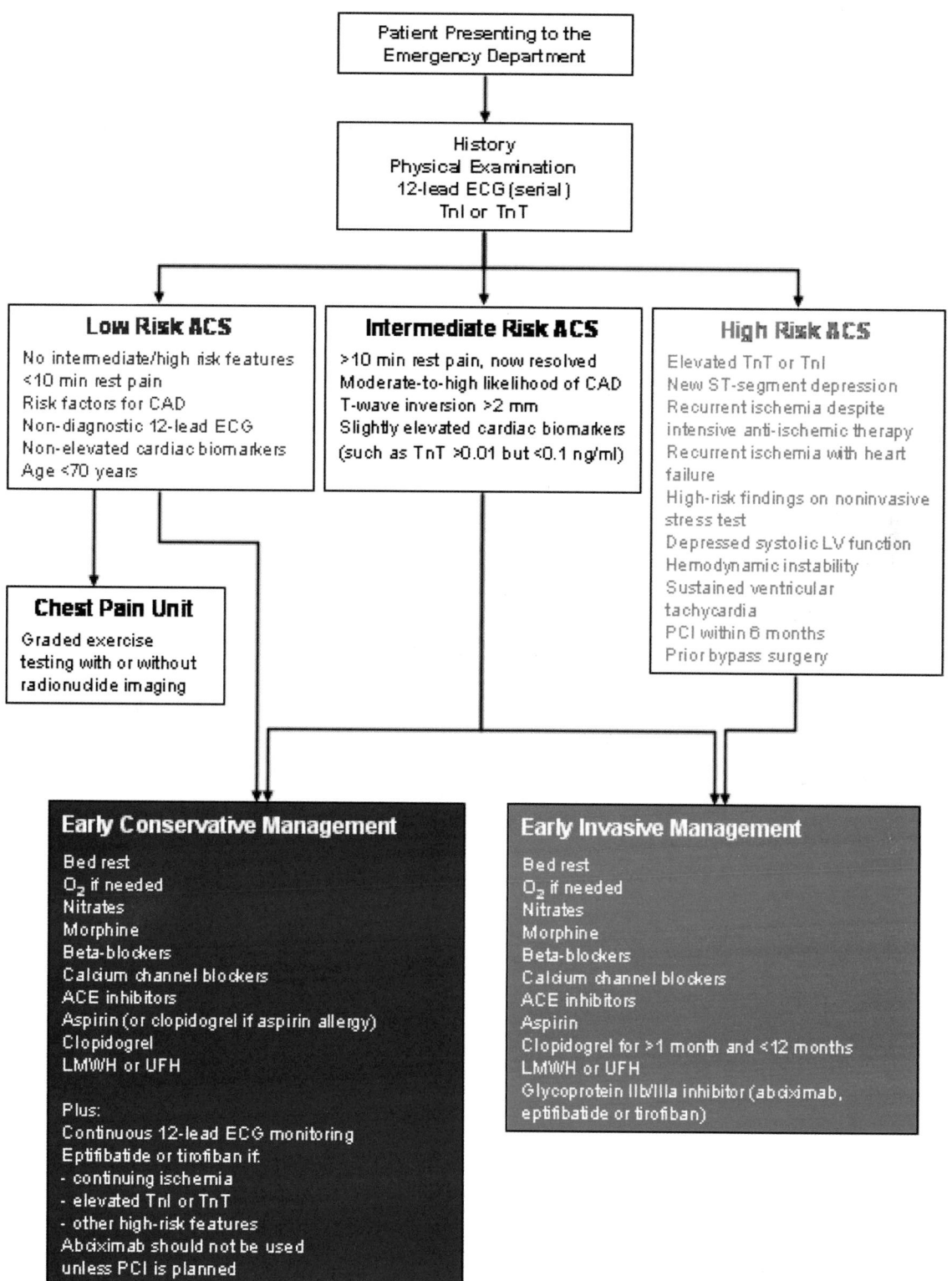

FIGURE 61-1. Management strategies in relation with short-term risk of death or nonfatal myocardial infarction in patients with unstable angina/non–ST-segment elevation myocardial infarction (UA/NSTEMI). ACE, angiotensin-converting enzyme; CAD, coronary artery disease; LMWH, low-molecular-weight heparin; LV, left ventricle; PCI, percutaneous coronary intervention; Tn, troponin; UFH, unfractionated heparin. *Source: Adapted from the AHA Practical Implementation of Guidelines for UA/NSTEMI in the Emergency Department. Gibler WB, Cannon CP, Blomkalns AL, et al. Practical implementation of the guidelines for unstable angina/non-ST-segment elevation myocardial infarction in the emergency department: a scientific statement from the American Heart Association Council on Clinical Cardiology (Subcommittee on Acute Cardiac Care), Council on Cardiovascular Nursing, and Quality of Care and Outcomes Research Interdisciplinary Working Group, in Collaboration with the Society of Chest Pain Centers. Circulation 2005;111:2699–2710.*

TABLE 61–2

Treatment for Unstable Angina/Non–ST-Segment Elevation Myocardial Infarction Patients: Rationale and Class of Recommendation[a]

TREATMENT	ANTIISCHEMIA	PREVENTION OF EVENTS	PREVENTION OF EVENTS AT SHORT-TERM FOLLOWUP	CLASS OF RECOMMENDATION[b]
Bedrest	C	—	—	I
Supplemental O$_2$	C	—	—	I[c]
Morphine sulfate	C	—	—	I
Nitrates	C	—	—	I
β Blockers	A	B	A	I
Calcium antagonists	B	B	—	II
Aspirin	—	A	A	I
Thienopyridine	B	B	B	I
Glycoprotein IIb/IIIa inhibitors	A	A	A	II
Unfractionated heparin	C	B	—	I
Low-molecular weight heparin	A	A	C	I
Direct anti-thrombin inhibitors	—	A	—	I
Revascularization	C	B	B	I

Level of evidence: level A: data derived from multiple randomized clinical trials or meta-analyses; level B: data derived from a single randomized trial or nonrandomized studies; level C: consensus opinion of the experts.
[a]See Chap. 11.
[b]Class of recommendation: Class I: conditions for which there is evidence that a given therapy is useful and effective; class II: conditions for which there is conflicting evidence and/or divergence about the efficacy/usefulness of a given treatment; class III: contraindications.
[c]In patients with signs of respiratory distress or arterial hypoxemia.
SOURCE: Modified from Bertrand ME, Simoons ML, Fox KA, et al. Management of acute coronary syndromes in patients presenting without persistent ST-segment elevation. Eur Heart J 2002;23:1809–1840.

within the previous 24 hours represents the only absolute contraindication to nitrate administration.[10] A limitation to continuous nitrate therapy is the phenomenon of tolerance to the hemodynamic effects of these drugs, which typically becomes evident after 24 hours of continuous therapy. When symptoms are controlled, intravenous nitrates should be replaced by nonparenteral alternatives. At the moment of therapy interruption, graded reduction in the dose of intravenous nitrates is advisable to avoid possible exacerbation of ischemic changes on ECG, which is observed in some cases after abrupt cessation of therapy.[11]

【 】 β BLOCKERS

The use of β blockers in patients with UA/NSTEMI is logical given prevailing concepts of the balance between myocardial oxygen supply and demand. The primary benefits of β blockers in the treatment of myocardial ischemia are a result of an effect of blockade of cardiac β$_1$-adrenergic receptors resulting in reductions in myocardial contractility, sinus node rate and atrioventricular node conduction velocity. Overall, these mechanisms act to reduce myocardial oxygen consumption.

Data supporting the use of β blockers in the acute setting are limited and come from small, randomized studies showing a 13 percent relative risk reduction in the rate of progression to an acute myocardial infarction (MI),[12] and a 29 percent relative risk reduction in death among high-risk individuals with threatened or evolving MI in comparison with placebo.[13] Nevertheless, current recommendations are to start a β blocker early in the management of patients with UA/NSTEMI, with an initial intravenous bolus followed by an oral regimen targeted to establish a resting heart rate between 50 and 60 beats/min. Table 61–3 describes possible β-blocker regimens that may be administered in UA/NSTEMI patients. No agent is more effective than another, except that β blockers with increased β$_1$ selectivity and without intrinsic sympathomimetic activity are preferable.

Advanced atrioventricular block, overt bronchospasm, or a history of frank asthma, severe LV dysfunction with congestive heart failure, marked bradycardia (heart rate <50 beats/min), or hypotension (systolic blood pressure <90 mmHg) represent contraindications to the use of β blockers. In cases of doubt, a short-acting cardioselective agent at a reduced dose (i.e., esmolol at 25 μg/kg/min intravenously) is preferable to the complete avoidance of a β blocker.[14]

TABLE 61–3

Therapeutic Regimens for Some β Blockers of Clinical Use in Unstable Angina/Non–ST-Segment Elevation Myocardial Infarction

β BLOCKER	STARTING DOSE	MAINTENANCE DOSE PO
Metoprolol	5–15 mg IV	50–200 mg × 2 times daily
Propanolol	0.5–1.0 mg IV	20–80 mg × 2 times daily
Atenolol	5–10 mg IV	50–200 mg daily
Esmolol	0.3–0.5 mg/kg/min IV	0.05–0.3 mg/kg/min IV

CALCIUM ANTAGONISTS

Calcium antagonists may be used to control ongoing or recurring ischemia-related symptoms in patients already receiving adequate doses of nitrates and β blockers, in patients who are unable to tolerate nitrates and/or β blockers, and in the subgroup of patients with variant angina.

By reducing cell transmembrane inward calcium flux, calcium antagonists produce a variable degree of vasodilation (at peripheral and coronary level), decreased myocardial contractility, atrioventricular block, and sinus node slowing. The combination of a decreased myocardial oxygen demand and improved myocardial flow justifies the use of calcium antagonists as antiischemic drugs.

Potential side effects include hypotension, bradycardia, atrioventricular block, and worsening heart failure. The combination of a β blocker and a heart-rate-limiting calcium antagonist is particularly likely to cause conduction disturbances, especially in elderly patients with underlying conduction system disease. Based on composition, calcium antagonists are classified into three subgroups: dihydropyridines (such as nifedipine), which are characterized by an intense peripheral arterial dilatory effect, but little or no atrioventricular or sinus node effects; benzothiazepines (such as diltiazem), which are responsible for prominent atrioventricular and sinus node effects and for some peripheral arterial dilatory effects; phenylalkylamines (such as verapamil), with a spectrum of effects similar to the benzothiazepines.[7]

A meta-analysis of comparative studies in patients with stable angina found calcium antagonists effective but inferior to β blockers in controlling anginal episodes and in preventing adverse events.[15] Consequently, calcium antagonists are indicated as a second-line therapeutic option for symptom control.[16,17] In particular, verapamil (80 to 160 mg × 3 times daily) and diltiazem (30 to 80 mg × 3 to 4 times daily) are often indicated in patients with contraindications to therapy with β blockers. Dihydropyridines (including amlodipine, 5 to 10 mg, and felodipine, 5 to 10 mg) should be preferred to benzothiazepines and phenylalkylamines in patients with severe LV dysfunction or conduction abnormalities.[18,19] However, particular cautions need to be adopted when prescribing rapid-release, short-acting dihydropyridines (e.g., nifedipine, 30 to 90 mg daily) in ACS. Controlled trials suggest increased adverse outcomes with the use of nifedipine alone in ACS patients, but a protective effect when this drug is administered to patients with adequate concurrent β blockade.[20,21]

MORPHINE SULFATE

Morphine sulfate (1 to 5 mg intravenously) is indicated in patients with persistent or recurrent symptoms *despite adequate antiischemic therapy*. The administration may be repeated every 5 to 30 minutes as needed to relieve symptoms. These recommendations are based exclusively on expert consensus, as there are no controlled clinical trials evaluating the efficacy

or safety of morphine in this population.[22] This drug combines potent analgesic and anxiolytic effects with beneficial hemodynamic effects (i.e., venodilation and an increased vagal tone resulting in a modest reduction in the myocardial oxygen demand). Hypotension may be severe in patients who are volume depleted. Nausea and vomiting may occur in up to 20 percent of treated patients and an antiemetic is frequently coadministered. The use of morphine may be limited by the occurrence of hypotension and/or bradycardia and it may rarely induce severe respiratory depression, usually responsive to naloxone (0.4 to 20 mg intravenously).

ANTITHROMBOTIC TREATMENT

Antithrombotic therapy in UA/NSTEMI patients is crucial to modify the disease course and to reduce the risk of progression to STEMI or death. This class of medications includes drugs of two major groups: (1) *antiplatelet agents,* such as aspirin, thienopyridines, and glycoprotein IIb/IIIa inhibitors; and (2) *antithrombin agents,* such as unfractionated heparin, low-molecular-weight heparin, and direct thrombin inhibitors (Fig. 61–2). In the individual patient, the number of medications and the intensity of antithrombotic treatment are based on global risk.

Of note, fibrinolytic agents have no significant beneficial effects in UA/NSTEMI (they might actually increase the risks) and are contraindicated in patients without STEMI.[23]

Aspirin

Aspirin should be started as soon as ACS is suspected (chew the first dose). This drug inhibits platelet aggregation by blocking the intraplatelet thromboxane A_2 pathway and, in patients with

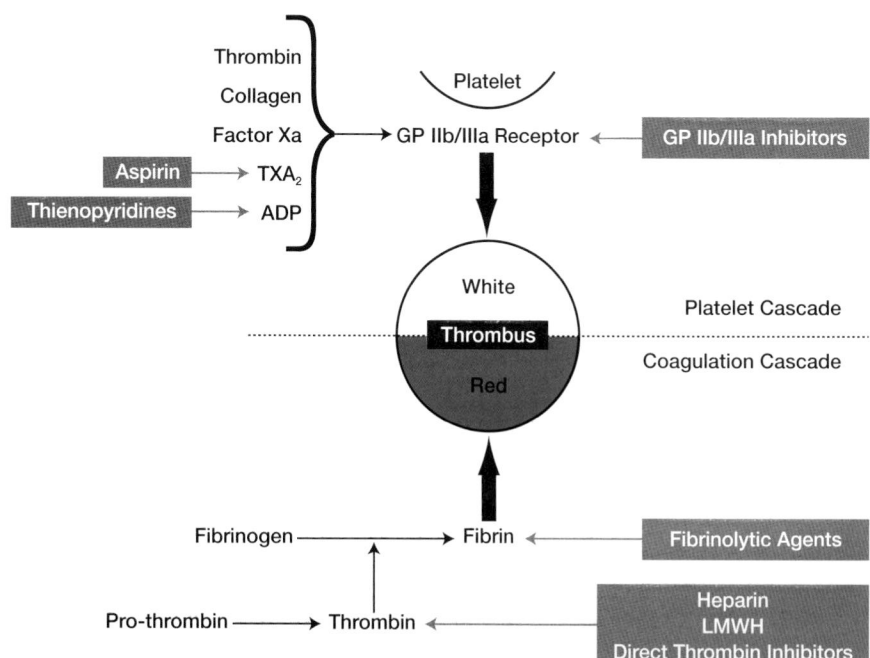

FIGURE 61–2. Role of platelet and coagulation cascades in the intracoronary thrombus formation. The site of action for antiplatelet, antithrombin, and fibrinolytic agents is reported. ADP, adenosine diphosphate; GP, glycoprotein; LMWH, low-molecular-weight heparin; TXA_2, thromboxane A_2. *Source: Adapted from Boersma E, Mercado N, Poldermans D, et al. Acute myocardial infarction. Lancet 2003;361:847–858.*

UA/NSTEMI, has been proved effective in significantly reducing the incidence of death and MI in short- and long-term followup studies.[12,24,25]

Current guidelines recommend that all patients with UA/NSTEMI initially receive 160 to 325 mg of aspirin, followed by 75 to 160 mg daily thereafter.[7] These low doses ensure inhibition of one of the major intraplatelet pathways without significantly increasing the risk of bleeding. The treatment should be continued indefinitely, unless there are specific contraindications, including well-defined intolerance to acetylsalicylic acid, active bleeding, hemophilia, and active peptic ulcer.

Thienopyridines

Clopidogrel and ticlopidine block the adenosine diphosphate (ADP) receptor normally expressed on platelets and are the only thienopyridines approved for antiplatelet therapy. Clopidogrel is currently the clinically preferred thienopyridine because of a more rapid onset of action and better safety profile than ticlopidine. The usefulness of ticlopidine is limited by potentially serious hematologic adverse events, including severe neutropenia and, rarely, thrombotic thrombocytopenia purpura.

Clopidogrel is indicated in patients with UA/NSTEMI who are unable to tolerate aspirin.[26] Because the mechanisms of the antiplatelet effects of aspirin and thienopyridines differ, a potential exists for additive benefit with their combination. The benefits of long-term association between aspirin and clopidogrel were demonstrated in the large-scale CURE (Clopidogrel in Unstable Angina to Prevent Recurrent Ischemic Events) trial, which showed a 20 percent relative risk reduction in the composite end point of cardiac death, nonfatal MI, or stroke when patients received the dual antiplatelet therapy for 9 to 12 months after an episode of UA/NSTEMI.[27] A clear increase in bleeding risk occurred as the daily dose of aspirin increased to more than 100 mg. Clopidogrel is also efficacious among patients with UA/NSTEMI who are undergoing percutaneous coronary intervention (PCI).[28,29]

Currently, recommendations are to add clopidogrel (300 mg loading dose followed by 75 mg daily) to low-dose aspirin (<100 mg daily) on admission of all UA/NSTEMI patients.[7] In these patients, clopidogrel therapy should be continued for up to 12 months. In patients who are taking clopidogrel in whom elective surgical revascularization is planned, the drug should be withheld, if possible, for at least 5 days so as to reduce the surgical risk of bleeding.

In recent years, considerable concern has been generated by the results of some ex vivo studies suggesting that atorvastatin attenuates the antiplatelet effects of clopidogrel, but this negative drug interaction has not been confirmed in subsequent clinical studies.[30]

Glycoprotein IIb/IIIa Inhibitors

Glycoprotein (GP) IIb/IIIa surface receptors are actively involved in the final common pathway leading to platelet aggregation (see Fig. 61–2). Various intravenous GPIIb/IIIa receptor inhibitors (with different pharmacokinetic and pharmacodynamic properties) have been studied, but only a monoclonal antibody fragment (abciximab, 0.25 mg/kg bolus plus infusion of 0.125 µg/kg/min

for 12 to 24 hours) and two small-molecule agents (eptifibatide, 180 g/kg bolus plus 2.0 µg/kg/min for 72 to 96 hours; and tirofiban, 0.4 µg/kg/min for 30 minutes plus 0.1 µg/kg/min for 48 to 96 hours) are approved for clinical use in ACS.

Available data strongly support the use of GPIIb/IIIa inhibitors in UA/STEMI patients managed with an early invasive strategy (see Fig. 61–1).[31,32] In patients who are undergoing an early conservative strategy, tirofiban and eptifibatide showed a more pronounced benefit in reducing the occurrence of adverse events when continuing ischemia, positive troponin level, or other high-risk features were present. However, in conservatively managed patients, an actual trend toward worse outcomes has been observed with abciximab therapy.

As a result, a GPIIb/IIIa inhibitor should be administered, in addition to aspirin and clopidogrel (plus heparin), to patients in whom PCI is planned (triple antiaggregation).[33] Eptifibatide and tirofiban are also indicated in UA/NSTEMI patients who are managed with a conservative strategy, but who have high-risk features. Abciximab is contraindicated for patients who are receiving only medical management without cardiac catheterization.

Treatment with a GPIIb/IIIa antagonist increases the risk of bleeding, which is typically mucocutaneous or involves the access site of vascular intervention. Thrombocytopenia is an unusual complication and may be observed in 0.5 percent of patients during administration of parenteral GPIIb/IIIa inhibitors.[34] A possible safe approach may be to withhold the drug administration until the coronary anatomy is established and revascularization is planned (infusion may be started immediately before PCI). Inhibition of platelet aggregation may also result in bleeding complications at the time of cardiac surgery. In contrast to abciximab, eptifibatide and tirofiban have a short half-life and, at the end of infusion, platelet aggregation recovery occurs in 4 to 8 hours (vs. 24 to 48 hours with abciximab). By withholding the infusion of eptifibatide or tirofiban immediately before surgery, platelet function should be partially recovered at the end of the procedure when hemostasis is necessary.[8]

Unfractionated Heparin

Unfractionated heparin (UFH) exerts its anticoagulant effect by accelerating the action of circulating antithrombin in the inactivation of thrombin, factor IXa and factor Xa (see Fig. 61–2). Therefore, it prevents thrombus propagation, but does not actually lyse existing thrombi.

It is interesting that, UFH was never evaluated in clinical trials that enrolled the number of patients or accumulated the number of events that would be required currently. Nevertheless, based on relatively small studies in selected populations, UFH is recommended in clinical practice guidelines.[7] Taken together, these studies on UFH indicate that its early administration is associated with a reduction in the progression to STEMI and death in patients with UA/NSTEMI.[35]

Anticoagulation with UFH should be added to aspirin and clopidogrel in UA/NSTEMI.[7,8] Most of the trials that evaluate the use of UFH in UA/NSTEMI have continued therapy for 2 to 5 days and optimal duration of therapy remains undefined. Heparin requires frequent monitoring of the activated partial thromboplastin time (aPTT). Clinical trials indicate that a weight-adjusted dosing regimen (60 to 70 U/kg at a 12 to 15 U/kg/h infusion rate) could provide more predictable anticoagulation than a fixed-dose regimen. Measurements of aPTT should be made 4 to 6 hours after any dosage change and UFH infusion rate adjusted until the aPTT is within the therapeutic level (1.5 to 2.5 times control or 60 to 80 seconds).

Serial hemoglobin/hematocrit and platelet measurements are necessary to monitor for heparin-induced thrombocytopenia (severe in 1 to 2 percent of cases) and autoimmune thrombocytopenia with thrombosis (<0.2 percent of cases).

Low-Molecular-Weight Heparin

Low-molecular-weight heparin (LMWH) is produced through depolymerization of the polysaccharide chains of heparin and is relatively more potent in inhibiting factor Xa than in the inactivation of thrombin (see Fig. 61–2). Distinct advantages of LMWH over UFH include a more predictable anticoagulant effect with once- or twice-a-day subcutaneous administration. LMWH does not usually require laboratory monitoring of activity. In addition, LMWH is associated with less-intense platelet activation and heparin-induced thrombocytopenia compared with UFH.

Two large trials, A to Z (Aggrastat to Zocor) and SYNERGY (Superior Yield of the New Strategy of Enoxaparin, Revascularization, and Glycoprotein IIb/IIIa Inhibitors), recently compared the safety and efficacy of enoxaparin with that of UFH in patients with UA/NSTEMI.[36,37] Overall, the results of these and four other ACS trials documented that enoxaparin provided a modest but significant reduction in the 30-day incidence of death or nonfatal MI (Fig. 61–3), with no significant differences in the rate of major bleeding.[38] In particular, LMWH treatment consistently showed benefit in the group of patients managed with an early conservative approach.

Based on these data, LMWH (specifically enoxaparin at 1 mg/kg subcutaneously every 12 hours) should be the preferred anticoagulant in UA/NSTEMI patients managed with an early conservative strategy.[7] On the other hand, because the anticoagulant effect of UFH can be more readily reversed than that of LMWH, UFH should be preferred in patients who are likely to undergo coronary bypass graft surgery within 24 hours.

Direct Thrombin Inhibitors

Direct thrombin inhibitors are able to specifically block thrombin without the need for any cofactor (i.e., antithrombin; see Fig. 61–2). These drugs produce a more predictable anticoagulant response than UFH.

The OASIS (Organization for the Assessment of Strategies for Ischemic Syndromes)-2 trial randomized 10,141 patients with UA/NSTEMI to a 72-hour infusion of either the direct antithrombin hirudin (0.4 mg/kg bolus, 0.15 mg/kg/h infusion) or UFH.[39] This study demonstrated a nonsignificant difference between hirudin and heparin in the primary outcome of cardiovascular death or MI at 7 days, with a tendency toward a benefit in the hirudin group. However, a secondary end point of cardiovascular death, MI or refractory angina at 7 days, was significantly reduced with hirudin. Compared with UFH, hirudin was associated with a significantly increased risk of major (but not life-threatening) bleeding. A pooled analysis of the OASIS, GUSTO (Global Utilization of Streptokinase and Tissue Plasminogen Activator for Occluded Arteries)-2B, and TIMI-9B trials showed superiority of hirudin compared with heparin for the prevention of death or MI at 30 to 35 days.[39] Recently, the ACUITY (Acute Catheterization and Urgent Intervention Triage Strategy) trial showed that in UA/NSTEMI patients who were undergoing early invasive management, the rates of ischemic events and bleeding were similar with the use of either the direct thrombin inhibitor bivalirudin (bolus of 0.1 mg/kg followed by 0.25 mg/kg/h infusion) or heparin when combined

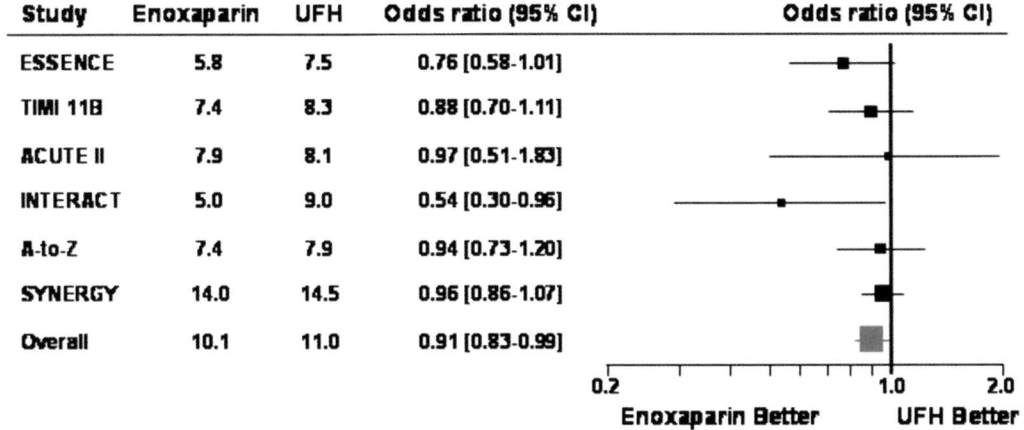

FIGURE 61–3. Effect of enoxaparin in comparison with unfractionated heparin (UFH) on composite efficacy end point of death or myocardial infarction at 30 days. Data derive from a meta-analysis of six trials (ESSENCE, TIMI-11B, ACUTE II, INTERACT, A to Z, and SYNERGY) enrolling a total of 21,946 patients with unstable angina/non–ST-segment elevation myocardial infarction and randomized to receive low-molecular-weight heparin (enoxaparin) or UFH. Black squares indicate odds ratios (ORs); horizontal lines, 95 percent confidence intervals (CIs). The size of each square reflects the statistical weight of a trial in calculating the OR. *Source: Adapted from Petersen JL, Mahaffey KW, Hasselblad V, et al. Efficacy and bleeding complications among patients randomized to enoxaparin or unfractionated heparin for antithrombin therapy in non–ST-segment acute coronary syndromes: a systematic overview. JAMA 2004;292:89–96.*

with the planned use of a GPIIb/IIIa inhibitor.[40] Interestingly, bivalirudin alone was shown to be as effective as the combination of heparin plus GPIIb/IIIa inhibitor, but with a significantly reduced frequency of major bleeding.

Overall, the data seem to support the superiority of direct thrombin inhibitors compared to UFH in UA/NSTEMI, particularly in the setting of patients who are managed with an early invasive strategy.

[ ] OTHER MEDICATIONS FOR EARLY MANAGEMENT OF UA/NSTEMI

In UA/NSTEMI, angiotensin-converting enzyme (ACE) inhibitors are recommended in the early management of patients with heart failure, but also in patients with left ventricular systolic dysfunction when hypertension persists despite treatment with nitroglycerin and β blockers.[41]

Statins should be administered early in the management of all ACS patients, with target levels of low-density lipoprotein (LDL) cholesterol particularly low (<100 mg/dL; see corresponding paragraph in the STEMI section below).[8]

[ ] UA/NSTEMI MANAGEMENT IN SUMMARY

After the diagnosis of UA/NSTEMI has been established, all patients should receive a baseline treatment including aspirin, LMWH (or UFH), clopidogrel, β blocker, and nitrates (see Fig. 61–1 and Table 61–2). To identify the subgroup of patients at high risk for subsequent events, initial risk stratification should be performed from clinical data, ECG, and troponins measurements. Infusion of GPIIb/IIIa inhibitors followed by coronary angiography within the hospitalization period is generally indicated in high-risk patients. Emergency angiography is performed in patients with hemodynamic instability or recurrent life-threatening arrhythmias.

Duration of treatment is variable for the different drugs and for some of them (e.g., heparin) is not well established. For the antiischemic medications (i.e., nitrates, β blockers, and calcium antagonists), the strongest evidence for a benefit in continuing the therapy after the initial control of ischemia-induced symptoms and signs has been shown for β blockers. Aspirin should be continued indefinitely. Guidelines recommend the administration of clopidogrel for at least 1 month (but less than 12 months).

In low-risk patients, a stress test (with or without imaging) to assess the probability and the severity of coronary artery disease should be performed after repeated negative troponins measurements have been obtained and before discharge. Based on test results, coronary angiography is often planned for patients in this group.

In all cases, an aggressive management of the classic risk factors must be implemented during hospitalization and continued during the followup.

ST-SEGMENT ELEVATION MYOCARDIAL INFARCTION

Optimal management of patients presenting with STEMI comprises varies therapeutic modalities, but it is mainly focused on the prompt access to a reperfusion therapy (either pharmacologic or mechanical) to restore flow in the occluded epicardial infarct-related artery. In STEMI patients, after the introduction of (in particular) fibrin-specific fibrinolytic agents and of primary PCI, mortality rates decreased significantly compared to the prefibrinolytic era.[42]

Because the benefits of reperfusion therapy in terms of myocardial salvage and prognosis are strictly time-dependent, it is crucial to start reperfusion therapy as early as possible after onset of symptoms and, ideally, within the initial 60 minutes ("golden hour") following symptom onset.[42,43]

[ ] PREHOSPITAL MANAGEMENT

In STEMI, the value of reducing delay to treatment depends both on the amount of time saved and on when it occurs, with the first 2 hours being the ones with the greatest biologic importance. In particular, transportation time is a key component of the final delay to reperfusion therapy. Thus, patients with STEMI (see Chap. 60) may benefit from the application of general strategies of prehospital chest pain evaluation and treatment (Fig. 61–4). In the prehospital setting, a 12-lead ECG should be undertaken in all patients with chest discomfort of suspected ischemic origin as this significantly reduces time to reperfusion.[44]

Early aspirin administration (162 to 325 mg) is indicated in all non–aspirin-allergic patients with symptoms suggestive of ACS.[45] Specifically designed trials demonstrate that prehospital initiation of fibrinolytic therapy reduces treatment delays by up to 1 hour and reduces mortality by 17 percent in comparison with fibrinoly-

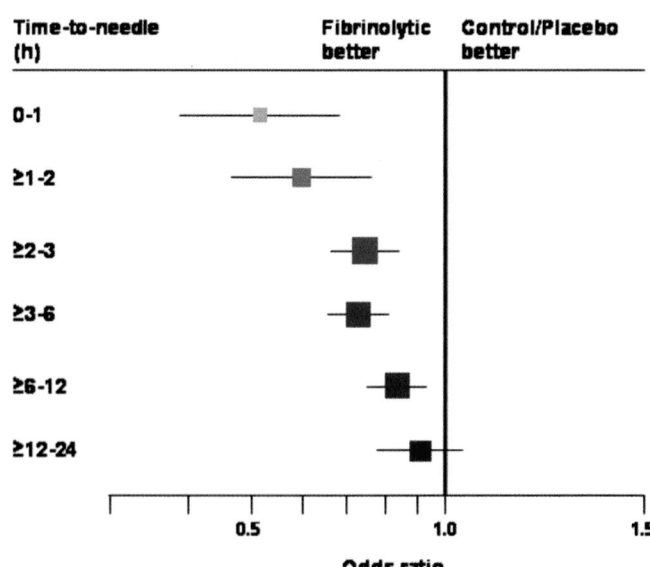

FIGURE 61–4. Influence of time-to-needle on the reduction of mortality in patients treated with fibrinolysis. Data referred to 22 randomized trials (N = 50,246 STEMI patients) that compared fibrinolytic therapy with placebo or control. Odds ratios (ORs) are plotted with 95 percent confidence interval (CI) and areas of blue squares are proportional to number of events. *Source: Adapted from Boersma E, Maas AC, Deckers JW, Simoons ML. Early thrombolytic treatment in acute myocardial infarction: reappraisal of the golden hour. Lancet 1996;348:771–777.*

tic therapy received in the hospital setting.[46] No significant safety risk has been demonstrated for prehospital fibrinolysis when compared with inhospital fibrinolysis. Prehospital fibrinolysis is beneficial, especially in rural areas, whereas transportation times tend to be shorter in urban areas.[47]

INITIAL MANAGEMENT IN THE EMERGENCY DEPARTMENT

Because the effectiveness of therapies for STEMI diminishes rapidly in the first several hours after onset of symptoms, it is crucial to establish effective guideline-based protocols for triaging and managing patients who present to the emergency department with symptoms suggestive of STEMI. The primary objective should be to reduce the delay from patient contact with the healthcare system to the initiation of fibrinolytic therapy to less than 30 minutes (or to less than 90 minutes when primary PCI is chosen).

A concise medical history should be obtained together with the execution of a focused physical examination. The 12-lead ECG is at the center of the therapeutic decision pathway; there is no evidence of benefit from fibrinolytic therapy in patients with normal ECG or nonspecific changes. In addition, because lethal ventricular arrhythmias may develop abruptly in patients with STEMI, all patients should be monitored electrocardiographically on arrival in the emergency department.

Measurement of serum biomarkers for cardiac damage should also be immediately performed as part of the management of STEMI patients, but the recommendation is that therapeutic decisions should not be unnecessarily delayed waiting for the results of blood tests (see Chap. 60).[43]

GENERAL MEASURES

To prevent physiologic deconditioning and deep venous thrombosis, current practice routinely suggests only a short period of bedrest (12 to 24 hours).

Supplemental oxygen (nasal cannula at 2 L/min) is generally administered to all patients suspected of having STEMI, but is especially recommended in cases with arterial oxygen saturation <90 percent.

Morphine sulfate (2 to 4 mg intravenously with increments of 2 to 8 mg repeated at 5- to 15-minute intervals) is the analgesic of choice for management of pain and anxiety (and consequent sympathetic drive) associated with ongoing myocardial ischemia/necrosis.[43]

Pain management should be directed toward acute relief of symptoms of ongoing myocardial ischemia and necrosis, as well as toward general relief of anxiety and apprehension, which can heighten pain perception.

NITRATES

Sublingual nitroglycerin (0.4 mg every 5 minutes for a total of 1.2 mg) is initially administered to alleviate ongoing ischemic discomfort and, in the majority of STEMI cases, it is followed by intravenous infusion of nitroglycerin (initial rate of 5 to 10 μg/min with increases of 5 to 20 μg/min until symptom relief or significant hypotension).[43] However, this is not the primary

therapeutic measure and should not delay initiation of fibrinolytic infusion.

Nitroglycerin may help in the control of hypertension and management of pulmonary congestion. Nitrates should be avoided in patients with hypotension (systolic blood pressure <90 mmHg), marked bradycardia or tachycardia, or who have used a phosphodiesterase inhibitor in the prior 24 to 48 hours (synergic hypotensive effects).

Patients with known or suspected infarction of the right ventricle should not receive nitrates. These patients are especially dependent on adequate right ventricular preload to maintain cardiac output.

ASPIRIN

As already discussed for UA/STEMI, aspirin forms an important part of the early management of all patients with suspected ACS. Aspirin should be given promptly, as soon as the diagnosis of STEMI has been made on the ECG, at a dose between 162 and 325 mg and continued indefinitely at a daily dose of 75 to 162 mg. In patients with STEMI, aspirin is highly effective in reducing mortality when employed either alone or, even more, in combination with fibrinolytic therapy (Fig. 61–5). In patients with true aspirin allergy, clopidogrel or ticlopidine may be substituted.

β BLOCKERS

β Blocker benefits in STEMI are a consequence of several well-established pharmacologic properties, including antiischemic and electrophysiologic effects. Recommendations for β-blocker use in STEMI are based on their demonstrated efficacy in improving survival and reducing reinfarction in several large randomized clinical trials. These benefits are observed whether or not reperfusion therapy had taken place and, as shown in the CAPRICORN trial (N = 1959 patients with LV dysfunction) in which patients were randomized to receive carvedilol (6.25 mg up to 25 mg twice daily) or placebo, are particularly evident in presence of moderate-to-severe LV dysfunction.[48] Also, large trials like the ISIS (International Study of Infarct Survival)-1 (atenolol 5 to 10 mg intravenously followed by oral atenolol 100 mg/d) and the MIAMI (metoprolol 15 mg intravenously followed by oral metoprolol 100 mg twice daily), revealed that reduction in mortality between patients given β blocker and those given placebo was already evident by the end of day 1 and remained sustained thereafter.[17,49] The randomized COMMIT trial of intravenous and then oral metoprolol therapy for the emergency treatment of STEMI involved nearly twice as many patients as all previous such trials combined.[96] The results did not show that metoprolol significantly reduced inhospital mortality in the overall population. In fact, while the metoprolol did produce a significant 15 to 20 percent proportional reduction in the risk of reinfarction and of ventricular fibrillation, overall these benefits were counterbalanced by an increased risk of developing cardiogenic shock, particularly in individuals who already had unstable hemodynamic conditions. Therapy was associated with a modest, but significant, reduction in mortality only in patients who were at low risk of developing shock.

Current guidelines recommend the administration of β-blocker therapy to all STEMI patients in whom there is no contraindica-

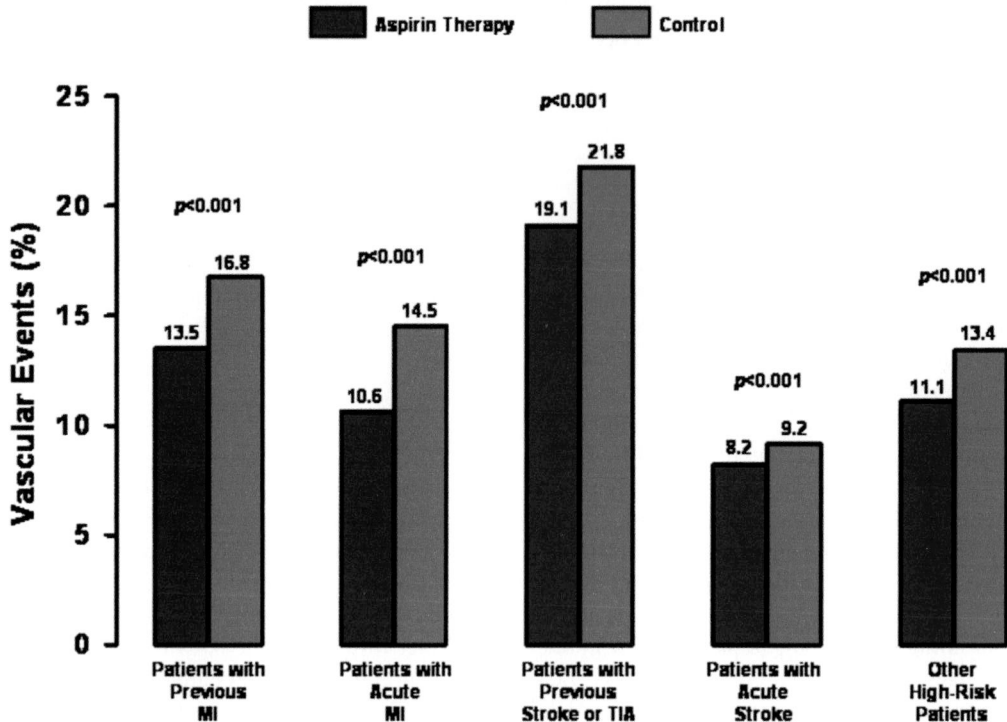

FIGURE 61–5. Effects of therapy with aspirin on the risk of vascular events (nonfatal myocardial infarction, non-fatal stroke, or death from vascular causes) in high-risk patients. The figure is based on the analysis of data derived from a systematic review of 287 studies comparing the efficacy of aspirin versus control in about 135,000 patients (Antithrombotic Trialists' Collaboration). MI, myocardial infarction; TIA, transient ischemic attack. *Source: Adapted from Patrono C, Garcia Rodriguez LA, Landolfi R, et al. Low-dose aspirin for the prevention of atherothrombosis. N Engl J Med 2005;353:2373–2383.*

tion to its administration. In patients with sinus tachycardia, β blockers should be given promptly and intravenously. Other than unstable hemodynamic conditions, relative contraindications to early intravenous β-blocker therapy include bradycardia, PR interval >0.24 seconds, advanced atrioventricular block, and active asthma or bronchospasm.

【 】 REPERFUSION THERAPY

Evidence exists that, regardless of whether reperfusion is achieved by fibrinolysis or PCI, expeditious restoration of flow in the obstructed infarct-related artery after the onset of symptoms in patients with STEMI is a key determinant of short- and long-term outcome.[50] Physicians can now choose from different pharmacologic reperfusion regimens based on the availability of diverse fibrinolytic agents in combination with antiplatelet and antithrombin drugs (Fig. 61–2).

【 】 FIBRINOLYTIC AGENTS

All of the fibrinolytic agents currently used or under investigation are plasminogen activators and are classified as fibrin-specific (e.g., streptokinase, anistreplase, urokinase) or non–fibrin-specific (e.g., alteplase, reteplase, tenecteplase; Table 61–4). Streptokinase (a β-hemolytic streptococcal isolate) still is the most frequently employed thrombolytic agent.

GISSI (Gruppo Italiano per lo Studio della Sopravvivenza nell'Infarto Miocardico)-1 and ISIS-2 are landmark studies of thrombolytic therapy that showed an approximate 25 percent reduction in 30-day

mortality in patients given streptokinase, administered as a short-term infusion, compared with patients given placebo.[51,52] However, this agent is able to achieve complete reperfusion (TIMI grade 3 flow) only in about one-third of treated patients and the induction of anti-streptokinase antibodies makes repeated administration impractical because of the high risk of allergic reactions. To overcome some of these limitations, fibrin-specific lytic agents produced with recombinant DNA technology have been successively introduced. The results of the GUSTO-I trial demonstrated that front-loaded or accelerated alteplase (100 mg infusion over 90 minutes, with over half of the dose within 30 minutes) was superior to streptokinase for both early and 1-year mortality reduction.[53] Further developments led to the introduction of agents (i.e., reteplase, tenecteplase, and lanoteplase) that can be administered as a single practical bolus. Two large mortality trials, GUSTO-III and ASSENT (Assessment of the Safety and Efficacy of a New Thrombolytic Regimen)-2, showed no superiority with reteplase, and equivalent results with tenecteplase, respectively, when compared with accelerated alteplase.[54,97] Fibrin-specific agents are easier to use, especially in a prehospital setting, but are more expensive compared to streptokinase and are associated to a certain increase in the incidence of intracranial hemorrhage.

【 】 INDICATIONS AND CONTRAINDICATIONS TO FIBRINOLYTIC THERAPY

It has been well established that fibrinolytic therapy provides a survival benefit for patients with STEMI by reducing infarct size and electrical heterogeneity of the myocardium. The efficacy of fibri-

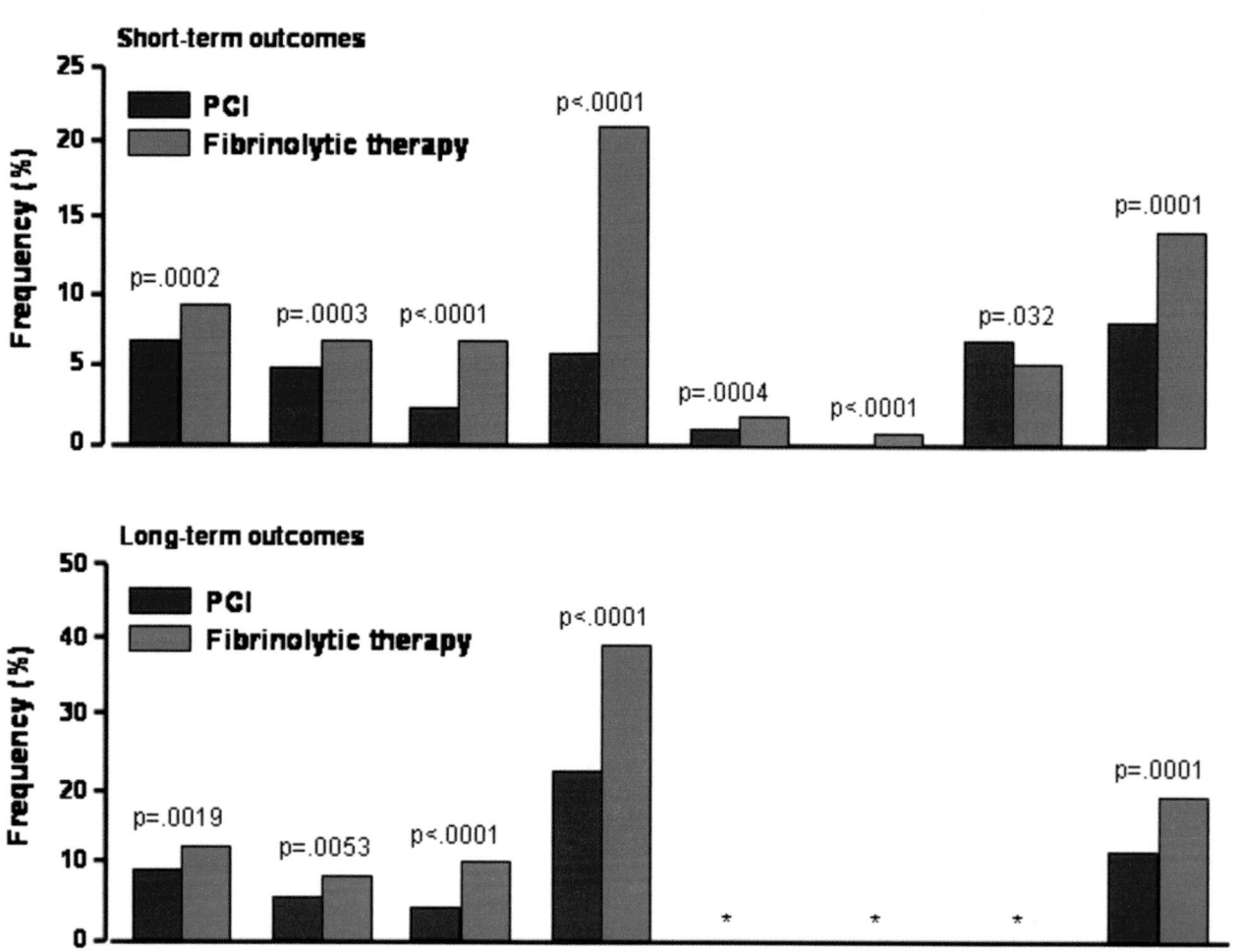

FIGURE 61-6. Short- and long-term clinical outcomes in individuals with ST-segment elevation myocardial infarction (STEMI) who were treated with primary percutaneous coronary intervention (PCI) or fibrinolytic therapy. Data are derived from 23 trials that randomly assigned patients with STEMI to primary PCI (plus stent in 12 trials) or fibrinolytic therapy. *Source: Adapted from Keeley EC, Boura JA, Grines CL. Primary angioplasty versus intravenous thrombolytic therapy for acute myocardial infarction: a quantitative review of 23 randomised trials. Lancet 2003;361:13–20.*

nolytic agents in lysing thrombus and improving prognosis diminishes with the passage of time. The greatest benefit occurs when therapy is given within the first 3 hours and up to 12 hours from the onset of symptoms.

Indications for fibrinolysis include symptoms of myocardial ischemia and ST-segment elevation greater than 0.1 mV in two contiguous leads or new (or presumably new) left bundle-branch block on the presenting ECG. The mortality benefit is greater in the set-

TABLE 61-4

Approved Fibrinolytic Agents for ST-Segment Elevation Myocardial Infarction Treatment

CHARACTERISTIC	STREPTOKINASE	ALTEPLASE	RETEPLASE	TENECTEPLASE
Dose	1.5×10^6 U in 30–60 min	Up to 100 mg in 90 min	2×10 U bolus	0.5 mg/kg bolus
Antigenicity	++	–	–	–
Fibrin specificity	–	++	+	+++
90-min patency	++	+++	++++	+++/++++
Mortality reduction	+	++	++	++
Hemorrhagic stroke	+	++	++	++
Cost	+	+++	+++	+++

ting of anterior STEMI, and is less significant in patients with inferior STEMI. In general, thrombolysis shows detrimental effects on prognosis in patients with only ST-segment depression on ECG, with an important exception represented by cases of true posterior MI (i.e., patients presenting with ST-segment depression in V_1 to V_4 leads associated with tall R waves in the right precordial leads).

As a result, fibrinolytic therapy should not be administered to currently asymptomatic patients whose initial symptoms of STEMI began more than 24 hours earlier or to patients with ST-segment depression (unless a true posterior MI is suspected). Major complications of fibrinolytic therapy include intracranial hemorrhage (affecting 5 to 10 of 1000 patients treated) and other moderate to severe bleeding that may or may not require transfusion. It is always important to evaluate the benefit of fibrinolysis in relation to the increased risk of bleeding associated with this therapy.

SELECTION OF REPERFUSION STRATEGY (FIBRINOLYSIS VERSUS PCI)

There is still controversy about which form of reperfusion therapy is superior in the various clinical settings and given the heterogeneity of STEMI patient profiles and availability of resources, it is difficult to produce a simple algorithm. Several issues should be considered when selecting the type of reperfusion therapy for the individual patient (Fig. 61–7). The availability of interventional cardiology facilities is certainly a key determinant. STEMI patients who present to a facility that lacks the capability for expert, prompt intervention with primary PCI (within 90 minutes of first medical contact) should undergo fibrinolysis unless contraindicated. In contrast, for facilities that can offer PCI, the literature suggests that this approach is superior to pharmacologic reperfusion provided it can be delivered expeditiously.[55]

Primary PCI results in fewer deaths, reinfarctions, and strokes than does pharmacologic reperfusion. The relative benefits of primary PCI can be attributed to more frequent achievement of normal antegrade coronary blood flow, resulting in greater myocardial salvage, together with avoidance of the life-threatening hemorrhagic complications of fibrinolysis. As a result, primary PCI became accepted as the preferred reperfusion modality when it can be done in a timely fashion. It is of note, that the level of experience of the interventional team influences differences in outcome and PCI reperfusion superiority is maintained only in centers with high volumes of primary PCI.

When transfer of the patient in a different facility is required for PCI, transportation time needs to be taken into account. Compared with a fibrinolytic agent, a PCI strategy may not reduce mortality when a delay greater than 1 to 2 hours is anticipated versus immediate administration of a lytic agent (Fig. 61–8).[56] The level of risk represents another element to consider in the definition of the reperfusion strategy. When the estimated mortality risk is high, as is the case in patients in cardiogenic shock, compelling evidence exists that favors a PCI strategy.[57]

Finally, the choice of reperfusion therapy is also affected by the patient's risk of bleeding. The higher the risk of bleeding with fibrinolytic therapy, the more strongly the decision should favor PCI (e.g., in low-weight elderly patients).

FACILITATED PCI

The treatment delay in transferring patients from noninterventional to interventional hospitals cannot always be adequately managed. This has stimulated interest in "facilitated PCI," consisting in a PCI performed after an initial pharmacologic regimen (i.e., full-dose fibrinolysis or a combination of reduced-dose fibrinolytic therapy and a GPIIb/IIIa inhibitor). Potential advantages of this approach include earlier time to reperfusion and greater procedural success rates.

Recent pooled analyses considered data from 17 trials comparing facilitated and primary PCI in 4504 patients with STEMI, with the inclusion of the largest of such studies, the ASSENT-4 PCI (full-dose tenecteplase before PCI; N = 1667).[98–100] This meta-analysis showed that facilitated PCI with GPIIb/IIIa inhibitors conferred no benefit over primary PCI, whereas the use of fibrinolytic-based regimens (alone or combined with GPIIb/IIIa inhibitors) was associated with higher risk for death, reinfarction, urgent revascularization, and major bleeding. These disappointing results might be in part explained by their largely being driven by the ASSENT-4 PCI data (open-label design). An important limitation to this study was that the bolus tenecteplase was given a median of 2.6 hours after the onset of symptoms and, in addition, the median time between bolus and PCI was particularly short (104 minutes). Assuming a delay of about 30 to 45 minutes between injection and recanalization of the infarct vessel, the

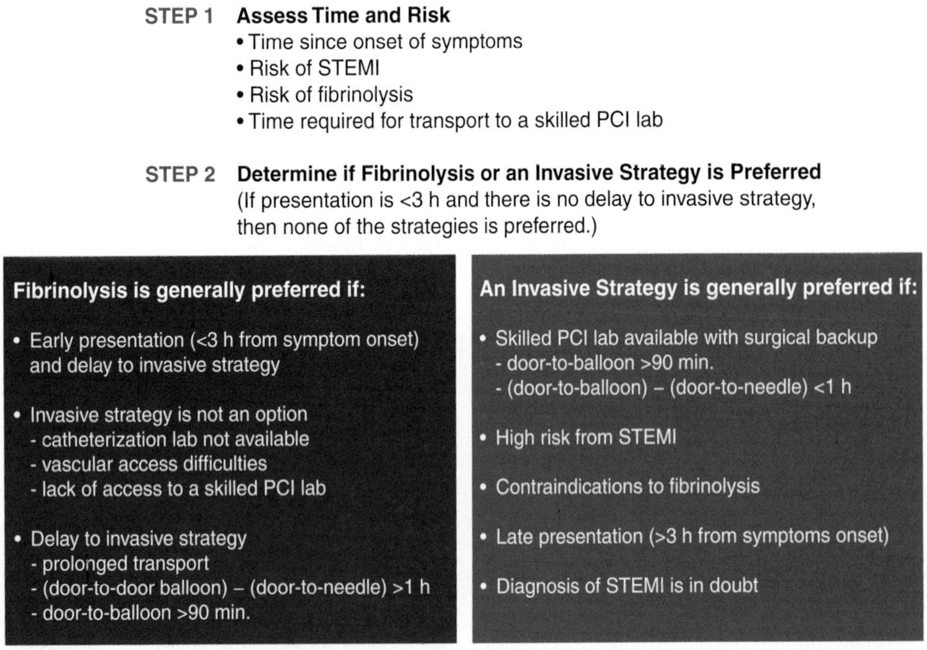

STEP 1 Assess Time and Risk
- Time since onset of symptoms
- Risk of STEMI
- Risk of fibrinolysis
- Time required for transport to a skilled PCI lab

STEP 2 Determine if Fibrinolysis or an Invasive Strategy is Preferred
(If presentation is <3 h and there is no delay to invasive strategy, then none of the strategies is preferred.)

Fibrinolysis is generally preferred if:
- Early presentation (<3 h from symptom onset) and delay to invasive strategy
- Invasive strategy is not an option
  - catheterization lab not available
  - vascular access difficulties
  - lack of access to a skilled PCI lab
- Delay to invasive strategy
  - prolonged transport
  - (door-to-door balloon) – (door-to-needle) >1 h
  - door-to-balloon >90 min.

An Invasive Strategy is generally preferred if:
- Skilled PCI lab available with surgical backup
  - door-to-balloon >90 min.
  - (door-to-balloon) – (door-to-needle) <1 h
- High risk from STEMI
- Contraindications to fibrinolysis
- Late presentation (>3 h from symptoms onset)
- Diagnosis of STEMI is in doubt

FIGURE 61–7. Assessment of reperfusion options in patients with STEMI. PCI, percutaneous coronary intervention. *Source: Adapted from Antman EM, Anbe DT, Armstrong PW, et al.[43]*

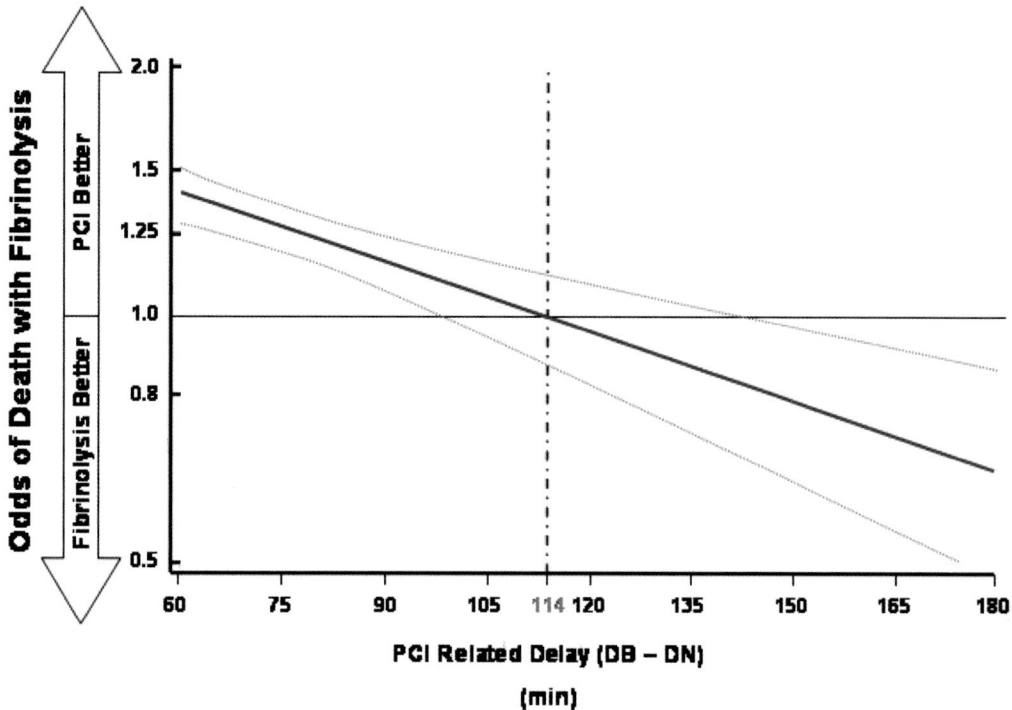

FIGURE 61–8. Treatment effect on death of reperfusion therapy with percutaneous coronary intervention (PCI) or fibrinolysis based on increasing PCI-related delay. Multivariable analysis was performed using data from 192,509 ST-segment elevation myocardial infarction (STEMI) patients at 645 National Registry of Myocardial Infarction (NRMI) hospitals. PCI-related delay (DB-DN time) was calculated by subtracting median door-to-needle time (DN) from median door-to-balloon time (DB). After correction for patient- and hospital-based factors, the time at which odds of death with PCI were equal to those for fibrinolysis occurred when the DB-DN time was approximately 114 minutes. *Source: Adapted from Pinto DS, Kirtane AJ, Nallamothu BK, et al. Hospital delays in reperfusion for ST-elevation myocardial infarction: implications when selecting a reperfusion strategy. Circulation 2006;114:2019–2025.*

time gain for reperfusion with facilitated PCI was probably short in many patients. More generally, the time-to-reperfusion shortening with facilitated PCI might occur in a time-independent phase of the mortality curve described in STEMI patients who were treated by reperfusion therapy. In conclusion, there is currently no evidence for the recommendation of facilitated PCI in STEMI patients.[58]

【 】 ANCILLARY THERAPY FOR STEMI

Together with reperfusion therapy, a series of other medications (ancillary therapy) are involved in the overall management of patients with STEMI. Ancillary therapy has the role to facilitate and maintain coronary reperfusion, limit the consequences of myocardial ischemia, enhance myocardial healing, and reduce the likelihood of recurrent events (see Table 61–5). A particular impact on the outcome of STEMI patients has been documented with the use of antithrombotic drugs, including antiplatelets and antithrombin agents.

Aspirin

Specific pharmacologic reperfusion strategies have been developed to combine fibrinolytic treatment with aggressive antiplatelet therapy. Treatment with a fibrinolytic agent only resolves the fibrin-rich red part of the thrombus, whereas the platelet-rich white part remains largely untouched (see Fig. 61–2). In addition, fibrinolysis induces the generation of free thrombin with intense activation of platelet aggregation.

Indications for administration of aspirin have been already discussed in the section on the initial management of STEMI patients in the emergency department. For the documented favorable effects on outcomes in ischemic patients, aspirin should be given to all patients with suspected STEMI as early as possible and continued indefinitely. Other treatments for STEMI are always additive and not alternative to aspirin, excepting in subjects with true aspirin allergy.

Thienopyridine

Clopidogrel is a good alternative to aspirin for antiplatelet therapy in subjects with clearly defined and objective hypersensitivity to aspirin (see Table 61–5).[43]

Currently, clopidogrel combined with aspirin is only recommended for patients with STEMI who undergo PCI with coronary stent implantation. However, new information on the value of adding clopidogrel to fibrinolysis and aspirin has been recently published. The CLARITY-TIMI (Clopidogrel as Adjunctive Reperfusion Therapy–Thrombolysis in Myocardial Infarction) 28 trial enrolled 3491 patients with STEMI treated with fibrinolytic agents and aspirin who were randomly assigned to additional placebo or clopidogrel (300-mg loading dose and 75 mg/d thereafter).[59] Clopidogrel use in this trial was associated with a significant reduction in the composite primary end point (death, reinfarction, and occlusion of the infarct-related artery) with no increase in the rate of bleeding. Similarly, the

TABLE 61–5

Indication for Fibrinolysis and Ancillary Therapy in ST-Segment Elevation Myocardial Infarction

	INDICATION IN STEMI

Fibrinolysis	• All patients without contraindications and presenting within 12 h from symptoms onset onto a facility without capability for expert, prompt primary PCI (time-to-balloon >90 min):
	    STEMI or new left bundle-branch block on ECG (*Class I*)ᵃ
	    ECG evidence for true posterior MI (*Class IIa*)
	• Patients without contraindications and presenting at 12–24 h from symptoms onset who have continuing ischemic symptoms and ST elevation on ECG (*Class IIa*)
	• Patients with only ST-segment depression on ECG except if a true posterior MI is suspected (*Class III*)
	• Asymptomatic patients presenting at more than 24 h from symptoms onset (*Class III*)

Aspirin	• All patients excluding those with confirmed aspirin allergy (*Class I*)
Thienopyridines	• Patients in whom PCI is planned and who are not at high risk for bleeding (clopidogrel for at least 1 month and up to 12 months; *Class I*) • Patients with aspirin allergy (clopidogrel; *Class IIa*)

Glycoprotein IIb/IIIa inhibitors	• Patients in whom primary PCI is planned:
	    Abciximab (*Class IIa*)
	    Tirofiban and eptifibatide (*Class IIb*)
	• Patients <75 years old, with anterior MI and no risk factors for bleeding even if referred for early angiography and PCI (abciximab plus half-dose reteplase or tenecteplase; *Class IIb*)
	• Patients >75 years old (abciximab plus half-dose reteplase or tenecteplase, *Class III*)

Unfractionated heparin	• Patients treated with non–fibrin-specific fibrinolytic agents who are at high risk for systemic emboli (*Class I*) • Patients treated with fibrin-specific fibrinolytic agents (*Class I*) • Patients undergoing PCI or surgical revascularization (*Class I*) • Patients receiving streptokinase (*Class IIb*)
Low-molecular-weight heparin	• As alternative to heparin in patients <75 years old and no renal dysfunction (enoxaparin plus full-dose fibrinolytic; *Class IIb*) • As alternative to heparin in patients >75 years old or with reduced renal function who are receiving fibrinolytic therapy (*Class III*)
Direct thrombin inhibitors	• As alternative to heparin in patients with known heparin-induced thrombocytopenia (bivalirudin plus full-dose streptokinase; *Class IIa*)

PCI, percutaneous coronary intervention; STEMI, ST-segment elevation myocardial infarction.
ᵃClass of recommendation: class I: conditions for which there is evidence that a given therapy is useful and effective; class II: conditions for which there is conflicting evidence and/or divergence about the efficacy/usefulness of a given treatment (class IIa: weight of evidence/opinion is in favor of usefulness/efficacy; class IIb: usefulness/efficacy is less-well established by evidence/opinion); class III: contraindications.
SOURCE: Based on ACC/AHA guidelines for the management of patients with STEMI.[43]

COMMIT randomly assigned 39,755 patients >75 years old with STEMI to aspirin alone versus aspirin plus clopidogrel (75 mg/dL).[96] Patients treated with clopidogrel had a lower rate of the composite end point (death, reinfarction, and stroke) and no increase in bleeding. All together these data suggest that patients with STEMI who are already being treated with fibrinolytic agents and aspirin should also receive clopidogrel.

Glycoprotein IIb/IIIa Inhibitors

To improve rates of achieving normal flow (TIMI 3) with pharmacologic reperfusion therapy, GPIIb/IIIa inhibitors have been tested in combination with fibrinolytic agents. Fibrinolytic therapy is associated with increased platelet activation and aggregation, and the antiplatelet action of GPIIb/IIIa inhibitors may diminish distal embolization of platelet aggregates.

The large-scale mortality study GUSTO-V tested full-dose reteplase (10 U × 2) compared with half-dose reteplase (5 U × 2) plus abciximab (0.25 mg/kg bolus and 0.125 μg/kg/min for 12 hours) in 16,588 STEMI patients.[60] Nonfatal reinfarction rates were reduced in the combination therapy group, as were other complications of STEMI (i.e., life-threatening arrhythmias, high-grade atrioventricular block, and septal or free-wall rupture), whereas there was no observed effect on the number of deaths. However, moderate-to-severe bleeding was significantly increased in the combined therapy group, with the excess bleeding risks concentrated in patients older than age 75 years. This lack of mortality benefit and excess bleeding risk with combination therapy was also found in the ASSENT-3 (half-dose tenecteplase plus abciximab plus reduced-dose UFH) and INTEGRITI (Integrilin and Tenecteplase in Acute Myocardial Infarction; reduced-dose tenecteplase plus eptifibatide) studies.[61,62]

Intravenous GPIIb/IIIa receptor inhibitors showed encouraging results on reducing adverse outcomes when used as supportive antiplatelet therapy in patients who were undergoing primary PCI (with or without stenting).[63] A recent meta-analysis (11 studies; N = 27,115 patients) investigated the value of adding abciximab to both pharmacologic and mechanical reperfusion.[64] Results showed that adjunctive abciximab therapy was associated with a significant reduction in 30-day reinfarction in patients with STEMI who were treated with either pharmacologic or mechanical reperfusion, whereas a significant reduction in short- and long-term mortality was observed only in patients who were undergoing primary PCI.

Current guidelines state that although this approach is not expected to bring any survival benefit, a combined pharmacologic therapy with abciximab and half-dose reteplase or tenecteplase may be considered in <75-year-old patients with no risk factors for bleeding for prevention of reinfarction and other complications of STEMI. In addition, considering the reported effects in reducing mortality rates, the administration of a GPIIb/IIIa inhibitor (abciximab, in particular) for a period of up to 12 months may be reasonable in STEMI patients when primary PCI is planned (see Table 61–5).

Unfractionated Heparin

During fibrinolysis, release of thrombin from the thrombus may contribute to a procoagulant state. Thus, fibrinolytic and antiplatelet therapy could be combined with antithrombin (or anticoagulant) therapy (see Fig. 61–2). However, the intensity of the induced procoagulant state is dependent on the type of fibrinolytic agent used, and a stronger rationale for using UFH exists in patients who are receiving fibrin-specific agents than in patients who are being treated with non–fibrin-specific agents. In fact, with non–fibrin-specific agents (i.e., streptokinase, anistreplase, and urokinase) the procoagulant increase in thrombin activity is partially compensated for by a certain anticoagulant activity, which is significantly less evident when fibrin-specific agents (i.e., alteplase, reteplase, and tenecteplase) are used.[65] Consequently, in patients who are treated with fibrinolytic therapy, recommendations for heparin therapy depend on the fibrinolytic agent used.

Overall, only weak evidence supports the value of UFH in improving outcomes in STEMI. The recommendation to administer UFH to STEMI patients undergoing reperfusion therapy with streptokinase is based on the results of trials demonstrating a small reduction in 30-day death and reinfarction rates by adding subcutaneous UFH (GISSI-2 and ISIS-3) or intravenous UFH (GUSTO-I) to the control regimen.[101–103] Intravenous UFH is currently recommended in patients who are being treated with non–fibrin-specific agents (streptokinase, anistreplase, urokinase) and who are at high risk for systemic emboli (i.e., large or anterior MI, atrial fibrillation, previous embolus, or known left ventricular thrombus).

Separately, a series of angiographic trials reported that intravenous UFH in conjunction with fibrin-specific alteplase leads to higher rates of infarct-related artery perfusion, with a demonstrable direct relation between duration of aPTT and likelihood of infarct-related artery perfusion. Consequently, UFH *should* be given intra-venously to patients who are undergoing reperfusion therapy with alteplase (or reteplase or tenecteplase) with dosing as follows: bolus of 60 U/kg (maximum: 4000 U) followed by an infusion of 12 U/kg/h (maximum: 1000 U) initially adjusted to maintain aPTT at 1.5 to 2.0 times control (approximately 50 to 70 seconds).[43] The aPTT measurement should be repeated 4 to 6 hours after each dose adjustment until it is in the target range and then daily thereafter.

Even when all these precautions are implemented, UFH therapy may be associated with a slight excess risk of bleeding. The appropriate duration of therapy with UFH is uncertain. After the first 48 hours of treatment, UFH may be discontinued in low-risk patients, but it should be continued in patients who are at high risk for coronary reocclusion. Heparin-induced thrombocytopenia may occur in 1 to 2 percent of patients and platelet counts should be monitored on alternate days in patients being treated with UFH.

Low-Molecular-Weight Heparin

LMWH has better pharmacologic properties than UFH, with important advantages for its use in clinical practice. A number of clinical trials, mostly conducted with enoxaparin and dalteparin, provide data that suggests LMWH may be an attractive alternative to UFH.[66–69] These studies consistently reported a lower rate of reocclusion of the infarct-related artery and of reinfarction in patients receiving LMWH compared to the placebo- or UFH-treated group. Important data has been provided by the ASSENT-3 trial, in which patients received tenecteplase and either UFH (bolus 60 U/kg; initial infusion 12 U/kg/h; duration of treatment equals 48 hours) or enoxaparin (bolus 30 mg; subcutaneous injections 1.0 mg/kg every 12 hours; treatment given for the duration of hospital stay).[104] Enoxaparin reduced 30-day mortality, inhospital reinfarction and inhospital recurrent ischemia, although no difference was noted in the composite end point when the two patient groups were compared at 1-year followup. Overall, enoxaparin was associated with a slight, nonsignificant increase in noncerebral bleeding complications, but the bleeding risk was significantly increased in patients older than age 75 years. Furthermore, patients with significant renal dysfunction were excluded from ASSENT-3; thus enoxaparin is currently not recommended for use in combination with fibrinolytics in patients with severe renal dysfunction.

A recent meta-analysis of studies involving STEMI patients (N = 7098) who were treated with aspirin and fibrinolytics evaluated the effects of adding LMWH or UFH to the therapy.[70] Pooled data indicate that compared with intravenous UFH, LMWH significantly reduced the risk of reinfarction but with no reduction in mortality (Fig. 61–9). LMWH therapy was associated with a significant increase of the risk of minor bleeding, with no difference in the overall risk of stroke.

Current guidelines state that LMWH might be considered an acceptable alternative to UFH as ancillary therapy for patients younger than age 75 years who are receiving fibrinolytic therapy, provided that significant renal dysfunction (serum creatinine >2.5 mg/dL in men or >2.0 mg/dL in women) is not present. Enoxaparin (30-mg IV bolus, followed by 1.0 mg/kg subcutaneously every 12 hours until hospital discharge) is the most studied regimen. These indications can be supported following the recent publication of the results from the EXTRACT (Enoxaparin and Thrombolysis Reperfusion for Acute Myocardial Infarction Treat-

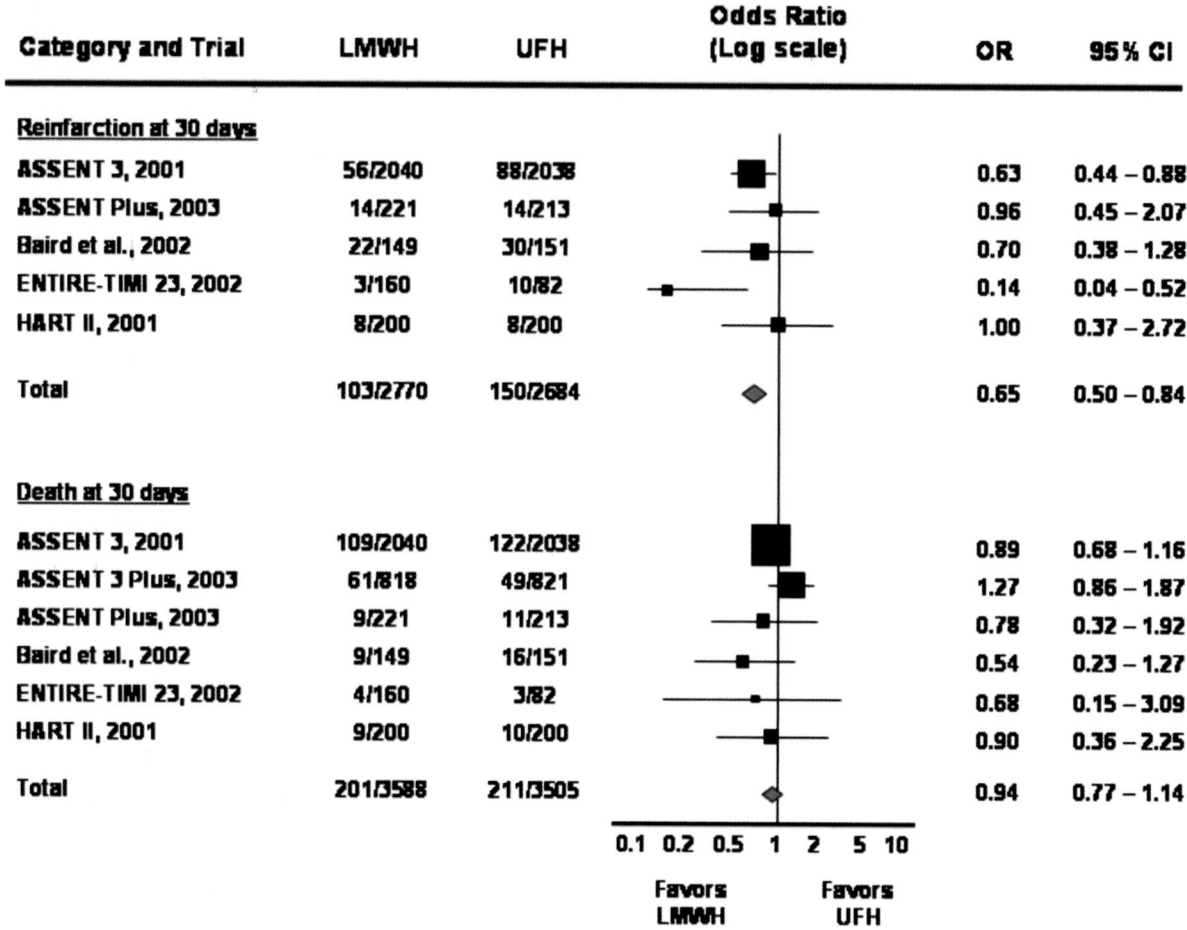

FIGURE 61–9. Comparison between low-molecular-weight heparin (LMWH) and unfractionated heparin (UFH) on the risk of reinfarction and death in ST-segment elevation myocardial infarction (STEMI) patients already treated with fibrinolytic and aspirin. Data are derived from five studies (ASSENT [Assessment of the Safety and Efficacy of a New Thrombolytic Regimen]-3, ASSENT-3 Plus, ASSENT Plus, Baird et al., ENTIRE-TIMI [Thrombolysis in Myocardial Infarction], and HART) involving a total of 7098 patients. CI, confidence interval; OR, odds ratio. *Source: Adapted from Eikelboom JW, Quinlan DJ, Mehta SR, et al. Unfractionated and low-molecular-weight heparin as adjuncts to thrombolysis in aspirin-treated patients with ST-elevation acute myocardial infarction: a meta-analysis of the randomized trials. Circulation 2005;112:3855–867.*

ment) TIMI-25 Trial.[71] In a population of more than 20,000 STEMI patients scheduled to undergo fibrinolysis and in comparison with standard therapy with UFH, enoxaparin (dosing strategy was adjusted according to the patient's age and renal function) was associated with a 17 percent relative risk reduction for the primary end point (death and recurrent MI).

Direct Thrombin Inhibitors

Molecules such as hirudin and bivalirudin (formerly known as *hirulog*) do not require the presence of antithrombin III to be active and therefore are defined as direct thrombin inhibitors.

In a meta-analysis of 11 trials with an overall enrollment of 35,000 patients presenting with STEMI, use of direct thrombin inhibitors (particularly of hirudin and bivalirudin) was associated with a significant reduction in the incidence of reinfarction compared with UFH, but with little impact on death.[72] Similar data were reported in the HERO (Hirulog and Early Reperfusion or Occlusion)-2 trial (N = 17,073 patients), which compared bivalirudin and UFH in patients presenting with STEMI and already treated with streptokinase.[73] Use of direct bivaliru-

din was not associated with an increase in the frequency of major bleeding, but the frequency of mild-to-moderate bleeding was greater compared to UFH.

Thus, in the circumstance of STEMI patients who receive fibrinolysis with streptokinase and have heparin-induced thrombocytopenia (which is uncommon), it is reasonable to consider bivalirudin as a useful alternative to UFH.

[ ] OTHER PHARMACOLOGIC MEASURES IN THE MANAGEMENT OF STEMI

Other medications may be part of the pharmacologic management of patients with a diagnosis of STEMI.

ACE Inhibitors

Drugs acting through an inhibition of the renin–angiotensin–aldosterone system (i.e., ACE inhibitors, angiotensin receptor blockers, and aldosterone antagonists) are frequently part of the pharmacologic strategy for the initial management of STEMI. ACE inhibitors competitively inhibit the ACE, a nonspecific enzyme involved in the conversion of the inactive angiotensin I into angiotensin II, and also inhibit kininase, an enzyme that catalyses the degradation of bradykinin and other potent vasodilator peptides. During chronic administration, inhibition of plasma ACE appears to be less important than inhibition of ACE in different tissues (i.e., vessels, kidney, and heart). ACE inhibitors decrease total vascular resistance with a reduction in cardiac hypertrophy and blood pressure in hypertensive patients, and a reduction in endothelial dysfunction in normotensive patients with coronary artery disease, diabetes, or congestive heart failure. In addition, the increase in the levels of kinins, prostacyclin, and nitric oxide in part may explain the vasodilator, antithrombotic and antiproliferative effects of ACE inhibitors. They reverse ventricular remodeling after MI principally by reducing ventricular preload/afterload, preventing the proliferative effects of angiotensin II and sympathetic nerve activity.[74]

Overall ACE inhibitors are generally well tolerated, but side effects include hypotension, dry cough (in 5 to 10 percent of treated patients), hyperkalemia, and acute renal failure (particularly in patients with renal artery stenosis). ACE inhibitors are contraindicated during pregnancy (teratogenic effects when administered during the II or III trimester).

The role of ACE inhibitors in the early phase of MI has been assessed in a number of clinical trials. In ISIS-4 (N = 58,050 patients with suspected acute MI), a significant 7 percent relative reduction was observed in 5-week mortality among patients randomly assigned to oral captopril (titrated up to 50 mg twice daily) compared to placebo, with the largest benefit observed among those with an anterior infarction or with heart failure.[105] In the GISSI-3 trial (N = 19,394 patients with either ST-segment elevation or depression), a significant reduction in 6-week mortality was observed in patients assigned to lisinopril (5-mg initial dose and then 10 mg daily) compared to open control.[75] A meta-analysis of these major trials along with 11 smaller studies that collectively enrolled more than 100,000 patients, revealed an absolute benefit of about 5 fewer deaths per 1000 patients treated among those who received the ACE inhibitor (see Fig. 61–10).[76] Most of the benefit was observed during the first week of treatment and was greater in high-risk groups, which included patients with anterior MI, heart failure, or left ventricular dysfunction. These data support a role for ACE inhibitors in the early phase of STEMI.

In the absence of hypotension or known contraindications to this class of medications, an oral ACE inhibitor (i.e., captopril, lisinopril, ramipril, zofenopril, enalapril, or quinapril) is indicated within the first 24 hours of STEMI, particularly in patients with anterior infarction, heart failure, or a left ventricular ejection fraction <0.40.[43]

In contrast, intravenous ACE inhibitors should be avoided in the early post-MI phase. A total of 6090 patients were randomized in the CONSENSUS (Cooperative New Scandinavian Enalapril Survival Study)-2 trial to receive intravenous enalapril or placebo within 24 hours of the onset of acute MI.[77] Mortality rates in the two groups at 1 and 6 months were not significantly different and the study was terminated early because of concern regarding adverse effects among elderly patients who experienced an early hypotensive reaction. Current recommendations state that intravenous ACE inhibitors should be avoided in STEMI patients until stable hemodynamic conditions are obtained.

Angiotensin II Type 1 Receptor Blockers

Angiotensin II type 1 receptor blockers (ARBs) offer an alternative means of blocking the renin–angiotensin system. Angiotensin II is produced by enzymes other than ACE, meaning that ACE inhibitors might be not able to block completely this peptide. In addition, ACE inhibitors inhibit bradykinin breakdown and bradykinin accumulation may cause some of the adverse effects of ACE inhibitors (i.e., cough, rash, and angioedema). Thus, an ARB, hypothetically, might be more effective or better tolerated than an ACE inhibitor. The use of ARBs has not been explored as thoroughly as ACE inhibitors in patients with STEMI.

The OPTIMAAL (Optimal Trial in Myocardial Infarction with the Angiotensin II Antagonist Losartan) and VALIANT (Valsartan in Acute Myocardial Infarction Trial) trials were designed to test for superiority or noninferiority of losartan (target dose 50 mg daily) or valsartan (target dose 160 mg twice daily), respectively, over captopril (titrated to 50 mg three times daily) on all-cause mortality in high-risk survivors of acute MI.[78,79] Globally, ARBs were as effective as captopril in reducing all-cause mortality. In VALIANT, the combination of valsartan and captopril treatment did not improve outcomes compared with the proven dose of captopril, but this combination significantly increased the rate of adverse events. Given the extensive randomized trials and routine clinical experience with ACE inhibitors, they remain the logical first agent for inhibition of the renin–angiotensin–aldosterone system in STEMI patients. However, ARBs are indicated in patients with depressed LV function or clinical heart failure who are intolerant to an ACE inhibitor.

Aldosterone Antagonists

Aldosterone blockade represents another means of inhibiting the renin–angiotensin–aldosterone system that has been tested in patients following STEMI.

Data supporting their use comes from heart-failure studies that enrolled a large proportion of patients with a history of MI. The RALES study included patients with advanced heart failure who were already being treated with ACE inhibitors who were randomized to either spironolactone (25 to 50 mg daily) or placebo. The study demonstrated a significant reduction in all-cause mortality with spironolactone.[80] The EPHESUS (Eplerenone Post-Acute Myocardial Infarction Heart Failure Efficacy and Survival Study) randomized 6632 post-MI patients with an ejection fraction <0.40, heart failure, or diabetes to receive eplerenone (target dose: 50 mg daily) or placebo in conjunction with routine indicated cardiac medications.[81] Although patients were already being managed with optimal therapy, eplerenone was associated with a significant reduction in overall mortality, cardiovascular mortality, and cardiac hospitalizations. The major risk associated with aldosterone blockade is hyperkalemia, particularly in patients with reduced renal function.

Thus, the RALES and EPHESUS studies support the long-term use of an aldosterone antagonist in patients with STEMI with associated heart failure and/or an ejection fraction of 0.40 or less. Significant renal dysfunction or hyperkalemia are contraindications to therapy with aldosterone blockers.

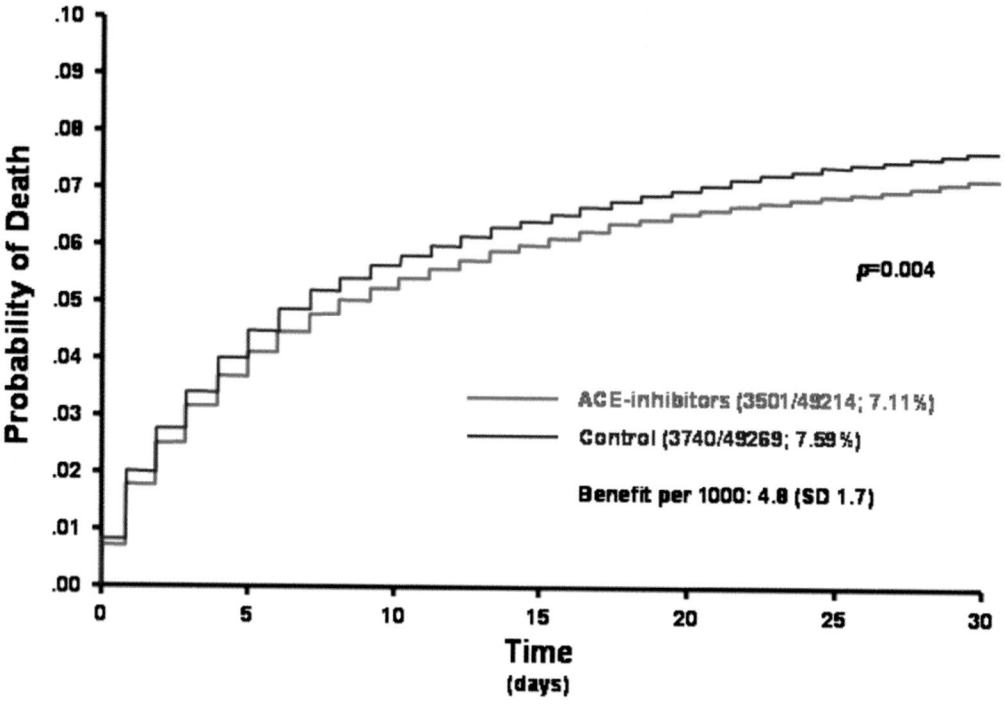

FIGURE 61-10. Effect of angiotensin-converting enzyme (ACE) inhibitor therapy on cumulative mortality at early follow-up in patients with acute myocardial infarction. Data are based on 98,496 patients from 4 randomized trials (CONSENSUS [Cooperative New Scandinavian Enalapril Survival Study]-II, GISSI [Gruppo Italiano per lo Studio della Sopravvivenza nell'Infarto Miocardico]-3, ISIS [International Study of Infarct Survival]-4, and CCS [Chinese Cardiac Study]-1). SD, standard deviation. *Source: Adapted from a report of the ACE Inhibitor Myocardial Infarction Collaborative Group. Circulation 1998;97:2202–2212.*

Glucose-Insulin-Potassium Infusion

The usefulness of metabolic modulation of the glucose–insulin axis in STEMI patients has been proposed for a long time, but it was only recently addressed through international randomized trials.

A meta-analysis of 16 trials of glucose-insulin-potassium (GIK) infusion versus control involving almost 5000 patients indicated a significant reduction in mortality risk with GIK infusion therapy.[82] Nevertheless, current guidelines recommend insulin infusion only to normalize blood glucose in STEMI patients, and no definitive indications regarding GIK have been formulated. The CREATE-ECLA trial, conducted in 470 centers worldwide, included 20,201 patients with STEMI who were randomly assigned to receive GIK infusion for 24 hours.[83] The results of this study revealed that high-dose GIK infusion has no impact on mortality in STEMI patients.

Magnesium Sulfate

Initial studies suggested a significant mortality benefit of magnesium infusion in STEMI, but this was not confirmed in the low-risk population of the ISIS-4 nor in the high-risk population enrolled in the MAGIC trial.[75,84] Thus, on the basis of the available evidence, there is no indication for the routine administration of intravenous magnesium to patients with STEMI.[43]

Magnesium sulfate can continue to be administered for repletion of documented electrolyte deficits and at a dosage of 1 to 2 mg bolus intravenously over 5 minutes, may be indicated for the treatment of life-threatening ventricular arrhythmias such as torsade de pointes.

Calcium Antagonists

Because of the associated reflex sympathetic activation (leading to an increase in myocardial oxygen demands) and of the tachycardia and hypotension (associated with a reduction in coronary perfusion pressure), use of immediate-release nifedipine is *contraindicated* in the treatment of STEMI.

Although the overall results of trials with verapamil showed no mortality benefits, subgroup analysis showed that in patients who were not candidates for a β-blocking agent and who had preserved LV function, immediate-release verapamil (initiated several days after STEMI) reduces the incidence of a composite end point of reinfarction and death.[85] Similarly, multiple studies suggest that patients with MI, preserved LV, and no evidence of heart failure may benefit from immediate-release diltiazem.[86,87] Therefore, in the absence of heart failure, ventricular dysfunction, or atrioventricular block, it is reasonable to give verapamil or diltiazem to STEMI patients in whom β blockers are ineffective or contraindicated for relief of ongoing ischemia.

Statins

There is growing evidence that statins, beyond their LDL cholesterol-lowering effects, possess so-called *pleiotropic effects* (e.g., plaque stabilization, antiinflammation, antithrombogenicity, enhanced arterial compliance, blood pressure reduction, modulation of endothelial function) that could affect outcomes for patients with cardiovascular disease.[88]

Several observational studies suggest a large reduction in mortality in patients with ACS who were treated with statins that were started prior to hospital discharge.[89] In contrast, a recent meta-analysis concluded that initiation of statin therapy within 14 days following onset of ACS does not reduce death, MI, or stroke as evaluated at 4-month followup.[90] This analysis included 12 studies that enrolled 13,024 patients who were randomized early after ACS to statin therapy (pravastatin, atorvastatin, fluvastatin, or simvastatin) or placebo/standard therapy. Additional studies evaluated the efficacy of an intensive statin therapy in ACS patients. The PROVE-IT (Pravastatin or Atorvastatin Evaluation and Infection Therapy) trial enrolled 4162 patients with a recent diagnosis of ACS (STEMI in one-third of the total) and demonstrated that an intensive (atorvastatin 80 mg daily, target LDL cholesterol <70 mg/dL) versus a moderate (pravastatin 40 mg daily, target LDL cholesterol <100 mg/dL) lipid-lowering strategy is more effective in reducing the incidence of death or major cardiovascular events.[91] Interestingly, a meta-analysis that included 17,963 patients enrolled in 13 randomized trials showed that early, intensive statin therapy for ACS decreases the rate of death and cardiovascular events over 2 years of followup, but that this benefit starts between 4 and 12 months, achieving statistical significance only by 12 months (Fig. 61–11). Even with this intensive lipid-lowering strategy the occurrence of severe adverse events (i.e., hepatitis and rhabdomyolysis) related to statins was extremely uncommon.

Current guidelines indicate a target LDL cholesterol level of <100 mg/dL in patients after STEMI and to reach this target, recommend the prescription of therapy with a statin at hospital discharge. However, the discussed arguments seem to provide a basis to start statin therapy prior to hospital discharge to achieve LDL cholesterol levels of at least less than 100 mg/dL and preferably less than 70 mg/dL in all patients with ACS.[92]

[ ] STEMI MANAGEMENT IN SUMMARY

The urgent priority in patients with a diagnosis of STEMI is to provide prompt and effective reperfusion for all those eligible.[86]

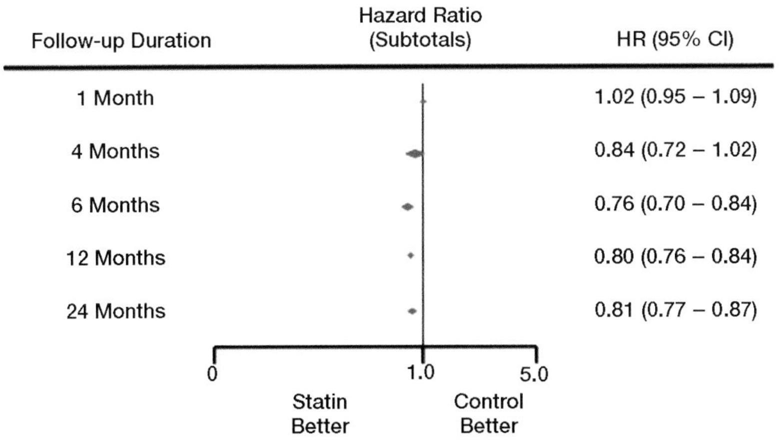

Apart from reperfusion therapy, some general measures (quick clinical evaluation, bedrest, ECG monitoring) and treatments (aspirin, nitrates, β blockers) are integral to an effective initial management of STEMI patients (see Table 61–5).

Current evidence indicates that primary PCI is superior to fibrinolysis if it can be delivered promptly and by expert operators. In many cases, fibrinolysis remains a convenient approach for STEMI treatment. Considering that most benefit is gained from reperfusion within the first 1 to 2 hours from symptom onset, fibrinolytic infusion should be started immediately after arrival in the emergency department, or even in the prehospital setting.

Various antithrombotic agents are employed to facilitate and maintain coronary reperfusion that is obtained either mechanically or pharmacologically. A combination of one or more antiplatelet drugs plus one antithrombin agent are generally prescribed as ancillary therapy. Aspirin and UFH (or LMWH) are routinely administered to all STEMI patients. Clopidogrel is recommended in patients treated by PCI or as alternative to aspirin in cases of aspirin allergy. Abciximab may also be given to patients who are receiving a half-dose of a fibrinolytic (reteplase or tenecteplase) or who are treated by PCI. The direct thrombin inhibitor bivalirudin is a valuable alternative to heparin in patients with heparin-induced thrombocytopenia.

Additional medications (e.g., statins, insulin, modulators of the renin–angiotensin–aldosterone system) may be part of an overall strategy for management of risk factors (e.g., dyslipidemia, diabetes, hypertension) and secondary prevention.

Patients with STEMI may experience heart failure, serious arrhythmias, or recurrent ischemia. All complications (including cardiogenic shock) need to be promptly recognized and treated.[93]

After the initial phase of patient management is completed, what further strategies to apply will depend mainly on the results provided by diagnostic tests applied to the evaluation of critical prognostic indicators such as infarct size and presence/extension of inducible ischemia.

Follow-up Duration	Hazard Ratio (Subtotals)	HR (95% CI)
1 Month		1.02 (0.95 – 1.09)
4 Months		0.84 (0.72 – 1.02)
6 Months		0.76 (0.70 – 0.84)
12 Months		0.80 (0.76 – 0.84)
24 Months		0.81 (0.77 – 0.87)

FIGURE 61–11. Early intensive statin therapy on cardiovascular events in acute coronary syndrome (ACS) patients: effects of duration of therapy. Plot refers to 13 randomized, controlled trials (N = 17,963) of statins begun within 14 days of hospitalization for ACS. CI, confidence interval; HR, hazard ratio. *Source: Adapted from Hulten E, Jackson JL, Douglas K, et al. The effect of early, intensive statin therapy on acute coronary syndrome: a meta-analysis of randomized controlled trials. Arch Intern Med 2006;166:1814–1821.*

REFERENCES

1. Sabatine MS, Antman EM. The thrombolysis in myocardial infarction risk score in unstable angina/non-ST-segment elevation myocardial infarction. *J Am Coll Cardiol* 2003;41:89S–95S.
2. Eagle KA, Lim MJ, Dabbous OH, et al. A validated prediction model for all forms of acute coronary syndrome: estimating the risk of 6-month postdischarge death in an international registry. *JAMA* 2004;291:2727–2733.
3. Antman EM, Cohen M, Bernink PJ, et al. The TIMI risk score for unstable angina/non-ST elevation MI. A method for prognostication and therapeutic decision making. *JAMA* 2000;284:835–842.
4. Gluckman TJ, Sachdev M, Schulman SP, Blumenthal RS. A simplified approach to the management of non-ST-segment elevation acute coronary syndromes. *JAMA* 2005;293:349–357.
5. Cannon CP, Weintraub WS, Demopoulos LA, et al. Comparison of early invasive and conservative strategies in patients with unstable coronary syndromes treated with the glycoprotein IIb/IIIa inhibitor tirofiban. *N Engl J Med* 2001;344:1879–1887.
6. Fox KA, Poole-Wilson PA, Henderson RA, et al. Interventional versus conservative treatment for patients with unstable angina or non-ST-elevation myocardial infarction: the British Heart Foundation RITA 3 randomised trial. Randomized Intervention Trial of unstable Angina. *Lancet* 2002;360:743–751.

7. Braunwald E, Antman EM, Beasley JW, et al. ACC/AHA guideline update for the management of patients with unstable angina and non-ST-segment elevation myocardial infarction—2002: summary article: a report of the American College of Cardiology/American Heart Association Task Force on Practice Guidelines (Committee on the Management of Patients With Unstable Angina). *Circulation* 2002;106:1893–1900.

8. Bertrand ME, Simoons ML, Fox KA, et al. Management of acute coronary syndromes in patients presenting without persistent ST-segment elevation. *Eur Heart J* 2002;23:1809–1840.

9. Curfman GD, Heinsimer JA, Lozner EC, Fung HL. Intravenous nitroglycerin in the treatment of spontaneous angina pectoris: a prospective, randomized trial. *Circulation* 1983;67:276–282.

10. Cheitlin MD, Hutter AM Jr, Brindis RG, et al. ACC/AHA expert consensus document. Use of sildenafil (Viagra) in patients with cardiovascular disease. American College of Cardiology/American Heart Association. *J Am Coll Cardiol* 1999;33:273–282.

11. Figueras J, Lidon R, Cortadellas J. Rebound myocardial ischaemia following abrupt interruption of intravenous nitroglycerin infusion in patients with unstable angina at rest. *Eur Heart J* 1991;12:405–411.

12. Yusuf S, Wittes J, Friedman L. Overview of results of randomized clinical trials in heart disease. II. Unstable angina, heart failure, primary prevention with aspirin, and risk factor modification. *JAMA* 1988;260:2259–2263.

13. Metoprolol in acute myocardial infarction. Mortality. The MIAMI Trial Research Group. *Am J Cardiol* 1985;56:15G–22G.

14. Mitchell RG, Stoddard MF, Ben-Yehuda O, et al. Esmolol in acute ischemic syndromes. *Am Heart J* 2002;144:E9.

15. Heidenreich PA, McDonald KM, Hastie T, et al. Meta-analysis of trials comparing β blockers, calcium antagonists, and nitrates for stable angina. *JAMA* 1999;281:1927–1936.

16. Pepine CJ, Faich G, Makuch R. Verapamil use in patients with cardiovascular disease: an overview of randomized trials. *Clin Cardiol* 1998;21:633–641.

17. Boden WE, Krone RJ, Kleiger RE, et al. Electrocardiographic subset analysis of diltiazem administration on long-term outcome after acute myocardial infarction. The Multicenter Diltiazem Post-Infarction Trial Research Group. *Am J Cardiol* 1991;67:335–342.

18. Goldstein RE, Boccuzzi SJ, Cruess D, Nattel S. Diltiazem increases late-onset congestive heart failure in postinfarction patients with early reduction in ejection fraction. The Adverse Experience Committee; and the Multicenter Diltiazem Postinfarction Research Group. *Circulation* 1991;83:52–60.

19. Opie LH, Yusuf S, Kubler W. Current status of safety and efficacy of calcium channel blockers in cardiovascular diseases: a critical analysis based on 100 studies. *Prog Cardiovasc Dis* 2000;43:171–196.

20. Furberg CD, Psaty BM, Meyer JV. Nifedipine. Dose-related increase in mortality in patients with coronary heart disease. *Circulation* 1995;92:1326–1331.

21. Tijssen JG, Kerkkamp HJ, Viersma JW, de Beijer JM, de Feijter PJ, Lubsen J. Nifedipine and metoprolol in suspected unstable angina. Treatment, observations, and outcome events. *Eur Heart J* 1987;8 Suppl H 35–48.

22. Meine TJ, Roe MT, Chen AY, et al. Association of intravenous morphine use and outcomes in acute coronary syndromes: results from the CRUSADE Quality Improvement Initiative. *Am Heart J* 2005;149:1043–1049.

23. Effects of tissue plasminogen activator and a comparison of early invasive and conservative strategies in unstable angina and non-Q-wave myocardial infarction. Results of the TIMI IIIB Trial. Thrombolysis in Myocardial Ischemia. *Circulation* 1994;89:1545–1556.

24. Lewis HD Jr, Davis JW, Archibald DG, et al. Protective effects of aspirin against acute myocardial infarction and death in men with unstable angina. Results of a Veterans Administration Cooperative Study. *N Engl J Med* 1983;309:396–403.

25. Collaborative meta-analysis of randomised trials of antiplatelet therapy for prevention of death, myocardial infarction, and stroke in high risk patients. *BMJ* 2002;324:71–86.

26. A randomised, blinded, trial of clopidogrel versus aspirin in patients at risk of ischaemic events (CAPRIE). CAPRIE Steering Committee. *Lancet* 1996;348:1329–1339.

27. Yusuf S, Zhao F, Mehta SR, Chrolavicius S, Tognoni G, Fox KK. Effects of clopidogrel in addition to aspirin in patients with acute coronary syndromes without ST-segment elevation. *N Engl J Med* 2001;345:494–502.

28. Mehta SR, Yusuf S, Peters RJ, et al. Effects of pretreatment with clopidogrel and aspirin followed by long-term therapy in patients undergoing percutaneous coronary intervention: the PCI-CURE study. *Lancet* 2001;358:527–533.

29. Fox KA, Mehta SR, Peters R, et al. Benefits and risks of the combination of clopidogrel and aspirin in patients undergoing surgical revascularization for non-ST-elevation acute coronary syndrome: the Clopidogrel in Unstable angina to prevent Recurrent ischemic Events (CURE) Trial. *Circulation* 2004;110:1202–1208.

30. Steinhubl SR, Akers WS. Clopidogrel-statin interaction: a mountain or a mole hill? *Am Heart J* 2006;152:200–203.

31. Brown DL, Fann CS, Chang CJ. Meta-analysis of effectiveness and safety of abciximab versus eptifibatide or tirofiban in percutaneous coronary intervention. *Am J Cardiol* 2001;87:537–541.

32. Boersma E, Harrington RA, Moliterno DJ, et al. Platelet glycoprotein IIb/IIIa inhibitors in acute coronary syndromes: a meta-analysis of all major randomised clinical trials. *Lancet* 2002;359:189–198.

33. Dalby M, Montalescot G, Bal dit Sollier C, et al. Eptifibatide provides additional platelet inhibition in non-ST-elevation myocardial infarction patients already treated with aspirin and clopidogrel. Results of the platelet activity extinction in non-Q-wave myocardial infarction with aspirin, clopidogrel, and eptifibatide (PEACE) study. *J Am Coll Cardiol* 2004;43:162–168.

34. Huxtable LM, Tafreshi MJ, Rakkar AN. Frequency and management of thrombocytopenia with the glycoprotein IIb/IIIa receptor antagonists. *Am J Cardiol* 2006;97:426–429.

35. Oler A, Whooley MA, Oler J, Grady D. Adding heparin to aspirin reduces the incidence of myocardial infarction and death in patients with unstable angina. A meta-analysis. *JAMA* 1996;276:811–815.

36. Blazing MA, de Lemos JA, White HD, et al. Safety and efficacy of enoxaparin vs unfractionated heparin in patients with non-ST-segment elevation acute coronary syndromes who receive tirofiban and aspirin: a randomized controlled trial. *JAMA* 2004;292:55–64.

37. Ferguson JJ, Califf RM, Antman EM, et al. Enoxaparin vs unfractionated heparin in high-risk patients with non-ST-segment elevation acute coronary syndromes managed with an intended early invasive strategy: primary results of the SYNERGY randomized trial. *JAMA* 2004;292:45–54.

38. Petersen JL, Mahaffey KW, Hasselblad V, et al. Efficacy and bleeding complications among patients randomized to enoxaparin or unfractionated heparin for antithrombin therapy in non-ST-segment elevation acute coronary syndromes: a systematic overview. *JAMA* 2004;292:89–96.

39. Effects of recombinant hirudin (lepirudin) compared with heparin on death, myocardial infarction, refractory angina, and revascularisation procedures in patients with acute myocardial ischaemia without ST elevation: a randomised trial. Organisation to Assess Strategies for Ischemic Syndromes (OASIS-2) Investigators. *Lancet* 1999;353:429–438.

40. Stone GW, McLaurin BT, Cox DA, et al. Bivalirudin for patients with acute coronary syndromes. *N Engl J Med* 2006;355:2203–2216.

41. Yusuf S, Pepine CJ, Garces C, et al. Effect of enalapril on myocardial infarction and unstable angina in patients with low ejection fractions. *Lancet* 1992;340:1173–1178.

42. Granger CB, Goldberg RJ, Dabbous O, et al. Predictors of hospital mortality in the global registry of acute coronary events. *Arch Intern Med* 2003;163:2345–2353.

43. Antman EM, Anbe DT, Armstrong PW, et al. ACC/AHA guidelines for the management of patients with ST-elevation myocardial infarction: a report of the American College of Cardiology/American Heart Association Task Force on Practice Guidelines (Committee to Revise the 1999 Guidelines for the Management of Patients with Acute Myocardial Infarction). *Circulation* 2004;110:e82–e292.

44. Curtis JP, Portnay EL, Wang Y, et al. The pre-hospital electrocardiogram and time to reperfusion in patients with acute myocardial infarction, 2000–2002: findings from the National Registry of Myocardial Infarction-4. *J Am Coll Cardiol* 2006;47:1544–1552.

45. Eisenberg MJ, Topal EJ. Prehospital administration of aspirin in patients with unstable angina and acute myocardial infarction. *Arch Intern Med* 1996;156:1506–1510.

46. Huber K, De Caterina R, Kristensen SD, et al. Pre-hospital reperfusion therapy: a strategy to improve therapeutic outcome in patients with ST-elevation myocardial infarction. *Eur Heart J* 2005;26:2063–2074.

47. Pedley DK, Bissett K, Connolly EM, et al. Prospective observational cohort study of time saved by prehospital thrombolysis for ST elevation myocardial infarction delivered by paramedics. *BMJ* 2003;327:22–26.

48. Dargie HJ. Effect of carvedilol on outcome after myocardial infarction in patients with left-ventricular dysfunction: the CAPRICORN randomised trial. *Lancet* 2001;357:1385–1390.

49. Randomised trial of intravenous atenolol among 16 027 cases of suspected acute myocardial infarction: ISIS-1. First International Study of Infarct Survival Collaborative Group. *Lancet* 1986;2:57–66.

50. Boersma E, Mercado N, Poldermans D, Gardien M, Vos J, Simoons ML. Acute myocardial infarction. *Lancet* 2003;361:847–858.

51. Effectiveness of intravenous thrombolytic treatment in acute myocardial infarction. Gruppo Italiano per lo Studio della Streptochinasi nell'Infarto Miocardico (GISSI). *Lancet* 1986;1:397–402.

52. Randomised trial of intravenous streptokinase, oral aspirin, both, or neither among 17,187 cases of suspected acute myocardial infarction: ISIS-2. ISIS-2 (Second International Study of Infarct Survival) Collaborative Group. *Lancet* 1988;2:349–360.

53. An international randomized trial comparing four thrombolytic strategies for acute myocardial infarction. The GUSTO investigators. *N Engl J Med* 1993;329:673–682.

54. A comparison of reteplase with alteplase for acute myocardial infarction. The Global Use of Strategies to Open Occluded Coronary Arteries (GUSTO III) Investigators. *N Engl J Med* 1997;337:1118–1123.

55. Andersen HR, Nielsen TT, Rasmussen K, et al. A comparison of coronary angioplasty with fibrinolytic therapy in acute myocardial infarction. *N Engl J Med* 2003;349:733–742.

56. Pinto DS, Kirtane AJ, Nallamothu BK, et al. Hospital delays in reperfusion for ST-elevation myocardial infarction: implications when selecting a reperfusion strategy. *Circulation* 2006;114:2019–2025.

57. Hochman JS, Sleeper LA, White HD, et al. One-year survival following early revascularization for cardiogenic shock. *JAMA* 2001;285:190–192.

58. Van de Werf F, Ardissino D, Betriu A, et al. Management of acute myocardial infarction in patients presenting with ST-segment elevation. The Task Force on the Management of Acute Myocardial Infarction of the European Society of Cardiology. *Eur Heart J* 2003;24:28–66.

59. Sabatine MS, Cannon CP, Gibson CM, et al. Addition of clopidogrel to aspirin and fibrinolytic therapy for myocardial infarction with ST-segment elevation. *N Engl J Med* 2005;352:1179–1189.

60. Topol EJ. Reperfusion therapy for acute myocardial infarction with fibrinolytic therapy or combination reduced fibrinolytic therapy and platelet glycoprotein IIb/IIIa inhibition: the GUSTO V randomised trial. *Lancet* 2001;357:1905–1914.

61. Efficacy and safety of tenecteplase in combination with enoxaparin, abciximab, or unfractionated heparin: the ASSENT-3 randomised trial in acute myocardial infarction. *Lancet* 2001;358:605–613.

62. Giugliano RP, Roe MT, Harrington RA, et al. Combination reperfusion therapy with eptifibatide and reduced-dose tenecteplase for ST-elevation myocardial infarction: results of the Integrilin and tenecteplase in acute myocardial infarction (INTEGRITI) Phase II Angiographic Trial. *J Am Coll Cardiol* 2003;41:1251–1260.

63. Montalescot G, Barragan P, Wittenberg O, et al. Platelet glycoprotein IIb/IIIa inhibition with coronary stenting for acute myocardial infarction. *N Engl J Med* 2001;344:1895–1903.

64. De Luca G, Suryapranata H, Stone GW, et al. Abciximab as adjunctive therapy to reperfusion in acute ST-segment elevation myocardial infarction: a meta-analysis of randomized trials. *JAMA* 2005;293:1759–1765.

65. Popma JJ, Califf RM, Ellis SG, et al. Mechanism of benefit of combination thrombolytic therapy for acute myocardial infarction: a quantitative angiographic and hematologic study. J Am Coll Cardiol 1992;20:1305–1312.

66. Simoons M, Krzeminska-Pakula M, Alonso A, et al. Improved reperfusion and clinical outcome with enoxaparin as an adjunct to streptokinase thrombolysis in acute myocardial infarction. The AMI-SK study. *Eur Heart J* 2002;23:1282–1290.

67. Ross AM, Molhoek P, Lundergan C, et al. Randomized comparison of enoxaparin, a low-molecular-weight heparin, with unfractionated heparin adjunctive to recombinant tissue plasminogen activator thrombolysis and aspirin: second trial of Heparin and Aspirin Reperfusion Therapy (HART II). *Circulation* 2001;104:648–652.

68. Kontny F, Dale J, Abildgaard U, Pedersen TR. Randomized trial of low molecular weight heparin (dalteparin) in prevention of left ventricular thrombus formation and arterial embolism after acute anterior myocardial infarction: the Fragmin in Acute Myocardial Infarction (FRAMI) Study. *J Am Coll Cardiol* 1997;30:962–969.

69. Wallentin L, Bergstrand L, Dellborg M, et al. Low molecular weight heparin (dalteparin) compared to unfractionated heparin as an adjunct to rt-PA (alteplase) for improvement of coronary artery patency in acute myocardial infarction-the ASSENT Plus study. *Eur Heart J* 2003;24:897–908.

70. Eikelboom JW, Quinlan DJ, Mehta SR, Turpie AG, Menown IB, Yusuf S. Unfractionated and low-molecular-weight heparin as adjuncts to thrombolysis in aspirin-treated patients with ST-elevation acute myocardial infarction: a meta-analysis of the randomized trials. *Circulation* 2005;112:3855–3867.

71. Antman EM, Morrow DA, McCabe CH, et al. Enoxaparin versus unfractionated heparin with fibrinolysis for ST-elevation myocardial infarction. *N Engl J Med* 2006;354:1477–1488.

72. Direct thrombin inhibitors in acute coronary syndromes: principal results of a meta-analysis based on individual patients' data. *Lancet* 2002;359:294–302.

73. White H. Thrombin-specific anticoagulation with bivalirudin versus heparin in patients receiving fibrinolytic therapy for acute myocardial infarction: the HERO-2 randomised trial. *Lancet* 2001;358:1855–1863.

74. Lopez-Sendon J, Swedberg K, McMurray J, et al. Expert consensus document on angiotensin converting enzyme inhibitors in cardiovascular disease. The Task Force on ACE-inhibitors of the European Society of Cardiology. *Eur Heart J* 2004;25:1454–1470.

75. GISSI-3: effects of lisinopril and transdermal glyceryl trinitrate singly and together on 6-week mortality and ventricular function after acute myocardial infarction. Gruppo Italiano per lo Studio della Sopravvivenza nell'infarto Miocardico. *Lancet* 1994;343:1115–1122.

76. Indications for ACE inhibitors in the early treatment of acute myocardial infarction: systematic overview of individual data from 100,000 patients in randomized trials. ACE Inhibitor Myocardial Infarction Collaborative Group. *Circulation* 1998;97:2202–2212.

77. Swedberg K, Held P, Kjekshus J, Rasmussen K, Ryden L, Wedel H. Effects of the early administration of enalapril on mortality in patients with acute myocardial infarction. Results of the Cooperative New Scandinavian Enalapril Survival Study II (CONSENSUS II). *N Engl J Med* 1992;327:678–684.

78. Dickstein K, Kjekshus J. Effects of losartan and captopril on mortality and morbidity in high-risk patients after acute myocardial infarction: the OPTIMAAL randomised trial. Optimal Trial in Myocardial Infarction with Angiotensin II Antagonist Losartan. *Lancet* 2002;360:752–760.

79. Pfeffer MA, McMurray JJ, Velazquez EJ, et al. Valsartan, captopril, or both in myocardial infarction complicated by heart failure, left ventricular dysfunction, or both. *N Engl J Med* 2003;349:1893–1906.

80. Pitt B, Zannad F, Remme WJ, et al. The effect of spironolactone on morbidity and mortality in patients with severe heart failure. Randomized Aldactone Evaluation Study Investigators. *N Engl J Med* 1999;341:709–717.

81. Pitt B, Remme W, Zannad F, et al. Eplerenone, a selective aldosterone blocker, in patients with left ventricular dysfunction after myocardial infarction. *N Engl J Med* 2003;348:1309–1321.

82. Yusuf S, Mehta SR, Diaz R, et al. Challenges in the conduct of large simple trials of important generic questions in resource-poor settings: the CREATE and ECLA trial program evaluating GIK (glucose, insulin and potassium) and low-molecular-weight heparin in acute myocardial infarction. *Am Heart J* 2004;148:1068–1078.

83. Mehta SR, Yusuf S, Diaz R, et al. Effect of glucose-insulin-potassium infusion on mortality in patients with acute ST-segment elevation myocardial infarction: the CREATE-ECLA randomized controlled trial. *JAMA* 2005;293:437–446.

84. Early administration of intravenous magnesium to high-risk patients with acute myocardial infarction in the Magnesium in Coronaries (MAGIC) Trial: a randomised controlled trial. *Lancet* 2002;360:1189–1196.

85. Effect of verapamil on mortality and major events after acute myocardial infarction (the Danish Verapamil Infarction Trial II--DAVIT II). *Am J Cardiol* 1990;66:779–785.

86. Gibson RS, Boden WE, Theroux P, et al. Diltiazem and reinfarction in patients with non-Q-wave myocardial infarction. Results of a double-blind, randomized, multicenter trial. *N Engl J Med* 1986;315:423–429.

87. The effect of diltiazem on mortality and reinfarction after myocardial infarction. The Multicenter Diltiazem Postinfarction Trial Research Group. *N Engl J Med* 1988;319:385–392.

88. Sposito AC, Chapman MJ. Statin therapy in acute coronary syndromes: mechanistic insight into clinical benefit. *Arterioscler Thromb Vasc Biol* 2002;22:1524–1534.

89. Aronow HD, Topol EJ, Roe MT, et al. Effect of lipid-lowering therapy on early mortality after acute coronary syndromes: an observational study. *Lancet* 2001;357:1063–1068.

90. Briel M, Schwartz GG, Thompson PL, et al. Effects of early treatment with statins on short-term clinical outcomes in acute coronary syndromes: a meta-analysis of randomized controlled trials. *JAMA* 2006;295:2046–2056.

91. Cannon CP, Braunwald E, McCabe CH, et al. Intensive versus moderate lipid lowering with statins after acute coronary syndromes. *N Engl J Med* 2004;350:1495–1504.

92. Hulten E, Jackson JL, Douglas K, et al. The effect of early, intensive statin therapy on acute coronary syndrome: a meta-analysis of randomized controlled trials. *Arch Intern Med* 2006;166:1814–1821.

93. Gibler WB, Cannon CP, Blomkalns AL, et al. Practical implementation of the guidelines for unstable angina/non-ST-segment elevation myocardial infarction in the emergency department: a scientific statement from the American Heart Association Council on Clinical Cardiology (Subcommittee on Acute Cardiac Care), Council on Cardiovascular Nursing, and Quality of Care and Outcomes Research Interdisciplinary Working Group, in Collaboration With the Society of Chest Pain Centers. *Circulation* 2005;111:2699–2710.

94. Roux S, Christeller S, Ludin E. Effects of aspirin on coronary reocclusion and recurrent ischemia after thrombolysis: a meta-analysis. *J Am Coll Cardiol* 1992:19:671–677.

95. Verheugt FW, Gersh BJ. Aspirin beyond platelet inhibition. *Am J Cardiol* 2002;90:39–41.

96. Chen ZM, Pan HC, Chen YP, et al. Early intravenous then oral metoprolol in 45,852 patients with acute myocardial infarction: randomised placebo-controlled trial. *Lancet* 2005;366:1622–1632

97. Van De Werf F, Adgey J, Ardissino D, et al. Single-bolus tenecteplase compared with front-loaded alteplase in acute myocardial infarction: the ASSENT-2 double-blind randomised trial. *Lancet* 1999;354:716–722.

98. Keeley EC, Boura JA, Grines CL. Comparison of primary and facilitated percutaneous coronary interventions for ST-elevation myocardial infarction: quantitative review of randomised trials. *Lancet* 2006;367:579–588.

99. Borden WB, Faxon DP. Facilitated percutaneous coronary intervention. *J Am Coll Cardiol* 2006;48:1120–1128.

100. Primary versus tenecteplase-facilitated percutaneous coronary intervention in patients with ST-segment elevation acute myocardial infarction (ASSENT-4 PCI): randomised trial. *Lancet* 2006;367:569–578.

101. An international randomized trial comparing four thrombolytic strategies for acute myocardial infarction. The GUSTO investigators. *N Engl J Med* 1993;329:673–682.

102. In-hospital mortality and clinical course of 20,891 patients with suspected acute myocardial infarction randomised between alteplase and streptokinase with or without heparin. The International Study Group. *Lancet* 1990;366:71–75.

103. ISIS-3: a randomised comparison of streptokinase vs tissue plasminogen activator vs anistreplase and of aspirin plus heparin vs aspirin alone among 41,299 cases of suspected acute myocardial infarction. ISIS-3 (Third International Study of Infarct Survival) Collaborative Group. *Lancet* 1992;339:753–770.

104. Efficacy and safety of tenecteplase in combination with enoxaparin, abciximab, or unfractionated heparin: the ASSENT-3 randomised trial in acute myocardial infarction. *Lancet* 2001;358:605–613.

105. ISIS-4: a randomised factorial trial assessing early oral captopril, oral mononitrate, and intravenous magnesium sulphate in 58,050 patients with suspected acute myocardial infarction. ISIS-4 (Fourth International Study of Infarct Survival) Collaborative Group. *Lancet* 1995;345:669–685.

CHAPTER (62)

Percutaneous Coronary Intervention

John S. Douglas, Jr. / Spencer B. King, III

The treatment of patients with coronary heart disease changed dramatically with the development of surgical coronary artery revascularization techniques in the 1970s, and with percutaneous coronary intervention (PCI) in the next decade, performed initially with balloon angioplasty and then, beginning in 1986, with metallic stents. Accelerated change occurred in the United States with the introduction of drug-eluting stents in 2003. This chapter addresses the development and contemporary use of catheter-based coronary artery intervention, including selection of patients and devices, procedural issues, results, complications, and future directions.

DEVELOPMENT OF BALLOON ANGIOPLASTY

Percutaneous transluminal coronary angioplasty (PTCA) was conceived and shepherded into worldwide acceptance by Andreas R. Gruentzig, but the stage was set by the pioneering work of Dotter and Judkins,[1] who, in 1964, mechanically dilated femoral arteries with a coaxial double-catheter system, and of Zeitler,[2] who applied this technique successfully in West Germany and introduced it to Gruentzig. After Gruentzig's development of a polyvinyl chloride balloon catheter with fixed maximal inflated diameters in 1974, modern balloon angioplasty evolved rapidly.[3–5] In September 1977, the first PTCA was performed in Zurich in a 37-year-old insurance salesman with severe angina pectoris and high-grade stenosis of the proximal left anterior descending (LAD) coronary artery.[6–8] Balloon angioplasty was successful in relieving the stenosis, and on the 10th and 23rd anniversaries of this landmark procedure, coronary arteriography revealed wide patency of the LAD and stress testing remained normal (Fig. 62–1).[9]

Following the report of Gruentzig's first five patients in 1978[10] and 50 patients in 1979,[11] worldwide interest in the technique was assured. Under the auspices of the National Heart, Lung, and Blood Institute (NHLBI), multicenter registries were formed to report experiences with the evolving technique of coronary angioplasty.[12,13] Development of an over-the-wire balloon catheter by Simpson et al.,[14] combined with advances in guidewire and balloon catheter technology, resulted in steerable balloon catheter systems capable of crossing and dilating heretofore unreachable coronary stenoses. The use of percutaneous revascularization (PCI) exceeded 130,000 procedures in the United States in 1986,

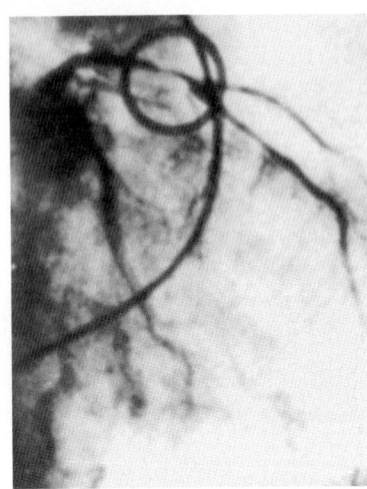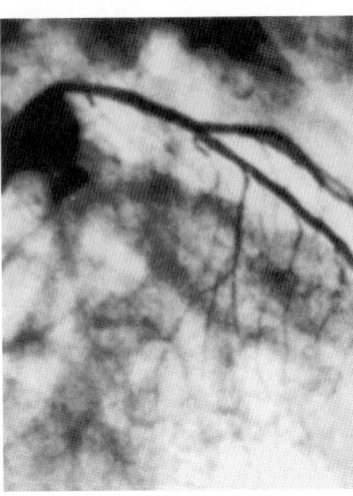

FIGURE 62–1. Right anterior oblique coronary arteriogram of the first patient who underwent transluminal coronary angioplasty on September 16, 1977 (*left*) and on September 16, 1987 (*right*). During this 10-year period, the patient remained completely asymptomatic, and the arteriogram at 10 years showed no narrowing in the coronary arteries. Subsequent angiographic followup at 23 years revealed continued patency of this first PTCA site.[9]

400,000 in 1995, and 1,000,000 in 1999, about a twofold dominance over the use of surgical revascularization.

RANDOMIZED TRIALS OF BALLOON ANGIOPLASTY

[ ] PTCA VERSUS MEDICAL THERAPY

The favorable results of observational studies reporting outcomes in single-vessel and multivessel diseased patients[15,16] led to a series of randomized trials comparing balloon angioplasty with medical therapy[17–25] and with coronary artery bypass graft (CABG).[26–32] The Angioplasty Compared to Medical Therapy Evaluation (ACME) trial, involving 212 patients with single-vessel disease and abnormal stress tests, revealed greater freedom from angina in the angioplasty group at 6 months (64 percent vs. 46 percent) as well as better treadmill performance. There was no difference in death or myocardial infarction (MI).[17] The second Randomized Intervention Treatment of Angina (RITA-2) trial randomized 1018 patients with stable angina to PTCA or medical therapy.[20] The majority had single-vessel disease, and 33 percent had two-vessel disease. Angina relief and treadmill performance were significantly better in the PTCA patients, but complications also were more frequent. At 5 years, death or myocardial infarction had occurred in 9.4 percent of PTCA patients, compared with in 7.6 percent of medically treated patients, and the mortality rates were similar. The recently reported, Fast Revascularization During Instability in Coronary Disease (FRISC II) study, the Treat Angina with Aggrastat and Determine Cost of Therapy with Invasive or Conservative Strategy–Thrombolysis in Myocardial Infarction (TACTICS-TIMI 18) and RITA-3 trials strongly supported an invasive approach which has become the treatment of choice for this patient subset.[22–25] (See Non–ST-Elevation Acute Coronary Syndromes below.)

In 341 mildly symptomatic patients (59 percent asymptomatic or class I; 40 percent class II) in the Atorvastatin Versus Revascu-

larization Treatment (AVERT) trial, PTCA was compared with aggressive lipid-lowering therapy (atorvastatin 80 mg).[21] At 18-month followup, angina relief was significantly better ($p < 0.009$) in the PTCA group, with 54 percent having improvement, versus 41 percent in the aggressive lipid-lowering group, but quality-of-life scores were similar, and there was a trend toward more events (primarily hospitalization for ischemia) in the PTCA group. In AVERT, stents were used in 30 percent of patients. This study suggests that in low-risk patients with no or mild symptoms, aggressive lipid lowering is as effective as PTCA with limited stenting in reducing subsequent ischemic events and emphasizes the importance of extending aggressive lipid lowering in all patients with obstructive coronary artery disease. The Medicine, Angioplasty, or Surgery Study (MASS-I) randomized 214 patients with stable angina, normal left ventricular function, and severe proximal LAD stenosis to bypass surgery (with left internal mammary artery [LIMA] graft), PTCA (without stent use), or medical therapy.[19] At 3 years, there was no difference in death or MI. Both revascularization strategies yielded better symptom relief, but subsequent procedures were more common in the PTCA group. In MASS-II, 611 patients with stable angina, multivessel disease, and preserved left ventricular (LV) function were randomized to medical therapy, CABG, or PTCA.[26] Symptom relief was better with PTCA and CABG than with medical therapy at 1 year. There was no difference in survival at 5 years, but there was less subsequent revascularization in the surgical group (3.5 percent) than in the medical group (24.2 percent) or PCI group (32.2 percent).[26,27]

[ ] PTCA VERSUS CABG

More than 5000 patients were randomized in trials comparing balloon angioplasty with CABG surgery (Table 62–1). Two of these trials were sponsored by the NHLBI and performed in the United States. The first, the Emory Angioplasty Versus Surgery Trial (EAST), was a single-center study,[28] whereas the larger Bypass Angioplasty Revascularization Investigation (BARI)[29] involved 18 centers. In-hospital mortality was similar for angioplasty and bypass surgery (approximately 1 percent) in these two studies of patients with multivessel disease, and 5-year survival also was similar. Repeat revascularization procedures, however, were more common in the angioplasty group, occurring in more than 50 percent of patients compared to 8 to 16 percent of CABG patients. Meta-analyses of eight randomized published trials comparing PTCA and CABG (BARI not included) reported no difference in mortality or MI at 1 year after angioplasty or CABG, but 18 percent of the angioplasty patients had required bypass surgery and 20 percent had an additional angioplasty, a significantly higher rate of repeat revascularization than in the surgery group.[30,31] This increased need for additional revascularization procedures in angioplasty patients, largely as a consequence of restenosis, eroded the initial cost advantage of angioplasty; by 3 years in the EAST study, angioplasty had been 95 percent as costly as bypass surgery[32] and at 8 years, total costs were $46,548 for CABG and $44,491 for PTCA ($p = 0.37$).[33] Importantly, however, the ability to undergo a low-risk initial CABG was preserved for the vast majority of PTCA patients.

TABLE 62–1

Trials Comparing PCI with CABG in Patients
with Multivessel Coronary Artery Disease

PCI alone vs. CABG
  EAST (Emory Angioplasty versus Surgery Trial)
  BARI (Bypass Angioplasty Revascularization Investigation)
  CABRI (Coronary Angioplasty vs. Bypass Revasculariza-
    tion Investigation)
  RITA (Randomized Intervention Treatment of Angina)
  GABI (German Angioplasty Bypass Surgery Investigation)
  ERACI (Argentine Randomized Study of Coronary
    Angioplasty)

PCI with stenting vs. CABG
  ARTS (Arterial Revascularization Therapies Study)
  SoS (Stent or Surgery)
  ERACI II
  MASS II (Medicine Angioplasty or Surgery Study)[a]
  AWESOME (Angina With Extremely Serious Operative
    Mortality Evaluation)[b]

PCI with drug-eluting stenting vs. CABG
  ARTS II
  FREEDOM (Future Revascularization Evaluation of
    Patients with Diabetes Mellitus: Optimal Management
    of Multivessel Disease)
  SYNTAX (Synergy Between Percutaneous Coronary Inter-
    vention with Taxus and Cardiac Surgery)

CABG, coronary artery bypass grafting; PCI, percutaneous coronary
intervention.
[a]In MASS II, 72 percent of patients received stents.
[b]In AWESOME, approximately 50 percent of patients received stents.

Considerable interest was generated by a subset analysis of treated diabetics in BARI. Among the 353 diabetics treated with insulin or oral hypoglycemic agents, 5-year survival was significantly better in patients who underwent surgery compared to patients who underwent PTCA (80.6 percent vs. 65.5 percent; p = 0.003).[34] Analysis of 7-year survival for all patients in BARI revealed for the first time a significantly better survival with CABG compared with PTCA-treated patients (84.4 percent vs. 80.9 percent; p = 0.0425). Although there was no difference in the survival of nondiabetics following PTCA and CABG, there was a poorer survival of treated diabetics revascularized with PTCA (55.7 percent vs. 76.4 percent for CABG; p = 0.0011).[35] Further analysis of treated diabetics in BARI revealed that the survival benefit with CABG was conferred only to those patients who received an internal mammary artery (IMA) graft. EAST, which initially showed no difference between PTCA and CABG in diabetics, at 8 years showed the same trend as BARI.[36] Development of new lesions, perhaps unrecognized, probably accounts for those events occurring many years after revascularization. Significantly poorer PTCA outcomes were also reported for insulin requiring diabetics in the Emory database.[37] In the BARI Registry where revascularization therapy of diabetics was chosen by the physician for patients with two- and three-vessel disease, there was no significant difference in cardiac morality even when adjusted for baseline differences.[38] In the Northern New England Observational Study, survival was en-

hanced by CABG in diabetics with three-vessel disease, but not in those with two-vessel disease.[39] Use of stents has been shown to reduce restenosis, and their use in trials of stents versus CABG, and in diabetic patients is discussed below. Caution should be exercised in the use of PTCA in diabetic patients with multivessel disease[40] and use of arterial grafts emphasized in diabetic patients.[41,42]

METALLIC CORONARY STENTS

Development of stainless steel intracoronary stents and, subsequently, drug-eluting stents, profoundly influenced interventional cardiology. The first coronary stents were implanted in patients in 1986 by Puel in Toulouse and Sigwart in Lausanne for restenosis prevention,[43,44] an unproven hypothesis at the time, whereas the initial implantation in a patient in the United States was performed by the authors at Emory University in 1987 in the setting of abrupt closure,[45,46] following encouraging results in a canine model by Roubin et al.[47] The initial European experience was with a self-expanding mesh stent, whereas the experience at Emory was with a balloon-mounted coil stent that was approved by FDA for abrupt or threatened closure in 1993. This stent made balloon angioplasty considerably safer by providing effective therapy for coronary dissections and reducing the need for emergency coronary bypass surgery, but the use of this stent, despite intensive anticoagulation with heparin and warfarin, was complicated by stent thrombosis in 5 to 10 percent of patients, and bleeding was a common complication.

【 】 METALLIC STENTS VERSUS PTCA

The device that revolutionized interventional cardiology was the Palmaz-Schatz stent (Johnson & Johnson Interventional Systems, Warren, NJ). On the basis of two carefully conducted randomized trials that showed reduced restenosis compared with balloon angioplasty,[48,49] this device was granted U.S. Food and Drug Administration (FDA) approval for marketing in 1994 for the elective treatment of de novo lesions in native coronary arteries. More than 100,000 implantations of this stent were performed in the first year of its availability. The interest in stenting was greatly heightened by a pivotal observation that complete stent expansion by high-pressure balloon inflation, confirmed by intravascular ultrasound, and with substitution of aspirin and ticlopidine for warfarin, yielded a very low stent thrombosis rate and fewer hemorrhagic complications.[50] A prospective, randomized trial of stent placement without ultrasound guidance comparing aspirin and ticlopidine with phenprocoumon (a warfarin derivative) revealed a low 30-day incidence of both cardiac events and bleeding in the aspirin-ticlopidine patients, supporting this simplified antithrombotic strategy.[51] These findings were confirmed and extended by (1) the Stent Anticoagulation Restenosis Study (STARS) investigation, which showed that aspirin and ticlopidine resulted in a lower rate of stent thrombosis than aspirin alone or a combination of aspirin and warfarin,[52] (2) by a multicenter comparison of aspirin and ticlopidine versus aspirin and oral anticoagulation in medium-risk and in high-risk patients showing better outcome with the simpler approach,[53,54] and (3) by a report suggesting that 14 days of ticlopidine and aspirin was adequate for prophylaxis against stent thrombosis in most patients.[55] However, rare reports of thrombotic thrombocytopenia purpura related to ticlopidine use accounting for at least 20 deaths[56,57] led most centers to abandon ticlopidine in favor of clopidogrel which was also an antagonist of platelet adenosine diphosphate (ADP) receptors with similar pharmacologic activity but with far fewer side effects.[58] Clopidogrel proved equal to ticlopidine in observational reports,[59] and in a randomized investigation, the Clopidogrel Aspirin Stent Interventional Cooperative Study (CLASSICS), it was observed that neutropenia, thrombocytopenia, or early discontinuation of the drug was more common in the ticlopidine group (9.1 percent vs. 2.9 percent) than in the clopidogrel group, which received 300 mg as a loading dose and 75 mg subsequently,[60] and that major cardiac events were similar at 1 month. Currently, most centers use a loading dose of 300 to 600 mg clopidogrel when prolonged pretreatment is not possible, plus aspirin 81 to 325 mg daily, and 75 mg clopidogrel plus aspirin for 3–12 months after stent implantation (see Adjunctive Strategies below for further discussion of clopidogrel therapy).

A number of randomized trials comparing stents and PTCA were conducted using dual antiplatelet therapy. The important Belgium Netherlands Stent II (BENESTENT II) study that randomized the heparin-coated Palmaz-Schatz stent and standard balloon angioplasty found better event-free survival at 12 months in the stent group (89 percent vs. 79 percent; $p = 0.004$), lower restenosis (16 percent vs. 31 percent; $p = 0.0008$), and $1020 in higher costs in stent patients at 1 year.[61] The Optimal Angioplasty Versus Primary Stenting (OPUS-1) trial randomized 479 patients to primary stenting or balloon angioplasty followed by provisional stenting only when necessary and reported that after 6 months the combined incidence of death, MI, and target-vessel revascularization was significantly lower in the primary stenting arm (6.1 percent vs. 14.9 percent; $p = 0.003$), and at 6 months primary stenting was slightly less expensive ($10,206 vs. $10,490).[62] This provocative study in which 99 percent of patients in the primary stent arm received a stent, compared with 37 percent of patients in the provisional stenting arm, supported routine stenting when the anatomy was appropriate as opposed to primary balloon angioplasty with stent backup. Routine stent implantation was also supported by the EPISTENT trial in which patients receiving stents plus abciximab had lower target-lesion revascularization (8.7 percent vs. 15 percent, $p <0.001$) and death (0.5 percent vs. 1.8 percent, $p <0.02$) than patients undergoing PTCA (with stent backup plus abciximab)[63] and by a meta-analysis of 29 published, randomized trials of routine stenting versus balloon angioplasty (with provisional stenting for inadequate results). This analysis, which involved 9918 patients, showed no difference in death, myocardial infarction, or the need for coronary bypass surgery but the need for repeat PCI, was reduced by routine stenting (odds ratio [OR] 0.59). Routine stenting resulted in the avoidance of a repeat procedure in approximately 5 patients per 100 treated.[64] A recently published observational trial of the use of bare-metal stents in more than 17,000 unselected patients confirmed a single-digit target-vessel revascularization rate of 8.4 percent.[65] Lesion subsets for which there was the most convincing data supporting stent implantation include native coronary arteries 3.0 to 4.0 mm in diameter, stenotic saphenous vein grafts, chronic total occlusions, restenotic lesions following nonstent intervention, and in the setting of acute myocardial infarction. Less-convincing data was

available for use of stents in bifurcations, vessel diameters ≤2.5 mm in diameter, long lesions, diffuse disease, ostial lesions, and in multivessel disease. The use of coronary stents was reviewed extensively in an American College of Cardiology Expert Consensus Document[66] and in other reports.[67–69]

[ ] METALLIC STENTS VERSUS CABG
Randomized Trials

The issue of whether to choose CABG or PCI in patients with multivessel disease must be guided by the long-term outcome of observational and randomized trials comparing bare-metal stents with bypass surgery and by ongoing trials comparing drug-eluting stents with CABG (see Table 62–1). Followup data from the Arterial Revascularization Therapies Study (ARTS), which randomized 1205 multivessel disease patients in 68 clinical centers to bare-metal stent or standard CABG, was reported. At 1, 3, and 5 years, there was no difference in death or MI; however, repeat interventions were higher in the stent group.[70–72] One-year survival free of death, MI, and reintervention was seen in 89.4 percent of the surgical group and in 75.2 percent of the stent group ($p <0.04$), but at 1 year, costs were higher for surgery (13,645 vs. 10,860 euros). The occurrence of late events in 25 percent of ARTS stented patients was approximately one-half the incidence observed following balloon angioplasty in multivessel disease in BARI, the European Coronary Angioplasty Versus Bypass Revascularization Investigations (CABRI), and EAST because of a reduced need for repeat revascularization in stented patients. As in BARI, the mortality rate of diabetic patients in ARTS was significantly higher than that of nondiabetics (6.3 percent vs. 3.1 percent; $p <0.01$).[72] In the smaller Argentine Randomized Study of Stents Versus CABG in Multivessel Disease (ERACI II), 450 patients were randomized, and at 18.5 months, survival was better in the stent group (97.4 percent vs. 92.5 percent; $p <0.015$) and freedom from MI was higher (96.9 percent vs. 92.5 percent; $p <0.017$), but repeat revascularization was needed more often in the stent group and costs were similar.[73] The Stent or Surgery (SOS) trial, conducted in 53 European and Canadian centers, randomized 500 multivessel disease patients to CABG and 488 to bare-metal stent, and at 1 year repeat revascularization was higher with stents (21 percent vs. 6 percent, $p <0.0001$).[74] The mortality at 5 years favored surgery (4.3 percent vs. 8.1 percent).[75] In the AWESOME (Angina With Extremely Serious Operative Mortality Evaluation) study, 454 high-surgical-risk patients with refractory ischemia were randomized to PCI (approximately one-half received stents) or CABG.[76] Survival and symptom relief were similar at 3 years, but repeat revascularization was more frequent in the stent group. At 5 years, in the AWESOME study, average total costs were $63,896 for PCI versus $84,364 for CABG patients—a difference of $18,732—and survival was at least as good, suggesting that PCI was the economically "dominant" strategy in high-risk patients.[77,78] A meta-analysis of 1533 patients from 4 randomized trials comparing bare-metal stents with CABG (patients from ARTS, SOS, ERACI II, and MASS-2) revealed no difference in MI, death, or stroke, but more repeat revascularizations were needed in stent-treated patients (18 percent vs. 4 percent; $p <0.001$; Fig. 62–2).[79] Both PCI and CABG are evolving and it is

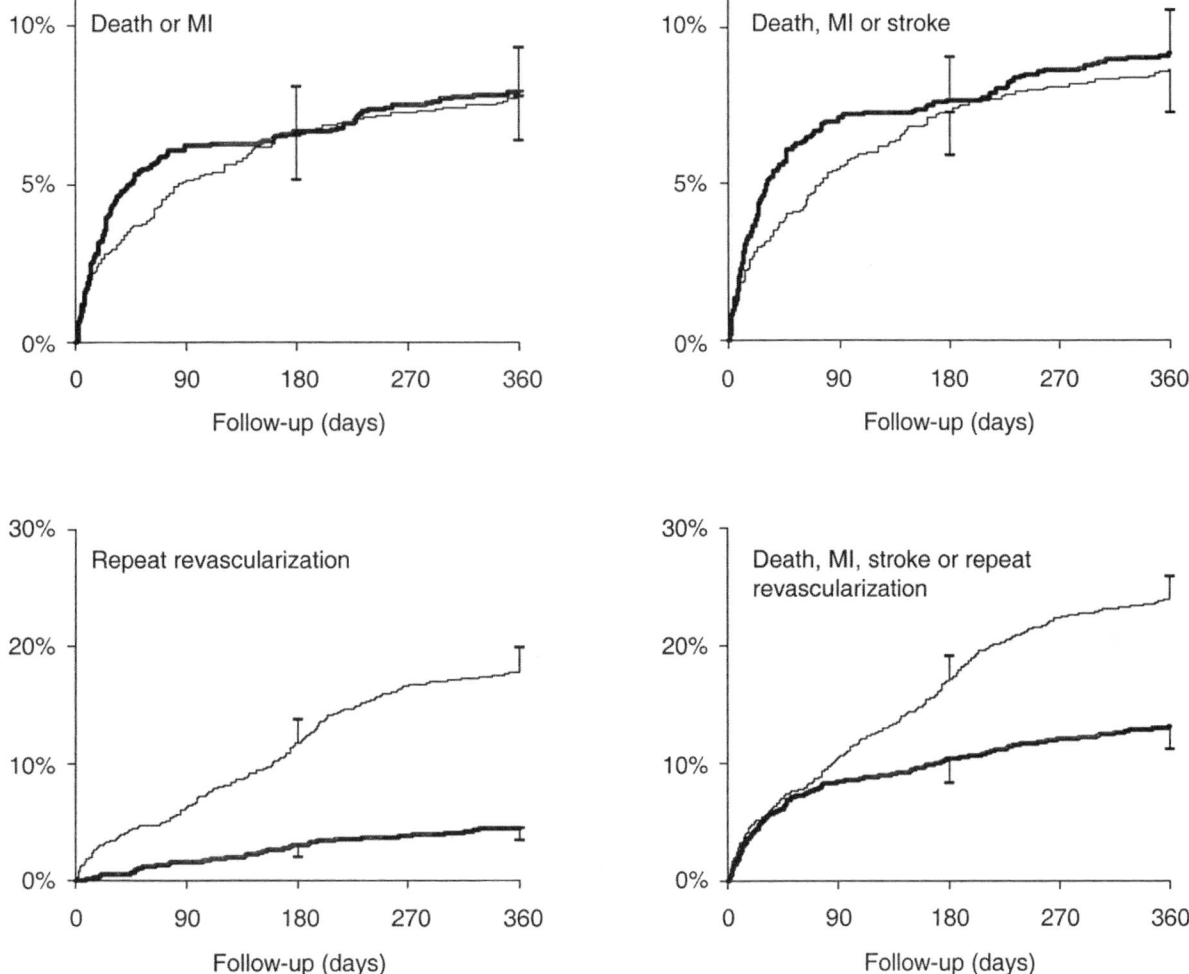

FIGURE 62–2. A meta-analysis of 1-year outcomes of patients from four randomized trials comparing bare metal stents with coronary bypass surgery (*bold line* represents CABG group). *Source: From Mercado N, Wijns W, Serruys PW, et al. One-year outcomes of coronary artery bypass graft surgery versus percutaneous coronary intervention with multiple stenting for multisystem disease: a meta-analysis of individual patient data from randomized clinical trials. J Thorac Cardiovasc Surg 2005;130:512–519, with permission.*

important to note that off-pump coronary surgery, IIb/IIIa platelet receptor inhibitors and, of course, drug-eluting stents were not used in these studies.

A meta-analysis of long-term followup of percutaneous intervention versus CABG in patients with multivessel disease was provocative and showed a lower 5-year mortality with surgery.[80] There were 1.9 fewer deaths per 100 patients in the surgical group. These trials showed an advantage for surgery that was not apparent at 1 or 3 years, but became significant at 5 and 8 years.

Observational Studies

Recently published data from registries in New York state permitted a comparison of outcomes of 59,314 patients with multivessel disease who were treated with metallic stents or CABG between January 1997 and December 2000.[81] Patients with prior revascularization, left main disease, or myocardial infarction within 24 hours were excluded. Patients selected for CABG were older, had more comorbidity, lower ejection fractions, and more severe coronary disease. After adjustment for baseline differences between CABG and stent-treated patients, there was a significantly higher likelihood of survival at 3 years with CABG in all anatomic sub-

groups (Fig. 62–3). The adjusted survival curves diverged quite early and continued to diverge over the 3-year followup period (Fig. 62–4). Repeat revascularization was required in only 4.9 percent of CABG patients, compared to 35.1 percent of stented patients (*p* <0.001). The disparity in mortality outcomes between the New York registry and the prior individual, randomized, controlled trials fueled the controversy regarding the optimal revascularization strategy for patients with multivessel disease. Should the "gold standard" randomized trials with their restricted inclusion criteria and small size guide our therapeutic decisions regarding an individual patient or should the larger, more inclusive observation registry data which must be corrected for fundamental baseline differences weigh more heavily?

DRUG-ELUTING STENTS: THE NEW DOMINANT STRATEGY

Although metallic stents conferred a significant advantage over balloon angioplasty both in reducing initial complications and late events, in-stent restenosis remained a major obstacle to wider application of percutaneous revascularization especially in

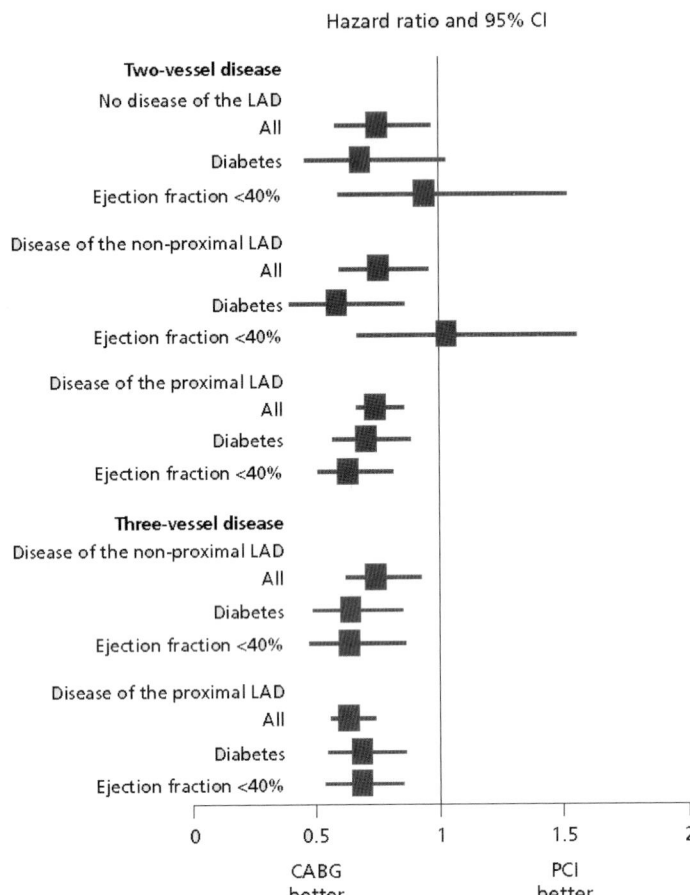

FIGURE 62–3. Mortality outcomes in subgroups in the New York registry study. *Source: From Hannan EL, Racz MJ, Walford G, et al. Long-term outcomes of coronary artery bypass grafting versus stent implantation. N Engl J Med 2005;352:2174–2183.*

complex lesions and clinical subsets where restenosis rates could approach and exceed 50 percent. Although one systemic drug trial aimed at reducing in-stent restenosis caused by neointimal hyperplasia was positive,[82] the most exciting strategy for restenosis prevention was the drug-eluting stent which combined mechanical scaffolding with local pharmacologic action.[67,83–88] Multiple agents were tested and the most promising had antiproliferative effects mediated by inhibiting the cell cycle. The agents which were applied to first-generation drug-eluting stents were sirolimus, an immunosuppressive macrolide antifungal agent which blocked the G1S phase of cellular replication, and paclitaxel an antimicrotubular agent that acted predominantly during the mitosis (M) phase (Fig. 62–5). Both agents decreased smooth muscle migration and proliferation and were shown to be effective in reducing restenosis in clinical trials when polymers were used to bind the agent to the stent. Other agents currently being evaluated are the sirolimus analogues zotarolimus and everolimus, which inhibit the cell cycle at the same point as sirolimus. The largest body of information and longest followup is with the sirolimus-eluting stent. Among 45 patients with de novo lesions in vessels 3.0 to 3.5 mm and lesion length <18 mm, there was no in-stent restenosis or stent thrombosis at 2 years and ultrasonography at 4 years revealed continued effectiveness.[88]

【 】 DRUG-ELUTING VERSUS BARE METALLIC STENTS

In RAVEL (Randomized Study with the Sirolimus Coated Bx Velocity Balloon-Expandable Stent in the Treatment of Patients with de novo Native Coronary Artery Lesions), 238 patients at 19 international centers were randomized to either bare-metal or sirolimus-eluting stent with 6-month angiographic followup in 89 percent.[89] The mean lesion length was 9.6 mm, 19 percent had diabetes, and approximately 40 percent had stable angina. No patient in the sirolimus-eluting stent group had restenosis of 50 percent or more of the luminal diameter, compared to 27 percent in the bare stent group (*p* <0.001) (Fig. 62–6). There were no stent thromboses and at 1 year the major cardiac event rates were 5.8 percent for the drug-eluting stent group and 20 percent for those treated with bare stents (*p* <0.001), a difference entirely attributable to more repeat revascularizations in the bare stent group. This result with relatively simple lesions was not achieved in the subsequent U.S. multicenter Sirolimus-coated Bx Velocity Balloon-expanded Stent in the Treatment of Patients with De Novo coronary lesions (SIRIUS) trial where 1058 patients with longer lesions (≥15 mm to ≤30 mm by visual estimate; actual length 14.4 mm by core lab) were randomized to receive a sirolimus coated or bare Bx Velocity stent.[90] In-stent restenosis was reduced from 35 percent with the bare stent to 3.2 percent (*p* <0.001) with sirolimus, but when the stent edges (5 mm proximal or distal to the stent) were included, the reduction was less but still quite significant (in-segment restenosis was reduced from 37 percent to 9 percent; *p* <0.001). Target-lesion revascularization was reduced from 17 percent to 4 percent (*p* <0.001) and major cardiac events from 19 percent to 7 percent (*p* <0.001). In addition to longer lesions in SIRIUS compared to RAVEL, there were more diabetics (25 percent vs. 19 percent) and more patients with other risk factors, such as hyperlipidemia and hypertension. Based on this favorable safety and efficacy data, the FDA approved the sirolimus-eluting stent for marketing in the United States in 2003. Figure 62–6 displays the results of additional trials using sirolimus-eluting stents.

Several clinical trials evaluating paclitaxel-coated stents have been reported. In TAXUS I, a safety trial involving 61 patients, there was no restenosis in the paclitaxel group and a 10 percent restenosis rate in the bare stent group (see Fig. 62–6).[91] In TAXUS II, an international efficacy trial, 536 patients were randomized to receive a bare 15-mm metal stent or one of two polymeric formulations of paclitaxel (slow and moderate release). Restenosis occurred in 2.3 percent of patients receiving slow-release paclitaxel stents, in 4.7 percent of patients in the moderate-release group (*p* <0.002 for both), and in 20 percent of patients with bare stents.[92] There was no increase in stent thrombosis or aneurysm formation in the paclitaxel groups. TAXUS IV, a pivotal U.S. trial in which 1314 patients were randomized to paclitaxel-coated or bare stents with angiographic and clinical followup, was designed to achieve FDA approval. Lesions were 10 to 28 mm in length and vessel size ranged from 2.5 to 3.75 mm. At 9 months, angiographic restenosis was reduced from 26.6 percent to 7.9 percent by use of drug-eluting stents. There was no differences in death, myocardial infarction (0.6 percent) or stent

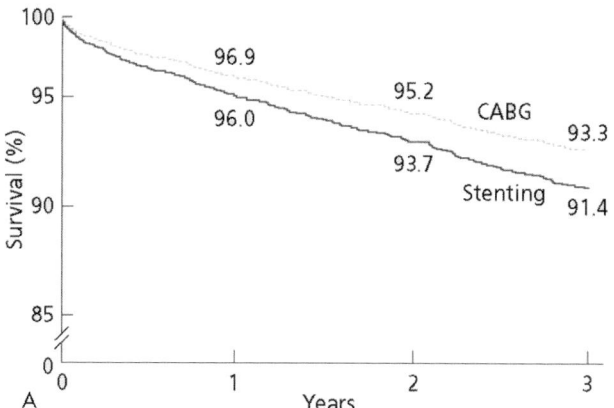

Two-vessel disease without disease of the LAD artery

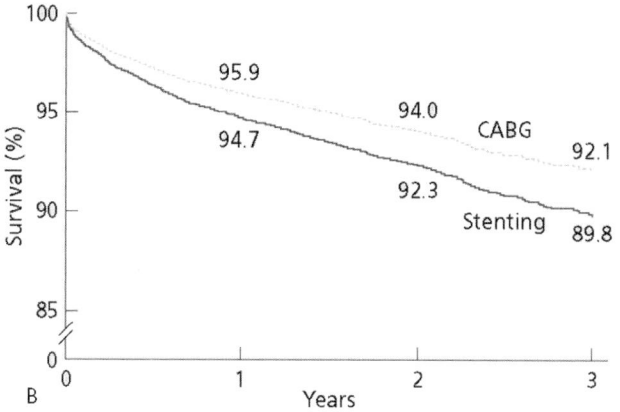

Two-vessel disease with disease of the proximal LAD artery

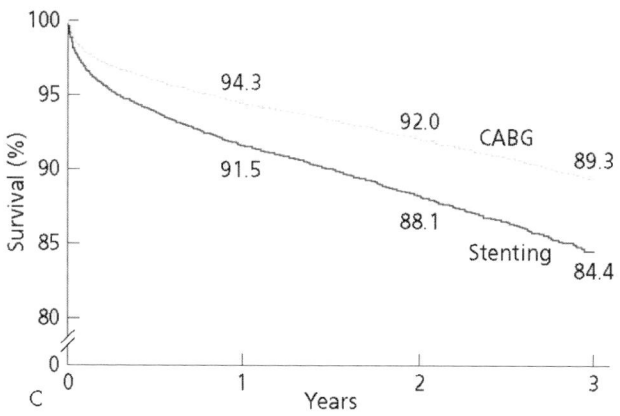

Three-vessel disease with disease of the proximal LAD artery

FIGURE 62–4. Adjusted Kaplan-Meier survival curves among New York patients with multivessel coronary artery disease. **A.** Patients with two-vessel disease without involvement of the left anterior descending (LAD) artery. **B.** Patients with two-vessel disease with involvement of the proximal LAD artery. **C.** Patients with three-vessel disease with involvement of the proximal LAD artery. Values and percentages at 1, 2, and 3 years adjusted for baseline characteristics. *Source: From Hannan EL, Racz MJ, Walford G, et al. Long-term outcomes of coronary artery bypass grafting versus stent implantation. N Engl J Med 2005;352:2174–2183, with permission.*

thrombosis (0.8 percent).[93] TAXUS III reported use of a paclitaxel-coated stent in 28 patients with in-stent restenosis, 8 of whom (29 percent) had subsequent adverse cardiac events[94] (see In-Stent Restenosis below).

Clinical trials to evaluate the Medtronic AVE ABT-578 eluting Driver stent, which eluted zotarolimus from a phosphorylcholine-delivery matrix, included the ENDEAVOR-1 safety trial, the randomized international ENDEAVOR-2 trial, and the randomized U.S. ENDEAVOR-3. ENDEAVOR-2, a 1197-patient randomized trial, showed that the zotarolimus-eluting stent was effective in reducing restenosis (13.2 percent compared to 35 percent for bare-metal stents; $p <0.001$) and target-vessel revascularization was significantly reduced,[95] from 11.8 percent to 4.6 percent ($p = 0.0001$). Early stent thrombosis occurred in 0.5 percent with the ENDEAVOR stent and 1.2 percent of bare-metal stents ($p = NS$) and late thrombosis was not seen. In both ENDEAVOR 1 and 2, the mean in-stent late loss was 0.62 mm, significantly higher than in trials of sirolimus- and paclitaxel-eluting stents. ENDEAVOR-3 is complete. Clinical trials using zotarolimus on the trilayer stent of tantalum and stainless steel (ZOMAXX-Abbott) are underway, as are trials using everolimus (FUTURE and SPIRIT). It should be remembered that most of the drug-eluting stent trials required a followup angiogram, which inflates the reintervention rate and widens the apparent advantage of drug-eluting stent.

Comparative Trials of Drug-Eluting Stents

A varying degree of suppression of intimal hyperplasia noted in observational and randomized trials suggested differences between drug-eluting stents and led to head-to-head comparative studies. In a 1353-patient randomized multicenter trial, sirolimus-eluting and paclitaxel-eluting stents were compared.[96] The primary end point, binary restenosis at 8 months was not different (9.6 percent vs. 11.1 percent; $p = 0.31$) and there was no difference in death, cardiac death, MI, target-lesion revascularization, or major adverse coronary events (MACE) at 8 months. Angiographically determined late loss was less for the sirolimus-eluting stent (0.09 mm vs. 0.31 mm; $p <0.001$).

In a two-center, randomized study of 1012 patients, outcomes were better with sirolimus-eluting stents than with paclitaxel-eluting stents with respect to in-segment restenosis (6.7 percent vs. 11.9 percent; $p = 0.02$), target-vessel revascularization (4.8 percent vs. 8.3 percent; $p = 0.02$), and late loss (0.19 mm vs. 0.32 mm; $p = 0.001$).[97] However, in two large registries, there were no differences in adverse cardiac events at 9 to 12 months.[98,99] In a meta-analysis of 6 trials that included 3669 patients, and in a two-center study of 1845 patients, odds ratios for angiographic restenosis were 0.68 and 0.60, respectively, favoring sirolimus-eluting stents.[100,101]

Preliminary data from SPIRIT II reported at the World Congress of Cardiology comparing the everolimus-eluting Xience Vision stent (Abbott) with the Taxus stent in 300 patients, revealed less in-stent late loss (0.11 mm vs. 0.36 mm; $p = 0.0001$) with nonsignificant differences in binary restenosis (1.3 percent vs. 3.5 percent) and MACE (2.7 percent vs. 6.5 percent).[102]

【 】 DRUG-ELUTING STENTS VERSUS CABG

The clear restenosis advantage of drug-eluting stents compared to bare-metal stents in most lesion and patient subsets has engendered an increasing use of these devices in patients with multivessel disease. However, randomized trial data are not available to guide the choice between PCI with drug-

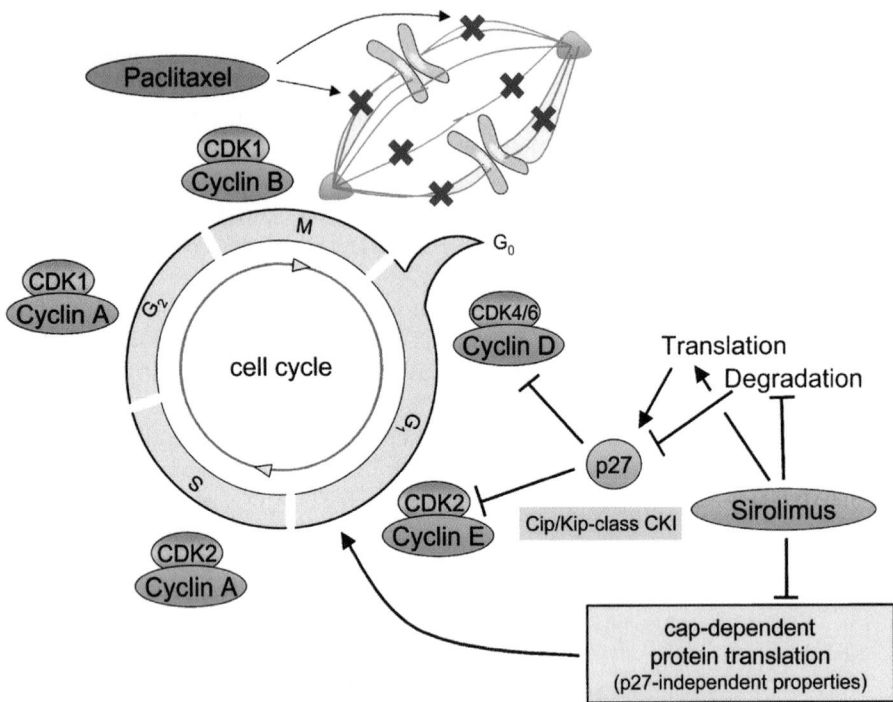

FIGURE 62–5. Schematic of the cell cycle and its regulatory mechanisms that are relevant for the inhibitory effect imposed by sirolimus (SRL) and paclitaxel (PTX). The cell cycle is regulated by the oscillating activities of cyclin/cyclin-dependent kinase (CDK) complexes. Cyclin-dependent kinase inhibitors (CKIs) negatively control the activity of distinct cyclin/CDK complexes. The CKIs of the Cip/Kip class are major regulators of the cell cycle in its initial stage, the G_1/S phase. Cip/Kip CKI include p21^{Cip1} and p27^{Kip1}, among others. Both are critical cell-cycle regulators in smooth muscle cells. P27^{Kip1} activity is regulated at the posttranscriptional level via protein stability and translation. Subsequent to binding its intracellular receptor FKBP12 (FK-506 binding protein), SRL inhibits the activity of mammalian target of rapamycin (mTOR). mTOR is a pivotal protein kinase that mediates mitogen-induced cell proliferation. The inhibition of mTOR by SRL attenuates p27^{Kip1} degradation, thus increasing p27^{Kip1} protein stability. Additionally, p27^{Kip1} protein translation may also be enhanced. Non–p27^{Kip1}-dependent mechanisms of mTOR that lead to stimulation of cap-dependent protein synthesis and are inhibited by SRL include p70^{S6K} and eIF4E activation, the latter via induction of eIF4E binding protein-1 (4EBP1). Paclitaxel impacts predominantly during cell division in the mitosis (M) phase of the cell cycle through centrosomal impairment, induction of abnormal spindles, and suppression of spindle microtubule dynamics. *Source: From Wessely R, Schörnig A, Kastati A. Sirolimus and paclitaxel on polymer-based drug-eluting stents. J Am Coll Cardiol 2006;47:708–714.*

eluting stents and CABG in multivessel disease patients. Observation data has been reported from the ARTS-II registry in which 607 multivessel disease patients who received an average of 3.7 sirolimus-eluting stents each were compared to the surgical and bare-metal stent arms of ARTS-1.[103,104] At 1 year, 89.5 percent of ARTS II patients were MACE-free, a better outcome than ARTS-1 CABG patients. Figure 62–7 shows the Kaplan-Meier curves comparing ARTS 1 and 2 and CABRI outcomes. However; repeat intervention was needed in only 4.1 percent of ARTS-1 CABG patients versus being needed in 8.5 percent (*p* 0.003) of ARTS-2 drug-eluting patients and in 12.6 percent of diabetics in ARTS 2.[105] Recently reported data from ERACI III indicating a 3.1 percent incidence of stent thrombosis at 18 months in 225 patients with multivessel disease is troubling,[106] as are reports of the importance of disease progression, a circumstance somewhat less relevant to the CABG-treated, multivessel disease patient.[107,108] The three ongoing randomized comparisons of PCI with drug-eluting stents and CABG for treatment of multivessel coronary disease will provide important guidance for future decision making (see Table 62–1).[109]

[ ] COST-EFFECTIVENESS OF DRUG-ELUTING STENTS

Drug-eluting stents reduce restenosis and the need for costly repeat revascularization procedures, but this benefit comes at a significantly higher initial price.[110] Two reports suggested that drug-eluting stents were cost-effective.[111,112] However, multiple factors influence this calculation, including the number of stents required and the effectiveness of the drug-eluting stent in avoiding the need for repeat intervention.[113–118] Subgroups in which a drug-eluting stent is most likely to be cost-effective compared to a bare-metal stent include diabetes, long lesions, small vessels, and perhaps those with lesions in left main, proximal LAD, saphenous vein grafts, or other sites at high risk of restenosis. As the number of lesions escalate, the cost-effectiveness of drug-eluting stents quickly erodes. The impact of this more expensive new technology is different for the payer, provider (i.e., hospital), and vendor.[113] Modeling of the ARTS II and ARTS CABG data suggests that the drug-eluting stent had an overall economic advantage.[116,118] Results of ongoing randomized trials are needed, however, to more fully address this issue.

[ ] PROBLEMS UNIQUE TO DRUG-ELUTING STENTS

Although clinical trials provide compelling evidence suggesting that the use of drug-eluting stents is safe and highly effective in reducing repeat revascularizations, recent studies reporting coronary endothelial dysfunction, coronary spasm, hypersensitivity reactions, stent fracture or malapposition, delayed healing, and late stent thrombosis, complications not reported with bare-metal stents, are worrisome.[119–134] In addition, the increased risk associated with nonresponsiveness to,[135,136] or premature discontinuation of, antiplatelet therapy, with a reported hazard ratio as high as 89.78,[127] may be unavoidable because of complications from required surgery or bleeding. Advanced age, lower socioeconomic status and inadequate counseling are also associated factors in patients who prematurely omit dual antiplatelet therapy.

ADJUNCTIVE STRATEGIES
[ ] PHARMACOTHERAPY
Thienopyridines

Clopidogrel inhibits platelet activation by irreversibly blocking the ADP (P_2Y_{12}) receptor. It has better tolerability, fewer side ef-

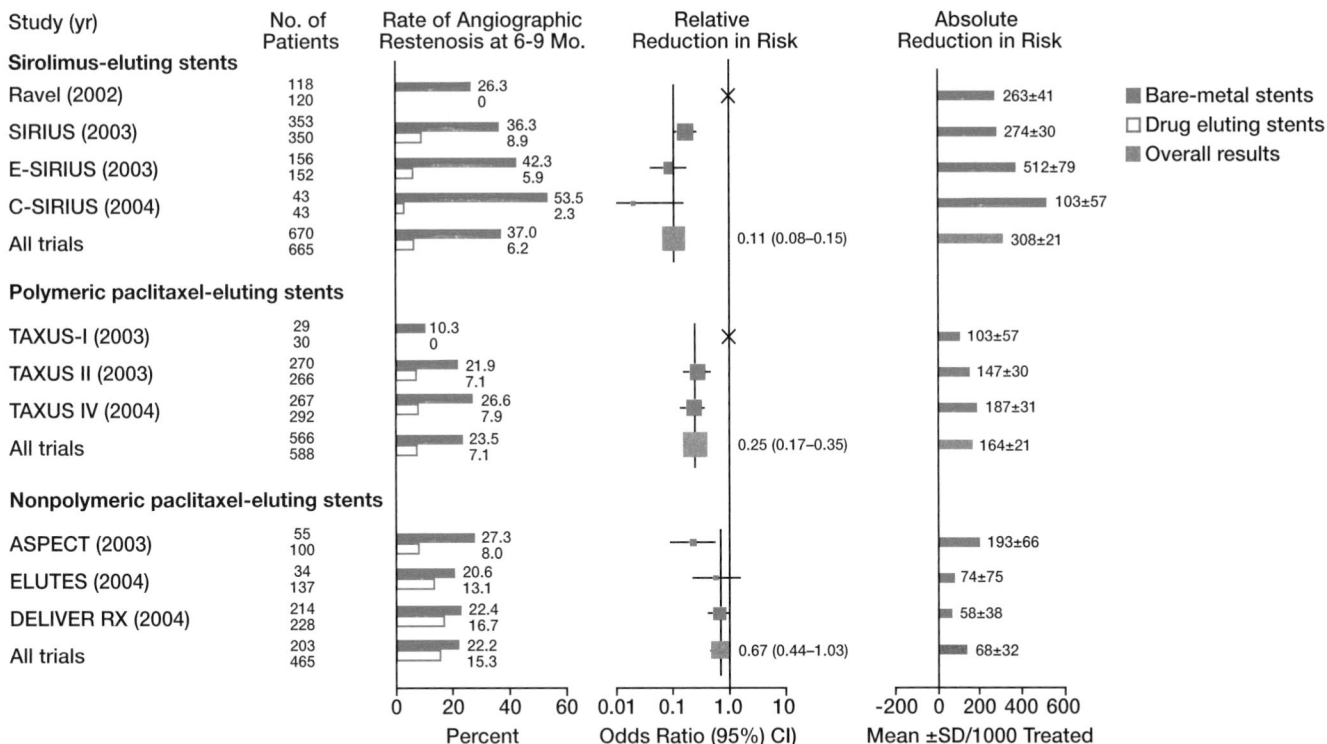

FIGURE 62–6. Results of selected trials of drug-eluting stents. *Source: From Serruys PW, Kutryk MJB, Ong ATL. Coronary artery stents. N Engl J Med 2006;354:483–495, with permission.*

fects, and is at least as effective as ticlopidine, and along with aspirin, is routinely administered prior to stent implantation.[69] Recent evidence supports its use in nonstent PCI as well.[137,138] Although initial clopidogrel doses of 600 mg are needed to produce potent inhibition of ADP-induced platelet aggregation within 2 hours,[139–141] a 300-mg loading dose is commonly used when longer pretreatment is possible and has been shown to produce maximal platelet inhibition within 24 hours with substantial inhibition at 15 hours.[142] A 600-mg loading dose of clopidogrel 2 hours before elective, low-risk stent implantation showed similar results to those obtained with the same dose of clopidogrel plus routine abciximab administration.[143] When tested in high-risk patients with non–ST-elevation acute coronary syndrome, the clopidogrel 600-mg loading dose alone was also as effective as clopidogrel plus abciximab in troponin-negative patients, but not in troponin-positive patients (adverse events: 18.3 percent clopidogrel alone compared to 13.1 percent clopidogrel plus abciximab; *p* = 0.02).[144] Following PCI, long-term (1 year) clopidogrel was associated with a 27 percent relative reduction in adverse ischemic events (*p* = 0.02) compared to 4 weeks of therapy.[145] These findings extended and amplified the similar findings of the PCI-CURE (Clopidogrel in Unstable Angina to Prevent Recurrent Ischemic Events) trial.[138] Major bleeding was not significantly increased at 1 year and clopidogrel therapy for 1 year was highly cost-effective.[146] Recent reports suggest that inadequate inhibition of platelet aggregation may occur in patients with higher body mass index[147] and that insensitivity to clopidogrel is

more common than previously thought. Both factors may contribute to periprocedural ischemic complications and stent thrombosis. Depending on the definition used, 10 to 15 percent of patients undergoing PCI are resistant to aspirin and 25 percent are resistant to clopidogrel. In addition, about half of aspirin-resistant patients have a lower response to clopidogrel, placing them at higher risk of periprocedural myonecrosis and stent thrombosis.[148–150] Reliable, standardized, bedside measures of resistance to dual antiplatelet therapy are not routinely available. Duration of dual antiplatelet therapy also has not been standard-

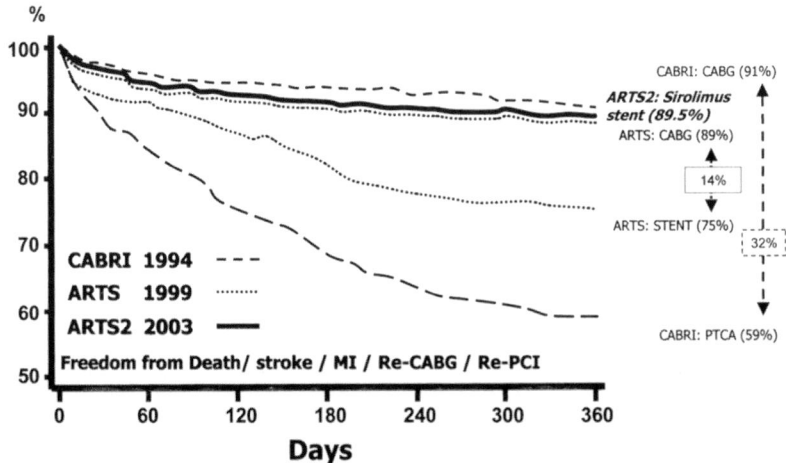

FIGURE 62–7 Comparison of outcomes from CABRI (balloon angioplasty), ARTS stent-treated patients, ARTS CABG-treated patients, and ARTS 2 patients treated with sirolimus-eluting stents. *Source: From Serruys PW,[104] with permission.*

ized, but U.S. and European guidelines and practice trends appear to support extension to 12 months following implantation of drug-eluting stents and 1 month following bare-metal stents in patients who do not have a high risk of bleeding. In patients recognized to be resistant to clopidogrel, an increased dose of 150 mg/d and/or addition of cilostazol may be considered.[69,82] The heightened risk of thrombosis because of a drug-eluting stent associated with premature discontinuation of dual antiplatelet therapy, especially in the setting of noncardiac surgery, deserves emphasizing.[127,128]

IIb/IIIa Platelet Receptor Inhibitors

Among the arrows in the quiver of the interventionalist are the potent platelet glycoprotein IIb/IIIa receptor inhibitors.[151–154] The first approved by the FDA, a monoclonal antibody, abciximab (ReoPro, Centocor, Malvern, PA), was shown to reduce ischemic complications and late clinical events in high-risk angioplasty.[155] The other IIb/IIIa receptor inhibitors approved by the FDA, are competitive inhibitors; eptifibatide (Integrilin, COR Therapeutics, San Francisco, CA) a peptide, and tirofiban (Aggrastat, Merck, White House Station, NJ) a small nonpeptide molecule. Each of these agents reduces a composite end point of death or nonfatal MI in the setting of coronary intervention and in acute coronary syndromes. Furthermore, in the EPIC trial, a subgroup of 555 patients with acute coronary syndromes treated with bolus abciximab and infusion had a significant reduction in mortality at 3 years.[156] A meta-analysis of 19 randomized trials of IIb/IIIa agents (20,137 patients) during PCI reported a significant and sustained decrease (20 to 30 percent) in the risk of death.[157] The relative risk reduction was similar in patients with and without acute MI and with and without stents. In a review of the use of the three FDA-approved IIb/IIIa receptor inhibitor agents in acute coronary syndromes, it was noted that they were each effective in reducing a composite end point of death or MI when administered prior to or at the time of percutaneous coronary intervention.[158] Contributing to their use was the favorable outcome of IIb/IIIa receptor inhibitor-treated patients in the Evaluation of Platelet IIb/IIIa Inhibitors of Stenting (EPISTENT) trial, in which abciximab therapy in patients undergoing stent implantation or balloon angioplasty was evaluated.[159,160] At 6 months, the incidence of a composite end point of death or MI was 5.6 percent in stented patients receiving abciximab, compared with 11.4 percent in patients receiving placebo ($p <0.001$) and 7.8 percent in patients treated with balloon angioplasty and abciximab. In diabetics, the combination of abciximab and stenting was associated with a lower rate of repeat target-vessel revascularization (8.1 percent) and this benefit persisted through 1-year followup. Previous reports indicate that abciximab did not prevent neointimal proliferation or reduce in-stent restenosis.[161] EPISTENT does, however, raise the question regarding whether all diabetic patients receiving stents should receive IIb/IIIa platelet inhibitors. A meta-analysis of diabetics in six large trials indicated that 30-day mortality following PCI was reduced by IIb/IIIa inhibitors from 4.0 percent to 1.2 percent ($p = 0.0002$).[162] In the CAPTURE trial, death or MI was significantly less frequent in patients with elevated baseline troponin who were treated with abciximab than in those patients who were treated with placebo (9.5 percent vs. 23.9 percent; $p =$

0.002), but not in troponin-negative patients (7.5 percent vs. 9.4 percent; $p = 0.47$).[163] Although there was no difference in death, MI, or urgent intervention in simple lesions, there was for complex lesions (19.1 percent for placebo vs. 11.5 percent for abciximab; $p = 0.03$). When flow in the culprit artery was less than TIMI grade 3 after angioplasty, the incidence of death and MI at 30 days was 11.5 percent with placebo and 4.1 with abciximab, supporting a role for abciximab in ameliorating the consequences of postprocedure slow flow. These observations that IIb/IIIa receptor inhibitors appear to be more effective in patients with refractory unstable angina, complex anatomy, and slow flow may help to determine the place of these agents.

The clinical effectiveness of eptifibatide, a short-acting heptapeptide was evaluated in 2064 patients undergoing nonurgent stent implantation. A double-bolus regimen of eptifibatide was compared to placebo with 48-hour and 30-day composite end points (death, MI, urgent target-vessel revascularization). There was a consistent treatment effect with a 35 percent reduction in adverse cardiac events (6.8 percent vs. 10.4 percent; $p = 0.003$).[164] In the ESPRIT (Enhanced Suppression of the Platelet IIb/IIIa Receptor with Integrilin Therapy) trial, high-risk patients (age >75 years, diabetes, positive biomarkers, recent MI, and unstable angina) treated with eptifibatide experienced a reduction in adverse events from 12 percent to 6 percent ($p <0.001$).[165]

The decision to use a IIb/IIIa platelet receptor in the era of high-dose clopidogrel pretreatment is complex and requires an assessment of the patient's risk of bleeding and ischemic complications with and without these agents. The patient who cannot receive the acute benefit of clopidogrel therapy because of allergy or intolerance should receive a IIb/IIIa receptor, a class I indication in the ACC *Guideline* statement.[69] Troponin-positive acute coronary syndrome patients were shown to have incremental benefit with abciximab plus high-dose clopidogrel compared to high-dose clopidogrel alone[166] and could reasonably be selected if bleeding risks permit. Although there is conflicting data with respect to the diabetic patient, the weight of evidence appears to support use of IIb/IIIa inhibitors, abciximab specifically.[167] In addition to analyzing the risk of bleeding, which is increased in women and those with renal insufficiency, recent evidence suggests there are subgroups, such as the elderly, in which efficacy of IIb/IIIa inhibitors may be attenuated.[168–170]

Thrombin Inhibitors

Unfractionated heparin (UFH) was the thrombin inhibitor used in the first two decades of PCI, and was the only thrombin inhibitor with a class I indication for routine use in the most recent PCI *Guidelines*.[69] The appearance of low-molecular-weight heparin (LMWH) as the antithrombin of choice in American College of Cardiologists/American Heart Association (ACC/AHA) *Unstable Angina Guidelines* (a class IIA recommendation), and FDA approval of three direct thrombin inhibitors for use in PCI, challenges the interventional cardiologist to provide optimal antithrombotic therapy for a diverse population of complex patients. Clearly, UFH has a number of disadvantages including nonlinear anticoagulant kinetics, a requirement for cofactor antithrombin III, an inability to inactivate clot-bound thrombin, platelet activation, stimulation of antibody formation, and a prothrombotic rebound phenomenon. It was generally recommended that anticoagulation for coronary angioplasty procedures with UFH be carried out with a weight-adjusted bolus of 70 to 100 IU per kg without IIb/IIIa inhibitors and 50 to 70 IU per kg with them. Monitoring of activated clotting time (ACT) was recommended to achieve an ACT target of approximately 300 seconds without IIb/IIIa inhibitors and 200 to 250 seconds when these agents were used. Several investigators have suggested that ACT targets with stent implantation can safely be reduced to 200 to 250 seconds to minimize hemorrhagic risks.[171,172] Postprocedural heparin infusions were generally not recommended because of increased bleeding.

LMWH (molecular weights of approximately 4000 to 6000 daltons) inactivates thrombin less than UFH and binds factor Xa more avidly with anti-IIa-to-anti-Xa ratios that vary from 1:2 to 1:4, depending on the LMWH agent used. LMWH is more bioavailable than UFH, is less inhibited by platelet factor-4, causes less thrombocytopenia, and its predictable anticoagulant effect eliminates to a degree the need for laboratory monitoring. The absence of easy monitoring of LMWH activity has been a stumbling block to broad acceptance of LMWH during PCI by interventionalists accustomed to readily available ACT monitoring of UFH. The ideal LMWH regimen for PCI has not been determined, although achieving an anti-Xa level of >0.5 IU/mL has been a suggested target,[173,174] and this was achieved in more than 97 percent of 242 patients with a 0.5 mg/kg intravenous bolus of enoxaparin, and PCI safety was preserved.[175] The Superior Yield of the New Strategy of Enoxaparin, Revascularization, and Glycoprotein IIb/IIIa Inhibitors (SYNERGY) study evaluated the efficacy of LMWH versus UFH plus IIb/IIIa inhibitors in high-risk patients. If PCI was performed within 8 hours of LMWH, no further LMWH was given. If the PCI was between 8 and 12 hours, a 0.3-mg/kg bolus of enoxaparin was given intravenously. The occurrence of major ischemic complications in patients receiving LMWH and UFH were similar.[176] In a meta-analysis of randomized studies comparing LMWH and UFH in patients undergoing PCI, there was no difference in ischemic events and a nonsignificant trend toward less major bleeding with LMWH.[177] A recently reported trial compared the safety of intravenous enoxaparin with UFH in real-world elective PCI with drug-eluting stents, frequent IIb/IIIa inhibitors (40 percent), and clopidogrel (94 percent). The trial noted a 31 percent reduction in major and minor bleeding with 0.5 mg/kg of enoxaparin compared to UFH ($p = 0.01$) and an insignificant reduction with a 0.75 mg/kg dose, indicating noninferiority compared to UFH.[178] Predictors of major or minor bleeding were use of IIb/IIIa inhibitors, age ≥75 years, and female sex. A slightly, but not significantly, higher death rate with the 0.5-mg dose of enoxaparin was unexplained. The study was underpowered for assessing ischemic events. The class IIa indication for LMWH as a reasonable alternative to UFH appears warranted pending further investigation.

The direct thrombin inhibitor (DTI) Hirulog (bivalirudin) was approved by the FDA in 2000 for high risk PCI whereas hirudin, argatroban and lepirudin are all FDA approved for heparin-induced thrombocytopenia. Advantages of DTI for PCI include the ease of monitoring their action with ACT measurement, their ability to inactivate clot-bound thrombin, and a favorable safety profile. In 4098 unstable angina patients randomized to UFH or bivalirudin, similar outcomes were reported on initial analysis, but

22 percent reduction ($p = 0.039$) in 7-day ischemic end points on reanalysis of isoenzyme samples and reduced bleeding was noted with bivalirudin.[179,180] In a more contemporary, stent-based, PCI experience, the Randomized Evaluation of Percutaneous Coronary Intervention Linking Angiomax To Reduced Clinical Events (REPLACE-1) trial, bivalirudin use (0.75 mg/kg bolus plus 1.75 mg/kg/h infusion during PCI) reduced adverse events and major bleeding compared to UFH.[181] In REPLACE-II, bivalirudin was compared to UFH plus abciximab, and was found not to be inferior to the more expensive alternative strategy.[182] In the Acute Catheterization and Urgent Intervention Triage Strategy Trial (ACUITY PCI) use of UFH plus a IIb/IIIa inhibitor (N = 2561) was compared to bivalirudin plus a IIb/IIIa inhibitor (N = 2609), and bivalirudin alone (N = 2619) in treatment of patients with acute coronary syndrome undergoing PCI.[183] At 30 days, adverse events (death, MI, ischemic revascularization, or major bleeding) occurred in 11.7 percent of patients receiving bivalirudin, 15.1 percent with bivalirudin plus IIb/IIIa inhibitor, and 13.5 percent UFH plus IIb/IIIa inhibitor ($p = 0.001$). This outcome was driven by more bleeding with IIb/IIIa inhibitors. An ischemia-related event rate of 8.4 percent occurred with UFH plus IIb/IIIa inhibitors, 8.9 percent for bivalirudin monotherapy and 9.4 percent in the bivalirudin plus IIb/IIIa arm. These differences were not significant. In the latest guideline statement, bivalirudin has a class IIa indication for use in low-risk patients who are undergoing elective PCI.[69] Together these studies suggest that DTI (primarily bivalirudin) administered during PCI are as effective in avoiding ischemic complications as UFH, or UFH plus IIb/IIIa in certain patient subsets but with less bleeding risk. It has been suggested that optimal antithrombin therapy for PCI in certain complex patient subgroups, such as those with a high risk of bleeding, renal failure, and heparin-induced thrombocytopenia, is perhaps best accomplished with a DTI, whereas those with troponin positivity, diabetes, thrombus-containing lesions, and ST elevation infarction, are probably best managed with an indirect thrombin inhibitor and IIb/IIIa platelet receptor inhibitor.[184] Further studies are needed to determine safety and efficacy of DTI combined with IIb/IIIa inhibitors, a combination associated with the highest risk of bleeding in ACUITY-PCI.

Other Peri-PCI Pharmacotherapy

At the time of PCI, or shortly thereafter, administration of a variety of therapeutic agents not directed at the clotting cascade or platelets are associated with improved patient outcomes. Preprocedural statin therapy is associated with a reduction in periprocedure myocardial injury[185–187] and improvement in survival at 30 days, 6 months, and 1 year after stenting, independent of patient characteristics.[188,189] Similarly, β-blocker therapy at the time of elective PCI is associated with reduced post-PCI myocardial infarction[190] and with a 1-year survival benefit (3.9 percent vs. 6.0 percent; $p = 0.0014$) independent of ventricular function, diabetic status, hypertension, or history of myocardial infarction.[191]

Intravascular Ultrasound

Although coronary angiography is the reference standard for the diagnosis of coronary artery disease, it has major limitations. Assessment of the significance of intermediate or indeterminant le-

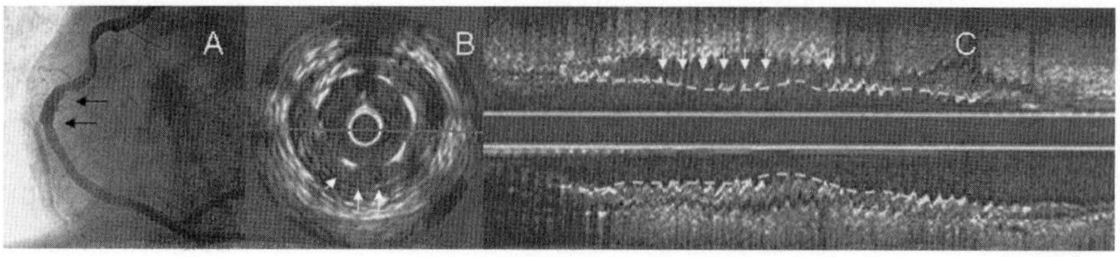

FIGURE 62–8. Coronary angiogram of the right coronary artery showing excellent patency. (**A**) Cross-sectional (**B**) and longitudinal (**C**) views of intravascular ultrasound indicate that the Cypher stent was not well apposed to the vessel well. This was not an example of poor stent expansion, however, as this study was performed 18 months after implantation and earlier IVUS studies showed good apposition. This is an example of late stent malapposition, which according to Hong et al.,[131] rarely leads to adverse cardiac events. However, this patient at 40 months after stent implantation developed stent thrombosis and had further increase in malapposition compared to the IVUS study at 18 months. *Source: From Feres F, Gosta R, Abizaid A. Very late thrombosis after drug-eluting stents. Catheter Cardiovasc Interv 2006;68:83–88, with permission.*

sions, plaque characterization, recognition of diffuse intimal thickening, accurate assessment of vessel dimensions and lesion extent are important pre-PCI determinations in which intravascular ultrasound (IVUS) greatly surpasses angiography. A minimal lumen cross sectional area between 3.0 and 4.0 mm^2 in major epicardial vessels, excluding left main, has a sensitivity and specificity exceeding 80 percent for predicting ischemia, while a left main minimal lumen diameter of 2.8 mm or minimal lumen area of 5.9 mm^2 indicates physiologic significance.[192–195] As stent underexpansion is the most common mechanism leading to failure in the drug-eluting stent era, IVUS can play an important role in identifying the calcified lesion best prepared with the use of rotational atherectomy and to insure optimal drug-eluting stent expansion, as well as stent apposition to the vessel wall (Fig. 62–8) and full lesion coverage.[196] It has been suggested that routine IVUS imaging during drug-eluting stent implantation is indicated in a number of high-risk patient subsets (renal failure, limitations to dual antiplatelet use, diabetes, poor LV function) and in high-risk lesion subsets (left main, bifurcations, ostial site, small vessels, long lesions, in-stent restenoses). In the authors' experience, clarification of the cause of all drug-eluting stent failures, either restenosis or stent thrombosis, by use of IVUS is essential to guide treatment decisions for further expansion of the underdeployed drug-eluting stent or dilation and additional drug-eluting stents for restenosis related to intimal hyperplasia. IVUS permits the identification of late stent malapposition (Fig. 62–8), a finding reported to occur in approximately 10 percent of drug-eluting stents overall, but more frequently in acute MI (32 percent) and chronic total occlusions (27 percent).[196,197] In addition, IVUS has identified drug-eluting stent strut fracture as an important mechanism for the development of focal in-drug-eluting stent restenosis accounting for about a third of these lesions.[134] Newly developed virtual histology IVUS, permitting classification of tissue into one of four phenotypes (fibrous, fibrofatty, necrotic core, or calcium), is a new addition to the diagnostic armamentarium of the interventionalist and is currently being studied.

Fractional Flow Reserve Measurements

Although intracoronary pressure gradients were used to evaluate lesions in the earliest days of percutaneous coronary intervention, it

was the combination of miniaturized pressure sensors and validation of fractional flow reserve measurements that permitted simple, reliable, and reproducible guidewire-based physiologic assessment of lesion severity during coronary interventional procedures[198] and provide the ability to determine coronary stenosis severity independent of baseline hemodynamics, blood pressure, and heart rate. A fractional flow reserve (FFR) of less than 0.75 was shown to be 100 percent specific, 88 percent sensitive, and 93 percent accurate in predicting ischemia,[199] and it was safe to defer PCI when FFR was ≥0.75.[200] This easily performed measurement of distal coronary and aortic pressure during maximal hyperemia allows one to also determine culprit stenoses in patients with multivessel disease and to evaluate ostial, left main coronary lesions, serial lesions, and side branch stenoses that may be ambiguous angiographically (Fig. 62–9). Measurement of FFR after stent deployment, has prognostic value regarding future adverse events. In the era of costly drug-eluting stent, FFR can be used to limit intervention only to flow limiting lesions and has been shown to be helpful in identifying lesions with low risk of restenosis (5 percent) with bare metal stent implantation obviating drug-eluting stent usage.[201] When FFR was used to assess left main stenoses in 54 patients, 30 patients with a FFR ≥0.75 were treated medically and after 3 years none had MI or death.[200] This adjunctive strategy, which can be safely performed in a few minutes, brings substantial value to the patient and is cost effective in many applications.

Embolic Protection

Sabor et al. called attention to the importance of microembolization during PCI when they studied 32 patients who died within 3 weeks, noting that more than 80 percent had histologic evidence of microembolization.[202] Subsequently, there has been increasing awareness of the importance of embolization in atherosclerotic vascular disease particularly during PCI in patients with acute coronary syndrome and saphenous vein graft lesions.[203] A variety of occlusion–aspiration and filter-based strategies have evolved for embolic protection during saphenous vein graft interventions, which reduce atheroembolic myocardial infarction by approximately 50 percent and constitute a class I indication in PCI guidelines. There has been limited application of embolic protection in native vessel PCI.

【 】 ATHEROABLATION, CUTTING BALLOON, THROMBECTOMY DEVICES

The directional atherectomy catheter developed by Simpson was, in 1990, the first nonballoon device approved for coronary intervention and the first to undergo randomized comparison with balloon angioplasty. In native coronary artery and saphenous vein graft lesions judged suitable for either procedure, however, the more costly directional atherectomy did not show a substantial advantage over balloon angioplasty. Additional trials using techniques to achieve optimal atherectomy (<20 percent residual stenosis) have been reported.[204,205] The randomized Balloon Versus

significantly different. Excimer laser angioplasty was approved by the FDA in 1992 for lesions that were not favorable for balloon angioplasty, but it has not been shown that this technology is superior to balloon angioplasty and most centers use it infrequently, primarily for treating in-stent restenosis, where it is safe and initially effective but has no proven superiority. In 1994, an additional atherectomy device, the Rotablator (Scimed/Boston Scientific, Maple Grove, MI) was approved for marketing by the FDA. The Rotablator's principal advantage is in the treatment of calcified and undilatable stenoses, but it has also been used to treat ostial and bifurcation lesions, rigid chronic occlusions, and in-stent restenosis, and to debulk prior to stenting. The main benefit of rotational atherectomy is to permit optimal stent expansion in calcified lesions; a secondary benefit is ease of stent insertion following rotablation. In 1999, a rheolytic thrombectomy device known as the AngioJet (POSSIS Medical, Inc., Minneapolis, MN) became available for treatment of intracoronary thrombus, and it has proved useful in the setting of acute coronary syndromes associated with large thrombi and in treatment of stent thrombosis. The Export (Medtronic-AVE, Santa Rosa, CA) and PRONTO (Vascular Solutions, Minneapolis, MN) catheters are much simpler aspiration catheters that have proved useful in removing intracoronary thrombus. The cutting balloon (Scimed, Boston Scientific, Maple Grove, MN), which consists of longitudinally mounted microsurgical blades on an angioplasty balloon, has been used for bifurcations, small vessels, ostial lesions, in-stent restenosis, and undilatable lesions with favorable clinical experience, but without convincing randomized trials that indicate incremental benefit. Use of the X-SIZER helical atherectomy device (Endicor Medical, San Clemente, CA) was first reported in 2002. This relatively simple device has promise for use in thrombus-associated lesions.

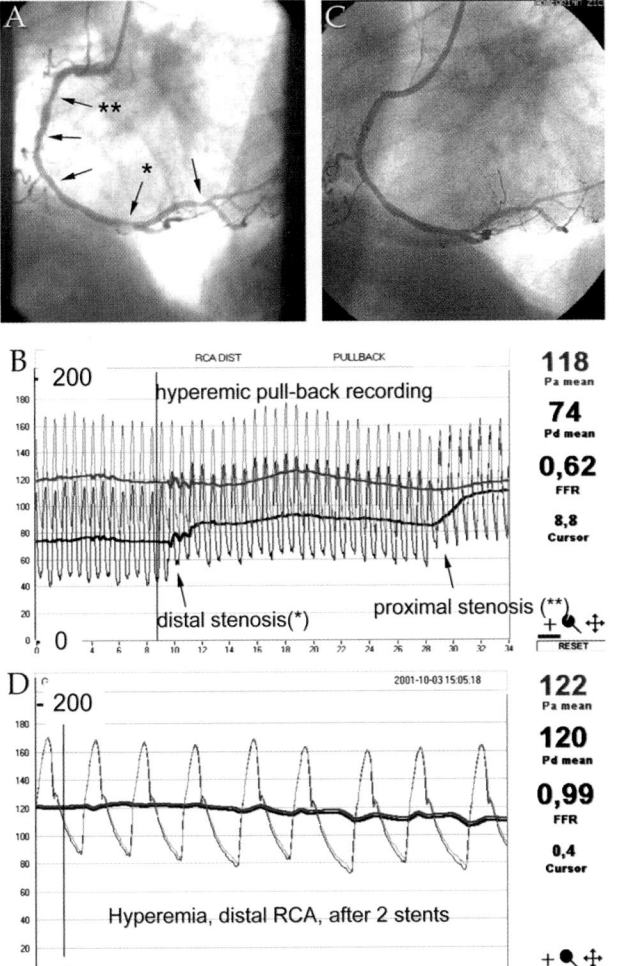

FIGURE 62–9. **A.** Right coronary artery of a 66-year-old man with recurrent angina who had stent implantation in the mid-right coronary artery 1 year previously and now has a positive nuclear scan in the inferior wall. The right coronary artery shows diffuse disease with five or more stenoses of intermediate severity (*arrows*). **B.** Fractional flow reserve (FFR) of the distal myocardium obtained at the most distal point of the arrow was 0.62. The pressure pullback curve at hyperemia showed that two mild plaques (indicated by the *asterisks*) were hemodynamically significant. The other regions did not have hemodynamically significant stenoses. **C** and **D.** Two stents were placed with improved angiograms and normalization of FFR. *Source: From Kern MJ, Lerman A, Bech J, et al. Physiological assessment of coronary artery disease in the cardiac catheterization laboratory: a scientific statement from the American Heart Association Committee on Diagnostic and Interventional Cardiac Catheterization Council on Clinical Cardiology. Circulation 2006;114:1321–1341, with permission.*

HYBRID REVASCULARIZATION

The hybrid approach incorporates drug-eluting stent implantation and minimally invasive coronary surgery, the combination of these adjunctive strategies permitting complete revascularization. Most commonly the LIMA is used to bypass the LAD coronary artery, and non-LAD coronary artery targets are stented.[207–210] This approach uses the best of the two revascularization worlds. The LIMA graft is a conduit that is "immune" to atherosclerosis which bypasses the atherosclerosis prone proximal LAD coronary artery segments and services the most important coronary vascular bed. Other vessels, typically treated with saphenous vein grafts, which offer no mortality advantage, receive durable drug-eluting stent. In most centers, the minimally invasive LIMA graft to the LAD coronary artery is performed first; stents may be deployed either during the same procedure using an operating room[210] fitted with radiologic imaging equipment or 1 or more days later as a staged procedure.[208] We have found this approach to be ideal for patients with complex LAD coronary artery disease (ostial, bifurcational, or diffuse proximal involvement), significant but noncritical left main disease, and diabetes where LIMA-to-LAD coronary artery may have a mortality advantage. Avoidance of a sternotomy and cardiopulmonary bypass, reduced bleeding, transfusion, and infection, and shortened hospitalization, all shown to apply in hybrids, hastens recovery. However, specialized surgical skills are necessary and long-term followup is not yet available.

Optimal Atherectomy Trial (BOAT) showed no increase in inhospital death, Q wave MI, or CABG with directional atherectomy, but a higher rate of non–Q-wave infarction occurred (16 percent vs. 6 percent; *p* <0.0001). Restenosis was lower in the atherectomy arm (31 percent vs. 39.8 percent; *p* = 0.016), but there was no difference in late clinical events. The Atherectomy Before MULTI-LINK Improves Luminal Gain and Clinical Outcomes (AMIGO) trial randomized 753 patients to directional coronary atherectomy plus stent or stent alone failed to show benefit of debulking prior to bare-metal stenting.[206] Thirty-day MACE (1.6 percent vs. 1.1 percent) and binary restenosis (24 percent vs. 20 percent) were not

HEMODYNAMICALLY SUPPORTED PCI

Although surgical revascularization is currently recommended for left main and certain equivalencies, comorbidities or poor left ventricular function may necessitate a high risk PCI. Intraaortic balloon pump counterpulsation is widely available but provides limited support and extracorporeal membrane oxygenation is impractical. The Tandem Heart Percutaneous Ventricular Assist device (CardiacAssist, Inc., Pittsburgh, Penn.) is a relatively simple centrifugal pump that provides sufficient hemodynamic support (up to 5.5 L/min) to sustain patients who are transiently without cardiac output and has been used to provide circulatory protection during high-risk PCI.[211] This device has also been used to salvage patients in cardiogenic shock by providing support during PCI or bridging the patient to another therapy (cardiac surgery, left ventricular assist device, transplantation).[212]

CLOSURE DEVICES

A variety of devices are currently available to close common femoral artery access sites following PCI. They permit earlier ambulation, enhance patient comfort, increase costs, and do not significantly alter overall access site complication rates. Rarely, infection or vascular compromise may occur and necessitate surgery. Patients not selected for closure devices include those with sterility issues (transferred patient with sheath in place or patients outside of the cardiac catheterization laboratory), or compromised immune system, or entry sites below the common femoral artery bifurcation.

INDICATIONS FOR CORONARY INTERVENTION

In general, when one is selecting percutaneous coronary intervention, there should be assurance that the operator can treat, with a high probability of success, the coronary lesion(s) accounting for the symptoms or signs of myocardial ischemia. Furthermore, the associated risk and durability of the revascularization should be acceptable as compared with bypass surgery or medical therapy during both early and long-term followup. The latter estimate requires consideration of the likelihood and consequences of abrupt vessel closure, stent thrombosis, restenosis, and incomplete revascularization. In addition, one cannot disregard the comparative costs of the initial intervention, its complications, the need for subsequent revascularization procedures, and the cost and potential risks associated with prolonged dual antiplatelet therapy. The American College of Cardiology/American Heart Association *Guidelines for Percutaneous Transluminal Coronary Angioplasty and Coronary Bypass Surgery* provide a detailed analysis of many of these issues.[41,69,213] Table 62–2 summarizes the *PCI Guideline* recommendations for patients with asymptomatic ischemia or classes I to III angina.

SELECTION OF PATIENTS
Single-Vessel Disease

Percutaneous revascularization is an attractive option for many symptomatic patients who are anatomically suitable and who have single-vessel coronary disease. It is important, however, to remem-

TABLE 62–2

Recommendations for PCI Adopted from the ACC/AHA/SCAI 2005 Guideline Update in Patients with Asymptomatic Ischemia or Class I to III Angina

Class IIa	One or more lesions in one or more vessels with high likelihood of success and low risk; vessels subtend large area of viable myocardium or produce moderate to severe ischemia (*level of evidence: B*); or a recurrent stenosis following PCI (*level of evidence: C*); or left main stenosis >50 percent in CABG-ineligible patient (*level of evidence: B*); or SVG lesions in poor candidate for reoperation (*level of evidence: C*).
Class IIb	Efficacy of PCI in multivessel disease patients with proximal LAD stenosis and diabetes or an abnormal left ventricle is less well established (*level of evidence: B*); PCI may be considered in non-LAD sites producing ischemia (*level of evidence: C*).
Class III	Small amount of myocardium at risk, absence of ischemia, low PCI success, mild symptoms unlikely to be ischemia, increased PCI risk, left main stenosis and eligible for CABG, <50 percent stenosis (*level of evidence: C*).

ACC, American College of Cardiology; AHA, American Heart Association; CABG, coronary artery bypass grafting; LAD, left anterior descending artery; PCI, percutaneous coronary intervention; SCAI, Society of Cardiac Angiography and Intervention; SVG, saphenous vein graft.

ber that there are few studies comparing PCI with surgery in this group of patients and none that show a statistically significant survival benefit of PCI compared with surgery or medical therapy. Of 7604 patients with single-vessel disease treated at Emory University Hospital with angioplasty between 1980 and 1991, angiographic success was 90 percent and complications were infrequent (Q-wave MI, 0.8 percent; emergency CABG, 1.7 percent; and death, 0.2 percent).[214] Among these patients with single-vessel disease, 1-, 5-, and 10-year survival was 99, 93, and 86 percent, respectively, whereas 80, 69, and 58 percent were PTCA-free and 92, 87, and 77 percent were CABG-free at 1, 5, and 10 years. In the Duke Data Bank experience, 5-year survival with angioplasty in single-vessel disease compared favorably with bypass surgery (95 vs. 93 percent with CABG).[215]

The ACME study showed that angioplasty in single-vessel disease can lead to improved quality of life compared with medical therapy at 6 months, with reduced angina and improved exercise performance out to 3 years.[17,216,217] The ACME data suggest that using the angioplasty techniques available at that time resulted in a slightly increased risk of acute complications (2 percent emergency CABG, 1 percent Q-wave MI) and repeat revascularization (23 percent vs. 9 percent) at 6 months, but no difference in late revascularization at 3 years.[217]

In the randomized Medicine, Angioplasty, or Surgery Study of isolated LAD coronary artery disease, there was no difference in MI or mortality at 5 years, but fewer late events in the surgery group.[218] In a relatively small, randomized trial of angioplasty and

IMA surgery for isolated disease of the LAD coronary artery, there was no difference in mortality or MI, but angioplasty patients had more repeat revascularizations (25 percent vs. 3 percent; *p* <0.01).[219] Clear superiority of stenting over balloon angioplasty for isolated LAD coronary artery disease was demonstrated in a randomized comparison of these strategies in 120 patients.[220] One-year rates of event-free survival were 87 percent after stenting and 70 percent after angioplasty (*p* = 0.04), and restenosis rates were 19 and 40 percent, respectively (*p* = 0.02).

When 220 patients with severe proximal LAD coronary artery stenosis were randomized to bare-metal stent implantation or minimally invasive bypass surgery, MACE was significantly higher following stenting (31 percent vs. 15 percent; *p* = 0.02).[221] The difference was predominately a result of repeat revascularizations for restenosis (29 percent vs. 8 percent; *p* = 0.003). Death or MI occurred in 3 percent of the stent group and in 6 percent of surgery patients (*p* = 0.50). In patients with single-vessel LAD coronary artery disease, coronary stenting with a bare-metal stent is cost-effective compared with medical therapy.[222,223] A study comparing drug-eluting stents with CABG or medical therapy in single-vessel disease has not been performed, but low restenosis and lower need for target-vessel revascularization make PCI with a drug-eluting stent a more durable and attractive strategy. Studies from the Cleveland Clinic analyzing the importance of repeat procedures in determining 2-year cardiac cost in the bare-metal stent era suggest that coronary intervention is more cost-effective than medical and surgical therapy when the probability of repeat procedures is low.[222] One would infer from this analysis that the presence of multiple or complex lesions, which are more likely to recur, may tilt the scale sufficiently to modify adversely the favorable comparative cost-effectiveness of percutaneous intervention in single-vessel disease. In the drug-eluting stent era, the need for additional drug-eluting stents quickly jeopardizes the cost-effectiveness of PCI, even in single-vessel disease.[111–117] In complex LAD coronary artery disease, minimally invasive CABG has considerable appeal.[224]

Multivessel Disease

A dramatic increase in the use of percutaneous intervention in multivessel disease, fueled by improved angioplasty technology and the drug-eluting stent, accounts for the growth in these procedures worldwide. *Rational selection of patients, however, requires a careful analysis of multiple issues, including a risk-to-benefit assessment of each ischemia-producing lesion, a projection of the possible completeness and durability of the physiologic revascularization, and an estimate of resource consumption compared with surgery and medical therapy.*

In general, as stated in *PTCA Guidelines*,[69,213] patients selected for intervention are symptomatic, have evidence of significant ischemia, need noncardiac surgery, are recovering from cardiac arrest or malignant arrhythmia, or have compelling anatomy. Patient preferences must be considered, because repeat interventions are an integral aspect of percutaneous intervention in multivessel disease. Candidacy for dual antiplatelet therapy is an important consideration. Complete revascularization, which the surgical experience has shown produces superior long-term results, is associated with fewer late interventions after angioplasty,[225] but it is not frequently attained because of the presence of total occlusions, non-

critical stenoses, and diffuse disease. In the 1985–1986 NHLBI PTCA Registry, complete revascularization was achieved in 19 percent of multivessel patients.[226]

Among 10,783 patients at Emory University Hospital who underwent coronary intervention, complete revascularization was achieved in 84 percent of patients with single-vessel disease and in 25 percent with two-vessel disease, but in only 5 percent with triple-vessel disease.[214] In EAST, 71 percent of index segments were revascularized in PTCA patients.[227] Culprit-lesion angioplasty is clearly an accepted strategy, but care must be taken to avoid significant residual ischemia after intervention. This approach was reflected in EAST, where revascularization was attempted in 96 percent of high-priority lesions in PTCA patients and in 99 percent of surgical patients. *High-priority lesions* were defined as 70 to 100 percent stenoses located proximally or in large vessels (2.5 mm). This strategy yielded similar 3-year EAST primary end points for CABG and PTCA, and an identical frequency of patients with all index segments free of severe stenosis of 70 to 100 percent (82 percent vs. 82 percent).[227] Published data from BARI indicated that planned incomplete revascularization was unrelated to 5-year risk of cardiac death or death/MI, but was related to risk of CABG.[228] Recently reported data from the New York state registry indicated incomplete revascularization, especially, chronic total occlusions, significantly influenced post-PCI mortality (see Chronic Total Occlusions below).

The risks of multivessel percutaneous coronary intervention are increased in the presence of unstable angina, advanced age, poor left ventricular function, extensive coronary artery disease, comorbid conditions, and female gender.[229] At Emory University Hospital, in-hospital mortality for one-, two-, and three-vessel disease was 0.2, 0.4, and 1.2 percent, respectively (*p* <0.0001), and emergency bypass surgery was needed in 1.7, 3.0, and 3.2 percent, respectively.[214] In general, the risk of intervention is directly related to the probability and consequences of abrupt closure or major atheroembolization. In multivessel disease, both are frequently higher, and impaired left ventricular function is commonly present. Application of stenting in multivessel percutaneous intervention has improved outcomes significantly.[230–232] The randomized ARTS trial (see Metallic Stents versus CABG above) revealed no differences in death or MI, but more repeat interventions at 5 years.[70–72] A meta-analysis of more than 1500 patients in 4 randomized trials comparing bare-metal stents with CABG (ARTS, SOS, ERACI II, MASS-2) also revealed no difference in MI, death, or stroke, but more repeat intervention with stent therapy (18 percent vs. 4 percent; *p* <0.001). However, a mortality advantage with CABG for all multivessel disease subsets was reported from the observational New York State registry (see above).[81] ARTS II, in which multivessel disease patients received Cypher stents, repeat intervention was reduced to 8.5 percent and outcomes rivaled those of ARTS I CABG patients (see Drug-Eluting Stents versus CABG above and Fig. 62–9).[105] Of concern, however, is the potential for adverse late events, including stent thrombosis in drug-eluting stent-treated multivessel-diseased patients, especially those in whom clopidogrel is discontinued. Stent thrombosis was reported in 3.1 percent in ERACI III.[106] Although the major randomized trials of PCI versus bypass surgery showed no overall difference in mortality on long-term followup, BARI reported that patients being treated for diabetes had significantly worse 5-year mortality with angioplasty compared with surgery (35 percent vs. 19 percent).[35] The BARI findings question the safety of PCI in the diabetic population, who frequently have diffuse multivessel disease, more frequent restenoses, more rapid disease progression, and in many cases, a reduced recognition of recurrent ischemia. ARTS extended this cautionary theme in multivessel diabetics with observations that stented diabetics had roughly twice the mortality of nondiabetics[72] and in ARTS II, diabetics required more reintervention.[105] Studies to analyze outcomes and cost effectiveness of the more expensive drug-eluting stents in multivessel disease are in progress (SYNTAX and FREEDOM).

Non–ST-Segment Elevation Acute Coronary Syndrome

With a conservative approach consisting of aspirin, unfractionated or low-molecular-weight heparin, nitrates, and β blockers, patients with non–ST-elevation acute coronary syndrome have a significant risk of death (6 percent), recurrent MI (11 percent), or coronary revascularization (50–60 percent) within the next year.[233] With the availability of IIb/IIIa inhibitors and coronary stents, outcomes of early PCI improved substantially[234] and the ACC/AHA *2002 Guidelines* recommended an early invasive therapy for patients with increased risk (Table 62–3).[233] Risk stratification was shown to be enhanced by quantitative ST-segment depression and multiple biomarkers.[235,236] Recently, reductions in periprocedural myonecrosis were documented with clopidogrel loading and pretreatment with a statin[185–187] and longer-term outcomes improved in acute coronary syndrome (ACS) patients treated with drug-eluting stent.[237] In non–ST-elevation ACS patients with elevated troponin who received 600 mg clopidogrel before the procedure, the addition of abciximab was associated with a 25 percent reduction in death, MI, or urgent target-vessel revascularization at 30 days,[166] but no benefit occurred with abciximab in troponin-negative patients. Two recent trials indicated benefit with the upstream use of IIb/IIIa inhibitors with respect to coronary flow and myocardial perfusion parameters[238] with optimal cost efficacy in high-risk patients.[239]

Seven studies involving 8375 patients and comparing early invasive therapy with a more conservative approach in the modern era of IIb/IIIa inhibitors, thienopyridines, and coronary stents were performed. A meta-analysis indicated that the invasive approach was associated with a 25 percent decrease in mortality ($p = 0.001$) and a significantly lower incidence of non fatal MI (7.6 percent vs. 9.1 percent; $p = 0.012$) and more than 30 percent less rehospitalization for unstable angina (Fig. 62–10).[240] With respect to the optimal timing of early invasive intervention, this meta-analysis demonstrated no incremental

TABLE 62–3

Early Invasive Strategy Is Recommended in Unstable Angina or Non–ST-Elevation Myocardial Infarction

Class I
Any of the high-risk indications
- Recurrent angina at rest or minimal activity despite therapy
- Elevated troponin
- New ST-segment depression
- Recurrent angina/ischemia with symptoms or signs of congestive heart failure or new or worsening mitral regurgitation
- Positive stress test
- Ejection fraction <40%
- Hemodynamic instability
- Sustained ventricular tachycardia
- Percutaneous coronary intervention within 6 months or prior coronary artery bypass grafting

SOURCE: From the 2002 ACC/AHA Unstable Angina Guidelines. Braunwald E, Antman EM, Beasley JW, et al.[233]

benefit of intervening within 24 hours (very early) compared to after 24 hours. In CRUSADE, it was reported that the delay imposed by weekend presentation did not increase adverse events,[241] but in SYNERGY, a time-to-catheterization of <6 hours was asso-

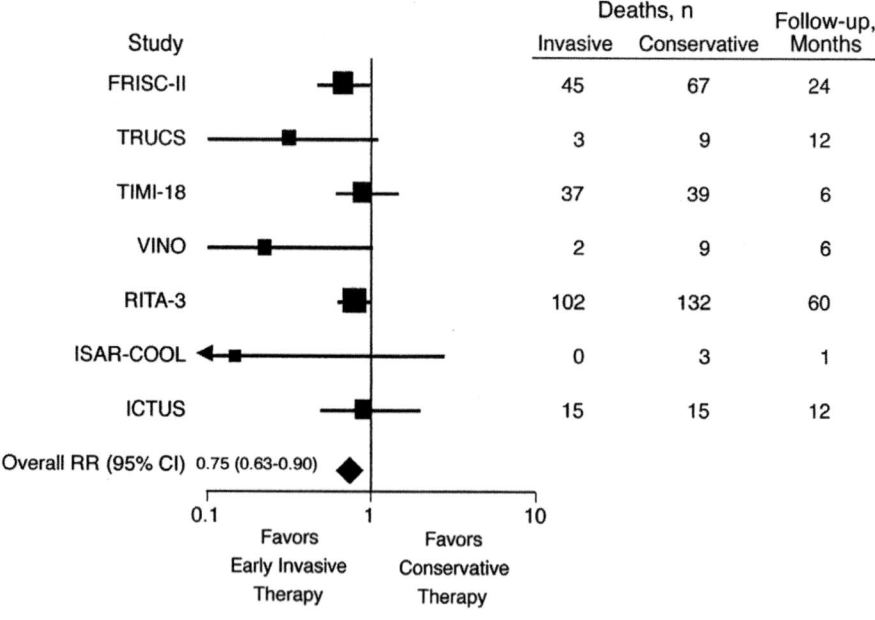

FIGURE 62–10. Relative risk of all-cause mortality for early invasive therapy compared with conservative therapy at a mean followup of 2 years. The results show a long-term survival benefit from early invasive therapy. CI, confidence interval; FRISC-II, Fragmin and Fast Revascularization During Instability in Coronary Disease; ICTUS, Invasive Versus Conservative Treatment in Unstable Coronary Syndromes Investigators; ISAR-COOL, Intracoronary Stenting With Antithrombotic Regimen Cooling Off; RITA-3, Randomized Intervention Trial of Unstable Angina; RR, relative risk; TIME-18, Thrombolysis In Myocardial Infarction-18; TRUCS, Treatment of Refractory Unstable Angina in Geographically Isolated Areas Without Cardiac Surgery; VINO, Value of First Day Coronary Angiography/Angiography in Evolving Non–ST-Segment Elevation Myocardial Infarction. *Source: From Bavry AA, Kumbhani DJ, Rassi AN, et al. Benefit of early invasive therapy in acute coronary syndromes. A meta-analysis of contemporary randomized clinical trials. J Am Coll Cardiol 2006;48:1319–1325, with permission.*

ciated with fewer ischemic events and no increased bleeding.[242] Very early intervention was also supported by the ISAR-Cool (Intracoronary Stenting With Antithrombotic Regimen Cooling Off) study in which 410 patients with non–ST-elevation ACS received aspirin, clopidogrel, heparin, and tirofiban, and were randomized to intervention within 6 hours or delayed intervention at 3 to 5 days. Very early intervention was associated with a 49 percent reduction in death or MI, all of which occurred prior to intervention.[243] These apparently discrepant results may be related to analysis of small subgroups, the long interval before intervention in ISAR-Cool, or other factors, such as differing indications to intervene in conservatively managed patients. Perhaps the clearest message is that there may be an advantage with very early intervention, but at present there are no advantages with waiting. Recent publications highlight methods to reduce complications in ACS syndromes. One emphasized that antiplatelet and antithrombotic agents are frequently overdosed: excess use (overdosing) of UFH in 33 percent, LMWH in 14 percent, and 27 percent of patients who were treated with IIb/IIIa inhibitors. Perhaps equally important, Peterson et al. noted that outcomes and compliance with ACC/AHA guidelines were closely linked; a 10 percent decrease in in-hospital mortality occurred with every 10 percent increase in guideline compliance.[244] This is a strong endorsement of ACC/AHA guidelines.

For information on ST-elevation myocardial infarction, see Chap. 56.

【 】 SELECTION OF LESIONS

Lesion Characteristics

The importance of coronary stenosis angiographic morphology in predicting the outcome of PCI was reflected in the early ACC/AHA *Guidelines* and the lesion classification was updated in each revision. In the ACC/AHA/SCAI (Society for Cardiac Angiography and Interventions) *2005 Guideline Update for PCI*, six high-risk lesion characteristics (type C) were recognized as important in the stent era. Four lesion classifications were suggested by considering the presence or absence of a type-C lesion and whether the vessel was patent or occluded (Table 62–4).[245–247] This classification was shown to provide improved prediction of success and complications compared to the old ACC/AHA lesion classification. Interestingly, thrombus, bifurcation, and left main do not appear, but remain important predictors of adverse outcome in the experience of the authors (see Left Main Coronary Lesions and Bifurcation Lesions below).

Left Main Coronary Lesions

Historically, the prognosis of patients with significant stenosis of the left main coronary treated medically has been poor. Data from the 1970s suggested a 3-year survival of only 50 percent. A Veterans Administration (VA) randomized trial and a meta-analysis of seven trials indicated a mortality benefit at 5 years with coronary bypass surgery. Subsequently, surgery became the recommended therapy in the United States for those who could undergo it. The first report of percutaneous intervention in unprotected left main coronary artery disease was by Andreas Gruentzig in 1978.[10] The early experience with balloon angioplasty was unfavorable, how-

TABLE 62–4

Society of Cardiac Angiography and Intervention Lesion Classification System: Characteristics of Class I to IV Lesions

Type I lesion (highest success expected, lowest risk)
(1) Does not meet criteria for C lesion
(2) Patent vessel

Type II lesions
(1) Meets any of these criteria for ACC/AHA C lesion
  Diffuse (greater than 2-cm length)
  Excessive tortuosity of proximal segment
  Extremely angulated segments, greater than 90 degrees
  Inability to protect major side branches
  Degenerated vein grafts with friable lesions
(2) Patent vessel

Type III lesions
(1) Does not meet criteria for C lesion
(2) Occluded vessel

Type IV lesions
(1) Meets any of these criteria for ACC/AHA C lesion
  Diffuse (greater than 2-cm length)
  Excessive tortuosity of proximal segment
  Extremely angulated segments, greater than 90 degrees
  Inability to protect major side branches
  Degenerated vein grafts with friable lesions
  Occluded for more than 3 months
(2) Occluded vessel

ACC, American College of Cardiology; AHA, American Heart Association.
SOURCE: From Krone RJ, Shaw RE, Klein LW, et al.[247]

ever, with the Mid-American Heart Institute reporting a 64 percent 3-year mortality in a collection of 127 cases with varying acuity.[248] With the approval of stents in 1994, unprotected left main coronary artery stenting was carried out increasingly in patients who were not excellent surgical candidates. In the Ultima registry, Ellis et al. reported on 107 such patients with a high 6-month mortality of 11 percent.[249] In several series, in-hospital mortality for left main coronary artery stenting was low, especially for those who were deemed acceptable candidates for CABG. Although acute results were favorable, Park et al. reported late outcomes with bare-metal stenting, noting a restenosis rate of 21 percent with 20 late deaths (7.4 percent).[250] Takagi et al. reported in 64 patients that at 5 months restenosis had occurred in 30 percent of patients and 16 percent had died.[251] These reports suggested that left main coronary artery stenting could be carried out with a high success rate initially in selected patients, but the long-term outcomes with bare-metal stents were inferior to CABG. These adverse, late, clinical outcomes, primarily death or MI, in patients following left main coronary artery stenting were apparently related to restenosis, a process that infrequently leads to these outcomes when it occurs outside the left main coronary artery.

Several registries demonstrated that applying drug-eluting stent technology to unprotected left main coronary artery lesions made restenosis rare for ostial and mid lesions, but significantly higher for distal left main coronary artery lesions that involved bifurcation lesions.[252–254] Restenosis at the ostium of the circumflex accounted for about one-half of restenoses and stent fracture has been described at this site. Target-vessel revascularization was needed in 2 to 13 percent of patients overall, and mid-term cardiac mortality for nonshock patients was 2 to 4 percent. Lee et al. compared 50 patients with drug-eluting stent treatment to 123 patients who underwent CABG during the same time period.[255] Sixty percent were treated with two stents. Procedural success was 98 percent for PCI and in-hospital mortality was low (2 percent compared to 5 percent with CABG; p = NS). Survival at 6 months was nonsignificantly better with PCI (96 percent vs. 87 percent). Mortality of left main coronary artery disease treated surgically at the Cleveland Clinic was 2.3 percent in-hospital and 11.3 percent at 1 year in 1998,[256] and similar in a more recent report.[257] Price et al.[258] reported angiographic followup in 50 patients, 94 percent of whom received kissing stents to treat left main coronary artery bifurcations. Procedural success was 100 percent and in-hospital mortality was zero. Followup angiography was performed at 3 and 9 months. Angiographic restenosis occurred in 23 percent of the stents that extended into the LAD coronary artery and in 35 percent of the circumflex stents (overall restenosis of 42 percent). The MACE occurrence rate (death, MI, revascularization) was 10 percent in-hospital and 42 percent, with a median followup of 9 months. Only 7 of 19 revascularizations were ischemia-driven and all were PCI. Chieffo et al. compared 107 drug-eluting stent-treated patients (74 percent had both branches stented) to 142 CABG-treated patients in a propensity analysis to adjust for baseline difference and reported no difference in outcome at 1 year.[259] Kim et al. reported on 116 patients with left main coronary artery bifurcation stenosis who were treated with sirolimus-eluting stents in the LAD coronary artery (N = 67) or both branches (N = 24); they found a lower restenosis with the simpler approach (5.3 percent vs. 24.4 percent; p = 0.024).[260] There were no incidences of death or MI at a median followup of 18.6 months and target-vessel revascularization was required in 6 patients. Valgimigli et al. compared 55 patients who were treated with sirolimus-eluting stents to 55 left main coronary artery disease patients who were treated with paclitaxel-eluting stents. They noted a similar MACE occurrence (25 percent vs. 29 percent, respectively) at a median followup of 660 days.[261]

In summary, the 6- to 12-month mortality of drug-eluting stent treatment of left main coronary artery disease of approximately 2 to 4 percent is similar to in-hospital mortality for CABG. Angiographic restenosis for ostial and mid left main coronary artery is ≤5 percent, but none of the strategies for the commonly required bifurcation stenting provide the durability of CABG. With two-stent approaches, there is an approximate 2 percent stent thrombosis rate and a 20 to 40 percent restenosis rate. This mandates angiographic surveillance at 3 months, and probably at 9 months, in order to detect and treat restenosis. Therefore, applications of this technology to good surgical candidates do not appear warranted for bifurcation left main coronary artery disease. In the less-common ostial or mid left main coronary artery disease, longer-term followup, out to 5 years, may be required before this strategy

is recommendable to all comers. ACC/AHA/SCAI *Guidelines* continue to recommend CABG for patients who are surgical candidates. Application of drug-eluting stents to treatment in left main coronary artery disease patients with higher surgical risk continues to be an option, but prolonged dual antiplatelet therapy and angiographic surveillance should be mandated.

Chronic Total Occlusions

Chronic total occlusions (CTOs; Fig. 62–11) are found in up to 30 percent of diagnostic angiograms, but accounted for only 5.7 percent of coronary interventions in the NHLBI Dynamic Registry in 2004 and only 71.4 percent of these selected cases were successful.[262] Similarly, in 419 consecutive patients in a multicenter Italian registry in 1999–2000, 77 percent were technically successful, and in-hospital MACE occurred in 5 percent (death, 0.3 percent; Q-wave MI, 0.4 percent; non–Q-wave MI, 4 percent; perforation, 2 percent).[263] At 1 year, patients with successful CTO therapy (90 percent received a bare-metal stent) had a lower occurrence of death or MI (1 percent vs. 7 percent; p = 0.005), less need for CABG (2 percent vs. 16 percent; p <0.0001), and greater freedom from angina (89 percent vs. 75 percent; p = 0.008). The importance of revascularizing CTOs in multivessel disease patients undergoing PCI was recently emphasized by Hannan et al. who reported that at 3 years, patients with an unopened CTO were 35 percent more likely to die.[264]

Fortunately, in the past few years, a better understanding of CTOs and strategies for successful PCI have evolved.[265–267] Stiffer, specially designed Japanese guidewires, the Safe Cross guidewire (IntraLuminal Therapeutics, Carlsbad, CA), coupling guidance with radiofrequency energy, and a helical screw-in microcatheter are examples of new technology to assist the PCI operator in passing a guidewire across the CTO into the true lumen of the distal vessel.[268,269] Use of local delivery of thrombolytic therapy to the CTO,[270] intravascular ultrasound guidance,[271] anchoring techniques to improve guide catheter support,[272] subintimal tracking and reentry,[273] antegrade and retrograde subintimal tracking,[274] and multislice computed tomography to characterize the CTO[275] are innovative new approaches to CTO PCI. These strategies increasingly permit successful PCI in spite of the traditional predictors of PCI failure in CTO lesions, which are chronicity, long occlusions, bridging collaterals, calcification, and side-branch location. Tapered CTOs, frequently possessing recanalized channels up to 200 μm and not visible on angiography, predict successful PCI.[276]

After successful recanalization, drug-eluting stent implantation significantly improves outcomes. In a prospective, randomized comparison of sirolimus-eluting stents versus bare-metal Bx Velocity stents in 200 patients, sirolimus-eluting stent-treated patients had lower in-segment restenosis (11 percent vs. 41 percent; p <0.001), and target-lesion revascularization (4 percent vs. 19 percent; p <0.001).[277] In a prospective, nonrandomized study of 308 patients (128 treated with sirolimus-eluting stents and 180 with paclitaxel-eluting stent) in 5 high-volume Asian centers, restenosis was infrequent with both stents (1.5 percent and 1.7 percent) as was MACE (2.3 percent and 2.2 percent).[278] Long-term outcome data is needed to fully understand CTO PCI with drug-eluting stent, but prospects appear bright.

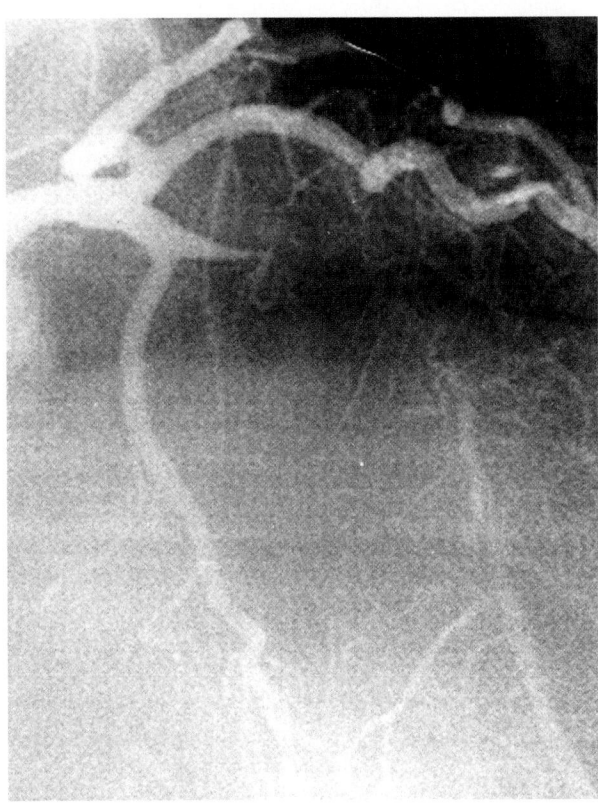
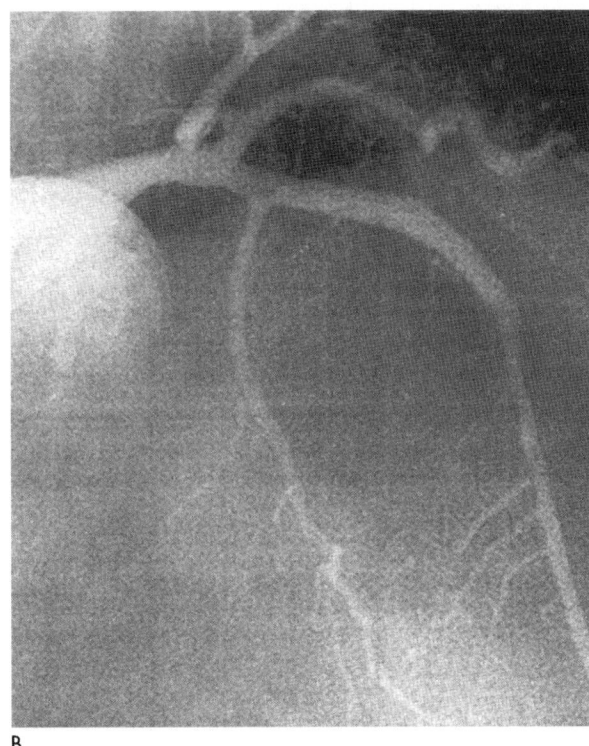

A   B

FIGURE 62–11. An 82-year-old man with disabling angina and an occluded LAD coronary artery of uncertain duration (**A,** right anterior oblique view). It was possible to recanalize the long LAD coronary artery occlusion (**B**) using a hydrophilic-coated stiff guidewire and balloon angioplasty followed by placement of two stents. A randomized, controlled trial demonstrated that drug-eluting stents are superior to bare-metal stents. *Source: From Suttorp MJ, Laarman GJ, Rahel BM, et al.*[277]

Bifurcation Lesions

Bifurcations have been the problem stepchild of PCI. They were recognized early to be problematic, were excluded from most formalized trials of balloon angioplasty, bare-metal stents, and drug-eluting stents, and remain a problem after almost 30 years. Compared to nonbifurcation lesions, bifurcations were found to be more complex (angulated, eccentric, ostial, tortuous) and have a higher need for repeat intervention.[279] To protect the side branch many bare-metal stent bifurcation techniques were developed (T-stenting, modified T-stenting, provisional T-stenting, Y- and V-stenting, and culotte stenting). None, however, proved superior to a single stent if side-branch patency was achieved with balloon dilation.[280] Using a strategy of provisional T-stenting with a bare-metal stent and final kissing balloon angioplasty with side-branch stenting in 34 percent of 186 consecutive patients, Brunel et al. reported very low inhospital MACE (3.2 percent) and a 16 percent need for target-vessel revascularization at 7 months.[281] Two randomized trials comparing two versus one sirolimus-eluting stent in treatment of bifurcations reported equal or better outcomes with one sirolimus-eluting stent.[282,283] In an attempt to overcome ostial side-branch restenosis, the "crush" technique was performed with suboptimal outcomes (stent thrombosis: procedural 1.3 percent, postprocedural 4.3 percent; restenosis: main branch 9 percent, side branch 25 percent).[284] Ormiston et al., in a Plexiglas bifurcation model, analyzed a number of bifurcation stent techniques finding

MLD to be at the crush site and the internal or reversed crush to have favorable outcome when finished with a main branch inflation (Fig. 62–12).[285,286] Sharma et al., in 200 consecutive patients with large vessels using a kissing stent approach with sirolimus-eluting stents, reported procedural success in all main branches and in 99 percent of side branches, low in-hospital and 30-day MACE (3 percent and 5 percent), and at 9 months target-vessel revascularization was needed in only 4 percent of patients.[287] In the Nordic Bifurcation Study, 413 patients were randomized to stenting of main branch (MB) or both (MB+SB [side branch]) with sirolimus-eluting stents.[288] The SB was stented in only 4.3 percent of the MB group and in 95 percent of MB+SB group. Final kissing balloon was performed in 74 percent of MB+SB patients and in 32 percent of MB patients. Biomarker elevation greater than three times the upper limit of normal occurred in 18 percent of MB+SB patients and in 8 percent of MB patients ($p = 0.01$). At 6 months, there was no difference in cardiac mortality (1 percent in both groups), target-vessel revascularization (1.9 percent in both groups), or stent thrombosis (1 patient). The simple approach of stenting the MB and optional stenting of the SB was recommended as the routine bifurcation stenting technique. We favor this approach and use of the internal crush technique may be preferred if the side branch must be stented. If there is uncertainty regarding the need to stent the side branch, measurement of fractional flow reserve is both safe and feasible. Koo et al. found that no side branch with <75 percent stenosis had FFR <0.75 and of 73 lesions with ≥75 percent steno-

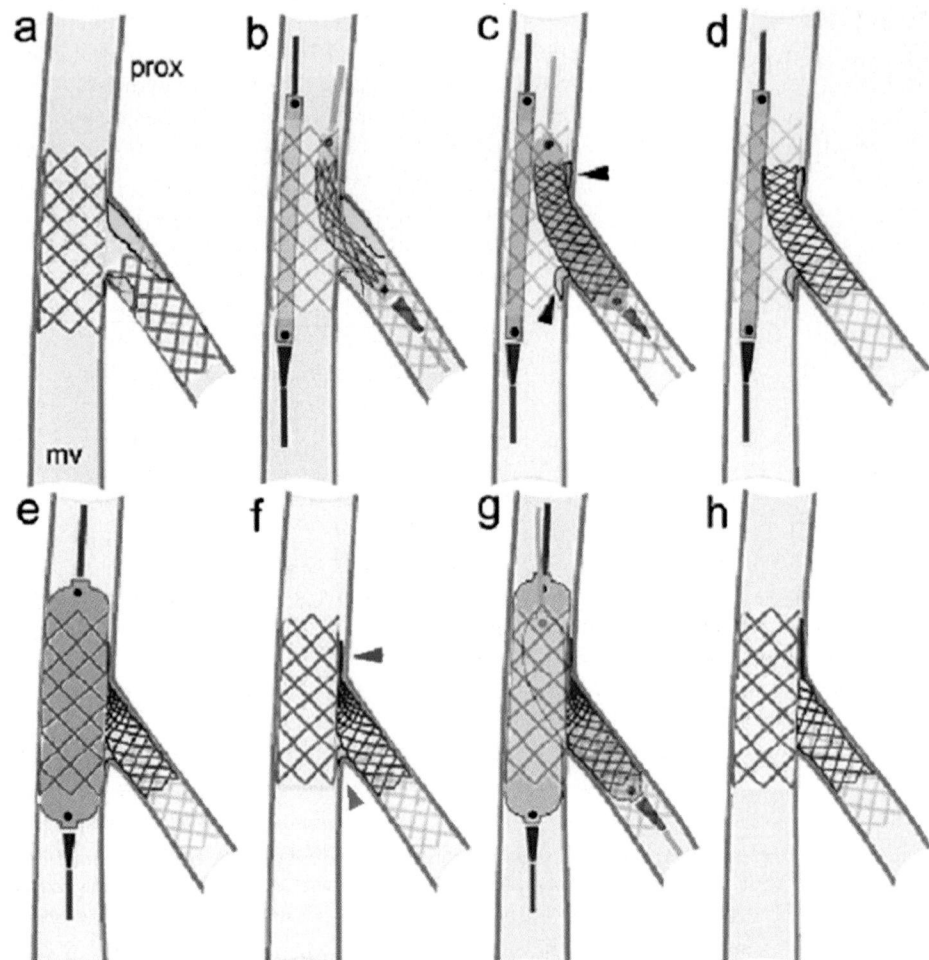

FIGURE 62–12. Schematic of the reversed crush technique. **A.** The stent is already deployed in the main vessel (*mv*), and the side branch (*sb*) has a severe ostial restenotic lesion. **B.** A stent is placed in the sb and a balloon of the same size or larger than the mv stent is positioned in the mv. **C** and **D.** After the stent is deployed, the balloon and wire are withdrawn. However, plaque shift may occur in the mv (*arrowheads*). **E.** The balloon within the mv is dilated, (**F**) and the stent is crushed (*blue arrowhead*). **G.** Kissing balloon postdilatation ensures optimal deployment of the stent with complete coverage of the carina (**H**). Ormiston et al. recommend finishing with a main branch inflation based on a Plexiglas model.[286] *Source: From Sianos G, Varma S, Hoge Q, et al. Bifurcation stenting with drug-eluting stents: illustration of the crush techniques. Catheter Cardiovasc Interv 2006;67:839–845, with permission.*

sis, only 20 (27 percent) were functionally significant.[289] Dedicated bifurcation stents are under development.

In-Stent Restenosis

In-stent restenosis, a new disease created by the explosion of bare-metal stent use in the early part of this decade, was almost entirely a result of intimal hyperplasia. The clinical presentation was exertional angina in 64 percent, unstable angina in 26 percent, and acute myocardial infarction in 10 percent of 1186 cases.[290,291] The treatment of these lesions was initially with balloon angioplasty, but results were adequate only in very focal lesions where target-vessel revascularization was needed in 19 percent, compared to 50 percent for lesions longer than 10 mm and extending beyond the stent and 83 percent for total occlusions.[292] Atheroablative strategies and routine bare-metal stent were not shown to improve outcomes. The use of intracoronary brachytherapy was shown to reduce restenosis from 50 to 60 percent to approximately 20 percent, but recently there

was reported evidence of a late target-vessel revascularization catch up.[293] Two randomized trials compared drug-eluting stent and brachytherapy, and the results were very similar, indicating that either sirolimus- or paclitaxel-eluting stents roughly halve the risk of restenosis compared to brachytherapy.[294,295] A meta-analysis of 1230 patients with bare-metal stent in-stent restenosis reported a markedly lower target-vessel revascularization (OR 0.35; *p* <0.001) and angiographic restenosis (OR 0.36; *p* = 0.001) with drug-eluting stent therapy.[296] The superiority of drug-eluting stent is a result of greater acute gain and similar or less late loss than with brachytherapy. Drug-eluting stents have become the dominant strategy for treatment of bare-metal stent restenosis. A pilot trial of 52 patients randomized to paclitaxel-coated or uncoated balloon dilation for treatment of bare-metal stent restenosis was notable, with lower restenosis in the coated balloon (5 percent vs. 43 percent; *p* = 0.002).[297] When restenosis occurs following placement of a drug-eluting stent, the pattern of the restenotic lesion predicts the outcome of PCI. Restenosis occurred in 18 percent with focal lesions and 51 percent with nonfocal lesions (*p* = 0.0001).[298] Very little information is available to guide therapy of an in-drug-eluting stent restenosis lesion. Cosgrove et al. reported that the rate of subsequent restenosis and target-lesion revascularization were similar when the same or different drug-eluting stent was used (restenosis in approximately 24 percent of same or different drug-eluting stent and target-vessel revascularization was 15 percent for both).[299] When restenosis occurs in a drug-eluting stent, stent underexpansion is the most common mechanism and should be searched for with IVUS and corrected.[196] Stent fracture-related restenosis is also a problem that can be recognized by IVUS.

Aortocoronary Graft Lesions

PCI of distal anastomotic stenoses of saphenous vein grafts (SVGs) and LIMA grafts occurring within a year of CABG is safe and associated with good long-term patency, whereas proximal SVG anastomotic and midgraft lesions have high recurrence rates, especially when long lesions are present. PCI of proximal and mid-LIMA grafts is rarely needed as this conduit is "immune" to atherosclerosis, but stent implantation has been performed successfully. Atheromatous SVG lesions begin to appear about 3 years after CABG, and PCI is frequently associated with periprocedural myocardial infarction caused by atheroembolization, a complication not prevented by IIb/

IIIa platelet receptor inhibitors.[300] Stent implantation was more effective than balloon angioplasty in SVG PCI in a randomized trial (6-month MACE 26 percent vs. 38 percent; $p = 0.05$).[301] Use of embolic protection with the PercuSurge Guardwire occlusion-aspiration strategy (Medtronic, Santa Rosa, CA) resulted in a 42 percent reduction in 30-day MACE in a randomized trial of 801 patients who were undergoing SVG stenting,[302] and use of a filter device produced comparable protection when 650 patients were randomized to the Filter-wire (Boston Scientific, Boston, MA) or Guardwire during SVG stent procedures.[303] When a Tri Active distal occlusion balloon with active flush and aspiration (Kensey Nash, Exton, PA) was compared to either the Guardwire or Filter-wire, MACE was similar (8.7 percent vs. 9.2 percent; $p = NS$).[304] Each of these filters and the Guardwire require several centimeters of normal SVG distal to the target site for placement of the filter or occlusion balloon. Proximal protection with the Proxis system (St. Jude, St. Paul, MN) is applicable when there is insufficient room beyond the target lesion for distal protection. The Proxis system had a MACE occurrence similar to either Filter-wire or Guardwire in a randomized trial (9.2 percent vs. 10 percent; $p = NS$).[305] Use of embolic protection during PCI of de novo SVG lesions is a class I indication in the ACC/AHA *Guideline Statement* and is cost-effective.[306,307] Webb reported that 39 percent of SVG lesions could be protected with a proximal or distal strategy, 18 percent with distal only, 20 percent with proximal only, and 23 percent with neither. It appears, based on work by Rogers et al., that the amount of embolic debris retrieved by proximal and distal strategies is similar,[308] but occlusion-aspiration devices would be more effective in retrieving vasoactive substances liberated by SVG stenting.[309] Treatment of no-reflow after stenting includes aspiration of the stagnant dye column, hemodynamic support if needed, and administration of microvascular dilators distally (nitroprusside, calcium channel blocker, or adenosine).[310] In a number of SVG PCI registries, use of drug-eluting stents has yielded superior outcomes to those reported with bare-metal stents. In a prospective, randomized trial, Vermeersch et al. showed that the sirolimus-eluting stent was superior to bare-metal stent with respect to late loss (0.46 vs. 0.93 mm; $p <0.0005$) and binary restenosis (5 percent vs. 37 percent; $p <0.0005$).[311] A high late cardiac event rate following SVG PCI related largely to nontarget progression, especially in diabetics,[312] mandates consideration of native vessel intervention, including CTO recanalization whenever possible and careful surveillance and aggressive lipid lowering of PCI-treated patients.

[ ] SELECTION OF DEVICES

Conventional balloon angioplasty is a simple, relatively low cost, and reasonably effective method of reducing coronary stenosis, but drug-eluting stents are being used with increasing frequency, as a result of favorable initial outcome and reduced restenosis. Patients selected for bare-metal stents include those judged to be unable or unwilling to be compliant with dual antiplatelet therapy, and patients with small (<2.5 mm) or large (>4 mm) vessels, known nonresponsiveness to aspirin or clopidogrel, or lesions with anticipated low probability of restenosis. Directional coronary atherectomy is rarely used in the United States; in Asia, it has been used to debulk and prevent plaque shift during left main coronary artery stenting. Rotational atherectomy is useful to pretreat calcified or lesions that cannot be dilated prior to stenting, but highly

angulated lesions or segments with myocardial bridging should be avoided. Additionally, care is needed in patients with reduced left ventricular function because regional ventricular dysfunction has been shown to persist for more than 2 hours after the procedure.

When large intracoronary thrombi are present, PCI is associated with increased complications. In one trial of an embolic protection strategy, presence of a thrombus was associated with a 10 percent incidence of no-reflow and a 3 percent mortality, and use of embolic protection was protective (OR 0.625; $p = 0.02$).[302] Alternatives include "dissolving" the thrombus (thrombolytic or prolonged treatment with an anti-thrombin ± IIb/IIIa inhibitor), thrombectomy (guide catheter, aspiration catheter, AngioJet, X-sizer), embolic protection or a combination of thrombectomy and embolic protection. Treatment of a SVG restenotic lesion is one of the few SVG PCI conditions where embolic protection is not required. Use of embolic protection in native vessel PCI has not been well studied.

PERFORMANCE OF CORONARY INTERVENTION

[ ] OPERATOR PROFICIENCY

Current guidelines recommend that cardiologists who wish to become competent in coronary intervention receive special training in diagnostic and therapeutic catheterization during an additional year after the standard fellowship training program and maintain skills by performance of 75 procedures per year.[69] Ideally, operators with an annual procedural volume <75 should only work at active centers (>600 procedures per year) with onsite cardiac surgery.

[ ] INTERVENTIONAL LABORATORY

Optimal conditions for performance of coronary angioplasty procedures require sophisticated imaging systems; trained personnel; a large inventory of dilation, thrombectomy, atherectomy, and stent hardware and software; and a variety of therapeutic safety nets to protect the patient when intervention fails or is complicated. Most studies suggest that laboratory procedural volume is important and inversely related to adverse procedural outcomes. The quality of the video image of the coronary arteries is an important determinant of PCI success. A freeze-frame storage and display capability is required for use during the procedure, as is a high-quality video replay with slow-motion and stop-frame capability. The ability to solve specific problems such as lesion eccentricity or rigidity, vessel tortuosity, and unusual position or orientation of the coronary ostia often depends on specific device characteristics. Consequently, it is necessary to have available dilating catheters, stents, atherectomy devices, guidewires, and guiding catheters in a variety of shapes and sizes. The ACC/AHA/SCAI PCI *2005 Guidelines* recommend that elective PCI be performed only in centers with cardiac surgery available for emergency situations.[69]

[ ] THE CORONARY INTERVENTIONAL PROCEDURE

Prior to coronary intervention, patients should receive an explanation of the procedure, including the operator's estimate of success, possible complications, risks, and benefits. A booklet and video-tape describing the procedure and an explanation by the nursing staff will help to reduce anxiety and ensure that both patient and family are well informed.

Dual antiplatelet therapy is used routinely, usually a 600-mg loading dose of clopidogrel unless pretreatment for several days has been performed. A platelet glycoprotein IIb/IIIa receptor antagonist is commonly used when there is perceived to be an increased risk (e.g., suspected or definite thrombus, troponin-positive acute coronary syndrome, complex lesion, diabetes, or multisite intervention). Once the patient is in the catheterization laboratory, electrocardiographic monitoring leads are applied, a peripheral intravenous line is started, and midazolam 1 mg, or an equivalent drug, is given intravenously. In most laboratories, a femoral approach is employed; use of a radial artery approach, however, is increasing. A thrombin inhibitor is administered. Patients with a history of allergy to contrast medium are premedicated with prednisone 40 to 60 mg orally the night before and the day of the procedure, and with diphenhydramine (Benadryl) 50 mg intravenously at the time of the procedure; a nonionic contrast agent is preferred.

Intracoronary stenting is conducted most often as a primary strategy, but may be used for suboptimal outcomes after balloon angioplasty or other interventions. Intravascular ultrasound and/or FFR measurement are commonly used to guide therapy. Deployment strategies vary depending on stent designs, as some are balloon-mounted and others are self-expanding. Stent deployment with a properly sized balloon is performed (usually to >12 atm) to expand the stent optimally throughout its length. When the operator is confident that the best possible result has been obtained, the procedure is ended. Puncture-site closure devices are used with increasing frequency. Creatine kinase and troponin determinations are performed. Because of the dehydrating effect of the osmotic load, most patients receive at least 1 L of intravenous fluids after the procedure. Delayed sheath removal is performed at 2 to 4 hours when the ACT is below 150 seconds.

RESULTS OF CORONARY INTERVENTION

In the last 5 years, angiographic success has been achieved in 95 percent of patients. With drug-eluting stents becoming the default strategy, intermediate- and long-term outcomes parallel the formal trials and registries of drug-eluting stent-treated patients (see Drug-Eluting Stents: The New Dominant Strategy above).

COMPLICATIONS

Patients undergoing coronary intervention are subject to the same complications encountered with the performance of coronary arteriography. In addition, because instrumentation of the atherosclerotic lesion takes place, coronary artery dissection, thrombus formation, and coronary artery spasm may occur, leading to occlusion of the coronary artery or of side branches arising from it. Atheroembolism may lead to MI in an otherwise successful procedure. Atheroembolic myocardial infarction has replaced occlusion of the treated artery as the most common serious complication of coronary intervention, and the availability of stents to treat dissection has reduced the need for emergency bypass surgery from 30 to 50 per 1000 in the 1980s to about 1 to 3 per 1000 in 2006 (Fig. 62–13).

Major complications include death, MI, emergency CABG, and stroke; important so-called *minor complications* consist of transient ischemia, bleeding, access site problems, renal insufficiency, arrhythmias, coronary perforation, stent embolization, aortic injury, and contrast reactions. Death, greatly influenced by clinical factors, occurred in 0.6 percent of patients in the 20-year Emory University Hospital experience. A variety of risk scores were developed to accurately predict risk of death incorporating factors such as age, gender, ejection fraction, hemodynamic status, and comorbidity.[313–315] Only recently has it been appreciated that even modest elevations of creatine kinase myocardial band and troponin are markers of myocardial necrosis, most commonly caused by atherembolism,[290,291] and even minor elevations have prognostic implications.[316] The latest ACC/AHA/SCAI PCI guideline assigns a class I indication for determination of creatine kinase myocardial band or troponin when ischemia is suspected and a class IIa indication for routine measurement after PCI. Stroke, an infrequent complication of coronary angiography and intervention, is almost always embolic, and immediate cerebral angiography and consideration of thrombolysis is indicated.[317] Major bleeding was reported in 4 to 7

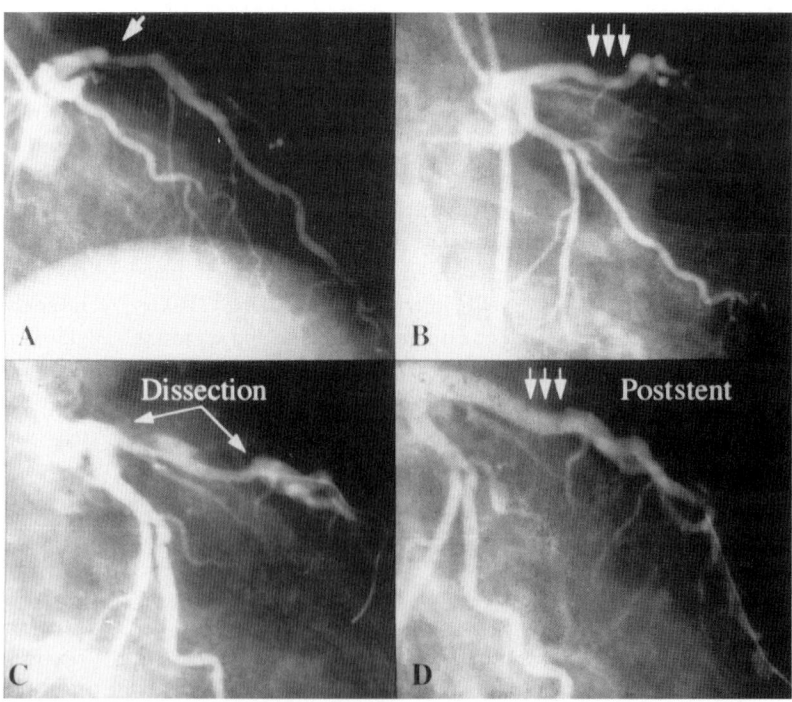

FIGURE 62–13. Complex stenosis of tortuous proximal left anterior descending coronary artery. **A.** Right anterior oblique, cranial angulation. **B.** Caudal angulation. Following an initial attempt at treatment of the lesion, a long dissection occurred. **C.** Prompt stent implantation stabilized the patient, preventing the need for emergency coronary artery bypass graft (CABG). **D.** Stents have reduced the need for emergency CABG to approximately 1 per 1000 patients undergoing PCI.

percent of patients in two recent clinical trials, adding a cost of $10,000 per event, or an average of $400 to the cost of every PCI.[318] Blood loss was most often from the femoral access site. Among 163 patients with retroperitoneal hemorrhage complicating PCI, 10 percent of whom died, retroperitoneal hemorrhage was independently associated with puncture superior to the inferior epigastric artery, female sex, Angio-Seal closure device, IIb/IIIa use, and acute MI presentation.[319]

Coronary perforation occurred in 1.4 percent of 5500 consecutive patients and the mortality rate was significantly higher in those treated with IIb/IIIa inhibitors (24 percent vs. 6 percent; $p = 0.02$).[320] In a more recent series of perforations, need for emergency surgery, but not mortality was associated with IIb/IIIa use.[321] Among 36 perforations observed during PCI in the period 1995 to 1999 at Christ Hospital, atheroablative strategies were more likely to lead to perforation (OR 16) and especially to severe perforation (OR 29).[322] In the current era, guidewire-induced perforations associated with IIb/IIIa use are an important cause of delayed cardiac tamponade, which occurs in 40 percent of cases at a mean time of 5 hours postprocedure.[323] For treatment of small distal guidewire-induced perforations, a number of approaches are used, including balloon inflation, coil embolization, thrombin, Gelfoam, organized thrombus, and platelets injected through an inflated balloon catheter, whereas more proximal balloon/stent-induced vessel perforation may require a covered stent.[324-326] Stent dislodgment and intracoronary embolization occurs rarely in the era of premounted stents and is usually related to inadequate predilation of a rigid lesion. A variety of retrieval techniques are described, but risk proximal vessel injury, whereas deployment at an unintended coronary site or advancement to the target after dilation is usually safer.[327] Aortic injury with dissection associated with aggressive guide catheter maneuvers is more common with right coronary interventions.[328]

Acute contrast-induced nephropathy requiring dialysis is a costly complication of coronary intervention, which occurred in 15 of 1828 (0.8 percent) patients and was associated with a high (33.8 percent) in-hospital mortality.[329] Independent predictors of contrast nephropathy included decreased baseline creatinine clearance, diabetes, and contrast dose (no dialysis was required in patients receiving less than 100 mL of contrast material). Adequate periprocedural hydration and limitation of contrast volume are the most important measures in high-risk patients. The use of the antioxidant acetylcysteine has been associated with a reduction in contrast nephropathy in some randomized trials; however, other studies have failed to show benefit. The use of the dopamine antagonist fenoldopam was not protective in a recently reported randomized trial. Two studies reported that sodium bicarbonate infusion was protective. It was suggested that an isoosmolar contrast agent may be preferred in patients who are at high risk for contrast nephropathy.[330] Hemofiltration, although invasive and costly, was effective in preventing contrast-induced nephropathy.[331]

Stent thrombosis in the bare-metal stent era occurred within 30 days in 0.9 percent of 6186 patients, resulting in a 20 percent mortality; coronary dissection, longer stents, and small vessels were predictive.[332] Among 2229 patients in the drug-eluting stent era, 0.6 percent experienced stent thrombosis within 30 days, and 0.7 percent experienced it between 30 days and 9 months, with a case fatality rate of 45 percent[127] (see Problems Unique to Drug-

Eluting Stents above). Independent predictors of stent thrombosis in this study of drug-eluting stents were premature antiplatelet therapy discontinuation (OR 89.78), renal failure (OR 6.49), bifurcation lesions (OR 6.42), diabetes (OR 3.71), and lower ejection fraction (OR 1.09 for each 10 percent decrease). These observations regarding late drug-eluting stent thrombosis were extended by Pfisterer et al. who compared outcomes of 746 patients who were randomized to bare-metal stents or drug-eluting stents. Pfisterer et al. reported death/MI at 7 to 18 months (when clopidogrel had been discontinued) was higher in drug-eluting stent-treated patients (4.9 percent vs. 1.3 percent).[333] Industry reports of a small increased risk of stent thrombosis after 1 year of 1 per 200 to 500 patient-years of followup also extended the observations regarding late drug-eluting stent thrombosis. These reports resulted in a special FDA panel meeting on drug-eluting stent safety in December 2006, with recommendations that patients and physicians be warned about this small but real increased risk of late stent thrombosis. A landmark study of almost 5000 patients with bare-metal stents or drug-eluting stents compared outcomes of patients between 6 months and 24 months (also 12 months and 24 months) after PCI, noting that drug-eluting stent-treated patients on clopidogrel had less death or death/MI than drug-eluting stent-treated patients who were not taking clopidogrel, whereas clopidogrel had no protective effect in bare-metal stent-treated patients.[334] The cause of these late events is the failure to heal and the inflammation associated with drug-eluting stents (Fig. 62–14). Recommendations that clopidogrel be continued for 1 year or longer must be balanced against a 1 percent major bleeding risk per year and enormous cost of lifelong clopidogrel. Prospective trials needed to guide therapy are underway.

POSTINTERVENTION THERAPY

The most recent ACC/AHA/SCAI PCI *Guideline* statement emphasizes the importance of behavior and risk factor modification, and institution of medical therapy for secondary prevention of atherosclerosis prior to hospital discharge. Recommendations should include dual antiplatelet therapy with aspirin and a thienopyridine, a statin aimed at a target low-density lipoprotein cholesterol of <100 mg/dL, optimal diabetes management, smoking cessation, weight control, regular exercise, and angiotensin-converting enzyme inhibitor therapy as recommended in the AHA/ACC consensus statement on secondary prevention. Preliminary data suggests that β blockade after successful elective PCI provides a mortality benefit.[190,191] The optimal duration of thienopyridine therapy is uncertain. The latest PCI guideline statement recommends that bare-metal stent-treated patients receive clopidogrel 75 mg daily for 1 month (2 weeks if there is an increased bleeding risk) and that drug-eluting stent-treated patients ideally receive clopidogrel for 12 months. A study from Duke University Hospital is supportive.[335]

FUTURE DIRECTIONS

With the new availability of second-generation drug-eluting stents, the future of coronary intervention appears bright. There

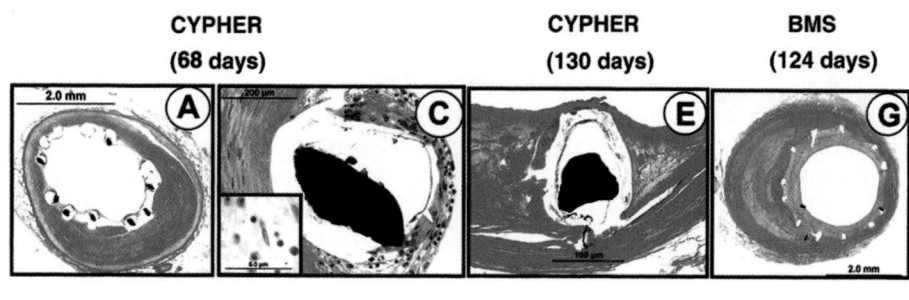

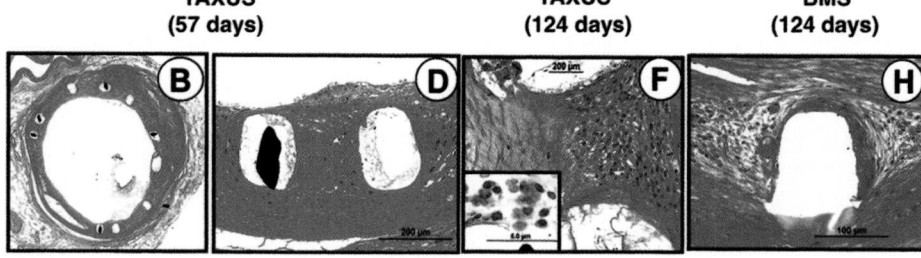

FIGURE 62–14. Histologic sections with hematoxylin and eosin (HE) stain from patent drug-eluting stents (DES) and bare-metal stents (BMS) from various time points. Coronary arteries with Cypher (**A**) and Taxus (**B**) stents at 68 and 57 days, respectively. High-powered views showing inflammatory infiltrate around Cypher struts (**C**) include eosinophils (inset Luna stain), whereas around the Taxus stent struts (**D**) there is a predominance of fibrin. At 130 and 124 days, respectively, there is a focal fibrin deposition and giant cell reaction seen around the Cypher stent (**E**), whereas in the Taxus stent (**F**) there is greater inflammation, including eosinophils (inset Luna stain). A BMS at 124 days is shown in **G** and **H**. *Source: From Joner M, Finn AV, Farb A, et al. Pathology of drug-eluting stents in humans: delayed healing and late thrombotic risk. J Am Coll Cardiol 2006;48:193–202, with permission.*

are, however, a number of problems to be solved. Needs include more optimal periprocedural and long-term antithrombotic therapy, antiproliferative agents that retard restenosis but permit rapid and healthy endothelialization, improved strategies for complex lesion subsets (bifurcations, CTO, SVG, left main coronary artery, small vessels, calcification, diffuse disease), embolic protection strategies suitable for native coronaries, and nonmetallic or absorbable stents that permit subsequent noninvasive MRI and CT angiography. It is hoped that the impediments related to the high cost of new strategies will be ameliorated by competitive forces in the market.

REFERENCES

1. Dotter CT, Judkins MP. Transluminal treatment of arteriosclerotic obstruction: description of a new technique and a preliminary report of its application. *Circulation* 1964;30:654–670.
2. Zeitler EJ, Schmidtke J, Schoop W. Die Perkutane Behandlung von Arteriellen Durchbluteungsstorungen der Estremiaten mit Katheter. *Vasa* 1973;2:401–404.
3. Gruentzig AR, Turina MI, Schneider JA. Experimental percutaneous dilatation of coronary artery stenosis [abstract]. *Circulation* 1985;54(Suppl II):II-81.
4. Gruentzig AR, Kumpe DA. Technique of percutaneous transluminal angioplasty with the Gruentzig balloon catheter. *AJR Am J Roentgenol* 1979;132:547–552.
5. Sheldon WC, Sones FM Jr. Stormy petrel of cardiology. *Clin Cardiol* 1994;17:405–407.
6. Hurst JW. History of cardiac catheterization. In: King SB III, Douglas JS Jr, eds. *Coronary Arteriography and Angioplasty.* New York: McGraw-Hill, 1985:1–9.
7. King SB III. Angioplasty from bench to bedside to bench. *Circulation* 1996;93:1621–1629.
8. King SB III. The development of interventional cardiology. *J Am Coll Cardiol* 2000;31(Suppl B):64B–88B.
9. Meier B. The first patient to undergo coronary angioplasty—23-year follow-up. *N Engl J Med* 2001;344:144–145.
10. Gruentzig A. Transluminal dilatation of coronary artery stenosis. *Lancet* 1978;1:263.
11. Gruentzig AR, Senning A, Siegenthaler WE. Nonoperative dilatation of coronary artery stenosis: Percutaneous transluminal coronary angioplasty. *N Engl J Med* 1979;301:61–68.
12. Kent KM, Bentivoglio LG, Block PC. Percutaneous transluminal coronary angioplasty: report from the Registry of the National Heart, Lung, and Blood Institute. *Am J Cardiol* 1982;49:2011–2020.
13. Detre K, Holubkov R, Kelsey S, et al. Percutaneous transluminal coronary angioplasty in 1985–1986 and 1977–1981: the National Heart, Lung, and Blood Institute Registry. *N Engl J Med* 1988;318:265–270.
14. Simpson JB, Baim DS, Robert EW, et al. A new catheter system for coronary angioplasty. *Am J Cardiol* 1982;49:1216–1222.
15. Cowley MJ, Vetrovec GW, DiSciascio G, et al. Coronary angioplasty of multiple vessels: short-term outcome and long-term results. *Circulation* 1985;72:1314–1320.
16. O'Keefe JH Jr, Rutherford BD, McConahay DR, et al. Multivessel coronary angioplasty from 1980–1989: procedural results and long-term outcome. *J Am Coll Cardiol* 1990;16:1097–1102.
17. Parisi AF, Folland ED, Hartigan P. A comparison of angioplasty with medical therapy in the treatment of single-vessel coronary artery disease. *N Engl J Med* 1992;326:10–16.
18. Boden WE, O'Rourke RA, Crawford MH, et al. Outcomes in patients with acute non–Q-wave myocardial infarction randomly assigned to an invasive as compared with a conservative management strategy. *N Engl J Med* 1998;338:1785–1792.
19. Hueb WA, Bellotti G, de Oliveira SA, et al. The Medicine, Angioplasty or Surgery Study (MASS): a prospective, randomized trial of medical therapy, balloon angioplasty or bypass surgery for single proximal left anterior descending artery stenoses. *J Am Coll Cardiol* 1995;26:1600–1605.
20. Coronary angioplasty versus medical therapy for angina: The Second Randomized Intervention Treatment of Angina (RITA-2) trial. *Lancet* 1997;350:461–468.
21. Pitt B, Waters D, Brown WV, et al. Aggressive lipid-lowering therapy compared with angioplasty in stable coronary artery disease. *N Engl J Med* 1999;341:70–76.
22. Wallentin L. Fast revascularization during instability in coronary artery disease (FRISC II): an early invasive versus early noninvasive strategy in unstable coronary artery disease. *J Am Coll Cardiol* 1999;34:1.
23. Fragmin and Fast Revascularization During Instability in Coronary Artery Disease Investigators. Invasive compared with non-invasive treatment in unstable coronary-artery disease: FRISC II prospective randomised multicentre study. *Lancet* 1999;354:708–715.
24. Cannon CP, Weintraub WS, Dempoulos LA, et al. Comparison of early invasive and conservative strategies in patients with unstable coronary syndromes treated with the glycoprotein IIb/IIIa inhibitor tirofiban. *N Engl J Med* 2001;344:1879–1887.
25. Fox KAA, Poole-Wilson PA, Henderson RA, et al. Interventional versus conservative treatment for patients with unstable angina or non-ST-elevation myocardial infarction: the British Heart Foundation RITA 3 randomised trial. *Lancet* 2002;360:743–751.
26. Hueb W, Soares PR, Gersh BJ, et al. The Medicine, Angioplasty, or Surgery Study (MASS-II): a randomized, controlled clinical trial of three therapeutic strategies for multivessel coronary artery disease: one-year results. *J Am Coll Cardiol* 2004;43:1743–1751.
27. Hueb W, Lopes N, Gersh BJ, et al. Five year follow-up of the Medicine, Angioplasty or Surgery Study (MASS II): a randomized clinical trial. *Circulation* 2007;(in press).
28. King SB III, Lembo NJ, Weintraub WS, et al. A randomized trial comparing coronary angioplasty with coronary bypass surgery. *N Engl J Med* 1994;331:1044–1050.

29. The Bypass Angioplasty Revascularization Investigation (BARI) Investigators. Comparison of coronary bypass surgery with angioplasty in patients with multivessel disease. *N Engl J Med* 1996;335:217–225.

30. Pocock SJ, Henderson RA, Rickards AF, et al. Meta-analysis of randomized trials comparing coronary angioplasty with bypass surgery. *Lancet* 1995;346:1184–1189.

31. Sim I, Gupta M, McDonald K, et al. A meta-analysis of randomized trials comparing coronary artery bypass grafting with percutaneous transluminal coronary angioplasty in multivessel coronary artery disease. *Am J Cardiol* 1995;76:1025–1029.

32. Weintraub WS, Mauldin PD, Becker E, et al. A comparison of the costs and quality of life after coronary angioplasty or coronary surgery for multivessel coronary artery disease: results from the Emory Angioplasty Versus Surgery Trial (EAST). *Circulation* 1995;92:2831–2840.

33. Weintraub WS, Becker ER, Mauldin PD, et al. Costs of revascularization over eight years in the randomized and eligible patients in the Emory Angioplasty Versus Surgery Trial (EAST). *Am J Cardiol* 2000;86:747–752.

34. The BARI Investigators. Influence of diabetes on 5-year mortality and morbidity in a randomized trial comparing CABG and PTCA in patients with multivessel disease: the Bypass Angioplasty Revascularization Investigation (BARI). *Circulation* 1997;96:1761–1769.

35. The BARI Investigators. Seven-year mortality in the Bypass Angioplasty Revascularization Investigation (BARI) by treatment and diabetic status. *J Am Coll Cardiol* 2000;35:1122–1129.

36. King SB III, Kosinski AS, Guyton RA, et al. Eight-year mortality in the Emory Angioplasty Versus Surgery Trial (EAST). *J Am Coll Cardiol* 2000;35:1116–1121.

37. Weintraub WS, Stein B, Kosinski A, et al. Outcome of coronary bypass surgery versus coronary angioplasty in diabetic patients with multivessel coronary artery disease. *J Am Coll Cardiol* 1998;31:10–19.

38. Detre KM, Guo P, Holubkov R, et al. Coronary revascularization in diabetic patients: a comparison of the randomized and observational components of the Bypass Angioplasty Revascularization Investigation (BARI). *Circulation* 1999;99:633–640.

39. Niles NW, McGrath PD, Malenka D, et al. Survival of patients with diabetes and multivessel coronary artery disease after surgical or percutaneous coronary revascularization: results of a large regional prospective study. *J Am Coll Cardiol* 2001;37:1008–1015.

40. Kuntz RE. Importance of considering atherosclerosis progression when choosing a coronary revascularization strategy: the diabetics-percutaneous transluminal coronary angioplasty dilemma. *Circulation* 1999;99:847–851.

41. Eagle KA, Guyton RA, Davidoff R, et al. ACC/AHA guidelines for coronary artery bypass graft surgery: executive summary and recommendations. A report of the American College of Cardiology/American Heart Association Task Force on Practice Guidelines (Committee to Revise the 1991 Guidelines for Coronary Artery Bypass Graft Surgery). *Circulation* 1999;100:1464–1480.

42. Hirotani T, Kameda T, Kumamoto T, et al. Effects of coronary artery bypass grafting using internal mammary arteries for diabetic patients. *J Am Coll Cardiol* 1999;34:532–538.

43. Sigwart U, Puel J, Mirkovitch V, et al. Intravascular stents to prevent occlusion and restenosis after transluminal angioplasty. *N Engl J Med* 1987;316:701–706.

44. Puel J, Joffre F, Rousseau H, et al. Endo-protheses coronanennes and auto-expansive dans la preventions des restenoses apres angioplastie transluminale. *Arch Mal Coeur* 1987;8:131–132.

45. Roubin GS, King SB III, Douglas JS Jr, et al. Intracoronary stenting during percutaneous transluminal coronary angioplasty. *Circulation* 1998;81(Suppl IV):IV-92–IV-100.

46. Hearn JA, King SB III, Douglas JS Jr, et al. Clinical and angiographic outcomes after coronary artery stenting for acute or threatened closure after percutaneous transluminal coronary angioplasty: initial results with a balloon-expandable, stainless steel design. *Circulation* 1993;88:2086–2096.

47. Roubin GS, Robinson KA, King SB, et al. Early and late results of intracoronary arterial stenting after coronary angioplasty in dogs. *Circulation* 1987;76:891–897.

48. Fischman DL, Leon MB, Baim DS, et al. A randomized comparison of coronary-stent placement and balloon angioplasty in treatment of coronary artery disease. *N Engl J Med* 1994;331:496–501.

49. Serruys PW, de Jaegere P, Kiemeneij F, et al. A comparison of balloon-expandable stent implantation with balloon angioplasty in patients with coronary artery disease. *N Engl J Med* 1994;331:489–495.

50. Colombo A, Hall P, Nakamura S, et al. Intracoronary stenting without anticoagulation accomplished with intravascular ultrasound guidance. *Circulation* 1995;91:1676–1688.

51. Schoemig A, Newmann FJ, Kastrati A, et al. A randomized comparison of antiplatelet and anticoagulant therapy after the placement of coronary artery stents. *N Engl J Med* 1996;334:1084–1089.

52. Leon MB, Baim DS, Popma JJ, et al. A clinical trial comparing three antithrombotic drug regimens after coronary artery stenting. *N Engl J Med* 1998;339:1665–1671.

53. Urban P, Macaya C, Rupprecht HJ, et al. Randomized evaluation of anticoagulation versus antiplatelet therapy after coronary stent implantation in high-risk patients: the Multicenter Aspirin and Ticlopidine Trial after Intracoronary Stenting (MATTIS). *Circulation* 1998;2126–2132.

54. Bertrand M, Legrand V, Boland J, et al. Randomized multicenter comparison of conventional anticoagulation versus antiplatelet therapy in unplanned and elective coronary stenting: the Full Anticoagulation Versus Aspirin and Ticlopidine (FANTASTIC) study. *Circulation* 1998;98:1597–1603.

55. Berger PB, Bell MR, Hasdai D, et al. Safety and efficacy of ticlopidine for only 2 weeks after successful intracoronary stent placement. *Circulation* 1999;99:248–253.

56. Steinhubl SR, Tan WA, Foody JM, et al. Incidence and clinical course of thrombotic thrombocytopenic purpura due to ticlopidine following coronary stenting. *JAMA* 1999;281:806–810.

57. Bennett CL, Davidson CJ, Raisch DW, et al. Thrombotic thrombocytopenic purpura associated with ticlopidine in the setting of coronary artery stents and stroke prevention. *Arch Intern Med* 1999;159:2524–2528.

58. Quinn MJ, Fitzgerald DJ. Ticlopidine and clopidogrel. *Circulation* 1999;100:1667–1672.

59. Moussa I, Oetgen M, Roubin G, et al. Effectiveness of clopidogrel and aspirin versus ticlopidine and aspirin in preventing stent thrombosis after coronary stent implantation. *Circulation* 1999;99:2364–2366.

60. Bertrand ME. Clopidogrel Aspirin Stent International Study (CLASSICS) trial. *J Am Coll Cardiol* 1999;34:7.

61. Serruys PW, van Hout B, Bonnier H, et al. Randomised comparison of implantation of heparin-coated stents with balloon angioplasty in selected patients with coronary artery disease (Benestent II). *Lancet* 1998;352:673–681.

62. Weaver WD. Late-breaking trials in interventional cardiology: optimal angioplasty versus primary stenting (OPUS). *J Am Coll Cardiol* 2003;34:1.

63. The EPISTENT Investigators. Randomized placebo-controlled trial to assess safety of coronary stenting with use of platelet glycoprotein IIb/IIIa blockage. *Lancet* 1998;352:87–92.

64. Brophy JM, Belisle P, Lawrence J. Evidence for use of coronary stents. *Ann Intern Med* 2003;138:777–786.

65. Yock CA, Isbill JM, King SB III. Bare-metal stent outcomes in an unselected patient population. *Clin Cardiol* 2006;29:352–356.

66. Holmes DR, Hirshfeld J, Faxon D, et al. ACC expert consensus document on coronary artery stents: document of the American College of Cardiology. *J Am Coll Cardiol* 1998;32:1471–1482.

67. Serruys PW, Kutryk MJB, Ong ATL. Coronary artery stents. *N Engl J Med* 2006;354:483–495.

68. Serruys PW, Unger F, Sousa JE, et al. for the Arterial Revascularization Therapies Study Group. Comparison of coronary artery bypass surgery and stenting for the treatment of multivessel disease. *N Engl J Med* 2001;344:1117–1124.

69. Smith SC Jr, Feldman TE, Hirschfeld JW, et al. ACC/AHA/SCAI 2005 guideline update for percutaneous intervention: a report of the American College of Cardiology/American Heart Association Task Force on the Guidelines (ACC/AHA/SCAI Writing Committee to Update the 2001 Guidelines for Percutaneous Coronary Intervention). *J Am Coll Cardiol* 2006;47:1–121.

70. Serruys PW, Unger F, Sousa JE, et al. for the Arterial Revascularization Therapies Study Group. Comparison of coronary artery bypass surgery and stenting for the treatment of multivessel disease. *N Engl J Med* 2001;344:1117–1124.

71. Serruys PW, Ong ATL, van Herwerden LA, et al. Five-year outcomes after coronary stenting versus bypass surgery for the treatment of multivessel disease. The final analysis of the Arterial Revascularization Therapies Study (ARTS) randomized trial. *J Am Coll Cardiol* 2005;46:575–581.

72. Serruys PW, Costa MA, Betriu A, et al. The influence of diabetes mellitus on clinical outcome following multivessel stenting or CABG in the ARTS trial. *Circulation* 1999;100(Suppl I):I-364.

73. Rodriquez A, Palacios IF, Navia J, et al. Argentine randomized study: coronary angioplasty with stenting versus coronary artery bypass surgery in patients with multiple vessel disease (ERACI II): 30-day and long-term follow-up results. *Circulation* 1999;100(Suppl I):I-234.

74. The SOS Investigators. Coronary artery bypass surgery versus percutaneous intervention with stent implantation in patients with multivessel coronary

artery disease (the Stent or Surgery Trial): a randomized controlled trial. *Lancet* 2002;360:965–970.

75. Booth J, Stables RH, Pepper J, et al. The Stent or Surgery trial: longer term followup. Presented at the European Society of Cardiology Scientific Sessions. Barcelona, Spain, August 2006.

76. Morrison DA, Sethi G, Sacks J, et al. Percutaneous coronary intervention versus coronary artery bypass graft surgery for patients with medically refractory myocardial ischemia and risk factors for adverse outcomes with bypass: a multicenter, randomized trial. Investigators for the Department of Veterans Affairs Cooperative Study #385 the Angina With Extremely Serious Operative Mortality Evaluation (AWESOME). *J Am Coll Cardiol* 2005;38:143–149.

77. Stroupe KT, Morrison DA, Glatky MA, et al. Cost-effectiveness of coronary artery bypass graft versus percutaneous coronary intervention for revascularization of high-risk patients. *Circulation* 2006;114:1251–1257.

78. Radford MJ. Percutaneous coronary intervention "dominates" coronary artery bypass graft surgery for high-risk patients. Good news for patients, a challenge for healthcare planners. *Circulation* 2006;114:1229.

79. Mercado N, Wijns W, Serruys PW, et al. One-year outcomes of coronary artery bypass graft surgery versus percutaneous coronary intervention with multiple stenting for multisystem disease: a meta-analysis of individual patient data from randomized clinical trials. *J Thorac Cardiovasc Surg* 2005;130:512–519.

80. Hoffman SN, TenBrook JA, Wolf M, et al. A meta-analysis of randomized controlled trials comparing coronary artery bypass graft with percutaneous transluminal coronary angioplasty: one to eight year outcomes. *J Am Coll Cardiol* 2003;41:1293–1304.

81. Hannan EL, Racz MJ, Walford G, et al. Long-term outcomes of coronary artery bypass grafting versus stent implantation. *N Engl J Med* 2005;352:12–21.

82. Douglas JS Jr, Holmes DR Jr, Kereiakes DJ, et al. Coronary stent restenosis in patients treated with cilostazol. *Circulation* 2005;112:2826–2832.

83. Sousa JE, Serruys PW, Costa MA. New frontiers in cardiology—drug-eluting stents: part I. *Circulation* 2003;107:2274–2279.

84. Sousa JE, Serruys PW, Costa MA. New frontiers in cardiology—drug-eluting stents: part II. *Circulation* 2003;107:2383–2389.

85. Sousa JE, Costa MA, Abizaid A, et al. Lack of neointimal proliferation after implantation of sirolimus-coated stents in human coronary arteries: a quantitative coronary angiography and three-dimensional intravascular ultrasound study. *Circulation* 2001;103:192–195.

86. Sousa JE, Costa MA, Abizaid AC, et al. Sustained suppression of neointimal proliferation by sirolimus-eluting stents: one-year angiographic and intravascular ultrasound follow-up. *Circulation* 2001;104:2007–2011.

87. Degertekin M, Serruys PW, Foley DP, et al. Persistent inhibition of neointimal hyperplasia after sirolimus-eluting stent implantation: long-term (up to 2 years) clinical, angiographic, and intravascular ultrasound follow-up. *Circulation* 2002;106:1610–1613.

88. Sousa JE, Costa MA, Abizaid A, et al. Four-year angiographic and intravascular ultrasound follow-up of patients treated with sirolimus-eluting stents. *Circulation* 2005;111:2326–2329.

89. Morice MC, Serruys PW, Sousa JE, et al. A randomized comparison of a sirolimus-eluting stent with a standard stent for coronary revascularization. The RAVEL trial. *N Engl J Med* 2002;346:1773–1780.

90. Moses JW, Leon MB, Popma JJ, et al. Sirolimus-eluting stents versus standard stents in patients with stenosis in a native coronary artery. *N Engl J Med* 2003;349:1315–1323.

91. Grube E, Siber MS, Hauptmann KE, et al. Prospective, randomized, double-blind comparison of NIRx stents coated with paclitaxel in a polymer carrier in de-novo coronary lesions compared with uncoated controls. *Circulation* 2001;104(Suppl):II-463.

92. Colombo A, Drzewiecki J, Banning A, et al. Randomized study to assess the effectiveness of slow- and moderate-release, polymer-based, paclitaxel-eluting stents for coronary artery lesions. *Circulation* 2003;108:788–794.

93. Stone GW, Ellis SG, Cox DA, et al. A polymer-based, paclitaxel-eluting stent in patients with coronary artery disease. *N Engl J Med* 2004;350:221–231.

94. Tanabe K, Serruys PW, Grube E, et al. TAXUS III Trial. In-stent restenosis treated with stent-based delivery of paclitaxel incorporated in a slow-release polymer formulation. *Circulation* 2002;107:559–564.

95. Fajadet J, Wijns W, Larrman G, et al. Randomized, double-blind, multicenter study of the endeavor zotarolimus-eluting phosphorylcholine-encapsulated stent for treatment of native coronary artery lesions: clinical and angiographic results of the ENDEAVOR II Trial. *Circulation* 2006;114:798–806.

96. Morice M, Colombo A, Meier B, et al. Sirolimus- vs. paclitaxel-eluting stents in de novo coronary artery lesions: the REALITY trial. *JAMA* 2006;295:895–904.

97. Windecker S, Remondino A, Eberli FR, et al. Sirolimus-eluting and paclitaxel-eluting stents for coronary revascularization. *N Engl J Med* 2005;353:653–662.

98. Ong AT, Serruys PW, Aoki J, et al. The unrestricted use of paclitaxel- versus sirolimus-eluting stents for coronary artery disease in an unselected population: one-year results for the Taxus-Stent Evaluated at Rotterdam Cardiology Hospital (T-SEARCH) registry. *J Am Coll Cardiol* 2005;45:1135–1141.

99. Simonton C, Brodie B, Cheek B, et al. for the STENT investigators. *Comparative Late Clinical Outcomes of Paclitaxel and Sirolimus-Eluting Coronary Stents in Diabetic Patients from a Large Prospective Multicenter Registry: Results from the Strategic Transcatheter Evaluation of New Therapies (STENT) Group.* Presented at American College of Cardiology's 55th Annual Scientific Session. Atlanta, GA; March 11–14, 2006.

100. Kastrati A, Dibra A, Eberle S, et al. Sirolimus-eluting stents vs. paclitaxel-eluting stents in patients with coronary artery disease; meta-analysis of randomized trials. *JAMA* 2005;294:819–825.

101. Kastrati A, Dibra A, Mehilli J, et al. Predictive factors of restenosis after coronary implantation of sirolimus- or paclitaxel-eluting stents. *Circulation* 2006;113:2293–2300.

102. Serruys PW, on behalf of the SPIRIT II investigators. *SPIRIT II Study: A Clinical Evaluation of the* XIENCE V *Everolimus-Eluting Coronary Stent System in the Treatment of Patients with De Novo, Native Coronary Artery Lesions.* World Congress of Cardiology 2006. Barcelona, Spain. September 5, 2006; Presentation 3415.

103. Serruys PW, for the ARTS-II Investigators. *ARTS-II: Arterial Revascularization Therapies Study Part II of the Sirolimus-Eluting Stent in the Treatment of Patients with Multivessel De Novo Coronary Artery Lesions. Late Breaking Clinical Trial.* Presented at the American College of Cardiology's 54th Annual Meeting. Orlando, FL: March 2005.

104. Serruys PW. Fourth Annual American College of Cardiology International Lecture: a journey in the interventional field. *J Am Coll Cardiol* 2006;47:1754–1758.

105. Macaya C, Garcia H, Serruys P, et al. Sirolimus-eluting stents versus surgery and bare metal stenting in the treatment of diabetic patients with multivessel disease—comparison between ARTS I and ARTS II. *Circulation* 2005;112:II-655.

106. Rodriguez AE, Mieres J, Fernandez-Pereira C, et al. Coronary stent thrombosis in current drug-eluting stent era: insights from ERACI III trial. *J Am Coll Cardiol* 2006;47:205–207.

107. Greenberg D, Bakhai A, Neil N, et al. Modeling the impact of patient and lesion characteristics on the cost-effectiveness of drug-eluting stents. *J Am Coll Cardiol* 2003;41 Suppl A:538A.

108. Glaser R, Selzer F, Faxon DP, et al. Clinical progression of incidental, asymptomatic lesions discovered during culprit vessel coronary intervention. *Circulation* 2005;111:143–149.

109. Klein LW. Are drug-eluting stents the preferred treatment for multivessel coronary artery disease? *J Am Coll Cardiol* 2006;47:22–26.

110. Greenberg D, Bakhai A, Cohen DJ. Can we afford to eliminate restenosis? Can we afford not to? *J Am Coll Cardiol* 2004;43:513–518.

111. Cohen DJ, Bakhai A, Shi C, et al. SIRIUS Investigators. Cost-effectiveness of sirolimus-eluting stents for treatment of complex coronary stenoses: results from the Sirolimus-Eluting Balloon Expandable Stent in the Treatment of Patients With De Novo Native Coronary Artery Lesions (SIRIUS) trial. *Circulation* 2004;110:508–514.

112. van Hout BA, Serruys PW, Lemos PA, et al. One year cost effectiveness of sirolimus-eluting stents compared with bare metal stents in the treatment of single native de novo coronary lesions: an analysis from the RAVEL trial. *Heart* 2005;91:507–512.

113. Vaitkus PT. Common sense, dollars and cents, and drug-eluting stents. *J Am Coll Cardiol* 2006;48:268–269.

114. Bakhai A, Stone GW, Mahoney E, et al. Cost effectiveness of paclitaxel-eluting stents for patients undergoing percutaneous coronary revascularization: results from the TAXUS-IV trial. *J Am Coll Cardiol* 2006;48:253–261.

115. Elezi S, Dibra A, Folkerts U, et al. Cost analysis from two randomized trials of sirolimus-eluting stents versus paclitaxel-eluting stents in high-risk patients with coronary artery disease. *J Am Coll Cardiol* 2006;48:262–267.

116. Ryan J, Cohen DJ. Will drug-eluting stents bankrupt the healthcare system? Are drug-eluting stents cost-effective? It depends on whom you ask. *Circulation* 2006;114:1736–1744.

117. Eisenberg MJ. Drug-eluting stents. The price is not right. *Circulation* 2006;114:1745–1754.

118. Cohen DJ. *Cost-effectiveness of DES in Multivessel Disease: Insights from ARTS I and ARTS II.* Presented at Transcatheter Therapeutics (TCT-2005). Washington, DC: 2005.

119. Hofma SH, van der Giessen WJ, van Dalen BM, Lemos PA, et al. Indication of long-term endothelial dysfunction after sirolimus-eluting stent implantation. *Eur Heart J* 2006;27:166–170.

120. Togni M, Windecker S, Cocchia R, et al. Sirolimus-eluting stents associated with paradoxic coronary vasoconstriction. *J Am Coll Cardiol* 2005;46:231–236.

121. Lerman A, Eckhout E. Coronary endothelial dysfunction following sirolimus-eluting stent placement: should we worry about it? *Eur Heart J* 2006;27:170–172.

122. Nebeker JR, Virmani R, Bennett CL, et al. Hypersensitivity cases associated with drug-eluting stents: a review of available cases from the Research on Adverse Drug Events and Reports (RADAR) project. *J Am Coll Cardiol* 2006;47:175–181.

123. Azarbal B, Currier JW. Allergic reactions after the implantation of drug-eluting stents. *J Am Coll Cardiol* 2006;47:182–183.

124. Virmani R, Guagliumi G, Farb A, et al. Localized hypersensitivity and late thrombosis secondary to a sirolimus-eluting stent. Should we be cautious? *Circulation* 2004;109:701–705.

125. Wheatcroft S, Byrne J, Thomas M, et al. Life-threatening coronary artery spasm following sirolimus-eluting stent deployment. *J Am Coll Cardiol* 2006;47:1911–1912.

126. Serru R, Penny WF. Endothelial dysfunction after sirolimus-eluting stent placement. *J Am Coll Cardiol* 2005;46:237–238.

127. Iakovou I, Schmidt T, Bonizzoni E, et al. Incidence, predictors, and outcome of thrombosis after successful implantation of drug-eluting stents. *JAMA* 2005;293:2126–2130.

128. McFadden EP, Stabile E, Regar E, et al. Late thrombosis in drug-eluting coronary stents after discontinuation of antiplatelet therapy. *Lancet* 2004;364:1519–1521.

129. Moreno R, Fernandez C, Hernandez R, et al. Drug-eluting stent thrombosis: results from a pooled analysis including 10 randomized studies. *J Am Coll Cardiol* 2005;45:954–959.

130. Joner M, Finn AV, Farb A, et al. Pathology of drug-eluting stents in humans: delayed healing and late thrombotic risk. *J Am Coll Cardiol* 2006;48:193–202.

131. Hong M, Mintz GS, Lee CW, et al. Late stent malapposition after drug-eluting stent implantation: an intravascular ultrasound analysis with long-term follow-up. *Circulation* 2006;113:414–419.

132. Kotani J, Awata M, Nanto S, et al. Incomplete neointimal coverage of sirolimus-eluting stents: angioscopic findings. *J Am Coll Cardiol* 2006;47:2108–2111.

133. Tsimikas S. Drug-eluting stents and late adverse clinical outcomes: lessons learned, lessons awaited. *J Am Coll Cardiol* 2006;47:2112–2115.

134. Lee SH, Pack J, Kim U, et al. Stent fracture is one of the leading causes of restenosis after sirolimus-eluting stent implantation. *Circulation* 2006;114(Suppl II):II-390.

135. Gurbel PA, Bliden KP, Hayes KM, et al. The relation of dosing to clopidogrel responsiveness and the incidence of high post-treatment platelet aggregation in patients undergoing coronary stenting. *J Am Coll Cardiol* 2005;45:1392–1396.

136. Gurbel PA, Lau WC, Bliden KP, et al. Clopidogrel resistance: implications for coronary stenting. *Curr Pharm Des* 2006;12:1261–1269.

137. Mehta S, Yusuf S, Peters R, et al. Effects of pretreatment with clopidogrel and aspirin followed by long-term therapy in patients undergoing percutaneous coronary intervention: the PCI-CURE study. *Lancet* 2001;358:527–533.

138. Berger PB, Steinubl S. Clinical implications of percutaneous coronary intervention-clopidogrel in unstable angina to prevent recurrent events (PCI-CURE) study—a U.S. perspective. *Circulation* 2002;106:2284–2287.

139. Pache J, Kastrati A, Mehilli J, et al. Clopidogrel therapy in patients undergoing coronary stenting: value of a high-loading dose regimen. *Catheter Cardiovasc Interv* 2002;55:436–441.

140. Kandzari DE, Berger PB, Kastrati A, et al. Influence of treatment duration with a 600 mg dose of clopidogrel before percutaneous coronary revascularization. *J Am Coll Cardiol* 2004;44:2133–2136.

141. Cuisset T, Frere C, Quilici J, et al. Benefit of a 600 mg loading dose of clopidogrel on platelet reactivity and clinical outcomes in patients with non–ST-segment elevation acute coronary syndrome undergoing coronary stenting. *J Am Coll Cardiol* 2006;48:1339–1345.

142. Steinhubl S, Berger PB, Brennan DM, et al. Optimal timing for the initiation of pretreatment with 300 mg clopidogrel before percutaneous coronary intervention. *J Am Coll Cardiol* 2006;47:939–943.

143. Kastrati A, Mehilli J, Schuhlen H, et al. A clinical trial of abciximab in elective percutaneous coronary intervention after pretreatment with clopidogrel. *N Engl Med* 2004;350:232–238.

144. Kastrati A, Mehilli J, Neumann F, et al. Abciximab in patients with acute coronary syndromes undergoing percutaneous coronary intervention after clopidogrel pretreatment: the ISAR-REACT 2 randomized trial. *JAMA* 2006;295;1531–1538.

145. Steinhubl SR, Berger PB, Mann JT III, et al. Early and sustained dual oral antiplatelet therapy following percutaneous coronary interventional: a randomized controlled trial. *JAMA* 2002;288:2411–2420.

146. Beinart SC, Kolm P, Veledar E, et al. Long-term cost effectiveness of early and sustained dual oral antiplatelet therapy with clopidogrel given for up to one year after percutaneous coronary intervention results: from the Clopidogrel for the Reduction of Events During Observation (CREDO) trial. *J Am Coll Cardiol* 2005;46:761–769.

147. Angiolillo DJ, Fernandez-ortiz A, Bernardo E, et al. Platelet aggregation varies according to Body Mass Index in patients undergoing coronary stent implantation. Should clopidogrel load-dose be weight adjusted? *Circulation* 2002;106:II-79.

148. Lev EI, Patel RT, Maresh KJ, et al. Aspirin and clopidogrel drug response in patients undergoing percutaneous coronary intervention: the role of dual drug resistance. *J Am Coll Cardiol* 2006;47:27–33.

149. Hochholzer W, Trenk D, Bestehorn H, et al. Impact of the degree of peri-interventional platelet inhibition after loading with clopidogrel on early clinical outcome of elective coronary stent placement. *J Am Coll Cardiol* 2006;48:1742–1750.

150. Wenaweser P, Dorffler-Melly J, Imboden K, et al. Stent thrombosis is associated with an impaired response to antiplatelet therapy. *J Am Coll Cardiol* 2005;45:1748–1752.

151. The PURSUIT Investigators. Inhibition of platelet glycoprotein IIb/IIIa with eptifibatide in patients with acute coronary syndromes. *N Engl J Med* 1998;339:436–443.

152. PRISM-PLUS Investigators. Inhibition of the platelet glycoprotein IIb/IIIa receptor with tirofiban in unstable angina and non–Q-wave myocardial infarction. *N Engl J Med* 1998;338:1488–1497.

153. The CAPTURE Investigators. Randomized placebo-controlled trial of abciximab before and during coronary intervention in refractory unstable angina: the CAPTURE study. *Lancet* 1997;349:1429–1435.

154. The EPILOG Investigators. Platelet glycoprotein IIb/IIIa receptor blockade and low-dose heparin during percutaneous coronary revascularization. *N Engl J Med* 1997;336:1689–1696.

155. The EPIC Investigators. Use of a monoclonal antibody directed against the platelet glycoprotein IIb/IIIa receptor in high-risk coronary angioplasty. *N Engl J Med* 1994;330:956–961.

156. Topol EJ, Ferguson JJ, Weisman HF, et al. Long-term protection from myocardial ischemic events after brief integrin beta$_3$ blockade with percutaneous coronary intervention. *JAMA* 1997;278:479–484.

157. Karvouni E, Katritsis DG, Ioannidis JPA. Intravenous glycoprotein IIb/IIIa receptor antagonists reduce mortality after percutaneous coronary interventions. *J Am Coll Cardiol* 2003;41:26–32.

158. Boersma E, Akkerhuis M, Theroux P, et al. Platelet glycoprotein IIb/IIIa receptor inhibition in non–ST-elevation acute coronary syndromes: early benefit during medical treatment only, with additional protection during percutaneous coronary intervention. *Circulation* 1999;100:2045–2048.

159. The EPISTENT Investigators. Randomized placebo-controlled and balloon angioplasty-controlled trial to access safety of coronary stenting with use of platelet glycoprotein-IIb/IIIa blockade. *Lancet* 1998;352:87–92.

160. Lincoff AM, Califf RM, Moliterno DJ, et al. Complementary clinical benefits of coronary artery stenting and blockade of platelet glycoprotein IIb/IIIa receptors. *N Engl J Med* 1999;341:319–327.

161. The ERASER Investigators. Acute platelet inhibition with abciximab does not reduce in-stent restenosis (ERASER study). *Circulation* 1999;100:799–806.

162. Roffi M, Chew DP, Mukherjee D, et al. Platelet glycoprotein IIb/IIIa inhibitors reduce mortality in diabetic patients with non–ST-segment-elevation acute coronary syndromes. *Circulation* 2001;104:2767–2771.

163. Hamm CW, Heeschen C, Goldman B, et al. Benefit of abciximab in patients with refractory unstable angina in relation to serum troponin T levels. *N Engl J Med* 1999;340:1623–1629.

164. The ESPRIT investigators. Novel dosing regimen of eptifibatide in planned stent implantation (ESPRIT): a randomized placebo-controlled trial. *Lancet* 2000;356:2037–2044.

165. Puma JA, Banko LT, Pieper KS, et al. Clinical characteristics predict benefits from eptifibatide therapy during coronary stenting: insights from the Enhanced Suppression of the Platelet IIb/IIIa Receptor with Integrilin Therapy (ESPRIT) trial. *J Am Coll Cardiol* 2006;47:715–718.

166. Kastrati A, Mehilli J, Neumann FJ, et al. Abciximab in patients with acute coronary syndromes undergoing percutaneous coronary intervention after

clopidogrel pretreatment. The ISAR-REACT 2 Randomized trial. *JAMA* 2005;295:1531–1538.

167. Tang WHW, Lincoff AM. Diabetes, coronary intervention, and platelet glycoprotein IIb/IIIa blockade. The triad revisited. *Circulation* 2004;110:3618–3620.

168. Colombo A, Stankovic G. The value of selectivity. *J Am Coll Cardiol* 2006;47:719–720.

169. Leopold JA. Small-molecule glycoprotein IIb/IIIa antagonist and bleeding risk in women. Too much of a good thing? *Circulation* 2006;114:1344–1346.

170. Ndrepepa G, Kastrati A, Mehilli J, et al. Age-dependent effect of abciximab in patients with acute coronary syndromes treated with PCI. *Circulation* 2006;114:2040–2046.

171. Chew DP, Bhatt DL, Lincoff MA, et al. Defining the optimal activated clotting time during percutaneous coronary intervention: aggregate results from 6 randomized, controlled trials. *Circulation* 2001;103:961–966.

172. Tolleson TR, O'Shea JC, Bittl JA, et al. Relationship between heparin anticoagulation and clinical outcomes in coronary stent intervention—observations from the ESPRIT Trial. *J Am Coll Cardiol* 2003;41:386–393.

173. Collet JP, Montalescot G, Lison L, et al. Percutaneous coronary intervention after subcutaneous enoxaparin pretreatment in patients with unstable angina pectoris. *Circulation* 2001;103:658–663.

174. Martin JL, Fry ETA, Serano A, et al. Pharmacokinetic study of enoxaparin in patients undergoing coronary intervention after treatment with subcutaneous enoxaparin in acute coronary syndromes. The PEPCI study. *Eur Heart J* 2001;22:143.

175. Choussat R, Montalescot G, Philippe J, et al. A unique, low dose of intravenous enoxaparin in elective percutaneous coronary intervention. *J Am Coll Cardiol* 2002;40:1943–1950.

176. Ferguson JJ, Califf RM, Antman EM, et al. Enoxaparin vs. unfractionated heparin in high-risk patients with non-ST segment elevation acute coronary syndromes managed with an intended early invasive strategy: primary results of the SYNERGY randomized trial. *JAMA* 2004;292:45–54.

177. Boretain M, Montalescot G, Bouzamondo A, et al. Low-molecular-weight vs. unfractionated heparin in percutaneous coronary intervention: a combined analysis. *Catheter Cardiovasc Interv* 2005;65:212–221.

178. Montalescot G, White HD, Gallo R, et al. Enoxaparin versus unfractionated heparin in elective percutaneous coronary intervention. *N Engl J Med* 2006;10:1006–1017.

179. Bittl JA, Strony J, Brinker JA, et al. Treatment with bivalirudin (Hirulog) as compared with heparin during coronary angioplasty for unstable or postinfarction angina. Hirulog Angioplasty Study Investigators. *N Engl J Med* 1995;333:764–769.

180. Bittl J, Chaitman B, Feit F, et al. Bivalirudin versus heparin during coronary angioplasty for unstable or postinfarction angina: final report reanalysis of the Bivalirudin Angioplasty Study. *Am Heart J* 2001;142:952–959.

181. Lincoff AM, Bittl JA, Kleiman NS, et al. The REPLACE I trial; a pilot study of bivalirudin versus heparin during percutaneous coronary intervention. *J Am Coll Cardiol* 2002;39:16a.

182. Lincoff AM, Bittl JA, Harrington RA, et al. Bivalirudin and provisional glycoprotein IIb/IIIa blockade compared with heparin and planned glycoprotein IIb/IIIa blockade during percutaneous coronary intervention. *JAMA* 2003;289:853–863.

183. Stone GW. Presentation TCT 2006.

184. Antman EM. Should bivalirudin replace heparin during percutaneous coronary interventions? *JAMA* 2003;289:903–905.

185. Herrmann J, Lerman A, Baumgart D, et al. Preprocedural statin medication reduces the extent of periprocedural non–Q-wave myocardial infarction. *Circulation* 2002;106:2180–2183.

186. Pasceri V, Parri G, Nusca A, et al. Randomized trial of atorvastatin for reduction of myocardial damage during coronary intervention: results from ARMYDA (Atorvastatin for Reduction of Myocardial Damage During Angioplasty) study. *Circulation* 2004;110:674–678.

187. Patti G, Chello M, Paseri V, et al. Protection from procedural myocardial injury by atorvastatin is associated with lower levels of adhesion molecules after percutaneous coronary intervention: results from the ARMYDA-CAMs (Atorvastatin for Reduction of Myocardial Damage during Angioplasty–Cell Adhesion Molecules) substudy. *J Am Coll Cardiol* 2006;48:1560–1566.

188. Chan AW, Bhatt DL, Chew DP, et al. Early and sustained survival benefit associated with statin therapy at the time of percutaneous coronary intervention. *Circulation* 2002;105:691–696.

189. Schomig A, Mehilli J, Holle H, et al. Statin treatment following coronary artery stenting and one-year survival. *J Am Coll Cardiol* 2002;40:854–861.

190. Uretsky BF, Schwarz ER, Osmana, et al. Intracoronary beta blockage during percutaneous coronary intervention: 30-day results of randomized angio-

plasty beta blocker intracoronary trial II. *Circulation* 2006;114(Suppl II):II-547.

191. Chan AW, Quinn MJ, Bhatt DL, et al. Mortality benefit of beta-blockade after successful elective percutaneous coronary intervention. *J Am Coll Cardiol* 2002;40:669–675.

192. Takagi A, Tsurumi Y, Ishii Y, et al. Clinical potential of intravascular ultrasound for physiological assessment of coronary stenosis: relationship between quantitative ultrasound tomography and pressure-derived fractional flow reserve. *Circulation* 1999;100:250.

193. Nishioka T, Amanullah AM, Luo H, et al. Clinical validation of intravascular ultrasound imaging for assessment of coronary stenosis severity: comparison with stress myocardial perfusion imaging. *J Am Coll Cardiol* 1999;33:1870.

194. Jasti V, Ivan E, Yalamanchili V, et al. Correlations between fractional flow reserve and intravascular ultrasound in patients with an ambiguous left main coronary artery stenosis. *Circulation* 2004;110:2831–2836.

195. Fassa AA, Wagatsuma K, Higano ST, et al. Intravascular ultrasound-guided treatment for angiographically indeterminant left main coronary artery disease. *J Am Coll Cardiol* 2005;45:204–211.

196. Mintz GS, Weissman NJ. Intravascular ultrasound in the drug-eluting stent era. *J Am Coll Cardiol* 2006;48:421–429.

197. Hong M, Mintz GS, Lee GW, et al. Late stent malapposition after drug-eluting stent implantation: an intravascular ultrasound analysis with long-term follow-up. *Circulation* 2006;113:313–419.

198. Pijls NH, van Son JA, Kirkeeide RL, et al. Experimental basis of determining maximum coronary, myocardial, and collateral blood flow by pressure measurements for assessing functional stenosis severity before and after percutaneous transluminal coronary angioplasty. *Circulation* 1993;87:1354.

199. Pijls NH, De Bruyne B, Peels K, et al. Measurements of fractional flow reserve to assess the functional severity of coronary artery stenoses. *N Engl J Med* 1996;334:1703.

200. Bech GJ, De Bruyne B, Pijls NH, et al. Fractional flow reserve to determine the appropriateness of angioplasty in moderate coronary stenosis: a randomized trial. *Circulation* 2001;103:2928.

201. Samady H, McDaniel MC, Veledar E, et al. Pre-stent fractional flow reserve and stent diameter predict optimal post-stent fractional flow reserve: implications for selection of drug-eluting stents. *Circulation* 2006;114(Suppl II):II-784.

202. Saber RS, Edwards WD, Bailey KR, et al. Coronary embolization after balloon angioplasty or thrombolytic therapy: an autopsy study of 32 cases. *J Am Coll Cardiol* 1993;22:1283–1288.

203. Topol EJ, Yadav JS. Recognition of the importance of embolization in atherosclerotic vascular disease. *Circulation* 2000;101:570–580.

204. Baim DS, Cutlip DE, Sharma SK, et al. Final results of the Balloon Versus Optimal Atherectomy Trial (BOAT). *Circulation* 1998;97:322–331.

205. Simonton CA, Leon MB, Baim DS, et al. "Optimal" directional coronary atherectomy: final results of the Optimal Atherectomy Restenosis Study (OARS). *Circulation* 1998;97:332–339.

206. Colombo A. Atherectomy Before MULTI-LINK Improves Luminal Gain and Clinical Outcomes (AMIGO): a comparison of coronary stenting with or without adjunctive directional coronary atherectomy. *J Am Coll Cardiol* 2002;40:4.

207. Murphy GJ, Bryan AJ, Angelini GD. Hybrid coronary revascularization in the era of drug-eluting stents. *Ann Thorac Surg* 2004;78:1861–1867.

208. Vassiliades TA, Douglas JS, Morris DC, et al. Integrated coronary revascularization with drug-eluting stents: immediate and seven-month outcome. *J Thorac Cardiovasc Surg* 2006;131:956–962.

209. Kiaii B, McClure RS, Rayman R, et al. A novel approach to integrated coronary artery revascularization using bivalirudin. *Circulation* (In press).

210. Damp J, Zhao DX, Greelish J, et al. Intra-operative completion angiography after CABG with immediate catheterization or surgical revision of defects: one year experience from the Vanderbilt Hybrid Catheterization and Operating Room. *Circulation* 2006;114(Suppl II):II:429.

211. Kar B, Forrester M, Gemmato C, et al. Use of the TandemHeart percutaneous ventricular assist device to support patients undergoing high-risk percutaneous coronary intervention. *J Invasive Cardiol* 2006;18:93–98.

212. Burkhoff D, O'Neill W, Brunckhorst C, et al. Feasibility study of the use of the TandemHeart percutaneous ventricular assist device for the treatment of cardiogenic shock. *Catheter Cardiovasc Interv* 2006;68:211–217.

213. Smith SC Jr, Dove JT, Jacobs AK, et al. ACC/AHA guidelines for percutaneous coronary intervention (revision of the 1993 guidelines for percutaneous transluminal coronary angioplasty). *J Am Coll Cardiol* 2001;37:2239.

214. Weintraub WS, King SB III, Douglas JS Jr, et al. Percutaneous transluminal coronary angioplasty as a first revascularization procedure in single, double,

and triple-vessel coronary artery disease. *J Am Coll Cardiol* 1995;26:142–151.

215. Mark DB, Nelson CL, Califf RM, et al. Continuing evaluation and therapy for coronary artery disease: initial results from the era of coronary angioplasty. *Circulation* 1994;89:2015–2025.

216. Strauss WE, Fortin T, Hartigan P, et al. A comparison of quality of life scores in patients with angina pectoris after angioplasty compared with after medical therapy: outcomes of a randomized clinical trial. *Circulation* 1995;92:1710–1719.

217. Giacomini JC, Parisi AF, Folland ED, et al. Three year follow-up of patients in the VA ACME trial. *Circulation* 1993;88(Suppl I):I-218.

218. Hueb WA, Soares PR, de Oliveiras A, et al. Five-year follow-up of the Medicine, Angioplasty, or Surgery Study (MASS): a prospective, randomized trial of medical therapy, balloon angioplasty, or bypass surgery for single proximal left anterior descending coronary artery stenosis. *Circulation* 1999;100(Suppl II):II-107–II-113.

219. Goy JJ, Eickhout E, Burnand B. Coronary angioplasty versus left internal mammary artery grafting for isolated proximal left anterior descending artery stenosis. *Lancet* 1994;343:1449–1454.

220. Versaci F, Gaspardone A, Fabrizio P, et al. A comparison of coronary artery stenting with angioplasty for isolated stenosis of the proximal left anterior descending coronary artery. *N Engl J Med* 1997;336:817–822.

221. Diegeler A, Thiele H, Falk V, et al. Comparison of stenting with minimally invasive bypass surgery for stenosis of the left anterior descending coronary artery. *N Engl J Med* 2002;347:561–566.

222. Ellis SG, Brown K, Howell G, et al. Two-year cardiac cost after cardiac catheterization: Profound impact of revascularization after first PTCA compared with initial medical or surgical therapy. *J Am Coll Cardiol* 1996;27(Suppl A):72A.

223. Brophy JM, Sleight P. Enthusiasm, reality, and cost-effectiveness analysis. *Heart* 1998;79:9–11.

224. Vassiliades TA, Rogers EW, Nielsen JL, et al. Minimally invasive direct coronary artery bypass grafting: intermediate-term results. *Ann Thorac Surg* 2000;70:1963–1065.

225. Cowley MJ, Vandermael M, Topol EJ. Is traditionally defined complete revascularization needed for patients with multivessel disease treated with elective coronary angioplasty? *J Am Coll Cardiol* 1993;22:1289–1297.

226. Bourassa MG, Holubkov R, Yeh W, et al. Strategy of complete revascularization in patients with multivessel coronary artery disease: a report from the 1985–1986 NHLBI PTCA Registry. *Am J Cardiol* 1992;70:174–178.

227. Zhao XQ, Brown BG, Stewart DK, et al. Effectiveness of revascularization in the Emory Angioplasty Versus Surgery Trial: A randomized comparison of coronary angioplasty with bypass surgery. *Circulation* 1996;93:1954–1962.

228. Kip KE, Bourassa MG, Jacobs AK, et al. Influence of pre-PTCA strategy and initial PTCA result in patients with multivessel disease: the Bypass Angioplasty Revascularization Investigation (BARI). *Circulation* 1999;100:910–917.

229. Ellis SG, Roubin GS, King SB III, et al. Angiographic and clinical predictors of acute closure after native vessel coronary angioplasty. *Circulation* 1988;77:372–379.

230. Laham RJ, Ho KL, Baim DS, et al. Palmaz-Schatz stenting: early results and one-year outcome. *J Am Coll Cardiol* 1997;30:180–185.

231. Moussa I, Reiners B, Moses J, et al. A long-term angiographic and clinical outcome of patients undergoing multivessel coronary stenting. *Circulation* 1997;96:3873–3979.

232. Hernandez-Antolin RA, Alfonso F, Goicolea J, et al. Results (>6 months) of stenting of >1 major coronary artery in multivessel coronary artery disease. *Am J Cardiol* 1999;84:147–151.

233. Braunwald E, Antman EM, Beasley JW, et al. ACC/AHA 2002 guidelines for the management of patients with unstable angina and non-st-segment elevation myocardial infarction. *J Am Coll Cardiol* 2002;40:1366–1374.

234. Sabatine MS, Morrow DA, Giugliano RP, et al. Implications of upstream GP IIb/IIIa inhibition and stenting in the invasive management of UA/NSTEMI: a comparison of TIMI IIIb and TACTICS-TIMI 18. *Circulation* 2001;104:II-549.

235. Westerhout CM, Fu Y, Lauer MS, et al. Short- and long-term risk stratification in acute coronary syndromes. The added value of quantitative ST-segment depression and multiple biomarkers. *J Am Coll Cardiol* 2006;48:939–947.

236. Giugliano RP, Braunwald E. The year in non-ST-segment elevation acute coronary syndromes. *J Am Coll Cardiol* 2006;48:386–395.

237. Moses JW, Mehran R, Nikolsky E, et al. Outcomes with the paclitaxel-eluting stent in patients with acute coronary syndromes: analysis from the TAXUS-IV trial. *J Am Coll Cardiol* 2005;45:1165–1171.

238. Bolognese L, Falsini G, Liistro F, et al. Randomized comparison of upstream tirofiban versus downstream high bolus dose tirofiban or abciximab on tissue-level perfusion and troponin release in high-risk acute coronary syndromes treated with percutaneous coronary interventions: the EVEREST trial. *J Am Coll Cardiol* 2006;47:522–528.

239. Glaser R, Glick HA, Hermann HC, et al. The role of risk stratification in the decision to provide upstream versus selective glycoprotein IIb/IIIa inhibitors for acute coronary syndromes: a cost-effective analysis. *J Am Coll Cardiol* 2006;47:529–537.

240. Bavry AA, Kumbhani DJ, Rassi AN, et al. Benefit of early invasive therapy in acute coronary syndromes. A meta-analysis of contemporary randomized clinical trials. *J Am Coll Cardiol* 2006;48:1319–1325.

241. Ryan JW, Peterson ED, Chen AY, et al. Optimal timing of intervention in non–ST-segment elevation acute coronary syndromes. Insights from the CRUSADE (Can Rapid risk stratification of Unstable angina patients Suppress Adverse outcomes with Early implantation of the ACC/AHA guidelines) Registry. *Circulation* 2005;112:3049–3057.

242. Tricoci P, Lokhnygina Y, Berdan LG, et al. Shortening time to cardiac catheterization is associated with improved outcomes among patients with non-ST-segment elevation acute coronary syndromes: Results from the Randomized Synergy Trial. *Circulation* 2006;114(Suppl II):II-421.

243. Neumann FJ, Kastrati A, Pogastsa-Murray G, et al. Evaluation of prolonged antithrombotic pretreatment ("cooling off" strategy) before intervention in patients with unstable coronary syndromes: a randomized controlled trial. *JAMA* 2003;290:1593–1599.

244. Peterson ED, Roe MT, Mulgund J, et al. Association between hospital process performance and outcomes among patients with acute coronary syndromes. *JAMA* 2006;295:1912–1920.

245. Zaaks SM, Allen JE, Calvin JE, et al. Value of the American College of Cardiology/American Heart Association stenosis morphology classification for coronary interventions in the late 1990s. *Am J Cardiol* 1998;82:43–49.

246. Krone RJ, Laskey WK, Johnson C, et al. A simplified lesion classification for predicting success and complications of coronary angioplasty. Registry Committee of the Society for Cardiac Angiography and Intervention. *Am J Cardiol* 2000;85:1179–1184.

247. Krone RJ, Shaw RE, Klein LW, et al. Evaluation of the American College of Cardiology/American Heart Association and the Society for Coronary Angiography and Interventions lesion classification system in the current "stent era" of coronary interventions (from the ACC-National Cardiovascular Data Registry). *Am J Cardiol* 2003;92:389–394.

248. O'Keefe JH, Hartzler GO, Rutherford BD, et al. Left main coronary angioplasty: early and late results of 127 acute and elective procedures. *Am J Cardiol* 1989;64:144–147.

249. Ellis SG, Tamai H, Nobuyoshi M, et al. Contemporary percutaneous treatment of unprotected left main coronary stenoses: initial results from a multicenter registry analysis 1994–1996. *Circulation* 1997;96:3867–3872.

250. Park SJ, Park SW, Hong MK, et al. Long-term (three-year) outcomes after stenting of unprotected left main coronary artery stenosis in patients with normal left ventricular function. *Am J Cardiol* 2003;91:12–16.

251. Takagi T, Stankovic G, Finci L, et al. Results and long-term predictors of adverse clinical events after elective percutaneous interventions in unprotected left main coronary artery. *Circulation* 2002;106:698–702.

252. Park SJ, Kim YH, Lee BK, et al. Sirolimus-eluting stent implantation for unprotected left main coronary artery stenosis: comparison with bare metal stent implantation. *J Am Coll Cardiol* 2005;45:351–356.

253. Chieffo G, Stankovic G, Bonizzoni E, et al. Early and mid-term results of drug-eluting stent implantation in unprotected left main. *Circulation* 2005;111:791–795.

254. Colombo A, Moses JW, Morice MC, et al. Randomized study to evaluate sirolimus-eluting stents implanted at coronary bifurcation lesions. *Circulation* 2004;109:1244–1249.

255. Lee MS, Kapoor N, Jamal F, et al. Comparison of coronary artery bypass surgery with percutaneous coronary intervention with drug-eluting stents for unprotected left main coronary artery disease. *J Am Coll Cardiol* 2006;47:864–870.

256. Ellis SG, Hill CM, Lytle BW. Spectrum of surgical risk for left main coronary stenoses: benchmark for potentially competing percutaneous therapies. *Am Heart J* 1998;135:335–338.

257. Sabik JF, Blackstone EH, Firstenberg MS, et al. A benchmark for evaluating innovative treatment of left main coronary disease. *Circulation* 2006;114(Suppl II):II-431.

258. Price MJ, Cristea E, Sawhney N, et al. Serial angiographic follow-up of sirolimus-eluting stents for unprotected left main coronary artery revascularization. *J Am Coll Cardiol* 2006;47:871–877.

259. Chieffo A, Morici N, Maisano F, et al. Percutaneous treatment with drug-eluting stent implantation versus bypass surgery for unprotected left main stenosis. A single-center experience. *Circulation* 2006;113:2542–2547.

260. Kim Y, Park S, Hong M, et al. Comparison of simple and complex stenting techniques in the treatment of unprotected left main coronary artery bifurcation stenosis. *Am J Cardiol* 2006;97:1597–1601.

261. Valgimigli M, Malagutti P, Aoki J, et al. Sirolimus-eluting versus paclitaxel-eluting stent implantation for the percutaneous treatment of left main coronary artery disease. A combined RESEARCH and T-SEARCH long-term analysis. *J Am Coll Cardiol* 2006;47:507–514.

262. Abbott JD, Kip KE, Vlachos HA, et al. Recent trends in the percutaneous treatment of chronic total coronary occlusions. *Am J Cardiol* 2006;97:1691–1696.

263. Olivari Z, Rubartelli P, Piscione F, et al. Immediate results and one-year clinical outcome after percutaneous coronary interventions in chronic total occlusions: data from a multicenter, prospective, observational study (TOAST-GISE). *J Am Coll Cardiol* 2003;41:1672–1678.

264. Hannan EL, Racz M, Holmes DR, et al. Impact of completeness of percutaneous coronary intervention revascularization on long-term outcomes in the stent era. *Circulation* 2006;113:2406–2412.

265. Stone GW, Kandzari DE, Mehran R, et al. Percutaneous recanalization of chronically occluded coronary arteries: a consensus document: part I. *Circulation* 2005;112:2364–2372.

266. Stone GW, Reifart NJ, Moussa I, et al. Percutaneous recanalization of chronically occluded coronary arteries: a consensus document: part II. *Circulation* 2005;112:2530–2537.

267. Douglas JS Jr. Percutaneous intervention in chronic total occlusions. In: King SB III, Yeung A, eds. *Interventional Cardiology*. New York: McGraw-Hill, 2007:385–391.

268. Baim DS, Braden G, Heuser R, et al. Utility of the Safe-Cross-guided radiofrequency total occlusion crossing system in chronic coronary total occlusions (results from the Guided Radio Frequency Energy Ablation of Total Occlusion Registry Study). *Am J Cardiol* 2004;94:853–858.

269. Tsuchikane E, Katoh O, Shinogami M, et al. First clinical experience of a novel penetration catheter for patients with severe coronary artery stenosis. *Catheter Cardiovasc Interv* 2005;65:368–373.

270. Abbas AE, Bewington SD, Dixon SR, et al. Intracoronary fibrin-specific thrombolytic infusion facilitates percutaneous recanalization of chronic total occlusions. *J Am Coll Cardiol* 2005;46:793–798.

271. Kimura BJ, Tsimikas S, Bhargava V, et al. Subintimal wire position during angioplasty of a chronic total coronary occlusion: detection and subsequent procedural guidance by intravascular ultrasound. *Cathet Cardiovasc Diagn* 1995;35:262–265.

272. Hirokami M, Saito S, Muto H. Anchoring techniques to improve guiding catheter support in coronary angioplasty of chronic total occlusions. *Catheter Cardiovasc Interv* 2006;67:366–371.

273. Colombo A, Mikhail GW, Michev I, et al. Treating chronic total occlusions using subintimal tracking and reentry: the STAR technique. *Catheter Cardiovasc Interv* 2005;64:407–411.

274. Surmely J, Tsuchikane E, Katoh, et al. New concept for CTO recanalization using controlled antegrade and retrograde subintimal tracking: the CART technique. *J Invasive Cardiol* 2006;18:334–338.

275. Mollet NR, Hoye A, Lemos PA, et al. Value of preprocedure multislice computed tomographic coronary angiography to predict the outcome of percutaneous recanalization of chronic total occlusions. *Am J Cardiol* 2005;95:240–243.

276. Katsuragawa M, Fujiwara H, Miyamae M, et al. Histologic studies in percutaneous transluminal coronary angioplasty for chronic total occlusion: comparison of tapering and abrupt types of occlusion and short and long occluded segments. *J Am Coll Cardiol* 1993;21:604.

277. Suttorp MJ, Laarman GJ, Rahel BM, et al. Primary stenting of totally occluded native coronary arteries II (PRISON II): a randomized comparison of bare metal stent implantation with sirolimus-eluting stent implantation for the treatment of total coronary occlusions. *Circulation* 2006;114:921–928.

278. Nakamura S, Murhasamy TS, Bae JH, et al. Comparison of efficacy and safety between sirolimus-eluting stent (Cypher) and paclitaxel-eluting stent (Taxus) on the outcome of patients with chronic total occlusions: Multicenter Registry of Asia. *J Am Coll Cardiol* 2005;45(Suppl A):48A.

279. Garot P, Lefevre T, Savage M, et al. Nine-month outcome of patients treated by percutaneous coronary interventions for bifurcation lesions in the recent era. A report from the Prevention of Restenosis With Tranilast and Its Outcomes (PRESTO) trial. *J Am Coll Cardiol* 2005;46:606–612.

280. Melikian N, DiMario C. Treatment of bifurcation coronary lesions: a review of current techniques and outcomes. *J Interv Cardiol* 2003;16:507–513.

281. Brunel P, Lefevre T, Darremont O, et al. Provisional T-stenting and kissing balloon in the treatment of coronary bifurcation lesions: results of the French Multicenter "TULIPE" Study. *Catheter Cardiovasc Interv* 2006;68:67–73.

282. Colombo A, Moses JW, Morice MC, et al. Randomized study to evaluate sirolimus-eluting stents implanted at coronary bifurcation lesion. *Circulation* 2004;109:1244–1249.

283. Delgado A, Ojeda S, Melian F, et al. Rapamycin-eluting stents for the treatment of bifurcated coronary lesions: a randomized comparison of a simple versus complex strategy. *Am Heart J* 2004;148:857–864.

284. Hoye A, Iakovou I, Ge L, et al. Long-term outcomes after stenting of bifurcation lesions with the "Crush" technique. Predictor of adverse outcome. *J Am Coll Cardiol* 2006;47:1949–1958.

285. Ormiston JA, Currie E, Webster MWI, et al. Drug-eluting stents for coronary bifurcation: insights into the crush technique. *Catheter Cardiovasc Interv* 2004;63:332–336.

286. Ormiston JA, Webster MWI, Jack SE, et al. Drug-eluting stents for coronary bifurcation: bench testing of provisional side-branch strategies. *Catheter Cardiovasc Interv* 2006;67:49–55.

287. Sharma SK. Simultaneous kissing drug-eluting stent technique for percutaneous treatment of bifurcation lesions in large-size vessels. *Cathet Cardiovasc Interv* 2005;65:10–16.

288. Steigen TK, Maeng M, Wiseth R, et al. Randomized study on simple versus complex stenting of coronary artery bifurcation lesions. The Nordic Bifurcation Study. *Circulation* 2006;114:1955–1961.

289. Koo B, Kang H, Youn T, et al. Physiologic assessment of jailed side branch lesions using fractional flow reserve. *J Am Coll Cardiol* 2005;46:633–637.

290. Chen, MS, John JM, Chew DP, et al. Bare metal stent restenosis is not a benign clinical entity. *Am Heart J* 2006;151:1260–1264.

291. Nayak AK, Kawamura A, Nesto RW, et al. Myocardial infarction as a presentation of clinical in-stent restenosis. *Circ J* 2006;70:1026–1029.

292. Mehan R, Dangas G, Abizaid AS, et al. Angiographic patterns of in-stent restenosis: classification and implications for long-term outcome. *Circulation* 1999;100:1872–1878.

293. Waksman R, Ajani AE, White RL, et al. Five-year follow-up after intracoronary radiation: results of a randomized clinical trial. *Circulation* 2004;105:2737–2740.

294. Stone GW, Ellis SG, O'Shaughnessy CD, et al. for the TAXUS V ISR Investigators. Paclitaxel-eluting stents vs. vascular brachytherapy for in-stent restenosis within bare-metal stents: the TAXUS V ISR randomized trial. *JAMA* 2006;295:1253–1263.

295. Holmes DR Jr, Teirstein P, Satler L, et al. For the SISR Investigators. Sirolimus-eluting stents vs. vascular brachytherapy for in-stent restenosis within bare-metal stents: the SISR randomized trial. *JAMA* 2006;295:1264–1273.

296. Dibra A, Kastrati A, Alfonso F, et al. Effectiveness of drug-eluting stents in patients with bare-metal in-stent restenosis. Meta-analysis of randomized trials. *J Am Coll Cardiol* 2007;48:1304–1309.

297. Scheller B, Hehrlein C, Bocksch W, et al. Treatment of coronary in-stent restenosis with a paclitaxel-coated balloon catheter. *N Engl J Med* 2006;355:2113–2124.

298. Cosgrave J, Melzi G, Biondi-Zoccai G, et al. Drug-eluting stent restenosis. The pattern predicts the outcome. *J Am Coll Cardiol* 2006;47:2399–2404.

299. Cosgrave J, Melzi G, Corbett S, et al. Repeat drug-eluting stent implantation for drug-eluting stent restenosis: the same or a different stent. *Circulation* 2006;114(Suppl II):II-698.

300. Roffi M, Mukherjee D, Chew DP, et al. Lack of benefit from intravenous platelet glycoprotein IIb/IIIa receptor inhibition as adjunctive treatment for percutaneous interventions of aortocoronary bypass grafts—a pooled analysis of five randomized clinical trials. *Circulation* 2002;106:3063–3067.

301. Savage MP, Douglas JS, Fischman DL, et al. Stent placement compared with balloon angioplasty for obstructed coronary bypass grafts. *N Engl J Med* 1997;337:740–747.

302. Baim DS, Wahr D, George B, et al. Randomized trial of distal embolic protection device during percutaneous intervention of saphenous vein aorto-coronary bypass grafts. *Circulation* 2002;105:1285–1290.

303. Stone GW, Rogers C, Hermiller J, et al. Randomized comparison distal protection with a filter-based catheter and a balloon occlusion and aspiration system during percutaneous intervention of diseased saphenous vein aorto-coronary bypass grafts. *Circulation* 2003;108:548–553.

304. Carrozza JP, Mumma M, Breall JA, et al. Randomized evaluation of the Tri-Activ Balloon-Protection flush and extraction system for the treatment of saphenous vein graft disease. *J Am Coll Cardiol* 2005;46:1677–1683.

305. Rogers C. Proximal protection during saphenous vein graft intervention using the Proxis embolic protective system: a randomized, prospective, multi-center clinical trial (PROXIMAL). Presented at TCT 2005. Washington, DC. *J Am Coll Cardiol* 2004;44:1801.

306. Cohen DJ, Murphy SA, Baim DS, et al. Cost-effectiveness of distal embolic protection for patients undergoing percutaneous intervention of saphenous vein bypass grafts: Results from the SAFER trial. *J Am Coll Cardiol* 2004;44:1801–1808.

307. Kong DF, Mark DB. Economic impact of new interventional therapies: are we asking the right questions? *J Am Coll Cardiol* 2004;44:1809–1811.

308. Rogers C, Huynh R, Seifert PA, et al. Embolic protection with filtering or occlusion balloons during saphenous vein graft stenting retrieves identical volumes and sizes of particulate debris. *Circulation* 2004;109:1735–1740.

309. Leineweber K, Bose D, Vogelsang M, et al. Intense vasoconstriction in response to aspirate from stented saphenous vein aortocoronary bypass grafts. *J Am Coll Cardiol* 2006;47:981–986.

310. Huang RI, Patel P, Walinsky P, et al. Efficacy of intracoronary nicardipine in the treatment of no-reflow during percutaneous coronary intervention. *Catheter Cardiovasc Interv* 2006;68:671–676.

311. Vermeersch P, Van Langenhove G, Covens C, et al. First randomized trial comparing sirolimus-eluting stents versus bare metal stents in severely diseased saphenous vein graft treatment six month clinical and angiographic outcome. *J Am Coll Cardiol* 2005;45(Suppl A):84A.

312. Ashfaq S, Ghazzal Z, Douglas JS, et al. Impact of diabetes on five-year outcomes after vein graft interventions performed prior to the drug-eluting stent era. *J Invasive Cardiol* 2006;18:100–105.

313. Wu C, Hannan EL, Walford G, et al. A risk score to predict in-hospital mortality for percutaneous coronary interventions. *J Am Coll Cardiol* 2006;47:654–660.

314. Weintraub WS. Evaluating the risk of coronary surgery and percutaneous coronary intervention. *J Am Coll Cardiol* 2006;47:669–671.

315. Singh M, Rihal CS, Lennon RJ, et al. A critical appraisal of current models of risk stratification for percutaneous coronary interventions. *Am Heart J* 2005;149:753–760.

316. Prasad A, Singh M, Lerman A, et al. Isolated elevation in troponin T after percutaneous coronary intervention is associated with higher long-term mortality. *J Am Coll Cardiol* 2006;48:1765–1770.

317. Presbitero P, Gasparini GL, Pagnotta P. Intra-arterial thrombolysis for left middle cerebral artery embolic stroke during coronary angiography. *Circulation* 2006;113:e64–e66.

318. O'Neill WW. Risk of bleeding after elective percutaneous coronary intervention. *N Engl J Med* 2006;355:10.

319. Ellis SG, Bhatt D, Kapadia S, et al. Correlates and outcomes of retroperitoneal hemorrhage complicating percutaneous coronary intervention. *Catheter Cardiovasc Interv* 2006;67:541–545.

320. Bajzer CT, Whitlow PL, Lincoff M, et al. Coronary perforation and pericardial tamponade risk in the abciximab era. *J Am Coll Cardiol* 1999;33:72A.

321. Fasseas P, Orford JL, Panetta CJ, et al. Incidence, correlates, management and clinical outcome of coronary perforation: analysis of 16,298 procedures. *Am Heart J* 2004;47:140–145.

322. Dippel EJ, Kereiakes DJ, Tramuta DA, et al. Coronary perforation during percutaneous coronary intervention in the era of abciximab platelet glycoprotein IIb/IIIa blockade: an algorithm for percutaneous management. *Catheter Cardiovasc Interv* 2001;52:279–286.

323. Fejka M, Dixon SR, Safian RD, et al. Diagnosis, management, and clinical outcome of cardiac tamponade complicating percutaneous coronary intervention. *Am J Cardiol* 2002;90:1183–1186.

324. Fischell TA, Carter AJ, Ashraf K, et al. Coronary artery rupture during balloon angioplasty, rescued with localized thrombin injection and coil embolization. *Catheter Cardiovasc Interv* 2006;68:254–257.

325. Petrie MC, Peels JOJ, Jessurun G. The role of covered stents: more than an occasional cameo? *Catheter Cardiovasc Interv* 2006;68:21–26.

326. Colombo A. Covered stents: no class I A indication but "thank God they still exist!" *Catheter Cardiovasc Interv* 2006;68:27–28.

327. Patterson M, Slagboom T. Intracoronary stent dislodgment: updated strategy enabled by the new generation of materials. *Catheter Cardiovasc Interv* 2006;67:386–390.

328. Dunning W, Kahn JK, Hawkins ET, et al. Iatrogenic coronary artery dissections extending into and involving the aortic root. *Catheter Cardiovasc Interv* 2000;51:387–393.

329. McCullough PA, Wolyn R, Rocher LL, et al. Acute contrast nephropathy after coronary intervention: Incidence, risk factors and relationship to mortality. *J Am Coll Cardiol* 1996;17(Suppl A):304A.

330. McCullough PA, Bertrand ME, Brinker JA, et al. A meta-analysis of the renal safety of isosmolar iodixanol compared with low-osmolar contrast media. *J Am Coll Cardiol* 2006;48:692–699.

331. Tepel M, Aspelin P, Lameire N. Contrast-induced nephropathy. A clinical and evidence-based approach. *Circulation* 2006;113:1799–1806.

332. Cutlip DE, Baim DS, Ho KK, et al. Stent thrombosis in the modern era: a pooled analysis of multicenter coronary stent clinical trials. *Circulation* 2001;103:1967–1971.

333. Pfisterer M, Brunner-LaRocca HP, Buser PT, et al. Late clinical events after clopidogrel discontinuation may limit the benefit of drug-eluting stents. *J Am Coll Cardiol* 2006;48:2584–2591.

334. Eisenstein EL, Anstrom KJ, King DF, et al. Clopidogrel use and long-term clinical outcomes after drug-eluting stent implantation. *JAMA* 2007;297:E1–E10.

335. Feres F, Gosta R, Abizaid A. Very late thrombosis after drug-eluting stents. *Catheter Cardiovasc Interv* 2006;68:83–88.

CHAPTER 63

Mechanical Interventions in Acute Myocardial Infarction

Bruce R. Brodie / William W. O'Neill

HISTORICAL OVERVIEW

Reperfusion therapy for acute myocardial infarction (AMI) had its inception with Fletcher and Tillet's initial treatise describing the use of intravenous thrombolytic therapy in thromboembolic disorders, including myocardial infarction.[1] Shortly after this, Boucek et al. published their observations using catheters to deliver fibrinolytic therapy to the aortic root of patients presenting with AMI,[2] and Favaloro et al. applied saphenous vein aortocoronary bypass surgery to patients presenting with acute infarction.[3] Two groups, one in Spokane, Washington, and one in Göttingen, Germany, performed emergency catheterization prior to surgical revascularization for AMI, and for the first time, knowledge of the coronary anatomy during AMI became available.[4,5] DeWood et al. described the high prevalence of total coronary occlusion in the early hours after acute transmural myocardial infarction, and defined the role of the electrocardiographic injury current in identifying a population of patients most likely to have acute total occlusion of the infarct artery and thus most likely to benefit from emergency revascularization.[6,7]

In 1978, Rentrop et al. performed emergency guidewire recanalization of an acute thrombotic coronary occlusion and subsequently reported on the first 13 patients with AMI treated with mechanical reperfusion.[8,9] These investigators also reported their results with selective catheter infusion of intracoronary streptokinase at the American Heart Association meetings in 1979, and the modern era of reperfusion therapy was born.[10] Once the works of DeWood and Rentrop were disseminated, enormous research interest in reperfusion therapy was generated in both Europe and the United States, and a number of randomized trials quickly followed. Khaja et al.[11]

first demonstrated the efficacy of intracoronary streptokinase administration in establishing coronary reperfusion, and the Western Washington investigators[12] documented improved survival in patients with AMI treated with intracoronary streptokinase therapy. Because of the necessity of selective coronary angiography for this treatment, it quickly became apparent that a severe residual stenosis persisted in most patients after successful thrombolysis. The Ann Arbor group demonstrated that balloon angioplasty could effectively treat the residual stenosis, and that this resulted in less recurrent ischemia and better preservation of ventricular function.[13] However, logistical constraints and the limited number of trained operators and catheterization facilities hindered the development of both intracoronary streptokinase and primary angioplasty as reperfusion strategies in the mid-1980s.

The large GISSI (Gruppo Italiano per lo Studio della Sopravvivenza nell'Infarto Miocardico) and ISIS (International Study of Infarct Survival)-2 trials,[14,15] published in 1984 and 1986, established the efficacy of intravenous streptokinase in improving survival in patients with AMI. Intravenous streptokinase with aspirin gained widespread use and became the standard of care as reperfusion therapy for AMI. Research interest soon focused on the development of new fibrin-specific thrombolytic drugs that could be administered intravenously. However, many investigators were still concerned about the severe underlying residual stenosis remaining after thrombolytic therapy, and three major randomized trials, the TAMI (Thrombolysis and Angioplasty in Myocardial Infarction), TIMI (Thrombolysis in Myocardial Infarction) II-A, and European Cooperative trials, were designed to determine the value of routine percutaneous transluminal coronary angioplasty (PTCA) after thrombolytic therapy.[16–18] These studies gave surprising and disappointing results. Not only was routine PTCA unnecessary, it appeared actually to be harmful, and angioplasty was mostly abandoned as an adjunct to thrombolytic therapy in the 1990s.

However, interest still persisted in the use of PTCA without antecedent thrombolytic therapy (primary PTCA). Large credit should be given to the pioneering work of Hartzler et al. in Kansas City, Kansas, who demonstrated the feasibility of primary PTCA.[19,20] At the same time, Brodie in Greensboro, North Carolina, and O'Neill and Grines in Royal Oak, Michigan, concluded that primary PTCA had been inadequately tested as a reperfusion modality.[21,22] These three groups joined forces and organized the original PAMI (Primary Angioplasty in Myocardial Infarction) study group. This group and investigators from the Zwolle group and the Mayo Clinic published the results of the first large randomized trials comparing primary PTCA with thrombolytic therapy in 1993.[23–25] These trials demonstrated superior outcomes with primary PTCA compared with thrombolytic therapy and established primary PTCA as a legitimate and competing reperfusion strategy for patients with AMI.

PRIMARY PERCUTANEOUS CORONARY INTERVENTION

Primary percutaneous coronary intervention (PCI) has become the preferred reperfusion strategy for ST-segment elevation myocardial infarction (STEMI) when it can be performed in a timely manner by experienced personnel.[26] This position from the American College of Cardiologists/American Heart Association (ACC/AHA) *Guidelines* is based on data from numerous randomized trials comparing primary PCI with fibrinolytic therapy.

[ ] COMPARISON OF OUTCOMES WITH PRIMARY PCI VERSUS FIBRINOLYTIC THERAPY
Comparison of Acute Clinical Outcomes

Keeley and Grines performed a meta-analysis of 23 randomized trials incorporating 7739 patients comparing primary PCI with

fibrinolytic therapy for STEMI.[27] Primary PCI was superior to fibrinolytic therapy in reducing short-term mortality (5.3 percent vs. 7.4 percent; $p = 0.0003$), nonfatal reinfarction (2.5 percent vs. 6.8 percent; $p < 0.0001$), stroke (1.0 percent vs. 2.0 percent; $p = 0.0004$), and the composite end point of death, nonfatal reinfarction, and stroke (8.2 percent vs. 14.3 percent; $p = 0.0001$; Fig. 63–1). These results were maintained at long-term followup and were independent of the type of thrombolytic agent used (streptokinase vs. fibrin-specific thrombolytics) and whether patients were transferred emergently for primary PCI. The incidence of intracranial hemorrhage was significantly less with primary PCI (0.05 percent vs. 1.1 percent; $p < 0.0001$), but the overall risk of major bleeding (mostly related to access site bleeding) was higher with primary PCI (6.8 percent vs. 5.3 percent; $p = 0.03$). The risk of access site bleeding with primary PCI appears to be less in more recent trials with better management of anticoagulation and earlier femoral artery sheath removal.

The survival benefit of primary PCI compared with fibrinolytic therapy reported in this meta-analysis was substantial (21 lives saved per 1000 patients treated) and is of similar magnitude to the survival benefit of fibrinolytic therapy compared with placebo reported by the Fibrinolytic Therapy Trialists' (FTT) Collaborative Group (19 lives saved per 1000 patients treated; Fig. 63–2).[28] The relative reduction in death and nonfatal reinfarction is similar across all subgroups of patients treated, including elderly patients, women, diabetics, patients with anterior or nonanterior infarction, patients with prior infarction, and patients classified as at low risk or not at low risk.[29] The greatest absolute benefit occurs in patients who are at highest risk, and several randomized trials have specifically evaluated these high-risk subgroups. The SHOCK (Should We Revascularize Occluded Coronaries for Cardiogenic Shock?) trial, which randomized 302 patients with cardiogenic shock to emergency revascularization versus medical stabilization, found a lower 6-month mortality with emergency revascularization (50 percent versus 63 percent; $p = 0.03$).[30] The survival benefit was especially pronounced in patients who were treated within 6 hours of symptom onset and was seen only in patients younger than age 75 years. Garcia et al. randomized 220 patients with anterior infarction to primary PCI versus alteplase and found substantially lower mortality with primary PCI (2.8 percent vs. 10.8 percent; $p = 0.02$).[31] Recently, Grines et al. reported results from SENIOR PAMI which randomized 481 elderly patients ($\geq$ 70 years old) to fibrinolytic therapy versus primary PCI.[32] The difference in the primary end point of death or stroke between groups did not reach statistical significance, but patients treated with PCI had a lower incidence of combined major adverse coronary event (MACE; death, reinfarction, or stroke) at 30 days (11.6 percent vs. 18 percent; $p = 0.05$). Patients $\geq$80 years old did not appear to benefit.

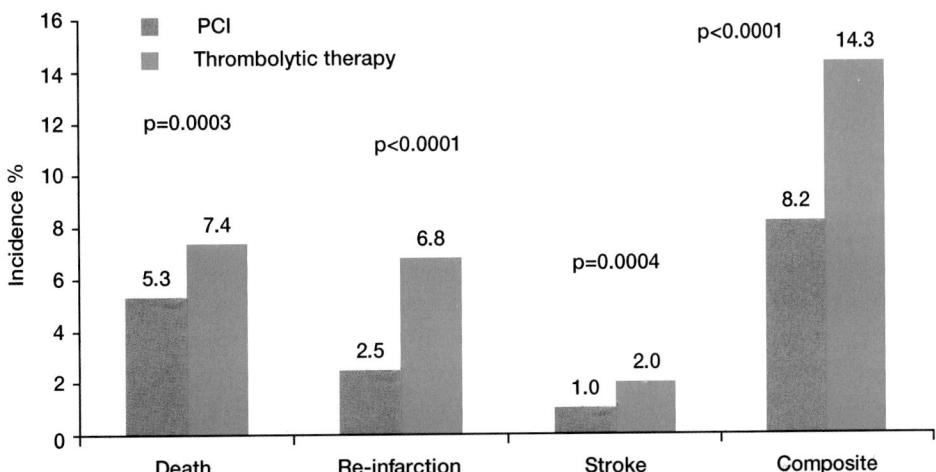

FIGURE 63–1. Meta-analysis of 23 randomized trials comparing short-term outcomes with primary percutaneous coronary intervention (PCI) versus thrombolytic therapy for acute myocardial infarction (AMI). *Source: Adapted from Keeley EC, Boura JA, Grines CL. Primary angioplasty vs. intravenous thrombolytic therapy for acute myocardial infarction, a quantitative review of 23 randomized trials. Lancet 2003;361:13–20, with permission.*

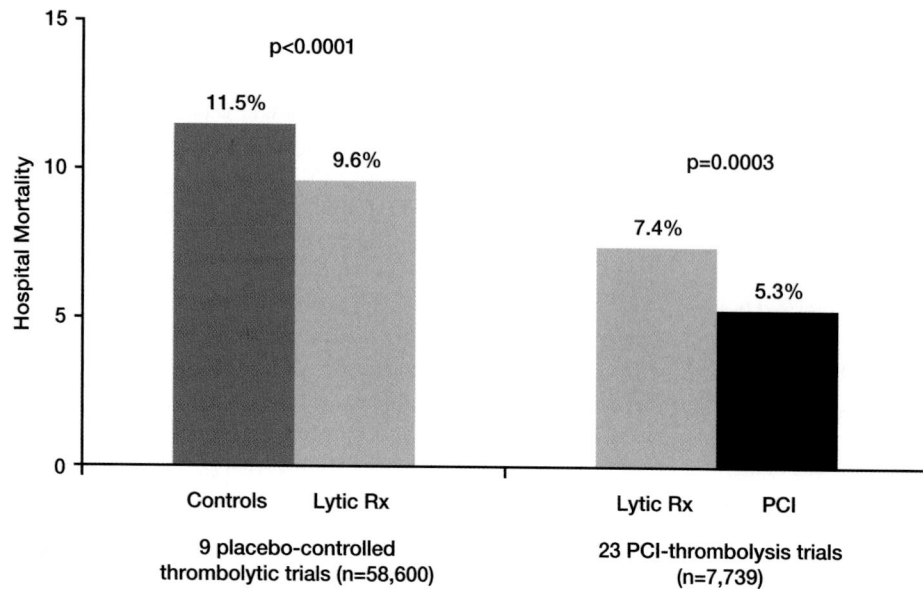

FIGURE 63–2. Comparison of mortality reduction with thrombolytic therapy versus placebo[28] and primary percutaneous coronary intervention (PCI) versus thrombolytic therapy.[27]

Comparison of Late Clinical Outcomes

The initial clinical benefit of primary PCI over fibrinolytic therapy in reducing death and reinfarction appears to be maintained at late followup. The PAMI investigators found that death or reinfarction was lower at 2 years with primary PCI than with fibrinolytic therapy (14.9 percent vs. 23.0 percent; p = 0.03; Fig. 63–3).[33] Similarly, the Zwolle investigators found lower mortality (13.4 percent vs. 23.9 percent; p = 0.01) and less reinfarction (6.2 percent vs. 21.9 percent; p <0.0001) with primary PCI than with streptokinase at 5 years.[34] Both studies found a lower frequency of hospital readmissions with primary PCI. Keeley's recent meta-analysis also showed that the initial benefit with primary PCI was maintained at late followup at 6 to 18 months.[27]

Comparison of Angiographic Outcomes

Primary PCI can achieve TIMI 3 flow in the infarct artery in >90 percent of patients[35,36] and has a clear advantage over thrombolytic therapy, which can achieve TIMI 3 flow in only approximately 54 percent of patients.[37,38] Achieving TIMI 3 flow has a major impact on short- and long-term mortality,[37] and the advantage of primary PCI in achieving high rates of TIMI 3 flow is likely responsible for much of the mortality advantage over fibrinolytic therapy. Indeed, there appears to be a tight inverse relationship between short-term mortality and the ability to achieve TIMI-3 flow with various thrombolytic

regimens and with primary PCI (Fig. 63–4).[23,35,37,39–43] Newer fibrinolytic strategies using combination therapy with low-dose thrombolytics and platelet glycoprotein IIb/IIIa inhibitors have shown improved TIMI-3 flow rates in small pilot trials,[38] but these rates are well below the TIMI-3 flow rates achieved with primary PCI, and they have not shown any mortality advantage in the large GUSTO (Global Utilization of Streptokinase and Tissue Plasminogen Activator for Occluded Arteries) V and ASSENT (Assessment of the Safety and Efficacy of a New Thrombolytic Regimen)-3 trials.[44,45]

Although achieving TIMI-3 flow in the *epicardial* coronary artery is important, optimal outcomes with reperfusion therapy also require optimum reperfusion of the microvasculature or optimum *myocardial* reperfusion. This is discussed under Distal Protection and Thrombectomy.

Late angiographic outcomes with primary PCI have been substantially improved with the use of stents.[35,43] With stenting, reocclusion occurs in 5 to 6 percent of patients, restenosis in 20 to 22 percent of patients, and target-vessel revascularization in 7 to 8 percent of patients. This may improve further with the use of drug-eluting stents (see Stents and Drug-Eluting Stents below). Following fibrinolytic therapy, late reocclusion of the infarct artery occurs in 20 to 28 percent of patients when adjunctive PCI is not employed.[46,47]

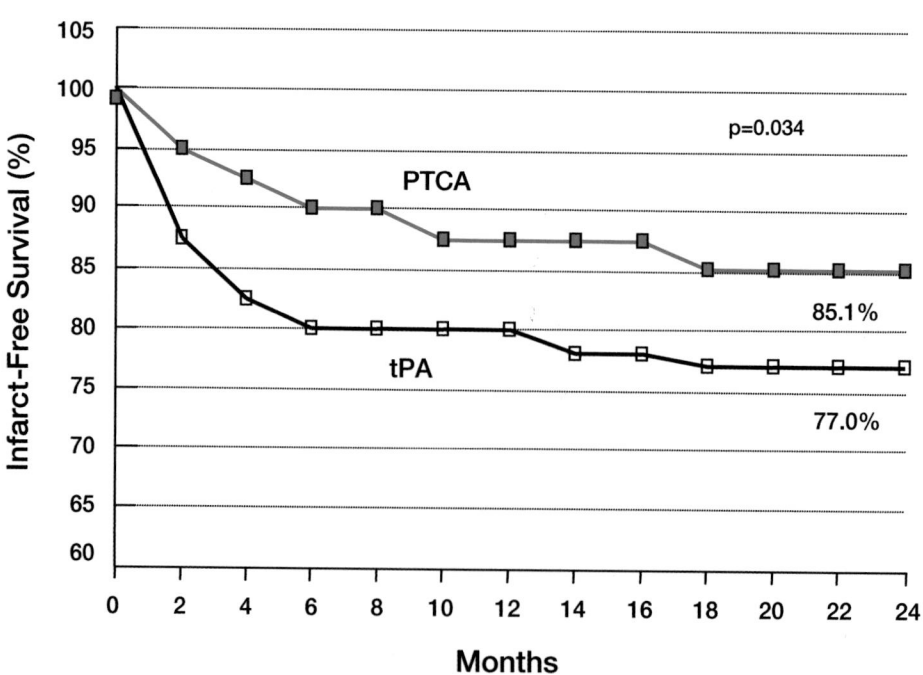

FIGURE 63–3. Actuarial infarction-free survival curves for patients with acute myocardial infarction treated with primary angioplasty (PTCA; *solid boxes*) versus tissue plasminogen activator (tPA; *open boxes*). Source: Reproduced with permission from Nunn CM, O'Neill WW, Rothbaum D, et al. Long-term outcome after primary angioplasty: report from the Primary Angioplasty in Myocardial Infarction (PAMI-1) trial. J Am Coll Cardiol 1999;33:640–646.

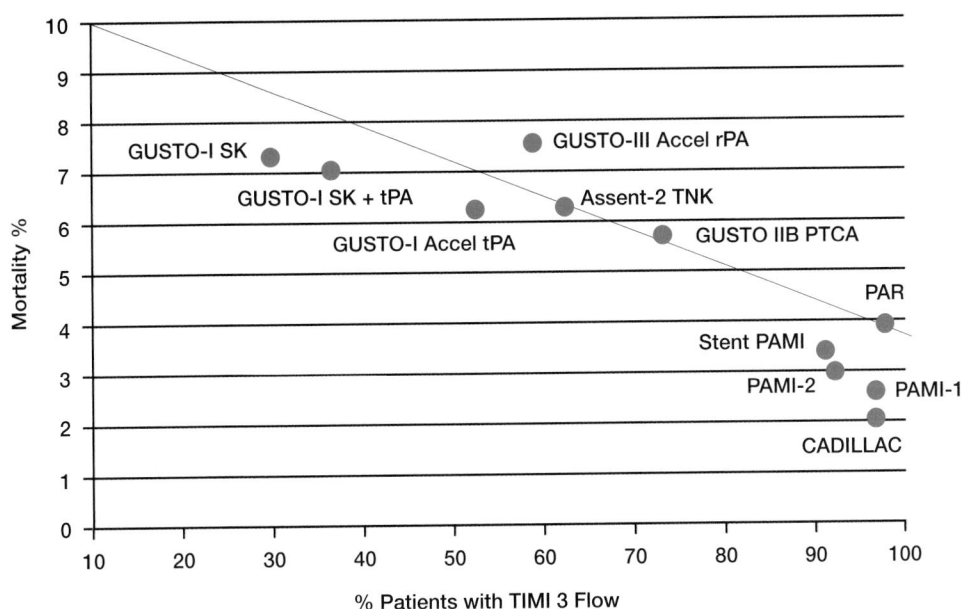

FIGURE 63–4. Relationship between short-term mortality and the frequency of achieving TIMI-3 flow measured acutely in the infarct artery in trials with thrombolytic therapy and primary PCI. The thrombolytic trials include GUSTO-I (Global Utilization of Streptokinase and Tissue Plasminogen Activator for Occluded Arteries), GUSTO-III, ASSENT-2 (Assessment of the Safety and Efficacy of a New Thrombolytic Regimen). The primary PCI trials include CADILLAC (Controlled Abciximab and Device Investigation to Lower Late Angioplasty Complications), PAMI-1 and -2 (Primary Angioplasty in Myocardial Infarction), Stent PAMI, PAR (Primary Angioplasty Registry) and GUSTO IIB. PTCA, percutaneous transluminal coronary angioplasty; rPA, reteplase; SK, streptokinase; TNK, tenecteplase; tPA, tissue plasminogen activator.

Comparison of Myocardial Salvage

Myocardial salvage following primary PCI and fibrinolytic therapy has been evaluated in direct comparisons using paired technetium-99m sestamibi scintigraphy.[48–50] These studies showed better myocardial salvage with primary PCI. Most recently, Schomig et al. found smaller infarct size and better myocardial salvage at all intervals of time to treatment with primary stenting versus fibrinolytic therapy (Fig. 63–5).[50] The greater myocardial salvage with primary PCI is probably related to higher frequency of TIMI-3 flow in the infarct artery, less reocclusion, and possibly better *myocardial* reperfusion.

〖 〗 ADJUNCTIVE THERAPIES WITH PRIMARY PCI

Mechanical reperfusion therapy has improved greatly since its introduction in the early 1980s as a result of increased operator experience, better equipment, and the introduction of new adjunctive therapies. The most important and widely studied of these adjunctive therapies have been glycoprotein IIb/IIIa platelet inhibitors, stents, distal protection, and thrombectomy.

Glycoprotein IIb/IIIa Platelet Inhibitors

Five large, randomized trials have evaluated abciximab as adjunctive therapy with primary PCI with STEMI and all have shown a reduction in the composite end point of death, reinfarction, or urgent target-vessel revascularization (TVR) at 30 days (Table 63–1).[35,51–54] These trials have been summarized in a recent meta-analysis.[55] The greatest benefit was seen in the ADMIRAL (Abciximab Before Direct Angioplasty and Stenting in Myocardial Infarction Regarding Acute and Long-term Follow-up) trial, in which abciximab was often given early, at the time of randomization before primary PCI.[52] In addition to better clinical outcomes, the ADMIRAL trial found improved infarct artery patency prior to PCI and improved left ventricular ejection fraction at 6 months with abciximab. However, a recent meta-analysis of small trials in which abciximab was given upfront prior to primary PCI (facilitated approach) showed no benefit in reducing mortality, reinfarction or urgent target revascularization.[56] The CADILLAC (Controlled Abciximab and Device Investigation to Lower Late Angioplasty Complications) trial showed improvement in 30-day outcomes with

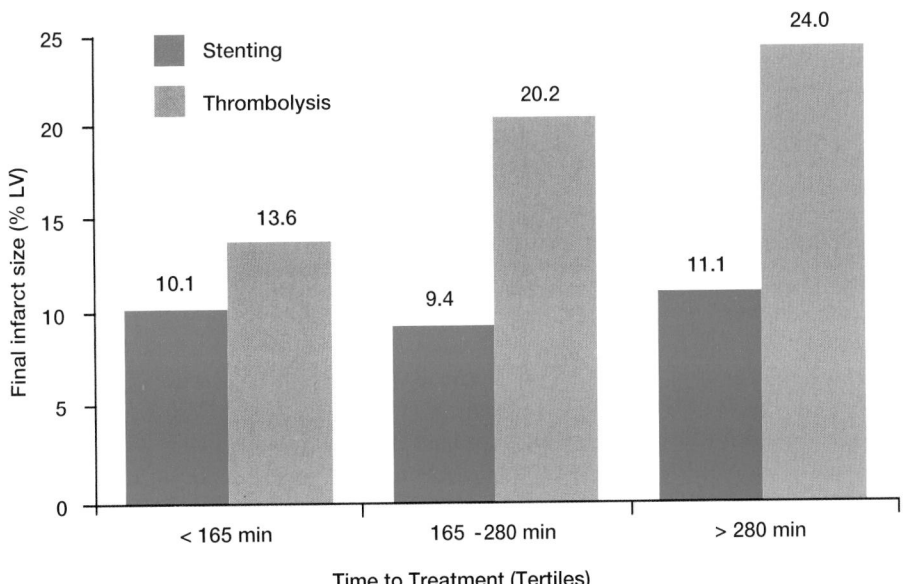

FIGURE 63–5. Comparison of final median infarct size measured by sestamibi imaging in patients with ST-segment elevation myocardial infarction treated with fibrinolysis versus primary percutaneous coronary intervention according to tertiles of time to treatment. *Source: Reproduced with permission from Schomig A, Ndrepepa G, Mehilli J, et al. Therapy-dependent influence of time-to-treatment interval on myocardial salvage in patients with acute myocardial infarction treated with coronary artery stenting or thrombolysis. Circulation 2003;108:1084–1088.*

TABLE 63–1

Randomized Trials Comparing 30-Day Outcomes with Abciximab versus Placebo with Primary PCI for Acute Myocardial Infarction

	ABCIXIMAB	PLACEBO	P VALUE
RAPPORT (n = 483)[51]			
Death	2.5%	2.1%	NS
Reinfarction	3.3%	4.1%	NS
Urgent TVR	1.7%	6.6%	0.006
Composite	5.8%	11.2%	0.03
ADMIRAL (n = 300)[52]			
Death	3.4%	6.6%	NS
Reinfarction	1.3%	2.6%	NS
Urgent TVR	1.3%	6.6%	0.02
Composite	6.0%	14.6%	0.01
ISAR-2 (n = 401)[53]			
Death	2.5%	4.5%	NS
Reinfarction	0.5%	1.5%	NS
Urgent TVR	3.0%	5.0%	NS
Composite	5.0%	10.5%	0.04
CADILLAC (n = 2082)[35]			
Death	1.9%	2.3%	NS
Reinfarction	0.8%	0.9%	NS
Urgent TVR	2.5%	4.4%	0.02
Stroke	0.1%	0.2%	NS
Composite	4.6%	7.0%	0.02
ACE (n = 400)[54]			
Death	3.5%	4.0%	NS
Reinfarction	0.5%	4.5%	0.01
Urgent TVR	0.5%	1.5%	NS
Stroke	0.0%	0.5%	NS
Composite	4.5%	10.5%	0.02

ACE, Abciximab and carbostent evaluation; ADMIRAL, Abciximab Before Direct Angioplasty and Stenting in Myocardial Infarction Regarding Acute and Long-Term Follow-Up; CADILLAC, Controlled Abciximab and Device Investigation to Lower Late Angioplasty Complications; ISAR, Intracoronary Stenting and Antithrombotic Regimen; PCI, percutaneous coronary intervention; RAPPORT, ReoPro and Primary PTCA Organization and Randomized Trial; TVR, target vessel revascularization.

abciximab, but most of the benefit of abciximab was seen in patients treated with PTCA alone (4.8 percent vs. 8.4 percent; p = 0.02), and was without benefit in stented patients (4.5 percent vs. 5.7 percent; p = NS).[35] There was no improvement in left ventricular ejection fraction at 7 months. Abciximab did reduce acute thrombosis in stented patients (0 vs. 1.0 percent; p = 0.03) as well as in all patients (0.4 percent vs. 1.4 percent; p = 0.01).

Currently, abciximab has a class IIa indication by ACC/AHA *Guidelines* for use with primary PCI for STEMI.[26] There are little data with eptifibatide or tirofiban. Because many of the trials showing benefit of abciximab with primary PCI were performed before the routine use of stents, and because the largest trial, CADILLAC, showed little benefit in stented patients, the role of

glycoprotein IIb/IIIa platelet inhibitors with primary PCI remains controversial. Although most trials have not shown an increased incidence of major bleeding with abciximab when used with primary PCI, bleeding is still a major problem when primary PCI is performed with unfractionated heparin, clopidogrel, and platelet glycoprotein IIb/IIIa inhibitors. The HORIZONS (Harmonizing Outcomes with Revascularization and Stents) trial will compare bivalirudin, a direct thrombin inhibitor, with unfractionated heparin plus glycoprotein IIb/IIIa inhibition in STEMI patients who are undergoing primary PCI in an effort to determine the optimum anticoagulant therapy.

Stents and Drug-Eluting Stents

The Stent PAMI trial first documented a clear benefit of stenting by comparing the heparin-coated Palmaz-Schatz stent with balloon angioplasty; stenting reduced restenosis, reocclusion, and the need for TVR after primary PCI for STEMI.[43] However, stented patients had lower TIMI-3 flow rates after PCI and a disturbing trend toward higher mortality at 1 year. The CADILLAC trial evaluated the role of stenting and platelet glycoprotein IIb/IIIa inhibition with abciximab in 2082 patients with STEMI who were treated with primary PCI.[35] Stented patients had a clear benefit over balloon angioplasty alone in reducing 6-month restenosis (22 percent vs. 41 percent; p <0.01), reocclusion (5.7 percent vs. 11.3 percent; p = 0.01), ischemic TVR (6.8 percent vs. 14.7 percent; p <0.001), and MACE (10.9 percent vs. 18.3 percent; p <0.001). In contrast to Stent PAMI, the CADILLAC trial, using the newer-generation MultiLink stent (Guidant Corporation), showed no degradation of TIMI flow post-stenting and no difference in 6-month mortality. Based on these data, stenting is recommended for routine use in eligible patients with STEMI who are treated with mechanical intervention.

Drug-eluting stents (DESs) have proven very effective in reducing restenosis and TVR compared with bare-metal stents (BMSs) following elective and urgent PCI, but their role in treating patients with STEMI who are undergoing primary PCI has not been established. There is concern that the incidence of stent thrombosis with DESs may be higher in the setting of STEMI, and the benefits of DESs may not be as great as with elective and urgent PCI, as the incidence of TVR is relatively low with the use of BMSs in patients with STEMI. Two recent randomized trials found conflicting results with DESs versus BMSs in STEMI. The TYPHOON (A Multi-center Randomized Trial Comparing Sirolimus-eluting Stents to Bare Metal Stents in Primary Angioplasty for Acute Myocardial Infarction) trial (n = 705) found less TVR with sirolimus-eluting stents versus BMSs (5.6 percent vs. 13.4 percent; p <0.001)[57] while the PASSION (Randomized Comparison of Paclitaxel-eluting Stent versus Conventional Stent in ST-elevation Myocardial Infarction) trial (n = 617) found no difference in target lesion revascularization between paclitaxel-eluting stents and BMSs (6.2 percent vs. 7.4 percent; *p* = 0.23).[58] In a large observational experience from the STENT Group, Brodie et al. found no significant difference in TVR between DESs (n = 520) and BMSs (n = 304; 3.9 percent vs. 5.3 percent; *p* = 0.38) and a low incidence of stent thrombosis with DESs (0.8 percent).[59] The HORIZONS trial will randomize 3400 patients who are undergoing primary PCI for STEMI to paclitaxel-eluting stents versus BMSs in a 3:1 ratio and may clarify the role of DES in patients with STEMI.

Distal Protection and Thrombectomy

Primary PCI is effective in restoring normal *epicardial* coronary flow (TIMI-3 flow) in more than 90 percent of patients with STEMI, but more than half of these patients will have suboptimal flow at the tissue level, as evidenced by poor angiographic blush scores or lack of complete electrocardiographic ST-segment resolution.[60–62] Although achieving TIMI-3 flow in the *epicardial* coronary artery is important, optimal outcomes with reperfusion therapy also require optimal reperfusion of the microvasculature or optimal *myocardial* reperfusion. There are numerous studies showing that patients with suboptimal myocardial reperfusion, as evidenced by abnormal myocardial blush or ST-segment resolution, have worse outcomes.[60–62]

The causes of abnormal myocardial reperfusion after primary PCI are not clear. One potential cause is distal embolization of thrombus and fragments of atherosclerotic plaque at the time of PCI, resulting in obstruction of the distal microcirculation. Several distal protection devices, including the PercuSurge System (Medtronic PercuSurge, Sunnyvale, CA) and the Filter Wire (Boston Scientific, Natick, MA), have been tested in clinical trials with the hope that distal protection will prevent distal embolization and will result in improved myocardial reperfusion and better outcomes. Initial small trials showed promising results, but the large EMERALD (Enhanced Myocardial Efficacy and Recovery by Aspiration of Liberalized Debris) trial showed no benefit with the Guardwire (PercuSurge System) in reducing infarct size or improving ST-segment resolution or myocardial blush despite retrieving visible thrombus or atheroma in >70 percent of patients.[36] The authors concluded that distal microembolization may not be important in the pathogenesis of impaired microvascular reperfusion.

A number of thrombectomy devices have been used as adjunctive therapy with primary PCI in an attempt to reduce distal embolization, improve mi-

crovascular reperfusion, and improve outcomes. Those that have been most thoroughly studied are the X-Sizer Catheter System (EndiCOR Medical, Inc., San Clemente, CA), several aspiration devices, and the AngioJet System (Possis Medical, Minneapolis, MN). There have been a number of small randomized trials evaluating thrombectomy with primary PCI and most,[63–68] but not all,[69,70] have shown improved surrogate end points (ST-segment resolution and myocardial blush, and in some cases, reduced infarct size) with thrombectomy (Tables 63–2 and 63–3).[71] However, the largest randomized trial, the AIMI (AngioJet Rheolytic Thrombectomy in Patients Undergoing Primary Angioplasty for Acute Myocardial Infarction) trial using the AngioJet, showed no benefit.[70] There was no difference in ST-segment resolution and myocardial blush, and, surprisingly, infarct size was slightly larger with the AngioJet. There was also an increased mortality in the AngioJet group, raising safety concerns. However, recent experience from several registries have documented the safety of the device.[72–76] The AIMI study investigators concluded that there is no indication for the routine use of rheolytic thrombectomy with primary PCI for STEMI.

Based on the results of the EMERALD and AIMI studies, there is general agreement that distal protection and thrombectomy are not indicated for routine use with primary PCI for STEMI. However, patients with large thrombus burden (Fig. 63–6) will fre-

TABLE 63–2

Randomized Trials with Aspiration Thrombectomy (AT) in ST-Segment Elevation Myocardial Infarction

	AT	CONTROL	P VALUE
REMEDIA TRIAL (DIVER) (*n* = 100)[65]			
Grade 2–3 blush	63%	45%	0.02
ST resolution ≥ 70%	58%	37%	0.03
DE LUCA ET AL. (DIVER) (*n* = 76)[66]			
Grade 3 blush	37%	13%	0.02
ST resolution >50%	82%	55%	0.02
Echo ESV (6 months)	75 mm	82 mm	0.001
Echo EDV (6 months)	138 mm	153 mm	0.001
NOEL ET AL. (EXPORT) (*n* = 50)[67]			
TIMI 3 flow	96%	89%	NS
CTFC	21	32	0.04
ST resolution ≥ 70%	50%	12%	0.01
MRI infarct size at 48 h %	12.90%	20.90%	0.04
KALTOFT ET AL. (RESCUE) (*n* = 215)[69]			
TIMI 3 flow	89%	88%	NS
CTFC	16	17	NS
ST resolution (median %)	62%	62%	NS
Myocardial salvage (sestamibi)	13%	18%	0.12
Final infarct size %	16%	9%	0.004

CTFC, corrected TIMI frame count; DIVER, Diver CE Catheter (eV3, Inc, Plymouth, Minn); EXPORT, Export Catheter (Medtronic, Inc, Minneapolis, Minn); RESCUE, Rescue Catheter (Boston Scientific, Natick, Mass); TIMI, Thrombolysis in Myocardial Infarction.

TABLE 63–3

Randomized Trials with Rheolytic Thrombectomy (RT) in ST-Segment Elevation Myocardial Infarction

	RT	CONTROL	P VALUE
ANTONIUCCI ET AL. (n = 100)[68]			
CTFC	18	23	0.03
ST resolution >50%	90%	72%	0.02
Infarct size at 1 mo. (sestamibi)	13.0%	21.2%	0.01
AIMI (n = 480)[70]			
TIMI 3 flow	92%	97%	0.02
CTFC	35	32	0.13
Grade 2–3 blush	49%	58%	0.06
ST Resolution ≥ 70%	60	68	0.14
Infarct Size at 14–28 days (sestamibi)	12.5%	9.8%	0.02

AIMI, AngioJet Rheolytic Thrombectomy in Patients Undergoing Primary Angioplasty for Acute Myocardial Infarction; CTFC, corrected TIMI frame count; TIMI, Thrombolysis in Myocardial Infarction.

quently have distal *macroembolization,* and studies have shown that *macroembolization* is harmful and leads to impaired myocardial reperfusion and worse clinical outcomes.[77] Therefore, until there are more data from new trials, it seems reasonable to perform adjunctive thrombectomy in patients with large thrombus burden prior to primary PCI.

【 】 THE ROLE OF CARDIAC SURGERY IN THE PRIMARY PCI STRATEGY

Not all patients with STEMI brought emergently to the cardiac catheterization laboratory undergo PCI.[39] Approximately 10 percent of patients are triaged to either medical treatment or are treated with coronary artery bypass graft (CABG) surgery as the primary reperfusion strategy (primary CABG). Patients may be selected for primary CABG when there is severe left main disease or severe multivessel coronary artery disease with preserved (TIMI-3) flow in the infarct artery, which allows time for transfer to the operating room. Patients may be selected for medical therapy for several reasons, such as no myocardial infarction (mistaken diagnosis), no significant stenosis in the infarct artery (resolution of spasm or thrombus), the infarct artery could not be identified, and, occasionally, unsuitable anatomy or a very small infarct artery.

Coronary artery bypass surgery may be performed emergently after failed angioplasty, urgently for reinfarction or recurrent ischemia, and electively for definitive treatment of left main or severe multivessel disease. In experienced centers, and with the availability of stents, emergency bypass surgery after failed PCI is rare (approximately 0.4 percent); the need for urgent bypass surgery for reinfarction or recurrent ischemia that cannot be managed with repeat PCI is also rare (0.1 percent).[43] Elective bypass surgery for treatment of residual coronary artery disease after initial successful primary angioplasty has been used in approximately 2 to 5 percent of patients.[43,78] Altogether, bypass surgery is performed in approximately 6 to 10 percent of patients with the primary angioplasty approach.[43,78] Considering the severity of illness of these patients, surgical mortality has been very acceptable (6.4 percent with emergency or urgent bypass surgery and 2.0 percent with elective bypass surgery in the PAMI-2 trial).[78]

Cardiac surgery is also indicated in patients with mechanical complications of STEMI. Those with ventricular septal rupture,

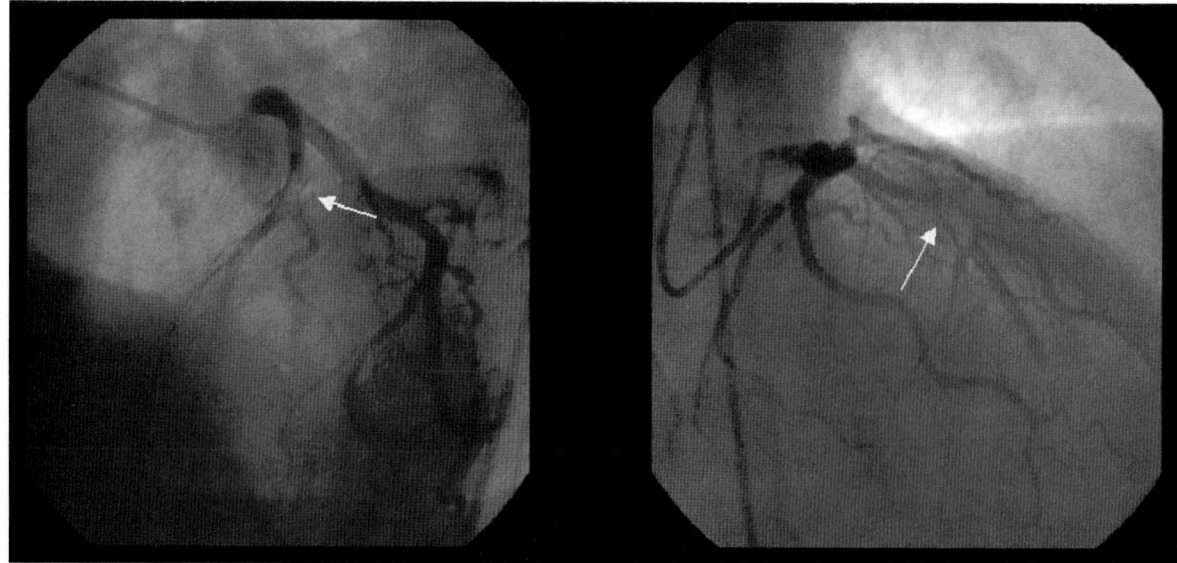

FIGURE 63–6. Coronary angiogram of a patient with an anterior wall myocardial infarction showing a large thrombus burden (*arrow*) in the proximal left anterior descending artery.

acute mitral regurgitation from papillary muscle rupture, and contained myocardial rupture with tamponade usually develop cardiogenic shock and have a very poor outcome without surgical intervention. These patients are candidates for emergent surgery.

TECHNICAL ASPECTS OF PRIMARY PCI

Treatment in the Emergency Department

When primary PCI is planned for patients with known or suspected STEMI, only a limited history and physical examination should be performed to avoid delays in initiating the catheterization procedure. Patients are given 325 mg of soluble chewable aspirin, 5000 U of unfractionated heparin, sublingual nitroglycerin, intravenous β blockers unless contraindicated, and supplemental oxygen, and are transported promptly from the emergency department to the catheterization laboratory. Clopidogrel 300 to 600 mg should also be given in the emergency department based on evidence from multiple trials[79–81] (although not specifically STEMI patients who were treated with primary PCI) and because the need for emergent CABG following primary PCI for STEMI is very low.

Cardiac Catheterization and Angiography

Femoral access is usually preferred because this allows for the use of larger devices if necessary and facilitates the use of adjunctive therapy such as intraaortic balloon pumping or transvenous pacing when indicated. An activated clotting time (ACT) is measured and additional heparin is given to prolong the ACT to >300 seconds or 200 to 300 seconds if platelet glycoprotein IIb/IIIa inhibitors are used. Left ventriculography should be performed prior to intervention, even in patients who are hemodynamically unstable, to assess the severity of ventricular and valvular dysfunction, help identify the infarct artery (if this is uncertain), and aid in making decisions regarding the necessity for adjunctive therapy, such as intraaortic balloon pumping and pulmonary artery catheter insertion. Occasionally, papillary muscle rupture, ventricular septal defect, or, rarely, even frank free wall rupture will be demonstrated when not previously suspected, prompting urgent surgery. Alternatively, demonstration of normal left ventricular function may raise early concerns of nonischemic diagnoses such as aortic dissection or pericarditis. A femoral venous sheath may be helpful in patients with occlusion of the right coronary artery to allow access for temporary transvenous pacing if necessary. In patients with hypotension or in patients who are hemodynamically unstable, placement of a pulmonary artery catheter is important to define and monitor hemodynamics. The use of a pulse oximeter to monitor oxygen saturation is also helpful. Following diagnostic coronary and left ventricular angiography, patients are triaged to the most appropriate therapy. Approximately 10 percent of patients who are undergoing emergency coronary angiography do not undergo primary angioplasty and are triaged to bypass surgery or medical therapy based on the criteria described earlier.

Primary PCI Procedure

If stenting is planned and clopidogrel had not been previously given, clopidogrel 300 to 600 mg is given prior to initiation of PCI. Primary PCI is generally performed with 6F standard guiding catheters and soft- or floppy-tipped 0.014-in steerable guidewires. The soft tip can almost always cross the soft, fresh thrombus (in contrast to a chronic total occlusion) and is less traumatic than stiffer wires. The guidewire is advanced well down the infarct artery to ensure that it is in the true lumen and not in a small side branch or under an intimal dissection, since navigation distal to the occlusion is usually done blindly. If the infarct-related artery is totally occluded, reperfusion will often be established after the occlusion is crossed with the guidewire. If not, it may be preferable to cross the occlusion with a balloon and then withdraw the balloon without inflating it (*Dottering* the lesion) to establish reperfusion. The more gradual reperfusion provided with the wire or Dottering technique may result in fewer reperfusion arrhythmias than immediate balloon inflation and also allows assessment of thrombus burden and the size of the distal vessel. Balloon angioplasty or stenting of the infarct lesion is performed with techniques similar to conventional PCI. No-flow (TIMI 0–1 flow) or slow-flow (TIMI 2 flow) may occur after successful opening of the epicardial infarct artery obstruction. This is generally caused by microvascular dysfunction from spasm, distal emboli, or endothelial injury and should be treated with intracoronary verapamil, adenosine, or nitroprusside, which often helps to improve flow. Intracoronary abciximab may also help with no-reflow. PCI is generally performed only on the infarct artery. Tandem lesions in the infarct vessel can be dilated, but dilating a noninfarct artery places too much myocardium acutely in jeopardy and is usually not recommended. Exceptions to this rule are sometimes made in patients with severe multivessel disease and refractory cardiogenic shock, and in patients with plaque rupture and critical obstruction in multiple vessels.

Catheterization Laboratory Complications

With increasing operator experience, improved equipment, and the availability of stents, major catheterization laboratory complications with primary PCI have become infrequent. Table 63–4 shows the acute complications from the Stent PAMI trial in nonshock patients.[43] Laboratory deaths and emergency bypass surgery for failed PCI are rare. Ventricular tachycardia or fibrillation, asystole and bradycardia (including second- and third-degree atrioventricular block), and hypotension are the most common complications and usually occur immediately after reperfusion. With increased operator experience and anticipation, these complications can usually be managed effectively, and often can be prevented.

Adjunctive Intraaortic Balloon Counterpulsation

The PAMI-2 trial evaluated the prophylactic use of intraaortic balloon pumping (IABP) in high-risk patients following primary PCI and found that it did not reduce the frequency of the primary end point of death, reinfarction, reocclusion of the infarct artery, or new congestive heart failure.[82] As a result of this and other data, IABP has not been recommended for prophylactic use in high-risk patients following primary PCI.[82,83] IABP is generally indicated prior to primary PCI in hemodynamically unstable patients with congestive heart failure or shock, in patients with mechanical complications of acute infarction, and in those whose anatomy is unsuitable for PCI as a bridge to surgery. There may also be a role for prophylactic IABP before primary angioplasty in selected high-risk patients to prevent hemodynamic deterioration.[84]

TABLE 63–4

Acute Catheterization Laboratory Complications with Primary PCI from the Stent PAMI Trial (Nonshock Patients)[43]

COMPLICATION	STENT (n = 451)	PTCA (n = 448)	COMBINED (n = 899)
Laboratory death	0.2%	0%	0.1%
Emergency bypass surgery	0.2%	0.2%	0.2%
Ventricular tachycardia/fibrillation[a]	3.1%	4.7%	3.9%
Cardiopulmonary resuscitation[b]	0.9%	0.4%	0.7%
Intubation	0.2%	0.7%	0.4%
Asystole/bradycardia[c]	9.3%	8.5%	8.9%
Sustained hypotension[d]	7.8%	8.3%	8.0%

PAMI, Primary Angioplasty in Myocardial Infarction; PCI, percutaneous coronary intervention; PTCA, percutaneous transluminal coronary angioplasty.
[a]Requiring electric cardioversion.
[b]Requiring chest compression.
[c]Requiring atropine or temporary pacing.
[d]Requiring vasopressors or intraaortic balloon counterpulsation.

After PCI Care

Postprocedure care has been standardized in a number of recent randomized trials.[35,36] Following the procedure, heparin is discontinued, unless there are other reasons to resume heparin, such as the need for IABP, severe left ventricular dysfunction with concern about left ventricular thrombus, or atrial fibrillation. If a femoral artery closure device is not used, the sheath is generally removed at 2 to 3 hours when the ACT is <170 seconds. If bivalirudin is used, the sheath is generally removed at 2 hours. Patients who are not at high risk can be transferred from the catheterization laboratory directly to the subacute unit (rather than the coronary care unit) and can be targeted for discharge on day 2 (day 0 = day of admission).[85] All patients without contraindications should be treated with aspirin indefinitely, clopidogrel 75 mg/d for 1 year, β blockers, and a statin. Angiotensin-converting enzyme (ACE) inhibitors should be used in patients with congestive heart failure, hypertension, or low ejection fraction (<40 percent). Patients who develop symptoms or electrocardiographic changes of recurrent ischemia or reinfarction should undergo emergency repeat catheterization and intervention if indicated.

[ ] TIME TO TREATMENT AND TRIAGE ISSUES

ACC/AHA *Guidelines* recommend primary PCI as the preferred reperfusion strategy for patients with STEMI if it can be performed promptly (within 90 minutes of recognition) by experienced operators.[26] Based on these guidelines, there has been a nationwide effort through the AHA and others to reduce door-to-balloon times to <90 minutes. Most hospitals with coronary interventional services, dedicated physicians, nursing and administrative leadership, and the establishment of detailed protocols, are able to meet these guidelines.[86,87]

The management of patients with STEMI presenting to hospitals without interventional services is more difficult. The results from randomized trials (predominantly from Europe) indicate that outcomes are better when patients with STEMI who present to nonprimary PCI hospitals are transferred promptly to an interventional facility for primary PCI compared with being given thrombolytic therapy at the local hospital (Table 63–5 and Fig.

63–7).[88–93] The additional treatment delays of primary PCI compared with fibrinolytic therapy (door-to-balloon time minus door-to-needle time) in these trials have ranged from 55 to 103 minutes. Unfortunately, in the United States, transfer delays are much longer than this. Recent data from the National Registry of Myocardial Infarction (NRMI) found median delays of 180 minutes from arrival at the noninterventional hospital to balloon inflation at the primary PCI hospital with only 4.2 percent of transferred patients achieving door-to-balloon times of <90 minutes.[94] Consequently, many patients presenting to nonprimary PCI hospitals in the United States may not be eligible for primary PCI because of the long potential treatment delays. There are currently nationwide and statewide efforts to reduce time to primary PCI. It has been shown that with well-defined goals, commitment from administrative and clinical leaders, standardized protocols, integrated systems of transfer, and data feedback to monitor progress, door-to-balloon times for patients presenting to noninterventional hospitals can be dramatically reduced and can approach and meet guidelines for timely treatment with primary PCI.[86,87] In addition, regionalization of STEMI care to interventional centers using coordinated emergency medical technician transport and in the field tele-transmitted ECGs, can markedly reduce transfer delays.

Another approach is to establish primary PCI services at hospitals without cardiac surgery on site. It has been demonstrated that primary PCI can be performed safely and effectively at community hospitals without onsite cardiac surgery when rigorous criteria are established.[95] The C-PORT (Atlantic Cardiovascular Patient Outcomes Research Team) trial evaluated primary PCI at hospitals with catheterization laboratories but without cardiac surgery or elective PCI.[96] Using skilled operators who perform PCI at nearby tertiary centers, the C-PORT investigators documented lower 6-month composite event rates of death, reinfarction, or stroke with primary PCI versus lytic therapy (12.4 percent vs. 19.9 percent; $p = 0.03$). Based on this randomized trial and other observational studies, the ACC/AHA *Clinical Guidelines* provide that primary PCI can be performed in such institutions when it is done by experienced operators with defined access to surgical facilities using rigorous protocols and proper case selection (class IIb indication).[26]

TABLE 63–5

Randomized Trials Comparing 30-Day Outcomes in Patients Transferred for Primary PCI versus Treated Locally with Thrombolytic Therapy

	DEATH	REINFARCTION	STROKE	COMPOSITE	P VALUE[a]	TREATMENT DELAY[b]
VERMEER (n = 150)[88]						
PCI	6.7%	1.3%	2.7%	10.7%	0.25	90 min
Alteplase	6.7%	9.3%	2.7%	18.7%		
PRAGUE-1 (n = 200)[89]						
PCI	6.9%	1.0%	0%	7.9%	0.005	88 min
Streptokinase	14.1%	10.1%	1.0%	23.2%		
AIR PAMI (n = 137)[90]						
PCI	8.4%	1.4%	0%	8.5%	0.33	104 min
Alteplase	12.1%	0%	4.5%	13.6%		
DANAMI-2 (n = 1572)[91]						
PCI	6.6%	1.6%	1.1%	8.0%	0.0004	61 min
Alteplase	7.5%	6.3%	2.0%	13.5%		
PRAGUE-2 (n = 850)[92]						
PCI	6.8%			8.4%	0.003	92 min
Streptokinase	10.0%			15.2%		

AIR PAMI, Air Primary Angioplasty in Myocardial Infarction; DANAMI, Danish Multicenter Randomized Study on Fibrinolytic Therapy versus Acute Coronary Angioplasty in Acute Myocardial Infarction; PRAGUE, Primary Angioplasty in Acute Myocardial Infarction Patients from General Community Hospitals Transported for Percutaneous Transluminal Coronary Angioplasty Units versus Emergency Thrombolysis.
[a]Compares composite end points.
[b]Treatment delay is the difference between symptom onset to balloon inflation with PCI and symptom onset to thrombolytic therapy.

Achieving door-to-balloon times of <90 minutes may not be possible in many situations at noninterventional hospitals, and recommendations regarding triage of patients with STEMI for fibrinolytic therapy versus transfer for primary PCI have been controversial. Boersma's meta-analysis of randomized trials comparing fibrinolytic therapy versus primary PCI suggested that primary PCI has a mortality advantage even with additional delays to PCI (door-to-balloon minus door-to-needle time) of up to 2 hours

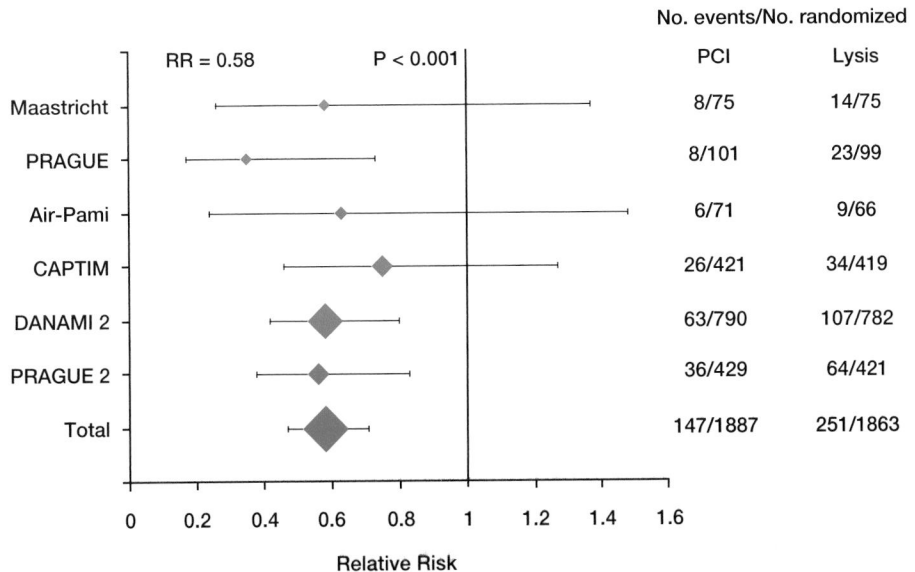

FIGURE 63–7. Relative risks for the composite of death/reinfarction/stroke comparing fibrinolytic therapy at noninterventional hospitals versus transfer for primary percutaneous coronary intervention (PCI) from several randomized trials. AIR PAMI, Air Primary Angioplasty in Myocardial Infarction; CAPTIM, Comparison of Angioplasty and Prehospital Thrombolysis in Acute Myocardial Infarction. *Source: Reproduced with permission from Dalby M, Bouzamondo A, Lechat P, Montalescot G.[93]*

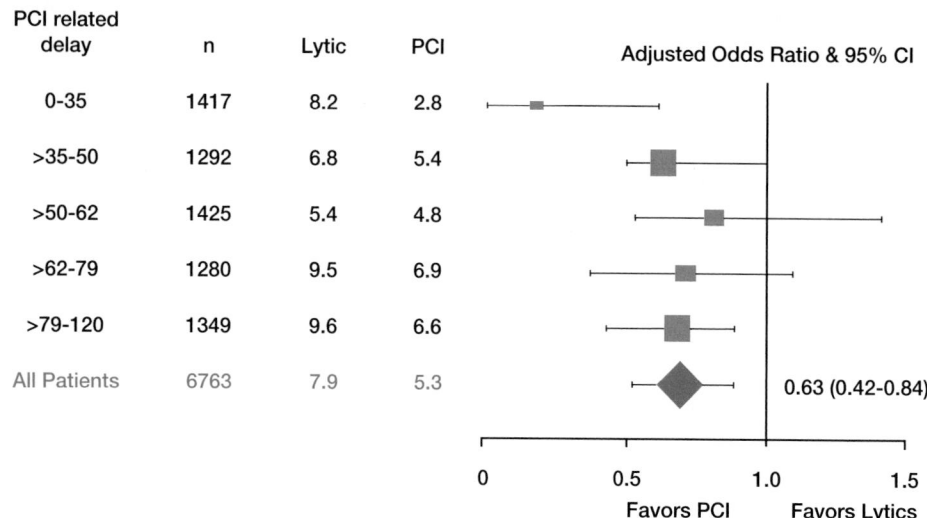

PCI related delay	n	Lytic	PCI
0-35	1417	8.2	2.8
>35-50	1292	6.8	5.4
>50-62	1425	5.4	4.8
>62-79	1280	9.5	6.9
>79-120	1349	9.6	6.6
All Patients	6763	7.9	5.3

0.63 (0.42-0.84)

Adjusted Odds Ratio & 95% CI

Favors PCI   Favors Lytics

FIGURE 63–8. Adjusted odds ratio (95 percent confidence intervals) for 30-day mortality in patients with ST-segment elevation myocardial infarction randomized to fibrinolytic therapy versus primary percutaneous coronary intervention (PCI) from 22 randomized trials according to PCI-related delay (door-to-balloon time minus door-to-needle time). *Source: Reproduced with permission from Boersma E and the PCAT-2 Trialists' Collaborative Group. Does time matter? A pooled analysis of randomized clinical trials comparing primary percutaneous coronary intervention and in-hospital fibrinolysis in acute myocardial infarction patients. Eur Heart J 2006;27:779–788.*

(Fig. 63–8).[97] Data evaluating the impact of treatment delays with primary PCI on mortality suggest that treatment delays impact mortality in patients presenting early after the onset of symptoms but have much less impact in patients presenting late after the onset of symptoms.[98–100] Currently, ACC/AHA guidelines recommend that patients with cardiogenic shock and patients who are ineligible for fibrinolytic therapy should be transferred for primary PCI. Decisions regarding triage of remaining STEMI patients should depend on an assessment of time and risk—time to presentation, time delay to PCI, risk of bleeding from fibrinolytic therapy, and risk of the STEMI. High-risk patients presenting early with long delays to primary PCI should preferentially be treated with fibrinolytic therapy, whereas patients presenting later should preferentially be transferred for primary PCI, even with longer delays to PCI.

There is hope that facilitated PCI (early pharmacologic reperfusion therapy followed by transfer for emergent PCI) may provide a solution to the problem of time delays with primary PCI. Unfortunately, recent trials with facilitated PCI have not shown benefit.[101] This is discussed in a later section (see Facilitated PCI below).

RESCUE PCI

With current fibrinolytic therapy, successful reperfusion (TIMI-3 flow) is achieved in only approximately 55 percent of patients.[37] Rescue PCI, the mechanical reopening of an occluded infarct artery after failed fibrinolysis, has been used as adjunctive therapy in an attempt to improve outcomes in patients with failed fibrinolysis. Rescue PCI should be differentiated from facilitated PCI (see Facilitated PCI below), which is the use of pharmacologic therapy followed by planned emergent PCI, regardless of whether the infarct artery is open or closed at initial angiography. Facilitated PCI is planned intervention, whereas rescue PCI is generally not planned. Initial experience with rescue PCI often showed

suboptimal procedural outcomes, but with the introduction of stents and platelet inhibitors procedural outcomes have improved, and there are now several randomized trials documenting improved outcomes with rescue PCI (Table 63–6).[102–104]

The RESCUE (Randomized Evaluation of Salvage Angioplasty with Combined Utilization of Endpoints) trial investigators randomized 151 patients with first anterior wall myocardial infarction who were treated with fibrinolytic therapy and who had an occluded infarct artery within 8 hours of symptom onset to rescue PCI versus conservative care.[102] The rescue PCI group had a lower composite event rate of death or congestive heart failure and better exercise left ventricular ejection fraction (43 percent vs. 38 percent; *p* = 0.04). These benefits occurred despite the fact that stents were not yet available and despite what the authors thought was a strong investigator bias not to randomize patients presenting very early in the course of their infarction. The MERLIN (Middlesbrough Early Revascularization to Limit Infarction) trial investigators randomized patients with STEMI and failed thrombolysis (<50 percent ST-segment resolution at 60 minutes) to rescue PCI versus conservative care.[103] There was no difference in 30-day mortality (the primary end point), but event-free survival was better with rescue PCI (*p* = 0.02). The REACT (Rescue Angioplasty Versus Conservative Treatment or Repeat Thrombolysis) trial randomized patients with STEMI and failed fibrinolysis (<50 percent ST-segment resolution at 90 minutes) to rescue PCI, repeat fibrinolysis, or conservative care.[104] Patients treated with rescue PCI had a lower incidence of the composite end point (death, reinfarction, stroke, or heart failure) than did patients treated with either repeat fibrinolytic therapy or conservative care.

Based on these data, acute angiography and rescue PCI, if indicated, should be considered in patients with STEMI who are thought to have failed thrombolysis, as evidenced by persistent chest pain, lack of resolution of ST-segment elevation, or hemodynamic compromise persisting for more than 90 minutes after treatment.

FUTURE DIRECTIONS

【 】 PREVENTING REPERFUSION INJURY

There is evidence that deleterious effects to the myocardium may occur at the time of reperfusion. The pathogenesis of this *reperfusion injury* (other than from distal embolization) is poorly understood but may be related to a complement-dependent inflammatory response, to the formation of oxygen free radicals, or other mechanisms. Studies evaluating agents to reduce reperfusion injury have generally been disappointing, but several recent studies

TABLE 63–6

Randomized Trials Evaluating Rescue PCI for Failed Fibrinolysis

	CONTROL	RESCUE PCI	REPEAT LYTICS	P VALUE
RESCUE TRIAL (n = 151)[102]				
Death	9.6%	5.1%		0.18
CHF	7.0%	1.3%		0.11
Death or CHF	16.6%	6.4%		0.05
MERLIN TRIAL (n = 136)[103]				
Death	19.3%	16.2%		0.60
Reinfarction	12.9%	5.4%		0.10
Stroke	1.6%	6.8%		0.20
TVR	22.6%	5.4%		0.003
CHF	38.7%	29.7%		0.30
Composite	62.9%	48.6%		0.09
REACT TRIAL (n = 427)[104]				
Death	12.8%	6.2%	12.7%	0.12
Reinfarction	8.5%	2.1%	10.6%	<0.01
Stroke	0.7%	2.1%	0.7%	0.63
CHF	7.8%	4.9%	7.0%	0.58
Composite	29.8%	15.3%	31.0%	<0.01

CHF, congestive heart failure; MERLIN, Middlesbrough Early Revascularization to Limit Infarction; PCI, percutaneous coronary intervention; REACT, Rescue Angioplasty versus Conservative Treatment or Repeat Thrombolysis; RESCUE, Randomized Evaluations of Salvage Angioplasty with Combined Utilization of Endpoints; TVR, target vessel revascularization.

have shown promise. Adenosine potentially can reduce reperfusion injury by suppressing free radical formation and by preventing neutrophil activation. AMISTAD I (Acute Myocardial Infarction Study of Adenosine) evaluated adenosine in STEMI patients who were treated with primary PCI or lytic therapy and found a 33 percent reduction in infarct size in patients with anterior wall infarction who were treated with adenosine but no benefit in inferior infarction.[105] AMISTAD II, which evaluated only patients with anterior wall infarction, found no benefit with adenosine in the primary end point of death or congestive heart failure at 6 months, but did find a trend toward smaller infarct size with adenosine (17 percent vs. 27 percent; $p = 0.07$) and a significantly smaller infarct size in the high-dose adenosine group (11 percent vs. 27 percent; $p = 0.02$).[106]

In another reperfusion injury trial (COMMA [Complement Inhibition in Myocardial Infarction Treated with Angioplasty]), the investigational complement inhibitor, pexelizumab (Alexian Pharmaceuticals and Proctor and Gamble), showed a mortality benefit in patients with STEMI who were treated with primary PCI.[107] This surprising result occurred despite no reduction in infarct size, and has raised questions regarding the potential mechanisms. The results of COMMA have stimulated the initiation of the large APEX trial, which was designed to evaluate the effect of pexelizumab on survival in patients with STEMI who were undergoing primary PCI. Unfortunately, the study was stopped early by the sponsor for financial reasons, and the study did not meet its primary end point.

The results of these clinical trials may be encouraging enough to warrant further investigation with adenosine and pexelizumab to reduce reperfusion injury.

[ ] SYSTEMIC HYPOTHERMIA

Numerous studies in experimental animal models of acute myocardial infarction have documented the effectiveness of systemic hypothermia initiated prior to reperfusion in reducing infarct size.[108,109] New technology has now made systemic hypothermia feasible in patients with STEMI. Current endovascular systems used for achieving systemic hypothermia deploy catheters with coils that are placed in the inferior vena cava via the femoral vein through which cold saline is circulated. These systems can provide rapid cooling and have been evaluated in patients with STEMI in the COOL MI (Hypothermia as an Adjunctive Therapy to PCI in Patients with Acute Myocardial Infarction) and ICE-IT (Intravascular Cooling Adjunctive to Percutaneous Coronary Intervention) trials.[110,111] Because of logistical problems resulting in delays in initiating cooling in both of these trials, many patients were not cooled to target temperatures prior to reperfusion, and neither of these trials met its primary end point—reduction in infarct size. However, both trials suggested that hypothermia reduced infarct size in patients with anterior infarction when cooling to target temperature was achieved prior to reperfusion. These results have encouraged the initiation of the COOL MI-2 Trial, which is evaluating the effects of systemic hypothermia on infarct size in patients with *anterior infarction* who are cooled to target temperatures prior to reperfusion.

[ ] FACILITATED PCI

The time delay required to initiate primary PCI has led to a great deal of interest in pharmacologic reperfusion combined with mechanical reperfusion, or facilitated PCI. Facilitated PCI is the use of pharmacologic reperfusion to establish reperfusion as rapidly as possible, followed by immediate PCI to maximize reperfusion and to stabilize the ruptured plaque with stenting when possible. The observation that patients with STEMI arriving at the catheterization laboratory for primary PCI who have an open versus a closed infarct artery on initial angiography have much better outcomes suggests that facilitated PCI may be beneficial.[112,113] Furthermore, there are a number of studies documenting that infarct artery patency and TIMI-3 flow rates are higher at initial angiography in patients treated with facilitated PCI compared with primary PCI alone.[114] Unfortunately, clinical results with facilitated PCI have been less encouraging. The ASSENT-4 PCI trial, which randomized patients to tenecteplase-facilitated PCI versus PCI alone, found a higher incidence of death, reinfarction, and stroke with facilitated PCI.[101] The potential benefit of facilitated PCI in this trial may have been compromised by the lack of use of potent platelet inhibitors in the facilitated group (either upstream clopidogrel or platelet glycoprotein IIb/IIIa inhibitors), the relatively long time to presentation in most patients, and the relatively short time from randomization to PCI in most patients. Despite these limitations, the data suggest that PCI and fibrinolytic therapy are not synergistic—that PCI performed shortly after fibrinolytic therapy is associated with worse outcomes, possibly because of platelet activation by fibrinolytic therapy. In a recent meta-analysis performed by Keeley and Grines, facilitated PCI using lytic therapy also was associated with higher rates of death, reinfarction, stroke, and bleeding compared with primary PCI alone.[114] Facilitated PCI using platelet IIb/IIIa inhibitors alone (without fibrinolytic therapy) resulted in no difference in outcomes or major bleeding. Facilitated PCI using combination therapy (half-dose lytics plus IIb/IIIa inhibitors showed no difference in outcomes but increased bleeding. Based on these data, facilitated PCI cannot be currently recommended as a reperfusion strategy. Facilitated PCI would be expected to help most in patients who present early after the onset of symptoms and in patients who have long delays to PCI. It is possible that facilitated PCI may be helpful in these patients when adequate platelet inhibition is used, but this remains to be proven in randomized trials. The FINESSE (Facilitated Intervention for Enhanced Reperfusion Speed to Stop Ischemic Events) trial, which is randomizing patients to facilitated PCI (with either half-dose reteplase plus abciximab or abciximab alone) versus primary PCI, will provide further data that may help define the role of facilitated PCI with STEMI.

CONCLUSIONS

Mechanical reperfusion therapy has become the preferred reperfusion strategy for patients with STEMI when it can be performed by skilled operators in a timely fashion.[26] Outcomes have improved with the use of stents, platelet inhibitors, and with increased experience, and there is promise that outcomes can become even better with new methods to enhance *myocardial* reperfusion and reduce reperfusion injury and with new anticoagulants and drug-eluting stents. Recent trends from the NRMI show that the frequency of use of primary PCI has increased, surpassing lytic therapy, but primary PCI is still only used to treat a minority of patients with STEMI. The major challenge for clini-

cians in the next decade will be to find ways to make prompt mechanical reperfusion more available. The American Heart Association has accepted this challenge and has launched a nationwide effort to reduce door-to-balloon times for patients presenting to interventional and noninterventional hospitals, with the goal of making primary PCI more available to patients with STEMI.

REFERENCES

1. Fletcher AP, Sherry S, Alkjaersig N, et al. The maintenance of a sustained thrombolytic state in man: II. Clinical observations on patients with myocardial infarction and other thromboembolic disorders. *J Clin Invest* 1959;38:1111.
2. Boucek RJ, Murphy WP Jr. Segmental perfusion of the coronary arteries with fibrinolysin in man following a myocardial infarction. *Am J Cardiol* 1960;6:525–533.
3. Favaloro RG, Effler DB, Cheanvechai C, et al. Acute coronary insufficiency (impending myocardial infarction and myocardial infarction): surgical treatment by saphenous vein graft technique. *Am J Cardiol* 1971;28:598–607.
4. Berg R, Everhart FJ, Duvoisin G, et al. Operation for acute coronary occlusion. *Am Surg* 1976;42(7):517–521.
5. Rentrop KP. Development and pathophysiological basis of thrombolytic therapy in acute myocardial infarction: Part II. 1977–1980. The pathogenetic role of thrombus is established by the Göttingen pilot studies of mechanical interventions and intracoronary thrombolysis in acute myocardial infarction. *J Intervent Cardiol* 1998;11(4):265–285.
6. DeWood MA, Spores J, Notske R, et al. Prevalence of total coronary occlusion during the early hours of transmural myocardial infarction. *N Engl J Med* 1980;303:897–902.
7. DeWood MA, Stifter WF, Simpson CS, et al. Coronary arteriographic findings soon after non–Q-wave myocardial infarction. *N Engl J Med* 1986;315:417–423.
8. Rentrop P, DeVivie ER, Karsch KR, et al. Acute coronary occlusion with impending infarction as an angiographic complication relieved by guide-wire recanalization. *Clin Cardiol* 1978;1:101–106.
9. Rentrop KP, Blanke H, Karsch KR, et al. Initial experience with transluminal recanalization of the recently occluded infarct-related coronary artery in acute myocardial infarction—comparison with conventionally treated patients. *Clin Cardiol* 1979;2:92–105.
10. Rentrop KP, Blanke H, Karsch KR, et al. Acute myocardial infarction: intracoronary application of nitroglycerin and streptokinase. *Clin Cardiol* 1979;2:354–363.
11. Khaja F, Walton JA Jr, Brymer JF, et al. Intracoronary fibrinolytic therapy in acute myocardial infarction: report of a prospective randomized trial. *N Engl J Med* 1983;308:1305–1311.
12. Kennedy JW, Ritchie JL, Davis KB, et al. Western Washington randomized trial of intracoronary streptokinase in acute myocardial infarction. *N Engl J Med* 1983;390:1477–1482.
13. O'Neill W, Timmis G, Bourdillon P, et al. A prospective randomized clinical trial of intracoronary streptokinase versus coronary angioplasty for acute myocardial infarction. *N Engl J Med* 1986;314:812–818.
14. Gruppo Italiano per lo Studio della Streptochinasi nell'Infarto Miocardico (GISSI). Effectiveness of intravenous thrombolytic treatment in acute myocardial infarction. *Lancet* 1986;1:397–402.
15. ISIS-2 Collaborative Group. Randomized trial of intravenous streptokinase, oral aspirin, both, or neither among 17,187 cases of suspected acute myocardial infarction. *Lancet* 1988;2(8607):349–360.
16. TIMI Research Group. Immediate vs delayed catheterization and angioplasty following thrombolytic therapy for acute myocardial infarction. *JAMA* 1988;260:2849–2858.
17. Topol EJ, Califf RM, George BS, et al. A randomized trial of immediate versus delayed elective angioplasty after intravenous tissue plasminogen activator in acute myocardial infarction. *N Engl J Med* 1987;317:581–588.
18. Simoons ML, Arnold AER, Betriu A, et al. Thrombolysis with tissue plasminogen activator in acute myocardial infarction: no additional benefit from immediate percutaneous coronary angioplasty. *Lancet* 1988;1:197–202.
19. Hartzler GO, Rutherford BD, McConahay DR, et al. Percutaneous transluminal coronary angioplasty with and without thrombolytic therapy for treatment of acute myocardial infarction. *Am Heart J* 1983;106:965–973.
20. O'Keefe JM, Rutherford BD, McConahay DR, et al. Early and late results of coronary angioplasty without antecedent thrombolytic therapy for acute myocardial infarction. *Am J Cardiol* 1989;64:1221–1230.

21. Brodie B, Weintraub R, Stuckey T, et al. Outcomes of direct coronary angioplasty for acute myocardial infarction in candidates and non-candidates for thrombolytic therapy. *Am J Cardiol* 1991;67:7–12.
22. O'Neill WW, Weintraub R, Grines CL, et al. A prospective, placebo-controlled, randomized trial of intravenous streptokinase and angioplasty versus lone angioplasty therapy of acute myocardial infarction. *Circulation* 1992;86:1710–1717.
23. Grines CL, Brown KF, Marco J, et al. A comparison of immediate angioplasty with thrombolytic therapy for acute myocardial infarction. *N Engl J Med* 1993;328:673–679.
24. Zijlstra F, Jan de Boer M, Hoorntje JCA, et al. A comparison of immediate coronary angioplasty with intravenous streptokinase in acute myocardial infarction. *N Engl J Med* 1993;328:680–684.
25. Gibbons RJ, Holmes ZR, Reeder GS, et al. Immediate angioplasty compared with the administration of a thrombolytic agent followed by conservative treatment for myocardial infarction. *N Engl J Med* 1993;328:685–691.
26. Antman EM, Anbe DT, Armstrong PW, et al. ACC/AHA guidelines for the management of patients with ST-elevation myocardial infarction—executive summary. *Circulation* 2004;110:588–636.
27. Keeley EC, Boura JA, Grines CL. Primary angioplasty vs. intravenous thrombolytic therapy for acute myocardial infarction, a quantitative review of 23 randomized trials. *Lancet* 2003;361:13–20.
28. Fibrinolytic Therapy Trialists' (FTT) Collaborative Group. Indications for fibrinolytic therapy in suspected acute myocardial infarction: collaborative overview of early mortality and major morbidity results from all randomized trials of more than 1000 patients. *Lancet* 1994;343:311–322.
29. Grines CL, Ellis S, Jones M, et al. Primary coronary angioplasty vs thrombolytic therapy for acute myocardial infarction: Long term follow up of ten randomized trials [abstract]. *Circulation* 1999;100(18):I-499.
30. Hochman JS, Sleeper LA, Webb JG, et al. Early revascularization in acute myocardial infarction complicated by cardiogenic shock. *N Engl J Med* 1999;341:625–634.
31. Garcia E, Elizaga J, Perez-Castellano N, et al. Primary angioplasty vs systemic thrombolysis in anterior myocardial infarction. *J Am Coll Cardiol* 1999;33:605–611.
32. Grines C. Senior PAMI. *A Prospective Randomized Trial of Primary Angioplasty and Thrombolytic Therapy in Elderly Patients with Acute Myocardial Infarction.* Presented at Transcatheter Therapeutics (TCT). Washington, DC: October 2005.
33. Nunn CM, O'Neill WW, Rothbaum D, et al. Long-term outcome after primary angioplasty: report from the Primary Angioplasty in Myocardial Infarction (PAMI-1) Trial. *J Am Coll Cardiol* 1999;33:640–646.
34. Zijlstra F, Hoorntje JCA, de Boer M-J, et al. Long-term benefit of primary angioplasty as compared with thrombolytic therapy for acute myocardial infarction. *N Engl J Med* 1999;341:1413–1419.
35. Stone GW, Grines CL, Cox DA, et al. Comparison of angioplasty with stenting, with or without abciximab, in acute myocardial infarction. *N Engl J Med* 2002;346:957–966.
36. Stone GW, Webb J, Cox DA, et al. Distal microcirculatory protection during percutaneous coronary intervention in acute ST-segment elevation myocardial infarction: a randomized controlled trial. *JAMA* 2005;293:1063–1072.
37. GUSTO Angiographic Investigators. The effects of tissue plasminogen activator, streptokinase, or both, on coronary artery patency, ventricular function, and survival after acute myocardial infarction. *N Engl J Med* 1993;329:1615–1622.
38. Antman EM, Giugliano RP, Gibson CM, et al. Abciximab facilitates the rate and extent of thrombolysis: Results of the thrombolysis in myocardial infarctions (TIMI) 14 trial. *Circulation* 1999;99:2720–2732.
39. O'Neill WW, Brodie BR, Ivanhoe R, et al. Primary coronary angioplasty for acute myocardial infarction (The Primary Angioplasty Registry). *Am J Cardiol* 1994;73:627–634.
40. GUSTO III Investigators. A comparison of reteplase with alteplase for acute myocardial infarction. The global use of strategies to open occluded coronary arteries. *N Engl J Med* 1997;337:1118–1123.
41. ASSENT-2 Investigators. Single-bolus tenecteplase compared with front-loaded alteplase in acute myocardial infarction: ASSENT-2 double-blind randomized trial. *Lancet* 1999;354:716–722.
42. The Global Use of Strategies to Open Occluded Coronary Arteries in Acute Coronary Syndromes (GUSTO IIb) Angioplasty Substudy Investigators. A clinical trial comparing primary coronary angioplasty with tissue plasminogen activator for acute myocardial infarction. *N Engl J Med* 1997;336:1621–1628.
43. Grines CL, Cox DA, Stone GW, et al. for the stent primary angioplasty in myocardial infarction study group. Coronary angioplasty with or without

stent implantation for acute myocardial infarction. *N Engl J Med* 1999;341:1949–1956.
44. The GUSTO V Investigators. Reperfusion therapy for acute myocardial infarction with fibrinolytic therapy or combination reduced fibrinolytic therapy and platelet glycoprotein IIb/IIIa inhibition: The GUSTO V randomised trial. *Lancet* 2001;357:1905–1914.
45. The ASSENT-3 Investigators. Efficacy and safety of tenecteplase in combination with enoxaparin, abciximab, or unfractionated heparin: ASSENT-3 randomised trial in acute myocardial infarction. *Lancet* 2001;358:605–613.
46. White HD, French JK, Hamer AW, et al. Frequent re-occlusion of patent infarct-related arteries between four weeks and one year: effects of anti-platelet therapy. *J Am Coll Cardiol* 1995;25:218–223.
47. Veen G, de Boer M-J, Zijlstra F, et al. Improvement in three-month angiographic outcome suggested after primary angioplasty for acute myocardial infarction (Zwolle Trial) compared with successful thrombolysis (APRICOT Trial). *Am J Coll Cardiol* 1999;84:763–767.
48. Schömig A, Kastrati A, Dirschinger J, et al. Coronary stenting plus platelet glycoprotein IIb/IIIa blockade compared with tissue plasminogen activator in acute myocardial infarction. *N Engl J Med* 2000;343:385–391.
49. Kastrati A, Mehilli J, Dirschinger J, et al. Myocardial salvage after coronary stenting plus abciximab vs fibrinolysis plus abciximab in patients with acute myocardial infarction: a randomized trial. *Lancet* 2002;359:920–925.
50. Schomig A, Ndrepepa G, Mehilli J, et al. Therapy-dependent influence of time-to-treatment interval on myocardial salvage in patients with acute myocardial infarction treated with coronary artery stenting or thrombolysis. *Circulation* 2003;108:1084–1088.
51. Brener SJ, Barr LA, Burchenal JEB, et al. Randomized placebo-controlled trial of platelet glycoprotein IIb/IIIa blockade with primary angioplasty for acute myocardial infarction. *Circulation* 1998;98:734–741.
52. Montalescot G, Barragan P, Wittenberg O, et al. Platelet glycoprotein IIb/IIIa inhibition with coronary stenting for acute myocardial infarction. *N Engl J Med* 2001;344:1895–1903.
53. Neumann FJ, Kastrati A, Schmitt C, et al. Effect of glycoprotein IIb/IIIa receptor blockade with abciximab on clinical and angiographic restenosis rate after the placement of coronary stents following acute myocardial infarction. *J Am Coll Cardiol* 2000;35:915–921.
54. Antoniucci D, Rodriguez A, Hempel A, et al. A randomized trial comparing primary infarct artery stenting with or without abciximab in acute myocardial infarction. *J Am Coll Cardiol* 2003;42:1879–1885.
55. De Luca G, Suryapranata H, Stone GW, et al. Abciximab as adjunctive therapy to reperfusion in acute ST-segment elevation myocardial infarction: a meta-analysis of randomized trials. *JAMA* 2005;293:1759–1765.
56. Keeley EC, Boura JA, Grines CL. Comparison of primary and facilitated percutaneous coronary interventions for ST-elevation myocardial infarction: quantitative review of randomised trials. *Lancet* 2006;367:579–588.
57. Spaulding C. *Final Results of the TYPHOON Study, a Multi-Center Randomized Trial Comparing the Use of Sirolimus-Eluting Stents to Bare Metal Stents in Primary Angioplasty for Acute Myocardial Infarction.* Presented at the American College of Cardiology Scientific Sessions. Atlanta, GA: March 2006.
58. Dirksen MT. *Randomized Comparison of Paclitaxel Eluting Stent Versus Conventional Stent in ST-Segment Elevation Myocardial Infarction: Results of the PASSION Trial.* Presented at the American College of Cardiology Scientific Sessions. Atlanta, GA: March 2006.
59. Brodie BR, Stuckey TD, Pulsipher M, et al. Stent thrombosis and target vessel revascularization following primary percutaneous coronary intervention with drug-eluting stents versus bare metal stents for ST elevation myocardial infarction: results from the STENT registry. *J Am Coll Cardiol* 2006;47(Suppl B):41B.
60. van't Hof AWJ, Liem A, Suryapranata H, et al. Angiographic assessment of myocardial reperfusion in patients treated with primary angioplasty for acute myocardial infarction. *Circulation* 1998;97:2302–2306.
61. van't Hof AWJ, Liem A, de Boer M-J, et al. Clinical value of 12-lead electrocardiogram after successful reperfusion therapy for acute myocardial infarction. *Lancet* 1997;350:615–619.
62. Brodie BR, Stuckey TD, Hansen C, et al. Relation between electrocardiographic ST-segment resolution and early and late outcomes after primary percutaneous coronary intervention for acute myocardial infarction. *Am J Cardiol* 2005;95:343–348.
63. Napodano M, Pasquetto G, Sacca S, et al. Intracoronary thrombectomy improves myocardial reperfusion in patients undergoing direct angioplasty for acute myocardial infarction. *J Am Coll Cardiol* 2003;42:1395–1402.
64. Lefevre T, Garcia E, Reimers B, et al. X-sizer for thrombectomy in acute myocardial infarction improves ST-segment resolution: results of the X-sizer

in AMI for negligible embolization and optimal ST resolution (X AMINE ST) trial. *J Am Coll Cardiol* 2005;46:246–252.

65. Burzotta F, Trani C, Romagnoli E, et al. Manual thrombus-aspiration improves myocardial reperfusion: the randomized evaluation of the effect of mechanical reduction of distal embolization by thrombus-aspiration in primary and rescue angioplasty (REMEDIA) trial. *J Am Coll Cardiol* 2005;46:371–376.

66. De Luca L, Sardella G, Davidson CJ, et al. Impact of intracoronary aspiration thrombectomy during primary angioplasty on left ventricular remodeling in patients with anterior ST-elevation myocardial infarction. *Heart* 2006;92(7):951–957.

67. Noel B, Morice MC, Lefevre T, et al. Thrombus-aspiration in acute ST elevation MI improves myocardial reperfusion. Results of the Export Study. Presented at Transcatheter Therapeutics, Washington, DC, 2005.

68. Antoniucci D, Valenti R, Migliorini A, et al. Comparison of rheolytic thrombectomy before direct infarct artery stenting versus direct stenting alone in patients undergoing percutaneous coronary intervention for acute myocardial infarction. *Am J Cardiol* 2004;93(8):1033–1035.

69. Kaltoft A, Bottcher M, Nielsen SS, et al. Routine thrombectomy in percutaneous coronary intervention for acute ST-segment elevation myocardial infarction: a randomized controlled trial. *Circulation* 2006;114:40–47.

70. Ali A, Cox D, Dib N, et al. Rheolytic thrombectomy with percutaneous coronary intervention for infarct size reduction in acute myocardial infarction: 30 day results from a multicenter randomized study. *J Am Coll Cardiol* 2006;48:244–252.

71. Brodie BR. Adjunctive thrombectomy with primary percutaneous coronary intervention for ST-elevation myocardial infarction: summary of randomized trials. *J Invasive Cardiol* 2006;18:24C–27C.

72. Chinnaiyan KM, Grines CL, O'Neill WW, et al. Safety of AngioJet thrombectomy in acute ST-segment elevation myocardial infarction: a large single center experience. *J Invasive Cardiol* 2006;18:17C21C.

73. Sherev DA, Shavelle DM, Abdelkarim M, et al. AngioJet rheolytic thrombectomy during rescue PCI for failed thrombolysis: a single center experience. *J Invasive Cardiol* 2006;18:12C–16C.

74. Sharma SK, Tamburrino F, Mares AM, Kini AS. Improved outcome with AngioJet thrombectomy during primary stenting in acute myocardial infarction patients with high-grade thrombus. *J Invasive Cardiol* 2006;18:8C–11C.

75. Simonton CA, Brodie B, Wilson H, et al. AngioJet experience from the multi-center STENT registry. *J Invasive Cardiol* 2006;18:22C–23C.

76. Sianos G, Papafaklis MI, Vaina S, et al. Rheolytic thrombectomy in patients with ST-elevation myocardial infarction and large thrombus burden. The Thoraxcenter experience. *J Invasive Cardiol* 2006;18:3C–7C.

77. Henriques JP, Zijlstra F, Ottervanger JP, et al. Incidence and clinical significance of distal embolization during primary angioplasty for acute myocardial infarction. *Eur Heart J* 2002;23:1112–1117.

78. Stone GW, Brodie BR, Griffin JJ, et al. for the PAMI-2 Investigators. The role of cardiac surgery in the hospital phase management of patients treated with primary angioplasty for acute myocardial infarction. *Am J Cardiol* 2000;85:1292–1296.

79. Mehta SR, Yusuf S, Peters RJ, et al. Effects of pretreatment with clopidogrel and aspirin followed by long-term therapy in patients undergoing percutaneous coronary intervention: the PCI-CURE study. *Lancet* 2001;358:527–533.

80. Steinhubl SR, Berger PB, Mann JT, et al. Early and sustained dual oral antiplatelet therapy following percutaneous coronary intervention: a randomized controlled trial. *JAMA* 2002;288:2411–2420.

81. Sabatine MS, Cannon CP, Gibson CM, et al. Effect of clopidogrel pretreatment before percutaneous coronary intervention in patients with ST-elevation myocardial infarction treated with fibrinolytics: the PCI-CLARITY study. *JAMA* 2005;294:1224–1232.

82. Stone GW, Marsalese D, Brodie BR. A prospective, randomized evaluation of prophylactic intra-aortic balloon counterpulsation in high risk patients with acute myocardial infarction treated with primary angioplasty. *J Am Coll Cardiol* 1997;29:1459–1467.

83. van't Hof AWJ, Liem AM, de Boer MJ, et al. A randomized comparison of intra-aortic balloon pumping after primary coronary angioplasty in high risk patients with acute myocardial infarction. *Eur Heart J* 1999;20:659–665.

84. Brodie BR, Stuckey TD, Hansen C, et al. Intra-aortic balloon counterpulsation before primary percutaneous transluminal coronary angioplasty reduces catheterization laboratory events in high risk patients with acute myocardial infarction. *Am J Cardiol* 1999;84:18–23.

85. Grines CL, Marsalese DL, Brodie BR, et al. Safety and cost-effectiveness of early discharge after primary angioplasty in low risk patients with acute myocardial infarction. *J Am Coll Cardiol* 1998;31:967–972.

86. Henry TD, Unger BT, Sharkey SW, et al. Design of a standardized system for transfer of patients with ST-elevation myocardial infarction for percutaneous coronary intervention. *Am Heart J* 2005;150:373–384.

87. Bradley EH, Curry LA, Webster TR, et al. Achieving rapid door-to-balloon times: how top hospitals improve complex clinical systems. *Circulation* 2006;113:1079–1085.

88. Vermeer F, Oude Ophuis AJ, van der Berg EJ, et al. Prospective randomized comparison between thrombolysis, rescue PTCA, and primary PTCA in patients with extensive myocardial infarction admitted to a hospital without PTCA facilities: a safety and feasibility study. *Heart* 1999;82(4):426–431.

89. Widimsky P, Groch L, Zelizko M, et al. Multi-center randomized trial comparing transport to primary angioplasty vs. immediate thrombolysis vs. combined strategy for patients with acute myocardial infarction presenting to a community hospital without a catheterization laboratory. *Eur Heart J* 2000;21:823–831.

90. Grines CL, Westerhausen DR Jr., Grines LL, et al. A randomized trial of transfer for primary angioplasty vs. on-site thrombolysis in patients with high-risk myocardial infarction: the air primary angioplasty in myocardial infarction study. *J Am Coll Cardiol* 2002;39:1713–1719.

91. Andersen HR, Nielsen TT, Rasmussen K, et al. A comparison of coronary angioplasty with fibrinolytic therapy in acute myocardial infarction. *N Engl J Med* 2003;349(8):733–742.

92. Widimsky P, Budesinsky T, Vorac D, et al. Long distance transport for primary angioplasty vs immediate thrombolysis in acute myocardial infarction. *Eur Heart J* 2003;24:94–104.

93. Dalby M, Bouzamondo A, Lechat P, Montalescot G. Transfer for primary angioplasty versus immediate thrombolysis in acute myocardial infarction. A meta-analysis. *Circulation* 2003;108:1809–1814.

94. Nallamothu BK, Bates ER, Herrin J, et al. Times to treatment in transfer patients undergoing primary percutaneous coronary intervention in the United States: National Registry of Myocardial Infarction (NRMI)-3/4 analysis. *Circulation* 2005;111;718–720.

95. Wharton TP Jr, Grines LL, Turco MA, et al. Primary angioplasty in acute myocardial infarction at hospitals with no surgery on-site (the PAMI-No SOS study) versus transfer to surgical centers for primary angioplasty. *J Am Coll Cardiol* 2004;43:1943–1950.

96. Aversano T, Aversano LT, Passamani E, et al. Thrombolytic therapy vs. primary percutaneous coronary intervention for myocardial infarction in patients presenting to hospitals without on-site cardiac surgery: a randomized control trial. *JAMA* 2002;287:1943–1951.

97. Boersma E and the PCAT-2 Trialists' Collaborative Group. Does time matter? A pooled analysis of randomized clinical trials comparing primary percutaneous coronary intervention and in-hospital fibrinolysis in acute myocardial infarction patients. *Eur Heart J* 2006;27:779–788.

98. Brodie BR, Hansen C, Stuckey TD, et al. Door-to-balloon time with primary percutaneous coronary intervention for acute myocardial infarction impacts late cardiac mortality in high-risk patients and patients presenting early after the onset of symptoms. *J Am Coll Cardiol* 2006;47:289–295.

99. Brodie BR, Stone GW, Cox DA, et al. Impact of treatment delays on outcomes of primary percutaneous coronary intervention for acute myocardial infarction: analysis from the CADILLAC trial. *Am Heart J* 2006;151(6):1231–1238.

100. Gersh BJ, Stone GW, White HD, et al. Pharmacological facilitation of primary percutaneous coronary intervention for acute myocardial infarction. Is the slope of the curve the shape of the future? *JAMA* 2005;293:979–986.

101. ASSENT-4 PCI Investigators. Primary versus tenecteplase-facilitated percutaneous coronary intervention in patients with ST-segment elevation acute myocardial infarction (ASSENT-4 PCI): randomised trial. *Lancet* 2006;367:569–578.

102. Ellis SG, da Silva ER, Heyndrickx G, et al. Randomized comparison of rescue angioplasty with conservative management of patients with early failure of thrombolysis for acute anterior myocardial infarction. *Circulation* 1994;90:2280–2284.

103. Sutton AGC, Campbell PG, Graham R, et al. A randomized trial of rescue angioplasty versus a conservative approach for failed fibrinolysis in ST-segment elevation myocardial infarction. *J Am Coll Cardiol* 2004;44:287–296.

104. Gershlick AH, Stephens-Lloyd A, Hughes S, et al. Rescue angioplasty after failed thrombolytic therapy for acute myocardial infarction. *N Engl J Med* 2005;353:2758–2768.

105. Mahaffey KW, Puma JA, Barbagelata NA, et al. Adenosine as an adjunct to thrombolytic therapy for acute myocardial infarction: Results of a multi-center randomized, placebo controlled trial: The acute myocardial infarction study of adenosine (AMISTAD) trial. *J Am Coll Cardiol* 1999;34(6):1711–1720.

106. Ross AM, Gibbons RJ, Stone GW, et al. A randomized double-blinded, placebo-controlled multicenter trial of adenosine as an adjunct to reperfusion in the treatment of acute myocardial infarction (AMISTAD-II). *J Am Coll Cardiol* 2005;45:1775–1780.

107. Granger CB, Mahaffey KW, Weaver D, et al. Pexelizumab, an anti-C5 complement antibody, as adjunctive therapy to primary percutaneous coronary intervention in acute myocardial infarction. *Circulation* 2003;108:1184–1190.

108. Hale SL, Dave RH, Kloner RA. Regional hypothermia reduces myocardial necrosis even when instituted after the onset of ischemia. *Basic Res Cardiol* 1997;92(5):351–357.

109. Miki T, Liu GS, Cohen MV, Downey JM. Mild hypothermia reduces infarct size in the beating rabbit heart: a practical intervention for acute myocardial infarction? *Basic Res Cardiol* 1998;93(5):372–383.

110. O'Neill WW. *Hypothermia as an Adjunctive Therapy to PCI in Patients with Acute Myocardial Infarction*. Presented at TCT (Transcatheter Therapeutics), Washington, DC: 2003.

111. Grines C. *Intravascular cooling adjunctive to percutaneous coronary intervention*. Presented at TCT (Transcatheter Therapeutics), Washington, DC: 2004.

112. Brodie BR, Stuckey TD, Hansen C, et al. Benefit of coronary reperfusion before intervention on outcomes after primary angioplasty for acute myocardial infarction. *Am J Cardiol* 2000;85:13–18.

113. Stone GW, Cox D, Garcia E, et al. Normal flow (TIMI-3) before mechanical reperfusion therapy is an independent determinant of survival in acute myocardial infarction: analysis from the primary angioplasty in myocardial infarction trials. *Circulation* 2001;104:636–641.

114. Keeley EC, Boura JA, Grines CL. Comparison of primary and facilitated percutaneous coronary intervention for ST-elevation myocardial infarction: quantitative review of randomized trials. *Lancet* 2006;367:579–588.

CHAPTER 64

Diagnosis and Management of Patients with Chronic Ischemic Heart Disease

Robert A. O'Rourke / Patrick T. O'Gara / Leslee J. Shaw / John S. Douglas, Jr.

Ischemic heart disease continues to be a major public health problem.[1] Chronic stable angina is the first indicator of ischemic heart disease in approximately 50 percent of patients. The reported annual incidence of angina is 213 per 100,000 people older than age 30 years. The number of patients with stable angina in the United States approximates 16.5 million, not including individuals who do not seek medical attention for their chest pain or who are shown to have a noncardiac cause of chest discomfort. Angina pectoris is a clinical syndrome that consists of discomfort or pain in the chest, jaw, shoulder, back, or arm. Typically it is precipitated or aggravated by exertion or emotional stress and relieved by nitroglycerin. Angina usually occurs in patients with coronary artery disease (CAD) affecting one or more large epicardial arteries. However, angina is often present in individuals with valvular heart disease, hypertrophic cardiomyopathy, and uncontrolled hypertension. It also occurs in patients with normal coronary arteries and myocardial ischemia caused by coronary artery spasm or endothelial dysfunction. The symptom of angina is often observed in patients with noncardiac disorders affecting the esophagus, chest wall, or lungs. An extensive discussion of the differential diagnosis of chest pain is included in Chap. 12 and Table 64–1.

HISTORICAL PERSPECTIVE

In 1768, William Heberden presented his classic description of angina pectoris in a lecture before the Royal College of Physicians; it was published in 1772.[2] This classic description was published again with minor changes in a chapter entitled "Pectoris Dolor" in his *Commentaries on the History and Cure of Diseases*, which was translated from the Latin and published by his son, also named William Heberden, in 1802.[3] The following quotation is from the original lecture:

There is a disorder of the breast, marked with strong and peculiar symptoms, considerable for the kind of danger belonging to it, and extremely rare, of which I do not recollect any mention among medical authors. The seat of it, and sense of strangling and anxiety, with which it is attended, may make it not improperly be called angina pectoris. Those who are afflicted with it are seized, while they are walking, and more particularly when they walk soon after eating, with a painful and most disagreeable sensation in the breast, which seems as if it would take their life away, if it were to increase or to continue: the moment they stand still all this uneasiness vanishes.

After it has continued some months, it will not cease so instantaneous upon standing still; and it will come on, not only when the persons are walking, but when they are lying down, and oblige them to rise up from their beds every night for many months together; and in one or two very inveterate cases it has been brought on by the motion of a horse or a carriage, and even by swallowing, coughing, going to stool or speaking, or by any disturbance of mind.

…but all the rest, whom I have seen, who are at least twenty, were men, and almost all above fifty years old, and most of them with a short neck, and inclining to be fat. When a fit of this sort comes on by walking, its duration is very short, as it goes off almost immediately upon stopping. If it comes on in the night, it will last an hour or two; and I have met one, in whom it once continued for several days, during all which time the patient seemed to be in imminent danger of death.

But the natural tendency of this illness be to kill the patients suddenly, yet unless it have a power of preserving a person from all other ails, it will easily be believed that some of those, who are afflicted with it, may die in a different manner, since this disorder will last, as I have known it more than once, near twenty years, and most usually attacks only those who are

TABLE 64–1

Clinical Classification of Angina

Typical angina (definite)
  1. Substernal chest discomfort with a characteristic quality and duration that is
  2. Provoked by exertion or emotional stress and
  3. Relieved by rest or nitroglycerin.
Atypical angina (probable)
  Meets two of the above characteristics.
Noncardiac chest pain
  Meets one or none of the typical anginal characteristics.

SOURCE: *Modified from Diamond GA, Staniloff HM, Forrester JS, et al. Computer-assisted diagnosis in the noninvasive evaluation of patients with suspected coronary disease. J Am Coll Cardiol 1983;1:444–455.*

above fifty years of age. I have accordingly observed one, who sunk under a lingering illness of a different nature.

The os sterni is usually pointed to as the seat of this malady, but it seems sometimes as if it was under the lower part of it, and at other times under the middle or upper part, but always inclining more to the left side, and sometimes there is with it a pain about the middle of the left arm.

The syndrome of angina pectoris was described as rare in textbooks of medicine in 1866 (Austin Flint) and 1892 (William Osler). Paul Dudley White wrote: "[Angina pectoris] was uncommon in my early professional years. But when the automobile came in the 1920s and the population at large became more prosperous and over nourished, the current epidemic of coronary heart disease, as shown mainly by the symptom angina pectoris, began and incidentally involved younger and younger men."[4] In the United States, the peak mortality rate from coronary heart disease (CHD) occurred about 1962 to 1965; since then, it has been decreasing steadily.

ETIOLOGY AND CLASSIFICATION

Coronary atherosclerosis (or atherothrombosis) is the cause of angina pectoris in most patients (see Chaps. 51 to 67). Many nonatherosclerotic causes of CAD (see Tables 12–1 and 64–1) can also produce angina pectoris or myocardial infarction. Other conditions particularly associated with angina pectoris include congenital coronary artery abnormalities (see Chap. 83), aortic stenoses (see Chap. 75), mitral stenoses with resulting severe right ventricular hypertension (see Chap. 77), hypertrophic cardiomyopathy (see Chap. 30), and systemic arterial hypertension (see Chap. 69).

Disorders in which angina occurs less frequently include aortic regurgitation (see Chap. 75), idiopathic dilated cardiomyopathy (see Chap. 29), and luetic heart disease. Mitral valve prolapse (see Chap. 76) rarely causes true angina pectoris. Certain conditions may alter the balance between myocardial oxygen supply–demand and precipitate or aggravate angina pectoris, including severe anemia, tachycardia, fever, hyperthyroidism, and Paget disease of bone.

The Canadian Cardiovascular Society Grading Scale (see Table 12–2) is commonly used to classify the severity of angina pectoris,

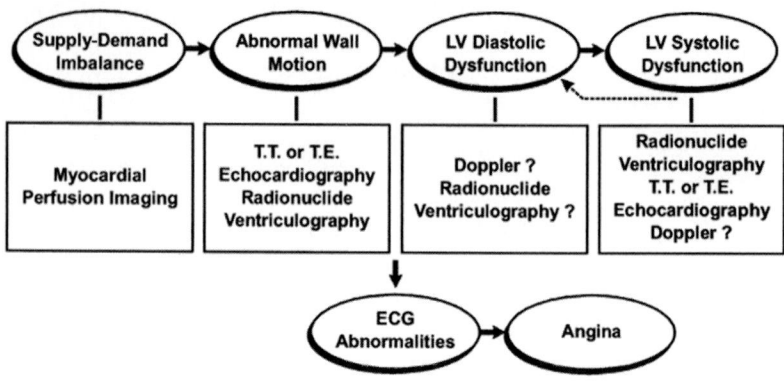

FIGURE 64–1. Sequence of events in the ischemic cascade plus noninvasive tests for detecting its presence. T.E., transesophageal; T.T., transthoracic.

with the most severe symptoms occurring at rest and the least severe only with excessive exercise.

DIAGNOSIS

【 】 HISTORY AND PHYSICAL EXAMINATION

The first step is to obtain a detailed description of the symptom complex in order to characterize the chest pain or discomfort. Five descriptors typically are considered: (1) location, (2) quality, (3) duration of the discomfort, (4) inciting factors, and (5) factors relieving the pain.[1]

The most commonly used classification scheme for chest pain divides patients into three groups: *typical angina, atypical angina,* and *noncardiac chest pain* (see Table 64–1).[5]

Angina is further labeled as *stable* when its characteristics are usually unchanged for 60 days (see Chaps. 54 and 57). The presence of *unstable angina* predicts a much higher short-term risk of an acute coronary event. *Unstable angina* is defined as angina that presents in one of three major ways: *rest angina, severe new-onset angina,* or *prior angina increasing in severity* (see Chap. 54). Recently, the acute coronary syndromes of unstable angina and non–ST-segment elevation myocardial infarction were linked together by their similar presentation and treatment (see Chap. 56).[6]

Usually, the discomfort of chronic stable angina pectoris is precipitated by physical activity, emotions, eating, or cold weather. Certain patients are able to describe accurately the extent and type of exercise at which they reproducibly experience their chest pain (see Chap. 12). Many patients will develop angina if they walk up a hill against a cold wind after a large meal. Emotions, particularly anger, excitation, and frustration, often precipitate angina in patients with CAD. Cigarette smoking induces chest discomfort or lowers the exertion threshold for angina in some patients. A history of cocaine use should be sought because it can precipitate myocardial ischemia with or without infarction by coronary vasoconstriction.

When stable angina pectoris develops, it often increases to a plateau over 10 to 30 seconds and usually disappears within minutes if the exertion is discontinued. Occasionally, the angina will disappear despite continued physical activity ("walk-through an-

gina"), which is attributed to the opening of collaterals. Most patients have discomfort that lasts only several minutes, sometimes up to 10 to 15 minutes, and rarely up to 30 minutes (see Chap. 12).

The discomfort of angina is most often located substernally or just to the left of the sternum. Some patients, in describing the discomfort, clench their fist over their upper sternum (Levine sign)—a sign of high diagnostic accuracy. Less often, angina is located over the precordium. The discomfort is rarely localized *only* to the apex of the heart. Nevertheless, angina can be located anywhere from the epigastrium to the neck; rarely, it may be located only in the neck, throat, arm, or back.

The pain often radiates down the arms or to the neck, jaw, teeth, shoulders, or back. Radiation to the left side is more common, but both sides can be involved. The radiation, characteristically down the ulnar aspect of the arm, is often described as numbness. Increased heat or humidity also may lower the exertional threshold at which angina occurs.

Disorders that increase the myocardial oxygen requirement (MVO_2) may exacerbate the occurrence of angina pectoris and sometimes may be associated with angina in the absence of moderate or severe CAD stenosis on coronary arteriography. Patients with stable angina may have many episodes of myocardial ischemia that are asymptomatic or silent. Also, myocardial ischemia may result in symptoms due to either systolic or diastolic left ventricular (LV) dysfunction without the characteristic chest discomfort. *Angina equivalent* symptoms usually are associated with exertion and are relieved by rest and nitroglycerin. *Exertional dyspnea* likely is caused by reduced diastolic LV compliance resulting from myocardial ischemia. *Exertional fatigue* or exhaustion probably results from an acute decrease in cardiac output caused by diminished systolic LV function and/or associated mitral regurgitation from transient papillary muscle dysfunction.

In general, when myocardial ischemia is produced, an *ischemic cascade* occurs. Regional diastolic and systolic dysfunction precede global diastolic and then systolic dysfunction, which in turn often occurs prior to changes in the electrocardiogram (ECG) and before the symptoms of angina pectoris (Fig. 64–1). Noninvasive testing is often useful in detecting ischemia (see below). The detection of LV diastolic dysfunction by Doppler mitral valve recording or by diastolic filling curves using radionuclide ventriculography has many limitations (see Chaps. 15 and 19). Although diaphoresis and alterations in blood pressure and heart rate may occur, the physical examination is often normal. An examination performed during an episode of pain, however, can be useful. A fourth (most common) or third heart sound, a mitral regurgitant systolic murmur, reversed splitting of the S_2, bibasilar pulmonary rates, or palpable ectopic cardiac impulses that disappear when the pain subsides are all predictive of CAD (see Chap. 12). Carotid sinus pressure often terminates anginal chest pain. Evidence of noncoronary atherosclerotic disease such as a carotid bruit, diminished pedal pulse, or abdominal aneurysm increases the likelihood of CAD. An elevated blood pressure, xanthomas, and retinal exudates point to the presence of CAD risk factors (see Chap. 12).

TABLE 64-2

Pretest Likelihood of CAD in Symptomatic Patients According to Age and Sex[a,b]

AGE, YEARS	NONANGINAL CHEST PAIN		ATYPICAL ANGINA		TYPICAL ANGINA	
	MEN	WOMEN	MEN	WOMEN	MEN	WOMEN
30–39	4	2	34	12	76	26
40–49	13	3	51	22	87	55
50–59	20	7	65	31	93	73
60–69	27	14	72	51	94	86

[a]Each value represents the percent with significant CAD on catheterization.
[b]Combined Diamond/Forrester and CASS data.
SOURCE: Modified from Gibbons RJ, Chatterjee K, Daley J, et al.[1]

[ ] CLINICAL ASSESSMENT OF THE LIKELIHOOD OF CAD

The clinicopathologic study performed by Diamond and Forrester[7] demonstrated that it is possible to predict the probability of CAD after the history and the physical examination. By combining data from several angiographic studies performed before 1980, they showed that simple clinical observations of pain type, age, and sex were powerful predictors of the probability of CAD.

The usefulness of this approach was confirmed subsequently in prospective studies at Duke and Stanford universities. In both men and women, the initial clinical characteristics most helpful in predicting CAD were determined. In these studies, age, sex, and pain type were the most powerful predictors (see Table 64–2). Smoking, Q waves, or ST-segment–T-wave changes on ECG, hyperlipidemia, and diabetes further strengthened the predictive abilities of these models.[1]

[ ] SPECIAL TESTS FOR DIAGNOSIS

Most special tests in patients with suspected stable angina are performed either to establish the diagnosis and/or to determine the risk for coronary events.[1] Table 64–2 indicates the likelihood for each gender by age and characteristics of the chest discomfort. It also indicates why women have more false-positive responses to ECG exercise testing than do men (see Chap. 14). Table 64–3 lists terms useful in the evaluation and selection of diagnostic tests for CAD. The Bayes theorem states that the pretest prevalence of disease influences the posttest likelihood of significant CAD (see Chap. 14). Figure 64–2 illustrates the impact of the Bayes theorem when evaluating several diagnostic tests for CAD. More accurate data on the sensitivity and specificity of noninvasive testing for diagnosis of CAD are provided in Chaps. 14, 16, 19, 20, and 21.

If an exercise ECG test was performed on a 55-year-old woman with atypical chest pain and a pretest likelihood for coronary disease of 0.46, a positive ECG stress test response would indicate her posttest likelihood for disease to be 0.86. However, if she had a positive thallium scan, her likelihood of disease would increase to 0.98. If her thallium scan was negative, the probability of disease would decrease to 0.63.

Diagnostic tests should be performed only when necessary to answer a specific clinical question. Thus a diagnostic test may be of limited additional diagnostic value in patients with either a very high (>0.90) or a very low (<0.10) pretest risk for CAD.[1]

Electrocardiogram and Chest Roentgenogram

A resting 12-lead ECG should be recorded in all patients with symptoms suggestive of angina; however, it will be normal in up to 50 percent of patients with chronic stable angina. ECG evidence of LV hypertrophy or ST-segment–T-wave changes consistent with myocardial ischemia favors the diagnosis of angina pectoris. Evidence of prior Q-wave myocardial infarction (MI) on the ECG makes CAD very likely. Patients with a completely normal resting ECG *rarely have* significant LV systolic dysfunction.[1]

TABLE 64-3

Glossary of Terms

True positive (TP): positive result in patient with disease
True negative (TN): negative result in patient without disease
False positive (FP): positive result in patient without disease
False negative (FN): negative result in patient with disease

Sensitivity: $\dfrac{TP}{TF + FP}$

Specificity: $\dfrac{TN}{TN + FP}$

Predictive value of a positive test: $\dfrac{TP}{TP + FP}$

Predictive value of a negative test: $\dfrac{TN}{TN + FN}$

Bayes theorem:

Probability of disease presence with a positive test =
$$\frac{\text{sensitivity} \times \text{prevalence}}{(\text{sensitivity} \times \text{prevalence}) + [(1 - \text{specificity}) \times (1 - \text{prevalence})]}$$

Probability of disease presence with a negative test =
$$\frac{(1 - \text{sensitivity}) \times \text{prevalence}}{[(1 - \text{sensitivity}) \times \text{prevalence} + [\text{specificity} \times (1 - \text{prevalence})]}$$

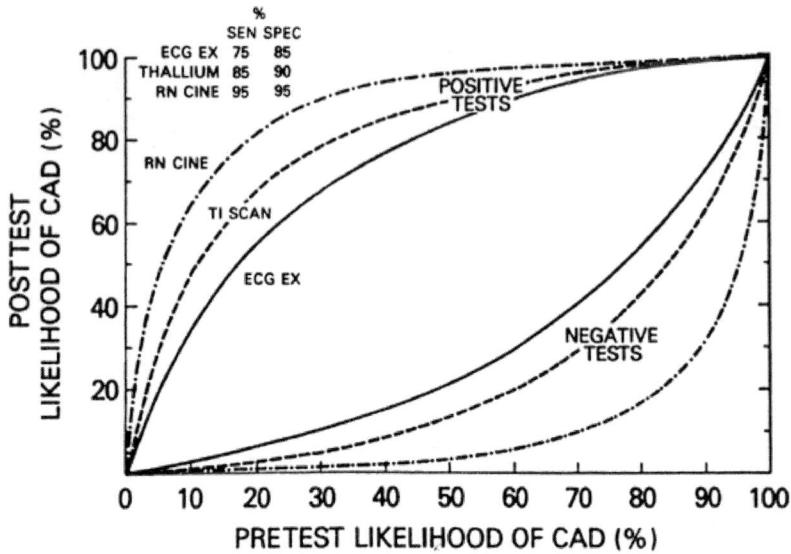

FIGURE 64–2. Probability of coronary artery disease (CAD). Comparison of ECG exercise testing (ECG EX), thallium perfusion imaging (TI Scan), and radionuclide cineangiography (RN CINE). Sensitivity (SEN) and specificity (SPEC) values are approximations derived from published series. *Source: From Epstein et al. Am J Cardiol 1980;46:491. Reproduced with permission from the publisher and authors.*

The presence of arrhythmias (e.g., atrial fibrillation or ventricular tachyarrhythmias) on the ECG in patients with chest pain also increases the probability of underlying CAD; however, these arrhythmias frequently are caused by other types of cardiac disease. Various degrees of atrioventricular (AV) block occur in patients with chronic CAD, but have a very low specificity for the diagnosis. Left anterior fascicular block, right bundle-branch block (RBBB), and left bundle-branch block (LBBB) are often present in patients with CAD and frequently indicate multivessel CAD, but are not specific.

An ECG obtained during chest pain is abnormal in approximately 50 percent of patients with angina and a normal resting ECG. Sinus tachycardia is frequent; bradyarrhythmias are less common. ST-segment elevation or depression establishes a high likelihood of angina and indicates ischemia at a low workload, suggesting an unfavorable prognosis. Many high-risk patients with severe episodes of angina need no further noninvasive testing. Coronary arteriography usually defines the severity of CAD and determines the necessity and feasibility of myocardial revascularization. In patients with ST-segment–T-wave depression or inversion on the resting ECG, pseudonormalization of these abnormalities during pain is another indicator that CAD is likely. The occurrence of tachyarrhythmias, AV block, left anterior fascicular block, or bundle branch block during chest pain also increases the probability of CHD and often leads to coronary arteriography.

The *chest roentgenogram* often is normal in patients with stable angina pectoris. Its usefulness as a routine test is *not* well established. It is more likely to be abnormal in patients with previous or acute MI, those with a noncoronary artery cause of chest pain, and those with noncardiac chest pain.

Coronary artery calcification increases the likelihood of symptomatic CAD. *Fluoroscopically detectable* coronary calcification is correlated with major vessel occlusion in 94 percent of patients *with* chest pain; however, the sensitivity of the test is less than 40 percent.

Electron-beam computed tomography (EBCT) and multislice tomography are being used with increasing frequency for screening asymptomatic individuals. However, the specificity of a positive result may be as low as 49 percent, and the predictive accuracy is less than 70 percent. The role of EBCT in CAD diagnosis and risk stratification continues to be controversial.[8] The most recent report of an American College of Cardiology/American Heart Association (ACC/AHA) expert consensus writing group does not recommend EBCT for *routine screening* of asymptomatic patients for CAD or for its use in most patients with chest pain.[9] It also is of limited use in detecting high-risk plaques[10] (see below). An updated report of the usefulness of EBCT and multislice tomograms has recently been published.[10a] The higher patient scores (75 percent of score adjusted for age) are associated with a worse prognosis.

Exercise ECG Stress Testing

Exercise ECG stress testing is a well-established procedure that has been in widespread clinical use for many decades.[11] Although usually a safe procedure, both MI and death occur at a rate of up to 1 per 2500 tests. Absolute contraindications include acute MI within 2 days, symptomatic cardiac arrhythmias causing hemodynamic compromise, symptomatic and severe aortic stenoses, symptomatic heart failure, acute pulmonary embolus or infarction, acute myocarditis or pericarditis, and acute aortic dissection.

For optimizing the information obtained, the protocol should be tailored to the individual patient, with exercise lasting at least 6 minutes.[12] Exercise capacity should be reported in estimated metabolic equivalents (METs) of exercise (1 MET is the standard basal oxygen uptake of 3.5 mL/kg/min) as well as in minutes.

The ECG, heart rate, and blood pressure should be monitored carefully and recorded during each stage of exercise, as well as during ST-segment abnormalities and chest pain, as detailed in Chap. 14.

Interpretation of the exercise ECG should include symptomatic response, exercise capacity, hemodynamic response, and ECG changes. The most important ECG abnormalities are ST-segment depression and ST-segment elevation (in leads without diagnostic Q waves) of greater than 1 mm for at least 60 to 80 milliseconds after the end of the QRS complex. Although exercise testing is often terminated when subjects reach a standard percentage (often 85 percent of age-predicted maximum heart rate), there is a *great variability* in maximum heart rate among individuals (see Chap. 16). Many stress testing laboratories still use approaches that are not up-to-date.

A meta-analysis of 147 published reports describing 24,074 patients who underwent both coronary angiography and exercise testing found wide variation in sensitivity and specificity (see Chap. 16). The mean sensitivity was 68 percent and the mean specificity 77 percent. In a prospective study of 814 men that minimized workup bias, sensitivity was 45 percent and specificity 85 percent.[12] Therefore, the true diagnostic value of the exercise ECG relates to its *relatively high specificity*. The modest sensitivity of the exercise ECG is generally lower than that of imaging procedures.[13]

To improve the clinical usefulness of exercise ECG testing in the diagnosis of CAD, a treadmill score[13] was developed, as well as a prognostic score that predicted 5-year survival using the amount of ST-segment depression, the degree of angina during exercise, and the duration of exercise (see Chap. 16).[14] Other methods employed include the ST/HR slope, calculated from linear regression of ST-segment depression against heart rate (HR) during peak exercise, and the simple ST/HR index, in which additional ST-segment depression is divided by the overall change in heart rate throughout the exercise period. The cost-effectiveness of these techniques remains unknown.

Diagnostic testing is most valuable when the pretest probability of obstructive CAD is intermediate. In these conditions, the test result has the largest effect on the posttest probability of disease and thus on clinical decisions. Intermediate probability has been defined arbitrarily as between 10 and 90 percent; this definition has been used in several reports, including the ACC/AHA *Exercise Test Guidelines*.[11]

Special issues in ECG exercise testing include the effect of digoxin on ST–T-wave changes, the usefulness of withholding β-blocking drugs when possible, changes in ST-segment depression in patients with LBBB or RBBB, changes in the exercise ECG in patients with LV hypertrophy on ECG with or without repolarization abnormalities, and the usefulness of ECG testing in patients with resting ST-segment depression; these are discussed in great detail in Chap. 16.[11]

Exercise-induced ST-segment depression usually occurs with LBBB and does not necessarily indicate ischemia.[15] However, in RBBB, ST-segment depression in the left chest leads (V_5 to V_6) or inferior leads (II and aVF) during exercise has the same significance as when the resting ECG is normal.

The difficulties of using exercise testing for diagnosing obstructive CAD in women have led to speculation that initial stress imaging may be preferable to standard ECG stress testing. However, *women with a completely normal resting ECG* do not have a greater incidence of false-positive tests than men.[1]

Rest Echocardiography

Echocardiography can be useful for establishing a diagnosis of CAD and in defining the consequences of CAD in selected patients with chronic stable angina (see Chap. 16).[1] However, most patients undergoing a diagnostic evaluation for angina do not need a resting echocardiogram.[1]

Chronic ischemic heart disease, with or without angina, can result in impaired systolic LV function. The extent and severity of regional and global abnormalities are important considerations in choosing appropriate medical or surgical therapy. Echocardiographic findings that may help establish the diagnosis of chronic ischemic heart disease include regional systolic wall-motion abnormalities, such as hypokinesis, akinesis, dyskinesis, and diminished segmental wall thickening.[16]

Mitral regurgitation demonstrated by Doppler echocardiography may result from global LV systolic dysfunction, regional papillary muscle dysfunction, scarring and shortening of the chordae tendineae, papillary muscle rupture, or other causes.[15]

Stress Imaging for Diagnosis

Patients who should undergo cardiac stress testing with imaging for the diagnosis of CAD as opposed to exercise ECG alone include those in the following categories: (1) complete LBBB, electronically paced ventricular rhythm, preexcitation syndromes, and other similar ECG conduction abnormalities; (2) patients who have greater than 1 mm of resting ST-segment depression, including those with LV hypertrophy or those taking drugs such as digitalis; (3) patients who are unable to exercise to a level high enough to give meaningful results on routine stress ECG (pharmacologic stress imaging should be considered); and (4) patients with angina who have undergone prior revascularization, in whom localization of ischemia, establishing the functional significance of lesions, and demonstrating myocardial viability are important considerations. In our experience, false-positive ECG tests often occur in patients with hypertension, no evidence of LV hypertrophy on the ECG, but LV hypertrophy by echocardiography. Stress imaging is used in most patients with a history of hypertension even when the resting ECG is normal.

Several methods can be used to induce stress, including exercise (treadmill or bicycle) and pharmacologic techniques (dobutamine or vasodilator drugs). When the patient can exercise to an appropriate level of cardiovascular stress for 6 to 12 minutes, exercise stress testing is generally preferred to pharmacologic stress.[1]

Myocardial Perfusion Imaging   In patients with suspected or known chronic stable angina, the largest accumulated experience in myocardial perfusion imaging (MPI) has been with the isotope thallium-201 (^{201}Tl); however, the available evidence indicates that the newer isotopes technetium-99m (^{99m}Tc) sestamibi and ^{99m}Tc tetrofosmin provide similar diagnostic accuracy (see Chap. 19). Thus, for the most part, these isotopes can be used interchangeably, with a similar diagnostic accuracy for CAD.[15]

MPI may use either planar or single-photon emission computed tomography (SPECT), visual analyses, or quantitative techniques (see Chap. 19). Quantification using horizontal or circumferential profiles may improve the test's sensitivity, especially in patients with single-vessel disease. For the less commonly used ^{201}Tl planar scintigraphy, average reported values of sensitivity and specificity (uncorrected for posttest referral bias) have been in the range of 83 and 88 percent, respectively, for visual analysis, and 90 and 80 percent, respectively, for quantitative analyses.[16] ^{201}Tl SPECT is generally more sensitive than planar imaging for diagnosing CAD, localizing hypoperfused vascular segments, identifying left anterior descending and left circumflex coronary artery stenoses, and accurately predicting multivessel CAD. The average sensitivity and specificity of exercise ^{201}Tl SPECT imaging (uncorrected for referral bias) are in the range of 89 and 76 percent, respectively, for qualitative analyses, and 90 and 70 percent, respectively, for quantitative analyses.[17]

Pharmacologic stress uses dipyridamole or adenosine-induced coronary vasodilatation as an adjunct to myocardial perfusion imaging. Dipyridamole planar scintigraphy has a high sensitivity (90 percent average) and acceptable specificity (70 percent average) for the detection of CAD. Dipyridamole SPECT with ^{201}Tl or ^{99m}Tc sestamibi is as accurate as planar imaging, and results of MPI during adenosine infusion are similar to those obtained with dipyridamole and exercise imaging (see Chap. 19). Evidence of CAD is demonstrated by redistribution defects comparing stress and resting scintigrams (ischemia), fixed defects at rest (scar), and LV dilation or lung uptake of isotope during stress (see Chap. 19).

Stress Echocardiography Stress echocardiography is based on the assessment of myocardial thickening during stress compared with baseline (see Chap. 16). Echocardiographic findings suggestive of myocardial ischemia include (1) decrease in wall motion in one or more LV segments with stress, (2) diminution in systolic wall thickening in one or more segments during stress, and (3) compensatory hyperkinesis in complementary (nonischemic) wall segments.[15] The use of digital acquisition and storage, as well as side-by-side display of cine loops of LV images acquired at rest and at different levels of stress, has improved efficiency and accuracy in interpretation of stress echocardiograms.[15]

In 36 studies that included 3210 patients, the reported overall sensitivities (uncorrected for referral bias) ranged from 70 to 97 percent. The average overall sensitivity was 85 percent for exercise echocardiography and 82 percent for dobutamine stress echocardiography. The reported sensitivity of exercise echocardiography for multivessel disease was higher (approximately 90 percent) than the sensitivity for single-vessel disease (approximately 79 percent). In this series of studies, specificity averaged approximately 86 percent for exercise echocardiography and 85 percent for dobutamine echocardiography.[15]

Pharmacologic stress echocardiography is best accomplished using dobutamine because it enhances myocardial contractile performance and wall motion, both of which can be evaluated directly by echocardiography (see Chap. 16). In 36 studies, average sensitivity and specificity (uncorrected for referral bias) of dobutamine stress echocardiography in the detection of CAD were 82 and 85 percent, respectively.[15] Additional information concerning the sensitivity of exercise imaging in patients receiving β blockers, the need for pharmacologic stress imaging in patients with LBBB, and the accuracy of myocardial perfusion and echocardiographic imaging in selected patient subgroups is included in Chaps. 16, 19, 20, and 21.

Echocardiography and MPI have complementary roles, and both add value to routine stress ECG under appropriate circumstances. The choice of which test to perform depends, importantly, on issues of local expertise, available facilities, and considerations of cost-effectiveness. Table 64–4 summarizes the comparative advantages of stress myocardial perfusion imaging and stress echocardiography.

Coronary Angiography for Diagnosis Direct referral for diagnostic coronary angiography in patients with chest pain is appropriate when noninvasive tests are contraindicated or likely to be inadequate because of the patient's illness, disability, or physical characteristics.[1] Many patients with obesity, chronic obstructive pulmonary disease, bronchospasm, and heart failure are likely to have suboptimal imaging tests; diagnostic coronary angiography provides accurate diagnostic information with minimal risk.

Patients with noninvasive tests that are abnormal but not clearly diagnostic often require clarification of an uncertain diagnosis by coronary angiography. In certain cases, a second noninvasive test (imaging modality) may be recommended for a patient with a low likelihood of CAD but an intermediate-risk treadmill result. Coronary angiography is likely to be most appropriate for a patient with a high-risk treadmill outcome.[1]

In individuals with symptoms consistent with but not diagnostic of stable angina, coronary angiography may be a necessity when the patient's occupation or activity could constitute a personal risk or a risk to others (e.g., pilots, firefighters, professional athletes).[1] When

TABLE 64–4

Comparative Advantages of Stress Echocardiography and Stress Radionuclide Perfusion Imaging in Diagnosis of Coronary Artery Disease

Advantages of stress echocardiography
1. Higher specificity
2. Versatility; more extensive evaluations of cardiac anatomy and function
3. Greater convenience/efficacy/availability
4. Lower cost

Advantages of stress perfusion imaging
1. Higher technical success rate
2. Higher sensitivity, especially for single-vessel coronary disease involving the left circumflex
3. Better accuracy in evaluating possible ischemia when multiple resting left ventricle wall-motion abnormalities are present
4. More extensive published database, especially in evaluation of prognosis

SOURCE: *From Gibbons RJ, Chatterjee K, Daley J, et al.[1]*

typical or atypical symptoms suggest stable angina and there is a high clinical probability of severe CAD, direct referral for coronary angiography may be indicated and cost-effective.[16] In diabetic patients, the diagnosis of chronic stable angina can be particularly difficult because of the absence of characteristic symptoms of myocardial ischemia caused by the autonomic and sensory neuropathies (see Chap. 90). Thus a lower threshold for coronary angiography is appropriate. Special groups for the consideration of coronary angiography include women, who more often have atypical chest discomfort, and the elderly, in whom symptoms are common but noninvasive testing may be difficult and comorbid conditions that mimic angina pectoris are frequent.[1] Coronary angiography is useful in patients in whom coronary artery spasm is suspected, in younger patients with signs or symptoms of myocardial ischemia possibly caused by coronary anomalies, in patients with a history of cocaine use, and in those who have survived sudden cardiac death or ventricular arrhythmias.[1] Table 64–5 lists the ACC/AHA recommendations concerning the value of coronary angiography. Coronary angiographic findings in patients with chronic stable angina are depicted in Fig. 64–3.

DIFFERENTIAL DIAGNOSIS

Table 64–1 lists the differential diagnoses of angina pectoris. Usually, the distinction is clear if an accurate history is obtained and a complete, accurate physical examination is performed, as discussed in Chap. 12.

PATHOPHYSIOLOGY

In patients with stable angina pectoris caused by atherosclerotic CAD, the correlation between the severity or extent of atherosclerosis and the magnitude of anginal symptoms is poor.[17] Also, no

TABLE 64–5

American College of Cardiology/American Heart Association Recommendations for Establishing the Diagnosis by Coronary Angiography

Class I
1. Patients with known or possible angina pectoris who have survived sudden cardiac death. *(Level of Evidence: A)[a]*

Class IIa
1. Patients with an uncertain diagnosis after noninvasive testing in whom the benefit of a more certain diagnosis outweighs the risk and cost of coronary angiography. *(Level of Evidence: B)*
2. Patients who cannot undergo noninvasive testing due to disability, illness, or morbid obesity *(Level of Evidence: B)*
3. Patients with an occupational requirement for a definitive diagnosis. *(Level of Evidence: B)*
4. Patients who by virtue of young age at onset of symptoms, noninvasive imaging, or other clinical parameters are suspected of having a nonatherosclerotic cause of myocardial ischemia (coronary artery anomaly, Kawasaki disease, primary coronary artery dissection, radiation-induced vasculoplasty). *(Level of Evidence: B)*
5. Patients in whom coronary artery spasm is suspected and provocative testing may be necessary. *(Level of Evidence: A)*
6. Patients with a high pretest probability of left main or three-vessel coronary artery disease. *(Level of Evidence: A)*

Class IIb
1. Patients with recurrent hospitalization for chest pain in whom a definite diagnosis is judged necessary. *(Level of Evidence: B)*
2. Patients with an overriding desire for a definitive diagnosis and a greater than low probability of coronary artery disease. *(Level of Evidence: B)*

Class III
1. Patients with significant comorbidity in whom the risk of coronary arteriography outweighs the benefits of the procedure. *(Level of Evidence: C)*
2. Patients with an overriding personal desire for a definitive diagnosis and a low probability of coronary artery disease. *(Level of Evidence: C)*

[a]Level of Evidence A, B, or C in Chap. 11 and Fig. 12–4.
SOURCE: From Gibbons RJ, Chatterjee K, Daley J, et al.[1]

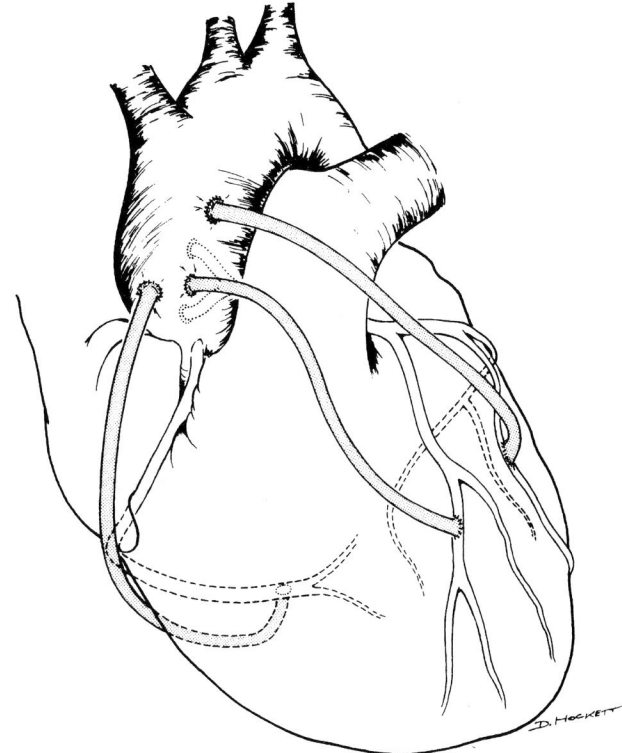

FIGURE 64–3. Usual insertion sites of vein grafts to coronary arteries. The proximal (aortic) anastomosis site of the graft to the right coronary artery is most anterior and usually the lowest. Grafts to the branches of the left coronary artery usually are inserted in a progressively higher and more posterolateral position. Variations frequently occur. *Source: From Tilkian AG, Daily EK. Cardiovascular Procedures: Diagnostic Techniques and Therapeutic Procedures. St. Louis: Mosby, 1986, with permission.*

myocardium (MVO_2). This imbalance may result in clinical manifestations of ischemia when MVO_2 demand exceeds the capacity of the coronary arteries to deliver an adequate supply of oxygen.

Atherosclerotic disease in either the epicardial coronary arteries or in the coronary microvasculature may cause an imbalance between supply and demand at even modest levels of exercise or increased cardiac work load. An understanding of the determinants of CBF and myocardial metabolic demand is important in the management of chronic ischemic heart disease.[1]

【 】 MYOCARDIAL OXYGEN DEMAND

The major relevant determinants of MVO_2 are heart rate, contractility, and systolic wall stress (Fig. 64–4). Heart rate is one of the most important determinants of MVO_2 and can be altered easily by medical therapy in most patients.

Myocardial contractility, partially reflected in the isovolumic rate of change of LV pressure (dP/dt), is a major determinant of MVO_2, but not usually a primary factor for therapeutic intervention. However, LV systolic wall stress is an important consideration in the medical treatment of angina pectoris.

According to the Laplace relationship, systolic wall stress (σ) is directly related to the LV systolic pressure (P) and radius (r) and inversely related to wall thickness (h): $\sigma = PR/h$. Thus, reducing systolic pressure afterload (i.e., treating hypertension) can decrease MVO_2. Decreasing preload by venodilation, and thus reducing LV

definite relation exists between the location of the chest discomfort and the site of the myocardial ischemia. Women have angina as the initial manifestation of CAD more commonly than men, who more often present with acute MI. The pathology of coronary atherosclerosis is discussed in detail in Chap. 57 and the nonatherosclerotic causes of CHD are detailed in Chap. 55.

Myocardial ischemia results from an imbalance between the supply of coronary blood flow (CBF) and the metabolic demands of the

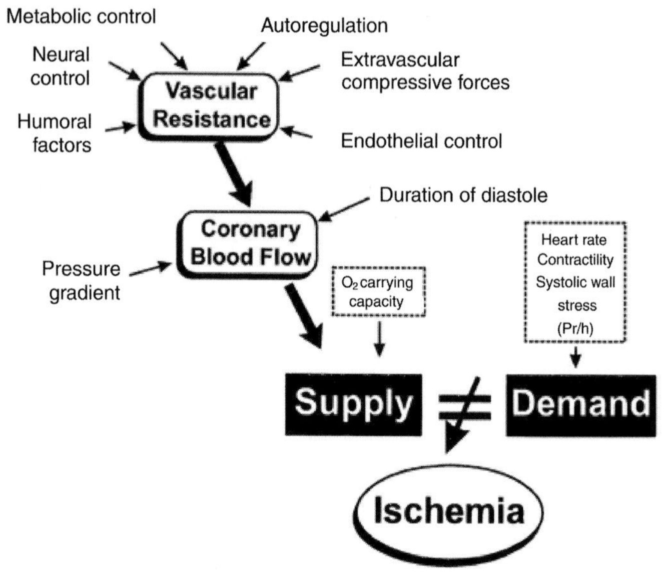

FIGURE 64–4. Factors controlling myocardial oxygen demand. h, Wall thickness; P, systolic pressure; r, radius. *Source: Modified from Ardehali A, Ports TA. Myocardial oxygen supply and demand. Chest 1990;98:699–705. Reproduced with permission from the publisher and authors.*

size and oxygen consumption, is an important mechanism for the efficacy of nitrate therapy in angina pectoris. Positive inotropic agents may actually decrease MVO_2 in patients with an enlarged left ventricle if the benefits of a diminished LV radius outweigh the negative results of increasing contractility.

❰ ❱ MYOCARDIAL OXYGEN SUPPLY

Oxygen supply to the myocardium depends on the oxygen-carrying capacity of the blood, and on CBF (see Fig. 64–4). Although a decrease in oxygen-carrying capacity (e.g., anemia) may contribute to the development or exacerbation of myocardial ischemia related to oxygen supply, ischemia usually results from inadequate CBF.

The arteriolar resistance vessels are normally the primary regulators of CBF because the epicardial arteries act more like conductance vessels and are relatively low-resistance conduits. Narrowing of the large coronary arteries transiently by vasospasm or permanently by obstructive lesions may increase the coronary artery resistance sufficiently to reduce CBF.

In the past decade, the pathophysiologic role of the coronary microvasculature has been recognized[18] either concomitantly with atherosclerotic narrowing of the large-conduit arteries or predominantly in anginal syndromes with normal epicardial arteries ("syndrome X").[19]

The determinants of CBF are relatively complex and include (1) metabolic control, (2) autoregulation, (3) extravascular compressive forces, (4) duration of diastole, (5) humoral agents composed of both circulating hormones and autocrine and paracrine factors produced within the arterial wall, particularly by the endothelium, (6) neural control, and (7) the difference between aortic diastolic pressure and right atrial pressure (i.e., the coronary perfusion pressure; see Fig. 64–4).

CBF is relatively constant, being autoregulated during perfusion pressures between 60 and 160 mmHg. Below a perfusion

pressure of 60 mmHg, vasodilator reserve disappears and blood flow is directly related to perfusion pressure. Experimentally, loss of vasodilator reserve occurs distal to lesions with an 85 percent decrease in diameter. A decrease in CBF, likely a result of vasoconstriction and loss of vasodilator reserve, has been observed despite an increase in blood pressure during cold pressor stimulation in patients with significant CAD.

Extravascular compressive forces—including intrapericardial, intramyocardial, and intraventricular pressures—are important in controlling CBF and account for 30 to 50 percent of the vascular resistance. Because intramyocardial and intraventricular pressures are maximal during systole and are exerted maximally on the subendocardium, LV subendocardial blood flow decreases during systole. Thus, subendocardial blood flow is most vulnerable whenever total blood flow is decreased or MVO_2 is increased and blood flow is limited. Because of the systolic compressive forces, the subendocardium is also critically dependent on the duration of diastole for its blood flow (see Chap. 54).

CBF is regulated by systemic hormones and by neural control mechanisms similar to those of other vascular beds. Angiotensin II is a coronary vasoconstrictor; β-adrenergic agonists dilate and α-adrenergic agonists constrict coronary arteries, although there are some regional differences in distribution of receptors in vessels of different sizes. Importantly, the integrated vasomotor response to the various vasoactive stimuli affecting a coronary artery or arteriole appears greatly influenced by the functional state of the endothelium (see Chap. 54).

❰ ❱ ENDOTHELIAL FUNCTION AND CORONARY VASOMOTOR CONTROL

The phenomenon of endothelium-dependent relaxation and the identification of endothelium-derived relaxing factor as nitric oxide are discussed in detail in Chap. 7. The defect in endothelial function in atherosclerotic epicardial coronary arteries that results in vasoconstriction in response to stimuli that normally cause vasodilation—such as acetylcholine, exercise, or cold pressor testing—is discussed in Chap. 54.

The majority view is that endothelium-dependent vasodilator mechanisms are predominant in nondiseased epicardial coronary arteries. Thus interventions such as exercise, mental stress, cold pressor testing, or even pacing-induced tachycardia, that normally induce increases in MVO_2 and flow, are associated with epicardial coronary artery dilatation that is partially endothelium-dependent and coupled to the increase in myocardial oxygen demand. The presence of even nonocclusive, early atherosclerosis appears to attenuate this vasodilator mechanism and results in prevailing constrictor forces.

The local infusion of the α-adrenergic agonist phenylephrine does not constrict normal coronary arteries of patients with intact endothelium-dependent dilatation. However, vasoconstriction occurs in even minimally diseased coronary arteries at low concentrations of phenylephrine. Thus, in CAD, there appears to be both loss of endothelium-dependent dilatation and enhanced vasoconstrictor sensitivity to catecholamines. This disordered vasomotor control is an important contributor to the variability in anginal threshold commonly observed in many patients.

THE MICROVASCULATURE AND CORONARY ISCHEMIA

The recognition of the likely importance of the coronary microvascular resistance vessels in the pathogenesis of angina pectoris resulted from studies of patients with angina-like chest pain and angiographically normal epicardial coronary arteries.[20]

The coronary etiology of the chest pain is supported by the frequent but not universal evidence of ischemia in these patients during exercise testing; many are found to have abnormal vasodilator reserve. Specifically in patients with angina and angiographically normal coronary arteries, endothelium-dependent vasodilatation of the resistance arteries is often diminished relative to controls.[21]

In contrast, the flow responses to the non–endothelium-dependent dilators, isosorbide dinitrate and papaverine, is no different between patients and controls, suggesting that the intrinsic vasodilator capacity of the resistance vessels is not defective. Similar defects in endothelium-dependent coronary vasodilation have been observed in LV hypertrophy associated with hypertension, another condition that may be associated with angina pectoris with normal coronary angiography.[21]

The histopathology of biopsy specimens from patients with normal epicardial coronaries but with anginal syndromes has demonstrated capillary narrowing with swollen endothelium encroaching on the lumen, as well as decreased capillary density relative to myocardial mass. Thus the coronary microvasculature can develop dysfunction of vasomotor control mechanisms and of endothelium-dependent vasodilation that may become clinically significant in the setting of increased MVO_2. The loss of vasodilator reserve and the actual constriction of resistance arterioles may induce ischemia and chest pain.

SPECTRUM OF PATHOPHYSIOLOGIC MECHANISMS ASSOCIATED WITH THE STABLE CORONARY ISCHEMIA SYNDROMES

Myocardial ischemia, primarily caused by microvascular abnormalities in the control of coronary vascular tone, partially explains the characteristics of stable angina syndromes. Fixed stenoses of an epicardial coronary artery, which may cause angina pectoris or anginal equivalents at a *relatively constant* threshold, also determine the spectrum of clinical symptoms. Most patients have a somewhat variable anginal threshold from day to day or even at different times of the day.

Interestingly, the same activity that causes chest discomfort in the early morning may not do so in the afternoon or evening. Yet, the patient may experience angina at a consistent level of exercise on protocol exercise testing because of the augmented MVO_2 that is a result of increases in heart rate, contractility, and blood pressure, and the associated increment in systolic wall stress. This phenomenon is explained by the presence of both flow-limiting epicardial coronary stenoses and associated episodic vasoconstriction. Maseri et al.[20] termed this phenomenon *mixed angina*. Myocardial ischemia is induced by both an increase in MVO_2 and a decrease in CBF. The site(s) of vasoconstriction may be at an epicardial stenosis, in the microvasculature, or at both locations. Figure 64–5 depicts the concept of a *variable flow reserve* that interacts with differing metabolic demands to produce intermittent ischemia.

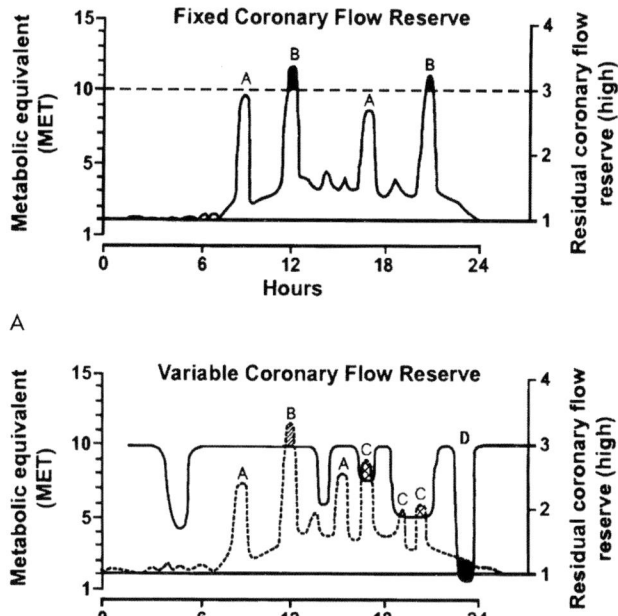

FIGURE 64–5. Concept of variable coronary flow reserve in the presence of variable atherosclerotic obstruction. —, Residual coronary flow reserve; - - -, variable atherosclerotic obstruction as measured by MET; A, episodes not associated with ischemia; B, ischemic episode occurring at levels of exercise exceeding threshold of residual coronary flow reserve; C, ischemic episodes occurring at lower levels of exercise when residual coronary flow is reduced; D, ischemic episodes occurring at rest in the presence of maximal reduction in residual coronary flow reserve. *Source: Modified from Cohn PF. Mechanisms of myocardial ischemia. Am J Cardiol 1992;70:14G–18G; and Maseri A. Role of coronary artery spasm in symptomatic and silent myocardial ischemia. J Am Coll Cardiol 1987;9:249–262. Reproduced with permission from the authors and publishers.*

In the stable anginal syndromes, the predominant vasoconstrictors are likely neural and hormonal, whereas in the unstable (acute) coronary syndromes, platelet and coagulation products, as well as inflammatory mediators are important contributors (see Chap. 54). Patients with predominantly vasoconstrictor pathophysiology in an epicardial vessel have been classified as having *vasospastic angina* or *Prinzmetal variant angina* (see Chap. 54).[22]

CELLULAR BASIS FOR THE CLINICAL MANIFESTATIONS OF ISCHEMIA

The cellular effects of myocardial ischemia are discussed in detail in Chapter 54. The rapid decreases in systolic function and diastolic compliance that are associated with creatine phosphate depletion and ionic shifts will increase LV end-diastolic pressure. Elevated pulmonary vascular pressures often stimulate mechanoreceptors and mediate the dyspnea response. Dyspnea may be associated with angina or may be present as an anginal equivalent in patients who do not develop chest discomfort.

The metabolic abnormalities as a result of ischemia cause cellular depolarization and the flow of electric currents between normal and ischemic areas that are reflected on the ECG. ST-segment depression reflecting decreased subendocardial perfusion is the most common ECG manifestation of ischemia in chronic stable angina during ambulatory recordings or exercise testing, and is usually not associated with complex or life-threatening ventricular arrhythmias. Exercise-induced ventricular ectopic activity is not a reliable predictor of cardiac events in asymptomatic persons.

[ ] THE CORONARY ISCHEMIA CASCADE

Studies in which hemodynamic and ECG recordings have been performed during spontaneous episodes of ischemia, either in unstable patients or during balloon inflation at coronary angioplasty, have provided insights into the sequential responses evoked at the onset of ischemia and are consistent with those described in animals undergoing acute coronary artery ligation (see Fig. 64–1).

After balloon inflation, impaired LV compliance occurs within a few seconds and is followed rapidly by systolic contractile dysfunction causing a decrease in LV ejection fraction of up to 30 percent within 10 seconds.[23] ECG changes occur at about 20 seconds, and angina, if it occurs, appears at between 25 and 30 seconds.

Considering this "ischemic cascade," there are likely to be episodes of ischemia that do not progress to angina. Because many patients do not perceive coronary ischemic pain or have high pain thresholds, the common occurrence of asymptomatic (silent) ischemia in individuals with CAD is not surprising.

Hemodynamic measurements and ECG recordings in patients with spontaneous or exercise-induced ischemia provide physiologic explanations for many of the classic clinical observations about angina.

As noted earlier, an anginal episode may be associated with new physical findings, particularly the development of an S_4 or of mitral regurgitation because of papillary muscle dysfunction.

[ ] CIRCADIAN RHYTHM OF CORONARY ISCHEMIA

The prevalence of MI, unstable angina, variant angina, and silent ischemia is greatest in the morning, during the first few hours after awakening, and the threshold for precipitating anginal attacks in patients with stable angina also appears to be lowest in the morning. Patients often develop ST-segment depression and angina at lower thresholds during exercise testing in the morning than later in the day. Studies with ambulatory ECG recordings have confirmed that the incidence of both painful and painless episodes of ST-segment depression is highest in the morning,[24] particularly in the first few hours after awakening (Fig. 64–6).

The diurnal variation in ischemic threshold is attributed to the endogenous rhythms of catecholamine secretion and to the sensitivity to coronary vasoconstrictors, both of which appear to peak in the morning. The increase in sympathetic nervous system activity is associated with increases in heart rate, blood pressure, contractility, and MVO_2. The lowered morning anginal threshold and the higher morning systolic blood pressure have *important therapeutic implications*. A decrease in the frequency of ischemia can be achieved by blunting the morning surge of β-adrenergic stimulation by the administration of β blockers. The control of hypertension by the *early morning use of antihypertensive drugs* is also important. In patients with recurrent morning angina, the use of nitroglycerin (NTG) soon after awakening may prevent angina in many instances.

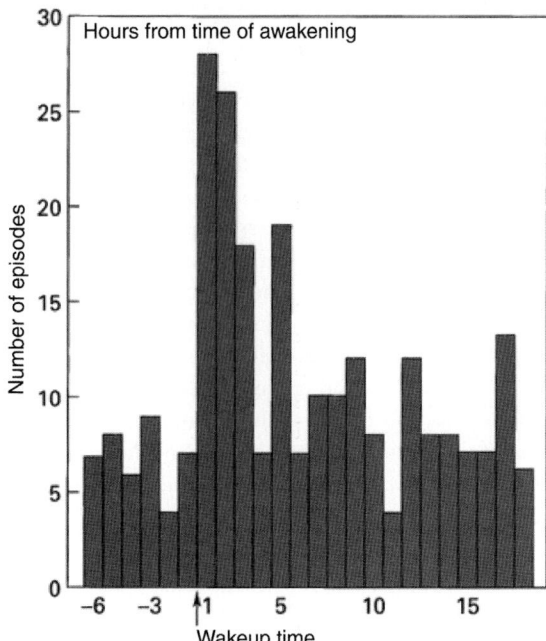

FIGURE 64–6. When the frequency of episodes is displayed hourly from the time of awakening, the peak activity occurs in the first and second hour after arising. *Source: From Rocco MB, Barry J, Campbell S, et al. Circadian variation of transient myocardial ischemia in patients with coronary artery disease. Circulation 1987;75:395–400. Reproduced with permission from the authors and publishers.*

[ ] MECHANISMS OF ANGINAL PAIN

Anginal pain is a useful warning, but it is often too insensitive. Its mechanism is discussed in detail in Chap. 12. Pain stimuli arise within the myocardium and most likely stimulate free nerve endings in or near small coronary vessels. Impulses travel in afferent unmyelinated or small myelinated cardiac sympathetic nerves through the upper five thoracic sympathetic ganglia to dorsal horn cells and through the spinothalamic tract of the thalamus and then to the cortex.

Integration and modification of these impulses occur at several levels, including the cerebral cortex. This modulation may also contribute importantly to the variability in anginal threshold. At the cortical level, psychosocial and cultural factors may alter the perception of pain. The radiation patterns of angina are determined by the levels of the thoracic spinal cord that share the sensory inputs from the heart and from somatic structures.

The nature of the stimuli causing angina has been poorly delineated. The causes are probably chemical, and several molecules—including kinins, serotonin, hydrogen ions, and inflammatory mediators—have been proposed. By contrast, adenosine, which is increased during ischemia, caused anginal-type pain during intravenous infusion in normal volunteers.

ASYMPTOMATIC (SILENT) ISCHEMIA IN STABLE CAD

The presence of unrecognized and painless myocardial infarction was mentioned by Herrick in 1912.[25] The frequent presence of extensive CAD and MI at autopsies of apparently asymptomatic persons was recognized later. Direct evidence of asymptomatic (silent) ischemia during ECG exercise testing and ambulatory ECG recording stimulated interest in this clinical entity.

PREVALENCE OF SILENT ISCHEMIA

Asymptomatic ischemic episodes may be present in patients with any of the ischemic coronary syndromes and may be observed in patients who are totally asymptomatic or who have chest discomfort with some episodes of ischemia but not with others. The prevalence of silent ischemic episodes approximates 40 percent in patients with chronic stable angina and in those with a history of instability. The incidence of asymptomatic ischemia occurring in individuals with extensive CAD has been estimated at 5 percent. ST-segment depression of 60 seconds or more on ambulatory ECG recordings is uncommon in patients with no evidence of CAD.[26]

The true prevalence of silent ischemia is difficult to determine and obviously will depend on age and the presence and extent of CAD. In the presence of CAD, however, it is apparent that episodes of asymptomatic ischemia are often more common than are painful episodes.

❚ ❚ SCREENING FOR SILENT ISCHEMIA

In the absence of symptoms, ambulatory ECG monitoring can reveal transient ST-segment depression suggestive of CAD. However, as indicated in the ACC/AHA *Guidelines for Ambulatory Electrocardiography*,[27] there is presently no evidence that ambulatory ECG monitoring provides reliable information concerning ischemia in asymptomatic subjects without known CAD.

In the absence of symptoms, cardiac computed tomography is sometimes used as a means of screening for CAD, either via the detection of coronary calcium or via the performance of coronary CT angiography. The use of cardiac CT for these purposes is highly controversial.[9] Available data are insufficient to support recommending cardiac CT for this indication to asymptomatic members of the general public. Some authorities recommend its performance for persons at intermediate risk by Framingham criteria as a means to target the intensity of treatment for primary prevention.[28] Appropriateness criteria for the performance of cardiac computed tomography for coronary calcium scoring were recently released by ACCF in collaboration with several imaging societies.[29] Physicians are often confronted with concerned, asymptomatic patients with abnormal findings on cardiac CT. In the absence of symptoms, such patients have a low probability of significant ischemic jeopardy and can often be managed medically with strict attention to primary prevention. The presence of severe coronary calcification on cardiac CT imaging is common in older individuals. Because the evidence supporting the value of additional testing after cardiac CT is scant, the ACC/AHA Committee on Chronic Stable Angina suggests that further testing be reserved for individuals with severe calcification, defined as a calcium score greater than the 75th percentile for age and gender-matched populations. Asymptomatic patients with abnormal findings on ambulatory ECG or cardiac CT who are able to exercise can be evaluated with exercise ECG testing, although the efficacy of exercise ECG testing in asymptomatic patients is not well established. Stress imaging procedures (i.e., either stress myocardial perfusion imaging or stress echocardiography) are generally not indicated as the initial stress test in most such patients. However, in patients with resting ECG abnormalities that preclude adequate interpretation of the exercise ECG, stress imaging procedures are preferable to the exercise ECG for the evaluation of severe coronary calcification on cardiac CT. If the baseline ECG shows right ventricular pacing, left ventricular hypertrophy, preexcitation, or greater than 1 mm of ST-segment depression, or if the patient is taking digoxin, exercise stress imaging procedures are preferred. In patients who are unable to exercise, pharmacologic stress imaging is indicated (see Chap. 11 and ACC/AHA/ASNC *Guidelines for the Clinical Use of Cardiac Radionuclide Imaging 2003*).

❚ ❚ PATHOPHYSIOLOGY OF SILENT ISCHEMIA

An obvious possible explanation for painful, as opposed to asymptomatic, ischemia is that the ischemia, and thus the noxious stimulus, is more severe in the former. The correlation between the duration and severity of an ischemic episode and the development of anginal pain in chronic stable angina, however, is only fair.[27] Symptomatic episodes last slightly longer and have a slightly higher frequency of severe ST-segment depression than do painless ones, but there is considerable overlap.

An alternative reason for lack of pain with myocardial ischemia is neurologic. Neuropathy with defective sensory afferent nerves definitely occurs in some patients and is particularly prevalent in diabetics (see Chap. 90). Modification of pain stimuli in the central nervous system (CNS) may contribute importantly to the variable expression of ischemic pain. This modulation may occur in spinal centers because transcutaneous nerve, esophageal, and dorsal column stimulation can increase anginal threshold. Modulation of pain-mediating afferent messages also may occur at supraspinal centers. Psychological or cultural factors also may affect pain perception. Subsets of patients with predominantly painless ischemic episodes tend to have a higher threshold and tolerance for painful stimuli than those who experience pain. Thus processing of pain signals in the CNS likely contributes to the variability of anginal threshold or to the absence of pain.

Diabetic patients have a relatively high incidence of painless MI and definite silent ischemic episodes as documented by exercise testing and ambulatory ECG recordings (see Chap. 90).

❚ ❚ CAUSES AND FUNCTIONAL CONSEQUENCES OF ASYMPTOMATIC ISCHEMIA

Ischemia caused by the increased MVO_2 associated with exercise testing is often silent. Ambulatory ECG recordings have provided insights into potential mechanisms of many episodes of painless or painful ischemia during daily living. The heart rate at the onset of ischemia is generally lower with ambulatory ECG recordings than with exercise testing. These observations suggest that coronary vasoconstriction likely contributes to many episodes of silent ischemia.

❚ ❚ CLINICAL IMPLICATIONS OF SILENT ISCHEMIA

Asymptomatic silent ischemia is a common component of both acute and chronic coronary artery syndromes. Thus it may have the same clinical importance as symptomatic ischemia. The important indicators of risk are the extent and severity of ischemia, regardless of how it is detected or manifest, and whether the disease is in a stable or unstable phase. Whether ECG monitoring for silent ischemia and changing therapy to decrease or eliminate it diminish morbidity and mortality in a cost-effective manner is unproven.

Therapeutically, it is appropriate to treat high-risk ischemia whether or not it is associated with pain. Persistent, severe ischemia despite medical therapy should lead to consideration of myocardial revascularization.

【 】 TREATMENT OF SILENT ISCHEMIA

Most medical or interventional strategies that reduce symptomatic ischemia will also reduce asymptomatic ischemia.[30] The available data from early clinical trials of the treatment of asymptomatic (silent) ischemia in stable CAD were recently summarized.[30] NTG is highly effective, and β blockers appear to be somewhat more effective than calcium antagonists. Calcium antagonists may be most effective in preventing ischemia occurring at lower heart rates, because coronary artery vasoconstriction may be a predominant factor in this situation. In patients with ischemic CAD, the total ischemic burden and not just symptoms may be the more appropriate therapeutic target.

RISK STRATIFICATION OF PATIENTS WITH CHRONIC ISCHEMIC HEART DISEASE

Risk stratification lies at the core of clinical decision making for patients with chronic ischemic heart disease. Over the past several decades, as the end points of therapeutic clinical trials have largely focused on reductions in cardiovascular morbidity and mortality, detection of risk based on ECG, physical findings, laboratory markers, or from noninvasive and invasive testing, have become critical to targeted strategies for optimizing antiischemic therapy. Thus, for the patient with an expected risk of coronary heart disease death of approximately 3 percent, the initiation of a therapy resulting in a 30 to 45 percent reduction in major adverse cardiovascular events can have a decided impact on patient outcome. This clinical management strategy that includes a focused strategy of risk detection and treatment, as well as careful followup for reassessment of risk, forms the basis for averting clinical risk and has resulted in the dramatic declines in cardiovascular mortality noted during the past several decades.[1]

To apply principles of risk stratification, the clinician must understand the basics of expected risk. Expected risk may be defined as the clinician's global estimate of a patient's likelihood of major adverse cardiovascular events (generally, cardiovascular death or nonfatal MI) over the near- (i.e., <1 year) and long-term (i.e., 3–5 years). Thus, for initial decision making, each patient must be assessed based on their baseline risk. Baseline risk is defined as their expected risk given their physical examination, ECG, and clinical history. In general, patients with chronic coronary disease have an annual risk of cardiovascular death or nonfatal MI that approaches 2 percent per year.[1] Comorbidity and disease extent and severity will accentuate a patient's baseline risk. That is, patients with few risk factors and less-extensive coronary disease (e.g., single-vessel

disease) would have an expected event risk of <2 percent per year, whereas the risk of patients with multivessel disease or those with extensive comorbidity could approach 3 to 5 percent per year.

The prognosis for the patient with chronic CHD is usually related to four patient factors.[1] *LV performance* is the strongest predictor of long-term survival in patients with CHD, and the ejection fraction (EF) is the most often used measure of the presence and the degree of LV dysfunction. The second predictive factor is the *anatomic extent and severity* of atherosclerotic involvement of the coronary arteries. The number of stenosed coronary arteries is the most common measure of this factor. The third patient factor affecting prognosis is evidence of a *recent coronary plaque rupture*, indicating a much higher short-term risk for cardiac death or nonfatal MI. Worsening clinical symptoms with unstable features are an important clinical marker of a complicated plaque. The fourth prognostic factor is *general health and noncoronary comorbidity*.[1] All of these mitigating factors will mediate the clinicians determination of a patient's baseline risk.

Serial reassessment of risk may be applied at predetermined intervals (e.g., every 2 years) or in a setting of clinical worsening (e.g., symptom instability). Signs of clinical worsening, including a change in anginal symptoms or other markers of disease progression, are harbingers of a change in baseline risk and decry the need for clinical reassessment. The specific indications for ischemic and anatomic testing are described elsewhere in this chapter. But suffice it to say for this preface that the next step in clinical reasoning is for the clinician to integrate findings from a patient's baseline risk assessment (e.g., 2 percent annual event risk) into the context of the extent and severity of ischemia, noting the array of diagnostic test modalities or given a reassessment of coronary anatomy and ventricular function. Low-risk findings are those without ischemia, normal ventricular function, or minimal angiographic disease. High-risk findings include severe or extensive ischemia, depressed LV function, as well as extensive angiographic disease. Thus, for the patient with chronic ischemic heart disease with a baseline risk of 2 percent per year, low-risk findings could decrease their expected risk to approximately 1 percent per year, whereas high-risk findings could accentuate their risk up to 3 to 5 percent per year. For this latter finding, the severity of noninvasive and invasive test findings prompts the intensity and timeliness of treatment decisions, with high-risk patients requiring intensive antiischemic therapies aimed at symptom amelioration and ensuing risk reduction. Thus, as we review the evidence in each section of this chapter, the clinician should apply these heuristics of risk stratification using this sequential pattern of risk detection, therapeutic risk reduction, and reassessment of risk (either routine or for clinical worsening).

【 】 HISTORY AND PHYSICAL EXAMINATION FOR PROGNOSIS

Useful information relative to *risk stratification* can be obtained from the history, including demographics such as age and gender, as well as a medical history focusing on hypertension, diabetes, hypercholesterolemia, smoking, peripheral vascular disease, and previous MI (see Chap. 51).

The physical examination can be useful in risk stratification by defining the presence or absence of signs that may alter the probability of *severe* CAD.[1] Useful physical findings include those suggesting vascular disease (abnormal fundi, decreased peripheral pulses, bruits), long-standing hypertension (high blood pressure, abnormal fundi), aortic valve stenoses or hypertrophic obstructive cardiomyopathy (systolic murmur, abnormal carotid arterial pulse, abnormal LV impulse), left-sided heart failure (third heart sounds, displaced LV impulse, bibasilar rales), and right-sided heart failure (elevated jugular venous pressure, hepatomegaly, ascites, peripheral edema).[1] Hubbard et al.[31] identified five clinical markers that independently predicted severe three-vessel and left main CAD—age, typical angina, diabetes, male gender, and prior MI—which were used to develop a five-point cardiac risk score.

[ ] ECG AND CHEST ROENTGENOGRAM FOR PROGNOSIS

Patients with chronic stable angina who have abnormalities on resting ECG are at greater risk than those with normal ECGs. Evidence of one or more prior MIs on ECG indicates a greater risk for cardiac events. The presence of Q waves in multiple ECG leads, often accompanied by an R wave in lead V_1 (posterior infarction), is commonly associated with a markedly reduced left ventricular ejection fraction (LVEF)—an important factor in the natural history of patients with CAD. Persistent ST-segment–T-wave inversions, particularly in leads V_1 to V_3, are associated with an increased prevalence of future coronary events and a poor prognosis.

On the chest roentgenogram, the presence of cardiomegaly, a LV aneurysm, or pulmonary venous congestion is associated with a poorer long-term prognosis than would apply to patients with a normal chest radiograph.

The presence of calcium in the coronary arteries on chest radiography or fluoroscopy in patients with symptomatic CAD suggests an increased risk of cardiac events. Although the presence and amount of coronary artery calcification by EBCT correlate *to some extent* with the severity of CAD, there is considerable patient variation.

[ ] NONINVASIVE TESTING FOR PROGNOSIS

Assessment of LV Function

LV global systolic function and volumes are important predictors of prognosis in patients with cardiac disease.[1] In patients with chronic CHD, LVEF measured at rest by either echocardiography (usually qualitative and less reliable) or radionuclide ventriculography (RVG) is predictive of long-term prognosis. As LVEF decreases, subsequent mortality increases; a resting ejection fraction of greater than 35 percent is associated with an annual mortality rate of more than 3 percent.[1]

Radionuclide LVEF may be measured at rest using a gamma camera, a ^{99m}Tc tracer, and first-pass or gated equilibrium blood pool angiography (RVG), or by gated SPECT perfusion imaging using a technetium-based isotope (see Chap. 19). LV diastolic function can also be estimated from RVG diastolic filling curves. LV systolic function can be measured by quantitative two-dimensional echocardiography (see Chap. 15), and LV diastolic function can be assessed by transmitral valve Doppler recording.

In patients with chronic stable angina and a history of previous MI, segmental wall-motion abnormalities are apparent not only in the zone(s) of prior infarction, but also in areas with ischemic "stunning" or "hibernation" of myocardium that are nonfunctional but still viable.[32] In patients with CHD, the presence, severity, and mechanism of mitral regurgitation can be detected reliably using transthoracic and transesophageal two-dimensional imaging and Doppler echocardiographic techniques (see Chap. 15).

Echocardiography is the definitive test for detecting intracardiac thrombi.[15] LV thrombi are most common in patients with stable angina pectoris who have significant LV wall-motion abnormalities. In patients with anterior and apical infarctions, the presence of LV thrombi denotes an increased risk of both embolism and death (see Chap. 53).

ECG Exercise Testing

Unless cardiac catheterization is clearly indicated, symptomatic patients with suspected or known CAD who have no confounding features on their resting ECG and are able to exercise usually should undergo exercise testing to assess the risk of future cardiac events (see Chap. 14).[1] Also, demonstration of exercise-induced ischemia is desirable for most patients who are being considered for revascularization.[32]

Several studies have shown that risk assessment in patients with a normal ECG who are not taking digoxin and who are physically capable should *usually* start with the exercise test (see Chap. 14).[1] In contrast, a stress-imaging technique should be used for patients with ECG evidence of LV hypertrophy, widespread resting ST-segment depression (>1 mm), complete LBBB, ventricular paced rhythm, or preexcitation.[12] The primary evidence that ECG exercise testing can be used to estimate prognosis and assist in management decisions consists of seven observational studies.[1,11] One of the strongest and most consistent prognostic markers is the *maximum exercise capacity*.

A second group of *prognostic markers* relates to exercise-induced ischemia (see Chap. 14). ST-segment depression and ST-segment elevation (in leads without pathologic Q waves) best summarize the prognostic information related to ischemia. Other variables are less powerful, including angina, the number of leads with ST-segment depression, the configuration of the ST-segment depression, and the duration of ST-segment deviation into the recovery phase.

The *Duke treadmill score* combines this information and provides a way to calculate risk.[33] This score equals the exercise time in minutes minus five times the peak ST-segment deviation during or after exercise (in millimeters) minus four times the angina index (which has a value of 0 if there is no angina, 1 if angina occurs, and 2 if angina is the reason for stopping the test). Among outpatients with suspected CAD, two-thirds of those with scores indicating low risk had a 4-year survival of 99 percent (average annual mortality of 0.25 percent); the 4 percent who had scores indicating high risk had a 4-year survival of 79 percent (average annual mortality rate of 5 percent; Table 64–6). Recent studies indicate that this approach is equally applicable in men and women.

Stress Imaging for Prognosis

Stress-imaging studies using radionuclide MPI techniques or two-dimensional echocardiography at rest and during stress are useful for risk stratification and determining the most effective treatment strategy for patients with chronic stable angina.[1] Whenever feasi-

TABLE 64–6

Survival According to Risk Groups Based on Duke Treadmill Scores

RISK GROUP (SCORE)	PERCENTAGE OF TOTAL	FOUR-YEAR SURVIVAL	ANNUAL MORTALITY (%)
Low (≥ + 5)	62	0.99	0.25
Moderate (–10 to + 4)	34	0.95	1.25
High (< –10)	4	0.79	5.0

SOURCE: From Gibbons RJ, Chatterjee K, Daley J, et al.[1]

ble, treadmill or bicycle exercise should be used as the most desirable forms of stress because exercise provides the most information concerning a patient's symptoms, cardiovascular function, and hemodynamic response during usual activity (see Chap. 19). The inability to perform a bicycle or exercise treadmill test has been shown to be a serious and negative prognostic factor for patients with chronic CAD.[1]

In patients unable to exercise adequately, various types of pharmacologic stress are commonly used for *risk stratification*. The type of pharmacologic stress selected will depend on specific patient factors, including the patient's heart rate and blood pressure, evidence of bronchospastic disease, the presence of LBBB or a pacemaker, and the likelihood of ventricular arrhythmias. Pharmacologic agents are often used to increase workload or cause an increase in overall CBF.

MPI is an important technique in the risk stratification of patients with CAD. Either planar (uncommonly) or SPECT imaging using ^{201}Tl or ^{99m}Tc perfusion tracers with images obtained during stress and at rest provides important information concerning the severity and location of functionally significant CAD (see Chap. 19).

Stress echocardiography is also used frequently for detecting the presence and amount of ischemia in patients with chronic stable angina. However, the amount of prognostic data obtained with this approach is less-well documented. Nevertheless, the presence or absence of inducible myocardial wall-motion abnormalities has useful predictive value in patients who are undergoing exercise or pharmacologic stress echocardiography. A negative stress echocardiographic study denotes a low cardiovascular event rate during followup.

Myocardial Perfusion Imaging for Prognosis

Normal poststress thallium scan results are highly predictive of a benign prognosis, even in patients with known CAD.[1] An analysis of 16 studies involving 3594 patients followed for an average of 29 months indicated a rate per year of cardiac death and MI of 0.9 percent, differing little from that of the general population.[34] In an often quoted prospective study of 5183 consecutive patients who were underwent myocardial perfusion imaging during stress and later at rest, patients with normal scans were at low risk (<0.5 percent per year) for the composite end point of cardiac death and MI during 642 ± 226 days of mean followup (see Chap. 19).[35]

The number, extent, and sites of abnormalities on stress MPI reflect the location and severity of functionally significant coronary artery stenoses (see Chap. 19). Lung uptake of ^{201}Tl on postexercise or pharmacologic stress images is an indicator of stress-

induced global LV dysfunction and is associated with pulmonary venous hypertension in the presence of multivessel CAD.[36] Transient poststress ischemic LV dilatation also correlates with severe two- or three-vessel CAD (see Chap. 19). SPECT may be more accurate than planar imaging for determining the size of defects, detecting particularly left circumflex CAD, and localizing abnormalities in the distribution of individual coronary arteries. However, more false-positive results are likely to result from photon attenuation during SPECT imaging.

The assessment of both myocardial perfusion and LV function at rest may help determine the extent and severity of CAD.[1] This combined information can be obtained by performing two separate exercise tests (e.g., stress MPI and stress RVG) or by combining the studies after a single exercise test (first-pass RVG) with ^{99m}Tc-based agents followed by MPI or by perfusion imaging using ECG gating. The use of ECG-gated ^{99m}Tc sestamibi SPECT imaging at rest and with exercise or pharmacologic stress provides important prognostic information concerning LVEF and the extent of reversible ischemia (see Chap. 19).

Pharmacologic stress perfusion imaging for risk stratification is preferable to *exercise perfusion* imaging in patients with LBBB.[1] Recently, 245 patients with LBBB underwent SPECT imaging with ^{201}Tl or ^{99m}Tc sestamibi during dipyridamole or adenosine stress.[1,36] The 3-year survival was 57 percent in the high-risk group, compared with 87 percent in the low-risk group ($p = 0.001$).

Stress Echocardiography for Prognosis

Stress echocardiography is both sensitive and specific for detecting inducible myocardial ischemia in patients with chronic stable angina.[15] Compared with standard exercise ECG treadmill testing, stress echocardiography provides additional clinical value for detecting and localizing myocardial ischemia. Several studies indicate that patients can be risk-stratified by the presence or absence of inducible wall-motion abnormalities on stress echocardiography.[1] The presence of ischemia on the exercise echocardiogram is independent and additive to clinical and exercise data in predicting cardiac events in both men and women.[1]

Coronary Angiography for Prognosis

The availability of powerful but expensive therapeutic strategies to reduce the long-term morbidity and mortality of CAD dictates that the patients most likely to benefit because of increased risk be defined. The assessment of cardiac risk and the need for further testing usually begins with simple, repeatable, and inexpensive use of the history and physical examination, which often leads to noninvasive or invasive testing, depending on outcome. Clinical risk factors are generally additive, and a crude estimate of 1-year mortality can be obtained from these variables. Methods for the accurate identification of vulnerable or high-risk plaques are lacking. However, magnetic resonance imaging (MRI) offers significant promise in this regard.[1]

Risk stratification of patients with chronic stable angina by stress testing with exercise or pharmacologic agents has been shown to permit the identification of groups of patients with low, intermediate, or high risk for subsequent cardiac events.[1]

The randomized trials of coronary artery bypass grafting (CABG) demonstrated that patients randomized to initial CABG had a lower mortality risk than those who were assigned to medical therapy only if they were at substantial risk (annual mortality risk >3 percent). Coronary angiography is appropriate for patients whose mortality risk is in this range. Table 64–7 lists the noninvasive test findings that identify high-risk patients. Patients identified as at high risk are generally referred for coronary arteriography

independent of their symptomatic status. Table 64–8 lists the ACC/AHA guidelines for risk stratification using coronary angiography in patients with stable angina.

TREATMENT OF ASYMPTOMATIC PATIENTS WITH KNOWN CAD AND CHRONIC STABLE ANGINA

Even in asymptomatic patients, aspirin and β blockers are recommended in those persons with prior MI. The data in support of these recommendations are detailed in the ACC/AHA *Guideline*

TABLE 64–7

Noninvasive Risk Stratification for Chronic Ischemic Heart Disease

High risk (greater than 3 % annual mortality rate)
1. Severe resting left ventricular dysfunction (LVEF <35%)
2. High-risk treadmill score (score ≤ −11)
3. Severe exercise left ventricular dysfunction (exercise LVEF <35%)
4. Stress-induced large perfusion defect (particularly if anterior)
5. Stress-induced multiple perfusion defects of moderate size
6. Large, fixed perfusion defect with left ventricle dilatation or increased lung uptake (thallium 201)
7. Stress-induced moderate perfusion defect with left ventricle dilatation or increased lung uptake (thallium 201)
8. Echocardiographic wall motion abnormality (involving greater than two segments) developing at low dose of dobutamine (≤10 mg/kg/min) or at a low heart rate (<120 beats/min)
9. Stress echocardiographic evidence of extensive ischemia

Intermediate risk (1% to <3% annual mortality rate)
1. Mild/moderate resting left ventricular dysfunction (LVEF = 35% to 49%)
2. Intermediate-risk treadmill score[a] (−11 < score <5)
3. Stress-induced moderate perfusion defect without left ventricle dilatation or increased lung intake (thallium 201)
4. Limited stress echocardiographic ischemia with a wall motion abnormality only at higher doses of dobutamine involving less than or equal to two segments

Low risk (less than 1% annual mortality rate)
1. Low-risk treadmill score (score ≥5)
2. Normal or small myocardial perfusion defect at rest or with stress
3. Normal stress echocardiographic wall motion or no change of limited resting wall motion abnormalities during stress

LVEF, left ventricular ejection fraction.
[a]Duke treadmill score; see text.
Source: From Gibbons RJ, Chatterjee K, Daley J, et al.[1]

TABLE 64–8

American College of Cardiology/American Heart Association Risk Stratification of Coronary Arteriography in Patients with Chronic Stable Angina[a]

Class I
1. Patients with disabling (CCS classes III and IV) chronic stable angina despite medical therapy. *(Level of Evidence: A)*
2. Patients with high-risk criteria on noninvasive testing regardless of anginal severity. *(Level of Evidence: A)*
3. Patients with angina who have survived sudden cardiac death or serious ventricular arrhythmia. *(Level of Evidence: A)*
4. Patients with angina and symptoms and signs of CHF. *(Level of Evidence: A)*
5. Patients with clinical characteristics that indicate a high likelihood of severe CAD. *(Level of Evidence: B)*

Class IIa
1. Patients with significant LV dysfunction (ejection fraction less than 45 %), CCS class I or II angina, and demonstrable ischemia but less than high-risk criteria on noninvasive testing. *(Level of Evidence: C)*
2. Patients with inadequate prognostic information after noninvasive testing. *(Level of Evidence: C)*

Class IIb
1. Patients with CCS class I or II angina, preserved LV function (ejection fraction greater than 45 %), and less than high-risk criteria on noninvasive testing. *(Level of Evidence: C)*
2. Patients with CCS class III or IV angina, which with medical therapy improves to class I or II. *(Level of Evidence: C)*
3. Patients with CCS class I or II angina but intolerance (unacceptable side effects) to adequate medical therapy. *(Level of Evidence: C)*

Class III
1. Patients with CCS class I or II angina who respond to medical therapy and who have no evidence of ischemia on noninvasive testing. *(Level of Evidence: C)*
2. Patients who prefer to avoid revascularization. *(Level of Evidence: C)*

CAD, coronary artery disease; CCS, Canadian Cardiovascular Society; CHF, congestive heart failure; LV, left ventricular.
[a]See Chap. 11 and Fig. 12–4.

for the Management of Patients with Acute Myocardial Infarction.[37] In the absence of prior MI, patients with documented CAD on the basis of noninvasive testing or coronary angiography probably also benefit from aspirin, although the data on this specific subset of patients are limited.

Several studies have investigated the potential role of β blockers in patients with asymptomatic ischemia demonstrated on exercise testing and/or ambulatory monitoring.[11,27] The data generally demonstrate a benefit from β-blocker therapy, but not all trials have been positive.

Lipid-lowering therapy in asymptomatic patients with documented CAD was demonstrated to decrease the rate of adverse ischemic events in the Scandinavian Simvastatin Survival Study (4S) trial, as well as in the CARE (Cholesterol and Recurrent Events) study and the Long-term Intervention with Pravastatin in Ischaemic Disease (LIPID) trial.

Angiotensin-converting enzyme (ACE) inhibitors are indicated in patients with CAD who have diabetes and/or systemic left ventricular dysfunction (see Chap. 51).

TREATMENT OF CHRONIC STABLE ANGINA

There are two major purposes in the treatment of stable angina. The first is to prevent MI and death and *thereby increase the quantity of life.* The second is to reduce symptoms of angina and the frequency and severity of ischemia, which should *improve the quality of life.* Therapy directed toward preventing death has the highest priority. The choice of therapy often depends on the clinical response to initial medical therapy, although some patients (and many physicians) prefer coronary revascularization in situations where either may be successful. It must be stressed that the pharmacologic treatment of chronic CAD has greatly improved and may even be superior to revascularization therapy for many patients.[38] Patient education, cost-effectiveness, and patient preference are important components in this decision-making process.

[ ] PHARMACOTHERAPY TO PREVENT MI

Antiplatelet Agents

Aspirin exerts an antithrombotic effect by inhibiting cyclooxygenase and synthesis of platelet thromboxane A_2. In the Physicians' Health Study, aspirin given on alternative days to asymptomatic individuals was associated with a decreased incidence of MI.[39] In the Swedish Angina Pectoris Aspirin Trial (SAPAT) in patients with stable angina, the addition of 75 mg of aspirin to sotalol resulted in a 34 percent reduction in primary outcome events of MI and sudden death, and a 32 percent decrease in secondary vascular events. A recent meta-analysis of 200,000 patients showed similar benefits of aspirin doses from 75 to 325 mg.[40]

Ticlopidine is a thienopyridine derivative that inhibits platelet aggregation induced by adenosine diphosphate and low concentrations of thrombin, collagen, thromboxane A_2, and platelet-activating factor. It has *not* been shown to decrease adverse cardiovascular events and may induce neutropenia and often thrombotic thrombocytopenic purpura.

Clopidogrel, also a thienopyridine derivative, is chemically related to ticlopidine, but it appears to possess a greater antithrombotic effect than ticlopidine. In a randomized trial that compared clopidogrel with aspirin in patients with previous MI, stroke, or peripheral vascular disease, clopidogrel was slightly more effective than aspirin in decreasing the combined risk of MI, vascular death, and ischemic stroke.[41]

More recently, investigators in the CHARISMA (Clopidogrel for High Atherothrombotic Risk and Ischemic Stabilization, Management and Avoidance) trial found a *nonsignificant trend* toward a reduction in the primary composite end point of cardiovascular death, MI, and stroke at 28 days (19.7 percent relative risk reduction, confidence interval [CI]: 13.3 to 43.1). Importantly, there was no difference in death and/or MI alone.[42]

The greater reduction in event rates with clopidogrel in the CURE (Clopidogrel in Unstable Angina to Prevent Recurrent Ischemic Events), PCI CURE (Percutaneous Coronary Intervention–Clopidogrel in Unstable Angina to Prevent Recurrent Ischemic Events), and CREDO (Clopidogrel for the Reduction of Events During Observation) studies cannot yet be applied to patients who are not undergoing revascularization.[43]

Aspirin, 75 to 325 mg/d, should be used routinely in all patients with acute and chronic ischemic heart disease and with and without clinical symptoms in the absence of contraindications. In those unable to take aspirin, clopidogrel may be used instead. Warfarin is the third choice.[44]

Antithrombotic Therapy

Disturbed fibrinolytic function after exercise appears to be associated with an increased risk of subsequent cardiovascular death in patients with chronic stable angina, providing the rationale for long-term antithrombotic therapy. In small placebo-controlled trials among patients with chronic stable angina, daily subcutaneous administration of low-molecular-weight heparin decreased the fibrinogen level and improved the exercise time to ST-segment depression. The clinical experience of such therapy, however, is extremely limited. The efficacy of newer antiplatelet and antithrombotic agents such as glycoprotein IIa/IIIb inhibitors and recombinant hirudin in the management of patients with chronic stable angina has not been established. Low-intensity oral anticoagulation with warfarin decreased the risk of ischemic events in a randomized trial of patients with risk factors for atherosclerosis but without symptoms of angina.

Lipid-Lowering Agents

Recent clinical studies have convincingly demonstrated that low-density lipoprotein (LDL)-lowering agents can decrease the risk of adverse ischemic events in patients with established CAD (see Chap. 51). In the 4S trial,[45] treatment with an beta-hydroxy-beta-methylglutaryl-coenzyme A (HMG-CoA) reductase inhibitor in patients with documented CAD (including stable angina) and a baseline total cholesterol concentration between 212 and 308 mg/dL was associated with a 30 to 35 percent reduction in both mortality rate and major coronary events. In the CARE study,[46] in men and women with previous MI and total cholesterol levels of less than 240 mg/dL and LDL-cholesterol levels of 115 to 174 mg/dL, treatment with an HMG-CoA reductase inhibitor (statin) was associated with a 24 percent reduction in risk for nonfatal MI. Thus lipid-lowering therapy should be recommended even in the presence of mild to moderate elevations of LDL cholesterol in patients with chronic stable angina. Recent studies and ongoing clinical trials, including the Heart Protection Trial,[47] suggest that a reduction of LDL-cholesterol below 100 mg/dL will further reduce cardiac events (see Chap. 51). Recent trials indicated that the lower LDL cholesterol level the greater the secondary prevention with a target of 70 mg/dL superior to <100 mg/dL (see Chap. 51), particularly for type 2 diabetes.

【 】 ANGIOTENSIN-CONVERTING ENZYME INHIBITORS

The potential cardiovascular protective effects of ACE inhibitors have been suspected for some time. As early as 1990, several randomized clinical trials showed that ACE inhibitors reduced the incidence of recurrent MI and that this effect could not be attributed to the effect on blood pressure alone (see Chap. 51).

The results of the Heart Outcomes Prevention Evaluation (HOPE) trial confirm that use of the ACE inhibitor ramipril (10 mg/d)[48] reduces the rate of cardiovascular death, MI, and stroke in patients who are at high risk or have vascular disease in the absence of heart failure.

Greater than 90 percent of ACE is tissue-bound, whereas only 10 percent of ACE is present in soluble form in the plasma. In nonatherosclerotic arteries, the majority of tissue ACE is bound to the cell membranes of endothelial cells on the luminal surface of the vessel walls, and there is a large concentration of ACE within the adventitial vasa vasorum endothelium. It is now well appreciated that atherosclerosis represents different stages of a process that is in large part mediated by the endothelial cell (Fig. 64–7). Thus,

in the early stage, ACE, with its predominant location for the endothelial cells, would be an important mediator of local angiotensin II and bradykinin levels that could have an important impact on endothelial function.

ACE inhibition shifts the balance of ongoing vascular mechanisms in favor of those promoting vasodilatory, antiaggregatory, antiproliferative, and antithrombotic effects (see Fig. 64–7).

The HOPE study was unique in that of the 9541 patients in this study, 3577 (37.5 percent) had diabetes. There was a significant reduction in diabetic complications, a composite for the development of diabetic nephropathy, need for renal dialysis, and laser therapy for diabetic retinopathy in those patients receiving ramipril. The Microalbuminuria, Cardiovascular, and Renal Outcomes (MICRO)-HOPE, a substudy of the HOPE study,[49] provided new clinical data on the cardiorenal therapeutic benefits of ACE inhibitor intervention in a broad range of middle-age patients with diabetes mellitus who are at high risk for cardiovascular events.

ACE inhibitors should be used as routine secondary prevention for patients with known CAD, particularly in type 2 diabetics.

In the ongoing Bypass and Revascularization Investigation (BARI) 2 Diabetes (2D) and Clinical Outcomes Utilizing Aggressive Drug Evaluation (COURAGE) trials, ACE inhibitors are prescribed for all diabetics with documented ischemic heart disease unless contraindicated. The ACE inhibitor used in the BARI-2D trial is quinapril (an agent with high lipophilicity and enzyme-binding capabilities—a tissue ACE).

【 】 ANTIANGINAL AND ANTIISCHEMIC THERAPY

Antianginal and antiischemic drug therapy consists of β-adrenoreceptor-blocking agents (β blockers), calcium antagonists, and ni-

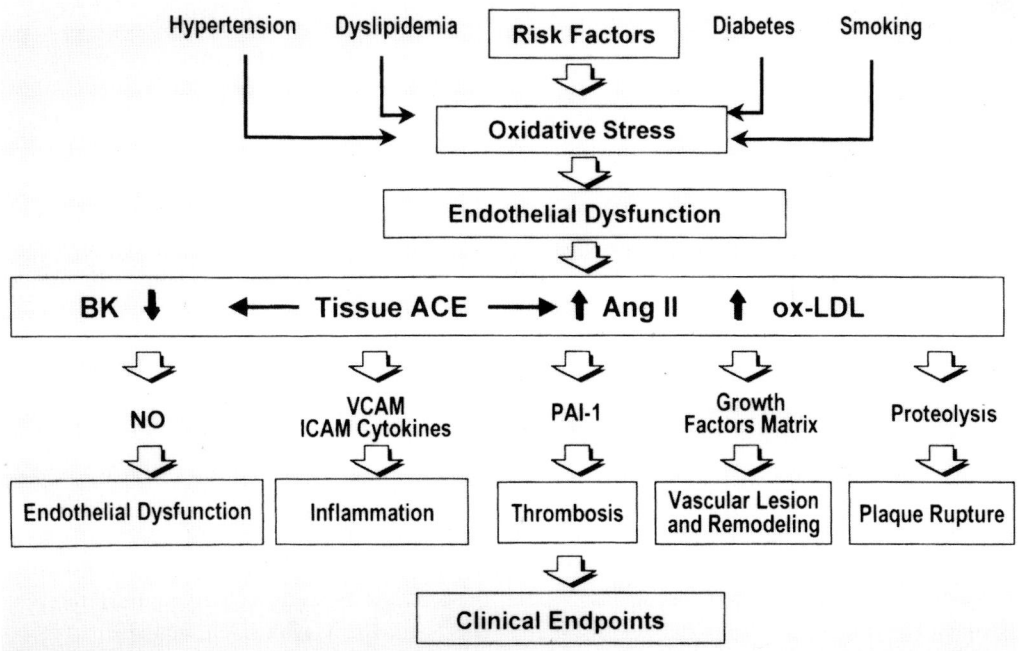

FIGURE 64–7. Interaction among the renin–angiotensin system, diabetes, and atherothrombosis. ACE, angiotensin-converting enzyme; Ang, angiotensin; BK, bradykinin; ICAM, intercellular adhesion molecule; NO, nitric oxide; ox-LDL, oxidized low-density lipoprotein; PAI, plasminogen activator inhibitor; VCAM, vascular cell adhesion molecule.

trates. Drug interactions are described in Chap. 94. There is a tendency for physicians to give *lower doses* of antianginal medications than those proven to be effective in clinical trials; higher doses and combined therapy are often not utilized in patients who could be "angina-free" if treated more appropriately; this is particularly true with β-blocker therapy. For example, the usual dose for angina is 50 to 200 mg of metoprolol twice daily.

β Blockers

The decrease in heart rate, contractility, arterial pressure, and usually LV wall stress with β blockers is associated with decreased MVO_2. A reduction in heart rate also increases diastolic coronary artery perfusion time, which may enhance LV perfusion.

All β blockers without intrinsic sympathetic activity appear to be equally effective in angina pectoris. In patients with chronic stable exertional angina, these agents decrease the heart rate–blood pressure product during exercise, and the onset of angina or the ischemic threshold during exercise is delayed or avoided.[1] In treating stable angina, it is essential that the dose of β blockers be adjusted to lower the resting heart rate to 60 beats or less per minute. In patients with severe angina, the heart rate can be reduced to less than 50 beats per minute if there are no symptoms associated with bradycardia and AV block does not develop (see Chap. 94). In patients with exertional angina, β blockers attenuate the increase in heart rate during exercise, which ideally should not exceed 75 percent of the heart rate response associated with the onset of ischemia. It is often useful for the patient to perform exercise (sit-ups, running in place) before and after the institution of β-blocker therapy. If the heart rate increase with exercise is not significantly reduced by therapy, the dose of the β blocker is inadequate. β Blockers are definitely effective in reducing exercise-induced angina. Three controlled studies comparing β blockers with calcium antagonists report equal efficacy in the treatment of chronic stable angina.

In the International Multicenter Angina Exercise (IMAGE) study,[50] both metoprolol and nifedipine were effective as monotherapy in increasing exercise time, although metoprolol was more effective than nifedipine. The combination therapy also significantly increased the exercise time to ischemia compared with either drug alone. The absolute contraindications to the use of β blockers are severe bradycardia, preexisting high-degree AV block, sick sinus syndrome, and severe, unstable LV failure (see Chap. 94). Asthma and bronchospastic disease, severe depression, and peripheral vascular disease are relative contraindications (see Chap. 94). Fatigue, inability to perform exercise, lethargy, insomnia, nightmares, worsening claudication, and impotence are frequently experienced side effects. Most patients with chronic CAD and diabetes can be treated with β blockers (see Chap. 90).

In patients with postinfarction stable angina and those who require antianginal therapy after revascularization, treatment with β blockers appears to be effective in controlling symptomatic and asymptomatic ischemic episodes. β Blockers are still the antiischemic drugs of choice in elderly patients with stable angina.[1]

β Blockers are frequently combined with nitrates for treating chronic stable angina. This combination of therapy appeared to be more effective in several studies than nitrates or β blockers alone.[51] β Blockers may also be combined with calcium antagonists. For combination therapy, slow-release dihydropyridine derivatives or new-generation long-acting dihydropyridine derivatives are the calcium antagonists of choice.[1]

Calcium Antagonists

These agents, also considered in Chap. 94, reduce the transmembrane flux of calcium by the calcium channels. There are three types of voltage-dependent calcium channels: L type, T type, and N type.

All calcium antagonists exert a negative inotropic effect, depending on dosage. In smooth muscle, calcium ions also regulate the contractile mechanism, and calcium antagonists reduce smooth muscle tension in the peripheral vascular bed, thus causing vasodilation. All the calcium antagonists cause dilatation of the epicardial conduit vessels and the arterial resistance vessels, the former being the primary mechanism for the beneficial effect of calcium antagonists for relieving vasospastic angina. Calcium antagonists also decrease MVO_2 demand, primarily by reducing the systemic vascular resistance and arterial pressure. The negative inotropic effect of calcium antagonists also decreases the MVO_2.

Randomized clinical trials comparing calcium antagonists and β blockers have demonstrated that calcium antagonists are *equally as effective* as β blockers in relieving angina and improving exercise time to onset of angina or ischemia.[1] The calcium antagonists are effective in reducing the incidence of angina in patients with vasospastic angina.[52]

In a *retrospective, case-controlled study* reported in patients with hypertension, treatment with immediate-acting nifedipine, diltiazem, and verapamil was associated with an increased risk of MI of 31 to 61 percent.[53] Although a subsequent meta-analysis of immediate-release and short-acting nifedipine in patients with MI and unstable angina reported a dose-related influence on excess mortality, further analysis of the published reports failed to confirm an increased risk of adverse cardiac events with calcium antagonists.[54] Importantly, long-acting calcium antagonists, including slow-release and long-acting dihydropyridine and nondihydropyridine derivatives, are effective in relieving symptoms in patients with chronic stable angina. They should be used in combination with β blockers when initial treatment with β blockers is not successful or as a substitute for β blockers when initial treatment leads to unacceptable side effects. Calcium blockers may decrease the incidence of coronary artery spasms, which β blockers do not. Many patients with two- or three-vessel CAD are asymptomatic on combined β-blocker and calcium antagonist therapy. Some have further improvement on triple therapy (combined β blocker, calcium antagonist, and long-acting nitrates). Further information concerning the potential side effects of the calcium antagonists is given elsewhere (see Chap. 94).

Nitroglycerin and Nitrates

Nitrates are endothelium-independent vasodilators that produce beneficial effects by both reducing the MVO_2 and improving CBF perfusion. The decreased MVO_2 results from the reduction of LV volume and arterial pressure primarily as a consequence of reduced preload. Nitroglycerin also exerts antithrombotic and antiplatelet effects in patients with stable angina.[1]

Nitrates dilate large epicardial arteries and collateral vessels. The vasodilating effect on epicardial coronary arteries with or without atherosclerotic CAD is beneficial in relieving coronary vasospasm in patients with vasospastic angina.

In patients with exertional stable angina, nitrates improve exercise tolerance, time to onset of angina, and time to ST-segment depression during treadmill exercise testing. In combination with β blockers or calcium antagonists, nitrates produce greater antianginal and antiischemic effects in patients with stable angina.[1]

The interaction between nitrates and sildenafil (Viagra) is discussed in detail elsewhere.[55] The coadministration of nitrates and sildenafil greatly increases the risk of potentially life-threatening hypotension.

The major problem with long-term use of nitroglycerin and long-acting nitrates is development of nitrate tolerance.[56] Tolerance develops not only to antianginal and hemodynamic effects but also to platelet antiaggregatory effects. The mechanism for development of nitrate tolerance remains unclear. For practical purposes, the administration of nitrates with an adequate nitrate-free interval (8 to 12 hours) appears to be the most effective method of preventing nitrate tolerance. Unfortunately, this means that patients with unpredictable episodes of myocardial ischemia should not be treated with nitrate therapy alone because they will be "unprotected" for part of each 24-hour day.

The primary consideration in the choice of pharmacologic agents for treatment of angina should be to *improve prognosis*. Aspirin and lipid-lowering therapies have been shown to reduce the risk of death and nonfatal myocardial infarction in both primary and secondary prevention trials. β Blockers also reduce cardiac events when used as secondary prevention in postinfarction patients and reduce mortality and morbidity among patients with hypertension. Nitrates have not been shown to reduce mortality with acute infarction or in patients with chronic CAD.

Table 64–9 lists the recommended drug therapy using calcium antagonists versus β blockers in patients with angina-associated conditions.

[ ] TREATMENT OF RISK FACTORS

The recommendations of the AHA for the treatment of risk factors are detailed in Chap. 51. *Interventions that reduce the incidence of CAD events include those that lead to declines in* (1) cigarette smoking, (2) LDL cholesterol, (3) systemic hypertension, (4) LV hypertrophy, and (5) thrombogenic factors (see Chap. 51).

The causal role of *LDL cholesterol* in the pathogenesis of atherosclerotic CAD has been affirmed by recent randomized, controlled clinical trials of lipid-lowering therapy. Several primary and secondary prevention trials have shown that the lowering of LDL cholesterol is associated with a reduced risk of CAD (see Chap. 51). Angiographic trials provide firm evidence linking cholesterol reduction to favorable trends in coronary anatomy.

Data from numerous observational studies indicate a continuous and graded relation between blood pressure and cardiovascular disease risk. Hypertension predisposes patients to coronary events both as a result of the direct vascular injury caused by increases in blood pressure and by its effects on the myocardium, including increased wall stress and MVO_2. CAD, diabetes, LV hypertrophy, heart failure, retinopathy, and nephropathy are indicators of increased cardiovascular disease risk in hypertensive patients. The target of therapy is a reduction in blood pressure to less than 130 mmHg systolic and less than 85 mmHg diastolic in patients with CAD and coexisting diabetes, heart failure, or renal failure.[57] In diabetics, an even lower blood pressure (<120 mmHg) appears to be of greater benefit.

Treatment of *hypertension* begins with nonpharmacologic means. When lifestyle modifications and dietary alterations adequately reduce blood pressure, pharmacologic intervention may be unnecessary (see Chap. 70).

When pharmacologic treatment is necessary (as is usually the case), β blockers or calcium antagonists may be especially useful in patients with hypertension and angina pectoris; however, short-acting calcium antagonists should not be used.[58]

Epidemiologic studies implicate *LV hypertrophy* as a risk factor for the development of MI, congestive heart failure, and sudden death. LV hypertrophy has also been shown to predict a poorer prognosis in patients with definite CAD. In the Framingham Heart Study, the subjects who demonstrated ECG evidence of LV hypertrophy regression on followup were at a substantially reduced risk for cardiovascular events.

Coronary artery thrombosis is a trigger of acute MI. Aspirin has been documented to reduce the risk for CHD in both primary and secondary prevention settings.[1] Elevated plasma fibrinogen levels predict CAD risk in prospective observational studies (see Chap. 51).

Interventions that are likely to reduce the incidence of CAD events include those that lead to declines in diabetes mellitus, LDL cholesterol, obesity, physical inactivity, and postmenopausal status (see Chap. 51).

Diabetes mellitus, which is defined as a fasting blood sugar level of more than 126 mg/dL,[59] is present in a significant minority of adult Americans. Data supporting an important role of diabetes mellitus as a risk factor for cardiovascular disease come from a number of observational settings. This is true for both type 1 and type 2 diabetes. Atherosclerosis accounts for 80 percent of all diabetic mortality (see Chaps. 51 and 90). The goal is to maintain a blood glucose hemoglobin A1c level of less than 7 percent and a blood glucose level of less than 140 mg/dL. In diabetic patients with hypertension, microalbuminuria, or decreased LV systolic function, ACE inhibitors appear to be indicated. This may apply to most diabetics with CAD.[1,60] Observational studies and clinical trials have demonstrated a strong inverse association between *HDL cholesterol* and CAD risk (see Chap. 51). This inverse relation is observed in both men and women and among asymptomatic persons as well as patients with established CAD.[1] The National Cholesterol Adult Treatment Panel III has defined a low high-density lipoprotein (HDL)-cholesterol level as less than 40 mg/dL.[59]

Obesity is a common condition associated with increased risk for CHD and mortality (see Chap. 51). New AHA guidelines for weight control have been published.[60]

Multiple randomized, controlled trials comparing exercise training with a "no exercise" control group have demonstrated a statistically significant improvement in exercise tolerance for the exercise group versus the control group.[1] The threshold for ischemia is likely to increase with exercise training because training reduces the heart rate–blood pressure product at a given submaximal exercise workload.[1]

Postmenopausal Hormonal Replacement Therapy

Both estrogenic and androgenic hormones produced by the ovary appear to be protective against the development of atherosclerotic cardiovascular disease. When hormonal production decreases in the perimenopausal period over several years, the risk of CAD rises in postmenopausal women. By age 75 years, the risk of atherosclerotic cardiovascular disease among men and women is equal. Women have an accelerated risk of developing CAD if they experience an early

TABLE 64–9

American College of Cardiology/American Heart Association Recommended Drug Therapy (Calcium Antagonist versus β Blocker) in Patients with Angina and Associated Conditions

CONDITION	RECOMMENDED TREATMENT AND ALTERNATIVE	AVOID
Medical conditions		
Systemic hypertension	β Blockers (calcium antagonists)	
Migraine or vascular headaches	β Blockers (verapamil or diltiazem)	
Asthma or chronic obstructive pulmonary disease with bronchospasm	Verapamil or diltiazem	β Blockers
Hyperthyroidism	β Blockers	
Raynaud syndrome	Long-acting slow-release calcium antagonists	β Blockers
Insulin-dependent diabetes mellitus	β Blockers (particularly if prior myocardial infarction) or long-acting slow-release calcium antagonists	
Non–insulin-dependent diabetes mellitus	β blockers or long-acting slow-release calcium antagonists	
Depression	Long-acting slow-release calcium antagonists	β blockers
Mild peripheral vascular disease	β Blockers or calcium antagonists	
Severe peripheral vascular disease with rest ischemia	Calcium antagonists	β Blockers
Cardiac arrhythmias and conduction abnormalities		
Sinus bradycardia	Long-acting slow-release calcium antagonists that do not decrease heart rate	β Blockers, diltiazem, verapamil
Sinus tachycardia (not caused by heart failure)	β Blockers	
Supraventricular tachycardia	Verapamil, diltiazem, or β blockers	
Atrioventricular block	Long-acting slow-release calcium antagonists that do not slow AV conduction	β Blockers, verapamil, diltiazem
Rapid atrial fibrillation (with digitalis)	Verapamil, diltiazem, or β blockers	
Ventricular arrhythmias	β Blockers	
Left ventricular dysfunction		
Congestive heart failure		
Mild (LVEF ≥40 %)	β Blockers	
Moderate to severe (LVEF <40 %)	Amlodipine or felodipine (nitrates)	Verapamil, diltiazem
Left-sided valvular heart disease		
Mild aortic stenosis	β Blockers	
Aortic insufficiency	Long-acting slow-release dihydropyridines	
Mitral regurgitation	Long-acting slow-release dihydropyridines	
Mitral stenosis	β Blockers	
Hypertrophic cardiomyopathy	β Blockers, nondihydropyridine calcium antagonist	Nitrates, dihydropyridine, calcium antagonists

AV, atrioventricular; LVEF, left ventricular ejection fraction.
SOURCE: From Gibbons RJ, Chatterjee K, Daley J, et al.[1]

menopause or abrupt onset of menopause through surgical removal or chemotherapeutic ablation of the ovaries. Loss of estrogen and the onset of menopause result in an increase in LDL cholesterol, a small decrease in HDL cholesterol, and, therefore, an increased ratio of total cholesterol to HDL cholesterol. Numerous epidemiologic studies suggest a favorable influence of estrogen replacement therapy on the primary prevention of CAD in postmenopausal women.

Based on the above, postmenopausal estrogen replacement has previously been advocated for both primary and secondary prevention of CAD in women. However, the first published randomized

trial of estrogen plus progestin therapy in postmenopausal women with known CAD did not show any reduction in cardiovascular events over 4 years of followup despite an 11 percent lower LDL cholesterol level and a 10 percent higher HDL-cholesterol level in those women receiving hormone replacement therapy.

The Women's Health Initiative, a randomized, controlled, primary prevention trial of estrogen plus progestin, found that the overall health risks of this therapy exceeded its benefits.[61] Thus, current information suggests that hormone replacement therapy in postmenopausal women does not reduce risk for major vascular events or coronary deaths in secondary prevention. Women who are taking hormone replacement therapy and who have vascular disease can continue this therapy if it is being prescribed for other well-established indications (e.g., osteoporosis) and no better alternative therapies are appropriate. There is, however, at the present time, no basis for adding or continuing estrogens in postmenopausal women with clinically evident CAD or cerebrovascular disease in an effort to prevent or retard progression of their underlying disease.

Other randomized trials of hormone replacement therapy in primary and secondary prevention of CAD in postmenopausal women are being conducted.[62] As their results become available over the next several years, this recommendation may require modification.

Interventions that may reduce the incidence of CAD events include those that lead to declines in psychosocial factors, triglycerides, lipoprotein(a), homocysteine, oxidative stress, and consumption of alcohol (see Chap. 51).

Triglyceride levels are predictive of CHD in a variety of observational studies and clinical settings. However, much of the association of triglycerides with CHD risk is related to other factors, including diabetes, obesity, hypertension, high LDL cholesterol, and low HDL cholesterol (see Chap. 51).[63]

Lipoprotein(a) is a lipoprotein particle that has been linked to CHD risk in observational studies. Elevated levels of lipoprotein(a) are largely genetically determined and found in 15 to 20 percent of patients with premature CHD. Increased *homocysteine* levels are associated with increased risk of CAD, peripheral arterial disease, and carotid disease.[1] Elevated homocysteine levels can occur as a result of inborn errors of metabolism such as homocystinuria, and they also can be increased by deficiencies of vitamin B_6, vitamin B_{12}, and folate, which are commonly seen in older patients (see Chap. 51).[1]

Extensive laboratory data indicate that oxidation of LDL cholesterol promotes and accelerates the atherosclerosis process. Observational studies have documented an association between dietary intake of antioxidant vitamins (vitamin C, vitamin E, and beta-carotene) and reduced risk for CHD. Observational studies repeatedly have shown an inverse relation of *moderate alcohol intake* to the risk of CHD events. However, excessive alcohol intake can promote many other medical problems that outweigh its beneficial effects on CHD risk.

Risk factors associated with increased risk but that cannot be modified, or when modified are unlikely to change the incidence of CHD events, include age, male gender, and a positive family history of premature CHD. The latter is defined as definite MI or sudden death before age 55 years in a father or other male first-degree relative, or before age 65 years in a mother or other female first-degree relative (see Chap. 51).[1]

MYOCARDIAL REVASCULARIZATION

There are currently two well-established revascularization approaches to treatment of chronic stable angina caused by coronary atherosclerosis. One is CABG surgery, in which segments of autologous arteries or veins are used to reroute blood around relatively stenotic segments of the proximal coronary artery. The other is percutaneous coronary intervention (PCI) using catheter-borne or laser techniques to open usually short areas of stenosis from within the coronary artery. These techniques are described in greater detail in Chapters 62 and 63. Revascularization is also potentially feasible with transthoracic (laser) myocardial revascularization in patients

in whom neither CABG nor PCI is feasible. Table 64–10 lists the recommendations of the American College of Cardiology/American Heart Association, American College of Physicians–American Society of Internal Medicine (ACC/AHA/ACP–ASIM) for revascularization with PCIs or CABG in patients with stable angina.

Patients with stable angina pectoris may be appropriate candidates for revascularization either by CABG surgery or PCI. In general, this is an individual decision to be made by the patient with knowledge of the advantages and disadvantages either of medical therapy alone or revascularization with either CABG or PCI.

There are two general indications for revascularization procedures: the presence of symptoms that are not acceptable to the patient either because of (1) restriction of physical activity and lifestyle as a result of limitations or side effects from medications, or (2) the presence of findings that indicate clearly that the patient would have a better prognosis with revascularization than with medical therapy. Considerations regarding revascularization are based on an assessment of the grade or class of angina experienced by the patient, the presence and severity of myocardial ischemia on noninvasive testing, the degree of LV function, and the distribution and severity of coronary artery stenoses.

A recent meta-analysis of three major large, multicenter, randomized trials of initial surgery versus medical management (performed in the 1970s) as well as other smaller trials confirms the surgical benefits achieved by surgery at 10 postoperative years for patients with three-vessel disease, two-vessel disease, or even one-vessel disease that included a severe stenosis of the proximal left anterior descending coronary artery (see Chap. 65).

The advantages of PCI for the treatment of CAD include a low level of procedure-related morbidity, a low procedure-related mortality rate in properly selected patients, a short hospital stay, early return to activity, and the feasibility of multiple procedures. However, PCI is not feasible in all patients; it remains accompanied by a significant incidence of restenosis, and there is an occasional need for emergency CABG surgery (see Chap. 62).

Three randomized studies have compared PCI with medical management alone for the treatment of chronic stable angina.[64-66] All these randomized studies of PCI versus medical management have involved patients at a low risk of mortality even with medical management and did not assess patients with moderate to severe CAD (see Chap. 62).

COURAGE Trial

In the COURAGE trial, 2287 patients with objective evidence of myocardial ischemia and significant CAD from 58 U.S. and Canadian centers were randomized: 1149 patients were assigned to PCI with optimal medical therapy and 1138 to optimal medical therapy alone. The primary outcome was all-cause mortality or nonfatal myocardial infarction during the 2.5- to 7.0-year (median: 4.6 years) followup (Fig. 64–8).[67]

There were 202 primary events in the PCI group and 199 events in the medical therapy group. The 4.6-year cumulative primary event rate was 18.3 percent in each group (hazard ratio [HR] for death or MI in the PCI group compared with the medical therapy group: 1.01; 95 percent confidence interval [CI], 0.83 to 1.23; $P = 0.90$; Fig. 64–9). Comparing the PCI and medical therapy groups, there were no differences in death, MI, or stroke (19.2 percent vs. 19.2 percent; HR 1.01; 95 percent CI 0.84 to 1.23; $P = 0.89$), hos-

TABLE 64–10

American College of Cardiology/American Heart Association/American College of Physicians–American Society of Internal Medicine Recommendations for Chronic Stable Angina[a]

Class I

1. CABG for patients with significant left main coronary disease. *(Level of Evidence: A)*
2. CABG for patients with three-vessel disease. The survival benefit is greater in patients with abnormal LV function (ejection fraction <50 %). *(Level of Evidence: A)*
3. CABG for patients with two-vessel disease with significant proximal left anterior descending CAD and either abnormal LV function (ejection fraction <50 %) or demonstrable ischemia on noninvasive testing. *(Level of Evidence: B)*
4. PCI for patients with two- or three-vessel disease with significant proximal left anterior descending CAD, who have anatomy suitable for catheter-based therapy, normal LV function, and who do not have treated diabetes. *(Level of Evidence: C)*
5. PCI or CABG for patients with one- or two-vessel disease CAD without significant proximal left anterior descending CAD, but with a large area of viable myocardium and high-risk criteria on noninvasive testing. *(Level of Evidence: B)*
6. CABG for patients with one- or two-vessel disease CAD without significant proximal left anterior descending CAD who have survived sudden cardiac death or sustained ventricular tachycardia. *(Level of Evidence: C)*
7. In patients with prior PCI, CABG, or PCI for recurrent stenosis associated with a large area of viable myocardium or high-risk criteria on noninvasive testing. *(Level of Evidence: B)*
8. PTCA or CABG for patients who have not been treated successfully by medical therapy and can undergo revascularization with acceptable risk. *(Level of Evidence: C)*

Class IIa

1. Repeat CABG for patients with multiple saphenous vein graft stenoses, especially when there is significant stenosis of a graft supplying the LAD. It may be appropriate to use PTCA for focal saphenous vein graft lesions or multiple stenoses in poor candidates for reoperative surgery. *(Level of Evidence: B)*
2. Use of PCI or CABG for patients with one- or two-vessel disease CAD without significant proximal LAD disease but with a moderate area of viable myocardium and demonstrable ischemia on noninvasive testing. *(Level of Evidence: B)*
3. Use of PCI or CABG for patients with one-vessel disease with significant proximal LAD disease. *(Level of Evidence: C)*

Class IIb

1. Compared with CABG, PCI for patients with two- or three-vessel disease with significant proximal left anterior descending CAD, who have anatomy suitable for catheter-based therapy, and who have treated diabetes or abnormal LV function. *(Level of Evidence: C)*
2. Use of PCI for patients with significant left main coronary disease who are not candidates for CABG. *(Level of Evidence: C)*
3. PCI for patients with one- or two-vessel disease CAD without significant proximal left anterior descending CAD, who have survived sudden cardiac death or sustained ventricular tachycardia. *(Level of Evidence: C)*

Class III

1. Use of PCI or CABG for patients with one- or two-vessel CAD without significant proximal left anterior descending CAD, who have mild symptoms that are unlikely caused by myocardial ischemia, or who have not received an adequate trial of medical therapy and
   a. Have only a small area of viable myocardium or *(Level of Evidence: C)*
   b. Have no demonstrable ischemia on noninvasive testing *(Level of Evidence: C)*
2. Use of PCI or CABG for patients with borderline coronary stenoses (50% to 60% diameter in locations other than the left main coronary artery) and no demonstrable ischemia on noninvasive testing. *(Level of Evidence: C)*
3. Use of PCI or CABG for patients with insignificant coronary stenosis (<50% diameter). *(Level of Evidence: C)*
4. Use of PCI in patients with significant left main coronary disease who are candidates for CABG. *(Level of Evidence: C)*

CABG, coronary artery bypass graft; CAD, coronary artery disease; LAD, left anterior descending coronary artery; LV, left ventricle; PCI, percutaneous coronary intervention; PTCA, percutaneous transluminal coronary angioplasty.
Note: PTCA is used in these recommendations to indicate PTCA or other catheter-based techniques, such as stents, atherectomy, and laser therapy. See classifications and levels of evidence in Chap. 11 and Table 12–8.
[a]See Chap. 11 and Fig 12–4.

pitalization for acute coronary syndrome (12.0 percent vs. 11 percent; HR 1.11; 95 percent CI 0.86 to 1.42; P = 0.43), or MI (12.3 percent vs. 11.8 percent; HR 1.09; 95 percent CI 0.85 to 1.39; P = 0.52). Thus, as an initial management strategy in symptomatic patients with stable CAD, PCI does not reduce death, MI, or other major cardiovascular events when added to optimal medical therapy.

Multiple trials have compared the strategy of an initial PCI with initial CABG surgery for treatment of multivessel CAD (see Chaps.

62 and 65). The results of all these trials show that early and late survival rates are equivalent for the PCI and CABG surgery groups. In the BARI trial, the subgroups of patients with treated diabetes had a significantly better survival rate with CABG surgery.[68] This was true, however, on post hoc analysis of the clinical variables, including diabetes, which was not a prerandomization blocking variable.

The randomized studies of invasive therapy for chronic angina have all excluded patients who developed recurrent angina after previous

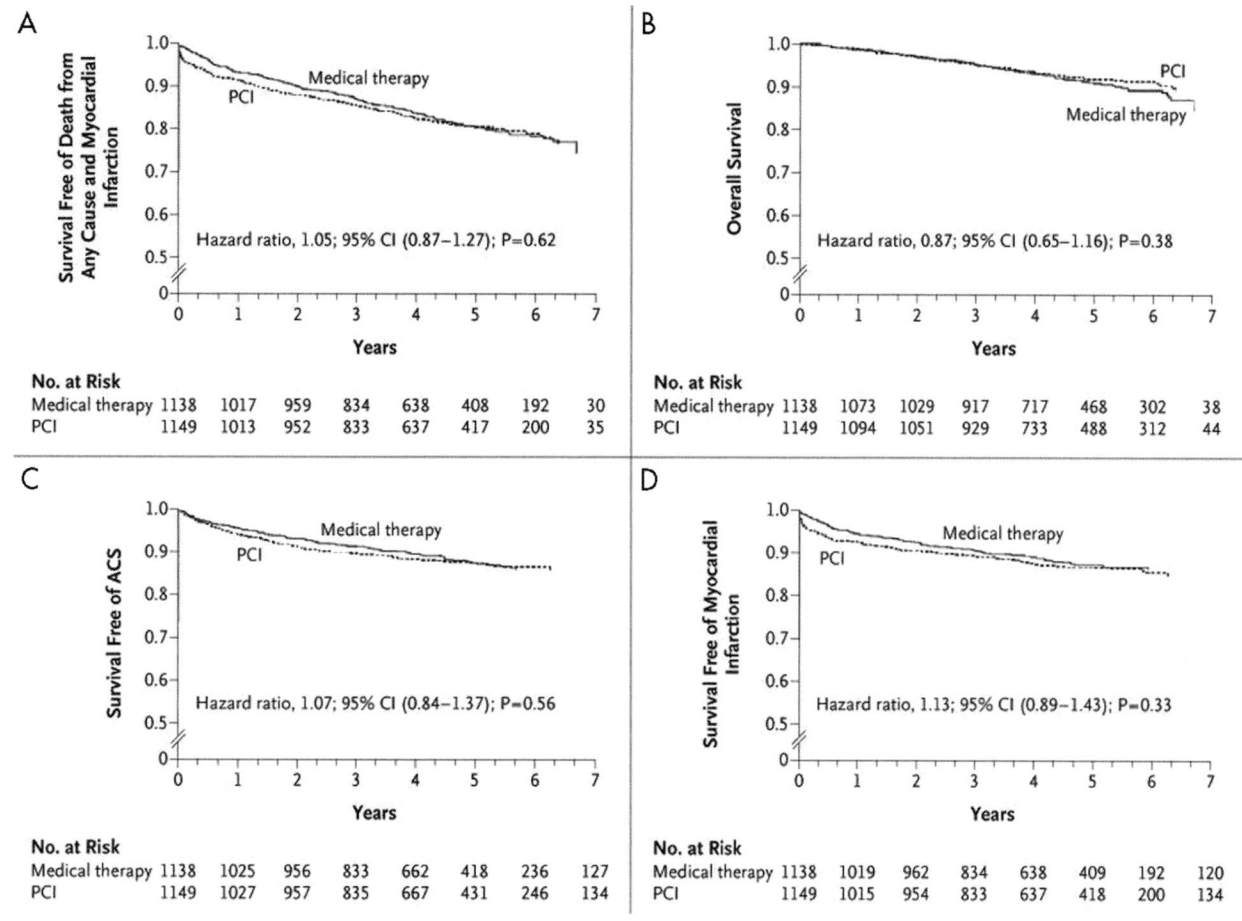

FIGURE 64-8. Kaplan–Meier survival curves. In panel **A**, the estimated 4.6-year rate of the composite primary outcome of death from any cause and non-fatal myocardial infarction was 19.0% in the PCI group and 18.5% in the medical therapy group. In panel **B**, the estimated 4.6-year rate of death from any cause was 7.6% in the PCI group and 8.3% in the medical therapy group. In panel **C**, the estimated 4.6-year rate of hospitalization for acute coronary syndromes (ACS) was 12.4% in the PCI group and 11.8% in the medical therapy group. In panel **D**, the estimated 4.6-year rate of acute myocardial infarction was 13.2% in the PCI group and 12.3% in the medical therapy group. *Source: Reprinted with permission from Boden WE, O'Rourke RA, Teo KK, et al.*[67]

CABG surgery. Few existing data define outcomes for risk-stratified groups of patients who develop recurrent angina after bypass surgery. Those that do indicate that patients with ischemia produced by late atherosclerotic stenoses in vein grafts are at a higher risk with medical management alone than those with ischemia produced by native-vessel disease.

OTHER THERAPIES IN PATIENTS WITH REFRACTORY ANGINA

Recent evidence has emerged regarding the relative efficacy, or lack thereof, of a number of techniques for the management of refractory chronic angina pectoris. These techniques should only be used in patients who cannot be managed adequately by medical therapy and who are not candidates for revascularization (interventional and/or surgical). Data are reviewed regarding three techniques: spinal cord stimulation, enhanced external counterpulsation, and laser transmyocardial revascularization.[1]

【 】 SPINAL CORD STIMULATION

The efficacy of spinal cord stimulation depends on the accurate placement of the stimulating electrode in the dorsal epidural space, usually at the C7-T1 level. A review of the literature reveals two small, randomized, clinical trials involving implanted spinal cord stimulators, one of which directly tested its efficacy. The authors concluded that spinal cord stimulation was effective in the treatment of chronic intractable angina pectoris and that its effect was exerted through an antiischemic action.[1]

【 】 ENHANCED EXTERNAL COUNTERPULSATION

This technique uses a series of cuffs that are wrapped around both of the patient's legs. Using compressed air, pressure is applied via the cuffs to the patient's lower extremities in a sequence synchronized with the cardiac cycle. Specifically, in early diastole, pressure is applied sequentially from the lower legs to the lower and upper thighs, to propel blood back to the heart. The procedure results in an increase in arterial blood pressure and retrograde aortic blood flow during diastole (diastolic augmentation). Treatment was relatively well tolerated and free of limiting side effects in most patients. However, the sample size in this study was relatively small.[1] (Two multicenter registry studies found the treatment to be generally well tolerated and efficacious; anginal symptoms were improved in approximately 75 to 80 percent of patients. However, additional clinical trial data are necessary before this technology can be recommended definitively.)

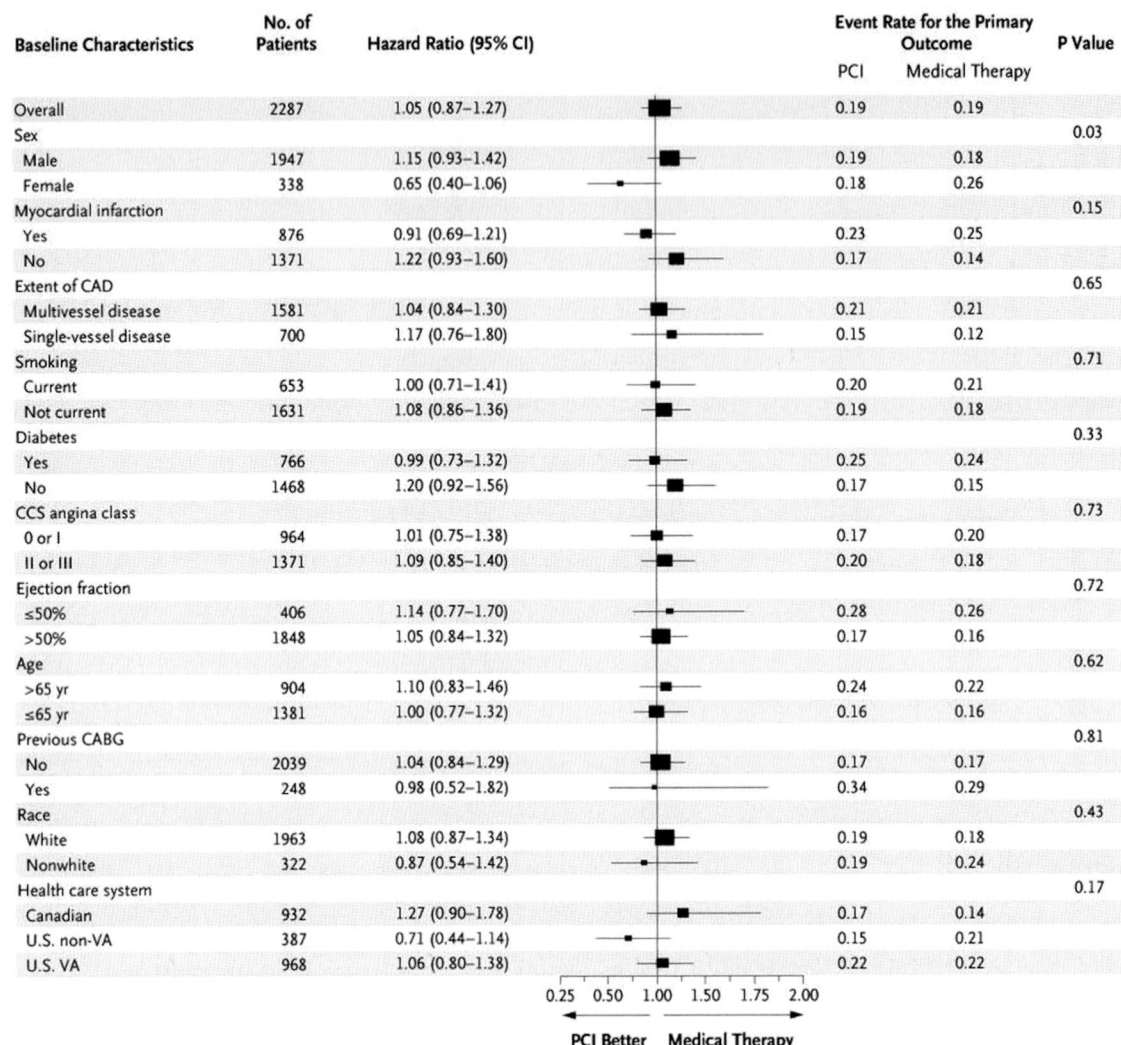

Baseline Characteristics	No. of Patients	Hazard Ratio (95% CI)		Event Rate for the Primary Outcome		P Value
				PCI	Medical Therapy	
Overall	2287	1.05 (0.87–1.27)		0.19	0.19	
Sex						0.03
Male	1947	1.15 (0.93–1.42)		0.19	0.18	
Female	338	0.65 (0.40–1.06)		0.18	0.26	
Myocardial infarction						0.15
Yes	876	0.91 (0.69–1.21)		0.23	0.25	
No	1371	1.22 (0.93–1.60)		0.17	0.14	
Extent of CAD						0.65
Multivessel disease	1581	1.04 (0.84–1.30)		0.21	0.21	
Single-vessel disease	700	1.17 (0.76–1.80)		0.15	0.12	
Smoking						0.71
Current	653	1.00 (0.71–1.41)		0.20	0.21	
Not current	1631	1.08 (0.86–1.36)		0.19	0.18	
Diabetes						0.33
Yes	766	0.99 (0.73–1.32)		0.25	0.24	
No	1468	1.20 (0.92–1.56)		0.17	0.15	
CCS angina class						0.73
0 or I	964	1.01 (0.75–1.38)		0.17	0.20	
II or III	1371	1.09 (0.85–1.40)		0.20	0.18	
Ejection fraction						0.72
≤50%	406	1.14 (0.77–1.70)		0.28	0.26	
>50%	1848	1.05 (0.84–1.32)		0.17	0.16	
Age						0.62
>65 yr	904	1.10 (0.83–1.46)		0.24	0.22	
≤65 yr	1381	1.00 (0.77–1.32)		0.16	0.16	
Previous CABG						0.81
No	2039	1.04 (0.84–1.29)		0.17	0.17	
Yes	248	0.98 (0.52–1.82)		0.34	0.29	
Race						0.43
White	1963	1.08 (0.87–1.34)		0.19	0.18	
Nonwhite	322	0.87 (0.54–1.42)		0.19	0.24	
Health care system						0.17
Canadian	932	1.27 (0.90–1.78)		0.17	0.14	
U.S. non-VA	387	0.71 (0.44–1.14)		0.15	0.21	
U.S. VA	968	1.06 (0.80–1.38)		0.22	0.22	

0.25 0.50 1.00 1.50 1.75 2.00

← PCI Better   Medical Therapy Better →

FIGURE 64–9. Subgroup analysis. The chart shows hazard ratios (*black squares*, sized in proportion to the number of subjects in a group), 95% CIs (*horizontal lines*), cumulative 4.6-year event rates for the composite primary outcome (death from any cause and nonfatal myocardial infarction) for the PCI group versus the medical therapy group for the specified subgroups, and p values for the interaction between the treatment effects and subgroup variables. *P* values were calculated with the use of the Wald statistic. There was no significant interaction between treatment and subgroup variables as defined according to the prespecified value for interaction (p <0.01), although there was a trend for interaction with respect to sex (p = 0.03). CCS, Canadian Cardiovascular Society; CABG, coronary-artery bypass grafting. *Source: Reprinted with permission from Boden WE, O'Rourke RA, Teo KK, et al.*[67]

[ ] LASER TRANSMYOCARDIAL REVASCULARIZATION

Another emerging technique for the treatment of more severe chronic stable angina refractory to medical or other therapies is laser transmyocardial revascularization (TMR). This technique has either been performed in the operating room (using a carbon dioxide or holmium:YAG laser) or by a percutaneous approach with a specialized (holmium:YAG laser) catheter. Eight prospective randomized clinical trials have been performed, two using the percutaneous technique and the other six using an epicardial surgical technique.[1]

Percutaneous TMR

The two randomized percutaneous TMR trials assessed parameters such as angina class, freedom from angina, exercise tolerance, and quality of life score. In general, these studies have shown improvements in severity of angina class, exercise tolerance, and quality of life, as well as increased freedom from angina.[1] However, percutaneous TMR technology has not been approved by the Food and Drug Administration; therefore, percutaneous TMR should still be considered an experimental therapy.

Surgical TMR

The surgical TMR technique also generally has been associated with improvement in symptoms in patients with chronic stable angina. The mechanism for improvement in angina symptoms is still controversial.[1] Three studies also assessed myocardial perfusion using thallium scans. Only one of these studies demonstrated an improvement in myocardial perfusion in patients who underwent TMR versus those continuing to receive only medical therapy. Despite the apparent benefit in decreasing angina symptoms, no definite benefit has been demonstrated in terms of increasing myocardial perfusion.[1]

A New Class of Antiangina Drugs: pFOX Inhibitors

The potential clinical usefulness of newer antianginal drugs currently being studied include the pFOX (partial fatty acid oxidation) inhibitor class of drugs, which partially inhibit fatty acid oxidation and improve cardiac efficiency. Clearly, the development of drugs that modulate myocardial metabolism, have the potential to reduce extent of myocardial ischemia and angina symptoms, yet have no clinically significant effects on heart rate, blood pressure, or coronary blood flow, are of considerable interest. Ranolazine has recently received U.S. Food and Drug Administration approval for patients with symptomatic, persistent angina despite optimal medical therapy. The biochemical rationale and progress in development of pFOX inhibitors is the result of approximately two decades of research.

The pFOX inhibitor drugs partially relieve the inhibition of pyruvate dehydrogenase through an inhibition of the enzyme sequence necessary for β-oxidation of free fatty acids in mitochondria (when there is sufficient residual oxygen supply to the myocardium to allow pyruvate oxidation). The reader is referred to several excellent reviews for a more detailed discussion of these concepts. The sustained-release formulation of ranolazine was tested for chronic angina in both the MARISA (Monotherapy Assessment of Ranolazine and Stable Angina) and CARISA (Combination Assessment of Ranolazine and Stable Angina) trials.[69,70]

The MARISA and CARISA studies indicate that ranolazine is a potentially effective drug to alleviate chronic angina in patients with moderately severe symptoms. The increase in exercise time with monotherapy or when combined with other antianginal drugs averaged about of 30 seconds with more marked improvements in individual patients. The average increase of 30 seconds over placebo approximates the magnitude of increase seen with β blockers or calcium channel antagonists when time-dependent placebo controls were used.

FOLLOWUP OF PATIENTS WITH CHRONIC STABLE ANGINA

Published evidence of the efficacy of specific strategies for the followup of patients with chronic stable angina on patient outcome is nonexistent. The ACC/AHA/ACP-ASIM guidelines[1] for the monitoring of symptoms and antianginal therapy during patient followup are as follows:

For the patient with successfully treated chronic stable angina, a followup evaluation every 4 to 12 months is appropriate. During the first year of therapy, evaluations every 4 to 6 months are recommended. After the first year of therapy, annual evaluations are recommended if the patient is stable and reliable enough to return for evaluation when anginal symptoms become worse or other symptoms occur.[1] At the time of followup, a general assessment of the patient's functional and health status and quality of life may reveal additional issues that affect angina. Symptoms that have worsened should follow reevaluation as outlined above. A detailed history of the patient's daily activity is critical because anginal symptoms may remain stable only because stressful activities have been eliminated.

A careful history of the characteristics of the patient's angina, including provoking and alleviating factors, must be repeated at each visit. Detailed questions should be asked about common drug side effects. The patient's adherence to the treatment program must be assessed.

The physical examination should be focused by the patient's history. Every patient should have his or her weight, blood pressure, and pulse noted. The jugular venous pressure, carotid pulse magnitude and upstroke, and presence or absence of carotid bruits should be noted. Pulmonary examination with special attention to rales, rhonchi, wheezing, and decreased breath sounds is required. A cardiac examination should note the presence of fourth and third heart sounds, a new or changed systolic murmur, the location of the LV impulse, and any change from previous examinations. Clearly, the vascular examination should identify any change in peripheral pulses and new bruits; the abdominal examination should identify hepatomegaly and the presence of any pulsatile mass suggesting an abdominal aortic aneurysm. The presence of new or worsening peripheral edema should be noted.

The American Diabetes Association recommends that patients not known to have diabetes should have a *fasting blood glucose* measured every 3 years and an annual measurement of glycosylated hemoglobin for individuals with established diabetes. Fasting blood work, 6 to 8 weeks after initiating lipid-lowering drug therapy, should include liver function testing and assessment of the cholesterol profile. This should be repeated every 8 to 12 weeks during the first year of therapy and at 4- to 6-month intervals thereafter.

An ECG should be repeated when medications affecting cardiac conduction are initiated or changed. A repeat ECG is indicated for a change in the anginal pattern, symptoms or finding suggestive of an arrhythmia or conduction abnormality, and near or frank syncope. There is no clear evidence showing that routine, periodic ECGs are useful in the absence of a change in history or physical examination.

In the absence of a change in clinical status, low-risk patients with an estimated annual mortality rate of less than 1 percent over each year of the interval do not require repeat stress testing for 3 years after the initial evaluation.[1] *Annual followup for noninvasive testing in the absence of a change in symptoms* has not been studied adequately; it may be useful in high-risk patients with an estimated annual mortality rate of greater than 5 percent. Followup testing should be performed in a stable high-risk patient only if the initial decision not to proceed with revascularization may change if the patient's estimated risk worsens. Patients with an immediate-risk (>1 and <3 percent) annual mortality rate are more problematic because of limited data. They may need testing at an interval of 1 to 3 years depending on the individual circumstances. Table 64–11 lists the ACC/AHA, ACP–ASIM recommendations for echocardiography, treadmill exercise testing, stress imaging studies, and coronary angiography during patient followup.

MANAGEMENT OF SPECIAL CATEGORIES
〖 〗 SYSTEMIC ARTERIAL HYPERTENSION

Patients with systemic arterial hypertension often have angina pectoris. In most patients, significant coronary atherosclerosis of the epicardial blood vessels is present, but some patients with systemic arterial hypertension may have angina pectoris, or even fatal MI, without significant obstruction of the large epicardial vessels. A major mistake is to send a patient for noninvasive testing when the pa-

TABLE 64–11

American College of Cardiology/American Heart Association/American College of Physicians–American Society of Internal Medicine Recommendations for Noninvasive Studies of Coronary Angiography during Patient Followup

Class I

1. Chest radiograph for patients with evidence of new or worsening congestive heart failure.
2. Assessment of LV ejection fraction and segmental wall motion in patients with new or worsening congestive heart failure or evidence of intervening MI by history or ECG.
3. Echocardiography for evidence of new or worsening valvular heart disease.
4. Treadmill exercise test for patients without prior revascularization who have a significant change in clinical status, are able to exercise, and do not have any of the ECG abnormalities listed below in number 5.
5. Stress imaging procedures for patients without prior revascularization who have a significant change in clinical status and are unable to exercise or have one of the following ECG abnormalities:
   a. Preexcitation (Wolff-Parkinson-White) syndrome.
   b. Electronically paced ventricular rhythm.
   c. More than 1 mm of rest ST-segment depression.
   d. Complete left bundle-branch block.
6. Stress imaging procedures for patients who have a significant change in clinical status and required a stress imaging procedure on their initial evaluation because of equivocal or intermediate-risk treadmill results.
7. Stress imaging procedures for patients with prior revascularization who have a significant change in clinical status.
8. Coronary angiography in patients with marked limitation of ordinary activity. (CCS class III despite maximal medical therapy.)

Class IIb

Annual treadmill exercise testing in patients who have no change in clinical status, can exercise, have none of the ECG abnormalities listed in number 5 above, and have an estimated annual mortality of >1%.

Class III

1. Echocardiography or radionuclide imaging for assessment of LV ejection fraction and segmental wall motion in patients with a normal ECG, no history of MI, and no evidence of congestive heart failure.
2. Repeat treadmill exercise testing in <3 years in patients who have no change in clinical status and an estimated annual mortality ≥1 % on their initial evaluation as demonstrated by one of the following:
   a. Low-risk Duke treadmill score (without imaging).
   b. Low-risk Duke treadmill score with negative imaging.
   c. Normal LV function and a normal coronary angiogram.
   d. Normal LV function and insignificant CAD.
3. Stress imaging procedures for patients who have no change in clinical status and a normal rest ECG, are not taking digoxin, are able to exercise, and did not require a stress imaging procedure on their initial evaluation because of equivocal or intermediate-risk treadmill results.
4. Repeat coronary angiography in patients with no change in clinical status, no change on repeat exercise testing or stress imaging, and insignificant CAD on initial evaluation.

CAD, coronary artery disease; CCS, Canadian Cardiovascular Society; LV, left ventricle; MI, myocardial infarction.
NOTE: See classifications and levels of evidence in Chap. 11 and Table 12–8.

tient's hypertension has not been treated. In many patients, treatment of the hypertension with a β blocker, calcium antagonist, or ACE inhibitor also will decrease MVO$_2$ and prevent the development of angina pectoris. In general, efforts should be made to control the blood pressure both at rest and during exercise. It is now known that many patients with an elevated systolic and/or diastolic blood pressure above the normal variation during exercise will develop severe fixed systemic arterial hypertension. Efforts should be made to control the blood pressure both at rest and during exertion.

CHRONIC OBSTRUCTIVE PULMONARY DISEASE/ ASTHMA

β Blockers should be avoided in the subset of patients who have true bronchospastic lung disease; in them, the use of nitrates and calcium antagonists is preferred. Because many of these patients receive medications for their pulmonary disease that may increase their heart rate or even produce supraventricular tachycardia, it is preferable to use a heart rate-slowing calcium antagonist such as diltiazem or verapamil.

ELDERLY PATIENTS

In general, elderly patients tolerate calcium antagonists better than β blockers. The presence of sinus tachycardia or atrial fibrillation is a relative contraindication to the selection of dihydropyridines such as nifedipine or amlodipine. In such patients, diltiazem or verapamil, or even a β blocker is preferable. On the other hand, β blockers, verapamil, and diltiazem can exacerbate AV block, and verapamil produces constipation in many elderly patients. Also, some elderly patients develop postural hypotension from short-acting nitrates.

PERIPHERAL VASCULAR DISEASE

Patients with peripheral vascular disease may have a worsening of their symptoms when they are treated with a nonselective β blocker, permitting unopposed α-induced vasoconstriction. Alternatively, the worsening symptoms may be the result of a decrease in arterial perfusion pressure. In general, it is preferable to treat patients with chronic stable angina who have peripheral vascular disease with nitrates and a calcium antagonist.

❪ ❫ DIABETES MELLITUS

Patients with chronic stable angina who have diabetes mellitus and insulin-induced hypoglycemic episodes should probably be treated with nitrates and calcium antagonists (see Chap. 90). If it is necessary to use a β blocker, a cardioselective agent should be chosen, because it is less likely to impair the recognition of and recovery from insulin-induced hypoglycemia. In most diabetics, cardioselective β blockers are well tolerated. The BARI-2D randomized clinical trial is evaluating the efficacy of *early* myocardial revascularization in diabetes with CAD.

❪ ❫ CHRONIC RENAL DISEASE

Although β blockers and calcium antagonists can normally be used effectively in patients with chronic angina and chronic renal insufficiency, careful monitoring may be necessary, because many β blockers and calcium antagonists are excreted primarily by the kidneys.

LONG-TERM MANIFESTATIONS OF CHRONIC ISCHEMIC HEART DISEASE

❪ ❫ HEART FAILURE

Patients with severe CAD that produces a loss of 20 percent or more of the myocardium or that results in a ventricular septal defect or severe mitral regurgitation may develop important LV failure. While there may be significant hypertrophy of the remaining myocytes and interstitium (see Chap. 24), the ventricle is unable to compensate completely and heart failure often results, with a decreased stroke volume and elevated diastolic filling pressures. Such a syndrome of heart failure may be clinically predominant and often more incapacitating than any symptom of angina pectoris.

Patients with severe LV dysfunction because of CAD have a poor prognosis. Usually it reflects permanent, irreversible loss of myocytes. In some patients, severe chronic CAD is associated with persistently impaired LV function at rest as a result of reduced CBF that can be partially or completely restored to normal either by improving blood flow (more common) or by reducing oxygen demand. This concept of "hibernating" myocardium is important because there can be significant improvement following good LV revascularization. Although this does not occur routinely, it must be considered before concluding that the LVEF of an individual patient is too low to consider revascularization surgery or that the etiology of the heart failure is not CHD. Myocardial perfusion imaging techniques, MRI, dobutamine echocardiography, and positron-emission tomography are useful in detecting myocardial viability.

The treatment of patients with heart failure as a consequence of CHD is the same as for most patients with combined systolic and diastolic LV failure and includes diuretics, an ACE inhibitor, digitalis, β blockers, and spironolactone.

Cardiac transplantation is also frequently performed for severe heart failure caused by CAD (see Chap. 27). A patient with heart failure who has a large LV aneurysm may benefit from aneurysmectomy if there is sufficient remaining functioning LV tissue. Similarly, heart failure because of severe mitral regurgitation sometimes can be improved significantly by corrective mitral valve surgery, which is often combined with myocardial revascularization. Mitral valve repair in patients with severe functional mitral regurgitation, with a reduced annular size, can improve symptoms considerably (see Chap. 76).

❪ ❫ CARDIAC ARRHYTHMIAS, CONDUCTION DISTURBANCES

Chronic ischemic heart disease causes many cardiac arrhythmias. Basic management of cardiac arrhythmias is discussed in Chap. 36. In general, β blockers should be employed whenever there is no strong contraindication, and type IC antiarrhythmic agents should be avoided unless the patient is symptomatic. In patients with atrial fibrillation, the ventricular response rate should be controlled with digoxin.

Patients with chronic atrial fibrillation also should be maintained on warfarin (international normalized ratio [INR] = 2 to 3) unless there is a contraindication, in which case aspirin (80 to 325 mg/d) should be used. Patients in heart failure who have atrial fibrillation may benefit from an effective atrial contraction restored by electrical cardioversion; unfortunately, large percentages revert to atrial fibrillation in the next few months.

❪ ❫ EMBOLIC DISEASE

Patients with ischemic disease are likely to have systemic emboli, particularly patients with a history of systemic embolus, chronic atrial fibrillation, ventricular aneurysm, a large dyskinetic or hypokinetic area of myocardium, or a severely depressed LVEF. Such patients should be considered for chronic, long-term, low-dose warfarin therapy (INR = 2 to 3).

CHEST PAIN WITH NORMAL CORONARY ARTERIES

The combination of chest pain with many of the features of angina pectoris—although frequently atypical—and normal epicardial coronary arteries at cardiac catheterization, was first described in the 1960s. The early studies identified many of the features of what was subsequently characterized as a syndrome: female predominance; frequent ischemic ST-segment changes on the exercise ECG; inconsistent relationship between ECG changes and metabolic or hemodynamic evidence of ischemia; and pain that may be very severe, prolonged, variable in location, precipitated by unusual events, and unresponsive to usual antiischemic therapy.

The term *syndrome X* was applied to this diagnostic combination in 1973; it is usually used to describe patients with the common features of angina-like pain and normal epicardial coronaries, but the term is also used to categorize groups that undoubtedly are heterogeneous.[71] The continued use of this term is unfortunate and has been discouraged,[72] especially as there is also a *metabolic syndrome X*—characterized by insulin resistance, hyperinsulinemia, and diabetes—that is associated with abnormal lipids, hypertension, and abdominal obesity (see Chap. 91). A more specific term, such as *angina with normal coronary arteriography*, is preferable.

REFERENCES

1. Gibbons RJ, Chatterjee K, Daley J, et al. American College of Cardiology/American Heart Association, American College of Physicians–American Society of Internal Medicine (ACC/AHA/ACP–ASIM) guidelines for the management of patients with chronic stable angina: a report of the ACC/AHA Task Force on Practice Guidelines (Committee on the Management of Patients with Chronic Stable Angina). *J Am Coll Cardiol* 2002;41:160–168.

2. Herberden W. Some account of disorder of the breast. *Med Trans R Coll Phys (Lond)* 1772;2:59–67.

3. Herberden W. *Commentaries on the History and Care of Disease.* London: T Payne, 1802.

4. White PD. Angina pectoris: historical background. In: Paul O, ed. *Angina Pectoris.* New York: Medcom Press, 1974:1.

5. Diamond GA, Staniloff HM, Forrester JS, et al. Computer-assisted diagnosis in the noninvasive evaluation of patients with suspected coronary disease. *J Am Coll Cardiol* 1983;1:444–455.

6. O'Rourke RA, Hochman JS, Cohen MC, et al. New approaches to diagnosis and management of unstable angina and non-ST-segment elevation myocardial infarction. *Arch Intern Med* 2001;161:674–682.

7. Diamond GA, Forrester JS. Analysis of probability as an aid in the clinical diagnosis of coronary artery disease. *N Engl J Med* 1979;300:1350–1358.

8. Wexler L, Brundage B, Crouse J, et al. Coronary artery calcification, pathophysiology, epidemiology, imaging methods and clinical implications. *Circulation* 1996;94:1175–1192.

9. O'Rourke R, Brundage B, Froelicher V, et al. American College of Cardiology/American Heart Association consensus document on electron beam computed tomography for the diagnosis of coronary artery disease (Committee on Electron Beam Computer Tomography). *Circulation* 2000;20:126–140.

10. Detrano RC, Duherty TM, Davies MJ, et al. Predicting coronary events with coronary calcium: pathophysiologic and clinical problems. *Curr Probl Cardiol* 2000;25:369–404.

10a. Greenland P, Bonow RO, Brundage BH, et al. ACCF/AHA Writing Committee to Update the 2000 Expert Consensus Document on Electron Beam Computed Tomography, developed in collaboration with the Society of Atherosclerosis Imaging and Prevention and the Society of Cardiovascular Computed Tomography. *J Am Coll Cardiol* 2007;49(3):378–402.

11. Gibbons RJ, Balady GJ, Bricker JT, et al. ACC/AHA 2002 guideline update for exercise testing: a report of the American College of Cardiology/American Heart Association Task Force on Practice guidelines (Committee on Exercise Testing). *J Am Coll Cardiol* 2002;41:160–168. American College of Cardiology website: http://www.acc.org/clinical/guidelines/exercise/exercise_clean.pdf. Last accessed October 17, 2002.

12. Froelicher VF, Lehmann KG, Thomas R, et al. The electrocardiographic exercise test in a population with reduced workup bias: diagnostic performance, computerized interpretation, and multivariable prediction. Veterans Affairs Cooperative Study in Health Services 016 (QUEXTA) Study Group, Quantitative Exercise Testing and Angiography. *Ann Intern Med* 1998;128:965–974.

13. Froelicher V, Shetler K, Ashley E. Better decisions through science: exercise testing scores. *Curr Probl Cardiol* 2003;28:595–620.

14. Mark DB, Shaw L, Harrell FE, et al. Prognostic value of a treadmill exercise score in outpatients with suspected coronary artery disease. *N Engl J Med* 1991;325:849–853.

15. Cheitlin MD, Armstrong WF, Aurigemma GP, et al. ACC/AHA/ASE 2003 guideline update for the clinical application of echocardiography. *J Am Coll Cardiol* 2003;42:954–970.

16. Klocke FJ, Baird MG, Lorell BH, et al. ACC/AHA/ASNC revision of the 1995 guidelines for the clinical use of cardiac radionuclide imaging. *J Am Coll Cardiol* 2003;42:1318–1333.

17. Douglas JS Jr, Hurst JW. Limitations of symptoms in the recognition of coronary atherosclerotic heart disease. In: Hurst JW, ed. *Update I. The Heart.* New York: McGraw-Hill, 1979:3.

18. Pupita G, Maseri A, Kaski JC, et al. Myocardial ischemia caused by distal coronary artery constriction in stable angina pectoris. *N Engl J Med* 1990;323:514–520.

19. Egashira K, Inou T, Hirooka Y, et al. Evidence of impaired endothelium-dependent coronary vasodilatation in patients with angina pectoris and normal coronary angiograms. *N Engl J Med* 1993;328:1659–1664.

20. Maseri A, Crea F, Kaski JC. Mechanisms of angina pectoris in syndrome X. *J Am Coll Cardiol* 1991;17:499–506.

21. Egashira K, Inou T, Hirooka Y, et al. Evidence of impaired endothelium-dependent coronary vasodilatation in patients with angina pectoris and normal coronary angiograms. *N Engl J Med* 1993;328:1659–1664.

22. Bortone AS, Hess OM, Eberli FR. Abnormal coronary vasomotion during exercise in patients with normal coronary arteries and reduced coronary flow reserve. *Circulation* 1991;83:26–37.

23. Sigwart U, Grbic M, Payot L, et al. Ischemic events during coronary artery balloon occlusion. In: Rutishauser W, Roskamm H, eds. *Silent Myocardial Ischemia.* Berlin: Springer-Verlag, 1984:29.

24. Rocco MB, Barry J, Campbell S, et al. Circadian variation of transient myocardial ischemia in patients with coronary artery disease. Circulation 1987;75:395–400.

25. Herrick JB. Clinical features of sudden obstruction of the coronary arteries. *JAMA* 1912;59:2015–2020.

26. Crawford NH, Bernstein SJ, DiMarco J, et al. ACC/AHA guidelines for ambulatory electrocardiography. *Circulation* 1999;34:912–948.

27. Crawford MH, Bernstein SJ, Deedwania PC, et al. ACC/AHA guidelines for ambulatory electrocardiography: a report of the American College of Cardiology/American Heart Association Task Force on Practice Guidelines (Committee to Revise the Guidelines for Ambulatory Electrocardiography): Developed in collaboration with the North American Society for Pacing and Electrophysiology. *J Am Coll Cardiol* 1999;34:912–948.

28. Greenland P, LaBree L, Azen SP, Doherty TM, Detrano RC. Coronary artery calcium score combined with Framingham score for risk prediction in asymptomatic individuals. *JAMA* 2004;291:210–215.

29. Hendel R, et al. *J Am Coll Cardiol* 2006. Available at http://www.cardiosource.com/guidelines/index.asp.

30. Davies RF, Goldberg AD, Forman S, et al. Asymptomatic Cardiac Ischemia Pilot (ACIP) study two-year follow-up: outcomes of patients randomized to initial strategies of medical therapy versus revascularization. *Circulation* 1997;95:2037–2043.

31. Hubbard BL, Gibbons RJ, Lapeyre AC, et al. Identification of severe coronary artery disease using simple clinical parameters. *Arch Intern Med* 1992;152(2):309–312.

32. Guidelines for percutaneous transluminal coronary angioplasty: a report of the American College of Cardiology/American Heart Association Task Force on Assessment of Diagnostic and Therapeutic Cardiovascular Procedures (Committee on Percutaneous Transluminal Coronary Angioplasty). *J Am Coll Cardiol* 1993;22(7):2033–2054.

33. Mark DB, Shaw L, Harrell FE, et al. Prognostic value of a treadmill exercise score in outpatients with suspected coronary artery disease. *N Engl J Med* 1991;325:849–853.

34. Brown KA. Prognostic value of thallium-201 myocardial perfusion imaging: a diagnostic tool comes of age. *Circulation* 1991;83:363–381.

35. Hachamovitch R, Berman DS, Shaw LJ, et al. Incremental prognostic value of myocardial perfusion single photon emission computed tomography for the prediction of cardiac death: differential stratification for risk of cardiac death and myocardial infarction [published erratum appears in *Circulation* 1999;98(2):190]. *Circulation* 1998;97(6):533–543.

36. Wagdy HM, Hodge D, Christian TF, et al. Prognostic value of vasodilator myocardial perfusion imaging in patients with left bundle-branch-block. *Circulation* 1998;97(16):1563–1570.

37. Ryan TJ, Antman EM, Brooks NH, et al. ACC/AHA guidelines for the management of patients with acute myocardial infarction: 1999 update: a report of the American College of Cardiology/American Heart Association Task force on Practice Guidelines (Committee on Management of Acute Myocardial Infarction). Available at http://www.acc.org/clinical/guidelines/nov96/1999/index.htm. Last accessed October 17, 2002.

38. O'Rourke R, Boden W, Weintraub W, et al. Medical therapy versus percutaneous coronary intervention: implications of the Avert Study and the Courage Trial. *Curr Pract Med* 1999;2(11):225–227.

39. Final report on the aspirin component of the ongoing Physicians' Health Study. Steering Committee of the Physicians' Health Study Research Group. *N Engl J Med* 1989;321:129–135.

40. O'Rourke RA. *Hurst's Online: Meta-Analysis of 200,000 Patients with Low/High ASA Doses.* (See website for references.)

41. Yusuf S, Zhao F, Mehta SR, et al. Effects of clopidogrel in addition to aspirin in patients with acute coronary syndromes without ST-segment-elevation. *N Engl J Med* 2001;345(7):494–502.

42. American Heart Association. *Updated American Heart Association Statement: Patient guidance based on results of the CHARISMA trial.* March 16, 2006. American Heart Association.

43. Khot UN, Nissen SE. Is CURE a cure for acute coronary syndromes? Statistical versus clinical significance. *J Am Coll Cardiol* 2002;40:218–219.

44. CAPRIE Steering Committee. A randomized, blinded trial of clopidogrel versus aspirin in patients at risk of ischemic events (CAPRIE). *Lancet* 1996;348(9038):1329–1339.
45. Pedersen T, Olsson A, Faergeman O, et al. Lipoprotein changes and reduction in the incidence of major coronary heart disease events in the Scandinavian Simvastatin Survival Study (4S). *Circulation* 1998;97:1453–1460.
46. Sacks FM, Pfeffer MA, Moye LA, et al. The effect of pravastatin on coronary events after myocardial infarction in patients with average cholesterol levels: Cholesterol and Recurrent Events Trial investigators. *N Engl J Med* 1996;335(14):1001–1009.
47. MRC/BHF heart protection study of cholesterol lowering with simvastatin in 20,536 high-risk individuals: a randomized placebo-controlled trial. *Lancet* 2002;360:7–22.
48. Yusef S, Sleight P, Pogue J, et al. Effects of an angiotensin-converting-enzyme inhibitor, ramipril, on cardiovascular events in high-risk patients. The Heart Outcomes Prevention Evaluation Study Investigators. *N Engl J Med* 2000;342:145–153.
49. Heart Outcomes Prevention Evaluation Study Investigators. Effects of ramipril on cardiovascular outcomes in people with diabetes mellitus: results of the HOPE study and MICRO-HOPE sub-study. *Lancet* 2000;355:253–259.
50. Savonitto S, Ardissiono D, Egstrup K, et al. Combination therapy with metoprolol and nifedipine versus monotherapy in patients with stable angina pectoris: results of the International Multicenter Angina Exercise (IMAGE) study. *J Am Coll Cardiol* 1996;27(2):311–316.
51. Waysbort J, Meshulam N, Brunner D. Isosorbide-5-mononitrate and atenolol in the treatment of stable exertional angina. *Cardiology* 1991;79(Suppl 2):19–26.
52. Pepine CJ, Feldman RL, Whittle J, et al. Effect of diltiazem in patients with variant angina: a randomized double-blind trial. *Am Heart J* 1981;101(6):719–725.
53. Psaty BM, Heckbert SR, Koepsell TD, et al. The risk of myocardial infarction associated with antihypertensive drug therapies. *JAMA* 1995;274(8):620–625.
54. Ad Hoc Subcommittee of the Liaison Committee of the World Health Organization and the International Society of Hypertension. Effects of calcium antagonists on the risks of coronary heart disease, cancer and bleeding. *J Hypertens* 1997;15:105–115.
55. Cheitlin MD, Hutter AM Jr, Brindis RG, et al. ACC/AHA expert consensus documents: use of sildenafil (Viagra) in patients with cardiovascular disease. *J Am Coll Cardiol* 1999;33:273–282.
56. Fung HL, Bauer JA. Mechanisms of nitrate tolerance. *Cardiovasc Drugs Ther* 1994;8(3):489–499.
57. The sixth report of the Joint National Committee on prevention, detection, evaluation, and treatment of high blood pressure. *Arch Intern Med* 1997;157(21):2413–2446.
58. Alderman MH, Cohen H, Roque R, Madhavan S. Effect of long-acting and short-acting calcium antagonist on cardiovascular outcomes in hypertensive patients. *Lancet* 1997;349(9052):594–598.
59. National Cholesterol Education Program. Third report of the expert panel on detection, evaluation, and treatment of high blood cholesterol in adults (Adult Treatment Panel III). *Circulation* 2002;106:3143–3421.
60. Eckel RH. Obesity and heart disease: a statement for healthcare professionals from the Nutrition Committee, American Heart Association. *Circulation* 1997;96(9):3248–3250.
61. Curb JD, McTiernan A, Heckbert SR, et al. Outcomes ascertainment and adjudication methods in the women's health initiative. *Ann Epidemiol* 2003;95:S122–S128.
62. Barrett-Connor E, Ensrud KE, Harper K, et al. Post hoc analysis of data from the Multiple Outcomes of Raloxifene Evaluation (MORE) trial on the effects of three years of raloxifene treatment on glycemic control and cardiovascular disease risk factors in women with and without type 2 diabetes. *Clin Ther* 2003;25(3):919–930.
63. Reaven GM. Insulin resistance and compensatory hyperinsulinemia: Role in hypertension, dyslipidemia, and coronary heart disease. *Am Heart J* 1991;121(4 pt 2):1283–1288.
64. Parisi AF, Folland ED, Hartigan P. A comparison of angioplasty with medical therapy in the treatment of single-vessel coronary artery disease: Veterans Affairs ACME Investigators. *N Engl J Med* 1992;326(1):10–16.
65. Coronary angioplasty versus medical therapy for angina: The second Randomised Intervention Treatment of Angina (RITA-2) trial. RITA-2 trial participants. *Lancet* 1997;350(9076):461–468.
66. Pitt B, Waters D, Brown WV, et al. Aggressive lipid-lowering therapy compared with angioplasty in stable coronary artery disease: Atorvastatin versus Revascularization Treatment Investigators. *N Engl J Med* 1999;341(2):70–76.
67. Boden WE, O'Rourke RA, Teo KK, et al. Optimal medical therapy with or without PCI for stable coronary disease. *N Engl J Med* 2007;356:1503–1516.
68. Comparison of coronary bypass surgery with angioplasty in patients with multivessel disease: the Bypass Angioplasty Revascularization Investigation (BARI) investigators [published erratum appears in *N Engl J Med* 1997;336(2):147]. *N Engl J Med* 1996;335(4):217–225.
69. Pepine CJ, Wolff AA. A controlled trial with a novel anti-ischemic agent, ranolazine, in chronic stable angina pectoris that is responsive to conventional antianginal agents. *Am J Cardiol* 1999;84:46–50.
70. Chaitman BR, Skettino S, DeQuattro V. Improved exercise performance on ranolazine in patients with chronic angina and a history of heart failure: the MARISA trial. *J Am Coll Cardiol* 2001;37(Suppl A):149A.
71. Cannon RO III, Canici PG, Epstein SE. Pathophysiological dilemma of syndrome X. *Circulation* 1992;85:883–892.
72. Kaplan MN. Syndromes X. Two too many. *J Am Coll Cardiol* 1992;69:1643–1644.

CHAPTER 65

Coronary Bypass Surgery

Joseph F. Sabik, 3rd / Bruce W. Lytle

Coronary bypass surgery—as a planned, consistent therapy for patients with angiographically documented coronary atherosclerosis—was begun by Sones, Favaloro, and colleagues in 1967. The fundamental concept behind bypass surgery was that the symptoms and clinical events of coronary artery disease are related to stenotic coronary lesions that can be identified by angiography, and if those lesions are bypassed, then those symptoms and clinical events become less common. Experience has shown that concept to be correct.

Effective bypass surgery relieves symptoms of angina, and early randomized trials demonstrated that it prolongs life expectancy of some subsets of patients with severe coronary artery disease (CAD). The arrival of this anatomic treatment for CAD, the most common cause of premature death in western countries, initiated a rapid growth in the personnel and medical infrastructure dedicated to bypass surgery. Along with the growth of bypass surgery came the development of endoluminal, or percutaneous coronary intervention (PCI) of CAD. Also, pharmacologic treatments for CAD have progressed rapidly, particularly in the last decade. The roles of these complementary therapies for treatment of CAD continue to evolve.

GRAFTS IN BYPASS SURGERY

【 】 SAPHENOUS VEIN GRAFTS

Early coronary bypass operations were based almost entirely on aorta-to-coronary reversed saphenous vein grafts (SVGs) (Fig. 65–1A). Al-

though patency of SVGs within the first postoperative year have been 80 to 90 percent, serial angiographic studies have demonstrated significant late (>5 postoperative years) attrition of initially successful SVGs that has ranged from 2 to 5 percent per year (Fig. 65–2).[1–4] Serial Cleveland Clinic Foundation studies found that of those SVGs patent within 5 years after operation, only 55 percent remained angiographically perfect 6 to 12 years after surgery.[1,2]

Much of late SVG failure is caused by intimal fibroplasia and vein graft atherosclerosis.[4,5] Vein graft atherosclerosis (VGA) is characterized by lipid infiltration of areas of intimal fibroplasia and is different in distribution and character than native coronary atherosclerosis. Native coronary artery atherosclerosis is a proximal, eccentric, and intermittent lesion that is covered by a fibrous cap. VGA is distributed throughout the length of vein grafts, is circumferential, not encapsulated, and extremely friable (Fig. 65–3). VGA is a dangerous lesion. Because of the friability and nonencapsulated nature of this lesion, embolization of atherosclerotic debris is a major risk during PCI and reoperations, and it is probable that spontaneous embolization occurs. The increased SVG attrition seen more than 5 years after operation appears to be in large part a result of VGA, and the presence of late stenoses in vein grafts predicts adverse clinical events.

Substantial progress has been made in extending the effectiveness of SVGs. Perioperative treatment with platelet inhibitors decreases SVG occlusion,[6,7] and lipid-lowering regimens, such as 3-hydroxy-3-methylglutaryl-coenzyme A (HMG-CoA) reductase

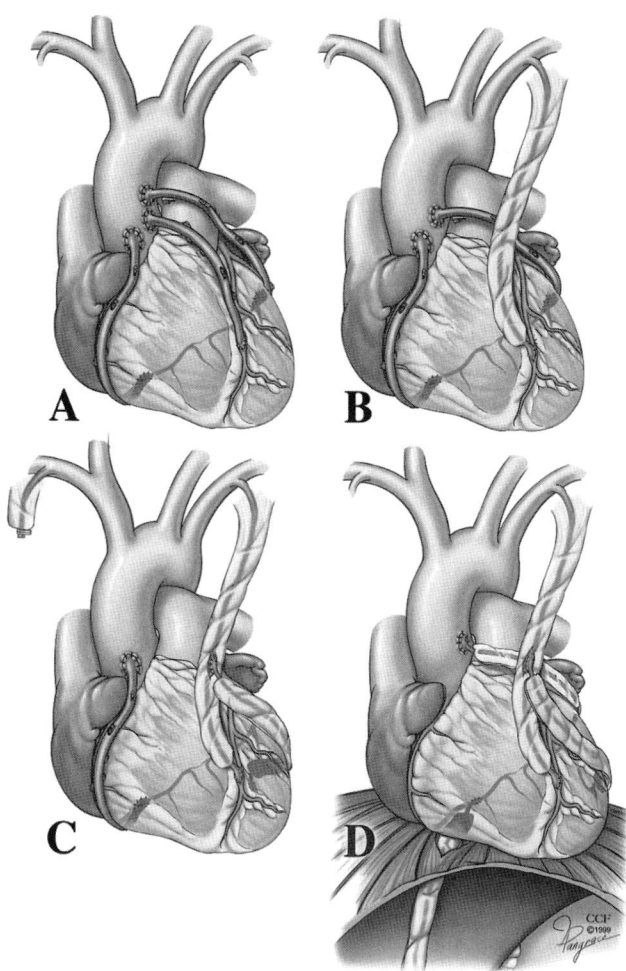

FIGURE 65–1. A. Most early coronary bypass operations involved only aorta-to-coronary saphenous vein grafts. **B.** The use of a LITA-to-LAD graft combined with vein grafts has become the standard bypass operation. **C.** Bilateral ITA grafting may be accomplished with a composite ITA graft. Here the RITA is anastomosed to the LITA–LAD graft and used as a graft to the circumflex coronary artery with an SVG used to graft the RCA. **D.** Total arterial revascularization is accomplished here with an aorta-to-coronary RITA-to-circumflex graft. The radial artery is used as a composite graft from the LITA to the diagonal coronary artery, the LITA is used as a graft to the LAD, and an in situ gastroepiploic graft to the RCA. ITA, internal thoracic artery; LAD, left anterior descending coronary artery; LITA, left internal thoracic artery; RCA, right coronary artery; RITA, right internal thoracic artery; SVG, saphenous vein graft.

inhibitors, or statins, decreases vein graft atherosclerosis and the risk of death and nonfatal myocardial infarction (MI).[8,9]

Despite the imperfections of SVGs, many SVGs provide substantial long-term benefit. Studies of patients more than 15 years after operation have shown approximately 50 percent of SVGs are still functioning.[10]

INTERNAL THORACIC ARTERY GRAFTS

The patency of internal thoracic artery (ITA) grafts is better than SVGs. More importantly, the late attrition rate of ITA grafts is extremely low (see Fig. 65–2).[1,2,11–14] Prospective angiography from the Bypass Angioplasty Revascularization Investigation (BARI) trial noted a 98 percent 1-year patency (<50 percent stenosis) for ITA grafts.[13] Because atherosclerosis of ITA grafts is rare, the 20-year patency rate of left internal thoracic artery (LITA)-to-left anterior descending (LAD) coronary artery grafts is still approximately 90 percent.[15] The most common cause of ITA graft failure is competition in blood flow through a native coronary artery that is only moderately stenotic (Fig. 65–4).[11] This may result in diffuse ITA narrowing or *string sign*.

The success of the LITA-to-LAD graft has led to the use of the right internal thoracic artery (RITA) as a bypass graft, usually simultaneously with the LITA (bilateral internal thoracic artery [BITA] grafting). The RITA has been used as an in situ graft and as a "free" graft, with the proximal anastomosis constructed either to the LITA (see Fig. 65–1C) or the aorta (see Fig. 65–1D). Patency of ITA grafts to circumflex or right coronary arteries have not been as good as patency of ITA grafts to the LAD (see Fig. 65–4).[2,11]

A strategy that greatly expands the capacity to achieve extensive revascularization with ITA grafts is composite arterial grafting, where the RITA is anastomosed to the LITA (Fig. 65–5).[16] Composite BITA grafting may be used to achieve arterial total revascularization.

CLINICAL IMPACT OF ITA GRAFTS

The high and stable patency of the LITA-to-LAD graft produces improved clinical outcomes. A large observational study by Loop et al. showed that patients who received a LITA-to-LAD graft (with or without SVGs to the Cx and right coronary artery [RCA] systems) had better survival, underwent fewer reoperations, and experienced fewer adverse cardiac events when compared to patients who received only SVGs (see Fig. 65–1B).[14] Followup data from the Cleveland Clinic show that the benefits of LITA-to-LAD grafting extend to 20 years after operation (Fig. 65–6). The LITA-to-LAD graft is the most effective and longest-lasting anatomic treatment of CAD known.

If one ITA graft is good, might two ITA grafts be better? BITA grafting has not become widespread because (1) it is technically more difficult, (2) diabetics are at increased risk of wound complications, and (3) outcomes for patients receiving LITA-to-LAD grafts are very good during the first postoperative decade. Despite the lack of widespread adoption of BITA grafting, several studies demonstrate that BITA grafting results in better survival and freedom from coronary reintervention, particularly during the second postoperative decade (Fig. 65–7).[17,18]

ALTERNATIVE ARTERIAL BYPASS GRAFTS

The gastroepiploic artery (GEA) has been successfully used as an in situ graft, usually to the RCA (see Fig. 65–1D). Suma reported 644 of 685 GEA grafts (94 percent) patent within 1 year and 43 of 52 previously patent grafts with persistent patency 5 to 10 years after operation.[19] GEA grafts are adversely effective by competitive flow and prone to spasm. The GEA is not a widely used graft because it is difficult to use.

The inferior epigastric artery has been used as a bypass graft with a 90 percent patency within 1 year of operation; 25 of 29 grafts studied by Buche et al. were patent 25 months after operation.[20] The inferior epigastric artery is useful as a composite arterial graft because it is relatively short.

The most widely used alternative arterial graft is the radial artery. It has the advantages of long length, large size, and a low

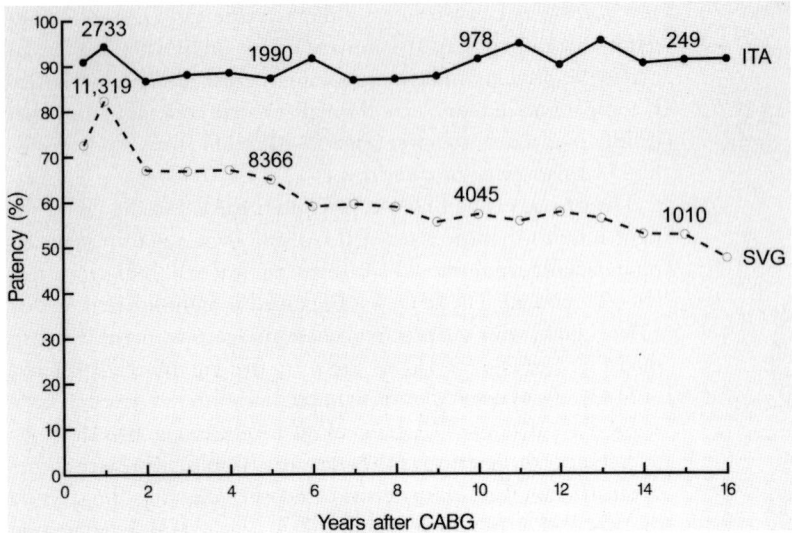

FIGURE 65–2. Internal thoracic artery (ITA) and saphenous vein graft (SVG) patency by year after coronary artery bypass grafting (CABG). Numbers represent number of grafts studied at corresponding year after CABG. *Source: Reprinted with permission from Sabik JF 3rd, Lytle BW, Blackstone EH, Houghtaling PL, Cosgrove DM. Comparison of saphenous vein and internal thoracic artery graft patency by coronary system. Ann Thorac Surg 2005;79(2):544–551.*

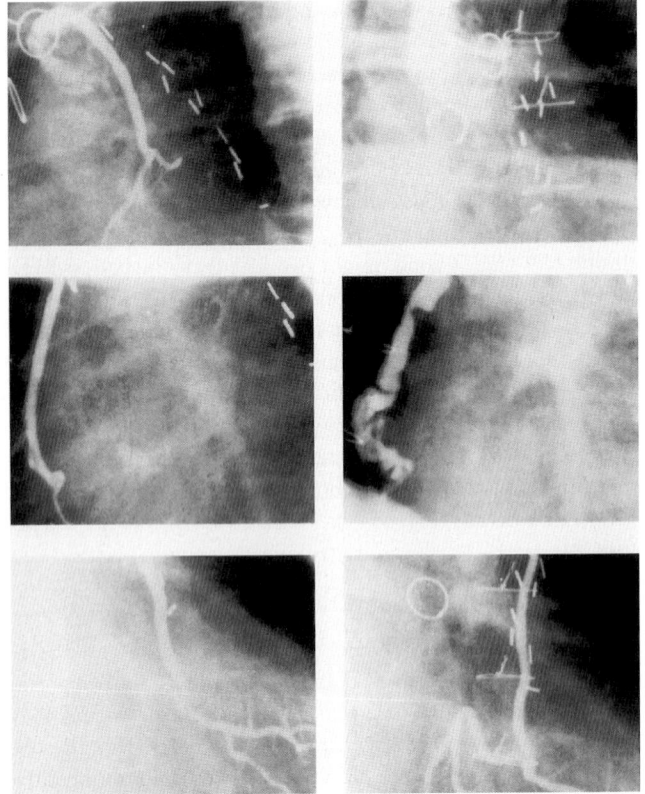

FIGURE 65–3. Angiographic anatomy 1 year after operation (*left*) showing patent vein grafts to the LAD and RCA and an ITA graft to the circumflex artery. Seven years later (*right*), the LAD vein graft is occluded, the RCA graft exhibits diffuse irregular stenoses characteristic of vein graft atherosclerosis, and the ITA graft is unchanged. ITA, internal thoracic artery; LAD, left anterior descending coronary artery; RCA, right coronary artery. *Source: Reprinted with permission from Lytle BW, Loop FD, Cosgrove DM, et al. Long-term (5 to 12 years) serial studies of internal mammary artery and saphenous vein coronary bypass grafts. J Thorac Cardiovasc Surg 1985;89:2548–2558.*

rate of complications associated with its use. Observational studies have demonstrated that 80 to 85 percent of radial artery grafts are patent at 5 years, and randomized comparisons of radial artery grafts to SVGs have noted similar patency at 1 year.[21,22] However, radial artery grafts may be superior to vein grafts if they are resistant to late graft atherosclerosis.

The clinical importance of total arterial revascularization is not yet certain. Total arterial revascularization can be achieved sometimes with only ITA grafts; however, for many patients, alternative arterial grafts are needed to complement the ITA grafts (see Fig. 65–1D). Bergsma et al. reported on a group of 256 selected patients with triple-vessel disease who were revascularized with two ITA grafts and a GEA graft. These relatively low-risk patients had good survival and low recurrence of angina.[23] If the radial artery is resistant to atherosclerosis, long-lasting total arterial revascularization will be more easily achievable.

EVOLUTION OF THE BYPASS SURGERY PATIENT POPULATION

In the early years of coronary artery bypass graft (CABG), patients were young, had limited CAD, good left ventricular (LV) function, and few comorbidities. Today the surgical population is older, has extensive CAD, and many comorbidities (Tables 65–1 and 65–2).[24] The bypass surgery population has changed for multiple reasons: (1) Improved technology and experience have made it possible to operate on more complex and sicker patients with reasonable risk; (2) the randomized trials demonstrated that the patients who derive the most benefit from CABG are those with left main or multivessel disease and abnormal LV function; (3) the population has been aging, and older patients have high expectations for their activity level; and (4) PCI provided an alternative treatment for patients with limited coronary lesions, removing many of those patients from being treated surgically.

CURRENT OPERATIVE STRATEGIES AND RISKS

STANDARD OPERATIVE STRATEGIES

Most CABG operations are performed via a median sternotomy with cardiopulmonary bypass (CPB). Aortic occlusion and cold potassium-based cardioplegia are used to achieve a combination of an immobile surgical field and myocardial protection. The development of effective cardioplegic arrest allowed major advances in the complexity of surgical revascularization to be carried out with a low risk of perioperative myocardial damage. Today, standard revascularization techniques most commonly involve the use of a single ITA graft to the LAD coronary artery (82 percent of patients in 2001, STS database), and SVGs to other coronary arteries (see Fig. 65–1B). More extensive use of ITA grafts has not become widespread, as only 3.7 percent of STS-reported patients received BITA grafts in 2001.

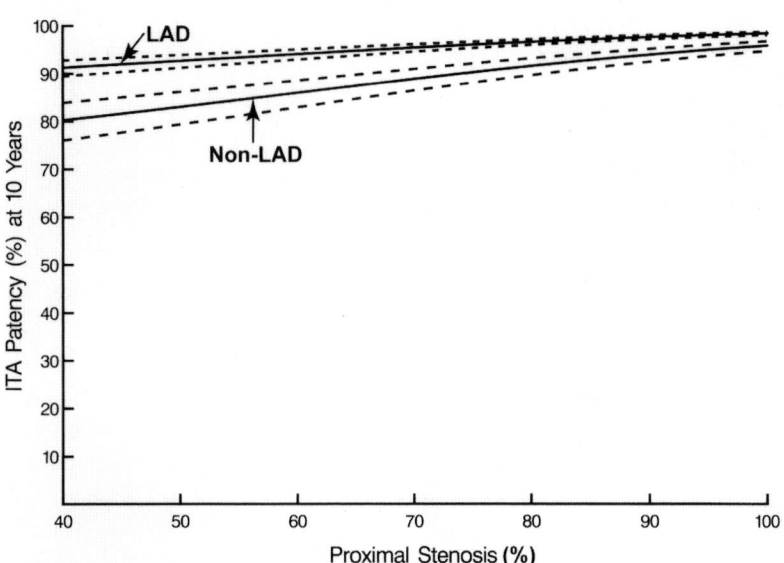

FIGURE 65–4. Internal thoracic artery (ITA) patency of left ITA to left anterior descending (LAD) and non-LAD coronary arteries at 10 years after coronary artery bypass grafting, by degree of proximal coronary artery stenosis. *Solid lines* represent estimates and *dashed lines* represent 70 percent confidence intervals. *Source: Reprinted with permission from Sabik JF 3rd, Lytle BW, Blackstone EH, et al. Does competitive flow reduce internal thoracic artery graft patency? Ann Thorac Surg 2003;76(5):1490–1496.*

【 】 DIFFERENTLY INVASIVE BYPASS SURGERY

Changes in operative techniques have been evolving that are designed to decrease the perioperative morbidity and possibly the mortality of bypass surgery. These new concepts include surgery through small incisions (minimally invasive bypass surgery) and operations performed without the use CPB (beating-heart or off-pump surgery). Small incisions have the advantage of patient preference, a decrease in the risk of major wound complications, and an early return to full activity. Off-pump surgery offers the possibility of decreasing CPB-related complications. An operation that combines both concepts involves preparation of a LITA graft through a small left thoracotomy, then an off-pump anastomosis to the LAD coronary artery under direct vision—the MIDCAB (minimally invasive direct coronary artery bypass) operation (Fig. 65–8). To achieve more extensive revascularization, some institutions have used the minimally invasive LITA-to-LAD graft strategy in combination with percutaneous stenting of other vessels, a "hybrid" approach. The outcomes of such alternative procedures have been reported as favorable by some authors, although others have noted imperfect early angiographic and clinical outcomes.[25]

A more common alternative strategy than small incision surgery is the use of a full median sternotomy incision without the use of CPB (Fig. 65–9).[26–30] Termed *off-pump, beating-heart,* or *OPCAB* (off-pump coronary artery bypass) surgery, this strategy was used for approximately 19 percent of STS-reported cases in 2001. The avoidance of CPB has many possible advantages, including decreasing the inflammatory response, avoiding activation of the coagulation system, maintaining pulsatile flow, decreasing myocardial ischemia, and decreasing the risk of micro- or macroembolization that might contribute to end-organ failure.

OPCAB offers real advantages in decreasing the risk of noncardiac complications for some subgroups of high-risk patients, including those with known atherosclerosis of the ascending aorta, previous neurologic events, and disorders of the coagulation system. For standard-risk patients, the advantages of OPCAB are less clear. Studies comparing OPCAB with on CPB revascularization have shown consistent advantage for OPCAB in blood use and intensive care unit stay.

A possible major disadvantage of OPCAB, and of all alternative revascularization strategies, is that the extent and effectiveness of revascularization might be compromised relative to that achieved via a median sternotomy, with CPB (cardiopulmonary bypass) and

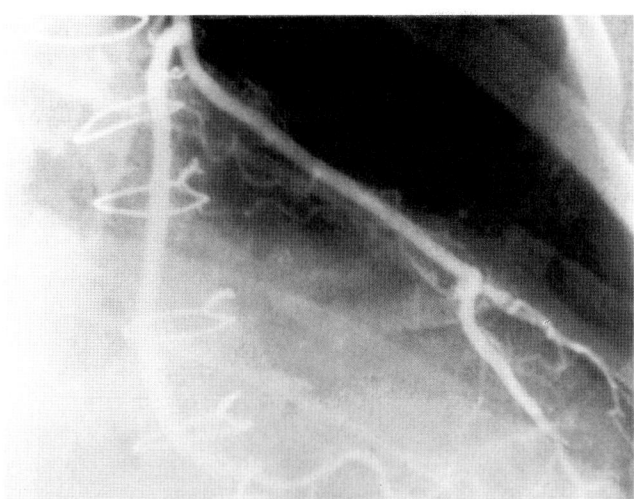

FIGURE 65–5. Early patency studies of composite internal thoracic artery grafts have been favorable. Here the left internal thoracic artery supplies the diagonal and left anterior descending vessels and the right internal thoracic artery the circumflex.

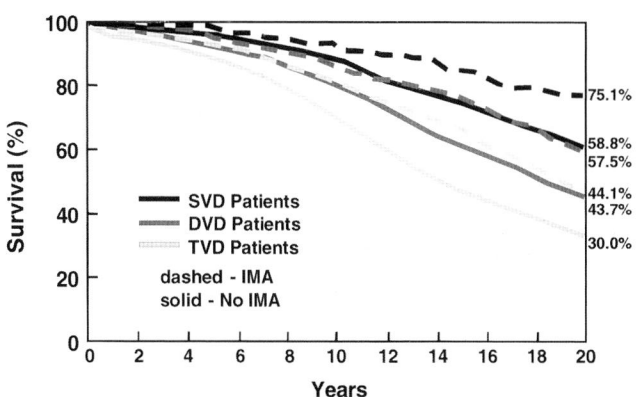

FIGURE 65–6. The 20-year followup of Cleveland Clinic Foundation patients from the years 1971 to 1974 shows superior survival rates for patients receiving left internal mammary artery (IMA) grafts compared with those receiving only vein grafts. These differences widen during the second postoperative decade. DVD, double-vessel disease; SVD, single-vessel disease; TVD, triple-vessel disease.

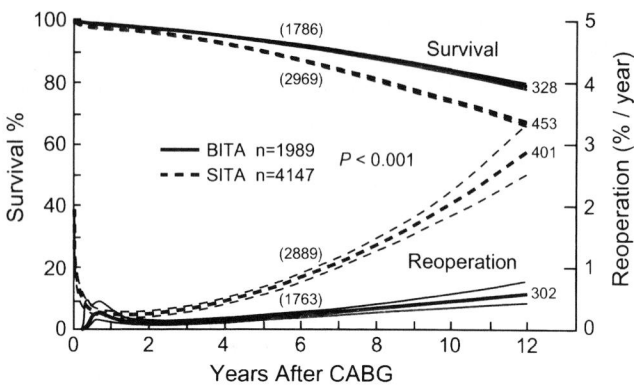

FIGURE 65–7. Comparison of survival and freedom from reoperation curves in propensity-matched patients who received bilateral internal thoracic artery (BITA) grafts and single internal thoracic artery (SITA) grafts with or without additional vein grafts. CABG, coronary artery bypass grafting. *Source: Reprinted with permission from Lytle BW, Blackstone EH, Loop FD, et al. Two internal thoracic artery grafts are better than one. J Thorac Cardiovasc Surg 1999;117:855–872.*

cardioplegic arrest. Early in the OPCAB learning experience, the revascularization disadvantages were real and consistent, but surgeons and OPCAB technologies have steadily improved, such that the gap between OPCAB and on-pump revascularization has narrowed. Today, OPCAB revascularization is still difficult in settings of calcified or intramyocardial coronary arteries, diffuse small vessel disease requiring multiple grafts, reoperations for patients with atherosclerotic vein grafts, severe cardiac hypertrophy, and a desire to achieve complex ITA and complete revascularization.

The ultimate fruition of differently invasive bypass surgery would be port-access, off-pump, multivessel revascularization with ITA grafts. Strategies similar to this have been attempted in small numbers of highly selected cases using robotics technology. The technological horizon includes mechanical suture devices and graft to coronary and aortic connectors—parallel technologies that may make robotic surgery more accurate and efficient.

Postoperative Medical Therapy

After coronary revascularization, patients should be treated with anti-platelet agents, lipid-lowering medication, and β blockers. Administration of antiplatelet agents after CABG improves both early (<1 month) and 1-year patency of SVGs,[6,7,31,32] and lipid-lowering therapy, with statins, decreases the rate of SVG atherosclerosis and lowers the risk of death and myocardial infarction.[8,9]

HOSPITAL MORTALITY

Hospital mortality for primary CABG has been reported to be approximately 1 to 4 percent. Hospital mortality in the voluntary countrywide STS database ranged from 2.69 to 2.37 percent during 1999 to 2001, and the New York State Registry (a compulsory registry with subsequent public disclosure) noted an inhospital mortality from 1998 to 2000 of 2.15 to 2.32 percent (Hannan EL, personal communication, 2003). Single-institution reviews have reported hospital mortality of 1 percent or less for elective surgery (Fig. 65–10).[26,33,34] Overall risks are associated with patient-related characteristics, and factors increasing the risk of CABG in multiple datasets have included acuity of operation, age, prior cardiac surgery, gender, LV ejection fraction, left main coronary artery stenosis, and number of coronary systems with >70 percent stenosis.[34] Acuity of operation, age, and previous surgery have had the greatest predictive value. Also identified have been 13 variables that have added some predictive value to the core variables: percutaneous transluminal coronary angioplasty (PTCA) during the same admission, MI less than 1 week prior to operation, angina, ventricular arrhythmia, congestive heart failure (CHF), mitral regurgitation, diabetes, cerebrovascular disease, peripheral vascular disease, chronic obstructive pulmonary disease (COPD), and elevated serum creatinine.

The use of historical data to elucidate the association of patient-, surgeon-, and institution-related variables with outcomes and to then predict outcomes for future patients is common. This *risk stratification* process has value for both physicians and patients in selecting

TABLE 65–1

Preoperative Clinical Characteristics for the First 1000 Patients per Year Undergoing Elective Primary Isolated Coronary Bypass Grafting

CLINICAL VARIABLE	1976	1982	1988	1994	1999	2002	2005[a]
Age (years, median)	55	59	64	64	66	67	65
Men (%)	89	84	78	75	73	71	72
Diabetes (%)	6	9	19	24	32	33	44
Age ≥70 years (%)	3	10	26	28	36	39	35
Single-vessel disease[b] (%)	15	8	3	9	10	10	5
Double-vessel disease[b] (%)	28	25	19	29	27	20	21
Triple-vessel disease[b] (%)	57	67	78	60	62	68	77
Left main coronary stenosis (≥50%) (%)	12	13	16	19	23	24	33
Left ventricular asynergy (%)	45	55	57	48	45	47	48

[a]For 2005 N = 651 (Cleveland Clinic Foundation).
[b]The terms *single-*, *double-*, and *triple-vessel disease* refer to the number of the three main coronary vessels (left anterior descending, circumflex, and right coronary arteries) that have stenoses ≥50%.

TABLE 65-2

Comparison of Isolated CABG Patient Characteristics 1990, 2000, 2005[a]

CHARACTERISTIC	1990	2000	2005	P VALUE
Age (years)	64 ± 10	65.2	65.1	<0.0001
EF	0.51 ± 0.14	50.6	50.7	0.008
Female	27	28.8	27.0	<0.0001
Diabetes mellitus	23	33.1	36.8	<0.0001
MI ≤21 days before CABG	12	23.9	26.9	<0.0001
Cardiogenic shock	1.61	1.7	2.0	<0.0001
Unstable angina	48	50.0	39.9	<0.0001
Left main disease	12	22.6	30.7	<0.0001
Previous cardiac surgery	7	9.4	6.4	<0.0001
Nonelective operation	18	42.0	50.9	<0.0001

CABG, coronary artery bypass grafting; EF, ejection fraction; IABP, intraaortic balloon pump; MI, myocardial infarction.
[a]Values are shown as percentages except for age and EF, which are shown as mean ± standard deviation.
SOURCE: *Edwards et al.*[24] *and Fall 2003 and Spring 2006 Data Analysis of The Society of Thoracic Surgeons National Adult Cardiac Surgery Database,*[25] *with permission.*

treatment and in the clarification of likely outcomes and complications. However, the risk-stratification process is imperfect, particularly when data from multiple institutions are combined. The setting in which bypass surgery is performed impacts outcomes.[35] According to Medicare data, the risks of CABG are less in high-volume centers and that those decreased risks are not based on patient selection.

One advantage of identifying characteristics that predict risk is that patients who are at extremely low risk may also be identified. For example, during the years 1995 to 1998, the STS database recorded 25,776 patients who underwent a primary elective bypass operation, had a LV ejection fraction of >50 percent, and did not have peripheral vascular disease, carotid disease, renal failure, a prior myocardial in-farction, or an intraaortic balloon pump. For those good-risk patients, 98 deaths occurred, for a 0.38 percent mortality rate (Edwards FH for the STS database, personal communication, 1999).

HOSPITAL MORBIDITY

PERIOPERATIVE MYOCARDIAL INFARCTION

The introduction of cardioplegic arrest increased the effectiveness of myocardial protection. Cardioplegia has a high concentration of po-

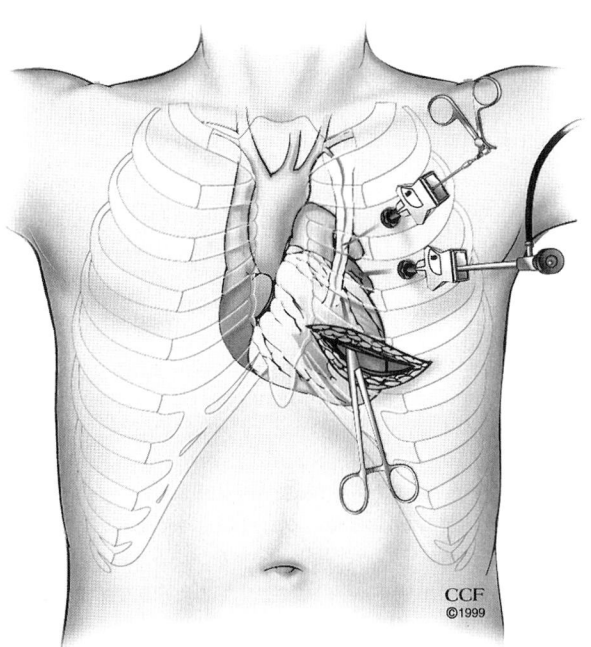

FIGURE 65-8. A small left anterior thoracotomy may be used to construct limited anastomosis without the use of cardiopulmonary bypass (CPB); with the use of percutaneous CPB, more vessels are accessible through this small incision. Endoscopic preparation of the left internal thoracic artery graft may be employed.

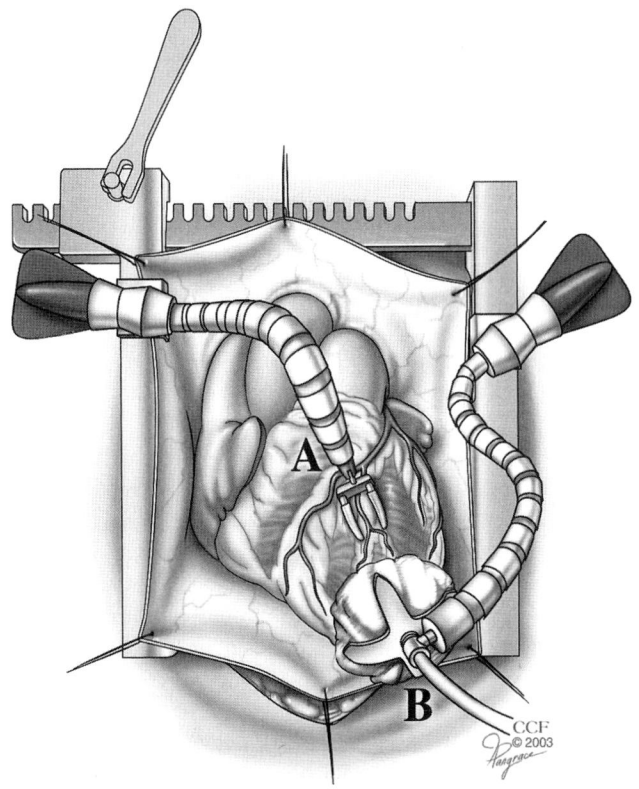

FIGURE 65-9. Myocardial stabilizers allow multivessel revascularization to be accomplished without cardiopulmonary bypass.

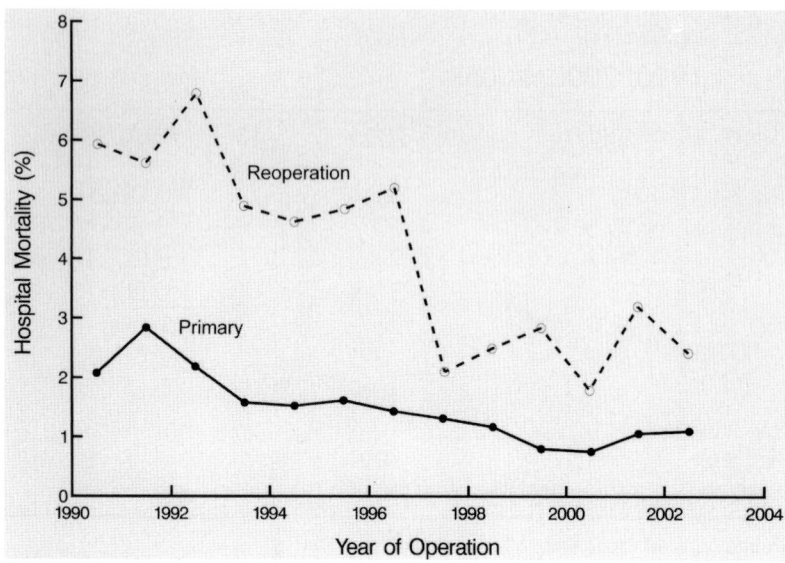

FIGURE 65–10. Hospital mortality after primary and reoperative coronary artery bypass grafting by year of operation. *Source: Reprinted with permission from Sabik JF, Blackstone EH, Houghtaling PL. Is reoperation still a risk factor in coronary artery bypass surgery? Ann Thorac Surg 2005;80:1719–1727.*[36]

tassium and is injected into the aortic root after aortic cross-clamping to arrest the heart and decrease energy consumption. Modifications of this basic strategy include addition of blood, addition of metabolic substrates, warming of some or all of the cardioplegic solution, and the delivery of cardioplegia retrograde through the coronary sinus. Retrograde delivery of cardioplegia provides more effective myocardial protection during reoperations, acute coronary ischemia, and if the aortic valve is insufficient.[36]

The metabolic environment created by cardioplegia appears to be sufficient for protection. When significant perioperative MI occurs, it is often based on anatomic causes, acute coronary occlusion, graft failure, incomplete revascularization, or embolization of atherosclerotic debris. Some comparative studies of OPCAB and CPBCAB have shown cardiac enzyme release to be decreased after OPCAB. However, the significance of these differences is not known, and studies of focal MI often have not shown differences.

[ ] NEUROLOGIC COMPLICATIONS

Neurologic complications of CABG include focal stroke (type I) and diffuse encephalopathy (type II). In a multicenter trial examining patients undergoing CPBCAB-type CABG, Roach et al. found that the total number of adverse neurologic events was 6.1 percent—type I (3.1 percent) and type II (3.0 percent). Focal strokes have multiple causes, including carotid or intracranial vascular disease, emboli from intracardiac thrombus, and atheroembolization from aorta manipulation at the time of CABG.[37–39] Multiple techniques are available to diminish the risk of stroke when aortic atherosclerosis is present, including alternative arterial cannulation sites, single aortic cross-clamping, circulatory arrest and aortic replacement, and OPCAB surgery. Two nonrandomized studies have cited a lower stroke risk with OPCAB compared with CPBCAB surgery, although a randomized trial of good-risk patients showed no differences in neurologic complications.[29,40,41] To be fully effective in avoiding neurologic compli-

cations, OPCAB strategies must avoid manipulation of an atherosclerotic aorta. This can be accomplished by using composite grafts from the ITAs and may be aided by graft to aortic connectors.

An issue that is currently unresolved is the degree of cognitive dysfunction associated with OPCAB and CPBCAB surgery. Cognitive dysfunction, particularly late out-of-hospital cognitive dysfunction, has been noted after bypass surgery but seems to improve over time. A randomized trial comparing OPCAB and CPBCAB showed no cognitive differences 1 year after surgery.

Symptomatic or asymptomatic carotid stenosis in patients undergoing CABG is associated with an increased early and late risk of stroke. Multiple management strategies have been used to decrease this risk. Staged procedures with carotid endarterectomy or carotid stenting performed first are safe but can be applied in very select patients with stable CAD. Staged operations with patients undergoing CABG first is associated with an increased risk of stroke in patients with severe carotid stenoses, patients with bilateral stenoses being at greatly increased risk.[42] Combined carotid endarterectomy and coronary surgery has been employed for many patients, but overall risks have been increased compared to those for patients undergoing isolated bypass surgery.

[ ] WOUND COMPLICATIONS

Deep sternal wound complications represent a serious adverse outcome and occur in 0.5 to 4 percent of cases, depending on patient selection. Obesity and diabetes have been associated with increased risk, but aggressive treatment of blood glucose levels with intravenous insulin may mitigate this. No study shows that the use of a single ITA graft increases the risk of sternal wound complications, but some authors have implicated bilateral ITA grafting, particularly for diabetic patients.[43] Dissection of the ITA as a skeletonized artery rather than a pedicle may leave collateral circulation to the sternum intact and diminish the impact of ITA use.[44]

[ ] LONG-TERM OUTCOMES AFTER BYPASS SURGERY

Survival after CABG is related to the patient's cardiac status at the time of operation, the bypass operation, progression of atherosclerosis, and noncardiac comorbidity. Recent followup of 8221 surgical patients from the CASS (Coronary Artery Surgery Study) registry documented overall survival of 96, 90, 74, 56, and 45 percent at 1, 5, 10, 15, and 18 postoperative years, respectively.[44] These figures are inferior to those for the age-sex-matched U.S. population and inferior to series of patients receiving ITA grafts at operation (see Fig. 65–7).

Patient-related variables have a strong impact on survival, and the longer the followup, the more important those variables become. Age is a major determinant of survival. However, elderly patients after CABG have better survival than age-matched controls, an effect that begins to be observed around age 60 years.

LV function, left main stenosis, proximal LAD coronary artery stenosis, and the number of stenotic coronary arteries are cardiac variables that decrease survival of CABG patients. Although survival of patients treated medically is dramatically influenced by these cardiac variables, surgery partially or totally negates their impact. In our study analyzing the impact of arterial revascularization, a proximal LAD coronary artery stenosis had no effect on late survival and left main disease, and the number of systems diseased had minor influence.[18] In no long-term study has bypass surgery completely obliterated the impact of abnormal LV function on late survival.

Risk factors for atherosclerosis—particularly cigarette smoking, hypercholesterolemia, hypertension, and diabetes—are associated with decreased survival. Smoking cessation after CABG returns the patient to a nonsmoker's prognosis.[45] Postoperative treatment with statins decreases the angiographic progression of atherosclerosis in SVG and coronary arteries and decreases the risk of late cardiac events, even for patients without hyperlipidemia.[8,9] Diabetes severe enough to require treatment is associated with decreased survival.

Operation-related variables also affect late outcome. As discussed previously, the surgical strategies of the LITA-to-LAD graft and bilateral ITA grafting incrementally improve late survival.[14,18] The impact of incomplete revascularization on late outcomes is of increasing importance with the emergence of PCI and minimally invasive bypass operations, strategies that may involve less complete revascularization. Definitions of *incomplete revascularization* have varied, and it is difficult to separate incomplete revascularization as a surgical strategy from incomplete revascularization as a marker of bad atherosclerosis. An observational study from the Cleveland Clinic identified incomplete revascularization as a risk factor for late death, an effect also noted by Weintraub et al.[46,47] A CASS registry study noted a strong negative effect of incomplete revascularization on the survival of CABG patients with abnormal LV function.[48]

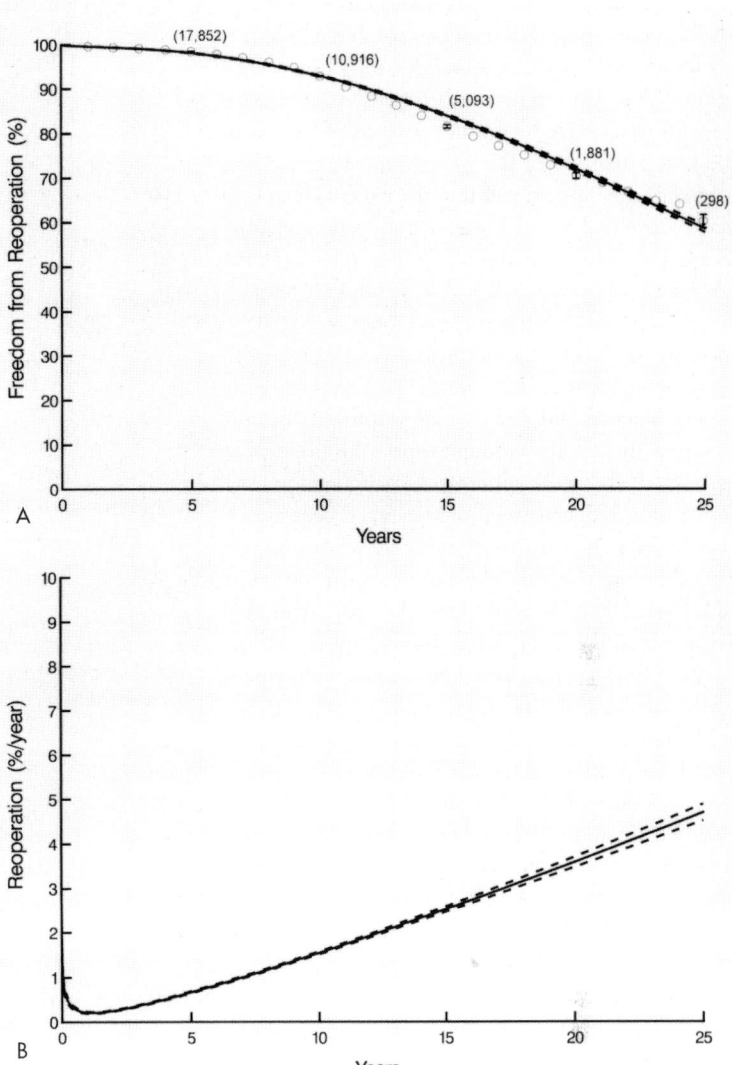

FIGURE 65–11. Occurrence of coronary reoperation after primary CABG. **A.** Predicted and actuarial estimates for freedom from reoperation. *Solid line* represents predicted estimates enclosed within *dashed* 70 percent confidence limits. *Symbols* represent actuarial estimates at yearly intervals, and *error bars* represent 70 percent confidence limits. *Numbers in parentheses* represent patient at risk. **B.** Instantaneous rate (hazard function) for coronary reoperation. *Dashed lines* are 70 percent confidence intervals. *Source:* Reprinted with permission from Sabik JF III, Blackstone EH, Gillinov AM, et al. Influence of patient characteristics and arterial grafts on freedom from coronary reoperation. J Thorac Cardiovasc Surg 2006;131:90–98.

REOPERATION

Atherosclerosis is a progressive disease, and some surgical patients will undergo reoperation because of graft failure, progression of atherosclerosis in native coronary arteries, or both. A recent observational study of 26,927 patients who had CABG from 1971 to 1997 noted a cumulative occurrence of reoperation of 1.6 percent, 7 percent, 18 percent, 28 percent, and 35 percent at 5, 10, 15, 20, and 25 years, respectively (Fig. 65–11).[49] Young age, diabetes, elevated lipids, severe symptoms, normal LV function, more extensive CAD, and not having an ITA graft were all factors that increased the likelihood of a reoperation.

Patients who are candidates for reoperation are different from those having primary CABG. Today, typical candidates for reoperation underwent primary CABG more than 10 years ago and had triple-vessel disease at that time. Their atherosclerosis is advanced and they have a higher prevalence of aortic atherosclerosis, left main stenosis, severe distal CAD, abnormal LV function, and

noncardiac atherosclerosis than patients undergoing primary surgery. They usually have the unique characteristics of having their myocardial blood supply dependent on ITA grafts (at risk for injury) or atherosclerotic vein grafts that create the possibility of coronary atheroembolism.

Few data are available that help to define the indications for reoperation, particularly for patients that are not severely symptomatic. Because the myocardium of reoperative candidates is usually jeopardized by vascular pathology that differs from that in native coronary artery atherosclerosis, generalizations from the randomized studies of patients without previous surgery are unwise. We examined outcomes for patients with prior surgery who developed recurrent ischemic syndromes in two observational studies. These studies showed that late stenoses in SVGs, caused by vein graft atherosclerosis, are dangerous lesions and predict a higher mortality than comparable native coronary lesions.[50] Comparing outcomes for patients with stenotic SVGs who underwent repeat surgery with those who were treated without initial reoperation, we found that patients with late stenoses in SVGs had better survival with surgery and that the patients who particularly benefited were those with an atherosclerotic SVG to the LAD coronary artery (Fig. 65–12).[51] Patients with a 50 percent LAD SVG stenosis had immediate and obvious benefit, but even those with a 20 to 50 percent stenosis had an improved survival rate with surgery when followed for 5 years. Patients with early vein graft stenoses did not have an improved late survival rate with surgery, although those who underwent reoperation had fewer symptoms at late followup.

In the past, reoperative coronary surgery was associated with an increased risk of mortality relative to primary operations. Within the last few years we have found that the risks are equivalent when patient-related variables are adjusted for.[33] This improvement in operative risk is likely related to experience in avoiding perioperative myocardial infarction.

In the reoperative CABG, emergency operation produces a large increase in risk. Definitions of *emergency* vary among studies, but the lesson is the same. In the STS database for 1997, mortality rates were 5.2 percent for elective, 7.4 percent for urgent, 13.5 percent for emergency, and 40.7 percent for *salvage* reoperations. Left main stenosis, advanced age, CHF, female gender, and number of stenotic vein grafts are other factors associated with increased risk.

The late outcomes after reoperation are slightly inferior to those after primary CABG. Loop et al. noted a 69 percent 10-year survival for 2429 hospital survivors of a first reoperation.[52] LV function was the variable having the strongest impact on survival. Reoperations tend to achieve less-perfect revascularization than primary procedures, and by 5 to 6 postoperative years, approximately 50 percent of reoperative patients have some angina, although it is severe in only a few.[53]

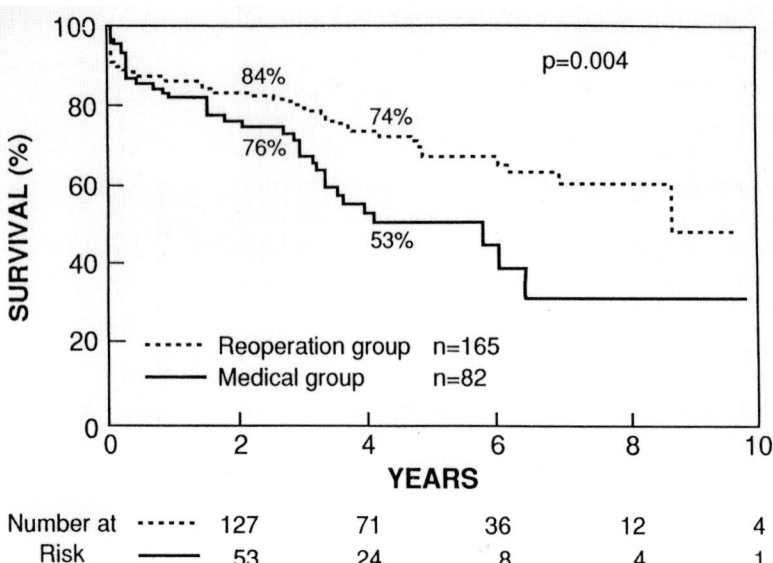

FIGURE 65–12. Patients with late (≥5 years after operation) stenoses in venous grafts to the LAD coronary artery have better survival with reoperation than with medical treatment. *Source: Reprinted with permission from Lytle BW, Loop FD, Taylor PC, et al. The effect of coronary reoperation on the survival of patients with stenoses in saphenous vein bypass grafts to coronary arteries. J Thorac Cardiovasc Surg 1993:105:605–614.*

COMPARATIVE TRIALS INVOLVING BYPASS SURGERY

For an invasive treatment of any disease to be widely applied, it must provide outcomes superior outcomes to those of less-invasive therapies. Since its inception, bypass surgery has been carefully scrutinized, and its status relative to alternative treatments such as medical therapy and PCI has been tested with randomized trials and nonrandomized comparisons. Randomized trials of widely differing treatments are difficult to perform. They are expensive, recruitment is difficult, and vast allowances must be made for changes in physician opinions and patient outcomes. The strength of randomized trials is that they eliminate bias in the selection of the initial treatment once the patient has been entered into the trial. However, they do not eliminate physician and patient bias at the point of entry into the trial, and in the randomized trials involving bypass surgery, only subsets of patients with CAD were el-

igible, and the majority of patients eligible to be randomized were not randomized. Also, randomized trials do not eliminate bias in the selection of further therapy once the initial therapy has been carried out. Nonrandomized trials have the disadvantage of bias in the selection of treatment but the advantage of inclusiveness. Therefore both randomized and nonrandomized trials provide information that is useful in the selection of therapies for patients with CAD.

【 】 TRIALS OF CABG VERSUS MEDICAL TREATMENT

During the 1970s, multicenter randomized trials of patients with chronic angina were initiated to test the effectiveness of CABG versus medical management. The most influential of these trials were the Veterans Administration Study of patients with Chronic Stable Angina (VA Study),[54] the European Coronary Surgery Study (ECSS),[55] and the CASS.[56,57] These trials randomized patients either to initial medical management or to initial treatment with CABG, and their primary emphasis was survival. In the two largest trials (ECSS and CASS), severely symptomatic patients were excluded from randomization. These trials showed that prompt CABG improved life expectancy of some patients, and those who benefited the most from surgery were patients at the highest risk of death without operation. Individual trials noted improved survival for patients with left main stenosis (≥50 percent), three-vessel disease with abnormal LV function (Fig. 65–13), and two- or three-vessel disease with a >75 percent stenosis in the proximal LAD coronary artery (Fig. 65–14). The clinical descriptors of an abnormal baseline ECG or a strongly positive exercise test helped to define patient subsets that experienced improved survival with CABG. A meta-analysis of randomized trials confirmed the observations of the individual trials but also showed a significant survival benefit for patients with triple-, double-, or even single-vessel disease that

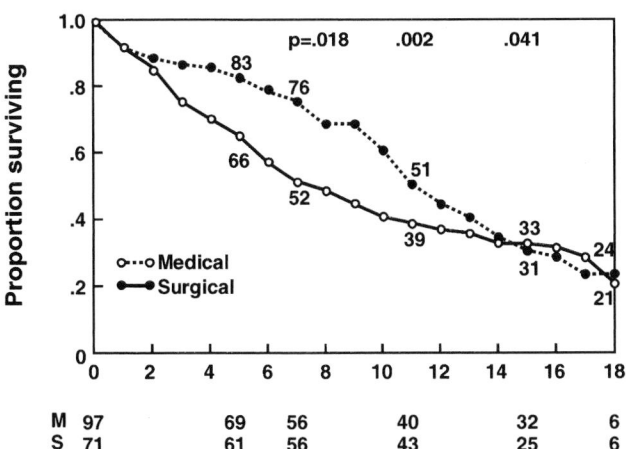

High Angiographic Risk

FIGURE 65–13. In the initial trial of bypass surgery versus medical management, the VA Study, patients with abnormal left ventricular function and three-vessel disease had a better survival rate with surgery. *Source: Reprinted with permission from The VA Coronary Artery Bypass Surgery Cooperative Study Group. Eighteen-year follow-up in the Veterans Affairs Cooperative Study of Coronary Artery Bypass Surgery for Stable Angina. Circulation 1992;86:121–130.*

included a proximal LAD stenosis regardless of whether they had normal or abnormal LV function.[58] For patients without a proximal LAD stenosis, surgery improved the survival only for those with left main stenosis or triple-vessel disease. The CABG patients had fewer symptoms and took fewer antianginal medications.

The degree of benefit in survival and freedom from recurrent symptoms achieved with initial CABG diminished with time. There were multiple reasons for this. First, the status of the surgically treated patients deteriorated because of late vein graft failure and the progression of native-vessel atherosclerosis. Few patients in these early trials received ITA grafts or were treated with platelet inhibitors or lipid-lowering agents, strategies that we now know significantly extend the benefits of surgery. Second, the status of the "medically treated" patients improved slightly because a large proportion of those patients "crossed over" and underwent bypass surgery, although they were still analyzed as part of the medically treated group. In the three major studies, 40 to 44 percent of the total medically treated patient population had undergone bypass surgery by 10 postoperative years, including 65 percent of patients with left main disease and 48 percent of those with three-vessel disease.[59] Finally, when all-cause mortality is the end point, any two survival curves will eventually meet at zero.

In all these trials, a minority of patients presenting for evaluation met the criteria for entry into the trial, and of those that met the criteria for entry, a minority were actually randomized. In the case of the CASS study, however, patients who were not randomized were prospectively followed in a nonrandomized registry that has provided useful information. Among the important conclusions from the CASS registry are that asymptomatic patients with 50 percent left main stenosis and those with left main equivalent (70 percent

stenosis of proximal LAD and circumflex vessels) have improved survival with CABG.[60,61] For severely symptomatic patients, bypass surgery improved the survival rates of those with three-vessel disease regardless of whether they had normal or abnormal LV function, even if they did not have severe proximal coronary artery stenoses.[62]

Outcomes for patients with unstable angina were tested in another VA trial. Patients with rest angina and abnormal LV function had greatly improved survival with initial surgery. Patients with progressive angina did not appear to have a worse survival rate if they were initially treated with medical therapy, but 19 percent of this group crossed over to surgery within 30 days of randomization; by 96 months, 45 percent had crossed over to surgery.[63]

There are modern comparative studies that show a persistent advantage for revascularization over modern medical therapy. First, the randomized three-armed MASS (Medicine, Angioplasty, or Surgery Study) trial (surgery versus PCI versus medicine) for the treatment of isolated LAD coronary artery stenosis showed that the surgically treated patients experienced fewer symptoms and cardiac events during a 5-year follow-up, although the low incidence of cardiac death was not different in the three groups.[64] Second, the Asymptomatic Cardiac Ischemia Pilot (ACIP) trial showed that good-risk patients with asymptomatic ischemia experienced better survival with initial revascularization (PCI or surgery) than with medical treatment alone.[65] Third, analysis of the Studies of Left Ventricular Dysfunction (SOLVD) trial involving high-risk patients (ejection fraction <35 percent) showed that patients with bypass surgery had a 26 percent lower mortality than those without revascularization.[66] Finally, a study of nonrandomized data from the Alberta (APPROACH) registry showed better-risk survival rates for surgically treated patients compared with those treated medically, the largest difference being noted in patients older than 70 years of age.[67]

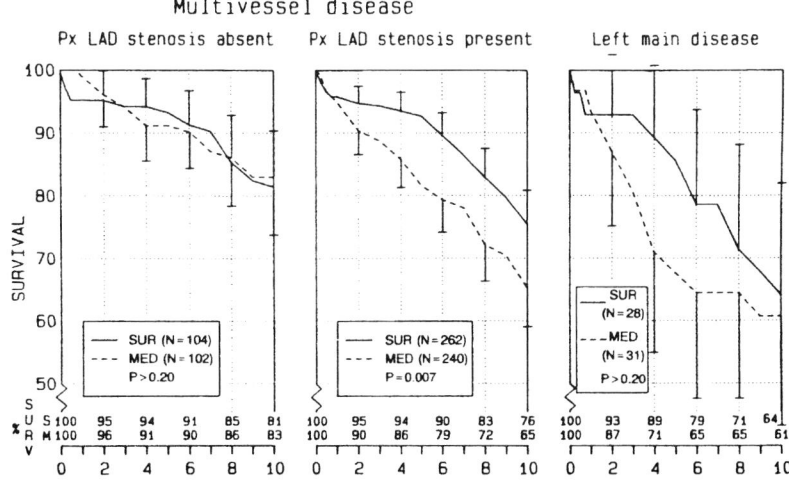

Multivessel disease

FIGURE 65–14. In the European Coronary Surgery Study, patients with multivessel disease and a proximal left anterior descending (LAD) coronary artery lesion (*center*) experienced an improved survival rate with surgery, whereas those without an LAD lesion (*left*) did not. Px, proximal. *Source: Reprinted with permission from Varnauskas E and the European Coronary Surgery Study Group. Twelve-year follow-up of survival in the randomized European Coronary Surgery Study. N Engl J Med 1988;319:332–337.*

[ ] BYPASS SURGERY VERSUS PCI

Randomized Trials

Fifteen randomized trials have compared patient outcomes of CABG to PCI: nine compared CABG to balloon angioplasty alone and six compared CABG to balloon angioplasty with stenting.[68–80] Except for the Angina With Extremely Serious Operative Mortality Evaluation (AWESOME) trial, the patients enrolled were relatively low risk, had no serious comorbidities, normal ventricular function, and mostly two-vessel coronary artery disease that was amenable to both CABG and PCI. In all but one of these studies, survival was similar in patients treated with either CABG or PCI. BARI found a survival advantage in patients treated with CABG. In BARI, CABG resulted in better survival than balloon angioplasty in medically treated diabetic patients who also had LITA grafting of their LAD coronary artery (Fig. 65–15). A consistent and important finding in these randomized trials was that CABG resulted in greater freedom from recurrent angina and need for repeat coronary intervention than PCI. PCI resulted in less-effective revascularization. In the studies comparing CABG to balloon angioplasty alone, balloon angioplasty resulted in a 4 to 10 times higher rate of coronary reintervention than CABG. In the randomized trials comparing CABG to balloon angioplasty with stenting, CABG similarly resulted in a lower need for coronary reintervention than PCI; however, the addition of stenting to balloon angioplasty reduced the need of coronary reintervention in the PCI group to half that observed in the earlier trials of CABG to balloon angioplasty alone.[81]

Although these randomized studies are often used to demonstrate survival equivalence of CABG and PCI in patients with multivessel CAD, the studies were not designed to detect a survival difference. The studies enrolled too few patients, the patients were too low risk, and followup was too short. First, to power the trials to detect a survival difference between CABG and PCI, 2000 to 4000 patients would needed to have been enrolled in both the CABG and PCI arms of the trials.[68] The randomized studies each only enrolled anywhere from 121 to 1829 total patients. The trials were grossly underpowered. Interestingly, a meta-analysis of 7964 patients from the randomized trials demonstrated a survival advantage for CABG over PCI.[81] Second, only the enrollment of patients known to derive a survival benefit from CABG over medical therapy could have shown a survival difference, but these patients (left main stenosis, LV dysfunction, LAD coronary artery stenosis, triple-vessel CAD) were usually not included. Less than half of the patients in the trials had LAD coronary artery stenosis or triple-vessel CAD. Instead, the trials enrolled mostly low-risk patients who do not derive a survival benefit from CABG over medical therapy. Therefore, the only way CABG could have prolonged survival compared to PCI, was if PCI was worse than medical therapy in prolonging survival. In addition, for these trials to be generalizable, the studies should have included patients who are similar to the population of patients having multivessel revascularization. Many subgroups of patients with multivessel CAD were excluded from enrollment, and only a small percentage of eligible patients were actually enrolled.[74] Third, for the randomized studies to detect a survival difference, followup should have been at least 5 years. In these 15 trials, followup was anywhere from for 1 to 8 years; however, it was usually 3 years or less. Many of the studies lacked adequate followup.

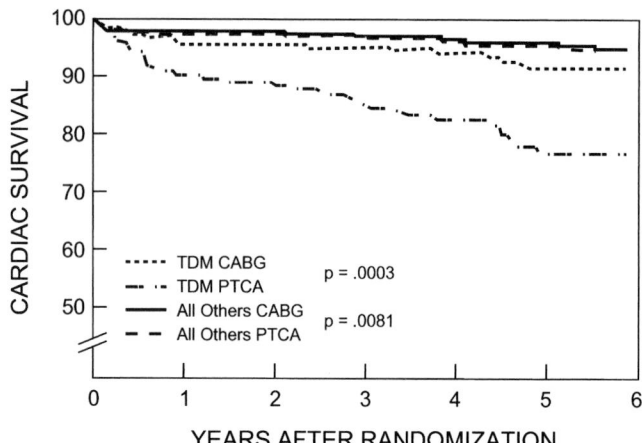

FIGURE 65–15. BARI trial patients with treated diabetes had worse survival following PTCA than following CABG (*p* = 0.003). Patients without diabetes had equivalent survival. CABG, coronary artery bypass grafting; PTCA, percutaneous transluminal coronary angioplasty. *Source: Reprinted with permission from BARI Investigators. Influence of diabetes on 5-year mortality and morbidity in a randomized trial comparing CABG and PTCA in patients with multivessel disease. Circulation 1997;96:1761–1769.*

Observational Studies

Several large observational studies have compared the outcomes of PCI to CABG.[82–85] Two large New York State registry studies identified angiographic subgroups of patients that derive a survival advantage from CABG over PCI.[82,83] In a study of 60,000 patients (30,000 CABG and 30,000 balloon angioplasty alone), patients with single- or double-vessel CAD that included the LAD coronary artery, and those with triple-vessel CAD (irrespective of whether the LAD coronary artery was involved) obtained a survival advantage with CABG. Patients with non-LAD coronary artery single-vessel disease derived a survival benefit with balloon angioplasty alone over CABG. In a later New York State registry study of 37,212 CABG and 22,101 balloon angioplasty with stenting patients, similar findings were observed. Patients with double- and triple-vessel CAD derived a survival benefit from CABG over balloon angioplasty with stenting (Fig. 65–16). An 18,481-patient study from Duke University reported similar findings. Patients with severe CAD (mostly triple-vessel CAD) had better survival with CABG than PCI.[85]

A weakness of observational studies is that patient selection is biased at the point of treatment. A factor determining whether patients are treated with PCI or CABG is diffuseness of CAD. Patients treated with CABG tend to have more extensive, diffuse CAD, whereas those treated with PCI tend to have more focal, discrete lesions. This treatment bias should decrease the long-term results of CABG in observational studies, and this bias against CABG makes the survival advantage found in these observational studies more impressive. Other strengths of these studies are the large numbers of patients included that power these studies to detect survival differences, and that they are representative of how CAD is actually treated.

The Future: Drug-Eluting Stents

Third-generation PCI and drug-eluting stents (DESs) promise to decrease the restenosis rate of PCI. Early reported data demon-

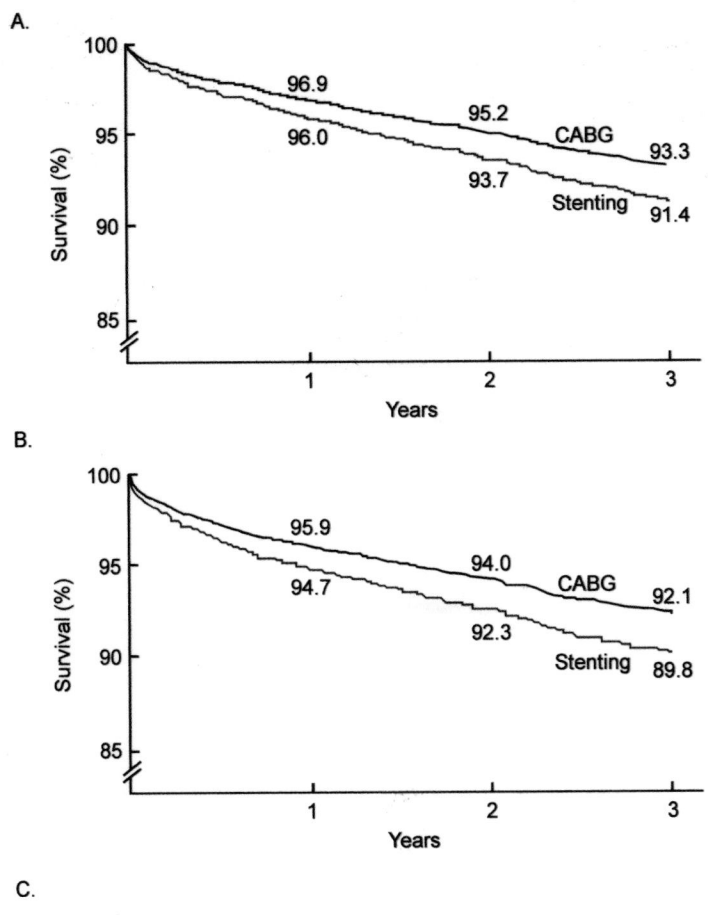

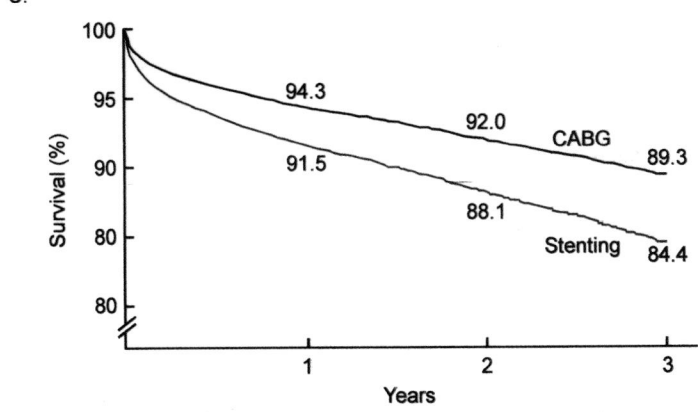

FIGURE 65–16. Adjusted survival among patients treated with stenting or coronary artery bypass grafting (CABG) by extent of coronary artery disease. *Source: Reprinted with permission from Hannan EL, Racz M.J, Walford G, et al. Long-term outcomes of coronary-artery bypass grafting versus stent implantation. N Engl J Med 2005;352(21):2174–2183.*

strated a 1-year restenosis rate of 10 percent or less for coronary arteries of 2.5 mm diameter. However, it is not known whether the lower restenosis rate observed with DESs will improve the survival of patients undergoing PCI; randomized and observational studies suggest that it will not.[82,83,86,87] A meta-analysis of 11 randomized trials comparing the outcomes of 5103 patients who were treated with either DESs or bare-metal stents (BMSs) did not find a survival difference despite there being a lower restenosis rate in the DES patients.[86] Previous observational studies did not find a survival difference in patients with or without restenosis after PCI.[87] Recent studies with longer followup have not found a survival

benefit of DESs over BMSs. Eighteen-month results from BASKET found a lower target-vessel revascularization in DESs than in BMSs, but no advantage in death or MI for DESs versus BMSs. Similarly, 5 year results from RAVEL demonstrated lower target-lesion revascularization in patients with DESs than in those with BMSs; however, the freedom from death or MI trended toward a benefit for BMSs.

Thus for patients with multivessel CAD, CABG appears to prolong survival, decrease recurrence of angina, and decrease the need for repeat coronary intervention. Although multiple randomized trials suggest that in patients with multivessel CAD, PCI and CABG result in similar survival, these studies were underpowered, lacked sufficient followup, and compared mostly low-risk patients who would not be expected to derive a survival benefit from CABG. Large, risk-adjusted observational studies clearly demonstrate that CABG results in better survival compared to PCI, particularly in patients with multivessel disease that includes the LAD coronary artery. Although DESs may lower the restenosis rate, the evidence suggests that this will not result in improved survival in patients undergoing PCI. The benefits of CABG over PCI may be a result of the difference in how PCI and CABG treat coronary artery disease. PCI treats only the stenosis *present* at the time of intervention, whereas CABG treats the stenosis *present* at the time of surgery and any additional stenoses that develop in the *future* proximal to the bypass graft.

INDICATIONS FOR BYPASS SURGERY
【 】 FOR PROGNOSIS

Patients who experience an improved survival rate with bypass surgery even in the absence of severe symptoms include those with a left main coronary stenosis of 50 percent or multivessel disease with a proximal LAD coronary artery lesion and abnormal LV function. In addition, patients with previous bypass surgery who have large amounts of myocardium in jeopardy should undergo reoperation even in the absence of severe symptoms. These situations are anatomic indications for surgery.[68] The worse the patient's symptoms and the worse the LV function, the stronger the survival benefit of surgery. Modern imaging allows the identification of patients with abnormal LV function and viable myocardium, a subset that appears to experience great benefit from surgery.[88]

For nondiabetic patients with multivessel disease, a proximal LAD coronary artery lesion, and normal LV function, revascularization should be recommended even without severe symptoms. For patients in this subgroup, midterm followup of good candidates for PCI appears to show equivalent survival as compared with surgery; the advantages and disadvantages of both revascularization strategies should be discussed with the patient. For diabetic patients with multivessel disease, data from multiple sources indicate an excess mortality associated with PCI; therefore surgery should be the first choice of revascularization for these patients.[89]

【 】 FOR SYMPTOM RELIEF

Patients without life-threatening CAD who are, however, symptomatic with angina, usually enjoy significant and persistent symptom relief after surgery. Before suggesting operation for symptom relief, ischemia in areas supplied by graftable vessels should be demonstrated. The choice of revascularization strategies is usually based on coronary vascular anatomy, the likelihood of complete revascularization with PCI, diabetic status, and patient preference.

TRANSMYOCARDIAL LASER REVASCULARIZATION

The concept of achieving myocardial revascularization by the creation of channels in the myocardium has been investigated since the 1950s, and the increasing population of patients with severe distal native-vessel atherosclerosis (usually occurring years after previous bypass surgery) who may not be well treated with either bypass surgery alone or PCI, has provided impetus to the search for such alternative revascularization strategies. Laser energy has been used to create such channels, and randomized clinical trials of transmyocardial laser revascularization (TMLR) versus medical management have been conducted involving patients with angina and severe CAD judged untreatable by conventional invasive means. Both CO_2 and holmium lasers have been tested; in both studies, more than 70 percent of TMLR patients noted improvement in angina at 1 year after surgery, compared with 13 to 32 percent improvement in the medically treated group ($p = 0.001$).[90] Five-year followup showed persistence of the benefit in the CO_2 study.[91] Survival data on the TMLR and medically treated patients were the same in both studies. Although there is some apparent benefit from TMLR, the mechanism of improvement is not clear (see Chap. 57). Autopsy studies have noted granulation tissue occluding the myocardial channels within a few days of operation, and anginal relief may not be immediate. Denervation and microcollateral stimulation have been suggested as possible mechanisms of angina relief. TMLR appears to have a role in revascularization, but currently does not appear to produce the degree or the consistency of improved myocardial perfusion that can be achieved when bypass surgery or PTCA is possible. The indications for TMLR are still in evolution.

REFERENCES

1. Lytle BW, Loop FD, Cosgrove DM, et al. Long-term (5 to 12 years) serial studies of internal mammary artery and saphenous vein coronary bypass grafts. *J Thorac Cardiovasc Surg* 1985;89(2):248–258.
2. Sabik JF 3rd, Lytle BW, Blackstone EH, et al. Comparison of saphenous vein and internal thoracic artery graft patency by coronary system. *Ann Thorac Surg* 2005;79(2):544–551; discussion 544–551.
3. Fitzgibbon GM, Kafka HP, Leach AJ, et al. Coronary bypass graft fate and patient outcome: angiographic follow-up of 5,065 grafts related to survival and reoperation in 1,388 patients during 25 years. *J Am Coll Cardiol* 1996;28:616–626.
4. Bourassa MG, Campeau L, Lesperance J. Changes in grafts and in coronary arteries after coronary bypass surgery. *Cardiovasc Clin* 1991;21(2):83–100.
5. Neitzel GF, Barboriak JJ, Pintar K, et al. Atherosclerosis in aortocoronary bypass grafts. Morphologic study and risk factor analysis 6 to 12 years after surgery. *Arteriosclerosis* 1986;6(6):594–600.
6. Gavaghan TP, Gebski V, Baron DW. Immediate postoperative aspirin improves vein graft patency early and late after coronary artery bypass graft surgery. A placebo-controlled, randomized study. *Circulation* 1991;83(5):1526–1533.
7. Goldman S, Copeland J, Moritz T, et al. Starting aspirin therapy after operation. Effects on early graft patency. Department of Veterans Affairs Cooperative Study Group. *Circulation* 1991;84(2):520–526.
8. The Post Coronary Artery Bypass Graft Trial Investigators. The effect of aggressive lowering of low-density lipoprotein cholesterol levels and low-dose anticoagulation on obstructive changes in saphenous-vein-coronary-artery bypass grafts. *N Engl J Med* 1997;336:153–162.
9. Flaker GC, Warnica JW, Sacks FM, et al. Pravastatin prevents clinical events in revascularized patients with average cholesterol concentrations. Cholesterol and Recurrent Events (CARE) Investigators. *J Am Coll Cardiol* 1999;34(1):106–112.
10. Lawrie GM, Morris GC Jr, Earle N. Long-term results of coronary bypass surgery. Analysis of 1698 patients followed 15 to 20 years. *Ann Surg* 1991;213(5):377–385; discussion 386–387.
11. Sabik JF 3rd, Lytle BW, Blackstone EH, et al. Does competitive flow reduce internal thoracic artery graft patency? *Ann Thorac Surg* 2003;76(5):1490–1496; discussion 1497.
12. Fitzgibbon GM, et al. Coronary bypass graft fate and patient outcome: angiographic follow-up of 5,065 grafts related to survival and reoperation in 1,388 patients during 25 years. *J Am Coll Cardiol* 1996;28(3):616–626.
13. Whitlow PL, Dimas AP, Bashore TM, et al. Relationship of extent of revascularization with angina at one year in the Bypass Angioplasty Revascularization Investigation (BARI). *J Am Coll Cardiol* 1999;34(6):1750–1759.
14. Loop FD, Lytle BW, Cosgrove DM, et al. Influence of the internal-mammary artery graft on 10-year survival and other cardiac events. *N Engl J Med* 1986;314:1–6.
15. Lytle BW, Cosgrove DM 3rd. Coronary artery bypass surgery. *Curr Probl Surg* 1992;29(10):733–807.
16. Tector AJ, Amundsen S, Schmahl TM, et al. Total revascularization with T grafts. *Ann Thorac Surg,* 1994;57(1):33–38; discussion 39.
17. Lytle BW, Blackstone EH, Sabik JF, et al. The effect of bilateral internal thoracic artery grafting on survival during 20 postoperative years. *Ann Thorac Surg* 2004;78(6):2005–2012; discussion 2012–2014.
18. Lytle BW, Blackstone EH, Loop FD, et al. Two internal artery grafts are better than one. *J Thorac Cardiovasc Surg* 1999;117:855–872.
19. Suma H, Isomura T, Horii T, et al. Late angiographic result of using the right gastroepiploic artery as a graft. *J Thorac Cardiovasc Surg* 2000;120(3):496–498.
20. Buche M, Schroeder E, Gurne O, et al. Coronary artery bypass grafting with the inferior epigastric artery. Midterm clinical and angiographic results. *J Thorac Cardiovasc Surg* 1995;109(3):553–559; discussion 559–560.
21. Acar C, Ramsheyi A, Pagny JY, et al. The radial artery for coronary artery bypass grafting: clinical and angiographic results at five years. *J Thorac Cardiovasc Surg* 1998;116(6):981–989.
22. Possati G, Gaudino M, Alessandrini F, et al. Midterm clinical and angiographic results of radial artery grafts used for myocardial revascularization. *J Thorac Cardiovasc Surg* 1998;116(6):1015–1021.
23. Bergsma TM, Grandjean JG, Voors AA, et al. Low recurrence of angina pectoris after coronary artery bypass graft surgery with bilateral internal thoracic and right gastroepiploic arteries. *Circulation* 1998;97(24):2402–2405.
24. Edwards FH, Clark RE, Schwartz M. Coronary artery bypass grafting: the Society of Thoracic Surgeons National Database Experience. *Ann Thorac Surg* 1994;57:12–19.
25. Diegeler A, Thiele H, Falk UF, et al. Comparison of stenting with minimally invasive bypass surgery for stenosis of the left anterior descending coronary artery. *N Engl J Med* 2002;347(8):561–566.
26. Sabik JF, Gillinov AM, Blackstone EH, et al. Does off-pump coronary surgery reduce morbidity and mortality? *J Thorac Cardiovasc Surg* 2002;124(4):698–707.
27. Calafiore AM, Teodori G, Giammarco G, et al. Multiple arterial conduits without cardiopulmonary bypass: early angiographic results. *Ann Thorac Surg* 1999;67(2):450–456.
28. Puskas JD, Thourani VH, Marshall JJ, et al. Clinical outcomes, angiographic patency, and resource utilization in 200 consecutive off-pump coronary bypass patients. *Ann Thorac Surg* 2001;71(5):1477–1483; discussion 1483–1484.
29. Nathoe HM, van Dijk D, Jansen EW, et al. A comparison of on-pump and off-pump coronary bypass surgery in low-risk patients. *N Engl J Med* 2003;348(5):394–402.
30. Angelini GD, Taylor FC, Reeves BC, et al. Early and midterm outcome after off-pump and on-pump surgery in Beating Heart Against Cardioplegic

Arrest Studies (BHACAS 1 and 2): a pooled analysis of two randomised controlled trials. *Lancet* 2002;359:1194–1199.

31. Chesebro JH, Clemens IP, Fuster V, et al. A platelet inhibitor drug trial in coronary artery bypass operations: benefit of perioperative dipyridamole and aspirin on early vein graft patency. *N Engl J Med* 1982:307:73–78.

32. Chesebro JH, Fuster V, Elveback LR, et al. Effect of dipyridamole and aspirin on late vein-graft patency after coronary bypass operations. *N Engl J Med* 1984;310:209–214.

33. Sabik JF 3rd, Blackstone EH, Houghtaling PL, et al. Is reoperation still a risk factor in coronary artery bypass surgery? *Ann Thorac Surg* 2005;80(5):1719–1727.

34. Jones RH, Hannan EL, Hammermeister KE, et al. Identification of preoperative variables needed for risk adjustment of short-term mortality after coronary artery bypass graft surgery. The Working Group Panel on the Cooperative CABG Database Project. *J Am Coll Cardiol* 1996;28(6):1478–1487.

35. Birkmeyer JD, Siewers AE, Finlayson EV, et al. Hospital volume and surgical mortality in the United States. *N Engl J Med* 2002;346(15):1128–1137.

36. Buckberg GD. Strategies and logic of cardioplegic delivery to prevent, avoid, and reverse ischemic and reperfusion damage. *J Thorac Cardiovasc Surg* 1987;93(1):127–139.

37. Roach GW, Kanchuger M, Mangano CM, et al. Adverse cerebral outcomes after coronary bypass surgery. Multicenter Study of Perioperative Ischemia Research Group and the Ischemia Research and Education Foundation Investigators. *N Engl J Med* 1996;335(25):1857–1863.

38. Hartman GS, Yao FS, Bruefach M III. Severity of aortic atheromatous disease diagnosed by transesophageal echocardiography predicts stroke and other outcomes associated with coronary artery surgery: a prospective study. *Anesth Analg* 1996;83(4):701–708.

39. Blauth CI, Cosgrove DM, Webb BW, et al. Atheroembolism from the ascending aorta. An emerging problem in cardiac surgery. *J Thorac Cardiovasc Surg* 1992;103(6):1104–1111; discussion 1111–1112.

40. Iaco AL, Contini M, Teodori G, et al. Off or on bypass: what is the safety threshold? *Ann Thorac Surg* 1999;68(4):1486–1489.

41. Van Dijk, D, Jansen EW, Hijman R, et al. Cognitive outcome after off-pump and on-pump coronary artery bypass graft surgery: a randomized trial. *JAMA* 2002;287(11):1405–1412.

42. Hertzer, NR, Loop FD, Beven EG, et al. Surgical staging for simultaneous coronary and carotid disease: a study including prospective randomization. *J Vasc Surg* 1989;9(3):455–463.

43. Loop FD, Lytle BW, Cosgrove DM, et al. J. Maxwell Chamberlain memorial paper. Sternal wound complications after isolated coronary artery bypass grafting: early and late mortality, morbidity, and cost of care. *Ann Thorac Surg* 1990;49(2):179–186; discussion 186–187.

44. Myers WO, Blackstone EH, Davis K, et al. CASS Registry long term surgical survival. Coronary Artery Surgery Study. *J Am Coll Cardiol* 1999;33(2):488–498.

45. Cavender JB, Rogers WJ, Fisher LD, et al. Effects of smoking on survival and morbidity in patients randomized to medical or surgical therapy in the Coronary Artery Surgery Study (CASS): 10-year follow-up. CASS Investigators. *J Am Coll Cardiol* 1992;20(2):287–294.

46. Cosgrove DM, Loop FD, Lytle BW, et al. Determinants of 10-year survival after primary myocardial revascularization. *Ann Surg* 1985;202(4):480–490.

47. Jones EL, Weintraub WS. The importance of completeness of revascularization during long-term follow-up after coronary artery operations. *J Thorac Cardiovasc Surg* 1996;112(2):227–237.

48. Bell MR, Gersh BJ, Schaff HV, et al. Effect of completeness of revascularization on long-term outcome of patients with three-vessel disease undergoing coronary artery bypass surgery. A report from the Coronary Artery Surgery Study (CASS) Registry. *Circulation* 1992;86(2):446–457.

49. Sabik JF, Blackstone EH, Gillinov AM, et al. Influence of patient characteristics and arterial grafts on freedom from coronary reoperation. *J Thorac Cardiovasc Surg* 2006;131:90–98.

50. Lytle BW, Loop FD, Taylor PC, et al. Vein graft disease: the clinical impact of stenoses in saphenous vein bypass grafts to coronary arteries. *J Thorac Cardiovasc Surg* 1992;103(5):831–840.

51. Lytle BW, Loop FD, Taylor PC, et al. The effect of coronary reoperation on the survival of patients with stenoses in saphenous vein bypass grafts to coronary arteries. *J Thorac Cardiovasc Surg* 1993;105(4):605–612; discussion 612–614.

52. Loop FD, Lytle BW, Cosgrove DM, et al. Reoperation for coronary atherosclerosis. Changing practice in 2509 consecutive patients. *Ann Surg* 1990;212(3):378–385; discussion 385–386.

53. Lytle BW, Loop FD, Cosgrove DM, et al. Fifteen hundred coronary reoperations. Results and determinants of early and late survival. *J Thorac Cardiovasc Surg* 1987;93(6):847–859.

54. Eleven-year survival in the Veterans Administration randomized trial of coronary bypass surgery for stable angina. The Veterans Administration Coronary Artery Bypass Surgery Cooperative Study Group. *N Engl J Med* 1984:311:1333–1339.

55. Varnauskas E. Twelve-year follow-up of survival in the randomized European Coronary Surgery Study. *N Engl J Med* 1988;319(6):332–337.

56. Passamani E, Davis KB, Gillespie MJ, et al. A randomized trial of coronary artery bypass surgery. Survival of patients with a low ejection fraction. *N Engl J Med* 1985;312(26):1665–1671.

57. Alderman EL, Bourassi MG, Cohen LS, et al. Ten-year follow-up of survival and myocardial infarction in the randomized Coronary Artery Surgery Study. *Circulation* 1990;82:1629–1646.

58. Yusuf S, Zucker D, Peduzzi P, et al. Effect of coronary artery bypass graft surgery on survival: overview of 10-year results from randomised trials by the Coronary Artery Bypass Graft Surgery Trialists Collaboration. *Lancet* 1994;344:563–570.

59. Rogers WJ, Coggin CJ, Gersh BJ, et al. Ten-year follow-up of quality of life in patients randomized to receive medical therapy or coronary artery bypass graft surgery. The Coronary Artery Surgery Study (CASS). *Circulation* 1990;82(5):1647–1658.

60. Taylor HA, Deumite NJ, Chaitman BR, et al. Asymptomatic left main coronary artery disease in the Coronary Artery Surgery Study (CASS) registry. *Circulation* 1989;79(6):1171–1179.

61. Caracciolo EA, Davis KB, Sopko G, et al. Comparison of surgical and medical group survival in patients with left main equivalent coronary artery disease. Long-term CASS experience. *Circulation* 1995;91(9):2335–2344.

62. Myers WO, Schaff HV, Gersh BJ, et al. Improved survival of surgically treated patients with triple vessel coronary artery disease and severe angina pectoris. A report from the Coronary Artery Surgery Study (CASS) registry. *J Thorac Cardiovasc Surg* 1989;97(4):487–495.

63. Sharma GV, Deupree RH, Khuri SF, et al. Coronary bypass surgery improves survival in high-risk unstable angina. Results of a Veterans Administration Cooperative study with an 8-year follow-up. Veterans Administration Unstable Angina Cooperative Study Group. *Circulation* 1991;84(5 Suppl):III260–III267.

64. Hueb WA, Soares PR, Almeida De Oliveira S, et al. Five-year follow-up of the Medicine, Angioplasty, or Surgery Study (MASS): a prospective, randomized trial of medical therapy, balloon angioplasty, or bypass surgery for single proximal left anterior descending coronary artery stenosis. *Circulation* 1999;100(19 Suppl):II107–II113.

65. Davies RF, Goldberg AD, Forman S, et al. Asymptomatic Cardiac Ischemia Pilot (ACIP) study two-year follow-up: outcomes of patients randomized to initial strategies of medical therapy versus revascularization. *Circulation* 1997;95(8):2037–2043.

66. Veenhuyzen G.D, Singh SN, McAreavey D, et al. Prior coronary artery bypass surgery and risk of death among patients with ischemic left ventricular dysfunction. *Circulation* 2001;104(13):1489–1493.

67. Graham MM, Ghali WA, Faris PD, et al. Survival after coronary revascularization in the elderly. *Circulation* 2002;105(20):2378–2384.

68. Eagle KA, Guyten RA, Davidoff R, et al. ACC/AHA 2004 guideline update for coronary artery bypass graft surgery: summary article. A report of the American College of Cardiology/American Heart Association Task Force on Practice Guidelines (Committee to Update the 1999 Guidelines for Coronary Artery Bypass Graft Surgery). *J Am Coll Cardiol* 2004;44(5):e213–e310.

69. The Bypass Angioplasty Revascularization Investigation (BARI) Investigators. Comparison of coronary bypass surgery with angioplasty in patients with multivessel disease. The Bypass Angioplasty Revascularization Investigation (BARI) Investigators. *N Engl J Med* 1996;335(4):217–225.

70. CABRI Trial Participants. First-year results of CABRI (Coronary Angioplasty Versus Bypass Revascularisation Investigation). *Lancet* 1995;346(8984):1179–1184.

71. King SB 3rd, Lembo NJ, Weintraub WS, et al. A randomized trial comparing coronary angioplasty with coronary bypass surgery. Emory Angioplasty Versus Surgery Trial (EAST). *N Engl J Med* 1994;331(16):1044–1050.

72. Hamm CW, Reimers J, Ischinger T, et al. A randomized study of coronary angioplasty compared with bypass surgery in patients with symptomatic multivessel coronary disease. German Angioplasty Bypass Surgery Investigation (GABI). *N Engl J Med* 1994;331(16):1037–1043.

73. Rodriguez A, Boullon F, Perez-Balino N, et al. Argentine randomized trial of percutaneous transluminal coronary angioplasty versus coronary artery

bypass surgery in multivessel disease (ERACI): in-hospital results and 1-year follow-up. ERACI Group. *J Am Coll Cardiol* 1993;22(4):1060–1067.

74. Bourassa MG, Roubin GS, Detre KM, et al. Bypass Angioplasty Revascularization Investigation: patient screening, selection, and recruitment. *Am J Cardiol* 1995;75(9):3C–8C.

75. Coronary angioplasty versus coronary artery bypass surgery: the Randomized Intervention Treatment of Angina (RITA) trial. *Lancet* 1993;341(8845):573–580.

76. Serruys PW, Unger F, Sousa JE, et al. Comparison of coronary-artery bypass surgery and stenting for the treatment of multivessel disease. *N Engl J Med* 2001;344(15):1117–1124.

77. Coronary artery bypass surgery versus percutaneous coronary intervention with stent implantation in patients with multivessel coronary artery disease (the Stent or Surgery trial): a randomised controlled trial. *Lancet* 2002;360(9338):965–970.

78. Rodriguez A, Bernardi V, Navia J, et al. Argentine Randomized Study: coronary angioplasty with stenting versus coronary bypass surgery in patients with multiple-vessel disease (ERACI II): 30-day and one-year follow-up results. ERACI II Investigators. *J Am Coll Cardiol* 2001;37(1):51–58.

79. Morrison DA, Sethi G, Sacks J, et al. Percutaneous coronary intervention versus coronary artery bypass graft surgery for patients with medically refractory myocardial ischemia and risk factors for adverse outcomes with bypass: a multicenter, randomized trial. Investigators of the Department of Veterans Affairs Cooperative Study #385: the Angina with Extremely Serious Operative Mortality Evaluation (AWESOME). *J Am Coll Cardiol* 2001;38(1):143–149.

80. Goy JJ, Kaufmann U, Goy-Eggenberger D, et al. A prospective randomized trial comparing stenting to internal mammary artery grafting for proximal, isolated de novo left anterior coronary artery stenosis: the SIMA trial. Stenting vs. Internal Mammary Artery. *Mayo Clin Proc* 2000;75(11):1116–1123.

81. Hoffman SN, TenBrook JA, Wolf MP, et al. A meta-analysis of randomized controlled trials comparing coronary artery bypass graft with percutaneous transluminal coronary angioplasty: one- to eight-year outcomes. *J Am Coll Cardiol* 2003;41(8):1293–1304.

82. Hannan EL, Racz MJ, Walford G, et al. Long-term outcomes of coronary-artery bypass grafting versus stent implantation. *N Engl J Med* 2005;352(21):2174–2183.

83. Hannan EL, Racz MJ, McCallister BD, et al. A comparison of three-year survival after coronary artery bypass graft surgery and percutaneous transluminal coronary angioplasty. *J Am Coll Cardiol* 1999;33(1):63–72.

84. Brener SJ, Lytle BW, Casserly IP, et al. Propensity analysis of long-term survival after surgical or percutaneous revascularization in patients with multivessel coronary artery disease and high-risk features. *Circulation* 2004;109(19):2290–2295.

85. Smith PK, Califf RM, Tuttle RH, et al. *Selection of Surgical or Percutaneous Coronary Intervention Provides Longevity Benefit that Varies with the Severity of Coronary Disease.* Presented at the Society of Thoracic Surgeons, 42nd Annual Meeting. 2006.

86. Babapulle MN, et al. A hierarchical Bayesian meta-analysis of randomised clinical trials of drug-eluting stents. *Lancet* 2004;364(9434):583–591.

87. Weintraub WS, Ghazzal ZM, Douglas JS Jr., et al. Long-term clinical follow-up in patients with angiographic restudy after successful angioplasty. *Circulation* 1993;87(3):831–840.

88. Allman KC, Shaw LJ, Hachamovitch R, et al. Myocardial viability testing and impact of revascularization on prognosis in patients with coronary artery disease and left ventricular dysfunction: a meta-analysis. *J Am Coll Cardiol* 2002;39(7):1151–1158.

89. Kip KE, Alderman EL, Bourassa MG, et al. Differential influence of diabetes mellitus on increased jeopardized myocardium after initial angioplasty or bypass surgery: bypass angioplasty revascularization investigation. *Circulation* 2002;105(16):1914–1920.

90. Allen KB, Dowling RD, Fudge TL, et al. Comparison of transmyocardial revascularization with medical therapy in patients with refractory angina. *N Engl J Med* 1999;341(14):1029–1036.

91. Horvath KA, Aranki SF, Cohn LH, et al. Sustained angina relief 5 years after transmyocardial laser revascularization with a CO(2) laser. *Circulation* 2001;104(12 Suppl 1):I81–I84.

CHAPTER (66)

Management of the Patient after Cardiac Surgery

Douglas C. Morris / Stephen D. Clements, Jr. / John Pepper

The initial management of most patients following cardiac surgery occurs in specialized intensive care units (ICUs). The unique pathophysiologic alterations associated with hypothermia and cardiopulmonary bypass (CPB) mandated that a specialized environment, including sophisticated electrophysiologic and hemodynamic monitoring and intensive attention and supervision by specially trained critical care nurses, be available. Although CPB is no longer universally applied in cardiac surgery (presently, at least one-third of bypass procedures are performed "off-pump"), the multiple management problems posed by cardiac patients continue to demand specialized treatment.

ROLE OF VASCULAR CANNULAS, LIFE SUPPORT, AND MONITORING IN THE IMMEDIATE POSTOPERATIVE PERIOD

The patient typically arrives in the ICU or postcardiac surgery recovery area from the operating room with the necessary apparatus for monitoring the following parameters: heart rate and rhythm; systemic arterial, central venous, pulmonary artery, and pulmonary artery occlusion pressures (PAOPs); cardiac output; urinary output; mediastinal drainage; body temperature; arterial oxygen saturation (SpO_2); mixed venous oxygen saturation (SvO_2) and end-tidal carbon dioxide ($ETCO_2$) tension.

Most of the apparatus attached to the patient on arrival in the ICU serves multiple purposes. A pulmonary artery catheter not only allows monitoring of pulmonary artery pressures but can also be used to estimate the filling pressure of the left ventricle, cardiac output, and body core temperature. The pulmonary artery catheter also allows for measurement of the SvO_2, which is used as an indirect index of tissue oxygenation. The peripheral arterial cannula provides a continuous pulse-wave tracing of systemic blood pressure and ready access to arterial blood sampling for laboratory analysis. Regular periodic assessments of arterial blood gases, especially after a major change in ventilator settings, are essential unless continuous $ETCO_2$ and SpO_2 by pulse oximetry are being monitored. $ETCO_2$ and SpO_2 are reliable in guiding the weaning of mechanical ventilation and removal of the endotracheal tube. Monitoring of these parameters has been used very effectively in "fast-track" protocols. Assessment of volume loss is based on chest and mediastinal tube drainage plus urine output. The endotracheal tube secured in the correct position with an appropriately inflated cuff is essential for positive-pressure ventilation of the lungs. Confirmation of bilateral breath sounds and absence of tracheal air leak versus cuff inflation should be made upon arrival in the ICU.

The endotracheal tube's position should be ascertained on the initial chest radiograph. The endotracheal tube also allows for suctioning of bronchial secretions and reduces (but does not eliminate) the risk of oropharyngeal and gastric reflux secretions entering the trachea and bronchi. The endotracheal tube can often be removed the evening of surgery if the patient is conscious, is able to protect the airway, has good ventilatory mechanics and muscle strength, and is able to take on the work of breathing. Most patients can have the pulmonary artery catheter removed within 12 to 24 hours if cardiovascular drug therapy is at minimum levels. The peripheral arterial cannula can be removed once cardiovascular function is satisfactory and the need for blood sampling is at a routine daily level. The urinary catheter is usually removed when the patient is ambulatory unless there is a vigorous diuresis or an increased risk of urinary retention. Chest tubes are generally removed when the total drainage is less than 100 mL per tube over 8 hours.

The primary factor that differentiates cardiac surgery from other forms of surgery is CPB. With such improvements in extracorporeal technology as membrane oxygenation, arterial blood filtration, and blood-sparing techniques, the noncardiac complications have been significantly reduced. Major improvements in myocardial protection coupled with changes in anesthetic and CPB techniques now frequently allow extubation within several hours of surgery.

The patient can often be safely and comfortably transferred from the ICU within the first 6 to 24 hours, a process that has been termed *fast tracking*.[1] Individuals undergoing "off-pump" procedures also have the potential for rapid recovery and early extubation and removal of catheters and chest tubes; they can be sitting up in the chair the next morning ready for transfer.

Fast tracking requires that the patient's status be characterized as follows: awake or easily aroused, neurologically intact, cooperative, and comfortable; stable, satisfactory hemodynamics; normothermia; satisfactory spontaneous ventilation; normal coagulation with minimal chest tube drainage; satisfactory urine output, electrolyte, and acid-base balance.[2]

EARLY POSTOPERATIVE MANAGEMENT

【 】 PATHOPHYSIOLOGIC CONSEQUENCES OF CARDIOPULMONARY BYPASS

The basic pathophysiology during the early postoperative period revolves around the following variables: transient left ventricular dysfunction, capillary leak, warming from hypothermia, mediastinal bleeding, and emergence from anesthesia.

Although improvements in surgical techniques, cardioplegia delivery, and other myocardial protection features achieved in the past decade were expected to lessen the likelihood of developing transient left ventricular systolic dysfunction following CPB, the reported prevalence of this complication (90 percent) did not change between 1979 and 1990.[3] This transient myocardial depression has been attributed by some authors to inadequate myocardial protection or the effects of cold cardioplegia, but the bulk of the evidence incriminates the inflammatory state induced by CPB as the primary causative factor.[4]

The inflammatory state induced by CPB involves platelet–endothelial cell interactions and vasospastic responses that result in low-flow states in the coronary circulation.[5] The inflammatory reaction causes vascular endothelial adhesion molecules to attract inflammatory cells that subsequently adhere to the vascular endothelium. These inflammatory cells mediate much of the subsequent injury by the release of oxygen free radicals or proteolytic enzymes. This release of oxygen free radicals in response to reperfusion injury is now generally accepted as the explanation for the transient postoperative ventricular dysfunction.[6,7] Whether the depressed ventricular function is caused by oxygen free radicals or the myocardial ischemia associated with cardioplegia, the expectation would be that "off-pump" coronary artery bypass graft (CABG) would reduce myocardial injury by reducing the inflammatory response. A significant attenuation of the inflammatory response has been demonstrated with the "off-pump" approach. It must be emphasized, however, that the inflammatory response is not totally eliminated as other factors, such as surgical trauma and anesthetic agents, contribute to this process. Better myocardial function in association with a reduction in systemic inflammation is substantiated by reduced creative kinase myocardial banding and better postoperative left ventricular function in the "off-pump" patients.[8] Depressed myocardial function seems to be unrelated to CPB time, number of coronary artery grafts, preoperative medications, or postoperative core temperature. Ventricular function is generally depressed by 2 hours and is at its worst at 4 to 5 hours after CPB. Significant recovery of function usually occurs by 8 to 10 hours, and full recovery is reached by 24 to 48 hours.[9] Systemic vascular resistance, while not rising immediately after surgery, increases as ventricular function worsens. This rise in systemic vascular resistance is likely secondary to reduced ventricular function and the need to maintain systemic blood pressure, and is not per se a major causative factor of depressed cardiac contractility. The confounding effect of vasopressor drugs used in an attempt to increase systemic blood pressure must be recognized.

The inflammation-mediated production of oxygen free radicals and release of proteolytic enzymes by neutrophils also damages the endothelial cells. The "gatekeeper" function of the endothelium is disturbed and capillary permeability increases, resulting in edema. The capillary leak syndrome may last from a few hours up to 1 to 2 days, depending to a large degree on the duration of CPB. When the capillary leak ceases and interstitial edema fluid is mobilized, intravascular volume overload is a threat.

Hypothermia predisposes the patient to cardiac arrhythmias, increases systemic vascular resistance, precipitates shivering (which increases O_2 consumption and CO_2 production), and impairs coagulation.[9] Hypothermia with the patient's core temperature below 95°F (35°C) frequently recurs after rewarming to 98.°F (37°C) at the end of CPB. This fall in core temperature reflects the loss of heat from the surgical field after CPB, exposure of the patient to ambient temperature, and incomplete rewarming of peripheral tissues, especially fat and muscle. If the patient is hypothermic upon arrival in the ICU, monitoring the temperature of noncore body sites such as a finger or toe can assure complete assessment of rewarming. Hypothermia causes peripheral vasoconstriction and contributes to the hypertension frequently seen after cardiac surgery. Furthermore, hypothermia causes a decrease in cardiac output by producing bradycardia along with the increase in vascular resistance. Most believe that the patient should be passively rewarmed by warm air (e.g., Bear Hugger) and that shivering should be eliminated by the administration of meperidine (25 to 50 mg) and muscle relaxants. As body temperature increases, the vasoconstriction and hypertension associated with hypothermia are replaced by vasodilatation, tachycardia, and hypotension. Volume loading during the rewarming process helps reduce the rapid swings in blood pressure. Vasopressors (e.g., norepinephrine) may be required to maintain an adequate systemic blood pressure. As the patient is rewarmed, large increases in O_2 consumption and CO_2 production can occur, with a consequent increase in demand on cardiovascular and pulmonary functions.[10]

Hypercarbia will cause catecholamine release, tachycardia, and pulmonary hypertension. If the patient cannot increase the cardiac output and O_2 delivery, venous hemoglobin desaturation and metabolic acidosis will result.

The commonly reported prevalence of severe postoperative bleeding (more than 10 U of blood transfused) following cardiac surgery is between 3 and 5 percent. While approximately half of the patients who undergo reoperation for excessive bleeding exhibit incomplete surgical hemostasis, the remainder bleed because of various acquired hemostatic defects, most often related to platelet dysfunction.[11] There is a reduced need for blood products in those patients operated upon without CPB. The factors that predispose to bleeding following CPB are residual heparin effect, platelet dysfunction (which may be intensified by preoperative drug therapy—e.g., aspirin, clopidogrel, and glycoprotein [GP] IIb/IIIa inhibitors), clotting-factor depletion, inadequate surgical hemostasis, hypothermia, and postoperative hypertension. CPB decreases both platelet count and function. Hemodilution causes platelet counts to fall rapidly to approximately 50 percent of preoperative values. Within minutes after instituting CPB, the bleeding time is prolonged and platelet aggregation impaired. The bleeding time usually normalizes by 2 to 4 hours after CPB. The platelet count usually requires several days to return to normal levels. While the exact mechanism responsible for the transient platelet dysfunction remains undefined, it appears to be related to contact of platelets with the synthetic surfaces of the extracorporeal oxygenator and to hypothermia. Reductions in the plasma concentrations of coagulation factors II, V, VII, IX, X, and XIII as a consequence of hemodilution occur during CPB, but these coagulation factors remain well above levels considered adequate for hemostasis and generally normalize within the first 12 hours after surgery. Moreover, while bleeding after CPB is often attributed to excessive fibrinolysis, the decrease in both plasminogen and fibrinogen levels during CPB is a result of hemodilution and not consumption.[11] Exploration for postoperative bleeding commonly identifies no localized site of bleeding but only diffuse oozing. Less frequently, a specific site such as an internal mammary pedicle will be identified.

Recombinant activated factor VIIa (NovoSeven) is a prohemostatic agent that may be considered in patients with life-threatening bleeding. Factor VIIa is thought to act locally at sites of vascular wall disruption. It binds to exposed tissue factor and generates thrombin sufficient to activate platelets. The agent is approved only for management of hemophilia A and B in the presence of inhibitors. It is not clear at what stage of intractable bleeding it should be used, but the safest approach is to administer after all other treatments (full-dose aprotinin, platelets, fresh-frozen plasma, and cryoprecipitate) have failed.[12]

MANAGEMENT OF COMMON POSTOPERATIVE SYNDROMES

【 】 VASOCONSTRICTION WITH HYPERTENSION AND BORDERLINE CARDIAC OUTPUT

Increased arteriolar resistance as a consequence of hypothermia and increased levels of circulating catecholamines, plasma renin, or angiotensin II is present in most postoperative cardiac patients. The usual criterion for pharmacologic lowering of blood pressure in postoperative patients is a mean arterial blood pressure 10 percent above the upper level of normal (>90 mmHg). Patients with a friable aorta or friable suture lines might be subjected to a lower mean arterial pressure to prevent dehiscence. The mean arterial blood pressure is monitored because it is most reflective of systemic vascular resistance. As the hypothermic patient is rewarmed, a short-acting vasodilator (nitroprusside, nitroglycerin, or nicardipine) can be infused intravenously to maintain mean arterial pressure at 80 to 90 mmHg. Intravascular volume should be maintained at a relatively high level (PAOP of 14 to 16 mmHg) in anticipation of vasodilation on rewarming and to enhance cardiac output and peripheral perfusion. If the cardiac index is marginal (2.0 to 2.2 L/min/m²), an inotropic drug should be administered in addition to the vasodilator.

【 】 VASODILATATION AND HYPOTENSION

This condition, which generally appears during rewarming, is most effectively prevented and best treated by fluid administration. There is a paucity of data indicating that any specific volume expander is better than another, although colloids remain in the intravascular space longer than crystalloid solutions. Fluid should be administered until cardiac output no longer increases or appropriate left ventricular filling pressures have been restored (PAOP approximately 14 to 16 mmHg for a normal ventricle, or 18 to 22 mmHg for a noncompliant ventricle).

If the systemic arterial pressure is inadequate despite fluid administration, vasoactive drugs become the mainstay of hemodynamic management. If the cardiac index is over 2.5 L/min/m², either dopamine in high doses or norepinephrine is preferable. Although the safety and efficacy of vasopressin seems established and endogenous vasopressin levels are depressed after CPB, vasopressin is not currently recommended as first-line therapy. Epinephrine produces visceral hypoperfusion and lactic acid production and, consequently, is not recommended as first-line therapy. If the cardiac index is marginal (less than 2.0 L/min/m²), an inotropic agent—either a β_1-adrenoceptor agonist (dobutamine) or a phosphodiesterase III inhibitor (milrinone)—is used to push the mixed venous or central venous oxygen saturation to greater than 70 percent. Each of these classes of inotropic agents increases myocardial oxygen demand and has the potential of causing arrhythmogenesis. Consequently, in some centers levosimendan is the preferred inotrope. This inotropic agent with vasodilatory activity is now approved in 31 countries. Regardless of the inotrope used, norepinephrine should be added if the mean arterial pressure remains below 60 mmHg.

In the critically ill patient, hemodynamic optimization is probably best achieved by measuring the SvO_2 in conjunction with the cardiac output. The central venous oxygen saturation ($ScvO_2$) can be used as a surrogate for the SvO_2; although the absolute values of the $ScvO_2$ and SvO_2 differ, the values tend to change in parallel over a wide range of hemodynamic conditions.

【 】 NORMAL VENTRICULAR SYSTOLIC FUNCTION AND LOW CARDIAC OUTPUT

This set of circumstances is often noted in small women with systemic hypertension and in patients undergoing aortic valve replacement for aortic stenosis. The likely explanation is diastolic dysfunction. The problem should be managed by volume expansion with the intent to elevate PAOP to levels as high as 20 to 25 mmHg if necessary, as long as right ventricular function is adequate to fill the left ventricle. Sinus rhythm and atrioventricular synchrony are essential and, if not present, should be restored. In the absence of other reasons for diastolic dysfunction, the possibility of cardiac compression from clots in the mediastinum and pericardial space should be considered. If volume expansion does not lead to hemodynamic improvement, transesophageal echocardiography should be used to establish or exclude the presence of clots or other causes of low output.

APPROACH TO POSTOPERATIVE CARDIOVASCULAR PROBLEMS

【 】 LOW-CARDIAC-OUTPUT SYNDROME

Satisfactory cardiac performance following cardiac surgery is usually indicated by a cardiac index greater than 2.2 L/min/m^2 with a heart rate below 100 beats per minute. Marginal cardiac function is present with a cardiac index between 2.0 and 2.2 L/min/m^2. A cardiac index below 2.0 L/min/m^2 is unacceptably low, and therapeutic intervention is indicated. Clinical signs of the adequacy or inadequacy of organ perfusion must be incorporated into any assessment of cardiac performance. It is also useful to measure the mixed venous oxygen saturation, as a subset of patients who are hypothermic may have a low cardiac index but an acceptable mixed venous oxygen tension.

Assessment

The most common causes of low cardiac output postoperatively are related to a decreased left ventricular preload. The decreased preload, in turn, can likely be attributed to hypovolemia (a result of bleeding or of vasodilatation as a consequence of warming or of drugs), cardiac tamponade, or right ventricular dysfunction. Alternative explanations for low cardiac output include decreased contractility caused by a preexisting low ejection fraction or to intra- or postoperative ischemia or infarction. Tachy- or bradyarrhythmias decrease cardiac output by reducing ventricular preload (e.g., decreased diastolic filling time, loss of atrial contraction or atrioventricular synchrony) or by reducing the number of effective

ventricular contractions per minute. Substantial increases in systemic vascular resistance (i.e., vasoconstriction) impede ventricular ejection and lower cardiac output. Vasodilatation from sepsis or anaphylaxis resulting in systemic hypotension can lead to reduced coronary blood flow and myocardial ischemia. Sepsis (an unlikely occurrence in the immediate postoperative period) is also associated with the production of myocardial depressant factors. Anemia may result in reduced blood viscosity (a major determinant of total peripheral resistance) leading to hypotension and decreased oxygen delivery to the heart. The hypotension in anemia, however, is most often caused by changes in effective blood volume rather than to the changes in viscosity.

Etiology and Management

The multiple variables constantly monitored usually provide sufficient clues as to the cause of low cardiac output. If there is no obvious noncardiac cause then the first step is to optimize the heart rate by either cardiac pacing or antiarrhythmic drugs. Postoperative myocardial performance is usually best at a rate of 90 to 100 beats/min. The next step is to increase preload until cardiac output is no longer increasing (PAOP of 15 to 18 mmHg). If these measures prove unsuccessful, pharmacologic intervention with inotropic agents, vasodilators, vasopressors, or a combination of these drugs must be considered. The selection of drugs should be based on the balance of their effects on heart rate, contractility, ventricular preload, and systemic vasculature resistance (Table 66–1). If the patient has circulatory collapse with low blood pressure (mean arterial pressure <55), vasopressors should be initial therapy. If the systemic blood pressure is marginal and there is an element of pulmonary congestion, therapy can begin with an inotropic agent. Phosphodiesterase inhibitors, such as amrinone and milrinone, may offer advantages for patients who were in heart failure preoperatively as β receptors may be downregulated and catecholamines may be less effective. If pulmonary congestion is the primary problem with satisfactory systemic arterial pressure, then vasodilators are beneficial. Intravenous nitroglycerin or nesiritide are options. Nesiritide, particularly, should not be used in patients with excessive diuresis, who are hypotensive, or who have signs of inadequate perfusion. Nitric oxide inhalation has been used in the setting of cardiogenic shock accompanied by pulmonary hypertension. The cost and complexity of administration are deterrents to its use. Sildenafil is increasingly used as an alternative to nitric oxide in the management of elevated pulmonary arterial pressures. The presence of elevated left- and right-sided filling pressures, a recent cessation of mediastinal drainage, and progressively increasing dosage requirements for inotropic drugs suggests tamponade, which should be relieved emergently.

【 】 HYPERTENSION

Management

A variety of medications are available for control of hypertension; the drug selected should depend on the hemodynamic status of the patient, the cardiovascular effects of the drug, and the patient's other medical problems. Systemic hypertension in the presence of a high left ventricular filling pressure and marginal cardiac output

TABLE 66–1

Medications Used in Low-Cardiac-Output Syndrome

MEDICATION	HEMODYNAMIC PROPERTIES	DOSAGE RANGE
Dopamine	Low dose—dopaminergic effect	1–5 µg/kg/min
	Moderate dose—inotropic effect	5–10 µg/kg/min
	High dose—vasopressor effect	10–20 µg/kg/min
Dobutamine	Positive inotropic agent	2–20 µg/kg/min
Epinephrine	Positive inotropic agent	1–4 µg/min
Milrinone	Positive inotropic agent	50 µg/kg, then 0.25–1 µg/kg/min
Isoproterenol	Potent inotropic agent Pronounced chronotropic effect	0.5–10 µg/min
Norepinephrine	Potent vasopressor effect; inotropic effect	1–100 µg/min
Phenylephrine	Potent vasopressor agent	10–500 µg/min
Vasopressin	Potent vasopressor agent; not first line therapy	0.01–0.04 µg/min

is most appropriately treated by an arterial vasodilator. Nitroprusside relaxes vascular smooth muscle in arterial resistance vessels (both systemic and pulmonary) and in venous capacitance vessels. The advantages of the drug are its very rapid onset and the rapid dissipation of its effects. The risks with this agent are rapid and excessive hypotension, production of a coronary steal syndrome by dilatation of the coronary resistance vessels, and the potential for either acute cyanide toxicity or thiocyanate toxicity with prolonged use.

Nitroglycerin is primarily a venous dilator, although it produces varying degrees of arterial vasodilatation, especially at high doses. Its major role in treating systemic hypertension is in the patient with high filling pressures and active myocardial ischemia. Nicar-

dipine is a potent systemic and coronary vasodilator without the risk of coronary steal, and it has no significant effect on the venous system. Although its onset of action is rapid (1 to 2 minutes), its elimination half-life is about 40 minutes. Unlike some calcium-channel blockers, this agent lacks a negative inotropic effect and has no effect on atrioventricular conduction.

When the hypertension is associated with a normal cardiac output and a relatively rapid sinus heart rate or a propensity toward dysrhythmias, a drug with negative inotropic and chronotropic properties is desirable. Esmolol is a cardioselective, ultrashort-acting β blocker, which also produces a rapid and titratable control of the blood pressure accompanied by a decrease in heart rate. The drug is usually tolerated satisfactorily by patients with a history of bronchospasm because of its relatively high selectivity for beta$_1$-type adrenergic receptors. It is not ideal for patients with impaired cardiac contractility, particularly in the presence of elevated filling pressures. Diltiazem is an arterial vasodilator that has a mild negative inotropic effect and a more potent negative chronotropic effect. Labetalol has both α- and β-blocking properties, as well as a direct vasodilatory effect. Its predominant effect is as a β blocker, especially in the intravenous form. The angiotensin-converting enzyme inhibitor enalaprilat can be administered intermittently by the intravenous route. This agent is usually reserved for the patient who is hemodynamically stable with either a normal or reduced cardiac output but with hypertension expected to persist (Table 66–2).

TABLE 66–2

Intravenous Antihypertensive Agents

DRUG	PEAK EFFECT	DURATION	DOSAGE
Nitroprusside	Immediate	2–5 min	0.3–1.0 µg/kg/min
Nitroglycerine	Immediate	2–5 min	5–100 µg/min infusion
Nicardipine	5–60 min	20–40 min	2.5 mg over 5 min; may repeat times 4 at 10-min intervals; infusion 2–15 mg/h
Esmolol	2–5 min	8–10 min	1-min loading infusion of 0.25–0.5 mg/kg; sustained infusion of 50–200 µg/kg/min
Enalaprilat	15–30 min	6 h or more	0.625–1.25 mg slowly over 5 min every 6 h
Hydralazine	15–20 min	3–4 h	5- to 10-mg bolus may be repeated every 15 min; up to total of 40 mg
Diltiazem	3–30 min	3 h	20- to 25-mg bolus may repeat; infusion of 10–20 mg/h
Verapamil	2–3 min	20–40 min	5- to 10-mg bolus; may repeat in 10 min; infusion of 3–25 mg/h
Labetalol	5–15 min	2–6 h	20-mg bolus over 2 min; then 40- to 80-mg boluses every 15 min until effect achieved (to total dose of 300 mg)

[ ] ARRHYTHMIAS

General Considerations and Sinus Tachycardia

The most common rhythm disturbance immediately after cardiac surgery is sinus tachycardia. This condition is appropriately treated by searching for and correcting the underlying cause (pain, anxiety, low cardiac output, anemia, fever, or β-blocker withdrawal). The second most common arrhythmia is ventricular ectopy. Again, an underlying cause such as myocardial ischemia, hypokalemia, hypomagnesemia, hypoxia, or administration of sympathomimetic drugs must be sought and corrected if possible. Occasionally repositioning of a ventricular pacemaker lead or a pulmonary artery catheter that slipped back into the right ventricle will stop the ectopy. It is also important to review the patient's preoperative record to determine if the patient had preexisting ectopy. Patients with chronic ventricular ectopy frequently have their ectopy exaggerated postoperatively. In the presence of active myocardial ischemia, pharmacologic suppression is advisable for complex ventricular ectopy. If suppression of ventricular ectopy seems necessary, the most effective agent is intravenous amiodarone. The drug should be administered through a three-phase infusion over the first 24 hours: 150 mg over 10 minutes, 300 mg over the next 6 hours, and a 0.5- to 1.0-mg/min infusion.

Ventricular Tachycardia and Fibrillation

After cardiac surgery, a few patients develop sustained ventricular tachycardia (either monomorphic or polymorphic) or ventricular fibrillation. These profound rhythm disturbances may develop in the absence of evidence of acute myocardial ischemia or infarction or electrolyte imbalance. In most cases, the patients have had previous myocardial infarction and have undergone "complete" revascularization, including regions likely to be nonviable. Reperfusion of these areas that probably include viable as well as nonviable myofibrils embedded in the healed infarct may lead to altered dispersion of repolarization. These changes support development of reentry arrhythmias.[13] The ventricular tachycardia in these patients uncommonly responds to lidocaine and usually requires amiodarone. In some instances, a combination of amiodarone and a β blocker is required. In a rare circumstance, aortic counterpulsation has seemed to be of benefit.

Every encounter with a wide complex tachycardia requires careful consideration as to the possibility of supraventricular tachycardia with aberrant conduction. In the presence of atrial fibrillation with a rapid ventricular response, right bundle-branch aberrant conduction often mimics ventricular tachycardia. Care must be given to avoid lidocaine in these situations, because it may result in an even more rapid ventricular rate. Wide complex tachyarrhythmias in the range of 250 to 300 beats/min should suggest the presence of an anomalous conduction pathway. The mechanism of this arrhythmia usually involves atrial flutter, with one-to-one conduction or atrial fibrillation with a very fast ventricular response involving an anomalous pathway. Once this is recognized, procainamide becomes the drug of choice, because it does have favorable therapeutic effects on the bypass track tissue. A more widely applied therapeutic approach is immediate electrical cardioversion, especially if the patient is already intubated and sedated. Lidocaine and verapamil should be avoided if the presence of an anomalous pathway is suspected (see Chap. 24).

Supraventricular Arrhythmias

The most common supraventricular dysrhythmias with the exception of sinus tachycardia are atrial fibrillation and atrial flutter. These rhythm disturbances occur in 10 to 30 percent of patients following cardiac surgery. The predominant predisposing factor in the development of atrial fibrillation is the patient's age. The prevalence of atrial fibrillation in postoperative cardiac patients younger than 40 years of age is as low as 3.7 percent, whereas the prevalence is at least 28 percent in patients older than 70 years of age. It is unclear whether the prevalence of postoperative atrial fibrillation is reduced by the "off-pump" approach. The evidence from observational and randomized studies is conflicting. Atrial fibrillation is most likely to appear on the second postoperative day. Within 1 to 3 days, 80 percent of these patients will return to sinus rhythm with only digoxin or β-blocker therapy.[14,15] The prophylactic use of β blockers has a protective effect against the development of atrial fibrillation or flutter. This beneficial effect has been demonstrated with any one of several β blockers, administered in low or high doses and started preoperatively or postoperatively. Neither digoxin nor verapamil has demonstrated effective prophylaxis against atrial fibrillation or flutter.[16]

Preoperative oral administration of amiodarone also reduces the prevalence of postoperative atrial fibrillation.[17] The major limitation to the widespread application of this prophylactic approach is the apparent need for a 7-day preoperative treatment period. An accelerated loading regimen over 1 to 2 days may be effective but is unproved. Intravenous infusions of either esmolol or diltiazem can be used to control the ventricular rate with atrial fibrillation or flutter. Esmolol is given as a 1-minute loading infusion of 0.25 to 0.5 mg/kg, followed by a sustained infusion of 50 to 200 µg/kg/min. Diltiazem is administered as a bolus of 20 to 25 mg (which may be repeated), followed by an infusion of 10 to 15 mg/h. Diltiazem is preferred in patients with impaired ventricular function. Atrial epicardial pacing wires provide the means of atrial pacing to convert some cases of atrial flutter to sinus rhythm. Short bursts (15 to 30 seconds) of atrial pacing at rates of 300 to 600 per minute may be effective in converting atrial flutter. Approximately 10 percent of patients with atrial fibrillation require electrical cardioversion to restore sinus rhythm. If hemodynamic compromise is present and aggravated by a supraventricular tachyarrhythmia, cardioversion should be used immediately rather than later.

Intravenous ibutilide (1 mg infused over 10 minutes to be repeated once if necessary) is the most effective pharmacologic means of converting recent-onset atrial flutter. The drug is much less effective (in the range of 30 to 50 percent) for conversion of recent-onset atrial fibrillation. The disadvantage of ibutilide is the propensity for causing torsade de pointes in 2 to 4 percent of patients.

Conduction Defects

The prevalence of intraventricular conduction abnormalities after coronary bypass surgery is reported to be from 1 to 45 percent, with approximately 10 percent being the most commonly reported frequency. The most common conduction defect is right bundle-branch block, which may be caused by selective sensitivity of the right bundle to the effects of hypothermia and the extracorporeal circulation process. Only approximately 5 percent of the patients are left with a permanent conduction abnormality, and the prognosis for these patients is no worse than it is for comparable patients with no conduction defect.[18] The development of high-degree (second- or third-degree) atrioventricular block is an indication for temporary pacing via epicardial pacing wires. Atrioventricular block is not as common as either bundle-branch block or fascicular block, but it does occur, especially after aortic valve surgery.

RESPIRATORY MANAGEMENT

Expected Respiratory Changes after Cardiac Surgery

Pulmonary problems are the most significant cause of morbidity following cardiac surgery. The problem ranges from subclinical function changes in most patients to full-blown acute respiratory distress syndrome in less than 2%. Splinting because of chest pain, phrenic nerve damage, cephalad displacement of the diaphragm by abdominal contents, and alveolar edema as a consequence of elevated left-heart filling pressures may all contribute to pulmonary dysfunction. Although an attenuated inflammatory response has been demonstrated following "off-pump" CABG, when compared with "on-pump" CABG, there appears to be a similar degree of postoperative lung dysfunction.

Atelectasis is the most common pulmonary complication, occurring in approximately 70 percent of patients following cardiac surgery with CPB. During CPB, the lungs are not perfused and are usually allowed to collapse. Once the lungs are reexpanded, a variable amount of atelectasis remains. The preponderance of atelectasis occurs in the left lower lobe because of its compression during cardiac surgery, the tendency to suction more thoroughly the right mainstem bronchus during blind nasoorotracheal suctioning, and the frequent surgical practice of opening the left pleural space to facilitate dissection of the left internal mammary artery.

After thoracotomy, both lung and chest wall compliance decrease significantly. The maximum decrease occurs at approximately 3 days, but the decrease persists to a lesser degree 6 or more days after sternotomy. Alterations in chest wall mechanics lead to a decrease in the forced expiratory volume in 1 second (FEV_1) and the functional residual capacity. The changes in the FEV_1 may persist for 6 weeks. In addition to these changes in flows and volumes, reduced inspiratory strength and uncoordinated rib cage expansion occur. These changes result in an increase in respiratory rate and a decrease in tidal volume, a decrease in respiratory efficiency, and an increase in oxygen cost of breathing. The atelectasis and decrease in lung volume result in ventilation: perfusion mismatch and shunting. The clinical manifestation is a decrease in arterial PO_2 and hemoglobin saturation.[19] Nitric oxide can be used as rescue therapy in the management of refractory hypoxemia.

Basic Concepts of Oxygenation and Alveolar Ventilation

The goals of mechanical ventilation are the maintenance of satisfactory arterial oxygenation and CO_2 removal. An SpO_2 >90 percent is considered acceptable, but it may be associated with a marginal PaO_2 (arterial oxygen partial pressure). A PaO_2 below 65 mmHg will result in a precipitous fall in the oxygen saturation of hemoglobin. The fraction of inspired oxygen (FiO_2) should be gradually decreased to 0.4 as tolerated, to minimize adsorption atelectasis and

pulmonary O_2 toxicity. Mechanical ventilation is also used to maintain alveolar ventilation, which regulates the arterial blood CO_2 tension ($PaCO_2$). Alveolar ventilation is regulated by controlling the tidal volume and the respiratory rate. Generally, the ventilator should maintain an exhaled minute ventilation of 6 to 8 L/min. Decreasing the tidal volume below 8 to 10 mL/kg may result in alveolar hypoventilation and atelectasis. Mild hypocarbia ($PaCO_2$ of 30 to 35 mmHg) is satisfactory immediately after surgery, but more profound respiratory alkalosis should be avoided because it leads to hypokalemia and a leftward shift of the oxygen–hemoglobin dissociation curve (decreased oxygen release to the tissues). Hypercarbia in the immediate postoperative period usually indicates that minute ventilation is inadequate. The problem can be rectified primarily by increasing the ventilator rate; in some cases it is appropriate to increase the tidal volume as well. Later, as the patient is weaned from the ventilator, hypercarbia may reflect opioid analgesia (a necessary side effect of satisfactory analgesia) or compensatory hypoventilation in response to a metabolic alkalosis, most likely as a result of excessivediuresis. Severe hypercarbia should raise a concern about mechanical problems such as ventilator malfunction, endotracheal tube malposition, or a pneumothorax. Occasionally, hypoxemia and even hypotension may develop in the mechanically ventilated patient because of a tension pneumothorax or hemothorax.

Ventilatory Weaning and Extubation

Ventilatory support should be reduced as tolerated when the cardiovascular system has become stable and the arterial oxygen tension is satisfactory (a PaO_2/FiO_2 ratio >300 mmHg with peak end-expiratory pressure of 5 cm H_2O). The patient should also be alert, normothermic, and have no active bleeding. Monitoring of SpO_2 and $ETCO_2$ is helpful and allows the weaning process to be done safely and expeditiously. Weaning should be discontinued if any of the following signs appear: SpO_2 <90; PaO_2 <60 mmHg; $ETCO_2$ >50 mmHg; $PaCO_2$ >55 mmHg; pH <7.30; a 10-mmHg rise in pulmonary artery pressure; respiratory rate >30 breaths/min; a 20-mmHg rise in systemic blood pressure; or a 20 beats/min rise in heart rate.[3]

Most patients require low to moderate doses of morphine or another opioid in order to tolerate the endotracheal tube. As long as the spontaneous ventilatory rate remains greater than 15 breaths/min, the patient will almost certainly be able to maintain adequate ventilation after the endotracheal tube is removed.

Bronchospasm

Severe bronchospasm during CPB is an unusual event, but it can occur. The most likely cause of this fulminant bronchospasm is activation of human C5a anaphylatoxin by the extracorporeal circulation. Other likely causes of bronchospasm in the postoperative period are cardiogenic pulmonary edema; simple exacerbation of preexisting bronchospastic disease triggered by instrumentation, secretions, or cold anesthetic gas; β-adrenergic blockers in susceptible individuals; and allergic reaction to protamine. The initial therapy of bronchospasm in the postoperative patient, once a diagnosis of heart failure is excluded, should be inhaled β₂ agonists (terbutaline, metaproterenol, albuterol) and/or inhaled cholinergic agents (ipratropium bromide or glycopyrrolate). In the inhaled form, these rather potent bronchodilators have minimal cardiovascular effects. In addition to their bronchodilator effect, these agents may augment mucociliary transport and aid in clearing secretions. A combination of β$_2$-agonists and cholinergic agents should be tried in the patient refractory to a single agent. Even more refractory bronchospasm requires either a short course of systemic steroids or intravenous aminophylline.

POSTOPERATIVE OLIGURIA AND RENAL INSUFFICIENCY

Etiology

The use of radiocontrast agents in the days immediately preceding cardiac surgery may embarrass renal function, as manifest by a rise in blood urea nitrogen and serum creatinine values. Following CPB, there is a substantial incidence of postoperative renal dysfunction (up to 30 percent) but a relatively low incidence of severe renal impairment requiring dialysis (1 to 5 percent). Renal blood flow and glomerular filtration rate are reduced by 25 to 75 percent during bypass, with partial but not complete recovery in the first day after CPB. This reduction in renal function is attributed to renal artery vasoconstriction, hypothermia, and loss of pulsatile perfusion during CPB. Angiotensin II levels are higher with nonpulsatile flow as compared to pulsatile flow. Although renal dysfunction cannot be consistently related to the systemic blood pressure and pump flow rate during nonpulsatile bypass, there is a definite relation between the incidence of postbypass renal dysfunction and the duration of CPB. In addition to the duration of CPB, the risk of developing postbypass renal failure seems to be a function of the patient's underlying renal function (also affected by age) and the perioperative circulatory status. The histologic changes that accompany renal impairment after cardiopulmonary bypass are characteristic of tubular necrosis. The tubular cells seem to be the most susceptible to acute reductions in renal perfusion.[20]

Management

There are three agents (so-called *renoprotective drugs*) that might be used during CPB to prevent an ischemic insult to the kidneys. Mannitol used in the CPB priming fluid may moderate ischemic insult, probably by volume expansion and hemodilution. It also initiates an osmotic diuresis, which prevents tubular obstruction and may serve as a free radical scavenger. Furosemide appears to improve renal blood flow when given during bypass. So-called *renal-dose* dopamine (1 to 2.5 µg/kg/min based on ideal body weight) may maintain renal blood flow and urine output. Once renal failure has developed, none of these drugs is likely to offer any beneficial effect. A megadose of furosemide (200 to 300 mg) may be tried, but if there is no diuretic response, it should not be repeated. Similarly, a single dose of mannitol (12.5 to 25 mg) either with or without furosemide could be tried, but it should not be repeated if there is no effect.

POSTOPERATIVE GASTROINTESTINAL DYSFUNCTION

Gastrointestinal Consequences of Cardiopulmonary Bypass

The gastrointestinal consequences of CPB appear to be minimal. Reviews of the subject report a 1 percent prevalence.[21,22] Most pa-

tients eat within 24 to 48 hours after an uncomplicated elective procedure. The limited investigations of the gastrointestinal tract after cardiac surgery have found a slight decrease in hepatic and pancreatic blood flow during cooling and rewarming on bypass and a decrease in gastric pH.[19,23] Transient elevations in liver function tests and hyperamylasemia may occur after cardiac surgery; the risk factors include long CPB time, multiple transfusions, and multiple valve replacements. Appearance of jaundice portends a poor prognosis.[24] Severe gastrointestinal complications are usually ischemic in nature and are often associated with a low-output syndrome.[19] The use of opioids as part of general anesthesia and postoperative pain management contributes to gastrointestinal dysfunction (cramping, ileus, and constipation) and to postoperative nausea and vomiting. The nausea and vomiting can be minimized by use of a naso- or orogastric tube to maintain gastric decompression intraoperatively and early in the postoperative period, with the additional benefit of improving thoracoabdominal compliance to positive-pressure ventilation. Occasionally acute cholelithiasis, appendicitis, diverticulitis, or bowel ischemia occur as acute abdominal problems.

POSTOPERATIVE METABOLIC DISORDERS

Potassium Imbalance

There are multiple factors that can produce large and rapid shifts in the serum potassium levels during and after CPB. The principal detrimental effects of these potassium shifts involve the electrical activity of the heart. The electrocardiographic signs of hyperkalemia and hypokalemia are described in Chap. 13. The electrocardiographic changes of hyperkalemia do not necessarily appear in the classic progressive manner; they are more related to the rate of rise in serum potassium rather than to the absolute serum concentration. The therapy of severe hyperkalemia should include counteracting the toxic cardiac effects of the elevated potassium with intravenous calcium gluconate or calcium chloride and lowering the serum level of potassium with sodium bicarbonate and/or administration of regular insulin and glucose. Hypokalemia is treated with the intravenous administration of KCl at a rate of no more than 10 to 15 mEq/h. The serum potassium rises approximately 0.1 mEq/L for each 2 mEq of KCl administered. Large doses of KCl should be administered by a central venous catheter because of the caustic effect of potassium on peripheral veins.

Hypomagnesemia

Hypomagnesemia is common following cardiac surgery using CPB. Magnesium mimics potassium in its effects on the electrical activity of the heart. The cause of the hypomagnesemia is unknown, but it is probably multifactorial. Many patients will be hypomagnesemic preoperatively because of the use of loop diuretics, thiazides, digoxin, or alcohol, and the effects of type 1 diabetes mellitus. Magnesium is usually lost in the urine during CPB. Patients with postoperative hypomagnesemia develop atrial and ventricular dysrhythmias more frequently and require more prolonged mechanical ventilatory support than do patients with normal magnesium levels.[25] Magnesium administration also seems to improve stroke volume and cardiac index in the early postoperative period.[26] Magnesium can be administered as magnesium sulfate (2 g in a 100-mL solution) to raise serum levels to 2 mEq/L.

Hyperglycemia

During CPB there is a rise in blood glucose levels. The elevation is modest during hypothermia and becomes more marked during rewarming. This rise in glucose is partly a result of increased glucose mobilization related to dramatic increases in cortisol, catecholamine, and growth hormone levels during CPB. Also, there is an apparent failure of insulin secretion, particularly during hypothermia, probably related to inhibition of the insulin secretory response by the elevated catecholamines. This blunting of the insulin response persists for the first 24 hours after surgery. These changes are exaggerated in the diabetic patient.[27] Insulin requirements are likely to be seven times greater than the preoperative requirements during the first 4 hours postoperatively. Furthermore, such insulin resistance is exacerbated by catecholamines, diuretics, and blood transfusions.[28] Hyperglycemia results in poorer wound healing, more infections complications, and overall worse outcome. Aggressive glycemic control improves the clinical outcomes. IV insulin infusion is appropriate for all type 1 diabetic patients and most type 2 diabetics. A variety of insulin infusion protocols have been published.

POSTOPERATIVE FEVER

Fever is a common occurrence in the postoperative patient. It is generally a consequence of pleuropericarditis, atelectasis, or phlebitis. A reasonable assumption in a patient with a core temperature <100.4°F (38°C) and no evidence of phlebitis or presence of a pericardial or pleural rub is that the source of the fever is atelectasis. The appropriate therapeutic approach is to encourage intensified efforts at incentive spirometry and coughing. Any fever >101.3°F (38.5°C) warrants blood, sputum, and urine cultures. A white blood cell count (total and differential) and a chest radiograph should also be obtained. Sternal wound infections occur in 0.4 to 5 percent of patients after sternotomy.[29–31] Multiple factors have been identified as increasing the risk of developing sternal wound infection. These include pneumonia, prolonged mechanical ventilation (especially with tracheostomy), emergency operations, postoperative hemorrhage with mediastinal hematoma, early reexploration, obesity, diabetes mellitus, and use of bilateral internal mammary grafts. The greatest risk for sternal infection seems to be in diabetic patients who receive bilateral internal mammary grafts.[30] Debate continues as to whether the most appropriate initial treatment is debridement and closure, or open packing and subsequent plastic surgical closure with a muscle flap.

Approximately 1 percent of patients who have had coronary artery bypass surgery experience leg wound infections that necessitate extra care. Leg infections seem to occur more frequently in obese women, especially if the thigh veins are harvested.[32]

NEUROLOGIC AND NEUROPHYSIOLOGIC DYSFUNCTION

Mechanism

The mechanisms thought to account for most cerebral injury during cardiac surgery are macroembolization of air; debris from aortic atheroma or left ventricular thrombus; microembolization of aggregates of granulocytes, platelets, and fibrin; and cerebral hypoperfusion. The total number of intraoperative microemboli, as well as the proportion of solid microemboli, has been demonstrated by transcranial Doppler ultrasound are reduced with "off-pump," as compared to "on-pump," CABG. Death or disabling stroke occurs in approximately 2 percent of patients, with another 3 percent experiencing transient or minor functional disability secondary to cerebral infarction. Focal neurologic deficits resulting from intraoperative events are usually noted within the first 24 to 48 hours after surgery.

Encephalopathy and Delirium

From 33 to 67 percent of patients can be documented to have a cognitive decline of variable duration following CABG. Despite the reduction in cerebral microemboli with "off-pump" CABG, initial trials failed to demonstrate a significant difference in cognitive decline with "off-pump" CABG. Although the appearance of encephalopathic symptoms likely reflects cerebral injury, other causes must be excluded, including drugs, sepsis, fever, hypoxemia, ethanol withdrawal, renal failure, and hyperosmolar state. Postoperative encephalopathic changes, varying from mild confusion and disorientation to protracted somnolence or agitation and hallucinations, may appear at any time during the hospital stay.[33] Studies of this condition have not identified any consistent risk factors, but advancing age, duration of CPB, and sleep deprivation are frequently associated. The prevalence of this condition has remained rather constant since the early days of cardiac surgery involving CPB, but there has been a shift in the clinical presentation. Currently, the condition seems to present with disorientation rather than with hallucinations, paranoid ideation, and the agitation that had been noted earlier.[33] Recognition of this entity is important because the family can be assured that the patient's mental status is likely to recover. Agitation and acute psychosis in these patients usually respond to intravenous haloperidol, 2 to 10 mg, repeated as needed to produce adequate sedation.

Brachial Plexopathy and Ulnar Nerve Dysfunction

Another serious neurologic complication of cardiac surgery is brachial plexopathy. This neurologic dysfunction, involving C8 and T1, usually results from mechanical trauma secondary to sternal retraction, but it may be caused by penetration by a posterior fractured segment of the first rib or injury during internal jugular cannulation. There is no specific therapy for this condition, and recovery can take as long as 6 months, with a few cases being permanent.[34] Ulnar nerve dysfunction may result from malpositioning of the upper extremities during surgery, which results in pressure being exerted on the ulnar nerve at the elbow.

REFERENCES

1. Aps C. Fast-tracking in cardiac surgery. *Br J Hosp Med* 1995;54:139–142.
2. Jindosi A, Aps C, Neville E, et al. Postoperative cardiac surgical care: an alternative approach. *Br Heart J* 1993;69:59–64.
3. Bojar RM. *Manual of Perioperative Care in Cardiac and Thoracic Surgery*, 2d ed. Boston: Blackwell Scientific, 1994.
4. Cameron D. Initiation of white cell activation during cardiopulmonary bypass: cytokines and receptors. *J Cardiovasc Pharmacol* 1996;27(Suppl 1):S1–S5.
5. Gold JP, Roberts AJ, Hoover EL, et al. Effects of prolonged aortic cross clamping with potassium cardioplegia on myocardial contractility in man. *Surg Forum* 1979;30:252–254.

6. Bolli R. Oxygen derived free radicals and postischemic myocardial dysfunction. *J Am Coll Cardiol* 1988;12:239–249.

7. Przyklenk K, Kloner RA. "Reperfusion injury" by oxygen derived radicals? *Circ Res* 1989;64:86–96.

8. Breisblatt WM, Stein KI, Wolfe CJ, et al. Acute myocardial dysfunction and recovery: a common occurrence after coronary bypass surgery. *J Am Coll Cardiol* 1990;15:1261–1269.

9. Keenan T, Abu-Omar Y, Taggart D. Bypassing the pump: changing practices in coronary artery surgery. *Chest* 2005;128:363–369.

10. Donati F, Maille JG, Blain R, et al. End-tidal carbon dioxide tension and temperature changes after coronary artery bypass surgery. *Can Anaesth Soc J* 1985;32:272–277.

11. Harker L, Malpass TW, Branson HE, et al. Mechanism of abnormal bleeding in patients undergoing cardiopulmonary bypass: acquired transient platelet dysfunction associated with selective alpha-granule release. *Blood* 1980;56:824–834.

12. Levi M, Peters M, Butler H. Efficacy and safety of recombinant factor VIIa for treatment of severe bleeding: a systematic review. *Crit Care Med* 2005;33:883–890.

13. Topol EJ, Lerman BB, Baughman KL, et al. De novo refractory ventricular tachyarrhythmias after coronary revascularization. *Am J Cardiol* 1986;57:57–59.

14. Leith JW, Thomson D, Baird DK, Harris PJ. The importance of age as a predictor of atrial fibrillation and flutter after coronary artery bypass grafting. *J Thorac Cardiovasc Surg* 1990;100:338–342.

15. Hashimoto K, Ilstrup DM, Schaff HV. Influence of clinical and hemodynamic variables on risk of supraventricular tachycardia after coronary artery bypass. *J Thorac Cardiovasc Surg* 1991;101:56–65.

16. Andrews TC, Reimold SC, Berlin JA, Antman EM. Prevention of supraventricular arrhythmias after coronary artery bypass surgery. A meta-analysis of randomized controlled trials. *Circulation* 1991;84(Suppl III):III-236–III-244.

17. Daoud EG, Strickberger SA, Man KC, et al. Preoperative amiodarone as prophylaxis against atrial fibrillation after heart surgery. *N Engl J Med* 1997;337:1785–1791.

18. Tuzcu EM, Emre A, Goormastic M, Loop FD. Incidence and prognostic significance of intraventricular conduction abnormalities after coronary bypass surgery. *J Am Coll Cardiol* 1990;16:607–610.

19. Sladden RN, Berkowitz DE. Cardiopulmonary bypass and the lung. In: Gravlee GP, Davis RF, Utley IR, eds. *Cardiopulmonary Bypass.* Baltimore: Williams & Wilkins, 1993:468–487.

20. Ramsey J. The respiratory, renal and hepatic systems: effects of cardiac surgery and cardiopulmonary bypass. In: Mora CT, ed. *Cardiopulmonary Bypass.* New York: Springer, 1995:147–168.

21. Hanks JB, Curtis SE, Hanks BB, et al. Gastrointestinal complications after cardiopulmonary bypass. *Surgery* 1982;92:394–400.

22. Welling RE, Rath R, Albers JE, Glaser RS. Gastrointestinal complications after cardiac surgery. *Arch Surg* 1986;121:1178–1180.

23. Mori A, Watanabe K, Onoe M, et al. Regional blood flow in the liver, pancreas, and kidney during pulsatile and nonpulsatile perfusion under profound hypothermia. *Jpn Circ J* 1988;52:219–227.

24. Collins JD, Bassendine MF, Ferner R, et al. Incidence and prognostic importance of jaundice after cardiopulmonary bypass surgery. *Lancet* 1983;1:1119–1123.

25. Aglio LS, Stanford GG, Maddi R, et al. Hypomagnesemia is common following cardiac surgery. *J Cardiothorac Anesth* 1991;5:201–208.

26. England MR, Gordon G, Salem M, Chernow B. Magnesium administration and dysrhythmias after cardiac surgery: a placebo-controlled, double-blind, randomized trial. *JAMA* 1993;269:2369–2370.

27. Frater RW, Oka Y, Kadish A, et al. Diabetes and coronary artery surgery. *Mt Sinai J Med* 1982;49:237–240.

28. Elliott MJ, Gill GV, Home PD, et al. A comparison of two regimens for the management of diabetes during open-heart surgery. *Anesthesiology* 1984;60:364–368.

29. Ulicny KS, Hiradzka SF. The risk factors of median sternotomy infection: a current review. *J Cardiac Surg* 1991;6:338–351.

30. Hazelrigg SR, Wellons HA, Schneider JA, Kolm P. Wound complications after median sternotomy: relationship to internal mammary grafting. *J Thorac Cardiovasc Surg* 1989;98:1096–1099.

31. Grossi EA, Esposito R, Harris LJ, et al. Sternal wound infections and use of internal mammary artery grafts. *J Thorac Cardiovasc Surg* 1991;102:342–347.

32. De Laria GA, Hunter JA, Goldin MD, et al. Leg wound complications associated with coronary revascularization. *J Thorac Cardiovasc Surg* 1981;81:403–407.

33. Breuer AC, Furlan AJ, Hanson MR, et al. Central nervous system complications of coronary artery bypass graft surgery: prospective analysis of 421 patients. *Stroke* 1983;14:82–87.

34. Shaw PJ, Bates D, Cartlidge NE, et al. Early neurological complications of coronary artery bypass surgery. *Br Med J* 1985;291(6506):1384-1387.

CHAPTER (67)

Rehabilitation of the Patient with Coronary Heart Disease

Ian Graham / Shirley Ingram / Noeleen Fallon /
Tora Leong / John Gormley / Veronica O'Doherty /
Vincent Maher / Suzanne Benson

This chapter presents an account of cardiac rehabilitation that reflects both American and European perspectives. We find that the distinction between prevention and rehabilitation is becoming obsolete. The sections on risk estimation and prevention guidelines are partly based on European data and complement Chap. 51 which provides much evidence from American sources. References 1–7 in Chap. 51 and Tables 51–1, 51–2, and 51–3 reflect current American guidance. It should be stressed that the main objectives and targets are in close agreement. Both stress the need for total risk estimation as a first step in implementing practical preventive measures (see Chap. 11).

INTRODUCTION

Atherosclerotic cardiovascular disease, particularly coronary heart disease and stroke, is now the largest cause of death across the world except in sub-Saharan Africa.[1] The creation of coronary care units in 1961 and associated advances in medical and nursing care are thought have been responsible for the fall in mortality in patients with myocardial infarction (MI) from 25 to 30 percent, to 18 percent in the prethrombolytic era of the mid 1980s[2] to as low as 10 percent by 1997.[2,3] More recently, the needs of the patient recovering from cardiac disease have received increased attention, resulting in the development of cardiac rehabilitation.

Substantial changes have occurred in our concepts of cardiac rehabilitation in recent years. In Eastern Europe, rehabilitation often involved inpatient assessment and care. In America and Western Europe, structured outpatient programs were favored. There was comparatively little communication between the disciplines of epidemiology, prevention, and rehabilitation, despite the fact that prevention requires advice on exercise, and rehabilitation involves risk factor management.

The differentiation between primary and secondary prevention may be challenged. Pathologic studies indicated decades ago that atherosclerosis, the underlying cause of coronary heart disease, starts in childhood, develops insidiously, and is generally advanced by the time that symptoms occur. A person with asymptomatic disease on carotid ultrasonography or coronary artery calcification on CT scanning should be managed no less vigorously than one who has had a clinical event.

Newer diagnostic tests for acute coronary syndromes have taught us the obvious—that myocardial infarction represents a continuum of damage and does not occur suddenly when cardiac enzymes reach "two times the upper limit of normal." Newer therapies mean that, at least for those who reach medical care in time, major heart muscle loss with consequent complications such as shock or heart failure with a high risk of death is becoming unusual.

The presentation of a person with angina or an acute coronary syndrome, or, indeed, coincidental asymptomatic disease, should trigger the initiation of a lifelong program of risk factor modification including physical exercise. Of course death is deferred, not prevented, and rehabilitation programs now tend to see both more young people with multiple risk factors and older persons who have developed heart failure. The increasing prevalence of obesity and premature glucose intolerance pose additional problems.

Although the definitions of cardiac rehabilitation are several, many would accept the simple definition of *return to normal life*. Prolonged hospital attendance may create medical dependency and impede rather than assist such a return. Increasingly, hospital-based cardiac rehabilitation programs are seeking to integrate with community- and home-based programs. This is easier in medical systems that promote integration of health services.

A major advance has been the realization that no one individual or discipline owns rehabilitation. Most current rehabilitation programs are multidisciplinary, with all members participating in both the planning and delivery of programs and having a sense of coownership.

HISTORY AND CHANGING CONCEPTS

The first attempt at cardiac rehabilitation was probably made by the Greek physician Asclepiades of Bithynia in 1124 B.C. There have been various reports through the centuries by people such as William Stokes who, in 1854, advocated "early mobilization and walking" for patients with heart disease. This view was contrary to the opinion of the early 20th century, which stressed the importance of absolute bedrest for 4 to 8 weeks. Advocating the need for long-term restrictive physical, social, and vocational measures led inevitably to the concept of the cardiac cripple.

It was not until the early 1950s that this practice was challenged. Levine and Lown demonstrated that sitting in a chair 7 days after the onset of acute coronary symptoms was safe and had physical and psychological benefits.[4] The finding that prolonged rest causes deconditioned responses to exercises led to the use of physical training to aid recovery.[5]

Concurrent with gradual changes from sedentary convalescence to early mobilization, the importance of risk factors and lifestyles in the genesis of coronary disease was realized and the concept of cardiac rehabilitation was born. The first structured rehabilitation program was pioneered in Israel in 1955.[6]

From these beginnings, cardiac rehabilitation has developed worldwide, but differs widely among countries, from highly structured inpatient programs to informal home-based programs. While there may be no ideal rehabilitation program, the majority of programs consist of regular outpatient exercise and educational programs. Comprehensive rehabilitation involves a multidisciplinary team comprising physician, nurse coordinator, cardiovascular nurses, physiotherapist, sports therapist, dietician, pharmacist, social worker, clinical psychologist, vocational advisor, occupational therapist, and as many other professionals as are available to the program. The rationale for such a team approach is that disability in the cardiac patient arises for a number of different reasons which may be medical, psychological, nutritional, or social, as well as from the underlying cardiac complaint. These are most effectively tackled by using the skills of health professionals in these areas. The traditional aims of cardiac rehabilitation are to restore patients to their rightful place in the social and family structure, to improve psychological well-being, and to improve prognosis through secondary prevention measures.

The delivery of the cardiac rehabilitation service depends on a partnership between the patient, family members, multidisciplinary team, and primary care services, as well as on geographic location, until such time as the patient has the ability to reclaim control of his or her healthy lifestyle. Cardiac rehabilitation is tailored to meet each patient's needs with individual assessment of risk, including age, gender, family history, diabetes, alcohol intake, dyslipidemia, hypertension, smoking, obesity, physical inactivity and psychological status. Delivered by the multidisciplinary team, cardiac rehabilitation comprises exercise prescription, educational sessions, medication advice, healthy eating guidelines, stress management and relaxation, behavioral change, smoking cessation and vocational counseling. By incorporating lifestyle management, the intention is to reduce the possibility of a subsequent cardiac event, slow or stop the progression of cardiovascular disease (CVD) and improve quality of life.[7]

RECOMMENDATIONS AND GUIDELINES

Cardiac rehabilitation and secondary prevention programs are now accepted as an integral component of the comprehensive care of patients with cardiovascular disease. Typically, cardiac rehabilitation includes exercise and educational programs with the aim of promoting the uptake and maintenance of appropriate physical activity and a healthier lifestyle so as to positively influence the individual's recovery, and as a means of secondary prevention. Since the 1980s a variety of working groups and committees have published guidelines and recommendations for cardiac rehabilitation.[8–12]

In 1982 the World Health Organization Expert Committee for the Prevention of Coronary Heart Disease recommended that planned preventive measures should be part of usual care for every coronary artery disease patient.[13] Cardiac rehabilitation was subsequently defined as:

> *The sum of activities required to influence favorably the underlying cause of the disease, as well as to ensure the patients the best possible physical, mental and social conditions so that they may by their own efforts preserve, or resume*

when lost, as normal a place as possible in the life of the community. Rehabilitation cannot be regarded as an isolated form of therapy but must be integrated with the whole treatment, of which it only forms one facet.[14]

The World Health Organization has summarized the medical goals of cardiac rehabilitation as:

1. The prevention of cardiac death;
2. A decrease in cardiac morbidity; and
3. The relief of symptoms such as angina and breathlessness.[14]

In 1995, the U.S. Department of Health and Human Services, Public Health Service, Agency for Health Care Policy and Research issued guidelines[8] that are still widely used, and which describe cardiac rehabilitation as:

Comprehensive long-term programs involving medical evaluation, prescribed exercise, cardiac risk factor modification, education, and counseling, designed to limit the physiological and psychological effect of cardiac illness, reduce the risk of sudden death or reinfarction, control cardiac symptoms, and enhance the psychological and vocational status of the individual patient.

In the 21st century, the Scottish Intercollegiate Guidelines Network (SIGN)[10] and European Society of Cardiology (ESC)[11] published guidelines with regard to evaluation and intervention in all aspects of cardiac rehabilitation. These initiatives were aimed to assist cardiac rehabilitation staff with the development of cardiac rehabilitation programs at European level. The SIGN guideline 57[10] states that:

Cardiac rehabilitation is the process by which patients with cardiac disease, in partnership with a multidisciplinary team of health professionals, are encouraged and supported to achieve and maintain optimal physical and psychosocial health.

The American Heart Association (AHA) consensus statement[9] on "core components" of cardiac rehabilitation recognizes the role cardiac rehabilitation has to play in risk factor management, defining specific goals for lifestyle targets; these have similarly been adopted by the ESC.[11] Physical activity is also strongly emphasized in the current European guidelines on cardiovascular disease prevention.[15]

PREVENTION AND REHABILITATION: WHAT'S THE DIFFERENCE?

The current European guidelines on cardiovascular disease prevention in clinical practice[15] give the highest priority to those with established cardiovascular disease. What priorities should be set given limited resources?

The priorities in terms of patient selection for cardiovascular disease prevention in clinical practice are:

1. Patients with established coronary heart disease, peripheral artery disease and cerebrovascular atherosclerotic disease.

2. Asymptomatic individuals who are at high risk of developing atherosclerotic disease because of:
   (a) multiple risk factors resulting in a 10-year risk of >5 percent now (or if extrapolated to age 60 years) for developing a fatal CVD event.
   (b) markedly raised levels of single risk factors: cholesterol >8 mmol/L (320 mg/dl), low-density lipoprotein (LDL) cholesterol >6 mmol/L (240 mg/dL), blood pressure >180/110 mmHg.
   (c) diabetes type 2 and diabetes type 1 with microalbuminuria.
3. Close relatives of:
   (a) patients with early onset atherosclerotic cardiovascular disease.
   (b) asymptomatic individuals who are at particularly high risk.
4. Other individuals encountered in routine clinical practice.

This confirms the realization that the aims of prevention and rehabilitation are the same. There is a trend to offer rehabilitation services to asymptomatic high risk persons. Such people can be identified by risk scoring systems such as those advocated in Chap. 51, or by using the European SCORE system (Figs. 67–1A and B), which illustrates graphically that, in most people, risk is the product of multiple interacting risk factors.

Risk factor targets for those at very high risk, which includes all who have had an atherosclerotic clinical event, in the European Guidelines[15] are as follows:

- No tobacco
- Make healthy food choices
- Be physically active
- Body mass index <25 kg/m^2
- Blood pressure <140/90 mmHg; <130/80 mmHg in diabetics
- Total cholesterol <175 mg/dL (4.5 mmol/L)
- LDL cholesterol <100 mg/dL (2.5 mmol/L)

RATIONALE: THE EVIDENCE BASE

Early randomized trials of cardiac rehabilitation after acute myocardial infarction show consistent trends toward a survival benefit among patients enrolled in cardiac rehabilitation programs. Meta-analyses of these randomized trials have calculated a significant 20 to 25 percent reduction in cardiovascular death, but no change in the occurrence of nonfatal reinfarction in patients assigned to medically supervised and prescribed exercise programs.[16,17] A more recent meta-analysis of exercise-based rehabilitation by Jolliffe et al. demonstrated a 27 percent decrease in all cause mortality with exercise only cardiac rehabilitation, and a 13 percent decrease with comprehensive cardiac rehabilitation, but could not conclude that exercise alone was significantly better than a comprehensive approach.[18] Total cardiac mortality was reduced by 31 percent with exercise-only cardiac rehabilitation and by 26 percent with comprehensive cardiac rehabilitation. The populations studied were male, middle-aged, and low risk, and therefore may not reflect the entire population suitable for cardiac rehabilitation. For example, those who present with comorbidities, are female, older, or of different ethnicity. The majority of these studies did not report details of medications or thrombolysis, which may have affected mortality rates.

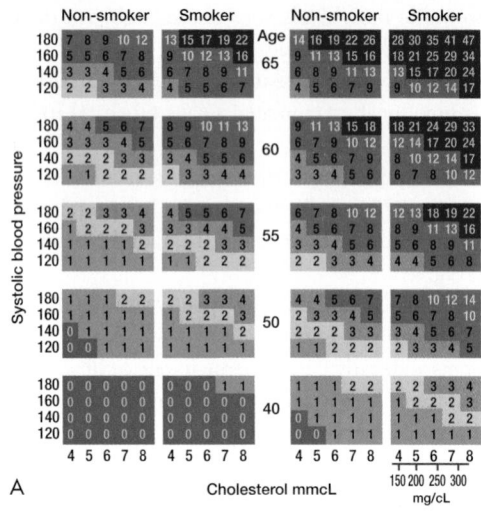

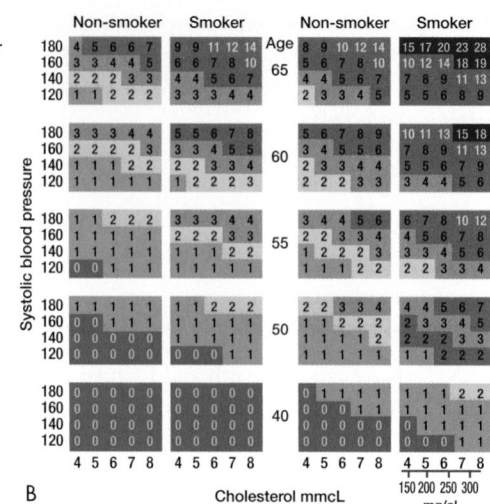

10-year risk of fatal CVD in high-risk regions of Europe by gender, age, systolic blood pressure, total cholesterol and smoking status.

10-year risk of fatal CVD in low-risk regions of Europe by gender, age, systolic blood pressure, total cholesterol and smoking status.

INSTRUCTIONS ON HOW TO USE THE CHART

- The low-risk chart should be used in Belgium, France, Greece, Italy, Luxembourg, Spain, Switzerland and Portugal; the high-risk chart should be used in all other countries of Europe.

- To estimate a person's total ten-year risk of CVD death, find the table for their gender, smoking status and age. Within the table find the cell nearest to the person's systolic blood pressure (mmHg) and total cholesterol (mmcL/L or mg/cL).

- The effect of lifetime exposure to risk factors can be seen by following the table upwards. This can be used when advising younger people.

- Low-risk individuals should be offered advice to maintain their low-risk status. Those who are at 5% risk or higher or will reach this level in middle age should be given maximal attention.

- To define a person's relative risk, compare their risk category with that of a nonsmoking person of the same age and gender, blood pressure <140/90 mmHg and total cholesterol <5 mmcL/L (190 mg/cL).

- The chart can be used to give some indications of the effect of changes from one risk category to another, for example, when the subject stops smoking or reduces other risk factors.

QUALIFIERS

Note that total CVD risk may be higher than indicated in the chart:

- as the person approaches the next age category

- in asymptomatic subjects with pre-clinical evidence of atherosclerosis (e.g., CT scan, ultrasonography)

- in subjects with a strong family history of premature CVD

- in subjects with low HDL cholesterol levels, with raised triglyceride levels, with impaired glucose tolerance and with raised levels of C-reactive protein, fibrinogen, homocysteine, apolipoprotein B or Lp(a).

- in obese and sedentary subjects.

FIGURE 67–1. A. SCORE chart for high-risk regions of Europe. **B.** SCORE chart for low-risk regions of Europe.

In a systematic review of randomized, controlled trials conducted up to March 2003, Taylor and coworkers found a decrease in all-cause mortality of 20 percent and a decrease in cardiac mortality of 26 percent with no significant differences between exercise-only cardiac rehabilitation and comprehensive cardiac rehabilitation. This analysis included more randomized, controlled trials from the thrombolysis era and the period of intensive lipid-lowering therapies.[19]

These meta-analyses suggest that reported mortality reductions associated with exercise-based rehabilitation may apply to both subjects with acute coronary syndromes and to those who have undergone revascularization. Psychological benefits, improved coronary blood flow, functional capacity, and reductions in risk factors and inducible ischaemia have also been reported.

BROAD PRINCIPLES OF CARDIAC REHABILITATION

Table 67–1 summarizes the indications and contraindications for cardiac rehabilitation. It will be appreciated that such lists are for guidance only and should be tempered by clinical judgement. Clearly, some of the listed contraindications, such as acute systemic illness, may be temporary.[20]

【 】 PHASES

Worldwide, cardiac rehabilitation is structured in different ways. The term *phase* is used to describe the varying timeframes after a cardiac event. There are four phases of cardiac rehabilitation in both Europe and United States (Table 67–2), but there are variations in the structure of these phases between the two continents. In some European countries, residential cardiac rehabilitation is the common practice for more complicated, disabled patients, and outpatient cardiac rehabilitation is used for more independent, lower-risk, and clinically stable patients.

Phase I traditionally begins on admission to the coronary care unit. The patient is reviewed by the cardiac rehabilitation team members. Individual risk factors are discussed and the patient is introduced to the concept of lifelong lifestyle changes. Pain and anxiety may impede effective communication and advice must be simple and repetitive. As soon as it is deemed safe, simple breathing and leg exercises are commenced with a program of gradual mobilization. The emphasis at this stage is to counteract the negative effects of deconditioning after a cardiac event rather than to promote training adaptations.[21] The patient may require intervention from other members of the multidisciplinary team at this stage, for example, the dietician, social worker, psychologist, or the smoking-cessation officer. This is an ideal opportunity to commence education and psychological support. Following discharge from the coronary care unit, the cardiac rehabilitation team continues patient education and counseling. A discharge plan is formulated taking into account individual needs such as return to work, medications, and exercise program. Prior to discharge, the patient might visit the rehabilitation gym and meet recovering patients.

Phase II usually consists of an educational program where exercise is prescribed by the physiotherapist and plans for the patient to attend phase III are consolidated. The patient may have ongoing review by various members of the multidisciplinary team for example, the dietician or psychologist at this stage.

Phase III usually consists of an 8- to 12-week program of structured or supervised exercise and education. When a 4-week program was compared to a usual care 10-week program, higher attendance in the 4-week group (96 percent vs. 84 percent) was noted. This suggests that brief and intense cardiac rehabilitation is acceptable to patients.[22] This phase involves the expertise of the multidisciplinary team and the commitment of the patient to attend the program. Traditionally, this program was always hospital based but community-led or independent programs are also available. In the United

TABLE 67–1

Clinical Indications and Contraindications for Inpatient and Outpatient Cardiac Rehabilitation

Indications
- Medically stable after myocardial infarction
- Stable angina
- Coronary artery bypass surgery
- Percutaneous transluminal coronary angioplasty
- Compensated congestive heart failure
- Cardiomyopathy
- Heart or other organ transplantation
- Other cardiac surgery including valvular and pacemaker insertion (including implantable cardioverter defibrillator)
- Peripheral vascular disease
- High-risk cardiovascular disease ineligible for surgical intervention
- Sudden cardiac death syndrome
- End-stage renal disease
- At risk for coronary artery disease, with diagnosis of diabetes mellitus, hyperlipidemia, hypertension, etc.
- Other patients who may benefit from structured exercise and/or patient education (based on physician referral and consensus of the rehabilitation team)

Contraindications
- Unstable angina
- Resting systolic blood pressure (>200 mmHg or diastolic >110 mmHg)
- Blood pressure drop of >20 mmHg with symptoms
- Severe aortic stenosis
- Acute systemic illness or fever
- Uncontrolled atrial or ventricular arrhythmias
- Uncontrolled tachycardia (>100 beats/min)
- Uncompensated congestive heart failure
- Third-degree heart block (without pacemaker)
- Active pericarditis or myocarditis
- Recent embolism
- Thrombophlebitis
- Resting ST displacement (>2 mm)
- Uncontrolled diabetes
- Orthopedic problems prohibiting exercise
- Other metabolic problems

Kingdom and Ireland, there are some home-based programs that are suited to the rural population who have too far a distance to travel to commit to a hospital-based program.

Phase IV is, ideally, the maintenance program in the form of a lifelong commitment to exercise and healthy nutrition.

THE COMPONENTS OF CARDIAC REHABILITATION

The mode in which cardiac rehabilitation is delivered may differ nationally and internationally but there are certain standard core

TABLE 67–2

Traditional Terminology for the Phases of Cardiac Rehabilitation

Phase I

Inpatient rehabilitation, usually lasting for the duration of hospitalization. It emphasizes a gradual, progressive approach to exercise and an education program that helps the patient understand the disease process, and initial preventive efforts to slow the progression of disease.

Phase II

Multifaceted safe physical activity to improve conditioning with continued behavior modification aimed at smoking cessation, weight loss, healthy eating, and other factors to reduce disease risk. Initiate an exercise prescription

Phase III

Supervised rehabilitation lasting 6 to 12 months. Establishes a prescription for safe exercise that can be performed at home or in a community service facility, such as a senior center or YMCA, and continues to emphasize risk-factor reduction.

Phase IV

Maintenance, indefinite

SOURCE: Adapted from Pasternak RC. Comprehensive rehabilitation of patients with cardiovascular disease. In: Braunwald E, Zipes D, Libby P, Bonow R, eds. Braunwald's Heart Disease, A Textbook of Cardiovascular Medicine, 7th ed. Philadelphia: Elsevier Saunders, 2004:1086.

components, outlined in Table 67–3, that have been adopted by Europe and the United States.

[ ] TARGET POPULATION

Traditionally, cardiac rehabilitation is offered to patients after uncomplicated myocardial infarction or post successful revascularization, that is, coronary artery bypass surgery or percutaneous intervention.[21] Demographic changes and advances in medical care have occurred that dictate cardiac rehabilitation, including for high-risk patients, many of whom have complicated cardiac histories. Elderly patients who have additional comorbidities, heart-failure patients, patients with implantable cardioverter defibrillators, and postcardiac transplantation make up the majority of this high-risk group. Insurance and reimbursement patterns differ in the United States and Europe, with little or none present in the United Kingdom and Ireland where the service is offered within the public hospital sector at no charge.

THE MULTIDISCIPLINARY COMPONENTS AND ROLES

All current recommendations on prevention and rehabilitation acknowledge that patient management should be based on an assessment of total risk. As the highest-risk individuals gain most from intervention, current European guidelines[15] define priorities for prevention as

well as for rehabilitation (Table 67–4). The various components addressed by cardiac rehabilitation programs may include:

- Behavior change
- Smoking
- Exercise
- Weight management
- Nutrition
- Lipids
- Blood pressure
- Psychosocial factors
- Cardiopulmonary resuscitation training

[ ] BEHAVIOR CHANGE

Strategies to make behavioral counseling more effective have been summarized,[15] and include:

- Developing a therapeutic alliance with the patient
- Gaining commitment from the patient to achieve lifestyle change
- Ensuring the patient understands the relationship between lifestyle and disease
- Helping the patient overcome barriers to lifestyle change
- Involving the patient in identifying the risk factor(s) to change
- Designing a lifestyle modification plan
- Using strategies to reinforce the patients' own capacity to change
- Monitoring progress of lifestyle change through followup contacts
- Involving other healthcare staff wherever possible

[ ] SMOKING

Cigarette smoking is the leading cause of preventable death.[23] Approximately 1.1 billion people smoke worldwide. This figure is expected to increase to more than 1.6 billion by 2025.[24] The causative relationship between smoking and cardiovascular disease is well established. Cigarette smoking is a major risk factor for the development of coronary artery disease and increases the risk of mortality and morbidity among people with established coronary artery disease.[7] There are a multitude of cardiovascular toxins in tobacco smoke, and Table 67–5 lists its effects on the cardiovascular system. Smoking cessation will reduce the subsequent risk of mortality by up to 9 percent in absolute terms.[24] Observational studies in postmyocardial infarction subjects suggest that this may be reflected as a halving of long-term mortality.

Cardiac rehabilitation is the ideal setting to promote smoking cessation. Educating patients about the association between smoking and heart disease in this vulnerable period may be the trigger to motivate smoking cessation. Numerous nonpharmacologic and pharmacologic agents are available to aid the patient and health professional with this campaign. Both group therapy and individual counseling to instigate behavioral change are useful in helping the patient to quit smoking. Nicotine replacement therapy in the form of transdermal patches, chewing gum, nasal spray, oral inhalers and sublingual tablets are safe and may augment this process.

Strategies that may help include the *five As*[15]:

- Ask: systematically identify all smokers at every opportunity
- Assess: determine the patient's degree of addiction and readiness to cease smoking

TABLE 67–3

Core Components of Cardiac Rehabilitation/Secondary Prevention Programs and Expected Outcomes

Initial evaluation
- Take medical history and perform physical examination
- Measure risk factors
- Obtain electrocardiograms at rest and during exercise
- Determine level of risk
- Assess occupational status and prepare vocational counseling

Management of lipid levels[a]
- Assess and modify diet, physical activity, and drug therapy
- Primary goal: LDL cholesterol <100 mg/dL
- Secondary goals: HDL cholesterol >45 mg/dL, triglycerides <200 mg/dL

Management of hypertension[a]
- Measure blood pressure on >2 visits
- If resting systolic pressure is >140 mmHg or diastolic pressure is >90 mmHg, recommend drug therapy
- Monitor effects of intervention in collaboration with primary care physician
- Goal: blood pressure <140/90 mmHg (or <130/85 mmHg if patient has diabetes or chronic heart or renal failure)

Cessation of smoking
- Document smoking status (never smoked, stopped smoking in remote past, stopped smoking recently or currently smokes)
- Determine patient's readiness to quit; if ready, pick date
- Offer nicotine-replacement therapy, bupropion, or both
- Offer behavioral advice and group or individual counseling
- Goal: long-term abstinence

Weight reduction
- Consider for patients with BMI >25 or waist circumference >40 inches (100 cm; in men), >35 inches (90 cm; in women), particularly if associated with hypertension, hyperlipidemia, or insulin resistance or diabetes
- Provide behavioral and nutritional counselling with follow-up to monitor progress in achieving goals
- Goal: loss of 5% to 10% of body weight and modification of associated risk factors with long-term adherence
- For newly detected diabetes, refer patient to primary care physician for evaluation and treatment
- Goals: normalization of fasting plasma glucose level (80 to 110mg/dL) or glycosylated hemoglobin level (<7.0%) and control of associated obesity, hypertension, and hyperlipidemia

Psychosocial management
- Identify psychosocial problems such as denial, depression, anxiety, social isolation, anger, and hostility by means of an interview, standardized questionnaire, or both
- Provide individual or group counselling, or both, for patients with clinically significant psychosocial problems
- Provide stress-reduction classes for all patients
- Provide family members intervention
- Goal: improvement of clinically significant psychosocial problems and acquisition of stress-management skills

Physical activity counseling and exercise training
- Assess current physical activity and exercise tolerance with monitored exercise stress test
- Identify barriers to increased physical activity
- Provide advice regarding increasing physical activity
- Develop an individualized regimen of aerobic and resistance training, specifying frequency, intensity, duration, and types of exercise
- Goals: increases in regular physical activity, strength, and physical functioning; more simply, at least 30 min of submaximal work or moderate exercise daily is recommended. Greater benefit however can be achieved by further increasing physical activity

[a]Targets in mmol would be low-density lipoprotein cholesterol <2.5 mmol/L, high-density lipoprotein cholesterol >1.2 mmol/L, triglycerides <2.2 mmol/L. European Guidelines do not define specific targets for high-density lipoprotein cholesterol and triglycerides. The European blood pressure target for diabetics is slightly more rigorous at <130/80 mm Hg.
SOURCE: Adapted from Balady GJ, Ades PA, Comoss P, et al.[9]

- Advise: urge strongly all smokers to quit
- Assist: agree on a smoking-cessation strategy including behavioral counseling, nicotine replacement therapy, and/or pharmacologic intervention
- Arrange a schedule of followup visits

【 】 EXERCISE

The evidence base for exercise-based and comprehensive cardiac rehabilitation programs was considered in Rationale: The Evidence Base. Meta-analyses suggest that both may be associated with a reduction in

TABLE 67–4

Main Objectives for Prevention in Patients with Established Cardiovascular Disease and in High-Risk People

No smoking
Make healthy food choices
Be physically active
Body mass index <25 kg/m²
Blood pressure <140/90 mmHg in most, <130/80 mmHg in particular groups
Low-density lipoprotein cholesterol <3 mmol/L (115 mg/dL) in most, <2.5 mmol/L (100 mg/dL) in particular groups
Good glycemic control in all persons with diabetes
Consider other prophylactic drug therapy in particular patient groups

TABLE 67–5

Effects of Smoking on Cardiovascular System

Free radicals oxidize low-density lipoprotein and cause endothelial injury
Stimulation of smooth muscle proliferation and cell migration to intima
Nicotine increases platelet adhesion to the endothelium
Nicotine increases fibrinogen levels (increased clotting)
↑ Lipids and harmful lipoproteins
↑ Insulin resistance → may cause diabetes mellitus
↓ Coronary artery blood flow by ↑ sympathetic nervous system
Nicotine causes release of adrenaline into blood stream and constriction of arterioles and veins
Hemoglobin binds to carbon monoxide reducing availability of O_2
Tar is a solid irritant linked with cancer

mortality after acute coronary syndromes and after revascularization procedures, and with other psychological and physical benefits.

Phase I (The Inpatient)

The major components of this inpatient stage are evaluation of the patients condition, an assessment of their motivation, risk-factor assessment, education, mobilization, and discharge planning.[12,17] It can be difficult for the healthcare professional to address all components adequately as the time spent in a medical facility may only be 4 to 7 days for a patient with an uncomplicated myocardial infarction. Exercise is gradually introduced on day 2 to the patient and the intensity of exercise up to discharge usually does not exceed 4 metabolic equivalents (METS). By day 4, the patient will have progressed to walking 5 to 10 minutes in the corridor three or four times per day.

Phase II (Postdischarge)

This is the period following discharge from the medical facility and prior to the commencement of the phase III/outpatient. The length of time between discharge and commencement of the phase III program varies between countries and facilities. Contact between the patient and the rehabilitation team can vary from a telephone call to home visits. Thus it is imperative that the patient has clear instructions on his or her individualized exercise prescription. The usual mode of exercise prescribed is walking on level ground initially. The intensity should be maintained at approximately 4 METS and heart rate should not exceed 20 beats/min above their resting heart rate, or a score of 11 to 12 on the rating of perceived exertion scale in the early stages. In practical terms, we advise patients to stay indoors for the first day or two as they may expect to feel somewhat fatigued and perhaps anxious. Uncomplicated cases are advised to increase their walking distance progressively to three to 3 miles (5 kilometers) daily after 4 to 6 weeks.

Phase III (Outpatient Exercise Program)

The aim of this phase of a cardiac rehabilitation program is to enable the patient to exercise safely in a structured environment and to understand the benefits of exercise. Prior to commencing an exercise program, it is usual for a patient to undergo a symptom-limited exercise stress test. Exercise testing can be used as either a

diagnostic or prognostic tool, or as a test of functional capacity. It is for the latter reason that exercise testing is most commonly used in cardiac rehabilitation. This information aids assessment for exercise prescription, return-to-work evaluation, and helps in an estimation of prognosis. Not all patients referred for cardiac rehabilitation may require an exercise test but the absence of a test may lead to an inappropriate exercise prescription.[25] Furthermore, there are many absolute and relative contraindications to exercise testing and these are shown in Table 67–6.

Current recommended intensities for the structured exercise in phase III (outpatient phase) are 60 to 75 percent of maximum heart rate (HR_{max}), or 40 to 60 percent of maximum heart rate reserve, corresponding to a score of 12 to 15 on the rating of perceived exertion scale. Although most accurately measured using a cardiac stress test, the most common way of calculating the HR_{max} is to subtract the patient's age from 220. The heart rate reserve is calculated by subtracting the resting heart rate from the HR_{max}. The duration of the program may vary from 8 to 12 weeks and patients attend two to three times per week. This is deemed sufficient to achieve both physiologic and psychosocial adaptations.[10] It is important to stress to participants that it is necessary to exercise on nonprogram days to achieve maximal potential.

The types of exercises used during the exercise program should promote total physical conditioning and should include treadmills, cycle and arm ergometers, stair climbers, and rowing machines.[20] These exercises are mainly aerobic in nature but resistance training can be used in low- to moderate-risk cardiac patients. It is, however, recommended that patients spend some time on aerobic-type exercises first before progressing to resistance exercise. This allows them to become used to monitoring their own exercise intensity.[10] The type and quantity of equipment available will depend on the resources available, the available space, and the number of patients in the group. It is usual for 8 to 10 patients of similar functional capacities to exercise together, but this number will vary depending on the patients' functional limitation and the availability of staff. A warmup period of approximately 15 minutes is followed by the exercise session lasting 30 to 35 minutes, and followed by a cool down period of 10 minutes.

TABLE 67-6

Absolute and Relative Contraindications to Exercise Testing (American College of Sports Medicine 2005)

Absolute contraindications
- Acute MI (within 2 days)
- High risk unstable angina
- Uncontrolled cardiac arrhythmias causing symptoms or hemodynamic compromise
- Acute endocarditis
- Symptomatic severe aortic stenosis
- Decompensated symptomatic heart failure
- Acute pulmonary embolus or pulmonary infarction
- Acute noncardiac disorder that may affect exercise performance or be aggravated by exercise (e.g., infection, renal failure, thyrotoxicosis)
- Relative acute myocarditis or pericarditis
- Physical disability that would preclude safe and adequate test performance

Relative contraindications
- Left main coronary stenosis or its equivalent
- Moderate stenotic valvular heart disease
- Electrolyte abnormalities
- Tachyarrhythmias or bradyarrhythmias
- Atrial fibrillation with uncontrolled ventricular rate
- Hypertrophic cardiomyopathy
- Mental impairment leading to inability to cooperate
- High-degree atrioventricular block
- Severe arterial hypertension (systolic blood pressure > 200 mmHg and diastolic >110 mmHg

Phase IV

Phase IV is when the patient exercises independently and maintains his or her lifestyle modifications. Increased physical activity and increased physical fitness positively influence cardiovascular health but exercise must be current, as previous physical activity does not confer protection. The change in exercise behavior achieved during phase III (outpatient) has to be lifelong and is not just for the duration of the phase III program. Adherence to long-term exercise may be assisted by means of organized exercise sessions in a community setting.

[ ] EXERCISE STRESS TESTING

The exercise stress test is both a practical and useful means of clinical evaluation. A standard graded-exercise stress test assesses the patients' ability to tolerate increasing intensities of exercise while monitoring symptomatic and hemodynamic response for abnormalities such as myocardial ischaemia or electrical instability.[20] According to a World Health Organization expert committee on cardiac rehabilitation, the primary purpose of an exercise test is to determine the responses of the individual to efforts a given levels and from this information to estimate probable performance in specific life and occupational situations.[26] Indications for exercise stress testing include diagnostic, prognostic, and therapeutic appli-

cations. The main aim of exercise testing in cardiac rehabilitation is to determine the target heart rate for exercise prescription. Exercise stress testing in cardiac rehabilitation is performed to measure the ischemic threshold, assess for arrhythmias, assess exercise tolerance, evaluate hemodynamic changes (i.e. blood pressure, heart rate), and observe for signs and symptoms of ischemia. Although the need for prephase III exercise testing has been questioned in the past,[27] the majority of guidelines recommend a graded exercise stress test for all patients participating in cardiac rehabilitation.

The most accurate method of assessing exercise capacity is by means of a maximal exercise test using gas analysis. In the context of cardiac rehabilitation, this is not usually feasible or necessary, so incremental tests, which provide an estimate of exercise capacity, are employed. The test is traditionally carried out using a treadmill or a cycle ergometer with monitoring of ECG, heart rate, and blood pressure. The rating of perceived exertion is also assessed as well as the individual's description of their levels of angina and dyspnea.

There are various protocols available for exercise testing and the choice should depend on the outcome and the clinical characteristics of the patient. The Bruce protocol is perhaps the most common protocol used, but the increments between each stage are quite large, so for old or deconditioned patients, protocols such as the Naughton may be more appropriate.[20] Treadmill testing mimics exercise that most individuals are familiar with—walking—and patients are more likely to achieve a higher oxygen uptake and peak heart rate using a treadmill. Patients can be fearful and may use the handrails, which can affect the estimation of exercise capacity. Because of the associated noise, blood pressure monitoring may be difficult during treadmill testing. Although unfamiliar to many patients, a cycle ergometer may be more appropriate for those with orthopedic conditions, and because there is less movement of the arms and thorax, blood pressure and ECG recordings may be easier.[25] The exercise test usually lasts for 8 to 12 minutes and is terminated when the patient either reaches exhaustion, or when the patient achieves a physiologic end point such as the maximal predicted heart rate in the case of a maximal test, or 75 percent of maximal predicted heart rate for a submaximal test. Table 67–7 lists other absolute and relative indications for terminating the test.

The workload for exercise training can be calculated from the exercise test, and for cardiac patients, the heart rate is the most common method used. There are three methods of using the heart rate, and these include the direct method, the percent of HR_{max}, and the heart rate reserve. In the direct method, the heart rate is plotted against oxygen consumption and the appropriate exercise intensity extrapolated. The percent of HR_{max} method uses 60 to 75 percent of the heart rate achieved during the exercise test which approximates to 40 to 60 percent of an individuals VO_2max (maximal oxygen consumption). In the heart rate reserve method, the resting heart rate is subtracted from the maximal heart rate to give the heart rate reserve. If an exercise prescription of 60 to 80 percent VO_2max is required, then 60 percent and 80 percent values of the heart rate reserve are calculated and the resting heart rate added to each value to give the training heart rate values.

Safety of Cardiac Rehabilitation

Physical activity reduces the incidence of atherosclerosis and cardiovascular disease. Nevertheless, vigorous exercise may acutely

TABLE 67–7

Indications for Terminating Exercise Testing (American Association of Cardiovascular Prevention and Rehabilitation)

Absolute indications

- Drop in systolic blood pressure of >10 mmHg from baseline blood pressure despite an increase in workload when accompanied by other evidence of ischemia
- Moderately severe angina
- Increasing nervous system symptoms (e.g., ataxia, dizziness, or near syncope)
- Signs of poor perfusion (cyanosis or pallor)
- Technical difficulties monitoring the ECG or systolic pressure
- Subject's desire to stop
- Sustained ventricular tachycardia
- ST elevation (+1.0 mm) in leads without diagnostic Q waves (other than V_1 or aVR)

Relative indications

- Drop in systolic blood pressure of >10 mmHg from baseline blood pressure despite an increase in workload in the absence of other evidence of ischemia
- ST or QRS changes such as excessive ST depression (>2 mm horizontal) or downsloping ST-segment depression) or marked axis shift
- Arrhythmias other than sustained ventricular tachycardia, including multifocal premature ventricular contractions (PVCs), triplets of PVCs, supraventricular tachycardia, heart block, or bradyarrhythmias
- Fatigue, shortness of breath, wheezing, leg cramps, or claudication
- Development of bundle-branch block or intraventricular tachycardia
- Increasing chest pain
- Hypertensive response (systolic blood pressure >250 mmHg and/or a diastolic blood pressure of >115 mmHg)

and transiently increase risk of sudden cardiac death and myocardial infarction. Individuals diagnosed with coronary artery disease are at the highest risk of experiencing a cardiac event during exercise. It has been estimated that vigorous exercise increases the risk of cardiac event 100 times in this population. Conversely, studies of cardiac events during cardiac rehabilitation document that risk of vigorous exercise in such supervised populations is low.[28]

Residual coronary ischaemia may occur with reduced supply and increased demand during exercise, the main threat being ventricular fibrillation. However, exercise training as a component of cardiac rehabilitation is safe with low reports of adverse coronary events. The incidence of cardiac arrest is 8.9 per 1 million patient hours, 3.4 per 1 million patient hours for myocardial infarction, and 1.3 per 1 million patient hours for death.[29] A 16-year followup of cardiac rehabilitation patients in one center demonstrated an incidence rate of 17.1 per 1 million patient hours of medically supervised exercise.[30] Risk is increased *when there is* ex-

tensive damage to the myocardium, residual ischemia, and ventricular arrhythmias on exercise. Therefore, staff supervising such exercise programs must be appropriately trained in advanced cardiac life support, with ECG monitoring available for those patients deemed to be at high risk.

WEIGHT MANAGEMENT

Obesity is a major public health problem throughout the developed world. Current data from individual national studies suggest that in European countries between 10 and 20 percent of men and 10 and 25 percent of women are obese.[31] Studies indicate that overweight, obesity, and excess abdominal fat are related to important coronary heart disease risk factors, including high levels of total cholesterol, LDL cholesterol, triglycerides, blood pressure, fibrinogen, and insulin, and low levels of high-density lipoprotein (HDL)-cholesterol.[32]

For overweight and obese patients with coronary heart disease, the combination of a reduced energy diet and increased physical activity are recommended. An energy deficit is most readily achievable through choice of foods low in total fat content, with a reduction in saturated fat being preferable. Further reductions in total energy intake can be achieved by reducing refined carbohydrate intake. A recent meta-analysis reported that a low-fat diet, high in protein and fiber-rich carbohydrates is more satiating than higher kilocalorie fatty foods.[33] However, popular or commercial high-protein weight-loss diets restrict consumption of healthy foods and do not provide the variety of foods needed to meet nutritional needs.[34]

Nutrition

Nutrition plays a pivotal role in the etiology and development of cardiovascular disease. Good evidence exists for a range of dietary measures that can make a favorable contribution to the secondary prevention of coronary artery disease.[35] Changes in the quantity and quality of dietary fat improve the lipid profile.[36] Blood pressure is lowered by reducing sodium intake[37] and by increasing potassium intake.[38] Advice that encourages consumption of a diet relatively lower in any one or more of fat, trans-fatty acids, saturated fatty acids, cholesterol, or sodium, or relatively higher in any one of fruit, vegetables, polyunsaturated fatty acids, monounsaturated fatty acids, fish, fiber, or potassium is likely to reduce the risk of cardiovascular disease.[39–42] Dietary therapy is additive to drug therapy and further reduces cardiovascular risk. Failure to adopt a cardioprotective diet may result in the need to use higher doses or combinations of medications.[43,44] A cardioprotective diet pattern has been developed for easy incorporation into cardiac rehabilitation programs. The cumulative advantage accruing from all food and nutrients in an integrated dietary pattern offers the prospect of a substantial reduction in risk of cardiovascular disease for individuals and populations.[45]

This dietary pattern (which is based on the Mediterranean diet) is as follows:

- Low in saturated fatty acids
- Low in trans-fatty acids
- Replace saturated fats with monounsaturated and polyunsaturated fats

- Omega 3 fatty acids—oily fish
- Replace some fat intake with soluble fiber
- Reduced salt
- Five or more portions of fruit and vegetables

There is insufficient evidence to recommend nutrition supplements of antioxidant vitamins, minerals, or trace elements for the treatment of cardiovascular disease. Although supplemental vitamin E may reduce the susceptibility of LDL cholesterol to oxidation, vitamin E supplements have no beneficial effects on cardiovascular events or mortality rates. Evidence shows that supplemental beta-carotene 20 g/d taken singly or in combination with vitamin E, may increase coronary heart disease mortality.[46] Fish or fish oil supplements may reduce the risk of sudden cardiac death.[47] Garlic can be used as part of a normal diet but there is insufficient evidence to recommend garlic supplements for the prevention or treatment of cardiovascular disease.[48] Folic acid supplements to reduce blood homocysteine levels have not yet been shown to reduce cardiovascular risk. Folate-rich foods, especially fortified grains and cereals, fruit, legumes, vegetables, and nuts should be included as part of a normal varied diet. Regular consumption of a small amount of alcohol may provide health benefits if there are no contraindications. The protective effect of alcohol is seen at doses as low as one standard drink every second day. The maximum intake should be limited to two standard drinks per day for women and three standard drinks per day for men.

Nutrition Intervention in Cardiac Rehabilitation Program

There is evidence to support the effectiveness of nutritional education in generating positive and long-lasting changes in the dietary habits of patients involved in cardiac rehabilitation.[49] Therefore, nutritional evaluation, counseling, and monitoring must occur as part of a comprehensive cardiac rehabilitation program.

Cardiac rehabilitation nutrition education is conducted over four phases to facilitate patient learning. It is unrealistic to expect sustained dietary change to result from a single nutrition education phase and patients can also find it difficult to absorb a large amount of information in a short period of time. Some patients may require more information/nutrition counseling than they can obtain in the context of a group program, for example:

- Patients with additional health needs (e.g., diabetes mellitus, obesity, chronic heart failure); and
- Patients from culturally and linguistically diverse backgrounds.

Structure of Nutrition Education Sessions

Phase 1: Coronary care unit/wards:

1. Each patient is seen individually as an in-patient or out-patient by the clinical nutritionist/dietitian. Diet history is taken and an individual dietary prescription is completed for the patient.
2. Full risk factor profile is recorded.
3. Anthropometric measurements including weight and height are taken.

Phase 2: Immediate postdischarge followup (4 to 6 weeks) to further assess risk factors and adherence to lifestyle change recommendations.

4. Patients are seen in out-patient department for anthropometry and motivational talk (cognitive behavioral therapy approach).
5. Food diaries are given to patients to complete at home for 5 days.

Phase 3: Structured cardiac rehabilitation program:

6. Patients attend two 1-hour nutrition talks.
7. Food diaries are collected and analyzed. Food diaries are returned and urgent areas for improvement are highlighted.

Phase 4: Postcardiac rehabilitation program to facilitate long-term maintenance of lifestyle changes.

8. Patients attend outpatient department for review, including anthropometry.

【 】 LIPIDS

Chapter 51 addresses the issues regarding hyperlipidemia in detail, based largely on the National Cholesterol Education Program Guidelines from the United States. Current Joint European Guidelines[15] are somewhat simpler and may be summarized. The European Guidelines firmly recommend the evaluation of total risk as the first step, resulting in the priorities defined earlier. In general, plasma cholesterol should be below 5 mmol/L (190 mg/dL) and LDL cholesterol below 3 mmol/L (115 mg/dL). For patients with established CVD or diabetes, treatment goals are lower: total cholesterol <4.5 mmol/L (175 mg/dL) and LDL-cholesterol <2.5 mmol/L (100 mg/dL). Treatment goals are not defined for HDL-cholesterol or triglycerides, but HDL-cholesterol of <1.0 mmol/L (40 mg/dL) in men and <1.2 mmol/L (46 mg/dL) in women, and fasting triglycerides >1.7 mmol/L (150 mg/dL) are markers of increased cardiovascular risk.

For subjects who do not reach lipid goals with dietary measures, therapy with statins will achieve this in the majority of cases (for the evidence base, see Chap. 51). Additional options include ezetimibe, nicotinic acid, fibrates, and bile-sequestering resins such as cholestyramine. On the premise that LDL-cholesterol must have been too high for an individual to sustain a myocardial infarction, many now prescribe statins for all persons who have had such an event.

In considering individual risk factors such as cholesterol or raised blood pressure, one should be aware of the necessity of managing all risk factors. The total risk approach also allows more options; for example, if a target cannot be reached for one factor because of drug side effects, it may be appropriate to try harder with other targets.

【 】 BLOOD PRESSURE

Hypertension is traditionally defined as the level of blood pressure above which intervention reduces risk, or the level of blood pressure where treatment with antihypertensive medication may be of more benefit than detriment.[50] There is evidence regarding the importance of blood pressure as a risk factor for cardiovascular disease and the importance of lifestyle measures and appropriate medication to treat and control hypertension.[15]

Hypertension is a common and potentially serious condition. If not diagnosed and treated appropriately, it can have devastating consequences for the individual, with increased risk of stroke, coronary heart disease, multiinfarct dementia, heart failure, and renal failure.[51] The decision to treat hypertension depends on the level of blood pressure, assessment of total CVD risk, and the presence or absence of target-organ damage.[15] The guidelines for treatment are based on European Society of Cardiology Third Joint Task Force recommendations on the prevention of cardiovascular disease in clinical practice (Fig. 67–2).

Management of Hypertension

It is well recognized that hypertensive vascular disease is a continuum with evidence of childhood disease progressing into adulthood. Genetic, environmental and coexisting risk factors influence the rapidity and progression of vascular changes within the blood vessel walls.[52] Proof of hypertension is required before embarking of lifelong treatment with medication, which may cause unwanted side effects. Because of the large physiologic variability in blood pressure readings, several separate recordings of an elevated blood pressure are required to diagnose hypertension.[53] Ambulatory blood pressure monitoring is advised if diagnosis is unclear. Contributing factors must be explored and ruled out.

Excessive alcohol consumption is associated with hypertension and it is important to rule it out to avoid commencing drug treatment for a self-induced problem.[51,53,54] Salt has a huge impact on hypertensive patients, particularly if they are salt sensitive.[51,54] The addition of salt and salt substitutes should not be encouraged. There is a direct link between increasing body weight and blood pressure levels, particularly if fat is centrally located. Obesity contributes to hypertension through its effect on the sympa-

thetic and renin–angiotensin–aldosterone systems. An 11-lb (5-kg) weight loss corresponds to a blood pressure reduction of 10/5 mmHg.[4] Referral to a dietician for expert advice is essential. Stress has a major effect on blood pressure and recognition and elimination of this factor may correct the hypertension.[52,54] All these issues can be addressed within a cardiac rehabilitation program. Secondary causes are rare, but blood pressure of 180/110 mmHg or higher, nondipping of blood pressure during 24-hour ambulatory blood pressure monitoring, or uncontrolled hypertension despite three medications may indicate this and warrant further investigations.

Lifestyle changes and patient education are paramount in the management of hypertension. They may lower blood pressure as much as drug monotherapy and may reduce the need for drug treatment. Such lifestyle measures include smoking cessation, regular exercise, weight reduction, and dietary advice.[50,55] These will also enhance the effects of antihypertensive drugs and demonstrate favorable influence overall cardiovascular risk.[53,54] The recommended DASH (Dietary Approaches to Stop Hypertension) diet (low in salt and saturated fat, and high in fiber, fruit, and vegetables) can as effectively lower blood pressure as can nondietary measures with maximum monotherapy.[56]

Effective implementation of nonpharmacologic measures requires knowledge, patience, enthusiasm, time, and resources. This is best undertaken by well-trained health professionals and an ideal location is cardiac rehabilitation. Patients need to have a clear understanding of their condition, the risks associated with hypertension, and the proven benefits of treatment.[50,56]

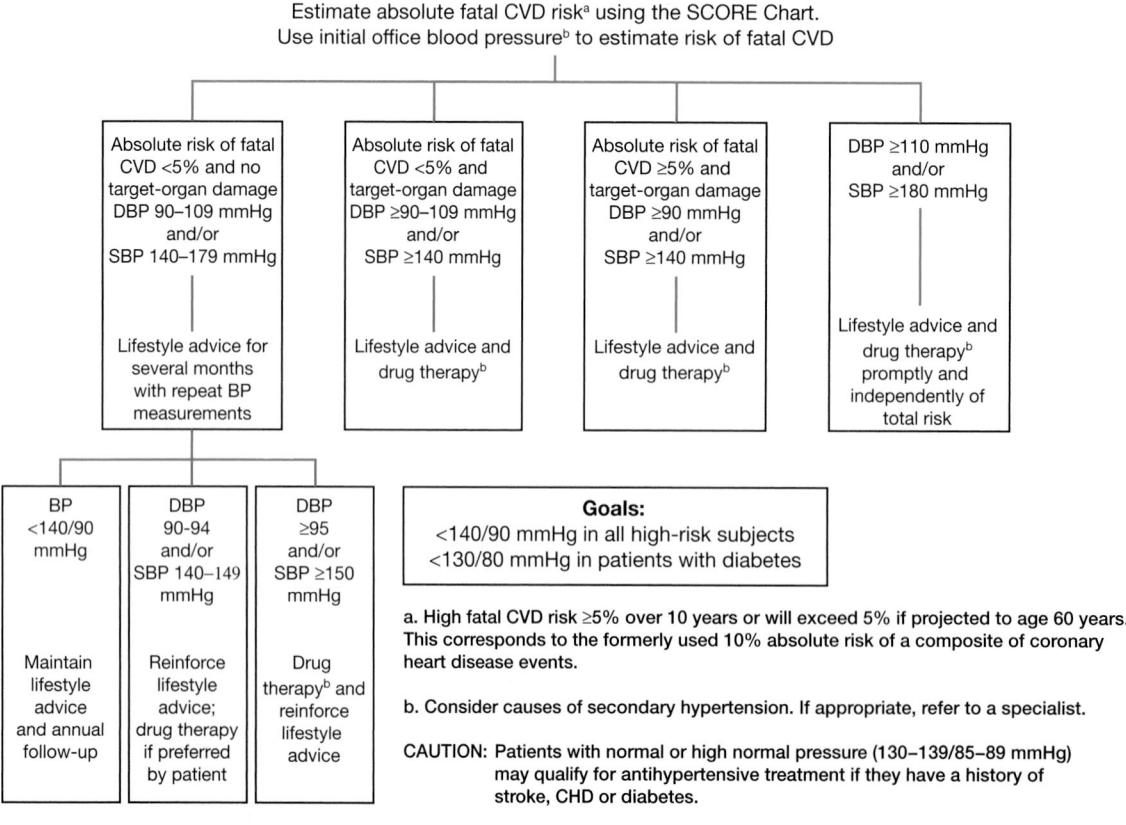

FIGURE 67–2. Guide to blood pressure management. BP, blood pressure; CHD, coronary heart disease; CVD, cardiovascular disease; DBP, diastolic blood pressure; SBP, systolic blood pressure.

If lifestyle changes have not resulted in adequate blood pressure control, drug therapy needs to be commenced. Drugs used in the treatment of hypertension should be capable of effectively lowering systolic and diastolic blood pressure, have a favorable tolerability and safety profile, and reduce cardiovascular morbidity and mortality.[15,55] Generally combination therapy is required to achieve desired blood pressure levels.[55] Choice of antihypertensive drug depends on the underlying cardiovascular disease, target-organ damage, additional vascular disease, and the presence of other cardiovascular risk factors.[15] Five classes of drugs currently meet the safety requirements for treatment of hypertension. These include diuretics, β blockers, angiotensin-converting enzyme inhibitors, calcium channel blockers, and angiotensin receptor blockers. Recently, the place of β-blocking agents as first-line agents has been questioned, but more important is effective control of blood pressure and total risk, however achieved. Additional medications may include aspirin and a statin, particularly in the rehabilitation setting where most subjects will be at high risk. Treatment is usually for life and this poses a major challenge to healthcare professionals to increase compliance of patients with their medication.[15]

Careful consideration should be given to the fact that in general clinical practice, hypertension is not well recognized, treated, or controlled. The *rule of halves* often applies, whereby half of the hypertensive patients are undiagnosed, with half of those known not treated and half of those treated not controlled.[51] It is essential that all patients diagnosed with hypertension are identified (*register*) and have regular follow up at clinics (*recall*) in order to check blood pressure control. Other risk factors are reviewed along with concordance with medications and tests to monitor target organs can be carried out or arranged (*review*). Finally, it is important to keep information accessible for staff for audit and research purposes (*record*).[53] Monitoring and subsequent treatment of hypertension should be as convenient as possible to encourage patients to take up this insurance against stroke and other cardiovascular diseases.

【 】 PSYCHOSOCIAL FACTORS

Psychosocial factors may impact on the occurrence and recurrence of coronary heart disease, and may affect rehabilitation. They are numerous and include anxiety and/or depression, personality issues (hostility, cynicism, mistrust), social isolation, anger and hostility, type D personality, lack of social support, chronic or subacute life stress (i.e., stress at work, high demands, limited decision making, low rewards), or accumulation of painful and difficult situations during a relatively short period of time.

Psychosocial stresses may lead to the maintenance of unhealthy lifestyle behaviors that promote atherosclerosis and impede rehabilitation. Pathophysiologic mechanisms with acute stress and intense emotion lead to sympathetic nervous system stimulation with an increase in heart rate and blood pressure, vasoconstriction, proarrhythmic potential, reduced endothelial dysfunction, endothelial injury, platelet activation, and/or hemostatic changes; all of the foregoing have the following clinical consequences: myocardial ischemia, arrhythmias, and the potential for thrombosis.

Psychological Insights and Support

The positive psychological effects of cardiac rehabilitation have been demonstrated, although the variety of instruments used to assess health-related quality of life makes quantitative analysis difficult.[18] Survivors of cardiac arrest, MI, or coronary artery bypass grafting and their families have many varied psychological and educational needs. Surviving a life-threatening event is a trauma for all involved. Initial management in the coronary care unit focuses on prevention of further arrhythmias and pain management. A tranquil atmosphere and reassuring, but not facile, staff are important. Emotional support is given by the coronary care unit nursing team, as fear of a cardiac arrest or death by both the patient and family is to be expected. This may manifest as anxiety, insomnia, or fear of leaving the hospital and of going home. The information given to the patient while they are in the hospital can be overwhelming, and cardiac rehabilitation provides a relaxed setting in which to provide the patient and family with ongoing education and support. Support groups may help.

Anxiety and Depression

Anxiety and depression are prevalent in both cardiac patients and their families, and are associated with increased morbidity and mortality. Although they may be normal responses following a cardiac event and a natural part of recovery following any life-threatening or stressful event, in excess they may seriously impede rehabilitation.

Anxiety can affect both short- and long-term recovery and after a cardiac event. It may relate more to how an individual responds to his or her condition than its severity. It may trigger a variety of physiologic responses, such as increased levels of circulating lipids, platelet and macrophage cell activation, increased heart rate, blood pressure, and myocardial oxygen demand—all of which have the potential to contribute to atherosclerosis and acute coronary syndromes. These responses have implications for the development of atherosclerosis, ischaemia, MI, or sudden death.

Depression during hospital admission for myocardial infarction is a significant predictor of long-term mortality and morbidity. Whereas most patients will suffer transient symptoms of a reactive depression after a life-threatening illness, a considerable number of patients after a MI exhibit persistent depression. A number of studies relate depression to poor prognosis for coronary heart disease in patients hospitalized for acute MI. Depression may confer about 2.5 times the risk for mortality.[57] Depression following an acute cardiac event can have a negative impact on adherence to medical treatments, including lifestyle changes, and the depressed patient is at greater risk of dropout from a cardiac rehabilitation program.

Although it has been recommended that depression should receive as much attention as diabetes mellitus as a risk factor for coronary heart disease prognosis, and that routine screening for depression should be performed,[58,59] it has proved difficult to demonstrate benefits from therapy. The SADHART study compared the efficacy and safety of the antidepressant medication, sertraline, and placebo for treatment of major depression after myocardial infarct or unstable angina[60] and the Enhancing Recovery in Coronary Heart Disease Patients (ENRICHD) study[61] examined survival rates and psychosocial treatments for 2481 patients with coronary heart disease. SADHART showed only modest outcome differences between treated patients and controls, and failed to address impact of treatment on clinical end points. ENRICHD found no significant difference in event-free survival between usual care and psychosocial intervention. There is a need therefore, to continue to identify and evaluate effective treatments for depression that may impact on clinical outcomes.

Assessment in Cardiac Rehabilitation

Psychological interventions are reported to be powerful, cost-effective methods of care.[62-66] Verification of such claims requires the development of objective and verifiable measurement tools. Contributions in this area have come from psychology and include instruments and procedures for the measurement of psychological adjustment, health-related quality of life, and other important psychological characteristics in chronic illness patients, as well as the development of psychologically based intervention programs for this population.[67]

Cardiac rehabilitation programs provide a valuable chance to assess cardiac patients for anxiety and depression and to provide interventions for those who need specialized care. There are many instruments available to cardiac rehabilitation professionals to assess anxiety and depression. The most practical method is the use of a self-report scale. Within psychology, psychometric robustness (which includes reliability and validity), sensitivity to change over time, brevity (which minimizes demands on patients), and a track record of having been used in past, well-designed studies, are some of the important hallmarks of good self-report measures for use in assessment, intervention and evaluation studies with chronic illness patients.[68] A commentary on these instruments is included in Appendix 67–1.

Psychosocial Intervention Programs

For patients with chronic illness or who are in the early stages of treatment, there is evidence from controlled treatment outcome studies that structured psychotherapeutic intervention programs can improve both psychological adjustment and quality of life.[69] Results of research on stress and coping, and practices rooted in cognitive behavior therapy provide the rationale for these programs. There is evidence that the use of active coping strategies, rather than avoidant coping strategies, may lead to positive psychological adjustment and an improved quality of life.

The principles of self-management programs, cognitive behavioral therapy, individual psychotherapeutic interventions, relaxation and stress management, mindfulness meditation, and social support in the context of cardiac rehabilitation are given in Appendix 67–2.

Cardiopulmonary Resuscitation Training for Relatives of Cardiac Patients

Sudden cardiac death is defined as "An unexpected death due to cardiac causes that occurs within 1 hour of symptom onset. *Cardiac arrest*, usually due to cardiac arrhythmias, is the term used to describe the sudden collapse, loss of consciousness, and loss of effective circulation that precedes biologic death."[70]

Recognition and treatment of these potentially lethal arrhythmias in the coronary care unit has reduced mortality; however, up to 75 percent of fatalities occur out of hospital.[71,72] Of these out-of-hospital cardiac arrests, it is estimated that up to 80 percent occur in the home with the spouse or family member being a witness.[73,74]

An important need identified by spouses of recovering cardiac patients is the need to learn what to do if their spouse has a cardiac arrest at home.[75] However, resuscitation of the cardiac patient by a relative is an emotive area and Dracup and coworkers have suggested that family members do not seek cardiopulmonary resuscitation (CPR) training on their own initiative and often will look to health professionals for advice.[76] Various professional bodies have made recommendations regarding CPR training for the relatives of cardiac patients. The American Heart Association endorsed CPR training of the lay public in 1971 and from 1992, the AHA guidelines recommend targeting courses to relatives and close friends of persons at risk. The AHA's *International Guidelines 2000* strongly recommends targeting family members of high-risk adult and pediatric patients, stating that:

> *Healthcare professionals should recommend CPR training for family members as part of the discharge teaching plan for high-risk patients. Persons caring for high-risk populations must be educated to recognize airway or cardiovascular emergencies and must be taught how to intervene appropriately and to contact the emergency medical system.*[77]

A feature of cardiac rehabilitation is education on the management of angina and on the signs and symptoms of myocardial infarction. Cardiac rehabilitation is an appropriate environment in which to enhance this education by providing CPR training. Research examining the effect of CPR training on the cardiac patient's spouse or family members suggests that receiving CPR training within a supportive environment such as cardiac rehabilitation poses no adverse psychological consequences for family members.[78] Patients are often excluded from this CPR training because of fears of the possible physiologic consequences.[79] Conversely, there may be negative psychological consequences for patients who are excluded from CPR training.[79] Prior research has shown[80,81] that cardiac patients appear to want to learn CPR; consequently, it is suggested that cardiac patients be involved in the training. Although cardiac patients are at high risk of cardiac arrest, this should not preclude them from having the ability to help others. Such patients live in the community as everyday citizens and many of them will have relatives with cardiovascular disease. It is recommend that cardiac patients be involved in CPR training as it poses them no adverse psychological consequences and may increase participation in CPR training by cardiac patients' relatives.[82] In this study, a higher percentage of significant others participated in the training when their relative (the cardiac patient) took part.

COMMON QUESTIONS: ASKED AND UNASKED

[ ] RETURNING HOME AND GOING BACK TO WORK

Admission to a hospital with an acute coronary syndrome is often a daunting and frightening experience with a major impact on a person's life. Often, the person feels immortal until admitted, then control is taken away and the person is, in effect, treated as a child. Just as they become accustomed to this, the patient is told that all is well and that the patient is to be discharged. It is hardly surprising that, following discharge from hospital, patients and their families may feel vulnerable. Worries and concerns about returning to work and normal everyday life are present at this time.

Cardiac rehabilitation and exercise training improves functional capacity and a patient's ability to perform most activities and job-related tasks.[12] This may not have the desired impact on a patient's return to work. Some of the factors that influence a patient's return to work include age, socioeconomic status, worksite and type of work, previous employment, cardiac event and any residual/long-term symptoms, employers, physicians, families, and the patient's attitudes. Few jobs today are too physically demanding for the patient with preserved ventricular function to undertake. Perhaps the most important factor in facilitating a return to work is the physician's unequivocal statement that this is medically acceptable and desirable, if this is the patient's wish.

It is not unusual for a patient to complete a rehabilitation program and yet be advised by a partner not to undertake lifting, even though the person may now be more fit than he or she was before hospital admission. This illustrates the importance of full communication with family members regarding the healing process and the safety of everyday physical tasks.

[ ] DRIVING A CAR

It is advisable not to drive a car for 4 weeks after a heart attack, and for 6 weeks after surgery, as the wired sternum may be at risk if a collision occurred.[21] Reaction time may be slower because of tiredness, the anesthetic, or weakness. At first patients are advised not to drive alone, in heavy traffic, or for long distances. If the patient is a driver of a heavy goods vehicle or passenger carrier, the patient is advised to inform the licensing authority before driving again.

[ ] SEXUAL ACTIVITY

Issues related to sexual activity need to be addressed by members of the cardiac rehabilitation team. Patients are often shy or embarrassed about such a discussion and are often worried about having sexual relations after a heart attack or heart surgery.

The heart rate achieved climbing up two flights of stairs equates to usual sexual activity.[83] If a patient can comfortably achieve this without getting chest pain or becoming breathless, then the patient is physically ready. The hemodynamic response increases in certain circumstances, such as sex with an unfamiliar partner or in unfamiliar circumstances, and after excessive alcohol or food consumption.[84] The most common problems that patients with cardiovascular disease experience are reduced libido, avoidance of sexual activity, and impotence. Sexual dysfunction may be the result of anxiety or depression, fear of causing another cardiac event, or the result of particular medications, such as diuretics or β blockers. Caution is recommended to those with erectile dysfunction. Patients with erectile dysfunction who are taking nitrates may not be prescribed sildenafil or similar medications that can cause severe hypotension.

Cardiac rehabilitation is an ideal setting to encourage the patient to resume normal sexual activity, and the ideal forum for patients to report if they are experiencing any problems. *The Sensuous Heart*[85] is an excellent guide for patients recovering from a heart attack or heart surgery. It is important for staff to have appropriate communication skills to provide support and understanding for this sensitive topic as it may have long-lasting consequences for patients and their families.

PRACTICAL IMPLEMENTATION

The lessons learned from multidisciplinary, nurse-led rehabilitation programs were recently developed and formalized through a European Society of Cardiology demonstration program called Euro-Action. This program is particularly suitable for hospitals that wish to establish a rehabilitation program, and also contains innovative ideas for anyone interested in rehabilitation It can be accessed at: www.escardio.org/initiatives/prevention/euroaction/general.

CONCLUSIONS

As the world's population ages, cardiac rehabilitation will need to be provided to a growing number of elderly patients, many of whom will have a variety of comorbidities.[7] Benzer and Oldridge have compared the vast medical and industrial resources that exist for medical imaging, drug therapy, and interventional cardiology to the "tiny" input into cardiac rehabilitation.[7]

Although mortality from cardiovascular diseases is on the decline, there is a dramatic rise in clinical conditions that will cause cardiovascular morbidity to increase further, these being obesity, diabetes mellitus, and the metabolic syndrome. While traditional cardiac rehabilitation focuses on secondary prevention, the future scope of cardiac rehabilitation needs to be broadened to encompass aspects of primary prevention, becoming centers for intensive lifestyle management for physical, medical, and psychological support and education. Preventing these chronic conditions from developing into acute and chronic cardiovascular disease would save lives and be cost-effective. It is recommended that future research evaluates cardiac rehabilitation expanding to fulfill this need.[12]

The nature of cardiac rehabilitation will need to change to accommodate primary prevention programs. Lower-risk patients will avail themselves of community settings and increasing numbers of higher-risk patients with increasing complex medical conditions will require supervised, monitored cardiac rehabilitation. As medical interventions and medications continue to lead to successful physical outcomes for cardiac patients, health-related quality of life is a vital component of cardiac rehabilitation that requires more research to evaluate the efficacy of cardiac rehabilitation.

REFERENCES

1. *Hurst's The Heart* 11th ed. New York: McGraw-Hill. 2004:1517–1527.
2. Acute myocardial infarction: pre-hospital and in-hospital management. The Task Force on the Management of Acute Myocardial Infarction of the European Society of Cardiology. *Eur Heart J* 1996;17(1):43–63.
3. Sloman J, Julian D. History and future of the coronary care unit. In: Thompson P, ed. *Coronary Care Manual*. New York: Churchill, 1997:4.
4. Levine SA, Lown B. The "chair" treatment of acute thrombosis. *Trans Assoc Am Physicians* 1951;64:316–327.
5. Horgan J, Bethell H, Carson P, et al. Working party report on cardiac rehabilitation. *Br Heart J* 1992;67(5):412–418.
6. Kellermann JJ, Levy M, Feldman S, Kariv I. Rehabilitation of coronary patients. *J Chronic Dis* 1967;20(10):815–821.
7. Benzer W, Oldridge N. Current concepts in cardiac rehabilitation medical considerations and outcomes evaluations. *J Clin Basic Cardiol* 2001;4(3):211–219.
8. Wenger NK, Froelicher ES, Smith LK, et al. Cardiac rehabilitation as secondary prevention. Agency for Health Care Policy and Research and National Heart, Lung, and Blood Institute. *Clin Pract Guidel Quick Ref Guide Clin* 1995(17):1–23.

9. Balady GJ, Ades PA, Comoss P, et al. Core components of cardiac rehabilitation/secondary prevention programs: a statement for healthcare professionals from the American Heart Association and the American Association of Cardiovascular and Pulmonary Rehabilitation Writing Group. *Circulation* 2000;102(9):1069–1073.

10. Scottish Intercollegiate Guidelines Network (SIGN). *Guideline 57, Cardiac Rehabilitation.* Available at: www.sign.ac.uk/guidelines/fulltext/57/section1.html.

11. Giannuzzi P, Saner H, Bjornstad H, et al. Secondary prevention through cardiac rehabilitation: position paper of the Working Group on Cardiac Rehabilitation and Exercise Physiology of the European Society of Cardiology. *Eur Heart J* 2003;24(13):1273–1278.

12. Leon AS, Franklin BA, Costa F, et al. Cardiac rehabilitation and secondary prevention of coronary heart disease: an American Heart Association scientific statement from the Council on Clinical Cardiology (Subcommittee on Exercise, Cardiac Rehabilitation, and Prevention) and the Council on Nutrition, Physical Activity, and Metabolism (Subcommittee on Physical Activity), in collaboration with the American association of Cardiovascular and Pulmonary Rehabilitation. *Circulation* 2005;111(3):369–376.

13. *Prevention of Coronary Heart Disease: Report of WHO Expert Committee.* Geneva: World Health Organization, 1982.

14. *Needs and Action Priorities in Cardiac Rehabilitation and Secondary Prevention in Patients with Coronary Heart Disease.* Geneva: World Heart Organization Regional Office for Europe, 1993.

15. De Backer G, Ambrosioni E, Borch-Johnsen K, et al. European guidelines on cardiovascular disease prevention in clinical practice: third joint task force of European and other societies on cardiovascular disease prevention in clinical practice (constituted by representatives of eight societies and by invited experts). *Eur J Cardiovasc Prev Rehabil* 2003;10(4):S1–S10.

16. Oldridge NB, Guyatt GH, Fischer ME, Rimm AA. Cardiac rehabilitation after myocardial infarction. Combined experience of randomized clinical trials. *JAMA* 1988;260(7):945–950.

17. O'Connor GT, Buring JE, Yusuf S, et al. An overview of randomized trials of rehabilitation with exercise after myocardial infarction. *Circulation* 1989;80(2):234–244.

18. Jolliffe J, Rees K, Taylor R, Thompson D, Oldridge N, Ebrahim S. Exercise-based rehabilitation for coronary heart disease. *Cochrane Database Syst Rev* 2006, Issue 3.

19. Taylor RS, Brown A, Ebrahim S, et al. Exercise-based rehabilitation for patients with coronary heart disease: systematic review and meta-analysis of randomized controlled trials. *Am J Med* 2004;116(10):682–692.

20. *American College of Sports Medicine Guidelines for Exercise Testing and Prescription,* 6th ed. Philadelphia: Lippincott Williams & Wilkins, 2000:166–167.

21. Woods S, Froelicher E, Adams S, Bridges E. *Cardiac Nursing,* 5th ed. Philadelphia: Lippincott Williams & Wilkins, 2005.

22. Hevey D, Brown A, Cahill A, Newton H, Kierns M, Horgan JH. Four-week multidisciplinary cardiac rehabilitation produces similar improvements in exercise capacity and quality of life to a 10-week program. *J Cardiopulm Rehabil* 2003;23(1):17–21.

23. Centers for Disease Control and Prevention. Annual smoking-attributable mortality, years of potential life lost, and economic costs—United States 1995–1999. *MMWR Morb Mortal Wkly Rep* 2002;51(14):300–303.

24. Camm A, Luscher T, Serruys P. *The ESC Textbook of Cardiovascular Medicine.* Oxford, UK: Blackwell, 2006: Chap 26.

25. *American Association of Cardiovascular and Pulmonary Rehabilitation (AACVPR) Guidelines for Rehabilitation Programmes,* 4th ed. Champaign IL: Human Kinetics, 2004.

26. *American College of Sports Medicine Guidelines for Exercise Testing and Prescription,* 6th ed. Philadelphia: Lippincott Williams & Wilkins, 2000:115.

27. McConnell TR, Klinger TA, Gardner JK, Laubach CA Jr, Herman CE, Hauck CA. Cardiac rehabilitation without exercise tests for post-myocardial infarction and post-bypass surgery patients. *J Cardiopulm Rehabil* 1998;18(6):458–463.

28. Cobb LA, Weaver WD. Exercise: a risk for sudden death in patients with coronary heart disease. *J Am Coll Cardiol* 1986;7(1):215–219.

29. Ades PA. Cardiac rehabilitation and secondary prevention of coronary heart disease. *N Engl J Med* 2001;345(12):892–902.

30. Franklin BA, Bonzheim K, Gordon S, Timmis GC. Safety of medically supervised outpatient cardiac rehabilitation exercise therapy: a 16-year follow-up. *Chest* 1998;114(3):902–906.

31. *Obesity in Europe: The Case for Action.* International obesity task force and the European Association for the Study of Obesity. London, 2002.

32. *Obesity: The Policy Challenges. The Report of the National Taskforce on Obesity 2005.* Department of Health, Ireland.

33. Astrup A, Ryan L, Grunwald GK, et al. The role of dietary fat in body fatness: evidence from a preliminary meta-analysis of ad libitum low-fat dietary intervention studies. *Br J Nutr* 2000;83(Suppl 1):S25–S32.

34. St Jeor ST, Howard BV, Prewitt TE, Bovee V, Bazzarre T, Eckel RH. Dietary protein and weight reduction: a statement for healthcare professionals from the Nutrition Committee of the Council on Nutrition, Physical Activity, and Metabolism of the American Heart Association. *Circulation* 2001;104(15):1869–1874.

35. Hooper L, Summerbell CD, Higgins JP, et al. Reduced or modified dietary fat for preventing cardiovascular disease. *Cochrane Database Syst Rev* 2001(3):CD002137.

36. Mensink RP, Zock PL, Katan MB, Hornstra G. Effect of dietary cis and trans fatty acids on serum lipoprotein(a) levels in humans. *J Lipid Res* 1992;33(10):1493–1501.

37. Hooper L, Bartlett C, Davey SM, Ebrahim S. Reduced dietary salt for prevention of cardiovascular disease. *Cochrane Database Syst Rev* 2003(1):CD003656.

38. Cappuccio FP, MacGregor GA. Does potassium supplementation lower blood pressure? A meta-analysis of published trials. *J Hypertens* 1991;9(5):465–473.

39. *Report of the Cardiovascular Review Group of the Committee of Medical Aspects of Food Policy number 46.* London: Department of Health, HMSO.

40. Thompson TG, Veneman AM. *Dietary Guidelines for Americans 2005.* United States Department of Health and Human Services and United States Department of Agriculture.

41. *Diet, Nutrition and the Prevention of Chronic Diseases. WHO Technical Report Series 916. Report of a Joint WHO/FAO Expert Consultation.* World Health Organization, 2003.

42. Lifestyle and risk factor management and use of drug therapies in coronary patients from 15 countries; principal results from EUROASPIRE II Euro Heart Survey Programme. *Eur Heart J* 2001;22(7):554–572.

43. Summary of the second report of the National Cholesterol Education Program (NCEP) Expert Panel on Detection, Evaluation, and Treatment of High Blood Cholesterol in Adults (Adult Treatment Panel II). *JAMA* 1993;269(23):3015–3023.

44. Executive summary of the third report of The National Cholesterol Education Program (NCEP) Expert Panel on Detection, Evaluation, and Treatment of High Blood Cholesterol in Adults (Adult Treatment Panel III). *JAMA* 2001;285(19):2486–2497.

45. de Lorgeril M, Renaud S, Mamelle N, et al. Mediterranean alpha-linolenic acid-rich diet in secondary prevention of coronary heart disease. *Lancet* 1994;343(8911):1454–1459.

46. Dietary supplementation with n-3 polyunsaturated fatty acids and vitamin E after myocardial infarction: results of the GISSI-Prevenzione trial. Gruppo Italiano per lo Studio della Sopravvivenza nell'Infarto miocardico. *Lancet* 1999;354(9177):447–455.

47. Singh RB, Niaz MA, Sharma JP, Kumar R, Rastogi V, Moshiri M. Randomized, double-blind, placebo-controlled trial of fish oil and mustard oil in patients with suspected acute myocardial infarction: the Indian experiment of infarct survival—4. *Cardiovasc Drugs Ther* 1997;11(3):485–491.

48. Jain AK, Vargas R, Gotzkowsky S, McMahon FG. Can garlic reduce levels of serum lipids? A controlled clinical study. *Am J Med* 1993;94(6):632–635.

49. Karvetti R, Hamalainen H. Long-term effects of nutrition education on myocardial infarction patients: a 10- year follow-up study. *Nutr Metab Cardiovasc Dis* 1993(3):185–192.

50. Beevers D. *Understanding Blood Pressure. Family Doctor Publications in association with the British Medical Association.* Oxon: 2001.

51. Clinical factfile: Pressure points. *World Ir Nurs.*

52. Maher V, Carey M, Markham C. Considerations in blood pressure management. *Heartwise* 2001;4(4):35–39.

53. Corzio J, Kennedy S. Managing cardiovascular risk factors. In: *Development in Cardiovascular Education,* 2nd ed. Glasgow: University of Glasgow, 2001.

54. Williams B, Poulter NR, Brown MJ, et al. British Hypertension Society guidelines for hypertension management 2004 (BHS-IV): summary. *BMJ* 2004;328(7440):634–640.

55. Golino P, Trimarco B. *Management of Arterial Hypertension Comparison Between American and European Guidelines.* Bologna, Italy: OSC Media, 2003.

56. Ibrahim W, Colwell N. Why BP control can fall short. *World Ir Nurs* 2005;13(8):44–45.

57. Lett H, Blumenthal J. Depression, exercise and coronary heart disease. *Heartwise* 2004;7(2):5–11.

58. Ziegelstein RC. Depression in patients recovering from a myocardial infarction. *JAMA* 2001;286(13):1621–1627.

59. Ziegelstein R. Depression and recovery from cardiac events. *Heartwise* 2004;7:19–20.

60. Glassman AH, O'Connor CM, Califf RM, et al. Sertraline treatment of major depression in patients with acute MI or unstable angina. *JAMA* 2002;288(6):701–709.

61. Berkman LF, Blumenthal J, Burg M, et al. Effects of treating depression and low perceived social support on clinical events after myocardial infarction: the Enhancing Recovery in Coronary Heart Disease Patients (ENRICHD) Randomized Trial. *JAMA* 2003;289(23):3106–3116.

62. Cummings N, Dorken H, Pallack M, Henke C. *Managed Mental Health Care, Medicaid, and Cost-Offset: The Impact of Psychological Services in the Hawaii-HCFA-Medicaid Project.* San Francisco: Foundation for Behavioral Health, 1993.

63. Glasgow RE, Wagner EH, Kaplan RM, Vinicor F, Smith L, Norman J. If diabetes is a public health problem, why not treat it as one? A population-based approach to chronic illness. *Ann Behav Med* 1999;21(2):159–170.

64. Kaplan RM. Two pathways to prevention. *Am Psychol* 2000;55(4):382–396.

65. Miller W. What really triggers health behaviour change? *Ann Behav Med* 2002;24(Suppl):xii.

66. Terris M. The development and prevention of cardiovascular disease risk factors: socioenvironmental influences. *Prev Med* 1999;29(6 Pt 2):S11–S17.

67. White C. *Cognitive Behaviour Therapy for Chronic Medical Problems.* Chichester: Wiley, 2001.

68. Bowling A. *Measuring Disease: A Review of Disease-Specific Quality of Life Measurement Scales,* 2nd ed. Philadelphia: Open University Press, 2001.

69. Seligman ME. The effectiveness of psychotherapy. The Consumer Reports study. *Am Psychol* 1995;50(12):965–974.

70. Chandler-Main C, Gerity D. *Sudden Cardiac Death and Cardiac Arrest,* 4th ed. Philadelphia: Lippincott Williams & Wilkins, 2000.

71. Holmberg M, Holmberg S, Herlitz J. Effect of bystander cardiopulmonary resuscitation in out-of-hospital cardiac arrest patients in Sweden. *Resuscitation* 2000;47(1):59–70.

72. Capewell S, MacIntyre K, Stewart S, et al. Age, sex, and social trends in out-of-hospital cardiac deaths in Scotland 1986–95: a retrospective cohort study. *Lancet* 2001;358(9289):1213–1217.

73. Herlitz J, Eek M, Holmberg M, Engdahl J, Holmberg S. Characteristics and outcome among patients having out of hospital cardiac arrest at home compared with elsewhere. *Heart* 2002;88(6):579–582.

74. Swor RA, Jackson RE, Compton S, et al. Cardiac arrest in private locations: different strategies are needed to improve outcome. *Resuscitation* 2003;58(2):171–176.

75. Moser DK, Dracup KA, Marsden C. Needs of recovering cardiac patients and their spouses: compared views. *Int J Nurs Stud* 1993;30(2):105–114.

76. Dracup K, Moser DK, Guzy PM, Taylor SE, Marsden C. Is cardiopulmonary resuscitation training deleterious for family members of cardiac patients? *Am J Public Health* 1994;84(1):116–118.

77. The AHA emergency cardiovascular programs. In: Stapleton E, Aufderheide T, Hazinski M, Cummins R, eds. *AHA Basic Life Support Instructor's Manual. Part 1, New Teaching Strategies for BLS Courses.* Deerfield, IL: Worldpoint ECC, 2000.

78. Dracup K, Moser DK, Taylor SE, Guzy PM. The psychological consequences of cardiopulmonary resuscitation training for family members of patients at risk for sudden death. *Am J Public Health* 1997;87(9):1434–1439.

79. Dracup K, Guzy PM, Taylor SE, Barry J. Cardiopulmonary resuscitation (CPR) training. Consequences for family members of high-risk cardiac patients. *Arch Intern Med* 1986;146(9):1757–1761.

80. Thoren AB, Axelsson A, Herlitz J. The attitude of cardiac care patients towards CPR and CPR education. *Resuscitation* 2004;61(2):163–171.

81. Thoren AB, Axelsson AB, Herlitz J. Possibilities for, and obstacles to, CPR training among cardiac care patients and their co-habitants. *Resuscitation* 2005;65(3):337–343.

82. Ingram S, Maher V, Bennett K, Gormley J. The effect of cardiopulmonary resuscitation training on psychological variables of cardiac rehabilitation patients. *Resuscitation* 2006;71(1):89–96.

83. Falk RH. The cardiovascular response to sexual activity: do we know enough? *Clin Cardiol* 2001;24(4):271–275.

84. Pasternak R. Comprehensive rehabilitation of patients with cardiovascular disease. In: Braunwald E, Zipes D, Libby P, Bonow R, eds. *Braunwald's Heart Disease, A Textbook of Cardiovascular Medicine,* 7th ed. Philadelphia: Elsevier Saunders 2004:1096.

85. Cambre S. *The Sensuous Heart.* Atlanta, GA: Pritchett & Hull Associates, 2005.

86. Zigmond AS, Snaith RP. The hospital anxiety and depression scale. *Acta Psychiatr Scand* 1983;67(6):361–370.

87. Derogatis L. *Manual for the Brief Symptom Inventory 18 (BSI 18).* Minnetonka, MN: National Computer Systems; 2001.

88. McNair D, Lorr M, Droppleman L. *POMS Profile of Mood States Manual.* Toronto, ON: MHS, 1992.

89. Spertus JA, Winder JA, Dewhurst TA, Deyo RA, Fihn SD. Monitoring the quality of life in patients with coronary artery disease. *Am J Cardiol* 1994;74(12):1240–1244.

90. Spertus JA, Winder JA, Dewhurst TA, et al. Development and evaluation of the Seattle Angina Questionnaire: a new functional status measure for coronary artery disease. *J Am Coll Cardiol* 1995;25(2):333–341.

91. Davis N. Carers' options and emotional responses following cardiac surgery: cardiac rehabilitation implications for critical care nurses. *Intensive Crit Care Nurs* 2000;16:66–75.

92. Roebuck A. Telephone support in the early post-discharge period following elective cardiac surgery: does it reduce anxiety and depression levels? *Intensive Crit Care Nurs* 1999;15:142–146.

93. Von Korff M, Gruman J, Schaefer J, Curry SJ, Wagner EH. Collaborative management of chronic illness. *Ann Intern Med* 1997;127(12):1097–1102.

94. Clark D, Fairburn C. *The Science and Practice of Cognitive Behaviour Therapy.* Oxford: Oxford University Press, 1997.

95. Fawzy FI, Fawzy NW. Group therapy in the cancer setting. *J Psychosom Res* 1998;45(3):191–200.

96. Watson JC, Greenberg LS. Alliance ruptures and repairs in experiential therapy. *J Clin Psychol* 2000;56(2):175–186.

97. Nolen-Hoeksema S. Responses to depression and their effects on the duration of depressive episodes. *J Abnorm Psychol* 1991;100(4):569–582.

98. Moser DK. Social support and cardiac recovery. *J Cardiovasc Nurs* 1994;9(1):27–36.

99. Moser DK, Dracup K. Impact of cardiopulmonary resuscitation training on perceived control in spouses of recovering cardiac patients. *Res Nurs Health* 2000;23(4):270–278.

100. Riegel BJ, Dracup KA. Does overprotection cause cardiac invalidism after acute myocardial infarction? *Heart Lung* 1992;21(6):529–535.

101. Evenson KR, Fleury J. Barriers to outpatient cardiac rehabilitation participation and adherence. *J Cardiopulm Rehabil* 2000;20(4):241–246.

102. Beach EK, Maloney BH, Plocica AR, et al. The spouse: a factor in recovery after acute myocardial infarction. *Heart Lung* 1992;21(1):30–38.

103. Drory Y, Florian V. Long-term psychosocial adjustment to coronary artery disease. *Arch Phys Med Rehabil* 1991;72(5):326–331.

104. Taylor S, Helgeson V, Reed G, Skokan L. Self-generated feelings of control and adjustment to physical illness. *J Soc Issues* 1991;47(4):91–109.

105. Moser DK, Dracup K. Psychosocial recovery from a cardiac event: the influence of perceived control. *Heart Lung* 1995;24(4):273–280.

106. Newens A, Bond S, McColl E. The experience of women during their partners' hospital stay after MI. *Nurs Stand* 1995;10(6):27–29.

107. Svedlund M, Danielson E, Norberg A. Men's experiences during the acute phase of their partners' myocardial infarction. *Nurs Crit Care* 1999;4(2):74–80.

108. O'Farrell P, Murray J, Hotz SB. Psychologic distress among spouses of patients undergoing cardiac rehabilitation. *Heart Lung* 2000;29(2):97–104.

APPENDIX 67–1

A Sample of Assessment Protocols Used in the Psychological Evaluation of Cardiac Rehabilitation Patients

PSYCHOLOGICAL ADJUSTMENT / MOOD DISTURBANCE

The 18-item version of the **Brief Symptom Inventory** (BSI 18)[87] and the short version of the **Profile of Mood States** (POMS-SF)[88] are particularly good measures of psychological adjustment. The BSI 18 has good criterion validity and is a highly reliable way of screening patients with clinically significant psychological adjustment problems. The POMS-SF is useful for detecting changes in mood states over time because of its high sensitivity to such changes.

HEALTH-RELATED QUALITY OF LIFE

Physical disability associated with having a chronic illness coupled with psychological mood disturbance problems combine to reduce the overall health-related quality of life of patients with chronic disease.[68] The self-report version of the **Psychological Adjustment to Illness Scale** (PAIS-SR)[87] is a well-established measure of health-related quality of life in chronic illness patients. It has good construct validity and covers the full range of areas relevant to overall quality of life, specifically: health-care orientation, vocational environment, domestic environment, sexual relationships, extended family relationships, social environment, and psychological distress.

The **Seattle Angina Questionnaire** (SAQ)[89,90] appears to be reliable and valid based on the testing to date. It also appears to be able to detect changes over time. The SAQ is a specific measure of functional status for patients with coronary artery disease. It covers clinically important dimensions: physical limitation, anginal stability, patient satisfaction with treatment and perception of heart disease.

APPENDIX 67–2

Self-Management and Psychosocial Programs

This appendix outlines the principles of self-management programs, cognitive behavioral therapy, individual psychotherapeutic interventions, relaxation and stress management, mindfulness meditation, and social support in the context of cardiac rehabilitation.

Self-Management Programs

For patients with chronic health problems, there has been a growing interest in "patient education" and "self-management programs." Self-management programs are distinct from simple patient education or skills training in that they are designed to allow people with chronic conditions to take an active part in the management of their own condition. Patients with chronic illness need not be mere recipients of care. They can become key decision makers in the treatment process. Managing chronic conditions involves behavioral and lifestyle changes, patients must be empowered to take a central role in their own care. There are a variety of models of both formal and informal self-management. Based on a literature review of more than 400 articles, Gruman and Von Korff (1996) proposed the following definition of self-management:

> Self-management involves (the person with the chronic health problem) engaging in activities that protect and promote mental health, monitoring and managing of symptoms and signs of illness, managing the impacts of illness on functioning, emotions, and interpersonal relationships, and adhering to treatment regimes.[93]

Cognitive Behavioral Therapy

It has been demonstrated that patients with mild levels of anxiety and depression can benefit from psychosocial interventions provided alongside exercise in cardiac rehabilitation. Cognitive behavioral therapy is practiced and taught in many cardiac rehabilitation programs so as to enable patients to regain control over adverse emotional events arising or exacerbated by the cardiac event. Solution-focused brief therapy is an intervention suited to patients who need to reanimate their latent strengths and talents, which may have been challenged by acquiring the label of cardiac patient. Cognitive behavior therapy offers a range of clinical techniques for enhancing active coping strategies,[94] some of which have been incorporated into patient-focused psychoeducational programs for newly diagnosed cancer patients. Effective programs include some or all of the following components: health education, stress management training, coping and problem-solving skills training, assertiveness and anger management skills training, and group support.[95] Outcome studies show that cognitive behavioral therapy works in a range of patient populations, although the ENRICHD study, discussed above, did not confirm that cognitive behavioral therapy had any impact on clinical outcomes for patients with coronary heart disease. The patients did report feeling less depressed and did score higher in health-related quality-of-life measures in the short-term. Long-term maintenance of relapse for depression and reduction in mortality rates remains a problem for clinicians treating patients with both depression and coronary heart disease.

(continued)

Self-Management and Psychosocial Programs *(continued)*

Individual Psychotherapeutic Interventions

Clinical counseling psychologists and psychotherapists attached to cardiac rehabilitation teams often assess patients for individual interventions, which can include cognitive behavior therapy, emotion-focused therapy,[96] interpersonal therapy, and psychodynamic therapy. Therapy is tailored to meet individual patient need responsiveness and requires specialist therapist input. Length of sessions are usually about 1 hour per week, and treatment can be brief and symptom focused (8 to 12 sessions) or longer term for patients with depression who do not respond well to group interventions (12 to 40 sessions). Research shows that duration of psychological therapy does impact on outcomes. A consistent finding across studies indicates that therapies of less than 8 sessions are unlikely to be effective and that 75 percent of clients show improvement by 26 sessions of therapy. Maintenance of change may however require up to 40 sessions.

Relaxation and Stress Management

Relaxation and stress management techniques are an integral component of any rehabilitation program. As an aid to relaxation, our cardiac rehabilitation department in the Adelaide & Meath Hospital, Dublin, Ireland, has developed a Progressive Muscular Relaxation CD that is available to all cardiac rehabilitation patients. The provision of a relaxation CD becomes, for patients, a constant link back to the positive motivational atmosphere of the rehabilitation program. Having a familiar voice from the program speaking on the tracks is further reinforcement for recreating the positivity of rehabilitation. Progressive Muscular Relaxation was chosen as the featured relaxation method, as this is proven to be the most effective in dealing with muscular tension, general anxiety, raised blood pressure, sleeping difficulties, muscular tension, and the like. Teaching the techniques should never be complicated, hence Progressive Muscular Relaxation, because the real challenge for patients is "buying" the need to keep practicing. The CD is introduced to patients only after they have learned how stress affects their hearts have learned how to do relaxation breathing and have seen the importance of becoming proactive about their own health.

Mindfulness Meditation

Teesdale et al., and later Williams et al., suggested that the skills learned from cognitive therapy training for individuals with depression may not necessarily be practiced and maintained by patients when they are in a recovery phase of depression. These patients depend on the presence of depression or negative automatic thought. Mindfulness (attentional) training in contrast can be practiced on a variety of thoughts, including those related to depression. It is also an intrinsically positive experience, which is more likely to reinforce continued practice. Finally it appears to be associated with a reduction in ruminative thinking, associated with more hopeless cognition.[97] Mindfulness training is about teaching individuals to be in full awareness of their thoughts and feelings from moment to moment. This is a training that turns patients toward thoughts and feelings, both positive and negative, rather than away, which may help them recognize and identify early signs of depressive feelings, and facilitate the seeking of preventative actions.

Social Support

Sudden onset of a cardiac illness is a major life event and impacts not only on the patient but also on the spouse and extended family. Social support has been expressed as "The comfort, assistance and/or information one receives through formal or informal contact with individuals or groups."[98]

Cardiac patients who live alone or who lack a source of emotional support face a significantly higher risk of recurrent MI, sudden death, and all-cause mortality than do patients with adequate sources of support.[99] Patients who receive more social support from family and friends than desired, who may even be considered "overprotected," experience less anxiety, depression, anger, and confusion, and a higher self-esteem at 4 months after MI.[100]

Social support can take many forms, from a close friend to older child; however, it is usually the female spouse who is associated with social support. Wives have a pivotal influence on lifestyle change and in promotion of heart healthy behaviors. A frequent reason given for nonattendance at cardiac rehabilitation programs is a lack of support from the spouse.[101] The spouse's ability to deal with the cardiac illness impacts on the family and also on the patient's adaptation to illness, both physical and emotional.[102]

Moser et al. state that although spousal support can be positive there can be a negative effect on social relationships.[99] A wife's perception of her husband's physical ability can influence recovery either positively or negatively. A spouse who does not have the resources to manage his or her own emotional distress cannot offer adequate support to a recovering partner. A key to improving a spouse's ability to provide support for his or her partner is helping the spouse manage his or her own emotional distress. Emotional distress following the onset of a serious illness is often thought to be the result of the perception of loss of control.[103]

(continued)

APPENDIX 67–2

Self-Management and Psychosocial Programs *(continued)*

Vicarious control has been described as the "Belief that others have some response that can reduce, modify, or terminate an aversive situation that affects the self."[104] During hospitalization the healthcare providers, doctors, nurses, and other staff assume this role. In the home situation, the spouse or family member may be seen as taking on this role. This can be a positive form of control when the patient is at his or her most vulnerable, but may reinforce the "invalid" status over the long-term. The perception by patients that family members felt in control after the cardiac event was one component of the perception of control felt by patients.[105]

In the literature, the majority of research on aspects of social support has been done on male MI or coronary artery bypass grafting patients and their female spouses.[106] There is a paucity of literature examining the male spouses' response to their wives' illness[107] or to other caregivers within the supportive network. The majority of studies examine the needs of the partner during the acute hospital and early discharge stages. Fewer studies exist that examine the family relationships during long-term recovery.[108]

The need for information seems to be the main requirement of spouses both during the acute event and throughout the recovery period in cardiac rehabilitation, especially as fear of reoccurrence and death are prevalent. For many spouses, worries about the future are important. O'Farrell et al. found that of 213 female spouses of patients undergoing cardiac rehabilitation, 66 percent were significantly distressed, and concerns about treatment, recovery, and prognosis were the most prevalent stressors.[108] It is vital, therefore, to invite and include the cardiac patients' significant family members or friends to participate in the rehabilitation process, from in-patient to long-term maintenance. Frequently, the time schedules of cardiac rehabilitation programs, that is, their being held during working hours, prohibit family participation. Evening sessions, family only groups, and choice must be considered to ensure the cardiac patients' significant family members or friends' inclusion.

PART 9

Systemic Arterial Hypertension

CHAPTER (68)

Epidemiology of Hypertension

Thomas G. Pickering / Gbenga Ogedegbe

Hypertension is a condition that can claim a number of firsts: It is the most common chronic condition in the United States; it is the number one reason for an office visit to a physician; it accounts for the most drug prescriptions; it is a major risk factor for heart disease and stroke, which are the first and third leading causes of death in the United States; and it is the number one attributable risk for death throughout the world.[1] At the same time, it is both preventable and treatable in the majority of patients. Despite these impressive statistics, hypertension continues to be neglected. It is not recognized as a condition worthy of specialist care, and only about one-third of hypertensive patients in the United States have their blood pressure controlled to target levels that have been proven in numerous studies to reduce the rates of heart attacks and strokes. In addition, although the death rates from these two conditions have been decreasing over the past 20 years, the rates of two others that are also consequences of hypertension—heart failure and chronic kidney disease—have been increasing. It gets worse yet: A major public health concern in the United States today is the epidemic of obesity, which has resulted in a major increase in the prevalence of type II diabetes, and which increases the risk of cardiovascular events to the same degree as a prior myocardial infarction, for which the most effective treatment is the aggressive reduction of blood pressure. So perhaps the worst single statistic relating to hypertension is that less than 25 percent of patients with diabetes have their blood pressure adequately controlled.

This chapter reviews the epidemiology of hypertension—what it is, and how it is classified; how common it is; who is affected by it; its consequences, and how they are affected by treatment; and the degree to which it is being controlled.

WHAT IS HYPERTENSION?

There is agreement that hypertension is a quantitative rather than a qualitative disease. The basis for this statement rests on a large number of epidemiologic studies showing that the distribution of blood pressure in the population is continuous, although the curve is skewed at the higher levels of blood pressure. This was not always accepted: In the 1950s there was a sharp debate between Sir George Pickering and Lord Robert Platt that played out in the correspondence section of the *Lancet*, and was subsequently assembled in a monograph.[2] Pickering took the view that the distribution of blood pressure in the population is continuous, and that there is no discernible separation between subjects with high blood pressure from those with normal blood pressure. Platt had data that indicated that there was a bimodal distribution, and that a hypertensive subpopulation could be distinguished from the normotensive majority, a dispute that could be summarized as "one hump or two?" The general consensus was that Pickering won, and that the unimodal distribution holds sway. This has important implications, first because it suggests that hypertension is unlikely to be the result of a single physiologic process or gene, and second, because it also suggests that any blood pressure level used to define hypertension is arbitrary.

❲ ❳ CLASSIFICATION AND SUBTYPES OF HYPERTENSION

There are several ways in which hypertension can be classified, which are helpful for its diagnosis and clinical management (Fig. 68–1). The two principal divisions are to classify it by its severity (the height of the blood pressure) and by its underlying cause (primary, or essential hypertension versus secondary hypertension). A third major component is age: the pathophysiology of hypertension in younger and older people is quite different.

❲ ❳ CLASSIFICATION BY SEVERITY

The original subdivision of hypertension according to its severity was "benign" and "malignant." While malignant hypertension carries a prognosis that is equivalent to other malignant diseases (if untreated), the term *benign* for less severe forms of hypertension is a misnomer, and is no longer used. Malignant hypertension is now relatively uncommon in Western countries, and somewhat surprisingly, it no longer features in the JNC 7 (Seventh Report of the Joint National Committee on Prevention, Detection, Evaluation and Treatment of High Blood Pressure) classification of hypertension,[1] which is the generally accepted classification in the United States. It still does occur, however, and is important because it requires urgent treatment, which can dramatically alter its natural history.

In most hypertensive patients both the systolic and diastolic pressure are raised, but there are circumstances in which only one of them is high. The most common circumstance is isolated systolic hypertension of the elderly, in which the pathophysiology is quite different from other types of hypertension, as described below. Systolic hypertension also occurs in young adults, but the mechanism is different. Isolated elevation of the diastolic pressure can also occur. Hypertension can also be situational: the tradi-

tional methods of classification have all been based on office or clinic blood pressure measurements, but with the wider use of out-of-office blood pressure measurement, it is increasingly recognized that office measurements may significantly over- or underestimate the blood pressure level during daily life. In most hypertensive patients the blood pressure is higher in the office than at other times, a phenomenon referred to as the *white coat effect*, and which is usually defined as the difference between the office pressure and the average daytime pressure.

❲ ❳ JNC 7 CLASSIFICATION

The JNC 7 classification[1] has continued the definition of hypertension as a blood pressure exceeding 140/90 mmHg for adults age 18 years or older. The classification is based on the average of two or more seated blood pressures, properly measured with well-maintained equipment, at each of two or more visits to the office or clinic. Hypertension has been divided into stages one and two, as shown in Table 68–1. JNC 7 has defined normal blood pressure as <120 and <80 mmHg. The intervening levels, 120 to 139 and 80 to 89 mmHg, are now defined as *prehypertension*, a group that has an intermediate level of risk and which may progress to definite hypertension.

Prehypertension

It is estimated that approximately 15 percent of blood pressure-related deaths from coronary heart disease occur in individuals with blood pressure in the prehypertensive range.[3] The main justification for JNC 7's concern about prehypertension was two publications from the Framingham Heart Study.[4,5] The first showed that people who have blood pressure in the high normal or prehypertensive range do have a higher risk of heart disease and stroke than do people with blood pressures below this level. They are also more likely to progress to real hypertension (above 140/90 mmHg).[4] The second paper stated that the lifetime risk of hypertension approaches 90 percent.[5] This is somewhat misleading, however, because the criterion for "hypertension" was a blood pressure above 140/90 mmHg or being put on antihypertensive treatment. Although a pressure above 140 mmHg in an older person predicts increased risk, there are no studies showing that treating systolic pressure between 140 and 160 mmHg in people older than age 65 years is beneficial. For the more relevant criterion of a

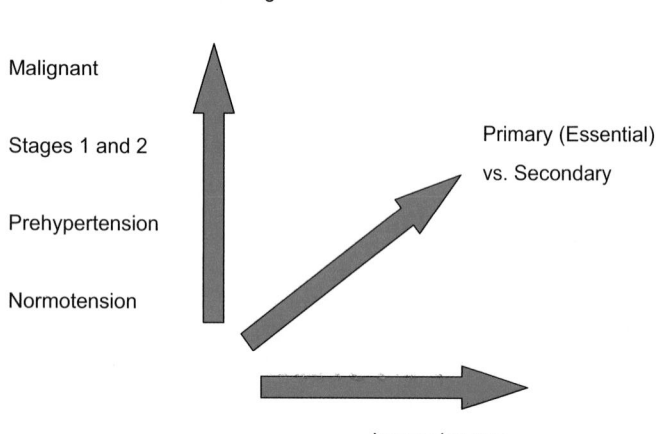

FIGURE 68–1. Three-dimensional classification of hypertension according to severity (height of the blood pressure [BP]), etiology (primary versus secondary), and age.

◗ TABLE 68–1

Classification of Hypertension (JNC 7)

BLOOD PRESSURE CLASSIFICATION	SYSTOLIC BLOOD PRESSURE[a] MMHG	DIASTOLIC BLOOD PRESSURE[a] MMHG
Normal	<120	<80
Prehypertension	120–139	80–89
Stage 1 hypertension	140–159	90–99
Stage 2 hypertension	≥160	≥100

[a]Classification determined by highest blood pressure category.

systolic pressure higher than 160 mmHg or being on treatment, the lifetime risk was closer to 70 percent for both men and women.

The numbers of prehypertensive individuals are huge: A recent analysis of the National Health and Nutritional Examination Surveys (NHANES) data found that 39 percent of adults over the age of 20 are normotensive, 31 percent prehypertensive, and 29 percent hypertensive.[6] The recommended treatment of prehypertension is lifestyle changes, but a recent study found that 2 years of antihypertensive drug treatment delayed the onset of hypertension after the treatment was discontinued.[7]

Malignant Hypertension

Malignant hypertension is diagnosed not only by the height of the blood pressure, but also by the manifestations of target organ damage, particularly retinal hemorrhages and papilledema. The critical pathologic change is the presence of fibrinoid necrosis in the arterial walls, which may be responsible for the manifestations such as hypertensive encephalopathy and impaired renal function.[8] Its importance lies in the fact that if untreated it has a 5-year survival rate of 1 percent.[9] It is still common in underdeveloped countries such as Nigeria,[10] and in western countries such as the United Kingdom it is typically seen in immigrants.[8] It can result from essential or secondary hypertension. Treatment of malignant hypertension has a dramatic effect on survival, and the first paper demonstrating the benefits of antihypertensive drugs was based on patients with malignant hypertension.[11]

Isolated Systolic Hypertension

In many older adults, systolic blood pressure tends to rise and diastolic to fall. When the average systolic blood pressure is ≥140 mmHg and diastolic blood pressure is <90 mmHg, the patient is classified as isolated systolic hypertensive. The increased pulse pressure (systolic-diastolic) and systolic pressure predict risk and determine treatment.[12] It is described further below.

Isolated Systolic Hypertension of the Young
In older children and young adults, often athletic males, a high systolic pressure in the brachial artery, but normal diastolic and mean pressures is not an uncommon finding.[13] The high systolic pressure may be the result of two changes: a high stroke volume and increased arterial stiffness. In contrast to essential hypertension which raises both systolic and diastolic pressures, peripheral resistance is not increased.[14]

Isolated Diastolic Hypertension

More commonly seen in some younger adults, the average systolic pressure remains <140 mmHg but the diastolic is ≥90 mmHg. Although diastolic pressure is generally thought to be the best predictor of risk in patients younger than age 50 years,[15] some prospective studies of isolated diastolic hypertension have indicated that the prognosis may be benign.[16] However, an analysis of data from the Framingham Heart Study concluded that isolated diastolic hypertension may evolve into systolic and diastolic hypertension.[17] Thus any patients in whom this diagnosis is made should be carefully followed.

White Coat Hypertension

In approximately 15 to 20 percent of people with stage 1 hypertension, blood pressure may only be elevated persistently in the presence of a healthcare worker, particularly a physician. When measured elsewhere, including while at work, the blood pressure is not elevated. When this phenomenon is detected in patients who are not taking medications, it is referred to as *white coat hypertension* or *isolated office hypertension*. The commonly used definition is a persistently elevated average office blood pressure of >140/90 mmHg and an average awake ambulatory reading of <135/85 mmHg.[18] Although it can occur at any age, it is more common in older men and women. White coat hypertension is the result of an exaggerated white coat effect, which may be a conditioned anxiety response.[19] Its magnitude can be reduced (but not eliminated) by the use of stationary oscillometric devices that automatically determine and analyze a series of blood pressures over 15 to 20 minutes with the patient in a quiet environment in the office or clinic. White coat hypertension is generally thought to have a relatively benign prognosis, although in some patients it may progress to definite sustained hypertension, and the risk may increase with long-term followup, for example, after more than 5 years.[20] Hence all patients need to be followed indefinitely with office and out-of-office measurements of blood pressure. Treatment with antihypertensive drugs may lower the office blood pressure but does not change the ambulatory measurement. This pattern of findings suggests that drug treatment of white coat hypertension is less beneficial than treatment of sustained hypertension.

Masked Hypertension

The mirror image of white coat hypertension, *masked hypertension* is defined as a normal office blood pressure (<140/90 mmHg) together with an elevated daytime pressure (>135/85 mmHg). It was recognized only relatively recently,[21] but is important because it is associated both with target-organ damage[22] and an adverse prognosis.[23] It has been detected both in subjects who have not been diagnosed or treated for hypertension and in patients on antihypertensive treatment.[23,24] In either case, the implications are the same: the prognosis is related to the out-of-office blood pressure more closely than to the office pressure. It has been detected using both ambulatory and home blood pressure monitoring.[25] Lifestyle can contribute to this; for example, alcohol, tobacco, caffeine consumption, and physical activity away from the clinic/office.

Pseudohypertension

In some elderly patients the peripheral muscular arteries become very rigid from advanced, and sometimes calcified, arteriosclerosis. Consequently, the cuff has to be at a higher pressure to compress them, so that a falsely high blood pressure is recorded. It is difficult to detect clinically, so these patients may be overdosed with antihypertensive medications, inadvertently resulting in orthostatic hypotension and other side effects. One noninvasive technique that has been described to detect orthostatic hypotension is the Osler maneuver, which is the ability to palpate the brachial or radial artery when a sphygmomanometer cuff is inflated to well above the systolic pressure (positive Osler sign). Unfortunately, the Osler maneuver is not a reliable screen for pseudohypertension: it may be positive in the absence of pseudohypertension in a third of patients.[26] It has been suggested that blood pressure recorded from the finger may be less susceptible to the increased rigidity of the larger arteries. Using a definition of a systolic pressure difference between the brachial artery and the finger of more than 30 mmHg, it has been estimated that 2.5 percent of subjects older than age 65 years may have pseudohypertension.[27]

Orthostatic or Postural Hypotension

This is defined as a reduction of systolic blood pressure of at least 20 mmHg or 10 mmHg in diastolic blood pressure within 3 minutes of quiet standing.[28] An alternative method is to detect a similar fall during head-up tilt at 60 degrees. This may be asymptomatic or accompanied by symptoms of lightheadedness, faintness, dizziness, blurred vision, and cognitive impairment.[29] If chronic the fall of blood pressure may be part of pure autonomic failure, or a complication of diabetes. The major life-limiting failure is inability to control the level of blood pressure, especially in those patients with orthostatic hypotension who concomitantly have supine hypertension. In these patients, there are great and swift changes in pressure so that the patients faint as a result of profound hypotension on standing and have very severe hypertension when supine. Often the heart rate is fixed as well. The supine hypertension subjects them to serious consequences such as left ventricular hypertrophy[30] and stroke.[30–32]

❚ ❘ CLASSIFICATION BY CAUSE

In more than 95 percent of cases of hypertension no single and reversible cause can be detected, and the terms *essential* and *primary* hypertension have been used. The former term was introduced because it was thought that a higher-than-usual level of blood pressure was needed to maintain perfusion of vital organs.

In approximately 5 percent of cases there is a definable cause of the hypertension. Table 68–2 shows a list adapted from JNC 7.[1] From an epidemiologic point of view, the two most important conditions on the list are chronic kidney disease and sleep apnea.

❘ TABLE 68–2

Secondary Forms of Hypertension

Condition
Chronic kidney disease
Renal artery stenosis
Cushing disease
Coarctation of the aorta
Drug-induced hypertension
Obstructive uropathy
Pheochromocytoma
Primary aldosteronism and other causes of mineralocorticoid excess
Sleep apnea
Thyroid/parathyroid disease

SOURCE: Adapted from Chobanian AV, Bakris GL, Black HR, et al. The Seventh Report of the Joint National Committee on Prevention, Detection, Evaluation, and Treatment of High Blood Pressure: the JNC 7 report. JAMA 2003;289(19):2560–2572.

Although chronic kidney disease is certainly a major cause of hypertension, it is often hard to decide whether the hypertension or the kidney disease came first, because a vicious cycle can develop where one condition exacerbates the other. In practice, however, this distinction is of little consequence, as most forms of chronic kidney disease are not reversible. The most common curable form of hypertension is renal artery stenosis, which has two principal causes: fibromuscular disease in children and young adults, and atherosclerosis in middle-age and older patients.

Sleep apnea is emerging as one of the major causes of hypertension that is of epidemiologic significance. A population survey that 2 percent of women and 4 percent of men have sleep apnea, which was defined as having an apnea–hypopnea index (AHI) score of 5 or more and daytime sleepiness.[33] The prevalence of an AHI of ≥5 increases with age, reaching a maximum prevalence in a population at about the age of 70 years.[34] Both sleep apnea and hypertension are common, and unsurprisingly there are many individuals who have both conditions. Furthermore, both are closely linked to obesity (particularly central obesity as seen in the metabolic syndrome), so there is a cluster of related syndromes: hypertension, sleep apnea, diabetes, and the metabolic syndrome. Thus approximately 60 percent of sleep apnea patients are hypertensive,[35] and, conversely, approximately 25 percent of hypertensive patients have sleep apnea.[36,37] One issue is the causal link between sleep apnea and hypertension. The largest study of this is the Sleep Heart Health Study, which is a prospective study of the relationship between sleep apnea and cardiovascular morbidity. In an initial cross-sectional study of 6132 subjects age 40 years or older,[38,39] there was a dose–response relationship between the AHI score and the prevalence of hypertension, although some of it was attributable to the effects of increased body mass index. The association between sleep apnea and hypertension was seen in both sexes, at older and younger ages, and among normal and overweight groups. In elderly patients with systolic hypertension, however, there appears to be no relationship between sleep apnea and hypertension.[40]

To establish that sleep apnea is an independent risk factor for the development of essential hypertension it is necessary to be able to demonstrate that it precedes and predicts the onset of hypertension, and that there is a dose–response relationship between the two. This was achieved most convincingly by the Wisconsin Sleep Cohort Study, which found a consistent dose–response relationship, even after controlling for age, sex, body mass index, and antihypertensive medications.[41,42]

❚ ❘ CLASSIFICATION BY AGE

There is a fundamental difference between the genesis of hypertension in young and older patients (Table 68–3). The most obvious difference is that in the younger patients, whatever the underlying etiology of the hypertension (with a few exceptions noted below) both systolic and diastolic pressure are raised, whereas in people older than age 60 years the diastolic pressure starts to fall (Fig. 68–2), but there is a marked increase of systolic pressure. The underlying hemodynamics are also different: in younger patients the characteristic changes are an increased peripheral resistance with a normal cardiac output, whereas in older patients the reason for the selective increase of systolic pressure is increased ar-

TABLE 68-3

Differences Between Hypertension in Younger and Older Patients

FACTOR	YOUNG (<60 YEARS)	OLD (>60 YEARS)
Blood pressure increase	Systolic and diastolic	Systolic
Major cause	Hormonal	Mechanical
Hemodynamic change	Increased peripheral resistance	Increased arterial stiffness
Sleep apnea	Yes	No
Treatment threshold	140/90 mmHg	160 mmHg systolic

terial stiffness. This has two consequences: first, when the left ventricle pumps into a stiffened aorta, there will be a higher systolic pressure because the stiffer vessel will be less able to accommodate the stroke volume. The second is that the velocity of the arterial pulse wave traveling out to the peripheral vessels will be increased. Just like a wave resulting from a stone dropped in a pool, the wave is reflected when it reaches the periphery, so that the pressure waves in the circulation will be a combination of the outgoing and reflected waves. In younger people, where the pulse wave velocity is low, the reflected wave arrives relatively late, and coincides with the diastolic downslope of the incident wave, so that it has no effect on the systolic or diastolic pressure. But in older individuals it returns earlier, and forms a second or late systolic peak, which augments the height of the systolic pressure. Another difference concerns the physiologic measurements: in younger patients the increased peripheral resistance is a result of active vasoconstriction that is mediated hormonally, particularly by the sympathetic nervous system and the renin–angiotensin system. In older patients with systolic hypertension, hormonal mediation is less important and the changes are mostly mechanical, for example, loss of elastin fibers in the media of the arterial wall.[43] The affected vessels (principally the aorta and central elastic vessels) dilate and stiffen. The effects of increased aortic stiffness may be bidirectional, that is, hypertension will itself increase arterial stiffness, so there may be a vicious cycle.[44] Sleep apnea, the hypertensive effects of which are thought to be mediated by the sympathetic nervous system, is related to hypertension in younger patients, but not to isolated systolic hypertension in the elderly. Sleep apnea is associated with hypertension in younger patients, but not with systolic hypertension in patients older than age 60 years.[40]

Treatment thresholds are also different. In younger patients it is clearly established that starting drug treatment when the pressure exceeds 140/90 mmHg is beneficial. This may also be true in older patients, but the clinical trials that have investigated the benefits of treatment have almost all used an initial systolic pressure of greater than 160 mmHg as an entry criterion, and have not lowered the pressure to below 140 or 150 mmHg.[45] Thus the benefits of treatment in older patients with systolic pressures below 160 mmHg remain unproven.

There is some evidence that in the very old (age 85 years or older) mortality may be higher in patients with the lowest blood pressures,[46] and that lowering the diastolic pressure with treatment may actually increase mortality.[47] The benefits or harm of treating very old patients is currently being evaluated.[48]

THE PREVALENCE OF HYPERTENSION

The NHANES, which has been studying the health of representative samples of Americans since 1960, has provided data on the changing prevalence of hypertension and its control. According to this, the prevalence of hypertension decreased somewhat between 1960 and 1991,[49] but the latest published analysis by the Centers for Disease Control and Prevention (CDC),[50] based on data obtained in the period 1999 to 2002, reported that the prevalence had increased by 3.6 percent, and that 28.6 percent of participants had hypertension (defined by a systolic pressure >140 mmHg, a diastolic >90 mmHg, or taking antihypertensive medications). When generalized to the entire U.S. population, this number translates to 58.4 million Americans (about 1 in 4) being hypertensive (Fig. 68–3). Factors associated with increased prevalence of hypertension included increasing age, obesity, and African American race. Another quarter of U.S. adults has a blood pressure in the prehypertension range, a systolic blood

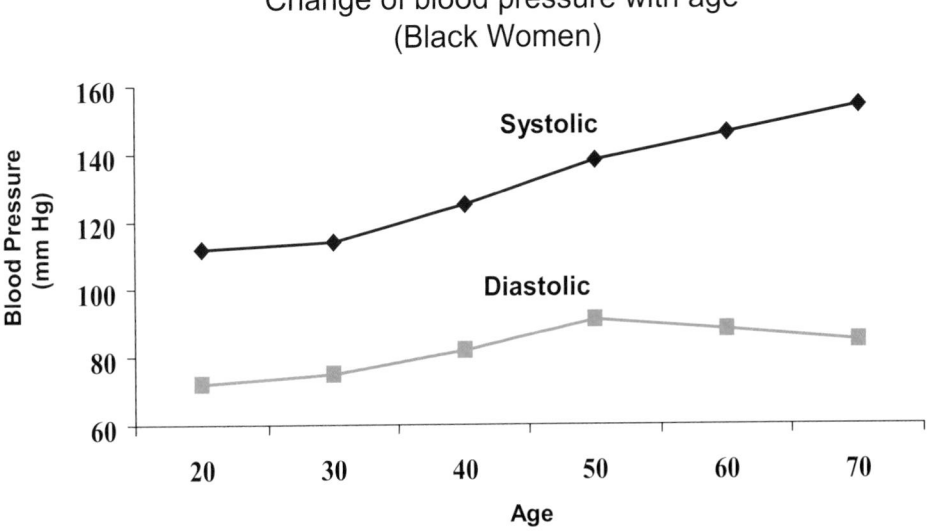

FIGURE 68-2. Changes of systolic and diastolic pressure with age in black women. Data from National Health and Nutritional Examination Surveys (NHANES). Note the decrease of diastolic pressure after age 50 years. *Source: Adapted from Burt VL, Whelton P, Roccella EJ, et al. Prevalence of hypertension in the U.S. adult population. Results from the Third National Health and Nutrition Examination Survey, 1988–1991. Hypertension 1995;25:3305–3313.*

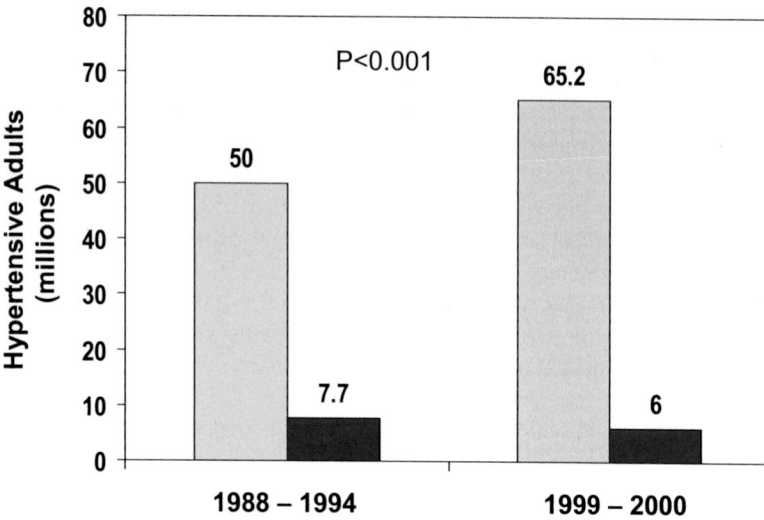

FIGURE 68–3. Increased prevalence of hypertension in the United States over a 10-year period. Data from National Health and Nutritional Examination Surveys (NHANES). *Pale bars* show prevalence of hypertension diagnosed by a blood pressure >140/90 mmHg or taking antihypertensive medications. *Dark bars* show prevalence of subjects with normal blood pressure on examination, but who had previously been diagnosed as hypertensive. *Source: Adapted from Centers for Disease Control and Prevention (CDC). Racial/ethnic disparities in prevalence, treatment, and control of hypertension—United States, 1999–2002. MMWR Morb Mortal Wkly Rep 2005;54:7–9.*

pressure of 120 to 139 mmHg, or diastolic blood pressure of 80 to 89 mmHg. The prevalence of hypertension rises progressively with age, such that more than half of all Americans age 60 years or older have hypertension.

Surveys in Europe show much higher rates of hypertension.[51] A comparison of seven European countries' data found the highest rate in Germany (55 percent) and the lowest in Italy (38 percent) with France, England, Spain, and Sweden all showing a prevalence between these two extremes. The prevalence in Canada is very similar to that in the United States (27 percent).[51] The reasons for these wide differences are unknown, but do not appear to be because of differences in measurements or sampling rates. In Egypt the rate is also approximately 25 percent, whereas in China, where much of the population is still rural, the rate is lower (14 percent), but is increasing rapidly.[52]

【 】 AFRICAN AMERICANS

In the United States, hypertension is significantly more prevalent in African Americans than in whites. In the most recent NHANES survey,[53] the prevalence in African American men was 38.6 percent, whereas in white men it was 29.6 percent; in women the prevalence was 44 percent for African Americans and 29.6 percent for whites (Fig. 68–4). A big issue here is whether the higher prevalence

is genetic or environmental. Although the prevalence is higher than in whites in other countries, for example, Brazil,[54] there is a large literature showing that the rates of hypertension in Africans living in traditional rural societies are relatively low, but increase markedly when they move to the cities.[55]

A huge effort has already been made to try to understand the reasons for the higher prevalence of hypertension in African Americans, almost all of which has made the underlying assumption that there is some genetically determined physiologic difference. So far, the results have been disappointing at best.[56] For one thing, it is becoming clear that, with rare exceptions, human hypertension is determined by several genes, and it is unlikely that genetic factors account for more than 50 percent of hypertension. A recent comparative study involving large surveys of blood pressure in populations of European versus African descent outside the United States indicated a lower range of hypertension prevalence in blacks (14 to 44 percent) than in whites (27 to 55 percent).[57] One of the most powerful pieces of evidence that environmental, particularly psychosocial, factors are important in the development of hypertension is a series of epidemiologic studies going back for many years, which have shown that when people move from a traditional tribal society to an urban westernized lifestyle, their blood pressure goes up. Many of these studies have been conducted in Africa, and hypertension is (or was) relatively rare in rural Africans. A good example is the Luo study from Kenya.[55] People who had moved to Nairobi had higher pressures than people living in the villages, even if they had only been in the city for a month. They also had higher heart rates, consistent with activation of the sympathetic nervous system. While these studies indicate that there is something pressor about our western lifestyle, they do not tell

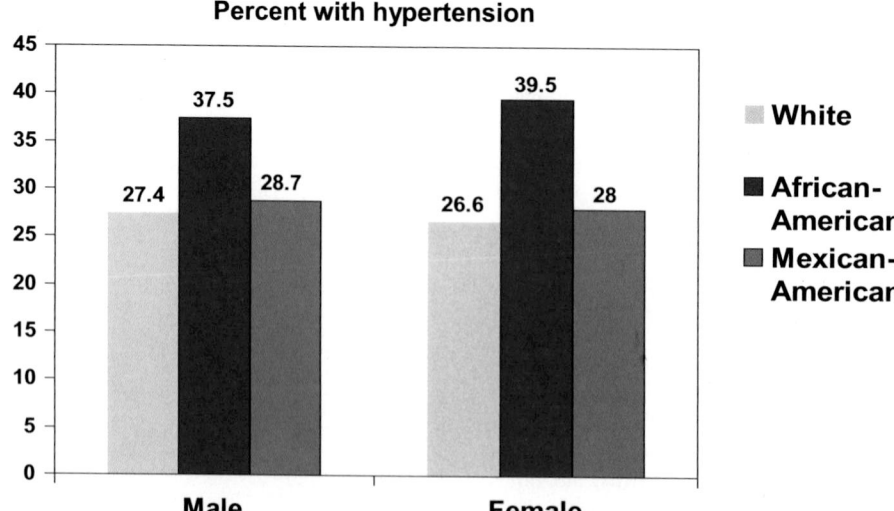

FIGURE 68–4. Prevalence of hypertension in U.S. men and women from three different ethnic groups. *Source: Adapted from Centers for Disease Control and Prevention (CDC). Racial/ethnic disparities in prevalence, treatment, and control of hypertension—United States, 1999–2002. MMWR Morb Mortal Wkly Rep 2005;54:7–9.*

us whether it is stress or diet that is more important (it is probably both). Studies from other countries also show that the higher blood pressures seen in blacks is not invariable. The Health Surveys for England (equivalent to the NHANES in the United States) found that the prevalence of hypertension was much higher in blacks than whites, even after controlling for potential mediators such as age, body mass index, and alcohol intake.[58] However another study conducted in English factory workers found no ethnic differences in blood pressure.[59] Socioeconomic status, which is strongly associated with ethnicity in the United States, affects the prevalence of hypertension, particularly in African Americans.[60] A series of classic studies conducted by Ernest Harburg in Detroit in the 1970s was the first to really get at this question.[61,62] He showed that blood pressure in African Americans living in the inner city was highest in those people living in the worst-off neighborhoods. A more recent analysis of the ARIC (Atherosclerosis Risk in Communities) study by Diez-Roux et al. found that "neighborhood" effects were independently related to blood pressure after controlling for other risk factors.[63] In four U.S. communities, people living in the neighborhoods with the lowest median house prices tended to have the highest blood pressure. This was most pronounced in the one community (Jackson, MI) that was largely African American.

【 】 HYPERTENSION IN HISPANICS

The fastest growing segment of the U.S. population is Hispanics or Latinos, who are overtaking African Americans as the largest minority group. Between 1980 and 1990 the Hispanic population increased by 39 percent, while the overall U.S. population increased by only 7 percent.[64] Many are recent immigrants, and they tend to be of relatively low socioeconomic status. If psychosocial factors are so important in determining the socioeconomic status gradient of disease, one might expect that Hispanics would also have higher mortality rates than whites. Surprisingly, this does not appear to be the case. According to the National Center for Health Statistics,[65] the age-adjusted death rates for heart disease are 121.9 per 100,000 for whites, 183.3 for African Americans, and 84.2 for Hispanics. For stroke, the corresponding figures are 23.3, 41.4, and 19.0, and for cancer 121.0, 161.2, and 76.1. Thus, for all these conditions the rates appear to be lower, not higher, for Hispanics.

There are two major subgroups of Hispanics in the United States: those from Mexico and Latin America, who are predominant in states such as Texas and California, and those of Caribbean origin, who are mostly in the Northeast and Florida. The literature on hypertension in Hispanics is both sparse and confusing. The gold standard for defining the prevalence of hypertension in different groups of the U.S. population is NHANES, which has now conducted four surveys that have included blood pressure measurement. Race/ethnicity is self-defined by necessity, and is classified into four groups: non-Hispanic whites, non-Hispanic Blacks, Mexican Americans, and "other groups." Non-Mexican American Hispanic whites and blacks are put in the last category. To obtain more reliable figures for differences between groups, each survey oversampled African Americans and Mexican Americans. The latest results, published in 2005,[50] were based on a survey conducted in 1999 and 2002, the results of which were compared with two earlier surveys (1988 to 1991 and 1991 to 1994). There were parallel ethnic differences in all three surveys, with non-Hispanic blacks (African Americans) having the highest prevalence of hypertension (40.5 percent in 1999 to 2002), and Mexican Americans the lowest (25.1 percent); whites were in the middle (27.4 percent). The lower rates in Mexican Americans cannot be attributed to better awareness or treatment of hypertension, as both measures were lower in them than in either of the other two groups: in 1999 to 2002 the percentages of hypertensive individuals who were on treatment were 55.4 percent for African Americans, 48.6 percent for whites, and only 34.9 percent for Mexican Americans.

Some early studies suggested that, despite higher rates of obesity and diabetes in Mexican Americans, they have a lower all-cause and cardiovascular mortality than whites,[66] leading to what has been called the *Hispanic paradox*. However, the most recent analysis from the San Antonio Heart Study found just the opposite, namely that mortality from cardiovascular disease is approximately 60 percent higher in Mexican Americans than whites.[67] This is the largest prospective study of Hispanics, so its findings command respect. The authors attribute the contrary findings of the earlier studies to underreporting of deaths in Mexican Americans.

There is very little published information about the prevalence of hypertension and cardiovascular disease in Caribbean Hispanics. One study that has begun to look at the issue is the Northern Manhattan Stroke Study (NOMAS),[64] which includes a high proportion of Caribbean Hispanics. In the control group, both hypertension and diabetes were more common in blacks and Hispanics than in whites: for hypertension the rates were 62 percent, 58 percent, and 43 percent, respectively. An interesting survey was conducted in Cuba,[68] where everyone can claim to be "Hispanic," but where there is also a mix of people of European origin (whites) and African origin (blacks). The prevalence of hypertension was only minimally higher in the blacks (46 percent) than in the whites (43 percent), which the authors attributed to the fact that socioeconomic differences between blacks and whites are much smaller in Cuba than in the United States. The ethnic difference was also small in comparison with the situation reported in Puerto Rico, where statistical adjustment for social class narrowed the gap between blacks and whites.[69]

【 】 OTHER RACIAL/ETHNIC GROUPS

There are also differences in the prevalence of hypertension in other ethnic groups. Hypertension tends to be relatively uncommon in Japanese Americans, while Filipinos have rates approaching those of African Americans.[70] In American Indians the prevalence of hypertension is similar to that of American whites, despite a higher prevalence of obesity.[71]

HYPERTENSION AND RISK

Data from numerous observational epidemiologic studies provide persuasive evidence of the direct relationship between blood pressure and cardiovascular disease. In a recent meta-analysis that aggregated data across 61 prospective observational studies that together enrolled 958,074 adults,[72] there were strong, direct relationships between average blood pressure and vascular mortality. These relationships were evident in middle-age and older individuals (Fig. 68–5). Importantly, there was no evidence of a blood pressure threshold; that is, vascular mortality increased progressively throughout the range of blood pressure, including the prehypertensive range, down to a systolic pressure of 115 mmHg and a diastolic of 75 mmHg. Between the ages of 40 and 70 years, each 20-mmHg increment of systolic pressure (and 10-mmHg of diastolic pressure) is associated with a doubling in the risk of stroke. The slope of the lines relating blood pressure and risk are shallower for older people.

【 】 WHICH MEASURE OF BLOOD PRESSURE IS MOST CLOSELY RELATED TO RISK?

A continuing debate in the field of hypertension is the relative importance of the different components of the arterial pressure wave in determining cardiovascular risk. There are four candidates: systolic, diastolic, pulse, and mean pressure. An additional issue is whether the traditional brachial artery pressure should be used, or the central aortic pressure. For many years the diastolic pressure reigned supreme, and most of the early

hypertension treatment trials used a high diastolic pressure as an entry criterion. This was reinforced by the publication of an analysis by MacMahon and coworkers[73] based on pooled data from 420,000 subjects, which showed a log-linear relationship between diastolic pressure and the risk of stroke and myocardial infarction. Although the importance of systolic pressure was never in doubt, it gained precedence over diastolic pressure with the publication of a series of epidemiologic studies showing not only that a high systolic pressure was the best predictor of risk in the elderly, but also that a low diastolic pressure was associated with increased risk.[74] An analysis by Franklin and coworkers[15] examined the Framingham Heart Study data and provided an elegant solution to this apparent paradox. In subjects younger than age 50 years the best predictor of risk was a high diastolic pressure, but in those older than age 60 years systolic pressure was the best predictor, and the relationship between diastolic pressure and risk was now negative, so that a low diastolic pressure was related to higher risk.

【 】 IS PULSE PRESSURE A BETTER PREDICTOR THAN SYSTOLIC PRESSURE?

It is well known that systolic pressure increases steadily with age, but after the age of 50 years diastolic pressure starts to fall. A number of studies suggest that pulse pressure may be the best predictor of risk in the elderly. In the JNC 7, however, which is

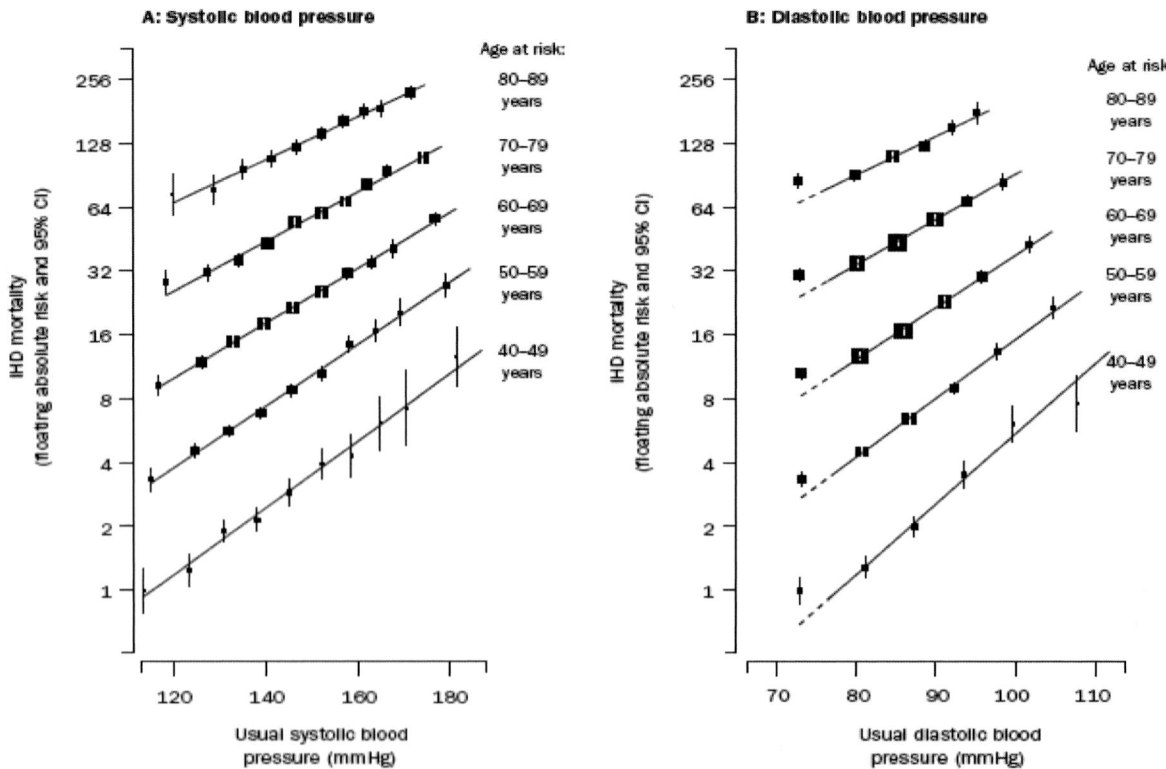

FIGURE 68–5. Relationships between systolic and diastolic pressure with deaths from coronary heart disease in 958,074 adults from the Prospective Studies Collaboration. IHD, ischemic heart disease. *Source: Reproduced with permission from Prospective Studies Collaboration. Age-specific relevance of usual blood pressure to vascular mortality: a meta-analysis of individual data for one million adults in 61 prospective studies. Lancet 2002;360:1903–1913.*

still the official guideline for the evaluation and management of hypertension,[1] there is no mention of pulse pressure as a predictor. If pulse pressure is the best predictor, a low diastolic pressure should be harmful, which seems to be in contradiction to the finding of a positive association between diastolic pressure and risk shown in Fig. 68–5, even for the oldest individuals. However, the explanation of the apparent paradox is that the relationship depends not just on diastolic pressure, but on its interaction with systolic pressure. This was clearly shown by an analysis of the Multiple Risk Factor Intervention Trial (MRFIT) data, which found that the highest-risk group was patients who had a systolic pressure above 160 mmHg and a diastolic pressure below 80 mmHg[75] (Fig. 68–6). Thus if the systolic pressure is normal, a low diastolic pressure in an elderly patient is quite harmless.[76]

This raises the issue whether pulse pressure should be the target in older patients. Not all studies that have compared the predictive powers of systolic versus pulse pressure in older patients have found that pulse pressure is superior,[77,78] and some of its apparent superiority may be a statistical artifact. Thus many of the studies expressed the risk in terms of a 10-mmHg change of pressure; because systolic pressure is always numerically greater than pulse pressure, this tends to attribute a greater predictive value to the latter. An analysis of the NHANES data[79] showed that the relative importance of pulse pressure diminishes if the standard deviations for the two measures are used. In practical terms, high-risk patients can be identified by a very high systolic pressure (e.g., >160 mmHg) and a very low diastolic pressure (e.g., <70 mmHg), without any specific reference to pulse pressure. There are no evidence-based guidelines relating to the treatment of a high pulse pressure. The trials examining the effects of treating systolic hypertension recruited patients largely on the basis of a high systolic pressure alone[80] or in combination with a diastolic pressure <90 or 95 mmHg.[81,82] In the Systolic Hypertension in China (Syst-China) study,[80] the pretreatment blood pressure was 170/86 mmHg, and the final pressure in the active treatment group was 150/81 mmHg. Thus the treatment had a greater effect on systolic than diastolic pressure, with a reduction of pulse pressure, and none of these trials lowered systolic pressure below 145 mmHg.[45] The best we have relating to treatment based on pulse pressure is an analysis of the Systolic Hypertension in the Elderly Program (SHEP) results, which found that the baseline pulse pressure did not influence the benefits of treatment.[83] However, it was also found that if the diastolic pressure on treatment was less than 70 mmHg, there was a significantly increased risk of cardiovascular events.

combination with a very high systolic pressure is associated with high risk. There are at least two explanations for this, which we may call *direct* and *indirect*. Taking the direct explanation first, it is possible that a very low diastolic pressure might impair coronary artery perfusion, which takes place during diastole. If this were the case, we should expect the adverse outcomes resulting from a low diastolic pressure to be ischemic cardiac events, but not strokes. The indirect explanation is that the low diastolic pressure is not harmful per se, but is a marker for generalized cardiovascular disease, or more particularly increased arterial stiffness. It is generally accepted that the age-related increase of systolic and decrease of diastolic pressure that is seen in the brachial artery is largely the result of accelerated wave reflection in stiff arteries.[84] There are some studies that have examined the relationship of pulse and diastolic pressure with specific outcomes. Millar and coworkers[85] analyzed the data from the MRC trial, and found that at low levels of diastolic pressure (below 90 mmHg), there was an increased risk of myocardial infarction (MI) (the J-curve phenomenon), whereas for strokes, the lowest risk was associated with the lowest diastolic pressure. Madhavan et al. also found that pulse pressure predicted MI.[76]

If the further reduction of an initially low diastolic pressure in patients with systolic hypertension is harmful, it would be desirable to have antihypertensive drugs that selectively reduce pulse pressure. Unfortunately, most of the currently available drugs have relatively little effect, which is reflected by the fact that the single most important factor associated with inability to reduce blood pressure to target levels is old age.[86] There are differences in the extent to which antihypertensive drugs lower pulse pressure relative to their effects on the other components: in elderly patients the greatest reductions of pulse pressure were seen with clonidine and hydrochlorothiazide, whereas atenolol had very little effect.[87]

[ ] CAN A LOW DIASTOLIC PRESSURE BE HARMFUL?

These findings are thus consistent with the idea that a very low diastolic pressure in

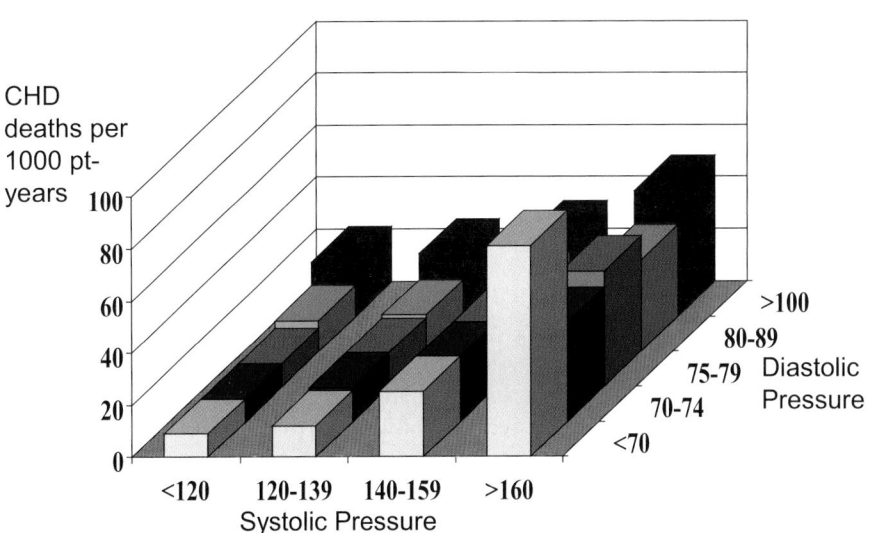

FIGURE 68–6. The interrelationships between systolic and diastolic pressure with deaths from coronary heart disease in the Multiple Risk Factor Intervention Trial. CHD, coronary heart disease; pt, patient. *Source: Reproduced with permission from Domanski M, Mitchell G, Pfeffer M, et al. Pulse pressure and cardiovascular disease-related mortality: follow-up study of the Multiple Risk Factor Intervention Trial (MRFIT). JAMA 2002;287:202677–202683.*

WHAT IS THE ROLE OF MEAN PRESSURE?

Mean pressure is another potential candidate as a risk marker. It is customarily defined as diastolic pressure plus one-third of the pulse pressure, but it is measured directly by oscillometric devices, although the numbers are rarely displayed. In an analysis of three intervention studies in elderly patients Blacher and coworkers[74] found that pulse pressure, but not mean pressure, predicted cardiovascular outcomes. However, in younger patients, mean pressure is more important. In two studies of younger patients, pulse pressure was the strongest predictor of coronary events,[76,85] whereas mean pressure was the best predictor of stroke.[88] This finding was confirmed by Verdecchia and coworkers in a study using ambulatory blood pressure monitoring.[89] One explanation for this finding may be that the patient with the high pulse pressure has increased arterial stiffness and is effectively being hit with a "double whammy": the high systolic pressure in the central aorta increases the afterload on the heart, and the low diastolic pressure impairs coronary perfusion. The reason why mean pressure is a better predictor of stroke may be that it is closer to diastolic than to systolic pressure, and many studies have shown that the relationship between diastolic pressure and stroke is steeper than for coronary events,[73] whereas no studies have shown that a very low diastolic pressure predicts stroke.

CENTRAL VERSUS PERIPHERAL ARTERIAL PRESSURE

The arterial pressure wave in the brachial artery looks very different from the waves recorded at more proximal sites, where the damage to target organs, such as the heart and brain, occurs, and it is now possible to estimate the central aortic pressure indirectly from measurements made noninvasively from peripheral sites such as the radial artery. In older patients with stiff arteries the central aortic systolic pressure is similar to the brachial pressure, whereas in younger subjects with compliant arteries, it is substantially lower.[84] As shown above, different drugs have different effects on pulse pressure, and recent studies show that similar differences occur in their effects on central pressure.[90] There are, however, many different methods for measuring arterial stiffness,[91] and there is disagreement as to which is the most reliable. Some have been shown to predict cardiovascular events,[92,93] and it is likely that such measurements will become part of routine clinical practice in the near future.

THE ADVERSE EFFECTS OF HYPERTENSION

Hypertension leads to adverse events in the brain, heart, and kidneys through two related mechanisms, both of which involve the effects of increased pressure on the arteries. The first is the effects on the structure and function of the heart and arteries, and the second is the acceleration of the development of atherosclerosis. The former is directly the result of the blood pressure, whereas the latter requires an interaction with other risk factors for cardiovascular disease, most importantly cholesterol. Thus strokes are closely related to the direct effects of blood pressure, whereas coronary heart disease is related to atherosclerosis, and the relationship between blood pressure and events is steeper for stroke than for coronary heart disease (CHD) events. In countries where cholesterol levels are low, such as Japan, strokes are common, but CHD events are not.[94]

CORONARY HEART DISEASE

The Prospective Studies Collaboration of 61 studies[72] found strong log-linear relationships between both systolic and diastolic pressure and the risk of CHD events in five deciles of age, ranging from 40 to 49 to 80 to 89, such that for each 20-mmHg increase of systolic pressure there was a twofold increase of risk over a range from 115 to 180 mmHg. For diastolic pressure, the risk doubled with a 10-mmHg increase over a range of 75 to 100 mmHg. There is an interactive effect between the various risk factors; thus the relationship between systolic pressure and CHD risk is much steeper in patients whose cholesterol is high than in patients in whom it is normal.[95] This relationship has been reported in several countries, although the slope of the line relating blood pressure and risk is shallower in countries where the overall risk of CHD is low, such as Japan.[96] Although it is well recognized that blood pressure is one of the three major risk factors for the development of CHD (the other two being high cholesterol and smoking), it has been claimed that CHD events often occur in patients who lack all of these risk factors. An analysis of three large prospective studies found that for both fatal and nonfatal myocardial infarctions, at least one of the big three was present in more than 90 percent of cases.[97]

The relationship between risk and blood pressure in individuals who have already had a myocardial infarction is different, and has been reported to be J-shaped for the first 2 years after the MI (i.e., there is a paradoxical increase of risk in those with the lowest blood pressure, e.g., below 110/70 mmHg), but with longer followup there is a positive relationship.[98] The increased mortality at lower levels of pressure may be an example of reverse causality; that is, the pressure is low because of extensive damage to the heart. A history of hypertension per se does not necessarily lead to an increased mortality after an MI, but it does predict reinfarction.[99]

The official recommendation for the treatment of hypertensive patients with coronary heart disease is that the target blood pressure should be 140/90 mmHg; whether further reduction is beneficial or harmful is controversial. The J-curve hypothesis was postulated on the basis of observations suggesting that if diastolic pressure was lowered below a certain level (about 85 mmHg) there was a paradoxical increase of events.[100] The proposed explanation was that because coronary artery perfusion occurs during diastole, excessive reduction in combination with diseased coronary arteries would result in ischemia. Subsequent work supported this idea, because the J-curve was seen for myocardial infarction but not with stroke, where the adage that the lower the blood pressure, the better still holds.[85] A recent analysis of the INVEST trial,[101] which compared two drug regimens in post-MI patients, confirmed that there was an increased risk of all-cause mortality and MI in patients whose diastolic pressure was below 75 mmHg (Fig. 68–7). Again there was no such relationship for strokes. Data from the Framingham Heart Study also support the idea of a J-curve phenomenon, but only in patients with previous myocardial infarctions and in the presence of a high systolic pressure as well as a low diastolic pressure.[102] This would be consistent with the results of the CAMELOT trial,[103] which randomized normotensive patients with documented CHD to amlodipine, enalapril, or placebo, and found that although both active drugs lowered the blood pressure, amlodipine resulted in a lower rate of recurrent events than either placebo or enalapril. The blood pressures at entry to the study were 129/78 mmHg, and there was a 5 mmHg reduction with treatment. Consequently, at the present time, it would seem prudent to avoid excessive reductions of diastolic pressure in patients with known CHD, particularly if the systolic pressure is high. In practice, this is a difficult task, because it is hard to lower systolic pressure without affecting diastolic pressure.

[ ] HEART FAILURE

Heart failure is now the leading cause of hospitalization for people age 65 years and older in the United States, and unlike other complications of hypertension, its prevalence has been increasing over the past 30 years.[104] For a 40-year-old man or woman, the "remaining lifetime risk" of developing heart failure is approximately 20 percent, a surprisingly high number; if subjects with known coronary heart disease are excluded, the risk is 11 percent in men and 15 percent in women.[105] Blood pressure is a major contributor to this: The risk is twice as high in hypertensive men as in normotensives, and three times as high in hypertensive women; 90 percent of new cases of heart failure in the

Framingham Heart Study had a history of previous hypertension.[106] This risk is much more strongly related to systolic than diastolic pressure.[107] Treatment of hypertension in older people reduces the incidence of heart failure by approximately 50 percent.[81] The good news is that the incidence of heart failure is now decreasing in women (but not men), while survival has improved in both sexes.[108]

In the last 10 years or so it has become apparent that approximately half of the patients who present with classic signs and symptoms of heart failure appear to have normal ventricular function, typically defined by the finding of an ejection fraction of more than 50 percent on echocardiography. This group has been variously described as having diastolic dysfunction, diastolic heart failure, or "heart failure with a normal ejection fraction." Diastolic heart failure is thought to be responsible for as many as 74 percent of cases of heart failure in hypertensive patients.[109] Despite this, it is rarely diagnosed in clinical practice, except by default. This is a problem because the symptoms, such as dyspnea and fatigue, are very nonspecific.

This condition, although undoubtedly of major importance, remains a murky area for several reasons. First, assessment of diastolic function is difficult, and ideally requires cardiac catheterization; although noninvasive measures are used, they are very nonspecific. Second, there are no reliable animal models of diastolic heart failure, Third, there are no treatments that are specifically aimed at improving diastolic function.

Two population-based studies compared the prognosis of systolic and diastolic failure. One[110] evaluated all 216 patients who were diagnosed with heart failure in Olmsted County, Minnesota in 1991. Of the patients who had their systolic function evaluated, the ejection fraction was normal in 43 percent. The prognosis was similar in the patients with diastolic and systolic failure. The second is the Framingham Heart Study,[111] where it was found that half of 73 heart-failure patients had normal systolic function—65 percent of whom were women—whereas 75 percent of patients with impaired systolic function and heart failure were men. Approximately 75 percent of both groups had a history of hypertension. Mortality was high in both groups, but higher in those with systolic heart failure.

Most discussions of the underlying causes of diastolic heart failure have only considered changes occurring in the heart itself. Nevertheless, the obvious primary change in hypertension is what is happening in the arterial circulation. It is generally accepted wisdom that the reason why hypertensive patients develop ventricular hypertrophy and heart failure is because the increased arterial pressure places an excessive burden on the heart, or afterload. Why should the same explanation not apply to diastolic heart failure? Patients with diastolic heart failure have been found to have stiffer aortas than normal,[112] which may result in accelerated wave reflection from the periphery, and a combined increase of central aortic systolic pressure and reduced diastolic pressure. The latter will lead to decreased coronary artery perfusion during diastole, and hence impair

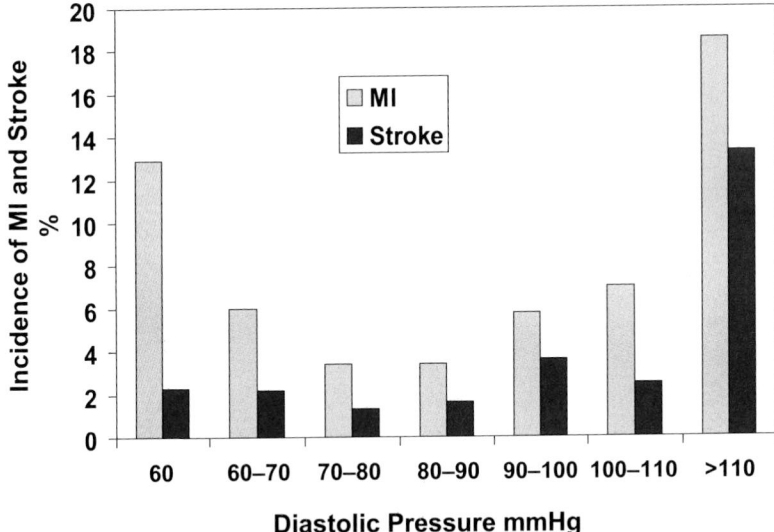

FIGURE 68–7. Relationship between diastolic pressure, recurrent myocardial infarction, and stroke in patients enrolled in the INVEST trial, all of whom had had a previous myocardial infarction (MI). *Source: Adapted from Messerli FH, Mancia G, Conti CR, et al. Dogma disputed: can aggressively lowering blood pressure in hypertensive patients with coronary artery disease be dangerous? Ann Intern Med 2006;144:12884–12893.*

myocardial relaxation. These and other findings have led some investigators to state that diastolic heart failure "has nothing to do with diastolic dysfunction at all."[113]

【 】 CEREBROVASCULAR DISEASE

Stroke is the third most common cause of death throughout the world after coronary heart disease and cancer. Approximately 80 percent of strokes are ischemic, 15 percent are hemorrhagic, and 5 percent are caused by subarachnoid hemorrhage.[114] As with coronary events, there is a strong log-linear relationship between both systolic and diastolic pressure and stroke, although the relationship is steeper for strokes than for CHD events, and much stronger for systolic than diastolic pressure.[115] Approximately 60 percent of patients who present with strokes have a past history of hypertension, and in those who are hypertensive, approximately 78 percent have not had their blood pressure adequately controlled.[116] Of all the risk factors for stroke, hypertension has the highest relative risk (4.0 between the ages of 40 and 50 years, falling to 2.0 at ages 70 to 80 years), and the highest population attributable risk (40 percent at ages 40 to 50 years, and 30 percent at ages 70 to 80 years).

In contrast with blood pressure, the relationship between cholesterol and stroke is weaker than that between cholesterol and CHD. The Prospective Studies Collaboration analyzed data from 45 prospective studies of 450,000 individuals, and found a fivefold difference in stroke risk over a range of diastolic pressure from 75 to 102 mmHg, but no relationship with cholesterol over a range from 4.7 to 6.5 mmol/L.[117] Paradoxically, however, there is strong evidence that statin drugs lower the risk of strokes in proportion to their lowering of low-density lipoprotein cholesterol,[118] and also that they can prevent recurrent strokes.[119] It is possible to construct risk equations for strokes just as for coronary heart disease. This has been done using the Framingham Heart Study and the Cardiovascular Heath Study.[120] Systolic pressure is the principal predictor variable, and others are serum creatinine, diabetes, left ventricular hypertrophy by ECG, age, atrial fibrillation, and history of heart disease.

The different subtypes of stroke have somewhat different relationships with blood pressure. A large proportion of cerebral infarcts are classified as lacunar infarcts, which are the result of lesions in small arteries penetrating the deeper layers of the cerebral cortex, and approximately 70 percent of patients who experience these are hypertensive.[121] The characteristic pathology is a destructive lesion of the vessel wall, termed *lipohyalinosis*, which is distinct from both atherosclerosis and the remodeling of arteries that occurs in other vascular beds. Infarcts of the large cranial and extracranial arteries are more related to atherosclerosis, and only 50 percent of patients with this type of stroke are hypertensive,[122] but it is still the most important risk factor.[123] Cardioembolic strokes are increasingly recognized, and atheromatous plaques that protrude from the aorta are an independent risk factor for ischemic strokes.[124] Cerebral hemorrhage also shows a very strong relationship with hypertension and, more particularly, with discontinuing antihypertensive medications.[123]

The decline in the death rate from strokes since the 1960s has received a lot of publicity, and because blood pressure is such an important risk factor for stroke, it is tempting to think that better hypertension control can take the credit. There are, however, reasons why this may not be the case. First, the decline of stroke mortality preceded the widespread use of antihypertensive medications.[122] Second, attempts to correlate the decline of mortality with improved blood pressure control rates have been unsuccessful,[125,126] suggesting that changes in socioeconomic status might be more important.

Blood pressure typically rises acutely after a stroke, and it is postulated that this helps to maintain cerebral perfusion in the infarct's "penumbra" zone.[116] This forms the rationale for avoiding excessive reduction of blood pressure immediately following a stroke.

Treatment of hypertension reduces stroke rates by 35 to 44 percent;[127] this has been shown in both younger patients with systolic and diastolic hypertension, and in older patients with isolated systolic hypertension.[81] It is not yet known if treatment of patients older than age 85 years is beneficial, but the preliminary findings from the HYVET (Hypertension in the Very Elderly Trial) suggest that it does.[48] There is general agreement that the reduction of blood pressure is more important than which drugs are used to lower it,[128] but there are some minor differences. Blockers are less effective than other drugs for preventing stroke,[129] and there is some evidence that angiotensin receptor blockers may be more effective.[130]

【 】 CHRONIC KIDNEY DISEASE

A Japanese study of nearly 100,000 men and women found a progressive relationship between the height of the blood pressure and the risk of developing end-stage renal disease during a 17-year followup period, such that there was an increased risk even in patients with high normal blood pressure, in comparison with those whose pressure was optimal (less than 120/80 mmHg).[131] Hypertensive patients whose blood pressure is not well controlled are more likely to show a deterioration of renal function.[132] A prospective analysis of the MRFIT study also found that blood pressure was closely related to the likelihood of developing end-stage renal disease, but for any level of pressure the risk was about twice as high in African Americans as in whites.[133] A study of post-MI patients found that there was a steep and linear relationship between glomerular filtration rate (GFR) and cardiovascular death.[134] In addition, hypertensive patients with mildly impaired renal function (estimated GFR <60 mL/min) have an increased prevalence of target-organ damage, such as left ventricular hypertrophy, increased carotid intima-media thickness, and microalbuminuria.[135] The importance of these considerations to cardiologists is, first, that chronic kidney disease (CKD) is an important consequence of hypertension, and, second, that it is associated with a marked increase in cardiovascular risk. In the case of patients on hemodialysis, the risk is 10 to 30 times higher than in the general population, and a task force of the American Heart Association has recommended that patients with CKD should be considered as being in the highest risk group for cardiovascular disease.[136] There are two main effects of CKD on the arteries: First, there is an increased prevalence of atherosclerosis, and it has been suggested that uremia accelerates atherogenesis[137]; second, there is remodeling of the arteries and increased stiffness, which has been related to increased mortality.[93]

As highlighted by JNC 7,[1] the dramatic decline in death rates from coronary heart disease and stroke that we have witnessed in the past 30 years has not been paralleled by any decline of end-stage renal disease, which has been showing a relentless increase.[1] Many of these incident cases have been attributed to poorly controlled hypertension, and the others mostly to diabetes. Renal disease and diabetes are the two conditions where JNC 7[1] and other guidelines, such as those from the National Kidney Foundation,[138,139] have proposed lower thresholds for treatment (130/80 mmHg vs. 140/90 mmHg) than in other hypertensive patients, so one would think that the relationship between blood pressure and clinical outcomes should be particularly tight in these conditions.

The only intervention study that has looked at the effects of aggressive antihypertensive treatment in both diabetes and CKD is the HOT (Hypertension Optimal Treatment) study,[140] which was designed to determine if reducing blood pressure to levels lower than in previous trials would produce a greater reduction of events (as predicted by epidemiologic studies). A second reason for the study was to test the J-curve hypothesis,[100] which stated that a more aggressive reduction of blood pressure would result in a paradoxical increase of events than more moderate reductions. The study recruited 18,790 hypertensive patients and randomized them to three groups with different target diastolic blood pressures: <90 mmHg, <85 mmHg, and <80 mmHg. The main conclusion of HOT was somewhere between these two extremes—there was no convincing evidence of additional benefit at the lowest levels of pressure, but also no evidence of harm. One reason why the results were less conclusive than hoped was that there was less separation of the three target levels of blood pressure than was expected. In diabetic patients, however, there was strong evidence that the lower the pressure, the lower the risk. These findings give strong support for the adoption of the lower target blood pressure in diabetes.

A much-less-publicized analysis of the HOT data looked at patients with CKD.[141] Of 18,597 patients in whom serum creatinine values were available at baseline, 2821 had an estimated GFR of less than 60 mL/min. These patients had an event rate during the 3.8 years of followup that was approximately twice as high as the rate in patients with normal renal function (GFR >60 mL/min), which was consistent with other studies showing that impaired renal function is an independent risk factor for cardiovascular disease.[136] The other finding of note was that aggressive reduction of blood pressure, in marked contrast to patients with diabetes, provided no additional benefit in reducing this risk, as shown in Fig. 68–8. Two other randomized controlled trials of patients with CKD, the AASK (African-American Study of Kidney Disease) and REIN-2 (Renoprotection in Patients with Nondiabetic Renal Disease) studies,[142] also

found that more aggressive blood pressure reduction conferred no additional benefit.[143] More recently, a secondary analysis of the AASK data reported that in one of the three drug groups (amlodipine), there was a reduction of one of the secondary end points in the lower blood pressure group.[144] The significance of this is unclear. A third trial, the MDRD (Modification of Diet and Renal Disease) study,[145] did, however, find that randomization to a lower target blood pressure (120/75 mmHg vs. 140/90 mmHg) was associated with a reduced likelihood of progression to renal failure and overall cardiovascular events. It is not clear why these studies have given discrepant results: the MDRD was the longest (6 years as opposed to 3 years for REIN-2 and 4 years for AASK), and it was only after 2 years that the protective effect became apparent. The cumulative probability curves of events for the two groups diverged after 2 years, but showed no further separation between 3 and 6 years.

If it is correct that blood pressure is such an important risk factor for the development of end-stage renal disease, it would be reasonable to suppose that it is also closely related to the incidence of cardiovascular events in patients with end-stage renal disease, as the vast majority of these patients are hypertensive, and cardiovascular disease is the leading cause of death. U.S. Renal Data System statistics[146] indicate that 45 percent of all deaths in patients on hemodialysis are from cardiovascular disease. Unfortunately, no clinical trials have investigated the consequences of treating hypertension in this population. There have been, however, at least 20 observational studies relating blood pressure and mortality in patients on hemodialysis, which were recently reviewed by Agarwal[147] and Pickering.[148] This series of observational studies showed that the usual relationship between systolic blood pressure

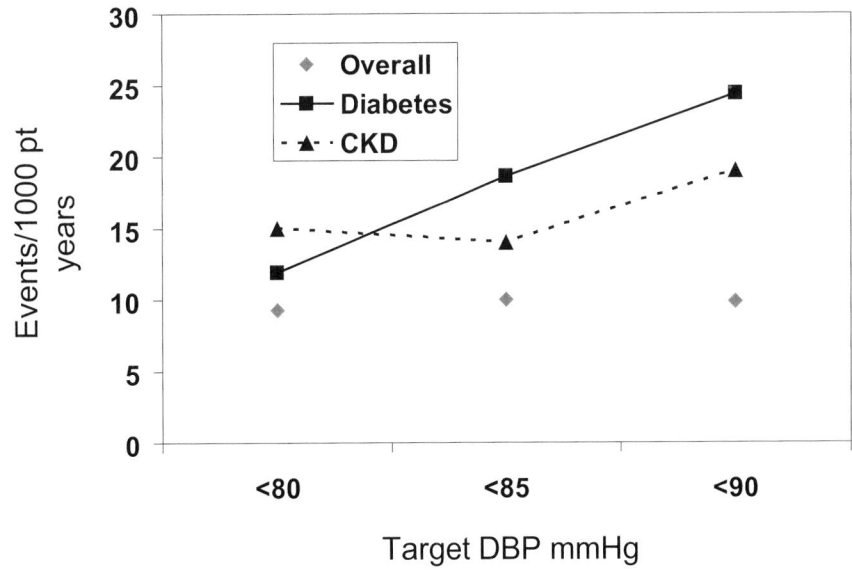

FIGURE 68–8. Relationship between cardiovascular events and achieved diastolic pressure in the HOT study for the overall population and for patients with diabetes and chronic kidney disease (CKD). DBP, diastolic blood pressure; pt, patient. *Source: Data from Hansson L, Zanchetti A, Carruthers SG, et al. Effects of intensive blood-pressure lowering and low-dose aspirin in patients with hypertension: principal results of the Hypertension Optimal Treatment (HOT) randomised trial. HOT Study Group. Lancet 1998;351:1755–1762; and Ruilope LM, Salvetti A, Jamerson K, et al. Renal function and intensive lowering of blood pressure in hypertensive participants of the Hypertension Optimal Treatment (HOT) study. J Am Soc Nephrol 2001;12:2218–2225.*

and risk is rarely found, and the actual relationship may be inverse (higher pressures being associated with lower risk),[149–151] absent,[152,153] or U-shaped (both extremes of blood pressure related to increased risk).[154,155] Although a limited number of these studies did conclude that patients with uncontrolled hypertension were at higher risk,[156,157] none of the studies showed the usual graded and curvilinear relationship between increased systolic blood pressure and risk that is so clearly seen in other populations.

PERIPHERAL VASCULAR DISEASE

Hypertension is a major risk factor for peripheral vascular disease. This is important for two reasons: first, it causes debilitating symptoms, and second, it is a marker of high risk for cardiovascular events.[158] The accepted definition is an ankle-brachial blood pressure index of less than 0.9 (the ratio between the systolic pressure in the ankle and the brachial artery). This test was performed in the latest NHANES examination, and in adults older than age 40 years, the prevalence was 4.3 percent.[159] It is strongly associated with the risk factors of atherosclerotic disease—blood pressure, smoking, cholesterol, diabetes, and, most importantly, age. In a study of the Framingham Offspring the strongest risk factor for peripheral vascular disease was age (odds ratio [OR]: 2.6 per 10 years), followed by hypertension (OR 2.2), and smoking (OR 2.0).[160] The ankle-brachial index predicts stroke more reliably than coronary heart disease.[161] The detection of peripheral vascular disease should prompt a search for atherosclerotic disease in other vascular beds, as 60 percent of patients with it have significant coronary disease, cerebrovascular disease, or both, whereas 40 percent of patients with coronary or cerebrovascular disease also have peripheral vascular disease.[162]

THE BENEFITS OF TREATING HYPERTENSION

It is well established that treating hypertension reduces the rate of strokes by 35 to 40 percent, coronary heart disease events by 20 to 25 percent, and congestive heart failure by up to 50 percent[1] (Table 68–4), and that the benefits of antihypertensive treatment are more closely related to the change of blood pressure than how it is lowered.[128,163] In a patient with stage 1 hypertension (blood pressure 140 to 159/90 to 99 mmHg) it has been estimated that a reduction of 12 mmHg over a 10-year period will prevent 1 death for every 11 patients treated.[1]

TABLE 68–4

Effects of Hypertension Treatment on Morbid Events

EVENT	AVERAGE PERCENT REDUCTION
Stroke	35–40%
Myocardial infarction	20–25%
Heart failure	50%

SOURCE: Adapted from Chobanian AV, Bakris GL, Black HR, et al. The Seventh Report of the Joint National Committee on Prevention, Detection, Evaluation, and Treatment of High Blood Pressure: the JNC 7 report. JAMA 2003;289:(19)2560–2572.

HYPERTENSION AWARENESS AND CONTROL

AWARENESS

The NHANES surveys, which have provided estimates of the prevalence of hypertension, have asked participants if they have been diagnosed as having hypertension. The proportion of hypertensive subjects who are aware of their condition has not shown any significant change over the past 10 years: in 1988 to 1991 it was 69.2 percent, and in 1999 to 2000 it was 68.9 percent.[164] Despite their lower rates of control (28 percent vs. 33.4 percent in whites), African Americans were more likely to be aware that they were hypertensive (73.9 percent vs. 69.5 percent).

In countries where healthcare systems are less-well developed, the level of awareness of hypertension is much lower. In China, 35.6 percent of city dwellers were aware of their condition in 1991, but only 13.9 percent of those living in rural areas were aware of their condition.[52]

CONTROL

The usual definition of blood pressure control is a level less than 140/90 mmHg. For the latest NHANES survey, the overall control rate in the United States in 1999 to 2000 was 31 percent, or 53.1 percent of those on antihypertensive treatment.[164] Thus there are about 40 million Americans with hypertension that is inadequately controlled. Although these figures are disappointing, there was a 6 percent increase in both the treatment and control rates from 1988 to 2000.[164] In the United States, approximately 52 percent of hypertensives are taking medications, whereas in the Europe the numbers are much lower: in Germany, where the prevalence of hypertension is very high (55 percent), only 26 percent of patients are taking antihypertensive medication.[51] In other countries it is even lower: in China, in 1991, the control rate was 4 percent in urban areas, and 1 percent in rural areas.[52] In Egypt, the control rate is 8 percent.[52]

Surveys based on healthcare programs rather than the general population give a more optimistic picture. The 2003 HEDIS (Health Plan Employer Data and Information Set) report stated that blood pressure control rates ranged from 58.6 percent for Medicaid to 62.2 percent for commercial plans, but studies based on ambulatory care practices have quoted figures in the range of 30 to 50 percent.[49] In clinical trials, control rates of up to 70 percent can be obtained;[165] the crucial ingredients here are likely to be the use of rigid treatment protocols and the fact that the participants are likely to be compliant.

For the majority of hypertensive patients, the target blood pressure is 140/90 mmHg, whereas in patients with diabetes or chronic kidney disease, the goal is 130/80 mmHg.[1] The proportion of diabetics who have their blood pressure controlled is approximately 20 to 25 percent,[49] a disappointingly low number in view of the fact that a reduction of blood pressure has such a dramatic impact on cardiovascular morbidity in diabetics. The situation in patients with kidney disease is equally dismal: in NHANES III, only 11 percent of hypertensive CKD patients were below 130/85 mmHg.[166]

The public health implications of poor blood pressure control are enormous. It has been estimated that controlling blood

TABLE 68-5

Factors Related to Poor Control of Hypertension

PATIENT	PHYSICIAN	HEALTH CARE SYSTEM
Older age	Therapeutic inertia	Poor availability of care
Resistant hypertension	Inappropriate choice of drugs	
Poor adherence	Lack of knowledge	
Poor access to care		

pressure to the JNC target levels could prevent 19 percent of CHD events in men and 31 percent in women.[167] Another study, using data from the United Kingdom, concluded that 20 to 35 percent of CHD events and 28 to 44 percent of strokes could be prevented.[168]

[ ] FACTORS RELATED TO POOR BLOOD PRESSURE CONTROL

There are multiple reasons, ranging from physiologic to societal, why blood pressure control is not better. They can be divided into three general categories: factors related to the patient, the healthcare provider, and the healthcare system. Table 68-5 lists some of the more important reasons.

It has been traditional to blame the patients for the poor rates of blood pressure control, on the grounds that they are not taking their prescribed medications. One survey found that 70 percent of doctors attributed treatment failures to poor compliance by their patients, while 81 percent of patients thought their compliance was good.[169] One recent report[170] notes that dropout rates for hypertension range from 11 to 15 percent in the first year, and increase to a range of 16 to 25 percent in the second year of treatment. By the end of 2 years, 25 to 33 percent of patients are no longer compliant with the treatment regimen. Thus, this report indicates that compliance decreases with years of treatment; because control of hypertension requires a lifelong adherence to medication, this is clearly an important factor in morbidity and mortality caused by sustained blood pressure elevations. Other recent reports replicate these results, indicating that approximately one-third of hypertensive patients maintain inadequate followup schedules.[171] In addition, several studies suggest that more than one-third of hypertensive patients are noncompliant with medication regimens.[172] In summary, compliance is a problem. Compliance is highly necessary for the control of hypertension, but continues to remain at relatively low levels.

Another major factor is therapeutic inertia, a concept that was first put on the map by Berlowitz and coworkers[86] who surveyed Veterans' Affairs (VA) clinics, and found that 40 percent of hypertensive patients had blood pressures in excess of 160/90 mmHg, despite an average of six annual visits. Increases in medications were prescribed in only 7 percent of visits. This state of affairs is not likely to be a result of doctors' ignorance about the goals of treatment. In a survey conducted at about the same time as the VA study, 97 percent of physicians knew that the goal blood pressure was 140/90 mmHg.[173] Knowledge does not necessarily dictate behavior, however. In another study of 21 primary care physicians in the United States[174] who were also familiar with the guidelines, the systolic pressure of their hypertensive patients was above 140 mmHg at 93 percent of visits. A more recent study[175] surveyed clinical records of 7253 hypertensive patients from family practices in the South, and quantified therapeutic inertia as the proportion of visits during which the blood pressure was more than 140 mmHg systolic or 90 mmHg diastolic, with no increase in medication. The main finding was a linear relationship between the therapeutic inertia scores and the degree of blood pressure control. For the highest quintile of therapeutic inertia (i.e., the least likely to increase antihypertensive medications) the control rate was 25 percent at the first visit, and 6 percent at the last visit. In contrast, for the lowest therapeutic inertia quintile the control rate increased from 53 percent to 75 percent.

In a recent review of blood pressure control rates in the United States, achieved both in different healthcare systems and in clinical trials, Krakoff[176] suggested four types of intervention that might improve national rates of control: providing education and feedback to providers (which would include attention to therapeutic inertia); making greater use of nonphysician providers; wider use of electronic medical records; and self-monitoring of blood pressure.

REFERENCES

1. Chobanian AV, Bakris GL, Black HR, et al. The seventh report of the Joint National Committee on Prevention, Detection, Evaluation, and Treatment of High Blood Pressure: the JNC 7 report. *JAMA* 2003;289(19):2560–2572.
2. Swales JD. *Platt versus Pickering. An Episode in Recent Medical History*. Cambridge: Keynes Press. British Medical Association, 1985.
3. Miura K, Daviglus ML, Dyer AR, et al. Relationship of blood pressure to 25-year mortality due to coronary heart disease, cardiovascular diseases, and all causes in young adult men: the Chicago Heart Association Detection Project in Industry. *Arch Intern Med* 2001;161(12):1501–1508.
4. Vasan RS, Larson MG, Leip EP, et al. Impact of high-normal blood pressure on the risk of cardiovascular disease. *N Engl J Med* 2001;345(18):1291–1297.
5. Vasan RS, Beiser A, Seshadri S, et al. Residual lifetime risk for developing hypertension in middle-aged women and men: the Framingham Heart Study. *JAMA* 2002;287(8):1003–1010.
6. Greenlund KJ, Croft JB, Mensah GA. Prevalence of heart disease and stroke risk factors in persons with prehypertension in the United States, 1999–2000. *Arch Intern Med* 2004;164(19):2113–2118.
7. Julius S, Nesbitt SD, Egan BM, et al. Feasibility of treating prehypertension with an angiotensin-receptor blocker. *N Engl J Med* 2006;354(16):1685–1697.
8. Edmunds E, Beevers DG, Lip GY. What has happened to malignant hypertension? A disease no longer vanishing. *J Hum Hypertens* 2000;14(3):159–161.
9. Keith NM, Wagener HP, Barker NW. Some different types of essential hypertension: their course and prognosis. *Am J Med Sci* 1939;196:332–343.
10. Kadiri S, Olutade BO. The clinical presentation of malignant hypertension in Nigerians. *J Hum Hypertens* 1991;5(4):339–343.
11. Harington M, Kincaid-Smith P, McMichael J. Results of treatment in malignant hypertension. A seven-year experience in 94 cases. *Br Med J* 1959;ii:969–980.
12. Franklin SS, Khan SA, Wong ND, Larson MG, Levy D. Is pulse pressure useful in predicting risk for coronary heart Disease? The Framingham heart study. *Circulation* 1999;100(4):354–360.
13. Pickering TG. Isolated systolic hypertension in the young. *J Clin Hypertens (Greenwich)* 2004;6(1):47–48.
14. McEniery CM, Yasmin, Wallace S, et al. Increased stroke volume and aortic stiffness contribute to isolated systolic hypertension in young adults. *Hypertension* 2005;46(1):221–226.

15. Franklin SS, Larson MG, Khan SA, et al. Does the relation of blood pressure to coronary heart disease risk change with aging? The Framingham Heart Study. *Circulation* 2001;103(9):1245–1249.

16. Pickering TG. Isolated diastolic hypertension. *J Clin Hypertens (Greenwich)* 2003;5(6):411–413.

17. Franklin SS, Pio JR, Wong ND, et al. Predictors of new-onset diastolic and systolic hypertension: the Framingham Heart Study. *Circulation* 2005;111(9):1121–1127.

18. Pickering TG, Hall JE, Appel LJ, et al. Recommendations for blood pressure measurement in humans and experimental animals: part 1: blood pressure measurement in humans: a statement for professionals from the Subcommittee of Professional and Public Education of the American Heart Association Council on High Blood Pressure Research. *Circulation* 2005;111(5):697–716.

19. Jhalani J, Goyal T, Clemow L, Schwartz JE, Pickering TG, Gerin W. Anxiety and outcome expectations predict the white coat effect. *Blood Press Monit* 2005;10(6):317–319.

20. Verdecchia P, Reboldi GP, Angeli F, et al. Short- and long-term incidence of stroke in white-coat hypertension. *Hypertension* 2005;45(2):203–208.

21. Pickering TG, Davidson K, Gerin W, Schwartz JE. Masked hypertension. *Hypertension* 2002;40(6):795–796.

22. Liu JE, Roman MJ, Pini R, et al. Cardiac and arterial target organ damage in adults with elevated ambulatory and normal office pressure. *Ann Intern Med* 1999;131:564–571.

23. Bjorklund K, Lind L, Zethelius B, Andren B, Lithell H. Isolated ambulatory hypertension predicts cardiovascular morbidity in elderly men. *Circulation* 2003;107(9):1297–1302.

24. Pierdomenico SD, Lapenna D, Bucci A, di Tommaso R, di Mascio R, Manente BM, et al. Cardiovascular outcome in treated hypertensive patients with responder, masked, false resistant and true resistant hypertension. *Am J Hypertens* 2005;18(11):1422–1428.

25. Bobrie G, Chatellier G, Genes N, et al. Cardiovascular prognosis of "masked hypertension" detected by blood pressure self-measurement in elderly treated hypertensive patients. *JAMA* 2004;291(11):1342–1349.

26. Belmin J, Visintin JM, Salvatore R, Sebban C, Moulias R. Osler's maneuver: absence of usefulness for the detection of pseudohypertension in an elderly population. *Am J Med* 1995;98(1):42–49.

27. Anzal M, Palmer AJ, Starr J, Bulpitt CJ. The prevalence of pseudohypertension in the elderly. *J Hum Hypertens* 1996;10(6):409–411.

28. Consensus statement of the definition of orthostatic hypotension, pure autonomic failure, and multiple system atrophy. *J Neurol Sci* 1996;144:218–219.

29. Jordan J, Biaggioni I. Diagnosis and treatment of supine hypertension in autonomic failure patients with orthostatic hypotension. *J Clin Hypertens (Greenwich)* 2002;4(2):139–145.

30. Vagaonescu TD, Saadia D, Tuhrim S, Phillips RA, Kaufmann H. Hypertensive cardiovascular damage in patients with primary autonomic failure. *Lancet* 2000;355(9205):725–726.

31. Toyry JP, Niskanen LK, Lansimies EA, Partanen KP, Uusitupa MI. Autonomic neuropathy predicts the development of stroke in patients with non-insulin-dependent diabetes mellitus. *Stroke* 1996;27(8):1316–1318.

32. Low PA, Opfer-Gehrking TL, McPhee BR, Fealey RD, Benarroch EE, Willner CL, et al. Prospective evaluation of clinical characteristics of orthostatic hypotension. *Mayo Clin Proc* 1995;70(7):617–622.

33. Young T, Palta M, Dempsey J, Skatrud J, Weber S, Badr S. The occurrence of sleep-disordered breathing among middle-aged adults. *N Engl J Med* 1993;328(17):1230–1235.

34. Young T, Shahar E, Nieto FJ, et al. Predictors of sleep-disordered breathing in community-dwelling adults: the Sleep Heart Health Study. *Arch Intern Med* 2002;162(8):893–900.

35. Silverberg DS, Oksenberg A, Iaina A. Sleep-related breathing disorders as a major cause of essential hypertension: fact or fiction? *Curr Opin Nephrol Hypertens* 1998;7(4):353–357.

36. Lavie P, Ben Yosef R, Rubin AE. Prevalence of sleep apnea syndrome among patients with essential hypertension. *Am Heart J* 1984;108(2):373–376.

37. Fletcher EC, DeBehnke RD, Lovoi MS, Gorin AB. Undiagnosed sleep apnea in patients with essential hypertension. *Ann Intern Med* 1985;103(2):190–195.

38. Nieto FJ, Young TB, Lind BK, et al. Association of sleep-disordered breathing, sleep apnea, and hypertension in a large community-based study. Sleep Heart Health Study. *JAMA* 2000;283(14):1829–1836.

39. O'Brien E, Mee F, Atkins N, O'Malley K. Accuracy of the SpaceLabs 90207 Novacor DIASYS 200 Del Mar Avionics Pressurometer IV and Takeda TM-2420 ambulatory systems according to British and American criteria. *J Hypertens* Suppl 1991;9(6):S332–S333.

40. Haas DC, Foster GL, Nieto FJ, et al. Age-dependent associations between sleep-disordered breathing and hypertension: importance of discriminating between systolic/diastolic hypertension and isolated systolic hypertension in the Sleep Heart Health Study. *Circulation* 2005;111(5):614–621.

41. Peppard PE, Young T, Palta M, Skatrud J. Prospective study of the association between sleep-disordered breathing and hypertension. *N Engl J Med* 2000;342(19):1378–1384.

42. Sega R, Cesana G, Costa G, Ferrario M, Bombelli M, Mancia G. Ambulatory blood pressure in air traffic controllers. *Am J Hypertens* 1998;11(2):208–212.

43. Nichols WW, O'Rourke MF. *McDonald's Blood Flow in Arteries*, 5th ed. London: Hodder Arnold, 2005.

44. Franklin SS. Arterial stiffness and hypertension: a two-way street? *Hypertension* 2005;45(3):349–351.

45. Bulpitt CJ. Controlling hypertension in the elderly. *QJM* 2000;93(4):203–205.

46. Mattila K, Haavisto M, Rajala S, Heikinheimo R. Blood pressure and five year survival in the very old. *BMJ* 1988;296(6626):887–889.

47. Langer RD, Criqui MH, Barrett-Connor EL, Klauber MR, Ganiats TG. Blood pressure change and survival after age 75. *Hypertension* 1993;22(4):551–559.

48. Bulpitt CJ, Beckett NS, Cooke J, et al. Results of the pilot study for the Hypertension in the Very Elderly Trial. *J Hypertens* 2003;21(12):2409–2417.

49. Wang TJ, Vasan RS. Epidemiology of uncontrolled hypertension in the United States. *Circulation* 2005;112(11):1651–1662.

50. Centers for Disease Control and Prevention (CDC). Racial/ethnic disparities in prevalence, treatment, and control of hypertension—United States, 1999–2002. *MMWR Morb Mortal Wkly Rep* 2005;54:7–9.

51. Wolf-Maier K, Cooper RS, Banegas JR, et al. Hypertension prevalence and blood pressure levels in 6 European countries, Canada, and the United States. *JAMA* 2003;289(18):2363–2369.

52. Whelton PK, He J, Muntner P. Prevalence, awareness, treatment and control of hypertension in North America, North Africa and Asia. *J Hum Hypertens* 2004;18(8):545–551.

53. Hertz RP, Unger AN, Cornell JA, Saunders E. Racial disparities in hypertension prevalence, awareness, and management. *Arch Intern Med* 2005;165(18):2098–2104.

54. Ribeiro AB, Ribeiro MB. Epidemiological and demographic considerations. Hypertension in underdeveloped countries. *Drugs* 1986;31(suppl 4):23–28.

55. Poulter NR, Khaw KT, Hopwood BE, et al. The Kenyan Luo migration study: observations on the initiation of a rise in blood pressure. *BMJ* 1990;300(6730):967–972.

56. Cooper R, Rotimi C. Hypertension in blacks. *Am J Hypertens* 1997;10(7 Pt 1):804–812.

57. Cooper RS, Wolf-Maier K, Luke A, et al. An international comparative study of blood pressure in populations of European vs. African descent. *BMC Med* 2005;3:2.

58. Primatesta P, Bost L, Poulter NR. Blood pressure levels and hypertension status among ethnic groups in England. *J Hum Hypertens* 2000;14:143–148.

59. Cruickshank JK, Jackson SH, Beevers DG, Bannan LT, Beevers M, Stewart VL. Similarity of blood pressure in blacks, whites and Asians in England: the Birmingham Factory Study. *J Hypertens* 1985;3(4):365–371.

60. Tyroler HA. Socioeconomic status in the epidemiology and treatment of hypertension. *Hypertension* 1989;13(5 Suppl):I94–I97.

61. Harburg E, Erfurt JC, Hauenstein LS, Chape C, Schull WJ, Schork MA. Socio-ecological stress, suppressed hostility, skin color, and black-white male blood pressure: Detroit. *Psychosom Med* 1973;35(4):276–296.

62. Harburg E, Erfurt JC, Chape C, Hauenstein LS, Schull WJ, Schork MA. Socioecological stressor areas and black-white blood pressure: Detroit. *J Chronic Dis* 1973;26(9):595–611.

63. Diez-Roux AV, Nieto FJ, Muntaner C, et al. Neighborhood environments and coronary heart disease: a multilevel analysis. *Am J Epidemiol* 1997;146(1):48–63.

64. Sacco RL, Boden-Albala B, Abel G, et al. Race–ethnic disparities in the impact of stroke risk factors: the northern Manhattan stroke study. *Stroke* 2001;32(8):1725–1731.

65. Cooper RS. Race, genes, and health—new wine in old bottles? *Int J Epidemiol* 2003;32(1):23–25.

66. Sorlie PD, Backlund E, Johnson NJ, Rogot E. Mortality by Hispanic status in the United States. *JAMA* 1993;270(20):2464–2468.

67. Hunt KJ, Resendez RG, Williams K, Haffner SM, Stern MP, Hazuda HP. All-cause and cardiovascular mortality among Mexican-American and non-Hispanic white older participants in the San Antonio Heart Study—evidence against the "Hispanic paradox." *Am J Epidemiol* 2003;158(11):1048–1057.

68. Ordunez-Garcia PO, Espinosa-Brito AD, Cooper RS, Kaufman JS, Nieto FJ. Hypertension in Cuba: evidence of a narrow black–white difference. *J Hum Hypertens* 1998;12(2):111–116.

69. Costas R Jr, Garcia-Palmieri MR, Sorlie P, Hertzmark E. Coronary heart disease risk factors in men with light and dark skin in Puerto Rico. *Am J Public Health* 1981;71(6):614–619.

70. Stavig GR, Igra A, Leonard AR. Hypertension among Asians and Pacific islanders in California. *Am J Epidemiol* 1984;119(5):677–691.

71. Howard BV, Lee ET, Yeh JL, et al. *Hypertension* in adult American Indians. The Strong Heart Study. *Hypertension* 1996;28(2):256–264.

72. Prospective Studies Collaboration. Age-specific relevance of usual blood pressure to vascular mortality: a meta-analysis of individual data for one million adults in 61 prospective studies. *Lancet* 2002;360:1903–1913.

73. MacMahon S, Peto R, Cutler J, et al. Blood pressure, stroke, and coronary heart disease. Part 1. Prolonged differences in blood pressure: prospective observational studies corrected for the regression dilution bias [see comments]. *Lancet* 1990;335(8692):765–774.

74. Blacher J, Staessen JA, Girerd X, et al. Pulse pressure not mean pressure determines cardiovascular risk in older hypertensive patients. *Arch Intern Med* 2000;160(8):1085–1089.

75. Domanski M, Mitchell G, Pfeffer M, et al. Pulse pressure and cardiovascular disease-related mortality: follow-up study of the Multiple Risk Factor Intervention Trial (MRFIT). *JAMA* 2002;287(20):2677–2683.

76. Madhavan S, Ooi WL, Cohen H, Alderman MH. Relation of pulse pressure and blood pressure reduction to the incidence of myocardial infarction. *Hypertension* 1994;23(3):395–401.

77. Miura K, Dyer AR, Greenland P, et al. Pulse pressure compared with other blood pressure indexes in the prediction of 25-year cardiovascular and all-cause mortality rates: The Chicago Heart Association Detection Project in Industry Study. *Hypertension* 2001;38(2):232–237.

78. Lawes CM, Bennett DA, Parag V, et al. Blood pressure indices and cardiovascular disease in the Asia Pacific region: a pooled analysis. *Hypertension* 2003;42(1):69–75.

79. Davidson KW, Haas DC, Shimbo D, Pickering TG, Jonas BS. Standardizing the comparison of systolic blood pressure vs pulse pressure for predicting coronary heart disease. *J Clin Hypertens (Greenwich)* 2006;8(6):411–413.

80. Liu L, Wang JG, Gong L, Liu G, Staessen JA. Comparison of active treatment and placebo in older Chinese patients with isolated systolic hypertension. Systolic Hypertension in China (Syst-China) Collaborative Group. *J Hypertens* 1998;16(12 Pt 1):1823–1829.

81. Prevention of stroke by antihypertensive drug treatment in older persons with isolated systolic hypertension. Final results of the Systolic Hypertension in the Elderly Program (SHEP). SHEP Cooperative Research Group. *JAMA* 1991;265(24):3255–3264.

82. Staessen JA, Fagard R, Thijs L, et al. Randomised double-blind comparison of placebo and active treatment for older patients with isolated systolic hypertension. The Systolic Hypertension in Europe (Syst-Eur) Trial Investigators. *Lancet* 1997;350(9080):757–764.

83. Somes GW, Pahor M, Shorr RI, Cushman WC, Applegate WB. The role of diastolic blood pressure when treating isolated systolic hypertension. *Arch Intern Med* 1999;159(17):2004–2009.

84. O'Rourke MF. From theory into practice: arterial haemodynamics in clinical hypertension. *J Hypertens* 2002;20(10):1901–1915.

85. Millar JA, Lever AF. Implications of pulse pressure as a predictor of cardiac risk in patients with hypertension. *Hypertension* 2000;36(5):907–911.

86. Berlowitz DR, Ash AS, Hickey EC, et al. Inadequate management of blood pressure in a hypertensive population. *N Engl J Med* 1998;339:1957–1963.

87. Cushman WC, Materson BJ, Williams DW, Reda DJ. Pulse pressure changes with six classes of antihypertensive agents in a randomized, controlled trial. *Hypertension* 2001;38(4):953–957.

88. Millar JA, Lever AF, Burke V. Pulse pressure as a risk factor for cardiovascular events in the MRC Mild Hypertension Trial. *J Hypertens* 1999;17(8):1065–1072.

89. Verdecchia P, Schillaci G, Reboldi G, Franklin SS, Porcellati C. Different prognostic impact of 24-hour mean blood pressure and pulse pressure on stroke and coronary artery disease in essential hypertension. *Circulation* 2001;103(21):2579–2584.

90. Williams B, Lacy PS, Thom SM, et al. Differential impact of blood pressure-lowering drugs on central aortic pressure and clinical outcomes: principal results of the Conduit Artery Function Evaluation (CAFE) study. *Circulation* 2006;113(9):1213–1225.

91. Van Bortel LM, Duprez D, Starmans-Kool MJ, et al. Clinical applications of arterial stiffness, Task Force III. Recommendations for user procedures. *Am J Hypertens* 2002;15(5):445–452.

92. Mattace-Raso FU, van der Cammen TJ, Hofman A, et al. Arterial stiffness and risk of coronary heart disease and stroke: the Rotterdam Study. *Circulation* 2006;113(5):657–663.

93. London GM, Blacher J, Pannier B, Guerin AP, Marchais SJ, Safar ME. Arterial wave reflections and survival in end-stage renal failure. *Hypertension* 2001;38(3):434–438.

94. Kato J, Aihara A, Kikuya M, et al. Risk factors and predictors of coronary arterial lesions in Japanese hypertensive patients. *Hypertens Res* 2001;24(1):3–11.

95. Neaton JD, Wentworth D. Serum cholesterol, blood pressure, cigarette smoking, and death from coronary heart disease. Overall findings and differences by age for 316,099 white men. Multiple Risk Factor Intervention Trial Research Group. *Arch Intern Med* 1992;152(1):56–64.

96. van den Hoogen PC, Feskens EJ, Nagelkerke NJ, Menotti A, Nissinen A, Kromhout D. The relation between blood pressure and mortality due to coronary heart disease among men in different parts of the world. Seven Countries Study Research Group. *N Engl J Med* 2000;342(1):1–8.

97. Greenland P, Knoll MD, Stamler J, et al. Major risk factors as antecedents of fatal and nonfatal coronary heart disease events. *JAMA* 2003;290(7):891–897.

98. Flack JM, Neaton J, Grimm R Jr, et al. Blood pressure and mortality among men with prior myocardial infarction. Multiple Risk Factor Intervention Trial Research Group. *Circulation* 1995;92(9):2437–2445.

99. Herlitz J, Bang A, Karlson BW. Five-year prognosis after acute myocardial infarction in relation to a history of hypertension. *Am J Hypertens* 1996;9(1):70–76.

100. Cruickshank JM, Thorp JM, Zacharias FJ. Benefits and potential harm of lowering high blood pressure. *Lancet* 1987;1(8533):581–584.

101. Messerli FH, Mancia G, Conti CR, et al. Dogma disputed: can aggressively lowering blood pressure in hypertensive patients with coronary artery disease be dangerous? *Ann Intern Med* 2006;144(12):884–893.

102. Kannel WB, Wilson PW, Nam BH, D'Agostino RB, Li J. A likely explanation for the J-curve of blood pressure cardiovascular risk. *Am J Cardiol* 2004;94(3):380–384.

103. Nissen SE, Tuzcu EM, Libby P, et al. Effect of antihypertensive agents on cardiovascular events in patients with coronary disease and normal blood pressure: the CAMELOT study: a randomized controlled trial. *JAMA* 2004;292(18):2217–2225.

104. Lloyd-Jones DM, Larson MG, Leip EP, et al. Lifetime risk for developing congestive heart failure: the Framingham Heart Study. *Circulation* 2002;106(24):3068–3072.

105. Lloyd-Jones DM. The risk of congestive heart failure: sobering lessons from the Framingham Heart Study. *Curr Cardiol Rep* 2001;3(3):184–190.

106. Levy D, Larson MG, Vasan RS, Kannel WB, Ho KK. The progression from hypertension to congestive heart failure. *JAMA* 1996;275(20):1557–1562.

107. Haider AW, Larson MG, Franklin SS, Levy D. Systolic blood pressure, diastolic blood pressure, and pulse pressure as predictors of risk for congestive heart failure in the Framingham Heart Study. *Ann Intern Med* 2003;138(1):10–16.

108. Levy D, Kenchaiah S, Larson MG, et al. Long-term trends in the incidence of and survival with heart failure. *N Engl J Med* 2002;347(18):1397–1402.

109. Vasan RS, Benjamin EJ, Levy D. Prevalence, clinical features and prognosis of diastolic heart failure: an epidemiologic perspective. *J Am Coll Cardiol* 1995;26(7):1565–1574.

110. Senni M, Tribouilloy CM, Rodeheffer RJ, et al. Congestive heart failure in the community: trends in incidence and survival in a 10-year period. *Arch Intern Med* 1999;159(1):29–34.

111. Vasan RS, Larson MG, Benjamin EJ, Evans JC, Reiss CK, Levy D. Congestive heart failure in subjects with normal versus reduced left ventricular ejection fraction: prevalence and mortality in a population-based cohort. *J Am Coll Cardiol* 1999;33(7):1948–1955.

112. Hundley WG, Kitzman DW, Morgan TM, et al. Cardiac cycle-dependent changes in aortic area and distensibility are reduced in older patients with isolated diastolic heart failure and correlate with exercise intolerance. *J Am Coll Cardiol* 2001;38(3):796–802.

113. Burkhoff D, Maurer MS, Packer M. Heart failure with a normal ejection fraction: is it really a disorder of diastolic function? *Circulation* 2003;107(5):656–658.

114. Warlow C, Sudlow C, Dennis M, Wardlaw J, Sandercock P. Stroke. *Lancet* 2003;362(9391):1211–1224.

115. Nielsen WB, Lindenstrom E, Vestbo J, Jensen GB. Is diastolic hypertension an independent risk factor for stroke in the presence of normal systolic blood pressure in the middle-aged and elderly? *Am J Hypertens* 1997;10(6):634–639.

116. Droste DW, Ritter MA, Dittrich R, et al. Arterial hypertension and ischaemic stroke. *Acta Neurol Scand* 2003;107(4):241–251.

117. Prospective Studies Collaboration. Cholesterol, diastolic blood pressure, and stroke: 13,000 strokes in 450,000 people in 45 prospective cohorts. *Lancet* 1995;346:1647–1653.

118. Amarenco P, Labreuche J, Lavallee P, Touboul PJ. Statins in stroke prevention and carotid atherosclerosis: systematic review and up-to-date meta-analysis. *Stroke* 2004;35(12):2902–2909.

119. Amarenco P, Bogousslavsky J, Callahan A III, et al. High-dose atorvastatin after stroke or transient ischemic attack. *N Engl J Med* 2006;355(6):549–559.

120. Lumley T, Kronmal RA, Cushman M, Manolio TA, Goldstein S. A stroke prediction score in the elderly: validation and Web-based application. *J Clin Epidemiol* 2002;55(2):129–136.

121. Fisher CM. Capsular infarcts: the underlying vascular lesions. *Arch Neurol* 1979;36(2):65–73.

122. Donnan GA, Thrift A, You RX, McNeil JJ. Hypertension and stroke. *J Hypertens* 1994;12(8):865–869.

123. Thrift AG, McNeil JJ, Forbes A, Donnan GA. Three important subgroups of hypertensive persons at greater risk of intracerebral hemorrhage. Melbourne Risk Factor Study Group. *Hypertension* 1998;31(6):1223–1229.

124. Di Tullio MR, Sacco RL, Savoia MT, Sciacca RR, Homma S. Aortic atheroma morphology and the risk of ischemic stroke in a multiethnic population. *Am Heart J* 2000;139(2 Pt 1):329–336.

125. Jacobs DR Jr, McGovern PG, Blackburn H. The U.S. decline in stroke mortality: what does ecological analysis tell us? *Am J Public Health* 1992;82(12):1596–1599.

126. Casper M, Wing S, Strogatz D, Davis CE, Tyroler HA. Antihypertensive treatment and U.S. trends in stroke mortality, 1962 to 1980. *Am J Public Health* 1992;82(12):1600–1606.

127. Goldstein LB, Adams R, Alberts MJ, et al. Primary prevention of ischemic stroke: a guideline from the American Heart Association/American Stroke Association Stroke Council: cosponsored by the Atherosclerotic Peripheral Vascular Disease Interdisciplinary Working Group; Cardiovascular Nursing Council; Clinical Cardiology Council; Nutrition, Physical Activity, and Metabolism Council; and the Quality of Care and Outcomes Research Interdisciplinary Working Group. *Circulation* 2006;113(24):e873–e923.

128. Staessen JA, Wang JG, Thijs L. Cardiovascular prevention and blood pressure reduction: a quantitative overview updated until 1 March 2003. *J Hypertens* 2003;21(6):1055–1076.

129. Lindholm LH, Carlberg B, Samuelsson O. Should beta blockers remain first choice in the treatment of primary hypertension? A meta-analysis. *Lancet* 2005;366(9496):1545–1553.

130. Schrader J, Luders S, Kulschewski A, et al. Morbidity and mortality after stroke, eprosartan compared with nitrendipine for secondary prevention: principal results of a prospective randomized controlled study (MOSES). *Stroke* 2005;36(6):1218–1226.

131. Tozawa M, Iseki K, Iseki C, Kinjo K, Ikemiya Y, Takishita S. Blood pressure predicts risk of developing end-stage renal disease in men and women. *Hypertension* 2003;41(6):1341–1345.

132. Vupputuri S, Batuman V, Muntner P, et al. Effect of blood pressure on early decline in kidney function among hypertensive men. *Hypertension* 2003;42(6):1144–1149.

133. Klag MJ, Whelton PK, Randall BL, Neaton JD, Brancati FL, Stamler J. End-stage renal disease in African-American and white men. 16-year MRFIT findings. *JAMA* 1997;277(16):1293–1298.

134. Anavekar NS, McMurray JJ, Velazquez EJ, et al. Relation between renal dysfunction and cardiovascular outcomes after myocardial infarction. *N Engl J Med* 2004;351(13):1285–1295.

135. Leoncini G, Viazzi F, Parodi D, et al. Mild renal dysfunction and subclinical cardiovascular damage in primary hypertension. *Hypertension* 2003;42(1):14–18.

136. Sarnak MJ, Levey AS, Schoolwerth AC, et al. Kidney disease as a risk factor for development of cardiovascular disease: a statement from the American Heart Association Councils on Kidney in Cardiovascular Disease, High Blood Pressure Research, Clinical Cardiology, and Epidemiology and Prevention. *Circulation* 2003;108(17):2154–2169.

137. Jungers P, Massy ZA, Nguyen KT, et al. Incidence and risk factors of atherosclerotic cardiovascular accidents in predialysis chronic renal failure patients: a prospective study. *Nephrol Dial Transplant* 1997;12(12):2597–2602.

138. K/DOQI clinical practice guidelines on hypertension and antihypertensive agents in chronic kidney disease. *Am J Kidney Dis* 2004;43(suppl):11–270.

139. K/DOQI clinical practice guidelines for cardiovascular disease in dialysis patients. *Am J Kidney Dis* 2005;45 suppl 3:S1–S75.

140. Hansson L, Zanchetti A, Carruthers SG, et al. Effects of intensive blood-pressure lowering and low-dose aspirin in patients with hypertension: principal results of the Hypertension Optimal Treatment (HOT) randomised trial. HOT Study Group . *Lancet* 1998;351(9118):1755–1762.

141. Ruilope LM, Salvetti A, Jamerson K, et al. Renal function and intensive lowering of blood pressure in hypertensive participants of the hypertension optimal treatment (HOT) study. *J Am Soc Nephrol* 2001;12(2):218–225.

142. Ruggenenti P, Perna A, Loriga G, et al. Blood-pressure control for renoprotection in patients with non-diabetic chronic renal disease (REIN-2): multicentre, randomised controlled trial. *Lancet* 2005;365(9463):939–946.

143. Wright JT Jr, Bakris G, Greene T, et al. Effect of blood pressure lowering and antihypertensive drug class on progression of hypertensive kidney disease: results from the AASK trial. *JAMA* 2002;288(19):2421–2431.

144. Contreras G, Greene T, Agodoa LY, et al. Blood pressure control, drug therapy, and kidney disease. *Hypertension* 2005;46(1):44–50.

145. Sarnak MJ, Greene T, Wang X, et al. The effect of a lower target blood pressure on the progression of kidney disease: long-term follow-up of the modification of diet in renal disease study. *Ann Intern Med* 2005;142(5):342–351.

146. U.S. Renal data system. Death rates by primary cause of death. 659. 2000. Bethesda. 2000 Annual Data Report, reference tables; table H 18. Ref Type: Report.

147. Agarwal R. Hypertension and survival in chronic hemodialysis patients—past lessons and future opportunities. *Kidney Int* 2005;67(1):1–13.

148. Pickering TG. Target blood pressure in patients with end-stage renal disease: evidence-based medicine or the emperor's new clothes? *J Clin Hypertens (Greenwich)* 2006;8(5):369–375.

149. Klassen PS, Lowrie EG, Reddan DN, et al. Association between pulse pressure and mortality in patients undergoing maintenance hemodialysis. *JAMA* 2002;287(12):1548–1555.

150. Foley RN, Parfrey PS, Harnett JD, Kent GM, Murray DC, Barre PE. Impact of hypertension on cardiomyopathy, morbidity and mortality in end-stage renal disease. *Kidney Int* 1996;49(5):1379–1385.

151. Goodkin DA, Bragg-Gresham JL, Koenig KG, et al. Association of comorbid conditions and mortality in hemodialysis patients in Europe, Japan, and the United States: the Dialysis Outcomes and Practice Patterns Study (DOPPS). *J Am Soc Nephrol* 2003;14(12):3270–3277.

152. Salem MM. *Hypertension* in the haemodialysis population: any relationship to 2-years survival? *Nephrol Dial Transplant* 1999;14(1):125–128.

153. Koch M, Thomas B, Tschope W, Ritz E. Survival and predictors of death in dialysed diabetic patients. *Diabetologia* 1993;36(10):1113–1117.

154. Lynn KL, McGregor DO, Moesbergen T, Buttimore AL, Inkster JA, Wells JE. *Hypertension* as a determinant of survival for patients treated with home dialysis. *Kidney Int* 2002;62(6):2281–2287.

155. Zager PG, Nikolic J, Brown RH, et al. "U" curve association of blood pressure and mortality in hemodialysis patients. Medical Directors of Dialysis Clinic, Inc. *Kidney Int* 1998;54(2):561–569.

156. Tomita J, Kimura G, Inoue T, et al. Role of systolic blood pressure in determining prognosis of hemodialyzed patients. *Am J Kidney Dis* 1995;25(3):405–412.

157. De Lima JJ, Vieira ML, Abensur H, Krieger EM. Baseline blood pressure and other variables influencing survival on haemodialysis of patients without overt cardiovascular disease. *Nephrol Dial Transplant* 2001;16(4):793–797.

158. Criqui MH, Langer RD, Fronek A, et al. Mortality over a period of 10 years in patients with peripheral arterial disease. *N Engl J Med* 1992;326(6):381–386.

159. Selvin E, Erlinger TP. Prevalence of and risk factors for peripheral arterial disease in the United States: results from the National Health and Nutrition Examination Survey, 1999–2000. *Circulation* 2004;110(6):738–743.

160. Murabito JM, Evans JC, Nieto K, Larson MG, Levy D, Wilson PW. Prevalence and clinical correlates of peripheral arterial disease in the Framingham Offspring Study. *Am Heart J* 2002;143(6):961–965.

161. Zheng ZJ, Sharrett AR, Chambless LE, et al. Associations of ankle-brachial index with clinical coronary heart disease, stroke and preclinical carotid and popliteal atherosclerosis: the Atherosclerosis Risk in Communities (ARIC) Study. *Atherosclerosis* 1997;131(1):115–125.

162. Hirsch AT, Haskal ZJ, Hertzer NR, et al. ACC/AHA 2005 guidelines for the management of patients with peripheral arterial disease (lower extremity, renal, mesenteric, and abdominal aortic): executive summary a collaborative report from the American Association for Vascular Surgery/Society for Vascular Surgery, Society for Cardiovascular Angiography and Interventions, Society for Vascular Medicine and Biology, Society of Interventional Radiology, and the ACC/AHA Task Force on Practice Guidelines (Writing Committee to Develop Guidelines for the Management of Patients With Peripheral Arte-

rial Disease) endorsed by the American Association of Cardiovascular and Pulmonary Rehabilitation; National Heart, Lung, and Blood Institute; Society for Vascular Nursing; TransAtlantic Inter-Society Consensus; and Vascular Disease Foundation. *J Am Coll Cardiol* 2006;47(6):1239–1312.

163. Blood Pressure Lowering Treatment Trialists' Collaboration. Effects of ACE inhibitors, calcium antagonists, and other blood-pressure-lowering drugs: results of prospectively designed overviews of randomised trials. *Lancet* 2000;355:1955–1964.

164. Hajjar I, Kotchen TA. Trends in prevalence, awareness, treatment, and control of hypertension in the United States, 1988–2000. *JAMA* 2003;290(2):199–206.

165. Black HR, Elliott WJ, Neaton JD, et al. Baseline characteristics and early blood pressure control in the CONVINCE trial. *Hypertension* 2001;37(1):12–18.

166. Coresh J, Wei GL, McQuillan G, et al. Prevalence of high blood pressure and elevated serum creatinine level in the United States: findings from the third National Health and Nutrition Examination Survey (1988–1994). *Arch Intern Med* 2001;161(9):1207–1216.

167. Wong ND, Thakral G, Franklin SS, et al. Preventing heart disease by controlling hypertension: impact of hypertensive subtype, stage, age, and sex. *Am Heart J* 2003;145(5):888–895.

168. He FJ, MacGregor GA. Cost of poor blood pressure control in the UK. 62,000 unnecessary deaths per year. *J Hum Hypertens* 2003;17(7):455–457.

169. Menard J, Chatellier G. Limiting factors in the control of BP. Why is there a gap between theory and practice? *J Hum Hypertens* 1995;9 Suppl 2:S19–S23.

170. Luscher TF, Vetter W. Adherence to medication. *J Hum Hypertens* 1990;4 Suppl 1:43–46.

171. Ballard DJ, Strogatz DS, Wagner EH, et al. Hypertension control in a rural southern community: medical care process and dropping out. *Am J Prev Med* 1988;4(3):133–139.

172. Nelson EC, Stason WB, Neutra RR, Solomon HS. Identification of the non-compliant hypertensive patient. *Prev Med* 1980;9(4):504–517.

173. Margolis KL, Rolnick SJ, Fortman KK, Maciosek MV, Hildebrant CL, Grimm RH Jr. Self-reported hypertension treatment beliefs and practices of primary care physicians in a managed care organization. *Am J Hypertens* 2005;18(4 Pt 1):566–571.

174. Oliveria SA, Lapuerta P, McCarthy BD, L'Italien GJ, Berlowitz DR, Asch SM. Physician-related barriers to the effective management of uncontrolled hypertension. *Arch Intern Med* 2002;162(4):413–420.

175. Okonofua EC, Simpson KN, Jesri A, Rehman SU, Durkalski VL, Egan BM. Therapeutic inertia is an impediment to achieving the Healthy People 2010 blood pressure control goals. *Hypertension* 2006;47(3):345–351.

176. Krakoff LR. Systems for care of hypertension in the United States. *J Clin Hypertens (Greenwich)* 2006;8(6):420–426.

CHAPTER 69

Pathophysiology of Hypertension

*John E. Hall / Joey P. Granger / Michael E. Hall /
Daniel W. Jones*

INTRODUCTION

More than 1 *billion* individuals worldwide, including 50 million Americans, have high blood pressures warranting some form of treatment.[1–4] Higher-than-optimal blood pressure is the number one attributable risk for death throughout the world and approximately 7.1 million deaths per year are attributed to uncontrolled hypertension.[3] As life expectancy increases, hypertension is becoming an even more important medical and public health issue as blood pressure rises with aging in industrialized countries. In the United States, 50 percent of people 60 to 69 years old, and approximately 75 percent of people 70 years and older, have hypertension.[1] In some isolated, nonindustrialized populations, however, blood pressure does not increase with increasing age and only a small fraction of the population develops hypertension. This suggests that predisposing environmental factors play a major role

in causing hypertension and that a rise in blood pressure with aging is not inevitable when these factors are absent.

A direct positive relationship between blood pressure and cardiovascular disease (CVD) risk has been observed in men and women of all ages, races, ethnic groups, and countries, regardless of other risk factors for CVD.[4] Observational studies indicate that death from CVD increases progressively and linearly as blood pressure rises above 115 mmHg systolic and 75 mmHg diastolic pressure.[3] For every 20 mmHg systolic or 10 mmHg diastolic increase in blood pressure there is a doubling of mortality from both ischemic heart disease and stroke in all age groups from 40 to 89 years old.[5] Despite major advances in our understanding of its pathophysiology and the availability of many drugs that can effectively reduce blood pressure in most hypertensive subjects, hypertension continues to be the most important modifiable risk factor for CVD.

CLASSIFICATION OF HYPERTENSION

Blood pressure is a variable quantitative trait with a normal distribution that is slightly skewed to the right. Although there is no clear level of blood pressure where cardiovascular disease begins to occur, a definition of hypertension, although somewhat arbitrary, is useful for making decisions about treatment. A commonly used blood pressure classification was proposed in 2003 by the Seventh Report of the United States Joint National Committee on Prevention, Detection, Evaluation, and Treatment of High Blood Pressure (JNC 7) (Table 69–1).[6] This classification is based on the average of two or more blood pressure readings after an initial screening visit, and is for individuals who are not on antihypertensive medication and who are not acutely ill. When systolic and diastolic blood pressures fall into different categories, the JNC 7 recommends that the higher category be selected to classify the person's blood pressure.

According to JNC 7 criteria, normal blood pressure is defined as a systolic blood pressure <120 mmHg and a diastolic blood pressure <80 mmHg. Persons with a systolic blood pressure between 120 and 139 mmHg or diastolic blood pressure between 80 and 89 mmHg are designated as having *prehypertension*. The diagnosis of hypertension is made by a confirmed systolic blood pressure ≥140 mmHg or a diastolic blood pressure ≥90 mmHg. Hypertension is further characterized into two stages according to the patient's level of systolic and diastolic blood pressure. Stage 1, the milder (systolic 140 to 159 mmHg and/or diastolic 90 to 99 mmHg) and most common form of hypertension, accounts for approximately 80 percent of hypertension. Stage 2 hypertension includes those with systolic blood pressure ≥160 mmHg and/or diastolic blood pressure ≥100 mmHg. Isolated systolic hypertension is defined as systolic blood pressure of ≥140 mmHg and diastolic blood pressure <90 mmHg and staged appropriately.

Using these definitions and including those who are taking antihypertensive medication, approximately 24 percent of the adult population in the United States has hypertension.[6] This percentage varies with (1) race, being higher in blacks (32 percent) and lower in whites (23 percent) and Mexican Americans (23 percent); (2) age, because systolic blood pressure rises throughout life in the United States, as well as in most industrialized countries, whereas diastolic blood pressure rises until age 55 to 60 years; (3) gender, with hypertension being more prevalent in men than in premenopausal women; (4) geographic patterns, with hypertension being more prevalent in the southeastern United States; and (5) socioeconomic status, which is inversely related to the prevalence, morbidity, and mortality rates of hypertension.

DEFINITION OF PRIMARY (ESSENTIAL) HYPERTENSION

Primary (essential) hypertension, which accounts for 95 percent of all cases of hypertension, has been traditionally defined as high blood pressure for which an obvious secondary cause (e.g., renovascular disease, aldosteronism, pheochromocytoma, or gene mutations) cannot be determined.

Although primary hypertension is a heterogeneous disorder, some of the main causes of high blood pressure in primary hypertension are known. For example, overweight and obesity may account for a much as 65 to 75 percent of the risk for primary hypertension, as discussed later in this chapter. Other factors, such as sedentary lifestyle, excess intake of alcohol or salt, and low potassium intake, are also known to increase blood pressure in many patients who are classified as having primary hypertension. Therefore, it is probably inappropriate to define primary hypertension as a rise in blood pressure without cause because identified causes can be found in many patients.[7,8]

This chapter discusses basic concepts of circulatory regulation, the physiologic mechanisms involved in short-term and long-term control of blood pressure, and the pathophysiologic changes in the major blood pressure control systems that can lead to a few types of secondary hypertension, as well as primary hypertension. We also review interactions between genetic and environmental factors that influence intermediate phenotypes such as sympathetic nerve system (SNS) activity, the renin–angiotensin system (RAS), endothelial factors, oxidative stress, and natriuretic hormones, which, in turn, influence vascular resistance, cardiac output, renal excretion of salt and water, and, therefore, blood pressure.

BASIC CONCEPTS OF CIRCULATORY CONTROL

CARDIAC OUTPUT AND TISSUE BLOOD FLOW REGULATION

A discussion of cardiac output regulation often begins with the well-known formula: *cardiac output = stroke volume × heart rate*.

TABLE 69–1

Classification of Blood Pressure for Adults Age 18 Years and Older According to JNC 7[a]

CATEGORY	SYSTOLIC BLOOD PRESSURE (MMHG)		DIASTOLIC BLOOD PRESSURE (MMHG)
Normal[b]	<120	and	<80
Prehypertension	120–139	and	81–89
Hypertension[c]			
Stage 1	140–159	or	90–99
Stage 2	≤160	or	≤100

JNC 7, Seventh Report of the United States Joint National Committee on Prevention, Detection, Evaluation, and Treatment of High Blood Pressure.
[a]This classification assumes that the patients are not taking antihypertensive drugs and are not acutely ill. When systolic and diastolic pressures fall into different categories, the higher category should be used to classify the individual's blood pressure status. Isolated systolic hypertension is defined as systolic blood pressure of ≥140 mmHg and diastolic blood pressure <90 mmHg and staged appropriately.
[b]Normal blood pressure with respect to cardiovascular disease risk is <120/80 mmHg. However, unusually low readings should be evaluated for clinical significance.
[c]Based on the average of two or more readings taken at each of two or more visits after an initial screening.
SOURCE: Chobanian AV, Bakris GL, Black HR, et al. Seventh report of the joint National Committee on Prevention, Detection, Evaluation, and Treatment of High Blood Pressure. Hypertension 2003;42:1206–1252.

This equation provides a conceptual framework that is adequate to describe the general determinants of cardiac pumping but it does not elucidate another major determinant of cardiac output—the venous return, or total tissue blood flow. To illustrate this point, consider the following question: *Which of the following changes in cardiac output would you expect to find 7 days after surgical reduction of kidney mass by 50 percent (removal of one kidney): an increase, a decrease, or no change?* The correct answer is a *decrease* in cardiac output. Why is cardiac output reduced by removal of a kidney when there has been no obvious effect on cardiac pumping ability or heart rate? This is not easy to comprehend if we think in a "cardiocentric" manner. However, the answer becomes obvious if we consider that cardiac output is, in the steady state, equal to the sum of the blood flows of all of the tissues.

Figure 69–1 illustrates the important relationship between cardiac output and tissue blood flow, and shows why removing a kidney, or any of other organ, reduces cardiac output. Removing one kidney decreases venous return to the heart by approximately 10 percent (assuming that total flow to both kidneys is approximately 20 percent of the cardiac output). There is very little change in blood volume because the remaining kidney is able to rapidly increase its excretion to match intake of water and electrolytes. A reduction in cardiac output would also be observed with amputation of an arm or a leg, or removal of any other tissue from the body. This example illustrates that cardiac output is determined not only by the function of the heart, but also by the peripheral circulation. Except when the heart is severely weakened and unable to adequately pump the venous return, cardiac output (total tissue blood flow) is determined mainly by the metabolic needs of the tissues and organs of the body, although intrinsic and neurohumoral mechanisms allow the heart to effectively accommodate changes in venous return.

This conceptual framework is very helpful in explaining changes in cardiac output during exercise (where metabolic activity and blood flow to skeletal muscles are increased), after eating a large meal (which increases metabolic activity and blood flow in the gastrointestinal system) and in pathophysiologic conditions such as hypertension where cardiac output is also determined largely by the metabolic demands of the tissues. In most circumstances, cardiac pumping ability plays a permissive role in determining the cardiac output.

Tissue Blood Flow Autoregulation and Cardiac Output

The importance of integrating the principles of tissue blood flow regulation in discussing cardiac output can be illustrated by consideration of the effects of vasodilators and vasoconstrictors. In most cases, cardiac output changes very little even when there are high levels of circulating vasoconstrictors (e.g., angiotensin II [ANG II]) or vasodilators (e.g., calcium channel blockers). If cardiac output regulation is the sum of all local blood flow regulations, why is cardiac output not significantly altered in these conditions?

To answer this question we must consider one of the most fundamental principles of circulatory function—the ability of each tissue to *autoregulate* its own blood flow according to the metabolic needs and other functions of the tissue.[9-11] Administration of a powerful vasoconstrictor, such as ANG II, may cause a transient decrease in cardiac output, but usually has little long-term effect if

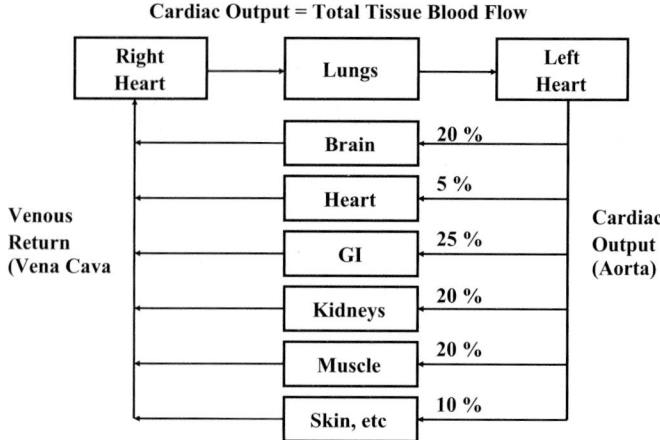

FIGURE 69–1. Relationship between cardiac output, peripheral blood flow regulation, and venous return.

it does not alter metabolic rate of the tissues. Likewise, most vasodilators cause only short-term changes in tissue blood flow and cardiac output if they do not alter tissue metabolism.

Therefore, to effectively explain cardiac output regulation, it is necessary to discuss the mechanisms that control blood flow in the different tissues. Local blood flow regulation, as is true for most physiologic control systems, involves short-term and long-term mechanisms. Acute control occurs within seconds or minutes as a result of constriction or dilation of the vasculature. After administration of a vasoconstrictor that does not alter metabolic rate of the tissues, there is a transient decrease in the supply of nutrients and oxygen to the tissues and an accumulation of metabolic waste products. This, in turn, causes vasodilation and a return of tissue blood flow toward normal. In some tissues where blood flow regulation is not determined mainly by metabolic needs, such as the kidney, some vasoconstrictors, such as ANG II, may cause a small, sustained decrease in blood flow that barely alters cardiac output. Other short-term controls, such as the *myogenic response*, also alter vascular resistance in response to changes in blood pressure and help to autoregulate blood flow in the different tissues.

Long-term blood flow regulation takes place over several days or weeks and involves structural changes in the blood vessels, such as thickening of vessel walls and decreased numbers of capillaries (rarefaction) in some tissues when blood pressure is chronically elevated. Together, the short-term and long-term mechanisms maintain the required levels of blood flow in each tissue to insure normal tissue function. Thus, in most physiologic conditions, excluding those associated with impaired cardiac pumping ability, the cardiac output reflects mainly the combined actions of the multiple control mechanisms for blood flows in the different tissues of the body.

In conditions such as heart failure or when large increases in cardiac output are needed to meet the metabolic demands of the body's tissues, such as exercise, the various factors that alter cardiac pumping also play a major role in regulating cardiac output regulation.

Blood Flow Regulation in Normotensive and Hypertensive Subjects

The main function of the circulation is to provide adequate blood flow to each tissue to meet its requirements. This is achieved by a combination of local tissue controls that regulate vascular tone as well as overall adjustments of the circulation that influence cardiac pumping and vascular tone.[11,12] For example, during intense exercise, local conditions (e.g., accumulation of metabolites or decreased levels of oxygen and nutrients) in the skeletal muscles cause intense vasodilation that permits adequate blood flow to match the increased metabolic requirements of the muscles. However, this also reduces peripheral vascular resistance that tends to decrease blood pressure. Normally, this is offset by multiple neurohumoral changes that tend to elevate the blood pressure.

If for some reason peripheral vasodilation continues for several days, such as occurs with anemia or with opening a large arteriovenous fistula, additional adjustments take place that cause salt and water retention by the kidneys and increased blood volume, or even hypertrophy of the heart if the stimulus lasts for several weeks. Thus, the multiple factors that control the circulation, including those that influence cardiac output, blood pressure, blood volume, and others, normally work in concert to provide adequate blood flow to the tissues of the body.

In hypertension, the same control mechanisms are also operative. However, one of the important characteristics of many, but not all, hypertensive patients is that they have increased total peripheral vascular resistance. Does this also mean that blood flow to the tissues is impaired? Excluding those hypertensive persons with heart failure or severe target-organ injury, the answer to this question is generally no. In most instances, blood flows in most tissues are approximately the same in normotensive and hypertensive subjects and are regulated at a level that is adequate to supply the needs of the tissues.[13] Thus, the hemodynamic pattern that is often (but not always) observed in nonobese subjects with essential hypertension is normal blood flow, normal oxygen consumption, and elevated vascular resistance.[13]

Cerebral blood flow, for example, shows a normal value of about 50 mL/min per 100 g/tissue weight in essential hypertension. Coronary blood flow is elevated in essential hypertension in proportion to the increase in myocardial hypertrophy. Blood flow per unit weight of heart muscle is usually normal, however, with a value of about 80 mL/min per 100 g/tissue weight. Splanchnic blood flow is slightly reduced in essential hypertension, having a typical value of about 750 mL/min/m^2 of surface area compared with about 800 mL/min/m^2 in normotensive subjects. Skin blood flow is also normal in essential hypertension.

Although resting skeletal muscle blood flow is, for the most part, normal in essential hypertension, several differences in blood flow regulation have been noted. For example, the ability of skeletal muscle blood vessels to dilate in some patients with essential hypertension is impaired and the minimal attainable vascular resistance is reduced.[14] This reduced blood flow "reserve" in hypertension is probably a result of structural limitations imposed by blood vessel hypertrophy and of endothelial dysfunction and impaired release of nitric oxide.

In general, the maximal level of exercise as quantified by oxygen uptake is depressed in proportion to the severity of hypertension. Arterial pressure is high before exercising and increases even further during exercise. In the presence of impaired vasodilation, elevated blood pressure boosts blood flow through the skeletal muscle but it also increases cardiac afterload, which limits both cardiac output and exercise performance. At each level of exercise below maximum, however, cardiac output and skeletal muscle blood flow are generally identical to flows seen in normotensive subjects.[13] These flows, however, are achieved at higher vascular resistances and higher blood pressures; the resistance and blood pressure effects cancel each other to yield a normal blood flow in most tissues.

In obese hypertensive patients, resting skeletal muscle blood flow per gram of tissue weight may be somewhat elevated compared to lean individuals; however, the increase in skeletal muscle blood flow that occurs in exercise is attenuated and the forearm reactive hyperemia after temporary occlusion of the brachial artery patients is less in obese than in lean normotensive subjects.[15] Thus, although obesity-associated hypertension may be associated with increased resting blood flow, flow reserve is often reduced.

In older hypertensive individuals, total tissue blood flow (i.e., cardiac output) is often reduced, compared to the flow in younger individuals. This is perhaps not surprising if one considers that lean muscle mass usually decreases with aging. Because cardiac output is a sum of all tissue blood flows, decreased muscle mass and decreased physical activity characteristic of older hypertensive patients also are associated with reduced cardiac output and decreased total body oxygen consumption.

Renal blood flow has been observed to be increased, normal, or decreased in essential hypertension.[16] These seemingly disparate observations, however, should be interpreted with regard to the special functional needs of the kidney and the conditions under which renal blood flow is studied. For example, increased dietary protein, high sodium intake, and excess weight gain all are associated with increased renal blood flow. Nephron loss, which can occur with prolonged, uncontrolled hypertension and diabetes, leads to reduction in renal blood flow. Impaired renal blood flow is also related to the etiology of hypertension in some individuals.

Importance of Arterial Pressure in Regional Blood-Flow Regulation

Adequate tissue blood flow in response to normal daily activities requires an adequate blood pressure. This is illustrated by the response to physical exercise in patients with autonomic dysfunction. As a person with normal autonomic reflexes begins to exercise, skeletal muscle vascular resistance is reduced whereas skeletal muscle blood flow and cardiac output increase markedly and blood pressure remains relatively constant. In persons with autonomic dysfunction, exercise also decreases skeletal muscle vascular resistance but blood pressure falls and muscle blood flow and cardiac output increase only modestly because of impaired autonomic reflexes. Therefore, exercise is not well tolerated and syncope often occurs.

When cardiac output is inadequate to meet normal tissue needs, as occurs in heart failure or severe hypovolemia, activation of the SNS, the RAS, and other hormonal factors produce vasoconstriction that may override normal flow regulation in some organs, such as skeletal muscle and skin. This keeps blood pressure from falling too low and provides adequate blood flow to the vital organs, especially the brain and the heart.

[ ] BASIC PRINCIPLES OF BLOOD PRESSURE REGULATION

The most important function of blood pressure is to provide the driving force that moves blood through the vascular system in order to supply the needs of the tissues. Consequently, the regulation of blood pressure is a complex physiologic function that depends on the integrated actions of multiple cardiovascular, renal, neural, endocrine, and local tissue control systems.

Blood pressure varies considerably throughout the day depending on the activity of the body, environmental influences, and the responses of these multiple blood pressure control systems. Hypertension is usually considered to be a disorder of the average level at which blood pressure is regulated, although there is increasing interest in other measures of blood pressure, including peak arterial pressure, lability of blood pressure, nighttime and daytime blood pressure, blood pressure responses to stress, and so forth. Many of the cardiovascular derangements associated with hypertension, such as cardiac and vascular hypertrophy, arise as compensatory mechanisms for the hypertension, and reducing blood pressure can largely reverse these changes if they have not progressed too far.

The multiple local control, hormonal, neural, and renal systems that regulate blood pressure are often discussed in terms of how they influence cardiac pumping or vascular resistance because of the well-known formula: *mean arterial pressure = cardiac output × total peripheral resistance*. This conceptual framework (with the addition of factors that influence vascular capacity and transcapillary exchange) is adequate to explain short-term blood pressure regulation, but is inadequate when discussing abnormalities of long-term blood pressure regulation, such as hypertension.

To illustrate this point let us consider the following question: *What changes in blood pressure, cardiac output, and extracellular fluid volume would you expect to find several days after a 50 percent increase in total peripheral vascular resistance (TPR) caused by closure of a large arteriovenous (A-V) fistula?* In this case, cardiac pumping ability is not directly altered and TPR is chronically increased by 50 percent. One might assume that blood pressure would also rise chronically if increased TPR is sustained. However, several days after closure of an A-V fistula there are no detectable changes in mean arterial pressure despite a sustained increase of TPR. Likewise, increasing TPR by amputation of a limb or hypothyroidism (which reduces metabolic rate of the tissues and increases vascular resistance), or decreasing TPR by creating an A-V fistula, anemia, or hyperthyroidism, fail to have a significant long-term effect on mean arterial pressure (Fig. 69–2). Why do these large chronic changes in TPR have no significant long-term effect on mean arterial pressure? To explain blood pressure regulation in these circum-

stances, we must introduce two other concepts: (1) time-dependency of blood pressure control mechanisms, and (2) the necessity of maintaining balance between intake and output of water and electrolytes, and the role of blood pressure in maintaining this balance.

Feedback Control Systems for Blood Pressure Are Time Dependent Blood pressure control systems are often considered as if they were static, and time dependency is usually not discussed. Short-term control mechanisms are often emphasized to a greater degree than long-term controls, probably because they have been studied much more extensively and are easier to explain, even though most cardiovascular disorders, including hypertension, involve abnormalities of long-term regulation.

If we examine the maximal feedback gain of several blood pressure controllers, it is obvious that their quantitative importance is highly time dependent. Figure 69–3 shows the response of some of the major control systems following a sudden change in blood pressure, as might occur with rapid blood loss. The degree of response of the different control systems can be expressed in terms of *feedback gain* of the system; the higher the gain, the greater the response. Three important neural control systems begin to function within seconds: (1) the arterial baroreceptors, which detect changes in blood pressure and send appropriate autonomic reflex signals back to the heart and blood vessels to return the blood pressure toward normal; (2) the chemoreceptors, which detect changes in oxygen or carbon dioxide in the blood and initiate autonomic feedback responses that influence blood pressure; and (3) the central nervous system, which responds within a few seconds to ischemia of the vasomotor centers in the medulla, espe-

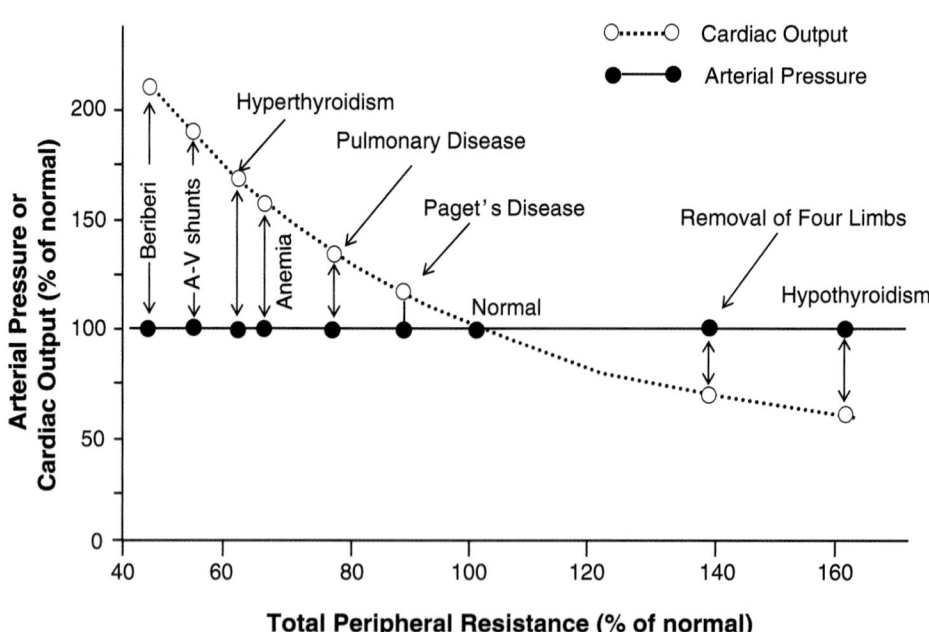

FIGURE 69–2. Failure of changes in total peripheral vascular resistance (TPR) to cause chronic changes in arterial pressure in several clinical conditions in which the kidneys are functioning normally. In each case there is a reciprocal relationship between TPR and cardiac output, but no long-term effect on arterial pressure. *Source: Redrawn from Guyton AC, Hall JE. Textbook of Medical Physiology, 11th ed. Philadelphia: Elsevier, 2006.*

cially when blood pressure falls below about 50 mmHg. Each of these nervous control mechanisms works rapidly and can have potent effects on blood pressure.

Within a few minutes or hours after a blood pressure disturbance, several additional control systems react, including (1) a shift of fluid from the interstitial spaces into the blood stream in response to decreased blood pressure (or a shift of fluid out of the blood into the interstitial spaces in response to increased blood pressure); (2) the RAS which is activated when blood pressure falls too low and suppressed when blood pressure increases above normal; (3) multiple vasodilators systems (not shown in the figure) that are suppressed when blood pressure decreases and stimulated when blood pressure rises above normal.

Most of the blood pressure regulators are *proportional* control systems. This means that they will correct a blood pressure abnormality only part of the way back toward the normal level, but never all the way back. The arterial baroreceptor reflex system, for example, has a proportional feedback gain of approximately 2.0 during acute changes in blood pressure and therefore buffers about two-thirds of a sudden change in the blood pressure.[11]

There is one blood pressure control system, the renal–body fluid feedback system, with *infinite feedback gain* if it is given enough time to operate.[16,17] Thus, the renal–body fluid feedback control mechanism does not stop functioning until the arterial pressure returns all the way back to its original control level, as discussed below.

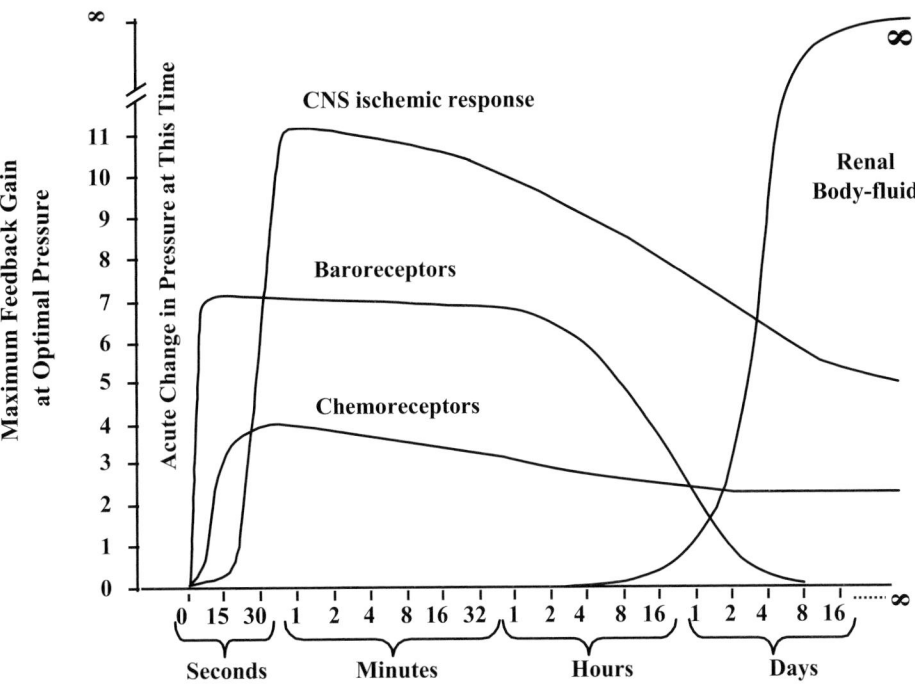

FIGURE 69-3. Time dependency of blood pressure control mechanisms. Approximate maximum feedback gains of various blood pressure control mechanisms at different time intervals after the onset of a disturbance to arterial pressure. *Source: Redrawn from Guyton AC, Hall JE. Textbook of Medical Physiology, 11th ed. Philadelphia: Elsevier, 2006, p. 230.*

【 】 THE RENAL–BODY FLUID FEEDBACK IS A DOMINANT MECHANISM FOR LONG-TERM BLOOD PRESSURE REGULATION

Figure 69–4 shows the conceptual framework for understanding long-term control of blood pressure by the renal–body fluid feedback mechanism. Extracellular fluid volume is determined by the balance between intake and excretion of salt and water by the kidneys. Even a temporary imbalance between intake and output can lead to a change in extracellular volume and potentially a change in blood pressure. Under steady-state conditions there must always be a precise balance between intake and output of salt and water; otherwise, there would be continued accumulation or loss of fluid leading to complete circulatory collapse within a few days. In fact, it is more critical to maintain salt and water balance than to maintain a normal level of blood pressure and, as discussed below, increased blood pressure is a means of regulating these balances in the face of impaired kidney function.

A key mechanism for regulating salt and water balance is pressure natriuresis and diuresis, the effect of increased blood pressure to raise sodium and water excretion.[18,19] Under most conditions this mechanism acts to stabilize blood pressure and body fluid volumes. For example, when blood pressure is increased above the renal setpoint, because of increased TPR or increased cardiac pumping ability, this also increases sodium and water excretion via pressure natriuresis if kidney function is not impaired. As long as fluid excretion exceeds fluid intake, extracellular fluid volume will continue to decrease, reducing venous return and cardiac output, until blood pressure returns to normal and fluid balance is reestablished.

An important feature of pressure natriuresis is that various hormonal and neural control systems can greatly amplify or blunt the basic effects of blood pressure on sodium and water excretion.[19] For example, during chronic increases in sodium intake only small changes in blood pressure are needed to maintain sodium balance in most people. One reason for this insensitivity of blood pressure to changes in salt intake is decreased formation of antinatriuretic hormones such as ANG II and aldosterone, which enhance the effectiveness of pressure natriuresis and allow sodium balance to be maintained with minimal increases in blood pressure. On the other hand, excessive activation of these antinatriuretic systems can reduce the effectiveness of pressure natriuresis, thereby necessitating greater increases in blood pressure to maintain sodium balance.

Another important feature of pressure natriuresis is that it continues to operate until blood pressure returns to the original setpoint. In other words, it acts as part of an *infinite gain* feedback

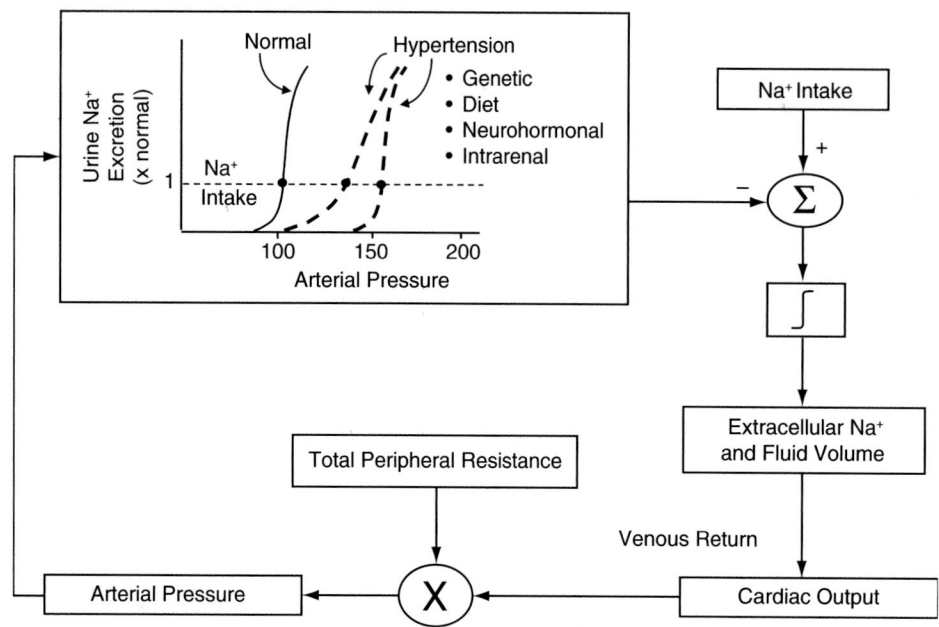

FIGURE 69–4. Block diagram showing the basic elements of the renal–body fluid feedback mechanism for long-term regulation of arterial pressure.

ther by directly increasing renal excretory capability (e.g., with diuretics), or by reducing extrarenal antinatriuretic influences (e.g., with RAS blockers) on the kidneys.

RENAL MECHANISMS OF HYPERTENSION

For more than 100 years severe kidney disease has been recognized as closely associated with hypertension. However, the importance of more subtle renal dysfunction in the pathogenesis of essential hypertension has not been as well appreciated, partly because there are no obvious renal defects in most patients with primary hypertension. Many of the measurements commonly used to evaluate kidney function, such as glomerular filtration rate (GFR), renal blood flow, serum creatinine, and sodium excretion are often within the normal range, at least in the early stages of hypertension. On the other hand, increased TPR is an obvious abnormality found in most patients with hypertension, leading many researchers to emphasize peripheral vasoconstriction as a cause of increased blood pressure. However, as discussed previously, increased peripheral vascular resistance in the absence of altered kidney function does not cause sustained hypertension.

An observation that points toward abnormal kidney function as a key factor in hypertension is that almost all forms of experimental hypertension, as well as all monogenic forms of human hypertension thus far discovered, are caused by obvious insults to the kidneys that alter renal hemodynamics or tubular reabsorption. For example, constriction of the renal arteries (e.g., Goldblatt hypertension), compression of the kidneys (e.g., perinephritic hypertension), or administration of sodium-retaining hormones (e.g., mineralocorticoids or ANG II) are all associated with either initial reductions in renal blood flow and GFR or increases in tubular reabsorption prior to development of hypertension. Likewise, in all known monogenic forms of human hypertension, the common pathway to hypertension appears to be increased renal tubular sodium reabsorption caused by mutations that directly increase renal electrolyte transport or the synthesis and/or activity of antinatriuretic hormones. As blood pressure rises, the initial renal changes are often obscured by compensations that restore kidney function toward normal. The rise in blood pressure then initiates a cascade of cardiovascular changes, including increased peripheral vascular resistance that may be more striking than the initial disturbance of kidney function. For this reason, the importance of renal dysfunction in causing hypertension has often been underestimated.

control system.[17] As far as we know, it is the only infinite gain feedback system for blood pressure regulation in the body, and it is this property which makes it a dominant long-term controller of blood pressure.

Figure 69–5 illustrates the infinite gain characteristic of the renal–body fluid feedback system. In this case, blood pressure is increased without a change in pressure natriuresis, as would occur with increased TPR because of closure of an A-V fistula, coarctation of the aorta *below* the kidneys (aortic coarctation *above* the kidneys causes marked hypertension), or other changes that increase peripheral vascular resistance without influencing renal vascular resistance. The peripheral constriction initially increases blood pressure from point A to point B, but the rise in blood pressure cannot be sustained; as long as pressure natriuresis is unaltered, sodium excretion will increase above intake, thereby reducing extracellular fluid volume until blood pressure eventually returns all the way back to normal. In fact, the normal blood pressure is the only point at which sodium and water balance can be maintained. Likewise, disturbances that decrease peripheral vascular resistance or alter cardiac function without influencing renal pressure natriuresis have no long-term effect on arterial pressure.[16,17]

Therefore, in all forms of human or experimental hypertension studied thus far, there is a shift of pressure natriuresis that appears to initiate and sustain the hypertension. In some cases, abnormal kidney function is caused by intrarenal disturbances that alter renal hemodynamics or increased tubular reabsorption. In other cases, the altered kidney function is caused by extrarenal disturbances, such as increased SNS activity or excessive formation of antinatriuretic hormones that reduce the kidney's ability to excrete sodium and water and eventually raise arterial pressure. Consequently, effective treatment of hypertension requires interventions that reset pressure natriuresis toward normal levels of blood pressure ei-

Although specific abnormalities of kidney function are difficult to identify in most patients with primary hypertension, the one aspect of kidney function that is abnormal in all types of experimental and clinical hypertension is renal pressure natriuresis.[16,18] The fact that a normal rate of sodium excretion (equal to sodium intake) is maintained in chronic hypertension despite elevated blood pressure, which would normally cause natriuresis and diuresis, indicates that pressure natriuresis is reset in hypertensive subjects.

Because tubular reabsorption and GFR are both approximately 100-fold greater than urinary excretion, relatively small changes in either of these variables can have large effects on urinary excretion. Any long-term reduction in GFR must be perfectly compensated for by mechanisms that either restore GFR or decrease tubular reabsorption if renal excretion is to be returned toward normal and sodium and fluid balance are maintained. Likewise, any chronic increase in tubular reabsorption must be compensated for by increased GFR or by a restoration of tubular reabsorption to normal. Otherwise, fluid retention would continue eventually causing circulatory collapse.

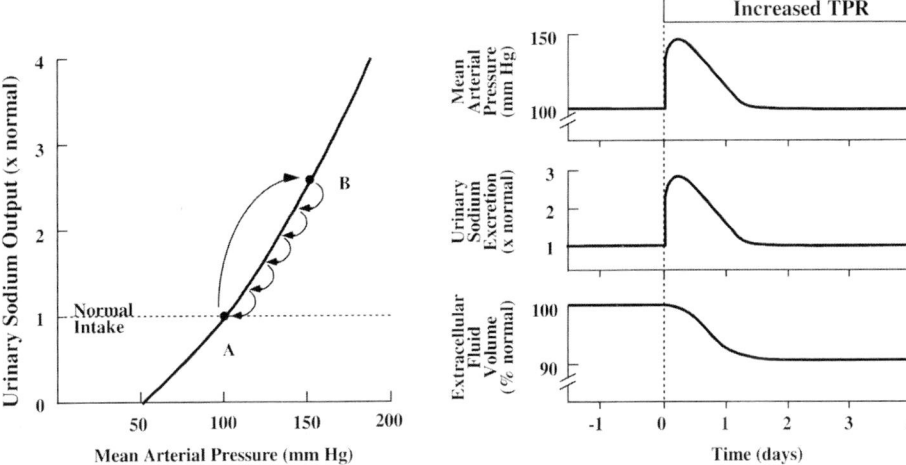

FIGURE 69–5. Long-term effects of increased total peripheral resistance (TPR), such as that caused by closure of a large arteriovenous fistula, with no change in the renal pressure natriuresis relationship. Blood pressure is initially increased from point A to point B, but elevated blood pressure cannot be sustained because sodium excretion exceeds intake, reducing extracellular fluid volume until blood pressure returns to normal and sodium balance is reestablished. *Source: Redrawn from Hall JE. The kidney, hypertension, and obesity. Hypertension 2003;41:625–633.*

If intrinsic renal mechanisms or neurohumoral adjustments are capable of returning renal excretion to normal in the face of insults to the kidneys, hypertension may not develop. However, the fact that hypertension occurs so frequently indicates that intrinsic renal mechanisms and neurohumoral controls may not be powerful enough to completely prevent alterations in renal excretion when there are major abnormalities of GFR or tubular reabsorption. In these instances, increased arterial pressure helps to maintain glomerulotubular balance and normal rates of sodium and water excretion, equal to intake, despite abnormal kidney function. The general types of renal abnormalities that can cause chronic hypertension include (1) increased preglomerular resistance, (2) decreased glomerular capillary filtration coefficient, (3) reduced numbers of functional nephrons, and (4) increased tubular reabsorption (see Table 69–1 and Fig. 69–6).

⟨ ⟩ HYPERTENSION CAUSED BY GENERALIZED INCREASES IN PREGLOMERULAR RESISTANCE

Examples of a generalized increase in preglomerular resistance are those caused by suprarenal aortic coarctation or constriction of one of the renal arteries and removal of the contralateral kidney (e.g., one-kidney, one-clip Goldblatt hypertension). Immediately after constriction of the renal artery or aortic coarctation, renal blood flow is reduced and there is a rapid rise in renin secretion and transient sodium retention. Within a few days, sodium excretion returns to normal and sodium balance is reestablished. If sodium intake is normal and adequate volume is available, renin secretion also returns to normal in the established phase of hypertension. At this point, most indices of renal function are nearly normal, including pressure distal to the stenosis if the constriction is not too severe. The rate at which renal function returns to normal and time course for development of hypertension depend the severity of the stenosis, the sodium intake, and the rate of ANG II formation.[17]

How do these experimental models of increased preglomerular resistance relate to human hypertension, other than the obvious conditions of aortic coarctation or renal artery stenosis? When Harry Goldblatt first introduced hypertension in dogs by constricting the main renal artery, his goal was to produce an experimental model that mimicked the pathologic changes found in human essential hypertension.[20] Goldblatt has previously noted that many hypertensive patients at autopsy had nephrosclerosis and hypothesized that essential hypertension might be caused by diffuse renal arteriolar sclerosis, particularly in preglomerular vessels. Presumably, functional or pathologic increases in preglomerular resistance at other sites besides the main renal arteries, such as the interlobular arteries or afferent arterioles, could increase blood pressure through the same mechanisms as activated by clipping the renal artery. For example, widespread structural increases in afferent arteriolar resistance (e.g., nephrosclerosis) or functional increases in resistance caused by excessive activation of the SNS or high levels of catecholamines (e.g., pheochromocytoma) would also cause hypertension through the same mechanisms as constriction of the main renal artery.

Some have questioned whether Goldblatt hypertension is relevant to human essential hypertension because of the observation that many hypertensive patients have no obvious indication of renal ischemia and have nearly normal renal blood flow and GFR. However, as previously discussed, there is little indication of renal ischemia even in experimental Goldblatt hypertension after compensatory increases in blood pressure have occurred.

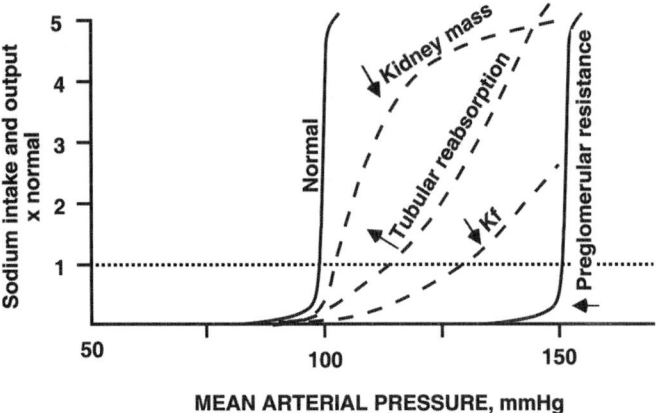

FIGURE 69–6. Steady-state relationships between arterial pressure and urinary sodium excretion and sodium intake for subjects with normal kidneys and four general types of renal dysfunction that cause hypertension: decreased kidney mass, increased reabsorption in distal and collecting tubules, reductions in glomerular capillary filtration coefficient (K_f), and increased preglomerular resistance. Note that increased preglomerular resistance causes *salt-insensitive* hypertension, whereas the other renal abnormalities cause *salt-sensitive* hypertension.

It is interesting to note that some patients with primary hypertension have the same characteristics seen in the one-kidney, one-clip Goldblatt model of hypertension, including nearly normal GFR and plasma renin activity, a parallel shift of pressure natriuresis to higher blood pressure, and a relatively salt-insensitive form of hypertension.[18,21] Indeed, studies in hypertensive patients show that drug therapy that decreases preglomerular resistance, such as calcium channel blockers, causes a parallel shift of pressure natriuresis toward lower blood pressure.[22] Thus, primary hypertension in some patients may be caused by functional or pathologic increases in preglomerular resistance. This is almost certainly the case in patients who have severe artherosclerotic lesions in the renal blood vessels.

[ ] HYPERTENSION CAUSED BY PATCHY INCREASES IN PREGLOMERULAR RESISTANCE

In the two-kidney, one-clip Goldblatt model of hypertension, or in patients with a stenosis in only one renal artery, there is a nonhomogeneous increase in preglomerular resistance with ischemia occurring in nephrons of the clipped/stenotic kidney, while nephrons in the contralateral nonclipped/nonstenotic kidney have increased single-nephron blood flow and GFR. The underperfused clipped kidney secretes large amounts of renin, whereas the untouched kidney secretes very little renin.[18,19]

An important distinction between a generalized increase in preglomerular resistance and patchy, nonhomogeneous increases in preglomerular resistance is the evolution of renal injury associated with hypertension. When there is a generalized, homogeneous increase in preglomerular resistance, the glomeruli are protected from the damaging effects of increased blood pressure. In the two-kidney, one-clip model, however, the glomeruli of the untouched kidney are subjected to the full effects of increased blood pressure. With prolonged hypertension, pathologic changes in the untouched kidney add to the impairment of overall renal excretory capability. At this stage, removal of the clipped kidney only par-

tially restores arterial pressure to normal. However, removal of the contralateral untouched kidney and unclipping the stenotic kidney normalizes blood pressure. Thus, chronic exposure to high blood pressure in the untouched kidney apparently causes structural changes as well as functional changes that contribute to the progression of hypertension in this model.

The relevance of experimental models of nonhomogeneous increases in preglomerular resistance to human hypertension is obvious in those cases in which there is stenosis of only one renal artery, with the contralateral kidney being initially unaffected. If the contralateral nonstenotic kidney eventually becomes injured as a result of being exposed to high blood pressure, this kidney may also contribute to the hypertension.

Some patients with essential hypertension may have patchy nephrosclerosis within each kidney also providing a clinical counterpart to the two-kidney, one-clip Goldblatt model of hypertension. In these instances, the ischemic nephrons secrete large amounts of renin and the nonischemic nephrons vasodilate and initially have increased single nephron GFR. The combined effects of hypertension and hyperfiltration, however, may eventually damage the nephrons that were initially nonischemic, leading to progressive nephron loss.

[ ] HYPERTENSION CAUSED BY DECREASED GLOMERULAR CAPILLARY FILTRATION COEFFICIENT

Reducing the glomerular capillary filtration coefficient (K_f) initially lowers GFR and sodium excretion while stimulating renin release and causing vasodilation of afferent arterioles via a macula densa feedback.[18,19] The sodium retention and increased ANG II formation raise arterial pressure, which then helps to restore GFR and renin release to normal. After these compensations, the main persistent abnormalities of kidney function are reduced filtration fraction, increased glomerular hydrostatic pressure, and increased renal blood flow.

Unfortunately, compensatory increases in blood pressure and glomerular hydrostatic pressure, which are needed to offset a fall in K_f and to restore sodium excretion to normal, may also lead to additional renal dysfunction over a period of years by causing further glomerular injury; this further reduces K_f and requires additional increases in blood pressure to maintain normal water and electrolyte balances. Such a sequence may initiate progressive kidney damage.

The clinical counterparts of this sequence may be found in hypertension caused by glomerulonephritis or by other conditions that cause thickening and damage to the glomerular capillary membranes, such as chronic diabetes mellitus.[23]

[ ] REDUCED NEPHRON NUMBER INCREASES SALT-SENSITIVITY OF BLOOD PRESSURE

A factor that contributes to salt sensitivity of blood pressure in some hypertensive patients is a loss of functional nephrons. Complete loss of nephrons (such as surgical reduction of kidney mass or unilateral nephrectomy) in the absence of other abnormalities usually does not lead to significant hypertension.[18,19] In contrast, loss of functional nephrons because of ischemia or infarction of renal tissue usually causes marked hypertension that is initially caused by increased renin secretion and then is eventually mediated by additional abnormalities, such as immunologic and renal injury, in the established phase of the hypertension.[24]

Considering the previous discussion, one might predict that reductions in nephron number should impair renal excretory capability and cause hypertension regardless of whether the loss was associated with renal ischemia. Yet, experimental studies show that surgical removal of large amounts of the kidney, to the point that uremia occurs, rarely causes severe hypertension as long as sodium intake is normal.[18,25] The reason hypertension does not develop is that overall glomerular filtration and tubular reabsorption capability are proportionally reduced so that balance between filtration and reabsorption can be maintained without major adaptive changes in blood pressure.

Reducing the number of functional nephrons, however, does make the kidneys very susceptible to additional insults that impair their function or to additional challenges of sodium homeostasis. Thus, hypertension associated with excess mineralocorticoids is much more severe after reducing kidney mass. Likewise, the kidney's ability to increase sodium excretion in response to the additional challenge of high sodium intake is accompanied by much larger increases in blood pressure when kidney mass is reduced.[18,19]

With the loss of entire nephrons, each surviving nephron must excrete greater amounts of sodium and water to maintain balance. This is achieved by increasing GFR and decreasing reabsorption in the remaining nephrons, resulting in increased sodium chloride delivery to the macula densa and suppression of renin release. This, in turn, impairs the kidney's ability to further decrease renin secretion during high sodium intake. Therefore, after loss of kidney mass blood pressure becomes very salt sensitive.

Nephron loss may also initiate compensatory changes that eventually damage the surviving nephrons.[23] For example, renal vasodilation and increased single nephron GFR can, over long periods of time, lead to glomerulosclerosis and reductions in K_f. These pathologic changes, in addition to the loss of functional nephrons, may eventually shift pressure natriuresis sufficiently to cause severe hypertension.

What is the relevance of experimental models produced by surgically removing kidney mass to human hypertension? With normal aging, especially after age 40 to 50 years, there is gradual nephron loss that is accelerated by renal diseases, such as glomerulonephritis, diabetes mellitus, or long-standing hypertension. Thus, even though hypertension may not begin with loss of nephrons, chronic elevations in glomerular pressure and other metabolic abnormalities that are often associated with hypertension may eventually cause glomerular injury and progressive nephron loss that amplifies the hypertension and makes blood pressure more salt-sensitive.

Nephron Loss by Partial Renal Infarction Causes Hypertension
The experimental model of surgical reduction of kidney mass discussed above should not be confused with the model of partial renal infarction hypertension produced by tying off branches of the renal artery, the so-called *5/6 ablation* model. This model is usually produced by removing one kidney and obstructing two of the three branches of the renal artery of the remaining kidney. In the

infarction model, hypertension develops even without a high sodium intake because of ischemia of the surviving nephrons, activation of the RAS, and immune-mediated injury of the kidney.[23,24] The 5/6 renal ablation hypertension is a model of severe patchy renal ischemia with characteristics similar to that described for the two-kidney, one-clip Goldblatt model or nonhomogeneous patchy glomerulosclerosis. The clinical counterpart of this model occurs with partial renal infarction caused by septic emboli, thrombus, trauma, or sometimes after corrective surgery for renal artery stenosis.

[ ] HYPERTENSION CAUSED BY INCREASED RENAL TUBULAR SODIUM REABSORPTION

Hypertension can also be caused by factors that raise renal tubular sodium reabsorption, such as excessive levels of mineralocorticoids or ANG II. The severity of hypertension depends on the degree to which tubular reabsorption is stimulated and on other factors, such as the functional kidney mass and sodium intake.[18,19] With loss of functional nephrons or high sodium intake, the hypertensive potency of mineralocorticoids or ANG II is greatly enhanced.

Increased Distal and Collecting Tubule Reabsorption Causes *Salt-Sensitive* Hypertension
One feature of hypertension caused by increased distal or collecting tubular reabsorption is that it is usually salt sensitive, with increased sodium intake exacerbating the hypertension. Increased reabsorption at sites beyond the macula densa, such as the distal tubules and collecting tubules, elicits chronic increases in sodium chloride delivery to the macula densa, which, in turn, suppress renin secretion.[16,18,19] The reduction of renin secretion to *very low* levels, characteristic of disorders associated with increased distal or collecting tubular reabsorption, prevents further suppression of ANG II formation during high sodium intake, making blood pressure salt sensitive.

Another feature of blood pressure caused by increased tubular reabsorption is that it is often associated with extracellular volume expansion. When increased tubular reabsorption is associated with marked peripheral vasoconstriction, such as occurs with very high levels of ANG II, the degree of volume expansion depends on the relative effects of the vasoconstrictor on the peripheral blood vessels and the renal blood vessels.[18,19] With severe peripheral vasoconstriction and decreased vascular capacitance, relatively small amounts of volume retention can lead to marked substantial hypertension.

Increased Proximal Reabsorption Causes *Salt-Insensitive* Hypertension
An increase in tubular reabsorption occurring prior to the macula densa (e.g., in the proximal tubules or loop of Henle) usually results in a salt-insensitive form of hypertension. Increased tubular reabsorption prior to the macula densa tends to increase renin secretion and elicits a compensatory renal vasodilation that raises GFR and renal plasma flow. However, as hypertension develops, macula densa sodium chloride delivery and renin secretion return to nearly normal, and the RAS is fully capable of responding to additional challenges such as increased sodium intake. Therefore, high sodium intake is accompanied by appropriate suppression of renin release and ANG II formation, which permits sodium balance to be maintained with only small increases in blood pressure.[16,18]

Nevertheless, the pressure natriuresis mechanism is shifted to higher blood pressure, parallel to the normal curve, and the severity of the hypertension depends on the degree to which reabsorption is increased in the proximal tubules and loops of Henle.

SALT-SENSITIVE AND SALT-INSENSITIVE HYPERTENSION

Salt sensitivity of blood pressure is a quantitative phenotype, rather than following a bimodal categorization of *salt-sensitive* or *salt-insensitive*, and there is considerable heterogeneity of blood pressure responses to changes in sodium intake in normotensive, as well as in hypertensive, individuals.[26]

Although various methods have been used to assess salt sensitivity, none are widely used in clinical practice. Most salt-sensitivity protocols involve relatively short-term changes in sodium intake, usually over a few days. Weinberger et al.[26] defined salt sensitivity as a 10 mmHg or greater change in mean blood pressure from the level measured after a 4-hour infusion of 2 L of normal saline compared to the level measured the morning after 1 day of a low-sodium (10 mmol) diet and administration of three doses of furosemide. With this definition, 51 percent of hypertensive and 26 percent of normotensive subjects were found to be salt sensitive.[26] However, there has been little effort to determine the repeatability of salt sensitivity in the same persons over long periods of time (years), and it is not known whether short-term blood pressure responses reliably predict the long-term effects of changes in salt intake.

From clinical observations it is clear that there are many demographic and pathophysiologic conditions associated with salt sensitivity. Older individuals are usually more salt sensitive than young people and African Americans are often more salt sensitive than whites. However, there are many exceptions to these generalizations and considerable heterogeneity exists in the blood pressure responses to changes in salt intake even in these populations.

Genetic factors independent of race have also been linked to salt sensitivity of blood pressure. For example, monogenic disorders that increase distal and collecting tubule sodium reabsorption or that cause excess secretion of sodium-retaining hormones (e.g., mineralocorticoids) cause salt-sensitive hypertension.[27] Also, diabetes mellitus, renal diseases that cause nephron loss, and abnormalities of the RAS are all associated with increased salt sensitivity of blood pressure.[19,28] All of these examples appear to share two common pathways to salt sensitivity of blood pressure: loss of functional nephrons or reduced responsiveness of the RAS.

Loss of Functional Nephrons Causes Salt-Sensitive Blood Pressure

As discussed previously, the effect of nephron loss to enhance salt-sensitivity is well established by experimental and clinical studies. Figure 69–7 shows the effect of surgically reducing kidney mass on salt sensitivity in dogs. As long as sodium intake was normal, surgical reduction of kidney mass by 25 percent, or even as much as 70 percent, did not markedly alter blood pressure.[25] However, after loss of kidney mass, blood pressure became exquisitely sensitive to changes in sodium intake and with high sodium intake, blood pressure rose by approximately 40 mmHg.

How is this experimental study conducted in dogs relevant to human hypertension? Even in normal, healthy people, there is a

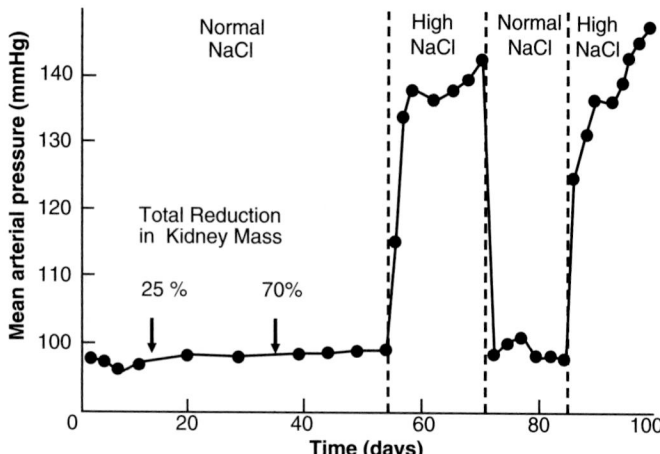

FIGURE 69–7. The effect of reducing kidney mass on salt sensitivity in dogs. Note that as long as sodium chloride intake was normal, surgical reduction of kidney mass by 25 or even 70 percent did not markedly alter arterial pressure. However, after loss of kidney mass, blood pressure became exquisitely sensitive to high sodium chloride intake. *Source: Redrawn from Langston JB, Guyton AC, Douglas BH, et al. Effect of changes in salt intake on arterial pressure and renal function in partially nephrectomized dogs. Circ Res 1963;12:508–512.*

years the average healthy individual typically has at least a 30 percent decrease in the number of nephrons, compared to a young adult, a factor that may contribute to the rise in blood pressure with age in industrialized societies. When there is underlying renal disease, hypertension, or diabetes, the loss of nephrons with aging is greatly exacerbated. Other, less-common causes of nephron loss include primary renal diseases such as glomerulonephritis, acquired renal disease caused by analgesic abuse, uncontrolled diabetes mellitus, and developmental causes because of poor maternal nutrition or placental ischemia.

Reduced Responsiveness of the RAS Causes Salt Sensitivity of Blood Pressure

Because the RAS is the most powerful hormonal system in the body for controlling sodium excretion, it plays a major role in determining salt sensitivity of blood pressure.[30] With high sodium intake, suppression of the RAS permits normal excretion of sodium and water without substantial increases in blood pressure. Conversely, activation of the RAS is a primary mechanism for preventing a reduction in blood pressure during low sodium intake.

Figure 69–8 shows the importance of changes in ANG II formation in maintaining blood pressure relatively constant during variations in salt intake from a very low level of 5 mmol/d up to 80, 240, and 500 mmol/d for 8 days at each level. In normal dogs, with a functional RAS, there were only small increases in blood pressure associated with this 100-fold range of sodium intakes.[31] However, when ANG II was infused at a low level that had initially no effect on blood pressure, but which prevented ANG II from being suppressed as sodium intake was raised, blood pressure became very salt sensitive. After blockade of ANG II formation, blood pressure also became salt sensitive, although pressure was maintained at a much lower level, especially when sodium intake was low.[31] Thus, one of the major functions of the RAS is to permit wide variations in intake and excretion of sodium without large fluctuations in blood pressure that would otherwise be needed to maintain sodium balance.

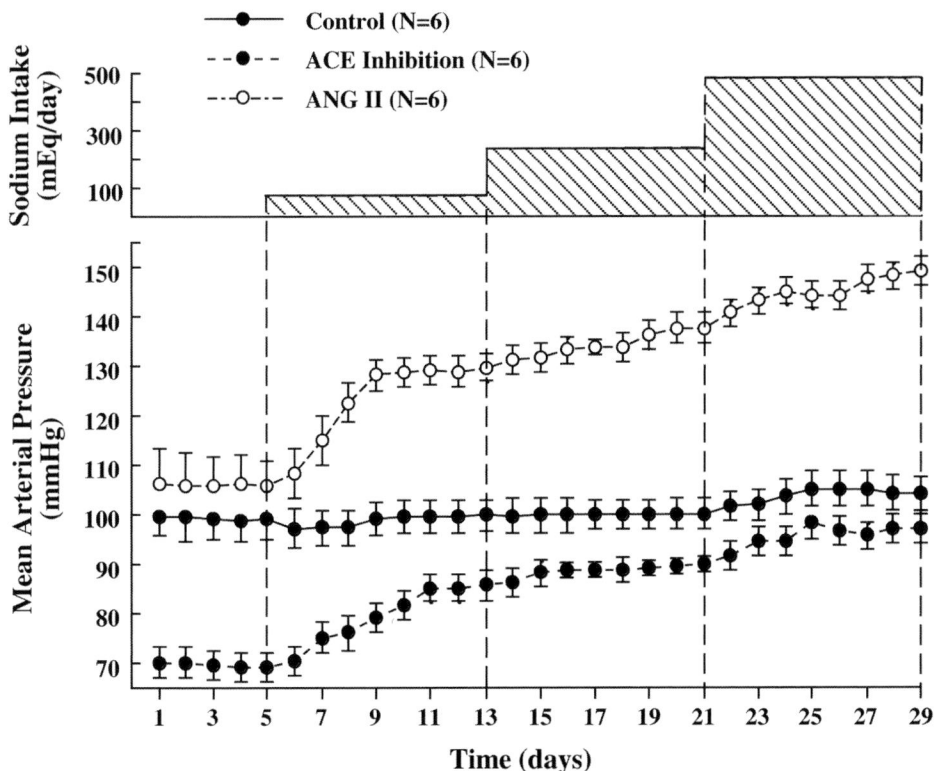

FIGURE 69–8. Changes in mean arterial pressure during chronic changes in sodium intake in normal control dogs, after ACE inhibition, or after ANG II infusion (5 ng/kg/min) to prevent ANG II from being suppressed when sodium intake was raised. *Source: Redrawn from Hall JE, Guyton AC, Smith MJ Jr, et al. Blood pressure and renal function during chronic changes in sodium intake: role of angiotensin. Am J Physiol 1980;239:F271–F280.*

What clinical conditions can lead to reduced responsiveness of the RAS? As discussed previously, focal nephrosclerosis or patchy preglomerular vasoconstriction, as occurs with renal infarction, leads to increased renin secretion in ischemic nephrons and very low levels of renin release by overperfused nephrons.[18,19,32] Thus, in ischemic, as well as overperfused, nephrons the ability to adequately suppress renin secretion during high salt intake is impaired.

Another cause of reduced responsiveness of the RAS is increased distal and collecting tubular sodium reabsorption, as occurs with mineralocorticoid excess or mutations that increase distal and collecting tubule reabsorption (e.g., Liddle syndrome). In these conditions, excess sodium retention causes almost complete suppression of renin secretion, resulting in an inability to further decrease renin release during high sodium intake. Consequently, blood pressure becomes very salt sensitive.

Not all renal abnormalities cause salt-sensitive hypertension. Some, such as generalized diffuse increases in preglomerular resistance, cause a parallel shift of pressure natriuresis and hypertension, but do not cause blood pressure to be salt sensitive. Salt sensitivity is not increased in this form of hypertension because the RAS system is fully capable of appropriate suppression during high sodium intake and sodium balance is maintained with minimal rises in blood pressure.

Salt-Sensitive Subjects May Have Greater Target-Organ Injury

What is the clinical significance of salt sensitivity besides the obvious fact that it provides insight into the pathogenesis of hypertension and it indicates which patients may benefit most from reduction of salt intake? Some studies suggest salt sensitivity also predicts

which patients are at greatest risk for hypertensive target-organ injury. Salt-sensitive forms of hypertension caused by increased distal tubular reabsorption, nephron loss, or inability to suppress ANG II formation are usually associated with glomerular hyperfiltration and increased glomerular hydrostatic pressure that is further amplified by the hypertension (Table 69–2)[19]; together the hypertension and renal hyperfiltration promote glomerular injury and may eventually cause loss of nephron function. Clinical studies support this concept and demonstrate that salt-sensitive individuals typically have an increase in glomerular hydrostatic pressure and albumin excretion when given a salt load, whereas salt-resistant individuals have lower glomerular hydrostatic pressure and less urinary albumin excretion.[33]

There is also evidence that salt-sensitive subjects may die earlier than individuals who are salt resistant. In a study by Weinberger et al. in which individuals were followed for more than 20 years, normotensive individuals with increased salt sensitivity died almost at the same rate as hypertensive individuals and much faster than salt-resistant individuals who were normotensive.[34] Whether this increased mortality was related to blood pressure effects of salt or to other effects is still unclear. It is also not known whether long-term high salt intake, lasting over many years, may cause a person who is initially "salt insensitive" to become "salt sensitive" as a consequence of gradual renal injury.

NEUROHUMORAL MECHANISMS OF HYPERTENSION

Although impaired renal pressure natriuresis plays a central role in all forms of experimental and human hypertension studied thus far, not all disorders of pressure natriuresis originate within the kidneys. Inappropriate activation of the multiple antinatriuretic hormone systems (e.g., ANG II, aldosterone) that normally regulate sodium excretion or a deficiency of natriuretic influences (e.g., atrial natriuretic peptide, nitric oxide) on the kidneys can impair renal pressure natriuresis and cause chronic hypertension. Likewise, excessive activation of the SNS plays a major role in elevating blood pressure in many hypertensive patients. The following sections discuss the multiple neural, hormonal, and autacoid mechanisms that contribute to long-term blood pressure regulation, their actions on the kidneys, and their potential roles in hypertension.

⟦ ⟧ THE SYMPATHETIC NERVOUS SYSTEM

The SNS is a major short-term and long-term controller of blood pressure. Sympathetic vasoconstrictor fibers are distributed to al-

TABLE 69-2

Renal Causes and Characteristics of Salt-Sensitive and Salt-Insensitive Hypertension

CAUSES	BLOOD PRESSURE	PRESSURE NATRIURESIS	RENAL BLOOD FLOW	GFR	PLASMA RENIN ACTIVITY	GLOMERULO-SCLEROSIS[a]
Salt-Sensitive Hypertension						
1. Decreased kidney mass	↑, ↔	Decreased slope	↓	↓	↓	Yes
2. Decreased glomerular capillary filtration coefficient (K_f)	↑	Decreased slope	↑	↓, ↔	↑, ↔	Yes
3. Increased distal and collecting tubule reabsorption	↑	Decreased slope	↑	↑	↓	Yes
Salt-Insensitive Hypertension						
1. Increased preglomerular resistance	↑	Parallel shift	↓, ↔	↓, ↔	↑, ↔	No
2. Increased reabsorption in proximal tubules and loops of Henle	↑	Parallel shift	↑	↑	↑, ↔	Yes

GFR, glomerular filtration rate.
[a]Glomerulosclerosis is predicted to occur secondary to hypertensive stimuli that cause chronic increases in glomerular hydrostatic pressure and/or hyperfiltration of surviving nephrons.

most all of regions of the vasculature, as well as to the heart, and activation of the SNS can raise blood pressure within a few seconds by causing vasoconstriction, increased cardiac pumping capability, and increased heart rate. Conversely, sudden inhibition of SNS activity can decrease blood pressure to as low as half normal within less than a minute. Therefore, changes in SNS activity, caused by various reflex mechanisms, central nervous system ischemia, or by activation of higher centers in the brain, provide powerful and rapid, moment-to-moment regulation of blood pressure.

The SNS also plays an important role in long-term regulation of blood pressure and in the pathogenesis of hypertension, in large part by activation of the renal sympathetic nerves.[35] There is extensive innervation of the renal blood vessels, the juxtaglomerular apparatus, and the renal tubules and excessive activation of these nerves causes sodium retention, increased renin secretion, and impaired renal pressure natriuresis.[35] Except for extreme circumstances, such as severe hemorrhage or other conditions associated with marked circulatory depression, activation of the renal sympathetic nerves is usually not great enough to cause marked reductions in renal blood flow or GFR. However, even mild increases of the renal sympathetic activity stimulate renin secretion and sodium reabsorption in multiple segments of the nephron, including the proximal tubule, the loop of Henle, and more distal segments.[35] Thus, the renal nerves provide a mechanism by which the various reflex mechanisms and higher central nervous system (CNS) centers can contribute to long-term regulation of blood pressure.

The preganglionic neurons that synapse with the renal sympathetic postganglionic fibers are located in the lower thoracic and upper lumbar segments of the spinal cord and receive multiple inputs from various regions of the brain, including the brainstem, the forebrain, and the cerebral cortex. These complex neural pathways provide multiple pathways by which neural reflexes and higher CNS centers can influence renal SNS activity and chronic regulation of blood pressure.[36,37]

Evidence for a role of the renal nerves in hypertension comes from multiple studies showing that renal denervation reduces blood pressure in several models of experimental hypertension.[35] For example, complete renal denervation attenuates the development of hypertension in spontaneously hypertensive rats[35] as well as in obese hypertensive dogs.[38] Renal denervation may also delay or attenuate increased blood pressure in several forms of experimental hypertension, although some studies have not found an important role for the renal nerves in various forms of secondary hypertension. In ANG II hypertension, for example, *decreased* renal sympathetic activity appears to attenuate the rise in blood pressure.[39]

Human primary hypertension, especially when associated with obesity, is often associated with increased renal sympathetic activity.[40] Although the mechanisms that cause activation of renal sympathetic nerves in primary hypertension or in most experimental models are still unclear, we will briefly discuss three that have attracted the interest of many researchers.

Resetting of Baroreceptor Reflexes in Hypertension

The importance of the arterial baroreceptors in buffering moment-to-moment changes in blood pressure is clearly evident in baroreceptor-denervated animals in which there is extreme variability of blood pressure associated with normal daily activities.[41] Although blood pressure increases to very high levels or falls to low levels throughout the day after baroreceptor denervation, the average 24-hour mean arterial pressure is not markedly altered.

The arterial baroreceptors clearly provide a powerful means for moment-to-moment regulation of arterial pressure, but their role in long-term blood pressure regulation is controversial. Some studies suggest that the baroreceptors are relatively unimportant in chronic regulation of blood pressure because they tend to reset within a few days to the level of blood pressure to which they are exposed.[41] In most forms of chronic hypertension, the arterial baroreflexes are reset to higher blood pressures. To the extent that resetting of baroreceptors occurs, this would attenuate their potency as a long-term controller of blood pressure.

Some experimental studies, however, suggest that the baroreceptors do not completely reset and therefore may contribute to long-term blood pressure regulation. With prolonged increases in arterial pressure, the baroreflexes may contribute to *reductions* in renal sympathetic activity and promote sodium and water excretion.[39] This, in turn, may attenuate the rise in arterial blood pressure. Thus, impairment of baroreflexes may contribute to increased lability of blood pressure in hypertension, but there is little evidence that baroreceptor dysfunction plays a major role in *causing* chronic hypertension. Instead, their primary role in hypertension, as in normotension, is to buffer changes in blood pressure from the set-point determined by renal pressure natriuresis.

Increased blood pressure lability associated with baroreflex dysfunction, however, is accompanied by periodic large increases in blood pressure that may cause gradual renal injury and eventually lead to chronic hypertension. Studies in experimental animals show, for example, that baroreceptor-denervated animals have significant structural changes in the kidneys, including glomerular injury.[42]

Does Chronic Stress Cause Hypertension by SNS Activation?

Acute physiologic stresses, including pain, exercise, exposure to cold, and mental stress, can all lead to increased SNS activity and transient hypertension. It is also widely believed, however, that chronic stress may lead to long-term increases in blood pressure. Support for this concept comes largely from a few epidemiologic studies showing that air traffic controllers, lower socioeconomic groups, and other groups who are believed to lead more stressful lives, also have increased prevalence of hypertension.[43] There is limited evidence, however, for a direct cause-and-effect relationship between psychosocial stress and chronic hypertension. Nevertheless, there is widespread belief by many researchers and by the general public that stress is an important cause of hypertension in humans.

Obesity

As discussed in more detail later, excess weight gain appears to be a major cause of human primary hypertension. The mechanisms responsible for obesity hypertension appear to be closely linked to increased renal SNS activity.[16,44] Obese persons have elevated SNS activity in various tissues, including the kidneys and skeletal muscle, as assessed by microneurography, tissue catecholamine spillover, and other methods.[16,40] Studies in experimental animals and humans indicate that combined α- and β-adrenergic blockade markedly attenuates the hypertension associated with obesity.[16,44,45] Moreover, the renal sympathetic efferent nerves mediate much of the chronic effects of SNS activation on blood pressure in obesity as bilateral renal denervation greatly attenuates the sodium retention and hypertension in obese dogs.[38] Thus, obesity increases renal sodium reabsorption, impairs pressure natriuresis, and causes hypertension in part by increasing renal SNS activity.

The mechanisms that increase renal SNS activity in obesity have not been fully elucidated although several potential mediators have been suggested including hyperinsulinemia, increased ANG II, activation of chemoreceptor-mediated reflexes associated with sleep apnea, and hyperleptinemia.[16,44] One of the most promising of these is increased leptin, a peptide secreted by adipocytes in proportion to the degree of adiposity. However, further studies are needed to determine the role of leptin and other potential pathways that increase renal SNS activity and raise blood pressure in human primary hypertension.

【 】 THE RENIN–ANGIOTENSIN SYSTEM

The RAS is perhaps the most powerful hormone system for regulating body fluid volumes and blood pressure as evidenced by the effectiveness of various RAS blockers in reducing blood pressure in normotensive and hypertensive subjects. Although the RAS has many components, its most important effects on blood pressure regulation are exerted by ANG II which participates in both short-term and long-term control of arterial pressure.

ANG II is a powerful vasoconstrictor and helps maintain blood pressure in conditions associated with acute volume depletion (e.g., hemorrhage), sodium depletion, or circulatory depression (e.g., heart failure). The long-term effects of ANG II on blood pressure, however, are closely intertwined with volume homeostasis through direct and indirect effects on the kidneys.

When the RAS is fully functional, the chronic renal pressure natriuresis curve is steep, and sodium balance can be maintained over a wide range of intakes with minimal changes in blood pressure (Fig. 69–9). One reason for the effectiveness of the normal pressure natriuresis mechanism is that ANG II levels are suppressed during high sodium intake and increased when sodium intake is restricted, thereby adjusting renal sodium excretion appropriately without the need to invoke large changes in blood pressure to maintain sodium balance.

Blockade of the RAS, with ANG II receptor blockers (ARBs) or angiotensin-converting enzyme (ACE) inhibitors, increases renal excretory capability so that sodium balance can be maintained at reduced blood pressure.[19] However, blockade of the RAS also reduces the slope of pressure natriuresis and makes blood pressure salt sensitive.[30] Thus, the effectiveness of RAS blockers in lowering blood pressure is greatly diminished by high salt intake and, in many patients, effectiveness is improved by the addition of a diuretic.

Inappropriately high levels of ANG II reduce renal excretory capability and impair pressure natriuresis, thereby reducing the slope and necessitating increased blood pressure to maintain sodium balance. The mechanisms mediating the potent antinatriuretic effects of ANG II include renal hemodynamic effects as well as direct and indirect effects to increase tubular reabsorption.[30]

ANG II-Mediated Efferent Arteriolar Constriction Attenuates Reductions in GFR When Renal Perfusion is Threatened

Physiologic activation of the RAS usually occurs as a compensation for conditions that cause underperfusion of the kidneys, such as sodium depletion or hemorrhage. The RAS acts in concert with other autoregulatory mechanisms, such as tubuloglomerular feedback (TGF) and myogenic activity, to maintain a relatively constant GFR when perfusion of the kidney is threatened.[19,30] In these cases, administration of ARBs or ACE inhibitors may actually reduce GFR further, even though renal blood flow is preserved. The impairment of GFR after RAS blockade is caused, in part, by inhibition of the constrictor effects of ANG II on efferent arterioles as well as reduced blood pressure.[30]

The vasoconstrictor effect of ANG II on efferent arterioles is most important when renal perfusion pressure is reduced to low levels, near the limits of autoregulation, or when other disturbances such as sodium depletion are superimposed on low perfusion pressure. Clinically, the constrictor effects of ANG II on efferent arterioles become especially important in patients with renal artery stenosis and/or sodium depletion or with heart failure who may have substantial decreases in GFR when treated with RAS blockers.[30]

The relatively weak constrictor action of ANG II on preglomerular vessels is related, in part, to selective protection of these vessels by autacoid mechanisms such as prostaglandins or endothelial-derived nitric oxide (NO). After blockade of prostaglandin synthesis or inhibition of NO, ANG II infusion causes marked constriction of preglomerular as well as postglomerular vessels.[30] When the ability of the kidneys to produce these autocoids is impaired by treatment with nonsteroidal antiinflammatory drugs or by chronic vascular disease (e.g., atherosclerosis), increased levels of ANG II may reduce GFR by constricting afferent arterioles.

Increased ANG II May Mediate Glomerular Injury in Overperfused Kidneys Although blockade of the vasoconstrictor effects of ANG II on the efferent arterioles may cause a further decline in GFR in ischemic nephrons, RAS blockade may be beneficial when nephrons are hyperfiltering, especially if ANG II is not appropriately suppressed. For example, in diabetes mellitus and in certain forms of hypertension associated with glomerulosclerosis and nephron loss, ANG II blockade, by decreasing efferent arteriolar resistance and arterial pressure, lowers glomerular hydrostatic pressure and attenuates glomerular hyperfiltration.[46,47] Clinical and experimental studies indicate that RAS blockers are more effective than other antihypertensive agents in preventing glomerular injury, even with similar reductions in blood pressure;[48–50] this appears to be partly caused by a greater reduction in glomerular hydrostatic pressure as a result of vasodilation of efferent arterioles after blockade of the RAS.

Do Nonhemodynamic Effects of ANG II Cause Target-Organ Injury?

It also has been suggested that ANG II causes injury to the kidneys and other organs through direct actions that pro-

mote vascular smooth muscle migration and proliferation, increased collagen formation, and production of extracellular matrix, in addition to its hemodynamic effect. Much of the evidence supporting this hypothesis comes from in vitro studies, often using supraphysiologic concentrations of ANG II. Although in vivo studies have demonstrated greater renal protective effects of RAS blockers compared to other antihypertensive drugs, decreases in glomerular hydrostatic pressure because of efferent arteriolar vasodilation may have contributed to these beneficial effects. In studies where blood pressure was measured very accurately, using 24-hour telemetry, the renal protective effects of RAS blockade appear to be largely a result of reductions in blood pressure.[51]

An observation that is difficult to reconcile with the concept that ANG II directly mediates target-organ injury, independent of blood pressure, is the finding that physiologic activation of the RAS is not associated with vascular or renal injury as long as the blood pressure is not elevated. For example, sodium depletion does not cause renal, cardiac or vascular injury despite marked increases in renal ANG II levels. Also, the clipped kidney of the two-kidney, one-clip Goldblatt model of hypertension is exposed to very high ANG II levels but is protected from increased arterial pressure by the clip on the renal artery and has no visible injury as long as the stenosis is not too severe. However, the nonclipped kidney, exposed to lower ANG II concentrations but higher blood pressure, has marked focal segmental glomerular sclerosis as well as tubulointerstitial changes characteristic of hypertension.[52] These observations suggest that the hemodynamic effects of ANG II are necessary for most of the vascular and renal injury that occur in ANG II-dependent hypertension.

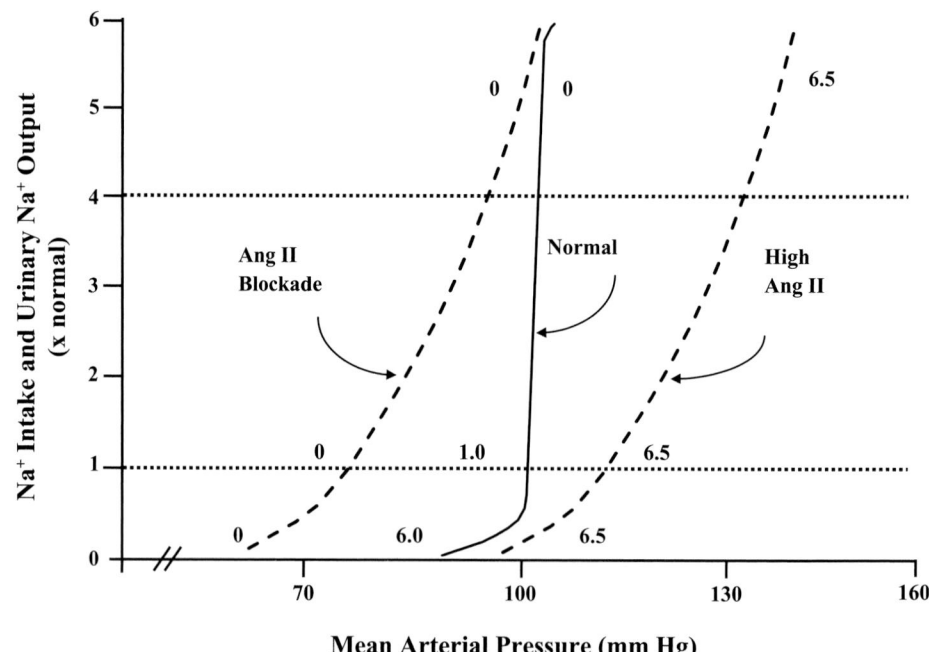

FIGURE 69–9. Steady-state relationships between arterial pressure and sodium intake and excretion under normal conditions with a fully functional renin–angiotensin system, after blockade of ANG II formation with an angiotensin-converting enzyme (ACE) inhibitor, and after ANG II infusion at a low dose to prevent ANG II levels from being suppressed when sodium intake was increased. The numbers in parentheses are estimated ANG II levels expressed as times normal. *Source: Redrawn from Hall JE, Guyton AC, Smith MJ Jr, et al. Blood pressure and renal function during chronic changes in sodium intake: role of angiotensin. Am J Physiol 1980;239:F271–F280.*

ANG II Stimulates Renal Tubular Sodium Reabsorption

ANG II increases renal tubular sodium reabsorption through stimulation of aldosterone secretion, by direct effects on epithelial transport, and by hemodynamic effects. ANG II-mediated constriction of efferent arterioles reduces renal blood flow and peritubular capillary hydrostatic pressure, and increases peritubular colloid osmotic pressure as a result of increased filtration fraction.[30] These changes, in turn, increase the driving force for fluid reabsorption across tubular epithelial cells. Reductions in renal medullary blood flow caused by efferent arteriolar constriction or by direct effects of ANG II on the vasa recta may also enhance reabsorption in the loop of Henle and collecting ducts.[30]

ANG II also directly stimulates proximal tubular sodium reabsorption. This effect occurs at very low ANG II concentrations and is mediated by actions on the luminal and basolateral membranes (Fig. 69–10).[30,46] ANG II stimulates the Na^+-H^+ antiporter on the luminal membrane and increases sodium-potassium-adenosine triphosphatase (ATPase) activity, as well as sodium bicarbonate cotransport on the basolateral membrane.[46,53] These effects appear to be partly a result of inhibition of an adenyl cyclase and increased phospholipase C activity.

Sodium reabsorption in the loop of Henle, macula densa, and distal nephron segments is also stimulated by ANG II. At physiologic concentrations, ANG II increases bicarbonate reabsorption in the loop of Henle and stimulates Na^+-K^+-2 Cl transport in the medullary thick ascending loop of Henle.[46,53] ANG II stimulates multiple ion transporters in the distal parts of the nephron, including H^+-ATPase activity, as well as epithelial sodium channel activity in the cortical collecting ducts.[46,53]

ANG II also amplifies TGF sensitivity by increasing ion transport in the macula densa epithelial cells.[53] The macula densa operates to maintain a relatively constant delivery of sodium chloride to the distal tubules by feedback regulation of afferent and efferent arteriolar resistances and, therefore, GFR. ANG II-mediated enhanced TGF sensitivity permits a decrease in distal sodium chloride delivery without compensatory increases in GFR via TGF. Decreased distal tubular NaCl delivery, caused by the multiple proximal tubule and vascular actions of ANG II, combines with other actions of ANG II on the distal nephron sites to reduce sodium excretion and exert powerful antinatriuretic effects. It is for this reason that ANG II is one of the most powerful sodium-retaining hormones in the body, and it exerts important effects on renal pressure natriuresis and long-term blood pressure regulation. Conversely, blockade of ANG II provides a means of enhancing renal excretory capability, thereby allowing sodium balance to be maintained at greatly reduced arterial blood pressures.

[ ] ALDOSTERONE

Aldosterone is a powerful sodium-retaining hormone and consequently has important effects on renal pressure natriuresis and blood pressure regulation. The primary sites of actions of aldosterone on sodium reabsorption are the principal cells of the distal tubules, cortical collecting tubules, and collecting ducts where aldosterone stimulates sodium reabsorption and potassium secretion. Aldosterone binds to intracellular mineralocorticoid receptors

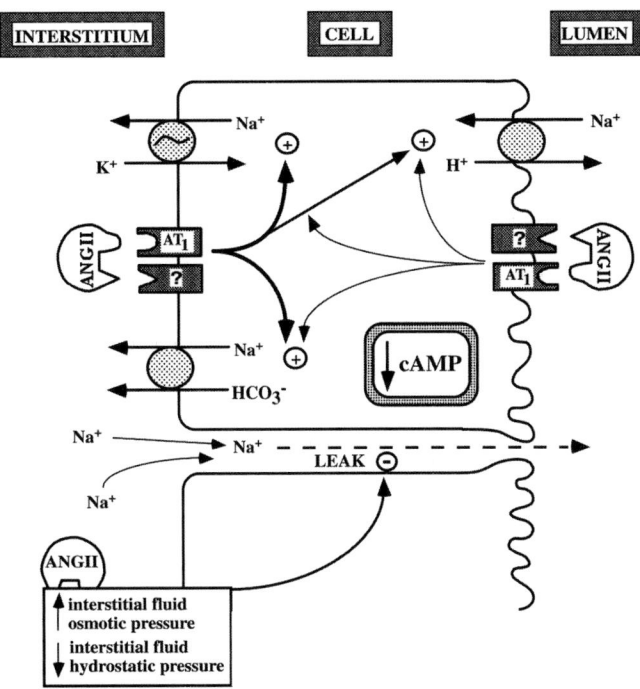

FIGURE 69–10. Angiotensin (ANG) II increases proximal tubular reabsorption by binding to receptors on the luminal and basolateral membranes and stimulating Na^+/H^+ antiporter, Na^+/HCO_3 cotransport, and Na^+/K^+ adenosine triphosphatase (ATPase) activity. ANG II also increases reabsorption by increasing interstitial fluid colloid osmotic pressure and decreasing interstitial fluid hydrostatic pressure. *Source: Redrawn from Hall JE, Brands MW, Henegar JR. Angiotensin II and long-term arterial pressure regulation: the overriding dominance of the kidney. J Am Soc Nephrol 1999;10:S258–S265.*

(MRs) and activates transcription by target genes which, in turn, stimulate synthesis or activation of the Na^+-K^+-ATPase pump on the basolateral epithelial membrane and activation of amiloride-sensitive sodium channels on the luminal side of the epithelial membrane.[54] These effects are termed *genomic* because they are mediated by activation of gene transcription and require 60 to 90 minutes to occur after administration of aldosterone.

Aldosterone also exerts rapid *nongenomic* effects on the cardiovascular and renal systems.[55,56] Aldosterone increases the sodium current in principal cells of the cortical collecting tubule through activation of the amiloride-sensitive channel and stimulates the Na^+-H^+ exchanger in a few minutes after application.[55,56] In vascular smooth muscle cells, aldosterone stimulates sodium influx by activating the Na^+-H^+ exchanger in less than 4 minutes. Acute aldosterone administration may rapidly reduce forearm blood flow in humans, although some investigators have found either no change or an increase in blood flow (see references 55 and 56 for review). The putative membrane receptor and the cell-signaling mechanisms responsible for these rapid nongenomic actions of aldosterone have not been identified, especially with physiologic levels of aldosterone. Thus, the importance of the nongenomic effects of aldosterone on long-term regulation of renal pressure natriuresis and blood pressure are still unclear.

The overall effects of aldosterone on renal pressure natriuresis are similar to those observed for ANG II. With low sodium intake, increased aldosterone helps prevent sodium loss and reductions in blood pressure. Conversely, during high sodium intake, suppression of aldosterone helps to prevent excessive sodium retention and attenuates an increase in blood pressure.

Excess aldosterone secretion reduces the slope of pressure natriuresis so that blood pressure becomes very salt sensitive. Consequently, increasing plasma aldosterone 6- to 10-fold causes marked hypertension when sodium intake is normal or elevated, but there is very little effect on blood pressure when sodium intake is low.[17,57]

The role of aldosterone and activation of MRs in human hypertension is a topic of renewed interest in recent years. Some investigators suggest that hyperaldosteronism or excess activation of MRs may be more common than previously believed, especially in patients with hypertension that is resistant to treatment with the usual antihypertensive medications. For example, the prevalence of primary aldosteronism is reported to be almost 20 percent among patients referred to specialty clinics for resistant hypertension. Many of these patients, however, are overweight or obese.[58]

Regardless of the prevalence of primary aldosteronism, there is emerging evidence that antagonism of MRs may provide an important therapeutic tool for preventing target-organ injury and reducing blood pressure in hypertension[58,59]; for example, antagonism of MR attenuated sodium retention, hypertension, and glomerular hyperfiltration in obese dogs fed a high-fat diet.[60] This finding was somewhat surprising in view of the fact that plasma aldosterone concentration was only slightly elevated in obesity. However, even mild increases of plasma aldosterone may increase blood pressure when accompanied by high sodium intake and volume expansion because aldosterone greatly enhances salt sensitivity of blood pressure.

In obese, insulin-resistant patients there may also be enhanced sensitivity to the effects of aldosterone because of increased abundance of epithelial sodium channels (ENaCs) which would amplify the effects of MR activation on sodium reabsorption and blood pressure. It is also possible that glucocorticoids may contribute to activation of the MRs in obese, insulin-resistant patients. Normally the MR is "protected" from activation by glucocorticoids as a consequence of the effects of 11β-hydroxysteroid dehydrogenase-2 (11β-HSD2) which converts active cortisol into inactive cortisone. Consequently, reductions in 11β-HSD2 in the renal tubules would lead to increased MR activation by cortisol, causing sodium retention, hypokalemia, and hypertension. Although studies in some experimental models of hypertension, such as the Dahl salt-sensitive rat, have shown reduced expression of 11β-HSD2 in the kidney, few studies have assessed the potential role of this mechanism in human hypertension.

【 】 THE ENDOTHELIN SYSTEM

Endothelin-1 (ET-1), the most powerful vasoconstrictor produced in humans, is derived from a 203-amino-acid peptide precursor, preproendothelin, which is cleaved after translation to form proendothelin.[61] A converting enzyme located within the endothelial cells cleaves proendothelin (or big endothelin) to produce the 21-amino-acid peptide, endothelin.[62–65]

Cardiovascular and Renal Effects of ET-1

ET-1 receptor binding sites have been identified throughout the body, with the greatest numbers of receptors in the kidneys and lungs.[62–65] Although the biochemical and molecular nature of en-

dothelin is well characterized, its physiologic importance in regulating renal and cardiovascular function has yet to be fully elucidated.[62–65] ET-1 can either elicit a hypertensive effect by activating endothelin type A (ET_A) receptors in the kidneys or an antihypertensive effect via endothelin type B (ET_B) receptor activation. Thus, the ability of ET-1 to influence blood pressure regulation is highly dependent on where ET-1 is produced and which ET receptor type is activated (Fig. 69–11).

Endothelin-1 produces vasoconstriction, impairs renal pressure natriuresis, and increases blood pressure via ET_A receptor activation. ET_A receptors are located primarily on vascular smooth muscle cells and are thought to mediate ET-1 vasoconstriction and cellular proliferation in various disease states.[62–65] Although ET_A receptors may play a role in certain forms of hypertension, they do not appear to have a major influence on cardiovascular and renal function under normal physiologic conditions.

ET-1, via ET_A receptor activation exerts multiple actions within the kidney that, if sustained chronically, could contribute to the development of hypertension and progressive renal injury. ET-1 decreases GFR and renal plasma flow through stimulation of vascular smooth muscle and mesangial cell contraction. Long-term effects of ET-1 on the kidney include stimulation of mesangial cell proliferation and extracellular matrix deposition, as well as vascular smooth muscle hypertrophy in renal resistance vessels.[62–64]

Expression of ET-1 is greatly enhanced in several animal models of severe hypertension with renal vascular hypertrophy and in models of progressive renal injury.[66–74] In addition, treatment with endothelin receptor antagonists attenuated the hypertension and small artery morphologic changes, and improved kidney function in these models.[68–72]

Role of ET-1 in Salt-Sensitive Hypertension

Several lines of evidence suggest that ET-1 may contribute to salt-sensitive hypertension. Dahl salt-sensitive (DS) rats placed on a high-sodium diet are characterized by attenuated pressure natriuresis, development of hypertension, extensive glomerulosclerosis, renal arteriolar, and tubular injury, as well as progressive renal injury. There is growing evidence that ET-1, acting via an ET_A receptor, may play a role in mediating the renal injury of DS hypertension. Prepro-ET-1 mRNA and vascular responsiveness to ET-1 are increased in the renal cortex of DS rats compared with Dahl salt-resistant (DR) rats and a positive correlation between ET-1 generation in the renal cortex and the extent of glomerulosclerosis has been reported in DS hypertensive rats.[67] Also supporting a role of ET-1 in DS hypertension is the finding that acute infusion of a nonselective ET_A-ET_B receptor antagonist directly into the renal interstitium improved renal hemodynamic and excretory function in DS rats but not in DR rats.[68] Moreover, chronic blockade of ET_A receptors attenuated the hypertension and proteinuria and ameliorated the glomerular and tubular damage associated with high salt intake in DS rats.[69] An important unanswered question is whether the beneficial effect of the ET_A blockade in reducing renal injury is mediated through lower blood pressure or through direct renal mechanisms.

Interaction between ET-1 and the RAS

Recent studies also suggest an important interaction between ET-1 and the RAS. Renal ET-1 synthesis is enhanced in various animal

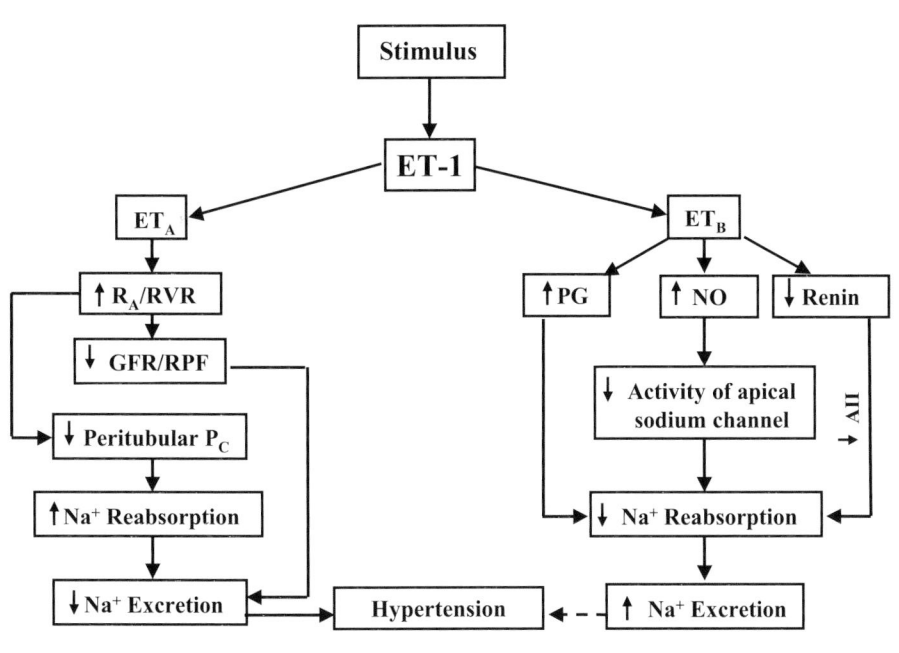

FIGURE 69–11. Summary of the pro- and antihypertensive actions of endothelin-1 (ET-1). The ability of ET-1 to influence blood pressure regulation and renal pressure natriuresis is highly dependent on where ET-1 is produced and which renal ET receptor type is activated. ET-1 can elicit a prohypertensive antinatriuretic effect by activating ET_A receptors in the kidneys. Activation of renal ET_A receptors increases renal vascular resistance (RVR), which decreases renal plasma flow (RPF) and glomerular filtration rate (GFR), and enhances sodium reabsorption by decreasing peritubular capillary hydrostatic pressure (Pc). The net effect of renal ET_A receptor activation is decreased sodium excretion and increased blood pressure. Conversely, ET-1 can elicit an antihypertensive natriuretic effect via ET_B receptor activation. Activation of the renal ET_B receptor leads to enhanced synthesis of nitric oxide (NO) and prostaglandin (PG) E_2 and suppression of the renin–angiotensin system. The net effect of renal ET_B receptor activation is increased sodium excretion and decreased blood pressure.

ductions in uterine perfusion pressure in pregnant rats. The role of ET-1 in mediating the cardiovascular and renal disorders in women with preeclampsia, however, is unknown.

Endothelin type B receptor activation causes vasodilation, enhances renal pressure natriuresis, and decreases blood pressure. While much attention has been given to ET_A receptor activation in the pathophysiology of cardiovascular and renal disease, recent studies indicate an important antihypertensive role for ET_B receptor.[79,80] The most compelling evidence for a major role of ET_B receptors in regulating renal function and blood pressure comes from reports that transgenic mice deficient in ET_B receptors develop a severe salt-sensitive hypertension and that pharmacologic antagonism of ET_B receptors produces significant hypertension in rats.[80,81]

Because ET_B receptors are located on multiple cell types throughout the body, including endothelial cells and renal epithelial cells, both intrarenal and extrarenal mechanisms could theoretically mediate the hypertension produced by chronic disruption of ET_B receptors. Bagnall et al. reported that ablation of ET_B receptors exclusively from endothelial cells produced endothelial dysfunction but did not cause hypertension.[82]

models of chronic ANG II-induced hypertension,[70–72] and the renal and hypertensive effects of ANG II in rats are markedly attenuated or completely abolished by ET_A receptor antagonists.[70–74] The quantitative importance of ET-1 in mediating the chronic hypertensive actions of ANG II may depend on the level of dietary sodium intake.

Possible Role of ET-1 in Preeclampsia

Preeclampsia is associated with hypertension, proteinuria, and endothelial dysfunction.[75,76] Because endothelial damage is a known stimulus for ET-1 synthesis, increases in the production of ET-1 and activation of ET_A receptors may participate in the pathophysiology of hypertension during preeclampsia. Alexander and coworkers found that renal expression of preproendothelin was significantly elevated in the renal medulla and the cortex in a rat model of preeclampsia induced by chronic reductions in uterine perfusion pressure.[77,78] Moreover, they reported that chronic administration of the selective ET_A receptor antagonist markedly attenuated the increase in blood pressure in pregnant rats with chronic reductions in uterine perfusion pressure. In sharp contrast to the response in reduced uterine perfusion pressure rats, ET_A receptor blockade had no significant effect on blood pressure in normal pregnant animal.[77] These findings suggest that ET-1 plays a major role in mediating the hypertension produced by chronic re-

In contrast to models of total ET_B receptor ablation, the blood pressure response to a high-salt diet was unchanged in endothelial cell-specific ET_B receptor knockouts compared to control mice. These findings suggest that ET_B receptors in nonendothelial cells are important for blood pressure regulation. Supporting this concept is the finding that collecting duct ET_B knockout (KO) mice on a normal sodium diet were hypertensive and that a high-sodium diet had worsened the hypertension.[83] These findings provide strong evidence that the intrarenal effect of ET_B receptor activation on the collecting duct is an important physiologic regulator that increases renal sodium excretion and reduces blood pressure.

Role of Endothelin in Human Hypertension

Although ET-1 clearly plays a significant role in the pathogenesis of some forms of experimental hypertension, especially salt-sensitive models, its role in human primary hypertension is unclear. Bosentan, a combined ET_A-ET_B receptor antagonist, significantly lowered blood pressure in a large, double-blind, clinical trial, indicating that endothelin system helps maintain blood pressure in human hypertension.[84] However, the magnitude of the blood pressure reduction by bosentan was almost the same as that observed in normotensive humans. Although this observation suggests that endothelin probably does not play a major role in raising blood pressure in most patients with essential hypertension, interpretation of the results is complicated by the fact that bosentan blocks both ET_A and ET_B receptors; blockade of the antihypertensive ET_B receptor may have masked an important role of endothelin in essential hypertension via ET_A receptor activation. Therefore, the importance of ET-1 in human essential hypertension deserves further investigation.

Role of Endothelin in Pulmonary Arterial Hypertension

Although the importance of ET-1 in human essential hypertension remains unclear, ET-1 appears to play an important role in pulmonary arterial hypertension (PAH). PAH is characterized by a progressive increase in pulmonary vascular resistance resulting from vascular remodeling, vasoconstriction, and cellular proliferation.[85] Depending on the severity of the disease, PAH may progress to right ventricular failure and death. Studies in animal models of PAH and in humans suggest that ET-1 plays an important role in mediating the vascular remodeling, vasoconstriction, and cellular proliferation associated with PAH.[85] Thus, ET-1 receptor antagonists have proven to be efficacious in treatment of patients with PAH.

【 】 NITRIC OXIDE

Tonic release of NO by the vascular endothelium plays a major role in regulating vascular function and long-term inhibition of nitric oxide synthase models causes sustained hypertension associated with increases in total peripheral resistance and impaired renal pressure natriuresis.[86] The magnitude of the increase in blood pressure during NO inhibition depends on the sodium intake, indicating that NO also regulates sodium balance and renal pressure natriuresis.

NO Enhancement of Pressure Natriuresis

The renal mechanisms whereby reductions in NO synthesis enhance pressure natriuresis can be divided into hemodynamic and tubular components, each of which may be modulated by processes that are intrinsic or extrinsic to the kidneys (Fig. 69–12). For example, reductions in NO synthesis may decrease renal sodium excretory function by increasing renal vascular resistance directly or by enhancing the renal vascular responsiveness to vasoconstrictors such as ANG II or norepinephrine.[86] Reductions in NO synthesis also increase renal tubular sodium reabsorption via direct effects on renal tubular transport and through changes in intrarenal physical factors, such as renal interstitial hydrostatic pressure and medullary blood flow.[86–90] Inhibition of NO synthesis reduces renal interstitial fluid hydrostatic pressure (RIHP) and urinary sodium excretion.[86] Stimulation of NO production normalizes the blunted pressure natriuretic response in DS rats as a result of improvement in the kidney's ability to generate increased RIHP in response to increased renal perfusion pressure.[86]

Most investigators attribute the alterations in RIHP to changes in flow and pressure in the renal medullary circulation.[88,89] Consistent with this hypothesis is the observation that acute infusion of an NO synthase inhibitor directly into the renal medulla significantly reduces papillary blood flow, RIHP, and urinary sodium and water excretion without affecting GFR or systemic arterial pressure.[88] Chronic renal medullary interstitial infusion of NO synthase inhibitors in conscious rats caused sustained reductions in medullary blood flow, sodium and water retention, and hypertension, which were reversed when the infusion was discontinued.[88] These findings suggest that reductions in medullary blood flow may be another important mechanism whereby inhibition of NO in the kidney leads to a hypertensive impairment of pressure natriuresis.

NO and the SNS

Several studies show that renal sympathetic nerve activity is suppressed following stimulation of NO production and increased after systemic administration of NO synthesis inhibitors. As changes in SNS activity are known to alter both renal hemodynamics and sodium reabsorption, changes in renal sympathetic activity may also contribute to the blunted pressure natriuresis observed in conditions of impaired NO production. However, not all studies support this concept[91] and the importance of interactions between NO and the SNS in long-term blood pressure control is still unclear.

NO Interacts with the RAS

Inhibition of NO production enhances renin release from juxtaglomerular cells directly as well as through a macula densa mediated mechanism.[92] Moreover, activation of the RAS accounts for a significant part of the hypertensive effects of impaired NO release.

Impaired NO Production Produces Salt-Sensitive Hypertension

Several lines of evidence suggest that NO plays an important role in the regulation of sodium balance and in the pathogenesis of salt-sensitive hypertension.[93] Increased renal NO production or

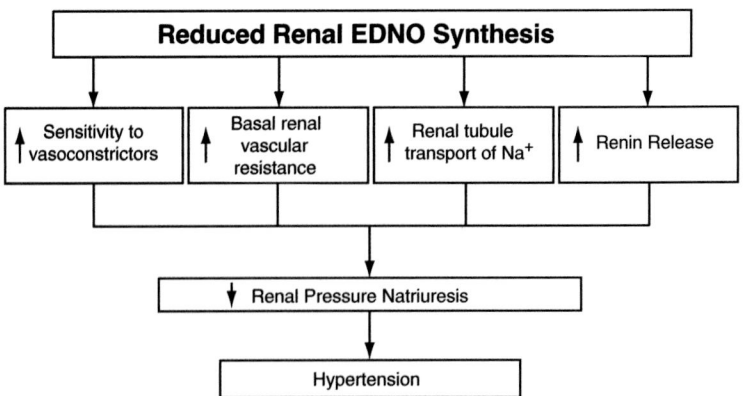

FIGURE 69–12. Renal mechanisms whereby reduced nitric oxide (NO) synthesis decreases pressure natriuresis and increases blood pressure. Decreased endothelial-derived nitric oxide (EDNO) synthesis impairs renal sodium excretory function by increasing basal renal vascular resistance, enhancing the renal vascular responsiveness to vasoconstrictors such as ANG II or norepinephrine, or activating the renin–angiotensin system. Reductions in NO synthesis also impair sodium excretory function either by directly increasing tubular reabsorption or by altering intrarenal physical factors, such as renal interstitial hydrostatic pressure or medullary blood flow.

release, as evidenced by increased urinary excretion of NO metabolites or the NO second messenger, cyclic guanosine monophosphate, has been reported to be essential for the maintenance of normotension during a dietary salt challenge. Prevention of this increase in renal NO production resulted in salt-sensitive hypertension.[93]

There is also evidence that NO synthesis is impaired in some vascular beds in human primary hypertension. The extent to which these changes are secondary to increased blood pressure or reflect important mechanisms for the pathogenesis of hypertension, however, remains unclear.

OXIDATIVE STRESS

Oxidative stress occurs when total oxidant production exceeds antioxidant capacity. Recent studies suggest that reactive oxygen species (ROS) may play a role in the initiation and progression of cardiovascular dysfunction associated with hyperlipidemia, diabetes mellitus, and hypertension.[94] In many forms of hypertension, the increased ROS appear to be derived mainly from nicotinamide adenine dinucleotide phosphate oxidases, which could serve as a triggering mechanism for uncoupling endothelial nitrous oxide synthase (NOS) by oxidants.[94]

ROS produced by migrating inflammatory cells and/or vascular cells have distinct effects on different cell types.[94] These effects include endothelial dysfunction, increased renal tubule sodium transport, cell growth and migration, inflammatory gene expression, and stimulation of extracellular matrix formation. ROS, by affecting vascular and renal tubule function, can also impair renal pressure natriuresis, alter systemic hemodynamics, and raise blood pressure (Fig. 69–13).[95–100]

Considerable evidence supports a role for ROS in various animal models of sodium-sensitive hypertension.[95–100] The DS rat, for example, has increased vascular and renal superoxide production and increased levels of H_2O_2. The renal expression of superoxide dismutase is decreased in the kidneys of DS rats, and long-term administration of Tempol, a superoxide dismutase mimetic, significantly decreases blood pressure and attenuates renal damage. Another salt-sensitive model, the stroke-prone spontaneously hypertensive rats, has elevated levels of superoxide and decreased total plasma antioxidant capacity. Superoxide production is also increased in the deoxycorticosterone acetate (DOCA)-salt hypertensive rat and treatment with apocynin, an nicotinamide adenine dinucleotide phosphate oxidase inhibitor, decreases arterial pressure.

The importance of oxidative stress in human hypertension is unclear. An imbalance between total oxidant production and the antioxidant capacity in human primary hypertension has been reported to occur in some but not all studies.[95] The equivocal findings in human studies are most likely a result of the difficulty of assessing oxidative stress in humans. However, most of the recent human studies have found that vitamin E and C supplementation has little or no effect on blood pressure.[95]

INFLAMMATORY CYTOKINES

Epidemiologic and experimental studies reveal an association between biochemical markers of systemic inflammation and cardiovascular disorders such as atherosclerosis, heart failure, and hyper-

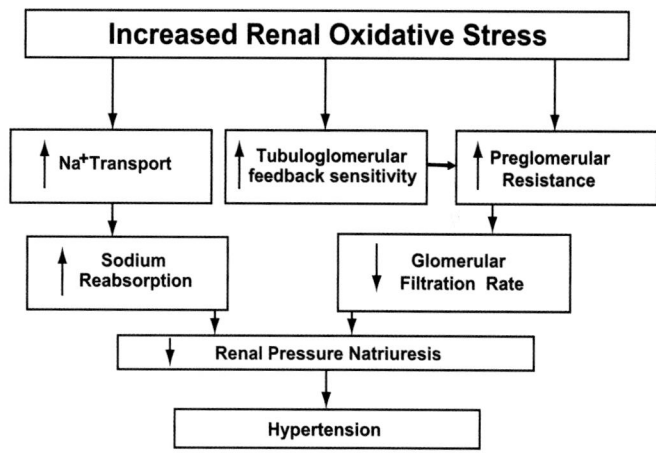

FIGURE 69–13. Renal mechanisms whereby reactive oxygen species impair pressure natriuresis and increase blood pressure. An increase in renal oxidative stress impairs renal pressure natriuresis by increasing renal vascular resistance or enhancing tubuloglomerular feedback, both of which decrease the glomerular filtration rate. Renal oxidative stress also reduces sodium excretion by direct effects to increase renal tubular reabsorption.

sion. Although significant progress has been made in understanding the role of inflammatory cytokines in pathogenesis of atherosclerotic disease, the quantitative importance of cytokines in the pathogenesis and progression of hypertension has yet to be fully elucidated.

Inflammatory Cytokines Interact with Important Blood Pressure Regulatory Systems Important blood pressure regulatory systems, such as the RAS and SNS, interact with the proinflammatory cytokines, such as interleukin (IL)-6 and tumor necrosis factor-α (TNF-α). The SNS stimulates the release of proinflammatory cytokines and sympathetic nerves may also serve as a source of cytokines.[101–105] There is also experimental evidence that proinflammatory cytokines may activate the sympathetic nervous system. ANG II enhances the synthesis of TNF-α and IL-6 and stimulates chemokine monocyte chemoattractant protein-1 and nuclear factor kappa B. ANG II also increases the production of ROS, including hydrogen peroxide, that participate in the process of inflammation.

Inflammatory Cytokines Interact with Endothelium-Derived Factors Proinflammatory cytokines also affect vascular function and endothelium-derived factors involved in the regulation of blood pressure. TNF-α and IL-6 induce both structural and functional alterations in endothelial cells. These cytokines enhance the formation of a number of endothelial cell substances, such as endothelin, reduce acetylcholine-induced vasodilatation, and destabilize the mRNA of endothelial nitric oxide synthase. Thus, endothelial dysfunction associated with many forms of hypertension may, in part, be mediated by proinflammatory cytokines.

Inflammatory Cytokines in Human and Experimental Hypertension Also supporting a potential role for cytokines in the regulation of blood pressure are findings that plasma levels of proinflammatory cytokines correlate with increased blood pressure in human hypertension and in some experimental animal models of hypertension.[106–108] Moreover, several recent studies have demonstrated that chronic increases in plasma cytokines, comparable to concentrations observed in the hypertension associated with preeclampsia, cause significant and sustained increases in blood pressure. For example, Alexander and coworkers[106] and LaMarca and coworkers[107] reported that a twofold elevation in the plasma levels of TNF-α significantly increased blood pressure and renal vascular resistance in pregnant rats. Orshal and coworkers[108] reported similar findings during IL-6 infusion for 5 days in pregnant rats. These studies are consistent with the hypothesis that increasing plasma levels of cytokines may contribute to pregnancy-induced hypertension.

A recent study by Lee and coworkers[109] also suggests that the hypertension caused by chronic ANG II excess may depend, at least in part, on the presence of IL-6. Mice with knockout of IL-6 had significantly lower blood pressure than wild-type mice during 2 weeks of ANG II infusion. Although these findings demonstrate a significant role for IL-6 in mediating the chronic hypertensive response to ANG II in mice, the importance of inflammatory cytokines in the pathogenesis and progression of the various forms of human hypertension is unclear and is currently an area of active investigation.

【 】 EICOSANOIDS

Eicosanoids are thought to be important regulators of vascular function, platelet aggregation, and sodium and water homeostasis.[110,111] Cyclooxygenase metabolizes arachidonic acid into prostaglandin (PG) G_2 and subsequently to PGH_2, which is then further metabolized by tissue-specific isomerases to PGs such as prostacyclin and thromboxane.

Although PGs play an important role in regulating vascular function in many vascular beds, the renal actions of PGs are thought to have a critical role in long-term blood pressure regulation under certain physiologic and pathophysiologic conditions. The kidneys produce many types of prostaglandins with multiple functions, including prostacyclin, thromboxane, 20-hydroxyeicosatetraenoic acid (20-HETE), and epoxyeicosatetraenoic acids (EETs), all of which have been reported to influence renal pressure natriuresis and blood pressure. However, the major renal prostaglandin controlling sodium excretion is probably PGE_2.[110] The largest production of PGE_2 occurs in the renal medulla with decreasing synthesis in the cortex. PGE_2 is synthesized and rapidly inactivated, and once synthesized, is released, not stored. Once released, PGE_2 inhibits sodium reabsorption by several mechanisms, including direct effects on the renal tubules.

Despite numerous reports that PGs may contribute to the natriuresis of acute physiologic perturbations, the importance of endogenous renal PGs in the long-term regulation of sodium balance under normal physiologic conditions remains unclear.[110] Increases in sodium intake have little or no effect on urinary PG excretion. In addition, nonspecific cyclooxygenase (COX) inhibitors do not affect sodium excretion or blood pressure responses to chronic alterations in dietary sodium intake. Thus, endogenous renal PGs may not play a major role in regulating sodium excretion during chronic changes in sodium intake.[110]

Even though long-term administration of PG synthesis inhibitors has very little effect on volume and/or blood pressure regulation under normal physiologic conditions, renal PGs may be important in pathophysiologic states associated with enhanced

activity of the RAS.[110] In vitro and in vivo studies indicate that renal PGs protect the preglomerular vessels from excessive ANG II-induced vasoconstriction.[110] In the absence of this protective mechanism, the renal vasculature could be exposed to the potent vasoconstrictor actions of ANG II in various conditions, such as sodium and volume depletion. This could, in turn, lead to significant impairment of renal hemodynamics and excretory function.

Inhibitors of the COX-2 enzyme reduce renal pressure natriuresis, cause vasoconstriction, and increase blood pressure. There are at least two distinct cyclooxygenases—COX-1 and COX-2.[111] COX-1 is called the *constitutive enzyme* because of its wide tissue distribution, whereas COX-2 has been termed as *inducible* because of its more restricted basal expression and its upregulation by inflammatory and/or proliferative stimuli.[111] Based on the concept that COX-1 performs cellular housekeeping functions for normal physiologic activity and COX-2 acts at inflammatory sites, it was initially hypothesized that the blood pressure and renal effects of nonsteroidal antiinflammatory drugs might be linked to COX-1 inhibition.[111] However, increasing experimental and clinical evidence indicates that COX-2 metabolites may play a role in the regulation of vascular and renal function under various physiologic and pathophysiologic conditions.[111]

Selective COX-2 inhibitors were designed to minimize gastrointestinal complications of traditional NSAIDs—adverse effects attributed to suppression of COX-1–derived PGE_2 and prostacyclin. Randomized controlled-outcome trials of inhibitors of COX-2 indicate that such compounds may elevate the risk of hypertension, myocardial infarction, and stroke, possibly by removing the protective action of prostacyclin in counteracting thrombogenesis, hypertension, and atherogenesis.[112]

Eicosanoids Produced by Cytochrome P450 Monooxygenase Metabolism of Arachidonic Acid Alter Vascular Function and Renal Pressure Natriuresis

In addition to the PGs generated via the COX pathway, other eicosanoids that affect vascular function and/or renal sodium transport are produced by cytochrome P450 (CYP) monooxygenase metabolism of arachidonic acid. CYP enzymes metabolize arachidonic acid primarily to 20-HETE and EETs. 20-HETE is a potent vasoconstrictor that may have an important role in regulation vascular tone and in autoregulation of renal blood flow.[113] 20-HETE and EETs also inhibit sodium reabsorption in the proximal tubule and thick ascending limb of the loop of Henle. Compelling evidence suggests that the renal production of CYP metabolites of arachidonic acid is altered in genetic and experimental models of hypertension and that this system contributes to the resetting of pressure natriuresis and the development of hypertension. In the spontaneously hypertensive rat, renal production of 20-HETE is increased and inhibitors of the formation of 20-HETE decrease blood pressure.[113] Blockade of 20-HETE synthesis also reduces blood pressure and improves renal function in DOCA-salt, ANG II–infused, and Lyon hypertensive rats.[113] In contrast, 20-HETE formation is reduced in the thick ascending limb of DS rats, which contributes to elevated sodium reabsorption.[113] Enhanced 20-HETE synthesis improves pressure natriuresis and lowers blood pressure in DS rats, whereas inhibitors of

20-HETE production promote the development of hypertension in Lewis rats.[113]

Studies in humans also suggest that CYP metabolites may play a role in sodium homeostasis. Urinary 20-HETE excretion is regulated by salt intake and is differentially regulated in salt-sensitive versus salt-resistant individuals.[114] Moreover, there appears to be a strong negative relationship between the excretion of 20-HETE and body mass index (BMI), suggesting that some factor related to obesity may be responsible for decreased synthesis or excretion of this eicosanoid in hypertension.[115] These observations support the possibility that attenuated renal production of 20-HETE could contribute to impaired renal pressure natriuresis in human hypertension, especially when associated with obesity. However, further mechanistic studies are needed to test the importance of 20-HETE in human hypertension.

[ ] ATRIAL NATRIURETIC PEPTIDE

Atrial natriuretic peptide (ANP) is a 28-amino-acid peptide synthesized and released from atrial cardiocytes in response to stretch. ANP is released from the atria and reduces vascular resistance while enhancing sodium excretion through extrarenal and intrarenal mechanisms.[110] ANP increases GFR but has little effect on renal blood flow. However, an increase in GFR is not a prerequisite for ANP to enhance sodium excretion. ANP may also inhibit renal tubular sodium reabsorption either directly by inhibiting active tubular transport of sodium or indirectly via alterations in medullary blood flow, physical factors, and intrarenal hormones.[110,116]

ANP Inhibits Renin and Aldosterone Secretion ANP has important actions at several sites of the RAS cascade.[110] Intrarenal or intravenous infusion of ANP reduces the renin secretion rate by a macula densa mechanism, and reductions in intrarenal ANG II levels likely contribute to ANP-induced natriuresis. When intrarenal levels of ANG II were prevented from decreasing, the natriuretic effects of ANP were blunted.[110]

ANP also decreases aldosterone release from the adrenal zona glomerulosa cells.[110] Two mechanisms for ANP-induced suppression of aldosterone release have been suggested: (1) a direct action on adrenal glomerulosa cells, and (2) reduced circulating levels of ANG II because of suppressed renin secretion.[110] Although the suppression of aldosterone release does not mediate the acute natriuretic responses to ANP, decreases in circulating levels of aldosterone could contribute to the long-term actions of ANP on sodium balance and blood pressure regulation.

ANP Plays a Role in Short- and Long-Term Volume Regulation Plasma levels of ANP are elevated in numerous physiologic conditions associated with enhanced sodium excretion.[110] Acute blood volume expansion consistently elevates circulating levels of ANP. Some, but not all, investigators report that chronic increases in dietary sodium intake also raise circulating levels of ANP. Infusions of exogenous ANP at rates that result in physiologically relevant plasma concentrations, comparable to those observed during volume expansion, elicit significant natriuresis, especially in the presence of other natriuretic stimuli, such as high renal perfusion pressure.[110] Long-term physiologic elevations in plasma ANP also enhance renal pressure natriuresis and reduce blood pressure.[117]

Blockade of the ANP System Produces Salt-Sensitive Hypertension The development of genetic mouse models that exhibit altered expression of ANP or its receptors (NPR-A, NPR-C) have provided compelling evidence for a role of ANP in chronic regulation of renal pressure natriuresis and blood pressure.[118] Transgenic mice overexpressing ANP are hypotensive relative to their wild-type littermates, whereas mice harboring functional disruptions of the ANP or NPR-A genes are hypertensive. ANP gene knockout mice develop salt-sensitive form of hypertension in association with failure to adequately suppress the RAS. These findings suggest that genetic deficiencies in ANP or its receptors could play a role in the pathogenesis of salt-sensitive hypertension.

SECONDARY CAUSES OF HYPERTENSION

In a small percentage of patients, the clinical features, history, and physical examination point to a specific cause of increased blood pressure and the hypertension is therefore said to be *secondary*. Some types of secondary hypertension have a definite genetic basis, whereas others are caused by cardiovascular diseases and target-organ injury associated with various disorders such as diabetes and kidney disease, and in some instances, hypertension can be caused by drugs or treatments that the patient receives. Nearly all forms of secondary hypertension, however, are characterized by impaired renal function or altered activity of the SNS or hormones that, in turn, impair the ability of the kidneys to excrete salt and water.

Table 69–3 lists some of the most frequently diagnosed causes of secondary hypertension, including those caused by drugs that either themselves raise blood pressure or exacerbate underlying disorders that contribute to hypertension. These drugs include nonsteroidal antiinflammatory drugs, oral contraceptive agents, glucocorticoids, and sympathomimetics that are used as cold remedies. This chapter discusses only a few of the more common causes of secondary hypertension.

[ ] RENOVASCULAR HYPERTENSION

Renovascular hypertension, although accounting for only 2 to 3 percent of all hypertension, is one of the most common causes of secondary hypertension. The pathophysiology of renovascular hypertension is related directly to the reduction in renal perfusion that occurs as a result of stenosis of the main renal artery, one of its branches, or stenosis/injury of other smaller preglomerular blood vessels and glomeruli. The majority of renal vascular lesions reflect either fibromuscular dysplasia or atherosclerosis.[119] The predominant lesion found in the main renal artery or its branches in patients older than 50 years of age is atherosclerotic disease. More subtle functional (constriction) or structural changes in smaller blood vessels (e.g., afferent arterioles, glomeruli), however, are difficult to detect clinically and can contribute to increased blood pressure.

Renovascular hypertension can be unilateral, involving only one kidney, or bilateral, and can result in a homogeneous or a nonhomogeneous ischemia of nephrons. As discussed earlier in the chapter, there are some important differences in the pathophysiology of homogeneous compared to nonhomogenous impairment of renal perfusion. Experimental counterparts of these two clinical forms of renovascular hypertension can be found in the one-kidney, one-clip and the two-kidney, one-clip models of Goldblatt hypertension, respectively.

One-Kidney, One-Clip Model of Goldblatt Hypertension, or Stenosis of a Single Remaining Kidney

In the one-kidney, one-clip model of Goldblatt hypertension, and in patients with stenosis of a single remaining kidney, there is a fairly homogeneous reduction in perfusion of all nephrons leading to an elevation of blood pressure that is proportional to the severity of the stenosis. In experimental one-kidney, one-clip Goldblatt hypertension, the blood pressure increases rapidly after clipping the renal artery and remains stable as long as the stenosis does not worsen. Moreover, blood pressure returns to normal when the stenosis is removed.

Renal artery constriction, if severe enough to reduce renal perfusion pressure below the range of autoregulation (approximately

TABLE 69–3

Some Secondary Causes of Hypertension

A. Renal parenchymal disease
  • Acute and chronic glomerulonephritis
  • Chronic nephritis (e.g., pyelonephritis, radiation)
  • Polycystic disease
  • Diabetic nephropathy
  • Hydronephrosis
  • Neoplasms
B. Renovascular
  • Renal artery stenosis/compression
  • Intrarenal vasculitis
  • Suprarenal aortic coarctation
C. Renoprival (renal failure, loss of kidney tissue)
D. Endocrine Disorders
  • Renin-producing tumors
  • Cushing syndrome
  • Primary aldosteronism
  • Pheochromocytoma (adrenal or extraadrenal chromaffin tumors)
  • Acromegaly
E. Pregnancy-induced hypertension
F. Sleep apnea
G. Increased intracranial pressure (brain tumors, encephalitis)
H. Exogenous hormones and drugs (partial list)
  • Glucocorticoids
  • Mineralocorticoids
  • Sympathomimetics
  • Tyramine-containing foods and monoamine oxidase inhibitors
  • Estrogen (e.g., oral contraceptive pills)
  • Apparent mineralocorticoid excess (e.g., licorice)
  • Nonsteroidal antiinflammatory drugs
  • Cyclosporine
  • Excess alcohol use
  • Drug abuse (e.g., amphetamines, cocaine)

70 mmHg), initially decreases renal blood flow, GFR, and sodium excretion, while increasing renin secretion. However, sodium excretion returns to normal and if sodium intake is normal and adequate volume is available, renin secretion also returns to nearly normal in the established phase of hypertension if the stenosis is not too severe.[18,120] At this point, the hypertension is stable and most indices of renal function are relatively normal, including pressure distal to the stenosis.

Increased ANG II accounts for most of the rapid increase in blood pressure after stenosis of the renal artery. However, even after blocking the RAS, blood pressure still increases (although more slowly) until renal perfusion pressure returns to nearly normal. This increase in renal perfusion pressure, at the expense of systemic arterial hypertension, permits normal excretion of sodium and water to be maintained. As long as the sodium intake is normal, activation of the RAS serves mainly to increase the rate at which blood pressure is elevated. In the established phase of hypertension, blockade of the RAS causes only small reductions in blood pressure, similar to the decreases observed in normal subjects after ANG II blockade.[121]

The importance of volume expansion in elevating blood pressure in one-kidney, one-clip Goldblatt hypertension depends on the sodium intake. With normal or high sodium intake, significant extracellular volume expansion occurs, whereas a low-sodium diet converts this model of hypertension from one that is volume dependent to one that is highly ANG II dependent. Thus, a combination of low-sodium diet and blockade of ANG II formation often normalizes blood pressure in one-kidney, one-clip Goldblatt hypertension.[122]

When the stenosis is severe and adequate renal perfusion cannot be restored even with increased systemic arterial pressure, renin secretion continues to increase, as does arterial pressure, leading eventually to malignant hypertension and renal failure. Thus, the ability to return renal perfusion pressure to normal, or nearly normal, by volume retention or activation of the RAS is critical to maintaining homeostasis when there is a stenosis of a single remaining kidney.

The same sequence as described above occurs when there are widespread homogeneous increases in preglomerular resistance caused by bilateral renal artery stenosis or aortic coarctation above both renal arteries.[18,21]

Two-Kidney, One-Clip Model of Goldblatt Hypertension (Nonhomogeneous Increases in Preglomerular Resistance)

In the two-kidney, one-clip model of Goldblatt hypertension, or in patients with nonhomogeneous increases in preglomerular resistance, the pathophysiology of hypertension is more complicated. Nonhomogeneous increases in preglomerular resistance can be a result of stenosis of one renal artery and normal perfusion of the contralateral kidney or of patchy increases in preglomerular resistance within the kidneys, with some nephrons being underperfused and others having normal or increased blood flow. Thus, these models of hypertension are characterized by underperfusion of some nephrons and normal or increased blood flow in adjacent nephrons or in the nonstenotic kidney.

In experimental models with unilateral renal artery stenosis, the increase in blood pressure is less predictable as long as the contralateral kidney does not become injured because of the hypertension. In this situation, the underperfused nephrons (or the entire underperfused kidney in the case of a unilateral renal artery stenosis) are exposed to reduced perfusion pressure, secrete increased amounts of renin, and excrete less sodium and water than kidneys with normal blood flow. In contrast, the nonischemic nephrons (or nonstenotic kidney) are exposed to increased renal perfusion pressure causing renin secretion to fall to very low levels and increasing sodium excretion above normal. However, even with increased perfusion pressure the function of the nonischemic nephrons (or unclipped, nonstenotic kidney) is impaired because of increased circulating levels of ANG II which exert an antinatriuretic effect and help to sustain hypertension.

The higher blood pressures experienced by the nonstenotic kidney may eventually cause damage to its nephrons. If sufficient damage occurs, unclipping the stenotic kidney (in the case of the experimental two-kidney, one-clip Goldblatt model) or repair of a unilateral renal artery stenosis in humans, may not completely normalize blood pressure. Thus, the contralateral, nonstenotic kidney in these instances may, because of injury, sustain increased blood pressure even after correction of the stenosis in the other kidney. However, correction of the stenosis plus nephrectomy of the nonstenotic kidney usually normalizes blood pressure.[123]

As discussed previously, the two-kidney, one-clip hypertension is *salt sensitive,* whereas the one-kidney, one-clip model is *salt insensitive.* The main reason for the differences in salt sensitivity relate to the reactivity of the RAS in these two models. In one-kidney, one-clip hypertension, renin secretion is normal after hypertension is established and high salt intake results in normal suppression of renin release. In two-kidney, one-clip hypertension, however, the stenotic kidney has a high level of renin secretion that cannot be adequately suppressed when salt intake is raised. The contralateral nonstenotic kidney already has suppressed renin secretion as a consequence of the high blood pressure and therefore cannot suppress renin secretion further when salt intake is raised. Thus, blood pressure in the two-kidney, one-clip model of Goldblatt becomes sensitive to increased salt intake because of impaired responsiveness of the RAS.

Administration of ACE inhibitors or ARBs as a treatment for renovascular hypertension may improve the structure and function of the nonstenotic kidney, but can also produce shrinkage of the stenotic kidney, resulting in fibrosis and deterioration of its function. This is partly a result of the fall in blood pressure, which may reduce renal perfusion pressure distal to the lesion to a level below the range of autoregulation. However, blockade of the RAS also causes vasodilation of efferent arterioles, which contributes to a decline in GFR in the stenotic kidney. In some patients with severe renal vascular lesions, administration of ACE inhibitors or ARBs may cause severe decreases in renal function, especially when there is also volume depletion because of concomitant use of diuretics. Therefore, renal function should be monitored frequently after administration of RAS inhibitors in patients suspected of having renovascular hypertension. Fortunately, these effects appear to be reversible upon cessation of ACE inhibition or ARB, and in many patients the beneficial effects of RAS blockade in reducing blood pressure can be achieved without precipitating further loss of kidney function.

【 】 ADRENAL CORTEX HYPERTENSION

Aldosterone normally exerts nearly 90 percent of the mineralocorticoid activity of the adrenocortical secretions. However, cortisol, the major glucocorticoid secreted by the adrenal cortex, can also provide significant amount of mineralocorticoid activity in some conditions. Aldosterone's mineralocorticoid activity is about 3000 times greater than that of cortisol, but the plasma concentration of cortisol is nearly 2000 times that of aldosterone. As discussed previously, the renal MR is normally protected from activation by cortisol as a result of the effects of 11β-HSD2, which converts active cortisol into inactive cortisone, but when activity of this enzyme is reduced or when cortisol levels are very high, the MR can be activated by cortisol.

Primary Aldosteronism (Conn Syndrome)

Primary aldosteronism, also called *Conn Syndrome* in honor of Jerome Conn who first described this condition in 1955, is the syndrome that results from hypersecretion of aldosterone in the absence of a known stimulus. The excess aldosterone secretion almost always comes from the adrenal cortex and is usually associated with a solitary adenoma or bilateral hyperplasia of the adrenal cortex. *Secondary aldosteronism* refers to increased aldosterone secretion that occurs secondary to a know stimulus, such as activation of the RAS. This is the most common form of aldosteronism seen in clinical practice and occurs in various conditions associated with stimulation of renin secretion, such as congestive heart failure, sodium depletion, or renal artery stenosis.[124]

Primary aldosteronism can occur as a result of an aldosterone-producing adenoma (APA) or because of unilateral or bilateral adrenal hyperplasia.[125] The effects of excess aldosterone were discussed earlier, but the most important with regard to chronic blood pressure regulation are increased sodium reabsorption and increased potassium secretion by the principal cells of the renal tubules. This leads to expansion of extracellular fluid volume, hypertension, suppression of renin secretion, hypokalemia, and metabolic alkalosis, hallmarks of primary aldosteronism. Most of these effects are highly salt sensitive and low sodium intake can greatly attenuate the hypertension and hypokalemia associated with primary aldosteronism.

Adrenal adenomas and bilateral adrenal hyperplasia account for more than 95 percent of primary aldosteronism. However, this is a rare form of hypertension, and in most studies of unselected patients, the classic form of primary aldosteronism was found in less than 1 percent of hypertensive patients.[124] Some adrenal glands in patients with primary aldosteronism may have varying degrees of hyperplasticity and the term *idiopathic hyperaldosteronism* (IHA) was coined to describe this condition. Clinically, APA and IHA are difficult to distinguish, although patients with APA often have more severe hypertension and hypokalemia compared to those with IHA.

The measurement of the aldosterone–renin ratio has been used is recent years in an attempt to define more subtle cases of primary aldosteronism.[125,126] This approach has lead to the suggestion that excess aldosterone secretion may account for as much as 5 to 10 percent of essential hypertension.[125] However, there is considerable debate about whether patients with an increased aldosterone–renin ratio truly have primary aldosteronism, as first described by

Conn. In many of these patients, the major reason for the increased aldosterone–renin ratio is the low level of renin, rather than excess aldosterone secretion.[124]

Increased Arterial Pressure and "Escape" from Sodium Retention during Hyperaldosteronism

Although aldosterone is one of the body's most powerful sodium-retaining hormones, sodium excretion eventually returns to match sodium intake even in patients with APA and very high levels of aldosterone. This "escape" from sodium retention is secondary to increases in extracellular fluid volume and arterial pressure, which in turn increases renal excretion of salt and water via the pressure natriuresis and diuresis mechanisms.[57] Thus, after the extracellular fluid volume increases 5 to 15 percent above normal, arterial pressure also increases 15 to 25 mmHg and this elevated blood pressure returns the renal output of salt and water to normal despite the excess aldosterone (Fig. 69–14). However, this escape occurs at the expense of hypertension, which lasts as long as the person is exposed to the high levels of aldosterone. The importance of pressure natriuresis in permitting aldosterone escape has been demonstrated experimentally by servocontrolling renal perfusion pressure; when renal perfusion pressure was servocontrolled, aldosterone infusion caused continued sodium retention and progressive increases in cumulative sodium balance and extracellular fluid volume, resulting in severe circulatory congestion and edema.[57] Failure of the kidneys to escape from aldosterone-induced sodium retention can also be observed in patients with heart failure who, because of a severely weakened heart, cannot increase arterial pressure sufficiently to reestablish salt and water balance.

Sustained Hypokalemia and Metabolic Alkalosis with Hyperaldosteronism

Excess aldosterone not only increases secretion of potassium ions by the principal cells of the renal tubules, but also stimulates transport of potassium from the extracellular fluid into most cells of the body. This shift of potassium from the extracellular to intracellular fluid accounts for a significant part of the hypokalemia that occurs with excess aldosterone secretion.

Excess aldosterone secretion also stimulates secretion of hydrogen ions in exchange for sodium in the intercalated cells of the renal cortical collecting tubules. This decreases the hydrogen ion concentration in the extracellular fluid causing metabolic alkalosis.

Patients with IHA often have a milder form of aldosteronism than those with APA, although there may be overlap in severity of the clinical features of these two groups.[124,125] In patients with APA, plasma aldosterone concentration is not usually increased in response to upright posture because of marked suppression of the RAS and insensitivity of the aldosterone-secreting adenoma to ANG II. In contrast, patients with IHA usually have a significant increase in aldosterone concentration during upright posture suggesting that adrenal sensitivity to ANG II is maintained.[125] These differences between IHA and APA in adrenal responsiveness to RAS activation have been used to discriminate these two forms of primary aldosteronism.[124]

Cushing Syndrome (Glucocorticoid Excess)

Cushing syndrome is a serious disorder characterized by excess glucocorticoids. Hypertension occurs in approximately 80 percent of patients with Cushing syndrome and is difficult to control.[127]

Cushing syndrome can be caused by either administration of excess cortisol (e.g., for treatment of various inflammatory disorders) or by excess endogenous cortisol secretion. The most common cause of endogenous cortisol excess is overproduction of adrenocorticotrophic hormone (ACTH) from a pituitary adenoma, a condition referred to as *Cushing disease*. The increased ACTH causes adrenal hyperplasia and stimulates cortisol secretion. Cushing disease can also occur as a result of ectopic secretion of ACTH by tumors outside the pituitary, such as an abdominal carcinoma.

ACTH-independent hypercortisolism can occur as a result of adenomas of the adrenal cortex. Primary overproduction of cortisol by the adrenal glands, independent of ACTH, accounts for approximately 20 to 25 percent of Cushing syndrome and is usually associated with suppressed ACTH levels caused by cortisol-induced feedback inhibition of ACTH secretion by the anterior pituitary gland. Administration of large doses of dexamethasone, a synthetic glucocorticoid, can be used to distinguish between ACTH-dependent and ACTH-independent Cushing syndrome. In patients with overproduction of cortisol because of an ACTH-secreting pituitary adenoma or hypothalamic–pituitary dysfunction, even large doses of dexamethasone usually do not suppress ACTH secretion. In contrast, patients with primary adrenal overproduction of cortisol (ACTH independent) usually have low or undetectable levels of ACTH. However, the dexamethasone test may occasionally give an incorrect diagnosis because some ACTH-secreting pituitary tumors respond to dexamethasone with suppression of ACTH secretion.

Glucocorticoids modulate a wide variety of cell processes and the precise mechanisms by which hypercortisolism causes hypertension are incompletely understood. One potential mechanism is activation of the MR; the high levels of cortisol in Cushing syndrome may simply overwhelm the ability of the renal 11β-HSD2 to convert active cortisol into inactive cortisone at the MR receptor, so that cortisol stimulates the MR and causes sodium retention, volume expansion, hypertension, and hypokalemia. High levels of cortisol also increase levels of angiotensinogen and may increase the responsiveness to various pressor stimuli, including ANG II and norepinephrine.[128]

Studies in experimental animals suggest that excess cortisol may also raise blood pressure through mechanisms that may be at least partially independent of activation of classical glucocorticoid or MR.[128] Most of the available evidence, however, suggests that sodium retention may play a key role, although the precise mechanisms that lead to sodium retention are incompletely understood. Regardless of the precise mechanisms of hypertension, the morbidity associated with cortisol excess is substantial, and the risk for death is largely a result of excess cardiovascular events, including heart attack and stroke.

Other Forms of Adrenocortical Hypertension

There are several other rare forms of adrenocortical hypertension, as discussed in Genetic Causes of Hypertension below. Some of these are genetic disorders and include familial hyperaldosteronism, glu-

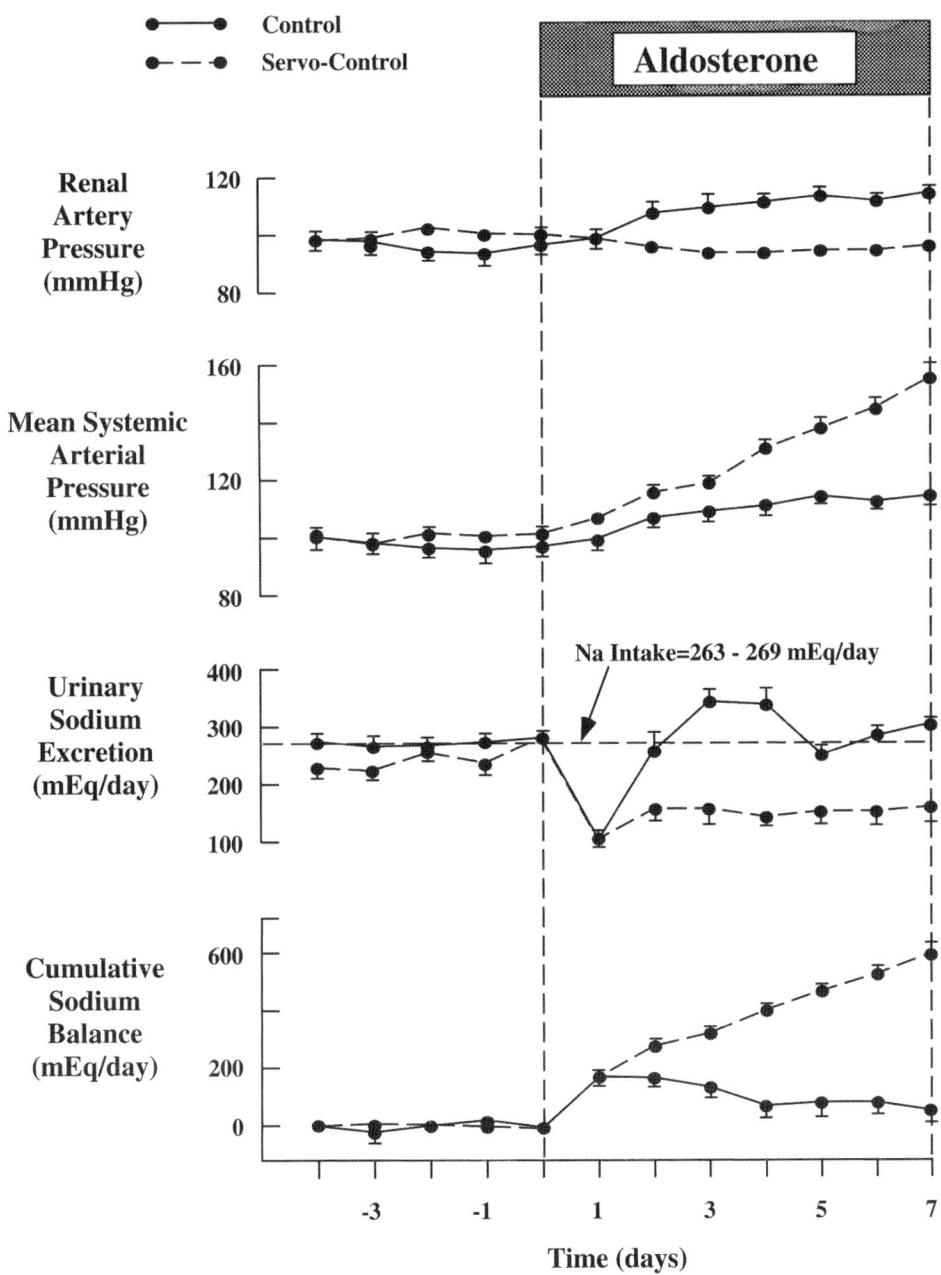

FIGURE 69–14. Effects of chronic aldosterone infusion when renal perfusion pressure was servo-controlled (*dashed lines*) or allowed to increase (*solid lines*). When real perfusion pressure was prevented from increasing, "escape" from sodium retention did not occur and cumulative sodium balance and systemic arterial pressure continued to increase. *Source: Redrawn from Hall JE, Granger JP, Smith MJ Jr, et al. Role of renal hemodynamics and arterial pressure in aldosterone "escape." Hypertension 1984;6(Suppl I):I183–I192.*

cocorticoid remediable aldosteronism, deoxycorticosterone-secreting tumors, and the syndrome of apparent mineralocorticoid excess where glucocorticoids activate the mineralocorticoid receptor because of a deficiency of 11β-HSD2. In each of these conditions, the clinical characteristics are similar to those observed with primary increases in aldosterone secretion caused by adrenal adenomas or idiopathic primary aldosteronism.

【 】 PHEOCHROMOCYTOMA

Pheochromocytoma is a rare form of secondary hypertension occurring in approximately 0.05 percent of hypertensive patients.[124,129]

Although rare, pheochromocytoma can provoke fatal hypertensive crises if unrecognized and untreated. Pheochromocytoma can arise from neuroectodermal chromaffin cells, which are part of the sympathoadrenal system. The chromaffin cells have the capacity to synthesize and store catecholamines and are normally found mainly in the adrenal medulla. Although most chromaffin cell tumors are found in the adrenal medulla, as many as 15 to 30 percent may be extraadrenal, located along the sympathetic chain or, rarely, in other sites.[124,129]

The symptoms and severity of hypertension associated with pheochromocytoma are highly variable, depending on the secretory pattern and amount of catecholamines released.[124,129,130] With tumors that continuously release large amounts of catecholamines, there may be sustained hypertension with few paroxysms, or sudden bursts of very high levels of blood pressure. Tumors that are less active may have cyclical release of catecholamines stores that induce paroxysms of hypertension.

The clinical presentation also depends on whether the predominant catecholamine that is secreted is norepinephrine or epinephrine. Norepinephrine produces α-adrenergically mediated vasoconstriction with diastolic hypertension, whereas epinephrine produces β-adrenergically mediated cardiac stimulation with mainly systolic hypertension and tachycardia, along with sweating, tremors, and flushing. Patients with predominantly epinephrine-secreting tumors sometimes have hypertension alternating with hypotension, and approximately 5 percent of patients with pheochromocytoma remain normotensive.[124]

Pheochromocytoma patients often have decreased blood volume, consistent with the potent effects of norepinephrine to cause peripheral vasoconstriction. This observation, and the finding that chronic excess catecholamines often increase sodium excretion, could be interpreted as evidence that the hypertensive effects of catecholamines are unrelated to any impairment of renal excretory capability. However, the natriuretic effect of catecholamines and volume contraction appear to be secondary to peripheral vasoconstriction, decreased vascular capacitance, and increased arterial pressure, which causes a pressure natriuresis.[15,18] Chronic intrarenal infusion of norepinephrine causes sustained hypertension, indicating important direct effects of catecholamines on the kidney to cause hypertension.

Figure 69–15 shows the relationship between blood pressure and sodium excretion after chronic intravenous infusion of norepinephrine, which has a relatively weak antinatriuretic effect but a powerful peripheral vasoconstrictor action. The antinatriuretic effect of norepinephrine shifts the pressure natriuresis curve to higher blood pressures, thereby necessitating a small increase in blood pressure to maintain sodium balance. However, because norepinephrine has a weak antinatriuretic effect, compared to its potent peripheral vasoconstrictor effect, arterial pressure initially increases above the renal setpoint for regulation of sodium balance and causes transient natriuresis. The sodium loss is transient because extracellular fluid volume decreases and arterial pressure eventually stabilizes at a point where sodium intake and output are balanced.

Orthostatic hypotension is common among patients with pheochromocytoma and is related not only to the reduction of blood volume but perhaps also to desensitization of adrenergic receptors secondary to the chronic excess of catecholamines.

Although a high level of circulating catecholamine is the ultimate cause of hypertension in pheochromocytoma, blood pressure is often only modestly correlated with the level of plasma catecholamines. However, the periodic burst of catecholamine release may cause moderate to severe hypertension and lead to target-organ injury. Consequently, diagnosis and effective treatment of pheochromocytoma is essential.

【 】 PREECLAMPSIA

Preeclampsia in women is characterized by hypertension and proteinuria. Progression of the disease may lead to eclampsia in which seizures develop in association with a high risk for fetal and maternal mortality. Despite being a leading cause of maternal death and a major contributor of maternal and perinatal morbidity, the mechanisms responsible for the pathogenesis of preeclampsia have not yet been fully elucidated. Hypertension associated with preeclampsia develops during pregnancy and remits after delivery, implicating the placenta as a central culprit in the disease.

Although numerous factors including genetic, immunologic, behavioral, and environmental factors have been implicated in the pathogenesis of preeclampsia, reduced uteroplacental perfusion as a result of abnormal cytotrophoblast invasion of spiral arterioles appears to play a key role.[131] Placental ischemia is thought to lead to widespread activation/dysfunction of the maternal vascular endothelium, which results in enhanced formation of endothelin, thromboxane, and superoxide, increased vascular sensitivity to ANG II, and decreased formation of vasodilators such as nitric oxide and prostacyclin. These endothelial abnormalities, in turn, cause hypertension by impairing renal function and increasing total peripheral resistance.[131,132]

Inflammatory cytokines such as IL-6 and TNF-α are thought to be important links between placental ischemia and cardiovascular and renal dysfunction.[131] Supporting a potential role of cytokines are findings that plasma levels of TNF-α and IL-6 are elevated in women with preeclampsia. Important blood pressure regulatory systems such as the RAS, sympathetic nervous system, and endothelial factors interact with proinflammatory cytokines such as IL-6 and TNF-α to raise blood pressure. Proinflammatory cytokines also affect vascular function and endothelium-derived factors involved in blood pressure regulation. Thus, endothelial dysfunction associated with preeclampsia may be mediated, at least in part, by cytokines.

Recent studies indicate that chronic reductions in placental perfusion in pregnant animals are associated with enhanced production

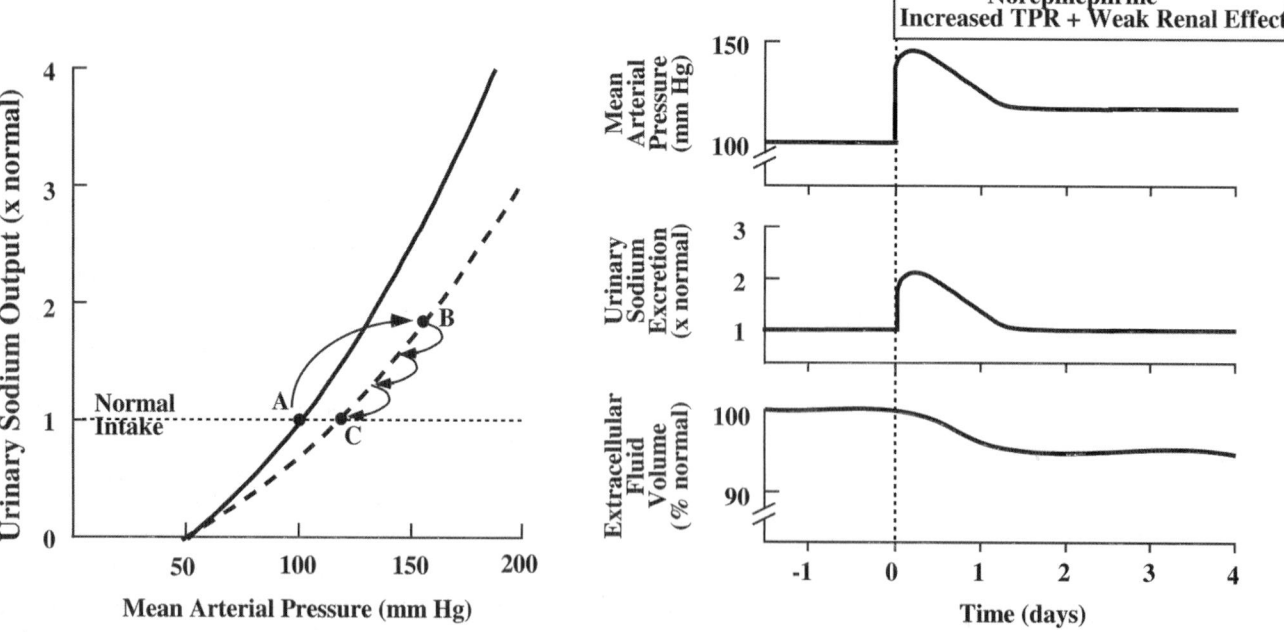

FIGURE 69–15. Long-term effects of norepinephrine, a powerful vasoconstrictor that has a relatively weak effect to impair pressure natriuresis. The normal curve (*solid line*) is compared with the vasoconstrictor curve (*dashed line*). Initially the vasoconstrictor raises blood pressure (from *point A* to *point B*) above the renal set point for sodium balance. Increased arterial pressure, however, causes a transient natriuresis and decreases extracellular fluid volume until blood pressure eventually stabilizes at a level (*point C*) at which sodium intake and output are balanced at a reduced extracellular fluid volume. *Source: Redrawn from Hall JE. The kidney, hypertension, and obesity. Hypertension 2003;41:625–633.*

of inflammatory cytokines, such as TNF-α and IL-6.[133–135] In addition, chronic infusion of either TNF-α or IL-6 into normal pregnant rats results in significant increases in blood pressure and a decrease in renal hemodynamics. TNF-α activates the endothelin system in placenta, renal, and vascular tissues, whereas IL-6 stimulates the renin–angiotensin system.[133–135] Collectively, these findings suggest that inflammatory cytokines play a role in causing hypertension in response to chronic reductions in uterine perfusion during pregnancy by activating multiple vasoactive pathways.

Although recent studies support a role for cytokines such TNF-α and IL-6 as potential mediators of endothelial dysfunction, identification of novel factors that link placental ischemia and maternal endothelial and vascular abnormalities in preeclampsia remains an important area of investigation. Recent studies in preeclamptic women have demonstrated increased soluble fms-like tyrosine kinase-1 (sFlt-1), a naturally occurring antagonist of circulating vascular endothelial growth factor and placental growth factor.[136] Increased sFlt-1 during preeclampsia is associated with decreased free vascular endothelial growth factor and free placental growth factor in the blood. Moreover, sFlt-1 administration to pregnant rats decreases free vascular endothelial growth factor and free placental growth factor in the blood and produces hypertension and proteinuria.[137]

Another novel placenta-derived factor, soluble endoglin (sEng), was recently implicated in pathogenesis of preeclampsia.[138] sEng, a TGF-β coreceptor, is elevated in preeclamptic women and falls after delivery. sEng causes hypertension in vivo and its effects in pregnant rats are amplified by coadministration of sFlt-1, leading to severe preeclampsia including the hemolysis, elevated liver enzymes, low platelets (HELLP) syndrome. sEng is thought to impair binding of TGF-β_1 to its receptors and downstream signaling, including effects on activation of endothelial nitric oxide synthase and vasodilation. These findings suggest that sEng may act in concert with sFlt-1 to induce severe preeclampsia.

Unfortunately, effective treatments for preeclampsia remain elusive. In light of the recent developments in our understanding of the pathophysiology of preeclampsia, treatment strategies aimed at improving endothelial dysfunction, safely lowering blood pressure, and reducing maternal and perinatal morbidity should be further explored.

GENETIC CAUSES OF HYPERTENSION

【 】 GENE VARIANTS AND HUMAN PRIMARY HYPERTENSION

With the development of superb tools for genetic studies and sequencing of the human genome, there has been great enthusiasm for the possibility that genetic causes of primary hypertension can be identified. Proponents of the genetic basis for primary hypertension have implied that the recent advances in genetics will offer unparalleled insights into the pathophysiology of hypertension and the development of more effective individualized treatments for hypertension. However, despite the expenditure of great financial resources and effort, there have been no clear successes in identifying genes that cause human primary hypertension. The success that has been achieved thus far has been limited to identification of monogenic forms of hypertension. A detailed discussion of this topic is beyond the scope of the chapter but Luft has dis-

cussed some reasons why the "geneticism of hypertension" approach has had limited success.[139]

When one considers the complexity of the multiple neural, hormonal, renal, and vascular mechanisms that contribute to short-term and long-term blood pressure regulation, it is perhaps unsurprising that finding a few variant genes (alleles) to account for a substantial portion of blood pressure variation has been difficult. The complexity of the problem is further amplified by the fact that genetic variation of blood pressure is unlikely caused by only single-gene variations, but also by polymorphic genetic differences, complex interactions among several genes, and interaction among genetic and environmental factors. The observation that increases in blood pressure do not occur with significant frequency in multiple populations living in nonindustrialized regions of the world suggests that environmental influences play a major role in the development of common forms of hypertension.

What is the evidence that gene variants play a major role in human primary hypertension? Multiple studies provide evidence that the closer the genetic relatedness, the greater the similarity of blood pressure.[140–143] For monozygotic twins (with genetic similarity of 100 percent), the correlation coefficient for systolic blood pressure has ranged from 0.5 to 0.8 (average: 0.6), for dizygotic twins it has ranged from 0.19 to 0.46 (average: 0.35), and for nontwin siblings (genetic similarity of around 50 percent) the correlation coefficient has averaged around 0.23. There is also a better correlation of blood pressure values in biologic children than in adopted children. However, the importance of shared family environment is also evident from the blood pressure correlations observed in genetically unrelated adopted siblings.

Comprehensive familial analyses that include other relatives in addition to twins suggest that environment may contribute to as much as 30 percent of blood pressure variance, and genetic factors may contribute 40 to 50 percent of blood pressure variance.[140–143] However, despite the use of sophisticated mathematical models for these calculations, the possibility of nonlinear gene–environmental interactions makes it difficult to quantify the precise roles of genes and environment in blood pressure variation.

Hypertension has been suggested to result from the additive effects of multiple variant genes acting in concert to elevate blood pressure. Each gene variant is presumed to have a relatively weak impact on blood pressure but may produce significant hypertension when they act together in the presence of the necessary environmental conditions. This *polygenic* model also applies to other complex diseases (such as diabetes or cancer) where multiple genes and environmental factors may play a role in the development of the disease.

Although the hypertension research literature is replete with studies showing associations of gene polymorphisms and blood pressure, the genetic alterations that contribute to primary hypertension remain unknown.[143,144] Most of these genetic studies have produced mixed results, even for widely studied polymorphisms such as the ACE insertion/deletion and angiotensinogen polymorphisms.[143,144] Polymorphisms and mutations in other genes such as α-adducin, atrial natriuretic factor, the insulin receptor, β_2-adrenergic receptor, calcitonin gene-related peptide, angiotensinase C, renin-binding protein, endothelin-1 precursor, G-protein β_3-subunit have also been associated with the development of hypertension in some studies;[139,143–145] however, all of these polymorphisms show weak associations, if any, with blood pressure, and many of the early studies showing statistically significant associations have not been confirmed. At best, the gene variations discovered thus far explain only a small part of the blood pressure variation found in humans.

MONOGENIC DISORDERS THAT CAUSE HYPERTENSION

At least 10 monogenic disorders have been identified that have either high blood pressure or low blood pressure as part of the phenotype.[146,147] Table 69–4 shows some of the monogenic disorders that are associated with high blood pressure. An interesting feature of these genetic disorders is that most of them affect either electrolyte transport in the renal tubule or the synthesis and/or activity of mineralocorticoid hormones. In all monogenic hypertensive disorders thus far, the final common pathway to hypertension appears to be increased sodium reabsorption and volume expansion. Monogenic hypertension, however, is rare and all of the known forms together account for less than 1 percent of human hypertension.

Familial Hyperaldosteronism Type I

Also called *glucocorticoid remediable aldosteronism*, familial hyperaldosteronism type I (FH-I) is inherited as an autosomal dominant trait caused by a chimeric gene derived from a meiotic mismatch and unequal crossing between the promoter of the 11β-hydroxylase (*CYP11B1*) controlled by the structural portion of the aldosterone synthase gene (*CYP11B2*).[148] This causes aldosterone secretion to be regulated by ACTH. Because ACTH is suppressed by glucocorticoids, administration of excess glucocorticoids is effective in reducing aldosterone secretion in patients with FH-I.

Patients with FH-I exhibit many of the same characteristics as those with primary aldosteronism, including high aldosterone, hypokalemia, volume expansion, metabolic alkalosis, and low plasma renin. Although some patients with FH-I have severe hypertension, others have only moderate hypertension or may even be normotensive.[149] The reasons for this wide range of blood pressure in patients are unclear but could be related to variable expression of the chimeric gene or to other differences in genetic background that would place their inherited blood pressure in the low or normal range in the absence of the FH-I mutation. The final blood pressure could therefore be the combined result of the low or normal inherited blood pressure, the hypertensive effect of the FH-I mutation, and other environmental factors, such as salt intake. When sodium intake is high, even moderate increases in aldosterone raise blood pressure, whereas low sodium intake markedly attenuates the hyperten-

TABLE 69–4

Known Genetic Causes of Hypertension

GENETIC DISORDER	AGE OF ONSET	PATTERN OF INHERITANCE	ALDOSTERONE LEVEL	SERUM POTASSIUM LEVEL	TREATMENT[a]
FH-I (GRA)[b]	2nd or 3rd decade	Autosomal dominant	High	Decreased in 50 percent of cases; marked decrease with thiazides	Glucocorticoids
FH-II[c]	Middle age	Autosomal dominant	High	Low to normal	Spironolactone, eplerenone
DOC oversecretion due to CAH[c,d]	Childhood	Autosomal recessive	Low	Low to normal	Glucocorticoids
Activating MR mutation exacerbated by pregnancy[e]	2nd or 3rd decade	Unknown	Low	Low to normal	Delivery of fetus
AME2[c,f]	Childhood	Autosomal recessive	Low	Low to normal	Spironolactone, dexamethasone
Liddle's syndrome[g]	3rd decade	Autosomal dominant	Low	Low to normal	Amiloride, triamterene
Gordon's syndrome[h]	2nd or 3rd decade	Autosomal dominant	Low	High	Thiazide diuretic, low-sodium diet

ACTH, adrenocorticotropic hormone; AME, apparent mineralocorticoid excess; CAH, congenital adrenal hyperplasia; DOC, deoxycorticosterone; FH-I, familial hyperaldosteronism type I; FH-II, familial hyperaldosteronism type II; GRA, glucocorticoid-remediable aldosteronism; MCR, mineralocorticoid receptor.
[a]Treatment for underlying mechanisms; other forms of treatment, including different antihypertensive medications, might be needed to adequately control blood pressure.
[b]Familial hyperaldosteronism.
[c]Excess production of non-aldosterone mineralocorticoids.
[d]Congenital adrenal hyperplasia, DOC-producing tumors.
[e]Because of increased activity of MCRs.
[f]Apparent mineralocorticoid excess caused by either licorice ingestion or ectopic ACTH secretion.
[g]Increased activity of sodium channels.
[h]Increased activity of Na-Cl cotransporter in the distal tubule.
SOURCE: Adapted from Garovic VD, Hilliard AA, Turner ST. Monogenic forms of low-renin hypertension. Nat Clin Pract Nephrol 2006; 2:624–630.

sive effects of excess aldosterone secretion. Patients with FH-I respond well to both thiazide diuretics and spironolactone.

Familial Hyperaldosteronism Type II

Familial hyperaldosteronism type II (FH-II) is a rare cause of hypertension in which the hypertension is caused by excessive secretion of aldosterone that is not suppressed by glucocorticoid administration, distinguishing it from FH-I.[150,151] Patients with FH-II have the same clinical symptoms as patients with primary hyperaldosteronism caused by bilateral adrenal hyperplasia. The genetic abnormality causing FH-II has been localized to chromosome 7p22.[151] Although hypertension in FH-II is unresponsive to glucocorticoids, spironolactone is effective in reducing blood pressure and correcting the metabolic disturbances.

Congenital Adrenal Hyperplasia

This disorder describes a group of syndromes caused by defects in cortisol biosynthesis.[152] Congenital adrenal hyperplasia is an autosomal recessive disorder. When 21-hydroxylase (CYP21A2) is deficient, the most common cause of congenital adrenal hyperplasia, patients are normotensive.[150,152] When 11β-hydroxylase (CYP11B1) and 17α-hydroxylase (CYP17) are deficient, production of deoxycorticosterone, which has mineralocorticoid activity, is increased, leading to hypertension. Defects in CYP11B1 and CYP17 cause inhibition of cortisol production with a subsequent reduction in feedback inhibition of ACTH secretion by the anterior pituitary and hypothalamus. Increased ACTH secretion then stimulates production of steroid precursors proximal to the blocked step, leading to excessive levels of deoxycorticosterone.

Both forms of congenital adrenal hyperplasia are associated with early onset hypertension and hypokalemia. Signs of androgen excess distinguish the two disorders: 11β-hydroxylase deficiency causes virilization in girls and precocious puberty in boys, whereas 17α-hydroxylase deficiency causes sex hormone deficiency, primary amenorrhea, and delayed sexual development in girls, and ambiguous genitalia in boys. Genetic diagnosis of both conditions relies on testing for mutations that either severely depress or abolish enzyme activity. Both conditions can be effectively treated by administering glucocorticoids that normalize ACTH secretion and ACTH-mediated buildup of cortisol precursors proximal to the enzymatic deficiency, including deoxycorticosterone.

Liddle's Syndrome

This is an autosomal dominant form of monogenic hypertension that results from mutations in the amiloride-sensitive ENaC. Several mutations that result in the elimination of 45 to 75 amino acids from the cytoplasmic carboxyl terminus of β- or γ-subunits of the channel have been reported. Mutations that increase ENaC activity, in turn, cause excessive distal and collecting tubule sodium reabsorption and hypertension.[150,153]

Liddle's syndrome is characterized by the early onset of hypertension with hypokalemia and suppression of plasma renin activity and aldosterone. The suppression of aldosterone and lack of responsiveness to MR antagonists differentiates this syndrome from primary aldosteronism. Both the hypertension and the hypokalemia vary in severity, depending on salt intake, and can be treated with amiloride or triamterene, specific inhibitors of the ENaC.

Apparent Mineralocorticoid Excess

Apparent mineralocorticoid excess is an autosomal recessive form of monogenic hypertension that results from a mutation in the renal-specific isoform of the 11β-hydroxysteroid dehydrogenase gene.[154] This enzyme normally converts cortisol to the inactive metabolite cortisone and "protects" the MR from being activated by cortisol. This is important because the renal epithelial MR receptor in the distal and collecting tubules has a similar affinity for aldosterone and cortisol, while cortisol concentrations are normally much higher than aldosterone. Deficiency of 11β-hydroxysteroid dehydrogenase allows the tubular MR to be occupied and activated by cortisol, causing sodium retention and volume expansion, low renin, low aldosterone, and a form of hypertension that is salt sensitive.

A nongenetic form of the apparent mineralocorticoid excess syndrome can be observed in persons ingesting large amounts of licorice, which contains glycyrrhetinic acid, an inhibitor of the enzyme 11β-hydroxysteroid dehydrogenase. Both forms of apparent mineralocorticoid excess are effectively treated with MR antagonists such as spironolactone or eplerenone.

Pseudohypoaldosteronism Type II

Also called Gordon's syndrome, pseudohypoaldosteronism type II is a rare mendelian form of hypertension that is salt sensitive and is associated with hyperkalemia (despite normal glomerular filtration rate), hyperchloremia, metabolic acidosis, and suppressed plasma renin and aldosterone levels. The disorder is caused by mutations in two genes encoding the serine/threonine protein kinases: WNK1 and WNK4.[155]

The phenotypes of excessive salt retention and hypertension are caused by loss of normal inhibition or to constitutive activation of the renal tubular NaCl cotransporter by mutant WNK1 or WNK4 genes; thiazide diuretics, which inhibit distal nephron NaCl reabsorption, are especially effective in reducing blood pressure in patients with pseudohypoaldosteronism type II. The mutant WNKs may also have a direct effect on ROMK1, the major potassium secretory channel in the distal nephron, as hyperkalemia is another major feature of pseudohypoaldosteronism type II.[150,155] The fact that hyperkalemia is invariably present in pseudohypoaldosteronism type II is often used to distinguish it from other monogenic forms of hypertension.

Mineralocorticoid Receptor Activating Mutation

This monogenic disorder is caused by a substitution of leucine for serine at codon 810 of the MR.[156] This mutation alters the shape and the specificity of the MR and eliminates the usual requirement for the 21-hydroxyl group of aldosterone to interact with the MR. This explains why other steroids, such as progesterone, activate the MR and why spironolactone, which is normally an antagonist of the MR, acts as an agonist for the MR in this disorder. Thus treatment of these patients with spironolactone or increased levels of progesterone, as occurs in pregnancy, worsens the sodium retention, hypokalemia, and hypertension.

PATHOPHYSIOLOGY OF PRIMARY (ESSENTIAL) HYPERTENSION

Widespread human primary (essential) hypertension appears to be a relatively modern disorder associated with industrialization and the ready availability of food. Nearly all studies of westernized, industrialized populations have demonstrated that blood pressure, and therefore the prevalence of hypertension, rises with age.[157] Hunter-gatherers living in nonindustrialized societies, however, rarely develop hypertension or progressive increases in systolic and mean pressures that occur in the majority of individuals living in industrialized societies.[157–159] This observation suggests that environmental factors play a major role in raising blood pressure in many patients with primary hypertension. This does not, however, imply that genetic factors are unimportant in primary hypertension. Genetic variation almost certainly is responsible for differences in baseline blood pressure that result in normal distribution of blood pressure in a population. When hypertension-producing environmental factors are added to the population baseline blood pressure, the normal distribution is shifted toward higher blood pressure. Moreover, variations in the impact of environmental factors flatten the blood pressure curve and cause even greater variability in the overall population blood pressure.

What are the elements of industrialized societies that cause blood pressure to rise in the majority of people as they age? How do they affect the physiologic controllers of blood pressure? As discussed earlier, many of the long-term blood pressure controllers either directly or indirectly influence renal function. In all patients with primary hypertension there is a resetting of renal pressure natriuresis so that sodium balance is maintained at higher blood pressures.[16,18] In some individuals, this resetting is related to increased renal tubular reabsorption, because of abnormalities intrinsic to the kidneys or to altered neurohumoral control of the kidneys.[16,19] In other instances, resetting of pressure natriuresis is associated with renal vasoconstriction and reductions in GFR, as a result of intrarenal mechanisms or of nervous and hormonal mechanisms acting on the kidneys.[16,19] After hypertension is established, many of these changes in kidney function are difficult to detect because increased blood pressure often returns renal function to normal.

Experimental, clinical, and population studies suggest some of the key environmental factors that affect blood pressure include excess weight gain, excess sodium intake, and excess alcohol intake.

[ ] OBESITY IS A MAJOR CAUSE OF PRIMARY HYPERTENSION

The prevalence of obesity has risen dramatically in the past two to three decades and has rapidly become the most important public health problem in most industrialized countries. Current estimates indicate that more than 1 *billion* people in the world are overweight or obese.[160,161] In the United States, more than 64 percent of adults are overweight and almost one-third of the adult population is obese with a BMI greater than 30.[162] Population studies show that excess weight gain is perhaps the best predictor we have for the development of hypertension, and the relationship between BMI and systolic and diastolic blood pressure appears to be nearly linear in diverse populations throughout the world.[163] Risk estimates from the Framingham Heart Study, for example, suggest that approximately 78 percent of primary hypertension in men and 65 percent in women can be ascribed to excess weight gain.[164] Clinical studies also indicate that weight loss is effective in reducing blood pressure in most hypertensive subjects and have also shown the effectiveness of weight loss in primary prevention of hypertension.[165,166]

One question often raised is why some overweight or obese persons are not hypertensive by the usual standards (i.e., blood pressure greater than 140/90 mmHg) if obesity is a major cause of hypertension. Perhaps this is not surprising if one considers that blood pressure is normally distributed, and accepts the assumption that excess weight gain shifts the frequency distribution of blood pressure toward higher levels. Although obesity increases the probability that a person's blood pressure will register in the hypertensive range, not all obese people will have a blood pressure greater than 140/90 mmHg (Fig. 69–16). However, even those obese individuals who are classified as "normotensive" have higher blood pressure than they would at a lower body weight. This assumption is supported by the fact that weight loss lowers blood pressure in normotensive as well as hypertensive obese subjects.[167]

Although the importance of obesity as a cause of primary hypertension is well established, the physiologic mechanisms by which excess weight gain alters renal function and raises blood pressure are only beginning to be elucidated. Table 69–5 summarizes some of the changes in hemodynamics, neurohumoral systems, and renal function that occur with excess weight gain in humans and experimental animals.

Effect on Tissue Blood Flow and Cardiac Output

Obesity is associated with expansion of extracellular fluid volume, as well as increased tissue blood flow and cardiac output.[168–171] Studies in experimental animals and in humans indicate that blood flow is increased in many tissues, including the heart, kidneys, gastrointestinal tract, and skeletal muscles.[168–171] Some of the increased flow is caused by tissue growth in organs in response to increased workload and the metabolic demands associated with obesity. However, obesity also causes a functional vasodilation,

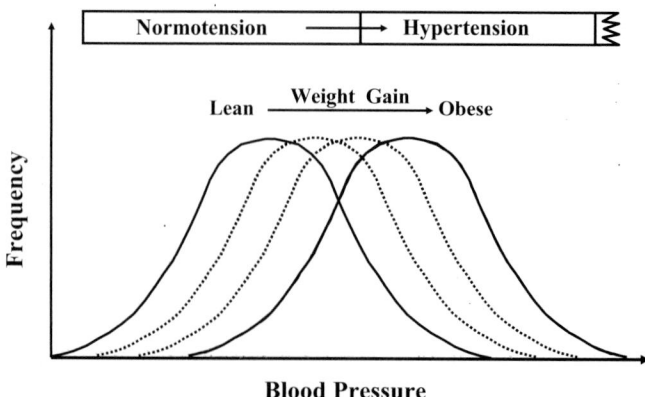

FIGURE 69–16. Effect of weight gain to shift the frequency distribution of blood pressure to higher levels. Not all obese subjects have blood pressures in the hypertensive range (>140/90 mmHg), but excess weight gain raises blood pressure above the baseline level for an individual.

perhaps as a consequence of an increased metabolic rate, higher oxygen consumption, and accumulation of vasodilator metabolites. Despite higher resting blood flows in many tissues, there also appears to be reduced blood flow "reserve" during exercise or during reactive hyperemia in obese, compared to lean, individuals.[15,171] There is also a decreased cardiac reserve in obesity despite higher resting cardiac outputs.

Mechanisms of Impaired Renal Pressure Natriuresis in Obesity Hypertension

Increased renal tubular sodium reabsorption appears to play a major role in initiating the rise in blood pressure associated with excess weight gain and obese individuals require higher-than-normal blood pressures to maintain sodium balance, indicating impaired renal pressure natriuresis. Three mechanisms appear to be especially important in mediating increased sodium reabsorption and impaired pressure natriuresis in obesity hypertension: (1) increased SNS activity, (2) activation of the RAS, and (3) physical compression of the kidneys by fat accumulation within and around the kidneys and by increased abdominal pressure (Fig. 69–17).

SNS Activation in Obesity Hypertension

Several observations indicate that increased SNS activity contributes to obesity hypertension[16,44]: (1) SNS activation, especially renal sympathetic activity, is increased in obese subjects; (2) pharmacologic blockade of adrenergic activity lowers blood pressure to a greater extent in obese, compared to lean, individuals; and (3) renal denervation markedly attenuates sodium retention and hypertension associated with a high-fat diet in experimental animals.

Increased SNS activity appears to be highly differentiated in obesity. For example, cardiac sympathetic activity does not appear to be substantially elevated, whereas SNS activity is usually increased in the kidneys and skeletal muscles of obese subjects.[172–174] Genetic factors may be important in modulating the SNS response to excess weight gain. In Pima Indians who have a high prevalence of obesity but a relatively low prevalence of hypertension, muscle SNS activity is lower than in whites and does not track well with adiposity.[175] In black men, SNS activity is higher and hypertension is more prevalent than in white men despite comparable levels of obesity.[176] In young, overweight, black women, adiposity is associated with sympathetic hyperactivity.[176] Factors such as differences in fat mass distribution may contribute to some of the racial variation in SNS responses to increasing adiposity. For reasons that are still unclear, abdominal obesity elicits a much greater sympathetic activation than does subcutaneous or lower body obesity.[177]

The mechanisms of SNS activation in obesity have not been fully elucidated, but as discussed earlier, one of the more promising candidates is hyperleptinemia (Fig. 69–18). Leptin is released from adipocytes and acts on the hypothalamus and other regions of the brain, such as the brainstem to reduce appetite and increase SNS activity.[44] In rodents, increasing plasma leptin concentration to levels comparable to those found in severe obesity not only increases SNS activity, but also raises blood pressure.[178,179] Moreover, the hypertensive effects of leptin are enhanced when NO synthesis is inhibited,[180] as often occurs in obese subjects with endothelial dysfunction.

Another observation that points toward leptin as a potential link between obesity and hypertension is the finding that leptin-deficient, obese mice and obese mice with mutations of the leptin receptor usually have little or no increase in blood pressure compared to their lean controls.[181] Similar results have been found in obese children with leptin gene mutations. Ozata and coworkers[182] reported that in young patients with homozygous missense mutations of the leptin gene there was no indication of hypertension despite early onset morbid obesity. These children also had decreased, rather than increased SNS activity, as well as postural hypotension and attenuated RAS responses to upright posture. Moreover, children with leptin gene mutations did not have hypertension despite having many other characteristics of the metabolic syndrome, including severe insulin resistance, hyperinsulinemia, and hyperlipidemia.[182] These observations are consistent with those observed in rodents and suggest that the functional effects of leptin appear to be important in linking obesity with SNS activation and hypertension.

Leptin's stimulatory effect on SNS activity appears to be mediated with interaction with other hypothalamic factors, especially the proopiomelanocortin pathway. Antagonism of the melanocortin 3/4 receptor (MC3/4-R) completely abolished leptin's chronic blood pressure effects.[183] The chronic hypertensive effects of leptin

TABLE 69–5

Hemodynamic, Neurohumoral, and Renal Changes in Experimental Obesity Caused by a High-Fat Diet and in Human Obesity

MODEL	ARTERIAL PRESSURE	HEART RATE	CARDIAC OUTPUT	RENAL SYMPATHETIC ACTIVITY	PLASMA RENIN ACTIVITY	NA+ BALANCE	RENAL TUBULAR REABSORPTION	GFR[a]	INSULIN RESISTANCE
Obese rabbits (high-fat diet)	↑	↑	↑	↑	↑	↑	↑	↑	↑
Obese dogs (high-fat diet)	↑	↑	↑	↑	↑	↑	↑	↑	↑
Obese humans	↑	↑	↑	↑	↑	↑	↑	↑	↑

[a]The glomerular filtration rate (GFR) changes refer to the early phases of obesity before major loss of nephron function has occurred.

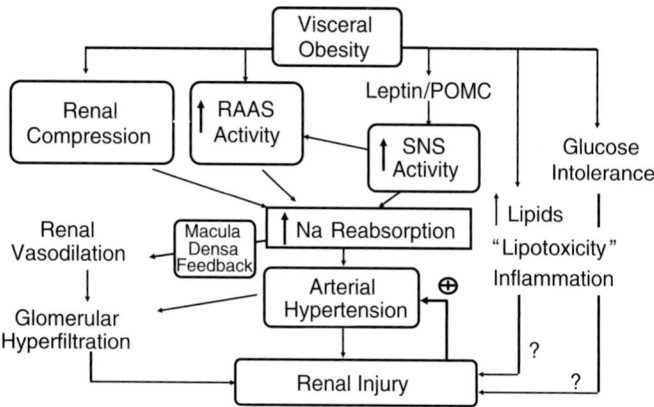

FIGURE 69–17. Summary of potential mechanisms by which obesity causes hypertension and renal injury. Visceral obesity increases blood pressure by activation of the sympathetic nervous system (SNS), the renin–angiotensin–aldosterone system (RAAS), and by physical compression of the kidneys from the fat surrounding the kidneys. SNS activation may be caused by, in large part, the effects of leptin, which acts on proopiomelanocortin (POMC) neurons in the hypothalamus and brainstem. Obesity-induced hypertension and glomerular hyperfiltration may cause renal injury, especially when combined with dyslipidemia and hyperglycemia. Renal injury then exacerbates the hypertension and makes it more difficult to control.

were also completely abolished in MC4-R knockout mice, suggesting that the MC4-R may mediate most of the effects of leptin to activate SNS activity.[184] However, the importance of the proopiomelanocortin pathway in regulating SNS activity and raising blood pressure in humans has not been elucidated.

Renin–Angiotensin–Aldosterone System Activation in Obesity

Obese individuals, especially those with visceral obesity, often have mild to moderate increases in plasma renin activity, angiotensinogen, ACE activity, ANG II, and aldosterone levels.[185,186] Activation of the RAS in obese subject occurs despite sodium retention, volume expansion, and hypertension, all of which would normally tend to suppress renin secretion and ANG II formation.

An important role for ANG II in stimulating renal sodium reabsorption and in mediating obesity hypertension is supported by studies in experimental animals demonstrating that ANG II receptor blockade or ACE inhibition blunts sodium retention, volume expansion, and increased blood pressure during the development of obesity.[187,188] Unfortunately, there have been no large-scale clinical studies comparing the effectiveness of RAS blockers in obese and lean hypertensive patients, although smaller clinical tri-

als have shown that both ARBs and ACE inhibitors are effective in lowering blood pressure in obese hypertensive patients.[189,190]

Increased aldosterone and MR activation also appear to contribute to obesity-induced hypertension. Antagonism of MR in obese dogs markedly attenuated sodium retention, hypertension, and glomerular hyperfiltration.[191] Moreover, this protection against hypertension occurred in spite of marked increases in plasma renin activity, suggesting that combined blockade of MR and ANG II might be especially effective in treating obesity hypertension. The observation that MR antagonism attenuated glomerular hyperfiltration may also have important implications for renal protection in obesity, although there are no studies, to our knowledge, that have directly tested this in obese humans. Administration of the MR antagonists does appear to provide significant antihypertensive benefit in resistant obese patients.[192] The reductions in blood pressure caused by MR antagonism in resistant obese patients occurred despite concurrent therapy with ACE inhibitor or ARB, calcium channel blocker, and thiazide diuretic, suggesting that MR activation in obesity can occur independently of ANG II–mediated stimulation of aldosterone secretion.

Renal Compression Caused by Visceral Obesity

Visceral obesity initiates several changes that may lead to compression of the kidneys, increased intrarenal pressures, impaired renal pressure natriuresis, and hypertension.[15] For example, intraabdomi-

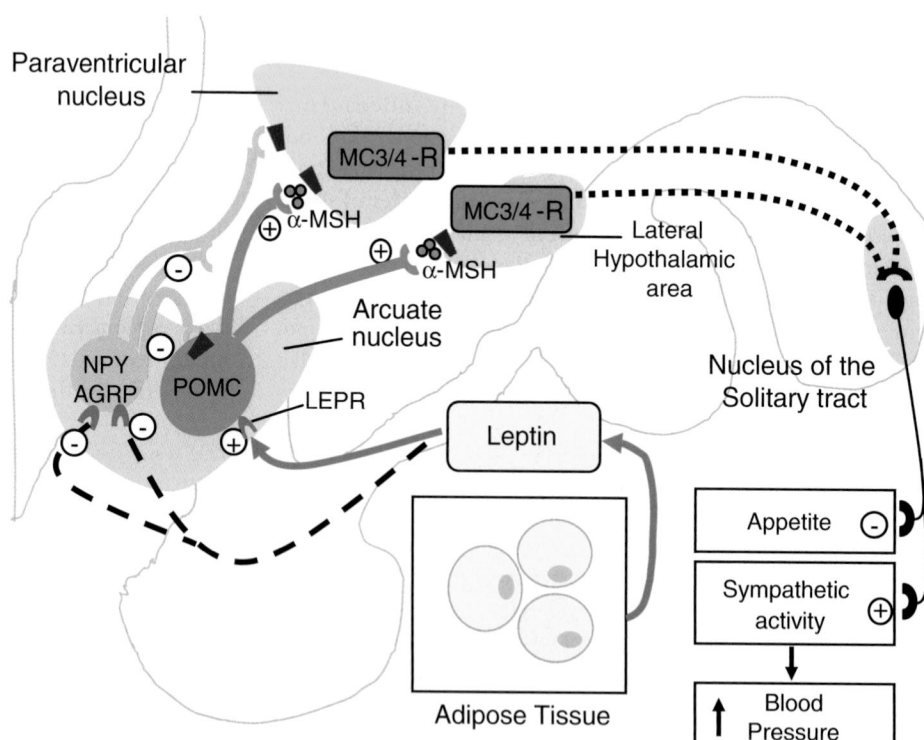

FIGURE 69–18. Possible links among leptin and its effects on the hypothalamus, sympathetic activation, and hypertension. Within the hypothalamus, one of the key pathways of leptin's action on appetite, SNS activity, and blood pressure is stimulation of the proopiomelanocortin (POMC) neurons in the arcuate nucleus. These neurons send projections to the paraventricular nucleus and lateral hypothalamus, releasing α-melanocyte–stimulating hormone (α-MSH), which then acts as an agonist for melanocortin 3/4-receptors (MC3/4-R). These neurons then send projections to the nucleus of the solitary tract to effect changes in appetite, SNS activity, and blood pressure. Leptin also suppresses the NPY/AGRP neurons, but their role in controlling SNS activity and blood pressure are still unclear.

nal pressure rises in proportion to the abdominal diameter, reaching levels as high as 35 to 40 mmHg in some individuals.[193] In addition, retroperitoneal adipose tissue often encapsulates the kidney and penetrates the renal hilum into the renal medullary sinuses, causing additional compression and increased intrarenal pressures.[194]

Obesity also causes changes in renal medullary histology and increased extracellular matrix that could exacerbate intrarenal compression and hypertension.[195] The increased intrarenal hydrostatic pressure may, in turn, cause compression of the loops of Henle and vasa recta, thereby increasing tubular sodium and water reabsorption. Although these physical changes in the kidneys cannot account for the initial increase in blood pressure that occurs with rapid weight gain, they may help to explain why abdominal obesity is much more closely associated with hypertension than subcutaneous obesity.[194,195]

Glomerular Injury and Nephron Loss in Obesity Hypertension

Obese patients often develop proteinuria, frequently in the nephrotic range that is followed by progressive loss of kidney function in a significant number of patients.[196] The most common types of renal lesions observed in renal biopsies are of obese subjects are focal and segmental glomerular sclerosis and glomerulomegaly.[197]

Animals placed on a high-fat diet for only a few weeks demonstrate significant structural changes in the kidneys, including enlargement of the Bowman space, glomerular cell proliferation, increased mesangial matrix, and increased expression of glomerular TGF-β.[198] These early changes occur with only modest hypertension, no evidence of diabetes, and only mild metabolic abnormalities that may be the precursors of more severe renal injury as obesity is sustained.

Population studies indicate that obesity is a major cause of renal disease even after adjustment for hypertension, diabetes, or preexisting renal disease.[199] Moreover, obesity also amplifies the effect of other primary renal insults, even those that are usually considered to be relatively benign, such as unilateral nephrectomy. Praga and coworkers[200] reported that of patients with a BMI greater than 30 who had undergone unilateral nephrectomy, 92 percent developed proteinuria or renal insufficiency, whereas only 12 percent of patients with a BMI less than 30 developed these disorders. Similar findings have also been reported for patients with immunoglobulin A nephropathy.[201] These observations indicate that obesity greatly exacerbates the loss of kidney function in patients with preexisting glomerulopathies and that weight loss may lessen the impact of renal injury from other causes.

The gradual loss of kidney function, as well as the hypertension and diabetes that commonly coexist with obesity, lead to progressive impairment of pressure natriuresis, increasing salt sensitivity, and greater increases in blood pressure (Fig. 69–19). Thus renal injury in obese subjects not only makes the hypertension more severe, but also more difficult to control with antihypertensive drugs.

[ ] WHAT IS THE ROLE OF METABOLIC SYNDROME/INSULIN RESISTANCE IN PRIMARY HYPERTENSION?

In 1988, Gerald Reaven hypothesized that insulin resistance and compensatory hyperinsulinemia are the underlying causes

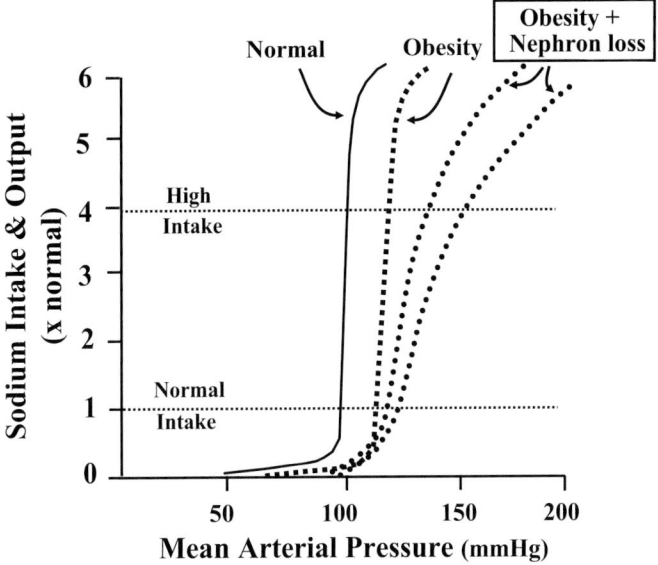

FIGURE 69–19. Effect of obesity to shift renal pressure natriuresis curve to higher arterial pressure. With chronic obesity lasting for many years, there may be a gradual loss of nephron function, further impairment of pressure natriuresis, increasing salt sensitivity, and higher arterial pressures.

of hypertension, hyperlipidemia, and diabetes, and thus are major causes of CVD.[202] He coined the term *syndrome X* to describe this cluster of CVD risk factors. Subsequently, many other investigators observed that dyslipidemia, hyperinsulinemia, and hyperglycemia often occurred concurrently with hypertension, leading to the proposal of a unique pathophysiologic condition that is now called the *metabolic syndrome*. Definitions of the metabolic syndrome have been proposed by the World Health Organization (WHO),[203] the Third Report of the National Cholesterol Education Program's Adult Treatment Panel (ATP III),[204] and other organizations.[205] All of these definitions include disordered glucose homeostasis or measures of insulin resistance, dyslipidemia, hypertension and obesity, as discussed in more detail in Chap. 91.

Questions have been asked about whether the diagnosis of metabolic syndrome has much clinical usefulness. Some researchers suggest that a defect in insulin action is the main cause of all the CVD risk factors that constitute the different versions of the metabolic syndrome.[206] Broadly defined, insulin resistance refers to a subnormal tissue response to a given concentration of insulin or an impairment of insulin's action of overall glucose homeostasis. However, the term *insulin resistance* can have several different meanings, depending on the methods of assessment and the type of abnormalities that cause impaired insulin action. For example, when insulin resistance is defined by fasting hyperinsulinemia, the most likely cause is impaired insulin-mediated suppression of hepatic glucose output.[207] However, when insulin resistance is defined by methods that assess the ability of insulin to increase glucose disposal (e.g., glucose tolerance test, euglycemic clamp), the most likely cause is decreased action of insulin on skeletal muscle glucose uptake.[207] Presently, it is not clear which of these measures of insulin resistance (if any) best predicts risk for CVD.

Recent analyses of the metabolic syndrome have questioned whether insulin resistance and hyperinsulinemia are, in fact, the underlying causes of this complex cluster of cardiovascular risk factors.[208] As discussed below, most of the available evidence indicates that insulin resistance and hyperinsulinemia, although clearly important features of the metabolic syndrome, are not directly involved in mediating hypertension.

Does Hyperinsulinemia Cause Hypertension in Humans?

Hyperinsulinemia, which occurs as a compensation for insulin resistance, is postulated to mediate increased blood pressure in essential hypertension via multiple mechanisms, such as stimulation of SNS activity and renal tubular sodium reabsorption.[202,209] Evidence supporting this hypothesis comes mainly from epidemiologic studies showing correlations between insulin resistance, hyperinsulinemia, and blood pressure, and from short-term studies indicating that insulin has renal and sympathetic effects that, if sustained, could theoretically raise blood pressure. For example, acute infusions of insulin cause modest sodium retention and increased SNS activity, and these observations have been extrapolated to infer that hyperinsulinemia may be an important cause of hypertension in insulin-resistant states such as obesity.[202,209] However, insulin also has vasodilator effects that tend to lower blood pressure and, as discussed earlier, results of short-term studies cannot be extrapolated to form an understanding of chronic hypertension.[210]

Chronic hyperinsulinemia, in the absence of obesity, does not raise blood pressure in either dogs or humans (see references 210 and 211 for reviews). For example, infusion of insulin for several weeks at rates that raised plasma insulin concentration above those found in obesity reduced, rather than increased, blood pressure as a consequence of the peripheral vasodilator effects of insulin.[212] Moreover, chronic insulin infusions did not raise blood pressure even when there was preexisting impairment of renal function caused by a 70 percent reduction of kidney mass.[212] Hyperinsulinemia also did not enhance the hypertensive effects of other pressor substances such as norepinephrine or ANG II.[210,212] Chronic hyperinsulinemia also did not raise blood pressure in insulin-resistant obese dogs that were resistant to the vasodilator effects of insulin.[213] Multiple studies in humans also have shown that chronic treatment with insulin injections does not raise blood pressure and patients with severe hyperinsulinemia as a result of insulinoma are not hypertensive.[211,214,215] These observations suggest that hyperinsulinemia per se is insufficient to cause chronic hypertension.

Does Insulin Resistance Cause Hypertension Independent of Hyperinsulinemia?

Insulin resistance has also been suggested to cause hypertension by raising total peripheral vascular resistance through mechanisms that are independent of hyperinsulinemia. One interesting hypothesis is that insulin's vasodilator action normally helps to prevent hypertension initiated by other stimuli and that decreased vascular sensitivity to insulin contributes to increased blood pressure in insulin-resistant individuals.[216]

It seems unlikely, however, that decreased action of a hormone that is primarily responsible for glucose regulation and that remains in relatively low concentrations except after meals would be capable of disrupting the multiple mechanisms that operate to maintain normal blood pressure. Moreover, there are several disorders associated with severe insulin resistance in humans and experimental animal models that are not associated with hypertension. For example, experimental models of obesity caused by mutations of the leptin gene or the leptin receptor, or by mutations of the MC4-R, have severe insulin resistance and many of the characteristics of the metabolic syndrome, but do not have increased blood pressure compared to wild-type controls.[181,184] Likewise, humans with leptin gene mutations have severe insulin resistance but no indication of SNS activation or hypertension.[182] These observations argue against a direct role for insulin resistance in causing hypertension.

Several reports indicate that antihyperglycemic agents that increase insulin sensitivity, such as the thiazolidinediones, also lower blood pressure. However, these drugs also influence the expression of multiple genes by binding to the peroxisome proliferator-activated receptor-γ (PPARγ) a nuclear receptor. Thiazolidinediones may also inhibit L-type calcium channels, and they reduce blood pressure in renovascular hypertension that is not associated with insulin resistance or hyperinsulinemia.[217–219] Therefore, it appears that the blood pressure-lowering effects of these drugs are not directly related to improvement of insulin sensitivity but to other actions.

Although a direct causal relationship between insulin resistance and hypertension has not been established, abnormalities of glucose and lipid metabolism associated with insulin resistance may, over a period of many years, lead to vascular and renal injury, and in this way contribute indirectly to increased blood pressure. For example, insulin normally decreases mobilization of fatty acids and promotes fat storage via multiple mechanisms, including inhibition of hormone-sensitive lipase, which decreases lipolysis of triglycerides and prevents release of fatty acids from adipocytes into the circulation. When adipocytes are resistant to insulin's actions, hormone-sensitive lipase activity is reduced, thereby decreasing lipid storage and increasing plasma concentration of fatty acids. These changes, if prolonged, could contribute to atherosclerosis and increased blood pressure, especially if the renal blood vessels and glomeruli are damaged. Also, resistance to insulin's actions on glucose homeostasis would cause glucose intolerance and hyperglycemia, which, if sustained, could cause glycosylation of glomerular proteins, increased production of extracellular matrix, and loss of nephron function. Progressive loss of kidney function, as discussed previously, could contribute to the development of hypertension. Thus, the metabolic disturbances associated with severe insulin resistance could exacerbate hypertension by causing renal injury, although the importance of these effects, in the absence of diabetes, is still unclear.

Does Hypertension Cause Insulin Resistance?

It also has been suggested that insulin resistance is secondary to vascular changes that occur in hypertension.[220] According to this concept, insulin resistance may occur as a result of increased peripheral vascular resistance, decreased tissue blood flow, and vascular rarefaction, which decrease the delivery of insulin and glucose and therefore impair glucose uptake in tissues such as skeletal muscle.[220] This hypothesis is intuitively pleasing because hypertension is often associated with increased peripheral vascular resistance and vascular rarefaction is common in long-standing hypertension. It is likely that tissue blood flow and substrate delivery can be important determinants of glucose uptake under some acute conditions, such as during transients of glucose disposal after a carbohydrate meal or glucose tolerance test. However, it is important to keep in mind the chronic nature of hypertension and that increased blood pressure and insulin resistance are both found under long-term, steady state conditions, not simply when the system is acutely challenged.

For the hemodynamic hypothesis of insulin resistance to be valid, at least two conditions must be met: (1) there must be a sustained reduction in tissue blood flow, or a failure of blood flow to increase appropriately at the sites at which insulin resistance occurs; and (2) reductions in tissue blood flow, to the levels observed in hypertension, must impair glucose uptake by the tissues. However, neither of these conditions occurs in most patients with essential hypertension. Although peripheral vascular resistance is elevated in hypertension, most tissues, including skeletal muscles, do not appear to be underperfused.[12,207] Also, multiple studies and mathematical models indicate that underperfusion of peripheral tissues cannot explain, quantitatively, chronic hyperinsulinemia observed under fasting conditions as long as the sensitivity of the liver to insulin is normal.[207] Also, mathematical models of glucose homeostasis suggest that mild tissue underperfusion, or the lack of vasodilation, does not account for impaired glucose homeostasis during hyperinsulinemic euglycemic clamp conditions.[207] Finally, most models of secondary hypertension, such as mineralocorticoid or renovascular hypertension, are characterized by increased peripheral vascular resistance and vascular rarefaction but are not associated with the development of insulin resistance (see references 207 and 211 for reviews). These observations indicate that hypertension per se is not a primary cause of insulin resistance.

Although insulin resistance and hypertension are often closely correlated, much of the available evidence suggests that this association is largely a consequence of the fact that obesity causes both insulin resistance and high blood pressure through parallel mechanisms. There is little doubt that obesity, especially visceral obesity, is a major cause of the entire cluster of CVD risk factors associated with the metabolic syndrome (Fig. 69–20).[205,207] Most patients with metabolic syndrome and insulin resistance are overweight or obese and the increasing prevalence of metabolic syndrome has closely paralleled the increasing prevalence of obesity. Importantly, all of the disorders associated with the metabolic syndrome can be reversed in most patients by weight loss.

Thus, although hypertension is a well-recognized component of the metabolic syndrome, there is little direct evidence that insulin resistance or hyperinsulinemia actually cause hypertension. Excess weight gain and visceral obesity appear to be the primary driving forces for all of the major disorders associated with the metabolic syndrome, including hypertension. Available evidence suggests that as much as 65 to 75 percent of primary (essential) hypertension may be attributed to excess weight gain.

Until effective antiobesity drugs are developed, the impact of obesity on hypertension and related cardiovascular, renal, and metabolic disorders is likely to become even more important in the future as the prevalence of obesity continues to increase. In the meantime, effective control of blood pressure is essential in treating patients with metabolic syndrome and preventing CVD.

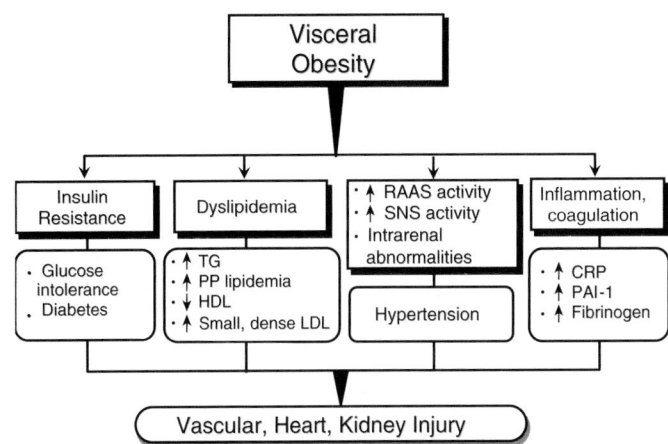

FIGURE 69–20. Cardiovascular, metabolic and renal disease associated with visceral obesity which appears to be a primary cause of all of cluster of CVD risk factors in the metabolic syndrome. CRP, C-reactive protein; HDL, high-density lipoprotein; LDL, low-density lipoprotein; PAI, platelet activator inhibitor; PP, postprandial; RAAS, renin–angiotensin–aldosterone system; SNS, sympathetic nervous system; TG, triglycerides.

Weight reduction is an essential first step in the effective management of most patients with metabolic syndrome and hypertension, and more emphasis should be placed on lifestyle modifications that help patients to maintain a healthier weight and prevent CVD.

REFERENCES

1. Burt VL, Whelton P, Roccella EJ, et al. Prevalence of hypertension in the U.S. adult population. Results from the Third National Health and Nutrition Examination Survey, 1988–1991. *Hypertension* 1995;25:305–313.
2. Hajjar I, Kotchen TA. Trends in prevalence, awareness, treatment, and control of hypertension in the United States, 1988–2000. *JAMA* 2003;290:199–206.
3. World Health Report 2002: Reducing risks, promoting healthy life. Geneva, Switzerland: World Health Organization, 2002. Available at: http://www.who.int/whr/2002.
4. Kearney PM, Whelton M, Reynolds K, et al. Global burden of hypertension: analysis of worldwide data. *Lancet* 2005;365(9455):217–223.
5. Lewington S, Clarke R, Qizilbash N, et al. Age-specific relevance of usual blood pressure to vascular mortality: a meta-analysis of individual data for one million adults in 61 prospective studies. Prospective Studies Collaboration. *Lancet* 2002;360:1903–1913.
6. Chobanian AV, Bakris GL, Black HR, et al. Seventh report of the Joint National Committee on Prevention, Detection, Evaluation, and Treatment of High Blood Pressure. *Hypertension* 2003;42:1206–1252.
7. Beilin LJ. The fifth Sir George Pickering memorial lecture: epitaph to essential hypertension: a preventable disorder of known aetiology? *J Hypertens* 1988;6:85–94.
8. Carretero OA, Oparil S. Essential hypertension. Part I. Definition and etiology. *Circulation* 2000;101:329–335.
9. Guyton AC, Coleman TG, Granger HJ. Circulation: overall regulation. *Annu Rev Physiol* 1972;34:13–46.
10. Hall JE. Integration and regulation of cardiovascular function. *Am J Physiol* 1999;277(6 Pt 2):S174–S186.
11. Guyton AC, Hall J E. *Textbook of Medical Physiology,* 11th ed. Philadelphia: Elsevier, 2006.
12. Guyton AC. Abnormal renal function and autoregulation in essential hypertension. *Hypertension* 1991;8(5 Suppl):III49–III53.
13. Coleman TG, Hall JE. Systemic hemodynamics and regional blood flow regulation. In Izzo JL, Black HR, eds. *Hypertension Primer: The Essentials of High Blood Pressure,* 2nd ed. American Heart Association, 1999:92–94.
14. Takeshita A, Mark AL. Decreased vasodilator capacity of forearm resistance vessels in borderline hypertension. *Hypertension* 1980;2:610–616.
15. Rocchini AP, Moorehead C, Katch V, et al. Forearm resistance vessel abnormalities and insulin resistance in obese adolescents. *Hypertension* 1992;19:615–620.
16. Hall JE. The kidney, hypertension, and obesity. *Hypertension* 2003;41:625–633.

17. Guyton AC. The surprising kidney–fluid mechanism for pressure control—its infinite gain! *Hypertension* 1990;16:725–730.

18. Guyton AC. Arterial pressure and hypertension. In: *Circulatory Physiology II*. Philadelphia: WB Saunders, 1980:1–564.

19. Hall JE, Guyton AC, Brands MW. Pressure-volume regulation in hypertension. *Kidney Int* 1996;49(Suppl 55):S35–S41.

20. Goldblatt H, et al. Studies on experimental hypertension. I. The production of persistent elevation of systolic blood pressure by means of renal ischemia. *J Exp Med* 1934;59:347–380.

21. Hall JE. Renal function in one-kidney, one-clip hypertension and low renin essential hypertension. *Am J Hypertens* 1991;4:523S–533S.

22. Kimura G, Brenner BM. The renal basis for salt sensitivity in hypertension. In: Laragh JH, Brenner BM, eds. *Hypertension: Pathophysiology, Diagnosis, and Management*. New York: Raven Press, 1995:1569–1588.

23. Brenner BM. Nephron adaptation to renal injury or ablation. *Am J Physiol* 1985;249:F324–F337.

24. Norman RA Jr, Galloway PG, Dzielak DJ, et al. Mechanisms of partial renal infarct hypertension. *J Hypertens* 1988;6:397–403.

25. Langston JB, Guyton AC, Douglas BH, et al. Effect of changes in salt intake on arterial pressure and renal function in partially nephrectomized dogs. *Circ Res* 1963;12:508–512.

26. Weinberger MH. Salt sensitivity of blood pressure in humans. *Hypertension* 1996;27:481–490.

27. Lifton RP. Molecular genetics of human blood pressure variation. *Science* 1996;272:676–680.

28. Johnson RJ, Rodriguez-Iturbe B, Nakagawa T, et al. Subtle renal injury is likely a common mechanism for salt-sensitive essential hypertension. *Hypertension* 2005;45:326–330.

29. Dunhill MS, Halley W. Some observations on the quantitative anatomy of the kidney. *J Pathol* 1973;110:113–161.

30. Hall JE. Control of sodium excretion by angiotensin II. Intrarenal mechanisms and blood pressure regulation. *Am J Physiol* 1986;250:R960–R972.

31. Hall JE, Guyton AC, Smith MJ Jr, et al. Blood pressure and renal function during chronic changes in sodium intake: role of angiotensin. *Am J Physiol* 1980;239:F271–F280.

32. Laragh JH. Nephron heterogeneity: clue to the pathogenesis of essential hypertension and effectiveness of angiotensin-converting enzyme inhibitor treatment. *Am J Med* 1989;87:2S–14S.

33. Campese VM. Salt sensitivity in hypertension. Renal and cardiovascular implications. *Hypertension* 1994;23:531–550.

34. Weinberger MH, Fineberg NS, Fineberg SE, et al. Salt sensitivity. Pulse pressure, and death in normal and hypertensive humans. *Hypertension* 2001;37:429–432.

35. DiBona GF. Neural control of the kidney: past, present, and future. *Hypertension* 2003;4:621–624.

36. Guyenet PG. The sympathetic control of blood pressure. *Nat Rev* 2006;7:335–346.

37. Dampney RAL, Horiuchi J, Killinger S, et al. Long-term regulation of arterial blood pressure by hypothalamic nuclei: some critical questions. *Clin Exp Pharmacol Physiol* 2005;32:419–425.

38. Kassab S, Kato T, Wilkins FC, et al. Renal denervation attenuates the sodium retention and hypertension associated with obesity. *Hypertension* 1995;25:893–897.

39. Lohmeier TE, Hildebrandt DA, Warren S, et al. Recent insights into the interactions between the baroreflex and the kidneys in hypertension. *Am J Physiol Regul Integr Comp Physiol* 2005;288:R828–R836.

40. Esler M. The sympathetic system and hypertension. *Am J Hypertens* 2000;13:99S–105S.

41. Cowley AW Jr. Long-term control of arterial blood pressure. *Physiol Rev* 1992;72:231–300.

42. Orfila C, Damase-Michel C, Lepert JC, et al. Renal morphological changes after sinoaortic denervation in dogs. *Hypertension* 1993;21:758–766.

43. Kaplan NM. *Clinical Hypertension*, 8th ed. Philadelphia: Lippincott William & Wilkins, 2002:89–92.

44. Hall JE, Hildebrandt DA, Kuo JJ. Obesity hypertension: role of leptin and sympathetic nervous system. *Am J Hypertens* 2001;14:103s–115s.

45. Wofford MR, Anderson DC, Brown CA, et al. Antihypertensive effect of alpha and beta adrenergic blockade in obese and lean hypertensive subjects. *Am J Hypertens* 2001;14:164–168.

46. Hall JE, Brands MW, Henegar JR. Angiotensin II and long-term arterial pressure regulation: the overriding dominance of the kidney. *Kidney Int* 1999;10:s258–s265.

47. Parving HH, Hommel E, Smidt UM. Protection of kidney function and decrease in albuminuria by captopril in insulin dependent diabetics with nephropathy. *BMJ* 1988;297:1086–1091.

48. Lewis EM, Hunsicker LG, Bain RP, et al. The effect of angiotensin-converting enzyme inhibition on diabetic nephropathy. *N Engl J Med* 1993;329:1456–1462.

49. Brenner BM, Cooper ME, de Zeeuw D, et al. RENAAL Study Investigators. Effects of losartan on renal and cardiovascular outcomes in patients with type 2 diabetes and nephropathy. *N Engl J Med* 2001;345:861–869.

50. Matsuaka M, Hymes J, Ichikawa I. Angiotensin in progressive renal diseases: theory and practice. *J Am Soc Nephrol* 1996;7:2025–2043.

51. Griffin KA, Abu-Amarah I, Picken M, et al. Renoprotection by ACE inhibition or aldosterone blockade is blood pressure-dependent. *Hypertension* 2003;41:201–206.

52. Eng E, Veniants M, Floege J, et al. Renal proliferative and phenotypic changes in rats with two-kidney, one-clip Goldblatt hypertension. *Am J Hypertens* 1994;7:177–185.

53. Hall JE, Granger JP. Regulation of fluid and electrolyte balance in hypertension: role of hormones and peptides. In: Battegay EJ, Lip GHY, Bakris GL, eds. *Hypertension: Principles and Practice*. Boca Raton, FL: Taylor & Francis, 2005:121–142.

54. Fuller PJ, Young MJ. Mechanisms of mineralocorticoid action. *Hypertension* 2005;46:1227–1235.

55. Funder, JW. The nongenomic actions of aldosterone. *Endocr Rev* 2005;26:313–321.

56. Wehling M, Kasmayr J, Theisen K. Rapid effects of mineralocorticoids on sodium-proton exchanger: genomic or nongenomic pathway? *Am J Physiol* 1991;260:E719–E726.

57. Hall JE, Granger JP, Smith MJ Jr, et al. Role of renal hemodynamics and arterial pressure in aldosterone "escape." *Hypertension* 1984;6(Suppl I):I183–I192.

58. Calhoun DA, Nishizaka MK, Zaman MA, et al. Hyperaldosteronism among black and white subjects with resistant hypertension. *Hypertension* 2002;40:892–896.

59. Krum H, Nolly H, Workman D, et al. Efficacy of eplerenone added to renin–angiotensin blockade in hypertensive patients. *Hypertension* 2002;40:117–123.

60. de Paula RB, da Silva AA, Hall JE. Aldosterone antagonism attenuates obesity-induced hypertension and glomerular hyperfiltration. *Hypertension* 2004;43:41–47.

61. Yanagisawa M, Kurihara H, Kimura S, et al. A novel potent vasoconstrictor peptide produced by vascular endothelial cells. *Nature* 1988;332:411–415.

62. Kohan D. Endothelins in the normal and diseased kidney. *Am J Kidney Dis* 1997;29:2–26.

63. Schiffrin EL. Endothelin: potential role in hypertension and vascular hypertrophy. *Hypertension* 1995;25:1135–1143.

64. Simonson MS, Dunn MJ. Endothelin peptides and the kidney. *Annu Rev Physiol* 1993;55:249–265.

65. Schiffrin EL. Vascular endothelin in hypertension. *Vascul Pharmacol* 2005;43:19–29.

66. Granger JP. Endothelin. *Am J Physiol Regul Integr Comp Physiol* 2003;285:R298–R301.

67. Kohan DE. The renal medullary endothelin system in control of sodium and water excretion and systemic blood pressure. *Curr Opin Nephrol Hypertens* 2006;15:34–40.

68. Kassab S, Novak J, Miller T, et al. Role of endothelin in mediating the attenuated renal hemodynamics in Dahl salt-sensitive hypertension. *Hypertension* 1997;30:682–686.

69. Kassab S, Miller M, Novak J, et al. Endothelin-A receptor antagonism attenuates the hypertension and renal injury in Dahl salt-sensitive rats. *Hypertension* 1998;31:397–402.

70. Alexander BT, Cockrell KL, Rinewalt AN, et al. Enhanced renal expression of preproendothelin mRNA during chronic angiotensin II hypertension. *Am J Physiol Regul Integr Comp Physiol* 2001;280:R1388–R1392.

71. Ballew JR, Fink GD. Role of ET-1$_A$ receptors in experimental ANG II-induced hypertension in rats. *Am J Physiol Regul Integr Comp Physiol* 2001;281:R150–R154.

72. d'Uscio LV, Moreau P, Shaw S, et al. Effects of chronic ET-1$_A$-receptor blockade in angiotensin II-induced hypertension. *Hypertension* 1997;29:435–441.

73. Perez del Villar C, Garcia Alonso CJ, Feldstein CA, et al. Role of endothelin in the pathogenesis of hypertension. *Mayo Clin Proc* 2005;80:84–96.

74. Sasser JM, Pollock JS, Pollock DM. Renal endothelin in chronic angiotensin II hypertension. *Am J Physiol Regul Integr Comp Physiol* 2002;283:R243–R248.

75. Granger JP, Alexander BT, Llinas MT, et al. Pathophysiology of hypertension during preeclampsia: linking placental ischemia with endothelial dysfunction. *Hypertension* 2001;38:718–722.

76. Khalil RA, Granger JP. Vascular mechanisms of increased arterial pressure in preeclampsia: lessons from animal models. *Am J Physiol Regul Integr Comp Physiol* 2002;283:R29–R45.

77. Alexander BT, Rinewalt AN, Cockrell KL, et al. Endothelin-A receptor blockade attenuates the hypertension in response to chronic reductions in uterine perfusion pressure. *Hypertension* 2001;37:485–489.

78. Granger JP, LaMarca BBD, Cockrell K, et al. Reduced uterine perfusion pressure (RUPP) model for studying cardiovascular-renal dysfunction in response to placental ischemia. *Methods Mol Med* 2006;122:383–392.

79. Gariepy CE, Cass DT, Yanagisawa M. Null mutation of endothelin receptor type B gene in spotting lET-1hal rats causes aganglionic megacolon and white coat color. *Proc Natl Acad Sci U S A* 1996;93:867–872.

80. Gariepy CE, Ohuchi T, Williams SC, et al. Salt-sensitive hypertension in endothelin-B receptor-deficient rats. *J Clin Invest* 2000;105:925–933.

81. Pollock DM, Pollock JS. Evidence for endothelin involvement in the response to high salt. *Am J Physiol Renal Physiol* 2001;281:F144–F150.

82. Bagnall AJ, Kelland NF, Gulliver-Sloan F, et al. Deletion of endothelial cell endothelin B receptors does not affect blood pressure or sensitivity to salt. *Hypertension* 2006;48:286–293.

83. Ge Y, Bagnall A, Stricklett P, et al. Collecting duct-specific knockout of the endothelin B receptor causes hypertension and sodium retention. *Am J Physiol Renal Physiol* 2006;291(6): F1274–1280.

84. Krum H, Viskoper RJ, Lacourciere Y, et al. The effect of an endothelin-receptor antagonist, bosentan, on blood pressure inpatients with essential hypertension. Bosentan Hypertension Investigators. *N Engl J Med* 1998;338:784–790.

85. Sahara M, Takahashi T, Imai Y, et al. New insights in the treatment strategy for pulmonary arterial hypertension. *Cardiovasc Drugs Ther* 2006;20(5):377–386.

86. Schnackenberg CG, Kirchner K, Patel A, et al. Nitric oxide, the kidney, and hypertension. *Clin Exp Pharmacol Physiol* 1997;24:600–606.

87. Ortiz PA, Garvin JL. Role of nitric oxide in the regulation of nephron transport. *Am J Physiol Renal Physiol* 2002;282:F777–F784.

88. Cowley AW Jr, Mori T, Mattson D, et al. Role of renal NO production in the regulation of medullary blood flow. *Am J Physiol Regul Integr Comp Physiol* 2003;284:R1355–R1369.

89. Granger JP, Alexander BT. Abnormal pressure natriuresis in hypertension: role of nitric oxide. *Acta Physiol Scand* 2000;168:161–168.

90. Nakamura T, Alberola A, Granger JP. Role of renal interstitial pressure as a mediator of sodium retention during blockade of endothelium derived nitric oxide hypertension. *Hypertension* 1993;21:956–960.

91. Granger JP, Novak J, Schnackenberg C, et al. Role of renal nerves in mediating the hypertensive effects of nitric oxide synthesis inhibition. *Hypertension* 1996;27:613–618.

92. Schnackenberg C, Tabor B, Strong M, et al. Intrarenal NO blockade enhances renin secretion rate by a macula densa mechanism. *Am J Physiol* 1997;272:R879–R886.

93. Sanders PW. Sodium intake, endothelial cell signaling, and progression of kidney disease. *Hypertension* 2004;43:142–146.

94. Taniyama Y, Griendling KK. Reactive oxygen species in the vasculature: molecular and cellular mechanisms. *Hypertension* 2003;42:1075–1081.

95. Wilcox CS. Reactive oxygen species: roles in blood pressure and kidney function. *Curr Hypertens Rep* 2002;4:160–166.

96. Manning RD Jr, Meng S, Tian N. Renal and vascular oxidative stress and salt-sensitivity of arterial pressure. *Acta Physiol Scand* 2003;179:243–250.

97. Reckelhoff JF, Romero JC. Role of oxidative stress in angiotensin-induced hypertension. *Am J Physiol Regul Integr Comp Physiol* 2003;284:R893–R912.

98. Romero JC, Reckelhoff JF. State-of-the-Art lecture. Role of angiotensin and oxidative stress in essential hypertension. *Hypertension* 1999;34:943–949.

99. Sedeek M, Alexander BT, Abram SR, et al. Role of oxidative stress in endothelin-induced hypertension in rats. *Hypertension* 2003;42:806–810.

100. Garvin JL, Ortiz PA. The role of reactive oxygen species in the regulation of tubular function. *Acta Physiol Scand* 2003;179:225–232.

101. Chae CU, Lee RT, Rifai N, et al. Blood pressure and inflammation in apparently healthy men. *Hypertension* 2001;38:399–403.

102. Conrad KP, Benyo DF. Placental cytokines and the pathogenesis of preeclampsia. *Am J Reprod Immunol* 1997;37:240–249.

103. Donners MM, Daemen MJ, Cleutjens KB, et al. Inflammation and restenosis: implications for therapy. *Ann Med* 2003;35:523–531.

104. Sattar N, McCarey DW, Capell H, et al. Explaining how "high-grade" systemic inflammation accelerates vascular risk in rheumatoid arthritis. *Circulation* 2003;108:2957–2963.

105. Siwik DA, Colucci WS. Regulation of matrix metalloproteinases by cytokines and reactive oxygen/nitrogen species in the myocardium. *Heart Fail Rev* 2004;9:43–51.

106. Alexander BT, Massey MB, Cockrell KL, et al. Elevations in plasma TNF in pregnant rats decreases renal nNOS and iNOS and results in hypertension. *Am J Hypertens* 2002;15:170–175.

107. LaMarca BB, Bennett WA, Alexander BT, et al. Hypertension produced by reductions in uterine perfusion in the pregnant rat. Role of tumor necrosis factor-α. *Hypertension* 2005;46:1022–1025.

108. Orshal JM, Khalil RA. Reduced endothelial NO-cGMP-mediated vascular relaxation and hypertension in IL-6-infused pregnant rats. *Hypertension* 2004;43:434–444.

109. Lee DL, Sturgis LC, Labazi H, et al. Angiotensin II hypertension is attenuated in interleukin-6 knockout mice. *Am J Physiol Heart Circ Physiol* 2006;290:H935–H940.

110. Knox FG, Granger JP. Control of sodium excretion: an integrative approach. In: Windhager E, ed. *Handbook of Renal Physiology.* New York: Oxford University Press, 1992:927–967.

111. Cheng HF, Harris RC. Cyclooxygenases, the kidney, and hypertension. *Hypertension* 2004;43:525–530.

112. Grosser T, Fries S, FitzGerald GA. Biological basis for the cardiovascular consequences of COX-2 inhibition: therapeutic challenges and opportunities. *J Clin Invest* 2006;116(1):4–15.

113. Roman RJ. P-450 metabolites of arachidonic acid in the control of cardiovascular function. *Physiol Rev* 2002;82:131–185.

114. Laffer CL, Laniado-Schwartzman M, Wang MH, et al. Differential regulation of natriuresis by 20-hydroxyeicosatetraenoic acid in human salt-sensitive versus salt-resistant hypertension. *Circulation* 2003;107:574–578.

115. Laffer CL, Laniado-Schwartzman M, Wang MH, et al. 20-HETE and furosemide-induced natriuresis in salt-sensitive essential hypertension. *Hypertension* 2003;41:703–708.

116. Vesely DL. Atrial natriuretic peptides in pathophysiological diseases. *Cardiovasc Res* 2001;51:647–658.

117. Granger JP, Opgenorth TJ, Salazar J, et al. Long-term hypotensive and renal effects of chronic infusions of atrial natriuretic peptide in conscious dogs. *Hypertension* 1986;8:II112–II116.

118. Melo LG, Steinhelper ME, Pang SC, et al. ANP in regulation of arterial pressure and fluid-electrolyte balance: lessons from genetic mouse models. *Physiol Genomics* 2000;3:45–58.

119. Garovic VD, Textor SC. Renovascular hypertension and ischemic nephropathy. *Circulation* 2005;112:1362–1374.

120. Bianchi G, Tenconi LT, Lucca R. Effect in the conscious dog of constriction of the renal artery to a sole remaining kidney on haemodynamics, sodium balance, body fluid volumes, plasma renin concentration and pressor responsiveness to angiotensin. *Clin Sci* 1970;38:741–766.

121. Bengis RG, Coleman TG. Antihypertensive effect of prolonged blockade of angiotensin formation in benign and malignant, one- and two-kidney Goldblatt hypertensive rats. *Clin Sci (Lond)* 1979;57:53–62.

122. Gavras H, Brunner HB, Vaughan ED, et al. Angiotensin-sodium interaction in blood pressure maintenance of renal hypertensive and normotensive rats. *Science* 1973;180:1369–1371.

123. Thurston H, Bing RF, Marks ES, et al. Response of chronic renovascular hypertension to surgical correction or prolonged blockade of the renin–angiotensin system by two inhibitors in the rat. *Clin Sci (Lond)* 1980;58:15–20.

124. Kaplan NM. *Clinical Hypertension,* 8th ed. Philadelphia: Lippincott William & Wilkins, 2002:89–92.

125. Young WF Jr. Primary aldosteronism—changing concepts in diagnosis and treatment. *Endocrinology* 2003;144:2208–2213.

126. Calhoun DA, Nishizaka MK, Zaman MA, et al. Hyperaldosteronism among black and white subjects with resistant hypertension. *Hypertension* 2002;40:892–896.

127. Fallo F, Paoletta A, Tona F, et al. Response of hypertension to conventional antihypertensive treatment and/or steroidogenesis inhibitors in Cushing's syndrome. *J Intern Med* 1993;234:595–598.

128. Whitworth JA, Mangos GJ, Kelly JJ. Cushing, cortisol, and cardiovascular disease. *Hypertension* 2000;36:912–916.

129. Manger WM. An overview of pheochromocytoma: history, current concepts, vagaries, and diagnostic challenges. *Ann N Y Acad Sci* 2006;1073:1–20.

130. Goldstein DS. Diagnosis and localization of pheochromocytoma. *Hypertension* 2004;43:907–910.

131. Granger JP, Alexander BT, Llinas MT, et al. Pathophysiology of preeclampsia: linking placental ischemia/hypoxia with microvascular dysfunction [review]. *Microcirculation* 2002;9(3):147–160.

132. Granger JP, LaMarca BBD, Cockrell K, et al. Reduced uterine perfusion pressure (RUPP) model for studying cardiovascular-renal dysfunction in response to placental ischemia. *Methods Mol Med* 2006;122:383–392.

133. LaMarca BB, Gadonski G, Cockrell K, et al. Endothelin type A receptor blockade attenuates TNF alpha-induced hypertension in pregnant rats. *Hypertension* 2005;46:1–5.

134. LaMarca BB, Bennett WA, Alexander BT, et al. Hypertension produced by reductions in uterine perfusion in the pregnant rat. Role of tumor necrosis factor-α. *Hypertension* 2005;46(4):1022–1025.

135. Gadonski G, LaMarca BB, Sullivan E, et al. Hypertension produced by reductions in uterine perfusion in the pregnant rat. Role of interleukin 6. *Hypertension* 2006; 48(4):711–716.

136. Lam C, Lim KH, Karumanchi SA. Circulating angiogenic factors in the pathogenesis and prediction of preeclampsia. *Hypertension* 2005;46(5):1077–1085.

137. Maynard SE, Min JY, Merchan J, et al. Excess placental soluble fms-like tyrosine kinase 1 (sFlt1) may contribute to endothelial dysfunction, hypertension, and proteinuria in preeclampsia. *J Clin Invest* 2003;111(5):649–658.

138. Venkatesha S, Toporsian M, Lam C, et al. Soluble endoglin contributes to the pathogenesis of preeclampsia. *Nat Med* 2006;12(6):642–649.

139. Luft FC. Geneticism of essential hypertension. *Hypertension* 2004;43:1155–1159.

140. Longini IM, Higgins MW, Minton PC, et al. Environmental and genetic sources of familial aggregation of blood pressure in Tecumseh, Michigan. *Am J Epidemiol* 1984;120:131–144.

141. Havlik RJ, Garrison RJ, Feinleib M, et al. Blood pressure aggregation in families. *Am J Epidemiol* 1979;110:304–312.

142. Cui J, Hopper JL, Harrap SB. Genes and family environment explain correlations between blood pressure and body mass index. *Hypertension* 2002;40:7–12.

143. Barlassina C, Lanzani C, Manunta P, et al. Genetics of essential hypertension: from families to genes. *J Am Soc Nephrol* 2002;13(Suppl 3):S155–S164.

144. Luft FC. Molecular genetics of human hypertension. *J Hypertens* 1998;16:1871–1878.

145. Williams RR, Hunt SC, Hopkins PN, et al. Tabulations and expectations regarding the genetics of human hypertension. *Kidney Int* 1994;45(Suppl 44):S57–S64.

146. Lifton RP, Gharavi AG, Geller DS. Molecular mechanisms of human hypertension. *Cell* 2001;104:545–556.

147. O'Shaughnessy KM, Karet FE. Salt handling and hypertension. *J Clin Invest* 2004;113:1075–1081.

148. Lifton RP, Dluhy RG, Powers M, et al. Hereditary hypertension caused by chimaeric gene duplications and ectopic expression of aldosterone synthase. *Nat Genet* 1992;2:66–74.

149. Dluhy RG, Lifton RP. Glucocorticoid-remediable aldosteronism (GRA): diagnosis, variability of phenotype and regulation of potassium homeostasis. *Steroids* 1995;60:48–51.

150. Garovic VD, Hilliard AA, Turner ST. Monogenic forms of low-renin hypertension. *Nat Clin Pract Nephrol* 2006;2:624–630.

151. Stowasser M, Gordon RD, Tunny TJ, et al. Familial hyperaldosteronism type II. five families with a new variety of primary aldosteronism. *Clin Exp Pharmacol Physiol* 1992;19:319–322.

152. Biglieri EG, Kater CE. Mineralocorticoids in congenital adrenal hyperplasia. *J Steroid Biochem Mol Biol* 1991;40:493–499.

153. Hansson JH, Nelson-Williams C, Suzuki H, et al. Hypertension caused by a truncated sodium channel gamma subunit: genetic heterogeneity of Liddle syndrome. *Nat Genet* 1995;11:76–82.

154. Mune T, Rogerson FM, Nikkila H, et al. Human hypertension caused by mutations in the kidney isozyme of 11 beta-hydroxysteroid dehydrogenase. *Nat Genet* 1995;10:394–399.

155. Wilson FH, Disse-Nicodeme S, Choate KA, et al. Human hypertension caused by mutations in WNK kinases. *Science* 2001;293:1107–1112.

156. Geller DS, Farhi A, Pinkerton N, et al. Activating mineralocorticoid receptor mutation in hypertension exacerbated by pregnancy. *Science* 2000;289:119–123.

157. Whelton PK. Epidemiology of hypertension. *Lancet* 1994;344:101–106.

158. He J, Klag MJ, Whelton PK, et al. Migration, blood pressure pattern, and hypertension: the Yi migrant study. *Am J Epidemiol* 1991;134:1085–1101.

159. Carvalho JJ, Baruzzi RG, Howard PF, et al. Blood pressure in four remote populations in the Intersalt Study. *Hypertension* 1989;14:238–246.

160. World Health Organization. *Controlling the Obesity Epidemic*, 2000. Accessed June 5, 2007 at: http://www.who.int/nutrition/topics/obesity/en/.

161. Yach D, Stuckler D, Brownell KD. Epidemiologic and economic consequences of the global epidemics of obesity and diabetes. *Nature Medicine* 2006;12:62–66.

162. Flegal KM, Carroll MD, Ogden CL, et al. Prevalence and trends in obesity among U.S. adults 1999–2000. *JAMA* 2002;288:1723–1727.

163. Jones DW, Kim JS, Andrew ME, et al. Body mass index and blood pressures in Korean men and women: the Korean National Blood Pressure Survey. *J Hypertens* 1994;12:1433–1437.

164. Garrison RJ, Kannel WB, Stokes J, et al. Incidence and precursors of hypertension in young adults: the Framingham Offspring Study. *Prev Med* 1987;16:234–251.

165. Jones DW, Miller ME, Wofford MR, et al. The effect of weight loss interventions on antihypertensive medication requirements in the Hypertension Optimal Treatment (HOT) study. *Am J Hypertens* 1999;12:1175–1180.

166. Stevens VJ, Obarzanek E, Cook NR, et al. Long-term weight loss and changes in blood pressure: results of the Trials of Hypertension Prevention, phase II. *Ann Intern Med* 2001;134(1):1–11.

167. Alexander J, Dustan HP, Sims EAH, et al. *Report of the Hypertension Task Force*, U.S. Department of Health, Education, and Welfare Publication 70–1631 (NIH). Washington, DC: U.S. Government Printing Office 61–77, 1979.

168. Hall JE, Brands MW, Dixon WN, et al. Obesity-induced hypertension: renal function and systemic hemodynamics. *Hypertension* 1993;22:292–299.

169. Carroll JF, Huang M, Hester RL, et al. Hemodynamic alterations in obese rabbits. *Hypertension* 1995;26:465–470.

170. Messerli FH, Christie B, DeCarvalho JG, et al. Obesity and essential hypertension. Hemodynamics, intravascular volume, sodium excretion and plasma renin activity. *Arch Intern Med* 1981;141:81–85.

171. Rocchini AP. The influence of obesity in hypertension. *News Physiol Sci* 1990;5:245–249.

172. Rumantir MS, Vaz M, Jennings GL, et al. Neural mechanisms in human obesity-related hypertension. *J Hypertens* 1999;17:1125–1133.

173. Esler M. The sympathetic system and hypertension. *Am J Hypertens* 2000;13:99s–105s.

174. Grassi G, Servalle G, Castaneo BM, et al. Sympathetic activity in obese normotensive subjects. *Hypertension* 1995;25:560–563.

175. Weyer C, Pratley RE, Snitker S, et al. Ethnic differences in insulinemia and sympathetic tone as links between obesity and blood pressure. *Hypertension* 2000;36(4):531–537.

176. Abate NI, Mansour YH, Arbique D, et al. Overweight and sympathetic activity in black Americans. *Hypertension* 2001;38:379–383.

177. Davy KP, Hall JE. Obesity and hypertension: two epidemics or one? *Am J Physiol Regul Integr Comp Physiol* 2004;286:R803–R813.

178. Shek EW, Brands MW, Hall JE. Chronic leptin infusion increases arterial pressure. *Hypertension* 1998;31:409–414.

179. Carlyle M, Jones OB, Kuo JJ, et al. Chronic cardiovascular and renal actions of leptin-role of adrenergic activity. *Hypertension* 2002;39:496–501.

180. Kuo J, Jones OB, Hall JE. Inhibition of NO synthesis enhances chronic cardiovascular and renal actions of leptin. *Hypertension* 2001;37:670–676.

181. Mark AL, Shaffer RA, Correia ML, et al. Contrasting blood pressure effects of obesity in leptin-deficient ob/ob mice and agouti yellow mice. *J Hypertens* 1999;17:1949–1953.

182. Ozata M, Ozdemir IC, Licinio J. Human leptin deficiency caused by a missense mutation: multiple endocrine defects, decreased sympathetic tone, and immune system dysfunction indicate new targets for leptin action, greater central than peripheral resistance to the effects of leptin, and spontaneous correction of leptin-mediated defects. *J Clin Endocrinol Metab* 1999;10:3686–3695.

183. daSilva AA, Kuo JJ, Hall JE. Role of hypothalamic melanocortin 3/4 receptors in mediating the chronic cardiovascular, renal, and metabolic actions of leptin. *Hypertension* 2004;43:1312–1317.

184. Tallam LS, da Silva AA, Hall JE. Melanocortin-4 receptor mediates chronic cardiovascular and metabolic actions of leptin. *Hypertension* 2006;48:58–64.

185. Engeli S, Sharma AM. The renin angiotensin system and natriuretic peptides in obesity associated hypertension. *J Mol Med* 2001;79:21–29.

186. Tuck ML, Sowers J, Dornfeld L, et al. The effect of weight reduction on blood pressure, plasma renin activity, and plasma aldosterone levels in obese patients. *N Engl J Med* 1981;304:930–933.

187. Robles RG, Villa E, Santirso R, et al. Effects of captopril on sympathetic activity, lipid and carbohydrate metabolism in a model of obesity-induced hypertension in dogs. *Am J Hypertens* 1993;6:1009–1019.

188. Boustany CM, Brown DR, Randall DC, et al. AT1-receptor antagonism reverses the blood pressure elevation associated with diet-induced obesity. *Am J Physiol Regul Integr Comp Physiol* 2005;289:R181–R186.

189. Reisen E, Weir M, Falkner B, et al. Lisinopril versus hydrochlorothiazide in obese hypertensive patients: a multicenter placebo-controlled trial. *Hypertension* 1997;30:140–145.

190. Grassi G, Seravalle G, Dell'Oro R, et al. Comparative effects of candesartan and hydrochlorothiazide on blood pressure, insulin sensitivity, and sympathetic drive in obese hypertensive individuals: results of the CROSS study. *J Hypertens* 2003;21:1761–1769.
191. de Paula RB, da Silva AA, Hall JE. Aldosterone antagonism attenuates obesity-induced hypertension and glomerular hyperfiltration. *Hypertension* 2004;43:41–47.
192. Goodfriend TL, Calhoun DA. Resistant hypertension, obesity, sleep apnea, and aldosterone: theory and therapy. *Hypertension* 2004;43:518–524.
193. Sugarman HJ, Windsor ACJ, Bessos MK, et al. Intra-abdominal pressure, sagittal abdominal diameter and obesity co-morbidity. *J Intern Med* 1997;241:71–79.
194. Hall JE, Henegar JR, Dwyer TM, et al. Is obesity a major cause of chronic renal disease? *Adv Ren Replace Ther* 2004;11:41–54.
195. Hall JE, Brands MW, Henegar JR. Mechanisms of hypertension and kidney disease in obesity. *Ann N Y Acad Sci* 1999;892:91–107.
196. Hall JE, Crook ED, Jones DW, et al. Mechanisms of obesity-associated cardiovascular and renal disease. *Am J Med Sci* 2002;324(3):127–137.
197. Kambham N, Markowitz GS, Valeri AM, et al. Obesity related glomerulopathy: an emerging epidemic. *Kidney Int* 2001;59:1498–1509.
198. Hall JE, Jones DW, Henegar J, et al. Obesity hypertension, and renal disease. In: Eckel RH, ed. *Obesity: Mechanisms and Clinical Management.* Philadelphia: Lippincott, Williams & Wilkins, 2003:273–300.
199. Hsu CY, McCulloch CE, Iribarren C, et al. Body mass index and risk for end-stage renal disease. *Ann Intern Med* 2006;144:21–28.
200. Praga M, Hernandez E, Herrero JC, et al. Influence of obesity on the appearance of proteinuria and renal insufficiency after unilateral nephrectomy. *Kidney Int* 2000;58:2111–2118.
201. Bonnet F, Deprele C, Sassolas A, et al. Excessive body weight as a new independent risk factor for clinical and pathological progression in primary IgA nephritis. *Am J Kidney Dis* 2001;37:720–727.
202. Reaven GM. Banting Lecture 1988. Role of insulin resistance in human disease. *Diabetes* 1988;37:1595–607.
203. Alberti KG, Zimmet PZ. Definition, diagnosis and classification of diabetes mellitus and its complications. Part 1: diagnosis and classification of diabetes mellitus provisional report of a WHO consultation. *Diabet Med* 1998;15:539–553.
204. Executive summary of the Third Report of the National Cholesterol Education Program (NCEP) Expert Panel on Detection, Evaluation, and Treatment of High Blood Cholesterol in Adults (Adult Treatment Panel III). *JAMA* 2001;285:2486–2497.
205. Alberti KG, Zimmet P, Shaw J. Metabolic syndrome—a new world-wide definition. A consensus statement from the International Diabetes Federation. *Diabet Med* 2006;23:469–480.
206. Reaven G. The metabolic syndrome: is this diagnosis necessary? *Am J Clin Nutr* 2006;83:1237–1247.
207. Hall JE, Summers RL, Brands MW, et al. Resistance to metabolic actions of insulin and its role in hypertension. *Am J Hypertens* 1994;7:772–788.
208. Kahn R, Buse J, Ferrannini E, et al. American Diabetes Association; European Association for the Study of Diabetes. The metabolic syndrome: time for a critical appraisal: joint statement from the American Diabetes Association and the European Association for the Study of Diabetes. *Diabetes Care* 2005;28:2289–2304.
209. Landsberg L, Krieger DR. Obesity, metabolism, and the sympathetic nervous system. *Am J Hypertens* 1989;2:125S–132S.
210. Hall JE, Brands MW, Zappe DH, et al. Cardiovascular actions of insulin: are they important in long-term blood pressure regulation? *Clin Exp Pharmacol Physiol* 1995;22:689–700.
211. Hall JE, Brands MW, Zappe DH, et al. Insulin resistance, hyperinsulinemia, and hypertension: causes, consequences, or merely correlations? *Proc Soc Exp Biol Med* 1995;208:317–329.
212. Hall JE, Brands MW, Mizelle HL, et al. Chronic intrarenal hyperinsulinemia does not cause hypertension. *Am J Physiol* 1991;260:F663–F669.
213. Hall JE, Brands MW, Zappe DH, et al. Hemodynamic and renal responses to chronic hyperinsulinemia in obese, insulin-resistant dogs. *Hypertension* 1995;25:994–1002.
214. Sawicki PT, Baba T, Berger M, et al. Normal blood pressure in patients with insulinoma despite hyperinsulinemia and insulin resistance. *J Am Soc Nephrol* 1992;3(4 Suppl):s64–s68.
215. Pontiroli AE, Alberetto M, Pozza G. Patients with insulinoma show insulin resistance in the absence of arterial hypertension. *Diabetologia* 1992;35:294–295.
216. Sowers JR. Insulin resistance and hypertension. *Mol Cell Endocrinol* 1990;74:C87–C89.
217. Dubey R, Zhang HY, Reddy SR, et al. Pioglitazone attenuates hypertension and inhibits growth of renal arterial smooth muscle in rats. *Am J Physiol* 1993;265:R726–R732.
218. Kurtz TW, Gardner DG. Transcription-modulating drugs. A new frontier in the treatment of essential hypertension. *Hypertension* 1998;32:380–386.
219. Zhang F, Sowers JR, Ram JL, et al. Effects of pioglitazone or calcium channels in vascular smooth muscle. *Hypertension* 1994;24:170–175.
220. Julius S, Gudbrandsson T, Jamerson K, et al. The hemodynamic link between insulin resistance and hypertension. *J Hypertens* 1991;9:983–986.

CHAPTER (70)

Diagnosis and Treatment of Hypertension

Arash Rashidi / Mahboob Rahman / Jackson T. Wright, Jr.

EVALUATION OF THE HYPERTENSIVE PATIENT

【 】 BLOOD PRESSURE MEASUREMENT

The current classification of blood pressure, described in the Seventh Report of the Joint National Committee on Prevention, Detection, Evaluation, and Treatment of High Blood Pressure (JNC 7), places patients in one of four categories (Table 70–1). To apply this classification in clinical practice, the blood pressure must be recorded accurately. But the measurement of blood pressure, although being one of the most important measurements in clinical medicine, is also among those with the greatest source of error. Intraarterial blood pressure can be measured directly by inserting a catheter into the lumen of an artery, but this method is impractical and is rarely employed in bedside examination except in intensive care units. The gold standard for clinical measurement of blood pressure is readings taken by a trained healthcare provider using a mercury sphygmomanometer. Aneroid and automated sphygmomanometers have increased in popularity over recent years. When used as a substitute for a mercury sphygmomanometer, a protocol for regular periodic calibration of the device should be in place.[1,2] Regardless of the device used, it is important to appreciate that blood pressure is a variable hemodynamic phenomenon, which is influenced by many factors. Therefore, the circumstances and procedures for blood pressure measurement must be standardized.

Blood pressure measurements can be taken in the clinic, at home, and by ambulatory blood pressure monitoring. To maintain its predictive value, blood pressure measurement should be standardized with trained observers following the established protocol. Tight clothing should be removed, the arm supported at heart level, and talking avoided during the measurement. Patients should be seated for at least 5 minutes in a chair (rather than on an examination table), with feet on the floor, in a quiet room before the measurement is made.[3–5] Cuffs of the appropriate size should be used such that the bladder encircles at least 80 percent of the upper arm and a width that is at least 40 percent of arm circumference. Using too small a cuff will lead to overestimation of blood pressure. The distal margin of the cuff should be at least 3 cm proximal to the antecubital fossa. The cuff should be inflated to a pressure about 30 mmHg above the point where the palpable pulse disappears. The mercury column should be deflated at 2 to 3 mm per second. The onset of phase I of the Korotkoff sounds (tapping sounds corresponding to the appearance of a palpable pulse) corresponds to systolic pressure. The disappearance of sounds (phase V) corresponds to diastolic pressure. The fifth phase should be used, except in situations in which the disappearance of sounds cannot reliably be determined because sounds are audible even after complete deflation of the cuff. This occurs in pregnant women, for example, in which case the fourth phase (muffling) may be used. At least two measurements spaced

TABLE 70–1

Classification of Blood Pressure for Adults

BLOOD PRESSURE CLASSIFICATION	SYSTOLIC BLOOD PRESSURE (MMHG)	DIASTOLIC BLOOD PRESSURE (MMHG)
Normal	<120	<80
Prehypertension	120–139	80–89
Stage 1 Hypertension	140–159	90–99
Stage 2 Hypertension	≥160	≥100

SOURCE: From Chobanian AV, Bakris GL, Black HR, et al. Seventh Report of the Joint National Committee on Prevention, Detection, Evaluation, and Treatment of High Blood Pressure. NIH Publication No. 04–5230. Available at: http://www.nhlbi.nih.gov/guidelines/hypertension/jnc7full.htm.

by 1 to 2 minutes apart should be taken. Blood pressure should be measured in both arms at the first visit to detect possible differences because of peripheral vascular disease; if present, the higher value should be used. Measurement of blood pressure in the standing position should be undertaken initially and periodically, especially in those who are at risk of postural hypotension.[6–8] Atrial fibrillation can make the measurement of blood pressure particularly difficult due to marked beat-to-beat variability. This is a particularly important consideration when using semiautomatic or automated devices. In such circumstances, multiple auscultatory readings are recommended.[7]

[ ] AMBULATORY BLOOD PRESSURE MEASUREMENT

Ambulatory blood pressure measurement is a noninvasive, fully automated technique in which multiple blood pressure measurements are recorded over an extended period of time, typically 24 hours. Several prospective studies have documented that the average level of ambulatory blood pressure predicts risk of morbid events better than clinic blood pressure. Normal ambulatory blood pressure values for adults (nonpregnant) are <135/85 mmHg while awake and <120/75 mmHg during the night.[8] The most common application of ambulatory blood pressure monitoring is to ascertain an individual's usual level of blood pressure outside the clinic setting, and thereby identify individuals with white-coat hypertension in whom there is a large discrepancy between clinic and home measurements. In addition to mean absolute levels of ambulatory blood pressure, certain diurnal ambulatory blood pressure patterns may predict blood pressure-related complications. Nighttime (asleep) blood pressure is usually lower than daytime blood pressure; individuals with a nondipping pattern (<10 percent blood pressure reduction from night to day) appear to be at increased risk for blood pressure-related complications compared with those with a normal dipping pattern. Other evidence suggests that the nighttime blood pressure may be the best predictor of cardiovascular risk. Other applications of ambulatory blood pressure monitoring are in patients with apparently refractory hypertension but little target-organ damage, sus-

pected autonomic neuropathy, patients with apparent drug resistance, hypotensive symptoms with antihypertensive medications, and episodic hypertension. Ambulatory blood pressure monitoring will also detect the presence of *masked hypertension*, defined as a normal clinic blood pressure and a high ambulatory blood pressure, which is the reverse of white-coat hypertension. Although the presence of masked hypertension is associated with increased cardiovascular risk, the therapeutic implications of this diagnosis remain uncertain at this time.[9,10]

[ ] HOME BLOOD PRESSURE MONITORING

Home blood pressure monitoring is a useful adjunct in the management of hypertension and is a practical option to assess differences between office and out-of-office blood pressure by eliminating the white-coat effect. Proper use of a validated and accurate device for home blood pressure measurement and adequate training are important in enhancing the value of self blood pressure measurement. Normal home blood pressure levels are lower than readings (<135/85 mmHg).[11,12] Home blood pressure monitoring also has been shown to improve compliance with antihypertensive medications and to be at least as good a predictor of cardiovascular risk as office-based blood pressure readings.

[ ] HISTORY AND PHYSICAL EXAMINATION AND LABORATORY EVALUATION

The three main goals of the initial evaluation of the hypertensive patient are to (1) assess the presence of target-organ damage related to hypertension, especially those that might influence choice of therapy, (2) determine the presence of other cardiovascular risk factors and disease, and (3) evaluate for possible underlying secondary causes of hypertension. These goals are usually accomplished by a thorough medical history, physical examination, and simple laboratory investigations.[8]

History

The key issues that need to be addressed in the history include:

- Duration, age of onset, and previous levels of high blood pressure;
- Previous antihypertensive therapy, its impact on blood pressure and adverse effects;
- Symptoms suggestive of secondary causes of hypertension (see Secondary Causes of Hypertension below);
- Lifestyle factors, such as dietary intake of fat, salt, alcohol, smoking, and physical activity, weight gain since early adult life;
- History of symptoms of neurologic dysfunction, heart failure, coronary heart disease, or peripheral arterial target-organ damage;
- Use of medications that influence blood pressure such as oral contraceptives, licorice, carbenoxolone, nasal drops, cocaine, amphetamines, steroids, nonsteroidal anti-inflammatory drugs, erythropoietin, and cyclosporine; and
- Presence of other cardiovascular risk factors.[13]

Physical Examination

In addition to blood pressure measurement, the physical examination should search for signs of secondary hypertension and for evidence of organ damage. During the physical examination note should be made of blood pressure, features of Cushing syndrome, tuberous sclerosis or skin stigmata of neurofibromatosis (suggesting possible pheochromocytoma), palpation of enlarged kidneys (polycystic kidney), auscultation of abdominal bruits (renovascular hypertension) and precordial murmurs (aortic coarctation or aortic disease), and diminished and delayed femoral pulses (aortic coarctation, aortic disease); these features all suggest secondary hypertension. Other signs, such as carotid bruits; motor or sensory defects; funduscopic abnormalities; abnormal cardiac rhythms; ventricular gallop; pulmonary rales; dependent edema; and absence, reduction, or asymmetry of pulses and cold extremities, may suggest end organ damage (Table 70–2).[13]

Laboratory Tests

Routine investigations before initiation of therapy include urine for protein and blood; serum creatinine (estimated glomerular filtration rate [GFR]) and electrolytes; fasting blood glucose; fasting lipid profile; and electrocardiogram (ECG). Generally, it is not necessary to do more extensive tests unless blood pressure control is not achieved or there are clinical or laboratory clues of secondary hypertension. An echocardiogram may be helpful in evaluating cardiac function in patients with cardiac symptoms or findings. Additional workup is guided by the clinical presentation in an individual patient, and the need to evaluate possible causes of secondary hypertension.

Risk Assessment

Increased cardiovascular risk across the whole range of BP is well described. However, the coexistence of other risk factors results in a significant increase in cardiovascular disease (CVD) risk associated with any blood pressure stratum. Those at highest absolute risk include people with multiple risk factors, those with diabetes who tend to demonstrate risk factor clustering, and those who have already suffered a cardiovascular event. Thus, during the evaluation, the key risk factors which need to be considered are age (>55 years male, >65 years female), family history of premature cardiovascular disease (age <55 in men, age <65 years in women), cigarette smoking, dyslipidemia, diabetes, obesity (body mass index >30 kg/m^2), reduced GFR (<60 mL/min), or presence of microalbuminuria. Online tools, such as those developed from the Framingham Study, can be used to quantify risk of cardiovascular disease.[14] Other risk factors have been proposed but remain to be confirmed (see Chaps. 52–55).

SECONDARY CAUSES OF HYPERTENSION

Secondary hypertension is said to be present when the hypertension results from a specific cause in contrast to the more common "primary" form ("essential" hypertension) in which no direct cause is known. The most common causes of secondary hypertension are renal artery stenosis, renal parenchymal disease, sleep apnea, primary aldosteronism, Cushing syndrome, and pheochromocytoma.[15–19] Table 70–3 summarizes the clinical clues suggesting secondary hypertension.

TABLE 70–2

Important Findings in Physical Examination That Might Help to Diagnose Secondary Hypertension or Find End-Organ Damage

	FINDING	SIGNIFICANCE
Vital sign	Pulse pressure >60 mmHg	↑ CVD risk
	Tachycardia	Hyperthyroid, pheochromocytoma, HF
Body habitus	Cushingoid	Cushing syndrome
Skin	Oral-facial tumors	MEN-2A/2B (pheochromocytoma)
	Neurofibromas, café-au-lait spots	Pheochromocytoma
Eyes	AV nicking, hemorrhages, exudates	Hypertensive retinopathy
Neck	Bruits	Carotid disease
	Thyroid	Hypothyroid MEN-2A
Chest wall	Rib bruits	Coarctation of aorta
	Post flank bruits	Renal artery stenosis
Lungs	Crackles, wheezes	Heart failure
Cardiac	Gallops, LVH, murmur	Heart failure, valvular disease
Abdomen	Palpable kidneys, bruit, epigastric and post	Polycystic kidneys, renal artery stenosis
Extremities	Diminished pulses,[a] femoral pulse-delay	Coarctation of aorta
	Bruits	Vascular damage

AV, atrioventricular; CVD, cardiovascular disease; HF heart failure; LVH, left ventricular hypertrophy; MEN, multiple endocrine neoplasia.
[a]Patients younger than age 35 years should have blood pressure measured in legs.

RENAL ARTERY STENOSIS

Renovascular hypertension occurs in 1 to 2 percent of the overall hypertensive population, but the prevalence may be as high as 10 percent in patients with resistant hypertension, and even higher in patients with accelerated or malignant hypertension. Clinical clues to renovascular disease include (1) onset of hypertension before age 30 years (especially without a family history) or recent onset of significant hypertension after age 55 years; (2) an abdominal bruit, particularly if it continues into diastole and is lateralized; (3) accelerated or resistant hypertension; (4) recurrent (flash) pulmonary edema; (5) renal failure of uncertain etiology, especially with a normal urinary sediment; (6) coexisting diffuse atherosclerotic vascular disease, especially in heavy smokers; or (7) acute renal failure precipitated by antihypertensive therapy, particularly angiotensin-converting enzyme (ACE) inhibitors or angiotensin receptor blockers (ARBs).[20] Fibromuscular dysplasia is a common cause of renovascular hypertension in younger patients, especially women between 15 and 50 years of age. On the other hand, atherosclerotic renal artery stenosis occurs in older persons, is bilateral

TABLE 70-3

Clinical and Laboratory Clues for Diagnosis of Secondary Hypertension

CAUSE	CLUES
Renovascular hypertension	Abrupt onset before age 30 years or worsening after age 55 years; renal artery diastolic or lateralizing bruit; resistance to therapy; sustained rise in creatinine after initiation of angiotensin-converting enzyme inhibitor, retinal hemorrhages, exudates, or papilledema; "flash" pulmonary edema
Renoparenchymal disease	Abnormal urinalysis (proteinuria, hematuria); elevated serum creatinine; abnormal renal ultrasonography
Sleep apnea	Obesity; gaspy nocturnal breathing with prominent snoring.
Primary aldosteronism	Unexplained hypokalemia, metabolic alkalosis
Cushing syndrome	Truncal obesity, acne, plethora, fat pads, striae, and bruising; hyperglycemia.
Pheochromocytoma	Labile blood pressure, paroxysms of, palpitations, pallor, perspiration, headache (pain)

SOURCE: *From Hall WD. Resistant hypertension, secondary hypertension, and hypertensive crises. Cardiol Clin 2002;20(2):281–289.*

in 35 to 50 percent of cases, and is associated with atherosclerosis of the coronary, carotid, and lower-extremity vessels. Hypertension in this setting is often resistant to standard therapy.[21]

Numerous invasive and noninvasive tests are available to screen for renal artery stenosis in appropriate patients.[22] Before starting any evaluation it is important to remember that screening tests or angiography are unlikely to benefit those patients who are judged not to be candidates for either surgery or angioplasty. In contrast, if fibromuscular dysplasia is suspected as the etiology of renal artery disease, it is best to proceed directly to renal angiography. The duplex ultrasonography test is noninvasive and safe in all age groups and in patients with impaired renal function. Serial followup examination after revascularization is advised. However, sensitivity and specificity of this measurement are operator dependent, and there can be significant false-negative or false-positive results as a consequence of the operator's inexperience or the presence of obesity or bowel gas.[23] The ACE-inhibitor renal scintiscan in which administration of oral captopril decreases the GFR of the affected kidney using the tracer ^{99}Tc-diethylenetriamine pentaacetic acid (DTPA) is a highly sensitive and specific nuclear imaging test that can be used to identify critical renal artery stenosis. The test lacks anatomic information about the renal arteries, and its accuracy is reduced in patients with impaired renal function.[24,25]

Three-dimensional gadolinium magnetic resonance angiography has been established as a reliable technique for detection and grading of renal artery stenosis. Using current software and digital subtraction techniques, the sensitivity and specificity of this test to diagnose renal artery stenosis exceeds 90 percent. Major disadvantages are related to costs false-positive artifacts related to respiration, peristalsis, and tortuous vessels, and inability to identify nonostial stenosis or stenoses in accessory renal arteries.[26] Renal angiography remains the gold standard for diagnosis. It provides information about the site and severity of stenoses and appropriate revascularization strategies. The need for contrast and its related complications limits its usefulness in patients with impaired renal function. Spiral computed tomography with angiography combines high sensitivity and high specificity. The use of carbon dioxide or gadolinium as contrast agents minimizes the risk of contrast-induced nephrotoxicity.

Treatment of renal artery stenosis is controversial. With the current armamentarium of antihypertensive drugs, satisfactory blood pressure control can be achieved, even in patients with renovascular hypertension. Invasive options to correct the stenosis include renal artery angioplasty with stent placement and surgical revascularization. Case series have reported that angioplasty can restore renal function[27,28] and prevent recurrent heart failure.[29] Comparative trials with medical therapy failed to confirm the beneficial findings,[30] but each trial was small and may have missed important treatment effects as a result of methodologic issues. Most atherosclerotic lesions are now treated initially by angioplasty with balloon-expandable stent placement.[31]

A multidisciplinary approach, including the participation of hypertension specialist, interventional radiology, and vascular surgery, is needed to review all options in a given patient. The central question is whether the benefits of renal revascularization on both blood pressure control and prevention of progressive renal injury outweigh the risks of the procedure. The use of various risk factors has been proposed to select patients who are likely to benefit from revascularization. Urinary protein excretion of at least 1 g/d, hyperuricemia; creatinine clearance of <40 mL/min; age older than 65 years; the presence of coronary artery disease, arterial occlusive disease of the legs, or cerebrovascular disease; and a resistance index of >80 in the segmental arteries of both kidneys, as measured by Doppler ultrasonography, are useful in identifying patients who are unlikely to benefit.[32,33]

【 】 SLEEP APNEA

Obstructive sleep apnea is a common medical condition characterized by abnormal collapse of the pharyngeal airway during sleep, causing repetitive arousals from sleep. It affects 4 percent of middle-aged men and 2 percent of middle-aged women.[34,35] Obstructive sleep apnea may occur in up to 50 percent of patients with hypertension.[36–43] The most common clinical presentation of obstructive sleep apnea is loud snoring, breathing pauses observed by the bed partner, and excessive daytime sleepiness. A formal sleep study usually is needed for diagnosis of obstructive sleep apnea and the determination of corrective interventions. There are several questionnaires that can be used in screening for this disorder.[44,45] Although there is consensus that continuous positive airway pressure treatment can reduce nocturnal blood pressure in patients with obstructive sleep apnea, the effect on daytime blood pressure is less clear. Selected patients may be candidates for oral appliances, uvulopalatopharyngoplasty, or other surgical procedures. Sleep apnea is associated with elevated aldosterone levels, and aldosterone antagonists have been used to treat sleep apnea-related hypertension.[46,47]

PRIMARY ALDOSTERONISM

Screening for hyperaldosteronism should be considered for at least the following patients: hypertensive patients with spontaneous hypokalemia (K+ less than 3.5 mmol/L); hypertensive patients with marked diuretic-induced hypokalemia (K+ less than 3.0 mmol/L); patients with hypertension refractory to treatment with three or more drugs; and hypertensive patients found to have an incidental adrenal adenoma.[48] Screening for hyperaldosteronism includes assessment of plasma aldosterone and plasma renin activity measured under standardized conditions, that is, the collection of morning samples taken from patients in a sitting position after resting at least 15 minutes. Antihypertensive drugs, with the exception of aldosterone antagonists may be continued before initial testing. The screening test is considered positive if the plasma aldosterone/renin activity ratio is greater than 550 pmol/L/ng/mL/h. The diagnosis of primary aldosteronism is established by demonstrating inappropriate autonomous hypersecretion of aldosterone after oral or IV saline loading.[48]

Primary aldosteronism may be caused by the presence of an adrenal adenoma or bilateral adrenal hyperplasia. Imaging with adrenal computed tomography scan or magnetic resonance imaging may help differentiate between the two conditions, although selective adrenal venous sampling may be needed. The treatment of confirmed unilateral aldosterone-producing adenoma is surgical removal of the affected adrenal gland, usually by laparoscopic adrenalectomy. Before pursuing the surgery, patients should be treated medically for 8 to 10 weeks to correct metabolic abnormalities and to control blood pressure. Medical treatment with aldosterone antagonists (spironolactone or eplerenone) should be considered for patients with adrenal hyperplasia, bilateral adenoma, or increased risk of perioperative complications. Amiloride is another alternative for the patient who is intolerant to spironolactone.[48]

CUSHING SYNDROME

Cushing syndrome results from excessive concentrations of circulating free glucocorticoids. Endogenous Cushing syndrome is more common in women; corticotropin-dependent causes account for approximately 80 to 85 percent of cases. Of these, 80 percent are caused by pituitary adenomas (Cushing disease), with the remaining 20 percent caused by ectopic corticotrophin syndrome (Cushing syndrome).[49–51] Cortisol excess predisposes to hypertension by salt retention and glucose intolerance. The presence of facial plethora, rounded face, decreased libido, menstrual irregularity, hirsutism, depression and emotional liability, thin skin in the young, easy bruising, and proximal weakness are clinical clues for Cushing syndrome. The 24-hour urinary free cortisol (>90 mg/d; sensitivity = 100 percent; specificity = 98 percent) is a useful screening test for Cushing syndrome. The single-dose (1-mg) overnight dexamethasone suppression test is equally sensitive but is a little less specific than the 24-hour urinary cortisol. Treatment of Cushing syndrome is either medical or surgical. Metyrapone, ketoconazole, and mitotane can all be used to lower cortisol by directly inhibiting synthesis and secretion in the adrenal gland.[52]

PHEOCHROMOCYTOMA

Patients with paroxysmal and/or severe sustained hypertension who are refractory to the usual antihypertensive therapy should be evaluated for pheochromocytoma. Presence of headaches, palpitations, sweating, panic attacks, pallor in a hypertensive patient are symptoms suggesting a possible pheochromocytoma. Triggering of hypertension by β blockers, monoamine oxidase inhibitors, micturition, or changes in abdominal pressure should also raise the suspicions for pheochromocytoma. It may also be present in some other rare conditions such as patients with hypertension and multiple endocrine neoplasias (MEN-2A/2B), von Recklinghausen neurofibromatosis, or von Hippel-Lindau disease. A 24-hour urinary metanephrine (cutoff point of >3.70 nmol/d) is highly sensitive and specific when done carefully, but urine collection is inconvenient and may be incomplete. Plasma metanephrines (metanephrine >0.66 nmol/L or normetanephrine >0.30 nmol/L) are easy to obtain, and may represent a good screening test for pheochromocytoma, especially if the patient is symptomatic or blood pressure is elevated. Because they have limited specificity (85 percent), a positive plasma metanephrine should be confirmed by the 24-hour urinary metanephrine-to-creatinine ratio (cutoff point of >0.354; specificity = 98 percent) before proceeding to anatomical localization of the tumor. Imaging studies commonly used to localize pheochromocytomas include CT scan and meta-iodobenzylguanidine (MIBG) scintigraphy, the latter is particularly useful when an extraabdominal focus is suspected. α Blockers (prazosin, doxazosin, phenoxybenzamine) should be used as first-line agents in suspected pheochromocytoma. Treatment of benign pheochromocytoma should be surgical resection. It is important not to use β blockers alone because the unopposed α activity will worsen the vasoconstriction, resulting in a further increase in blood pressure. Thus, β blockers should generally be withheld until surgery is performed, unless there are arrhythmias present and adequate α blockade has been achieved. Perioperative care of the patient with pheochromocytoma requires administration of intravenous fluids to ensure adequate volume expansion to avoid shock after tumor removal, and phentolamine hydrochloride as needed for severe hypertension. For patients with inoperable or metastatic malignant pheochromocytoma, blood pressure and adrenergic symptoms may be controlled with α-adrenergic blockade plus beta-blockade and/or tyrosine hydroxylase inhibition with metyrosine.

TREATMENT OF ESSENTIAL HYPERTENSION

Hypertension is the most important preventable cause of premature death[53] and treatment should focus on achieving the recommended blood pressure goal. The benefits of antihypertensive therapy for the prevention of cardiovascular and renal mortality and morbidity are well established.[8] The best evidence demonstrating benefit comes from clinical outcome trials assessing the effect of drug treatment. However, there are recent data relating a reduction in clinical outcomes with lifestyle changes. For most patients, reduction to <140 mmHg for the systolic blood pressure and <90 mmHg for the diastolic blood pressure are the recommended goals of most guideline panels, with lower goals (<130/80 mmHg) recommended in those with diabetes and chronic kidney disease (see Table 70–7 later in this chapter). Observational studies suggest benefit at lower blood pressures. However, these need to be confirmed by specific randomized outcome trials.

Lifestyle Modification

Recent controlled trials have confirmed that lifestyle changes can lower blood pressure.[58–61] Clear verbal and written guidance on lifestyle measures should be provided for all hypertensive patients and those with prehypertension (see Table 70–1). Lifestyle interventions reduce the need for drug therapy, enhance the antihypertensive effects of drugs, and favorably influence overall CVD risk.[8] Conversely, failure to adopt these measures may attenuate the response to antihypertensive drugs.

Lifestyle changes for patients with high blood pressure includes weight reduction, dietary changes (notably reduction of salt intake), moderation of alcohol intake, cessation of smoking, and aerobic exercise (Table 70–4). Weight loss of as little as 10 lbs (4.5 kg) reduces blood pressure and/or prevents hypertension in a large proportion of overweight persons. A diet rich in fruits, vegetables, and low-fat dairy products with a reduced content of dietary cholesterol as well as saturated and total fat (DASH [Dietary Approaches to Stop Hypertension] diet) is helpful in lowering blood pressure.[62] The DASH diet is also rich in potassium and calcium. Patients should be instructed in methods to reduce dietary salt to <6 g/d.[63] Regular aerobic physical activity such as brisk walking at least 30 minutes per day most days of the week should become part of the hypertensive patient's life. Alcohol intake should be limited to no more than 1 oz (30 mL) of ethanol, the equivalent of two drinks, per day in most men, and no more than 0.5 oz of ethanol (one drink) per day in women and lighter weight persons. For overall cardiovascular risk reduction, patients should be strongly counseled to stop smoking.

Pharmacology of Available Antihypertensives

There are nine classes of drugs available for the treatment of hypertension (Table 70–5).

Diuretics are a critical part of the antihypertensive armamentarium. They can be separated based on their mechanism of action.

Thiazide-Type Diuretics
Thiazide-type diuretics inhibit the Na-Cl cotransporter in the distal tubule to reduce extracellular

volume and cardiac output. Diuresis is essential to their antihypertensive action, and their antihypertensive efficacy can be antagonized by high salt intake. Diuresis does not fully explain their long-term blood pressure reduction and these drugs do cause some vasodilatation.[64] Other proposed antihypertensive mechanisms of these agents include activation of Ca^{2+}-activated K^+ channels and alteration of vascular smooth muscle cytosolic pH by inhibiting vascular carbonic anhydrase. Hydrochlorothiazide and chlorthalidone are the most commonly prescribed agents of this class in the United States. Chlorthalidone has 1.5 to 2.0 times the potency of hydrochlorothiazide.[65] Indapamide, at the recommended doses produces less hypokalemia, although at higher doses it behaves similar to other thiazides. Thiazide diuretics were the primary agents used in the initial studies that demonstrated the benefit of blood pressure reduction in patients with hypertension. With the exception of metolazone and indapamide, most thiazide diuretics lose their antihypertensive effectiveness when the GFR declines to <30 to 40 mL/min.

Most side effects of thiazide-type diuretics are related to fluid and electrolyte abnormalities. Hypokalemia, hyponatremia, hypochloremia, hypomagnesemia, metabolic alkalosis, hypercalcemia, and hyperuricemia are among the side effects, and serum electrolyte levels should be monitored at regular intervals. Diuretics can also increase blood glucose and lipids (each approximately 5 mg/dL). The effect of anticoagulants, uricosuric medications, sulfonylureas, and insulin

---

TABLE 70–4

Lifestyle Modifications to Prevent and Manage Hypertension

MODIFICATION	RECOMMENDATION	APPROXIMATE SYSTOLIC BLOOD PRESSURE REDUCTION (RANGE)
Weight reduction	Maintain normal body weight (body mass index 18.5–24.9 kg/m²)	5–20 mmHg/ 10 kg
Adopt DASH (Dietary Approaches to Stop Hypertension) eating plan	Consume a diet rich in fruits, vegetables, and low-fat dairy products with a reduced content of saturated and total fat	8–14 mmHg
Dietary sodium reduction	Reduce dietary sodium intake to no more than 100 mmol/d (2.4 g sodium or 6 g sodium chloride)	2–8 mmHg
Physical activity	Engage in regular aerobic physical activity such as brisk walking (at least 30 minutes per day, most days of the week).	4–9 mmHg
Moderation of alcohol consumption	Limit consumption to no more than 2 drinks (e.g., 24 oz beer, 10 oz wine, or 3 oz 80-proof whiskey) per day in most men and to no more than 1 drink per day in women and lighter weight persons	2–4 mmHg

SOURCE: Adapted from Chobanian AV, Bakris GL, Black HR, et al. Seventh Report of the Joint National Committee on Prevention, Detection, Evaluation, and Treatment of High Blood Pressure. NIH Publication No. 04–5230. Available at: http://www.nhlbi.nih.gov/guidelines/hypertension/jnc7full.htm.

TABLE 70-5

Antihypertensive Drug Classes[a]

CLASS	DRUG (TRADE NAME)	USUAL DOSE RANGE IN MG/D	USUAL DAILY FREQUENCY[a]
Thiazide diuretics			
	chlorothiazide (Diuril)	125–500	1–2
	chlorthalidone (generic)	12.5–25	1
	hydrochlorothiazide (Microzide, HydroDIURIL[b])	12.5–50	1
		2–4	1
	polythiazide (Renese)	1.25–2.5	1
	indapamide (Lozol[b])	0.5–1.0	1
	metolazone (Mykrox)	2.5–5	1
	bendroflumethiazide	2.5–10	1–2
	metolazone (Zaroxolyn)		
Loop diuretics			
	bumetanide (Bumex[b])	0.5–2	2
	furosemide (Lasix[b])	20–80	2
	torsemide (Demadex[b])	2.5–10	1
Potassium-sparing diuretics			
	amiloride (Midamor[b])	5–10	1–2
	triamterene (Dyrenium)	50–100	1–2
Aldosterone receptor blockers			
	eplerenone (Inspra)	50–100	1–2
	spironolactone (Aldactone[b])	25–50	1
β Blockers			
	atenolol (Tenormin[b])	25–100	1
	betaxolol (Kerlone[b])	5–20	1
	bisoprolol (Zebeta[b])	2.5–10	1
	metoprolol (Lopressor[b])	50–100	1–2
	metoprolol extended release (Toprol XL)	50–100	1
	nadolol (Corgard[b])	40–120	1
	propranolol (Inderal[b])	40–160	2
	propranolol long-acting (Inderal LA[b])	60–180	1
	timolol (Blocadren[b])	20–40	2
	Nebivolol (Nebilet[c])	5	1
β Blockers with intrinsic sympathomimetic activity			
	acebutolol (Sectral[b])	200–800	2
	penbutolol (Levatol)	10–40	1
	pindolol (generic)	10–40	2
Combined α and β blockers			
	carvedilol (Coreg[c])	12.5–50	2
	labetalol (Normodyne, Trandate[b])	200–800	2
ACEIs			
	benazepril (Lotensin[b])	10–40	1
	captopril (Capoten[b])	50–200	2
	enalapril (Vasotec[b])	50–40	1–2
	fosinopril (Monopril)	10–40	1
	lisinopril (Prinivil, Zestril[b])	10–40	1
	moexipril (Univasc)	7.5–30	1
	perindopril (Aceon)	4–8	1
	quinapril (Accupril)	10–80	1
	ramipril (Altace)	2.5–20	1
	trandolapril (Mavik)	1–4	1

(continued)

TABLE 70–5

Antihypertensive Drug Classes^a *(continued)*

CLASS	DRUG (TRADE NAME)	USUAL DOSE RANGE IN MG/D	USUAL DAILY FREQUENCY^a
Angiotensin II antagonists			
	candesartan (Atacand)	8–32	1
	eprosartan (Teveten)	400–800	1–2
	irbesartan (Avapro)	150–300	1
	losartan (Cozaar)	25–100	1–2
	olmesartan (Benicar)	20–40	1
	telmisartan (Micardis)	20–80	1
	valsartan (Diovan)	80–320	1–2
Calcium channel blockers—nondihydropyridines			
	diltiazem extended release (Cardizem CD, Dilacor XR, Tiazac^b)	180–420	1
	diltiazem extended release (Cardizem LA)	120–540	1
	verapamil immediate release (Calan, Isoptin^b)	80–320	2
	verapamil long acting (Calan SR, Isoptin SR^b)	120–480	1–2
	verapamil (Covera HS, Verelan PM)	120–360	1
CCBs—Dihydropyridines			
	amlodipine (Norvasc)	2.5–10	1
	felodipine (Plendil)	2.5–20	1
	isradipine (Dynacirc CR)	2.5–10	2
	nicardipine sustained release (Cardene SR)	6–120	2
	nifedipine long-acting (Adalat CC, Procardia XL)	30–60	1
	nisoldipine (Sular)	10–40	1
α_1 Blockers			
	doxazosin (Cardura)	1–16	1
	prazosin (Minipress^b)	2–20	2–3
	terazosin (Hytrin)	1–20	1–2
Central α_2 agonists and other centrally acting drugs			
	clonidine (Catapres^b)	0.1–0.8	2
	clonidine patch (Catapres-TTS)	0.1–0.3	1 wkly
	methyldopa (Aldomet^b)	250–1000	2
	reserpine (generic)	0.1–0.25	1
	guanfacine (Tenex^b)	0.5–2	1
Direct vasodilators			
	hydralazine (Apresoline^b)	25–100	2
	minoxidil (Loniten^b)	2.5–80	1–2
Renin inhibitor			
	Aliskiren^d	50–600	1

^aIn some patients treated once daily, the antihypertensive effect may diminish toward the end of the dosing interval (trough effect). Blood pressure should be measured just prior to dosing to determine if satisfactory blood pressure control is obtained. Accordingly, an increase in dosage or frequency may need to be considered. These dosages may vary from those listed in the *Physicians' Desk Reference*, 61st ed. (2007).
^bAvailable in generic preparations.
^cLicense may only exist in some countries.
^dPending FDA approval.
SOURCE: Adapted from Chobanian AV, Bakris GL, Black HR, et al. Seventh Report of the Joint National Committee on Prevention, Detection, Evaluation, and Treatment of High Blood Pressure. NIH Publication No. 04–5230. Available at: http://www.nhlbi.nih.gov/guidelines/hypertension/jnc7full.htm.

may be diminished by thiazides. Conversely, they can increase the effect of diazoxide, loop diuretics, digitals, lithium, nonsteroidal antiinflammatory drugs (NSAIDs), and bile acid sequestrants. The hyponatremia can be concerning, especially in the elderly.

Loop Diuretics Loop diuretics inhibit Na-K-2Cl transport in the thick ascending limb of the loop of Henle and include furosemide, bumetanide, ethacrynic acid, and torsemide. Because of their short half-life, they are less effective than thiazide-type diuretics in lowering blood pressure in patients with normal renal function when prescribed once or twice daily. In those with estimated GFR <30–40 mL/min/1.73 m², their use is essential to achieve blood pressure goals. They are also usually required for volume control in those requiring vasodilators, especially minoxidil. Most adverse reactions are related to electrolyte abnormalities, that is, extracellular volume depletion, hypokalemia, hyponatremia, hypochloremic alkalosis, hyperuricemia, and hyperglycemia. Increased Mg and Ca excretion may lead to hypomagnesemia and hypocalcemia. NSAIDs and probenecid blunt the effect of loop diuretics and thiazide diuretics have synergic effects with loop diuretics.

Potassium-Sparing Diuretics The potassium-sparing diuretics triamterene and amiloride inhibit the renal epithelial Na channels and cause small increases in NaCl excretion. They are relatively weak diuretics and rarely used as a single agent in the treatment of hypertension or edema. They are useful in preventing diuretic-induced hypokalemia when prescribed with other diuretics. The most serious side effect of this class of diuretics is hyperkalemia. Use with NSAIDs, ACE inhibitors, ARBs, β blockers and in diabetic hypertensives with or without nephropathy increases the risk of this side effect.

Antagonists of Mineralocorticoid Receptors These are another class of potassium-sparing diuretics. Mineralocorticoids bind to the mineralocorticoid receptor to cause salt and water retention and increase the excretion of potassium and H⁺. The two available mineralocorticoid antagonist are spironolactone and eplerenone. Mineralocorticoid antagonists, often in combination with thiazides or loop diuretics, are effective in treating hypertension. They are particularly useful in the treatment of primary aldosteronism. The major adverse effects of these agents include hyperkalemia, hypertriglyceridemia, and antiandrogen effects like breast pain, gynecomastia, and sexual dysfunction in males. Eplerenone is more selective for the mineralocorticoid receptor than the spironolactone and less likely to produce antiandrogenic effects.

Calcium Channel Blockers Calcium channel blockers (CCBs) inhibit calcium entry into vasculature smooth muscle through the voltage-sensitive L-type Ca^{2+} channels, resulting in vasodilation of coronary and peripheral arteries. Two subclasses of calcium channel blockers, dihydropyridines (DHPs; e.g., nifedipine) and non-

dihydropyridines (non-DHP; e.g., verapamil and diltiazem) are available (see Table 70–5). They have similar antihypertensive efficacy but differ in their effect on cardiac contractility, vasodilation, and atrioventricular conduction. Non-DHP CCBs, like the β blockers, substantially reduce contractility and atrioventricular nodal conduction. Thus, they are appropriate when β blockers are not anticipated to be needed for blood pressure lowering (i.e., for those patients expected to require four or fewer antihypertensives). They are inappropriate for the patient with significant left ventricular dysfunction or atrioventricular block. Unlike the DHP-CCBs, they are less likely to produce headache, edema, and palpitations. The non-DHP CCB, verapamil relaxes gastrointestinal smooth muscle, making it more likely to cause constipation. In the older hypertensive, and in other individuals who are predisposed to this condition, diltiazem is the non-DHP of choice. A common mistake in dosing diltiazem for hypertension is to use lower (antianginal) doses. Typical antihypertensive doses of diltiazem range from 180 to 540 mg/d.

The DHP-CCBs are potent arteriolar vasodilators and especially effective in the more resistant patient as their antihypertensive action and side-effect profile complements that of β blockers when used together. They have little effect on cardiac conduction and contractility. Both felodipine and amlodipine have demonstrated their safety in hypertensives with systolic dysfunction in heart failure trials.

The most common side effect of the DHP-CCBs include headache, flushing, and dose-dependent peripheral edema. The edema results from precapillary arteriolar dilatation and transudation of fluid from the vascular compartments into dependent tissues rather than from fluid retention; it does not respond well to treatment with diuretics.

β Blockers β Blockers lower blood pressure predominantly by inhibiting β₁-adrenergic receptors. Thus, they reduce cardiac output by decreasing cardiac contractility and heart rate. Renin release and the generation of angiotensin II is also inhibited by this mechanism.[64] In addition, β blockers are reported to alter baroceptor sensitivity, downregulate peripheral adrenergic receptors, and increase prostacyclin biosynthesis. They are particularly beneficial in hypertensive patients with coronary disease and heart failure (Table 70–6). *They are less effective in lowering blood pressure in black*

TABLE 70–6

Compelling Indications for Individual Drug Classes

COMPELLING INDICATION	RECOMMENDED DRUGS					
	DIURETIC	BB	ACEI	ARB	CCB	ALDO ANT
Heart failure	✕	✕	✕	✕		✕
Postmyocardial infarction		✕	✕			✕
High coronary disease risk	✕	✕	✕		✕	
Diabetes	✕	✕	✕	✕	✕	
Chronic kidney disease			✕	✕		
Recurrent stroke prevention	✕		✕			

ACEI, angiotensin-converting enzyme inhibitor; Aldo ANT, aldosterone antagonist; ARB, angiotensin receptor blocker; BB, β blocker; CCB, calcium channel blocker.
SOURCE: Adapted from Chobanian AV, Bakris GL, Black HR, et al. Seventh Report of the Joint National Committee on Prevention, Detection, Evaluation, and Treatment of High Blood Pressure. NIH Publication No. 04–5230. Available at: http://www.nhlbi.nih.gov/guidelines/hypertension/jnc7full.htm.

patients and in the elderly unless accompanied by the use of diuretics or calcium channel blockers. β Blockers with intrinsic sympathomimetic activity properties may be useful in patients requiring β blockade who develop bradycardia or vasoconstrictor symptoms (e.g., claudication). β Blockers with α blocker properties show faster onset of blood pressure lowering and less effect on blood glucose and lipids.[66] Despite the pharmacokinetic and pharmacodynamic differences among various β blockers, they have similar clinical antihypertensive efficacy, and the additional properties have not been shown to offer added benefits on clinical outcomes.

Inhibitors of the Renin–Angiotensin System Pharmacologic inhibition of the renin–angiotensin system (RAS) can occur by inhibiting the formation of angiotensin II (ACE inhibitors or by blocking its receptor (ARBs). They are specifically indicated in hypertensive patients with heart failure and chronic kidney disease. ACE inhibitors also are useful in hypertensive patients following a large myocardial infarction and in combination with thiazide-type diuretics after a stroke (see Table 70–6). A new class of RAS inhibitors, the renin inhibitors, will soon be released in the United States. RAS inhibitors, like the β blockers, are less effective in lowering blood pressure, and they are less effective in preventing cardiovascular events in black hypertensive patients (see Ethnicity section below). Generally, ACE inhibitors and ARBs are well tolerated, and the incidence of side effects is low. Although rare, angioedema can occur at any time during treatment and occurs more frequently in blacks. Cough occurs in up to 25 percent of patients (also increased in blacks). ARBs (and presumably renin inhibitors) are reasonable alternatives for patients with ACE inhibitor-associated cough. Generally, it is recommended to avoid ARBs in patients with a history of ACE inhibitor-related angioedema, although there are case reports of this being done safely.

α Blockers The α blockers prazosin, terazosin, and doxazosin block the activation of the vasoconstricting $α_1$-adrenoreceptors. They are indicated for add-on therapy with other agents for blood pressure control. Additional properties include alleviation of some of the symptoms of benign prostatic hypertrophy. Postural hypotension is often a problem, especially with the initiation of therapy, rapid dosage titration, and with shorter-acting prazosin.

$α_2$ Agonists Central $α_2$ agonists include methyldopa, clonidine, guanabenz, and guanfacine, and stimulate central nervous system $α_2$ receptors to reduce central nervous system sympathetic outflow. The antihypertensive efficacy of these agents diminish with time when given as monotherapy. Their effect is enhanced by concomitant diuretic, vasodilator, or CCB administration. They are less effective when prescribed with other sympatholytics or with inhibitors of the renin–angiotensin system. Clonidine is useful in treating hypertensive urgencies and emergencies. The most common side effects include sedation, dry mouth, and, fatigue. Liver dysfunction and a Coombs-positive hemolytic anemia can be seen with methyldopa.

Vasodilators Short-acting direct arterial vasodilators such as hydralazine and minoxidil have been largely replaced by better tolerated and more effective drugs such as the CCBs. However, minoxidil is a powerful vasodilator, which is generally used to treat

resistant hypertension. Hirsutism, fluid retention, which can result in pericardial effusion/tamponade and heart failure, are the major side effects of these medications, and can occur in the absence of careful monitoring and attention to fluid status.

Drug Therapy of Hypertension

The number of patients with hypertension by itself, without other cardiovascular risk factors or target-organ damage, is small. However, few of these conditions specifically include or exclude one class over another (see Table 70–6). Thus the uncomplicated hypertensive can be defined as one without a specific indication for a specific class of antihypertensive (compelling indication). The overriding goal of treating the patient with uncomplicated hypertension is to lower systolic blood pressure consistently to <140 mmHg and diastolic blood pressure to <90 mmHg.[6–8,13,55,57] In most hypertensive patients, achieving the goal blood pressure requires lifestyle modification and drug therapy. Furthermore, multiple drugs are required in most patients to achieve the recommended blood pressure goals. In patients whose blood pressure is more than 20 mmHg above their blood pressure goal, most guideline panels recommend initiating multiple drug therapy either as individual agents or using combination agents (Table 70–7).

Factors determining initial antihypertensive drug selection include blood pressure lowering-efficacy, availability of favorable clinical outcome data, tolerability, presence of concomitant diseases such as diabetes or target-organ damage (chronic kidney disease, coronary artery, heart failure), and cost of drugs. Blood pressure-lowering efficacy is similar across drug classes, except for reduced efficacy with ACE inhibitors, ARBs, and β blockers in black patients unless combined with a diuretic or CCB. Placebo-controlled, double-blind, tolerability studies demonstrate little difference in tolerability aside from those predicted by the drug's mechanism of action (e.g., bronchospasm with β blockers, orthostatic hypotension with α blockers, cough with ACE inhibitors, edema with DHP-CCBs, and urinary urgency with short-acting diuretics).[67,68] Although all classes except ARBs and renin inhibitors have members at generic prices, diuretics continue to be the least-expensive drugs.

The placebo-controlled outcome trials have demonstrated cardiovascular disease (including renal disease and stroke) reduction with nearly all classes of antihypertensive agents. Beginning in the late 1990s, results of studies comparing different classes of antihypertensive agents on clinical outcomes became available (Table 70–8). With few exceptions, benefit from the various regimens on reducing clinical outcomes correlated with degree of blood pressure lowering rather than specific drug characteristics. Thiazide-type diuretics, introduced in the early 1950s have been the most studied, most recommended, and most cost-effective of all the antihypertensive drug classes. They remain unsurpassed by any other antihypertensive class in preventing clinical outcomes (Table 70–8).

The metabolic effects, especially the increase in glucose with thiazide diuretics compared to other agents like ACE inhibitors, have raised concerns about the risk of type II diabetes with the long-term use of thiazide diuretics. The questions about the significance of the metabolic effects of available agents prompted the multiple clinical outcomes trials in the 1990s that compared antihypertensives with differing metabolic effects to determine

TABLE 70–7

Summary of Major Available Guidelines for Treatment of Hypertension

GUIDELINE	INITIAL DRUG OF CHOICE IN UNCOMPLICATED HTN	INITIAL DRUG OF CHOICE IN PATIENTS WITH DM	HAS INITIATION WITH COMBINATION BEEN SUPPORTED?	BLOOD PRESSURE TREATMENT GOAL IN HIGH RISK POPULATION	
				DM	CKD
Australian Hypertension Management Guide[54]	All antihypertensive medications can be used based on cardiovascular risk profile.	ACEIs and ARBs	Yes	<130/85 mmHg	<130/85 mmHg and if proteinuria is more than 1 g/d the blood pressure goal is <125/75 mmHg
Canadian Recommendations for the Management of Hypertension[55]	Diuretics, β blockers and ACEIs, ARBs, and CCBs	ACEIs and ARBs or thiazide diuretics	Yes	<130/80 mmHg	130/80 mmHg and if proteinuria is more than 1 g/d the blood pressure goal is <125/75
European Society of Hypertension European Society of Cardiology[13]	All major classes including diuretics, β blockers, CCBs, ACEIs, and ARBs	ARBs	Yes	<130/80 mmHg	—
The British Hypertension Society Guidelines[7]	<u><55 y/o and non-blacks:</u> ACEIs/ARBs or β blockers <u>>55 y/o or blacks:</u> Diuretics or CCBs	ACEIs and ARBs	Yes	<130/80 mmHg	—
The Seventh Report of the Joint National Committee (JNC 7)[56]	Diuretics	Combination of medications which should an be an ACEI- or ARB-based regimen	Yes	<130/80 mmHg	<130/80 mmHg
World Health Organization (WHO) International Society of Hypertension (ISH) statement on management of hypertension[6]	Diuretics	ACEIs and ARBs	Yes	<130/80 mmHg	<130/80 mmHg
NICE Guidelines[57]	<u><55 y/o and non-blacks:</u> ACEIs/ARBs or β blockers <u>>55 y/o or blacks:</u> Diuretics or CCBs	ACEIs and ARBs	Yes	—	—

ACEI, angiotensin-converting enzyme inhibitor; ARB, angiotensin receptor blocker; CCB, calcium channel blocker; CKD, chronic kidney disease; DM, diabetes mellitus; HTN, hypertension; y/o, years old.

whether the differences correlated with differences in clinical outcomes, especially coronary events. In the ALLHAT (Antihypertensive and Lipid-lowering Treatment to Prevent Heart Attack Trial), the 4-year rate of new-onset diabetes with the diuretic chlorthalidone was 11.6 percent, compared with 9.8 percent for the CCB and 8.1 percent for the ACE inhibitor, although the mean difference in fasting glucose between the diuretic and ACEI was approximately 5 mg/dL and approximately 8 mg/dL between the diuretic and α blocker. Despite the differences in glucose levels, diabetes incidence, and comparable changes in cholesterol, the 5-year end

TABLE 70–8

Comparative Effect of Antihypertensive Drug Classes on Cardiovascular Outcomes in the Major Hypertension Outcome Trials

TRIAL	DESIGN	POPULATION	TREATMENT GROUPS	OUTCOME
ALLHAT trial[69,70]	PRDB	42,418	1- Chlorthalidone 2- Lisinopril 3- Doxazosin 4- Amlodipine	Chlorthalidone was superior to doxazosin and lisinopril but not to amlodipine
ANBP2 trial[71]	PROBE	6083	1- ACEI (enalapril recommended) 2- Diuretic (hydrochlorothiazide recommended)	Overall no difference between the groups; in males, ACEIs were superior to diuretic
ASCOT-BPLA trial[72]	PROBE	19,257	1- Amlodipine adding perindopril 2- Atenolol adding bendroflumethiazide	Amlodipine base treatment was superior to atenolol base treatment
CAPPP trial[73]	PROBE	10,985	1- Captopril 2- β Blocker and/or diuretic	No difference between groups
CONVINCE trial[74]	PRDB	16,602	1- Verapamil 2- Hydrochlorothiazide or atenolol	No difference between the groups
INSIGHT trial[75]	RRDB	6321	1- Nifedipine 2- Coamilozide (hydrochlorothiazide plus amiloride)	No difference between the groups
LIFE trial[76]	PRDB	9193	1- Losartan 2- Atenolol	Losartan was superior to atenolol
NORDIL trial77	PRDB	11,000	1- Diltiazem 2- β Blocker and/or diuretic	Diltiazem is not superior to β blocker and/or diuretic
STOP-2 trial[73]	PROBE	6614	1- Dihydropyridine calcium channel blocker (felodipine or isradipine) 2- β Blocker or diuretic	No difference between the groups
VALUE[78]	PROBE	15,525	1- ARB 2- DHP-CCB	ARB not superior to DHP-CCB

ACEI, angiotensin-converting enzyme inhibitor; ARB, angiotensin receptor blocker; DHP-CCB, dihydropyridine–calcium channel blocker; PRDB, prospective, randomized, double-blind design; PROBE, prospective, randomized, open-label, masked end point assessment design.

point data demonstrated that chlorthalidone performed as well as (or better) than doxazosin, amlodipine, and lisinopril in reducing cardiovascular disease rates. These are consistent with data from other studies (Fig. 70–1).[79,80]

Although one study with up to 16 years of followup suggested an increase in cardiovascular disease rates in new-onset diabetics, the study did not show this to be related to diuretic therapy.[81] The metabolic differences between antihypertensives in clinical trials such as ALLHAT, VALUE, and STOP-2 with up to 8 years of followup have not been associated with differences in cardiovascular or cerebrovascular events.[73,78,82,83] The small differences in glucose levels between antihypertensive agents are likely overwhelmed by other differences between agents, especially blood pressure lowering, even if the differences result in the more individuals crossing the threshold defining diabetes.

The findings to date confirm that in the patient with uncomplicated hypertension, as well as in the patient with diabetes without nephropathy, initial therapy with "newer therapies" (e.g. ACEIs, CCBs, and ARBs) are effective, but not more effective than older agents (thiazide-type diuretics and β blockers) at reducing stroke, coronary heart disease morbidity or mortality, or all-cause mortal-

ity.[84] The caveats to this general conclusion are that recent studies indicate that β blockers are less effective than ARBs and CCBs in preventing cardiovascular disease outcomes, and in older studies they were less effective than thiazide-type diuretics.[71,72,74,76,85] CCB-based therapy appears less protective than other agents (except α blockers) in preventing the development of heart failure, but may be slightly more beneficial in stroke prevention.[83] There are compelling indications for specific drug classes in those with hypertension and specific target-organ damage (see Table 70–6).

In summary, given their low cost and unsurpassed efficacy, thiazide diuretics remain the drug of first choice in uncomplicated hypertensive patients—regardless of gender, age, or race—to be included in most antihypertensive drug regimens. This is consistent with the recommendation of most guideline panels, including JNC 7, although the recommendations of some panels continue to show concern over the metabolic consequences of these agents (see Table 70–7). ACE inhibitors, ARBs, and CCBs followed by β blockers are reasonable choices to be added to the regimen for blood pressure control or as an alternative in the patient who cannot tolerate a diuretic, although a CCB would be the preferred alternative in blacks. In the absence of heart failure or renal disease,

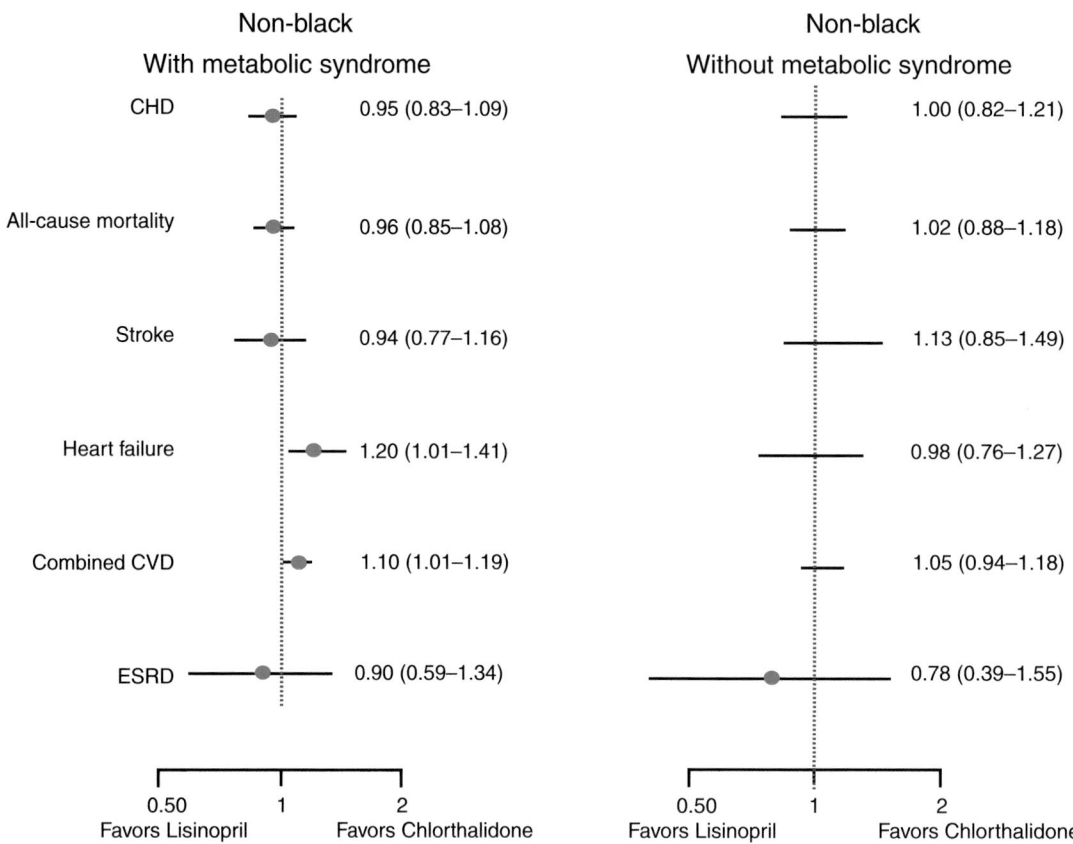

FIGURE 70–1. Lisinopril/chlorthalidone. *Source: Adapted from Wright JT Jr, Dunn JK, Cutler JA, et al. Outcomes in hypertensive black and nonblack patients treated with chlorthalidone, amlodipine, and lisinopril. JAMA 2005;293:131595–131608.*

inhibitors of the renin–angiotensin system have shown little advantage in clinical trials over diuretics (or CCBs) in preventing cardiovascular disease and are not indicated as an initial therapy in blacks.

Importantly, the major goal of therapy is to reduce the blood pressure below the blood pressure goal. In the overwhelming majority of patients, this will require multiple agents. After the initial drug selection, drugs should be added to the regimen in a rational manner taking advantage of complementary mechanisms of action and concomitant clinical condition(s). To facilitate patients achieving their blood pressure goal, nearly all guideline panels support the initiation of treatment with two or more antihypertensive medications to achieve the blood pressure goals in most of the patients when blood pressure is more than 20/10 mmHg above goal. Patients with indications for specific agents should obviously have these included in the regimen.

SPECIAL POPULATIONS

【 】 ELDERLY

The prevalence of hypertension is high, 60 to 80 percent, in populations older than 65 years of age. Systolic blood pressure rises and

diastolic blood pressure declines after ages 50 to 55 years in both normotensive and untreated hypertensive subjects.[86,87] Thus hypertension in older hypertensive patients is characterized by elevated systolic and pulse pressure, and these parameters are also the major predictors of outcome in this population.[87,88] In older hypertensives, measuring standing blood pressure becomes important because of the increased risk of orthostatic hypotension and the greater need for agents that may aggravates this condition. In addition, in those with acute worsening of their hypertension or onset of the disease after age 50 years, greater attention to the possibility of secondary hypertension should be considered.

Despite the strongest evidence supporting the benefit of treatment of hypertension being noted in older patients, they are the group least likely to be treated to their blood pressure goal. Similar to the other patients, lifestyle modification is effective and the cornerstone of treatment in older populations.[89] Drug selection and the blood pressure goal in the elderly is similar to that in younger populations, but there are a few special considerations in these patients. Starting medication doses should be lower than in younger patients and blood pressure reduction should be more gradual. Most older hypertensives achieve their diastolic blood pressure goal, and it is the systolic blood pressure goal that is more challenging. Multiple antihypertensives are required to achieve this goal in a population that already requires multiple medications for other conditions. The best evidence and most guidelines recommend the inclusion of a thiazide diuretic as one agent in the regimen. A CCB is a reasonable alternative at an increased cost and with less protection against heart failure. A long-acting thiazide (chlorthalidone or metolazone) may be considered in patients who note urgency with shorter-acting agents like hydrochlorothiazides.

[ ] DIABETIC HYPERTENSION

Diabetes is highly prevalent in hypertensive patients, and when they occur together, places the patient at markedly higher risk for complications of both diseases. More than 35 percent of hypertensives have diabetes, and approximately 75 percent of diabetics are either on medications or have a blood pressure higher than the recommended goal of 130/80 mmHg. In more than half of diabetics, their blood pressures are >140/90 mmHg.[90] Appropriate treatment of hypertension in diabetic patients is aimed at minimizing the effects of these disorders on cardiovascular and kidney disease outcomes, although retinopathy benefits from aggressive antihypertensive therapy.[91]

Diabetes is the leading cause of end-stage renal disease in the United States in all ethnic/race subgroups. Elevated blood pressure is associated with greater risk of end-stage renal disease, and blood pressure lowering slows the progression of renal disease. Multiple studies of renal outcomes have demonstrated that blood pressure lowering using either an ACE inhibitor or an ARB will slow the progression of both type 1 and 2 diabetic renal disease.[92–95] In hypertensive patients with diabetes and renal disease, an ACE inhibitor or an ARB should be included in the regimen. Nearly every patient with renal insufficiency will require a diuretic to lower blood pressure, especially to the recommended goal of <130/80 mmHg. In the ALLHAT, one of the few renal outcome studies able to address this question, there was no loss of protection against renal disease progression when a diuretic-based regimen was compared with one containing an ACE inhibitor, even in participants with diabetes.[96] Several studies suggest that CCBs are less effective in preventing renal outcomes than either an ACE inhibitor or ARB.[92,97]

The most common complication and leading cause of death in the diabetic is cardiovascular disease. Several clinical trials have also demonstrated cardiovascular benefit with "aggressive" blood pressure lowering in diabetic patients. In fact, the increased risk associated with diabetes in the presence of hypertension and available observational and clinical trial evidence in diabetic patients were sufficiently convincing to justify most guideline panels to recommend a lower blood pressure goal in the diabetic than in the nondiabetic patient (see Table 70–7).

For patients with diabetes and hypertension, the recommended blood pressure goal is <130/80 mmHg. Clinical trial evidence was provided by the HOT (Hypertension Optimal Treatment) study to define the diastolic blood pressure goal of <80 mmHg in diabetic patients. The systolic blood pressure goal of <130 mmHg appears to be mostly based on observational data showing a linear relationship between systolic blood pressure and cardiovascular outcomes starting at a systolic blood pressure <120 mmHg. Clinical trials provide evidence of benefit for achieved systolic blood pressures as low as 144 mmHg in the UKPDS (United Kingdom Prospective Diabetes Study) and 138 mmHg in the HOT trial in diabetics.[98,99] The ongoing Action to Control Cardiovascular Risk in Diabetes (ACCORD) study comparing a blood pressure goal of <120 mmHg systolic versus a target of <140 mmHg systolic should provide the definitive answer in this high-risk group.

Although ACE inhibitors and ARBs are significantly better than other antihypertensive classes in slowing progression of diabetic renal disease, they do not appear to have an advantage over thiazide diuretics or CCBs in the prevention of cardiovascular disease. Thus, most antihypertensive agents are now recommended in diabetics without nephropathy or albuminuria (see Table 70–6).

[ ] ETHNICITY

Ethnic and racial differences in hypertension prevalence, severity, and response to therapy have been reported.[100–102] Hypertension is more common and severe in black populations than in white populations, and its onset begins at an earlier age. It is less common and less severe in Mexican Americans and Native Americans, but blood pressure control rates are generally lower. Reasons for the ethnic differences in hypertension are unknown. Clinical evaluation and diagnostic testing is similar regardless of ethnicity. Because a major screening criteria for secondary hypertension is based on hypertension severity and resistance, the higher prevalence and severity of essential hypertension in blacks means a higher percentage of evaluations will not be positive, making screening more challenging. In addition, despite a higher prevalence of left ventricular hypertrophy, the ECG is less specific for detecting left ventricular hypertrophy in blacks with false-positive rates up to 40 percent.[103,104]

In general, the treatment of hypertension is similar for all demographic groups, but socioeconomic factors may present barriers to blood pressure control in some ethnic groups. African Americans demonstrate somewhat reduced blood pressure lowering in response to monotherapy with β blockers, ACE inhibitors, or ARBs, compared to diuretics or CCBs. These differential responses are largely eliminated by drug combinations that include adequate doses of a diuretic or CCB. ACE inhibitors were less effective in preventing many major clinical outcomes (including heart failure, stroke, and coronary events) than diuretics in black participants on ACE inhibitors in the ALLHAT trial (Fig. 70–2). Less benefit in cardiovascular event reduction was also seen in the small black cohort (n = 533) in the LIFE trial with the ARB losartan (Fig. 70–2). Thus, thiazide diuretics (or CCBs) are preferred over RAS-blocking agents in black patients. Where compelling indications (i.e., heart failure or renal disease) have been identified for prescribing RAS-blocking agents (either ACE inhibitors or ARBs) or β blockers, these compelling indications should be applied equally to black patients. In addition, because of the severity of hypertension in this population, RAS blockers will usually be required (added to diuretics and CCBs) to achieve the blood pressure goal.[95]

[ ] RENAL DISEASE

Hypertension is well-recognized as a risk factor for progression of renal disease.[105] Consequently, the goals of treatment of hypertension in chronic kidney disease are both to slow decline in renal function and to reduce risk for cardiovascular disease. Current Kidney Disease Outcomes Quality Initiative (K/DOQI) *Clinical Practice Guidelines on Hypertension and Antihypertensive Agents in Chronic Kidney Disease* and also JNC 7 recommend a goal blood pressure of 130/80 mmHg

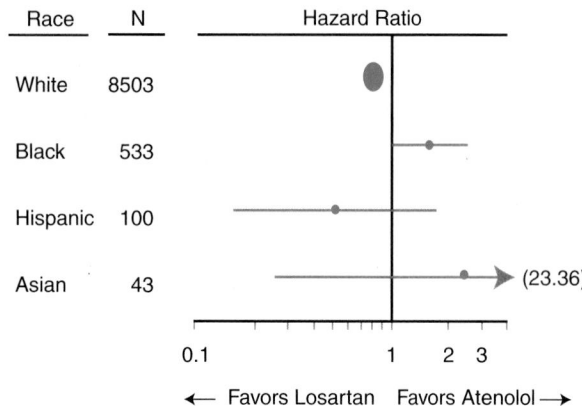

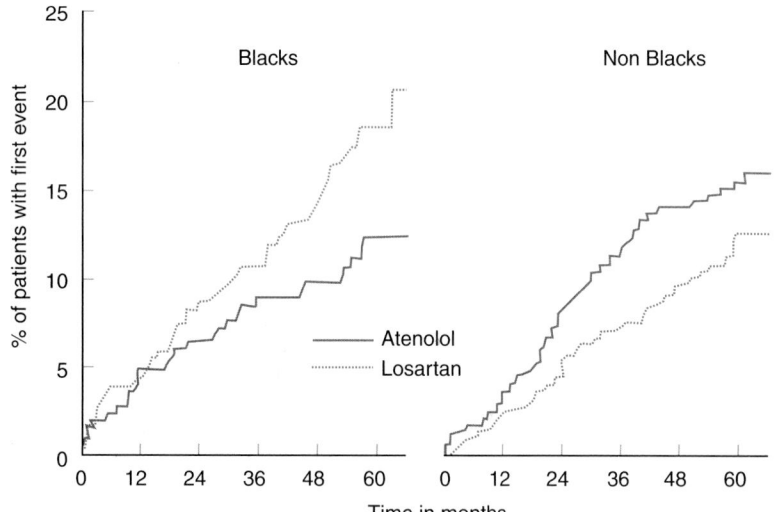

FIGURE 70–2. Results of primary composite end point in LIFE by ethnic group. The dots *(top)* represent the hazard ratio; dot size is proportional to the number of patients for each ethnic group, as shown to the left. The line through each dot corresponds to the 95% confidence interval. *Source: From Julius S, Alderman MH, Beevers G, et al. J Am Coll Cardiol 2004;43:1047–1055.*

in patients with chronic kidney disease. These guidelines are based on epidemiologic data showing the relationship between hypertension and renal/cardiovascular outcomes, and secondary analyses of clinical trial data showing a beneficial effect of lower blood pressure levels on prevention of renal and cardiovascular disease. Patients with proteinuria >1g/d have been shown to benefit from an even lower blood pressure goal (<125/75 mmHg).

Several studies show that inhibition of the renin–angiotensin axis is superior to conventional antihypertensive therapy in slowing decline in renal function in patients with diabetic nephropathy and proteinuria.[97] Consequently, patients with diabetic kidney disease or nondiabetic kidney disease with a total protein/creatinine ratio of 200 mg/g or greater should be treated with an ACE inhibitor or ARB; a diuretic and other agents should be added as necessary to reach the target blood pressure.

[ ] HYPERTENSION DURING PREGNANCY

Hypertension occurring during pregnancy falls into four major classifications[106]:

1. Chronic hypertension is the presence of hypertension before the 20th week of gestation or persistent hypertension for longer than 12 weeks postpartum.
2. Gestational hypertension (also called *transient hypertension*) refers to elevated blood pressure first detected after 20 weeks of gestation without proteinuria, and
3. Preeclampsia-eclampsia (also called *pregnancy-induced hypertension*) is defined by new onset of hypertension with a systolic blood pressure ≥140 mmHg or a diastolic blood pressure ≥90 mmHg after 20th week of gestation in a previously normotensive woman, which is accompanied by more than 300 mg proteinuria in 24 hours.
4. Preeclampsia superimposed on underlying hypertension.

For management and counseling purposes, chronic hypertension in pregnancy is also categorized as either low risk or high risk (Fig. 70–3). The patient is considered to be at low risk when she has mild essential hypertension without any organ involvement.

Women with low-risk chronic hypertension without superimposed preeclampsia usually have a pregnancy outcome similar to that in the general obstetric population. Initiation of therapy is usually considered in women without end-organ damage if systolic blood pressure exceeds 160 mmHg or diastolic pressure exceeds 110 mmHg.[106,107]

In women with end-organ damage, it is desirable to keep the blood pressure below 140/90 mmHg. ACEIs and ARBs are contraindicated, and should be discontinued as soon as pregnancy is detected. Women of childbearing potential should be counseled about the teratogenic potential of these agents.

If drug therapy is necessary, methyldopa (250 mg twice daily orally, maximum dose 4 g/d) has a long track record of safety and efficacy in pregnant patients, and is often the initial drug of choice. Hydralazine and β blockers, such as labetalol (100 mg twice daily orally, maximum dose 800 mg every 8 hours) can also be used. Atenolol, a β blocker without α-blocking properties, is associated with lower placental and fetal weight at delivery when used early in pregnancy.[107–109]

Preeclampsia occurs in approximately 5 percent of pregnancies. It is associated with significant maternal and fetal risk. The major decisions in the management are obstetrical ones regarding timing of delivery. In preeclamptic hypertension, the reasonable goal for systolic and diastolic blood pressures are 140 to 155 mmHg and 90 to 105 mmHg, respectively.

[ ] HYPERTENSION ASSOCIATED WITH SOLID-ORGAN TRANSPLANTATIONS

Hypertension is common is patients who undergo solid organ transplantation, and is associated with increased risk for cardiovascular morbidity and graft loss.[110] Preexisting hypertension may be exacerbated by use of calcineurin inhibitors, corticosteroids, and progressive chronic kidney disease. Treatment goals are similar to the goals for the general population, including lower blood pressure goals

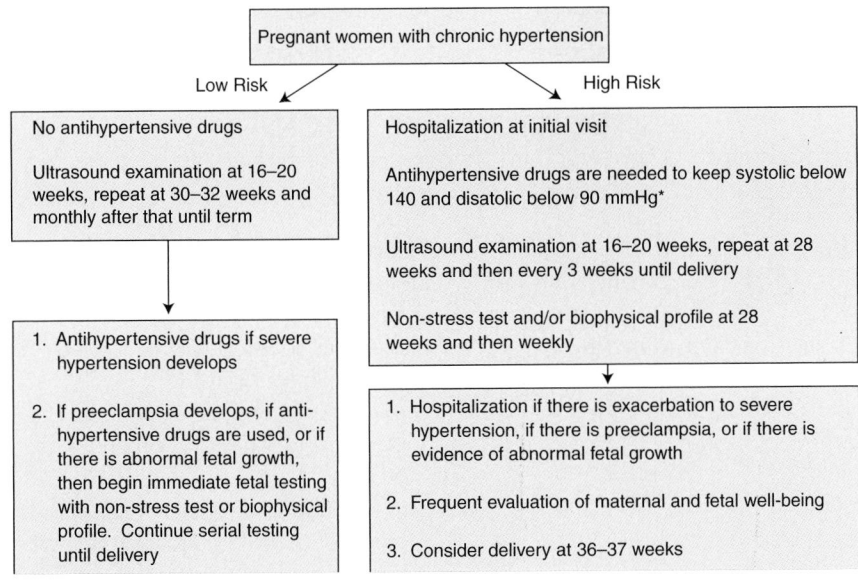

FIGURE 70–3. Algorithm for the management of pregnant women with chronic hypertension. *Source: From Sibai BM. Chronic hypertension in pregnancy. Obstet Gynecol 2002;100:369-377.*

(<130/80 mmHg) in patients with diabetes and chronic kidney disease. Although there are few prospective clinical trials to guide choice of antihypertensive therapy in transplantation patients, dihydropyridine calcium channel blockers are commonly used because of their pharmacologic property to antagonize calcineurin-mediated vasoconstriction.[111] It is important to consider any possible interactions with immunosuppressive therapy when initiating antihypertensive drug therapy in transplantation patients.

[ ] HYPERTENSIVE EMERGENCIES AND URGENCIES

Hypertensive emergency is defined by acute and rapidly evolving end-organ damage, such as aortic dissection, heart failure, symptomatic coronary heart disease, progressive renal disease, stroke, or cerebral dysfunction associated with significant hypertension. Although there is no blood pressure threshold for the diagnosis of hypertensive emergency, most end-organ damage is noted with systolic blood pressures exceeding 220 mmHg or diastolic blood pressures exceeding 120 mmHg. The condition is usually related to an acute exacerbation of chronic hypertension, as seen with the development of a secondary cause of hypertension, or the rapid progression of target-organ damage with previously asymptomatic uncontrolled hypertension. In these patients, immediate but monitored reduction, often accomplished with parenteral medications, is essential to prevent long-term damage. Controlling blood pressure within hours is desirable and usually requires admission to a monitored or critical care setting.

Hypertensive urgency is defined by a markedly elevated blood pressure, usually in the same range seen in a hypertension emergency, but without the rapid progression of target-organ damage. If the patient is asymptomatic or clinically stable, the patient can be managed as an outpatient with close followup within days. Blood pressure lowering is essential, but the reduction can be achieved over a period of days without an intensive monitoring setting, usually with oral medications. In fact, there is evidence

that the rapid reduction of blood pressure in asymptomatic hypertension may precipitate adverse outcomes.[112] Hypertension urgencies most often results from inadequate treatment of chronic severe hypertension.

The initial assessment of hypertensive crisis is straightforward. A history and physical examination will rapidly direct further investigation to the involved organs. Appropriate chemistry measurements and ECG are available widely. Urine toxicology for cocaine metabolites is helpful in select populations. Plain chest radiographs are useful for assessing volume status and cardiac size and are a first screen for aortic dissection.

The treatment of hypertensive urgencies and emergencies depends on the judgement of how rapidly the blood pressure must be lowered in addition to the selection of an appropriate antihypertensive therapy. Because of the lack of proven benefit and potential risk with rapid blood pressure lowering, most cases of hypertension urgencies can be treated with aggressive but gradual improvement in blood pressure control. In addition to timely control of blood pressure, emergency care should emphasize the thoughtful initiation of long-term therapy and appropriate followup care. Therapy should begin with two oral agents. If the condition is caused by anxiety, pain, use of sympathomimetics or cocaine, or by withdrawal states such as alcohol or discontinuation of antihypertensive medications, addressing the underlying condition is the first priority. Patients hospitalized with hypertensive urgencies can be treated in a nonintensive care unit setting with oral medications over 24 to 48 hours.

In the case of acute organ damage (hypertension emergency), admission to a monitored or intensive care setting should be considered and treatment with intravenous medications. The goal of therapy is prompt but gradual reduction in blood pressure. The most reasonable goal is to lower the mean arterial pressure by approximately 25 percent within 2 hours, and to 160/100 mmHg by 6 hours.

Multiple medications are available for the treatment of hypertension crisis (Table 70–9). Sodium nitroprusside is the drug of choice for most hypertensive emergencies because it has an immediate onset of action and can be titrated quickly and accurately. The duration of effect is 1 to 2 minutes. Thiocyanate levels must be followed in patients who have hepatic or renal insufficiency to prevent toxic buildup.

Parenteral labetalol is another first-line agent for hypertensive emergency. Its onset of action is within 5 to 10 minutes, and the duration of action is about 3 to 6 hours. Labetalol can be used safely in most patients, but caution should be exercised in patients who have severe bradycardia, congestive heart failure, or bronchospasm.

Nicardipine is a calcium-channel blocker administered parenterally by continuous infusion for hypertensive crises. The onset of action of this drug is 5 to 10 minutes, and the duration of action is 1 to 4 hours. Nicardipine is contraindicated in patients with heart failure.

Esmolol is a cardioselective β blocker with a short duration of action. It reduces systolic blood pressure and mean arterial pressure, as well as heart rate, cardiac output, and stroke volume. There is a notable decrease in myocardial oxygen consumption. Peak effects are gen-

TABLE 70–9

Medical Treatment for Management of Hypertension Crises

AGENT	DOSE	ONSET OF ACTION	PRECAUTIONS
Parenteral Vasodilators			
Sodium nitroprusside	0.25–10 μg/kg/min IV infusion	Immediate	Thiocyanate toxicity with prolonged use
Nitroglycerin	5–100 μg/min IV infusion	2–5 min	Headache, tachycardia, tolerance
Nicardipine	5–15 mg/h IV infusion	1–5 min	Protracted hypotension after prolonged use
Fenoldopam mesylate	0.1–0.3 μg/kg/min IV infusion	1–5 min	Headache, tachycardia, increased intraocular pressure
Hydralazine	5–10 mg as IV bolus or 10–40 mg IM repeat q4–6h	10 min IV 20 min IM	Unpredictable and excessive falls in pressure; tachycardia; angina exacerbation
Enalaprilat	0.625–1.25 mg q6h IV bolus	15–60 min	Unpredictable and excessive falls in pressure; acute renal failure in patients with bilateral renal artery stenosis
Parenteral Adrenergic Inhibitors			
Labetalol	20–80 mg as slow IV injection q10min, or 0.5–2 mg/min IV as infusion	5–10 min	Bronchospasm, heart block, orthostatic hypotension
Metoprolol	5 mg IV q10min × 3 doses	5–10 min	Bronchospasm, heart block, heart failure, exacerbation of cocaine-induced myocardial ischemia
Esmolol	500 μg/kg IV over 3 min then 25–100 mg/kg/min as IV infusion	1–5 min	Bronchospasm, heart block, heart failure
Phentolamine	5–10 mg IV bolus q5–15 min	1–2 min	Tachycardia, orthostatic hypotension

SOURCE: From Victor R. Arterial hypertension. In Goldman L, Cecil Textbook of Medicine, 22nd ed. Philadelphia: W.B. Saunders, 2004:361, with permission from Elsevier Company.

erally seen within 6 to 10 minutes after a bolus dose, and the effects resolve 20 minutes after discontinuing the infusion.

Fenoldopam is the first selective dopamine-1 receptor agonist approved for in-hospital short-term management of severe hypertension up to the first 48 hours of treatment. Fenoldopam is a good choice in these patients because of the improvement in renal perfusion, diuresis, and lack of production of toxic metabolites. Tolerance develops to fenoldopam after 48 hours.

In patients with hypertension and myocardial ischemia, intravenous nitroglycerin is effective in reducing both systemic vascular resistance and improving coronary perfusion. β Blockers and CCBs may also be useful; both can decrease blood pressure while improving myocardial oxygenation. Acute pulmonary edema that is precipitated by hypertension is best treated with sodium nitroprusside. The concomitant venous and arterial dilation improve forward flow and cardiac output.

Aortic dissection is the most dramatic and most rapidly fatal complication of severe hypertension. Mortality rates from aortic dissection remain high. Systolic blood pressure should be decreased as rapidly as possible to 100 to 110 mmHg or lower. This reduction is best achieved with a combination of β blockers and intravenous vasodilators such as sodium nitroprusside. Therapy for acute aortic dissection aims to reduce stress on the aortic wall by lowering both blood pressure and heart rate and,

consequently, the change in blood pressure versus time (dP/dt). Because sodium nitroprusside can cause reflex tachycardia, therapy with β-blocking agents should be started beforehand.

RESISTANT HYPERTENSION

Resistant hypertension is the failure to reach goal blood pressure in patients who are adhering to full doses of an appropriate three-drug regimen that includes a diuretic. Clinicians should systematically explore reasons why the patient may not be at goal blood pressure. Blood pressure measurement issues such as isolated office (white-coat) hypertension, positioning the patient on the examination table rather than a chair for measurement, and the use of a smaller-than-required cuff should be considered. The presence of pseudohypertension should be considered, particularly in patients with marked hypertension in the absence of target-organ damage.

An important cause of refractory hypertension is poor compliance or adherence to therapy. Other causes include excess sodium intake, volume overload from kidney disease, inadequate diuretic therapy, inadequate doses or inappropriate combinations of antihypertensive drug therapy, and excessive alcohol use. Some concomitant medications may interfere with blood pressure control; these include nonsteroidal antiinflammatory drugs, cyclooxygenase-2 inhibitors, cocaine, amphetamines, other illicit drugs, sympathomimetics (decongestants, anorectics), oral contraceptives, adrenal steroids, cyclosporine and tacrolimus, erythropoietin, licorice (including some chewing tobacco), and selected over-the-counter dietary supplements. After eliminating and reversing these contributing factors, secondary causes should be considered as discussed above.

Because volume overload is common among such patients, the most important therapeutic maneuver is generally to add or increase diuretic therapy. More than 60 percent of patients with resistant hypertension may respond to this approach. If the glomerular filtration rate is below 30 mL/min, loop diuretics should be used instead of thiazide diuretics. Short-acting loop diuretics, such as furosemide or bumetanide, should be given two or three times per day. Longer-acting loop diuretics, such as torsemide (at 2.5 to 5.0 mg), may also be considered.[113]

Hypertension is a major clinical problem across the world. With the increasing availability of cheap generic drugs, a major goal for the cardiovascular physician is to identify and to treat as many patients as possible.

REFERENCES

1. Pickering TG, Hall JE, Appel LJ, et al. Recommendations for blood pressure measurement in humans and experimental animals: part 1: blood pressure measurement in humans: a statement for professionals from the Subcommittee of Professional and Public Education of the American Heart Association Council on High Blood Pressure Research. *Hypertension* 2005;45(1):142–161.

2. Beevers G, Lip GY, O'Brien E. ABC of hypertension. Blood pressure measurement. Part I—sphygmomanometry: factors common to all techniques. *BMJ* 2001;322(7292):981–985.

3. Peters GL, Binder SK, Campbell NR. The effect of crossing legs on blood pressure: a randomized single-blind cross-over study. *Blood Press Monit* 1999;4(2):97–101.

4. Netea RT, Bijlstra PJ, Lenders JW, Smits P, Thien T. Influence of the arm position on intra-arterial blood pressure measurement. *J Hum Hypertens* 1998;12(3):157–160.

5. Netea RT, Smits P, Lenders JW, Thien T. Does it matter whether blood pressure measurements are taken with subjects sitting or supine? *J Hypertens* 1998;16(3):263–268.

6. Whitworth JA. 2003 World Health Organization (WHO)/International Society of Hypertension (ISH) statement on management of hypertension. *J Hypertens* 2003;21(11):1983–1992.

7. Williams B, Poulter NR, Brown MJ, et al. Guidelines for management of hypertension: report of the fourth working party of the British Hypertension Society, 2004-BHS IV. *J Hum Hypertens* 2004;18(3):139–185.

8. Chobanian AV, Bakris GL, Black HR, et al. Seventh report of the Joint National Committee on Prevention, Detection, Evaluation, and Treatment of High Blood Pressure. *Hypertension* 2003;42(6):1206–1252.

9. Pickering TG, Hall JE, Appel LJ, et al. Recommendations for blood pressure measurement in humans and experimental animals: part 1: blood pressure measurement in humans: a statement for professionals from the Subcommittee of Professional and Public Education of the American Heart Association Council on High Blood Pressure Research. *Circulation* 2005;111(5):697–716.

10. Pickering TG, Shimbo D, Haas D. Ambulatory blood-pressure monitoring. *N Engl J Med* 2006;354(22):2368–2374.

11. O'Brien E. Ambulatory blood pressure measurement is indispensable to good clinical practice. *J Hypertens Suppl* 2003;21(2):S11–S18.

12. Yarows SA, Julius S, Pickering TG. Home blood pressure monitoring. *Arch Intern Med* 2000;160(9):1251–1257.

13. 2003 European Society of Hypertension-European Society of Cardiology guidelines for the management of arterial hypertension. *J Hypertens* 2003;21(6):1011–1053.

14. Wilson PW, D'Agostino RB, Levy D, Belanger AM, Silbershatz H, Kannel WB. Prediction of coronary heart disease using risk factor categories. *Circulation* 1998;97(18):1837–1847.

15. Textor SC. Ischemic nephropathy: where are we now? *J Am Soc Nephrol* 2004;15(8):1974–1982.

16. Freel EM, Connell JM. Mechanisms of hypertension: the expanding role of aldosterone. *J Am Soc Nephrol* 2004;15(8):1993–2001.

17. Baguet JP, Hammer L, Levy P, et al. Night-time and diastolic hypertension are common and underestimated conditions in newly diagnosed apnoeic patients. *J Hypertens* 2005;23(3):521–527.

18. Barzon L, Fallo F, Sonino N, Boscaro M. Development of overt Cushing's syndrome in patients with adrenal incidentaloma. *Eur J Endocrinol* 2002;146(1):61–66.

19. Hall WD. Resistant hypertension, secondary hypertension, and hypertensive crises. *Cardiol Clin* 2002;20(2):281–289.

20. Vashist A, Heller EN, Brown EJ Jr, Alhaddad IA. Renal artery stenosis: a cardiovascular perspective. *Am Heart J* 2002;143(4):559–564.

21. Simon G. What is critical renal artery stenosis? Implications for treatment. *Am J Hypertens* 2000;13(11):1189–1193.

22. Canzanello VJ, Textor SC. Noninvasive diagnosis of renovascular disease. *Mayo Clin Proc* 1994;69(12):1172–1181.

23. Hansen KJ, Tribble RW, Reavis SW, et al. Renal duplex sonography: evaluation of clinical utility. *J Vasc Surg* 1990;12(3):227–236.

24. Mann SJ, Pickering TG. Detection of renovascular hypertension. State of the art, 1992. *Ann Intern Med* 1992;117(10):845–853.

25. Pedersen EB. Angiotensin-converting enzyme inhibitor renography. Pathophysiological, diagnostic and therapeutic aspects in renal artery stenosis. *Nephrol Dial Transplant* 1994;9(5):482–492.

26. Postma CT, Joosten FB, Rosenbusch G, Thien T. Magnetic resonance angiography has a high reliability in the detection of renal artery stenosis. *Am J Hypertens* 1997;10(9 Pt 1):957–963.

27. Logan AG, Steinhardt MI. Restoration of renal function by unilateral percutaneous transluminal dilatation of stenosed renal artery. *Can Med Assoc J* 1980;122(8):910–912.

28. Rimmer JM, Gennari FJ. Atherosclerotic renovascular disease and progressive renal failure. *Ann Intern Med* 1993;118(9):712–719.

29. Pickering TG, Herman L, Devereux RB, et al. Recurrent pulmonary oedema in hypertension due to bilateral renal artery stenosis: treatment by angioplasty or surgical revascularisation. *Lancet* 1988;2(8610):551–552.

30. Ritz E, Mann JF. Renal angioplasty for lowering blood pressure. *N Engl J Med* 2000;342(14):1042–1043.

31. Leertouwer TC, Gussenhoven EJ, Bosch JL, et al. Stent placement for renal arterial stenosis: where do we stand? A meta-analysis. *Radiology* 2000;216(1):78–85.

32. Radermacher J, Chavan A, Bleck J, et al. Use of Doppler ultrasonography to predict the outcome of therapy for renal-artery stenosis. *N Engl J Med* 2001;344(6):410–417.

33. Radermacher J, Haller H. The right diagnostic work-up: investigating renal and renovascular disorders. *J Hypertens Suppl* 2003;21(2):S19–S24.

34. Young T, Palta M, Dempsey J, Skatrud J, Weber S, Badr S. The occurrence of sleep-disordered breathing among middle-aged adults. *N Engl J Med* 1993;328(17):1230–1235.

35. Duran J, Esnaola S, Rubio R, Iztueta A. Obstructive sleep apnea-hypopnea and related clinical features in a population-based sample of subjects aged 30 to 70 yr. *Am J Respir Crit Care Med* 2001;163(3 Pt 1):685–689.

36. Kales A, Bixler EO, Cadieux RJ, et al. Sleep apnoea in a hypertensive population. *Lancet* 1984;2(8410):1005–1008.

37. Fletcher EC, DeBehnke RD, Lovoi MS, Gorin AB. Undiagnosed sleep apnea in patients with essential hypertension. *Ann Intern Med* 1985;103(2):190–195.

38. Lavie P, Ben Yosef R, Rubin AE. Prevalence of sleep apnea syndrome among patients with essential hypertension. *Am Heart J* 1984;108(2):373–376.

39. Nieto FJ, Young TB, Lind BK, et al. Association of sleep-disordered breathing, sleep apnea, and hypertension in a large community-based study. Sleep Heart Health Study. *JAMA* 2000;283(14):1829–1836.

40. Peppard PE, Young T, Palta M, Skatrud J. Prospective study of the association between sleep-disordered breathing and hypertension. *N Engl J Med* 2000;342(19):1378–1384.

41. Lavie P, Herer P, Hoffstein V. Obstructive sleep apnoea syndrome as a risk factor for hypertension: population study. *BMJ* 2000;320(7233):479–482.

42. Bixler EO, Vgontzas AN, Lin HM, Ten Have T, Leiby BE, Vela-Bueno A, et al. Association of hypertension and sleep-disordered breathing. *Arch Intern Med* 2000;160(15):2289–2295.

43. Quan SF, Howard BV, Iber C, Kiley JP, Nieto FJ, O'Connor GT, et al. The Sleep Heart Health Study: design, rationale, and methods. *Sleep* 1997;20(12):1077–1085.

44. Netzer NC, Stoohs RA, Netzer CM, Clark K, Strohl KP. Using the Berlin Questionnaire to identify patients at risk for the sleep apnea syndrome. *Ann Intern Med* 1999;131(7):485–491.

45. Chervin RD, Murman DL, Malow BA, Totten V. Cost-utility of three approaches to the diagnosis of sleep apnea: polysomnography, home testing, and empirical therapy. *Ann Intern Med* 1999;130(6):496–505.
46. Goodfriend TL, Calhoun DA. Resistant hypertension, obesity, sleep apnea, and aldosterone: theory and therapy. *Hypertension* 2004;43(3):518–524.
47. Calhoun DA, Nishizaka MK, Zaman MA, Harding SM. Aldosterone excretion among subjects with resistant hypertension and symptoms of sleep apnea. *Chest* 2004;125(1):112–117.
48. Hemmelgarn BR, Zarnke KB, Campbell NR, et al. The 2004 Canadian Hypertension Education Program recommendations for the management of hypertension: part I—blood pressure measurement, diagnosis and assessment of risk. *Can J Cardiol* 2004;20(1):31–40.
49. Ilias I, Torpy DJ, Pacak K, Mullen N, Wesley RA, Nieman LK. Cushing's syndrome due to ectopic corticotropin secretion: twenty years' experience at the National Institutes of Health. *J Clin Endocrinol Metab* 2005;90(8):4955–4962.
50. Isidori AM, Kaltsas GA, Pozza C, et al. The ectopic adrenocorticotropin syndrome: clinical features, diagnosis, management, and long-term follow-up. J Clin *Endocrinol Metab* 2006;91(2):371–377.
51. Wajchenberg BL, Mendonca BB, Liberman B, et al. Ectopic adrenocorticotropic hormone syndrome. *Endocr Rev* 1994;15(6):752–787.
52. Newell-Price J, Bertagna X, Grossman AB, Nieman LK. Cushing's syndrome. *Lancet* 2006;367(9522):1605–1617.
53. Ezzati M, Lopez AD, Rodgers A, Vander HS, Murray CJ. Selected major risk factors and global and regional burden of disease. *Lancet* 2002;360(9343):1347–1360.
54. National Heart Foundation. *Hypertension Management Guide for Doctors 2004*. Heart Foundation, 2003.
55. Bolli P, Myers M, McKay D. Applying the 2005 Canadian Hypertension Education Program recommendations: 1. Diagnosis of hypertension. *CMAJ* 2005;173(5):480–483.
56. Chobanian AV, Bakris GL, Black HR, et al. The Seventh Report of the Joint National Committee on Prevention, Detection, Evaluation, and Treatment of High Blood Pressure: the JNC 7 report. *JAMA* 2003;289(19):2560–2572.
57. National Collaborating Centre for Chronic Conditions. *Hypertension: Management of Hypertension in Adults in Primary Care: Partial Update, 2006*. London; Royal College of Physicians, 2006.
58. Sacks FM, Svetkey LP, Vollmer WM, et al. Effects on blood pressure of reduced dietary sodium and the Dietary Approaches to Stop Hypertension (DASH) diet. DASH-Sodium Collaborative Research Group. *N Engl J Med* 2001;344(1):3–10.
59. Hagberg JM, Park JJ, Brown MD. The role of exercise training in the treatment of hypertension: an update. *Sports Med* 2000;30(3):193–206.
60. Xin X, He J, Frontini MG, Ogden LG, Motsamai OI, Whelton PK. Effects of alcohol reduction on blood pressure: a meta-analysis of randomized controlled trials. *Hypertension* 2001;38(5):1112–1117.
61. He J, Whelton PK. Effect of dietary fiber and protein intake on blood pressure: a review of epidemiologic evidence. *Clin Exp Hypertens* 1999;21(5–6):785–796.
62. Appel LJ, Moore TJ, Obarzanek E, et al. A clinical trial of the effects of dietary patterns on blood pressure. DASH Collaborative Research Group. *N Engl J Med* 1997;336(16):1117–1124.
63. Appel LJ, Espeland MA, Easter L, Wilson AC, Folmar S, Lacy CR. Effects of reduced sodium intake on hypertension control in older individuals: results from the Trial of Nonpharmacologic Interventions in the Elderly (TONE). *Arch Intern Med* 2001;161(5):685–693.
64. Hoffman BB. Therapy of hypertension. In: Brunton LL, Lazo JS, Parker KL, eds. *The Pharmacological Basis of Therapeutics*. New York: McGraw-Hill, 2006:845–868.
65. Carter BL, Ernst ME, Cohen JD. Hydrochlorothiazide versus chlorthalidone: evidence supporting their interchangeability. *Hypertension* 2004;43(1):4–9.
66. Bakris GL, Fonseca V, Katholi RE, et al. Metabolic effects of carvedilol vs metoprolol in patients with type 2 diabetes mellitus and hypertension: a randomized controlled trial. *JAMA* 2004;292(18):2227–2236.
67. Materson BJ, Reda DJ, Cushman WC, et al. Single-drug therapy for hypertension in men. A comparison of six antihypertensive agents with placebo. The Department of Veterans Affairs Cooperative Study Group on Antihypertensive Agents. *N Engl J Med* 1993;328(13):914–921.
68. Neaton JD, Grimm RH Jr, Prineas RJ, et al. Treatment of Mild Hypertension Study. Final results. Treatment of Mild Hypertension Study Research Group. *JAMA* 1993;270(6):713–724.
69. The ALLHAT Officers and Coordinators for the ALLHAT Collaborative Research Group. Major outcomes in high-risk hypertensive patients random-

ized to angiotensin-converting enzyme inhibitor or calcium channel blocker vs diuretic: the Antihypertensive and Lipid-Lowering Treatment to Prevent Heart Attack Trial. *JAMA* 2002;288(23):2981–2997.
70. Diuretic versus alpha-blocker as first-step antihypertensive therapy: final results from the Antihypertensive and Lipid-Lowering Treatment to Prevent Heart Attack Trial (ALLHAT). *Hypertension* 2003;42(3):239–246.
71. Wing LM, Reid CM, Ryan P, et al. A comparison of outcomes with angiotensin-converting enzyme inhibitors and diuretics for hypertension in the elderly. *N Engl J Med* 2003;348(7):583–592.
72. Dahlof B, Sever PS, Poulter NR, et al. Prevention of cardiovascular events with an antihypertensive regimen of amlodipine adding perindopril as required versus atenolol adding bendroflumethiazide as required, in the Anglo-Scandinavian Cardiac Outcomes Trial-Blood Pressure Lowering Arm (ASCOT-BPLA): a multicentre randomised controlled trial. *Lancet* 2005;366(9489):895–906.
73. Hansson L, Lindholm LH, Ekbom T, et al. Randomised trial of old and new antihypertensive drugs in elderly patients: cardiovascular mortality and morbidity the Swedish Trial in Old Patients with Hypertension-2 study. *Lancet* 1999;354(9192):1751–1756.
74. Black HR, Elliott WJ, Grandits G, et al. Principal results of the Controlled Onset Verapamil Investigation of Cardiovascular End Points (CONVINCE) trial. *JAMA* 2003;289(16):2073–2082.
75. Brown MJ, Palmer CR, Castaigne A, et al. Morbidity and mortality in patients randomised to double-blind treatment with a long-acting calcium-channel blocker or diuretic in the International Nifedipine GITS study: Intervention as a Goal in Hypertension Treatment (INSIGHT). *Lancet* 2000;356(9227):366–372.
76. Dahlof B, Devereux RB, Kjeldsen SE, et al. Cardiovascular morbidity and mortality in the Losartan Intervention For Endpoint reduction in hypertension study (LIFE): a randomised trial against atenolol. *Lancet* 2002;359(9311):995–1003.
77. Hansson L, Hedner T, Lund-Johansen P, et al. Randomised trial of effects of calcium antagonists compared with diuretics and beta-blockers on cardiovascular morbidity and mortality in hypertension: the Nordic Diltiazem (NORDIL) study. *Lancet* 2000;356(9227):359–365.
78. Julius S, Kjeldsen SE, Weber M, et al. Outcomes in hypertensive patients at high cardiovascular risk treated with regimens based on valsartan or amlodipine: the VALUE randomised trial. *Lancet* 2004;363(9426):2022–2031.
79. Mancia G. The association of hypertension and diabetes: prevalence, cardiovascular risk and protection by blood pressure reduction. *Acta Diabetol* 2005;42(Suppl 1):S17–S25.
80. Stump CS, Hamilton MT, Sowers JR. Effect of antihypertensive agents on the development of type 2 diabetes mellitus. *Mayo Clin Proc* 2006;81(6):796–806.
81. Verdecchia P, Reboldi G, Angeli F, et al. Adverse prognostic significance of new diabetes in treated hypertensive subjects. *Hypertension* 2004;43(5):963–969.
82. Wright JT Jr, Dunn JK, Cutler JA, et al. Outcomes in hypertensive black and nonblack patients treated with chlorthalidone, amlodipine, and lisinopril. *JAMA* 2005;293(13):1595–1608.
83. Turnbull F. Effects of different blood-pressure-lowering regimens on major cardiovascular events: results of prospectively-designed overviews of randomised trials. *Lancet* 2003;362(9395):1527–1535.
84. Neal B, MacMahon S, Chapman N. Effects of ACE inhibitors, calcium antagonists, and other blood-pressure-lowering drugs: results of prospectively designed overviews of randomised trials. Blood Pressure Lowering Treatment Trialists' Collaboration. *Lancet* 2000;356(9246):1955–1964.
85. Medical Research Council trial of treatment of hypertension in older adults: principal results. MRC Working Party. *BMJ* 1992;304(6824):405–412.
86. Franklin SS, Gustin W, Wong ND, et al. Hemodynamic patterns of age-related changes in blood pressure. The Framingham Heart Study. *Circulation* 1997;96(1):308–315.
87. Azizi F, Rashidi A, Ghanbarian A, Madjid M. Is systolic blood pressure sufficient for classification of blood pressure and determination of hypertension based on JNC-VI in an Iranian adult population? Tehran lipid and glucose study (TLGS). *J Hum Hypertens* 2003;17(4):287–291.
88. Franklin SS, Larson MG, Khan SA, et al. Does the relation of blood pressure to coronary heart disease risk change with aging? The Framingham Heart Study. *Circulation* 2001;103(9):1245–1249.
89. Whelton PK, Appel LJ, Espeland MA, et al. Sodium reduction and weight loss in the treatment of hypertension in older persons: a randomized controlled trial of nonpharmacologic interventions in the elderly (TONE). TONE Collaborative Research Group. *JAMA* 1998;279(11):839–846.
90. Stults BJRE. Management of hypertension in diabetes. *Diabetes Spectrum* 2006;19(1):25–31.

91. Clinical practice recommendations 2005. *Diabetes Care* 2005;28 Suppl 1:S1–S79.

92. Lewis EJ, Hunsicker LG, Clarke WR, et al. Renoprotective effect of the angiotensin-receptor antagonist irbesartan in patients with nephropathy due to type 2 diabetes. *N Engl J Med* 2001;345(12):851–860.

93. Lewis EJ, Hunsicker LG, Bain RP, Rohde RD, for the Collaborative Study Group. The effect of angiotensin-converting-enzyme inhibition on diabetic nephropathy. *N Engl J Med* 1993;329:1456–1462.

94. Brenner BM, Cooper ME, de Zeeuw D, et al. Effects of losartan on renal and cardiovascular outcomes in patients with type 2 diabetes and nephropathy. *N Engl J Med* 2001;345(12):861–869.

95. Bakris GL, Weir MR, Shanifar S, et al. Effects of blood pressure level on progression of diabetic nephropathy: results from the RENAAL study. *Arch Intern Med* 2003;163(13):1555–1565.

96. Rahman M, Pressel S, Davis BR, et al. Renal outcomes in high-risk hypertensive patients treated with an angiotensin-converting enzyme inhibitor or a calcium channel blocker vs a diuretic: a report from the Antihypertensive and Lipid-Lowering Treatment to Prevent Heart Attack Trial (ALLHAT). *Arch Intern Med* 2005;165(8):936–946.

97. Wright JT Jr, Bakris G, Greene T, et al. Effect of blood pressure lowering and antihypertensive drug class on progression of hypertensive kidney disease: results from the AASK trial. *JAMA* 2002;288(19):2421–2431.

98. Tight blood pressure control and risk of macrovascular and microvascular complications in type 2 diabetes: UKPDS 38. UK Prospective Diabetes Study Group. *BMJ* 1998;317(7160):703–713.

99. Hansson L. The Hypertension Optimal Treatment study and the importance of lowering blood pressure. *J Hypertens Suppl* 1999;17(1):S9–S13.

100. Douglas JG, Bakris GL, Epstein M, et al. Management of high blood pressure in African Americans: consensus statement of the Hypertension in African Americans Working Group of the International Society on Hypertension in Blacks. *Arch Intern Med* 2003;163(5):525–541.

101. Oparil S, Wright JT Jr. Ethnicity and blood pressure. *J Clin Hypertens (Greenwich)* 2005;7(6):357–364.

102. Rachidi A, Rahman M, Wright JTJ. Which drug should be used to treat patients with uncomplicated essential hypertension. *Curr Opin Nephrol Hypertens* 2006;15:303–308.

103. Lee DK, Marantz PR, Devereux RB, Kligfield P, Alderman MH. Left ventricular hypertrophy in black and white hypertensives: standard electrocardiographic criteria overestimate racial differences in prevalence. *JAMA* 1992;267:3294–3299.

104. Okin PM, Wright JT, Nieminen MS, et al. Ethnic differences in electrocardiographic criteria for left ventricular hypertrophy: the LIFE study. *Am J Hypertens* 2002;15(8):663–671.

105. K/DOQI clinical practice guidelines for chronic kidney disease: evaluation, classification, and stratification. *Am J Kidney Dis* 2002;39(2 Suppl 1):S1–S266.

106. Report of the National High Blood Pressure Education Program Working Group on High Blood Pressure in Pregnancy. *Am J Obstet Gynecol* 2000;183(1):S1–S22.

107. Sibai BM. Chronic hypertension in pregnancy. *Obstet Gynecol* 2002;100(2):369–377.

108. Montan S, Ingemarsson I, Marsal K, Sjoberg NO. Randomised controlled trial of atenolol and pindolol in human pregnancy: effects on fetal haemodynamics. *BMJ* 1992;304(6832):946–949.

109. Lydakis C, Lip GY, Beevers M, Beevers DG. Atenolol and fetal growth in pregnancies complicated by hypertension. *Am J Hypertens* 1999;12(6):541–547.

110. Ojo AO. Cardiovascular complications after renal transplantation and their prevention. *Transplantation* 2006;82(5):603–611.

111. Textor SC, Canzanello VJ, Taler SJ, et al. Cyclosporine-induced hypertension after transplantation. *Mayo Clin Proc* 1994;69(12):1182–1193.

112. Aggarwal M, Khan IA. Hypertensive crisis: hypertensive emergencies and urgencies. *Cardiol Clin* 2006;24(1):135–146.

113. Moser M, Setaro JF. Clinical practice. Resistant or difficult-to-control hypertension. *N Engl J Med* 2006;355(4):385–392.

PART 10 Cardiopulmonary Disease

CHAPTER (71)

Pulmonary Hypertension

Lewis J. Rubin

Pulmonary hypertension is a hemodynamic abnormality common to a variety of conditions that is characterized by increased right ventricular (RV) afterload and work. The clinical manifestations, natural history, and reversibility of pulmonary hypertension depend heavily on the nature of the pulmonary vascular lesions and the etiology and severity of the hemodynamic disorder. For example, subacute or chronic hypoxia predominantly causes increased muscularization of the small muscular pulmonary arteries and arterioles with the intima relatively intact. Relief of the hypoxia improves or occasionally reverses the process with little or no pathologic residue.[1,2] In contrast, the lesions of systemic sclerosis (scleroderma), mostly confined to the intima of the small pulmonary arteries and arterioles, are usually progressive and irreversible. Unlike these two examples, which spare the pulmonary capillary bed, the pulmonary capillaries are the primary site of involvement in pulmonary capillary hemangiomatosis.[3] Because of its large capacity, its great distensibility, its low resistance to blood flow, and the modest amounts of smooth muscle in the small arteries and arterioles, the *pulmonary circulation is not predisposed to become hypertensive*. When total cross-sectional area is decreased by destruction or obliteration of lung tissue or occlusive lesions in the resistance vessels, pulmonary arterial pressures increase. The degree of pulmonary hypertension that develops is a function of the amount of the pulmonary vascular tree that has been eliminated. Pulmonary hypertension is usually secondary to cardiac or pulmonary disease. Although idiopathic pulmonary artery hypertension

(IPAH; formerly known as primary pulmonary hypertension) is uncommon, it is well recognized as a distinctive clinical entity in which intrinsic pulmonary vascular disease is free of the complicating features of pulmonary hypertension contributed by diseases of the heart and/or lungs. Mild pulmonary hypertension can exist for a lifetime without becoming evident clinically. For example, native residents at high altitude, in whom mild to moderate pulmonary hypertension is a natural result of sustained exposure to hypoxia, can adapt and function normally. When pulmonary hypertension does become manifest clinically, the symptoms tend to be nonspecific (Table 71–1).

DEFINITIONS

Pulmonary *arterial* hypertension (PAH) can be either acute or chronic. The acute form is usually a result of either pulmonary embolism (see Chap. 72) or the adult respiratory distress syndrome. This chapter deals with *chronic* pulmonary arterial hypertension.

Pulmonary *venous* hypertension usually is encountered as a consequence of left ventricular (LV) dysfunction or mitral valve disease. Occasionally, it may occur in the course of fibrosing mediastinitis. Only rarely is the entity known as pulmonary venoocclusive disease encountered. Even though pulmonary hypertension may be confined, at the outset, to the pulmonary veins (e.g., acute mitral regurgitation), sooner or later pulmonary arterial hyperten-

TABLE 71–1

TABLE 71–1

Symptoms of Pulmonary Artery Hypertension

Dyspnea	Palpitations
Fatigue	Orthopnea
Dizziness	Cough
Syncope	Hoarseness
Chest pain	

sion supervenes. The hallmarks of pulmonary venous hypertension are pulmonary congestion and edema. For practical purposes, pulmonary venous hypertension exists when pulmonary venous (or left atrium [LA]) pressure rises above approximately 15 mmHg.

Cor pulmonale signifies the presence of pulmonary hypertension and cardiac dysfunction in the setting of diseases affecting the structure or function of the lung.[4] Pulmonary hypertension in patients with chronic lung disease tends to be less severe than in connective tissue diseases, chronic thromboembolic disease, or IPAH. Pulmonary hypertension may be severe, however, in some patients with interstitial lung disease.

NORMAL PULMONARY CIRCULATION

[ ] STRUCTURE

Immediately before birth, pulmonary and systemic arterial blood pressures are near equal and about 70/40 mmHg, with a mean of 50 mmHg. Immediately after birth, with closure of the ductus arteriosus and initiation of ventilation, pulmonary arterial pressure falls rapidly to about one-half of systemic levels. Thereafter, pulmonary arterial pressures gradually decrease over several weeks to reach adult levels.[5]

In some neonates, the normal pulmonary hypertension of the fetus fails to recede normally, generally as a result of either a developmental anomaly or a relentless increase in pulmonary vascular tone. In such infants, the persistent pulmonary hypertension and RV failure may become life-threatening. Surgical intervention or temporizing measures, such as the use of inhaled nitric oxide (NO) or extracorporeal membrane oxygenation, may be useful in reversing the pulmonary vascular abnormalities.[6]

In the normal adult at sea level, the small muscular arteries and arterioles in the lungs are thin-walled and contain very little smooth muscle. In contrast, in the fetus or the adult who has lived under hypoxic conditions (e.g., native residents at high altitude), the media of the arterioles are thickened, and the muscle extends distally into precapillary vessels that are ordinarily devoid of muscle; that is, the precapillary vessels undergo "remodeling."[7]

[ ] ENDOTHELIUM AND ENDOTHELIUM–SMOOTH MUSCLE INTERACTIONS

In addition to its role as a semipermeable barrier between blood and interstitium, the endothelium provides many biologically important functions, the net effect of which is the processing of blood flowing through the lungs. Among these functions are the

synthesis, uptake, storage, release, and metabolism of vasoactive substances; transduction of blood-borne signals; modulation of coagulation and thrombolysis; regulation of cell proliferation; engagement in the local inflammatory and proliferative reactions to injury; involvement in immune reactions; and angiogenesis (see Chap. 4). Some of the enzymes involved in these processes, such as the angiotensin-converting enzyme, are found on the surface of endothelial cells; others, such as 5-nucleotidase, are found within the cell. Hence it is appropriate to regard the endothelium as an organ with diverse metabolic and endocrine functions, one that is unique because of its strategic location as a continuous, monolayered lining of blood vessels throughout the body. Importantly, the lungs contain the largest expanse of endothelium in the body.

The cells that make up the monolayered endothelial lining communicate not only with each other by anatomic junctions and bridges but also with the underlying smooth muscle by way of biologically active substances. This interaction participates in regulating normal vasomotor tone as well responding to the administration of vasoactive substances. Thus damage to the lining cells, proliferation of the intima, or hypertrophy of the smooth muscle will each upset the normal interplay.

[ ] HEMODYNAMICS

For the adult pulmonary circulation, the definition of *normal* depends on the altitude. Table 71–2 compares the normal pulmonary hemodynamics of adults residing at sea level and above sea level. At *sea level,* a cardiac output of 5 to 6 L/min is associated with a pulmonary arterial pressure of about 20/12 mmHg, with a mean of about 15 mmHg. At an altitude of 15,000 ft, the same level of blood flow is associated with somewhat higher pressures (see Table 71–2). Pulmonary arterial pressures also tend to increase somewhat with age.

A pressure drop of only 5 to 10 mmHg between the pulmonary artery and left atrium accompanies the cardiac output of 5 to 6 L/min (see Table 71–2). Determination of pulmonary vascular resistance (PVR), calculated as the ratio of the difference in mean pres-

TABLE 71–2

Values for Normal Pulmonary Circulation at Sea Level and High Altitude

	SEA LEVEL	ALTITUDE (~15,000 FT)
Pulmonary arterial pressure (P_{PA}), mmHg	20/12, 15	38/14, 25
Cardiac output (Q), L/min	6	6
Left atrial pressure (P_{LA}), mmHg	5	5
Pulmonary vascular resistance (PVR),[a] (mmHg/L)/min (R units)	1.7	3.3

[a]$PVR = \dfrac{P_{PA} - P_{LA}}{Q} = \dfrac{15 - 5}{6} = 1.67$ R units. To convert R units to CGS (centimeter-gram-second) units (dynes • s/cm⁵), multiply R units by 80.

sure at the two ends of the pulmonary vascular bed (pulmonary arterial pressure minus LA pressure) divided by the cardiac output (see Table 71–2), is a practical clinical tool for assessing the hemodynamic state of the pulmonary circulation and for distinguishing between active and passive changes in the pulmonary resistance vessels (e.g., the effect of administering a vasodilator agent to a patient with pulmonary hypertension). In practice, because the LA may not be readily accessible, pulmonary artery wedge pressure is generally substituted for LA pressure.

Another approach to defining certain characteristics of the pulmonary arterial tree and its behavior—that is, elastic properties and geometry—is the calculation of pulmonary arterial input impedance. This approach has more physiologic than clinical value. It takes into account the pulsatile nature of pulmonary arterial pressures and flow. Like vascular resistance, it is defined as a ratio. But instead of a ratio involving *mean* pressures and blood flow, the ratio uses the amplitudes of pulsatile pressure to oscillatory flow near the beginning of the pulmonary artery at a particular frequency. Values for the ratio are obtained by resolving mathematically the pulsatile pressure and flow curves into their sinusoidal components.

The PVR has proved useful in assessing the state of the normal and abnormal pulmonary circulation, but reliance on the calculated resistance must be done with caution. For example, pulmonary vascular resistance may decrease despite an *increase* in pulmonary artery pressure if cardiac output increases to a greater degree as a result of a drug-induced primary effect on cardiac contractility or heart rate with little direct effect on pulmonary vasomotor tone. It is unlikely that this pattern of hemodynamic response will be beneficial. Also, a clinical shortcut, such as the substitution in the numerator of the pulmonary arterial pressure for the pressure *drop* between the pulmonary artery and LA, may be useful empirically but deprives the calculation of any physiologic meaning. Finally, the clinical significance of a value calculated for PVR depends heavily on the implications of the hemodynamic changes on the work of the RV. For example, the same decrease in calculated PVR brought about by two different pulmonary vasodilators may affect the work of the RV differently: Should one agent elicit a *decrease* in pulmonary arterial pressure along with an *increase* in cardiac output (an ideal response), it is more apt to be of long-term benefit than another agent that, while increasing the cardiac output, fails to decrease the pulmonary arterial pressure.

In the normal lung, a considerable increase in cardiac output, that is, two to three times that at rest, generally increases pulmonary arterial pressure by only a few millimeters of mercury. On the other hand, in pulmonary hypertensive states, in which the distensibility and recruitability of the pulmonary vascular bed are restricted by disease, pulmonary arterial pressure increases along with even small increments in pulmonary blood flow. Changes in pulmonary blood volume are much more subtle than changes in blood pressure or flow in their hemodynamic effects; they are also much more difficult to quantify. Clinical clues can be helpful in recognizing that the pulmonary blood volume has increased. Often a fullness of the pulmonary vascular pattern on the chest radiograph along with evidences of interstitial edema suggest that pulmonary blood volume has increased acutely. In chronic mitral stenosis or LV failure, the pulmonary blood volume is not only increased but is also redistributed toward the apices of the lungs, that is, *cephalization* (see Chap. 15).

Autonomic innervation of the pulmonary vascular tree plays a lesser role in modulating vasomotor tone than do local stimuli, particularly hypoxia. Indeed, hypoxia can exert its pulmonary pressor effect in the denervated lung. The mechanism by which hypoxia exerts its local pressor effect is not fully characterized but appears to involve altered smooth muscle cell membrane ion channel activity.[2] Acidosis potentiates the hypoxic pressor effect. Hypercapnia also exerts a pulmonary pressor effect, presumably by way of the local acidosis that it generates, but it is less powerful than hypoxia as a pulmonary vasoconstrictor agent.

PULMONARY HYPERTENSION: GENERAL FEATURES

CLINICAL MANIFESTATIONS

Pulmonary hypertension is a final common hemodynamic consequence of multiple etiologies and diverse mechanisms. As noted earlier, most cases of pulmonary hypertension are secondary (Table 71–3). Among the underlying causes of pulmonary hypertension are mechanical compression and distortion of the resistance vessels of the lungs (e.g., by diffuse pulmonary fibrosis), hypoxic vasoconstriction (e.g., in severe obstructive airways or diffuse parenchymal diseases), intravascular obstruction (e.g., thromboemboli or tumor emboli), and combinations of mechanical and vasoconstrictive influences. The significance of pulmonary hypertension, however, is that the increased afterload compromises RV function. Once pulmonary arterial pressures reach systemic levels, RV failure becomes inevitable.

SPECIAL STUDIES

The "gold standard" for the diagnosis of pulmonary hypertension is right-heart catheterization. This technique enables the direct determination of right atrial and ventricular pressures, pulmonary arterial pressure, pulmonary artery wedge pressure (as an approximation of pulmonary venous pressure), pulmonary blood flow (cardiac output), and the responses of these parameters to interventions (vasodilators, oxygen, exercise). However, the skilled clinician can often suspect pulmonary hypertension on the basis of the assessment of an elevated jugular venous pressure pulsation and a loud P_2 (see Chap. 12). PVR can be calculated from the measurements and samples obtained during cardiac catheterization (see Table 71–2). As a rule, noninvasive methods are less reliable and less informative.

Chest Radiography

The findings on the chest radiograph depend on the duration of the pulmonary hypertension and its etiology (see Chap. 15). The characteristic findings of pulmonary hypertension are enlargement of the pulmonary trunk and hilar vessels in association with attenuation (pruning) of the peripheral pulmonary arterial tree (Fig. 71–1). Right-sided heart enlargement can best be detected radiographically on the lateral view as fullness in the retrosternal airspace. In secondary pulmonary hypertension, changes in the lungs (e.g., hyperinflation, fibrosis) and in the position of the heart and diaphragm often mask the radiologic changes of pulmonary hy-

TABLE 71–3

Nomenclature and Classification of Pulmonary Hypertension

Diagnostic Classification
1. Pulmonary arterial hypertension
   1.1 Idiopathic
       Familial
   1.2 Related to
      (a) Connective tissue disease
      (b) Congenital systemic to pulmonary shunts
      (c) Portal hypertension
      (d) HIV infection
      (e) Drugs/toxins
         (1) Anorexigens
         (2) Other
      (f) Persistent pulmonary hypertension of the newborn
      (g) Other
2. Pulmonary venous hypertension
   2.1 Left-side atrial or ventricular heart disease
   2.2 Left-side valvular heart disease
   2.3 Extrinsic compression of central pulmonary veins
      (a) Fibrosing mediastinitis
      (b) Adenopathy/tumors
   2.4 Pulmonary venoocclusive disease/ pulmonary capillary hemangiomatosis
   2.5 Other
3. Pulmonary hypertension associated with disorders of the respiratory system and/or hypoxemia
   3.1 Chronic obstructive pulmonary disease
   3.2 Interstitial lung disease
   3.3 Sleep-disordered breathing
   3.4 Alveolar hypoventilatory disorders
   3.5 Chronic exposure to high altitude
   3.6 Neonatal lung disease
   3.7 Alveolar-capillary dysplasia
   3.8 Other
4. Pulmonary hypertension caused by chronic thrombotic and/or embolic disease
   4.1 Thromboembolic obstruction of proximal pulmonary arteries
   4.2 Obstruction of distal pulmonary arteries
      (a) Pulmonary embolism (thrombus, tumor, ova and/or parasites, foreign material)
      (b) In situ thrombosis
      (c) Sickle cell disease
5. Pulmonary hypertension as a consequence of disorders directly affecting the pulmonary vasculature
   5.1 Inflammatory
      (a) Schistosomiasis
      (b) Sarcoidosis
      (c) Other

pertension. Contrast angiography has a role in the workup for pulmonary hypertension when chronic thromboembolic disease, which may be treated surgically, is suspected.[8]

The Electrocardiogram

The electrocardiogram (ECG) can disclose hypertrophy of the right ventricle and is more reliable in nonrespiratory etiologies than in obstructive airways disease or parenchymal lung disease (see Chap. 13).

Echocardiography

The amount of reliable information obtained by Doppler and two-dimensional echocardiography depends greatly on the commitment of individual clinics to standardizing and perfecting these noninvasive techniques (see Chap. 16). In general, echocardiographic techniques have proved useful in providing a measure of right ventricle thickness as an index of RV hypertension. Estimates of the level of pulmonary hypertension can be obtained by determining regurgitant flows across the tricuspid valves using continuous-wave Doppler echocardiography.[9] In patients in whom the pulmonic valve has been visualized, its behavior during the cardiac cycle has also been used to estimate the level of pulmonary arterial pressure. Echocardiography is an attractive alternative to repeated cardiac catheterization in following the course of the disease and assessing the effects of therapeutic interventions in some patients (see Chap. 16).

Lung Scans

Ventilation–perfusion scans are of most value in the diagnosis and exclusion of pulmonary thromboembolic disease (see Thromboembolic Disease below; also Chap. 72).

Radionuclide Studies

The response of the RV ejection fraction to exercise can be assessed using radionuclide angiography. Scintigraphy using thallium-201 also has been useful in detecting hypertrophy of the right ventricle caused by pulmonary hypertension (see Chap. 19).

Lung Biopsy

The sampling of lung tissue by open thoracotomy or thoracoscopy is rarely helpful in identifying the etiology of the pulmonary hypertension—for example, in the setting of suspected pulmonary vasculitis. Furthermore, the procedure carries substantial risk in these hemodynamically compromised individuals. Attempts to predict responsiveness to vasodilators on the basis of lung biopsy have had limited success.[10]

SECONDARY PULMONARY HYPERTENSION

Cardiac and/or respiratory diseases are the most common causes of secondary pulmonary hypertension. Cardiac disease leads to pulmonary hypertension by increasing pulmonary blood flow (e.g., large left-to-right shunts) or by increasing pulmonary venous pressure (e.g., LV failure). Almost invariably, secondary influences such as intimal proliferation in the pulmonary resistance vessels add a component of obstructive pulmonary vascular disease.[11] In respiratory disease, the predominant mechanism for the pulmonary hypertension is an increase in resistance to pulmonary blood flow arising from perivascular parenchymal changes coupled with

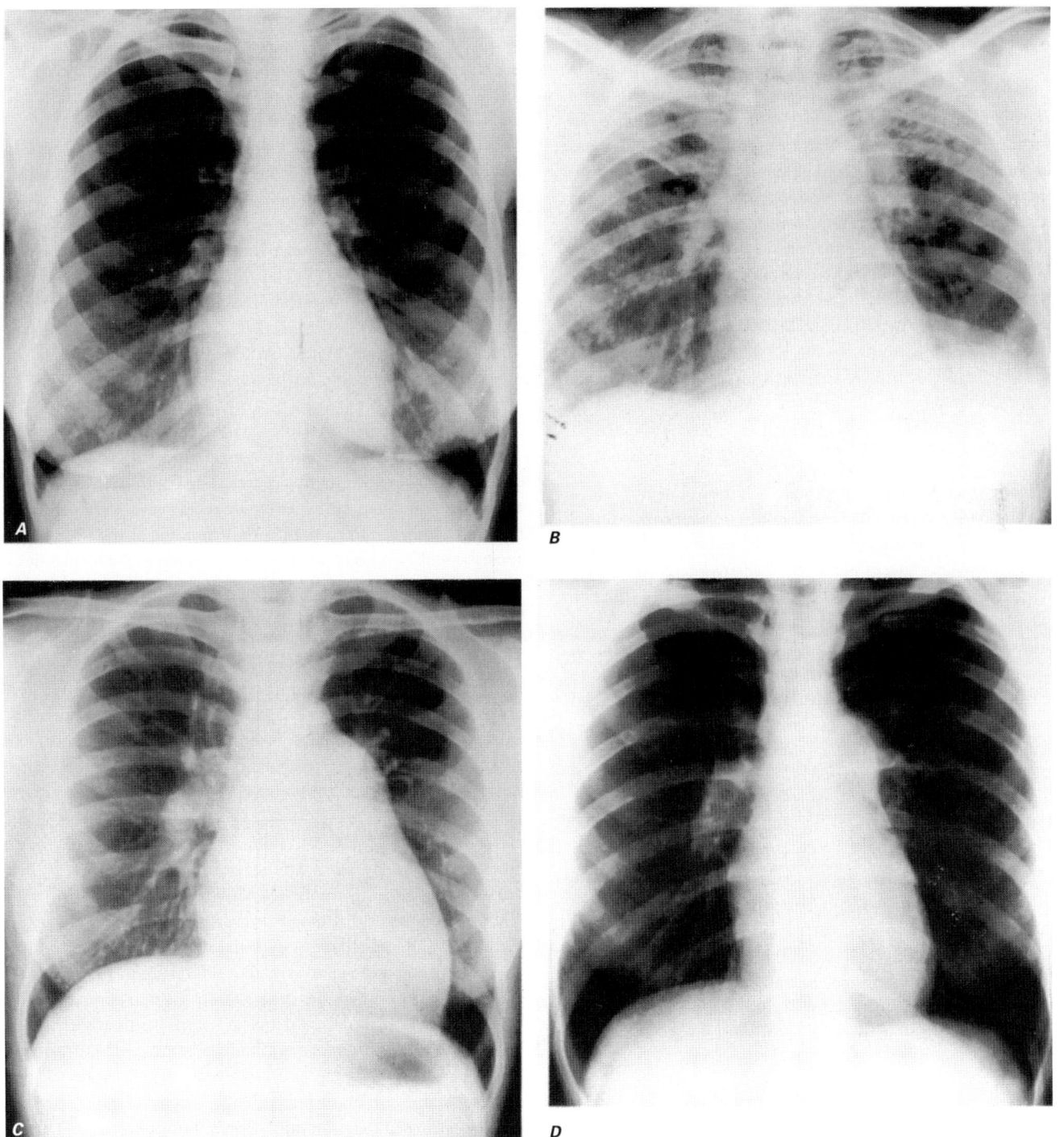

FIGURE 71-1. Cardiac silhouette in four patients with severe pulmonary hypertension on admission to the hospital. **A, B.** Primary pulmonary hypertension showing different stages in the evolution of right-sided heart failure. **C.** Widespread pulmonary fibrosis. **D.** Systemic lupus erythematosus proven by lung biopsy. This radiograph is indistinguishable from that of idiopathic pulmonary artery hypertension.

pulmonary vasoconstriction and remodeling because of hypoxia. In pulmonary thromboembolic disease, clots in various stages of organization and affecting pulmonary vessels of different size increase resistance to blood flow.[12]

【 】 CARDIAC DISEASE

The mechanisms of pulmonary hypertension usually are quite different in acquired disorders of the left side of the heart than in those of congenital heart disease.

Acquired Disorders of the Left Side of the Heart

LV failure is the most common cause of pulmonary hypertension. Among the various etiologies, myocardial disorders and lesions of the mitral and aortic valves predominate. Both categories of lesions lead to an increase in pulmonary venous pressure that, in turn, evokes an increase in pulmonary arterial pressure. Presumably, the increase in pulmonary arterial pressure is reflex in origin. In time, three types of morphologic changes supervene: (1) occlusive intimal and medial changes not only in pulmonary venules and veins, but also in the precapillary vessels; (2) perivascular interstitial edema and fibrosis that, under the influence of gravity, cause vascular and perivascular changes to be most marked in the dependent portions of the lungs; and (3) occlusion of small pulmonary vessels by emboli or thrombi when the right ventricle fails and cardiac output decreases. Chap. 26 discusses the medical management of myocardial failure. The treatment of congenital heart disease and of mitral valvular disease is usually mechanical (e.g., surgical or balloon mitral valvuloplasty). The prospect for relief of the pulmonary venous hypertension, as by mitral valve commissurotomy or replacement, depends on the reversibility of the pulmonary vascular and perivascular lesions.

Although LV failure is the most common cause of RV failure, the level of pulmonary hypertension that accompanies LV failure rarely is sufficient to account for the RV failure. RV failure, secondary to LV failure, is usually attributed in part to failure of the muscle in the shared ventricular septum.

Congenital Heart Disease

Pulmonary hypertension is part of the natural history of many types of congenital heart disease and is often a major determinant of the clinical course, the feasibility of surgical intervention, and the outcome (see Chap. 83). The major cause of pulmonary hypertension in congenital heart disease is an increase in blood flow, an increase in resistance to blood flow, or, most often, a combination of the two. In congenital heart disease with right-to-left shunting (systemic hypoxemia), pulmonary vasoconstriction because of mixed venous hypoxemia may add to the resistance to blood flow. Erythrocytosis, acting by way of increased viscosity and propensity to thrombosis, also contributes to the increase in resistance. Although the increase in pulmonary vascular tone elicited by hypoxia contributes to the increase in PVR, the predominant resistance is offered by anatomic changes in the walls of the small muscular arteries and arterioles. Patients with congenital heart disease and pulmonary hypertension who become pregnant are at increased risk of sudden death, both in the course of delivery and in the immediate postpartum period, because of acute exacerbations of pulmonary hypertension and right ventricular decompensation that may result from intravascular volume shifts and worsening hypoxemia caused by atelectasis, infection, thromboembolism, and other factors.

Vasodilators are rarely helpful in diminishing heightened pulmonary vasomotor tone in the setting of congenital cardiac defects. Caution is required in administering vasodilators to such patients because of the potential to increase right-to-left shunting by reducing systemic vascular resistance to a greater degree than its pulmonary counterpart. Phlebotomy, with replacement of fluid (e.g., plasma or albumin) is helpful in congenital cyanotic heart disease in which severe hypoxemia has evoked a large increase in red cell mass. Once again, caution is required to avoid depletion of iron stores and a reduction in the circulating blood volume.

Thromboembolic Disease

Thromboembolic disease is a form of occlusive pulmonary vascular disease that may be acute or chronic. In the United States and Europe, clots originating in peripheral veins represent a common cause of chronic occlusive pulmonary vascular disease. Elsewhere in the world, other intravascular particulates may cause pulmonary vascular occlusive disease. For example, in Egypt, where schistosomiasis is endemic, pulmonary vascular disease stemming from ova lodged in

pulmonary vessels and hypersensitivity reactions to the organism (usually situated outside the lungs) is common. In some parts of Asia, filariasis is reputed to be an important cause of pulmonary hypertension. Tumor emboli to the lungs from extrapulmonary sites (e.g., the breast) can cause pulmonary hypertension by invading the adjacent minute vessels of the lungs. Intravenous drug use may be associated with talc or cotton fiber embolism to the lungs, which can result in a granulomatous pulmonary arteritis.

The *syndromes of thromboembolic pulmonary hypertension* can be categorized according to the segments of the pulmonary arterial tree that are primarily affected: (1) small (muscular pulmonary arteries and arterioles), (2) intermediate arteries, and (3) large central arteries. Some overlap is inevitable because clots lodged in large vessels are fragmented by the churning motion of the heart, and both the parent clot and its derivatives tend to move peripherally for final lodging.

Occlusion of Small Muscular Arteries and Arterioles by Organized Thrombi
At autopsy, small thrombi, predominantly recent in origin, are commonplace in the small pulmonary vessels of patients with pulmonary hypertension who have developed heart failure preterminally. In contrast is the syndrome of widespread pulmonary vascular occlusion by organized thrombi in the small pulmonary arteries and arterioles. Once attributed to multiple pulmonary emboli, these lesions are now regarded as organized, in situ thrombi.[12] The syndrome is rare and indistinguishable during life from idiopathic pulmonary artery hypertension except by lung biopsy. However, histologic identification of these lesions serves little purpose in management. After a ventilation–perfusion scan has excluded chronic proximal thromboembolism (see below), treatment consists of long-term anticoagulation using warfarin or related agents, antiplatelet agents, or both to prevent further clotting.

Occlusion of Intermediate Pulmonary Arteries by Emboli
This syndrome is by far the most common of the three.[12] It is thought to be caused by multiple emboli released from vessels in the upper legs and thighs that progressively amputate the pulmonary arterial tree. Ventilation–perfusion scans and selective angiography demonstrate the pulmonary vascular occlusion, although both studies tend to underestimate the degree of obstruction compared with direct inspection of the vascular tree at surgery or postmortem (see Chap. 72). The major therapeutic concern in these patients is to exclude chronic proximal pulmonary thromboembolism (see below) and to prevent recurrent thromboemboli. Treatment involves the use of anticoagulants of the warfarin type and antiplatelet agents.

Chronic Proximal Pulmonary Thromboembolism
In some patients who have survived large to massive pulmonary emboli, resolution fails to occur, and the clots become organized and incorporated into the walls of the major pulmonary arteries, leading to pulmonary hypertension (Fig. 71–2). Overwhelming the capacity of the local fibrinolytic mechanisms also allows the clot to propagate, to obstruct large segments of the pulmonary vascular bed, and to decrease the compliance of the central pulmonary vessels. By the time the diagnosis is made, the obstructing lesions in the central pulmonary arteries have become an integral part of the vascular wall through the processes of endothelialization and recanalization.[12]

The importance of recognizing *proximal* pulmonary thromboembolism as a cause of pulmonary hypertension is the possibility of relieving

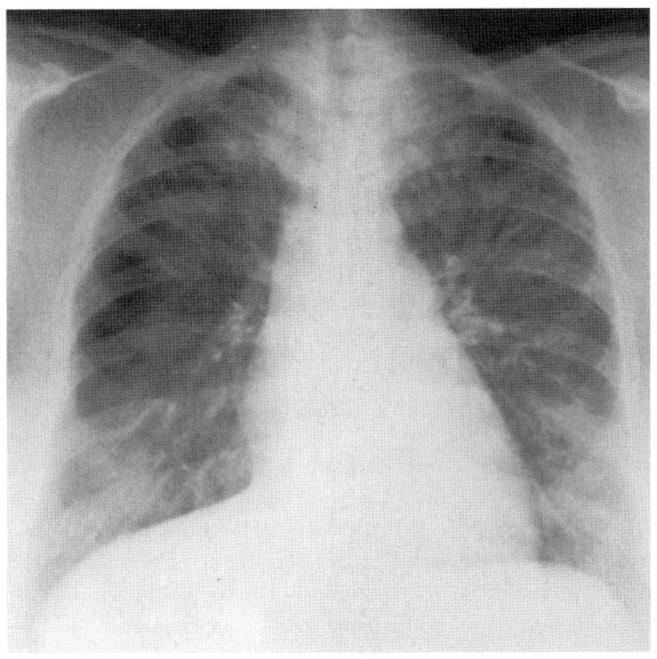

A

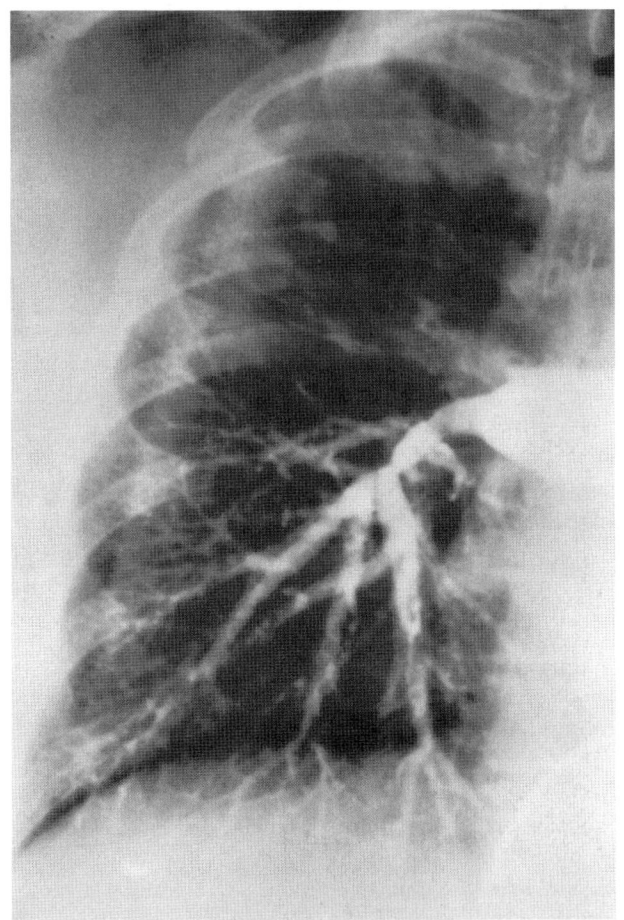

B

FIGURE 71-2. Pulmonary hypertension as a result of an organized clot in central pulmonary arteries. Dramatic relief after pulmonary thromboendarterectomy. **A.** Chest radiograph. The right upper lobe is strikingly hypoperfused, and the vasculature on the left is quite prominent, reflecting redirection of the pulmonary blood flow to open vessels. **B.** Angiogram. The flow to the right upper lung is interrupted by the large central clot.

the pulmonary hypertension by surgical intervention, that is, by pulmonary thromboendarterectomy. Ventilation–perfusion lung scanning is the critical diagnostic test. As a rule, patients with proximal pulmonary thromboembolism show two or more segmental perfusion defects. If the perfusion defects are segmental or larger, selective pulmonary angiography is called for to define the location, extent, and number of pulmonary vascular occlusions.[13,14] Cardiac catheterization for selective pulmonary angiography also enables hemodynamic assessment. Fiberoptic angioscopy, helical computed tomographic scanning, and magnetic resonance imaging may be helpful in defining the lesions of proximal thromboembolic pulmonary hypertension (see Chap. 72).[15]

Surgery is advocated for patients with pulmonary hypertension who have persistent clots in lobar or more proximal pulmonary arteries after at least 6 months of anticoagulation. Thromboendarterectomy is done using a median sternotomy and deep hypothermic cardiopulmonary bypass with intermittent periods of circulatory arrest. Postoperatively, hemodynamic improvement is often quite dramatic.[8,14] Reperfusion pulmonary edema can be a severe complication immediately after the obstruction has been relieved. In experienced hands, mortality is approximately 5 percent. After the operation, patients are placed on lifelong anticoagulants. A filter is usually placed in the inferior vena cava to further prevent recurrence.

【 】 RESPIRATORY DISEASES AND DISORDERS

In addition to intrinsic pulmonary diseases, disturbances in respiratory muscle function or in the control of breathing also can cause pulmonary hypertension. Among the intrinsic lung diseases are those affecting the airways (e.g., chronic bronchitis), as well as those affecting the parenchyma (i.e., emphysema, pulmonary fibrosis). Among the ventilatory disorders are the syndromes of alveolar hypoventilation caused by respiratory muscle weakness and sleep-disordered breathing.

Intrinsic Diseases of the Lungs and/or Airways

Diseases that affect the parenchyma of the lungs or the tracheobronchial tree can elicit pulmonary hypertension in different ways, depending on the underlying disease (Fig. 71–3). In obstructive

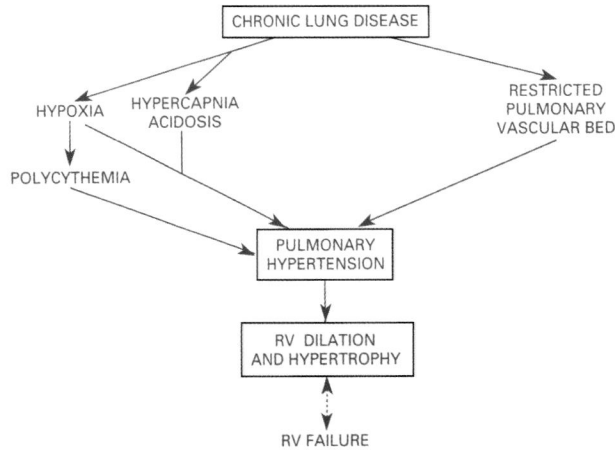

FIGURE 71-3. The evolution of right ventricular (RV) failure in chronic obstructive airways disease (chronic bronchitis and emphysema; chronic obstructive pulmonary disease). The factors on the left arise primarily from the bronchitis; those on the right from emphysema.

airways disease, ventilation–perfusion abnormalities cause vasoconstriction because of arterial hypoxemia. In diffuse fibrosis, several mechanisms act in concert: loss of vascular surface area because of lung destruction, loss of vascular compliance because of hyperinflation-induced vascular compression, and vascular remodeling caused by hypoxic vasoconstriction.

Interstitial Fibrosis

Pulmonary sarcoidosis, asbestosis, and idiopathic and radiation-induced fibrosis commonly cause widespread pulmonary fibrosis that result in cor pulmonale. Dyspnea and tachypnea dominate the clinical picture of interstitial fibrosis; cough is rarely prominent. Usually, severe pulmonary hypertension occurs toward the end of the illness, when hypoxemia and hypercapnia are present at rest (see Fig. 71–1).

Systemically administered vasodilators have no proven place in treating the pulmonary hypertension associated with interstitial fibrosis and may worsen intrapulmonary gas exchange. Recent experience with inhaled vasodilators, such as the prostacyclin analogue iloprost, is encouraging and suggests the possibility of producing selective pulmonary vasodilator and/or antiproliferative effects in this population.[16] Oxygen therapy, particularly during daily activity or sleep, can be important in attenuating the hypoxic pulmonary pressor response. Glucocorticoids and other potent immunosuppressive agents are the mainstay of therapy and often effect some symptomatic relief. The advent of lung transplantation has widened greatly the therapeutic horizons for dealing with widespread interstitial fibrosis.

Chronic Obstructive Airways Disease

Chronic bronchitis and emphysema (chronic obstructive pulmonary disease [COPD]) are the most common causes of cor pulmonale in patients with intrinsic pulmonary disease.[17,18] Cystic fibrosis is an example of a mixed airways and parenchymal lung disease in which pulmonary hypertension plays a significant role in outcome.

Cor pulmonale is encountered in two different settings: *acutely* in the setting of decompensation, which is often caused by an acute respiratory infection, and *chronically*, when progressive lung disease and worsening gas exchange lead to unremitting vascular remodeling.

The gold standard for diagnosing pulmonary hypertension in patients with COPD is right-heart catheterization. Noninvasive studies, such as echocardiography, have proved useful in some centers.[19,20] RV enlargement, the cardinal sign of pulmonary hypertension, can be difficult to discern in obstructive airways disease because of hyperinflation and cardiac rotation.[21] Once suspicion is raised that the clinical picture of RV failure stems from gas exchange abnormalities, an arterial blood sample will confirm that the PO_2 is low (PO_2 <50 mmHg) and the PCO_2 is high (PCO_2 >50 mmHg). Derangement in gas exchange to this degree is rare in LV failure unless overt pulmonary edema is present.

ECG evidence of RV hypertrophy is also often equivocal in patients with chronic obstructive airways disease (chronic bronchitis and emphysema, COPD) because of rotation and displacement of the heart, widened distances between electrodes and the cardiac surface, and the predominance of right-sided heart dilatation over hypertrophy. Be-

cause of these limitations, standard ECG criteria for RV enlargement apply in about one-third of patients with COPD who have cor pulmonale at autopsy. Consecutive changes in the ECG are often more useful than a single ECG in detecting RV overload. As the arterial PO_2 drops to abnormal levels (e.g., <60 to 70 mmHg while awake), T waves tend to become inverted, biphasic, or flat in the right, precordial leads (V_1 to V_3); the mean electrical axis of the QRS shifts 30 degrees or more to the right of the patient's usual axis; ST segments become depressed in leads II, III, and aVF; and right bundle-branch block (incomplete or complete) often appears. These changes tend to reverse as arterial oxygenation improves (see Chap. 13).

In the patient with COPD with acute cor pulmonale precipitated by a bout of bronchitis or pneumonia, the goal of therapy is to maintain tolerable levels of arterial oxygenation while waiting for the upper respiratory infection to subside. Considerable improvement also may be accomplished even in the individual who has chronic pulmonary hypertension by sustained (>18 h/d) breathing of oxygen-enriched air. Once the RV has failed, inotropic agents should be used cautiously because of the threat of arrhythmias posed by arterial hypoxemia and respiratory acidosis. Moreover, after adequate oxygenation has been achieved, the need for digitalis and diuretics often decreases because the hemodynamic burden on the RV decreases. Even though acute cor pulmonale is largely reversible, each bout appears to leave behind a slightly higher level of pulmonary hypertension after recovery.[17]

Arterial blood gas composition is the therapeutic compass to the control of pulmonary hypertension in COPD. The degree of hypoxia may be underestimated by blood sampling while the patient is awake and at rest, as hypoxemia is more marked during sleep and with physical activity. Determinations of the oxygen saturation during sleep or with ambulation using pulse oximetry are helpful in optimally prescribing supplemental oxygen.

Polycythemia is rarely severe enough to be a serious problem in cor pulmonale associated with bronchitis and emphysema; when it is present, it is usually indicative of suboptimal use of supplemental oxygen. Vasodilators recently have been tried in various types of secondary pulmonary hypertension, including that caused by COPD.[22] They may aggravate arterial hypoxemia by exaggerating ventilation–perfusion abnormalities. To date, the safest and most effective approach to pulmonary vasodilatation in obstructive lung disease with arterial hypoxemia is the use of supplemental oxygen.[22]

Connective Tissue Diseases

Pulmonary vascular disease is an important component of certain connective tissue diseases, most commonly systemic lupus erythematosus (SLE), the scleroderma spectrum of diseases, and dermatomyositis (see Chap. 88).[23] The lesions may take the form of interstitial inflammation and fibrosis, obliterative disease, or vasculitis, either singly or in combination. Although pulmonary hypertension can complicate many connective tissue diseases, it has been documented most often in SLE and progressive systemic sclerosis (scleroderma) and its variant syndromes. The possibility has been raised that IPAH is an inflammatory, or autoimmune, disease. The high frequency of both collagen-vascular disease and IPAH in women and the occurrence of Raynaud phenomenon in up to 20 percent of patients with IPAH has been used as additional evidence.[24] Finally, there is a high incidence of positive serologic tests for antibodies (antinuclear antibody, anti-Ku), particularly in women with IPAH.

The lungs and pleura are frequently involved in SLE, with a reported frequency of up to 70 percent. Patients with pulmonary hypertension and SLE are predominantly women; most of these patients also exhibit Raynaud phenomenon.

The histopathologic lesions in these patients resemble those of IPAH. Pulmonary hypertension in these patients may originate in thrombi secondary to the hypercoagulable state caused by lupus anticoagulant or anticardiolipin antibodies in the blood. Unfortunately, treatment of pulmonary hypertension associated with SLE using either anticoagulants or pulmonary vasodilators has had only modest success. However, patients with active pulmonary vasculitis may either improve or stabilize their vascular disease with immunosuppressive agents.

In progressive systemic sclerosis (scleroderma) and its variants, such as the CREST (*c*alcinosis, *R*aynaud syndrome, *e*sophageal involvement, *s*clerodactyly, and *t*elangiectasia) syndrome, and in overlap syndromes (e.g., mixed connective tissue disease), the incidence of pulmonary vascular disease is estimated to be between 20 and 40 percent. In these patients, pulmonary hypertension is the cause of considerable morbidity and mortality.[25] The pulmonary vascular disease may be independent of pulmonary or other visceral disease. As in the case of SLE, the pathology of these lesions is often indistinguishable from that of IPAH. Newer therapies, such as continuous intravenous epoprostenol, endothelin receptor antagonists, and phosphodiesterase type-5 inhibitors, have been shown to improve hemodynamics and exercise tolerance.[26]

Alveolar Hypoventilation in Patients with Normal Lungs

In patients who hypoventilate despite normal lungs (alveolar hypoventilation), the primary pathogenetic mechanism is alveolar hypoxia potentiated by respiratory acidosis.[27] These abnormal alveolar and arterial blood gases play the same role in eliciting pulmonary hypertension in patients with alveolar hypoventilation as in those in whom the abnormal alveolar and blood gases are the result of ventilation–perfusion abnormalities. In individuals with normal lungs, the alveolar hypoventilation generally originates from an inadequate ventilatory drive (e.g., after encephalitis or in central sleep apnea), covert obstruction of the upper airways (e.g., in obstructive sleep apnea), an ineffective chest bellows (e.g., after poliomyelitis or polymyositis), lungs entrapped by neoplasm or fibrosis (e.g., in trapped lung caused by asbestosis), or in morbid obesity.

Regardless of etiology, whether pulmonary hypertension will occur in patients with alveolar hypoventilation and normal lungs depends on the whether there is sufficient alveolar and arterial hypoxia to raise pulmonary arterial pressures considerably. In the sleep apnea syndromes, severe arterial hypoxemia and pulmonary hypertension that develop initially only during sleep may become self-perpetuating and carry over into wakefulness, although pulmonary hypertension tends to be mild and only occurs in those with severe disturbances in respiration during sleep.[28]

For the patient with alveolar hypoventilation with combined respiratory and cardiac (RV) failure, the highest therapeutic priority is to improve oxygenation. Assisted ventilation, particularly during sleep (e.g., continuous positive airway pressure), may be particularly helpful in improving oxygenation and reducing hypercapnia. Pharmacologic therapy is rarely needed for patients with alveolar hypoventilation because of the efficiency of assisted ventilation coupled with oxygen therapy in promoting pulmonary vasodilatation.

IDIOPATHIC PULMONARY ARTERY HYPERTENSION

【 】 DEFINITION

IPAH is a disorder intrinsic to the pulmonary vascular bed that is characterized by sustained elevations in pulmonary artery pressure and vascular resistance that generally lead to RV failure and death.[24] The diagnosis of IPAH requires the exclusion on clinical grounds of other conditions that can result in pulmonary artery hypertension (see Table 71–3).[29] IPAH is a rare disease, with an incidence of 1 to 2 per million.[30] Its prevalence is approximately 0.1 to 0.2 percent of all patients who come to autopsy.

The clinical diagnosis of IPAH rests on three different types of evidence: (1) clinical, radiographic, and ECG manifestations of pulmonary hypertension; (2) hemodynamic features consisting of abnormally high pulmonary arterial pressures and PVR in association with normal left-sided filling pressures and a normal or low cardiac output; and (3) exclusion of the causes of secondary pulmonary hypertension.

Certain associations of PAH have attracted interest because of their prospects for shedding light on some etiologies. These include anorexigen-induced pulmonary hypertension, familial pulmonary hypertension, human immunodeficiency virus (HIV) infection-associated pulmonary hypertension, and portal-pulmonary hypertension.[29–32] In each of these, the clinical findings and the histologic appearance of the lungs at autopsy are identical to those characterizing the sporadic form of IPAH. This diversity in associations underscores the likelihood that so-called IPAH is the final common expression of heterogeneous etiologies.

【 】 GENERAL FEATURES

After puberty, females predominate, those between 10 and 40 years of age being most often affected. Before puberty, no sex difference is discernible. The typical picture of a patient with IPAH is that of a young woman who develops one or more of the symptoms listed in Table 71–1 without discernible cause. Gender and age are sometimes useful in distinguishing clinically between the likelihood of IPAH and pulmonary thromboembolic disease. The latter generally favors men, particularly in their later years.[24]

Prior to the modern therapeutic era, the median survival of patients was predictable on the basis of the New York Heart Association's functional classification: 6 months for class IV, 2 to 2.5 years for class III, and 6 years for classes I and II. Unless interrupted by sudden death, which occurs in approximately 10 percent of patients, the course terminates in intractable RV failure.[33]

【 】 ETIOLOGY

The common denominator in the pathogenesis of IPAH appears to be injury to the layers of the vascular wall of the small muscular pulmonary arteries and arterioles.[34] The intima of these vessels proliferates, perhaps in response to injury, so that the endothelium changes from a single flat layer to a piled-up projection that narrows the caliber of the vascular lumen. Also, both the media and the adventitia of the affected vessels undergo hypertrophy.[35]

The primary site of injury in IPAH remains uncertain. An intrinsic defect in ion channel function and calcium homeostasis in vascular smooth muscle has been implicated.[36] Other studies show that endothelial function is disturbed, leading to altered production or handling of a variety of endothelium-derived vasoactive substances, including endothelin, nitric oxide, and prostacyclin.[34] These abnormalities, coupled with altered platelet-endothelial interactions that predispose to intravascular thrombosis and release of growth factors, lead to an inexorable course of enhanced vascular reactivity, proliferation and remodeling, and progressive obliterative vasculopathy. Diverse etiologies seem to be capable of eliciting PAH[37] (Table 71–4). For example, ingestion of the anorexigens fenfluramine and its isomer dexfenfluramine has been demonstrated to markedly increase the risk of PAH[30]; ingestion of toxic oil elicited an outbreak of pulmonary hypertension in Spain[38]; and HIV infection also has been implicated.[31]

An epidemic of PAH in Europe between 1967 and 1970 that was linked to the use of aminorex, an anorectic agent, raised the prospect of hereditary predisposition, because only 1 in 1000 who took the drug developed pulmonary hypertension. More recently, the fenfluramines have been associated with both severe pulmonary hypertension and valvular heart disease.[30,39] The toxic oil epidemic in Spain has reinforced the concept of individual susceptibility to pulmonary vasotoxic agents.[38]

In recent years, an increasing number of patients have been identified in whom PAH is genetically linked.[40] In these individuals, the hereditary pattern is that of autosomal dominance with incomplete penetrance. The gene responsible for familial disease recently has been identified as the *BMPR2* (bone morphogenetic

protein receptor 2) gene, a member of the transforming growth factor- family.[41] One major insight provided by the families with familial pulmonary hypertension is the diversity of pulmonary vascular lesions in members of the same family.[40]

PATHOLOGY

The evolution of IPAH depends on progressive attenuation of the pulmonary arterial tree, which gradually increases PVR to the point of eliciting RV strain and failure. The seat of the disease is in the small pulmonary arteries (between 40 and 100 μm in diameter) and arterioles. The obliterative lesions can affect one or more layers of these vessels. In some instances, medial hypertrophy predominates; in others, it is the intima that proliferates. In addition, evidence of inflammation may be present (Fig. 71–4).[35]

Histologic examination of the lung identifies a constellation of pulmonary precapillary lesions that are consistent with the clinical diagnosis of PAH—that is, plexiform lesions, angiomatoid lesions, concentric intimal fibrosis, and necrotizing arteritis. The pathologist is often hard pressed to distinguish between organized clots in small vessels that initiate the pulmonary hypertension and those that result from the obliterative pulmonary vascular disease. Recent clots in small pulmonary arteries and arterioles are common at autopsy in patients with IPAH, particularly when the RV has failed and cardiac output falls. Although similar clots may not have initiated the pulmonary hypertension process in IPAH, it seems reasonable that more often they are complicating features that aggravate and exaggerate pulmonary vascular obstruction.

PATHOPHYSIOLOGY

The hemodynamic hallmarks of IPAH in the resting patient were indicated earlier: a combination of a high pulmonary arterial pressure, a normal or low cardiac output, and a normal LA or pulmonary artery wedge pressure. Calculated PVR is high, generally leading to the logical conclusion that the resistance vessels, that is, the small muscular arteries and arterioles, are the predominant sites of vascular obstruction. During exercise, as cardiac

TABLE 71–4

Suggested Mechanisms for Idiopathic Pulmonary Artery Hypertension

PROPOSED MECHANISM	EVIDENCE
Early/sustained vaso-constriction kinetics	Altered smooth muscle cell calcium
	Endothelial dysfunction
Genetic predisposition	Familial disease with gene locus identified
	Susceptibility with exposures, e.g., anorexigens, HIV, portal hypertension
Pulmonary thrombosis/embolism	Widespread occlusion of arteries/arterioles
	Altered endothelial–platelet interaction
Autoimmune disease	Raynaud phenomenon and antinuclear antibodies common; female gender predilection

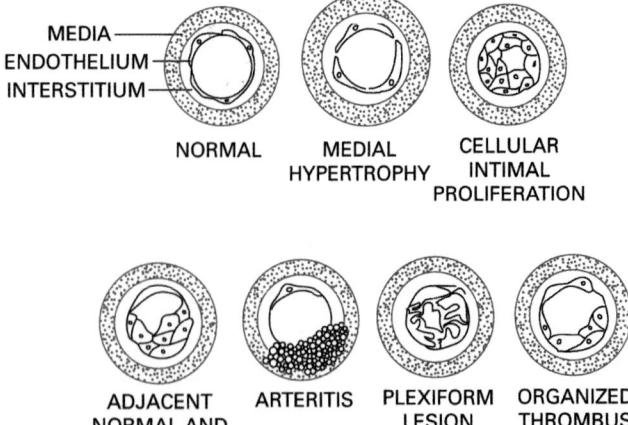

FIGURE 71–4. Vascular lesions in idiopathic pulmonary artery hypertension. The plexiform lesion, once believed to be the histologic hallmark of idiopathic pulmonary artery hypertension, has emerged as only one feature of a constellation of lesions.

output increases, pulmonary arterial pressures increase further; the increments in pressure in the pulmonary hypertensive circuit are much more striking than in the normotensive pulmonary circulation, owing to the inability of the existing vasculature to dilate or recruit unused vessels to accommodate the rise in pulmonary blood flow.

Pulmonary vasodilators are currently administered acutely for testing the responsiveness of the pulmonary circulation.[29] Among these, inhaled NO and intravenous prostacyclin or adenosine have become the gold standards. Several clinical and hemodynamic changes are sought as desirable end points: (1) improvement in exercise tolerance and in the quality of life, attributable to an increase in cardiac output, which, in turn, improves oxygen delivery to peripheral organs and tissues; (2) a decrease in the level of pulmonary arterial hypertension, with evidence of regression of RV hypertrophy and or dilatation; and (3) a decrease in calculated PVR; optimally, this decrease should entail an increase in cardiac output (with minimal increase in heart rate) accompanied by a substantial decrease in pulmonary arterial pressure. Because pulmonary vasodilators are also systemic vasodilators, pulmonary vasodilatation must be effected without evoking undue systemic hypotension and tachycardia.

The combination of right-heart catheterization and vasodilator testing is particularly useful not only for defining the hemodynamic state of the patient but also in providing a hemodynamic baseline for future invasive and noninvasive studies, such as serial echocardiograms.

【 】 CLINICAL PICTURE

In its early stages, the disease is difficult to recognize. In the sporadic case, the first clue is often an abnormal chest radiograph (see Fig. 71–1) or ECG indicative of RV hypertrophy (Fig. 71–5). Both are late manifestations. The existence of RV enlargement is generally confirmed by echocardiography. By the time these changes appear, however, pulmonary hypertension is moderate to severe. Initial complaints—particularly easy fatigability and dyspnea—tend to be discounted, that is, attributed to being "out of shape," except when the index of suspicion is high, as with a history of ingestion of anorectic agents or of familial pulmonary hypertension (see Table 71–1).

When the disease is advanced, increasing nonspecific discomfort progressively reduces the activities of daily life. Dyspnea, particularly during physical activity, becomes incapacitating. Some patients develop an anginal type of chest pain along with breathlessness. Other common symptoms are weakness, fatigue, and exertional or postexertional syncope (see Table 71–1). Infrequently, an en-

larged pulmonary artery causes hoarseness because of compression of the left recurrent laryngeal nerve. In time, right-heart failure develops.

Patients with severe pulmonary hypertension seem vulnerable to sudden death. Death has occurred unexpectedly during normal activities, cardiac catheterization, and surgical procedures and after the administration of anesthetic agents. The mechanisms of sudden death are not clear and may include arrhythmias or acute pulmonary thromboembolism. It was noted earlier that as far as clinical manifestations and physical examination are concerned, IPAH has an advantage over secondary pulmonary hypertension in that signs and symptoms of underlying cardiac or respiratory disease do not obscure its manifestations. On physical examination, the jugular venous pulse usually shows a prominent *a* wave. RV hypertrophy causes a heave along the left sternal border, and a distinct systolic impulse is palpable over the region of the main pulmonary artery (see Chap. 12). The pulmonic component of the second sound is markedly accentuated, the second heart sound is narrowly split, and an ejection sound is heard in the pulmonic area. Often a fourth heart sound emanating from the hypertrophied RV is heard at the lower left sternal border. The murmur of tricuspid regurgitation is best heard along the sternal border with the patient in the supine position and can be accentuated with inspiration In some patients, a midsystolic murmur is audible at the pulmonic area; as pulmonary arterial pressures approximate systemic arterial levels, the murmur of pulmonary valvular regurgitation often appears.

The onset of RV failure is accompanied by jugular venous distension and a gallop (S_3); inspiration intensifies the gallop. The liver becomes enlarged and tender, and hepatojugular reflux can be elicited. Hydrothorax and ascites may be seen as RV failure progresses.

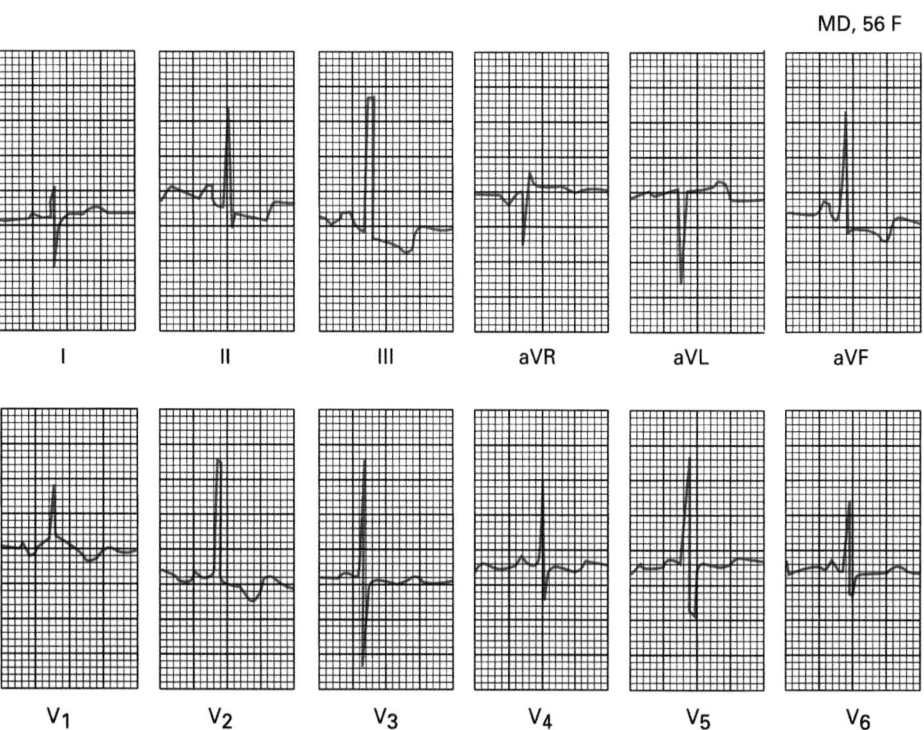

MD, 56 F

FIGURE 71–5. ECGs in patients with idiopathic pulmonary artery hypertension and cor pulmonale.

SPECIAL STUDIES

Direct determination of pulmonary circulatory pressures by right-heart catheterization is the only way to definitively establish the diagnosis of pulmonary hypertension; however, other studies that are less direct can strongly suggest that it is present. Because the diagnosis of IPAH is one of exclusion, a number of tests are undertaken, usually in the hope of identifying a more treatable disease.[37]

Chest Radiography and Electrocardiography

In the early stages, the chest radiograph is generally normal. Later it shows cardiac enlargement in association with enlargement of the pulmonary trunk, while the peripheral pulmonary arterial branches are attenuated; the lung fields appear oligemic (see Fig. 71–1). Although fullness of the central pulmonary arterial trunks and peripheral "pruning" are distinctive, appearances vary somewhat from patient to patient in accord with the level and pace of the pulmonary hypertension and the age of the patient. Radiographic evidence of RV enlargement usually becomes overt only late in the course of the pulmonary hypertension (see Chap. 15). The ECG usually shows right axis deviation, RV hypertrophy, and, usually, right atrial enlargement (see Chap. 13).

The Echocardiogram

Transthoracic echocardiography confirms the enlargement and hypertrophy of the right atrium and right ventricle, tricuspid regurgitation, and pulmonic valvular regurgitation. At the same time, left ventricle structure and function are normal. The magnitude of the velocity of the tricuspid regurgitant jet using Doppler techniques can provide a noninvasive estimate of RV peak systolic pressure. On occasion, transesophageal echocardiography is helpful to search for intracardiac shunts or other congenital abnormalities.

Lung Scans

Lung scans are particularly helpful in suggesting the possibility of large, long-standing organized clots in the major pulmonary arteries that may be amenable to surgical removal (thromboendarterectomy). The lung scan in IPAH fails to disclose major perfusion defects. Angiography is done in cases where the scan is equivocal. Scanning over the brain or kidneys may disclose the presence of an intracardiac or intrapulmonary right-to-left shunt.

Right-Sided Heart Catheterization

Cardiac catheterization is invaluable in quantifying the hemodynamic abnormalities, in excluding cardiac causes of pulmonary arterial hypertension, and in assessing the hemodynamic responses of the heart and pulmonary circulation to vasodilator agents.[29]

DIAGNOSIS

The diagnosis of IPAH rests on two pillars: (1) the detection of pulmonary hypertension and (2) the exclusion of known causes of high pulmonary arterial pressure. The history is of utmost importance. Before categorizing pulmonary hypertension as "idiopathic," due regard must be paid to the exclusion of known etiologies (see Table 71–3), particularly thromboembolic disease and connective tissue disorders. Account also should be taken of the

likelihood of familial disease. Pulmonary function tests are useful in excluding diffuse pulmonary disorders, particularly interstitial lung disease. Serologic testing can point the way to covert connective tissue disorders and occult HIV infection. Abnormal liver function tests can signal the coexistence of portal and pulmonary hypertension. The value of cardiac catheterization in eliminating acquired or congenital heart disease was indicated earlier. Unfortunately, by the time pulmonary hypertension complicating heart disease is recognized, the anatomic lesions are often too far advanced for the obliterative pulmonary vascular disease to be reversible with corrective surgery.

TREATMENT

Treatment of IPAH initially focused on the use of vasodilators in the hope that an increase in pulmonary vascular tone contributed importantly to the high pulmonary arterial pressures. Although the bulk of the pulmonary vascular obstruction was clearly anatomic, vasodilators offered the prospect not only of decreasing pulmonary arterial pressures somewhat, and therefore the hemodynamic burden on the RV, but also of prompting reversibility of the anatomic lesions. Unfortunately, the use of vasodilators, which could affect the systemic as well as the pulmonary circulation, led to progressive disenchantment with one agent after another.

The situation has changed considerably during the past decade. The introduction of acute vasodilator testing for responsiveness has shown that fewer than 10 percent of patients manifest heightened pulmonary vasomotor tone as the cause of pulmonary hypertension. An optimal "responder" to acute testing manifests an increase in cardiac output along with a decrease in pulmonary arterial pressure to near-normal levels with no undue effect on systemic arterial pressure. Calcium channel blocking agents that can be taken orally may maintain those patients who were highly responsive during acute testing at lower pulmonary arterial pressures. A landmark development for patients who failed to satisfy the criteria for a good hemodynamic response to acute vasodilator testing was the demonstration that such patients respond to continuous infusion of epoprostenol. Indeed, a substantial number of such patients have been treated in this way for years or have used continuous intravenous epoprostenol as a transition to transplantation or newer drug therapies. During this evolution, heart–lung and then lung transplantation became increasingly feasible and available, although the donor supply is still a limiting factor. More recently, the development of oral medications that block the receptors for endothelin or that augment the effects of endogenous nitric oxide by inhibiting phosphodiesterase type-5 (the enzyme responsible for breakdown of cyclic guanosine monophosphate) have been shown to be effective therapy and may obviate the need for prostanoid therapy in many severely afflicted patients. Alternative forms of delivery of longer-acting prostacyclin analogues, including subcutaneous and aerosolized medications, have also been developed and may obviate the need for parenteral prostanoid therapy in many patients.

As a result of these advances, a patient with PAH has several therapeutic options. However, none of these modalities is free of complications. The oral calcium channel blocking agents must generally be administered in large doses that are often accompanied by undesirable side effects.[42] Endothelin receptor antagonists can cause hepatic injury. The continuous infusion of prostacyclin runs the risks of a permanently placed intravenous catheter.[43,44] Transplantation offers the substitution of immunosuppression and its attendant risk of infection as a better option than chronic cor pulmonale and RV failure.[45] Despite the limitations of each of these therapeutic modalities, together they provide a graduated therapeutic approach that has provided, at each stage, a better quality of life for many individuals with PAH.

Drugs That Block Calcium Transport

The designation *calcium channel blocker* refers to a heterogeneous group of agents of different structural, pharmacologic, and electrophysiologic properties. The agents in this category currently receiving the most clinical attention as potential pulmonary vasodilators are nifedipine, diltiazem, and amlodipine.

These drugs may have significant direct negative inotropic effects, although this may not become manifest clinically if reflex sympathetic stimulation of the heart is present. They are used for therapy of patients who manifest acute vasoreactivity when tested with short-acting agents under hemodynamic monitoring. Sustained-release preparations are preferred, with the dosage generally titrated to the maximal tolerable level based on avoiding untoward systemic effects, that is, hypotension, headache, dizziness, and flushing. Considerable caution is necessary in administering the higher dosages, however, because side effects can occur precipitously and be life-threatening.

A trial of calcium channel blockers orally should be preceded by use of testing of acute vasoreactivity using one or more of three agents: (1) inhaled NO, in concentrations of 10 to 40 ppm for 5 to 10 minutes; (2) prostacyclin (prostaglandin I_2, epoprostenol, Flolan), administered intravenously in increasing doses (starting dose of 1 to 2 ng/kg/min followed by successive increments every 15 minutes of 2 ng/kg/min until a maximal dose of 12 ng/kg/min is reached or until side effects preclude further increases); and (3) adenosine (50–200 µg/kg/min). Only patients who manifest substantial reductions in PVR (usually to values below 5 to 6 mmHg/L/min), resulting from a fall in pulmonary artery pressure without systemic hypotension and accompanied by an unchanged or increased cardiac output, are considered candidates for chronic therapy with oral calcium channel antagonists.

Prostacyclin and Its Analogues
Epoprostenol (Flolan, prostacyclin, prostaglandin I_2), a metabolite of arachidonic acid, and its analogues continue to be a major focus of attention as treatments for a variety of forms of pulmonary hypertension. The pulmonary endothelium elaborates prostacyclin into the bloodstream, where it has a short biologic half-life (2 to 3 minutes). In principle, it is attractive for the treatment of pulmonary hypertension on several accounts: (1) it is a pulmonary vasodilator, (2) it inhibits platelet aggregation, and (3) it inhibits proliferation of vascular smooth muscle. Unfortunately, it suffers the disadvantage of requiring continuous intravenous infusion, which is accomplished using portable pumps.[43,44] Treprostinil, a longer-acting prostacyclin analogue, is approved for continuous subcutaneous or intravenous use. Aerosolized iloprost, another stable prostacyclin analogue that has received regulatory approval for the treatment of PAH, is effective when administered six to nine times daily.[16,46]

Endothelin Receptor Antagonists
Endothelin (ET) is a potent mitogen and vasoconstrictor that is produced in excess by the hypertensive pulmonary endothelium. Circulating levels of endothelin are increased in patients with PAH, and the magnitude of elevation correlates with survival. Bosentan (Tracleer), an orally active dual ET_A and ET_B receptor antagonist, improves hemodynamics and exercise tolerance and delays the time to clinical worsening in PAH.[47] Although the drug is generally well tolerated, liver function must be monitored monthly as it produces significant hepatic dysfunction in approximately 5 percent of patients. Selective ET_A receptor antagonists have also recently been investigated in PAH but remain investigational at this time.

Nitric Oxide
NO is synthesized in endothelial cells from one of the guanidine nitrogens of L-arginine by the enzyme NO synthase. It has proved to be the endothelium-derived relaxing factor that contributes to the low initial tone of the pulmonary circulation. It has the advantage of other vasodilators of selectively relaxing pulmonary vessels without affecting systemic arterial pressure. It is currently being used as a test of vasoreactivity in a wide variety of pulmonary hypertensive states and also has been used to control pulmonary hypertension in the syndrome of persistent pulmonary hypertension in the newborn.[48–50]

Sildenafil, which enhances nitric oxide activity by inhibiting phosphodiesterase type-5, the enzyme responsible for catabolism of cyclic guanosine monophosphate, also was recently approved for the treatment of PAH.

Anticoagulants
Since 1984, when Fuster and coworkers,[51] in a retrospective study, showed that long-term survival was improved in patients with IPAH by anticoagulant therapy (warfarin in low doses), the use of anticoagulants has been incorporated into the therapeutic regimens of patients with PAH. This practice is supported by the high incidence of antemortem clots found at autopsy in the small pulmonary arteries and arterioles of patients with IPAH. Moreover, in a nonrandomized trial that separated "responders" from "nonresponders" to calcium channel blockers, survival was significantly better in those given warfarin than in those who were not anticoagulated.[42] The usual goal of anticoagulation is to achieve and maintain an international normalized ratio (INR) of 2 to 2.5.[52]

Atrial Septostomy

Blade–balloon atrial septostomy has been performed in patients with severe RV pressure and volume overload refractory to maximal medical therapy.[53] The goal of this approach is to decompress the overloaded right heart and improve systemic output of the underfilled left ventricle. Improvements in exercise function and signs of severe right-heart dysfunction, such as syncope and ascites, have been observed. Because the creation of an interatrial communication will result in an increased venous admixture, worsening hypoxemia is an expected outcome. The size of the septostomy that is created should be monitored carefully to achieve the ideal balance of optimizing systemic oxygen transport and reducing right-heart filling pressures without overfilling a noncompliant left ventricle or producing extreme degrees of venous admixture.

Lung Transplantation

Fewer than 10 percent of patients with IPAH, and even fewer with other forms of PAH, are responsive to long-term oral vasodilator therapy. Of the remainder, approximately 75 percent maintain sustained clinical improvement with the newer oral therapies or long-term inhaled, continuous intravenous or subcutaneous prostanoid therapy. When pulmonary hypertensive disease has progressed, or threatens to progress, to the stage of RV failure, the physician and patient are left with few therapeutic options other than lung transplantation. Lung transplantation is currently being done at specialized centers and is almost invariably handicapped by a shortage of donor lungs, which can lead to long delays. Single- or double-lung transplantation has largely replaced heart–lung transplantation. Hemodynamic improvement is often dramatic,[54] but transplantation for PAH poses both a considerable surgical risk and the prospect of opportunistic infections that accompany lifelong immunosuppression.[55] Rejection phenomena, notably bronchiolitis obliterans, are the major limiting factor to prolonged survival. The median survival after lung transplantation is approximately 3 years.[45]

PROGNOSIS

The diagnosis of PAH carries with it a poor prognosis unless medical or surgical therapy succeeds in decreasing PVR. Although sudden death accounts for 10 to 15 percent of all PAH-related deaths, the prognosis is largely determined by the severity of pulmonary hypertension and right-heart dysfunction and the hemodynamic and clinical response to therapy.[33]

PULMONARY VENOOCCLUSIVE DISEASE AND PULMONARY CAPILLARY HEMANGIOMATOSIS

These are the least common of all types of unexplained pulmonary hypertension.[56] Not infrequently, the patient is thought to have IPAH until manifestations inconsistent with pulmonary precapillary disease, such as pulmonary congestion and edema or severe hypoxemia, redirect attention to the vascular bed distal to the arterioles. The pathogenetic mechanism of pulmonary venoocclusive disease (PVOD) is unknown, but the disease may begin as an inflammatory-thrombotic process in the small pulmonary veins and venules and end in fibrous obliteration of the venous and venular lumens. Presumably as a secondary phenomenon, the distal pulmonary arterial tree also develops obstructive lesions that are generally proliferative ("reactive") rather than inflammatory in nature; the intervening capillary bed is generally normal. The pulmonary venoocclusive lesions have been attributed to an inflammatory response to vascular injury, followed by thrombosis and scarring. Among the postulated etiologies are viral illness, chemotherapy, toxins, autoimmune disease, and mediastinal fibrosis.[35]

Both PVOD and capillary hemangiomatosis can be familial. When the pulmonary hypertension is suspected of originating distal to the pulmonary capillary bed, mitral valve disease, myocardial dysfunction, or even LA myxoma has a greater likelihood of being the cause than does PVOD.

CLINICAL PICTURE

Predominantly children and young adults are affected, but the age has ranged from infancy to 48 years. Clinical suspicion of this disorder generally arises when a patient with congested and edematous lungs proves to have a normal mitral valve and left ventricle.

The cardinal signs are dyspnea and fatigue on exertion in conjunction with evidence of pulmonary hypertension; the pulmonary venous rather than pulmonary arterial etiology is suggested by radiologic evidence of postcapillary pulmonary hypertension without evidence of involvement of the left side of the heart (Fig. 71–6A). Pleural effusions are common. Cyanosis, syncope, hemoptysis, and finger clubbing have been inconsistent findings. Moderate to severe hypoxemia, caused by intrapulmonary shunting through the abnormal capillary network, is a hallmark of capillary hemangiomatosis. Rarely, systemic embolization may occur.

HEMODYNAMICS

Cardiac catheterization discloses a high pulmonary arterial pressure with a normal pulmonary wedge and LV end-diastolic pressure. Although one might expect the pulmonary wedge pressure to be elevated, the reason that it is usually normal is as follows: Inflation of the balloon at the tip of a pulmonary artery catheter creates a downstream "stop-flow" phenomenon that extends to same diameter veins, and therefore generally gives a satisfactory estimate

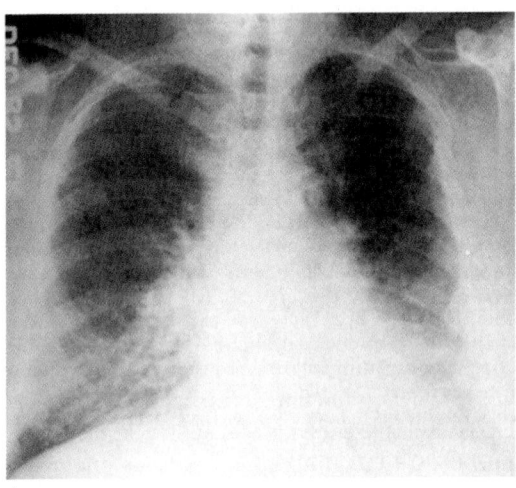

A

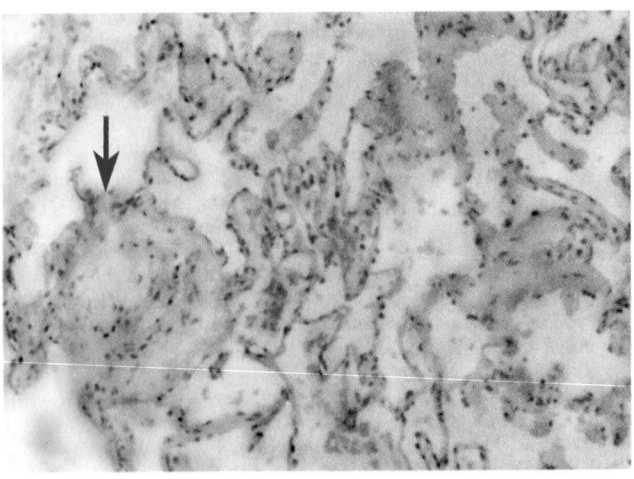

B

FIGURE 71–6. Pulmonary venoocclusive disease (PVOD) proven by open lung biopsy. **A.** Chest radiography. Pulmonary interstitial edema is marked at both bases. **B.** Lung biopsy. In addition to obliterative pulmonary venular disease, the pulmonary arterioles (*arrow*) showed intimal proliferation and medical hypertrophy. *Source: Courtesy of Dr. G. G. Pietra.*

of left atrial or end-diastolic LV pressure. When epoprostenol is administered to a patient with PVOD, an acute pulmonary edema pattern may ensue, resulting from increasing pulmonary blood flow in the face of downstream vascular obstruction.[44,57] This response, when present, is virtually diagnostic of PVOD. Patients with capillary hemangiomatosis may experience worsening hypoxemia with epoprostenol, attributable to increased shunting through the low-resistance capillary meshwork.

PATHOLOGY

At autopsy, both lungs are involved. The lungs are the seat of congestion, edema, and focal fibrosis, which may become extensive. The venous lesions may be more marked in one region than in another. Although both the small pulmonary arteries and the small pulmonary veins are affected, the lesions are different (see Fig. 71–6B). Most striking are the morphologic changes in the pulmonary veins and venules, which are narrowed or occluded by intimal proliferation and fibrosis; up to 95 percent of the veins and venules may be affected in this way, but complete occlusion is uncommon. Bronchial veins and bronchopulmonary anastomoses share in the occlusive process. Hypertrophy in the walls of the pulmonary arteries may be quite striking. PVOD, to varying degrees, may also coexist with capillary hemangiomatosis. Thrombi in the pulmonary arteries are common.[35]

TREATMENT

Medical management has been disappointing, because the lesions generally are irreversible. An occasional patient has been reported to do well with medical therapy, although most experienced clinicians consider both PVOD and capillary hemangiomatosis to be contraindications to the use of oral medications or intravenous epoprostenol. The usual duration of life after recognition ranges from a few weeks in infants to several years in adults, with 7 years being the maximum. The treatment of choice is probably lung transplantation.

REFERENCES

1. Hales CA. Physiological function of hypoxic pulmonary vasoconstriction. In: JX-J Yuan, ed. *Hypoxic Pulmonary Vasoconstriction.* Boston: Kluwer Academic, 2004:3–14.
2. Olschewski A, Weir EK. Hypoxic pulmonary vasoconstriction and hypertension. In: Peacock AJ, Rubin LJ, eds. *Pulmonary Circulation.* London: Arnold/Oxford University Press, 2004:33–44.
3. Thurlbeck WM. Pulmonary capillary hemangiomatosis as a rare cause of pulmonary hypertension. *Pathol Res Pract* 1996;192:298–299.
4. Budev MM, Arroliga AC, Wiedemann HP, Matthay RA. Cor pulmonale: an overview. *Semin Respir Crit Care Med* 2003;24(3):233–244.
5. Harris P, Heath D. The structure of the normal pulmonary blood vessels after infancy. In: Harris P, Heath D, eds. *The Human Circulation: Its Form and Function in Health and Disease.* Edinburgh: Churchill-Livingstone, 1986:30–47.
6. Kinsella JP, Abman SH. Recent developments in the pathophysiology and treatment of persistent pulmonary hypertension of the newborn. *J Pediatr* 1995;126:853–864.
7. Morrell NW, Jeffery TK. Pulmonary vascular remodeling. In: Peacock AJ, Rubin LJ, eds. *Pulmonary Circulation.* London: Arnold/Oxford University Press, 2004:45–61.
8. Fedullo PF, Auger WR, Kerr KM, Rubin LJ. Chronic thromboembolic pulmonary hypertension. *N Eng J Med* 2001;345:1465–1472.
9. McGoon M, Gutterman D, Steen V, et al. Screening, early detection and diagnosis of pulmonary arterial hypertension. *Chest* 2004;126:14S–34S.
10. Palevsky HI, Schloo BL, Pietra GG, et al. Primary pulmonary hypertension: vascular structure, morphometry, and responsiveness to vasodilator agents. *Circulation* 1989;80:1207–1221.
11. Tuder RM, Zaiman AL. Pathology of pulmonary vascular disease. In: Peacock AJ, Rubin LJ, eds. *Pulmonary Circulation.* London: Arnold/Oxford University Press, 2004:25–32.
12. Williamson TL, Kim NH, Rubin LJ. Chronic thromboembolic pulmonary hypertension. *Prog Cardiovasc Dis* 2002;45:203–212.
13. Coulden R. State-of-the-art imaging techniques in chronic thromboembolic pulmonary hypertension. *Proc Am Thorac Soc* 2006;3:577–583.
14. Jamieson SW, Kapelanski DP, Sakakibara N, et al. Pulmonary endarterectomy: experience and lessons learned in 1500 cases. *Ann Thorac Surg* 2003;76:1457–1464.
15. Kim NH. Assessment of operability in chronic thromboembolic pulmonary hypertension. *Proc Am Thorac Soc* 2006;3:584–588.
16. Olschewski H, Ardeschir H, Walmrath D, et al. Inhaled prostacyclin and iloprost in severe pulmonary hypertension secondary to lung fibrosis. *Am J Respir Crit Care Med* 1999;160:600–603.
17. Weitzenblum E. Chronic cor pulmonale. *Heart* 2003;89:225–230.
18. Kessler R, Faller R, Weitzenblum E, et al. Natural history of pulmonary hypertension in a series of 131 patients with chronic obstructive pulmonary disease. *Am J Respir Crit Care Med* 2001;164:219–224.
19. Matthay RA, Shub C. Imaging techniques for assessing pulmonary artery hypertension and right ventricular performance with special reference to COPD. *J Thorac Imaging* 1990;5:47–67.
20. Rubin LJ, Badesch DB. Evaluation and management of the patient with pulmonary arterial hypertension. *Ann Intern Med* 2005;143:282–292.
21. Maeda S, Katsura H, Chida K, et al. Lack of correlation between P pulmonale and right atrial overload in chronic obstructive airways disease. *Br Heart J* 1991;65:132–136.
22. Ghofrani HA, Voswinckel R, Reichenberger F, et al. Hypoxia- and non-hypoxia-related pulmonary hypertension—established and new therapies. *Cardiovasc Res* 2006;72:30–40.
23. Fagan KA, Badesch DB. Pulmonary hypertension associated with connective tissue disease. *Prog Cardiovasc Dis* 2002;45:225–234.
24. Rich S, Dantzker DR, Ayres SM, et al. Primary pulmonary hypertension: a national prospective study. *Ann Intern Med* 1987;107:216–223.
25. Kawut SM, Taichman DB, Archer-Chicko CL, Palevsky HI, Kimmel SE. Hemodynamics and survival in patients with pulmonary arterial hypertension related to systemic sclerosis. *Chest* 2003;123:344–350.
26. Galie N, Seeger W, Naeije R, et al. Comparative analysis of clinical trials and evidence-based treatment algorithm in pulmonary arterial hypertension. *J Am Coll Cardiol* 2004;43:81S–88S.
27. Bady E, Achkar A, Paschal S, et al. Pulmonary arterial hypertension in patients with sleep apnoea syndrome. *Thorax* 2000;55:934–939.
28. Atwood CW, McCrory D, Garcia JGN, Abman SH, Ahearn GS. Pulmonary artery hypertension and sleep-disordered breathing. *Chest* 2004;126:72S–77S.
29. Rubin LJ. Primary pulmonary hypertension. *N Eng J Med* 1997;336:111–117.
30. Abenhaim L, Moride Y, Brenot F, et al. Appetite-suppressant drugs and the risk of primary pulmonary hypertension. *N Engl J Med* 1996;335:609–616.
31. Speich R, Jenni R, Opravil M, et al. Primary pulmonary hypertension in HIV infection. *Chest* 1991;100:1268–1271.
32. Kuo PC, Plotkin JS, Rubin LJ. Distinctive clinical features of portopulmonary hypertension. *Chest* 1997;112:980–986.
33. D'Alonzo GE, Barst RJ, Ayres SM, et al. Survival in patients with primary pulmonary hypertension. *Ann Intern Med* 1991;115:343–349.
34. Humbert M, Morrell NW, Archer SL, et al. Cellular and molecular pathobiology of pulmonary arterial hypertension. *J Am Coll Cardiol* 2004;43:13S–24S.
35. Pietra G, Capron C, Stewart S, et al. Pathologic assessment of vasculopathies in pulmonary hypertension. *J Am Coll Cardiol* 2004;43:25S–32S.
36. Yuan JXJ, Aldinger AM, Juhaszova M, et al. Dysfunctional voltage-gated K^+ channels in pulmonary artery smooth muscle cells of patients with primary pulmonary hypertension. *Circulation* 1998;98:1400–1406.
37. Gaine SP, Rubin LJ. Primary pulmonary hypertension. *Lancet* 1998;353:719–725.
38. Lopez-Sendon J, Sanchez MAG, De Juan MJM, Coma-Canella I. Pulmonary hypertension in the toxic oil syndrome. In: Fishman AP, ed. *The Pulmonary Circulation: Normal and Abnormal.* Philadelphia: University of Pennsylvania Press, 1990:385–396.
39. Connolly HD, Crary JL, McGoon MD, et al. Valvular heart disease associated with fenfluramine-phentermine. *N Engl J Med* 1997;337:581–588.

40. Loyd J, Newman J. Familial primary pulmonary hypertension: clinical patterns. *Am Rev Respir Dis* 1984;129:194–197.

41. The International PPH Consortium, Lane KB, Machado RD, Pauciulo MW, et al. Heterozygous germ line mutations in BMPR2 encoding a TGF-beta receptor, cause familial primary pulmonary hypertension. *Nat Genet* 2000;26:81–84.

42. Sitbon O, Humbert M, Jais X, et al. Long-term response to calcium channel blockers in idiopathic pulmonary arterial hypertension. *Circulation* 2005;111:3105–3111.

43. McLaughlin VV, Shillington A, Rich S. Survival in primary pulmonary hypertension: the impact of epoprostenol therapy. *Circulation* 2002;106:1477–1482.

44. Sitbon O, Humbert M, Nunes H, et al. Long-term intravenous epoprostenol infusion in primary pulmonary hypertension: prognostic factors and survival. *J Am Coll Cardiol* 2002;40:780–788.

45. Olsson JK, Zamanian RT, Feinstein JA, Doyle RL. Surgical and interventional therapies for pulmonary arterial hypertension. *Semin Respir Crit Care Med* 2005;26:417–428.

46. Olschewski H, Simonneau G, Galie N, et al. Inhaled iloprost for severe pulmonary hypertension. *N Engl J Med* 2002;347:322–329.

47. Rubin LJ, Badesch DB, Barst RJ, et al. Bosentan therapy for pulmonary arterial hypertension. *N Engl J Med* 2002;346:896–903.

48. Sitbon O, Brenot F, Denjean A, et al. Inhaled nitric oxide as a screening vasodilator agent in primary pulmonary hypertension: a dose–response study and comparison with prostacyclin. *Am J Respir Crit Care Med* 1995;151:384–389.

49. Krasuski RA, Warner JJ, Wang A, et al. Inhaled nitric oxide selectively dilates pulmonary vasculature in adult patients with pulmonary hypertension, irrespective of etiology. *J Am Coll Cardiol* 2000;36:2204–2211.

50. Roberts JD, Fineman JR, Morin FC, et al. Inhaled NO and PPHN. *N Eng J Med* 1997;336:605–610.

51. Fuster V, Steele PM, Edwards WD, et al. Primary pulmonary hypertension: natural history and the importance of thrombosis. *Circulation* 1984;70:580–585.

52. Badesch DB, Abman SH, Ahearn GS, et al. Medical therapy for pulmonary arterial hypertension: ACCP evidence-based clinical practice guidelines. *Chest* 2004;126; 35S–62S.

53. Sandoval J, Gaspar J, Pulido T, et al. Graded balloon dilation atrial septostomy in severe primary pulmonary hypertension. A therapeutic alternative for patients nonresponsive to vasodilator treatment. *J Am Coll Cardiol* 1998;32(2):297–304.

54. Galie N, Torbicki A, Barst R, et al. Guidelines on diagnosis and treatment of pulmonary arterial hypertension. *Eur Heart J* 2004;25:2243–2278.

55. Doyle RL, McCrory D, Channick RN, Simonneau G, Conte J. Surgical treatments/interventions for pulmonary arterial hypertension. *Chest* 2004;126:63S–71S.

56. Mandel JME, Hales CA. Pulmonary veno-occlusive disease. *Am J Respir Crit Care Med* 2000;162(5):1964–1973.

57. Davis LL, deBoisblanc BP, Glynn CE, et al. Effect of prostacyclin on microvascular pressures in a patient with pulmonary veno-occlusive disease. *Chest* 1995;108:1754–1756.

CHAPTER (72)

Pulmonary Embolism

Peter F. Fedullo

INTRODUCTION

Approximately 100,000 patients in the United States die each year directly as a consequence of acute pulmonary embolism (PE), with another 100,000 deaths occurring in patients with concomitant disease in whom PE contributes significantly to their demise.[1,2] Three-month mortality in unselected patients with acute PE is as high as 15 percent.[3] Although a number of patients die of comorbidities that predisposed them to the thromboembolic event, a substantial number of patients die from PE within an hour of presentation, before the diagnosis can be confirmed and therapy initiated, or because the diagnosis was overlooked.[4] Autopsy studies have repeatedly documented the high frequency with which PE has gone unsuspected and undetected.[5] Despite advances in diagnostic imaging tests and therapeutic interventions, PE remains underdiagnosed and prophylaxis continues to be dramatically underused.

Over the past decade, a number of vauable insights into the natural history of venous thrombosis and pulmonary embolism have enhanced our diagnostic and therapeutic approach. One such insight is the awareness that patients hospitalized for medical problems face a thromboembolic risk similar to their surgical counterparts. Another is an understanding of the substantial thromboembolic recurrence risk among patients with idiopathic or unprovoked venous thrombosis.[6] Yet another insight is the awareness that the presence of right ventricular dysfunction in the setting of pulmonary embolism may be associated with an increased risk of adverse consequences, including subsequent cardiovascular collapse and death.[7] Anticoagulation with heparin as a "bridge" to warfarin is still considered the standard treatment for PE. The spectrum of anticoagulant drugs has been expanded recently. Low-molecular-weight heparins (LMWHs) have been shown to be effective and safe for both treatment and for prevention of VTE, particularly in hospitalized medical patients. Fondaparinux, a new pentasaccharide, is very effective in a fixed low dose in preventing venous thromboembolism (VTE) after orthopedic and abdominal surgery, and has been demonstrated in clinical trials to be as effective as LMWH and unfractionated heparin for the initial treatment of patients with deep venous thrombosis and pulmonary embolism. The promise of oral direct thrombin inhibitors, which can be administered in a fixed dose, remains unrealized.

RISK FACTORS AND PATHOGENESIS OF VENOUS THROMBOEMBOLISM

In 1856, Virchow proposed his triad of factors leading to intravascular coagulation, including stasis, vessel wall injury, and hypercoagulability. Risk factors for deep venous thrombosis (DVT) are based on these processes (Table 72–1). The overwhelming majority of emboli originate from the deep veins of the lower extremities, although any venous bed can be involved. Although thrombi may form at any point along the vein wall, most originate in valve pockets. The veins of the calf are the most common site of origin, with subsequent extension of the clot prior to embolization.[8] Eventually, the thrombus may expand to fill the vessel entirely, with both retrograde and proximal extension. If embolization does not occur, the thrombosis can partially or completely resolve via three mechanisms: recanalization, organization, and lysis. Postthrombotic syndrome occurs in 20 to 50 percent of patients and involves chronic pain, swelling, edema, and skin changes, which reduce quality of life and incur significant healthcare costs.[9]

ACQUIRED RISK FACTORS

Frequently, more than one risk factor for venous thrombosis is present; knowledge of these risk factors provides the rationale for both prophylaxis and clinical suspicion. Comorbidities enhance the risk of VTE. In the DVT FREE prospective registry of 5451 patients with ultrasound-confirmed DVT, the most common co-

TABLE 72–1
Risk Factors for Venous Thromboembolism

Acquired factors
  Age older than 40
  Prior history of venous thromboembolism
  Prior major surgical procedure
  Trauma
  Hip fracture
  Immobilization/paralysis
  Venous stasis
  Varicose veins
  Congestive heart failure
  Myocardial infarction
  Obesity
  Pregnancy/postpartum period
  Oral contraceptive therapy
  Cerebrovascular accident
  Malignancy
  Severe thrombocythemia
  Paroxysmal nocturnal hemoglobinuria
  Antiphospholipid antibody syndrome (including lupus anticoagulant)
Inherited factors
  Antithrombin III deficiency
  Factor V Leiden (activated protein C resistance)
  Prothrombin gene (G20210A) defect
  Protein C deficiency
  Protein S deficiency
  Dysfibrinogenemia
  Disorders of plasminogen
  Hyperhomocysteinemia

morbidities were arterial hypertension (50 percent), surgery within 3 months (38 percent), immobility within 30 days (34 percent), cancer (32 percent), and obesity (27 percent).[10]

Although studies to date have yielded inconsistent results, long automobile or airplane trips appear to be risk factors for VTE. The proportion of subjects who develop acute PE during or after airplane travel appears to be associated with other thrombotic risk factors, such as the presence of the factor V Leiden mutation or the use of oral contraceptive agents, and correlates with the flight distance. The risk of PE significantly increases with a flight distance >3107 miles (5000 km) or a duration >8 hours.[11]

Obesity merits further investigation, because recent studies implicate obesity as a risk factor for VTE, particularly in the United States, where obesity represents a major health issue.[12,13] The Nurses' Health Study explored risk factors for PE in women and found that a body mass index ≥29 kg/m² was an independent risk factor.[14] The Framingham Study has confirmed that obesity is a risk factor for PE, particularly in women.[15] In addition to increased venous stasis, obesity may also increase the risk for VTE as a consequence of elevated plasma levels of certain clotting factor such as fibrinogen, factor VII, and plasminogen activator inhibitor-1, and as a result of platelet activation caused by enhanced lipid peroxidation.[16–19]

An abundance of literature documents that the risk of venous thromboembolism increases with age, with a relative risk for those 70 years of age approximately 25-fold greater than the risk for those 20 to 29 years of age.[20] Age also appears to increase mortality because of PE, and PE is suspected less commonly prior to death in the elderly patient.[4,21]

Prior VTE substantially increases the risk of subsequent events. Surgical patients with a previous history of VTE who do not receive prophylaxis develop postoperative DVT in more than 50 percent of cases.[22] Surgery itself significantly enhances the risk. Patients who are undergoing general surgery without additional risk factors develop DVT in nearly 20 percent of cases if neither pharmacologic nor mechanical prophylaxis is applied.[23] Patients who are undergoing lower-extremity orthopedic procedures such as total hip or total knee replacement develop DVT in more than 50 percent of cases.[24] Prophylactic anticoagulation may be initiated either prior to surgery or shortly thereafter to prevent the development of intraoperative and early postoperative thrombosis. These orthopedic settings have been comprehensively investigated, prompted by the increasing use of LMWH. Spinal surgery, pelvic surgery, and neurosurgery place patients at a particularly high risk for VTE.

Trauma, particularly of the lower extremities and pelvis, heightens the risk of DVT. PE has been identified at autopsy in as many as 60 percent of patients with lower-extremity fractures, and mortality has been attributed to PE in as many as 50 percent of patients dying after hip fracture.[25,26] The incidence of VTE increases with time after the traumatic event. Autopsy-confirmed PE in patients surviving for less than 24 hours after trauma has been demonstrated in 3.3 percent, increasing to 5.5 percent in patients surviving up to 7 days. Pulmonary emboli occurred in 18.6 percent of patients surviving for a longer period.[27]

Upper-extremity DVT has become more important because of an increasing use of pacemakers, implantable defibrillators, and long-term, indwelling, central venous catheters.[28] Symptomatic PE can originate from upper-extremity thrombi, although this appears much less common than embolization from lower-extremity DVT. Upper-extremity DVT poses the risk of superior vena cava syndrome and loss of vascular access.[29] Effort-related, upper-extremity axillosubclavian thrombosis (Paget-Schroetter syndrome) may occur spontaneously or be associated with an underlying thrombophilic tendency, and may result in significant, long-term functional impairment.[30]

Epidemiologic analyses, as well as autopsy data, suggest that patients with cardiac disease are predisposed to VTE.[4] Although myocardial infarction without anticoagulation is associated with a significant incidence of DVT, more recent therapeutic strategies for acute coronary syndromes have had a beneficial impact.[31] Large, placebo-controlled acute myocardial infarction trials indicate that the use of thrombolytic therapy reduces the incidence of VTE.[32,33]

Cancer clearly augments the risk of VTE, although the precise pathogenesis of thromboembolism in cancer is not well understood. Numerous mechanisms, including intrinsic tumor procoagulant activity and extrinsic factors such as chemotherapeutic agents and indwelling access catheters, contribute to this process. The thrombophilic tendency associated with cancer is often amplified by clinical factors such as patient weakness and immobility. An analysis based on data from PIOPED (Prospective Investigation of Pulmonary Embolism Diagnosis) found that of 399 patients with PE, 73 (18.3 percent) had cancer.[4] Pancreatic, lung, gastric, genitourinary tract, and breast malignancies are associated with a particularly high risk of DVT and PE. About half of all cancer patients and approximately 90 percent of those with metastases exhibit abnormalities of one or more coagulation parameters.[34,35] Following the administration of various chemotherapeutic agents, changes in the levels of coagulation factors, suppression of anticoagulant and fibrinolytic activity, and direct endothelial damage have been documented clinically and experimentally.[36] Hormonal therapy, particularly tamoxifen in breast cancer adjuvant therapy, is also associated with an increased risk of thromboembolism, particularly when combined with chemotherapy.[37] Neutropenia and sepsis, which often accompany chemotherapeutic regimens, often necessitate hospitalization and bedrest, which contributes further to the risk of VTE. A subsequent malignancy has been reported to occur within 2 to 3 years in approximately 5 to 10 percent of patients presenting with idiopathic venous thrombosis.[38] Although an aggressive search for cancer does not appear to be warranted in patients presenting with idiopathic DVT, recent data suggests that a limited approach (abdominal/pelvic CT, mammography, sputum cytology) may be cost-effective.[39]

Pregnancy and the postpartum period are the most common settings in which women younger than age 40 years acquire thromboembolic disease. Venous thrombosis develops in these settings three to six times more often than in age-matched women not on oral contraceptives.[40] Although DVT appears to be more common in the third trimester and postpartum than prior to delivery, the risk is considerable throughout pregnancy.[41] Cesarean section further augments the risk. Oral contraceptives are associated with an increased relative risk of venous thromboembolism, although the absolute risk (approximately 1 to 3 cases per 10,000 woman-years) remains small.[40] Third-generation agents (agents containing desogestrel or gestodene as the progestogen component) appear to cause acquired resistance to activated protein C

and double the risk of VTE.[42,43] Oral contraceptive use should be avoided by women with protein C, protein S, and antithrombin III deficiency, as well as those who are homozygous carriers of the factor V Leiden mutation. Results from a clinical trial evaluating hormonal replacement therapy indicated that such therapy increased the incidence of VTE in women 45 to 64 years of age. Best available evidence suggests a two- to fourfold increased relative risk of venous thromboembolism among oral hormonal replacement therapy users compared to nonusers.[40,44] The risk of VTE also appears to be highest during the first year of exposure to hormonal replacement.[45] It has not been clearly established that previous use increases the risk.[46] Although such therapy is associated with quality-of-life benefits in women who require postmenopausal symptom control, physicians must balance this benefit against the risk of venous thromboembolism, cardiovascular disease, and breast cancer before prescribing hormonal replacement therapy. Whether routine screening should be performed prior to the initiation of oral contraceptive agents or hormonal replacement therapy remains controversial.[47] Given the low absolute risk, especially among users of oral contraceptive agents, the general consensus is that such an approach would not be cost-effective.[48]

[ ] INHERITED RISK FACTORS

Inherited thrombophilias result in variable degrees of VTE risk.[49,50] Antithrombin III deficiency was first described in 1965, and was the first inherited trait associated with thrombophilia. Functional and quantitative abnormalities of protein C and protein S were subsequently described. The factor V Leiden mutation, a single base mutation (substitution of A for G at position 506), is a far more common genetic polymorphism associated with activated protein C resistance. It is present in approximately 4 to 6 percent of European populations, but is less common among those of Asian, Indian, or African descent.[51,52] The relative risk of a first idiopathic DVT among men heterozygous for the mutation is three- to sevenfold higher than that of those not affected.[52] This genetic mutation is also a risk factor for recurrent pregnancy loss, probably because of placental thrombosis.[53] Oral contraceptive use in patients with heterozygous factor V Leiden mutation is associated with a tenfold higher risk of VTE.[54]

Another, less frequent thrombophilic mutation has been identified in the 3′ untranslated region of the prothrombin gene (substitution of A for G at position 20210).[43] This mutant allele is present in 2 to 4 percent of the general population and causes increased levels of prothrombin.[55] This prothrombin gene defect increases the risk of DVT by a factor of 2.7 to 3.8.[55,56] It appears that carriers of both factor V Leiden and the prothrombin G20210A defect have an increased risk of recurrent DVT after a first episode and are candidates for lifelong anticoagulation.[57]

Homocysteine has potential thrombogenic effects, including injury to vascular endothelium and antagonism of the synthesis and function of nitric oxide.[58] Coexisting hyperhomocysteinemia has been shown to increase the risk for thrombosis in patients with factor V Leiden.[59] However, the thermolabile methylenetetrahydrofolate reductase gene variant is not independently associated with thrombosis, emphasizing that the precise role of homocysteine in venous thrombosis is unclear. Thus, interactions between the genetic factors (defects in enzymes) that control homocysteine metabolism and nutritional factors (folate, vitamin B$_6$, and vitamin B$_{12}$ deficiencies) that affect homocysteine metabolism warrant additional investigation with regard to VTE.[60]

Recently, elevated levels of clotting factors VII, VIII, IX, XI, and XII have been associated with an increased risk for venous thrombosis. In particular, elevated factor VIIIc levels have been demonstrated to be a strong and independent risk factor for both acute and recurrent venous thrombosis.[61,62]

PATHOPHYSIOLOGY OF ACUTE PULMONARY EMBOLISM

GAS-EXCHANGE ABNORMALITIES

The effect of PE on oxygenation and hemodynamics depends on the extent of obstruction of the pulmonary vascular bed and the severity of underlying cardiopulmonary disease.[7,63–65] Hypoxemia develops in the preponderance of patients with PE and has been attributed to various mechanisms, including intrapulmonary or intracardiac right-to-left shunting, elevated alveolar dead space, ventilation–perfusion (V/Q) inequality, and decreases in the mixed venous O$_2$ level, thereby magnifying the effect of the normal venous admixture. The two latter mechanisms are proposed to account for the majority of hypoxemia and hypocarbia associated with acute embolism. Shunt can occur as a consequence of atelectasis related to loss of surfactant, alveolar hemorrhage, or from bronchoconstriction related to regional areas of hypocarbia. Hypoxemia leads to an increase in sympathetic tone, with systemic vasoconstriction, and may actually increase venous return with augmentation of stroke volume, at least initially, if there is no significant underlying cardiac or pulmonary pathology already present.

HEMODYNAMIC ALTERATIONS

The hemodynamic effects of embolism are related to three factors: the degree of reduction of the cross-sectional area of the pulmonary vascular bed, the preexisting status of the cardiopulmonary system, and the physiologic consequences of both hypoxic and neurohumorally mediated vasoconstriction.[7,63–65] Obstruction of the pulmonary vascular bed by embolism acutely increases the workload on the right ventricle, a chamber ill-equipped to deal with high-pressure load. In patients without preexisting cardiopulmonary disease, obstruction of less than 20 percent of the pulmonary vascular bed results in a number of compensatory events that minimize adverse hemodynamic consequences. Recruitment and distension of pulmonary vessels occur, resulting in a normal or near-normal pulmonary artery pressure and pulmonary vascular resistance; cardiac output is maintained by increases in the right ventricular stroke volume and increases in the heart rate. As the degree of pulmonary vascular obstruction exceeds 30 to 40 percent, increases in pulmonary artery pressure and modest increases in right atrial pressure occur. The Frank-Starling mechanism maintains right ventricular stroke work and cardiac output. When the degree of pulmonary artery obstruction exceeds 50 to 60 percent, compensatory mechanisms are overcome, cardiac output begins to fall, and right atrial pressure increases dramatically. With

acute obstruction beyond this amount, the right heart dilates, right ventricular wall tension increases, right ventricular ischemia may develop, the cardiac output falls, and systemic hypotension develops. In patients without prior cardiopulmonary disease, the maximal mean pulmonary artery pressure capable of being generated by the right ventricle appears to be 40 mmHg. The correlation between the extent of pulmonary vascular obstruction and the pulmonary vascular resistance appears to be hyperbolic, reflecting at its lower end the expansible nature of the pulmonary vascular bed, and at its upper end, the precipitous decline in cardiac output that may occur as the right ventricle fails.[66,67]

The hemodynamic response to acute pulmonary embolism in patients with preexisting cardiopulmonary disease may be considerably different.[64] Patients with prior cardiopulmonary disease demonstrate degrees of pulmonary hypertension that are disproportionate to the degree of pulmonary vascular obstruction. As a result, severe pulmonary hypertension may develop in response to a relatively small reduction in pulmonary artery cross-sectional area. Thus, evidence of right ventricular hypertrophy (rather than right ventricular dilatation) associated with a mean pulmonary artery pressure in excess of 40 mmHg should suggest an element of chronic pulmonary hypertension resulting from a potentially diverse group of etiologic possibilities (e.g., chronic thromboembolic pulmonary hypertension, left ventricular failure, valvular disease, right-to-left cardiac shunts).

DIAGNOSIS OF DEEP VENOUS THROMBOSIS AND PULMONARY EMBOLISM

HISTORY AND PHYSICAL EXAMINATION

The presence of erythema, warmth, pain, swelling, and/or tenderness are not specific for DVT but suggest the need for further evaluation. PE must always be considered when unexplained dyspnea is present. Pleuritic chest pain and hemoptysis are also common in PE. Coughing may be present, and while sometimes caused by PE, it more commonly occurs with bronchitis or pneumonia. Anxiety and light-headedness are symptoms that may be caused by PE but may also be caused by a number of other entities that result in hypoxemia or hypotension. Severe dyspnea and syncope are the principal symptoms that may suggest massive, life-threatening PE.[68,69] Tachypnea and tachycardia are the most common signs of PE, but they are also nonspecific. A pleural rub or accentuated pulmonic component of the second heart sound may suggest PE, but can also be explained by other disorders. With embolism of sufficient magnitude to cause right ventricular dysfunction, a murmur of tricuspid regurgitation, systemic hypotension, or jugular venous distension might be present.

A major advance in the diagnostic approach to both venous thrombosis and pulmonary embolism has been a transition from a technique-oriented approach to one that utilizes Bayesian analysis. In doing so, the pretest probability of the disease, calculated independently of a particular test result through either empiric means or through a standardized prediction rule, is calculated. This pretest probability aids in the selection and interpretation of further diagnostic tests to create a posttest probability of the disease. This posttest probability can then be used as a basis for clinical decision making. For pulmonary embolism, three such scores have been developed and validated. Wells and coworkers prospectively tested a rapid seven-item bedside assessment to estimate the clinical pretest probability for PE.[70] An alternative scoring system, the Geneva score, involved seven variables and required gas exchange and radiographic information.[71] Recently, a revised Geneva score requiring eight clinical variables without gas exchange or radiographic information was validated and published.[72] Although such scoring systems have not proven to be more accurate than implicit assessment, they do provide a means of standardization that compensates for variability in physician experience and judgment.

[ ] DIFFERENTIAL DIAGNOSIS

PE may mimic a large spectrum of diseases. The most common differential diagnoses are chronic lung disease, asthma, congestive heart failure, pneumonia, acute myocardial infarction, aortic dissection, primary pulmonary hypertension, chronic thromboembolic hypertension, pericarditis, cancer, pneumothorax, costochondritis, musculoskeletal pain, and anxiety states.

[ ] NONIMAGING STUDIES FOR PULMONARY EMBOLISM

D-Dimer

The plasma D-dimer is a specific derivative of cross-linked fibrin. Measurement of circulating plasma D-dimer has been comprehensively evaluated as a diagnostic test for acute VTE.[73] A normal enzyme-linked immunosorbent assay (ELISA) is highly sensitive in excluding PE and DVT. When an ELISA D-dimer level is below an established cutoff level, the sensitivity and negative predictive value for VTE are ≥98 percent, respectively.[73] In another prospective analysis, 76 (96 percent) of 79 patients with high-probability ventilation–perfusion scans had elevated D-dimer levels.[74] Thus, increased levels of cross-linked fibrin degradation products are an indirect but suggestive marker of intravascular thrombosis, indicating endogenous fibrinolysis. An increased D-dimer level is nonspecific for PE and may be seen with advancing age and in patients with various diseases, including infections and other inflammatory states, cancer, myocardial infarction, the postoperative state, and second- and third-trimester pregnancies.

It is important to recognize that the usefulness of D-dimer testing in inpatients is limited as a result of comorbidities in this population that elevate D-dimer levels.

Arterial Blood Gas Analysis

Although hypoxemia is common in acute PE, some patients, particularly young individuals without underlying cardiopulmonary disease, may have a normal PaO_2 (arterial oxygen partial pressure). In a retrospective study of hospitalized patients with PE, the PaO_2 was greater than 80 mmHg in 29 percent of patients who were younger than 40 years old, compared with 3 percent in the older group.[68] However, the alveolar-arterial (A-a) difference was elevated in all patients. An important tenet should be that unexplained hypoxemia, particularly in the setting of risk factors for DVT, suggests the possibility of PE.

Electrocardiography

ECG findings in acute PE are generally nonspecific and include T-wave changes, ST-segment abnormalities, incomplete or complete right bundle-branch block, right axis deviation in the extremity leads, and clockwise rotation of the QRS vector in the precordial leads. The changes that do occur are likely caused by right-heart dilatation. Approximately 20 percent of patients with PE have no electrocardiographic changes. Therefore, the ECG cannot be relied upon to rule in or rule out PE, though ECG proof of a clear alternative diagnosis, such as myocardial infarction, is useful when PE is among the possible diagnoses. The "classic" $S_1 Q_3 T_3$ pattern described by McGinn and White in 1935 in seven patients with acute cor pulmonale secondary to PE was subsequently demonstrated to be present in approximately 10 percent of PE cases.[75,76] In patients without underlying cardiac or pulmonary disease from the Urokinase Pulmonary Embolism Trial (UPET), ECG abnormalities were documented in 87 percent of patients with proven PE.[77] These findings were not specific for PE, however. In this clinical trial, 26 percent of patients with massive or submassive PE and 32 percent of those with massive PE had manifestations of acute cor pulmonale, such as the $S_1 Q_3 T_3$ pattern, right bundle-branch block, a P-wave pulmonale, or right axis deviation. The low frequency of specific ECG changes associated with PE was confirmed in the PIOPED study.[68]

Despite its lack of diagnostic accuracy, ECG may be helpful in predicting adverse clinical outcomes in patients with PE. It was recently suggested that a T-wave inversion in V_2 or V_3 is the most frequent ECG sign of massive PE.[78] In another PE study, both the pseudoinfarction pattern (Qr in V_1) (Fig. 72–1) and T-wave inversion in V_2 were closely related to the presence of right ventricular dysfunction and were independent predictors of adverse clinical outcome.[79] In a recent trial, an abnormal electrocardiogram at presentation proved to be an independent predictor of an adverse outcome, although no individual abnormality appeared capable of predicting such an outcome after being adjusted for the patients' clinical symptoms and findings on admission, and for the presence of preexisting cardiac or pulmonary disease.[80]

[ ] IMAGING STUDIES FOR PULMONARY EMBOLISM

Chest Radiography

The chest radiograph is abnormal in the majority of patients with PE, but the findings are nonspecific and often subtle. Atelectasis, cardiomegaly, pulmonary infiltrates, small pleural effusions, and mild elevation of a hemidiaphragm may be present.[68,81] Classic radiographic evidence of pulmonary infarction (Hampton hump) or decreased vascularity (Westermark sign) are suggestive but uncommon. A normal chest radiograph in the presence of significant dyspnea and hypoxemia without evidence of bronchospasm or anatomic cardiac shunt is strongly suggestive of PE. In most situations, however, the chest radiograph cannot be used to definitively diagnose or exclude PE. Although exclusion of other processes such as pneumonia, congestive heart failure, pneumothorax, or rib fracture (which may cause symptoms similar to acute PE) is im-

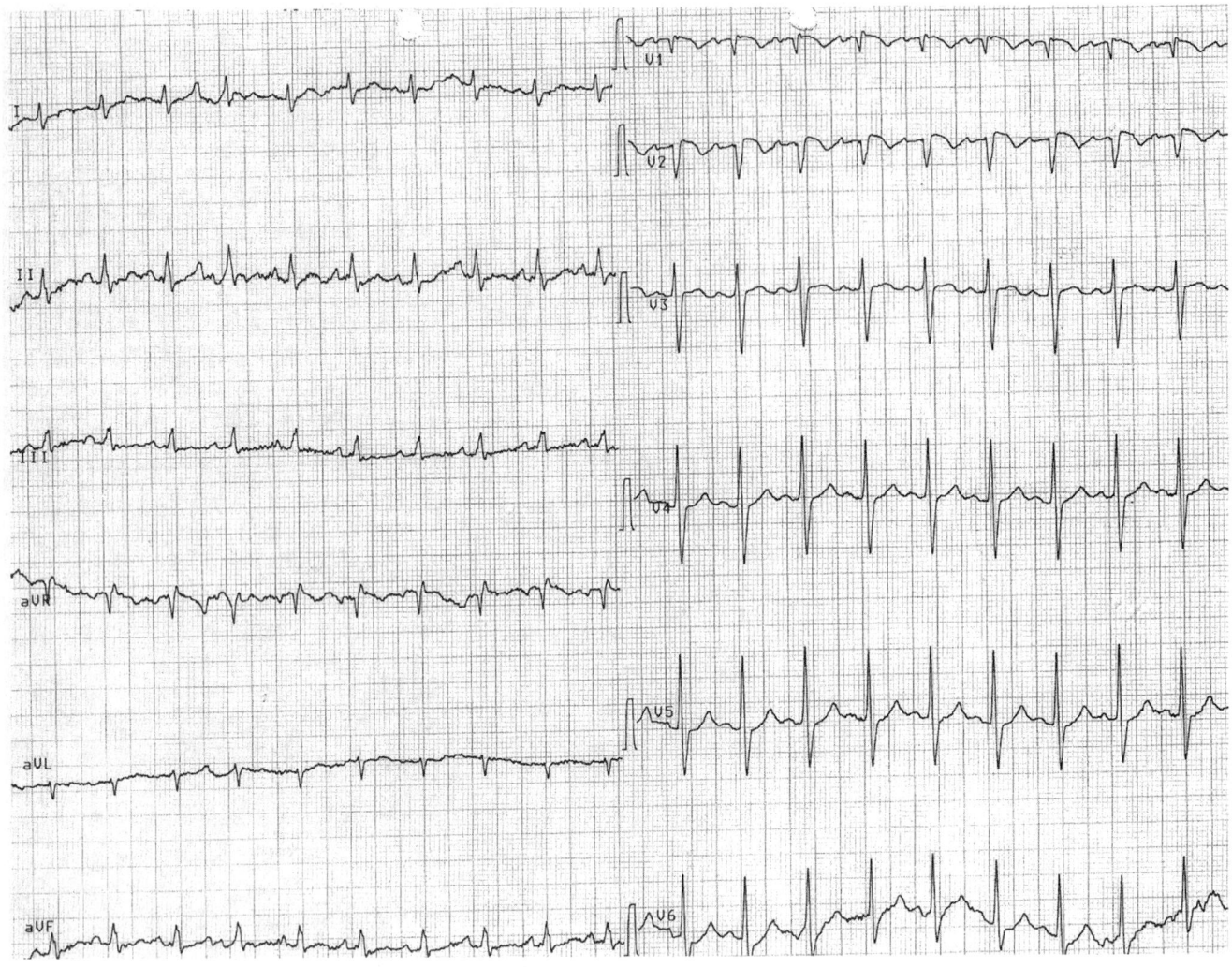

FIGURE 72–1. Twelve-lead ECG from a 54-year-old man with massive pulmonary embolism (PE) and cardiogenic shock. Several signs of right ventricular strain are present: sinus tachycardia with a heart rate of 100 beats/min; right axis deviation; SI SII SIII; clockwise rotation of QRS vector in the precordial leads; Qr in V$_1$; and T-wave inversion in V$_2$.

portant, it is important to recognize that PE often coexists with other underlying lung diseases.

Computed Tomography of the Chest

Contrast-enhanced computed tomography (CT) of the chest has become the most useful imaging test in patients with clinically suspected acute PE.

First-generation scanners have poor resolution in the segmental pulmonary arteries and a limited sensitivity for subsegmental clots. However, they appear to predict a benign clinical course over the ensuing 3 months.[82]

Second-generation scanners involve continuous movement of the patient through the scanner with concurrent scanning by a constantly rotating gantry and detector system.[83–89] A helix of projecting data is obtained. Continuous volume acquisitions can be obtained during a single breath. Rapid scans can be obtained, facilitating imaging in critically ill patients.

The latest generation of multidetector-row CT scanners (Figs. 72–2 and 72–3) permits image acquisition of the entire chest with 1-mm or submillimeter resolution with a breathhold of less than 10 seconds.[90,91]

Limitations of chest CT in early clinical studies included poor visualization of horizontally oriented vessels in the right middle lobe and lingula because of volume averaging.[84] The peripheral areas of the upper and lower lobes may be inadequately scanned, and the presence of intersegmental lymph nodes may result in false-positive studies. Multiplanar reconstructions in coronal, sagittal, or oblique planes aid in distinguishing lymph nodes from emboli. CT is capable of revealing emboli in the main, lobar, or segmental pulmonary arteries with >90 percent sensitivity and specificity.[84–88] However, for subsegmental emboli, the sensitivity and specificity are lower. The incidence of isolated subsegmental emboli with first- and second-generation scanners appears to be approximately 6 to 30 percent.[89] When CT is being used for PE diagnosis, it should be incorporated into an overall diagnostic strategy that includes pretest probability, D-dimer testing, and perhaps ultrasound examination of the deep veins.[90,91] An additional advantage is evaluating a patient for the entire spectrum of VTE in one imaging session by scanning the legs and pelvis, as well as the lungs.

Outcome studies have demonstrated that embolism can be safely excluded using a clinical assessment tool, D-dimer testing, and computed tomography except in those patients who present

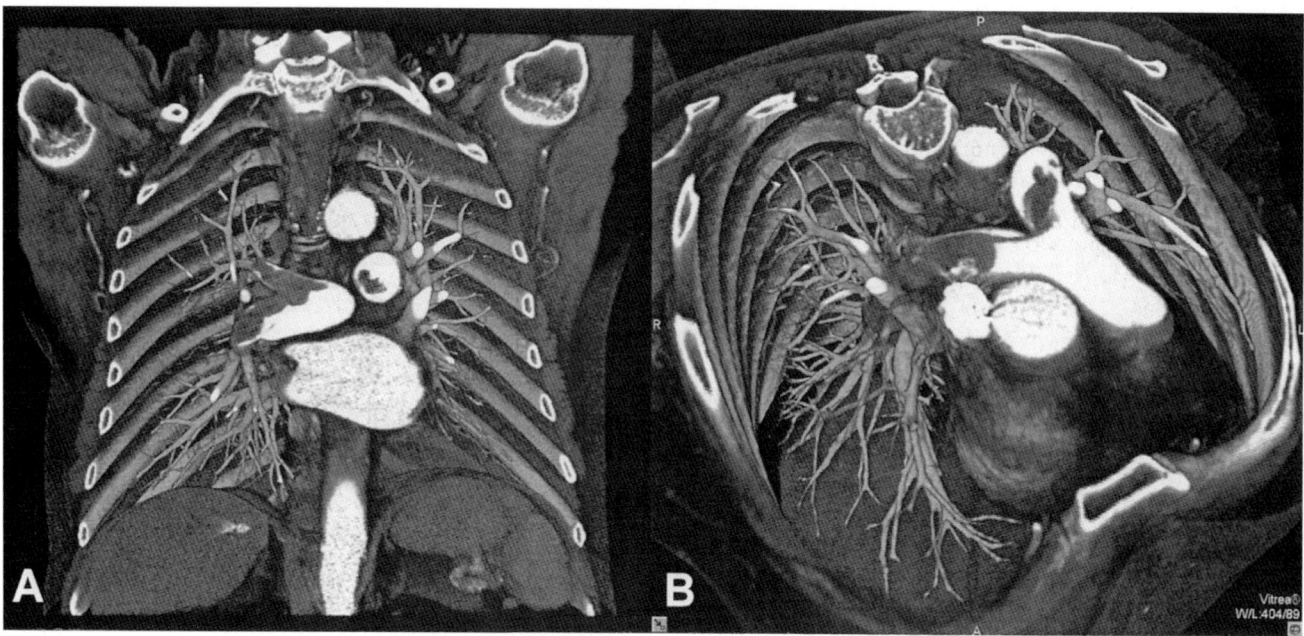

FIGURE 72–2. Contrast-enhanced 16-slice computed tomography in a 72-year-old man with extensive, acute central pulmonary embolism showing a "saddle embolus" (*arrows*) extending into both central pulmonary arteries. Colored volume rendering technique seen from an anterocranial (**A**) and anterior (**B**) perspective allows intuitive visualization of location and extent of embolism.

with a high clinical likelihood of embolism.[92–95] In the recently published PIOPED II trial, the sensitivity of computed tomography was 83 percent, a finding somewhat at odds with published outcome data.[95] PIOPED II did confirm the usefulness of clinical assessment in that the negative predictive value of a normal CT scan was 96 percent in patients with a low probability of embolism, 89 percent for those with an intermediate probability, but only 60 percent in those with a high-probability scan finding.

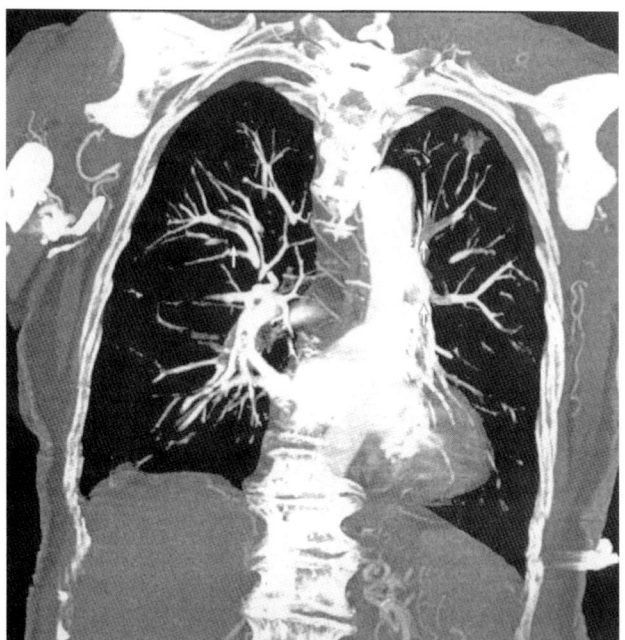

FIGURE 72–3. Contrast-enhanced 16-slice computed tomography (coronal reconstruction) in a 63-year-old man with multiple segmental pulmonary emboli (*arrows*). As an incidental finding, the examination also revealed a focal lung lesion in the left upper lobe, which was later confirmed to be stage I small cell lung cancer.

Normal results on CT scanning, therefore, appear capable of excluding embolism in embolic suspects with low or intermediate probabilities of the disease. In embolic suspects with a high probability of embolism and a negative CT angiogram, additional diagnostic testing should be considered. As demonstrated in the initial PIOPED trial, a negative V/Q scan or contrast pulmonary angiogram would achieve this end.[96] Sequential, noninvasive, lower-extremity examinations in patients with adequate cardiopulmonary reserve, although not confirming that embolism did not occur, would render the probability of recurrence unlikely. Alternatively, additional testing should be considered in patients with a low clinical probability of embolism and a CT scan that is suggestive but not clearly diagnostic of embolism as the positive predictive value of CT scanning under this circumstance in PIOPED II was only 58 percent.[95]

Another important advantage of chest CT is the concomitant ability to define nonvascular and vascular structures such as airway, parenchymal, and pleural abnormalities; lymphadenopathy; and cardiac and pericardial disease. This is very important for rapid detection of alternative diagnoses (e.g., aortic dissection, pneumonia, pericardial tamponade) in patients with acute "chest syndromes" in the emergency setting. The intravenous contrast agent may precipitate renal failure in patients with renal insufficiency. Those patients with a history of allergy to contrast agents should receive preprocedure treatment with steroids.

Ventilation–Perfusion Scanning

V/Q scanning has been the pivotal diagnostic test for suspected PE for many years. Chest CT has now virtually replaced lung scanning.

Ventilation–perfusion scanning is nondiagnostic in up to 70 percent of patients with suspected PE. Normal and high-probability scans are considered diagnostic. A normal perfusion scan excludes the diagnosis of PE with enough certainty that further diagnostic testing is unnecessary.

In the PIOPED study, the usefulness of lung scanning combined with clinical assessment of patients with suspected PE was prospectively evaluated.[96] Patients with PE had scans that were of high, intermediate, or low probability, but so did most individuals without PE. Although the specificity of high-probability scans was 97 percent, the sensitivity was only 41 percent. Of interest, 33 percent of patients with intermediate-probability scans and 12 percent of those with low-probability scans were diagnosed definitively with PE by pulmonary arteriography. Forty percent of low-probability scans in the presence of high clinical suspicion were followed by documentation of PE at angiography. When the clinical suspicion of PE was considered very high, the positive predictive value of high-probability scans for PE was 96 percent. In patients with nondiagnostic lung scans, further diagnostic testing for PE should be undertaken.

Pulmonary Angiography

Standard contrast pulmonary arteriography is the established "gold standard" imaging test for the diagnosis of PE. The risk of subsequent VTE in patients with a negative test and without anticoagulation is less than 2 percent. Two referee readers from the PIOPED study agreed on the presence or absence of subsegmental emboli in only 66 percent of cases.[97] In another study, using selective pulmonary arteriography, there was excellent agreement on main, lobar, and segmental emboli, but only 13 percent agreement on subsegmental emboli.[98]

Technique　Prior to injecting contrast agents into the pulmonary artery, optimal recording of right-heart pressure tracings is important. If pressure curves "wedge" in the main pulmonary arteries, massive PE should be suspected. If the mean pulmonary artery pressure exceeds 40 mmHg, preexisting pulmonary hypertensive disorders, including chronic thromboembolic pulmonary hypertension, should be included in the differential diagnosis. A reduced amount of contrast agent is recommended in patients with right-heart failure and extremely high pulmonary artery pressures.

A pigtail catheter is preferred because it permits a high contrast injection rate with optimal images and side holes for contrast that maximize safety. At least two views of each lung should be obtained. The standard procedure includes the ipsilateral posterior oblique and the anteroposterior or ipsilateral anterior oblique view.

The primary sign for PE is an intraluminal filling defect in an arterial branch or cutoff of a branch with the visualized tail of the embolus (Fig. 72–4). Secondary signs of PE are decreased abrupt occlusion of a vessel, oligemia or avascularity of a segment, a prolonged arterial phase with slow filling and emptying of veins, and tortuous peripheral vessels.

In chronic pulmonary hypertension, the pulmonary arteries are pouched and contain organized thrombi with usually concave edges. Bands and webs within the arteries may be present. Lobar and segmental vessels may show abrupt narrowing or occlusion.

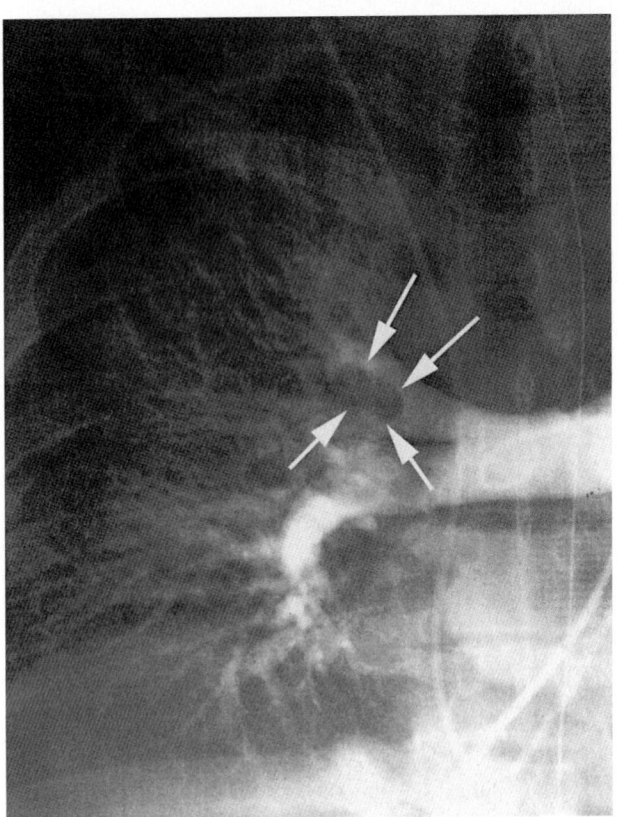

FIGURE 72–4. Selective conventional angiography of the right pulmonary artery in a 67-year-old woman with acute onset of dyspnea and chest pain, an elevated D-dimer enzyme-linked immunosorbent assay (ELISA) level, and an inconclusive ventilation–perfusion scan. The right-upper-lobe artery is obstructed with visualization of the tail of the embolus in the proximal right-upper-lobe artery.

Magnetic Resonance Imaging

Gadolinium-enhanced magnetic resonance (MR) angiography is also being used to evaluate clinically suspected PE.[99,100] In a clinical trial comparing MR with chest CT, the average sensitivity of chest CT for five observers was 75 percent and of MR 46 percent.[101] The average specificity of chest CT was 89 percent, compared with 90 percent for MR. A more recent study showed that when MR is performed under optimal conditions, it appears to be highly sensitive and specific even for segmental PE in comparison to pulmonary angiography.[102] MR has several attractive advantages over chest CT, including excellent sensitivity and specificity for the diagnosis of DVT and no requirement of ionizing radiation or iodinated contrast agents. Furthermore, MR technology also allows assessment of left and right ventricular size and function—potentially important for the risk stratification of PE patients. Use of the technique has been hampered by cost, required scanning time in relationship to CT, and availability of scanners.

Echocardiography

Transthoracic echocardiography has emerged as a potentially important tool for risk assessment and treatment guidance in patients with acute PE. The presence of right ventricular dysfunction on a baseline echocardiogram in normotensive patients appears to represent an independent predictor of an adverse outcome or early death.[3,103–107] However, approximately 40 percent of normotensive patients with symptomatic pulmonary embolism will have echocardiographic evidence of right ventricular dysfunction and it remains controversial whether all such patients, the majority of whom will do well with conventional therapy, should be subjected to the risks of thrombolytic therapy.

Technique Right ventricular systolic dysfunction in routine clinical practice is semiquantitatively assessed by examination of the right ventricular free wall motion using a four-point scale: normal/near-normal right ventricular function and mild, moderate, or severe right ventricular dysfunction. Patients with severe right ventricular dysfunction may show regional wall motion abnormalities of the right ventricle known as the *McConnell sign*: evidence of severe hypokinesis of the right ventricular free wall combined with preserved systolic contraction of the right ventricular apex.[108]

Right ventricular dilatation is an indirect sign of right ventricular pressure overload in the setting of acute PE. The ratio of right ventricular to left ventricular size should be measured using M-mode echocardiography in the parasternal long-axis view at the level between the mitral valve and the papillary muscle. An alternative is to measure the size ratio of both ventricles in the apical four-chamber view at the level of the atrioventricular valves (Fig. 72–5B). A ratio of right ventricular to left ventricular size of ≥1 in the apical four-chamber view and ≥0.5 in the parasternal long-axis view indicates right ventricular dilation. In patients with severe right ventricular pressure overload, a constant shift of the interventricular septum toward the left ventricle or a paradoxical (systolic) septal movement toward the left ventricle may be observed. In the parasternal short-axis view, a constant shift of the septum to the left side often causes a "D-shaped" left ventricle (Fig. 72–5C). Further indirect signs of right ventricular dysfunction are systolic pulmonary artery hypertension manifested by an increased tricuspid regurgitant velocity >2.6 m/s and reduced inspiratory collapse of a dilated inferior vena cava because of elevated central venous pressure.

Echocardiography is also useful to diagnose a patent foramen ovale in patients with suspected paradoxical embolism, directly visualizing thrombi in the main pulmonary artery (Fig. 72–5D), right-heart chambers, and vena cava.[109,110]

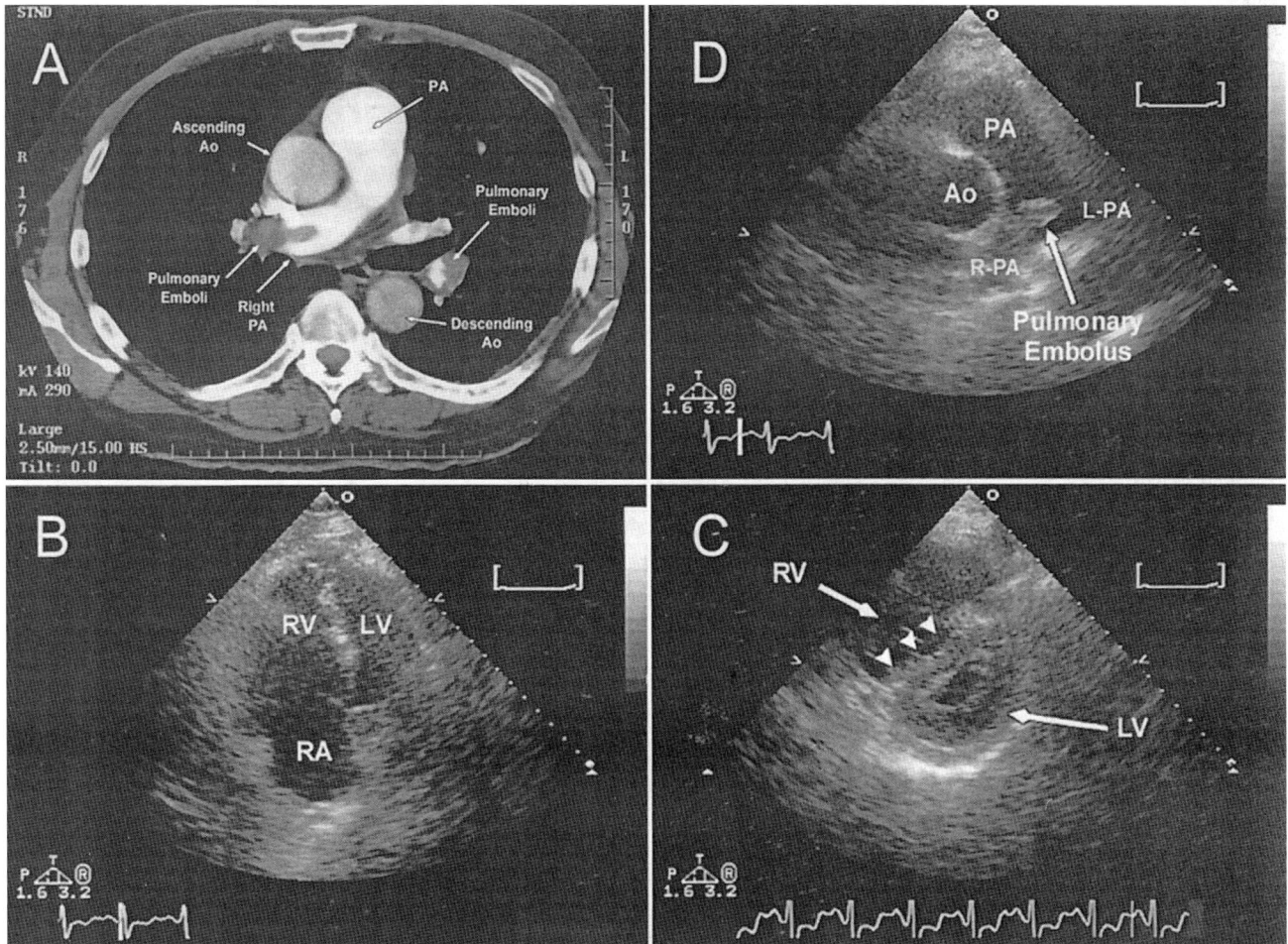

FIGURE 72–5. Chest computed tomography and echocardiographic findings in a 55-year-old man with submassive PE. **A.** Chest computed tomogram demonstrating multiple segmental emboli, including a central embolus in main pulmonary artery and extending into right pulmonary artery. **B.** Transthoracic apical four-chamber view with severe right ventricular dilatation. **C.** Transthoracic parasternal short-axis view showing flattening of interventricular septum ("D-shaped" left ventricle, *arrowheads*). **D.** Transthoracic short-axis view demonstrating the central clot in the main and right pulmonary arteries. Ao, aorta; L-PA, left pulmonary artery; LV, left ventricle; PA, pulmonary artery; RA, right atrium; R-PA, right pulmonary artery. *Source: From Clark RK, Bednarz J, Spencer KT, Lang RM. Acute pulmonary embolism. Circulation 2000;102: 2441, with permission.*

【 】 IMAGING STUDIES FOR DEEP VENOUS THROMBOSIS

A number of diagnostic techniques can be used to evaluate the patient with suspected DVT. Compression ultrasound (duplex ultrasonography) is the most common technique used in the United States and in many other areas of the world. Impedance plethysmography is used at some centers, and a number of important clinical trials have been performed utilizing this now outdated technique. Magnetic resonance imaging (MRI) appears to have some important advantages, but it has not generally been used as a first-line test because of cost and lack of availability. CT venography used alone or in conjunction with CT angiography appears to have a sensitivity and specificity equivalent to that of duplex ultrasonography, but exposes the patient to additional radiation. Contrast venography remains the gold standard, but it is performed infrequently in view of the accuracy of ultrasound. Each diagnostic technique has advantages and limitations. Although diagnostic algorithms may be suggested for suspected DVT, these are institution-specific, depending on resources and available expertise with certain techniques.

Ultrasonography

Compression ultrasound with venous imaging is a portable, accurate, and widely available diagnostic technique for DVT.[111] The primary criterion to diagnose DVT by ultrasound is the noncompressibility of the vein. Combined with a Doppler reading, this technique is referred to as *duplex ultrasonography*. Ultrasound technology has been further improved by the development of color duplex instrumentation that displays Doppler frequency shifts as color superimposed on the grayscale image. The color duplex images display both mean blood-flow *velocity*, expressed as a change in hue or saturation, and *direction* of blood flow, displayed as red or blue. Ultrasound imaging techniques can also identify or suggest the presence of pathology other than DVT such as Baker cysts, hematomas, lymphadenopathy, arterial aneurysms, superficial thrombophlebitis, and abscesses.[112] The sensitivity and specificity of ultrasound for symptomatic proximal DVT has been well above 90 percent in most recent clinical trials.[113,114] There are limitations, including insensitivity for asymptomatic DVT (less than 50 percent), operator dependence, the inability to accurately distinguish acute from chronic DVT in symptomatic patients, and insensitivity for calf vein thrombosis.[115–117] Compared with other technologies, ultrasound is relatively inexpensive and is the preferred diagnostic modality for symptomatic suspected proximal DVT.

Ultrasound is considered diagnostic for PE if it confirms DVT in patients with PE symptoms. However, approximately 50 percent of patients with CT-confirmed embolism will have no imaging evidence of lower-extremity venous thrombosis.[118] Thus, embolism cannot safely be ruled out in patients with suspected PE on the basis of a negative lower extremity duplex ultrasound. In patients with suspected embolism and a negative multidetector-row computed tomographic examination of the chest, the addition of duplex ultrasonography appears to only minimally increase diagnostic yield.

Contrast Venography

Contrast venography is a costly and invasive procedure that may result in superficial phlebitis or hypersensitivity reactions, but it is generally safe and accurate. Although contrast venography is the gold standard for DVT diagnosis, it is now rarely performed except in clinical trials because of its higher sensitivity in detecting asymptomatic thrombi than duplex ultrasonography.[119] DVT is usually diagnosed with compression or Doppler ultrasonography, which is widely available, noninvasive, and accurate. Alternative diagnostic approaches are contrast CT and MRI.

Venography is performed whenever noninvasive testing is nondiagnostic or impossible to perform or during interventional procedures such as catheter-directed thrombolysis, catheter embolectomy, percutaneous angioplasty, or insertion of an inferior vena caval filter.

Impedance Plethysmography

Impedance plethysmography has been used in patients who presented with suspected acute DVT but is rarely obtained in the era of ultrasound.

Magnetic Resonance Imaging

MRI has clear advantages as a diagnostic test for suspected DVT and appears to be an accurate, noninvasive alternative to venography.[120,121] A major feature of this technique is excellent resolution of the inferior vena cava and pelvic veins.[99,100] Preliminary experience with MRI suggests that it is at least as accurate as contrast venography or ultrasound imaging and more sensitive than ultrasound for pelvic vein and calf-limited thrombosis.[121–123] Simultaneous bilateral lower-extremity imaging can be accomplished, and MRI appears to accurately distinguish acute from chronic DVT. This technique is also useful in differentiating other entities such as cellulitis or a Baker cyst from acute DVT. As with many other diagnostic techniques, its usefulness depends to a certain degree on the experience of the reader.

DIAGNOSTIC STRATEGY

The overall diagnostic approach depends on the hemodynamic presentation of the patient. While rapid diagnosis and therapeutic intervention is required in patients with shock and suspected massive PE, there is sufficient time to obtain imaging tests in hemodynamically stable patients with suspected PE.

【 】 PATIENTS WITH SUSPECTED PULMONARY EMBOLISM AND SHOCK

In patients with hypotension or cardiogenic shock associated with suspected massive PE, rapid initiation of therapy is potentially lifesaving. The definition of massive pulmonary embolism should be based on hemodynamic considerations rather than purely anatomic considerations.[7] Irrespective of the degree of vascular obstruction, patients with pulmonary embolism who present with shock have a mortality rate that approaches 30 percent, whereas those suffering a cardiopulmonary arrest have a mortality rate that approximates 70 percent. Time-consuming imaging tests often can be avoided when emergency bedside echocardiography is available. In patients with suspected massive PE and evidence of severe acute right ventricular dysfunction on the echocardiogram, thrombolysis or embolectomy may be rapidly initiated. A caveat to this general recommendation exists in patients presenting with decompensated right-heart failure caused by nonembolic forms of pulmonary hypertension. Clues to the chronic nature of the right ventricular dysfunction would be a history of chronic rather than acute dyspnea, the presence of right ventricular hypertrophy rather than simple dilatation, or estimated pulmonary artery systolic pressures by echocardiogram greater than approximately 70 mmHg.

【 】 PATIENTS WITH SUSPECTED PULMONARY EMBOLISM WITHOUT SHOCK

Pulmonary embolism cannot be excluded without objective testing. The history, physical examination, and diagnostic studies, such as a chest radiograph, electrocardiogram, or arterial blood gas analysis, can raise or lower the clinical suspicion of embolism but are incapable of excluding or confirming it unless a clearly identifiable condition (e.g., pneumothorax) is identified to account for the patient's complaints. Noninvasive strategies have been investigated and algorithms constructed capable of confirming or excluding the diagnosis of embolism under most circumstances.

In all emergency room or other outpatients, the clinical pretest probability for PE should be calculated by implicit assessment or, preferably, through a standardized technique.[70–72] A highly sensitive plasma D-dimer assay such as an ELISA should be obtained. Unless the pretest probability is high, pulmonary embolism can be excluded by a D-dimer result below the assay-specific cutoff level. In patients with elevated D-dimer levels or a high clinical probability of embolism, spiral chest CT should be obtained (Fig. 72–6). In patients with significant impairment of renal function, pregnancy, or allergy to contrast agents, lower-extremity duplex study, or ventilation–perfusion scanning may be preferred as the primary chest imaging test. A V/Q scan can also be performed in patients with a nondiagnostic or negative chest CT when the clinical suspicion of PE persists. A normal V/Q is capable of excluding the diagnosis, whereas a high-probability scan is capable of confirming the diagnosis in patients with a high or intermediate probability of disease. If a high clinical suspicion for PE persists, pulmonary angiography can be performed. This strategy is safe and requires pulmonary angiography in less than 10 percent of patients.[125]

The approach to a hospitalized patient with suspected embolism is different. At the present time, the safe exclusion of embolism in inpatients using a clinical prediction rule and D-dimer result remains to be established. D-Dimer testing has little clinical utility in inpatients because of its poor specificity. Clinical findings suggestive of embolism may be misleading as a result of comorbid conditions, and translation of a standardized clinical prediction rule validated in outpatients to an inpatient population is problematic. A negative CT angiogram coupled with a negative lower-extremity duplex ultrasound can exclude embolism under most circumstances. In those patients with a high clinical suspicion, es-

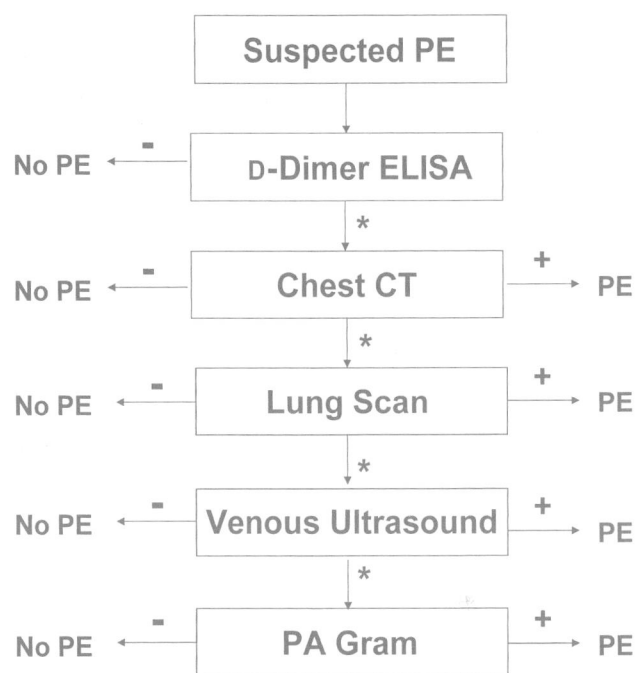

FIGURE 72–6. Diagnostic strategy for patients with suspected pulmonary embolism (PE) without shock. In this strategy, chest computed tomography is used as the principal imaging test. *Further testing should be considered if the test is inconclusive or negative, with a persistent suspicion of PE.

pecially those with limited cardiopulmonary reserve, pulmonary angiography may be required.

The amount of contrast required for CT scanning (100 to 150 mL) poses a substantial risk of radiocontrast-induced nephropathy for patients with preexisting renal disease (serum creatinine approximately 2 mg/dL or creatinine clearance <60 mL/min), especially when it is associated with diabetes mellitus.[126] In such patients, a strategy using duplex ultrasonography and V/Q scanning would appear prudent, followed by selective conventional pulmonary angiography should the noninvasive techniques not yield a diagnosis. Although multiple pharmacologic agents have been used, only periprocedural hydration, the use of nonionic, iso-osmolar contrast agents, and perhaps N-acetylcysteine are of proven benefit in preventing dye nephropathy.[127]

Given the potential risk of radiation exposure to the fetus, a diagnostic approach that limits that exposure during pregnancy is warranted. Therefore, duplex ultrasonography is an appropriate initial diagnostic approach. If ultrasonography is negative, the evaluation should proceed based on the clinical probability assessment and using V/Q scanning as the next diagnostic technique. This recommendation may change in the future based on studies that demonstrate equivalent fetal radiation exposure from V/Q and current generation CT scanners.[128] The reproductive toxicity of contrast agents remains to be completely established.

At the present time, embolism can be safely excluded in patients with a low or intermediate probability of embolism by a normal, highly-sensitive D-dimer assay, a normal or near-normal ventilation–perfusion scan, a negative CT angiogram, or a negative contrast angiogram. In patients with a high probability of embolism, clinical outcome appears to be acceptable following a negative CT angiogram and lower-extremity duplex examination, but definitive exclusion requires either a normal ventilation–perfusion scan or a negative contrast pulmonary angiography. Under this circumstance, clinical judgment must come into play with the risk of possible recurrence balanced against the risk of additional diagnostic procedures.[124]

Embolism can be confirmed in patients with an intermediate or high probability of embolism by a high probability ventilation–perfusion scan, a positive CT angiogram, or a positive lower-extremity duplex examination. In patients with a low probability of embolism, pulmonary angiography is required unless a CT angiogram is convincingly positive.[124]

PREVENTION OF VENOUS THROMBOEMBOLISM

[ ] BACKGROUND

Prophylaxis for DVT is effective.[129] A substantial reduction in the incidence of DVT can be accomplished when individuals at risk receive appropriate preventive care; however, such measures appear to be grossly underused. A review of the use of prophylaxis for DVT in 16 Massachusetts hospitals revealed that prophylaxis was administered to only 44 percent of high-risk patients in teaching hospitals and to only 19 percent of high-risk patients in nonteaching hospitals.[130] The frequency of prophylaxis ranged from 9 to 56 percent among hospitals. Another retrospective analysis revealed that only 97 of 250 patients (39 percent) at *very high risk* for DVT received any form of prophylaxis and that only 64 of these 97 (66 percent) received appropriate regimens.[131] A recent review confirmed that prophylaxis can be administered safely with major bleeding complications occurring in only 0.2 percent of surgical patients.[132]

Prophylaxis can be pharmacologic or nonpharmacologic. Pharmacologic prophylaxis options include unfractionated heparin, LMWH, fondaparinux, and warfarin.[133–137] Aspirin has a slight benefit but not enough to be used as a standard therapy to prevent VTE.[138] LMWHs are increasingly used in clinical practice for both prevention and treatment of established VTE. The LMWH preparations are advantageous in that they produce a more predictable dose–response and are administered subcutaneously only once or twice daily (without monitoring), depending on the preparation.[139] Early ambulation whenever possible is always recommended in postoperative patients.

[ ] GENERAL MEDICAL PATIENTS

Prophylactic measures to prevent VTE are not widely implemented among patients with medical illness. In the DVT FREE Registry of 5451 DVT patients, 59 percent of those who did not receive prophylaxis were medical patients.[10] Recent trials have demonstrated that medical patients have a thrombosis risk equivalent to that of moderate-risk surgical patients and that the use of prophylaxis can significantly reduce the rate of venous thromboembolic events with an acceptable rate of bleeding.[140–142]

Patients should be stratified according to DVT risk, and certain prophylactic measures are more appropriate for some patients than for others. The intensity of a prophylactic regimen should take into account the relative risk for thrombosis. Generally, low-dose anticoagulation with standard, unfractionated heparin or LMWH is indicated in medical or surgical patients who are deemed to be at risk for DVT. When standard heparin is used for prophylaxis in general medical patients, 5000 U given subcutaneously every 8 to 12 hours is generally adequate. LMWHs have also been studied in general medical patients. In a large, double-blind, randomized, clinical study comparing two different doses of subcutaneous LMWH (enoxaparin) delivered once daily to acutely ill medical patients, the higher dose (40 mg) proved effective and the lower dose (20 mg) was no better than placebo.[140] The incidence of DVT was 5.5 percent in the former group and 14.9 percent in the latter group.

When prophylactic anticoagulation is contraindicated, mechanical devices, such as gradual vascular compression stockings or intermittent pneumatic compression stockings, are used. Anticoagulation together with pneumatic compression is appropriate in patients who are deemed to be at exceptionally high risk or who have multiple risk factors for DVT.

[ ] GENERAL SURGICAL PATIENTS

In general surgical patients, a number of prophylactic strategies have been employed. An overview of the results of randomized trials in surgical patients demonstrated the substantial benefit of DVT prophylaxis.[143] In this review of more than 70 randomized trials involving 16,000 patients, it was found that perioperative use of subcutaneous heparin could prevent about half of all embolic events and about two-thirds of all episodes of venous thrombosis. In a large meta-analysis, the value of prophylaxis to reduce the incidence of DVT was confirmed; it was also suggested that intermittent pneumatic compression plus the use of gradient compression stockings may result in the lowest incidence of postoperative DVT.[143] Other combined treatments were associated with lower rates than heparin alone and appear appropriate in patients who are at exceptionally high risk for DVT. For those patients undergoing minor operations who are younger than age 40 years and who have no additional risk factors for DVT, no prophylaxis other than early ambulation is recommended. Older patients who are undergoing major operations without additional risk factors should receive either standard unfractionated heparin, LMWH, or intermittent pneumatic compression. When additional risk factors are present in the latter group, standard heparin every 8 hours or LMWH should be administered. Enoxaparin has been approved by the U.S. Food and Drug Administration (FDA) for prophylaxis in patients undergoing elective abdominal surgery (40 mg subcutaneously once daily). A second preparation, dalteparin, has also been approved in the United States for once-daily use as prophylaxis for elective abdominal surgery.

[ ] OTHER HIGH-RISK PATIENTS

Enoxaparin has been approved by the FDA for prophylaxis against DVT in patients who are undergoing elective total hip or knee replacement. The approved dosing regimens are 30 mg subcutaneously twice daily initiated within 12 to 24 hours after surgery (rarely used) and 40 mg once daily initiated preoperatively (commonly used). The duration of prophylaxis depends on whether the patient is ambulatory and on additional risk factors (Fig. 72–7).

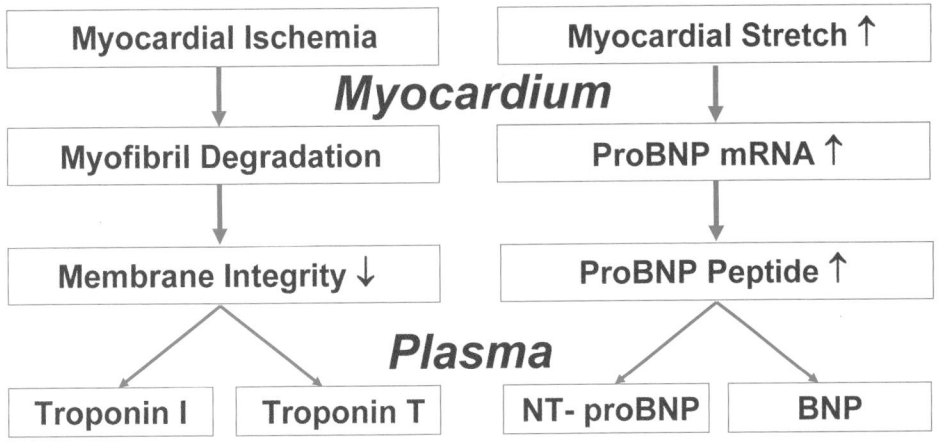

FIGURE 72–7. Mechanism of cardiac biomarker release in patients with acute pulmonary embolism. Right ventricular pressure overload with increased myocardial shear stress are responsible for myocardial synthesis and secretion of natriuretic peptides. Troponin release is a result of myocardial ischemia and microinfarction (see also the discussion under Pathophysiology of Acute Pulmonary Embolism, Hemodynamic Alterations above).

MANAGEMENT

【 】 RISK STRATIFICATION

Echocardiography

Transthoracic echocardiography is the most important tool for risk stratification in PE because right ventricular dysfunction on the echocardiogram is a powerful and independent predictor of mortality.[3] From a prognostic point of view, echocardiography helps to classify PE into three groups: (1) low-risk PE (no right ventricular dysfunction) with a hospital mortality of <4 percent, (2) submassive PE (right ventricular dysfunction and a preserved systemic arterial pressure) with a hospital mortality of 5 to 10 percent, and (3) massive PE (right ventricular dysfunction and cardiogenic shock) with a hospital mortality of approximately 30 percent.[144] A limitation of echocardiography is its limited avail-

ability on a 24-hour, 365 days per year basis, as well as its cost. Another problem is occasional poor imaging quality of the right ventricle, particularly in obese patients or those with chronic lung disease.

Cardiac Biomarkers

Troponins and natriuretic peptides are similarly accurate in identifying low-risk PE patients (Figs. 72–8 and 72–9).[145,146] The negative predictive value for inhospital death is high for the biomarker assays (Table 72–2). The cutoff levels for troponins are the lower detection limits for myocardial ischemia reported by the manufacturer. In one clinical trial, the cutoff level for the brain natriuretic peptide triage assay to predict a benign clinical outcome in PE patients was lower (<50 pg/mL) than the "congestive heart failure" cutoff level of 90 pg/mL.[147]

At present, elevated cardiac biomarkers or CT findings cannot be recommended to independently guide treatment decisions. In hemodynamically stable PE patients with evidence of right ventricular enlargement, or an extensive thrombus burden on CT scanning, or those with an increased troponin and/or brain natriuretic peptide level, further risk stratification with echocardiography should be considered. In patients with biomarker levels below the assay-specific cutoff, echocardiography will not add prognostic information. At the present time, risk stratification techniques appear most useful in identifying a low-risk population in whom outpatient management might be considered and in selecting those at risk who might be at risk for he-

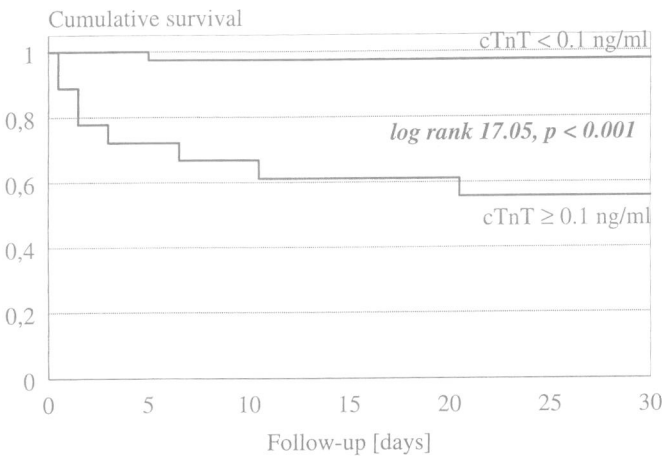

FIGURE 72–8. Cumulative survival rate at 30 days in patients with acute pulmonary embolism according to the level of troponin T. A level >0.1 ng/mL identifies patients at high risk for adverse clinical outcome. *Source: From Giannitsis E, Muller-Bardorff M, Kurowski V, et al. Independent prognostic value of cardiac troponin T in patients with confirmed pulmonary embolism. Circulation 2000;102:211–217, with permission.*

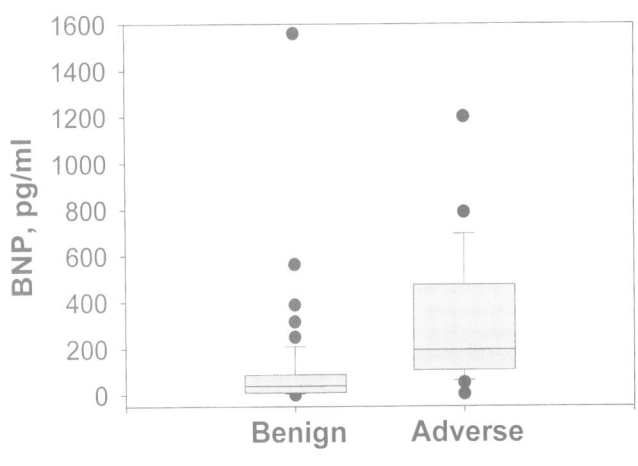

FIGURE 72–9. Brain natriuretic peptide (BNP) levels (median, confidence interval, and outliers) in patients with acute pulmonary embolism according to clinical outcome. Although BNP levels between patients with benign and adverse outcome overlap, the negative predictive value for the absence of adverse outcomes for BNP triage levels <50 pg/mL was 97 percent. *Source: From Kucher N, Printzen G, Doernhoefer T, et al. Low pro-brain natriuretic peptide levels predict benign clinical outcome in acute pulmonary embolism. Circulation 2003;107:1576–1578, with permission.*

TABLE 72–2

Cardiac Biomarkers and Inhospital Death in Patients with Pulmonary Embolism

EMBOLISM BIOMARKER	ASSAY	CUTOFF LEVEL	TEST + %	NPV %	PPV %
cTnI	Centaur, Bayer[129]	0.07 ng/mL	41	98	14
cTnT	Elecsys, Roche[129]	0.04 ng/mL	37	97	12
cTnT	TropT, Roche[131]	0.10 ng/mL	32	97	44
cTnT	Elecsys, Roche[140]	0.09 ng/mL	11	99	34
cTnT	Elecsys, Roche[130]	0.01 ng/mL	50	100	25
BNP	Shionoria, CIS[141]	21.7 pmol/L	33	99	17
BNP	Triage, Biosite[134]	50 pg/mL	58	100	12
NT-proBNP	Elecsys, Roche[135]	500 pg/mL	58	100	12

BNP, brain natriuretic peptide; cTnI, cardiac troponin I; cTnT, cardiac troponin T; NPV, negative predictive value; NT-proBNP, N-terminal pro-brain natriuretic peptide; PPV, positive predictive value.

modynamic deterioration and for whom close, inpatient surveillance would be indicated.

[ ] ANTICOAGULATION

Standard Unfractionated Heparin

When intravenous unfractionated heparin is instituted, the activated partial thromboplastin time (aPTT) should be aggressively followed at 6-hour intervals until it is consistently in the therapeutic range of 1.5 to 2.0 times control values.[148] Heparin can be administered by several protocols, but a weight-based approach substantially enhances the chances of attaining the therapeutic range quickly. Heparin can be administered as an intravenous bolus of 5000 U followed by a maintenance dose of at least 30,000 U every 24 hours by continuous infusion.[149] This aggressive approach decreases the risk of subtherapeutic anticoagulation and, although excessive levels are sometimes achieved initially, bleeding complications do not appear to be increased.[149] An alternative regimen consisting of a bolus of 80 U/kg followed by 18 U/kg/h has been recommended.[150,151] Subsequent adjusting of the heparin dose should also be weight based (Table 72–3). Warfarin therapy may be initiated as soon as the aPTT is therapeutic, and heparin should be maintained until a therapeutic international normalized ratio (INR) of 2.0 to 3.0 has overlapped with a therapeutic aPTT for 2 consecutive days. This initial anticoagulation approach applies to both acute DVT and PE. If a contraindication to anticoagulation exists, noninvasive testing over 10 to 14 days should be performed to detect possible extension into the popliteal vein.[152,153]

Although therapeutic dosing of heparin traditionally has used intravenous therapy with aPTT monitoring, a recent study examined the safety and efficacy of subcutaneous administration without monitoring in inpatients and outpatients presenting with either venous thrombosis or pulmonary embolism.[154] In this study, an initial subcutaneous dose of 333 U/kg of unfractionated heparin was administered followed by 250 U/kg every 12 hours. Fixed dose, unmonitored unfractionated heparin proved to be as effective and safe as low-molecular-weight heparin for the initial treatment of patients with venous thrombosis and pulmonary embolism.

The spectrum of upper-extremity venous thrombosis is variable and includes patients with peripherally and centrally placed intravenous catheters, as well as those with underlying malignancy. Patients with documented upper-extremity DVT should be anticoagulated.[155] Prophylactic anticoagulation in patients with long-term indwelling catheters should also be instituted.[156,157] Effort-related upper-extremity venous thrombosis (Paget-Schroetter syndrome) usually affects young, active men and is related to extrinsic compression of the subclavian vein at the thoracic inlet.[158] A multidisciplinary approach to management is often required to avoid long-term consequences including recurrence, embolism, and symptomatic sequelae.

TABLE 72–3

Nomogram for Heparin Therapy in Acute Venous Thromboembolism

The initial heparin dose is 80 U/kg bolus, then 18 U/kg/h. Subsequent dose modifications, based on aPTT as follows:

aPTT		HEPARIN DOSE ADJUSTMENT
SECONDS	TIMES CONTROL	
<35	<1.2	80 U/kg bolus, then increase by 4 U/kg/h
35 to 45	1.2 to 1.5	40 U/kg bolus, then increase by 2 U/kg/h
46 to 70	1.5 to 2.3	No change
71 to 90	2.3 to 3	Decrease infusion rate by 2 U/kg/h
>90	>3	Hold infusion 1 h, then decrease rate by 3 U/kg/h

aPTT, activated partial thromboplastin time.
SOURCE: American College of Chest Physicians Guidelines: Hyers TM, Agnelli G, Hull RD, et al. Antithrombotic therapy for venous thromboembolic disease. Chest 1998;114:561S–578S; and Raschke RA, Reilly BM, Guidry JR, et al. The weight-based heparin dosing nomogram compared with a "standard care" nomogram. Ann Intern Med 1993;119:874.

TABLE 72–4

A Comparison of Low-Molecular-Weight Heparin with Unfractionated Heparin

CHARACTERISTIC	UFH	LMWH
Mean molecular weight	12,000–15,000	4000–6000
Protein binding	Substantial	Minimal
Anti-Xa activity	Substantial	Substantial
Anti-IIa activity	Substantial	Minimal
Platelet inhibition	Substantial	Minimal
Vascular permeability	Moderate	None
Microvascular permeability	Substantial	Minimal
Elimination (predominant)	Hepatic/macrophages	Renal

LMWH, low-molecular-weight heparin; UFH, unfractionated heparin.

Low-Molecular-Weight Heparin

Mechanisms of Action and Pharmacology LMWHs are being increasingly used for acute VTE. These agents differ in a number of respects from standard, unfractionated heparin (Tables 72–4 and 72–5). A major advantage of these preparations over unfractionated heparin is substantially enhanced bioavailability.

Clinical Trials and Indications Numerous clinical trials have demonstrated the efficacy and safety of LMWHs for treatment of acute proximal DVT, using recurrent symptomatic VTE as the primary outcome measure.[159–165] Treatment with LMWHs is more convenient for the patient and the nursing staff for several reasons. A continuous intravenous line is not required, as these agents can be administered once or twice per day subcutaneously at fixed therapeutic doses, usually without laboratory monitoring.

In certain settings, therapy can be monitored by measuring anti-Xa levels.[166] Prophylactic doses of LMWH usually result in anti-Xa levels of 0.1 to 0.3 U/mL. The therapeutic target peak anti-Xa level drawn 4

TABLE 72–5

Potential Advantages of Low-Molecular-Weight Heparins over Unfractionated Heparin

Efficacy: comparable or superior[a]
Safety: comparable or superior[b]
Bioavailability: superior
Subcutaneous administration
Once- or twice-daily dosing
No laboratory monitoring[c]
Less phlebotomy
Earlier ambulation
Home therapy in certain patient subsets

[a]Based on objectively documented recurrence rates in clinical trials.
[b]Based on rates of major and minor bleeding in clinical trials.
[c]In certain patient populations (significant obesity, renal insufficiency), monitoring is suggested.

hours after administration should be in the range of 0.6 to 1 U/mL. The peak anti-Xa level is useful for monitoring heparin therapy under the following circumstances: (1) a baseline elevated aPTT because of antiphospholipid antibodies or other circulating anticoagulants in patients being treated with unfractionated heparin; (2) extremes of body weight (<40 kg and >150 kg); (3) renal failure or insufficiency (creatinine clearance <30 mL/min); (4) pregnancy; and (5) the occurrence of an unexpected bleeding or clotting event during therapy.

In two large, randomized (Canadian and European) trials, therapy with LMWH was compared with that using standard weight-based unfractionated heparin.[159,160] The LMWH patients were treated entirely as outpatients or continued at home after a brief hospitalization. The outpatient LMWH regimens proved safe and effective. Three meta-analyses examined the use of LMWH compared with unfractionated heparin in the initial treatment of acute proximal DVT.[167–169] Although there was overlap among the clinical trials included in the analyses, they have helped to confirm the efficacy and safety of LMWH for the treatment of established DVT. Both enoxaparin and tinzaparin are FDA-approved for use in the United States for treatment of established DVT in the outpatient setting or for DVT (with or without PE) in the inpatient setting. Dalteparin is approved for prevention of venous thrombosis and pulmonary embolism. Unlike regimens for prophylaxis, in which fixed dosing is used, a weight-based dosing regimen is employed for treatment of established VTE with both agents. In addition to being more convenient, the LMWH preparations appear to be cost-effective, particularly when outpatient therapy is used.[169] Table 72–6 lists

TABLE 72–6

Doses of Low-Molecular-Weight Heparin (LMWH) for Prevention and Treatment of Venous Thromboembolism

LMWH	PREVENTION	TREATMENT
Enoxaparin	30 mg q12h or 40 mg qd	1 mg/kg bid, 1.5 mg/kg qd[a]
Dalteparin	2500 to 5000 Xa U qd	200 Xa U/kg qd
Tinzaparin	75 Xa U/kg qd	175 Xa U/kg qd
Nadroparin	41 to 62 U/kg qd	<50 kg: 4100 Xa U q12h 50 to 75 kg: 6150 Xa U q12h >70 kg: 9200 Xa U q12h
Reviparin	4200 Xa U qd	35 to 45 kg: 3500 Xa U q12h 46 to 60 kg: 4200 Xa U q12h >60 kg: 6300 Xa U q12h
Ardeparin	50 Xa U/kg q12h	Not evaluated

[a]Enoxaparin is the only LMWH approved for use in the United States for established DVT. It is indicated in patients who present with DVT (with or without concomitant pulmonary embolism [PE]). A dose of either 1.5 mg/kg or 1 mg/kg q12h has proven effective for inpatients with DVT ± PE. Outpatient studies have been with 1 mg/kg q12h. It would appear highly likely that the once-daily dose would be adequate for outpatients, particularly as these patients tend to be stable and *may* have smaller thrombotic burdens.

some of the different LMWH products and their prophylaxis and treatment regimens.

In patients with symptomatic embolism, LMWH appears at least as effective as intravenous unfractionated heparin as a "bridge" to warfarin.[170] Extended 3-month treatment as monotherapy without warfarin for symptomatic acute PE is feasible and shortens the duration of hospitalization compared with that of patients receiving standard treatment.[171]

Complications of Heparin

Heparin-Induced Thrombocytopenia
Heparin-induced thrombocytopenia typically develops 5 or more days after the initiation of heparin therapy and occurs in 5 to 10 percent of patients.[172–174] If a patient is placed on heparin for VTE and the platelet count progressively decreases either by 50 percent or to 100,000/mm^3 or less, heparin therapy should be discontinued. Although the risk of heparin-induced thrombocytopenia appears to be lower with LMWH, it is important for clinicians to realize that heparin-induced thrombocytopenia can occur with the use of either form of heparin.[175]

Prolonged administration of unfractionated heparin may cause asymptomatic osteopenia, osteoporosis, and, rarely, pathologic bone fractures. After discontinuation of heparin, bone metabolism by densitometry usually improves within a year. LMWHs should not be given for at least 12 hours prior to placement of an epidural catheter because of the risk of epidural or spinal hematoma, which can cause permanent paraplegia.

Warfarin

Warfarin therapy should be initiated with concomitant unfractionated heparin or LMWH; otherwise, the first few days of warfarin administration may lead to a paradoxical prothrombotic state because of rapid depletion of proteins C and S. The procoagulant effect of warfarin can be inhibited by overlapping heparin with warfarin for at least 5 days.

Ordinarily, the initial dose should be 10 mg for 2 days, with monitoring performed daily. A standardized nomogram has been developed and can be used to make dose adjustments based on INR values obtained on days 3 and 5.[176] The initial dose should be lowered for debilitated, malnourished, and elderly patients.[176,177] A few patients have extremely low daily warfarin dose requirements of 1 to 2 mg, with an increased bleeding risk because of cytochrome P450 (CYP)2C9 variant alleles.[178]

In carefully selected patients, self-management of warfarin therapy using INR measurement with "point of care" devices may be effective and safe.[179]

Adverse Effects of Warfarin
Warfarin has a narrow therapeutic window, and the risk of bleeding increases with increasing INR. A large retrospective survey of more than 42,000 patients who were taking vitamin K antagonists suggested that an INR of 2.2 to 2.3 has the highest benefit-to-risk ratio.[180] In this study, a twofold increase in the hazard of mortality per unit INR elevation greater than 2.5 was observed. Risk factors for warfarin-related bleeding include hepatic disease, renal dysfunction, alcoholism, drug interactions, trauma, cancer, and history of gastrointestinal bleeding. The risk of bleeding is greatest in the first month after initiation of anticoagulation.[181]

Major bleeding can routinely be treated with vitamin K, cryoprecipitate, or fresh-frozen plasma. In patients with excessive INR values without bleeding, withholding one or two doses of warfarin with administration of oral vitamin K 2.5 mg is an effective strategy.

Rare complications of warfarin are skin necrosis and cholesterol microembolization, causing the "purple toes" syndrome by enhancing crystal release from ulcerated plaques.[182]

Reliable contraception is mandatory in women of childbearing potential because warfarin is teratogenic, particularly during weeks 6 to 12 of gestation.[183]

Optimal Duration and Intensity of Anticoagulation

The duration of outpatient anticoagulation for patients with venous thromboembolism remains controversial. Patients with a clearly defined initial predisposition, whose initial thromboembolic risk factors have resolved and whose ventilation–perfusion scan and noninvasive lower-extremity testing have normalized, can be managed with a 3-month course of anticoagulation. Patients without a clearly defined initial predisposition to thromboembolism and those with persistent ventilation–perfusion scan defects or abnormal lower-extremity test results should be treated for 6 months or more. This is especially true if the initial event was symptomatic embolism rather than venous thrombosis. The risk of both thrombotic and embolic recurrence appears to be considerably higher in patients who initially present with embolism than in patients who initially present with venous thrombosis alone.[184] Finally, certain patients, such as those with recurrent spontaneous episodes of venous thromboembolism, an irreversible clinical risk factor, combined thrombophilic tendencies, antithrombin III deficiency, or the presence of a lupus anticoagulant, should be treated with an indefinite period of anticoagulation even though such a strategy is associated with an increased risk of bleeding complications.

【 】 VENA CAVA INTERRUPTION

In patients with established VTE in whom heparin therapy cannot be continued, inferior vena cava (IVC) filter placement can be undertaken to prevent lower-extremity thrombi from embolizing to the lungs. The essential indications for filter placement include contraindications to anticoagulation, recurrent embolism while on adequate therapy, and significant bleeding complications during anticoagulation.[185] Filters are sometimes placed in the setting of anatomically massive PE when it is believed that any further emboli might be lethal.[185]

Although IVC filters can be potentially lifesaving by preventing early recurrence of pulmonary embolism, patients with filters appear to be at higher short-term and long-term risk for recurrent venous thromboembolism.[186–188] Consequently, anticoagulation is generally continued when a filter is placed unless it is contraindicated. A number of filter devices exist, but the Greenfield filter design is the most widely used. These devices can be inserted via the jugular or femoral vein. Possible mechanisms of IVC filter failure include filter migration; improper filter positioning, allowing thrombi to bypass the filter; and formation of thrombosis proximal to the filter or on the proximal tip of the filter with subsequent embolization. Rare complications include clinically significant perforation of the IVC, migration to the

TABLE 72–7

Relative Risk of Inhospital Death for Thrombolysis versus Heparin Alone in the Pulmonary Embolism Trials

STUDY	HEPARIN/THROMBOLYSIS		RELATIVE RISK (95% CONFIDENCE INTERVAL)
	N/N	MORTALITY (N/N)	
UPET, 1973[77]	78/82	7/6	0.82 (0.29–2.32)
Tibbutt, 1974[199]	17/13	1/0	0.43 (0.02–9.74)
Ly, 1978[200]	11/14	2/1	0.39 (0.04–3.79)
Marini, 1988[194]	10/20	0/0	—
PIOPED, 1990[96]	4/9	0/1	1.50 (0.07–30.59)
Levine, 1990[195]	25/33	0/1	2.29 (0.10–54.05)
PAIMS 2, 1992[197]	16/20	1/2	1.60 (0.16–16.10)
Goldhaber, 1993[198]	55/46	2/0	0.24 (0.01–4.84)
Jerjes-Sanchez, 1995[196]	4/4	4/0	0.11 (0.01–1.57)
MAPPET-3, 2002[85]	138/118	3/4t	1.56 (0.36–6.83)
Metaanalysis	358/359	20/15	0.75 (0.39–1.44)

heart, and displacement of the filter during insertion. Rarely, these devices may erode into the wall of the IVC. Occasionally, IVC obstruction caused by thrombosis at the filter site may occur. Deaths as a consequence of filter placement are extraordinarily uncommon. The use of temporary filters can obviate the problems associated with permanent filter insertion.[189] Four different retrievable vena caval filters have received approval for temporary insertion (Günther tulip filter, ALN filter, recovery filter, OptEase filter). Temporary filters have been placed in individuals who were deemed at extremely high risk for DVT yet unable to receive anticoagulant prophylaxis, such as certain trauma patients.[190] Depending on the filter type, retrievable filters can be removed within weeks to months of placement or can remain permanently if necessary because of a trapped large thrombus or a persistent contraindication to anticoagulation.[189]

[ ] THROMBOLYTIC THERAPY

Systemic Thrombolysis

The use of thrombolytic agents in acute pulmonary embolism remains controversial.[191,192] Although thrombolytic therapy does appear to accelerate the rate of thrombolysis, there is no convincing evidence to suggest that it decreases mortality, increases the ultimate extent of resolution when measured at 7 days, reduces thromboembolic recurrence rates, improves symptomatic outcome, or decreases the incidence of thromboembolic pulmonary hypertension.[193] The role of thrombolytic therapy in pulmonary embolism should be limited to those circumstances in which an accelerated rate of thrombolysis may be considered lifesaving; that is, in patients with pulmonary embolism who present with hemodynamic compromise, patients who develop hemodynamic compromise during conventional therapy with heparin, and patients with embolism associated with intracavitary right-heart thrombi. At the present time, the finding of right ventricular dysfunction on echocardiography in the absence of hemodynamic instability should not serve as a justification for routine thrombolytic therapy.

There are only 10 randomized PE trials of thrombolysis versus heparin to date, with a total of 717 patients with varying severity of PE.[77,107,194–200] In an overview, there is a trend toward mortality reduction with thrombolysis (Table 72–7).

None of the thrombolytic agents have been shown to be superior to the others. FDA-approved thrombolytic agents include recombinant tissue plasminogen activator, streptokinase, and urokinase. Table 72–8 presents thrombolytic regimens for the treatment of PE. Primary contraindications for thrombolytic therapy include medical conditions that increase the possible risk of bleeding complications, such as recent bleeding, surgery, stroke, or gastrointestinal hemorrhage.[201] Absolute and relative contraindications to thrombolysis are listed in *The Task Force on Pulmonary Embolism Guidelines* from the European Society of Cardiology.[144]

Heparin should be withheld until the thrombolytic infusion is completed. The aPTT is then determined and heparin is initiated without a loading dose if this value is less than twice the upper limit of normal. If the aPTT exceeds this value, the test is repeated every 4 hours until it is safe to proceed with heparin.

The use of systemic thrombolytic therapy for DVT without PE is even more controversial than its use in patients with symptomatic PE. Thrombolysis may be associated with a reduction in postphlebitic syndrome when used for acute DVT, but at the cost of an increased risk of bleeding.[202] It is reasonable to consider systemic thrombolytic therapy in patients with proximal occlusive DVT associated with significant swelling and symptoms when there are no contraindications.

Local Thrombolysis

For acute PE, the peripheral intravenous route is the primary method of drug delivery. A number of investigators have em-

TABLE 72–8

Regimens for Systemic Thrombolytic Therapy in Pulmonary Embolism

LYTIC AGENT	DOSE REGIMEN
Streptokinase	Loading dose: 250,000 U IV Continuous infusion: 100,000 U/h for 24 h
Urokinase	Loading dose: 2000 U/lb IV over 10 min Continuous infusion: 2000 U/lb/h for 12–24 h
Alteplase (tPA)	Loading dose: none Continuous infusion: 100 mg over 2 h
Reteplase	1. Bolus: 10 U IV 2. Bolus: 10 U IV after 30 min

tPA, tissue plasminogen activator.

ployed standard or low-dose intrapulmonary arterial thrombolytic infusions in order to deliver a high concentration of drug in close proximity to the clot.[203–205]

The potential benefits of intrapulmonary dosing remain theoretical; there have been no controlled trials demonstrating a safety or efficacy benefit of intrapulmonary over systemic thrombolysis.

【 】 CATHETER FRAGMENTATION AND EMBOLECTOMY

Interventional thrombus fragmentation with or without embolectomy is an alternative to systemic thrombolysis or surgical embolectomy. If the bleeding risk is not exceedingly high, catheter fragmentation may be combined with local or systemic thrombolysis. Most of the devices appear to be effective, safe, and potentially lifesaving in the presence of large "fresh" clots. However, none of the devices has been investigated in a large controlled trial, and all commercially available devices have important limitations (Table 72–9).

【 】 SURGICAL EMBOLECTOMY

Acute embolectomy might be considered in patients with hemodynamically massive pulmonary embolism or right-heart thrombus who have an absolute contraindication to anticoagulant or thrombolytic therapy, in patients who have suffered a cardiopulmonary arrest (although the mortality associated with embolectomy in those who have experience arrest is far higher than those who have not), in patients with impending paradoxical embolism, and in patients in whom aggressive medical therapy, including the use of thrombolysis, has proven ineffective.

【 】 SUPPORTIVE MEASURES

When massive PE associated with hypotension and/or severe hypoxemia is suspected, supportive treatment is immediately initi-

TABLE 72–9
Catheter Fragmentation and Embolectomy Devices for Pulmonary Embolism

DEVICE	MECHANISM	RISK/ DISADVANTAGE
Greenfield catheter[209]	Suction embolectomy	Ineffective for older clots
Pigtail catheter[210]	Fragmentation via pigtail catheter rotation	Distal microembolization
Amplatz device[211] ("clot buster")	Clot maceration via high-speed impeller rotation	Distal microembolization, hemolysis
Angioget[212]	Embolectomy via high-pressure saline injection (Venturi effect)	Ineffective for older clots
Hydrolyzer[213]	Embolectomy via rheolytic effect	Ineffective for older clots

ated. Intravenous saline can be infused rapidly, but caution is recommended. Excess fluid can result in further right ventricular dilatation, increased right ventricular wall tension, and a decreased cardiac output that may result in right ventricular ischemia.[7] Dopamine or norepinephrine appear to be the favored choices of vasoactive therapy in massive PE and should be administered if the blood pressure is not rapidly restored.[206] Death from massive PE results from right ventricular failure, and dobutamine has been recommended by some as a means by which to augment right ventricular output.[207–208] A vasopressor, such as norepinephrine combined with dobutamine, might offer optimal results. Mechanical ventilation may be instituted to decrease systemic oxygen demands or to manage respiratory failure. Intubation in the setting of a decompensated right ventricle, however, is fraught with risk. Premedications may cause systemic vasodilatation, whereas positive pressure ventilation may abruptly reduce preload and cardiac output.

CHRONIC THROMBOEMBOLIC PULMONARY HYPERTENSION

In a few patients with acute PE, the residual thromboembolic burden is sufficiently extensive to cause thromboembolic pulmonary hypertension.[209–210] Estimates of the incidence of thromboembolic pulmonary hypertension range from 0.5 percent to 3.8 percent following an initial episode of embolism and 13.4 percent following recurrent episodes of venous thromboembolism.[211–213] Approximately 30 percent of patients who develop chronic thromboembolic pulmonary hypertension have no documented history of acute DVT or PE, and this feature greatly impedes the diagnosis. Anticardiolipin antibodies or a lupus anticoagulant have been detected in approximately 10 percent of patients and elevated factor VIII levels detected in 40 percent.[214] No other defined thrombophilic or fibrinolytic abnormality has been encountered in this population.

As in other forms of pulmonary hypertension, progressive exertional dyspnea and exercise intolerance are characteristic. Later in the course of the disease, exertional chest pain, presyncope or syncope may occur. Diagnostic delay, particularly in the absence of a history of acute venous thromboembolism, occurs commonly.

The chest radiograph usually reveals right ventricular enlargement and enlarged main pulmonary arteries. ECG changes are consistent with right ventricular hypertrophy. Arterial blood gases generally reveal hypoxemia with a widened A-a gradient, although some patients may demonstrate only exercise-induced hypoxemia. Echocardiography documents the presence of pulmonary hypertension, as well as right ventricular hypertrophy.

Ventilation–perfusion lung scanning represents a simple, noninvasive means of differentiating disorders of the peripheral pulmonary vascular bed from those of the central vascular bed. In chronic thromboembolic disease, at least one segmental or larger mismatched perfusion defect is present. In disorders of the distal pulmonary vascular bed, perfusion scans either are normal or exhibit a "mottled" appearance characterized by subsegmental defects. Mismatched segmental or larger defects in patients with pulmonary hypertension may also arise from other processes that result in obstruction of the central pulmonary arteries or veins, such as pulmonary artery sarcoma, large-vessel pulmonary vasculitides, extrinsic vascular compression by mediastinal adenopathy or fibrosis, and pulmonary venoocclusive disease.[215] A variety of CT abnormalities have been described in patients with chronic thromboembolic disease including right-sided cardiac enlargement, enlargement of the pulmonary arteries, a mosaic perfusion pattern, intraluminal thrombus, subpleural densities, and dilated bronchial arteries.[216] The absence of these findings, however, cannot absolutely exclude the diagnosis (Fig. 72–10).

Following acute embolism, stable hemodynamics are achieved within 6 to 8 weeks.[217] Consequently, to avoid the possible development of a secondary, small-vessel arteriopathy that ultimately contributes to the elevation in pulmonary vascular resistance and which is not amenable to surgical correction, there is no need to delay evaluation beyond 3 months. Right-heart catheterization and contrast pulmonary arteriography are performed to establish the diagnosis with certainty and to determine operability. The angiographic findings in chronic thromboembolic pulmonary hypertension are distinct from those encountered in acute embolism and considerable experience is required for accurate angiographic interpretation (Fig. 72–11). Although anticoagulation should be instituted and IVC filters are recommended in patients with chronic thromboembolic pulmonary hypertension, the only means by which to alleviate symptoms and improve survival is with surgery. The University of California at San Diego has been the leading center for the evaluation and surgical therapy of chronic thromboembolic hypertension in more than 2000 patients.[218]

The majority of patients who undergo thromboendarterectomy exhibit a pulmonary vascular resistance >300 dyne · s · cm⁻⁵. At centers reporting their experience with thromboendarterectomy surgery, preoperative pulmonary vascular resistance is typically in the range of 700 to 1100 dyne · s · cm⁻⁵. At this level of pulmonary hypertension, patient impairment at rest and with exercise can be considerable. Patients without substantially altered pulmonary hemodynamics, such as those with involvement of one main pulmonary artery, those with unusually vigorous lifestyle expectations, and those who live at altitude, may also be considered for surgery to alleviate the exercise impairment associated with their high dead-

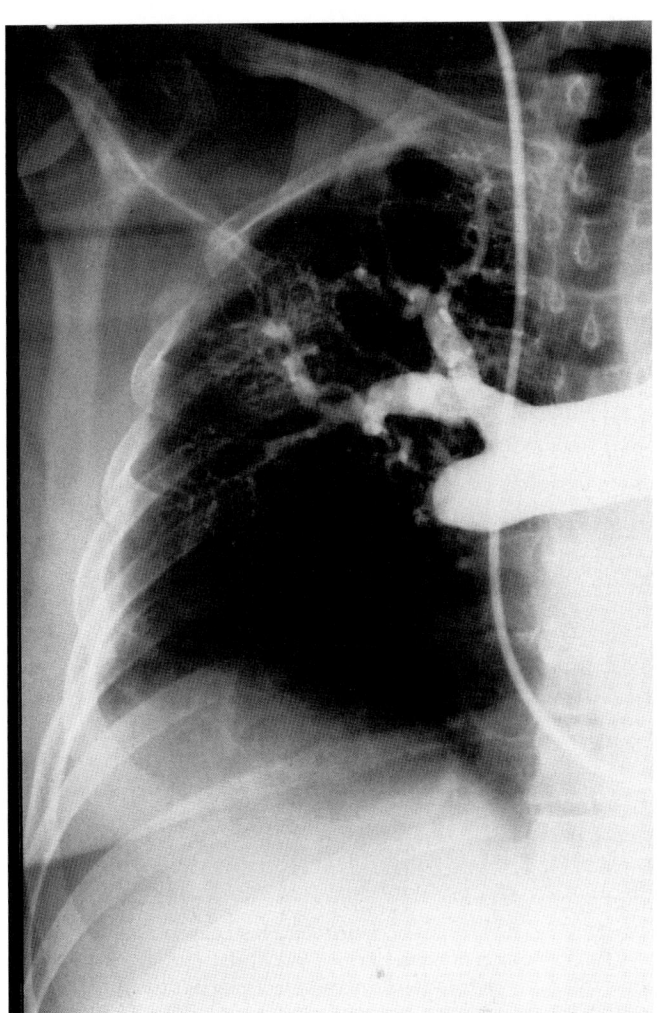

FIGURE 72–11. Representative right-sided pulmonary angiogram in a patient with chronic thromboembolic pulmonary hypertension demonstrating classic "pouch" defect with absent flow to right middle and lower lobes.

space and minute ventilatory demands. Surgery also is offered to patients with normal pulmonary hemodynamics, or with only mild levels of pulmonary hypertension at rest, who develop significant levels of pulmonary hypertension with exercise.

Pulmonary thromboendarterectomy is performed via median sternotomy on cardiopulmonary bypass with periods of deep hypothermic circulatory arrest and is technically quite distinct from pulmonary embolectomy for acute embolic disease. The procedure is a true endarterectomy, which requires careful dissection of chronic endothelialized material from the native intima to restore pulmonary arterial patency (Fig. 72–12).

The overall mortality, which has continued to improve, is now less than 5 percent with the major causes of mortality related to reperfusion lung injury and residual pulmonary hypertension.[219] In patients with a preoperative pulmonary vascular resistance less than 1000 dynes · s · cm⁻⁵, mortality has declined to the range of 1 to 2 percent.[218] In published series, the mean reduction in pulmonary vascular resistance has approximated 70 percent and a pulmonary vascular resistance in the range of 200 to 350 dyne · s · cm⁻⁵ can be achieved.[219] A corresponding improvement in right ventricular function determined by echocardiography, gas exchange, exercise capacity, and quality of life also has been reported.

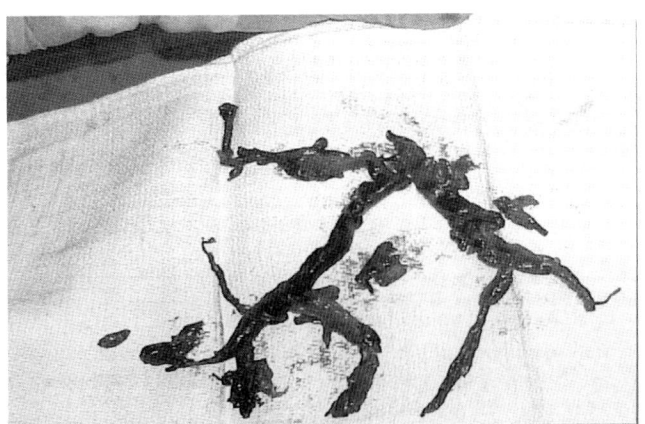

FIGURE 72–10. Extensive clot was removed from a 58-year-old patient with massive pulmonary embolism and shock who had a benign clinical course following emergency embolectomy on cardiopulmonary bypass.

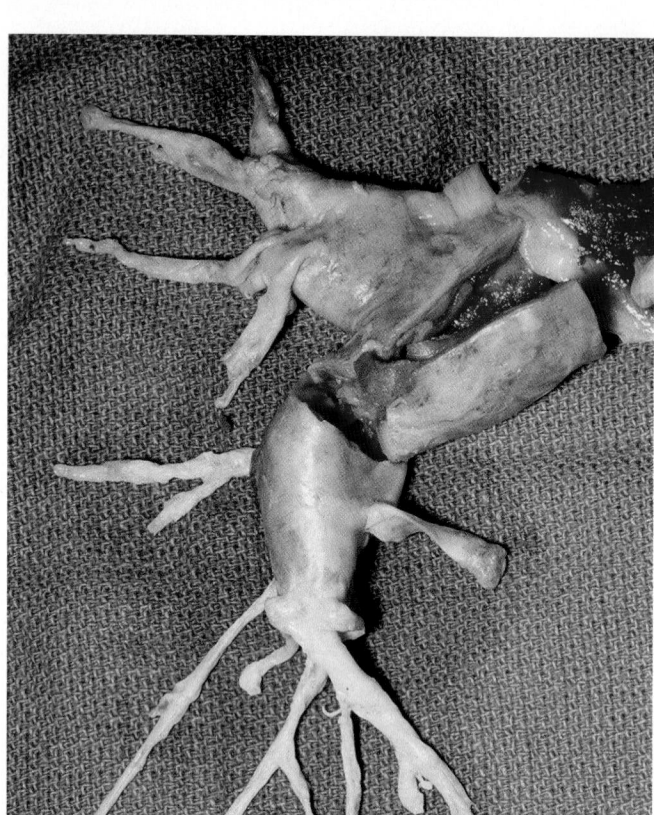

FIGURE 72–12. Example of chronic thromboembolic material obtained from the right pulmonary artery at the time of pulmonary thromboendarterectomy. Note the chronic fibrotic material that must be meticulously dissected from native intima to achieve optimal outcome.

Patients who are not deemed to be candidates for thromboendarterectomy either because of the distal nature of their pulmonary vascular obstruction or because of the presence of a severe, secondary arteriopathy, may be eligible for lung transplantation or may benefit from medical therapy.[220] Medical therapy has also been used as a therapeutic bridge prior to thromboendarterectomy in patients with severe pulmonary hypertension or right ventricular failure, although a beneficial effect on mortality has not yet been demonstrated. Medical therapy has also been used in patients with residual pulmonary hypertension following thromboendarterectomy.[28]

ACKNOWLEDGMENTS

With thanks to Nils Kucher and Victor F. Tapson for their contribution to the previous edition of this chapter.

REFERENCES

1. Anderson FA, Wheeler HB. Venous thromboembolism: risk factors and prophylaxis. *Clin Chest Med* 1995;16:235–251.
2. Dalen JE, Alpert JS. Natural history of pulmonary embolism. *Prog Cardiovasc Dis* 1975;17:257–270.
3. Goldhaber SZ, Visani L, De Rosa M. Acute pulmonary embolism: clinical outcomes in the International Cooperative Pulmonary Embolism Registry (ICOPER). *Lancet* 1999;353:1386–1389.
4. Carson JL, Kelley MA, Duffy A, et al. The clinical course of pulmonary embolism. *N Engl J Med* 1992;326:1240–1245.
5. Lindblad B, Eriksson A, Bergquist D. Autopsy-verified pulmonary embolism in a surgical department: analysis of the period from 1951 to 1988. *Br J Surg* 1991;78:849–852.
6. Goldhaber SZ. Prevention of recurrent idiopathic venous thromboembolism. *Circulation* 2004;110(24 Suppl 1):IV20–IV24.
7. Wood KE. Major pulmonary embolism: review of a pathophysiologic approach to the golden hour of hemodynamically significant pulmonary embolism *Chest* 2002;121:877–905.
8. Cotton LT, Clark C. Anatomical localization of venous thrombosis. *Ann R Coll Surg Engl* 1965;36:214–224.
9. Kahn SR. The post-thrombotic syndrome: the forgotten morbidity of deep venous thrombosis. *J Thromb Thrombolysis* 2006;21:41–48.
10. Goldhaber SZ, Tapson VF, for the DVT FREE Steering Committee. A prospective registry of 5451 patients with confirmed deep vein thrombosis. *Am J Cardiol* 2004;93:259–262.
11. Aryal KR, Al-Khaffaf H. Venous thromboembolic complications following air travel: what's the quantitative risk. A literature review. *Eur J Vasc Surg* 2006;31;187–199.
12. Flegal KM, Carroll MD, Ogden CL, et al. Prevalence and trends in obesity among U.S. adults, 1999–2000. *JAMA* 2002;288:1723–1727.
13. Freedman DS, Khan LK, Serdula MK, et al. Trends and correlates of class 3 obesity in the United States from 1990 through 2000. *JAMA* 2002;288:1758–1761.
14. Goldhaber SZ, Grodstein F, Stampfer MJ, et al. A prospective study of risk factors for pulmonary embolism in women. *JAMA* 1997;277:642–645.
15. Goldhaber SZ, Savage DD, Garrison RJ, et al. Risk factors for pulmonary embolism. The Framingham Study. *Am J Med* 1983;74:1023–1028.
16. Primrose JN, Davies JA, Prentice CR, et al. Reduction in factor VII, fibrinogen and plasminogen activator inhibitor-1 activity after surgical treatment of morbid obesity. *Thromb Haemost* 1992;68:396–399.
17. Sundell IB, Nilsson TK, Ranby M, et al. Fibrinolytic variables are related to age, sex, blood pressure, and body build measurements: a cross-sectional study in Norsjo, Sweden. *J Clin Epidemiol* 1989;42:719–723.
18. Landin K, Stigendal L, Eriksson E, et al. Abdominal obesity is associated with an impaired fibrinolytic activity and elevated plasminogen activator inhibitor-1. *Metabolism* 1990;39:1044–1048.
19. Davi G, Guagnano MT, Ciabattoni G, et al. Platelet activation in obese women: role of inflammation and oxidant stress. *JAMA* 2002;288:2008–2014.
20. Stein PD, Hull RD, Kayali F, et al. Venous thromboembolism according to age; the impact of an aging population. *Arch Intern Med* 2004:2260–2265.
21. Goldhaber SZ, Hennekens CH, Evans DA, et al. Factors associated with correct antemortem diagnosis of major pulmonary embolism. *Am J Med* 1982;73:822–826.
22. Kakkar VV, Howe CT, Nicolaides AN, et al. Deep vein thrombosis of the legs: is there a "high risk" group? *Am J Surg* 1970;120:527–530.
23. Clagett GP, Reisch JS. Prevention of venous thromboembolism in general surgical patients: results of a meta-analysis. *Ann Surg* 1988;208:227–240.
24. Clagett GP, Anderson FA Jr, Geerts W, et al. Prevention of venous thromboembolism. *Chest* 1998;114:531S–560S.
25. Fisher M, Michele A, McCann W. Thrombophlebitis and pulmonary infarction associated with fractured hip. *Clin Res* 1963;11:407.
26. Fitts WT Jr, Lehr HB, Bitner RL, et al. An analysis of 950 fatal injuries. *Surgery* 1964;56:663–668.
27. Coon WW. Risk factors in pulmonary embolism. *Surg Gynecol Obstet* 1976;143:385–390.
28. Joffe HV, Kucher N, Tapson VF, Goldhaber SZ. Upper-extremity deep venous thrombosis. A prospective registry of 592 patients. *Circulation* 2004:110;1605–1611.
29. Joffe HV, Goldhaber SZ. Upper-extremity deep vein thrombosis. *Circulation* 2002;106:1874–1880.
30. Haire WD. Arm vein thrombosis. *Clin Chest Med* 1995;16:341.
31. Handley AJ, Emerson PA, Fleming PR. Heparin in the prevention of deep vein thrombosis after myocardial infarction. *Br Med J* 1972;2:436–438.
32. Gruppo Italiano per lo Studio della Streptochinasi nell'Infarto Miocardico (GISSI). Effectiveness of intravenous thrombolytic treatment in acute myocardial infarction. *Lancet* 1986;1:397–402.
33. ISIS-2 Collaborative Group. Randomized trial of IV streptokinase, oral aspirin, both or neither among 17,187 cases of suspected acute myocardial infarction. *Lancet* 1988;2:349–360.
34. Rickles FR, Levine MN, Edwards RL. Hemostatic alterations in cancer patients. *Cancer Metastasis Rev* 1992;11:291–311.
35. Carroll VA, Binder BR. The role of the plasminogen activation system in cancer. *Semin Thromb Hemostas* 1999;25:183–198.

36. Lee AYY, Levine MN. The thrombophilic state induced by therapeutic agents in the cancer patient. *Semin Thromb Hemost* 1999;25:137–146.

37. Decensi A, Maisonneuve P, Rotmensz N, et al. Effect of tamoxifen on venous thromboembolic events in a breast cancer prevention trial. *Circulation* 2005;111:650–656.

38. Sorensen HT, Mellemkjaer L, Steffensen FH, et al. The risk of a diagnosis of cancer after primary deep venous thrombosis or pulmonary embolism. *N Engl J Med* 1993;38:1169–1173.

39. Di Nisio M, Otten HM, Piccioli A, et al. Decision analysis for cancer screening in idiopathic venous thrombosis. *J Thromb Haemost* 2005;3:2391–2396.

40. Gomes MPV, Deitcher SR. Risk of venous thromboembolic disease associated with hormonal contraceptives and hormone replacement therapy. *Arch Intern Med* 2004;164:1965–1976.

41. Toglia MR, Weg JG. Current concepts: venous thromboembolism during pregnancy. *N Engl J Med* 1996;335:108–114.

42. Weiss N. Third-generation oral contraceptives: how risky? *Lancet* 1995;346:1570.

43. World Health Organization Collaborative Study of Cardiovascular Disease and Steroid Hormone Contraception. Venous thromboembolic disease and combined oral contraceptives: results of international multicentre case-control study. *Lancet* 1995;346:1575–1582.

44. Daly E, Vessey MP, Hawkins MM, et al. Risk of venous thromboembolism in users of hormone replacement therapy. *Lancet* 1996;348:977–980.

45. Jick H, Derby LE, Wald Myers M, et al. Risk of hospital admission for idiopathic venous thromboembolism among users of postmenopausal estrogens. *Lancet* 1996;348:981–983.

46. Grodstein F, Stampfer MJ, Goldhaber SZ, et al. Prospective study of exogenous hormones and risk of pulmonary embolism in women. *Lancet* 1996;348:983–987.

47. Wu O, Robertson L, Twaddle S, et al. Screening for thrombophilia in high-risk situations: a meta-analysis and cost-effectiveness analysis. *Br J Haematol* 2005;131:80–90.

48. Wu O, Robertson L, Langhorne P, et al. Oral contraceptives, hormone replacement therapy, thrombophilias and the risk of venous thromboembolism: a systematic review. *Thromb Haemost* 2005;94:17–25.

49. Anderson FA, Spencer FA. Risk factors for venous thromboembolism. *Circulation* 2003;107:9–16.

50. Simioni P, Tormene D, Spiezia L, et al. Inherited thrombophilia and venous thromboembolism. *Semin Thromb Hemost* 2006;32:700–708.

51. Ridker PM, Miletich JP, Hennekens CH, Buring JE. Ethnic distribution of factor V Leiden in 4047 men and women. Implications for thromboembolic screening. *JAMA* 1997;277:1305–1307.

52. Ridker PM, Hennekens CH, Lindpainter K, et al. Mutation in the gene coding for coagulation factor V and the risk of myocardial infarction, stroke, and venous thrombosis in apparently healthy men. *N Engl J Med* 1995;332:912.

53. Kujovich JL. Thrombophilia and pregnancy complications. *Am J Obstet Gynecol* 2004;191:412–424.

54. Vandenbroucke JP, Rosing J, Bloemenkamp KW, et al. Oral contraceptives and the risk of venous thrombosis. *N Engl J Med* 2001;344:1527–1535.

55. Poort SR, Rosendaal FR, Reitsma PH, et al. A common genetic variation in the 3-untranslated region of the prothrombin gene is associated with elevated plasma prothrombin levels and an increase in venous thrombosis. *Blood* 1996;88:3698–3703.

56. Hillarp A, Zoller B, Svensson PJ, Dahlback B. The 20210A of the prothrombin gene is a common risk factor among Swedish outpatients with verified deep venous thrombosis. *Thromb Haemost* 1997;78:990–992.

57. De Stefano V, Martinelli I, Mannucci PM, et al. The risk of recurrent deep venous thrombosis among heterozygous carriers of both factor V Leiden and the G20210A prothrombin mutation. *N Engl J Med* 1999;341:801–806.

58. D'Angelo A, Selhub J. Homocysteine and thrombotic disease. *Blood* 1997;90:1–11.

59. Ridker PM, Hennekens CH, Selhub J, et al. Interrelation of hyperhomocysteinemia, factor V Leiden, and risk of future venous thromboembolism. *Circulation* 1997;95:1777–1782.

60. Undas J, Brozek J, Szczeklik A. Homocysteine and thrombosis: from basic science to clinical evidence. *Thromb Haemost* 2005;94:907–915.

61. Kraaijenhagen RA, in't Anker PS, Koopman MM, et al. High plasma concentration of factor VIIIc is a major risk factor for venous thromboembolism. *Thromb Haemost* 2000;83:5–9.

62. Kyrle PA, Minar E, Hirschl M, et al. High plasma levels of factor VIII and the risk of recurrent thromboembolism. *N Engl J Med* 2000;343:457–462.

63. McIntrye KM, Sasahara AA. Hemodynamic and ventricular response to pulmonary embolism. *Prog Cardiovasc Dis* 1974;17:175–180.

64. McIntrye KM, Sasahara AA. The hemodynamic response to pulmonary embolism in patients without prior cardiopulmonary disease. *Am J Cardiol* 1971;17:288–294.

65. Elliott CG. Pulmonary physiology during pulmonary embolism. *Chest* 1992;101:163S–171S.

66. Azarian R, Wartski M, Collignon MA, et al. Lung perfusion scans and hemodynamics in acute and chronic pulmonary embolism. *J Nucl Med* 1997;38:980–983.

67. McIntyre KM, Sasahara AA. The ratio of pulmonary artery pressure to pulmonary vascular obstruction. *Chest* 1997;71:692.

68. Stein PD, Terrin ML, Hales CA, et al. Clinical, laboratory, roentgenographic, and electrocardiographic findings in patients with acute pulmonary embolism and no pre-existing cardiac or pulmonary disease. *Chest* 1991;100:598–603.

69. Stein PD, Henry JW. Clinical characteristics of patients with acute pulmonary embolism stratified according to their presenting syndromes. *Chest* 1997;112:974–979.

70. Wells PS, Anderson DR, Rodger M, et al. Derivation of a simple clinical model to categorize patients' probability of pulmonary embolism: increasing the models utility with the SimpliRED D-dimer. *Thromb Haemost* 2000;83:416–420.

71. Wicki J, Perneger TV, Junod AF, et al. Assessing clinical probability of pulmonary embolism in the emergency ward. *Arch Intern Med* 2001;161:92–97.

72. Le Gal G, Righini M, Roy P-M, et al. Prediction of pulmonary embolism in the emergency department: the revised Geneva Score. *Ann Intern Med* 2006;144:165–171.

73. Stein PD, Hull RD, Patel KC, et al. D-Dimer for the exclusion of acute venous thrombosis and pulmonary embolism: a systematic review. *Ann Intern Med* 2004;140:589–602.

74. Rowbotham BJ, Egerton-Vernon J, Whitaker AN, et al. Plasma cross-linked fibrin degradation products in pulmonary embolism. *Thorax* 1990;45:684–687.

75. McGinn S, White PD. Acute cor pulmonale resulting from pulmonary embolism. *JAMA* 1935;104:1473–1480.

76. Sokolow M, Katz LN, Muscovitz AN. The electrocardiogram in acute pulmonary embolism. *Am Heart J* 1940;19:166–184.

77. The Urokinase Pulmonary Embolism Trial. A national cooperative study. *Circulation* 1973;47(Suppl II):1–108.

78. Ferrari E, Imbert A, Chevalier T, et al. The ECG in pulmonary embolism. Predictive value of negative T waves in precordial leads: 80 case reports. *Chest* 1997;111:537–543.

79. Kucher N, Walpoth N, Wustmann K, et al. QR in V_1—an ECG sign associated with right ventricular dysfunction and adverse clinical outcome in pulmonary embolism. *Eur Heart J* 2003;24:1113–1119.

80. Geibel A, Zehender M, Kasper W, et al. Prognostic value of the ECG on admission in patients with acute pulmonary embolism. *Eur Respir J* 2005;25:843–848.

81. Elliott CG, Goldhaber SZ, Visani L, DeRosa M. Chest radiographs in acute pulmonary embolism. Results from the International Cooperative Pulmonary Embolism Registry. *Chest* 2000;118:33–38.

82. van Strijen MJ, de Monye W, Schiereck J, et al. Single-detector helical CT as the primary diagnostic test in suspected pulmonary embolism: a multicenter clinical management study of 510 patients. *Ann Intern Med* 2003;138:307–314.

83. Remy-Jardin M, Remy J. Spiral CT angiography of the pulmonary circulation. *Radiology* 1999;212:615–636.

84. Remy-Jardin M, Remy J, Wattinne L, Giraud F. Central pulmonary thromboembolism: diagnosis with spiral volumetric CT with the single-breath-hold technique: comparison with pulmonary angiography. *Radiology* 1992;185:381–387.

85. Remy-Jardin M, Remy J, Deschildre F, et al. Diagnosis of pulmonary embolism with spiral CT. Comparison with pulmonary angiography and scintigraphy. *Radiology* 1996;200:699–706.

86. Goodman LR, Curtin JJ, Mewissen MW, et al. Detection of pulmonary embolism in patients with unresolved clinical and scintigraphic diagnosis: helical CT versus angiography. *AJR Am J Roentgenol* 1995;164:1369–1374.

87. Teigen CL, Maus TP, Sheedy PF, et al. Pulmonary embolism: diagnosis with contrast-enhanced electron-beam CT and comparison with pulmonary angiography. *Radiology* 1995;194:313–319.

88. van Rossum AB, Pattynama PM, Treurniat FE, et al. Spiral CT angiography for detection of pulmonary embolism: validation in 124 patients. *Radiology* 1995;197(P):303.

89. van Rossum AB, Treurniat FE, Kieft GJ, et al. Role of spiral volumetric computed tomographic scanning in the assessment of patients with clinical suspi-

cion of pulmonary embolism and an abnormal ventilation perfusion scan. *Thorax* 1996;51:23–28.

90. Schoepf UJ, Holzknecht N, Helmberger TK, et al. Subsegmental pulmonary emboli: improved detection with thin-collimation multi-detector row spiral CT. *Radiology* 2002;222:483–490.

91. Schoepf UJ, Goldhaber SZ, Costello P. Spiral computed tomography for pulmonary embolism. *Circulation* 2004;109:2160–2167.

92. Perrier A, Roy PM, Sanchez O, et al. Multi-detector row computed tomography in acute pulmonary embolism. *N Engl J Med* 2005;352:1760–1768.

93. Quiroz R, Kucher N, Zou KH, et al. Clinical validity of a negative computed tomography scan in patients with suspected pulmonary embolism: a systematic review. *JAMA* 2005;293:2012–2017.

94. van Belle A, Buller HR, Huisman MV, et al. Effectiveness of managing suspected pulmonary embolism using an algorithm combining clinical probability, D-dimer testing, and computed tomography. *JAMA* 2006;295:172–179.

95. Stein PD, Fowler SE, Goodman LR, et al. Multidetector computed tomography for pulmonary embolism. *N Engl J Med* 2006;354:2317–2327.

96. The PIOPED Investigators. Value of the ventilation/perfusion scan in acute pulmonary embolism. Results of the prospective investigation of pulmonary embolism diagnosis. *JAMA* 1990;263:2753–2759.

97. Stein PD, Athanasoulis C, Alavi A, et al. Complications and validity of pulmonary angiography in acute pulmonary embolism. *Circulation* 1992;85:462–468.

98. Quinn MF, Lundell CJ, Klotz TA, et al. Reliability of selective pulmonary arteriography in the diagnosis of acute pulmonary embolism. *AJR Am J Roentgenol* 1987;149:469–471.

99. Meaney JFM, Weg JG, Chenevert TL, et al. Diagnosis of pulmonary embolism with magnetic resonance angiography. *N Engl J Med* 1997;336:1422–1427.

100. Tapson VF. Pulmonary embolism—new diagnostic approaches. *N Engl J Med* 1997;336:1449–1451.

101. Sostman HD, Layish DT, Tapson VF, et al. Prospective comparison of helical CT and MR imaging in clinically suspected acute pulmonary embolism. *J Magn Reson Imaging* 1996;6:275.

102. Oudkerk M, van Beek EJ, Wielopolski P, et al. Comparison of contrast-enhanced magnetic resonance angiography and conventional pulmonary angiography for the diagnosis of pulmonary embolism: a prospective study. *Lancet* 2002;359:1643–1647.

103. Goldhaber SZ. Echocardiography in the management of pulmonary embolism. *Ann Intern Med* 2002;136:691–700.

104. Miniati M, Monti S, Pratali L, et al. Value of transthoracic echocardiography in the diagnosis of pulmonary embolism: results of a prospective study in unselected patients. *Am J Med* 2001;110:528–535.

105. Grifoni S, Olivotto I, Cecchini P, et al. Short-term clinical outcome of patients with acute pulmonary embolism, normal blood pressure, and echocardiographic right ventricular dysfunction. *Circulation* 2000;101:2817–2822.

106. Ribeiro A, Lindmarker P, Johnsson H, et al. Pulmonary embolism: one-year follow-up with echocardiography Doppler and five-year survival analysis. *Circulation* 1999;99:1325–1330.

107. Konstantinides S, Geibel A, Heusel G, et al. Heparin plus alteplase compared with heparin alone in patients with submassive pulmonary embolism. *N Engl J Med* 2002;347:1143–1150.

108. Ricou F, Nicod PH, Moser KM, Peterson KL. Catheter-based intravascular ultrasound imaging of chronic thromboembolic pulmonary disease. *Am J Cardiol* 1991;67:749–752.

109. Konstantinides S, Geibel A, Kasper W, et al. Patent foramen ovale is an important predictor of adverse outcome in patients with major pulmonary embolism. *Circulation* 1998;97:1946.

110. Goldhaber SZ. Echocardiography in the management of pulmonary embolism. *Ann Intern Med* 2002;136:691–700.

111. Zierler BK. Ultrasonography and the diagnosis of venous thromboembolism. *Circulation* 2004;109:I-9–I-14.

112. Borgstede JP, Clagett GE. Types, frequency, and significance of alternative diagnoses found during duplex Doppler venous examinations of the lower extremities. *J Ultrasound Med* 1992;11:85–89.

113. Lensing AW, Levi MM, Buller HR, et al. Diagnosis of deep-vein thrombosis using an objective Doppler method. *Ann Intern Med* 1990;113:9–13.

114. White R, McGahan JP, Daschbach MM, Hartling MM. Diagnosis of deep-vein thrombosis using duplex ultrasound. *Ann Intern Med* 1989;111:297–304.

115. Cronan JJ, Leen V. Recurrent deep venous thrombosis: limitations of ultrasound. *Radiology* 1989;170:739–742.

116. Killewich LA, Bedford GR, Beach KW, Strandness DE. Diagnosis of deep venous thrombosis: a prospective study comparing duplex scanning to contrast venography. *Circulation* 1989;79:810–814.

117. Davidson BL, Elliott CG, Lensing AWA. Low accuracy of color Doppler ultrasound in the detection of proximal leg vein thrombosis in asymptomatic high-risk patients. *Ann Intern Med* 1992;117:735–738.

118. Mac Gillavry MR, Sanson BJ, Buller HR, Brandjes DP. Compression ultrasonography of the leg veins in patients with clinically suspected pulmonary embolism: is a more extensive assessment of compressibility useful? *Thromb Haemost* 2000;84:973–976.

119. Rabinov K, Paulin S. Roentgen diagnosis of venous thrombosis in the leg. *Arch Surg* 1972;104:134.

120. Fraser DG, Moody AR, Morgan PS, et al. Diagnosis of lower-limb deep venous thrombosis: a prospective blinded study of magnetic resonance direct thrombus imaging. *Ann Intern Med* 2002;136:89–98.

121. Evans AJ, Tapson VF, Sostman HD, et al. The diagnosis of deep venous thrombosis: a prospective comparison of venography and magnetic resonance imaging. *Chest* 1992;102:120S.

122. Witty LA, Tapson VF, Evans AJ, et al. MRI versus ultrasound: a radiologic and clinical evaluation of DVT. *Am Rev Respir Dis* 1993;147: A998.

123. Burke B, Sostman HD, Carroll BA, Witty LA. The diagnostic approach to deep venous thrombosis: which technique? *Clin Chest Med* 1995;16:253–268.

124. Roy P-M, Colombet I, Durieux P, et al. Systematic review and meta-analysis of strategies for the diagnosis of suspected pulmonary embolism. *BMJ* 2005;331:259–268.

125. Musset D, Parent F, Meyer G, et al. Diagnostic strategy for patients with suspected pulmonary embolism: a prospective multicentre outcome study. *Lancet* 2002;360:1914–1920.

126. Tepel M, Aspelin P, Lameire N. Contrast-induced nephropathy: a clinical and evidence-based approach. *Circulation* 2006;113:1799–1806.

127. Schrader R. Contrast-material induced renal failure: an overview. *J Interv Cardiol* 2005;18:427–433.

128. Hurwitz LM, Yoshizumi T, Reiman RE, et al. Radiation dose to the fetus from body MDCT during gestation. *AJR Am J Roentgenol* 2006;186:871–876.

129. Collins R, Scrimgeour A, Yusuf S, Peto R. Reduction in fatal pulmonary embolism and venous thrombosis by perioperative administration of subcutaneous heparin. *N Engl J Med* 1988;318:1162–1173.

130. Anderson FA Jr, Brownell W, Goldberg RJ, et al. Physician practices in the prevention of venous thromboembolism. *Ann Intern Med* 1991;115:591–595.

131. Bratzler DW, Raskob GE, Murray CK, et al. Underuse of venous thromboembolism prophylaxis for general surgery patients: physician practices in the community hospital setting. *Arch Intern Med* 1998;158:1909–1912.

132. Leonardi MJ, McGory ML, Ko CY. The rate of bleeding complications after pharmacologic deep venous thrombosis prophylaxis. A systematic review of 33 randomized trials. *Arch Surg* 2006;141:790–799.

133. Prevention of fatal postoperative pulmonary embolism by low doses of heparin. An international multicentre trial. *Lancet* 1975;2:45–51.

134. Collins R, Scrimgeour A, Yusuf S, Peto R. Reduction in fatal pulmonary embolism and venous thrombosis by perioperative administration of subcutaneous heparin: overview of results of randomized trials in general, orthopedic, and urologic surgery. *N Engl J Med* 1988;318:1162.

135. Lassen MR, Bauer KA, Eriksson BI, Turpie AG. Postoperative fondaparinux versus preoperative enoxaparin for prevention of venous thromboembolism in elective hip-replacement surgery: a randomised double-blind comparison. *Lancet* 2002;359:1715–1720.

136. Bounameaux H, Perneger T. Fondaparinux: a new synthetic pentasaccharide for thrombosis prevention. *Lancet* 2002;359:1710–1711.

137. Colwell CW, Collis DK, Paulson R, et al. Comparison of enoxaparin and warfarin for the prevention of venous thromboembolic disease after total hip arthroplasty. Evaluation during hospitalization and three months after discharge. *J Bone Joint Surg Am* 1999;81-A:932.

138. Antithrombotic Trialists' Collaboration. Collaborative meta-analysis of randomised trials of antiplatelet therapy for prevention of death, myocardial infarction, and stroke in high-risk patients. *BMJ* 2002;324:71–86.

139. Tapson VF, Hull R. Management of venous thromboembolic disease: the impact of low-molecular-weight heparin. *Clin Chest Med* 1994;16:281–294.

140. Samama MM, Cohen AT, Darmon JY, et al. A comparison of enoxaparin with placebo for the prevention of venous thromboembolism in acutely ill medical patients. *N Engl J Med* 1999;341:793–800.

141. Leizorovicz A, Cohen AT, Turpie AG, et al. Randomized, placebo-controlled trial of dalteparin for the prevention of venous thromboembolism in acutely ill medical patients. *Circulation* 2004;110:874–879.

142. Cohen AT, Davidson BL, Gallus AS, et al. Efficacy and safety of fondaparinux for the prevention of venous thromboembolism in older acute medical patients: randomized placebo controlled trial. *BMJ* 2006;332:325–329.

143. Colditz GA, Tuden RL, Oster G. Rates of venous thrombosis after general surgery: combined results of randomised clinical trials. *Lancet* 1986;2:143.

144. Guidelines on diagnosis and management of acute pulmonary embolism. Task Force on Pulmonary Embolism, European Society of Cardiology. *Eur Heart J* 2000;21:1301–1336.

145. Janata K, Holzer M, Laggner AN, et al. Cardiac troponin T in the severity assessment of patients with pulmonary embolism: cohort study. *BMJ* 2003;326:312–313.

146. ten Wolde M, Tulevski II, Mulder JW, et al. Brain natriuretic peptide as a predictor of adverse outcome in patients with pulmonary embolism. *Circulation* 2003;107:2082–2084.

147. Kucher N, Printzen G, Goldhaber SZ. Prognostic role of brain natriuretic hormone in acute pulmonary embolism. *Circulation* 2003;107:2545–2547.

148. Hull RD, Raskob GE, Hirsh J, et al. Continuous intravenous heparin compared with intermittent subcutaneous heparin in the initial treatment of proximal vein thrombosis. *N Engl J Med* 1986;315:1109–1114.

149. Hull R, Raskob G, Rosenbloom D, et al. Optimal therapeutic level of heparin therapy in patients with venous thrombosis. *Arch Intern Med* 1992;152:1589–1595.

150. Raschke RA, Reilly BM, Guidry JR, et al. The weight-based heparin dosing nomogram compared with a "standard care" nomogram. *Ann Intern Med* 1993;119:874.

151. Hyers TM, Agnelli G, Hull RD, et al. Antithrombotic therapy for venous thromboembolic disease. *Chest* 1998;114:561S–578S.

152. Lagerstedt CI, Olsson C-G, Fagher BO, Oqvist BW. Need for long-term anticoagulant treatment in symptomatic calf-vein thrombosis. *Lancet* 1985;2:515–518.

153. Moser KM, Le Moine JR. Is embolic risk conditioned by location of deep venous thrombosis? *Ann Intern Med* 1981;94:439–444.

154. Kearon C, Ginsberg JS, Julian JA, et al. Comparison of fixed-dose weight-adjusted unfractionated heparin and low-molecular-weight heparin for acute treatment of venous thromboembolism. *JAMA* 2006;296:935–942.

155. Prandoni P, Polistena P, Bernardi E, et al. Upper extremity deep vein thrombosis. *Arch Intern Med* 1997;157:57–62.

156. Randolph AG, Cook DJ, Gonzalez CA, et al. Benefit of heparin in central venous and pulmonary artery catheters: a meta-analysis of randomized controlled trials. *Chest* 1998;113:165–171.

157. Klerk CP, Smorenburg SM, Buller HR. Thrombosis prophylaxis in patient populations with a central venous catheter: a systematic review. *Arch Intern Med* 2003;163:1913–1921.

158. Hicken GJ, Ameli FM. Management of subclavian-axillary vein thrombosis: a review. *Can J Surg* 1998;41:13–25.

159. Levine M, Gent M, Hirsh J, et al. A comparison of low-molecular-weight heparin administered primarily at home with unfractionated heparin administered in the hospital for proximal deep vein thrombosis. *N Engl J Med* 1996;334:677–681.

160. Koopman MM, Prandoni P, Piovella F, et al. Low-molecular-weight heparin versus heparin for proximal deep vein thrombosis. *N Engl J Med* 1996;334:682–687.

161. A Collaborative European Multicentre Study. A randomized trial of subcutaneous low-molecular-weight heparin (CY216) compared with intravenous unfractionated heparin in the treatment of deep vein thrombosis. *Thromb Haemost* 1991;65:251–256.

162. Hull RD, Raskob GE, Pineo GF, et al. Subcutaneous low-molecular-weight heparin compared with continuous intravenous heparin in the treatment of proximal-vein thrombosis. *N Engl J Med* 1992;326:975–983.

163. Prandoni P, Lensing AWA, Buller HR, et al. Comparison of subcutaneous low-molecular-weight heparin with intravenous standard heparin in proximal deep vein thrombosis. *Lancet* 1992;339:441–445.

164. Simonneau G, Charbonnier B, Decousus H, et al. Subcutaneous low-molecular-weight heparin compared with continuous intravenous unfractionated heparin in the treatment of proximal deep vein thrombosis. *Arch Intern Med* 1993;153:1541–1546.

165. Lindmarker P, Holmstrom M, Granqvist S, et al. Fragmin once daily subcutaneously in a fixed dose compared with continuous intravenous unfractionated heparin in the treatment of deep venous thrombosis. *Thromb Haemost* 1993;69:648.

166. Duplaga BA, Rivers CW, Nutescu E, et al. Dosing and monitoring of low molecular weight heparins in special populations. *Pharmacotherapy* 2001;21:218–234.

167. Lensing AWA, Prins MH, Davidson BL, Hirsh J. Treatment of deep venous thrombosis with low-molecular-weight heparins: a meta-analysis. *Arch Intern Med* 1995;155:601–607.

168. Leizorovicz A, Simonneau G, Decousus H, Boissel JP. Comparison of efficacy and safety of low molecular weight heparins and unfractionated heparin in initial treatment of deep venous thrombosis. *BMJ* 1994;309:299–304.

169. O'Brien B, Levine M, Willan A, et al. Economic evaluation of outpatient treatment with low-molecular-weight heparin for proximal vein thrombosis. *Arch Intern Med* 1999;159:2298–2304.

170. Simonneau G, Sors H, Charbonnier B, et al. A comparison of low-molecular-weight heparin with unfractionated heparin for acute pulmonary embolism. *N Engl J Med* 1997;337:663.

171. Beckman JA, Dunn K, Sasahara AA, Goldhaber SZ. Enoxaparin monotherapy without oral anticoagulation to treat acute symptomatic pulmonary embolism. *Thromb Haemost* 2003;89:953–958.

172. Greinacher A, Warkentin TE. Recognition, treatment, and prevention of heparin-induced thrombocytopenia: review and update. *Thromb Res* 2006;118:165–176.

173. Amiral J, Bridey F, Dreyfus M, et al. Platelet factor 4 complexed to heparin is the target for antibodies generated in heparin-induced thrombocytopenia. *Thromb Haemost* 1992;68:95–96.

174. Visentin GP, Ford SE, Scott JP, Aster RH. Antibodies from patients with heparin-induced thrombocytopenia/thrombosis are specific for platelet factor 4 complexed with heparin or bound to endothelial cells. *J Clin Invest* 1994;93:81–88.

175. Warkentin TE, Levine MN, Hirsh J, et al. Heparin-induced thrombocytopenia in patients treated with low-molecular-weight heparin or unfractionated heparin. *N Engl J Med* 1995;332:1330–1335.

176. Kovacs MJ, Rodger M, Anderson DR, et al. Comparison of 10-mg and 5-mg warfarin initiation nomograms together with low-molecular-weight heparin for outpatient treatment of acute venous thromboembolism: a randomized, double-blind, controlled study. *Ann Intern Med* 2003;138:714–719.

177. Joffe HV, Goldhaber SZ. Effectiveness and safety of long-term anticoagulation of patients ≥ 90 years of age with atrial fibrillation. *Am J Cardiol* 2002;90:1397–1398.

178. Higashi MK, Veenstra DL, Kondo LM, et al. Association between CYP2C9 genetic variants and anticoagulation-related outcomes during warfarin therapy. *JAMA* 2002;287:1690–1698.

179. Sawicki PT. A structured teaching and self-management program for patients receiving oral anticoagulation. *JAMA* 1999;281:145.

180. Oden A, Fahlen M. Oral anticoagulation and risk of death: a medical record linkage study. *BMJ* 2002;325:1073–1075.

181. White RH, Beyth RJ, Zhou H, Romano PS. Major bleeding after hospitalization for deep-venous thrombosis. *Am J Med* 1999;107:414–424.

182. Egred M, Rodrigues E. Purple digit syndrome and warfarin-induced skin necrosis. *Eur J Intern Med* 2005;15:294–295.

183. Toglia M, Weg JG. Venous thromboembolism during pregnancy. *N Engl J Med* 1996;335:108.

184. Eichinger S, Weltermann A, Minar E, et al. Symptomatic pulmonary embolism and the risk of recurrent venous thromboembolism. *Arch Intern Med* 2004;164:92–96.

185. Greenfield LJ. Vena caval interruption and pulmonary embolectomy. *Clin Chest Med* 1984;5:495–505.

186. White RH, Zhou H, Kim J, Romano PS. A population-based study of the effectiveness of inferior vena cava filter use among patients with venous thromboembolism. *Arch Intern Med* 2000;160:2033–2041.

187. Decousus H, Leizorovicz A, Parent F, et al. A clinical trial of vena caval filters in the prevention of pulmonary embolism in patients with proximal deep-vein thrombosis. *N Engl J Med* 1998;338:409–415.

188. The PREPIC Study Group. Eight-year follow-up of patients with permanent vena cava filters in the prevention of pulmonary embolism. *Circulation* 2005;112:416–422.

189. Dentali F, Ageno W, Imberti D. Retrievable vena caval filters: clinical experience. *Curr Opin Pulm Med* 2006;12:304–309.

190. Rosenthal D, Wellons ED, Levitt AB, et al. Role of prophylactic temporary vena cava filters placed at the ICU bedside under intravascular ultrasound guidance in patients with multiple trauma. *J Vasc Surg* 2004;40:958–964.

191. Agnelli G, Becattini C, Kirschstein T. Thrombolysis vs. heparin in the treatment of pulmonary embolism: a clinical outcome-based meta-analysis. *Arch Intern Med* 2002;162:2537–2541.

192. Dalen JE. The uncertain role of thrombolytic therapy in the treatment of pulmonary embolism. *Arch Intern Med* 2002:162:2521–2523.

193. Dalen JE, Alpert JS, Hirsh J. Thrombolytic therapy for pulmonary embolism. Is it effective? Is if safe? When is it indicated? *Arch Intern Med* 1997;157:2550–2556.

194. Marini C, Di Ricco G, Rossi G, et al. Fibrinolytic effects of urokinase and heparin in acute pulmonary embolism: a randomized clinical trial. *Respiration* 1988;54:162–173.

195. Levine M, Hirsh J, Weitz J, et al. A randomized trial of a single bolus dosage regimen of recombinant tissue plasminogen activator in patients with acute pulmonary embolism. *Chest* 1990;98:1473–1479.

196. Jerjes-Sanchez C, Ramirez-Rivera A, de Lourdes Garcia M, et al. Streptokinase and heparin versus heparin alone in massive pulmonary embolism: a randomized controlled trial. *J Thromb Thrombolysis* 1995;2:227–229.

197. Dalla-Volta S, Palla A, Santolicandro A, et al. PAIMS 2: Alteplase combined with heparin versus heparin in the treatment of acute pulmonary embolism. Plasminogen activator Italian multicenter study 2. *J Am Coll Cardiol* 1992;20:520–526.

198. Goldhaber SZ, Haire WD, Feldstein ML, et al. Alteplase versus heparin in acute pulmonary embolism: randomised trial assessing right-ventricular function and pulmonary perfusion. *Lancet* 1993;341:507–511.

199. Tibbutt DA, Davies JA, Anderson JA, et al. Comparison by controlled clinical trial of streptokinase and heparin in treatment of life-threatening pulmonary embolism. *Br Med J* 1974;1:343–347.

200. Ly B, Arnesen H, Eie H, et al. A controlled clinical trial of streptokinase and heparin in the treatment of major pulmonary embolism. *Acta Med Scand* 1978;203:465–470.

201. Kanter DS, Mikkola KM, Patel SR, et al. Thrombolytic therapy for pulmonary embolism. Frequency of intracranial hemorrhage and associated risk factors. *Chest* 1997;111:1241.

202. Rogers LQ, Lutcher CL. Streptokinase therapy for deep vein thrombosis: a comprehensive review of the literature. *Am J Med* 1990;88:389–395.

203. Leeper KV Jr, Popovich J Jr, Lesser BA, et al. Treatment of massive acute pulmonary embolism. The use of low doses of intrapulmonary arterial streptokinase combined with full doses of systemic heparin. *Chest* 1988;93:234–240.

204. The UKEP study. Multicentre clinical trial on two local regimens of urokinase in massive pulmonary embolism. *Eur Heart J* 1987;8:2–10.

205. Verstraete M, Miller GAH, Bounameaux H, et al. Intravenous and intrapulmonary recombinant tissue-type plasminogen activator in the treatment of acute massive pulmonary embolism. *Circulation* 1988;77:353–360.

206. Tapson VF, Witty LA. Massive pulmonary embolism: diagnostic and therapeutic strategies. *Clin Chest Med* 1996;16:329.

207. Jardin F, Genevray B, Brunney D, Margairaz A. Dobutamine: a hemodynamic evaluation in pulmonary embolism shock. *Crit Care Med* 1985;13:1009–1012.

208. Manier G, Castaing Y. Influence of cardiac output on oxygen exchange in acute pulmonary embolism. *Am Rev Respir Dis* 1992;145:130–136.

209. Hoeper M, Mayer E, Simonneau G, Rubin LJ. Chronic thromboembolic pulmonary hypertension. *Circulation* 2006;113:2011–2020.

210. Fedullo PF, Auger WR, Kerr KM, Rubin LJ. Chronic thromboembolic pulmonary hypertension. *N Engl J Med* 2001;345:1465–1472.

211. Pengo V, Lensing AWA, Prins MH, et al. Incidence of chronic thromboembolic pulmonary hypertension after pulmonary embolism. *N Engl J Med* 2004;2257–2264.

212. Miniati M, Monti S, Bottai S, et al. Survival and restoration of pulmonary perfusion in a long-term follow-up of patients after acute pulmonary embolism. *Medicine (Baltimore)* 2006;85:253–262.

213. Becattini C, Agnelli G, Pesavento R, et al. Incidence of chronic thromboembolic pulmonary hypertension after a first episode of pulmonary embolism. *Chest* 2006;130:172–175.

214. Lang I, Kerr K. Risk factors for chronic thromboembolic pulmonary hypertension. *Proc Am Thorac Soc* 2006;3:568–570.

215. Bailey CL, Channick RN, Auger WR, et al. "High probability" perfusion scan in pulmonary venoocclusive disease. *Am J Resp Crit Care Med* 2000;162:1974–1978.

216. Heinrich M, Uder M, Tscholl D, et al. CT scan findings in chronic thromboembolic pulmonary hypertension. Predictors of hemodynamic improvement after pulmonary thromboendarterectomy. *Chest* 2005;127:1606–1613.

217. Ribeiro A, Lindmarker P, Johnsson H, et al. Pulmonary embolism. One-year follow-up with echocardiography Doppler and five-year survival analysis. *Circulation* 1999;99:1325–1330.

218. Jamieson SW, Kapelanski DP, Sakakibara N, et al. Pulmonary endarterectomy: experience and lessons learned in 1,500 cases. *Ann Thorac Surg* 2003;76:1457–1464.

219. Fedullo PF, Auger WR, Kerr KM, Kim NH. Chronic thromboembolic pulmonary hypertension. *Semin Respir Crit Care Med* 2003;24:273–286.

220. Bresser P, Pepke-Zaba J, Jais X, et al. Medical therapies for chronic thromboembolic pulmonary hypertension. An evolving treatment paradigm. *Proc Am Thorac Soc* 2006;3:594–600.

CHAPTER (73)

Chronic Cor Pulmonale

E. Clinton Lawrence / Kenneth L. Brigham

DEFINITION

The term *pulmonary heart disease* (i.e., cor pulmonale) refers to cardiac dysfunction resulting from altered structure or function of the lungs. Because the lungs are interposed in the cardiovascular circuit between the right ventricle and left side of the heart, alterations in lung structure or function will selectively affect the right side of the heart.

Cor pulmonale has been variably defined. Some definitions provide a useful classification of disease for clinicians, whereas others are based more on alterations in organ structure and function. The best general definition of the term *cor pulmonale* remains the one articulated in 1963 by an expert committee appointed by the director general of the World Health Organization (WHO): *chronic cor pulmonale* is "hypertrophy of the right ventricle resulting from diseases affecting the function and/or structure of the lung, except when these pulmonary alterations are the result of diseases that primarily affect the left side of the heart or congenital heart disease."[1]

Acute dilatation of the right ventricle of the heart, that is, acute cor pulmonale, is a disorder in which the right ventricle is dilated and the muscular wall is stretched thin. This is most often the result of massive pulmonary embolism as described in Chap. 72. The chronic form of the disorder, the principal subject of this chapter, is characterized by right ventricular (RV) hypertrophy with eventual dilatation and right side of the heart failure.

The right ventricle is ill suited to excessive mechanical demands, being adapted to pump blood through the normally low-resistance, high-capacitance lung circulatory bed. R.T.H. Laennec, in his *Treatise on Diseases of the Chest* published early in the 19th century, gives an elegant description of the gross anatomy of cardiac dilatation and hypertrophy, including findings limited to the right ventricle (in fact, his tour de force elegantly describes the gross pathology of virtually every lung disease).[2]

The final common pathophysiologic event that causes chronic cor pulmonale is chronically increased resistance to blood flow through the pulmonary circulation leading to pulmonary arterial hypertension (PAH; see Chap. 71). Unlike systemic hypertension, PAH is difficult to diagnose clinically so that pulmonary vascular pressures may be elevated for prolonged periods before the disorder is recognized. In fact, dysfunction of the right ventricle (i.e., cor pulmonale) is often recognized as the initial clinical diagnosis in patients with either primary or secondary PAH. Newer noninvasive techniques can provide more information about pulmonary circulatory function than in the past. However, suspecting PAH early in its course still depends largely on the skill of the experienced clinician.

Although lung disorders that cause chronic cor pulmonale can be classified in many ways, this chapter uses a classification that is based on the mechanism by which the disorder increases pulmonary vascular resistance.

INCIDENCE

Estimates of the incidence of chronic cor pulmonale, as well as estimates of morbidity and even mortality directly attributable to right-heart dysfunction secondary to lung disease, are difficult to obtain. It is difficult to separate epidemiologic data relevant to cor pulmonale from the lung disease that is its primary cause. In addition, a definitive diagnosis most often requires invasive diagnostic procedures, often at a time when treating the lung disease is the most paramount clinical issue. However, the magnitude of the clinical problem can be appreciated from data on chronic obstructive pulmonary disease (COPD), undoubtedly the most common cause of cor pulmonale.

The estimated total prevalence of COPD in the world is currently 400 million individuals. In 1999, there were 713,000 hospital discharges with a diagnosis of COPD in the United States, a discharge rate of 25.9 per 10,000 population. In the United States, there were 123,550 deaths caused by COPD in the year 2000.[3] According to a WHO report, COPD accounted for 4.8 percent of all deaths in the United States in 1998. Worldwide, the problem is even more dramatic. WHO estimates that COPD accounted for 4.73 percent of all deaths in member nations (Table 73–1). Thus, for every 100,000 people in the world, 43 died of COPD in 2001.[3]

WHO estimates that up to 14 percent of patients with COPD suffer from secondary PAH, whereas RV dysfunction has been found in up to 66 percent of patients with end-stage lung disease referred for lung transplantation evaluation.[3,4] However, the incidence of severe pulmonary hypertension in COPD is 5 percent or less.[5,6] The fraction of patients with right side of the heart dysfunction resulting from secondary PAH is unknown. A study from the United Kingdom estimates that 0.3 percent of the population had both an arterial oxygen tension less than 55 mmHg and clear evidence of airways obstruction by pulmonary function testing.[7]

These data would predict 60,000 subjects in England and Wales at serious risk for secondary PAH.[7] Again, the number of these subjects who had cor pulmonale cannot be determined.

It is clear from the available epidemiologic data that diseases predisposing to cor pulmonale are an enormous health problem throughout the world. Undoubtedly cor pulmonale is a major contributor to the morbidity and mortality in these diseases.

ETIOLOGIES

Diseases that affect lung structure and function can increase pulmonary vascular resistance either directly or indirectly through effects on the lungs' gas exchange function. Any cause of persistent PAH of sufficient magnitude and duration can cause cor pulmonale.

PAH is discussed in detail in Chap. 71. However, an understanding of where the causes of PAH fit in a pathophysiologic schema that relates lung dysfunction to dysfunction of the RV is essential for understanding cor pulmonale. Table 73–2 presents a pathophysiologic classification of potential causes of chronic cor pulmonale.

A classification of this sort is somewhat arbitrary. In fact, there is enormous overlap in mechanisms in virtually all of the diseases listed in Table 73–2. It is probably more accurate to consider the various basic mechanisms as interacting, with the eventual outcome of a remodeling of the pulmonary vascular bed, resulting in a largely irreversible increase in pulmonary vascular resistance. Fig. 73–1 illustrates this concept.

PATHOPHYSIOLOGY OF INCREASED PULMONARY VASCULAR RESISTANCE

【 】 PERSISTENT PULMONARY VASOCONSTRICTION

The lung has the daunting task of removing carbon dioxide from and reoxygenating all of the blood destined for the systemic circulation. For the lung to perform its principal function of gas exchange efficiently, it must not only maintain the integrity of the vast gas exchange surface that brings blood into intimate contact with air, but must match the amount of blood perfusing with the amount of air ventilating each gas exchange unit. This matching of ventilation and

TABLE 73–1

Worldwide Mortality Attributable to Chronic Obstructive Pulmonary Disease (COPD)

WHO REGION	TOTAL POPULATION	TOTAL DEATHS	COPD DEATHS	COPD PERCENT OF TOTAL DEATHS	DEATHS PER 100,000
Africa	655,476,000	10,680,871	116,045	1.09	17.7
The Americas	837,967,000	5,910,811	221,682	3.75	26.5
Eastern Mediterranean	493,091,000	4,156,667	88,318	2.12	17.9
Europe	874,178,000	9,702,763	284,581	2.93	32.6
Southeast Asia	1,559,810,000	14,466,690	614,555	4.25	39.4
Western Pacific	1,701,689,000	11,636,373	1,347,093	11.58	79.2
Total	6,122,211,000	56,554,175	2,672,274	4.73	43.6

SOURCE: World Health Organization. Consultation on the Development of a Comprehensive Approach for the Prevention and Control of Chronic Respiratory Diseases.[3]

TABLE 73–2

Pathophysiologic Classification of Diseases of the Lungs That Can Cause Cor Pulmonale

PRINCIPAL PATHOPHYSIOLOGIC MECHANISM	DISEASE ENTITY
Persistent vasoconstriction	• High-altitude dwellers • Hypoventilation syndromes • Chest deformities • ? Idiopathic pulmonary hypertension
Loss of cross-sectional area of the vascular bed	• Thromboembolic disease • Emphysema • Lung resection • Fibrotic lung diseases • Cystic fibrosis
Obstruction of large vessels	• Extrinsic compression of pulmonary veins • Fibrosing mediastinitis • Adenopathy/tumors • Pulmonary venoocclusive disease
Chronically increased blood flow	• Eisenmenger syndrome
Vascular remodeling	• Primary pulmonary hypertension • Secondary pulmonary hypertension • Collagen vascular diseases • Cystic fibrosis

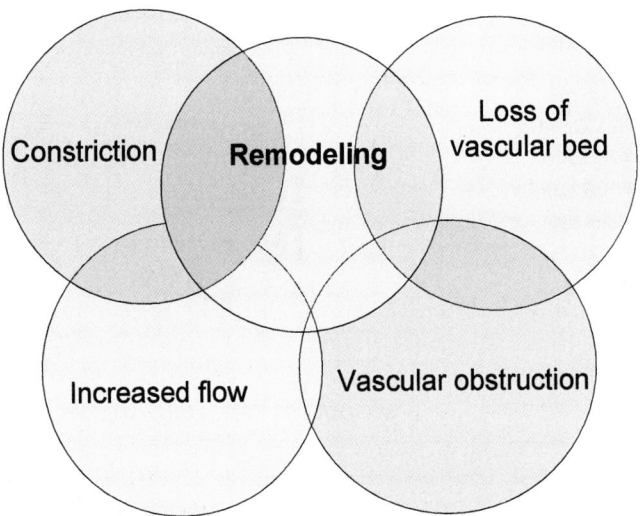

FIGURE 73–1. Interactions among pathophysiologic mechanisms of pulmonary hypertension.

perfusion is accomplished primarily by the unique property of pulmonary vessels to constrict when exposed to a hypoxic environment (systemic vessels dilate in response to hypoxia). The mechanism responsible for transducing hypoxic pulmonary vasoconstriction remains unclear but may involve local generation of reactive oxygen species that affect smooth muscle ion channels.[8] Because laminar flow of blood through tubes is governed by the Poiseuille law (i.e., resistance to flow is inversely proportional to vessel radius to the fourth power), this is a very sensitive mechanism. Small changes in resistance vessel diameter can have major effects on perfusion.

Viewed teleologically, hypoxic pulmonary vasoconstriction must be a local phenomenon. To optimize gas exchange, blood flow needs to be selectively reduced to areas of lung that are poorly ventilated (and thus hypoxic). Because the normal pulmonary vascular bed has a very large capacitance and a reserve of capacity to exchange carbon dioxide and oxygen, blood shunted away from poorly ventilated areas will be shunted to well-ventilated areas and thus contribute arterialized blood to the systemic blood supply with essentially no increase in overall pul-

monary vascular resistance in the normal lung. The diagram in Fig. 73–2 illustrates this phenomenon.[9]

But what if all (or a very large fraction) of the lung is hypoxic? In that case, there will be global constriction of the resistance vessels in the lung circulation with an obligatory increase in pulmonary vascular resistance and PAH. The purest clinical example of this is the persistent PAH (and cor pulmonale) that develops in people who are living at a high enough altitude so that ambient air is deficient in oxygen because of the low barometric pressure.[10] Alveolar hypoventilation resulting either from decreased central ventilatory drive or from physical distortions of the lung relative to the ventilatory apparatus because of deformities of the chest can also result in hypoxia. If hypoxia is sufficiently extensive, the normal hypoxic vasoconstrictive response will result in PAH. That chronic hypoventilation can result in cor pulmonale is graphically illustrated in drawings of the "fat boy" in Charles Dickens' *Pickwick Papers,* who is generally said to have suffered from obesity-hypoventilation (thus pickwickian) syndrome. The peripheral edema characteristic of right side of the heart failure is evident in both Dickens' elegant description and in the classic illustration.[11] The current epidemic of obesity in the United States makes recog-

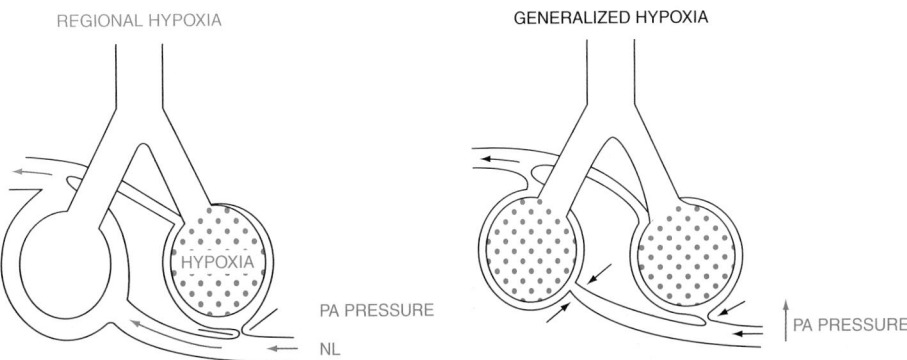

FIGURE 73–2. Illustration of the pulmonary hemodynamic consequences of alveolar hypoxia. Local hypoxia causes local vasoconstriction, matching perfusion to alveolar ventilation. Generalized hypoxia causes global vasoconstriction resulting in pulmonary hypertension. NL, normal lung. *Source: Reproduced with permission from Brigham KL, Newman JH. The pulmonary circulation.[9]*

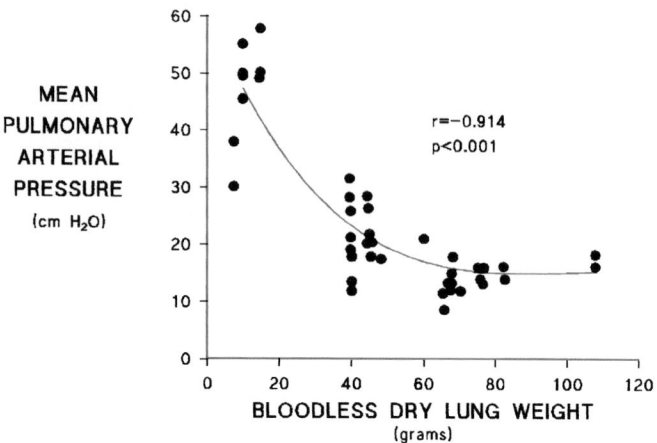

FIGURE 73–3. Effects of resecting progressively more lung tissue on pulmonary artery pressure in anesthetized sheep. About half of the lung tissue can be removed before pulmonary artery pressure rises at rest. When sufficient tissue has been removed to cause pressure to increase, pulmonary artery pressure becomes a steep function of the amount of lung tissue perfused. *Source: Reproduced with permission from Snapper JR, Harris, TR, Brigham, KL. Effect of changing lung mass on lung water and permeability-surface area in sheep. J Appl Physiol 1982;52:1591–1597.*

nition of this entity especially important and may well result in an increasing incidence of the syndrome.[12]

[ ] LOSS OF CROSS-SECTIONAL AREA OF THE PULMONARY VASCULAR BED

Resistance to blood flow through the pulmonary vasculature depends on the radius of individual resistance vessels and on the total cross-sectional area of the vascular bed. If the area of the vascular bed is sufficiently decreased, then PAH will develop.

Although it is clear that resistance to flow should increase if the total amount of vascular bed is decreased, the relationship for the lungs is not linear, at least in situations where the remaining lung vessels are intrinsically normal. The large capacitance of the normal lung vascular bed allows large reductions in the amount of the bed that is perfused without an increase in resistance. The clearest example of the direct effects of reducing the size of the vascular bed is with lung resection. Fig. 73–3 is from a group of studies in animals in which careful measurements of pulmonary hemodynamics were made with the lungs intact and following resection of different amounts of lung tissue.[13] The total lung mass could be decreased by half before there was any increase in pulmonary artery pressure. That observation is consistent with clinical experience with lung resection in humans. If the unresected lung is essentially normal, a total pneumonectomy does not result in PAH at rest. Once the capacitance of the pulmonary vascular bed is exceeded, there is a steep relation between pulmonary artery pressure and the amount of vascular bed. Following pneumonectomy in humans, PAH on exercise may occur because of increased pulmonary blood flow in a vascular bed with little remaining capacitance.[14]

In the most common clinical settings in which there is loss of lung vessels, the remaining perfused vessels are either functionally or structurally abnormal. For example, destruction of lung parenchyma with COPD reduces the area of the vascular bed, but there may be vasoconstriction in the perfused bed as a result of an ab-

normal ventilatory pattern. Pulmonary emboli directly obstruct lung vessels, but even patent vessels may be constricted because of release of humoral mediators. In addition, chronic pulmonary embolic disease can result in structural remodeling of the pulmonary vascular bed with irreversible PAH and cor pulmonale.[15]

Pulmonary artery pressure in patients with COPD increases with exercise even though resting pulmonary artery pressure may be normal. Fig. 73–4 shows data from studies in patients with COPD and a range of resting pulmonary artery pressures.[16] Pressure during exercise was a steep function of resting pressure, although exercise increased pressure even in subjects with normal resting pressures indicating loss of pulmonary vascular capacitance. In the compromised vascular bed, hemodynamic reserve is lost so that physiologic changes such as local hypoxic vasoconstriction or increased pulmonary blood flow, which are easily accommodated in the normal lung circulation, result in increased afterload to the right ventricle, the proximate cause of cor pulmonale.

[ ] OBSTRUCTION OF LARGE PULMONARY VESSELS

The most common cause of acute cor pulmonale is occlusion of the large proximal pulmonary artery by a massive embolus. However, large pulmonary vessels may also be compromised more insidiously by disorders of the mediastinum.

Direct compression of either pulmonary arteries or veins can result from enlarging mediastinal lymph nodes or mediastinal tumors. In addition, the rare but devastating disorder, fibrosing mediastinitis, can enmesh large pulmonary arteries or veins (or bronchi) in an inexorably advancing mass of connective tissue with progressive occlusion.[17] Occlusion of the main pulmonary artery imposes a direct resistance against which the right ventricle must pump, analogous physiologically to stenosis of the pulmonary valve or hypertrophic stenosis of the pulmonary outflow tract of the right ventricle. If progression of the obstruction is sufficiently slow, chronic cor pulmonale can be a principal clinical pic-

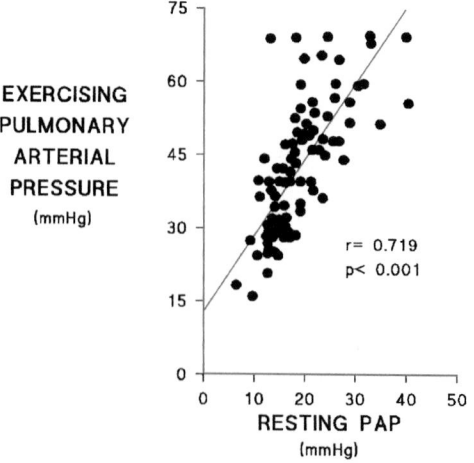

FIGURE 73–4. Pulmonary artery pressures at rest and exercise in a group of patients with chronic obstructive pulmonary disease and a wide range of resting pressures. In this group of subjects, pulmonary artery pressure (PAP) during exercise was a steep function of resting pressure. *Source: Reproduced with permission from Weitzenblum E. Chronic cor pulmonale. BMJ 2003;89:225–230.*

ture in the presence of normal lungs. Obstruction of pulmonary veins will also elevate overall pulmonary vascular resistance, but in this case the lung microvasculature will bear the brunt of the pressure increase. The consequences for the pulmonary circulation and the right side of the heart are analogous to those of either the left side of the heart failure or mitral valve stenosis. Depending on the chronicity and pace of the obstruction, cor pulmonale may result.

CHRONICALLY INCREASED PULMONARY BLOOD FLOW

Although the definition of cor pulmonale given earlier excludes congenital heart disease, chronically increased flow through the pulmonary circulation results in functional and structural alterations in the pulmonary vascular bed, and these changes in the lung come to dominate the pathophysiology. This clinical situation develops most often as a result of an abnormal shunting of blood from the left side of the circulation back to the right side, bypassing the systemic circulation (e.g., septal defects). In order to maintain blood supply to systemic organs, the right side of the heart must pump a larger volume of blood per unit time (the shunted blood in addition to the systemic venous return).

Increased flow through pulmonary vessels causes remodeling of the lung circulation and progressive PAH. The remodeling process involves apparently direct effects of increased flow on expression of several factors that alter the structure of the vessels. Studies in animal models with chronically increased pulmonary blood flow demonstrate increased expression of vascular endothelial growth factor and its receptors, transforming growth factor-β) and the cell growth promoters, tenascin-C and matrix metalloproteinase, in muscular vessels.[18–20] Increased linear shear stress imposed on cultured pulmonary vascular endothelial cells induces cytoskeleton remodeling and other endothelial cell alterations.[21] Endothelial dependent pulmonary vascular relaxation is also compromised in experimentally induced increased pulmonary blood flow,[22] so that loss of normal homeostatic mechanisms for maintaining low pulmonary vascular resistance may contribute to the development of persistent PAH in this circumstance.

The ultimate result of persistent increased pulmonary blood flow and the worsening PAH is reversal of flow through the shunt. As pulmonary vascular resistance increases, right side of the heart pressures rise, finally reaching levels approaching systemic pressures, reversing the pressure gradient and forcing blood to flow through the shunt from the right side of the circulation to the left. Clinically, this condition is termed *Eisenmenger complex*[23] (see Chaps. 82 and 83). Although patients with this syndrome appear to tolerate high right-sided pressures better than patients with PAH from other causes do, eventually right side of the heart failure, cor pulmonale, occurs.

PULMONARY VASCULAR REMODELING

A low baseline resistance to blood flow, a large vascular capacitance, and the ability to create flow heterogeneities in order to match perfusion to ventilation are all essential to normal function of the lung circulation. Structural remodeling of the pulmonary arterial circulation that occurs in several lung diseases resulting in PAH compromises each of these essential characteristics.

The clearest example of vascular remodeling in the lungs is the unusual disorder, idiopathic pulmonary arterial hypertension (IPAH; formerly primary PAH), which occurs as both a familial, inherited, and a sporadic disorder (see Chap. 71). The etiology of this progressive fatal disease remains unknown, although an inherited abnormality in the gene encoding bone morphogenic protein receptor-2 (a member of the transforming growth factor-β receptor superfamily) is apparently responsible for the disease in at least some families (see Chap. 9).[24,25] Exactly how this genetic predisposition fits into the pathogenesis of PAH is not yet clear. Remodeling also occurs in secondary PAH with functional consequences such as those in the primary form of the disease. For example, pulmonary complications of collagen vascular diseases include remodeling of the lung vasculature[26] (see Chap. 88); vascular remodeling is a feature of COPD as well.[27]

Much has been learned about how remodeling of the pulmonary arterial circulation occurs from studies in animals in which pulmonary vascular resistance is elevated chronically by various experimental interventions. Remodeling is a complex process that, anatomically, includes hypertrophy of smooth muscle in arterial resistance vessels, extension of vascular smooth muscle peripherally to previously nonmuscular arteries, and loss of microvascular bed resulting from intimal proliferation.[28] These structural changes act in concert to increase resistance to blood flow through the lung circulation. In addition, in some forms of persistent PAH, there is a tonic vasoconstrictive component that compounds the problem.[29]

RESPONSE OF THE RIGHT CARDIAC VENTRICLE TO INCREASED PULMONARY VASCULAR RESISTANCE

NORMAL RIGHT VENTRICULAR STRUCTURE AND FUNCTION

Mechanical demands on the right ventricle under normal conditions are minimal compared to demands on the left ventricle because the work required to pump blood through the low resistance, low impedance lung circulation is a fraction of that required to perfuse the high pressure systemic circulation. The structure of the right ventricle compared to the left ventricle reflects the difference in their physiologic requirements. Fig. 73–5 shows a cross section through a normal heart.[30] The left ventricle is symmetrical with a thick muscular wall. In contrast, the RV wall is much thinner and the cavity is crescent shaped, because the convexity of the septum bulges toward the right. Both the geometry of the two ventricles and the mass of their muscular walls reflect their different functions. The symmetrical, thick-walled left ventricle is suited to generating high outflow pressures, whereas the thin-walled, asymmetric right ventricle is not.

Fig. 73–6 compares the responses of the normal right and left ventricles to increased afterload in an experimental preparation.[31] When aortic pressure is increased (i.e., increased afterload to the left ventricle), there is a marked increase in stroke work, but stroke volume is maintained. However, RV stroke volume decreases as a steep function of increasing pulmonary artery pressure (i.e., increased afterload to the right ventricle) with only a modest increase in stroke work. Note that the degree of elevation of pulmo-

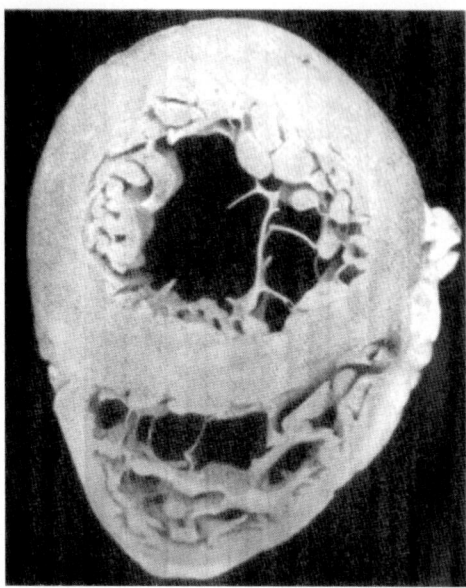

FIGURE 73–5. A cross section of a gross specimen of a normal heart illustrating a thick-walled, spherical left ventricle contrasted to a thin-walled, crescent-shaped right ventricle. *Source: Reprinted with permission from Rappaport E. Cor pulmonale. In: Murray J, Nadel J, eds. Textbook of Respiratory Medicine, 3rd ed. Philadelphia: W.B. Saunders, 2000:1635.*

nary artery pressure in the studies depicted in Fig. 73–6 were modest, well below those in both primary and secondary PAH in humans.

█ █ REMODELING OF THE RIGHT VENTRICLE: STRUCTURE AND FUNCTION

The right ventricle dilates enough with even modest acute increases in afterload that its effectiveness as a pump is compromised; this results in failure of the right side of the heart—*acute cor pulmonale.* However, with prolonged increases in pulmonary artery pressure that are not high enough initially to precipitate RV failure, the right ventricle, like the left ventricle, undergoes hypertrophy. Fig. 73–7, a cross section of a gross specimen of a heart from a patient who died of PAH,[30] should be compared to the normal heart in Fig. 73–5. The grossly thickened myocardium and massively enlarged trabeculae carneae are exactly as described by Laennec.[2] In this advanced case, it is not difficult to imagine that the right ventricle could sustain pulmonary artery pressures as high as systemic arterial pressures.

However, the robust appearance of the hypertrophied ventricle is misleading; the complex process of hypertrophy is not entirely adaptive. As the right ventricle hypertrophies in response to a chronic pressure load, several alterations occur that result in less-

efficient function. Such changes include loss of cardiac myocytes[32] and myocardial edema followed by fibrosis.[33] In addition, the hypertrophied ventricle becomes stiff, resulting in an increase in end-diastolic RV pressure that compromises endocardial perfusion and creates a mismatch of myocardial oxygen demand and supply.

In addition to these pathologic changes at the organ level, hypertrophy is accompanied by changes in the architecture and mechanical function of individual cardiac myocytes. Alterations, such as subcellular relocation of critical cell proteins,[34] alterations in microtubules,[35] changes in calcium handling,[36] and depressed sarcomere contraction,[37] occur in experimental RV hypertrophy and are likely important parts of the pathogenesis of cor pulmonale in humans.

As RV hypertrophy progresses, failure of its pump function with either persistence of increased pulmonary artery pressure or acute increases resulting from altered status of the underlying lung disease is increasingly likely. The sequence of events is initial dilatation of the hypertrophied ventricle, an elevation in RV end-diastolic pressure resulting in increased systemic venous pressure, and clinically apparent peripheral edema. In patients with COPD, bouts of increasing respiratory failure, and hypoxemia may result in acute worsening of RV function and peripheral edema that is a transient function of the severity of the respiratory failure, resolving if treatment of the lung disease is effective. Fig. 73–8 shows data from a study of nine patients with COPD who had right side of the heart catheterizations while they were edema free and during an episode of exacerbation of their lung disease and cor pulmonale.[38] During an acute episode of respiratory decompensation, decreased arterial oxygenation was accompanied by marked increases in pulmonary artery pressure and in RV end-diastolic pressure, reflecting worsening RV failure. Interestingly, acute edematous episodes in patients with COPD are not invariably accompanied by increased RV end-diastolic pressure, so that factors other than RV failure may be responsible for peripheral edema in those cases.[38]

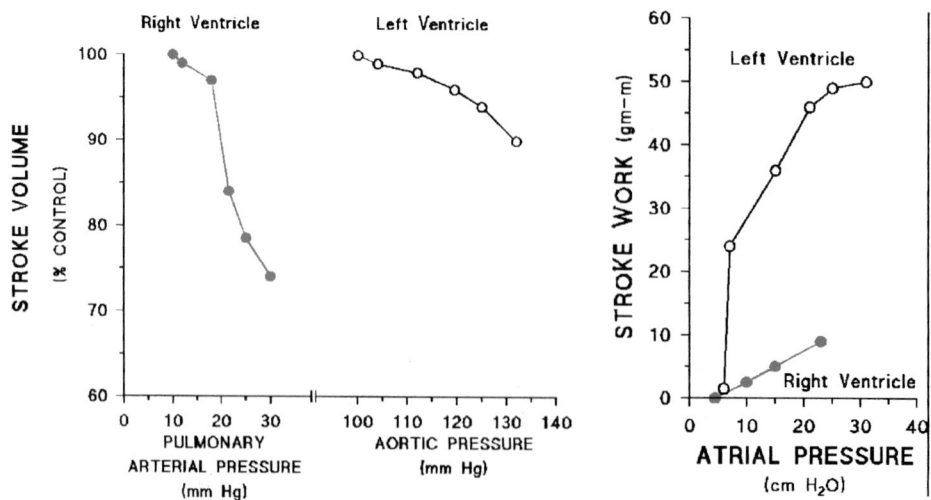

FIGURE 73–6. Responses of the right and left ventricles to experimental increases in afterload to each ventricle contrasting responses of the two ventricles. *Source: Reproduced with permission from Macnee W. Pathophysiology of cor pulmonale in chronic obstructive pulmonary disease. Am J Respir Crit Care Med 1994;150:833–852.*

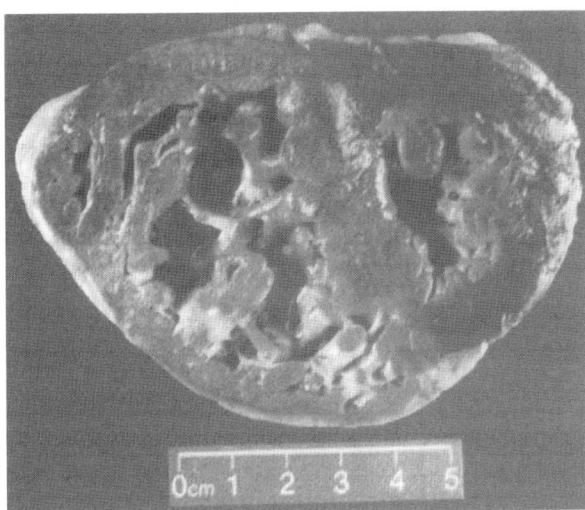

FIGURE 73–7. Cross section of a gross specimen of a heart from a patient who died of pulmonary hypertension illustrating selective marked hypertrophy of the right ventricle. *Source: Reproduced with permission from Macnee W. Pathophysiology of cor pulmonale in chronic obstructive pulmonary disease. Am J Respir Crit Care Med 1994;150:833–852.*

There may also be primary abnormalities in the RV that account for the unique clinical features of Eisenmenger syndrome. One study reported extensive evaluations of ventricular morphology in patients with Eisenmenger complex, a group with "pre-Eisenmenger" syndrome (i.e., ventricular septal defect with left-to-right shunting), and fetuses with healthy hearts.[39] They found the same ventricular morphology in all groups—a flat ventricular septum and equal thickness of the right and left ventricular free walls—concluding that the usual regression of right ventricle wall thickness subsequent to birth does not occur in the presence of large shunts so that the right ventricle retains function even with increased mechanical demand. In adults with severe PAH as a result of Eisenmenger syndrome, the right ventricle may be functionally devoid of sympathetic innervation, contributing to eventual ventricular failure.[40]

In addition to the structural and functional alterations in the right ventricle that occur with hypertrophy, other systemic factors can adversely affect function either by directly affecting cardiac muscle or by exaggerating RV afterload. Generalized hypoxia, regardless of the cause, will exaggerate PAH, imposing increased mechanical demand on the right ventricle. Increased blood viscosity secondary to polycythemia that develops as a response to chronic hypoxemia will exaggerate the increased afterload resulting from PAH. Hypercapnia and the resulting acidemia appear to affect the myocardium directly, compromising the ability of the ventricle to increase work in response to increased afterload.[31] Thus, either hypoventilation syndromes with chronic hypercapnia and acidosis or acute elevations in carbon dioxide that occur with acute exacerbations

in patients with COPD will challenge the reserve of the right side of the heart while increasing the mechanical demand.

CLINICAL MANIFESTATIONS

【 】 SYMPTOMS

Although cor pulmonale may result from many different pulmonary diseases, the cardinal symptom is shortness of breath, especially with exertion, with progression over months to years.[41] However, shortness of breath is virtually universal with all disorders of the cardiopulmonary system and thus does not serve to differentiate primary pulmonary disorders from secondary RV dysfunction. Other nonspecific symptoms of cor pulmonale include fatigue, palpitations, atypical chest pain, swelling of the lower extremities, dizziness, and even syncope. In essence, the symptoms of cor pulmonale are those of PAH (see Chap. 71). However, complaints consistent with Raynaud phenomena suggest either an underlying connective tissue disorder or IPAH; a history of liver disease suggests the possibility of portal PAH; and a history of previous pulmonary emboli and/or deep venous thrombosis may indicate chronic thromboembolic PAH (see Chap. 72).

PHYSICAL EXAMINATION

The physical findings in cor pulmonale are a combination of those of the underlying pulmonary disease and those of PAH (see Chap. 12). Thus pursed lip breathing, hyperresonant chest, and diminished breath sounds with prolonged expiratory phase are characteristic of emphysema, whereas coarse "Velcro" rales with small lung volumes, dullness to percussion, egophony, and clubbing are seen in many interstitial lung diseases. Telangiectasias of the skin may be present with either cirrhosis of the liver or CREST (calci-

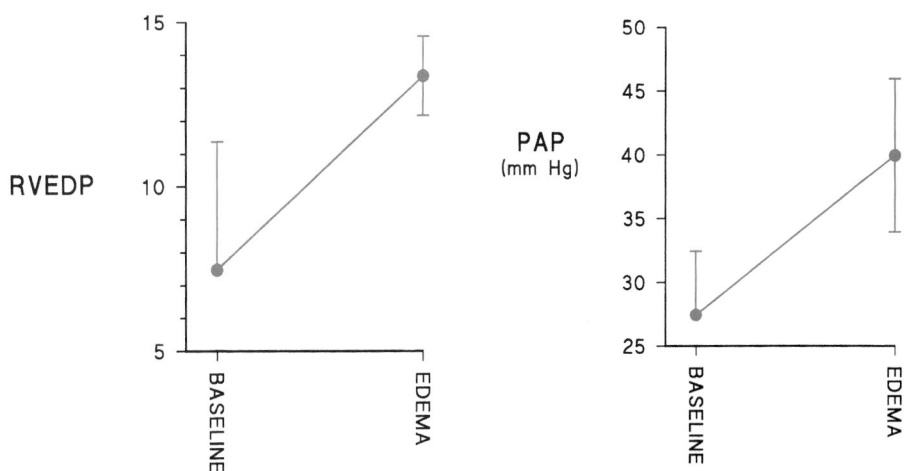

FIGURE 73–8. Right ventricular end-diastolic pressure (RVEDP) and pulmonary artery pressure (PAP) in a group of patients with chronic obstructive pulmonary disease measured at a time when they were free of peripheral edema and repeated during an episode of worsening pulmonary symptoms associated with peripheral edema. Elevated right-sided pressures are evidence of cor pulmonale. *Source: Weitzenblum E, Apprill M, Oswald M, et al. Pulmonary hemodynamics in patients with chronic obstructive pulmonary disease before and during an episode of peripheral edema. Chest 1994;105:1377–1382.*

nosis cutis, Raynaud phenomenon, esophageal motility disorder, sclerodactyly, and telangiectasia) syndrome; patients with the latter disorder may exhibit tightening of the skin circumorally and of the fingers (sclerodactyly), often with digital ulcerations and even loss of distal portions of digits. Arthritic changes may be seen with connective tissue diseases but are most pronounced with rheumatoid arthritis.

The physical findings of PAH may not be present until the disease process is far advanced. However, an increased pulmonic component of the second heart sound (P_2), as demonstrated by splitting of S_2 over the cardiac apex with inspiration, is a reliable sign of PAH and cor pulmonale.[42] With progression of the disease process, one may appreciate a left parasternal (RV) lift, murmurs of tricuspid regurgitation, pulmonic flow and regurgitation (Graham Steele) murmurs, and prominent "A" waves in jugular venous pulsations. With decompensated cor pulmonale (RV failure), distension of jugular neck veins, a tender liver with hepatojugular reflux, peripheral edema, and ascites often ensue, usually accompanied by right-sided S_3 and often by S_4 gallops (see Chap. 12).

【 】 ELECTROCARDIOGRAM

Electrocardiographic abnormalities, when present, are helpful in establishing a diagnosis of cor pulmonale, whereas the absence of such findings does not exclude the diagnosis.[43] Characteristic findings in advanced cor pulmonale include tall, peaked P waves anteriorly (i.e., "P pulmonale"), and rightward axis and prominent R waves in early V leads producing an R/S ratio greater than 1 in lead V_1 and a R/S ratio less than 1 in V_5 to V_6 (i.e., "RVH"). However, the triad of "$S_1 Q_3 T_3$" indicative of RV strain are more commonly found (see Chap. 13).

【 】 CHEST RADIOGRAPH

Characteristic findings on chest radiograph are those of PAH (see Chap. 15) and include cardiomegaly on the posteroanterior view with the lateral view showing the normally clear retrosternal airspace obscured by the enlarged right ventricle. Additional findings include a right main pulmonary artery greater than 16 mm in diameter and left main pulmonary artery prominence below the aortic knob, with "pruning" of the peripheral vasculature (Fig. 73–9).[44] However, some of these changes can be masked or minimized with the severe hyperinflation that accompanies end-stage emphysema or the smaller lung volumes and severe fibrotic changes seen in certain interstitial lung diseases.

【 】 ECHOCARDIOGRAM

Transthoracic echocardiography (TTE) is helpful both in detecting the presence of RV dysfunction and in excluding cau-

sation from left ventricular (LV) disease processes, mitral valve disease, congenital heart defects, or global disorders of the myocardium (see Chap. 16). The findings of cor pulmonale with two-dimensional echocardiography include RV dilatation and/or hypertrophy, and diminished function.[45] Whenever tricuspid regurgitation is present, Doppler studies can estimate RV, and therefore pulmonary artery, systolic pressure in millimeters of mercury from the velocity (v) of the regurgitant jet by the formula

$$PAPs = (v^2 \times 4) + CVP$$

where PAPs is pulmonary artery systolic pressure and CVP is central venous pressure.[46] Occasionally, pulmonic regurgitation is present permitting estimation of pulmonary artery diastolic pressure.

DIAGNOSTIC EVALUATION

【 】 STRATEGY

Figure 73–10 shows the diagnostic approach that ultimately leads to the finding of chronic cor pulmonale. The initial and most basic evaluation should include the history, physical examination, electrocardiogram (ECG), and chest radiograph (posteroanterior and lateral). When the initial evaluation suggests some disorder of the cardiopulmonary system, a TTE with two-dimensional and color Doppler modes is indicated. These echocardiographic studies allow assessment of the global myocardium, the left ventricle, and the heart valves, and with the intravenous infusion of agitated saline "bubbles" or color Doppler, also may detect intracardiac shunts (see Chap. 16). Echocardiographic evidence of RV dysfunction and/or PAH in the absence of the aforementioned abnormalities is often sufficient to make a diagnosis of cor pulmonale. In some cases, TTE immediately after exercise will reveal RV dysfunction not readily apparent on resting studies.[47]

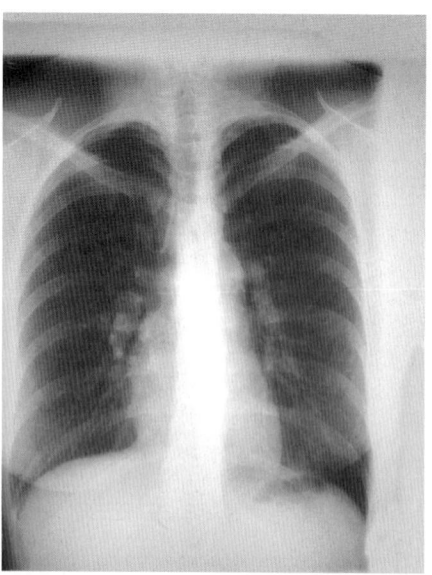 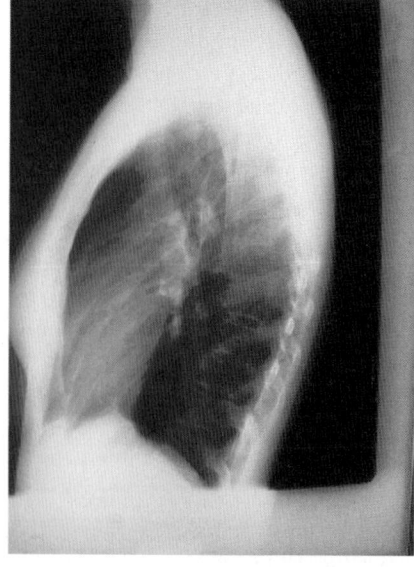

FIGURE 73–9. Chest radiographs from a patient with primary pulmonary hypertension. The posteroanterior view shows prominent central pulmonary arteries with relative oligemia (pruning) of peripheral vessels, whereas the lateral view demonstrates the enlarged right ventricle filling the retrosternal airspace.

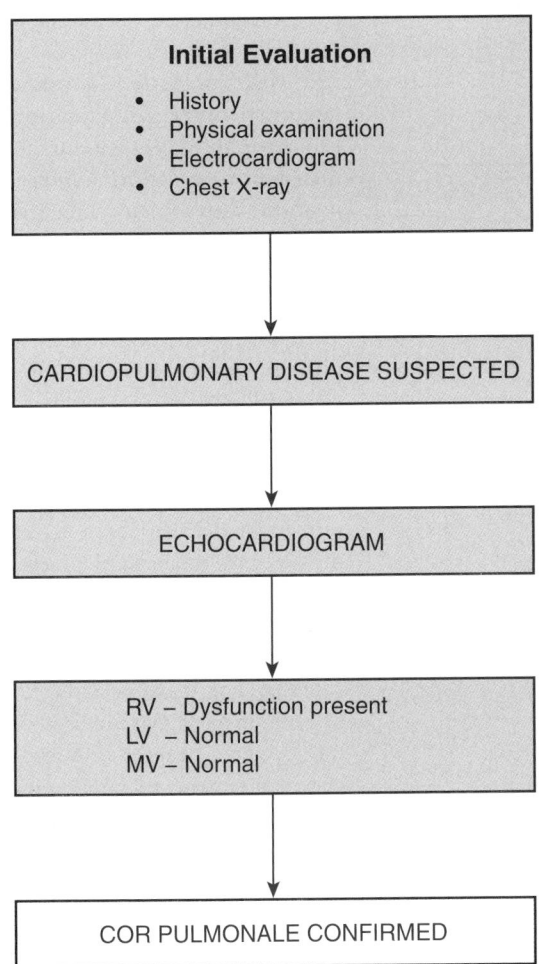

FIGURE 73–10. Diagnostic evaluation. Algorithm of process leading to a diagnosis of chronic cor pulmonale. LV, left ventricle; MV, mitral valve; RV, right ventricle.

Although right heart catheterization may eventually be required for confirmation and more complete assessment of pulmonary hemodynamics, the immediate question to be addressed is the cause of the RV dysfunction. As shown in Fig. 73–11, the possibility of acute and/or chronic pulmonary thromboembolic disease must be addressed by either rapid sequence spiral contrast computed tomography (CT) of the chest (i.e., "pulmonary embolism protocol"), radionuclide ventilation–perfusion lung scanning, or pulmonary arteriography. Supplemental studies may include bilateral lower-extremity Doppler ultrasound examination and measurements of blood D-dimer levels. Whenever there is concern for acute thromboembolism, immediate anticoagulation with intravenous heparin is indicated while diagnostic studies are being obtained.

When life-threatening pulmonary emboli have been excluded, attention is turned to evaluation of pulmonary or systemic causes for the RV dysfunction. Pulmonary function studies should include spirometry with flow-volume loops, lung volumes by plethysmography, diffusion capacity for carbon monoxide, and arterial blood gases. High-resolution CT scanning of the chest may be helpful in evaluation of interstitial lung disorders and may obviate the need for open lung biopsy. Should the history suggest the pos-

sibility of sleep-disordered breathing (e.g., severe snoring with periods of apnea, daytime somnolence), a formal sleep study should be ordered. Hypoxia related to underlying lung pathology, altered respiratory drive, or sleep-disordered breathing can be readily assessed by pulse oximetry at rest and with exercise, whereas overnight monitoring of oxygen saturation may be performed at home. Serologic studies should include screening for connective tissue diseases with antinuclear antibody and rheumatoid factor levels; antibodies to the HIV virus should be measured in at-risk individuals. Whenever liver disease is expected, antibodies to hepatitis A, B, and C should be measured in addition to standard liver function studies.

If all of the preceding studies are nonrevealing, by exclusion the diagnosis is IPAH, which is discussed in Chap. 71.

【 】 DIFFERENTIAL DIAGNOSIS

The differential diagnosis of chronic cor pulmonale is the same as that for PAH, except that by definition left-sided myocardial or valvular diseases have been excluded. Although the diagnostic possibilities are extensive, they may be considered for clinical purposes as caused by disorders of (1) lung parenchyma, (2) lung vasculature, (3) systemic disorders, or (4) hypoxic vasoconstriction. The diagnostic strategies outlined in Figs. 73–10 and 73–11 are taken from American College of Chest Physicians (ACCP) guidelines[48–49] and will narrow the diagnostic possibilities to the most likely etiology.

【 】 SPECIAL DIAGNOSTIC STUDIES

Transesophageal Echocardiogram

In clinical situations where TTE cannot adequately evaluate either the mitral valve or atrial septum, transesophageal echocardiogram views may provide valuable information (see Chap. 16). The finding of severe mitral stenosis or regurgitation or an atrial septal defect may lead to surgical correction of these processes with resolution or improvement in PAH and cor pulmonale.

Right Heart Catheterization

In experienced hands, TTE, with or without a transesophageal echocardiogram study, in concert with available clinical information, is sufficient to make a diagnosis of cor pulmonale. Formal catheterization of the right side of the heart with oxygen saturation determinations at various levels may be performed to determine whether congenital heart defects, such as ventricular or atrial septal defects, or patent ductus arteriosus are present and to exclude stenosis of the pulmonic valve or pulmonary arteries. Right-heart catheterization also permits direct measurement of pulmonary artery pressures. Essential data obtained include right atrial, right ventricle, pulmonary artery, and pulmonary capillary wedge pressures; pulmonary and systemic vascular resistance; and cardiac output and cardiac index. In addition to the diagnostic and prognostic information thus obtained, the hemodynamic effects of selective pulmonary vasodilators can be assessed.

Cardiac Magnetic Resonance Imaging

Although echocardiography is excellent for assessing RV function, cardiac MRI may be even more sensitive.[50] Cardiac MRI studies

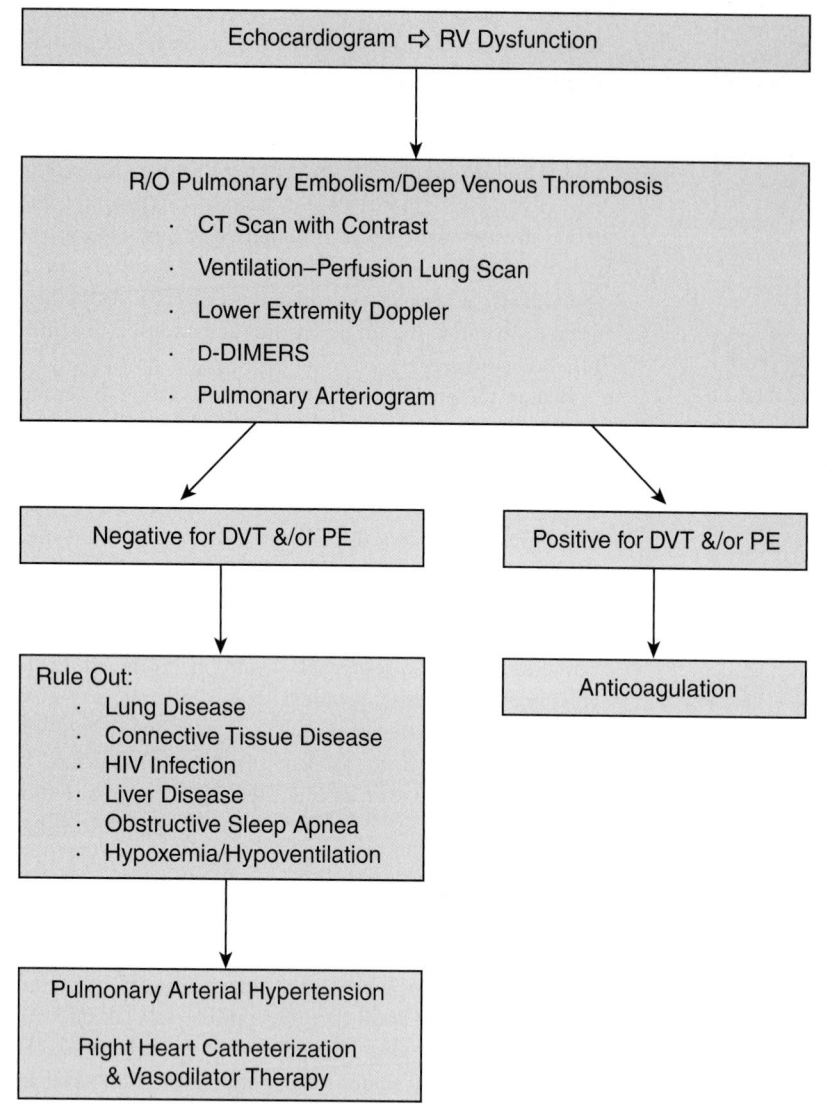

FIGURE 73–11. Evaluation of cor pulmonale. Algorithm of clinical approach to patients with chronic cor pulmonale. DVT, deep venous thrombosis; PE, pulmonary embolism; RV, right ventricular.

provide such exquisite detail of the heart chambers and valves that serial cardiac catheterizations may be avoided in many instances (see Chap. 21).

TREATMENT

【 】 SUPPLEMENTAL OXYGEN THERAPY

Regardless of the underlying disease leading to cor pulmonale, alveolar hypoxia will aggravate and compound the pathologic process through compensatory regional pulmonary vasoconstriction. In recognition of this fact, Medicare criteria for supplemental oxygen are less stringent for patients with cor pulmonale, requiring a PaO$_2$ (arterial oxygen partial pressure) <59 mmHg or SaO$_2$ (arterial oxygen saturation) <89 percent for patients with cor pulmonale versus a PaO$_2$ <55 mmHg or SaO$_2$ <88 percent for other patients. It is imperative that every patient with cor pulmonale be assessed as to the patient's need for supplemental oxygen therapy. The need for supplemental

oxygen should be assessed at least by measuring oxygen saturation at rest and with ambulation; monitoring for nocturnal oxygen desaturation is appropriate in those patients who remain normoxic with ambulation and in those whose history suggest sleep-disordered breathing. Long-term oxygen therapy does extend life for patients with COPD.[51]

Supplemental oxygen may be supplied in various ways but most easily via nasal cannula in liters per minute sufficient to maintain SaO$_2$ >90 percent and/or PaO$_2$ >60 mmHg. It is important that portable oxygen be prescribed so that patients can remain as mobile and active as their conditions permit. Humidification of the home oxygen delivery helps alleviate the drying effect of oxygen delivered via nasal cannula. The maximal rate of delivery of home oxygen systems is about 6 L/min; selected patients with greater oxygen requirements may maintain higher levels of SaO$_2$ when oxygen is delivered via a transtracheal catheter.

【 】 GENERAL MEASURES

Useful adjuncts in the treatment of cor pulmonale include diuretics, systemic anticoagulation, supplemental oxygen, and perhaps digitalis.[52] Patients often respond well to a combination of a loop diuretic, such as furosemide, and the potassium-sparing diuretic spironolactone. Anticoagulation with warfarin has proven beneficial in patients with IPAH,[53] and is often used in patients with cor pulmonale resulting from COPD. Although similar data are not available for other causes of PAH and cor pulmonale, warfarin therapy is generally recommended unless a relative contraindication exists (e.g., history of bleeding varices, liver dysfunction, or hemoptysis). In contrast to full anticoagulation that is proper for treating known thromboembolic disease or other cardiac disorders, the recommended international normalized ratio range is 1.5 to 2.5 for PAH and cor pulmonale as prophylaxis. The value of digitalis in the treatment of cor pulmonale is controversial, but in the circumstance of decompensated RV failure, it may have some value. Digitalis, calcium channel blockers, and warfarin have comprised the "conventional" treatment arm in studies comparing conventional versus specific pulmonary vasodilators in addition to conventional treatment for IPAH.[54]

【 】 DISEASE-SPECIFIC THERAPY

The following information is taken from ACCP guidelines,[55] which are currently under revision (see Chap. 11).

Because cor pulmonale by definition results from some pulmonary process, it follows that treatment of the underlying disease, if successful, should improve the function of the RV. Unfortunately, medical treatment for most established diseases of the lungs, such as COPD, idiopathic pulmonary fibrosis, and cystic fibrosis, may at best slow progression of the disease process, and in most instances, is merely symptomatic. *Smoking cessation* and avoidance of exposure to secondary smoke is critically important for all patients; indeed, patients with COPD who are able to stop smoking have improved survival as compared to those COPD patients who continue to smoke.[56] Immunosuppressive therapy is often administered to patients with connective tissue diseases and those with interstitial lung disorders, although only a minority of patients in the latter category responds. Idiopathic pulmonary fibrosis is a particularly difficult disorder to treat. Although reports of improvements in pulmonary function and oxygenation in patients who are receiving γ-interferon injections thrice weekly[57,58] have engendered hope in both patients and physicians, some patients receiving γ-interferon have fared less well.[59] Supplemental oxygen therapy is specific therapy when hypoxemia without parenchymal lung disease is the cause of cor pulmonale. Hypoxemia resulting from sleep-disordered breathing may be alleviated by use of positive pressure (continuous positive airway pressure or bilevel positive airway pressure) masks along with supplemental oxygen for obstructive sleep apnea, by central nervous system stimulants for central sleep apnea, and by weight reduction for the obesity–hypoventilation syndrome. Hypoxemia with resultant cor pulmonale as a consequence of neuromuscular disorders may respond to supplemental oxygen along with nocturnal ventilation using positive pressure masks, negative pressure body suits, or mechanical ventilation delivered through a tracheostomy tube. However, none of the aforementioned "specific treatments" is curative and cor pulmonale usually progresses over time.

Chronic thromboembolic PAH with cor pulmonale is treated with lifelong anticoagulation using warfarin; placement of an inferior vena cava filter is recommended. Patients with clots in more central pulmonary vessels may benefit from thromboendarterectomy (see Chap. 72), which may be curative.

【 】 PULMONARY VASODILATOR/ REMODELING THERAPY

A number of pulmonary vasodilator agents are available for the treatment of cor pulmonale caused by pulmonary arterial hypertension. PAH and cor pulmonale resulting from other processes, such as left-sided heart or valve disease, disorders of respiration and/or hypoxemia, or chronic thromboembolic disease, would not be expected to respond to pulmonary vasodilator therapy, and such therapy is generally not approved and is often contraindicated. In some instances, however, a pulmonary vasoconstrictor component coexists such that a trial of specific pulmonary vasodilator therapy may be warranted. Some patients with sarcoidosis present with PAH and cor pulmonale disproportionate to the degree of parenchymal disease and may respond to pulmonary vasodilators.[60] Patients with chronic thromboembolic PAH and cor pulmonale may partially respond to pulmonary vasodilator therapy, indicating a component of vasoconstriction in the smaller pulmonary vessels.[61]

A variety of pulmonary vasodilator agents have been used in the treatment of PAH and cor pulmonale. There was initial enthusiasm for calcium channel blockers in the 1990s when Rich et al. demonstrated that those patients with IPAH who responded acutely to high doses of diltiazem or verapamil, as demonstrated by >20 percent reduction in mean pulmonary artery pressure and pulmonary vascular resistance ("responders"), had an excellent prognosis over 5 years compared to the group of "nonresponders."[53] However, these data applied only to patients with IPAH and the percentage of long-term responders now appears to be less than 10 percent of patients referred to centers specializing in the treatment of PAH.[62] Thus calcium channel blockers have only a minor role in the treatment of patients with most forms of cor pulmonale.

The medical treatment of IPAH and other forms of PAH has been transformed by continuous intravenous infusion of *prostacyclin and its analogues (epoprostenol, prostaglandin, Flolan).*[54] Prostacyclin has relatively specific vasodilatory effects on the pulmonary microvasculature along with antiplatelet effects; over time it may also promote vascular remodeling.[63] Prostacyclin is the "gold standard" in the medical treatment of IPAH, but is ineffective in the larger group of patients with severe COPD or interstitial pulmonary fibrosis or when hypoxemia is the cause for PAH. Prostacyclin may also be administered subcutaneously,[64] orally,[65] or by inhalation,[66] albeit with less effect than the intravenous route (see also Chap. 71).

Endothelin receptor blockers are another class of drugs for the treatment of PAH. The endothelin receptor blockers prevent the binding of the potent vasoconstrictor endothelin-1 (ET-1) to its receptors on pulmonary vascular smooth muscle cells, thereby producing vasodilatation of the pulmonary vascular bed. There is one currently commercially available endothelin receptor blockers, bosentan (Tracleer), which blocks the binding of endothelin to its A and B receptors (ET_A, ET_B).[67] Bosentan has proven effective in improving the pulmonary hemodynamics and functional class of patients with PAH. There are additional endothelin receptor blockers in clinical trials that selectively block ET_A. The receptor ET_A regulates vasoconstriction, whereas ET_B regulates the inflammatory and fibroproliferative actions of ET-1.

Oral sildenafil was recently found effective in pulmonary arterial hypertension (PAH) and approved by the U.S. Food and Drug Administration (FDA) for this indication as Revatio.[68]

Initially, specific treatment of pulmonary hypertension focused on the vasodilator properties of available agents. More recently, however, attention has focused on the possibility that the long-term treatment effects may be more a result of vascular remodeling; that is, reversal of the fibroproliferative process within the vascular wall and lumen. In two differing animal models of PAH, inhibition of the receptor for platelet-derived growth factor begun 28 days after initiation of disease resulted in nearly complete reversal of PAH and RV hypertrophy.[69] Moreover, significantly increases in the platelet-derived growth factor receptor was found in lung tissue of PAH patients. The inhibitor used, STI571 (imatinib), is commercially available as Gleevec for the treatment of chronic myelogenous leukemia, and has been used successfully in one case of refractory PAH.[70] These exciting data have led to clinical trials testing the safety and efficacy of Gleevec in PAH. Thus, specific targeting of the vascular fibroproliferative process of PAH may greatly improve the outcomes of PAH patients.

[ ] LUNG TRANSPLANTATION

Lung transplantation has become an accepted form of treatment for a variety of end-stage lung and pulmonary vascular diseases. Indeed, the first successful lung transplant was actually a combined heart–lung transplant performed for PAH and cor pulmonale in 1981 at Stanford University. As the discipline of lung transplantation has evolved over the past two decades, heart–lung transplantation has been supplanted by single or bilateral lung transplantation,[71] with bilateral lung transplantation becoming the transplantation procedure of choice for IPAH.[72] In fact, unless the PAH is totally reversed with medical therapy, bilateral lung transplantation offers the *only* definitive treatment for cor pulmonale. One argument in favor of combined heart–lung transplantation for PAH was concern that the extremely dilated and hypocontractile right ventricle of advanced cor pulmonale was irreversibly damaged. However, studies show that the right ventricle almost immediately begins to diminish in size with improved contractility following lung transplantation with restoration of more normal pulmonary vascular resistance.[73] The recuperative abilities of the right ventricle are described in Fig. 73–12, which shows a patient with primary PAH and New York Heart Association (NYHA) class IV right-sided heart failure who received a bilateral lung transplant at Emory University Hospital. The transthoracic echocardiogram demonstrated severe right ventricle dilatation and hypocontractility 2 months prior to the transplant procedure, which was markedly improved at 2 months posttransplant.

PROGNOSIS

The prognosis for patients with chronic cor pulmonale may be most quantitatively assessed by review of the natural history of IPAH before there was effective treatment, as documented in the National Institutes of Health Registry begun in the 1970s.[74] The median survival was 2.8 years, with 1-, 3-, and 5-year survival of 65, 50, and 33 percent, respectively. However, the initial hemodynamic data from right side of the heart catheterization identified sub-

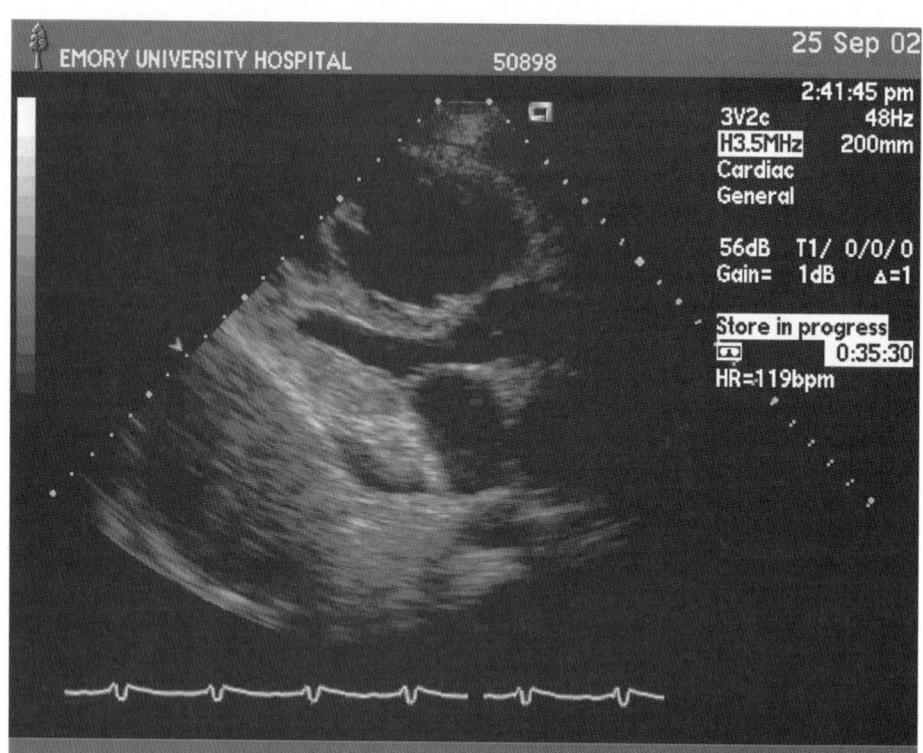

A

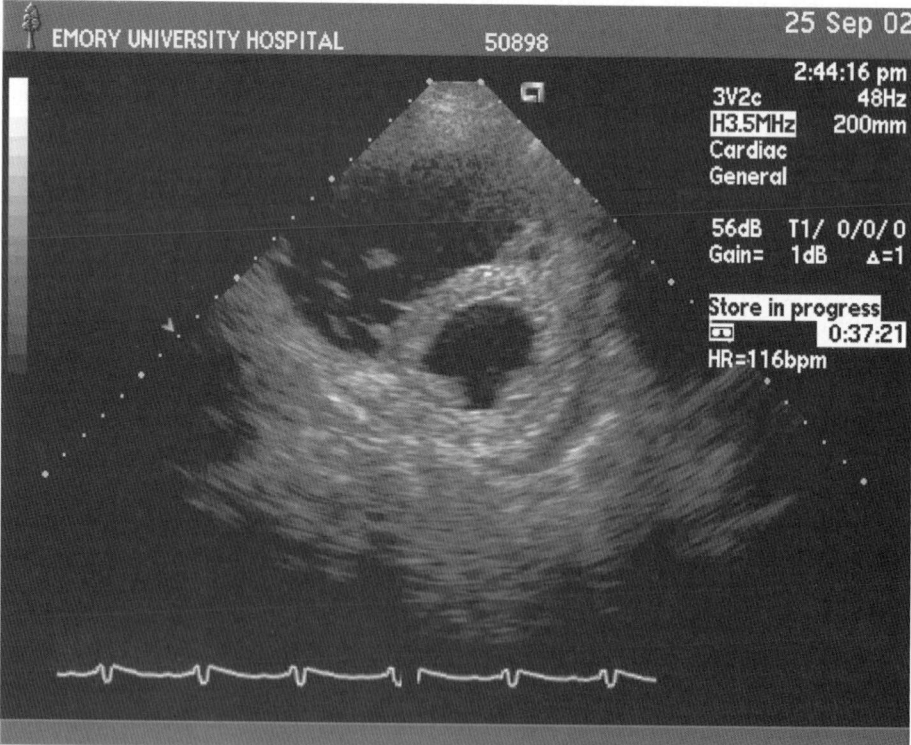

B

FIGURE 73–12. Resolution of chronic cor pulmonale by lung transplantation. Panels **A** to **C** represent echocardiographic findings 2 months prior to bilateral lung transplantation in a patient with primary pulmonary hypertension. Panels **D** to **F** represent echocardiographic findings 2 months following transplant. Panels **A** and **D** depict the horizontal long axis; panels **B** and **E** show the short axis; panels **C** and **F** represent the apical four-chamber view. Note the diminution in right ventricle size, resolution of right ventricle impingement on the left ventricle with normalization of left ventricle size following transplant.

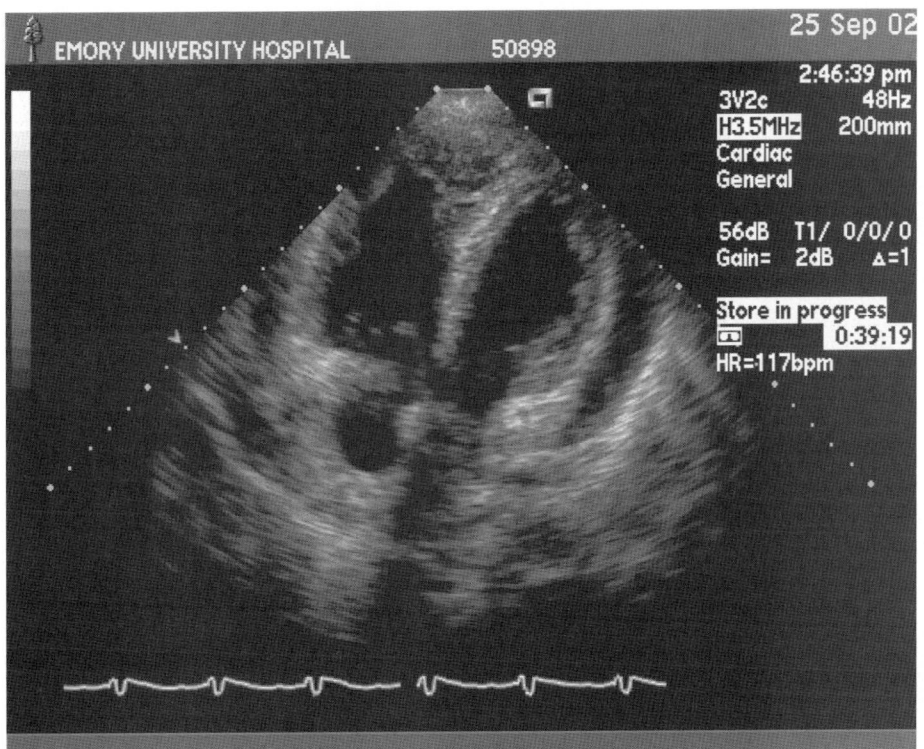

C

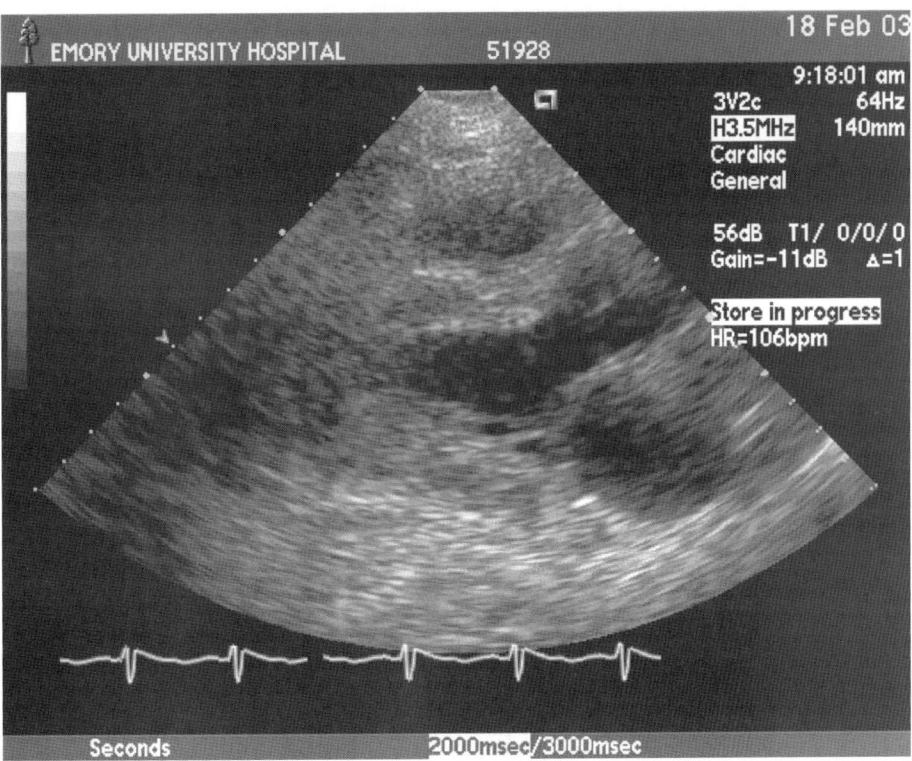

D

FIGURE 73–12. *(continued)*

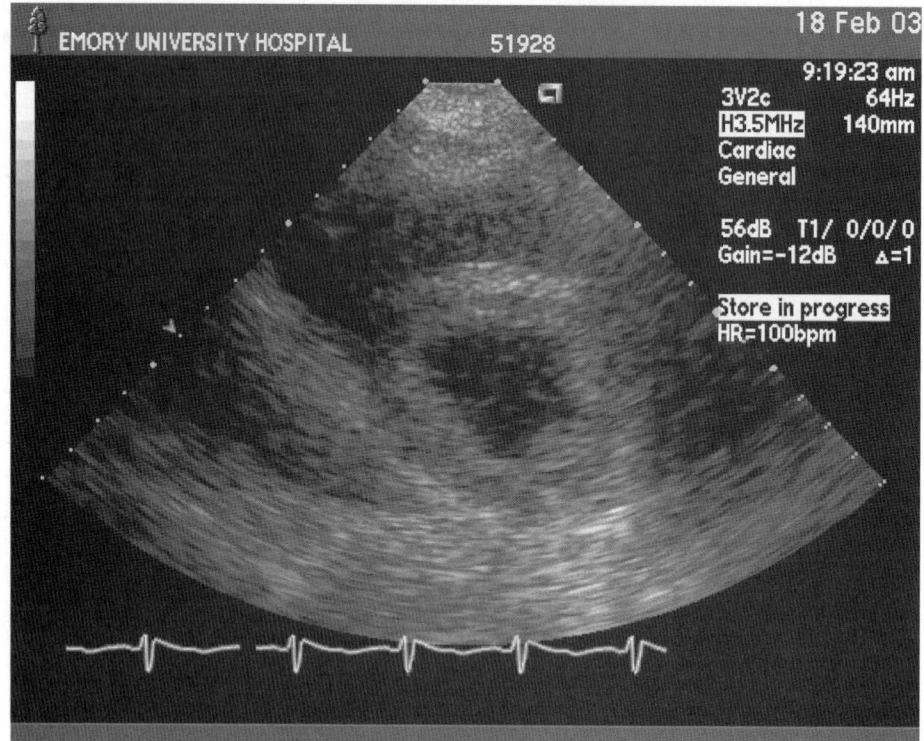

E

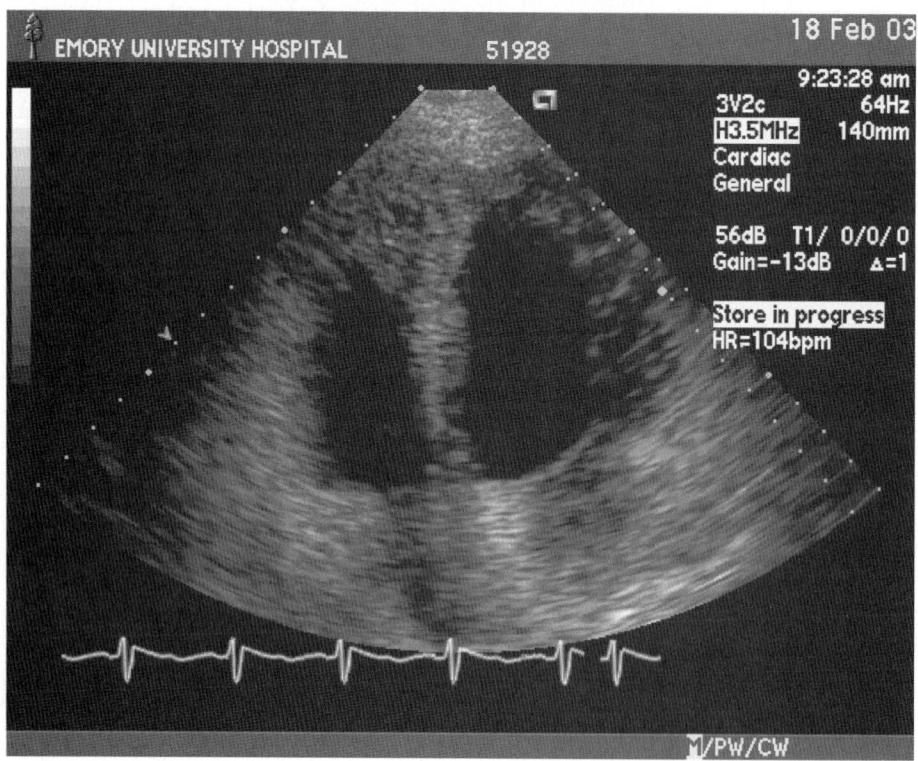

F

FIGURE 73–12. (continued)

groups with greater likelihood of death. Subjects at greatest risk were those with systemic levels of mean pulmonary artery pressure (>85 mmHg), cardiac index <2.0 L/min/m^2, and/or mean right atrial pressure >20 mmHg. Moreover, clinical assessment by NYHA functional class was highly predictive of outcome with median survival for patients in classes I and II at 58.6 months, class III at 31.5 months, and class IV at 6 months. Treatment of IPAH with continuous intravenous infusion of prostacyclin (Flolan), which is indicated for treatment of NYHA classes III and IV patients, has roughly doubled survival.[75]

Patients with cor pulmonale resulting from COPD have a greater likelihood of dying than do similar patients with COPD alone.[76] Although information is not readily available for other disease processes resulting in cor pulmonale, clinical experience strongly supports the notion that cor pulmonale, regardless of etiology, is an independent risk factor for earlier demise.

REFERENCES

1. World Health Organization. Chronic cor pulmonale. A report of the expert committee. *Circulation* 1963;27:594–598.
2. Laennec RTH. *A Treatise on Diseases of the Chest.* London: T. and G. Underwood, 1821.
3. World Health Organization. *Consultation on the Development of a Comprehensive Approach for the Prevention and Control of Chronic Respiratory Diseases.* Geneva: WHO, 2001:6.
4. Vizza CD, Lynch JP, Ochoa LL, et al. Right and left ventricular dysfunction in patients with severe pulmonary disease. *Chest* 1998;113:576–583.
5. Scharf SM, Iqbal M, Keller C, et al. Hemodynamic characterization of patients with severe emphysema. *Am J Respir Crit Care Med* 2002;166:314–322.
6. Chaouat A, Bugnet A, Kadaoui N, et al. Severe pulmonary hypertension and chronic obstructive pulmonary disease. *Am J Respir Crit Care Med* 2005;172:189–194.
7. Williams BT, Nicholl JP. Prevalence of hypoxaemic chronic obstructive lung disease with reference to long-term oxygen therapy. *Lancet* 1985;I:369–372.
8. Moudgil R, Michelakis ED, Archer SL. Hypoxic pulmonary vasoconstriction. *J Appl Physiol* 2005;98(1):390–403.
9. Brigham KL, Newman JH. The pulmonary circulation. In: *Basics of Respiratory Disease.* New York: Am Thorac Soc 1979;5:15–19.
10. Reeves JT, Weil JV. Chronic mountain sickness: a view from the crow's nest. *Adv Exp Med Biol* 2001;502:419–437.
11. Dickens C. *The Works of Charles Dickens: The Pickwick Papers.* Boston: Houghton, Osgood: 1879.
12. Olson AL, Zwillich C. The obesity hypoventilation syndrome. *Am J Med* 2005;118(9):948–956.
13. Snapper JR, Harris, TR, Brigham, KL. Effect of changing lung mass on lung water and permeability-surface area in sheep. *J Appl Physiol* 1982;52:1591–1597.
14. Van Miegham W, Demedts M. Cardiopulmonary function after lobectomy or pneumonectomy for pulmonary neoplasm. *Respir Med* 1989;83:199.
15. Fedillo PF, Auger WR, Channick RN, et al. Chronic thromboembolic pulmonary hypertension. *Clin Chest Med* 1995;16:353–374.
16. Weitzenblum E. Chronic cor pulmonale. *BMJ* 2003;89:225–230.
17. Loyd JE, Tillman BF, Atkinson, JB, et al. Mediastinal fibrosis complicating histoplasmosis. *Medicine (Baltimore)* 1988;67:295–310.
18. Mata-Greenwood E, Meyrick B, Soifer SJ, et al. Expression of VEGF and its receptors FLT-1 and FLK-1/KDR are altered in lambs with increased pulmonary blood flow and pulmonary hypertension. *Am J Physiol Lung Cell Mol Physiol* 2003;285:L209–L221.
19. Mata-Greenwood E, Meyrick B, Fineman JR, et al. Alterations in TGF-β$_1$ expression in lambs with increased pulmonary blood flow and pulmonary hypertension. *Am J Physiol Lung Cell Mol Physiol* 2003;285(1):L209–L221.
20. Jones PL, Chapados R, Baldwin HS, et al. Altered hemodynamics controls matrix metalloproteinase activity and tenascin-C expression in neonatal pig lung. *Am J Physiol Lung Cell Mol Physiol* 2002;282:L26–35.
21. Birukov KG, Birukova AA, Dudek SM, et al. Shear stress-mediated cytoskeletal remodeling and cortactin translocation in pulmonary endothelial cells. *Am J Respir Cell Mol Biol* 2002;26:453–464.
22. Vitvvitsky EV, Griffin JP, Collins MH, et al. Increased pulmonary blood flow produces endothelial cell dysfunction in neonatal swine. *Ann Thorac Surg* 1998;66:1372–1377.
23. Berman EB, Barst RJ. Eisenmenger's syndrome: Current management. *Prog Cardiovasc Dis* 2002;45:129–138.
24. Lane KB, Machado RD, Pauciulo MW, et al. Heterozygous germline mutations in BMPR2 encoding a TGF-beta receptor, cause familial primary pulmonary hypertension. The International PPH Consortium. *Nat Genet* 2000;26:81–84.
25. Thomas AQ, Gaddipati R, Newman JH, et al. Genetics of primary pulmonary hypertension. *Clin Chest Med* 2001;22:477–491.
26. Fagan KA, Badesch DB. Pulmonary hypertension associated with connective tissue disease. *Prog Cardiovasc Dis* 2002;45:225–234.
27. Naeije R, Barbera JA. Pulmonary hypertension associated with COPD. *Crit Care* 2001;5(6)286–289.
28. Meyrick B, Reid L. Pulmonary hypertension. Anatomic and physiologic correlates. *Clin Chest Med* 1983;4:199–217.
29. Perkett EA, Brigham KL, Meyrick B. Continuous air embolization into sheep causes sustained pulmonary hypertension and increased pulmonary vasoreactivity. *Am J Pathol* 1988;132:444–454.
30. Rappaport E. Cor pulmonale. In: Murray J, Nadel J, eds. *Textbook of Respiratory Medicine,* 3rd ed. Philadelphia: W.B. Saunders, 2000:1635.
31. Macnee W. Pathophysiology of cor pulmonale in chronic obstructive pulmonary disease. *Am J Respir Crit Care Med* 1994;150:833–852.
32. Yamamoto S, Sawada K, Shimomura H, et al. On the nature of cell death during remodeling of the hypertrophied human myocardium. *J Mol Cell Cardiol* 2000;32:161–175.
33. Davis KL, Laine GA, Geissler HJ, et al. Effects of myocardial edema on the development of myocardial interstitial fibrosis. *Microcirculation* 2000;7:269–280.
34. Ecarnot-Laubriet A, De Luca K, Vandroux D, et al. Downregulation and nuclear relocation of MLP during the progression of right ventricular hypertrophy induced by chronic pressure overload. *J Mol Cell Cardiol* 2000;32:2385–2395.
35. Sato H, Nagai T, Kuppuswamy D, et al. Microtubule stabilization in pressure overload cardiac hypertrophy. *J Cell Biol* 1997;139:963–973.
36. Kuramochi T, Honda M, Tanaka K, et al. Calcium transients in single myocytes and membraneous ultrastructures during the development of cardiac hypertrophy and heart failure in rats. *Clin Exp Pharmacol Physiol* 1994;21:1009–1018.
37. Hamrell BB, Dey SK. Sarcomere shortening velocity in pressure overload hypertrophied rabbit right ventricular myocardium at physiological sarcomere lengths. *J Mol Cell Cardiol* 1993;25:1483–1500.
38. Weitzenblum E, Apprill M, Oswald M, et al. Pulmonary hemodynamics in patients with chronic obstructive pulmonary disease before and during an episode of peripheral edema. *Chest* 1994;105:1377–1382.
39. Hopkins WE, Waggoner AD. Severe pulmonary hypertension without right ventricular failure: the unique hearts of patients with Eisenmenger syndrome. *Am J Cardiol* 2002;89:34–38.
40. Hirose Y, Ishida Y, Hayashida K, et al. Viable but denervated right ventricular myocardium: a case of Eisenmenger reaction. *Cardiology* 1997;88:609–612.
41. Rich S, Dantzker D, Ayres S, et al. Primary pulmonary hypertension: a national prospective study. *Ann Intern Med* 1987;107:216–223.
42. Rappaport E. Cor pulmonale. In: Murray F, Nadel J, eds. *Textbook of Respiratory Medicine,* 3rd ed. Philadelphia: W.B. Saunders, 2000:1631–1648.
43. Ahearn GS, Tapson VF, Rebeiz A, et al. Electrocardiography to define clinical status in primary pulmonary hypertension and pulmonary arterial hypertension secondary to collagen vascular disease. *Chest* 2002;122(2):524–527.
44. Fraser RG, Paré JAP, Paré PD, et al. Pulmonary hypertension and edema. In: Fraser WD, ed. *Diagnosis of Diseases of the Chest,* 3rd ed. Philadelphia: W.B. Saunders, 1990:1823–1968.
45. Jardin F, Dubourg O, Bourdarias JP. Echocardiographic pattern of acute cor pulmonale. *Chest* 1997;111(1):209–217.
46. Berger M, Haimowitz A, Van Tosh A, et al. Quantitative assessment of pulmonary hypertension in patients with tricuspid regurgitation using continuous wave Doppler ultrasound. *J Am Coll Cardiol* 1985;2:359–365.
47. Bossone E, Avelar E, Bach DS, et al. Diagnostic value of resting tricuspid regurgitation velocity and right ventricular ejection flow parameters for the detection of exercise induced pulmonary arterial hypertension. *Int J Cardiovasc Imaging* 2000;6:429–436.
48. Rubin LJ. Diagnosis and management of pulmonary arterial hypertension: ACCP evidence-based clinical practice guidelines. *Chest* 2004;126(1 Suppl):4s–6s.

49. Rubin LJ. Diagnosis and management of pulmonary arterial hypertension: ACCP evidence-based clinical practice guidelines. *Chest* 2004;126(1 Suppl):7s–10s.

50. Saba TS, Foster J, Cockburn M, et al. Ventricular mass index using magnetic resonance imaging accurately estimates pulmonary artery pressure. *Eur Respir J* 2002;6:1519–1524.

51. Cranston JM, Crockett AJ, Moss JR, et al. Domiciliary oxygen for chronic obstructive pulmonary disease. *Cochrane Database Syst Rev* 2005;(4):CD001744.

52. Rubin L. Primary pulmonary hypertension. *N Engl J Med* 1997;336(2):111–117.

53. Rich S, Kaufmann E, Levy PS. The effect of high doses of calcium-channel blockers on survival in primary pulmonary hypertension. *N Engl J Med* 1992;327(2):76–81.

54. Barst R, Rubin L, Long W, et al. A comparison of continuous intravenous epoprostenol (prostacyclin) with conventional therapy for primary pulmonary hypertension. *N Engl J Med* 1996;334(5):296–301.

55. Badesch DB, Abman SH, Ahearn GS, et al. Medical therapy for pulmonary arterial hypertension: ACCP evidence-based clinical practice guidelines. *Chest* 2004;126(1 Suppl):35s–62s.

56. Anthonisen NR, Skeans MA, Wise RA, et al. The effects of a smoking cessation intervention on 14.5-year mortality. *Ann Intern Med* 2005;142:233–239.

57. Ziesche R, Hofbauer E, Wittmann K, et al. A preliminary study of long-term treatment with interferon gamma-1b and low-dose prednisolone in patients with idiopathic pulmonary fibrosis. *N Engl J Med* 1999;341(17):1264–1269.

58. Bajwa EK, Ayas NT, Schulzer M, et al. Interferon-γ1b therapy in idiopathic pulmonary fibrosis. *Chest* 2005;128:203–206.

59. Honoré I, Nunes H, Groussard O, et al. Acute respiratory failure after interferon-γ therapy of end-stage pulmonary fibrosis. *Am J Respir Crit Care Med* 2003;167:953–957.

60. Preston IR, Klinger JR, Landzberg MJ, et al. Vasoresponsiveness of sarcoidosis-associated pulmonary hypertension. *Chest* 2001;120(3):866–872.

61. Dantzker DR, Bower JS. Partial reversibility of chronic pulmonary hypertension caused by pulmonary thromboembolic disease. *Am Rev Respir Dis* 1981;124(2):129–131.

62. Sitbon O, Humbert M, Jas X, et al. Long-term response to calcium channel blockers in idiopathic pulmonary arterial hypertension. *Circulation* 2005;111:3105–3111.

63. Archer S, Rich S. Primary pulmonary hypertension: a vascular biology and translational research "work in progress." *Circulation* 2000;28:2781–2791.

64. Simonneau G, Barst RJ, Galie N, et al. Continuous subcutaneous infusion of treprostinil, a prostacyclin analogue, in patients with pulmonary arterial hypertension. *Am J Respir Crit Care Med* 2002;165:800–804.

65. Galie N, Humbert M, Vachiery JL, et al. Effects of beraprost sodium, an oral prostacyclin analogue, in patients with pulmonary arterial hypertension: a randomized, double-blind, placebo-controlled trial. *J Am Coll Cardiol* 2002;39(9):1496–1502.

66. Olschewski H, Simonneau G, Galie N, et al. Inhaled iloprost for severe pulmonary hypertension. *N Engl J Med* 2002;347(5):322–329.

67. Channick R, Simonneau G, Sitbon O, et al. Effects of the dual endothelin-receptor antagonist bosentan in patients with pulmonary hypertension: a randomized placebo-controlled study. *Lancet* 2001;358(9288):1119–1123.

68. Galiè N, Ghofrani HA, Torbicki A, et al. Sildenafil citrate therapy for pulmonary arterial hypertension. *N Engl J Med* 2005;353(20):2148–2157.

69. Schmeruly RT, Dony E, Ghofrani HA, et al. Reversal of experimental pulmonary hypertension by PDGF inhibition. *J Clin Invest* 2005;115(10):2811–2821.

70. Ghofrani HA, Seeger W, Grimminger F. Imatinib for the treatment of pulmonary arterial hypertension. *N Eng J Med* 2005;353(13):1412–1413.

71. Mendeloff EN, Meyers BF, Sundt TM, et al. Lung transplantation for pulmonary vascular disease. *Ann Thorac Surg* 2002;73(1):209–217.

72. Conte JV, Borja MJ, Patel CB, et al. Lung transplantation for primary and secondary pulmonary hypertension. *Ann Thorac Surg* 2001;72(5):1673–1679.

73. Katz WE, Gasior TA, Quinlan JJ, et al. Immediate effects of lung transplantation on right ventricular morphology and function of patients with variable degrees of pulmonary hypertension. *J Am Coll Cardiol* 1996;27(2):384–391.

74. D'Alonzo GE, Barst RJ, Ayres SM, et al. Survival in patients with primary pulmonary hypertension. *Ann Intern Med* 1991;115(5):343–349.

75. Barst RJ, Rubin LJ, McGoon MD, et al. Survival in primary pulmonary hypertension with long-term continuous intravenous prostacyclin. *Ann Intern Med* 1994;121(6):409–415.

76. Incalzi RA, Fuzo L, De Rosa M, et al. Electrocardiographic signs in chronic cor pulmonale: A negative prognostic finding in chronic obstructive pulmonary disease. *Circulation* 1999;99(12):1600–1605.

PART (11) Valvular Heart Disease

CHAPTER (74)

Acute Rheumatic Fever

Bongani M. Mayosi / Jonathan R. Carapetis

Acute rheumatic fever (ARF) is a multisystem autoimmune disease resulting from infection with group A streptococcus. Episodes of ARF tend to recur in the same individual unless preventive measures are instituted, and each recurrence increases the chance of long-term damage to the heart valves—that is, rheumatic heart disease (RHD). Now uncommon in the developed world, ARF and RHD remain a major public health problem in developing countries and in some poor, mainly indigenous populations in wealthy countries.

EPIDEMIOLOGY

The incidence of ARF began to decline in developed countries toward the end of the 19th century and by the second half of the 20th century ARF had become rare in most affluent populations. This decline is attributed to more hygienic and less crowded living conditions, better nutrition, improved access to medical care, and, to a lesser extent, the advent of antibiotics in the 1950s. However, according to the World Health Organization (WHO), approximately 500,000 individuals acquire ARF each year, of whom 97 percent are in developing countries where the incidence of ARF exceeds 50 per 100,000 children per year. Epidemiologic data from many developing countries are poor and these are very likely to be underestimates. Much higher rates of 80 to 500 per 100,000 have been documented in careful studies in the indigenous populations of Australia and New Zealand.[1] By contrast, the incidence of ARF in industrialized countries is less than 10 per 100,000 children.[1,2] There have been several outbreaks of ARF in middle-class populations in the intermountain region of the United States since the mid-1980s, associated with mucoid strains of group A streptococcus, particularly of M type 18.[3]

The peak incidence of ARF occurs in those ages 5 to 15 years, with a decline thereafter such that cases are rare in adults older than age 35 years.[1] First attacks are rare in the very young; only 5 percent of first episodes arise in children younger than age 5 years and the disease is almost unheard of in those younger than age 2 years.[4] Recurrent attacks are most frequent in adolescence and young adulthood, and are diagnosed infrequently after age 45 years.

ARF is equally common in males and females, but RHD is more common in females. Whether this trend is a result of innate susceptibility, increased exposure to group A streptococcus because of greater involvement of women in child rearing, or reduced access to preventive medical care for females is unclear.[1] No association with ethnic origin has been found. There is some evidence that between 3 and 6 percent of any population is susceptible to ARF.[5]

PATHOGENESIS

Epidemiologic and immunologic evidence clearly implicates group A -hemolytic streptococcus in the initiation of the disease in a susceptible host. Most patients with ARF have elevated titers of antistreptococcal antibodies. Outbreaks of ARF usually follow epidemics of streptococcal pharyngitis. Adequate treatment of streptococcal pharyngitis reduces the incidence of subsequent ARF and appropriate antimicrobial prophylaxis prevents recurrences after initial attacks.[6,7]

It has generally been considered that certain strains of group A streptococcus are more prone to result in ARF, and this "rheumatogenicity" was thought to be a feature of strains belonging to certain M serotypes. More recent studies suggest that rheumatogenicity may not be serotype specific. The long-held opinion that only streptococcal pharyngitis, and not streptococcal skin infections such as impetigo, may be followed by ARF has also been challenged.[8] Studies in populations where ARF is common find no definite association between group A streptococcal sequence type and site of infection or ability to cause disease.[9,10] Thus the distinction between rheumatogenic and nonrheumatogenic strains, and between those trophic for the skin or throat, is considered by some to become blurred in areas where ARF is common and multiple different group A streptococcal strains circulate within small populations.[1]

Host factors have been considered to be important ever since familial clustering was reported last century. Associations between disease and human leukocyte antigen (HLA) class II alleles have been identified, but the alleles associated with susceptibility or protection differ depending on the population investigated.[11] High concentrations of circulating mannose-binding lectin and polymorphisms of transforming growth factor-β_1 and immunoglobulin genes also are associated with ARF.[12–14]

Certain B-cell alloantigens are expressed to a greater level in patients with ARF or RHD than controls, with family members having intermediate expression, suggesting that these antigens are markers of inherited susceptibility. The best characterized is D8/17, which is associated with ARF and RHD in several populations worldwide.[15] Further investigation is needed before B-cell alloantigen markers can be used to identify individuals with, or at risk for, ARF or RHD. There is, as yet, no specific investigation that reliably identifies individuals who are at risk of ARF or who will develop chronic rheumatic valvular heart disease.

The molecular mimicry theory holds that antibodies or cellular immune responses directed against group A streptococci cross-react with epitopes on host tissue.[16] Streptococcal M protein and a carbohydrate streptococcal antigen (*N*-acetylglucosamine in group A carbohydrate) share epitopes with cardiac myosin and valve tissue. There is no myosin in cardiac valves, the main site of human cardiac damage, but it is known that laminin in valvular basement membrane is recognized by T cells against myosin and the M protein. Antibodies to valve tissue cross-react with *N*-acetylglucosamine in group A carbohydrate.[1] In an animal model, antibodies that caused chorea bound to both the carbohydrate antigen and mammalian lysoganglioside.

The exact mechanism of the initial insult is unclear. Subsequent damage appears to be caused by T-cell and macrophage infiltration, which persists for years after the initial event.[11] The pathologic lesion of ARF is the Aschoff body, a granulomatous lesion containing T and B cells, macrophages, large mononuclear cells, multinucleated giant cells and polymorphonuclear leukocytes in the myocardium (Fig. 74–1).[17]

CLINICAL PRESENTATION

The protean manifestations of this condition were well described in the middle of the last century. The Jones criteria, established in 1944 and modified and updated subsequently (Table 74–1), are the current "gold-standard" for diagnosis.[18,19] Revisions of the Jones criteria have increased specificity but decreased sensitivity. Overreliance on the Jones criteria in areas where ARF is common may result in missed diagnoses and failure to provide secondary prophylaxis to deserving patients.

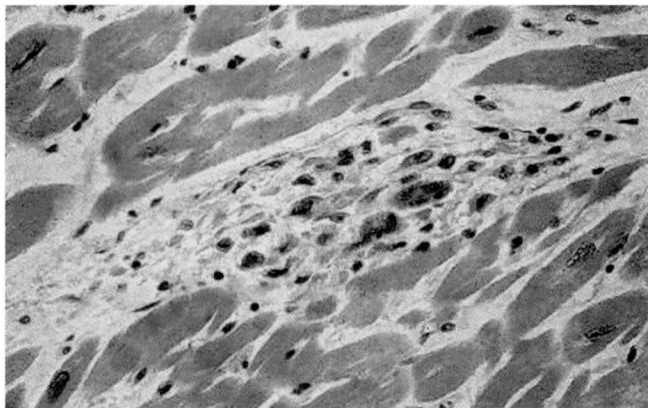

FIGURE 74–1. Aschoff body. A myocardial Aschoff body that is characterized by a nodular aggregate of large mononuclear and multinuclear cells. *Source: Reproduced with permission from Binotto MA, Guilherme L, Tanaka AC. Rheumatic fever. Images Paediatr Cardiol 2002;11:12–25.*

The disease usually has an acute febrile onset and variable combinations of arthritis and arthralgia, carditis, chorea, and skin manifestations.

[ ] ARTHRITIS AND ARTHRALGIA

The classical description is of a polyarthritis affecting large joints, with the lower-limb joints involved first, and involvement of each joint overlapping to give the impression that the process "migrates." The arthritis of ARF responds promptly to antiinflammatories and thus the classical presentation may be uncommon where self-medication with readily available NSAIDs or their prescription before the diagnosis is considered or confirmed is common. Monoarticular arthritis is recognized to be important in populations where ARF is common.

The differential diagnosis of polyarticular arthritis in children and adolescents is wide (Table 74–2).[20] Poststreptococcal reactive arthritis is diagnosed in patients who have an arthritis that is not typical of ARF but who recently had streptococcal infection. This condition is said to occur after a shorter latent period than ARF, responds less well to antiinflammatories, may be associated with renal manifestations, and evidence of carditis is usually not seen. The distinction between poststreptococcal reactive arthritis and ARF is unclear and many would recommend that a diagnosis of poststreptococcal reactive arthritis not be made in populations in which ARF is common.[1,20] Even if the diagnosis is considered it is appropriate to offer a period of secondary penicillin prophylaxis as for episodes of ARF in such populations.[20]

[ ] CARDITIS

Carditis is the single most important component of the disease in determining prognosis. Pathologically, ARF produces a pancarditis with involvement of the pericardium, myocardium and endocardium. Clinical manifestations may vary widely and range from subclinical to life-threatening. Pericarditis may manifest with typical pericardial pain and a friction rub. Auscultation may reveal new murmurs or changing murmurs. The commonest valvular lesion is mitral regurgitation causing an apical pansystolic murmur. Aortic regurgitation is less common. Stenotic lesions are uncommon in the early stages of the disease, but a transient apical mid-

TABLE 74-1

2002–2003 WHO Criteria for Diagnosis of Acute Rheumatic Fever and Rheumatic Heart Disease

DIAGNOSTIC CATEGORIES	CRITERIA
1. Primary episode of rheumatic fever.	Two major[a] or one major and two minor[b] manifestations plus evidence of a preceding group A streptococcal infection.[c]
2. Recurrent attack of rheumatic fever in a patient without established rheumatic heart disease.	As for a primary episode of rheumatic fever.
3. Recurrent attack of rheumatic fever in a patient with established rheumatic heart disease	Two minor manifestations plus evidence of a preceding group A streptococcal infection.
4. Rheumatic chorea	Other major manifestations or evidence of group A streptococcal infection are not required because these are delayed manifestations of streptococcal infection.
5. Insidious onset rheumatic carditis	
6. Chronic valve lesions of rheumatic heart disease, i.e., patients presenting for the first time with pure mitral stenosis or mixed mitral valve disease with or without aortic valve disease.	Do not require any other criteria to be diagnoses as having rheumatic heart disease.

[a]Major manifestations: carditis, polyarthritis, chorea, erythema marginatum, and subcutaneous nodules.
[b]Minor manifestations: clinical—fever, polyarthralgia; electrocardiogram–prolonged PR interval; laboratory—elevated acute phase reactants (erythrocyte sedimentation rate, white cell count, C-reactive protein).
[c]Supporting evidence of a preceding streptococcal infection within the last 45 days: elevated or rising antistreptolysin-O or other streptococcal antibody, or a positive throat culture, or rapid antigen test for group A streptococci, or recent scarlet fever.
SOURCE: WHO Technical Report Series No. 923.[19]

diastolic murmur (Carey-Coombs) may occur in association with the murmur of mitral regurgitation.

Severe valvular inflammation, particularly if it occurs on a background of preexisting rheumatic valvular disease, may produce life-threatening heart failure. Atrioventricular conduction delay, which is common, rarely produces clinical symptoms but is an important and helpful diagnostic clue.

【 】 CHOREA

Sydenham chorea may be associated with other manifestations of ARF but may also be the sole expression of the disease. It is a neurologic disorder characterized by involuntary, purposeless, rapid, and abrupt movements associated with muscular weakness and emotional lability. The abnormal movements disappear during sleep.

Mild chorea may best be demonstrated by asking the patient to squeeze the examiner's hand. This results in repetitive irregular squeezes labeled as "the milking sign." Emotional lability manifests in personality changes with inappropriate behavior, restlessness, and outbursts of anger or crying.[20]

【 】 SKIN MANIFESTATIONS

Older descriptions of ARF were prominently illustrated with pictures of patients with large rheumatic subcutaneous nodules, although this

manifestation is rare in recent reports of the disease. The nodules generally appear later in the course of the disease after several weeks of illness and are seen most commonly in patients with carditis. They are firm and painless, the overlying skin is not inflamed and may vary in size from a few millimeters to several centimeters. They are most commonly located over bony surfaces or tendons and best detected by palpating actively to seek them over elbows, wrists, knees, occiput, and spinous processes of the vertebrae.

Erythema marginatum is a nonitchy, evanescent rash that is pink or slightly red, and which affects the trunk predominantly. The rash extends centrifugally and the skin in the center returns toward normal (Fig. 74–2). The rash may be fleeting and disappear within hours. It may be brought out by a warm bath or shower. It is reported to be found in only 4 to 15 percent of cases and may be difficult to detect in dark-skinned patients.

Many other clinical features occur in patients with ARF, including abdominal pain (occasionally severe enough to have warranted laparotomy in the past), malaise, anemia, epistaxis, rapid sleeping pulse rate, and tachycardia out of proportion to the fever. These signs and symptoms are frequent in many other illnesses and thus are not useful diagnostically.

DIAGNOSIS AND INVESTIGATIONS

There is no definitive laboratory test for ARF and diagnosis is based on a combination of clinical manifestations and laboratory evidence of previous streptococcal infection. The Jones and WHO criteria (see Table 74–1) require two major or one major and two

TABLE 74-2

Differential Diagnosis[a] of Polyarthritis in Children and Adolescents

Acute rheumatic fever
Other autoimmune disease
Septic arthritis
Poststreptococcal reactive arthritis
Infective endocarditis
Lyme disease
Lymphoma/leukemia
Viral arthropathy
Sickle cell disease

[a]Excludes presentations with chorea.

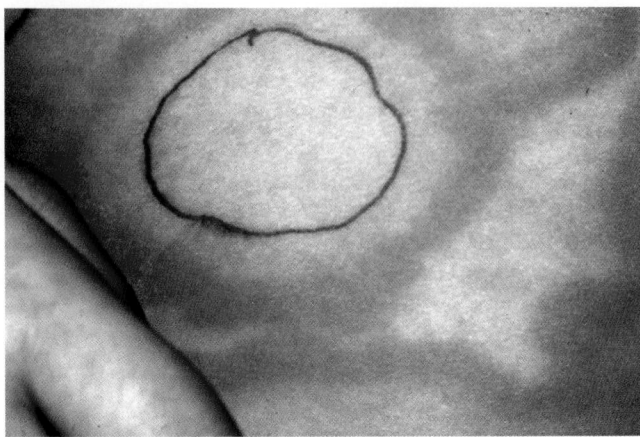

FIGURE 74–2. Erythema marginatum. Erythema marginatum on the trunk of an 8-year old Caucasian boy. The pen mark shows the location of the rash approximately 60 minutes previously. *Source: Photo kindly provided by Professor Mike South, Royal Children's Hospital, Melbourne, Australia. Published in a chapter for the textbook Infectious Diseases, edited by Cohen and Powderly.*

minor manifestations to be present, plus evidence of antecedent group A streptococcal infection to establish the diagnosis in an initial episode.[18,19]

There has been concern that strict application of the Jones criteria may result in underdiagnosis particularly in the case of recurrent episodes.[20] During recurrence of rheumatic activity in a patient with preexisting RHD the carditis may precipitate heart failure but may not be possible to diagnose because of lack of information on previous cardiac findings or because valve replacement surgery has been performed. The new WHO criteria thus recommend that a diagnosis of a recurrence of ARF in a patient with preexisting RHD is possible on the basis of minor manifestations and evidence of recent streptococcal infection (see Table 74–1).[19]

Doctors should recognize that the published criteria are guidelines, and are particularly useful in epidemiologic investigations where diagnostic rigor is essential. It is appropriate for clinical judgment to be applied and to supersede guidelines, particularly in parts of the world where ARF remains common.[20]

Evidence of preceding streptococcal infection may be demonstrated by increased or rising antistreptolysin-*O* titer, or other streptococcal antibodies, or a positive throat swab culture, or rapid antigen test for group A β-hemolytic streptococci. Serology may be difficult to interpret in populations in which streptococcal infection is common. Absolute values may be unreliable. Variation in normal antibody titers is well recognized to be related to age and geographical location.

Laboratory investigations are otherwise nonspecific and usually unhelpful diagnostically, but as markers of disease activity they may be a useful guide when tapering and stopping antiinflammatory therapy. Inflammatory markers such as C-reactive protein and erythrocyte sedimentation rate are usually elevated. Modest normochromic normocytic anaemia of chronic inflammation is frequent.

The electrocardiogram may be unhelpful apart from reflecting sinus tachycardia. Prolongation of the PR interval serves as a useful minor criterion and a clinically helpful clue, which may be particularly relevant in recurrences where previous electrocardiograms are available. During sinus tachycardia the PR interval usually shortens, and even modest prolongation is abnormal in the face of tachycardia.

Clinical evaluation is central to the diagnosis of ARF and echocardiography is not widely available in populations in which the disease is common. It is, however, becoming more widely available, which brings with it both advantages and disadvantages. Used correctly by experienced clinicians echocardiography is an excellent tool that may prevent overdiagnosis of ARF by excluding physiologic flow murmurs and undetected congenital heart disease.[19]

TREATMENT

[ ] MANAGEMENT OF THE ACUTE EPISODE

The aims of treatment of ARF are to suppress the inflammatory response so as to minimize cardiac damage, to provide symptomatic relief, and to eradicate pharyngeal streptococcal infection.[20] Patients are usually hospitalized and the long-standing recommendation of bedrest or chair rest is appropriate if heart failure is present. Ambulation is usually started once fever has subsided and joint pain and heart failure are controlled.

Although evidence of active infection is unusual during the acute phase, it is recommended that patients receive a single dose of benzathine penicillin or a 10-day course of penicillin-V (or erythromycin if penicillin allergic) to curtail exposure to streptococcal antigens. After completion of the course, secondary prophylaxis should be commenced.

Antiinflammatory agents, including salicylates and corticosteroids in appropriate dose provide dramatic improvement in symptoms such as arthritis and fever soon after starting treatment. Doses of aspirin of 80 to 100 mg/kg/d in children and 4 to 8 g/d in adults may be needed initially. The usual dose of prednisone or prednisolone is 1 to 2 mg/kg/d. There is no good evidence that steroids are superior to aspirin in terms of altering the natural history of the disease.[21] Some believe that they do result in more rapid resolution of carditis and can be lifesaving, but this is unproven.[22] Antiinflammatory agents are usually used in high dose for about 2 weeks and then decreased by approximately 20 percent each week, depending on clinical response and laboratory measurement of inflammatory markers. When tapering steroids it is recommended to overlap with aspirin to prevent the rebound of disease.

Patients with severe heart failure require usual antifailure treatment. When carditis complicated by marked valvular regurgitation causes severe hemodynamic compromise, valve surgery is lifesaving and should not be delayed by trials of antiinflammatory medication.[23] Valve replacement rather than repair is the preferred option under these circumstances, but must be performed by a surgeon experienced in rheumatic valvular surgery.[20]

[ ] PREVENTION

Primary prevention refers to antibiotic treatment of group A streptococcal pharyngitis to prevent subsequent attacks of ARF. A single intramuscular injection of 600,000 or 1.2 million units of benzathine penicillin (depending on weight) or 10 days of penicillin V is advised (Table 74–3). Efforts at primary prevention are confounded by the fact that many patients who develop ARF are not aware of preceding sore throat, there are no simple specific clinical signs diagnostic of streptococcal pharyngitis, and throat swabs and

TABLE 74–3

Prevention of Acute Rheumatic Fever

AGENT	DOSE	ROUTE	DURATION
Primary Prevention			
Benzathine penicillin G	≥27 kg: 1.2 million units <27 kg: 600,000 units	IM injection	Once
Penicillin V	Children 250 mg, ×2–3/d Adults 500 mg, ×2–3/d	Oral	10 days
Erythromycin estolate (if penicillin allergy)	20–40 mg/kg/d ×2–4/d (max 1 g/d)	Oral	10 days
Secondary Prevention (prevention of recurrent attacks)			
Benzathine penicillin G	≥30 kg: 1.2 million units (<30 kg: 600,000 units) every 2–4 weeks[a]	IM injection	
Penicillin V	250 mg ×2/d	Oral	
Erythromycin	250 mg ×2/d	Oral	

[a]Duration of secondary prophylaxis depends on history of carditis and if valvular involvement persists.

cultures are expensive. However, antibiotic treatment for suspected streptococcal sore throat, with the diagnosis made on clinical grounds, is effective in reducing the occurrence of subsequent attacks of ARF by 70 to 80 percent.[6] It has been suggested that this approach may be affordable for developing countries as a strategy for preventing ARF,[6] although there are few examples of the success of this strategy in reducing overall ARF incidence.[1]

Secondary prevention, the long-term administration of antibiotics to prevent recurrences, is of proven benefit and is cost-effective.[7] Benzathine penicillin 600,000 or 1.2 million units intramuscularly every 4 weeks is the standard recommendation.[19] An injection once every 2 or 3 weeks is more effective but may be more difficult to implement.[7] Oral penicillin V 250 mg orally twice daily is preferred by some practitioners particularly in very thin patients who are on warfarin anticoagulation after valve replacement surgery when deep intramuscular injections may be undesirable.[20] However, no studies have compared oral penicillin V with intramuscular benzathine penicillin in the prevention of rheumatic fever.

Prophylaxis has been advised until age 21 years or for at least 5 years after the last attack of ARF, whichever is longer. The WHO points out that it is not possible to generalize, and duration of secondary prophylaxis should be individualized taking into account factors influencing risk of recurrence (see Table 74–3).[19] Lifelong prophylaxis is recommended for patients with severe valve disease or after valve replacement surgery.[19]

PROGNOSIS

Rheumatic fever is said to be a disease that "licks the joints and bites the heart."[20] This underlines the fact that cardiac involvement is the most serious manifestation of ARF. ARF may be associated with severe heart failure, which may be life-threatening if appropriate medical and surgical therapy is not instituted. The failure to put patients with ARF on antibiotic prophylaxis to prevent future attacks leads to repeated episodes of ARF, scarring of the heart valves, chronic valvular heart disease, heart failure, and death, usually before middle age.

REFERENCES

1. Carapetis J, McDonald M, Wilson NJ. Acute rheumatic fever. *Lancet* 2005;366:155–168.
2. Lennon D. Rheumatic fever, a preventable disease? The New Zealand experience. In: Martin DR, Tagg JR, eds. *Streptococci and Streptococcal Diseases: Entering the New Millennium*. Porirua: Institute of Environmental Science and Research, 2000:503–512.
3. Veasy LG, Tani LY, Daly JA, et al. Temporal association of the appearance of mucoid strains of *Streptococcus pyogenes* with a continuing high incidence of rheumatic fever in Utah. *Pediatrics* 2004;113:e168–e172.
4. Tani LY, Veasy LG, Minich LL, at al. Rheumatic fever in children younger than 5 years: is the presentation different? *Pediatrics* 2003;112:1065–1068.
5. Carapetis JR, Currie BJ, Mathews JD. Cumulative incidence of rheumatic fever in an endemic region: a guide to the susceptibility of the population? *Epidemiol Infect* 2000;124:239–244.
6. Robertson KA, Volmink JA, Mayosi BM. Antibiotics for the primary prevention of acute rheumatic fever: a meta-analysis. *BMC Cardiovasc Disord* 2005;5:11.
7. Manyemba J, Mayosi BM. Intramuscular penicillin is more effective than oral penicillin in secondary prevention of rheumatic fever—a systematic review. *S Afr Med J* 2003;93:212–218.
8. McDonald M, Currie BJ, Carapetis JR. Acute rheumatic fever: a chink in the chain that links the heart to the throat? *Lancet Infect Dis* 2004;4:240–245.
9. Bessen DE, Carapetis JR, Beall B, et al. Contrasting molecular epidemiology of group A streptococci causing tropical and nontropical infections of the skin and throat. *J Infect Dis* 2000;182:1109–1116.
10. Pruksakorn S, Sittisombut N, Phornphutkul C, et al. Epidemiological analysis of non–M-typeable group A *Streptococcus* isolates from a Thai population in northern Thailand. *J Clin Microbiol* 2000;38:1250–1254.
11. Guilherme L, Fae K, Oshiro SE, et al. Molecular pathogenesis of rheumatic fever and rheumatic heart disease. *Expert Rev Mol Med* 2005;7:1–15.
12. Berdeli A, Celik HA, Ozyurek R, et al. Involvement of immunoglobulin FcgammaRIIA and FcgammaRIIIB gene polymorphisms in susceptibility to rheumatic fever. *Clin Biochem* 2004;37:925–929.
13. Chou HT, Chen CH, Tsai CH, et al. Association between transforming growth factor-beta1 gene C-509T and T869C polymorphisms and rheumatic heart disease. *Am Heart J* 2004;148:181–186.
14. Schafranski MD, Stier A, Nisihara R, et al. Significantly increased levels of mannose-binding lectin (MBL) in rheumatic heart disease: a beneficial role for MBL deficiency. *Clin Exp Immunol* 2004;138:521–525.

15. Khanna AK, Buskirk DR, Williams RCJ, et al. Presence of a non-HLA B cell antigen in rheumatic fever patients and their families as defined by a monoclonal antibody. *J Clin Invest* 1989;83:1710–1716.

16. Bisno AL, Brito MO, Collins CM. Molecular basis of group A streptococcal virulence. *Lancet Infect Dis* 2003;3:191–200.

17. Binotto MA, Guilherme L, Tanaka AC. Rheumatic fever. *Images Paediatr Cardiol* 2002;11:12–25.

18. Guidelines for the diagnosis of rheumatic fever. Jones criteria, 1992 update. Special Writing Group of the Committee on Rheumatic Fever, Endocarditis, and Kawasaki Disease of the Council on Cardiovascular Disease in the Young of the American Heart Association. *JAMA* 1992;268:2069–2073.

19. WHO Technical Report Series No. 923. *Rheumatic Fever and Rheumatic Heart Disease: Report of a WHO Expert Panel, Geneva 29 October –1 November 2001.* Geneva: WHO, 2004.

20. Cilliers AM, Manyemba J, Saloojee H. Anti-inflammatory treatment for carditis in acute rheumatic fever. *Cochrane Database Syst Rev* 2003;2:CD003176.

21. Cilliers A. Treating acute rheumatic fever. *BMJ* 2003;327:631–632.

22. Essop MR, Nkomo V. Rheumatic and nonrheumatic valvular heart disease: epidemiology, management, and prevention in Africa. *Circulation* 2005;112:3584–3591.

23. Monya-Tambi I, Robertson KR, Volmink JA, et al. Acute rheumatic fever. *Lancet* 2005;366:1355.

CHAPTER 75

Aortic Valve Disease

Shahbudin H. Rahimtoola

Rheumatic heart disease is not the most important cause of valve disease in the developed countries. Mitral valve prolapse and congenital aortic valve disease are the most common valvular lesions. Most patients with severe valve disease are considered candidates for surgery. Echocardiography/Doppler ultrasound has a very important role in the diagnosis and followup of these patients. Cardiac catheterization/angiography remains an extremely important diagnostic procedure that is needed in almost all patients considered for interventional therapy.

AORTIC VALVE STENOSIS

Aortic stenosis (AS) is obstruction to outflow of blood from the left ventricle (LV), which may be at the valve, above the valve (supravalvular), or below the valve (subvalvular).[1] Supravalvular AS is a congenital lesion. Subvalvular AS results either from a congenital discrete fibromuscular obstruction or from a muscular obstruction (hypertrophic cardiomyopathy).

【 】 ETIOLOGY

A heritable component was documented in the Utah Population Database of 2,237,324 individuals. The familial relative risk of

death for age <65 years was four times higher in first-degree relatives of those with aortic valve disease.[2]

The most common causes of AS are congenital, rheumatic, and calcific (degenerative).[1] Calcific AS is seen in patients 35 years of age or older and is the result of calcification of a congenital or rheumatic valve or of a normal valve. Other causes of AS[1] are rare (Table 75–1). At the present time, calcific AS in the older patient is the most common valve lesion requiring aortic valve replacement (AVR).[1,3] Among patients younger than age 70 years, congenital bicuspid valve accounted for one-half of the surgical cases; "degenerative" changes were the cause in 18 percent.[4] In those age 70 years or older, degenerative changes accounted for almost one-half of the surgical cases and a congenital bicuspid valve accounted for approximately one-quarter of the cases (Fig. 75–1).

"Degenerative" or calcific AS is an atherosclerotic disorder. The mechanism is a "response to injury," similar to what has been described for vascular atherosclerosis. The evidence for this etiology and the mechanism can be summarized as follows: (1) animals fed a high-cholesterol diet develop atherosclerotic lesions on the aortic valve (AV)[5]; (2) those animals who were also fed atorvastatin showed markedly lower lesions (Fig. 75–2)[5]; (3) risk factors for calcific AS are similar to those that promote the development of vascular atherosclerosis[4]; (4) there is evidence of inflammation

TABLE 75–1

Etiology of Aortic Valve Stenosis

I. Congenital
II. Acquired
  A. Rheumatic
  B. Calcific (degenerative/autoimmune)
  C. Rare causes
    1. Obstructive infective vegetations
    2. Homozygous type II hyperlipoproteinemia
    3. Paget disease of bone
    4. Systemic lupus erythematosus
    5. Rheumatoid involvement
    6. Ochronosis (alkaptonuria)
    7. Irradiation

(Fig. 75–3)[6–8]; (5) the early lesion is an atherosclerotic plaque[9]; (6) calcified AV have all the markers of bone formation[9–10]; and (7) the low-density lipoprotein coreceptor (Lrp 5/Wnt3 signaling pathway) is upregulated to a greater extent in the calcified AV than in the "degenerative" mitral valve.[11]

PATHOLOGY

In congenital AS, the valve may be unicuspid, bicuspid, or tricuspid, depending on the patient's age.[1] In patients younger than age 15 years, more than 80 percent of stenotic valves are either unicuspid or bicuspid and 15 to 20 percent are tricuspid.[12] In patients ages 15 to 65 years, 60 percent are bicuspid, 10 percent are unicuspid, and 25 to 30 percent are tricuspid.[12] In patients 65 years of age or older, 90 percent of the valves are tricuspid and 10 percent are bicuspid. Unicuspid valves produce severe obstruction in infancy. Congenital bicuspid valves can produce severe obstruction to LV outflow after the first few years of life.[1] The valvular abnormality produces turbulent flow, which traumatizes the leaflets and eventually leads to fibrosis, rigidity, and calcification of the valve. In a congenitally abnormal tricuspid aortic valve, the cusps are of unequal size and have some degree of commissural fusion; the third cusp may be diminutive. Eventually, the abnormal structure leads to changes similar to those seen in a bicuspid valve, and significant LV outflow obstruction often results. In calcific AS, early changes show chronic inflammatory cell infiltrate (macrophages and T lymphocytes), lipids in lesions and in adjacent fibrosa, and thickening of fibrosa with collagen and elastin.[4] These patients also have a higher incidence of risk factors for coronary atherosclerosis.[13]

Rheumatic AS results from adhesions and fusion of the commissures and cusps. The leaflets and the valve ring become vascularized, which leads to retraction and stiffening of the cusps. Calcification occurs, and the aortic valve orifice is reduced to a small triangular or round opening, which is frequently regurgitant as well as stenotic.

Importantly, the heart exhibits other evidence of rheumatic heart disease, namely, involvement of the mitral valve and presence of Aschoff nodules in the myocardium.

The LV is concentrically hypertrophied.[14] The hypertrophied cardiac muscle cells are increased in size, with their transverse diameters ranging from 15 to 70 μm (normal: 10 to 15 μm). There is an increase of connective tissue[15,16] and a variable amount of fibrous tissue (collagen fibrils) in the interstitial tissue. Usually, the cardiac muscle cells do not degenerate in patients with AS. Myocardial ultrastructural changes[1] may account for the LV systolic dysfunction that occurs late in the disease; such changes include unusually large nuclei, loss of myofibrils, accumulation of mitochondria, large cytoplasmic areas devoid of contractile material, and proliferation of fibroblasts and collagen fibers in the interstitial space. Subclinical calcific emboli are commonly found in calcific AS if diligently sought at autopsy.

PATHOPHYSIOLOGY

With reduction in the *aortic valve area* (AVA), energy is dissipated during the transport of blood from the LV to the aorta. The AVA has to be reduced by approximately 50 percent of normal before a measurable gradient can be demonstrated in humans.[17] When a pressure gradient develops between the LV and the ascending aorta, LV pressure rises; aortic pressure remains within the normal range until end-stage heart failure occurs. The relationship of AVA to cardiac output and pressure gradient is discussed in Chap. 17. As LV pressure rises, ventricular wall stress increases, which leads to impaired LV function. Hypertrophy develops in proportion to increased intraventricular pressure, and myocardial stress remains normal.[18] *Thus, the major compensatory mechanism by which the heart copes with LV outflow obstruction is left ventricular hypertrophy (LVH).* LV mass in patients with severe AS undergoing AVR averages 229 g/m² (normal: 105 g/m²)[16]; LV volume is within the normal range,[18] and so there is a considerable thickening of the LV wall.

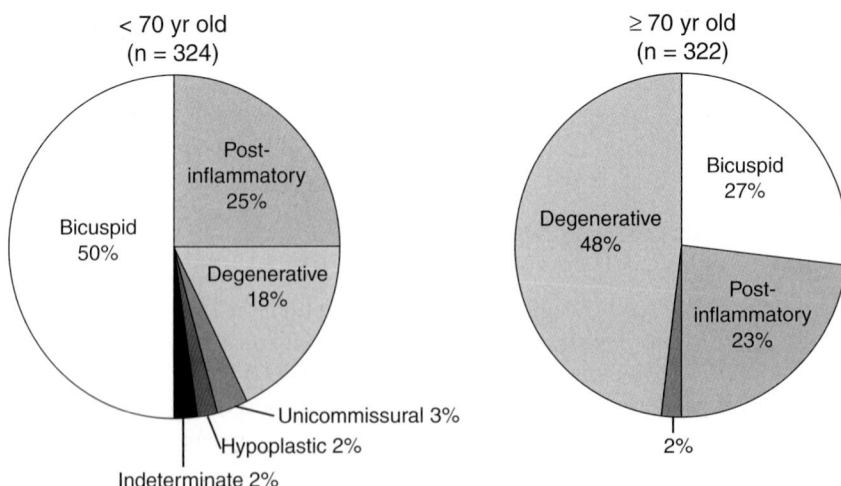

FIGURE 75–1. Etiology of aortic stenosis in patients younger than age 70 years (*left panel*); congenital bicuspid valve accounted for one-half of the surgical cases. In those age 70 years or older (*right panel*), "degenerative" changes accounted for almost one-half of the surgical cases. *Source: From Passik CS, Ackerman DM, Pluth JR, et al. Temporal changes in the causes of aortic stenosis: a surgical pathological study of 646 cases. Mayo Clin Proc 1987;62:119–123, with permission.*

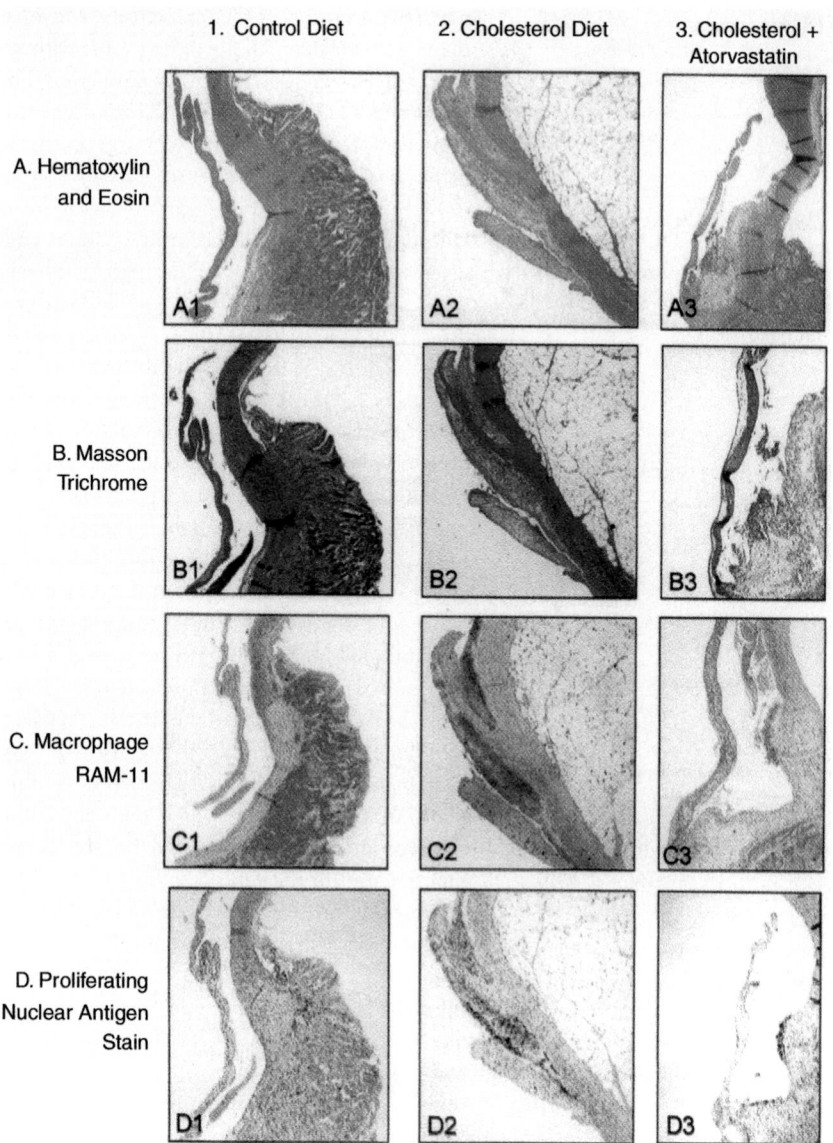

1. Control Diet   2. Cholesterol Diet   3. Cholesterol + Atorvastatin

A. Hematoxylin and Eosin

B. Masson Trichrome

C. Macrophage RAM-11

D. Proliferating Nuclear Antigen Stain

FIGURE 75–2. The normal aortic valve surface is thin and intact, with a smooth endothelial layer in the spongiosa layer of the valve (**A1, B1**) and there are no macrophages or proliferation (**C1, D1**). On the cholesterol diet, foam cells converged to form a large, lipid-laden lesion on the valve leaflet (**A2**) collagen is formed and is stained blue (**B2**), foam cells stained positive for macrophage (**C2**) and there is a marked increased in myofibroblast proliferation cell nuclear antigen staining (**D2**). Animals on cholesterol diet and treated with atorvastatin had a marked decrease (**A3 to D3**) in the abnormal findings seen in animals on only the cholesterol diet (**A2 to D2**). *Source: From Rajamannan NM, Subramanian M, Springett M, et al. Atorvastatin inhibits hypercholesterolemia-induced cellular proliferation and bone matrix production in the rabbit aortic valve. Circulation 2002;105:2660–2265.*

LVH, that is, greater amounts of LVH in spite of similar degrees of severity of AS.[22] They have "supernormal" LV systolic pump function (high LV ejection fraction) and a small, thick-walled chamber with lower end-systolic wall stress.

LV systolic pump function is determined by myocardial (muscle) function and by a combination of LV afterload and preload. Thus, impaired LV systolic pump function (as measured by ejection fraction) may be the result of afterload preload mismatch,[23] impaired myocardial function, or both. LV systolic pump function is normal in most patients with severe AS. When LVH alone is inadequate to overcome the outflow obstruction, the LV uses the Frank-Starling mechanism (preload reserve) to maintain systolic pump function. When the preload reserve is no longer adequate, a reduction of LV systolic pump function occurs (Fig. 75–4). In AS, major use of the preload reserve is not a good compensatory mechanism. Even small increases in LV volume may result in major increases in LV end-diastolic pressure because the LV is on the very steep portion of its diastolic pressure-volume curve, and the corresponding increase in mean LA pressure produces pulmonary edema. Thus, clinical heart failure may be a result of either LV diastolic dysfunction in the presence of normal LV systolic function or impaired myocardial function producing LV systolic dysfunction, with or without associated LV diastolic dysfunction. Eventually, pulmonary artery, right ventricular, and right atrial pressures are elevated. Peripheral edema results from increases in systemic venous pressure and salt and water retention.

In most patients with AS, cardiac output is in the normal range and initially increases normally with exercise. Later, as the severity of AS increases progressively, the cardiac output remains within the normal range at rest, but, on exercise, it no longer increases in proportion to the amount of exercise undertaken or does not increase at all (fixed cardiac output). With the development of heart failure, there is a reduction in the resting cardiac output and a tachycardia. As a result, stroke volume may be so lowered that it results in a small gradient across the LV outflow tract in spite of severe AS. As the patient's age increases, there is a progressive decrease of cardiac output with exercise and a progressive increase of LV end-diastolic pressure at equal levels of AVA. This may be related only to LV diastolic dysfunction and is most marked in the older patient.[24]

In severe AS, myocardial oxygen needs are increased (Fig. 75–5). Total coronary blood flow is increased because of the severe LVH; however, coronary blood flow per 100 g of LV mass is reduced.[25] As a result, blood flow to the subendocardium is inadequate at rest;[26] and because coronary vasodilator reserve is reduced,[27] myocardial blood flow is also reduced further, relative to need, on exercise. Coronary blood flow is diminished because of a reduced coronary perfusion pressure (the elevated LV end-diastolic pressure

The diastolic properties of the LV are affected in AS.[19,20] This diastolic abnormality results from a combination of impaired myocardial relaxation with altered chamber compliance, because the LVH per se offers increased resistance to filling, and from increased myocardial stiffness because of structural alterations.[20] As a result, LV end-diastolic pressure is elevated. Powerful left atrial (LA) contraction produces the required LV filling and results in an elevated LV end-diastolic pressure (atrial booster pump function).[21] The necessary LV filling and fiber length to achieve an adequate stroke volume are achieved by LA systole, which occupies only a small part of the cardiac cycle. In patients 60 years of age or older, a higher percentage of women (41 percent) than men (14 percent) have "excessive"

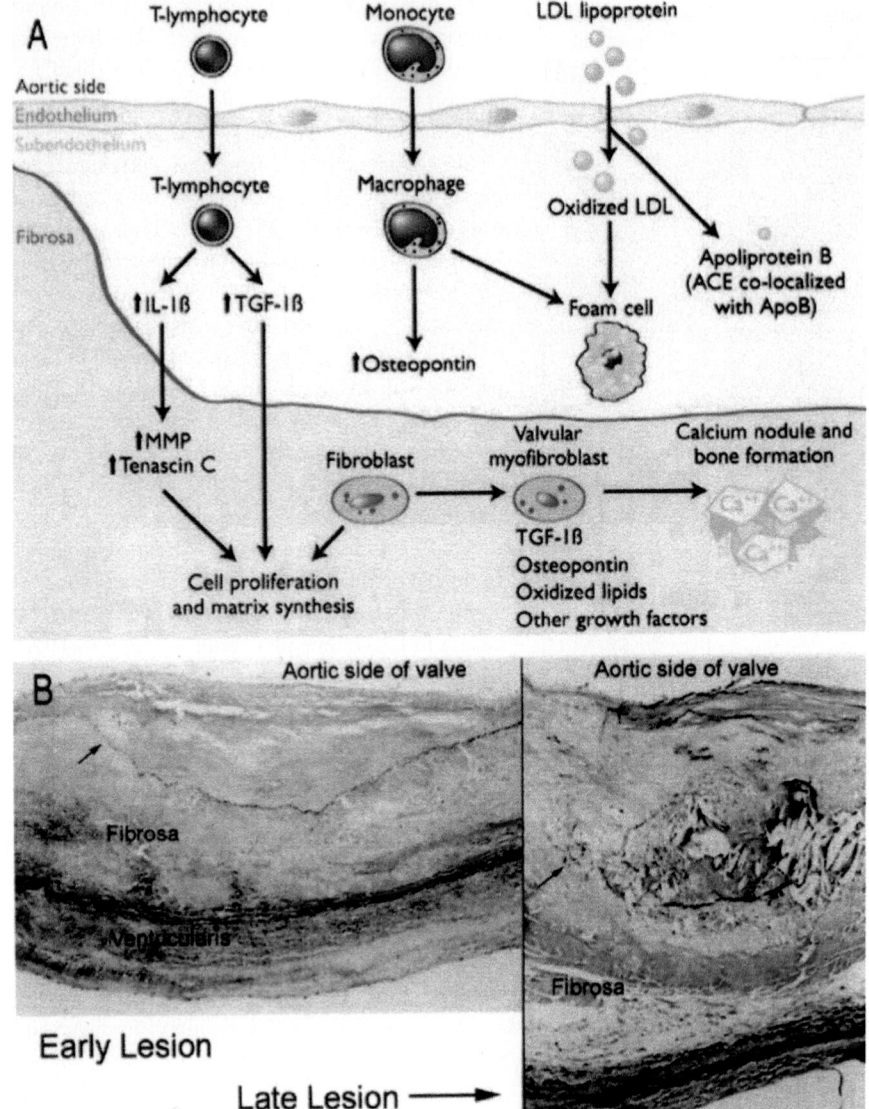

FIGURE 75-3. **A.** Potential pathways depicting calcific aortic valve disease. ACE, angiotensin-converting enzyme; IL, interleukin; LDL, low-density lipoprotein; MMP, matrix metalloproteinase; TGF, transforming growth factor. **B.** Histologic findings in early and late lesions of calcific aortic valve disease. In early lesion, *arrow* indicates displacement of normal subendothelial elastic lamina. In late lesion, *arrow* indicates elastic lamina is displaced and fragmented. (Verhoeff-van Gieson stain, original magnification ×100.) *Source: From Freeman RV, Otto CM. Spectrum of calcific aortic valve disease: pathogenesis, disease progression, and treatment strategies. Circulation 2005;111:3316–3326.*

may have a history of rheumatic fever. Most patients with valvular AS, including some with severe valve stenosis, are asymptomatic. The symptoms of AS are angina pectoris, syncope, exertional presyncope, dyspnea (on exertion, orthopnea, paroxysmal nocturnal dyspnea, pulmonary edema), and the symptoms of heart failure. Once symptoms occur in a patient with severe AS, the life span of the patient is very short without surgical treatment. Sudden cardiac death is stated to occur in 5 percent of patients with AS. It occurs only in those with severe valve stenosis, most of whom have had some cardiac symptoms before the fatal episode. Typical angina pectoris occurs with or without associated CAD (see Fig. 75–3).

Syncope is the result of reduced cerebral perfusion. Syncope occurring on effort is caused by either systemic vasodilatation in the presence of a fixed or inadequate cardiac output, an arrhythmia, or both.[28–30] Syncope at rest is usually caused by a transient ventricular tachyarrhythmia, from which the patient recovers spontaneously. Other possible causes of syncope include transient atrial fibrillation or transient AV block, during which the ventricle is deprived of the powerful atrial booster pump function and/or the ventricular rate is slow.

Dyspnea on exertion, orthopnea, paroxysmal nocturnal dyspnea, and pulmonary edema result from varying degrees of pulmonary venous hypertension. Systemic venous congestion with enlargement of the liver and peripheral edema result from increased systemic venous pressure and salt and water retention. There is an increased incidence of gastrointestinal arteriovenous malformations.[1] As a result, these patients are susceptible to gastrointestinal hemorrhage and anemia. Bleeding can be caused by an acquired defect in the structure of von Willebrand factor.[31] Calcific systemic embolism may occur.[1]

lowers the diastolic aortic–LV pressure gradient) and also because the hypertrophied myocardium compresses the coronary arteries as they traverse the myocardium to supply blood to the subendocardium (systolic "milking" of intramural arteries). As a result, patients may have classic angina pectoris even in the absence of *coronary artery disease* (CAD) (see Chap. 12). Associated obstructive CAD further increases the imbalance between myocardial oxygen needs and supply (see Fig. 75–3).

【 】 CLINICAL FINDINGS
History

Patients with congenital valve stenosis may give a history of a murmur since childhood or infancy; those with rheumatic stenosis

Physical Findings

There is a spectrum of physical findings in patients with AS, depending on the severity of the stenosis, stroke volume, LV function, and the rigidity and calcification of the valve (Table 75–2). The arterial pulse rises slowly, taking a longer time than normal to reach peak pressure, and the peak is reduced (*parvus et tardus*)[32]; the pulse pressure may be narrowed. The anacrotic notch on the upstroke is best appreciated in the carotid arteries. The more severe the valve stenosis, the lower the anacrotic notch on the arterial pulse (see Chap. 12). A systolic thrill may be felt in the carotid arteries. The jugular venous pulse is normal unless the patient is in heart failure. In the absence of heart failure, the heart size is normal. The cardiac impulse is heaving and sustained in character, and there may be a palpable fourth heart sound (S_4). An aortic systolic thrill is often

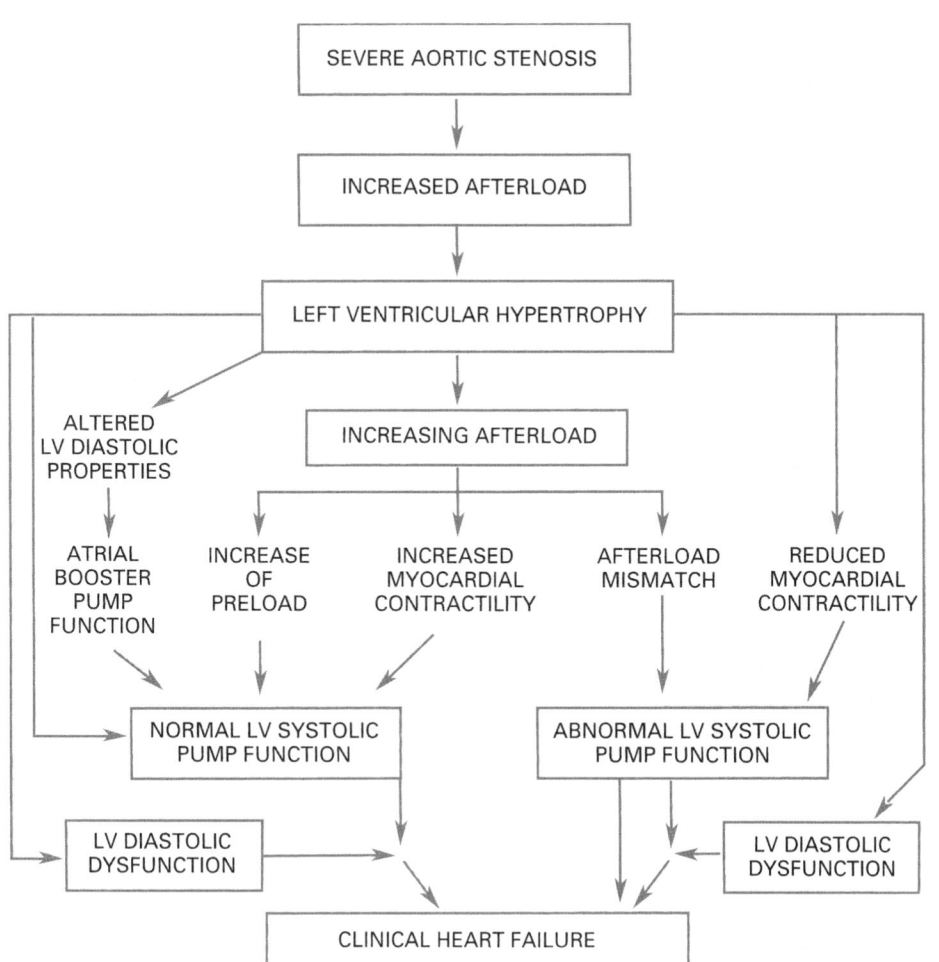

FIGURE 75–4. Illustration of some aspects of the pathophysiology in severe aortic stenosis (see text). The heart responds to aortic stenosis by hypertrophy, and left ventricular (LV) systolic pump function remains normal. LV hypertrophy may alter the LV diastolic properties. As a result, LV end-diastolic pressure is elevated, but powerful atrial contraction produces the required LV filling and fiber length (atrial booster pump function). As LV afterload continues to increase, the LV uses two additional compensatory mechanisms, namely, increase of preload and increase of myocardial contractility. Both of these help maintain normal LV systolic pump function. When the limit of the preload reserve has been reached (afterload mismatch) or myocardial contractility is reduced, LV systolic pump function becomes abnormal. Clinical heart failure is usually a result of abnormal LV systolic pump function; diastolic dysfunction may also be present in some patients. Clinical heart failure in those with normal LV systolic pump function is a result of LV diastolic dysfunction. *Source: Copyright by S.H. Rahimtoola. Rahimtoola SH. Aortic stenosis. In: Rahimtoola SH, ed. Atlas of Heart Diseases: Valvular Heart Disease, vol 11. Philadelphia: Current Medicine, 1997:7.1–7.26.*

present at the base of the heart. In 80 to 90 percent of adult patients with severe AS, there is an S_4 gallop sound, a midsystolic ejection murmur that peaks late in systole, and a single second heart sound (S_2) because A_2 and P_2 are superimposed or A_2 is absent or soft. There is often a faint early diastolic murmur of minimal aortic regurgitation (AR). In the young patient with valvular AS, a systolic ejection sound (systolic ejection click) initiates the systolic murmur but later tends to disappear as AS becomes severe (see Chap. 12). The systolic ejection click is more commonly heard in patients with a bicuspid AV. The S_2 may be paradoxically split because of late A_2, and there may be no early diastolic murmur. In many patients, particularly the older patients, the systolic ejection murmur is atypical, may be soft, is described as a seagull sound (or musical, or cooing), and may be heard only at the apex of the heart (Gallavardin phenomenon). In the presence of heart failure, the jugular venous pressure is often increased, the LV is dilated, a third heart sound is present, and the systolic murmur may be very soft or absent. Thus, the clinical features on physical examination may resemble those of heart failure from a variety of causes, such as dilated cardiomyopathy, rather than AS (see Chap. 12).

Severe valvular AS is common in patients 60 years of age or older.[33] The clinical features in many of these patients tend to be somewhat different.[33] Systemic hypertension is present in approximately 20 percent of the patients, half of whom have moderate or severe systolic and diastolic hypertension. A fifth of the patients first present in heart failure. The male-to-female ratio is 2:1. Because of thickening of the arterial wall and its associated lack of distensibility, the arterial pulse rises normally or even rapidly, and the pulse pressure is wide. The S_2 is either absent or single. As noted earlier, the murmur may be high pitched and musical and may radiate from the base to the apex, or may be heard best at the apex, mimicking mitral regurgitation.

The three most important signs indicating AS is severe in the older patients are late peaking of ejection systolic murmur, S_2 that is single or A_2 that is paradoxical, and the ejection systolic murmur is a seagull sound that is not frequently heard but is very specific.

Specific Clinical Syndrome (Heyde Syndrome)

Of 3.8 million patients discharged from public hospitals in the Republic of Ireland, the incidence of gastrointestinal bleeding in the presence of AS was 0.9 percent (odds ratio [OR] 4.5; [95 percent confidence interval [CI] of 3.0 to 6.8; *p* value <0.0001).[8] Patients who have bleeding from endoscopically proven dysplasia may also have severe deficiency of high-molecular-weight multimers of von Willebrand factor.[31] In patients with this deficiency after valve replacement, the deficiency may normalize postoperatively and bleeding may not be recurrent.[31] Bleeding recurs after surgery in a proportion of patients.

Chest Radiograph

The characteristic finding is a normal-sized heart with a dilated proximal ascending aorta ("poststenotic" dilation). Calcium in the aortic valve can often be seen on the lateral film. In the current era,

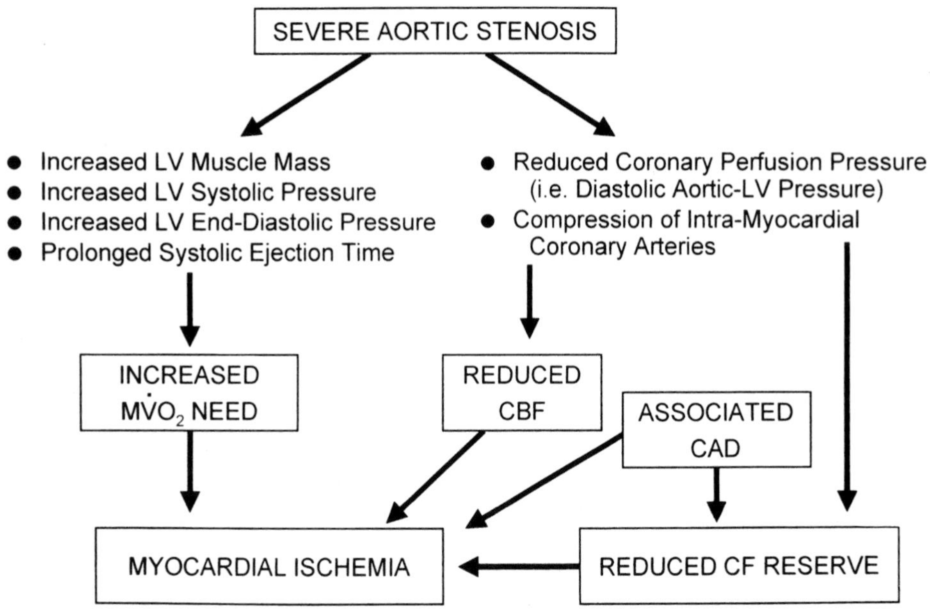

FIGURE 75–5. In severe aortic stenosis (AS), myocardial oxygen needs are increased because of increased muscle mass (hypertrophy), increases in left ventricle (LV) pressures, and prolongation of the systolic ejection time. Total coronary blood flow is increased; however, coronary blood flow per 100 g of LV mass is reduced because of a reduction in diastolic aortic–LV pressure gradient and "systolic milking" of the coronary arteries in the hypertrophied LV as they traverse the myocardium from the epicardium to the endocardium to supply the subendocardial myocardial region. Thus, these patients may have myocardial ischemia, particularly in the subendocardial region. Coronary vasodilator reserve (i.e., the ability of the coronary blood flow to increase with vasodilatation) is also significantly reduced, and thus the myocardial ischemia can be markedly exacerbated on effort. Associated obstructive coronary artery disease can be expected to further exacerbate the myocardial ischemia. CAD, coronary artery disease; CBF, coronary blood flow; CF, coronary flow; MVO$_2$, maximal venous oxygen. *Source: Copyright by S.H. Rahimtoola. Rahimtoola SH. Aortic stenosis. In: Rahimtoola SH, ed. Atlas of Heart Diseases: Valvular Heart Disease, vol 11. Philadelphia: Current Medicine, 1997:7.1–7.26.*

calcification is most easily recognized on two-dimensional echocardiography. Calcium in the aortic valve is the hallmark of AS in adults 40 to 45 years of age.[1] In patients age $\geq$ 45 years, the diagnosis of severe AS is doubtful if there is no calcium in the aortic valve. The presence of calcium, however, does not necessarily mean that the valve is stenotic or that the AS is severe. In patients with heart failure, the cardiac size is increased because of dilatation of the LV and LA; the lung fields show pulmonary edema and pulmonary venous congestion with redistribution of blood flow. In the presence of heart failure, the right ventricle and the right atrium may be dilated (see Chap. 14).

Electrocardiogram

The *electrocardiogram* (ECG) in severe AS shows LVH with or without secondary ST–T-wave changes. It is important to recognize, however, that in approximately 10 to 15 percent of patients with severe AS, LVH cannot be appreciated on the ECG. In fact, the ECG may be entirely normal in some of these patients. The P-wave abnormality ($p \geq 0.12$ seconds) of LA enlargement and/or hypertrophy and/or conduction delay is present in more than 80 percent of patients.[1] The ECG may show left bundle-branch block, right bundle-branch block with left or right axis deviation, or, occasionally, isolated right bundle-branch block.[34] In some patients, the conduction abnormality results from aortic valve

TABLE 75–2

Physical Examination of Patients with Varying Severity of Aortic Valve Stenosis

	MILD	MODERATE	SEVERE + NORMAL LV FUNCTION	SEVERE + LV DYSFUNCTION	SEVERE + HEART FAILURE[a]
Arterial pulse	Normal	Slowly rising	*Parvus et tardus*	*Parvus et tardus*	Small volume
Jugular venous pulse	Normal	Normal	Normal	Normal	±
Carotid thrill	±	±	±	±	±
Cardiac impulse	Normal	Heaving	Heaving, sustained palpable *a* wave	Heaving	Heaving or reduced
Precordial thrill	±	±	Usually ++	±	–
Auscultation					
S$_4$	–	±	++	+	–
S$_3$	–	–	–	±	+
ESS	+	±	–	–	–
Peak of ESM	Early systole	Midsystole	Late systole	Late to midsystole, soft	Midsystole, soft or absent
S$_2$	Normal	Normal or single	Single or paradoxical	Single	Single

ESM, ejection systolic murmur; ESS, ejection systolic sound; LV, left ventricular; S$_2$, second heart sound; S$_3$, third heart sound (diastolic gallop); S$_4$, fourth heart sound (presystolic gallop).
[a]There may be signs of mitral and tricuspid regurgitation and of pulmonary hypertension.

calcification extending into the specialized conducting tissue, which may even produce heart block. The patients are usually in sinus rhythm. The presence of atrial fibrillation indicates the presence of associated mitral valve disease, CAD, or heart failure secondary to aortic valve disease. Atrial fibrillation is relatively common in the older patients with calcific AS, probably because of the increased presence of associated diseases (see Chap. 12).

[ ] LABORATORY INVESTIGATIONS
Echocardiography/Doppler Ultrasound

Echocardiography/Doppler (echo/Doppler) ultrasound (see Chap. 16) is an extremely important and useful noninvasive test and should be used in every instance. On the echocardiogram, the aortic valve leaflets normally are barely visible in systole. In the presence of a bicuspid aortic valve, eccentric valve leaflets may be seen (see below). The aortic valve leaflets may appear to be thickened as a result of calcification and/or fibrosis; however, the older patient without valve stenosis may also have thickened cusps. The aortic valve may have a reduced opening, but this also occurs in other conditions in which the cardiac output is reduced. The LVH often results in thickening of both the interventricular septum and the posterior LV wall. The LV cavity size is normal. All these abnormalities are better appreciated on two-dimensional echocardiography. When LV systolic function is impaired, the LV and LA are dilated and the percentage of dimensional shortening is reduced.

M-mode, or two-dimensional echocardiography, is not always a reliable technique for assessing the severity of AS. The presence of normal movement of thin aortic leaflets on the echocardiogram, however, is strong evidence against severe AS in adults. Echo/Doppler, when properly applied, is extremely useful for estimating the valve gradient and AVA noninvasively.[35,36] When compared with results obtained at cardiac catheterization, the standard error of the estimate of mean gradient in the best laboratories is 10 mmHg.[37] Thus, the mean gradient by Doppler can be expected to be within ±20 mmHg (95 percent CI) of that obtained at catheterization.[37] Similarly, the AVA will be within ±0.3 cm² of that obtained at cardiac catheterization.[37] A study of 156 patients compared AVA obtained by cardiac catheterization with that obtained by Doppler ultrasound.[38] Of 125 patients with AVA ≥0.8 cm² at cardiac catheterization, 36 patients (29 percent) had a Doppler-estimated AVA ≥0.9 cm². In all seven patients with AVA >1.0 cm² by cardiac catheterization, Doppler-estimated AVA was 1.0 cm²; the findings in these seven patients must be interpreted cautiously because they were likely to be a highly selected subgroup. Table 75-3 shows the criteria for assessing severity of AS based on Doppler-obtained gradients. In a study of 636 patients studied by cardiac catheterization, no single aortic valve gradient was found to be both sensitive and specific for severe AS.[39] A mean gradient of ≥50 mmHg or a peak gradient ≥60 mmHg were "specific," with a 90 percent or more positive predictive value. It was not possible to find a lower limit with 90 percent negative predictive value.[39] Thus, a mean gradient of <50 mmHg is compatible with mild, moderate, or severe AS.

Transesophageal echo/Doppler ultrasound is very useful in defining an aortic valve abnormality and in assessing its severity when an adequate examination cannot be obtained with the transthoracic technique.

TABLE 75-3

Suggested Conservative Guidelines for Relating Severity of Aortic Stenosis to Doppler Gradients in Adults

PEAK GRADIENT, MMHG	MEAN GRADIENT, MMHG	SEVERE AS
≥80	≥70	Highly likely
60–79	50–69	Probable
<60	<50	Uncertain

A SUGGESTED GRADING OF THE DEGREE OF AORTIC STENOSIS

AORTIC STENOSIS	AVA (CM²)[a]	AVA INDEX (CM²/M²)[a]
Mild	>1.5	>0.9
Moderate	>1.0–1.5	>0.6–0.9
Severe[b]	≤1.0	≤0.6

AS, aortic stenosis; AVA, aortic valve area.
[a]By echocardiogram/Doppler or by cardiac catheterization.
[b]Patients with AVAs that are at borderline values between the moderate and severe grades (0.9–1.1 cm²; 0.55–0.65 cm²/m²) should be considered individually.
SOURCE: Adapted from Rahimtoola SH. Perspective on valvular heart disease: update II. In: Knoebel S, ed. An Era in Cardiovascular Medicine. New York: Elsevier, 1991:45–70, with permission.

Electron-Beam Computed Tomography

Electron-beam computed tomography detects AV calcium in less than 20 percent of cases of AS. The sensitivity and specificity of electron-beam computed tomography for detecting "degenerative" AV disease was 24 percent and 94 percent, respectively.[8]

Multislice Computed Tomography and Cardiac Magnetic Resonance

Neither of these tests has been shown to be superior to echo/Doppler for the diagnosis of and assessing severity of AS (see Chap. 20).[7,8]

Myocardial Viability

Please see Chronic Aortic Regurgitation section.

Cardiac Catheterization and Angiography

Cardiac catheterization remains the standard technique to assess the severity of AS "accurately." This is done by measuring simultaneous LV and ascending aortic pressures and measuring cardiac output by either the Fick principle or the indicator dilution technique. Obtaining simultaneous LV and ascending aortic pressures using a double-lumen catheter is liable to produce severe errors[7]; using two catheters is the ideal, is preferable, and is essential in those with mean gradients <50 mmHg. It is important to calculate the AVA (see Chap. 16).[39] AS can be considered to be severe when the AVA is 1.0 cm² or less or the AVA index is 0.6 cm²/m² or less (see Table 75-3).[37] The state of LV systolic pump function can be quantitated by measuring LV end-diastolic and end-systolic vol-

TABLE 75–4

Aortic Valve Disease: Indications for Coronary Arteriography

Patients ≥35 years
Patients <35 years
    Left ventricular dysfunction
    Symptoms or signs suggesting CAD
    Two or more risk factors for premature CAD (excluding gender)

CAD, coronary artery disease.
SOURCE: From Rahimtoola SH. Perspective on valvular heart disease: update II. In: Knoebel S, ed. An Era in Cardiovascular Medicine. New York: Elsevier 1991:45–70, with permission.

umes and ejection fraction. *It must be recognized that the ejection fraction may underestimate myocardial function in the presence of the increased afterload of severe AS.*

The presence of CAD and its site and severity can be estimated only by selective coronary angiography (Table 75–4). The incidence of associated CAD will vary considerably, depending on the prevalence of CAD in the population.[37] It was reported to be 50 percent in patients with AS and 20 percent in patients with AR.[37] In general, in persons 50 years of age or older, it is approximately 50 percent (Table 75–5).[40–42]

Natriuretic Peptides

Natriuretic peptide levels are increased in patients with aortic and mitral valve heart disease, and in those with systolic and/or diastolic overload. The levels are higher in those who later become symptomatic, and are increased further with increasing New York Heart Association (NYHA) functional classes, decreasing left ventricular ejection fraction (LVEF), and increasing LA pressure.[7,8]

Gated Blood Pool Radionuclide Scans

Gated blood pool radionuclide scans provide information on ventricular function similar to that provided by two-dimensional echocardiography and LV cineangiography. These studies are of value in the patient in whom LV cineangiography is unsuccessful and echocardiographic studies are suboptimal.

Exercise Tests

It is usually recommended that exercise tests of any kind not be undertaken by patients with severe AS unless there is a specific reason for such studies. Exercise tests in these patients may precipitate ventricular tachyarrhythmias and ventricular fibrillation,[29] particularly if they have significant associated CAD. If there is doubt about the severity of AS and concern that the patient's symptoms may not be caused by AS, it is

usually wise to document the absence of severe AS and of associated CAD before performing an exercise test. Occasionally, in a patient with severe AS who denies all symptoms, a closely monitored exercise test by experienced and skilled physicians may be needed to assess exercise capacity, but should usually *only* be undertaken after exclusion of associated significantly obstructive CAD.

Ambulatory Electrocardiogram Recording

Ambulatory ECG recordings may be needed occasionally in a patient suspected of having an arrhythmia or painless ischemia (see Chap. 41).

Provocative Diagnostic Test

Occasionally, the severity of the AS may be in doubt in a patient because of a small mean aortic valve gradient. The AS may be severe or mild to moderate, and the calculated AVA may be very small because of severe stenosis or because the small stroke volume only opens the valve to a limited extent; thus, the AVA will be determined to be small even on echo/Doppler ultrasound. Infusion of an inotropic agent such as dobutamine, which results in increases of cardiac output (and of stroke volume) and heart rate (and of shortening of systolic ejection time), usually helps one make a correct diagnosis. In these circumstances, it is important to measure cardiac output and LV and aortic pressures simultaneously and meticulously, both before and during dobutamine infusion,[43,44] because with dobutamine, systemic vascular resistance may increase or decrease, and in patients with associated CAD, myocardial ischemia may be induced, all of which may have different effects on the gradient.[6] Whether the AS is mild or severe, the gradient increases with dobutamine infusion; however, in mild AS the AVA increases significantly, but in severe AS the AVA does not increase or increases minimally (approximately 10 percent). In a prospective study of 136 patients, those who had an increase of LV stroke volume (obtained from echo/Doppler) of ≥20 percent (group A) had the best survival after AVR, and it was much better

TABLE 75–5

Isolated Aortic Valve Replacement: Incidence of Associated Coronary Artery Disease

	VA CO-OP STUDY[a]	MAYO CLINIC[b]	MGH[c] (80–89 YEARS)
Total number of patients	643	618	64
Patients with coronary artery disease	312	321	37
%	49%	52%	58%
1 VD	17%	22%	27%
2 VD	17%	14%	19%
3 VD	15%	17%	13%
Additional LMCAD	—	5%	3%

LMCAD, left main coronary artery disease; MGH, Massachusetts General Hospital; VA, Veterans Administration; VD, vessel disease.
[a]Sethi GK, et al.[40]
[b]Mullany CJ, et al.[41]
[c]Levinson JR, et al.[42]

than for those who had no AVR.[45] However, in those with an increase of LV stroke volume of <20 percent (group B), the survival after AVR was also better than in those who had no AVR. In subgroup B (LV stroke volume increase of <20 percent), the survival after AVR was worse than for patients in the subgroup A who had AVR, and the survival with no AVR was similar to that of the patients who had no AVR in subgroup A. It is possible that tests of myocardial viability and of cardiac magnetic resonance for presence of and extent of previous myocardial infarction (MI) may be of help (see Chronic Aortic Regurgitation section).

[ ] CLINICAL DECISION MAKING

There are a number of steps involved in clinical decision making in patients with valvular heart disease (Table 75–6).[37] The first is a complete clinical evaluation, which includes history, physical examination, ECG, and chest radiography. Next, disease of all cardiac valves, ventricular function, hemodynamic effects, as well as CAD, other cardiovascular disease, and disease of other organs, should be diagnosed and the severity assessed. Before proceeding to additional testing, it is important to list the questions to be answered and to be reasonably certain that these questions need to be answered. The tests that are most likely to provide these answers *in the clinician's own institution* should then be performed, with the following criteria kept in mind: reliability, accuracy, lowest risk to patient, and reasonable (lowest) cost. The results of the tests should be reviewed as they become available, and an overall evaluation/assessment of the patient and, finally, recommendations regarding management should be made.

In a prospective, blinded study of consecutive patients with valvular heart disease, the sensitivity and specificity of diagnosis of AS and the accuracy of assessment of severity of AS were determined (Table 75–7).[46] This study revealed the following important points: (1) Clinical evaluation was sensitive, highly specific, and reasonably accurate in diagnosing AS and was highly accurate in assessing its severity when AS was moderate or severe. This emphasizes the importance of a thorough clinical evaluation of the patient. (2) Echo/Doppler ultrasound improved the accuracy of this assessment to only a certain extent because of the limitations of gradients obtained by Doppler echocardiogram.[47] (3) The reason clinical evaluation and echo/Doppler do not have a 100 percent specificity is the occasional inability in a patient to distinguish mild AS from turbulence across a normal or slightly diseased aortic valve. (4) Both clinical evaluation and echo/Doppler ultrasound are excellent in diagnosing the AS as being at least moderate or severe. (5) An important difficulty in diagnosis by clinical evaluation and by echo/Doppler is in not being able to separate accurately all patients with moderate AS from those with severe AS.

[ ] NATURAL HISTORY AND PROGNOSIS

Valvular AS is frequently a progressive disease, its severity increasing over time.[1,43,47] The factors that control this progression and the time it takes for severe outflow obstruction to develop are unknown; however, it is possible that in the older patient, AS may progress at a faster rate than it does in the younger patient. In a study of 142 patients with "mild" stenosis (catheterization-proven AVA >1.5 cm^2),[48] the rate of progression to severe stenosis was 8 percent in 10 years, 22 percent in 20 years, and 38 percent in 25 years. At 25 years, 38 percent still had mild AS (Table 75–8). The

> **TABLE 75–6**
>
> **Steps in Clinical Decision Making for Patients with Valvular Heart Disease**

1. Perform a complete clinical evaluation
   History
   Physical examination
   Electrocardiogram
   Chest radiograph film
2. Diagnose and assess severity of disease
   All valves
   Ventricular function
   Hemodynamic effects
   Coronary artery disease
   Other cardiovascular disease
   Effects on other body organs
   Other organ diseases
3. List questions that need answering
4. Be reasonably certain these questions need to be answered
5. Perform test(s) most likely to provide these answers in one's own institution with the following criteria:
   Reliability
   Accuracy
   Lowest risk to patients
   Reasonable (or lowest) cost
6. Review results of test(s)
7. Make an overall assessment of patient
8. Make recommendations regarding management

SOURCE: From Rahimtoola SH. Perspective on valvular heart disease: update II. In: Knoebel S, ed. An Era in Cardiovascular Medicine. New York: Elsevier 1991:45–70, with permission.

> **TABLE 75–7**
>
> **Clinical Decision Making Using Clinical Evaluation and Echo/Doppler in Patients with Aortic Stenosis**

	AFTER CLINICAL EVALUATION (%)	AFTER ECHO/ DOPPLER (%)
Diagnosis of aortic stenosis		
Sensitivity	78	100
Specificity	92	92
Accuracy of diagnosis		
All levels of severity	48	65
Moderate or severe aortic stenosis	100	100

SOURCE: From Kotlewski A, Kawanishi DT, McKay CR, et al. The relative value of clinical examination, echocardiography with Doppler and cardiac catheterization with angiography in the evaluation of aortic valve disease. In: Bodnar E, ed. Surgery for Heart Valve Disease. London: ICR 1990:66–72, with permission.

TABLE 75–8

Natural History of Mild[a] Aortic Stenosis (n = 142)

	10 YEARS	20 YEARS	25 YEARS
Mild	88%	63%	38%
Moderate	4%	15%	25%
Severe	8%	22%	38%

[a]Mild stenosis is defined here as an aortic valve area >1.5 cm².
SOURCE: From Horstkotte D, Loogen F. The natural history of aortic valve stenosis. Eur Heart J 1988;9(Suppl E):57–64, with permission.

duration of the asymptomatic period after the development of severe AS is also unknown; some data suggest that it may be less than 2 years.

Several recent studies[49–51] have examined the "natural history" of severe AS (Table 75–9). There is a wide range of events over the years, which may be explained by several factors:

1. Doppler velocities of ≥4 m/s may represent moderate and severe AS;
2. In two of the studies, 15 to 20 percent of patients had early AVR and these patients had more severe AS as judged by gradients and/or AVAs;
3. In the Otto study[50] 50 percent of patients were subsequently shown to have significant obstructive CAD. In the other two studies, the incidence of associated CAD is unknown; and
4. In the Pellikka study,[49] only "cardiac" death is reported. (Also see Surgery below for longer followup data.)

However, the limitations of gradients and of aortic peak velocity obtained by Doppler ultrasound should be considered.[47] In the Amato study of 66 patients with AVA ≤1.0 cm² and no associated CAD, the incidence of sudden death and events was high (Table 75–10).[52] The overwhelming majority of adults with severe AS who are seen by cardiologists have symptoms.

Severe disease in adults is lethal, particularly if the patient is symptomatic, with a prognosis that is worse than for many forms of neoplastic disease.[37,53] The 3-year mortality is approximately 36 to 52 percent; the 5-year mortality is approximately 52 to 80 percent; and the 10-year mortality is 80 to 90 percent.[37,43] A study of elderly patients (average age: 77 years) showed 1- and 3-year mortalities were 44 and 75 percent, respectively.[43] With the onset of severe symptoms (angina, syncope, or heart failure), the average life expectancy is 2 to 3 years (Table 75–11).[48,53] Almost all patients with heart failure are

dead in 1 to 2 years.[48,53] A combination of symptoms is much more ominous, a sign of a greatly reduced survival. Sudden death, like syncope, occurs in the presence of severe AS. Its exact incidence is difficult to determine, but may be approximately 5 percent.[53] Most, but not all, of these patients have had some cardiac symptoms before the fatal episode; at times, the only symptom has been exertional presyncope. Patients with aortic valve "sclerosis" have an approximately 50 percent increase in cardiovascular mortality and myocardial infarction.[54] This incidence is lower than it is in patients with AS, and aortic sclerosis appears to be a marker for vascular atherosclerosis.

Table 75–12 outlines the major factors influencing outcome in patients with valvular heart disease.

[ ] MANAGEMENT

All patients with AS need antibiotic prophylaxis against infective endocarditis (see Chap. 85). Those in whom the valve lesion is of rheumatic origin need additional prophylaxis against recurrence of rheumatic fever (see Chap. 74). Patients with mild or moderate stenosis rarely have symptoms or complications and do not need any specific medical therapy (Table 75–13). In mild stenosis, the patient should be encouraged to lead a normal life. Those with moderate AS should avoid moderate to severe physical exertion and competitive sports. Atrial fibrillation in patients with mild or moderate AS should be reverted rapidly to sinus rhythm. In severe AS, reversion to sinus rhythm often becomes a matter of some urgency.

The role of statins in the prevention and/or slowing of progression of calcific AS is, at present, under intensive investigaton.[55]

Surgery

Operation should be advised for the symptomatic patient who has severe AS. In young patients, if the valve is pliable and mobile, simple commissurotomy or valve repair may be feasible; the operative mortality is <1 percent.[56] It will relieve outflow obstruction to a major degree. In such patients, catheter balloon valvuloplasty (CBV) is the procedure of choice in experienced and skilled centers. Both of these are palliative procedures that postpone AVR for many years. Older patients and even young patients with calcified, rigid valves need AVR. The natural history of symptomatic patients with severe AS is dismal (i.e., a 10-year mortality of 80 to 90 percent), but there is good outcome after AVR, particularly in patients without any comorbid cardiac and noncardiac conditions. Given the unknown natural history of the asymptomatic patient with severe AS, which may not be benign,[37] it is reasonable to recommend AVR even to

TABLE 75–9

"Natural History" of Asymptomatic Patients with Aortic Stenosis

AUTHOR (REF. #)	NO. PATIENTS	AGE (YEARS)	AVR WITHIN 3 MONTHS	DEATH	DEATH + AVR
Pellikka et al.[49]	143	70	30 (21 %)	10 ± 4 %	26 ± 6 %[a]
Otto et al.[50]	26	63 ± 16	1 (4 %)	—	79 ± 18 %
Rosenhek et al.[51]	128	[b]	22 (17 %)	9 ± 3 %	44 ± 5 %

AVR, aortic valve replacement.
[a]Cardiac death.
[b]AVR within 3 months: n = 22, age 57 ± 9 years.
Others: n = 106, age 71 ± 12 years, p < 0.001.

TABLE 75-10

Natural History of 66 Asymptomatic Patients with Severe Aortic Stenosis (AVA ≥1.0 cm²) and No Coronary Artery Disease

FOLLOW-UP MONTHS[a]	SUDDEN DEATH (SD)	EVENT RATE (SD; SYMPTOMS)
6	3/66 (4.5 %)	29 ± 6 %
12	—	43 ± 6 %
18	4/66 (6.2 %)	57 ± 6 %
24	—	62 ± 6 %

[a]Average followup = 7.8 months.

SOURCE: From Amato MCM, Moffa PJ, Werner K et al. Treatment decision in asymptomatic aortic stenosis: role of exercise testing. Heart 2001;86:381–386.

the asymptomatic patient. There is, however, no consensus about AVR in all asymptomatic patients; it is clearly indicated in those undergoing surgery for CAD, aorta or other valve disease, in those with LV dysfunction, and/or with associated CAD (Table 75–14).[57] A more recent, long-term followup of the Pellikka study of asymptomatic patients with AS, showed the mortality in those who subsequently became symptomatic was 21.7 percent versus 77.7 percent in those who had AVR versus no AVR, and in those who remained asymptomatic, it was 28 percent versus 57 percent in those who had AVR versus no AVR.[58]

In one database the operative mortality of AVR was approximately 4 percent, and for AVR and coronary bypass surgery, it was 6.8 percent.[59] In patients without associated CAD, heart failure, or other comorbid factors, it may be 1 to 2 percent in centers with experienced and skilled staff,[41,43,60] and in those needing coronary artery bypass surgery (CABG) it may be 2 to 4 percent. In the STS database, for patients in NYHA functional classes I, II, III, and IV, it was 1.25 percent, 1.81 percent, 3.69 percent, and 7.05 percent, respectively.[60] Patients with associated CAD should have CABG at the same time as AVR because it results in a lower operative and late mortality (Table 75–15).[41] The operative mortality in octogenarians or in those who are older is much higher: 6 percent for iso-

TABLE 75-11

Average Survival of Symptomatic Patients with Severe Aortic Stenosis

	AUTOPSY DATA (YEARS)[a]	POST CARDIAC CATHETERIZATION (MONTHS)[b]
Overall	3	23
Angina	5	45
Syncope	3	27
Heart failure	<2	11

[a]From Ross J Jr, Braunwald E. Aortic stenosis. Circulation 1968;36(Suppl IV):61–67.

[b]From Horstkotte D, Loogen F. The natural history of aortic valve stenosis. Eur Heart J 1988;9(Suppl E):57–64.

TABLE 75-12

Major Factors Influencing Outcome in Patients with Valvular Heart Disease

LV dysfunction and its magnitude
Duration of LV dysfunction
Degree of LV dilatation
Greater NYHA functional class
Older age
Associated CAD
Previous myocardial infarction
Comorbid conditions
  Cardiac
  Non-cardiac

CAD, coronary artery disease; LV, left ventricle; NYHA, New York Heart Association.

SOURCE: Copyright S.H. Rahimtoola.

lated AVR and 10 percent for those undergoing AVR and associated coronary bypass surgery;[55] again in centers with experienced and skilled staff it is lower, at 3 and 6 percent, respectively.

In severe AS, AVR results in an improvement of survival (Fig. 75–6),[48,61] even in those with normal preoperative LV function. LV function remains normal postoperatively if perioperative myocardial damage has not occurred.[16,35,62,63] LVH regresses toward normal[62,63]; after 2 years, the regression continues at a slower rate for up to 8 to 10 years after AVR.[63] In those with excessive LVH preoperatively,[22] the LVH may regress slowly or not at all. These patients may have persistent severe LV diastolic dysfunction, which may be a difficult clinical problem both in the early postoperative period and after hospital discharge. Their clinical picture subsequently resembles that of patients with hypertrophic cardio-

TABLE 75-13

Medical Treatment of Patients with Aortic Valve Stenosis

I. Antibiotic prophylaxis
  A. Infective endocarditis (See Chap. 85)
  B. Recurrent rheumatic carditis (See Chap. 74)
II. Restriction of activities
  A. Severe exercise
  B. Competitive sports
III. Arrhythmias
  A. Prevent and/or control
  B. Restore sinus rhythm, if possible
IV. Cardiac medications (only if essential)
  A. Avoid negative inotropic and proarrhythmic agents if possible
  B. Diuretics—use cautiously
  C. Arteriolar and venodilators—use cautiously
V. Followup of asymptomatic patients
  A. Mild aortic stenosis: every 2–5 years
  B. Moderate aortic stenosis: every 6–12 months
  C. Develop symptoms: immediate

SOURCE: Copyright S.H. Rahimtoola.

TABLE 75–14

Severe Aortic Valve Stenosis: Indications for Surgery

I. All symptomatic patients
  A. LV function normal: as soon as possible
  B. LV dysfunction: urgent
  C. Heart failure: emergent
II. Asymptomatic patients
  A. Patients undergoing surgery for CAD, aorta, other valves
  B. Associated significantly obstructed CAD
  C. LV dysfunction
  D. Progressive decline of LVEF
  E. Marked or excessive LVH:
    1. ≥11–12 mm in smaller people, e.g., women
    2. ≥13-14 mm in larger people, e.g., men
  F. Patients aged ≥60–65 years
  G. "Very" severe AS ≤0.7 cm^2; 0.4 cm^2/m^2
  H. Others:
    1. Abnormal response to exercise
     a. Hypotension/no or minimal increase of blood pressure
     b. Ischemia
     c. LV dysfunction
     d. Arrhythmias
    2. Arrhythmias
     a. Ventricular/atrial tachyarrhythmias
     b. A-V block >1° AVB

AVB, atrioventricular block; CAD, coronary artery disease; EF, ejection fraction; LV, left ventricular; LVH, left ventricular hypertrophy.
SOURCE: Copyright © by Shahbudin H. Rahimtoola.

myopathy without outflow obstruction, and they may have to be treated as such. Surviving patients are functionally improved.

After AVR, the 10-year survival is 50 percent or better and the 15-year survival is 33 percent or better.[57] Approximately 40 percent of the late deaths are not related to the prosthesis but to associated cardiac abnormalities and other comorbid conditions.[57] Thus, the late survival will vary in different subgroups of patients, for example, in those with fewer or no comorbid conditions, sur-

vival will be very much better. Older patients (≥65 years) have a relative 10-year survival (actual survival compared to an age- and gender-matched person in the population) after AVR that is significantly better than that of those who are younger (<65 years): 94 versus 81 percent (Fig. 75–7).[64]

Care should be exercised in the interpretation of operative and late mortality (see Chap 79).

Heart Failure

Patients who present with heart failure should be hospitalized and treated with digitalis and diuretics, and should undergo surgery as soon as possible (Table 75–16). *Angiotensin-converting enzyme* (ACE) inhibitors should be used cautiously, if at all. The patient must be monitored and *hypotension* avoided; a "significant" fall in blood pressure is an indication to discontinue or reduce the dose of ACE inhibitor. If heart failure does not respond satisfactorily and rapidly to medical therapy, surgery becomes a matter of considerable urgency. CBV can be an important bridge procedure in selected critically ill patients.[65] Although it usually improves the patients' hemodynamics and makes them better candidates for valve replacement, in approximately 5 percent of patients, severe AR is produced that may necessitate emergent AVR. AVR in patients with AS and heart failure can be performed at an operative mortality of 10 percent or less.[43,66] Although this is higher than it is in patients not in heart failure, the risk is justified because late survival in those who survive the operation is excellent and is far superior to that which can be expected with medical therapy; the 7-year survival of patients who survive operation is 84 percent.[67] The survival is lower in those with associated CAD.[66] The impaired LV function improves in all such patients provided that there has been no perioperative myocardial damage; it becomes normal in two-thirds of the patients (Fig. 75–8).[68] In some patients the improvement is less marked.[66] This is more likely in those with longer duration of preoperative LV dysfunction and in those with associated CAD. In addition, the operative survivors are functionally much improved. LV hypertrophy and dilatation (if present preoperatively) regress toward normal. Despite the excellent results of AVR in patients with severe AS who are in heart failure, it is important to recognize that surgery should *not* be delayed until heart failure develops. Patients with severe AS, mean gradient ≥ 30 mmHg, and LV ejection fraction ≤0.35 have a

TABLE 75–15

Aortic Valve Replacement (AVR) Operative Mortality and Late Survival: Effect of Coronary Bypass Surgery (CBS)

	1982–1983	1967–1976					
	OPERATIVE MORTALITY (%)	OPERATIVE MORTALITY (%)	ALL PATIENTS (%)	1 VD (%)	2 VD (%)	3 VD (%)	LMCAD (%)
AVR + no CAD	1.4	4.5	63	—	—	—	—
AVR + CAD + CBS	4.0	6.3	49	38	28	34	11
AVR + CAD + no CBS	9.4	10.3	36	65	22	13	1

CAD, coronary artery disease; LMCAD, left main coronary artery disease; VD, vessel disease.
SOURCE: From Mullany CJ, Elveback ER, Frye RL, et al. Coronary artery disease and its management: influence on survival in patients undergoing AVR. J Am Coll Cardiol 1987;10:66–72, with permission.

higher operative mortality; however, the survivors have an improvement in LV function and functional class.[69,70] For patients who have severe AS, heart failure and "severe" pulmonary hypertension have a high operative mortality and poor late survival; however, this is still better than it is for those who have only medical treatment.[71]

Up to 6 percent of the older patients present in cardiogenic shock.[72] The hospital mortality in such patients is very high, almost 50 percent. After hospital discharge, the subsequent mortality is also very high if the patients have not had their stenosis relieved.[72] Thus, these patients need to be treated aggressively with medical therapy using hemodynamic monitoring; they need emergent surgery. CBV may be used as a "bridge" procedure[65] (Table 75–17) or a hybrid procedure percutaneous coronary intervention (PCI) for CAD followed by AVR.[73,74] Table 75–18 lists the American College of Cardiologists/American Heart Association (ACC/AHA) recommendations.[75]

Recently it was suggested that patients with heart failure can be treated with intravenous nitroprusside to increase cardiac output and titrated to produce mean arterial pressure between 60 and 70 mmHg. The cardiac index is said to have increased from 1.60 ± 0.35 to 2.52 ± 0.55 L/mim/m^2,[76] however, the study is seriously flawed because (1) cardiac output was measured by the Fick principle but body oxygen consumption was not measured[6]; (2) there was only a very small reduction of pulmonary artery wedge pressure; and (3) the 30-day mortality was 24 percent, probably because of marked reduction of perfusing pressure, and thus, of myocardial blood flow (see above). This compares very poorly with a 25 percent mortality at 7 years of those who were treated with digoxin, diuretics, and very early AVR ± CABG.[67] Intravenous nitroprusside is likely to be helpful in patients with associated severe (or possibly moderate) systemic hypertension. Table 75–16 shows a suggested management strategy.

Asymptomatic AS in Patients Undergoing CABG

Patients who are undergoing CABG may have associated AS. There is a need to compare the expected outcomes (survival + comorbidities) of isolated CABG plus subsequent AVR at a later date, if necessary, to initial AVR + CABG. One review[77] determined the outcome of initial AVR + CABG in those with mild and moderate AS was not favorable (see Table 75–17). The review also suggested that because the progression of AS may be rapid in those who are borderline between moderate and severe AS and there is a variability in calculating AVA of perhaps 10 percent, patients in the borderline range should be considered for combined

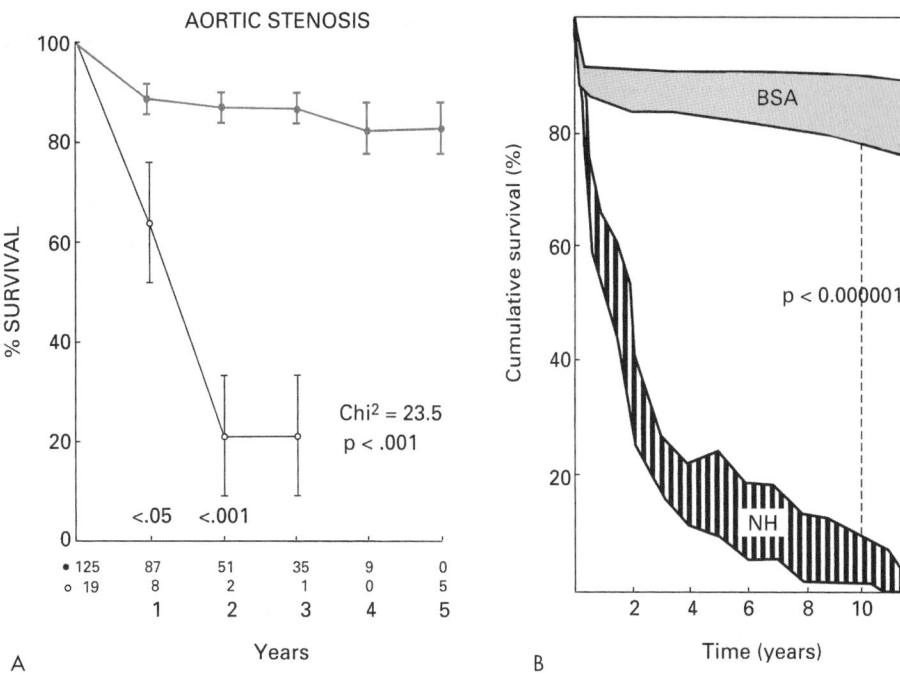

FIGURE 75–6. There are no prospective randomized trials of aortic valve replacement (AVR) in severe aortic stenosis, and there are unlikely to be any in the near future. Two studies have compared the results of AVR with medical treatment during the same time period in symptomatic patients with normal left ventricular systolic pump function. **A.** Patients who had AVR (*closed circles*) had a much better survival than did those treated medically (*open circles*). **B.** Patients who were treated with AVR (body surface area, BSA) had a better survival than did those treated medically (natriuretic hormone, NH). These differences in survival between those treated medically and those treated surgically are so large that there is a great deal of confidence that AVR significantly improves the survival of those with severe AS. *Source: (A) From Shwarz F, Banmann P, Manthey J, et al. The effect of aortic valve replacement on survival. Circulation 1982;66:1105–1110, with permission. (B) From Horstkotte D, Loogen F. The natural history of aortic valve stenosis. Eur Heart J 1988;9(Suppl E):57–64, with permission.*

CABG and AVR, initially in those with AVA ≤1.2 cm^2 (AVA index ≤0.8 cm^2/m^2) provided (1) there is appropriate skill and experience at one's institution; (2) one inserts a prosthetic heart valve with known favorable outcome data up to 15 to 20 years; and (3) one can insert a prosthetic heart valve that would not necessitate use of lifetime of warfarin therapy.

Catheter Balloon Valvuloplasty

In calcific AS, the average increase in AVA after CBV is 0.3 cm^2 and the final AVA usually averages 0.8 cm^2; consequently, many patients continue to have severe AS.[65,72] The 30-day, 1-year, and 3-year mortalities average 14, 35, and 71 percent, respectively. In the older patient (average age: 78 ± 9 years) with calcific AS,[72] the mortality rate was similar to the natural history of this lesion. This technique (CBV) may be indicated[65] as a bridge procedure in those who need emergent noncardiac surgery, and in other selected subgroups (see Table 75–18). CBV is the procedure of choice in young patients who have pliable, noncalcified valves with commissural fusion.

"Guideline" Recommendations

Tables 75–19 and 75–20 show the recommendations of the ACC/AHA *Practice Guidelines*.[75] Guidelines *are not* and *should not* be the law. Application of these guidelines to clinical practice should be based on the following principles: (1) Classes I and III apply to

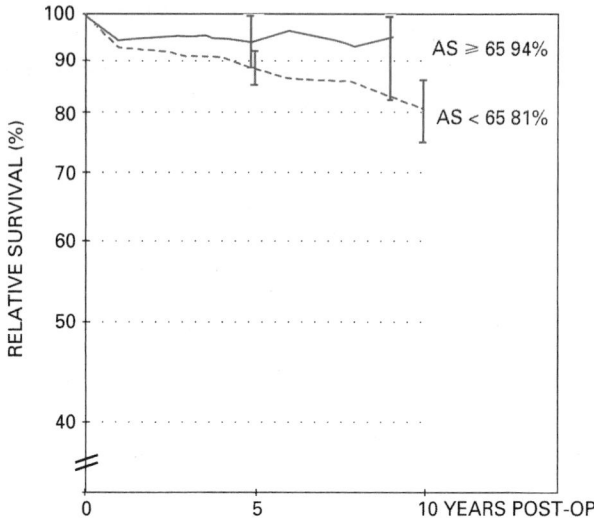

FIGURE 75–7. Data from the Karolinska Institute in Sweden provided an interesting perspective on the long-term survival of patients ages ≥65 years after aortic valve replacement (AVR). The Institute examined the relative survival; that is, compared the survival of the patient who had undergone AVR with another age- and sex-matched person in the same population. Patients <65 years of age had a relative survival of 81 percent, significantly lower than 100 percent. In contrast, patients ages ≥65 years who underwent AVR had a relative survival of 94 percent at the end of 10 years—not significantly different from 100 percent. These data indicate that (1) survival following AVR for aortic stenosis (AS) in patients ages ≥65 years is identical to an age- and sex-matched individual in the population who does not have AS and (2) the late relative survival of patients ≥65 years is much better than that of patients ≤65. *Source: From Lindblom D, Lindblom U, Qvist J, et al. Long-term relative survival rates after heart AVR. J Am Coll Cardiol 1990;15:566–573, with permission.*

all patients in these classes unless there are specific clinical circumstances not to do so; (2) class II applies to patients in this class, depending on the clinical conditions of the patients and the skill and experience at the individual medical center.

TABLE 75–16

MANAGEMENT OF PATIENTS WITH SEVERE AORTIC STENOSIS IN CLINICAL HEART FAILURE

Need for urgent/emergent AVR CABG
Up to 48 hours (48 hours) window for medical therapy before AVR
   Right balloon flotation catheter (± arterial line) for measurement of cardiac output (CO) and pulmonary artery (PA) and PA wedge pressures
Digitalis, diuretics
IV dobutamine, if necessary, to increase CO
ACEI, use very cautiously, must avoid hypotension
"Quick" coronary arteriography on way to operating room and hemodynamic study if AS severity is uncertain. Both may need to be performed day before study.
Patients with severe AS + CAD
Consider Hybrid Procedure (PCI followed by AVR)

ACEI, angiotensin-converting enzyme inhibitors; AS, aortic stenosis; AVR, aortic valve replacement; CABG, coronary artery bypass graft; CAD, coronary artery disease; PCI, percutaneous coronary intervention.
Source: Copyright S. H. Rahimtoola.

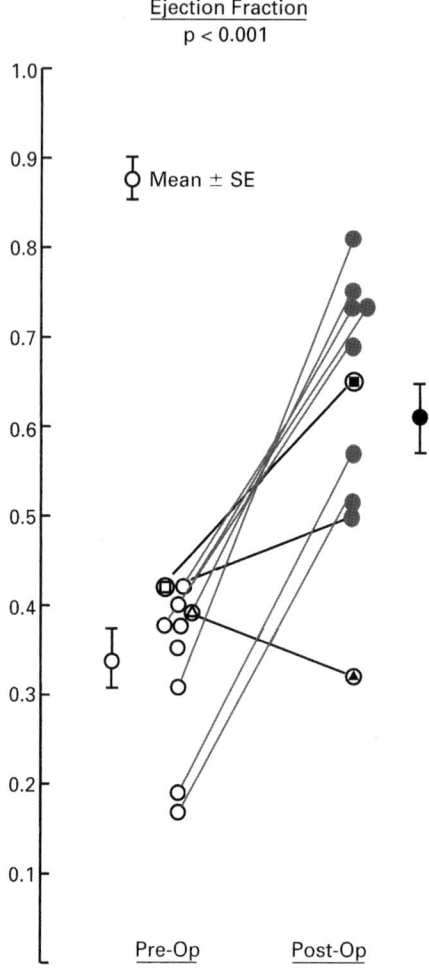

Ejection Fraction
$p < 0.001$

◭ Peri-Op MI and late CHB
◉ Post-Op Perivalvular Aortic Incompetence

FIGURE 75–8. Examination of changes in left ventricular ejection fraction in each individual patient. In those who had aortic stenosis with left ventricular systolic dysfunction and clinical heart failure, the left ventricular ejection fraction after aortic valve replacement (AVR) increased from 0.34 to 0.63. All but one patient showed an improvement in left ventricular ejection fraction. The only patient who showed a deterioration in ejection fraction suffered a perioperative MI and had complete heart block. The only patient who showed only a small increase in ejection fraction had had a myocardial infarct prior to AVR. Note that ejection fraction normalized in two-thirds of the patients, and in the two patients with the lowest ejection fraction (0.18 and 0.19), the ejection fraction normalized in both. These data indicate that there is probably no lower limit of ejection fraction at which time these patients become inoperable. This also indicates that the lower the ejection fraction, the more urgent the need for AVR. SE, standard error. *Source: From Smith N, McAnulty JH, Rahimtoola SH. Severe aortic stenosis with impaired left ventricular function and clinical heart failure: results of AVR. Circulation 1978;58:255–264, with permission.*

Percutaneous Transcatheter Prosthetic Heart Valve Insertion

The first human implantation of an aortic prosthetic heart valve was described in 2002.[78] In 2005, the various cardiologic and cardiac surgical societies in the United States and the U.S. Food and Drug Administration recommended this as an experimental procedure at the present time.[79]

TABLE 75–17

Expected Outcomes after 10 Years of a Policy of Initial CABG + AVR for Mild and Moderate AS[a]

	SEVERE CAD AND MILD AS: 100 PATIENTS	SEVERE CAD AND MODERATE AS: 100 PATIENTS
To eliminate		
Late AVR	9	46[b,c]
Deaths from late AVR	2	7
Results in		
Unnecessary AVR	91	54
Excess deaths	29	24

AS, aortic stenosis; AVR, aortic valve replacement; CABG, coronary artery bypass graft; CAD, coronary artery disease.
[a]Morbidity associated with prosthetic heart valve was not evaluated in the outcomes.
[b]Probably an overestimate.
[c]For exceptions see text.
SOURCE: From Rahimtoola S.H. Should asymptomatic patients with mild or moderate aortic stenosis undergo valve replacement at time of coronary artery bypass graft surgery? Heart 2001;85:337–341.

ACUTE AORTIC REGURGITATION

ETIOLOGY

The two most common causes of acute AR are infective endocarditis and prosthetic valve dysfunction.[80] Other causes include dissection of the aorta, systemic hypertension, and trauma.[81] AR associated with dissection of the aorta indicates that the dissection involves the ascending aorta down to the aortic valve annulus and root. AR associated with systemic hypertension is usually mild and transient; it is associated with severe elevation of aortic pressure, and, when the systemic hypertension is controlled, the AR usually disappears unless permanent changes have occurred in the aortic valve annulus and root or valve leaflets.

PATHOPHYSIOLOGY

The LV diastolic pressure–volume relationship plays a very important role in the pathophysiology of acute AR (Fig. 75–9).[82,83] Two features should be considered[80]: (1) Because the ability of the LV to dilate acutely is limited, the volume overload of acute AR produces a rapid increase of LV diastolic pressure (curve B in Fig. 75–9). (2) The LV diastolic pressure–volume relationship before the onset of acute AR. If the LV is already stiff or less compliant than normal from an associated lesion (e.g., AS or systemic hypertension), the LV diastolic pressure will rise more precipitously as a result of the volume overload of acute AR (curve A in Fig. 75–9) than if the LV were normal (curve B in Fig. 75–9). In comparison, if the LV is somewhat dilated from a previous lesion—for example, mild AR (curve C in Fig. 75–9)—initially the LV pressure will rise more gradually with acute AR, but may subsequently rise to the same high levels as that seen with a normal or stiff LV.

Acute AR that is mild produces little or no hemodynamic abnormality, for example, when associated with systemic hypertension. Increasing severity of AR produces greater degrees of hemodynamic abnormalities, and severe AR often produces the clinical picture of "heart failure."

TABLE 75–18

Suggested Indications for Catheter Balloon Valvuloplasty in Patients with Severe Calcific Aortic Valve Stenosis[a]

I. "Bridge" procedure to eventual AVR
   A. Cardiogenic shock
   B. Moderate to severe heart failure
   C. Emergent/urgent need for noncardiac therapeutic procedures (e.g., operation)
II. Patient with limited life span
   A. Noncardiac reasons (e.g., carcinoma)
   B. Cardiac reason(s) other than aortic stenosis
III. Others
   A. Patient at extremely high risk for AVR
   B. AVR not desirable for noncardiac reasons or cardiac causes other than aortic stenosis
   C. Patient refuses surgery
IV. Rare
   A. "Therapeutic test": patients with small stroke volume and small valve gradient, with valve stenosis suspected to be severe but severity in doubt even after provocative diagnostic tests

AVR, aortic valve replacement.
[a]Caution should be exercised in recommending this procedure in asymptomatic patients.
SOURCE: Adapted from Rahimtoola SH. Catheter balloon valvuloplasty for severe calcific aortic stenosis: limited role. J Am Coll Cardiol 1994; 23:1076–1078, with permission.

Acute AR that is severe results in a large volume of regurgitant blood; therefore, the volume of blood in the LV in diastole is increased. In an acute situation, the LV end-diastolic volume can only increase mildly (no more than 20 to 30 percent) and the LV diastolic pressure–volume relationships are particularly important. The LV systolic pump function is initially normal (Fig. 75–10). The increased

TABLE 75–19

Indications for Aortic Balloon Valvotomy

Class IIb
   1. Aortic balloon valvotomy might be reasonable as a bridge to surgery in hemodynamically unstable adult patients with AS who are at high risk for AVR. (Level of Evidence: C)
   2. Aortic balloon valvotomy might be reasonable for palliation in adult patients with AS in whom AVR cannot be performed because of serious comorbid conditions. (Level of Evidence: C)
Class III
   1. Aortic balloon valvotomy is not recommended as an alternative to AVR in adult patients with AS. (Level of Evidence: C)

AS, aortic stenosis; AVR, aortic valve replacements.
SOURCE: Bonow RO, Carabello B, Chatterjee K, et al. ACC/AHA Guidelines on the management of patients with valvular heart disease: A report of the ACC/AHA Task Force or practice guidelines 2006. Available at: www.acc.org, e26.

TABLE 75–20

INDICATIONS FOR AORTIC VALVE REPLACEMENT (AVR) IN AORTIC STENOSIS (AS)

Class I
  1. AVR is indicated for symptomatic patients with severe AS. (Level of Evidence: B)
  2. AVR is indicated with severe AS undergoing artery bypass graft surgery (CABG). (Level of Evidence: B)
  3. AVR is indicated with severe AS undergoing surgery on the aorta or other heart valves. (Level of Evidence: B)
  4. AVR is indicated with severe AS and left ventricular systolic dysfunction. (Level of Evidence: C)

Class IIa
  1. AVR is reasonable for patients with moderate AS undergoing CABG or surgery on the aorta or other heart valves (see Section 3.7 on combined multiple valve disease, and Section 10.4 on AVR in patients undergoing CABG). (Level of Evidence B).
  2. AVR may be considered for adults with severe asymptomatic AS if there is a high likelihood of rapid progression (such as previous rate of progression). (Level of Evidence: C)
  3. AVR may be considered in patients undergoing CABG who have mild AS when there is evidence, such as moderate-severe valve calcification, that progression may be rapid. (Level of Evidence: C)
  4. AVR may be considered for asymptomatic patients with extremely severe AS (AVR less than 0.6 cm^2, mean gradient greater than 60 mmHg, and jet velocity greater than 5.0 m/s) when the patient's expected operative mortality is 1.0 percent or less. (Level of Evidence: C)

Class III
  1. AVR is not useful for the prevention of sudden death in asymptomatic patients with severe AS who have none of the findings listed under the Class IIa/IIb recommendations. (Level of Evidence: B)

SOURCE: Bonow RO, Carabello B, Chatterjee K, et al. ACC/AHA Guidelines on the management of patients with valvular heart disease: a report of the ACC/AHA Task Force or practice guidelines 2006. Available at: www.acc.org, e24.

LV diastolic pressure results in increases in mean LA and pulmonary venous pressures and produces varying degrees of pulmonary edema.[80] The normal LV systolic pump function in the presence of LV dilatation results in an increase of LV stroke volume. A large percentage of the LV stroke volume is returned to the LV in diastole; as a result, however, the forward stroke volume is reduced. The LV uses two mechanisms: an increase of myocardial contractility and, importantly, a compensatory tachycardia to maintain an adequate forward cardiac output. As a result, the forward cardiac output may be appropriate initially. If the compensatory mechanisms are inadequate, forward cardiac output is reduced. Pulmonary edema, with or without an adequate cardiac output, produces the picture of clinical heart failure.[84] Subsequently, LV systolic pump function may become abnormal; when that occurs, the pulmonary edema is further increased and the forward cardiac output is further reduced, leading to more severe manifestations of heart failure.

tients may have peripheral signs of infective endocarditis (see Chap. 85), a history of trauma, or severe chest pain of aortic dis-

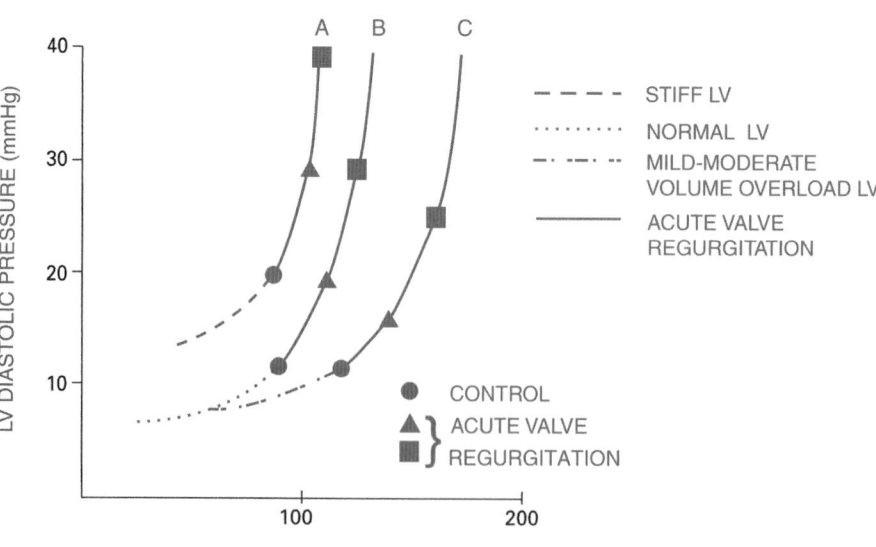

FIGURE 75–9. The left ventricular (LV) diastolic pressure–volume relationship in acute valve regurgitation. The volume overload of acute aortic regurgitation (AR) produces a rapid increase of LV diastolic pressure in a patient with a normal LV diastolic pressure–volume relationship prior to the acute AR (*curve B*). The LV diastolic pressure will rise more or less precipitously as a result of the volume overload of acute AR, depending on whether the LV is already stiff (*curve A*) or is somewhat dilated from a previous volume overload (*curve C*). *Source: From Rahimtoola SH. Management of heart failure in valve regurgitation. Clin Cardiol 1992;15(Suppl I):22–27, with permission.*

[ ] CLINICAL FINDINGS
History and Physical Findings

The clinical presentations are those relating to preexisting disorders that have caused the acute AR. For example, pa-

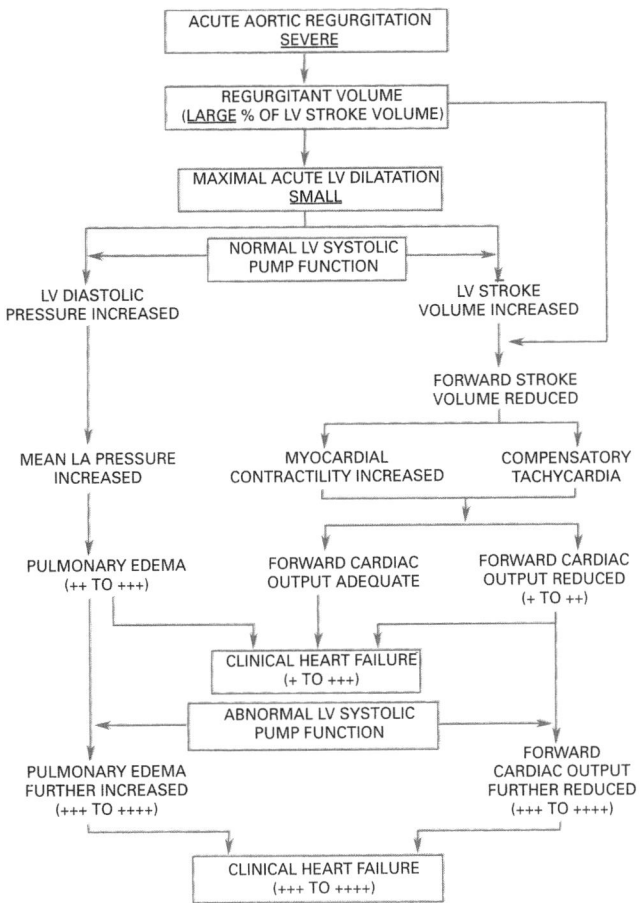

FIGURE 75-10. Pathophysiology of acute severe aortic regurgitation (AR). Acute AR that is severe results in a large volume of regurgitant blood; consequently, the volume of blood in the left ventricle (LV) in diastole is increased. In an acute situation, the LV end-diastolic volume can only increase mildly (no more than 20 to 30 percent) and the LV diastolic pressure–volume relationships are particularly important (see Fig. 75–1). The subsequent findings are dependent on LV systolic pump function, LV diastolic pressure–volume relationship, myocardial contractile state, and compensatory tachycardia (see text for details). LA, left atrium. *Source: Copyright by S.H. Rahimtoola. Rahimtoola SH. Aortic regurgitation. In: Rahimtoola SH, ed. Atlas of Heart Diseases: Valvular Heart Disease, vol 11. Philadelphia: Current Medicine, 1997:7.1–7.26.*

section. The other clinical presentations are those related to the AR itself. If the AR is mild, the patient is usually asymptomatic. In the symptomatic patient, the symptoms are those of heart failure.

On physical examination, the symptomatic patient with acute severe AR usually has a tachycardia. The arterial pulse shows an increased rate of rise of pressure. Systolic pressure is usually normal unless there is very severe heart failure; however, the diastolic pressure is in the normal range or may be decreased. The pulse pressure is usually normal. Thus, although the classic peripheral signs of chronic, severe AR are often absent, an important diagnostic clue is the rapid rate of rise of arterial pressure. The usual clinical signs of heart failure may be present. On examination of the precordium, the LV impulse is normal or slightly displaced to the left; it is usually hyperkinetic unless LV systolic dysfunction is present. The first heart sound is soft, and the second heart sound is often single and is soft. If pulmonary hypertension is present, P_2 is loud and there is a loud S_3 gallop sound; an S_4 gallop sound is absent. The clinical sine qua non of AR is the AR murmur, an early or im-

mediate, blowing, decrescendo, diastolic murmur beginning after A_2 that is best heard with the diaphragm of the stethoscope. Having the patient sit up and lean forward with the breath held in expiration facilitates the audibility of the murmur in difficult cases. The murmur may be short and soft if the ascending aortic pressure equalizes with LV pressure in early or mid-diastole. An Austin Flint murmur, if present, occurs in presystole and/or mid-diastole (see Chap. 12).

An important clinical picture in intravenous drug abusers[80] includes (1) a peripheral arterial pulse that has a rapid rate of rise and fall, even though the pulse pressure is small; (2) the telltale signs of intravenous drug abuse; (3) sinus tachycardia; and (4) "normal" heart size with pulmonary edema on chest radiograph.

Chest Radiograph

The chest radiograph shows a "normal" heart size with pulmonary edema; however, some enlargement of all cardiac chambers and the main pulmonary artery may be present. The aorta is not dilated unless aortic annular/root disease or dissection of the aorta is the cause of the acute AR. The aorta may also be dilated in the older patient and/or in patients with an associated disease such as systemic hypertension. The lungs may show the signs of infected pulmonary emboli if there is associated tricuspid valve endocarditis.

Electrocardiogram

The ECG often shows nonspecific ST–T-wave changes and a sinus tachycardia; however, it may be normal. The ECG may show signs that are usually found in the associated causative disorder (e.g., LVH with ST–T-wave changes in patients with severe hypertension). The ECG may show a variety of conduction abnormalities (atrioventricular and bundle branch block), including heart block, which, in the presence of infective endocarditis, is a sign of paravalvular or myocardial abscess.

❚ ❘ NATURAL HISTORY AND PROGNOSIS

The natural history of this condition is variable. If the AR is mild to moderate in severity, these patients are likely to do well with medical therapy. Eventually, the changes of chronic AR will be seen. In patients with severe AR, the natural history depends on whether or not they have heart failure.[80] If heart failure is present, which is common, the prognosis is very poor without AVR unless the heart failure can be very easily controlled with medical therapy.

❚ ❘ MANAGEMENT
Diagnosis of Aortic Regurgitation

In most instances, the diagnosis can be made by clinical evaluation. The diagnosis by physical examination in an acutely ill patient who is in extremis may be difficult.

Transthoracic echo/Doppler ultrasound is an important and valuable noninvasive procedure that should be used in every instance. It will demonstrate the AR and its severity, and will provide useful information about the size and function of the LV and other valvular and cardiac abnormalities. If the transthoracic method is inadequate, the transesophageal method should be used, which is usually essential in those with infective endocarditis (see Chaps. 16 and 85).

Echocardiography shows the diastolic flutter of the anterior leaflet of the mitral valve. In addition, the echocardiogram may show vegetations on the aortic valve, prolapse of an aortic valve leaflet into the LV in diastole, and premature mitral valve closure. The mitral valve may be seen to open for only a short time because the stroke volume is limited. Occasionally, the aortic valve leaflets were totally destroyed and none are seen on the echocardiogram. Doppler ultrasound demonstrates the AR and an estimate of its severity.

Cardiac catheterization and angiography, including coronary arteriography, show the abnormal physiology described, and aortography shows gross AR. These modalities may be needed to make the diagnosis and are usually indicated before surgical intervention. Coronary arteriography is indicated in the appropriate patient (see Table 75–4). In the extremely ill patient, there is often a need for clinical judgment regarding which tests are essential. Other tests may be needed in very special circumstances.

Diagnosis of the Etiology of Acute Aortic Regurgitation

The diagnosis of the etiology is usually made during the clinical evaluation. Additional laboratory tests will be needed to confirm the diagnosis; for example, blood cultures in those with suspected infective endocarditis. Echo/Doppler ultrasound examination is also extremely valuable in diagnosing the underlying lesion. Its widespread availability and comparative ease of use, especially in the very acutely ill patient, make it the noninvasive procedure of choice. The availability of biplane and omniplane transesophageal probes should further enhance its value as a diagnostic tool.

Cardiac magnetic resonance has a very high specificity for the diagnosis of dissection of the aorta[85,86] and, if available, should be used in all hemodynamically stable patients if the diagnosis has not already been made. The availability of biplane or omniplane transesophageal echocardiography improves the specificity and diagnostic accuracy of transesophageal echocardiography. Angiography is also an effective and time-honored method of diagnosing dissection of the aorta.

In summary, clinical evaluation is available in all institutions; echo/Doppler ultrasound is available in almost all institutions. The use of the other tests depends on the availability of equipment and the skill and experience of personnel using the equipment for this purpose at each institution.

Bedside Hemodynamic Monitoring

In acute disorders affecting the LV, there may be a phase lag between the rise in pulmonary venous pressure and the appearance of pulmonary edema on the chest radiographic film. As a result, the reliability of the chest radiography in demonstrating the presence and severity of elevated LA pressure initially is less than satisfactory in the acutely ill patient.[81,87] If the assessment of LA pressure is made by physical examination and chest radiography, a significant number of errors may be made in these patients with an acute cardiac problem. Therapeutic decisions based on incorrect assessments may result in significant problems. The optimization of filling pressures and cardiac output may not be made accurately in acute heart failure without measuring their actual values. Thus use of a balloon flotation catheter for bedside hemodynamic monitoring is required in most, if not all, acutely ill patients with acute AR.

Treatment

Treatment of heart failure is directed toward reducing pulmonary venous pressure and increasing cardiac output. In all patients, treatment is also directed toward correcting or controlling the etiologic disease/disorder and/or the altered pathophysiologic state (Table 75–21).[80,84]

Intravenous nitroprusside for an acute, severe condition is useful and important in the management of these patients.[88] Combined arteriolar and venous dilators will produce a reduction of LA v wave and mean LA pressure. They produce a reduction in LV end-diastolic and end-systolic volumes, and an increase in LV ejection fraction. The regurgitant fraction and regurgitant volume are reduced; as a result, the forward stroke volume and cardiac output are increased.[88] Digitalis therapy is of significant benefit in the management of heart failure. The combination of various agents (vasodilators, diuretics, and digitalis) tends to produce the maximum benefit in an individual patient; intravenous nitroprusside is often necessary in the acutely ill patient.

Surgical therapy (valve replacement/valve repair or appropriate surgery for dissection of the aorta) is the cornerstone of the most definitive therapy currently available for heart failure in these patients. Fig. 75–11 outlines the management of the patient with heart failure or suspected heart failure).[80,84] If the AR is due to *dissection of the aorta,* the need for cardiac surgery is an emergency, even if the regurgitation is mild or moderate, because AR indicates

TABLE 75–21

Treatment of Heart Failure in Acute Valve Regurgitation

I. Correct or control altered pathophysiologic state
  A. Reduce pulmonary venous pressure
    1. Diuresis
    2. Vasodilation
    3. Control heart rate and maintain sinus rhythm (digitalis, cardioversion, antiarrhythmics)
  B. Increase cardiac output
    1. Reduction of valve regurgitation (vasodilators)
    2. Inotropic stimulation (digitalis, dobutamine)
  C. Improve left ventricular systolic dysfunction
    1. Reduce pulmonary venous pressure
    2. Increase cardiac output
    3. Angiotensin-converting enzyme inhibitors
II. Correct or control underlying disease or disorder
  A. Antibiotics for infective endocarditis
  B. Pharmacologic therapy for systemic hypertension
  C. Surgery for valve regurgitation in infective endocarditis, prosthetic valve dysfunction, dissection of the aorta, trauma

SOURCE: From Rahimtoola SH. Management of heart failure in valve regurgitation. Clin Cardiol 1992;15(Suppl I):22–27, with permission.

ACUTE SEVERE VALVE REGURGITATION

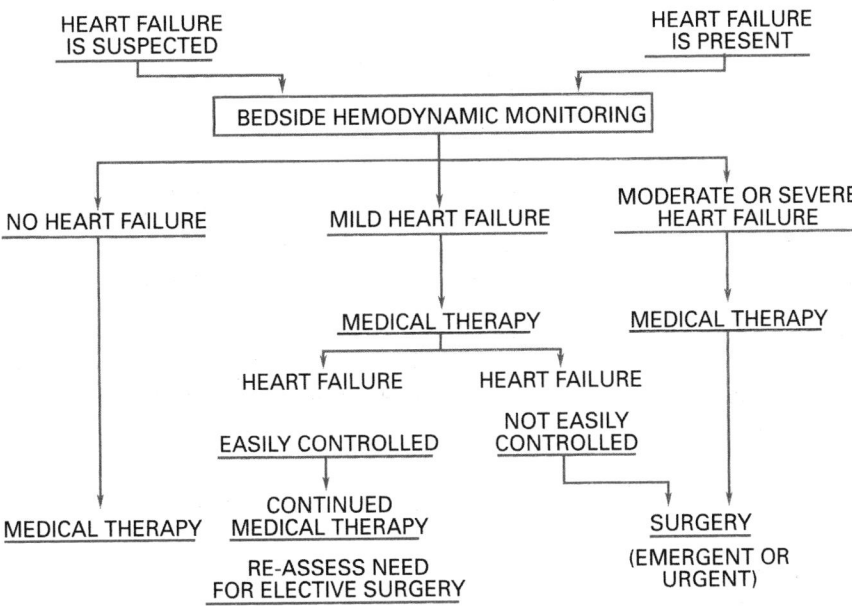

FIGURE 75–11. Role of bedside hemodynamic monitoring in acute aortic regurgitation (AR). All patients with acute AR probably should have this procedure. If the AR is mild and there are no significant hemodynamic abnormalities, then the balloon flotation catheter can be withdrawn. In comparison, if the AR is moderate to severe and there are significant hemodynamic abnormalities, then the balloon flotation catheter is left in place to guide therapy in the management of these acutely ill patients. If the hemodynamic abnormalities are mild, the patient is treated medically. If these abnormalities are easily controlled, medical therapy is continued and periodic reassessments are made to assess the need for elective surgery. If the hemodynamic abnormalities are not easily corrected or the hemodynamic abnormalities initially are moderate to severe, then surgery is undertaken either emergently or urgently. *Source: From Rahimtoola SH. Management of heart failure in valve regurgitation. Clin Cardiol 1992;15(Suppl I):22–27, with permission.*

involvement of the ascending aorta down to the region of the aortic valve annulus and root. The outcome of the patient with heart failure due to infective endocarditis is very poor with medical therapy but is improved with AVR.[8,88] The indications for surgery in *infective endocarditis* are listed in Table 75–22.[85] Infective endocarditis caused by special organisms (e.g., fungi) can only rarely be controlled by pharmacologic therapy alone, and surgery is almost always needed.[37,89] In these and some other conditions, valve surgery may be needed even if the AR is only mild or moderate. It must be recognized, however, that in 90 to 95 percent of patients needing surgery for endocarditis, the indication for valve surgery is heart failure. When the heart failure is a result of *prosthetic valve dysfunction* or *trauma*, the need for surgery can be an emergency, an urgent situation, or an elective procedure. Prosthetic heart valves are inherently stenotic. When regurgitation is superimposed, it produces a pressure plus volume overload on the LV that the ventricle may not handle very well acutely. Furthermore, AR may be a sign of bioprosthetic valve degeneration or prosthetic endocarditis; in both conditions, prosthetic AVR is usually needed even if the AR is mild to moderate (see Chap. 79). Trauma may result in AR from damage to valve leaflets or aortic annulus and root or from dissection of the aorta. If trauma produces dissection of the aorta and AR, the need for surgery may be an emergent one.

In some instances, heart failure can be controlled completely with pharmacologic therapy, and the LV and LA are able to dilate and adapt to the volume overload; in such instances, surgical ther-

apy may be delayed, perhaps for a considerable period.

CHRONIC AORTIC REGURGITATION

【 】 ETIOLOGY

In North America, the most common cause of chronic, isolated severe AR is aortic root and annular dilatation that is presumably the result of medial disease. Other common causes include a congenital (bicuspid) valve, previous infective endocarditis, and rheumatic disease.[1,84] Chronic AR also occurs in association with a variety of other diseases (Table 75–23). Between 40 and 60 percent of the surgically removed valves from patients with isolated severe AR are classified as idiopathic. Half of these (or 20 to 30 percent of all the valves removed) show histologic criteria of myxomatous degeneration.[90]

【 】 PATHOLOGY

During systole the aortic root and annulus expands by an increase of 14 to 16 percent of the diameter (twice the radius).[91] This causes the commissural attachments to spread apart, initiating the opening of the valves. These movements are continued during LV systole, which produces the forward motion of the blood. The length of the free edge of the cusps equals the diameter of the aortic root and annulus, or roughly one-third of the perimeter. Therefore, dilatation of the aortic root and annulus, if it is not accompanied by an enlargement of the cusps, results in AR.[91]

TABLE 75–22

Indications for Surgery in Infective Endocarditis

Congestive heart failure
Infection
    Uncontrolled by antibiotic therapy
    Fungal
    Usually with staphylococcal infection of aortic or mitral valves
    Serratia
    Usually with gram-negative bacillary infection
Recurrent septic systemic emboli despite adequate antibiotic therapy
Perivalvular and myocardial abscesses
Structural damage to valve in association with other catastrophes (e.g., ruptured sinus of Valsalva)
Very large mobile vegetation

SOURCE: From Rahimtoola SH. Perspective on valvular heart disease: update II. In: Knoebel S, ed. An Era in Cardiovascular Medicine. New York: Elsevier 1991:45–70, with permission.

TABLE 75-23

Etiology of Chronic Aortic Valve Regurgitation

Aortic root dilatation
Congenital bicuspid valve
Previous infective endocarditis
Rheumatic
In association with other diseases
  Congenital lesions, e.g., supravalvular or discrete sub-
    valvular aortic stenosis, ventricular septal defect, and
    aneurysm of the sinus of Valsalva
  Connective tissue disease, e.g., Marfan syndrome, ·
    osteogenesis imperfecta, and Ehlers-Danlos syndrome
  Autoimmune diseases, e.g., ankylosing spondylitis, rheu-
    matoid arthritis, and systemic lupus erythematosus
  Various forms of aortitis and arteritis, e.g., giant cell
    arteritis and Takayasu disease
  Syphilis

Depending on the cause, the valve cusps may show thickening, shortening, commissural lesions, or calcification.[1] Regardless of the cause, the LV is dilated and hypertrophied; some of the largest ventricles have been described in association with chronic severe AR. Little pockets may be seen in the LV outflow tract. These are pouches out of the endocardial lining formed by the regurgitant jets striking the LV.

The myocardium is hypertrophied, with replication of sarcomeres in series, elongation of fibers, and wall thickening. The wall is not thickened as much as it is in patients with AS.

Ultrastructural changes in the myocardial cells are similar to those seen in AS; an important difference, however, is the frequent presence of degenerated cardiac muscle cells in patients with severe AR.[1] Cardiac muscle cells with mild degeneration show focal myofibrillar lysis, with preferential loss of thick myofilament and focal proliferation of tubules of the sarcoplasmic reticulum. Moderately degenerated muscle cells show a marked decrease in the number of myofibrils and T tubules, and proliferation of sarcoplasmic reticulum, mitochondria, or both. Severely degenerated muscle cells usually are present in areas of marked fibrosis; they are often atrophic, have thickened basement membranes, and have lost their intercellular connections. These degenerated cardiac muscle cells may represent the ultrastructural basis for impaired LV function, which is seen more commonly in severe AR than it is in severe AS.

Nodules on the outer surface of the anterior leaflet of the mitral valve have been described in patients with rheumatoid arthritis and ankylosing spondylitis (see Chap. 88).

【 】 PATHOPHYSIOLOGY

In chronic as opposed to acute AR, the AR becomes severe over time; consequently, the LV diastolic pressure–volume relationships are different from those seen in acute AR (see Fig. 75–9). If the AR is mild to moderate, the LV end-diastolic volume is increased moderately, the LV diastolic pressure–volume curve is moved to the right (Fig. 75–12, *curve B*) of normal (Fig. 75–12, *curve A*), and the LV diastolic pressure is usually normal. In severe AR, the LV dia-

stolic pressure–volume curves are moved further to the right (Fig. 75–12, *curves C* and *D*). If the LV systolic pump function is normal, the LV end-diastolic volume can be quite large without significant elevation of LV end-diastolic pressure (Fig. 75–12, *curve C*). If the LV diastolic volume increases further, however, the LV diastolic pressures will be increased. If LV systolic pump dysfunction supervenes, the LV diastolic pressure–volume curve (Fig. 75–12, *curve D*) relationships are moved even further to the right, with quite marked LV dilatation and increases in LV diastolic pressure.

The increase of LV end-diastolic volume[92] is a result of the regurgitant volume (and is proportional to the amount of regurgitation) and LV systolic dysfunction. The increase in end-diastolic volume is proportional to the increase of regurgitant volume. As LV systolic dysfunction supervenes and increases in severity, for any severity of regurgitant volume the LV end-diastolic volume increases further in an attempt to maintain LV stroke volume (see Fig. 75–12).

Severe chronic AR results in a large regurgitant volume (a large percentage of LV stroke volume). The LV responds by dilating (average LV end-diastolic volume in patients undergoing surgery was 205 mL/m²)[18]; the dilatation is proportional to the amount of the regurgitant volume (see Fig. 75–11). The subsequent large LV stroke volume produces LV systolic hypertension. Both of these increase LV wall stress (afterload), which can result in an impairment of LV function. The heart responds by becoming hypertrophied (average LV mass in patients undergoing valve surgery was 222 g/m²),[18] and LV systolic pump function remains normal. There is also an alteration of the LV diastolic pressure–volume relationship (Fig. 75–13). As a result, some patients with normal LV systolic pump function become symptomatic[93] because of the abnormal LV diastolic function (see Fig. 75–12).

In AR, the LV is ejecting against systemic resistance, and the myocardial tension that is developed to open the aortic valve and

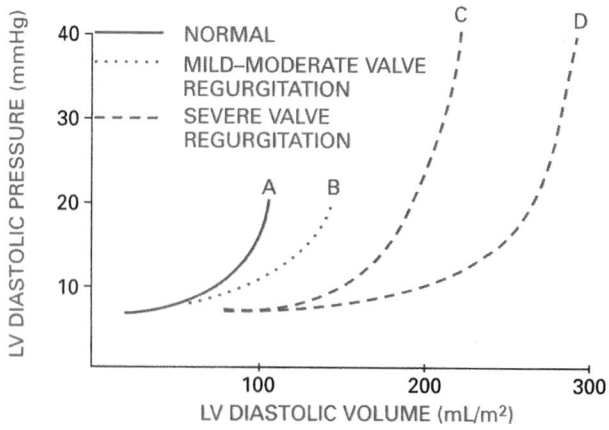

FIGURE 75–12. In chronic aortic regurgitation (AR) as opposed to acute AR, the AR becomes severe over time; consequently, the left ventricular (LV) diastolic pressure–volume (P–V) relationships are different from those seen in acute AR (see Fig. 75–9). If the AR is mild to moderate, the LV diastolic P–V curve is moved to the right (*curve B*). In severe AR, the LV diastolic P–V curves are moved further to the right, depending on whether the LV systolic pump function is normal (*curve C*) or abnormal (*curve D*). Source: From Rahimtoola SH. Management of heart failure in valve regurgitation. *Clin Cardiol* 1992;15(Suppl I):22–27, with permission.

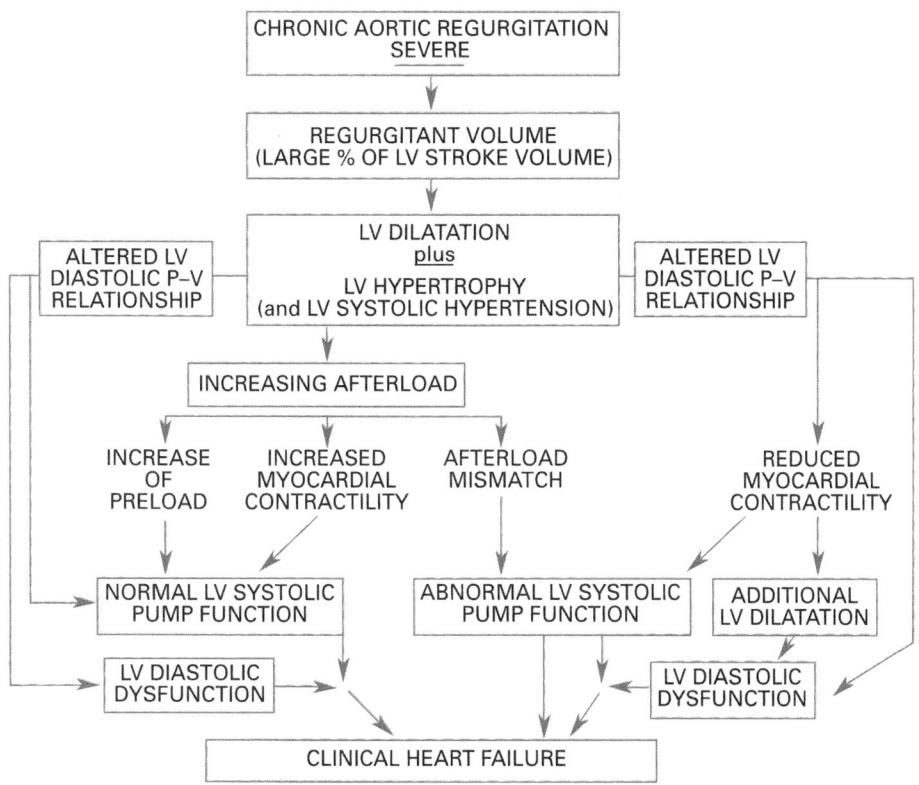

FIGURE 75–13. Severe chronic aortic regurgitation results in a large regurgitant volume (a large percentage of left ventricular [LV] stroke volume). The LV responds by dilating; the subsequent large LV stroke volume results in the production of LV systolic hypertension. There is an alteration of the LV diastolic pressure–volume (P–V) relationship. However, some patients with normal LV systolic pump function become symptomatic because of the abnormal LV diastolic function. As LV afterload (a result of LV dilatation, hypertrophy, and systolic hypertension) continues to increase, the LV uses two additional compensatory mechanisms (i.e., increase of preload and an increase of myocardial contractility). Both of these help maintain normal LV systolic pump function. When the limit of preload reserve has been reached (afterload mismatch) and/or myocardial contractility is reduced, LV systolic pump function becomes abnormal. The additional LV dilatation also results in further alteration of the LV diastolic P–V relationship. Clinical heart failure is usually a result of the abnormal LV systolic pump function; diastolic dysfunction may also be present in some patients. Clinical heart failure in those with normal LV systolic pump function is a result of LV diastolic dysfunction. *Source: Copyright by S.H. Rahimtoola. From Rahimtoola SH. Aortic regurgitation. In: Rahimtoola SH, ed. Atlas of Heart Diseases: Valvular Heart Disease, vol 11. Philadelphia: Current Medicine, 1997:7.1–7.26.*

eject the huge stroke volume is great. This contrasts with another volume-overload lesion, mitral regurgitation, in which there is a low-resistance chamber into which the LV is also emptying (the LA). Thus, for the same degree of regurgitant volume, afterload is higher in AR.

As LV afterload (a combination of LV dilatation, LVH, and systolic hypertension) continues to increase, the LV uses two additional compensatory mechanisms, namely, increase of preload and an increase of myocardial contractility. Both of these help maintain normal LV systolic pump function.

When the limit of preload reserve has been reached (afterload mismatch)[23] and/or myocardial contractility is reduced, LV systolic pump function becomes abnormal. At this stage, correction of AR will result in normalization or marked improvement of LV systolic function. The additional LV dilatation also results in further alteration of the LV diastolic pressure–volume relationship (see Fig. 75–10). Clinical heart failure is usually a result of the abnormal LV systolic pump function. In patients with normal LV systolic pump function,

clinical heart failure is a result of LV diastolic dysfunction.

Because of the leak of blood from the ascending aorta to the LV in diastole, the aortic diastolic pressure is reduced. The large LV stroke volume (a combination of forward stroke volume and regurgitant volume) results in elevation of the aortic systolic pressure, and thus the pulse pressure is considerably increased. Reduction or normalization of aortic systolic pressure is suggestive of LV systolic dysfunction in these patients.

LV stroke volume in AR consists of the forward stroke volume (blood delivered to the body tissues and the heart), which, multiplied by heart rate, makes up the forward cardiac output and the regurgitant volume (the volume of blood that regurgitates back to the LV). In the early stages, even in severe AR, the forward cardiac output and LV ejection fraction are normal at rest. During exercise, as in normal individuals, the systemic vascular resistance is decreased[94] and the heart rate is increased, which reduces the length of diastole. Both these factors reduce the regurgitant volume, and forward stroke volume and cardiac output are increased during exercise.[94] Thus, the ejection fraction on exercise is related to both the myocardial contractile state[95] and the fall in systemic vascular resistance.[94] Accordingly, a decline in ejection fraction on exercise cannot be used as a specific marker of LV function in these patients unless the change in systemic vascular resistance has also been measured. A fall of normal resting ejection fraction to less than 0.50 on exercise, however, correlates with reduced total body oxygen consumption and increased LA pressure during exercise.[94,96]

Further impairment of LV function produces demonstrable abnormalities at rest; there is a further increase in LV end-diastolic volume, which helps to maintain forward stroke volume. The resting LV ejection fraction is reduced, and mean LA pressure begins to increase. Even at this stage, the forward cardiac output may be maintained in the normal range. The increases in LA pressure may produce various grades of pulmonary edema. Finally, in the state of severe heart failure, the ejection fraction may be low, LV end-diastolic volume is large, and LV end-diastolic pressure is greatly increased and is associated with increases in LA, pulmonary, right ventricular, and right atrial pressures. Forward cardiac output is no longer normal. An increase in systemic venous pressure in association with salt and water retention produces engorgement of systemic organs (e.g., the liver), as well as peripheral edema.

In severe AR, myocardial oxygen needs are increased because of increases in LV diastolic and systolic volumes, LV muscle mass (hy-

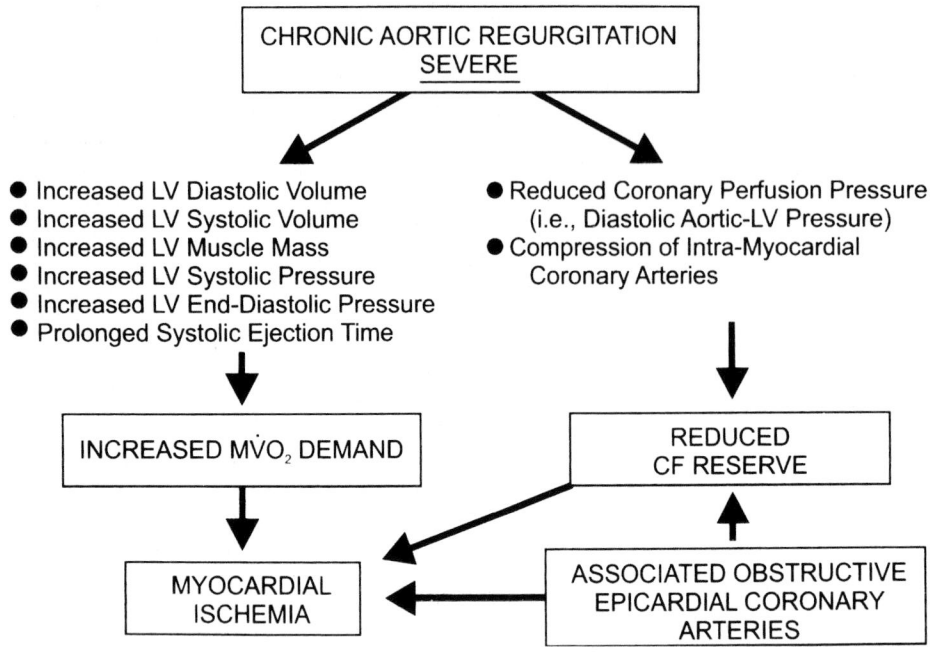

FIGURE 75–14. In severe aortic regurgitation, myocardial oxygen needs are increased. Total coronary blood flow is increased, but coronary reserve (i.e., the ability of the coronary blood flow to increase with vasodilatation) is significantly reduced, probably because of a reduced diastolic aortic–left ventricular (LV) pressure gradient and compression (systolic milking) of intramyocardial coronary arteries. Therefore, myocardial ischemia is often present on stress in these patients. Associated obstructive coronary artery disease can be expected to further exacerbate the myocardial ischemia. CF, coronary flow; MVO$_2$, myocardial oxygen. *Source: Copyright by S.H. Rahimtoola. From Rahimtoola SH. Aortic regurgitation. In: Rahimtoola SH, ed. Atlas of Heart Diseases: Valvular Heart Disease, vol 11. Philadelphia: Current Medicine, 1997:7.1–7.26.*

pertrophy), and LV pressures, as well as by prolongation of systolic ejection time. Total coronary blood flow is increased. Coronary reserve, the ability of the coronary blood flow to increase with vasodilatation, however, is significantly reduced,[97–99] probably because of a reduced diastolic aortic–LV pressure gradient and compression of intramyocardial coronary arteries (systolic "milking" of intramural arteries); consequently, myocardial ischemia is often present on stress in these patients.[97–99] Some patients with severe AR may complain of angina pectoris on effort even in the absence of epicardial CAD. Associated obstructive CAD can be expected to exacerbate further the myocardial ischemia (Fig. 75–14).

【 】 CLINICAL FEATURES

History

Patients with mild to moderate AR usually do not have symptoms that can be attributed to the heart. Even patients with severe AR may be asymptomatic. They may complain of pounding of the head or palpitations, which result from their awareness of the beating of a dilated LV that undergoes a large volume change in systole, during either sinus beats or postectopic beats. The main symptoms of severe AR result from elevated pulmonary venous pressures and include dyspnea on exertion, orthopnea, and paroxysmal nocturnal dyspnea. When heart failure occurs, patients complain of fatigue and weakness. Angina pectoris occurs in 20 percent of such patients and may be present even if the coronary arteries are normal. Angina associated with syphilitic AR may be a

result of associated ostial stenosis of the coronary arteries. In such patients, angina often occurs at rest and is difficult to control.

Physical Examination

A variety of interesting but not very useful clinical signs may be present in patients with chronic severe AR. These include the *de Musset sign* (bobbing of the head with each heartbeat), the *Traube sign* (pistol-shot sound heard over the femoral artery), the *Duroziez sign* (systolic murmur over the femoral artery when it is compressed proximally and diastolic murmur when it is compressed distally), and the *Quincke pulse* (capillary pulsations that can be detected by pressing a glass slide on the patient's lip or transmitting a light through the patient's fingertips).

The arterial pulse is characteristic and consists of an abrupt distension with a rapid rise and a quick collapse (*Corrigan pulse*). The arterial pulse may be bisferious, a double impulse during systole. The systolic arterial pressure is increased (in severe AR it averages 145 to 160 mmHg), the diastolic pressure is reduced (in severe AR it averages 45 to 60 mmHg), and the Korotkoff sounds persist down to 0 mmHg. Even in such instances, however, the recorded intraarterial pressure rarely falls below 30 mmHg. The vasoconstriction that occurs in the presence of heart failure may result in some elevation of the arterial diastolic pressure and should not be interpreted as an improvement in severity of AR. Similarly, LV systolic dysfunction can produce a fall of systolic blood pressure that should not be considered to be an improvement of the AR. The fall of systolic pressure along with elevation of diastolic pressures tends to normalize the pulse pressure. The jugular venous pressure is normal except in heart failure and in those rare instances in which the greatly dilated ascending aorta obstructs the superior vena cava.

On inspection, the chest may rock and the cardiac impulse may be visible. The cardiac impulse is hyperdynamic (Table 75–24). There may be a systolic thrill at the base of the heart, over the carotids, and in the suprasternal notch. This results from a large LV stroke volume across a diseased aortic valve. A diastolic thrill signifies severe AR. S$_1$ is usually soft because the mitral valve leaflets are close to each other at the onset of systole, or there may be premature mitral valve closure. This is exaggerated if the PR interval is prolonged. The S$_2$ is usually single because the aortic valve does not close properly or because the LV ejection time is prolonged and the P$_2$ may not be heard. Often, a systolic ejection murmur, which is sometimes very loud, is present. The clinical sine qua non of AR is an early or immediate, blowing, decrescendo diastolic murmur beginning after A$_2$. It is best heard with the diaphragm of the stethoscope at the left sternal border or, in difficult instances,

TABLE 75–24

Physical Examination of Patients with Varying Severity of Chronic Aortic Valve Regurgitation

	MILD	MODERATE	SEVERE	SEVERE + LEFT VENTRICULAR SYSTOLIC DYSFUNCTION	SEVERE + HEART FAILURE + LEFT VENTRICULAR SYSTOLIC DYSFUNCTION
Arterial pulse	Normal	Corrigan + to + +	Corrigan + + +	Corrigan + +	Corrigan +
Arterial pressure					
Systolic	Normal	Increased + to + +	Increased + + +	Increased + +	Normal/+
Diastolic	Normal	Decreased + to + +	Decreased + + + to + + + +	Decreased + + to + + +	Decreased +
Pulse pressure	Often normal	Increased + to + +	Increased + + + to + + + +	Increased + + to + + +	Increased +
Cardiac impulse	Often normal	Hyperdynamic	Very hyperdynamic visible ± chest may rock	Hyperdynamic	May be hypodynamic
Precordial thrill					
Systolic	–	±	±	±	–
Diastolic	–	–	±	±	–
Auscultation					
S_4	–	–	–	–	–
S_1	Normal	Often soft	Soft	Soft	Soft
S_2	Normal	Normal or single	Often single	Often single	Often single
S_3	–	+	+ + to + + +	+ + +	+ + +
ESM	±	+	+ to + +	+ to + +	+
AoDM	+	+ +	+ + + to + + + +	+ + to + + +	+ to + +
Austin Flint murmur	–	–	±	–	–

–, absent; + + + +, most prominent; ±, present or absent; AoDM, aortic diastolic murmur; ESM, ejection systolic murmur; S_1 and S_2, first and second heart sounds; S_3, third heart sound (diastolic gallop); S_4, fourth heart sound (presystolic gallop).

by having the patient sit up and lean forward and by auscultating with the respiration held at the end of a deep expiration. In severe AR, the murmur may be holodiastolic. When it is soft, its intensity can be increased by having the patient perform isometric exercise, for example, a handgrip, which increases aortic diastolic pressure. At times, this murmur is better heard along the right sternal border, which should draw attention to the possibility that the cause of the AR is aortic root and annular disease (see Chap. 12). Classically, rupture of the sinus of Valsalva into the right side of the heart chambers produces a continuous murmur.

In many patients with severe AR, an Austin Flint murmur[100] (see Chap. 12) is present in presystole and/or mid-diastole. Two inferences can be drawn from the presence of an Austin Flint murmur: (1) it signifies that the AR is severe; and (2) it requires that associated mitral stenosis be excluded. The most helpful sign at the bedside is the response of the murmur to the inhalation of amyl nitrite. The vasodilatation produced by amyl nitrite increases forward flow, reduces the regurgitant volume, and results in the Austin Flint murmur becoming much softer or disappearing. In comparison, the increased cardiac output and tachycardia accentuate or increase the murmur of mitral stenosis. Alternatively, echocardiography can easily demonstrate the presence of organic mitral stenosis.

With severe LV dilatation and/or LV systolic dysfunction, secondary mitral regurgitation may be present with the characteristic holosystolic murmur. Heart failure may be associated with pulmonary congestion or edema, pulmonary hypertension, right ventricular enlargement, tricuspid regurgitation, elevated jugular venous pressure, hepatomegaly, and peripheral edema (see Chap. 12).

Chest Radiography

The LV is increased in size, resulting in an increase in the cardiothoracic ratio. Because the upper limit of normal of the cardiothoracic ratio is 0.49, many patients with increased LV size have an enlarged LV volume and may still have a cardiothoracic ratio within the normal range. A better noninvasive quantification of LV size can be obtained by echocardiography. The ascending aorta is dilated throughout, and there may be calcium in the aortic valve. With increased filling pressures in the later stages, there might be evidence of an enlarged LA and an increased LA and pulmonary venous pressure, which are manifested in the pulmonary vascular shadows by a redistribution of blood flow, pulmonary congestion, and pulmonary edema. In the presence of heart failure, enlargement of the right atrium and superior vena cava may be appreciated. Calcification that is limited to the ascending aorta is strongly suggestive of luetic aortitis.

Electrocardiogram

The ECG shows LVH with or without associated secondary ST–T-wave changes. In a small percent of patients, ECG evidence of LVH is absent in spite of severe AR. Conduction abnormalities, such as atrioventricular block or left or right bundle-branch block with or without axis deviation, may be present. The PR interval may be prolonged, particularly in patients with ankylosing spondylitis. The rhythm is usually sinus. The presence of atrial fibrillation should make one suspect the presence of associated mitral valve disease or heart failure.

Echocardiography

The sign of AR on echocardiography is diastolic fluttering of the anterior leaflet of the mitral valve. Echocardiography can easily exclude the presence of associated mitral stenosis. LV dimensions are increased, and if LV function is normal, the percent of dimensional shortening is normal. The increase in LV dimensions caused by volume overload, results in separation between the open anterior leaflet of the mitral valve and the endocardial surface of the interventricular septum (septal-E point separation). In AR, as in other volume-overload lesions, the response in mild volume overload is an elongation of the heart. Because M-mode echocardiography takes a pencil look at the short axis of the heart, LV dimensions by M-mode echocardiography may appear to be normal. In such patients, two-dimensional echocardiography is much superior to the M-mode technique for assessing LV volumes and systolic function. A dilated ascending aorta can be detected on echocardiography, as can an enlarged LA. Aortic valve vegetations suggest infective endocarditis. Some other conditions can easily be detected by echocardiography—for example, prolapse of the aortic leaflet into the LV in diastole.

Doppler ultrasound is essential for diagnosing and assessing the severity of AR. When using Doppler, there is a high incidence of "false-positive" (physiologic) trivial regurgitation. There is also an overlap between the various grades of severity of assessment of AR by Doppler when compared with angiography (see Chap. 16).

Transesophageal echocardiography is a useful technique when transthoracic echocardiogram is unsatisfactory and, in certain instances, when identifying the anatomy of the valve leaflets and aortic root and annulus. It is essential to evaluate if the valve is suitable for repair, especially in patients suspected of having infective endocarditis. Echo/Doppler ultrasound is also very useful for assessing disease of other valves.

Cardiac Catheterization and Angiography

Cardiac catheterization allows the measurement of intracardiac and intravascular pressures and cardiac output, both at rest and during exercise, and can demonstrate the changes described in Pathophysiology above. In addition, other valvular disease—for example, mitral stenosis, aortic stenosis, and mitral regurgitation—can be excluded. LV angiography demonstrates enlarged LV volumes and allows the calculation of LV volumes and LV ejection fraction. Angiography performed with injection of contrast medium in the ascending aorta demonstrates AR and allows a semi-quantitative assessment of the degree of AR. In addition, the angiogram demonstrates the dimensions of the aortic root and the state of the ascending aorta. The indications for selective coronary angiography are the same as for aortic stenosis (see Table 75–4).

Gated Blood Pool Radionuclide Scans

Gated blood pool radionuclide scans also allow the measurement of LV volumes and ejection fraction. The scans also allow measurement of LV ejection fraction on exercise and on serial studies. It is also possible to quantify the amount of AR.

Treadmill Exercise Test

A treadmill exercise test provides an objective assessment of the degree of functional impairment and documentation of arrhythmias related to exertion. In some patients, however, the exercise test may remain normal despite deterioration of LV function.

Ambulatory Electrocardiogram Recording

Ambulatory ECG recording may be needed occasionally in a patient suspected of having an arrhythmia (see Chap. 41).

Cardiac Magnetic Resonance

Cardiac magnetic resonance can demonstrate AR but is rarely needed clinically (see Chap. 21).

Viability Testing

In selected patients with valve disease especially in those with LV dysfunction it may be necessary to diagnose and quantify the extent of myocardial infarction by cardiac magnetic resonance, as well as the extent of hibernating myocardium.[101]

【 】 CLINICAL DECISION MAKING

Please see the equivalent section Aortic Valve Stenosis above.

Table 75–25 shows the sensitivity, specificity, and accuracy of diagnosis of chronic AR.[46] The following should be noted: (1) The sensitivity, specificity, and accuracy of diagnosing AR after clinical evaluation are good but not quite as good as in AS. (2) Echo/Dop-

TABLE 75–25

Clinical Decision Making Using Clinical Evaluation versus Echo/Doppler in Patients with Aortic Regurgitation (AR)

	AFTER CLINICAL EVALUATION (%)	AFTER ECHO/ DOPPLER (%)
Diagnosis of AR		
Sensitivity	66	79
Specificity	76	74
Accuracy of diagnosis		
All levels of severity	43	57
Moderate or severe AR	91	100

SOURCE: Kotlewski A, Kawanishi DT, McKay CR, et al. The relative value of clinical examination, echocardiography with Doppler and cardiac catheterization with angiography in the evaluation of aortic valve disease. In: Bodnar E, ed. Surgery for Heart Valve Disease. London: ICR 1990:66–72, with permission.

pler ultrasound improves these criteria to a greater extent than it does in AS. (3) The difficulties lie in accurately distinguishing patients with mild[102] AR from healthy individuals and those with moderate AR and in distinguishing between moderate AR and severe AR. (4) Both clinical evaluation and echo/Doppler ultrasound are excellent aids for diagnosing AR as moderate or severe. The single most important sign of severe chronic AR is an enlarged LV which increases proportionally to the severity of AR (see Fig. 75–13 and Pathophysiology above).

[ ] NATURAL HISTORY AND PROGNOSIS

Patients with mild AR that does not progress should have a normal life expectancy. Their major risk is the development of infective endocarditis and further valve destruction. Patients with moderate AR, if their disease does not progress, would be expected to have a life expectancy that is reasonably close to the normal range. The disease does progress, however, and mortality at the end of 10 years appears to be approximately 15 percent.

A recent study shows that the time from diagnosis of rheumatic carditis/AR to development of symptoms is 30 years; that is, there is very long asymptomatic period.[103]

Patients with severe AR are known to have a long asymptomatic period before the condition is discovered. In asymptomatic patients with normal LV function at rest, symptoms and/or LV dysfunction (and/or sudden death) develops at the rate of approximately 3 to 6 percent per year.[104] The predictor of development of symptoms is LV systolic dysfunction at rest.[104] In patients with normal LV systolic function at rest (Table 75–26), the predictors of development of LV systolic dysfunction and/or symptoms are an increased LV size (LV dimension at end-diastole of ≥70 mm and at end-systole of ≥50 mm,[104–107] and LV end-diastolic volume index of ≥150 mL/m²)[106] and abnormal LV ejection fraction on exercise of ≤0.50.[106] In small people, for example, in women,[107] these values are too large and have to be corrected for body size. The corrected dimensions for end-diastole and end-systole are 35 mm/m² and 25 mm/m², respectively.[107] Sudden

TABLE 75–26

Chronic Severe Aortic Regurgitation: Asymptomatic + Normal Left Ventricle (LV) Function at Rest

		LIKELIHOOD OF SYMPTOMS OR LV DYSFUNCTION OR DEATH (% PER YEAR)
LV end-diastolic dimension	≥70 mmᵃ	10
	<70 mm	2
LV end-systolic dimension	≥50 mmᵃ	19
	40–49 mm	6
	<40 mm	0

ᵃWhen corrected for body size the values are ≥35 mm/m² and ≥25 mm/ m²; please see text.
SOURCE: *From Bonow RO, Lakatos E, Maron BJ, et al. Serial long-term assessment of the natural history of asymptomatic patients with chronic aortic regurgitation and normal left ventricular systolic function. Circulation 1991;84:1625–1635, with permission.*

death in asymptomatic patients appears to occur only in those with a massively dilated LV (LV end-diastolic dimension of ≥80 mm).[105] It is likely that LV dysfunction first appears on exercise and later also at rest; eventually, heart failure ensues. Severe symptoms, however, may occur even when LV systolic pump function is normal at rest. The 5-year mortality of symptomatic patients with severe AR is approximately 25 percent, and the 10-year mortality averages 50 percent.[108] Once symptoms occur in patients with AR, it is likely that the rate of deterioration will be rapid. Most patients with angina are dead within 4 years.[109] The 2- to 3-year mortality of those with heart failure is 50 to 70 percent. In a study of older patients, the mortality was 4.7 percent per year; in the symptomatic patients, it was 9.4 percent per year;[110] and in the asymptomatic patients, it was 2.8 percent per year, which was not significantly different from age- and gender-matched individuals in the population. In the symptomatic patient, those in the NYHA classes III and IV had an annual mortality of 24.6 percent per year, whereas in the class II patient, it was 6.3 percent per year. In asymptomatic patients with a LV ejection fraction <0.55, the annual mortality was 5.8 percent per year, whereas in patients with a LV end-systolic dimension >25 mm/m², it was 7.8 percent per year.[110]

Table 75–12 outlines the major factors that influence outcome in patients with valvular heart disease.

[ ] MANAGEMENT

All patients with AR need antibiotic prophylaxis to prevent infective endocarditis. Patients with AR of a rheumatic origin need antibiotic prophylaxis to prevent recurrences of rheumatic carditis. Patients with syphilitic AR need a course of antibiotics to treat syphilis.

Patients with mild AR need no specific therapy (see Table 75–23). They do not need to restrict their activities and can lead a normal life. Patients with moderate AR also usually need no specific therapy. These patients, however, should avoid heavy physical exertion, competitive sports, and isometric exercise.

In asymptomatic patients with severe AR and normal LV systolic function,[111,112] a calcium channel blocking agent, long-acting nifedipine, produced significant reductions in blood pressure and LV end-diastolic volume, and mass and major increases in LV ejection fraction at the end of 1 year. Almost all patients completed the trial. A prospective randomized trial in *asymptomatic* patients with *normal LV systolic* function (Padua trial)[113] showed that at the end of 6 years, 34 ± 6 percent of patients treated with digoxin developed LV systolic dysfunction and/or symptoms, and thus needed AVR, compared with 15 ± 3 percent of patients who were treated with long-acting nifedipine (*p* <.001; Fig. 75–15); 89 percent (23 of 26) of those who needed AVR had developed LV systolic dysfunction with or without symptoms; only 3 had become symptomatic without developing LV systolic dysfunction. Accordingly, all asymptomatic patients with severe AR and normal LV systolic function should be treated with a vasodilator (the calcium antagonist long-acting nifedipine) unless there is a contraindication to its use.

A recent trial (Barcelona trial) failed to show a beneficial effect of nifedipine in patients with AR.[114] There are at least four problems with this trial[115]: (1) Patients were in a prospective study of

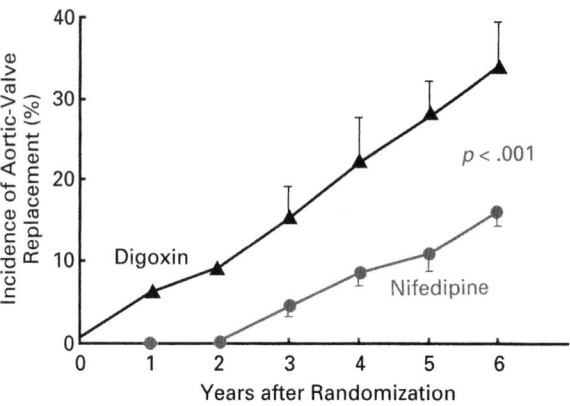

FIGURE 75–15. The role of long-term nifedipine therapy in asymptomatic patients with severe aortic regurgitation (AR) and normal left ventricular (LV) systolic pump function was evaluated in 143 asymptomatic patients in a prospective randomized trial. By actuarial analysis, at 6 years, 34 ± 6 percent of patients in the digoxin group underwent aortic valve replacement (AVR), versus 15 ± 3 percent of those in the nifedipine group (p <.001). This randomized trial demonstrates that long-term vasodilator therapy with nifedipine reduces and/or delays the need for AVR in asymptomatic patients with severe AR and normal LV systolic pump function. *Source: From Scognamiglio R, Rahimtoola SH, Fasoli G, et al. Nifedipine in asymptomatic patients with severe aortic regurgitation and normal left ventricular function. N Engl J Med 1994;331:689–695, with permission.*

long duration and did not have AVR and were then entered into the trial. (2) The diastolic blood pressure was 78 ± 11 mmHg (in the Padua trial it was 60 ± 8 mmHg) and the LV end-diastolic volume was 94 ± 27 mL/m^2 (in the Padua trial it was 126 ± 16 mL/m^2), which data indicate that many patients in the Barcelona trial[114] did not have severe AR. (3) There were only 32 patients in the nifedipine group, of which 7 (22 percent) dropped out at 2 ± 7 months; thus, there was only a very small number of patients in the trial. (4) Nifedipine (not long-acting) 20 mg was given every 12 hours and there was no change in blood pressure.

The role of nifedipine in patients with moderate AR has not been studied. In view of its beneficial effects in severe AR, long-acting nifedipine could be used in selected patients with moderate AR if there are no contraindications to its use. The value of an ACE inhibitor is not well documented. Moreover, there are no published data to show that ACE inhibitor therapy reduces the need for valve surgery. In brief, ACE inhibitors are not of proven benefit in asymptomatic patients with AR and normal LV systolic function.

Table 75–27 gives the followup for asymptomatic patients with severe AR and normal LV systolic function.

Symptomatic patients with severe AR need medical and surgical treatment. Medical treatment (Table 75–28) consists of the administration of digitalis, diuretics, and vasodilators. Digitalis is clearly indicated in patients with symptoms. The need for and benefits of this therapy in asymptomatic patients are not well documented. Diuretics are of value when the LA pressure is elevated and in the presence of heart failure.

Long-term hydralazine therapy in symptomatic patients results in significant benefit in only 20 to 35 percent of patients.[37] Those patients who are likely to benefit cannot be predicted. Vasodilators are indicated in patients who refuse surgery or who are not operative candidates for any reason.

TABLE 75–27

Followup for Asymptomatic Patients with Severe Aortic Regurgitation and Normal Left Ventricle (LV) Systolic Function

Monitor
  Symptoms
  LV dysfunction[a]
  Progressive decrease of
    Exercise capacity
    LV systolic function[a]
  Progressive increase of LV size[a]

[a]These are best done by high-quality echocardiographic/Doppler studies, ideally performed every 6 months.
Source: Copyright S.H. Rahimtoola.

Vasodilators are also indicated for short-term therapy in patients awaiting AVR to optimize their hemodynamics (reduce filling pressures and increase cardiac output) and thus reduce their operative risks. If LV systolic function is normal, they can be given long-acting nifedipine. If they have abnormal LV systolic function, they should be treated with digitalis and ACE inhibitors; diuretics and hydralazine, with or without nitrates, can be used if needed. Small doses of hydralazine (50 mg) are without therapeutic effect in AR, and larger doses (≥100 mg) need to be given only twice daily[116]; the twice-daily regimen reduces the incidence of side effects but is not a good choice for long-term followup because by 6 months up to 50 percent of patients develop significant side effects. Hydralazine should be started in small doses and gradually increased, depending on patient tolerance of the drug.

Vasodilators are of considerable short-term benefit in patients in NYHA functional classes III and IV or heart failure. All such patients need digitalis, diuretics, and ACE inhibitors. In patients in NYHA functional class IV with heart failure, vasodilators should ideally be started after the institution of bedside hemodynamic monitoring, that is, measurement of pulmonary artery wedge pressure and cardiac output with the use of balloon flotation catheters. Hemodynamic monitoring accurately identifies patients who need the therapy, since clinical judgments can be wrong. It establishes whether arterial dilators alone will suffice or whether additional venodilators are needed. Finally, it provides information on the optimum dosage of vasodilator therapy. After the initial hemodynamic measurements are made, arterial dilators are given in progressively increasing dosage until an optimum effect on cardiac output has been obtained. If cardiac output does not show any further increase but LA pressure is still very high, additional venodilator therapy should be given. If the patient is very ill or the hemodynamic abnormalities are marked, intravenous therapy (e.g., sodium nitroprusside) is the vasodilator of first choice. In this situation, intravenous vasodilator therapy should be used only with bedside hemodynamic monitoring. Inotropic agents, such as dobutamine, may be needed to improve LV function and increase cardiac output. Low-dose dopamine may be of value to increase urinary output.

Patients with severe chronic AR need valve surgery. The correct timing of surgical therapy is now better defined but is not fully clarified. AVR should be performed before irreversible LV dys-

TABLE 75-28

Medical Treatment of Patients with Aortic Regurgitation

I. Antibiotic prophylaxis
  A. Infective endocarditis
  B. Recurrent rheumatic carditis
II. Restriction of activities (moderate/severe AR)
  A. Severe exercise
  B. Competitive sports
III. Arrhythmias
  A. Prevent and/or control
  B. Restore sinus rhythm, if possible
IV. Cardiac medications
  A. Asymptomatic, normal LV function
    1. Mild AR: None
    2. Moderate AR: ? Nifedipine long-acting
    3. Severe AR: Nifedipine long-acting
  B. Severe AR symptomatic (while waiting for surgery)
    1. Normal LV function: Nifedipine long-acting
    2. LV dysfunction: Digitalis
                    ACE inhibitors
                    Hydralazine ± nitrates,
                      if needed
                    Diuretics, if needed
                    Dobutamine, if needed
  C. Severe AR + heart failure:
    Digitalis, diuretics, ACE inhibitors
    Hydralazine + nitrates
    IV nitroprusside, if IV therapy needed
    Dobutamine, if needed
V. Followup of asymptomatic patient
  A. Mild AR: Every 2–5 years
  B. Moderate AR: Every 1–2 years
  C. Severe AR: Every 6–12 months
  D. Develop symptoms: Early or immediate

ACE, angiotensin-converting enzyme; AR, aortic regurgitation; LV, left ventricle.
Source: Copyright by S.H. Rahimtoola.

TABLE 75-29

Chronic Severe Aortic Regurgitation: Indications for Surgery[a]

I. Symptomatic patients
  A. LV function normal: as soon as possible
  B. LV dysfunction: urgent
  C. Heart failure: emergent
  D. Individualize if
    1. Very severe LV dysfunction (LVEF ≤0.20)
    2. Severe LV dilatation (LVEDD ≥80 mm with severe LV dysfunction; LVEDVI ≥300 mL/m^2)
    3. Small RgV (RgV/EDV ≤0.14)
II. Asymptomatic patients
  A. LV systolic dysfunction (LVEF ≤0.50–0.54)
  B. Normal LV systolic function
    1. Associated cardiovascular diseases requiring surgery
      a. CAD
      b. Other valve disease
      c. Ascending aortic aneurysm
    2. Large LV
      LVEDD ≥70; ≥35 mm/m^2
      LVESD ≥50–55 mm; ≥25–27 mm/m^2
      LVEDVI ≥150 mL/m^2
      PLUS PA wedge on exercise ≥20–22 mmHg
    3. Progressive changes in LV size and function
      Increase of LVEDD and/or LVESD
      Decrease of LVEF

CAD, coronary artery disease; EDD, end-diastolic dimension; EDVI, end-diastolic volume index; EDV, end-diastolic volume; EF, ejection fraction; LV, left ventricular; PAW, pulmonary artery wedge; RgV, regurgitant volume.
[a]Valve replacement/valve repair.
Source: Copyright by S.H. Rahimtoola.

function occurs. The major problem, however, is identifying the precise point at which LV dysfunction will occur. Here, two major difficulties are encountered: (1) patients may already have impaired LV systolic pump function at rest when they first present or at the time of the first symptom, and (2) patients with severe symptoms may have normal LV systolic pump function. Patients may be in NYHA functional class III (symptoms with less than ordinary activity) with a normal LV ejection fraction,[93] or they may be in NYHA functional class I (asymptomatic) with a reduced LV ejection fraction.[93,117] A reduced LV ejection fraction demonstrated by two-dimensional echocardiography and/or radionuclide ventriculography is the best noninvasive indicator of depressed LV systolic function.

Decisions about AVR should be based on the clinical functional class and on the LV ejection fraction at rest (Table 75–29).[118] Patients with chronic severe AR who are symptomatic (NYHA functional classes II to IV) need valve replacement. The benefit from

AVR has been demonstrated even when the LV ejection fraction is 0.25 or less.[119] As opposed to AS, in which there is no lower level of ejection fraction that indicates inoperability, it is likely that some patients with AR and a very low ejection fraction become inoperable. This level has not been precisely defined but may be about 0.15 or less. There is a need to individualize the need for AVR in those with very severe LV systolic dysfunction at rest (LV ejection fraction <0.20), in those with very severe LV dilatation (LV end-diastolic volume index ≥300 mL/m^2),[120] and in those with a small regurgitant volume with a ratio of regurgitant volume to end-diastolic volume of 0.14.[121] Data indicate that patients with severe AR, LV end-diastolic dimension on echocardiography of ≥80 mm, and mild to moderate reduction of LV ejection fraction (mean: 0.43) can obtain benefit from AVR.[122] Postoperatively, they are symptomatically improved, LV ejection fraction increases, and LV size is reduced; the 5- and 10-year survivals are 87 and 71 percent, respectively.

Patients who are in NYHA functional class I (asymptomatic) and who have a reduced ejection fraction at rest should be offered AVR. If the ejection fraction is normal at rest, one should consider AVR in NYHA functional class I patients if they have severe obstructive CAD and/or need surgery for other valve disease (see Table 75–28). It is suggested that patients undergo an

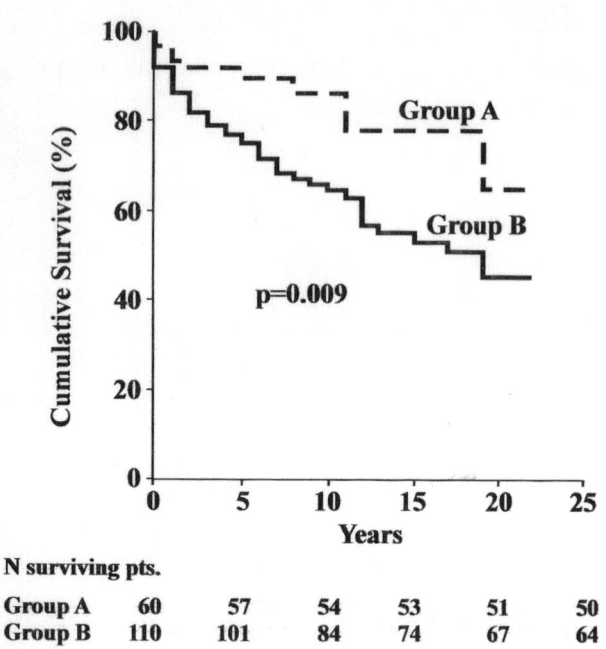

FIGURE 75-16. Survival in group A patients, that is, those who had early surgery according to *Guideline* recommendations, was significantly better than those who had it "too late." Source: From Tornos P, Sambola A, Permanyta-Miralda G, et al. Long-term outcome of surgically treated aortic regurgitation. J Am Coll Cardiol 2006;47:1012–1017.

exercise test during right side of the heart catheterization if the LV is large (LV end-diastolic volume ≥150 mL/m² and LV internal dimension on M-mode echocardiography of ≥70 mm [≥25 mm/m²] at end-diastole and ≥50 mm [≥25 mm/m²] at end-systole) and/or the LV ejection fraction shows a new, persistent reduction to 0.54 to 0.60; if the patients have reduced exercise capacity on treadmill testing; or if ambulatory ECG monitoring demonstrates ventricular tachyarrhythmias. AVR is recommended if the pulmonary artery wedge pressure during exercise increases more than 20 to 24 mmHg. Patients with associated significant CAD should have coronary bypass surgery performed at the time of valvular surgery (see Aortic Valve Stenosis above and Table 75–15).

A recent study evaluated long-term outcome of early surgery (group A; n = 60) according to *Guideline* recommendations (asymptomatic with a LVEF <50 percent or with LV end-diastolic diameter >70 mm and LV end-systolic diameter >50 mm; or in NYHA functional class II) or "too late" (NYHA functional classes III and IV). The survival in groups A and B at 10 years was 86 ± 5 percent versus 64 ± 5 percent and at 15 years was 78 ± 7 percent versus 53 ± 6 percent, respectively (*p* = 0.009)[123] (Fig. 75–16). AVR, with or without associated coronary bypass surgery for obstructive CAD, can be performed at many surgical centers with an operative mortality of 5 percent or lower. In many centers with appropriate skill and experience in patients with none or few comorbidities, the operative mortality can be ≤2 percent, and for AVR + CABG it can be ≤4 percent. If AVR is successful and uncomplicated, LV volume and LVH regress but do not return to normal; the beneficial effects on LV size, volume, and mass continue to be seen for as long as 5 years after surgery.[63,124,125] Impaired LV systolic pump function improves postoperatively in 50 percent or more of patients[119]; this improvement is more likely to occur if LV dysfunction has been present preoperatively for 12 months or less, and in this subgroup LV ejection fraction usually normalizes.[105] Even if LV systolic pump function does not improve, there is a reduction in end-diastolic volume and LVH;[119] from a cardiac point of view, this is advantageous to the patient. The 5-year survival of patients undergoing AVR in severe AR is 85 percent (this figure includes operative and late cardiac deaths).[118] The 5-year survival of patients with a LV ejection fraction of ≥0.45 is 87 percent, versus 54 percent in patients with an ejection fraction of <0.45.[118] Late survival after valve replacement for chronic severe AR is best predicted by variables indicative of LV systolic pump function. In the future, it is possible that selected patients may eventually need to have valve repair rather than AVR for AR (see Chap. 79).

Care should be exercised in the interpretation of the data on operative or late mortality (see Chap. 79).

Table 75–30 provides the recommendations of the ACC/AHA *Practice Guidelines* for AVR in AR.[75] Guidelines are *not* and should *not* be the *law*. Application of such guidelines to clinical practice should be based on the following principles: (1) NYHA classes I and III apply to all patients in these classes unless there is a specific clinical circumstance not to do so; (2) NYHA class II applies to patients in this class depending on the clinical conditions of the patients and the skill and experience at the individual medical center.

BICUSPID AORTIC VALVE IN ADULTS

Although a bicuspid aortic valve (BAV) is a congenital lesion (see Chap. 82), its clinical importance is largely in adults. An excellent recent review article pointed out that the earliest description of the BAV is attributed to Leonardo de Vinci who, more than 400 years ago, sketched the bicuspid variant of the aortic valve.[126]

【 】 PREVALENCE AND INCIDENCE

In a prospective study of all 817 children (400 males, 417 females, age 10 years) in a valley with 41,432 inhabitants, echocardiography of the children showed BAV in 0.5 percent.[127] Prevalence in boys was 0.75 percent, and in girls it was 0.24 percent; the ratio of incidence in boys-to-girls was 3:1.

A review of seven necropsy studies showed the incidence of BAV ranged from 0.5 percent to 1.39 percent.[128]

【 】 HEREDITY

In one study of 309 probands and relatives, echocardiography showed BAV in 74 (prevalence 24 percent and heritability [h₂] of 89 percent); BAV and/or other cardiovascular malformation was present in 97 (prevalence 31 percent, h₂ 75 percent).[129] The authors concluded that (1) the high heritability of BAV suggests that in their study population, BAV is "almost entirely genetic"; and (2) the inheritance of BAV is likely a result of mutations in

TABLE 75–30

Indications for Aortic Valve Replacement in Aortic Regurgitation

Class I

1. AVR is indicated for symptomatic patients with severe AR irrespective of LV systolic function. *(Level of Evidence: B)*
2. AVR is indicated for asymptomatic patients with chronic severe AR and LV systolic dysfunction (ejection fraction 0.50 or less) at rest. *(Level of Evidence: B)*
3. AVR is indicated for patients with chronic severe AR while undergoing CABG or surgery on the aorta or other heart valves. *(Level of Evidence: B)*

Class IIa

1. AVR is reasonable for asymptomatic patients with severe AR with normal LV systolic function (ejection fraction greater than 0.50) but with severe LV dilation (end-diastolic dimension greater than 75 mm or end-systolic dimension greater than 55 mm). *(Level of Evidence B)*

Class IIb

1. AVR may be considered in patients with moderate AR while undergoing surgery on the ascending aorta. *(Level of Evidence: C)*
2. AVR may be considered in patients with moderate AR while undergoing CABG. *(Level of Evidence: C)*
3. AVR may be considered for asymptomatic patients with severe AR and normal LV systolic function at rest (ejection fraction greater than 0.50) when the degree of LV dilatation exceeds (end-diastolic dimension of 70 mm or end-systolic dimension of 50 mm when there is evidence of progressive LV dilation, declining exercise tolerance, or abnormal hemodynamic responses to exercise. *(Level of Evidence: C)*

Class III

1. AVR is not indicated for asymptomatic patients with mild, moderate, or severe AR and normal LV systolic function at rest (ejection fraction greater than 0.50) when degree of dilatation is not moderate or severe (end-diastolic dimension less than 70 mm, end-systolic dimension less than 50 mm). *(Level of Evidence: B)*

AR, aortic regurgitation; AVR, aortic valve replacement; CABG, coronary artery bypass graft; LV, left ventricle.
SOURCE: Bonow RO, Carabello B, Chatterjee K, et al. ACC/AHA guidelines on the management of patients with valvular heart disease: report of the ACC/AHA Task Force or practice guidelines 2006. www.acc.org, e37.

diverse genes with dissimilar inheritance patterns in families. The incidence of familial recurrence of BAV is approximately 9 percent. Inheritance is most likely with an autosomal-dominant inheritance pattern with reduced penetrance.[130] Consequently, screening with echocardiography is recommended for first-degree relatives of patients with BAV.

ABNORMALITIES IN ANEURYSMAL TISSUE OF BAV

Marfan syndrome is known to be a genetic disorder caused by a mutation in the fibrillin gene.[131] The study by Nataatmadja et al. of BAV and Marfan syndrome (Fig. 75–17)[131] showed (1) cystic medial necrosis without inflammatory infiltrate in tissues of both groups. (2) Immunohistochemical study of cultured BAV and of Marfan syndrome vascular smooth muscle cell (VSMC) showed intracellular accumulation and reduction of extracellular distribution of fibrillin, fibronectin, and tenascin. (3) The VSMC of both groups showed no increase in expression of fibrillin, fibronectin, or tenascin and an increased expression of matrix metalloproteinase-2 in Marfan syndrome (see Chap. 88).[131,132] (4) There was a fourfold increase in loss of cultured VSMC in serum-free medium for 24 hours of 32 ± 4 percent of patients with BAV and of 27 ± 8 percent of patients with Marfan syndrome versus the occurrence in controls of 7 ± 5 percent (p <0.05). These data suggest the presence of a fundamental cellular abnormality in the thoracic aorta of patients with BAV.[133] Other studies have also shown a reduction of fibrillin and an increase of matrix metalloproteinase-2 in the walls of aneurysms associated with BAV.[127,128]

AORTIC DILATATION IN BAV

The dimensions of the aortic root are larger in children[134] with BAV than in children with tricuspid AV; and also larger than in young adults. There is a progression of aortic dilation in adults with BAV. In a study of 68 patients with BAV,[135] mean age 44 years, at an average followup of 47 months, an increase was seen at the sinus of Valsalva (mean: 1.9 mm; 95 percent CI: 1.3 to 2.5), at the sinotubular junction (mean: 1.6 mm; 95 percent CI: 0.8 to 2.3), and at the proximal ascending aorta (mean: 2.7 mm; 95 percent CI: 1.9 to 3.6). Progression of aortic dilatation occurred irrespective of baseline BAV function.

PATHOLOGIC FEATURES

The anatomy of the BAV usually includes one large cusp (caused by fusion of two cusps) and a central raphe that is identifiable in most patients with BAV. The raphe does not contain valve tissue.[136] Frequently, the left and right coronary cusps are the larger with fused commissures (raphe) and the coronary arteries tend to arise from the front of the cusps in which a raphe is present. The left main coronary artery is short and the coronary circulation tends to be left dominant.[137,138] Fig. 75–18 shows an echocardiographic-anatomic correlation in 115 patients.[139] The pattern is very variable; in 1135 children, pattern A was seen in 70 percent, and in a surgical series of 542 cases,[140] 86 percent had pattern A. The calcification process that occurs in BAV is similar in its cellular and molecular mechanisms to the processes involved in calcific AS of tricuspid AV,[141] but is accelerated.

ASSOCIATED CONGENITAL CARDIOVASCULAR MALFORMATIONS

Table 75–31 identifies the more common associated cardiovascular malformations. Coarctation of the aorta may be "simple" (iso-

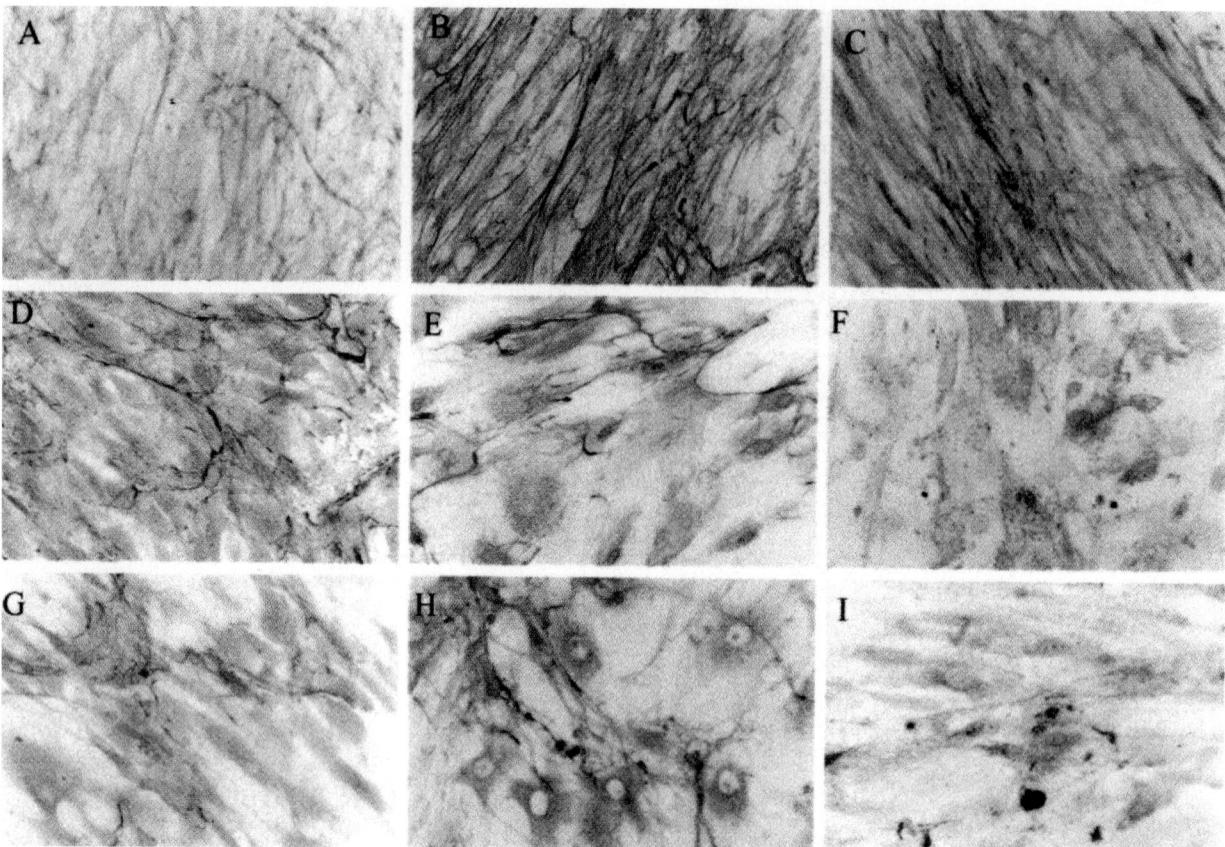

FIGURE 75–17. Cultured control vascular smooth muscle cells (**A** to **C**), Marfan syndrome (**D** to **F**), and bicuspid aortic valve (**G** to **I**). Immunohistochemistry using antibodies against fibrillin (**A,D,G**), fibronectin (**B,E,H**), and tenascin (**C,F,I**). Magnification × 250. *Source: From Nataatmadja M, West M, West J, et al. Abnormal extracellular matrix protein transport associated with increased apoptosis of vascular smooth muscle cells in Marfan's syndrome and bicuspid aortic valve thoracic aortic aneurysms. Circulation 2003;108 Suppl II:329–334.*

lated defect) or "complex" (associated with other intracardiac or extracardiac defects). BAV should be looked for in patients who have a patent ductus arteriosus. Ventricular septal defect is the most common congenital defect in children and occurs in 30 percent. Perimembranous ventricular septal defect with partial aortic leaflet prolapse into the defect causes AR. Left coronary dominance is common (see above) and many coronary artery anomalies have been reported.[142]

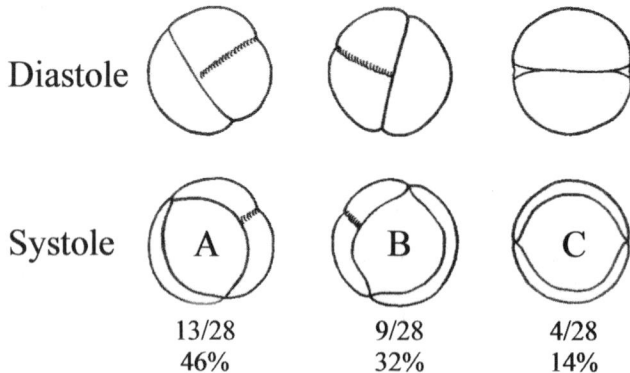

FIGURE 75–18. The morphologic pattern noted on parasternal short axis echocardiography of 28 patients with bicuspid aortic valve. *Source: From Brandenburg RO, Tajik AJ, Edwards WD, et al. Accuracy of 2-dimensional echocardiographic diagnosis of congenital bicuspid aortic valve: echocardiographic-anatomic correlation in 115 patients. Am J Cardiol 1983;51:1469–1473.*

Diastole / Systole

A 13/28 46% B 9/28 32% C 4/28 14%

COMPLICATIONS

Table 75–32 lists the complications associated with BAV. Infective endocarditis is a frequent problem partly because patients with BAV are often unaware of their disease and, thus, have not been advised about antibiotic prophylaxis for prevention of infective endocarditis.

SYMPTOMS

There are no specific symptoms of BAV, only those that are a result of associated malformations or complications (see Tables 75–31 and 75–32).

TABLE 75–31

Balloon Aortic Valvuloplasty and Associated Congenital Cardiovascular Lesions

Coarctation of the aorta[a]
Patent ductus arteriosus[a]
Coronary arteries anatomic variants[a]
Supravalvular aortic stenosis/Williams syndrome
Mitral valve malformations (parachute valve, etc.)
Shone Syndrome
Turner Syndrome

[a]An associated lesion that is more commonly seen in adults.

TABLE 75-32

Complications Associated with Balloon Aortic Valvuloplasty

Aortic stenosis
Aortic regurgitation
Aortic root/ascending aortic dilatation/aneurysm
Ascending aortic dissection
Infective endocarditis

[ ] PHYSICAL EXAMINATION

A functionally normal BAV may have an ejection sound (systolic ejection click) that may be followed by an early peaking systolic flow murmur. The ejection sound is a reflection of the sudden cephalad movement of the dome-shaped bicuspid valve in systole and generally correlates with valve leaflet mobility.[143] The ejection sound diminishes as the valve cusps become more immobile and stenotic and in the presence of moderate or severe AR. The ejection sound is often loudest at the apex and lower sternal edge but usually radiates to the base. A systolic murmur that radiates to the right sternal border is rarely innocent. The differential diagnosis of an ejection sound includes a small perimembranous ventricular septal defect with a septal aneurysm, mitral/tricuspid valve prolapse, and mild valvar pulmonary stenosis.

[ ] ELECTROCARDIOGRAM

There are no specific findings and is usually normal except for findings of associated malformations and complications.

[ ] CHEST RADIOGRAPHY

There are no specific findings. If there is a right parasternal convex shadow consistent with ascending aorta, the aortic root is dilated and BAV should be suspected.

[ ] ECHOCARDIOGRAM (TWO-DIMENSIONAL, M-MODE, AND DOPPLER)

An echocardiogram is the usual manner in which the diagnosis is made (see Chap. 16). Once the diagnosis is made in adults, it is very *important* to look for the associated abnormalities, especially coarctation of the aorta, patent ductus arteriosus, ventricular septal defect, and coronary artery variants, and complications by quantifying the severity of AS, AR (see above and Chap. 15), and ascending aorta dilatation by measuring the dimensions at the aortic annulus, sinotubular junction, and ascending aorta. Also evaluate whether aortic dissection and vegetations are present. If transthoracic echocardiography is inadequate, transesophageal echocardiography must be performed.

[ ] COMPUTED TOMOGRAPHY/CARDIAC MAGNETIC RESONANCE

If the echocardiographic images are not optimal, CT and/or cardiac magnetic resonance should be performed (see Chaps. 19 and 20).

TABLE 75-33

Recommendations in Patients with Bicuspid Aortic Valve with Dilated Ascending Aorta

Class I
1. Patients with known bicuspid aortic valves should undergo an initial transthoracic echocardiogram to assess diameter of the aortic root and ascending aorta. *(Level of Evidence: B)*
2. Cardiac magnetic resonance or cardiac computed tomography is indicated in patients with bicuspid aortic valves when morphology of the aortic root or ascending aorta cannot be assessed accurately by echocardiography. *(Level of Evidence: C)*
3. Patients with bicuspid aortic valves and dilatation of the aortic root or ascending aorta (diameter greater than 4 cm*) should undergo serial evaluation of aortic root/ ascending aorta size and morphology by echocardiography, cardiac magnetic resonance, or computed tomography on a yearly basis. *(Level of Evidence: C)*
4. Surgery to repair the aortic root or replace the ascending aorta is indicated in patients with bicuspid aortic valves if the diameter of the aortic root or ascending aorta is greater than 5.0 cm* or if the rate of increase in diameter is 0.5 cm/year or greater. *(Level of Evidence: C)*
5. In patients with bicuspid valves undergoing AVR because of severe AS or AR (see Sections 3.1.7. and 3.2.3.8.), repair of the aortic root or replacement of the ascending aorta is indicated if the diameter of the aortic root or ascending aorta is greater than 4.5 cm.* *(Level of Evidence: C)*

Class IIa
1. It is reasonable to give β-adrenergic blocking agents to patients with bicuspid valves and dilated aortic roots (diameter greater than 4.0 cm*) who are not candidates for surgical correction and who do not have moderate to severe AR. *(Level of Evidence: C)*
2. Cardiac magnetic resonance or cardiac computed tomography is indicated in patients with bicuspid aortic valves when aortic root dilatation is detected by echocardiography to further quantify severity of dilatation and involvement of ascending aorta. *(Level of Evidence: B)*

*Consider lower threshold values for patients with small stature.
AR, aortic regurgitation; AS, aortic stenosis; AVR, aortic valve replacement.
SOURCE: ACC/AHA Guidelines. Bonow RO, Carabello B, Chatterjee K, et al. ACC/AHA Guidelines on the management of patients with valvular heart disease: A report of the ACC/AHA Task Force or practice guidelines 2006. Available at: www.acc.org, e40.

[ ] MANAGEMENT

1. The serious nature and expected outcomes of patients with BAV should be discussed with the patient and appropriate family members.
2. Echocardiography should be recommended, and its importance emphasized, for first-degree relatives of the patients to detect BAV and/or ascending aorta dilatation.

3. Antibiotic prophylaxis for prevention for infective endocarditis is very important (see Chap. 85). It should also be prescribed for delivery of a pregnant mother because it is not possible to know in advance if she will have vaginal tears or need an episiotomy.

4. β Blockers are helpful in Marfan syndrome to slow the rate of dilatation of the ascending aorta (see Chap. 88). Considering the similarity of pathologic findings in the ascending aorta in the two conditions, it is reasonable to recommend long-term β-blocker therapy, if there are no contraindications to this use, to patients with a dilated aorta that is not yet in the range of needing surgery (see Chap. 105). Its role in those with a normal-size aorta needs to be evaluated.

5. AVR is needed for AS and AR according to recommendations for AVR in these two conditions (see above).

6. If patients have ascending aortic dilation that needs surgery (diameter of ≥5.0 to 5.5 cm) but have no or only mild valve disease, a valve-sparing operation should be performed. Valve-sparing operations in patients with BAV, compared to patients with tricuspid valve, have a lower rate of AR grade ≥II and of reoperation up to 8 years of followup.[144]

7. In patients who have had AVR but who do not have a dilated ascending aorta, the ascending aorta should be screened at regular intervals because progression is more common in patients with BAV than in patients with tricuspid AV.[145]

8. The Ross principle for AVR should be avoided, if possible (see Chap. 79). If a Ross principle is planned, it should be explained to the patient that the procedure is more complex, progressive dilatation of the autograft occurs, there is a significant risk of AR, and reoperation is a very much more complex procedure.

9. Patients with BAV need lifelong close followup, both before and after surgery.

Table 75–33 lists the ACC/AHA recommendations.[75]

REFERENCES

1. Rahimtoola SH. Aortic valve disease. In: Fuster V, Alexander RW, O'Rourke RA, eds. *Hurst's The Heart,* 10th ed. New York: McGraw Hill, 1998:1667–1695.
2. Horne BD, Camp NJ, Muhlestin JB, et al. Evidence for a heritable component in death resulting from aortic and mitral valve disease. *Circulation* 2004;110:3143–3148.
3. Passik CS, Ackerman DM, Pluth JR, et al. Temporal changes in the causes of aortic stenosis: a surgical pathological study of 646 cases. *Mayo Clin Proc* 1987;62:119–123.
4. Otto CM, Knusisto J, Reichenbach D, et al. Characterization of the early lesion of "degenerative" valvular aortic stenosis: historical and immunohistochemical studies. *Circulation* 1994;90:844–853.
5. Rajamannan NM, Subramanian M, Springett M, et al. Atorvastatin inhibits hypercholesterolemia-induced cellular proliferation and bone matrix production in the rabbit aortic valve. *Circulation* 2002;105:2660–2265.
6. Rahimtoola SH. The year in valvular heart disease. *J Am Coll Cardiol* 2004;43:491–504.
7. Rahimtoola SH. The year in valvular heart disease. *J Am Coll Cardiol* 2006;47:427–439.
8. Rahimtoola SH. The year in valvular heart disease. *J Am Coll Cardiol* 2005;45:111–122.
9. Freeman RV, Otto CM. Spectrum of calcific aortic valve disease: pathogenesis, disease progression, and treatment strategies. *Circulation* 2005;111:3316–3326.
10. Rajamannan NM, Subramaniam M, Rickard D, et al. Human aortic valve calcification is associated with an osteoblast phenotype. *Circulation* 2003;107:2181–2184.
11. Caira FC, Stock SR, Gleason TG, et al. Human degenerative valve disease is associated with up-regulation of low-density lipoprotein receptor-related protein 5 receptor mediated bone formation. *J Am Coll Cardiol* 2006;47:1707–1712.
12. Roberts WC. The structural basis of abnormal cardiac function: a look at coronary, hypertensive, valvular, idiopathic myocardial, and pericardial heart disease. In: Levine JJ, ed. *Clinical Cardiovascular Physiology.* New York: Grune & Stratton, 1976.
13. Stewart BF, Siscovick P, Lind B, et al. Clinical factors associated with calcific aortic valve disease. *J Am Coll Cardiol* 1997;29:630–634.
14. Kennedy JW, Twiss RD, Blackmon JR, et al. Quantitative angiography: III. Relationships of left ventricular pressure, volume, and mass in aortic valve disease. *Circulation* 1968;38:838–845.
15. Bonow RO. Left ventricular structure and function in aortic valve disease. *Circulation* 1989;79:966–969.
16. Krayenbuehl HP, Hess OM, Monrad ES, et al. Left ventricular myocardial structure in aortic valve disease before, intermediate, and later after AVR. *Circulation* 1989;79:744–755.
17. Tobin JR Jr, Rahimtoola SH, Blundell PE, et al. Percentage of left ventricular stroke work loss: a simple hemodynamic concept for estimation of severity in valvular aortic stenosis. *Circulation* 1967;35:868–879.
18. Pantely G, Morton MJ, Rahimtoola SH. Effects of successful, uncomplicated AVR on ventricular hypertrophy, volume, and performance in aortic stenosis and aortic incompetence. *J Thorac Cardiovasc Surg* 1978;75:383–391.
19. Hess OM, Ritter M, Schneider J, et al. Diastolic stiffness and myocardial structure in aortic valve disease before and after replacement. *Circulation* 1984;69:855–865.
20. Hess OM, Villari B, Krayenbuehl HP. Diastolic dysfunction in aortic stenosis. *Circulation* 1993;87(Suppl IV):73–76.
21. Stott DK, Marpole DGF, Bristow JD, et al. The role of LA transport in aortic and mitral stenosis. *Circulation* 1970;41:1031–1041.
22. Carroll JD, Carroll EP, Feldman T, et al. Sex-associated differences in left ventricular function in aortic stenosis of the elderly. *Circulation* 1992;86:1099–1107.
23. Ross J Jr. Afterload mismatch and preload reserve: a conceptual framework for the analysis of ventricular function. *Prog Cardiovasc Dis* 1976;18:255–264.
24. Bache RJ, Wang Y, Jorgensen CR. Hemodynamic effects of exercise in isolated valvular aortic stenosis. *Circulation* 1971;44:1003.
25. Johnson LL, Sciacca RR, Ellis K, et al. Reduced left ventricular myocardial blood flow per unit mass in aortic stenosis. *Circulation* 1978;57:582–590.
26. Vinten-Johansen J, Weiss HR. Oxygen consumption in subepicardial and subendocardial regions of the canine LV. The effect of experimental acute valvular aortic stenosis. *Circ Res* 1980;46:139–145.
27. Marcus ML, Doty DB, Horatzka LF, et al. Decreased coronary reserve: a mechanism for angina pectoris in patients with aortic stenosis and normal coronary arteries. *N Engl J Med* 1982;307:1362–1366.
28. Grech ED, Ramsdale DR. Exertional syncope in aortic stenosis: evidence to support inappropriate left ventricular baroreceptor response. *Am Heart J* 1991;121:603–606.
29. Schwartz LS, Goldfischer J, Sprague GJ, et al. Syncope and sudden death in aortic stenosis. *Am J Cardiol* 1969;23:647–658.
30. Kulbertus HE. Ventricular arrhythmias, syncope and sudden death in aortic stenosis. *Eur Heart J* 1988;9(Suppl E):51–52.
31. Sadler JE. Aortic stenosis, von Willebrand factor, and bleeding. *N Engl J Med* 2003;349:323–325.
32. Wood P. Aortic stenosis. *Am J Cardiol* 1958;1:553–571.
33. Murphy ES, Lawson RM, Starr A, et al. Severe aortic stenosis in the elderly: state of left ventricular function and result of AVR on ten-year survival. *Circulation* 1981;64(Suppl II):184–188.
34. Thompson R, Mitchell A, Ahmed M, et al. Conduction defects in aortic valve disease. *Am Heart J* 1979;98:3–10.
35. Skjaerpe T, Hegrenaes L, Hatle L. Noninvasive estimation of valve area in patients with aortic stenosis by Doppler ultrasound and two-dimensional echocardiography. *Circulation* 1985;72:810–815.
36. Currie PJ, Seward JB, Reeder GS, et al. Continuous-wave Doppler echocardiographic assessment of severity of calcific aortic stenosis: a simultaneous Doppler-catheter correlative study in 100 adult patients. *Circulation* 1985;71:1162–1169.
37. Rahimtoola SH. Perspective on valvular heart disease: update II. In: Knoebel S, ed. *An Era in Cardiovascular Medicine.* New York: Elsevier, 1991:45–70.
38. Roger VL, Tajik AJ, Reeder GS, et al. Effect of Doppler echocardiography on utilization of hemodynamic cardiac catheterization in the preoperative evaluation of aortic stenosis. *Mayo Clin Proc* 1996;71:141–149.
39. Griffith MJ, Carey C, Coltart DJ, et al. Inaccuracies of using aortic valve gradients alone to grade severity of aortic stenosis. *Br Heart J* 1989;62:372–378.

40. Sethi GK, Miller DC, Sonchek J, et al. Clinical, hemodynamic and angiographic predictors of operative mortality in patients undergoing single AVR. *J Thorac Cardiovasc Surg* 1987;93:884–887.

41. Mullany CJ, Elveback ER, Frye RL, et al. Coronary artery disease and its management: Influence on survival in patients undergoing AVR. *J Am Coll Cardiol* 1987;10:66–72.

42. Levinson JR, Akins CW, Buckley MJ, et al. Octogenarians with aortic stenosis: outcome after aortic valve replacement. *Circulation* 1989;80(Suppl 1):49–56.

43. Connolly HM, Rahimtoola SH. Indications for surgery in aortic valve disease. In: Yusuf S, Cairus JA, Canu AJ, et al., eds. *Evidence-Based Cardiology.* London: BMJ Books, 2003;767–781.

44. Nishimura RA, Grahtham JA, Connolly HM, et al. Low output, low-gradient aortic stenosis in patients with depressed left ventricular systolic function. The clinical utility of the dobutamine challenge in the catheterization laboratory. *Circulation* 2002;106:809–813.

45. Monin J-L, Quéré JP, Mouchi M, et al. Long-gradient aortic stenosis: operative risk stratification and predictors for long-term outcome. A multicenter study using dobutamine stress hemodynamics. *Circulation* 2003;108:319–324.

46. Kotlewski A, Kawanishi DT, McKay CR, et al. The relative value of clinical examination, echocardiography with Doppler and cardiac catheterization with angiography in the evaluation of aortic valve disease. In: Bodnar E, ed. *Surgery for Heart Valve Disease.* London: ICR, 1990:66–72.

47. Rahimtoola SH. Prophylactic AVR for mild aortic valve disease at time of surgery for other cardiovascular disease? NO. *J Am Coll Cardiol* 1999;33:2009–2015.

48. Horstkotte D, Loogen F. The natural history of aortic valve stenosis. *Eur Heart J* 1988;9(Suppl E):57–64.

49. Pellikka P, Nishimura R, Bailey K, et al. The natural history of adults with asymptomatic, hemodynamically significant aortic stenosis. *J Am Coll Cardiol* 1990;15:1012–1017.

50. Otto CM, Burwash JG, Legget ME, et al. Prospective study of asymptomatic valvular aortic stenosis: clinical, echocardiographic, and exercise predictors of outcome. *Circulation* 1997;95:2262–2270.

51. Rosenhek R, Bindar T, Porenta G, et al. Predictors of outcome in severe, asymptomatic aortic stenosis. *N Engl J Med* 2000;343:611–617.

52. Amato MCM, Moffa PJ, Werner K, et al. Treatment decision in asymptomatic aortic stenosis: role of exercise testing. *Heart* 2001;86:381–386.

53. Ross J Jr, Braunwald E. Aortic stenosis. *Circulation* 1968;36(Suppl IV):61–67.

54. Otto CM, Lind BK, Kitzman DW, et al. Association of aortic valve sclerosis with cardiovascular mortality and morbidity in the elderly. *N Engl J Med* 1999;341:142–147.

55. Liebe V, Breuckmann M, Borggrefe M, et al. Statin therapy of calcific stenosis: hype or hope? *Eur Heart J* 2006;27:773–778.

56. Kirklin JW, Barratt-Boyes BG. Congenital valvular aortic stenosis. In: *Cardiac Surgery.* New York: Wiley, 1986:972–988.

57. Hammermeister KL, Sethi GK, Henderson WG, et al. Outcomes 15 years after valve replacement with a mechanical valve or bioprosthetic valve: report of the Veterans Affairs Randomized Trial. *J Am Coll Cardiol* 2000;36:1152–1158.

58. Pellikka PA, Sarano ME, Nishimura RA, et al. Outcome of 622 adults with asymptomatic hemodynamically significant aortic stenosis during follow-up. *Circulation* 2005;111:3290–3295.

59. Edwards FH, Peterson Ed, Coombs LP, et al. Prediction of operative mortality after valve replacement surgery. *J Am Coll Cardiol* 2001;37:885–892.

60. Society of Thoracic Surgery Database 1997: Internet.

61. Shwarz F, Banmann P, Manthey J, et al. The effect of aortic valve replacement on survival. *Circulation* 1982;66:1105–1110.

62. Rahimtoola SH. Valvular heart disease: a perspective. *J Am Coll Cardiol* 1983;1:199–215.

63. Monrad ES, Hess OM, Murakami T, et al. Time course of regression of left ventricular hypertrophy after aortic valve replacement. *Circulation* 1988;77:1345–1355.

64. Lindblom D, Lindblom U, Qvist J, et al. Long-term relative survival rates after heart AVR. *J Am Coll Cardiol* 1990;15:566–573.

65. Rahimtoola SH. Catheter balloon valvuloplasty for severe calcific aortic stenosis: a limited role. *J Am Coll Cardiol* 1994;23:1076–1078.

66. Connolly HM, Oh JK, Orszulak TA, et al. AVR for aortic stenosis with severe left ventricular dysfunction: prognostic indicators. *Circulation* 1997;95:2395–2400.

67. Rahimtoola SH, Starr A. Valvular surgery. In: Braunwald E, Mock M, Watson J, eds. *Congestive Heart Failure: Current Research and Clinical Applications.* Orlando, FL: Grune & Stratton, 1982:89–93.

68. Smith N, McAnulty JH, Rahimtoola SH. Severe aortic stenosis with impaired left ventricular function and clinical heart failure: results of AVR. *Circulation* 1978;58:255–264.

69. Connolly HM, Oh JK, Schaff HV, et al. Severe aortic stenosis with low transvalvular gradient and severe left ventricular dysfunction. Result of aortic valve replacement in 52 patients. *Circulation* 2000;101:1940–1946.

70. Rahimtoola SH. Severe aortic stenosis with low systolic gradient. The good and bad news. *Circulation* 2000;101:1892–1894.

71. Malouf JF, Enriquez-Serrano M, Pellikka PA, et al. Severe pulmonary hypertension in patients with severe aortic stenosis: clinical profile and prognostic implications. *J Am Coll Cardiol* 2002;40:789–795.

72. Otto CM, Mickel MC, Kennedy JW, et al. Three-year outcome after balloon aortic valvuloplasty: Insights into prognosis of valvular aortic stenosis. *Circulation* 1994;89:642–650.

73. Byrne JG, Leacche M, Unic D, et al. Staged initial percutaneous coronary intervention followed by valve surgery ("hybrid approach") for patients with complex coronary and valve disease. *J Am Coll Cardiol* 2005;45:14–18.

74. Meier MA, Deeb M, Chetui S, et al. Acute ad long term outcomes of percutaneous coronary intervention prior aortic valve replacement. *J Am Coll Cardiol* 2005;45 Suppl A:351A.

75. Bonow RO, Carabello B, Chatterjee K, et al. ACC/AHA guidelines on the management of patients with valvular heart disease: a report of the ACC/AHA Task Force or practice guidelines 2006. Available at: www.acc.org.

76. Knot UN, Navarro GM, Popovic ZB, et al. Nitroprusside in critically ill patients with left ventricular dysfunction and aortic stenosis. *N Engl J Med* 2003;348:1756–1763.

77. Rahimtoola SH. Should asymptomatic patients with mild or moderate aortic stenosis undergo valve replacement at time of coronary artery bypass graft surgery? *Heart* 2001;85:337–341.

78. Cribier A, Eltchaninoff H, Bash A, et al. Percutaneous transcatheter implantation of an aortic valve prosthesis for calcific aortic stenosis. First human case description. *Circulation* 2002;106:3006–3008.

79. Vassiliades TA Jr, Block PC, Cohn LH, et al. The clinical development of percutaneous heart valve therapy. *J Am Coll Cardiol* 2005;45:1554–1560.

80. Rahimtoola SH. Recognition and management of acute aortic regurgitation. *Heart Dis Stroke* 1993;2:217–221.

81. Rahimtoola SH. Valvular heart disease. In: Stein J, ed. *Internal Medicine,* 4th ed. St. Louis: Mosby-Year Book, 1994:202–234.

82. Belenkie I, Rademaker A. Acute and chronic changes after aortic valve damage in the intact dog. *Am J Physiol* 1981;241:H95–H103.

83. Welch GH Jr, Braunwald E, Sarnoff SJ. Hemodynamic effects of quantitatively varied experimental aortic regurgitation. *Circ Res* 1957;5:546–551.

84. Rahimtoola SH. Aortic regurgitation. In: Rahimtoola SH, ed. *Atlas of Heart Diseases: Valvular Heart Disease,* vol 11. Philadelphia: Current Medicine, 1997:7.1–7.26.

85. Rahimtoola SH. Management of heart failure in valve regurgitation. *Clin Cardiol* 1992;15(Suppl I):22–27.

86. Cigarroa JE, Isselbacher EM, De Sanctis RW, et al. Diagnostic imaging in the evaluation of suspected aortic dissection: old standards and new directions. *N Engl J Med* 1993;328:35–43.

87. Kostuk W, Barr JW, Simon AL, Ross J Jr. Correlations between the chest film and hemodynamics in acute myocardial infarction. *Circulation* 1973;48:624–632.

88. Chatterjee K, Parmley WW, Swan HJC, et al. Beneficial effects of vasodilator agents in severe mitral regurgitation due to dysfunction of subvalvular apparatus. *Circulation* 1973;48:684–690.

89. Richardson JV, Karp RB, Kirklin JW, et al. Treatment of infective endocarditis: a 10-year comparative analysis. *Circulation* 1978;58:589–597.

90. Tonnemacher D, Reid CL, Kawanishi DT, et al. Frequency of myxomatous degeneration of the aortic valve as a cause of isolated aortic regurgitation severe enough to warrant AVR. *Am J Cardiol* 1987;60:1194–1196.

91. Antunes M. Repair for acquired valvular heart disease. In: Rahimtoola SH, ed. *Atlas of Heart Diseases: Valvular Heart Disease*, vol 11. Philadelphia: Current Medicine, 1997:12.1–12.23.

92. Miller GAH, Kirklin JW, Swan HJC. Myocardial function and left ventricular volumes in acquired valvular insufficiency. *Circulation* 1965;31:374–384.

93. Karaian CH, Greenberg BH, Rahimtoola SH. The relationship between functional class and cardiac performance in patients with chronic aortic insufficiency. *Chest* 1985;88:553–557.

94. Kawanishi DT, McKay CR, Chandraratna PAN, et al. Cardiovascular response to dynamic exercise in patients with chronic symptomatic mild-to-moderate and severe aortic regurgitation. *Circulation* 1986;73:62–72.

95. Shen WF, Roubin GS, Choong CY-P, et al. Evaluation of relationship between myocardial contractile state and left ventricular function in patients with aortic regurgitation. *Circulation* 1985;71:31–38.

96. Boucher CA, Wilson RA, Kanarek DJ, et al. Exercise testing in asymptomatic or minimally symptomatic aortic regurgitation: relationship of left ventricular ejection fraction to left ventricular filling pressure during exercise. *Circulation* 1983;67:1091–1100.

97. Falsetti HL, Carroll RJ, Cramer JA. Total and regional myocardial blood flow in aortic regurgitation. *Am Heart J* 1979;97:485–493.

98. Uhl GS, Boucher CA, Oliveros RA, et al. Exercise-induced myocardial oxygen supply-demand imbalance in asymptomatic or mildly symptomatic aortic regurgitation. *Chest* 1981;80:686–691.

99. Nittenburg A, Foult JM, Antony I, et al. Coronary flow and resistance reserve in patients with chronic aortic regurgitation, angina pectoris, and normal coronary arteries. *J Am Coll Cardiol* 1988;11:478–486.

100. Schaefer RA, McAnulty JH, Starr A, et al. Diastolic murmurs in the presence of Starr-Edwards mitral prosthesis: with emphasis on the genesis of the Austin Flint murmur. *Circulation* 1975;51:402–409.

101. Rahimtoola SH, LaCanna G, Ferrari R. Hibernating myocardium. Another piece of the puzzle falls into place. *J Am Coll Cardiol* 2006;47:978–980.

102. Rahimtoola SH. Drug induced valvular heart disease: here we go again. Will we do better this time? *Mayo Clinic Proc* 2002;77:1275–1277.

103. Tarasoutchi F, Grinberg M, Spina GS, et al. Ten-year clinical laboratory follow-up after application of a symptom-based therapeutic strategy to patients with severe chronic aortic regurgitation of predominant rheumatic etiology. *J Am Coll Cardiol* 2003;41:1316–1324.

104. Bonow RO, Carabello B, de Leon AC Jr, et al. ACC/AHA guidelines for the management of patients with valvular heart disease: a report of the American College of Cardiology/American Heart Association Task Force on Practice Guidelines (Committee on Management of Patients with Valvular Heart Disease). *J Am Coll Cardiol* 1998;32:1486–1588.

105. Bonow RO, Lakatos E, Maron BJ, et al. Serial long-term assessment of the natural history of asymptomatic patients with chronic aortic regurgitation and normal left ventricular systolic function. *Circulation* 1991;84:1625–1635.

106. Siemienczuk D, Greenberg B, Morris C, et al. Chronic aortic insufficiency: factors associated with progression to AVR. *Ann Intern Med* 1989;110:587–592.

107. Klodas E, Enrique-Sarano M, Tajik AJ, et al. Surgery for aortic regurgitation in women: Contrasting indications and outcomes compared with men. *Circulation* 1996;94:2472–2478.

108. Rapaport E. Natural history of aortic and mitral valve disease. *Am J Cardiol* 1975;35:221–227.

109. McKay CR, Rahimtoola SH. Natural history of aortic regurgitation. In: Gaasch WH, Levine HJ, eds. *Chronic Aortic Regurgitation*. Boston: Kluwer Academic, 1980:1–17.

110. Dujardin KS, Enriquez-Sarano M, Schaff HV, et al. Mortality and morbidity of aortic regurgitation in clinical practice: A long-term follow-up study. *Circulation* 1999;99:1851–1857.

111. Scognamiglio R, Rasoli G, Ponchia A, et al. Long-term nifedipine unloading therapy in asymptomatic patients with chronic severe aortic regurgitation. *J Am Coll Cardiol* 1990;16:424–429.

112. Rahimtoola SH. Vasodilator therapy in chronic severe aortic regurgitation. *J Am Coll Cardiol* 1990;16:430–432.

113. Scognamiglio R, Rahimtoola SH, Fasoli G, et al. Nifedipine in asymptomatic patients with severe aortic regurgitation and normal left ventricular function. *N Engl J Med* 1994;331:689–695.

114. Evangelista A, Tornos P, Sambola A, et al. Long-term vasodilator therapy in patients with severe aortic regurgitation. *N Engl J Med* 2005;353:1342–1349.

115. Rahimtoola SH. Vasodilators in aortic regurgitation [letter]. *N Engl J Med* 2006;354:301–302.

116. McKay CR, Nanna M, Kawanishi DT, et al. Importance of internal controls, statistical methods, and side effects in acute vasodilator trials: a study of hydralazine kinetics in patients with aortic regurgitation. *Circulation* 1985;72:865–872.

117. Borer JS, Bonow RO. Contemporary approach to aortic and mitral regurgitation. *Circulation* 2003;108:2432–2438.

118. Greves J, Rahimtoola SH, McAnulty JH, et al. Preoperative criteria predictive of late survival following AVR for severe aortic regurgitation. *Am Heart J* 1981;101:300–308.

119. Clark DG, McAnulty JH, Rahimtoola SH. Valve replacement in aortic insufficiency with left ventricular dysfunction. *Circulation* 1980;61:411–421.

120. Taniguchi K, Nakano S, Hirose H, et al. Preoperative left ventricular function: Minimal requirement for successful late results of AVR for aortic regurgitation. *J Am Coll Cardiol* 1987;10:510–518.

121. Levine HJ, Gaasch WH. Ratio of regurgitant volume to end-diastolic volume: A major determinant of ventricular response to surgical correction of chronic volume overload. *Am J Cardiol* 1983;52:406–410.

122. Klodas E, Enriquez-Sarano M, Tajik AJ, et al. Aortic regurgitation complicated by extreme left ventricular dilation: long-term outcome after surgical correction. *J Am Coll Cardiol* 1996;27:670–677.

123. Tornos P, Sambola A, Permanya-Miralda G, et al. Long-term outcome of surgically treated aortic regurgitation. *J Am Coll Cardiol* 2006;47:1012–1017.

124. Gaasch WH, Carroll JD, Levine HJ, et al. Chronic aortic regurgitation: prognostic value of left ventricular end-systolic dimension and end-diastolic radius/thickness ratio. *J Am Coll Cardiol* 1983;1:775–782.

125. Bonow RO, Dodd JT, Maron BJ, et al. Long-term serial changes in left ventricular function and reversal of ventricular dilatation after AVR for chronic aortic regurgitation. *Circulation* 1988;78:1108–1120.

126. Braverman AC, Güven H, Beardslee MA, et al. The bicuspid aortic valve [review]. *Curr Prob in Cardiol* 2005;30:461–522.

127. Bassco C, Boschello M, Perrone C, et al. An echocardiographic survey of primary school children for bicuspid aortic valve. *Am J Cardiol* 2004;93:661–663.

128. Cripe L, Andelfinger G, Martin LJ, et al. Bicuspid aortic valve is heritable. *J Am Coll Cardiol* 2004;44:138–143.

129. Huntington K, Hunter A, Chau K. A prospective study to assess the frequency of familial clustering of congenital bicuspid aortic valve. *J Am Coll Cardiol* 1997;30:1809–1812.

130. Connolly HM. Comments in Reference 126, page 479.

131. Nataamadja M, West M, West J, et al. Abnormal extracellular matrix protein transport associated with increased apoptosis of vascular smooth muscle cells in Marfan's syndrome and bicuspid aortic valve thoracic aortic aneurysms. *Circulation* 2003;108 Suppl II:329–334.

132. Boyum J, Fellinger EK, Schmoker JD, et al. Matrix metalloproteinase activity in thoracic aneurysms associated with bicuspid and tricuspid aortic valves. *J Thorac Cardiovasc Surg* 2004;127:686–691.

133. Fedax PWM, de Sa MPL, Verma S, et al. Vascular matrix remodeling in patients with bicuspid aortic valve malformations: implications for aortic dilatation. *J Thorac Cardiovasc Surg* 2003;126:797–806.

134. Morgan-Hughes GJ, Roobottom CA, Owens PE, et al. Dilatation of the aorta in pure, severe, bicuspid aortic valve stenosis. *Am Heart J* 2004;147:736–740.

135. Ferencik M, Pape LA. Changes in size of ascending aorta and aortic valve function with time in patients with congenitally bicuspid aortic valves. *Am J Cardiol* 2003;92:43–46.

136. Pomerance A. Pathogenesis of aortic stenosis and its relation to age. *Br Heart J* 1972;34:569–574.

137. Murphy ES, Rösch J, Rahimtoola SH. The frequency and significance of coronary arteria dominance in isolated aortic stenosis. *Am J Cardiol* 1977;39:505–509.

138. Hutchins GM, Nazarian IH, Bulkley BH. Association of left dominant coronary arterial system with congenital bicuspid aortic valve. *Am J Cardiol* 1978;42:57–59.

139. Brandenburg RO, Tajik AJ, Edwards WD, et al. Accuracy of 2 dimensional echocardiographic diagnosis of congenital bicuspid aortic valve: echocardiographic-anatomic correlation in 115 patients. *Am J Cardiol* 1983;51:1469–1473.

140. Sabet HY, Edward WD, Tazelaar HD, et al. Congenitally bicuspid aortic valves: A surgical pathology study of 542 cases and a literature review of 2,715 additional cases. *Mayo Clin Proc* 1999;74:14–26.

141. Wallby L, Janerot-Sjöberg B, Steffensen J, et al. T lymphocyte infiltration in non-rheumatic aortic stenosis: A comparative descriptive study between tricuspid and bicuspid aortic valves. *Heart* 2002;88:348–351.

142. Tejada JG, Albarran A, Hernandez F, et al. Anomalous coronary artery origin associated with bicuspid aortic valve. *J Thoracic Cardiovasc Surg* 2001;122:842–843.

143. Perloff JK. *The Clinical Recognition of Congenital Heart Disease*, 4th ed. Philadelphia: W.B. Saunders, 1994.

144. Aicher D, Langer F, Kissinger A, et al. Valve-sparing aortic root replacement in bicuspid aortic valves: a reasonable operation? *J Thorac Cardiovasc Surg* 2004;128:662–668.

145. Yasuda H, Nakatani S, Stugaard M, et al. Failure to prevent progressive dilatation of ascending aorta by aortic valve replacement in patients with bicuspid aortic valve: comparison with tricuspid valve. *Circulation* 2003;108 Suppl II:291–294.

CHAPTER 76

Mitral Valve Regurgitation Including the Mitral Valve Prolapse Syndrome

Robert A. O'Rourke / Louis J. Dell'Italia

MITRAL REGURGITATION

【 】 NORMAL MITRAL STRUCTURE AND FUNCTION

The mitral valve is a complex structure formed by four elements.[1]

1. The annulus is asymmetrical, with a fixed portion (corresponding to the anterior leaflet) shared with the aortic annulus and a dynamic portion (corresponding to the posterior leaflet) that represents most of the circumference of the annulus.
2. The two leaflets are asymmetrical; the anterior has the greater length of tissue but occupies a smaller portion of the circumference of the annulus than does the posterior portion.
3. The chordae join each papillary muscle to the corresponding commissure and the adjoining halves of both leaflets and maintain the two leaflets in a position allowing coaptation.
4. The two papillary muscles and the adjacent wall attach the mitral apparatus to the left ventricle. Mitral valve closing during systole is normally ensured, first by a large area of coaptation between leaflets allowing high-friction resistance to abnormal valve movement, and second by the systolic position to the anterior leaflet parallel to the direction of blood flow.[2]

【 】 MITRAL REGURGITATION

In Western society, the most common causes of chronic mitral regurgitation (MR) are ischemic heart disease and myxomatous de-generation of the valve, resulting in prolapse (often not as part of the mitral valve prolapse syndrome), ruptured chordae, and/or partial flail leaflet.[2] Patients with chronic severe degenerative MR and symptoms of heart failure and/or left ventricular (LV) dysfunction are clearly candidates for mitral valve repair or replacement. However, the indications for such surgery in asymptomatic patients, especially those with normal LV function falls within recommended guidelines,[3,4] remains controversial, especially considering data demonstrating structural and biochemical *abnormalities in the valve itself* that may affect the durability and longevity of the repaired valve. Also, there is an uncertainty about the ability of vasodilator therapy to obviate or delay the need for surgery in asymptomatic patients with chronic MR. These controversial issues are compounded by the difficulty in determining the transition to irreversible LV dysfunction and, thus, the timing for optimal surgical intervention.

Etiology and Mechanism

MR is often referred to as *organic,* if there is an intrinsic valve disease, or *functional,* if the valve is structurally normal but leaks as a result of an extravalvular abnormality, such as an alteration in LV chamber geometry and/or dilatation of the mitral annulus that adversely affects normal coaptation of the mitral valve leaflets during systole (Table 76–1). Ischemic MR may be organic (ruptured or ischemic papillary muscle) and/or functional because of LV chamber dilatation. Nonischemic MR may be organic (e.g., rheumatic) or functional (e.g., dilated cardiomyopathy).

TABLE 76–1

Mitral Regurgitation Mechanisms

ETIOLOGY	MECHANISM	ECHOCARDIOGRAPHIC APPEARANCE
Rheumatic	Retraction	Thickened chordae/leaflets
Lupus erythematosus	Thickening	Normal or restricted motion
Anticardiolipin syndrome		
Carcinoid		
Ergot lesions		
Postradiation		
Degenerative	Prolapsed leaflets	Prolasping/flail leaflets
Marfan syndrome	Ruptured chords	Redundant tissue
Ehlers-Danlos syndrome		Ruptured chords
Traumatic mitral regurgitation		
Ischemic (infarction)	Ruptured papillary muscle	Flail leaflet
Myocardial disease	Dilatation of annulus	Normal leaflets
Ischemic (chronic)	Traction anterior leaflet	Reduced motion of leaflets
Cardiomyopathies		
Infiltrative disease	Thickened leaflet	Thickened leaflet
Hypereosinophilic syndrome	Loss of coaptation	Reduced motion
Endomyocardial fibrosis		
Hurler disease		
Endocarditis	Destructive lesions	Perforations
		Flail leaflets
Congenital	Cleft leaflet	Cleft leaflet
	Transposed valve	Tricuspid valve

Rheumatic Disease

Rheumatic MR in most cases, is associated with stenosis and fusion of the commissures (Fig. 76–1). Severe rheumatic MR requiring surgical correction still occurs frequently in developing countries but rarely occurs in developed countries.[2] The underlying lesion is retractile fibrosis of leaflets and chordae, causing loss of coaptation. The secondary dilatation of the mitral annulus tends to further decrease the contract between leaflets. Elongated or ruptured chordae are infrequent.

Degenerative Mitral Regurgitation

Mitral annular calcification is a common autopsy finding, especially in the elderly population, is accelerated by the association with hypertension, aortic stenosis, and diabetes, and is also associated with connective tissue diseases such as Marfan and Hurler syndromes (Fig. 76–2). Although it is usually of little functional consequence, it can be a cause of severe MR, and in some severe cases, it can cause inflow obstruction that may require surgical management.[3]

Degenerative MR is often associated with valve prolapse, an abnormal movement of the leaflets into the left atrium (LA) during systole caused by inadequate chordal support (elongation or rupture) and excessive valvular tissue. In Western countries, mitral prolapse represents the most frequent causes leading to surgery for severe MR.[2] Myxomatous degeneration is the pathologic substrate of mitral valve prolapse, characterized by redundant, floppy leaflets and associated with progressive MR.[5] Heart valves have a complex, layered architecture and highly specialized, functionally adapted cells and extracellular matrix (ECM). As in other tissues, turnover of the valvular ECM depends on a dynamic balance between synthesis and degradation. In most tissues, degradation of the ECM occurs through the action of matrix metalloproteinases (MMPs) and other proteases, especially in those within inflammatory cells. Myxomatous valves have significant thickening and highly abnormal layered architecture and ECM components.[5] In particular, interstitial cells in myxomatous leaflets exhibited features of activated myofibroblasts, expressed elevated levels of MMPs (Fig. 76–3) and other proteolytic enzymes and cytokines, and were significantly increased in number in the spongiosa.[6] It is unproven whether high proteolytic activity and cell activation in the mitral leaflets are causal or whether regurgitation and abnormal mechanical stress induce matrix remodeling as a reactive mechanism. Patients with severe MR caused by mitral valve prolapse, who are asymptomatic or minimally symptomatic with normal ventricular performance, can be expected to progress to surgical indications at an annual rate of 10.3 percent.[7]

To date, chromosomal loci 11, 13, and 16 have been identified with mitral valve prolapse.[8–10] Chromosome 13 compromises a class of genes, the glypican family, that could induce the phenotype of mitral valve prolapse. This family of genes, in particular glypican 5 and 6, encode for the cell surface heparin sulfate proteoglycans, which serve as ligand for adhesion and several growth factors that collectively could increase glycosaminoglycans in myxomatous valves.[11] In a mouse model of Marfan syndrome, fibrillin-1-deficient mice were associated with postnatal mitral valve architecture that

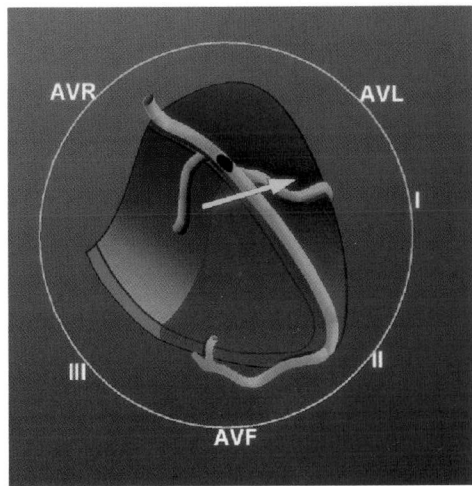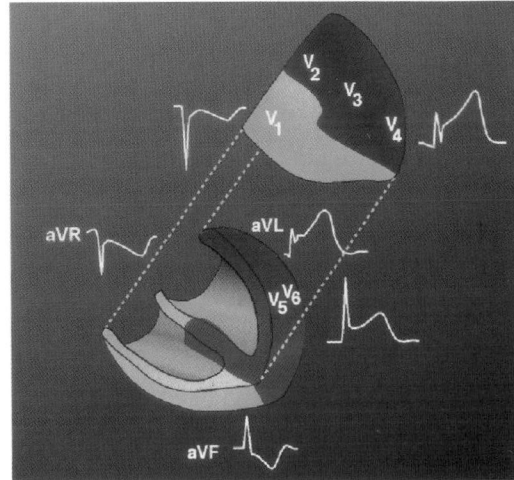

FIGURE 76–1. Anatomic example of rheumatic mitral regurgitation. Note the thickening of the leaflet and chordae and the retraction of the mitral tissue. *Source: Courtesy of W.D. Edwards.*

correlated with in vivo echocardiographic demonstration of mitral valve prolapse with leaflet elongation and valve thickening at 9 months of age.[12] Mitral valves had increased cell proliferation, decreased apoptosis, and increased transforming growth factor (TGF)-α signaling with increased cytokine activation. TGF-α antagonism in vivo reversed the valve phenotype, suggesting a cause-and-effect relationship. Thus, there is much evidence that mitral valve prolapse is the final common pathway for a variety of genetic disorders that weaken the connective tissue of the valve, leading to elongation, thickening, and, often, degeneration.[13]

Myxomatous mitral valve specimens from patients had up to 10 percent more water content and 30 to 150 percent higher glycosaminoglycan concentrations than normal.[14] Studies of the collagen content reported a decrease per weight, suggesting that the mechanical load-bearing capabilities of collagen were distributed over a larger area (Fig. 76–3). Furthermore, there was a shift from type I to type II collagen, which has less mechanical strength. Mitral valves from patients with congestive heart failure also had 60 percent more glycosaminoglycan content than normal mitral valves.[15] These findings suggest that increased stretch on the mitral valvular apparatus in heart failure contributes to matrix remodeling; consequently, functional mitral regurgitation secondary to idiopathic and ischemic dilated cardiomyopathy may not be purely functional but has a component of structural mitral valvular remodeling.[16]

Mechanical properties of myxomatous leaflets and chordae from patients demonstrate that myxomatous leaflets were more extensible and half as strong as normal valve tissue, suggesting that the abnormal stresses engendered by progressive stretching of enlarged leaflets and inherent weakness in part also as result of catabolic enzymes (Fig. 76–4) are synergistic in valve degeneration, possibly following, as well as preceding, valve repair.[17] Most notably, myxoid chordae failed at loads

one-half of those of normal chordae.[17] Thus chordal rupture is the main indication for repair of myxoid mitral valves. These findings also suggest that chordal preservation should be carried out with caution, as myxoid chordae are clearly abnormal with compromised mechanical strength. Nevertheless, 7 years after repair, the incidence of severe regurgitation remains low (29 percent), with good clinical outcome and low reoperation rates after repair (93 to 96 percent freedom at 10 years).[18–20] However, a published study in 242 patients receiving mitral valve repair for degenerative valve regurgitation reported that freedom from nontrivial MR (>1/4) was 94.3 ± 1.6 percent at 1 month, 58.6 ± 4.9 percent at 5 years, and 27.2 ± 8.6 percent at 7 years. Freedom from severe MR (>2/4) was 98.3 ± 0.9 percent at 1 month, 82.8 ± 3.8 percent at 5 years, and 71.1 ± 7.4 percent at 7 years.[21] This is not surprising because genetic evidence suggests that myxoid changes are not entirely acquired and that genetic determinants are at least responsible for

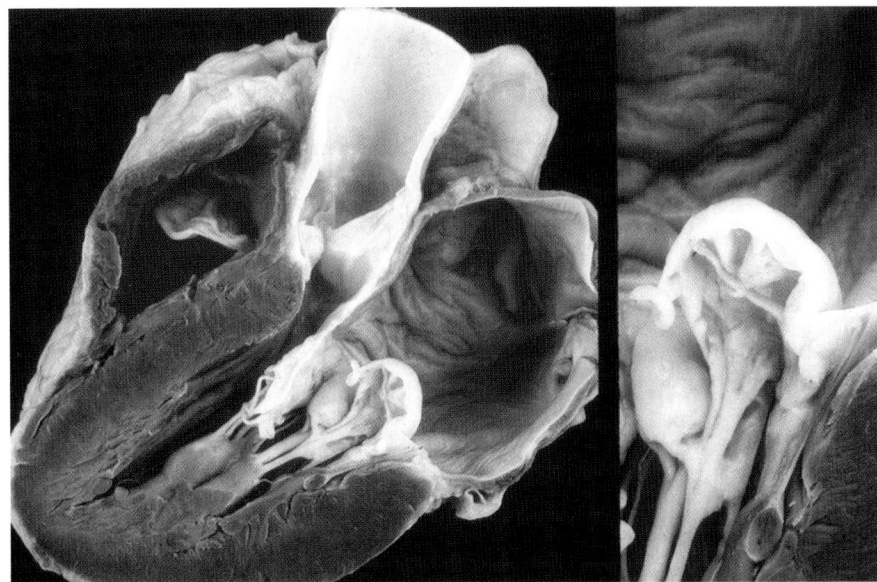

FIGURE 76–2. Anatomic example of a flail posterior leaflet with ruptured chord. On the right of the picture, close-up view of the ruptured chord. Otherwise the left atrium is enlarged and the valvular tissue normal. *Source: Courtesy of W.D. Edwards.*

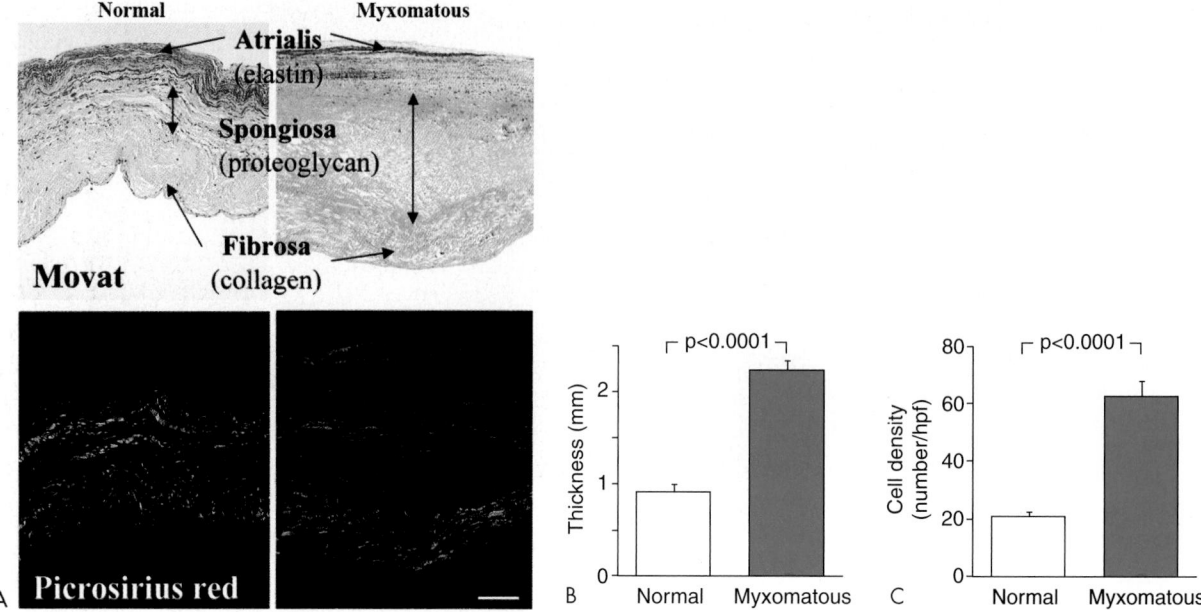

FIGURE 76–3. Morphologic features of normal and myxomatous mitral valves. **A.** Normal mitral valves (*left*) and valves with myxomatous degeneration (*right*). Myxomatous valves have an abnormal layered architecture: loose collagen in fibrosa, expanded spongiosa strongly positive for proteoglycans, and disrupted elastin in atrialis (*top*). *Top,* Movat pentachrome stain (collagen stains yellow; proteoglycans, blue-green; and elastin, black). *Bottom,* Picrosirius red staining viewed under polarized light detected disruption and lower birefringence of collagen fibers in myxomatous leaflets. Bar = 200 μm. Magnification ×100. **B.** Quantitative analysis of valve thickness, demonstrating thickening of myxomatous valves. **C.** Increased density of interstitial cells in myxomatous spongiosa. Bars represent SEM (standard error of mean).

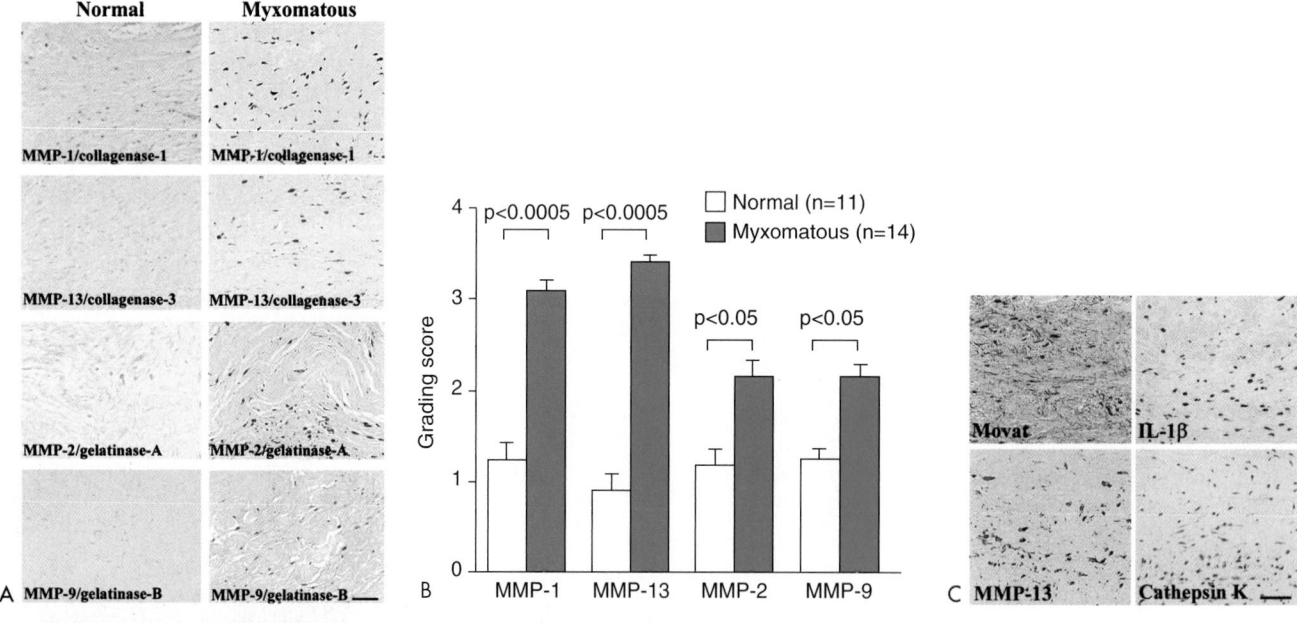

FIGURE 76–4. Expression of catabolic enzymes in myxomatous valves. **A.** Strong expression of MMP-1, MMP-13, MMP-2, and MMP-9 in interstitial cells of spongiosa of myxomatous valves compared with normal valves. Bar = 50 μm. Magnification ×400. **B.** Semiquantitative analysis of MMPs immunohistochemically demonstrated elevated levels of proteolytic enzymes, especially collagenases (MMP-1 and MMP-13), in myxomatous valves compared with normal valves. Bars represent SEM (standard error of mean). **C.** Typical area of myxomatous degeneration with loose collagen and fragmented elastin (Movat stain) colocalized with accumulation of interstitial cells immunoreactive for interleukin (IL)-1β, MMP-13, and cathepsin K. Bar = 50 μm. Magnification ×400. **D.** Immunofluorescent double-labeling for catabolic enzymes (Texas red;red) and IL-1ββ (FITC;green) showed coexpression of MMP-13 and IL-1ββ (*top*) and cathepsin S and IL-1ββ (*bottom*) in myxomatous spongiosa. Bar = 50 μm. Magnification ×400.

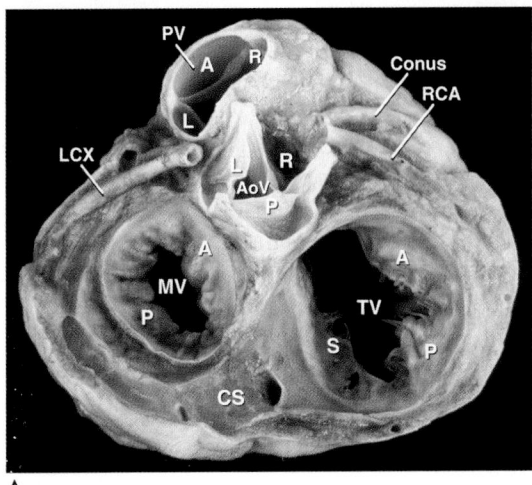
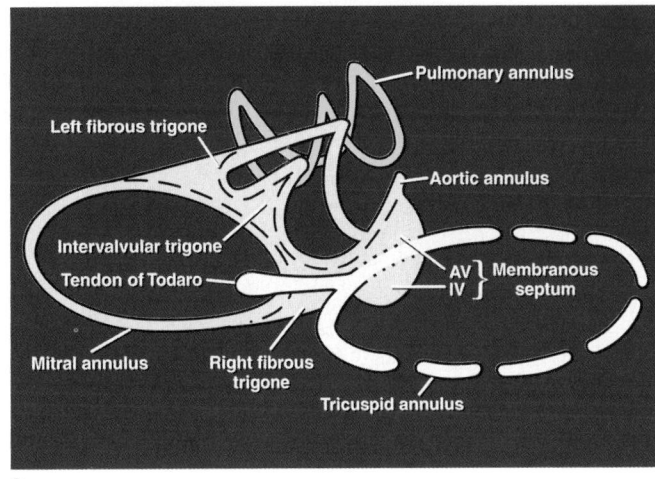

FIGURE 76–5. Anatomic example of mitral regurgitation caused by endocarditis. Note the vegetations of the anterior leaflet and the ruptured chords. *Source: Courtesy of W.D. Edwards.*

permanent cellular alterations in these valves.[22] Thus data suggest that the durability of a successful mitral reconstruction for degenerative mitral valve disease is not constant, and this should be taken into account when asymptomatic patients are offered early mitral valve repair.

Infective Endocarditis

Infective endocarditis accounts for approximately 5 percent of cases of severe MR. Vegetations may produce mild MR by interposition between leaflets. Severe endocarditic MR is usually related to ruptured chordae and less frequently to destruction of mitral tissue involving either the leaflet's edges or a perforation (Fig. 76–5). Surgery for severe mitral regurgitation traditionally has been recommended after complete course of antibiotic therapy. However, persistent pulmonary edema or large vegetations with systemic emboli may require surgery prior to a complete course of antibiotics. Studies demonstrate that mitral valve repair can be accomplished with excellent long-term results and a low recurrence of mitral regurgitation.[23–25]

Ischemic and Functional Mitral Regurgitation

Ischemic and functional MR, as a consequence of LV wall dysfunction secondary to ischemia, scarring, aneurysm, cardiomyopathy, or myocarditis, have in common both the same mechanism and that the coaptation of intrinsically normal leaflets is incomplete. However, MR may be determined more by localized LV deformation than by the systolic function. Studies using real-time three-dimensional echocardiography in humans with MR demonstrated that the pattern of mitral valve (MV) deformation from the medial to the lateral side was asymmetrical in ischemic MR, whereas it was symmetrical in nonischemic MR of cardiomyopathy.[26] This study supports the hypothesis that the geometry of the MV related to unilateral papillary displacement (regional LV dysfunction) is different from that related to bilateral displacement (global LV dysfunction), as each papillary muscle distributes the chordae only to the ipsilateral half of both leaflets. These types of MR are usually responsive to vasodilators or improvement of ischemia, which, presumably, is a result of a reversal of adverse LV geometry. However, patients undergoing coronary artery bypass

grafting for ischemic cardiomyopathy (left ventricular ejection fraction [LVEF] ≤30 percent) had a worse long-term prognosis with a moderate amount of MR prior to surgery.[27] In one study, moderate MR did not reliably resolve with coronary bypass grafting and was not associated with the preoperative extent of coronary artery disease or LV dysfunction.[28] Structural abnormalities in mitral valves of patients with congestive heart failure may prevent an improvement in LV size.[15] Thus, it may be advisable to consider mitral valvular repair in addition to coronary artery bypass grafting in patients whose valves appear thickened and elongated prior to surgery. Rupture of papillary muscle produces MR because of the flail leaflet, and in 80 percent of cases involves the posteromedial papillary muscle, and is most often associated with infarction of the adjacent ventricular wall.[29] It is the rarest form of heart rupture and of ischemic MR. Complete rupture is rapidly fatal without surgery, and partial- or single-head rupture of the papillary muscle more often allows emergency surgery[29] (Fig. 76–6).

Other Causes of Mitral Regurgitation

Clinically significant MR may be found in (1) *connective tissue disorders* such as Marfan syndrome, Ehlers-Danlos syndrome, pseudoxanthoma elasticum, osteogenesis imperfecta, Hurler disease, systemic lupus erythematosus, and anticardiolipin syndrome; (2) penetrating or nonpenetrating *cardiac trauma;* (3) *myocardial disease*—hypertrophic cardiomyopathy, amyloidosis, or sarcoidosis; (4) *endocardial lesions* caused by hypereosinophilic syndrome, endocardial fibroelastosis, carcinoid tumors, ergot toxicity, radiation toxicity, diet or drug toxicity[30]; (5) *congenital* lesions such as cleft mitral valve isolated or associated with persistent atrioventricular canal, corrected transposition with or without Ebstein abnormality of the left atrioventricular valve; and (6) *cardiac tumors.*

⟦ ⟧ HEMODYNAMICS OF MITRAL REGURGITATION

The abnormal coaptation of the mitral leaflets creates a *regurgitant orifice* during systole. The systolic pressure gradient between the

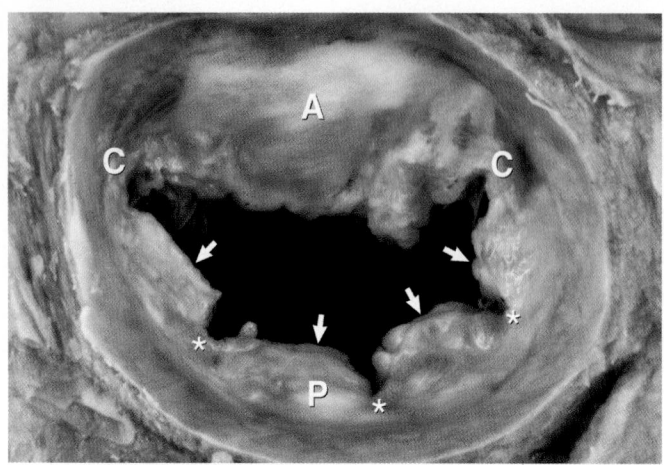

FIGURE 76–6. Anatomic example of a ruptured posterior papillary muscle. Note the normal valvular tissue otherwise. *Source: Courtesy of W.D. Edwards.*

LV and LA is the driving force of the regurgitant flow, which results in a *regurgitant volume*. This regurgitant volume represents a percentage of the total ejection of the LV and may be expressed as the *regurgitant fraction*. The regurgitant volume creates a volume overload by entering the LA in systole and the LV in diastole, thereby creating a unique hemodynamic stress by inducing a low-pressure form of volume overload as a result of ejection into the LA. Moderate MR is said to be present when the regurgitant fraction is in the range of 30 to 50 percent; severe MR is defined as a regurgitant fraction >50 percent.

The determinants of mitral regurgitant volume are best understood in the context of the orifice equation. This equation, based on the Torricelli principle, states that flow through an orifice varies by the square root of the pressure gradient across that orifice:

$$MRV = MROA \cdot C \cdot T_S \cdot \sqrt{LVP - LAP}$$

where MRV = mitral regurgitant volume, MROA = mitral regurgitant orifice area, C = constant, T_S = time or duration of systole, LVP = LV mean systolic pressure, and LAP = left atrial mean systolic pressure. In many if not most patients with MR, the regurgitant orifice area is dynamic with variations that are dependent on LV geometry. The systolic pressure gradient across the valve can also vary dramatically. These two determinants of regurgitant volume are the primary therapeutic targets in patients with MR.

The pressure gradient between the LV and atrium begins with mitral closure (simultaneous to S_1) and persists after closure of the aortic valve (S_2) until the mitral valve opens.[31] Thus, timing of regurgitant flow is determined by that of the regurgitant orifice and is most often holosystolic. Regurgitant flow and orifice area (OA) have been shown to vary throughout systole in distinct patterns characteristic of the underlying mechanism of mitral regurgitation.[32] In functional regurgitation in dilated cardiomyopathy, there was a constant decrease in OA throughout systole.[33] In mitral valve prolapse, OA was small in early systole, increasing substantially in midsystole, and decreasing mildly during LV relaxation.[34] In rheumatic MR, there was a roughly constant regurgitant OA during most of systole.

The dynamic changes in OA during systole that differ across various MR etiologies may help explain the response to therapy in chronic MR. Afterload reduction has not been shown to be uniformly effective in patients with chronic MR using standard vasodilators or agents that block rennin angiotensin system components,[35] but many vary depending on the underlying etiology of MR.[36] The observed efficacy of angiotensin-converting enzyme (ACE) inhibitor in papillary muscle dysfunction or dilated cardiomyopathy produces a decrease in LV size and improved LV geometry and thereby regurgitant OA as a result of afterload reduction. In contrast, ACE inhibitors were ineffective in reducing LV volumes in patients with structural valve disease caused by rheumatic heart disease or mitral annular calcification, which was attributed to an inability of these agents to decrease the relatively "fixed" mitral regurgitant OA that characterizes these conditions. ACE inhibitors were similarly ineffective in mitral valve prolapse, a condition in which preload or afterload reduction may actually increase the degree of prolapse and subsequently the severity of MR.

【 】 DEGREE AND CONSEQUENCES OF REGURGITATION

The degree of volume overload depends on three factors: the area of the regurgitant orifice, the regurgitant gradient, and the regurgitant duration. The volume overload is usually less severe in mitral than in aortic regurgitation (AR), despite a usually larger regurgitant gradient and orifice that is in part related to a shorter duration of MR during the cardiac cycle in mitral than in AR. However, another important consideration is related to the unique loading conditions of MR, where the LV is intrinsically unloaded in both early and late systole by ejection into the low-pressure LA; whereas in AR, the excess volume is ejected into the high-pressure aorta. Taken together, the inherent differences in the hemodynamics of the volume overload reflect the lower LV mass and mass-to-volume ratio in patients with MR as compared to AR.[37]

The height of the LA V wave and, more generally, left atrial pressure is mainly determined by left atrial compliance.[38] In acute MR, the LA is less compliant than it is in chronic MR and the MR produces a marked increase in LA pressure. The atrial V wave, in turn, decreases the ventriculoatrial gradient and, thus, for any effective regurgitant orifice, tends to limit the regurgitant volume. When MR becomes chronic, the LA dilates, and the V wave is less prominent and does not limit the regurgitant volume; the LA pressure may be normal even with severe MR at rest.[39] However, a study of patients with ischemic and nonischemic heart failure (LV ejection fraction <25 percent) and mild-to-moderate MR, there was an increase in exercise-induced changes in MR severity that correlated with maximal oxygen consumption (VO_2max) and increases in pulmonary capillary wedge pressure, end-diastolic and end-systolic sphericity indexes, and with mitral valvular coaptation distance.[40] There are numerous studies demonstrating the importance of resting right ventricular (RV) ejection fraction in determining exercise capacity and morbidity and mortality after mitral valve repair or replacement in patients with chronic MR. The effect on resting RV function reflects chronic passive pulmonary congestion of MR that may not be impressive at rest but may increase in severity during mild-to-moderate exercise.

【 】 LEFT VENTRICULAR FUNCTION

Effects on Myocardial Oxygen Consumption

The volume overload of chronic MR produces an eccentric pattern of hypertrophy manifested by a decrease in the LV mass-to-volume ratio in response to the increase in diastolic load, as systolic load is facilitated by ejection into the low-pressure LA. Moreover, the marked increase in LV end-diastolic volume, that over time outstrips the increase in LV mass, produces an increase in stress-volume area that is equivalent to dogs with pure pressure overload, suggesting a similar myocardial oxygen consumption.[41] In patients, the severity of MR, determined by LV volumes, related to the decreased LV creatine phosphate-to-adenosine triphosphate ratios,[29] suggests that bioenergetic abnormalities occur in the dilated LV in spite of "normal" LV ejection fraction.

Effects on Diastolic Function

Patients with MR may remain compensated without symptoms of congestive heart failure for many years. The eccentricity index, which relates the relative sizes of the long and short axes, demonstrated progressive LV sphericity over time that was greatest during the early rapid filling phase and a near fourfold increase in the transmitral pressure gradient. In patients, chronic MR caused the pressure-dimension and volume curve to shift to the right as myocardial stiffness was unchanged (Fig. 76–7).[29] However, as the LV fails in patients with chronic MR, the chamber stiffness and pressure–volume curve is shifted toward a less-compliant ventricle.[42]

Much has been studied regarding the role of the profibrotic response in the course of pressure overload. In contrast, hearts with volume overload undergo a continual state of remodeling of the ECM that opposes excess collagen deposition, in spite of increased cardiac renin–angiotensin system (RAS) expression. Indeed, in human hearts, there is a greater increase in steady-state mRNA for collagen I and collagen III in the pressure overload of aortic valvular stenosis as compared to the volume overload of AR. In addition, in the dog model of MR, there is upregulation of the intracardiac RAS, decreased LV wall thickness-to-diameter ratio, increased MMP activity, and dissolution of the collagen weave within 2 weeks and lasting for 5 months after induction of MR.[31] These findings are consistent with the contention that less ECM allows for the necessary LV chamber enlargement and compliance characteristics in volume overload. However, the loss of ECM attachments to myocytes may foster the slippage of cells and collections of cells that compromise the laminar structure of the heart, resulting in further LV dilation and subsequent failure.

Effects on Systolic Function

It is difficult to measure contractility of the LV, particularly in the case of MR because the definition of end-systole and end-ejection has been used interchangeably to assess LV performance based on the assumption that timing of these events is nearly coincident. However, studies in animals and in humans[43] clearly demonstrate that end-ejection, defined as minimum ventricular volume, dissociates from end-systole in MR because of the shortened time to LV end-systole in association with preserved time to end-ejection (minimum volume) as a result of the low impedance ejection presented by the LA (Fig. 76–8). Thus, the load-dependent ejection

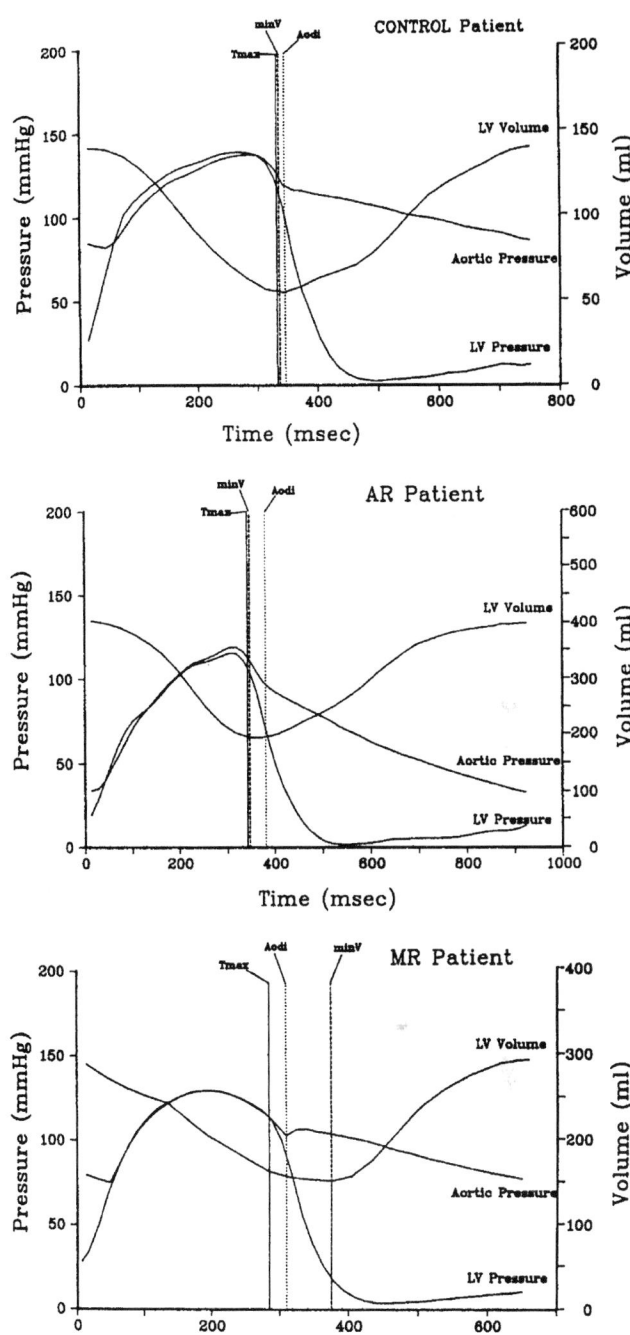

FIGURE 76–7. Shows the LV pressure–volume relationships in a control patient, a patient with aortic regurgitation, and a patient with mitral regurgitation.

or shortening phase indices of function, such as LVEF and velocity of circumferential shortening, can be normal and mask significant myocardial dysfunction in the setting of MR. For this reason it is not surprising that an LVEF value of 60 percent is considered the lower limit for timing for mitral valve surgery in MR.

Ejection fraction is dependent upon preload and afterload. Plotting ejection fraction against afterload provides a better index of contractile function than ejection fraction alone. As an alternative to ejection fraction, end-systolic volume or dimension is relatively independent of preload and varies linearly with afterload.

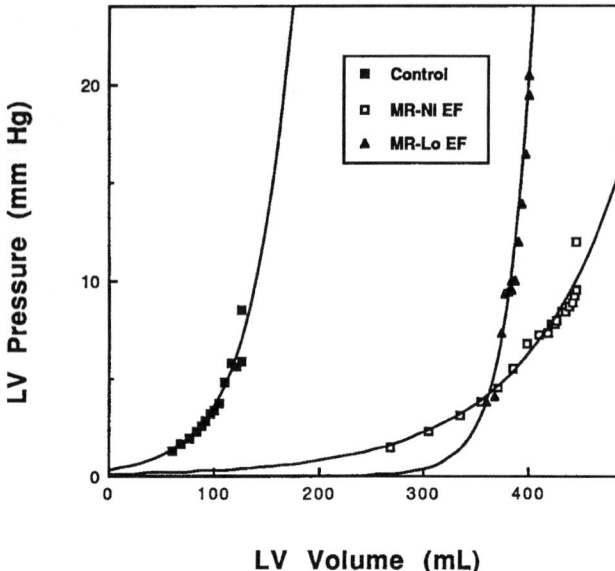

FIGURE 76–8. Shows the LV diastolic pressure–volume relationships in a control patient, two patients with MR one of whom had normal LVEF, and another patient who had reduced LVEF.

The slope of this relation describes the end-systolic pressure-stress and volume-dimension relation or systolic elastance. An analysis of LV chamber elastance in patients with chronic MR supported the concepts that contractile function is impaired in some patients with long-term MR and a normal LVEF. However, use of this methodology in patients is potentially hazardous because it requires invasive hemodynamic monitoring and manipulation of blood pressure to alter loading conditions.

End-systolic wall stress is a better index of afterload because it accounts for ventricular geometry, which is especially important in the case of the spherically dilated heart with MR. A relatively high end-systolic volume for a given end-systolic wall stress indicates relatively less ventricular shortening for a given afterload, thus depressed myocardial contractility. In patients having surgery for severe MR, the end-systolic stress-to-end-systolic volume ratio separated patients with a good prognosis for valve replacement. The incorporation of a wall-stress determination adds complementary physiologic and prognostic data to LV end-systolic dimension and volume and LVEF in the assessment of MR.

NEUROHORMONAL ACTIVATION

The adrenergic nervous system provides inotropic support for the overloaded heart and may represent an important mechanism of compensation in the course of MR because Starling (preload) reserve is called upon as an early compensatory mechanism. Indeed, there was a positive relation between norepinephrine release rates (an index of sympathetic activity) with increasing end-systolic dimension and decrease in LV performance in patients with chronic MR.[44] In addition, B-type natriuretic peptide (BNP) activation in organic MR independently predicts adverse events and is directly related to the LV end-systolic volume index.[44] However, increased catecholamine release has also been documented in patients with chronic MR early in disease process. Other studies also demonstrate

a decrease in LV myocardial β-adrenergic receptor density that was related to the severity of symptoms and LV dysfunction. It is of great interest that β-adrenergic blockade treatment of MR dogs improved LV chamber function and ECM preservation,[42] as well as improved isolated cardiomyocyte contractile function and an increase in the number of contractile elements within cardiomyocytes.[31] Tumor necrosis factor-α (TNF-α) is a proinflammatory cytokine that activates MMPs and is increased in the myocardium in response to stretch. TNF-α is elevated in the plasma of patients with congestive heart failure and in the plasma of patients with aortic stenosis and MR. Furthermore, in patients with chronic MR, increased TNF-α expression in the myocardium and plasma is related to the extent of LV dilatation. Moreover, correction of the LV volume overload state with MV repair leads to reversal of TNF-α expression and reverse LV remodeling. These findings suggest that TNF-α may play a key role in inflammatory-mediated changes in the ECM that results in progressive LV dilatation in patients with chronic MR.

CLINICAL PRESENTATION

Primary MR often is initially diagnosed based on a finding of a systolic murmur in an asymptomatic patient. However, the nature and severity of symptoms with MR are related to its severity, which, in turn, is related to the presence of pulmonary hypertension, coronary artery disease, atrial fibrillation, and associated valvular disease. Fatigue and mild dyspnea on exertion are the usual symptoms and are rapidly improved by rest. The administration of diuretics and progressive self-limitation of physical activity may prevent the occurrence of more severe symptoms. Severe dyspnea on exertion or, more rarely, paroxysmal nocturnal dyspnea, frank pulmonary edema, or even hemoptysis may be observed later in the course of the disease. Such severe symptoms may be triggered by a new onset of atrial fibrillation, an increase in degree of MR, the occurrence of endocarditis or ruptured chordae, or a change in LV compliance or function.

With severe MR of *acute onset,* symptoms are usually more dramatic with pulmonary edema or congestive heart failure, but will progressively subside with administration of a diuretic, afterload reduction, and increased LA compliance with time. A syndrome of sudden onset of atypical chest pain and dyspnea may occur with abrupt chordal rupture. Sudden death as the initial presentation of MR as a consequence of flail leaflet is 1 to 2.5 percent over 6 years and is related to LV systolic dysfunction, leaflet redundancy, severe MR, and associated comorbid conditions. Rupture of papillary muscle in the setting of acute myocardial infarction usually has a dramatic presentation, with cardiogenic shock or a severe pulmonary edema. Pulmonary edema may also be observed in transient severe papillary muscle dysfunction.

Physical Examination

In addition to the following material, see Chap. 12.

Blood pressure is usually normal. Carotid upstroke is brisk. Cardiac palpation may show laterally displaced, diffuse, and brief apical impulse with enlarged LV. An apical thrill is characteristic of severe MR. The left sternal border lift is observed with RV dilatation and may be difficult to distinguish from the left atrial lift because of the dilated, expansive LA, which is more substernal and lower. S_1 is included in the murmur and is usually normal but may be increased in rheumatic disease. S_2 is usually normal but may be paradoxically split if the LV ejection time is markedly shortened. The presence of a third heart sound (S_3) is directly related to the volume of the regurgitation in patients with organic MR. It is often associated with an early diastolic rumble caused by the increased mitral flow in diastole even without mitral stenosis. The S_3 and diastolic rumble are low-pitched sounds and may be difficult to detect without careful auscultation in the left lateral decubitus position. The S_3 increases with expiration. In ischemic-functional MR, S_3 corresponds more often to restrictive LV filling. An atrial gallop (S_4) is heard mainly in MR of recent onset and in ischemic or functional MR in sinus rhythm. Midsystolic clicks are markers of valve prolapse (see Mitral Valve Prolapse Syndrome below).

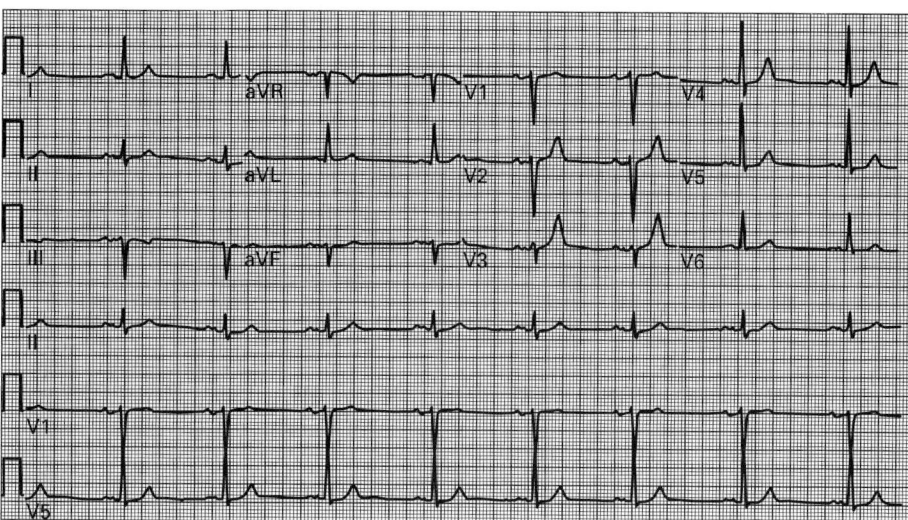

FIGURE 76–9. Electrocardiogram of a patient with severe mitral regurgitation. Note left atrial enlargement, as indicated by notched P waves (lead I and rhythm strip lead II).

The hallmark of MR is the systolic murmur, most often holosystolic, including first and second heart sounds. Only a careful examination beginning at the base of the heart to identify the second heart sound and progressing toward the apex will allow clear recognition of the nature of the murmur. The murmur is of the blowing type but may be harsh, especially in valve prolapse. The maximum intensity is usually at the apex, and it may radiate to the axilla in rheumatic or anterior leaflet prolapse, affecting primarily the anterior leaflet. In posterior leaflet prolapse, the jet is usually superiorly and medially directed and the murmur radiates toward the base of the heart. The murmur may be heard in the back, in the neck, and sometimes on the skull. In the cases where the murmur radiates to the base, it may be difficult to distinguish from the murmur of aortic stenosis or obstructive cardiomyopathy, and pharmacologic maneuvers showing that the murmur decreases with amyl nitrite and increases with methoxamine strongly suggest MR. Murmur intensity does not increase with postextrasystolic beats and usually parallels the degree of MR, but in myocardial infarction, severe MR may be totally silent. Murmurs of shorter duration usually correspond to mild MR; they may be mid or late systolic in mitral valve prolapse or early systolic in functional MR.

Electrocardiogram

The most frequent feature of MR is atrial fibrillation, which was found in approximately 50 to 60 percent of earlier series and is now present in approximately 50 percent of surgically corrected MR.[45] Patients in sinus rhythm may present with signs of left atrial enlargement (Fig. 76–9). LV hypertrophy is more rarely seen and may be associated with secondary ST-T abnormalities. RV hypertrophy is uncommon. The ECG, especially in acute MR, may be entirely normal, whereas ischemic MR may manifest Q waves or ST-T wave changes.

Chest Roentgenogram

Cardiomegaly may be present in chronic MR or in ischemic or functional MR (Fig. 76–10). LA body and appendage dilatation is frequent, but giant LA is rare and is usually seen in severe mixed valve disease. Although valvular calcifications are rare, annular calcification, seen as a C-shaped density below the posterior leaflet, is frequent. Because LA pressure is frequently normal even with severe MR, signs of pulmonary hypertension or pulmonary edema are rarely observed.

Doppler Echocardiography

Doppler echocardiography (see Chap. 16) in MR characteristically reveals a high-velocity jet in the LA during systole, and the severity of the regurgitation is a function of the distance from the valve that the jet can be detected. Most centers grade regurgitation as mild, moderate, or severe using a combination of color-flow, con-

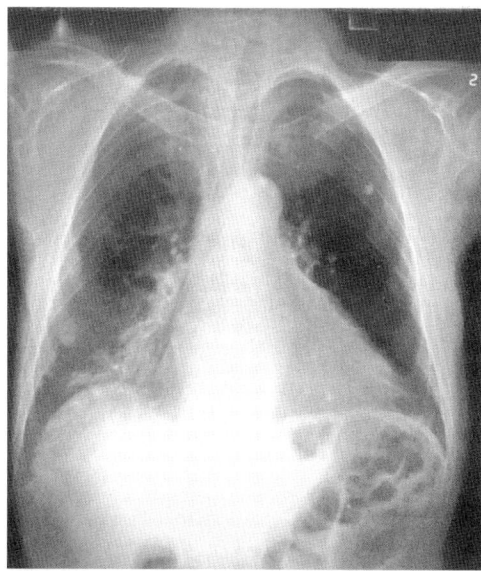

FIGURE 76–10. Chest roentgenogram of a patient with severe mitral regurgitation. Note the cardiomegaly and enlargement of the left atrial body and appendage.

tinuous, and pulsed-wave Doppler imaging. Area of the mitral jet >8 cm² indicates severe MR. However, jet area is significantly affected by the cause of the MR, which, in some cases, can produce an eccentric jet that limits the accuracy of this approach. Another method of determining MR severity uses the vena contracta defined as the narrowest cross-sectional area of the regurgitant jet by color-flow Doppler. Although Doppler echocardiography provides several methods of quantifying regurgitation, none have been shown to predict clinical outcome.

Echocardiography

The most important aspect of echocardiography is the quantification of LV end-diastolic and end-systolic dimensions, wall thickness, and ejection fraction and fractional shortening. M-mode diameter or volume can assess the LA size by two-dimensional echocardiography. However, the LVEF may be normal in the setting of myocardial dysfunction, resulting in postoperative LV dysfunction, even in the absence of clinical symptoms prior to surgery. For this reason, clinical management requires periodic imaging studies to detect changes, especially in the end-systolic dimension. Surgery should be considered when LVEF is <60 percent and LV end-systolic dimension is >45 mm.[35] One study demonstrated that the preoperative exercise echocardiographic LVEF and LV end-systolic volume were the best predictors of postoperative LV dysfunction in patients with minimal symptoms prior to surgery.

Evaluation of the valvular leaflets is an important part of the echocardiographic examination. *Rheumatic MR* is characterized by thickening of the leaflets and chordae. The posterior leaflet has reduced mobility, whereas the anterior leaflet may be doming if commissural fusion is associated. In *degenerative MR*, prolapse is observed with the passage of valvular tissue beyond the annulus plane in the long-axis view (Fig. 76–11). The valve leaflets are diffusely thickened leaflets and excessive valvular tissue and increased echogenicity of the annulus is consistent with mitral annular calcification. Flail segments can appear as complete eversion of the segment with or without the small floating echo of ruptured chordae (Fig. 76–12).

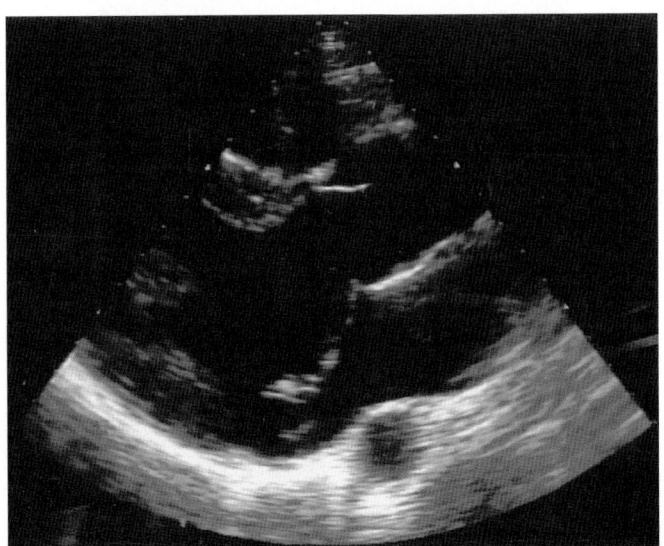

FIGURE 76–11. Echocardiogram of a bileaflet mitral valve prolapse seen from the parasternal long-axis view.

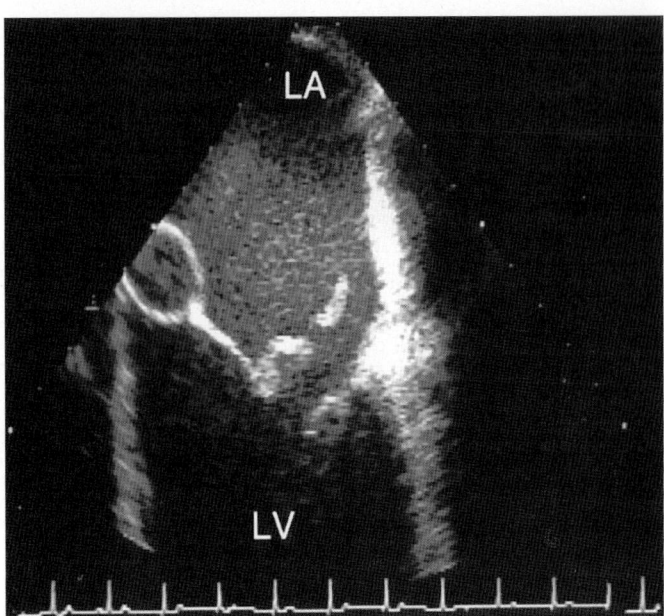

FIGURE 76–12. Transesophageal echocardiography (*horizontal plane*) of a flail anterior leaflet. The ruptured chord is seen at the tip of the anterior leaflet.

In ischemic or functional MR, the finding of a dilated annulus is nonspecific and annular descent is reduced. The features of ischemic heart disease may be observed as regional wall motion abnormalities. The leaflet tissue is normal. The mitral tenting caused by the abnormal traction by the principal chordae on the anterior leaflet reduces the area of coaptation of the two leaflets, allowing for a central jet of MR. With papillary muscle rupture, MR is a result of the flail leaflet. The diagnosis is based on visualization of a small mass of muscle, which is attached to chordae and floats freely during the cardiac cycle.

Transesophageal echocardiography provides superior imaging quality to transthoracic echocardiography (see Chap. 16). However, its incremental value is notable only when the transthoracic information is suboptimal or incomplete and when questions arise regarding the feasibility of valve repair the presence of endocarditis or other associated complications. It is also used on a large scale intraoperatively to monitor the results of valve repair with loading conditions matched to a baseline study performed at the beginning of the surgical procedure.

Radionuclide Studies

Radionuclide angiography can be used to estimate the LV end-diastolic and end-systolic volume, as well as the RV and LVEF. The detection of exercise-induced LV dysfunction can be helpful in the asymptomatic patient. A comparison of the stroke counts measured over the RV and LV allows the calculation of a regurgitant fraction in the absence of tricuspid and pulmonary regurgitation. Recent guidelines also suggest that the RV ejection fraction response to exercise may be an important determinant, in addition to LV size and function, in timing for valve surgery.

Cardiac Catheterization

Cardiac catheterization is used to assess hemodynamic status, the severity of MR, LV function, and coronary anatomy. The large V wave of the pulmonary wedge pressure is more frequent in acute MR than it is in chronic MR, but can be observed in other diseases, such as ventricular septal defect or heart failure with reduced left atrial compliance without MR (Fig. 76–13). Selective LV cineangiography provides a clinically useful assessment of MR severity, qualitatively grading the degree of opacification of the LA and pulmonary veins. Quantitation of MR regurgitant volume and regurgitant fraction can be obtained by comparing the angiographic stroke volume to the forward stroke volume, calculated by the Fick method. LV function can be assessed using quantitative angiography; using high-fidelity pressure recording provides important information on LV elastance and LV chamber stiffness in patients with MR. Obstructive coronary atherosclerosis continues to be frequent even in the absence of angina, and coronary angiography is ordinarily performed in patients older than 40 to 50 years of age.

【 】 NATURAL HISTORY

In patients with primary MR, there may be a period of several years without symptoms. In a prospective study of 300 patients

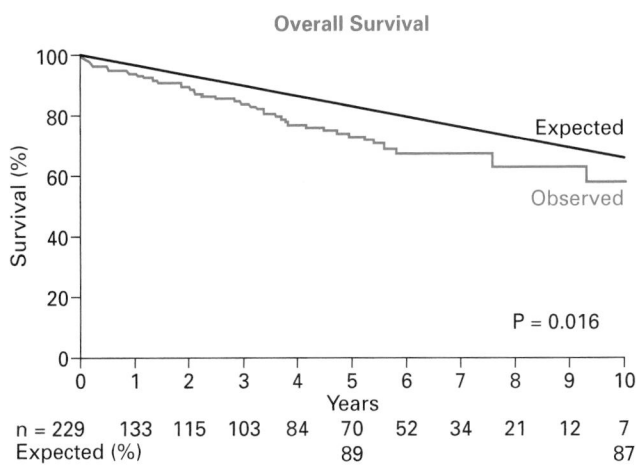

FIGURE 76–14. Survival with medical treatment of patients diagnosed with mitral regurgitation caused by flail leaflets. Note the excess mortality in comparison to the expected survival. *Source: Reprinted by permission of the New England Journal of Medicine from Ling H, Enriquez-Sarano M, Seward J, et al. Clinical outcome of mitral regurgitation due to flail leaflets. N Engl J Med 1996;335:1417–1423. Copyright 1996, Massachusetts Medical Society.*

with MR, rate of symptom onset was 2 to 4 percent per year. Morbidity in patients with severe MR is also high. Of patients who are initially asymptomatic, approximately 10 percent per year develop symptoms, which may be hastened by atrial fibrillation. In patients with flail leaflets 10 years after diagnosis, heart failure occurred in 63 percent and permanent atrial fibrillation in 30 percent of those initially in sinus rhythm (Fig. 76–13). Also at 10 years, 90 percent of the patients had either died or undergone surgery, confirming that in these patients surgery is almost unavoidable (Fig. 76–14). In summary, at 10 years, survival was 57 percent (Fig. 76–15) and sudden death in patients with MR caused by flail leaflets occurred at a rate of 1.8 percent per year.

In another recent study, mortality was 22 percent at 5 years in patients with severe MR. A major independent determinant of

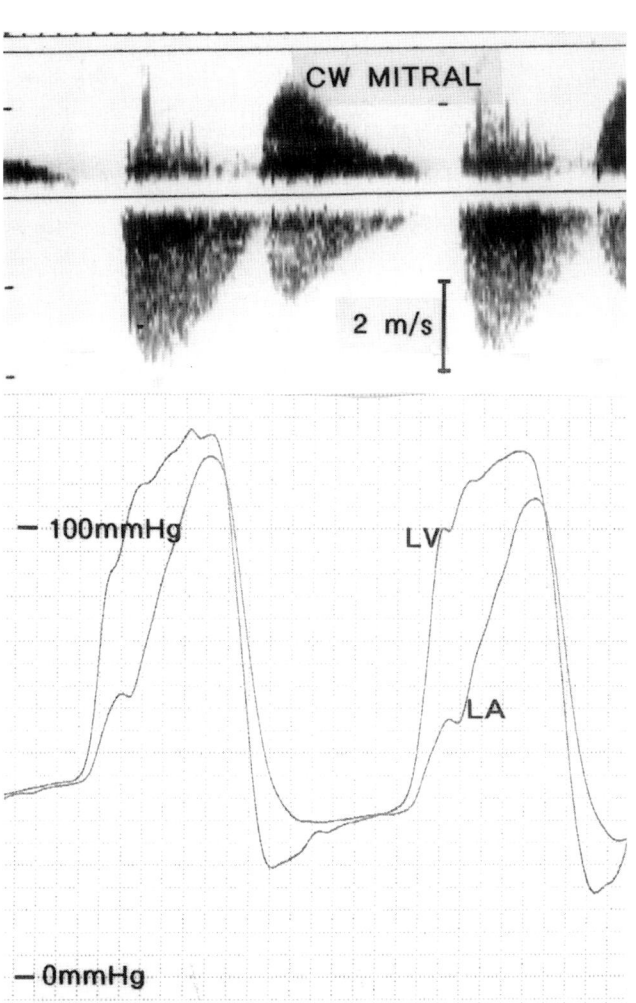

FIGURE 76–13. Simultaneous recording of left ventricular and left atrial pressures and continuous-wave Doppler in a patient with severe mitral regurgitation. Note the large V wave on the left atrial pressure recording, with a triangular shape of the mitral regurgitant jet obtained by continuous-wave Doppler. *Source: Courtesy of Rick Nishimura, Mayo Clinic.*

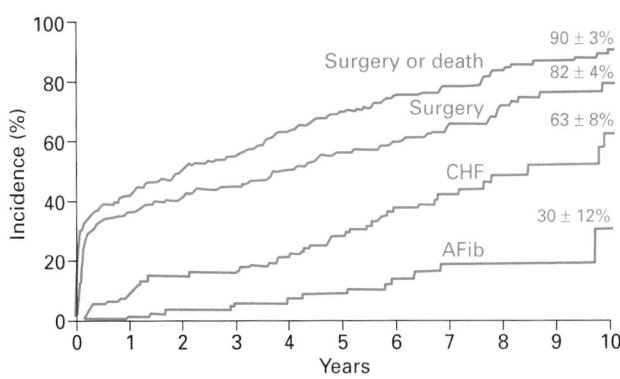

FIGURE 76–15. Cardiac morbidity with medical treatment in patients diagnosed with mitral regurgitation caused by flail leaflets. Afib, atrial fibrillation; CHF, congestive heart failure. *Source: Reprinted by permission of the New England Journal of Medicine from Ling H, Enriquez-Sarano M, Seward J, et al. Clinical outcome of mitral regurgitation due to flail leaflets. N Engl J Med 1996;335:1417–1423. Copyright 1996, Massachusetts Medical Society.*

survival was regurgitant orifice area, which was associated with 58 percent survival when ≥0.4 cm². Based on these studies from the Mayo Clinic experience, Enriquez-Saramo has championed early repair in the setting of severe MR, as postponing surgery seemed to expose the patient to unnecessary risk. However, a drawback to these studies is that these patients were followed by their individual physicians without documentation of adherence to currently accepted guidelines for periodic evaluation of LV size and function. A recent study from a single center reported a good perioperative and postoperative outcome in asymptomatic patients with severe degenerative MR when intervention was determined by the onset of symptoms or currently recommended American College of Cardiologists/American Heart Association (ACC/AHA) guidelines for LV size,[46] LV function and pulmonary hypertension (see Chap. 11). Consequently, prophylactic surgery for all patients with asymptomatic severe degenerative MR is not recommended.[46] Table 76–2 lists some of the determinants of outcome.

【 】 MANAGEMENT

Medical Treatment

Prevention of infective endocarditis using the appropriate prophylaxis is necessary in patients with MR (see Chap. 85). Young patients with rheumatic MR should receive rheumatic fever prophylaxis. In patients with atrial fibrillation (see Chap. 37) control is achieved using digoxin and/or β blockers. Long-term maintenance of sinus rhythm after cardioversion in patients with severe MR or enlarged LA is usually not possible in patients who are treated medically. However, return to sinus rhythm after surgery is possible in patients with atrial fibrillation of short duration. Oral anticoagulation should be used in patients with atrial fibrillation.

Although vasodilators are successfully used to increase forward output and decrease LV filling pressure in patients with acute MR and dilated cardiomyopathy, the hemodynamic effects are less clear in patients with primary mitral valve disease. Studies to date report conflicting results regarding the benefits of chronic ACE inhibitor therapy in patients with MR of heterogeneous etiologies. In concordance with these clinical studies, reports from two independent laboratories demonstrate that blockade of the RAS fails to improve LV function and remodeling in a canine model of MR.[47] The canine model of MR is characterized by an absence of fibrosis, activation of MMPs, and by dissolution of the fine collagen weave. As RAS blockade is antifibrotic, it may have accentuated this process resulting in loss of the fine collagen weave that destroys the structural support of the ECM that is necessary for maintenance of normal LV chamber geometry and for the translation of forces from individual cardiomyocytes to the LV chamber. β_1-Adrenergic blockade treatment of MR dogs improved LV chamber remodeling and ECM preservation and decreased norepinephrine release into the cardiac interstitium, as well as improved isolated cardiomyocyte contractile function and an increase in the number of contractile elements within cardiomyocytes. Insights from the canine model of MR, coupled with a lack of conclusive clinical data on treatment, provide a strong rationale for a well-designed clinical trial of β-receptor blockade in patients with MR that incorporates information on LV size and function, and especially clinical outcome.[48]

TABLE 76–2

Determinants of Outcome

UNOPERATED PATIENTS	OPERATED PATIENTS
Symptoms	Age
Pulmonary hypertension	Preoperative symptoms
LV end-diastolic volume	Coronary disease
AV-O$_2$ difference	End-systolic dimensions
Ejection fraction	Ejection fraction
	LA size
	Valve repair

AV, atrioventricular; LA, left atrial; LV, left ventricular.

Surgical Treatment

In most patients requiring surgery, the most relevant question is the timing of the surgical indication, which is influenced by the natural history of MR and by the outcome after surgical correction of MR. Table 76–2 lists the determinants of outcome. The 2006 American College of Cardiology and American Heart Association guidelines[3] for timing of surgery suggest that surgery should be considered in patients with chronic asymptomatic severe MR when LV end-systolic dimension is ≥45 mm (normal: <40 mm) and LVEF is ≤60 percent (normal: 65 percent; Table 76–3). The recent study by the group

TABLE 76–3

American College of Cardiology/American Heart Association Guidelines for Surgery for Nonischemic Severe Mitral Regurgitation

Class I (evidence and/or general agreement that surgery is useful and effective)
Symptoms cause by MR (acute or chronic)
Asymptomatic patients with severe MR and mild-moderate LV dysfunction defined as an
   —Ejection fraction 30–60% **and**
   —End-systolic dimension 45–55 mm

Class IIa (conflicting evidence and/or divergence of opinion but the weight of evidence/opinion favors surgical intervention)
Asymptomatic patients with normal LV function and
   —Atrial fibrillation **or**
   —Pulmonary hypertension (>50 mmHg at rest of >60 mmHg with exercise)
Asymptomatic patients with
   —Ejection fraction 50–60% **or**
   —End-systolic dimension 45–55 mm
Severe left ventricular dysfunction (ejection fraction <30% and/or end-systolic dimension >55 mm) if chordal preservation is highly likely

LV, left ventricular; MR, mitral regurgitation.

from University of Vienna demonstrates that adherence to these guidelines results in good perioperative and postoperative outcomes but requires careful followup.[49] These guidelines were validated by another large prospective study from the Sakakibara Heart Institute in Tokyo.[49] Importantly, these investigators found that the incidence of postoperative LV dysfunction (defined as LVEF <50 percent) was high in patients with LVEF <55 percent (38 percent) or LV end-systolic dimension ≥40 mm (23 percent), although a markedly reduced preoperative ejection fraction (<50 percent) is associated with a high late mortality. In patients with severe MR and an ejection fraction <30 percent or an end-systolic dimension >55 mm should be considered for surgery if it is highly likely that a valve repair can be performed. However, valve repair remains highly controversial in dilated cardiomyopathy. In the patient with ischemic heart disease and MR, revascularization can improve MR, and valve repair and/or annuloplasty should be considered on a case-by-case basis. This may gain more support in view of the recent studies demonstrating structural abnormalities in valve leaflets of patients with dilated ischemic and nonischemic cardiomyopathies. However, cardiac resynchronization therapy reduces functional MR in patients with LV dysfunction.[50,51] Thus, the mechanism of functional mitral regurgitation appears to be a multifactorial process that involves structural valvular changes, LV dyssynchrony, and LV geometry that may be a global as well as a regional problem. A recent study in a well-characterized sheep model of myocardial infarction found that transplantation of autologous skeletal myoblasts into the inferior scar improved moderate MR by decreasing tethering distance and improving LVEF and wall motion score resulting in better coaptation of mitral valve leaflets. In the future, such a procedure may provide an important adjunct to valve repair in ischemic functional MR. Finally, the preliminary results of percutaneous transseptal approach to mitral valve repair has recently been reported in patients with degenerative MR.[52] The preliminary results of this phase 1 trial suggest that the procedure can be performed safely with a reduction in MR and this approach is now being tested in a multicenter trial (EVEREST II [Endovascular Valve Edge-to-Edge Repair Study]).

Postoperative Outcome

Mitral valve repair offers several advantages, including avoidance of long-term anticoagulation and, most importantly, preservation of the continuity between the mitral annulus and papillary muscles. This annular–papillary muscle continuity helps maintain normal left LV geometry and systolic function. When annular–papillary muscle continuity is preserved, ejection fraction typically remains stable or improves after mitral surgery, in contrast to a decline by an average of 10 ejection fraction units when this continuity is disrupted. The average operative mortality for mitral valve repair is 1 to 2 percent, compared to 5 to 10 percent with valve replacement. Age and the existence of coronary artery disease are important predictors of survival. Mitral valve repair has a low rate of reoperation for recurrent MR with an event-free survival ranging from 80 to 90 percent at 5 to 10 years in published series. However, considering the inherent

structural abnormalities of the valve of degenerative MR and the data in patients with valve repair, the durability of a successful mitral reconstruction for degenerative mitral valve disease is not constant. This should be taken into account when asymptomatic patients are offered early mitral valve repair, especially when LV functional dimensions are within accepted guidelines for observational treatment.

Atrial fibrillation when present preoperatively usually persists postoperatively—unless it is of brief duration—but the excess risk caused by this arrhythmia appears modest, although it requires anticoagulation. In the patient with MR and atrial fibrillation, some centers now advocate a concurrent atrial procedure to restore sinus rhythm and prevent recurrent atrial fibrillation.[53] Late risk of thromboembolism after mitral replacement for MR is not different from it as in other mitral valve diseases. Differences in thromboembolic risk after valve repair and valve replacement have been variably estimated but appear to favor valve repair. In addition, anticoagulation is recommended permanently following valve repair only if atrial fibrillation persists; the occurrence of bleeding is less common than it is when following prosthetic replacement.

MITRAL VALVE PROLAPSE SYNDROME

The syndrome of mitral valve prolapse (MVP) is the most common form of valvular heart disease, occurring in 0.6 to 2.4 percent of the population, thus being more common than a bicuspid aortic valve. The incidence of MVP and risk of complications range greatly, depending on the criteria used for its diagnosis,[1,2] as well as the patient population studied.[53-57]

These may differ importantly in a referral population as compared with community patients. They do not appear to differ by ethnicity. Studies of native American Indian tribes show the same prevalence as other general populations when screened using contemporary criteria.[58] MVP is genetically heterogenous and is inherited as an autosomal dominant trait that exhibits both sex- and age-dependent penetrance.[59] The discovery of genes involved in the pathogenesis of this common disorder is critical to understanding its diversity in presentation.[60] Clinically, patients with MVP exhibit fibromyxomatous changes in one or both of the mitral leaflets that result in superior displacement of the leaflets into the LA. MVP is typically a diagnosis commonly detected by cardiac auscultation with one or more systolic clicks and/or a mid-to-late systolic murmur detected on a careful physical examination. Often the auscultatory complex is the only clinical manifestation of cardiac disease, and many patients are asymptomatic. MVP is likely overdiagnosed in many patients by examiners who misidentify the auscultatory findings and/or overread the two-dimensional echocardiograms.

Midsystolic clicks were first described in the late 19th century and originally were attributed to a pericardial or extracardiac etiology. Subsequently, late-systolic murmurs were recognized in apparently healthy people to be associated with a benign natural history. Thus, the murmur also was considered to be extracardiac in origin.

In 1961, Reid[61] suggested that the midsystolic click and the late-systolic murmur were a result of mitral regurgitation. In

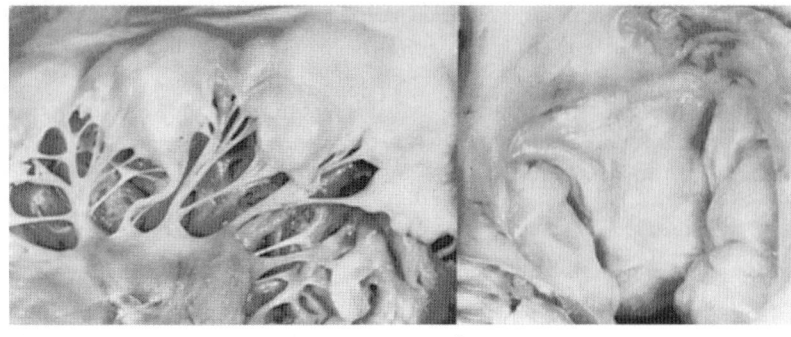

FIGURE 76–16. Myxomatous mitral valve. **A.** The opened mitral valve shows characteristic interchordal hooding and redundancy of the leaflets. **B.** The unopened mitral valve viewed from the LA side shows extensive scalloping that is characteristic of a myxomatous mitral valve. *Source: From Lukas RV Jr and Edwards JE.[64] Reproduced with permission from the publisher and authors.*

1963, Barlow and coworkers[62] confirmed this hypothesis by LV cineangiography. Subsequently, intracardiac phonocardiogram studies documented the mitral valve origin of a systolic click and late-systolic murmur.

During the past 40 years, considerable new data obtained from pathologic studies, echocardiography, and cineventriculography have demonstrated that this common syndrome is associated with prolapse of one or both mitral valve leaflets into the atrium during LV systole.

Recognition of MVP (also known as the *systolic click–late systolic murmur syndrome*) is often difficult because of the extreme variability of its clinical manifestations and the diminishing auscultatory skills of physicians who often default the physical examination in lieu of noninvasive diagnostic testing. It is, however, an important cause of incapacitating chest pain and refractory arrhythmias in certain patients. The abnormal components of the mitral valve apparatus are a potential site for endocarditis, and some patients, particularly males 60 to 80 years old, can develop severe MR as a result of ruptured chordae tendineae.

TABLE 76–4

Classification of Mitral Valve Prolapse

Primary mitral valve prolapse
  Familial
  Nonfamilial
  Marfan syndrome
  Other connective tissue diseases
Mitral valve prolapse without myxomatous proliferation
  Coronary artery disease
  Rheumatic heart disease
  Cardiomyopathies
  "Flail" mitral valve leaflets
Normal variant labeled as mitral valve prolapse
  Inaccurate auscultation
  "Echocardiographic heart disease"

【 】 DEFINITION, ETIOLOGY, AND TIMING

MVP refers to the systolic billowing of one or both mitral leaflets into the LA, with or without MR. MVP often occurs as a clinical entity with no or only mild MR, but it is frequently associated with unique clinical characteristics when compared with the other causes of MR.[63–65] Importantly, MVP is the most common cause of significant MR and the most frequent substrate for mitral valve endocarditis in the United States.[1] The mitral valve apparatus is a complex structure composed of the mitral annulus, valve leaflets, chordae tendineae, papillary muscles, and the supporting LV, left atrium, and aortic walls[1] (Fig. 76–16). Disease processes involving any one or more of these components may result in dysfunction of the valvular apparatus and prolapse of the mitral leaflets toward the LA during systole when LV pressure exceeds LA pressure.

The complexity of the mitral valve apparatus explains the presence of secondary prolapse in many conditions that affect one or more components of the apparatus (e.g., ruptured mitral chordae). There is, however, considerable evidence that a disorder of the mitral valve leaflets exists in which there are specific pathologic changes causing redundancy of the mitral leaflets and their prolapse into the LA during systole. This is the primary form of MVP (Table 76–4).

In *primary* MVP, there is interchordal hooding as a result of leaflet redundancy that involves both the rough and clear zones of the involved leaflets[64] (Fig. 76–17). The height of the interchordal hooding usually exceeds 4 mm and involves at least one-half of the anterior leaflet or at least two-thirds of the posterior leaflet. The basic anatomic feature seen by microscopy in primary MVP is the marked proliferation of the *spongiosa,* the delicate myxomatous connective tissue between the *atrialis* (a thick layer of collagen and elastic tissue forming the atrial aspect of the leaflet) and the *fibrosa,* or *ventricularis,* which is composed of dense layers of collagen and forms the basic support of the leaflet.[64] In primary MVP, myxomatous proliferation of the acid mucopolysaccharide-containing spongiosa tissue causes focal interruption of the fibrosa. Secondary effects of the primary MVP syndrome include fibrosis of the surfaces of the mitral valve leaflets, thinning and/or elongation of chordae tendineae, and ventricular friction lesions.

Fibrin deposits often form at the mitral valve–LA angle.

The primary form of MVP may be familial, where it appears to be inherited as an autosomal dominant trait with varying penetrance.[65] Several chromosomal abnormalities have been identified in certain patients with primary MVP, which often occurs in isolated cases.[66] Primary MVP occurs with increasing frequency in patients with Marfan syndrome, where it is usually present, and in other inherited connective tissue diseases such as Ehlers-Danlos syndrome,[67] pseudoxanthoma elasticum,[68] and osteogenesis imperfecta.[69] Polycystic kidney disease is associated with a 25 percent prevalence of MVP. Marfan syndrome is a heritable disorder of connective tissue caused by a defect in fibrillin protein encoded by the fibrillin gene on chro-

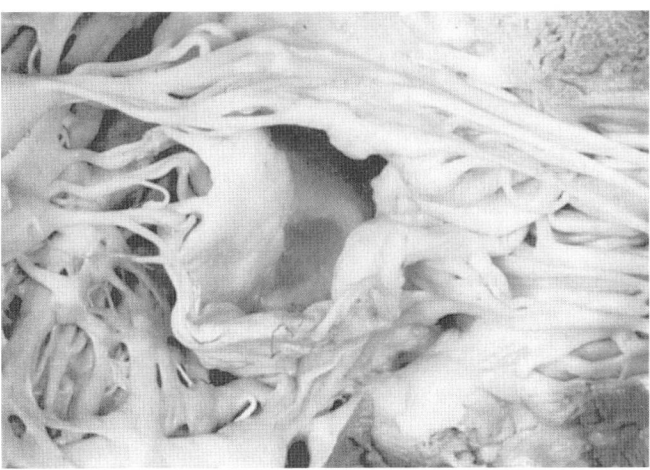

FIGURE 76–17. Myxomatous mitral valve with ruptured posterior leaflet chordae. The central part of the posterior leaflet (*lower center*) shows fragments of ruptured chordae. The intact chordae are elongated, and the leaflets show redundancy and fibrous thickening. *Source: From Edwards F. Pathology of mitral incompetence. In: Silver MD, ed. Cardiovascular Pathology. New York: Churchill Livingstone, 1983. Reproduced with permission from the publisher and authors.*

mosome 15 at 15-q20 (see Chap. 88). Because fibrillin is diffuse, Marfan syndrome affects skeletal, ocular, cardiovascular, skin, pulmonary, and central nervous systems. Many observers have speculated that primary MVP syndrome represents a generalized disorder of connective tissue. Thoracic skeletal abnormalities such as straight thoracic spine and pectus excavatum are commonly associated with this syndrome. The mitral valve undergoes differentiation between the 35th and 42nd days of fetal life, when the vertebrae and thoracic cage are beginning chondrification and ossification.[70] Any adverse factors in this period can affect both the mitral valve and the bones of the thoracic cage. It is postulated that the MVP syndrome is a connective tissue disorder resulting from fetal exposure to toxic substances during the early part of pregnancy.[71,72]

Others suggest that MVP is a result of defective embryogenesis of cell lines of mesenchymal origin. The increased prevalence of primary MVP in patients with von Willebrand disease and other coagulopathies, primary hypomastia, and various connective tissue diseases is used to support this concept.

In other instances of echocardiographic excessive systolic prolapse of one or both mitral leaflets into the LA, myxomatous proliferation of the spongiosa portion of the mitral valve leaflet is absent. Tei and coworkers[73] were able to produce de novo echocardiographic evidence of MVP, often with MR, in closed-chest dogs undergoing transient coronary artery occlusion; MVP was attributed to relative displacement of ischemic papillary muscles. Also, serial studies in patients with known ischemic heart disease occasionally have documented unequivocal MVP following an acute coronary syndrome that was documented to be absent prior to the acute coronary syndrome. In most patients with coronary artery disease (CAD) and MVP, however, the two entities are coincident but unrelated.

Other studies[74,75] indicate that MR caused by MVP may result from postinflammatory changes, including those following rheumatic fever. In histologic studies of surgically excised valves, fibrosis with vascularization and scattered infiltration of round cells, including lymphocytes and plasmacytes, was found *without myxomatous proliferation* of the spongiosa.[74] With rheumatic carditis, the anterior mitral leaflet is more likely to prolapse.[75]

MVP has been observed in patients with hypertrophic cardiomyopathy, in whom posterior MVP may result from a disproportionately small LV cavity, altered papillary muscle alignment, or a combination of factors.[72] Occasionally, the pathologic changes of primary MVP are present. When present, ventricular wall motion abnormalities usually disappear when the mitral valve is repaired or replaced.[76] In MVP patients, atrial septal defects, pulmonary hypertension, anorexia nervosa, dehydration, or straight back syndrome may be secondary to the relatively small size of the LV in this disorder, resulting in a mitral apparatus that is relatively large and redundant.[74] However, atrial septal defect may be associated with primary MVP.[20] Atrial septal aneurysms were considered more likely to occur in MVP patients but a review of patients from the Framingham Study did not demonstrate an increase in the prevalence of atrial septal aneurysms.[77] Patients with primary and secondary MVP must be distinguished from those with normal variations on cardiac auscultation or echocardiography. Other auscultatory findings may be misinterpreted as midsystolic clicks or late-systolic murmurs. Patients with mild to moderate billowing of one or more nonthickened leaflets toward the LA with the leaflet coaptation point on the ventricular side of the mitral annulus and no or minimal MR by Doppler echocardiography are probably normal.

PATHOPHYSIOLOGY

In patients with MVP, there is frequently LA and LV enlargement, depending on the presence and severity of MR. The supporting apparatus is often involved, and in patients with connective tissue syndromes such as Marfan syndrome, the mitral annulus is usually dilated, sometimes calcified, and does not decrease its circumference by the usual 30 percent during LV systole. The hemodynamic effects of mild to moderate MR are similar to those from other causes of MR.

Many studies suggest an increased prevalence of autonomic nervous system dysfunction in patients with primary MVP. In 1979, Gaffney and coworkers[78] reported reduced heart rate slowing with intravenous phenylephrine and an abnormal diving reflex heart rate response in patients with MVP as compared with age-matched controls. Patients with MVP had less lower-extremity pooling of blood in response to lower-body negative pressure. Increased vagal tone and prolonged QT intervals on the ECG are more common in patients with MVP. Measurements of serum and 24-hour urine epinephrine and norepinephrine levels are often increased in patients with symptomatic MVP as compared with controls.[79] Patients with MVP often have an increased heart rate and contractility response to intravenous isoproterenol. An increased incidence of high-affinity β receptors in the lymphocytes of patients with MVP has been reported, as well as greater-than-usual increases in cyclic adenosine monophosphate with isoproterenol stimulation as compared with normal individuals.[80] Patients with MVP often have postural phenomena such as orthostatic tachycardia and hypotension. Low intravascular volume and/or an abnormality in the renin–aldosterone axis may contribute to the orthostatic changes.

[ ] ASSOCIATED CONDITIONS

Tricuspid valve prolapse, with similar interchordal hooding and histologic evidence of mucopolysaccharide proliferation and collagen dissolution, occurs in approximately 40 percent of patients with MVP.[64] Pulmonic valve prolapse occurs in approximately 10 percent, and aortic valve prolapse in 2 percent, of patients with MVP.[64] The frequent findings of thoracic skeletal abnormalities in patients with MVP were noted earlier. There is an increased incidence of secundum atrial septal defect in patients with MVP (but not of atrial septal aneurysms) and an increased incidence of MVP in patients with atrial septal defects. An increased incidence of left-sided atrioventricular bypass tracts and supraventricular tachycardias also occurs in patients with MVP.[81]

[ ] CLINICAL MANIFESTATIONS

Symptoms

The diagnosis of MVP is most commonly made by cardiac auscultation in asymptomatic patients or by echocardiography performed for some other purpose. The patient may be evaluated because of a family history of cardiac disease or, occasionally, may be referred because of an abnormal resting ECG. Some patients consult their physicians because of one or more of the common symptoms that occur in patients with this syndrome. The most common presenting complaint is *palpitation*. The source of palpitation is usually ventricular premature beats, but various supraventricular arrhythmias are also frequent, and the most common sustained tachycardia is paroxysmal reentry supraventricular tachycardia. Ventricular tachycardia occurs in some patients; others have symptomatic bradyarrhythmias. Palpitation is often reported by patients at a time when continuous long-term ECG recordings show no arrhythmias.

Chest pain is a frequent complaint of patients with MVP. In most patients without coexisting ischemic heart disease, it is atypical (occurring at rest or exercise and is sharp, nonradiating, and prolonged in duration) and rarely resembles classic angina pectoris. In some patients it is recurrent and can be incapacitating. The etiology is unknown; rarely, it may represent true myocardial ischemia produced by abnormal tension on the papillary muscles and supporting ventricular wall by the prolapsing mitral leaflets. Coronary artery spasm has been reported in patients with MVP, but it is unlikely to be the cause of most episodes of atypical chest pain as there rarely is ECG ST-segment elevation.[82]

Dyspnea and *fatigue* are frequent symptoms in patients with MVP, including many without severe MR. Objective exercise testing often fails to show impaired exercise tolerance, and some patients exhibit distinct episodes of hyperventilation. Neuropsychiatric complaints occur in certain patients with MVP. Some have panic attacks (see Chap. 95), and others have frank manic-depressive syndromes. Transient cerebral ischemic episodes occur with increased incidence in patients with MVP, and some patients develop stroke syndromes.[83] Amaurosis fugax, homonymous field loss, and retinal artery occlusion have been reported; occasionally,

the visual loss persists.[84–86] These signs likely are a consequence of embolization of platelets and fibrin deposits that occur on the atrial side of the mitral valve leaflets.[87] *It is important to note that both MVP and panic attacks occur relatively frequently. Accordingly, the occurrence of the two syndromes in the same individual would be expected to occur frequently by chance, rather than panic attacks necessarily being part of the primary MVP syndrome.*

Physical Examination

The presence of thoracic skeletal abnormalities may suggest the diagnosis of MVP, the most common being scoliosis, pectus excavatum, straightened thoracic spine, and narrowed anteroposterior diameter of the chest.

The principal cardiac auscultatory feature of this syndrome is the midsystolic click, a high-pitched sound of short duration (see Chap. 12). The click may vary considerably in intensity and location in systole according to LV loading conditions and contractility. It results from the sudden tensing of the mitral valve apparatus as the leaflets prolapse into the LA during systole. Multiple systolic clicks may be generated by different portions of the mitral leaflets prolapsing at varying times during systole.[88] The major differentiating feature of the midsystolic click of MVP from that from other causes (e.g., ventricular septal aneurysms, atrial myxomas, or pericarditis) is that its timing during systole may be altered by maneuvers that change hemodynamic conditions.

The midsystolic click is frequently followed by a late-systolic murmur, usually medium- to high-pitched and most audible at the apex. Occasionally, the murmur has a musical or honking quality. The character and intensity of the murmur also vary with loading conditions, from brief and almost inaudible to holosystolic and loud (Fig. 76–18).

Dynamic auscultation is often useful for establishing the clinical diagnosis of the MVP syndrome (see Chap. 12) (Table 76–5). Changes in the LV end-diastolic volume lead to changes in the timing of the midsystolic click and murmur. When end-diastolic volume is decreased, the critical LV volume is achieved earlier in systole, and the click–murmur complex occurs shortly after the first heart sound (Fig. 76–19). In general, any maneuver that decreases the end-diastolic LV volume, increases the rate of ventricular contraction, or decreases the resistance to LV ejection of blood causes prolapse to occur earlier in systole, the systolic click and murmur moving toward the first heart sound. By contrast, any maneuver that augments the LV systolic volume, reduces myocardial contractility, or increases LV afterload lengthens the time from the onset of systole to the initiation of MVP; the systolic click and/or murmur moving toward S_2. Maneuvers that cause the click and/or murmur to occur earlier in systole include standing from the supine position, submaximal isometric handgrip exercise, the Valsalva maneuver, and amyl nitrite inhalation. Those that cause the click and murmur to move toward S_2 include squatting from the upright position and maneuvers that slow the heart rate.

Electrocardiogram

The ECG typically is normal in patients with MVP. The most common abnormality noted is the presence of ST-T-wave depression or T-wave inversion in the inferior leads (III, aV_F) (Fig. 76–20).

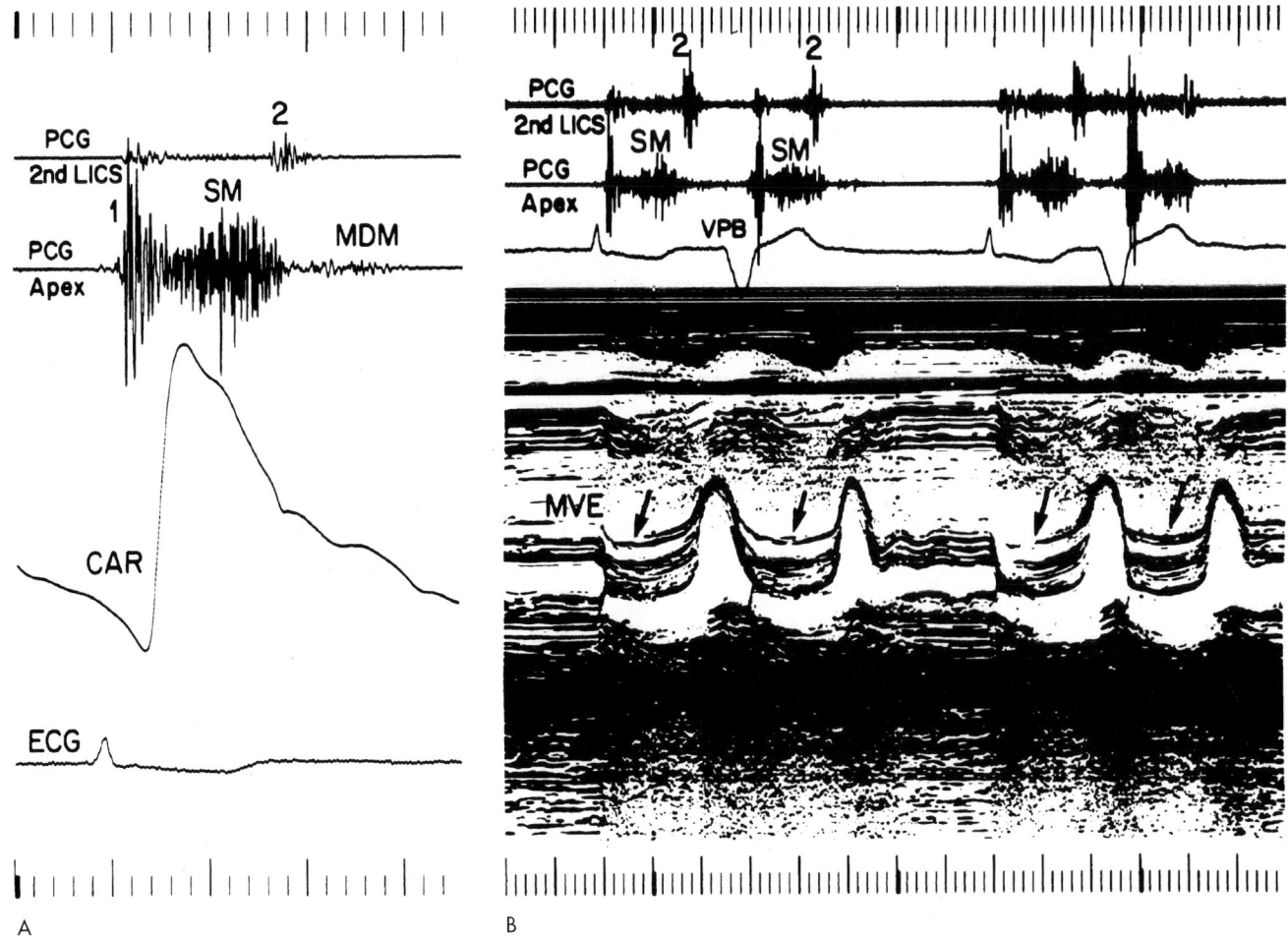

FIGURE 76–18. Phonocardiogram and echocardiogram in mitral valve prolapse. **A.** The phonocardiogram shows a high-frequency holosystolic murmur (HSM) with late-systolic accentuation. A low-frequency middiastolic murmur (MDM) is present at the apex. **B.** The echocardiogram demonstrates a hammock-shaped systolic motion of the valve leaflets. The rhythm is atrial fibrillation with bigeminy. *1*, first heart sound; *2*, second heart sound; *MVE*, mitral valve echogram. *Source: Courtesy of Dr. Ernest Craige.*

These changes may reflect ischemia of the inferior wall as a result of traction on the posteromedial papillary muscle by the prolapsing mitral leaflets. Sometimes ST-T-wave changes are present only during interventions that induce prolapse earlier in systole. More

unusual ECG changes include prominent U waves, peaked T waves in the midprecordial leads, and QT prolongation.

MVP is associated with an increased incidence of false-positive exercise ECG results especially in females. Myocardial perfusion imaging with thallium or technetium sestamibi has been useful for differentiating false from true abnormal exercise ECG findings in patients with MVP (see Chap. 19).

Although arrhythmias may be observed on the resting ECG or during treadmill or bicycle exercise, they are detected more reliably by continuous long-term ECG recordings (see Chap. 41). The reported incidence of documented arrhythmias is higher in patients with MVP, ranging from 40 to 75 percent. Most arrhythmias detected, however, are not life-threatening. Patients with ST-T-wave changes in the inferior ECG leads have a higher incidence of serious ventricular arrhythmias on ambulatory recordings.

Echocardiography

Echocardiography (see Chap. 16) is the most useful noninvasive test for defining MVP. The M-mode echocardiographic definition of MVP includes 2 mm or more of posterior dis-

TABLE 76-5

Response of the Murmur of Mitral Valve Prolapse to Interventions

INTERVENTION	TIMING	INTENSITY
Standing upright	←	↑
Recumbant	→	↓ or 0
Squatting	→	↓ or 0
Hand-grip	←	±
Valsalva	←	±
Amyl nitrite	±	↑

↑ = increase; ↓ = decrease; 0 = no change; ± = variable; ← = earlier; → = later.

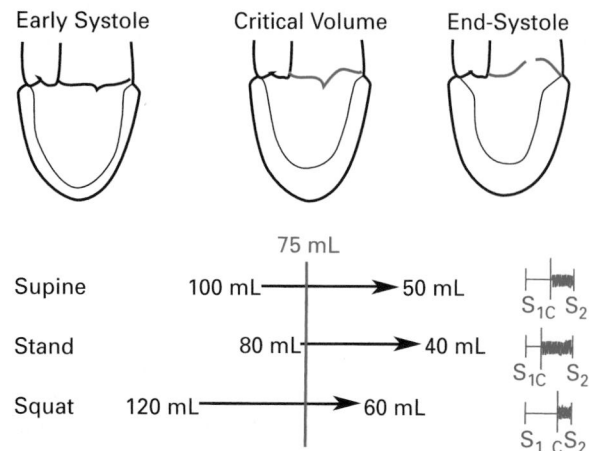

FIGURE 76–19. The effect of LV volume on the timing of MVP and the accompanying murmur. In the upper panel, three phases of LV systole are illustrated. In early systole, there is coaptation of the leaflets and no prolapse; when a critical ventricle volume of 75 mL is reached, valve prolapse commences and progresses until the end of systole. In the lower panel, three body positions are indicated; the corresponding change in volume and timing of the click–murmur are shown. The critical volume for prolapse remains constant. When the critical volume occurs earlier, the onset of the click–murmur is earlier. When the critical volume occurs later, the onset of the click–murmur is later. *Source: From Crawford MH, O'Rourke RA. In: Isselbacher KJ, et al., eds. Harrison's Principles of Internal Medicine, 9th ed. New York: McGraw-Hill, 1980:91–105. Reproduced with permission from the publisher, editors, and authors.*

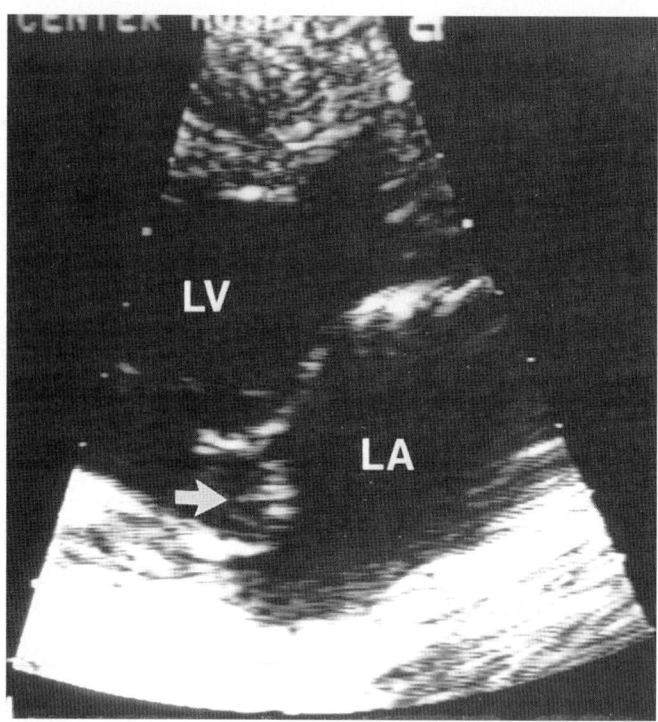

FIGURE 76–20. A parasternal two-dimensional echocardiographic view showing prolapse of a redundant posterior mitral leaflet toward the left atrium during systole. LA, left atrium; LV, left ventricle.

placement of one or both leaflets or holosystolic posterior "hammocking" of more than 3 mm (see Fig. 76–18). On two-dimensional echocardiography, systolic displacement of one or both mitral leaflets, particularly when they coapt on the LA side of the annular plane, in the parasternal long-axis view indicates a high likelihood of MVP (see Fig. 76–20). Disagreement persists concerning the reliability of an echocardiographic diagnosis of MVP when observed only in the apical four-chamber view. The diagnosis of MVP is even more certain when the leaflet thickness is greater than 5 mm during ventricular diastole. Leaflet redundancy is often associated with an enlarged mitral annulus and elongated chordae tendineae. On Doppler velocity recordings, the presence or absence of MR is an important consideration. MVP is more likely when the MR is detected as a high-velocity jet midway or more posterior in the LA.

At present, there is no consensus on the two-dimensional echocardiographic criteria for MVP. Because echocardiography is a tomographic cross-sectional technique, no single view can be considered diagnostic. The parasternal long-axis view permits visualization of the medial aspect of the anterior mitral leaflet and middle scallop of the posterior leaflet. If the findings of prolapse are localized to the lateral scallop in the posterior leaflet, they would be best visualized by the apical four-chamber view.[88–90] All available echocardiographic views should be used, with the provision that anterior leaflet billowing alone in the four-chamber apical view is not diagnostic of prolapse; however, a displacement of the posterior leaflet or the coaptation point in any view, including the apical views, suggests the diagnosis of prolapse. The echocardiographic criteria for MVP should include struc-

tural changes such as leaflet thickening, redundancy, annular dilatation, and chordal elongation.

Patients with echocardiographic criteria for MVP but without evidence of thickened or redundant leaflets or definite MR are more difficult to classify. If such patients have auscultatory findings typical of MVP, the echocardiogram confirms the diagnosis. In contrast, a patient with typical auscultatory findings but a negative echocardiogram likely also has MVP; in the past, as many as 10 percent of patients with MVP have had a nondiagnostic echocardiographic study. Currently, this percentage is less because of more accurate studies. In clinical practice, a false diagnosis of MVP occurs too frequently. The use of echocardiography as a screening test for MVP in patients with and without symptoms who have no systolic click or murmur on serial, carefully performed auscultatory examinations *is not recommended*.[90] The likelihood of finding MVP in such patients is extremely low. Most patients with or without symptoms who have negative dynamic cardiac auscultation and "mild mitral valve prolapse" by echocardiography should not be diagnosed as having MVP. Table 76–6 lists recommendations for echocardiography in MVP.

Echocardiography is useful for defining LA and LV size and function and the extent of mitral leaflet redundancy, as well as for detecting associated lesions such as secundum atrial septal defect. Doppler echocardiography also is helpful for the detection and *semiquantitation* of MR. Serial echocardiograms are often useful for following patients with murmurs, as quantitation of MR by examination alone is more difficult. In a carefully performed study comparing auscultatory findings with echocardiographic results in patients with clinical evidence of MVP, the amount of billowing of

TABLE 76–6

American College of Cardiology/American Heart Association Recommendations for Echocardiography in Mitral Valve Prolapse[a]

INDICATIONS	CLASS
1. Diagnosis, assessment of hemodynamic severity of mitral regurgitation (MR), leaflet morphology, ventricular compensation in patients with physical signs of mitral valve prolapse (MVP).	I
2. To exclude MVP in patients who have been given the diagnosis where there is no clinical evidence to support the diagnosis.	I
3. To exclude MVP in patients with first-degree relatives with known myxomatous valve disease.	IIa
4. Risk stratification in patients with physical signs of MVP with no or mild regurgitation.	IIa
5. To exclude MVP in patients in the absence of physical findings suggestive of MVP and a positive family history.	III
6. Routine repetition of echocardiography in patients with MVP with no MR and no changes in clinical signs or symptoms.	III

[a]See Chap. 11.
SOURCE: Reproduced with permission from ACC/AHA clinical practice guidelines for valvular heart disease. J Am Coll Cardiol 1998;32:1486–1588.

one or both mitral leaflets into the LA, the level of the leaflets' coaptation point, and the presence or absence of moderate or severe MR were each important considerations in deciding on the likelihood of MVP.[76]

Chest Roentgenogram

Posteroanterior and lateral chest radiograph films usually show normal cardiopulmonary findings. The skeletal abnormalities described earlier can be seen.[70] When severe MR is present, both LA and LV enlargement often result. Various degrees of pulmonary venous congestion are evident when failure of the left side of the heart results. Acute chordal rupture with a sudden increase in the amount of MR may present as pulmonary edema without obvious LV or LA dilatation. Calcification of the mitral annulus may be seen, particularly in adults with Marfan syndrome (see Chap. 15).

Myocardial Perfusion Scintigraphy

Exercise myocardial perfusion imaging with thallium or technetium sestamibi has been recommended as an adjunct to exercise ECG for determining the presence or absence of coexistent myocardial ischemia in patients with MVP.[90] Most MVP

patients *with clinical evidence of CAD* have an abnormal exercise scintigram. In comparison, a negative scintigram in these patients neither excludes ischemia as the basis for the chest pain nor does it completely exclude CAD as the etiology (see Chap. 19).

Cardiac Catheterization

Cardiac catheterization is rarely used as a diagnostic technique for MVP. Also, contrast ventriculography is unnecessary for determining LV function because it usually can be quantitated by two-dimensional echocardiogram or radionuclide ventriculography. Although contrast cineventriculography is often useful for assessing the severity of MR, cardiac catheterization and angiography are used more commonly in patients with MVP to exclude CAD. Intracardiac pressures and cardiac output are usually normal in uncomplicated MVP; however, these measurements become progressively more abnormal as MR becomes more severe.

LV cineangiography usually confirms the presence of MVP.[63] The right anterior oblique projection is best for observing prolapse of the three scallops of the posterior leaflet. Prolapse is defined as the bowing of the leaflets beyond a line drawn from the anterior aortic prominence to the base of the heart where the posteromedial papillary muscle attaches in the right anterior oblique view. The left anterior oblique view is necessary for the adequate evaluation of prolapse of the anterior leaflet.

LV wall motion is usually normal in patients with primary MVP, but some patients show abnormal contraction patterns in the absence of CAD.[63] These contraction abnormalities usually represent indentation of the LV at the point of attachment of the papillary muscles; it is attributed to abnormal traction on the papillary muscles and buckling of the ventricular wall. Patients with the most severe prolapse more commonly exhibit misshapen ventricular cavities during systole, and wall motion abnormalities frequently disappear after successful mitral valve replacement or repair.

Electrophysiologic Testing

The indications for electrophysiologic testing in a patient with MVP are the same as other patients (i.e., recurrent unexplained syncope, sudden death survivors, symptomatic complex ventricular ectopy, and the presence of preexcitation syndromes) (see Chap. 42). Upright tilt studies with monitoring of blood pressure and rhythm may be valuable in patients with light-headedness or syncope and in diagnosing autonomic dysfunction (see Chap. 42).

【 】 NATURAL HISTORY, PROGNOSIS, AND COMPLICATIONS

In most patient studies, the MVP syndrome is associated with a benign prognosis.[45,62,91–93] However, some of these results were affected by the maxim "a disease is particularly benign if you use a false positive" (Fig. 76–21). The age-adjusted survival rate for both males and females with MVP is similar to that in patients

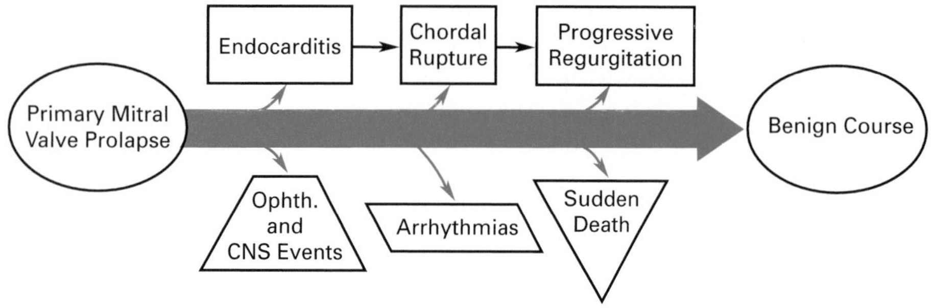

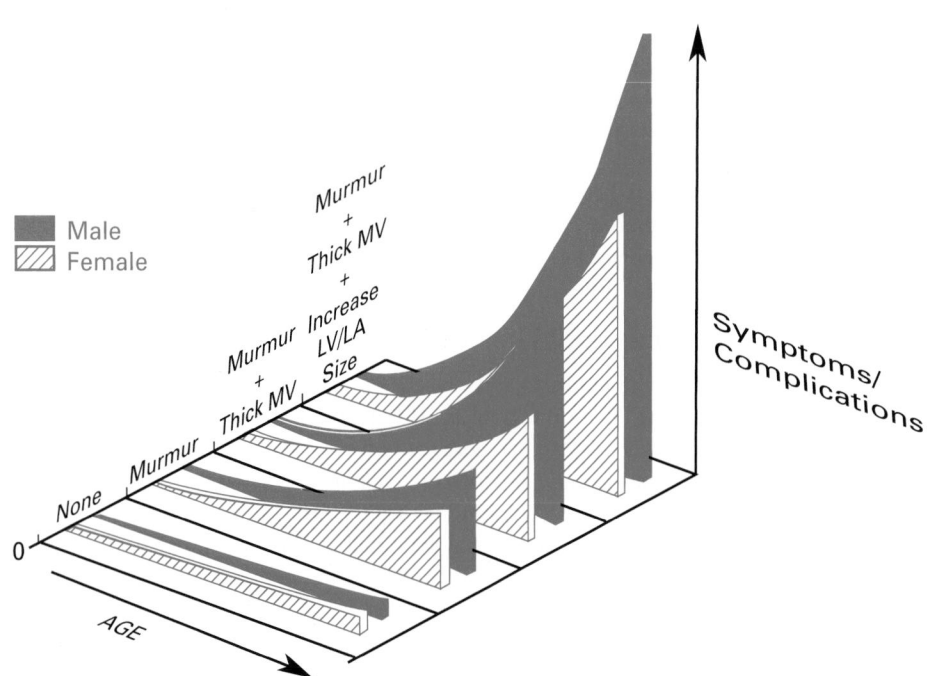

FIGURE 76-21. The course and possible complications of MVP. In most patients, the MVP syndrome is associated with a benign prognosis. CNS, central nervous system; Ophth, ophthalmologic. *Source: From Crawford MH, O'Rourke RA. In: Isselbacher KJ, et al, eds. Harrison's Principles of Internal Medicine, 9th ed. New York: McGraw-Hill, 1980:91–105. Reproduced with permission from the publisher, editors, and authors.*

without this common clinical entity. Gradual progression of MR in patients with mitral prolapse, however, might result in progressive dilatation of the LA and LV. LA dilatation often results in atrial fibrillation, and moderate to severe MR eventually results in LV dysfunction and the development of heart failure. Pulmonary hypertension may occur with associated right ventricular dysfunction. In some patients, after a prolonged asymptomatic interval, the entire process may enter an accelerated phase as a result of LA and LV dysfunction, atrial fibrillation, and in certain instances, ruptured mitral valve chordae. The lat-

ter occurs more commonly in males and with increasing age.[64]

Long-term prognostic studies suggest that complications occur most commonly in patients with a mitral systolic murmur, thickened redundant mitral valve leaflets, or increased LV or LA size[45,88,93] (Figs. 76–21 and 76–22 and Table 76–7).

In a prospective followup study of 237 asymptomatic or minimally symptomatic patients with documented MVP, sudden death occurred in 6 patients.[43] In a multivariant analysis of the echocardiographic findings, the presence or absence of redundant mitral valve leaflets by M-mode echocardiography was the only variable associated with sudden death. Ten patients sustained a cerebral embolic event, 6 of whom were in atrial fibrillation with LA enlargement. These data were confirmed in a retrospective two-dimensional echocardiographic study of 456 patients with MVP.[88] Complications or a history of complications was more prevalent in those with leaflet thickening and redundancy than in those without leaflet thickening. The incidence of stroke, however, was similar in the two groups. Long-term followup studies in patients with MVP associated with a floppy, myxomatous mitral valve permit several conclusions.[64] Serious complications occur in some patients with MVP, predominantly in those with diagnostic auscultatory findings. Also, redundant mitral valve leaflets and increased LV size are associated with a greater frequency of serious complications. Finally, men and people older than 50 years of age are at increased risk of complications, including severe MR requiring surgery.

Sudden death is the least-common complication of MVP (Table 76–8). Although infrequent, the highest incidence of sudden death has been reported in the familial form of MVP. Some of these patients have QT prolongation. Also, patients with MVP who have severe autonomic dysfunction and excessive vagotonia causing bradyarrhythmias and asystole have been reported.[98,99] Because arrhythmias are the usual cause of sudden death, it seems prudent to obtain ambulatory ECG recordings in MVP patients at highest risk. Many believe that patients with ECG ST-T-wave changes are more likely to have complex ventricular arrhythmias.[64] Certainly, patients with symptoms sug-

FIGURE 76-22. The relations between cardiac structure, age, and complications in the MVP syndrome. Patients with MVP, typical auscultatory findings, thickening of the valve leaflets, and LV or LA enlargement are at risk of developing complications. When two or more of these findings are present, the likelihood of complications is highest. By contrast, the absence of these features can be used to identify patients with MVP who have an exceedingly low risk. In general, complications increase with age and are more common in males than in females. *Source: From Boudoulas H, Reynolds JC, Mazzaferri E, Wooley CF. Metabolic studies in mitral valve prolapse syndrome. Circulation 1980;61:1200–1205. Reproduced with permission from the publisher and authors.*

TABLE 76–7

Use of Echocardiography for Risk Stratification in Mitral Valve Prolapse

STUDY	NO. OF PATIENTS	FEATURES EXAMINED	OUTCOME	p
Nishimura et al., 1985[55]	237	MV leaflet ≥5 mm	↑ Sum of sudden death, endocarditis and cerebral embolus	p <0.02
		LVID ≥60 mm	↑ MVR (26 vs. 3.1%)	p <0.001
Zuppiroli et al., 1994[94]	119	MV leaflet >5 mm	↑ Complex ventricular arrhythmia	p <0.001
Babuty et al., 1994[95]	58	Undefined MV thickening	No relation to complex ventricular arrhythmias	NS
Takamoto et al., 1991[96]	142	MV leaflet ≥3 mm redundant, low echo density	↑ Ruptured chordae (48 vs. 5%)	NS
Marks et al., 1989[88]	456	MV leaflet ≥5 mm	↑ Endocarditis (3.5 vs. 0%)	p <0.02
			↑ Moderate-severe MR (11.9 vs. 0%)	p <0.02
			↑ Stroke (7.5 vs. 5.8)	NS
Chandraratna et al., 1984[97]	86	MV leaflets >1.5 mm	↑ Cardiovascular abnormalities (60 vs. 6%) (Marfan syndrome, TVP, MR, dilated descending aorta)	p <0.001

LVID, left ventricular internal diameter; MR, mitral regurgitation; MV, mitral valve; MVR, mitral valve replacement; TVP, tricuspid valve prolapse.
SOURCE: Reproduced with permission from ACC/AHA guidelines for the clinical application of echocardiography. Circulation 1997;95:1686–1744 (updated 2003).

gestive of arrhythmias or who have arrhythmias noted during physical examination or on the resting ECG should be evaluated further.

Infective endocarditis is a serious complication of MVP, and MVP is the leading predisposing diagnosis in most series of patients reported with endocarditis.[64,100] Because the absolute incidence of endocarditis is extremely low for the entire MVP population, there has been much debate concerning the risk of

endocarditis in MVP.[101] Although there is general agreement that MVP patients with murmurs and/or thickened redundant valves confirmed by echocardiography or cineangiography should receive antibiotic prophylaxis, some authorities state that patients with isolated systolic clicks and no murmurs do not need antibiotic prophylaxis for endocarditis.[102] However, the dynamic nature of MVP, with variable physical findings on

TABLE 76–8

Mitral Valve Complications in 102 Hearts with Primary Mitral Valve Prolapse

	NO.	PERCENT
Sudden death	0	0
Primary rupture of chordae	7	7
Bacterial endocarditis	7	7
Mitral valve regurgitation	18	18
Primary rupture of chordae	(7)	—
Bacterial endocarditis	(4)	—
Severe prolapse	(4)	—
Entrapped chordae	(3)	—
Fibrin deposits	4	4

SOURCE: Modified from Lucas RV Jr, Edwards JE. The floppy mitral valve. Curr Probl Cardiol 1982;7:1–48.

TABLE 76–9

Recommendations for Antibiotic Endocarditis Prophylaxis for Patients with Mitral Valve Prolapse Undergoing Procedures Associate with Bacteremia

INDICATION	CLASS
1. Patients with characteristic systolic click–murmur complex	I
2. Patients with isolated systolic click and echo evidence of mitral valve prolapse (MVP), and mitral regurgitation (MR)	I
3. Patients with isolated systolic click, echo evidence of high-risk MVP	IIa
4. Patients with isolated systolic click and no or equivocal evidence of MVP	III

SOURCE: Reproduced with permission from ACC/AHA guidelines for the clinical application of echocardiography. Circulation 1997;95:1686–1744 (updated 2003).

TABLE 76–10

Recommendations for Aspirin and Oral Anticoagulants in Mitral Valve Prolapse

INDICATION	CLASS
1. Aspirin therapy for cerebral transient ischemic attacks (TIAs)	I
2. Warfarin therapy for patients in atrial fibrillation with age ≥65 years, hypertension, mitral regurgitation (MR) murmur, or history of heart failure	I
3. Aspirin therapy for patients in atrial fibrillation <65 years old with no history of MR, hypertension, or heart failure	I
4. Warfarin therapy for poststroke patients	I
5. Warfarin therapy patients for TIAs despite aspirin therapy	IIa
6. Aspirin therapy in poststroke patients with contraindications to anticoagulants	IIa
7. Aspirin therapy for patients in sinus rhythm with echocardiographic evidence of high-risk mitral valve prolapse	IIb

SOURCE: Reproduced with permission from ACC/AHA guidelines for the clinical application of echocardiography. Circulation 1997;95:1686–1744 (updated 2003).

TABLE 76–11

Mitral Stenosis: Results of Mitral Valve Replacement in 33 Patients

	MITRAL STENOSIS	
	PRE-MVR	POST-MVR
LV end-diastolic pressure mmHg	11 ± 5	12 ± 6
Mean PA wedge pressure, mmHg	36 ± 15	28 ± 14[a]
Mean systolic PA pressure, mmHg	54 ± 24	42 ± 22[b]
Cardiac index, L/min/m^2	2.1 ± 1.5	2.3 ± 0.6
LV EDVI, mL/m^2	79 ± 18	72 ± 24
LV ESVI mL/m^2	41 ± 13	39 ± 21
LV ejection fraction	0.48 ± 0.10	0.47 ± 0.14
Mitral regurgitant volume, mL	—	—
Regurgitant volume/end-diastolic volume	—	—
Mitral valve gradient, mmHg	15 ± 7	8 ± 3[a]
Mitral valve area, cm^2	12 ± 0.4	1.8 ± 0.6[a]

EDVI, end-diastolic volume index; ESVI, end-systolic volume index; LV, left ventricular; MVR, mitral valve replacement; PA, pulmonary artery.
[a]p <.001.
[b]p <.01 comparing PA pressure before and after mitral valve replacement.
SOURCE: Crawford MH et al.[76]

different examinations, makes it difficult to make judgments based on the presence or absence of a systolic murmur. With the increasing use of color-flow Doppler echocardiography studies, MR often has been observed in patients in whom no murmur is heard.[103] Table 76–9 lists recommendations for antibiotic endocarditis prophylaxis for patients with MVP undergoing procedures associated with bacteremia.

Progressive MR occurs frequently in patients with longstanding MVP (see Mitral Regurgitation section above). Fibrin emboli are responsible in some patients for visual problems consistent with involvement of the ophthalmic or posterior cerebral circulation. Several studies report an increased likelihood of cerebral vascular accidents of various types in patients younger than age 45 years who have MVP than what would have been expected in a similar population without MVP. Consequently, it is recommended that antiplatelet drugs such as aspirin be administered to patients who have MVP and suspected cerebral nervous system emboli. However, neither antiplatelet drugs nor anticoagulants should be prescribed routinely for patients with MVP because the incidence of embolic phenomena is very low. Table 76–10 lists recommendations for aspirin and oral anticoagulants in MVP.

It is important to avoid the incorrect diagnosis of MVP syndrome. This mistake is especially likely to occur in patients with neuropsychiatric symptoms, in whom an incorrect diagnosis of MVP is made based on the ECG. Such an improper diagnosis can form the foundation of a chronic, often disabling cardiac neurosis. Even if the diagnosis of MVP is properly made, it is not necessarily correct to attribute neuropsychiatric symptoms to the MVP.

【 】 TREATMENT

Most patients with MVP are asymptomatic and lack the high-risk profile described earlier. These patients with mild or no symptoms and findings of milder forms of prolapse should be assured of a benign prognosis. A normal lifestyle and regular exercise are encouraged.[64] For most patients in whom the *diagnosis of MVP is definite,* antibiotic prophylaxis is recommended for the prevention of infective endocarditis while undergoing procedures associated with bacteremia. Patients with MVP and palpitation associated with sinus tachycardia or mild tachyarrhythmias, as well as patients with chest pain, anxiety, or fatigue, often respond to therapy with β blockers.[64,104] However, the cessation of catecholamine stimulants such as caffeine, alcohol, cigarettes, and certain drugs might be sufficient to control symptoms.

Orthostatic symptoms are best treated with volume expansion, preferably by liberalizing fluid and salt intake. Mineralocorticoid therapy might be needed in severe cases, and wearing

TABLE 76-12

Recommendations for Percutaneous Mitral Balloon Valvotomy

INDICATION	CLASS
1. Symptomatic patients (NYHA functional class II, III, or IV), moderate or severe MS (mitral valve area ≤1.5 cm²),ᵃ and valve morphology favorable for percutaneous balloon valvotomy in the absence of left atrial thrombus or moderate to server MR	I
2. Asymptomatic patients with moderate or severe MS (mitral valve area ≤1.5 cm²),ᵃ a and valve morphology favorable for percutaneous balloon valvotomy who have pulmonary hypertension (pulmonary artery systolic pressure >50 mmHg at rest of 60 mmHg with exercise) in the absence of left atrial thrombus or moderate to severe MR	IIa
3. Patients with NYHA functional class III–IV symptoms, moderate or severe MS (mitral valve area ≤1.5 cm²),ᵃ and a nonpliable calcified valve who are at high risk for surgery in the absence of left atrial thrombus or moderate to severe MR	IIa
4. Asymptomatic patients, moderate or severe MS (mitral valve area ≤1.5 cm²) and valve morphology favorable for percutaneous balloon valvotomy who have new onset of atrial fibrillation in the absence of left atrial thrombus or moderate to severe MR	IIb
5. Patients in NYHA functional class III–IV, moderate or severe MS (MVA ≤1.5 cm²),ᵃ and a nonpliable calcified valve who are low-risk candidates for surgery	IIb
6. Patients with mild MS	III

MR, mitral regurgitation; MS, mitral stenosis; MVA, mitral valve area; NYHA, New York Heart Association.
ᵃThe committee recognizes that there may be variability in the measurement of mitral valve area and that the mean transmitral gradient, pulmonary artery wedge pressure, and pulmonary artery pressure at rest of during exercise should also be taken into consideration.
SOURCE: Reproduced with permission from ACC/AHA Guidelines.[108]

support stockings may be beneficial. In sudden-death survivors and those patients with symptomatic complex arrhythmias, specific antiarrhythmic therapy should be guided by monitoring techniques, including electrophysiologic testing when indicated (see Chap. 42).

Daily aspirin therapy in a dose of 80 to 325 mg/d (see Table 76–10) is recommended for MVP patients with documented focal neurologic events. Such patients also should avoid cigarettes and oral contraceptives. Some clinicians use long-term anticoagulant therapy with warfarin in poststroke patients with prolapse, particularly when symptoms occur on aspirin therapy.

Restriction from competitive sports is recommended only when moderate LV enlargement, LV dysfunction, uncontrolled tachyarrhythmias, long QT interval, unexplained syncope, prior sudden-death survival, or aortic root enlargement are present, individually or in combination.

The familial occurrence of MVP should be explained to the patient and is particularly important in those with associated diseases who are at greater risk for complications. Screening relatives can identify high-risk individuals and potentially prevent some complications. There is no contraindication to pregnancy based on the diagnosis of MVP alone.

Patients with severe MR with symptoms and/or impaired LV systolic function require cardiac catheterization studies and evaluation for mitral valve surgery. The thickened, redundant mitral valve often can be repaired rather than replaced, with a low operative mortality and excellent long-term results.[104–106] Followup studies also suggest lower thromboembolic and endocarditis risk than with prosthetic valves.

Asymptomatic low-risk patients with MVP and no significant MR can be evaluated clinically every 2 to 3 years. Echocardiography has been suggested every 5 years in such patients to help determine the natural history and the likelihood of complications. Patients with MVP who have high-risk characteristics, including those with moderate to severe MR, should be followed more frequently, even if no symptoms are present. Avierinos and coworkers[56] reported a widely heterogenous natural history of asymptomatic MVP in community patients depending on the presence of risk factors that were able to separate high- from low-risk groups.

Surgical Considerations

(See also Surgical Treatment under Mitral Regurgitation above.)

Management of the patient with MVP may require valve surgery, particularly in those who develop a flail mitral leaflet as a result of rupture of the chordae tendineae or their marked elongation. Most of these valves can be repaired successfully by surgeons experienced with mitral valve repair, especially when the posterior leaflet valve is predominantly affected (Table 76–11). Symptoms of heart failure, the severity of MR, the presence or absence of atrial fibrillation, LV systolic function, LV end-diastolic and end-systolic volumes, and pulmonary artery pressure (rest and exercise) all influence the decision to recommend mitral valve surgery. Recommendations for surgery in patients with MVP and MR are the same as for those with other forms of nonischemic severe MR and include class II to class IV symptoms, LVEF less than 60 percent, and/or marked increases in LV end-diastolic and end-systolic volumes. If mitral valve repair is likely to be successful, severe MR with mild symptoms or atrial fibrillation is an appropriate reason for surgical referral.

There is considerable controversy as to whether elderly patients with severe mitral regurgitation who are truly asymptomatic should be operated on at a site where surgical expertise and mitral valve repair are favorable. These have been discussed in detail elsewhere.[107–109] Table 76–12 lists recommendations for percutaneous mitral balloon valvotomy.

REFERENCES

1. Roberts WC, Perloff JK. Mitral valve disease. A clinicopathologic survey of the conditions causing the mitral valve to function abnormally. *Ann Intern Med* 1972;77(6):939–975.

2. Olson L, Subramanian R, Ackermann D, et al. Surgical pathology of the mitral valve: a study of 712 cases spanning 21 years. *Mayo Clin Proc* 1987;62:22–34.

3. Bonow RO, Carabello B, Chattegee, K, et al. ACC/AHA guidelines for the management of patients with valvular heart disease. *J Am Coll Cardiol* 2006;48:1–148.

4. Fuster V, Ryden LE, Asinger RW, et al. ACC/AHA guidelines for the management of patients with valvular heart disease. *J Am Coll Cardiol* 2001;38:1231–1265.

5. Tamura K, Fukuda Y, Ishizaki M, et al. Abnormalities in elastic fibers and other connective-tissue components of floppy mitral valve. *Am Heart J* 1995;129:1149–1158.

6. Rabkin E, Aikawa M, Stone JR, et al. Activated interstitial myofibroblasts express catabolic enzymes and mediate matrix remodeling in myxomatous heart valves. *Circulation* 2001;104:2525.

7. Avierinos JF, Gersh BJ, Melton LJ, et al. Natural history of asymptomatic mitral valve prolapse in the community. *Circulation* 2002;106:1355–1360.

8. Nesta F, Leyne M, Yosef C, et al. New locus for autosomal dominant mitral valve prolapse on chromosome 13: clinical insights from genetic studies. *Circulation* 2005;112:2022–2030.

9. Disse S, Abergel E, Berrebi A, et al. Mapping of a first locus for autosomal dominant myxomatous mitral-valve prolapse to chromosome 16p11.2-p12.1. *Am J Hum Genet* 1999;65:1242–1251.

10. Freed LA, Acierno JS, Dai D, et al. A locus for autosomal dominant mitral valve prolapse on chromosome 11p15.4. *Am J Hum Genet* 2003;72:1551–1559.

11. Roberts R. Another chromosomal locus for mitral valve prolapse: close but no cigar. *Circulation* 2005;112:1924–1926.

12. Ng C, Cheng A, Myers L, et al. TGF-β-dependent pathogenesis of mitral valve prolapse in a mouse model of Marfan syndrome. *J Clin Invest* 2004;114:1586–1591.

13. Weyman A, Scherrer-Crosbie M. Marfan syndrome and mitral valve prolapse. *J Clin Invest* 2004;114:1543–1546.

14. Grand-Allen KJ, Griffin BP, Ratliff NB, Cosgrove DM, Vesley I. Glycosaminoglycan profiles of myxomatous mitral leaflets and chordae the severity of mechanical alterations. *J Am Coll Cardiol* 2003;42:271–277.

15. Grande-Allen K, Borowski A, Troughton R, et al. Apparently normal mitral valves in patients with heart failure demonstrate biochemical and structural derangements. *J Am Coll Cardiol* 2005;45:54–61.

16. O'Brien F, Fishbein D. Mitral valve abnormalities in congestive heart failure. *J Am Coll Cardiol* 2005;45:62–63.

17. Barber JE, Kasper FK, Ratliff NB, et al. Mechanical properties of myxomatous mitral valves. *J Thorac Cardiovasc Surg* 2001;122:955–962.

18. Barber JE, Ratliff NB, Cosgrove DM, et al. Myxomatous mitral valve chordae. I. Mechanical properties. *J Heart Valve Dis* 2001;10:320–324.

19. Gillinov AM, Cosgrove DM, Blackstone EH, et al. Durability of mitral valve repair for degenerative disease. *J Thorac Cardiovasc Surg* 1998;116:734–743.

20. David TE, Omran A, Armstrong S, et al. Long-term results of mitral valve repair for myxomatous disease with and without chordal replacement with expanded polytetrafluoroethylene sutures. *J Thorac Cardiovasc Surg* 1998;115:1279–1286.

21. Flameng W, Herijgers P, Bogaerts K. Recurrence of mitral valve regurgitation after mitral valve repair in degenerative valve disease. *Circulation* 2003;107:1609–1611.

22. Glesby MJ, Pyeritz RE. Association of mitral valve prolapse and systemic abnormalities of connective tissue: a phenotypic continuum. *JAMA* 1989;262:523–528.

23. Doukas G, Oc M, Alexiou C, Sosnowski AW, Samani NJ, Spyt TJ. Mitral valve repair for active culture positive infective endocarditis. *Heart* 2006;92:361–363.

24. Zegdi R, Debieche M, Latremouille C, et al. Long-term results of mitral valve repair in active endocarditis. *Circulation* 2005;111:2532–2536.

25. Livesey SA. Mitral valve reconstruction in the presence of infection. *Heart* 2006;92:289–290.

26. Kwan J, Shiota T, Agler DA, et al. Geometric differences of the mitral apparatus between ischemic and dilated cardiomyopathy with significant mitral regurgitation. Real-time three-dimensional echocardiography study. *Circulation* 2003;107:1135–1140.

27. Di Mauro M, Giammarco G, Vitolla G, et al. Impact of no-to-moderate mitral regurgitation on late results after isolated coronary artery bypass grafting in patients with ischemic cardiomyopathy. *Ann Thorac Surg* 2006;81:2128–2134.

28. Lam K, Gillinov M, Blackstone EH, et al. Importance of moderate ischemic mitral regurgitation. *Ann Thorac Surg* 2005;79:462–470.

29. Tallaj J, Wei CC, Hankes GH, et al. Beta-adrenergic receptor blockade attenuates angiotensin II-mediated catecholamine release into the cardiac interstitium in mitral regurgitation. *Circulation* 2003;108:225–230.

30. Connolly H, Crary J, McGoon M, et al. Valvular heart disease associated with fenfluramine-phentermine. *N Engl J Med* 1997;337:581–588.

31. Mehta RH, Supiano MA, Oral H, et al. Relation of systemic sympathetic nervous system activation to echocardiographic left ventricular size and performance and its implication in patients with mitral regurgitation. *Am J Cardiol* 2000;86:1193–1197.

32. Schwammenthal E, Chen C, Benning F, et al. Dynamics of mitral regurgitant flow and orifice area. Physiologic application of the proximal flow convergence method: clinical data and experimental testing. *Circulation* 1994;90:307–322.

33. Yiu SF, Enriquez-Sarano M, Tribouilloy C, et al. Determinants of the degree of functional mitral regurgitation in patients with systolic left ventricular dysfunction. *Circulation* 2000;102:1400–1406.

34. Enriquez-Sarano M, Sinak L, Tajik A, et al. Changes in effective regurgitant orifice throughout systole in patients with mitral valve prolapse: a clinical study using the proximal isovelocity surface area method. *Circulation* 1995;92:2951–2958.

35. Borer J, Bonow R. Contemporary approach to aortic and mitral regurgitation. *Circulation* 2003;108:2432–2438.

36. Gaasch WH, Aurigemma G. Inhibition of the renin–angiotensin system and left ventricular adaptation to mitral regurgitation [editorial]. *J Am Coll Cardiol* 2002;39:1380–1381.

37. Wisenbaugh T, Spann J, Carabello B. Differences in myocardial performance and load between patients with similar amounts of chronic aortic versus chronic mitral regurgitation. *J Am Coll Cardiol* 1984;3:916–923.

38. Grose R, Strain J, Cohen M. Pulmonary arterial V waves in mitral regurgitation: clinical and experimental observations. *Circulation* 1984;69:214–222.

39. Lapu-Bula R, Robert A, Van Craeynest D, et al. Contribution of exercise-induced mitral regurgitation to exercise stroke volume and exercise capacity in patients with left ventricular systolic dysfunction. *Circulation* 2002;106:1342–1344.

40. Carabello BA, Nakano K, Corin W, et al. Left ventricular function in experimental volume overload hypertrophy. *Am J Physiol* 1989;256:H974–H81.

41. Corin WJ, Murakami T, Monrad ES, et al. Left ventricular passive chamber properties in chronic mitral regurgitation. *Circulation* 1991;83:797–807.

42. Starling M, Kirsch M, Montgomery D, Gross M. Impaired left ventricular contractile function in patients with long-term mitral regurgitation and normal ejection fraction. *J Am Coll Cardiol* 1993;22:239–250.

43. Detaint D, Messika-Zeitoun D, Avierinos J-F, et al. B-type natriuretic peptide in organic mitral regurgitation. Determinants an impact on outcome. *Circulation* 2005;111:2391–2397.

44. Grigioni F, Enriquez-Sarano M, Ling L, et al. Sudden death in mitral regurgitation due to flail leaflet. *J Am Coll Cardiol* 1999;34:2078–2085.

45. Nishimura RA, McGood MD, Shub C, et al. Echocardiographically documented mitral-valve prolapse: long-term follow-up of 237 patients. *N Engl J Med* 1985;313:1305–1309.

46. Enriquez-Sarano M, Avierinos J, Messika-Zeitoun D, et al. Quantitative determinant of the outcome of asymptomatic mitral regurgitation. *N Engl J Med* 2005;352:875–883.

47. Bonow RO, Carabello B, de Leon AC Jr, et al. ACC/AHA Clinical Practice Guidelines for Valvular Heart Disease 2006;48:1–148.

48. Sakagoshi N, Nakano S, Taniguchi K, et al. Relation between myocardial beta-adrenergic receptor and left ventricular function in patients with left ventricular volume overload due to chronic mitral regurgitation with and without aortic regurgitation. *Am J Cardiol* 1991;68:81–84.

49. Matsumara T, Ohtaki E, Tanaka K, et al. Echocardiographic prediction of left ventricular dysfunction after mitral valve repair for mitral regurgitation as an indicator to decide the optimal timing of repair. *J Am Coll Cardiol* 2003;42:458–463.

50. Breithardt OA, Stellbrink C, Herbots L, et al. Cardiac resynchronization therapy can reverse abnormal myocardial strain distribution in patients with heart failure and left bundle branch block. *J Am Coll Cardiol* 2003;42:486ñ494.

51. Kanzaki H, Bazaz R, Schwartzman D, et al. A mechanism for immediate reduction in mitral regurgitation after cardiac resynchronization therapy: insights from mechanical activation strain mapping. *J Am Coll Cardiol* 2004;44:1619ñ1625.

52. Feldman T, Wasserman HS, Herrmann HC, et al. Percutaneous mitral valve repair using the edge-to-edge technique. Six-month results of the EVEREST phase I clinical trial. *J Am Coll Cardiol* 2005;46:2134–2140.

53. Handa N, Schaff HV, Morris JJ, et al. Outcome of valve repair and the cox maze procedure for mitral regurgitation and associated atrial fibrillation. *J Thorac Cardiovasc Surg* 1999;118:628–635.

54. Freed LA, Benjamin EJ, Levy D, et al. Mitral valve prolapse in the general population: The benign nature of echocardiographic features in the Framingham Heart Study. *J Am Coll Cardiol* 2002:40(7).

55. Nishimura R, McGoon MD. Perspectives on mitral-valve prolapse. *N Engl J Med* 1999;341:48–58.

56. Avierinos J-F, Gersh BJ, Melton LJ, et al. Natural history of asymptomatic mitral valve prolapse in the community. *Circulation* 2002;106:1355–1361.

57. St. John Sutton M, Weyman AE. Mitral valve prolapse prevalence and complications. *Circulation* 2002;106:1305–1307.

58. Devereux RB, Jones EC, Roman MJ, et al. Prevalence and correlates of mitral valve prolapse in a population-based sample of American Indians: the Strong Heart Study. *Am J Med* 2001;111:679–685.

59. Freed LA, Acierno JS Jr, Dai D, et al. A locus for autosomal dominant mitral valve prolapse on chromosome 11p15.4. *Am J Hum Genet* 2003;72(6):1551–1559.

60. Chou HT, Shi YR, Hsu Y, Tsai FJ. Association between fibrillin-l gene exon 15 and 27 polymorphisms and risk of mitral valve prolapse. *J Heart Valve Dis* 2003;12(4):475–481.

61. Reid JV. Mid-systolic clicks. *S Afr Med J* 1961;35:353–357.

62. Barlow JB, Pocock WA, Marchand P, Denny M. The significance of late systolic murmurs. *Am Heart J* 1963;66:443–452.

63. O'Rourke RA, Crawford MH. The systolic click-murmur syndrome: Clinical recognition and management. *Curr Probl Cardiol* 1976;1(1):1.

64. Lucas RV Jr, Edwards JE. The floppy mitral valve. *Curr Probl Cardiol* 1982;7:1–48.

65. Devereux RB. Recent developments in the diagnosis and management of mitral valve prolapse. *Curr Opin Cardiol* 1995;10:107–116.

66. Savage DD, Garrison RJ, Devereux RB, et al. Mitral valve prolapse in the general population: I. Epidemiologic features: The Framingham Study. *Am Heart J* 1983;106:571–576.

67. Leier CV, Call TD, Fulkerson PK, Wooley CF. The spectrum of cardiac defects in the Ehlers-Danlos syndrome, types I and III. *Ann Intern Med* 1980;92:171–178.

68. Lebwohl MG, Distefano D, Prioleau PG, et al. Pseudoxanthoma elasticum and mitral valve prolapse. *N Engl J Med* 1982;307:228–231.

69. Schwartz T, Gotsman MS. Mitral valve prolapse in osteogenesis imperfecta. *Isr J Med Sci* 1981;17:1087–1088.

70. Bon Tempo CP, Ronan JA Jr. Radiographic appearance of the thorax in systolic click: late systolic murmur syndrome. *Am J Cardiol* 1975;36:27–31.

71. Crawford MH, O'Rourke RA. Mitral valve prolapse syndrome. In: Isselbacher KJ, Adams RD, Braunwald E, et al., eds. *Update I. Harrison's Principles of Internal Medicine*. New York: McGraw-Hill, 1981:91–152.

72. O'Rourke RA. The syndrome of mitral valve prolapse. In: Albert JA, ed. *Valvular Heart Disease*. New York: Lippincott-Raven; 1999:157–182.

73. Tei C, Sakamaki T, Shah PM, et al. Mitral valve prolapse in short-term experimental coronary occlusion: a possible mechanism of ischemic mitral regurgitation. *Circulation* 1983;68:183–189.

74. Tomaru T, Uchida Y, Mohri N. Post-inflammatory mitral and aortic valve prolapse: a clinical and pathological study. *Circulation* 1987;76:68–76.

75. Lembo NJ, Dell'Italia LJ, Crawford MH, et al. Mitral valve prolapse in patients with prior rheumatic fever. *Circulation* 1988;77:830–836.

76. Crawford MH, O'Rourke RA. Mitral valve prolapse: a cardiomyopathic state? *Prog Cardiovasc Dis* 1984;27:133–139.

77. Lax D, Eicher M, Goldberg SJ. Mild dehydration induces echocardiographic signs of mitral valve prolapse in healthy females with prior normal cardiac findings. *Am Heart J* 1992;124:1533–1540.

78. Gaffney FA, Karlsson ES, Campbell W, et al. Autonomic dysfunction in women with mitral valve prolapse. *Circulation* 1979;59:894–899.

79. Boudoulas H, Reynolds JC, Mazzaferri E, Wooley CF. Metabolic studies in mitral valve prolapse syndrome. *Circulation* 1980;61:1200–1205.

80. Anwar A, Kohn SR, Dunn JF, et al. Altered beta-adrenergic receptor function in subjects with symptomatic mitral valve prolapse. *Am J Med Sci* 1991;302:89–97.

81. Santos AD, Puthenpurakal MK, Ahmad H, et al. Orthostatic hypotension: a commonly unrecognized cause of symptoms in mitral valve prolapse. *Am J Med* 1981;71:746–750.

82. Sabom MB, Curry RC Jr, Pepine CJ, et al. Ergonovine testing for coronary artery spasm in patients with angiographic mitral valve prolapse. *Catheter Cardiovasc Diagn* 1978;4:265–274.

83. Barnett HJM, Jones MW, Boughner DR, Kostuck WJ. Cerebral ischemic events associated with prolapsing mitral valve. *Arch Neurol* 1976;33:777–782.

84. Barletta GA, Gagliardi R, Benvenuti L, Fantini F. Cerebral ischemic attacks as a complication of aortic and mitral valve prolapse. *Stroke* 1985;16:219–223.

85. Barnett HJM, Boughner DR, Taylor DW, et al. Further evidence relating mitral valve prolapse to cerebral ischemic event. *N Engl J Med* 1980;302:139–144.

86. Petty GW, Orencia AJ, Khandheria BK, Whisnant JP. A population-based study of stroke in the setting of mitral valve prolapse: risk factors and infarct subtype classification. *Mayo Clin Proc* 1994;69:632–634.

87. Wilson LA, Keeling PW, Malcolm AD, et al. Visual complications of mitral leaflet prolapse. *Br Med J* 1977;2:86–88.

88. Marks AR, Choong CY, Sanfilippo AJ, et al. Identification of high-risk and low-risk subgroups of patients with mitral valve prolapse. *N Engl J Med* 1989;320:1031–1036.

89. Shah PM. Echocardiographic diagnosis of mitral valve prolapse. *J Am Soc Echocardiogr* 1994;7(3 Pt 1):286–293.

90. Bonow RO, Carabello B, De Leon AC Jr, et al. ACC/AHA guidelines for the management of patients with valvular heart disease. *J Am Coll Cardiol* 1998;32:1486–1588.

91. Allen H, Harris A, Leatham A. Significance and prognosis of an isolated late systolic murmur: a 9- to 22-year follow-up. *Br Heart J* 1974;36:525–532.

92. Mills P, Rose J, Hollingsworth J, et al. Long-term prognosis of mitral valve prolapse. *N Engl J Med* 1977;297:13–18.

93. Düren DR, Becker AE, Dunning AJ. Long-term follow-up of idiopathic mitral valve prolapse in 300 patients: A prospective study. *J Am Coll Cardiol* 1988;11:42–47.

94. Zuppiroli A, Mori F, Favilli S, et al. Arrhythmias in mitral valve prolapse: relation to anterior mitral leaflet thickening, clinical variables, and color Doppler echocardiographic parameters. *Am Heart J* 1994;128:919–927.

95. Babuty D, Cosnay P, Breuillac JC, et. al. Ventricular arrhythmia factors in mitral valve prolapse. *Pacing Clin Electrophysiol* 1994;17:1090–1099.

96. Takamoto T, Nitta M, Tsujibayashi T, et al. The prevalence and clinical features of pathologically abnormal mitral valve leaflets (myxomatous mitral valve) in the mitral valve prolapse syndrome: an echocardiographic and pathological comparative study. *J Cardiol Suppl* 1991;25:75–86.

97. Chandraratna PA, Nimalasuriya A, Kawanishi D, et al. Identification of the increased frequency of cardiovascular abnormalities associated with mitral valve prolapse by two-dimensional echocardiography. *Am J Cardiol* 1984;54:1283–1285.

98. Cheitlin MD, Armstrong WF, Aurigemma GP, et al. ACC/AHA guidelines for the clinical application of echocardiography. *Circulation* 2003;108:1146–1162.

99. Cosgrove DM, Stewart WJ. Mitral valvuloplasty. *Curr Probl Cardiol* 1989;14:359–415.

100. Kirklin JW. Mitral valve repair for mitral incompetence. *Mod Concepts Cardiovasc Dis* 1987;56:7–11.

101. Marshall CE, Shappel SD. Sudden death and the ballooning posterior leaflet syndrome: detailed anatomic and histochemical investigation. *Arch Pathol* 1974;98:134–138.

102. Clemens JD, Horwitz RI, Jaffe CC, et al. A controlled evaluation of the risk of bacterial endocarditis in persons with mitral valve prolapse. *N Engl J Med* 1982;307:776–781.

103. Devereux RB, Frary CJ, Kramer-Fox R, et al. Cost-effectiveness of infective endocarditis prophylaxis for mitral valve prolapse with or without a mitral regurgitant murmur. *Am J Cardiol* 1994;74:1024–1029.

104. Galloway AC, Colvin SB, Baumann FG, et al. Current concepts of mitral valve reconstruction for mitral insufficiency. *Circulation* 1988;78:1087–1098.

105. Cheitlin MD. The timing of surgery in mitral and aortic valve disease. *Curr Probl Cardiol* 1987;12:75–149.

106. Cosgrove DM, Stewart WJ. Mitral valvuloplasty. *Curr Probl Cardiol* 1989;14:359–415.

107. Detaint D, Sundt TM, Nkomo VT, et al. Surgical correction of mitral regurgitation in the elderly. *Circulation* 2006;114:265–272.

108. Bonow R, Carabello B, DeLeon A, et al. ACC/AHA guidelines for the management of patients with valvular heart disease. *Circulation* 1998;98:1949–1984.

109. St. John Sutton MG, Gorman RC. Surgery for asymptomatic severe mitral regurgitation in the elderly: early surgery or wait and watch? *Circulation* 2006;258–260.

CHAPTER 77

Mitral Valve Stenosis

Shahbudin H. Rahimtoola

ETIOLOGY

Mitral stenosis (MS), an obstruction to blood flow between the left atrium (LA) and the left ventricle (LV), is caused by abnormal mitral valve function. In virtually all adult patients, the cause of MS is previous rheumatic carditis.[1] Approximately 60 percent of patients with rheumatic mitral valve disease do not give a history of rheumatic fever or chorea, and approximately 50 percent of patients with acute rheumatic carditis do not eventually have clinical valvular heart disease. Other causes of MS are all uncommon or rare.[2] Congenital MS is uncommon. MS, usually rheumatic, in association with atrial septal defect is called *Lutembacher syndrome*. A rare cause of MS is massive mitral valve annular calcification. This process occurs most frequently in elderly patients and produces MS by limiting leaflet motion. When stenosis is present, it is usually mild in degree. Other causes of obstruction to LA outflow include a LA myxoma, massive LA ball thrombus, and cor triatriatum, in which a congenital membrane is present in the LA.

PATHOLOGY

Acute rheumatic carditis is a pancarditis involving the pericardium, myocardium, and endocardium. In temperate climates and developed countries, there is usually a long interval (averaging 10 to 20 years) between an episode of rheumatic carditis and the clinical presentation of symptomatic MS. In tropical and subtropical climates and in less-developed countries, the latent period is often shorter, and MS may occur during childhood or adolescence (see Chap. 74).

The pathologic hallmark of rheumatic carditis is an Aschoff nodule. The most common lesion of acute rheumatic endocarditis is mitral valvulitis. In this condition the mitral valve has vegetations along the line of closure and the chordae tendineae. Mitral regurgitation (MR) may be present during an acute episode of rheumatic carditis.

MS is usually the result of repeated episodes of carditis alternating with healing and is characterized by the deposition of fibrous tissue. MS may result from fusion of the commissures, cusps, or chordae, or a combination of these.[2] Ultimately, the deformed valve is subject to nonspecific fibrosis and calcification. Lesions along the line of closure result in fusion of the commissures and contracture and thickening of the valve leaflets. The chordal lesions manifest as shortening and fusion of these structures. The combination of commissural fusion, valve leaflet contracture, and fusion of the chordae tendineae results in a narrow, funnel-shaped orifice, which restricts the flow of blood from the LA to the LV. The rapidity with which patients become symptomatic may depend on the number and severity of repeated bouts of rheumatic valvulitis. Frequently, the rheumatic episodes are not clinically apparent.

In pure MS, the LV is usually normal, but there may be evidence of previous carditis with deposition of fibrous tissue. The

LA is enlarged and hypertrophied as a consequence of LA hypertension. Mural thrombi are often found in the LA, particularly if atrial fibrillation has been present. Calcification of the mitral valve frequently also involves the mitral annulus.

PATHOPHYSIOLOGY

The pathophysiologic features of MS all result from obstruction of the flow of blood between the LA and the LV. With reduction in the valve area, energy is lost to friction during the transport of blood from the LA to the LV. Accordingly, a pressure gradient is present across the stenotic valve. The relation between valve areas, cardiac output, flow period, and average diastolic gradient between the LA and the LV is defined by the formula of Gorlin and Gorlin (see Chap. 16).

It is readily apparent that maintaining cardiac output when the valve area is small requires a large gradient and thus an elevated LA pressure. Similarly, an increased demand for cardiac output, such as occurs during exercise or pregnancy, results in an increase in gradient and high LA pressures. More subtle is the effect of the length of the diastolic flow period on the relation between cardiac output and gradient. The time available for systole is that part of the cardiac cycle occupied by isovolumic contraction and relaxation or by ejection. As the heart rate increases, the total amount of time spent during systole increases despite a reduction in the systolic time per beat.[3] *Thus, time available for diastole decreases as the heart rate increases.* Because blood can flow through the mitral valve only during diastole, the flow rate is inversely proportional to the duration of the flow period at a constant stroke volume. Of course, a higher flow rate results in a greater loss of energy to friction and requires a larger gradient and higher LA pressures. It is important to remember that the gradient from LA to LV is a function per beat, not per minute. Thus, the gradient is dependent on the stroke volume and the diastolic filling time, as well as the LV diastolic pressure.

The pressure gradient between the LA and the LV, which increases markedly with increased heart rate or cardiac output, is responsible for LA hypertension. The LA gradually enlarges and hypertrophies. Pulmonary venous pressure rises with LA pressure increase and is passively associated with an increase in pulmonary arterial (PA) pressure (Fig. 77–1). In up to 20 percent of patients, the pulmonary vascular resistance is also elevated,[4] which further increases PA pressure. PA hypertension results in *right ventricular* (RV) hypertrophy and RV enlargement. The changes in RV function eventually result in *right atrial* hypertension and enlargement and systemic venous congestion; frequently, tricuspid regurgitation also occurs. In a small percentage of patients, there may be regional or global LV systolic dysfunction, the cause or causes of which are not fully understood.[5–7]

Pulmonary venous hypertension alters lung function in several ways. Distribution of blood flow in the lung is altered, with a relative increase in flow to the upper lobes, and, therefore, in physiologic dead space. Pulmonary compliance generally decreases with increasing pulmonary capillary pressure, increasing the work of breathing, particularly during exercise. Chronic changes in the pulmonary capillaries and pulmonary arteries include fibrosis and thickening. These changes protect the lungs from the transudation

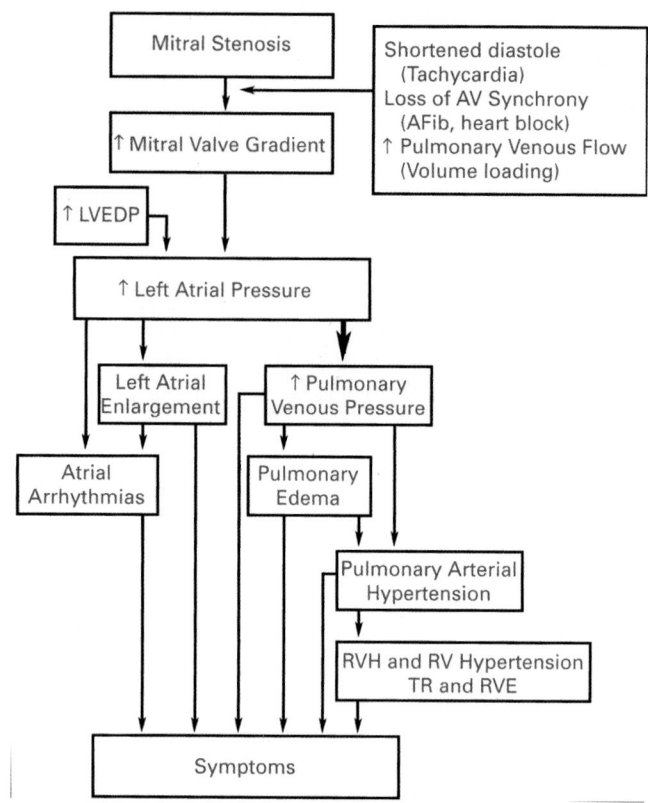

FIGURE 77–1. Pathophysiology of mitral stenosis. Mitral stenosis results in a diastolic pressure gradient from the left atrium (LA) to the left ventricle (LV). The actual gradient is dependent on the mitral valve area and the mitral valve *flow per diastolic second.* As a result, there is an elevation of LA pressure and as well as of pulmonary venous pressure. Physiologic and pathologic changes, such as tachycardia and atrial fibrillation (AFib), shorten diastole and may also result in loss of effective atrial contraction. Pregnancy, volume loading, and left-to-right shunts (at ventricular and aortopulmonary levels), which increase pulmonary venous flow, will increase the mitral valve gradient as well as LA and pulmonary venous pressures. An increased LV diastolic pressure will also result in further increase of LA pressure. An elevated LA pressure has several important effects, including enlargement of the left atrium, atrial arrhythmias, and an increase of pulmonary venous pressure. Pulmonary venous hypertension may result in pulmonary edema and pulmonary arterial (PA) hypertension. PA hypertension and right ventricular (RV) hypertension results in RV hypertrophy (RVH) and may result in tricuspid regurgitation (TR) and RV enlargement (RVE). All of these changes contribute to producing symptoms. In addition, a fixed or even reduced cardiac output will also contribute to the symptomatic state of the patient. LVEDP, left ventricular end-diastolic pressure. *Source: Reprinted with permission from Kawanishi DT, Rahimtoola SH. Mitral stenosis. In: Rahimtoola SH, ed. Valvular Heart Disease II. St. Louis: Mosby, 1996:8.1–8.24.*

of fluid into the alveoli (alveolar pulmonary edema). Indeed, it is not uncommon to find patients with severe MS whose resting PA wedge pressure (indirect LA pressure) exceeds 25 to 30 mmHg. Capillary and alveolar thickening, which help protect against pulmonary edema, further add to the abnormalities of ventilation and perfusion. Pulmonary vascular changes cause an elevated pulmonary vascular resistance.

In some patients with high pulmonary vascular resistance and right ventricle (RV) dysfunction, cardiac output may be low. The body maintains oxygen consumption by extracting more oxygen from the arterial blood, and the mixed venous oxygen content falls. The hemoglobin-O_2 dissociation curve is shifted to the right, facilitating the unloading of oxygen from hemoglobin to the tissues. The reduced cardiac output may result in a *surprisingly small gradient* across the mitral valve despite severe stenosis. Although pulmonary congestion may be less striking in these patients, the cardiac output does not increase normally with exercise, and, typically, the patients are severely limited by fatigue.

Long-standing MS with severe PA hypertension and resultant RV dysfunction may be accompanied by chronic systemic venous hypertension. Tricuspid regurgitation is frequently present, even in the absence of intrinsic disease of this valve. Functional pulmonic regurgitation may also be present. Dependent edema formation and visceral congestion directly reflect elevated systemic venous pressure and salt and water retention. Chronic passive congestion in the liver leads to central lobular necrosis and eventually to cardiac cirrhosis.

CLINICAL FINDINGS

【 】 HISTORY

An asymptomatic interval is usually present between the initiating event of acute rheumatic fever and the presentation of symptomatic MS (averaging 10 to 20 years).[4,8] During this interval, the patient feels well (Table 77–1). Initially, there is little or no gradient at rest, but with increased cardiac output, LA pressure rises and exertional dyspnea develops. As mitral valve obstruction increases, dyspnea occurs at lower work levels. The progression of disability is so subtle and so protracted that patients may adapt by circumscribing their lifestyles.

As obstruction progresses, the patients note orthopnea and paroxysmal nocturnal dyspnea that apparently results from redistribution of blood to the thorax on assuming the supine position. With severe MS and elevated pulmonary vascular resistance, fatigue rather than dyspnea may be the predominant symptom. Dependent edema, nausea, anorexia, and right-upper-quadrant pain reflect systemic venous congestion resulting from elevated systemic venous pressure and salt and water retention.

Palpitations are a frequent complaint in patients with MS and may represent frequent premature atrial contractions or paroxysmal atrial fibrillation and flutter. Of patients with severe symptomatic MS, 50 percent or more have chronic atrial fibrillation. Paroxysmal atrial fibrillation may produce pulmonary edema in some patients with MS. The acute increase in LA pressure that produces pulmonary edema results both from a decrease in the diastolic flow period caused by increased heart rate and from a loss of atrial transport function.

Systemic embolism, a frequent complication of MS, may result in stroke, occlusion of extremity arterial supply, occlusion of the aortic bifurcation, and visceral or myocardial infarction. Atrial fibrillation, increasing age of the patient, increasing LA size, and a previous history of embolism are associated with an increased incidence of systemic embolism (Table 77–2).[4]

Hemoptysis may result from a variety of causes. It is usually a result of increased pulmonary venous pressure. Sputum may be bloodstained with paroxysmal nocturnal dyspnea, pink frothy sputum may result from rupture of alveolar capillaries associated with acute pulmonary edema or from pulmonary infarction caused by pulmonary embolism, or hemoptysis may be severe and profuse (pulmonary apoplexy). The latter results from rupture of thin-walled, dilated bronchial veins, and although usually not fatal, it may be life-threatening because of aspiration pneumonia or massive hemorrhage. The edematous bronchial mucosa is more likely to be associated with chronic bronchitis, especially in cold and wet climates; it can also result in bloodstained sputum. Exertional chest pain, typical of angina pectoris, may be present in some patients with severe MS even if the coronary arteries are normal. Severe PA hypertension has been postulated as a cause. Infective endocarditis is an uncommon complication of pure MS.

Progression of symptoms in MS is generally slow but relentless. Thus, a sudden change in symptoms rarely reflects a change in valve obstruction. Rather, there is usually a noncardiac precipitating event or paroxysmal atrial fibrillation. Fever, pregnancy, hyperthyroidism, and noncardiac surgery, all of which increase cardiac output, can precipitate decompensation in patients with moderate to severe MS.

【 】 PHYSICAL FINDINGS

During the latent, presymptomatic interval, incidental physical findings may be normal or may provide evidence of mild MS. Frequently, the only characteristic finding noted at rest will be a loud

TABLE 77–1

Symptoms Associated with Mitral Stenosis

On exertion
  Dyspnea, wheezing, cough
  Fatigue
  Diminished activity/or pace of activity
  Palpitations
  Feeling faint, presyncope, syncope
At rest
  Cough, wheezing
  Paroxysmal nocturnal dyspnea
  Orthopnea
  Hemoptysis
  Hoarseness (Ortner syndrome)
From complications of mitral stenosis (see Table 77–2)

SOURCE: Copyright S.H. Rahimtoola.

TABLE 77–2

Complications of Mitral Stenosis

Arrhythmias
  Atrial flutter/fibrillation
Embolism
  Systemic—cerebral, coronary, abnormal, peripheral, pulmonary
Acute pulmonary edema
Pulmonary arterial hypertension
Right ventricular hypertrophy/dilatation
Tricuspid regurgitation
Clinical heart failure
Left ventricular dysfunction
Chest pain/angina
Infective endocarditis

SOURCE: Copyright by S.H. Rahimtoola.

S_1 and a presystolic murmur. A short diastolic decrescendo rumble may be heard only with exercise. In patients with symptomatic stenosis, the findings are more obvious, and careful physical examination usually leads to the correct diagnosis (see Chap. 11).

The general appearance of the patient in MS is usually normal. The MS facies, characterized by malar flush (pinkish-purple patches on the cheeks),[4] is uncommon and is caused by peripheral cyanosis, which is usually associated with a low cardiac output, systemic vasoconstriction, and severe PA hypertension. Tachypnea may be present if LA pressure is high. The arterial pulse is normal except for irregularity in atrial fibrillation and is of low volume when cardiac output is reduced. All peripheral pulses should be carefully examined because of the frequency of systemic embolism. The jugular venous pressure may be normal or may show evidence of elevated right atrial pressure. A prominent *a* wave is a result of RV hypertension and hypertrophy or of associated tricuspid stenosis. A prominent *v* wave is caused by tricuspid regurgitation. Atrial fibrillation produces an irregular venous pulse with absent *a* waves. The chest findings may be normal or may reveal signs of pulmonary congestion with rales or pleural fluid (dullness and absent breath sounds). Marked LA enlargement may produce egophony at the tip of the left scapula.

The precordium is usually unremarkable on inspection. On palpation, the apical impulse should be normal tapping (palpable mitral valve closure or RV forming the cardiac apex). An abnormal LV impulse suggests disease other than isolated MS. A diastolic thrill is usually felt only when the patient is examined in the left lateral position. When PA hypertension is present, a sustained RV lift along the left sternal border and pulmonic valve closure may be palpable.

On auscultation in the supine position, the only abnormality appreciated may be the accentuated S_1, which is caused by flexible valve leaflets and the wide closing excursion of the valve leaflets (see Chap. 11).[9] Failure to examine the patient in the left lateral position accounts for most of the missed diagnoses of symptomatic MS. The diastolic rumble is heard best with the bell of the stethoscope applied at the apical impulse. Nevertheless, the murmur may be localized, and the region around the apical impulse also should be auscultated. The *opening snap* (OS) occurs when the movement of the domed mitral valve into the LV is suddenly stopped.[9] It is heard best with the diaphragm and is often most easily appreciated midway between the apex and the left sternal border. In this intermediate region, the S_1, the pulmonary component of the second heart sound (P_2), and the OS can be identified. Figs. 77–2 and 77–3 illustrate the auscultatory signs of MS in sinus rhythm and in atrial fibrillation.

The OS occurs after the LV pressure falls below LA pressure in early diastole. When LA pressure is high, as in severe MS, the snap occurs earlier in diastole (see Fig. 77–2). The converse is true with mild MS. The interval between A_2 and the OS varies from 40 to 120 milliseconds. Although the OS is present in most cases of MS, it is absent in patients with stiff, fibrotic, or calcified leaflets. Thus, absence of the OS in severe MS suggests that mitral valve replacement rather than commissurotomy may be necessary.

The low-pitched diastolic rumble follows the OS and is best heard with the bell of the stethoscope. In some patients with low cardiac output or mild MS, brief exercise, such as sit-ups or walking, is adequate to increase flow and bring out the murmur. The murmur is low-pitched, rumbling, and decrescendo. In general, the more severe the MS, the longer the murmur (see Fig. 77–2).

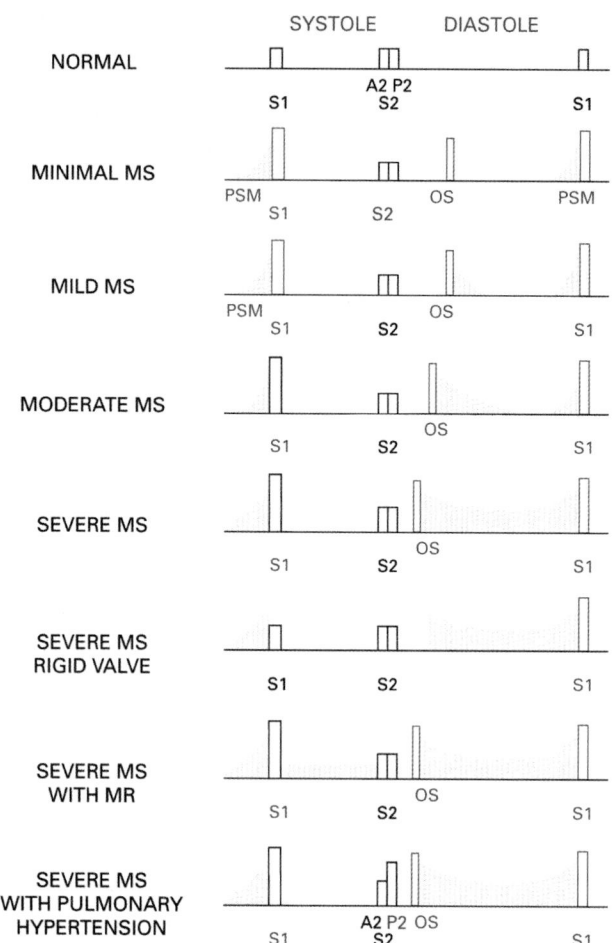

FIGURE 77-2. Auscultatory signs of mitral stenosis (MS) in patients with sinus rhythm are illustrated. These include a presystolic murmur, loud first heart sound (S_1), an opening snap (OS), and a middiastolic murmur (low-pitched, decrescendo diastolic rumble, and rumbling murmur). These signs may be accentuated or at times may be heard only by placing the patient in the left lateral decubitus position. Importantly, these signs are helpful in assessing the severity of the MS; as the MS becomes more severe, the S_2-OS interval is shortened and the length of the middiastolic rumble is increased. In mild OS, the S_2-OS interval is long and the diastolic murmur is short. In moderate MS, the S_2-OS interval is shorter, and although the diastolic murmur is longer at rest, there is usually a gap between the end of the murmur and the onset of the presystolic murmur. In severe MS, the S_2-OS interval is short (usually 0.04 to 0.06 seconds) and the diastolic murmur is a full-length murmur. With PA hypertension, P_2 is increased in intensity. In the presence of a rigid mitral valve (with or without calcification), S_2 is soft, and the OS is usually not heard. A holosystolic murmur of mitral regurgitation may be present. *Source: Adapted and modified from Kawanishi DT, Rahimtoola SH. Mitral stenosis. In: Rahimtoola SH, ed. Valvular Heart Disease II. St. Louis: Mosby, 1996:8.1–8.24. Copyright by S.H. Rahimtoola.*

Presystolic accentuation of the murmur occurs in sinus rhythm and has been reported even in atrial fibrillation. In the latter situation, a brief "presystolic" accentuation is caused by the narrowing of the mitral orifice produced by ventricular systole before the final, complete closure of the mitral valve and the mitral component of S_1. A diastolic rumble is not diagnostic of MS and may be heard with increased flow across a normal mitral valve—for example, in ventricular septal defect with a large left-to-right shunt.

The two most important auscultatory signs of severe MS are a short A_2-OS interval (usually 40 to 60 msec) and a full-length diastolic rumble. The A_2-OS interval may be longer if there is associ-

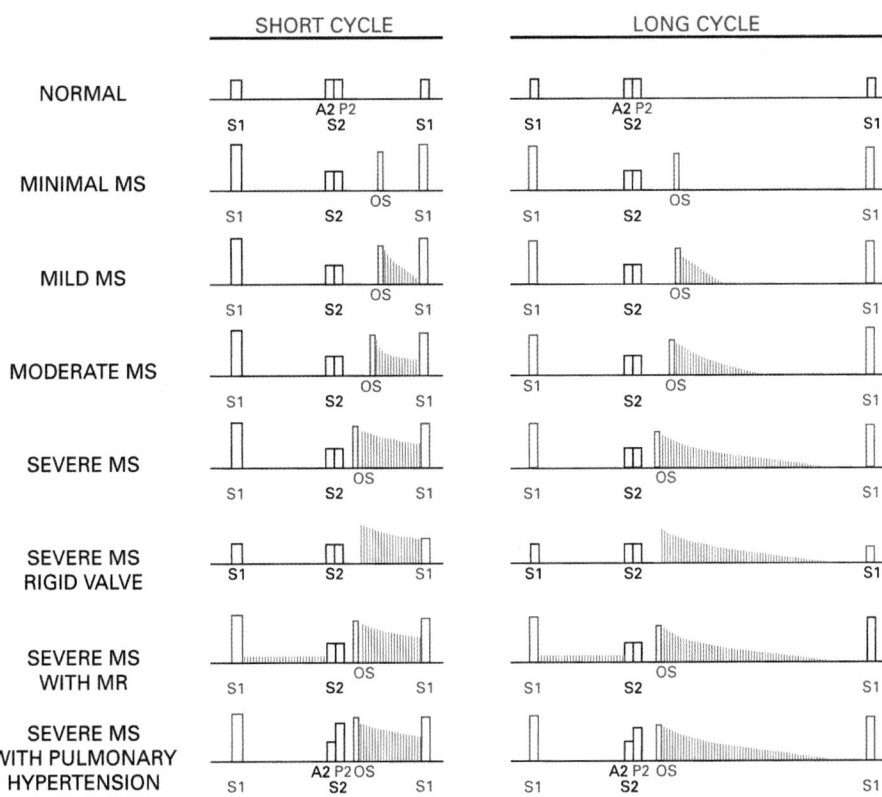

FIGURE 77–3. Auscultatory signs of mitral stenosis (MS) in atrial fibrillation are illustrated. The presystolic murmur is absent. The loud S₁ and the opening snap (OS) are still heard. In the short cycles, the duration of diastole is short and the middiastolic rumble occupies the whole of diastole (*left panel*). In the long cycles (*right panel*), the length of middiastolic murmur is related to the severity of MS. As the MS becomes more severe, the length of this murmur is increased. In atrial fibrillation, with a slow ventricular response and very long R-R intervals, the middiastolic rumble may not occupy the whole diastolic period and the presystolic murmur is usually absent. Thus, one may get the impression that the MS is moderate rather than severe. Increasing the heart rate—for example, with brief physical exertion—may produce more characteristic auscultatory findings. Alternatively, when the ventricular rate in atrial fibrillation is rapid or in short cycles, the auscultatory findings may suggest a more severe degree of MS than is really the case (*left panel*). *Source: Adapted and modified from Kawanishi DT, Rahimtoola SH. Mitral stenosis. In: Rahimtoola SH, ed. Valvular Heart Disease. II. St. Louis: Mosby, 1996:8.1–8.24. Copyright 1996 by S.H. Rahimtoola.*

ated moderate to severe aortic regurgitation (AR), and the OS may be absent when the mitral valve is rigid. The diastolic murmur may not be full-length in severe MS if the stroke volume is low and there is no tachycardia.

Systolic murmurs also may be heard in association with the murmur of MS. A blowing, holosystolic murmur at the apex suggests associated MR; whereas a systolic blowing murmur heard best at the lower left sternal border that increases with inspiration usually signifies tricuspid regurgitation. The Graham Steell murmur is a high-pitched diastolic decrescendo murmur of pulmonic regurgitation caused by severe PA hypertension. In most patients with MS, such a murmur usually indicates AR instead. In general, a left-sided S₃ is incompatible with severe MS, with the possible exception of concomitant severe AR and/or significant LV systolic dysfunction. If an S₃ and a rumble are present, MR is usually the predominant lesion (see Chap. 12).

❬ ❭ ROENTGENOGRAM

The posteroanterior and lateral chest films are often so typical that experienced clinicians can make the tentative diagnosis from them. The thoracic cage is normal. The lung fields show evidence of elevated pulmonary venous pressure. Blood flow is more evenly redistributed to the upper lobes, resulting in apparent prominence of upper-lobe vascularity. Increased pulmonary venous pressure results in transudation of fluid into the interstitium. Accumulation of fluid in the interlobular septa produces linear streaks in the bases, which extend to the pleura (Kerley B lines).[10] Interstitial fluid may also be seen as perivascular or peribronchial cuffing (Kerley A lines). With transudation of fluid into the alveolar spaces, alveolar pulmonary edema is seen. These changes are not specific for MS but represent long-standing elevated LA pressure. Chronic hemosiderin deposition can result in an interstitial radiodensity that does not resolve after the relief of stenosis. PA hypertension results in enlargement of the main pulmonary artery and right and left main pulmonary arteries.

The cardiac silhouette usually does not show generalized cardiomegaly, but the LA is invariably enlarged. This is manifest in the posteroanterior chest film by a density behind the right atrial border (double atrial shadow), prominence of the LA appendage on the left side of the heart border between the main pulmonary artery and LV apex, and elevation of the left main bronchus. The lateral film shows the LA bulging posteriorly. The LV silhouette is normal. The RV may be enlarged if PA hypertension has been present. RV enlargement is usually noted by filling of the retrosternal space, but this is an unreliable sign in adults. The combination of a normal-sized LV, enlarged LA, and pulmonary venous congestion should immediately raise the possibility of MS. Mitral valve calcification is occasionally seen on the plain chest film (see Chap. 15).

❬ ❭ ELECTROCARDIOGRAM

The *electrocardiogram* (ECG) is not usually as helpful as the chest radiograph. Patients in sinus rhythm may have a widened P wave caused by interatrial conduction delay and/or prolonged LA depolarization. Classically, the P wave is broad and notched in lead II and biphasic in lead V₁; it measures 0.12 seconds or more. Atrial fibrillation is common. LV hypertrophy is almost never present unless there are associated lesions. RV hypertrophy may be present if PA hypertension is marked (see Chap. 12).

❬ ❭ CLINICAL INDICATIONS OF SEVERE MITRAL STENOSIS

Some clinical features make it virtually certain that MS is severe. These clinical features include (1) moderate to severe PA hypertension as indicated by clinical and ECG evidence of RV hypertrophy or PA hypertension or both, and/or (2) moderate to severe elevation of LA pressure as indicated by orthopnea, a short P_2-OS interval, a diastolic rumble that occupies the whole length of a long diastolic interval in patients with atrial fibrillation, and pulmonary edema on the chest radiograph. In both these clinical circumstances, one must be certain that there is no other cause for elevated LA pressure and that LA hypertension is not caused mainly by a correctable transient elevation of LV diastolic pressure.

LABORATORY TESTS

【 】 ECHOCARDIOGRAPHY/DOPPLER ULTRASOUND

Echocardiography/Doppler ultrasound is both sensitive and specific for MS when adequate studies are done (see Chap. 16).[11,12] False-positive and false-negative results are uncommon. Doppler studies provide an estimate of mitral valve area (MVA) that is within ± 0.4 cm^2 (prior to interventional therapy) of that obtained by cardiac catheterization.[13] The echographic findings of MS reflect the loss of normal valve function (see Chap. 16).

Echocardiography is of great value in patients with equivocal signs and in patients with gross PA hypertension to differentiate MS from an Austin Flint murmur of AR, and in the rare patient with "silent" MS. When transthoracic echocardiography is unsatisfactory, transesophageal echocardiography is a useful technique to assess LA thrombus, the anatomy of the mitral valve and subvalvular apparatus, and to assess the suitability of the patient for catheter balloon commissurotomy (CBC) or surgical valve repair.

Echocardiography/Doppler ultrasound is a most useful test in MS and should be performed in all patients. It is essential to determine suitability of the valve for commissurotomy and/or repair and to determine the likely result. Table 77–3 lists the essential information that should obtained.[14] Noninvasive assessment of MVA, when compared to that obtained by the Gorlin formula,

TABLE 77–3

Assessment of Patient with Mitral Stenosis

Clinical[a]
  History
  Physical examination:
    Loud S$_1$
    A2–OS interval, length of MDM
    Loud P2, RVH
Chest radiograph
  Pulmonary edema (congestive, interstitial, alveolar)
  Enlargement of LA and other cardiac chambers
ECG
  Rhythm
  LA enlargement
  RV and LV "hypertrophy"
Echocardiogram/Doppler (blood pressure at time of study must be recorded)
M-mode
  LV and LA dimensions absolute and corrected for BSA
Two-dimensional/Doppler
  MVA (Doppler half-time, planimetry)
  Mitral valve morphology
    Score
    Ca^{2+} in one or both commissures
  LA thrombus
  MR severity
  PA pressure
  Mean MVG
  LV volumes, measured LV ejection fraction
  Other valve lesions
Transesophageal echocardiography, if necessary

Treadmill test
  Assessment of exercise capacity, if necessary
Cardiac catheterization/angiography
  MVA
  Mean PA wedge/LA pressure
  PA pressures: systolic, diastolic, mean
  Mean MVG
  Cardiac output/cardiac index
  Pulmonary and systemic vascular resistances
  MR severity
  LV volumes and EF
  Right-heart pressures
  Other valve lesions
Coronary arteriography
  Patients ages ≥35 years
  Patients ages <35 years
  LV dysfunction
  Symptoms or signs suggestive of CAD
  One or more risk factors for premature CAD (excluding gender)

BSA, body surface area; CAD, coronary artery disease; EF, ejection fraction; LA, left atrial; LV, left ventricular; MDM, middiastolic murmur; MR, mitral regurgitation; MVA, mitral valve area; MVG, mitral valve gradient; OS, opening snap; PA, pulmonary atrial; RVH, right ventricular hypertrophy.
[a]The important tests are bold.

SOURCE: From Rahimtoola SH, Durairaj A, Mehra A, Nuno I. Current evaluation and management of patients with mitral stenosis. Circulation 2002;106:1183–1188.

was better by real-time three-dimensional echocardiography than by any other echocardiography/Doppler methods.[15]

[ ] CARDIAC CATHETERIZATION/ ANGIOGRAPHY

In most patients with disabling symptoms from presumed MS, right and left side of the heart catheterization should be performed as part of a preoperative assessment. Simultaneous measurement of cardiac output and the gradient between the LA and the LV and calculation of valve area remain the "gold standard" for assessing the severity of MS (see Chap. 16). LV angiography assesses the competence of the mitral valve, an important determinant of operability for mitral commissurotomy. Quantification of LV function provides a useful prognostic indicator of operative and late survival and of the expected functional result. Aortic valve function should be evaluated in all patients. Selective supraventricular aortography should be performed in all patients unless there is a contraindication. Tricuspid valve function can be assessed when there is a question of coexisting lesions. In certain circumstances, for example, in a patient with suspected severe MS who has a small gradient and mildly elevated LA pressure, dynamic exercise in the catheterization laboratory with measurement of mitral valve gradient, cardiac output, LA, and PA pressures can be extremely useful. Another example is a patient with significant symptoms in whom the findings at rest suggest moderate (or even mild) MS. Selective coronary arteriography establishes the site, severity, and extent of coronary artery disease and should be performed in patients with angina, in those with LV dysfunction, in those with risk factors for coronary artery disease, and in those 35 years of age or older who are being considered for interventional therapy. Table 77–3 lists the essential information that should be obtained.[14]

[ ] OTHER INVESTIGATIONS

In most clinical situations, other investigations are not needed. Occasionally, a treadmill exercise test to evaluate functional capacity may be very useful clinically, for example, when a patient denies symptoms in spite of severe hemodynamic abnormalities.

CLINICAL DECISION MAKING

In a prospective, blinded study of consecutive patients with valvular heart disease, the sensitivity and specificity of diagnosis of MS by clinical evaluation was 86 and 87 percent, respectively. The accuracy of diagnosis of MS for moderate to severe stenosis was 92 percent by clinical evaluation and 97 percent by echocardiography/Doppler ultrasound.[16] This emphasizes the importance of a thorough clinical evaluation. The principal difficulty with both clinical evaluation and echocardiography/Doppler ultrasound is being able to accurately separate in all instances mild from moderate MS and moderate from severe MS (see also Aortic Stenosis section in Chap. 75).

NATURAL HISTORY AND PROGNOSIS

The population presenting with MS is changing because of the sharp decline in the incidence of acute rheumatic fever in the past

40 years (see Chap. 74). Native-born American citizens with symptomatic MS are presenting at an older age. Young adults in the third and fourth decades with symptomatic MS are more likely to come from low socioeconomic backgrounds and from the inner city or to be immigrants, particularly from the Middle East, Latin America, Africa, and Asia. Therefore, the latent period between acute rheumatic fever and symptomatic MS is variable and appears to be related to the presence of repeated streptococcal infection. Women with MS outnumber men by almost two to one. The most important feature of the asymptomatic interval is the susceptibility to repeated bouts of both rheumatic valvulitis and streptococcal infection. The mechanism for the progression from no symptoms to mild to severe symptoms is progressive stenosis of the mitral valve.

With the onset of exertional dyspnea and fatigue, the valve area is usually reduced to one-half to one-third its normal size. Further small reductions in valve area markedly obstruct flow and result in symptoms with minimal exertion. The interval from initial mild symptoms to disabling symptoms may be 10 years. During this time, the patient is at some risk of death (see below). Permanent injury may result from atrial fibrillation with rapid ventricular rate, resulting in pulmonary edema, and from systemic embolus. Unfortunately, it is not possible to predict who is at risk of embolism. When late New York Heart Association (NYHA) functional class II or functional class III symptoms are present, the valve area is usually 1.0 cm^2 or less (in an occasional patient the valve area is 1.2 or 1.3 cm^2), and both rest and exercise hemodynamics are deranged. Further small reductions in valve area result in symptoms at rest (see Chap. 12).

The 10-year survival of patients with MS who are asymptomatic is approximately 84 percent and that of those who are mildly symptomatic is 34 to 42 percent.[17–19] The 10-year survival of patients who are moderately or severely symptomatic and who do not have therapy is 40 percent or less, and the survival at 20 years is less than 10 percent.[17–19] Patients in NYHA functional class IV have a very poor survival without treatment:[17] 42 percent at 1 year and 10 percent or less at 5 years. All are dead by 10 years.

MANAGEMENT

MS can be prevented through two approaches primary and secondary (Table 77–4). Although the incidence of infective endocarditis is low in isolated MS, all patients exposed to bacteremia should receive appropriate prophylaxis against infective endocarditis (see Chap. 85). Family and vocational planning should be considered. Women with this disease should consider bearing children before symptoms occur, since pregnancy is usually well tolerated with mild MS. Occupations that require strenuous exertion in middle age and later should probably be avoided if possible. In patients with moderate or severe MS, activities such as strenuous exercise and competitive sports should be restricted.[9]

When patients reach the symptomatic threshold, medical treatment may be of benefit (see Table 77–4). Medical therapy is directed to (1) prevention or control of arrhythmia, the most common of which is atrial fibrillation, (2) anticoagulation, and (3) treatment of elevated pulmonary venous pressure, LV systolic dysfunction, and heart failure. Followup times are shown in the following algorithms[14]:

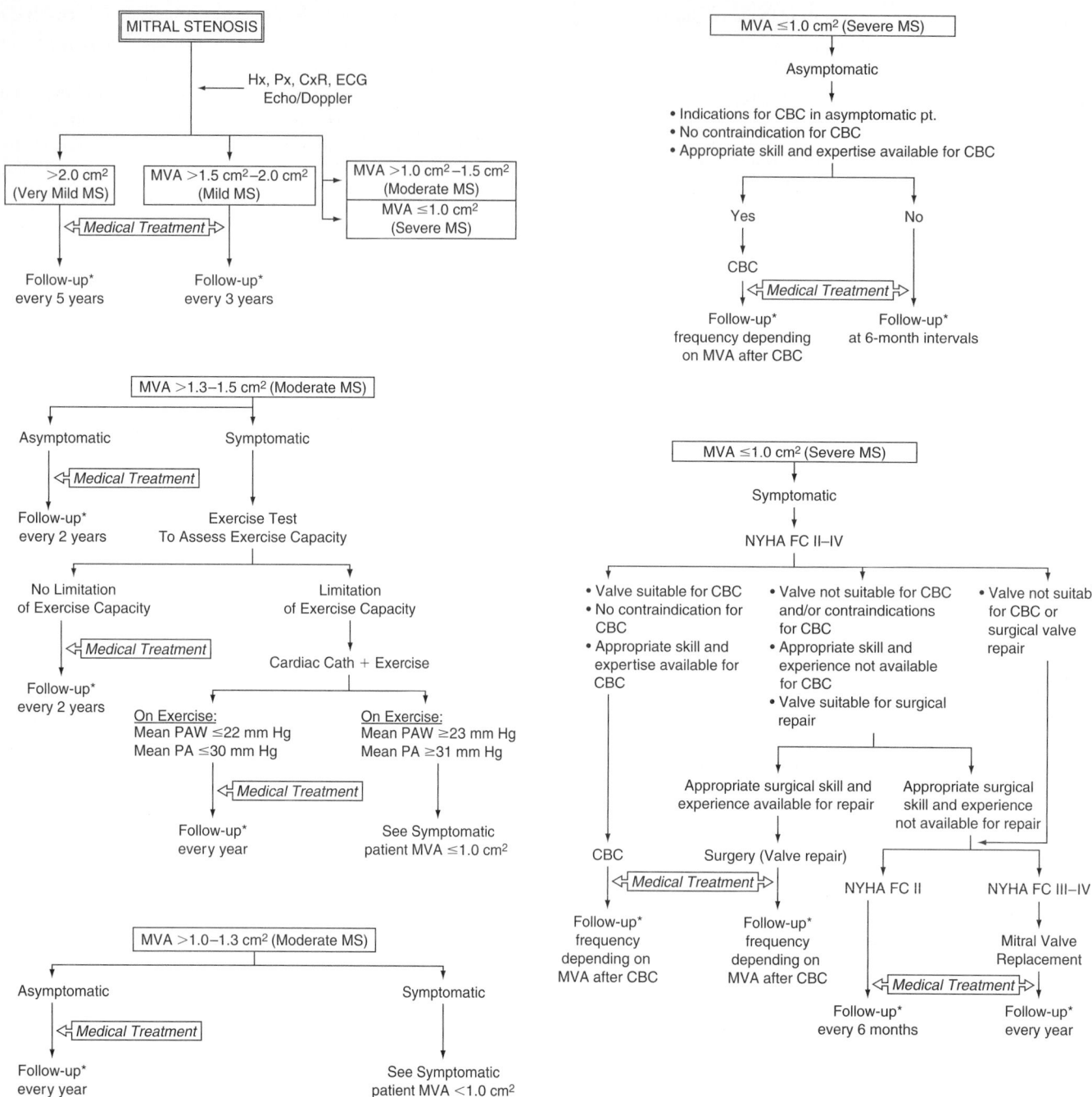

ALGORITHMS

Source: From Rahimtoola SH, Durairaj A, Mehra A, Nuno I. Current evaluation and management of patients with mitral stenosis. Circulation 2002;106:1183–1188.

[ ] INTERVENTIONAL THERAPY

Interventional therapy is usually performed in patients with severe MS (MVA ≤1.0 cm²) and occasionally in symptomatic patients with moderate MS (MVA >1.0 to 1.3 cm²). Patients with moderate MS (MVA >1.3 to 1.5 cm²) usually do not need interventional therapy. MVA >1.5 to 2.0 cm² is considered mild MS, and MVA >2.0 cm² is very mild MS.

Detailed management strategies are shown in the algorithms above. Followup times in the algorithms relate to when patients are seen by a cardiologist. Patients should be seen sooner by a cardiologist if there is any change in their condition. When seen by a car-diologist, patients should have a history, physical examination, ECG, chest radiography, and echocardiogram/Doppler. Patients should be seen at more frequent intervals by the primary care physician, family practitioner, internist, or cardiologist, at which times only a history, physical examination, ECG, and chest radiography are performed.

[ ] CATHETER BALLOON COMMISSUROTOMY

CBC is the procedure of choice if indicated (see algorithms) and if there are no contraindications (Table 77–5). In the United States,

TABLE 77-4

Medical Treatment of Mitral Stenosis

Antibiotic prophylaxis
  Recurrent rheumatic fever
  Infective endocarditis
Restrict activities (moderate/severe mitral stenosis)
  Severe exercise
  Competitive sports
Arrhythmias
  Prevent or control
  Atrial fibrillation/flutter
    Control ventricular rate
    Anticoagulation: start with IV heparin and warfarin;
      when INR is 2 to 3 discontinue heparin
  Restore sinus rhythm
Cardiac medications
  Warfarin anticoagulation: INR at 2 to 3
    Atrial fibrillation/supraventricular arrhythmias
    Systemic emboli
    LA thrombus
    Pulmonary emboli
    LV Systolic dysfunction
  Elevated pulmonary venous pressure: diuretics[a]
  "Heart failure"
    Pulmonary congestion: diuretics[a]
    Pulmonary edema: diuretics,[a] venodilators if necessary[a]
    LV systolic dysfunction: digitalis, ACE inhibitors
    Elevated systemic venous pressure and fluid retention:
      digitalis, diuretics, ACE inhibitors; β blockers (second
      generation) after patients are stabilized and there is
      LV systolic dysfunction.
Followup (see algorithms 1 to 5)[14]

ACE, angiotensin-converting enzyme; INR, international normalized ratio; LA, left atrial; LV, left ventricular.
[a]Use judiciously; patients with severe mitral stenosis need an elevated LA pressure to maintain adequate LV filling and cardiac output.
SOURCE: From Rahimtoola SH, Durairaj A, Mehra A, Nuno I. Current evaluation and management of patients with mitral stenosis. Circulation 2002;106:1183–1188.

TABLE 77-5

Contraindications (Absolute/Relative to Catheter Balloon Commissurotomy for Mitral Stenosis)

Related to valve
  • Mitral regurgitation that is truly 3+ to 4+
  • Thrombus in left atrium
  • Unfavorable valve morphology
    High score (MGH 9–16; USC 3–4)
    Commissural calcium
  • Mild mitral stenosis
Related to medical center
  • Lack of appropriate procedural skill and experience
Need for open heart surgery
  • Coronary artery bypass surgery
  • Other valve surgery
  • Ascending aorta surgery for
    Aneurysm
    Dilatation (≥5.5 cm)
    Annular ectasia
Procedural difficulties related to transseptal puncture
  • Severe tricuspid regurgitation
  • Huge right atrium
  • Distorted/displaced atrial septum
  • Venous problems
    Femoral-Iliac veins obstructed or thrombosed
    Inferior vena cava: Obstructed or thrombosed
    Drainage into azygos vein
Severe kyphoscoliosis (thoracic/abdominal)

SOURCE: From Rahimtoola SH, Durairaj A, Mehra A, Nuno I. Current evaluation and management of patients with mitral stenosis. Circulation 2002;106:1183–1188.

CBC is most commonly performed using the Inoue balloon. CBC is the procedure of choice because of the following:

1. Hospital mortality in the last 10 years is close to 0.[20,21]
2. The success rate is >95 percent.[20]
3. The MVA increases to an average of 1.9 to 2.0 cm². [20–22]
4. There are reductions of mitral valve gradient and LA (PA wedge) and PA pressures, and an increase of cardiac output.
5. Sixty percent of patients improve to NYHA functional class I and 30 percent to functional class II.[20,21]

The improvement has been objectively documented by exercise tests.[21] Good immediate results are obtained in approximately 89 percent of patients.[20] In a nonrandomized study in the 1950 to 1960s, closed mitral commissurotomy showed an improved survival rate in symptomatic patients (NYHA functional classes II and III–IV) when compared to medical therapy[18] (Fig. 77–4),

and in randomized trials the results of CBC versus closed surgical commissurotomy or surgical "repair" by open procedures are similar.[22] Followup to 10 years after CBC shows very good event-free survival (Fig. 77–5). There were no deaths up to 7 years of followup, and the event rate (mitral valve replacement or repeat CBC) was 10 percent[21] in patients who, after CBC, had a MVA >1.5 cm² and mean PA wedge pressure of 18 mmHg (Fig. 77–5). The 10-year results are also very good—event-free survival (freedom from cardiovascular deaths, mitral valve replacement, repeat CBC, and NYHA functional class I or II) is 56 ± 4 percent and those with good immediate result is 61 ± 5 percent (Fig. 77–6).[20] A study of 879 patients after CBC with a mean followup of 4.2 ± 3.7 years (range: 0.5 to 15 years) showed that the hospital mortality was 1.9 percent; the incidence of inhospital mitral valve replacement was 3.3 percent and mortality was 13 percent; mitral valve replacement and repeat CBC were needed in 27.7 percent and 6.4 percent of patients, respectively; and 47.2 percent of patients had events. Fig. 77–7 shows the event-free survival on the basis of mitral valve score.[23] CBC performed during pregnancy, if necessary, can produce good hemodynamic results in the mother and with no damage to the fetus/baby if appropriate precautions are taken and the procedure is performed by skilled and experienced interventionalists.[24]

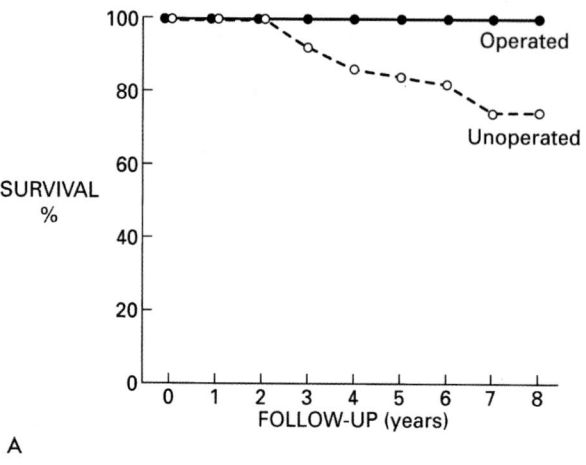

COMPARISON OF 33 OPERATED &
66 UNOPERATED PATIENTS WITH MITRAL STENOSIS
(MILD GROUP : Class II)

A

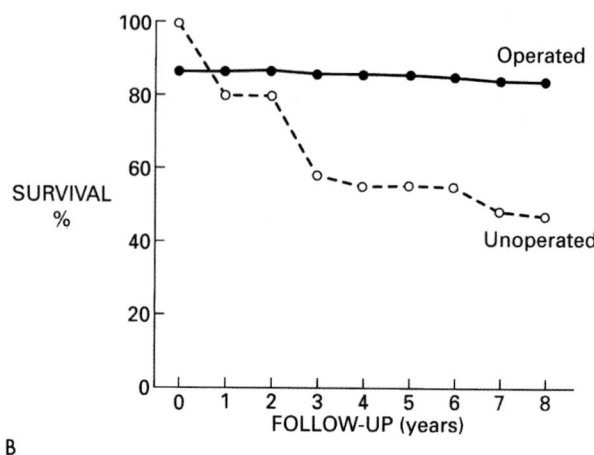

COMPARISON OF 67 OPERATED &
34 UNOPERATED PATIENTS WITH MITRAL STENOSIS
(SEVERE GROUP : Class III & IV)

B

FIGURE 77–4. Comparison of survival of patients with New York Heart Association functional class II symptoms **(A)** and class III and IV symptoms as a result of mitral stenosis **(B)**.[18] Survival of patients treated medically (unoperated) is indicated by the broken line and those with surgical closed mitral commissurotomy (operated) by the solid line. In patients treated by surgical commissurotomy, there were no operative or late deaths in those with mild symptoms and no late deaths in those with class III and IV symptoms. There is a clear improvement in survival in operated patients. The 5-year mortality with medical treatment alone in those with class III and IV symptoms approaches 50 percent; with surgery, there is no appreciable mortality following recovery from the procedure. *Source: From Roy SB, Gopinath N. Mitral stenosis. Circulation 1968;38(Suppl V):68–76.*

【 】 MITRAL VALVE REPAIR

If the valve is suitable for CBC but there are contraindications for CBC, surgical valve repair is the procedure of choice, if appropriate skill and experience is available.

【 】 CBC VERSUS MITRAL VALVE REPLACEMENT

MVAs after mitral valve replacement (MVR) and CBC are similar. There is a reduction of mean PA wedge and mean PA systolic pressures and of mitral valve gradient as well as an increase of MVA (Table 77–6); operative mortality is 2 to 7 percent,[22,25–27] prosthesis-related mortality averages 2.5 percent per year (range: 2 to 3 percent per year), and prosthesis-related complications average 5

percent per year (range: 2 to 6 percent per year).[22,24] Use of a mechanical valve necessitates use of anticoagulant therapy with its resultant problems and complications. The insertion of a bioprosthesis to avoid anticoagulation-related problems and complications is associated with structural valve deterioration. In young people (16 to 40 years of age), structural valve deterioration begins at 2 to 3 years and is >60 percent at 10 years. Even in people ages 41 to 60 years bioprosthesis is associated with high structural valve deterioration (up to 50 percent), and 50 percent of the late mortality is a consequence of structural valve deterioration.

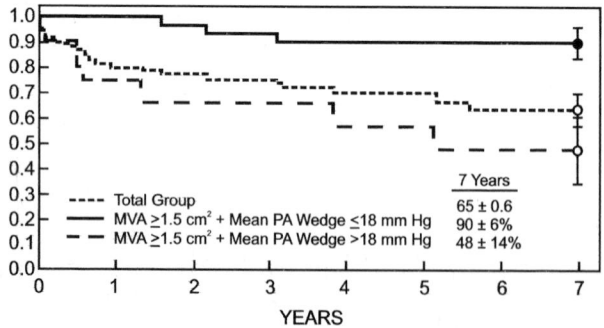

Event Free Survival
(Survival without MVR, Repeat CBC)

Orrange SE et al. Circulation 1997;95:382-389

FIGURE 77–5. Good event-free survival up to 7 years after catheter balloon commissurotomy (CBC). MVR, mitral valve replacement Source: From Orrange SE, Kawanish DT, Lopez BM, et al. Actuarial outcome after catheter balloon commissurotomy in patients with mitral stenosis. Circulation 1997;95:382–389.

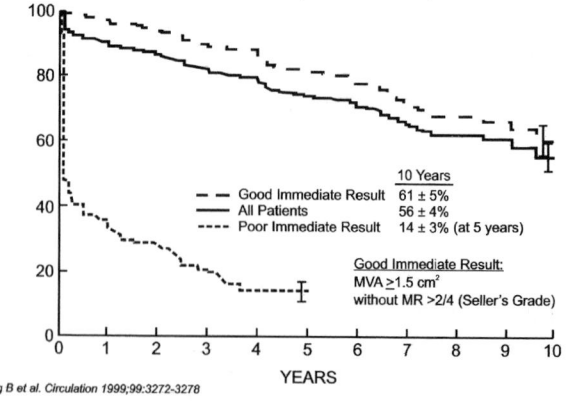

"Good Functional Results"
(Freedom from CV deaths, MVR, Repeat dilatation, & NYHA FC I or II)

Iung B et al. Circulation 1999;99:3272-3278

FIGURE 77–6. Good functional results up to 10 years after catheter balloon commissurotomy. MVA, mitral valve area; MVR, mitral valve replacement; NYHA FC, New York Heart Association functional class. *Source: From Iung B, Garbanz E, Michand P, et al. Late results of percutaneous mitral commissurotomy in a series of 1024 patients: analysis of late clinical deterioration: frequency, anatomic findings, and predictive factors. Circulation 1999;99:3272–3278.*

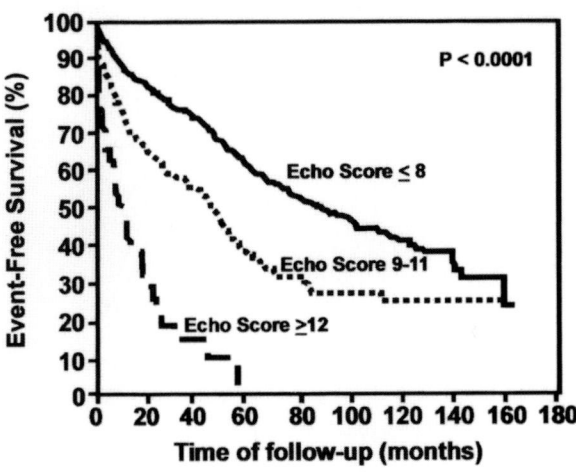

Echo Score	Successful PMV*	Event-free Survival
≤ 8	79%	38% at 12 yrs.
9-11	54%	39% at 5 yrs.
≥ 12	36%	10% at 4 yrs.

*Post-CBC: MVA ≥1.5cm² and MR <3 Seller's grade

FIGURE 77-7. Event-free survival on the basis of echo score. CBC, catheter balloon commissurotomy; MR, mitral regurgitation; MVA, mitral valve area; MVR, mitral valve replacement; PMV, percutaneous mitral balloon valvuloplasty. *Source: Adapted from Palacios IF, Sanchez PL, Itarvell LC, et al. Which patients benefit from percutaneous mitral balloon valvuloplasty? Prevalvuloplasty and postvalvuloplasty variables that predict long-term outcome. Circulation 2002;105:1465–1471.*

【 】 MITRAL VALVE REPLACEMENT

MVR is usually recommended in patients who are in NYHA functional class III and IV (see algorithm) because of the previously listed increased mortality and morbidity associated with MVR. MVR should also be considered in patients who are in NYHA functional class II who have moderate or severe pulmonary hypertension and in those who are in NYHA functional class I (asymptomatic) if they have a moderate or severe increase of pulmonary vascular resistance.

It is important to recognize that if the conditions exist for CBC and/or surgical valve repair, then performing MVR is inappropri-ate because MVR is associated with a higher hospitalization rate and late mortality, as well as a higher complication rate related to the prosthesis.

【 】 INDICATIONS FOR CATHETER BALLOON COMMISSUROTOMY IN ASYMPTOMATIC PATIENTS WITH MITRAL STENOSIS

In patients selected for CBC, the MVA should be ≤1.0 cm² or >1.0 to 1.5 cm², the valve should be suitable for CBC, there should be no contraindications for CBC, and appropriate skill

TABLE 77-6

Mitral Stenosis: Results of Mitral Valve Replacement in 33 Patients

	MITRAL STENOSIS	
	PRE-MVR	POST-MVR
LV end-diastolic pressure, mmHg	11 ± 5	12 ± 6
Mean PA wedge pressure, mmHg	36 ± 15	28 ± 14[a]
Mean systolic PA pressure, mmHg	54 ± 24	42 ± 22[b]
Cardiac index, L/min/m²	2.1 ± 1.5	2.3 ± 0.6
LV EDVI, mL/m²	79 ± 18	72 ± 24
LV ESVI, mL/m²	41 ± 13	39 ± 21
LV ejection fraction	0.48 ± 0.10	0.47 ± 0.14
Mitral regurgitant volume, mL	—	—
Regurgitant volume/end-diastolic volume	—	—
Mitral valve gradient, mmHg	15 ± 7	8 ± 3[a]
Mitral valve area, cm²	12 ± 0.4	1.8 ± 0.6[a]

EDVI, end-diastolic volume index; ESVI, end-systolic volume index; LV, left ventricular; MVR, mitral valve replacement; PA, pulmonary artery.
[a]*p* <.001.
[b]*p* <.01 comparing before and after mitral valve replacement artery.
Source: Crawford MH, Souchek J, Oprian CA, et al. Determinants of survival and left ventricular performance following mitral valve replacement. Circulation 1990;81:1173–1181.

TABLE 77-7

Recommendations for Percutaneous Mitral Balloon Valvotomy

INDICATION	CLASS
1. Percutaneous mitral balloon valvotomy is effective for symptomatic patients (NYHA functional class II, III, or IV), with moderate or severe MS (see Table 77-4) and valve morphology favorable for percutaneous balloon valvotomy in the absence of left atrial thrombus or moderate to severe MR. *(Level of Evidence: A)*	I
2. Percutaneous mitral balloon valvotomy is effective for asymptomatic patients with moderate or severe MS (see Table 77-4) and valve morphology favorable for percutaneous mitral balloon valvotomy who have pulmonary hypertension (pulmonary artery systolic pressure greater than 50 mmHg at rest or 60 mmHg with exercise) in the absence of left atrial thrombus or moderate to severe MR. *(Level of Evidence: C)*	I
3. Percutaneous mitral balloon valvotomy is reasonable for patients with moderate or severe MS (see Table 77-4) who have a nonpliable calcified valve in NYHA functional class III-IV, and who are either not candidates or at high risk for surgery. *(Level of Evidence: C)*	IIa
4. Percutaneous mitral balloon valvotomy may be considered for asymptomatic patients with moderate or severe MS (see Table 77-4) and valve morphology favorable for percutaneous balloon valvotomy who have new onset atrial fibrillation in the absence of left atrial thrombus or moderate to severe MR. *(Level of Evidence: C)*	IIb
5. Percutaneous mitral balloon valvotomy may be considered for symptomatic patients with valve area greater than 1.5 cm² if there is evidence of hemodynamically significant MS based on pulmonary artery systolic pressure greater than 60 mmHg, pulmonary wedge pressure of 25 mmHg or greater, or mean mitral valve gradient greater than 15 mmHg during exercise. *(Level of Evidence: C)*	IIb
6. Percutaneous mitral balloon valvotomy may be considered for patients with moderate or severe MS who have a non-pliable calcified valve and are in NYHA functional class III-IV as an alternative to surgery.	IIb
7. Percutaneous mitral balloon valvotomy is not indicated for patients with mild MS. *(Level of Evidence: C)*	III
8. Percutaneous mitral balloon valvotomy should not be performed in patients with moderate to severe MR or left atrial thrombus. *(Level of Evidence: C)*	

MR, mitral regurgitation; MS, mitral stenosis; MVA, mitral valve area; NYHA, New York Heart Association.
Source: Bonow RO, Carabello B, Chatterjee K, et al. ACC/AHA 2005 Guidelines on the Management of Patients with Valvular Heart Disease: A Report of the ACC/AHA Task Force on Practice Guidelines 2006. Available at: www.acc.org, e50.

TABLE 77-8

Indications for Surgery for Mitral Stenosis

INDICATION	CLASS
1. Mitral valve surgery (repair if possible) is indicated in patients with symptomatic (NYHA functional class III-IV) moderate or severe MS (see Table 77-4) when (1) PMBV is unavailable, or (2) PMBV is contraindicated because of left atrial thrombus despite anticoagulation or concomitant moderate to severe mitral regurgitation is present, or (3) when valve morphology is not favorable for PMBV in a patient with acceptable operative risk. *(Level of Evidence: B)*	I
2. Symptomatic patients with moderate to severe MS (see Table 77-4) who also have moderate to severe MR should receive MV replacement, unless valve repair is possible at the time of surgery. *(Level of Evidence: C)*	I
3. MV replacement is reasonable for patients with severe MS (see Table 77-4) and severe pulmonary hypertension (pulmonary artery systolic pressure greater than 60 to 80 mmHg) with NYHA functional class I-II symptoms who are not considered candidates for percutaneous balloon valvotomy or surgical MV repair. *(Level of Evidence: C)*	IIa
4. MV repair may be considered for asymptomatic patients with moderate or severe MS (see Table 77-4) who have had recurrent embolic events on adequate anticoagulation and have valve morphology favorable for repair. *(Level of Evidence C)*	IIb
5. MV repair for MS is not indicated for patients with mild MS. *(Level of Evidence C).*	III
6. Closed commissurotomy should not be performed in patients undergoing MV repair; open commissurotomy is the preferred approach. *(Level of Evidence C)*	

MR, mitral regurgitation; MS, mitral stenosis; NYHA, New York Heart Association; PMBV, percutaneous mitral balloon valvuloplasty.
Source: Bonow RO, Carabello B, Chatterjee K, et al. ACC/AHA 2005 Guidelines on the Management of Patients with Valvular Heart Disease: A Report of the ACC/AHA Task Force on Practice Guidelines 2006. Available at: www.acc.org, e53-e54.

and experience for CBC should be available. The indications are PA hypertension, episodic acute pulmonary edema, atrial fibrillation or flutter (paroxysmal/permanent), embolism (systemic/pulmonary), no thrombus in the LA or inferior vena cava, and patient should not be contemplating pregnancy and occupations that pose high risk to the patient or public.

Guidelines

Tables 77–7 and 77–8 list the recommendations of the American College of Cardiology and the American Heart Association *Practice Guidelines*.[28,29] Guidelines are *not* and should *not* be the law. Application of guidelines to clinical practice should be based on the following principles: (1) classes I and III apply to all patients in these classes unless there is a specific clinical circumstance contradicting this, and (2) class II applies to patients in this class depending on the clinical condition of the patient and the skill and experience at the individual medical center.

REFERENCES

1. Rahimtoola SH. Valvular heart disease. In: Stein J, ed. *Internal Medicine,* 4th ed. St. Louis: Mosby-Year Book, 1994:202–234.
2. Kawanishi DT, Rahimtoola SH. Mitral stenosis. In: Rahimtoola SH, ed. *Valvular Heart Disease II.* St. Louis: Mosby, 1996:8.1–8.24.
3. Selzer A. Effects of atrial fibrillation upon the circulation in patients with mitral stenosis. *Am Heart J* 1960;59:518–526.
4. Wood P. An appreciation of mitral stenosis: part 1. Clinical features. *BMJ* 1954;1:1051–1063. An appreciation of mitral stenosis: part 2. Investigations and results. *BMJ* 1954;1:1113–1124.
5. Gash AK, Carabello BA, Cepin D, Spann JE. Left ventricular ejection performance and systolic muscle function in patients with mitral stenosis. *Circulation* 1983;77:148–154.
6. Gaasch WH, Folland ED. Left ventricular function in rheumatic mitral stenosis. *Eur Heart J* 1991;12(Suppl B):66–69.
7. Mohan JC, Khalilullah M, Arora R. Left ventricular intrinsic contractility in pure rheumatic mitral stenosis. *Am J Cardiol* 1989;64:240–242.
8. Bowe JC, Bland EF, Sprague HB, White PD. The course of mitral stenosis without surgery: 10 and 20 year perspective. *Ann Intern Med* 1960;52:741–749.
9. Barrington WW, Bashore T, Wooley CE. Mitral stenosis: mitral dome excursion at M$_1$ and the mitral opening snap — the concept of reciprocal heart sounds. *Am Heart J* 1988;115:1280–1290.
10. Melhem RE, Dunbar JD, Booth RW. The "B" lines of Kerley and left atrial size in mitral valve disease: their correlation with mean atrial pressure as measured by left atrial puncture. *Radiology* 1991;76:65–69.
11. Khandheria BK, Tajik AJ, Reeder GS, et al. Doppler color flow imaging: a new technique for visualization and characterization of the blood flow jet in mitral stenosis. *Mayo Clin Proc* 1986;61:623–630.
12. Reid CL, Chandraratna PAN, Kawanishi DT, et al. Influence of mitral valve morphology on double-balloon catheter balloon valvuloplasty in patients with mitral stenosis: an analysis of factors predicting immediate and 3-month results. *Circulation* 1989;80:515–524.
13. Rahimtoola SH. Perspective on valvular heart disease: an update. *J Am Coll Cardiol* 1989;14:1–23.
14. Rahimtoola SH, Durairaj A, Mehra A, Nuno I. Current evaluation and management of patients with mitral stenosis. *Circulation* 2002;106:1183–1188.
15. Zamorano J, Cordeiro P, Sugeng L, et al. Real-time three dimensional echocardiography for rheumatic mitral valve stenosis evaluation: an accurate and novel approach. *J Am Coll Cardiol* 2004;43:2091–2096.
16. Kawanishi DT, Kotlewski A, McKay CR, et al. The relative value of clinical examination, echocardiography with Doppler and cardiac catheterization with angiography in the evaluation of mitral valve disease. In: Bodnar E, ed. *Surgery for Heart Valve Disease.* London: ICR Publishers, 1990:73–78.
17. Olesen KH. The natural history of 271 patients with mitral stenosis under medical treatment. *Br Heart J* 1962;24:349–357.
18. Roy SB, Gopinath N. Mitral stenosis. *Circulation* 1968;38(Suppl V):68–76.
19. Rowe JC, Bland EF, Sprague HB, White P. The course of mitral stenosis without surgery: ten- and twenty-year perspectives. *Ann Intern Med* 1960;52:741–749.
20. Iung B, Garbanz E, Michand P, et al. Late results of percutaneous mitral commissurotomy in a series of 1024 patients: analysis of late clinical deterioration: frequency, anatomic findings, and predictive factors. *Circulation* 1999;99:3272–3278.
21. Orrange SE, Kawanishi DT, Lopez BM, et al. Actuarial outcome after catheter balloon commissurotomy in patients with mitral stenosis. *Circulation* 1997;95:382–389.
22. Bonow RO, Carabello B, de Leon AC Jr, et al. ACC/AHA guidelines for the management of patients with valvular heart disease. *J Am Coll Cardiol* 1998;32:1486–1588.
23. Palacios IF, Sanchez PL, Itarvell LC, et al. Which patients benefit from percutaneous mitral balloon valvuloplasty? Prevalvuloplasty and postvalvuloplasty variables that predict long-term outcome. *Circulation* 2002;105:1465–1471.
24. Sivadasanpillai H, Srinivasan A, Sivasubramoniam S, et al. Long-term outcome of patients undergoing mitral valvotomy in pregnancy. *Am J Cardiol* 2005;95:1504–1506.
25. Fuster V, Ryden LE, Asinger RW, et al. ACC/AHA guidelines for the management of patients with valvular heart disease. *J Am Coll Cardiol* 2001;38:1231–1265.
26. Hammermeister K, Sethi GK, Henderson WG, et al. Outcomes 15 years after valve replacement with a mechanical vs. bioprosthetic valve: final report of the VA randomized trial. *J Am Coll Cardiol* 2000;36:1152–1158.
27. Kirklin JW, Barratt-Boyes BG. Mitral valve disease: with or without tricuspid valve disease. In: *Cardiac Surgery.* New York: Wiley, 1986:972–988.
28. Crawford MH, Souchek J, Oprian CA, et al. Determinants of survival and left ventricular performance following mitral valve replacement. *Circulation* 1990;81:1173–1181.
29. Bonow RO, Carabello B, Chatterjee K, et al. *ACC/AHA 2005 Guidelines on the Management of Patients with Valvular Heart Disease: A Report of the ACC/AHA Task Force on Practice Guidelines 2006.* Available at: www.acc.org.

CHAPTER 78

Tricuspid Valve, Pulmonary Valve, and Multivalvular Disease

Pravin M. Shah

TRICUSPID VALVE DISEASE

The tricuspid valve disease is often secondary to, or in association with, mitral or aortic valve disease or left ventricular (LV) disease, and receives less attention as compared to the primary left-sided disease. It is frequently labeled as "the forgotten valve" because surgical correction is often ignored. Appropriate treatment of the tricuspid valve disease, even when secondary to left heart diseases, may improve long-term functional outcome.

【 】 NORMAL VALVE ANATOMY

The tricuspid valve is the most apically (or caudally) placed valve with largest orifice among the four valves. The tricuspid valve apparatus includes leaflets or cusps, chordae and papillary muscles, and tricuspid annulus, in addition to the right atrium and right ventricle.

Annulus

The tricuspid annulus is oval in shape and when dilated becomes more circular. The annular orifice area is approximately 20 percent larger than to the mitral annulus area, with a major diameter being 3.0 to 3.5 cm in the adult. The larger orifice provides for the inflow to occur at a lower velocity and lower pressure drop. Both early and late diastolic velocities are lower than the mitral inflow. The annulus expands in diastole and constricts in midsystole.[1]

Leaflets

In general, the tricuspid valve has three distinct leaflets described as septal, anterior, and posterior. The septal and the anterior leaflets are larger. The posterior leaflet is smaller and appears to be of lesser functional significance because it may be imbricated without impairment of valve function. The septal leaflet is in immediate proximity of the membranous ventricular septum, and its extension provides a basis for spontaneous closure of the perimembranous ventricular septal defect. The anterior leaflet is attached to the anterolateral margin of the annulus and is often voluminous and sail-like in the Ebstein anomaly.

Papillary Muscles and Chordae

There are three sets of smaller papillary muscles, each set being composed of up to three muscles. The chordae tendineae arising from each set are inserted into two adjacent leaflets. Thus, the anterior set chordae insert into half of septal and half of anterior leaflets. The medial and posterior sets are similarly related to adjacent valve leaflets.

【 】 NORMAL VALVE FUNCTION

The diastolic valve opening with expansion of the annular orifice provides for unimpeded inflow. Although systolic narrowing of the orifice is intended to result in effective valve closure; some degree of valvular regurgitation with color Doppler imaging is quite common. Nearly 50 to 60 percent of young adults exhibit mild tricuspid regurgitation (TR). A smaller proportion of normal adults, up to 15 percent, have moderate TR.

TRICUSPID VALVE DISEASE

Tricuspid valve disease or dysfunction is generally classified as primary (i.e. intrinsic) valve pathology or secondary.[2,3] The latter is secondary to left-heart disease and resulting right ventricular hypertension, dilatation, and dysfunction. It is also described as *functional* TR.

Etiology of Primary Tricuspid Valve Disease

1. Congenital
   - Cleft valve in association with AV canal defect
   - Ebstein anomaly
   - Congenital tricuspid stenosis
   - Tricuspid atresia
2. Rheumatic valve disease, generally in association with rheumatic mitral disease
3. Infective endocarditis
4. Carcinoid heart disease
5. Toxic (e.g., Phen-Fen valvulopathy or methysergide valvulopathy)
6. Tumors (e.g., myxoma)
7. Iatrogenic—pacemaker lead trauma
8. Trauma—blunt or penetrating injuries
9. Degenerative—tricuspid valve prolapse

Etiology of Secondary or Functional Tricuspid Valve Disease

1. Right ventricular dilatation
2. Right ventricular hypertension (i.e., pulmonary hypertension)
3. Right ventricular dysfunction with cardiomyopathy, myocarditis, or chronic right ventricular hypertension
4. Segmental dysfunction secondary to ischemia or infarction of the right ventricle, endomyocardial fibrosis, arrhythmogenic right ventricular dysplasia.

The common causes of right ventricular (RV) hypertension, dilatation and failure are from left-heart disease in form of advanced mitral, aortic and left ventricular myocardial disorders. Thus, TR is most commonly secondary to conditions affecting the left heart, and is caused by annular dilatation and leaflet tethering.

Clinical Presentations

The functional derangement may be in form of (1) pure or predominant tricuspid stenosis, (2) pure or predominant tricuspid regurgitation, or (3) mixed.

Symptoms Generally the symptoms of left heart disease predominate in those with secondary tricuspid valve disease. The symptoms specific to advanced tricuspid valve disease are related to (a) decreased cardiac output, for example, fatigue; (b) right atrial hypertension, for example, liver congestion resulting in right upper quadrant discomfort, or gut congestion with symptoms of dyspepsia, indigestion, or fluid retention with leg edema and ascites. It may be emphasized that significant tricuspid valve (TV) disease may not be associated with any symptoms until a late stage of the disease involving progressive RV dysfunction.

Physical Signs These include signs related to tricuspid valve disease and those secondary to chronic venous congestion, that is, leg edema, ascites.

Tricuspid stenosis results in characteristic changes in the jugular venous pulse in form of a slow V to Y descent and prominent "a" waves. The liver is enlarged with a firm edge, and pulsatile in presystole. Auscultation reveals a low-to-medium-pitched diastolic rumble with inspiratory accentuation. This is usually localized to the lower sternal border (see Chap. 12).[4]

TR results in the jugular venous pulse exhibiting prominent C-V wave or systolic wave. There is often a parasternal lift from right ventricular enlargement.[5,6] The liver shows systolic pulsations, is enlarged and often tender. The cardiac auscultation reveals a soft early or holosystolic murmur which is augmented with inspiratory effort (Carvallo sign). A systolic honk may be present with tricuspid valve prolapse.[7] Substantial TR may exist without the classic ausculatory findings.

Laboratory Diagnosis

Electrocardiogram There are no specific markers of tricuspid valve (TV) disease, although the following clues may be present: (1) right ventricular (RV) hypertrophy and "strain" with right axis duration and (2) right atrial enlargement with prominent P waves.

Chest Radiograph Cardiomegaly associated with prominent right-heart borders may be noted. There are no specific findings to suggest a diagnosis of tricuspid valve disease.

Echocardiography Two-dimensional echocardiogram with spectral and color-flow Doppler evaluation provides the most accurate and comprehensive laboratory test in evaluation of TV disease (Fig. 78–1).[8] The TV morphology helps differentiate primary from secondary TR.[9] The right-heart chamber enlargement is best visualized in apical four-chamber and subcostal views, although accurate quantitation of chamber size and ejection fraction are problematic. An indirect measure of RV ejection fraction is based on systolic displacement of the tricuspid annulus using M-mode recording.[10] Tissue Doppler imaging of the annulus provides similar correlation between systolic velocity and RV function.

The TV morphology is best assessed using the parasternal tricuspid inflow view, apical and subcostal four-chamber views, and parasternal short axis view. Abnormal structure and function of the valve provides an insight into the likely underlying etiology. The functional or secondary tricuspid regurgitation is characterized by annular dilatation, the extent of which may determine its severity.

Quantitation of valve lesion is obtained using spectral and color-flow Doppler approaches. Tricuspid stenosis is detected by presence of flow acceleration on the atrial side of the valve and turbulence downstream with the RV inflow. The severity of tricuspid stenosis is based on mean and end-diastolic gradients measured using continuous wave Doppler recordings. The normal mean gradi-

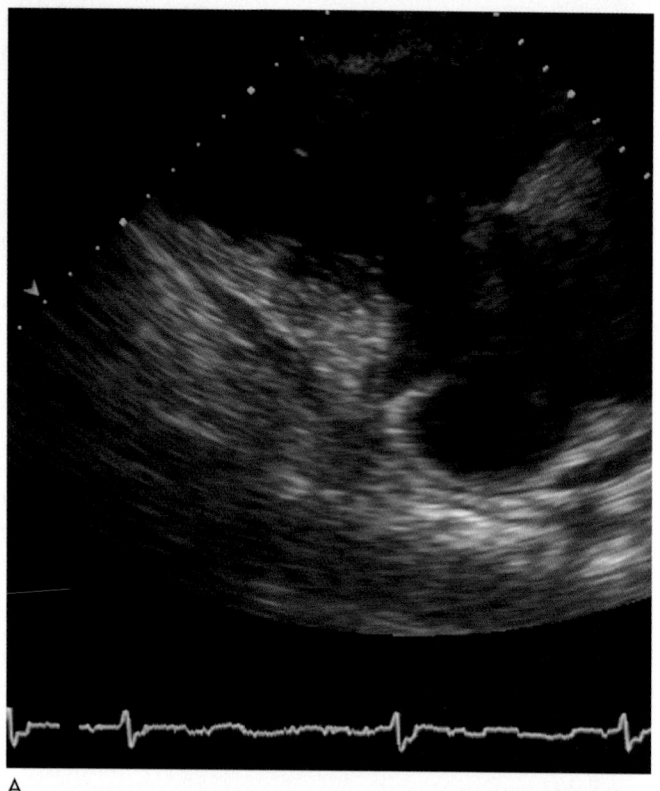

A

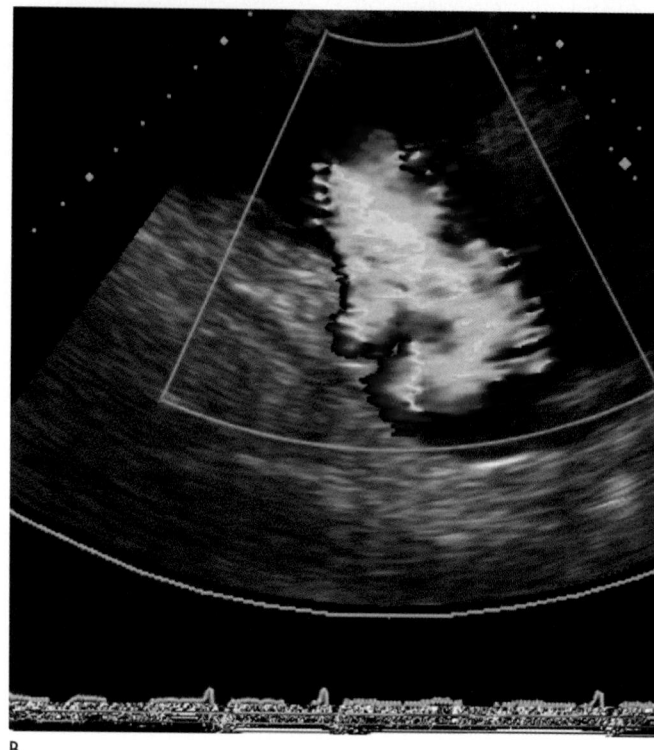

B

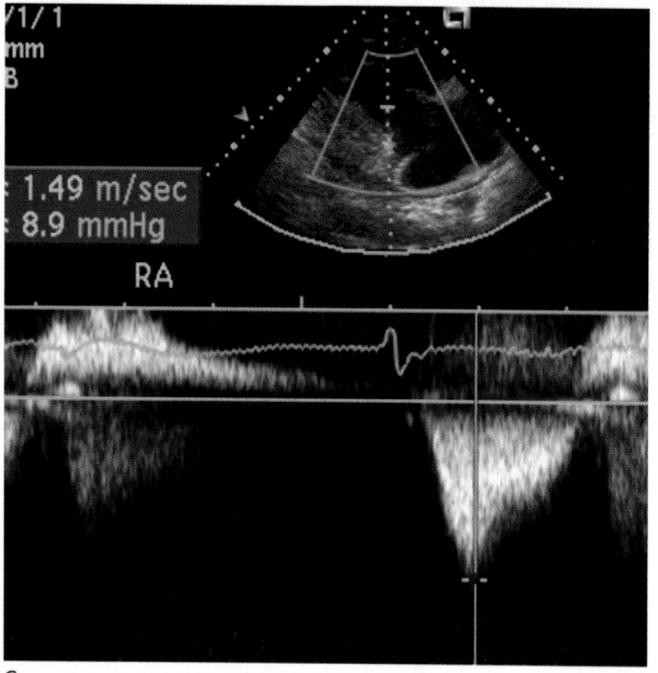

C

FIGURE 78–1. Severe secondary tricuspid regurgitation caused by extreme tethering of the tricuspid valve without intrinsic leaflet pathology. **A.** The right ventricular inflow view from parasternal transducer location shows markedly tethered valve in late systole. **B.** The color Doppler image shows flow accelerating and severe tricuspid regurgitation jet without turbulence. **C.** The continuous wave Doppler shows early peaking systolic profile associated with high right atrial pressure, which was estimated to be 25 mmHg. The peak TR velocity is measured at 9 mmHg and thus indicates right ventricular systolic pressure to be 34 mmHg (9 + 25).

ent is less than 2 mmHg and end-diastolic gradient is nearly zero. Significant stenosis of the TV may be present with a mean gradient of 3 to 5 mmHg and end-diastolic gradient of 1 to 3 mmHg. The use of pressure half time to estimate TV area and of two-dimensional echo-based planimetry of the tricuspid orifice have not been documented and are rarely, if ever, used. TR is detected using color Doppler imaging. Its severity may be semiquantitated based on extent of the regurgitation jet penetration into the right atrium and inferior vena cava. The jet of the mild TR occupies up

to 2 cm into the right atrium, whereas the jet of moderate regurgitation extends deeper (3 to 5 cm) into the atrium but does not exhibit systolic reversal in hepatic or caval flow. However, with severe TR there is consistent systolic flow reversal in the hepatic vein using pulsed Doppler approach. A more quantitative assessment of TR may be obtained by using flow acceleration, proximal isovelocity surface area methods and width of the vena contracta (see Chap. 16). A simpler approach is based on measuring the proximal isovelocity surface area radius. For the simpler method, the aliasing scale is adjusted at approximately one-twelfth of the peak regurgitation velocity (normally less than 3.0 m/s). The proximal isovelocity surface area radius at this adjusted aliasing scale of 1 to 4 mm indicates mild regurgitation, 5 to 8 mm moderate regurgitation, and greater than 9 mm severe regurgitation. The width of vena contracta greater than 7.0 mm is an additional indicator of severe regurgitation.

A spectral display of TR velocity is obtained using the continuous wave Doppler approach generally from RV inflow view, short-axis view or four-chamber view. The peak velocity used to estimate RV systolic pressure is calculated as follows: RV systolic pressure = 4 × peak TR velocity + RA (right atrial) pressure (see Chap. 16).

The right atrial pressure is assumed as 7 to 10 mmHg, but may also be estimated based on the inferior vena cava size, and its change with a sniff test.

The estimated RV systolic pressure correlates well with that measured at cardiac catheterization. However, the upper limit of measured peak systolic pressure using the Doppler approach is 40 mmHg rather than the 30 mmHg measured directly. This discrepancy is partly a result of respiratory variations and assumed right atrial pressure, which may vary by 3 to 5 mmHg from the measured mean atrial pressure. It must be emphasized the magnitude of the velocity does not indicate severity of regurgitation, but rather the height of RV systolic pressure.

Thus, a peak velocity between 3.0 and 3.9 m/s indicates moderate and in excess of 4.0 m/s severe pulmonary hypertension even if the TR severity is mild and vice versa. The shape of the velocity profile gives considerable hemodynamic information. An early peak with rapid deceleration indicates equalization of RV and right atrial pressures in late systole, generally from a large CV wave.

Transesophageal Echocardiography Transthoracic echocardiography is often of diagnostic quality because the tricuspid valve and the RV are closer to the anterior chest wall and several parasternal, apical, and subcostal views are used to image these structures. However, transesophageal echocardiography is indicated for better anatomic definitions of the valve lesions or precise measurement of the tricuspid annulus. The assessment of severity of tricuspid stenosis or TR is generally more accurate with transthoracic echocardiography. This is especially true in the intraoperative setting, where severity of TR may be underestimated as a result of lowered pulmonary vascular resistance from the anesthetic agents.

In the intraoperative setting, transesophageal echocardiography is especially used for measuring the tricuspid annulus diameter. This is done in the midesophageal four-chamber view and a plane perpendicular (90 degrees) to it.

Cardiac Catheterization and Selective Angiography Prior to the advent of diagnostic echocardiography, cardiac catheterization was used to confirm the presence and severity of tricuspid stenosis. It was recognized that simultaneous recordings of right atrial and RV diastolic pressures was needed for accurate assessment because the pressure gradients are small and there is considerable respiratory variation in the pressure wave forms. The diagnosis of TR posed a greater challenge, as selective angiography into the RV would often distort the tricuspid valve. The pressure wave forms in the right atrium showed the characteristic prominent systolic V wave with rapid descent only in the most severe cases. Diagnostic

cardiac catheterization should rarely, if ever, be undertaken for the diagnosis or quantitation of tricuspid valve disease alone.

Treatment

The management is guided by underlying etiology and pathology of the TV. Because functional or secondary TR in association with left-heart disorders is the more common, its management is emphasized here. The commonly encountered primary conditions with TV disease in adults is considered separately.

Secondary or Functional Tricuspid Regurgitation The treatment is often guided by the type and severity of the left-heart disease, which determines the clinical presentation. In nearly all cases of secondary TR, the timing and approach of surgical or interventional treatment is guided by the underlying mitral, aortic, and/or LV disease. The medical management—consisting of digitalis, diuretics, and angiotensin-converting enzyme inhibitors—may ameliorate functional TR associated with chronic congestive heart failure.

Mitral Valve Disease with Secondary Tricuspid Regurgitation The treatment of predominant severe mitral stenosis consists of percutaneous balloon valvuloplasty, open surgical mitral valve repair, or surgical mitral valve replacement (see Chap. 77). The treatment of mitral valve stenosis alone will in most patients result in a decline in pulmonary artery pressures which continues over 6 to 12 months.[11,12] The associated functional TR, depending on its severity, may impair improvement in cardiac output despite relief of the mitral valve obstruction, especially in early postoperative phase. TR often improves with a progressive decrease in pulmonary hypertension. However, in some patients the severity of tricuspid regurgitation fails to regress and remains an important factor in the long-term clinical outcome. These patients will often exhibit persistent right-heart failure with low cardiac output.[13] Most surgeons prefer to perform tricuspid valve annuloplasty at the time of mitral valve surgery. The established indication for tricuspid valve annuloplasty is the presence of moderate or severe TR. This must generally be determined by transthoracic echocardiogram. Intraoperative transesophageal echocardiography is less reliable for this assessment as the general anesthesia agents will cause an underestimation of TR because of their effects on pulmonary and systemic vascular resistances. There is suggestion that tricuspid annuloplasty should also be considered when the tricuspid annulus shows significant dilatation in order to prevent late occurrence of clinically significant TR.[14] The tricuspid annulus in a normal adult has maximum diameter of less than 3.5 cm. When this measurement *exceeds 4.0 cm*, tricuspid annuloplasty at the time of the mitral valve surgery should be undertaken. The latter adds a little more time to the surgery and may provide improved long-term outcome. It is important to emphasize that even as this practice of surgical tricuspid annuloplasty for annular dilatation is commonly practiced, it is not based on prospective randomized trials. There are basically two major approaches to tricuspid annuloplasty. DeVega annuloplasty consists of purse string suture around the annulus to reduce its circumference.[15–17] This is effective in early postoperative period but loses its efficacy over a few months. A more lasting reduction in the tricuspid annulus with improved functional regurgitation is achieved by using tricuspid band or ring annuloplasty. A restoration of the tricuspid annulus diameter to 3.0 cm permits improved valve coaptation and reduction of function tricuspid regurgitation.

The treatment of predominant or pure mitral regurgitation is guided by underlying etiology (see Chap. 76). The commonly encountered degenerative mitral valve disease, which is also classified under different terms such as *mitral valve prolapse*, lends itself to successful mitral valve repair in more than 85 percent of cases. The approach to undertaking tricuspid valve annuloplasty is similar to that described above. However, severe pulmonary hypertension is not a feature in most cases, unlike those with severe mitral stenosis. The practice of tricuspid annuloplasty for improved long-term outcome and preventing late occurrence of significant TR, although currently advocated, remains to be proven. The surgical management of ischemic or dilated cardiomyopathy related mitral regurgitation is not well established. However, a late recurrence rate of TR is reported to be common with an implication that tricuspid annuloplasty should be undertaken as a preemptive measure.

【 】 COMMON PRIMARY TRICUSPID VALVE DISEASES

Rheumatic Tricuspid Valve Disease

Rheumatic involvement of the tricuspid valve is far less common than the mitral and the aortic valves. Isolated rheumatic tricuspid valve disease is rare. However, clinically significant tricuspid valve disease, in association with mitral and/or aortic valve disease, is reported between 10 and 20 percent of patients. The tricuspid valve is thickened and the leaflets are contracted with fibrosis. Commissural fusion is often present. The resulting clinical syndrome is one of mixed stenosis and regurgitation. The murmur of tricuspid stenosis is heard along the lower left sternal border and is louder with inspiration (see Chap. 12). The opening snap is not often heard. A systolic murmur of TR is often soft, medium pitched and also increases with inspiration. Inspiratory increase in jugular venous pressure is common and simulates the Kussmaul sign in constrictive pericarditis. However, the jugular venous pulse with rheumatic tricuspid valve stenosis and regurgitation fails to show rapid "y" descent. The echocardiographic appearance of thickened distorted valve establishes a correct diagnosis.

Treatment of rheumatic TV disease consists of valve repair with annuloplasty when the valve dysfunction is not severe. However, in presence of severe disease, valve replacement with a low profile mechanical or a bioprosthetic valve is indicated. The mechanical valve in the tricuspid position has a high risk of complications such as thrombosis and infection. In general, the tissue valve is preferred despite a risk of late structural failure in younger subjects. Tricuspid valve balloon valvuloplasty has been advocated for predominant stenosis with mixed results. A common consequence is an aggravation of TR.

Infective Endocarditis

Infective endocarditis of the tricuspid valve is not uncommon among drug addicts using intravenous drugs. It may also be observed in patients with long-term intravenous lines (Fig. 78-2; see Chap. 85).

The clinical presentation is one of general systematic symptoms such as fever, weight loss, anemia, and fatigue, or of pulmonary embolism, or of right-heart failure with hepatic congestion, peripheral edema and ascites. The diagnostic confirmation is made by echocardiographic lesions suggestive of vegetations and positive blood cultures.

Treatment of drug addicts with infective endocarditis is especially challenging. A prosthetic valve is at a great risk of recurrent infection as the intravenous drug use is resumed. Surgical excision of the infected tricuspid valve has been attempted with some initial success, but poor long term outcome. This condition among IV drug users continues to be a difficult management problem.

Carcinoid Heart Disease

Carcinoid tumors arising in the intestinal tract with secondary liver metastases are commonly associated valvular pathology (see Chap. 89). The most commonly affected valve is the tricuspid valve followed by the pulmonary valve (Fig. 78-3). The left-sided cardiac valves are spared unless a right-to-left shunt through patent foramen ovale or atrial septal defect is present. Occasionally, the left-sided heart valves may be affected when primary carcinoid tumor is in the lung.

The pathology of the valve consists of thickening with fibrosis and markedly restricted motion. The valve leaflets are held partially open during systole and diastole. The opening results in obstructed inflow. Thus, there are signs of tricuspid stenosis and regurgitation, with the latter predominating.

The clinical features are those of the carcinoid tumor and right-heart failure. The echocardiographic appearance of the thickened restricted valve leaflets is quite characteristic. Color-flow Doppler reveals wide open tricuspid regurgitation often with laminar regurgitant flow into a large right atrium. Spectral Doppler tracing with continuous wave Doppler shows a characteristic pattern of early peaking profile suggestive of marked elevation of right atrial pressure.

Treatment is directed toward the primary tumor and tricuspid valve replacement for severely damaged valve; however, balloon dilatation of tricuspid and pulmonary valves has also been attempted.[18]

Traumatic Tricuspid Regurgitation

The trauma may be external, such as blunt chest wall injury with disruption of chordal structures (Fig. 78-4). Internal trauma is generally iatrogenic resulting from damage with pacemaker lead, a stiff guide wire or radiofrequency ablation for treatment of arrhythmias. The TR resulting from a pacemaker lead either may be from perforation of a leaflet or its restriction. It is often unrecognized as the functional consequences are slow to develop and the regurgitation is often progressive.

Treatment is based on recognition of the etiology of regurgitation. Transthoracic and transesophageal echocardiography provide important clues. Although the valve pathology is often repairable, the timing of surgery will be determined by clinical evidence of severe regurgitation before development of deterioration of RV function or elevations in liver enzymes.

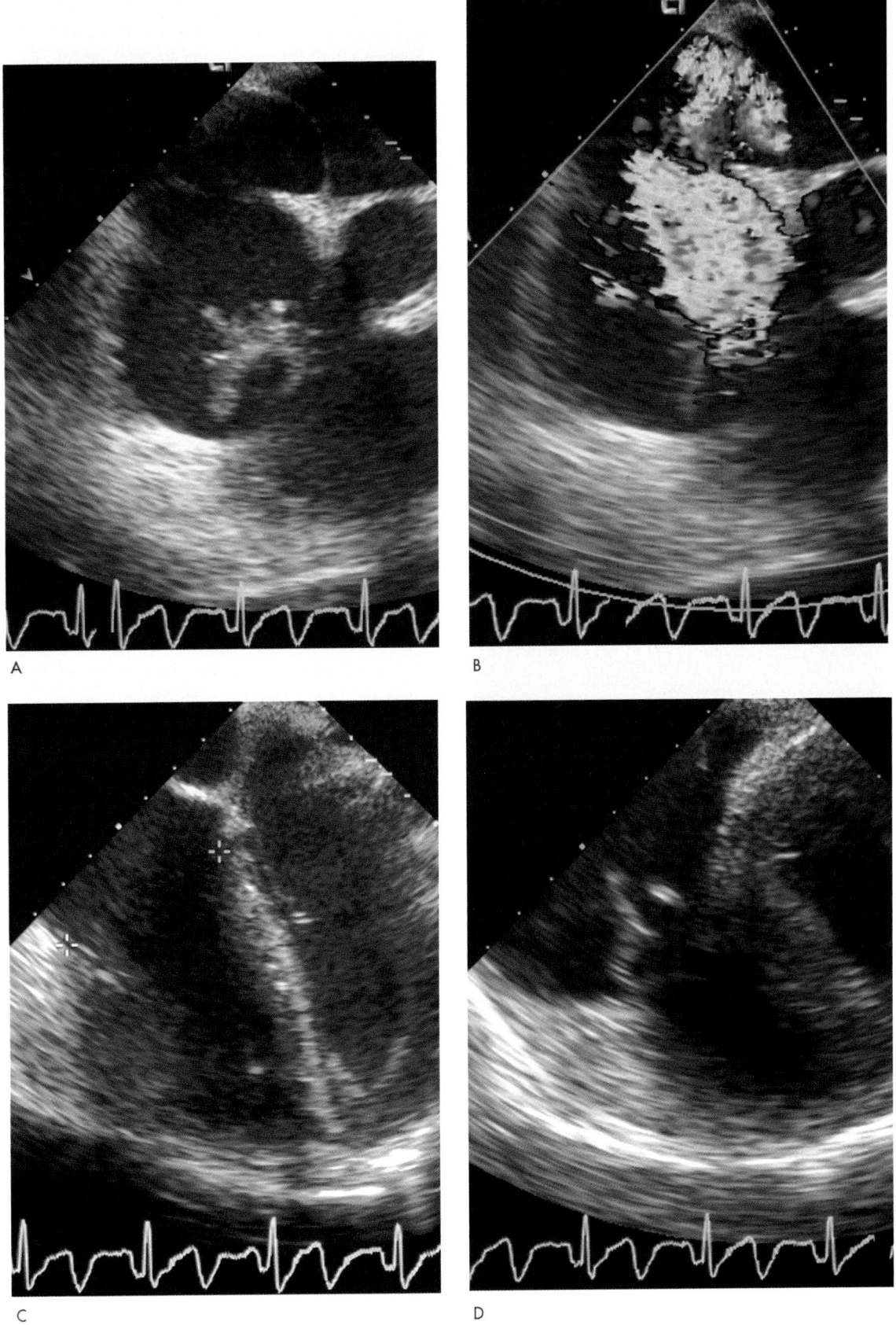

FIGURE 78–2. Tricuspid valve endocarditis in a 35-year-old male with positive blood cultures growing *Staphylococcus aureus*. Intraoperative transesophageal echocardiography shows salient features before and after tricuspid valve (TV) replacement. **A.** Large irregular vegetation prolapsing into the right atrium in systole. **B.** Severe tricuspid regurgitation (TR) associated with TV endocarditis. **C.** Tricuspid annulus measures 4.5 cm and is markedly dilated as a consequence of right ventricular and right atrial dilatation. **D.** The anterior TV leaflet is flail. *(continued)*

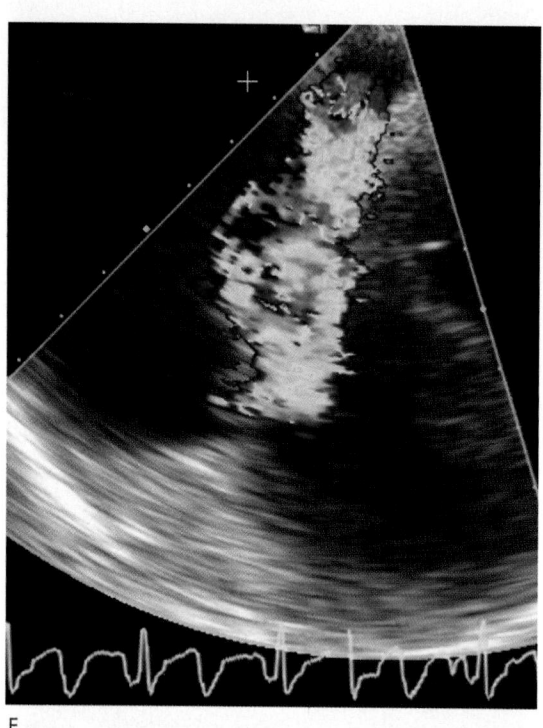

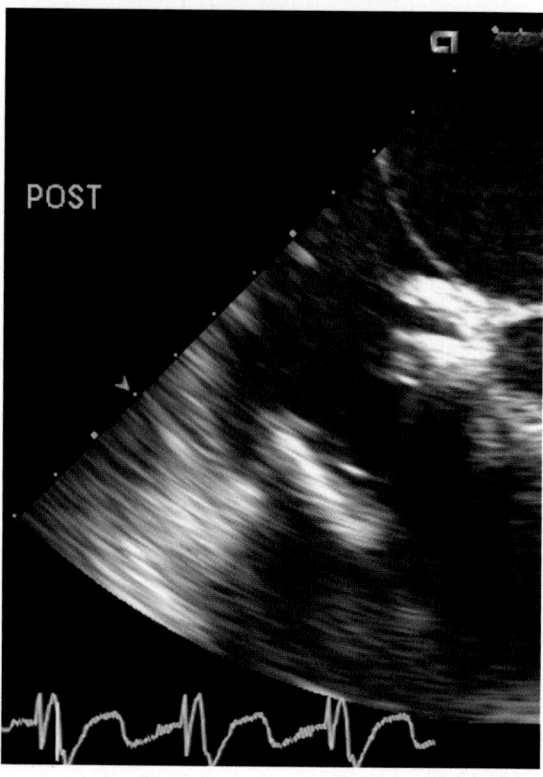

POST

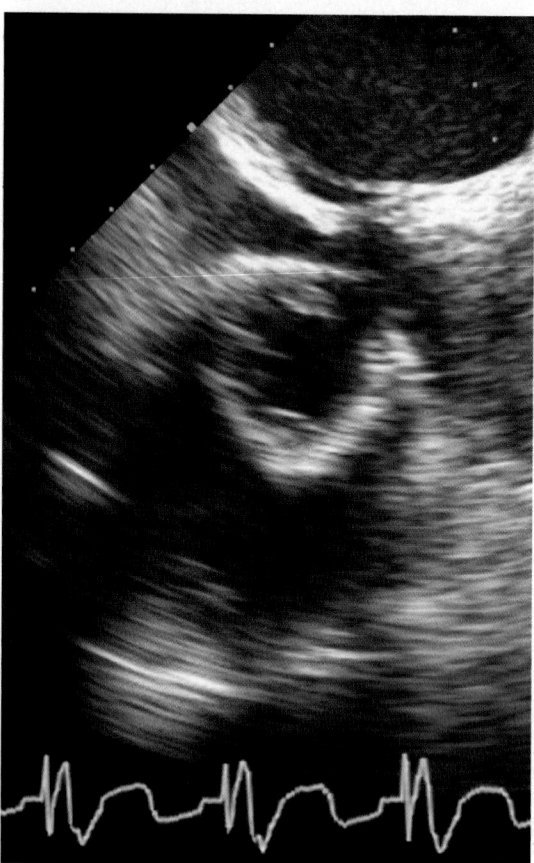

E

F

G

FIGURE 78–2. *(continued)* Tricuspid valve endocarditis in a 35-year-old male with positive blood cultures growing *Staphylococcus aureus*. Intraoperative transesophageal echocardiography shows salient features before and after tricuspid valve (TV) replacement. **E.** The TR jet is deflected into the coronary sinus as a result of flail TV. **F** and **G.** A bioprosthesis is placed in the tricuspid valve position shown in short axis and four-chamber views.

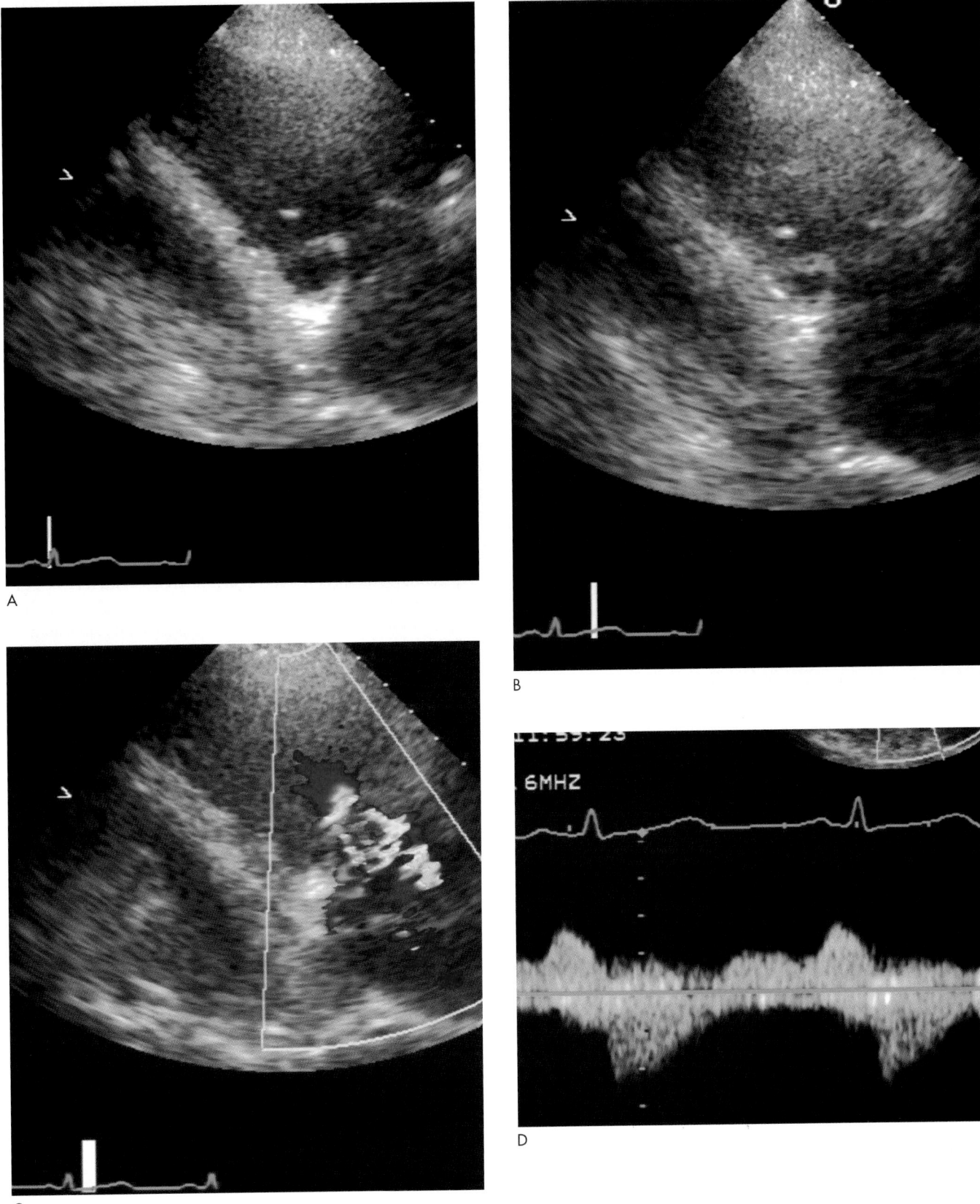

FIGURE 78–3. The echocardiographic images in 48-year-old male with carcinoid heart disease. **A.** End-diastolic frame showing tricuspid valve in open position. **B.** The tricuspid valve in the end-systolic frame is in partially open position. **C.** This characteristic valve restriction results in severe tricuspid regurgitation. **D.** The continuous wave Doppler shows several characteristic features. The systolic velocity of early peak and rapid deceleration indicate high right atrial pressure. The diastolic velocity with slow early deceleration and a prominent presystolic flow is consistent with some degree of tricuspid stenosis.

Ebstein Anomaly

The Ebstein anomaly is a congenital lesion that may first be detected at an adult age, with milder cases living up to the sixth decade (see Chap. 82). The characteristic features are apical displacement of the septal leaflet of the tricuspid valve, a large, sail-like anterior leaflet that results in atrialization of the RV inflow. Functionally, a variable degree of TR is observed. The right-heart chambers are markedly dilated. A right-to-left shunt at atrial level may be present if atrial septal defect coexists. The clinical presentation is marked by cardiomegaly involving right-heart chambers, quiet precordium with a soft systolic murmur, abnormal ECG with wide QRS complex, and short PR internal. Symptomatic supraventricular arrhythmias are common. The ECG exhibits a diagnostic apical displacement of the septal and anterior tricuspid leaflets with a large, sail-like anterior leaflet. Moderate low velocity TR may be observed.[19]

Treatment ranges from medical management in milder forms of the disease to valve repair or valve replacement in more advanced symptomatic patients.[20,21]

Tricuspid Valve Prolapse

Degenerative "myxomatous" mitral valve prolapse is associated with tricuspid valve prolapse in 30 to 40 percent of patients. In most cases there are no distinctive physical signs (see Chap. 12). Echocardiography reveals billowing of septal and anterior leaflets. The associated TR is generally mild. Rarely, spontaneous chordae rupture may result in severe regurgitation (see Fig. 78–4). When moderate or severe TR with dilatation of the annulus accompanies severe mitral regurgitation with degenerative mitral valve disease, the management consists of tricuspid valve annuloplasty in addition to mitral valve repair (Table 78–1).

PULMONARY VALVE DISEASE

Apart from congenital lesions involving the pulmonary valve and/or the RV infundibulum, pulmonary valve disease as an acquired condition in the adult is extremely rare (see Chap. 93). The pulmonary valve is the least commonly involved in an infectious process such as rheumatic fever and bacterial endocarditis. It may be pathologically affected in carcinoid heart disease with resulting stenosis and regurgitation.

【 】 ETIOLOGY

1. Congenital
   • Pulmonary Valve Stenosis
   • Pulmonary Atresia
   • Congenital Bicuspid Valve
   • Infundibular Pulmonary Stenosis
   • Idiopathic Dilatation of Pulmonary Artery
2. Acquired
   • Rheumatic
   • Infective Endocarditis
   • Carcinoid Heart Disease
   • Pulmonary Hypertension
   • Iatrogenic as following Ross operation
Table 78–2 lists the guidelines for managing these patients.

【 】 CLINICAL PRESENTATION

Bedside examination may provide important clues. Pulmonary valve stenosis is associated with characteristic auscultatory findings depending on severity.[22,23] Mild stenosis is characterized by a systolic ejection click and short early systolic murmur. With progressive severity, the murmur gets louder longer and peaks later in systole. The ejection click is often more prominent in expiration. This seemingly paradoxical behavior of the pulmonary ejection click is explained by an inspiratory increase in RV end-diastolic pressure, which opens the valve in late diastole and, hence, absence of systolic ejection click during inspiratory phase. Thus, ejection click may be absent in the most severe stenosis where RV end-diastolic pressure is consistently above the pulmonary arterial pressures. The behavior of the second heart sound is also of diagnostic importance. In milder cases the pulmonary component of second heart sound (P_2) is delayed, but retains further widening with inspiration (see Chap. 12). As stenosis increases in severity, the pulmonary component becomes softer and the murmur in the very severe cases spills past aortic component and the pulmonary component is inaudible.

Clinical assessment of pulmonary regurgitation is often more challenging. A high-pitched diastolic murmur following a prominent P_2 may be evident in patients with pulmonary regurgitation secondary to pulmonary hypertension. This murmur is often described as the Graham Steell murmur and may be erroneously interpreted to indicate aortic regurgitation as they both may be heard best along the left sternal border. Mild or even moderate pulmonary regurgitation may be present without an audible murmur.

Clinical assessment of infundibular pulmonary stenosis reveals a systolic murmur peaking in late systole and well-preserved, but delayed, P_2.

【 】 LABORATORY TESTS

Evidence of right-heart chamber enlargement is shown by 12-lead ECG and chest radiography. The echocardiogram provides diagnostic and quantitative assessment of pulmonary valve stenosis, infundibular pulmonary stenosis, and pulmonary regurgitation (see Chap. 16). The pulmonary valve morphology shows doming and incomplete opening in presence of pulmonary valve stenosis. Although the valve cusps are normal in infundibular stenosis, a characteristic midsystolic closure and prominent presystolic "a" wave are often diagnostic clues. The pulmonary artery and branches are dilated in pulmonary hypertension, idiopathic pulmonary artery dilatation and in severe pulmonary regurgitation. In rare cases of pulmonary valve endocarditis, a mobile vegetation may be observed (see Chap. 85). Hypertrophied and dynamic RV infundibulum are characteristic for infundibular stenosis, be it congenital or associated with hypertrophic cardiomyopathy. The spectral Doppler and color-flow Doppler reveal high-velocity turbulent flow in the main pulmonary artery in patients with pulmonary valve stenosis, and a late-peaking, high-velocity flow with turbulence in the RV outflow tract are noted in infundibular pulmonary stenosis. Trivial or mild pulmonary regurgitation are normal findings in most children, as well as adults. However, moderate and severe regurgitation are associated with RV volume overload and subsequent dilatation and dysfunction. The pulmonary regurgitation velocity waveform provides a unique insight into pressure difference be-

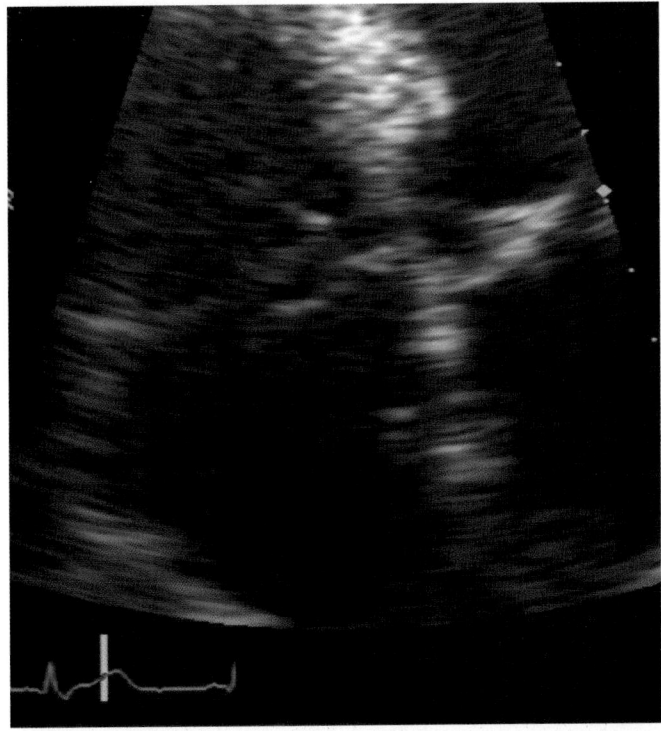

A

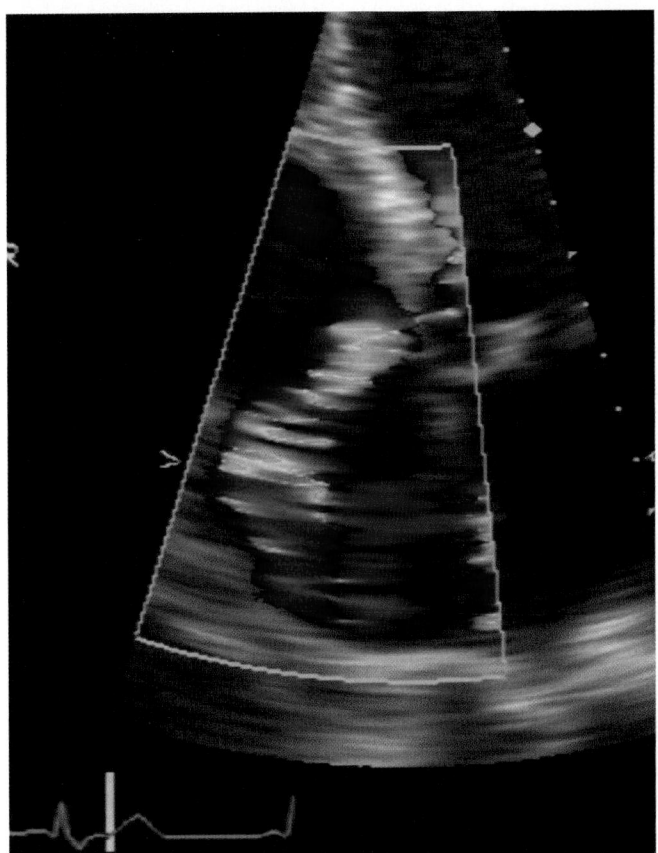

B

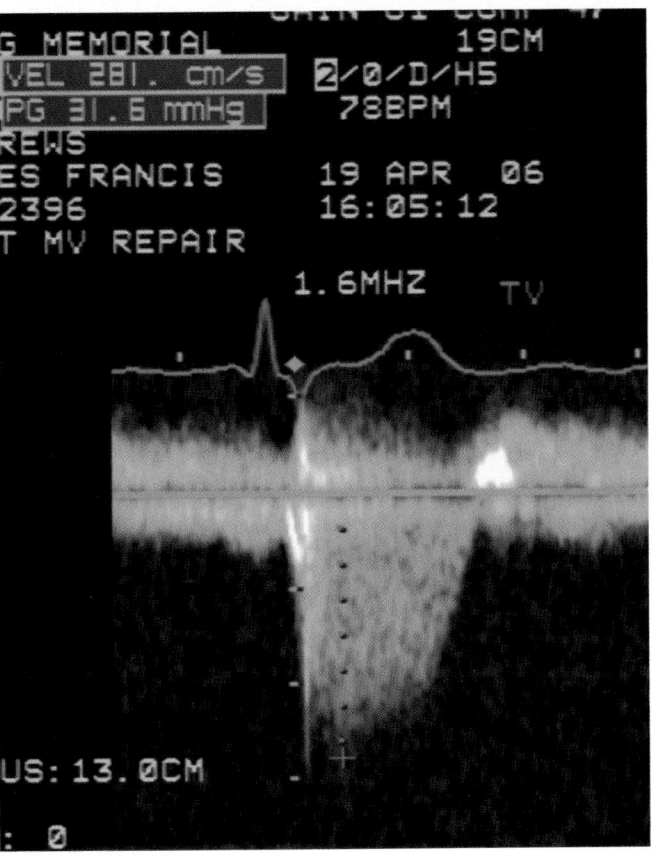

C

FIGURE 78–4. A 56-year-old male with mitral valve prolapse exhibited spontaneous rupture of the tricuspid valve. **A.** The flail septal leaflet of the tricuspid valve (TV) is shown in systole. **B.** The resulting eccentric tricuspid regurgitation (TR) jet directed laterally because of flail TV. **C.** The continuous wave Doppler recording of the TR jet with a peak systolic gradient between right ventricle and right atrial of 32 mmHg. The inferior vena cava was measured at 2.5 cm and showed no discernible collapse, indicating estimated right atrial pressure of 20 mmHg. Thus, the right ventricular systolic pressure is estimated as 52 mmHg.

TABLE 78-1

2006 American College of Cardiology/American Heart Association (ACC/AHA) Guidelines for Management of Patients with Valvular Heart Disease[a]

Management

Class I

TV repair is beneficial for severe TR in patients with MV disease requiring MV surgery. (Level of Evidence: B)

Class IIa

1. TV replacement or annuloplasty is reasonable for severe primary TR when symptomatic. (Level of Evidence: C)

2. TV replacement is reasonable for severe TR secondary to diseased/abnormal tricuspid valve leaflets not amenable to annuloplasty or repair. (Level of Evidence: C)

Class IIb

Tricuspid annuloplasty may be considered for less-than-severe TR in patients undergoing MV surgery when there is pulmonary hypertension or tricuspid annular dilatation. (Level of Evidence: C)

Class III

1. TV replacement or annuloplasty is not indicated in asymptomatic patients with TR whose pulmonary artery systolic pressure is less than 60 mmHg in the presence of a normal MV. (Level of Evidence: C)

2. TV replacement or annuloplasty is not indicated in patients with mild primary TR. (Level of Evidence: C)

MV, mitral valve; TR, tricuspid regurgitation; TV, tricuspid valve.
[a]See also Chap. 11.

tween pulmonary artery and RV during diastole. Because RV diastole pressure equilibrates with right atrial pressure in absence of tricuspid stenosis, an estimation of pulmonary arterial diastolic pressure is obtained using the end-diastolic velocity of pulmonary regurgitation and size of the inferior vena cava, which is used to estimate right atrial pressure.

[ ] CARDIAC CATHETERIZATION AND SELECTIVE ANGIOGRAPHY

Diagnostic right-heart catheterization is useful to measure pulmonary artery pressures and pulmonary wedge pressure, and to calculate pulmonary vascular resistance. These are useful to differentiate and quantify precapillary and postcapillary pulmonary arterial hypertension. Although quantification of pulmonary valve stenosis is generally made using echo Doppler methods, catheter-based measurements before and after pulmonary balloon valvotomy are used to evaluate successful dilatation of the stenotic pulmonary valve. Selective angiography is less useful for diagnostic or therapeutic interventions.

[ ] TREATMENT

Mild or even moderate pulmonary valve stenosis and regurgitation do not result in RV overload and may require no specific treatment other than prophylaxis for bacterial endocarditis.

TABLE 78-2

2006 American College of Cardiology/American Heart Association (ACC/AHA) Guidelines for the Management of Patients with Valvular Heart Disease

Evaluation of Pulmonic Stenosis in Adolescents and Young Adults

Class I

1. An ECG is recommended for the initial evaluation of pulmonic stenosis in adolescent and young adult patients, and serially every 5 to 10 years for followup examinations. (Level of Evidence: C)

2. Transthoracic Doppler echocardiography is recommended for the initial evaluation of pulmonic stenosis in adolescent and young adult patients, and serially every 5 to 10 years for followup examinations. (Level of Evidence: C)

3. Cardiac catheterization is recommended in the adolescent or young adult with pulmonic stenosis for evaluation of the valvular gradient if the Doppler peak jet velocity is greater than 3 meter per second (estimated peak gradient greater than 36 mmHg) and balloon dilatation can be performed if indicated. (Level of Evidence: C)

Class III

Diagnostic cardiac catheterization is not recommended for the initial diagnostic evaluation of pulmonic stenosis in adolescent and young adult patients. (Level of Evidence: C)

Indications for Balloon Valvotomy in Pulmonic Stenosis

Class I

1. Balloon valvotomy is recommended in adolescent and young adult patients with pulmonic stenosis who have exertional dyspnea, angina, syncope, or presyncope and a right ventricle (RV)-to-pulmonary artery peak-to-peak gradient greater than 30 mmHg at catheterization. (Level of Evidence: C)

2. Balloon valvotomy is recommended in asymptomatic adolescent and young adult patients with pulmonic stenosis and RV-to-pulmonary artery peak-to-peak gradient greater than 40 mmHg at catheterization. (Level of Evidence: C)

Class IIb

Balloon valvotomy may be reasonable in asymptomatic adolescent and young adult patients with pulmonic stenosis and an RV-to-pulmonary artery peak-to-peak gradient 30 to 39 mmHg at catheterization. (Level of Evidence: C)

Class III

Balloon valvotomy is not recommended in asymptomatic adolescent and young adult patients with pulmonic stenosis and RV-to-pulmonary artery peak-to-peak gradient less than 30 mmHg at catheterization. (Level of Evidence: C)

[a]See also Chap. 11.

Moderately severe and severe pulmonary valve stenosis are currently treated by percutaneous balloon valvotomy (see Chap. 82).[24–26] Surgical valvotomy is rarely needed. Similarly, severe pulmonary regurgitation in absence of pulmonary hypertension may require valve replacement in order to prevent irreversible right ventricular damage from long-standing volume overload and dilatation.[27] A bioprosthetic valve is generally used. Recent advances in percutaneous valve replacement to treat severe pulmonary regurgitation are noteworthy. A long-term efficacy of this approach remains to be proven.

MULTIVALVULAR DISEASE

Several etiologies, including rheumatic disease, infective endocarditis, and degenerative myxomatous valve disease, tend to affect more than one valve. The combination of valve involvement is often asymptomatic, with one valve having dominant dysfunction and other valves being less severely affected. There are special diagnostic and therapeutic challenges that arise when more than one valve is diseased. The aortic and mitral valve diseases may coexist or the mitral and tricuspid. The aortic and tricuspid valve combination is less common and the pulmonary valve is the least-often affected in multivalvular diseases.

[ ] AORTIC STENOSIS AND MITRAL STENOSIS

This combination is most commonly caused by rheumatic heart disease but may also be noted in degenerative calcific disease in the elderly. It offers special diagnostic and therapeutic challenges.

Diagnostic Challenges

The murmur of mitral stenosis may not be easily discerned in presence of severe aortic valve stenosis. The loud systolic murmur of aortic stenosis is also heard at the apex and hypertrophied left ventricle may mask the diastolic rumble of mitral stenosis. Similarly, the low cardiac output resulting from severe mitral stenosis may result in underestimation of the severity of aortic stenosis as the resulting gradient is low. The echocardiogram exhibits pathology in both valves, and the severity of mitral stenosis based on pressure half time is unaffected by aortic stenosis. The peak and mean gradients are underestimated because of reduced cardiac output.

Therapeutic Dilemma

Percutaneous balloon valvotomy for mitral stenosis may result in increased cardiac output and acute LV failure may develop when the severity of aortic stenosis has not been recognized. The appropriate treatment consists of aortic valve replacement and mitral valve repair or replacement.

[ ] AORTIC STENOSIS AND MITRAL REGURGITATION

This combination is not uncommon.

Diagnostic Challenge

The separate systolic murmurs of the two lesions may not be distinguished, as the apically transmitted murmur of aortic stenosis (Gallavardin sign) is often of higher pitch (see Chap. 12). Similarly, the systolic murmur associated with posterior leaflet prolapse may be transmitted to the base. Echocardiography provides accurate assessment of underlying valvular pathology, although severity of mitral

regurgitation is overestimated owing to high intraventricular systolic pressure secondary to severe aortic stenosis.

Therapeutic Dilemma

A decision to surgically treat mitral regurgitation while undertaking aortic valve replacement is often difficult. If the mitral valve has intrinsic pathology that lends itself to repair, such as mitral valve prolapse, the decision is made to undertake the mitral valve surgery prior to replacing the aortic valve. However, the dilemma occurs when the mitral regurgitation is mild or moderate without intrinsic mitral valve pathology. One is tempted to leave the mitral valve alone with a consideration that a decrease in LV systolic pressure will result in reduction in mitral regurgitation, avoiding higher morbidity and mortality of double-valve replacements. If the mitral valve needs to be replaced for persistent mitral regurgitation after the aortic valve has been replaced, it provides a technical challenge. It is generally preferable to perform the mitral surgery prior to aortic valve replacement.

[ ] AORTIC REGURGITATION AND MITRAL STENOSIS

Diagnostic Challenge

The clinical signs of aortic regurgitation are often masked owing to a low cardiac output in severe mitral stenosis. The LV enlargement is less pronounced. The quantitation of mitral stenosis by pressure half-time using Doppler echocardiography may result in underestimation of its true severity. Alternate methods to assess severity should be employed.

Therapeutic Dilemma

Treatment of mitral stenosis may unmask the severity of aortic regurgitation resulting in LV decompensation. The appropriate treatment for both severe lesions requires aortic valve replacement and mitral valve repair or replacement. However, if the aortic regurgitation by color-flow Doppler or by selective angiography is thought to be mild or mild to moderate, it may be tolerated without a need for valve replacement.

[ ] AORTIC REGURGITATION AND MITRAL REGURGITATION

Diagnostic Challenge

When both aortic and mitral valves are incompetent, the LV overload and decompensation are manifest early. The timing of surgery is often determined by size and function of the LV.

Therapeutic Dilemma

The mitral valve repair or replacement must precede the aortic valve replacement for technical reasons.

[ ] MITRAL AND TRICUSPID VALVE DISEASE

This may be seen with rheumatic etiology or the tricuspid regurgitation may be secondary to annular enlargement. Both lesions have to be identified and surgical correction attempted.

REFERENCES

1. Tei C, Pilgrim JP, Shah PM, et al. The tricuspid valve annulus: study of size and motion in normal subjects and in patients with tricuspid regurgitation. *Circulation* 1982;66(3):665–671.

2. Waller BF, Moriarty AT, Eble JN, et al. Etiology of pure tricuspid regurgitation based on anular circumference and leaflet area: analysis of 45 necropsy patients with clinical and morphologic evidence of pure tricuspid regurgitation. *J Am Coll Cardiol* 1986;7:1063–1074.

3. Waller BF, Howard J, Fess S. Pathology of tricuspid valve stenosis and pure tricuspid regurgitation—part III. *Clin Cardiol* 1995;18:225–230.

4. Wooley CF, Fontana ME, Kilman JW, et al. Tricuspid stenosis: atrial systolic murmur, tricuspid opening snap, and right atrial pressure pulse. *Am J Med* 1985;78:375–384.

5. Pellegrini A, Colombo T, Donatelli F, et al. Evaluation and treatment of secondary tricuspid insufficiency. *Eur J Cardiothorac Surg* 1992;6:288–296.

6. Kratz J. Evaluation and management of tricuspid valve disease. *Cardiol Clin* 1991;9:397–407.

7. Tei C, Shah PM, Tanaka H. Phonographic-echographic documentation of systolic honk in tricuspid prolapse. *Am Heart J* 1982;103(2):294–295.

8. Tei C, Shah PM, Cherian G, et al. Echocardiographic evaluation of normal and prolapsed tricuspid valve leaflets. *Am J Cardiol* 1983;52(7):796–800.

9. Rivera JM, Vandervoort PM, Vazquez de Prada JA, et al. Which physical factors determine tricuspid regurgitation jet area in the clinical setting? *Am J Cardiol* 1993;72:1305–1309.

10. Kaul S, Tei C, Hopkins JM, Shah PM. Assessment of right ventricular function using two-dimensional echocardiography. *Am Heart J* 1984;107(3):526–531.

11. Skudicky D, Essop MR, Dareli P. Efficacy of mitral balloon valvotomy in reducing the severity of associated tricuspid valve regurgitation. *Am J Cardiol* 1994;73:209–211.

12. Skudicky D, Essop MR, Dareli P. Efficacy of mitral balloon valvotomy in reducing the severity of associated tricuspid valve regurgitation. *Am J Cardiol* 1994;73:209–211.

13. Sagie A, Schwammenthal E, Newell JB, et al. Significant tricuspid regurgitation is a marker for adverse outcome in patients undergoing percutaneous balloon mitral valvuloplasty. *J Am Coll Cardiol* 1994;24:696–702.

14. Dreyfus GD, Corbi PJ, Chan KM, et al. Secondary tricuspid regurgitation or dilatation: which should be criteria for surgical repair? *Ann Thorac Surg* 2005;79:127–132.

15. De Paulis R, Bobbio M, Ottino G, et al. The De Vega tricuspid annuloplasty; perioperative mortality and long term follow-up. *J Cardiovasc Surg (Torino)* 1990;31:512–517.

16. Aoyagi S, Tanaka K, Hara H, et al. Modified De Vega's annuloplasty for functional tricuspid regurgitation—early and late results. *Kurume Med J* 1992;39:23–32.

17. Peltola T, Lepojarvi M, Ikaheimo, et al. De Vega's annuloplasty for tricuspid regurgitation. *Ann Chir Gynaecol* 1996;85:40–43.

18. Onate A. Alcibar J, Inguanzo R, Pena N, Gochi R. Balloon dilation of tricuspid and pulmonary valves in carcinoid heart disease. *Tex Heart Inst J* 1993;20:115–119.

19. Attie F, Rosas M, Rijlaarsdam M, et al. The adult patient with Ebstein anomaly; outcome in 72 unoperated patients. *Medicine (Baltimore)* 2000;79;27–36.

20. Scully HE, Armstrong CS. Tricuspid valve replacement: fifteen years of experience with mechanical prostheses and bioprostheses. *J Thorac Cardiovasc Surg* 1995;109:1035–1041.

21. Choi JB, Kim HK, Yoon HS, et al. Partial annular plication for atrioventricular valve regurgitation. *Ann Thorac Surg* 1995;59:891–895.

22. Nadas As, Ellison RC, Weidman WH. Report from the Joint Study on the Natural History of Congenital Heart Defects. *Circulation* 1977;56 Suppl I:I1–I87.

23. O'Fallon WM, Weidman WH. Long-term follow-up of congenital aortic stenosis, pulmonary stenosis and ventricular septal defect: report from the Second Joint Study on the Natural History of Congenital Heart Defects (NHS-2). *Circulation* 1993;87 Suppl I:I1–I126.

24. Kan JS, White RI Jr, Mitchell SE, et al. Percutaneous balloon valvuloplasty: a new method for treating congenital pulmonary-valve stenosis. *N Engl J Med* 1982;307:540–542.

25. Kaul UA, Singh B, Tyagi S, et al. Long-term results after balloon pulmonary valvoplasty in adults. *Am Heart J* 1993;126:115–115.

26. Chen CR, Cheng TO, Huang T, et al. Percutaneous balloon valvuloplasty for pulmonic stenosis in adolescents and adults. *N Engl J Med* 1996;335:21–25.

27. Discigil B, Dearani JA, Puga FJ, et al. Late pulmonary valve replacement after repair of tetralogy of Fallot. *J Thorac Cardiovasc Surg* 2001;121:344–351.

CHAPTER 79

Prosthetic Heart Valves: Choice of Valve and Management of the Patient

Shahbudin H. Rahimtoola / YingXing Wu /
Gary L. Grunkemeier / Albert Starr

PROSTHETIC HEART VALVES

There are two classes of prosthetic heart valves (PHVs): mechanical prostheses, with rigid, manufactured occluder and biologic or tissue valves. There are several types of mechanical valves and of tissue valves obtained from another species, porcine and bovine pericardium. Table 79–1 lists the Food and Drug Administration (FDA)-approved PHVs. To approve a PHV, the FDA requires studies with (1) ≥ 800 valves of followup and (2) the upper confidence limit of the incidence of complications should be less than twice the objective performance criteria (OPC). The OPC was determined by the FDA, which were calculated to allow an alpha error of 5 percent (p <0.05) and a beta error of 20 percent (power of 80 percent).[1,2] OPC are complication rates for critical complications, representing averages that were achieved by the best currently used valves at that time (Table 79–2).[3] Some of the PHV are shown in Figs. 79–1 to 79–5.

MECHANICAL VALVES

Mechanical valves are durable but have the problem of thrombogenicity. The first successful PHV, which led to long-term survivors, used a ball-in-cage design and was introduced in 1960.[4,5] The ball-in-cage PHV that has endured until today is the Starr-Edwards valve models A1200/A1260 and M6120 that were introduced in 1965 and have been virtually unchanged since then (called "Current").[6]

BIOLOGIC VALVES

Biologic valves have low thrombogenicity but have the problem of structural valve deterioration (SVD). *Bioprosthesis* (heterograft or xenograft) is a term that was introduced by Carpentier[7] for nonviable valves of biologic origin, such as the porcine and pericardial valves. Glutaraldehyde sterilizes valve tissue, renders these valves bioacceptable, and stabilizes the collagen cross-links for durability; its use for tissue preservation was pioneered by Carpentier et al.[8] Bioprostheses are mounted on rigid or flexible stents (stented) to which the leaflets and the sewing ring are attached. Nonstented versions are also available (stentless).

Other biologic valves are homografts and the autograft. A *homograft* (or allograft) valve is transplanted from another human, is obtained at autopsy, and was first used in the early 1960s.[9,10] Both stentless porcine valves and homografts that are

TABLE 79–1

FDA-Approved Prosthetic Heart Valves

Mechanical
  Ball and Cage
    Starr-Edwards
  Single Disc
    Medtronic Hall
    Medical Inc. Omniscience
  Bileaflet
    St. Jude Medical
    CarboMedics
    ATS Open Pivot
    On-X
Bioprosthesis
  Stentless Porcine
    Medtronic Hancock Standard
    Medtronic Hancock Modified Orifice
    Carpentier-Edwards Standard
    Carpentier-Edwards Duraflex
    Medtronic Hancock II
    Medtronic Mosaic
    Carpentier-Edwards Supra-annular
    St. Jude Medical Biocor Supra-annular
  Stentless Porcine
    St. Jude Medical Toronto SPV
    Medtronic Freestyle
    Edwards Prima Plus
  Pericardial
    Carpentier-Edwards Perimount
    Carpentier-Edwards Magna

SOURCE: U.S. Food and Drug Administration. Available at: http://www.accessdata.fda.gov/scripts/cdrh/cfdocs/cfPMA/pma.cfm.

TABLE 79–2

FDA Objective Performance Criteria (OPC) for Mechanical and Biological Heart Valves

MORBIDITY	OPC, %/YEAR	
	MECHANICAL	BIOLOGICAL
Structural deterioration	—	—
Nonstructural dysfunction:		
All leaks	1.2	1.2
Major	0.6	0.6
Valve thrombosis	0.8	0.2
Thromboembolism	3.0	2.5
Bleeding:		
All bleeding	3.5	1.4
Major bleeding	1.5	0.9
Prosthetic valve endo-carditis	1.2	1.2

SOURCE: Adapted from Draft Replacement Heart Valve Guidance. Rockville, MD: Prosthetic Devices Branch, Division of Cardiovascular, Respiratory and Neurological Devices, Office of Device Evaluation, Center of Devices and Radiological Health, Food and Drug Administration. October 14,1994.

Cox regression,[15] and multivariable parametric models.[16] The effectiveness of these statistical methods in comparing results from different series, however, is limited by the lack of standardization in definitions and followup methods.

made for aortic valve replacement (AVR) can be implanted in the subcoronary position, aortic root and mini root replacement with part of the donor aortic wall inserted within the host aorta. The latter two techniques need reimplantation of the coronary arteries. The pulmonary *autograft* introduced in 1967 by Ross[11] consists of an autotransplant of the pulmonary valve for AVR and the pulmonary valve is replaced by an aortic or pulmonary homograft or a bioprosthesis, and thus uses double-valves to solve a single-valve problem. It is a technically much-more-demanding procedure that also requires reimplantation of the coronary arteries. Variations of the procedure that were developed by Yacoub and David are different from what Ross described, and, thus, Ross believes it should be called the Ross principle.[12]

GUIDELINES FOR REPORTING CLINICAL RESULTS

The reporting of clinical results of heart valves has evolved since the first successful implants in 1960. As long-term experience accumulated, the need to analyze time-related events resulted in the use of actuarial analysis,[13] constant hazard ("linearized") rates,[14]

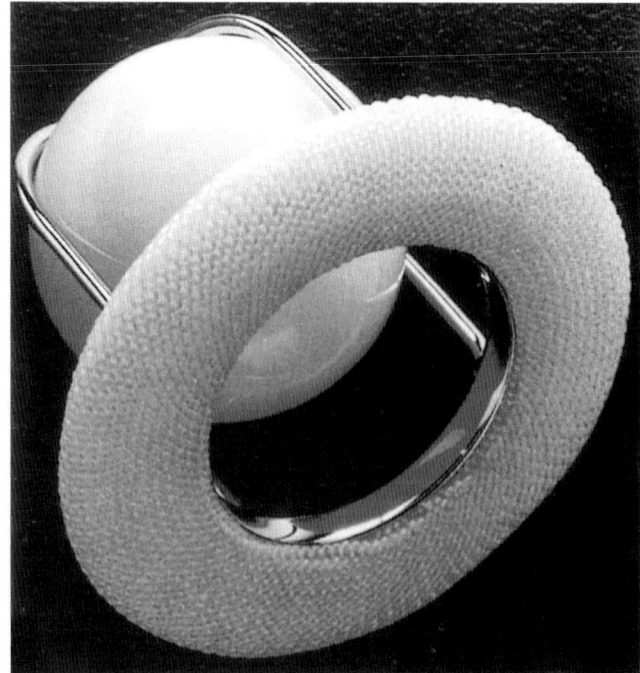

FIGURE 79–1. Starr-Edwards caged ball valve. The ball is a silicone rubber polymer, impregnated with barium sulfate for radiopacity, which oscillates in a cage of cobalt-chromium alloy. When the valve opens, blood flows through the circular primary orifice and a secondary orifice between the ball and the housing. In the aortic position, there is a tertiary orifice between the ball and the aortic wall.

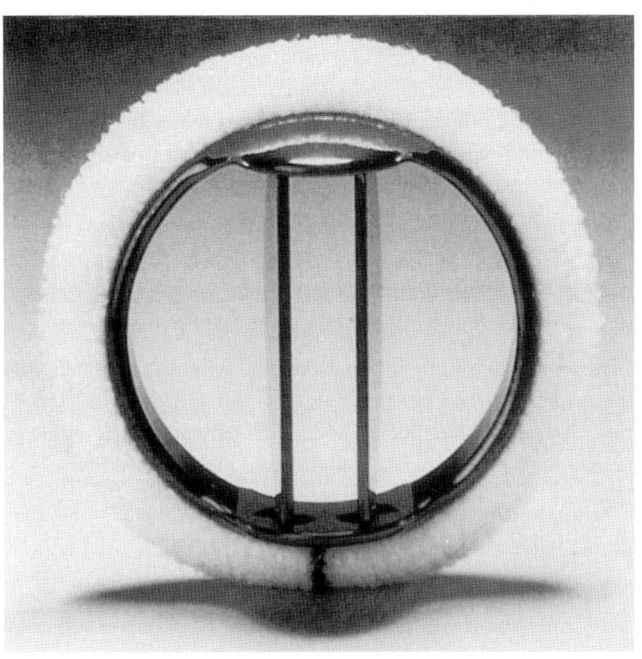

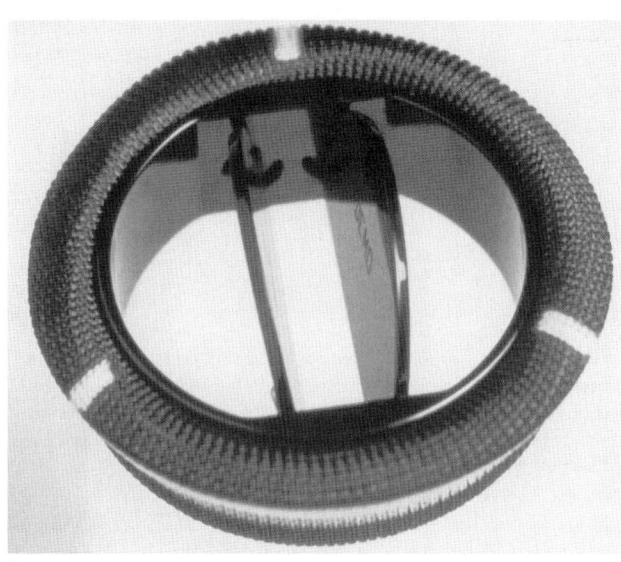

A   B

FIGURE 79-2. Bileaflet valves. The St. Jude Medical valve (**A**) has leaflets that open to an angle of 85 degrees from the plane of the orifice and travel from 55 to 60 degrees to the fully closed position, depending on valve size. The original version, whose housing did not rotate within the sewing ring, has been supplemented by a model that does rotate for intraoperative adjustment. The Carbomedics valve (**B**) has flat leaflets that open to 78 to 80 degrees and close at an angle of 25 degrees with the horizontal and has a carbon-coated surface on the sewing ring to inhibit thrombus formation.

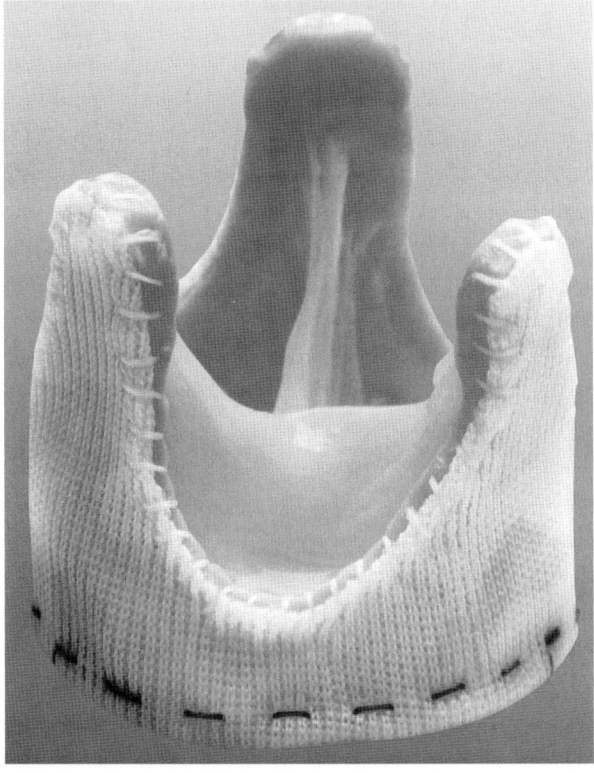

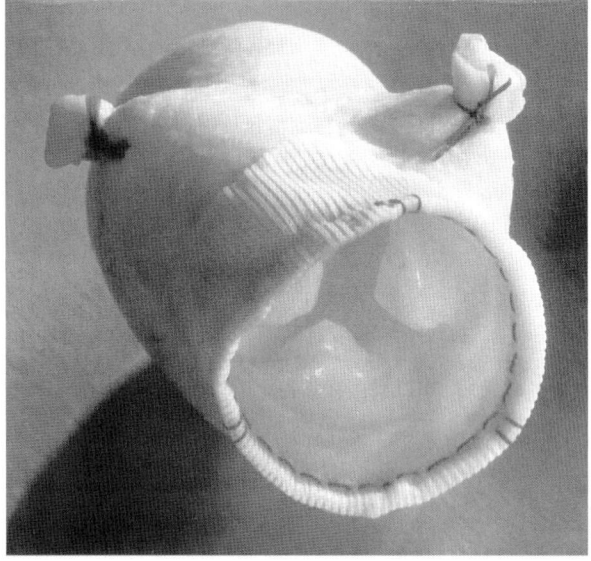

A   B

FIGURE 79-3. St. Jude Toronto SPV (**A**) and Medtronic Freestyle (**B**) stentless porcine valves. The Toronto SPV is designed to be used as a subcoronary valve replacement. The Freestyle can be implanted using any of the methods of implantation used for homografts: subcoronary implantation of the valve alone, aortic root replacement, or cylinder (root) inclusion.

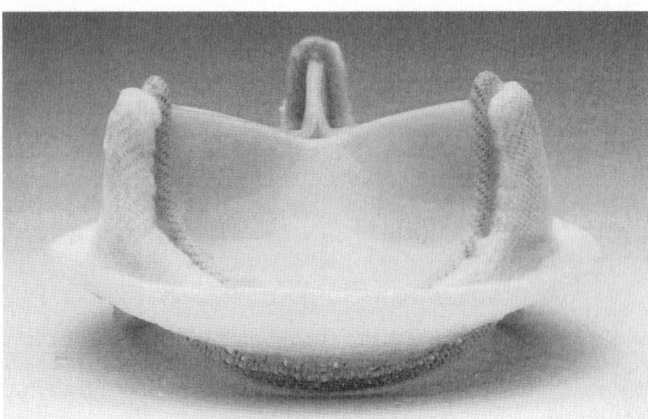

FIGURE 79–4. The Carpentier-Edwards Perimount pericardial bioprosthesis uses a method of mounting the leaflets to the stent, which does not depend on retaining stitches passed through the pericardium—a design weakness of previous pericardial valves. Instead, the leaflets are anchored behind the stent pillars.

[ ] AMERICAN ASSOCIATION FOR THORACIC SURGERY/SOCIETY OF THORACIC SURGEONS GUIDELINES FOR CLINICAL REPORTING

Standards that specified which complications should be collected and how they should be defined were proposed by a joint committee of the American Association for Thoracic Surgery and the Society of Thoracic Surgeons in 1988, and were revised in 1996[17] as follows:

1. *Structural valvular deterioration,* or any change in function of an operated valve resulting from an intrinsic abnormality that causes stenosis or regurgitation.
2. *Nonstructural dysfunction,* a composite category that includes any abnormality that results in stenosis or regurgitation of the operated valve that is not intrinsic to the valve itself, exclusive of thrombosis and infection. This includes inappropriate sizing, which is called *valve prosthesis–patient mismatch (VP-PM).*[18]
3. *Valve thrombosis* is any thrombus, in the absence of infection, attached to or near an operated valve that occludes part of the blood flow path or that interferes with the function of the valve.
4. *Embolism* is any embolic event that occurs in the absence of infection after the immediate perioperative period. These include any new, temporary or permanent, focal, or global neurologic deficits and peripheral embolic events; emboli proven to consist of nonthrombotic material are excluded.
5. *Bleeding* is any episode of major internal or external bleeding that causes death, hospitalization, or permanent injury (e.g., vision loss) or requires transfusion. This applies to all patients, whether or not they are taking anticoagulant or antiplatelet drugs.
6. *Operated valvular endocarditis* is any infection involving an operated valve. Morbidity associated with active infection—such as valve thrombosis, thrombotic embolus, bleeding event, or paravalvular leak—is included under this category but is not included in other categories of morbidity.

The *consequences* of the preceding morbid events include reoperation, valve-related mortality, sudden unexpected unexplained death, cardiac death, total deaths, and permanent valve-related impairment.

The assumption of constant risk for heart valve complications, as embodied by the OPC formulation, is only an approximation; but if operative events are excluded and followup is of sufficient length, this approximation may be acceptable. However, patients with a disabling stroke and their families do not particularly care if the event occurred operatively or later; therefore, all events must be included in long-term followup results.

CHOICE OF PROSTHETIC HEART VALVE

The choice of a PHV for an individual patient has to take into account known patient outcomes (survival and complications) with use of a particular PHV. The known patient outcomes are influenced by *factors* related to publications and to patients.

[ ] FACTORS RELATING TO PUBLISHED DATA

The wide variations in reported complications described below with even the use of the same model of PHV is a result of many different problems, which include the following:

1. *Reporting center*—medical and surgical variables, postoperative medical management, method, frequency and thoroughness of followup, definitions of complications.
2. Problems with *data analysis*[19,20]—many patient-related factors are known to influence thromboembolism,[21,22] stroke rates in patients with atrial fibrillation and in the elderly are equal to those observed in prosthetic valve series,[23] and standardized definitions[17] were not in effect or were not employed when many of the available series were reported.
3. *Published data*—these reports describe only a small fraction of the valves implanted and are probably not a representative subset. Several types of bias can affect reported results. As exam-

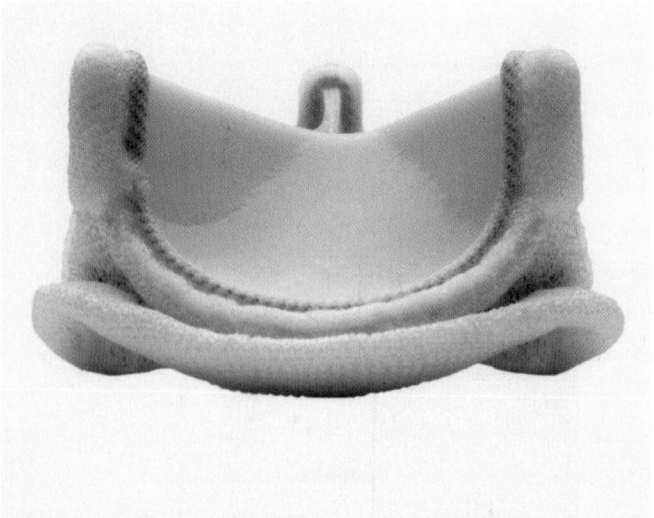

FIGURE 79–5. The Carpentier-Edwards Perimount Magna pericardial aortic bioprosthesis is constructed with a durable Elgiloy wire stent, has a compact and flexible sewing ring, and unsurpassed supra-annular construction. These features allow for a one-size-larger valve to be placed in a given patient's annulus. Because of its larger prosthetic heart valve area, this valve is of greater importance especially in the small valve sizes. *Source: Print of figure provided by Edwards Lifesciences.*

ples, selection bias occurs in the collection and analysis of data and the decision to report them[19]; publication bias is described by the fact that published series tend to be those with the best or worst, but not typical results.[24]

[ ] PATIENT-RELATED FACTORS

An initial review in 1988 concluded that patient comorbid conditions were one of the most important factors in determining patient's outcomes including operative and late mortality (Table 79–3) and other valve-related complications.[21]

Special care must also be exercised in interpreting data on operative mortality and late mortality because both are influenced by the valvular conditions and the patient's comorbidities, both cardiac and noncardiac (Table 79–4). Average mortalities from even large databases, such as Medicare, Society of Thoracic Surgeons[25] multicenter data, and even those from large-volume centers, do not necessarily provide detailed analyses of results, taking into account the appropriateness of the patients and adequate baseline data, including comorbidities and their combinations.[21,25,26] Similarly, large-volume centers do not necessarily provide the best outcomes compared to those from smaller-volume centers because they may have more complex cases referred to them, and in all centers, including large-volume centers, the skill and experience of individual surgeons and of surgical teams is a very important determinant of outcomes.

A subsequent review[27] of a large number of published reports concerning the performance of prosthetic heart valves reveals a widespread of results for every complication for every valve indicating that *patient-related factors* are very important determinants of complications of PHV.[21,27] In 172 series of heart valves covering 335,485 valve-years accumulated by 63,531 valves, the event rates ranged from 0 to 7.5 percent per year for thromboembolism; from 0 to 0.6 percent per year for thrombosis; from 0 to 9.3 percent per year for bleeding; from 0 to 1.7 percent per year for infection; and from 0 to 2.8 percent per year for paravalvular leak.[27] Caution must be exercised in directly comparing event rates among valves for many reasons, including the simplifications involved in the use of linearized rates, varying definitions of complications (many of

these reports predate the standardized definitions), and differences in patient characteristics between series.[21,27]

The 10- to 15-year mortality rates after AVR and mitral valve replacement (MVR) are high. The range is large, even with the use of the same brand of PHV, indicating the importance of factors other than the type of PHV.[28] Table 79–4 lists the risk factors for late mortality.

[ ] RANDOMIZED TRIALS

In view of the above known difficulties one has to carefully evaluate data from randomized trials. Although randomized trials provide ideal internal validity or valve-specific comparison within centers, they may lack external validity or generalizability to patients outside the study.[29] Randomized trials of heart valves can also have logistic and financial problems.[30,31] Consequently, the number of randomized studies of valves is small, and those that exist are of necessity of small size, thus these data must be interpreted along with those from high-quality observational studies that are carefully and properly analyzed.

Two small randomized trials compared two mechanical valves. The St. Louis trial randomized 156 patients,[32] mean age 80 years, to receive the St. Jude (n = 80) or the Medtronic hall (n = 76) PHV for MVR between 1986 and 1997. The operative mortality was 11.2 percent versus 13.1 percent. At 10 years there was no significant difference in survival or in events between the two PHV outcomes except for reoperation, which was 0 percent for the St. Jude versus 21 percent for the Medtronic Hall (*p* = 0.01).

A larger trial from London, UK[33] randomized 387 patients to receive the St. Jude or Starr-Edwards PHV between December 1991 and June 1997; 267 patients had AVR and 122 had MVR. At the end of 8 years survival and event-free survival with the two valves was almost identical after AVR and after MVR (Fig. 79–6).

TABLE 79–3

Factors That Influence Valve Surgery

Results of valve surgery with regard to
- Survival
- Complications
- Valve function
- Cardiac function
- Functional class

Are dependent on
- Patient-related factors[a]
- Type of surgery
- Type of prosthesis
- Healthcare delivery factors

[a]Now called *comorbid conditions*.
SOURCE: *Rahimtoola SH. Lessons learned about the determinants of the results of valve surgery. Circulation 1988;78:1503–1507.*

TABLE 79–4

Factors Influencing Operative and Late Mortality after PHV[a]

- Decade of age
- Other valve disease
- Complications of PHV
- Comorbid conditions
  - Cardiac
    LV dysfunction, heart failure, NYHA functional class III and IV, CAD, myocardial infarction, CABG, arrhythmias (e.g., atrial fibrillation), pulmonary hypertension
  - Noncardiac
    Impaired renal function (creatinine clearance), renal dialysis, diabetes, hypertension, dyslipidemia, metabolic syndrome, smoking, liver disease, lung disease (e.g., COPD)

CABG, coronary artery bypass graft; CAD, coronary artery disease; COPD, chronic obstructive pulmonary disease; LV, left ventricle; NYHA, New York Heart Association; PHV, prosthetic heart valve.
[a]For operative (30-day mortality) additional factors include emergency surgery > urgent > elective; previous cardiac surgery; perioperative myocardial infarction; duration of the operation and of aortic cross clamp time.
SOURCE: *Copyright S.H. Rahimtoola.*

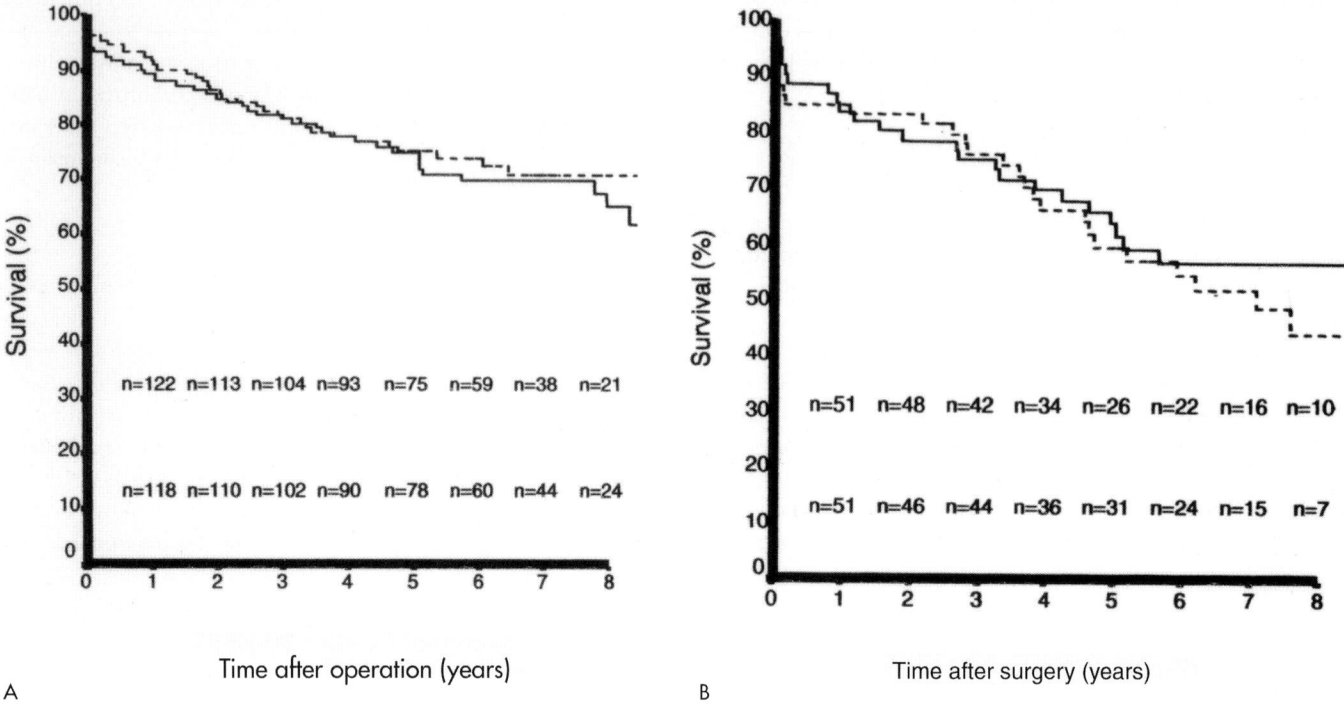

FIGURE 79–6. Survival after aortic valve replacement (AVR) (**A**) and mitral valve replacement (MVR) (**B**) with Starr-Edwards and St. Jude Medical prosthetic heart valves. Dashed lines, St. Jude Medical; solid lines, Starr-Edwards. *Source: From Murday AJ, Hochstitzky A, Mansfield J, et al. A prospective controlled trial of St. Jude versus Starr-Edwards aortic and mitral valve prosthesis. Ann Thorac Surg 2003;76:66–73, with permission.*

Two large randomized trials have compared patient outcomes with use of a mechanical valve (Delrin ring, tilting disk, Bjork-Shiley) and a porcine valve (Hancock or Carpentier-Edwards).

Edinburgh Heart Valve Trial

A total of 541 men and women were randomized between 1975 and 1979; 211 had AVR, 261 had MVR, and 61 had AVR plus MVR.[34] The average followup was 12 years. The major findings were as follows: (1) there was a trend toward an improved survival with the Bjork-Shiley valve ($p = 0.08$). (2) Reoperation rates were low and nonsignificant at 5 years, but at 12 years there was a higher reoperation rate with the porcine valve than with the mechanical valve (AVR 22.6 ± 5.7 percent vs. 4.2 ± 2.1 percent, $p <0.01$; MVR 43.1 ± 6.0 percent vs. 9.9 ± 3.2 percent, $p <0.001$). Younger patients were more likely to require reoperation, with "relative risk of reoperation increasing 55 percent for each 10 years, continuously over the whole range of ages studied." (3) The incidence of thromboembolism and of endocarditis were not statistically significantly different. (4) The bleeding rate was higher with the mechanical valve than with the porcine valve after AVR (32.6 ± 6.1 percent vs. 9.7 ± 4.7 percent, $p <0.001$) but not after MVR (24.5 percent vs. 24.5 percent). (5) There was no instance of SVD with the Bjork-Shiley valve. (6) SVD of the porcine valve began at about 5 to 6 years after MVR and at about 7 to 8 years after AVR. A subsequent report from the Edinburgh Trial,[35] with a mean followup of 18 years, showed that at 20 years there was no difference in survival, embolism, or endocarditis between the two valve types. The incidence of reoperation was higher with the porcine valve and bleeding was higher in those who had received the Bjork-Shiley valve. Survival at 20 years with the original PHV was much lower with the porcine valve than with the mechanical valve (Table 79–5).

Department of Veterans Affairs Trial

A total of 575 men were randomized between 1997 and 1982; 394 had AVR and 181 had MVR.[36]

Followup was up to 18 years; average followup was 15 years (Table 79–6). The principal long-term findings were as follows: (1) after AVR, use of the mechanical valve resulted in a lower mortality (66 ± 3 percent vs. 79 ± 3 percent, $p = 0.02$; Fig. 79–7) and a lower reoperation rate (10 ± 3 percent vs. 29 ± 5 percent, $p = 0.004$). The difference became apparent after 10 years, indicating the need for followup at ±15 years. The mortality after MVR was similar (81 percent vs. 79 percent). (2) After AVR, approximately 40 percent of the mortality was related to the PHV. After MVR, 44 percent of the mortality with mechanical valve and 57 percent of the mortality with bioprosthesis were related to the PHV. (3) There was *no* SVD with the mechanical valve. (4) Primary valve failure occurred mainly in patients who were younger than age 65 years (Table 79–6). It began at about 5 to 6 years after MVR and at about 7 to 8 years after AVR. Its incidence was higher after MVR (44 ± 8 percent vs. 23 ± 5 percent). (5) More than 10 years of followup was needed to determine the incidence and deleterious effects of SVD with use of porcine valve (Fig. 79–7). The primary valve failure rate between bioprosthesis and mechanical valve was not significantly different in those age 65 years or older after AVR. (7) Use of a bioprosthetic valve resulted in a lower bleeding rate. (8) There were no significant differences between the two valve types with regard to other valve-related complications, including thromboembolism and all complications (Table 79–7).

TABLE 79–5

Twenty-Year Outcome Data from Edinburgh Heart Valve Trial

	AVR			MVR		
	MECHANICAL	PORCINE	*p* VALUE	MECHANICAL	PORCINE	*p* VALUE
Survival						
All survivors	28.4 (4.4)	31.3 (4.7)	0.57	22.4 (3.8)	18.4 (3.6)	0.41
With original prosthesis	7.5 (4.3)	13.7 (3.6)	0.025	20.7 (7.5)	3.1 (3.1)	0.002
Without major event	15.2 (3.5)	8.1 (3.0)	0.34	17.2 (7.0)	3.1 (3.1)	0.018
Valve-related events						
Reoperation	7.4 (3.0)	56.2 (8.4)	<0.0001	13.4 (3.9)	77.6 (6.7)	<0.0001
All bleeding	61.1 (7.6)	42.4 (12.1)	0001	53.1 (8.2)	37.2 (0.9)	0.39
Major bleeding	8 (7.1)	32.0 (12.6)	0.021	47.3 (8.5)	9.5 (4.1)	0.044

AVR, aortic valve replacement; MVR, mitral valve replacement.
Source: Adapted from Oxenham H, Bloomfield P, Wheatley DJ et al. Twenty year comparison of a Bjork-Shiley mechanical heart valve with porcine bioprostheses. Heart 2003;89:715–721.

Major Differences between the Edinburgh and Department of Veterans Affairs Trials

The bleeding rate in the Edinburgh Heart Valve trial was 2 to 2.5 percent per year with the mechanical valve and 0.9 to 2 percent per year with the porcine valve.[34,35] After MVR the bleeding rates with a mechanical and porcine valve were not different, probably because many patients with porcine valves needed anticoagulation for other reasons, most likely atrial fibrillation. The exact reasons for the high bleeding rate in the Department of Veterans Affairs trial are not clear.[28] In the Department of Veterans Affairs trial it was recommended that prothrombin time should be maintained at 2.0 to 2.5 times control,[28] which is excessive anticoagulation. Also, some patients with porcine valves were anticoagulated and all bleeding episodes were included because it is not possible to separate bleeding caused by anticoagulation from that as a result of other causes.

The Department of Veterans Affairs trial had 87 percent more patients undergoing isolated AVR and 31 percent fewer patients undergoing isolated MVR than the Edinburgh Heart Valve Trial. These differences may account for differences in outcomes, especially with regard to mortality.

[ ] STRUCTURAL VALVE DETERIORATION

Mechanical Valves

The SVD of currently used mechanical valves is extremely low and remarkable, given the harsh biologic environment in which the valve must perform. For example, SVD of the Starr-Edwards valve is virtually zero after 38 years of followup; there were 6 cases in over 1 million patient-years of followup for a rate of 0.0005 percent per year. In the Starr series of "current" valves there was no SVD up to 35 to 40 years of followup (Fig. 79–8).[6] In the Edinburgh and Department of Veterans Affairs trials there were no instances of SVD with the Delrin ring Bjork-Shiley PHV.

Biologic Valves

Figure 79–9 shows the data on freedom from SVD for series of *porcine* and *pericardial bioprostheses* and *homografts*. The mean age

of patients in the older series is about 50 years. The durability of the Carpentier-Edwards pericardial valve appears superior to that of porcine valves (Fig. 79–9 and Table 79–8). The patients in the Carpentier-Edwards pericardial valve series were older than patients in previous series of porcine valves, and it is unknown to what extent this resulted in the improvement in their durability. However, more recent studies show the rate of SVD of the Carpentier-Edwards PHV is much lower than with porcine PHV.[37–39]

SVD with *homografts* is not, in general, better than with porcine bioprostheses (see Fig. 79–9). A study from Palka et al.[40] of 570 patients ages 48 ± 16 years showed the incidence of SVD detected by Doppler echocardiography at 6.8 years after aortic valve replacement was 72.1 percent.[40] A recent study has shown that in age groups ≤ 50 years, 50 to 60 years and >60 years at time of PHV, the incidence of SVD of homografts was similar to that of Carpentier-Edwards pericardial valves;[41] however, the followup of patients with homograft PHV was of shorter duration.

The pulmonary *autograft* is considered an "excellent" aortic valve substitute, for young patients. However, data from one center, which is the only one with followup for longer than 10 years, showed 48.5 percent freedom from reoperation at 19 years[42] and, after *excluding* patients from three hospitals, 85 percent freedom from reoperation

TABLE 79–6

Primary Valve Failure at 15 Years

AORTIC VALVE REPLACEMENT WITH PORCINE BIOPROSTHESIS

• Mechanical valve	0% ± 0%	*p* = 0.00001
• Bioprosthesis	23% + 5%	
• Age <65 years	26% ± 6%[a]	
• Age ≥65 years	9% ± 6%[b,c]	

[a]Versus mechanical valve *p* = 0.001.
[b]Versus mechanical valve *p* = 0.16.
[c]Not structural value deterioration.
Source: Adapted from DVA trial. Hammermeister KE, Sethi GK, Henderson WC, et al.[36]

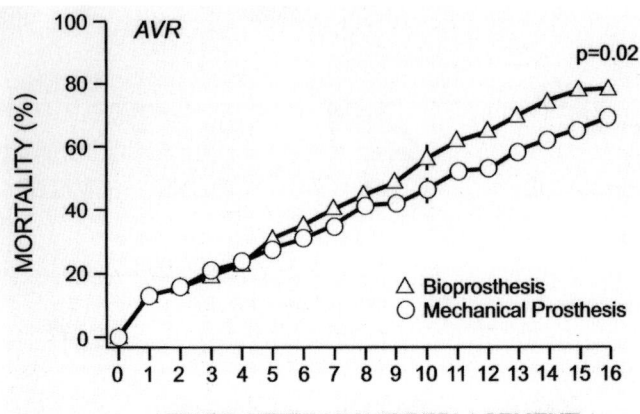

FIGURE 79–7. Mortality after aortic valve replacement (AVR) with the Bjork-Shiley and porcine valves from the Department of Veterans Affairs trial. *Source: From Hammermeister KE, Sethi GK, Henderson WC, et al. Outcomes 15 years after valve replacement with a mechanical versus bioprosthetic valve: final report of the Veterans Administration trial. J Am Coll Cardiol 2000;36:1152–1158.*

at 20 years.[43] A recent study of 91 patients (ages 27 ± 10 years) had a followup of 4.0 ± 1.9 years (range: 1 to 8 years).[44] At 7 years, the incidence of aortic dilatation was 58 ± 8 percent, the incidence of autograft regurgitation was 25 ± 8 percent, and the incidence of reoperation was 15 ± 10 percent. To evaluate complications of this procedure fully, problems with the valve used to replace the pulmonary valve must be combined with complications of the pulmonary autograft itself. In one study of 144 patients,[45] at a mean followup of 4 years, 15 (10 percent) patients had developed peak gradient across the homograft in the pulmonary position measured by magnetic resonance imaging of ≥ 30 mmHg (mean: 46 ± 18 mmHg) and 4 had to be reoperated. At 7 years, pulmonary homograft stenosis was 20.3

percent and reoperation rate was 3.3 percent. SVD of the pulmonary homograft is "clinically important"[45] and is an early postoperative inflammatory reaction to the pulmonary autograft that leads to extrinsic compression and/or shrinkage.[45] In small children this problem may be mitigated by use of the diseased aortic valve in the pulmonary position within a pericardial tube (unpublished data from Starr Wood Children's Cardiac Center).

【 】 SUMMARY

Table 79–9 lists the factors that need to be considered when choosing a PHV.

1. Mechanical valves are durable. Thus the question of which type of mechanical valve to use is dependent on other issues, for example, cause of insertion, experience, and physician preference, in FDA-approved PHV with known good outcomes ≥ 10 years on followup.
2. Homografts have a similar rate of SVD as bioprostheses, involve a more complex surgical procedure that is very much more complex at reoperation and perioperative myocardial infarction,[46] and are more expensive than bioprostheses. The main use for homografts is in patients with acute, active infective endocarditis[47] with a complication, such as an abscess; however, this does not imply its exclusive use in these clinical situations.
3. The benefits of the Ross principle in adults still needs to be proven.[28]
4. The most frequent issue in clinical decision making is whether to choose a mechanical or bioprosthetic PHV. The choice is based on balancing the disadvantages of these two types of PHV: anticoagulants and its complications with use of mechanical valve versus SVD and its complications with use of a bioprosthesis.[28] Figure 79–10 shows the recommendations based on age (and therefore rate of SVD) and ability to take

TABLE 79–7

Probability of Death from Any Cause, Any Valve-Related Complication, and Individual Valve-Related Complications 15 Years after Randomization

OUTCOME EVENT	AORTIC VALVE REPLACEMENT			MITRAL VALVE REPLACEMENT		
	MECHANICAL	BIOPROSTHETIC	p	MECHANICAL	BIOPROSTHESIS	p
	n = 198	n = 196		n = 88	n = 93	
Death from any cause	66 ± 3%[a]	79 ± 3%	0.02	81 ± 4%	79 ± 4%	0.30
Any valve-related complication	65 ± 4%	66 ± 5%	0.26	73 ± 6%	81 ± 5%	0.56
Systemic embolism	18 ± 4%	18 ± 4%	0.66	18 ± 5%	22 ± 5%	0.96
Bleeding	51 ± 4%	30 ± 4%	0.0001	53 ± 7%	31 ± 6%	0.01
Endocarditis	7 ± 2%	15 ± 5%	0.45	11 ± 4%	17 ± 5%	0.37
Valve thrombosis	2 ± 1%	1 ± 1%	0.33	1 ± 1%	1 ± 1%	0.95
Perivalvular regurgitation	8 ± 2%	2 ± 1%	0.09	17 ± 5%	7 ± 4%	0.05
Reoperation	10 ± 3%	29 ± 5%	0.0004	25 ± 6%	50 ± 8%	0.15
Primary valve failure	0 ± 0%	23 ± 5%	0.0001	5 ± 4%	44 ± 8%	0.0002

n, Number of patients randomized.
[a]Values given are actuarial percentages ± standard error.
NOTE: *p* values are for differences between mechanical and porcine valves.
SOURCE: *From Hammermeister KE, Sethi GK, Henderson WC, et al. Outcomes 15 years after valve replacement with a mechanical versus bioprosthetic valve: final report of the Veterans Administration trial. J Am Coll Cardiol 2000;36:1152–1158.*

A

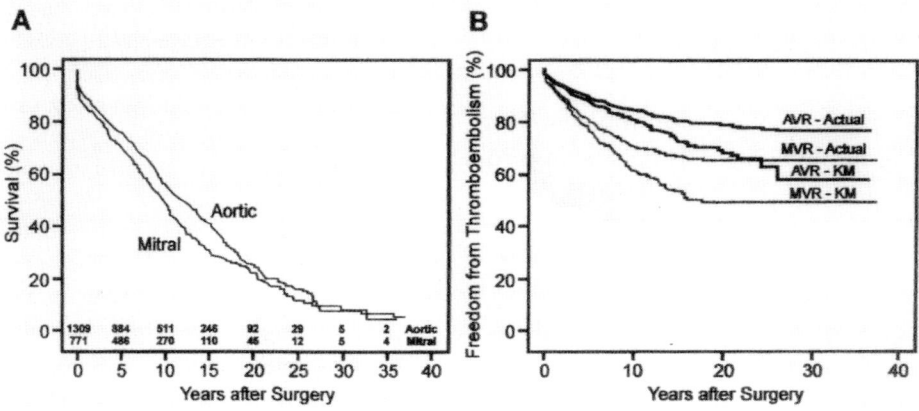

FIGURE 79-8. A. Actuarial survival curves after aortic valve replacement (AVR) and mitral valve replacement (MVR) in the "current" Starr-Edwards valves. **B.** Kaplan-Meier (KM) actuarial and actual freedom from thromboembolism after AVR and MVR with "current" valve. *Source: From Gao G, Wu YX, Grunkemeier GL, et al. Forty-year survival with the Starr-Edwards heart valve prosthesis. J Heart Valve Dis 2004;13:91–96.*

SPECIAL CIRCUMSTANCES

Renal Failure

The Society of Thoracic Surgeons Database shows that the operative mortality of valve replacement in patients on dialysis ranges from 17 to 22 percent and of valve replacement plus coronary artery bypass graft ranges from 25 to 37 percent.[25] The Renal Data System study of 5858 patients on renal dialysis[50] showed the mortality with mechanical and bioprosthetic PHV was similar; at 1, 2, 3, 5, and 10 years it was approximately 45, 60, 72, 85, and 95 percent, respectively. Approximately half of the deaths were from a cardiac cause; the nature of the cardiac cause was not provided nor was the incidence of SVD.

warfarin anticoagulant therapy.[28] Table 79–10 lists the American College of Cardiologists/American Heart Association (ACC/AHA) recommendations.[48] It must be *emphasized* that all such recommendations cannot apply to each and every patient because there are exceptions, and several factors that must be considered are shown in Table 79–9.

5. The choice between the two types of bioprosthesis (pericardial vs. porcine) indicates a superiority of the pericardial valves because of a lower rate of SVD. Even the newer porcine valves have a SVD rate that is similar to the older porcine valve and is higher than that seen with the pericardial valve (see Fig. 79–8). In addition, better hemodynamics, that is smaller gradients and PHV areas in the in vitro studies and larger PHV areas in patient studies, indicate a superiority of the pericardial valve.[28,38,39]

6. Octogenarians have a much better 5-year survival with bioprostheses than with a mechanical valve after AVR (81.7 percent vs. 56.7 percent, *p* = 0.02).[49]

Certain issues need to be emphasized when choosing a PHV.

1. The randomized trials and data with the Starr-Edwards valve show that the mechanical valves are durable[6,34–36] in FDA-approved valves, with "good" outcome results at followup of ≥ 10 years.

2. The Department of Veterans Affairs randomized trial[36] showed that after AVR approximately 60 percent of deaths and after MVR approximately 40 to 60 percent of the deaths are not caused by the PHV, again emphasizing the importance of a patient's comorbid conditions in determining patient outcomes (see Fig. 79–10).[21,13,27]

Furthermore, the very high mortality that is as high as or higher than that of medical therapy emphasizes that the important issue is not choice of PHV but selection of patients for PHV insertion.

Young Women

For a young woman who needs a PHV and who is planning a subsequent pregnancy, the choice is between a mechanical PHV and a bioprosthesis because the incidence of SVD with a homograft is similar

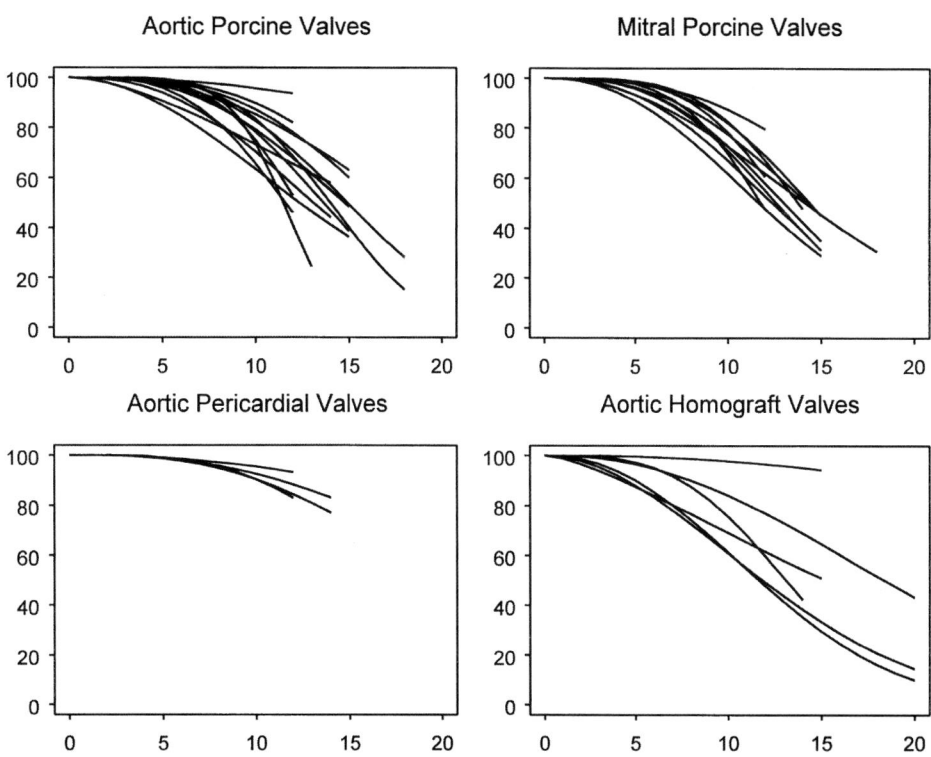

FIGURE 79-9. Structural valve deterioration (SVD) with four types of biologic valves. The vertical axes represent freedom from SVD; horizontal axes represent years after implant. These followup data relate to studies with minimum followup to 400 valve years and conform to FDA requirements for each location of valve. *Source: From Grunkemier GL, Li H-H, Starr A, et al. Long-term performance of heart valve prostheses. Curr Prob Cardiol 2000;25:75–154.*

TABLE 79–8

Fourteen-Year Results with Carpentier-Edwards Pericardial Valve

		FDA-MANDATED PATIENTS[a] (n = 267) ACTUARIAL (%)
Thromboembolism/thrombosis		19 ± 4
Anticoagulant-related bleeding		6 ± 2
Endocarditis/sepsis		7 ± 2
Valve dysfunction		70 ± 4
Explant because of structural valve deterioration:	Total	15 ± 3
	≤ 65 years of age	24 ± 5
	> 65 years of age	4 ± 2
Mortality:	Total	60 ± 3.1
	Valve-related	21 ± 3.2

[a]FDA approval was based on 719 patients at 7 years.
SOURCE: *Data from FDA-mandated longer followup of selected patients are from Frater RWM, Furlong P, Cosgrove DM, et al. Long-term durability and patient functional status of the Carpentier-Edwards Perimount pericardial bioprosthesis in the aortic position. J Heart Valve Dis 1998;7:48–53.*

to that of a bioprosthesis. The incidence of SVD and of other complications with the Ross principle in patients in their 20s is not low. In addition, the results with the autograft data (Ross principle) beyond 10 years are conflicting. Moreover, reoperation on autografts and homografts is very complex and a very-much-more-demanding procedure. The main disadvantage with mechanical PHV is the need for warfarin and of consequent warfarin embryopathy, which is low (0 to 3 percent) with close monitoring of warfarin therapy.[51] With bioprostheses the incidence of early SVD during pregnancy and shortly after delivery is as high as 24 percent, and at 10 years it is 55 to 57 percent; moreover, the operative mortality of reoperation for SVD is 3.8 to 8.7 percent.[51] Discontinuing warfarin and substituting intravenous unfractionated heparin in the first 6 to 12 weeks and the last 2 weeks of pregnancy reduces the incidence of warfarin embryopathy and of bleeding in the mother and baby during delivery. The data with low-molecular-weight heparin remains to be defined. The choice of PHV should be a joint decision by the *patient*, cardiologist, and cardiac surgeon (Fig. 79–11).[51]

VALVE REPAIR

[ ] MITRAL VALVE

When practicable, mitral valve repair is preferable to replacement. Mitral valve repair also provides good results for treating infective endocarditis[52] and for valve problems, even in elderly patients.[53] It has been suggested that it improves survival; however, there are problems associated with the comparisons (see Chap. 76).[21]

The weakness of valve repair is durability. The 10-year actuarial reoperation rate is reported to be 15 percent in nonrheumatic mitral disease.[54] The reoperation rate for patients with rheumatic mitral disease varies from 25 percent at 5 years[55] to 17 percent at 10 years in a large series in which calcium debridement[56] and anterior leaflet procedures were performed.[57] The reoperation rate at 10 years was

24 percent for patients younger than 20 years of age, and 9 percent at 10 years for patients older than 20 years of age.[58]

The longest followup with median followup of 17 years (range: 1 to 29 years) after mitral valve repair for mitral valve prolapse performed from 1970 to 1984 is from Carpentier's group,[59] which excluded patients with ischemic heart disease and those with associated cardiac or vascular procedures (Fig. 79–12). The hospital mortality was 1.9 percent (95 percent confidence interval [CI] 0.5 to 5.7 percent). The 20-year mortality was 53 percent for the whole group (95 percent CI 45 to 61 percent); in those with only posterior leaflet involvement mortality was 54 percent, for anterior leaflet involvement was 54 percent and for involvement of both leaflets 50 percent. The reoperation rate at 20 years for posterior leaflet involvement was 3.1 percent, for anterior leaflet involvement it was 13.8 percent, and for both leaflets involvement was 17.4 percent. There is another study of mitral valve repair for mitral regurgitation largely caused by degenerative mitral valve.[60] At 5 years, the survival of those without atrial fibrillation was 93 percent (95 percent CI 90 to 97 percent) versus 73 percent (95 percent CI 64 to 82 percent) for patients with atrial fibrillation; patients with atrial fibrillation had many comorbid conditions.[57] However, on multivariate analysis the only predictor of inferior survival was poor left ventricular function, which was assessed *subjectively* from echocardiograms and left ventricular angiograms.

The longest followup (up to 29 years) after mitral valve reconstructive surgery for rheumatic mitral regurgitation performed from 1970 to 1994 is also from Carpentier's group,[61] which excluded patients with associated valve lesions, organic tricuspid valve lesions, and those with coronary artery disease (Fig. 79–13); the hospital mortality was 2 percent. At 20 years, survival was 82 ± 18 percent and reoperation rate was 45 percent; the incidence of atrial fibrillation in patients who were in New York Heart Associa-

TABLE 79–9

Decision for Choice of Prosthetic Heart Valve

Factors to be considered
  Age of the patient
  Comorbid conditions
    Cardiac
    Noncardiac
  Expected life span of patient
  Long-term known outcomes with prosthetic heart valve
  Skill and experience with procedure(s) and prosthetic
    heart valve at the Medical Center and of Physicians
  Patient's "wishes"
  Other extenuating circumstances

SOURCE: *Copyright by S. H. Rahimtoola.*

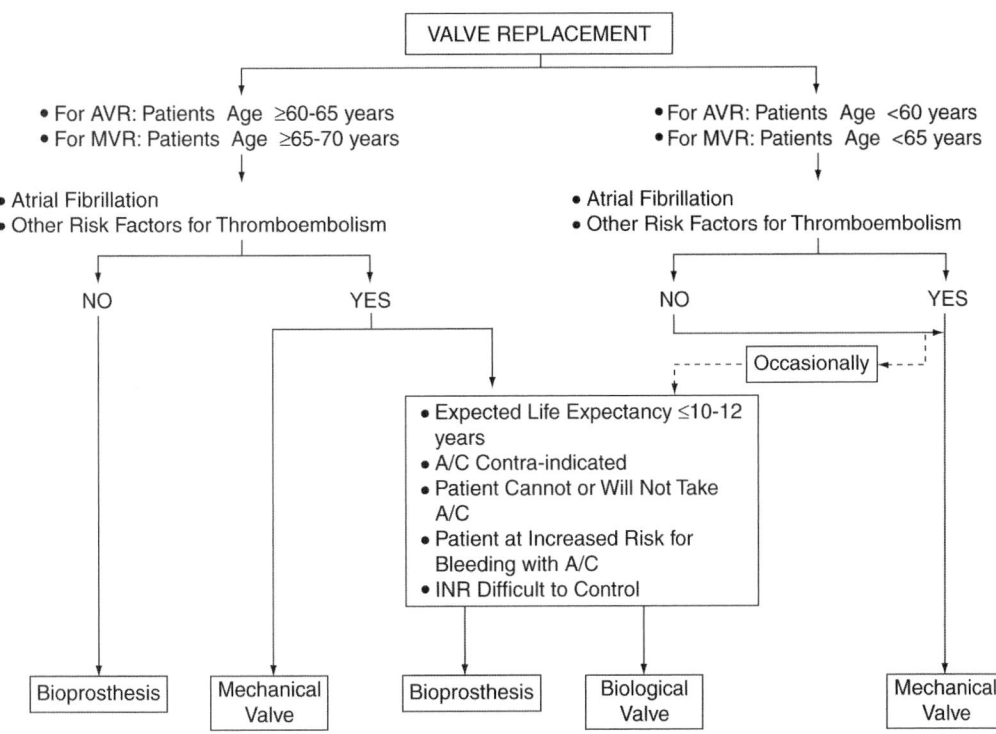

FIGURE 79–10. Suggested recommendation for choice of prosthetic heart valves based on age of the patient and the presence of risk factors. A/C, anticoagulation with warfarin; AVR, aortic valve replacement; INR, internationalized ratio; MVR, mitral valve replacement. *Source: From Rahimtoola SH.[28]*

tion (NYHA) functional classes I and II was 53 and 96 percent, respectively. Early results of aortic valve repair have been published, but further followup is needed to assess the long-term results.

Mitral valve repair is often feasible if patients are operated very early in the course of infective endocarditis. The feasibility of mitral valve repair ranges from 37 percent to 81 percent.[62,63] The hospital mortality was 3 percent.[62–64] The incidence of reoperation was 1.8 percent and at 10 years was 9 percent.[64] Survival at 1 year was 93 percent, at 5 years ranged from 91 percent to 96 percent, and at 10 years ranged from 61 percent to 80 percent.[62–64]

AORTIC VALVE

At one medical center between 1986 and 2001, 1410 patients had surgery for severe aortic regurgitation of whom 160 (11 percent) had AVrep.[65] There was one operative death (0.6 percent), and two patients required early re-repair; at a mean interval of 2.8 years 10 percent had re-operation. At seven years, survival was 89 percent and re-operation on the AV was 15 percent. At another center AVrep was performed in 57 percent of patients undergoing surgery for aortic regurgitation.[66] Hospital mortality was 3.9 percent; re-operation for recurrent AR was 3.3 percent. In patients with isolated repair, isolated root repair, and a combination of both, at 5 years the incidence of aortic regurgitation grade II or higher was 19 percent, 16 percent, and 6 percent, respectively; the incidence of reoperation was 7 percent, 5 percent, and 2 percent, respectively. The difference in these two reports are probably best explained by differences in the patient population.

MANAGEMENT OF PATIENTS WITH PROSTHETIC HEART VALVES

Patients who have undergone valve replacement are *not* cured; they still have serious heart disease. They have exchanged native valvular disease for prosthetic valvular disease and must be followed with great care.[67] The clinical course of patients with prosthetic heart valves is influenced by several factors.

VENTRICULAR DYSFUNCTION

Despite relief of valvular obstruction or regurgitation, some patients fail to improve after valve replacement or even deteriorate because of ventricular dysfunction. The cause of dysfunction may be carditis associated with rheumatic disease, myocardial degeneration and fibrosis from long-standing pressure or volume overload, ischemic damage at the time of valve replacement, coronary artery disease (CAD), or other associated diseases such as systemic hypertension or idiopathic dilated cardiomyopathy. Perioperative myocardial damage is an important cause of postoperative ventricular dysfunction.

OTHER CARDIAC LESIONS

Cardiac diseases affecting primarily one valve often affect other valves, the conduction system, the coronary arteries, and the pulmonary vasculature. With the exception of pulmonary hypertension and functional tricuspid regurgitation, these disorders usually do not improve after isolated valve replacement. Rheumatic disease typically affects both mitral and aortic valves but not necessarily with the same severity at the same time. Therefore, patients who have mitral valve replacement may subsequently, years later, require aortic valve replacement, or vice versa. Calcification of the aortic and mitral valve annuli may extend to the conduction system. High-degree or complete atrioventricular block may occur at the time of surgery or during the late postoperative period, requiring pacemaker implantation. CAD is very common in the age range of patients requiring valve replacement; preoperative coro-

TABLE 79–10

Major Criteria for Aortic Valve Selection

Class I

1. A mechanical prosthesis is recommended for aortic valve replacement (AVR) in patients with a mechanical valve in the mitral or tricuspid position. *(Level of Evidence: C)*
2. A bioprostheses is recommended for AVR in patients of any age who will not take warfarin or who have major medical contraindications to warfarin therapy. *(Level of Evidence: C)*

Class IIa

1. Patient preference is a reasonable consideration in the selection of aortic valve operation and valve prosthesis. A mechanical prosthesis is reasonable for AVR in patients less than 65 who do not have a contraindication for anticoagulation. A bioprosthesis is reasonable for AVR in patients under 65 years of age who elect to receive this valve for lifestyle considerations after detailed discussions of the risk of anticoagulation versus the likelihood that a second AVR may be necessary in the future. *(Level of Evidence: C)*
2. A bioprosthesis is reasonable for AVR in patients age 65 years or older without risk factors for thromboembolism. *(Level of Evidence: C)*
3. Aortic valve re-replacement with a homograft is reasonable for patients with active prosthetic valve endocarditis. *(Level of Evidence: C)*

Class IIb

1. A bioprosthesis might be considered for AVR in a woman of childbearing age. *(Level of Evidence: C)*

SOURCE: *From Bonow RO, Carabello B, Chatterjee K, et al. ACC/AHA 2005 Guidelines on the Management of Patients with Valvular Heart Disease: A Report of the ACC/AHA Task Force on Practice Guidelines 2006. Available at: www.acc.org.*

nary arteriography is important in those age 35 years or older (see Chap. 75).[67] Coronary bypass surgery of technically suitable vessels should be performed at the time of valve surgery if the patients have associated significant CAD.

【 】 PROSTHESIS-RELATED PROBLEMS

The incidence of problems with each prosthesis (Table 79–11) was discussed earlier. *Operative mortality* is related to advanced patient

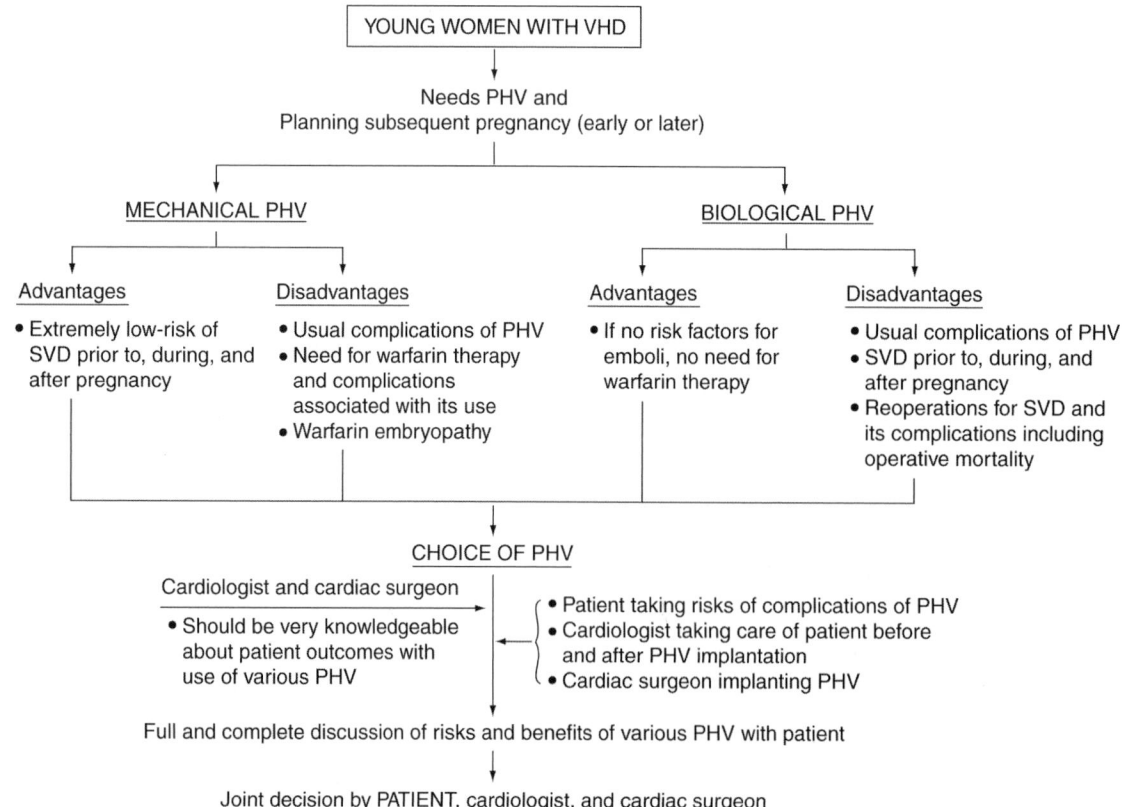

FIGURE 79–11. Factors to be considered in the choice of prosthetic heart valves (PHV) for young women with valvular heart disease (VHD). SVD, structural valve deterioration. *Source: From Hung L, Rahimtoola SH. Prosthetic heart valve and pregnancy. Circulation 2003;107:1240–1246.*

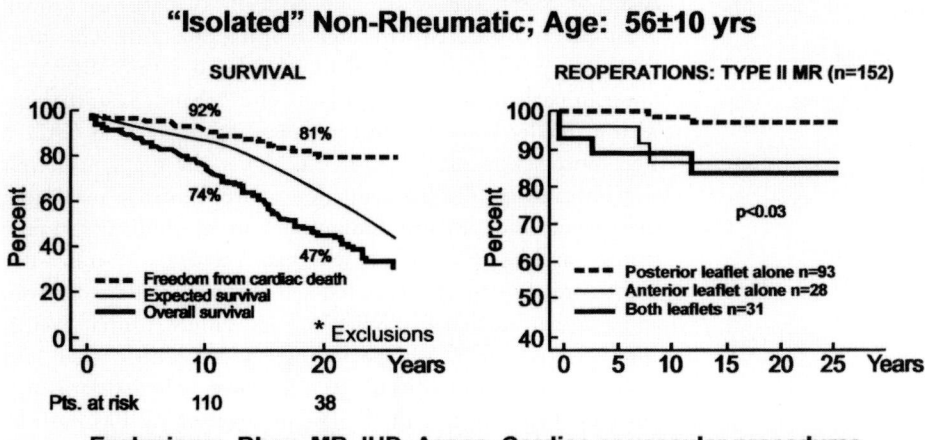

FIGURE 79-12. Mitral valve repair for mitral regurgitation (MR). Survival at 10 and 20 years and freedom from cardiac death (*left panel*). Reoperations according to leaflet prolapse (*right panel*). IHD, ischemic heart disease; Rheu. MR, rheumatic mitral regurgitation. *Source: From Braunberger E, Deloche A, Berrebi A, et al. Very long-term results (more than 20 years) of valve repair with Carpentier's techniques in non-rheumatic mitral valve insufficiency. Circulation 2001;104(Suppl 1):8–11.*

age and other factors (see Table 79–4). Coronary bypass surgery performed at the same time as valve replacement increases the operative mortality by 50 to 100 percent, which, nevertheless, is still not high, but associated CAD, if not bypassed, significantly increases both the operative and 10-year mortality.[68]

The risk of *prosthetic endocarditis* is approximately 3 percent in the first year and 0.5 percent in subsequent years. Infections in the early postoperative period (from 2 to 12 months) are a result of hospital-based organisms. Despite therapy, the infections are difficult to cure and have a high mortality (approximately 80 percent);[69,70] early reoperation is usually recommended. The mortality rate from late postoperative infection (2 to 12 months or later) is approximately 40 percent;[69] about half the patients can be treated successfully with medications alone. The infected valve should be replaced in patients who do not respond to medical treatment or for other reason (see Chap. 85). The importance of adequate antibiotic prophylaxis for the prevention of endocarditis cannot be overemphasized; the prevention and treatment of prosthetic valve endocarditis are discussed in Chap. 85.

Long-term anticoagulant therapy is associated with *bleeding* episodes. The management of antithrombotic therapy is discussed in Chap. 85.

Prosthetic dehiscence is the result of sutures pulling out of the cardiac tissues. It may result from infection, inadequate surgical technique, or diseased cardiac tissue (e.g., edema, necrosis, or calcification).

SVD is mainly a problem with biologic valves. With currently approved mechanical PHVs, SVD is comparatively rare. SVD of biologic PHVs results from leaflet deterioration or calcification; progressive prosthetic regurgitation and/or

stenosis is the rule. Bioprostheses failure is greater in young patients, in elderly with chronic renal insufficiency, and in the mitral position. In young patients (average age: <60 years), failure of mitral prostheses usually starts at 5 to 7 years and of aortic prostheses at 8 to 10 years. The incidence of SVD of aortic PHV in those age 60 to 65 years,[28,36] and of mitral PHV in those age 65 to 70 years, is low.[28] Preoperative lipid levels and other predictors of atherosclerosis do not appear to be predictors of SVD for aortic and mitral bioprostheses.

Red blood cells are fractured by turbulence and contact with foreign surfaces. Some degree of *hemolysis* is present with all mechanical prostheses but not with bioprostheses. Important hemolysis, however, may occur with a perivalvular leak or severe prosthetic obstruction regardless of prosthesis type. Serum lactic dehydrogenase is usually the simplest and most reliable index of hemolysis to follow in patients with prosthetic valves. A sudden increase in lactic dehydrogenase may indicate prosthesis dysfunction, perivalvular leak, or cloth tear. Iron and folate therapy usually correct the anemia. PHV replacement may be required for severe, refractory hemolytic anemia.

Important *systemic embolization* is an unfortunate complication of prosthetic valve replacement (see Chap. 80).

Thrombosed PHV occurs mainly with mechanical valves[38,39,71] but does occur with bioprostheses. There are no perfect test(s) for accurate diagnosis of this potentially lethal condition and clinical judgement is often necessary. Patients who have pannus plus thrombus should have surgery. For right-heart PHV thrombus, thrombolytics should be used initially, and if unsuccessful, surgery is usually necessary. For thrombosed left-heart PHV, surgery is indicated in those with pannus, thrombus plus

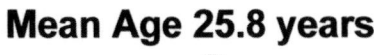

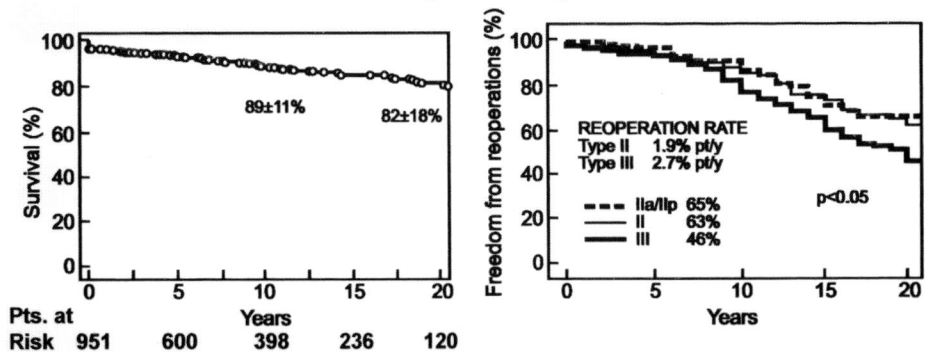

FIGURE 79-13. Mitral valve (MV) repair of patients with rheumatic mitral regurgitation (Rheu. MR). Actuarial survival after MV repair is shown in the *left panel*. Freedom from reoperation after MV repair of patients with Rheu. MR is shown in *right panel*. *Source: From Chauvand S, Fuzellier JF, Berrebi A, et al. Long-term (29 years) results of reconstructive surgery in rheumatic mitral insufficiency. Circulation 2001;104(Suppl I):12–15.*

TABLE 79-11

Major Complications of Valve Replacement

1. Operative mortality
2. Perioperative myocardial infarction
3. Prosthetic endocarditis
4. Prosthetic dehiscence
5. Prosthetic dysfunction
   a. Obstruction: usually thrombotic, occasionally caused by item 3, 4, or 8
   b. Regurgitation
   c. Hemolysis
   d. Structural failure
6. Thromboemboli
7. Hemorrhage with anticoagulant therapy
8. Valve prosthesis–patient mismatch
9. Prosthetic replacement often caused by item 3,4, or 5, occasionally caused by item 6,7, or 8
10. Late mortality, including sudden, unexplained death

SOURCE: Rahimtoola SH. Valvular heart disease: a perspective. J Am Coll Cardiol 1983;3:199–215. Reproduced with permission of the publisher and author.

pannus, large thrombus (diameter ≥ 1.0 cm^2) patients who are in NYHA functional classes III and IV and if thrombolytic therapy is unsuccessful. Thrombolytic therapy is indicated in those with small thrombus (area <0.8 cm^2) and in patients in NYHA functional classes I and II; surgery is not available for patients with severe comorbid conditions, including multisystem organ failure. Both surgery and thrombolytic therapy are associated with complications and both therapies provide the best results in patients who are in NYHA functional classes I and II.

No PHV currently used has an effective orifice as large as that of the native valve; consequently, VP-PM[18,72] occurs. *Almost all patients with prosthetic heart valves have mild-to-moderate stenosis; a few have severe stenosis.* Patients with aortic PHV have obstruction to left ventricular outflow (similar to aortic stenosis), and patients with mitral PHV have obstruction to left atrial emptying (similar to mitral stenosis). This is most important in a large patient in whom a prosthesis that is considered "small" in relation to body size must be placed for technical reasons. The resulting VP-PM (Table 79-12) contributes to incomplete relief of symptoms. The long-term effect of VP-PM can be expected to lead to long-term effects similar to those of

aortic or mitral stenosis.[73–76] In critically ill patients, a small prosthesis is associated with high hospital mortality. The long-term (5- to 10-year) survival in those with severe VP-PM is lower in patients with a larger body size[74] than it is in patients with a smaller body size and in those with associated CAD.[74] The more severe the VP-PM, the higher the gradient at rest and on exercise, the less reduction of left ventricle mass, and the greater the physical limitation and morbidity.[76] In one study,[73] at 15 years, patients who had received a 19-mm valve had poorer functional class, less left ventricle mass reduction, and a higher incidence of VP-PM, heart failure, cardiac events, and valve-related death, including sudden death, than did those patients who received a 21-mm valve. A higher late mortality has been documented.[77] The presence of VP-PM must be considered when patients with prosthetic heart valves are advised concerning activity. A method to predict the expected severity of VP-PM has been described.[76]

Reoperation to replace a prosthetic heart valve is a serious complication. It is usually required for moderate-to-severe prosthetic dysfunction and dehiscence, prosthetic valve endocarditis, and, occasionally, recurrent thromboembolism, severe recurrent bleeding from anticoagulant therapy, or VP-PM.

Late cardiac death may result from ventricular dysfunction, other cardiac lesions, or prosthesis-related causes. Late sudden death is not uncommon. It may result from a bradyarrhythmia; a tachyarrhythmia that is often associated with ventricular dysfunc-

TABLE 79-12

Valve Prosthesis–Patient Mismatch

AORTIC VALVE		
SEVERITY OF STENOSIS AND OF VP-PM AFTER AVR	VALVE AREA (CM^2/M^2)	CLINICAL STATUS
Mild	>0.9	Asymptomatic
Moderate	>0.6 to 0.9	Asymptomatic (symptoms with associated conditions)
Severe	≤0.6	Asymptomatic or symptomatic[a]
MITRAL VALVE		
SEVERITY OF MITRAL VALVE STENOSIS AND OF VP-PM AFTER MVR	VALVE AREA (CM^2)	CLINICAL STATUS
Very mild	>2.0 cm^2	Asymptomatic
Mild	>1.5 to 2.0	Asymptomatic
Moderate	1.1 to 1.5	Usually asymptomatic, some symptomatic
Severe	≤1.0 cm^2	Asymptomatic or symptomatic[b]

AVR, aortic valve replacement; MVR, mitral valve replacement; VP-PM, valve prosthesis–patient mismatch.
[a]Symptoms: angina, syncope, dyspnea, heart failure, sudden death.
[b]Symptoms associated with left atrial and pulmonary arterial hypertension and low/reduced cardiac output and their consequences.
SOURCE: From Rahimtoola SH. Choice of prosthetic heart valve in adult patients. J Am Coll Cardiol 2003;41:893–904.

tion, prosthetic dysfunction, or mismatch; coronary artery disease; or a combination of these.

【 】 MANAGEMENT

All patients with PHV need appropriate antibiotics for prophylaxis against infective endocarditis (see Chap. 85). Patients with rheumatic heart disease continue to need antibiotics as prophylaxis against the recurrence of rheumatic carditis (see Chap. 74). Adequate antithrombotic therapy is needed for appropriate patients (see Chap. 80). During the first 4 to 6 weeks after surgery, the physician and surgeon jointly manage the patient, directing their attention toward relieving postoperative discomfort, readjusting cardiac medications, and instituting anticoagulation if not contraindicated. A graduated plan of activity is started that, usually, enables the patient to return to full activity in 4 to 6 weeks.

Several syndromes are peculiar to the postoperative period. The *postperfusion syndrome* usually appears in the third or fourth postoperative week. It is characterized by fever, splenomegaly, and atypical lymphocytes; it is benign and self-limited. The *postpericardiotomy syndrome* is characterized by fever and pleuropericarditis. It usually develops in the second or third postoperative week, but can appear as late as 1 year after surgery and sometimes recurs. Although this syndrome is usually self-limited, most patients benefit from taking antiinflammatory drugs, such as aspirin or indomethacin; a short course of glucocorticoids is also occasionally required. Even though the pericardium is left open at the end of surgery, *cardiac tamponade* has been known to occur during the first 6 weeks and needs to be relieved. Usually, anticoagulants have been given and the fluid is hemorrhagic.

The 4- to 6-week postoperative visit is critical, because by this time the patient's physical capabilities and expected improvement in functional capacity can usually be assessed. At this time, the physician should assemble essential records and data for the subsequent office followup, including the preoperative history, physical examination, chest roentgenogram, electrocardiogram and indication for surgery, preoperative echocardiographic/Doppler ultrasound and cardiac catheterization/angiographic reports, surgeon's operative report, postoperative complications, and hospital discharge summary. *The prosthesis model, serial number, and size should be recorded.*

The workup on this visit should include an interval or complete initial history and physical examination, electrocardiogram, chest radiography, echocardiography/Doppler, complete blood cell count, and measurement of electrolytes, lactate dehydrogenase, and international normalized ratio (INR) if indicated (Table 79–13). The examination's main focus is on signs that relate to functioning of the prosthesis or suggest the presence of a myocardial, conduction, or valvular disorder. The auscultatory findings to expect with some normally functioning prostheses have been described.[78] Severe perivalvular mitral regurgitation can be inaudible on physical examination, a fact to remember when considering possible causes of functional deterioration in a patient.

The interval between routine followup visits depends on the patient's needs. Anticoagulant regulation usually does not require office visits.

Multiple noninvasive tests have emerged for assessing valvular and ventricular function. Fluoroscopy can reveal abnormal rocking of a dehiscing prosthesis or limitation of the occluder if the latter is

TABLE 79–13

Suggestions for Followup Strategy of Patient with Prosthetic Heart Valves

Indication

History, physical examination, ECG, chest radiograph, echocardiogram/Doppler, complete blood count, serum chemistries, and INR (if indicated) at first postoperative outpatient evaluation.[a,b]

Radionuclide angiography/CMR to assess LV function if result of echocardiography/Doppler is unsatisfactory.

CMR to assess native and PHV function if results of echocardiography/Doppler is unsatisfactory.

Routine followup visits at yearly intervals with earlier reevaluations for change in clinical status.

Routine serial echocardiograms at time of annual followup visit at 5 years after bioprosthetic MVR and at 8 years after bioprosthetic AVR even in the absence of change in clinical status.

Other tests, if indicated.

AVR, aortic valve replacement; CMR, cardiovascular magnetic resonance; INR, international normalized ratio; LV, left ventricle; MVR, mitral valve replacement; PHV, prosthetic heart valve.
[a]This evaluation should be performed 4 to 6 weeks after hospital discharge. In some settings, the outpatient echocardiogram may be difficult to obtain; if so, an inpatient echocardiogram may be obtained before hospital discharge.
[b]An echocardiogram/Doppler study at 6 to 12 months is essential for proper assessment of severity of valve prosthesis–patient mismatch.
SOURCE: Copyright by S. H. Rahimtoola.

opaque, as well as strut fracture of a Bjork-Shiley valve. Radionuclide angiography, to assess ventricular function, is performed if the same data cannot be obtained by echocardiography.

Echocardiography/Doppler is the most useful noninvasive test. It provides information about prosthesis stenosis or regurgitation, valve area, assessment of other valve diseases, pulmonary hypertension, atrial size, left ventricle hypertrophy, left ventricle size and function, and pericardial effusion or thickening. It is essential at the first postoperative visit because it allows an assessment of the effects and results of surgery and serves as a baseline for comparison should complications and/or deterioration occur later. Subsequently, it is performed as is needed; we recommend that in both symptomatic and asymptomatic patients it be performed at 1- to 2-year intervals. In patients with a bioprostheses in the mitral position, it is essential that Doppler echocardiography be performed at 5 years and annually thereafter, and in patients with a bioprostheses in the aortic position, that it be performed at 8 years and annually thereafter, because of the increasing incidence of bioprosthetic SVD.[35,36]

Figure 79–14 describes management of the patient with PHV who becomes pregnant.[51]

"Heart failure" after valve replacement may be the result of (1) preoperative left ventricular dysfunction that improved partially or not at all, (2) perioperative myocardial damage, (3) progression of other valve disease, (4) complications of PHV, or (5) associated heart disease such as CAD and systemic arterial hypertension.

Any patient with a prosthetic heart valve who does not improve after the surgery or who later shows deterioration of functional ca-

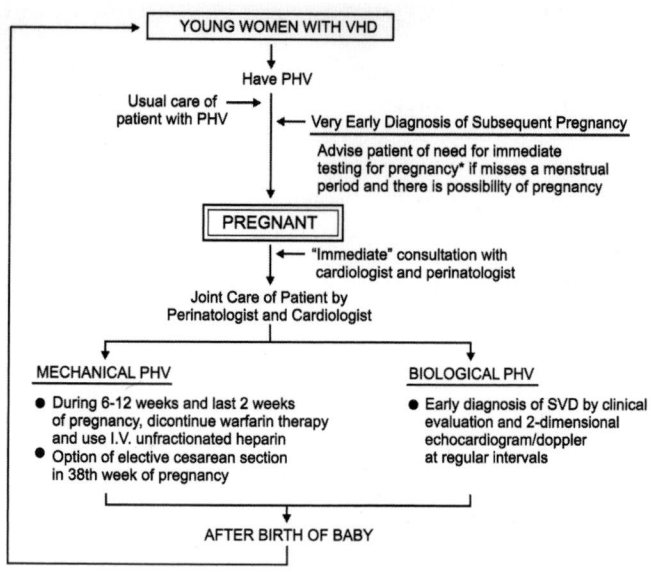

FIGURE 79–14. Management of the patient with prosthetic heart valve who becomes pregnant. PHV, prosthetic heart valve; SVD, structural valve deterioration; VHD, valvular heart disease. *Source: From Hung L, Rahimtoola SH. Prosthetic heart valve and pregnancy. Circulation 2003;107;1240–1246.*

pacity should undergo appropriate testing to determine the cause. Such studies are also usually necessary for patients who require reoperation for any cause. The indications for reoperating on a patient with prosthetic valve endocarditis were discussed earlier. A patient in stable condition, without prosthetic valve endocarditis, can usually undergo reoperation with only a slightly greater risk than that of the initial surgery. For the patient with catastrophic dysfunction, surgery is clearly indicated and urgent.

REFERENCES

1. Johnson DM, Sapirstein W. FDA's requirements for in-vivo performance data for prosthetic heart valves. *J Heart Valve Dis* 1994;3:350–356.
2. Grunkemeier GL, Anderson WN Jr. Clinical evaluation and analysis of heart valve substitute. *J Heart Valve Dis* 1998;7:163–169.
3. *Draft Replacement Heart Valve Guidance.* Rockville, MD: Prosthetic Devices Branch, Division of Cardiovascular, Respiratory and Neurological Devices, Office of Device Evaluation, Center of Devices and Radiological Health, Food and Drug Administration. October 14, 1994.
4. Harken D, Soroff HS, Taylor WJ. Partial and complete prosthesis in aortic insufficiency. *J Thorac Cardiovasc Surg* 1960;40:744–762.
5. Starr A, Edwards M. Mitral replacement: clinical experience with a ball valve prosthesis. *Ann Surg* 1961;154:726–740.
6. Gao G, Wu YX, Grunkemeier GL, et al. Forty-year survival with the Starr-Edwards heart valve prosthesis. *J Heart Valve Dis* 2004;13:91–96.
7. Carpentier A, Dubost C. From xenograft to bioprostheses. In: Ionescu MI, Ross DN, Wooler GH, eds. *Biological Tissue in Heart Valve Replacement.* London: Butterworth,1971:515–541.
8. Carpentier A, Lemaigre G, Robert L. Biological factors affecting long-term results of valvular homografts. *J Thorac Cardiovasc Surg* 1969;58:467–483.
9. Ross DN. Homograft replacement of the aortic valve. *Lancet* 1962;2:487.
10. Barratt-Boyes BG. Homograft aortic valve replacement in aortic incompetence and stenosis. *Thorax* 1964;19:131–135.
11. Ross DN. Replacement of aortic and mitral valves with a pulmonary autograft. *Lancet* 1967;2:956–958.
12. Ross DN. The pulmonary autograft: the Ross principle (or Ross procedural confusion). *J Heart Valve Dis* 2000;9:174–175.
13. Duvoisin GE, Brandenburg RO, McGoon DC. Factors affecting thromboembolism associated with prosthetic heart valves. *Circulation* 1967;35(4 Suppl):I70–I76.
14. Stinson EB, Griepp RB, Oyer PE, et al. Long-term experience with porcine xenografts. *J Thorac Cardiovasc Surg* 1977;73:54–63.
15. Grunkemeier GL, Macmanus Q, Thomas DR, et al. Regression analysis of late survival following mitral valve replacement. *J Thorac Cardiovasc Surg* 1978;75:131–138.
16. Blackstone EH, Naftel DC, Turner ME Jr. The decomposition of time varying hazard into separate phases, each incorporating a separate stream of concomitant information. *J Am Stat Assoc* 1986;81:615–624.
17. Edmunds LH Jr, Clark RE, Cohn LH, et al. Guidelines for reporting morbidity and mortality after cardiac valvular operations. *J Thorac Cardiovasc Surg* 1996;112:708–711.
18. Rahimtoola SH. The problem of valve prosthesis-patient mismatch. *Circulation* 1978;58:20–24.
19. Sackett DL. Bias in analytic research. *J Chronic Dis* 1979;32:51–63.
20. Rahimtoola SH. Valvular heart disease: a perspective. *J Am Coll Cardiol* 1983;3:199–215.
21. Rahimtoola SH. Lessons learned about the determinants of the results of valve surgery. *Circulation* 1988;78:1503–1507.
22. Edmunds LH Jr. Thrombotic and bleeding complications of prosthetic heart valves. *Ann Thorac Surg* 1987;44:430–445.
23. Bamford J, Warlow C. Stroke and TIA in the general population. In: Butchart EG, Bodnar E, eds. *Thrombosis, Embolism and Bleeding.* London: ICR, 1992:3–15.
24. Berlin JA, Begg CB, Louis TA. An assessment of publication bias using a sample of published clinical trials. *J Am Stat Assoc* 1989;84:381–392.
25. Edward FH, Peterson ED, Coombs LP, et al. Prediction of operative mortality after valve replacement surgery. *J Am Coll Cardiol* 2001;37:885–892.
26. Rahimtoola SH. The next generation of prosthetic heart valves needs a proven record of patient outcomes at ≥ 15 to 20 years. *J Am Coll Cardiol* 2003;42:1720–1721.
27. Grunkemier GL, Li H-H, Starr A, et al. Long-term performance of heart valve prostheses. *Curr Prob Cardiol* 2000;25:75–154.
28. Rahimtoola SH. Choice of prosthetic heart valve in adult patients. *J Am Coll Cardiol* 2003;41:893–904.
29. Kramer MS, Shapiro SH. Scientific challenges in the application of randomized trials. *JAMA* 1984;252:2739–2745.
30. Rahimtoola SH. Some unexpected lessons from large multicenter randomized clinical trials. *Circulation* 1985;72:449–455.
31. Grunkemeier GL, Starr A. Alternatives to randomization in surgical studies. *J Heart Valve Dis* 1992;1:142–151.
32. Fiore AC, Barner HB, Swartz MT, et al. Mitral valve replacement: Randomized trial of St. Jude and Medtronic Hall Prostheses. *Ann Thorac Surg* 1998;66:707–713.
33. Murday AJ, Hochstitzky A, Mansfield J, et al. A prospective controlled trial of St. Jude versus Starr Edwards aortic and mitral valve prosthesis. *Ann Thorac Surg* 2003;76(1):66–73.
34. Bloomfield P, Wheatley DJ, Prescott RJ, et al. Twelve-year comparison of a Bjork-Shiley mechanical heart valve with porcine bioprostheses. *N Engl J Med* 1991;324:573–579.
35. Oxenham H, Bloomfield P, Wheatley DJ, et al. Twenty year comparison of a Bjork-Shiley mechanical heart valve with porcine bioprostheses. *Heart* 2003;89:715–721.
36. Hammermeister KE, Sethi GK, Henderson WC, et al. Outcomes 15 years after valve replacement with a mechanical versus bioprosthetic valve: final report of the Veterans Administration trial. *J Am Coll Cardiol* 2000;36:1152–1158.
37. Frater RWM, Furlong P, Cosgrove DM, et al. Long-term durability and patient functional status of the Carpentier-Edwards Perimount pericardial bioprosthesis in the aortic position. *J Heart Valve Dis* 1998;7:48–53.
38. Rahimtoola SH. The year in valvular heart disease. *J Am Coll Cardiol* 2005;45:111–122.
39. Rahimtoola SH. The year in valvular heart disease. *J Am Coll Cardiol* 2006;47:427–439.
40. Palka P, Havrocks S, Lange A, et al. Primary aortic valve replacement with cryopreserved aortic allograft. An echocardiographic follow-up study of 570 patients. *Circulation* 2002;105:61–66.
41. Smedira NG, Blackstone EH, Roselli EE, et al. Are allografts the biologic valve of choice for aortic valve replacement in non-elderly patients? Comparison of explantation for structural valve deterioration of allograft and pericardial prosthesis. *J Thorac Cardiovasc Surg* 2006;131:558–564.
42. Matsuki O, Okita Y, Almeida RS, et al. Two decades' experience with aortic valve replacement with pulmonary autograft. *J Thorac Cardiovasc Surg* 1988;95:705–711.
43. Ross D, Jackson M, Davies J. Pulmonary autograft aortic valve replacement: long-term results. *J Cardiac Surg* 1991;6(Suppl 4):529–533.

44. Luciani GB, Casali G, Favaro A, et al. Fate of aortic root late after Ross operation. *Circulation* 2003;108 Suppl II:61–67.

45. Carr-White GS, Kilner PJ, Hon JFK, et al. Incidence, location, pathology, and significance of pulmonary homograft stenosis after the Ross operation. *Circulation* 2001;104(Suppl I):16–20.

46. Byrne JG, Karavas AN, Mihaljevic T, et al. Role of cryopreserved homograft in isolated elective aortic valve replacement. *Am J Cardiol* 2003;91:616–619.

47. Wilhelm MJ, Tavakoli R, Schneeberger K, et al. Cryopreserved aortic viable homograft for active aortic endocarditis. *Ann Thorac Surg* 2005;79:67–71.

48. Bonow RO, Carabello B, Chatterjee K, et al. *ACC/AHA 2005 Guidelines on the Management of Patients with Valvular Heart Disease: A Report of the ACC/AHA Task Force on Practice Guidelines 2006.* Available at: www.acc.org.

49. Chiappini B, Camarri N, Loforte A, et al. Outcome after aortic valve replacement in octogenarians. *Ann Thorac Surg* 2004;78:85–89.

50. Herzog CA, Ma JZ, Collins AJ. Long-term survival of dialysis patients in the United States with prosthetic heart valves. Should ACC/AHA practice guidelines on valve selection be modified? *Circulation* 2002;105:1336–1341.

51. Hung L, Rahimtoola SH. Prosthetic heart valve and pregnancy. *Circulation* 2003;107;1240–1246.

52. Hendren WG, Morris AS, Rosenkranz ER, et al. Mitral valve repair for bacterial endocarditis. *J Thorac Cardiovasc Surg* 1992;103:124–128; discussion 128–129.

53. Jebara VA, Dervanian P, Acar C, et al. Mitral valve repair using Carpentier techniques in patients more than 70 years old: early and late results. *Circulation* 1992;86(Suppl II):53–59.

54. Aoyagi S, Tanaka K, Kawara T, et al. Long-term results of mitral valve repair for non-rheumatic mitral regurgitation. *Cardiovasc Surg* 1995;3:387–392.

55. Skoularigis J, Sinovich V, Joubert G, et al. Evaluation of the long-term results of mitral valve repair in 254 young patients with rheumatic mitral regurgitation. *Circulation* 1994;90(Suppl II):167–174.

56. Grossi EA, Galloway AC, Steinberg BM, et al. Severe calcification does not affect long-term outcome of mitral valve repair. *Ann Thorac Surg* 1994;58:685–687.

57. Grossi EA, Galloway AC, LeBoutillier M III, et al. Anterior leaflet procedures during mitral valve repair do not adversely influence long-term outcome. *J Am Coll Cardiol* 1995;25:134–136.

58. Duran CM, Gometza B, Saad E. Valve repair in rheumatic mitral disease: an unsolved problem. *J Cardiac Surg* 1994;9(Suppl 2):282–285.

59. Braumberger E, Deloche A, Berrebi A, et al. Very long-term results (more than 20 years) of valve repair with Carpentier's techniques in non-rheumatic mitral valve insufficiency. *Circulation* 2001;104(Suppl I):8–11.

60. Lim E, Barlow CW, Hosseinpour AR, et al. Influence of atrial fibrillation on outcome following mitral valve repair. *Circulation* 2001;104(Suppl I):59–63.

61. Chauvand S, Fuzellier JF, Berrebi A, et al. Long-term (29 years) results of reconstructive surgery in rheumatic mitral insufficiency. *Circulation* 2001;104(Suppl I):12–15.

62. Wilhelm MJ, Tavakoli R, Schneeberger K, et al. Surgical treatment of infective mitral valve endocarditis. *J Heart Valve Dis* 2004;13:754–759.

63. Iung B, Rousseau-Pizaiaud J, Cormier B, et al. Contemporary results of mitral valve repair for infective endocarditis. *J Am Coll Cardiol* 2004;43:386–392.

64. Zegdi R, Debiéche M, Latrémonille C, et al. Long-term results of mitral valve repair for infective endocarditis. *J Am Coll Cardiol* 2004;43:386–392.

65. Minakata K, Schaff HV, Zehr KJ, et al. Is repair of aortic valve regurgitation a safe alternative to valve replacement? *J Thorac Cardiovasc Surg* 2004;127:645–653.

66. Langer F, Aircher D, Kissinger A, et al. Aortic valve repair using a differentiated surgical strategy. *Circulation* 2004;110 Suppl II:67–73.

67. Rahimtoola SH. Valvular heart disease. In: Stein J, ed. *Internal Medicine*, 4th ed. *Cardiology.* St. Louis: Mosby-Year Book, 1994:202–234.

68. Mullany CJ, Elveback LR, Frye RL, et al. Coronary artery disease and its management: influence on survival in patients undergoing aortic valve replacement. *J Am Coll Cardiol* 1987;10:66–72.

69. Kloster FE. Infective prosthetic valve endocarditis. In: Rahimtoola SH, ed. *Infective Endocarditis.* New York: Grune & Stratton, 1978:291–305.

70. Douglas JL, Cobbs CG. Prosthetic valve endocarditis. In: Kaye D, ed. *Infective Endocarditis,* 2d ed. New York: Raven Press, 1992:375–396.

71. Rahimtoola SH. The year in valvular heart disease. *J Am Coll Cardiol* 2006;47:427–439.

72. Rahimtoola SH, Murphy E. Valve prosthesis-patient mismatch: a long-term sequela. *Br Heart J* 1981;45:331–335.

73. Milano AD, DeCarlo M, Mecozzi G, et al. Clinical outcome in patients with 19 mm and 21 mm aortic prosthesis. Comparison at long-term follow-up. *Ann Thorac Surg* 2002;73:37–43.

74. Hé GW, Grunkemeier GL, Gately HL, et al. Up to thirty year survival after aortic valve replacement in the small aortic root. *Ann Thorac Surg* 1995;59:1056–1062.

75. Connolly HM, Oh JK, Schaff HV, et al. Severe aortic stenosis with low transvalvular gradient and severe left ventricular dysfunction: Result of valve replacement in 52 patients. *Circulation* 2000;101:1940–1946.

76. Pibarot P, Dumesnil JG. Hemodynamic and clinical impact of prosthesis–patient mismatch in the aortic valve position and its prevention. *J Am Coll Cardiol* 2000;36:1131–1141.

77. Mohty-Echahidi D, Malouf JF, Girard SE, et al. Impact of prosthesis-patient mismatch on long-term survival in patients with small St. Jude Medical mechanical prosthesis in the aortic position. *Circulation* 2006;113:420–426.

78. Vongpatawasin W, Hillis LD, Lange RA. Prosthetic heart valves. *N Engl J Med* 1996;335:407–416.

CHAPTER 80

Antithrombotic Therapy for Valvular Heart Disease

John H. McAnulty / Shahbudin H. Rahimtoola

Bleeding is a risk with all antithrombotic agents, but the frequency and consequences of a stroke make drug therapy appropriate in many patients with valve disease.[1,2] This is particularly true in patients with prosthetic heart valves, but is also true in patients with native valve disease accompanied by comorbid conditions associated with thromboemboli (Table 80–1).

ANTITHROMBOTIC DRUGS AND VALVE DISEASE

Warfarin, aspirin, unfractionated heparin, and thrombolytic agents are the only antithrombotic agents currently recommended for preventing or treating thromboemboli related to valve disease. There are no prospective randomized clinical trials comparing the efficacy or safety of these or of low-molecular-weight heparin as they are used for the purpose of preventing thromboemboli in valve-disease patients. Reports describe thrombosis, emboli, bleeding, (and in the case of pregnancy, teratogenicity and maternal and fetal death) with each. This is true with both native and prosthetic valve disease, and is true with their use for the "special clinical situations" described below. Therefore, clinical judgment is required in each case.

There are even less data on newer drugs, such as the 2B-3A platelet inhibitors, the thienopyridine agents (e.g., clopidogrel), and the direct thrombin and factor Xa inhibitors. These drugs are increasingly being used for other clinical syndromes, and may be used in patients who also require antithrombotic therapy for heart valve disease. Increased bleeding is likely, although not yet well de-

fined. Individual clinical decisions will be required; some of which are addressed in this chapter.

NATIVE VALVE DISEASE

Patients with native valve disease require antithrombotic therapy only in the presence of an associated stroke *risk factor* (Fig. 80–1). The two most common associated risk factors are atrial fibrillation and left ventricular (LV) systolic dysfunction.

【 】 RISK FACTORS FOR THROMBOEMBOLI
Atrial Fibrillation

In six large, prospective, randomized trials assessing the value of antithrombotic therapy for primary stroke prevention in patients with nonvalvular, constant or paroxysmal, atrial fibrillation, the embolic rate (essentially a stroke) was 3 to 8 percent per year in the placebo or untreated patients (see Chap. 37, Atrial Fibrillation). Warfarin therapy reduced the stroke rate to 0.5 to 2 percent per year.[3] "Nonvalvular" is not well defined in these trials as individuals with "insignificant" valve disease were included; however, patients with mitral stenosis or prosthetic heart valves (PHVs) were excluded. When an individual with native value disease has associated intermittent or continuous atrial fibrillation, clinical trial data can be used to assess stroke risk and direct treatment guidelines.[3–7] In summary, warfarin is recommended

TABLE 80-1

Valve Disease and Antithrombotic Therapy

1. Prevention of thromboemboli should be addressed each time a patient with valve disease is seen.
2. Lifelong antithrombotic therapy is required in patients with atrial fibrillation (paroxysmal or persistent).
3. Warfarin therapy is required in all patients with a mechanical prosthesis (See Table 80–2).
4. Antithrombotic therapy should be started early after valve surgery.
5. Warfarin should be avoided in the first trimester of pregnancy.
6. Antithrombotic therapy should be individualized during noncardiac surgery and cardiovascular procedures (See Table 80–4).

in any atrial fibrillation patient who has had a systemic embolus. It is also recommended in those with two or more of the following: diabetes mellitus, a history of hypertension, coronary artery disease, congestive heart failure, and older than age 75 years. Those with none or only one of them can reasonably be given aspirin 325 mg/d as an alternative.

Left Ventricular Dysfunction

Systemic or pulmonary thromboemboli occur at a rate greater than 5 percent per year in patients with LV systolic dysfunction unrelated to valve disease, but antithrombotic therapy is not of proven value in preventing or reducing the systemic embolic rate.[8,9] Nevertheless, because the risk is sufficiently high, warfarin (international normalized ratio [INR] 2 to 3) may be used if the LV ejection fraction (EF) is ≤ 0.30, or aspirin (325 mg daily) may be used if warfarin use is judged to be associated with an increased risk or is impractical. Less is known about the stroke risk with diastolic dysfunction. Given its frequent occurrence with hypertension, it's possible that this is one of the explanations for the association of hypertension and strokes.

Previous Thromboemboli

A thromboembolic event defines patients who are at high risk for having a recurrent event in clinical situations unrelated to native valve disease (e.g., in patients with atrial fibrillation or with a PHV).[3,10,11] It is unclear whether this is true in patients with native valve disease, but lifelong warfarin therapy should be considered if there are no contraindications to its use.

Hypercoagulable Conditions

Hypercoagulable states clearly increase the risk of venous thrombosis (see Chap. 108). The most common are the factor V Leiden and prothrombin gene mutations; defects in protein C, protein

S, or antithrombin; and many malignancies. Less is known about their effect on the incidence of thromboemboli related to valve disease, but their presence is a reason to more strongly consider anticoagulation.

Other Potential Thromboemboli Risk Factors

Beyond an assessment of left ventricular systolic function, the use of transthoracic and transesophageal echocardiography to determine which patients are at risk of thromboemboli is not yet well defined. Left atrial enlargement or thrombi, a patent foramen ovale, an atrial septal aneurysm, or spontaneous echo contrast are occasional findings of concern. The value of treatment based on these findings is unproven.

Antithrombotic Treatment Regimens for Native Valve Disease

Antithrombotic therapy is recommended *only* in the presence of *risk factors* (see Fig. 80–1).[2] The following treatment regimes are appropriate:

- Warfarin (INR 2–3) for previous thromboemboli, LV dysfunction (LVEF ≤ 0.30), hypercoagulable states that usually require treatment with this drug.
- Warfarin (INR 2–3) or aspirin (325 mg) for atrial fibrillation if valve lesion is other than mitral stenosis.

PROSTHETIC HEART VALVES

In patients with *mechanical* PHVs, the risk of stroke exceeds 10 percent per year in patients not taking warfarin.[11] With warfarin use, the risk of thromboemboli is 1 to 3 percent per year.[12–15] In patients in sinus rhythm with *biologic* PHVs, the risk of an embolus is approximately 0.6 to 0.7 percent per year when patients are not on warfarin therapy.[16,17] Most studies show that the risk of embolism is greater with a PHV in the mitral position (mechanical or biologic) than it is with a valve in the aortic position.[16–18]

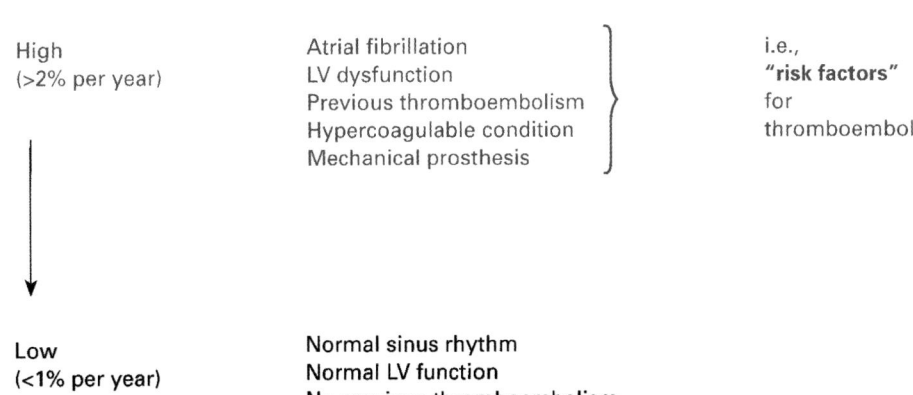

FIGURE 80–1. Risk of thromboembolism. Clinical variables define valve disease patients as being at high or low risk of thromboembolic events. LV, left ventricle.

With either type of PHV or valve location, the risk of emboli is probably higher in the first few days and months after valve insertion,[16] that is, before the valve ring is fully endothelialized.

ANTITHROMBOTIC TREATMENT FOR MECHANICAL PROSTHETIC HEART VALVES

All patients with a mechanical PHV require warfarin (Table 80–2).[2,17–22] It is frequently difficult to maintain a patient at a relatively fixed level of anticoagulation because of changes in the absorption of medication, the effects of various foods and medications, and changes in liver function. Therefore, in clinical practice, the patient is maintained within a certain therapeutic range. This can be optimized through a program of patient education and close surveillance by an experienced healthcare professional.

The INR in patients with a mechanical aortic valve prosthesis should be maintained between 2.0 and 3.0.[2] It should be maintained at 2.5 to 3.5 in those with a mitral prosthesis. The INR should be between 2.5 and 3.5 in those with a previous embolus and in those with multiple risk factors. The tilting-disk valves are more thrombogenic than others, and the INR may be increased to between 3 and 4.5, but this is associated with an increased risk of bleeding.[21]

The addition of *low-dose aspirin* (50 to 100 mg/d) to warfarin therapy is suggested because it further decreases the risk of thromboembolism without increasing the incidence of major bleeds in most patients.[2,23–26] A metanalysis[25] showed with the addition of aspirin to anticoagulants, the odds ratio (± 95 percent confidence interval) of thromboembolic events was 0.39 (0.28 to 0.56; *p* <0.001), the odds ratio of mortality was 0.55 (0.40 to 0.77; *p* <0.001), and the odds ratio of major bleeding was 1.66 (1.18 to 2.34; *p* = 0.005; Fig. 80–2).

In one randomized trial,[26] patients with a St. Judes medical mitral valve were assigned to oral anticoagulants (INR 2.5 to 3.5) or oral anticoagulants plus aspirin (200 mg/d). An observed reduction in thromboemboli in the aspirin-added group was a result of

a reduction in minor thromboemboli (8.2 vs. 20.8 percent; *p* = 0.007), and the reduction in major thromboemboli was not significant (0.9 vs. 4.1 percent).[21] This study is compatible with the view that if aspirin is added to warfarin, only low-dose aspirin (80 to 100 mg) should be used and that there is a need for clinical judgment when recommending the addition of aspirin.

The thromboembolic risk is increased early after the insertion of any PHV. Heparin therapy should be initiated within the first 24 to 48 hours of surgery if there is no contraindication to its use, and the *activated partial thromboplastin time* (aPTT) maintained at a "therapeutic effect" level (Table 80–3) until warfarin therapy has achieved the recommended INR level.[2,16]

ANTITHROMBOTIC TREATMENT FOR BIOLOGIC VALVES

Because of an increased risk of thromboemboli during the first 3 months after implantation of a biologic PHV, early anticoagulation with heparin and then warfarin is indicated.[2,16] After 3 months, the biologic valve can be treated in the same way as is done for patients with native valve disease (see Antithrombotic Treatment Regimens for Native Valve Disease above), and warfarin can be discontinued in approximately two-thirds of patients with biologic valves[2,15] if there are no associated stroke risk factors.

SPECIAL CLINICAL SITUATIONS
ALTERED NATIVE VALVES

Valve disease is treated increasingly by interventional catheter techniques or surgical valve repair. The recommendations given for treatment of native valve disease would seem most applicable in such patients; that is, antithrombotic treatment depends on associated stroke risk factors. Data on thrombotic complications af-

TABLE 80–2

Antithrombotic Therapy—Prosthetic Heart Valves[a]

	MECHANICAL PROSTHETIC VALVES			BIOLOGIC PROSTHETIC VALVES		
	WARFARIN INR 2–3	WARFARIN INR 2.5–3.5	ASPIRIN 50–100 MG	WARFARIN INR 2–3	WARFARIN INR 2.5–3.5	ASPIRIN 50–100 MG
First 3 months after valve replacement		+	±		+	±
After first 3 months						
Aortic valve						
Aortic valve	+		±			+
Aortic valve + risk factor[b]	+		+	+		
Aortic valve + embolus[c]		+	+	+		+
Mitral valve		+	±			+
Mitral valve + risk factor		+	+		+	±
Mitral valve + embolism[c]		+	+		+	+

± Clinical judgment very important for addition of aspirin therapy; INR, international normalized ratio.
[a]Depending on the clinical status of patient, antithrombotic therapy must be individualized (see special situations in text).
[b]Risk factors (see Fig. 80–1): atrial fibrillation, Left ventricle dysfunction, and hypercoagulable state.
[c]Embolus = previous thromboembolism.
NOTE: In an individual patient, there is a need for clinical judgment ± if aspirin is added to warfarin therapy.

Thromboemboli

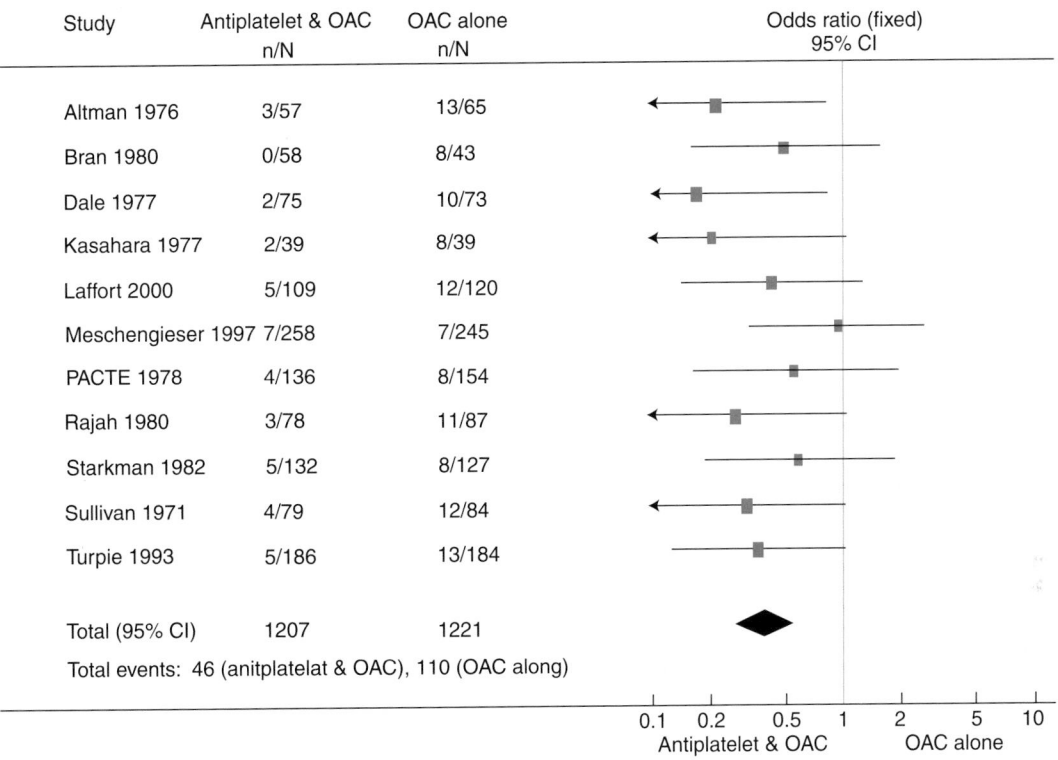

Study	Antiplatelet & OAC n/N	OAC alone n/N	Odds ratio (fixed) 95% CI
Altman 1976	3/57	13/65	
Bran 1980	0/58	8/43	
Dale 1977	2/75	10/73	
Kasahara 1977	2/39	8/39	
Laffort 2000	5/109	12/120	
Meschengieser 1997	7/258	7/245	
PACTE 1978	4/136	8/154	
Rajah 1980	3/78	11/87	
Starkman 1982	5/132	8/127	
Sullivan 1971	4/79	12/84	
Turpie 1993	5/186	13/184	
Total (95% CI)	1207	1221	

Total events: 46 (anitplatelat & OAC), 110 (OAC along)

0.1 0.2 0.5 1 2 5 10

Antiplatelet & OAC   OAC alone

Major Bleeding

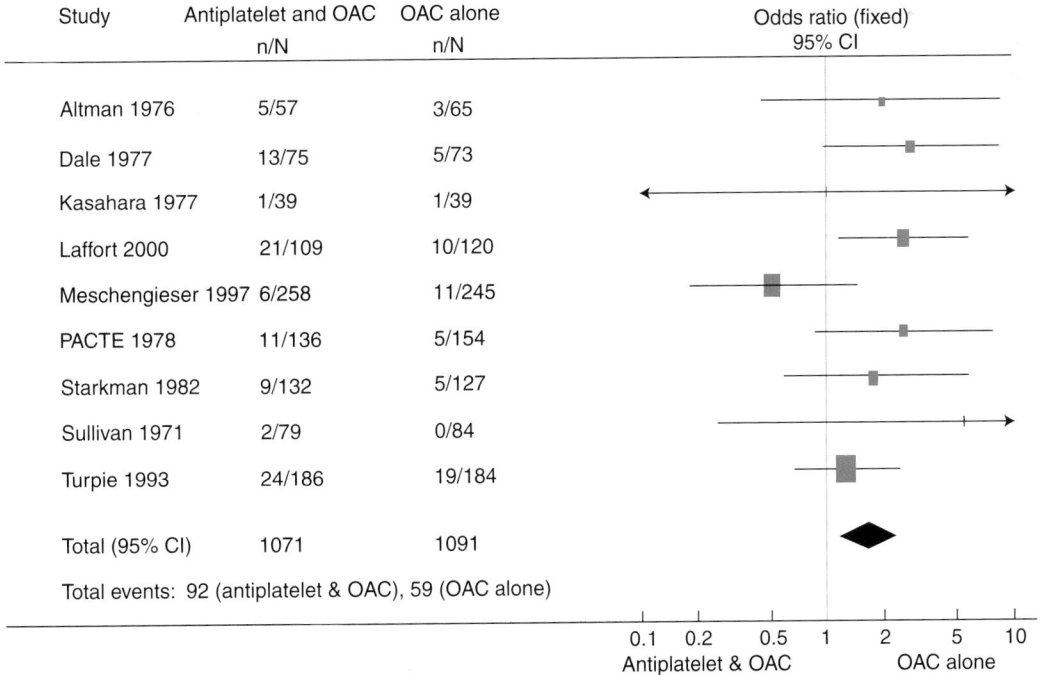

Study	Antiplatelet and OAC n/N	OAC alone n/N	Odds ratio (fixed) 95% CI
Altman 1976	5/57	3/65	
Dale 1977	13/75	5/73	
Kasahara 1977	1/39	1/39	
Laffort 2000	21/109	10/120	
Meschengieser 1997	6/258	11/245	
PACTE 1978	11/136	5/154	
Starkman 1982	9/132	5/127	
Sullivan 1971	2/79	0/84	
Turpie 1993	24/186	19/184	
Total (95% CI)	1071	1091	

Total events: 92 (antiplatelet & OAC), 59 (OAC alone)

0.1 0.2 0.5 1 2 5 10

Antiplatelet & OAC   OAC alone

FIGURE 80–2. Mechanical heart valves. Odds ratios for thromboemboli (*top*) and for major bleeding (*bottom*) are depicted for comparison of treatment with an antiplatelet agent in combination with an oral anticoagulant (OAC) versus an OAC alone. *Source: Data from meta-analysis by Little SH and Massel SR.*[25]

TABLE 80–3

"Therapeutic Effect" of Heparin

Unfractionated heparin	An aPTT at 8 h after a dose that has been calibrated[a] to reflect a heparin level of 0.35 to 0.70 anti-Xa units
LMW heparin	An aPTT at 8 h after a dose that has been calibrated[a] to reflect a heparin level of 0.7 to 1.1 anti-Xa units

aPTT, activated partial thromboplastin time; LMW, low-molecular-weight.
[a]Calibration of aPTT to heparin levels is performed in each clinical laboratory; thus the time (number of seconds) of the aPTT reflecting the "therapeutic effect" levels will vary.
During pregnancy, aPTT levels do not accurately reflect heparin levels. Factor anti-Xa levels should be 0.4 to 0.7 at 8 hours after a dose of unfractionated heparin and 0.7 to 1.1 at 10 hours after LMW heparin. LMW heparin has not been proven as effective treatment for prosthetic valves during pregnancy.

ter the Ross procedure are limited, but the risk seems low and the recommendations for a biologic valve seem reasonable.[27]

SURGERY AND DENTAL CARE

The risk of increased bleeding during a procedure performed with a patient on antithrombotic therapy has to be weighed against the increased risk of a thromboembolism caused by stopping the therapy. The risk of stopping warfarin can be estimated and is relatively low if the drug is withheld for only a few days. As an example, and using a *worst-case scenario* (e.g., a patient with a mechanical prosthesis and previous thromboemboli), the risk of a thromboembolus in a patient off warfarin could be as high as 10 to 20 percent per year. Thus, if the therapy were stopped for 3 days, the risk of an embolus would be 3/365 times 0.10 to 0.20, which equals 0.08 to 0.16 percent. There are theoretical concerns that stopping the drug and then reinstituting it might result in hypercoagulability with a thrombotic "rebound." An increase in markers for activation of thrombosis with abrupt discontinuation of warfarin therapy has been observed, but it is not clear that these increase the clinical risk of thromboembolism.[28–30] In addition, when reinstituting warfarin therapy, there are theoretical concerns of a hypercoagulable state caused by suppression of proteins C and S before the drug affects the thrombotic factors. Although the risks are hypothetical, they are reasons to treat individuals at very high risk with heparin therapy until the INR returns to the desired range.

Although antithrombotic therapy must be individualized, some generalizations apply (Table 80–4). For procedures where bleeding is unlikely or would be inconsequential if it occurred, antithrombotic therapy should not be stopped. This can apply to surgery on the skin, dental prophylaxis, or simple treatment for dental caries. Eye surgery, in particular surgery for cataracts or glaucoma, is usually associated with very little bleeding; many ophthalmologists do not alter antithrombotic therapy.[31,32]

When bleeding is likely or its potential consequences are severe, antithrombotic treatment should be altered.

If a patient is taking aspirin, it should be discontinued 7 to 10 days before the procedure and restarted as soon as it is considered safe by the surgeon or dentist.

For most patients taking warfarin, the drug should be stopped 72 hours before the procedure to achieve an INR of ≤1.5. Unless postop-

TABLE 80–4

Antithrombotic Therapy at the Time of Surgery

I. Usual approach
  A. If patient on warfarin
    Stop 72 h before procedure
    Restart on day of procedure or after control of active bleeding
  B. If patient on aspirin
    Stop 1 week before procedure
    Restart the day after procedure or after control of active bleeding
II. Unusual circumstances
  A. Very high risk of thrombosis if off warfarin[a]
    Stop warfarin 72 h before procedure
    Start heparin 48 h before procedure[b]
    Stop heparin 6 h before procedure
    Restart heparin within 24 h of procedure and continue until warfarin can be restarted and the INR is 2–3
  B. Surgery complicated by postoperative bleeding
    Start heparin as soon after surgery as deemed safe and maintain aPTT of 60–80 s until warfarin restarted and the INR is 2–3
  C. Very low risk from bleeding[c]
    Continue antithrombotic therapy

aPTT, activated partial thromboplastin time; INR, international normalized ratio.
[a]Clinical judgment: consider this approach if recent thromboembolus or if three risk factors are present.
[b]Heparin can be given in outpatient setting before and after surgery.
[c]For example, local skin surgery, dental prophylaxis, and treatment for caries.

erative hemorrhage occurs, warfarin can be restarted within 24 hours after the procedure. Admission to the hospital or a delay in discharge to give heparin is usually unnecessary.[28–30] Deciding who is at very high risk of thrombosis and thus should require "bridging" with heparin until warfarin can be reinstated, may be difficult; clinical judgment is required. Heparin can usually be reserved for patients who have had a recent thromboembolism (arbitrarily within 1 year), patients with demonstrated thrombotic problems when previously off therapy, and patients with two or more risk factors (see Fig. 80–2). When used, heparin should be started 24 hours after warfarin is stopped (i.e., 48 hours before surgery) and stopped 6 to 12 hours before the procedure. Heparin should be restarted as early after surgery as bleeding stability allows and the aPTT maintained at a "therapeutic level" (see Table 80–4) until warfarin is restarted and the desired INR can be achieved. Home administration and management of heparin (and warfarin) can be arranged to minimize time in the hospital.

Low-molecular-weight heparin is even more easily utilized outside of the hospital. One prospective (nonrandomized)[33] and one retrospective study[34] have evaluated the use of low-molecular-weight heparin for "bridging" warfarin anticoagulation therapy before and after surgery. Both showed reasonable freedom from adverse clinical effects in the postoperative period, even in PHV patients. Being a relatively new therapy, low-molecular-weight heparin is being scrutinized more carefully than older antithrombotic drugs.[34] While recommended for "bridging," a lack of randomized studies and manufacturer package warnings are reasons to individualize therapy.

[ ] CARDIAC CATHETERIZATION AND ANGIOGRAPHY

Neither antiplatelet therapy nor heparin need be stopped for these procedures. Cardiac catheterization can be performed with a patient taking warfarin, but, preferably, the drug should be stopped 72 hours before the procedure and restarted after the procedure on the same day.[35] If a patient is at very high risk of thromboembolism, heparin should be started 48 hours before the procedure and continued until warfarin is restarted and the desired INR is achieved. If the catheterization procedure is to include a transseptal puncture (especially in a patient who has not had previous opening of the pericardium), patients should be off all antithrombotic therapy and the INR should be <1.2.[35]

[ ] CORONARY ARTERY STENTS IN PATIENTS WITH VALVE DISEASE

Stent insertion complicates antithrombotic therapy. A thienopyridine agent, usually clopidogrel, is required for at least 30 days (6 to 12 months for a sirolimus-coated stent) for optimal prevention of in-stent thrombosis.[36,37] Clopidogrel has no proven efficacy in preventing thromboemboli in patients with PHV, so continuation of warfarin is recommended in patients with mechanical protheses. If these patients are also on aspirin (along with warfarin) it would seem prudent that it be stopped given concerns of bleeding, but this is unproved. Patients with tissue valves taking aspirin should continue that drug after stent insertion.

[ ] PREGNANCY

Indications for antithrombotic therapy are not altered by pregnancy but treatment regimens have to be adjusted.[38] This is because of risks to fetal development but also because of concerns about fetal and maternal bleeding. The incidence of a warfarin caused embryopathy is 3 to 25 percent when the drug is taken in the first 3 months (particularly weeks 6 to 12). It can essentially be eliminated by avoiding warfarin during this time and possibly be using doses of less than 5 mg/d.[39] Heparin does not cross the placenta, but like warfarin, can be ineffective or cause maternal bleeding. Given these concerns, in the pregnant women requiring anticoagulant for her valve, it is recommended that she use heparin for the first 3 months and then switch to warfarin (Fig. 80–3). At 1 to 3 weeks before labor and delivery, when it can be predicted, she should switch back to heparin. The return to heparin is with the hope of better control of maternal bleeding with labor and delivery, should it occur, and to prevent fetal hem-

orrhage as the baby will be anticoagulated if the mother is taking warfarin. If the mother has a PHV, use of low-molecular-weight heparin should be individualized for the reasons outlined in the previous discussion of "bridging."

[ ] THERAPY AT THE TIME OF A THROMBOEMBOLIC EVENT

Acute Management

Data and opinions about optimal timing for initiating or continuing anticoagulants in patients in whom an embolus is the presumed cause of a stroke are conflicting.[2,40–42] Ideally, treatment would be started immediately to prevent recurrence of an embolus, but the early use of heparin (within 72 hours) is associated with a 15 to 25 percent chance of converting a nonhemorrhagic stroke into a hemorrhagic stroke.[42] The risk of early recurrent emboli is less than 5 percent.[41] On balance, it seems preferable to withhold therapy for at least 72 hours. If a computed tomography (CT) scan at that time reveals little or no hemorrhage, heparin should be administered to maintain an aPTT at the lower end of the therapeutic level until warfarin, started at the same time, results in the desired INR. If the CT scan demonstrates significant hemorrhage, antithrombotic therapy should be withheld until the

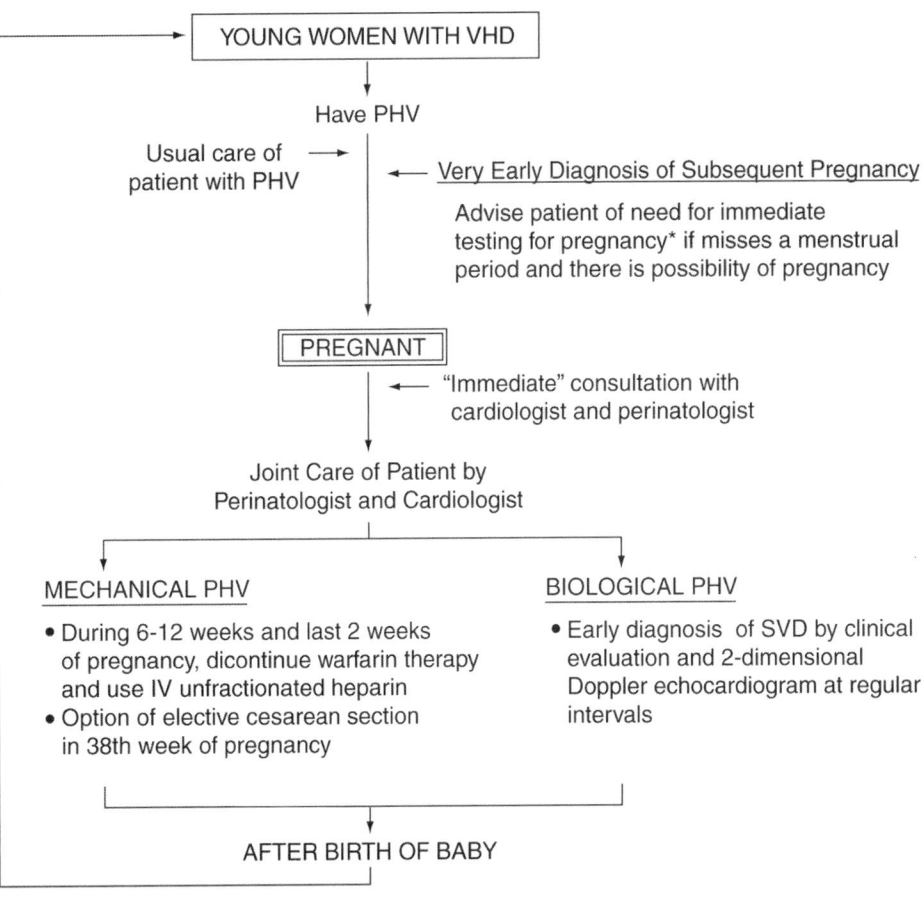

FIGURE 80–3. Management of a woman with a prosthetic heart valve (PHV) at time of pregnancy. SVC, structural valve deterioration; VHD, valvular heart disease. *Source: From Hung L, Rahimtoola SH. Prosthetic heart valve and pregnancy. Circulation 2003;107:1240–1246.*

bleed is treated or has stabilized (7 to 14 days). Anticoagulation can then be started as just described.

Long-Term Management

If the embolic event occurs when a patient is *off* antithrombotic therapy, long-term warfarin therapy is required. If the embolic event occurs while the patient is *on* adequate antithrombotic therapy with the following parameters, the therapy should be altered as follows[2]:

- If on warfarin-INR 2 to 3: increase dose to achieve an INR of 2.5 to 3.5
- If on warfarin-INR 2.5 to 3.5: add aspirin 50 to 100 mg/d
- If on warfarin with INR 2.5 to 3.5, plus aspirin 80 to 100 mg/d: aspirin dose may also need to be increased to 325 mg/d
- If on aspirin 325 mg/d: switch to warfarin-INR 2 to 3

Embolism occurring after this medical approach should lead to consideration of possible valve surgery if the valve is the likely source of the thrombus.

[ ] EXCESSIVE ANTICOAGULATION

In most patients with INR above the therapeutic range, excessive anticoagulation can be managed by withholding warfarin and following the level of anticoagulation with serial INR determinations. Excessive anticoagulation (INR >5) greatly increases the risk of hemorrhage. However, rapid decreases in INR that lead to INR falling below the therapeutic level may increase the risk of thromboembolism.

Patients with PHVs with an INR of 5 to 10 who are not bleeding can be managed by the following: (1) hospitalization with administration of oral vitamin K; (2) withholding warfarin and administering (2.5 mg) daily until the INR returns to an acceptable range. Warfarin therapy can then be restarted and dose adjusted appropriately to ensure that INR is in the therapeutic range. In emergency situations, the use of fresh-frozen plasma is preferable to high-dose vitamin K_1, especially *parenteral vitamin K_1*, because use of the latter increases the *risks of overcorrection to a hypercoagulable state and of anaphylaxis*.

Human recombinant factor (rFVIIa), dose 15 to 19 μg/kg body weight, has been used to reverse critically prolonged INR and bleeding complications safely and rapidly. Indications include an INR >10 in high-risk persons, clinical hemorrhage, and at time of life-sparing diagnostic and therapeutic procedures.[43]

[ ] THERAPY AT THE TIME OF A BLEED

With significant bleeding, antithrombotic therapy should be stopped and, if the patient is at risk, drug effects should be reversed.[2] If possible, the cause of bleeding should be corrected and antithrombotic therapy restarted as soon as possible. If this is not possible, treatment decisions are difficult. In patients with a mechanical prosthesis or multiple risk factors for thromboemboli, acceptance of intermittent bleeding with acute management for the bleeds may be necessary. In valve patients who are at lower risk of emboli or in whom the role of antithrombotic treatment is less clear (e.g., LV dysfunction), it may be optimal to withhold chronic

therapy or, if a patient is on warfarin, to switch to aspirin. With mechanical PHVs, consideration should be given to replacing the mechanical valve with a biologic valve in some patients (e.g., in those who have had multiple, large, life- or organ-threatening bleeds).

[ ] THROMBOSIS OF PROSTHETIC HEART VALVES

PHV obstruction is caused by thrombus in approximately 50 percent, pannus in 10 percent, and pannus plus thrombus in 40 percent of cases. The cause may be difficult to determine and requires knowledge of the clinical presentation (result of valve obstruction) and findings on Doppler echocardiography, including transesophageal echocardiography. Pannus is tissue ingrowth; therefore, thrombolytic therapy is ineffective and if obstruction is severe, valve replacement is indicated.

If a patient has a thrombotic obstruction of a right-sided PHV, thrombolytics are the first choice of therapy as they are successful in 80 to 100 percent of treated patients.[44,45]

Left-sided PHV thrombosis (aortic and mitral) is more serious. With use of thrombolytics, studies show a mortality of 2 to 16 percent depending on New York Heart Association (NYHA) functional status, thromboembolism in 12 to 15 percent, major bleeding in 5 percent, and nondisabling bleeding in 14 percent. Thrombolysis was ineffective in 16 to 29 percent, and thrombosis was recurrent in 11 to 20 percent.[45–48] Best results were obtained in patients who are in NYHA functional classes I and II and who have a "small" thrombus.

Surgical replacement of the thrombosed PHV is associated with a mortality of 10 to 60 percent. Again, best results are obtained in patients who are NYHA functional classes I and II.

[ ] ANTITHROMBOTIC THERAPY IN THE PATIENT WITH ENDOCARDITIS

Data on starting or stopping antithrombotic therapy in a patient with endocarditis are conflicting as noted in a recent review.[49] In balance, we recommend the following: If a patient with valve disease develops endocarditis while on antithrombotic therapy, the medication should be continued (see Chap. 85). If the patient presents with or develops an embolic event involving the central nervous system, therapy should be stopped as described earlier for acute embolic events.[41,42] Additionally, the issue of whether or not the embolus is caused by thrombus or infected vegetation should be addressed. If thrombus is likely, the chronic anticoagulation program will also require alteration.

REFERENCES

1. Rahimtoola SH. Lessons learned about the determinants of the results of valve surgery. *Circulation* 1988;78:1503–1506.
2. Bonow RO, Carabello B, Chatterjee K, et al. ACC/AHA 2006 guidelines for the management of patients with valvular heart disease: a report of the American College of Cardiology/American Heart Association Task Force on Practice Guidelines (Writing Committee to Revise the 1998 Guidelines for the Management of Patients With Valvular Heart Disease): developed in collaboration with the Society of Cardiovascular Anesthesiologists: endorsed by the Society for Cardiovascular Angiography and Interventions and the Society of Thoracic Surgeons. *Circulation* 2006;114(5):e84–e231.

3. Aguilar M, Hart R. Antiplatelet therapy for preventing stroke in patients with non-valvular atrial fibrillation and no previous history of stroke or transient ischemic attacks. *Cochrane Database Syst Rev* 2005;(4):CD001925.

4. Fuster V, Ryden LE, Cannon DS, et al. ACC/AHA/ESC 2006 guidelines for the management of patients with atrial fibrillation: a report of the American College of Cardiology/American Heart Association Task Force on Practice Guidelines and the European Society of Cardiology Committee for Practice Guidelines (Writing Committee to Revise the 2001 Guidelines for the Management of Patients with Atrial Fibrillation). *J Am Coll Cardiol* 2006;48(4):e149–e246.

5. Gage BF, Waterman AD, Shannon W, et al. Validation of clinical classification schemes for predicting stroke: results from the National Registry of Atrial Fibrillation. *JAMA* 2001;285(22):2864–2870.

6. Singer DE, Albers GW, Dalen JE, et al. Antithrombotic therapy in atrial fibrillation: the Seventh ACCP Conference on Antithrombotic and Thrombolytic Therapy. *Chest* 2004;126(3 Suppl):429S–456S.

7. Cooper NJ, Sutton AJ, Lu G, et al. Mixed comparison of stroke prevention treatments in individuals with nonrheumatic atrial fibrillation. *Arch Intern Med* 2006;166(12):1269–1275.

8. Al-Khadra AS, Salem DN, Rand WM, et al. Warfarin anticoagulation and survival: a cohort analysis from the studies of left ventricular dysfunction. *J Am Coll Cardiol* 1998;31:749–753.

9. Hunt SA, Abraham WT, Chin MH, et al. ACC/AHA 2005 guideline update for the diagnosis and management of chronic heart failure in the adult: a report of the American College of Cardiology/American Heart Association Task Force on Practice Guidelines (Writing Committee to Update the 2001 Guidelines for the Evaluation and Management of Heart Failure): developed in collaboration with the American College of Chest Physicians and the International Society for Heart and Lung Transplantation: endorsed by the Heart Rhythm Society. *Circulation* 2005;112(12):e154–e235.

10. Starr A, Grunkemeier GL. Recurrent thromboembolism: significance and management. In: Butchart EG, Bodnar E, eds. *Thrombosis, Embolism and Bleeding*. London: ICR, 1992:402–415.

11. Blackstone EH. Analyses of thrombosis, embolism and bleeding as time-related outcome events. In: Butchart EG, Bodnar E, eds. *Thrombosis, Embolism and Bleeding*. London: ICR, 1992:445–463.

12. Remadi JP, Baron O, Roussel C, et al. Isolated mitral valve replacement with St. Jude medical prosthesis: long-term results: a follow-up of 19 years. *Circulation* 2001;103(11):1542–1545.

13. Bloomfield P, Wheatley DJ, Prescott RJ, et al. Twelve-year comparison of a Bjork-Shiley mechanical heart valve with porcine bioprostheses. *N Engl J Med* 1991;324:573–579.

14. Hammermeister KE, Sethi GK, Henderson WG, et al. Outcomes 15 years after valve replacement with a mechanical versus bioprosthetic valve. *J Am Coll Cardiol* 2000;36:1152–1158.

15. Grunkemeier GL, Li H-H, Naftel DC, et al. Long-term performance of heart valve prosthesis. *Curr Probl Cardiol* 2000;25:73–156.

16. Geras M, Chesebro JH, Fuster V, et al. High risk of thromboemboli early after bioprosthetic cardiac valve replacement. *J Am Coll Cardiol* 1995;25:1111–1119.

17. Stein PD, Alpert JS, Bussey HI, et al. Antithrombotic therapy in patients with mechanical or biological prosthetic heart valves. *Chest* 2001;119:220S–227S.

18. Cannegieter SC, Rosendaal FR, Wintzen AR, et al. Optimal oral anticoagulant therapy in patients with mechanical heart valves. *N Engl J Med* 1995;333:11–17.

19. Saour JN, Sieck JO, Mamo LAR, et al. Trial of different intensities of anticoagulation in patients with prosthetic heart valves. *N Engl J Med* 1990;322:428–432.

20. Hylek EM, Skates SJ, Sheehan MA, et al. An analysis of the lowest effective intensity of prophylactic anticoagulation for patients with nonrheumatic atrial fibrillation. *N Engl J Med* 1996;335:540–546.

21. Acar J, Iung B, Boissel JP, et al. AREVA. Multicenter randomized comparison of low-dose versus standard-dose anticoagulation in patients with mechanical prosthetic heart valves. *Circulation* 1996;94:2107–2112.

22. Rahimtoola SH. Choice of prosthetic heart valve in adult patients. *J Am Coll Cardiol* 2003;41:893–904.

23. Turpie AG, Gent M, Laupacis A, et al. A comparison of aspirin with placebo in patients treated with warfarin after heart-valve replacement. *N Engl J Med* 1993;329:524–529.

24. Altman R, Rouvier J, Gurfinkel E, et al. Comparison of high-dose with low-dose aspirin in patients with mechanical heart valve replacement treated with oral anticoagulant. *Circulation* 1996;94:2113–2116.

25. Little SH, Massel DR. Antiplatelet and anticoagulation for patients with prosthetic heart valves. *Cochrane Database Syst Rev* 2003(4):CD003464.

26. Laffort P, Rondant R, Roques X, et al. Early and long-term (one-year) effects of the association of aspirin and oral anticoagulant on thrombi and morbidity after replacement of the mitral valve with the St. Jude Medical prosthesis. *J Am Coll Cardiol* 2000;35:739–746.

27. Chambers JC, Somerville J, Stone S, et al. Pulmonary autograft procedure for aortic valve disease: long-term results of the pioneer series. *Circulation* 1997;96(7):2206–2214.

28. Tinker JH, Tarhan S. Discontinuing anticoagulant therapy in surgical patients with cardiac valve prostheses: observations in 180 operations. *JAMA* 1978;239:738–739.

29. Bryan AJ, Butchart EG. Prosthetic heart valves and anticoagulant management during non-cardiac surgery. *Br J Surg* 1995;82:577–578.

30. Kearon C, Hirsh J. Current concepts: management of anticoagulation before and after elective surgery. *N Engl J Med* 1997;336(21):1506–1511.

31. Katz J, Feldman MA, Bass EB, et al. Risks and benefits of anticoagulant and antiplatelet medication use before cataract surgery. *Ophthalmology* 2003;110(9):1784–1788.

32. Kovacs MJ, Kearon C, Rodger M, et al. Single-arm study of bridging therapy with low-molecular-weight heparin for patients at risk of arterial embolism who require temporary interruption of warfarin [see comment]. *Circulation* 2004;110(12):1658–1663.

33. Spyropoulos AC, Jenkins P, Bornikova L, et al. Costs and clinical outcomes associated with low-molecular-weight heparin vs unfractionated heparin for perioperative bridging in patients receiving long-term oral anticoagulant therapy. *Chest* 2004;125(5):1642–1650.

34. FDA Med Watch. *2002 Safety Information*. [Internet] 2006 [cited August 3, 2006].

35. Morton MJ, McAnulty JH, Rahimtoola SH, et al. Risks and benefits of postoperative cardiac catheterization in patients with ball-valve prostheses. *Am J Cardiol* 1977;40:870–875.

36. Schomig A, Neumann F, Kastrati A, et al. A randomized comparison of antiplatelet and anticoagulant therapy after the placement of coronary-artery stents. *N Engl J Med* 1998;339:1084–1089.

37. Martin L, Baim D, Jeffrey P, et al. A Clinical trial comparing three antithrombotic-drug regimens after coronary artery stenting. *N Engl J Med* 1998;339:1665–1671.

38. Hung L, Rahimtoola SH. Prosthetic heart valve and pregnancy. *Circulation* 2003;107:1240–1246.

39. Vitale N, DeFeo M, DeSanto LS, et al. Dose-dependent fetal complications of warfarin in pregnant women with mechanical heart valves. *J Am Coll Cardiol* 1999;33(6):1637–1641.

40. Chamorro A, Vila N, Saiz A, et al. Early anticoagulation after large cerebral embolic infarction: a safety study. *Neurology* 1995;45:861–865.

41. Sherman DG, Dyken ML, Gent M, et al. Antithrombotic therapy for cerebrovascular disorders. An update. *Chest* 1995;108(4 Suppl):444S–456S.

42. Wijdicks EF, Schieviak W, Brown R, et al. The dilemma of discontinuation of anticoagulation therapy for patients with intracranial hemorrhage and mechanical heart valves. *Neurosurgery* 1998;42(4):769–773.

43. Deveras RA, Kessler CM. Reversal of warfarin-induced excessive anticoagulation with recombinant human factor VIIa concentrate. *Ann Intern Med* 2002;137(11):884–888.

44. Hurrell DG, Schaff HV, Tajik AJ. Thrombolytic therapy for obstruction of mechanical prosthetic valves. *Mayo Clinic Proc* 1996;71:604–613.

45. Roudaut R, Lafitte S, Roudaut MF, et al. Fibrinolysis of mechanical prosthetic valve thrombosis: a single-center study of 127 cases. *J Am Coll Cardiol* 2003;41(4):653–658.

46. Lengyel M, Fuster V, Keltai M, et al. Guidelines for management of left-sided prosthetic valve thrombosis: a role for thrombolytic therapy. Prosthetic valve thrombosis. *J Am Coll Cardiol* 1997;30:1521–1526.

47. Özkan M, Kaymaz C, Kirma C, et al. Intravenous thrombolytic treatment of mechanical prosthetic valve thrombosis: a study using serial transesophageal echocardiography. *J Am Coll Cardiol* 2000;35:1881–1889.

48. Shaprina Y, Herz I, Vatini M, et al. Thrombolysis is an effective and safe therapy in stuck bileaflet mitral valves in the absence of high-risk thrombi. *J Am Coll Cardiol* 2000;35:1874–1880.

49. Sexton D, Hart R. Anticoagulant and antiplatelet therapy in patients with infective endocarditis. *Up to Date Online*, 2006.

PART 12 Congenital Heart Disease

CHAPTER 81

Cardiovascular Diseases Caused by Genetic Abnormalities

Ali J. Marian / Ramon Brugada / Robert Roberts

ESSENTIALS OF GENETIC DISORDERS

Genetic factors play a significant role in all cardiovascular disorders (see also Chap. 5). Genetic defects are responsible for malformations of the heart and blood vessels, which account for the largest number of human birth defects. The estimated incidence of congenital heart disease is approximately 1 percent of all live births.[1] The prevalence is estimated to be 10-fold higher among stillbirths.[2] Genetic defects are also responsible for familial cardiovascular disorders, such as cardiomyopathies and the long QT (LQT) syndrome as well as nonfamilial and complex phenotypes, such as atherosclerosis and common forms of hypertension. Molecular genetics in conjunction with cytogenetics provide the opportunity to decipher the genetic basis and pathogenesis of cardiovascular diseases. Given the rapid pace of genetic discoveries, it is expected that genetic diagnosis and screening will become incorporated into standard practice in the near future. It is thus imperative that cardiologists understand the basis for genetic disorders and the medical and ethical implications of genetics.

[ ] BASIS FOR GENETIC TRANSMISSION

All hereditary information is transmitted through DNA, a linear polymer composed of purine (adenine, guanine) and pyrimidine (cytosine, thymine) bases. The gene is the basic hereditary unit. It consists of a distinct fragment of DNA, which encodes a specific polypeptide (protein). There are about 35,000 genes in the human genome.[3] Each individual has two copies of each gene, called *alleles*. The genes are localized in a linear sequence along 23 pairs of chromosomes, including 22 pairs of autosomes (chromosomes 1 to 22) and 1 pair of sex chromosomes, X and Y. Females have two X chromosomes, whereas males carry one X and one Y chromosome. Each parent contributes one of each chromosome pair (the members of the pair are referred to as *homologous chromosomes*) and thus one copy of each gene. The site at which a gene is located on a particular chromosome is referred to as the *genetic locus*. A given gene always resides at the same genetic locus on a particular chromosome, so the loci on homologous chromosomes are identical. However, alleles residing at these loci may be identical or different, leading to *homozygous* (identical alleles) and *heterozygous* (two different alleles present at the locus) states.

The genetic information is encoded by the linear sequence of the four bases of the DNA. Translation of this information into protein is through a translational code passed on through messenger ribonucleic acid (mRNA). Each unit of three bases, referred to as a *codon*, encodes a specific amino acid. The transcribed mRNA serves as the template that determines sequence of the amino acids in the resulting polypeptide. Both autosomal alleles are usually transcribed into mRNA and translated into protein. However, expression of a gene can be restricted to specific cells and organs or regulated during a developmental stage because of regulation by cell- and tissue-specific transcription factors. In cells that carry two X chromosomes, only one X is active and the other X is silent after early embryogenesis.

[ ] CLASSIFICATION OF GENETIC DISORDERS

In general, DNA nucleotide sequences remain stable during transmission to offspring. Nonetheless, occasional base sequence changes

do occur, which are referred to as *mutations*. Mutations represent stable, heritable alterations in DNA. Somatic mutations, however, are not heritable. A number of mutagenic factors—such as environmental agents, radiation, chemicals, and errors by the DNA synthetic and editing enzymes—can induce mutations. Mutations can involve a visible alteration at the level of the chromosome (chromosomal abnormalities), which can result in the deletion or translocation of a portion of the chromosome, whereby several genes are often eliminated or altered. In contrast, mutations can be restricted to minor alterations in the DNA sequence, which vary from the substitution of a single nucleotide to that of the deletion or addition of multiple nucleotides. Thus, hereditary and congenital diseases are conventionally classified into three broad categories: (1) chromosomal abnormalities, (2) single-gene or monogenic disorders, and (3) polygenic disorders or complex traits.

Chromosomal Abnormalities

Each human cell has two copies of each chromosome (*diploids*) and each chromosome has two arms, referred to as the long, or "q," and the short, or "p," arms. The arms of the chromosomes meet at a primary constriction referred to as the *centromere*. Mutations typically occur during meiosis when chromosomes separate. Mutations can involve large deletions, duplications, translocations, rearrangements, and aneuploidy (too few or too many chromosomes). Chromosomal abnormalities are relatively common during embryonic life and lead to spontaneous abortion, often during the first trimester of pregnancy. However, a significant number of fetuses with chromosomal abnormalities survive. Chromosomal aberrations, numerical or structural, occur in approximately 1 in 150 liveborn infants.[4] Most diseases caused by chromosomal abnormalities are detected in the neonates or infants because of involvement of many genes causing phenotypes that are easily diagnosed on physical examination. Chromosomal abnormalities often lead to structural heart defects and are found in 5 to 13 percent of liveborn children with congenital heart disease.[1]

The usual cause for gain of a chromosome is nondisjunction because of failure of a homologous pair of chromosomes to separate during meiosis. When an additional copy of the chromosome is added during fertilization, three copies of the same chromosome (or only one copy) are found in the new zygote instead of the chromosome pair. Two of the most common chromosomal disorders causing heart disease in the adult, namely Down syndrome (trisomy 21) and Turner syndrome (XO), are both commonly caused by nondisjunction. Chromosomal rearrangements occur when a chromosome breaks and rejoins within itself incorrectly, which can result in an inversion of the genetic material. Inversion occurs when a chromosome breaks at two points and the intermediate segment reunites in inverted orientation. Typically, there is no apparent phenotype in persons carrying an inversion, but their offspring may have severe abnormalities due to the disruption in chromosome pairing that can take place during meiosis. Isochromes are formed when two short or long arms join with loss of the other arm. Chromosomal translations occur when breaks arise in two chromosomes that are reunited after exchange of segments. Chromosome duplications or gains of chromosomal material may also be associated with phenotypic abnormality, but most commonly, they cause no obvious aberration.

Chromosome deletions are large deletions (equal to or greater than 10^6 base pairs) that commonly lead to loss of a large amount of DNA and loss or disruption of multiple genes. Consequently, a series of phenotypes in a single individual may be present as a result of interruptions in a series of genes within the loci of a single chromosome.

Single-Gene Disorders

A single-gene disorder is an inherited disease that can be caused by a mutation in a single gene. Single-gene disorders show a mendelian pattern of inheritance. They are classified as autosomal dominant, autosomal recessive, or X-linked (dominant or recessive). The majority of monogenic diseases exhibit an autosomal dominant mode of inheritance. Therefore, in a given family, approximately half of the members are affected. Monogenic disorders with an autosomal recessive inheritance are caused by mutations in both copies of the gene. Therefore, in a given family only 25 percent of the offspring exhibit the phenotype, 50 percent carry the mutation, and 25 percent are normal. In X-linked inheritance, males exhibit the disease and females are usually free of the phenotype but carry the mutation. However, if the mutation involves a major protein, the effect of the mutation may be dominant and females can exhibit the clinical phenotype. In diseases caused by mitochondrial DNA mutations, inheritance is from the mother (no male-to-male transmission), because mitochondrial DNA is predominantly inherited from the ovum.

Only a fraction of cardiovascular disorders is monogenic. The DNA mutation gives rise to a change in the corresponding amino acids of the encoded protein and exerts its deleterious effects via functional alterations. A change in even one amino acid located in a critical domain of the protein can enhance the function (gain-of-function mutation) or impair the function (loss-of-function mutation), with a concomitant change in the phenotype. On average, a mutation occurs every 10^6 cell divisions or once every 200,000 years. Only mutations occurring in the gametes are transmitted.

In single-gene disorders, although the presence of the causal mutations is necessary for the development of the disease, other factors also affect the phenotypic expression of the disease. Modifier genes (the genetic background of the affected subjects) and the environmental factors are major determinants of phenotypic expression of a single-gene disorder.

Polygenic Disorders

Polygenic or complex traits are caused by an assortment of interactions among variants of many genes and nongenetic factors. Therefore, in this setting, the presence of a single variant may not be sufficient to cause a disease, nor will its absence prevent development of the disease. Polygenic disorders account for the majority of the cardiovascular diseases, including atherosclerosis, essential hypertension, obesity, and diabetes mellitus. In polygenic diseases, multiple genes interact to induce the disorder or to provide an increased risk of developing it. Changes involving a single nucleotide are distributed throughout the human genome with a frequency of about 1 per 300 base pairs (bp).[5,6] These changes, referred to as *single nucleotide polymorphisms* (SNPs; see Chap. 5), account for most interindividual differences such as height and weight, susceptibility to disease, clinical outcome, and response to therapy (pharmacogenetics).

There are over 12 million validated SNPs in the human genome (see http://www.ncbi.nlm.nih.gov/projects/SNP/). Putatively functional SNPs, which are those located in the regulatory and coding regions or splice junctions, can affect expression or function of the encoded proteins. Therefore, they are likely to exert biologic and clinical effects. The effects could confer protection against or susceptibility toward a complex phenotype. In rare instances, SNPs located in introns or intergenic regions could affect susceptibility to disease.[7] Commonly, a large number of genetic variants are involved in the etiology of a complex disease. Therefore, each particular variant accounts for a very small fraction of the risk (genotype-related risk). Because of involvement of multiple gene variants on the same or different chromosome are involved in the pathogenesis of a polygenic disease, inheritance of the disease does not follow a classic mendelian pattern. Therefore, there is a lack of cosegregation of a candidate gene variant (allele) with inheritance of the phenotype. Consequently, it is often difficult to map and establish the causality of a genetic variant in susceptibility to a complex trait. Additional experiments are usually required to establish the causality. Mapping of the genes for complex traits is discussed in Chap. 9.

▌ ▐ CLASSIFICATION OF MUTATIONS

Most human diseases exhibit *genetic heterogeneity*, defined as being caused by different genes and mutations causing the same phenotype. The heterogeneity may arise from multiple mutations in one gene (*allele heterogeneity*) or in two or more genes (*locus heterogeneity*). Within any one family, however, there is one causal gene and mutation in all affected members; only rarely are two different causal mutations or genes transmitted for the same disease. A good example is familial hypertrophic cardiomyopathy (HCM), which involves more than a dozen different genes (locus heterogeneity) with multiple mutations in each (allelic heterogeneity). Mutations can involve a microscopically visible alteration, such as deletion or translocation of a portion of the chromosome (chromosomal abnormalities), or a minute change in the DNA sequence, such as alteration of one purine or pyrimidine base. Mutations involving only a single nucleotide are known as *point mutations* and are responsible for 70 percent or more of all adult single-gene disorders. A point mutation may be a substitution of one nucleotide for another, changing the amino acid sequence (*missense mutation*); or it may change from encoding an amino acid to become a stop codon, which will truncate the protein (*truncated* or *nonsense mutation*); or it may eliminate a stop codon so the protein is elongated (*elongated mutant*). Finally, it may change the codon without changing the amino acid sequence (*synonymous mutation*). All genes during transcription and translation are read from 5′ to 3′ orientation, with each triplet of bases (*codon*) coding for a specific amino acid. If a nucleotide is deleted (*deletion*) or an additional one is inserted (*insertion*), it will shift the reading frame. The resulting protein would be entirely different (*frameshift mutation*) and usually nonfunctional. If a purine nucleotide is substituted for a pyrimidine or vice versa, the mutation is referred to as a *transversion*. If purine or pyrimidine substitutes for another purine or pyrimidine, respectively, it is called a *transition*. Other mutations may result from the deletion or addition of several nucleotides. In one form of myotonic dystrophy, for example, a triplet repeat of several thousand nucleotides in length is inserted into the 3′ end of the gene. Another type of mutation is known as a *gene conversion,* where two genes interact and part of the nucleotide sequence of one gene becomes incorporated into that of the other. Mutations in genes exert their deleterious effects via a structural alteration of the protein that has functional consequences, as noted.

[ ] GENETIC PENETRANCE AND EXPRESSIVITY

The percentage of individuals within a family who have inherited the causal mutation and have one or more features of the disease is referred to as the *penetrance.* Penetrance is an all-or-none phenomenon. Any manifestation, however minute, indicates that the gene has penetrance in that individual. *Nonpenetrance* refers to lack of any observable phenotype. This feature is to be distinguished from *expressivity,* which refers to the variable nature of the clinical phenotype, such as the severity. Thus, by definition, to have expressivity, the trait must be penetrant. Numerous genetic and environmental factors can affect expression of a gene, making it nearly impossible to determine which factor is most important in a specific individual or disease. Table 81–1 shows these factors.

[ ] PATTERNS OF INHERITANCE

Inherited disorders caused by a single abnormal gene are transmitted to offspring in a predictable fashion termed *mendelian transmission.* As previously noted, each individual has two copies of each gene, referred to as alleles, one transmitted from each parent. Per Mendel's first law, each of the two alleles, located on separate chromosomes, segregates independently and is transmitted unchanged to offspring. Thus the chance of inheriting the mother's allele versus the father's is 50 percent. Mendel's second law states that genes on the same chromosome also assert themselves independently through the process of crossover between segments of chromosomes (discussed below). The greater the distance between two loci, the more likely they are to be separated during genetic transmission. Mutant genes located on any of the 22 autosomal pairs or the 2 sex chromosomes may produce phenotypes inherited by simple patterns classified as autosomal (dominant or recessive) or X-linked, respectively. The terms *dominant inheritance* and *recessive inheritance* refer to characteristics of the phenotype. Dominant inheritance implies that a person with one copy of a mutant allele and one copy of the normal allele develops the phenotype associated with the mutant allele. Recessive traits, on the other hand, require both alleles to be mutant in order to produce a phenotype.

Autosomal Dominant Inheritance

Dominant disorders are those exhibiting a phenotype in heterozygous individuals, as noted. Males and females are equally affected, and offspring of an affected heterozygote have a 50 percent chance of inheriting the mutant allele. In a sporadic case, the mutation occurs de novo and in one of the germ lines of parents (typically sperm). By definition, it is absent in the somatic cells of parents. Autosomal dominant inheritance can be misdiagnosed as sporadic if there is low expressivity in the phenotypically normal parent carrying the mutant allele or if extramarital paternity has occurred. Table 81–2 lists the features characteristic of autosomal dominant inheritance.

Autosomal Recessive Inheritance

Autosomal recessive phenotypes are clinically apparent when the patient carries two mutant alleles (i.e., is homozygous) at the locus responsible for the disease (Fig. 81–1). The disease-causing gene is found on one of the 22 autosomes. Thus, both males and females are equally affected. Clinical uniformity is typical and disease onset generally occurs early in life. Recessive disorders are more commonly diagnosed in childhood than are dominant diseases. On average, only 1 in 4 children (25 percent) will be affected (see Table 81–2).

X-Linked Inheritance

X-linked inherited disorders are caused by defects in genes located on the X chromosome. Because females have two X chromosomes, they may carry either one mutant allele (heterozygote) or two mutant alleles (homozygote). The trait may therefore display dominant or recessive expression. Males have a single X chromosome (and one Y chromosome). Consequently, a male is expected to display the full syndrome whenever he inherits the abnormal gene from his mother. Hence, the terms *X-linked dominant* and *X-linked recessive* apply only to the expression of the gene in females. Because a male must pass on his Y chromosome to all male offspring, he cannot pass on a mutant X allele to his sons. Therefore, no male-to-male transmission in X-linked disorders can occur. On the other hand, a male must contribute his one X chromosome to all daughters (see Fig. 81–1). All females receiving a mutant X chromosome are known as *carriers,* and those who become affected clinically with the disease are known as *manifesting female carriers.* Table 81–2 lists the characteristic features of X-linked inheritance. Examples of X-linked disorders of the heart include X-linked cardiomyopathy, Barth syndrome, and Duchenne, Becker, and Emery-Dreifuss muscular dystrophies.

Mitochondrial Inheritance

Spermatocytes contribute few or no mitochondria to the zygote. The entire mitochondrial DNA in an embryo is derived from the mitochondria already present in the cytoplasm of the oocyte.

[ ] TABLE 81–1

Factors Affecting the Phenotype in Genetic Disorders

1. Causal genes and mutations
2. Modifier genes (genetic background)
3. Age
4. Gender
5. Exogenous or environmental factors
6. Maternal factors
7. Epigenetic alterations (such as DNA methylation)
8. Posttranscriptional and posttranslation modifications
9. Gene–gene (epistasis) and gene–environmental interactions

Thus, phenotypes caused by mitochondrial DNA mutations demonstrate only maternal inheritance (see Fig. 81–1). Table 81–2 lists the characteristic features of mitochondrial inheritance.

OVERVIEW OF GENE MAPPING AND MUTATION DETECTION

CHROMOSOMAL MAPPING IN SINGLE-GENE DISORDERS

Until the 1980s, identification of a disease-causing gene without knowing the causal protein was nearly impossible. For the majority of diseases, neither the defect nor the protein was known. Technical advances that made chromosomal mapping feasible include (1) computerized linkage analysis, (2) development of highly informative DNA markers spanning the entire genome, and (3) detection of markers by polymerase chain reaction (PCR). The 46 chromosomes of the human genome contain 3.2 billion bp of DNA. To locate a particular gene, one must first map the chromosomal locus, which requires knowledge of certain chromosomal landmarks, referred to as *DNA markers*. A DNA marker is a polymorphic sequence of DNA with a known chromosomal position, which can be detected by analyzing an individual's DNA (discussed in detail below). Markers are now available that span each chromosome at intervals of not more than 4 million base pairs (Mbp) on all chromosomes (a set of approximately 800 markers). Genetic distance is measured in terms of centimorgans (cM), named after the geneticist T.H. Morgan. One cM approximates 1 million bp (Mbp). Markers like genes have two alleles in a given individual and are transmitted to offspring according to Mendel's law, with the individual being heterozygous or homozygous for that marker. If a marker is homozygous, it is not informative for genetic linkage. When all of the markers are placed together on each chromosome and the genetic distance between them is estimated, a *genetic map* is produced. Several maps of more than 5000 highly informative markers that span the entire genome have been developed.[8]

Identification of a particular locus is made possible by showing that the causal gene of interest is in close proximity to a DNA marker on the same chromosome, a method referred to as *genetic linkage analysis*. A fundamental requirement for linkage analysis is a family in which the disease of interest is transmitted to offspring over at least two and preferably three generations. At least six affected individuals are required for analyzing cosegregation of DNA markers with inheritance of the disease, although a larger number of affected individuals is preferable.

The homologous pairs of chromosomes are assorted, and one from each parent is transmitted to the offspring by chance. Each gene, allele, or marker is transmitted independently. Thus the odds of any two genes (or a marker and a gene) being coinherited is 50 percent (chance alone). Even genes on the same chromosome are transmitted independently by the mechanism of crossover between homologous chromosomes (Fig. 81–2), unless they are in close physical proximity to each other. In the latter case, they cosegregate together. Homologous recombination provides for continual mixing of the genes during every meiosis. It is the predominant reason why no two individuals have the same genotype for DNA markers unless they are identical twins. Prior to meiosis, the two homologous chromosomes come to-

TABLE 81–2

Characteristic Features of Patterns of Inheritance

A. Autosomal dominant transmission
 1. Each affected individual has an affected parent unless the disease occurred because of a new mutation or the heterozygous parent has low expressivity.
 2. Equal proportions (i.e., 50–50) of normal and affected offspring are likely to be born to an affected individual.
 3. Normal children of an affected individual bear only normal offspring.
 4. Equal proportions of males and females are affected.
 5. Both sexes are equally likely to transmit the abnormal allele to male and female offspring, and male-to-male transmission occurs.
 6. Vertical transmission through successive generations occurs.
 7. Delayed age of onset.
 8. Variable clinical expression.
B. Autosomal recessive transmission
 1. Parents are clinically normal (in alternate generations) but genetically are heterozygotes.
 2. Alternate generations are affected, with no vertical transmission.
 3. Both sexes are affected with equal frequency.
 4. Each offspring of heterozygous carriers has a 25 percent chance of being affected, a 50 percent chance of being an unaffected carrier, and a 25 percent chance of inheriting only normal alleles.
C. X-linked transmission
 1. No male-to-male transmission.
 2. All daughters of affected males are carriers.
 3. Sons of carrier females have a 50 percent risk of being affected and daughters have a 50 percent chance of being carriers.
 4. Affected homozygous females occur only when an affected male and carrier female have children.
 5. The pedigree pattern in X-linked recessive traits tends to be oblique because of the occurrence of the trait in the sons of normal carriers but not in the sisters of affected males (i.e., uncles and nephews affected).
D. Mitochondrial transmission
 1. Equal frequency and severity of disease for each sex.
 2. Transmission through females only, with offspring of affected males being unaffected.
 3. All offspring of affected females may be affected.
 4. Extreme variability of expression of disease within a family (may include apparent nonpenetrance).
 5. Phenotype may be age-dependent.
 6. Organ mosaicism is common.

gether and form bridges (*chiasmata*) such that segments of equal proportion are exchanged between them, giving rise to crossover between homologous regions of various genes. In genetic parlance, crossing over is referred to as *recombination*. The loci occupy the same chromo-

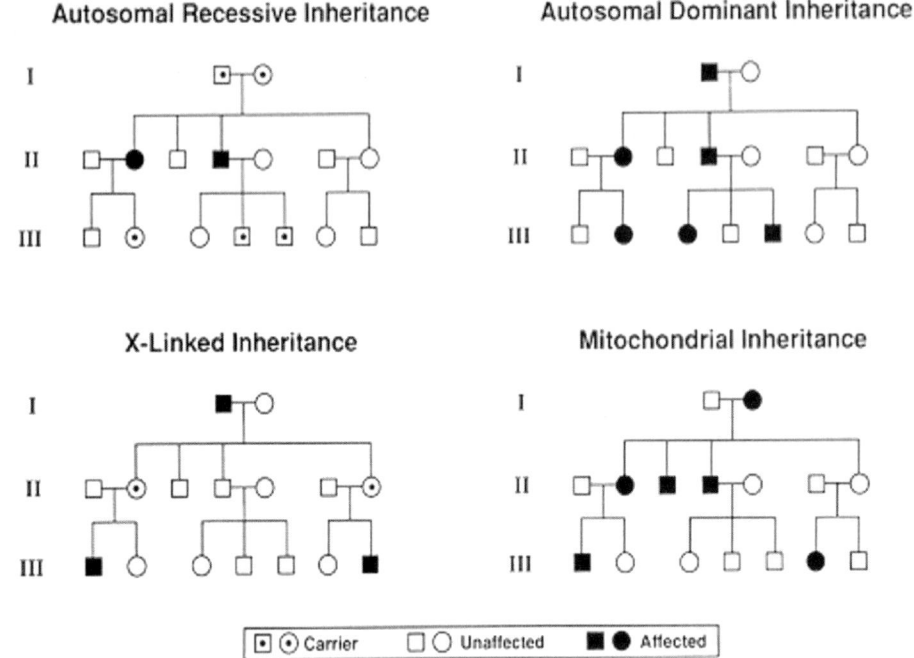

Autosomal Recessive Inheritance

Autosomal Dominant Inheritance

X-Linked Inheritance

Mitochondrial Inheritance

⊡ ⊙ Carrier   □ ○ Unaffected   ■ ● Affected

FIGURE 81–1. This typical set of pedigrees outlines the usual inheritance patterns for autosomal dominant and recessive traits, X-linked inheritance, and mitochondrial inheritance. *Squares* signify males; *circles* signify females. Filled-in circles and squares are affected females and males, respectively.

somal position on the homologous chromosome on which they are combined as they had on their original homologous chromosome. There is no net loss of chromosomal material or genes, but crossover leads to a constant intermixing of the chromosomes such that no two offspring will ever be identical. Crossovers occur only between homologous chromosomes. On average, there are 33 crossovers between homologous chromosome pairs per meiosis.

Family History and Evaluation

The most important part of an evaluation for genetic disease is the family history. First, this may give clues to the diagnosis of a particular phenotype and inheritance patterns within an individual family. For instance, an individual's ethnic background may suggest the need for specific types of genetic screening, such as for hemoglobinopathies in individuals of African or Mediterranean ancestry or for Tay-Sachs disease in individuals of eastern European (Ashkenazi) Jewish ancestry. The individual with the medical problem who brought the family to the attention of the physician is referred to as the *proband* or *propositus* (*proposita* for females) or index case. Information should generally be collected on all individuals who are first-, second-, or third-degree relatives of the proband. First-degree relatives of the proband are the parents and children. Second-degree relatives are aunts and

uncles, grandparents, and grandchildren of the proband. Third-degree relatives are first cousins, great aunts and uncles, great-grandparents, and great-grandchildren. A pedigree chart (see Fig. 81–1) is then generated. This information should include medical problems and pregnancies. If relatives are deceased, the age at death and the cause of death should be recorded. With a pedigree chart and specific family information, general questions are asked, including whether other family members have the same or similar problems. Information about various types of birth defects, mental retardation, early infant deaths, miscarriages, stillbirths, or other diseases or handicaps in the family is sought. With some disorders, there may be a variability of a particular condition (i.e., clinical heterogeneity), even within a family. For example, with a possible diagnosis of HCM, one should ask about premature death or syncope. A pregnancy history may provide information to support a possible teratogenic exposure. The date of the last menstrual period, whether the pregnancy was planned, whether contraception was used immediately prior to pregnancy, the time when the pregnancy was recognized, and when the mother sought prenatal care should be noted. Problems during the pregnancy—such as bleeding, spotting, cramping, fevers, rashes, or illnesses; drug exposures (both prescribed and nonprescribed), alcohol intake, or "recre-

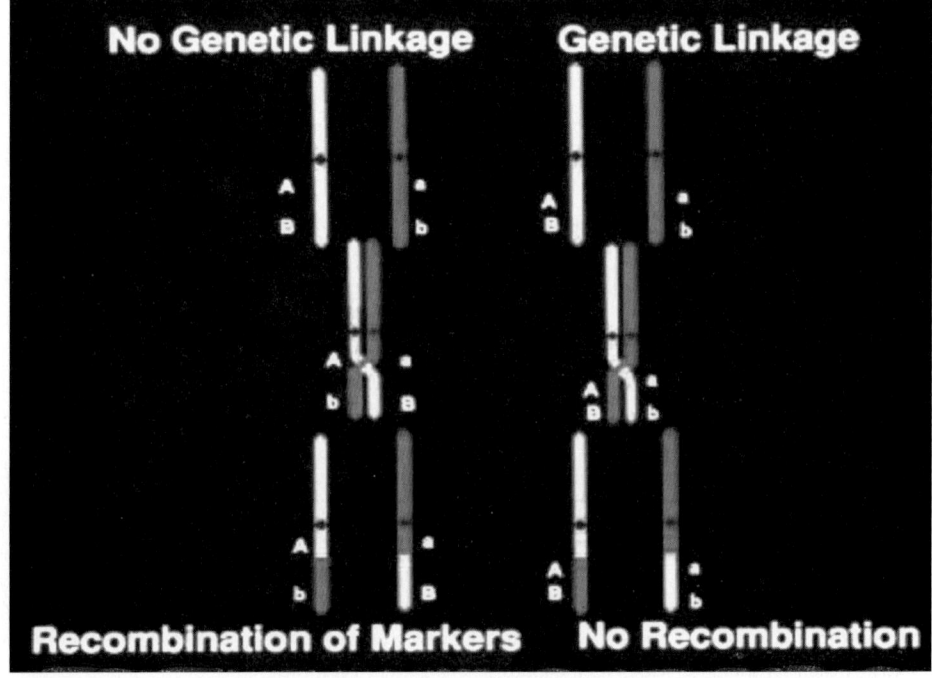

FIGURE 81–2. Linkage analysis. Loci A (disease locus) and B (DNA marker locus) are located in close proximity with minimal chance of crossover between them. Thus, even when crossover occurs between homologous segments of chromosomes during meiosis, A and B loci cosegregate together and thus are considered genetically linked.

ational" drug use; and exposures to potent chemicals in the workplace or while involved in various hobbies—should be explored. Pregnancy and family histories can then be used in conjunction with the findings on physical examination to derive a potential etiologic diagnosis and to plan for further diagnostic studies. The term *etiologic diagnosis* should suggest whether a specific cardiac defect is familial (by family history), genetic but not familial (sporadic), teratogenic (by pregnancy history), or multifactorial. Prognosis and recurrence risk are linked strongly to an accurate diagnosis and its probable etiology. In sum, accurate phenotypic characterization is essential for all genetic studies.

Concept of Genetic Linkage Analysis

Despite the independent assortment of chromosomes and genes during meiosis, genes (alleles) on two or more loci are often coinherited because they are so close together that a chiasmatic bridge does not form between them. Two loci coinherited more than 50 percent of the time are considered genetically linked. To map the chromosomal locus responsible for a causal gene, DNA markers that are evenly distributed across the chromosomes are selected. DNA is collected from all members of a family (normal and affected) and genotyped for the selected markers. If a DNA marker is coinherited with the phenotype in the affected individuals, the chromosomal locus where the DNA marker resides is in close physical proximity to the locus of the causal gene. This is referred to as *genetic linkage* between the disease (causal gene) and the DNA marker. Figure 81–2 illustrates the concept of linkage analysis. Shown in the left panel is an illustration of genetic linkage between a locus for a DNA marker and that of a disease that is inherited in a mendelian dominant fashion. The locus, designated with an "A," carries the allele responsible for the disease. The corresponding locus, "a," on the homologous chromosome has the allele that codes for the same protein but has not undergone a mutation and is thus the normal allele. The loci designated "B" and "b" represent alleles of a DNA marker of known location that has nothing to do with the disease. In the right panel, the disease and the marker loci are so close that they tend to be coinherited within the family. In contrast, in the left panel, the "A" and "b" loci are so far apart that recombination and crossover occur between the two markers; thus they segregate independently. The calculation necessary to prove definitively that genetic linkage does or does not exist between a DNA marker and a disease-related locus is sophisticated and requires advanced computer programs. The odds for and against linkage are calculated. Linkage exists if the odds in favor of linkage are at least 1000:1. Commonly, the logarithm of the odds, referred to as the *LOD score* (log of the odds), is used and a LOD score of 3 or greater indicates linkage. A LOD score of 2 (i.e., 10^2 or 100:1 odds against linkage) excludes the linkage. The likelihood of two genes being separated by recombination increases in proportion to the distance between them. The distance between a marker and a disease-causing gene when genetically linked is quite variable and may be anywhere from 1 to 50 Mbp but is usually within 1 to 10 Mbp. Thus, the inherent resolution of genetic linkage analysis is not better than 1 Mbp.

It is possible on the basis of linkage analysis alone to construct a chromosomal map of all of the DNA markers, with the distance between the various markers estimated in centimorgans. This is a complex calculation derived from the number of recombinations between the DNA markers during meioses. The recombination frequency between two markers, two genes, or a gene and a marker is the ratio of the number of crossover events to the total number of meioses. The

lower the recombination frequency between the locus of a DNA marker and that of a disease-causing gene, the closer those two are in physical distance on the chromosome. However, despite the close physical proximity of the loci of the DNA marker and the disease-causing gene, recombination still may occur. The extent to which recombination does occur reflects roughly the physical distance between the two loci. The recombination fraction (or *theta*) is used to develop a means of estimating the genetic distance (in centimorgans) between genetically linked loci. A recombination frequency or crossover of 1 percent between two loci, whether occupied by two genes or one gene and a DNA marker, reflects a physical distance of approximately 1 cM between them. For a marker and a gene separated by 1 cM, this means the chance of a crossover between them during meiosis is only 1 percent; thus, the chance of their being coinherited is 99 percent. This is a statistically derived genetic map, however, and the distances are only approximate.

Identification of the Gene and Mutation

Once the chromosomal location of a gene has been mapped, the first technique in attempting to identify the gene is referred to as the positional *candidate gene approach*. Although there are only about 30,000 genes in the genome, more than 100,000 expressed sequenced tags (ESTs) have been mapped. ESTs are unique DNA sequences of 100 to 200 bp, each of which is believed to represent a portion of the expressed sequences of a gene. These genes and ESTs are available through a worldwide network of databases in the United States, Europe, and Japan that is updated on a daily basis.

The known candidate genes or their representative ESTs are amplified, usually by PCR, to determine whether there is a mutation that segregates with the disease. If none of the candidate genes in the region is shown to have a mutation that cosegregates with the disease, it may be necessary to clone the region. This approach is referred to as *positional cloning*, so named because a region is cloned knowing only its position relative to the genetically linked DNA markers. Positional cloning is usually unnecessary as most genes in the human genome have been mapped and identified. However, if attempted, it is necessary to reduce the region (containing the gene) to 1 cM or less. It is often necessary to expand the family with the hope of finding crossovers such that DNA markers common to all affected would span only a short distance (<1 cM). The cloned genes or PCR-amplified DNA is then analyzed, commonly by direct sequencing, for the presence of the mutation. To strengthen the causality, the mutation must be shown to cosegregate with the disease and not with the unaffected members in the family. In addition, it is crucial to show that the variant is absent in large number of normal individuals and hence, it is not a polymorphism. Finally, to establish the causality, in vivo and in vitro functional studies are necessary. Table 81–3 summarizes the approach to chromosomal mapping of hereditary diseases by linkage analysis and subsequent isolation of the gene.

【 】 CHROMOSOMAL MAPPING IN POLYGENIC DISORDERS

The simplest and most commonly used approach is allelic association study, whereby an association between a variant or a haplotype with a particular phenotype is explored.[9] Two variations of the approach include candidate gene and genomewide allelic association studies. Re-

TABLE 81-3

Steps Involved in Chromosomal Mapping Gene Identification

1. Identification of a family with a familial disease.
2. Collection of clinical data from the family.
3. Clinical assessment to provide an accurate diagnosis of the disease using a consistent and objective criterion to separate normal individuals from those affected and from those who are indeterminate or unknown.
4. Collection of blood samples for immediate DNA analysis and development of lymphoblastoid cell lines for a renewable source of DNA.
5. Development of a family pedigree.
6. DNA analysis for markers of known chromosomal loci that span the human genome in an attempt to find a marker locus linked to the disease.
7. Identification of the gene.
8. Identification of mutation(s) causing the disease.
9. Demonstration of a causal relationship between the mutant gene and the disease.
10. Development of a convenient test to screen for the mutation.

cently, a haplotype-map of the human genome was developed, which is expected to facilitate mapping of the susceptibility genes for complex traits.[10,11] Susceptibility genes for complex traits also could be mapped through analysis of segregation of polymorphic DNA markers with a phenotype in related individuals. The principle behind the techniques of genomewide search is based on the likelihood of sharing a susceptibility allele between the two relatives with the phenotype. Chapter 9 discusses chromosomal mapping of the genes for complex phenotypes.

GENETIC COUNSELING PRINCIPLES

Genetic counseling should provide information about the diagnosis, possible etiology, and prognosis of a disease. In addition, psychosocial issues, reproductive options, and the availability of prenatal diagnosis should be discussed. Genetic counseling should be nondirective, providing information in a nonjudgmental, unbiased manner. The family should then be able to make decisions based on medical information in the context of their religious, moral, cultural, and social backgrounds and their financial situation. Although a genetic counselor may occasionally feel frustrated with a specific couple's decision, an effective counselor does not let personal biases interfere with the counseling role. Conflicts leading to major ethical issues and disputes may arise, however, and may be particularly apparent regarding issues of nonpaternity, sex selection, pregnancy termination, and selective nontreatment of malformed infants. Couples have many potential reproductive options, but not all may be acceptable religiously or culturally. Nevertheless, potential options should be mentioned in a sensitive manner. A common misunderstanding among families in genetic counseling is the issue of prenatal diagnosis and its relationship to abortion. Prenatal diagnosis does not imply that a parent should or would terminate the pregnancy. In many circumstances the information from prenatal diagnosis may help to reassure a couple that their risk of having another

handicapped child is, in fact, much lower than expected. Conversely, if defects are found, the subspecialist may use more diagnostic approaches to make rational decisions about medical management of the infant prior to or immediately after delivery.

The accelerated pace of progress in gene discovery, molecular medicine, and molecular diagnostics has begun to allow for improved genetic counseling and portends the possibility of future genetic therapy. As knowledge about the genetic basis of disease grows, however, so does the potential for discriminatory health insurance policies to exclude individuals who are at risk for an illness or to charge prohibitively high rates on the basis of predetermined illness. For this reason planners of the Human Genome Project recognized the need to protect individuals who volunteer for genetic study as well as those diagnosed by molecular methods in the future. Also for this reason, the National Institutes of Health–Department of Energy Working Group on Ethical, Legal, and Social Implications of the Human Genome Project was developed. Congress has passed a bill prohibiting companies from using DNA analysis to assess genetic risk as a basis for hiring. Only 11 states, however, prohibit the use of DNA analysis to determine who should get medical insurance or whether they qualify for high- or low-risk premiums.

CARDIOVASCULAR ABNORMALITIES CAUSED BY CHROMOSOMAL DEFECTS

Table 81–4 lists chromosomal defects that cause cardiovascular abnormalities. The most common chromosomal defects are described briefly below.

TURNER SYNDROME

Turner syndrome is characterized by a constellation of findings that result from partial or complete monosomy of the X chromosome.[12] It is the most common chromosomal abnormality in females, with an incidence of 1 per 2500 to 3000 liveborn girls, which corresponds to approximately 2 million cases worldwide.[13] It is characterized by cardiovascular anomalies, short stature, low-set ears, excess nuchal skin, broad chest with widely spaced nipples, peripheral lymphedema, and ovarian dysgenesis. Cardiac abnormalities are common, with a prevalence estimated to be between 23 and 40 percent.[13] The most common cardiovascular abnormalities are bicuspid aortic valve, which is present in 10 to 20 percent, and coarctation of aorta, present in 10 percent of the adult cases. The prevalence of these abnormalities is higher in children. Less-common cardiovascular anomalies include aortic stenosis, systemic hypertension, mitral valve prolapse, conduction defects, partial anomalous venous drainage, and ventricular septal defect (VSD). Aortic dilatation and dissection, partly because of concomitant hypertension, also occur (see also Chap. 12). Women with Turner syndrome are more susceptible to aortic aneurysms and ischemic heart disease.[13,14] Patients with Turner syndrome should undergo periodic cardiovascular evaluation, including 12-lead ECG and echocardiography.

Turner syndrome is caused by complete or partial absence of an X chromosome. The most common karyotype is monosomy X (45,X).[12] Approximately 5 to 10 percent of the cases have duplication of the long arm of one X (46,X,i[Xq]) and the rest have mosaicism.[12] The pathogenesis of Turner syndrome is not fully understood. It likely entails haploinsufficiency of genes (located on the X chromosome) that, un-

TABLE 81–4

Partial List of Chromosomal Abnormalities Associated with Heart Disease

CHROMOSOME DEFECTS	SYNDROMES	CARDIAC PHENOTYPE
45X	Turner syndrome	Coarctation of the aorta, ASD, aortic stenosis
Trisomy 5		Interrupted aortic arch
Trisomy 13	Patau syndrome	CHD, VSD
Trisomy 18	Edwards syndrome	CHD, VSD
Partial trisomy 20q		Dextrocardia
Trisomy 21	Down syndrome	CHD, ASD, VSD, PDA
Trisomy 22		VSD
Partial tetrasomy 22	Schmid-Fraccaro syndrome	CHD
		Anomalous pulmonary venous return
Deletion 4p	Wolf-Hirschhorn syndrome	CHD
Deletion 7q11.23	Williams syndrome	CHD, supravalvular aortic stenosis, hypertension, MVP
Deletion paternal 15q11	Prader-Willi syndrome	CHD
Deletion 17p	Miller Dieker syndrome	CHD, ASD
Deletion 22q11	CATCH-22, DiGeorge, and velocardiofacial syndromes	CHD
Rearrangement 5p15.1–3	Cri du chat	CHD
Recombination chromosome 8	San Luis Valley syndrome	Tetralogy of Fallot

ASD, atrial septal defect; CHD, congenital heart disease; MVP, mitral valve prolapse; PDA, patent ductus arteriosus; VSD, ventricular septal defect.

der normal conditions, escape inactivation. Inactivation of one copy of the X chromosome during early embryogenesis is partial and several genes escape inactivation. Specific genes that account for cardiovascular phenotype in Turner syndrome are unknown. *SHOX* (short stature homeobox-containing gene) or *PHOG* (pseudoautosomal homeobox-containing osteogenic gene), which encode two isoforms of a homeodomain protein, are considered responsible for the short stature in Turner syndrome.[13] Zinc finger protein X and zinc finger protein Y genes (*ZFX/ZFY*), which are involved in sex-determination, are also candidates genes for Turner syndrome.[15]

[ ] DOWN SYNDROME

Down syndrome, or trisomy 21, is a major cause of mental retardation and congenital heart disease, with a characteristic set of facial and physical features. The incidence of Down syndrome is approximately 1 in 700 livebirths, affecting more than 350,000 individuals in the United States alone.[16] The risk of having a liveborn with Down syndrome increases with maternal age. It is estimated at 1 in 1000 at age 30 years and 10-fold higher at age 45 years.[17] The recurrence rate in the offspring is approximately 1 percent. Clinical manifestations include congenital anomalies of

the heart and gastrointestinal tract, epicanthal folds, flattened facial profile, small and rounded ears, upslanted palpebral fissures, excess nuchal skin, and brachycephaly. An increased risk of leukemia, immune system defects, and an Alzheimer-like dementia are associated with Down syndrome. Cardiac abnormalities are present in approximately half of the cases.[18,19] The most common cardiac abnormalities are atrioventricular canal defect and isolated VSD, which occur in 45 and 35 percent of cases, respectively.[18,19] Isolated secundum atrial septal defect (ASD) is present in 8 percent and tetralogy of Fallot in 5 percent of cases (see also Chap. 12).[18]

Down syndrome is caused by trisomy 21. It is full trisomy in 95 percent, chromosomal translocation in 2 percent, and mosaic in 3 percent.[19,20] The vast majority of errors in meiosis leading to trisomy 21 are of maternal origin and occur during the first meiosis in two-thirds and during second meiosis in one-fifth of the cases. The exact causal genes responsible for the cardiovascular defects are unknown. However, four Down Syndrome Critical Regions (DSCRs) have been mapped.[21–24] DSCR1 encompasses an area of approximately 5 million bp and about 20 genes.[21] DNA markers in this region are associated with mental retardation and most of the facial features of the syndrome.[21] Among the candidate genes is *DSCR1*, which is abundantly expressed in the heart and brain.[25] It is a candidate for cardiac anomalies and mental retardation.[25]

The pathogenesis of Down syndrome is unknown. Down syndrome is considered a contiguous gene syndrome.[16] It is expected to involve increased expression of multiple contiguous genes. Overexpression of *DSCR1*, a product of DSCR, is shown in the brains of patients with Down syndrome.[26] *DSCR1* encodes calcipressin 1, which functions through direct binding and inhibition of calcineurin A, the catalytic subunit of the Ca^{2+}/calmodulin-dependent serine threonine protein phosphatase (PP2B).[26] Calcineurin dephosphorylates nuclear factor of activated T cells (NFAT), which leads to its nuclear localization and induction of gene expression.[27] Inhibition of calcineurin by *DSCR1* is expected to increase levels of phosphorylated NFAT and reduce nuclear localization of NFAT and NFAT-mediated gene expression. Inhibition of calcineurin by *DSCR1* is likely to be one of the multiple mechanisms involved in the pathogenesis of Down syndrome.[28]

[ ] EDWARDS SYNDROME

Edwards syndrome, or trisomy 18, is the second most common trisomy, with a prevalence of approximately 1 in 4000 to 8000 livebirths.[20] The majority of the infants die within a couple of weeks and approximately 10 percent survive more than a year.[29] The syndrome is characterized by anomalies of the heart and microcephaly with a prominent occiput, a narrow forehead, low-set and malformed ears, micrognathia, clefting of the lip and palate, clenched hand with overlapping digits, rocker-bottom feet, and various hernias.[20] Cardiovascular anomalies are present in approximately 90 percent of the cases. They include VSD, ASD, patent ductus arteriosus (PDA), pulmonary stenosis, tetralogy of Fallot, transposition of the great arteries, bicuspid aortic valve, dysplastic valves, and coarctation of the aorta.[18,20] Full trisomy occurs in more than 85 percent, chromosomal translocation in 3 percent, and mosaicism in 5 percent of cases.[20] The causal gene(s) for the cardiovascular anomalies remain unknown.

[ ] PATAU SYNDROME

Patau syndrome, or trisomy 13, is a rare disorder with an incidence of 1 per 5000 to 1 in 20,000 livebirths and a high early mortality.[20] Approximately 50 percent of the affected infants die within the first month and 85 percent within first year of life.[20] Patau syndrome is characterized by cardiac, urogenital, craniofacial, and central nervous system anomalies. Specific anomalies include microcephaly with sloping forehead, microphthalmia, cleft lip and palate, overlapping fingers with postaxial polydactyly, and renal abnormalities, including polycystic kidney disease. Cardiac abnormalities are present in approximately 80 percent of the cases. They include VSD, ASD, PDA, pulmonary stenosis, coarctation of the aorta, dextrocardia, and truncus arteriosus.[18,20]

Patau syndrome is caused by nondisjunction of chromosome 13 during meiosis in the vast majority of cases and rarely by translocation. Five percent of the cases are mosaic. The causal genes for cardiovascular anomalies in trisomy 13 are unknown.

[ ] DIGEORGE (CATCH-22) AND VELOCARDIOFACIAL SYNDROMES

DiGeorge and velocardiofacial syndromes are autosomal dominant congenital anomalies caused by hemizygous microdeletion of a large segment of the long arm of chromosome 22 (22q11). The deletion leads to anomalies of multiple organs including the heart and facial bones. The prevalence is approximately 1 in 4000, accounting for approximately 15 percent of all congenital heart defects.[30,31] The term CATCH-22 denotes cardiac, abnormal facies, thymic hypoplasia, cleft palate, hypocalcemia (as a result of parathyroid hypoplasia), and the 22nd chromosome. A diverse array of congenital heart defects including tetralogy of Fallot, interrupted aortic arch, truncus arteriosus, and PDA have been described. Tetralogy of Fallot is the most common abnormality.[30] Patients with velocardiofacial syndromes exhibit craniofacial anomalies, cleft palate, and a variety of cardiac abnormalities, such as aortic arch anomalies, tetralogy of Fallot, and VSD. Cardiac valves and the myocardium are usually spared.

DiGeorge syndrome is caused by microdeletion of approximately 3 Mbp of DNA encompassing approximately 30 genes.[30] Mutation analysis of the candidate genes in the region have led to identification of mutations in TBX1, which encodes a T-box transcription factor.[32] TBX1 is critical for embryogenesis of aortic and pulmonary outflow tracts. Loss-of-function mutations in TBX1 result in haploinsufficiency. The downstream target genes of TBX1 and the pathways involved in the pathogenesis of cardiac phenotype are mostly unknown.

Another candidate gene is UFD1L, which encodes a protein involved in degradation of ubiquitinated proteins. It is expressed during the embryogenesis of cell lines typically associated with DiGeorge syndrome. Similarly, UFD1L is expressed in association with the conotruncus and the fourth embryologic aortic arch. A large deletion in human transcription factor UFD1L in a single patient with a phenotype similar to that of DiGeorge syndrome has been identified.[33] Deletion of Ufd1L in mice produced some of the typical cardiac phenotypes that result from defective development of the fourth branchial arch.[34] However, several other studies have excluded mutations in UFD1L in patients with DiGeorge syndrome.[35] Other genes, such as ZNF74, which encodes a zinc-finger transcription factor, also have been implicated in the pathogenesis of DiGeorge syndrome.[36] However, the causal role remains to be established.

GENETIC BASIS OF SPECIFIC CONGENITAL HEART DISEASES

A significant number of congenital heart diseases occur in isolation and are not part of complex phenotypes as observed in chromosomal abnormalities. Recently, the causal genes for several congenital heart diseases have been identified. Preliminary studies depict a common theme in the pathogenesis of isolated congenital heart defects, which implicate deficiency of several transcriptional factors that regulate cardiac gene expression during embryogenesis. However, there is considerable phenotypic, locus, and allelic heterogeneity.

[ ] SUPRAVALVULAR AORTIC STENOSIS

Supravalvular aortic stenosis is an autosomal dominant disease characterized by discrete narrowing of the ascending aorta above the level of the sinus of Valsalva. It commonly occurs as a phenotype of Williams syndrome (or Williams-Beuren syndrome) in conjunction with mental retardation in some, and exceptional talents in others, hypercalcemia, characteristic facial appearance, and stenosis of other major arteries. The prevalence of supravalvular aortic stenosis is estimated to be 1 in 25,000 livebirths.

The gene responsible for supravalvular aortic stenosis was initially mapped to chromosome 7q11.23 and subsequently identified as ELN, encoding elastin.[37] Almost all cases of isolated supravalvular aortic stenosis are caused by ELN mutations, which comprise a variety of point and deletion mutations.[38] Mutations result in elastin deficiency, which in the vascular system leads to inelasticity of the vessel wall and subsequent fibrosis as a result of an altered stress–strain relation (elastin arteriopathy). Thus, haploinsufficiency underlies the pathogenesis of supravalvular aortic stenosis.

Patients with Williams syndrome may exhibit additional cardiovascular phenotypes, including pulmonary arterial stenosis, aortic and mitral valve abnormalities, and tetralogy of Fallot.[39] In 98 percent of cases of Williams syndrome the deletion mutation includes 1.5 Mbp of DNA comprising ELN and another 20 contiguous genes. Contribution of these genes to pathogenesis of specific phenotypes in Williams syndrome remains unknown.

[ ] FAMILIAL ATRIAL SEPTAL DEFECT

ASD is among the most common congenital heart diseases, with an estimated incidence of 1 in 1000 livebirth.[1] ASD is usually sporadic. However, familial ASD with an autosomal dominant mode of inheritance also have been described.[40,41] Individuals with ASD are commonly asymptomatic until the third or fourth decades. Common symptoms are palpitations, commonly caused by supraventricular arrhythmias, and symptoms associated with pulmonary hypertension and right-sided volume overload resulting in left-to-right shunt. Uncorrected ASD can lead to heart failure and premature death in the fourth or fifth decade of life.

The first gene identified for familial ASD is *NKX2–5 (CSX1)*, which is the human homologue of *Nkx2.5* in mouse and *tinman* in *Drosophila melanogaster*.[42] The gene is located on 5q35 and encode NKX2.5, a predominantly cardiac-specific transcription factor that regulates expression of several cardiac genes.[43] A multiplicity of mutations have been described in patients with secundum ASD and conduction defects.[42,44] Mutations often result in haploinsufficiency. Point mutations in the DNA binding domain reduce the affinity of NKX2.5 for the promoter regions and hence, decreases expression of cardiac-specific genes.[45] The spectrum of clinical phenotypes caused by mutations in NKX2.5 extends beyond secundum ASD and comprises VSDs, tetralogy of Fallot, subvalvular aortic stenosis, pulmonary atresia, and others.[46]

The second causal gene for familial ASD with an autosomal dominant mode of inheritance is *GATA4* on chromosome 8p22–23.[47] The mutations diminish DNA-binding affinity and transcriptional activity of GATA4 transcription factor and blocks its physical interaction with TBX5, another transcription factor involved in the pathogenesis of congenital heart disease.[47]

The third causal gene for familial ASD is *MYH6*, which is located in chromosome 14q12 and encodes myosin heavy chain 6.[48] A missense mutation in *MYH6* in a family with atrial fibrillation mapped to 14q12 locus has been identified.[48] The MYH6 protein is expressed at high levels in atrial tissues and plays an important role in formation of interatrial septum.[48]

[ ] HOLT-ORAM SYNDROME

Holt-Oram syndrome is a rare autosomal dominant inherited disorder characterized by anomalies of the heart and upper extremities, hence the name *hand–heart syndrome* (see also Chap. 12).[49] The most common congenital heart defects are ASD and VSD followed by conduction system abnormalities and atrial fibrillation.[50] Less-common cardiac abnormalities include truncus arteriosus, mitral valve defect, PDA, and tetralogy of Fallot.[50] Anomalies of the upper limb vary from mild malformation of the carpal bones to phocomelia, but upper limb preaxial radial abnormalities are commonly present.[50]

Mutations in *TBX5* on chromosome 12q24, which codes for transcription factor TBX5, are responsible for the cardiac and skeletal abnormalities in Holt-Oram syndrome.[50,51] A number of mutations have been described and most are nonsense, frameshift, or splice-junction abnormalities. The proposed molecular mechanism is haploinsufficiency, resulting in reduced expression level of TBX5. Haploinsufficiency because of truncation or frameshift mutations results in severe birth defects in the heart and hands, whereas point mutations predominantly affect either hand or heart development.[52] Mutations in the 5′ end of the gene exhibit a preponderance of cardiac abnormalities with mild skeletal abnormalities, and those in the 3′ end lead to severe skeletal and mild cardiac abnormalities.

[ ] ELLIS–VAN CREVELD SYNDROME

Ellis–van Creveld syndrome is an autosomal recessive skeletal dysplasia, which is associated with congenital heart disease in the majority of cases. Skeletal anomalies include short limbs, short ribs, postaxial polydactyly, and dysplastic nails and teeth. ASD and common atrium are the typical cardiac anomalies present in two-thirds of the cases (see also Chap. 12).

The gene responsible for Ellis–van Creveld syndrome was mapped to chromosome 4p16.1[53] near an area proximal to the *FGFR3* gene, which is known to cause hypochondroplasia and achondroplasia. Subsequently splice donor, truncation, and missense mutations in a novel gene, *EVC*, were identified.[54] Mutations in *EVC* account for approximately 20 percent of the cases of Ellis–van Creveld syndrome.[55] Recently, mutations in a second gene, named *EVC2*, for Ellis–van Creveld syndrome were identified.[55] The pathogenesis of Ellis–van Creveld syndrome remains unknown.

[ ] FAMILIAL PATENT DUCTUS ARTERIOSUS OR CHAR SYNDROME

PDA can occur as a sole cardiac anomaly or in conjunction with other congenital heart disease. Familial PDA with an autosomal dominant inheritance has been described in patients with Char syndrome. Char syndrome is a congenital disease that was first described by Florence Char in 1978, which is characterized by a constellation of facial dysmorphism, fifth-finger middle phalangeal hypoplasia, and PDA. Variation of this syndrome is associated with bicuspid aortic valve, distinctive facial appearance, polydactyly, and fifth-finger clinodactyly. The predominant clinical features are those of PDA, which include symptoms and signs of left-heart failure and pulmonary hypertension.

The gene responsible for Char syndrome in two families was recently mapped to chromosome 6p12–21.[56] Subsequently mutations in the *TFAP2B*, which encodes a neural crest-related helix-span-helix transcription factor, were identified.[57] These findings suggest that Char syndrome results from derangement of neural crest-cell derivatives.[57] A second locus for familial PDA has been mapped to a 3 cM interval on chromosome 12q24.[58] The causal gene remains unknown.

[ ] NOONAN AND LEOPARD SYNDROMES

Noonan syndrome is an uncommon autosomal dominant disorder characterized by dysmorphic facial features, HCM, pulmonic stenosis, mental retardation, and bleeding disorders.[59] Leopard syndrome (*l*entigines, *e*lectrocardiographic conduction abnormalities, *o*cular hypertelorism, *p*ulmonic stenosis, *a*bnormal genitalia, retardation of growth, and *deafness*) is an allelic variant of the Noonan syndrome.[59] Pulmonic stenosis and HCM are the primary cardiac phenotypes. Others include atrioventricular septal defects, aortic coarctation, ASD, mitral valve defects, PDA, and fibroelastosis. Noonan syndrome is also seen in conjunction with cardiofaciocutaneous syndrome and other congenital abnormalities, such as neurofibromatosis (see also Chap. 12).

Noonan syndrome is sporadic in half of the cases and an autosomal dominant disease in the other half. The gene responsible for autosomal dominant Noonan and Leopard syndromes was mapped to chromosome 12q22 and subsequently identified as encoding protein-tyrosine-phosphatase, nonreceptor type 11 (*PTPN11*).[60,61] With the exception of deletion of amino acid glycine 60, all mutations in *PTPN11* are missense mutations.[59] Most mutations are recurrent and localized to exons 3, 7, 8, and 13.[59] The N308D mutation is the most common and accounts for approximately 25 percent of the cases.[59] Overall, mutations in *PTPN11* are found in approximately two-thirds of the cases of Noonan syndrome.[59]

Mutations are located in interacting portions of the amino-terminal src-homology 2 (N-SH2) and protein-tyrosine-phosphatase (PTP) domains.[60,61] Both gain-of-function and dominant-negative mechanisms have been implicated in the pathogenesis of Noonan syndrome caused by *PTPN11* mutations.

[ ] FAMILIAL MYXOMA SYNDROME (CARNEY COMPLEX)

Myxomas are the most common cardiac tumors and are generally sporadic. Myxomas are familial with an autosomal dominant mode of inheritance in approximately 10 percent of cases (see also Chap. 85).[62] Familial myxoma commonly occurs as a part of Carney complex with the constellation of cardiac myxoma, endocrine disorders, and skin pigmentation.[63] LAMB (*l*entigines, *a*trial myxoma, *m*ucocutaneous myxoma, *b*lue nevi) and NAME (*n*evi, *a*trial myxoma, *m*yxoid neurofibromata, *e*phelides) syndromes are considered variants of Carney complex. Atrial, ventricular, and skin myxomas, endocrine tumors and disorders, such as Cushing syndrome, and skin lesions, such as lentiginosis, are part of the phenotypic expression of Carney complex. Clinical features of atrial myxoma may include fever, arthralgia, dyspnea, diastolic rumble, tumor plop, and systemic embolisms.

Carney complex exhibits locus heterogeneity, and at least two loci on chromosome 17q24 and 2p16 have been mapped.[64,65] The majority of familial cardiac myxomas (Carney complex) are caused by mutations in the *PRKRA1A* gene on chromosome 17q24.[66] It encodes the α-regulatory subunit of cyclic adenosine monophosphate (cAMP)-dependent protein kinase. Frameshift mutations in *PRKRA1A* result in haploinsufficiency, which suggests that the *PRKRA1A* functions as a tumor-suppressor gene. Recently, a missense mutation in the perinatal myosin heavy-chain gene (*MYH8*) was identified in members of a family with Carney complex and trismus-pseudocamptodactyly syndrome.[67]

[ ] SITUS INVERSUS

Situs inversus is a reversal of the asymmetric anatomic position of visceral organs. In situs inversus totalis, all visceral organs are reversed in a mirror-image manner. It is part of the immotile cilia syndrome (primary ciliary dyskinesia). Kartagener syndrome is situs inversus, bronchiectasis, and male sterility. Most cases of situs inversus are sporadic. Autosomal recessive, autosomal dominant, and X-linked forms have been reported.

Situs inversus, as a component of immotile cilia syndrome, such as that in Kartagener syndrome, is caused by mutations in dyneins.[68] Dyneins are large proteins with adenosine triphosphatase (ATPase) activity that interact with intermediary filaments to produce energy and motion. Mutations in dynein axonemal intermediate chain 1 (*DNAI1*) on chromosome 9p13-p21, dynein axonemal heavy chain 5 (*DNAH5*) on chromosome 5p, and dynein axonemal heavy chain type 11 (*DNAH11*) on chromosome 7p21 have been found in patients with primary ciliary dyskinesia (and situs inversus).[68–70]

Situs inversus has also been mapped to chromosome Xq26.2. Mutations in *ZIC3*, encoding a zinc-finger protein of the cerebellum, are associated with situs ambiguus in male and situs solitus or inversus in females.[71] Other causal genes for right-left axis abnormality include *CFC1* on chromosome 2, *LEFTB* (also known as *LEFTY2*) and *ACVR2B,* encoding activin receptor IIB.[72,73]

[ ] ALAGILLE SYNDROME (ARTERIOHEPATIC DYSPLASIA)

This is an autosomal dominant disorder characterized by anomalies of the right side of the heart and developmental abnormalities of eyes, skeleton, and kidney. Cardiac abnormalities are present in approximately 70 percent of cases; the most common is diffuse pulmonary artery stenosis. Others include hypoplastic pulmonary circulation, pulmonary atresia, tetralogy of Fallot, coarctation of aorta, secundum ASD, PDA, and VSD.[74] The most common causal gene is Jagged-1 gene (*JAG1*), located on chromosome 20p12.[75,76] Deletion or point mutations in *JAG1* are found in approximately 90 percent of the patients with Alagille syndrome. JAG1 is a cell surface protein that is a ligand for the Notch receptor. The Notch intercellular signaling pathway mediates cell fate decisions during development. The proposed molecular mechanism is haploinsufficiency leading to defective cell adhesions. Recently, mutations in *NOTCH2* were found in those who did not have JAG1 mutations.[77] Collectively, the findings indicate Alagille syndrome is disease of Notch signaling pathway.

GENETIC DISEASES OF CARDIAC MUSCLE

The term *cardiomyopathy* denotes an exclusive group of disorders in which the primary defect is in the myocardium, affecting cardiac myocyte structure and/or function. The primary defect, however, does not need to be exclusive to the heart. It can also involve other tissues and organs, as in cardiomyopathies arising from metabolic disorders and mitochondrial myopathies. Myocardial dysfunction can also occur because of systemic, infiltrative, toxic, and endocrine disorders; coronary atherosclerosis; and valvular pathologies. In such conditions, the primary defect is not in the myocardium. Thus, myocardial involvement is considered secondary. Recently, the Council on Clinical Cardiology, Heart Failure and Transplantation Committee of the American Heart Association provided the following definition for cardiomyopathies: "Cardiomyopathies are a heterogeneous group of diseases of the myocardium associated with mechanical and/or electrical dysfunction that usually (but not invariably) exhibit inappropriate ventricular hypertrophy or dilatation and are due to a variety of causes that frequently are genetic"[78] (see Chap. 75).

Cardiomyopathies are classified according to their phenotypic characteristics into four groups: hypertrophic, dilated, restrictive, and arrhythmogenic right ventricular cardiomyopathy. Phenotypic classification, while clinically convenient and useful, does not sufficiently reflect the molecular and genetic basis of cardiomyopathies. Future classification of cardiomyopathies is expected to be based on our understanding of their molecular pathogenesis.

【 】 GENETIC BASIS OF HYPERTROPHIC CARDIOMYOPATHY

HCM is a relatively common autosomal dominant disease diagnosed clinically by the presence of unexplained cardiac hypertrophy.[79] Commonly, a left ventricular wall thickness of 13 mm or greater, in the absence of hypertension or valvular heart disease, is used to define HCM. The prevalence of HCM is approximately 1 in 500 in young adults.[80] It is likely higher in the elderly population because of age-dependent penetrance.

Cardiac hypertrophy, the clinical hallmark of HCM, is asymmetric in approximately two-thirds of the cases with predominant involvement of the interventricular septum (Fig. 81–3). Hence the term *asymmetric septal hypertrophy* is used to describe this condition. Rarely, hypertrophy is restricted to apex of the heart (apical

HCM). Morphologically, the left ventricular cavity is small and left ventricular ejection fraction, a measure of global systolic function, is increased. However, more sensitive indices of myocardial function show impaired contraction and relaxation.[81] Diastolic function is commonly impaired, leading to an increased left ventricular end-diastolic pressure and thus, frequently, to symptoms of heart failure (see Chap. 77).

Patients with HCM exhibit protean clinical manifestations ranging from minimal or no symptoms to severe heart failure. The clinical manifestations often do not develop until the third or fourth decade of life, but the onset is variable. The majority of patients are asymptomatic or mildly symptomatic. Predominant symptoms include dyspnea, chest pain, palpitations, and/or syncope. Severe systolic heart failure is uncommon. It occurs in a small fraction of patients in whom the disease evolves into a dilated cardiomyopathy (DCM) phenotype.[82] In contrast, cardiac diastolic function is usually impaired and left ventricular end-diastolic pressure is elevated. A dynamic left ventricular outflow is present in approximately 25 percent of the patients. It could contribute to mitral regurgitations and symptoms of heart failure. Cardiac arrhythmias, in particular atrial fibrillation and nonsustained ventricular tachycardia, are relatively common and are associated with adverse clinical outcome.[83,84] Wolff-Parkinson-White (WPW) syndrome is present in a small percentage of patients with HCM. Its presence suggests the possibility of a phenocopy, typically a glycogen storage disease.[85–88]

Syncope is a serious symptom. It is often a result of serious cardiac arrhythmias and associated with an increased risk of sudden cardiac

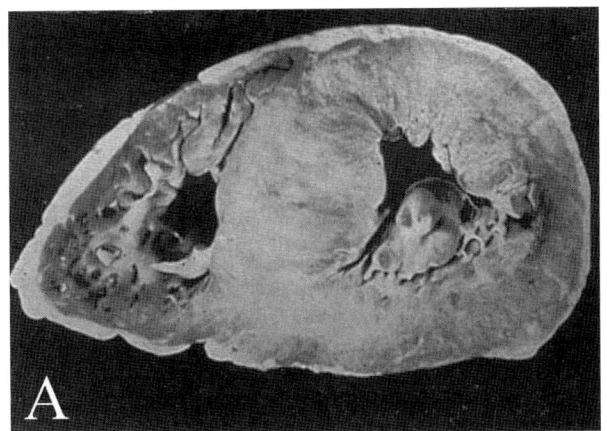
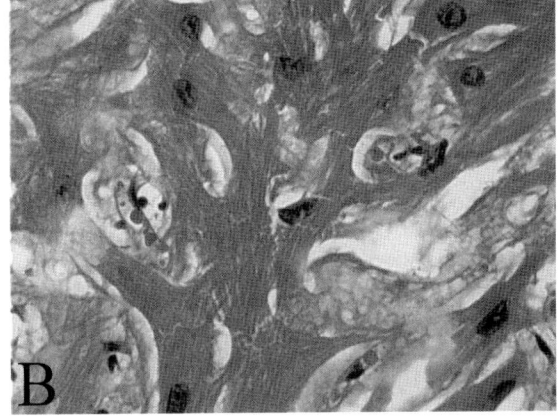
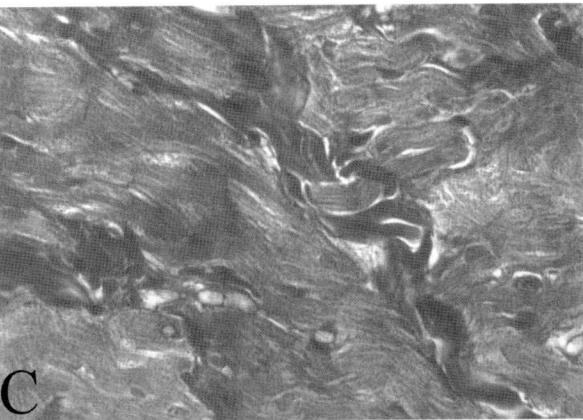

FIGURE 81–3. Main pathologic features of hypertrophic cardiomyopathy. **A.** Gross cardiac hypertrophy with predominant involvement of the interventricular septum and a small left ventricular cavity. **B.** Myocyte disarray and hypertrophy. **C.** Interstitial fibrosis.

TABLE 81–5

Potential Risk Factors for SCD in Patients with HCM

Established risk factors
  Prior episode of aborted SCD
  Family history of SCD (more than 1 victim of SCD)
    {1147}
  Causal mutations, including double mutations
    {156,176,180,15,336,371,377,698,138}
  Modifier genes (genetic background) {20}
  History of syncope {1144} {179}
  Severe cardiac hypertrophy {124,1144} {1153}
  Sustained and repetitive nonsustained ventricular tachy-
    cardia {179}
Less-established risk factors
  Outflow tract gradient {2069}
  Histologic phenotypes (interstitial fibrosis and myocyte
    disarray) {809}
  Early onset of clinical manifestations (young age) {1147}
  Abnormal blood pressure response to exercise {1147}
  Presence of myocardial ischemia

HCM, hypertrophic cardiomyopathy; SCD, sudden cardiac death.

death (SCD).[89–91] HCM, although uncommon, is the most common cause of SCD in young, competitive athletes.[92,93] It accounts for almost half of all cases of SCD in athletes younger than 35 years of age in the United States.[92,93] SCD is often the first and tragic manifestation of HCM in young apparently healthy individuals.[92,93] Table 81–5 lists the factors associated with an increased risk of SCD.[94] Overall, in the assessment of the risk of SCD, combination of all known risk factors should be considered.[91] In the absence of major risk factors for SCD, HCM has a relatively benign course with an estimated annual mortality of about 1 percent in the adult population.[95–97] Apical HCM, characterized by giant T wave inversion in the precordial leads on the electrocardiogram, is also a relatively benign disease.[98,99]

The pathologic hallmark of HCM is cardiac myocyte disarray.[100] It is defined as malaligned, distorted, and often short and hypertrophic myocytes oriented in different directions (see Fig. 81–3). Myocyte disarray often comprises more than 20 percent of the ventricle, as opposed to <5 percent of the myocardium in the normal hearts.[100–102] It is more prominent in the interventricular septum, but commonly is found throughout the myocardium.[100,102] Other pathologic features of HCM include myocyte hypertrophy, interstitial fibrosis, thickening of media of intramural coronary arteries, and sometimes malpositioned mitral valve with elongated leaflets. Cardiac hypertrophy, interstitial fibrosis, and myocyte disarray are associated with the risk of SCD, mortality and morbidity in patients with HCM.[103–106] Other pathologic features of HCM include thickening of the media of intramural coronary arteries, abnormal positioning of the mitral valve apparatus, and elongated mitral valve leaflets.

Molecular Genetics of Hypertrophic Cardiomyopathy

HCM is a genetically heterogeneous disease with an autosomal dominant mode of inheritance. Approximately two-thirds of pa-

tients have a family history of HCM.[107,108] In the remainder, the disease is sporadic. Familial and sporadic cases both are caused by mutations in contractile sarcomeric proteins.[109] In sporadic cases, mutations are de novo and could be transmitted to the offspring of the index cases.[110,111] Because hypertrophy is a common response of the heart to all forms of injury or stimuli, a phenotype of hypertrophy in the absence of an increased external load could also occur because of mutations in nonsarcomeric proteins. As such, unexplained cardiac hypertrophy, which clinically denotes HCM, could also occur in storage disorders,[112] metabolic disorders,[113] mitochondrial diseases,[114] and triplet repeat syndromes,[115] as well as congenital heart diseases.[60] Although the gross phenotype is similar, the pathogenesis of HCM caused by different classes of mutant proteins, at least in part, could differ. Therefore, such conditions are considered phenocopy (diseases mimicking HCM).

Causal Genes and Mutations The pioneering works of Christine and Jonathan Seidman have led to elucidation of the molecular genetic basis of HCM. In 1990, an arginine-to-glutamine substitution at codon 403 (R403Q) in the β-myosin heavy chain (MHC) was identified as the first causal mutation.[116] Since then, more than 300 different mutations in a dozen genes encoding sarcomeric proteins have been identified (Table 81–6). Consequently, HCM (excluding phenocopy) is considered a disease of contractile sarcomeric proteins (Fig. 81–4).[117] Systematic screening of sarcomeric genes suggests that mutations in *MYHC* and *MYBPC3*, which encode β-MHC and myosin-binding protein C (MBP-C), respectively, are the most common causes of human HCM, accounting for approximately half of all cases.[118–120] Mutations in *TNNT2* and *TNNI3*, encoding cardiac troponin T and I, respectively, are relatively uncommon, each accounting for approximately 5 percent of the HCM cases.[120–122] Thus, mutations in *MYH7*, *MYBPC3*, *TNNT2*, and *TNNI3* collectively account for approximately two-thirds of all HCM cases. A small fraction of HCM cases are caused by mutations in genes encoding α-tropomyosin (*TPM1*), titin (*TTN*), cardiac α-actin (*ACTC*), telethonin (*TCAP*), and essential and regulatory light chains (*MYL3* and *MYL2*, respectively).[117,123–128] Finally, rare mutations in cardiac troponin C (*TNNC1*), α-MHC (*MYH6*), myosin light chain kinase (*MYLK2*), phospholamban (*PLN*), and caveolin 3 (*CAV3*) have been reported in patients with HCM.[129–133] Overall, the causal genes and mutations for approximately 75 percent of HCM cases have been identified. The remainder are yet to be identified or are a result of genes inducing a phenocopy.

More than 100 different mutations in the β-MHC, a major component of thick filaments in sarcomeres, have been identified. The majority are missense mutations, localized in the globular head of the myosin molecule. Codons 403 and 719 are potential hot spots for mutations.[134,135] Missense, deletion, and insertion/deletion mutations in the rod and tail regions have also been described but are uncommon.[136–140] Overall, the frequency of each particular *MYHC* mutation is relatively low and most mutations are private. Accordingly, a founder effect (sharing of a common ancestor) is uncommon.

Mutations in *MYBPC3* account for approximately 30 percent of all HCM cases. Mutations are scattered throughout the gene without a particular predilection.[119,141–144] Unlike mutations in *MYHC*, a significant proportion of *MYBPC3* mutations are dele-

TABLE 81-6

Causal Genes for Hypertrophic Cardiomyopathy (Sarcomeric Genes)

GENE	SYMBOL	LOCUS	FREQUENCY	PREDOMINANT MUTATIONS
β-Myosin heavy chain	MYH7	14q12	~30%	Missenses
Myosin binding protein-C	MYBPC3	11p11.2	~30%	Splice-junction and insertion/deletion
Cardiac troponin T	TNNT2	1q32	~5%	Missenses
Cardiac troponin I	TNNI3	19p13.2	~5%	Missense and deletion
α-Tropomyosin	TPM1	15q22.1	~5%	Missenses
Essential myosin light chain	MYL3	3p21.3	<5%	Missenses
Regulatory myosin light chain	MYL2	12q23–24.3	<5%	Missense and 1 truncation
Cardiac α-actin	ACTC	15q11	<5%	Missense mutations
Titin	TTN	2q24.1	<5%	Missense mutations
Telethonin (Tcap)	TCAP	17q2	Rare	Missense mutations
α-Myosin heavy chain	MYH6	14q1	Rare	Missense and rearrangement mutations (association)
Cardiac troponin C	TNNC1	3p21.3–3p14.3	Rare	Missense mutations (association)
Cardiac myosin light peptide kinase	MYLK2	20q13.3	Rare	Point mutations (association)
Caveolin 3	CAV3	3p25	Rare	Point mutations (association)
Phospholamban	PLN	6p22.1	Rare	Point mutations (association)

tion/insertion or splice-junction mutations.[119] Insertion/deletion mutations could result in frameshift and truncation of the MBP-C protein. The mutant protein harbors severe structural and functional defects or become degraded. The frequency of each particular mutation is relatively low and a founder effect is uncommon.

Mutations in *TNNT2* are relatively common causes of human HCM, accounting for approximately 5 percent of all cases.[117,122,123,145,146] More than 20 mutations in *TNNT2* have been described, and codon 92 is considered a hot spot for mutations.[117,145,146] The majority of the mutations are missense, but deletion mutations that involve splice donor sites and could lead to truncated proteins also have been described.[117]

Mutations in *TNNI3* are also relatively uncommon and estimated to account for about 5 percent of all HCM cases.[120,121,147,148] Mutations in other components of thin and thick filaments are uncommon causes of HCM and collectively account for approximately 5 percent of all HCM cases. Mutations in other sarcomeric genes, namely *TPM1, TNNC1, TTN, ACTC, MYL3*, and *MYL2*, are very uncommon, and those in *MYH6*, myosin light chain kinase, SERCA2A, and phospholamban are rare.

Modifier Genes and Polymorphisms

A remarkable feature of HCM is the presence of considerable variability in its phenotypic expression, whether it is the degree of cardiac hypertrophy or the risk of SCD. The molecular basis of such vari-

ability is not fully known. It is probably partly because of the diversity of the causal genes and mutations, which impart a spectrum of functional and structural defects.[149] In addition, the presence of multiple mutations, detected in a small fraction of patients, is associated with a severe phenotype.[150,151] Environmental factors, such as competitive sports and exercise could potentially contribute to the phenotypic expression of HCM.[152,153] However, there is insufficient data to support their contributions to the phenotype.

The presence of considerable phenotypic variability among affected members of different families with identical causal muta-

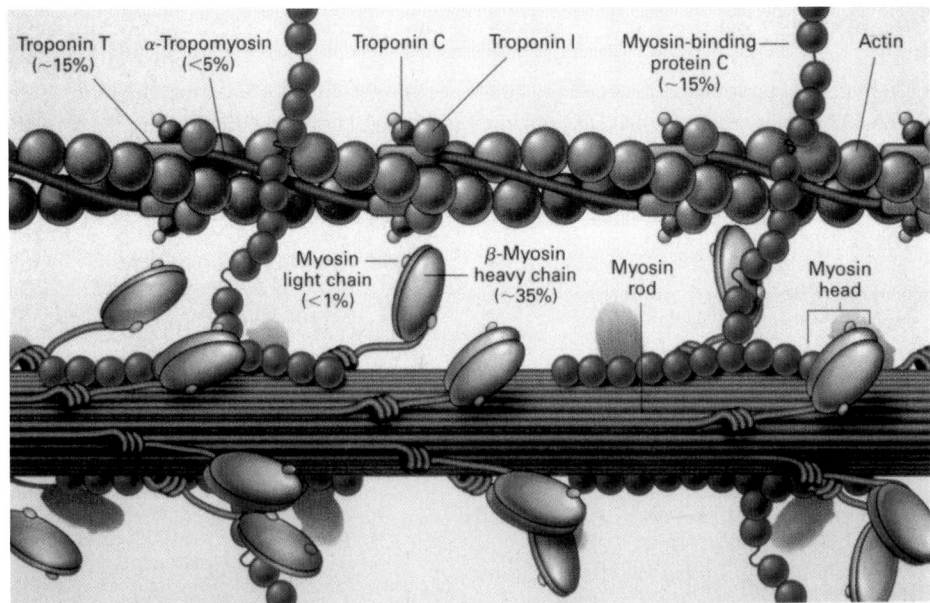

FIGURE 81-4. Schematic representation of sarcomeric proteins involved in cardiomyopathies.

tions emphasizes the significance of the genetic background to phenotypic expression of HCM. Genes other than the causal genes that affect the phenotype are referred to as the "modifier" genes. Unlike the causal genes, modifier genes are neither necessary nor sufficient to cause HCM.[154] However, they influence the severity of cardiac hypertrophy, risk of SCD, and expression of other cardiac phenotypes in HCM. DNA polymorphisms, including putatively functional SNPs, that is, SNPs located in the coding or regulatory regions or splice junctions, in genes involved in cardiac hypertrophy are the prime candidates. The identity of the modifier genes for HCM and the magnitude of their effects remain largely unknown. The specific modifier genes in HCM are largely unknown. Two modifier loci have been mapped and several genes have been implicated.[155] A modifier locus also has been mapped in a genetically engineered mouse model.[156] Functional variants of genes coding for the components of the renin-angiotensin-aldosterone system are the most extensively studied candidates. *ACE*, encoding angiotensin-I converting enzyme 1 (ACE-1) was the first gene implicated as a modifier of cardiac phenotype in human HCM.[157] ACE-1 catalyzes conversion of angiotensin I to angiotensin II and inactivates bradykinin, both of which are biologically active agents with opposing effects on cardiac growth and cellular proliferation.[158] *ACE* contains more than 30 different polymorphisms, which contribute to interindividual variation in plasma, tissue, and cellular levels of ACE-1.[159] The most commonly studied *ACE* polymorphism is an insertion (I) or deletion (D) of a 287-bp Alu repeat in intron 16. The I/D polymorphism, probably because of being in LD with other functional SNPs, is associated with variation in plasma, cellular, and tissue levels of ACE-1 in a codominant manner (DD > ID > II).[159]

ACE I/D polymorphism has been associated with the severity of cardiac hypertrophy and risk of SCD in HCM in most, but not all, studies.[157,160–166] The DD genotype is more common in HCM families with a high incidence of SCD, as compared to those with a low incidence, and is associated with the severity of cardiac hypertrophy.[157,160] The observed association is gene-dose dependent, consistent with the biologic effect of the I/D variants on plasma and tissue levels of ACE.[160] An interaction between the modifying effect of the I/D genotypes and the underlying causal mutations also has been reported.[161,166]

Variants of endothelin-1 (*EDN1*), tumor necrosis factor-α (*TNF-α*), angiotensinogen (*AGT*), angiotensin II receptor 1 (*AGTR1*), and platelet-activating factor acetylhydrolase (*PLA2G7*) have been associated with the severity of the cardiac hypertrophy.[167–169] The results, however, have been inconsistent, partly because of the small sample size of the studies, population characteristics, and presence of confounders that are common in SNP-association studies.[170]

Molecular Genetics of HCM Phenocopy

Mutations in nonsarcomeric proteins can cause a phenotype grossly similar to HCM, referred to as a *phenocopy*.[112] The distinction between true HCM and HCM phenocopy is important as the pathogenesis, as well as histologic phenotypes, of the two conditions differ. Table 81–7 provides a partial list of HCM phenocopy. The prevalence of HCM phenocopy is not precisely known. Given the prevalence of each particular HCM phenocopy, it is expected that phenocopy to comprise approximately 5 to 10 percent of the cases with the clinical diagnosis of HCM.[112] A prototypic example of HCM phenocopy is Fabry disease, an X-linked lysosomal storage disease.[171,172] Fabry disease is present in approximately 3 percent of the cases with the clinical diagnosis of HCM in adult population.[173] The phenotype results from deficiency of α-galactosidase A (α-Gal A), also known as ceramide trihexosidase.[174] The deficiency of the enzyme results in deposits of glycosphingolipids in multiple organs, including the heart. The causal gene is *GLA* on chromosome Xq22, which codes for lysosomal hydrolase α-Gal A protein.[174] The phenotype is characterized by angiokeratoma, renal insufficiency, proteinuria, neuropathy, transient ischemic attack, stroke, anemia, corneal deposits and cardiac hypertrophy.[174] Cardiac hypertrophy, which is often indistinguishable from the true HCM, is associated with high QRS voltage, conduction defects, and cardiac arrhythmias. Other cardiac phenotypes include valvular regurgitation, coronary artery disease, myocardial infarction, and aortic annular dilatation.[173,175] The disease predominantly affects males. Female carriers could exhibit a milder form.[175] The diagnosis is established by measuring α-Gal A levels and activity in leukocytes. Fabry could be treated with enzyme replacement therapy using human α-Gal A (agalsidase α) or recombinant human α-Gal A (agalsidase β).[171,172,176,177]

Glycogen storage disease caused by mutations in *PRKAG2* gene is another HCM phenocopy.[85–88] Cardiac hypertrophy results predominantly from storage of glycogen in myocytes. The gene encodes the γ₂ regulatory subunit of adenosine monophosphate (AMP)-activated protein kinase (AMPK), which is considered the

TABLE 81–7

Genes Known to Cause Hypertrophic Cardiomyopathy Phenocopy

GENE	GENE SYMBOL	CHROMOSOME	FREQUENCY
Protein kinase A, γ subunit	*PRKAG2*	7q22–q31.1	1–2%
α-Galactosidase A {2468}	*GLA*	Xq22	3%
Unconventional myosin 6	*MOY6*	6q12	Rare
Lysosome-associated membrane protein 2	*LAMP2*	Xq24	1–2%
Mitochondrial genes	*MTTG, MTTI*	MtDNA	Rare
Frataxin (Friedreich ataxia)	*FRDA*	9q13	Rare
Myotonin protein kinase (Myotonic dystrophy)	*DMPK, DMWD*	19q13	Uncommon
Protein tyrosine phosphatase, nonreceptor type 11	*PTPN11*	12q24	Uncommon, higher in children

energy biosensor of the cell. Mutations in *PRKAG2* lead to cardiac hypertrophy, conduction defects, and WPW.[85-87]

HCM phenocopy also occurs in trinucleotide repeat syndromes, a group of genetic disorders caused by expansion of naturally occurring trinucleotide repeats.[178] HCM phenocopy occurs in Friedreich ataxia, an autosomal recessive neurodegenerative disease caused by expansion of GAA repeat sequences in the intron of *FRDA*.[179]

HCM phenocopy also occurs in patients with Noonan syndrome. The phenotype is characterized by dysmorphic facial features, pulmonic stenosis, mental retardation, bleeding disorders and cardiac hypertrophy. Leopard syndrome is an allelic variant of Noonan syndrome. Noonan syndrome is an autosomal dominant disorder caused by mutations in gene-encoding protein-tyrosine-phosphatase, nonreceptor type 11 (*PTPN11*) in approximately half of the cases, as discussed earlier (see Noonan and Leopard Syndromes above).[60,61]

Metabolic diseases also cause HCM phenocopy. Refsum disease, Pompe disease (glycogen storage disease type II), Danon disease, Niemann-Pick disease, Gaucher disease, hereditary hemochromatosis, and CD36 deficiency are examples of metabolic disorders that cause HCM phenocopy.[180-183] Defective mitochondrial oxidative phosphorylation pathways also causes HCM phenocopy. Kearns-Sayre syndrome is a mitochondrial disease characterized by a triad of progressive external ophthalmoplegia, pigmentary retinopathy, and cardiac conduction defects, and less frequently HCM phenocopy.[114]

Gene Expression in Hypertrophic Cardiomyopathy

In keeping with the diversity of cardiac phenotypes in HCM, expression levels of a variety of genes, in response to the mutant protein, are altered. Expression of genes encoding contractile sarcomeric proteins, cytoskeletal proteins, ion channels, intracellular signaling transducers, proteins maintaining the reduction–oxidation state, and those involved in transcriptional and translation machinery are changed.[184,185] Expression levels of the markers of "secondary" cardiac hypertrophy, such as skeletal α-actin, isoforms of myosin light chain, and brain natriuretic factor are upregulated.[184] Upregulation of markers of secondary cardiac hypertrophy suggest that hypertrophy in HCM is also a "secondary" phenotype. Accordingly, common pathways are involved in induction of cardiac hypertrophy in genetic and acquired forms. The diversity of molecular phenotype is in accord with the diversity of pathologic and clinical phenotypes in HCM that encompass not only hypertrophy and disarray but also interstitial fibrosis and others.

Determinants of Cardiac Phenotype in Hypertrophic Cardiomyopathy

Collective data from genotype–phenotype correlation studies indicate that mutations exhibit highly variable clinical, ECG, and echocardiographic manifestations and that no particular phenotype is mutation specific.[186] Observational data show cardiac hypertrophy accelerates during puberty and adolescence in patients with HCM.[187] The finding suggests growth factors contributes to expression of cardiac hypertrophy. Similarly, experimental and clinical studies suggest cardiac hypertrophy, the clinical hallmark of HCM, is a compensatory phenotype and likely to be modulated

by a large number of genetic and nongenetic factors.[188] Overall, the final phenotype in HCM is determined not only by the causal mutations but also by the effects of modifier genes, environmental factors, epigenetic and epistatic factors, and posttranscriptional and posttranslational modifications of the proteins.

Impact of Causal Genes and Mutations Causal genes and mutations are the primary determinant of expressivity of cardiac phenotype, including the severity of hypertrophy and the risk of SCD.[118,119,136,146,189-193] Collectively, the data suggest gene- and mutation-specific effects. In general, mutations in *MYH7* are associated with an early onset, extensive hypertrophy and a high incidence of SCD, which are variable among different *MYH7* mutations.[189,190,192,194] *MYH7* mutations are considered major prognosticators in HCM (Fig. 81–5). Topography of the mutations and their impact on β-MHC protein function are likely to be important determinants of the severity of cardiac hypertrophy as well as the risk of SCD. However, it is important to note that there is a significant degree of variability, which is partly independent of the causal mutations and partly reflects the effects of modifier genes. Given the relatively low frequency of each causal mutation, results of genotype–phenotype correlation studies have had limited utility. Consistent correlations have been observed for only a few mutations, such as R403Q and R719W, which are associated with a high incidence of SCD and severe hypertrophy (Fig. 81–5).[189,195] In contrast, G256Q and L908V are associated with a benign and Q930L with an intermediate prognosis.[189,190]

The phenotype in the majority of patients with *MYBPC3* mutations is relatively mild. Commonly, the age of onset of clinical symptoms is late, the degree of cardiac hypertrophy is relatively mild, and the incidence of SCD is low.[119,141,192] Accordingly, the penetrance, although age dependent, is relatively low. Thus, a normal physical examination, electrocardiogram (ECG), and echocardiogram have low negative predictive value in early life. The clinical phenotype often develops in the fifth or sixth decades of life. It may be unmasked by the presence of concomitant hypertension. Indeed, hypertensive HCM of the elderly could be a form of

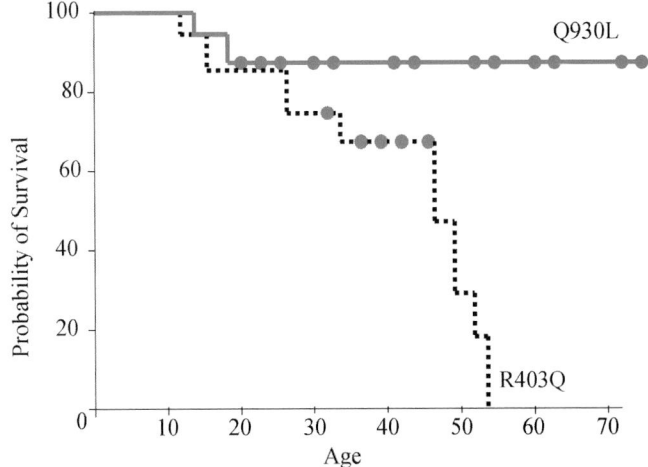

FIGURE 81–5. Kaplan-Meier survival curves in patients with hypertrophic cardiomyopathy. Survival curves in two families with two different mutations, namely arginine-to-glutamine substitution at amino acid 403 (R403Q) and glutamine-to-lysine change at amino acid 930 (Q930L) in the *MYH7* are shown.

HCM caused by mutations in *MYBPC3* and unmasked by hypertension.[141] Nonetheless, there is a significant degree of variability in the phenotypic expression of HCM caused by *MYBPC3*, as "malignant" mutations, associated with severe hypertrophy and a high incidence of SCD, also have been described.[119]

The risk of SCD in HCM caused by mutations in *MYH7* and *MYBPC3* is partially reflective of the severity of hypertrophy.[149] Mutations associated with mild hypertrophy generally carry a relatively benign prognosis and those with severe hypertrophy indicate a high incidence of SCD. This is in contrast to HCM caused by mutations in *TNNT2*, which is characterized by mild cardiac hypertrophy, a high incidence of SCD, and extensive myocyte disarray.[106,146] Inadequate genotype–phenotype correlation data are available regarding mutations in *TNNI3, TPM1, TNNC1, TTN, ACTC, MYL3,* and *MYL2.*

It is important to note that the results of genotype–phenotype correlation studies are subject to a large number of confounding factors, including the small size of the families, small number of families with identical mutations, low frequency of each mutation, phenotypic variability, homozygosity for the causal mutations or compound mutations, and the influence of modifier genes and the environmental factors.[154,196,197] Collective data indicate that mutations exhibit highly variable clinical, ECG, and echocardiographic manifestations, and no particular phenotype is mutation specific.[186]

Impact of Modifier Genes and Polymorphisms Expression of cardiac hypertrophy in HCM is modulated by interactions between the causal mutations, modifier genes, environmental factors, and epigenetic elements, as well as posttranscriptional and posttranslational modifications of proteins.[188] Given the complexity of cardiac hypertrophy, a large number of genes are likely to modify phenotypic expression of HCM, each contributing a small fraction of the phenotype.

ACE I/D polymorphism, which is the most commonly studied polymorphism in HCM,[157,160–166] accounts for approximately 5 percent of the total variability of left ventricular mass in genetically unrelated populations, and for approximately 10 to 15 percent in members of the same family.[160] Similarly, contributions of other potential modifier genes appears to be small.[167–169]

Impact of Environmental Factors Evidence for the effect of environmental factors on cardiac phenotypes in HCM in humans, while expected, is circumstantial. Experimental data in animal models of HCM have not shown consistent effects.[152,153,198] Because hypertrophy is considered a secondary phenotype, one could speculate that heavy physical exercise, particularly isometric exercise, could stimulate the development of severe hypertrophy in HCM. Although there is no direct evidence in humans, the common finding of HCM in young competitive athletes who succumb to SCD suggests heavy physical exercise may worsen the cardiac phenotypes.

Pathogenesis of Hypertrophic Cardiomyopathy

As the diversity of the causal mutations suggests, there is no single initial defect common to all mutations (Table 81–8). The diversity of the clinical phenotypes, such as hypertrophic, dilated, or restrictive cardiomyopathy arising from mutations in the same gene fur-

TABLE 81–8

Initial Defects Caused by Mutations in Sarcomeric Proteins

1. Mechanical defect
   Impaired actomyosin interaction
   Impaired cardiac myocyte and myofibril contractile performance
2. Biochemical defects
   Impaired Ca^{2+} affinity of myofibrillar force generation
3. Bioenergetics
   Impaired myofibrillar adenosine triphosphatase activity
4. Structural defects
   Impaired sarcomere assembly
   Impaired subcellular localization of sarcomeric proteins
   Altered stoichiometry

ther adds to the complexity of the pathogenesis. Topography of the causal mutation is likely to be important, as the initial defect is likely to be domain, but not protein, specific. Mutations located in a specific functional domain of a given protein are expected to confer similar initial defects. Given that each sarcomeric protein could have multiple functions, usually as a result of having multiple domains, mutations in the same protein could impart various initial defects.

The causal mutation initiates a series of molecular events, which begins with alteration of the molecular structure and function of the protein (see Table 81–8). Because the majority of mutant sarcomeric proteins differ from the wild type only by a single amino acid (missense mutations), the mutant proteins incorporate into the sarcomere, albeit sometimes inefficiently.[199] Following incorporation, mutant sarcomeric proteins exert diverse functional defects, such as alterations in myofibrillar Ca^{2+} sensitivity and ATPase activity.[200–204] Functional phenotypes lead to activation of secondary molecules, which are largely unknown but expected to include activating of many intracellular signaling pathways. The secondary molecular phenotype mediate induction of the morphologic and histologic phenotypes. Accordingly, hypertrophy and fibrosis are considered secondary phenotypes because of activation of intermediary molecular phenotypes (Fig. 81–6).

Many HCM mutations involve deletions or truncations that are considered null alleles because of the possible expression of unstable mRNA and proteins.[138,205] Whether haploinsufficiency causes HCM by altering the stoichiometry of the sarcomeric proteins remains unknown. Myocyte dropout caused by apoptosis also has been implicated in animal models.[206] However, the significance of myocyte apoptosis in the pathogenesis of human HCM remains to be established. Regardless of the initial primary defect, cardiac hypertrophy, the clinical hallmark of HCM, is considered a compensatory phenotype. Evidence suggesting the compensatory nature of cardiac hypertrophy includes upregulation of expression of molecular markers of secondary cardiac hypertrophy, such as atrial and brain natriuretic peptides,[184,207,208] endothelin-1,[209] transforming growth factor β_1 (TGFβ_1), and insulin-like growth factor 1 (IGF-1).[210] The predominant involvement of the left ventricle and its frequent absence in the low-pressure right ventricle, despite

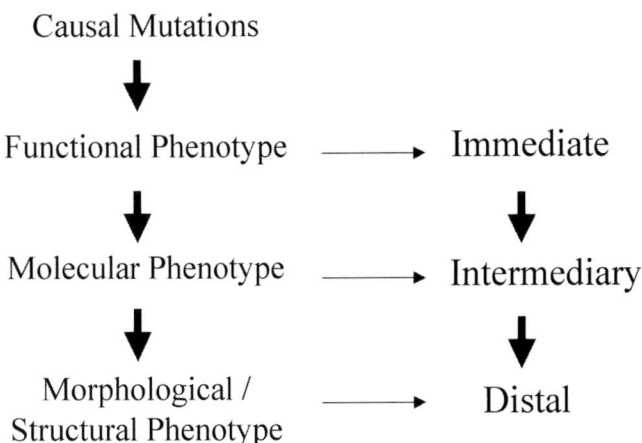

Causal Mutations

Functional Phenotype ⟶ Immediate

Molecular Phenotype ⟶ Intermediary

Morphological / Structural Phenotype ⟶ Distal

FIGURE 81–6. Sequence of phenotype characterization in the pathogenesis of cardiomyopathies.

equal expression of mutant sarcomeric protein in both, suggest contribution of the environment to the development of hypertrophy. Furthermore, variation in hypertrophic response because of the genetic background, its absence early on in life, and its attenuation through pharmacologic interventions, at least in animal models, supports the secondary nature of hypertrophy.[211,212] The primary impetus for hypertrophy is not well defined. It is likely to involve activation of myofibrillar signaling pathways in response to increased cell mechanical stress, altered moiety of the mutant proteins for the signaling molecules and/or altered Ca^{2+} homeostasis.

Potential New Therapeutic Interventions

Current pharmacologic interventions in HCM are empiric (class IIa).[79] None of the current pharmacologic agents has been shown to induce regression of hypertrophy, fibrosis, and disarray, which are associated with increased mortality and morbidity (class IIb).[103,104] Currently, there is no suitable method to correct the underlying genetic defect. Therefore, the emphasis has been on prevention, reversal, and attenuation of the phenotype through pharmacologic interventions aimed at blockade of intermediary molecular phenotypes. Recent studies have shown potential clinical usefulness of angiotensin II receptor blockers, beta-hydroxy-beta-methylglutaryl-coenzyme A (HMG-CoA) reductase inhibitors and antioxidants in prevention, attenuation and reversal of cardiac phenotypes in animal models of HCM (class IIb).[211–214] For example, blockade of angiotensin II receptor 1 in cardiac troponin T-Q92 transgenic mice reduced interstitial collagen volume, expression levels of collagen α_1 (I) mRNA, and $TGF\beta_1$ protein to normal levels.[213] Treatment with HMG-CoA reductase inhibitors also has been shown to prevent and attenuate cardiac phenotype in a transgenic rabbit model of human HCM.[211,212] Treatment with simvastatin, a pleiotropic HMG-CoA reductase inhibitor, reduced left ventricular mass, wall thickness, and collagen volume fraction in the β-MHC-Q403 transgenic rabbit model of human HCM.[211] In addition, indices of left ventricular filling pressure were improved significantly. Similarly, administration of atorvastatin prevented the development of cardiac hypertrophy in the same transgenic rabbit model.[212] Treatment with antioxidant N-acetylcysteine reversed interstitial fibrosis in a mouse model of HCM.[214] Calcineurin inhibitors, while effective in atten-

uation of experimental cardiac hypertrophy,[215] were found to worsen cardiac phenotype in an α-MHC mouse model of HCM.[200] Pretreatment with diltiazem, an L-type Ca^{2+} channel blocker, prevented the exaggerated cardiac hypertrophic response to calcineurin inhibitors in the α-MHC mouse model.[200] Collectively, the results in genetically engineered animal models raise the possibility of pharmacologic interventions to prevent, attenuate, and reverse evolving cardiac phenotype in HCM. Clinical trials in humans are needed to determine potential salutary effects of HMG-CoA reductase inhibitors, angiotensin II blockers, and N-acetylcysteine in human patients with HCM.

【 】 GENETIC BASIS OF DILATED CARDIOMYOPATHY

DCM is a primary disease of the myocardium that manifests by dilatation of the left ventricular along with a gradual decline in contractility. The diagnosis is based on a left ventricular ejection fraction of <0.45 and a left ventricular end-diastolic diameter >2.7 cm/m^2. It has a prevalence of 40 cases per 100,000 individuals and an incidence of 5 to 8 cases per 100,000 persons.[216] Patients with DCM are often asymptomatic in the early stages but gradually develop symptoms and signs of heart failure, syncope, cardiac arrhythmias, and SCD. Thus, a normal history and physical examination in a subject at risk, particularly in the early decades of life, does not exclude DCM. A significant number of affected relatives of patients with DCM are asymptomatic and are diagnosed for the first time on additional testing (such as an echocardiogram).[217] A family history of DCM is present in approximately half of all index cases with idiopathic DCM.[217,218] In the remainder, DCM is considered sporadic. Familial DCM is commonly inherited as an autosomal dominant disease,[217] which clinically manifests during the third and fourth decades of life.

An X-linked DCM is suspected when only male members of a family exhibit symptoms and signs of DCM and there is no male-to-male transmission. Three common forms of X-linked DCM have been identified, including Duchenne and Becker muscular dystrophies, Emery-Dreifuss syndrome, and Barth syndrome. DCM also occurs in multiorgan disorders, such as mitochondrial DNA mutations, triplet repeat syndromes, and metabolic disorders.

Molecular Genetics of Dilated Cardiomyopathy

DCM is an extremely heterogeneous disease, as indicated by the heterogeneity of the mapped loci and genes for familial DCM (Table 81–9). The predominant mode of inheritance is autosomal dominant; however, autosomal recessive and X-linked DCM also occur. Several causal genes for autosomal dominant DCM have been identified.[219] Several causal genes encode sarcomeric proteins, which are also known to cause HCM.[220] Thus, despite the contrasting phenotypes of HCM and DCM, mutations in sarcomeric genes can cause either of the phenotype. Because many of the known causal genes for DCM involve the myocyte cytoskeleton, DCM has been considered to be a disease of cytoskeletal proteins. However, mutations in proteins other than the cytoskeletal proteins also can cause DCM.

Causal Genes and Mutations The gene encoding cardiac α-actin (ACTC) was the first causal gene identified for autosomal

TABLE 81-9

Causal Genes for Dilated Cardiomyopathy (DCM)

GENE	SYMBOL	LOCUS	INHERITANCE	MUTATIONS/FREQUENCY/CONTEXT
Sarcomeric/Cytoskeletal				
Cardiac α-actin	ACTC	15q11–14	Autosomal dominant	Missense/uncommon; also causes HCM
β-Myosin heavy chain	MYH7	14q11–13	Autosomal dominant	Missense/~5 percent; also causes HCM
Cardiac troponin T	TNNT2	1q32	Autosomal dominant	Missense/uncommon; also causes HCM
α-Tropomyosin	TPM1	15q22.1	Autosomal dominant	Missense/rare; also causes HCM
Cypher/ZASP (LIM domain binding 3)	LDB3	10q22.3-q23.2	Sporadic and familial	
Titin	TTN	2q24.1	Autosomal dominant	Missense/uncommon; also causes HCM
Telethonin (T-cap)	TCAP	17q12		
Cytoskeletal				
α-Sarcoglycan	SGCA	17q21	Autosomal dominant	Limb–girdle muscular dystrophy
β-Sarcoglycan	SGCB	4q12	Autosomal dominant	
δ-Sarcoglycan	SGCD	5q33–34	Autosomal dominant Autosomal recessive	
Dystrophin	DMD	Xp21	X-linked	Muscular dystrophy
Muscle LIM protein	MLP (CSRP3)	11q15.1	Autosomal dominant	Rare, founder effect in families described
Intermediary Filaments				
Desmin	DES	2q35	Autosomal dominant	Also causes RCM and desminopathies
αB-crystallin	CRYAB	11q35		Desminopathy
Nuclear Proteins				
Lamin A/C	LMNA	1q21.2	Autosomal dominant	DCM, conduction defect, muscular dystrophy, lipodystrophy, insulin resistance
Emerin	EMD	Xq28	X-linked	
Vinculin	VCL	10q22.1-q23	Sporadic	Metavincluin isoform
Cell Junction Molecules				
Desmoplakin	DSP	6p23–25	Autosomal recessive	Also causes ARVC
Unknown				
Taffazin (G4.5)	TAZ	Xq28	X-linked	Ventricular noncompaction
		1q32		
		2q14–22		
		2q31		
		3p22–25		
		6q23–24		
		9q13–22		
		10q21–23	Autosomal dominant	
		7p12.1–7q21		

ARVC, arrhythmogenic right ventricular cardiomyopathy; DCM, dilated cardiomyopathy; HCM, hypertrophic cardiomyopathy; RCM, restrictive cardiomyopathy.

dominant DCM.[221] Subsequently, mutations in genes encoding additional components of the sarcomere, namely *MYH7, TNNT2, TTN,* and *TCAP* were found in patients with DCM.[219,220,222] Because mutations in *ACTC, MYH7,* and *TNNT2* are also known to cause HCM, these findings point to the commonality of the genetic basis of DCM and HCM. The diversity of the phenotype may reflect the topography of the causal mutations on the protein as well as the genetic background of the individuals.

Mutations in cytoskeletal proteins—namely, delta sarcoglycan,[223] beta sarcoglycan,[224] metavinculin,[225] and dystrophin[226]—are also im-

portant causes of DCM. Mutations in alpha sarcoglycan (adhalin) cause an autosomal recessive form of DCM that occurs in conjunction with limb-girdle muscular dystrophy.[224] Recently, a mutation in muscle LIM protein (MLP) was identified in several related families with DCM.[222] MLP interacts with telethonin, a titin-interacting protein, and colocalizes with it to the Z disk. Mutations in another Z disk protein named ZASP or Cypher or LIM domain binding protein 3 (LDB3) also have been identified in patients with DCM.[227,228] These findings, together with the results of studies in the LIM-deficient mouse model, implicate the Z disk is a mechanosensor for cardiac myocytes. Furthermore, rare mutations in *ABCC9*, which encodes the regulatory SUR2A subunit of the cardiac K(ATP) channel, have been identified in patients with DCM.[229] Mutant SUR2A proteins show aberrant redistribution of conformations in the intrinsic adenosine triphosphate (ATP) hydrolytic cycle and induce abnormal K(ATP) channel phenotypes.[229]

An intriguing causal gene for familial DCM is the lamin A/C gene,[230,230] which encodes a nuclear envelope protein. The observed phenotype resulting from mutations in the rod domain of lamin A/C is progressive conduction disease, atrial arrhythmias, heart failure, and SCD. Moreover, mutations in the intermediary filament desmin and its associated protein alphaB-crystallin have been identified in patients with DCM.[231,232] Often such mutations lead to a phenotype of cardiac and skeletal myopathy that is referred to as *desmin-related myopathy.*[232] Collectively, these findings suggest that mutations affecting the integrity of the sarcomeric, cytoskeleton, and Z disk proteins are the main causes of DCM.

Duchenne and Becker Muscular Dystrophies

The phenotype is characterized by progressive degeneration of muscle function. It commonly manifests itself as mild but progressive skeletal myopathy, early contractures, and cardiomyopathy. The incidence of Duchenne/Becker muscular dystrophy is 1 in 3500 newborn males.[233] Duchenne muscular dystrophy is a severe form and Becker muscular dystrophy a milder form of the disease. The disease commonly manifests itself during the first or second decades of life in male patients. Female family members are commonly spared. However, they may exhibit a mild phenotype, typically late in life. Cardiac involvement includes progressive atrioventricular block, arrhythmia, loss of P-wave amplitude on the ECG, atrial standstill, DCM, akinesis/dyskinesis of the posterobasal wall of the left ventricle, and SCD. Often, DCM is the primary feature of Duchenne and Becker muscular dystrophies. Approximately 90 percent of patients will eventually develop DCM.[234] Death often occurs by the third decade of life.

The gene responsible for Duchenne and Becker muscular dystrophies is dystrophin, located on Xp21, which encodes a large cytoskeletal protein.[235] A variety of point, deletion, and insertion mutations or gene rearrangements in dystrophin have been described.[226,234] Approximately two-thirds of the mutations are either deletions or duplications. DCM can also occur in the absence of skeletal myopathy. Mutations leading to a frameshift induce a severe form, while missense mutations often lead to a mild form of the disease. Mutations in the 5′ region of the dystrophin gene can cause DCM without skeletal involvement.[236]

Emery-Dreifuss Muscular Dystrophy

It is an X-linked degenerative disorder characterized by mild but progressive skeletal and cardiac myopathy.[237,238] Clinical features include muscle weakness and atrophy, flexion deformities of the elbows, and mild pectus excavatum. Cardiac phenotypes include cardiomyopathy, arrhythmia, SCD, conduction defects, loss of P-wave amplitude on the ECG, and atrial standstill.[239]

The causal gene is *EMD*, which encodes emerin. Emerin is located along the nuclear rim of many cell types. It is a member of the nuclear lamina-associated protein family.[240]

Barth Syndrome

DCM is also a major phenotypic component of the Barth syndrome, another X-linked disorder. The characteristic phenotype of Barth syndrome includes skeletal and cardiac myopathy, neutropenia, and abnormal mitochondria. Barth syndrome is caused by point, deletion, and splice-junction mutations in the tafazzin (*TAZ*) or G4.5 gene, located on Xq28.[241]

Modifier Genes and Mutations

The phenotype of DCM is determined not only by the causal mutations but also by the modifier genes and the environmental factors. Genetic studies to identify the modifier genes for DCM are largely restricted to SNP-association studies and have limitations similar to those described for HCM. Several potential candidates, including *ACE*, have been identified. None has been established to modify cardiac phenotypes in DCM. A modifier locus in a calsequestrin mouse model of DCM has been mapped.[242]

Genotype–Phenotype Correlation in Dilated Cardiomyopathy

There is no large-scale systematic study to delineate the impact of causal and modifier genes and mutations on the DCM phenotype. Therefore, the available genotype–phenotype data may be specific to a family or small number of families. Overall, a diverse array of phenotypes caused by mutations in different genes is observed in DCM families. Typically, mutations in cardiac α-actin, β-MHC, and cardiac troponin T (cTnT) cause DCM without other phenotypes, such as conduction defects or deafness.[220] In contrast, mutations in the rod domain of lamin A/C cause DCM in conjunction with progressive conduction defects, atrial arrhythmias, and SCD.[230] Mutations in the lamin A/C gene can also cause an autosomal-dominant form of Emery-Dreifuss syndrome.[243] Mutations in desmin and alphaB-crystallin genes are commonly associated with skeletal myopathy as well as DCM with unique pathologic features, a phenotype referred to as the *desmin-related myopathy.*[244] Mutations in the dystrophin gene commonly lead to skeletal and cardiac myopathy. The severity of the myopathic phenotype is partly determined by the type of mutation. Those that are frameshift mutations—for example, insertion or deletion of a single base—cause a severe form, whereas missense mutations often lead to a mild form of DCM and muscular dystrophy. Mutations in the 5′ region of the dystrophin gene can cause DCM without skeletal involvement.[236]

Cardiac involvement is quite common in triplet repeat syndromes and includes DCM, conduction disorders, and arrhythmia. Prevalence of cardiac involvement increases with advancing age, and approximately three-quarters of adult patients exhibit conduction defects, such as first-degree atrioventricular block and intraventricular conduction defects.[245] There is also a direct relationship between the severity of the disease and the severity of cardiac involvement and the number of CTG repeats.[245]

Pathogenesis of Dilated Cardiomyopathy

Mutations in cardiac α-actin, β-myosin heavy chain, cardiac troponin T, and cytoskeletal proteins are expected to impart a dominant-negative effect on transmission of the contractile force to the extracellular matrix proteins.[220,221] Identification of mutations in *MLP*, *LDB3*, and *TCAP* emphasize the significance of the Z disk in maintaining normal cardiac function.[222,227,228] Similarly, identification of mutations in the dystrophin-associated protein complex as causes of DCM signifies the role of sarcolemma in the pathogenesis of DCM.[223] Mutations in the dystrophin gene lead to decreased expression levels of dystrophin, a major cytoskeletal protein in skeletal and cardiac muscles. Decreased levels of dystrophin are expected to impair mechanical coupling and myocyte shortening.[236] The molecular pathogenesis of other X-linked DCMs because of mutations in *EMD* and *TAZ* is unknown.

Pathogenesis of DCM resulting from mutations in desmin and alphaB-crystallin involves deposition of desmin and alphaB-crystallin aggregates in the myocardium.[246] Molecular pathogenesis of DCM caused by mutations in lamin A/C or emerin remain largely unknown. It is likely to involve disruption of integrity of the cytoskeleton. The pathogenesis of cardiomyopathies in patients with the triplet repeat syndromes is also unclear. Expansion of the CTG (CUG in mRNA) repeats in the genes responsible for triplet repeat syndromes could indirectly affect transcription, transport, splicing, and translation of mRNAs of cardiac genes.[178]

[ ] GENETIC BASIS OF ARRHYTHMOGENIC RIGHT VENTRICULAR CARDIOMYOPATHY/DYSPLASIA

Arrhythmogenic right ventricular cardiomyopathy (ARVC) is an uncommon cardiomyopathy with characteristic clinical and pathologic features.[247–249] The clinical phenotype comprises ventricular arrhythmias, primarily originating from the right ventricle, SCD, and heart failure.[247,249,250] The pathologic phenotype is characterized by the gradual replacement of the cardiac myocytes by adipocytes and fibrosis (Fig. 81–7).[247,250] A comprehensive approach for the diagnosis of ARVC has been developed by the European Society of Cardiology and the Scientific Council on Cardiomyopathies of the International Society and Federation of Cardiology.[251]

The disease often has a "concealed" stage, which is characterized by minor ventricular arrhythmias and subtle pathologic findings. It is followed by symptomatic ventricular arrhythmias and gradual progression to right-heart failure and, finally, global cardiac failure.[250]

Electrocardiographic features include the characteristics and yet uncommon epsilon wave, depolarization and repolarization abnormalities in the right precordial leads, and ventricular arrhythmias originating from the right ventricle.[249,250]

ARVC is an important cause of SCD in apparently healthy individuals.[247,252–254] In the U.S. population, it accounts for 3 to 4 percent of SCD associated with physical activity in the young athletes.[92] In some reports, ARVC was found in up to 25 percent of the cases of nontraumatic SCD.[252–255,255] Collectively, the data suggests ARVC is an important cause of SCD in the young competitive athletes.

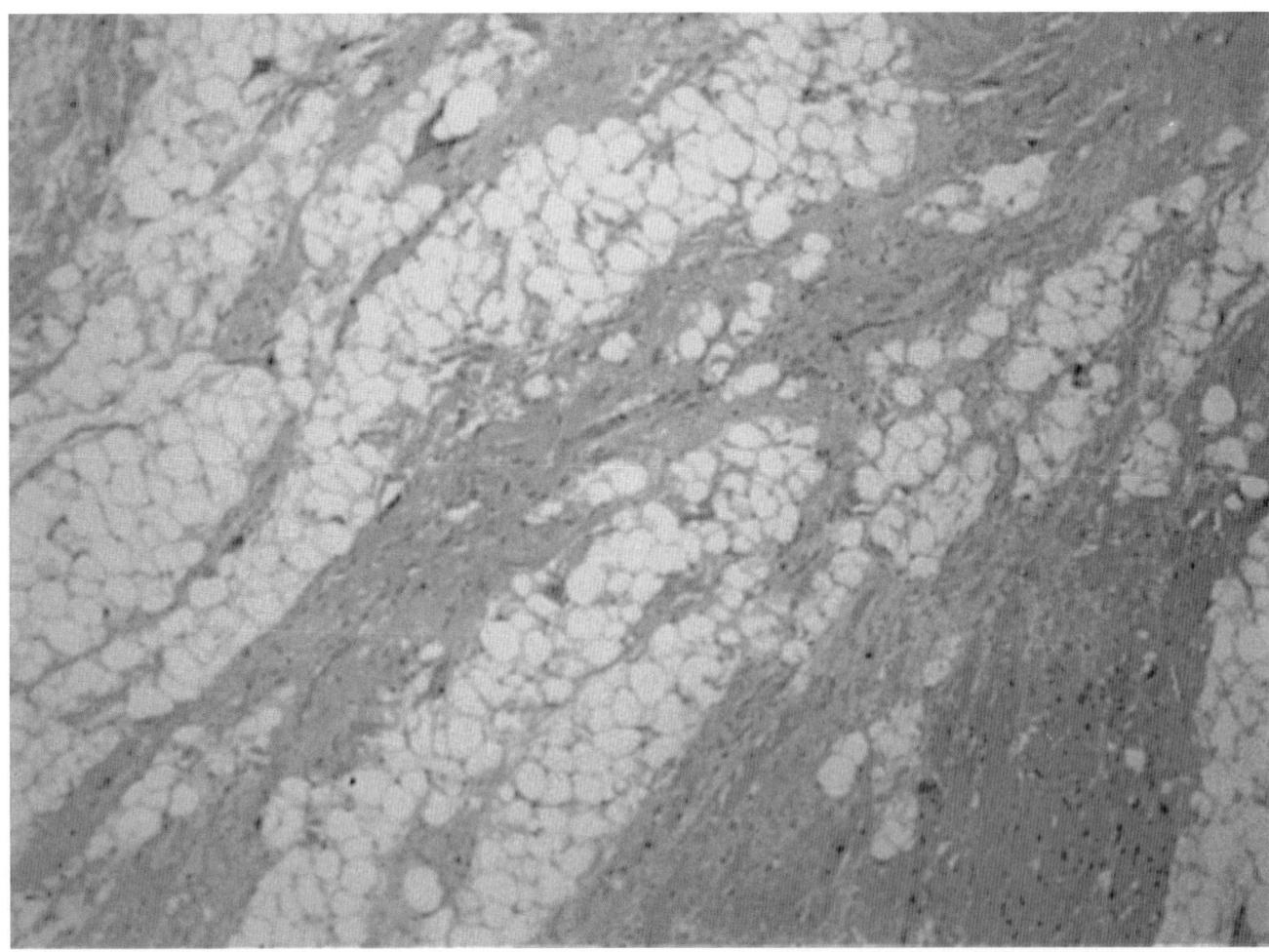

FIGURE 81–7. Histologic features of arrhythmogenic right ventricular dysplasia. Fibrofatty infiltrate in the right ventricle is shown.

ARVC Phenocopy

The presence of myocardial fat alone is distinct from ARVC. Significant fatty infiltration of the myocardium could be present in normal individuals, particularly in elderly.[256,257] Cor adiposum (fatty infiltration of the myocardium) is distinguished from true ARVC by the absence of right ventricular myocardial thinning, myocyte atrophy and apoptosis, patchy fibroadipocytic replacement of myocytes, predominantly in the right ventricle, and lymphocytic myocarditis.[256] Right ventricular dilatation, fibrosis, myocyte atrophy, and excess adipocytes have been observed in patients with Becker muscular dystrophy, Emery-Dreifuss muscular dystrophy, and myotonic dystrophy.[250] The distinction between muscular dystrophies and ARVC is usually not problematic because of the skeletal involvement in muscular dystrophies.

Idiopathic right ventricular outflow tract tachycardia and stress-induced (catecholaminergic) polymorphic ventricular tachycardia, caused by mutations in cardiac ryanodine receptor (RYR2), often present with arrhythmias resembling those in ARVC.[258,259] The absence of structural or histologic cardiac abnormalities suggests phenocopy and not true ARVC.[250]

Molecular Genetics of Arrhythmogenic Right Ventricular Cardiomyopathy/Dysplasia

ARVC is a genetic disease that is estimated to be familial in approximately 30 to 50 percent of the cases.[248] The most common mode of inheritance is autosomal dominant. Recessive forms in conjunction with keratoderma and woolly hair (Naxos disease) or with predominant involvement of the left ventricle (Carvajal syndrome) also have been described and referred to as *cardiocutaneous syndrome*.[260,261]

The genetic basis of ARVC is partially known. Chromosomal loci have been mapped (Table 81–10).[262–268] Mutations in *DSP*, *JUP*, *PKP2*, and *DSG2*, encoding desmosomal proteins desmoplakin (DP), plakoglobin (PG), plakophilin 2 (PKP2), and desmoglein 2 (DSG2) have been identified (Table 81–10).[260,269–272] Mutations in *PKP2* appear to be the most common causes of ARVC, accounting for approximately 20 percent of the cases.[269,272]

Mutations in *DSG2* and *DSP* each account for approximately 10 to 15 percent of the cases of ARVC.[272] The majority of causal mutations cause frameshift and hence, are expected to lead to premature termination of the proteins.

The causal gene for an autosomal recessive form of ARVC, palmoplantar keratoderma, and peculiar woolly hairs (Naxos syndrome), is *JUP*, which encodes plakoglobin.[260] Plakoglobin is also a desmosome protein and, along with desmoplakin, anchors intermediate filaments to desmosomes. The phenotype was described first in a family from the island of Naxos in Greece, and was mapped to 17q21. Mutational analysis detected a 2-bp deletion in *JUP*, which encodes PG, a major component of desmosomes and adherens junctions. Another recessive form of ARVC is Carvajal syndrome, which is a cardiocutaneous syndrome with predominant involvement of the left ventricle.[261] It is caused by mutations in *DSP*.

Recently, a point mutation in the 5 untranslated region (UTR) of *TGFB3* gene was identified in a family mapped to 14q24.3.[273] Whether this point mutation in the 5UTR is a true causal mutation or simply a DNA marker remains to be established.[274]

Mutations in *RYR2* cause catecholaminergic polymorphic ventricular tachycardia, which was initially considered a variant of ARVC. However, it is now considered a distinct phenotype because of the absence of fibrofatty infiltration in the myocardium.[250,258,259]

Pathogenesis of Arrhythmogenic Right Ventricular Cardiomyopathy

The molecular pathogenesis of ARVC is unknown. Infection and inflammation,[257,275,276] apoptosis,[277] myocyte transdifferentiation,[278] and myocyte detachment[250] have been proposed. Apoptosis has been detected in autopsy specimens collected from patients with ARVC.[279,280] However, apoptosis alone does not explain the mechanism for fibrofatty infiltration of the myocardium. Experimental data suggests suppression of the canonical Wnt signaling by PG is a mechanism for the pathogenesis of ARVC.[281] Accordingly, mutations in desmosomal protein impair desmosome assem-

TABLE 81–10

Chromosomal Loci and Causal Genes for Arrhythmogenic Right Ventricular Dysplasia

	CHROMOSOME	SYMBOL	PROTEIN	FUNCTION
ARVC1[a]	14q24.3	TGFβ3	Transforming growth factor-β 3	Mitotic and trophic factor
ARVC2[a]	14q42.2-q43	RYR2	Ryanodine receptor 2	Calcium channel
ARVC3	1q12-q22			
ARVC4	2q32.1			
ARVD5	3p23			
ARVD6	10p12-p14			
ARVD7	10q22			
ARVC8	6p24	DSP	Desmoplakin	Desmosomes
ARVC9	12p11	PKP2	Plakophilin 2	Desmosomes
	18q12.1	DSG2	Desmoglein 2	Desmosomes
Naxos disease	17q21	JUP	Plakoglobin	Desmosomes

[a]Phenocopy. *RYR2* mutations cause catecholaminergic polymorphic ventricular tachycardia and not true arrhythmogenic right ventricular cardiomyopathy.

bly and lead to excess free (unincorporated) PG and PKP2, which can translocate into the nucleus. Nuclear PG and PKP2, because of structural similarities to β-catenin, the effector of the canonical Wnt signaling, compete with β-catenin for binding to Wnt core protein complex, resulting in suppression of the canonical Wnt signaling. The latter leads to enhanced fibroadipogenesis and myocyte apoptosis, which are the characteristic findings in human ARVC.[281]

GENETIC BASIS OF RESTRICTIVE CARDIOMYOPATHY

Restrictive cardiomyopathy (RCM) is a heart-muscle disease characterized by severely enlarged atria as a result of elevated right and left ventricular filling pressures, normal or reduced ventricular volumes, and, usually, preserved global systolic function.[282] The clinical manifestations are those of heart failure, often with predominance of right-sided signs and symptoms. The age of onset of the disease is variable, and the prognosis is relatively poor. RCM can occur because of systemic infiltrative disorders, such as amyloidosis and sarcoidosis, and storage diseases, such as Fabry disease.[282] Although such disorders are also genetic in etiology, RCM in such disorders is an indirect consequence, and not a primary myocardial abnormality.

Molecular Genetics of Restrictive Cardiomyopathy

Familial RCM with an autosomal dominant form of inheritance in conjunction with skeletal myopathy and atrioventricular conduction defects have been described.[283–285] Two causal genes for RCM—DES,[286] encoding desmin, and TNNI,3,[287] encoding cardiac troponin I—have been identified. Desmin is an intermediary filament that is also involved in desminopathies involving skeletal muscles as well as the heart. Mutations in TNNI3, which are known to cause HCM and DCM, also cause RCM.[287] RCM also occurs in patients with Noonan syndrome,[288] which is caused by mutations in the protein tyrosine phosphatase, nonreceptor type II.[60] The pathogenesis of RCM remains largely unknown.

GENETIC BASIS OF CARDIOMYOPATHIES IN TRINUCLEOTIDE REPEAT SYNDROMES

Trinucleotide repeat syndromes are a group of genetic disorders caused by expansion of naturally occurring GC-rich triplet repeats in genes.[178,289] The group comprises more than 10 different diseases, including myotonic muscular dystrophy and Huntington disease.[178,289] Cardiac involvement is common in several forms of triplet repeat syndromes and is a major determinant of morbidity and mortality.[178] The phenotype commonly includes DCM, HCM, conduction disorders, and arrhythmias. Average life expectancy of the affected individuals is about 30 to 40 years.

Genetic Basis of Cardiomyopathies in Myotonic Dystrophy

Myotonic dystrophy (DM) is an autosomal dominant disorder with highly variable penetrance.[115] The estimated prevalence of DM is approximately 1 in 8000 in the North American population.[115,245] It is the most common form of muscular dystrophy in adults. DM commonly manifests itself as progressive degeneration of muscles and myotonia, cardiomyopathy, conduction defects, male-pattern baldness, infertility, premature cataracts, mental retardation, and endocrine abnormalities.[115,245] Cardiomyopathy is a common phenotypic manifestation of myotonic DM.[245] Cardiac conduction defects, such as first-degree atrioventricular block and intraventricular conduction defects, are present in approximately three-quarters of adult patients.[245]

Mutations in two genes have been identified for DM, including expansion of CTG (CUG in mRNA) trinucleotide repeats in the 3' untranslated region of DM protein kinase (DMPK), located on chromosome 19q3.[290–292] The number of CTG repeats in normal individuals varies between 5 and 37. It expands from 50 to more than several thousand in patients with DM.[115] Expansion of the repeats can interfere with DMPK transcription, RNA processing, and/or translation, resulting in decreased levels of expression of DMPK protein. Several proteins that bind to the trinucleotide repeats have been identified including CUGBP1, ETR3-like factors (CELFs), and muscle blind-like (MBNL) proteins.[293] Increased activities of these proteins affect splicing and processing of several mRNAs, including splicing of cTnT.[294] The length of the CTG repeats often correlates with the severity of clinical phenotypes, including conduction defects and cardiomyopathy.[295]

The second gene responsible for DM is zinc finger protein 9 (ZNF9), located on 3q21.[296] Expansion of a CCTG tetranucleotide repeats in intron 1 of ZNF9 leads to expression of abnormal RNA, which binds and alter activities of RNA-binding proteins. Increased activities of RNA-binding proteins affect splicing and expression of multiple target genes, resulting in the subsequent multiorgan phenotype.

Genetic Basis of Cardiomyopathies in Friedreich Ataxia

Friedreich ataxia (FRDA) is an autosomal recessive neurodegenerative disease. It primarily involves the central and peripheral nervous system and less frequently manifests as cardiomyopathy and occasionally as diabetes mellitus.[179] FRDA is caused by the expansion of the GAA trinucleotide repeats in intron 1 of FRDA.[179] The encoded protein is frataxin, which is a soluble mitochondrial protein with 210 amino acids. Cardiac involvement can manifest as either DCM or HCM. The severity of clinical manifestations of FRDA also correlates with the size of the repeats.[297] The pathogenesis of cardiomyopathies in FRDA is likely to involve impaired iron homeostasis and increased oxidative stress.[289]

GENETIC BASIS OF CARDIOMYOPATHIES IN METABOLIC DISORDERS

Metabolic cardiomyopathies encompass a group of disorders in which there is the primary metabolic abnormality in the heart (Table 81–11). This metabolic abnormality also may involve other organs; however, cardiac involvement is direct and not a consequence of secondary changes in other organs. Secondary involvement of the myocardium in systemic metabolic disorders is not considered a metabolic cardiomyopathy.

A prototype of metabolic cardiomyopathies is glycogen storage disease type II (glycogenosis type II or Pompe disease). Pompe dis-

TABLE 81-11

Examples of Causal Genes for Metabolic Cardiomyopathies

PROTEIN	SYMBOL	LOCUS	FREQUENCY	MUTATIONS/PHENOTYPE
AMP-activated protein kinase, γ2 regulatory subunit	PRKAG2	7q35-q36	Rare	Point and insertion mutations, HCM, WPW, and conduction defect
Acid maltase gene			Rare	Pompe disease, DCM, HCM, conduction defects
Phytanoyl-CoA hydroxylase	PAHX or PHYH		Rare	DCM, HCM, and conduction defects

AMP, adenosine monophosphate; CoA, coenzyme A; DCM, dilated cardiomyopathy; HCM, hypertrophic cardiomyopathy; WPW, Wolff-Parkinson-White syndrome.

ease is an autosomal recessive disorder caused by deficiency of α-1,4-glucosidase (acid maltase), which degrades α-1,4 and α-1,6 linkages in glycogen, maltose, and isomaltose.[181] Deficiency of the enzyme leads to storage of glycogen in lysosomal membranes. Phenotypic expression of Pompe disease includes HCM, DCM, conduction defects, and muscular hypotonia. The cause is mutations in the acid maltase gene. Mutations lead to deficiency of acid α-glucosidase. A high-protein diet and recombinant acid α-glucosidase have been used effectively to treat this disorder.[298]

Mutations in the gene encoding the AMP-activated γ2 noncatalytic subunit of protein kinase A (PRKAG2) have been identified in families with HCM and WPW syndrome.[85–87] AMP-activated kinase is a biosensor of the cellular energy state. Cardiac involvement varies from a predominant phenotype of preexcitation and conduction abnormalities to a predominant phenotype of cardiac hypertrophy.[85,87] Nonetheless, the primary phenotype appears to be a deposit of glycogen in the myocardium, which is responsible for cardiac enlargement as well as facilitated atrioventricular (AV) conduction.[88]

Refsum disease is an autosomal recessive disorder characterized clinically by a tetrad of retinitis pigmentosa, peripheral neuropathy, cerebellar ataxia, and elevated protein levels in the cerebrospinal fluid.[299] Cardiac involvement includes ECG abnormalities, which are common. Cardiac hypertrophy and heart failure are uncommon. Mutations in the gene encoding phytanoyl-coenzyme A (CoA) hydroxylase (PAHX or PHYH) are responsible for Refsum disease.[180] Mutations reduce the enzymatic activity and lead to accumulation of phytanic acid, an unusual branched-chain fatty acid in tissues and body fluids.[113]

Cardiac involvement in patients with mucopolysaccharidosis, Niemann-Pick disease, Gaucher disease, hereditary hemochromatosis, and CD36 deficiency have also been described (reviewed in Ref. 183).

[ ] GENETIC BASIS OF CARDIOMYOPATHIES IN MITOCHONDRIAL DISORDERS

Cardiomyopathies are common in patients with mitochondrial disorders. Mitochondrial cardiomyopathy exhibits a matrilineal transmission. Because nuclear genes encode for proteins that primarily regulate mitochondrial function, mutations in nuclear DNA can also cause mitochondrial myopathies. Mitochondrial DNA is a circular double-stranded genome of approximately 16.5 kb, encoding 13 polypeptides of the respiratory chain complexes I,

III, IV, and V subunits; 28 ribosomal RNAs; and 22 tRNAs (transfer ribonucleic acids). Mutations in mitochondrial oxidative phosphorylation pathways often result in a complex phenotype involving multiple organs, including the heart.[300] Cardiac involvement can lead to hypertrophy as well as dilatation. Each mitochondrion has multiple copies of its own DNA and each cell contains thousands of mitochondria. Therefore, mutations result in a significant degree of heteroplasmy, which increases over time as the mitochondria multiply. In general, approximately 80 to 90 percent of mitochondrial DNA must mutate in order to affect mitochondrial function and lead to a clinical phenotype.[301]

Kearns-Sayre syndrome is a mitochondrial disease caused by sporadically occurring mutations in mitochondrial DNA.[114] Kearns-Sayre syndrome is characterized by a triad of progressive external ophthalmoplegia, pigmentary retinopathy, and cardiac conduction defects.[114] The classic cardiac abnormality in Kearns-Sayre syndrome is conduction defects; however, DCM and HCM are also often observed, but at a lower frequency.

L-Carnitine deficiency is a cause of mitochondrial myopathy resulting from mutations in nuclear DNA. The phenotype is characterized by skeletal myopathy, congestive heart failure, abnormalities of the central nervous system and liver, and, rarely, HCM.[183,302] Carnitine is an important component of fatty acid metabolism and is necessary for the entry of long-chain fatty acids into mitochondria. Mutations in the chromosomal gene encoding solute carrier family 22, member 5 (SLC22A5), or OCTN2 transporter impair transport of carnitine to mitochondria and cause systemic carnitine deficiency.[302] Similarly, mutations in genes encoding enzymes involved in the transfer and metabolism of carnitine can cause carnitine deficiency. The list includes carnitine mitochondrial carnitine palmitoyltransferase I (CATI or CPT-1), located in the outer mitochondrial membrane; carnitine-acylcarnitine translocase (SLC25A20), located in the inner membrane; and carnitine palmitoyl transferase 2 (CPT-2).

Mutations in acyl-CoA dehydrogenase also impair mitochondrial fatty acid oxidation and can lead to cardiomyopathy.[183,303] The clinical manifestations are remarkable for cardiac hypertrophy with diminished systolic function, fasting hypoglycemia, inadequate ketotic response to hypoglycemia, hepatic dysfunction, skeletal myopathy, and SCD.[183,303] The majority of cases of medium-chain acyl-CoA dehydrogenase deficiency are caused by substitution of glutamic acid for lysine in the mutant protein, whereas the molecular genetic basis of short-chain acyl-CoA dehydrogenase deficiency is more heterogeneous.

GENETIC DISEASES OF CARDIAC RHYTHM AND CONDUCTION

Cardiac rhythm and conduction abnormalities could occur as the primary phenotypes of genetic disorders or secondary phenotypes resulting from genetic diseases that primarily affect structure of the heart. In general, cardiac arrhythmias and conduction defects result from abnormalities in three main families of proteins: contractile sarcomeric proteins, such as that in HCM; the cytoskeletal proteins, which are responsible for DCM; and the ion channels and their regulators, which are responsible for familial arrhythmias and conduction defects.[304] As discussed earlier, there is significant phenotypic overlap as mutations in the same gene could cause a variety of cardiac rhythm and conduction disorders. This is best exemplified by mutations in sodium channel SCN5A, which could cause long QT syndrome, Brugada syndrome, and familial conduction disease.[305] Therefore, a simplistic classification of genetic disorders is considered preliminary and some of the key genetic findings used to risk-stratify for SCD or arrhythmias are based on studies in only few families. Table 81–12 summarizes the list of genetic disorders in which the primary phenotype is cardiac arrhythmias and conduction defects.

[ ] ION CHANNELOPATHIES AS THE BASIS FOR CARDIAC ARRHYTHMIAS AND CONDUCTION DEFECTS

Ion channels, crucial units in cardiac excitability, are glycoproteins embedded in the membrane of the cardiac myocytes, which allow flux of ions in and out of the cell to modulate the electrical gradient. Many different ion channels are orderly activated to give rise to the electrical current that will ultimately be responsible for the development of the myocyte excitability. This is a complex process and requires a very well controlled ionic balance to prevent arrhythmogenesis.

The α subunit of the cardiac sodium channel gene, SCN5A, which is responsible for the phase 0 of the cardiac action potential, has been studied extensively during the past 5 years. SCN5A was first cloned and characterized in 1995 and localized to 3p21.[306] The gene is comprised of 28 exons that code

for a 2016 amino-acid protein. It contains four homologous domains (DI to DIV), each of which contains six membrane-spanning segments (S1 to S6).[304] In 1995, Wang et al. linked mutations in the SCN5A to long QT syndrome,[307] a disease characterized by prolongation of the QT interval and sudden death at a young age. Subsequently, mutations in SCN5A were

TABLE 81–12

Genetic Disorders Causing Cardiac Arrhythmias in the Absence of Structural Heart Disease (Primary Rhythm Disorders)

	RHYTHM	INHERITANCE	LOCUS	GENE
Supraventricular				
Atrial fibrillation	AF	AD	10q22	—
		AD	11p15	KCNQ1
		AD	21q22	KCNE2
		AD	11q13	KCNE3
		AD	17q23	KCNJ2
		AD	12p13	KCNA5
		AD	1q21	GJA5
		AD	6q14–16	—
		AR	5p13	—
Atrial standstill	SND, AF	AD	3p21	SCN5A
Sick sinus syndrome	SND	AD	15q24	HCN4
		AR	3p21	SCN5A
Absent sinus rhythm	SND, AF	AD	—	—
WPW	AVRT	AD	—	—
Familial PJRT	AVRT	AD	—	—
Conduction Disorders				
PCCD	AVB	AD	19q13	—
			3p21	SCN5A
Ventricular				
LQT syndrome (RW)	TdP	AD		
LQT1			11p15	KCNQ1
LQT2			7q35	HERG
LQT3			3p21	SCN5A
LQT4			4q25	ANKB
LQT5			21q22	minK
LQT6			21q22	MiRP1
LQT7			17q23	KCNJ2
LQT8			12p13	CACNA1C
LQT syndrome (JLN)	TdP	AR	11p15	KCNQ1
			21q22	minK
SQT syndrome	VF	AD		
SQT1			7q35	HERG
SQT2			11p15	KCNQ1
SQT3			17q23	KCNJ2
Catecholaminergic PVT	VT	AD	1q42	RYR2
		AR	1p13-p11	CASQ2
Brugada syndrome	VT/VF	AD	3p21	SCN5A

AD, autosomal dominant; AF, atrial fibrillation; AR, autosomal recessive; AVB, atrioventricular block; AVRT, atrioventricular reentrant tachycardia; JLN, Jervell and Lange-Nielsen; LQT, long QT; PCCD, progressive cardiac conduction defect; PJRT, paroxysmal junctional reentrant tachycardia; RW, Romano-Ward; SND, sinus node dysfunction; TdP, torsade de pointes; VF, ventricular fibrillation; VT, ventricular tachycardia; WPW, Wolff-Parkinson-White syndrome.

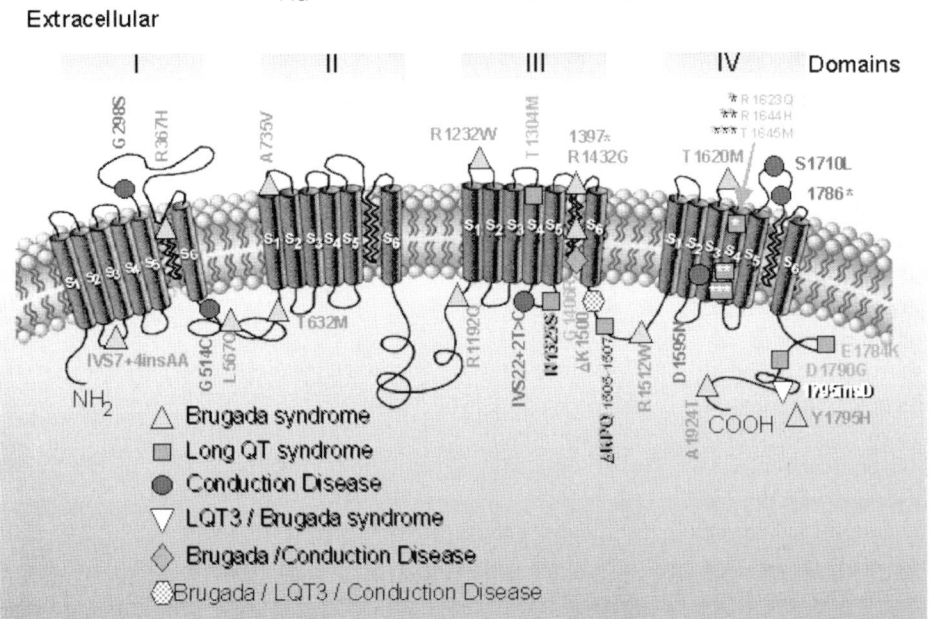

FIGURE 81-8. Schematic structure of I_{Na} sodium channel (SCN5A) and phenotypes arising from mutations in *SCN5A*.

linked to idiopathic ventricular fibrillation,[308] the Brugada syndrome,[305] progressive conduction defect,[309] sudden infant death syndrome (SIDS),[310] and sudden unexpected death syndrome (SUDS).[311] The latter is a phenotype identified two decades ago in Southeast Asia that was causing sudden death in males, usually at night.[311] Figure 81–8 shows the phenotypes arising from mutations in SCN5A.

[ ] BRUGADA SYNDROME AND ITS VARIANTS

Brugada syndrome is identified by characteristic ECG pattern consisting of right bundle-branch block and ST-segment elevation in V_1 to V_3 (Fig. 81–9) and sudden death at a young age.[312] It was described originally in 1992 based on electrocardiographic pattern and occurrence of syncope or sudden death episodes in patients with a structurally normal heart.[312] The episodes of syncope and sudden death are caused by fast polymorphic ventricular tachycardia.[312,313]

Brugada syndrome often manifests in subjects in the third or fourth decades of life, and occasionally in infants as SIDS.[310] Recent studies suggest SUDS, which is prevalent in Southeast Asia, is a form of Brugada syndrome. SUDS is estimated to affect up to 1 percent of the population and it is the most common cause of death in young males in Thailand.[314] Death often occurs at night and more commonly in male subjects (male-

to-female ratio is 10:1). Electrocardiographically, the disease is identical to Brugada syndrome. As in Brugada syndrome, mutations in SCN5A are responsible for SUDS and biophysical data indicates a nonworking SCN5A or accelerated inactivation.[311]

Genetics of the Brugada Syndrome

SCN5A was identified as the first, and thus far the only, causal gene for Brugada syndrome in 1998.[308] More than 60 different mutations in *SCN5A* have been identified that collectively account for approximately 25 percent of all cases with Brugada syndrome. As in many other genetic disorders, Brugada syndrome also exhibit locus heterogeneity and a second locus on chromosome 3 has been mapped.[315] However, the causal gene has not been identified yet.

Mutations of *SCN5A* can lead to a large spectrum of phenotypes, including Brugada syndrome, LQT3, isolated progressive cardiac conduction defect, idiopathic ventricular fibrillation, atrial standstill, and SUDS.[305] The phenotypes are all considered allelic variants, caused by mutations in *SCN5A*. Electrocardiographic, clinical, genetic and biophysical data have clarified the relationship between these phenotypes. The distinction between the LQT3 and Brugada syndromes is difficult to ascertain in some cases and one family has been described manifesting the phenotype of both Brugada and long QT3 syndrome.[316] Likewise, progressive conduction disease and Brugada syndrome have been described in members of a single family.[317] Collectively, these data suggests mutations in

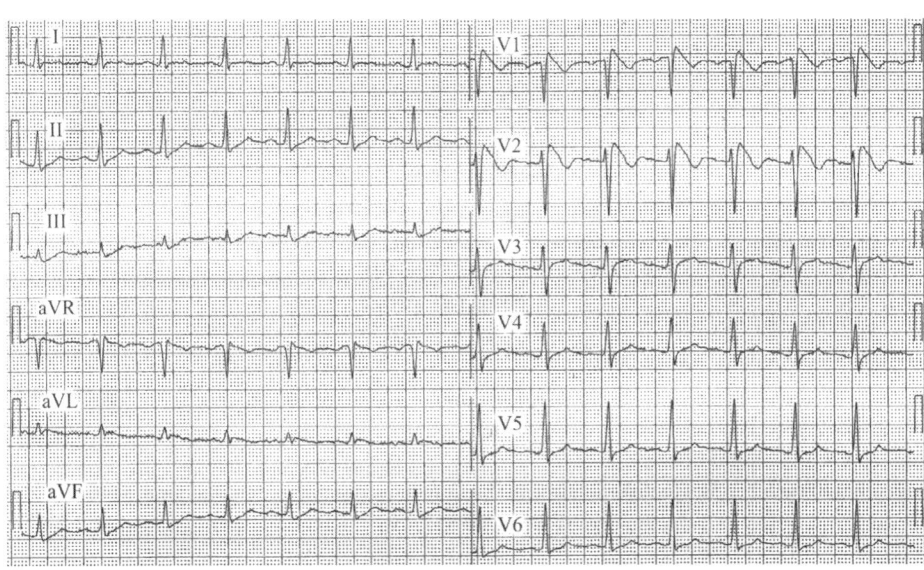

FIGURE 81-9. Typical electrocardiogram of Brugada syndrome. Note the pattern resembling a right bundle-branch block and the ST elevation in leads V_1 to V_2.

SCN5A cause variable phenotypic manifestations that span Brugada syndrome, LQT3 and progressive conduction defects (see Fig. 81–6).

Pathogenesis of Brugada Syndrome

The identification of mutations in *SCN5A* in patients with Brugada syndrome suggests decreased availability of sodium ions could shift the ionic balance in favor of I_{to} during phase 1 of the action potential. Biophysical characterization of mutations in *SCN5A* suggests that mutations decrease the Na^{1+} current availability by two main mechanisms: decreased expression of the mutant channel or acceleration of inactivation of the channel. In addition, the alteration in the ionic currents that worsen at higher temperatures has been implicated for certain mutations, such as the T1620M.[318] The clinical relevance of this mechanism is corroborated by the observation of several cases of ventricular fibrillation during febrile illnesses in patients with Brugada syndrome. Compared to LQT3, the pathogenesis of the Brugada syndrome could be considered a mirror image. Biophysical data indicates that LQT3 mutations cause a delayed inactivation of the channel,[304] which is exactly the opposite as in Brugada syndrome, where there is an accelerated inactivation.[318]

Genotype–Phenotype Correlation in Brugada Syndrome

Limited data is available regarding the correlation between genotypes and phenotype in patients with Brugada syndrome. This may partly reflect very recent identification of the first causal gene, phenotypic variability of *SCN5A* and allelic and locus heterogeneity of Brugada syndrome. It has been suggested that electrocardiographic parameters, such as longer conduction intervals (PQ and HV) on baseline ECG could distinguish the carriers of sodium channel mutations from the noncarriers.[319]

【 】 LONG QT SYNDROME

LQT syndrome is a disease of ventricular repolarization identified by the prolongation of the QT interval on ECG.[304] It is characterized by syncopal episodes, malignant ventricular arrhythmias and ventricular fibrillation. The majority of patients with the LQT syndrome are asymptomatic. However, approximately one-third present with syncope or aborted malignant ventricular arrhythmias including torsade de pointes, which is the most typical ventricular arrhythmia in LQT syndrome. SCD is relatively common. Prognosis of the symptomatic cases, if untreated is poor. Approximately one-fifth of patients who present with syncope and remain untreated die within 1 year and 50 percent die within 10 years.

The LQT syndrome is either acquired, which is iatrogenic and commonly induced by drugs, or congenital. A common cause of the acquired disease is the use of medications such as antiarrhythmics, antidepressants, and phenothiazines (Table 81–13). In addition, electrolyte imbalance, such as hypokalemia, hypomagnesemia, and hypocalcemia, especially in the presence of predisposing medications, could cause LQT syndrome.

Two patterns of inheritance have been described in the congenital LQT syndrome: (1) autosomal recessive disease, described by

TABLE 81–13

Selected Medications Associated with Prolonged QT Interval

Antiarrhythmic drugs
  Quinidine
  Procainamide hydrochloride
  Disopyramide phosphate
  Sotalol hydrochloride
  Amiodarone
  Ibutilide fumarate
  Dofetilide
  Propafenone
Anesthetics/antiasthmatics
  Droperidol
  Adrenaline
Antibiotics
  Clarithromycin
  Erythromycin
  Pentamidine
  Trimethoprim-sulfamethoxazole
  Ketoconazole
  Fluconazole
Antihistamines
  Terfenadine
  Diphenhydramine
Antihyperlipidemic
  Probucol
Central nervous system active drugs
  Droperidol
  Haloperidol
  Pimozide
  Risperidone
Gastrointestinal stimulants
  Cisapride

Jervell and Lange Nielsen in 1957, which is associated with deafness and (2) autosomal dominant disease, described by Romano and Ward, which is not associated with deafness and is more common than the recessive form.

The pathogenesis of LQT syndrome could be summarized as mutations in K^{1+} channel resulting in inadequate opening and decreased potassium outward current. While mutations in Na^{1+} channels lead to inadequate closure of the channels and excessive sodium inward currents. The ensuing result is inadequate maintenance of electrical gradient (loss of function) during an action potential and prolongation of the QT interval.

Autosomal Dominant LQT Syndrome (Romano-Ward Syndrome)

The first locus for the autosomal dominant disease was mapped to chromosome 11 in 1991.[320] Since then 7 loci have been mapped and 6 genes identified (see Table 81–12). All encode proteins that are responsible for automaticity of the electrical activity in the cardiac cells. Mutations cause a disruption in the formation of the channels, altering the cardiac action potential and creating a voltage gradient especially at the ventricular level, which is responsible for reentrant arrhythmias.

LQT Syndrome 1   The causal gene for LQT1 is the *KVLQT1* (or *KCNQ1*), which encodes a voltage-gated potassium channel α subunit and is strongly expressed in the heart.[321] It consists of 16 exons spanning 400 kb, which form 6 transmembrane segments. It coassembles with the β subunit min K (KCNE1) to form the slow-activating potassium current I_{Ks}. Mutations in this gene disrupt the normal function of the protein causing a decrease in the potassium current. Several mutations have been described in *KCNQ1* to date.

LQT Syndrome 2   LQT2 gene is HERG ("human ether-a-go-go related" gene), which was isolated in 1994 from hippocampus and named human ether-a-go-go related gene because of its homology to *Drosophila* "ether-a-go-go" gene. The gene is localized on chromosome 7q35-q36. It contains 16 exons spanning an approximately 55 Kb of genomic sequence. It encodes a protein that forms six transmembrane segments.[322] The protein is responsible for the rapidly activating delayed rectifier potassium current I_{Kr} after coassembly with MIRP1 (KCNE2). As in the case of LQT1, mutations in *HERG* cause an abnormal protein with a resulting loss of potassium current.

LQT Syndrome 3   The causal gene is *SCN5A*, located on chromosome 3 and encodes for the cardiac sodium channel.[307] Mutations in *SCN5A* also cause Brugada syndrome and progressive conduction system disease, as discussed earlier. Electrophysiologic studies following expression of the mutant proteins in xenopus oocytes indicate a gain of function mutations evidenced by delayed inactivation and persistent leaking of sodium ions after phase 0 of the action potential.

LQT Syndrome 4   A locus for a French family with 65 affected members with LQT and sinus node dysfunction was mapped to 4q25-q27 in 1995.[323] Very recently, the causal gene was identified as *ANKB* (also known as *ANK2*), which encodes ankyrin-B.[324] Mutations in ankyrin B disrupt cellular localization of the sodium pump, the sodium/calcium exchanger and inositol-1,4,5-triphosphate receptors, reduce their expression levels and affect Ca^{2+} signaling in adult cardiac myocytes. This finding suggest that not only mutations in ion channels causes cardiac arrhythmias but also mutations in proteins associated with ion channels, such as ankyrin B could induces a similar phenotype.

LQT Syndrome 5   *MinK* (minimal potassium ion channel), located on chromosome 21q22.1-q22.2, is the causal gene. It contains 3 exons. MinK coassembles with KVLQT1 to form the cardiac I_{Ks} channel.[321] Mutations in this gene have been identified as causing both the autosomal dominant and autosomal recessive disease.

LQT Syndrome 6   LQT6 is caused by mutations in *KCNE2* or MirP1 (minK-related peptide). It is mapped to 21q22.1, next to minK, arrayed in opposite direction. KCNE2 assembles with HERG to form the I_{Kr} current.[325] Mutations in *KCNE2* decrease potassium current availability, with slower activation.

LQT Syndrome 7   Andersen syndrome is a rare autosomal dominant inherited disorder characterized by constellation of periodic paralysis, cardiac arrhythmias, long QT, and dysmorphic features such as short stature, scoliosis, clinodactylism, hypertelorism, low-set or slanted ears, micrognathia, and broad forehead.[326] The causal gene is *KCNJ2*, located on chromosome 17q23. It encodes the inward rectifier potassium channel Kir2.1, expressed in skeletal and cardiac muscles. Kir2.1 is a strong inward rectified channel that prevents passage of any current at potential greater than 40 mV. Electrophysiologic studies indicate the mutant protein exerts a dominant negative effect on Kir2.1 function with an ultimate decrease in potassium current.

LQT Syndrome 8   LQT8, also known as Timothy syndrome, is characterized by the presence of facial dysmorphic features, syndactyly, small teeth, mental retardation and severe QT prolongation. Mutations in *CACNA1C*, encoding for the α subunit of L-type calcium channel have been identified as responsible for the syndrome. The mutations cause a gain of function defect, increasing the inward current and prolonging the action potential.[327]

Autosomal Recessive LQT Syndrome (Jervell and Lange-Nielsen Syndrome)

The autosomal recessive forms of the LQT syndrome have been linked to mutations in the genes encoding I_{Ks} current, namely KVLQT1 and minK.[328] For the LQT phenotype, which is also associated with sensorineuronal deafness, to express, the patients must inherit a mutation from both parents. Consequently, it is less common than the Romano-Ward syndrome but is associated with a more malignant course and a longer QT interval. The phenotype could also arise in recessive forms when different mutations in the same gene are inherited from the parents (compound heterozygote).

Genotype–Phenotype Correlation in LQT Syndrome

Given the availability of a large number of families with the LQT syndrome, several genotype–phenotype correlation studies have been performed to identify the genetic determinants of triggering events, electrocardiographic phenotype and response to therapy. The studies predominantly, encompass the three most common forms of LQT syndrome—LQT1, LQT2, and LQT3—and have significant limitations inherent to genotype–phenotype correlation studies described earlier. Despite their limitations, characteristic features have emerged that could guide the analysis of the patients toward a specific genetic defect (Table 81–14).[329] In general, individuals with LQT1 exhibit symptoms during physical activity, such as swimming and have a T wave of long duration on ECG. Individuals with LQT2 usually develop symptoms related to auditory stimuli and the T wave is small or notched. In contrast, subjects with LQT3 are symptomatic during sleep and the ECG shows a very late T wave with a prolonged ST segment.

Mutations also carry prognostic significance and in all three groups (LQT1, 2, and 3) there is a correlation between cardiac events and the QT interval. In general, patients with LQT1 and LQT2 have a higher risk of cardiac events than patients with LQT3. The latter despite having less events, has a relatively higher

TABLE 81-14

Genotype–Phenotype Correlation in Long-QT Syndromes

PHENOTYPE	GENE	T WAVE	TRIGGER
LQT1	KCNQ1	Early onset, broad-base T	Emotion, swimming
LQT2	HERG	Low amplitude	Auditory
LQT3	SCN5A	Late T, normal amplitude	Sleep

mortality, which indicates higher lethality of the events.[330] In addition, response to drug therapy seems to correlate with the genotype (class IIa). While β blockers are considered the first line of therapy in patients with LQT1, they have not been shown to be beneficial in patients with LQT3, who have a slower heart rate (class IIa). Preliminary data suggest LQT3 patients might benefit from Na^{1+} channel blockers, such as mexiletine, but long-term data is not yet available (class IIb).[331]

Induced or Acquired Long QT Syndrome

Induced or acquired long QT is iatrogenic, caused by a long list of medications (see Table 81–13) and electrolyte abnormalities. A large number of factors determine the risk of developing long QT syndrome in an individual in response to drug therapy. They include bioavailability of the drug, the interaction with other medications that affect the same repolarizing current and the presence of SNPs. SNPs play a major role in determining pharmacodynamics and pharmacokinetics of drugs and, thus, the risk of LQT syndrome. The final effect on the repolarization will depend on the so-called *repolarizing reserve*, or the degree of alteration that the ionic currents can sustain before repolarization is compromised. Any combination of genetic and environmental factors (drug, electrolyte abnormalities) that decrease this "repolarization reserve" below a safe threshold will place the individual at risk of arrhythmia.[332]

Epidemiologic studies have led to identification of mutations and SNPs in genes known to cause LQT syndrome. These SNPs are typically silent until unmasked by the use of I_{Kr} blockers. Thus, one may consider these subjects as those with unexpressed congenital LQT syndrome.[333] Recent identification of a common SNP that predisposes to induced arrhythmias in the African American population serves as an example.[333] A recent study has provided the first link of the usefulness of genomewide association studies in the identification of genes modulating cardiac repolarization. Genetic variants in the *NOS1AP*, encoding nitric oxide synthase 1, have been associated with a variation of 1.5 percent of the QT interval in the population.[334]

SHORT QT SYNDROME

The short QT syndrome is a newly described disease characterized by the presence of shortening of the QT interval on ECG and clinically by episodes of syncope, paroxysmal atrial fibrillation and/or life-threatening cardiac arrhythmias. Short QT syndrome usually affects young and healthy individuals with no structural heart disease. It may be present in sporadic cases, as well as in families. It was originally described in 2000.[335] In 2003, a link was provided between the short QT syndrome and familial sudden

death with the first clinical report of two families with short QT syndrome and a high incidence of SCD.[336]

Clinical Manifestations

Most patients with short QT syndrome have a history of familial sudden death and/or atrial fibrillation, short refractory periods and inducible ventricular fibrillation at electrophysiologic study.[335,336] The age at onset of clinical manifestations could be extremely young. Malignant forms of short QT syndrome responsible for neonatal SCD have been attributed to SIDS.[336]

The characteristic sign for the disease is the presence of a very short QT interval on ECG. The T wave remains upright and the interval between the peak and end of the T wave is not prolonged. The appearance of a well-separated U wave has also been reported in several cases. It is difficult to define the normal QT interval as the correcting equations have several limitations. Nevertheless, at a heart rate of 60 beats/min, the uncorrected QT interval is usually higher than 360 milliseconds.[337] From the data shown in the familial forms of the short QT syndrome, it is probably reasonable to postulate that the presence of a QT of <330 should raise high suspicion about the disease. The severity of the clinical manifestations of short QTs is highly variable, ranging from asymptomatic to atrial fibrillation, recurrent syncope to sudden death.

Molecular Genetics and Electrophysiology

Genetics and biophysical analysis have provided important information regarding the pathophysiologic mechanisms that cause the short QT syndrome. Short QT syndrome, as are the majority of primary familial electrical diseases, is caused by mutations in genes encoding cardiac ion channels. Three genes have so far been discovered thereby proving that the disease is genetically heterogeneous.[338–340]

Short QT Syndrome 1 *KCNH2* expresses a protein that makes up the channel responsible for the rapidly activating outward K+ current involved in phase 3 repolarization. The protein is often referred to as HERG. The first genetic basis for the disease was obtained with the identification of two different missense mutations in the same residue in KCNH2 in three unrelated families.[338,341] Both mutations resulted in the substitution of asparagine for lysine at codon 588 (N588K), an area at the outer mouth of the channel pore.

Analysis of the current generated after transferring the mutated channels into human mammalian cells showed that the mutation abolished the inactivation of the channels thus, resulting in an increased developing current. The biophysical analysis therefore showed that the mutation induced a "gain of function" in I_{Kr} current thus causing a shortening of the action potential.[338]

The presence of paroxysmal atrial fibrillation in some affected individuals and especially in one of the families as the only clinical manifestation suggested that the increased heterogeneity would also be present at the atrial level and could be responsible for the arrhythmia.

Short QT Syndrome 2 The *KCNQ1* gene encodes a subunit of the proteins responsible for the slowly activating delayed outward

K+ current. A missense mutation in this gene causing short QT syndrome was first identified by Bellocq et al. in a 70-year-old individual who suffered ventricular fibrillation and had a QT interval of 290 milliseconds after resuscitation.[339] He was not inducible at electrophysiologic study and had no cardiac structural abnormalities. A second mutation in KCNQ1 was identified in a baby girl born at 38 weeks after induction of delivery that was prompted by bradycardia and irregular rhythm.[342] The ECG revealed atrial fibrillation with slow ventricular response and short QT interval.

Biophysical analysis showed that both mutations were leading to a gain of function in the outward current that explains the short QT syndrome phenotype.

Short QT Syndrome 3

The third form of short QT syndrome has been linked to mutations in the *KCNJ2* gene, which codes for the channel protein responsible for the inward rectifier current.[340] The proband and her father with the mutation both displayed short QT intervals of 315 and 320 milliseconds, respectively. ECG recordings showed asymmetrical T waves with an abnormally rapid terminal phase. When expressed in Chinese Hamster Ovary cells, the mutated channels generated electrical currents that did not rectify (decreased) as much as the normal channels in their functional positive range of potentials (80 mV to 30 mV). Such a range of voltages corresponds to the very end of phase 3 repolarization and to phase 4. Simulation of the effects of the mutated channels on the morphology of the ventricular action potential showed a selective speeding of late repolarization, thus shortening significantly the action potential duration at 90 percent repolarization.

Phenotype–Genotype Correlation

Robust genotype–phenotype correlation data are not yet available for short QT syndrome. The disease is clinically highly heterogeneous, as indicated by the fact that in the three families with the same mutation.[338,341] There is a tremendous variation in symptoms and presentation.

Treatment Strategy

Preliminary data show that there may be effective pharmacologic therapy for this disease (class IIb).[343,344] However, the high incidence of SCD warrants the implantation of an intracardiac cardioverter-defibrillator, especially in individuals with aborted sudden death.

Because QT shortening is likely caused by an increase in the outward current, it was suggested that blocking the current with class III antiarrhythmic drugs (known to increase the QT interval) could be a potential therapeutic approach for the treatment of short QT syndrome (class IIb). More recently, in a clinical study, Gaita et al. showed that treatment with quinidine prolonged the QT interval, decreased inducibility, and, therefore, had the potential to be an effective therapy for these patients (class IIb).[343] Clinical followup in one family with paroxysmal atrial fibrillation indicates that the episodes respond well to treatment with class Ic agent propafenone (class IIb).[341]

[ ] PROGRESSIVE FAMILIAL HEART BLOCK

Familial heart block is autosomal dominant progressive disease of cardiac conduction system characterized by initial development of bundle branch block and gradual progression to complete heart block. Two forms have been recognized. In type I, the onset is early and the disease is rapidly progressive. In type II, the onset is later in life and commonly the QRS complex is narrow and AV nodal block predominates. Clinical features of the disease include syncope, SCD, and Stokes-Adams attacks. A locus was identified in a large family of Portuguese descent on chromosome 19q13.[345] The gene has not been identified yet. As discussed earlier, mutations in *SCN5A* have been shown in some families with familial heart block.[317] In addition, AV block in conjunction with congenital heart disease, such as ASD (NKX2.5 mutations), and DCM (lamin A/C mutations) have been described; these were discussed earlier.

[ ] CATECHOLAMINERGIC POLYMORPHIC VENTRICULAR TACHYCARDIA

Ryanodine receptors are responsible for release the calcium from the sarcoplasmic reticulum and are activated by the incoming calcium, therefore they are Ca^{2+}-activated Ca^{2+} channel. Mutations in ryanodine receptors (*RYR2*) have been shown to cause a phenotype electrically resembling ARVC (phenocopy),[346] as discussed earlier, and familial polymorphic ventricular tachycardia.[346]

Familial polymorphic ventricular tachycardia is an autosomal-dominant inherited disease with a mortality rate of approximately 30 percent by the age of 30 years. Phenotypically, it is characterized by runs of bidirectional and polymorphic ventricular tachycardia in response to vigorous exercise in the absence of evidence of structural myocardial disease.

A recessive form of familial polymorphic ventricular tachycardia also has been described and mapped to 1p13.3-p11.[347] Mutation screening identified a missense mutation in calsequestrin 2 (*CASQ2*) as responsible for the disease. CASQ2 is involved in the same pathway as RYR2 to control calcium release from the sarcoplasmic reticulum.

[ ] SICK SINUS SYNDROME

Sick sinus syndrome is characterized by the occurrence of sinus bradycardia, sinus arrest, and chronotropic incompetence. Sinus node dysfunction has been linked to loss of function mutations in *HCN4*,[348,349] and in recessive form to *SCN5A*.[350] HCN4 contributes to native f-channels in the sinoatrial node, the natural cardiac pacemaker region. In 2006, a loss of function defect in HCN4 was also linked to familial sinus bradycardia.[351]

[ ] FAMILIAL ATRIAL FIBRILLATION

Atrial fibrillation in the absence of known causes of secondary atrial fibrillation may be a familial disorder. The mode of inheritance is autosomal dominant. The first gene was localized to chromosome 10q22–24,[352] and, subsequently, genetic heterogeneity was established. The first causal gene for familial atrial fibrillation was identified as the *KCNQ1*, which is also responsible for LQT1 syndrome. The mutation for atrial fibrillation is a gain of function mutation, in contrast to the loss of function mutations observed in patients with LQT1.[353] A link between *KCNE2*,[354] *KCNE3*,[355] *KCNJ2*,[356] and *KCNA5*[357] with atrial fibrillation has confirmed the role of mutations in channels responsible for potassium currents in the development of atrial fibrillation. New loci have been identified—6q14–16[358] and 5p13[359]—but the genes have remained elusive. Recently, somatic mutations in *GJA5* in atrial tissues of a subset of patients with idiopathic atrial fibrillation were identified.[360] The gene encodes gap junction protein connexin 40, which is involved in electrical conduction in the myocardium.

【 】 MONOMORPHIC VENTRICULAR TACHYCARDIA

A somatic point mutation (F200L) in the inhibitory subunit 2 of G protein α was identified in a patient with sustained monomorphic ventricular tachycardia that was unresponsive to vagal maneuvers and adenosine.[361] The mutation was present in cardiac tissue at the arrhythmogenic locus and was shown to increase intracellular cAMP concentration and inhibit suppression of cAMP by adenosine.

【 】 FAMILIAL WOLFF-PARKINSON-WHITE SYNDROME

Familial WPW syndrome is a rare syndrome with autosomal dominant mode of inheritance. It occurs in isolation or in conjunction with other disorders, such as HCM and Pompe disease. It is characterized by evidence of preexcitation on electrocardiogram, palpitation, and syncope as a result of supraventricular arrhythmias. The phenotype of WPW in conjunction with HCM and conduction defect was found in patients with mutations in *PRKAG2*, as discussed earlier.[86,362,363] It has also been reported in patients with Pompe disease caused by mutations in α-1,4-glucosidase,[181] in patients with HCM caused by mutations in *TNNI3* and *MYBPC3*, and in Leber hereditary optic neuropathy, which is caused by mutations in mitochondrial DNA.[364]

GENETIC BASIS OF CARDIAC DISEASE IN CONNECTIVE TISSUE DISORDERS

【 】 MARFAN SYNDROME

Marfan syndrome is a primary disorder of connective tissue characterized by cardiovascular, ocular, and skeletal abnormalities.[365] There is significant variability in the clinical manifestations of Marfan syndrome, but the predominant features are progressive dilatation of the aortic root, aortic aneurysm, dissection, and aortic and mitral valve regurgitation. The estimated incidence of Marfan syndrome is 1 per 5000 population.[366] The age of onset of clinical manifestations of Marfan syndrome is variable, but cardiac phenotypes commonly occur in the third or fourth decades of life. Aortic dissection is the leading cause of premature death in patients with Marfan syndrome. In addition to cardiovascular abnormalities, marfanoid habitus (increased height, disproportionately long limbs and digits), lens dislocation or subluxation, arachnodactyly, thoracic abnormalities, and increased joint laxity are common clinical features (see also Chap. 88).

Genetic Basis of Marfan Syndrome

Marfan syndrome is an autosomal dominant disease that exhibits locus and allelic heterozygosity. The first causal gene to be identified is the *FBN1,* which is located on 15q15.23 and encodes fibrillin.[366,367] Fibrillin is a cysteine-rich protein with a molecular mass of 350 kDa; it is the major component of extracellular microfibrils in both elastic and nonelastic connective tissues. More than 600 nonrecurring unique mutations in *FBN1* have been described that encompass missense, nonsense, and deletion mutations, as well as abnormal splicing or exon skipping.[368] Mutations are spread throughout most of the gene, and the frequency of each particular mutation is relatively low, which makes screening for mutations tedious.

There is a significant variability in the phenotypic expression of Marfan syndrome. The phenotypic variability may be partly caused by locus and allelic heterogeneity and partly by the effect of modifier genes and perhaps environmental factors. The clinical spectrum varies from ectopia lentis in the absence of any other phenotype to neonatal Marfan syndrome and premature death, often within the first 2 years of life. Mutations inducing premature termination of the protein result in approximately a 50 percent reduction in the level of fibrillin and more frequent ocular manifestations.

A phenocopy or a variant of Marfan syndrome is congenital "contractural arachnodactyly." It is characterized by severe kyphoscoliosis, generalized osteopenia, flexion contractures of the fingers, abnormally shaped ears, and, less frequently, mitral regurgitation and congenital heart disease. Recently, point mutations in the *FBN2* gene have been described as causes of contractural arachnodactyly.[369] *FBN2* mutations clustered in limited regions alter amino acids in the calcium-binding consensus sequence in the EGF-like domains. Mutations affect either the conserved cysteine residues or residues of the calcium-binding consensus sequence of the cbEGF motifs, and often result in premature termination of the protein. In addition, mutations in TGFβ receptor 1 (*TGFBR1*) and TGFβ receptor 2 (*TGFBR2*) have been identified in individuals with Marfan-like syndrome.[370]

The pathogenesis of Marfan syndrome entails decreased expression levels of the fibrillin protein and reduced deposition of fibrillin in vascular adventitia, which results in weakening of the adventitia and aneurysm formation. Recently, increased TGFβ signaling was detected in mouse model of aortic aneurysm.[371] Treatment with a angiotensin II receptor blocker, known to inhibit TGFβ, prevented aortic aneurysm formation in this mouse model.[371]

【 】 EHLERS-DANLOS SYNDROME

Ehlers-Danlos syndrome (EDS), a relatively uncommon disorder, encompasses a group of conditions characterized by increased elasticity of the skin and connective tissue diseases (see also Chap. 84).[365,372] The classic form of EDS is characterized by joint hypermotility and fragile, bruisable skin that heals with peculiar "cigarette-paper" scars. Other clinical features include translucent elasticity of the skin, mitral valve prolapse, spontaneous rupture and aneurysm of large arteries, kyphoscoliosis, atrophic scars, and hematomas in the joint areas, especially in the knees and elbows. In the severe form, spontaneous rupture of the intestines and arteries is common. In the benign form, the only manifestations may be hyperextensibility of joints and easy bruisability. The age of onset of clinical manifestations is variable and ranges from childhood to late adulthood.

Genetic Basis of Ehlers-Danlos Syndrome

EDS has several different forms that are inherited in three different patterns of transmission—autosomal dominant, autosomal recessive, and X-linked recessive.[365,372] Cardiovascular abnormalities are more common in forms I and IV and include congenital malformations, such as tetralogy of Fallot, atrial septal defects, and valvular abnormalities such as mitral and tricuspid valve prolapse.[365]

Mutations in genes encoding collagen components are responsible for EDS.[372] For example, Ehlers-Danlos type IV, which is considered the most malignant form because of proneness to spontaneous rupture of the bowel and large arteries and a high incidence of pregnancy-related complications, is caused by mutations in *COL3A1*.[373] The gene is located on 2q31 and encodes type III procollagen. Cardiac manifestations include aortic and coronary artery aneurysms with a high incidence of rupture. Some case of EDS type I are caused by mutations in *COL5A2*, coding for collagen α-2(V), and *COL1A1*, encoding collagen α-1(I).[365] EDS is considered a primary disorder of collagen deficiency. Point and deletion mutations lead to either deficiency of collagen-processing enzymes, haploinsufficiency or expression of dominant-negative collagen α chains. Consequently, there is decreased collagen synthesis and loss of connective tissue resiliency.

[ ] ELLIS–VAN CREVELD SYNDROME

This syndrome is discussed above, in the text concerning congenital heart diseases.

[ ] CUTIS LAXA

Cutis laxa comprises a heterogeneous group of acquired and genetic disorders characterized by redundant, wrinkled, loose, sagging skin that slowly returns to normal after stretching. Cardiac manifestations include pulmonic stenosis, aortic aneurysms, and right-sided heart failure. Vessels are very tortuous, resembling corkscrews on the angiogram.

Autosomal dominant, autosomal recessive, and X-linked forms have been described, and mutations in the elastin gene (*ELN*) have been identified in the autosomal dominant form.[374] A homozygous missense mutation in the fibulin-5 (*FBLN5*) gene has been identified as responsible for the recessive form.[375]

[ ] PSEUDOXANTHOMA ELASTICUM

Pseudoxanthoma elasticum is a genetic disorder characterized by dermatologic, ocular, and cardiovascular abnormalities resulting from degeneration of the elastic fibers. Manifestations include pseudoxanthoma, especially in areas of the neck and axillae, angioid streaks in the optic fundus, and gastrointestinal hemorrhagic and occlusive disease. Cardiovascular abnormalities include calcification of the peripheral arteries, with resulting intermittent claudication, coronary artery disease, mitral valve prolapse, and hypertension.

Recently, mutations in the ATP-binding cassette (ABC) transporter gene (*ABCC6*) on chromosome 16p13 were identified as the cause of pseudoxanthoma elasticum.[376] The exact biologic function of ABCC6 protein and the mechanism(s) by which mutations in ABCC6 cause pseudoxanthoma elasticum are unknown.

[ ] OSTEOGENESIS IMPERFECTA

Osteogenesis imperfecta comprises a heterogeneous class of connective tissue disorders characterized by bone fragility. Bone fragility results from defective collagen synthesis, which leads to decreased bone mass, disturbed organization of bone tissue, and altered bone geometry (size and shape). Cardiovascular abnormalities include valvular lesions, such as mitral and aortic regurgitation, and an increased fragility of the blood vessels.

Mutations in one of the two genes encoding type I collagen, namely *COL1A1* and *COL1A2*, have been identified as the cause.[377,378]

GENETIC DISORDERS OF THE PULMONARY CIRCULATION

[ ] FAMILIAL PRIMARY PULMONARY HYPERTENSION

Primary pulmonary hypertension (PPH) is diagnosed when mean resting pulmonary artery blood pressure is greater than 25 mmHg in the absence of known secondary causes such as lung disease or pulmonary venous congestion secondary to heart failure (see also Chap. 62). Dyspnea is the most common symptom. It is the first symptom in 60 percent of the cases.[379] Other clinical manifestations include exercise intolerance, fatigue, cyanosis, syncope, and SCD.[380] Clinical manifestations often start in the third and fourth decades of life and are about twice as common in females.[379] Median survival is about 3 years.[381] Prevalence is 1 to 2 per 1,000,000 individuals.[380]

PPH is a familial disease with an autosomal dominant mode of inheritance in 5 to 10 percent of the cases.[379,382] PPH is a genetically heterogenous disease. Mutations in bone morphogenic protein receptor type II (*BMPR2*), mapped to chromosome 2q31–33, is responsible for approximately 50 percent of the familial PPH and 10 to 15 percent of the sporadic cases.[380,382–385] The spectrum of mutations includes nonsense and frameshift mutations, expected to produce dysfunctional protein. Bone morphogenic protein (BMP) receptor is a cell-surface receptor that belongs to the transforming growth factor β (TGFβ) family.[385] Binding of ligands to BMPR2 activates signaling through Smad molecules. Mutations in another member of the TGFβ receptor family, namely, activin-receptor–like kinase 1 (*ALK1*), are responsible for a small fraction of familial PPH.[386] Finally, an association between serotonin transporter (5-HTT) SNPs and pulmonary hypertension has been documented.[387]

The pathogenesis of pulmonary hypertension caused by mutations in *BMPR2* includes haploinsufficiency, wherein defective TGFβ signaling via Smad molecules results in proliferation of smooth muscle cells and reduced apoptosis.[385,388,389] Molecular pathogenesis of PPH as a consequence of mutations in *ALK1* and serotonin transporter also entails smooth muscle cell proliferation.

MONOGENIC LIPID DISORDERS

The majority of common dyslipidemias are complex traits caused by interaction of multiple genes and environmental factors. SNPs in a variety of genes encoding protein components of cholesterol and fatty acid biosynthesis have been implicated in susceptibility to dyslipidemia; these are discussed elsewhere (see Chap. 43). Monogenic forms of dyslipidemias are described briefly below.

【 】 FAMILIAL HYPERCHOLESTEROLEMIA

Familial hypercholesterolemia (FH) is an autosomal dominant disorder with a prevalence of 1 in 500 in the mild form and in 1 in 100,000 people in its severe form. It is characterized by severely elevated plasma levels of low-density lipoprotein cholesterol (LDL-C) (type IIa hyperlipidemia) and premature atherosclerosis.[390] Plasma levels of total cholesterol are in the range of 300 to 400 mg/dL in affected heterozygous individuals, and greater than 500 mg/dL in homozygous subjects. The affected individuals develop severe atherosclerosis involving multiple vascular territories, tendon xanthomata, and corneal arcus. Subjects homozygous for the causal mutations exhibit clinical atherosclerosis in the first or second decades of life and heterozygous subjects in the fourth or fifth decades. These patients often suffer from ischemic symptoms and/ or cardiac events requiring revascularization procedures very early in life (see also Chap. 43).

The causal gene is *LDLR*, which is located on chromosome 19p13.[391] It encodes LDL-C receptors. More than 1000 point, deletion, and splice mutations have been identified in patients with FH. Approximately 60 percent of the mutations are missense mutations, 20 percent are minor rearrangements, 13 percent are major rearrangements, and 7 percent are splice-junction mutations.[392] Mutations cause FH by perturbing the function of LDL-C receptors. Mutations could affect synthesis and targeting to the cell membrane, binding of the receptor to LDL-C, internalization of the receptor following binding to LDL-C, and recycling of the receptors. The ensuing biologic effect is impaired removal of apolipoprotein B (apoB) and apoE from the circulation.[391] Mutations affect LDL-C receptor function to variable degrees, leading to variable clinical manifestations.[393] In general, there is an inverse correlation between plasma levels of LDL-C and the level of residual LDLR activity. Mutations that completely inactivate the receptors lead to severe premature atherosclerosis in childhood. Frameshift mutations by markedly altering the structure of the LDL-C receptors cause severe phenotype. In contrast, mutations that partially inactivate the receptors cause mild to moderate hypercholesterolemia. Thus the development and severity of coronary atherosclerosis vary according to causal mutations, that is, residual LDL-C receptor activity. Genetic background, diet, environmental factors, and epigenetic factors are also likely to contribute to the phenotype.

【 】 FAMILIAL DEFECTIVE APOLIPOPROTEIN B100

Familial defective apolipoprotein B100 (FDB) is an autosomal dominant disease, expressed as increased plasma levels of LDL-C and very low-density lipoprotein C (VLDL-C).[394,395] Phenotypically it is similar to heterozygous FH and includes premature coronary artery disease and tendon xanthoma, in addition to elevated plasma levels of LDL-C. However, the LDL receptor activity is normal in these individuals. FDB is a relatively common disorder, with an estimated frequency of 1 in 1000 people, but the preva-

lence varies worldwide. The frequency of the mutation varies in different regions of the world.

The causal gene is *APOB*, located on chromosome 2q24.[396] The causal mutation involves amino acid 3500 in >99 percent of the cases, with the predominant mutation being R3500Q and, rarely, R3500W.[394–396] Mutations decrease the affinity of LDL receptors for apolipoprotein B, which result in accumulation of VLDL-C and LDL-C in the plasma and blood vessels.

【 】 AUTOSOMAL DOMINANT HYPERCHOLESTEROLEMIA TYPE 3

The phenotype is characterized by severely elevated plasma LDL-C levels and is similar to that in FH and FDB. The causal gene is *PCSK9*, which encodes proprotein convertase subtilisin/kexin type 9, also known as neural apoptosis-regulated convertase (NARC1).[397] Pathogenesis of autosomal dominant hypercholesterolemia type 3 involves enhanced degradation of the LDL receptors by PCSK9.[398] It is also noteworthy that SNPs in *PCSK9* are also associated with plasma LDL-C levels and risk of coronary artery disease in the general population.[399,400]

【 】 AUTOSOMAL RECESSIVE HYPERCHOLESTEROLEMIA

Autosomal recessive hypercholesterolemia is a rare disease with a phenotype similar to FH. The causal gene is *ARH*, which encodes a novel adaptor protein.[401] The pathogenesis of the phenotype involves impaired clearance of plasma LDL-C, despite normal activity of LDL receptors.

【 】 HYPOBETALIPOPROTEINEMIA

Hypobetalipoproteinemia, or abetalipoproteinemia, is a rare disease characterized by extremely low plasma levels of apolipoprotein B, total cholesterol, and LDL-C.[402,403] high-density lipoprotein cholesterol (HDL-C) levels are high and atherosclerosis is very uncommon. The phenotype often presents in childhood with failure to thrive, fat malabsorption, celiac disease, vitamin A and E deficiency, ataxia, demyelination of the central nervous system, and low plasma LDL-C levels.[403] Sporadic and familial cases with an autosomal dominant mode of inheritance have been reported. A causal gene is *MTTP* on chromosome 4q22–24, which encodes the microsomal triglyceride transfer protein.[404,405] MTTP is a heterodimer of a unique large subunit and the protein disulfide isomerase, which catalyzes the transport of triglyceride, cholesteryl ester, and phospholipid from phospholipid surfaces. Mutations encode truncated nonfunctional protein, thus leading to very low levels of apolipoprotein B, LDL-C, and total cholesterol.[405]

Familial hypobetalipoproteinemia also can arise because of truncation mutations in *APOB*.[406] It is also a rare disorder characterized by very low plasma levels of LDL-C and total cholesterol.[403]

Another form of hypobetalipoproteinemia is chylomicron retention disease, which is an autosomal dominant disease characterized by the selective absence of apoB-48.[403] Chylomicrons are absent in plasma of the affected individuals after a fat-containing meal. The phenotype is characterized by steatorrhea, growth retardation, malnutrition and acanthocytosis. The causal gene is *SARA2* located on chromosome 5q31.[407] The encoded protein is involved in intracellular trafficking of proteins in COP-coated vesicles.[407]

[ ] FISH-EYE DISEASE

Fish-eye disease is a rare autosomal dominant condition caused by deficiency of lecithin:cholesterol acyltransferase (LCAT).[408,409] The *LCAT* gene is located on chromosome 16q22.1 and codes for a protein involved in the synthesis from prealphalipoprotein A1 and conversion of HDL_3 to HDL_2 cholesterol. Deficiency of LCAT leads to premature coronary atherosclerosis, proteinuria, anemia, renal failure, and corneal opacification.

[ ] TANGIER DISEASE

Tangier disease is an autosomal codominant disease characterized by the virtual absence of HDL-C and very low plasma levels of apolipoprotein AI. Deposition of cholesteryl esters results in characteristic hypertrophic orange-colored tonsils, hepatosplenomegaly, and premature coronary artery disease.[410] Mutations in the ATP-binding cassette transporter (*ABCA1*) gene cause Tangier disease and familial hypoalphalipoproteinemia, its allelic variant.[411–414] *ABCA1* gene is located on chromosome 9q31 and codes for an mRNA of 6783 bp and a protein of 2261 amino acids.[411,413,414] ABCA1 is a transmembrane protein with 12 transmembrane domains. It acts as a flippase at the plasma membrane, stimulating cholesterol and phospholipid efflux to apolipoprotein AI and HDL-C.[410] Normally, ABCA1 transports free cholesterol to the extracellular space where it binds to apolipoprotein AI synthesized by the liver and forms nascent HDL particles from VLDL. In the absence of ABCA1, free cholesterol is not transported extracellularly and lipid-poor apolipoprotein AI rapidly degrades. Common polymorphisms in the *ABCA1* gene have been associated with coronary atherosclerosis in the general population.[415–417]

MONOGENIC FORMS OF HYPERTENSION

The predominant form of hypertension is essential hypertension, which accounts for 95 percent of all cases. Hypertension is a complex phenotype caused by the interactions of multiple genes and environmental factors. Several genes, in particular those coding for the components of the renin–angiotensin–aldosterone system, have been implicated in essential hypertension.[418–420] They are discussed in Chap. 61; only monogenic forms of hypertension are described briefly here.[421]

[ ] GLUCOCORTICOID-REMEDIABLE ALDOSTERONISM

Glucocorticoid-remediable aldosteronism is a rare autosomal dominant disorder and the first described familial form of hyperaldosteronism.[420] It is caused by a chimeric mutation that joins the promoter region of the 11β-hydroxylase (*CYP11B1*) gene to the coding region of the aldosterone synthase (*CYP11B2*) gene.[422] The new chimeric gene, located on chromosome 8q24, lacks the negative feedback regulation imparted by angiotensin II. The promoter of the fusion gene, which is made up of the 5′ fragment of *CYP11B1* gene, is responsive to adrenocorticotropic hormone. Thus expres-

sion of aldosterone remains unchecked, and excess aldosterone synthesis leads to the retention of sodium and salt and consequent hypertension. Glucocorticoid-remediable aldosteronism responds to treatment with glucocorticoids, which suppress the production of adrenocorticotropic hormone. Alternatively, treatment with mineralocorticoid receptor blockers also controls the hypertension.

[ ] APPARENT MINERALOCORTICOID EXCESS

Apparent mineralocorticoid excess is a rare autosomal recessive disease of peripheral metabolism of cortisol. Clinical manifestations of apparent mineralocorticoid excess, in addition to hypertension, include hypokalemia, low plasma renin activity, and responsiveness to spironolactone. There are two types of apparent mineralocorticoid excess, defined on the basis of severity of the biochemical phenotype. Both clinical variants are caused by mutations in the *HSD11B2* gene on chromosome 16q22, which encodes 11β-hydroxysteroid dehydrogenase II.[423,424] The enzyme is responsible for the peripheral conversion of biologically active cortisol to inactive cortisone. Point mutations in *HSD11B2* reduce or abolish the activity of 11β-hydroxysteroid dehydrogenase in the conversion of cortisol to cortisone. Thus, cortisol accumulates, leading to retention of salt and fluid through activation of mineralocorticoid receptors and hypertension.[424] Accordingly, patients with apparent mineralocorticoid excess respond to blockade of mineralocorticoid receptors.

[ ] LIDDLE SYNDROME

Liddle syndrome is a rare autosomal dominant disease characterized by hypertension, hypokalemic metabolic alkalosis, low plasma renin activity, and suppressed aldosterone secretion.[425] The phenotype usually develops early in life and hypertension is frequently severe. The first gene identified was the *SCNN1B*, located on locus 16p12, which encodes the β subunit of the amiloride-sensitive Na^{1+} channel.[425] The renal epithelial Na^{1+} channel has three subunits: α, β, and γ. Subsequently mutations in the γ subunit of epithelial sodium channels were also identified.[426] The mutations activate the channel (gain-of-function mutations) and lead to sodium retention and hypertension.

[ ] PSEUDOHYPOALDOSTERONISM TYPE II

Pseudohypoaldosteronism type II, also known as the Gordon hyperkalemia–hypertension syndrome, is a rare autosomal dominant disorder characterized by hypertension and hyperkalemia early in life, mild hyperchloremia, metabolic acidosis, and suppressed plasma renin activity. Two causal genes for pseudohypoaldosteronism type II—*WNK4* on chromosome 17q21 and *WNK1* on chromosome 12p—have been identified.[427] *WNK4* and *WNK1* encode serine-threonine kinases expressed in the distal nephron.[427] Missense and deletion mutations exert a gain-of-function effect, increasing the expression levels of the proteins in the kidney and leading to increased renal salt reabsorption and reduced renal K+ excretion.[427]

REFERENCES

1. Hoffman JIE, Kaplan S. The incidence of congenital heart disease. *J Am Coll Cardiol* 2002;39:1890–1900.

2. Hoffman JI. Incidence of congenital heart disease: II. Prenatal incidence. *Pediatr Cardiol* 1995;16:155–165.

3. Venter JC, Adams MD, Myers EW, et al. The sequence of the human genome. *Science* 2001;291:1304–1351.

4. Pinar H. Postmortem findings in term neonates. *Semin Neonatol* 2004;9:289–302.

5. Wang DG, Fan JB, Siao CJ, et al. Large-scale identification, mapping, and genotyping of single-nucleotide polymorphisms in the human genome. *Science* 1998;280:1077–1082.

6. Cargill M, Altshuler D, Ireland J, et al. Characterization of single-nucleotide polymorphisms in coding regions of human genes. *Nat Genet* 1999;22:231–238.

7. De Gobbi M, Viprakasit V, Hughes JR, et al. A regulatory SNP causes a human genetic disease by creating a new transcriptional promoter. *Science* 2006;312:1215–1217.

8. Murray JC, Buetow KH, Weber JL, et al. A comprehensive human linkage map with centimorgan density. Cooperative Human Linkage Center (CHLC). *Science* 1994;265:2049–2054.

9. Lander ES, Schork NJ. Genetic dissection of complex traits. *Science* 1994;265:2037–2048.

10. Gabriel SB, Schaffner SF, Nguyen H, et al. The structure of haplotype blocks in the human genome. *Science* 2002;296:2225–2229.

11. The International HapMap Consortium. A haplotype map of the human genome. *Nature* 2005;437:1299–1320.

12. Sybert VP, McCauley E. Turner's syndrome. *N Engl J Med* 2004;351:1227–1238.

13. Elsheikh M, Dunger DB, Conway GS, et al. Turner's syndrome in adulthood. *Endocr Rev* 2002;23:120–140.

14. Gravholt CH, Juul S, Naeraa RW, et al. Morbidity in Turner syndrome. *J Clin Epidemiol* 1998;51:147–158.

15. Schneider-Gadicke A, Beer-Romero P, Brown LG, et al. ZFX has a gene structure similar to ZFY, the putative human sex determinant, and escapes X inactivation. *Cell* 1989;57:1247–1258.

16. Korenberg JR, Chen XN, Schipper R, et al. Down syndrome phenotypes: the consequences of chromosomal imbalance. *Proc Natl Acad Sci U S A* 1994;91:4997–5001.

17. Hook EB, Cross PK, Schreinemachers DM. Chromosomal abnormality rates at amniocentesis and in live-born infants. *JAMA* 1983;249:2034–2038.

18. Hyett J, Moscoso G, Nicolaides K. Abnormalities of the heart and great arteries in first trimester chromosomally abnormal fetuses. *Am J Med Genet* 1997;69:207–216.

19. Stoll C, Alembik Y, Dott B, et al. Study of Down syndrome in 238,942 consecutive births. *Ann Genet* 1998;41:44–51.

20. Hill LM. The sonographic detection of trisomies 13, 18 and 21. *Clin Obstet Gynecol* 1996;39:831–850.

21. Fuentes JJ, Pritchard MA, Planas AM, et al. A new human gene from the Down syndrome critical region encodes a proline-rich protein highly expressed in fetal brain and heart. *Hum Mol Genet* 1995;4:1935–1944.

22. Nakamura A, Hattori M, Sakaki Y. A novel gene isolated from human placenta located in Down syndrome critical region on chromosome 21. *DNA Res* 1997;4:321–324.

23. Vidal-Taboada JM, Sanz S, Egeo A, et al. Identification and characterization of a new gene from human chromosome 21 between markers D21S343 and D21S268 encoding a leucine-rich protein. *Biochem Biophys Res Commun* 1998;250:547–554.

24. Nakamura A, Hattori M, Sakaki Y. Isolation of a novel human gene from the Down syndrome critical region of chromosome 21q22.2. *J Biochem (Tokyo)*. 1997;122:872–877.

25. Fuentes JJ, Pritchard MA, Planas AM, et al. A new human gene from the Down syndrome critical region encodes a proline-rich protein highly expressed in fetal brain and heart. *Hum Mol Genet* 1995;4:1935–1944.

26. Fuentes JJ, Genesca L, Kingsbury TJ, et al. DSCR1 overexpressed in Down syndrome, is an inhibitor of calcineurin-mediated signaling pathways. *Hum Mol Genet* 2000;9:1681–1690.

27. Molkentin JD. Calcineurin and beyond : cardiac hypertrophic signaling. *Circ Res* 2000;87:731–738.

28. Harris CD, Ermak G, Davies KJ. Multiple roles of the DSCR1 (Adapt78 or RCAN1) gene and its protein product calcipressin 1 (or RCAN1) in disease. *Cell Mol Life Sci* 2005;62:2477–2486.

29. Carter PE, Pearn JH, Bell J, et al. Survival in trisomy 18. Life tables for use in genetic counselling and clinical paediatrics. *Clin Genet* 1985;27:59–61.

30. De Decker HP, Lawrenson JB. The 22q11.2 deletion: from diversity to a single gene theory. *Genet Med* 2001;3:2–5.

31. Devriendt K, Fryns JP, Mortier G, et al. The annual incidence of DiGeorge/velocardiofacial syndrome. *J Med Genet* 1998;35:789–790.

32. Yagi H, Furutani Y, Hamada H, et al. Role of TBX1 in human del22q11.2 syndrome. *Lancet* 2003;362:1366–1373.

33. Yamagishi H, Garg V, Matsuoka R, et al. A molecular pathway revealing a genetic basis for human cardiac and craniofacial defects. *Science* 1999;283:1158–1161.

34. Lindsay EA, Botta A, Jurecic V, et al. Congenital heart disease in mice deficient for the DiGeorge syndrome region. *Nature* 1999;401:379–383.

35. Wadey R, McKie J, Papapetrou C, et al. Mutations of UFD1L are not responsible for the majority of cases of DiGeorge syndrome/velocardiofacial syndrome without deletions within chromosome 22q11. *Am J Hum Genet* 1999;65:247–249.

36. Aubry M, Demczuk S, Desmaze C, et al. Isolation of a zinc finger gene consistently deleted in DiGeorge syndrome. *Hum Mol Genet* 1993;2:1583–1587.

37. Curran ME, Atkinson DL, Ewart AK, et al. The elastin gene is disrupted by a translocation associated with supravalvular aortic stenosis. *Cell* 1993;73:159–168.

38. Morris CA, Mervis CB. Williams syndrome and related disorders. *Annu Rev Genomics Hum Genet* 2000;1:461–484.

39. Sawada K, Mizoguchi K, Hishida A, et al. Point mutation in the alpha-galactosidase A gene of atypical Fabry disease with only nephropathy. *Clin Nephrol* 1996;45:289–294.

40. Benson DW, Sharkey A, Fatkin D, et al. Reduced penetrance, variable expressivity, and genetic heterogeneity of familial atrial septal defects. *Circulation* 1998;97:2043–2048.

41. Pease WE, Nordenberg A, Ladda RL. Familial atrial septal defect with prolonged atrioventricular conduction. *Circulation* 1976;53:759–762.

42. Schott JJ, Benson DW, Basson CT, et al. Congenital heart disease caused by mutations in the transcription factor NKX2–5. *Science* 1998;281:108–111.

43. Tanaka M, Chen Z, Bartunkova S, et al. The cardiac homeobox gene Csx/Nkx2.5 lies genetically upstream of multiple genes essential for heart development. *Development* 1999;126:1269–1280.

44. Benson DW, Silberbach GM, Kavanaugh-McHugh A, et al. Mutations in the cardiac transcription factor NKX2.5 affect diverse cardiac developmental pathways. *J Clin Invest* 1999;104:1567–1573.

45. Kasahara H, Lee B, Schott JJ, et al. Loss of function and inhibitory effects of human CSX/NKX2.5 homeoprotein mutations associated with congenital heart disease. *J Clin Invest* 2000;106:299–308.

46. Landsberg RL, Sero JE, Danielian PS, et al. The role of E2F4 in adipogenesis is independent of its cell cycle regulatory activity. *Proc Natl Acad Sci U S A* 2003;100:2456–2461.

47. Garg V, Kathiriya IS, Barnes R, et al. GATA4 mutations cause human congenital heart defects and reveal an interaction with TBX5. *Nature* 2003;424:443–447.

48. Ching YH, Ghosh TK, Cross SJ, et al. Mutation in myosin heavy chain 6 causes atrial septal defect. *Nat Genet* 2005;37:423–428.

49. Huang T. Current advances in Holt-Oram syndrome. *Curr Opin Pediatr* 2002;14:691–695.

50. Bruneau BG, Logan M, Davis N, et al. Chamber-specific cardiac expression of Tbx5 and heart defects in Holt-Oram syndrome. *Dev Biol* 1999;211:100–108.

51. Basson CT, Bachinsky DR, Lin RC, et al. Mutations in human TBX5 cause limb and cardiac malformation in Holt-Oram syndrome. *Nat Genet* 1997;15:30–35.

52. Basson CT, Huang T, Lin RC, et al. Different TBX5 interactions in heart and limb defined by Holt-Oram syndrome mutations. *Proc Natl Acad Sci U S A* 1999;96:2919–2924.

53. Polymeropoulos MH, Ide SE, Wright M, et al. The gene for the Ellis-van Creveld syndrome is located on chromosome 4p16. *Genomics* 1996;35:1–5.

54. Ruiz-Perez VL, Ide SE, Strom TM, et al. Mutations in a new gene in Ellis-van Creveld syndrome and Weyers acrodental dysostosis. *Nat Genet* 2000;24:283–286.

55. Ruiz-Perez VL, Tompson SW, Blair HJ, et al. Mutations in two nonhomologous genes in a head-to-head configuration cause Ellis-van Creveld syndrome. *Am J Hum Genet* 2003;72:728–732.

56. Satoda M, Pierpont ME, Diaz GA, et al. Char syndrome, an inherited disorder with patent ductus arteriosus, maps to chromosome 6p12-p21. *Circulation* 1999;99:3036–3042.

57. Satoda M, Zhao F, Diaz GA, et al. Mutations in TFAP2B cause Char syndrome, a familial form of patent ductus arteriosus. *Nat Genet* 2000;25:42–46.

58. Mani A, Meraji SM, Houshyar R, et al. Finding genetic contributions to sporadic disease: A recessive locus at 12q24 commonly contributes to patent ductus arteriosus. *Proc Natl Acad Sci U S A* 2002;99:15054–15059.

59. Tartaglia M, Gelb BD. Noonan syndrome and related disorders: genetics and pathogenesis. *Annu Rev Genomics Hum Genet* 2005;6:45–68.:45–68.

60. Tartaglia M, Mehler EL, Goldberg R, et al. Mutations in PTPN11 encoding the protein tyrosine phosphatase SHP-2 cause Noonan syndrome. *Nat Genet* 2001;29:465–468.

61. Tartaglia M, Kalidas K, Shaw A, et al. PTPN11 mutations in Noonan syndrome: molecular spectrum, genotype-phenotype correlation, and phenotypic heterogeneity. *Am J Hum Genet* 2002;70:1555–1563.

62. Farah MG. Familial cardiac myxoma. A study of relatives of patients with myxoma. *Chest* 1994;105:65–68.

63. Rodriguez de la Concepcion ML, Yubero P, Iglesias R, et al. Lithium inhibits brown adipocyte differentiation. *FEBS Lett* 2005;579:1670–1674.

64. Casey M, Mah C, Merliss AD, et al. Identification of a novel genetic locus for familial cardiac myxomas and Carney complex. *Circulation* 1998;98:2560–2566.

65. Stratakis CA, Carney JA, Lin JP, et al. Carney complex, a familial multiple neoplasia and lentiginosis syndrome. Analysis of 11 kindreds and linkage to the short arm of chromosome 2. *J Clin Invest* 1996;97:699–705.

66. Casey M, Vaughan CJ, He J, et al. Mutations in the protein kinase A R1alpha regulatory subunit cause familial cardiac myxomas and Carney complex. *J Clin Invest* 2000;106:R31-R38.

67. Veugelers M, Bressan M, McDermott DA, et al. Mutation of perinatal myosin heavy chain associated with a Carney complex variant. *N Engl J Med* 2004;351:460–469.

68. Bartoloni L, Blouin JL, Pan Y, et al. Mutations in the DNAH11 (axonemal heavy chain dynein type 11) gene cause one form of situs inversus totalis and most likely primary ciliary dyskinesia. *Proc Natl Acad Sci U S A* 2002;99:10282–10286.

69. Pennarun G, Escudier E, Chapelin C, et al. Loss-of-function mutations in a human gene related to Chlamydomonas reinhardtii dynein IC78 result in primary ciliary dyskinesia. *Am J Hum Genet* 1999;65:1508–1519.

70. Olbrich H, Haffner K, Kispert A, et al. Mutations in DNAH5 cause primary ciliary dyskinesia and randomization of left-right asymmetry. *Nat Genet* 2002;30:143–144.

71. Gebbia M, Ferrero GB, Pilia G, et al. X-linked situs abnormalities result from mutations in ZIC3. *Nat Genet* 1997;17:305–308.

72. Kosaki K, Bassi MT, Kosaki R, et al. Characterization and mutation analysis of human LEFTY A and LEFTY B, homologues of murine genes implicated in left-right axis development. *Am J Hum Genet* 1999;64:712–721.

73. Kosaki R, Gebbia M, Kosaki K, et al. Left-right axis malformations associated with mutations in ACVR2B, the gene for human activin receptor type IIB. *Am J Med Genet* 1999;82:70–76.

74. McElhinney DB, Krantz ID, Bason L, et al. Analysis of cardiovascular phenotype and genotype-phenotype correlation in individuals with a JAG1 mutation and/or Alagille syndrome. *Circulation* 2002;106:2567–2574.

75. Li L, Krantz ID, Deng Y, et al. Alagille syndrome is caused by mutations in human Jagged1 which encodes a ligand for Notch1. *Nat Genet* 1997;16:243–251.

76. Oda T, Elkahloun AG, Pike BL, et al. Mutations in the human Jagged1 gene are responsible for Alagille syndrome. *Nat Genet* 1997;16:235–242.

77. McDaniell R, Warthen DM, Sanchez-Lara PA, et al. NOTCH2 mutations cause Alagille syndrome, a heterogeneous disorder of the notch signaling pathway. *Am J Hum Genet* 2006;79:169–173.

78. Maron BJ, Towbin JA, Thiene G, et al. Contemporary definitions and classification of the cardiomyopathies: an American Heart Association Scientific Statement from the Council on Clinical Cardiology, Heart Failure and Transplantation Committee; Quality of Care and Outcomes Research and Functional Genomics and Translational Biology Interdisciplinary Working Groups; and Council on Epidemiology and Prevention. *Circulation* 2006;113:1807–1816.

79. Maron BJ. Hypertrophic cardiomyopathy: a systematic review. *JAMA* 2002;287:1308–1320.

80. Maron BJ, Gardin JM, Flack JM, et al. Prevalence of hypertrophic cardiomyopathy in a general population of young adults. Echocardiographic analysis of 4111 subjects in the CARDIA study. Coronary Artery Risk Development in (Young) Adults. *Circulation* 1995;92:785–789.

81. Nagueh SF, McFalls J, Meyer D, et al. Tissue Doppler imaging predicts the development of hypertrophic cardiomyopathy in subjects with subclinical disease. *Circulation* 2003;108:395–398.

82. Biagini E, Coccolo F, Ferlito M, et al. Dilated-hypokinetic evolution of hypertrophic cardiomyopathy: prevalence, incidence, risk factors, and prog-

83. Olivotto I, Cecchi F, Casey SA, et al. Impact of atrial fibrillation on the clinical course of hypertrophic cardiomyopathy. *Circulation* 2001;104:2517–2524.

84. Monserrat L, Elliott PM, Gimeno JR, et al. Non-sustained ventricular tachycardia in hypertrophic cardiomyopathy: an independent marker of sudden death risk in young patients. *J Am Coll Cardiol* 2003;42:873–879.

85. Gollob MH, Green MS, Tang AS, et al. Identification of a gene responsible for familial Wolff-Parkinson-White syndrome. *N Engl J Med* 2001;344:1823–1831.

86. Gollob MH, Seger JJ, Gollob TN, et al. Novel PRKAG2 mutation responsible for the genetic syndrome of ventricular preexcitation and conduction system disease with childhood onset and absence of cardiac hypertrophy. *Circulation* 2001;104:3030–3033.

87. Blair E, Redwood C, Ashrafian H, et al. Mutations in the gamma(2) subunit of AMP-activated protein kinase cause familial hypertrophic cardiomyopathy: evidence for the central role of energy compromise in disease pathogenesis. *Hum Mol Genet* 2001;10:1215–1220.

88. Arad M, Benson DW, Perez-Atayde AR, et al. Constitutively active AMP kinase mutations cause glycogen storage disease mimicking hypertrophic cardiomyopathy. *J Clin Invest* 2002;109:357–362.

89. Kofflard MJ, ten Cate FJ, van der Lee C, et al. Hypertrophic cardiomyopathy in a large community-based population: Clinical outcome and identification of risk factors for sudden cardiac death and clinical deterioration. *J Am Coll Cardiol* 2002.

90. Nienaber CA, Hiller S, Spielmann RP, et al. Syncope in hypertrophic cardiomyopathy: multivariate analysis of prognostic determinants. *J Am Coll Cardiol* 1990;15:948–955.

91. Elliott PM, Poloniecki J, Dickie S, et al. Sudden death in hypertrophic cardiomyopathy: identification of high risk patients. *J Am Coll Cardiol* 2000;36:2212–2218.

92. Maron BJ, Shirani J, Poliac LC, et al. Sudden death in young competitive athletes. Clinical, demographic, and pathological profiles. *JAMA* 1996;276:199–204.

93. McKenna W, Deanfield J, Faruqui A, et al. Prognosis in hypertrophic cardiomyopathy: role of age and clinical, electrocardiographic and hemodynamic features. *Am J Cardiol* 1981;47:532–538.

94. Marian AJ. On predictors of sudden cardiac death in hypertrophic cardiomyopathy. *J Am Coll Cardiol* 2003;41:994–996.

95. Cannan CR, Reeder GS, Bailey KR, et al. Natural history of hypertrophic cardiomyopathy. A population-based study, 1976 through 1990. *Circulation* 1995;92:2488–2495.

96. Maron BJ, Olivotto I, Spirito P, et al. Epidemiology of hypertrophic cardiomyopathy-related death: revisited in a large non-referral-based patient population. *Circulation* 2000;102:858–864.

97. Nugent AW, Daubeney PEF, Chondros P, et al. Clinical features and outcomes of childhood hypertrophic cardiomyopathy: results from a national population-based study. *Circulation* 2005;112:1332–1338.

98. Sakamoto T, Tei C, Murayama M, et al. Giant T wave inversion as a manifestation of asymmetrical apical hypertrophy (AAH) of the left ventricle. Echocardiographic and ultrasono-cardiotomographic study. *Jpn Heart J* 1976;17:611–629.

99. Eriksson MJ, Sonnenberg B, Woo A, et al. Long-term outcome in patients with apical hypertrophic cardiomyopathy. *J Am Coll Cardiol* 2002;39:638–645.

100. Hughes SE. The pathology of hypertrophic cardiomyopathy. *Histopathology* 2004;44:412–427.

101. Maron BJ, Roberts WC. Quantitative analysis of cardiac muscle cell disorganization in the ventricular septum of patients with hypertrophic cardiomyopathy. *Circulation* 1979;59:689–706.

102. Maron BJ, Anan TJ, Roberts WC. Quantitative analysis of the distribution of cardiac muscle cell disorganization in the left ventricular wall of patients with hypertrophic cardiomyopathy. *Circulation* 1981;63:882–894.

103. Shirani J, Pick R, Roberts WC, et al. Morphology and significance of the left ventricular collagen network in young patients with hypertrophic cardiomyopathy and sudden cardiac death. *J Am Coll Cardiol* 2000;35:36–44.

104. Spirito P, Bellone P, Harris KM, et al. Magnitude of left ventricular hypertrophy and risk of sudden death in hypertrophic cardiomyopathy. *N Engl J Med* 2000;342:1778–1785.

105. Varnava AM, Elliott PM, Baboonian C, et al. Hypertrophic cardiomyopathy: histopathological features of sudden death in cardiac troponin T disease. *Circulation* 2001;104:1380–1384.

106. Varnava AM, Elliott PM, Mahon N, et al. Relation between myocyte disarray and outcome in hypertrophic cardiomyopathy. *Am J Cardiol* 2001;88:275–279.

107. Greaves SC, Roche AH, Neutze JM, et al. Inheritance of hypertrophic cardiomyopathy: a cross sectional and M-mode echocardiographic study of 50 families. *Br Heart J* 1987;58:259–266.

108. Maron BJ, Nichols PF, III, Pickle LW, et al. Patterns of inheritance in hypertrophic cardiomyopathy: assessment by M-mode and two-dimensional echocardiography. *Am J Cardiol* 1984;53:1087–1094.

109. Marian AJ. Clinical and molecular genetic aspects of hypertrophic cardiomyopathy. *Curr Cardiol Rev* 2005;1:53–63.

110. Watkins H, Anan R, Coviello DA, et al. A de novo mutation in alpha-tropomyosin that causes hypertrophic cardiomyopathy. *Circulation* 1995;91:2302–2305.

111. Watkins H, Thierfelder L, Hwang DS, et al. Sporadic hypertrophic cardiomyopathy due to de novo myosin mutations. *J Clin Invest* 1992;90:1666–1671.

112. Arad M, Maron BJ, Gorham JM, et al. Glycogen storage diseases presenting as hypertrophic cardiomyopathy. *N Engl J Med* 2005;352:362–372.

113. Jansen GA, Ofman R, Ferdinandusse S, et al. Refsum disease is caused by mutations in the phytanoyl-CoA hydroxylase gene. *Nat Genet* 1997;17:190–193.

114. Ashizawa T, Subramony SH. What is Kearns-Sayre syndrome after all? *Arch Neurol* 2001;58:1053–1054.

115. Korade-Mirnics Z, Babitzke P, Hoffman E. Myotonic dystrophy: molecular windows on a complex etiology. *Nucleic Acids Res* 1998;26:1363–1368.

116. Geisterfer-Lowrance AA, Kass S, Tanigawa G, et al. A molecular basis for familial hypertrophic cardiomyopathy: a beta cardiac myosin heavy chain gene missense mutation. *Cell* 1990;62:999–1006.

117. Thierfelder L, Watkins H, MacRae C, et al. Alpha-tropomyosin and cardiac troponin T mutations cause familial hypertrophic cardiomyopathy: a disease of the sarcomere. *Cell* 1994;77:701–712.

118. Charron P, Dubourg O, Desnos M, et al. Clinical features and prognostic implications of familial hypertrophic cardiomyopathy related to the cardiac myosin-binding protein C gene. *Circulation* 1998;97:2230–2236.

119. Erdmann J, Raible J, Maki-Abadi J, et al. Spectrum of clinical phenotypes and gene variants in cardiac myosin-binding protein C mutation carriers with hypertrophic cardiomyopathy. *J Am Coll Cardiol* 2001;38:322–330.

120. Richard P, Charron P, Carrier L, et al. Hypertrophic cardiomyopathy: distribution of disease genes, spectrum of mutations, and implications for a molecular diagnosis strategy. *Circulation* 2003;107:2227–2232.

121. Mogensen J, Murphy RT, Kubo T, et al. Frequency and clinical expression of cardiac troponin I mutations in 748 consecutive families with hypertrophic cardiomyopathy. *J Am Coll Cardiol* 2004;44:2315–2325.

122. Torricelli F, Girolami F, Olivotto I, et al. Prevalence and clinical profile of troponin T mutations among patients with hypertrophic cardiomyopathy in Tuscany. *Am J Cardiol* 2003;92:1358–1362.

123. Van Driest SL, Ellsworth EG, Ommen SR, et al. Prevalence and spectrum of thin filament mutations in an outpatient referral population with hypertrophic cardiomyopathy. *Circulation* 2003;108:445–451.

124. Satoh M, Takahashi M, Sakamoto T, et al. Structural analysis of the titin gene in hypertrophic cardiomyopathy: identification of a novel disease gene. *Biochem Biophys Res Commun* 1999;262:411–417.

125. Mogensen J, Klausen IC, Pedersen AK, et al. Alpha-cardiac actin is a novel disease gene in familial hypertrophic cardiomyopathy. *J Clin Invest* 1999;103:R39–R43.

126. Flavigny J, Richard P, Isnard R, et al. Identification of two novel mutations in the ventricular regulatory myosin light chain gene (MYL2) associated with familial and classical forms of hypertrophic cardiomyopathy. *J Mol Med* 1998;76:208–214.

127. Andersen PS, Havndrup O, Bundgaard H, et al. Myosin light chain mutations in familial hypertrophic cardiomyopathy: phenotypic presentation and frequency in Danish and South African populations. *J Med Genet* 2001;38:E43.

128. Hayashi T, Arimura T, Itoh-Satoh M, et al. Tcap gene mutations in hypertrophic cardiomyopathy and dilated cardiomyopathy. *J Am Coll Cardiol* 2004;44:2192–2201.

129. Hayashi T, Arimura T, Ueda K, et al. Identification and functional analysis of a caveolin-3 mutation associated with familial hypertrophic cardiomyopathy. *Biochem Biophys Res Commun* 2004;313:178–184.

130. Minamisawa S, Sato Y, Tatsuguchi Y, et al. Mutation of the phospholamban promoter associated with hypertrophic cardiomyopathy. *Biochem Biophys Res Commun* 2003;304:1–4.

131. Hoffmann B, Schmidt-Traub H, Perrot A, et al. First mutation in cardiac troponin C, L29Q, in a patient with hypertrophic cardiomyopathy. *Hum Mutat* 2001;17:524.

132. Carniel E, Taylor MRG, Sinagra G, et al. α-Myosin heavy chain: a sarcomeric gene associated with dilated and hypertrophic phenotypes of cardiomyopathy. *Circulation* 2005;112:54–59.

133. Davis JS, Hassanzadeh S, Winitsky S, et al. The overall pattern of cardiac contraction depends on a spatial gradient of myosin regulatory light chain phosphorylation. *Cell* 2001;107:631–641.

134. Anan R, Greve G, Thierfelder L, et al. Prognostic implications of novel beta cardiac myosin heavy chain gene mutations that cause familial hypertrophic cardiomyopathy. *J Clin Invest* 1994;93:280–285.

135. Dausse E, Komajda M, Fetler L, et al. Familial hypertrophic cardiomyopathy. Microsatellite haplotyping and identification of a hot spot for mutations in the beta-myosin heavy chain gene. *J Clin Invest* 1993;92:2807–2813.

136. Tesson F, Richard P, Charron P, et al. Genotype-phenotype analysis in four families with mutations in the beta-myosin heavy chain gene responsible for familial hypertrophic cardiomyopathy. *Hum Mutat* 1998;12:385–392.

137. Nakajima-Taniguchi C, Matsui H, Eguchi N, et al. A novel deletion mutation in the beta-myosin heavy chain gene found in Japanese patients with hypertrophic cardiomyopathy. *J Mol Cell Cardiol* 1995;27:2607–2612.

138. Marian AJ, Yu QT, Mares A, Jr, et al. Detection of a new mutation in the beta-myosin heavy chain gene in an individual with hypertrophic cardiomyopathy. *J Clin Invest* 1992;90:2156–2165.

139. Cuda G, Perrotti N, Perticone F, et al. A previously undescribed de novo insertion-deletion mutation in the beta myosin heavy chain gene in a kindred with familial hypertrophic cardiomyopathy. *Heart* 1996;76:451–452.

140. Blair E, Redwood C, de Jesus OM, et al. Mutations of the light meromyosin domain of the beta-myosin heavy chain rod in hypertrophic cardiomyopathy. *Circ Res* 2002;90:263–269.

141. Niimura H, Bachinski LL, Sangwatanaroj S, et al. Mutations in the gene for cardiac myosin-binding protein C and late-onset familial hypertrophic cardiomyopathy. *N Engl J Med* 1998;338:1248–1257.

142. Bonne G, Carrier L, Bercovici J, et al. Cardiac myosin binding protein-C gene splice acceptor site mutation is associated with familial hypertrophic cardiomyopathy. *Nat Genet* 1995;11:438–440.

143. Carrier L, Bonne G, Bahrend E, et al. Organization and sequence of human cardiac myosin binding protein C gene (MYBPC3) and identification of mutations predicted to produce truncated proteins in familial hypertrophic cardiomyopathy. *Circ Res* 1997;80:427–434.

144. Watkins H, Conner D, Thierfelder L, et al. Mutations in the cardiac myosin binding protein-C gene on chromosome 11 cause familial hypertrophic cardiomyopathy. *Nat Genet* 1995;11:434–437.

145. Forissier JF, Carrier L, Farza H, et al. Codon 102 of the cardiac troponin T gene is a putative hot spot for mutations in familial hypertrophic cardiomyopathy. *Circulation* 1996;94:3069–3073.

146. Watkins H, McKenna WJ, Thierfelder L, et al. Mutations in the genes for cardiac troponin T and alpha-tropomyosin in hypertrophic cardiomyopathy. *N Engl J Med* 1995;332:1058–1064.

147. Kimura A, Harada H, Park JE, et al. Mutations in the cardiac troponin I gene associated with hypertrophic cardiomyopathy. *Nat Genet* 1997;16:379–382.

148. Kokado H, Shimizu M, Yoshio H, et al. Clinical features of hypertrophic cardiomyopathy caused by a Lys183 deletion mutation in the cardiac troponin I gene. *Circulation* 2000;102:663–669.

149. Abchee A, Marian AJ. Prognostic significance of beta-myosin heavy chain mutations is reflective of their hypertrophic expressivity in patients with hypertrophic cardiomyopathy. *J Investig Med* 1997;45:191–196.

150. Van Driest SL, Vasile VC, Ommen SR, et al. Myosin binding protein C mutations and compound heterozygosity in hypertrophic cardiomyopathy. *J Am Coll Cardiol* 2004;44:1903–1910.

151. Blair E, Price SJ, Baty CJ, et al. Mutations in cis can confound genotype-phenotype correlations in hypertrophic cardiomyopathy. *J Med Genet* 2001;38:385–388.

152. Konhilas JP, Watson PA, Maass A, et al. Exercise can prevent and reverse the severity of hypertrophic cardiomyopathy. *Circ Res* 2006;98:540–548.

153. Stauffer BL, Konhilas JP, Luczak ED, et al. Soy diet worsens heart disease in mice. *J Clin Invest* 2006;116:209–216.

154. Marian AJ. Modifier genes for hypertrophic cardiomyopathy. *Curr Opin Cardiol* 2002;17:242–252.

155. Chen SN, Czernuszewicz GZ, Lu Y, et al. Two novel modifier loci for human hypertrophic cardiomyopathy map to chromosomes 8q12 and 10p13 [abstract]. *Circulation* 2005;112:II-412.

156. Semsarian C, Healey MJ, Fatkin D, et al. A polymorphic modifier gene alters the hypertrophic response in a murine model of familial hypertrophic cardiomyopathy. *J Mol Cell Cardiol* 2001;33:2055–2060.

157. Marian AJ, Yu QT, Workman R, et al. Angiotensin-converting enzyme polymorphism in hypertrophic cardiomyopathy and sudden cardiac death. *Lancet* 1993;342:1085–1086.

158. Yamazaki T, Komuro I, Yazaki Y. Role of the renin-angiotensin system in cardiac hypertrophy. *Am J Cardiol* 1999;83:53H–57H.

159. Rigat B, Hubert C, Alhenc-Gelas F, et al. An insertion/deletion polymorphism in the angiotensin I-converting enzyme gene accounting for half the variance of serum enzyme levels. *J Clin Invest* 1990;86:1343–1346.

160. Lechin M, Quinones MA, Omran A, et al. Angiotensin-I converting enzyme genotypes and left ventricular hypertrophy in patients with hypertrophic cardiomyopathy. *Circulation* 1995;92:1808–1812.

161. Tesson F, Dufour C, Moolman JC, et al. The influence of the angiotensin I converting enzyme genotype in familial hypertrophic cardiomyopathy varies with the disease gene mutation. *J Mol Cell Cardiol* 1997;29:831–838.

162. Pfeufer A, Osterziel KJ, Urata H, et al. Angiotensin-converting enzyme and heart chymase gene polymorphisms in hypertrophic cardiomyopathy. *Am J Cardiol* 1996;78:362–364.

163. Yoneya K, Okamoto H, Machida M, et al. Angiotensin-converting enzyme gene polymorphism in Japanese patients with hypertrophic cardiomyopathy. *Am Heart J* 1995;130:1089–1093.

164. Yamada Y, Ichihara S, Fujimura T, et al. Lack of association of polymorphisms of the angiotensin converting enzyme and angiotensinogen genes with nonfamilial hypertrophic or dilated cardiomyopathy. *Am J Hypertens* 1997;10:921–928.

165. Osterop AP, Kofflard MJ, Sandkuijl LA, et al. AT1 receptor A/C1166 polymorphism contributes to cardiac hypertrophy in subjects with hypertrophic cardiomyopathy. *Hypertension* 1998;32:825–830.

166. Perkins MJ, Van Driest SL, Ellsworth EG, et al. Gene-specific modifying effects of pro-LVH polymorphisms involving the renin-angiotensin-aldosterone system among 389 unrelated patients with hypertrophic cardiomyopathy. *Eur Heart J* 2005;26:2457–2462.

167. Brugada R, Kelsey W, Lechin M, et al. Role of candidate modifier genes on the phenotypic expression of hypertrophy in patients with hypertrophic cardiomyopathy. *J Investig Med* 1997;45:542–551.

168. Patel R, Lim DS, Reddy D, et al. Variants of trophic factors and expression of cardiac hypertrophy in patients with hypertrophic cardiomyopathy. *J Mol Cell Cardiol* 2000;32:2369–2377.

169. Yamada Y, Ichihara S, Izawa H, et al. Association of a G994 --> T (Val279 --> Phe) polymorphism of the plasma platelet-activating factor acetylhydrolase gene with myocardial damage in Japanese patients with nonfamilial hypertrophic cardiomyopathy. *J Hum Genet* 2001;46:436–441.

170. Marian AJ. On genetics, inflammation, and abdominal aortic aneurysm: can single nucleotide polymorphisms predict the outcome? *Circulation* 2001;103:2222–2224.

171. Wilcox WR, Banikazemi M, Guffon N, et al. Long-term safety and efficacy of enzyme replacement therapy for Fabry disease. *Am J Hum Genet* 2004;75:65–74.

172. Eng CM, Guffon N, Wilcox WR, et al. Safety and efficacy of recombinant human alpha-galactosidase A—replacement therapy in Fabry's disease. *N Engl J Med* 2001;345:9–16.

173. Sachdev B, Takenaka T, Teraguchi H, et al. Prevalence of Anderson-Fabry disease in male patients with late onset hypertrophic cardiomyopathy. *Circulation* 2002;105:1407–1411.

174. Desnick RJ, Brady R, Barranger J, et al. Fabry Disease, an under-recognized multisystemic disorder: expert recommendations for diagnosis, management, and enzyme replacement therapy. *Ann Intern Med* 2003;138:338–346.

175. Chimenti C, Pieroni M, Morgante E, et al. Prevalence of Fabry disease in female patients with late-onset hypertrophic cardiomyopathy. *Circulation* 2004;110:1047–1053.

176. Schiffmann R, Murray GJ, Treco D, et al. Infusion of alpha-galactosidase A reduces tissue globotriaosylceramide storage in patients with Fabry disease. *Proc Natl Acad Sci U S A* 2000;97:365–370.

177. Frustaci A, Chimenti C, Ricci R, et al. Improvement in cardiac function in the cardiac variant of Fabry's disease with galactose-infusion therapy. *N Engl J Med* 2001;345:25–32.

178. Cummings CJ, Zoghbi HY. Trinucleotide repeats: mechanisms and pathophysiology. *Annu Rev Genomics Hum Genet* 2000;1:281–328.

179. Palau F. Friedreich's ataxia and frataxin: molecular genetics, evolution and pathogenesis. *Int J Mol Med* 2001;7:581–589.

180. Mihalik SJ, Morrell JC, Kim D, et al. Identification of PAHX, a Refsum disease gene. *Nat Genet* 1997;17:185–189.

181. Raben N, Plotz P, Byrne BJ. Acid alpha-glucosidase deficiency (glycogenosis type II, Pompe disease). *Curr Mol Med* 2002;2:145–166.

182. Charron P, Villard E, Sebillon P, et al. Danon's disease as a cause of hypertrophic cardiomyopathy: a systematic survey. *Heart* 2004;90:842–846.

183. Guertl B, Noehammer C, Hoefler G. Metabolic cardiomyopathies. *Int J Exp Pathol* 2000;81:349–372.

184. Lim DS, Roberts R, Marian AJ. Expression profiling of cardiac genes in human hypertrophic cardiomyopathy: insight into the pathogenesis of phenotypes. *J Am Coll Cardiol* 2001;38:1175–1180.

185. Hwang JJ, Allen PD, Tseng GC, et al. Microarray gene expression profiles in dilated and hypertrophic cardiomyopathic end-stage heart failure. *Physiol Genomics* 2002;10:31–44.

186. Marian AJ. On genetic and phenotypic variability of hypertrophic cardiomyopathy: nature versus nurture. *J Am Coll Cardiol* 2001;38:331–334.

187. Maron BJ, Spirito P, Wesley Y, et al. Development and progression of left ventricular hypertrophy in children with hypertrophic cardiomyopathy. *N Engl J Med* 1986;315:610–614.

188. Marian AJ. Pathogenesis of diverse clinical and pathological phenotypes in hypertrophic cardiomyopathy. *Lancet* 2000;355:58–60.

189. Watkins H, Rosenzweig A, Hwang DS, et al. Characteristics and prognostic implications of myosin missense mutations in familial hypertrophic cardiomyopathy. *N Engl J Med* 1992;326:1108–1114.

190. Fananapazir L, Epstein ND. Genotype-phenotype correlations in hypertrophic cardiomyopathy. Insights provided by comparisons of kindreds with distinct and identical beta-myosin heavy chain gene mutations. *Circulation* 1994;89:22–32.

191. Epstein ND, Cohn GM, Cyran F, et al. Differences in clinical expression of hypertrophic cardiomyopathy associated with two distinct mutations in the beta-myosin heavy chain gene. A 908Leu—Val mutation and a 403Arg—Gln mutation [see comments]. *Circulation* 1992;86:345–352.

192. Charron P, Dubourg O, Desnos M, et al. Genotype-phenotype correlations in familial hypertrophic cardiomyopathy. A comparison between mutations in the cardiac protein-C and the beta-myosin heavy chain genes. *Eur Heart J* 1998;19:139–145.

193. Kubo T, Kitaoka H, Okawa M, et al. Lifelong left ventricular remodeling of hypertrophic cardiomyopathy caused by a founder frameshift deletion mutation in the cardiac myosin-binding protein C gene among Japanese. *J Am Coll Cardiol* 2005;46:1737–1743.

194. Van Driest SL, Jaeger MA, Ommen SR, et al. Comprehensive analysis of the beta-myosin heavy chain gene in 389 unrelated patients with hypertrophic cardiomyopathy. *J Am Coll Cardiol* 2004;44:602–610.

195. Marian AJ, Mares A Jr, Kelly DP, et al. Sudden cardiac death in hypertrophic cardiomyopathy. Variability in phenotypic expression of beta-myosin heavy chain mutations. *Eur Heart J* 1995;16:368–376.

196. Ho CY, Lever HM, DeSanctis R, et al. Homozygous mutation in cardiac troponin T: implications for hypertrophic cardiomyopathy. *Circulation* 2000;102:1950–1955.

197. Jeschke B, Uhl K, Weist B, et al. A high risk phenotype of hypertrophic cardiomyopathy associated with a compound genotype of two mutated beta-myosin heavy chain genes. *Hum Genet* 1998;102:299–304.

198. Geisterfer-Lowrance AA, Christe M, Conner DA, et al. A mouse model of familial hypertrophic cardiomyopathy. *Science* 1996;272:731–734.

199. Yang Q, Sanbe A, Osinska H, et al. A mouse model of myosin binding protein C human familial hypertrophic cardiomyopathy. *J Clin Invest* 1998;102:1292–1300.

200. Fatkin D, McConnell BK, Mudd JO, et al. An abnormal Ca(2+) response in mutant sarcomere protein-mediated familial hypertrophic cardiomyopathy. *J Clin Invest* 2000;106:1351–1359.

201. Chandra M, Rundell VL, Tardiff JC, et al. Ca(2+) activation of myofilaments from transgenic mouse hearts expressing R92Q mutant cardiac troponin T. *Am J Physiol Heart Circ Physiol* 2001;280:H705–H713.

202. Harada K, Potter JD. Familial hypertrophic cardiomyopathy mutations from different functional regions of troponin T result in different effects on the pH and Ca^{2+} sensitivity of cardiac muscle contraction. *J Biol Chem* 2004;279:14488–14495.

203. Heller MJ, Nili M, Homsher E, et al. Cardiomyopathic tropomyosin mutations that increase thin filament Ca^{2+} sensitivity and tropomyosin N-domain flexibility. *J Biol Chem* 2003;278:41742–41748.

204. Yanaga F, Morimoto S, Ohtsuki I. Ca^{2+} sensitization and potentiation of the maximum level of myofibrillar ATPase activity caused by mutations of troponin T found in familial hypertrophic cardiomyopathy. *J Biol Chem* 1999;274:8806–8812.

205. Rottbauer W, Gautel M, Zehelein J, et al. Novel splice donor site mutation in the cardiac myosin-binding protein-C gene in familial hypertrophic car-

diomyopathy. Characterization of cardiac transcript and protein. *J Clin Invest* 1997;100:475–482.

206. Tardiff JC, Factor SM, Tompkins BD, et al. A truncated cardiac troponin T molecule in transgenic mice suggests multiple cellular mechanisms for familial hypertrophic cardiomyopathy. *J Clin Invest* 1998;101:2800–2811.

207. Derchi G, Bellone P, Chiarella F, et al. Plasma levels of atrial natriuretic peptide in hypertrophic cardiomyopathy. *Am J Cardiol* 1992;70:1502–1504.

208. Hasegawa K, Fujiwara H, Doyama K, et al. Ventricular expression of brain natriuretic peptide in hypertrophic cardiomyopathy. *Circulation* 1993;88:372–380.

209. Hasegawa K, Fujiwara H, Koshiji M, et al. Endothelin-1 and its receptor in hypertrophic cardiomyopathy. *Hypertension* 1996;27:259–264.

210. Li RK, Li G, Mickle DA, et al. Overexpression of transforming growth factor-beta1 and insulin-like growth factor-I in patients with idiopathic hypertrophic cardiomyopathy. *Circulation* 1997;96:874–881.

211. Patel R, Nagueh SF, Tsybouleva N, et al. Simvastatin induces regression of cardiac hypertrophy and fibrosis and improves cardiac function in a transgenic rabbit model of human hypertrophic cardiomyopathy. *Circulation* 2001;104:317–324.

212. Senthil V, Chen SN, Tsybouleva N, et al. Prevention of cardiac hypertrophy by atorvastatin in a transgenic rabbit model of human hypertrophic cardiomyopathy. *Circ Res* 2005;97(3):285–292.

213. Lim DS, Lutucuta S, Bachireddy P, et al. Angiotensin II blockade reverses myocardial fibrosis in a transgenic mouse model of human hypertrophic cardiomyopathy. *Circulation* 2001;103:789–791.

214. Marian AJ, Senthil V, Chen SN, et al. Antifibrotic effects of antioxidant N-acetylcysteine in a mouse model of human hypertrophic cardiomyopathy mutation. *J Am Coll Cardiol* 2006;47:827–834.

215. Sussman MA, Lim HW, Gude N, et al. Prevention of cardiac hypertrophy in mice by calcineurin inhibition. *Science* 1998;281:1690–1693.

216. Manolio TA, Baughman KL, Rodeheffer R, et al. Prevalence and etiology of idiopathic dilated cardiomyopathy (summary of a National Heart, Lung, and Blood Institute Workshop). *Am J Cardiol* 1992;69:1458–1466.

217. Mestroni L, Rocco C, Gregori D, et al. Familial dilated cardiomyopathy: evidence for genetic and phenotypic heterogeneity. Heart Muscle Disease Study Group. *J Am Coll Cardiol* 1999;34:181–190.

218. Kasper EK, Agema WR, Hutchins GM, et al. The causes of dilated cardiomyopathy: a clinicopathologic review of 673 consecutive patients. *J Am Coll Cardiol* 1994;23:586–590.

219. Burkett EL, Hershberger RE. Clinical and genetic issues in familial dilated cardiomyopathy. *J Am Coll Cardiol* 2005;45:969–981.

220. Kamisago M, Sharma SD, DePalma SR, et al. Mutations in sarcomere protein genes as a cause of dilated cardiomyopathy. *N Engl J Med* 2000;343:1688–1696.

221. Olson TM, Michels VV, Thibodeau SN, et al. Actin mutations in dilated cardiomyopathy, a heritable form of heart failure. *Science* 1998;280:750–752.

222. Knoll R, Hoshijima M, Hoffman HM, et al. The cardiac mechanical stretch sensor machinery involves a Z disc complex that is defective in a subset of human dilated cardiomyopathy. *Cell* 2002;111:943–955.

223. Tsubata S, Bowles KR, Vatta M, et al. Mutations in the human delta-sarcoglycan gene in familial and sporadic dilated cardiomyopathy. *J Clin Invest* 2000;106:655–662.

224. Barresi R, Di Blasi C, Negri T, et al. Disruption of heart sarcoglycan complex and severe cardiomyopathy caused by beta sarcoglycan mutations. *J Med Genet* 2000;37:102–107.

225. Olson TM, Illenberger S, Kishimoto NY, et al. Metavinculin mutations alter actin interaction in dilated cardiomyopathy. *Circulation* 2002;105:431–437.

226. Arbustini E, Diegoli M, Morbini P, et al. Prevalence and characteristics of dystrophin defects in adult male patients with dilated cardiomyopathy. *J Am Coll Cardiol* 2000;35:1760–1768.

227. Vatta M, Mohapatra B, Jimenez S, et al. Mutations in Cypher/ZASP in patients with dilated cardiomyopathy and left ventricular non-compaction. *J Am Coll Cardiol* 2003;42:2014–2027.

228. Arimura T, Hayashi T, Terada H, et al. A cypher/ZASP mutation associated with dilated cardiomyopathy alters the binding affinity to protein kinase C. *J Biol Chem* 2004;279:6746–6752.

229. Bienengraeber M, Olson TM, Selivanov VA, et al. ABCC9 mutations identified in human dilated cardiomyopathy disrupt catalytic KATP channel gating. *Nat Genet* 2004;36:382–387.

230. Fatkin D, MacRae C, Sasaki T, et al. Missense mutations in the rod domain of the lamin A/C gene as causes of dilated cardiomyopathy and conduction-system disease. *N Engl J Med* 1999;341:1715–1724.

231. Li D, Tapscoft T, Gonzalez O, et al. Desmin mutation responsible for idiopathic dilated cardiomyopathy. *Circulation* 1999;100:461–464.

232. Perng MD, Muchowski PJ, van Den IJ, et al. The cardiomyopathy and lens cataract mutation in alphaB-crystallin alters its protein structure, chaperone activity, and interaction with intermediate filaments in vitro. *J Biol Chem* 1999;274:33235–33243.

233. Brooks AP, Emery AE. The incidence of Duchenne muscular dystrophy in the southeast of Scotland. *Clin Genet* 1977;11:290–294.

234. Finsterer J, Stollberger C. The heart in human dystrophinopathies. *Cardiology* 2003;99:1–19.

235. Malhotra SB, Hart KA, Klamut HJ, et al. Frame-shift deletions in patients with Duchenne and Becker muscular dystrophy. *Science* 1988;242:755–759.

236. Muntoni F, Wilson L, Marrosu G, et al. A mutation in the dystrophin gene selectively affecting dystrophin expression in the heart. *J Clin Invest* 1995;96:693–699.

237. Emery AE. Emery-Dreifuss syndrome. *J Med Genet* 1989;26:637–641.

238. Emery AE. Emery-Dreifuss muscular dystrophy—a 40-year retrospective. *Neuromuscul Disord* 2000;10:228–232.

239. Emery AEH. Muscular dystrophy into the new millennium. *Neuromuscul Disord* 2002;12:343–349.

240. Bione S, Maestrini E, Rivella S, et al. Identification of a novel X-linked gene responsible for Emery-Dreifuss muscular dystrophy. *Nat Genet* 1994;8:323–327.

241. D'Adamo P, Fassone L, Gedeon A, et al. The X-linked gene G4.5 is responsible for different infantile dilated cardiomyopathies. *Am J Hum Genet* 1997;61:862–867.

242. Suzuki M, Carlson KM, Marchuk DA, et al. Genetic modifier loci affecting survival and cardiac function in murine dilated cardiomyopathy. *Circulation* 2002;105:1824–1829.

243. Bonne G, Mercuri E, Muchir A, et al. Clinical and molecular genetic spectrum of autosomal dominant Emery-Dreifuss muscular dystrophy due to mutations of the lamin A/C gene. *Ann Neurol* 2000;48:170–180.

244. Dalakas MC, Park KY, Semino-Mora C, et al. Desmin myopathy, a skeletal myopathy with cardiomyopathy caused by mutations in the desmin gene. *N Engl J Med* 2000;342:770–780.

245. Phillips MF, Harper PS. Cardiac disease in myotonic dystrophy. *Cardiovasc Res* 1997;33:13–22.

246. Bova MP, Yaron O, Huang Q, et al. Mutation R120G in alphaB-crystallin, which is linked to a desmin-related myopathy, results in an irregular structure and defective chaperone-like function. *Proc Natl Acad Sci U S A* 1999;96:6137–6142.

247. Corrado D, Basso C, Thiene G, et al. Spectrum of clinicopathologic manifestations of arrhythmogenic right ventricular cardiomyopathy/dysplasia: a multicenter study. *J Am Coll Cardiol* 1997;30:1512–1520.

248. Corrado D, Fontaine G, Marcus FI, et al. Arrhythmogenic right ventricular dysplasia/cardiomyopathy: need for an international registry. Study Group on Arrhythmogenic Right Ventricular Dysplasia/Cardiomyopathy of the Working Groups on Myocardial and Pericardial Disease and Arrhythmias of the European Society of Cardiology and of the Scientific Council on Cardiomyopathies of the World Heart Federation. *Circulation* 2000;101:E101–E106.

249. Lemola K, Brunckhorst C, Helfenstein U, et al. Predictors of adverse outcome in patients with arrhythmogenic right ventricular dysplasia/cardiomyopathy: long-term experience of a tertiary care centre. *Heart* 2005;91:1167–1172.

250. Sen-Chowdhry S, Syrris P, McKenna WJ. Genetics of right ventricular cardiomyopathy. *J Cardiovasc Electrophysiol* 2005;16:927–935.

251. McKenna WJ, Thiene G, Nava A, et al. Diagnosis of arrhythmogenic right ventricular dysplasia/cardiomyopathy. Task Force of the Working Group Myocardial and Pericardial Disease of the European Society of Cardiology and of the Scientific Council on Cardiomyopathies of the International Society and Federation of Cardiology. *Br Heart J* 1994;71:215–218.

252. Tabib A, Loire R, Chalabreysse L, et al. Circumstances of death and gross and microscopic observations in a series of 200 cases of sudden death associated with arrhythmogenic right ventricular cardiomyopathy and/or dysplasia. *Circulation* 2003;108:3000–3005.

253. Shen WK, Edwards WD, Hammill SC, et al. Sudden unexpected nontraumatic death in 54 young adults: a 30-year population-based study. *Am J Cardiol* 1995;76:148–152.

254. Corrado D, Thiene G, Nava A, et al. Sudden death in young competitive athletes: clinicopathologic correlations in 22 cases. *Am J Med* 1990;89:588–596.

255. Furlanello F, Bertoldi A, Dallago M, et al. Cardiac arrest and sudden death in competitive athletes with arrhythmogenic right ventricular dysplasia. *Pacing Clin Electrophysiol* 1998;21:331–335.

256. Burke AP, Farb A, Tashko G, et al. Arrhythmogenic right ventricular cardio-myopathy and fatty replacement of the right ventricular myocardium: are they different diseases? *Circulation* 1998;97:1571–1580.

257. Shirani J, Berezowski K, Roberts WC. Quantitative measurement of normal and excessive (cor adiposum) subepicardial adipose tissue, its clinical signifi-cance, and its effect on electrocardiographic QRS voltage. *Am J Cardiol* 1995;76:414–418.

258. Tiso N, Stephan DA, Nava A, et al. Identification of mutations in the cardiac ryanodine receptor gene in families affected with arrhythmogenic right ven-tricular cardiomyopathy type 2 (ARVD2). *Hum Mol Genet* 2001;10:189–194.

259. Priori SG, Napolitano C, Tiso N, et al. Mutations in the cardiac ryanodine receptor gene (hRyR2) underlie catecholaminergic polymorphic ventricular tachycardia. *Circulation* 2001;103:196–200.

260. McKoy G, Protonotarios N, Crosby A, et al. Identification of a deletion in plakoglobin in arrhythmogenic right ventricular cardiomyopathy with pal-moplantar keratoderma and woolly hair (Naxos disease). *Lancet* 2000;355:2119–2124.

261. Kaplan SR, Gard JJ, Carvajal-Huerta L, et al. Structural and molecular pathology of the heart in Carvajal syndrome. *Cardiovasc Pathol* 2004;13:26–32.

262. Rampazzo A, Nava A, Erne P, et al. A new locus for arrhythmogenic right ventricular cardiomyopathy (ARVD2) maps to chromosome 1q42-q43. *Hum Mol Genet* 1995;4:2151–2154.

263. Rampazzo A, Nava A, Danieli GA, et al. The gene for arrhythmogenic right ventricular cardiomyopathy maps to chromosome 14q23-q24. *Hum Mol Genet* 1994;3:959–962.

264. Severini GM, Krajinovic M, Pinamonti B, et al. A new locus for arrhyth-mogenic right ventricular dysplasia on the long arm of chromosome 14. *Genomics* 1996;31:193–200.

265. Rampazzo A, Nava A, Miorin M, et al. ARVD4 a new locus for arrhyth-mogenic right ventricular cardiomyopathy, maps to chromosome 2 long arm. *Genomics* 1997;45:259–263.

266. Ahmad F, Li D, Karibe A, et al. Localization of a gene responsible for arrhythmogenic right ventricular dysplasia to chromosome 3p23. *Circulation* 1998;98:2791–2795.

267. Melberg A, Oldfors A, Blomstrom-Lundqvist C, et al. Autosomal dominant myofibrillar myopathy with arrhythmogenic right ventricular cardiomyopa-thy linked to chromosome 10q. *Ann Neurol* 1999;46:684–692.

268. Coonar AS, Protonotarios N, Tsatsopoulou A, et al. Gene for arrhyth-mogenic right ventricular cardiomyopathy with diffuse nonepidermolytic palmoplantar keratoderma and woolly hair (Naxos disease) maps to 17q21. *Circulation* 1998;97:2049–2058.

269. Gerull B, Heuser A, Wichter T, et al. Mutations in the desmosomal protein plakophilin-2 are common in arrhythmogenic right ventricular cardiomyop-athy. *Nat Genet* 2004;36:1162–1164.

270. Norgett EE, Hatsell SJ, Carvajal-Huerta L, et al. Recessive mutation in des-moplakin disrupts desmoplakin-intermediate filament interactions and causes dilated cardiomyopathy, woolly hair and keratoderma. *Hum Mol Genet* 2000;9:2761–2766.

271. Alcalai R, Metzger S, Rosenheck S, et al. A recessive mutation in des-moplakin causes arrhythmogenic right ventricular dysplasia, skin disorder, and woolly hair. *J Am Coll Cardiol* 2003;42:319–327.

272. Pilichou K, Nava A, Basso C, et al. Mutations in desmoglein-2 gene are asso-ciated with arrhythmogenic right ventricular cardiomyopathy. *Circulation* 2006;113:1171–1179.

273. Beffagna G, Occhi G, Nava A, et al. Regulatory mutations in transforming growth factor-beta3 gene cause arrhythmogenic right ventricular cardiomy-opathy type 1. *Cardiovasc Res* 2005;65:366–373.

274. Nattel S, Schott JJ. Arrhythmogenic right ventricular dysplasia type 1 and mutations in transforming growth factor [beta]3 gene regulatory regions: a breakthrough? *Cardiovasc Res* 2005;65:302–304.

275. Pinamonti B, Miani D, Sinagra G, et al. Familial right ventricular dysplasia with biventricular involvement and inflammatory infiltration. Heart Muscle Disease Study Group. *Heart* 1996;76:66–69.

276. Grumbach IM, Heim A, Vonhof S, et al. Coxsackievirus genome in myocar-dium of patients with arrhythmogenic right ventricular dysplasia/cardiomy-opathy. *Cardiology* 1998;89:241–245.

277. Mallat Z, Tedgui A, Fontaliran F, et al. Evidence of apoptosis in arrhyth-mogenic right ventricular dysplasia. *N Engl J Med* 1996;335:1190–1197.

278. d'Amati G, di Gioia CR, Giordano C, et al. Myocyte transdifferentiation: a possible pathogenetic mechanism for arrhythmogenic right ventricular car-diomyopathy. *Arch Pathol Lab Med* 2000;124:287–290.

279. Runge MS, Stouffer GA, Sheahan RG, et al. Morphological patterns of death by myocytes in arrhythmogenic right ventricular dysplasia. *Am J Med Sci* 2000;320:310–319.

280. Nishikawa T, Ishiyama S, Nagata M, et al. Programmed cell death in the myocardium of arrhythmogenic right ventricular cardiomyopathy in children and adults. *Cardiovasc Pathol* 1999;8:185–189.

281. Garcia-Gras E, Lombardi R, Giphart MJ, et al. Suppression of canonical Wnt/catenin signaling by nuclear plakoglobin recapitulates phenotype of arrhythmogenic right ventricular cardiomyopathy. *J Clin Invest* 2006;116:2012–2021.

282. Kushwaha SS, Fallon JT, Fuster V. Restrictive cardiomyopathy. *N Engl J Med* 1997;336:267–276.

283. Arbustini E, Morbini P, Grasso M, et al. Restrictive cardiomyopathy, atrio-ventricular block and mild to subclinical myopathy in patients with desmin-immunoreactive material deposits. *J Am Coll Cardiol* 1998;31:645–653.

284. Fitzpatrick AP, Shapiro LM, Rickards AF, et al. Familial restrictive cardiomy-opathy with atrioventricular block and skeletal myopathy. *Br Heart J* 1990;63:114–118.

285. Aroney C, Bett N, Radford D. Familial restrictive cardiomyopathy. *Aust N Z J Med* 1988;18:877–878.

286. Zachara E, Bertini E, Lioy E, et al. Restrictive cardiomyopathy due to desmin accumulation in a family with evidence of autosomal dominant inheritance. *G Ital Cardiol* 1997;27:436–442.

287. Mogensen J, Kubo T, Duque M, et al. Idiopathic restrictive cardiomyopathy is part of the clinical expression of cardiac troponin I mutations. *J Clin Invest* 2003;111:209–216.

288. Cooke RA, Chambers JB, Curry PV. Noonan's cardiomyopathy: a non-hypertrophic variant. *Br Heart J* 1994;71:561–565.

289. Gatchel JR, Zoghbi HY. Diseases of unstable repeat expansion: mechanisms and common principles. *Nat Rev Genet* 2005;6:743–755.

290. Mahadevan M, Tsilfidis C, Sabourin L, et al. Myotonic dystrophy mutation: an unstable CTG repeat in the 3 untranslated region of the gene. *Science* 1992;255:1253–1255.

291. Brook JD, McCurrach ME, Harley HG, et al. Molecular basis of myotonic dystrophy: expansion of a trinucleotide (CTG) repeat at the 3 end of a tran-script encoding a protein kinase family member. *Cell* 1992;68:799–808.

292. Fu YH, Pizzuti A, Fenwick RG Jr, et al. An unstable triplet repeat in a gene related to myotonic muscular dystrophy. *Science* 1992;255:1256–1258.

293. Timchenko LT, Miller JW, Timchenko NA, et al. Identification of a (CUG)n triplet repeat RNA-binding protein and its expression in myotonic dystro-phy. *Nucleic Acids Res* 1996;24:4407–4414.

294. Philips AV, Timchenko LT, Cooper TA. Disruption of splicing regulated by a CUG-binding protein in myotonic dystrophy. *Science* 1998;280:737–741.

295. Groh WJ, Lowe MR, Zipes DP. Severity of cardiac conduction involvement and arrhythmias in myotonic dystrophy type 1 correlates with age and CTG repeat length. *J Cardiovasc Electrophysiol* 2002;13:444–448.

296. Liquori CL, Ricker K, Moseley ML, et al. Myotonic dystrophy type 2 caused by a CCTG expansion in intron 1 of ZNF9. *Science* 2001;293:864–867.

297. Bit-Avragim N, Perrot A, Schols L, et al. The GAA repeat expansion in intron 1 of the frataxin gene is related to the severity of cardiac manifestation in patients with Friedreich's ataxia. *J Mol Med* 2001;78:626–632.

298. Amalfitano A, McVie-Wylie AJ, Hu H, et al. Systemic correction of the mus-cle disorder glycogen storage disease type II after hepatic targeting of a modi-fied adenovirus vector encoding human acid-alpha-glucosidase. *Proc Natl Acad Sci U S A* 1999;96:8861–8866.

299. Wierzbicki AS, Lloyd MD, Schofield CJ, et al. Refsum's disease: a peroxisomal dis-order affecting phytanic acid alpha-oxidation. *J Neurochem* 2002;80:727–735.

300. Simon DK, Johns DR. Mitochondrial disorders: clinical and genetic features. *Annu Rev Med* 1999;50:111–127.

301. Williams RS. Canaries in the coal mine: mitochondrial DNA and vascular injury from reactive oxygen species. *Circ Res* 2000;86:915–916.

302. Longo N, Amat di San FC, Pasquali M. Disorders of carnitine transport and the carnitine cycle. *Am J Med Genet C Semin Med Genet* 2006;142:77–85.

303. Kelly DP, Strauss AW. Inherited cardiomyopathies. *N Engl J Med* 1994;330:913–919.

304. Roden DM, Lazzara R, Rosen M, et al. Multiple mechanisms in the long-QT syndrome. Current knowledge, gaps, and future directions. The SADS Foun-dation Task Force on LQTS. *Circulation* 1996;94:1996–2012.

305. Brugada R, Roberts R. Brugada syndrome: why are there multiple answers to a simple question? *Circulation* 2001;104:3017–3019.

306. George AL Jr, Varkony TA, Drabkin HA, et al. Assignment of the human heart tetrodotoxin-resistant voltage-gated Na+ channel alpha-subunit gene (SCN5A) to band 3p21. *Cytogenet Cell Genet* 1995;68:67–70.

307. Wang Q, Shen J, Splawski I, et al. SCN5A mutations associated with an inherited cardiac arrhythmia, long QT syndrome. *Cell* 1995;80:805–811.

308. Chen Q, Kirsch GE, Zhang D, et al. Genetic basis and molecular mechanism for idiopathic ventricular fibrillation. *Nature* 1998;392:293–296.

309. Schott JJ, Alshinawi C, Kyndt F, et al. Cardiac conduction defects associate with mutations in SCN5A. *Nat Genet* 1999;23:20–21.

310. Priori SG, Napolitano C, Giordano U, et al. Brugada syndrome and sudden cardiac death in children. *Lancet* 2000;355:808–809.

311. Vatta M, Dumaine R, Varghese G, et al. Genetic and biophysical basis of sudden unexplained nocturnal death syndrome (SUNDS), a disease allelic to Brugada syndrome. *Hum Mol Genet* 2002;11:337–345.

312. Brugada P, Brugada J. Right bundle branch block, persistent ST segment elevation and sudden cardiac death: a distinct clinical and electrocardiographic syndrome. A multicenter report. *J Am Coll Cardiol* 1992;20:1391–1396.

313. Brugada J, Brugada R, Brugada P. Right bundle-branch block and ST-segment elevation in leads V1 through V3: a marker for sudden death in patients without demonstrable structural heart disease. *Circulation* 1998;97:457–460.

314. Nademanee K, Veerakul G, Nimmannit S, et al. Arrhythmogenic marker for the sudden unexplained death syndrome in Thai men. *Circulation* 1997;96:2595–2600.

315. Weiss R, Barmada MM, Nguyen T, et al. Clinical and molecular heterogeneity in the Brugada syndrome: a novel gene locus on chromosome 3. *Circulation* 2002;105:707–713.

316. Bezzina C, Veldkamp MW, van Den Berg MP, et al. A single Na(+) channel mutation causing both long-QT and Brugada syndromes. *Circ Res* 1999;85:1206–1213.

317. Kyndt F, Probst V, Potet F, et al. Novel SCN5A mutation leading either to isolated cardiac conduction defect or Brugada syndrome in a large French family. *Circulation* 2001;104:3081–3086.

318. Dumaine R, Towbin JA, Brugada P, et al. Ionic mechanisms responsible for the electrocardiographic phenotype of the Brugada syndrome are temperature dependent. *Circ Res* 1999;85:803–809.

319. Smits JP, Eckardt L, Probst V, et al. Genotype-phenotype relationship in Brugada syndrome: electrocardiographic features differentiate SCN5A-related patients from non-SCN5A-related patients. *J Am Coll Cardiol* 2002;40:350–356.

320. Keating M, Atkinson D, Dunn C, et al. Linkage of a cardiac arrhythmia, the long QT syndrome, and the Harvey ras-1 gene. *Science* 1991;252:704–706.

321. Barhanin J, Lesage F, Guillemare E, et al. K(V)LQT1 and lsK (minK) proteins associate to form the I(Ks) cardiac potassium current. *Nature* 1996;384:78–80.

322. Sanguinetti MC, Jiang C, Curran ME, et al. A mechanistic link between an inherited and an acquired cardiac arrhythmia: HERG encodes the IKr potassium channel. *Cell* 1995;81:299–307.

323. Schott JJ, Charpentier F, Peltier S, et al. Mapping of a gene for long QT syndrome to chromosome 4q25–27. *Am J Hum Genet* 1995;57:1114–1122.

324. Mohler PJ, Schott JJ, Gramolini AO, et al. Ankyrin-B mutation causes type 4 long-QT cardiac arrhythmia and sudden cardiac death. *Nature* 2003;421:634–639.

325. Abbott GW, Sesti F, Splawski I, et al. MiRP1 forms IKr potassium channels with HERG and is associated with cardiac arrhythmia. *Cell* 1999;97:175–187.

326. Plaster NM, Tawil R, Tristani-Firouzi M, et al. Mutations in Kir2.1 cause the developmental and episodic electrical phenotypes of Andersen's syndrome. *Cell* 2001;105:511–519.

327. Splawski I, Timothy KW, Decher N, et al. Severe arrhythmia disorder caused by cardiac L-type calcium channel mutations. *Proc Natl Acad Sci U S A* 2005;102:8089–8096.

328. Neyroud N, Tesson F, Denjoy I, et al. A novel mutation in the potassium channel gene KVLQT1 causes the Jervell and Lange-Nielsen cardioauditory syndrome. *Nat Genet* 1997;15:186–189.

329. Schwartz PJ, Priori SG, Spazzolini C, et al. Genotype-phenotype correlation in the long-QT syndrome: gene-specific triggers for life-threatening arrhythmias. *Circulation* 2001;103:89–95.

330. Zareba W, Moss AJ, Schwartz PJ, et al. Influence of genotype on the clinical course of the long-QT syndrome. International Long-QT Syndrome Registry Research Group. *N Engl J Med* 1998;339:960–965.

331. Roden DM. Pharmacogenetics and drug-induced arrhythmias. *Cardiovasc Res* 2001;50:224–231.

332. Camm AJ, Janse MJ, Roden DM, et al. Congenital and acquired long QT syndrome. *Eur Heart J* 2000;21:1232–1237.

333. Splawski I, Timothy KW, Tateyama M, et al. Variant of SCN5A sodium channel implicated in risk of cardiac arrhythmia. *Science* 2002;297:1333–1336.

334. Arking DE, Pfeufer A, Post W, et al. A common genetic variant in the NOS1 regulator NOS1AP modulates cardiac repolarization. *Nat Genet* 2006;38:644–651.

335. Gussak I, Brugada P, Brugada J, et al. Idiopathic short QT interval: a new clinical syndrome? *Cardiology* 2000;94:99–102.

336. Gaita F, Giustetto C, Bianchi F, et al. Short QT syndrome: a familial cause of sudden death. *Circulation* 2003;108:965–970.

337. Schulze-Bahr E, Breithardt G. Short QT interval and short QT syndromes. *J Cardiovasc Electrophysiol* 2005;16:397–398.

338. Brugada R, Hong K, Dumaine R, et al. Sudden death associated with short-QT syndrome linked to mutations in HERG. *Circulation* 2004;109:30–35.

339. Bellocq C, van Ginneken AC, Bezzina CR, et al. Mutation in the KCNQ1 gene leading to the short QT-interval syndrome. *Circulation* 2004;109:2394–2397.

340. Priori SG, Pandit SV, Rivolta I, et al. A novel form of short QT syndrome (SQT3) is caused by a mutation in the KCNJ2 gene. *Circ Res* 2005;96:800–807.

341. Hong K, Bjerregaard P, Gussak I, et al. Short QT syndrome and atrial fibrillation caused by mutation in KCNH2. *J Cardiovasc Electrophysiol* 2005;16:394–396.

342. Hong K, Piper DR, Diaz-Valdecantos A, et al. De novo KCNQ1 mutation responsible for atrial fibrillation and short QT syndrome in utero. *Cardiovasc Res* 2005;68:433–440.

343. Gaita F, Giustetto C, Bianchi F, et al. Short QT syndrome: pharmacological treatment. *J Am Coll Cardiol* 2004;43:1494–1499.

344. Wolpert C, Schimpf R, Giustetto C, et al. Further insights into the effect of quinidine in short QT syndrome caused by a mutation in HERG. *J Cardiovasc Electrophysiol* 2005;16:54–58.

345. Brink PA, Ferreira A, Moolman JC, et al. Gene for Progressive Familial Heart Block Type I Maps to Chromosome 19q13. *Circulation* 1995;91:1633–1640.

346. Laitinen PJ, Brown KM, Piippo K, et al. Mutations of the cardiac ryanodine receptor (RyR2) gene in familial polymorphic ventricular tachycardia. *Circulation* 2001;103:485–490.

347. Lahat H, Pras E, Olender T, et al. A missense mutation in a highly conserved region of CASQ2 is associated with autosomal recessive catecholamine-induced polymorphic ventricular tachycardia in Bedouin families from Israel. *Am J Hum Genet* 2001;69:1378–1384.

348. Ueda K, Nakamura K, Hayashi T, et al. Functional characterization of a trafficking-defective HCN4 mutation, D553N, associated with cardiac arrhythmia. *J Biol Chem* 2004;279:27194–27198.

349. Schulze-Bahr E, Neu A, Friederich P, et al. Pacemaker channel dysfunction in a patient with sinus node disease. *J Clin Invest* 2003;111:1537–1545.

350. Benson DW, Wang DW, Dyment M, et al. Congenital sick sinus syndrome caused by recessive mutations in the cardiac sodium channel gene (SCN5A). *J Clin Invest* 2003;112:1019–1028.

351. Milanesi R, Baruscotti M, Gnecchi-Ruscone T, et al. Familial sinus bradycardia associated with a mutation in the cardiac pacemaker channel. *N Engl J Med* 2006;354:151–157.

352. Brugada R, Tapscott T, Czernuszewicz GZ, et al. Identification of a genetic locus for familial atrial fibrillation. *N Engl J Med* 1997;336:905–911.

353. Chen YH, Xu SJ, Bendahhou S, et al. KCNQ1 gain-of-function mutation in familial atrial fibrillation. *Science* 2003;299:251–254.

354. Yang Y, Xia M, Jin Q, et al. Identification of a KCNE2 gain-of-function mutation in patients with familial atrial fibrillation. *Am J Hum Genet* 2004;75:899–905.

355. Zhang DF, Liang B, Lin J, et al. [KCNE3 R53H substitution in familial atrial fibrillation.]. *Chin Med J (Engl)*. 2005;118:1735–1738.

356. Xia M, Jin Q, Bendahhou S, et al. A Kir2.1 gain-of-function mutation underlies familial atrial fibrillation. *Biochem Biophys Res Commun* 2005;332:1012–1019.

357. Olson TM, Alekseev AE, Liu XK, et al. Kv1.5 channelopathy due to KCNA5 loss-of-function mutation causes human atrial fibrillation. *Hum Mol Genet* 2006;15:2185–2191.

358. Ellinor PT, Shin JT, Moore RK, et al. Locus for atrial fibrillation maps to chromosome 6q14–16. *Circulation* 2003;107:2880–2883.

359. Oberti C, Wang L, Li L, et al. Genome-wide linkage scan identifies a novel genetic locus on chromosome 5p13 for neonatal atrial fibrillation associated with sudden death and variable cardiomyopathy. *Circulation* 2004;110:3753–3759.

360. Gollob MH, Jones DL, Krahn AD, et al. Somatic mutations in the connexin 40 gene (GJA5) in atrial fibrillation. *N Engl J Med* 2006;354:2677–2688.

361. Lerman BB, Dong B, Stein KM, et al. Right ventricular outflow tract tachycardia due to a somatic cell mutation in G protein subunitalphai2. *J Clin Invest* 1998;101:2862–2868.

362. Van Wagoner DR. Electrophysiological remodeling in human atrial fibrillation. *Pacing Clin Electrophysiol* 2003;26:1572–1575.

363. Westenskow P, Splawski I, Timothy KW, et al. Compound mutations: a common cause of severe long-QT syndrome. *Circulation* 2004;109:1834–1841.

364. Nikoskelainen EK, Savontaus ML, Huoponen K, et al. Pre-excitation syndrome in Leber's hereditary optic neuropathy. *Lancet* 1994;344:857–858.

365. Abdelmalek NF, Gerber TL, Menter A. Cardiocutaneous syndromes and associations. *J Am Acad Dermatol* 2002;46:161–183.

366. Collod-Beroud G, Boileau C. Marfan syndrome in the third millennium. *Eur J Hum Genet* 2002;10:673–681.

367. Dietz HC, Cutting GR, Pyeritz RE, et al. Marfan syndrome caused by a recurrent de novo missense mutation in the fibrillin gene. *Nature* 1991;352:337–339.

368. Robinson PN, Booms P, Katzke S, et al. Mutations of FBN1 and genotype-phenotype correlations in Marfan syndrome and related fibrillinopathies. *Hum Mutat* 2002;20:153–161.

369. Putnam EA, Zhang H, Ramirez F, et al. Fibrillin-2 (FBN2) mutations result in the Marfan-like disorder, congenital contractural arachnodactyly. *Nat Genet* 1995;11:456–458.

370. Mizuguchi T, Collod-Beroud G, Akiyama T, et al. Heterozygous TGFBR2 mutations in Marfan syndrome. *Nat Genet* 2004;36:855–860.

371. Habashi JP, Judge DP, Holm TM, et al. Losartan, an AT1 antagonist, prevents aortic aneurysm in a mouse model of Marfan syndrome. *Science* 2006;312:117–121.

372. Mao JR, Bristow J. The Ehlers-Danlos syndrome: on beyond collagens. *J Clin Invest* 2001;107:1063–1069.

373. Superti-Furga A, Gugler E, Gitzelmann R, et al. Ehlers-Danlos syndrome type IV. A multi-exon deletion in one of the two COL3A1 alleles affecting structure, stability, and processing of type III procollagen. *J Biol Chem* 1988;263:6226–6232.

374. Tassabehji M, Metcalfe K, Hurst J, et al. An elastin gene mutation producing abnormal tropoelastin and abnormal elastic fibres in a patient with autosomal dominant cutis laxa. *Hum Mol Genet* 1998;7:1021–1028.

375. Loeys B, Van Maldergem L, Mortier G, et al. Homozygosity for a missense mutation in fibulin-5 (FBLN5) results in a severe form of cutis laxa. *Hum Mol Genet* 2002;11:2113–2118.

376. Bergen AA, Plomp AS, Schuurman EJ, et al. Mutations in ABCC6 cause pseudoxanthoma elasticum. *Nat Genet* 2000;25:228–231.

377. Cohn DH, Byers PH, Steinmann B, et al. Lethal osteogenesis imperfecta resulting from a single nucleotide change in one human proalpha 1(I) collagen allele. *Proc Natl Acad Sci U S A* 1986;83:6045–6047.

378. Lamande SR, Dahl HH, Cole WG, et al. Characterization of point mutations in the collagen COL1A1 and COL1A2 genes causing lethal perinatal osteogenesis imperfecta. *J Biol Chem* 1989;264:15809–15812.

379. Rich S, Dantzker DR, Ayres SM, et al. Primary pulmonary hypertension. A national prospective study. *Ann Intern Med* 1987;107:216–223.

380. Runo JR, Loyd JE. Primary pulmonary hypertension. *Lancet* 2003;361:1533–1544.

381. D'Alonzo GE, Barst RJ, Ayres SM, et al. Survival in patients with primary pulmonary hypertension. Results from a national prospective registry. *Ann Intern Med* 1991;115:343–349.

382. Newman JH, Wheeler L, Lane KB, et al. Mutation in the gene for bone morphogenetic protein receptor II as a cause of primary pulmonary hypertension in a large kindred. *N Engl J Med* 2001;345:319–324.

383. Machado RD, Pauciulo MW, Thomson JR, et al. BMPR2 haploinsufficiency as the inherited molecular mechanism for primary pulmonary hypertension. *Am J Hum Genet* 2001;68:92–102.

384. Lane KB, Machado RD, Pauciulo MW, et al. Heterozygous germline mutations in BMPR2 encoding a TGF-beta receptor, cause familial primary pulmonary hypertension. The International PPH Consortium. *Nat Genet* 2000;26:81–84.

385. Loscalzo J. Genetic clues to the cause of primary pulmonary hypertension. *N Engl J Med* 2001;345:367–371.

386. Trembath RC, Thomson JR, Machado RD, et al. Clinical and molecular genetic features of pulmonary hypertension in patients with hereditary hemorrhagic telangiectasia. *N Engl J Med* 2001;345:325–334.

387. Eddahibi S, Humbert M, Fadel E, et al. Serotonin transporter overexpression is responsible for pulmonary artery smooth muscle hyperplasia in primary pulmonary hypertension. *J Clin Invest* 2001;108:1141–1150.

388. Rabinovitch M. Linking a serotonin transporter polymorphism to vascular smooth muscle proliferation in patients with primary pulmonary hypertension. *J Clin Invest* 2001;108:1109–1111.

389. Rudarakanchana N, Flanagan JA, Chen H, et al. Functional analysis of bone morphogenetic protein type II receptor mutations underlying primary pulmonary hypertension. *Hum Mol Genet* 2002;11:1517–1525.

390. Rader DJ, Cohen J, Hobbs HH. Monogenic hypercholesterolemia: new insights in pathogenesis and treatment. *J Clin Invest* 2003;111:1795–1803.

391. Goldstein JL, Sobhani MK, Faust JR, et al. Heterozygous familial hypercholesterolemia: failure of normal allele to compensate for mutant allele at a regulated genetic locus. *Cell* 1976;9:195–203.

392. Soutar AK. Update on low density lipoprotein receptor mutations. *Curr Opin Lipidol* 1998;9:141–147.

393. Jansen AC, van Wissen S, Defesche JC, et al. Phenotypic variability in familial hypercholesterolaemia: an update. *Curr Opin Lipidol* 2002;13:165–171.

394. Rauh G, Keller C, Kormann B, et al. Familial defective apolipoprotein B100: clinical characteristics of 54 cases. *Atherosclerosis* 1992;92:233–241.

395. Vrablik M, Ceska R, Horinek A. Major apolipoprotein B-100 mutations in lipoprotein metabolism and atherosclerosis. *Physiol Res* 2001;50:337–343.

396. Soria LF, Ludwig EH, Clarke HRG, et al. Association between a specific apolipoprotein B mutation and familial defective apolipoprotein B-100. *Proc Natl Acad Sci U S A* 1989;86:587–591.

397. Abifadel M, Varret M, Rabes JP, et al. Mutations in PCSK9 cause autosomal dominant hypercholesterolemia. *Nat Genet* 2003;34:154–156.

398. Maxwell KN, Fisher EA, Breslow JL. Overexpression of PCSK9 accelerates the degradation of the LDLR in a post-endoplasmic reticulum compartment. *Proc Natl Acad Sci U S A* 2005;102:2069–2074.

399. Chen SN, Ballantyne CM, Gotto AM Jr, et al. A common PCSK9 haplotype, encompassing the E670G coding single nucleotide polymorphism, is a novel genetic marker for plasma low-density lipoprotein cholesterol levels and severity of coronary atherosclerosis. *J Am Coll Cardiol* 2005;45:1611–1619.

400. Cohen JC, Boerwinkle E, Mosley TH Jr, et al. Sequence variations in PCSK9 low LDL, and protection against coronary heart disease. *N Engl J Med* 2006;354:1264–1272.

401. Garcia CK, Wilund K, Arca M, et al. Autosomal recessive hypercholesterolemia caused by mutations in a putative LDL receptor adaptor protein. *Science* 2001;292:1394–1398.

402. Gregg RE, Wetterau JR. The molecular basis of abetalipoproteinemia. *Curr Opin Lipidol* 1994;5:81–86.

403. Hooper AJ, van Bockxmeer FM, Burnett JR. Monogenic hypocholesterolaemic lipid disorders and apolipoprotein B metabolism. *Crit Rev Clin Lab Sci* 2005;42:515–545.

404. Sharp D, Blinderman L, Combs KA, et al. Cloning and gene defects in microsomal triglyceride transfer protein associated with abetalipoproteinaemia. *Nature* 1993;365:65–69.

405. Narcisi TM, Shoulders CC, Chester SA, et al. Mutations of the microsomal triglyceride-transfer-protein gene in abetalipoproteinemia. *Am J Hum Genet* 1995;57:1298–1310.

406. Fouchier SW, Sankatsing RR, Peter J, et al. High frequency of APOB gene mutations causing familial hypobetalipoproteinaemia in patients of Dutch and Spanish descent. *J Med Genet* 2005;42:e23.

407. Jones B, Jones EL, Bonney SA, et al. Mutations in a Sar1 GTPase of COPII vesicles are associated with lipid absorption disorders. *Nat Genet* 2003;34:29–31.

408. Funke H, von Eckardstein A, Pritchard PH, et al. A molecular defect causing fish eye disease: an amino acid exchange in lecithin-cholesterol acyltransferase (LCAT) leads to the selective loss of alpha-LCAT activity. *Proc Natl Acad Sci U S A* 1991;88:4855–4859.

409. Klein HG, Santamarina-Fojo S, Duverger N, et al. Fish eye syndrome: a molecular defect in the lecithin-cholesterol acyltransferase (LCAT) gene associated with normal alpha-LCAT-specific activity. Implications for classification and prognosis. *J Clin Invest* 1993;92:479–485.

410. Tall AR, Wang N. Tangier disease as a test of the reverse cholesterol transport hypothesis. *J Clin Invest* 2000;106:1205–1207.

411. Bodzioch M, Orso E, Klucken J, et al. The gene encoding ATP-binding cassette transporter 1 is mutated in Tangier disease. *Nat Genet* 1999;22:347–351.

412. Brooks-Wilson A, Marcil M, Clee SM, et al. Mutations in ABC1 in Tangier disease and familial high-density lipoprotein deficiency. *Nat Genet* 1999;22:336–345.

413. Rust S, Rosier M, Funke H, et al. Tangier disease is caused by mutations in the gene encoding ATP-binding cassette transporter 1. *Nat Genet* 1999;22:352–355.

414. Remaley AT, Rust S, Rosier M, et al. Human ATP-binding cassette transporter 1 (ABC1): genomic organization and identification of the genetic

defect in the original Tangier disease kindred. *Proc Natl Acad Sci U S A* 1999;96:12685–12690.

415. Lutucuta S, Ballantyne CM, Elghannam H, et al. Novel polymorphisms in promoter region of atp binding cassette transporter gene and plasma lipids, severity, progression, and regression of coronary atherosclerosis and response to therapy. *Circ Res* 2001;88:969–973.

416. Brousseau ME, Bodzioch M, Schaefer EJ, et al. Common variants in the gene encoding ATP-binding cassette transporter 1 in men with low HDL cholesterol levels and coronary heart disease. *Atherosclerosis* 2001;154:607–611.

417. Cohen JC, Kiss RS, Pertsemlidis A, et al. Multiple rare alleles contribute to low plasma levels of HDL cholesterol. *Science* 2004;305:869–872.

418. Jeunemaitre X, Soubrier F, Kotelevtsev YV, et al. Molecular basis of human hypertension: role of angiotensinogen. *Cell* 1992;71:169–180.

419. Luft FC. Hypertension as a complex genetic trait. *Semin Nephrol* 2002;22:115–126.

420. Lifton RP, Gharavi AG, Geller DS. Molecular mechanisms of human hypertension. *Cell* 2001;104:545–556.

421. Toka HR, Luft FC. Monogenic forms of human hypertension. *Semin Nephrol* 2002;22:81–88.

422. Pascoe L, Curnow KM, Slutsker L, et al. Glucocorticoid-suppressible hyperaldosteronism results from hybrid genes created by unequal crossovers between CYP11B1 and CYP11B2. *Proc Natl Acad Sci U S A* 1992;89:8327–8331.

423. Mune T, Rogerson FM, Nikkila H, et al. Human hypertension caused by mutations in the kidney isozyme of 11 beta-hydroxysteroid dehydrogenase. *Nat Genet* 1995;10:394–399.

424. Li A, Tedde R, Krozowski ZS, et al. Molecular basis for hypertension in the "type II variant" of apparent mineralocorticoid excess. *Am J Hum Genet* 1998;63:370–379.

425. Scheinman SJ, Guay-Woodford LM, Thakker RV, et al. Genetic disorders of renal electrolyte transport. *N Engl J Med* 1999;340:1177–1187.

426. Hansson JH, Nelson-Williams C, Suzuki H, et al. Hypertension caused by a truncated epithelial sodium channel gamma subunit: genetic heterogeneity of Liddle syndrome. *Nat Genet* 1995;11:76–82.

427. Wilson FH, Disse-Nicodeme S, Choate KA, et al. Human hypertension caused by mutations in WNK kinases. *Science* 2001;293:1107–1112.

CHAPTER 82

Congenital Heart Disease in Children and Adolescents

David R. Fulton

INCIDENCE AND ETIOLOGY

The incidence of congenital heart disease in the United States is approximately 8 per 1000 livebirths.[1,2] Many infants who are born alive with cardiac defects have anomalies that do not represent a threat to life, at least during infancy. Almost one-third of those infants, or 2.6 per 1000 livebirths, however, have critical disease, which is defined as a malformation severe enough to result in cardiac catheterization, cardiac surgery, or death within the first year of life.[3] Today, with early detection and proper management, the majority of infants with critical disease can be expected to survive the first year of life.[3] Most who now survive infancy will join the increasingly large cohort of adults with congenital heart disease.

ACKNOWLEDGMENTS: The author would like to thank previous authors of this chapter, including Dr. Jesse Edwards, Dr. Willis Williams, and Dr. William Plauth, for their contributions to past editions, which we continue to use in this edition. In particular, special credit must be given to Dr. Michael Freed who authored many previous editions of this chapter and who provided invaluable guidance in preparation of this chapter.

Estimates of the incidence of specific lesions vary, depending on whether the data are drawn from infants or older children and whether the diagnosis is based on clinical, echocardiographic, catheterization, surgical, or postmortem studies.[1-4] The incidence in other countries is remarkably similar to that reported for the United States.[5,6] Despite these differences in case material, except for bicuspid aortic valve and mitral valve prolapse, it is apparent that ventricular septal defect (VSD) is the most common malformation, occurring in 28 percent of all patients with congenital heart disease (Table 82–1).

Among 2251 infants with critical congenital heart disease in the New England Regional Infant Cardiac Program,[3] 53.7 percent were male. Certain defects, however, are more much common in one sex than in the other. Aortic stenosis occurs more often in boys (4:1), and atrial septal defects (ASDs) occur more frequently in girls (2.5:1).

Although earlier theories concerning the etiology of congenital heart diseases suggested that most defects were multifactorial—that is, the malformations are caused by a combination of a hereditary predisposition (presumably caused by abnormalities in the genetic code) and an environmental trigger[7]—more recent advances in molecular biology suggest that a much higher percentage are caused by point mutations.[8]

Some abnormalities are caused by chromosomal aberrations (see Chap. 81). Trisomy 21 (Down syndrome) is highly associated with complete atrioventricular (AV) canal, VSDs, and tetralogy of Fallot, and children with Turner syndrome (XO chromosome) frequently have coarctation of the aorta. Other anomalies are caused by teratogens: VSD in fetal alcohol syndrome, Ebstein's anomaly in a fetus with prenatal exposure to lithium, and patent ductus arteriosus (PDA) in mothers who contracted rubella during the first trimester are examples.

TABLE 82–1

Incidence of Specific Congenital Heart Defects

DEFECT	PERCENTAGE OF CASES[a] (AVERAGED)
Ventricular septal defect (VSD)	28.3
Pulmonary stenosis	9.5
Patent ductus arteriosus	8.7
VSD with pulmonary stenosis[b]	6.8
Atrial septal defect, secundum	6.7
Aortic stenosis	4.5
Coarctation of aorta	4.2
Atrioventricular canal[c]	3.5
Transposition of the great arteries	3.4
Aortic atresia	2.4
Truncus arteriosus	1.6
Tricuspid atresia	1.2
Anomalous pulmonary venous connection	1.1
Double-outlet right ventricle	0.8
Pulmonary atresia without VSD	0.3

[a]Total number of cases = 103,590.
[b]Includes tetralogy of Fallot.
[c]Includes partial and complete.
SOURCE: Data from references 1–3, 5, and 6.

Some syndromes are inherited as single-gene defects and have congenital heart disease as one of their manifestations. Holt-Oram syndrome, an association of radial limb abnormalities and ASDs, is caused by an abnormality of a T-box transcription factor Tbx5, and the cardiofacial syndrome, associated with abnormalities of the conotruncus, resulting in a high proportion of infants born with truncus arteriosus or interrupted aortic arch, is a result of a deletion on chromosome 22 (22q11).[9]

It is clear now that a higher proportion of congenital heart disease than previously thought is caused by single-gene defects and that the same malformation may be caused by mutant genes at different loci.[8] With increasing knowledge of molecular mechanisms, it seems inevitable that the etiology and pathogenesis of congenital heart disease will be clarified increasingly in the years ahead.

FETAL CIRCULATION AND THE TRANSITION TO NEONATAL AND ADULT CIRCULATION

The fetus obtains all metabolic necessities, including oxygen, from the placenta. The fetal circulation is an adaptation to allow most of the right ventricular output to bypass the lungs and instead to perfuse the placenta. Most of the understanding of this adaptation comes from more than 40 years of research,[10-18] primarily on fetal lambs. The fetal circulation is arranged in parallel fashion rather than in series, with mixing at the atrial (foramen ovale) and great vessel (ductus arteriosus) levels (Fig. 82–1). Normally, systemic venous blood enters the right atrium via the superior or inferior vena cava. From the inferior vena cava, blood is diverted by the crista dividens through the foramen ovale into the left atrium, so that approximately 27 percent of combined ventricular output reaches the left ventricle, with the remainder passing through the tricuspid valve to the right ventricle. This left atrial flow mixes with a small volume of pulmonary venous return to enter the left ventricle and the ascending aorta. Most of this output perfuses the coronary arteries, head, and upper body vessels, with a small proportion crossing the aortic arch to the descending aorta. Right ventricular output enters the main pulmonary artery, where approximately 90 percent (59 percent of combined ventricular output) is diverted through the ductus arteriosus to the descending aorta. Thus, approximately two-thirds of the combined cardiac output passes through the right side of the heart and one-third passes through the left side of the heart.

The oxygen saturation of fetal blood is considerably lower than that in a newborn or infant because of the placenta's less efficient oxygen exchange compared with that the lungs (Fig. 82–2). The blood with the highest saturation (approximately 70 percent) is that returning from the placenta. As described above, some of this higher-saturation blood is diverted across the foramen ovale, so that saturation on the left side of the heart (65 percent) is somewhat higher than it is on the right side (55 percent). As a result, lower-saturation blood (some 55 percent) passes preferentially through the ductus arteriosus to the placenta, thus increasing the efficiency of oxygen pickup. The presence of high levels of fetal hemoglobin with a greater than normal affinity for oxygen hemoglobin promotes more efficient placental oxygen exchange related to a leftward shift of the oxygen dissociation curve.

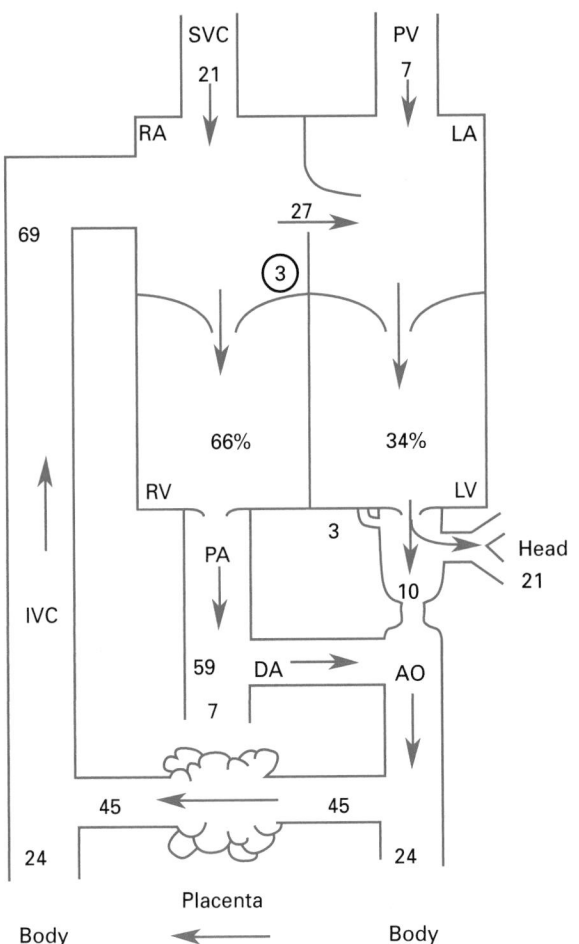

FIGURE 82–1. The course of the circulation in a late-gestation fetal lamb. *The numbers represent the percentage of combined ventricular output.* Some of the return from the inferior vena cava (IVC) is diverted by the crista dividens in the right atrium (RA) through the foramen ovale into the left atrium (LA), where it meets the pulmonary venous return (PV), passes into the left ventricle (LV), and is pumped into the ascending aorta. Most of the ascending aortic flow goes to the coronary, subclavian, and carotid arteries, with only 10 percent of combined ventricular output passing through the aortic arch (indicated by the narrowed point in the aorta) into the descending aorta (AO). The remainder of the inferior vena cava flow mixes with the return from the superior vena cava (SVC) and coronary veins, passes into the right atrium and right ventricle (RV), and is pumped into the pulmonary artery (PA). Because of the high pulmonary resistance, only 7 percent passes through the lungs (PV), with the rest going into the ductus arteriosus (DA) and then to the *descending aorta (AO)*, the placenta, and the lower half of the body. *Source: From Freed MD. Fetal and transitional circulation. In: Fyler DC, ed.[5] Reproduced with permission from the publisher and author.*

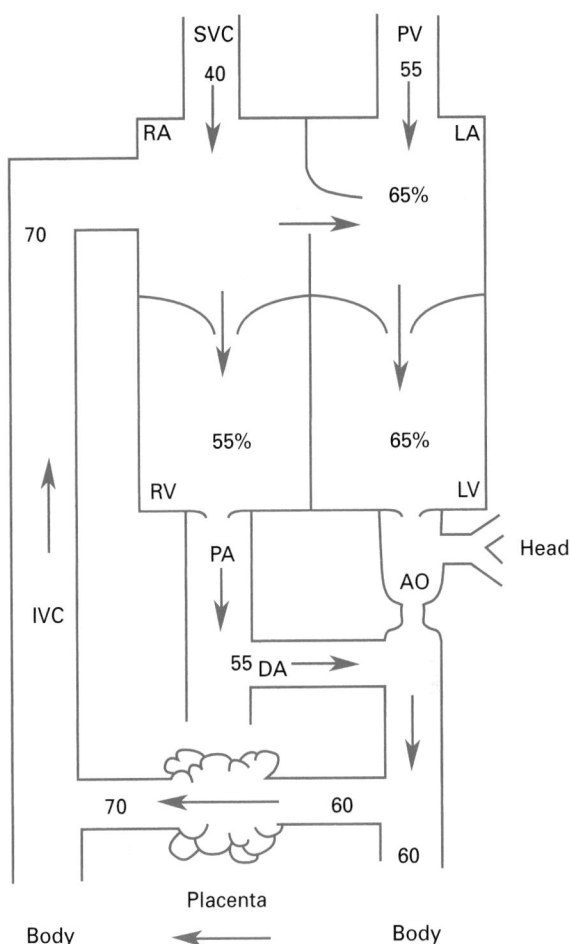

FIGURE 82–2. The numbers indicate the percent of oxygen saturation in a late-gestation lamb. The oxygen saturation is highest in the inferior vena cava, representing that primarily from the placenta. The saturation of blood in the heart is slightly higher on the left side than on the right side. The abbreviations in this diagram are the same as those in Fig. 82–1. *Source: From Freed MD. Fetal and transitional circulation. In: Fyler DC, ed.[5] Reproduced with permission from the publisher and author.*

The wide communication at the atrial level (foramen ovale) allows for near equalization of atrial and ventricular end-diastolic pressures. Similarly, at the great vessel level, the nonrestrictive ductus arteriosus allows equalization of systolic pressures in the aorta and the pulmonary artery and, in the absence of aortic or pulmonic stenosis, at the ventricular level (Fig. 82–3).

Within a few moments after birth, the circulatory physiology must switch rapidly from the placenta to the lung as the target organ for oxygen exchange. Failure of any one of a number of a complex series of pulmonary and cardiac events may result in cerebral or generalized hypoxemia, with lasting damage or death. With the onset of spontaneous respiration, the lungs expand and the pul-

monary arterioles, which have been vasoconstricted, dilate. The reduction in pulmonary vascular resistance results from both simple physical expansion of the lung with the onset of respiration and the vasodilation of the pulmonary resistance vessels, probably partly as a result of the high level of oxygen in alveolar gas. Simultaneously, the placenta is removed from the circulation either by clamping the umbilical cord or by constriction of the umbilical arteries. This sudden increase in systemic vascular resistance and drop in pulmonary vascular resistance causes blood leaving the right ventricle to enter the lung rather than the ductus arteriosus. The subsequent increase in pulmonary venous return to the left atrium increases left ventricular end-diastolic and left atrial pressure, shutting the flap valve of the foramen ovale against the edge of the cristae dividens, reversing the right-to-left atrial level shunt. In the presence of a lower pulmonary vascular resistance than systemic vascular resistance, some left-to-right (aorta to pulmonary artery) shunting occurs through the ductus arteriosus. The mechanism for closure of the ductus arteriosus is not completely understood. The increased level of oxygen probably causes vasoconstriction of the ductus' musculature, but there are strong suggestions that a reduction in circulating prostaglandins of the E series plays a

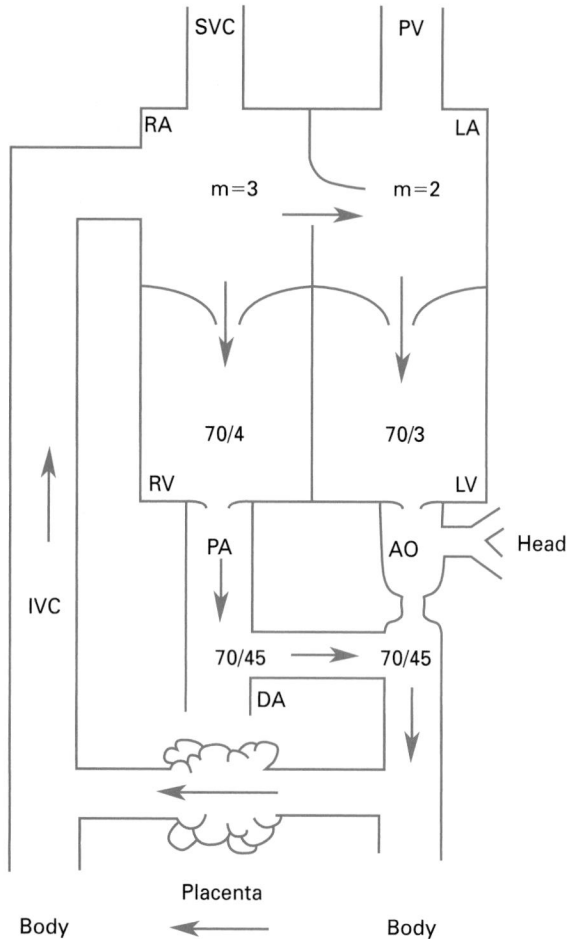

FIGURE 82–3. The numbers indicate the pressures observed in late-gestation lambs. Because large communications between the atrium and the great vessels are present, the pressures on both sides of the heart are virtually identical. The abbreviations are the same as those in Fig. 82–1. *Source: From Freed MD. Fetal and transitional circulation. In: Fyler DC, ed.[5] Reproduced with permission from the publisher and author.*

role. Within 3 or 4 days, the biochemical closure becomes irreversible, when cellular necrosis of the endothelium leads to obliteration of the lumen. The pulmonary artery pressure drops to approximately half systemic levels within a day or so but requires another 2 to 6 weeks to decrease to adult levels.

The structure and hemodynamics of the fetal circulation have significant consequences in a neonate with congenital heart disease.[19] The parallel circulation with connections at the atrial and great vessel level allows a wide variety of congenital cardiac malformations to exist while still maintaining placental oxygen exchange and tissue delivery. For example, atresia of the tricuspid or mitral valve, while devastating after birth, does not have a significant effect in utero. Furthermore, since the right ventricle performs two-thirds of the cardiac work before birth, the left ventricle is underloaded, possibly explaining why heart failure is not uncommonly seen with congenital defects. Because the normal flow across the aortic isthmus is relatively low (only approximately 10 percent of combined ventricular output), this area is especially vulnerable to small changes in flow across the foramen ovale. A somewhat small foramen may result in left-sided hypoplasia, which is almost always associated with narrowing (coarctation) or atresia (interruption) at the distal transverse aorta just proximal to ductal insertion.

Because the pulmonary blood flow in utero is less than 10 percent of combined ventricular output and increases four to five times at birth, anomalies that obstruct POD may be masked in utero under conditions of low POD. Finally, the low circulating levels of oxygen before birth (Po_2 26 to 38 mmHg and saturation at 50 to 60 percent) may account for the relative level of comfort observed in infants with cyanotic heart disease. These infants may do well, at least in the short run, with a Po_2 of 30 mmHg and an aortic saturation of 50 percent—levels that would lead to cerebral and cardiac anoxia, acidosis, and death within a few minutes in an older child or adult.

PERSISTENCE OF FETAL CIRCULATION

Persistence of fetal circulation[20,21] or persistent pulmonary hypertension in a newborn results in right-to-left shunting through the patent foramen ovale and/or PDA. It occurs most commonly in full-term infants. Severe hypoxia usually is manifest in the first few hours of life with tachypnea and metabolic acidosis, and a chest roentgenogram shows diminished vascular flow but no evidence of pulmonary parenchymal disease. Physical examination may reveal a parasternal heave, a loud second heart sound, and a systolic murmur.

Polycythemia, transient myocardial ischemia from hypoglycemia, and cyanotic congenital cardiac defects must be excluded. A higher oxygen level in the right radial artery than a subdiaphragmatic site confirms right-to-left shunting through the ductus arteriosus. Echocardiography and Doppler evaluation are of the utmost importance to rule out structural heart disease, especially total anomalous pulmonary venous connection. The initial treatment[21] includes an increase in the inspired oxygen level and correction of acidosis with hyperventilation or infusion of sodium bicarbonate when necessary. Diminishing the partial pressure of carbon dioxide can lower the pulmonary resistance diminishing the right-to-left shunt. Reduction of pulmonary vascular resistance with inhaled nitric oxide is a useful adjunct to other therapies.[22] Treatment of severe disease with extracorporeal membrane oxygenation is valuable in a significant number of patients.[23] Similar hemodynamic alterations also may be seen in newborns with parenchymal lung disease.

COMPLICATIONS OF CONGENITAL HEART DISEASE

Table 82–2 lists the complications associated with congenital heart disease.

CONGESTIVE HEART FAILURE

Heart failure is a potentially lethal complication of congenital heart disease and occurs in more than 80 percent of infants who have malformations severe enough to require cardiac catheterization or surgery within the first year of life.[24] The onset is usually within the first 6 months of life; it is rarely found after 1 year of age without a serious intercurrent problem such as infective endocarditis, pneumonia, or anemia.

Heart failure within the first 12 to 18 hours of life is usually a result of malformations that involve pressure or volume overload independent of pulmonary flow, as occurs with severe valvular regurgitation or a systemic arteriovenous fistula. Rarely, myocarditis may produce failure

TABLE 82–2

Complications of Congenital Heart Disease in Children

Congestive heart failure	Growth retardation
Hypoxemia	Pulmonary vascular disease

from the time of birth, as may congenital complete heart block or supraventricular tachycardia. Other causes in this age group include primary cardiomyopathy, severe polycythemia, anemia and depressed myocardial contractility resulting from neonatal asphyxia, hypocalcemia, hypoglycemia, or sepsis. *A majority of full-term infants presenting with severe heart failure during the remainder of the first week have critical obstruction to systemic arterial flow, which, in virtually all cases, is unmasked by narrowing or closure of the ductus arteriosus.* Examples are aortic atresia, coarctation of the aorta, interruption of the aortic arch, and critical aortic stenosis. *During the second week of life, aortic atresia and coarctation remain the most common causes of heart failure, but left ventricular volume overload from VSD, transposition of the great arteries with a VSD, and truncus arteriosus make their appearance.* These malformations present as the pulmonary vascular resistance falls, increasing the left-to-right shunt. *Statistically, VSD is the most frequent cause of congestive failure, followed by transposition, coarctation, complete AV canal, and PDA.*

The most common symptom of congestive heart failure is tachypnea with grunting, gasping breathing, or breathlessness with feeding. Observation of an undisturbed infant reveals nasal flaring and subcostal or intercostal retractions. A respiratory rate consistently above 60 is to be expected, and rates in the range of 90 to 100 are not uncommon. Poor weight gain from diminished intake and increased work of breathing is the rule. Cool, moist skin, a diminished and rapid arterial pulse, and hepatic enlargement are common accompanying signs. A gallop rhythm, pulmonary rales, and wheezing may be present. It may be difficult to distinguish the pulmonary findings of heart failure from those of pneumonia or bronchiolitis; indeed, many infants develop heart failure during an intercurrent pulmonary infection. Edema, if present, is usually found in the periorbital area and on the dorsa of the feet and hands. Cardiac enlargement is confirmed by chest roentgenography. Infants with malformations such as coarctation of the aorta and total anomalous pulmonary venous connection—abnormalities that usually are not characterized by an impressive murmur—are sometimes referred only after weeks of tachypnea and failure to thrive, when a chest roentgenogram taken to explore the possibility of lung disease has revealed cardiac enlargement.

When a sizable systemic-to-pulmonary communication exists in a premature infant, usually as a result of a PDA, signs of heart failure are often associated with signs of ventilatory failure.

【 】 HYPOXEMIA

Table 82–3 lists the sequelae of hypoxemia. *Cyanosis,* a bluish tinge to the color of the skin caused by the presence of at least 3 to 5 g/dL of reduced hemoglobin, is frequently the initial sign of congenital heart disease in an infant. It may also be an early sign of pulmonary, central nervous system, metabolic disease or methemoglobinemia. Prompt distinction between cardiac and noncardiac cyanosis, usually by echo-

cardiography, is extremely important, as palliation with PGE_1 infusion followed by early surgical intervention has improved survival.

Hypoxia leading to cyanosis in congenital heart disease may be caused by heart failure with pulmonary edema and pulmonary venous desaturation and/or intracardiac right-to-left shunting. The hypoxia that is either a result of heart failure or of lung disease with ventilation–perfusion mismatch usually responds dramatically to oxygen administration, whereas hypoxia that is caused by cyanotic defects does not. Because many infants are relatively anemic during the first few months of life (with a hemoglobin concentration of 10.4 to 12 g/dL), cyanosis may be subtle, despite significant decreases in arterial PO_2. When cyanosis has been present in older children for several months, the distal tips of the fingers and toes become hyperemic. Eventually, the capillary end loop dilation causes *clubbing* of the fingers and toes with a loss of the normal angle of the base of the nail and fingers. Also, with long-standing hypoxemia, the production of red blood cells increases to maintain the oxygen-carrying capacity of the blood (*polycythemia*). The increased hemoglobin concentration at any given oxygen saturation will result in more reduced hemoglobin, thus exaggerating the cyanosis.

The central nervous system may be the target organ of cerebrovascular accidents or brain abscess. *Brain abscess* is probably caused by bacteremia, primarily with mouth organisms that cross from the venous system to the arterial system from right-to-left shunting. The incidence seems to be directly related to arterial saturation and occurs mostly in older children and adolescents.[26]

Cerebrovascular accidents are directly caused by hypoxemia or indirectly in children who are polycythemic presumably secondary to sludging.[27] The former group usually consists of infants younger than 2 years of age who are anemic and thus may have markedly reduced oxygen levels. The latter group consists of children or young adults who are polycythemic and have sludging or in situ microthrombosis. Interestingly, because iron deficiency leads to decreased deformity of red cells, sludging may occur with modest levels of polycythemia (hematocrit 55 to 60 percent) in the presence of iron deficiency. With hematocrits in the range of 65 percent or higher, increased viscosity may lead to a cerebrovascular accident. Maintaining a proper level of hemoglobin has a salutary effect on hemodynamics and oxygen delivery in the presence of significant hypoxemia.[28,29] Other systems may also be affected by hypoxemia or polycythemia. In older adolescents, the increase in hemoglobin breakdown may result in hyperuricemia and can precipitate a secondary form of gout.[30]

Disturbances in hemostasis also occur with polycythemia. Coagulation factors are commonly abnormal in patients with hematocrits in excess of 60 percent.[31] Actual platelet counts may be normal but can be increased initially in some patients, with subsequent decreases related to persistent and worsening desaturation. There is evidence of shortened platelet survival time in patients with cyanotic heart disease.[32] Laboratory evaluation of coagulation status requires that cor-

TABLE 82–3

Sequelae of Hypoxemia

Cyanosis	Exercise intolerance
Clubbing	Hypoxic spells
Polycythemia	Brain abscess
Squatting	Cerebrovascular accidents

rection be made for the diminished volume of plasma and for the volume of anticoagulant used in blood samples, so as to avoid false results. Hematologic management of adults with cyanotic congenital heart disease requires special experience and knowledge.[33]

The major consequences of cyanosis can be avoided in many instances, although differences in intelligence have been demonstrated between cyanotic and acyanotic children.[34]

【 】 RETARDATION OF GROWTH AND DEVELOPMENT

Children with severe cardiac malformations frequently exhibit retardation of growth and development, with height and weight near or below the third percentile or weight 20 percentile points below the mean percentile for height.[35]

Growth retardation is most severe among children with overt cyanosis and those with large left-to-right shunts that cause heart failure. Heart failure tends to cause a greater reduction of weight than of height. Skeletal retardation, reflected by bone age, usually occurs with height and weight retardation and, among children with cyanotic heart disease, correlates with the severity of hypoxemia.

Other factors contribute to growth retardation, including insufficient caloric intake, dyspnea, frequent infections, psychological disturbances, malabsorption, and hypermetabolism. Among infants with severe congenital heart disease recognized within the first year of life, there is a significantly increased incidence of subnormal birth weight, intrauterine growth retardation, and major extracardiac anomalies.[3] Finally, a relatively small number of children have associated syndromes known to be characterized by growth retardation, such as rubella and Noonan, Turner, and Down syndromes. Growth retardation related primarily to congenital heart disease usually responds to surgical correction or palliation, with an impressive acceleration of growth and a return toward normal.

Although cardiac surgery is seldom recommended on the basis of growth failure alone, decelerated growth should be recognized early and, until proved otherwise, considered an index of the severity of heart disease. In general, the more successful the surgery, the less will be the retardation of growth and development, with its sequelae of physical, psychological, and intellectual problems.[36]

【 】 PULMONARY ARTERIAL HYPERTENSION AND PULMONARY VASCULAR OBSTRUCTIVE DISEASE

Pulmonary arterial hypertension (PAH) and pulmonary vascular obstructive disease (PVOD) are serious complications of congenital heart disease. PAH usually results from direct transmission of systemic arterial pressure to the right ventricle or pulmonary arteries via a large communication. Less frequently, it is caused by severe obstruction to blood flow through the left side of the heart at the pulmonary venous level or beyond. PVOD refers to a process involving structural and developmental changes in the smaller muscular arteries and arterioles of the lung that gradually diminishes and eventually destroys the ability of the pulmonary vascular bed to transport blood from the larger pulmonary arteries to the pulmonary veins without an abnormal elevation of proximal pulmonary arterial pressure.

Pulmonary resistance (R_p) may be as high as 8 to 10 Wood units immediately after birth, but falls rapidly throughout the first week of life. Indexed Wood units, as a measure of resistance to flow across either the pulmonary or the systemic vascular bed, are obtained by dividing the mean pressure difference (in millimeters of mercury) across the pulmonary or systemic vascular beds by the blood flow index (expressed in liters per minute per square meter) across those respective beds. By 6 to 8 weeks, it usually has reached the normal adult level (1 to 3 Wood units). These changes are accompanied by a gradual dilatation of the smaller followed by the larger muscular pulmonary arteries. In the weeks and months that follow, a thinning of the muscular walls occurs, with the growth of existing arteries and the development of new arteries and arterioles. The latter process contributes more than 90 percent of the smaller or intraacinar pulmonary arterial vessels present in older children and adults.[37]

Increased pulmonary arterial pressure has an adverse effect on the normal maturation of the pulmonary vascular bed. Such pressure encourages a persistence of the thick muscular medial layer present in the smaller pulmonary arteries of term newborns, stimulates an extension of smooth muscle into smaller and more peripheral arteries than normal for age, and retards the growth of existing acinar arteries and the development of new ones.

In the presence of a large systemic-to-pulmonary communication, pulmonary arterial pressures remain at or near systemic levels, with the result that the diminution in pulmonary muscle mass and pulmonary resistance is less rapid and of a lesser magnitude than in a normal infant. Nevertheless, the diminution is usually sufficient to permit a large pulmonary blood flow and, as a result, congestive failure by the end of the first month. Exceptions are found among infants with a large systemic-to-pulmonary communication but with alveolar hypoxia—a stimulus for pulmonary vasoconstriction—in whom there is less than normal involution of the medial musculature and a diminution in pulmonary vascular resistance. Clinically, this is expressed by the lower incidence of congestive failure observed among infants with large VSDs born and living at high altitude. It is also seen in some children with Down syndrome, and a large VSD or AV canal who may hypoventilate or have upper airway obstruction. Rarely, an infant will maintain a very high pulmonary vascular resistance in the face of an anatomically large systemic-to-pulmonary communication without evidence of significant hypoxemia or acidemia and remain free of the signs and symptoms of congestive failure. Conversely, in a premature infant in whom the medial muscle mass is less at birth than it is in a full-term infant, the fall in pulmonary vascular resistance is usually much more rapid than normal.

Chronic PAH, increased flow, or both produce a characteristic series of histologic changes in the smaller pulmonary arteries and arterioles originally described and graded by Heath and Edwards (grades I through VI below; Fig. 82–4)[38] and by Rabinovitch[37] (grades A through C below):

- Grade I: medial hypertrophy
- Grade II: concentric or eccentric cellular intimal proliferation
- Grade III: relatively acellular intimal fibrosis with occlusion of the smaller pulmonary arteries and arterioles
- Grade IV: progressive, generalized dilatation of the distal muscular arteries and the appearance of plexiform lesions, complex vascular structures composed of a network or plexus of proliferating endothelial tissue, frequently accompanied by thrombus, within a dilated thin-walled sac
- Grade V: thinning and fibrosis of the media superimposed on the plexiform lesions

- Grade VI: necrotizing arteritis within the media
- Grade A: extension of muscle into normally nonmuscular peripheral arteries with or without a mild increase in medial wall thickness of normally muscular arteries (less than 1.5 times normal)
- Grade B: extension of muscle as described above with an even greater increase in medial wall thickness of normally muscular arteries (mild: 1.5–2 × normal; severe: >2 × normal)
- Grade C: changes seen in grade B (severe) but with a decreased arterial concentration relative to alveoli (mild: ≥^{1}/$_2$ normal; severe: <^{1}/$_2$ normal)
- Grades A and B are partitions of Heath-Edwards grade I and may be seen with large left-to-right shunts with (B) or without increased pressure (A). Grade C criteria may be found with grades I and II, are invariable with grade III, and usually preclude a complete return to normal of pulmonary arterial pressures and resistance despite successful surgical correction of the systemic-to-pulmonary communication.

Estimation of pulmonary vascular resistance from data obtained at cardiac catheterization remains the most widely used means of assessing the state of the pulmonary vascular bed. Hypoxemia from oversedation, atelectasis, or pneumonitis at the time of study should be scrupulously avoided. If pulmonary vascular resistance is elevated, responsiveness to vasodilation induced by the inhalation of 100 percent oxygen, the pulmonary arterial administration of prostacyclin, or the inhalation of nitric oxide should be tested.[39]

Values of R_p ≤3 Wood units are considered normal. The status of the pulmonary vasculature also can be expressed as a ratio of pulmonary vascular resistance to systemic vascular resistance (R_p/R_s). *Pulmonary/systemic resistance ratios less than 0.2:1 are considered normal.*

As pulmonary vascular resistance increases, pulmonary blood flow generally decreases. Eventually, a point is reached where surgical closure of the defect will produce only a small diminution of blood flow, a proportionately small decrease in pulmonary arterial pressure, and no significant change in the factors contributing to the progression of vascular disease. At this point surgery usually is not recommended, as the benefits are minimal and closure of the defect may eliminate a useful "blow-off" for increasing resistance. *An R_p/R_s ratio of 0.7:1 or an R_p of 11 Wood units with a pulmonary-to-systemic blood flow ratio of 1.5:1 is the criterion generally used to define this situation.* Without surgery, these patients survive as examples of

the Eisenmenger syndrome, in which $R_p ≥ R_s$ and at least some right-to-left shunting occurs at rest or with exercise. Some of these patients can survive for several decades and lead productive lives, with relatively mild symptoms and few limitations.[40]

The decision regarding surgery for patients with less-severe PVOD is a clinical one. The higher the calculated resistance, the greater the structural changes in the pulmonary vasculature (as judged by lung biopsy or quantitative pulmonary arterial wedge angiography), and the older the patient with any given level of elevated resistance or grade of structural change, the less likely it is that the outcome of surgery will be satisfactory.[37]

The prevention of PVOD requires the identification of the patients at risk—that is, all patients with a systemic-to-pulmonary communication and a pulmonary arterial systolic pressure higher than half the systemic arterial systolic pressure. Also included are all patients with transposition, regardless of pressure or flow, with the possible exception of those with severe pulmonary stenosis. Ideally, all patients at risk should undergo correction of the lesion or protection of the pulmonary arterial bed within the first year of life unless there is proof that the pulmonary arterial systolic pressure has fallen

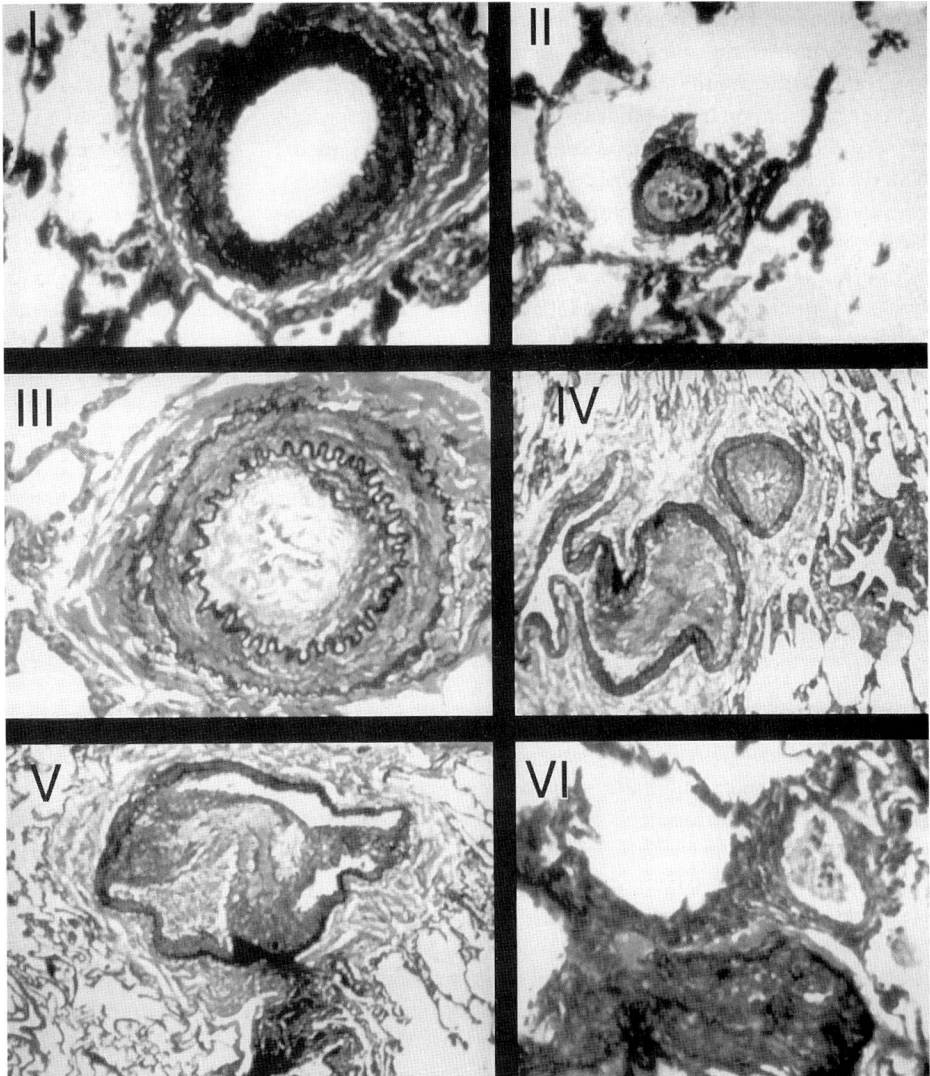

FIGURE 82–4. Pulmonary vascular changes by the Heath and Edwards criteria (see text). Grades 1 to 6 are represented by panels I to VI, respectively.

to or is less than half the systemic systolic pressure among those with normally related great arteries. Among patients with transposition with a large VSD or patent ductus arteriosus, action must be taken within the first 3 months of life.

【 】 LONG-TERM PROBLEMS WITH SURGICALLY CORRECTED DEFECTS

With advances in the surgical treatment of congenital heart defects, more patients are living to adulthood. This discussion of potential long-term problems is intended for those who follow these children after surgery and through adult life[41] (see Chaps. 74 and 83). Residua, sequelae, and complications result from most surgical procedures for congenital heart defects. A residual part of the original defect, such as mitral prolapse in repaired ASD, may purposefully not have been approached surgically. Some sequelae are unavoidable consequences of the intervention, such as pulmonary regurgitation after balloon dilation valvuloplasty or surgical valvotomy. There are also complications that occur as unexpected but related events after successful surgery, such as late complete heart block. When viewed with these possibilities in mind, only surgical ligation or coil occlusion of a PDA is likely to result in no long-term problems.

Most patients have residual murmurs after surgery for congenital heart defects. Determination of the origin of these murmurs and evaluation of the severity of the hemodynamic abnormalities they represent are important. Noninvasive diagnostic tools, especially two-dimensional echocardiography and Doppler, are often useful. The risk of infective endocarditis to patients persists after surgery, with the exception of those who have undergone patent ductus ligation or division or repair of an ASD or VSD in whom there is no residual shunt. Patients in whom it has been necessary to place an artificial valve are at increased risk of endocarditis.[42,43]

There are specific problems related to some of the more common defects. For those with repaired ASDs, VSDs, and AV (canal) septal defects, a residual shunt may be present, but ordinarily it is small and not hemodynamically significant. Those with repaired AV canal defects may have important AV valve regurgitation. Repaired coarctation of the aorta can gradually become narrowed again, or patients may develop systemic hypertension. Intervention for valvular pulmonary stenosis usually results in mild residual stenosis and regurgitation, which are well tolerated and have little tendency to progress with time. The natural history of valvular aortic stenosis after intervention is not as benign.[44,45] Significant regurgitation must be avoided, so the initial results may not be as good in terms of the severity of residual stenosis. In addition, because aortic stenosis tends to worsen with time, proper followup is mandatory for these patients.

Few patients enter adulthood with the continued problem of cyanosis, as those with defects amenable to surgical correction should have had surgery well before this time. Only patients with complex and irreparable defects and those with pulmonary vascular disease should experience problems of cyanosis during the adult years. Particularly important among these patients is management of any attendant psychosocial problems (employment, insurability,[46] and learning disabilities) and difficulties related to pregnancy.[47] Those who have had surgery for cyanotic defects are more likely to have sequelae and complications. Some degree of exercise intolerance is not unusual in this group of patients, and exercise stress testing aids in their management.[48]

Dysrhythmias are particularly common among these patients. *In patients who have had intraventricular repairs, most commonly for tetralogy of Fallot, late complete heart block and serious ventricular arrhythmias can occur and may result in sudden death.*[49] This risk appears to be highest in those who had transient complete heart block at the time of surgery and who develop right bundle-branch block with left anterior hemiblock after surgery. Extensive intraatrial surgical procedures for transposition of the great arteries also frequently lead to dysrhythmias, most commonly sick sinus syndrome with brady-tachyarrhythmias and atrial flutter, with a high incidence of sudden death.[50] Ambulatory 24-hour ECG monitoring (see Chap. 41), stress testing (see Chap. 14), and intracardiac electrophysiologic studies[51] are important in following patients who have had complex repairs. Atrial enlargement after the Fontan operation has resulted in atrial flutter and/or fibrillation, which are frequently therapeutically challenging.[52]

Serious ventricular dysfunction[53] and venous obstruction also may occur. Despite intraatrial baffle repairs for transposition of the great arteries, the anatomic right ventricle must perform systemic work leading to potential compromise of ventricular performance.[54] In addition, these repairs may lead to pulmonary and/or systemic venous obstruction. Atriopulmonary and more recently cavopulmonary connections for the repair of tricuspid atresia and many types of univentricular hearts frequently leave an anatomically abnormal ventricle as the systemic ventricle. In this group of patients, the absence of a ventricle on the pulmonary side of the circulation results in elevated systemic venous pressure, systemic venous hypertension, and possible protein-losing enteropathy.[55]

Finally, some children have had repairs with synthetic prostheses. Because artificial valves cannot keep pace with somatic growth of the child, long-term stability is critical. Conduits with or without valves placed at surgery can degenerate or become obstructive. *Bioprosthetic valves undergo accelerated fibrosis and calcification in patients younger than about 30 to 35 years of age.* In spite of these problems, the majority of patients who reach adulthood after surgical repair of congenital defects are relatively asymptomatic; they can and do lead productive lives.

INTRACARDIAC COMMUNICATIONS BETWEEN THE SYSTEMIC AND PULMONARY CIRCULATIONS, USUALLY WITHOUT CYANOSIS

【 】 VENTRICULAR SEPTAL DEFECT

Pathology and Incidence

A VSD is the most common congenital cardiac anomaly. It may be an isolated defect or part of a complex malformation. Approximately 80 percent of these defects are paramembranous but may extend into the inlet, trabecular, or outlet sections of the muscular septum. Less common are conal septal or subarterial doubly committed defects (5 to 7 percent), inlet defects lying beneath the septal leaflet of the tricuspid valve in the region of the atrioventricular canal (5 to 8 percent), and defects in the muscular septum that may be in the inlet, trabecular, or outlet area (Fig. 82–5).[56] Multiple muscular defects are not infrequently seen.

The incidence of VSDs is about 2 per 1000 livebirths, and its prevalence among school-age children has been estimated as 1 per 1000, constituting about one-quarter of the congenital cardiac malformations in combined series (see Table 82–1). Males and females are affected equally.

VSDs may be isolated or associated with other congenital cardiac abnormalities. Malformations associated with VSD are, in order of decreasing frequency, (1) coarctation of the aorta, (2) additional shunts, most commonly ASD and PDA, (3) intracardiac obstructions such as subpulmonary or subaortic stenosis, mitral stenosis, and anomalous muscle bundle of the right ventricle, and (4) incompetent atrioventricular valves.

Abnormal Physiology

The consequences of a VSD depend on the size of the defect and the pulmonary vascular resistance. A small defect offers a large resistance to flow. There is no elevation of right ventricular or pulmonary arterial pressure, and the left-to-right shunt may be so small that it can be detected only by two-dimensional imaging with Doppler color-flow mapping or selective left ventricular angiography. This type of defect imposes little physiologic burden on the heart, although patients are always at risk for infective endocarditis. A defect of moderate size permits a difference between the right and left ventricular systolic pressures but may allow a large left-to-right shunt with resulting left atrial hypertension and dilatation and left ventricular volume overload. The development of pulmonary vascular disease among these patients is unusual but possible.

When the effective area of the defect is large (equal to or greater than the aortic valve orifice), the defect offers virtually no resistance to flow and systolic pressures are present in the ventricles, the aorta, and the pulmonary artery. The relative resistance of the two vascular beds directly governs the proportion of blood entering the two circulations. At birth, pulmonary vascular resistance is high and there is little if any left-to-right shunt despite the presence of a large defect. This resistance to flow gradually falls over the first few weeks of life, permitting a progressively greater amount of blood to flow through

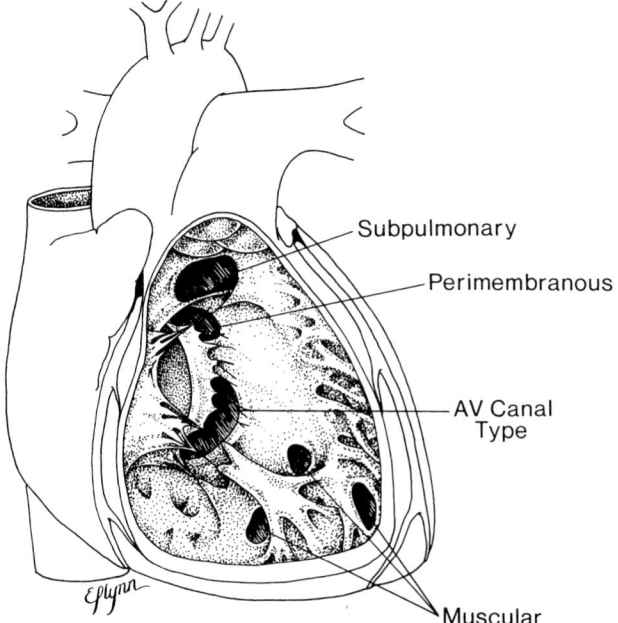

FIGURE 82–5. Different types of ventricular septal defects when viewed from the right ventricle. *Source: From Freed MD. Fetal and transitional circulation. In: Fyler DC, ed.[5] Reproduced with permission from the publisher and author.*

the defect, through the lungs, and back to the left atrium and left ventricle. In most infants, the left ventricular volume overload eventually leads to left ventricular "failure" with elevated left ventricular end-diastolic and left atrial pressures and pulmonary congestion.

History Infants or children with a small isolated defect are asymptomatic. The murmur of a small defect may be detected within the first 24 to 36 hours of life, as the very restrictive opening permits the normal rapid fall in pulmonary arterial resistance and pressures. In term infants born at sea level with a large VSD, clinical deterioration may occur at any time from about 3 to 12 weeks after birth. In premature infants, in whom the less-well-developed pulmonary vascular hypertrophy regresses more rapidly, failure frequently is noted at 1 to 4 weeks. Parents describe tachypnea, grunting respirations, and fatigue, particularly with feedings. Weight gain is slow, and excessive sweating is common.

Physical Examination A child with a small defect is comfortable. With moderate holes, a systolic thrill at the lower left sternal border is common. If the defect is small, the pulmonary artery pressure is normal, so the second heart sound is not accentuated. The systolic murmur along the lower left sternal border is characteristically holosystolic but may be limited to early or midsystole. This latter feature suggests a defect in the muscular septum rather than the membranous septum.

Infants with large defects, large left-to-right shunt, and PAH tend to be restless, irritable, and underweight. Moderate respiratory distress may be present. Both the right and the left ventricular systolic impulses are impressively hyperdynamic to palpation. A thrill at the lower left sternal border is common. The second heart sound is narrowly split, with a loud, frequently palpable pulmonary component. Third heart sound gallops at the apex are common. Characteristically, the systolic murmur is holosystolic at the lower left sternal border and is accompanied by a middiastolic rumble of grade 2 to 3 intensity at the apex, with the latter indicating a pulmonary-to-systemic blood flow ratio ($\dot{Q}_p/\dot{Q}_s$) of 2:1 or greater. Hepatic enlargement can be identified below the right costal margin. Pulmonary rales may be heard with severe failure.

With the passage of time, one may observe signs of a diminishing left-to-right shunt with an improved rate of weight gain, less dyspnea, diminution of the precordial hyperactivity, and disappearance of the apical diastolic flow rumble. This clinical improvement may be a result of the defect becoming smaller, the development of subvalvular pulmonary stenosis with little or no appreciable change in the size of the defect, or, most worrisome, the development of PVOD with continued severe PAH. With developing subpulmonary stenosis, the systolic murmur radiates more and more impressively to the upper left sternal border and the second heart sound becomes more widely split, with a progressive diminution in the intensity of the pulmonary component. Decreased flow resulting from pulmonary vascular disease is characterized by a gradual reduction in the intensity and duration of the systolic murmur, more narrow splitting of the second heart sound, and marked accentuation of the pulmonary component.

The clinical picture of advanced pulmonary vascular disease secondary to a congenital left-to-right shunt, or Eisenmenger syndrome, is that of a relatively comfortable older child, adolescent, or young adult with mild cyanosis and clubbing in whom one finds a prominent *a* wave in the jugular venous pulse, a mild right ventricular lift, and a second heart sound that is narrowly split or virtually single with a very loud, usually palpable pulmonary component. An early pulmonary systolic ejection sound reflecting dilatation of the main pulmonary artery may be present, and there may be no systolic murmur at all. In older adolescents and adults, an early diastolic murmur of pulmonary regurgitation or a holosystolic murmur of tricuspid regurgitation may appear.

Chest Roentgenogram In the presence of a small defect, the heart's size and shape and the pulmonary blood flow are barely altered. With large defects, there is moderate to marked enlargement of the heart, with prominence of the main pulmonary arterial segment and impressive overcirculation in the peripheral lung fields. The left atrium is dilated unless an associated ASD is present, allowing decompression of the left atrium. With increasing pulmonary vascular disease, there is diminution in heart size toward normal, while the central pulmonary arteries remain dilated. The peripheral pulmonary arterial markings become attenuated, and a "pruned" effect is produced in the outer third of the lung fields.

Electrocardiogram With a small defect, one can expect the normal progression of the mean QRS axis from right to left and the normal gradual decrease of the prominent right ventricular voltages characteristic of newborns. The left ventricular forces remain within normal limits or become slightly augmented as a reflection of the mild left ventricular volume overload. With large defects, the mean QRS axis tends to remain oriented to the right and there is little or no regression in right ventricular voltage. The left ventricular forces gradually increase, resulting in a pattern of biventricular hypertrophy within the first few weeks of life. Left atrial enlargement is usually present, as is right atrial enlargement. With the development of pulmonary vascular disease or significant pulmonary stenosis, the mean QRS axis tends to remain oriented to the right; there is no regression in right ventricular voltage, but the evidence of left ventricular and left atrial hypertrophy lessens or disappears.

Echocardiogram Two-dimensional imaging can distinguish an uncomplicated VSD from more complex malformations and is capable of imaging most defects directly when multiple transducer positions are used. The addition of pulsed-wave Doppler with color-flow mapping permits the identification of small, multiple, muscular, and other less easily visualized defects. The position and size of the opening can be determined as well as its relationships to the aorta, pulmonary artery, and AV valves. Continuous-wave Doppler echocardiography can predict the systolic right ventricular pressure from the difference between the systolic pressure measured by a blood pressure cuff, if there is no aortic stenosis, and the Doppler gradient (Fig. 82–6). In the absence of associated pulmonic stenosis, the right ventricular systolic pressure provides an estimate of the pulmonary artery pressure. Right ventricular systolic pressure also can be estimated by measuring the right ventricular to right atrial systolic pressure gradient across the tricuspid valve in the presence of tricuspid regurgitation.[57]

Cardiac Catheterization Though cardiac catheterization is performed infrequently in infants with isolated VSDs, these studies show an increase in oxygen saturation at the right ventricular level, reflecting the left-to-right ventricular shunt. With small defects, the right ventricular and pulmonary arterial systolic pressures are normal. With large defects, these pressures are at or near systemic levels, and the mean left atrial pressure may be elevated to the range of 10 to 15 mmHg.

Selective left ventricular angiography in the anteroposterior, lateral, and oblique views with craniocaudal angulation are used to establish

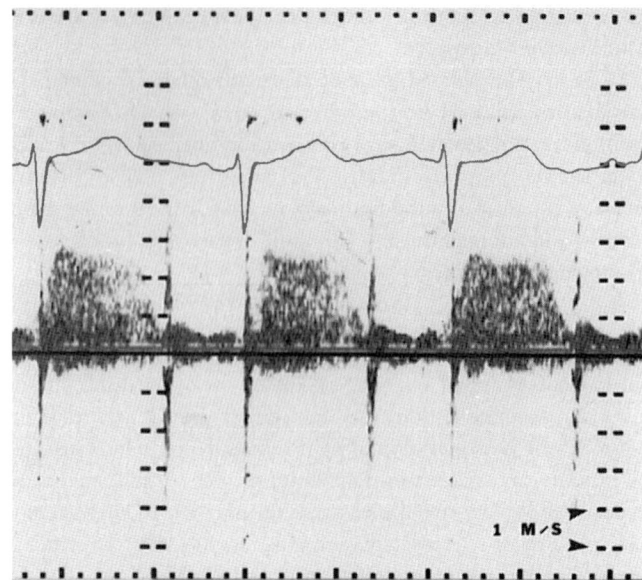

FIGURE 82–6. Continuous-wave Doppler with spectral display from the left lower sternal border of a child with a ventricular septal defect that demonstrates holosystolic turbulence with peak velocity = 2.8 m/s across the defect, compatible with an instantaneous systolic pressure difference of 31 mmHg between the right and left ventricles.

the spatial relations of the great arteries to each other, to the ventricles and also to determine the exact site, size, and number of septal defects (Fig. 82–7). Aortography is helpful in eliminating the possibility of an associated ductus arteriosus or unsuspected coarctation of the aorta if the arch cannot be well imaged by echocardiography.

Natural History and Prognosis

Fortunately, the majority of VSDs are small and do not present a serious clinical problem. Approximately 25 percent of these small defects close spontaneously by 18 months, 50 percent by 4 years, and 75 percent by 10 years.[58] A spontaneous closure rate approaching 45 percent within the first 12 to 14 months has been observed among infants with an uncomplicated paramembranous or muscular VSD in the neonatal period.[59] Even large defects tend to become smaller, but the likelihood of eventual spontaneous closure is much lower (probably in the range of 60 percent if judged large at 3 months of age, and only 50 percent if it is still large at 6 months).[58]

Congestive failure is an almost inevitable complication of a large VSD. Approximately 80 percent of infants with large defects require hospitalization by age 4 months.[3] The risk of death with congestive failure is in the range of 11 percent. Significant subvalvular pulmonary stenosis develops in approximately 3 percent of these individuals and may progress to right-to-left shunting at the ventricular level. Associated pulmonary arterial hypertension is generally reversible in the first 12 months of life; thereafter, it becomes progressively less likely to regress. Infants and children with a pulmonary systolic pressure in excess of 50 percent of the systemic arterial systolic pressure beyond the first year of life are at risk for this complication.[60] A very small number of infants with large VSDs maintain a high level of pulmonary vascular resistance throughout the first year of life and remain almost entirely free of symptoms of heart failure. In these patients, irreversible pulmonary vascular disease may develop without the usual and expected clinical signs and symptoms described above.

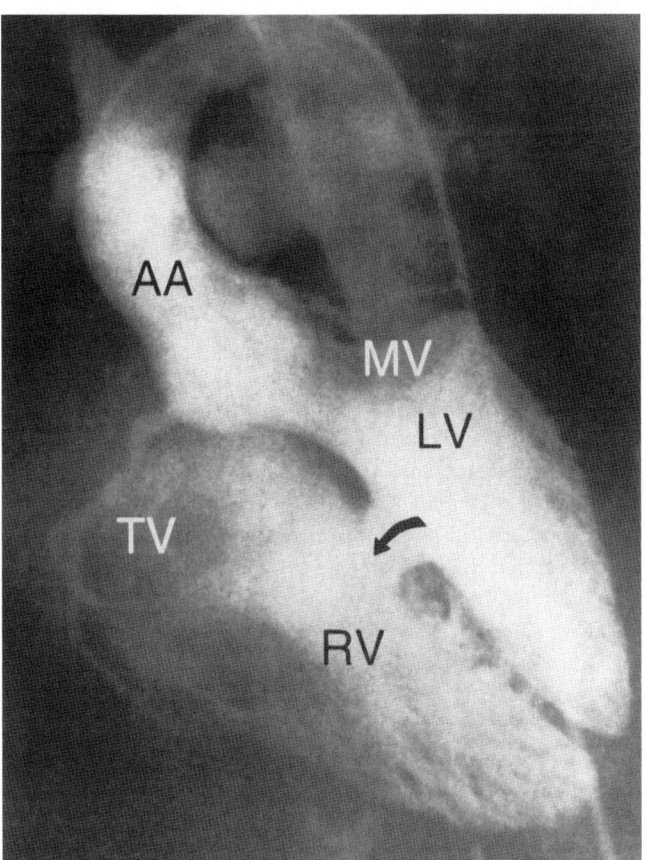

FIGURE 82-7. Multiple trabecular ventricular septal defects (VSDs). Retrograde left ventriculogram, four-chamber projection, profiles the mitral and tricuspid valves and the midtrabecular VSD (*arrow*). Additional VSDs closer to the apex are more anterior in location and are not profiled in this projection. AA, ascending aorta; LV, left ventricle; MV, mitral valve; RV, right ventricle; TV, tricuspid valve. *Source: From Lock JE, Keane JF, Perry SB. Diagnostic and Interventional Catheterization in Congenital Heart Disease, 2d. ed. Boston: Kluwer, 2000. Reproduced with permission from the publisher and authors.*

A small number of children, 0.6 percent in a large group of carefully followed patients, develop aortic regurgitation as a result of prolapse of the right, the posterior, or both aortic valve leaflets into the defect.[61] This complication is more prevalent among males than females, in a ratio of 2:1, and seems particularly likely to occur with defects of the subpulmonary type, but is also seen with perimembranous VSDs. Shunt size appears not to be related to the development of this complication. The characteristic aortic diastolic murmur may appear at any time between ages 6 months and 20 years. Regurgitation is usually progressive, sometimes rapidly so, and predisposes these individuals to infective endocarditis.

The risk of infective endocarditis in patients with an uncomplicated VSD that is managed medically lies somewhere between 4 and 10 percent for the first 30 years of life.[62] The development of aortic regurgitation more than doubles this risk. Attempts at surgical closure of the defect with or without aortic regurgitation reduce the risk to less than half that of unoperated patients.[63]

Medical Management

The basis of the medical management of children with VSDs is an understanding that defects frequently narrow and may close spontaneously. Approximately 70 percent of small VSDs probably close.[58] Even large muscular defects may get significantly smaller, and up to 25 percent of them will become hemodynamically insignificant if one can wait long enough. Nevertheless, significant complications can occur, and the decision whether to proceed with medical or surgical management must be reevaluated constantly.

For children with a large VSD, the first decision point usually occurs before 8 to 12 weeks of age. Infants with large septal defects generally develop significant left-to-right shunts as the pulmonary resistance drops. Congestive heart failure ensues with tachypnea, tachycardia, and difficulty feeding. Digoxin and diuretics are occasionally useful, but if the left-to-right shunt is very large, feeding may be problematic. For children who cannot gain weight of at least 15 g per day (30 g per day is normal) in whom no other cause is found for failure to thrive, surgical repair is indicated. Occasionally, in marginal cases, increasing the caloric density of the formula from 20 calories per ounce to as much as 32 calories per ounce may promote weight gain, which often requires 150 kcal/kg or more on a daily basis. In children unable to take more than 10 to 12 ounces per day, however, caloric supplementation is unlikely to be sufficient and surgical repair is necessary.

The second decision point in children who do thrive occurs between 9 and 12 months of age. Children with unrestrictive or mildly restrictive VSDs have pulmonary artery hypertension that may lead to irreversible pulmonary vascular obstructive disease. If the pulmonary artery pressure is elevated at 9 to 12 months of age, surgery is indicated to prevent this serious life-shortening complication. In some children, the high-pitched nature of the murmur, the normal pulmonary component of the second heart sound, the absence of right ventricular hypertrophy on ECG, and the large intraventricular pressure gradient on echocardiography support the presence of normal pulmonary artery pressure. Infrequently, in children in whom the signs, symptoms, and laboratory findings are ambiguous or conflicting, cardiac catheterization may be necessary to assure that the pulmonary artery pressure is normal and that pulmonary vascular obstructive disease is not a risk.

The third decision point occurs somewhere between 5 to 10 years of age. Although the defect has not caused failure to thrive or pulmonary hypertension, it may still produce a significant left-to-right shunt, causing a volume overload of the left ventricle. Eventually, heart failure is possible, and some clinicians recommend surgical closure during childhood if there is a significant volume overload. There is no firm number that suggests a dangerous level of left ventricular volume overload. Some centers close the VSD when the pulmonary-to-systemic flow ratio (measured by cardiac catheterization, radionuclide angiography, echocardiography, or magnetic resonance imaging) is more than 2:1. Others use significant left atrial and left ventricular dilation by echo. A minority of centers do not recommend surgical closure as long as the pulmonary artery pressure is normal as there are few adults with a VSD who develop late congestive heart failure.

Unfortunately, not all patients with a large defect are encountered during the first or second year of life, when it is possible to prevent injury to the pulmonary vascular bed. If significant PAH is allowed to persist, one can expect progression to irreversible pulmonary obstructive disease. For this reason, with late presentation, *prompt surgical closure of defects is recommended in all individuals older than the age of 2 years if the pulmonary arterial systolic pressure is greater than half the systemic arterial systolic pressure, the mean pulmonary pressure exceeds 25 mmHg, or the R_p/R_s ratio is higher than 0.3:1.* With severe pulmonary vascular disease, a point eventually is reached where the risk of death at operation or in the months or years immediately after the operation as a result of progressive vascular disease more than offsets the possible benefits from surgical closure. At present, surgery is recommended if the calculated R_p is less than 10 Wood units/m^2 or the R_p/R_s ratio is 0.7:1, provided that the $\dot{Q}_p/\dot{Q}_s$ ratio is still 1.5:1. In adults, the upper limit of pulmonary vascular resistance for surgery is approximately 10 Wood units. Patients in whom the defect is judged clinically to be small at 6 months of age may be reexamined at 1- or 2-year intervals to reassure the patient and family, reemphasize the importance of antibiotic protection against infective endocarditis, document further narrowing or closure of the defect, and (in a very small number of patients) detect the first signs of aortic valve prolapse.

In patients with Eisenmenger complex,[40] stamina is limited by systemic arterial hypoxemia and, in some, right-sided heart failure. Complications to be anticipated include syncope, hemoptysis, brain abscess, hyperuricemia, and congestive failure. Pregnancy, with a maternal mortality of 30 to 60 percent, and oral contraceptives are contraindicated. Transient symptomatic relief from extreme polycythemia (usually >65 percent) may be achieved with careful erythropheresis. Travel to or living at high altitudes is poorly tolerated, and supplemental oxygen should be provided and used during air travel. A recent study reports that the average age of death for individuals with Eisenmenger complex related to VSD is 43 years, with heart failure the cause of death in the majority.[64.]

The risk of congenital heart disease for a subsequent sibling of a single affected child is on the order of 1 to 2 percent. The risk to a newborn of a parent with VSD increases to 3 percent.[65] Pregnancy in the presence of a small defect and normal pulmonary vascular resistance does not appear to carry an increased risk to the patient or infant, although precautions against infective endocarditis should be taken.

Surgical Management

Previously, banding of the pulmonary artery to reduce pulmonary blood flow and pressures played an important role in the management of congestive heart failure and the prevention of PVOD. Now that surgical closure of VSDs in infancy is nearly uniformly successful, banding is used rarely. Complications of pulmonary arterial banding include deformity of the pulmonary arteries and/or pulmonary valve, progressive right ventricular hypertrophy with loss of ventricular compliance, and the development of subaortic left ventricular outflow tract obstruction.

VSDs are closed using cardiopulmonary bypass with cardioplegic arrest and moderate systemic hypothermia. Total circulatory arrest or minimal perfusion with profound hypothermia (64.4°F [18°C]) is sometimes necessary in infants who weigh less than 5 kg (11 lb).[66,67] Perimembranous VSDs may be exposed through the right atrium and the tricuspid valve orifice. A transverse or longitudinal right ventriculotomy may be necessary for closure of high conal septal defects associated with aortic valve leaflet prolapse.

Care is required to prevent injury to the AV node near the ostium of the coronary sinus and to the bundle of His as it courses inferiorly, passing on the left side of the ventricular septum near the posterocaudal margin of the septal defect. Intraoperative transesophageal echocardiography with Doppler color-flow assessment can be used for the detection of significant residual shunting or previously unsuspected problems that may be corrected in the operating room.

Results from primary surgical closure of VSDs are generally excellent. Surgical mortality is less than 1 percent in centers with extensive experience, when surgery is performed during the early months of life prior to the evolution of PVOD. Operative risk should be even lower in older children if the pulmonary vascular resistance remains low. The pulmonary vascular bed responds favorably when the systemic-to-pulmonary shunt is eliminated before age 2 years. Normal life expectancy and functional capabilities should be anticipated postoperatively. Survival 25 years after the closure of a VSD is approximately 95 percent.[67] The mortality rate is unquestionably higher among patients who are operated on with R_p >7 Wood units. In such cases, surgeons have employed fenestrated patch closure, which retains a restrictive ventricular communication to provide a "pop-off" right-to-left shunt postoperatively. In the setting of suprasystemic pulmonary artery pressure, the physiologic intent is to maintain systemic cardiac output while reducing the potential for right ventricular failure.

The surgical repair of a multiple muscular VSD has been more problematic. The highly trabecular right ventricular septal surface can make the localization of all the defects difficult. A new approach has achieved successful closure from a right ventricular apical infundibulotomy.[68,69] Devices now approved by the U.S. Food and Drug Administration (FDA) are available to close these defects in the catheterization laboratory.

Between February 1989 and July 2004, 170 attempts at transcatheter closures were performed at Children's Hospital in Boston, with no deaths and minimal morbidity resulting from catheter-related events. By echocardiography, 83 percent of the defects were closed or had trivial residual leaks.[70] More recently, devices specifically designed to close perimembranous VSDs have been used in experimental protocols. Good closure rate and significant reduction in shunt size has been reported, but the potential for adverse events will require more data to determine the benefit relative to surgical closure.[71] In a novel approach, closure of muscular septal defects using devices has been accomplished during surgical repair in so-called *hybrid procedures*, both for isolated muscular VSDs and for those found in combination with other complex lesions.[72]

【 】 ATRIAL SEPTAL DEFECT
Definition

An ASD is a communication between the atria at the septal level. It is to be distinguished from a patent foramen ovale, which may persist into adulthood.

Pathology

ASDs are usually sufficiently large to allow free communication between the atria. They may be subdivided according to anatomic location (Fig. 82–8).[73]

Anatomic Types

Defect at the Fossa Ovalis (Ostium Secundum) This defect classically involves the region of the fossa ovalis and is the most common type (70 percent; see Fig. 82–8A and C).[73,74] Atrial septal tissue separates the inferior edge of the defect from the AV valves. Associated partial anomalous pulmonary venous connections are not uncommon, with one or more of the right pulmonary veins draining into the right atrium or one of its tributaries. Mitral valve prolapse is present in some cases.

Partial Atrioventricular Canal Defects Defects of the AV septum, which lies inferior to the fossa ovalis, constitute approximately 20 percent of ASDs and are part of a complex malformation known as *common atrioventricular canal defects*, which are considered below (see Fig. 82–8D).

Sinus Venosus Defects These defects, accounting for approximately 6 percent of the total, appear to represent a biatrial connection of the superior vena cava (or, in rare instances, the inferior vena cava), which straddles the otherwise normal intact atrial septum. Also involved is an anomalous termination of one or more of the right-sided pulmonary veins either into the vena cava or into the right atrium near its junction with the vena cava (Fig. 82–8B).

Coronary Sinus Defects A coronary sinus defect is an uncommon type of ASD located in the position normally occupied by the ostium of the coronary sinus. This defect is part of a developmental complex consisting of the absence of the coronary sinus and entry of the left superior vena cava directly into the left atrium.

Conditions Common to All Anatomic Types The right atrial and ventricular chambers, as well as the central pulmonary arteries, become enlarged. When pulmonary hypertension intervenes, it usually does not do so before the third decade. The earliest lesion is cellular fibrous intimal thickening in the proximal segments of arterioles.

The pulmonary arterial pressure then rises, followed by the development of medial hypertrophy of muscular arteries and the appearance of plexiform lesions. The right ventricular wall hypertrophies, and atherosclerosis may occur in the major pulmonary arteries. Saccular aneurysm and thrombosis with dissecting aneurysm or rupture may occur (see Pulmonary Arterial Hypertension and Pulmonary Vascular Obstructive Disease above). In the final state, the pulmonary vascular bed may be difficult to distinguish from that in VSD with PVOD.

Abnormal Physiology

Usually there is no resistance to blood flow across the defect and no significant pressure difference between the two atria. A left-to-right shunt of blood occurs (Fig. 82–9) because (1) the right atrial system is more distensible than the left, (2) the tricuspid valve is normally more capacious than the mitral valve, and (3) the thinner-walled right ventricular chamber more readily accommodates a larger volume of blood at the same filling pressure than does the left ventricle. A large left-to-right shunt may be found in a neonate or young infant before the right ventricular compliance has had time to change appreciably from that of the left ventricle. Presumably, this shunt occurs because a rapid fall in pulmonary vascular resistance encourages a larger right ventricular stroke volume, a smaller end-systolic volume, and hence an increased ability of the right ventricle to accept a larger volume of blood during the diastolic filling phase of the cardiac cycle.[75] The pulmonary arterial system undergoes normal maturation after birth, with most patients tolerating the large volume load on the right ventricle and pulmonary

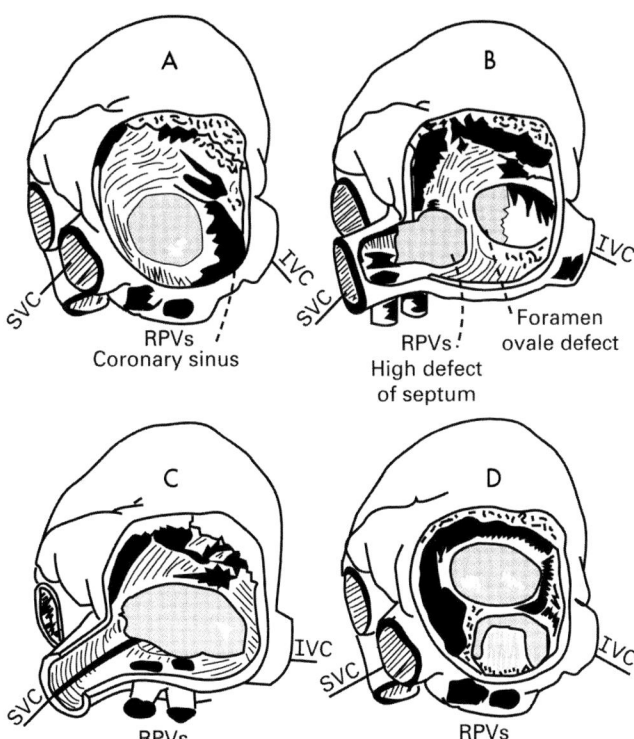

FIGURE 82–8. Types of interatrial communications. **A.** Large ostium secundum type of atrial septal defect. **B.** So-called *sinus venosus* type of defect—one high in the atrial septum associated with anomalous connection of the right superior pulmonary vein to the junctional area of the superior vena cava and right atrium. **C.** Very large ostium secundum type of atrial septal defect with absence of the posterior rim. **D.** Partial form of common atrioventricular canal with cleft mitral valve. IVC, inferior vena cava; RPVs, right pulmonary veins; SVC, superior vena cava. *Source: From Lewis FJ, Winchell P, and Bashour FA.[67] Copyright 1957, American Medical Association. Reproduced with permission from the publisher and authors.*

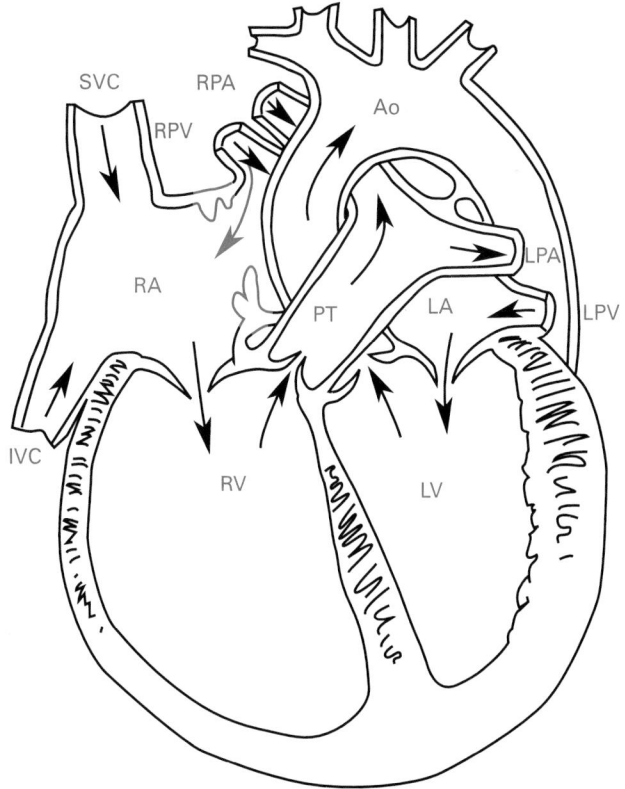

FIGURE 82–9. Atrial septal defect at fossa ovalis with left-to-right shunt. Ao, aorta; IVC, inferior vena cava; LA, left atrium; LPA, left pulmonary artery; LPV, left pulmonary vein; LV, left ventricle; PT, main pulmonary arterial trunk; RA, right atrium; RPA, right pulmonary artery; RPV, right pulmonary vein; RV, right ventricle; SVC, superior vena cava. *Source: From Edwards JE.[74] Reproduced with permission from the publisher and author.*

circuit quite well for many years. With the development of pulmonary vascular disease and PAH, the left-to-right shunt decreases, largely because of the increased thickness and decreased compliance of the right ventricle. In some patients, this process continues until there is eventually shunt reversal, with arterial desaturation and cyanosis.

Clinical Manifestations

ASD is found in approximately 6 percent of children who survive beyond the first year of life with congenital heart disease.[5] *If one excludes mitral valve prolapse and a congenitally bicuspid aortic valve, it is the most common form of congenital heart disease among adults.*

ASDs are more common among females, with a female-to-male ratio of approximately 2:1. The mode of transmission is best explained in most instances on a multifactorial basis, in which the risk would be approximately 2.5 percent for first-degree relatives of a single affected family member. However, examples of autosomal dominant transmission are recognized[76] either as an isolated entity associated with severe AV conduction disturbances or with upper extremity malformations, as in the Holt-Oram syndrome. Examples of mendelian autosomal recessive transmission are found in the Ellis–van Creveld syndrome.

History The majority of these children are considered asymptomatic but probably most have some mild diminution of stamina, because it is not unusual for the patient or the parents to comment on the increased endurance that follows surgical correction. Symptoms of mild fatigue and dyspnea tend to be recognized in the late teens and early twenties, and at least three-quarters of these individuals will be symptomatic as adults. Congestive heart failure is rare in childhood, but a small percentage may have heart failure in the first year of life. Failure becomes more common again in the fourth and fifth decades of life, and is usually associated with the onset of arrhythmias.[77]

Physical Examination Many of these children have a slender habitus, but normal growth and development are the rule. Prominence of the left anterior chest is common, and a hyperdynamic right ventricular systolic lift usually can be felt. Looking at the jugular venous pulse demonstrates that the *v* wave is equal to the *a* wave instead of revealing the normal *a* wave predominance. The first heart sound may be slightly accentuated at the lower left sternal border. The two components of the second heart sound are characteristically widely split, with the interval of splitting fixed despite expiration or the Valsalva maneuver. The pulmonary component of the second heart sound may be accentuated even in the absence of PAH. With increasing pulmonary arterial pressure and resistance, the interval between the aortic and pulmonary components of the second heart sound narrows and the pulmonary component becomes louder, but the lack of respiratory influence on the interval between the two components persists. A midsystolic crescendo–decrescendo murmur of grades 2 to 3 intensity is heard at the left upper sternal border, reflecting increased right ventricular stroke volume and relative pulmonary stenosis. A low- to medium-pitched early diastolic murmur over the lower left sternal border, denoting increased diastolic flow across the tricuspid valve, is present in most individuals with large shunts (see Chap. 78). Cyanosis and clubbing reflect right-to-left shunting. In this setting, the murmurs of tricuspid and pulmonary regurgitation are not uncommon.

Chest Roentgenogram Mild to moderate cardiac enlargement and prominence of the main and branch pulmonary arteries are characteristic. The absence of left atrial displacement of the barium-filled esophagus in the lateral view helps distinguish ASD from large left-to-right shunts at other levels (Fig. 82–10).

Electrocardiogram An rsR⁺ pattern over the right precordium indicating mild right ventricular conduction delay or mild right ventricular hypertrophy is characteristic though not pathognomonic of secundum-type ASD. A qR pattern in this lead is indicative of right ventricular hypertrophy related to right ventricular volume overload. The mean QRS axis in the frontal plane is 90 degrees or greater in 60 percent of patients. Left-axis deviation is common in primum-type ASD. Abnormal leftward *p* axis is often present in sinus venosus-type ASD. Atrial fibrillation and atrial flutter are usually limited to adults.

Echocardiogram M-mode studies reflect volume overload of the right side of the heart with increased right atrial and right ventricular dimensions and paradoxical ventricular septal motion. Two-dimensional and Doppler echocardiography with color-flow mapping (see Chap. 75) permits identification and visualization of secundum, AV canal, and sinus venosus defects. Visualization of anomalous draining pulmonary veins is slightly more difficult. The transesophageal approach offers excellent images for those patients in whom the transthoracic approach is inadequate.[78] Recently three-dimensional (3D) echocardiograms have been shown to provide excellent images of the atrial defects (Fig. 82–11).

Cardiac Catheterization There is a significant increase in oxygen saturation in the blood samples drawn from the right atrium, right ventricle, and pulmonary artery compared with those obtained from the superior or inferior vena cava. Pulmonary arterial and right ventricular systolic pressures are normal or only slightly elevated. A systolic pressure gradient of up to 20 mmHg across the right ventricular outflow tract is accepted as being secondary to flow rather than to anatomic obstruction. The right and left atrial mean and phasic pressures are virtually identical, with little if any elevation above normal (mean pressure gradient <3 mmHg) unless there are associated abnormalities.

Natural History and Prognosis

Defects of the secundum type usually go undetected in the first year or two of life because of the lack of symptoms and the unimpressive auscultatory findings. A soft systolic murmur is the usual reason for referral. Symptoms become more common in persons in their late teens and twenties, and by age 40 years, the majority of these individuals are symptomatic, some severely so.[81] Pulmonary vascular disease with serious pulmonary hypertension begins to make its appearance in persons in their early twenties. *It affects approximately 15 percent of young adults, particularly women, and may be rapidly progressive, especially with pregnancy.* The incidence of atrial fibrillation or flutter also increases with each decade and is closely linked to the onset of congestive failure. Heart failure is the most common cause of death among patients without intervention. Other causes of death include pulmonary embolism or thrombosis, paradoxical emboli, brain abscess, and infection.

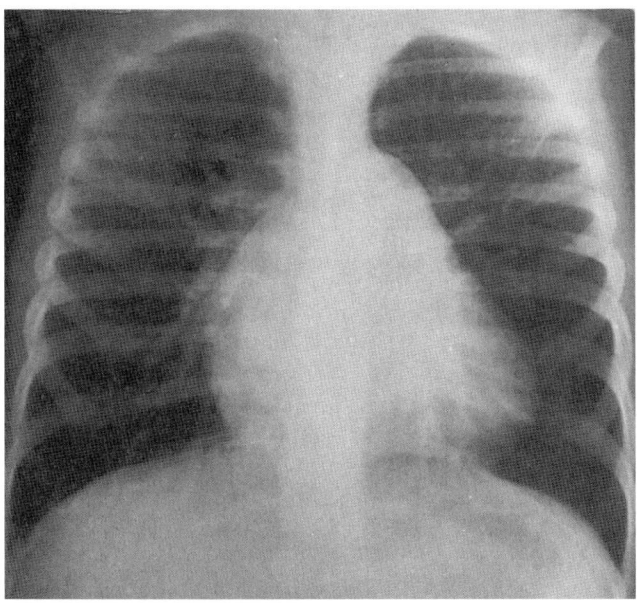
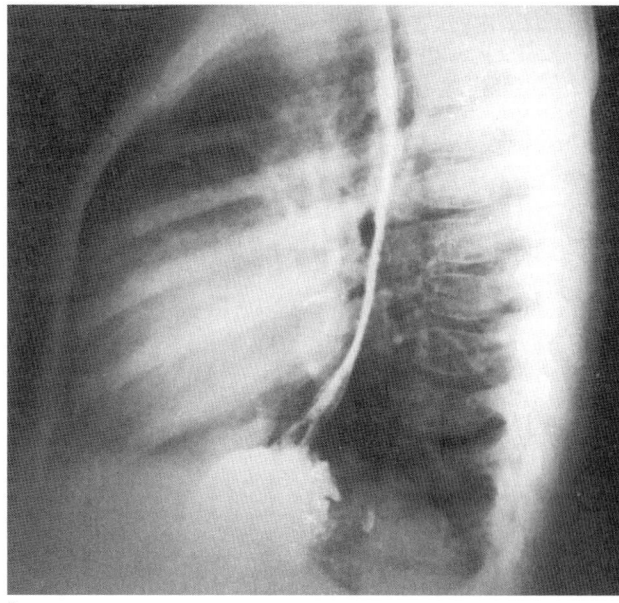

A

B

FIGURE 82–10. Chest roentgenogram of a 4-year-old child with a secundum atrial septal defect, a large left-to-right shunt, and normal pulmonary arterial pressures. **A.** Frontal. **B.** Lateral. Right ventricular enlargement (seen in the lateral view) accompanies prominence of the main pulmonary arterial segment and increased blood flow. No left atrial dilation is present.

Medical Management

The few infants who present with symptoms of congestive failure can be treated with anticongestive therapy. If the defect is uncomplicated and the symptoms persist, surgical closure is advised without further delay. For asymptomatic infants and children, closure is recommended just before entry into school. Restrictions of activity or exercise are unnecessary. If the physical, laboratory, and echocardiographic findings are completely characteristic, preoperative catheterization is unnecessary. Closure is recommended if the defect is associated with right ventricular volume overload on echocardiography. In those with pulmonary hypertension, closure is recommended for patients with $\dot{Q}_p/\dot{Q}_s$ ratios >1.5:1 by catheterization provided that the systemic arterial saturation is >92 percent and total R_p <15 Wood units.[82] Closure is prudent before pregnancy or the use of contraceptives in view of the tendency to develop rapidly progressive PVOD in this setting. Transcatheter closure of centrally located secundum ASDs in older infants, children, and adults using various devices appears to be an acceptable alternative to surgical closure and is now the preferred method in many centers.[83–86] *Infective endocarditis is rare, and antibiotic coverage at times of possible bacteremia is recommended only if associated mitral valve disease is suspected.*

Surgical Management

Defects of the interatrial septum are exposed through the lateral wall of the right atrium. Ostium secundum (fossa ovalis) defects are frequently closed by direct suturing; very large defects or those with tenuous margins are closed with a patch, usually glutaraldehyde-treated autologous pericardium. Anomalous pulmonary veins are sought along the posterolateral aspect of the superior or inferior vena cava and from within the right atrium before closure of the defect. Sutures are placed with care along the posterior rim of the inferior vena caval

orifice to prevent the creation of a tunnel from the inferior vena cava into the left atrium, which would cause postoperative hypoxemia.

High ASDs of the sinus venosus type, which are often associated with anomalous drainage of one or more right pulmonary veins into the superior vena cava, are corrected by means of the placement of a pericardial or tubular Dacron patch from above the abnormally draining vein or veins down to and around the ASD (Fig. 82–12). Pulmonary venous blood thus is diverted through the ASD into the left atrium. Pericardial gusset enlargement of the superior vena cava at the cavoatrial junction may be required. Anomalous right pulmonary veins draining to the right atrium are diverted into the left atrium by placement of a patch baffle well anterior and to the right of

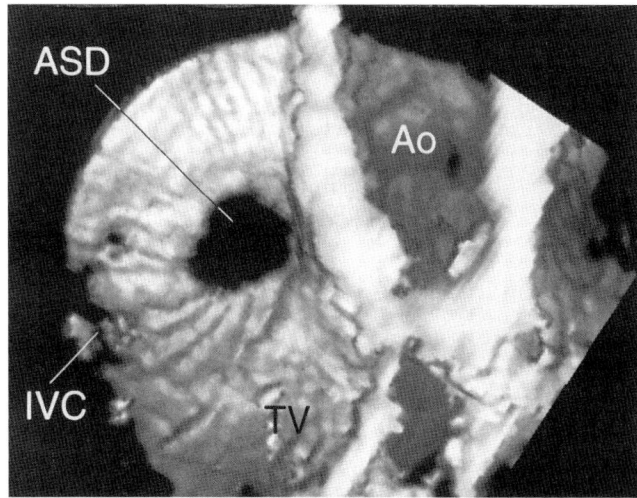

FIGURE 82–11. Three-dimensional echocardiogram of a secundum atrial septal defect (ASD). This is a right atrial en-face view that shows the size, shape, and position of the defect in relation to the right atrial septal surface. Ao, aortic valve; IVC, inferior vena cava; TV, tricuspid valve. *Source: Courtesy of Dr. Gerry Marx.*

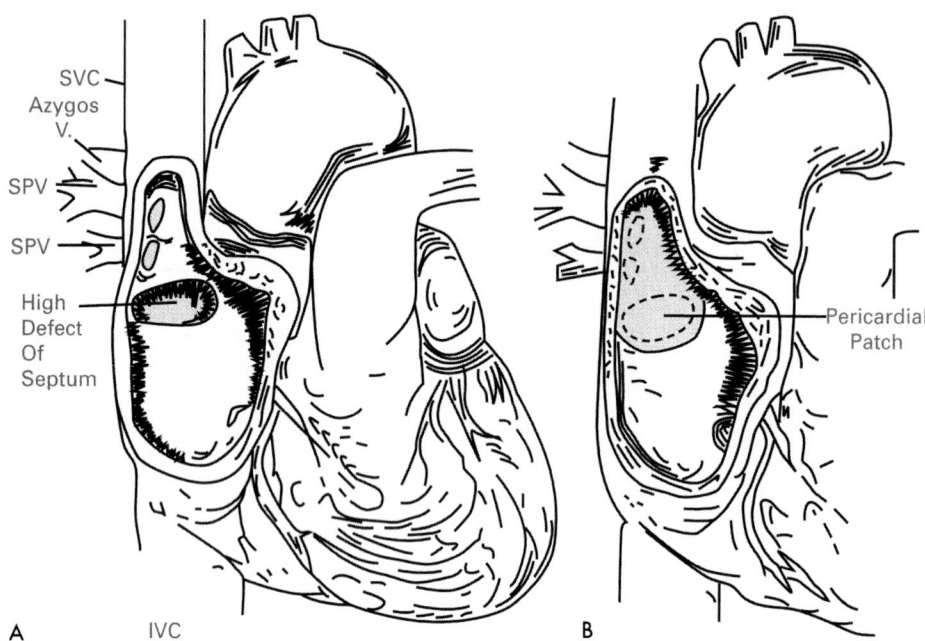

FIGURE 82–12. A. Sinus venosus type of atrial septal defect, with its constantly accompanying anomalous pulmonary venous connection of superior pulmonary vein (SPV) to superior vena cava (SVC). **B.** Repair is accomplished with a pericardial patch placed to divert pulmonary venous blood across the defect into the left atrium and to divert superior vena caval blood to the right atrium. IVC, inferior vena cava. *Source: This illustration appeared originally in the first edition of The Heart, in 1966, and again in all subsequent editions. It is reproduced here by courtesy of Dr. John W. Kirklin, Birmingham, Alabama.*

the pulmonary vein orifices. The risks of surgery are minimal (less than 0.5 percent), with virtually all these children home by the fourth postoperative day.

In adults, clinical benefit after closure of ASDs can be anticipated even in those with significant physiologic compromise,[87] but mortality is higher than it is in the young and the magnitude of improvement is less certain. Nonetheless, closure of ASDs is advised even when R_p approaches 15 Wood units because of the excessive morbidity and mortality associated with a persistent interatrial communication.[88] *Morbidity in adults and the low risk of surgical closure in young children mandate closure in the preschool or preadolescent years.*

Although life-threatening complications after closure of ASDs in children are rare, transient postoperative atrial arrhythmias and postpericardiotomy syndrome with pericardial effusions occasionally are seen. The long-term prognosis for a normal life expectancy and functional capability is excellent for patients who have closure of an uncomplicated ASD during the first two decades of life.

Interventional Closure of ASD

Many centers are using devices to close atrial septal defects in the cath lab.[83–86] This approach avoids potential surgical complications, reduces the length of hospitalization, and eliminates the midline sternotomy scar. Several devices are in various phases of investigation under FDA protocol. Although not universally successful in closure of defects, device placement has achieved good results, particularly for those lesions with a sufficient circumferential rim of tissue. However, despite persistent shunting in ASDs with insufficient rims, late closure has approximated the early results found with ASDs having sufficient tissue. The uncertainty of long-term morbidity remains with regard to potential for rhythm disturbance and

device erosion, so that longitudinal followup of each device is mandatory.

【 】 PARTIAL ANOMALOUS PULMONARY VENOUS CONNECTION

Pathology

In partial anomalous pulmonary venous connection, one or more—but not all—of the pulmonary veins enter the right atrium or its venous tributaries. An ASD is usually present, but the atrial septum is rarely intact. Although there are many patterns of anomalous pulmonary venous connection, the four most common, in order of decreasing frequency, are (1) pulmonary veins from the right upper and/or middle lobe to the superior vena cava, usually with a sinus venosus ASD; (2) all the right pulmonary veins to the right atrium, usually in the polysplenia syndrome; (3) all the right pulmonary veins to the inferior vena cava, entering this systemic vein just above or below the diaphragm; and (4) the left upper or both left pulmonary veins to an anomalous vertical vein draining to the left brachiocephalic vein.

When the right pulmonary veins are connected to the inferior vena cava, the atrial septum may be intact. This venous anomaly may be isolated or may be part of the *scimitar syndrome*. That syndrome includes hypoplasia of the right lung, bronchial abnormalities, anomalous systemic pulmonary arterial supply to the right lung from branches of the descending thoracic and/or abdominal aorta, and dextroposition of the heart.

Clinical Manifestations

In an old autopsy series, partial anomalous pulmonary venous connection occurred in 0.6 percent of 801 cases,[89] a much higher incidence than clinically suspected, suggesting that many cases may not be recognized during life. There is no sex predilection. Approximately 15 percent of all ASDs have this coexisting anomaly; however, in the case of the sinus venosus type, the association is in the range of 85 percent.

History When partial anomalous pulmonary venous connection coexists with an ASD, the symptoms, as well as the other clinical manifestations, are indistinguishable from those of an isolated ASD. Isolated, uncomplicated anomalous connection of a single pulmonary vein usually goes undetected clinically, as in this circumstance only approximately 20 percent of the pulmonary venous flow returns to the right atrium or its tributaries. When the entire venous return from one lung or two pulmonary veins is connected anomalously, approximately 65 percent of the pulmonary venous flow returns to the right side of the heart and the symptoms are similar to those of an ASD with a comparable increase in pulmonary blood flow.

Physical Examination The findings are the same as those in patients with an ASD with the exception that *the two components of the second heart sound, though usually widely split, move normally with respiration if the atrial septum is intact.*

Chest Roentgenogram Right ventricular enlargement, pulmonary arterial dilatation, and increased pulmonary blood flow are characteristic when more than one pulmonary vein connects anomalously. With anomalous connection of the right pulmonary veins to the inferior vena cava, the pulmonary venous pattern may assume a crescent-shaped or scimitar curve in the right lower lung field along the right lower heart border (scimitar).

Electrocardiogram The ECG is normal (in the case of anomalous connection of a single pulmonary vein) or reflects volume overload of the right side of the heart, as was described above under Atrial Septal Defect.

Echocardiogram If more than one pulmonary vein drains anomalously, the volume is usually sufficient to produce the characteristic pattern of right ventricular diastolic overload. Failure to visualize an atrial septal with two-dimensional imaging and color-flow mapping from a subcostal coronal or high right-sided parasternal longitudinal view should arouse suspicion of anomalous venous return. A variety of views supplemented by color-flow mapping may be necessary to identify the anomalous connection.[90]

Cardiac Catheterization Anomalously connected pulmonary veins may be entered directly with the venous catheter. Selective biplane angiograms in these vessels will document their site of connection. Left-to-right shunting with partial anomalous pulmonary venous connection and an intact atrial septum is usually small or moderate and may go undetected by oximetry techniques. Selective indicator dilution curves in the right and left pulmonary arteries with systemic arterial sampling can detect the lung with the anomalous pulmonary venous connection, and selective biplane angiograms in the pulmonary arterial branches will visualize these connections.

Natural History and Prognosis

Patients with partial anomalous pulmonary venous connection with ASD appear to follow a course similar, if not identical, to that of patients with an isolated ASD. When the atrial septum is intact, the course depends primarily on the volume of pulmonary venous blood returning to the right side of the heart. Rarely, PVOD may be found even in the presence of a single anomalously connected pulmonary vein and an intact atrial septum.[91]

Increasing left atrial pressure caused by mitral valve disease or diminished left ventricular compliance will, in the course of time, encourage redistribution of pulmonary arterial blood flow to the portion of the lung drained by the more compliant right atrium. Thus, patients who were initially asymptomatic with a modest volume of anomalous pulmonary venous return in youth may become symptomatic and even develop heart failure in adult life.

Medical Management

Asymptomatic patients with small shunts require no treatment. Those with symptoms, larger pulmonary blood flows, congestive failure, or PAH require surgical correction. With an intact atrial septum, precise preoperative identification of the site of the anomalous venous connection is essential. Long-term followup in patients who have not had surgery is indicated to detect increasing flow or the appearance of PAH.

Surgical Management

Anomalous connection of a right pulmonary vein or veins to the superior vena cava usually is associated with a sinus venosus ASD (see Fig. 82–12; see Atrial Septal Defect: Surgical Management above). Partial anomalous pulmonary veins draining to the superior vena cava, inferior vena cava, or right atrium are repaired by diversion through the ASD into the left atrium, using a patch baffle. Isolated left-sided anomalous pulmonary veins draining to the left ascending vertical vein or the left superior vena cava are detached and anastomosed directly to the left atrial appendage. Long-term morbidity and mortality are minimal among patients with uncomplicated partial pulmonary venous connections, equivalent to those observed after closure of an ASD.

【 】 COMMON ATRIOVENTRICULAR CANAL DEFECTS

Definition

AV canal defects are characterized by defects in isolation or combination including an ASD in the lowermost part of the atrial septum (ostium primum), a cleft of the mitral valve (either alone or in combination with a cleft of the tricuspid valve), or VSD. In the most severe form (complete AV canal defect), there is a large ostium primum ASD, a large VSD in the upper muscular septum and a common AV valve straddling the ventricular septum. The condition appears to result from incomplete growth of the AV endocardial cushions and the AV septum.

Pathology

The ostium primum type of ASD is characterized by a crescent-shaped upper border with no septal tissue forming the lower border. The lower aspect of the defect is bounded by the atrial surfaces of the AV valves and, in the complete type (see Complete Type below), in part by the upper edge of the ventricular septum. A small amount of septal tissue separates the defect from the posterior atrial wall.

Anatomic Types

Variations occur with respect to the nature of the AV valves. Rogers and Edwards first introduced the terms *partial* and *complete* to describe these types.[92]

Partial Type The ostium primum ASD is associated with a "cleft" in the anterior mitral leaflet or, probably more accurately, a septal commissure between the superior and inferior leaflets of the left AV valve (see Figs. 82–8D and 82–13).[74] The tricuspid valve is not cleft or shows a minor central deficiency. The ventricular aspects of the anterior mitral valve elements are fused to the upper edge of the deficient ventricular septum, precluding an interventricular communication. If there is no atrial septal tissue or if the atrial septum is so rudimentary that it produces a common chamber involving both atria, the term *common atrium* or *single atrium* is applied.

Complete Type The complete type of common AV canal is characterized by failure of partitioning of the primitive canal into separate AV orifices. The orifice between the atria and the ventricles is

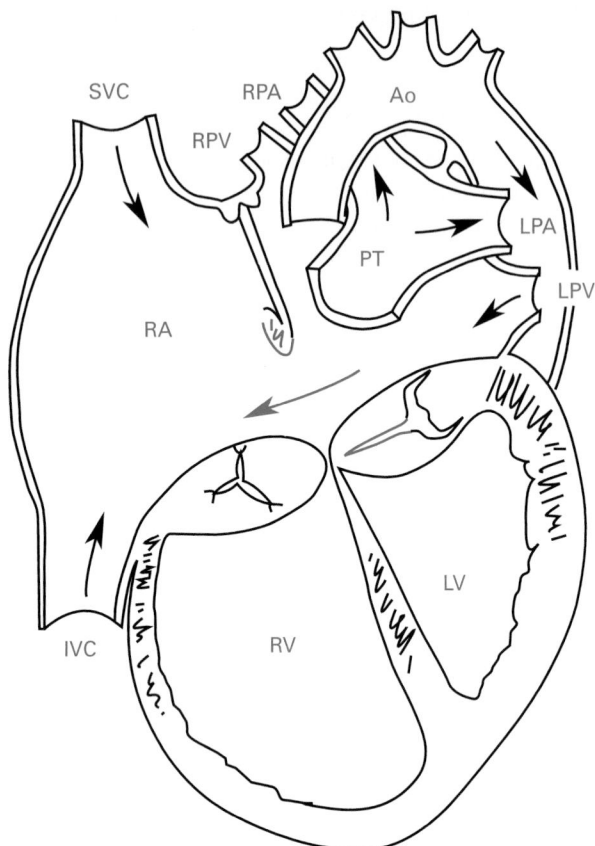

FIGURE 82–13. Common atrioventricular canal of the partial type. The mitral valve shows a cleft in its anterior leaflet, while the tricuspid valve is undisturbed. Ao, aorta; IVC, inferior vena cava; LPA, left pulmonary artery; LPV, left pulmonary vein; LV, left ventricle; RPA, right pulmonary artery; RPV, right pulmonary vein; SVC, superior vena cava. *Source: From Edwards JE.[74] Reproduced with permission from the publisher and author.*

guarded by a common valve with the anterior leaflet derived from the ventral AV endocardial cushion and represents the anterior halves of the anterior mitral and septal tricuspid leaflets. The posterior leaflet originates from the dorsal AV endocardial cushion and represents the posterior halves of the anterior mitral and septal tricuspid leaflets.

Usually, considerable space exists between the anterior and posterior leaflets above and the ventricular septum below; thus, in most cases of the complete type, there is free communication between the ventricles.

Rastelli et al.[86] subdivided the complete variety into three subgroups—types A, B, and C—on the basis of the structure of the common anterior leaflet and its chordal attachments to the ventricular septum and/or papillary muscles (Fig. 82–14). Considering the posterior common leaflet, there is variation among the three types in regard to the presence or absence of subdivision and whether the posterior leaflet is attached to the ventricular septum by chordae or by an imperforate membrane.

Variations from the classic types of AV canal defects are recognized, the most common being the AV canal type of isolated VSD, isolated ostium primum ASD without malformed AV valves, and isolated cleft of the anterior mitral or septal tricuspid valve leaflets.

Associated Conditions

In the asplenia syndrome, the complete variety is almost universal; with polysplenia, it occurs in about one-quarter of cases.[94] An ASD of

the secundum type is present in about half of these cases. A double orifice of the mitral valve may be associated with the incomplete type, and tetralogy of Fallot may be associated with the complete type.

Abnormal Physiology

If the communication at the ventricular level is large, the right ventricular and pulmonary artery pressures will be elevated. These patients are similar to those with large VSDs. Patients with a communication at the atrial level usually have only normal or slightly elevated systolic pressures in the right side of the heart and a large pulmonary blood flow, as in the secundum type of ASD. Defects in the tricuspid valve, mitral valve, or both may result in severe regurgitation or direct shunting of blood from the left ventricle to the right atrium.

Clinical Manifestations

Approximately 3 percent of infants and children with congenital heart disease have AV canal defects. The majority, some 60 to 70 percent, have the complete form with the female-to-male ratio being approximately 1.3:1. Well over half of patients with the complete form have associated Down syndrome. Among children with Down syndrome, 45 percent have some form of congenital heart disease, with malformations of the type involving the AV canal comprising approximately 50 percent of these abnormalities.[95]

History Only if the mitral valve is incompetent do the symptoms of patients with partial AV canal differ from those associated with a secundum type of ASD. The complete form of AV canal or the partial form connected with significant mitral regurgitation may be associated with poor weight gain, easy fatigue, tachypnea, repeated respiratory infections, and congestive heart failure. Patients with complete AV canal are almost invariably very sick.

Physical Examination The findings with a partial defect are those of an ASD. If the cleft anterior mitral leaflet is incompetent, the findings of mitral regurgitation also will be present. The physical findings with the complete AV canal defect are those of a very large VSD, usually with full-blown congestive failure. The murmur of mitral regurgitation may not be heard or recognized as such.

Chest Roentgenogram Overall cardiac enlargement that is out of proportion to the degree of pulmonary plethora or a cardiac silhouette, suggesting combined ventricular dilatation, may serve to distinguish an uncomplicated secundum ASD from a primum defect with significant mitral regurgitation. Marked cardiac enlargement and severe pulmonary overcirculation are features of the complete AV canal defect.

Electrocardiogram One of the most helpful diagnostic features in distinguishing individuals with AV canal defects from those with isolated ASDs or VSDs is the characteristic superior orientation of the mean QRS axis in the frontal plane, with a right bundle-branch delay in the precordial leads. Between 92 and 95 percent of both types of canal have a QRS axis lying between 0 and 150 degrees. The patterns of atrial and ventricular hypertrophy reflect the underlying hemodynamic abnormalities.

Echocardiogram Two-dimensional echocardiography is capable of visualizing the extent of septal defects and, with Doppler study and

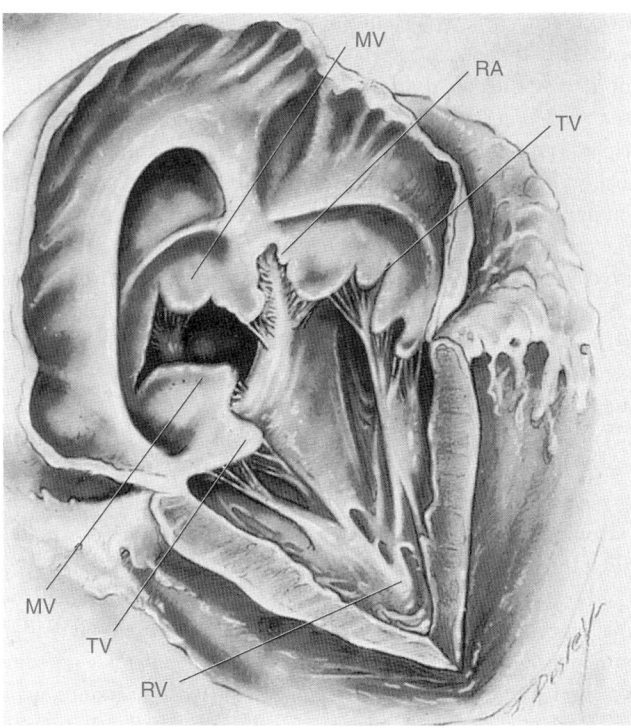

FIGURE 82–14. Complete form of common atrioventricular canal type A. The common anterior leaflet has a recognizable mitral valve component (MV) and tricuspid valve component (TV). In type B, not illustrated, those components are attached by chordae to a papillary muscle in the right ventricle. In type C, not illustrated, the common anterior leaflet is a single unit without any attachment to the underlying ventricular septum. Type A is most amenable to repair. RA, right atrium; RV, right ventricle. *Source: From Rastelli GC, Ongley PA, Kirklin JW, and McGoon DC.[93] Reproduced with permission from the publisher and authors.*

color-flow mapping, left-to-right shunting at the atrial and/or ventricular level and associated mitral and/or tricuspid valvular regurgitation (Fig. 82–15). The anatomic features of the anterior AV leaflet and its connections may be visualized with sufficient clarity to permit subdivision of complete AV canal defects into types A, B, and C (see Fig. 82–14). Straddling AV valves, a double-orifice mitral valve, single papillary muscles, and hypoplasia or outflow obstruction of the right or left ventricle also can be determined with this technique.[96]

Cardiac Catheterization Cardiac catheterization is rarely performed if the echocardiogram is characteristic and if the history, clinical examination, and echo suggest a large left-to-right shunt and low pulmonary resistance. When it is performed, a significant increase in oxygen saturation between the superior vena cava and the right atrium is present. A right ventricular or pulmonary arterial systolic pressure in excess of 60 percent of the systemic systolic pressure favors the presence of a complete canal. With a large communication between the two ventricles below the AV valves, the right ventricular, pulmonary arterial, and systemic arterial systolic pressures are virtually identical. Left ventricular angiography in the frontal view demonstrates the "gooseneck deformity" of the left ventricular outflow tract that is characteristic of AV canal malformations and allows a semiquantitative assessment of the degree of mitral regurgitation and shunting from the left ventricle to the right atrium. The left anterior oblique view with craniocaudal angulation is recommended for visualizing the interventricular defect and judging the extent of ventricular septal deficiency. Aortography will confirm the presence of a PDA.

Natural History and Prognosis

Partial defects without significant mitral regurgitation follow a course similar to that described for the secundum type of septal defects. An exception would be the greater likelihood of infective endocarditis because of the mitral valve deformity. Moderate or severe mitral regurgitation produces heart failure with resulting symptoms and growth retardation. Infants with a complete AV canal without protective pulmonary stenosis quickly develop and continue to have congestive failure until the course is altered by death, the development of PVOD, or surgical intervention.

Medical Management

Children with an uncomplicated partial defect are managed in the same manner as children with an uncomplicated ASD. Those who are symptomatic should undergo early surgical closure of the primum ASD and plication of the cleft in the septal commissure of the left AV ("mitral") valve. The few patients with significant residual mitral regurgitation after surgery are managed medically until mitral valve replacement is appropriate. Those without symptoms are repaired before they start school with the recent trend favoring intervention within the first 2 years.

The approach to an infant with complete AV canal is the same as that for an infant with a large VSD but is tempered by the knowledge that spontaneous improvement is very unlikely except at the expense of the pulmonary vascular bed. Repair is recommended by 6 months of age or earlier with intractable heart failure. Elevation of pulmonary vascular resistance in the first year of life warrants surgical intervention without delay.

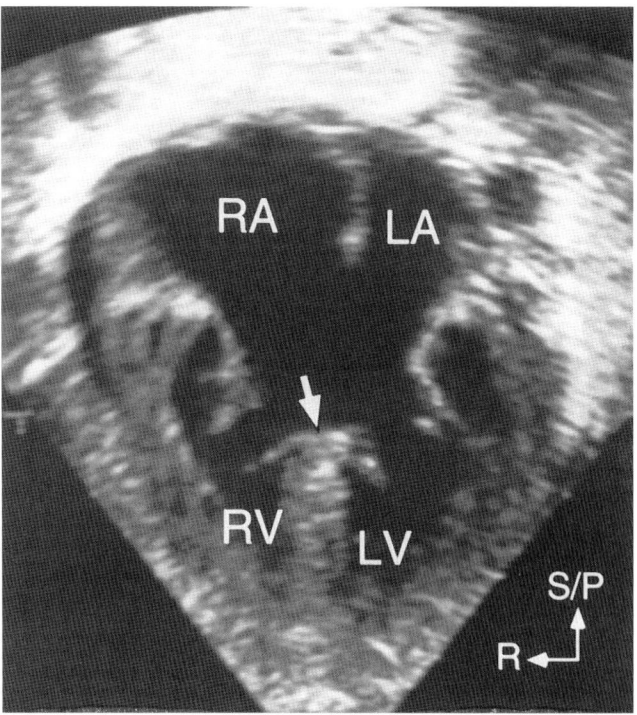

FIGURE 82–15. Apical four-chamber view of complete common atrioventricular canal. Note the large deficiency of both atrial and ventricular septa as well as apical displacement of the AV valves. The *arrow* points to the attachment of the inferior bridging leaflet to the ventricular septal crest. LA, left atrium; LV, left ventricle; RA, right atrium; RV, right ventricle. *Source: From Levine J and Geva T.[96] Reproduced with permission from the publisher and authors.*

With regard to genetic counseling, the risk of a subsequent sibling having heart disease in the presence of a single affected family member is in the range of 2 percent; it is probably higher for the offspring of an affected parent, particularly if that parent is the mother.[97] Concordance for AV canal defects among affected siblings or offspring is much higher than it is with other forms of congenital heart disease and approaches 90 percent.

Surgical Management

The remarkable clinical improvement that follows anatomic repair of complete common AV septal defects in infancy encourages correction early in the first year of life.[98] Banding of the pulmonary artery in a critically ill infant with a large ventricular defect was used in the past but has been replaced by operative repair in most centers. The specifics of repair are dictated by anatomic detail: individual variation is considerable (Fig. 82–16), but the creation of a competent, nonstenotic left-sided AV ("mitral") valve is essential for an acceptable early and long-term prognosis.

A patch is usually sutured to the right side of the ventricular septum to obliterate the interventricular communication. The anterior and posterior components of the common valve are divided, and the mitral valve is sutured to the patch at an appropriate level. The "cleft"

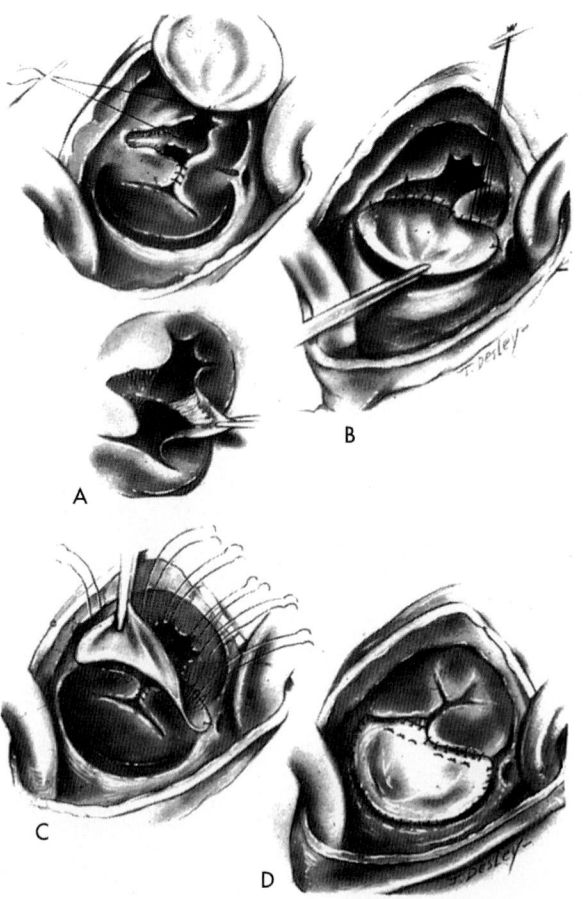

FIGURE 82–16. Steps in the repair of the complete form of common atrioventricular canal, type A. **A** and **B.** A pericardial patch is sutured to the ventricular septum. **C** and **D.** The anterior leaflet of the mitral valve is reconstructed and attached to the patch. A portion of the tricuspid leaflet is attached to the patch. *Source: From Rastelli GC, Ongley PA, Kirklin JW, and McGoon DC.[86] Reproduced with permission from the publisher and authors.*

between the left anterior and posterior leaflets is sutured to provide competence without the creation of stenosis. Prosthetic valve implantation rarely is required during primary anatomic repair.[99] The right-sided AV ("tricuspid") apparatus, although less critical to survival, is repaired using the same principles. The interatrial communication is usually closed with a separate piece of pericardium to minimize hemolysis in the presence of residual mitral regurgitation.[99] Mitral valve competence is assessed by gentle distension of the left ventricle with cold saline and more recently transesophageal echocardiography.

A partial AV canal is repaired through a right atriotomy. The cleft may be closed with a few simple interrupted sutures to encourage inversion and coaptation of the leaflet margins. The ASD usually is closed with a pericardial patch.

Permanent complete heart block once contributed substantially to early mortality and morbidity but is now rare. Patients undergoing repair of a partial AV canal should be observed for the possible development of subaortic left ventricular outflow tract obstruction caused by redundant or residual endocardial cushion tissue.

In-hospital mortality after correction of a complete AV canal in infancy ranges from 3 to 10 percent;[100,101] the highest mortality is encountered during the first few months of life in infants with severe AV valve regurgitation, elevated pulmonary vascular resistance, hypoplasia of the left or right ventricle, or other cardiac malformations. At Children's Hospital in Boston, 191 children with a median age of 4.6 months were repaired between January 1990 and December 1998, with an operative mortality of 1.5 percent. Reoperation was necessary in 22 patients (11.7 percent), at a mean of 20 months later—18 for residual mitral regurgitation and 4 for left ventricular outflow tract obstruction.[102] Successful correction of a complete AV canal can be accomplished despite associated tetralogy of Fallot, double-outlet ventricle, and other complex anomalies.[99]

EXTRACARDIAC COMMUNICATIONS BETWEEN THE SYSTEMIC AND PULMONARY CIRCULATIONS, USUALLY WITHOUT CYANOSIS

〖 〗 PATENT DUCTUS ARTERIOSUS

Definition

Patent ductus arteriosus, the most common type of extracardiac shunt, represents persistent patency of the vessel that normally connects the pulmonary arterial system and the aorta in a fetus (Fig. 82–17).

Pathology

The ductus arteriosus usually closes within 2 or 3 days after birth and becomes the *ligamentum arteriosum*, but it may remain patent for several months prior to spontaneous closure. It courses from the origin of the left pulmonary artery below to the lower aspect of the aortic arch just beyond the level of origin of the left subclavian artery above. The recurrent branch of the left vagus nerve hooks around its lateral and inferior aspects. Constriction of the ductus postnatally involves a complex interaction of increased partial pressure of oxygen, decreased circulating prostaglandin E_2 (PGE_2), decreased PGE_2 ductal receptors, and decreased pressure within the ductus. Subsequent vessel-wall hypoxia of the ductus promotes further closure through inhibition of prostaglandin and nitric oxide within the ductal wall.[103] Exogenous PGE_1 has been used extensively to keep the ductus open postnatally,[104] and indomethacin, a prostaglandin inhibitor, can close the ductus in many premature infants in whom persistent patency is disadvantageous.[105]

Abnormal Physiology

Patients with PDA may be divided into groups according to whether the vascular resistance through the ductus is low, moderate, or high. The resistance of the ductus is related not only to its cross-sectional area but also to its length. In patients with a very small ductus that offers high resistance, the flow across the ductus is relatively small. The extra volume of work on the left ventricle is small, and the pulmonary pressure and resistance are not elevated. Patients with only moderate resistance in the ductus have some increase in pulmonary artery pressure, with a moderately greater volume of shunting across the ductus.

In patients with a large patent ductus, the aorta and pulmonary artery are essentially in free communication; the systolic pressure in the pulmonary artery is equal to that in the aorta. Left ventricular volume overload results from recirculation through the lungs, with pulmonary congestion resulting from increased pulmonary flow and/or left ventricular failure. The left ventricle compensates by dilation followed in many cases by hypertrophy, and the pulmonary vasculature may respond to the high pressure (see Pulmonary Arterial Hypertension above). The right ventricle is subjected to a pressure load.

If the pulmonary resistance equals or exceeds the resistance of the systemic circulation, there is right-to-left shunting from the pulmonary artery to the aorta, resulting in hypoxemia, especially in the lower body and legs.

Clinical Manifestations

History
The history of the mother's pregnancy and of perinatal events may provide clues associated with a high incidence of PDA, such as exposure to rubella in the first trimester in a nonimmunized mother. PDA is also more common in premature infants, especially those with birth asphyxia or respiratory distress.[106]

Symptoms
Symptoms are usually restricted to patients with large shunts that produce heart failure or with other complicating problems, such as respiratory distress in a premature infant. The symptoms related to heart failure were discussed above. Heart failure is most likely to develop in the first few weeks or months of life. If it does not appear during infancy, it is unlikely to occur before the third decade. Growth may be affected in those with large shunts and failure. The clinical presentation in a premature infant is usually very different from that in a full-term infant, particularly in one with a birth weight under 1.5 kg (3.3 lb), who is more likely to have moderate to severe respiratory distress. In these infants, the clinical features of respiratory distress occur very early following delivery requiring mechanical ventilatory support. The inability to wean from the ventilator over the next several days or initial improvement followed by increasing ventilatory or oxygen requirements are signs that a PDA may be aggravating the clinical status.

Physical Examination
In a full-term infant or child with PDA, there is frequently a systolic thrill over the pulmonary artery and in the suprasternal notch. The peripheral pulses are generally brisk and bounding, especially with the larger shunts secondary to runoff from the aorta to the pulmonary artery in diastole. A patient with elevated pulmonary vascular resistance and a right-to-left shunt will have "dif-

ferential cyanosis," with cyanosis and clubbing of the toes but not the fingers, related to shunting of hypoxemic blood from the pulmonary artery into the descending aorta. The apical impulse may be increased or displaced in those with large shunts. The right ventricular impulse is increased in a premature infant with respiratory distress and in infants and children with significant pulmonary hypertension. The typical murmur is a continuous or "machinery" murmur best heard at the left upper sternal border and below the left clavicle. It is usually a rough murmur with eddy sounds, which are helpful in making the diagnosis, and it peaks at or near the second heart sound. In patients with at least a moderate shunt, there is a middiastolic rumble at the apex as a result of relative mitral stenosis from increased flow across the mitral valve. The second heart sound may be difficult to hear because of the continuous murmur, but it is usually normal. The pulmonary component is accentuated in those with pulmonary hypertension.

Chest Roentgenogram
Findings on chest roentgenography are also dependent on the magnitude of the shunt. In patients with a small shunt, the chest roentgenogram is normal. With larger shunts, the left atrium and left ventricle are enlarged. Increases in pulmonary arterial flow on radiograph parallel the magnitude of the shunt. In the presence of heart failure, there are signs of pulmonary edema. In older patients who have developed Eisenmenger physiology, the only abnormality may be marked prominence of the central pulmonary arteries, with rapid tapering to the periphery of the lung fields.

Electrocardiogram
With a small shunt the ECG is normal. Left atrial hypertrophy is probably the most common abnormality

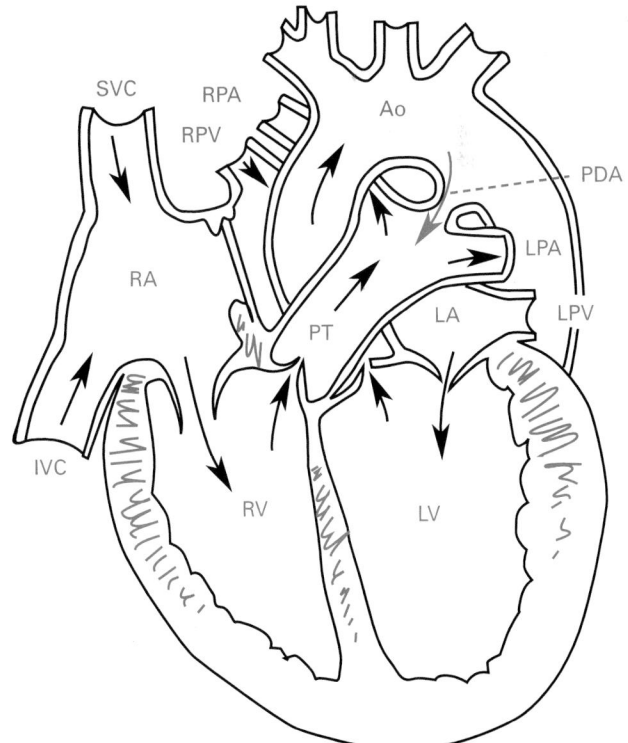

FIGURE 82–17. Patent ductus arteriosus (PDA). Ao, aorta; IVC, inferior vena cava; LA, left atrium; LPA, left pulmonary artery; LPV, left pulmonary vein; LV, left ventricle; PT, main pulmonary arterial trunk; RA, right atrium; RPA, right pulmonary artery; RPV, right pulmonary vein; RV, right ventricle; SVC, superior vena cava. *Source: From Edwards JE.[93] Reproduced with permission from the publisher and author.*

found, but left ventricular hypertrophy of the volume overload type, with deep Q waves and increased R-wave voltage in the left precordial leads, is also common as the shunt's size increases and left ventricular dilation occurs. Right ventricular hypertrophy is seen with pulmonary hypertension.

Echocardiogram In medium to large shunts, there is left atrial enlargement, and the left ventricular end-diastolic dimension and mean velocity of circumferential fiber shortening are increased significantly. Small shunts can be detected with color-flow Doppler imaging with a typical spectral flow pattern in the pulmonary artery, whereas a larger ductus can be visualized with two-dimensional echocardiography alone. Occasionally, a trivial amount of flow is seen through the ductus as an incidental finding in those with or without associated heart disease.

Cardiac Catheterization In patients with typical, uncomplicated PDA, cardiac catheterization is unnecessary unless closure in the catheterization lab is contemplated. When catheterization is performed, the catheter usually passes preferentially from the left pulmonary artery into the descending aorta except when the ductus is too small. The saturation is increased in the pulmonary artery compared with the right atrium and ventricle to a degree relative to the size of the shunt. The pulmonary arterial and right ventricular pressures are elevated in those with a large ductus. The pulmonary vascular resistance is elevated in older patients who have developed changes in the pulmonary vascular bed. These patients also have diminished saturation in the descending aorta once the pulmonary resistance reaches a level that will reverse the shunt. Aortography will opacify the ductus and pulmonary arteries.

Natural History and Prognosis

The complications related to PDA include infective endarteritis, heart failure, and pulmonary hypertension with vascular damage. Infection of the ductus is a risk regardless of ductal size, increasing with the length of survival. The development of a mycotic aneurysm has the potential to compress the recurrent laryngeal nerve, embolize septic material to the lungs, or rupture. Calcification of the ductal wall is common in adults. In patients with large shunts, heart failure can cause significant morbidity and mortality, particularly in a premature and young infant, and sudden death can occur. Progressive damage to the pulmonary vascular bed can occur in some, but it rarely occurs to an irreversible degree in the first year of life. Once irreversible damage occurs, premature death in late adolescence or early adulthood can be anticipated.

With improved echo technology, children without associated heart disease are identified with a trivial amount of flow through a very small (<1 mm) patent ductus. Frequently, the shunt is too small to produce an audible murmur. The natural history of this echo-Doppler–discovered ductus arteriosus without clinical findings is unknown, but most think it is benign as cardiologists have not noted patients with endarteritis in a "silent" ductus.

Medical Management

Interruption of flow through the PDA is the ultimate goal of management. For those in heart failure, usually premature infants, medical management with diuretics and fluid restriction may play a role, but the ultimate aim is closure to prevent heart failure, reduce respi-

ratory insufficiency, promote growth in infants, and prevent infective endarteritis and pulmonary vascular disease in older children.

For premature infants, treatment with indomethacin is usually the first-line therapy.[107] Successful closure depends on both the dosage and the timing of treatment, although the major determinants seem to be birth weight and gestational age. Because of ductal recurrence, serial treatment regimens may be necessary, especially in those weighing less than 1000 g at birth. There is increasing evidence that the administration of "prophylactic" indomethacin in infants weighing less than 1000 g at birth may be associated with a higher closure rate and a better outcome, but reopening of the ductus still occurs frequently.[108] Indomethacin therapy has been associated with an increased bleeding tendency resulting from platelet dysfunction, decreased urine output secondary to renal dysfunction, and necrotizing enterocolitis.[105] Ibuprofen has achieved closure rates equivalent to that of indomethacin with less renal toxicity[109] but questions remain related to the potential for chronic lung disease and pulmonary hypertension.

For premature infants whose PDA fails to close with indomethacin or for term infants with a persistent PDA, closure has been recommended. If the PDA is large, there is usually a large left-to-right shunt with congestive heart failure. In these infants, the indication for closure is heart failure and usually failure to thrive. Even in the absence of these indications, when a large PDA is associated with PAH, closure is recommended to prevent PVOD. In children with a smaller PDA with an audible murmur but no evidence of significant hemodynamic embarrassment, closure usually is recommended because of the incidence of bacterial endarteritis, in the range of 30 percent over a lifetime. For children with a PDA without a heart murmur, which usually is discovered incidentally when an echocardiogram is performed for other reasons, closure remains controversial.

Surgical and Interventional Catheter Closure

Surgery for a persistent PDA was first reported more than 60 years ago. The safety and efficacy of this procedure, even in very young children, are well established, with risks that are very low (well under 1 percent), with success of interruption almost universal. The PDA is exposed and mobilized through a small left thoracotomy in the fourth intercostal space. Ductus obliteration is accomplished by division or ligation. A short, broad, or thin-walled ductus is divided between vascular clamps. The ends are closed with a continuous suture. A long, narrow, thick-walled ductus can be divided or ligated with two or three sutures spaced a few millimeters apart. The suture ligatures at each end are anchored superficially in the ductus wall to prevent migration and assure thrombosis and obliteration.

The fragile, thin-walled PDA of a premature infant is obliterated by gentle ligation with a thick suture to minimize disruption or, if small, by occlusion using metallic surgical clips. Some surgeons prefer extrapleural exposure. Ligation in the neonatal intensive care unit, avoiding transport to the operating room, is common. Transport from a remote intensive care unit to a cardiac surgical unit for ductus ligation on a "day-stay" basis is also efficacious.[110] Ductus obliteration offers clinical improvement in infants weighing as little as 500 g, with minimal operative risk, a reduced incidence of necrotizing enterocolitis, a reduced duration of intubation, and improvement in late survival.

Closure of a PDA in an adult requires particular caution; calcification and rigidity of the ductus wall complicate clamping. Placement of a Dacron patch over the aortic orifice of the ductus from within the aorta may be advisable.[111]

Recently, less-invasive video-assisted thoracscopic surgery has been used for PDA closure. Among 230 patients, 1 had minimal residual flow and another had persistent dysfunction of the recurrent laryngeal nerve. There were no deaths, transfusions, or chylothoraces. The mean operating time was 20 minutes, and the hospital stay was 2 days.[112] At Children's Hospital in Boston, this procedure has been applied to premature infants as small as 575 g, with discharge from the hospital the day after the procedure in full-term infants and children.[113]

The PDA can be closed by interventional catheterization techniques. In 1971, Portsmann and Wierny introduced a rather complex methodology to plug a PDA by using a transarterial and transvenous approach employing very large catheters.[114] Subsequently, Rashkind and Cuaso introduced, and others have since popularized, the use of a double-umbrella device to plug a PDA,[115] but the large size of the delivery sheath of the Rashkind device made it inapplicable to young and very small children. Gianturco coils—thin metallic wires glossed with Dacron that assume a coil configuration when released from a catheter—have become an attractive alternative (Fig. 82–18). They can be delivered through relatively small catheters and have been found to be quite effective, although their usefulness is limited in those younger than 8 months of age with PDAs that are no greater than 3.5 or 4.0 mm at the narrowest point.[116] In the others using these coils, the results have been very promising, with a 90 percent success rate. Newer devices to occlude the ductus are being introduced that will likely obviate the need for surgical closure in the not distant future.

With several highly successful, low-risk, inexpensive, and minimally traumatic procedures available to close a persistent PDA in a neonate, child, adolescent, or adult without pulmonary vascular disease, local experience should guide the preferred option in an individual child.

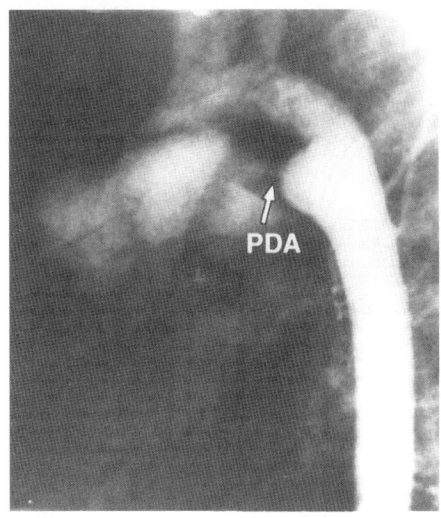 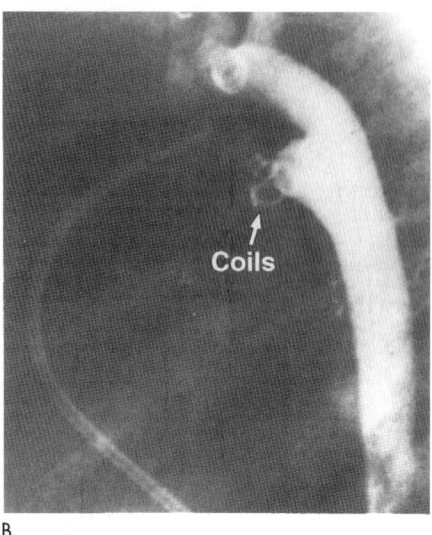

FIGURE 82–18. Lateral angiogram showing coil occlusion of a patent ductus arteriosus (PDA). **A.** Small PDA allows shunting from descending aorta to pulmonary artery. **B.** Shunting is eliminated by a coil placed in the ductus arteriosus. *Source: Courtesy of John F. Keane, MD.*

[ ] SINUS OF VALSALVA FISTULA

Pathology

Sinus of Valsalva fistula is uncommon; it also is referred to as *aortic sinus aneurysm.* Because of an assumed intrinsic weakness at the union of the aorta with the heart, the aortic media may separate from the aortic annulus and retract upward. The structure that lies between becomes aneurysmal and may rupture to form a fistula. The usual sites of the defects are the posterior (noncoronary) sinus aneurysms that rupture through the atrial septal wall into the right atrium (Fig. 82–19A) and those of the right sinus that rupture into the right ventricular infundibulum (Fig. 82–19B).[117] The aneurysm is represented by a colored pouch with multiple perforations in the wall. The principal associated condition is a supracristal VSD in cases with aneurysms of the right sinus (approximately 50 percent).

Clinical Manifestations

Sinus of Valsalva fistulas are most common in adults.[118] When the rupture is secondary to bacterial endocarditis, evidence of a preceding infection is found. If the rupture occurs slowly, a small fistulous tract into the right atrium or ventricle develops and presents as the recent onset of a small left-to-right shunt. With sudden rupture, there is usually a tearing pain in the midchest associated with dramatically rapid development of pulmonary congestion caused by the sudden onset of a large shunt. Characteristically, the murmur is loud and continuous but is heard lower on the chest than is the murmur of PDA. A to-and-fro murmur rather than a continuous one may be heard at times. The apical impulse is hyperdynamic, and the pulse pressure is widened. VSD may complicate the clinical picture. Echocardiography or cardiac catheterization will confirm the level of the shunt. A pressure difference across the right ventricular outflow tract may be present if the right sinus is involved. Aortography or Doppler echocardiography[119] will confirm the diagnosis.

Natural History and Prognosis

With slow rupture and a small shunt, the major risk is infective endocarditis or extension of the rupture with an increasing shunt. With a large shunt, the heart failure is usually rapidly progressive and may result in a quick demise. A few patients seem to stabilize in this situation.

Medical Management

Appropriate cultures should be drawn and antibiotics started if endocarditis is suspected. Treatment of heart failure should be instituted rapidly. *Because of the natural history, all patients should have this condition corrected surgically.*

Surgical Management

Aneurysms or fistulas from the noncoronary or right coronary sinuses are repaired through the aortic root while the patient is supported on total cardiopulmonary bypass with moderate hypothermia, using techniques similar to those employed for aortic valve replacement. The aortic valve leaflets, the margins of the aneurysm, and the coronary arterial orifices must be visualized precisely. Aneurysms of the noncoronary sinus can be repaired through the right atrium; those arising from the right coronary si-

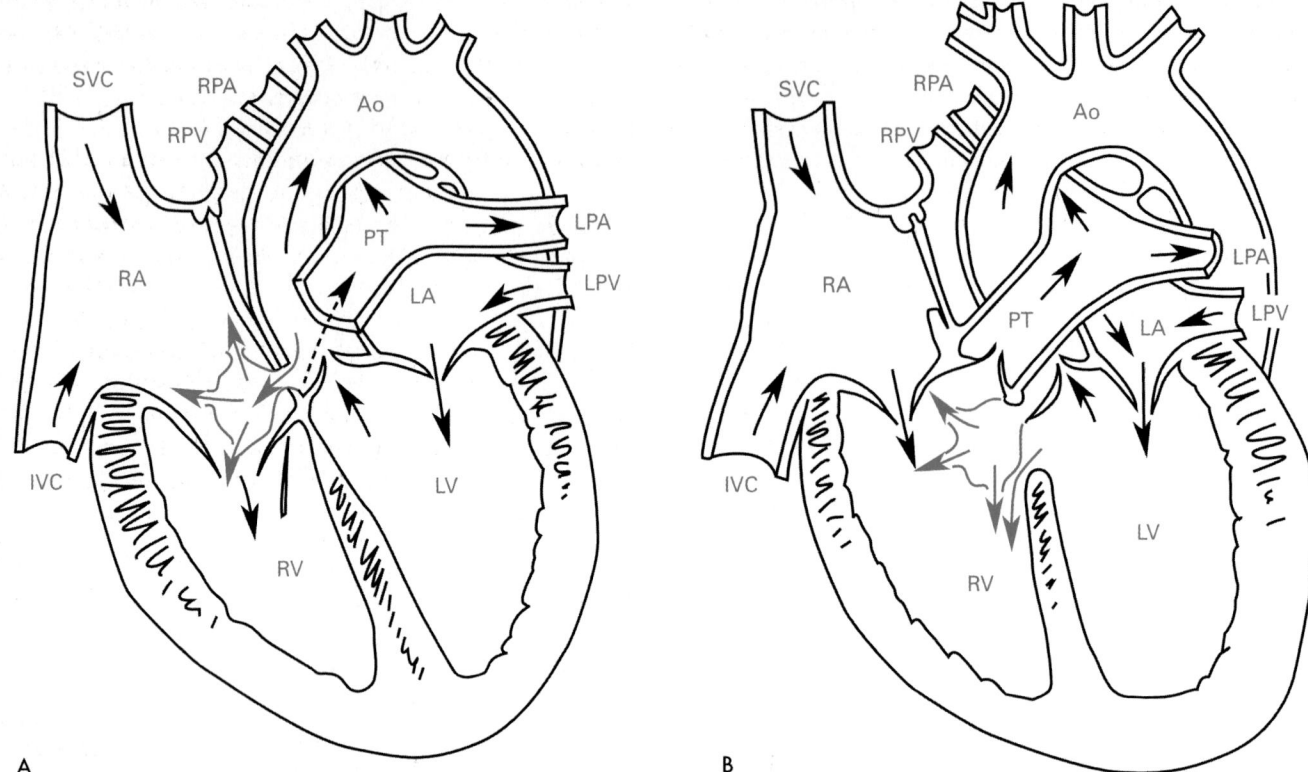

FIGURE 82–19. Sinus of Valsalva fistula. **A.** Aneurysm involves the posterior sinus and ruptures into the right atrium. **B.** Aneurysm involves the right aortic sinus and ruptures into the right ventricle. A ventricular septal defect is commonly associated, as illustrated. Ao, aorta; IVC, inferior vena cava; LA, left atrium; LPA, left pulmonary artery; LPV, left pulmonary vein; LV, left ventricle; PT, main pulmonary arterial trunk; RA, right atrium; RPA, right pulmonary artery; RPV, right pulmonary vein; RV, right ventricle; SVC, superior vena cava. *Source: From Edwards JE.[74] Reproduced with permission from the publisher and author.*

nus are accessible through the right ventricle. In most cases, the orifice of the aneurysmal fistula is surgically obliterated using a Dacron patch. In a recent series of 129 patients, reparative methods included plication (47 percent), patch repair (40 percent), and aortic root replacement (12 percent). Sixty percent of those patients needed aortic valve replacement at the same time.[118]

A conal, or supracristal (type I), VSD must be sought and closed through either the aortic valve or the right ventricular outflow tract when an aneurysm of the right coronary sinus extends into the right ventricle. Surgical results are usually quite good. In the large series cited above, the operative survival was 96 percent, with no late deaths in an average of 5.9 years of followup.[119]

VALVULAR AND VASCULAR MALFORMATIONS OF THE LEFT SIDE OF THE HEART WITH RIGHT-TO-LEFT, BIDIRECTIONAL, OR NO SHUNT

【 】 COARCTATION OF THE AORTA

Pathology

Coarctation of the aorta is a discrete narrowing of the distal segment of the aortic arch. The characteristic lesion is a deformity of the media of the aorta that involves the anterior, superior, and posterior walls and is represented by a curtain-like infolding of the wall that causes the lumen to be narrowed and eccentric.[120] In infants, the lesion lies either opposite the ductus or in a preductal location. In adolescents and adults, it is usually at the ligamentum arteriosum. An aberrant right

subclavian artery may be associated. In rare cases, the narrowing lies proximal to the origin of the left common carotid artery or involves a segment of the abdominal aorta. The principal cardiac abnormality is left ventricular hypertrophy. In some infants, left ventricular endocardial fibroelastosis may be associated. Tubular hypoplasia of the distal aortic arch and isthmus is very common, especially with associated cardiac abnormalities involving left heart obstruction.[121] The proximal aorta may show a moderate degree of cystic medial necrosis. Beyond the coarctation, the lining may show a localized jet lesion. Prominent collaterals are characteristic in older infants, children, and adolescents. They may be divided into anterior and posterior systems, with the anterior system originating with the internal mammary arteries and making use of the epigastric arteries in the abdominal wall to supply the lower extremities. The posterior system involves parascapular arteries connected with the posterior intercostal arteries and carries blood to the distal aortic compartment principally for supply of the abdominal viscera. The anterior spinal artery, receiving branches from the proximal and distal compartments of the aorta, is also dilated and tortuous.

Associated Conditions

The most commonly associated defects are tubular hypoplasia of the aortic arch, PDA, VSD, and aortic stenosis (valvular and/or subvalvular). A bicuspid aortic valve is present in 46 percent of autopsy cases.[120]

Abnormal Physiology

In most instances, both the systolic and diastolic arterial pressures above the coarctation are elevated. Below the coarctation, the systolic pressure is lower than that in the upper extremities, and the diastolic pressure is usually near or only slightly below the normal range. The mechanism of upper extremity hypertension appears to involve the increased resistance to aortic flow produced by the coarctation itself, the decreased capacity and distensibility of the vessels into which the left ventricle ejects, and humoral factors.[122]

Clinical Manifestations

Coarctation of the aorta occurs in approximately 4 percent of all infants and children with congenital heart disease and is the predominant lesion in approximately 8 percent of infants presenting with critical heart disease in the first year of life. It ranks behind only VSD, D-transposition of the great arteries, and tetralogy of Fallot.[3] Among all individuals born with coarctation, approximately half present within the first month or two of life with heart failure. Approximately 50 percent of infants so admitted have uncomplicated coarctation; the remaining half can be expected to have at least one complicating cardiac abnormality. VSD is the most common (64 percent), followed by left ventricular outflow tract obstruction (31 percent).[123] The timing of ductal tissue constriction in terms of both ductal closure and perhaps aortic constriction appear to play a decisive role in the onset or worsening of symptoms in most of these patients. The male-to-female ratio is approximately 3:1 for isolated coarctation but is only 1.1:1 for complicated coarctation. Approximately 45 percent of children with Turner syndrome have coarctation.

History The clinical picture in a symptomatic infant is one of dyspnea, difficulty in feeding, and poor weight gain. Older children are for the most part asymptomatic, although a few complain of mild fatigue, dyspnea, or symptoms of claudication of the lower extremities when running.

Physical Examination In a symptomatic infant, signs of congestive heart failure are characteristic. A gallop rhythm is common, and a murmur from associated defects or from the coarctation itself (posteriorly in the interscapular area) may be heard. Frequently, these murmurs are either inaudible or nondescript on admission and become characteristic only when congestive failure is brought under control. Prominent arterial pulsations may be visible in the suprasternal notch and carotid arteries, and the left ventricular impulse is forceful. An early systolic ejection click at the apex suggests the presence of a bicuspid aortic valve. The murmur from the coarctation is medium-pitched, systolic, and blowing in quality. It is best heard posteriorly in the interscapular area, usually with some degree of radiation to the left axilla, apex, and anterior precordium. Low-pitched, continuous murmurs of collateral circulation may be heard over the chest wall, particularly posteriorly, but seldom before adolescence. A short middiastolic rumble at the apex without clinical evidence of mitral disease is relatively common.

The characteristic systolic blood pressure difference between the upper and lower extremities may be difficult to appreciate or measure in infants with severe congestive failure or with a large VSD or PDA. With improved hemodynamic compensation, pulses in the upper extremities become readily palpable. The femoral pulses remain weak, delayed, or absent. In these very young infants, it is important to assess the brachial and carotid pulses. Weak or absent pulses in all sites are more characteristic of critical aortic stenosis or aortic atresia.

In older children and adults, the radial arterial pulses are typically strong; those in the femoral arteries are diminished, delayed, or absent. A repeatedly measured systolic or mean pressure difference between the upper and lower extremities greater than 10 mmHg is diagnostic. The pulse pressure in the leg is reduced, and in some patients no pressure can be measured by auscultation or Doppler. Approximately one-third of older children have hypertension. Some patients have only a mild pressure difference between the arms and the legs at rest but a much larger difference during treadmill exercise. A systolic pressure difference between the two arms suggests that the origin of one subclavian artery is at or below the obstruction, for example, aberrant right subclavian from the descending aorta.

In light of the simplicity of measuring blood pressure in the upper and lower extremities of children and the importance of early detection, it is concerning that approximately 95 percent of children and adolescents with coarctation are referred by pediatricians and other healthcare providers to a pediatric cardiologist for evaluation of a murmur and/or hypertension.[124]

Chest Roentgenogram For a symptomatic infant, the pattern is one of impressive cardiac enlargement and venous congestion. In an older and asymptomatic child, the heart's size is generally at the upper limits of normal with a left ventricular prominence. A figure-three configuration of the left margin of the aorta at the level of the coarctation may be seen in overpenetrated films, with the upper curve formed by the slightly dilated aorta just above the coarctation, the central indentation by the coarctation itself, and the lower curve by the poststenotic dilatation below the coarctation. Notching of the inferior margin of the ribs by tortuous intercostal arteries acting as collaterals is seldom present before 7 or 8 years of age.

Electrocardiogram The ECG of a symptomatic infant reflects right or biventricular hypertrophy during the first 3 months of life. T-wave inversion in the left precordial leads is common. In older children, the ECG is usually normal or may indicate mild left ventricular and left atrial hypertrophy.

Echocardiogram Two-dimensional echocardiographic imaging of the aortic arch from the suprasternal notch permits visualization of the coarctation and detection of anatomic variations such as isthmic or transverse arch hypoplasia. The precordial and subxiphoid views are of great value in assessing the presence and severity of associated defects. Doppler flow studies are helpful for diagnostic confirmation. In infants with heart failure, left ventricular dilation and decreased contractility are common. The severity of the coarctation can be evaluated by Doppler gradients and the diminished pulsatile flow in the abdominal aorta.

Cardiac Catheterization Study of symptomatic infants characteristically reveals left atrial and left ventricular hypertension and a significant systolic pressure difference between the left ventricle and the femoral artery, particularly if the coarctation is isolated. In the presence of a large VSD and PDA, the left ventricular hypertension and the systolic pressure difference between the left ventricle and the femoral artery are less impressive and may not exist at all related to a nonrestrictive PDA supplying perfusion to the descending aorta. Every attempt should be made to define the nature and severity of associated defects. Imaging is recommended in older children to demonstrate the exact site and length of the coarctation as well as to show unusual features of the collateral circulation that may be of importance to the surgeon. Magnetic resonance imaging is an excellent, and in most instances, the preferable alternative to angiography for demonstrating the site and length of the coarctation (Fig. 82–20).

Natural History and Prognosis

Approximately one-half of infants admitted with heart failure within the first weeks of life have coarctation without significant associated defects.[123] The majority of these infants respond well to medical management and, if no repair is performed, reach a stage at 2 or 3 years of age where they are indistinguishable from asymptomatic children of the same age whose coarctation is first detected during a routine physical examination. Upper extremity hypertension usually increases during the first several months of life and then tends to diminish again as collateral circulation improves, while signs of failure diminish at the same time. For infants with severe failure and any serious associated defects, balloon dilation or surgery provides virtually the only chance of survival.

The consequences of persistent hypertension in an individual who has not undergone surgery appear in the second and third decades in the form of severe hypertension, aortic rupture, or intracranial hemorrhage from an aneurysm of the circle of Willis. Heart failure often complicated by mitral or aortic valve disease, a dissecting aneurysm of the aorta, or atherosclerosis presents in the fourth decade. The risk of endocarditis on the aortic or mitral valves or endarteritis at the site of coarctation appears to be spread relatively evenly over the years. The average age of death of patients who survive childhood with coarctation without surgery is 34 years.[124,125]

Medical Management

Vigorous medical treatment is indicated for infants with severe heart failure. A newborn with severe failure may experience dramatic relief from the intravenous infusion of PGE_1 to reopen the closing ductus, which provides perfusion to the descending aorta.[104] Prompt correction of the coarctation is recommended for all infants with one or more associated defects and for all infants with isolated coarctation. Inotropic support with dopamine or dobutamine should be initi-

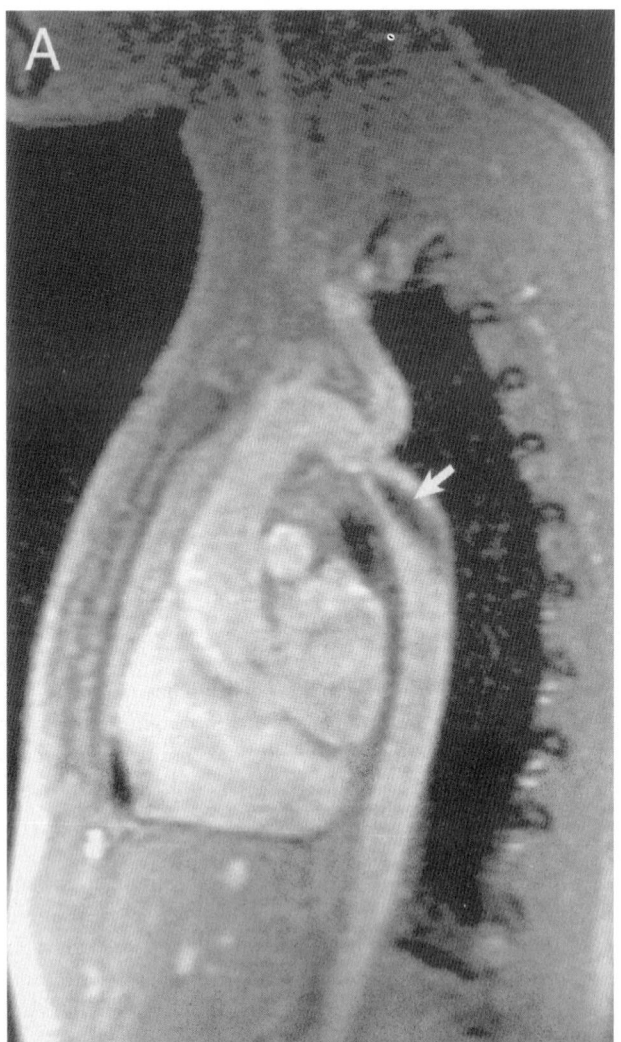
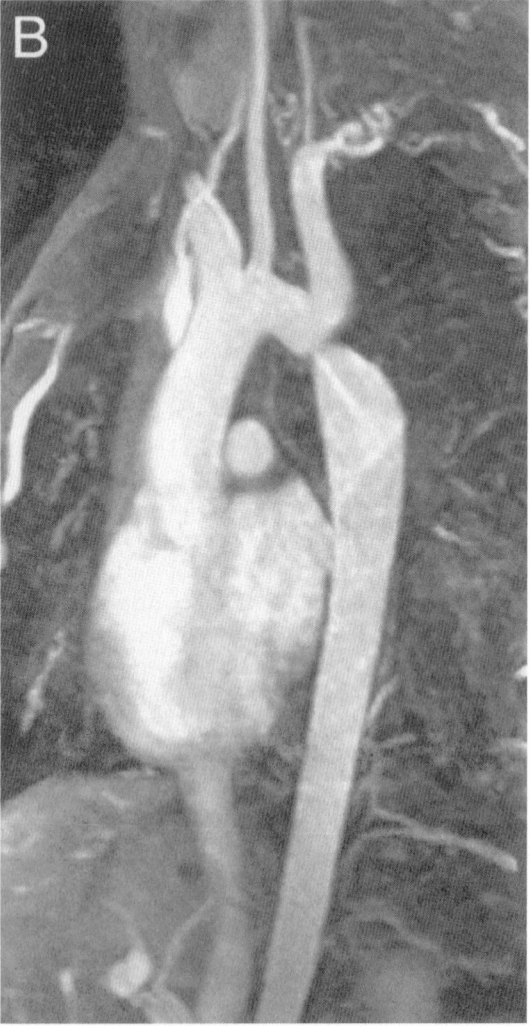

FIGURE 82–20. MRI evaluation of coarctation of the aorta. **A.** Systolic frame from a cine magnetic resonance sequence showing a turbulent jet at the coarctation site (*arrow*). **B.** Gadolinium-enhanced three-dimensional magnetic resonance angiography subvolume maximal intensity projection image of the aorta. *Source: From Geva T, Sahn DJ, Powell AC. Magnetic resonance imaging of congenital heart disease in adults. Prog Pediatr Cardiol 2003;17:21–39. Reproduced with permission of the authors and publisher.*

ated to augment diminished left ventricular function. Correction of metabolic acidosis should occur prior to surgical intervention.

Catheter Intervention

The timing and type of correction of isolated discrete coarctation of the aorta remain a topic of some dispute. There is general agreement that all children with heart failure should be repaired after a brief period of stabilization and treatment. Because balloon dilation of native coarctation in infants younger than 6 months of age has had an unacceptable restenosis rate of up to 75 percent,[126] most cardiologists would consider surgical repair as the favored approach. For older infants and children without heart failure, timing for intervention has been somewhat variable. Given the potential for restenosis in younger patients following surgery, intervention was often deferred until beyond 1 year of age.[127] With emergence of balloon dilation angioplasty as a method for improvement of residual gradients following surgery, many centers are less reluctant to proceed with surgical repair under 1 year of age for gradients >20 mmHg, systemic hypertension or marked collateral formation regardless of measured gradient.

For those patients with coarctation initially identified after 1 year of age, the preferred approach is not yet clear. It appears that balloon dilation angioplasty can achieve a reduction in gradient similar to that following surgery. Although reports of long-term followup are lacking, a randomized study comparing outcomes of a small population of children undergoing balloon dilation versus surgery for native coarctation, showed no difference between the two groups with regard to resting blood pressure, residual gradient, exercise performance and need for repeat interventions.[128] There was a significant increase in the frequency of aneurysm formation in those undergoing angioplasty (35 percent) compared with the surgical group (0 percent). The approach as to when to intervene for aneurysm remains unclear, though the use of covered stents may provide a reasonable long-term option for such patients. In addition to aneurysm formation, catheterization can cause femoral arterial damage related to the use of large catheters.

Currently, there is general agreement that symptomatic children younger than 6 months of age should be repaired surgically, and those who develop significant recurrent stenosis at any age should undergo balloon dilation or stent placement. The optimal therapy for the treatment of native coarctation in children older than 1 year of age remains somewhat controversial. For balloon dilation, immediate success (defined as an increase in the coarctation diameter with a residual gradient of less than 20 mmHg) occurs in a large percentage of patients.[129] However, long-term gradient relief after angioplasty has been somewhat less than that with surgery. Restenosis rates in the intermediate term seem to be directly related to the age at dilation, with 85 percent of neonates, 35 percent of infants, and 10 percent of children older than 2 years of age developing restenosis.[126] Repeat dilation is almost invariably successful, and many advocate this approach even if it requires two dilations rather than a one-step surgical approach. In older children, a stent can be placed if the balloon dilation fails (Fig. 82–21). In selected older children and adults, stent deployment has been very successful, with an average reduction in the gradient from 25 to 5 mm in 32 patients at Children's Hospital in Boston.[130] Complications have usually been related to associated diseases, although small aneurysms at the site of dilation have been reported in approximately 5 percent of cases. Trauma to the femoral artery, related to the use of large catheters, is not uncommon.

Patients who have had coarctation repair must be followed indefinitely. Residual hypertension is prevalent in many, even when repair is completed in infancy.[131] For those with significant recoarctation expressed as a systolic pressure gradient of 20 mmHg or more at rest, balloon angioplasty and/or stent placement are recommended. Repeat surgery for recurrent coarctation is rarely necessary. Occasionally, patients with insignificant or small residual resting gradients manifest abnormal upper extremity hypertension and significant gradients with exercise These patients should probably undergo balloon angioplasty and stent placement with pharmacologic control of their hypertension if present at rest or unmasked with exercise.

Surgical Management

The coarctation is exposed and mobilized through a left posterolateral thoracotomy. It is usually possible to resect the narrow segment and restore continuity with a direct end-to-end anastomosis (Fig. 82–22). When the narrowed segment is longer, repair by subclavian flap aortoplasty or, rarely, a tubular vascular prosthesis to bridge the gap between the two ends of the aorta may be necessary. In adults with a relatively inelastic or calcified aorta, a tubular vascular prosthesis can be used to bypass the unresected coarctation or the site of a previous repair. Dacron patch repair of coarctation has an unacceptably high incidence of late aneurysm formation and is no longer advised.[132] Tension-free suture lines are essential. Postoperative bleeding, chylothorax, paraplegia, and injury to the phrenic and recurrent laryngeal nerves remain potential complications.[133] Although long-term surgical results of those undergoing surgery in childhood are generally excellent, a large number of patients experience late hypertension.[134]

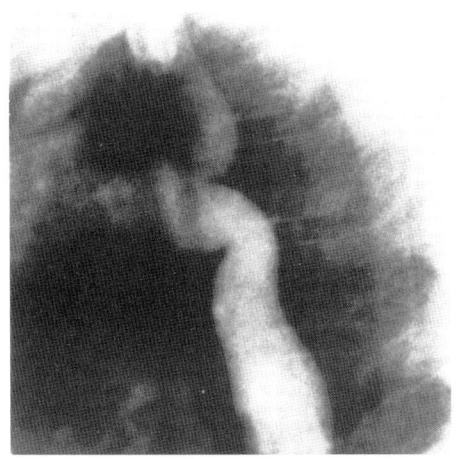 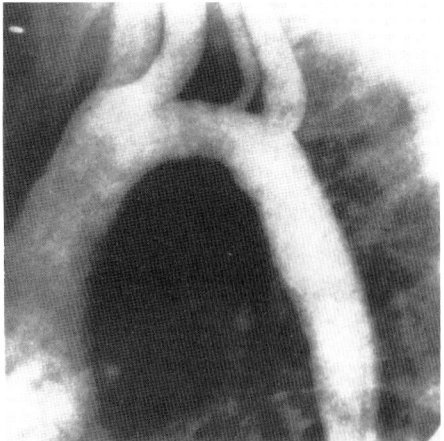

Pre   Post

FIGURE 82–21. Repair of coarctation with a stent. *Left panel:* Coarctation caused by kink with anterior indentation. *Right panel:* Narrowing eliminated with stent. *Source: Courtesy of Audrey Marshall, MD.*

If a significant VSD is also present, some surgeons prefer to place a pulmonary arterial band at the time of coarctation repair during infancy. The VSD may then be repaired electively during the next several months, when the heart failure is well controlled. Primary repair of the VSD shortly after or simultaneously with coarctation repair is an alternative that has gained favor among many surgical groups.[135]

Adequacy of collateral circulation to the spinal cord is crucial for the safe repair of coarctation. A rise in proximal systemic arterial pressure of more than 20 mmHg when the aorta is clamped above the coarctation suggests a marginal collateral circulation. Mild systemic hypothermia is a simple and useful adjunct, and monitoring of somatosensory cortical evoked potentials may warn of an impending ischemic insult to the spinal cord.[136] Postoperative paradoxical hypertension is common between the second and fifth postoperative days and may contribute to the *postcoarctation syndrome,* in which ileus, abdominal pain, mesenteric vasculitis, and visceral infarction can occur. This syndrome is rarely encountered if the postoperative blood pressure is maintained within the normal range for age with sodium nitroprusside, blockers, or angiotensin-converting enzyme inhibitors.

Operative mortality for infants with isolated coarctation is in the range of 0 to 3 percent,[128,133,135] but it is 10 percent or higher when other cardiovascular defects are present. Excellent results have been reported among low-birth-weight infants.[137] Subsequent deaths are uncommon in surviving infants with isolated coarctation but are more likely in those with complicated associated defects.

Long-Term Clinical Course

Patients who have had coarctation repair must be followed indefinitely. Residual hypertension is prevalent in many, even when repair is completed in infancy.[131] For patients with significant recoarctation, expressed as a systolic gradient of 20 mmHg or more at rest, balloon angioplasty and/or stent placement are recommended. Repeat surgery for recurrent coarctation is rarely necessary. Occasionally, patients with insignificant or small residual resting gradients manifest abnormal upper extremity hypertension and significant gradients with exercise.[124]

【 】 VALVULAR AORTIC STENOSIS

Definition

Aortic stenosis is defined as subtotal obstruction of varying severity in the channel of left ventricular outflow. In order of decreasing frequency, the sites of obstruction by congenital lesions are (1) valvular, (2) subvalvular, and (3) supravalvular (see Chap. 66).

Pathology

Most commonly, the aortic valve is bicuspid with two commissures, one or both of which are fused to varying degrees. A third rudimentary commissure, or raphe, is frequently present in the larger of the leaflets. The valve opening is eccentric. Less frequently encountered is a unicuspid, unicommissural, or noncommissural valve in which the orifice is often slit-like, at first glance suggesting a bicuspid valve. Uncommonly, a true dome is present, resembling the valve of congenital isolated pulmonary stenosis. Rarely, the valve is tricuspid, with fusion of one or more of the three commissures. When survival to adult life occurs, calcification may appear in the valvular tissue, leading to rigidity of the valve. Poststenotic dilation of the ascending aorta occurs in all cases to some degree. Coarctation of the aorta is the most common associated anomaly.

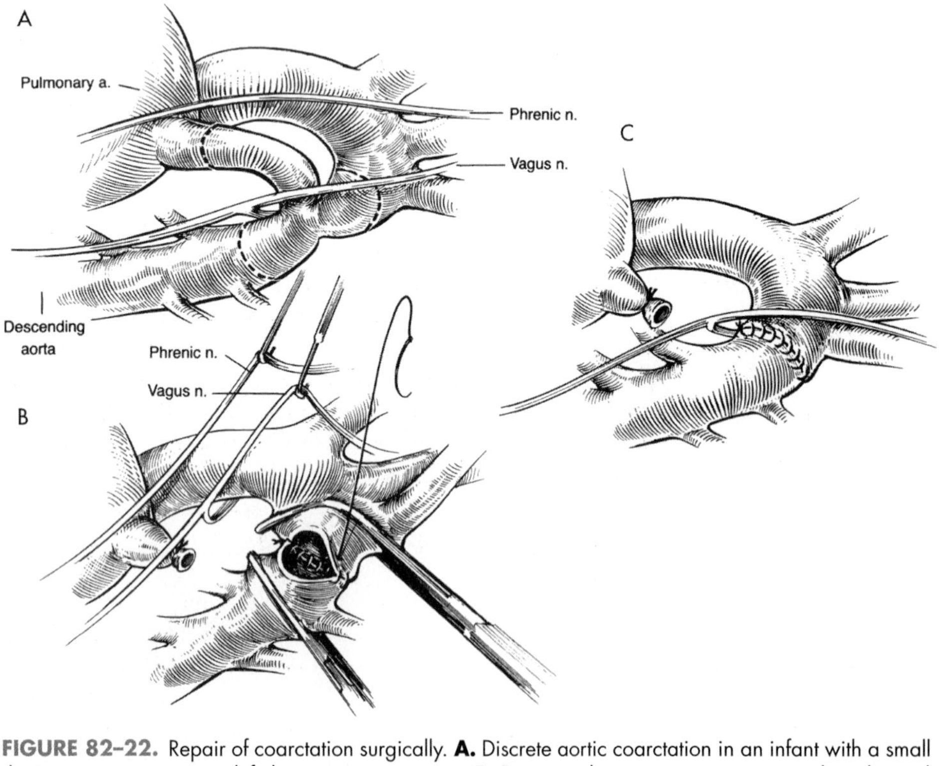

Abnormal Physiology

The hemodynamics of congenital valvular aortic stenosis are similar to those of acquired aortic stenosis except that a persistent PDA or stretched foramen ovale in the immediate postnatal period may lessen the severity of pulmonary edema by diverting blood away from the left ventricle.

Severity usually is judged by the peak systolic pressure gradient (PSPG) across the aortic valve and the calculated aortic valve area determined at cardiac catheterization. In the presence of a normal cardiac output, a PSPG ≥ 75 mmHg or an aortic valve area <0.5 cm^2/m^2 is considered severe, a PSPG between 50 and 75 mmHg or a valve area between 0.5 and 0.8 cm^2/m^2 is considered moderate, and a PSPG <50 mmHg or a valve area >0.9 cm^2/m^2 is considered mild (see Chaps. 17 and 66).

FIGURE 82–22. Repair of coarctation surgically. **A.** Discrete aortic coarctation in an infant with a small ductus arteriosus seen via left thoracotomy exposure. **B.** Repair technique using resection with end-to-end anastomosis. **C.** Complete repair. *Source: From Castaneda AR, Jonas RA, Mayer JE Jr, Hanley FL.*[66] *Reproduced with permission from the publisher and author.*

Clinical Manifestations

Approximately 7 percent of infants and children with congenital heart disease have aortic stenosis in one of its several forms, approximately 80 percent of which is valvular. Valvular stenosis is much more common among males than females, with a male-to-female ratio of 4:1.

History The detection of a systolic murmur leads to the discovery of this malformation in most patients, the vast majority of whom are asymptomatic. Easy fatigue, dyspnea, syncope, and angina suggest severe obstruction, but severe obstruction may exist in the absence of any symptoms. Sudden death may occur from this malformation, but in most such cases death is preceded by either symptoms or ECG changes. Infants with critical stenosis from birth present with congestive failure within 2 weeks and represent true emergencies. A similar small number of patients with less critical but severe obstruction are detected over the course of the next 4 to 6 months.

Physical Examination The arterial blood pressure and quality of the peripheral arterial pulses of older infants and children are usually normal. A measured pulse pressure <20 mmHg suggests severe stenosis. The cardiac apical impulse may be forceful and sustained; a systolic thrill along the right upper sternal border and over the carotid arteries is present in most of these patients. The absence of a thrill suggests a PSPG below 30 mmHg. Paradoxical splitting of the second heart sound is rare and associated with very severe obstruction or coexisting myocardial disease. An early systolic ejection click at the apex is characteristic and serves to distinguish valvular aortic stenosis from other forms of left ventricular outflow tract obstruction. The classic auscultatory finding is a harsh systolic crescendo-decrescendo murmur that is loudest at the right upper sternal border, with radiation into the carotid arteries and down the left sternal border to the apex (see Chap. 12). Among infants with critical obstruction and low cardiac output, there may be no palpable peripheral pulses and no distinctive murmur until implementation of anticongestive therapy.

Chest Roentgenogram The heart's overall size is normal, but infants with failure will have generalized cardiac enlargement and varying degrees of pulmonary edema. Poststenotic dilatation of the ascending aorta is characteristic.

Electrocardiogram Left ventricular hypertrophy, as indicated by voltage criteria in the left precordial leads, is seldom helpful in distinguishing patients with severe obstruction from those with mild to moderate obstruction. However, diminished anterior forces in the right precordial leads and a deep SV_1 ≥30 mm suggest severe stenosis, as does absence of the Q wave in V_6. Fifty percent of patients with severe obstruction have a flat, biphasic, or inverted T wave in V_6 (Fig. 82–23). However, severe, and even critical, obstruction may be present with none of the ECG abnormalities mentioned above. Monitoring of the ST segment in leads V_5 through V_7 during cautious exercise testing appears to be a reliable method of detecting children with a gradient exceeding 50 mmHg who may be at risk for sudden death.[138] Symptomatic infants may show right, left, or biventricular hypertrophy, frequently with T-wave inversion over the left precordium.

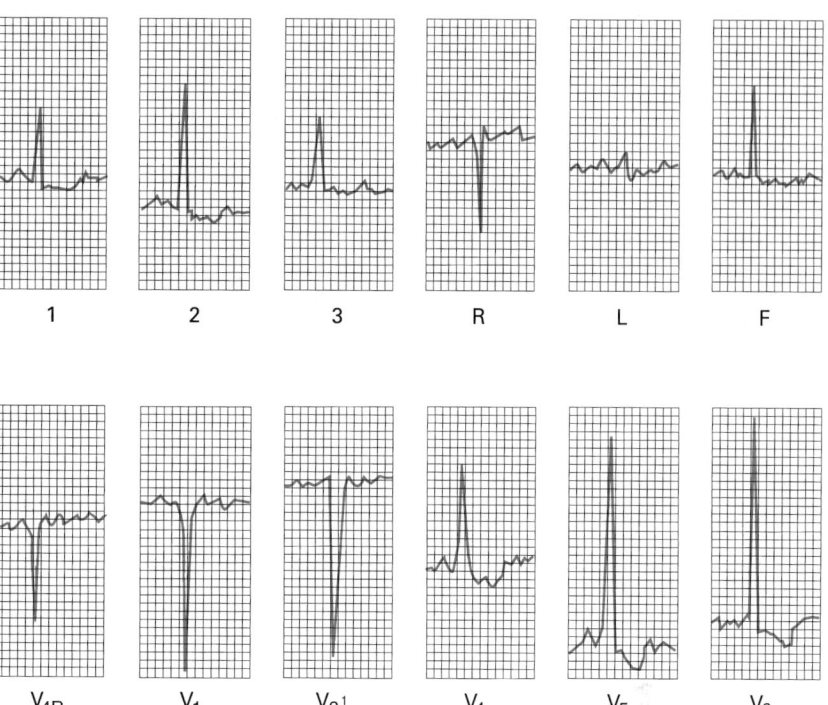

FIGURE 82–23. Electrocardiogram from an 8-year-old boy with valvular aortic stenosis and a 94 mmHg peak systolic pressure gradient. The small anterior QRS forces, abnormally large posterior forces, absent Q waves in leads V_5 and V_6, and abnormal T waves and ST segments reflect severe left ventricular systolic pressure overload with ischemia.

Echocardiogram Continuous-wave Doppler echocardiography guided by two-dimensional echocardiographic imaging predicts very accurately the peak instantaneous and mean systolic pressure gradient across discrete forms of left ventricular outflow tract obstruction (see Chap. 17; Fig. 82–24). The mean gradients appear to correlate well with peak-to-peak gradients measured at catheterization.[139] Two-dimensional echocardiography can distinguish the exact site of obstruction and identify hypoplasia of the left ventricle, mitral valve annulus, or aortic root to a degree that precludes survival.[140,141]

Cardiac Catheterization In general, catheterization is performed only when intervention is anticipated. Infants symptomatic with severe aortic obstruction often have a left-to-right shunt through a stretched foramen ovale, PAH, and a right-to-left shunt through a PDA. A marked increase in left ventricular end-diastolic pressure is usually present. The PSPG between the left ventricle and the central aorta should be documented whenever possible. If left ventricular output is markedly diminished, this gradient may be relatively small even in the presence of severe obstruction. Left ventricular angiography will confirm the site of obstruction and outline the size of the left ventricular cavity (Fig. 82–25A).

In older infants and children, pressures on the right side of the heart are usually normal. Simultaneous recording of central aortic and left ventricular pressures or a pressure tracing upon catheter withdrawal from the left ventricle to the aorta, coupled with an accurate estimate of cardiac output, is necessary for reliable assessment of severity. Left ventricular angiography will document the site of obstruction. The aortic leaflets are typically thickened and domed, with a central or eccentric jet of contrast material entering the ascending aorta. Poststenotic dilatation is characteristic. Supra-

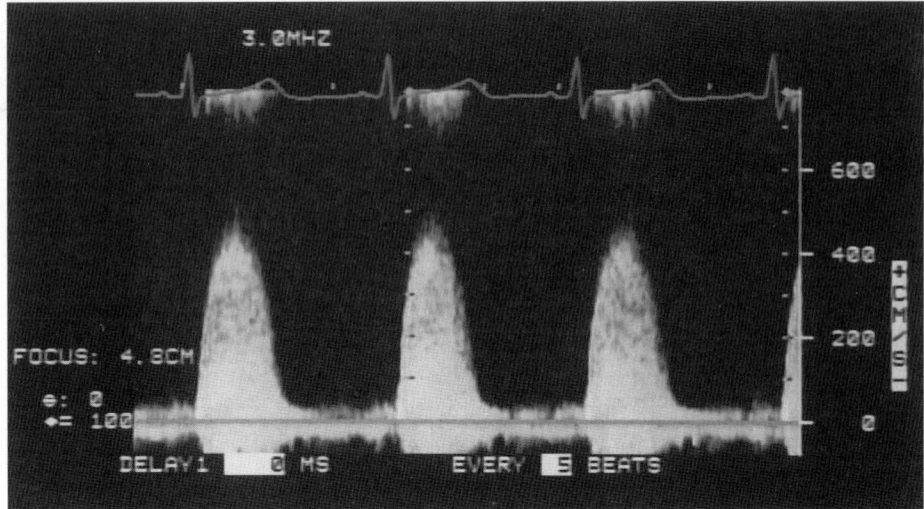

FIGURE 82–24. Doppler interrogation in the ascending aorta in a patient with valvular aortic stenosis. The peak velocity of 4.8 m/s correlates with a maximum instantaneous gradient of 92 mmHg across the aortic valve.

valvular aortography is recommended to assess the presence and severity of aortic regurgitation.

Natural History and Prognosis

About half the infants born with severe valvular aortic stenosis require hospitalization within the first week of life. Not uncommonly, the murmur is mistaken for that of a VSD. Heart failure beyond infancy and before adolescence is not seen without the presence of complicating factors. Symptomatic infants require prompt relief of obstruction by balloon valvuloplasty, the procedure of choice. The presence of endocardial fibroelastosis, papillary muscle necrosis, associated intra- and extracardiac deformities, and a small left ventricular cavity contribute incremental risk for mortality. Survivors may have significant aortic regurgitation, but the majority can be managed medically, or with aortic valvuloplasty or valve replacement, for those with severe regurgitation.

Most infants beyond the newborn period and children with mild aortic valvular stenosis (PSPG at catheterization <25 mmHg or a Doppler mean pressure gradient <25 mmHg) remain stable, with only a 21 percent likelihood of progression in severity and the need for intervention within the subsequent 25 years. For patients with a PSPG between 25 and 49 mmHg, the likelihood of significant progression rises to 41 percent, and with a PSPG >50 mmHg, it rises to 71 percent.[44] Patients with a PSPG >50 mmHg are at risk for serious ventricular arrhythmias and sudden death. Infective endocarditis on the aortic valve (see Chap. 85) poses an extremely serious complication in the form of systemic arterial emboli and serious, even catastrophic, aortic regurgitation with congestive failure, shock, and death.[63]

Medical and Surgical Management

Infants with the characteristic murmur detected in the first weeks of life should be evaluated very carefully to be certain the obstruction is not severe and does not become severe in the next few weeks or months.[142] Those who develop heart failure should have intervention without delay. In a critically ill neonate, intravenous PGE_1 infusion to open the ductus may provide temporary relief of pulmonary edema.

Beyond infancy, a yearly plan of reexamination with careful questioning regarding symptoms and an ECG, an echocardiogram with Doppler assessment of the mean and maximum pressure gradient every year or two, exercise testing, and 24-hour ECG monitoring about every 3 years should suffice to prevent progression from going unrecognized. Indications for cardiac catheterization for gradient assessment and possible balloon dilation include the appearance of symptoms or syncope, decreased anterior forces with an $SV_1 \geq 30$ mm or flattening or inversion of the T wave in V_6 in the resting ECG, abnormal ST-T segments on exercise testing, or a Doppler estimated maximum instantaneous gradient of >65 mmHg or mean gradient >40 mmHg.

Catheter-based balloon valvuloplasty has become the preferred alternative to surgery. In skilled hands, it can provide effective reduction of the transvalvular gradient while producing only a mild increment in aortic regurgitation in most instances.[143–145] Elective balloon dilation is recommended if the PSPG is >50 mmHg at catheterization with aortic regurgitation mild or nonexistent. For a neonate with critical valvular obstruction, some centers continue to rely on surgical intervention, but catheter balloon valvuloplasty has become a very competitive alternative and in the author's institution is the procedure of choice for these very sick infants.

Early studies and more recent experience suggest that the balloon diameter should not exceed that of the valve ring, and most centers now use balloons that are 85 to 90 percent of the diameter of the aortic annulus. The balloon is inflated to a pressure of 4 to 6 atm until the "waist" produced by the stenotic valve has been abolished (see Fig. 82–25B). Transient arrhythmias are seen occasionally, but apart from creating aortic regurgitation, other complications are uncommon.

In older children, the results are usually quite good, with a reduction of the peak gradient of approximately 60 percent, a mortality rate under 2 percent, and a complication rate of about 3 percent.[143,144] In neonates, the results are more problematic, probably because of severity and complexity of disease, unstable conditions, and the size of the patient, with 14 percent early mortality in one series with an improving trend (4 percent) in the most recent 8 years. Reintervention (usually repeat balloon dilation) was necessary in 62 percent within 5 years.[146]

When surgical intervention is required for critical aortic stenosis during infancy, the heart is exposed through a median sternotomy and the aortic valve visualized through the ascending aorta during a brief period of low-flow perfusion with mild hypothermia. Standard cardiopulmonary bypass, mild hypothermia, and cardioplegia are used in older children.[147] The surgeon must discriminate between true commissures and abnormal raphes, because incision of the latter produces intolerable aortic valvular regurgitation. Relief of valvular stenosis is accomplished with a carefully placed incision in the middle of each fused, but well-supported, true commissure.

A conservative attitude is essential during operation for aortic stenosis in an infant or small child. Mild valvular regurgitation almost always occurs consequent to commissurotomy but is usually well tolerated. Moderate residual stenosis is preferred to intolerable aortic

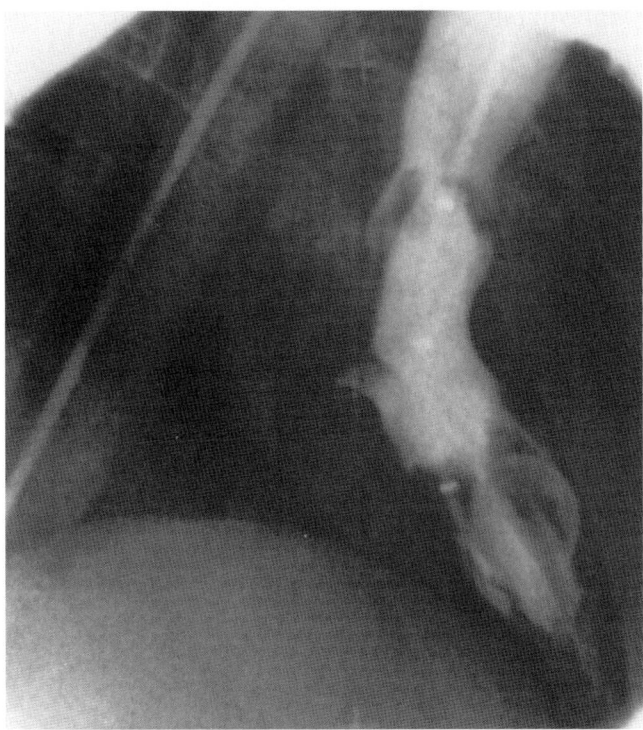
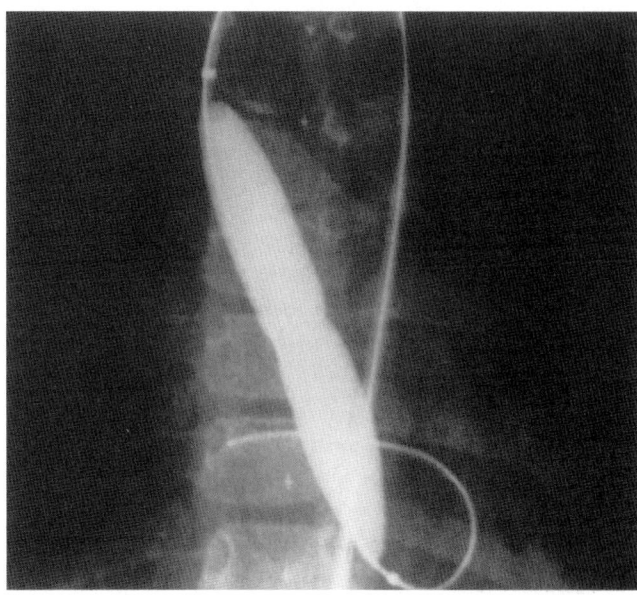

A B

FIGURE 82-25. Balloon aortic valvuloplasty. **A.** Left ventricular angiogram showing a domed, thickened aortic valve with fusion of the right and left commissures. **B.** Balloon dilation using a retrograde technique. A waist is demonstrated in the midportion of the balloon before full inflation. *Source: From Lock JE, Keane JF, Perry SB. Diagnostic and Interventional Catheterization in Congenital Heart Disease, 2d ed. Boston: Kluwer, 2000:151. Reproduced with permission from the publisher and authors.*

valvular regurgitation, especially in infants in whom valve implantation is technically difficult. If valve replacement is necessary in an infant or small child, use of the autograft pulmonary valve in the aortic position offers the attractive possibility of continuing growth of this neoaortic valve, which may parallel that of the patient.[148] The risk of operation is high in critically ill infants, in the range of 10 to 15 percent, particularly in those with a low ejection fraction, high left ventricular end-diastolic pressure, endocardial fibroelastosis, marked heart failure, or features of left ventricular hypoplasia.[149] Morbidity after aortic valvotomy in an older child is rare, and the likelihood of relief of left ventricular outflow tract obstruction and survival is good. The Natural History Study of Congenital Heart Defects, reporting on 133 children who underwent aortic commissurotomy after the age of 2 years, found that only 27 percent required a second operation in the subsequent 20 years, with 78 percent of those operations consisting of valve replacement. Aortic regurgitation was the indication for operation in 14 percent of those with valve replacements.[44]

Relief of aortic valve obstruction, whether by balloon valvuloplasty or surgical valvotomy, is palliative rather than curative. Gradual restenosis is the rule, with almost one-third of infants who undergo valvotomy requiring a second operation, usually valve replacement, within the next two decades. Aortic regurgitation, a well-recognized complication of valvuloplasty, valvulotomy, and/or infective endocarditis, may require surgical intervention as well. Endocarditis is a serious and lifelong hazard, with an incidence among patients followed for 20 years of approximately 5 percent, a mortality rate of just over 25 percent, and a predilection for patients in the second rather than the first decade of life and with PSPGs >50 mmHg.[44,63]

Secondary valvulotomy by balloon or surgery for recurrent or residual stenosis can be attempted, but calcification and restenosis eventually necessitate aortic valve replacement in almost all those requiring surgery on the aortic valve in infancy or childhood. A small aortic annulus severely limits the relief of left ventricular hypertension unless one resorts to the Konno operation, in which the annulus is divided; the upper ventricular septum resected, creating a VSD; patching the VSD with prosthetic material; and replacing the valve (a homograft or pulmonary autograft) into the enlarged annulus. The ascending aorta and anterior right ventricular wall are reconstructed using a prosthetic graft; in the case of an autograft, the main pulmonary artery and pulmonary valve are replaced with a cryopreserved pulmonary homograft.[150] *Children with more than mild aortic stenosis are restricted from strenuous organized athletics, isometric exercises, and activities that require a good deal of stamina and produce shortness of breath.*[151]

Fetal Intervention

More recently, some investigators have been using balloon valvuloplasty in the fetuses diagnosed with aortic stenosis and a small left ventricle. The conceptual goal is to provide improved antegrade flow through the left ventricular outflow tract facilitating left ventricular chamber growth. With sufficient growth, the object is to avoid a univentricular repair following delivery. Although the experience has been limited to a small number of centers, the largest reported group includes 20 of 26 fetuses who had a technically successful aortic valve dilation with improved antegrade flow. Twelve had at least mild aortic regurgitation. Surprisingly, all fetuses with moderate or severe aortic regurgitation had returned to no more than mild aortic regurgitation by 8 weeks from the intervention. Four of 20 infants had a two-ventricle circulation; the remainder underwent a stage I Norwood procedure. Longer-term followup is needed to determine if the success in achieving a two-ventricle circulation can be extended.[152]

【 】 SUPRAVALVULAR AORTIC STENOSIS

Pathology

The obstruction in the ascending aorta includes the following three types: (1) hourglass (discrete), (2) hypoplastic (diffuse), and (3) membranous. Associated obstructions in the pulmonary trunk, peripheral pulmonary arteries, and branches of the aortic arch are common.[153] Hypertrophy of the coronary arterial walls and premature coronary atherosclerosis have been described.[154]

Clinical Manifestations

Supravalvular stenosis may be familial, associated with characteristic facies and mental retardation, sporadic, or (rarely) the result of congenital rubella. All forms may be and usually are associated with varying degrees of peripheral or branch pulmonary arterial stenosis. The familial form is transmitted as an autosomal dominant trait with variable expression (see Chap. 12). Mental retardation is not present, and there are no characteristic facial features.[155] Supravalvular aortic stenosis associated with mental retardation, frequently called *Williams syndrome,* is associated with a high and prominent forehead, epicanthal folds, underdevelopment of the bridge of the nose and mandible, and a broad, overhanging upper lip. It is caused by a deletion of the elastin gene on chromosome 7 and can now be identified by fluorescent in situ hybridization studies. It has been linked with idiopathic hypercalcemia of infancy, but hypercalcemia is not present in the majority of patients recognized beyond infancy.

The symptoms of supravalvular aortic stenosis are similar to those of subvalvular aortic stenosis. Patients with the familial form usually have a distinctive family history but one that seldom emerges in its entirety on initial questioning. The physical findings are also similar to those of subvalvular aortic stenosis, although a systolic blood pressure difference may be recorded between the two arms on occasion, with the right-arm pressure being greater than that of the left (Coanda effect).[157] Chest roentgenography and ECG are not distinctive unless associated pulmonary arterial stenosis leads to right ventricular hypertrophy. Echocardiography can identify the narrowed aortic lumen just above the aortic valve and provide an estimate of the severity of the obstruction by the Doppler-derived instantaneous pressure gradient.

At cardiac catheterization, a systolic pressure gradient can be demonstrated just above the aortic valve by careful pullback. Supravalvular aortography or left ventricular angiography will visualize the supravalvular narrowing (Fig. 82–26). Pressure recordings in the branch pulmonary arteries should be obtained; in the presence of any significant stenoses, pulmonary arterial angiography should be performed. Narrowing at the branch points of major arteries (e.g., coronary, carotid, mesenteric, renal) is occasionally seen.

Natural History and Prognosis

The sequence of progressive obstruction, the appearance of symptoms and ECG changes, and the possibility of sudden death appear to apply for supravalvular aortic stenosis as well as for valvular aortic stenosis. Infective endocarditis represents a threat to these patients throughout life.

Management

The indications for cardiac catheterization and followup are the same as those for valvular aortic stenosis. Noninvasive imaging frequently suffices, but angiography may be necessary to evaluate the gradient and rule out arterial narrowing. Surgery is usually recommended if the gradient across the narrowing exceeds 40 mmHg.

Discrete supravalvular aortic stenosis is relieved by one or more incisions through the narrow segment of the ascending aorta, usually at the level of the sinotubular ridge at the top of the commissures. Incisions are extended well down into the aortic sinuses. Ridges of obstructing fibrous tissue are excised. The aorta is enlarged by the insertion of a gusset of prosthetic vascular graft material or pericardium to increase the circumference.[147] A favorable outcome can be anticipated postoperatively in most patients with supravalvular aortic stenosis if the abnormality of the arterial wall is localized[158]; however, despite angioplasty, deficiency of growth of the more distal segments of the aorta persists.[159] Intimal obstruction of the coronary arterial ostia may require debridement, dilation, or even saphenous vein or internal mammary bypass grafting.

Diffuse tubular hypoplasia of the ascending aorta is a technically challenging problem that is associated with a higher mortality rate and usually poor postoperative hemodynamic results.

【 】 SUBVALVULAR AORTIC STENOSIS

Pathology

Three classic varieties of subvalvular aortic stenosis involve the left ventricular outflow tract: the discrete, tunnel, and muscular types. The discrete type is characterized by a localized fibrous encirclement of the left ventricular outflow tract a short distance below the aortic valve (Fig. 82–27) or fibromuscular tissue that extends onto the mitral leaflet and may also attach to the aortic cusps. The tunnel type involves hypoplasia of the aortic annulus and a channel with a fibrous lining in the subjacent left ventricular outflow tract.[160,161] The muscular type also is known as *hypertrophic cardiomyopathy* (or idiopathic hypertrophic subaortic stenosis) and is discussed in Chap. 30. More than half these patients have associated malformations, of which PDA, VSD, or coarctation are the most common.

Clinical Manifestations

Discrete stenosis is more common among males, with a male/female ratio of approximately 2.5:1. In the isolated forms, the majority of patients are referred because of the detection of a murmur that not uncommonly is mistaken initially for that of a VSD. The symptoms have the same implications as they do for valvular aortic stenosis. The physical examination is similar to that of valvular aortic stenosis with two exceptions: an early systolic ejection click is not heard, and an early diastolic murmur of aortic regurgitation is present in approximately one-half of these patients. The roentgenographic features and ECG are also similar to those of valvular aortic stenosis except for the absence of poststenotic dilatation of the ascending aorta. Two-dimensional echocardiography permits excellent visualization of the anatomy of the obstruction. An estimate of the systolic pressure gradient can be obtained from Doppler echocardiographic studies.

When catheterization is performed, a careful pullback pressure tracing across the left ventricular outflow tract will document the severity of the gradient and establish the site of the obstruction.

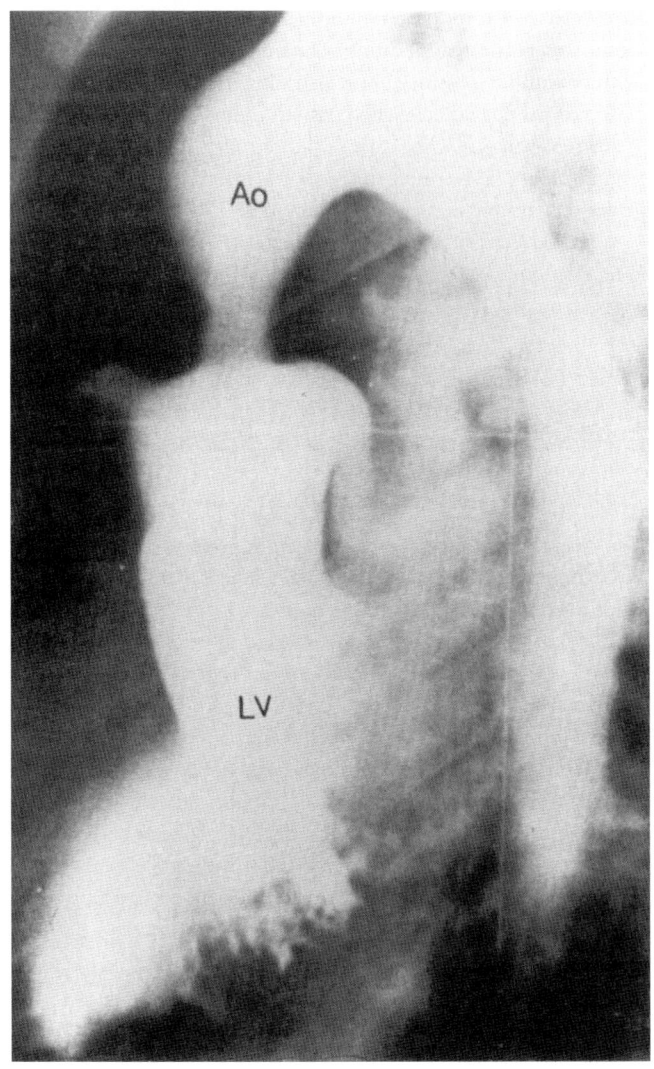

A

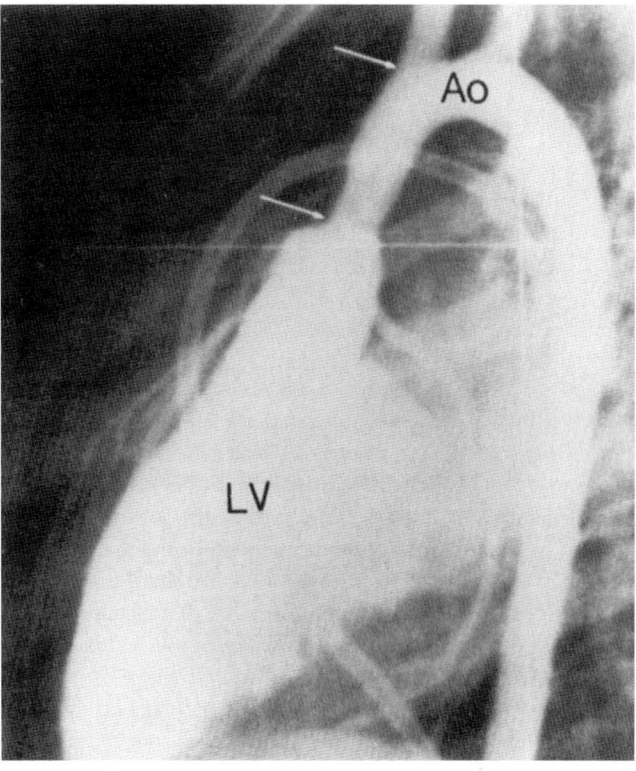

B

FIGURE 82-26. A. Supravalvular aortic stenosis, discrete type. The stenotic segment is located immediately above the aortic sinuses of Valsalva. The distal ascending aorta (Ao) is normal in size. LV, left ventricle. **B.** Supravalvular aortic stenosis, diffuse type. Narrowing in the ascending aorta begins above the aortic valve (*lower arrow*) and extends throughout the ascending aortic segment to the origin of the brachiocephalic vessels (*upper arrow*). In this patient, the aortic arch and descending aorta also appear hypoplastic. *Source: Keane JF, Fellows KE, La Farge G, et al. The surgical management of discrete and diffuse supravalvular aortic stenosis. Circulation 1976;54:112–117. Reproduced with permission from the publisher and authors.*

Left ventricular biplane angiography will outline the nature of the obstruction. Aortography is recommended to evaluate the degree of aortic regurgitation.

Natural History and Prognosis

Severe heart failure in infancy is unusual and, if present, is almost invariably associated with complicating defects.[160] The obstruction is progressive in most instances, sometimes rapidly so. In one study, 75 percent of patients showed an increase of 25 mmHg or more in a 5-year period.[162] The cause of the progression is not known, but an intriguing theory suggests that distorted anatomy increases shear stress, leading to a stimulation of growth factors and cellular proliferation.[163] Associated aortic regurgitation also tends to be progressive and appears to result from damage due to the jet of blood through the obstruction, with secondary thickening and deformity of the valve leaflets. The results of surgery depend on the extent of involvement of the left ventricular outflow tract, with the best results being obtained in patients with a thin,

discrete subvalvular membrane. The least-satisfactory results occur in patients with tunnel obstruction.

Management

Medical management is similar to that of patients with valvular aortic stenosis, but surgery for the discrete type is usually recommended for pressure gradients ≥30 mmHg because of the possibility of progression of obstruction and the likelihood of progressive aortic valvular deformity and regurgitation.[164] At least one report suggests, however, that surgical intervention does not change the progression of aortic regurgitation.[165] Continued followup for assessment of reobstruction and progression of aortic regurgitation and for reemphasis of the precautions against infective endocarditis is essential in all patients.[166]

Subvalvular fibromuscular (membranous) left ventricular outflow tract obstruction is exposed through the aortic root, as was described for aortic valvular stenosis (see Fig. 82–27). Small, half-circle needles and sutures or hooks are placed into the abnormal fibromuscular tissue, pulling it into view for precise excision from

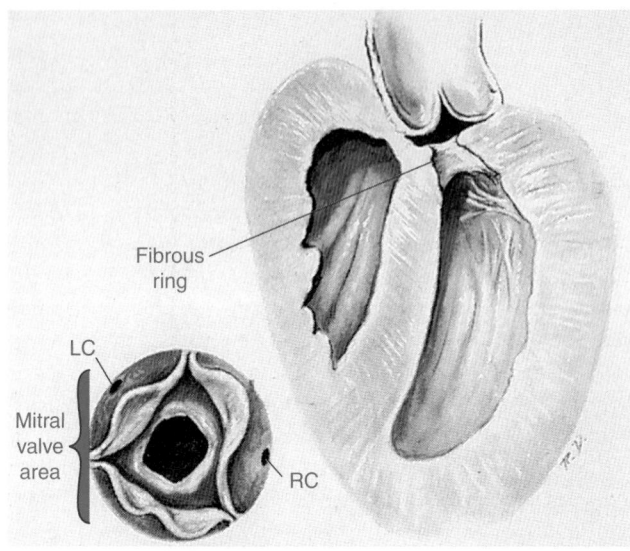

FIGURE 82–27. Localized subvalvular aortic stenosis. Obstruction is immediately upstream from the aortic valve. LC and RC, left and right coronary arteries. *Source: From Kirklin and Ellis.[167] Reproduced with permission from the publisher and authors.*

the underlying ventricular septum and the anterior mitral valve leaflet. The area of the bundle of His, which is usually just beneath the anterior commissure between the right and noncoronary leaflets, is avoided. An additional septal myectomy or myotomy beneath and to the left of the commissure between the right and left leaflets may be required if secondary hypertrophy is significant. Immediate and early operative outcome is generally good, but *residual, recurrent, and progressive subaortic obstruction occurs in up to 25 percent of these patients, requiring long-term followup.*[167,168]

Diffuse tunnel obstruction in the left ventricular outflow tract poses a difficult technical problem that requires aortoseptoplasty, reconstruction of the left ventricular outflow (Konno operation or a modification of it).[150,164]

BICUSPID AORTIC VALVE
Pathology

Classically, the two cusps are oriented anteriorly and posteriorly, with the anterior or conjoined cusp being the larger. A raphe, or ridge, is present along the aortic aspect of the larger cusp, running from the aortic wall to the free edge of the cusp. The most common associated condition of significance is coarctation of the aorta. The most common complication is calcification of the valve. *In approximately 85 percent of cases of calcific aortic stenosis in patients younger than age 70 years, the valve is congenitally bicuspid.* Aortic regurgitation from prolapse of the larger cusp is a less common complication and is usually not evident until adolescence or adult life.

Clinical Manifestations

The incidence in the general population approaches 2 percent; therefore, it is the most common congenital abnormality of the heart or great vessels except possibly for mitral valve prolapse (see Chap. 68). This condition serves as the substrate for further changes including stenosis from fibrosis and deposition of calcium, regurgitation, infective endocarditis, aortic root dilatation, and dissec-

tion.[169] It is also found commonly among patients with isolated or dominant aortic regurgitation, patients with infective endocarditis with or without a history of predisposing heart disease, and in otherwise normal individuals who come to the physician's attention incidentally. Patients with uncomplicated bicuspid aortic valve are asymptomatic. The incidence among males is approximately 2.5 times that among females (see Chap. 68).

The characteristic feature is auscultatory and consists of an early systolic ejection click, which is best heard at the apex and does not vary with respiration. A soft, early, or midsystolic murmur is frequently present at the right upper sternal border. Less commonly, a soft murmur of aortic regurgitation may be heard. Two-dimensional echocardiography with adequate images can identify the bicuspid valve with a high degree of sensitivity and diagnostic accuracy.

Natural History and Prognosis

The majority of congenitally bicuspid aortic valves are nonobstructive at birth; but with the passage of time, a few of these valves become fibrotic, less mobile, and more obstructive, eventually becoming the site of calcium deposition, primarily among individuals between ages 15 and 65 years. Important calcium deposition is unusual before age 30 years, whereas grossly visible deposits of calcium are present in the valves of virtually all patients with severe stenosis beyond that age. A much smaller number of individuals born with a bicuspid aortic valve develop isolated aortic regurgitation. In approximately one-third, this is the result of fibrosis, prolapse, or retraction of one or both of the leaflets; in the remainder, regurgitation results from infective endocarditis on an apparently functionally normal bicuspid valve (see Chap. 81).

CONGENITAL MITRAL REGURGITATION
Pathology

Mitral regurgitation may be due to a primary valve abnormality or secondary to a more complex defect (see Common Atrioventricular Canal Defects above). There are a variety of rare primary malformations, including isolated cleft, fenestration, and double orifice. Mitral regurgitation also occurs frequently with conditions that cause left ventricular dilatation and failure.

Clinical Manifestations

Poor growth, frequent respiratory infections, and failure occur with significant mitral regurgitation. The physical findings are generally similar to those with mitral regurgitation of other causes (see Chap. 12). There may be a prominent left precordial bulge if cardiomegaly has been present from infancy. The systolic murmur may radiate to the base of the heart. Left atrial and left ventricular enlargement correlate with the degree of volume overload. Echocardiography with Doppler color-flow mapping will demonstrate these as well as left ventricular function and the severity of regurgitation. The specific defect may be outlined, such as an isolated cleft or a double-orifice valve. Findings at cardiac catheterization substantiate the hemodynamic alterations.

Natural History and Prognosis

Mild and even moderate mitral regurgitation may be well tolerated, but severe regurgitation leads to progressive deterioration. Endocarditis is a risk.

Management

Vigorous medical treatment of heart failure and infections is warranted. Every attempt should be made to control symptoms to a degree that will allow growth in infants. In infants and young children, only those with very severe and uncontrollable failure are subjected to surgery. In adolescents, continued symptoms justify surgery. Afterload reduction with an angiotensin-converting enzyme blocker may be tried. Surgery is indicated for heart failure or deteriorating left ventricular function.

At surgery, the valve and its apparatus are inspected carefully. In many cases a valvuloplasty is possible, but occasionally replacement may be necessary. Currently, the St. Jude medical prosthesis is often used. Lifelong anticoagulation with warfarin (see Chap. 54) is required. With body growth, replacement with a larger prosthesis may be difficult, and no good annular enlarging operation exists.

VALVULAR AND VASCULAR MALFORMATIONS OF THE RIGHT SIDE OF THE HEART WITH RIGHT-TO-LEFT, BIDIRECTIONAL, OR NO SHUNT

【 】 PULMONARY STENOSIS WITH INTACT VENTRICULAR SEPTUM

Pathology

Valvular pulmonary stenosis with an intact ventricular septum is usually characterized by a dome-shaped stenosis of the pulmonary valve and less commonly by dysplasia of the valve. The valve may be unicuspid, bicuspid, or tricuspid. The annulus may also be narrow. The pulmonary trunk exhibits poststenotic dilatation. In adult patients, calcification of the valve may appear.

In pulmonary valvular dysplasia, the annulus of the valve may be abnormally narrow, but the most dramatic changes are related to the cusps, of which three are identifiable. The cusps are exceedingly thickened by mucoid and dense connective tissue.[170] Concentric hypertrophy of the right ventricle is present, with its extent reflecting the degree of obstruction at the valve level. *The hypertrophy of the infundibular musculature may cause secondary infundibular stenosis.*

Less commonly, there may be isolated subvalvular pulmonary stenosis caused by infundibular narrowing or an anomalous muscle bundle across the middle of the right ventricle.[171] Both types may be associated with a VSD.

Isolated supravalvular pulmonary stenosis, or pulmonary arterial coarctations, may also occur. From angiographic studies, these are classified into four types: (1) *localized stenosis with poststenotic dilatation*, (2) *segmental stenosis*, (3) *diffuse hypoplasia*, and (4) *multiple peripheral stenoses*. The stenosis may be localized to any segment of the pulmonary arterial system. The process is unilateral in about one-third of cases and bilateral in two-thirds. Pulmonary arterial stenosis is commonly (approximately 75 percent), although not universally, associated with other cardiovascular abnormalities, such as tetralogy of Fallot. It also may be seen as a sequela of congenital rubella or with Williams, Noonan,[172] LEOPARD (lentigines, electrocardiographic, ocular, pulmonary, abnormal, retardation, and deafness), or Alagille syndrome.

Abnormal Physiology

There is a pressure difference during systole between the main right ventricular cavity and the pulmonary artery. The area of the pulmonary valve orifice is normally 2 cm^2/m^2; it is about 0.5 cm^2 at birth and increases in size with body growth. In general, the effective valve area must be decreased about 60 percent before there is a hemodynamically significant obstruction to flow. PSPG may reach 150 to 240 mmHg in severe cases. The degree of obstruction is assessed by the peak and mean systolic pressure gradients and the amount of flow across the valve. In neonates, severe stenosis can be associated with a relatively small pressure difference if the flow is very low as a result of right ventricular failure. If pulmonary flow is normal, patients with PSPG at rest <40 mmHg have mild stenosis and patients with PSPG >75 mmHg have severe stenosis. When the pulmonary stenosis is severe, the right ventricle may fail and the cardiac output may be decreased at rest; this is associated with elevation of both the right ventricular end-diastolic pressure and the right atrial mean pressure. This may cause the foramen ovale to open and allow shunting of blood from the right atrium to the left atrium, resulting in arterial oxygen desaturation and cyanosis. In most adolescent or adult patients with significant pulmonary stenosis, the resting cardiac output is within normal limits but usually does not increase normally during exercise. In contrast, younger children may be able to increase cardiac output during exercise even with significant obstruction.[138,173]

Clinical Manifestations

Pulmonary stenosis is one of the most common congenital heart defects and accounts for approximately 10 percent of patients in most large study populations (see Table 82–1). The stenosis is at the level of the pulmonary valve in most instances, but it can occur within the right ventricle, in the pulmonary arteries, or in a combination of the two. Infants with severe stenosis with patency of the foramen ovale may have right-to-left shunting.

History Most infants and children are asymptomatic, but a small percentage with very severe obstruction manifest symptoms, usually mild fatigue or shortness of breath with exertion. Young infants with critical obstruction present with cyanosis if there is a patent foramen ovale or ASD. Squatting and syncope are rare in childhood.[174]

Physical Examination Patients with a dysplastic valve and occasional supravalvular stenosis have consistent noncardiac abnormalities in a familial syndrome described by Noonan,[172] with short stature, hypertelorism, ptosis, low-set ears, and mental retardation. In older patients with valvular pulmonary stenosis, cyanosis is uncommon except with severe obstruction and an atrial communication. Hepatomegaly and the murmur of tricuspid regurgitation may be present with severe obstruction. With at least moderate obstruction, a prominent *a* wave is seen on examination of the jugular venous pulse. A systolic thrill in the suprasternal notch and at the left upper sternal border is present with significant obstruction unless there is isolated subvalvular stenosis. The right ventricular parasternal impulse becomes increasingly forceful with more severe obstruction. *An early systolic click with expiration that disappears with inspiration heard at the left upper sternal border is the hallmark of valvular stenosis unless the obstruction is severe or the valve is dysplastic.* A click is not present with isolated stenosis at other levels. As the obstruction increases in severity, the pulmonary component of the second heart sound becomes progressively softer and more delayed, becoming inaudible when the right ventricular pressure reaches systemic levels or greater. The second heart sound is normal or accentuated with supravalvular stenosis. A fourth heart sound is heard if the obstruction is severe. The characteristic systolic murmur is harsh, crescendo–decrescendo in shape, and best heard at the left upper sternal border with radiation toward the left clavicle. The murmur radiates more to the axilla and back with supravalvular stenosis. The duration of the murmur and the timing of peak intensity correlate well with the severity of obstruction. With mild to moderate stenosis, the murmur peaks in midsystole and ends at or before the aortic component of the second heart sound. In patients with severe stenosis, the murmur peaks late in systole and extends beyond the aortic component of the second heart sound (see Chap. 12).[174]

Chest Roentgenogram   Most patients have a normal or only slightly increased heart size, primarily of the right ventricle. Significant enlargement is seen with critical obstruction and is an ominous sign. Characteristically, the main and proximal left pulmonary arteries are prominent as a result of poststenotic dilatation when the stenosis is valvular. This finding may be absent with very severe obstructions, with a dysplastic valve, in very young infants, or with stenosis above or below the valve. The pulmonary vascular pattern is normal in most of these patients, but the vascularity is diminished in those with a right-to-left shunt at the atrial level.

Electrocardiogram   Right ventricular forces in the anterior precordial leads correlate reasonably well with the degree of obstruction.[174] They are normal or demonstrate mild hypertrophy with an rsR⁺ pattern if there is mild obstruction. With severe stenosis, there is right axis deviation and right atrial hypertrophy as well as very tall pure R waves in the anterior precordial leads. The presence of a qR pattern in these leads is almost always a sign of very severe obstruction. Those with a dysplastic valve frequently have a superior QRS axis.

Echocardiogram   Two-dimensional imaging allows identification of the level of obstruction, and Doppler studies provide an excellent measure of severity. Shunting at the atrial level also can be evaluated.[175]

Cardiac Catheterization   Diagnostic catheterizations are rarely necessary, but data obtained before balloon dilation demonstrate an elevated right ventricular systolic pressure with a distinct systolic pressure difference across the narrowed segment, as demonstrated by slow withdrawal of the catheter from the distal pulmonary arterial branches to the proximal right ventricle. Simultaneous measurement of systemic arterial and right ventricular pressures with measurement of flow is necessary to assess severity accurately. The right ventricular end-diastolic pressure and right atrial a wave may be elevated. Systemic oxygen saturation is diminished only in those with more severe obstruction and a patent foramen ovale or, less commonly, a true ASD. A left-to-right shunt at the atrial level is detected in some patients with mild to moderate obstruction. With valvular stenosis, right ventricular angiography demonstrates thickened and doming valve leaflets and a jet of contrast material entering the dilated pulmonary artery (Fig. 82–28A). Doming is not characteristic of the dysplastic valve. Infundibular subvalvular narrowing caused by muscular hypertrophy may occur secondary to the valvular stenosis, or rarely as an isolated anomaly. Isolated anomalous muscle bundles in the right ventricle also may be seen. Pulmonary arterial angiography best demonstrates the sites of obstruction with supravalvular stenoses. Ventricular volume studies have demonstrated depressed ventricular function in patients with right-to-left shunts. Balloon dilation is discussed below under Management.

Natural History and Prognosis

The clinical course of valvular stenosis is favorable in most patients with mild to moderate obstruction. In a national cooperative study,[176] 86 percent of patients had no significant increase in their pressure gradients over a 4- to 8-year interval. Those with a significant increase were younger than 4 years of age and had at least moderate stenosis initially. Progression during the period of growth seems to be the likely explanation for most of the increases, but a few patients developed subvalvular muscular hypertrophy, which increased the obstruction. Even mild obstruction may progress significantly in some infants during the first year of life. The prognosis of those with severe obstruction without intervention is poor, especially in the case of infants with critical obstruction. With severe obstruction, right ventricular damage and dysfunction can ensue over the years, and heart failure or arrhythmias can cause premature death in adults.[177] Tricuspid regurgitation also may result. Obstruction of the subvalvular type frequently increases with time, whereas supravalvular stenosis usually does not progress. Brain abscess can occur if a right-to-left shunt is present. Infective endocarditis with vegetations on the valve, pulmonary arterial wall, or infundibular region is also a risk. The children originally followed and treated as part of the national cooperative study cited above[174,176] were reevaluated 15 to 25 years later.[178] Among the 580 patients alive at the completion of the previous study, new data were available on 464 (78.4 percent). The probability of 25-year survival was 95.7 percent compared with an expected age- and sex-matched control group survival of 96.6 percent. Ninety-seven percent were asymptomatic. Although cardiac catheterization studies were not repeated, clinical examination and echocardiography at followup suggested no pulmonary stenosis in 2 percent, mild stenosis in 93 percent, moderate stenosis in 3 percent, and severe stenosis in only 1 percent. Pulmonary regurgitation was present in 40 percent, usually secondary to surgical valvotomy. Endocarditis was uncommon, as were ventricular arrhythmias.

Management

Management obviously depends on the severity of obstruction. For those with mild to moderate valvular pulmonary stenosis, periodic reexamination is indicated to detect any evidence of progression, with more frequent evaluation for those under 1 year of age. Measures to treat heart failure should be instituted in an infant with critical stenosis, but prompt intervention is mandatory. Cyanosis or a right ventricular systolic pressure well above systemic levels also is an indication for prompt intervention. Intervention is warranted in older children when the gradient exceeds 75 mmHg and is clearly not indicated when the gradient is less than 25 mmHg. *In the intermediate group, there is still some controversy, but general practice suggests valvuloplasty when the gradient exceeds 40 mmHg, although objective data to support therapy at this level are lacking.* Balloon valvuloplasty has replaced surgical therapy as a first approach. Through the femoral vein, a balloon catheter is advanced across the valve and inflated to about 120 percent of the size of the pulmonary annulus, ripping the domed valve and thus relieving the obstruction (see Fig. 82–28B).

The Valvuloplasty and Angioplasty of Congenital Anomalies Registry published the combined results on 822 children.[179] Valvuloplasty resulted in improvement in most children with valvular obstruction, reducing the gradient from 71 ± 33 mmHg to 28 ± 24 mmHg. Valvuloplasty is, unsurprisingly, less effective in children with a dysplastic

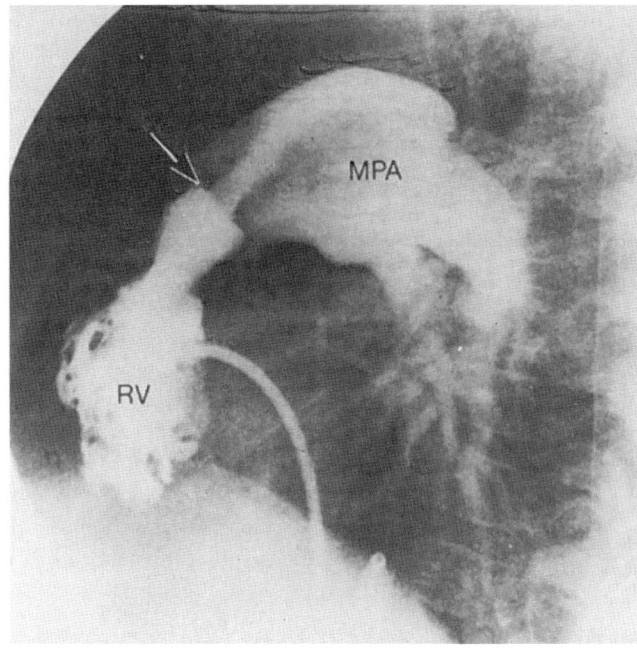

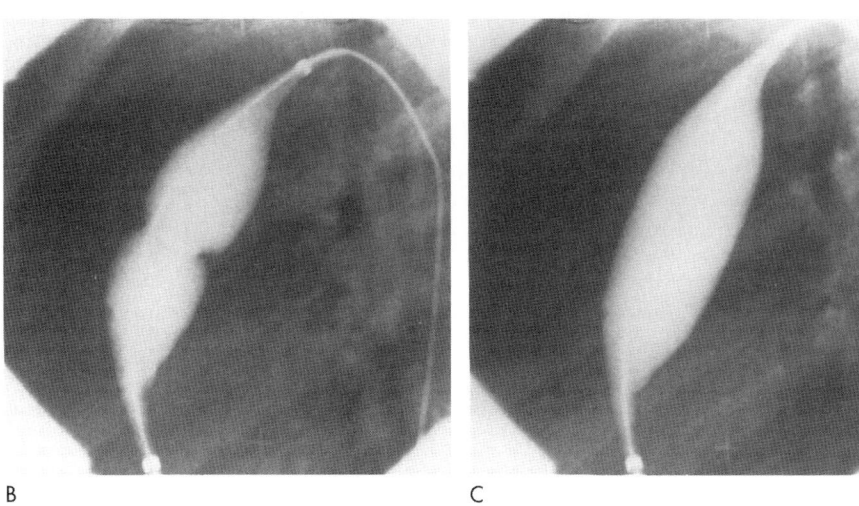

FIGURE 82–28. A. Lateral view of a right ventricular (RV) angiogram demonstrating the typical features of valvular pulmonary stenosis with doming of the pulmonary valve (*arrow*) and a narrow jet of contrast entering the dilated main pulmonary artery (MPA). **B.** An 18-mm balloon is inflated across the 14-mm annulus. A moderate waist is seen at 1 atm of pressure. **C.** The waist is eliminated at 4 atm. *Source: From Lock JE, Keane JF, Perry SB. Diagnostic and Interventional Catheterization in Congenital Heart Disease, 2nd ed. Boston: Kluwer, 2000. Reproduced with permission from the publisher and authors.*

The risk of death after pulmonary artery dilation is higher than that after dilatation of the valve. In the large collaborative study cited above, the death rate was 3 percent, although a more recent study found a mortality rate less than 1 percent among 400 cases.[186]

Surgical Management

Operation rarely is indicated for isolated pulmonary valvular stenosis; balloon valvuloplasty is virtually always successful in eliminating a clinically significant obstruction. A thickened, immobile, dysplastic pulmonary valve, however, is best treated by complete surgical excision (valvectomy). A small annulus is augmented with a pericardial or Dacron gusset.[187]

Subvalvular pulmonary stenosis is relieved through a right ventriculotomy, a main pulmonary arteriotomy, or a right atriotomy. Hypertrophic parietal and septal muscle bands constituting the fibrous orifice of the os infundibulum and obstructing moderator bands or muscle bundles within the body of the right ventricle are excised. Care is exercised to avoid injury to major coronary arterial branches. Usually, the ventriculotomy can be closed either by direct suturing or by augmenting the outflow tract with a patch of pericardium or Dacron to prevent constriction. A small patch that does not extend across the annulus compromises right ventricular function minimally. Larger patches to the pulmonary arterial bifurcation probably impair ventricular performance but may be necessary when there is associated annular or main pulmonary arterial hypoplasia. When possible, excision from the pulmonary artery or the right atrium is preferred to avoid ventricular injury. Excellent relief of right ventricular outflow tract obstruction can be expected after resection. Mortality and significant morbidity are rare.

pulmonary valve.[180,181] Complications were uncommon (5 in 822, or 0.6 percent), including two deaths. Valvuloplasty also has been performed in critical neonatal pulmonary stenosis with cyanosis caused by right-to-left shunting at the atrial level with a high success rate.[181,182] Subvalvular obstruction is less amenable to dilatation.

Peripheral pulmonary stenosis is amenable to dilatation, although the results are frequently less dramatic because of the multiple areas of stenosis and the fact that the complications, including pulmonary artery rupture, are more common.[183,184] Recently, stents have been used, with promising results, in those with peripheral pulmonary artery stenosis in an attempt to keep open vessels that recoil back to normal size after the balloon is deflated.[185,185] For those in whom isolated subvalvular stenosis or associated defects exist or in whom balloon dilatation has failed, surgical intervention is recommended.

Stenoses of main or extraparenchymal branch pulmonary arteries can be relieved by pericardial, synthetic, or homograft aortic or pulmonary arterial patches if the obstruction is proximal. Proximal coarctations in the larger portion of the arterial tree are more readily corrected than are those in small distal branches beyond the bifurcation of either the right or the left pulmonary artery, where results are poor.[188] In these instances, catheter balloon angioplasty, although certainly not without risk, offers nonsurgical relief of obstruction even in the small pulmonary arterial branches and should be considered the procedure of choice for distal pulmonary arterial stenoses.[184] Prophylaxis against infective endocarditis is recommended for all patients whether or not surgery is performed, although the risks seem to be lower than they are with many other congenital anomalies.

TETRALOGY OF FALLOT

Pathology

Tetralogy of Fallot is characterized by biventricular origin of the aorta above a large VSD (Fig. 82–29), obstruction to pulmonary blood flow, and right ventricular hypertrophy. Fibrous continuity of the aortic origin and the anterior mitral valve is maintained. The right ventricular infundibulum lies anterior to the position of the VSD and is bounded by the anterior and septal walls anteriorly and medially; the posterior wall is said to be a vertical crista supraventricularis or displaced conus septum.[189] The right ventricular infundibulum is a distinctive channel, but the caliber varies widely from only mild obstruction to atresia. Usually, it exhibits a significant degree of stenosis and is usually the dominant site of the obstruction to pulmonary flow that is characteristic of tetralogy. The pulmonary valve is often malformed, usually being either bicuspid or unicuspid. The valve may contribute to pulmonary stenosis, but uncommonly is it the only site of significant obstruction to pulmonary flow. Characteristically, the pulmonary trunk is thin-walled and its lumen is more narrow than normal, but usually it is wider than either the right ventricular infundibulum or the orifice of the pulmonary valve. The aorta is wider than normal, its change in cal-iber being roughly inversely proportional to that of the pulmonary trunk. The foramen ovale is frequently patent in patients of all ages. In all cases of tetralogy with significant pulmonary obstruction, it is common for collateral branches to the lungs to arise from the aorta.

There is invariably a large malalignment VSD. Anterior, middle, or apical muscular defects are also present in up to 5 percent of children seen as infants. Many close spontaneously, but if corrective surgery is to be performed successfully, they must be evaluated.

Coronary artery abnormalities are not uncommon. The anterior descending coronary artery in the interventricular septum may arise from the right instead of the left coronary artery. Although physiologically unimportant preoperatively, the course across the right ventricular outflow tract makes the usual site of right ventriculotomy and outflow patch unavailable during reparative surgery, frequently necessitating a conduit to "jump over" the vessel. Previously, angiography was mandatory to establish the anatomy of the coronary circulation, but echocardiography with Doppler color flow is sufficient to detail the distribution of the proximal coronary circulation in most cases.

Associated Conditions

The condition most commonly associated with tetralogy of Fallot is right aortic arch (about 30 percent).[190] A persistent left superior vena cava has been described in 10.6 percent of cases. When an associated ASD exists, this anomaly is referred to as *pentalogy of Fallot.* The ductus arteriosus may be absent, present unilaterally on either the right or the left side, or bilateral.

Abnormal Physiology

Because the VSD is large, with an area about as great as that of the aortic valve, both ventricles and the aorta have essentially the same systolic pressures. The most important hemodynamic factor is the ratio between the resistance to flow into the aorta and the resistance to flow across the right ventricular infundibulum. If the stenosis is not severe and resistance to right ventricular outflow is not large, the pulmonary flow may be more than twice the systemic flow, and the arterial oxygen saturation may be normal (acyanotic tetralogy of Fallot). However, the resistance to the pulmonary flow may be increased markedly, causing right-to-left shunting, arterial desaturation, and subsequent polycythemia. When the pulmonary stenosis is very severe, collateral vessels from the systemic arteries to the distal pulmonary arteries sustain pulmonary blood flow. The drugs, heart rate, or maneuvers that increase myocardial contractility or decrease right ventricular volume increase infundibular obstruction, often partially dynamic. In addition, the infundibular hypertrophy may increase gradually over time. As the systolic pressure in the right ventricle cannot exceed that in the left ventricle because of the large VSD, the right ventricle is "protected" from excessive pressure and work, and so heart failure is uncommon.

Hypercyanotic episodes (spells) in patients with tetralogy are of uncertain origin. It is likely that some episodes are caused by unusual hyperactivity of muscular fibers in the right ventricular outflow tract that produce or exaggerate the infundibular stenosis, increasing pulmonary resistance and thus increasing the right-to-left shunting. Some spells may be caused by a decrease in peripheral resistance and systemic arterial pressure, which also may cause the right-to-left shunt to increase and pulmonary blood flow to decrease.

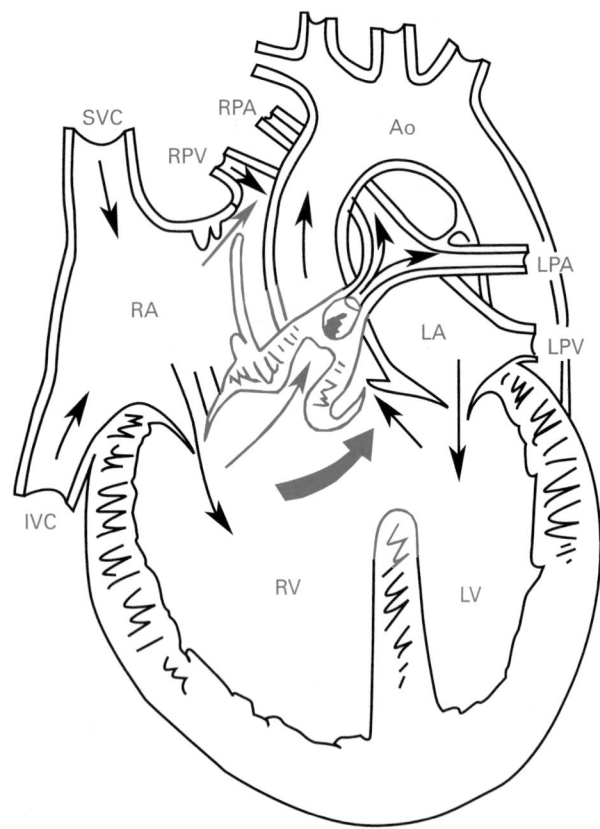

FIGURE 82–29. Classic tetralogy of Fallot. There are infundibular and pulmonary valvular stenoses. There is also right-to-left shunting at the atrial level. Ao, aorta; IVC, inferior vena cava; LA, left atrium; LPA, left pulmonary artery; LPV, left pulmonary vein; LV, left ventricle; RA, right atrium; RPA, right pulmonary artery; RPV, right pulmonary vein; RV, right ventricle; SVC, superior vena cava. *Source: From Edwards JE.[74] Reproduced with permission from the publisher and author.*

Clinical Manifestations

Tetralogy of Fallot is the most common congenital cardiac defect that causes cyanosis. Tetralogy with an associated ASD, or pentalogy of Fallot, is not distinguishable clinically. For a discussion on the hypoxemia and the consequences in tetralogy, see Complications of Congenital Heart Disease: Hypoxemia earlier in this chapter.

History Most of these patients are diagnosed by prenatal ultrasonography or because they present in the first days or weeks of life with a heart murmur. If the right ventricular obstruction is severe, cyanosis is present at birth and is exacerbated when the ductus closes. If the obstruction is milder, the infant may be acyanotic with left-to-right flow through the VSD and occasionally may develop heart failure. In this group, gradually increasing right ventricular obstruction may reduce the left-to-right shunt; eventually, when infundibular resistance and pulmonary resistance exceed systemic resistance, right-to-left shunting develops and cyanosis results.

Dyspnea with exertion occurs commonly in toddlers and older children with unrepaired defects. Attacks of suddenly increasing cyanosis associated with hyperpnea, or hypoxic spells,[191] are common between ages 2 months and 2 years. There are many precipitating events, including infection, exertion, and summer heat. They occur most often in the morning, with increasing irritability. The frequency and duration vary widely, but prolonged episodes can lead to syncope, seizures, and death. Squatting with exercise is common from 1.5 to 10 years of age in those who have not previously undergone repair. These problems are becoming uncommon as an increasing number of children receive early repair.

Physical Examination Growth is usually normal unless cyanosis is extreme. Clubbing of the fingers and toes occurs after 3 months of age and is proportional to the level of cyanosis.

Increased right ventricular activity is observed. A systolic thrill may be palpable at the left midsternal border, with a harsh midsystolic murmur in that location. Softer murmurs signal more severe obstruction and are common when presentation is in the newborn period or during hypoxic spells. The murmur ends before the second heart sound, which is characteristically single. A continuous murmur is heard if a PDA or large collateral vessels are present. An early systolic ejection sound at the left sternal border and apex is uncommon; its presence suggests primarily valvular pulmonary stenosis.

Chest Roentgenogram The total heart size is usually normal on chest roentgenography, but right ventricular enlargement is present in the lateral view. The aorta arches to the right in many cases. Pulmonary flow is diminished. The pulmonary segment is concave and the apex is elevated, giving the *coeur en sabot* (boot-shaped) contour. A very young infant may have only diminished pulmonary flow.

Electrocardiogram In tetralogy of Fallot, the mean QRS axis of the ECG is usually to the right, between +90 and +210 degrees. There is right ventricular hypertrophy, with a tall R wave in the right precordial leads and a deep S wave in the left leads. Some of these patients have right atrial hypertrophy.

Echocardiogram Two-dimensional echocardiography can delineate the anatomic components of tetralogy prenatally[192] or after birth.[193] Anomalies of the coronary arteries can be demonstrated and associated defects excluded.

Hematologic and Other Laboratory Studies Before surgical repair oximetry and measurement of hemoglobin and hematocrit should be measured; pulse oximetry should be performed at initial evaluation and periodically thereafter for determination of the degree of polycythemia and the early detection of anemia relative to the degree of cyanosis. The latter is common, especially in those younger than 2 years of age, and may predispose a patient to cerebrovascular accidents. Platelet counts and clotting studies may be advisable in older, unrepaired patients with marked polycythemia, particularly if a surgical procedure is planned. Serum uric acid levels should be measured if polycythemia is severe and of long standing.

Cardiac Catheterization In most centers, the quality of echocardiography (especially in neonates or infants) is sufficiently diagnostic to outline the right ventricular and proximal pulmonary artery anatomy, rule out additional muscular VSDs, and establish the proximal coronary circulation. As a consequence, diagnostic cardiac catheterization and angiography are less commonly performed preoperatively than they were in the past in children with tetralogy of Fallot.

In those in whom the study is performed, the right ventricular systolic pressure is equal to the pressure in the left ventricle and aorta. If the pulmonary artery can be entered, the pressure will be normal or low. The level or levels of obstruction can be evaluated by careful pullback to the right ventricle. Caution should be observed if the pulmonary artery is entered, as the catheter may critically reduce the pulmonary flow and cause a hypoxic episode. Systemic arterial oxygen saturation is reduced because of right-to-left shunting from the right to the left ventricle. If a patent foramen ovale or ASD is present, there may be an additional right-to-left or bidirectional shunt at the atrial level. Selective biplane right ventricular angiography will demonstrate levels of obstruction, continuity and size of the pulmonary arteries, and size and position of the ventricular defect. If this is not demonstrated by echocardiography or aortography, selective coronary arteriography should be performed on all patients preoperatively to demonstrate the coronary arterial pattern.[194] Magnetic resonance imaging (MRI) provides excellent images of the pulmonary artery anatomy particularly in the case of diminutive pulmonary vessels or discontinuous pulmonary arteries (Fig. 82–30).

Medical Management

Although the definitive treatment of tetralogy of Fallot is surgical, medical management plays a role before surgery and in the postoperative period. For a severely cyanotic newborn, prostaglandin administration is of benefit[104] to keep the ductus open until surgery can be done. Before surgery, the hematocrit and hemoglobin should be monitored and iron-deficiency anemia should be treated promptly to prevent strokes. Fever or other illness that would lead to dehydration and possible thrombotic complications should be treated promptly.

Hypoxic spells in an infant should be treated initially by placing the infant in the knee-chest position and administering a high concentration of oxygen and morphine sulfate. If acidosis is present and does not correct spontaneously and promptly, intravenous sodium bicarbonate and an α-adrenergic agonist should be given. Propranolol may be useful in preventing hypoxic spells.[195]

Bacterial endocarditis is a serious complication, especially in those who have had a systemic-to-pulmonary artery shunt. Meticulous care should be taken to maintain good dental hygiene, and prophylactic antibiotics at times of predictable risk are mandatory.

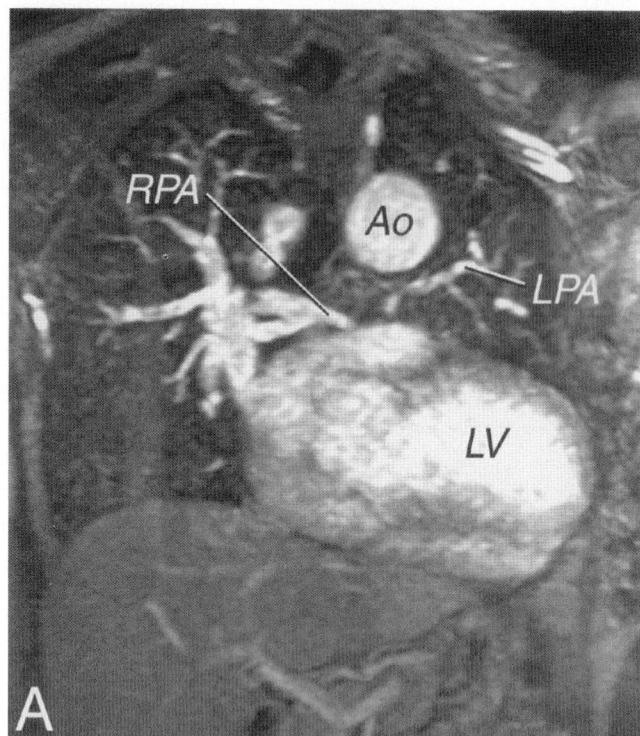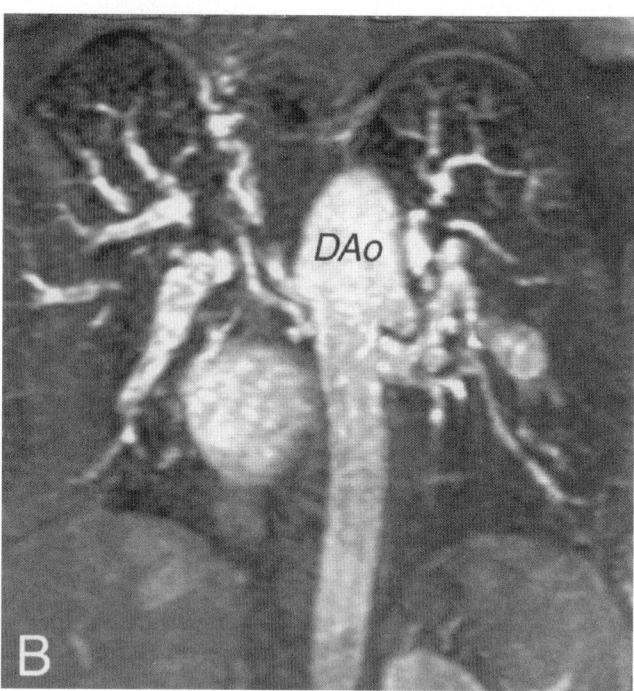

FIGURE 82–30. Preoperative MRI in a 33-year-old woman with tetralogy of Fallot, pulmonary atresia, and discontinuous pulmonary arteries. **A.** Gadolinium-enhanced three-dimensional magnetic resonance angiograph subvolume maximal intensity projection (MIP) in the coronal plane showing discontinuity between the right pulmonary artery (RPA) and the left pulmonary artery (LPA). **B.** Subvolume MIP image of the descending aorta (DAo) showing multiple aortopulmonary collaterals. *Source: From Geva T, Sahn DJ, Powell AC. Magnetic resonance imaging of congenital heart disease in adults. Prog Pediatr Cardiol 2003;17:21–39. Reproduced with permission of the authors and publisher.*

Surgical Management

Historically, the approach to tetralogy of Fallot has been either palliation or corrective surgery. The introduction of an aorta-to-pulmonary artery shunt for the treatment of tetralogy of Fallot[196] truly can be called the beginning of effective treatment for pediatric cardiovascular disease. When open heart surgery was initiated in the 1950s, tetralogy of Fallot was among the first lesions to be corrected.[197] Over the years, the age at which corrective surgery can be performed has dropped, so that in most centers primary repair is the procedure of choice at any age. Palliation, when it is now performed, almost inevitably involves a modified Blalock-Taussig shunt that interposes a graft between the subclavian artery and the ipsilateral pulmonary artery, usually on the side opposite the aortic arch.[198] Even in the perinatal period, the placement of a 4-mm tube will result in satisfactory palliation for a year in more than 90 percent of infants.

Surgical correction for those with pulmonary stenosis involves closing the VSD, usually through a right ventriculotomy, resecting infundibular muscle, and, if the infundibulum, pulmonary valve, and main pulmonary artery are hypoplastic, using a pericardial patch to open the narrowed area. Care must be taken to avoid heart block while closing the VSD and avoid cutting a major branch of the coronary artery. If a patent foramen ovale is present, it usually is left open to allow decompression in the perioperative period.[114] If a true ASD is present (pentalogy of Fallot), it should be closed to avoid left-to-right shunting once the right ventricle has recovered from the perioperative insult.[199] Tetralogy of Fallot and pulmonary atresia with good-sized pulmonary arteries are usually repaired by closing the VSD and interposing a conduit, frequently an aortic homograft, between the right ventricle and

the pulmonary artery.[200,201] If this procedure is performed prior to 7 or 8 years of age, as is usually the case, replacement of the conduit is to be expected secondary to somatic growth. Tetralogy of Fallot and hypoplastic and/or discontinuous pulmonary arteries call for an individualized approach that frequently involves balloon dilation with cutting balloons or stenting[116] of hypoplastic vessels, and unifocalization of discontinuous vessels, with the intent to complete eventual repair with a conduit closing the VSD.[202] In cases where pulmonary artery stenosis has been resistant to dilation with high pressure balloons, cutting balloon therapy has been shown to increase efficacy of dilation.[203] Operative and early mortality rates for repair of tetralogy of Fallot are now quite low in most centers. Kirklin and coworkers[198] in the early 1980s reported mortality rates of 1.6 percent with operations at 5 years of age to 4.1 percent at 1 year of age. At Children's Hospital in Boston, there was a 4.2 percent mortality rate among 330 children younger than 1 year of age who were operated on between 1973 and 1990, with a mortality rate of only 2.5 percent in the past 6 years of the study (1984–1990).[199] Late complications have included residual peripheral pulmonary stenosis, a small incidence of residual VSDs, and, rarely, aortic regurgitation. MRI is an excellent adjunct to echocardiography for assessment of residual anatomic abnormalities, especially with respect to the distal pulmonary arterial architecture (Fig. 82–31). The long-term survivors have had atrial or, more commonly, ventricular arrhythmias and continue to be at risk for infective endocarditis. An increasingly large cohort of young adults with pulmonary regurgitation have required pulmonary valve replacement although the indications and timing of surgery still need to be determined.[204]

Long-term surgical results have been promising. Physicians at the Mayo Clinic, the first center to use the pump oxygenator to repair tetralogy of Fallot in the 1950s, have reported a minimum 30-year follow-up of the 162 30-day survivors of surgery.[205] The 32-year actuarial survival rate was 86 percent, with subgroup survival rates of those who were younger than 5 years old, 5 to 7 years old, and 8 to 11 years old at the time of surgical repair of 90, 93, and 91 percent, respectively.[119] Late sudden death from cardiac causes occurred in 10 patients during the 32-year period. The performance of some previous palliative operation (Waterston or Pott's shunts) but not a palliative Blalock-Taussig shunt was associated with higher mortality. Similar results were found in a German study of 490 survivors of tetralogy of Fallot repair between 1958 and 1977.[120] With earlier surgery and less use of palliative procedures, it is anticipated that the surgical results will be even better for children born in the 1980s and 1990s and beyond.

〖 〗 EBSTEIN'S ANOMALY

Pathology

In Ebstein's anomaly, the anterior leaflet of the tricuspid valve is attached normally to the annulus, but varying portions of the posterior and septal leaflets are displaced downward, being attached to the ventricular wall below the annulus. The proximal part of the right ventricle is thin-walled and continuous with the right atrium. The functional right ventricle is small and made up of the apical and infundibular portions of the right ventricle. An additional common finding is that the papillary muscles and chordae are highly malformed, with great variation in the manner of attachment of the two involved leaflets to the right ventricular wall. Commonly, multiple direct attachments of valvular tissue to the right ventricular mural endocardium occur.[207,208]

An interatrial communication is present in most cases, usually taking the form of a patent foramen ovale. Continuity of right atrial and right ventricular myocardial tissues, in addition to the usual connections by way of the main conduction pathways, has been observed. *The presence of Ebstein's anomaly has been associated with maternal lithium use during pregnancy, although the risk ratio remains unclear.*[209]

Abnormal Physiology

Ebstein's anomaly results in obstruction to right ventricular filling because of a decrease in the size of the right ventricle, part of which is incorporated into the huge right atrium. The deformed tricuspid valve also frequently is associated with tricuspid regurgitation with a right-to-left shunt through the foramen ovale. In the perinatal period, when the pulmonary vascular resistance is high, the tricuspid regurgitation may be severe. This results in increased right atrial pressure and, when the patent foramen ovale is open, severe cyanosis. As

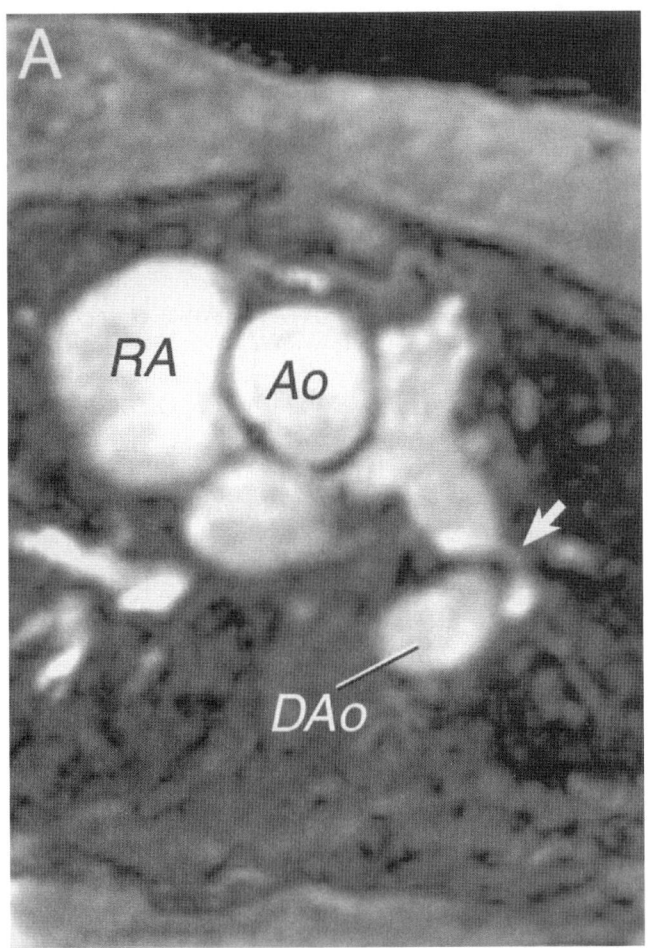

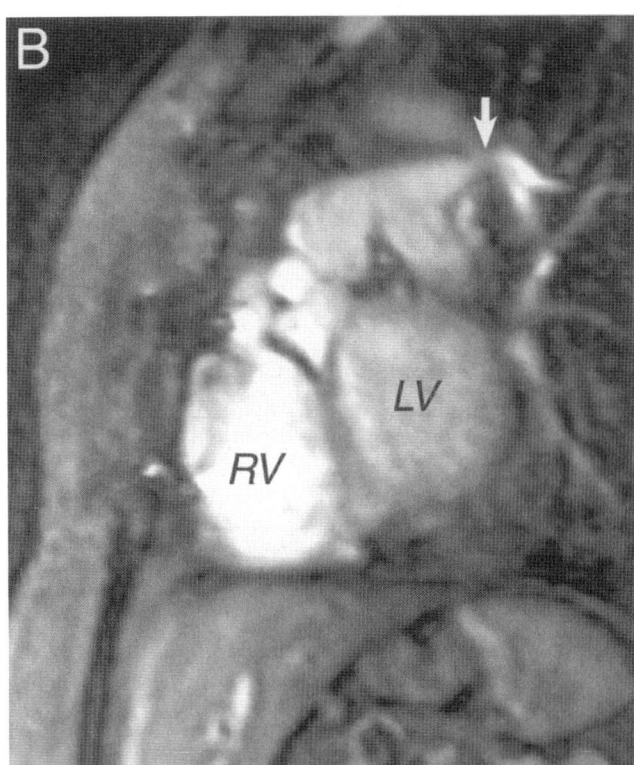

FIGURE 82–31. Postoperative MRI after tetralogy of Fallot repair in a patient with a previous Potts shunt. **A.** Gadolinium-enhanced three-dimensional magnetic resonance angiograph subvolume maximal image projection (MIP) in the axial plane showing severe left pulmonary artery stenosis (*arrow*) at the site of the previous Potts shunt. **B.** Oblique sagittal subvolume MIP image showing the superoinferior aspect of the left pulmonary artery stenosis (*arrow*). Ao, aortic artery; DAo, descending aortic artery; LV, left ventricle; RA, right atrium; RV, right ventricle. *Source: From Geva T, Sahn DJ, Powell AC. Magnetic resonance imaging of congenital heart disease in adults. Prog Pediatr Cardiol 2003;17:21–39. Reproduced with permission of the authors and publisher.*

the pulmonary vascular resistance falls, the right-to-left shunting is decreased and hypoxemia improves. In older children, right-sided heart failure with edema and/or ascites may develop.

Clinical Manifestations

History Approximately one-half of reported patients develop symptoms of cyanosis and right-sided heart failure in early infancy. The remainder present with dyspnea on exertion, palpitations from supraventricular arrhythmias, a murmur, or an abnormal chest roentgenogram,[122] but with no symptoms in early childhood or because of gradual progression of symptoms through late childhood or adult life.[210] The most common symptom is dyspnea on exertion. The spectrum of exercise intolerance has been described.[211] Palpitations resulting from supraventricular tachyarrhythmias occur in 20 to 30 percent of these children. Occasionally, syncope occurs as a result of arrhythmia or low cardiac output if the atrial septum is intact.

Physical Examination A newborn with elevated pulmonary vascular resistance usually has severe cyanosis. In older infants and children, cyanosis and clubbing are mild. Only a small percentage of children do not have an ASD or patent foramen ovale and thus are not cyanotic. The precordium is generally quiet even in those with striking cardiomegaly. The liver is enlarged, and the jugular venous pulse may be elevated. The holosystolic murmur of tricuspid regurgitation is heard at the lower left sternal border and may be accompanied by a "scratchy" diastolic murmur of tricuspid stenosis. The first heart sound is split and loud, and the second heart sound is widely and persistently split. Loud third and fourth heart sounds are usual, especially in older patients.

Chest Roentgenogram Heart size, as shown by chest roentgenography, varies, but the cardiac silhouette may be very large because of the dilated right atrium. In those with cyanosis, pulmonary blood flow is diminished correspondingly.

Electrocardiogram Giant, peaked P waves are common, along with a prolonged PR interval and right ventricular conduction delay or complete right bundle branch block. In approximately 10 percent of these patients, the pattern of Wolff-Parkinson-White syndrome (with a short PR interval and slurring of the initial QRS forces or a delta wave) is seen.[210]

Echocardiogram Two-dimensional echocardiography is very helpful in the diagnosis (Fig. 82–32), identifying the lesion, depicting the degree of displacement of the tricuspid valve into the right ventricle, and assessing the severity of the tricuspid regurgitation. In neonates, evaluation of the pulmonary valve usually allows a distinction between anatomic pulmonary atresia from absence of opening of the valve caused by severe tricuspid regurgitation and high pulmonary vascular resistance.[212]

Cardiac Catheterization There is a higher than usual risk associated with cardiac catheterization because of the frequency of rhythm disturbances. Proper precautions and prompt use of cardioversion when necessary minimize this risk. In most cases, echocardiography and color-flow Doppler evaluation are sufficient, and catheterization is rarely performed in the modern era. When done, there is usually right-to-left shunting at the atrial level. Right atrial hypertension is present. The characteristic right ventricular pressure recording is not obtained until the catheter is advanced to the apex or outflow tract. An intracar-

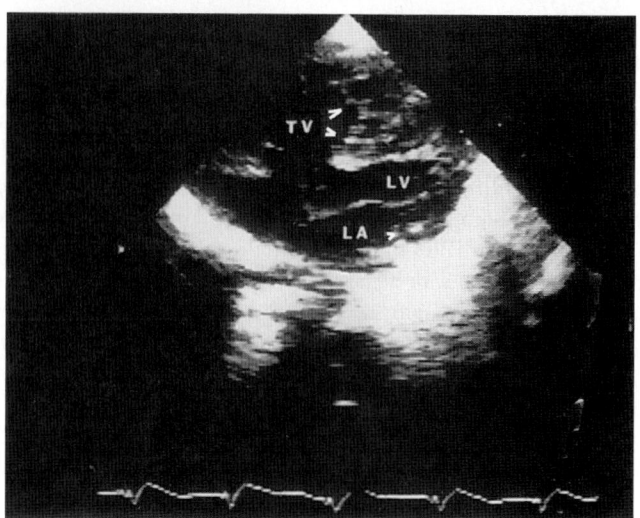

FIGURE 82–32. Two-dimensional echocardiogram in parasternal view in a patient with Ebstein anomaly of the tricuspid valve (TV). Numerous attachments of the tricuspid valve (*arrowheads*) to the interventricular septum and right ventricular apex are seen. LA, left atrium; LV, left ventricle.

diac ECG demonstrates, on pullback from the right ventricle, an area where the ECG is ventricular but the pressure is atrial in contour.[213] This method is not infallible, but it provides good evidence of tricuspid displacement with an "atrialized" portion of the right ventricle.

Natural History and Prognosis

The natural history varies greatly with the severity of the abnormality. In a study of 50 patients who presented in the neonatal period, 9 (18 percent) died in the perinatal period, with late deaths in another 15 (30 percent; 9 from hemodynamic deterioration, 5 sudden, and 1 noncardiac), for a 10-year actuarial survival of 61 percent.[214] In a study that included more children who presented after the perinatal period, the probability of survival was 50 percent at 47 years of age.[215] Predictors of poor outcome were New York Heart Association class III or IV, cardiothoracic ratio >65 percent, and atrial fibrillation. In a review of 72 unoperated adults with isolated Ebstein's anomaly followed from the age of 25 years, 41 percent were alive 20 years later. Though parameters predicting outcome were multifactorial, the ratio of septal leaflet displacement to ventricular septal length correlated well with survival.[216] Our own data at Children's Hospital in Boston is better; in those with a primary diagnosis of Ebstein's disease, the 10-year survival is approximately 85 percent.[217]

For women who survive into adulthood without significant arrhythmias or cyanosis, successful pregnancy with good fetal outcome is possible.[218]

Medical Management

Medical therapy varies depending on the severity of disease and the age at presentation. For patients who present with cyanosis in the perinatal period, procrastination until the pulmonary vascular resistance has decreased may be the best strategy. For those who are severely hypoxemic, maintaining the patency of the ductus with PGE_1 may be lifesaving. Reducing the pulmonary vascular resistance with nitric oxide may reduce right-to-left shunting and improve oxygenation.[219] Persistence of severe cyanosis beyond 1 week of age suggests pulmonary stenosis or pulmonary atresia in addition to Ebstein's deformity of the tricuspid valve.

For children with arrhythmias, an electrophysiologic study may be indicated. For those with disabling or life-threatening arrhythmias, radiofrequency ablation has been performed, with initial success rates of approximately 80 percent, but recurrences in 30 percent of patients.[220] In older children who develop right-sided heart failure, digoxin and diuretics may be tried, although this level of deterioration is usually an indication for surgical intervention.

Surgical Management

The surgical management of Ebstein's disease remains problematic. In the perinatal period, when the pulmonary vascular resistance is high, watchful waiting is probably the best approach. If the child remains severely hypoxemic (saturations <75 percent) after the pulmonary vascular resistance falls, palliation with a Blalock-Taussig shunt to improve pulmonary blood flow may be sufficient to relieve hypoxemia and should allow growth to an age at which other procedures can be considered.[221] For older children in whom hypoxemia remains a significant problem, three approaches have been used. The first is a Glenn anastomosis connecting the superior vena cava to the right pulmonary artery, allowing blood from the inferior vena cava to enter the right atrium and ventricle to the pulmonary artery.[222] A more definitive procedure that eliminates hypoxemia is used primarily for children with single ventricle; however, the modified Fontan is now applied in this situation as well. In this approach, the tricuspid valve is oversewn and the patent foramen ovale closed, diverting all systemic venous return to the pulmonary arteries bypassing the right heart.[223] In a small group of patients, this has been done with success.

The more common approach has been tricuspid valve reconstruction or replacement, usually with a bioprosthesis. Among 189 patients operated on at the Mayo Clinic over a period of almost 20 years, there were 12 hospital deaths (6.3 percent) and an additional 10 late deaths. Among those followed more than 1 year after operation, more than 90 percent were in New York Heart Association class I or II.[224] A review of the Mayo Clinic experience with biologic valve replacement demonstrated a 93 percent survival at 10 years with 81 percent freedom from operation.[225] More recently, other approaches have been suggested, including reconstruction of the normally shaped right ventricle with repositioning of the displaced leaflet of the tricuspid valve at the normal level[226] and reimplantation of the tricuspid valve leaflets with a vertical plication of the atrialized portion of the right ventricle to reduce its size (Fig. 82–33).[227] Intermediate-term results in severely ill neonates using improved techniques are encouraging.[228] *Although the newer approaches seem promising in small numbers of patients in the short run, many patients with the milder form of the disease can live well into adulthood*[135]; *consequently, indications for the newer operations in patients who are asymptomatic or only mildly limited remain problematic.*[229]

ABNORMALITIES OF THE PULMONARY VENOUS CONNECTIONS

【 】 TOTAL ANOMALOUS PULMONARY VENOUS CONNECTION

Pathology

When all pulmonary veins terminate in a systemic vein or the right atrium, the term *total anomalous pulmonary venous connection* or *return* is applied (Fig. 82–34). This occurs in about 1 in 17,000 live-births. Usually the pulmonary veins leave the lung and then join a chamber-like confluence posterior to the left atrium, the common pulmonary vein. Normally this chamber becomes incorporated into the developing left atrium. If this connection is not made in utero, one of the primitive embryologic vessels persist to drain the flow from the lungs and leads to the anomalous termination after birth. Less commonly, two or more vessels lead to multiple sites of termination.

If the left cardinal vein persists, drainage flows superiorly into the innominate vein and then to the superior vena cava and right atrium or inferiorly into a persistent left superior vena cava and coronary sinus to the right atrium. If the right cardinal vein persists, drainage is to the superior vena cava, the azygos vein, or the right atrium directly. These types are sometimes referred to collectively as supracardiac or supradiaphragmatic drainage and are almost never associated with pulmonary venous obstruction.[230] If the site of termination is infradiaphragmatic, with connection to the portal venous system or the inferior vena cava, the anomalous vein leaves the confluence of pulmonary veins and descends into the abdomen along the esophagus to join the ductus venosus, the portal vein, or the left gastric vein. *Pulmonary venous obstruction is present in virtually all cases of infradiaphragmatic connection.*[230]

In all cases of total anomalous pulmonary venous connection, there is a patent foramen ovale. The atrium and ventricle of the left side are small in comparison with the right-sided chambers but are within normal limits in regard to absolute size. In the absence of asplenia or polysplenia syndromes, associated anomalies are not common.

Abnormal Physiology

In this anomaly, all the blood from both the pulmonary and systemic circulation eventually returns to the right atrium. In neonates with the connection below the diaphragm, the increase in pulmonary flow as the pulmonary resistance decreases after birth cannot be accommodated and the obstruction to flow causes a marked increase in pulmonary venous pressure, resulting in a very high pulmonary vascular resistance. If the ductus arteriosus is still open, the pulmonary vascular resistance exceeds systemic vascular resistance with a right-to-left shunt at the ductal level. When the ductus closes, the increased pulmonary resistance results in increased right ventricular pressure. As the right ventricle fails and right atrial pressure increases, the resulting right-to-left shunt at the atrial level may cause profound hypoxemia.

In older children with unobstructed damage above the diaphragm (supracardiac), the pulmonary resistance is usually low, facilitating a high pulmonary flow. With mixing of all pulmonary and systemic flow in the right atrium, the oxygen saturation is usually relatively high, resulting in physiology similar to that of an ASD and mild cyanosis.[231]

Clinical Manifestations

Total Anomalous Pulmonary Venous Connection with Pulmonary Venous Obstruction Neonates with total anomalous pulmonary venous connection below the diaphragm who have pulmonary venous obstruction present with cyanosis, which may be severe, and tachypnea. Symptoms frequently develop beyond 12 hours of age, allowing differentiation from respiratory distress syndrome. In addition to tachypnea, feeding difficulties and heart failure are seen.

The physical findings are usually unimpressive. The heart is not hyperactive, and thrills are absent. The second heart sound may be split, with an increased pulmonary component. Significant murmurs are uncommon.

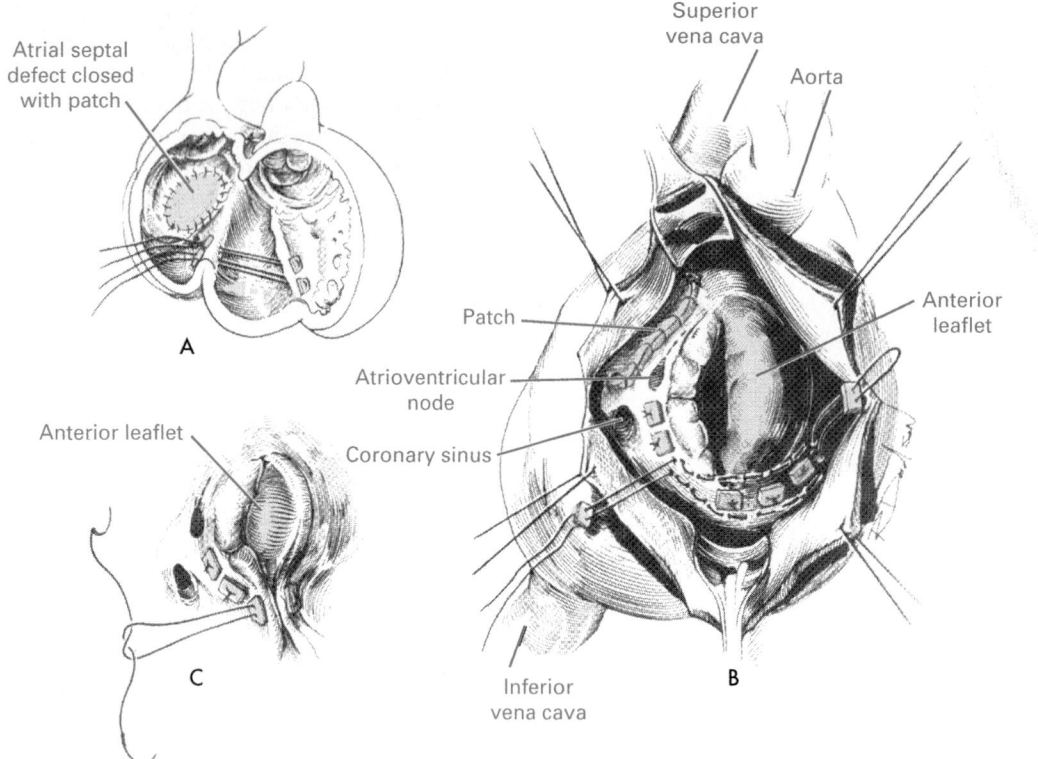

FIGURE 82–33. Danielson repair of the Ebstein malformation. **A.** Anterior cutaway drawing. The atrial septal defect is closed securely with a patch. Pledgeted sutures are placed to position the posterior leaflet at the annulus and imbricate the "atrialized" right ventricular chamber. **B** and **C.** Drawing of the right atrium showing the annuloplasty suture passed through two pledgets. Tying of this suture reduces dilation of the tricuspid valve so that the large anterior leaflet can meet the two smaller cusps and constitute a functional, essentially monocusp valve.

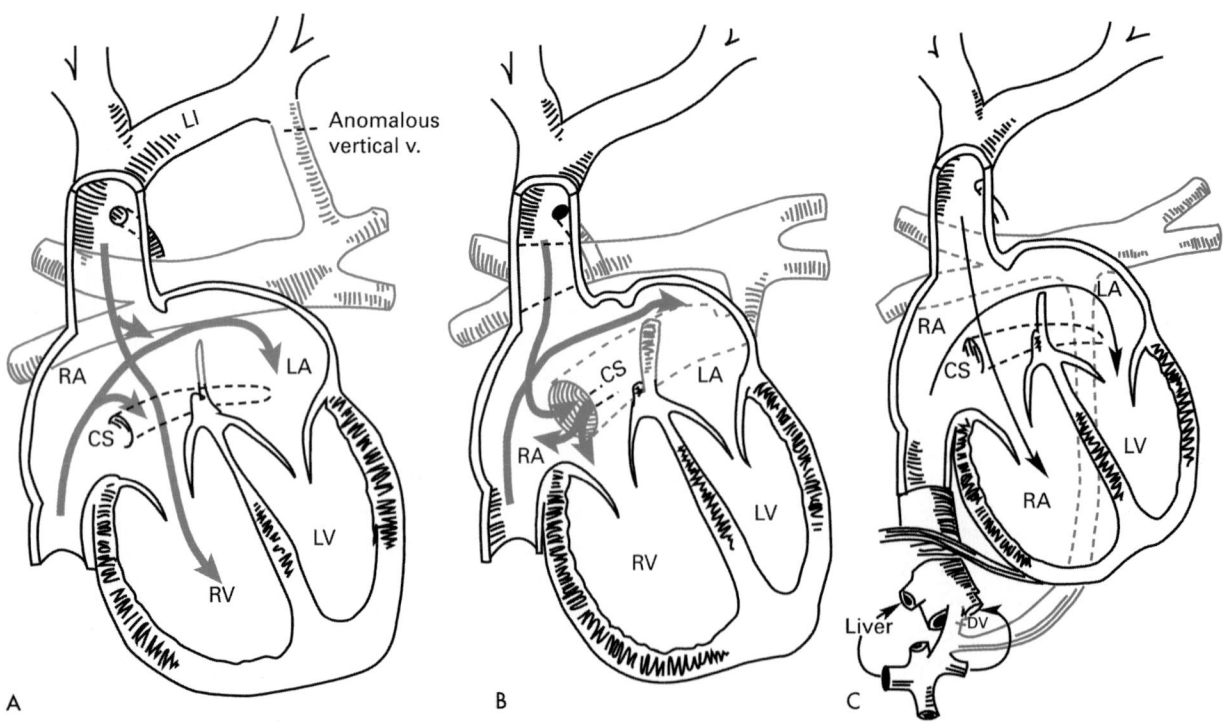

FIGURE 82–34. Three common types of total anomalous pulmonary venous connection. **A.** Total anomalous pulmonary venous connection to the left brachiocephalic (innominate) vein (LI). **B.** Total anomalous pulmonary venous connection to the coronary sinus (CS). **C.** Total anomalous pulmonary venous connection of the infradiaphragmatic type to the ductus venosus (DV). LA, left atrium; LV, left ventricle; RA, right atrium; RV, right ventricle.

Total Anomalous Pulmonary Venous Connection without Pulmonary Venous Obstruction

These patients are usually asymptomatic at birth, although some may develop transient tachypnea. Presentation typically occurs during the first year of life. Some of these children have tachypnea and feeding difficulties, with frequent respiratory infections. Cyanosis often is mild and may not be clinically apparent. Other children may be asymptomatic and present with a heart murmur.

The cardiac examination is similar to that of an ASD with increased right-sided flow. The right ventricular impulse is usually hyperactive. The jugular venous pulse is elevated, and hepatomegaly appears early. There is a diffuse and hyperdynamic right ventricular impulse. The second heart sound is split and relatively fixed; the loudness of the pulmonary component may be increased. There is usually a grade 2 or 3 midsystolic flow murmur at the left sternal border. At the lower sternal border, there is a middiastolic rumble and prominent third and fourth heart sounds. Rales may be heard over the lung fields, and periorbital edema is common. A continuous murmur rarely may be heard over the common venous channel.

Chest Roentgenogram

With the unobstructed types, the heart is enlarged with increased pulmonary flow. Pulmonary edema is uncommon. In patients with return to the left innominate vein, there may be a characteristic bulging of the superior mediastinum bilaterally, producing a "snowman" or figure-of-eight, contour. With obstructed types, the heart size is nearly normal; there is very marked pulmonary edema, which may give a granular appearance to the lungs, making differentiation from respiratory distress syndrome difficult in a newborn.

Electrocardiogram

There is right axis deviation and right atrial and right ventricular hypertrophy. Commonly, there is a qR pattern in the right precordial leads.

Echocardiogram

Echocardiography with color-flow Doppler is specific in defining the anomaly and the site of drainage.[232] The right side of the heart is enlarged when the venous return is unobstructed with increased flow. Although the right-sided chambers may dwarf the left heart, the left heart is usually of normal size. With obstructed return, there is evidence of severe pulmonary hypertension. Mixed drainage can be best visualized by MRI (Fig. 82–35).

Cardiac Catheterization

If echocardiography and MRI are inconclusive in delineating the site or sites of the pulmonary venous connection, catheterization may be necessary. There is an increase in oxygen saturation at the level of the abnormal connection, with similar saturations in the remainder of the chambers on both sides of the heart. Pulmonary arterial pressure is elevated to a variable degree, but it may be above systemic pressure if there is marked pulmonary venous or pulmonary vascular obstruction. Pulmonary capillary wedge pressures are elevated in proportion to the degree of venous obstruction. The atrial communication may rarely be obstructive,[231] if it is, balloon atrial septostomy may be helpful. Pulmonary arteriography usually will show the anomalous venous connection. Angiography in the common venous channel, if entered, will outline its course and any sites of obstruction optimally.

Natural History and Prognosis

The natural history varies depending on the degree of obstruction of egress of blood from the pulmonary veins.[231] Those who

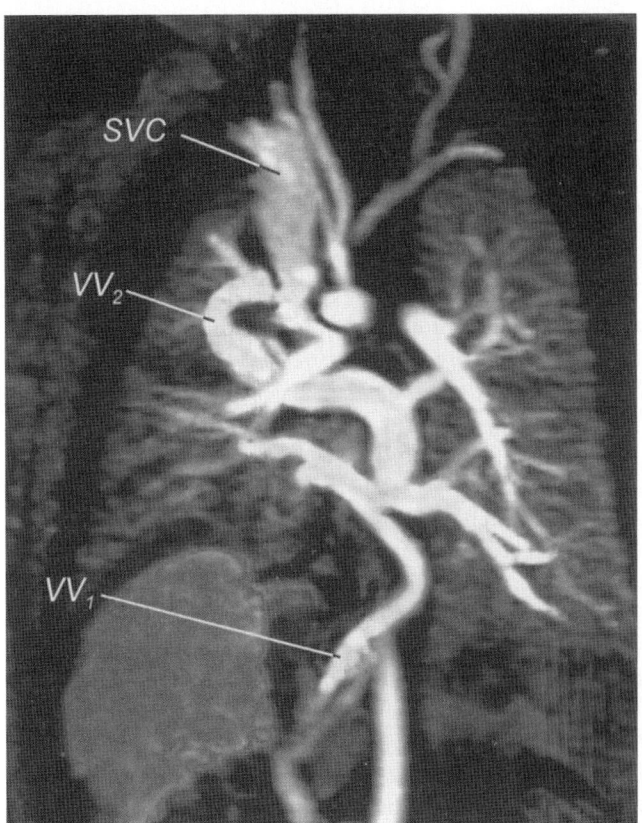

FIGURE 82–35. Maximal intensity projection coronal plane image of gadolinium-enhanced three-dimensional magnetic resonance angiogram in a newborn with obstructed mixed type total anomalous venous connection. There is infradiaphragmatic connection by means of a vertical vein (VV-1) to the portal vein, as well as supracardiac stenotic connection to the right superior vena cava (SVC) via an additional vertical vein (VV-2). *Source: Figure courtesy of Tal Geva, MD.*

present in the perinatal period with severe cyanosis and respiratory distress, usually with pulmonary venous drainage below the diaphragm, represent a medical emergency and will die without early surgery.

Those with supracardiac drainage and some degree of obstruction and pulmonary hypertension are sufficiently tachypneic that feeding is problematic, and they fail to gain weight at a normal rate. They tolerate respiratory infections poorly and occasionally need emergency surgery for respiratory failure.[233]

Those without pulmonary venous obstruction have large left-to-right shunts and mild cyanosis but may have no or minimal symptoms at rest or exercise. If corrective surgery is not performed, they are at risk for pulmonary vascular disease.

Medical Management

For neonates with severe cyanosis and respiratory disease, oxygen, a respirator, and PGE_1 can be used to temporize but survival is dependent on early surgery. For neonates with mild pulmonary hypertension and failure to thrive, surgery usually is performed semielectively. For neonates without pulmonary hypertension who present with murmurs and findings similar to those of an atrial septal defect, surgery is more elective but little is gained by waiting, and more centers are advocating early repair in this group as well.[234]

Surgical Management

Correction of total anomalous pulmonary venous connection requires (1) creation of a large communication between the left atrium and the pulmonary venous system, (2) obliteration of the anomalous pulmonary venous connection to the systemic circulation, and (3) closure of the associated interatrial communications.[234]

Supracardiac anomalous connection to the innominate vein and infracardiac connections to the portal venous system or the inferior vena cava are corrected by the creation of a wide anastomosis between the posterior aspect of the left atrium and the common transverse pulmonary vein. The stretched foramen ovale is closed. The ascending or descending anomalous pulmonary venous connection to the systemic circulation is ligated, as is the PDA.

Anomalous pulmonary venous connection to the coronary sinus is repaired by creating a large fenestration in the common wall between the coronary sinus and the left atrium. The coronary sinus is diverted into the left atrium by the placement of an intracardiac patch, which also closes the interatrial communication.

Total anomalous pulmonary venous connection to the right atrium is repaired by excision of the atrial septum and placement of a patch that diverts the opening of the anomalous pulmonary venous connection into the left atrium Mixed forms of total anomalous pulmonary venous connection pose particular technical difficulties that require individualized operations. Mortality rates are slightly higher after early repair of symptomatic neonates with mixed types of total anomalous pulmonary venous connections. Although the results of repair of total anomalous pulmonary venous connection without obstruction in an older child have always been quite good, until recently neonates with obstructed total venous return have been problematic. In the 1960s and early 1970s, the surgical mortality rate exceeded 50 percent.[235] Between 1970 and 1980, surgical techniques improved and the mortality rate was reduced to 10 to 20 percent.[236] Recent surgical results show continued improvement, with a 5 percent mortality among 108 children who underwent reparative surgery at Children's Hospital in Boston between 1988 and 2002.[237] Late survival has been quite good, with 98 percent surviving a median of 87 months in another study.[238]

After a satisfactory operative course, the prognosis has been excellent in those in whom a large common pulmonary vein can be attached to the back wall of the left atrium with a relatively large anastomosis. For those initially with obstructed total anomalous pulmonary venous return, the left atrium may be small and the anastomosis may be more difficult. Late obstruction of one or more pulmonary veins has been seen. When present, the obstruction can be approached by balloon dilation, stent placement, or repeat surgery.[239]

MALPOSITION OF THE CARDIAC STRUCTURES
【 】 DEFINITION AND TERMINOLOGY

The *segmental approach* to the diagnosis of complex congenital heart disease[240] provides an orderly, effective method for determining the anatomic and hemodynamic interrelationships of the cardiac chambers, valves, and great vessels. For this approach to be better understood, certain definitions are helpful. Positioning of viscera is described as situs solitus, inversus, or ambiguus. In *situs solitus* (S), the distribution of all the organs is recognized as normal—for example, a left-sided stomach and spleen, a predominantly right-sided liver, a trilobed right lung, and a bilobed left lung. In *situs inversus (totalis)* (I), the organs show a perfect mirror image in regard to left and right to that of situs solitus. Anteroposterior relations are not disturbed. When neither situs solitus nor situs inversus can be identified, *situs ambiguus* (A) is said to be present. This usually applies in cases of asplenia or polysplenia.

Almost exclusively, the *atria follow the body situs* and are so designated (morphologic right atrium to the right of the left atrium in atrial situs solitus and to the left of the left atrium in atrial situs inversus). The AV canal consists of the tricuspid valve, the mitral valve, and the septum of the AV canal and connects the atrial portion with the ventricular portion of the heart. As a rule, *each AV valve is part of the specific ventricle into which it leads.* The valve situs may be solitus, inversus, or ambiguus.

The alignment or type of AV or ventriculoarterial (VA) connection addresses the issue of what flows into what. The connection may be described at the AV or VA level as concordant (e.g., right atrium to right ventricle, left ventricle to aorta) or discordant (e.g., right atrium to left ventricle, left ventricle to pulmonary artery) or may be considered an arrangement that requires a special description. In the case of AV alignment in which the atria are not lateralized, the alignment would be ambiguous. In the univentricular heart, the designation would be double-inlet, absent right, or absent left AV connection. Special descriptions in the case of VA alignment or type of VA connection include double-outlet and single-outlet VA connection. The mode of connections, either AV or VA, addresses the structural makeup of the connecting segments: the AV canal and the infundibulum or conus. The mode of AV connection may be normal, common, stenotic, imperforate, atretic, double-orifice, overriding, straddling, or unguarded. The mode of VA connection may be expressed in terms of the position and development of the conus or infundibulum, which, although normally incorporated into the right ventricle, is not an intrinsic part of the true right ventricle. It may be described as subpulmonary, subaortic, very deficient, or bilaterally present or absent.[241]

The position of the ventricles may be described by the terms *d loop* and *l loop*. When the morphologic right ventricle lies to the right of the morphologic left ventricle, the ventricular portion of the heart is said to exhibit a d loop (D). The ventricles are said to be noninverted or in the solitus position. When the ventricular relations are reversed, l loop (L) is said to be present. The ventricles are inverted or in the inversus position. *These relationships are independent of the visceral or atrial situs as well as the position of the heart or its chambers within the chest.*

The great arteries may deviate from the usual with respect to both their anteroposterior and lateral (left-to-right) relationships. In solitus (S) or *normally related great arteries* (NRGAs), the aortic origin lies to the right of and posterior to the position of the pulmonary valve. In the inversus (I) relationship, the anteroposterior relationships are not disturbed but the aortic origin lies to the left of the pulmonary arterial origin. In *transposition of the great arteries* (TGA), the aorta arises from the anatomic right ventricle, the pulmonary artery arises from the anatomic left ventricle, and usually the aortic origin is more anterior than that of the pulmonary artery.

When the aortic origin lies to the right of the pulmonary origin, the transposition is called *dextro-* or *d-transposition* (d-TGA) (see the discussion of complete transposition of the great arteries, below). When the aortic origin lies to the left of the pulmonary origin, *levotransposition* (l-TGA) is said to be present (see the section on congenitally corrected transposition, below).

When the abnormal relationship of the great arteries is neither complete nor corrected transposition, the term *malposition of the great arteries* (MGA) may be used. Malpositions are designated as d-MGA or l-MGA, depending on the laterality in the relation between the origins of the two great arteries. Within this group are found examples of the abnormal VA alignment, where one great artery arises from the appropriate ventricle and the other great artery also arises from the same (or inappropriate) ventricle. These are examples of *double-outlet right ventricle* (DORV) or *double-outlet left ventricle* (DOLV). Also included is the arterial malposition termed *anatomically corrected malposition* (ACM). This is characterized by the great arteries having a normal VA alignment (concordant), but with the aorta anterior to the pulmonary artery by virtue of an abnormal mode of VA connection: the presence of a well-developed conus lying beneath both the aorta and the pulmonary artery or only beneath the aorta. The route for the flow of blood in ACMs may be normal or abnormal, depending on the AV alignment.[241]

[ ] THE SEGMENTAL APPROACH TO DIAGNOSIS

The segmental, or step-by-step, approach is a valuable tool for arriving at the correct diagnosis in patients with complex congenital heart disease and is independent of cardiac position. In order, one determines (1) the locations of the right and left atria and their venous connections, (2) the location of the right and left ventricles and their alignment with the atria, (3) the mode of connection of the AV valves to the ventricles, (4) the position of the great arteries and their alignment with the ventricles, and (5) the location and status of the infundibulum. In addition, one must search for associated malformations between and within each of these segments.

Determining atrial situs can be accomplished in most instances by taking advantage of the high degree of abdominal visceroatrial concordance. With abdominal situs solitus (S), the liver is on the right and the right atrium almost invariably is on the right as well; with abdominal situs inversus (I), the liver is on the left and the right atrium almost invariably is on the left. With abdominal situs ambiguus (A), the liver may be placed almost symmetrically across the midline and the atria may be located normally or inverted or both atria may have morphologic characteristics of either the right atrium or the left atrium (see Fig. 12–4). A symmetric liver is found in approximately 60 percent of patients with situs ambiguus. Lateralization of the liver, which is evident in the remainder, may simulate either situs solitus or situs inversus.

When both atria have characteristics of a right atrium,[242] *dextroisomerism,* or "bilateral right-sidedness," is said to be present. This situation is usually, though not invariably, accompanied by asplenia. When both atria have characteristics of a left atrium, *levoisomerism,* or "bilateral left-sidedness," is said to exist. This usually, but again not invariably, is accompanied by polysplenia.

Bronchial situs, as determined by overpenetrated chest roentgenogram or bronchial tomography, is an excellent predictor of atrial situs, but the most accurate technique appears to be two-dimensional echocardiography with Doppler color-flow mapping. The hepatic portion of the inferior vena cava, which almost always enters the morphologic right atrium, usually can be identified easily, as can the connections and structural details of the superior vena cava, coronary sinus, pulmonary veins, atrial septum, and atrial appendages.

Additional clinical clues to atrial situs may be obtained from the ECG, where a superior and leftward orientation of the P-wave vector suggests levoisomerism and polysplenia. Howell-Heinz and Howell-Jolly bodies in the peripheral blood smear are characteristic of dextroisomerism or asplenia.

For determination of the AV, ventricular, and VA relationships, high-quality two-dimensional echocardiography with Doppler color-flow mapping, and occasionally MRI or biplane angiography is essential. Symbols used to designate the combination or sequence of segments are arranged in order as follows: (1) the visceroatrial or bronchoatrial situs, (2) the ventricular loop, and (3) the relations of the great arteries. These may be included within parentheses and preceded by abbreviations that indicate the VA alignment, for example, TGA, DORV, or single ventricle (SV). Associated malformations such as VSD, pulmonary stenosis, and straddling tricuspid valve may be listed after the parentheses. Thus, the typical or usual transposition of the great arteries with situs solitus, d-ventricular loop, and aorta arising from the right ventricle and to the right of the pulmonary artery, with an intact ventricular septum (IVS), would be designated TGA (SDD), IVS. The designation for typical corrected transposition (TGA) with situs solitus (S), l-ventricular loop (L), aorta arising from the morphologic right ventricle and lying to the left of the pulmonary artery (L), with VSD and pulmonary stenosis (PS), would be TGA (SLL), VSD, PS. This designation would apply to transposition with situs solitus, whether the heart lay in the right or left chest (dextrocardia or levocardia, respectively). It should be noted that the description of the position of the heart within the chest would offer no additional information referable to the intracardiac anatomy or great vessel alignment.[240]

[ ] LEVOCARDIA, DEXTROCARDIA, AND MESOCARDIA

The position of the cardiac apex indicates a condition of levocardia, dextrocardia, or mesocardia. The term *isolated levocardia* is applied to all left-sided hearts with situs inversus or situs ambiguous, and a description of the visceroatrial situs should follow. Dextrocardia with complete situs inversus occurs in approximately 2 per 10,000 livebirths. *The incidence of congenital heart disease is relatively low among these individuals and is estimated to be approximately 3 percent.* Dextrocardia with situs solitus or situs ambiguus is considerably less common and occurs in perhaps 1 in 20,000 livebirths. The incidence of congenital heart disease is extremely high in this situation, however, probably in the range of 90 percent or greater. Approximately 50 percent of patients with dextrocardia and heart disease have situs solitus, and the remainder, perhaps 30 percent, have situs ambiguus.[141] An l-ventricular loop is found in the majority of patients with dextrocardia regardless of situs but is most common, as one might expect, among patients with situs inversus, in whom it approaches 80 percent. Cardiac malformations usually, although not invariably, are severe and complex. The most common lesions and their approximate frequency are as follows: transposition of the great arteries, 50 to 75 percent; double-outlet right ventricle, 10 to 18 percent; VSD, 60 to 80 percent; single ventricle, 15 to 40 percent; and pulmonary stenosis or atresia, 70 to 80 percent.[141] Polysplenia or asplenia is found in about one-third of patients with dextrocardia and almost invariably with situs ambiguus. Kartagener syndrome—the triad of situs inversus, sinusitis, and bronchiectasis—results from impaired ciliary movement. It is present in approximately

20 percent of patients with dextrocardia and situs inversus totalis.[142] The incidence of isolated levocardia has been estimated at approximately 0.6 per 10,000 livebirths. It is estimated that more than 90 percent of affected individuals have associated heart disease. Situs inversus is present in approximately 15 percent, and the remainder have situs ambiguus, with the ratio of asplenia to polysplenia or accessory spleens being from 2.5:1 to 1.5:1. The associated defects are comparable in complexity and severity to those associated with dextrocardia. *Mesocardia* may exist as a variant position of the normal heart or a variant position of dextrocardia or isolated levocardia.

Medical and Surgical Management

Medical management of patients with cardiac malposition is similar to that of patients with normally located hearts, with the exceptions of continuous daily antibiotic coverage and pneumococcal vaccine for patients with asplenia and the particular attention to detail that is necessary to establish the correct diagnosis in individuals with unusual and complex malformations. Surgical management differs in the technical considerations imposed by the malposition of the heart itself, the frequency of occurrence of the l-ventricular loop, and the variability of the intracardiac conduction system.

【 】 DEXTROTRANSPOSITION OF THE GREAT ARTERIES

Definition

In this condition, the aorta and the pulmonary artery are misplaced in relation to the ventricular septum, with the aorta arising from the right ventricle and the pulmonary artery arising from the left ventricle (discordant VA connection). It is the most common of the cyanotic lesions occurring in approximately 1 in 4000 livebirths.

Pathology

In the majority of cases, there are situs solitus of the atria and viscera (S) and concordance of the AV connection and the right ventricle lies to the right of the left ventricle (D loop; Fig. 82–36). The aorta lies to the right of the pulmonary arterial origin (d-transposition) and is anterior. Of the communications between the two sides of the circulation, a narrow patent foramen and PDA are common in very young infants. In our experience, the ventricular septum is intact in approximately half these patients, and another 10 percent have only a very small VSD. The remainder have a large VSD or multiple VSDs.[244]

Pulmonary stenosis of significance is very uncommon among neonates with an intact ventricular septum but develops with the passage of time in approximately one-third of patients in whom the right ventricle continues to be the systemic ventricle. In most cases it is mild and usually though not invariably the result of a bulging of the ventricular septum into the left ventricular outflow area. Approximately one-third of patients with a large VSD have significant left ventricular outflow tract obstruction (pulmonary stenosis). Causes of this obstruction include leftward malalignment of the infundibular septum, the presence of a membranous collar or ridge encircling the left ventricular outflow tract, anomalous adhesion of the anterior mitral leaflet to the ventricular septum, stenotic deformity of the pulmonary valve, and, rarely, an aneurysm of endocardial tissue related to the VSD.[245]

The coronary arteries usually arise from the two aortic sinuses adjacent to the pulmonary trunk—the "facing sinuses"—with the most common arrangement being the right coronary artery arising from the rightward sinus and the left coronary artery, with its anterior descending and circumflex branches, arising from the leftward sinus. Hypertensive pulmonary vascular disease may occur at an inordinately early age, even in patients with an intact ventricular septum and initially low left ventricular pressures. Three-quarters or more of patients with d-transposition, situs solitus, and D [TGA (SDD)] loop either have no significant associated cardiac defects or relatively simple malformations in the form of VSD, ASD, PDA, or pulmonary stenosis. The remainder have more complicated lesions and are not discussed in this section.

Abnormal Physiology

The systemic and pulmonary circulations are arranged so that the systemic venous return is conducted back to the systemic arterial system and the pulmonary venous return is directed to the pulmonary arterial system, with no obligatory mixing or interchange. For survival, there must be communication between the two circulations in the form of a patent foramen ovale, a PDA, or a VSD. The hemodynamics are dependent on the combination of defects present and particularly on the amount of mixing between the systemic and pulmonary circulations. The right ventricle is the systemic ventricle with concomitant pressure.

Clinical Manifestations

Approximately 3 to 4 percent of children with recognized congenital heart disease have transposition of the great arteries (see Table 82–1). Males are more commonly affected than females, in a male-to-female ratio between 2:1 and 3:1.

History Among infants with an intact ventricular septum, very early, severe, and progressive cyanosis is the presenting sign, making its clinical appearance within the first hour in more than half, and by the end of the first 24 hours in more than 60 percent of neonates so affected.[3] In a very few, a persistent PDA in combination with an incompetent foramen ovale or a small VSD permits survival for several weeks, but narrowing or closure of any of the three communications produces critical hypoxemia. In infants with transposition and a sizable VSD the presentation includes severe heart failure and minimal cyanosis by the end of the first month. Infants with a large VSD and severe pulmonary stenosis present within the first days of life with cyanosis, whereas those with more moderate stenosis tend to show cyanosis and mild heart failure somewhat later within the first month.

Physical Examination Among infants with an intact ventricular septum, the most prominent feature is intense cyanosis. Tachypnea and mild dyspnea are present. The right ventricular lift is forceful, and the first sound is usually loud at the lower left sternal border. In most patients, the second heart sound splits normally, confirming the presence of two semilunar valves, although the pulmonary valve closure is softer because it is posterior to the aorta. Murmurs are seldom impressive or distinctive. Signs of heart failure are absent unless the infant is beyond the first week of life and a large PDA is present. Infants with a large VSD appear thin, with mild cyanosis or a grayish pallor. Breathing is labored, and both the right and left ventricular impulses are hyperactive. A thrill is uncommon. A systolic murmur

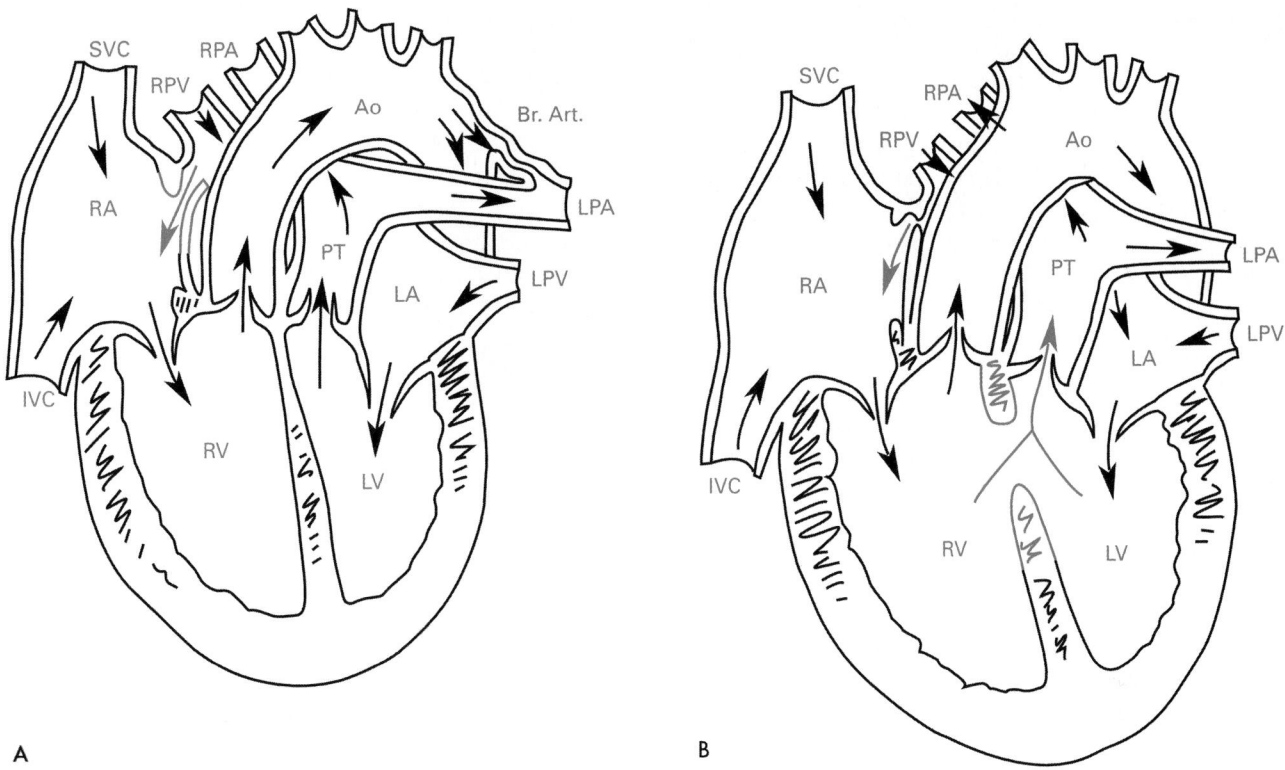

A   B

FIGURE 82–36. Complete d-transposition of the great arteries. **A.** With intact ventricular septum. A patent foramen ovale and enlarged bronchial arteries (Br. Art.) are present. **B.** With ventricular septal defect and without pulmonary stenosis. Ao, aorta; LA, left atrium; LPA, left pulmonary artery; LPV, left pulmonary vein; LV, left ventricle; PT, main pulmonary arterial trunk; RA, right atrium; RPA, right pulmonary artery; RPV, right pulmonary vein; RV, right ventricle; SVC, superior vena cava.

at the lower left sternal border is usually present but is seldom loud or holosystolic. A gallop rhythm and a diastolic flow rumble at the apex are typical. Infants and children with VSD and significant pulmonary stenosis are very cyanotic.

Chest Roentgenogram With an intact ventricular septum, the size of the heart and pulmonary vascularity appear normal or at the upper limits of normal during the first week. Later, a narrow base caused by the displaced pulmonary artery may give rise to the characteristic "egg-on-side" contour. Impressive cardiomegaly, pulmonary plethora, and this characteristic contour are more common during the second week and beyond. With a large VSD, marked cardiac enlargement involving all chambers, impressive pulmonary plethora, and the egg-on-side contour are present. With significant pulmonary stenosis, the heart resembles that of a patient with tetralogy of Fallot, but it is usually slightly larger and the pulmonary vascularity is less diminished than one would expect for a comparable degree of clinical cyanosis. A right aortic arch is present in 4 to 16 percent of these patients.

Electrocardiogram If the ventricular septum is intact, the ECG may reveal tall or peaked P waves by the second or third day of life; however, clearly abnormal right ventricular forces are usually not apparent until the latter part of the first week. The persistence of an upright T wave in leads V_1 and V_{3R} beyond 4 days of age provides an early clue that the right ventricular systolic pressure is at systemic levels. An older infant will have abnormal right axis deviation and marked right ventricular hypertrophy. A large VSD with a large pulmonary blood flow will usually produce biatrial and biventricular hypertrophy. If pulmonary blood flow is reduced toward normal—whether by significant pulmonary stenosis, pul-

monary arterial banding, or severe PVOD—the pattern becomes one of right ventricular and right atrial hypertrophy.

Echocardiogram Two-dimensional study with Doppler color-flow mapping is the diagnostic procedure of choice. The pulmonary artery can be seen arising from the left ventricle, and the aorta from the right ventricle (Fig. 82–37A). The presence or absence of VSDs, anomalies of the AV connections, the status of the left ventricular outflow tract, and the coronary arterial pattern can be identified. Magnetic resonance imaging is rarely required in the perinatal period.

Cardiac Catheterization A cardiac catheterization may be necessary to evaluate the coronary artery pattern and to perform a balloon atrial septostomy. Systemic arterial oxygen desaturation is present in all these patients. The pulmonary arterial oxygen saturation is invariably higher than the systemic arterial saturation. The right ventricular systolic pressure will be at systemic levels; the left ventricular pressure also will be at systemic levels if a large VSD, ductus arteriosus, or marked pulmonary stenosis is present. A wide pressure difference between the two ventricles or between the two atria indicates an intact or virtually intact ventricular or atrial septum, but the lack of such a gradient certainly does not guarantee the presence of an adequate opening at either level. Selective ventricular angiography will document the diagnosis and the associated defects (see Fig. 82–37B). The coronary arterial pattern should be established if it is not visible by echocardiography. *All newborns with transposition who are not immediately going to the operating room can benefit from balloon atrial septostomy at catheterization by virtue of the increased mixing of the pulmonary and systemic venous circulations and the decompression of the left atrium.*

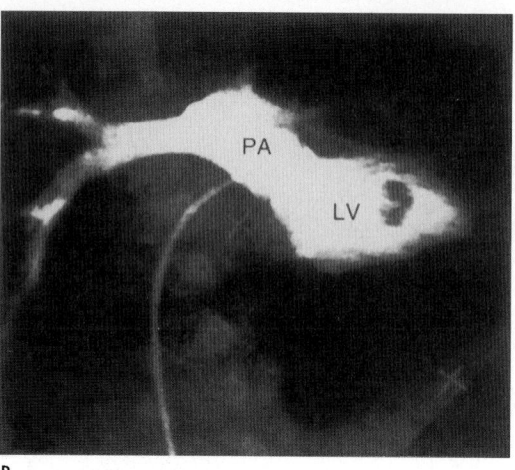

FIGURE 82–37. A. Two-dimensional echocardiogram. The left ventricle leads to a bifurcating great vessel (pulmonary artery [PA]), confirming transposition. **B.** Anterolateral projection of an angiogram in the smooth-walled left ventricle (LV). The dye is ejected into the pulmonary artery.

Natural History

Historically, without balloon septostomy or surgical intervention, 50 percent of infants with transposition die within the first month and 90 percent die within the first year of life.[247] Those with an intact ventricular septum die very early from hypoxemia. Those with a large VSD usually live somewhat longer, but the majority die in the first months of heart failure; the few survivors have severe PVOD. Those with a large VSD and pulmonary stenosis have the best outlook, but the average life expectancy is barely 5 years.

Medical Management

The first step in the treatment of infants with an intact ventricular septum is to provide adequate systemic arterial oxygen saturation. This end point is reached by creating a large interatrial opening with balloon atrial septostomy and augmenting systemic-to-pulmonary arterial shunting via the ductus using intravenous PGE_1 infusion.[247] The latter maneuver is supported by intubation in anticipation of prostaglandin-related apnea. An adequate atrial septostomy is marked by a sustained increase in the systemic arterial oxygen saturation above 60 percent and verified by two-dimensional echocardiography. If the response PGE_1 is unsatisfactory and if the interatrial opening is small by echocardiography, the alternatives are to perform a balloon atrial septectomy or to proceed directly with corrective surgery in the form of the arterial switch operation.

Surgical Management

Initial management of transposition (prior to the 1980s) involved an atrial switch by the Senning or Mustard technique. These earlier atrial switch operations, such as the Mustard and Senning procedures, are prone to residual abnormalities such as pulmonary stenosis and PVOD as well as complications that result from surgery, including residual intraatrial baffle leaks, systemic and/or pulmonary venous obstruction, and arrhythmias. Late sudden death has been described in approximately 3 percent of survivors, probably from arrhythmias. Finally, right ventricular dysfunction with or without progressive tricuspid regurgitation has been documented in some of the older survivors raising the question of whether the right ventricle can function adequately as the systemic arterial ventricle beyond adolescence and early

adult life.[31] Cardiac transplantation has been required in some (see Chap. 83).

Although complications have been problematic for some, long-term followup of the group as a whole has been good. The Toronto experience is the oldest and largest. Among 534 children who underwent a Mustard procedure since 1962, there were 52 early deaths (9.7 percent). Survival at 5 years was 89 percent, and at 20 years it was 76 percent.[50] In a study from New Zealand of 113 hospital survivors of surgery performed between 1964 and 1982, survival at 10, 20, and 28 years was 90, and 80 percent, respectively, with 76 percent of survivors being classified as New York Heart Association class I.[248] There has been less long-term follow-up of survivors of the "Senning" type of atrial repair. In a study of 100 patients, the actuarial survival at 13 years was 90 percent for those with simple transposition and 78 percent survival for those with complex disease.[249]

Arterial switch repair is now the preferred surgical alternative to the atrial inversion procedures for a neonate with an intact ventricular septum and for a slightly older infant with a large VSD and without significant structural pulmonary stenosis (Fig. 82–38). Arterial switching should be performed within the first 2 to 3 weeks of life, before left ventricular systolic pressure falls significantly below that of the right ventricle. For infants beyond 3 weeks of age, if the ratio of left ventricular to right ventricular pressure has fallen below 0.60, a pulmonary arterial band may be applied with or without a systemic-to-pulmonary arterial shunt. The arterial switch operation may be performed approximately 1 week later. Most patterns of coronary arterial origin and course appear to be amenable to the operation, and infants as small as 2.0 kg may be repaired successfully. In some centers, the surgical risks have been reduced to 5 to 10 percent[250,251] or less, although the surgical mortality continues to be higher in other centers.[234] Short- and medium-term prognosis is good, with a 10- and 15- year actuarial survival of 88 percent among 1200 patients who had an arterial switch at one institution between 1982 and 1999,[253] but longer-term studies are awaited. Exercise performance analyzed in a small group of patients following arterial switch has shown excellent cardiopulmonary capacity.[254] The most common postoperative problem has been stenosis at the pulmonary artery or, less commonly, at the aortic anastomotic site.[255] When severe, it has usually been amenable to balloon dilation or stenting.[256] Although aortic regurgitation related to neoaortic root dilation has been viewed as a long-term potential problem, an intermediate followup study has shown a small likelihood for development of hemodynamically significant regurgitation.[257]

Rhythm concerns, common with the atrial switch have been less common (thus far) with most patients having sinus rhythm (91.7 percent), with significant ectopy uncommon (1.7 percent).[258]

For infants with transposition, a large VSD, and pulmonary hypertension, the arterial switch technique with VSD closure must be carried out within the first 2 months of life to prevent severe PVOD. Infants with a large VSD and severe pulmonary stenosis may be palliated with a systemic-to-pulmonary arterial shunt and repaired in later infancy or early childhood,[186] although some centers are doing

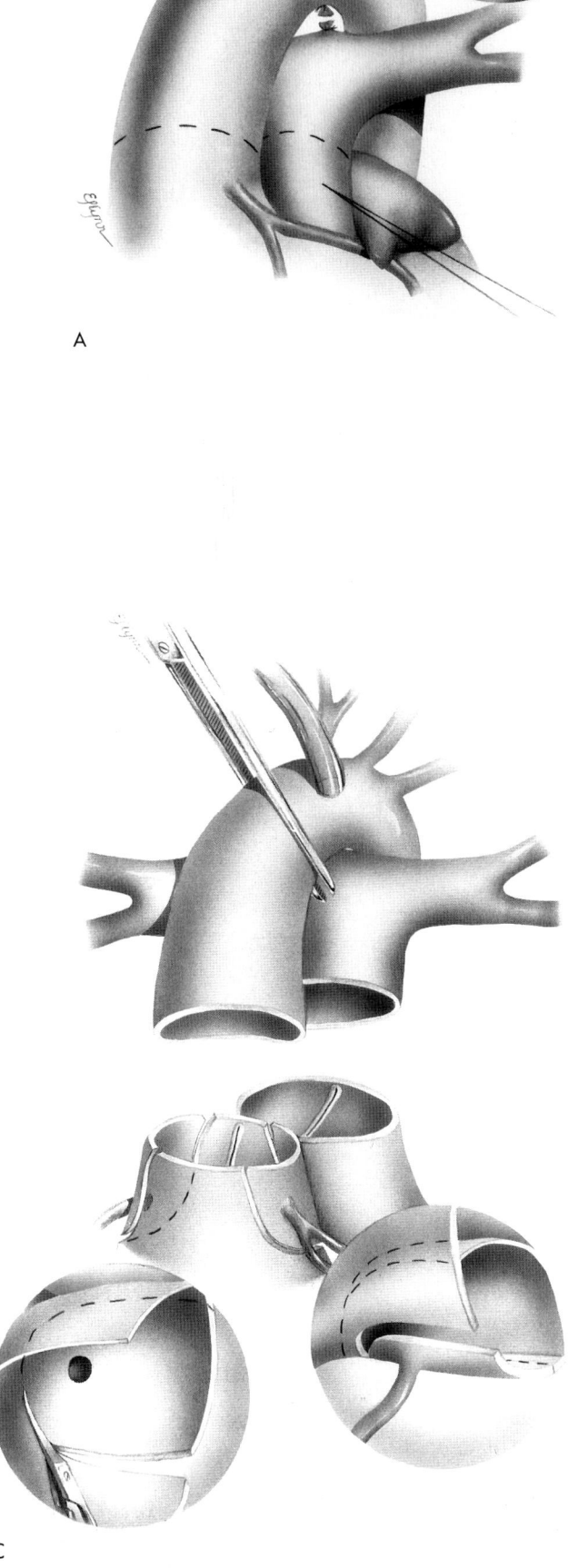

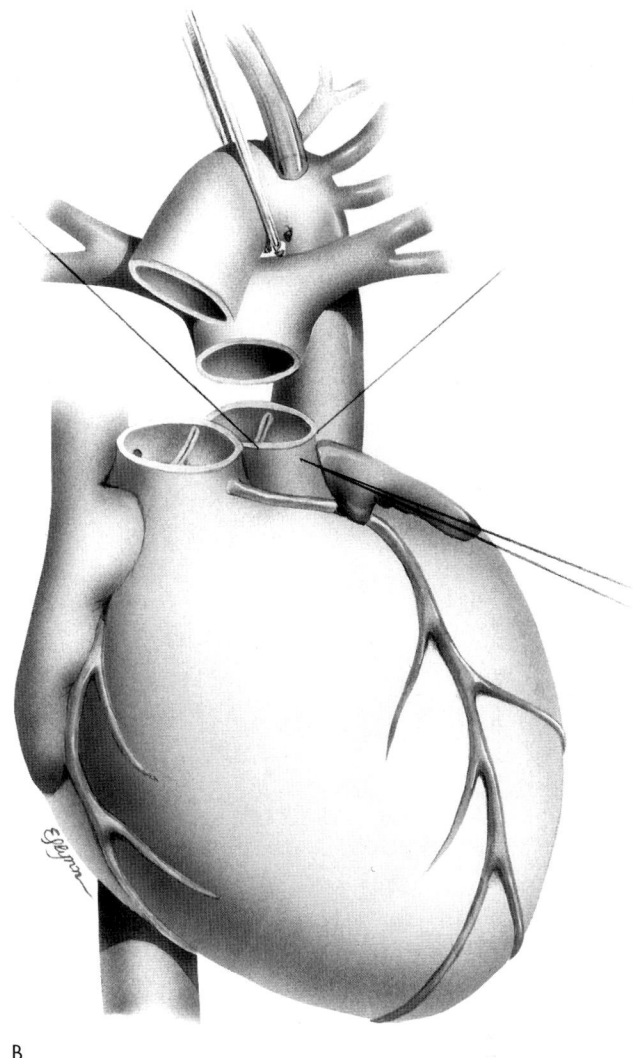

FIGURE 82–38. Surgical technique of the arterial switch operation. **A.** Aortic cannula is positioned distally in the ascending aorta, the ductus arteriosus is divided between suture ligatures, and the branch pulmonary arteries are dissected out to the hilum to provide adequate mobility for anterior translocation. The broken lines represent the levels of transection of the aorta and the main pulmonary artery. Marking sutures are placed in the anticipated sites of coronary transfer. **B.** Transection of the great arteries. The left ventricular outflow tract, neoaortic valve, and coronary arteries are inspected thoroughly. **C.** The coronary arterial buttons are excised from the free edge of the aorta to the base of the sinus of Valsalva. **D.** The coronary buttons are anastomosed to V-shaped excisions made in the neoaorta. **E.** The pulmonary artery is brought anterior to the aorta (Lecompte maneuver). Anastomosis of the proximal neoaorta is shown. **F** and **G.** The coronary donor sites are filled with autologous pericardial patches. A single U-shaped patch (**F**) or two separate patches (**G**) may be used. **H.** Completed anastomosis of the proximal neopulmonary artery and the distal pulmonary artery. *Source: Modified from Castaneda AR. Anatomic correction of transposition of the great arteries at the arterial level. In: Sabiston DC Jr, Spencer FC, eds. Surgery of the Chest, 5th ed. Philadelphia: WB Saunders, 1990. Reproduced with permission from the publisher and authors.*

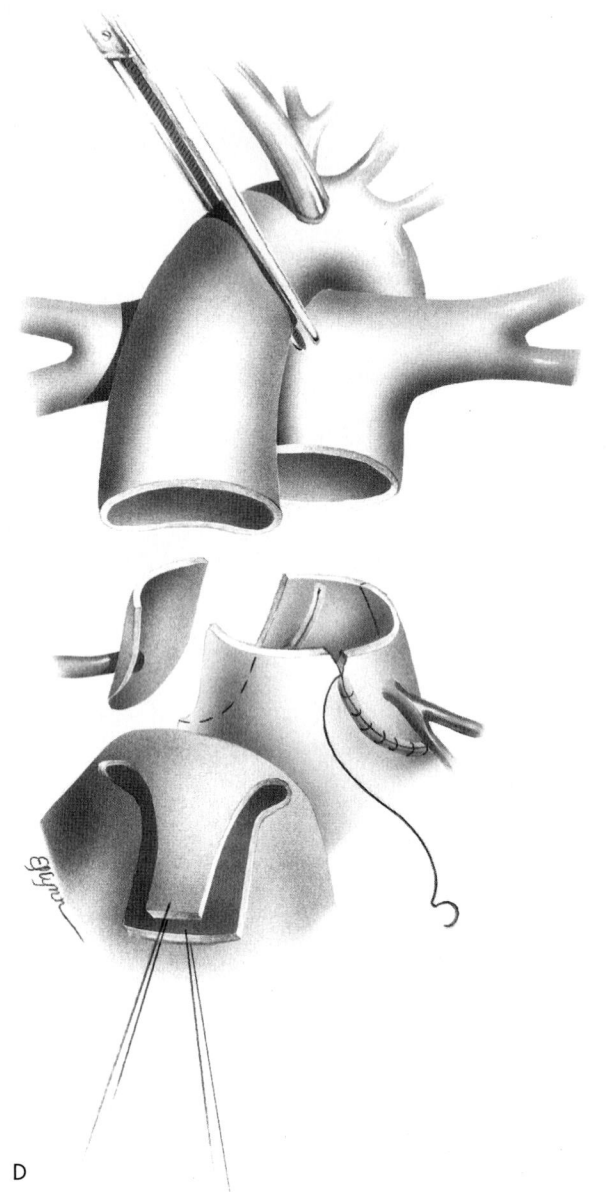

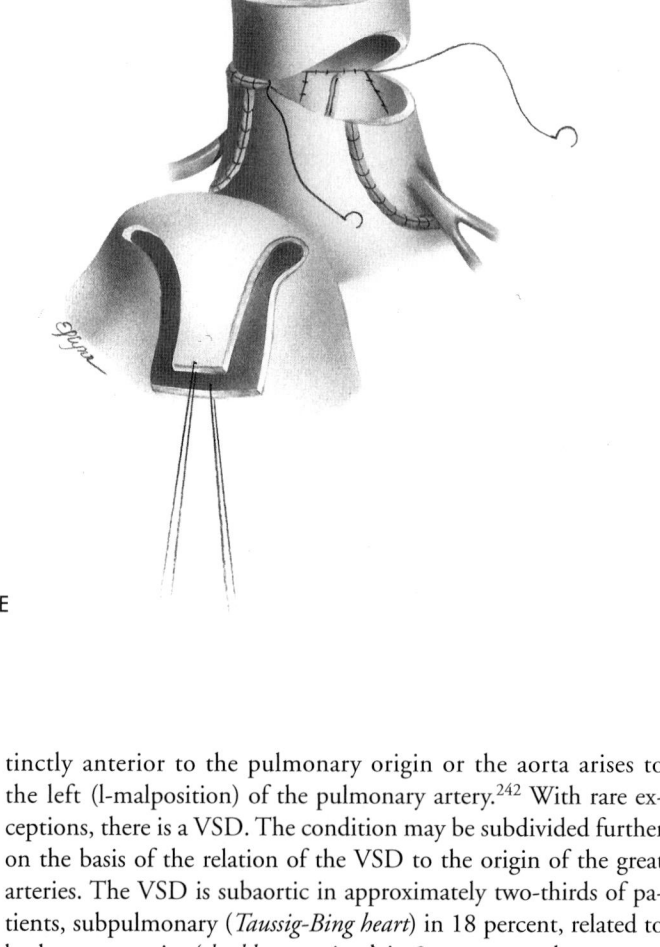

E

D

FIGURE 82-38. *(Continued)*

reparative surgery in infancy.[259] Finally, the severe hypoxemia present in older children or adults with a large VSD and severe PVOD may be reduced by an intraatrial repair performed as a palliative procedure, with no attempt at closure of the VSD.[260]

DOUBLE-OUTLET RIGHT VENTRICLE

Pathology

In this malformation, more than 50 percent of the semilunar valve orifices of both great arteries arise from the morphologic right ventricle. In most cases, the ventricles display a D loop, and the pulmonary arterial origin is normally positioned, arising from a conus above the right ventricle. The aorta also arises from the right ventricle above conal tissue. The two semilunar valves are at about the same level, and there is no fibrous continuity between the semilunar and mitral valves (Fig. 82–39).

In most cases, the aortic origin is to the right (d-malposition) of the pulmonary arterial origin, with the two vessels in a side-by-side relationship. Uncommonly, the aortic origin is dis-

tinctly anterior to the pulmonary origin or the aorta arises to the left (l-malposition) of the pulmonary artery.[242] With rare exceptions, there is a VSD. The condition may be subdivided further on the basis of the relation of the VSD to the origin of the great arteries. The VSD is subaortic in approximately two-thirds of patients, subpulmonary (*Taussig-Bing heart*) in 18 percent, related to both great arteries (*doubly committed*) in 3 percent, and remote or unrelated to either great artery in approximately 7 percent.[261]

Associated Conditions

Pulmonary stenosis occurs in more than half of these cases, with the condition usually resulting from a narrow subpulmonary conus. Atrial septal defects, subaortic stenosis, and coarctation of the aorta are also relatively common, with the latter particularly associated with the subpulmonary defect. Obstruction at the mitral valve may be observed in about one-fifth of cases of double-outlet right ventricle. Mitral valve straddling of the VSD and varying degrees of left ventricular hypoplasia also are encountered.

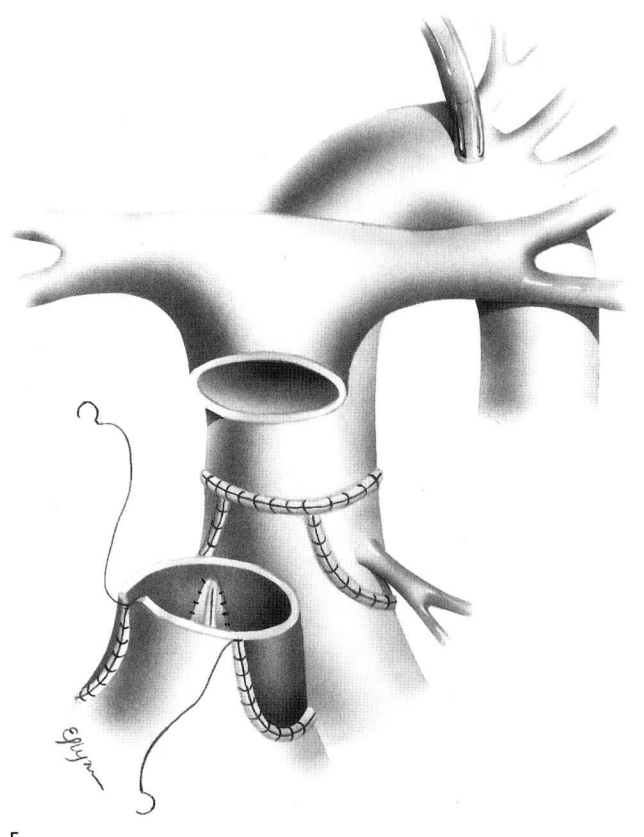

F

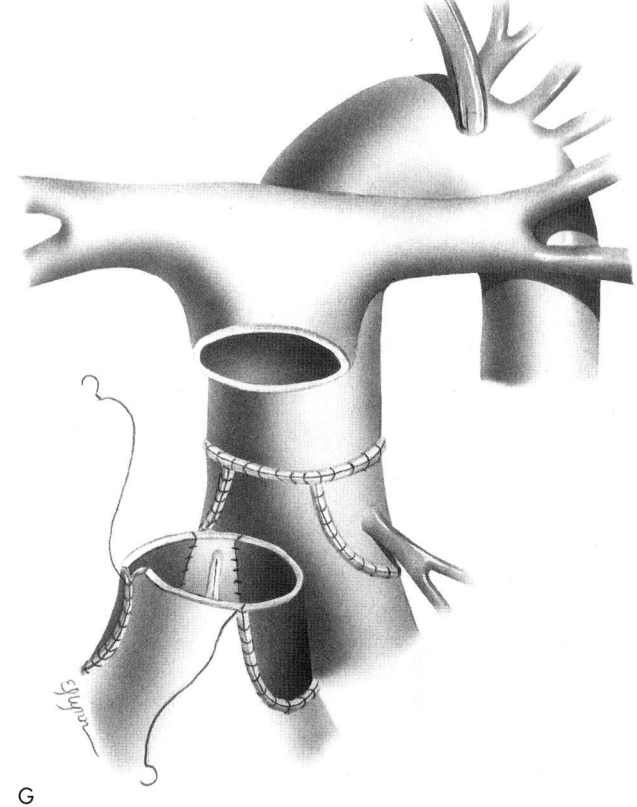

G

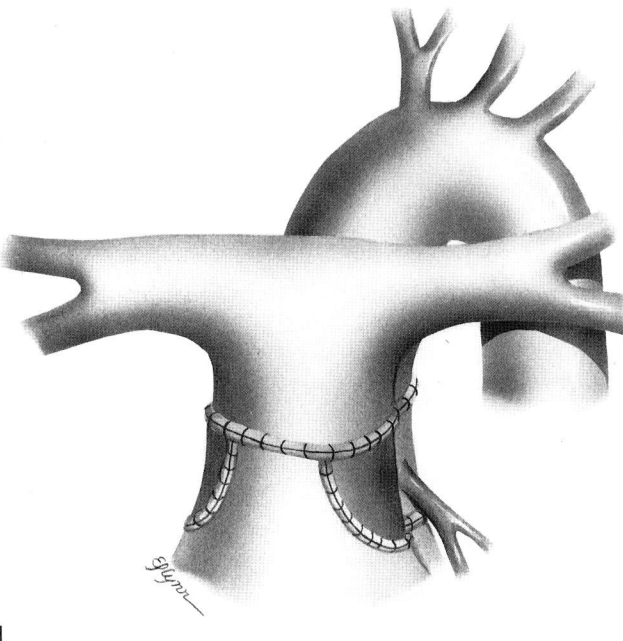

H

FIGURE 82–38. *(Continued)*

Clinical Manifestations

Double-outlet right ventricle, or origin of both great arteries from the right ventricle, is a relatively rare malformation that is found in less than 1 percent of patients with congenital heart disease. It is of considerable importance, however, because its clinical and laboratory features frequently resemble those of more common and more easily correctable malformations. Double-outlet right ventricle reflects the relationship of the great vessels to the ventricular septum; the presen-

tation and treatment of children with this condition depend on the associated anomalies.

History and Physical Examination Patients with a subaortic VSD without pulmonary stenosis (see Fig. 82–39A) have clinical findings that mimic a large isolated VSD. Heart failure appears within a few weeks of birth; cyanosis is seldom described. Those with a subaortic VSD and pulmonary stenosis (see Fig. 82–39B) usually present after the newborn period and follow a course similar to that of patients with

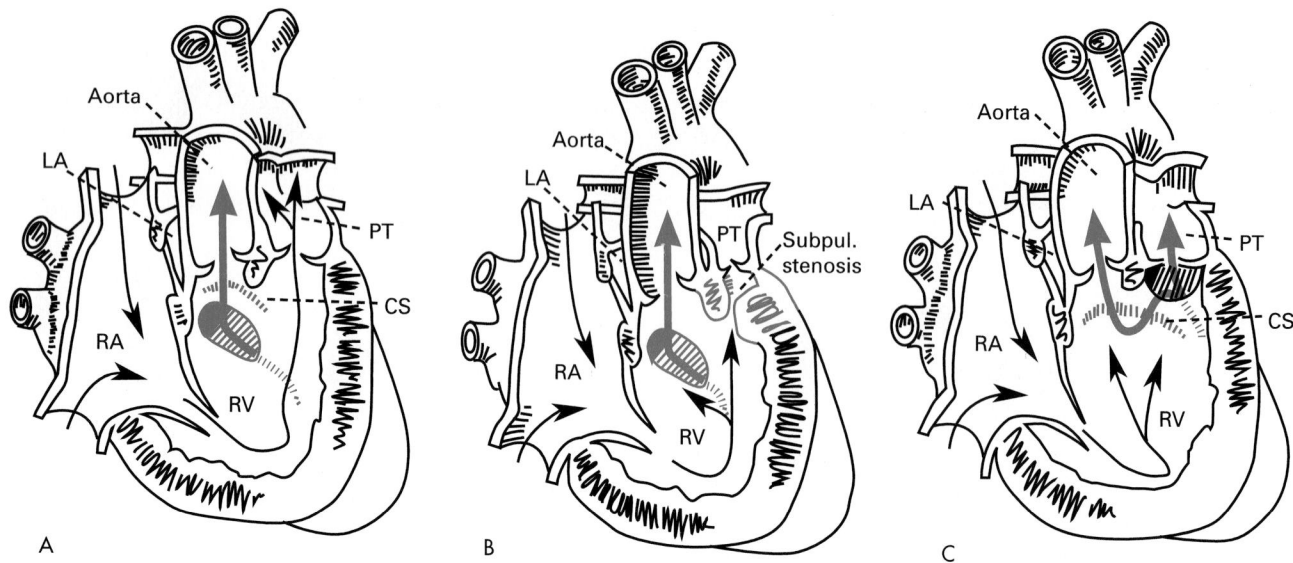

FIGURE 82–39. Double-outlet right ventricle. **A.** With subaortic ventricular septal defect without pulmonary stenosis. **B.** With subaortic ventricular septal defect and subpulmonary stenosis (Subpul. stenosis). **C.** With subpulmonary, supracristal ventricular septal defect. The so-called *Taussig-Bing complex*. CS, crista supraventricularis; LA, left atrium; PT, main pulmonary arterial trunk; RA, right atrium; RV, right ventricle.

tetralogy of Fallot. Patients with a subpulmonary defect without pulmonary stenosis and transposed great arteries (see Fig. 82–39C), the Taussig-Bing malformation, resemble patients with transposition of the great arteries and a large VSD without pulmonary stenosis. The findings are those of severe heart failure without cyanosis.

Chest Roentgenogram Cardiomegaly with pulmonary overperfusion is characteristic of all types of this anomaly without pulmonary stenosis. Double-outlet right ventricle with subaortic VSD and pulmonary stenosis resembles tetralogy of Fallot with a small heart and narrowed base of the heart. In the case of subpulmonary VSD without pulmonary stenosis, the pulmonary artery usually lies beside, rather than posterior to, the aorta; this clearly visible, dilated main pulmonary artery may permit distinction of this malformation from transposition, which it mimics so closely.

Electrocardiogram Right-axis deviation and right atrial and right ventricular hypertrophy are characteristic of double-outlet right ventricle.[261,262]

Echocardiogram Two-dimensional echocardiography is very useful in demonstrating the anatomic components and associated defects.[153]

Cardiac Catheterization When needed, a catheterization demonstrates an increase in oxygen saturation at the right ventricular level. The pulmonary arterial saturation is lower than that of the aorta in patients with a subaortic VSD and is invariably higher than that of the aorta in those with a subpulmonary septal defect and transposition physiology. Left ventricular systolic pressure may be higher than right pressure if the VSD is small and restrictive. Selective right and left ventricular biplane angiography and an aortogram are recommended if the echocardiogram is insufficient to demonstrate the ventricular great vessel.

Natural History and Prognosis

The clinical course of each variety of double-outlet right ventricle is determined by the associated defects. Without surgical intervention, those with an unguarded pulmonary artery either die in infancy with congestive failure or develop PVOD. Spontaneous narrowing or closure of the VSD may occur and leaves the left ventricle at increased pressure. Clinically, this may result in dyspnea, increasing intensity of the systolic murmur, and progressive left ventricular hypertrophy on the ECG. Patients with pulmonary stenosis tend to have progressive obstruction and cyanosis.

Medical Management

Vigorous treatment of heart failure is required for those without pulmonary stenosis. Almost all cases are best treated with surgical palliation or correction in infancy. If there is pulmonary hypertension, banding or, more commonly, correction should be done by 2 to 3 months of age. Patients with ventricular hypoplasia, mitral stenosis, straddling AV valve, or a remote VSD are usually not candidates for biventricular repair, and initial palliation should prepare the child for a modification of the Fontan operation. Whether or not corrective surgery has been performed, all patients with the left ventricular output passing through the VSD should be observed carefully for the possibility of spontaneous narrowing and obstruction at that site.

Surgical Management

Great variability exists in the morphologic spectrum of double-outlet right ventricle. Although primary total repair of most forms of double-outlet right ventricle is now performed and preferred in infancy, palliation (pulmonary arterial banding, repair of aortic coarctation, atrial septal excision, or the creation of a systemic arterial-to-pulmonary arterial or systemic venous-to-pulmonary arterial shunt) to adjust pulmonary blood flow and thus preserve the pulmonary vascular bed, ventricular function, and AV valve competence may be considered in complex variants.

In all forms of double-outlet ventricle, the relation of the VSD to the great arteries and the magnitude of ventricular outflow tract obstruction dictate management. Surgical correction requires (1) obliteration of the interventricular communication, (2) relief of pulmonary stenosis when present, (3) diversion of oxygenated pulmonary venous blood to the aorta, and (4) diversion of hypoxemic systemic venous blood to the pulmonary artery.[263] When the VSD is committed to the aorta, a Dacron semiconduit or tunnel-shaped patch is placed to obliterate the interventricular communication while the left ventricular blood is diverted through the VSD to the aorta. Pulmonary stenosis is corrected by a valvotomy, with excision of obstructive muscle bundles and placement of a transannular patch when necessary. Otherwise, an extracardiac conduit is placed between the right ventricle and the pulmonary artery.[264,265]

When the great arteries are transposed or the VSD is not committed to the aorta, the arterial switch operation, using the concepts of Jatene and Le Compte, permits patch closure of the VSD, directing left ventricular blood into the neoaorta.[266] Further consideration of repair of double-outlet right ventricle associated with more complex defects is beyond the scope of this discussion. For a patient who is not a candidate for biventricular repair because of hypoplasia of a ventricle or a straddling AV valve, initial palliation should prepare the child for a modification of the Fontan operation.

In a 10-year review of repair of double-outlet right ventricle in 73 patients,[245] early mortality was 11 percent, with an overall actuarial survival estimate at 8 years of 81 percent. Twenty-six percent required reoperation, and there was one death; 79 percent of the operative survivors required no restriction of physical activity, and 83 percent required no cardiac medications.

In a 20-year review of 124 patients from a single center, the 15-year survival varied between 90 and 96 percent, depending on the associated lesions, with a freedom from reoperation of 87 to 100 percent, except in the group with conduits where 28 percent required reoperation for enlargement of the conduits, presumably as a consequence of somatic growth.[267]

[ ] CORRECTED TRANSPOSITION OF THE GREAT ARTERIES

Definition

AV discordance and VA discordance form the characteristics of corrected transposition.

Pathology

Usually situs solitus is present, but the ventricles are inverted (an L loop). The great arteries are transposed and in the l position, so that the pulmonary artery arises posteriorly from the right-sided morphologic left ventricle and the l-transposed aorta arises anteriorly from the left-sided right ventricle (SLL; Fig. 82–40). If situs inversus is present, the segmental pattern is IDD. Along with the ventricular inversion, there is AV valvular inversion. The two coronary arteries arise from the right and left (posteriorly facing) sinuses, with the right-sided coronary artery giving off the anterior descending and circumflex branches.[268]

Associated Conditions

Rarely, no associated conditions are present and the circulation is normal. In the majority of cases (approximately 75 percent), a VSD is present. It may be in any location, but a perimembranous subpulmonary defect is most common.

The inverted left-sided systemic tricuspid valve frequently shows some degree of abnormality, usually leading to incompetence. The most common abnormality is an Ebstein-like displacement of the

septal and posterior leaflets, but dysplasia, clefts, and straddling of the ventricular septum have also been described.

Pulmonary atresia or stenosis is present in approximately 40 percent of cases, usually associated with a VSD. This obstruction is usually subvalvular, is only rarely valvular, and may characteristically result from attachments of accessory mitral valve tissue.

Clinical Manifestations

Corrected transposition is an uncommon malformation, occurring in slightly fewer than 1 percent of children with congenital heart disease. The importance of this anomaly lies in its frequent association with serious AV conduction disturbances, the intracardiac malformations, and the medical and surgical implications of the ventricular inversion. The clinical picture is determined primarily by the associated anomalies. At least one-third of these patients can be expected to develop complete AV block if followed for a 20-year period.[269]

History A slow, irregular heart rate often is detected in utero, and 10 percent of patients with congenital complete block prove to have corrected transposition. Patients with a large VSD without pulmonary stenosis usually present within the first month or so of life with symptoms indistinguishable from those of infants with a large VSD. Patients with VSD and pulmonary stenosis may present with cyanosis similar to tetralogy of Fallot.

Physical Examination The murmur of left AV valve regurgitation may be best heard either at the apex or at the lower left sternal border. Most of these patients have a murmur of VSD or pulmonary stenosis. Occasionally, an inordinately accentuated second heart sound at the upper left sternal border suggests the presence of PAH, although in reality it represents a loud aortic valve closure resulting from the anterior and superior displacement of the aorta valve.

Chest Roentgenogram A straight or gently curved convex upper left heart border representing the contour of the transposed ascending aorta is characteristic and is most easily recognized in patients with a VSD and pulmonary stenosis.

Electrocardiogram Varying degrees of AV conduction delay are present in almost one-third of these patients. The initial forces of ventricular depolarization are characteristically oriented anteriorly and to the left, with Q waves in the right precordial leads and not in leads I, V_5, and V_6 resulting from depolarization of the septum from the left side (right ventricle) to the right side (left ventricle). With normal or nearly normal pressure in the systemic venous morphologic left ventricle, a QS pattern in the right and an RS pattern in the left precordial leads are usual.

Echocardiogram Using a segmental approach, two-dimensional echocardiography permits identification of the anatomic components and associated defects.[270] The MRI is also diagnostic.

Cardiac Catheterization When diagnostic catheterization is performed, the morphologic left ventricle is entered from the right atrium; in the presence of a VSD, the catheter may cross the defect, traverse the morphologic right ventricle, and enter the ascending aorta in the position normally occupied by the pulmonary artery. Entry into the medially placed pulmonary artery with the use of flow-guided catheters permits successful entry for the measurement of pressure. Selective

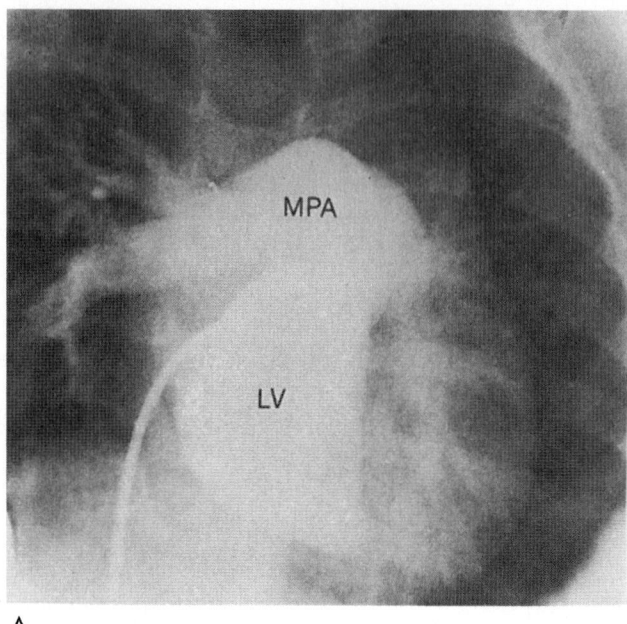
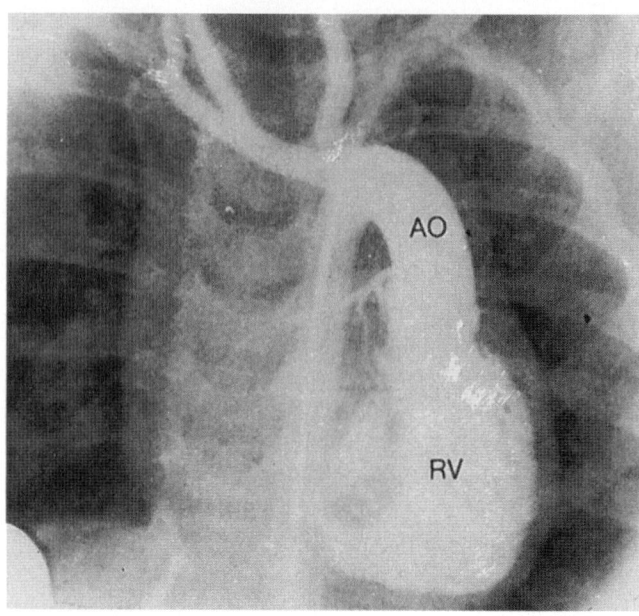

FIGURE 82–40. A. Posteroanterior view of the left ventricular (LV) angiogram in a child with corrected transposition of the great arteries. The main pulmonary artery (MPA) arises from the smooth-walled left ventricle, which receives the systemic venous blood. **B.** Posteroanterior view of the right ventricular angiogram (RV). The ascending aorta (AO) arises to the left of the pulmonary artery from the more heavily trabeculated right ventricle, which receives the pulmonary venous blood. The ventricular septum, seen here perpendicular to the frontal plane, is intact.

angiography in both ventricles will outline the defects. The ventricular septum usually lies in the anteroposterior plane, and frequently a VSD may be imaged best angiographically in the frontal view (see Fig. 82–40). Gentle manipulation of the catheter within the heart is indicated, as the production of varying degrees of transient AV block is not uncommon; in rare instances, the block may prove permanent.

Natural History and Prognosis

The clinical course is determined primarily by the severity of the associated defects. It is estimated that approximately 1 percent of individuals with corrected transposition have an otherwise normal heart. Even with complicating anomalies, survival to adulthood is possible,[271,272] although exercise performance is frequently markedly abnormal.[273] A number of affected females have carried pregnancies to term, but the potential for concurrent cardiac complications suggests the need for care delivery by physicians familiar with the condition.[274] Heart failure associated with a large VSD has been the most common cause of death, with most fatalities occurring within the first year of life. AV conduction abnormalities tend to be progressive, and complete AV block may appear at any age. Similarly, left AV valve regurgitation may present at any age and significantly alters the long-term outcome. Finally, the morphologic right ventricle may not be capable of sustaining adequate cardiac output over a normal life span.[272,276]

Medical Management

Management of corrected transposition includes the treatment of heart failure, cyanosis, and AV block and the prevention of infective endocarditis. Patients with severe pulmonary hypertension or congestive heart failure should undergo early banding of the pulmonary artery or repair of the defect. Patients with a VSD, severe pulmonary stenosis, and cyanosis benefit from systemic-to-pulmonary artery shunting procedures or total correction. Those with congenital block may require prompt pacemaker therapy. Patients with significant left AV valve re-

gurgitation require valve replacement. Regularly scheduled followup examinations are recommended to detect progressive AV conduction disorders and the progression or late appearance of left AV valve incompetence. Antibiotic coverage as protection against infective endocarditis is recommended, as is the introduction of an afterload reduction agent for AV valve regurgitation.[277]

Surgical Management

The conventional approach has been correction of the underlying lesion, closure of an isolated VSD, or closure of the VSD and a conduit from the left (pulmonary) ventricle to the pulmonary artery in those with l-TGA, VSD, and pulmonary stenosis.[278] Unfortunately, this approach has led to suboptimal results because of the high incidence of complete heart block, increasing left AV valve regurgitation, and right systemic ventricular dysfunction and heart failure.[275] Despite recent advances, operative mortality rates for VSD or VSD and pulmonary stenosis or atresia remain in the range of 4 to 15 percent, with postoperative heart block in the range of 14 to 33 percent.[279,280] Actuarial survival among 123 patients operated on at Children's Hospital in Boston from 1963 to 1996 was 84 percent, 75 percent, 68 percent, and 61 percent at 1, 5, 10, and 15 years, respectively.[281] Replacement of the regurgitant left AV valve at the first sign of progressive ventricular dysfunction has been recommended to preserve ventricular function but has been of limited utility.[282]

In view of the suboptimal results with the standard procedures, more innovative approaches have been suggested.[283] The "double-switch" procedure, an arterial switch procedure creating transposition physiology followed by concomitant atrial switch reversing the flow again, is a much more complex operation but has the advantage of using the left ventricle as the systemic ventricle and converting the problematic tricuspid valve to a systemic venous AV valve.

For those with corrected transposition, a VSD, and pulmonary stenosis, the VSD can be closed in a way that diverts the left ventricle into the aorta and the right ventricle via a conduit into the pulmonary artery. Because this also would create transposition physiology, an atrial switch is also performed. Early results are promising, with a 98 percent survival among 40 patients operated on and followed a median of 24 months,[284] an early mortality of 5.6 percent, and a 1- and 9-year actuarial survival of 94 percent and 90 percent, respectively, among 54 patients at another center.[285]

【 】 SINGLE VENTRICLE

Definition

The univentricular heart, or single ventricle, is characterized by the entire flow from the two atria being carried directly through the left and/or right AV valves into the single ventricular chamber. The double-inlet type of AV connection may take the form of either one common or two separate AV valves; straddling of one AV valve sometimes is included. The VA connections may be concordant (pulmonary artery from right ventricle and aorta from left ventricle), discordant (pulmonary artery from left ventricle and aorta from right ventricle), double-outlet (both great arteries from either the left or the right ventricle), or single-outlet (atresia of one great artery). Alternatively, one of the AV valves may be atretic. This is associated with normally related great vessels or transposition of the great arteries.

Pathology

A common type of single ventricle is associated with tricuspid atresia in which the ventricle has the morphology of a left ventricle. There may be normally related great vessels (type I; 65 percent), d-transposition of the great arteries (type II; 30 percent), or l-transposition (type III; 5 percent). Depending on the size of the ventricular communication with the hypoplastic right ventricle, there may be pulmonary atresia (A), pulmonary stenosis (B), or no pulmonary stenosis (C).

In a large series,[286] about two-thirds were type I, and of these about two-thirds had pulmonary stenosis (IB). Among the one-third with transposition, the most common variety is without pulmonary outflow obstruction (IIC). L transposition accounts for less than 5 percent in almost all series of children with tricuspid valve atresia.

When the mitral valve is severely stenotic or atretic, the left ventricle and aorta are usually hypoplastic or atretic (hypoplastic left heart syndrome). In this situation, the right ventricle is the predominant ventricle. Depending on the severity of the left-sided hypoplasia, the ascending aorta and aortic arch are usually hypoplastic as well. When there is one large atrioventricular valve or when both AV valves are present, the valve may straddle the ventricular septum, producing one large ventricle and one small ventricle (Fig. 82–41). The most common situation (65 to 70 percent of cases) is that in which the dominant ventricular chamber has the trabecular pattern of a left ventricle and communicates through an opening, the bulboventricular foramen, with a rudimentary right ventricle.[287] The VA connection is discordant (transposition of the great arteries) in about 90 percent of these patients. In about 20 percent of cases, the dominant ventricle shows the trabecular features of a right ventricle and the rudimentary chamber shows those of a left ventricle. The majority of these patients have a double-outlet VA connection from the main chamber, and a smaller number have a single-outlet connection with pulmonary atresia.[287] In 10 to 14 percent, neither ventricular sinus can be identified; this is the so-called primitive ventricle.

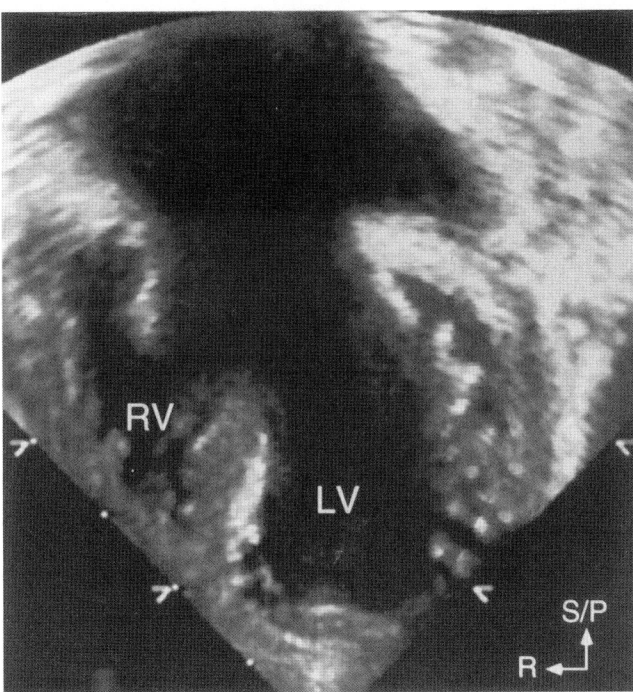

FIGURE 82–41. A malaligned atrioventricular canal with a large left ventricle (LV) and small right ventricle (RV). This would be repaired by a single ventricle approach (Fontan). *Source: From Levine and Geva.[96] Reproduced with permission from the publisher and authors.*

The term *Holmes heart,* which is of historical interest, refers to a double-inlet left ventricle with situs solitus, normally related arteries (SDS), an absent right ventricular sinus, and a subpulmonary infundibular outlet chamber communicating with the left ventricle via a restrictive bulboventricular foramen.[288]

Associated Conditions

Pulmonary stenosis or atresia is common. Subaortic stenosis and coarctation of the aorta occurs in association with l-transposition and may result from a narrow bulboventricular foramen. In patients with tricuspid or mitral atresia, an atrial communication is present.

Clinical Manifestations

This complex and challenging malformation is relatively rare. The clinical picture is determined largely by the associated defects, among which pulmonary stenosis or atresia, which is present in a little more than half of the patients, and obstruction to aortic flow are the most important.

All these patients have some degree of systemic hypoxemia because of mixing of the two sides of the circulation. If pulmonary stenosis or atresia is present, the presenting symptom is usually cyanosis. Without pulmonary stenosis, the presentation is usually heart failure at 2 to 6 weeks of age as the pulmonary resistance falls. For those with subaortic stenosis and/or coarctation of the aorta, failure can occur within the first days of life as the ductus arteriosus closes. Physical examination depends on the combination of lesions present, but systolic ejection murmurs and a single second heart sound are very common.

Chest Roentgenogram Almost all these patients have at least some degree of cardiac enlargement. Those with little or no pulmonary stenosis generally have very large hearts with marked pulmonary plethora. Only patients with very severe pulmonary stenosis or atresia show a nearly normal heart size and diminished pulmonary arterial blood flow.

Electrocardiogram

Evidence of right or left ventricular hypertrophy is common, depending on which ventricle predominates.

Echocardiography

Two-dimensional echocardiography with Doppler color-flow studies can identify the morphologic and functional features of this malformation that are necessary to establish the diagnosis and formulate a plan for clinical management.[289] In complex patients, MRI may be helpful.

Cardiac Catheterization

A degree of systemic arterial oxygen desaturation is present in all these patients, although the severity appears to be related mainly to the volume of pulmonary blood flow. Careful recording of intracardiac and arterial pressures is essential to detect significant or potentially significant obstruction to blood flow across either AV valve, across the atrial septum, or between the ventricle and the aorta or pulmonary artery. The morphologic features of the ventricle, the relation of the aorta and the pulmonary artery, and other features can be established with high-quality selective ventricular angiography, using specially angled views to supplement conventional views.[290]

Natural History and Prognosis

Because by definition only one ventricle is "usable," treatment must be aimed at preserving the anatomy, physiology, and function, allowing this single ventricle to support the circulation and establishing diversion of the systemic venous return directly to the lungs without a second ventricular chamber.

These patients usually present as newborns with cyanosis, congestive failure, or a combination of both. Those in whom pulmonary arterial pressure and blood flow are increased require surgery to prevent death from congestive heart failure or progressive PVOD. Patients with severe pulmonary stenosis or atresia require systemic-to-pulmonary arterial shunting procedures. Among patients with univentricular heart, there is a propensity for the development of subaortic obstruction[291] and AV valve regurgitation.[292] Both threaten ventricular compliance and diminish the likelihood of successful long-term palliation.[293] Survivors are subject to the threats of infective endocarditis, brain abscess, and progressive PVOD.

Medical Management

Early recognition and identification of patients with these complex defects are important so that successful palliative surgical procedures can be carried out for the relief of congestive failure or cyanosis. PGE$_1$ is useful in neonates with ductal-dependent defects.[104] An adequate interatrial communication is essential for those with mitral or tricuspid atresia. For those with pulmonary stenosis or atresia, a Blalock-Taussig shunt can be lifesaving. Ventricular function and AV valvular competence are preserved by early creation of a bidirectional modified Glenn anastomosis (superior vena cava to undivided pulmonary artery).[294] Subaortic stenosis or obstruction at the bulboventricular foramen can be bypassed by anastomosis of the proximal pulmonary artery to the lateral aspect of the ascending aorta while pulmonary blood flow is delivered to the distal pulmonary arterial tree through a systemic arterial or systemic venous shunt.[295,296] Digitalis and diuretics may be necessary for patients with continuing heart failure. Care should be taken

that anemia or severe polycythemia does not develop and that these patients are protected adequately against infective endocarditis. The pulmonary vascular bed must be protected and ventricular function and compliance carefully preserved if more definitive procedures are to be considered.

Surgical Management

Medical management without surgical treatment gives dismal results with only 42 percent of children surviving to 1 year of age.[3] Long-term palliation of children with a single ventricle is usually a three-stage approach: (1) initial palliation in the perinatal period, (2) a bidirectional Glenn at 6 to 18 months of age, and (3) a modified Fontan at 1 to 3 years of age. For complex problems, a heart transplant soon after birth has been suggested.[297]

Initial palliation for patients with univentricular AV connections requires adjustment of pulmonary blood flow with a pulmonary arterial band when it is excessive or the creation of a shunt when it is diminished. The modified Blalock-Taussig shunt is preferred in neonates. Relief of aortic stenosis and the creation of an adequate atrial communication are frequently necessary as well. The prognosis is affected adversely by a single ventricle of the right ventricular type,[298] the evolution of AV valvular regurgitation,[292] or subaortic obstruction.[299]

Ventricular function and AV valvular competence are preserved by early creation of a bidirectional modified Glenn anastomosis, in which the superior vena cava is divided with the caudad portion patched closed; the cephalad portion is sutured to the top of the right pulmonary artery. If pulmonary atresia is not present, the main pulmonary artery is closed.[300] Subaortic stenosis or obstruction at the bulboventricular foramen can be palliated by anastomosis of the proximal pulmonary artery to the lateral aspect of the ascending aorta, while pulmonary blood flow is delivered to the distal pulmonary arterial tree through a systemic arterial or systemic venous shunt (the Damus-Kaye-Stansel operation). Other surgical options for the relief of subaortic obstruction are direct enlargement of the bulboventricular foramen (VSD), the modified Norwood operation,[296] and the arterial switch operation.[295] Initially some types of single ventricle were repaired by dividing the common chamber into the right and left ventricles. This approach has largely been abandoned because of unacceptably high initial mortality resulting from problems in connecting the ventricles to the appropriate great vessels without interfering with the atrioventricular valves and the high incidence of complete heart block. The current approach is a modification of the principle suggested by Fontan and Baudet[301]—to bypass the right side of the heart, directing systemic venous blood directly to the pulmonary arteries, and allowing the single functioning ventricular chamber to pump blood to the systemic circulation. First, if it has not been done already, a bidirectional Glenn anastomosis is constructed (see above), and then an intraatrial tunnel is constructed to divert the inferior vena caval blood to the caudad portion of the superior vena cava, which then is connected to the underside of the right pulmonary artery (Figs. 82–42 and 82–43). A fenestration in the baffle is sometimes used to decompress the right side in the perioperative period. Recently, instead of tunneling within the atrium, an external conduit has been used between the inferior vena cava and the right pulmonary artery ligating the inferior vena cava–right atrial junction. The single ventricle is thus relieved of the burden of the volume overload and

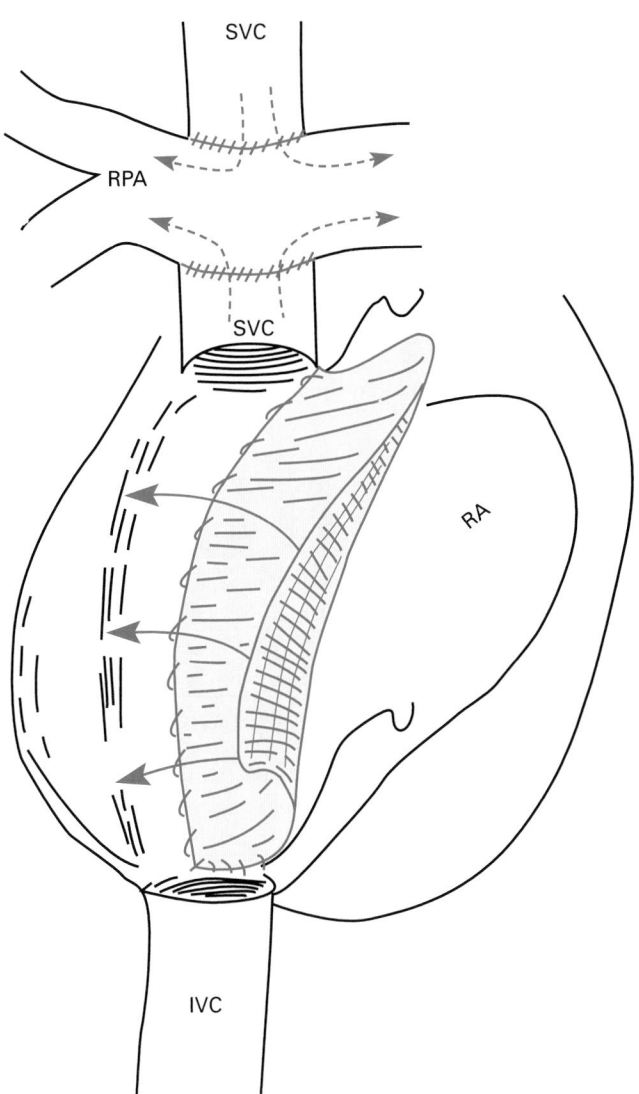

FIGURE 82-42. The modified Fontan operation. The superior vena cava (SVC) is divided. The cephalad portion is anastomosed to the superior aspect of the right pulmonary artery (RPA), and an intraatrial baffle is constructed from the inferior vena cava (IVC) to the superior vena cava along the lateral wall of the right atrium (RA). The caudad portion of the SVC then is connected to the inferior aspect of the right pulmonary artery.

ventricular hypertrophy required to maintain the pulmonary circulation and is asked only to deliver systemic cardiac output.[301]

The surgical risks depend on patient selection. For those with complex forms of single ventricle and patients with elevated pulmonary pressure or resistance, ventricular dysfunction, or atrioventricular valve regurgitation, the risks are increased. For those without risk factors and with tricuspid atresia or double-inlet left ventricle, the risks are less than 5 percent.[302] Even for those with some risk factors or with more complex disease, the mortality at some centers is less than 10 percent.[302,303]

For children with hypoplastic left heart syndrome, the survival from the three-stage procedure (initial Norwood, bidirectional Glenn, and Fontan) during the 1980s and early 1990s is approximately 50 percent.[304] Our data from 1995 to 2002 was better, with a survival of approximately 75 percent,[305] similar to other centers which report a survival rate as high as 76 percent.[284] Birth weight less than 2.5 kg (5.5 lb) and the presence of cardiac or noncardiac anomalies are risk factors associated with early mortality.[306] There does not

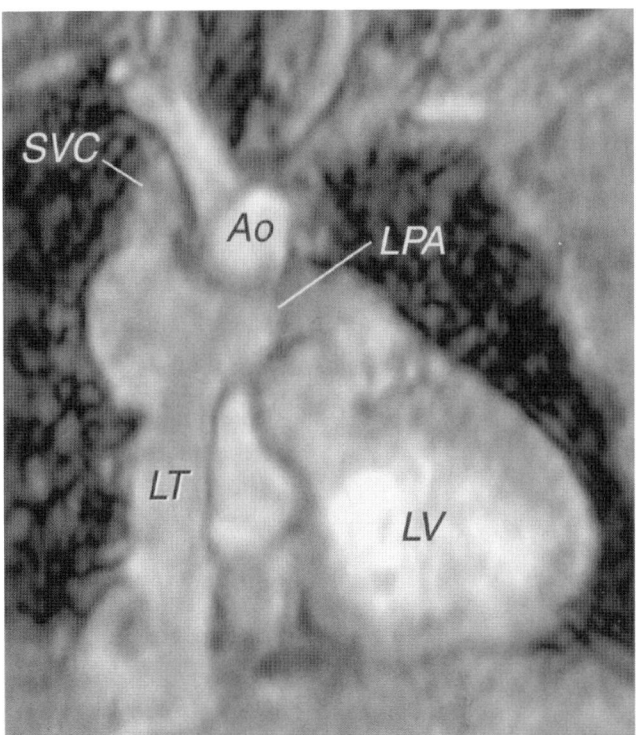

FIGURE 82-43. Cine MRI in a patient with a lateral tunnel (LT) and total cavopulmonary anastomosis. Ao, aorta; LPA, left pulmonary artery; LV, left ventricle; SVC, superior vena cava. *Source: From Geva T, Sahn DJ, Powell AC. Magnetic resonance imaging of congenital heart disease in adults. Prog Pediatr Cardiol 2003;17:21–39. Reproduced with permission of the authors and publisher.*

seem to be any significant difference in survival in centers that use the three-stage anatomic "repair" from primary heart transplantation in the perinatal period at 36 months of age.[304]

Quality and length of life are clearly improved, but persistent problems (AV valvular regurgitation, systemic embolization, limitation of exercise tolerance, protein-losing enteropathy, atrial arrhythmias, and deterioration of ventricular function) occur with a frequency of approximately 1 percent per year.[302] For patients with progressive deterioration, cardiac transplantation is recommended.

CONGENITAL ABNORMALITIES OF THE CORONARY ARTERIAL CIRCULATION

【 】 CORONARY ARTERIOVENOUS FISTULA

Pathology

A coronary arteriovenous fistula is a fistulous communication between a coronary artery and a cardiac chamber, the coronary sinus, or the pulmonary trunk (Fig. 82-44). The site of origin may involve any of the epicardial coronary arteries. *The right coronary artery is the site of origin in somewhat over half the cases, and the two most common sites into which the fistula feeds are a pulmonary artery and the right ventricle.* Although solitary communication is the rule, there may be multiple sites of termination. The artery or arteries feeding the fistula are grossly enlarged and tortuous. Saccular aneurysms may develop in segments of dilated vessels; such aneurysms usually are observed in adults and frequently show calcification of the wall.

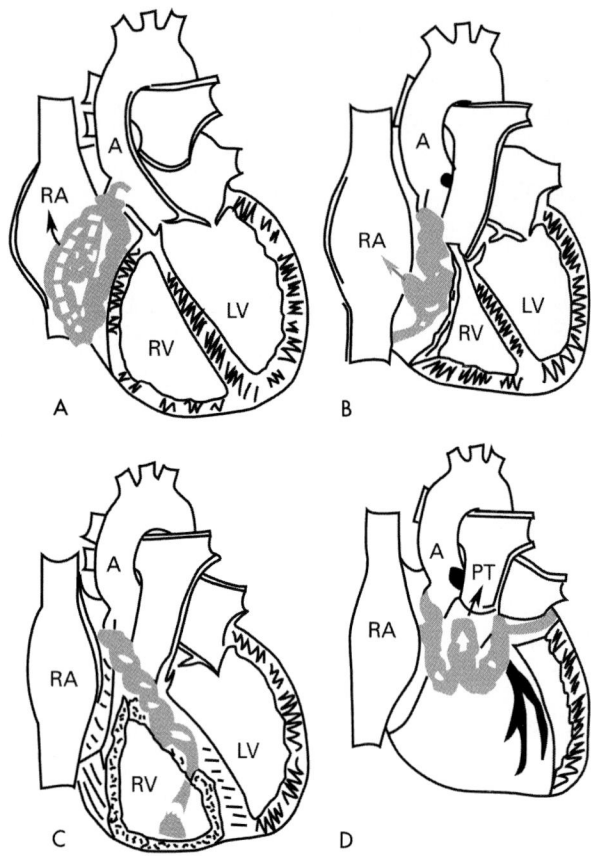

FIGURE 82–44. Anomalous communications of coronary arteries. **A.** Right coronary artery communicates with coronary sinus. **B.** Right coronary artery communicates with right atrium (RA). **C.** Anomalous communication of right coronary artery with right ventricle (RV). **D.** Two coronary arteries arise from the aorta (A) and make collateral communication with accessory coronary artery arising from pulmonary trunk (PT). LV, left ventricle.

Clinical Manifestations

Many patients with a coronary arteriovenous fistula are asymptomatic.[307,308] With increasing use of echocardiography tiny fistulous connections may be seen as an incidental finding. A conservative approach to these tiny connections is indicated as up to one-quarter of them may close spontaneously.[309] In some, the magnitude of the shunt into the right side of the heart is great enough to cause congestive heart failure, with a tendency for this to occur in early infancy or after 40 years of age. The classic finding is that of a continuous murmur with an unusual location, as it is loudest over the fistula. It may have a louder diastolic component, especially if communication is with the right ventricle. In those with large shunts, there may be cardiomegaly and increased pulmonary flow shown by chest roentgenography and right ventricular hypertrophy shown by ECG. Transthoracic echocardiography is usually diagnostic in children[310]; transesophageal studies may be necessary in adults. At cardiac catheterization, an increase in oxygen saturation may be encountered, usually in the right atrium or right ventricle, if the shunt is large enough. Selective coronary arteriography will demonstrate the involved coronary artery and the site of entry of the fistula. The most common complication is infective endocarditis, but thrombosis, myocardial ischemia, and rupture may occur.

Management

Except for very small fistulas, closure is recommended, because the flow tends to increase with age and these patients are at risk for infective endocarditis, congestive heart failure, and myocardial ischemia. Until relatively recently, closure was invariably surgical. Occasionally, closure was done without a coronary bypass by placing obliterating mattress sutures across the fistula beneath the coronary artery as it passes over the surface of the heart.[311] More commonly, cardiopulmonary bypass is preferred for safe exposure of large or multiple fistulas, such as those entering the right atrium near the junction of the superior vena cava and the right atrium, those arising from the artery to the sinoatrial node, and those between the left coronary artery and the left ventricle.[312] The orifice of the fistula is obliterated by direct suture or the placement of a Dacron or pericardial patch. Fistulas have been closed from within the open coronary artery; the artery is then repaired by direct suturing. Surgical mortality should be minimal[312]; the long-term results have been favorable.[313]

Fistulas have been closed by interventional catheterization techniques. Armsby and associates[314] attempted to close fistulas in 33 patients (35 procedures); Gianturco coils were used in 28 procedures, a double-umbrella was used in 6 procedures, and a Grifka vascular closure device was used in 1 procedure. Twenty-seven fistulas were completely occluded. In six patients with multiple fistulas, no attempt at closure was made in the catheterization laboratory and the patients were referred for surgery. This "noninvasive" technique seems to be applicable to some children and adults with coronary AV fistulas, although long-term followup is necessary to be certain that the fistulas do not recur.

[ ] ORIGIN OF THE LEFT CORONARY ARTERY FROM THE PULMONARY ARTERY

Pathology and Pathophysiology

In this anomaly, the left coronary artery arises from the pulmonary artery rather than from the aorta (Fig. 82–45). In the perinatal period, the pulmonary artery pressure is high and the left coronary is perfused with venous blood. Problems arise when the pulmonary resistance and pulmonary artery pressure fall and the diastolic pressure is insufficient to perfuse the left ventricular myocardium. In the absence of collateral vessels from the right coronary, left ventricular ischemia and, eventually, infarction of the left ventricular wall and papillary muscles occur. This, in turn, leads to congestive heart failure, usually by 3 to 8 weeks of age.

In a small group of children, extensive collaterals between the right coronary (arising normally from the aorta) and the left system develop. Perfusion via the right may be sufficient to oxygenate the left ventricular myocardium so that no ischemia develops. Over time, the higher perfusion pressure in the aorta may allow a left-to-right shunt into the pulmonary artery through the right and then the left coronary system. Eventually this may lead to a "steal" of blood from the myocardium into the lower-resistance pulmonary circuit.

Clinical Manifestations

The clinical spectrum and mode of presentation in patients with this abnormality vary.[307,308,315,316] The majority of patients present at 6 to 12 weeks of age. Acute episodes of irritability, profuse cold sweating, pallor (possibly due to angina), and respiratory distress occur, with evidence of heart failure. Less often, these patients present at an older age with mitral regurgitation and heart failure. A few reach adolescence or adulthood with no or relatively few symptoms other than occasional exertional angina or palpitations. Sudden death may be the first and only sign of this condition.

On physical examination, the heart is enlarged, with an abnormal left ventricular apex impulse. Other signs of failure are usually present. Pallor and clammy skin are common. In some patients, a soft, continuous murmur is heard at the upper left sternal border. This murmur is more prominent in older patients, presumably because of the development of a more extensive collateral circulation. The murmur of mitral regurgitation may be heard at the apex, radiating to the axilla; however, in young infants with heart failure, there can be a surprising degree of regurgitation without a distinctive murmur.

In patients with heart failure, the chest roentgenogram typically shows marked enlargement of the heart with posterior displacement of the esophagus by a large left atrium. There is pulmonary edema, and there may be atelectasis of the left lower lobe because of bronchial compression. Those with good collaterals and no left ventricular failure may have a normal radiograph.

In the infant group, the ECG demonstrates the pattern of anterolateral infarction, with deep Q wave in leads I and aV$_L$, and abnormal R-wave progression across the precordium. Arrhythmias are common. The echocardiogram shows marked enlargement of the left atrium and ventricle with little or no left ventricular wall motion. The origin of the coronary artery can be imaged, and flow can be seen toward the pulmonary artery instead of toward the heart.[317] Myocardial perfusion imaging with thallium-201[318] and, more recently, MRI can help distinguish an infarcted myocardium from myocardium "at risk." At cardiac catheterization, there may be an increase in saturation in the pulmonary artery if there is enough retrograde flow. There is usually some pulmonary hypertension, with very elevated pulmonary wedge pressure. Aortography or selective right coronary arteriography demonstrates the collateral circulation filling the left coronary artery retrograde, with at least faint opacification of the main pulmonary artery.

Management

The natural history and prognosis are related by the modes of presentation. Those who present in infancy die without surgical intervention. Medical management is aimed at control of congestive heart failure and arrhythmias before a surgical procedure.

Four approaches have been used for surgical repair. The first approach, which is of historical interest only, is ligation of the left coronary artery to eliminate the coronary artery-to-pulmonary artery shunt that acts as a coronary artery steal. Many children benefited from this procedure, but there continued to be myocardial ischemia, and late sudden death was not eliminated. The second approach was to tunnel the coronary artery inside the pulmonary artery to the wall of the aorta and create an aortopulmonary window.[319] This usually required an external roofing of the pulmonary artery to allow egress of flow from the right ventricle. Although this surgical approach has the advantage of making a two-coronary system, a high proportion of children developed supravalvular pulmonary stenosis at the site of the intrapulmonary artery tunnel.

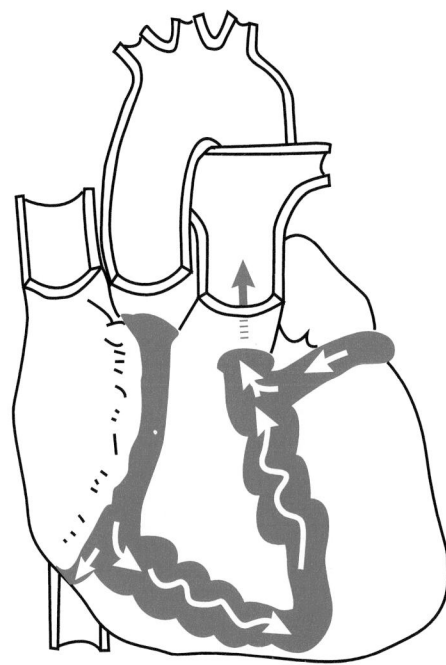

FIGURE 82–45. Anomalous origin of the left coronary artery from the pulmonary trunk. With time, wide collaterals develop between the two coronary systems so that right coronary arterial blood is shunted into the left coronary system and then into the pulmonary trunk.

This procedure is now rarely used. More recently, as coronary artery reimplantation has become more common in the arterial switch operation for transposition of the great arteries, surgeons have removed the anomalous coronary artery with a button of pulmonary artery and reimplanted it onto the aorta.[320] Finally, in a few older patients, saphenous vein grafting or internal mammary artery implantation has been used.[321]

The late results after surgery have been quite good.[320,322] The congestive heart failure frequently improves, the heart becomes smaller, the left ventricular shortening fraction improves, and mitral regurgitation tends to regress. Interestingly, the infarction pattern on ECG with deep anterolateral Q waves frequently disappears, suggesting that the poor function is due to extreme ischemia rather than infarction (hibernating myocardium).[323]

REFERENCES

1. Mitchell SC, Korones SB, Berendes HW. Congenital heart disease in 56,109 births. Incidence and natural history. *Circulation* 1971;43:323.
2. Hoffman JI, Christianson R. Congenital heart disease in a cohort of 19,502 births with long-term follow-up. *Am J Cardiol* 1978; 42:641.
3. Fyler DC. Report of the New England Regional Infant Cardiac Program. *Pediatrics* 1980 65:375.
4. Perry LW, Neill CA, Ferencz C, et al. Infants with congenital heart disease: The cases. In: Ferencz C, Rubin JD, Loffredo CA, Magee CA, eds. *Epidemiology of Congenital Heart Disease: The Baltimore-Washington Infant Study 1981–1989.* Mount Kisco, NY: Futura; 1993: 33–61.
5. Fyler DC. *Nadas' Pediatric Cardiology.* Philadelphia: Hanley & Belfus; 1992.
6. Keith JD. Prevalence, incidence and epidemiology. In: Keith JD, Rowe RD, Vlad P, eds. *Heart Disease in Infancy and Childhood,* 3d ed. New York: Macmillan; 1978:3.
7. Nora JJ. Causes of congenital heart diseases: Old and new modes, mechanisms, and models. *Am Heart J* 1993;125:1409.
8. Belmont JW. Recent progress in the molecular genetics of congenital heart defects. *Clin Genet* 1998;54:11.
9. Hall JG. Catch 22. *J Med Genet* 1993;30:801.

10. Dawes GS. *Foetal and Neonatal Physiology: A Comparative Study of the Changes at Birth.* Chicago: Year Book; 1968.

11. Lind J, Wegelius C. Human fetal circulation: Changes in the cardiovascular system at birth and disturbances in the postnatal closure of the foramen ovale and ductus arteriosus. *Cold Spring Harb Symp Quant Biol* 1954;19:109.

12. Rudolph AM, Heymann MA. The circulation of the fetus in utero. Methods for studying distribution of blood flow, cardiac output and organ blood flow. *Circ Res* 1967;21:163.

13. Rudolph AM, Heymann MA. Circulatory changes during growth in the fetal lamb. *Circ Res* 1970;26:289.

14. Rudolph AM, Heymann MA. Cardiac output in the fetal lamb: The effects of spontaneous and induced changes of heart rate on right and left ventricular output. *Am J Obstet Gynecol* 1976;124:183.

15. Teitel DF, Iwamoto HS, Rudolph AM. Effects of birth-related events on central blood flow patterns. *Pediatr Res* 1987;22:557.

16. Coceani F, Olley PM. Role of prostaglandins, prostacyclin, and thromboxanes in the control of prenatal patency and postnatal closure of the ductus arteriosus. In: Heymann MA, ed. *Prostaglandins in the Perinatal Period.* New York: Grune & Stratton; 1980:109.

17. Rudolph AM. Fetal and neonatal pulmonary circulation. *Annu Rev Physiol* 1979;41:383.

18. Fineman JR, Soifer SJ, Heymann MA. Regulation of pulmonary vascular tone in the perinatal period. *Annu Rev Physiol* 1995;57:115.

19. Heymann MA, Rudolph AM. Effects of congenital heart disease on fetal and neonatal circulations. *Prog Cardiovasc Dis* 1972;15:115.

20. Levin DL, Heymann MA, Kitterman JA, et al. Persistent pulmonary hypertension of the newborn infant. *J Pediatr* 1976;89:626.

21. Fox WW, Duara S. Persistent pulmonary hypertension in the neonate: Diagnosis and management. *J Pediatr* 1983;103:505.

22. Kinsella JP, Abman SH. Recent developments in inhaled nitric oxide therapy of the newborn. *Curr Opin Pediatr* 1999;11:121.

23. UK collaborative randomised trial of neonatal extracorporeal membrane oxygenation. UK Collaborative ECMO Trail Group. *Lancet* 1996;348:75.

24. Talner NS. Heart failure. In: Emmanouilides GC, Riemenschneider TA, Gutgesell HP, eds. *Moss and Adams Heart Disease in Infants, Children and Adolescents,* 5th ed. Baltimore: Williams & Wilkins;1995:1746.

25. Seguchi M, Nakazawa M, Momma K. Effect of enalapril on infants and children with congestive heart failure. *Cardiol Young* 1992;2:14–19.

26. Fischbein CA, Rosenthal A, Fischer EG, et al. Risk factors of brain abscess in patients with congenital heart disease. *Am J Cardiol* 1974;34: 97.

27. Phornphutkul C, Rosenthal A, Nadas AS, Berenberg W. Cerebrovascular accidents in infants and children with cyanotic congenital heart disease. *Am J Cardiol* 1973;32:329.

28. Beekman RH, Tuuri DT. Acute hemodynamic effects of increasing hemoglobin concentration in children with a right to left ventricular shunt and relative anemia. *J Am Coll Cardiol* 1985;5:357.

29. Gidding SS, Stockman JA III. Effect of iron deficiency on tissue oxygen delivery in cyanotic congenital heart disease. *Am J Cardiol* 1988;61:605.

30. Ross EA, Perloff JK, Danovitch GM, et al. Renal function and urate metabolism in late survivors with cyanotic congenital heart disease. *Circulation* 1986;73:396.

31. Henriksson P, Varendh G, Lundstrom NR. Haemostatic defects in cyanotic congenital heart disease. *Br Heart J* 1979;41:23.

32. Waldman JD, Czapek EE, Paul MH, et al. Shortened platelet survival in cyanotic heart disease. *J Pediatr* 1975;87:77.

33. Territo MC, Rosove MH, Perloff JK. Cyanotic congenital heart disease: Hematologic management, renal function, and urate metabolism. In: Perloff JK, Child JS, eds. *Congenital Heart Disease in Adults.* Philadelphia: Saunders; 1991:93.

34. Aram DM, Ekelman BL, Ben Shachar G, Levinsohn MW. Intelligence and hypoxemia in children with congenital heart disease: Fact or artifact? *J Am Coll Cardiol* 1985;6:889.

35. Cameron JW, Rosenthal A, Olson AD. Malnutrition in hospitalized children with congenital heart disease. *Arch Pediatr Adolesc Med* 1995;149:1098.

36. Schuurmans FM, Pulles-Heintzberger CF, Gerver WJ, et al. Long-term growth of children with congenital heart disease: A retrospective study. *Acta Paediatr* 1998;87:1250.

37. Rabinovitch M. Pathophysiology of pulmonary hypertension. In: Emmanouilides GC, Riemensschneider TA, Allen HD, Gutgesell HP, eds. *Moss and Adams Heart Disease in Infants, Children, and Adolescents,* 5th ed. Baltimore: Williams & Wilkins, 1995:1659.

38. Heath D, Edwards JE. The pathology of hypertensive pulmonary vascular disease: A description of six grades of structural changes in the pulmonary arteries with special reference to congenital cardiac septal defects. *Circulation* 1958;18:533.

39. Turanlahti MI, Laitinen PO, Sarna SJ, Pesonen E. Nitric oxide, oxygen, and prostacyclin in children with pulmonary hypertension. *Heart* 1998;79:169.

40. Nihill MR. Clinical management of patients with pulmonary hypertension. In: Emmanouilides GC, Riemenschneider TA, Allen HD, Gutgesell HP, eds. *Moss and Adams Heart Disease in Infants, Children and Adolescents,* 5th ed. Baltimore: Williams & Wilkins; 1995:1695.

41. Gersony WM. Long-term follow-up of operated congenital heart disease. *Cardiol Clin* 1989;7:915.

42. Freed MD. Infective endocarditis in the adult with congenital heart disease. *Cardiol Clin* 1993;11:589.

43. Morris CD, Reller MD, Manasse VD. Thirty-year incidence of infective endocarditis after surgery for congenital heart defect. *JAMA* 1998;279:599.

44. Keane JF, Driscoll DJ, Gersony WM. Second natural history study of congenital heart defects: Results of treatment of patients with aortic valvular stenosis. *Circulation* 1993;87:I16–I27.

45. McEllhinney DB, Lock JE, Keane JF et al. Left heart growth, function, and reintervention after balloon aortic valvuloplasty for neonatal aortic stenosis. *Circulation* 2005;111:451.

46. Hart EM, Garson A Jr. Psychosocial concerns of adults with congenital heart disease. Employability and insurability. *Cardiol Clin* 1993;11: 711.

47. Schmaltz AA, Neudorf U, Winkler UH. Outcome of pregnancy in women with congenital heart disease. *Cardiol Young* 1999;9:88.

48. Strong WB. Introduction: Pediatric cardiology exercise testing. *Pediatr Cardiol* 1999;20:1.

49. Chandar JS, Wolff GS, Garson A Jr, et al. Ventricular arrhythmias in postoperative tetralogy of Fallot. *Am J Cardiol* 1990;65:655.

50. Gelatt M, Hamilton RM, McCrindle BW, et al. Arrhythmia and mortality after the Mustard procedure: A 30-year single-center experience. *J Am Coll Cardiol* 1997;29:194.

51. Khairy P, Landzberg MJ, Gatzoulis MA et al. Value of programmed electrical stimulation after repair of tetralogy of Fallot: a multicenter study. *Circulation* 2004;109:1994.

52. Fishberger SB, Wernovsky G, Gentiles TL, et al. Factors that influence the development of atrial flutter after the Fontan operation. *J Thorac Cardiovasc Surg* 1997;113:80.

53. Moreau GA, Graham TP Jr. Clinical assessment of ventricular function after surgical treatment of congenital heart defects. *Cardiol Clin* 1989;7:439.

54.. Turina MI, Siebenmann R, von Segesser L, et al. Late functional deterioration after atrial correction for transposition of the great arteries. *Circulation* 1989;80:I1162–I1167.

55. Mertens L, Hagler DJ, Sauer U, et al. Protein-losing enteropathy after the Fontan operation: An international multicenter study. PLE study group. *J Thorac Cardiovasc Surg* 1998;115:1063.

56. Graham TP, Gutgesell HP. Ventricular septal defects. In: Emmanouilides GC, Riemenschneider TA, Allen HD, Gutgesell HP, eds. *Moss and Adams Heart Disease in Infants, Children, and Adolescents,* 5th ed. Baltimore: Williams & Wilkins; 1995:724.

57. Van den Bosch, Ten Harkel DJ, McGhie JS. Feasibility and accuracy of real-time 3-dimensional echocardiographic assessment of ventricular septal defects. *J Am Soc Echocardiog* 2006;19:7.

58. Alpert BS, Cook DH, Varghese PJ et al. Spontaneous closure of small ventricular septal defects: Ten-year follow-up. *Pediatrics* 1979;63:204.

59. Trowitzsch E, Braun W, Stute M et al.. Diagnosis, therapy, and outcome of ventricular septal defects in the 1st year of life: A two-dimensional colour-Doppler echocardiography study. *Eur J Pediatr* 1990;149:758.

60. Weidman WH, Blount SG Jr, DuShane JW, et al. Clinical course in ventricular septal defect. *Circulation* 1977;56:156.

61. Rhodes LA, Keane JF, Keane JP, et al. Long follow-up (to 43 years) of ventricular septal defect with audible aortic regurgitation. *Am J Cardiol* 1990;66:340.

62. Gersony WM, Hayes CJ. Bacterial endocarditis in patients with pulmonary stenosis, aortic stenosis, or ventricular septal defect. *Circulation* 1977;56:I84.

63. Gersony WM, Hayes CJ, Driscoll DJ, et al. Bacterial endocarditis in patients with aortic stenosis, pulmonary stenosis, or ventricular septal defect. *Circulation* 1993;87:I121.

64. Cantor WJ, Harrison DA, Moussadji JS, et al. Determinants of survival and length of survival in adults with Eisenmenger syndrome. *Am J Cardiol* 1999;84:677.

65. Driscoll DJ, Michels VV, Gersony WM, et al. Occurrence risk for congenital heart defects in relatives of patients with aortic stenosis, pulmonary stenosis, or ventricular septal defect. *Circulation* 1993;87:I114.

66. Castaneda AR, Jonas RA, Mayer JE, Hanley FL. *Cardiac Surgery of the Neonate and Infant.* Philadelphia: Saunders; 1994.

67. Moller JH, Patton C, Varco RL, Lillehei CW. Late results (30 to 35 years) after operative closure of isolated ventricular septal defect from 1954 to 1960. *Am J Cardiol* 1991;68:1491.

68. Stellin G, Padalino M, Milanesi O, et al. Surgical closure of apical ventricular septal defects through a right ventricular apical infundibulotomy. *Ann Thorac Surg* 2000;69:597–601.

69. Myhre U, Duncan BW, MeeRB et al. Apical right ventriculotomy for closure of apical ventricular septal defects. *Ann Thorac Surg* 2004; 78:204-208.

70. Knauth AL, Lock JE, Perry SB et al. Transcatheter device closure of congenital and postoperative residual ventricular septal defects. *Circulation* 2004;110:501.

71. Fu YC, Bass J, Amin Z et al. Transcatheter closure of perimembranous ventricular spetal defects using the new Amplatzer membranous VSD occluder: results of the U.S. phase I trial. *J Am Coll Cardiol* 2006;47: 319.

72. Bacha EA, Cao QL, Galantowicz ME et al. Multicenter experience with perventricular device closure of muscular ventricular septal defects. *Pediatr Cardiol* 2005; 26:169-175.

73. Lewis FJ, Winchell P, Bashour FA. Open repair of atrial septal defects: Results in sixty-three patients. *JAMA* 1957;165:922.

74. Edwards JE. Classification of congenital heart disease in the adult. In: Roberts WC, ed. *Congenital Heart Disease in Adults*. Philadelphia: Davis; 1979:1.

75. Mahoney LT, Truesdell SC, Krzmarzick TR, Lauer RM. Atrial septal defects that present in infancy. *Am J Dis Child* 1986;140:1115–1118.

76. Benson DW, Sharkey A, Fatkin D, et al. Reduced penetrance, variable expressivity, and genetic heterogeneity of familial atrial septal defects. *Circulation* 1998;97:2043.

77. Murphy JG, Gersh BJ, McGoon MD, et al. Long-term outcome after surgical repair of isolated atrial septal defect. Follow-up at 27 to 32 years. *N Engl J Med* 1990;323:1645.

78. Seward JB, Tajik AJ. Transesophageal echocardiography in congenital heart disease. *Am J Card Imaging* 1990;4:215.

79. Dall'Agata A, McGhie J, Taams MA, et al. Secundum atrial septal defect is a dynamic three-dimensional entity. *Am Heart J* 1999;137:1075.

80. Acar P, Dulac Y, Roux D, et al. Comparison of transthoracic and transesophageal three-dimensional echocardiography for assessment of atrial septal defect diameter in children. *Am J Cardiol* 2003;91:500.

81. Hamilton WT, Hattajee CE, Dalen JE, et al. Atrial septal defect secundum: Clinical profile with physiologic correlates. In: Roberts WC, ed. *Adult Congenital Heart Disease*. Philadelphia: Davis; 1987:395.

82. Steele PM, Fuster V, Cohen M, et al. Isolated atrial septal defect with pulmonary vascular obstructive disease—Long-term follow-up and prediction of outcome after surgical correction. *Circulation* 1987;76: 1037.

83. Prieto LR, Foreman CK, Cheatham JP, Latson LA. Intermediate-term outcome of transcatheter secundum atrial septal defect closure using the Bard Clamshell Septal Umbrella. *Am J Cardiol* 1996;78:1310.

84. Masura J, Lange PE, Wilkinson JL, et al. US/International multicenter trial of atrial septal catheter closure using the Amplatzer Septal Occluder: Initial results (abstr). *Am J Cardiol* 1998;131:57A.

85. Zamora R, Rao PS, Lloyd TR, et al. Intermediate-term results of phase I Food and Drug Administration trials of buttoned device occlusion of secundum atrial septal defects. *J Am Coll Cardiol* 1998;31:674.

86. Omeish A, Hijazi ZM. Transcatheter closure of atrial septal defects in children & adults using the Amplatzer Septal Occluder. *J Intervent Cardiol* 2001;14:37.

87. Brochu MC, Baril JF, Dore A et al. Improvement in exercise capacity in asymptomatic and mildly asymptomatic adults after atrial septal defect percutaneous closure. *Circulation* 2002;106:1821.

88. St.John Sutton MG, Tajik AJ, McGoon DC. Atrial septal defect in patients ages 60 years or older: Operative results and long-term postoperative follow-up. *Circulation* 1981;64:402.

89. Healy JE Jr. An anatomic survey of anomalous pulmonary veins: Their clinical significance. *J Thorac Cardiovasc Surg* 1952;23:433.

90. Silverman NH. Anomalous pulmonary venous connections. In: Silverman NH, ed. *Pediatric Echocardiography*. New York: Williams & Wilkins; 1993:179.

91. Saalouke MG, Shapiro SR, Perry LW et al.. Isolated partial anomalous pulmonary venous drainage associated with pulmonary vascular obstructive disease. *Am J Cardiol* 1977;39:439.

92. Rogers HM, Edwards JE. Incomplete division of the atrioventricular canal with patent interatrial foramen primum (persistent common cardioventricular ostium): Report of five cases and review of the literature. *Am Heart J* 1948;36:28.

93. Rastelli GC, Ongley PA, Kirklin JW et al. Surgical repair of the complete form of persistent common atrioventricular canal. *J Thorac Cardiovasc Surg* 1968;55:299.

94. Rose V, Izukawa T, Moes CA. Syndromes of asplenia and polysplenia. A review of cardiac and non-cardiac malformations in 60 cases withspecial reference to diagnosis and prognosis. *Br Heart J* 1975;37:840.

95. Lacro RV. Dysmorphology. In: Fyler DC, ed. *Nadas' Pediatric Cardiology*. Philadelphia: Hanley & Belfus; 1992:37.

96. Levine J, Geva T. Echocardiographic assessment of common atrioventricular canal. *Prog Pediatr Cardiol* 1999;10:137.

97. Nora JJ, Nora AH. Maternal transmission of congenital heart diseases: New recurrence risk figures and the questions of cytoplasmic inheritance and vulnerability to teratogens. *Am J Cardiol* 1987;59:459.

98. Stellin G, Vida VL, Milanesi O et al. Surgical treatment of complete A-V canal defects in children before 3 months of age. *Eur J Cardiothorac Surg* 2003;23:187.

99. Kirklin JW. Atrioventricular canal defect. In: Kirklin JW, Barratt-Boyes BG, eds. *Cardiac Surgery*, 2d ed. New York: Churchill Livingstone, 1993:693.

100. Hanley FL, Fenton KN, Jonas RA, et al. Surgical repair of complete atrioventricular canal defects in infancy. Twenty-year trends. *J Thorac Cardiovasc Surg* 1993;106:387.

101. Alexi-Meskishvili V, Ishino K, Dahnert I, et al. Correction of complete atrioventricular septal defects with the double-patch technique and cleft closure. *Ann Thorac Surg* 1996;62:519.

102. Daebritz S, del Nido PJ. Surgical management of common atriventricular canal. *Prog Pediatr Cardiol* 1999;10:161.

103. Clyman RI. Ibuprofen and patent ductus arteriosus. *N Engl J Med* 2000;343:728.

104. Freed MD, Heymann MA, Lewis AB, et al. Prostaglandin E1 infants with ductus arteriosus-dependent congenital heart disease. *Circulation* 1981;64:899.

105. Gersony WM, Peckham GJ, Ellison RC, et al. Effects of indomethacin in premature infants with patent ductus arteriosus: Results of a national collaborative study. *J Pediatr* 1983;102:895.

106. Siassi B, Blanco C, Cabal LA et al. Incidence and clinical features of patent ductus arteriosus in low-birthweight infants: A prospective analysis of 150 consecutively born infants. *Pediatrics* 1976;57:347.

107. Varvarigou A, Bardin CL, Beharry K, et al. Early ibuprofen administration to prevent patent ductus arteriosus in premature newborn infants. *JAMA* 1996;275:539.

108. Narayanan M, Cooper B, Weiss H et al. Prophylactic indomethacin: Factors determining permanent ductus arteriosus closure. *J Pediatr* 2000;136:330.

109. Ohlsson A, Walia R, Shah S. Ibuprofen for the treatement of patent ductus arteriosus in preterm and/or low birth weight infants. Cochrane Database Syst Rev. 4:CD003481, 2005.

110. Satur CR, Walker DR, Dickinson DF. Day case ligation of patent ductus arteriosus in preterm infants: A 10 year review. *Arch Dis Child* 1991;66:477.

111. Bell Thomson J, Jewell E, Ellis FH Jr et al. Surgical technique in the management of patent ductus arteriosus in the elderly patient. *Ann Thorac Surg* 1990;30:80.

112. Laborde F, Folliguet T, Batisse A, et al. Video-assisted thoracoscopic surgical interruption: The technique of choice for patent ductus arteriosus. Routine experience in 230 pediatric cases. *J Thorac Cardiovasc Surg* 1995;110:1681.

113. Burke RP, Wernovsky G, van der Valde M, et al. Video-assisted thoracoscopic surgery for congenital heart disease. *J Thorac Cardiovasc Surg* 1995;109:499.

114. Postmann W, Wierny L. Percutaneous transfemoral closure of the patent ductus arteriosus—An alternative to surgery. *Semin Roentgenol* 1981;16:95–102.

115. Rashkind WJ, Cuaso CC. Transcatheter closure of patent ductus arteriosus. *Pediatr Cardiol* 1979;1:3.

116. Shim D, Fedderly RT, Beekman RH III, et al. Follow-up of coil occlusion of patent ductus arteriosus. *J Am Coll Cardiol* 1996;28:207.

117. Sakakibara S, Konno S. Congenital aneurysm of the sinus of Valsalva: Anatomy and classification. *Am Heart J* 1962;63:405.

118. Takach TJ, Reul GJ, Duncan JM, et al. Sinus of Valsalva aneurysm or fistula: Management and outcome. *Ann Thorac Surg* 1999;68:1573.

119. Shaffer EM, Snider AR, Beekman RH, et al. Sinus of Valsalva aneurysm complicating bacterial endocarditis in an infant: Diagnosis with two-dimensional and Doppler echocardiography. *J Am Coll Cardiol* 1987;9:588.

120. Clagett OT, Kirklin JW, Edwards JE. Anatomic variations and pathologic changes in 124 cases of coarctation of the aorta. *Surg Gynecol Obstet* 1954;98:103.

121. Bharati S, Lev M. The surgical anatomy of the heart in tubular hypoplasia of the transverse aorta (preductal coarctation). *J Thorac Cardiovasc Surg* 1986;91:79.

122. Gardiner HM, Celermajer DS, Sorensen KE, et al. Arterial reactivity is significantly impaired in normotensive young adults after successful repair of aortic coarctation in childhood. *Circulation* 1954;89:1745.

123. Beekman RH. Coarctation of the aorta. In: Emmanouilides GC, Riemenschneider TA, Allen HD, Gutgesell HP, eds. *Moss and Adams Heart Disease in Infants, Children, and Adolescents*, 5th ed. Baltimore: Williams & Wilkins; 1995:1111.

124. Ing FF, Starc TJ, Griffiths SP et al. Early diagnosis of coarctation of the aorta in children: A continuing dilemma. *Pediatrics* 1996;98:378.

125. Campbell M. Natural history of coarctation of the aorta. *Br Heart J* 1970;32:633.

126. Fletcher SE, Nihill MR, Grifka RG, et al. Balloon angioplasty of native coarctation of the aorta: Midterm follow-up and prognostic factors. *J Am Coll Cardiol* 1995;25:730.

127. Zehr KJ, Gillinov AM, Redmond JM, et al. Repair of coarctation of the aorta in neonates and infants: A thirty-year experience. *Ann Thorac Surg* 1995;59:33.

128. Covley CG, Orsmond GS, Feola P, et al. Long-term, randomized comparison of balloon angioplasty and surgery for native coarctation of the aorta in childhood. *Circulation* 2005;111:3347-3348

129. Ovaert C, McCrindle BW, Nykanen D, et al. Balloon angioplasty of native coarctation: Clinical outcomes and predictors of success. *J Am Coll Cardiol* 2000;35:988.

130. Kreutzer J, Perry SB. Stents. In: Lock JE, Keane JF, Perry SB, ed. *Diagnostic and Interventional Catheterization in Congenital Heart Disease*, 2d ed. Boston: Kluwer; 2000:221.

131. O'Sullivan JJ, Derrick G, Darnell R. Prevalence of hypertension in children after early repair of coarctation of the aorta: A cohort study using casual and 24 hour blood pressure measurement. *Heart (British Cardiac Society)* 2000;88:163.

132. Parks WJ, Ngo TD, Plauth WH Jr, et al. Incidence of aneurysm formation after Dacron patch aortoplasty repair for coarctation of the aorta: Long-term results and assessment utilizing magnetic resonance angiography with three-dimensional surface rendering. *J Am Coll Cardiol* 1995;26:266.

133. Kirklin JW, Barratt-Boyes BG. Coarctation of the aorta and interrupted aortic arch. In: Kirklin JW, Barratt-Boyes BG, eds. *Cardiac Surgery*, 2d ed. New York: Churchill Livingstone; 1993:1263.

134. Toro-Salazar OH, Steinberger J, Thomas W, et al. Long-term follow-up of patients after coarctation of the aorta repair. *Am J Cardiol* 2002;89:541.

135. Quaegebeur JM, Jonas RA, Weinberg AD, et al. Outcomes in seriously ill neonates with coarctation of the aorta. A multiinstitutional study. *J Thorac Cardiovasc Surg* 1994;108:841.

136. Pollock JC, Jamieson MP, McWilliam R. Somatosensory evoked potentials in the detection of spinal cord ischemia in aortic coarctation repair. *Ann Thorac Surg* 1986;41:251.

137. Bacha EA, Almodovar M, Wessel DL, et al. Surgery for coarctation of the aorta in infants weighing less than 2 kg. *Ann Thorac Surg* 2001;71:1260.

138. Driscoll DJ, Wolfe RR, Gersony WM, et al. Cardiorespiratory responses to exercise of patients with aortic stenosis, pulmonary stenosis, and ventricular septal defect. *Circulation* 1993;87:I102.

139. Bengur AR, Snider AR, Serwer GA et al. Usefulness fo Doppler mean gradient in evaluation of children with aortic valve stenosis and comparison to gradient at catheterization. *Am J Cardiol* 1989; 64:756.

140. Silverman NH. *Pediatric Echocardiography.* New York: Williams & Wilkins; 1993.

141. Rhodes LA, Colan SD, Perry SB, et al. Predictors of survival in neonates with critical aortic stenosis. *Circulation* 1991;84:2325.

142. Yetman AT, Rosenberg HC, Joubert GI. Progression of asymptomatic aortic stenosis identified in the neonatal period. *Am J Cardiol* 1995;75:636.

143. McCrindle BW. Independent predictors of immediate results of percutaneous balloon aortic valvotomy in children. Valvuloplasty and Angioplasty of Congenital Anomalies (VACA) Registry Investigators. *Am J Cardio* 1996;77:286.

144. Moore P, Egito E, Mowrey H, et al. Midterm results of balloon dilation of congenital aortic stenosis: Predictors of success. *J Am Coll Cardiol* 1996;27:1257.

145. McElhinney DB, Lock JE, Keane JF et al. Left heart growth, function and reintervention after balloon aortic valvuloplasty for neonatal aortic stenosis. *Circulation* 2005;111:451.

146. Egito ES, Moore P, O'Sullivan J, et al. Transvascular balloon dilation for neonatal critical aortic stenosis: Early and midterm results. *J Am Coll Cardiol* 1997;29:442–447.

147. Kirklin JW, Barratt-Boyes BG. Congenital aortic stenosis. In: Kirklin JW, Barratt-Boyes BG, eds. *Cardiac Surgery*, 2d ed. New York: Churchill Livingstone; 1993:1195.

148. Elkins RC, Knott-Craig CJ, Ward KE, et al. The Ross operation in children: 10-year experience. *Ann Thorac Surg* 1998;65:496.

149. Hawkins JA, Minich LL, Tani LY, et al. Late results and reintervention after aortic valvotomy for critical aortic stenosis in neonates and infants. *Ann Thorac Surg* 1998;65:1758.

150. Najm HK, Coles JG, Black MD, et al. Extended aortic root replacement with aortic allografts or pulmonary autografts in children. *J Thorac Cardiovasc Surg* 1999;118:503.

151. Graham TP Jr, Bricker JT, James FW et al. . 26th Bethesda conference: Recommendations for determining eligibility for competition in athletes with cardiovascular abnormalities. Task Force 1: Congenital heart disease. *J Am Coll Cardiol* 1994;24:867.

152. Marshall AC, Tworetzky W, Bergerson L et al. Aortic valvuloplasty in the fetus: technical characteristics of successful balloon dilation. *J Pediatr* 2005;146:535.

153. Fyler DC. Aortic outflow abnormalities. In: Fyler DC, ed. *Nadas' Pediatric Cardiology.* Philadelphia: Hanley & Belfus; 1992:506.

154. van Son JA, Edwards WD, Danielson GK. Pathology of coronary arteries, myocardium, and great arteries in supravalvular aortic stenosis. Report of five cases with implications for surgical treatment. *J Thorac Cardiovasc Surg* 1994;108:21.

155. Ensing GJ, Schmidt MA, Hagler DJ, et al. Spectrum of findings in a family with nonsyndromic autosomal dominant supravalvular aortic stenosis: A Doppler echocardiographic study. *J Am Coll Cardiol* 1989;13:413.

156. Zalzstein E, Moes CA, Musewe NN, Freedom RM. Spectrum of cardiovascular anomalies in Williams-Beuren syndrome. *Pediatr Cardiol* 1991;12:219.

157. French JW, Guntheroth WG. An explanation of asymmetric upper extremity blood pressures in supravalvular aortic stenosis: The Coanda effect. *Circulation* 1970;42:31.

158.. van Son JA, Danielson GK, Puga FJ, et al. Supravalvular aortic stenosis. Long-term results of surgical treatment. *J Thorac Cardiovasc Surg* 1994;107:103.

159. English RF, Colan SD, Kanari PM et al. Growth of the aorta in children with William's syndrome: does surgery make a difference? *Pediatr Cardiol* 2003;24:566.

160. Wright GB, Keane JF, Nadas AS, et al. Fixed subaortic stenosis in the young: Medical and surgical course in 83 patients. *Am J Cardiol* 1983;52:830.

161. Choi JY, Sullivan ID. Fixed subaortic stenosis: Anatomical spectrum and nature of progression. *Br Heart J* 1991;65:280.

162. Freedom RM, Pelech A, Brand A, et al. The progressive nature of subaortic stenosis in congenital heart disease. *Int J Cardiol* 1985;8:137.

163. Cape EG, Vanauker MD, Sigfusson G, et al. Potential role of mechanical stress in the etiology of pediatric heart disease: Septal shear stress in subaortic stenosis. *J Am Coll Cardiol* 1997;30:247.

164. Drinkwater DC, Laks H. Surgery for subvalvular aortic stenosis. *Prog Pediatr Cardiol* 1994;3:189.

165. Giuffre RM, Ryerson LM, Vanderkooi OG et al. Surgical outcome following treatment of isolated subaortic obstruction. *Adv Ther* 2004;21:322.

166. Maginot KR, Williams RG. Fixed subaortic stenosis. *Prog Pediatr Cardiol* 1994;3:141.

167. Kirklin JW, Ellis FH Jr. Surgical relief of diffuse subvalvular aortic stenosis. *Circulation* 1961;24:739.

168. de Vries AG, Hess J, Witsenburg M, et al. Management of fixed subaortic stenosis: A retrospective study of 57 cases. *J Am Coll Cardiol* 1992;19:1013.

169. Braverman AC. Bicuspid aortic valve and associated aortic wall abnormalities. *Curr Opin Cardiol* 1996;11:501.

170. Koretzky ED, Moller JH, Korns ME, et al. Congenital pulmonary stenosis resulting from dysplasia of valve. *Circulation* 1969;40:43.

171. Li MD, Coles JC, McDonald AC. Anomalous muscle bundle of the right ventricle. Its recognition and surgical treatment. *Br Heart J* 1978;40:1040.

172. Noonan JA. Hypertelorism with Turner phenotype. A new syndrome with associated congenital heart disease. *Am J Dis Child* 1968;116:373.

173. Stone FM, Bessinger FB Jr, Lucas RV Jr, Moller JH. Pre- and postoperative rest and exercise hemodynamics in children with pulmonary stenosis. *Circulation* 1974;49:1102.

174. Ellison RC, Freedom RM, Keane JF, et al. Indirect assessment of severity in pulmonary stenosis. *Circulation* 1977;56:I14.

175. Lima CO, Sahn DJ, Valdes-Cruz LM, et al. Noninvasive prediction of transvalvular pressure gradient in patients with pulmonary stenosis by quantitative two-dimensional echocardiographic Doppler studies. *Circulation* 1983;67:866.

176. Nugent EW, Freedom RM, Nora JJ, et al. Clinical course in pulmonary stenosis. *Circulation* 1977;56:I38.

177. Mody MR. The natural history of uncomplicated valvular pulmonic stenosis. *Am Heart J* 1975;90:317.

178. Hayes CJ, Gersony WM, Driscoll DJ, et al. Second natural history study of congenital heart defects. Results of treatment of patients with pulmonary valvular stenosis. *Circulation* 1993;87:I28.

179. Stanger P, Cassidy SC, Girod DA, et al. Balloon pulmonary valvuloplasty: Results of the Valvuloplasty and Angioplasty of Congenital Anomalies Registry. *Am J Cardiol* 1990;65:775.

180. Marantz PM, Huhta JC, Mullins CE, et al. Results of balloon valvuloplasty in typical and dysplastic pulmonary valve stenosis: Doppler echocardiographic follow-up. *J Am Coll Cardiol* 1988;12:476.

181. Ali Khan MA, al Yousef S, Huhta JC, et al. Critical pulmonary valve stenosis in patients less than 1 year of age: Treatment with percutaneous gradational balloon pulmonary valvuloplasty. *Am Heart J* 1989;117:1008.

182. Ladusans EJ, Qureshi SA, Parsons JM, et al. Balloon dilatation of critical stenosis of the pulmonary valve in neonates. *Br Heart J* 1990;63:362.

183.. Kan JS, Marvin WJ Jr, Bass JL, et al. Balloon angioplasty—Branch pulmonary artery stenosis: Results from the Valvuloplasty and Angioplasty of Congenital Anomalies Registry. *Am J Cardiol* 1990;65:798.

184. O'Laughlin MP. Catheterization treatment of stenosis and hypoplasia of pulmonary arteries. *Pediatr Cardiol* 1998;19:48.

185. Bergerson L, Gauvreau K, Lock JE et al. Recent results of pulmonary arterial angioplasty: The differences between proximal and distal lesions. *Cardiol Young* 2005;15:597.

186. Baker C, McGowen F, Lock J, Keane J. Management of pulmonary artery trauma due to balloon dilation. *J Am Coll Cardiol* 1998;31:57A.

187. Vancini M, Roberts K, Silove E, Singh S. Surgical treatment of congenital pulmonary stenosis due to dysplastic leaflets and small valve annulus. *J Thorac Cardiovasc Surg* 1980;79:464.

188. McGoon MD, Fulton RE, Davis GD, et al. Systemic collateral and pulmonary artery stenosis in patients with congenital pulmonary valve atresia and ventricular septal defect. *Circulation* 1977;56:473.

189. Becker AE, Connor M, Anderson RH. Tetralogy of Fallot: A morphometric and geometric study. *Am J Cardiol* 1975;35:402–412.

190. Rao BN, Anderson RC, Edwards JE. Anatomic variations in the tetralogy of Fallot. *Am Heart J* 1971;81:361–371.

191. Morgan B, Guntheroth W, Bloom R, Fyler D. A clinical profile of paroxysmal hyperpnea in cyanotic congenital heart disease. *Circulation* 1965;31:66–69.

192. Kleinman CS, Weinstein EM, Talner NS et al Fetal echocardiography—applications and limitations. *Ultrasound Med Biol* 1984;10:747–55.

193. Hagler DJ, Tajik AJ, Seward JB, et al. Wide-angle two-dimensional echocardiographic profiles of conotruncal abnormalities. *Mayo Clin Proc* 1980;55:73–82.

194. Formanek A, Nath PH, Zollikofer C, Moller JH. Selective coronary arteriography in children. *Circulation* 1980;61:84–95.

195. Ponce FE, Williams LC, Webb HM, et al. Propranolol palliation of tetralogy of Fallot: Experience with long-term drug treatment in pediatric patients. *Pediatrics* 1973;52:100–108.

196. Blalock A, Taussig H. The surgical treatment of malformations of the heart in which there is pulmonary stenosis or pulmonary atresia. *JAMA* 1945;128:129.

197. Lillehei C, Cohen M, Warden H. Direct vision intracardiac surgical correction of the tetralogy of Fallot, pentalogy of Fallot, and pulmonary atresia defects: Report of the first 10 cases. *Ann Surg* 1955;142:418–442.

198. Kirklin JW, Blackstone EH, Kirklin JK, et al. Surgical results and protocols in the spectrum of tetralogy of Fallot. *Ann Surg* 1983;198:251–265.

199. Castaneda A, Jonas R, Mayer J, Hanley F. Tetralogy of fallot. In: Castaneda A, Jonas R, Mayer J, Hanley F, eds. *Cardiac Surgery of the Neonate and Infant*. Philadelphia: Saunders; 1994:215.

200. Rastelli GC, Wallace RB, Ongley PA. Complete repair of transposition of the great arteries with pulmonary stenosis. A review and report of a case corrected by using a new surgical technique. *Circulation* 1969;39:83–95.

201. Perron J, Moran AM, Gauvreau K, et al. Valved homograft conduit repair of the right heart in early infancy. *Ann Thorac Surg* 1999;68:542–548.

202. Kreutzer J, Perry SB, Jonas RA, et al. Tetralogy of Fallot with diminutive pulmonary arteries: preoperative pulmonary valve dilation and transcatheter rehabilitation of pulmonary arteries. *J Am Coll Cardiol* 1996;27:1741–1747.

203. Bergersen LJ, Perry SB, Lock JE. Effect of cutting balloon angioplasty on resistant pulmonary artery stenosis. *Am J Cardiol* 2003;91:185–189.

204. Geva T. Indications and timing of pulmonary valve replacement after tetralogy of Fallot repair. *Semin Thorac Cardiovasc Surg: Pediatr Card Surg Ann* 2006;9:11–22.

205. Murphy JG, Gersh BJ, Mair DD, et al. Long-term outcome in patients undergoing surgical repair of tetralogy of Fallot. *N Engl J Med* 1993;329:593–599.

206. Nollert G, Fisclein T, Bouterwek S, et al. Long-term survival in patients with repair of tetralogy of Fallot: 36-year follow-up of 490 survivors of the first year after surgical repair. *J Am Coll Cardiol* 1977;30:1374–1383.

207. Lev M, Liberthson RR, Joseph RH, et al. The pathologic anatomy of Ebstein's disease. *Arch Pathol Lab Med* 1970;90:334–343.

208. Schreiber C, Cook A, Ho SY, et al. Morphologic spectrum of Ebstein's malformation: Revisitation relative to surgical repair. *J Thorac Cardiovasc Surg* 1999;117:148–155.

209. Cohen LS, Friedman JM, Jefferson JW, et al. A reevaluation of risk of in utero exposure to lithium. *JAMA* 1994;271:146–150.

210. Watson H. Natural history of Ebstein's anomaly of tricuspid valve in childhood and adolescence. An international co-operative study of 505 cases. *Br Heart J* 1974;36:417–427.

211. Driscoll DJ, Mottram CD, Danielson GK. Spectrum of exercise intolerance in 45 patients with Ebstein's anomaly and observations on exercise tolerance in 11 patients after surgical repair. *J Am Coll Cardiol* 1988;11:831–836.

212. Roberson DA, Silverman NH. Ebstein's anomaly: Echocardiographic and clinical features in the fetus and neonate. *J Am Coll Cardiol* 1989; 14:1300–1307.

213. Hernandez F, Richkind R, Cooper H. The intracavitary electrocardiogram in the diagnosis of Ebstein's anomaly. *Am J Cardiol* 1958;1: 181–190.

214. Celermajer DS, Cullen S, Sullivan ID, et al. Outcome in neonates with Ebstein's anomaly. *J Am Coll Cardiol* 1992;19:1041–1046.

215. Gentles TL, Calder AL, Clarkson PM, Neutze JM. Predictors of long-term survival with Ebstein's anomaly of the tricuspid valve. *Am J Cardiol* 1992;69:377–381.

216. Attie F, Rosas M, Rijlaarsdam M, et al. The adult patient with Ebstein anomaly. Outcome in 72 unoperated patients. *Medicine* 2000;79: 27–36.

217. Keane J F, Fyler DC. Tricuspid valve problems. In Keane JF, Lock JE, Fyler DC, eds. *Nadas' Pediatric Cardiology* (2nd ed.). Philadelphia: Saunders Elsevier; 2006: 761.

218. Donnelly JE, Brown JM, Radford DJ. Pregnancy outcome and Ebstein's anomaly. *Br Heart J* 1991;66:368–371.

219. Kulik TJ. Inhaled nitric oxide in the management of congenital heart disease. *Curr Opin Cardiol* 1996;11:75–80.

220. Reich JD, Auld D, Hulse E, et al. The Pediatric Radiofrequency Ablation Registry's experience with Ebstein's anomaly. Pediatric Electrophysiology Society. *J Cardiovasc Electrophysiol* 1998;9:1370–1377.

221. Starnes VA, Pitlick PT, Bernstein D, et al. Ebstein's anomaly appearing in the neonate. A new surgical approach. *J Thorac Cardiovasc Surg* 1991;101:1082–1087.

222. Marianeschi SM, McElhinney DB, Reddy VM, et al. Alternative approach to the repair of Ebstein's malformation: Intracardiac repair with ventricular unloading. *Ann Thorac Surg* 1998;66:1546–1550.

223. van Son JA, Falk V, Black MD, et al. Conversion of complex neonatal Ebstein's anomaly into functional tricuspid or pulmonary atresia. *Eur J Cardiothorac Surg* 1998;13:280–284.

224. Danielson GK, Driscoll DJ, Mair DD, et al. Operative treatment of Ebstein's anomaly. *J Thorac Cardiovasc Surg* 1992;104:1195–1202.

225. Kiziltan HT, Theodoro DA, Warnes CA, et al. Late results of bioprosthetic tricuspid valve replacement in Ebstein's anomaly. *Ann Thorac Surg* 1998;66: 39–45.

226. Carpentier A, Chauvaud S, Mace L, et al. A new reconstructive operation for Ebstein's anomaly of the tricuspid valve. *J Thorac Cardiovasc Surg* 1988;96:92–101.

227. Quaegebeur JM, Sreeram N, Fraser AG, et al. Surgery for Ebstein's anomaly: The clinical and echocardiographic evaluation of a new technique. *J Am Coll Cardiol* 1991;17:722–728.

228. Knott-Craig CJ, Overholt ED, Ward KE, et al. Repair of Ebstein's anomaly in the symptomatic neonate: An evolution of technique with 7-year follow-up. *Ann Thorac Surg* 2002;73:1786–1792.

229. Radford DJ, Graff RF, Neilson GH. Diagnosis and natural history of Ebstein's anomaly. *Br Heart J* 1985;54:517–522.

230. Lucas RV Jr, Lock JE, Tandon R, Edwards JE. Gross and histologic anatomy of total anomalous pulmonary venous connections. *Am J Cardiol* 1988;62:292–300.

231. Gathman GE, Nadas AS. Total anomalous pulmonary venous connection: Clinical and physiologic observations of 75 pediatric patients. *Circulation* 1970;42:143–154.

232. Chin AJ, Sanders SP, Sherman F, et al. Accuracy of subcostal two-dimensional echocardiography in prospective diagnosis of total anomalous pulmonary venous connection. *Am Heart J* 1987;113: 1153–1159.

233. Newfeld EA, Wilson A, Paul MH, Reisch JS. Pulmonary vascular disease in total anomalous pulmonary venous drainage. *Circulation* 1980;61:103–109.

234. Castaneda AR, Jonas RA, Mayer JE, Hanley FL. *Cardiac Surgery in the Neonate and Infant*. Philadelphia: Saunders; 1994.

235. Behrendt DM, Aberdeen E, Waterson DJ, Bonham-Carter RE. Total anomalous pulmonary venous drainage in infants. I. Clinical and hemodynamic findings, methods, and results of operation in 37 cases. *Circulation* 1972;46:347–356.

236. Norwood WI, Hougen TJ, Castaneda AR. Total anomalous pulmonary venous connection: Surgical considerations. *Cardiovasc Clin* 1981;11: 353–364.

237. Keane JF, Fyler DC. Total anomalous pulmonary venous return. In Keane JF, Lock JE, Fyler DC, eds. *Nadas' Pediatric Cardiology* (2nd ed.) Philadelphia: Saunders Elsevier; 2006:773.

238. Bando K, Turrentine MW, Ensing GJ, et al. Surgical management of total anomalous pulmonary venous connection. Thirty-year trends. *Circulation* 1996;94:II12–II26.

239. Lacour-Gayet F, Zoghbi J, Serraf AE, et al. Surgical management of progressive pulmonary venous obstruction after repair of total anomalous pulmonary venous connection. *J Thorac Cardiovasc Surg* 1999; 117:679–687.

240. Van Praagh R, Weinberg P, Smith S. Malpositions of the heart. In: Adams F, Emmanouilides G, Riemenschneider T, eds. *Moss' Heart Disease in Infants, Children, and Adolescents*. Baltimore: Williams & Wilkins; 1989:530.

241. Van Praagh R. Segmental approach to diagnosis. In: Fyler D, ed. *Nadas' Pediatric Cardiology*. Philadelphia: Hanley & Belfus; 1992:27.

242. Van Praagh S, Santini F, Sanders S. Cardiac malpositions with special emphasis on visceral heterotaxy (asplenia and polysplenia syndromes). In: Fyler D, ed. *Nadas' Pediatric Cardiology*. Philadelphia: Hanley & Belfus; 1992:589.

243. Rooklin AR, McGeady SJ, Mikaelian DO, et al. The immotile cilia syndrome: A cause of recurrent pulmonary diseases in children. *Pediatrics* 1980;66:526–531.

244. Fulton DR, Flyer DC D. D-transposition of the great arteries. In: Keane JF, Lock JE Fyler D, eds. *Nadas' Pediatric Cardiology* (2nd ed). Philadelphia: Saunders Elsevier; 2006:645.

245. Wernovsky G. Transposition of the great arteries. In: Allen HD, Gutgesell HP Clarked Driscoll DJ, eds. *Moss and Adams Heart Disease in Infants, Children, and Adolescents*, 6th ed. Philadelphia: Lippincott Williams & Wilkins; 2001:1027.

246. Yoo S, Burrows P, Moes C. Evaluation of coronary arterial patterns in complete transposition by laidback aortography. *Cardiol Young* 1996; 6:149–155.

247. Liebman J, Cullum L, Belloc NB. Natural history of transposition of the great arteries. Anatomy and birth and death characteristics. *Circulation* 1969;40:237–262.

248. Wilson NJ, Clarkson PM, Barratt-Boyes BG, et al. Long-term outcome after the mustard repair for simple transposition of the great arteries. 28-year follow-up. *J Am Coll Cardiol* 1998;32:758–765.

249. Kirjavainen M, Happonen JM, Louhimo I. Late results of Senning operation. *J Thorac Cardiovasc Surg* 1999;117:488–495.

250. Wernovsky G, Mayer JE Jr, Jonas RA, et al. Factors influencing early and late outcome of the arterial switch operation for transposition of the great arteries. *J Thorac Cardiovasc Surg* 1995;109:289–301.

251. Pretre R, Tamisier D, Bonhoeffer P, et al. Results of the arterial switch operation in neonates with transposed great arteries. *Lancet* 2001;357:1826–1830.

252. Gutgesell HP, Massaro TA, Kron IL. The arterial switch operation for transposition of the great arteries in a consortium of university hospitals. *Am J Cardiol* 1994;74:959–960.

253. Losay J, Touchot A, Serraf A, et al. Late outcome after arterial switch operation for transposition of the great arteries. *Circulation* 2001;104:I126.

254. Mahle WT, McBride MG, Paridon SM. Exercise performance after the arterial switch operation for D-transposition of the great arteries. *Am J Cardiol* 2001;87:753–758.

255. Williams WG, Quaegebeur JM, Kirklin JW, Blackstone EH. Outflow obstruction after the arterial switch operation: A multi-institutional study. Congenital Heart Surgeons Society. *J Thorac Cardiovasc Surg* 1997;114:975–987.

256. Nakanishi T, Matsumoto Y, Seguchi M, et al. Balloon angioplasty for postoperative pulmonary artery stenosis in transposition of the great arteries. *J Am Coll Cardiol* 1993;22:859–866.

257. Marino BS, Wernovsky G, McElhinney DB, et al. Neo-aortic valvar function after the arterial switch. *Cardiol Young* 2006;16:481–489.

258. Hovels-Gurich HH, Seghaye MC, Ma Q, et al. Long-term results of cardiac and general health status in children after neonatal arterial switch operation. *Ann Thorac Surg* 2003;75:935–943.

259. Castaneda AR, Jonas RA, Mayer JE, Hanley FL. *Cardiac Surgery of the Neonate and Infant*. Philadelphia: Saunders; 1994.

260. Sagin-Saylam G, Somerville J. Palliative Mustard operation for transposition of the great arteries: Late results after 15–20 years. *Heart* 1996;75:72–77.

261. Hagler D. Double-outlet right ventricle and Double Outlet Left ventricle In In: Emmanouilides G, Allen H, Gutgesell H, Clark EB and Driscoll DJ eds. *Moss and Adams Heart Disease in Infants, Children, and Adolescents,* 6th ed. Philadelphia: Lippincott Williams & Wilkins; 2001:1102–1128.

262. Snider AR, Serwer G. *Echocardiography in Pediatric Heart Disease.* Chicago: Year Book; 1990.

263. Kirklin J, Barratt-Boyes B. Double outlet right ventricle. In: Kirklin J, Barratt-Boyes B, eds. *Cardiac Surgery,* 2d ed. New York: Churchill Livingstone; 1993:1469.

264. Aoki M, Forbess JM, Jonas RA, et al. Result of biventricular repair for double-outlet right ventricle. *J Thorac Cardiovasc Surg* 1994;107: 338–349.

265. Belli E, Serraf A, Lacour-Gayet F, et al. Surgical treatment of subaortic stenosis after biventricular repair of double-outlet right ventricle. *J Thorac Cardiovasc Surg* 1996;112:1570–1578.

266. Mavroudis C, Backer CL, Muster AJ, et al. Taussig-Bing anomaly: Arterial switch versus Kawashima intraventricular repair. *Ann Thorac Surg* 1996;61:1330–1338.

267. Brown JW, Ruzmetov M, Okada Y, et al. Surgical results in patients with double outlet right ventricle: a 20-year experience. *Ann Thorac Surg* 2001;72:1630–1635.

268. Freedom R. Congenitally corrected transposition of the great arteries: Definitions and pathologic anatomy. *Pediatr Cardiol* 1999;10:3–16.

269. Fischbach P, Law I, Serwer G. Congenitally corrected I-transposition of the great arteries: Abnormalities of atrioventricular conduction. *Prog Pediatr Cardiol* 1999;10:37–43.

270. Snider A, Serwer G, Ritter S. Abnormalities in ventricular connection. In: Snider A, Serwer G, Ritter S, eds. *Echocardiography in Pediatric Heart Disease.* St. Louis: Mosby; 1990:317–323.

271. Connelly MS, Liu PP, Williams WG, et al. Congenitally corrected transposition of the great arteries in the adult: Functional status and complications. *J Am Coll Cardiol* 1996;27:1238–1243.

272. Graham TP Jr, Bernard YD, Mellen BG, et al. Long-term outcome in congenitally corrected transposition of the great arteries: A multi-institutional study. *J Am Coll Cardiol* 2000;36:255–261.

273. Fredriksen PM, Chen A, Veldtman G, et al. Exercise capacity in adult patients with congenitally corrected transposition of the great arteries. *Heart (British Cardiac Society)* 2001;85:191–195.

274. Therrien J, Barnes I, Somerville J. Outcome of pregnancy in patients with congenitally corrected transposition of the great arteries. *Am J Cardiol* 1999;84:820–824.

275. Lundstrom U, Bull C, Wyse RK, Somerville J. The natural and "unnatural" history of congenitally corrected transposition. *Am J Cardiol* 1990;65:1222–1229.

276. Cowley C, Rosenthal A. Congenitally corrected transposition of the great arteries: The systemic right ventricle. *Prog Pediatr Cardiol* 1999;10:31–35.

277. Warnes CA. Congenitally corrected transposition: The uncorrected misnomer. *J Am Coll Cardiol* 1996;27:1244–1245.

278. Kirklin J, Barratt-Boyes B. Congenitally corrected transposition of the great arteries. In: Kirklin J, Barratt-Boyes B, eds. *Cardiac Surgery.* New York: Churchill Livingstone; 1993:1511.

279. Sano T, Riesenfeld T, Karl TR, Wilkinson JL. Intermediate-term outcome after intracardiac repair of associated cardiac defects in patients with atrioventricular and ventriculoarterial discordance. *Circulation* 1995;92:II272–II278.

280. Termignon JL, Leca F, Vouhe PR, et al. "Classic" repair of congenitally corrected transposition and ventricular septal defect. *Ann Thorac Surg* 1996;62:199–206.

281. Hraska V, Duncan BW, Mayer JE Jr, et al. Long-term outcome of surgically treated patients with corrected transposition of the great arteries. *J Thorac Cardiovasc Surg* 2005;129:182–191.

282. van Son JA, Danielson GK, Huhta JC, et al. Late results of systemic atrioventricular valve replacement in corrected transposition. *J Thorac Cardiovasc Surg* 1995;109:642–652.

283. Ilbawi MN, DeLeon SY, Backer CL, et al. An alternative approach to the surgical management of physiologically corrected transposition with ventricular septal defect and pulmonary stenosis or atresia. *J Thorac Cardiovasc Surg* 1990;100:410–415.

284. Duncan BW, Mee RB, Mesia CI, et al. Results of the double switch operation for congenitally corrected transposition of the great arteries. *Eur J Cardiothorac Surg* 2003;24:11–19.

285. Langley SM, Winlaw DS, Stumper O, et al. Midterm results after restoration of the morphologically left ventricle to the systemic circulation in patients with congenitally corrected transposition of the great arteries. *J Thorac Cardiovasc Surg* 2003;125:1229–1241.

286. Rosenthal A, Dick M. Tricuspid atresia. In: Emmanouilides G, Riemenschneider T, Allen H, Gutgesell H, eds. *Moss and Adams Heart Disease in Infants, Children, and Adolescents,* 5th ed. Baltimore: Williams & Wilkins; 1995:902.

287. Hagler D, Edwards W. Univentricular atrioventricular connection. In: Emmanouilides G, Riemenschneider T, Allen H, Gutgesell H, eds. *Moss and Adams Heart Disease in Infants, Children and Adolescents,* 5th ed. Baltimore: Williams & Wilkins; 1995:1278.

288. Dobell AR, Van Praagh R. The Holmes heart: Historic associations and pathologic anatomy. *Am Heart J* 1996;132:437–445.

289. Silverman N. *Pediatric Echocardiography.* Baltimore: Williams & Wilkins; 1993.

290. Freedom R, Culham J, Moes C. *Angiocardiography of Congenital Heart Disease.* New York: Macmillan; 1989.

291. George B, Kaplan S. Single ventricle and subaortic obstruction. *Prog Pediatr Cardiol* 1994;3:167–176.

292. Moak JP, Gersony WM. Progressive atrioventricular valvular regurgitation in single ventricle. *Am J Cardiol* 1987;59:656–658.

293. Donofrio MT, Jacobs ML, Norwood WI, Rychik J. Early changes in ventricular septal defect size and ventricular geometry in the single left ventricle after volume-unloading surgery. *J Am Coll Cardiol* 1995;26:1008–1015.

294. Mainwaring R, Lamberti J, Moore J. The bidirectional Glenn and Fontan procedures: Integrated management of the patient with a functionally single ventricle. *Cardiol Young* 1996;6:198–207.

295. van Son JA, Reddy VM, Haas GS, Hanley FL. Modified surgical techniques for relief of aortic obstruction in [S,L,L] hearts with rudimentary right ventricle and restrictive bulboventricular foramen. *J Thorac Cardiovasc Surg* 1995;110:909–915.

296. Norwood WI, Lang P, Hansen DD. Physiologic repair of aortic atresia-hypoplastic left heart syndrome. *N Engl J Med* 1983;308:23–26.

297. Bailey LL, Nehlsen-Cannarella SL, Doroshow RW, et al. Cardiac allotransplantation in newborns as therapy for hypoplastic left heart syndrome. *N Engl J Med* 1986;315:949–951.

298. Mayer JE Jr, Bridges ND, Lock JE, et al. Factors associated with marked reduction in mortality for Fontan operations in patients with single ventricle. *J Thorac Cardiovasc Surg* 1992;103:444–451.

299. Matitiau A, Geva T, Colan SD, et al. Bulboventricular foramen size in infants with double-inlet left ventricle or tricuspid atresia with transposed great arteries: Influence on initial palliative operation and rate of growth. *J Am Coll Cardiol* 1992;19:142–148.

300. Jacobs ML, Rychik J, Rome JJ, et al. Early reduction of the volume work of the single ventricle: The hemi-Fontan operation. *Ann Thorac Surg* 1996;62:456–461.

301. Fontan F, Baudet E. Surgical repair of tricuspid atresia. *Thorax* 1971; 26:240–248.

302. Cetta F, Feldt RH, O'Leary PW, et al. Improved early morbidity and mortality after Fontan operation: The Mayo Clinic experience, 1987 to 1992. *J Am Coll Cardiol* 1996;28:480–486.

303. Petrossian E, Reddy VM, McElhinney DB, et al. Early results of the extracardiac conduit Fontan operation. *J Thorac Cardiovasc Surg* 1999;117:688–696.

304. Jacobs ML, Blackstone EH, Bailey LL. Intermediate survival in neonates with aortic atresia: A multi-institutional study. The Congenital Heart Surgeons Society. *J Thorac Cardiovasc Surg* 1998;116: 417–431.

305. Lang P, Fyler DC. Hypoplastic left heart syndrome, mitral atresia and aortic atresia. In Keane JF, Lock JE, Fyler DC, eds. *Nadas' Pediatric Cardiology* (2nd ed.). Philadelphia: Saunders Elsevier; 2006:715.

306. Gaynor JW, Mahle WT, Cohen MI, et al. Risk factors for mortality after the Norwood procedure. *Eur J Cardiothorac Surg* 2002;22:82–89.

307. Tkebuchava T, Von Segesser LK, Vogt PR, et al. Congenital coronary fistulas in children and adults: Diagnosis, surgical technique and results. *J Cardiovasc Surg (Torino)* 1996;37:29–34.

308. Vavuranakis M, Bush CA, Boudoulas H. Coronary artery fistulas in adults: Incidence, angiographic characteristics, natural history. *Cathet Cardiovasc Diagn* 1995;35:116–120.

309. Sherwood MC, Rockenmacher S, Colan SD, et al. Prognostic significance of clinically silent coronary artery fistulas. *Am J Cardiol* 1999;83:407–411.

310. Velvis H, Schmidt KG, Silverman NH, Turley K. Diagnosis of coronary artery fistula by two-dimensional echocardiography, pulsed Doppler ultrasound and color flow imaging. *J Am Coll Cardiol* 1989; 14:968–976.

311. Urrutia-S CO, Falaschi G, Ott DA, Cooley DA. Surgical management of 56 patients with congenital coronary artery fistulas. *Ann Thorac Surg* 1983;35:300–307.

312. Mavroudis C, Backer CL, Rocchini AP, et al. Coronary artery fistulas in infants and children: A surgical review and discussion of coil embolization. *Ann Thorac Surg* 1997;63:1235–1242.

313. Blanche C, Chaux A. Long-term results of surgery for coronary artery fistulas. *Int Surg* 1990;75:238–239.

314. Armsby LR, Keane JF, Sherwood MC, et al. Management of coronary artery fistulae. Patient selection and results of transcatheter closure. *J Am Coll Cardio* 2002;39:1026–1032.

315. Hurwitz RA, Caldwell RL, Girod DA, et al. Clinical and hemodynamic course of infants and children with anomalous left coronary artery. *Am Heart J* 1989;118:1176–1181.

316. Wesselhoeft H, Fawcett JS, Johnson AL. Anomalous origin of the left coronary artery from the pulmonary trunk. Its clinical spectrum, pathology, and pathophysiology, based on a review of 140 cases with seven further cases. *Circulation* 1968;38:403–425.

317. Schmidt KG, Cooper MJ, Silverman NH, Stanger P. Pulmonary artery origin of the left coronary artery: Diagnosis by two-dimensional echocardiography, pulsed Doppler ultrasound and color flow mapping. *J Am Coll Cardiol* 1988;11:396–402.

318. Gutgesell HP, Pinsky WW, DePuey EG. Thallium-201 myocardial perfusion imaging in infants and children. Value in distinguishing anomalous left coronary artery from congestive cardiomyopathy. *Circulation* 1980;61:596–599.

319. Takeuchi S, Imamura H, Katsumoto K, et al. New surgical method for repair of anomalous left coronary artery from pulmonary artery. *J Thorac Cardiovasc Surg* 1979;78:7–11.

320. Cochrane AD, Coleman DM, Davis AM, et al. Excellent long-term functional outcome after an operation for anomalous left coronary artery from the pulmonary artery. *J Thorac Cardiovasc Surg* 1999;117:332–342.

321. el Said GM, Ruzyllo W, Williams RL, et al. Early and late result of saphenous vein graft for anomalous origin of left coronary artery from pulmonary artery. *Circulation* 1973;48:2–6.

322. Rein AJ, Colan SD, Parness IA, Sanders SP. Regional and global left ventricular function in infants with anomalous origin of the left coronary artery from the pulmonary trunk: Preoperative and postoperative assessment. *Circulation* 1987;75:115–123.

323. Rahimtoola SH. Concept and evaluation of hibernating myocardium. *Annu Rev Med* 1999;50:75–86.

CHAPTER (83)

Congenital Heart Disease in Adults

Jamil A. Aboulhosn / John S. Child

The incidence of moderate and severe forms of congenital heart disease (CHD) is 6 per 1000 livebirths. If bicuspid aortic valves are included, the incidence rises to 19 per 1000 livebirths.[1] Without early medical or surgical treatment, the majority of patients with complex CHD would not survive to adulthood.[2] Surgical and medical advances over the past 60 years have dramatically altered the once bleak prognosis of patients with CHD. In the current era, more than 85 percent of patients with CHD survive to reach adulthood and most live productive and functional lives.[3,4] Many patients have undergone surgical interventions that were once thought to be curative. With the exception of early surgical ligation of a patent ductus arteriosus, a surgical "cure" for CHD without operative sequelae or need for reoperation does not exist.[5]

Adults with operated and unoperated CHD require long-term followup. This long-term care should include cardiologists with experience in, or who specialize in, adult CHD. Diagnostic and treatment errors by cardiologists inexperienced in complex CHD can be minimized by improved understanding of the pathophysiology, hemodynamics, and prognosis of various lesions. Patient referral to regional adult CHD experts is encouraged so as to facilitate specialized counseling and management. These patients also face a variety of psychosocial issues, including self-image problems, difficulties in acquiring and maintaining health and life in-

surance, exercise and activity limitations, and issues of sexuality, contraception, and reproduction.

Specialized adult CHD centers are a relatively recent development. Requirements include close collaboration between adult and pediatric cardiologists, cardiac surgeons, nurse specialists and consultants. Training and research are of pivotal importance. The development of management, research and training guidelines over the past decade is a major step forward for the field of adult congenital heart disease.[6-9] Another encouraging development is the establishment of the Adult Congenital Heart Association in the United States, a patient-initiated association, is a nonprofit organization that seeks to improve the quality of life and extend the lives of adults with CHD.

MEDICAL CONSIDERATIONS

Many adults with CHD have not had, or may never require, surgical intervention. The most common defects incidentally encountered in adulthood are small ventricular or atrial septal defects, mild pulmonary stenosis, bicuspid aortic valves, and mitral valve prolapse (Table 83–1). Less common, but more complex conditions include nonrestrictive central shunts with right-to-left shunt rever-

TABLE 83-1

Unoperated Congenital Cardiac Defects Commonly Encountered in Adulthood

DEFECT	CYANOSIS	ENDOCARDITIS RISK
Mild pulmonary valve stenosis	No	Intermediate
Peripheral pulmonary stenosis	No	Intermediate
Bicuspid aortic valve	No	Intermediate/high
Mild subaortic stenosis	No	Intermediate
Mild supravalvar aortic stenosis	No	Intermediate
Small atrial septal defect	No	Low
Small ventricular septal defect	No	High
Small patent ductus arteriosus	No	High
Mitral valve prolapse	No	Low/intermediate
Atrioventricular septal defect	±	Intermediate/high
Marfan syndrome	No	Intermediate/high
Ebstein anomaly	±	Intermediate/high
Congenitally corrected transposition of the great arteries	±	Intermediate/high
Eisenmenger syndrome	+	High

sal resulting in the cyanotic Eisenmenger syndrome. Most patients require long-term followup to monitor for disease progression and to reinforce the need for diligent dental care and antibiotic prophylaxis against infective endocarditis. Women of childbearing age and men wishing to father children should be informed of the risks of pregnancy and the increased risk of congenital heart disease in their progeny. An increasing number of patients who underwent palliative or corrective operations in childhood are reaching adulthood (Table 83–2). Many patients are under the false impression that they are "cured" and are lost to followup until symptoms bring them back to medical attention. These patients should be monitored on a regular basis for progression of disease and need for re-operation. Some patients require repeat operations in adulthood.

【 】 HEMODYNAMICS

Progressive myocardial dysfunction with resultant heart failure is a leading cause of morbidity and mortality in patients with CHD. Patients may present with left, right, biventricular, or univentricular failure in the face of pressure and/or volume overload often in the presence of hypoxia secondary to coexistent pulmonary vascular disease. Intrinsic myocardial abnormalities may result in restrictive diastolic properties, leading to a chronic low cardiac output state, volume overload, congestive hepatopathy, ascites, and protein losing enteropathy. Complications of restrictive cardiomyopathy are often progressive and difficult to manage, cardiac transplantation is the ultimate therapeutic option. Physical examination includes thorough assessment of volume status with specific attention to the jugular venous filling pressure and waveform. Pulmonary hypertension or ventricular filling abnormalities are often accompanied by an amplified A wave in the jugular venous pulse. Right-sided atrioventricular valve regurgitation may result in an amplified jugular venous V wave proportional to the severity of regurgitation.

Percussion and palpation of the liver to evaluate for pulsatility and degree of hepatomegaly is recommended. Doppler echocardiography is indispensable for noninvasive evaluation of hemodynamics and shunt fractions.[10,11] Invasive cardiac catheterization is reserved for the patients with inadequate acoustic windows that limit the usefulness of transthoracic echocardiography or for patients whose pulmonary vascular resistance or chamber pressures must be measured.

Operations to palliate or repair congenital cardiovascular lesions were originally devised to address physiologic issues, specifically to increase or diminish the supply of blood to the pulmonary circulation. The early era of congenital cardiac surgery was marked by giant leaps forward in the physiologic treatment of lesions. For example, patients with pulmonary atresia or single ventricle underwent placement of an arteriopulmonary shunt, a wave of surgical innovation initiated by the famed Blalock-Taussig shunt, initially performed in 1945 (Fig. 83–1).[12] Another example is the atrial switch operation for correction of complete transposition of the great arteries (Fig. 83–2) in which deoxygen-

TABLE 83-2

Operated Congenital Cardiac Defects Commonly Encountered in Adulthood

DEFECT	ENDOCARDITIS RISK
Aortic valve repair/replacement	High
Pulmonary valve repair/replacement	Intermediate/high
Repaired tetralogy of Fallot	Intermediate/high
Atrial septal defect	Low
Ventricular septal defect	Low
Atrioventricular septal defect	Low/intermediate
Complete transposition status post Mustard or Senning	Intermediate
Complex cardiac malpositions s/p correction	Intermediate/high
Total anomalous pulmonary venous return	Low
Pulmonary atresia with intact ventricular septum	High
Single ventricle s/p Glenn or Fontan operation	Low/intermediate
Ebstein anomaly	Intermediate/high
Coarctation of the aorta	Intermediate
Mitral valve disease	Intermediate/high

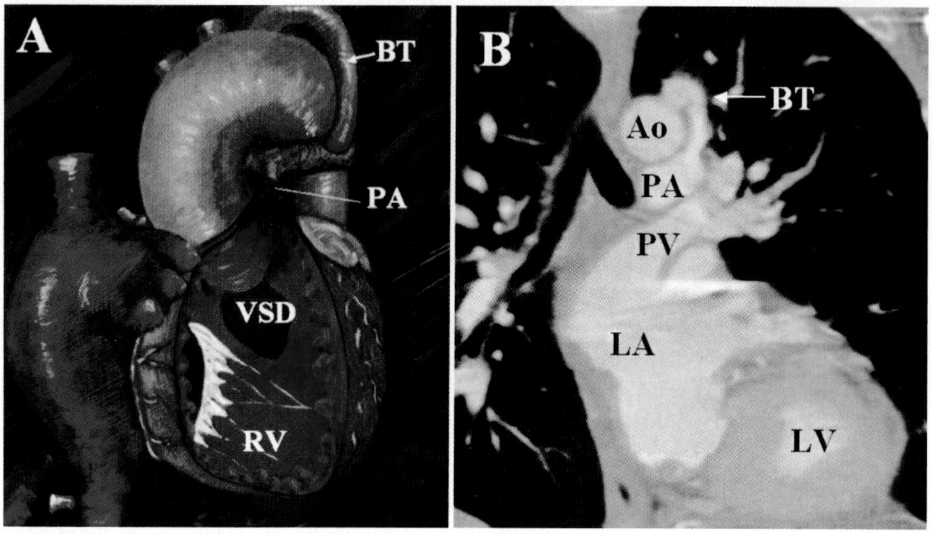

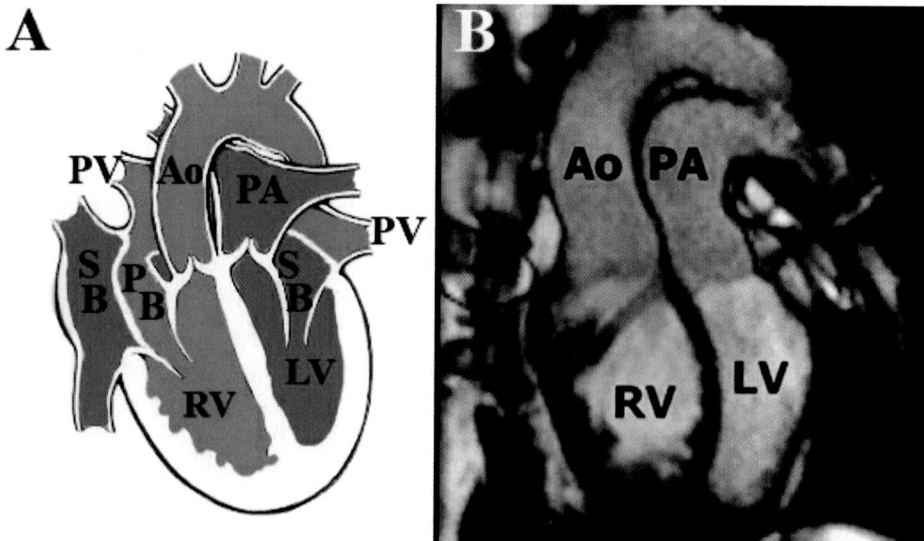

FIGURE 83–1. **A.** Classic left Blalock-Taussig (BT) shunt consisting of a direct attachment of the divided left subclavian artery to the left pulmonary artery in a patient with tetralogy of Fallot with pulmonary atresia (PA) and a large nonrestrictive ventricular septal defect (VSD). The right ventricle is labeled (RV). **B.** CT-angiogram (ECG-gated 64-slice CT) of a 53-year-old female with a double-inlet left ventricle and pulmonary atresia viewed from the coronal (frontal) projection. A classic left BT shunt diverts systemic blood flow from the aorta (Ao) to the pulmonary artery (PA) via a divided left subclavian artery. The left superior pulmonary vein (PV), left atrium (LA), and left ventricle (LV) are labeled.

Eventually, progressive right ventricular dilation and elevated filling pressures, particularly if ventriculotomy scars coexist, may create the substrate for ventricular arrhythmias. Medical therapy for heart failure in patients with congenital heart disease is adopted from the extensive evidence-based literature in patients with ischemic and nonischemic cardiomyopathies. There is a paucity of prospective randomized data evaluating heart failure therapies in patients with CHD. The renin–angiotensin system may not play as deleterious a role in certain subsets of patients with CHD as compared to those with ischemic and nonischemic cardiomyopathies. For example, patients with systemic right ventricles with depressed systolic function do not demonstrate increased angiotensin levels and therefore do not appear to derive demonstrable intermediate-term benefit from the use of angiotensin-converting enzyme (ACE) inhibitors or angiotensin receptor blockers.[15] β Blockers may retard the progression of ventricular dysfunction and decrease the likelihood of arrhythmias.[16] Diuretics have not been rigorously evaluated in patients with CHD.

ated blood is redirected by the atrial baffle from the cavae to the left ventricle and thereafter to the pulmonary arterial circulation. The oxygenated pulmonary venous blood returns to the systemic right ventricle. These operations are successful in diverting blood flow to improve or correct physiology, but do not normalize anatomy or optimize hemodynamics. Patients with systemic right ventricles or those with single ventricles are especially susceptible to deteriorating ventricular function. The heterogeneous morphology and loading conditions for these ventricles suggest that standard indices of ventricular function, namely echo or other imaging derived ejection fraction, may not be as useful in identifying the highest risk subsets. Elevations of serum brain natriuretic peptide (BNP) may help identify patients with increased ventricular wall tension often accompanied by ventricular enlargement and dysfunction.[13] Atrial and ventricular arrhythmias increase in frequency and severity as ventricular function deteriorates and themselves lead to further decreases in cardiac output. Medical and surgical interventions are aimed at preservation of function and prevention of arrhythmias.

Postoperative residual defects may be a major cause of progressive deterioration decades after surgery. Severe chronic pulmonary regurgitation may be well tolerated for decades following surgery.[14]

FIGURE 83–2. **A.** Valentine diagram of the cardiac anatomy in a patient with d-transposition of the great arteries who has undergone the Mustard or Senning atrial switch operation. Deoxygenated blood (blue) returning from the vena cavae is redirected via a systemic venous baffle (SB) to the left ventricle (LV) and thereafter into the transposed pulmonary artery (PA). Oxygenated blood (red) returning from the lungs via the pulmonary veins (PV) is redirected via a pulmonary venous baffle (PB) to the systemic right ventricle (RV) and then to an anterior and rightward aorta (Ao). **B.** A cine-MRI image of a patient with d-transposition of the great arteries as viewed from a left lateral projection. The right ventricle (RV) is anterior and is hypertrophied and moderately dilated. Note that the interventricular septum bows to the left in diastole consistent with right ventricular pressure overload. The aorta (Ao) emerges from the RV and is anterior to the pulmonary artery (PA) which emerges from a thin-walled left ventricle (LV).

【 】 CYANOSIS

Cyanosis may be a consequence of decreased pulmonary blood flow or admixture of desaturated systemic venous blood with pulmonary venous blood. Decreased pulmonary blood flow may be caused by pulmonary stenosis or atresia (e.g., unrepaired tetralogy of Fallot). Cyanosis with pulmonary vascular disease may be caused by unrepaired central shunts (Eisenmenger syndrome) or concomitant idiopathic pulmonary with an atrial septal defect (ASD).[17]

The *Eisenmenger complex* refers to a reversed shunt (right to left) in the presence of a nonrestrictive ventricular septal defect (VSD; Fig. 83–3). Eisenmenger syndrome refers to various lesions leading to pulmonary vascular disease and a reversed central shunt. During the first few years of life, the small muscular pulmonary artery branches are capable of relaxing and the defect can be closed with a subsequent gradual fall in pulmonary vascular resistance. After 2 to 3 years, reactive intimal fibrosis begins to obliterate the lumen of the muscular arteries, and they no longer respond to vasodilating agents. Patients with trisomy 21 (Down syndrome) are especially susceptible to developing pulmonary vascular disease.[18] Cyanosis with pulmonary vascular disease and shunt reversal causes decreased exercise capacity (Fig. 83–4).[19,20]

Death usually occurs by the fourth decade of life, although some people survive into the seventh decade. Patients with unrepaired truncus arteriosus and those with single ventricle morphology have a poorer prognosis than patients with nonrestrictive VSD (Eisenmenger complex).[21] Causes of death include pulmonary hemorrhage, pulmonary arterial thrombosis, pulmonary artery dissection, ventricular arrhythmias, and ventricular failure. All cyanotic patients are at risk for infective endocarditis. Patients with cyanotic CHD demonstrate an antiatherogenic substrate and are less susceptible to atherosclerotic heart disease then noncyanotic controls.[22–24] The coronary arterial tree is markedly dilated with tortuous extramural coronary arteries and a well developed microcirculation within the myocardium.[23,24] Serum lipid levels are low in cyanotic patients and remain

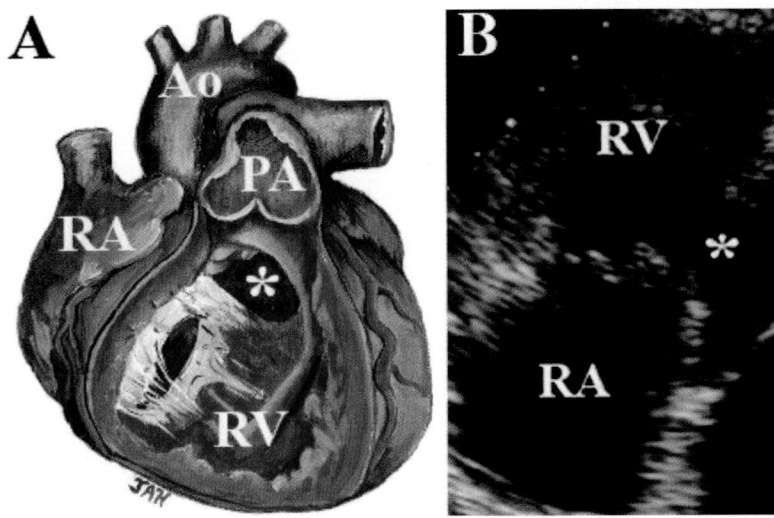

FIGURE 83–3. A. A patient with Eisenmenger complex, which is characterized by a nonrestrictive ventricular septal defect (VSD; *asterisk*). The right ventricle (RV) is hypertrophied and the main pulmonary artery (PA) is dilated and has evidence of atheroma formation. Also labeled are the right atrium (RA) and the aorta (Ao). **B.** Transthoracic echocardiographic image, apical four-chamber view of a patient with Eisenmenger complex. There is a large nonrestrictive VSD (*asterisk*). The RV is enlarged and hypertrophied. The left ventricle (LV) and left atrium (LA) are labeled.

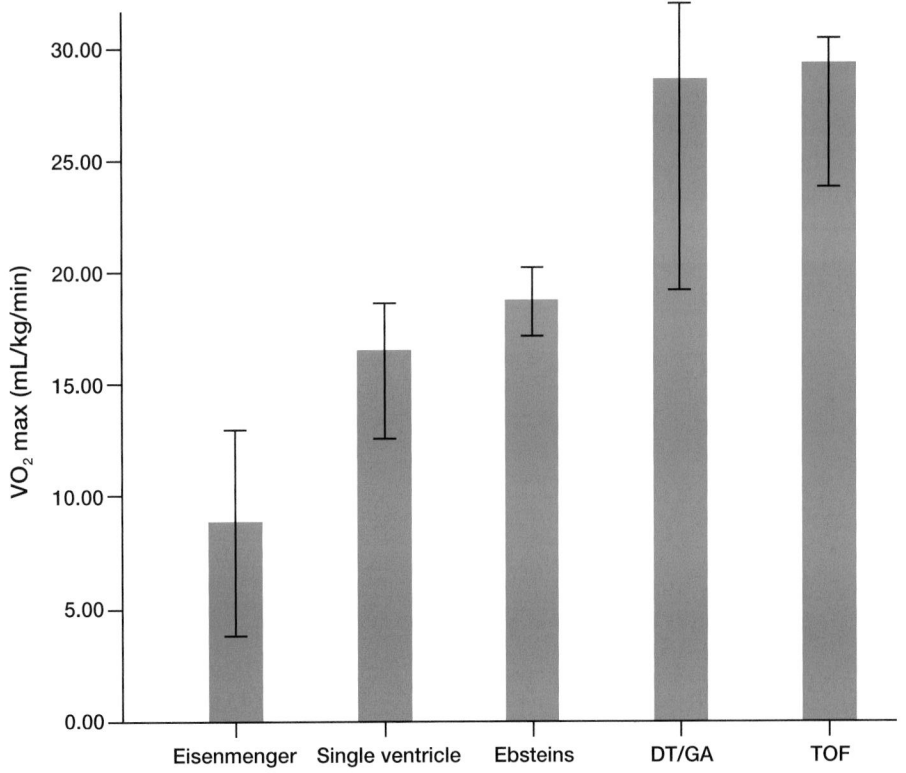

FIGURE 83–4. Distribution of maximum oxygen consumption (VO$_2$max) in 78 adults with various types of congenital heart disease followed at the Ahmanson/UCLA Adult Congenital Heart Disease Center. Surgically repaired patients with tetralogy of Fallot (TOF) and patients with d-transposition of the great arteries (DTGA) who have undergone an atrial switch operation performed significantly better than other subgroups. Patients with Eisenmenger syndrome had a mean VO$_2$max of less than 10 mL/kg/min, which was significantly lower than the VO$_2$max of any other subgroup.

low despite correction of cyanosis. The antiatherogenic state of these patients is further characterized by elevated bilirubin levels, increased nitric oxide (NO) production by vascular endothelial cells, and low platelet levels incurring less thrombotic risk.[22,25] Patients with chronic cyanosis also develop defective hemostasis from abnormalities in platelet function and in the coagulation and fibrinolytic systems.[26,27] The pulmonary arterial circulation is not spared from atherosclerosis and thrombosis.[28] Cardiac computed tomography quantifies calcium deposition in the pulmonary arterial tree; calcium being a surrogate marker for atherosclerosis (Fig. 83–5). Pulmonary artery luminal in situ thrombosis is common. Chronic anticoagulation increases the risk of pulmonary hemorrhage, particularly with thrombocytopenia, and should be avoided unless the patient has other definitive indications (e.g., atrial fibrillation or deep venous thrombosis).[21]

Chronic cyanosis leads to secondary erythrocytosis. Risk of symptomatic hyperviscosity is low with a hemoglobin level <20 g/dL. Symptoms include headache, dizziness, fatigue, and blurry vision. Phlebotomy may improve symptoms but should be reserved for patients who do not improve with hydration.[29] Phlebotomies should be minimized (regardless of the hemoglobin level) because they cause iron deficiency and microcytic, less-deformable red blood cells that do not pass easily through the microcirculation, thereby increasing the risk of stroke.[26,27,30] Hyperuricemia is common because of the increased red blood cell turnover and decreased renal excretion of uric acid; urate nephropathy is rare, as are tophaceous deposits within the soft tissue of the elbows or digits (Fig. 83–6).

Patients with right-to-left shunts are at risk for paradoxical emboli leading to cerebrovascular accidents, renal impairment, or myocardial infarction. Septic emboli can cause cerebral abscesses and should be considered in the cyanotic patient with fever and neurologic symptoms. Air filters should be used with intravenous lines and chronic indwelling venous catheters should be avoided. Anticoagulation may be considered in patients who must have chronic indwelling lines. Promising advances have occurred over the past decade in the treatment of pulmonary hypertension. The Breathe-5 trial, a prospective randomized clinical trial, revealed in

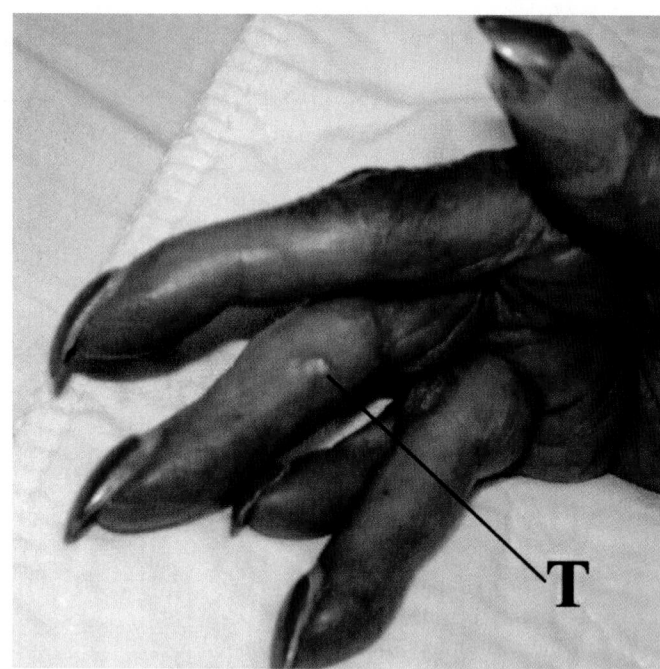

FIGURE 83–6. A 59-year-old female with pulmonary hypertension, a large ASD, cyanosis, and hyperuricemia. Note the cyanosis and clubbing of the digits. A tophaceous urate deposit (T) is noted on the middle phalanx of the second digit.

Eisenmenger syndrome that bosentan (a nonselective endothelin antagonist) decreased pulmonary and systemic vascular resistance, increased pulmonary blood flow, and increased 6-minute walk distance over a period of 16 weeks.[31] Serum BNP is a prognostic marker in systolic and diastolic heart failure, as well as pulmonary hypertension. Serum BNP is elevated in patients with Eisenmenger syndrome; an outpatient level ≥250 pg/mL in clinically euvolemic patients predicts impending heart failure admission or death.[32]

INFECTIVE ENDOCARDITIS

Patients with CHD (corrected or uncorrected) are often at risk for developing infective endocarditis (see Tables 83–1 and 83–2). Guidelines from the European Society of Cardiology and the American Heart Association's (AHA) *Special Report on Prevention of Infective Endocarditis* place patients with prosthetic valves, cyanosis, systemic or pulmonary artery conduits, and previous endocarditis into a "high-risk" subgroup.[33,34] Most other CHD conditions are at "moderate risk" with the exception of patients that have undergone surgical repair of atrial septal defect, ventricular septal defect, or patent ductus arteriosus (without residua beyond 6 months) who are considered "low risk" (provided there are no sequelae, e.g. aortic valve prolapse and/or aortic regurgitation). For moderate or high risk patients antibiotic prophylaxis is required for dental procedures. Other procedures requiring prophylaxis include respiratory, genitourinary, or gastrointestinal procedures. Those at risk for developing bacterial endocarditis should maintain the best oral health possible to reduce potential sources of bacterial seeding. A survey questionnaire of 102 adults with congenital heart disease found that patients' knowledge of their underlying condition, endocarditis risk, and prevention measures was inadequate.[35] There is an underrecognized

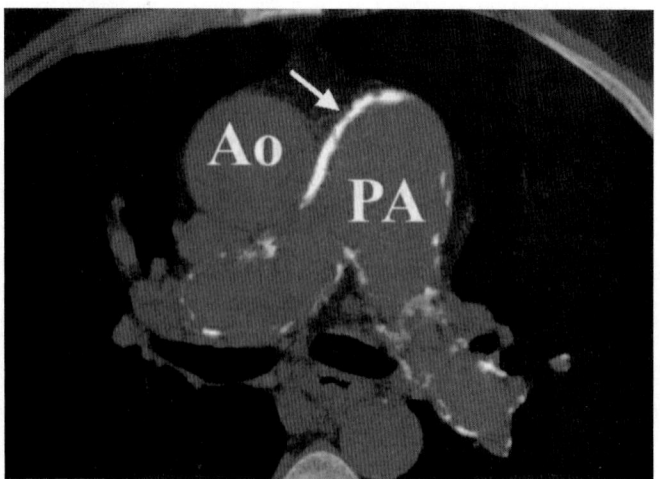

FIGURE 83–5. Noncontrast computed tomography (CT) scan of a 60-year-old man with Eisenmenger complex, demonstrating extensive white calcium deposits (*arrow*) within the walls of the pulmonary artery (PA) and branch pulmonary arteries. The ascending aorta (Ao) is labeled. Note the relative paucity of calcium in the walls of the aorta as compared to the PA.

risk of bacteremic infective endocarditis in patients who acquire tattoos or body piercings.[36] Patient education is of paramount importance. Patients should carry an information card that identifies endocarditis risk category. Symptoms of endocarditis may be subtle, including low-grade fever, malaise, fatigue, and headache. Diagnosis of endocarditis should be entertained in CHD patients with unexplained fever or malaise. Echocardiography is an integral tool in the diagnosis and followup of patients with infective endocarditis.[37] Transesophageal echocardiography is recommended in cases with high clinical suspicion but equivocal or negative findings on transthoracic echocardiography or when a prosthetic valve or conduit is involved.[38] Injudicious use of antibiotics without prior blood cultures often makes the culprit organism more difficult to culture and appropriate treatment delayed or more difficult. A 2005 AHA Scientific Statement delineates recommendations for the diagnosis and management of infective endocarditis.[37]

【 】 ELECTROPHYSIOLOGIC PROBLEMS

Arrhythmias and conduction defects are common in operated and unoperated CHD and have a major impact on survival and quality of life. The principles for diagnosis and treatment of arrhythmias are similar to those in patients with anatomically normal hearts, with some notable exceptions. Atrial rhythm disturbances that may be benign and well tolerated with a rate control strategy in a structurally normal heart may be poorly tolerated in complex congenital heart disease. This is exemplified by patients with functional single ventricle who have undergone total cavopulmonary (Fontan) connection in whom atrial tachyarrhythmias result in deleterious hemodynamics, decreased cardiac output, and functional deterioration despite adequate rate control.[39] Bradyarrhythmias are common in certain subsets (e.g., congenitally or surgically corrected transposition of the great arteries). The clinical significance of arrhythmias is greatly dependent on the hemodynamic context in which they occur.

Sinus node dysfunction (SND) is common in adults with CHD. Surgically corrected ASDs, particularly sinus venosus type are at increased risk of postoperative SND because of the proximity of the ASDs to the sinus node.[40] Uncorrected ASDs causing right atrial volume overload and right atrial stretch undergo a process of electrical remodeling with increases in effective refractory period, conduction delay at the crista terminalis, and SND. Conduction delay at the crista terminalis persists beyond ASD closure and may contribute to the long-term atrial arrhythmia substrate.[41] Surgeries that involve extensive atrial reconstruction (e.g., Senning or Mustard atrial switch operation for complete transposition of the great arteries; see Fig. 83–2) are particularly prone to SND. A retrospective study of 137 patients after Mustard or Senning operation revealed nearly 50 percent of patients had SND; the presence of SND did not influence mortality.[42] Frequency of SND is increased after corrective surgery for tetralogy of Fallot, placement of cavopulmonary shunt, and numerous other congenital heart operations. High grade atrioventricular (AV) node block is a well-recognized problem in congenitally corrected transposition of the great arteries; many patients are first diagnosed in adulthood when they present with heart block. Injury to the AV node and ventricular conduction tissue may result from surgery for lesions such as ventricular septal defect, tetralogy of Fallot, and mitral or tricuspid

valve repair or replacement. Transient complete AV block in the postoperative period carries prognostic significance, especially if the induced block is below the bundle of His.[43] Postoperative right bundle-branch block is frequent after right ventriculotomy and is likely secondary to transsection of distal Purkinje fibers and postsurgical scarring creating an area of slowed conduction and a substrate for reentrant ventricular arrhythmias.[44,45] Bradycardia has been postulated as the cause of death in some conditions but tachyarrhythmia is the more likely culprit. Bradycardia is a well recognized substrate for initiation of tachycardia.[46] Pacemaker implantation in asymptomatic SND or conduction system disease is controversial because the arrhythmia is benign in most cases. Patients who are asymptomatic with low levels of activity may become symptomatic with greater levels of exertion. ECG-stress testing identifies patients with chronotropic incompetence leading to decreased exercise capacity. Pacemaker implantation may be challenging in patients with complex underlying or post-operative anatomy.[47] Choice of pacemaker depends on the specific indication. In patients with isolated SND, a single atrial lead suffices. Single-site ventricular pacing causes dyssynchrony and progressive dysfunction; a problem that may be ameliorated by multisite ventricular pacing.[48]

Atrial tachyarrhythmias are common in patients who have undergone atrial surgery and in patients in whom atrioventricular valve disease or shunts lead to atrial volume and/or pressure overload. Scar-mediated reentrant atrial flutter is a common theme after many forms of atrial reconstruction. The various modifications of the Fontan operation are a response to the high incidence of poorly tolerated atrial tachyarrhythmias after right atrial-to-pulmonary artery Fontan repairs (Fig. 83–7).[39,49] Cardioversion should be carried out promptly to restore sinus rhythm; maintenance antiarrhythmic medications may be necessary. Surgical cryoablation and transvenous catheter ablation aided by electroanatomic mapping can be useful as therapeutic interventions in atrial tachyarrhythmias.[50–52] Electroanatomic mapping and radiofrequency ablation in CHD represent some of the most challenging procedures because of the complex pre- and postsurgical anatomy, chamber dilation, variable anatomy of the conduction system, and presence of intracardiac scars.

Ventricular arrhythmias occur in a variety of settings, particularly after tetralogy of Fallot repairs. The first generation of intracardiac repairs were performed via anterior ventriculotomy and frequently included placement of a transannular patch. This technique relieved the outflow tract obstruction but caused pulmonary regurgitation. The adverse hemodynamic effects of severe pulmonary regurgitation may become evident. After two or more decades, the right ventricle dilates, wall stress increases, and systolic and diastolic dysfunction ensue. Ventricular tachycardia (VT) may arise from the region of the transannular patch or ventriculotomy site. Programmed ventricular stimulation induced monomorphic or polymorphic VT is of prognostic importance.[53] In 793 patients with repaired tetralogy of Fallot followed for 21 years, VT occurred in 4.2 percent and sudden cardiac death occurred in 2 percent of patients.[14] QRS width on ECG has additive prognostic value; 88 percent of patients with VT and 63 percent of patients with sudden death had a QRS duration >180 milliseconds (see Fig. 83–15A).[14] The presence of VT (spontaneous or induced, monomorphic or polymorphic) in moderate/severe pulmonary regurgitation dictates

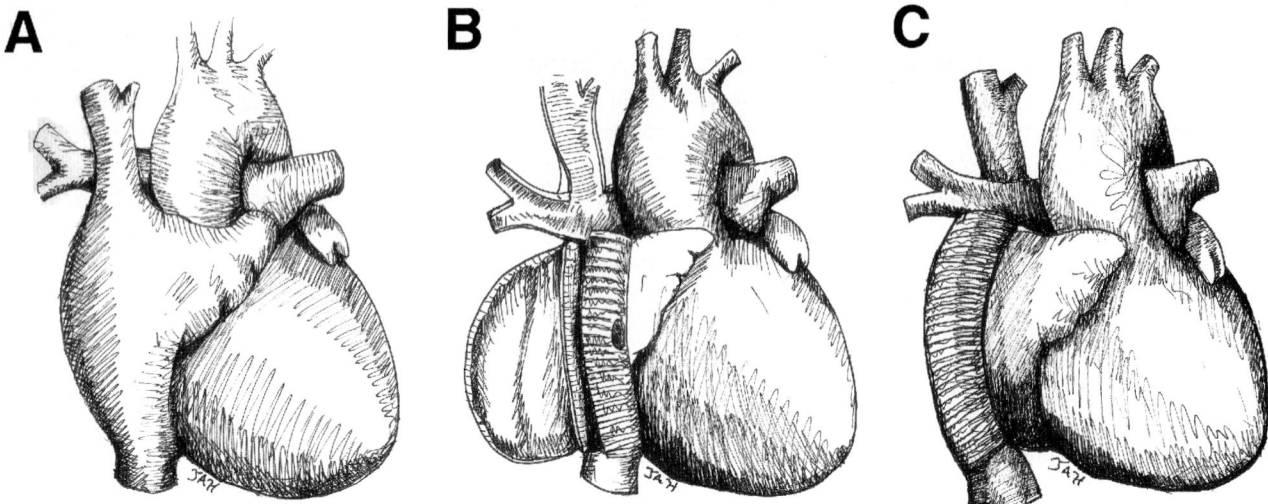

FIGURE 83–7. Various modifications of the Fontan operation. **A.** Right atrial-to-pulmonary artery Fontan connection with the right atrial appendage directly sutured to the main pulmonary artery in a patient with tricuspid and pulmonary atresia. **B.** The lateral-tunnel Fontan in which a synthetic material (e.g., Gore-Tex) is used to extend a tunnel along the inside lateral wall of right atrium to the right pulmonary artery (RPA) and the superior vena cava (SVC) is sutured directly to the right pulmonary artery. Note the fenestration in the wall of the synthetic conduit allowing right-to-left shunting and depressurization of the lateral tunnel at the expense of systemic desaturation. **C.** Extracardiac Fontan is the current standard. The entire right atrium is bypassed by a synthetic graft from the inferior vena cava directly to the RPA. The SVC is sutured directly to the RPA.

pulmonary valve replacement and ventricular scar excision. Transvenous radiofrequency ablation is feasible in patients with repaired tetralogy of Fallot who have VT and do not require valve or conduit replacement.[54–56] Transvenous defibrillator placement may be considered in those who continue to have inducible VT or spontaneous VT despite ablation or surgical repair. Prophylactic antiarrhythmic therapy has not demonstrated efficacy in asymptomatic patients. Identification of asymptomatic individuals at risk for VT or sudden cardiac death remains a challenge. A wide QRS (>180 milliseconds) on the surface ECG is a marker for increased risk but has low predictive accuracy in individual cases.[57] Further refinements in risk stratification are necessary and may involve electrophysiologic testing, exercise testing, evaluation of ventricular late potentials using signal-averaged ECG, heart rate variability, and presence of repolarization abnormalities.[58–60]

【 】 PREGNANCY

An increasing number of women with complex congenital heart disease survive into adulthood as a result of the surgical advancements of the past five decades. Thus, an increasing number of women with complex congenital heart disease reach childbearing age and are capable of reproducing. Pregnancy counseling is mandatory for all patients. Maternal and fetal risks of pregnancy and transmitted risk of congenital heart disease should be discussed, preferably prior to pregnancy. Evaluation includes a detailed medical and social history with specific attention to functional capacity, an important prognostic determinant of maternal and fetal outcomes.[61,62] Among risk factors for adverse outcomes, advanced New York Heart Association (NYHA) functional class and history of heart failure are well recognized. The detrimental effects of smoking include increases in systemic vascular resistance, systemic blood pressure, pulmonary artery pressure and vascular resistance, atrial pressures, heart rate, and arrhythmias.[63,64] Impaired ventricular function is associated with adverse maternal and fetal outcomes.[61,62]

The maternal cardiovascular system undergoes a myriad of changes during pregnancy that include a doubling of intravascular volume and cardiac output accompanied by a fall in systemic vascular resistance. Obstructive lesions are less well tolerated than regurgitant lesions or shunts. Severe aortic valve stenosis may be well tolerated if left ventricular function is not impaired.[62] Once left ventricular systolic function deteriorates, pregnancy becomes hazardous; the maternal mortality rate with a depressed ejection fraction and severe aortic stenosis is 5.9 percent.[62] Patients with severe pulmonary regurgitation and decreased subpulmonary ventricular function are at increased risk for adverse outcomes.[61] Heart failure and arrhythmia are major complications of pregnancy in patients with various congenital heart diseases. Patients who have undergone the Fontan operation tolerate pregnancy well but have increased risk of miscarriage.[65] Patients with repaired tetralogy of Fallot, depressed right ventricular function, and severe pulmonary regurgitation, are at an increased risk of adverse events.[66] Thirteen percent of patients have cardiac complications. Decreased left ventricular systolic function and pulmonary hypertension are similarly correlated with poor maternal and fetal outcomes.

Patients with cyanosis face the most problems in carrying a fetus to term and pregnancy is strongly advised against (Table 83–3).[67] The incidence of early spontaneous abortion is proportional to the severity of cyanosis. In a study by Presbitero et al., only 12 percent of pregnancies in women with an oxygen saturation less than 85 percent resulted in livebirths.[67] Eisenmenger syndrome carries a 50 percent risk of maternal mortality.[68] There is scant data on the best way to manage a patient seen late in pregnancy when safe termination is infeasible. Vaginal delivery is generally preferable because it results in less blood loss than cesarean delivery. It is our practice at the Ahmanson/UCLA Adult Congenital Heart Disease Center to

TABLE 83–3

Fetal Outcome in Cyanotic Congenital Heart Disease and Its Relation with Maternal Cyanosis

HEMOGLOBIN (G/DL)[a]	PREGNANCY (NO.)	LIVEBIRTHS (NO.)	LIVEBORN (%)
≤16	28	20	71
17–19	40	18	45
≥20	26	2	8
ARTERIAL OXYGEN SATURATION (%)[b]	PREGNANCY (NO.)	LIVEBIRTHS (NO.)	LIVEBORN (%)
≤85	17	2	12
85–89	22	10	45
≥90	13	12	92

[a]Hemoglobin level unknown in two pregnancies.
[b]Arterial oxygen saturation unknown in 44 pregnancies.
SOURCE: From Presbitero P, Somerville J, Stone S, et al. Pregnancy in cyanotic congenital heart disease: outcome of mother and fetus. Circulation 1994;89:2673–2676. Reproduced with permission from the publisher and authors.

advise our cyanotic patients against becoming pregnant and advise pregnancy termination if this is acceptable to the patient.

Patients with tissue abnormalities of the aorta, the worst extreme being Marfan syndrome, are at increased risk of aortic dissection or rupture if the ascending aorta is dilated (>40 mm).[69,70] Bicuspid aortic valves, independent of degree of valvular stenosis, demonstrate abnormalities of the ascending aorta media, a substrate for increased risk. β Blockers, usually well tolerated in the peripartum period, may decrease the risk of aortic dissection or rupture. Severe valvular aortic stenosis places both mother and fetus at risk as the fall in systemic vascular resistance and large volume shifts during pregnancy and postpartum results in exaggerated valve gradients and increased filling pressure.[71] Minimization of vascular volume and resistance alterations can be accomplished by avoidance of large intravenous volume infusions, avoidance of anesthetics known to decrease systemic vascular resistance, and adequate pain control to blunt increases in systemic blood pressure. Patients with severe aortic stenosis and congestive heart failure may require balloon valvuloplasty but balloon dilatation of a calcified aortic valve can lead to severe poorly tolerated aortic regurgitation. Pregnant patients with heavily calcified valves and significant aortic regurgitation who are in congestive heart failure or are hemodynamically unstable, may require surgical valve placement and cesarean delivery of the fetus.[72]

Management of pregnant women with mechanical valve prostheses is challenging for a number of reasons. Pregnant women are inherently hypercoagulable and the risk of valve thrombosis is increased, thus necessitating appropriate anticoagulation.[73,74] Oral warfarin accomplishes this task well, but it is teratogenic, especially in the first trimester.[75] Unfractionated heparin can be given subcutaneously twice a day or as a continuous intravenous infusion; even with meticulous control there is still an increased risk of valve thrombosis.[73,76] Subcutaneous low-molecular-weight heparin is more effective but requires frequent anti-Xa level monitoring.[73] Some authors have advocated the use of low-dose warfarin

throughout pregnancy because of the low risk of teratogenicity provided the dose is <5 mg/d.[74]

Hemodynamic deterioration during and following labor can be minimized by avoidance of rapid volume and/or pressure shifts. Planned induction 1 to 2 weeks before the expected term minimizes the risk of spontaneous labor and delivery. Invasive hemodynamic monitoring has not been shown to favorably effect outcomes and is often reserved for the highest risk subsets. Vaginal delivery is recommended unless there are obstetric contraindications. The use of antibiotics for endocarditis prophylaxis following rupture of membranes is controversial yet most cardiologists recommend antibiotics under these circumstances for patients at intermediate or high risk for developing infective endocarditis (see Tables 83–1 and 83–2).

GENETIC COUNSELING

CHD is the leading cause of birth defects and noninfectious mortality in the first year of life.[77] The etiology of CHD is multifactorial; genetic and environmental factors each may play an important role. Chemical teratogens (e.g., retinoic acid or lithium) or viral infections (e.g., rubella) are known to increase the risk of CHD. Genetic factors include increased incidence of CHD in patients with chromosomal abnormalities. Most defects are not part of a syndrome and most patients have no family history of CHD. Seemingly sporadic cases of CHD have an increased likelihood of CHD recurrence in subsequent pregnancies, supporting a genetic predisposition; 8 percent of CHD cases are caused by inherited genetic abnormalities.[78] In 6640 pregnancies with a first-degree family history of CHD, the incidence of CHD in pregnancies referred because of sibling CHD and paternal CHD was 2 to 3 percent.[79] There was a similar incidence of CHD for pregnancies referred because of maternal CHD (2.9 percent) or paternal CHD (2.2 percent). In 1094 patients with CHD, risk of CHD in the offspring of mothers with CHD was 5.7 percent versus 2.2 percent for fathers with CHD.[80] This study did challenge the polygenic basis for all forms of congenital heart disease by demonstrating that atrioventricular septal defect is a single-gene defect and tetralogy of Fallot is a polygenic disorder with a small number of interacting genes. The risk of recurrence of CHD increases with the number of affected siblings or relatives.[81] The molecular mechanisms leading to CHD are complex and the causes of the cardiac malformations observed in humans are still unclear.

DIAGNOSTIC CATHETERIZATION AND IMAGING

Cardiac catheterization with angiocardiography, the historical "gold standard" for hemodynamic and anatomic diagnosis of CHD, is challenged by the current array of noninvasive imaging techniques.

Transthoracic echocardiography with spectral Doppler and color-flow imaging is the most widely used and cost-effective tool for diagnostic imaging. Two-dimensional (and now three-dimensional) echocardiography is portable and provides a plethora of anatomic and functional data quickly, at relatively low cost without radiation. Continuous, pulse wave, and color-flow Doppler add incremental value for quantifying valvar pathology, estimating intracardiac pressure gradients, and diastolic parameters. Tissue Doppler quantitates myocardial velocities and ventricular electromechanical synchrony. Tissue Doppler and speckle tracking for determination of ventricular strain and torsion provide information regarding ventricular systolic and diastolic function.[82] The Achilles heel of transthoracic echocardiography is difficult image acquisition in some patients (e.g., obese patients or those

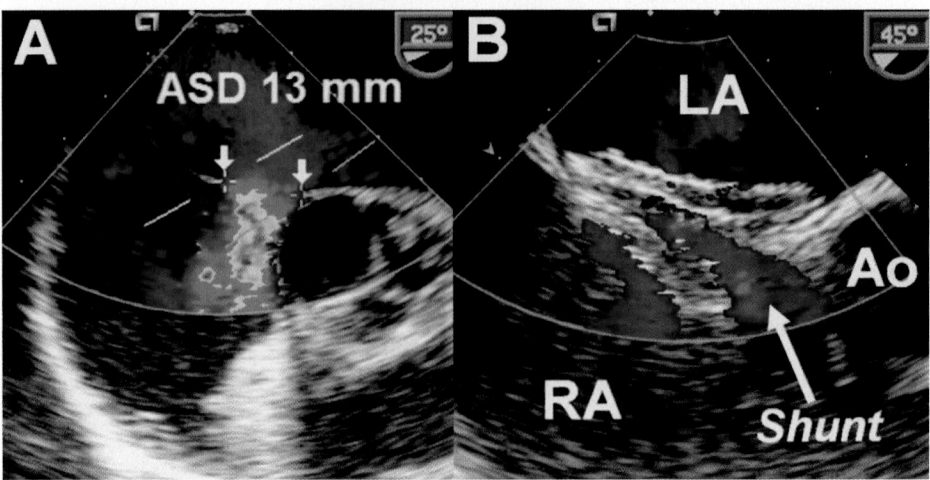

FIGURE 83–8. A. Transesophageal two-dimensional echocardiography with color-flow Doppler demonstrating a 13-mm secundum atrial septal defect (ASD) with a thin posterior rim and an absent anterior (retroaortic) rim. Note the left-to-right shunt (blue color-flow Doppler signal) across the ASD. **B.** The same patient following ASD closure of the ASD with an Amplatzer Septal Occluder. A small central left-to-right shunt (*white arrow*) from the left atrium (LA) to the right atrium (RA) is a common finding following device closure. The shunt usually resolves within a few weeks as the device endothelializes. Ao, aorta.

with chest wall abnormalities). Posterior cardiac structures, such as pulmonary veins, are often inadequately visualized. Transesophageal echocardiography overcomes the hurdles of transthoracic echocardiography for visualization of pulmonary venous anatomy, atrial anatomy, AV valve morphology, ventricular outflow tract lesions, and vegetations or thrombi. Intraoperative transesophageal echocardiography is particularly helpful during repair of congenital defects. In parallel with the decreasing need for diagnostic catheterization, there has been a dramatic increase in the number of transcatheter cardiac interventions in patients with CHD.[83] The majority of secundum ASDs can now be closed via transcatheter delivery of a closure device (Fig. 83–8). The success of percutaneous transcatheter closure of ASDs is contingent on proper patient selection.[84] Transesophageal echocardiography is widely used to assess the size, shape, and rim adequacy of ASDs, as well as to exclude the presence of atrial thrombi or anomalous pulmonary venous connection.

Cardiovascular magnetic resonance imaging (MRI) provides incremental anatomic and functional data in CHD. Magnetic resonance angiography (MRA) is invaluable in identifying the size, course, and degree of obstruction of medium to large vascular structures. Velocity mapping and flow quantification provide hemodynamic data, such as the volume of pulmonary valve regurgitation per cardiac cycle.[85] Gradient echocardiography cine-MRI provides information regarding ventricular systolic and diastolic wall motion, segmental strain, and ventricular volumes.[86,87] Myocardial fibrosis detected by late gadolinium enhancement MRI is common in patients with repaired tetralogy of Fallot.[88] The degree of late gadolinium enhancement is related to adverse clinical markers, including ventricular dysfunction, exercise intolerance, neurohormonal activation, and arrhythmia. MRA of the coronary arteries is feasible, however, imaging beyond the proximal coronary tree is suboptimal. Metallic structures, such as stents or valves, alter the local magnetic field and result in artifacts limiting the usefulness of MRI in this subset of patients. The presence of a permanent pacemaker or defibrillator is considered a relative contraindication for cardiac MRI.

Cardiac computed tomography (CT) is a widely used method for defining anatomy. ECG-gated electron beam and multidetector CT provide tomographic two-dimensional data that can be sculpted into three-dimensional images, thus clarifying complex anatomy. MRI tomographic images can similarly be reconstructed into three-dimensional structures. Computed tomography angiography (CTA) is gaining acclaim and experiencing exponential growth because of its capability to visualize the coronary arterial tree, with a high sensitivity, specificity, and negative predictive value for identifying obstructive coronary disease.[89] CTA has another advantage in that it does not require as much specialized training and technical knowledge as MRI. For these reasons, CT angiography is set to become the method of choice for noninvasive cardiovascular angiography in community practice, whereas cardiac MRI remains confined to specialized regional centers despite certain advantages of MRI over CT, such as the lack of radiation exposure and superiority in the provision of functional information. Moreover, cardiac CT can be performed in the presence of metallic structures or pacemakers.

Cardiac catheterization with angiocardiography remains the gold standard method for identifying anatomy, quantifying shunts, and measuring hemodynamics. Although the less-invasive methods described above often obviate the need for invasive evaluation, there are circumstances that necessitate invasive evaluation. These include cases in which the noninvasive techniques give inconsistent or conflicting data, and cases where exact pressures and resistances must be measured. For example, patients with single-ventricle physiology may be candidates for the Fontan operation if certain hemodynamic and functional criteria are met (Table 83–4).

【 】 STRESS TESTING

Exercise and pharmacologic stress testing provides prognostic information regarding maximum exercise capacity, cardiopulmonary reserve, and chronotropic capacity.[19,90] Exercise capacity is generally depressed in adults with congenital heart disease, and most drastically

TABLE 83-4

Criteria for Performance of the Fontan Operation at the Ahmanson-UCLA Adult Congenital Heart Disease Center

Morphologic criteria
Single ventricle with pulmonary stenosis/atresia
A hypoplastic ventricle that precludes biventricular repair
Hemodynamic criteria
Pulmonary arterial mean pressure <15 mmHg
Pulmonary arterial mean pressure up to 22 mmHg if $Q_p:Q_s$ >2:1 or if aortic saturation reaches 85%, provided the pulmonary vascular resistance is <4–5 Wood units × m2
Normal or mildly decreased ventricular systolic function (LV ejection fraction ≥50%, RV ejection fraction ≥40%)
No more than mild atrioventricular valve regurgitation
Ventricular end-diastolic pressure ≤12 mmHg

TABLE 83-5

Discriminating Gas Exchange Measurements during Exercise in Patients with Cyanotic Congenital Heart Disease

Low peak VO_2
Low AT
Reduced phase I VO_2
Increased ventilatory response to exercise (V_E/VCO_2)
Immediate worsening of hypoxemia at start of exercise

AT, anaerobic threshold; VCO_2, venous carbon dioxide production; V_E, minute ventilation; VO_2, volume of oxygen consumption.

so in patients with Eisenmenger syndrome (see Fig. 83–4). Cardiopulmonary exercise testing adds incremental diagnostic and prognostic information in patients with CHD. Maximum oxygen consumption (VO_2max) is decreased in patients with CHD (see Fig. 83–4). Poor exercise capacity identifies adult CHD patients who are at risk for hospitalization or death. Cyanotic patients with right-to-left shunts fail to demonstrate a normal increase in pulmonary blood flow with exercise. The systemic arterial resistance decreases with no appreciable change in pulmonary arterial resistance resulting in worsening cyanosis. Chemoreceptors located at the bifurcation of the internal and external carotid arteries detect this hypoxia, and via a complex feedback mechanism involving the respiratory control centers of the brain stem, increase the minute ventilation resulting in hyperventilation during exercise (Table 83–5). Ventilatory response to exercise is abnormal across the spectrum of CHD but is most markedly abnormal in cyanotic patients irrespective of pulmonary arterial hypertension. An increased ratio of minute ventilation to CO_2 production (volume of expired gas [V_E]/carbon dioxide elimination [VCO_2]) slope is a strong exercise predictor of death in noncyanotic CHD patients.[20] Submaximal exercise capacity as measured by six minute walk distance is used widely and is of prognostic importance in patients with pulmonary arterial hypertension and correlates closely with peak oxygen consumption (VO_2).

PSYCHOSOCIAL ASPECTS

As the patient with congenital heart disease makes the transition from adolescence to adulthood it is imperative that the patient understand the nature and implications of his or her heart problem and what interventions have or need to be performed. Appropriate advice and guidance should be available regarding employment, insurance, socialization, contraception, and exercise.

❚ ❱ EMPLOYMENT

Most operated and unoperated patients can be gainfully employed. Patients with simple forms of CHD, such as isolated ven-

tricular septal defect, pulmonary stenosis, or aortic valve stenosis, often achieve higher levels of education than the national standards.[91] In Holland, adults with complex CHD had reduced job participation compared with patients with mild CHD (59 percent vs. 76 percent employed).[92] Many receive disability benefits or experience career problems or job handicaps. Adults with CHD are at a disadvantage when applying for employment because of the tendency of some employers to consider the potential for future deterioration of an applicant with a "known heart problem."

Restrictions for employment do exist for certain jobs in which the safety of others is the direct responsibility of the patient with CHD. It is the task of the CHD specialist to estimate the risk of acute disability or sudden cardiac death in such patients. Low risk rates are defined in only a small subset of patients with CHD.[93]

❚ ❱ INSURANCE

Adults with CHD are significantly more likely to have difficulty obtaining life insurance.[94] This problem is compounded by the limited long-term survival data for specific CHD subtypes. Vonder Muhl et al. discuss this problem and provide a summary of mortality data and predictors of adverse outcomes in various subsets of CHD along with practical tips for patients and physicians to assist with the insurance application process.[95] In general, insurance policies are restrictive and patients with CHD are frequently insured at higher rates or not at all.[96] Transition from adolescence to adulthood is difficult enough for many with CHD and is often more difficult with cessation of health insurance under a parent's policy. As a result, the patient must seek a new policy, which often excludes benefits for treatment of the congenital cardiovascular condition. Moons et al. showed that patients with CHD incur a considerably higher expense than age- and sex-matched controls. This difference was accounted for by a minority of patients with dilated left ventricles, decreased functional capacity, females, and older patients.[97]

❚ ❱ PSYCHOSOCIAL DEVELOPMENT

Utens et al. compared the occurrence of behavioral and emotional problems in 166 young adults long-term after surgical correction to the occurrence in age-matched controls.[98] No relationship was found between cardiac diagnosis and problem behaviors in CHD adults. Moreover, no relationship was found between IQ scores and problem behaviors. Psychosocial problems can occur in patients with CHD, manifesting in excessive psychologic stress that is not related to the clinical severity of the original cardiac defect.[99] In a study by Ternestedt et al., two cohorts of patients who were operated on before the age of 15 years, one for tetralogy of Fallot and the other for ASD, were queried 20 and 30 years after surgical repair regarding their quality of life.[100] There was no connection between quality of life and functional capacity. Multiple questionnaire-based studies have demonstrated that the severity of the heart disease is not necessarily congruent with estimated quality of life, which suggests that patients develop coping strategies during childhood and adolescence.

Although most patients with CHD appear well adjusted, many believe that they are different from their peers and suffer from fear of isolation and low self-esteem; feelings that are compounded by exercise limitation, surgical scars, and parental overprotection. A number of large longitudinal series of patients with repaired tetralogy of Fallot have demonstrated that suicide is a common cause of late death, ranging in frequency from 4.8 percent to 10 percent.[101–103] Psychosocial anxiety and neurotic behavior may be avoided by early repair in childhood.[104] Anxieties about sexuality, relationships, and reproduction are common and often prove difficult to adequately discuss with the physician in a busy clinic setting; such issues are more thoroughly dealt with by a multispecialty team, which might include a psychologist, social worker, and nurse practitioner. Psychological support should be considered as one of the most important aspects in long-term care of patients with CHD.

The impact of CHD on intellectual development appears more dependent on lesion type and severity than on psychosocial issues. Although cyanosis is associated with mild intellectual impairment, it is unclear whether early repair of cyanotic lesions, such as tetralogy of Fallot, results in improved intellectual function.[105,106] Neurodevelopmental outcomes in patients with single-ventricle physiology who have undergone the Fontan operation are in the normal range, but performance on examinations of IQ are lower than in the general population.[107]

【 】 CONTRACEPTION

Advice regarding contraception should be available to adolescent and adult patients with CHD.[108] Unfortunately, contraceptive advice to patients with CHD is often inadequate or incorrect.[109] When giving family planning advice, it is important to weigh the risk of pregnancy (if the affected patient is a woman), risk of CHD in the fetus, and the risk of contraception. Understanding the normal physiology of pregnancy and its impact on various CHD subtypes is essential (see Pregnancy above). Contraceptive advice should be tailored to the individual in terms of their medical, social, and educational conditions. Sterilization is an effective form of contraception reserved for patients who are at very high risk of adverse events with pregnancy. Laparoscopic sterilization requires general anesthesia, placing the cyanotic patient at significant risk for operative mortality.[30] Hormonal contraception with low-dose estrogen is generally safe and effective.[110] Combined estrogen and progesterone formulations have a lower contraceptive efficacy, carry a risk of thromboembolic complications, and are best avoided in patients with previous thromboembolic events and in patients who are at high risk of thromboembolic events (e.g., pa-

tients with Fontan connection and sluggish venous flow).[111,112] They are also inappropriate for patients with congestive heart failure because of the tendency for fluid retention. Barrier methods, such as diaphragm or condom, are generally safe but less effective and can only be relied upon in the motivated patients. Intrauterine contraceptive devices are effective, however, they are associated with an increased risk of pelvic inflammatory disease.

EXERCISE AND SPORTS

The physical and mental benefits of exercise are established. Participation in sports is important for the normal socialization of children and adolescents. Patients with CHD often have diminished exercise capacity (see Fig. 83–4).[19] Reduced exercise capacity may reflect both the limitations of the underlying cardiovascular condition and of the deconditioning from adopting a sedentary lifestyle. Inappropriate avoidance of exercise is often reinforced by protective parents, or recommended by physicians who are unsure of the cardiovascular risk associated with a specific condition and choose to err on the side of short-term caution.

The 26th Bethesda Conference on exercise in cardiovascular disease provided exercise recommendations for this population.[113] In patients with simple, repaired CHD, exercise capacity is normal and the risk of exercise is minimal. At the other extreme are patients with pulmonary vascular disease and cyanosis in whom exercise capacity is severely limited. Exercise results in almost immediate worsening of hypoxia because of the fall in systemic arterial resistance and increased shunting of deoxygenated blood away from the pulmonary alveolar bed. These patients should be advised to avoid isometric exercise and confine themselves to mild isotonic exercise. All recommendations should take into account the individual's cardiovascular defect, functional capacity, hemodynamic status, and the form of exercise contemplated. Formal exercise testing helps delineate functional capacity. Cardiopulmonary exercise testing adds incremental diagnostic and prognostic value in patients with CHD.[19] Stress echocardiographic imaging is useful in determining ventricular and valvar function, and estimating pressure gradients with exercise.

SURGICAL AND INTERVENTIONAL CONSIDERATIONS

【 】 REOPERATIONS

Reoperations in adults with congenital heart disease are common and provide particular challenges.[114] The risks of reoperation are greater than for the primary procedures, often requiring careful entry into the chest with extensive dissection of scar tissue and longer cardiopulmonary bypass times and greater use of blood products.[115] Careful preoperative planning should include an in-depth understanding of the underlying cardiovascular anatomy and the alterations caused by previous surgical intervention. Computed tomography or magnetic resonance angiography may be used to determine the anatomic relationships and quantify the proximity of the heart to the sternum. Sternal entry is particularly risky when a high pressure ventricle, great artery, or conduit lies immediately posterior to the sternum. Moreover, these imaging modalities help identify arterial and venous collateral vessels that may need to be ligated during the course of reoperation.

[ ] INEVITABLE REOPERATION

Childhood repair of congenital heart defects that involved insertion of prosthetic valves or conduits often require reoperation. The prostheses used in the infant or child are often too small for the adult patient or they have undergone degeneration resulting in stenosis or regurgitation. Development of conduit obstruction is influenced by the type and size of the conduit as well as the timing of the original operation.[116] In the minority of patients with tetralogy of Fallot and pulmonary atresia, transannular patch placement is usually not possible and instead a valved conduit is placed from the right ventricle to the distal pulmonary trunk or confluence of the right and left pulmonary arteries. For all conduits, calcification and obstruction remain significant complications. Transthoracic echocardiography with Doppler is a valuable tool for monitoring ventricular size and function, as well as the conduit peak instantaneous and mean pressure gradient. Right-sided and anterior conduits are often not well visualized by transthoracic echocardiography and may require further imaging with CTA or MRA. Diagnostic cardiac catheterization and angiography may be needed when the degree of stenosis is unclear or there is conflicting noninvasive data. The consequences of chronic pressure overload, specifically on the right ventricle, are chamber dilation, decreased systolic function, and diastolic dysfunction. These deleterious consequences increase the risk of surgery and may not be fully reversible. Careful monitoring of ventricular size and function by transthoracic echocardiography is paramount in identifying these processes early in their course to avoid irreversible damage. Serial stress echocardiography is especially useful in estimating exercise-induced gradients, determining ventricular function with exercise, and quantifying functional capacity. Reoperation is usually indicated if the right ventricular pressure is 75 percent of the systemic pressure, if there is evidence of deteriorating ventricular function, or if functional capacity is declining.

[ ] RESIDUAL AND RECURRENT DEFECTS

Residual or recurrent defects affect long-term prognosis and attention should be paid to their presence following operative repair. As previously noted, patients with tetralogy of Fallot who have undergone early intracardiac repair with placement of a transannular patch inevitably develop pulmonary regurgitation. This represents the most common indication for reoperation in adults.[117] Indications for pulmonary valve replacement include progressive right ventricular dilation, decreasing systolic function, presence of arrhythmias, and decreasing exercise tolerance.[118]

[ ] STAGED REPAIR

In patients with complex congenital heart disease, specifically cyanotic lesions, definitive "correction" may not be possible until the anatomy and physiology have been optimized by one or more "palliative" procedures (e.g., tetralogy of Fallot with pulmonary atresia and multiple aortopulmonary collaterals). These patients frequently require complex "unifocalization" of aortopulmonary

collaterals, consisting of incorporation of these collaterals into a pericardial tube that receives arterial blood via a surgically created arterial shunt.[119] Although unifocalization alone has failed to show a mortality benefit, it is used as the first step in a staged repair that subsequently leads to surgical pulmonary artery connection and insertion of a conduit from the right ventricle to the pulmonary artery with concomitant VSD closure.[120,121] A one-stage repair combining unifocalization and total intracardiac repair may be an option in selected patients.[122]

Other situations in which definitive repair is delayed include patients with single-ventricle physiology who often undergo early placement of palliative arteriopulmonary shunts and pulmonary artery banding. Thereafter, these patients often undergo partial (Glenn) or total (Fontan) cavopulmonary connection if they fulfill the stringent criteria for this operation (see Table 83–4).

[ ] HEART AND HEART–LUNG TRANSPLANTATION

Heart and heart–lung (block) transplantation are ultimate therapeutic options in patients who continue to deteriorate with optimal medical therapy with no good reparative surgical options. Despite often complex anatomy, multiple previous thoracotomies, adhesions, and coexistent pulmonary vascular disease, orthotopic heart transplantation is associated with good outcomes.[123,124] Lung transplantation with repair of the cardiac defect or heart–lung transplantation for Eisenmenger syndrome has had limited success.[30,125] Given advancement in the medical treatment of pulmonary hypertension, plus the limited survival of these operations, only the sickest patients who fail to stabilize or improve on pulmonary arterial vasodilator therapy are referred for transplantation.

[ ] NONCARDIAC SURGERY

An awareness of the significance of various repaired or unrepaired congenital lesions is imperative for the safe management during and following noncardiac surgery. The anesthetic and bleeding risks encountered for cardiovascular operations also apply to noncardiac surgery. Many with CHD have increased risk for arrhythmias that may be exacerbated by sympathomimetic agents and elevated catecholamine levels. Anesthetic agents that depress ventricular function must be used with care. Patients with poor cardiac function or Fontan connections have prolonged circulation time and may not respond as quickly to intravenous agents as will other patients. This should be taken into account when monitoring the effect of anesthetics and titrating medication doses. The surgeon must also be aware of the potential presence of a pacemaker or defibrillator and pacing leads that may affect the safety of electric cautery. Infective endocarditis prophylaxis is often indicated (see Tables 83–1 and 83–2). With pulmonary vascular disease, general anesthesia may result in a sudden fall in systemic vascular resistance and hypotension.[126] Avoidance of vasodilating anesthetic agents is recommended. Cyanotic patients often have impaired hemostasis with bleeding disorders. Particle filters on intravenous lines in intracardiac shunts are imperative to prevent systemic embolization. The safety of noncardiac surgery is greatly increased when procedures are performed by physicians familiar with these issues in conjunction with consultation by an adult CHD specialist.

[ ] TRANSCATHETER INTERVENTIONS

Major advances in percutaneous transcatheter interventions have been made over the past 25 years in the field of congenital heart disease. In 1976, King and Mills published the first report of transcatheter closure of an ASD.[127] Since then, improved device, imaging, and catheterization technologies and techniques have brought interventional cardiology to the forefront as a therapeutic intervention that may delay or obviate surgery. The advances in noninvasive cardiovascular imaging, specifically echocardiography, MRI, and CT, have made diagnostic cardiac catheterization and angiocardiography necessary in a shrinking pool of patients. These include patients who have undergone the Fontan operation or those in whom noninvasive evaluation has resulted in ambiguous or conflicting results. Adult congenital cardiac catheterizations today are often performed solely for reparative or palliative transcatheter interventions. Interventional catheterization has largely replaced surgery as the treatment of choice for a number of congenital cardiovascular conditions, including, secundum ASD, coarctation of the aorta, patent ductus arteriosus, and pulmonary artery or valve stenosis.[83] Technologies for percutaneous valve replacement are under intense clinical evaluation and results are encouraging.[128,129] Careful patient selection and imaging are imperative to the safety and success of transcatheter procedures. Noninvasive imaging helps clarify anatomy prior to intervention and can be used as a means of monitoring for sequelae or complications. For example, MRI and CT are excellent tools for defining two- and three-dimensional vascular anatomy and are ideal for imaging of the aorta after transcatheter stent deployment (Fig. 83–9). The preprocedural images are key to defining lesion anatomy and to precisely identifying neighboring structures that may be affected by the intervention.

[ ] ELECTROPHYSIOLOGIC AND DEVICE-BASED THERAPIES

The past two decades have seen the explosive growth of electrophysiology as a major diagnostic and interventional field in cardiology. Adults with congenital heart disease are often plagued by a plethora of electrophysiologic problems, namely, supraventricular tachyarrhythmias, ventricular tachycardia, and various forms of bradycardia. Therefore, the dizzying technical advancements in invasive electrophysiologic diagnostics and interventions have been of enormous benefit to patients with operated and unoperated congenital heart disease. Diagnostic electrophysiologic testing is recommended in symptomatic patients or in those in whom arrhythmias can be detected by electrocardiographic monitoring.[130]

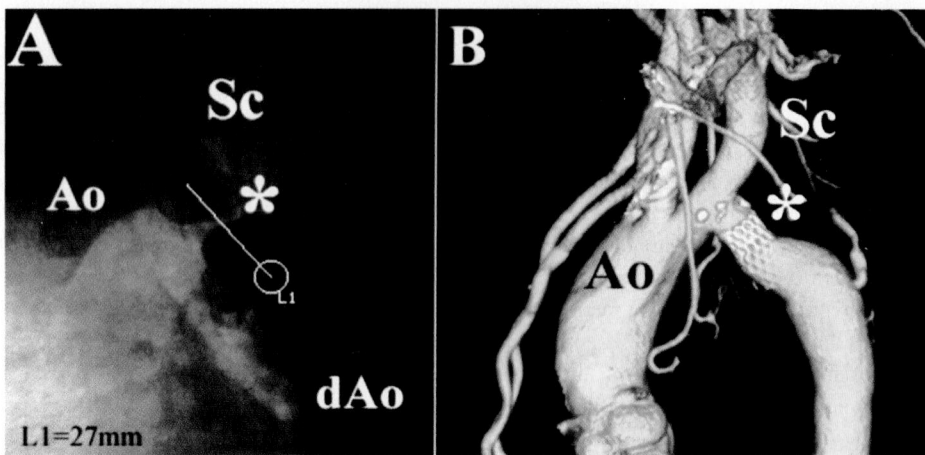

FIGURE 83–9. A. Invasive transcatheter cineangiography of a patient with severe coarctation of the aorta (*) viewed from the left anterior oblique projection. A "pigtail" catheter with side holes has been advanced from the descending aorta (dAo) to the aortic arch (Ao). L1 (27 mm) is the estimated length of stent needed to relieve the stenosis without "jailing" the dilated left subclavian artery (Sc). **B.** ECG-gated cardiovascular CT angiogram with three-dimensional reconstruction also viewed from the left anterior oblique projection. This study was performed on the same patient 6 months following stent deployment (*). The stent appears widely patent and does not intrude on the ostium of the left subclavian artery (Sc).

Transcatheter radiofrequency ablation is successful in the treatment of many supraventricular tachycardias but may be deferred in favor of surgical cryoablation in a patient requiring surgical intervention for other reasons (e.g., pulmonary valve replacement in a patient with tetralogy of Fallot). Transcatheter radiofrequency ablation is less successful in the treatment of ventricular tachycardia originating from ventriculotomy or transannular patch scar sites but should be attempted in a patient who does not require surgical valve or conduit replacement.[54,56] Transvenous defibrillator placement should be considered in patients who continue to have inducible ventricular arrhythmias or spontaneous symptomatic ventricular arrhythmias despite radiofrequency ablation or surgical repair (Fig. 83–10).[131] Electrical resynchronization via multisite ventricular pacing has demonstrated efficacy in patients with various forms of cardiomyopathy and dyssynchronous ventricular contraction. Approximately 4 to 9 percent of patients with complete or congenitally corrected transposition of the great arteries are eligible for resynchronization therapy based on degree of heart failure symptoms, ventricular systolic function, and QRS duration.[132] Initial clinical results have been favorable, but the small number of studies and the heterogeneous patient populations make definitive conclusions difficult. However, resynchronization therapy in appropriate candidates appears to improve ventricular function and clinical status.[133–135]

SPECIFIC LESIONS
[ ] ATRIAL SEPTAL DEFECT

ASDs occur in one-third of adults with congenital heart disease (Fig. 83–11). Secundum ASD present in the area of the fossa ovalis and account for 75 percent of defects. Ostium primum defects associated with endocardial cushion defects and inlet type ventricular septal defects occur in 20 percent of cases. Sinus venosus de-

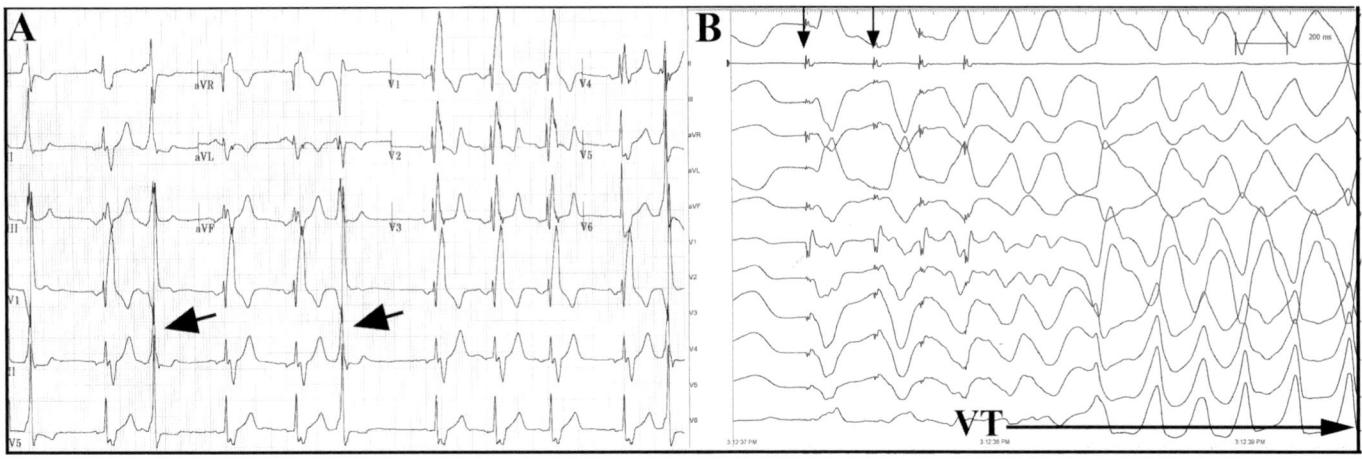

FIGURE 83-10. A. A 12-lead surface electrocardiogram of a patient with tetralogy of Fallot 23 years status post intracardiac repair with transannular patch placement who presented with syncope. The patient is in a low atrial rhythm and has a right bundle-branch block, measuring 185 milliseconds in duration. The *black arrows* indicate frequent premature ventricular complexes. **B.** Intracardiac electrogram recorded during right ventricular programmed stimulation (*small, vertical black arrows*). This pacing train initiates rapid and poorly hemodynamically tolerated ventricular tachycardia (VT).

fects (usually superior) occur in 5 percent of patients. The rarest is the coronary sinus ASD. Associated lesions include pulmonary stenosis, ventricular septal defect, mitral valve abnormalities, as well as syndromes such as Down syndrome and Holt-Oram syndrome. Most cases of ASD are sporadic but familial cases of ASD have been reported.

Natural History

ASDs often go unrecognized for two or more decades because of the indolent clinical course and benign findings on physical examination. The ECG usually demonstrates a characteristic RSR complex and a rightward QRS axis in secundum-type defects and left axis deviation in patients with primum ASD. Although survival into adulthood is the rule, life expectancy is not normal in the unrepaired patient, with mortality increasing by 6 percent per year after age 40 years.[136,137] Progressive dyspnea on exertion and palpitations frequently present in adulthood as a result of increasing right-sided chamber enlargement, pulmonary hypertension, right ventricular failure, tricuspid regurgitation, and atrial arrhythmias. The degree of left-to-right shunt augments with age as left ventricular compliance decreases and systemic arterial resistance increases. Paradoxical embolism is a rare complication. Risk of infective endocarditis is low unless there is coexistent valvar disease (Tables 83–1 and 83–2).

Management and Results

Direct surgical suture of small defects and patch closure of larger defects has been performed for more than 40 years and is efficacious and safe provided the pulmonary arterial resistance is not severely elevated.[138,139] Closure of small defects (<1 cm) in asymptomatic patients who are diagnosed after 25 years of age is controversial, given the absence of demonstrable difference in clinical outcomes between medically and surgically treated patients followed for over 20 years.[140] A retrospective study by Konstantinides et al. of 179 patients diagnosed after the age of 40 years with a Q_p/Q_s (pulmonary-to-systemic blood flow ratio) of 1.5:1 or greater demonstrated improved survival and functional capacity

over a 10-year period in the surgically corrected versus medically managed patients (95 percent vs. 84 percent).[141] Predictors of increased mortality in the surgical group included older age at operation, symptoms of heart failure, Q_p/Q_s >2.5:1, pulmonary artery systolic pressure >40 mmHg, and pulmonary vascular resistance >1.6 Wood units. Supraventricular arrhythmias occurred with similar frequency. However, the operations carried out in this study

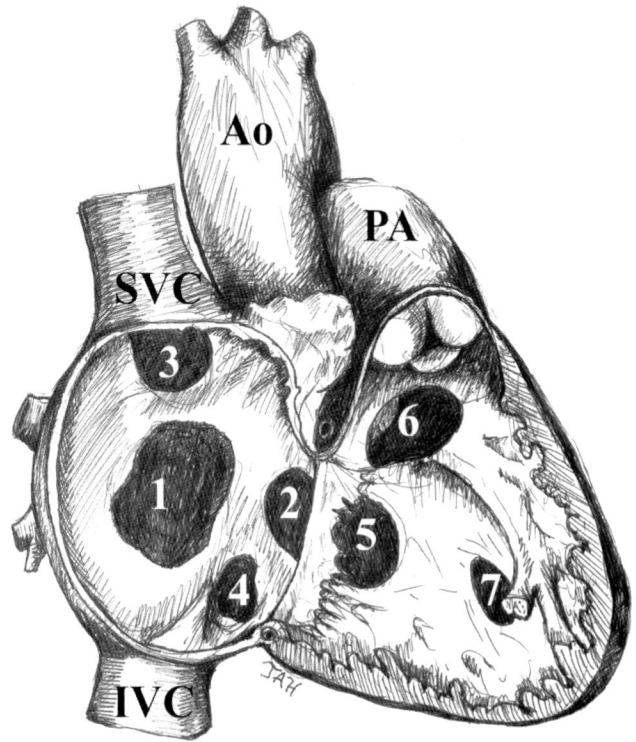

FIGURE 83-11. The various types of atrial (ASD) and ventricular (VSD) septal defects. The heart is viewed from a right anterior oblique projection and the right ventricular and right atrial free walls have been removed. 1. Secundum type ASD. 2. Primum type ASD. 3. Superior sinus venosus ASD. 4. Coronary sinus ASD. 5. Inlet type VSD. 6. Perimembranous VSD. 7. Muscular type VSD. Also labeled are the superior (SVC) and inferior (IVC) vena cavae, the aorta (Ao), and the pulmonary artery (PA).

did not include atrial arrhythmia surgery (maze or Cox-maze procedures) which is known to decrease arrhythmia recurrence in patients undergoing surgical ASD closure.[142] A prospective randomized study by Attie et al. of surgical versus medical management of ASD in 241 patients >40 years of age did not demonstrate similar survival advantages over 7 years of followup.[143] However, the incidence of nonfatal complications was reduced by surgical defect closure, leading the authors to conclude that surgical closure should be performed in all patients with an ASD and pulmonary artery systolic pressure <70 mmHg and Q_p/Q_s >1.6:1. The exclusion of patients with severe pulmonary hypertension may be obviated by pulmonary artery vasodilator therapy that may reduce pulmonary arterial pressure and resistance permitting shunt closure in these patients.[144] Severe pulmonary hypertension represents the coincidence of idiopathic pulmonary hypertension or pulmonary hypertension secondary to another process (e.g., scleroderma) and ASD.[17] Unlike patients with large nonrestrictive central shunts (e.g., VSD) who experience pulmonary hypertension from birth and develop pulmonary vascular disease within the first few years, those with large ASD of similar shunt magnitude do not necessarily develop severe pulmonary hypertension or the onset of pulmonary hypertension is delayed into late adulthood. That being said, a large ASD may well contribute to the development of pulmonary hypertension, but is rarely the sole cause of severe pulmonary vascular disease in a cyanotic patient. Patients with trisomy 21 (Down syndrome) may develop accelerated pulmonary vascular disease in the presence of ASD.

Advancements in device design and catheterization technology have led to the availability of a variety of transcatheter occlusion devices (see Fig. 83–11).[145,146] Transcatheter device closure compares favorably with surgical closure in terms of efficacy and is associated with shorter hospital stays and fewer postprocedural complications.[147] Appropriate patient selection is imperative and may be accomplished via a variety of noninvasive and/or invasive imaging methods.[148–151] Complications include device embolization, aortic root or atrial wall perforation, cardiac tamponade, thrombus formation, device erosion into the aortic root, atrial dysrhythmias, and infective endocarditis.[83] The use of platelet inhibitors for at least 6 months following device closure is recommended to decrease the risk of device thrombosis.[152] Transesophageal echocardiography is often performed within 4 weeks of device placement to identify thrombus formation. The long-term outcomes of device closure using the Amplatzer septal occluder are excellent as evidenced by no deaths and minimal complications in 151 patients followed for 6.5 years after ASD closure.[153]

【 】 VENTRICULAR SEPTAL DEFECT

Isolated VSD is the most commonly encountered form of congenital heart disease in the pediatric population (see Fig. 83–11). This is not the case in the adult population for three reasons.

1. Most children in the western world who have hemodynamically significant defects are diagnosed and undergo repair in childhood because they develop signs and symptoms of left ventricular enlargement and failure.
2. Small unrepaired perimembranous or muscular VSDs often spontaneously decrease in size or close with age. However,

small VSDs initially encountered in adulthood (age >20 years) are unlikely to close spontaneously.
3. Large nonrestrictive defects that are not surgically corrected within the first 2 years of life result in pulmonary vascular disease and increased mortality in childhood (see Fig. 83–3).

Consequently, the spectrum of isolated residual VSDs encountered in the adult patient usually consists of:

1. Small restrictive defects or defects that have closed partially. The pulmonary vascular resistance is not significantly elevated and the left-to-right shunt magnitude is mild (Q_p/Q_s ≤1.5:1). The intensity of the precordial holosystolic murmur is inversely related to the size of the defect, therefore, a disturbingly loud and harsh precordial holosystolic murmur in a patient with VSD should be viewed as a reassuring sign, not a cause for alarm.
2. Large nonrestrictive defects in cyanotic patients who have developed the Eisenmenger complex, with systemic pulmonary vascular resistance and shunt reversal (right to left).
3. Patients with moderately restrictive defects (Q_p/Q_s ≥1.6:1 and ≤2:1) who have not undergone closure. These patients often have mild to moderate pulmonary hypertension.
4. Patients who have had their defects closed in childhood. These patients may have VSD patch leaks that may be identified by careful color and two-dimensional Doppler scanning of the entire interventricular septum during echocardiographic examination.

Natural History

Small, restrictive defects of the muscular or perimembranous septum may be watched conservatively without need for operative intervention. Lifelong infective endocarditis prophylaxis is mandatory to minimize the otherwise high risk of infection (see Table 83–1). Six percent of small perimembranous defects develop aortic valve prolapse; resultant aortic regurgitation may be progressive.[154] The prolapsing aortic valve cusp may partially or completely close the VSD. Aortic valve repair or replacement may be necessary in patients with aortic regurgitation who develop exertional symptoms or progressive left ventricular dilation.[73] In a long-term followup registry, the overall survival rate was 87 percent for all patients with unoperated VSD.[155] In small defects (Q_p/Q_s <1.5 and low pulmonary artery pressure), the survival rate was 96 percent at 25 years; moderate and large defects fare worse with 25 year survival of 86 percent and 61 percent. With cyanosis, 25-year survival was 41.7 percent.

With a large, nonrestrictive VSD, pulmonary vascular disease develops soon after birth with abnormal vascular remodeling; if the VSD is not surgically repaired, obliterative pulmonary vascular disease results.[156] Systemic pulmonary vascular resistance results in a balanced bidirectional or right-to-left shunt and cyanosis. Survival is decreased in these patients, although with proper medical care and protection against certain risks (e.g., dehydration or endocarditis), survivors have been reported into the seventh decade.[30] Patients develop compensatory erythrocytosis appropriate to the decreased systemic oxygen saturation from right to left shunting of deoxygenated blood. Phlebotomy is not warranted unless patients develop symptoms of hyperviscosity (headache, visual changes) refractory to hydration.

Management and Results

Small, restrictive defects ($Q_p/Q_s \leq 1.5{:}1$ and low pulmonary artery pressure) are generally asymptomatic and should be managed conservatively and followed regularly.[155] Patients should be instructed in dental and skin care and infective endocarditis prophylaxis during bacteremic procedures. Small defects with aortic valve prolapse and aortic regurgitation may be repaired to avoid progressive aortic regurgitation.[157] Larger defects may be repaired in the absence of severe pulmonary hypertension and severely elevated pulmonary vascular resistance (>10 Wood units/m²), which incurs a high perioperative risk.[158,159] Postoperative life expectancy is not normal but has improved over the past 50 years with improved surgical techniques and experience. Postoperative conduction defects are common but complete heart block is rare in the current era. Postoperative risk of infective endocarditis is low (see Table 83–2). Transcatheter device occlusion of muscular and perimembranous VSD is feasible and early trials demonstrate a good safety and efficacy profile.[160,161] Complete heart block has been noted to occur in approximately 1 percent of patients.[161]

【 】 ATRIOVENTRICULAR SEPTAL DEFECTS

Atrioventricular septal defect is an umbrella term for endocardial cushion defects representing a spectrum of lesions involving the atrial and ventricular septum, atrioventricular valves, and the left ventricular outflow tract. Defects are classified into "partial" or "complete" forms. The "partial" form may be a primum ASD but no VSD (see Fig. 83–11). The "complete" form includes both a primum ASD and an inlet VSD (see Fig. 83–11). Deficiency of the inlet ventricular septum plus abnormalities of the AV valves (overriding, straddling, and/or cleft) produces an elongated left ventricular outflow tract described as a "goose neck" on left ventriculography. Subaortic stenosis is a common association often caused by chordal attachments of the cleft anterior mitral valve to the left ventricular outflow septum, may also occur de novo following surgical repair, as a result of a discrete fibrous membrane (Fig. 83–12).

Natural History

Approximately 5 percent of infants with congenital heart disease have AV septal defect, with two-thirds of patients having the "complete" form.[162] Trisomy 21 (Down syndrome) and other chromosomal abnormalities are frequently associated. The natural history of "partial" AV septal defect is dependent on the size of the defect; in many ways, primum ASDs behave in a similar manner to secundum ASD (see earlier). In Down syndrome, accelerated pulmonary vasculopathy may result in pulmonary hypertension at an earlier age. Mitral valve regurgitation, caused by a cleft (see Fig. 83–12), if present, leads to greater left-to-right shunt magnitude and earlier signs of pulmonary hypertension and heart failure. Complete defects unrepaired in childhood frequently develop severe pulmonary hypertension and shunt reversal characteristic of the Eisenmenger syndrome.

Management and Outcomes

Surgical repair involves patch closure of the primum ASD and VSD closure in patients with the "complete" form of AVSD. Cleft mitral valve repair should restore valvar competence without stenosis, assessment of which can be verified with intraoperative transesophageal echocardiography.[163,164] Percutaneous ASD closure of a primum defect is contraindicated given the close proximity of the defect to the tricuspid and mitral valves and the coronary sinus. Surgical mortality is 15 percent in the first 30 days postoperatively.[165] Adverse predictors of mortality include the "complete" type of AVSD, presence of pulmonary hypertension, and absence of cleft mitral valve repair. Late survival after operation in 121 patients was 80 percent at 1 year, 78 percent at 10 years, and 65 percent at 20 years. Freedom from reoperation was 91 percent at 1 year, 79 percent at 10 years, and 76 percent at 20 years. Mitral valve regurgitation necessitating valve repair or replacement was the most frequent indication for reoperation.

【 】 TETRALOGY OF FALLOT

The most common cyanotic congenital heart malformation and one of the first complex lesions to be successfully repaired, tetralogy of Fallot occurs in 7 to 10 percent of children with congenital heart disease. The four characteristic findings are (1) malaligned ventricular septal defect, (2) right ventricular outflow and/or pulmonary valve/artery stenosis or atresia, (3) dextroposed overriding aorta, and (4) right ventricular hypertrophy. In the modern era, early surgical repair, consisting of VSD closure and alleviation of right ventricular outflow obstruction, has gained favor over early palliation followed by intracardiac repair. Surgical outcomes are excellent and dramatically improve prognosis. However, these patients are not "cured" and are at significant risk of developing subsequent electrical and hemodynamic problems. Advances in imaging, medical therapy, electrophysiology, device/resynchronization

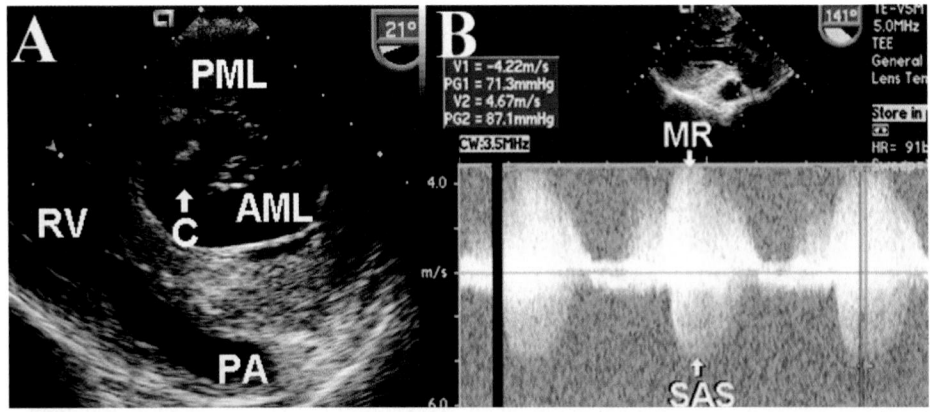

FIGURE 83–12. A. Transesophageal two-dimensional echocardiographic image as viewed from the transgastric view, demonstrating a cleft (C) in the anterior mitral leaflet (AML). Also labeled are the posterior mitral leaflet (PML), the right ventricle (RV), and the main pulmonary artery (PA). **B.** Continuous-wave Doppler across the mitral valve and left ventricular outflow tract (LVOT) performed from the transgastric position, demonstrating mitral regurgitation (MR) through the cleft AML and severe subaortic stenosis (SAS) with a maximum velocity of 4.67 m/s, caused by chordal attachments from the AML to the LVOT.

therapy, and percutaneous intervention provide the clinician with a number of therapeutic options.

Unoperated History

Unoperated history determined by the severity of obstruction to right ventricular outflow. Sixty-six percent of unoperated patients live to the age of 1 year, 49 percent to age 3 years, 24 percent to age 10 years, and only 3 percent of patients reach 40 years of age.[166] The chance of survival is greatly diminished when complete pulmonary atresia is present. Complications of right-to-left shunting include cyanosis, erythrocytosis, thrombocytopenia, and an increased risk of paradoxical emboli and cerebral abscess formation. Patients are at high risk for developing infective endocarditis (see Table 83–1). Malignant ventricular arrhythmias and congestive heart failure are major causes of death.

Management and Results

Since the successful clinical palliative Blalock-Taussig shunt in 1945, survival and quality of life for tetralogy of Fallot has improved dramatically, one of the great accomplishments for cardiovascular medicine in the 20th century (see Fig. 83–1). Surgical palliation with systemic-to-pulmonary arterial shunts increases blood flow to the pulmonary arteries. Palliative surgery was followed by intracardiac repair that included VSD closure and relief of the right ventricular outflow obstruction. Surgical techniques have evolved since the early intracardiac repairs of the 1960s. Deleterious hemodynamic and electrical effects of pulmonary regurgitation and ventriculotomy scars have spurred efforts to ensure pulmonary valvar competence and minimize ventricular incisions. Surgical repair now confers an 85 percent survival into adulthood in the United States.[167] The technique used for repair depends on the level and extent of right ventricular (RV) outflow obstruction.[168] Simple pulmonary valvar stenosis with a nondysplastic, well-developed pulmonary valve requires the least-extensive surgery, consisting of VSD closure and pulmonary valvotomy. More diffuse or more severe outflow tract stenoses necessitate a more extensive reconstruction of the RV outflow tract or complete bypass of the RV outflow tract by placement of a valved conduit. First-generation intracardiac repairs were performed via a large anterior ventriculotomy and frequently included incision of the pulmonary valve annulus and placement of a transannular pericardial or synthetic patch. This technique resulted in free pulmonary regurgitation. Pulmonary regurgitation, thought to have minimal adverse clinical consequences, results in adverse hemodynamic effects over time. The right ventricle dilates and wall stress increases. The right ventricular outflow tract in the region of the transannular patch becomes dyskinetic, causing turbulence and energy loss. The tricuspid annulus frequently dilates and tricuspid regurgitation often occurs. Additionally, the right ventricle develops "restrictive" diastolic properties that further compromise energy-efficient hemodynamics.[169] Ventricular arrhythmias are likely to occur under such conditions. Programmed ventricular stimulation resulting in monomorphic or polymorphic ventricular tachycardia is of prognostic importance in these patients.[53] Ventricular tachycardia occurs in 4.2 percent and sudden cardiac death in 2 percent of patients.[14] Transventricular and transannular repair are associated with ventricular tachycardia and sudden cardiac death. QRS width on the surface electrocardio-

gram has additive prognostic value, 88 percent of patients with ventricular tachycardia and 63 percent of patients with sudden death had a QRS duration ≥180 milliseconds.[14] Patients frequently have a right bundle-branch block that results from early injury from surgical VSD closure and ventriculotomy followed by subsequent QRS lengthening secondary to right ventricular dilation. A right ventricular-to-pulmonary artery valved conduit may develop progressive conduit stenosis. Atrial arrhythmias are a cause of morbidity and confer a worse prognosis in patients with repaired tetralogy of Fallot.[14] Atrioventricular block may occur following initial repair and is usually the result of damage to the conduction system at or below the bundle of His incurred during VSD closure. These patients require implantation of a permanent pacemaker. Chronic right ventricular pacing is known to lead to deterioration of biventricular function and dyssynchronous ventricular contraction. Biventricular resynchronization may improve dyssynchrony and increase cardiac output.[170,171] Left ventricular systolic and diastolic dysfunction may occur in the presence of severe pulmonary regurgitation. A decrease in left ventricular ejection fraction is ominous.[172] Approximately 1 in 10 patients will require subsequent reoperation for right ventricular outflow repair, conduit replacement, or pulmonary valve replacement.[173] Every effort should be made by the surgeon to excise the ventriculotomy scar tissue that serves as the source of reentrant ventricular arrhythmias. Reoperation carries a low perioperative risk of mortality.[117]

【 】 PULMONARY STENOSIS

Isolated pulmonary valve stenosis, common in adults with congenital heart disease, is typically characterized by a trileaflet valve with fused commissures. The exception is Noonan syndrome, in which a dysplastic and stenotic pulmonary valve is commonly present. Right ventricular hypertrophy and excessive hypertrophy of the infundibulum occurs in response to right ventricular pressure overload. Isolated infundibular stenosis is rare as is isolated supravalvar stenosis.

Natural History

Survival into adulthood is usual. Severe pulmonary stenosis (peak gradient ≥40 mmHg) that is uncorrected may result in progressive right ventricular hypertrophy, dilation, and symptoms of right-heart failure. Moderate or mild pulmonary stenosis generally does not progress and is well tolerated.

Management and Outcomes

Mild and moderate degrees of pulmonary stenosis (peak gradient ≤40 mmHg) are well tolerated and generally do not require surgical or percutaneous intervention.[73] Patients with severe pulmonary stenosis (peak gradient ≥40 mmHg) should undergo percutaneous or surgical intervention to reduce the severity of the stenosis, even if asymptomatic.[73]

Surgical valvotomy for isolated pulmonary stenosis has been successfully and safely performed for 50 years. Perioperative and late results are excellent, especially if surgery is performed in the first two decades of life. Severe pulmonary regurgitation may result when pulmonary valvectomy or transannular patching are performed (usually for dysplastic valves or narrowed annulus). The use of trans-

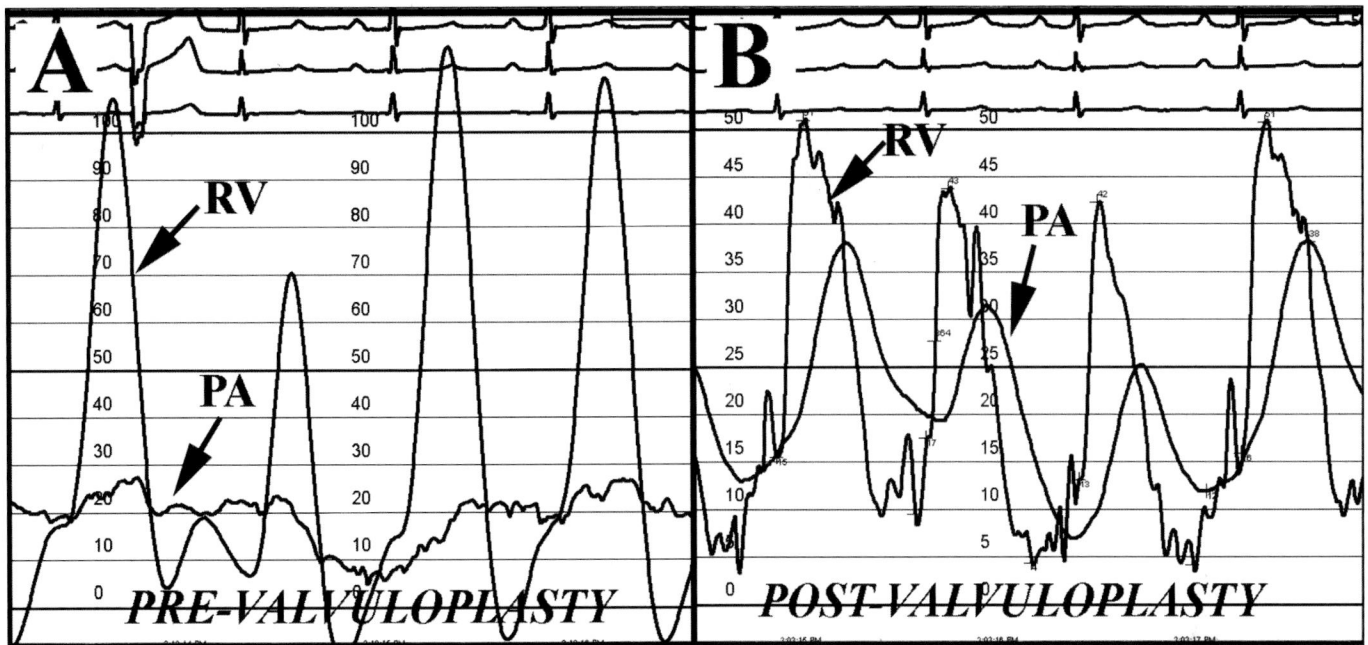

FIGURE 83-13. A. Simultaneous transcatheter pressure recordings in the right ventricle (RV) and pulmonary artery (PA) in a 47-year-old female with unoperated isolated severe pulmonary valve stenosis preballoon valvuloplasty. Note that the right ventricular systolic pressure exceeds 100 mmHg except on the beat following an interpolated premature ventricular complex. Also note the absence of systolic deflections on the PA pressure waveform, indicative of severe valvar PS. The maximum pressure gradient between the RV and PA at times exceeds 100 mmHg. **B.** Simultaneous RV and PA pressure tracings following transcatheter balloon valvuloplasty, demonstrating a lower RV systolic pressure (40 to 50 mmHg) and an increase in PA pressure with clear systolic deflections indicating resolution of severe stenosis. The patient has a residual gradient of 15 to 20 mmHg, consistent with mild stenosis.

catheter balloon valvuloplasty has made surgical valvotomy unnecessary in most cases of isolated valvar stenosis (Fig. 83–13).[174,175] The immediate and midterm results of balloon valvuloplasty in mobile nondysplastic pulmonary valvar stenosis are favorable. Subvalvar infundibular hypertrophy often results in a dynamic subvalvar gradient across the infundibulum that may increase following valvuloplasty because of the relief of downstream obstruction. β Blocker therapy prior to and following valvuloplasty helps decrease this dynamic gradient and avoid the rare, but catastrophic, severe infundibular stenosis characterizing the "suicide ventricle."

〖 〗 LEFT VENTRICULAR OUTFLOW TRACT OBSTRUCTION

Left ventricular outflow tract obstructions (LVOTOs) may occur at the subvalvar, valvar, or supravalvar levels, and may present alone or in association with other levels of obstruction.[176] LVOTOs cause increased left ventricular (LV) afterload, and, if severe and untreated, result in hypertrophy and eventual LV dilatation and failure. LVOTO is congenital in the majority of patients younger than age 50 years in the United States; some variants of subaortic obstruction are the exception. Patients with LVOTO are at high risk for infective endocarditis (see Table 83–1). Fixed subaortic stenosis (SAS) may be the result of a discrete fibrous membrane, a muscular narrowing, or a combination. The obstruction may be focal or more diffuse, resulting in a tunnel leading out of the left ventricle. The discrete form of fibromuscular SAS is most frequently encountered, but the tunnel type lesions are associated with a greater degree of stenosis. In some patients with atrioventricular septal defects and cleft mitral valve, abnormal accessory

mitral valve tissue or chords may cause SAS (see Fig. 83–12). A bicuspid aortic valve (BAV) is present in 23 percent of patients.[177] SAS may also present as part of a complex of obstructive lesions, as in the Shone complex, which frequently includes parachute mitral valve, mitral stenosis, BAV, and coarctation of the aorta. Thirty-seven percent of patients with SAS also may have concomitant VSDs of the perimembranous type.[177]

BAV is one of the most common congenital cardiovascular malformations, with an estimated incidence of 1 to 2 percent. BAV may be inherited and family clusters have revealed inheritance patterns are autosomal dominant with variable penetrance. Variants of BAV range from a nearly trileaflet bicommissural valve with mild cuspal inequality to a unicuspid unicommissural valve. Ascending aortic wall histology reveals medial abnormalities that are similar but less advanced than those of the Marfan syndrome. Aortic dilatation above a stenotic BAV is not just "poststenotic"; several studies clearly demonstrate that dilatation and histologic abnormalities of the ascending aorta in BAV occur even without valvar stenosis or regurgitation.[178]

Supravalvar aortic stenosis, the rarest type of LVOTO, is defined by a focal or diffuse narrowing starting at the sinotubular junction and often involving the entire ascending aorta. Supravalvar aortic stenosis is frequently associated with Williams-Beuren syndrome, a multisystem disorder with an autosomal dominant inheritance pattern.

Natural History

Absent left ventricular hypertrophy, dilatation, or failure, intervention in subaortic stenosis may be safely deferred; there should be careful lifelong followup for symptoms and stenosis progression. Aortic regurgitation may result from damage to the valve by the turbulent flow caused by SAS. The clinical course may be progressive with increasing obstruction and progression of aortic regurgitation in the majority of untreated patients. The primary hemodynamic effect is increased LV afterload. Patients with SAS are at risk for infective endocarditis, which frequently involves the aortic valve. Even without endocarditis, once the Doppler derived left ventricular outflow tract peak instantaneous gradient reaches ≥50 mmHg, there is an increased risk of moderate to severe aortic regurgitation.[179]

BAV disease is gradually progressive in most cases. Abnormal folding and creasing of the valve leaflets throughout the cardiac cycle, extended areas of valve contact, turbulent flow, and restricted motion lead to valve damage, scarring, calcification with resultant stenosis and regurgitation.[180] Turbulent flow into the ascending aorta plus the medial abnormalities lead to progressive dilation and risk of rupture or dissection. Atherosclerotic changes have been identified in BAV similar to those seen with calcific trileaflet stenosis; the presence of dyslipidemia may be associated with accelerated progression of BAV stenosis.[181,182] Aortic stenosis is the most common complication of BAV. Patients with a mobile BAV have an ejection sound best heard at the apex. This ejection sound is present until valve calcification restricts mobility. Echocardiographic sclerosis can be seen as early as the second decade of life, and thickening and calcification usually is present by the fourth decade; only 15 percent have a normally functioning BAV in the fifth decade.[183] BAV predisposes patients to the development of aortic regurgitation; progression of regurgitation occurs via several mechanisms, in most cases directly correlated with the degree of aortic root dilatation. Other mechanisms include leaflet prolapse, degeneration, and retraction. Infective endocarditis may cause leaflet destruction and perforation along with intimal dissection; sudden worsening of aortic regurgitation is poorly tolerated hemodynamically and is a surgical emergency. Aortic dissection is an infrequent but deadly complication. The ascending aorta in patients with BAV gradually dilates at a mean 0.9 mm/y.[184] The risk of dissection in patients with BAV is estimated to be five to nine times that of the general population and is highest in cases with concomitant coarctation.[185,186] Patients with a BAV and ≥45 mm aortic root diameter should be referred for surgical aortic root wrapping or replacement.[73]

In supravalvar aortic stenosis, 50 percent of patients have concomitant aortic valve abnormalities, usually a BAV.[187] A poorly distensible sinotubular junction causes leaflet thickening and damage with resultant regurgitation and stenosis. Subaortic stenosis occurs in 16 percent of cases.[188] Impaired coronary perfusion may be a result of aortic valve leaflet adhesion to the narrowed sinotubular junction restricting diastolic filling of the coronary arteries and the coronary arteries are subjected to elevated systolic pressures leading to dilatation, tortuosity, and accelerated atherosclerosis.

Management and Results

Surgical resection, the intervention of choice for SAS, is usually via a transaortic approach with discrete membrane excision and/or blunt dissection in focal SAS with focal septal myomectomy. Surgical mortality is low and complications are minimal.[189] Tunnel-type SAS is surgically challenging and often necessitates the Konno-Rastan procedure to reconstruct the left ventricular outflow tract.[190] Concomitant aortic valve repair is performed if aortic regurgitation severity is significant. SAS recurs in up to 37 percent of cases following surgical resection (tunnel-type SAS recurred in 71 percent of patients vs. a 14.7 percent recurrence rate for discrete SAS over 6 years of followup).[177] Because the presence of an immediate postoperative gradient of >10 mmHg led to progressive recurrent SAS in 75 percent of patients, attention must be paid to the excision of all abnormal tissue and removal of the membrane from the anterior mitral leaflet. Progressive aortic regurgitation may develop despite relief of SAS. Percutaneous balloon dilation of a fixed focal stenosis causes short-term improvement in the gradient and may be considered for palliation of SAS.[191]

There are currently no proven medical therapies that alter the course of aortic stenosis or regurgitation in patients with BAV. β Blockers can delay the progression of ascending aortic dilation.[73] Aortic regurgitation may benefit from ACE inhibitors, hydralazine, or calcium channel blockers, but a randomized prospective trial of enalapril or nifedipine versus placebo in severe aortic regurgitation revealed no differences in regurgitant volume, left ventricular size, or ejection fraction over 7 years of followup.[192] Once severe symptomatic aortic valve stenosis develops, surgical intervention is indicated.[73] Balloon valvuloplasty may safely decrease the gradient and improve symptoms in those without a calcified valve. Surgical repair or replacement is indicated for patients with severe stenosis (peak instantaneous Doppler velocity of ≥4 m/s) who are symptomatic.[73] Surgery should also be considered in those with less-severe stenosis who have moderate or severe aortic valve regurgitation or a dilated ascending aorta. Asymptomatic patients with severe BAV stenosis who desire to become pregnant or to exercise more vigorously should also be considered for surgery. Severe aortic regurgitation with symptoms, severe aortic root enlargement or left ventricular dilation and decreased ejection fraction should be operated.[73] Valve repair has shown promising results and should be considered if the valve is not calcified.[73,193] If valve replacement is needed, bioprosthetic valves are generally preferred in patients older than age 65 years, in women of childbearing age wishing to avoid warfarin, and in patients refusing to take or allergic to warfarin. Mechanical prostheses have superior durability in patients who can tolerate warfarin. The Ross procedure has been used successfully in patients with BAV and is usually the favored technique in patients with infective endocarditis.[194] Following the Ross procedure, patients are at risk for developing neoaortic dilatation, progressive aortic regurgitation, neopulmonary homograft regurgitation, and myocardial ischemia.

Supravalvar aortic stenosis may require surgical enlargement of the narrowed sinotubular region and adjacent ascending aorta in the presence of symptoms or a mean pressure gradient of ≥50 mmHg. Surgical relief of obstruction consists of excision of a focal stenosis with end-to-end anastomosis of the ascending aorta, patch enlargement of the sinotubular junction, or more complex aortoplasty involving patch placement into two or more sinuses of Valsalva. The Ross procedure has also been used to replace the aortic root in patients with concomitant aortic valve disease. Balloon angioplasty of supravalvar aortic stenosis does not result in relief of obstruction and risks aortic dissection or rupture.

[ ] COARCTATION OF THE AORTA

Coarctation of the aorta in the adult is usually a discrete narrowing at the ligamentum arteriosum, but diffuse forms may involve the arch or isthmus. Coarctation of the aorta occurs in 7 percent of patients with congenital heart disease and there is a small male predominance of 1.5:1. The descending aorta immediately distal to the segment of coarctation is often aneurysmal. A BAV is present in about half of cases. Intracranial aneurysms, often in the circle of Willis, have been detected in up to 10 percent of patients.[195] Adult unoperated patients present with systemic arterial hypertension in the upper extremities.

Natural History

Unoperated survival is poor; median survival is 35 years.[196] Patients die of congestive heart failure, aortic dissection or rupture, complications of infective endocarditis, or intracranial hemorrhage.

Management and Results

Excision of the narrowed segment and end-to-end anastomosis of the paracoarctation aorta is the preferred initial repair. Subsequent modifications in surgical technique include the use of prosthetic overlay grafts, subclavian patch aortoplasty, and prosthetic tube grafts from the ascending to the descending aorta in patients with complete interruption (Fig. 83–14). Percutaneous balloon angioplasty with stenting for primary coarctation is an attractive option in selected patients (see Fig. 83–9). Stent implantation is preferable to angioplasty alone and has excellent long-term outcomes.[197,198]

Patients with successfully treated coarctation often continue to have systemic arterial hypertension despite the absence of significant residual coarctation. Late repair (>14 years of age) is associated with higher rates of hypertension and decreased survival. Patients with hypertension after late repair are at an increased risk for developing heart failure, atherosclerosis, stroke, and progressive aortic disease.

[ ] COMPLETE TRANSPOSITION OF THE GREAT ARTERIES

Complete transposition of the great arteries (TGA) refers to a ventriculoarterial discordance characterized by medial transposition of the aorta which arises anteriorly and rightward from a morphologic right ventricle and the pulmonary artery arises posteriorly and leftward from a morphologic left ventricle. The aorta is anteriorly dextroposed and emerges from a normally located right ventricle while the pulmonary artery is posteriorly levoposed to emerge from the left ventricle (see Fig. 83–2). As a result, the systemic and pulmonary arterial circulations run in parallel, not in series, poorly oxygenated blood enters the aorta, and survival depends on the delivery of oxygenated blood to the systemic circulation via a left-to-right shunt. Other anomalies often coexist (e.g., ventricular septal defect and LVOTO).

Natural History

Surgical intervention in infancy is imperative for survival; most adults with this condition have undergone prior intervention. Patients with large, nonrestrictive shunts may survive into adulthood, but often develop congestive heart failure and pulmonary vascular disease in childhood.

Management and Results

Balloon atrial septostomy in the infant with TGA allows enough left-to-right shunting of oxygenated blood to keep the patient alive. The Senning operation (initially published in 1959) followed by the Mustard operation (1964), involved redirection of atrial blood via baffles to deliver oxygenated pulmonary venous blood to the systemic right ventricle and deoxygenated systemic venous blood to the pulmonary left ventricle (see Fig. 83–2). The main difference between these two is that the Senning operation uses atrial and septal tissue to create the baffles, whereas the Mustard operation uses extrinsic materials (e.g., pericardium). Long-term followup demonstrates an 80 percent 28-year survival with the majority of survivors in NYHA class I.[199] The Senning operation is associated with improved long-term survival.[200] Atrial arrhythmias occur over time, with sinus node dysfunction and inci-

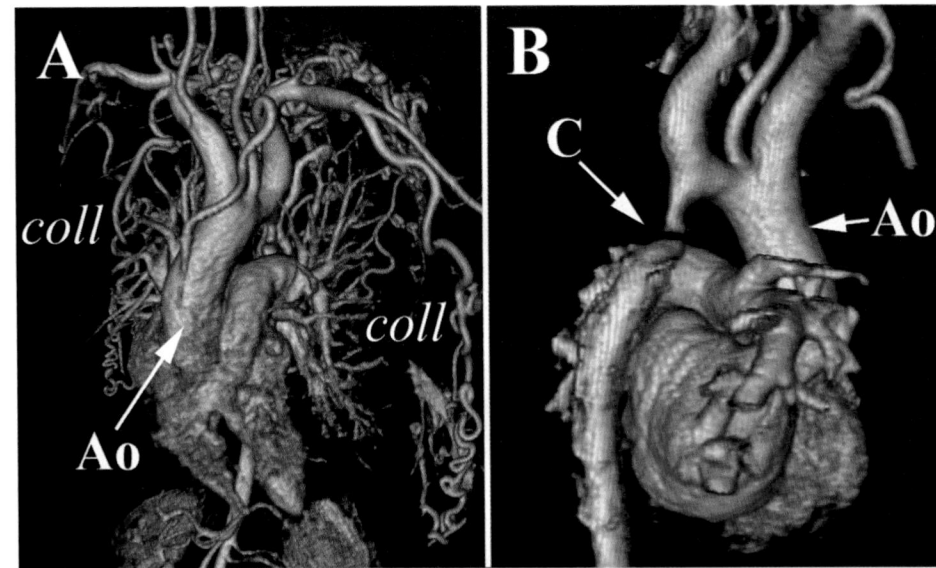

FIGURE 83–14. A. A 54-year-old female with interruption of the aorta. Three-dimensional surface rendered reconstruction of cardiac magnetic resonance angiogram as viewed from a right anterior oblique and cranial projection. The ascending aorta (Ao) is moderately dilated, as are the arch vessels. A plethora of bypassing collaterals (coll) are present. Adult unoperated patients present with systemic arterial hypertension in the upper extremities. A normal patient should have a 5- to 10-mmHg increase in systolic blood pressure in the lower extremities as compared to the upper extremities. Absence of this increase or presence of a decrease in the lower extremities should arouse suspicion of coarctation. **B.** Right lateral projection with collaterals removed during the editing and three-dimensional rendering process. Complete interruption (C) of the aorta is evident.

sional reentrant atrial arrhythmias as frequent long-term complications. Patients may show evidence of chronotropic incompetence with exercise and may benefit from pacemaker insertion. Reentrant atrial tachyarrhythmias often result in deleterious, poorly tolerated hemodynamics, and increased risk of sudden cardiac death (especially in the presence of right ventricular dysfunction).[201] Sudden death occurs in up to 15 percent of patients, usually during exercise.[199,201] Pulmonary or systemic venous baffle obstruction occurs occasionally and can usually be treated with transcatheter angioplasty and stenting. Baffle leaks are more common but are rarely significant and only 1 to 2 percent require intervention for cyanosis or volume overload. Progressive systemic right ventricular failure is a problem long-term. Angiotensin-converting enzyme or receptor inhibition does not improve exercise performance or decrease serum BNP levels.[15,202] This may be explained by lack of activation of the renin–angiotensin system and the presence of another, yet unidentified, mechanism for progressive systemic right ventricular dysfunction and impaired exercise capacity. β-Blocker therapy may be beneficial in halting adverse ventricular remodeling and improving exercise duration.[203]

The late complications cited above for atrial switch operations led to the increasing acceptance of the arterial switch (Jatene operation) as the operation of choice.[204] This procedure consists of anatomic correction by transection of the aorta and pulmonary artery at a level above the valve sinuses with detachment of the coronary arteries from the aorta. Then the positions of the transected great arteries are reversed so that the "neoaorta" emerges from the left ventricle and the "neopulmonary" artery emerges from the right ventricle. The coronary arteries are sutured into place in the neoaorta. Coronary ischemia and segmental wall motion abnormalities may occur.[205] This technically challenging surgery has certain advantages over the atrial switch operations; namely, the left ventricle is the systemic ventricle and the incidence of arrhythmias is lower.[206] Some authors advocate performing the arterial switch operation after "conditioning" the left ventricle with pulmonary artery banding in patients with a previous Mustard or Senning repair. The existing literature indicates a significant surgical mortality and inconsistent left ventricular response to "conditioning" if the arterial switch is performed after childhood.[207,208] The long-term outcomes of the arterial switch operation are now becoming available and the results are encouraging. The 10-year survival rate is 88 percent in patients without associated lesions such as VSDs, in whom the operative mortality is higher and the long-term survival is decreased.[209] Although neoaortic valve regurgitation occurs in approximately 15 percent of patients, only a minority of patients require reoperation for this problem. Neopulmonary artery stenosis or branch pulmonary artery stenosis occurs in a minority of patients and may require transcatheter or operative intervention. Coronary anomalies related to reimplantation, surgical manipulation, and distortion have been reported, and late deaths as a consequence of coronary events may occur in a minority of patients.[210]

CONGENITALLY CORRECTED TRANSPOSITION OF THE GREAT ARTERIES

Congenitally corrected transposition of the great arteries is characterized by atrioventricular and ventriculoarterial discordance. From a circulatory oxygenation standpoint these patients are "congenitally corrected", essentially "two wrongs make a right", and the pulmonary and systemic circulations run in series not in parallel as with d-TGA. There is ventricular inversion and the respective atrioventricular valves follow the ventricles. Therefore, the right ventricle is transposed to the left and the tricuspid valve goes with it. The left atrium empties into the right ventricle which then pumps to the leftward and usually anterior aorta (Fig. 83–15). The left ventricle and mitral valve are dextroposed and the pulmonary artery emerges posteriorly from the left ventricle. Less than 10 percent of patients are free of associated abnormalities, which include VSD (membranous or muscular) in up to 80 percent, pulmonic stenosis (valvar or subvalvar) in up to 70 percent, and tricuspid valve abnormalities (usually Ebstein) in 33 percent.[211]

Natural History

In the minority of patients without associated defects, unoperated survival into adulthood is common and survival into the eighth and ninth decades of life has been reported. There is an increased incidence of atrioventricular conduction problems and complete heart block with age.[212] Complete heart block may be present from birth (in approximately 10 percent) and has been reported to develop in 2 percent of patients per year. Systemic morphologic right ventricular dysfunction and congestive heart failure occur in more than 50 percent of patients with associated lesions by age 45 years.[212] Systemic atrioventricular valve abnormalities are common (Ebstein-like); regurgitation occurs in more than 80 percent of such adults. Subpul-

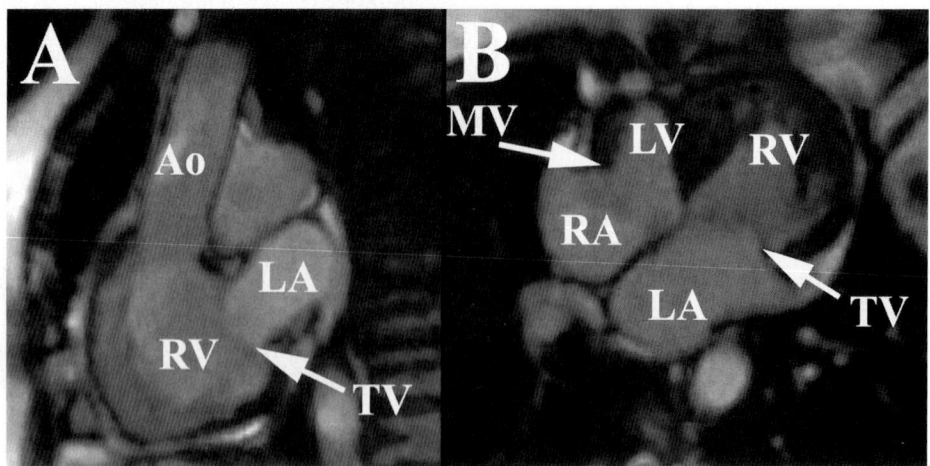

FIGURE 83–15. A. Cine-MRI of a 62-year-old female with congenitally corrected transposition of the great arteries (CCTGA) as viewed from a sagittal (lateral) projection. Note the left atrium (LA) is connected to the transposed right ventricle (RV) via a tricuspid valve (TV). The aorta (Ao) emerges anteriorly from the RV. **B.** Axial cut (four-chamber view). Note that the morphologic smooth walled left ventricle (LV) is dextroposed, thin walled, and not dilated. The right atrium (RA) empties into the LV via the mitral valve (MV). The morphologic RV is transposed to the left along with the TV.

monary left ventricular dysfunction occurs less often but may be present in up to 20 percent of patients. Aortic regurgitation of some degree is present in 25 percent of adults, but seldom requires surgical intervention.

Management and Results

Systemic atrioventricular (tricuspid) valve regurgitation is common and progressive and cause morphologic right ventricular dysfunction. Early surgical intervention in patients with severe tricuspid regurgitation to prevent systemic ventricular dysfunction is often warranted and associated with improved long-term outcomes. A combination of pulmonic stenosis and ventricular septal defect may cause cyanosis from right-to-left shunting. Surgical repair consists of VSD closure and pulmonary valvotomy or replacement, frequently accompanied by subinfundibular muscle bundle resection. Alternative surgical strategies involving the "double-switch" operation have been

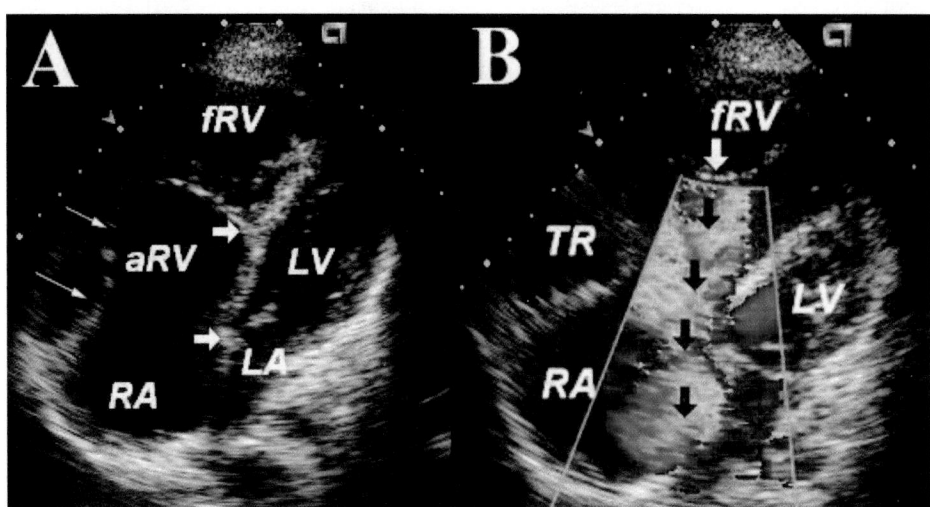

FIGURE 83–16. A. Ebstein anomaly of the tricuspid valve, in the apical four-chamber view by transthoracic two-dimensional echocardiography. Note the marked apical displacement of the septal leaflet of the tricuspid valve from the level of the true annulus (large, horizontal *white arrows*). The anterior leaflet of the tricuspid valve (small *white arrows*) is long and redundant and has attachments to the free wall. The functional right ventricle (fRV) is small as much of the right ventricular inflow is "atrialized" (aRV). **B.** Color-flow Doppler through the tricuspid valve in systole demonstrating severe regurgitation (TR) starting at the apically displaced septal leaflet and directed medially (*black arrows*). The right atrium (RA), left ventricle (LV), and left atrium (LA) are also labeled.

described. This surgery involves a Mustard/Senning-type atrial redirection along with a Jatene-style great arterial switch. Patients with pulmonic stenosis or atresia and a VSD may undergo a modification of the double-switch operation by baffling of morphologic left ventricular outflow through the VSD to the leftward and anterior aorta and placement of a conduit from the morphologic right ventricle to the pulmonary artery. Pacemaker placement is indicated for patients with Mobitz type 2 or complete heart block.

【 】 EBSTEIN ANOMALY OF THE TRICUSPID VALVE

The Ebstein anomaly is characterized by apical displacement of the septal leaflet of the tricuspid valve into the right ventricular cavity (Fig. 83–16). The right ventricle is divided into a proximal "atrialized" portion and a distal "functional" portion. The effective volume of the functional right ventricle is often small. The anterior leaflet is usually excessively long and may have attachments to the right ventricular free wall. The "atrialized" portion of the right ventricle is usually thin because of congenital absence of myocardium. The effective right atrium (including the atrialized portion of the right ventricle) is invariably large and becomes more so in the presence of tricuspid regurgitation, which is a very common occurrence. An atrial septal defect or patent foramen ovale is present in more than one-third of cases. Other associated lesions include pulmonary stenosis, VSD, and patent ductus arteriosus.

Natural History

Patients presenting in infancy represent the worst end of the spectrum with severe tricuspid regurgitation and a high incidence of associated abnormalities such as pulmonary stenosis or atresia. Patients surviving into adulthood without surgical valve repair or replacement may develop cyanosis (because of right-to-left shunting across an ASD or patent foramen ovale), dyspnea and fatigue (as a consequence of decreased cardiac output), or palpitations. In adolescents and adults, palpitations secondary to atrial arrhythmia are common. Ventricular preexcitation may involve more than one accessory pathway (endocardial or epicardial), which are often challenging to map and ablate from an intravascular approach. Up to 20 percent of unoperated patients may die from heart failure and approximately 5 percent may die suddenly, presumably from atrial or ventricular arrhythmias.[213] Heart failure results from right ventricular dysfunction and tricuspid regurgitation and may be exacerbated by left ventricular fibrosis and dysfunction.

Management and Results

Most surgical approaches consist of some form of repair (or replacement if repair is not feasible) of the tricuspid valve, often accompanied by atrial/ventricle plication, and closure of an interatrial communication. Valve repair may not be feasible in severe forms of the Ebstein anomaly if the anterior leaflet is adherent to the right ventricular endocardium with almost complete atrialization of the right ventricle; valve replacement is a good option. Surgery in patients with poor right ventricular function can be improved if the right ventricle is unloaded by a concomitant cavopulmonary (Glenn) shunt. In the most severe cases with near-complete absence of a functioning right ventricle, a univentricular repair with Fontan palliation may be necessary. Intraoperative cryoablation (modified MAZE) and division of accessory pathway/s is recommended at the time of valve repair or replacement.[214] Surgical mortality was 13 percent in a multicenter analysis; young age at the time of operation as the only multivariate risk factor.[215] Long-term survival and functional capacity of operated patients is good.[216]

REFERENCES

1. Hoffman JI, Kaplan S, et al. The incidence of congenital heart disease. *J Am Coll Card* 2002;39(12):1890–1900.

2. Macmahon B, McKeown T, Record RG. The incidence and life expectation of children with congenital heart disease. *Br Heart J* 1953;15(2):121–129.

3. Moller JH, Taubert KA, Allen HD, Clark EB, Lauer RM. Cardiovascular health and disease in children: current status. A Special Writing Group from the Task Force on Children and Youth, American Heart Association. *Circulation* 1994;89(2):923–930.

4. Warnes CA, Liberthson R, Danielson GK, et al. Task force 1: the changing profile of congenital heart disease in adult life. *J Am Coll Cardiol* 2001;37(5):1170–1175.

5. Stark J. Do we really correct congenital heart defects? *J Thorac Cardiovasc Surg* 1989;97(1):1–9.

6. Engelfriet P, Tijssen J, Kaemmerer H, et al. Adherence to guidelines in the clinical care for adults with congenital heart disease: the Euro Heart Survey on adult congenital heart disease. *Eur Heart J* 2006;27(6):737–745.

7. Williams RG, Pearson GD, Barst RJ, et al. Report of the National Heart, Lung, and Blood Institute Working Group on research in adult congenital heart disease. *J Am Coll Cardiol* 2006;47(4):701–707.

8. Murphy DJ Jr, Foster E. ACCF/AHA/AAP recommendations for training in pediatric cardiology. Task force 6: training in transition of adolescent care and care of the adult with congenital heart disease. *J Am Coll Cardiol* 2005;46(7):1399–1401.

9. Child JS, Collins-Nakai RL, Alpert JS, et al. Task force 3: workforce description and educational requirements for the care of adults with congenital heart disease. Care of the adult with congenital heart disease. Presented at the 32nd Bethesda Conference, Bethesda, MD, October 2–3, 2000. *J Am Coll Cardiol* 2001;1994;37(5):1183–1187.

10. Friedberg MK, Rosenthal DN. New developments in echocardiographic methods to assess right ventricular function in congenital heart disease. *Curr Opin Cardiol* 2005;20(2):84–88.

11. Lytrivi ID, Lai WW, Ko HH, Nielsen JC, Parness IA, Srivastava S. Color Doppler tissue imaging for evaluation of right ventricular systolic function in patients with congenital heart disease. *J Am Soc Echocardiogr* 2005;18(10):1099–1104.

12. Blalock A, Taussig HB. Landmark article May 19, 1945: the surgical treatment of malformations of the heart in which there is pulmonary stenosis or pulmonary atresia. By Alfred Blalock and Helen B. Taussig. *JAMA* 1984;251(16):2123–2138.

13. Oosterhof T, Tulevski, II, Vliegen HW, Spijkerboer AM, Mulder BJ. Effects of volume and/or pressure overload secondary to congenital heart disease (tetralogy of Fallot or pulmonary stenosis) on right ventricular function using cardiovascular magnetic resonance and B-type natriuretic peptide levels. *Am J Cardiol* 2006;97(7):1051–1055.

14. Gatzoulis MA, Balaji S, Webber SA, et al. Risk factors for arrhythmia and sudden cardiac death late after repair of tetralogy of Fallot: a multicentre study. *Lancet* 2000;356(9234):975–981.

15. Dore A, Houde C, Chan KL, et al. Angiotensin receptor blockade and exercise capacity in adults with systemic right ventricles: a multicenter, randomized, placebo-controlled clinical trial. *Circulation* 2005;112(16):2411–2416.

16. Bruns LA, Chrisant MK, Lamour JM, et al. Carvedilol as therapy in pediatric heart failure: an initial multicenter experience. *J Pediatr* 2001;138(4):505–511.

17. Wood P. The Eisenmenger syndrome or pulmonary hypertension with reversed central shunt. *Br Med J* 1958;(5099):755–762.

18. Lindberg L, Olsson AK, Jogi P, Jonmarker C. How common is severe pulmonary hypertension after pediatric cardiac surgery? *J Thorac Cardiovasc Surg* 2002;123(6):1155–1163.

19. Diller GP, Dimopoulos K, Okonko D, et al. Exercise intolerance in adult congenital heart disease: comparative severity, correlates, and prognostic implication. *Circulation* 2005;112(6):828–835.

20. Dimopoulos K, Okonko DO, Diller GP, et al. Abnormal ventilatory response to exercise in adults with congenital heart disease relates to cyanosis and predicts survival. *Circulation* 2006;113(24):2796–2802.

21. Niwa K, Perloff J, Kaplan S, Child JS, Miner PD. Eisenmenger syndrome in adults: ventricular septal defect, truncus arteriosus, univentricular heart. *J Am Coll Cardiol* 1999;34(1):223–232.

22. Fyfe A, Perloff JK, Niwa K, Child JS, Miner PD. Cyanotic congenital heart disease and coronary artery atherogenesis. *Am J Cardiol* 2005;96(2):283–290.

23. Chugh R, Perloff JK, Fishbein M, Child JS. Extramural coronary arteries in adults with cyanotic congenital heart disease. *Am J Cardiol* 2004;94(10):1355–1357.

24. Perloff JK. The coronary circulation in cyanotic congenital heart disease. *Int J Cardiol* 2004;97(Suppl 1):79–86.

25. Dedkov EI, Perloff JK, Tomanek RJ, Fishbein MC, Gutterman DD. The coronary microcirculation in cyanotic congenital heart disease. *Circulation* 2006;114(3):196–200.

26. Rosove MH, Perloff JK, Hocking WG, Child JS, Canobbio MM, Skorton DJ. Chronic hypoxaemia and decompensated erythrocytosis in cyanotic congenital heart disease. *Lancet* 1986;2(8502):313–315.

27. Ammash N, Warnes CA. Cerebrovascular events in adult patients with cyanotic congenital heart disease. *J Am Coll Cardiol* 1996;28(3):768–772.

28. Aboulhosn J, Castellon YM, Shao E, Siegerman C, Ratib O, Child JS. *Quantification of Pulmonary Artery Calcium Deposits in Patients with Primary and Secondary Pulmonary Hypertension Using Computed Tomography.* Oral abstract presented at the Western Regional Tri-society conference, Carmel, CA, 2006.

29. Perloff JK, Rosove MH, Child JS, Wright GB. Adults with cyanotic congenital heart disease: hematologic management. *Ann Intern Med* 1988;109(5):406–413.

30. Daliento L, Somerville J, Presbitero P, et al. Eisenmenger syndrome. Factors relating to deterioration and death. *Eur Heart J* 1998;19(12):1845–1855.

31. Galie N, Beghetti M, Gatzoulis MA, et al. Bosentan therapy in patients with Eisenmenger syndrome: a multicenter, double-blind, randomized, placebo-controlled study. *Circulation* 2006;114(1):48–54.

32. Aboulhosn J, Castellon Y, Rao S, Miner PD, Houser L, Child JS. *Serum Brain Natriuretic Peptide Predicts Adverse Clinical Events in Adults with Eisenmenger's Syndrome.* American Heart Association Scientific Sessions, oral abstract presentation, 2006.

33. Horstkotte D, Follath F, Gutschik E, et al. Guidelines on prevention, diagnosis and treatment of infective endocarditis executive summary; the task force on infective endocarditis of the European society of cardiology. *Eur Heart J* 2004;25(3):267–276.

34. Dajani AS, Taubert KA, Wilson W, et al. Prevention of bacterial endocarditis. Recommendations by the American Heart Association. *JAMA* 1997;277(22):1794–1801.

35. Cetta F, Warnes CA. Adults with congenital heart disease: patient knowledge of endocarditis prophylaxis. *Mayo Clin Proc* 1995;70(1):50–54.

36. Cetta F, Graham LC, Lichtenberg RC, Warnes CA. Piercing and tattooing in patients with congenital heart disease: patient and physician perspectives. *J Adolesc Health* 1999;24(3):160–162.

37. Baddour LM, Wilson WR, Bayer AS, et al. Infective endocarditis: diagnosis, antimicrobial therapy, and management of complications: a statement for healthcare professionals from the Committee on Rheumatic Fever, Endocarditis, and Kawasaki Disease, Council on Cardiovascular Disease in the Young, and the Councils on Clinical Cardiology, Stroke, and Cardiovascular Surgery and Anesthesia, American Heart Association: endorsed by the Infectious Diseases Society of America. *Circulation* 2005;111(23):e394–e434.

38. Cheitlin MD, Armstrong WF, Aurigemma GP, et al. ACC/AHA/ASE 2003 guideline update for the clinical application of echocardiography: summary article: a report of the American College of Cardiology/American Heart Association Task Force on Practice Guidelines (ACC/AHA/ASE Committee to Update the 1997 Guidelines for the Clinical Application of Echocardiography). *Circulation* 2003;108(9):1146–1162.

39. Alphonso N, Baghai M, Sundar P, Tulloh R, Austin C, Anderson D. Intermediate-term outcome following the Fontan operation: a survival, functional and risk-factor analysis. *Eur J Cardiothorac Surg* 2005;28(4):529–535.

40. Bolens M, Friedli B. Sinus node function and conduction system before and after surgery for secundum atrial septal defect: an electrophysiologic study. *Am J Cardiol* 1984;53(10):1415–1420.

41. Morton JB, Sanders P, Vohra JK, et al. Effect of chronic right atrial stretch on atrial electrical remodeling in patients with an atrial septal defect. *Circulation* 2003;107(13):1775–1782.

42. Dos L, Teruel L, Ferreira IJ, Rodriguez-Larrea J, et al. Late outcome of Senning and Mustard procedures for correction of transposition of the great arteries. *Heart* 2005;91(5):652–656.

43. Bonatti V, Agnetti A, Squarcia U. Early and late postoperative complete heart block in pediatric patients submitted to open-heart surgery for congenital heart disease. *Pediatr Med Chir* 1998;20(3):181–186.

44. Vetter VL, Horowitz LN. Electrophysiologic residua and sequelae of surgery for congenital heart defects. *Am J Cardiol* 1982;50(3):588–604.

45. Misaki T, Tsubota M, Watanabe G, et al. Surgical treatment of ventricular tachycardia after surgical repair of tetralogy of Fallot. Relation between intraoperative mapping and histological findings. *Circulation* 1994;90(1):264–271.

46. Hoffmann E, Sulke N, Edvardsson N, et al. New insights into the initiation of atrial fibrillation: a detailed intraindividual and interindividual analysis of the spontaneous onset of atrial fibrillation using new diagnostic pacemaker features. *Circulation* 2006;113(16):1933–1941.

47. Warfield DA, Hayes DL, Hyberger LK, Warnes CA, Danielson GK. Permanent pacing in patients with univentricular heart. *Pacing Clin Electrophysiol* 1999;22(8):1193–1201.

48. Vollmann D, Luthje L, Schott P, Hasenfuss G, Unterberg-Buchwald C. Biventricular pacing improves the blunted force-frequency relation present during univentricular pacing in patients with heart failure and conduction delay. *Circulation* 2006;113(7):953–959.

49. Fontan F, Baudet E. Surgical repair of tricuspid atresia. *Thorax* 1971;26(3):240–248.

50. de Groot NM, Zeppenfeld K, Wijffels MC, et al. Ablation of focal atrial arrhythmia in patients with congenital heart defects after surgery: role of circumscribed areas with heterogeneous conduction. *Heart Rhythm* 2006;3(5):526–535.

51. Magnin-Poull I, De Chillou C, Miljoen H, Andronache M, Aliot E. Mechanisms of right atrial tachycardia occurring late after surgical closure of atrial septal defects. *J Cardiovasc Electrophysiol* 2005;16(7):681–687.

52. Triedman JK, DeLucca JM, Alexander ME, Berul CI, Cecchin F, Walsh EP. Prospective trial of electroanatomically guided, irrigated catheter ablation of atrial tachycardia in patients with congenital heart disease. *Heart Rhythm* 2005;2(7):700–705.

53. Khairy P, Landzberg MJ, Gatzoulis MA, et al. Value of programmed ventricular stimulation after tetralogy of Fallot repair: a multicenter study. *Circulation* 2004;109(16):1994–2000.

54. Horton RP, Canby RC, Kessler DJ, et al. Ablation of ventricular tachycardia associated with tetralogy of Fallot: demonstration of bidirectional block. *J Cardiovasc Electrophysiol* 1997;8(4):432–435.

55. Furushima H, Chinushi M, Sugiura H, et al. Ventricular tachycardia late after repair of congenital heart disease: efficacy of combination therapy with radiofrequency catheter ablation and class III antiarrhythmic agents and long-term outcome. *J Electrocardiol* 2006;39(2):219–224.

56. Papagiannis J, Kanter RJ, Wharton JM. Radiofrequency catheter ablation of multiple haemodynamically unstable ventricular tachycardias in a patient with surgically repaired tetralogy of Fallot. *Cardiol Young* 1998;8(3):379–382.

57. Kugler JD. Predicting sudden death in patients who have undergone tetralogy of Fallot repair: is it really as simple as measuring ECG intervals? *J Cardiovasc Electrophysiol* 1998;9(1):103–106.

58. McLeod KA, Hillis WS, Houston AB, et al. Reduced heart rate variability following repair of tetralogy of Fallot. *Heart* 1999;81(6):656–660.

59. Brili S, Aggeli C, Gatzoulis K, et al. Echocardiographic and signal averaged ECG indices associated with non-sustained ventricular tachycardia after repair of tetralogy of Fallot. *Heart* 2001;85(1):57–60.

60. Cheung MM, Weintraub RG, Cohen RJ, Karl TR, Wilkinson JL, Davis AM. T-wave alternans threshold late after repair of tetralogy of Fallot. *J Cardiovasc Electrophysiol* 2002;13(7):657–661.

61. Khairy P, Ouyang DW, Fernandes SM, Lee-Parritz A, Economy KE, Landzberg MJ. Pregnancy outcomes in women with congenital heart disease. *Circulation* 2006;113(4):517–524.

62. Siu SC, Sermer M, Colman JM, et al. Prospective multicenter study of pregnancy outcomes in women with heart disease. *Circulation* 2001;104(5):515–521.

63. Walsh RA. Effects of maternal smoking on adverse pregnancy outcomes: examination of the criteria of causation. *Hum Biol* 1994;66(6):1059–1092.

64. Nicolozakes AW, Binkley PF, Leier CV. Hemodynamic effects of smoking in congestive heart failure. *Am J Med Sci* 1988;296(6):377–380.

65. Drenthen W, Pieper PG, Roos-Hesselink JW, et al. Pregnancy and delivery in women after Fontan palliation. *Heart* 2006;92(9):1290–1294.

66. Veldtman GR, Connolly HM, Grogan M, Ammash NM, Warnes CA. Outcomes of pregnancy in women with tetralogy of Fallot. *J Am Coll Cardiol* 2004;44(1):174–180.

67. Presbitero P, Somerville J, Stone S, Aruta E, Spiegelhalter D, Rabajoli F. Pregnancy in cyanotic congenital heart disease. Outcome of mother and fetus. *Circulation* 1994;89(6):2673–2676.

68. Gleicher N, Midwall J, Hochberger D, Jaffin H. Eisenmenger's syndrome and pregnancy. *Obstet Gynecol Surv* 1979;34(10):721–741.

69. Rossiter JP, Repke JT, Morales AJ, Murphy EA, Pyeritz RE. A prospective longitudinal evaluation of pregnancy in the Marfan syndrome. *Am J Obstet Gynecol* 1995;173(5):1599–1606.

70. Elkayam U, Ostrzega E, Shotan A, Mehra A. Cardiovascular problems in pregnant women with the Marfan syndrome. *Ann Intern Med* 1995;123(2):117–122.

71. Siu SC, Sermer M, Harrison DA, et al. Risk and predictors for pregnancy-related complications in women with heart disease. *Circulation* 1997;96(9):2789–2794.

72. Tzankis G, Morse DS. Cesarean section and reoperative aortic valve replacement in a 38-week parturient. *J Cardiothorac Vasc Anesth* 1996;10(4):516–518.

73. Bonow RO, Carabello BA, Kanu C, et al. ACC/AHA 2006 guidelines for the management of patients with valvular heart disease: a report of the American College of Cardiology/American Heart Association Task Force on Practice Guidelines (writing committee to revise the 1998 Guidelines for the Management of Patients With Valvular Heart Disease): developed in collaboration with the Society of Cardiovascular Anesthesiologists: endorsed by the Society for Cardiovascular Angiography and Interventions and the Society of Thoracic Surgeons. *Circulation* 2006;114(5):e84–e231.

74. Elkayam U, Bitar F. Valvular heart disease and pregnancy: part II. prosthetic valves. *J Am Coll Cardiol* 2005;46(3):403–410.

75. Schaefer C, Hannemann D, Meister R, et al. Vitamin K antagonists and pregnancy outcome. A multi-centre prospective study. *Thromb Haemost* 2006;95(6):949–957.

76. Salazar E, Izaguirre R, Verdejo J, Mutchinick O. Failure of adjusted doses of subcutaneous heparin to prevent thromboembolic phenomena in pregnant patients with mechanical cardiac valve prostheses. *J Am Coll Cardiol* 1996;27(7):1698–1703.

77. Hoffman JI, Kaplan S. The incidence of congenital heart disease. *J Am Coll Cardiol* 2002;39(12):1890–1900.

78. Nora JJ, Nora AH. The evolution of specific genetic and environmental counseling in congenital heart diseases. *Circulation* 1978;57(2):205–213.

79. Gill HK, Splitt M, Sharland GK, Simpson JM. Patterns of recurrence of congenital heart disease: an analysis of 6,640 consecutive pregnancies evaluated by detailed fetal echocardiography. *J Am Coll Cardiol* 2003;42(5):923–929.

80. Burn J, Brennan P, Little J, et al. Recurrence risks in offspring of adults with major heart defects: results from first cohort of British collaborative study. *Lancet* 1998;351(9099):311–316.

81. Gelb BD. Recent advances in the understanding of genetic causes of congenital heart defects. *Front Biosci* 2000;5:D321–D333.

82. Amundsen BH, Helle-Valle T, Edvardsen T, et al. Noninvasive myocardial strain measurement by speckle tracking echocardiography: validation against sonomicrometry and tagged magnetic resonance imaging. *J Am Coll Cardiol* 2006;47(4):789–793.

83. Schneider DJ, Levi DS, Serwacki MJ, Moore SD, Moore JW. Overview of interventional pediatric cardiology in 2004. *Minerva Pediatr* 2004;56(1):1–28.

84. Du ZD, Hijazi ZM, Kleinman CS, Silverman NH, Larntz K. Comparison between transcatheter and surgical closure of secundum atrial septal defect in children and adults: results of a multicenter nonrandomized trial. *J Am Coll Cardiol* 2002;39(11):1836–1844.

85. Reid SA, Walker PG, Fisher J, et al. The quantification of pulmonary valve haemodynamics using MRI. *Int J Cardiovasc Imaging* 2002;18(3):217–225.

86. Strugnell WE, Slaughter RE, Riley RA, Trotter AJ, Bartlett H. Modified RV short axis series--a new method for cardiac MRI measurement of right ventricular volumes. *J Cardiovasc Magn Reson* 2005;7(5):769–774.

87. Hu Z, Metaxas D, Axel L. In vivo strain and stress estimation of the heart left and right ventricles from MRI images. *Med Image Anal* 2003;7(4):435–444.

88. Babu-Narayan SV, Goktekin O, Moon JC, et al. Late gadolinium enhancement cardiovascular magnetic resonance of the systemic right ventricle in adults with previous atrial redirection surgery for transposition of the great arteries. *Circulation* 2005;111(16):2091–2098.

89. Mollet NR, Cademartiri F, van Mieghem CA, et al. High-resolution spiral computed tomography coronary angiography in patients referred for diagnostic conventional coronary angiography. *Circulation* 2005;112(15):2318–2323.

90. Dimopoulos K, Okonko DO, Diller GP, et al. Abnormal ventilatory response to exercise in adults with congenital heart disease relates to cyanosis and predicts survival. *Circulation* 2006;113(24):2796–2802.

91. Weidman W, Lenfant C, Hayes C. *The Report of the Natural History Study of Congenital Heart Defects: a 20 Year Follow-Up.* Paper presented at the 61st Scientific Session of the American Heart Association. Washington, DC, 1988.

92. Kamphuis M, Vogels T, Ottenkamp J, Van Der Wall EE, Verloove-Vanhorick SP, Vliegen HW. Employment in adults with congenital heart disease. *Arch Pediatr Adolesc Med* 2002;156(11):1143–1148.

93. Deanfield JE. Adult congenital heart disease with special reference to the data on long-term follow-up of patients surviving to adulthood with or without surgical correction. *Eur Heart J* 1992;13 Suppl H:111–116.

94. Crossland DS, Jackson SP, Lyall R, et al. Life insurance and mortgage application in adults with congenital heart disease. *Eur J Cardiothorac Surg* 2004;25(6):931–934.

95. Vonder Muhll I, Cumming G, Gatzoulis MA. Risky business: insuring adults with congenital heart disease. *Eur Heart J* 2003;24(17):1595–1600.

96. Celermajer DS, Deanfield JE. Employment and insurance for young adults with congenital heart disease. *Br Heart J* 1993;69(6):539–543.

97. Moons P, Siebens K, De Geest S, Abraham I, Budts W, Gewillig M. A pilot study of expenditures on, and utilization of resources in, health care in adults with congenital heart disease. *Cardiol Young* 2001;11(3):301–313.

98. Utens EM, Bieman HJ, Verhulst FC, Meijboom FJ, Erdman RA, Hess J. Psychopathology in young adults with congenital heart disease. Follow-up results. *Eur Heart J* 1998;19(4):647–651.

99. Brandhagen DJ, Feldt RH, Williams DE. Long-term psychologic implications of congenital heart disease: a 25-year follow-up. *Mayo Clinic Proc* 1991;66(5):474–479.

100. Ternestedt BM, Wall K, Oddsson H, Riesenfeld T, Groth I, Schollin J. Quality of life 20 and 30 years after surgery in patients operated on for tetralogy of Fallot and for atrial septal defect. *Pediatr Cardiol* 2001;22(2):128–132.

101. Nollert G, Fischlein T, Bouterwek S, Bohmer C, Klinner W, Reichart B. Long-term survival in patients with repair of tetralogy of Fallot: 36-year follow-up of 490 survivors of the first year after surgical repair. *J Am Coll Cardiol* 1997;30(5):1374–1383.

102. Rosenthal A, Behrendt D, Sloan H, Ferguson P, Snedecor SM, Schork A. Long-term prognosis (15 to 26 years) after repair of tetralogy of Fallot: I. Survival and symptomatic status. *Ann Thorac Surg* 1984;38(2):151–156.

103. Lillehei CW, Varco RL, Cohen M, et al. The first open heart corrections of tetralogy of Fallot. A 26–31 year follow-up of 106 patients. *Ann Surg* 1986;204(4):490–502.

104. Baer PE, Freedman DA, Garson A Jr. Long-term psychological follow-up of patients after corrective surgery for tetralogy of Fallot. *J Am Acad Child Psychiatry* 1984;23(5):622–625.

105. Oates RK, Simpson JM, Cartmill TB, Turnbull JA. Intellectual function and age of repair in cyanotic congenital heart disease. *Arch Dis Child* 1995;72(4):298–301.

106. Aram DM, Ekelman BL, Ben-Shachar G, Levinsohn MW. Intelligence and hypoxemia in children with congenital heart disease: fact or artifact? *J Am Coll Cardiol* 1985;6(4):889–893.

107. Forbess JM, Visconti KJ, Bellinger DC, Jonas RA. Neurodevelopmental outcomes in children after the Fontan operation. *Circulation* 2001;104(12 Suppl 1):I127–I132.

108. Canobbio MM. Contraception for the adolescent and young adult with congenital heart disease. *Nurs Clin North Am* 2004;39(4):769–785.

109. Leonard H, O'Sullivan JJ, Hunter S. Family planning requirements in the adult congenital heart disease clinic. *Heart* 1996;76(1):60–62.

110. Bonnar J. Coagulation effects of oral contraception. *Am J Obstet Gynecol* 1987;157(4 Pt 2):1042–1048.

111. Fraser IS. Progestogens for contraception. *Aust Fam Physician* 1988;17(10):882–885.

112. Swan L, Hillis WS, Cameron A. Family planning requirements of adults with congenital heart disease. *Heart* 1997;78(1):9–11.

113. 26th Bethesda Conference: recommendations for determining eligibility for competition in athletes with cardiovascular abnormalities. January 6–7, 1994. *J Am Coll Cardiol* 1994;24(4):845–899.

114. Dore A, Glancy DL, Stone S, Menashe VD, Somerville J. Cardiac surgery for grown-up congenital heart patients: survey of 307 consecutive operations from 1991 to 1994. *Am J Cardiol* 1997;80(7):906–913.

115. Stellin G, Vida VL, Padalino MA, Rizzoli G. Surgical outcome for congenital heart malformations in the adult age: a multicentric European study. *Semin Thorac Cardiovasc Surg Pediatr Card Surg Annu* 2004;7:95–101.

116. Mohammadi S, Belli E, Martinovic I, et al. Surgery for right ventricle to pulmonary artery conduit obstruction: risk factors for further reoperation. *Eur J Cardiothorac Surg* 2005;28(2):217–222.

117. Oechslin EN, Harrison DA, Harris L, et al. Reoperation in adults with repair of tetralogy of Fallot: indications and outcomes. *J Thorac Cardiovasc Surg* 1999;118(2):245–251.

118. Geva T. Indications and timing of pulmonary valve replacement after tetralogy of Fallot repair. *Semin Thorac Cardiovasc Surg Pediatr Card Surg Annu* 2006:11–22.

119. Puga FJ, Leoni FE, Julsrud PR, Mair DD. Complete repair of pulmonary atresia, ventricular septal defect, and severe peripheral arborization abnormalities of the central pulmonary arteries. Experience with preliminary unifocalization procedures in 38 patients. *J Thorac Cardiovasc Surg* 1989;98(6):1018–1028; discussion 1028–1019.

120. d'Udekem Y, Alphonso N, Norgaard MA, et al. Pulmonary atresia with ventricular septal defects and major aortopulmonary collateral arteries: unifocalization brings no long-term benefits. *J Thorac Cardiovasc Surg* 2005;130(6):1496–1502.

121. Carotti A, Albanese SB, Di Donato RM. Unifocalization and repair of pulmonary atresia with ventricular septal defect and major aortopulmonary collateral arteries. *Acta Paediatr Suppl* 2006;95(452):22–26.

122. Abella RF, De La Torre T, Mastropietro G, Morici N, Cipriani A, Marcelletti C. Primary repair of pulmonary atresia with ventricular septal defect and

major aortopulmonary collaterals: a useful approach. *J Thorac Cardiovasc Surg* 2004;127(1):193–202.

123. Speziali G, Driscoll DJ, Danielson GK, et al. Cardiac transplantation for end-stage congenital heart defects: the Mayo Clinic experience. Mayo Cardiothoracic Transplant Team. *Mayo Clin Proc* 1998;73(10):923–928.

124. Bernstein D, Naftel D, Chin C, et al. Outcome of listing for cardiac transplantation for failed Fontan: a multi-institutional study. *Circulation* 2006;114(4):273–280.

125. Choong CK, Sweet SC, Guthrie TJ, et al. Repair of congenital heart lesions combined with lung transplantation for the treatment of severe pulmonary hypertension: a 13-year experience. *J Thorac Cardiovasc Surg* 2005;129(3):661–669.

126. Ammash NM, Connolly HM, Abel MD, Warnes CA. Noncardiac surgery in Eisenmenger syndrome. *J Am Coll Cardiol* 1999;33(1):222–227.

127. Mills NL, King TD. Nonoperative closure of left-to-right shunts. *J Thorac Cardiovasc Surg* 1976;72(3):371–378.

128. Khambadkone S, Coats L, Taylor A, et al. Percutaneous pulmonary valve implantation in humans: results in 59 consecutive patients. *Circulation* 2005;112(8):1189–1197.

129. Khambadkone S, Bonhoeffer P. Percutaneous pulmonary valve implantation. *Semin Thorac Cardiovasc Surg Pediatr Card Surg Annu* 2006:23–28.

130. Zipes DP, DiMarco JP, Gillette PC, et al. Guidelines for clinical intracardiac electrophysiological and catheter ablation procedures. A report of the American College of Cardiology/American Heart Association Task Force on Practice Guidelines (Committee on Clinical Intracardiac Electrophysiologic and Catheter Ablation Procedures), developed in collaboration with the North American Society of Pacing and Electrophysiology. *J Am Coll Cardiol* 1995;26(2):555–573.

131. Winters SL, Packer DL, Marchlinski FE, et al. Consensus statement on indications, guidelines for use, and recommendations for follow-up of implantable cardioverter defibrillators. North American Society of Electrophysiology and Pacing. *Pacing Clin Electrophysiol* 2001;24(2):262–269.

132. Diller GP, Okonko D, Uebing A, Ho SY, Gatzoulis MA. Cardiac resynchronization therapy for adult congenital heart disease patients with a systemic right ventricle: analysis of feasibility and review of early experience. *Europace* 2006;8(4):267–272.

133. Dubin AM, Janousek J, Rhee E, et al. Resynchronization therapy in pediatric and congenital heart disease patients: an international multicenter study. *J Am Coll Cardiol* 2005;46(12):2277–2283.

134. Pham PP, Balaji S, Shen I, Ungerleider R, Li X, Sahn DJ. Impact of conventional versus biventricular pacing on hemodynamics and tissue Doppler imaging indexes of resynchronization postoperatively in children with congenital heart disease. *J Am Coll Cardiol* 2005;46(12):2284–2289.

135. Khairy P, Fournier A, Thibault B, Dubuc M, Therien J, Vobecky SJ. Cardiac resynchronization therapy in congenital heart disease. *Int J Cardiol* 2006;109(2):160–168.

136. Perloff JK. Ostium secundum atrial septal defect—survival for 87 and 94 years. *Am J Cardiol* 1984;53(2):388–389.

137. Campbell M. Natural history of atrial septal defect. *Br Heart J* 1970;32(6):820–826.

138. Kirklin JK, Barratt-Boyes B. *Cardiac Surgery*. New York: Wiley, 1986.

139. Morriss JH, McNamara DG. Residuae, sequelae, and complications of surgery for congenital heart disease. *Prog Cardiovasc Dis* 1975;18(1):1–25.

140. Shah D, Azhar M, Oakley CM, Cleland JG, Nihoyannopoulos P. Natural history of secundum atrial septal defect in adults after medical or surgical treatment: a historical prospective study. *Br Heart J* 1994;71(3):224–227; discussion 228.

141. Konstantinides S, Geibel A, Olschewski M, et al. A comparison of surgical and medical therapy for atrial septal defect in adults. *N Engl J Med* 1995;333(8):469–473.

142. Kobayashi J, Yamamoto F, Nakano K, Sasako Y, Kitamura S, Kosakai Y. Maze procedure for atrial fibrillation associated with atrial septal defect. *Circulation* 1998;98(19 Suppl):II399–II402.

143. Attie F, Rosas M, Granados N, Zabal C, Buendia A, Calderon J. Surgical treatment for secundum atrial septal defects in patients >40 years old. A randomized clinical trial. *J Am Coll Cardiol* 2001;38(7):2035–2042.

144. Schwerzmann M, Zafar M, McLaughlin PR, Chamberlain DW, Webb G, Granton J. Atrial septal defect closure in a patient with "irreversible" pulmonary hypertensive arteriopathy. *Int J Cardiol* 2006;110(1):104–107.

145. Banerjee A, Bengur AR, Li JS, et al. Echocardiographic characteristics of successful deployment of the Das Angel Wings atrial septal defect closure device: initial multicenter experience in the United States. *Am J Cardiol* 1999;83(8):1236–1241.

146. Walsh KP, Tofeig M, Kitchiner DJ, Peart I, Arnold R. Comparison of the Sideris and Amplatzer septal occlusion devices. *Am J Cardiol* 1999;83(6):933–936.

147. Du ZD, Koenig P, Cao QL, Waight D, Heitschmidt M, Hijazi ZM. Comparison of transcatheter closure of secundum atrial septal defect using the Amplatzer septal occluder associated with deficient versus sufficient rims. *Am J Cardiol* 2002;90(8):865–869.

148. Abdel-Massih T, Dulac Y, Taktak A, et al. Assessment of atrial septal defect size with 3D-transesophageal echocardiography: comparison with balloon method. *Echocardiography* 2005;22(2):121–127.

149. Mazic U, Gavora P, Masura J. The role of transesophageal echocardiography in transcatheter closure of secundum atrial septal defects by the Amplatzer septal occluder. *Am Heart J* 2001;142(3):482–488.

150. AboulHosn J, French WJ, Buljubasic N, Matthews RV, Budoff MJ, Shavelle DM. Electron beam angiography for the evaluation of percutaneous atrial septal defect closure. *Catheter Cardiovasc Interv* 2005;65(4):565–568.

151. Aboulhosn J, Shavelle DM, Matthews R, French WJ, Buljubasic N, Budoff MJ. Images in cardiology: Electron beam angiography of percutaneous atrial septal defect closure. *Clin Cardiol* 2004;27(12):702.

152. Franke A, Kuhl HP. The role of antiplatelet agents in the management of patients receiving intracardiac closure devices. *Curr Pharm Des* 2006;12(10):1287–1291.

153. Masura J, Gavora P, Podnar T. Long-term outcome of transcatheter secundum-type atrial septal defect closure using Amplatzer septal occluders. *J Am Coll Cardiol* 2005;45(4):505–507.

154. Corone P, Doyon F, Gaudeau S, et al. Natural history of ventricular septal defect. A study involving 790 cases. *Circulation* 1977;55(6):908–915.

155. Kidd L, Driscoll DJ, Gersony WM, et al. Second natural history study of congenital heart defects. Results of treatment of patients with ventricular septal defects. *Circulation* 1993;87(2 Suppl):I38–I51.

156. Hall SM, Haworth SG. Onset and evolution of pulmonary vascular disease in young children: abnormal postnatal remodelling studied in lung biopsies. *J Pathol* 1992;166(2):183–193.

157. Ogino H, Miki S, Ueda Y, et al. Surgical management of aortic regurgitation associated with ventricular septal defect. *J Heart Valve Dis* 1997;6(2):174–178.

158. Cartmill TB, DuShane JW, McGoon DC, Kirklin JW. Results of repair of ventricular septal defect. *J Thorac Cardiovasc Surg* 1966;52(4):486–501.

159. Mattila S, Kostiainen S, Kyllonen KE, Tala P. Repair of ventricular septal defect in adults. *Scand J Thorac Cardiovasc Surg* 1985;19(1):29–31.

160. Fu YC, Bass J, Amin Z, et al. Transcatheter closure of perimembranous ventricular septal defects using the new Amplatzer membranous VSD occluder: results of the U.S. phase I trial. *J Am Coll Cardiol* 2006;47(2):319–325.

161. Masura J, Gao W, Gavora P, et al. Percutaneous closure of perimembranous ventricular septal defects with the eccentric Amplatzer device: multicenter follow-up study. *Pediatr Cardiol* 2005;26(3):216–219.

162. Talner CN. Report of the New England Regional Infant Cardiac Program, by Donald C. Fyler, MD, Pediatrics, 1980;65(Suppl):375–461. *Pediatrics* 1998;102(1 Pt 2):258–259.

163. Fraisse A, Massih TA, Kreitmann B, et al. Characteristics and management of cleft mitral valve. *J Am Coll Cardiol* 2003;42(11):1988–1993.

164. Al-Hay AA, Lincoln CR, Shore DF, Shinebourne EA. The left atrioventricular valve in partial atrioventricular septal defect: management strategy and surgical outcome. *Eur J Cardiothorac Surg* 2004;26(4):754–761.

165. Boening A, Scheewe J, Heine K, et al. Long-term results after surgical correction of atrioventricular septal defects. *Eur J Cardiothorac Surg* 2002;22(2):167–173.

166. Bertranou EG, Blackstone EH, Hazelrig JB, Turner ME, Kirklin JW. Life expectancy without surgery in tetralogy of Fallot. *Am J Cardiol* 1978;42(3):458–466.

167. Murphy JG, Gersh BJ, Mair DD, et al. Long-term outcome in patients undergoing surgical repair of tetralogy of Fallot. *N Engl J Med* 1993;329(9):593–599.

168. Aboulhosn J, Child JS. Management after childhood repair of tetralogy of Fallot. *Curr Treat Options Cardiovasc Med* 2006;8(6):474–483.

169. Sachdev MS, Bhagyavathy A, Varghese R, Coelho R, Kumar RS. Right ventricular diastolic function after repair of tetralogy of Fallot. *Pediatr Cardiol* 2006;27(2):250–255.

170. Kirsh JA, Stephenson EA, Redington AN. Images in cardiovascular medicine. Recovery of left ventricular systolic function after biventricular resynchronization pacing in a child with repaired tetralogy of Fallot and severe biventricular dysfunction. *Circulation* 2006;113(14):e691–e692.

171. Zimmerman FJ, Starr JP, Koenig PR, Smith P, Hijazi ZM, Bacha EA. Acute hemodynamic benefit of multisite ventricular pacing after congenital heart surgery. *Ann Thorac Surg* 2003;75(6):1775–1780.

172. Ghai A, Silversides C, Harris L, Webb GD, Siu SC, Therrien J. Left ventricular dysfunction is a risk factor for sudden cardiac death in adults late after repair of tetralogy of Fallot. *J Am Coll Cardiol* 2002;40(9):1675–1680.

173. Cesnjevar R, Harig F, Raber A, et al. Late pulmonary valve replacement after correction of Fallot's tetralogy. *Thorac Cardiovasc Surg* 2004;52(1):23–28.

174. Kan JS, White RI Jr., Mitchell SE, Gardner TJ. Percutaneous balloon valvuloplasty: a new method for treating congenital pulmonary-valve stenosis. *N Engl J Med* 1982;307(9):540–542.

175. Rome JJ. Balloon pulmonary valvuloplasty. *Pediatr Cardiol* 1998;19(1):18–24; discussion 25–16.

176. Aboulhosn J, Child JS. Left ventricular outflow obstruction: subaortic stenosis, bicuspid aortic valve, supravalvar aortic stenosis, and coarctation of the aorta. *Circulation* 2006;114(22):2412–2422.

177. Brauner R, Laks H, Drinkwater DC Jr, Shvarts O, Eghbali K, Galindo A. Benefits of early surgical repair in fixed subaortic stenosis. *J Am Coll Cardiol* 1997;30(7):1835–1842.

178. Gurvitz MZ, Chang RK, Ramos FJ, Allada V, Child JS, Klitzner TS. Variations in adult congenital heart disease training in adult and pediatric cardiology fellowship programs. *J Am Coll Cardiol* 2005;46(5):893–898.

179. McMahon CJ, Gauvreau K, Edwards JC, Geva T. Risk factors for aortic valve dysfunction in children with discrete subvalvar aortic stenosis. *Am J Cardiol* 2004;94(4):459–464.

180. Robicsek F, Thubrikar MJ, Cook JW, Fowler B. The congenitally bicuspid aortic valve: how does it function? Why does it fail? *Ann Thorac Surg* 2004;77(1):177–185.

181. Chan KL, Ghani M, Woodend K, Burwash IG. Case-controlled study to assess risk factors for aortic stenosis in congenitally bicuspid aortic valve. *Am J Cardiol* 2001;88(6):690–693.

182. Mautner GC, Mautner SL, Cannon RO 3rd, Hunsberger SA, Roberts WC. Clinical factors useful in predicting aortic valve structure in patients >40 years of age with isolated valvular aortic stenosis. *Am J Cardiol* 1993;72(2):194–198.

183. Roberts WC. The congenitally bicuspid aortic valve. A study of 85 autopsy cases. *Am J Cardiol* 1970;26(1):72–83.

184. Ferencik M, Pape LA. Changes in size of ascending aorta and aortic valve function with time in patients with congenitally bicuspid aortic valves. *Am J Cardiol* 2003;92(1):43–46.

185. Nistri S, Sorbo MD, Marin M, Palisi M, Scognamiglio R, Thiene G. Aortic root dilatation in young men with normally functioning bicuspid aortic valves. *Heart* 1999;82(1):19–22.

186. Roberts CS, Roberts WC. Dissection of the aorta associated with congenital malformation of the aortic valve. *J Am Coll Cardiol* 1991;17(3):712–716.

187. McElhinney DB, Petrossian E, Tworetzky W, Silverman NH, Hanley FL. Issues and outcomes in the management of supravalvar aortic stenosis. *Ann Thorac Surg* 2000;69(2):562–567.

188. Sharma BK, Fujiwara H, Hallman GL, Ott DA, Reul GJ, Cooley DA. Supravalvar aortic stenosis: a 29-year review of surgical experience. *Ann Thorac Surg* 1991;51(6):1031–1039.

189. van Son JA, Schaff HV, Danielson GK, Hagler DJ, Puga FJ. Surgical treatment of discrete and tunnel subaortic stenosis. Late survival and risk of reoperation. *Circulation* 1993;88(5 Pt 2):II159–II169.

190. Rastan H, Koncz J. Aortoventriculoplasty: a new technique for the treatment of left ventricular outflow tract obstruction. *J Thorac Cardiovasc Surg* 1976;71(6):920–927.

191. de Vries AG, Hess J, Witsenburg M, Frohn-Mulder IM, Bogers JJ, Bos E. Management of fixed subaortic stenosis: a retrospective study of 57 cases. *J Am Coll Cardiol* 1992;19(5):1013–1017.

192. Evangelista A, Tornos P, Sambola A, Permanyer-Miralda G, Soler-Soler J. Long-term vasodilator therapy in patients with severe aortic regurgitation. *N Engl J Med* 2005;353(13):1342–1349.

193. Odim J, Laks H, Allada V, Child J, Wilson S, Gjertson D. Results of aortic valve-sparing and restoration with autologous pericardial leaflet extensions in congenital heart disease. *Ann Thorac Surg* 2005;80(2):647–653; discussion 653–644.

194. Luciani GB, Favaro A, Casali G, Santini F, Mazzucco A. Ross operation in the young: a ten-year experience. *Ann Thorac Surg* 2005;80(6):2271–2277.

195. Connolly HM, Huston J 3rd, Brown RD Jr, Warnes CA, Ammash NM, Tajik AJ. Intracranial aneurysms in patients with coarctation of the aorta: a prospective magnetic resonance angiographic study of 100 patients. *Mayo Clin Proc* 2003;78(12):1491–1499.

196. Campbell M. Natural history of coarctation of the aorta. *Br Heart J* 1970;32(5):633–640.

197. Chessa M, Carrozza M, Butera G, et al. Results and mid-long-term follow-up of stent implantation for native and recurrent coarctation of the aorta. *Eur Heart J* 2005;26(24):2728–2732.

198. Shah L, Hijazi Z, Sandhu S, Joseph A, Cao QL. Use of endovascular stents for the treatment of coarctation of the aorta in children and adults: immediate and midterm results. *J Invasive Cardiol* 2005;17(11):614–618.

199. Wilson NJ, Clarkson PM, Barratt-Boyes BG, et al. Long-term outcome after the mustard repair for simple transposition of the great arteries: 28-year follow-up. *J Am Coll Cardiol* 1998;32(3):758–765.

200. Lange R, Horer J, Kostolny M, et al. Presence of a ventricular septal defect and the Mustard operation are risk factors for late mortality after the atrial switch operation: thirty years of follow-up in 417 patients at a single center. *Circulation* 2006;114(18):1905–1913.

201. Kammeraad JA, van Deurzen CH, Sreeram N, et al. Predictors of sudden cardiac death after Mustard or Senning repair for transposition of the great arteries. *J Am Coll Cardiol* 2004;44(5):1095–1102.

202. Hechter SJ, Fredriksen PM, Liu P, et al. Angiotensin-converting enzyme inhibitors in adults after the Mustard procedure. *Am J Cardiol* 2001;87(5):660–663 A611.

203. Giardini A, Lovato L, Donti A, et al. A pilot study on the effects of carvedilol on right ventricular remodelling and exercise tolerance in patients with systemic right ventricle. *Int J Cardiol* 2006;114:241–246.

204. Jatene AD, Fontes VF, Paulista PP, et al. Successful anatomic correction of transposition of the great vessels. A preliminary report. *Arq Bras Cardiol* 1975;28(4):461–464.

205. Rouine-Rapp K, Rouillard KP, Miller-Hance W, et al. Segmental wall-motion abnormalities after an arterial switch operation indicate ischemia. *Anesth Analg* 2006;103(5):1139–1146.

206. Aseervatham R, Pohlner P. A clinical comparison of arterial and atrial repairs for transposition of the great arteries: early and midterm survival and functional results. *Aust N Z J Surg* 1998;68(3):206–208.

207. Poirier NC, Yu JH, Brizard CP, Mee RB. Long-term results of left ventricular reconditioning and anatomic correction for systemic right ventricular dysfunction after atrial switch procedures. *J Thorac Cardiovasc Surg* 2004;127(4):975–981.

208. Mee RB. Severe right ventricular failure after Mustard or Senning operation. Two-stage repair: pulmonary artery banding and switch. *J Thorac Cardiovasc Surg* 1986;92(3 Pt 1):385–390.

209. Losay J, Touchot A, Serraf A, et al. Late outcome after arterial switch operation for transposition of the great arteries. *Circulation* 2001;104(12 Suppl 1):I121–I126.

210. Losay J, Touchot A, Serraf A, et al. Late outcome after arterial switch operation for transposition of the great arteries. *Circulation* 2001;104(90001):121I–126I.

211. Lundstrom U, Bull C, Wyse RK, Somerville J. The natural and "unnatural" history of congenitally corrected transposition. *Am J Cardiol* 1990;65(18):1222–1229.

212. Graham TP Jr, Bernard YD, Mellen BG, et al. Long-term outcome in congenitally corrected transposition of the great arteries: a multi-institutional study. *J Am Coll Cardiol* 2000;36(1):255–261.

213. Celermajer DS, Bull C, Till JA, et al. Ebstein's anomaly: presentation and outcome from fetus to adult. *J Am Coll Cardiol* 1994;23(1):170–176.

214. Theodoro DA, Danielson GK, Porter CJ, Warnes CA. Right-sided maze procedure for right atrial arrhythmias in congenital heart disease. *Ann Thorac Surg* 1998;65(1):149–153; discussion 153–154.

215. Sarris GE, Giannopoulos NM, Tsoutsinos AJ, et al. Results of surgery for Ebstein anomaly: a multicenter study from the European Congenital Heart Surgeons Association. *J Thorac Cardiovasc Surg* 2006;132(1):50–57.

216. Kiziltan HT, Theodoro DA, Warnes CA, O'Leary PW, Anderson BJ, Danielson GK. Late results of bioprosthetic tricuspid valve replacement in Ebstein's anomaly. *Ann Thorac Surg* 1998;66(5):1539–1545.

PART 13 Pericardial Diseases and Endocarditis

CHAPTER 84

Pericardial Disease

Brian D. Hoit

ANATOMY OF THE PERICARDIUM

The pericardium is composed of visceral and parietal components. The visceral pericardium is a mesothelial monolayer that adheres firmly to the epicardium, reflects over the origin of the great vessels, and—together with a tough, fibrous coat—envelops the heart as the parietal pericardium (Fig. 84–1). The pericardial space is enclosed between these two serosal layers and normally contains up to 50 mL of a plasma ultrafiltrate, the pericardial fluid. Pericardial reflections around the great vessels tether the pericardium superiorly and result in the formation of two potential spaces: the oblique and transverse sinuses. Superior and inferior pericardiosternal and diaphragmatic ligaments limit displacement of the pericardium and its contents within the chest and neutralize the effects of respiration and change of body position. The phrenic nerves are embedded in the parietal pericardium and, for this reason, are vulnerable to injury during pericardial resection.

Histologically, the pericardium is composed predominantly of compact collagen layers interspersed with elastin fibers. The abundance and orientation of the collagen fibers are responsible for the characteristic viscoelastic mechanical properties of the pericardium. For example, the pressure–volume relation of the pericardium is nonlinear; that is, the relation is initially flat (producing little to no change in pressure for large changes in volume) and develops a "bend" or "knee" at a critical pressure, which terminates in a steep slope (producing large changes in pressure for small changes in volume) (Fig. 84–2). In addition, the pericardium is anisotropic; that is, it stretches more in the short axis than in the long axis.

PHYSIOLOGY OF THE PERICARDIUM

The pericardium is not essential for life; no adverse consequences follow congenital absence or surgical removal of the pericardium.

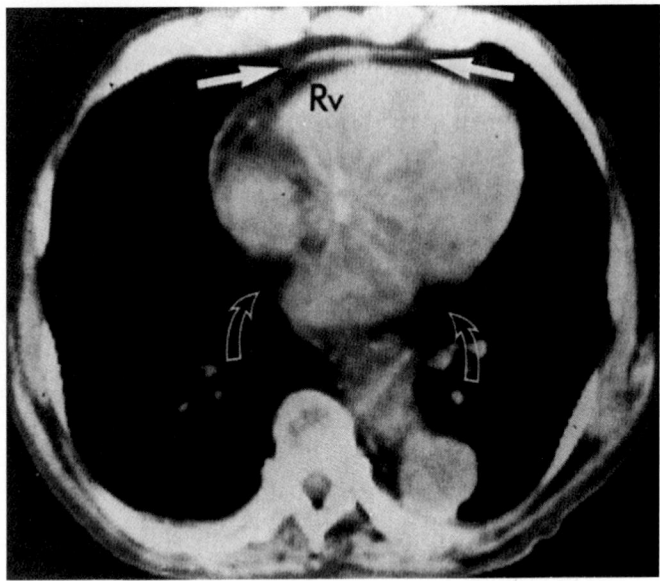

FIGURE 84–1. CT scan shows the normal pericardium as a thin, curvilinear line (*open arrows*). The increased thickening over the anterior surface of the heart (*solid arrows*) is probably an artifact from transmitted right ventricular pulsations. *Source: From Moncada R, Baker M. In: Higgins CB, ed. CT of the Heart and Great Vessels. Mt. Kisco, NY: Futura, 1983:292. Reproduced with permission.*

However, the pericardium serves many important (although subtle) functions (Table 84–1). It limits distension of the cardiac chambers and facilitates interaction and coupling of the ventricles and atria.[1] Thus, changes in pressure and volume on one side of the heart can influence pressure and volume on the other side. Limitation of cardiac filling volumes by the pericardium may also limit cardiac output and oxygen delivery during exercise.[1] The pericardium also influences quantitative and qualitative aspects of ventricular filling; the thin-walled right ventricle (RV) and atrium are more subject to the influence of the pericardium than is the more resistant, thick-walled left ventricle (LV).

Although the magnitude and importance of pericardial restraint of ventricular filling at physiologic cardiac volumes remain controversial, there is general agreement that pericardial reserve volume (i.e., the difference between unstressed pericardial volume and cardiac volume) is relatively small and that pericardial influences become significant when the reserve volume is exceeded. This may occur with rapid increases in blood volume and in disease states characterized by rapid increases in heart size (e.g., acute mitral and tricuspid regurgitation, pulmonary embolism, RV infarction). In contrast, chronic stretching of the pericardium results in "stress relaxation"; this explains why large but slowly developing effusions do not produce tamponade. In addition, the pericardium adapts to cardiac growth by "creep" (i.e., an increase in volume with constant stretch) and cellular hypertrophy.

The pericardium serves a variety of other important functions. It prevents excessive torsion and displacement of the heart, minimizes friction with surrounding structures, and is an anatomic barrier to the spread of infection from contiguous structures. The thin layer of pericardial fluid reduces friction on the epicardium and equalizes gravitational, hydrostatic, and inertial forces over the surface of the heart; transmural cardiac pressures therefore do not change during acceleration or differ regionally within cardiac

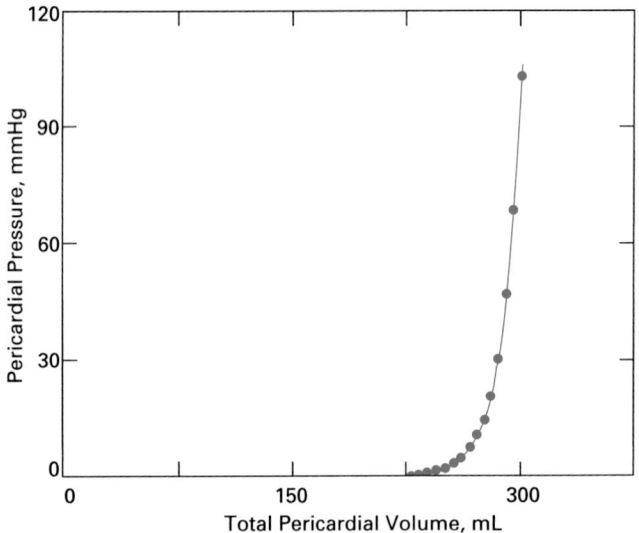

FIGURE 84–2. Pericardial pressure-volume relation in a dog. *Source: From Holt JP. The normal pericardium. Am J Cardiol 1970;26:455. Reproduced with permission.*

chambers. The pericardium also has immunologic, vasomotor, paracrine, and fibrinolytic activities.[2] The mesothelium of the pericardium is metabolically active and produces prostaglandin E_2, eicosanoids, and prostacyclin; these substances modulate sympathetic neurotransmission and myocardial contractility and may influence epicardial coronary arterial tone. Epicardial mesothelial cells may modulate myocyte structure and function and gene expression. The level of brain natriuretic peptide (BNP) in the pericardial fluid is a more sensitive and accurate indicator of ventricular volume and pressure than is either plasma BNP or atrial natriuretic factor; it may play an autocrine–paracrine role in heart failure.[3] Finally, the pericardial space has been used as a vehicle for drug delivery and gene therapy; studies using radiolabeled growth factors indicate that substances more consistently and reproduc-

TABLE 84–1

Functions of the Pericardium

Mechanical
  Effects on chambers
    Limits short-term cardiac distention
    Facilitates cardiac chamber coupling and interaction
    Maintains pressure-volume relation of the cardiac chambers and output from them
    Maintains geometry of left ventricle
  Effects on whole heart
    Lubricates, minimized friction
    Equalizes gravitation and inertial, hydrostatic forces
    Mechanical barrier to infection
Immunologic
Vasomotor
Fibrinolytic
Modulation of myocyte structure and function and gene expression
Vehicle for drug delivery and gene therapy

ibly gain access to the coronary arteries via pericardial fluid than via endoluminal delivery.[4]

PATHOLOGY OF THE PERICARDIUM

In view of the pericardium's simple structure, clinicopathologic processes involving it are understandably few; indeed, pericardial heart disease includes only pericarditis (an acute, subacute, or chronic fibrinous, "noneffusive," or exudative process) and its complications, tamponade and constriction (an acute, subacute, or chronic adhesive, fibrocalcific response), and congenital lesions. However, despite a limited number of clinical syndromes, the pericardium is affected by virtually every category of disease, including infectious, neoplastic, immune–inflammatory, metabolic, iatrogenic, traumatic, and congenital etiologies. Thus, the physician is likely to encounter patients with pericardial disease in a variety of settings, either as an isolated phenomenon or as a complication of a variety of systemic disorders, trauma, or certain drugs. In these settings, pericardial involvement may be overshadowed by extracardiac manifestations and difficult to recognize.

Treatment of pericardial disease is also challenging in that there is a paucity of randomized, placebo-controlled trials (level of evidence A) from which appropriate therapy may be selected and important clinical decisions assisted. Table 84–2 summarizes European Society of Cardiology[5] guidelines.

The remainder of this chapter reviews pericarditis and its sequelae, pericardial effusions, cardiac tamponade and constrictive pericarditis, and congenital diseases of the pericardium.

ACUTE PERICARDITIS

Acute fibrinous or dry pericarditis is a syndrome characterized by typical chest pain, a pathognomonic pericardial friction rub, and specific ECG changes. Table 84–3 lists many of the conditions associated with acute pericarditis. The following description refers to viral and idiopathic pericarditis without significant effusion. Specific forms of pericardial heart disease are reviewed below.

TABLE 84–2

Summary of the European Society of Cardiology Guidelines on the Diagnosis and Management of Pericardial Heart Disease

	INDICATION	EVIDENCE
Acute pericarditis		
NSAIDs	Class I	Level B
Colchicine[a]	Class IIa	Level B
Systemic corticosteroids[b]	Class IIa	Level B
Chronic pericarditis		
Balloon pericardiotomy or pericardiectomy[c]	Class IIb	Level B
Recurrent pericarditis		
Colchicine	Class I	Level B
Systemic corticosteroids[d]	Class IIa	Level C
Pericardiectomy[e]	Class IIa	Level B
Pericardial effusion		
Pericardiocentesis for cardiac tamponade	Class I	Level B
Pericardiocentesis for smaller effusions	Class IIa	Level B
Analysis of pericardial fluid		
Pericardial fluid and blood for bacteria	Class I	Level B
PCR, ADA, IFγ, lysozyme for tuberculosis	Class I	Level B
PCR, in situ hybridization for virus	Class IIa	Level B
Serum viral titers	Class IIb	Level B
Pericardial chemistry (specific gravity, protein, LDH, glucose)	Class IIb	Level B
Specific forms of pericarditis		
Corticosteroids for TB pericarditis	Class IIb	Level A
Pericardiocentesis for tamponade and large effusions unresponsive to dialysis	Class IIa	Level B
Pericardiocentesis for large neoplastic effusions	Class I	Level B
Diagnostic pericardiocentesis in suspected neoplastic effusion	Class IIa	Level B
Intrapericardial instillation of cytotoxic/sclerosing agent for neoplastic pericarditis	Class IIa	Level B
Radiation Rx for control of effusions in patients with radiosensitive tumors	Class IIa	Level B
Percutaneous balloon pericardiotomy for malignant effusions	Class IIa	Level B
Pleuropericardiotomy to drain malignant effusions	Class IIb	Level C
Surgical therapy of chylous effusion resistant to diet and pericardiocentesis	Class I	Level B
Thyroid hormone for effusion secondary to myxedema	Class I	Level B

[a]For initial attack and prevent of recurrences.
[b]For connective tissue disease-associated, autoreactive, and uremic effusions.
[c]For frequent and symptomatic recurrences.
[d]For recurrent pericarditis in patients in poor general condition or in frequent crises.
[e]For frequent, highly symptomatic recurrences resistant to medical therapy.
Abbreviations: PCR, polymerase chain reaction; ADA, adenosine deaminase; IFγ, interferon gamma. LDH, lactate dehydrogenase.
SOURCE: Reprinted with permission from Hoit BD. In Antman E, ed. Cardiovascular Therapeutics, 3rd ed. Philadelphia: Saunders Elsevier, 2007:787.

【 】 HISTORY

Acute pericarditis typically produces sharp retrosternal pain that radiates to the trapezius ridge and is aggravated by lying down and relieved by sitting up; its onset is frequently heralded by a pro-

<table>
<tr><td>

TABLE 84–3

Causes of Pericardial Heart Disease

Idiopathic
Infectious
  Bacterial (*Pneumococcus, Streptococcus, Staphylococcus, Haemophilus influenzae,* gram-negative rods, *Brucella melitensis, Francisella tularensis, Legionella pneumophilia, Neisseria gonorrhoeae, Neisseria meningitidis, Borrelia burgdorferi* [Lyme disease], *Mycoplasma*)
  Viral (coxsackievirus, echovirus, adenovirus, varicella, influenza, cytomegalovirus, HIV, hepatitis B, mumps, infectious mononucleosis)
  Mycobacterial (*Mycobacterium tuberculosis, Mycobacterium avium-intracellulare*)
  Fungal (*Histoplasma, Coccidioidomycosis, Blastomyces, Candida albicans, Nocardia, Actinomyces*)
  Protozoal (*Toxoplasma, Echinococcus,* amebae)
  AIDS-associated
Neoplastic
  Primary (mesothelioma, fibrosarcoma)
  Secondary (breast, lung, melanoma, lymphoma, leukemia)
Immune/inflammatory
  Connective tissue diseases (rheumatoid arthritis, systemic lupus erythematosus, scleroderma, acute rheumatic fever, dermatomyositis, mixed connective tissue disease, Wegener's granulomatosis)
  Arteritis (temporal arteritis, polyarteritis nodosa, Takayasu's arteritis)
  Acute myocardial infarction and post myocardial infarction (Dressler syndrome)
  Postcardiotomy
  Posttraumatic
Metabolic
  Nephrogenic
  Aortic dissection
  Myxedema
  Amyloidosis
  Iatrogenic
  Radiation injury
  Instrument/device trauma (implantable defibrillators, pacemakers, catheters)
  Drugs (hydralazine, procainamide, daunorubicin, isoniazid, anticoagulants, cyclosporine, methysergide, phenytoin, dantrolene, mesalazine)
  Cardiac resuscitation
Traumatic
  Blunt trauma
  Penetrating trauma
  Surgical trauma
Congenital
  Pericardial cysts
  Congenital absence of pericardium
  Mulibrey nanism

</td></tr>
</table>

drome of fever, malaise, and myalgia (Fig. 84–3). The pain of pericarditis is often worse with inspiration and is difficult to distinguish from pleurisy; in some cases, the pain is indistinguishable from that of myocardial infarction. The quality, severity, and location of pain vary greatly, and chest pain may be absent in acute pericarditis, especially in early pericarditis complicating myocardial infarction or cardiac surgery and in uremic pericarditis.

PHYSICAL FINDINGS

The hallmark of acute pericarditis is the pericardial friction rub; because of its superficial, creaky, or scratchy character, it often is likened to the sound of walking on dry snow or the squeak of a leather saddle (see Fig. 84–3). Rubs are heard anywhere over the precordium but most often between the lower left sternal edge and the cardiac apex; they are usually heard best with the diaphragm of the stethoscope applied firmly and with respiration suspended. Most pericardial friction rubs are independent of the respiratory cycle, but on occasion they are louder during inspiration. The pericardial rub may be confined to ventricular systole but most often includes a component during atrial systole and occasionally during ventricular diastolic filling, resulting in biphasic and triphasic rubs, respectively. Biphasic rubs must be distinguished from murmurs of mixed aortic valve disease, and monophasic rubs are often mistaken for systolic murmurs. Frequent examinations are necessary to detect a rub because of its evanescent nature; pericardial fluid does not prevent a friction rub.

In uncomplicated pericarditis, the jugular venous pressure usually remains normal. Ventricular third and fourth heart sounds indicate coexisting myocardial disease. The history and physical examination are also helpful in recognizing complications and in identifying underlying diseases associated with pericarditis. Depending on the etiology, there may be fever and other signs of inflammation or systemic illness.

ELECTROCARDIOGRAPHY

The ECG may either confirm the clinical suspicion of pericardial disease or first alert the clinician to the presence of pericarditis (Fig. 84–4). Serial tracings may be needed to distinguish the ST-segment elevations caused by acute pericarditis from those caused by acute myocardial infarction (MI) or normal early repolarization. The ST-T-wave changes in acute pericarditis are diffuse and have characteristic evolutionary changes. In the first stage, ST-segment elevations (which differ from ischemic ST-segment elevations by their upward concavity and seldom exceed 5 mm in height) typically occur within a few hours of the onset of chest pain and persist for hours or days. Depression of the PR segment (except in lead aVR) occurs in this stage and differentiates acute pericarditis from early repolarization variants. In the second stage, the ST segments return to baseline; at this point, the T waves may appear normal or exhibit a loss of amplitude. In the third stage, tracings show inversion of T waves. T-wave inversions may persist indefinitely, particularly with tuberculous, uremic, or neoplastic pericarditis. The ECG normalizes in the variably present fourth stage. In a typical case of acute pericarditis, the approximate time frame for these ECG changes is 2 weeks. However, only about 50 percent of patients wit[h acute pericarditis display all four ECG

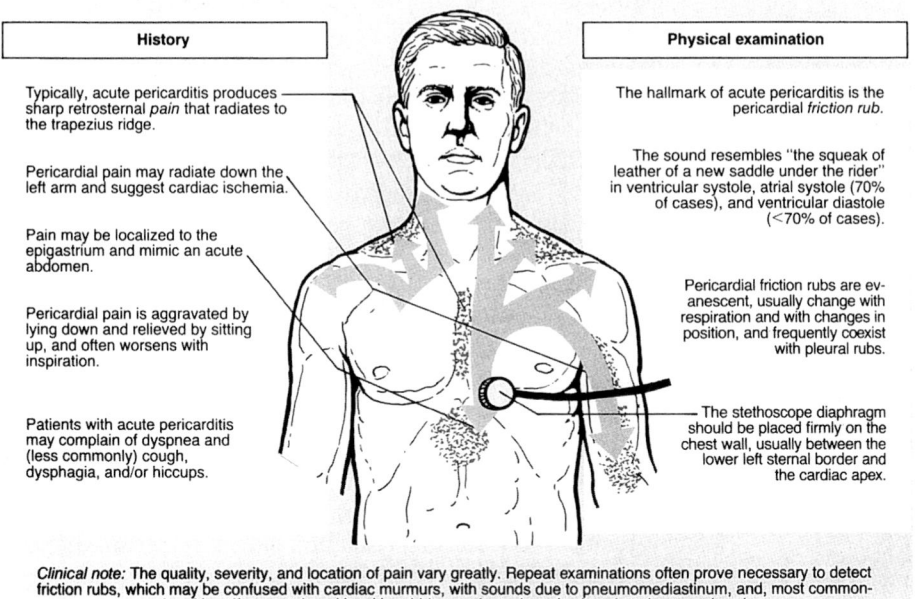

CLINICAL FEATURES OF ACUTE PERICARDITIS
A prodrome of fever, malaise, and myalgia may herald the chief complaint of chest pain.

History

Typically, acute pericarditis produces sharp retrosternal *pain* that radiates to the trapezius ridge.

Pericardial pain may radiate down the left arm and suggest cardiac ischemia.

Pain may be localized to the epigastrium and mimic an acute abdomen.

Pericardial pain is aggravated by lying down and relieved by sitting up, and often worsens with inspiration.

Patients with acute pericarditis may complain of dyspnea and (less commonly) cough, dysphagia, and/or hiccups.

Physical examination

The hallmark of acute pericarditis is the pericardial *friction rub.*

The sound resembles "the squeak of leather of a new saddle under the rider" in ventricular systole, atrial systole (70% of cases), and ventricular diastole (<70% of cases).

Pericardial friction rubs are evanescent, usually change with respiration and with changes in position, and frequently coexist with pleural rubs.

The stethoscope diaphragm should be placed firmly on the chest wall, usually between the lower left sternal border and the cardiac apex.

Clinical note: The quality, severity, and location of pain vary greatly. Repeat examinations often prove necessary to detect friction rubs, which may be confused with cardiac murmurs, with sounds due to pneumomediastinum, and, most commonly, with artifacts produced by skin rubbing against a loosely placed stethoscope head.

FIGURE 84–3. Clinical features of acute pericarditis: history and physical examination. *Source: From Hoit BD. Acute pericarditis: diagnosis and differential diagnosis. Hosp Pract 1991;27:23–43. Reproduced with permission.*

stages, and variations are very common. Atrial arrhythmias complicate 5 to 10 percent of cases of acute pericarditis.

The ST-segment elevation seen in acute pericarditis can usually be distinguished from that of acute MI by the absence of Q waves, the upwardly concave ST segments, and the absence of associated T-wave inversions. The acute ST-segment elevation of the Prinzmetal variant of angina is more transitory and is associated with ischemic pain. Although the ST-segment elevation in the early repolarization variant (common in young individuals, especially blacks, athletes, and psychiatric patients) may simulate the ECG of acute pericarditis, the former is distinguished by the absence of PR-segment depression and evolutionary ST-T-wave changes.

IMAGING AND LABORATORY STUDIES

In uncomplicated acute pericarditis, the chest radiograph is generally normal. However, an enlarged cardiac silhouette may be evident because of a moderate or large pericardial effusion (Fig. 84–5). The chest radiograph may provide evidence of tuberculosis, fungal disease, pneumonia, or neoplasm.

Echocardiographic identification of pericardial effusion confirms the clinical diagnosis of acute pericarditis (Fig. 84–6), but a patient with purely fibrinous acute pericarditis often has a normal echocardiogram. Echocardiography estimates the volume of pericardial fluid, identifies cardiac tamponade, suggests the basis of pericarditis, and documents associated acute myocarditis with congestive heart failure.

Nonspecific blood markers of inflammation, such as the erythrocyte sedimentation rate and the white blood cell count, usually increase in cases of acute pericarditis. Patients with extensive epicarditis occasionally have increases in serum cardiac isoenzymes suggestive of acute MI. In one series, nearly half of all patients presenting with acute, idiopathic pericarditis had increased serum troponin I levels, half of which were within the range considered diagnostic for acute myocardial infarction.[6] Although no significant coronary artery disease was detected in any of the patients who ultimately underwent coronary angiography, acute myocardial infarct should remain high on the differential diagnosis in this setting, as more than half of the patients with elevated troponin I presented with concurrent ST-segment elevation on ECG.

THERAPY FOR ACUTE PERICARDITIS

Hospitalization is warranted for many patients who present with an initial episode of acute pericarditis (particularly with moderate or large effusions) to determine the etiology and observe for cardiac tamponade; close followup is important in the remainder. Establishing the exact cause of acute pericarditis is an important aspect of management, but considerable judgment must be exercised in deciding whether and how to investigate the possibility of concomitant systemic disease.

An extensive evaluation is generally unnecessary in a young, previously healthy

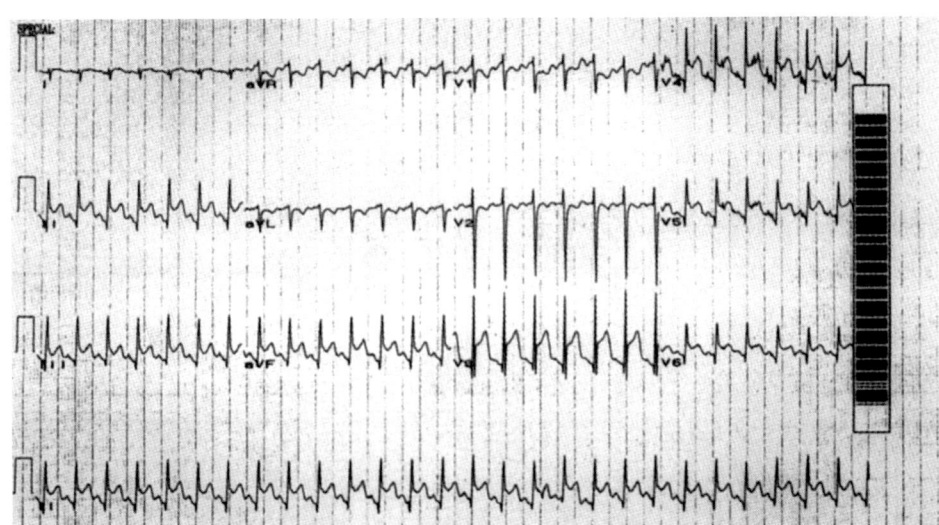

FIGURE 84–4. Twelve-lead electrocardiogram from a patient with acute pericarditis. *Source: From Hoit BD. Pericardial disease and pericardial heart disease. In: O'Rourke RA, ed. Stein's Internal Medicine, 5th ed. St. Louis: Mosby-Year Book, 1998:273. Reproduced with permission.*

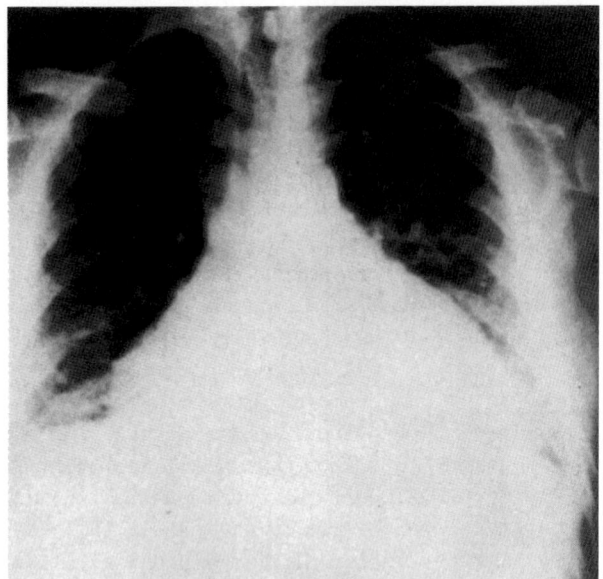

FIGURE 84-5. Chest radiograph of a patient with a large pericardial effusion. Note the "flask-shape" appearance of the cardiac silhouette. *Source: From Hoit BD. Imaging the pericardium. Cardiol Clin 1990;8:588. Reproduced with permission.*

adult who presents with a viral syndrome, typical pericardial chest pain, and a pericardial friction rub. Despite the availability of polymerase chain reaction (PCR) and histochemistry for etiolopathogenetic classification, most cases of viral pericarditis are recognized long after the period of viral activity, making a specific etiologic diagnosis and the need for antiviral chemotherapy unnecessary. Depending on the history and symptoms at presentation, trauma, myocarditis, systemic lupus erythematosus (SLE), and/or purulent pericarditis require consideration in younger patients. In older adults, myocardial infarction, tuberculosis, and especially neoplastic disease should be considered.

Acute pericarditis usually responds to oral nonsteroidal antiinflammatory agents (NSAIDs, e.g., aspirin [acetylsalicylic acid (ASA)] 650 mg every 3 to 4 hours or ibuprofen 300 to 800 mg ev-

ery 6 hours]. Prophylaxis against gastrointestinal bleeding with histamine-2 antagonists or proton pump inhibitors is warranted, particularly in those at high risk or that require longer durations of treatment. Cumulative anecdotal data suggest that colchicine (1 mg/d, with or without a 2-mg loading dose), either as a supplement to the use of NSAIDs or as monotherapy, is effective for the acute episode, is well-tolerated, and may prevent recurrences.

Chest pain is usually alleviated in 1 to 2 days, and the friction rub and ST segment elevation resolve shortly thereafter. Most mild cases of idiopathic and viral pericarditis are adequately treated with 1 to 4 days of treatment; however, the duration of therapy is variable and patients should be treated until an effusion, if present, has resolved. The intensity of therapy is dictated by the distress of the patient, and narcotics may be required for severe pain. Some cases necessitate steroid therapy (prednisone 60 to 80 mg/d) for a week to control pain, with the dosage tapered carefully on an individual basis thereafter. However, corticosteroids should be avoided unless there is a specific indication (such as connective tissue disease, autoreactive, or uremic pericarditis) because they enhance viral multiplication and may result in recurrences when the dosage is tapered; colchicine may be a useful adjunct in this situation. Importantly, tuberculous and pyogenic pericarditis should be excluded before steroid therapy is initiated. Intrapericardial instillation of triamcinolone (300 mg/m²) avoids systemic side effects and is highly effective.[7] Patients in whom pericarditis represents one manifestation of systemic illness (such as sepsis, uremia, connective tissue disease, or neoplasia) should, in addition to palliative and supportive treatment, also receive therapy directed toward the primary disorder.

RECURRENT PERICARDITIS

Recurrent or relapsing acute pericarditis is one of the most distressing disorders of the pericardium for both patient and physician; it may occur with or without pericardial effusion and is occa-

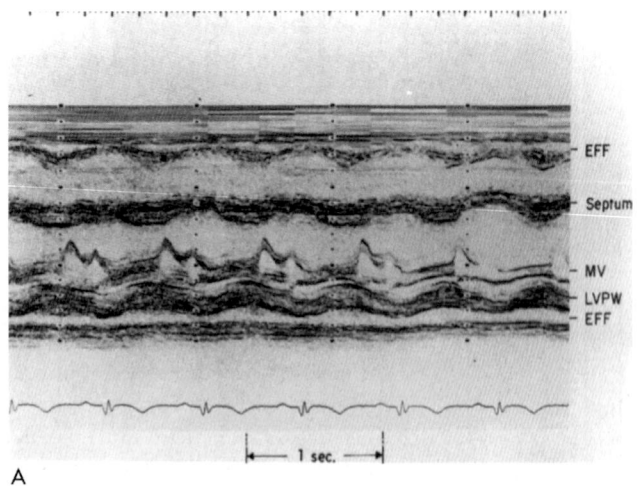

A

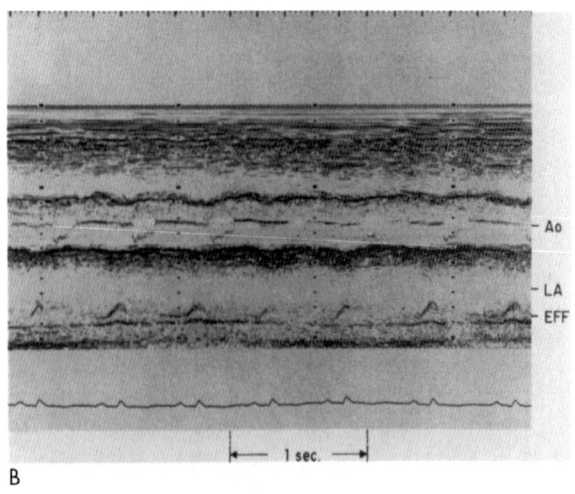

B

FIGURE 84-6. M-mode echocardiograms of pericardial effusion (EFF). **A.** The effusion appears as an echo-free space posterior to the left ventricular posterior wall (LVPW). Note that parietal pericardium has relatively flat motion throughout the cardiac cycle. MV, mitral valve. **B.** Pericardial effusion behind the left atrium (LA). Note the exaggerated motion of the posterior left atrial wall. *Source: From Hoit BD. Imaging the pericardium. Cardiol Clin 1990;8:588. Reproduced with permission.*

sionally associated with pleural effusion or parenchymal pulmonary lesions. Atypical features, such as the absence of symptoms, offer challenges for diagnosis, and require close followup and emotional support. Recurrences occur with highly variable frequency over a course of many years. The reasons for recurrence are unclear, but the phenomenon suggests that acute pericarditis itself may represent or generate an autoimmune process. Recurrences may be spontaneous (i.e., occurring at varying intervals after discontinuation of drug), but more commonly are "incessant," associated with discontinuation or tapering doses of antiinflammatory drugs. When associated with pericardial effusion, recurrent pericarditis can rarely cause cardiac tamponade.

Painful recurrences of pericarditis may respond to NSAIDs but commonly require corticosteroids. Once steroids are administered, dependency and the development of steroid-induced abnormalities are potential sequelae. Prednisone is begun at a high dose (60 to 80 mg/d) for at least 4 weeks and tapered slowly over the next 3 months.[8] When necessary, the risks of long-term steroids should be minimized by using the lowest possible dose, alternate-day therapy, combinations with nonsteroidal drugs, or colchicine (1 to 2 mg/d). In the most difficult cases, relapse occurs every time the dose of prednisone is reduced below 5 to 20 mg/d. When this occurs, the patient should be maintained for several weeks on the lowest suppressive dose before the next taper commences. In addition to its use as an adjunct to corticosteroid therapy, colchicine may be used as monotherapy for the prevention of recurrent pericarditis.[9] Most authors recommend 1 mg/d PO for at least 1 year with a gradual taper; the need for a loading dose of 2–3 mg p.o. is unsettled. Intrapericardial administration of triamcinolone (300 mg/m^2) has been shown to relieve symptoms in patients with recurrent autoreactive myopericarditis[7]; and azathioprine (50 to 100 mg/d) has also been used to prevent recurrent episodes.[8] Although encouraging results have been reported in a series of patients who underwent pericardiectomy for recurrent pericarditis, pericardiectomy may simply abbreviate rather than terminate the painful recurrences.[1] Thus, pericardiectomy should be considered only when repeated attempts at medical treatment have clearly failed.

PERICARDIAL EFFUSION

【 】 ETIOLOGY

Accumulation of transudate, exudate, or blood in the pericardial sac, a common complication of pericardial disease, should be sought in all patients with acute pericarditis.

Pericardial effusions are reported to be associated with heart failure, valvular disease, and myocardial infarction in 14, 21, and 15 percent of cases, respectively.[10] Hydropericardium results from elevated right atrial pressure and limited venous and lymphatic drainage from the pericardium. Although this is the usual explanation for effusions associated with heart failure and LV hypertrophy, recurrent bloody effusions that can be attributed only to congestive heart failure may occur.

Pericardial effusions are very common after cardiac surgery. In 122 consecutive patients studied before and serially after cardiac surgery, effusions were present in 103 patients; the majority appeared by postoperative day 2, reached their maximum size by postoperative day 10, and usually resolved without sequelae within the first postop-

erative month.[11] However, large effusions or effusions causing pericardial tamponade are uncommon following cardiothoracic surgery. In one retrospective survey of more than 4500 postoperative patients, only 48 were found to have moderate or large effusions by echocardiography; of those, 36 met diagnostic criteria for tamponade.[12] Use of preoperative anticoagulants, valve surgery, and female gender were all associated with a higher incidence of tamponade.

Symptoms and physical findings of significant postoperative pericardial effusions are frequently nonspecific, and echocardiographic detection and echo-guided pericardiocentesis, when necessary, are safe and effective; prolonged catheter drainage reduces the recurrence rate.[13] Pericardial effusions in cardiac transplant patients are associated with an increased incidence of acute rejection.

Chronic effusive pericarditis is an entity of unknown etiology that may be associated with large, asymptomatic effusions. Many conditions that cause pericarditis (e.g., uremia, tuberculosis, neoplasia, connective tissue disease) produce chronic pericardial effusions.

【 】 NATURE OF THE PERICARDIAL FLUID

Characteristics of the pericardial fluid other than culture and cytology are usually too nonspecific to be of diagnostic value. However, in one retrospective series, one-fifth of the patients had a specific etiologic diagnosis that had implications for management and prognosis.[14] Moreover, in certain situations, it is mandatory to determine the nature of the pericardial fluid. For example, in patients with neoplastic disease, it is important to determine whether pericardial effusion indicates invasion of the pericardium or a complication of radiation therapy. Cytologic examination of the fluid is also important in cases in which the primary tumor has not been identified clearly. In cases of bacterial or other nonviral infections, it becomes necessary to discover whether the pericardial effusion is exudative and to culture pericardial fluid; this is particularly important when tuberculous or fungal pericarditis is suspected. Transudative effusions (hydropericardium) occur in heart failure and other states associated with chronic salt and water retention (including pregnancy), and exudative effusions occur in a large number of the infectious and inflammatory causes of pericarditis. Although frank hemorrhagic effusions suggest recent intrapericardial bleeding, sanguineous and serosanguineous effusions occur in many infectious and inflammatory disorders. In certain disorders, the nature of the pericardial fluid has greater diagnostic value. For example, chylous pericarditis implies injury or obstruction to the thoracic duct, and cholesterol pericarditis is either idiopathic or associated with hypothyroidism, rheumatoid arthritis, or tuberculosis.

【 】 DIAGNOSTIC STUDIES

The etiology of a pericardial effusion is difficult to determine on historical or clinical grounds. In one series of 322 patients admitted to a tertiary care hospital with at least moderate effusions, the cause of the effusion was attributed to a preexisting medical condition in 192 patients. In the remaining patients, those with inflammatory signs were more likely to have acute idiopathic pericarditis; those without inflammatory signs or tamponade were more likely to have chronic, idiopathic effusions; and those presenting with tamponade but without inflammatory signs were more likely to have a malignant effusion.[15]

Specific diagnoses are possible using visual, cytologic, and immunologic analysis of the pericardial effusion and pericardioscopic-guided biopsy.[10] Observations using these techniques have suggested that (1) fibrin strands and neovascularization are common in inflammatory pericardial diseases; (2) the etiology of viral pericarditis can be established by using a variety of methods, such as in situ hybridization, microneutralization, and PCR; (3) combined analysis of the cytology in the effusion and epicardial biopsy are most important and pericardial biopsy is often inconclusive; and (4) viral and autoreactive effusions are associated with high titers of antimyolemmal and antisarcolemmal antibodies and in vitro cardiocytolysis of isolated rat heart cells.

There are clinical situations in which it is unnecessary to obtain pericardial fluid for analysis. For example, when pericardial effusion is found in a patient with typical viral or idiopathic pericarditis, pericardiocentesis should not be considered unless the effusion fails to respond to antiinflammatory treatment or cardiac tamponade develops. Similarly, when a patient undergoing chronic hemodialysis develops pericardial effusion, examination of pericardial fluid is needed only when the clinical course suggests a different etiology or when hemodynamic compromise is suspected.

Imaging Studies

Echocardiography is the procedure of choice for the diagnosis of pericardial effusion. Although flask-shaped enlargement of the cardiac silhouette on chest radiography occurs with a moderate or large pericardial effusion (see Fig. 84–5), differentiation of large effusions from cardiac dilatation often is difficult or impossible. In contrast, the relative contributions of cardiac enlargement and pericardial effusion to overall cardiac enlargement and the relative roles of tamponade and myocardial dysfunction to altered hemodynamics can be evaluated with echocardiography. Attention to technical detail results in excellent sensitivity and specificity. The diagnostic feature on M-mode echocardiography is the persistence of an echo-free space between parietal and visceral pericardium throughout the cardiac cycle (see Fig. 84–6). Separations that are observed only in systole represent clinically insignificant accumulations. Two-dimensional (2D) echocardiography (Fig. 84–7) has superior spatial orientation and allows delineation of the size and distribution of pericardial effusion, as well as detection of loculated fluid. As the amount of pericardial fluid increases, fluid distributes from the posterobasilar LV apically and anteriorly, and then laterally and posteriorly to the left atrium. Pericardial effusions are described as small, moderate, or large based on the size of the echo-free space seen between the parietal and visceral pleurae on two-dimensional echocardiography. Fluid adjacent to the right atrium is an early sign of pericardial effusion. Frond-like, band-like, or shaggy intrapericardial echoes should alert one to the possibility of a difficult and potentially less therapeutic pericardiocentesis (Fig. 84–8), but have little value in identifying the cause of the effusion. Epicardial fat tissue is more prominent anteriorly but may appear circumferentially, thus mimicking effusion (lipid envelope). Fat is slightly echogenic and tends to move in concert with the heart, two characteristics that help distinguish it from an effusion, which is generally echolucent and motionless. In addition to its mimicry, pericardial fat accumulation is a source of bioactive molecules, is significantly associated with obesity-related in-

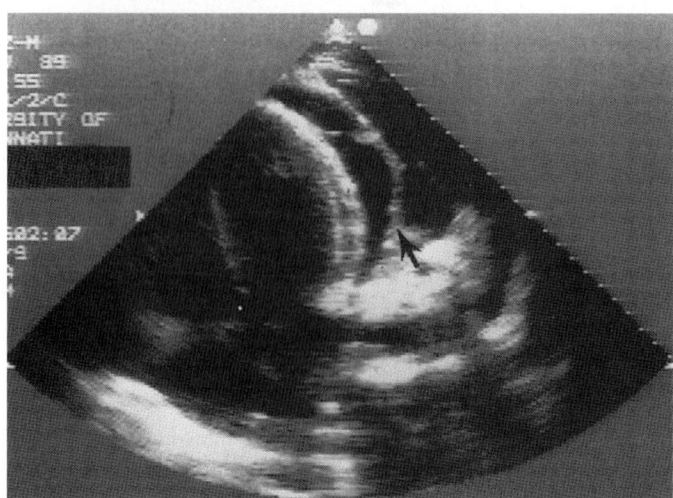

FIGURE 84–7. Two-dimensional echocardiogram from a patient with pleural and pericardial effusions. The thickness of the pericardium (*arrow*) can be appreciated in this patient. *Source: From Hoit BD. Imaging the pericardium. Cardiol Clin 1990;8:596. Reproduced with permission.*

sulin resistance and is a coronary risk factor in a population of Japanese men.[16]

Pericardial effusions are easily detected by computed tomography (Fig. 84–9). The size, geometry, and distribution of pericardial effusions can be obtained with this technique, and the attenuation coefficients for blood, exudate, chyle, and serous fluid are generally sufficiently characteristic to identify the nature of the effusion. Computed tomography may be useful in estimating the hematocrit of the pericardial effusion,[17] identifying loculated and atypically loculated pericardial effusions, and in guiding pericardiocentesis. Loculated and recurrent pericardial effusions can be

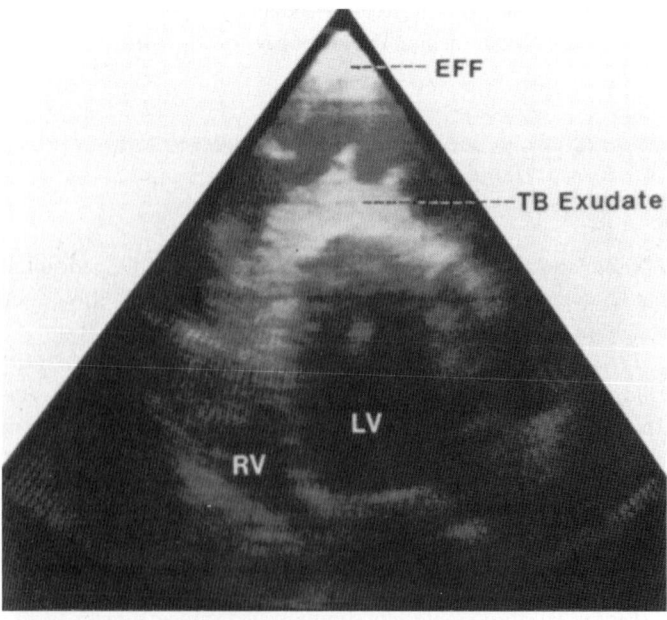

FIGURE 84–8. Two-dimensional echocardiogram from a patient with tuberculous pericarditis. Note the thickened pericardium with shaggy exudate that bridges a large pericardial effusion (EFF). *Source: From Hoit BD. Imaging the pericardium. Cardiol Clin 1990;8:590. Reproduced with permission.*

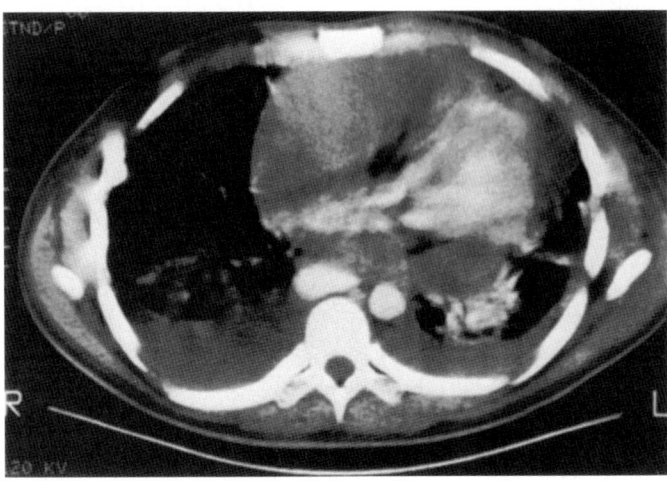

FIGURE 84-9. Computed tomographic scan from a patient with a large pericardial effusion. Note the compression of contrast-filled cardiac chambers. *Source: From Hoit BD. Imaging the pericardium. Cardiol Clin 1990;8:590. Reproduced with permission.*

treated safely and effectively with video-assisted thoracoscopic pericardial fenestration.

Magnetic resonance imaging (MRI) detects pericardial effusion with high sensitivity and provides an estimate of pericardial fluid volume; in addition, it effectively detects loculated pericardial effusion and pericardial thickening. Inflamed pericardium and adhesions have high signal intensity relative to pericardial fluid and myocardium, providing a potential means of identifying the nature of the effusion.

TREATMENT OF PERICARDIAL EFFUSION

Drainage of a pericardial effusion is usually unnecessary unless purulent pericarditis is suspected or cardiac tamponade supervenes, although pericardiocentesis is sometimes needed to establish the etiology of a hemodynamically insignificant pericardial effusion. Persistent (greater than 3 months) large or progressive effusion, particularly when the cause is uncertain, also warrants pericardiocentesis.[18] However, routine drainage of a large pericardial effusion without tamponade or suspected purulent pericarditis has a low diagnostic yield (7 percent) and no clear therapeutic benefit.[19] Anticoagulants should be discontinued temporarily, if possible, to reduce the risk of cardiac tamponade. In patients on chronic oral anticoagulation, heparin should be used, as its effect can be reversed rapidly. Large effusions may respond to nonsteroidal antiinflammatory drugs, corticosteroids, or colchicine.[9] Specific treatment for pericardial effusion is considered below (see Specific Forms of Pericardial Heart Disease).

CARDIAC TAMPONADE

Cardiac tamponade is a hemodynamic condition characterized by equal elevation of atrial and pericardial pressures, an exaggerated inspiratory decrease in arterial systolic pressure (pulsus paradoxus), and arterial hypotension. Arterial hypotension is generally a late sign in chronic effusions, and occasionally a heightened sympathoadrenal state produces systemic hypertension. As intrapericar-dial pressure rises, venous pressures increase to maintain cardiac filling and prevent collapse of the cardiac chambers. Although the absolute intracardiac pressures are elevated, the transmural pressures—that is, cavitary diastolic pressure minus pericardial pressure—are practically zero or even negative. The greatly reduced preload is responsible for the fall in cardiac output and, when compensatory mechanisms are exhausted, arterial pressure decreases.

CLINICAL FEATURES

Cardiac tamponade may be acute or chronic and should be viewed hemodynamically as a continuum ranging from mild (pericardial pressure lower than 10 mmHg) to severe (pericardial pressure higher than 15 to 20 mmHg). Mild cardiac tamponade is frequently asymptomatic, whereas moderate tamponade and especially severe tamponade produce precordial discomfort and dyspnea.

Tamponade may be so sudden that the patient does not complain of symptoms; in less drastic circumstances, patients with acute cardiac tamponade may complain of severe shortness of breath accompanied by chest tightness and dizziness. The venous pressure is greatly elevated, and the systemic arterial pressure is severely depressed. Pulsus paradoxus can usually be appreciated but may be absent when hypotension is extreme. In striking contrast to the elevation of venous pressure, arterial hypotension, and pulsus paradoxus, cardiac pulsations often are impalpable (Beck's triad). In the most severe cases, consciousness may be impaired, and except for the raised venous pressure, such patients appear to be in hypovolemic shock.

When cardiac tamponade complicates a diagnostic procedure, vague discomfort, generalized uneasiness, and precordial pain are common. Fluoroscopy shows an enlarged cardiac silhouette and diminished pulsations.

Cardiac tamponade should be suspected in a victim of recent chest trauma who appears to be in shock, especially when the venous pressure is elevated. When circumstances are deemed life-threatening, an immediate therapeutic trial of rapid infusion of fluid and diagnostic pericardiocentesis should be attempted. Otherwise, pericardiocentesis should be delayed until the presence of significant pericardial fluid can be demonstrated by prompt echocardiography. An exception to this rule occurs when tamponade complicates diagnostic procedures; in this instance, when pressures are being monitored and fluoroscopy is available, the diagnosis can safely be established without echocardiographic confirmation.

Other causes of acute tamponade are cardiac rupture complicating acute MI and rupture of a dissecting hematoma of the proximal aorta. Although successful pericardiocentesis may relieve aortic tamponade and increase hemorrhage, a limited pericardiocentesis is reasonable if cardiac tamponade is severe enough to be considered a threat to survival. Cardiac tamponade is an uncommon but potentially lethal complication of percutaneous coronary intervention. In one review of more than 25,000 interventions at a single center over a 7-year period, the incidence of tamponade was only 0.12 percent, but the in-hospital mortality rate was 42 percent.[20] The use of atheroablative therapy was associated with a higher incidence of tamponade than angioplasty and stenting alone. Finally, after cardiac surgery, dyspnea and fatigue should raise the suspicion of tamponade; in these instances, the effusion is often loculated, and echocardiographic and hemodynamic findings may be unreliable.

A large number of diseases may be associated with more slowly developing cardiac tamponade. In these instances, symptoms may be a result of the underlying illness, the culpable pericardial disease, and/or the tamponade itself. Many patients with inflammatory pericarditis give a history of prodromal fever, myalgia, and arthralgia, and patients with neoplastic disease may have symptoms associated with the neoplasm and its treatment. The symptoms of cardiac compression include rapidly progressive dyspnea accompanied by fullness or tightness in the chest, occasionally with dysphagia; pericardial pain is often absent. The course may be less rapid, allowing time for an increase in abdominal girth and the rapid onset and progression of edema.

[ ] PATHOPHYSIOLOGY

Elevated intrapericardial pressure exerted on the heart throughout the cardiac cycle, with only slight momentary relief when intrapericardial pressure falls (owing to the decrease in cardiac volume during ventricular ejection), is responsible for the pathophysiologic findings of cardiac tamponade. To understand the relationship between venous and pericardial pressures in cardiac tamponade, it is useful to review the normal biphasic pattern of venous return. A surge of venous return at the onset of ventricular ejection is accompanied by a small reduction in intrapericardial pressure. A second surge of venous return occurs in early diastole, when the tricuspid valve opens and atrial pressure decreases. In contrast, the venous return in cardiac tamponade is unimodal and is confined to ventricular systole; in severe cardiac tamponade, venous return is halted in diastole, at a time when cardiac volume and intrapericardial pressure are maximal. Pericardial pressure and right atrial pressure are elevated above normal and are equal to each other (Fig. 84–10). The inspiratory fall in intrathoracic pressure is transmitted to the pericardial space, which preserves the normal inspiratory increase in systemic venous return (the Kussmaul sign is absent).

Although systolic ventricular function is often supernormal, unrelieved extreme tamponade becomes fatal when venous pressure cannot increase to equal the pericardial pressure and maintain circulation. In severe cases, diminution of myocardial perfusion is aggravated by direct compression of the epicardial coronary arteries, abnormal transmyocardial distribution of blood flow, and, as a result, impaired ventricular systolic function.

Pulsus Paradoxus

In healthy individuals, systolic blood pressure may decline by as much as 10 mmHg during quiet inspiration. Pulsus paradoxus is an exaggeration of this normal physiologic response. A number of normal and abnormal mechanisms combine to create pulsus paradoxus in cardiac tamponade. Inspiratory augmentation of systemic venous return in cardiac tamponade increases the volume of the right side of the heart at the expense of the left side. The volume of the left side of the heart is decreased, in part by bulging of the intraventricular septum from right to left (changing the size, shape, and compliance of the LV) and in part by increased transmural pericardial pressure (decreasing pulmonary venous return). However, the inspiratory expansion of the volume of the right side of the heart and the transit time of the resulting augmented right-heart stroke volume are important in the genesis of

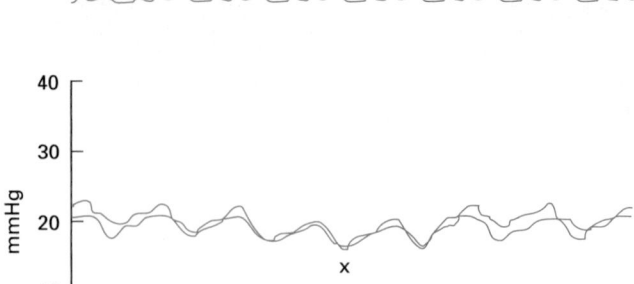

FIGURE 84–10. Simultaneous right atrial and pericardial pressures from a patient with severe cardiac tamponade. The pressures are elevated and equal to one another, and only the X descent on the right atrial tracing is present; the Y descent is absent. The pressures fall normally during inspiration. *Source: From Shabetai R. Diseases of the pericardium. In: Alexander WA, Schlant R, Fuster V, et al., eds. Hurst's The Heart, 9th ed. New York: McGraw-Hill; 1998:2179. Reproduced with permission.*

pulsus paradoxus. In addition, the negative thoracic pressure produced by inspiration is transmitted to the aorta, increasing LV afterload and reducing stroke volume. LV stroke volume falls more sharply than normal in response to decreased ventricular filling in cardiac tamponade because the small ventricle is operating on the steep ascending limb of the Starling curve. Finally, inspiratory traction by the diaphragm on the taut pericardium, reflex changes in vascular resistance and cardiac contractility, and increased respiratory effort owing to pulmonary congestion contribute to the genesis of pulsus paradoxus.

[ ] PHYSICAL FINDINGS

Physical findings are dictated by both the severity of cardiac tamponade and the time course of its development. Careful inspection of the jugular venous pulse waveform is essential for the diagnosis, although the venous pressure may be normal in early tamponade, whereas extreme elevations of venous pressure may go unrecognized in a recumbent or semirecumbent patient. Compression of the heart by pericardial fluid results in a characteristic loss of the atrial Y descent, but because of the decrease in intrapericardial pressure that occurs during ventricular ejection, the systolic atrial filling wave and the X descent are maintained. The Kussmaul sign, a failure of venous pressure to decrease during inspiration, is a sign of constriction and is generally not seen in pure cardiac tamponade.

An inspiratory decline of systolic arterial pressure exceeding 10 mmHg (pulsus paradoxus) may be detected with palpation of an arterial pulse, such as the femoral or brachial artery, and quantified by using sphygmomanometry by subtracting the pressure at which Korotkoff sounds are heard only during expiration from the pressure at which sounds are heard through the respiratory cycle. The origin of the paradoxical pulse is complex and multifactorial, and pulsus paradoxus is neither sensitive nor specific for cardiac tamponade. Nevertheless, in the appropriate clinical setting, pulsus paradoxus is a key finding that signifies cardiac tamponade, and its presence should be sought diligently.

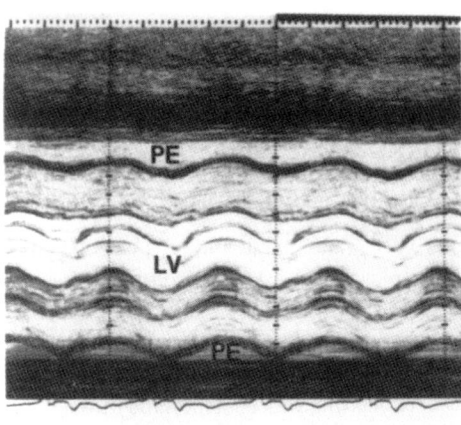
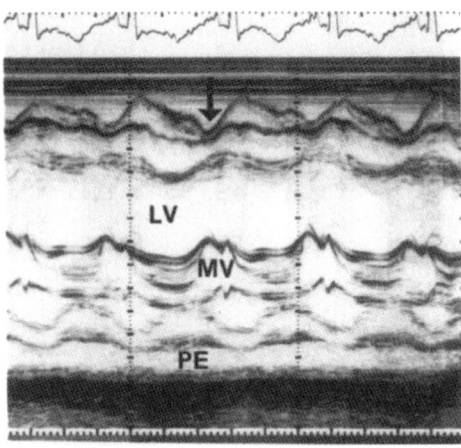

FIGURE 84–11. M-mode echocardiograms of pericardial effusion. The effusion (PE) appears as an echo-free space surrounding the heart. The effusion on the left does not cause cardiac compression. The effusion on the right demonstrates right ventricular diastolic collapse (*arrow*), evident as abnormal motion of the anterior free wall of the right ventricle that occurs after the mitral valve (MV) opens. LV, left ventricle. *Source: From Hoit BD. Pericardial disease and pericardial heart disease. In: O'Rourke RA, ed. Stein's Internal Medicine, 5th ed. St. Louis: Mosby-Year Book, 1998:273. Reproduced with permission.*

【 】 DIAGNOSTIC AND IMAGING STUDIES

Low voltage on the ECG and/or electrical alternans should suggest cardiac tamponade. However, electrical alternans is insensitive, occurring in approximately 20 percent of instances. When effusion is massive, the heart swings freely within the pericardial sac and acquires a pendular, rotary motion that is associated with electrical alternans. When tamponade is suspected, an echocardiogram should be obtained unless even a brief delay might prove life-threatening. During inspiration, a greater-than-normal increase in RV dimension and decrease in LV dimension occur in many cases of tamponade. These respiratory changes also accompany other conditions associated with pulsus paradoxus, such as chronic obstructive pulmonary disease and pulmonary embolism. Diastolic collapse of the RV, which is recognized as an abnormal posterior motion of the anterior RV wall during diastole (Fig. 84–11), signifies that pericardial pressure exceeds early diastolic RV pressure—that is, that transmural RV diastolic pressure is negative. Although this sign is a relatively sensitive and specific marker for tamponade, RV diastolic collapse is sensitive to alterations in ventricular loading conditions and may not be seen in the presence of RV hypertrophy. In addition, collapse of the right heart chamber occurs with smaller collections of fluid and higher pericardial pressures when there is coexisting LV dysfunction. Late diastolic right atrial collapse is virtually 100 percent sensitive for tamponade but is less specific (Fig. 84–12). Duration of right atrial collapse exceeding one-third of the cardiac cycle increases specificity without sacrificing sensitivity. Posterior loculated effusions after cardiac surgery may produce left atrial and LV diastolic collapse. Transesophageal echocardiography may be valuable in the detection and treatment of unusual cases of cardiac tamponade. In patients with unexplained hypotension who are undergoing transesophageal echocardiography, a diagnosis of a nonventricular limitation to cardiac output was associated with improved survival in the intensive care unit compared with a diagnosis of ventricular disease or hypovolemia/low systemic vascular resistance.[21]

During cardiac tamponade, tricuspid and pulmonary flow velocities measured by Doppler echocardiography (Fig. 84–13) increase markedly with inspiration, and flow velocities in the mitral and aortic valves decrease significantly compared with normal control patients and patients with asymptomatic effusions. Changes in the pattern of venous flow (reflecting the predominance of systolic flow) and exaggerated respiratory variations of venous flow velocities (Fig. 84–14) are also seen in cardiac tamponade. It is important to remember that clinically significant tamponade is a clinical diagnosis and "echocardiographic signs of tamponade" are not by themselves an indication for pericardiocentesis. Although the absence of any cardiac chamber collapse has a high negative predictive value (92 percent), the positive predictive value is reduced (58 percent); and although positive and negative predictive values are high (82 and 88 percent, respectively) for abnormal right-sided venous flows (i.e., systolic predominance and expiratory diastolic reversal), they are not evaluable in more than one-third of patients.[22]

【 】 CARDIAC CATHETERIZATION

The diagnosis of cardiac tamponade is confirmed by right-heart catheterization. The right atrial, pulmonary capillary wedge, and pulmonary artery diastolic pressures are elevated, usually between 10 and 30 mmHg, and are equal within 4 to 5 mmHg (Fig. 84–15). Pericardial pressure is elevated and is equal to right atrial pressure; the degree of elevation is related to both the severity of tamponade and the patient's intravascular volume status

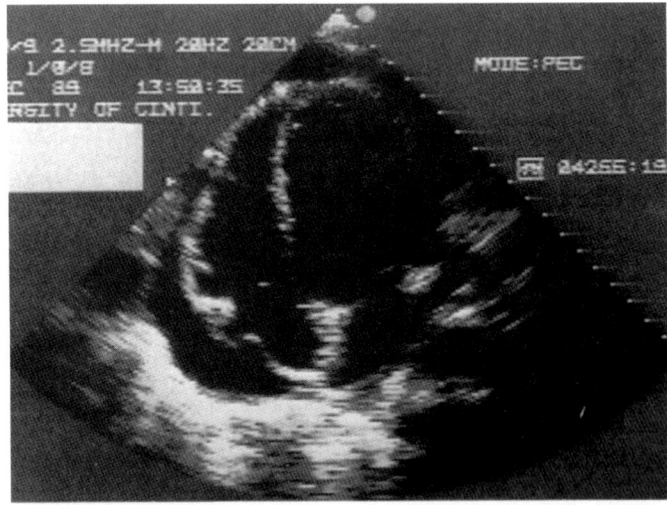

FIGURE 84–12. Two-dimensional echocardiogram in the apical four-chamber view. During late diastole, there is inversion of the lateral wall of the right atrium. *Source: From Hoit BD. Imaging the pericardium. Cardiol Clin 1990;8:593. Reproduced with permission.*

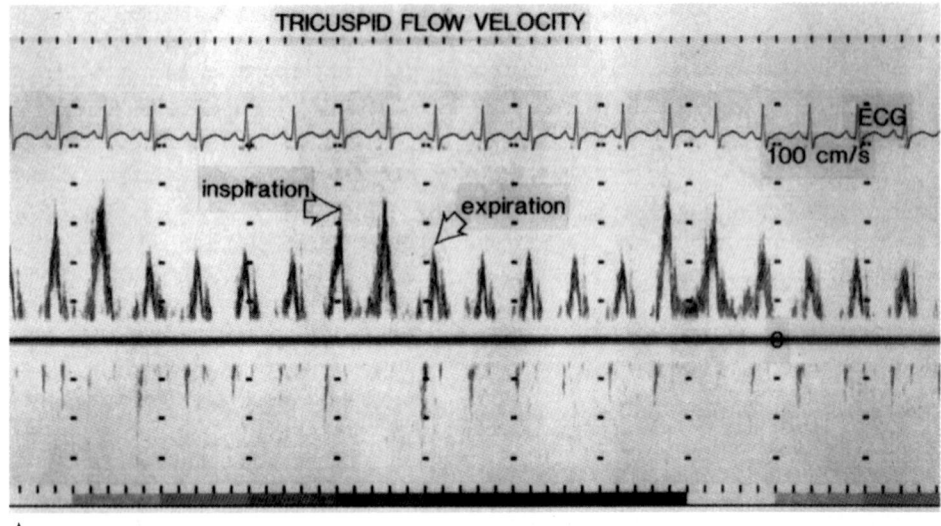

A

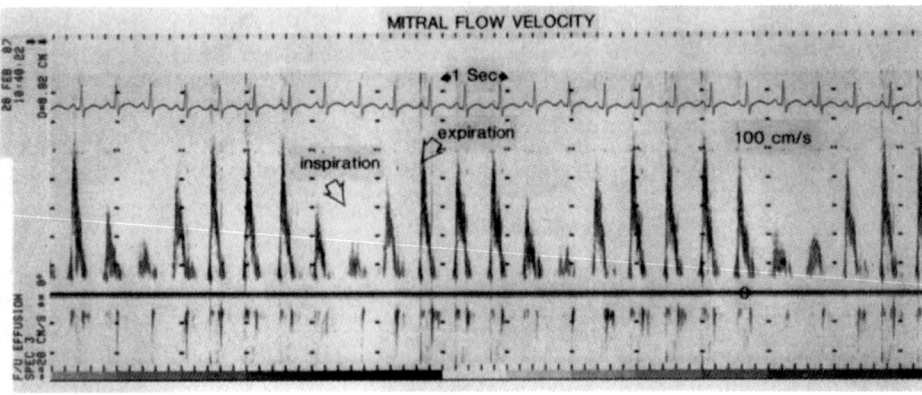

B

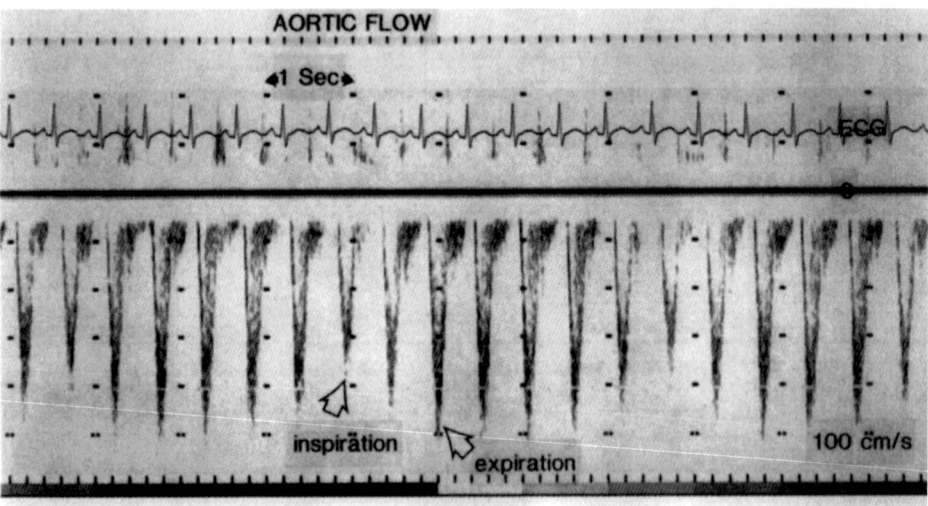

C

FIGURE 84–13. Doppler echocardiogram in a patient with cardiac tamponade. Note the inspiratory increase of tricuspid flow velocities (**A**) and the expiratory increase of mitral (**B**) and aortic (**C**) flow velocities. *Source: From Hoit BD. Imaging the pericardium. Cardiol Clin 1990;8:594. Reproduced with permission.*

diastolic dip and plateau (i.e., the "square root" sign) characteristic of pericardial constriction is seen in tamponade.

MANAGEMENT OF CARDIAC TAMPONADE

Removal of small amounts of pericardial fluid (about 50 mL) produces considerable symptomatic and hemodynamic improvement because of the steep pericardial pressure–volume relationship. Unless there is concomitant cardiac disease or coexisting constriction (i.e., effusive–constrictive pericarditis), removal of all the pericardial fluid normalizes pericardial, atrial, ventricular diastolic, and arterial pressures and cardiac output.

Mild or low-pressure tamponade (i.e., when the venous pressure is less than 10 cm of water, arterial blood pressure is normal, and pulsus paradoxus is absent), particularly when the etiology is idiopathic, viral, or when responsive to specific therapy (e.g., thyroid hormone), does not require pericardiocentesis. In contrast, hyperacute tamponade (usually resulting from cardiac trauma) necessitates immediate pericardiocentesis as an initial triage measure. However, the majority of patients falls between these two extremes and will require pericardial drainage. Either surgical means (via subxiphoid incision, video-assisted thoracoscopy, or thoracotomy) or percutaneous means (with a needle or balloon catheter) accomplishes the pericardial drainage.[23]

Unless the situation is immediately life-threatening, pericardiocentesis should be performed by experienced staff in a facility equipped for hemodynamic monitoring. The advantages of needle pericardiocentesis include the ability to perform careful hemodynamic measurements and relatively simple logistic and personnel requirements. The safety of the procedure has been improved by using 2D echo guidance, with a 1.2% major complication rate in 1127 cases over 21 years.[24] A catheter can be advanced over a guidewire into the pericardial space and remain there for several days; sclerosing agents, steroids, urokinase, and specific chemotherapeutic agents may be given through the catheter.

Drainage of the pericardial fluid using a catheter minimizes trauma, allows measurement of pericardial pressure and instillation of drugs into the pericardium, and helps prevent (but does not guarantee) reaccumulation of pericardial fluid. Extended (3 ± 2

(Fig. 84–16). The right atrial and wedge pressure tracings reveal an attenuated or absent Y descent. Cardiac output is reduced, and systemic vascular resistance is elevated. Equal elevation of diastolic pressures may also be seen with dilated cardiomyopathy and with RV infarction. Neither the Kussmaul sign nor the early ventricular

CONTROL

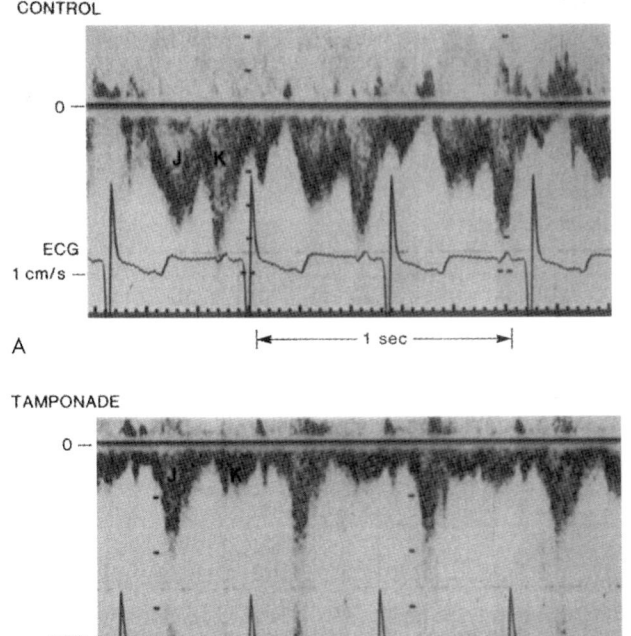

FIGURE 84–14. Doppler echocardiograms of pulmonary venous flow velocity from a dog before (**A**) and after (**B**) creation of cardiac tamponade. Note the predominance of systolic flow after tamponade. J, systolic flow; K, diastolic flow on control flow velocity (**A**). *Source: From Hoit BD. Imaging the pericardium. Cardiol Clin 1990;8:595. Reproduced with permission.*

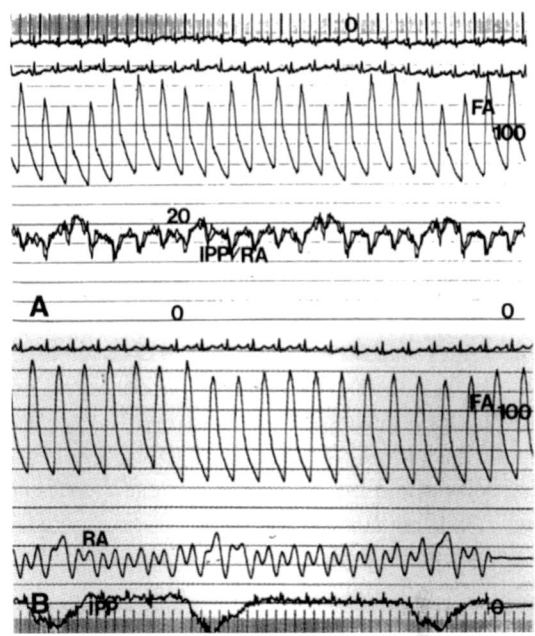

FIGURE 84–15. Hemodynamic record from a patient with cardiac tamponade before (**A**) and after (**B**) pericardiocentesis. **A.** Pulsus paradoxus is evident from the femoral artery (FA) pressure tracing. Note the absent Y descent on the right atrial (RA) tracing and the equal and elevated RA and pericardial (IPP) pressures. **B.** After removal of pericardial fluid, pericardial and right atrial pressures decrease and the pulsus paradoxus disappears. *Source: Courtesy of Noble O. Fowler, MD. From Hoit BD. Pericardial disease and pericardial heart disease. In: O'Rourke RA, ed. Stein's Internal Medicine, 5th ed. St. Louis: Mosby-Year Book, 1998:273. Reproduced with permission.*

days) catheter drainage is associated with a trend toward lower recurrence rates over a nearly 4-year follow up.[25] Generally speaking, drainage should continue until the volume of the aspirated volume is less than 25 mL/d; recurrent tamponade, particularly with hemorrhagic effusions, should be sought. Dilute heparin or fibrinolytic agents may be instilled in the catheter to prevent clotting.

Although pericardiocentesis may provide effective relief, percutaneous balloon pericardiotomy, subxiphoid pericardiotomy, or the surgical creation of a pleuropericardial or peritoneal–pericardial window may be required. The safety and efficacy of subxiphoid pericardiostomy was found to be superior to percutaneous drainage in both benign and malignant effusions. The authors of the latter study recommended that percutaneous needle drainage be reserved for patients with hemodynamic instability.[26]

Open surgical drainage offers several advantages, including complete drainage, access to pericardial tissue for histopathologic and microbiologic diagnoses, the ability to drain loculated effusions, and the absence of traumatic injury resulting from blind placement of a needle into the pericardial sac. The choice between needle pericardiocentesis and surgical drainage depends on institutional resources and physician experience, the etiology of the effusion, the need for diagnostic tissue samples, and the prognosis of the patient. Needle pericardiocentesis is often the best option when the etiology is known and/or the diagnoses of tamponade is in question, and surgical drainage is optimal when the presence of tamponade is certain but the etiology is unclear. Pericardiocentesis is ill-advised when there is less than 1 cm of effusion, loculation, or evidence of fibrin and adhesion. It should be recognized that

surgical approaches (subxiphoid pericardiotomy and thoracoscopic drainage) can be performed using local anesthesia with little attendant morbidity. Irrespective of the method of retrieval, pericardial fluid should be sent for hematocrit and cell count; glucose; Gram, Ziehl-Nielsen, and fungal smears; viral, bacterial and fungal culture; and cytology. Depending on the clinical circumstances, cytology, tumor markers and carbohydrate antigens (for suspected malignant disease), and adenosine deaminase, interferon-γ, pericardial lysozyme, and PCR analysis (for suspected tuberculosis) should be obtained.

Recurrent effusions may be treated by repeat pericardiocentesis, sclerotherapy with tetracycline, surgical creation of a pericardial window, or pericardiectomy. Subtotal pericardiectomy is preferred when the patient is expected to survive for more than 1 year. A pleuropericardial window is usually created in patients with malignant effusions, and pericardiectomy may be required for recurrent effusions in dialysis patients. The approach to surgical pericardiectomy depends on the clinical scenario.[27] In acute life-threatening situations, in high-risk patients, and for diagnostic purposes, the subxiphoid approach is generally used. For primarily effusive disease, a left anterior thoracotomy is generally performed, whereas a median sternotomy is the incision of choice with constrictive disease. Video-assisted thoracoscopic pericardiectomy (VATS) is an alternative to open thoracotomy, but it requires general anesthesia and single-lung ventilation and thus is unsuitable for patients with poor pulmonary reserve. In critically ill patients, a pericardial window may be created percutaneously with a balloon catheter.

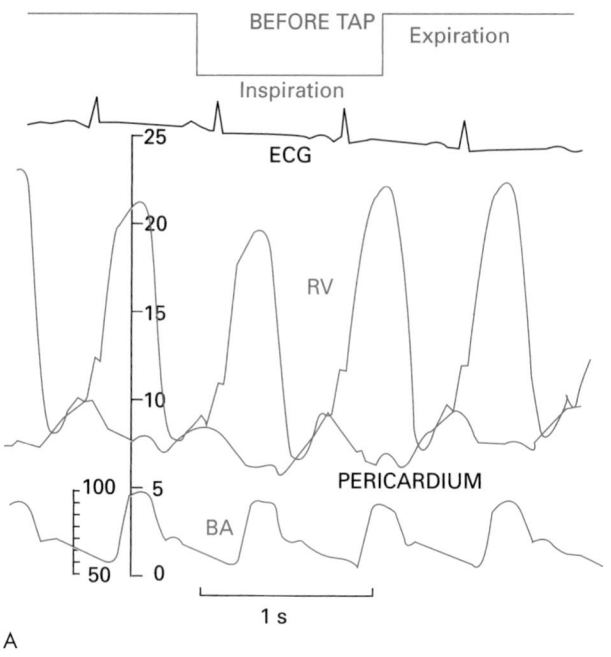

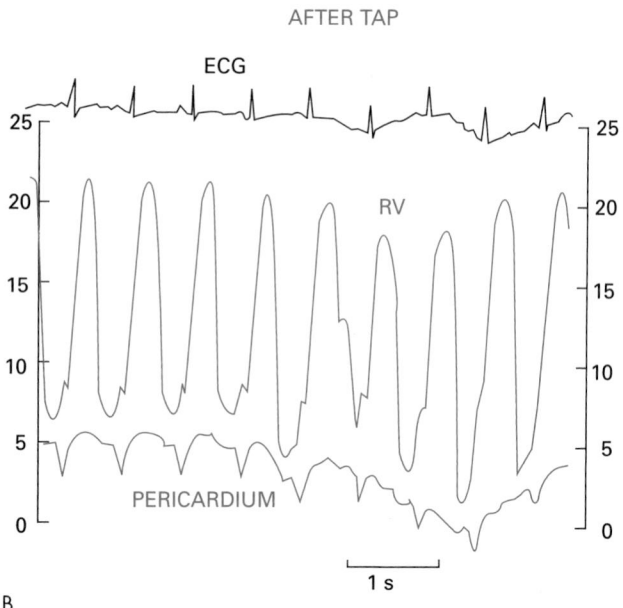

FIGURE 84–16. A. Low-pressure cardiac tamponade. Right ventricular (RV) diastolic pressure is only slightly elevated but is equal to pericardial pressure. Hypotension and pulsus paradoxus are absent. **B.** After pericardiocentesis, pericardial pressure is consistently lower than ventricular diastolic pressure. *Source: From Shabetai R. Diseases of the pericardium. In: Alexander WA, Schlant R, Fuster V, et al, eds. Hurst's The Heart, 9th ed. New York: McGraw-Hill, 1998:2185. Reproduced with permission.*

CONSTRICTIVE PERICARDITIS

Constrictive pericarditis is a condition in which a thickened, scarred, and often calcified pericardium limits diastolic filling of the ventricles. Although it is commonly thought that a normal pericardial thickness excludes the diagnosis of constrictive pericarditis, 28 percent of 143 surgically confirmed cases had normal pericardial thickness on CT scan, and 18 percent had normal thickness on histopathologic examination.[28] Acute pericarditis from most causes may eventuate in constrictive pericarditis, but the most common antecedents are idiopathic conditions, cardiac trauma and surgery, tuberculosis and other infectious diseases, neoplasms (particularly lung and breast), radiation therapy, renal failure, and connective tissue diseases. Rare causes include Dressler syndrome, sarcoidosis, Whipple disease, amyloidosis, and dermatomyositis. "Mulibrey" nanism is a hereditary form of constrictive pericarditis that is associated with abnormalities of the *mu*scle, *liver, br*ain, and *eyes.*

【 】 CLINICAL FEATURES

Constrictive pericarditis resembles the congestive states caused by myocardial disease and chronic liver disease. Patients generally complain of fatigue, dyspnea, weight gain, abdominal discomfort, nausea, increased abdominal girth, and edema. Although symptoms usually develop over years, they progress over a period of months in patients with subacute constrictive pericarditis after trauma, cardiac surgery, and mediastinal irradiation and may develop acutely and resolve spontaneously during the course of pericarditis (see Syndromes of Constrictive Pericarditis below).

【 】 PHYSICAL FINDINGS

Physical findings include ascites, hepatosplenomegaly, edema, and, in long-standing cases, severe wasting. This general appearance often leads to an erroneous diagnosis of hepatic cirrhosis. However, misdiagnosis is avoided through a careful examination of the neck veins. In constrictive pericarditis, the venous pressure is elevated and displays deep Y, and often deep X, descents. The venous pressure fails to decrease with inspiration (Kussmaul sign), but frank inspiratory swelling of the neck veins is uncommon. The Kussmaul sign lacks specificity, as it is seen also in cases of restrictive cardiomyopathy, RV failure and infarction, and tricuspid stenosis. The heart is often normal in size; when it is not, enlargement is modest. A pericardial knock that is similar in timing to the third heart sound is pathognomonic but occurs infrequently. Pulsus paradoxus may occur with associated pericardial effusion (effusive–constrictive pericarditis). Except in severe cases, the arterial blood pressure is normal.

【 】 DIAGNOSTIC AND IMAGING STUDIES

Low QRS voltage, nonspecific T-wave changes, and P mitrale are common, but the ECG findings are nonspecific (Fig. 84–17). Atrial fibrillation is seen in approximately one-third of cases, and atrial flutter is seen less often, although the exact percentage of atrial arrhythmias depends on the duration of constriction.

The cardiac silhouette may be normal or enlarged. Pericardial calcification is present in less than half the cases seen in the United States and Europe. Pericardial calcification may be seen with chronic adhesive pericarditis in the absence of constriction, but then it is usually less dense and has a more patchy distribution (Fig. 84–18).

Pericardial thickening and calcification and abnormal ventricular filling produce characteristic changes on the M-mode echocardiogram. Increased pericardial thickness is suggested by parallel

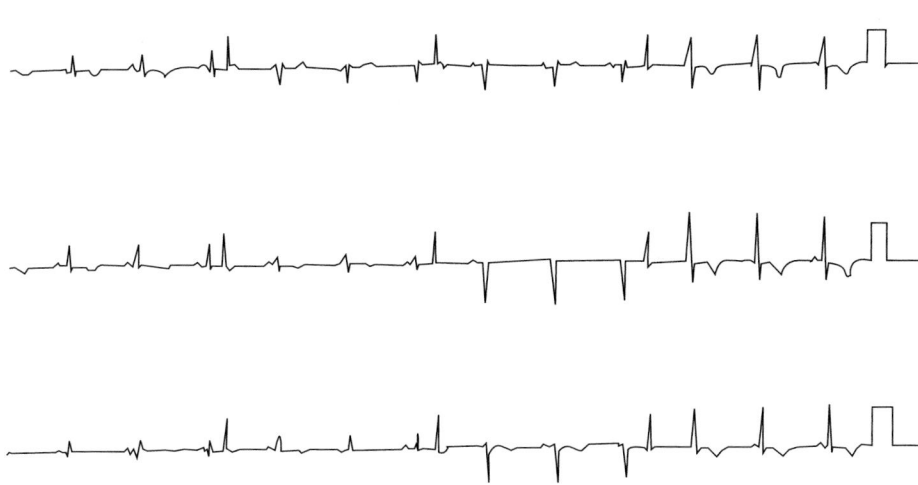

FIGURE 84–17. Electrocardiogram of a patient with tuberculous constrictive pericarditis showing widespread inversed polarity of the T waves. Leads are mounted in the conventional sequence. *Source: From Shabetai R. Diseases of the pericardium. In: Alexander WA, Schlant R, Fuster V, et al, eds. Hurst's The Heart, 9th ed. New York: McGraw-Hill, 1998:2188. Reproduced with permission.*

motion of the epicardium and parietal pericardium, which are separated by a relatively echo-free space at least 1 mm thick. Echocardiographic correlates of the hemodynamic abnormalities of constrictive pericarditis include flattening of the LV posterior wall endocardium, abnormal septal motion, and, occasionally, premature opening of the pulmonary valve (Fig. 84–19). These findings, which reflect abnormal filling of the ventricles, are insensitive and subtle and lack the specificity to be clinically useful. Although no sign or combination of signs on M-mode echocardiography is diagnostic of constrictive pericarditis, a normal study virtually rules out the diagnosis.

More recently, Doppler tissue imaging has been used in the diagnosis of constrictive pericarditis, and may be particularly useful in differentiating between constrictive pericarditis and restrictive cardiomyopathy (see Chap. 31). The myocardial velocity gradient of the LV posterior wall is significantly lower during rapid ventricular filling and ejection in patients with restrictive cardiomyopathy than in healthy controls or in individuals with constrictive pericarditis.[29] Mitral annular velocity is also reduced in patients with restrictive cardiomyopathy compared to those with constrictive pericarditis, and this relationship is evident in the absence of significant respiratory variation in early diastolic filling—a prominent feature of constrictive pericarditis.[30] CT is a highly accurate method of evaluating pericardial thickness and therefore plays an essential role in the diagnosis and management of constrictive disease (Fig. 84–20). The normal pericardium is identified as a 1- to 2-mm curvilinear line of soft-tissue density, whereas in constrictive pericarditis, the parietal pericardium is 4 to 20 mm thick. Failure to visualize the posterolateral LV wall on dynamic CT suggests myocardial fibrosis or atrophy and is associated with a poor surgical outcome. Because of the close physiologic similarities of constrictive pericarditis and restrictive cardiomyopathy, increased pericardial thickness detected by tomographic scanning is the most reliable means of distinguishing between the two disorders, as normal pericardial thickness excludes most cases of constrictive pericarditis. CT also is useful in planning pericardiectomy because of its ability to define the distribution of pericardial thickening.

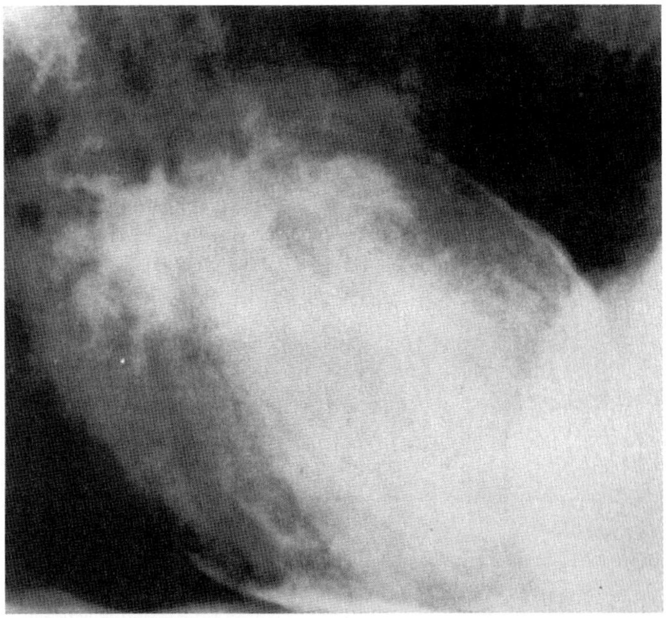

Accurate definition of pericardial thickness and its distribution also is possible with MRI (Fig. 84–21).[31] Unlike CT, ECG gating is necessary for adequate visualization, resolution is not quite as good, and calcification is difficult to distinguish from fibrosis. However, the diagnostic accuracy in identifying surgically confirmed constrictive pericarditis is excellent.

【 】 CARDIAC CATHETERIZATION

Cardiac catheterization is used to confirm the clinical suspicion of pericardial disease, uncover occult constriction, diagnose effusive–constrictive disease, and identify associated coronary, myocardial, and valvular disease. Endomyocardial biopsy is sometimes necessary to exclude restrictive cardiomyopathy, which shares many hemodynamic abnormalities with constrictive pericarditis.

【 】 DIFFERENCES BETWEEN CONSTRICTIVE PERICARDITIS AND CARDIAC TAMPONADE

The waveform of venous pressure in constrictive pericarditis differs from that in cardiac tamponade. In constrictive pericarditis, cardiac volume is determined by the thickened, rigid pericardium, and the heart is unable to exceed this volume, which is attained near the end of the first third of diastole. During ejection, venous return commences unimpeded; therefore the normal systolic surge of

FIGURE 84–18. Calcification of the pericardium seen on a lateral chest radiograph in a patient with chronic constrictive pericarditis. *Source: Courtesy of Ralph Shabetai, MD. From Hoit BD. Imaging the pericardium. Cardiol Clin 1990;8:595. Reproduced with permission.*

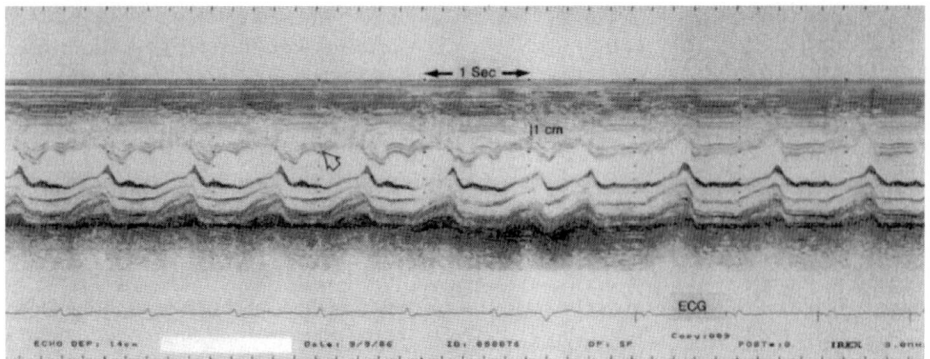

FIGURE 84–19. M-mode echocardiogram from a patient with constrictive pericarditis. An abrupt posterior motion of the septum begins after the onset of atrial systole. This atrial systolic notch is not seen on premature or paced beats. Note also the thickened pericardium and flat posterior wall in middle and late diastole. *Source: From Tei C, Child JS, Tanaka H, et al. Atrial systolic notch on the interventricular septum echogram: an echocardiographic sign of constrictive pericarditis. J Am Coll Cardiol 1983;1:908. Reproduced with permission.*

venous return is preserved. Cardiac compression remains insignificant at end systole (unlike cardiac tamponade), so that when the tricuspid valve opens, blood fills the ventricles at a supernormal rate. Thus, in constrictive pericarditis, the venous return is biphasic, but with a diastolic component greater than or equal to the systolic component.

Unlike the case in cardiac tamponade, the intrapericardial space is obliterated in constrictive pericarditis. As a result, during inspiration, the decreased intrathoracic pressure is not transmitted to the heart, venous pressure does not fall, and systemic venous return fails to increase. Another important distinction from cardiac tamponade is that early diastolic filling is faster than normal in constrictive pericarditis; consequently, the ventricular diastolic pressure is characterized by a dip in early diastole (Fig. 84–22). By the end of the rapid-filling phase, the ventricles are completely filled and the ventricular diastolic pressure remains unchanged and elevated for the remainder of diastole.

In contrast to cardiac tamponade, early diastolic filling in constrictive pericarditis is unrestrained, and only at the end of the first third of diastole does the stiff pericardium abruptly restrict ventricular filling. As a result, ventricular pressure falls rapidly in early diastole and subsequently rises abruptly to an elevated level, where it remains until the next ventricular systole. End-diastolic ventricular pressures and mean atrial pressures are elevated and nearly equal (within 5 mmHg), and end-diastolic volumes and, consequently, stroke volume and cardiac output are reduced. These pathophysiologic changes are responsible for the hemodynamic and physical findings that characterize constrictive pericarditis.

Pulsus paradoxus is much less common in constrictive pericarditis than it is in cardiac tamponade because, in constrictive pericarditis, inspiratory increases in venous return and in the volume of the right side of the heart seldom occur, and the position of the ventricular septum relative to the two ventricles is not as dramatically altered. Systolic LV function is usually unimpaired in both constrictive pericarditis and cardiac tamponade. Long-standing calcific constrictive pericarditis may invade the myocardium and coronary vessels, leading to conduction disturbances and impaired ventricular function.

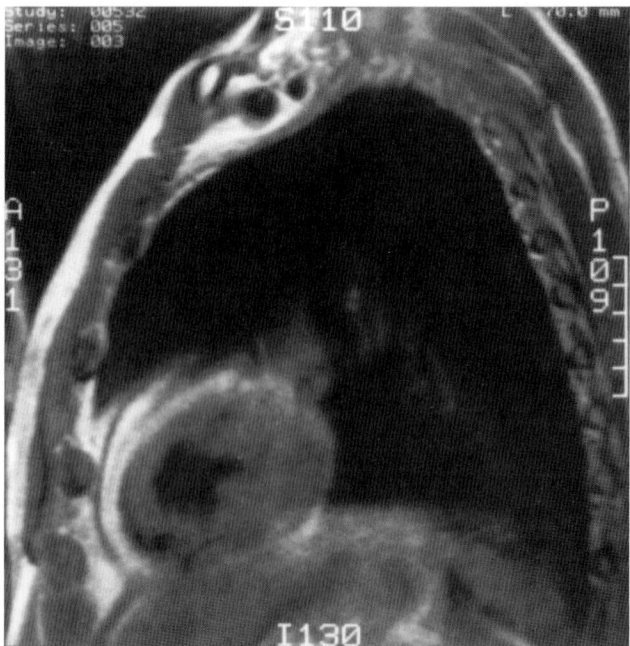

FIGURE 84–21. MRI scan (spin-echo image) from a patient with constrictive pericarditis. The pericardium is viewed as a line of low signal intensity (*black*) sandwiched between higher-intensity epicardial and pericardial fat (*white*). Note the regional variation of pericardial thickness, which is normally 1 to 2 mm. *Source: From Hoit BD. Pericardial disease and pericardial heart disease. In: O'Rourke RA, ed. Stein's Internal Medicine, 5th ed. St. Louis: Mosby-Year Book, 1998:273. Reproduced with permission.*

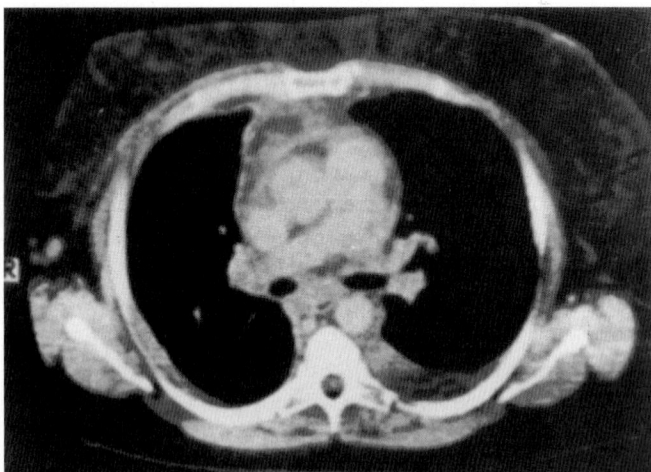

FIGURE 84–20. Computed tomogram from a patient with constrictive pericarditis. The diffusely thickened pericardium is bordered by low-intensity epicardial and mediastinal fat. *Source: Courtesy of Dr. N.O. Fowler. From Hoit BD. Imaging the pericardium. Cardiol Clin 1990;8:597. Reproduced with permission.*

SYNDROMES OF CONSTRICTIVE PERICARDITIS

Classic *chronic constrictive pericarditis* is encountered less frequently than it was in the past, whereas *subacute constrictive pericarditis* is becoming more common. In the latter syndrome, constriction occurs weeks to months after the inciting injury, pericardial calcification is uncommon, and the course may span a matter of weeks to a few years. *Postoperative constrictive pericarditis* is an important cause of constriction, with a reported incidence of 0.2 percent[32]; this incidence is surprisingly low considering that the pericardium is subject to cellular injury and is exposed to proinflammatory substances such as blood and local hypothermia.

Occult constrictive pericarditis requires a fluid challenge for detection. In the first series reported, the patients complained of nondescript chest pain, for which they underwent cardiac catheterization and coronary arteriography. Although hemodynamic studies revealed normal basal atrial and ventricular pressures, the right atrial pressure waveform assumed the characteristics of constrictive pericarditis and the diastolic pressures in the two ventricles became equal after a rapid infusion (10 minutes) of approximately 1 L of saline solution. Histologic examination confirmed the surgical findings of a thickened and fibrosed pericardium. However, rapid, large fluid challenges at cardiac catheterization should be administered with caution; furthermore, the induction of typical hemodynamic changes should seldom if ever be considered by itself as an indication for pericardiectomy. In asymptomatic patients, maximal O_2 consumption should be quantified, jugular venous pressure carefully estimated, and liver function tests measured. Increasing jugular venous pressure, the need for diuretic therapy, evidence of hepatic insufficiency, and reduced exercise tolerance indicate the need for surgery.

Localized constrictive pericarditis is rare, but occasionally a localized band constricts the inflow or outflow region of one or more of the cardiac chambers. The clinical picture then simulates valve disease or venous obstruction. Evidence of *transient (acute) constriction* may occur in approximately 15 percent of patients with acute effusive pericarditis.[33] Doppler-detected constrictive physiology resolved without pericardiectomy in 36 of 212 patients studied retrospectively after an average of approximately 8 weeks at Mayo Clinic.[34] Thus before one proceeds with pericardiectomy, the possibility that pericardial constriction may be reversible and amenable to medical therapy should be considered.

MANAGEMENT OF CONSTRICTIVE PERICARDITIS

Pericardiectomy is the definitive treatment for constrictive pericarditis but is unwarranted either in very early constriction or in

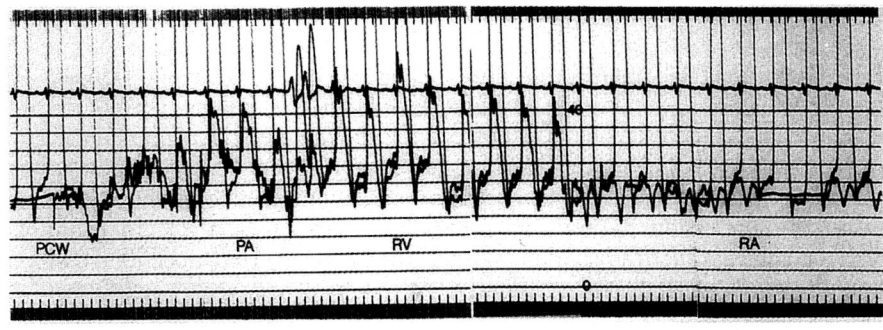
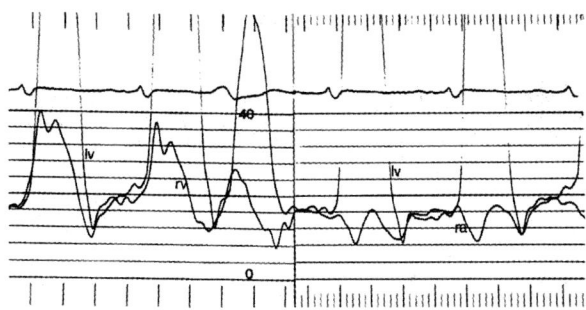

FIGURE 84–22. Hemodynamic record of a patient with surgically proven constrictive pericarditis. *Top.* Slow-paper-speed recording of high-gain left ventricular (LV) pressure and simultaneous right heart pullback from pulmonary capillary wedge (PCW) to pulmonary artery (PA), right ventricle (RV), and right atrium (RA). *Bottom.* Fast-paper-speed recording of LV and simultaneous RV and RA pressure tracings. Note the increased and equal atrial and diastolic pressures, the prominent X and Y descents on the RA tracing, and the dip and plateau on the RV and LV tracings during longer diastoles. *Source: Courtesy of Peter J. Engel, MD. From Hoit BD. Pericardial disease and pericardial heart disease. In: O'Rourke RA, ed. Stein's Internal Medicine, 5th ed. St. Louis: Mosby-Year Book, 1998:273. Reproduced with permission.*

severe, advanced disease (functional class IV), when the risk of surgery is excessive (30 to 40 percent mortality) and the benefits are diminished. Involvement of the visceral pericardium also increases the surgical risk. Symptomatic relief and normalization of cardiac pressures may take several months after pericardiectomy; they occur sooner when the operation is carried out before the disease is too chronic and when the pericardiectomy is almost complete. Complete or extensive pericardial resection is desirable, as recurrences may be seen more frequently in patients who have undergone partial versus complete resection of the pericardium. In highly selected patients, orthotopic transplantation may be considered. Constriction may be transitory with a course lasting weeks to a few months in patients recovering from acute effusive pericarditis. Thus it is sensible that patients with subacute constrictive pericarditis who are hemodynamically stable be given a trial of conservative management for 2 to 3 months until it is clear that the constrictive process is permanent before pericardiectomy is recommended.

Pericardiectomy is commonly carried out via a median sternotomy, although some surgeons prefer a thoracotomy. Despite a decline in the risk of mortality, the risk remains 5 to 15 percent. The risk is increased by heavy calcification and involvement of the visceral pericardium. LV systolic dysfunction may occur after decortication of a severely constricted heart. Although this condition may require treatment for several months, it usually resolves completely.

Recent data suggest that despite reduced perioperative mortality, the late survival of contemporary patients after pericardiectomy is inferior to that of an age- and sex-matched group of historical controls. The long-term outcome was predicted by three variables in a recent stepwise logistic regression analysis; specifically, the prognosis was worse with increasing age and New York Heart Association (NYHA) class and a postirradiation etiology.[35] In another study, age, renal dysfunction, pulmonary hypertension, left ventricular dysfunction, and hyponatremia were independent adverse predictors.[36]

Medical therapy of constrictive pericarditis plays a small but important role. In some patients, constrictive pericarditis resolves either spontaneously or in response to various combinations of NSAIDs, steroids, and antibiotics. Specific antibiotic (e.g., antituberculous) therapy should be initiated before surgery and continued afterward. Diuretics and digoxin (in the presence of atrial fibrillation) are useful in patients who are not candidates for pericardiectomy because of their high surgical risk. Preoperative diuretics should be used sparingly with the goal of reducing, not eliminating, elevated jugular pressure, edema, and ascites. Postoperatively, diuretics should be given if spontaneous diuresis does not occur; the central venous pressure may take weeks to months to return to normal after pericardiectomy. The LVEF may decrease postoperatively, only to return to normal months later. In the interim, digoxin, diuretics, and vasodilators may be useful.

Prevention consists of appropriate therapy for acute pericarditis and adequate pericardial drainage. Although instillation of fibrinolytics (urokinase 400,000 U per instillation to 1,600,000 U; streptokinase 250,000 IU per instillation to 1,000,000 IU) is promising, corticosteroids are often ineffective.[37]

EFFUSIVE–CONSTRICTIVE PERICARDITIS

Effusive–constrictive pericarditis occurs when pericardial fluid accumulates between the thickened, fibrotic parietal pericardium and visceral pericardium. Neoplasia, chest irradiation, infection (including TB where endemic), idiopathic pericarditis, and connective tissue diseases are common antecedents. Transient effusive–constrictive pericarditis may complicate chemotherapy. The hemodynamic features are those of cardiac tamponade before, and constrictive pericarditis after, pericardiocentesis. Thus, removal of pericardial fluid fails to lower atrial and ventricular diastolic pressures, but the previously attenuated or absent atrial Y descent becomes prominent (Fig. 84–23).

Effusive–constrictive pericarditis is relatively uncommon; in a series of 190 patients undergoing pericardiocentesis for cardiac tamponade, the disorder was diagnosed in 15 (8 percent).[38] The diagnosis was defined by a failure of the right atrial pressure to fall by 50 percent or to a level below 10 mmHg after pericardiocentesis. In these patients, constriction was clinically suspect in 7; symptoms were usually present for less than 3 months, right-heart failure was evident in all, evidence of acute pericarditis was noted in 7, pulsus paradoxus was noted in 10, and pericardial calcification was present in none.

Noninvasive imaging is not useful in the diagnosis of effusive–constrictive pericarditis.[39] The clinical course of effusive–constrictive disease is related to the etiology of the pericardial disease and the patient's general condition.[38] If surgery is required, a technically difficult visceral pericardiectomy must be performed.[39]

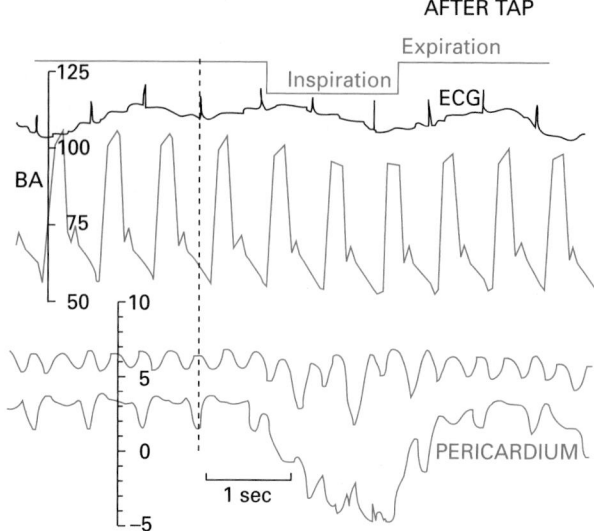

FIGURE 84–23. Recording from a patient with effusive-constrictive pericarditis caused by lung cancer. The tracings were obtained during the pericardiocentesis; right atrial pressure elevation persists, and there are prominent X and Y descents without respiratory variation. *Source: From Shabetai R. The Pericardium. New York: Grune & Stratton, 1981:273. Reproduced with permission.*

SPECIFIC FORMS OF PERICARDIAL HEART DISEASE

【 】 IDIOPATHIC PERICARDITIS

(See also Acute Pericarditis above.)

Acute pericarditis is most often idiopathic and is typically a self-limited disease lasting 2 to 6 weeks. Small pericardial effusions occur commonly, but cardiac tamponade is unusual. Heart failure caused by associated myocarditis and constrictive pericarditis are uncommon. These complications usually can be detected by clinical and echocardiographic evaluation. The clinical course and prognosis of individuals with pericarditis are otherwise determined largely by the presence and nature of any underlying disease.

【 】 INFECTIOUS PERICARDITIS

Viral Pericarditis

Viral pericarditis is the most common infectious type, although a definitive diagnosis from acute and convalescent (3 weeks) viral neutralizing antibodies is generally not helpful in a sporadic case of pericarditis. Viral isolation from pericardial fluid and in situ hybridization techniques have been used to identify a specific etiology.[10] However, viral infection is often presumed rather than proved, and many cases are classified as idiopathic. Common viral infections causing acute pericarditis are those resulting from echovirus and coxsackievirus; however, a great many different viruses may cause pericarditis (see Table 84–3).

Bacterial Pericarditis

Bacterial (purulent) pericarditis is most often caused by streptococci, staphylococci, and gram-negative rods; *Haemophilus influ-*

enzae is an important cause in children.[40] The increasing frequency of cardiac surgery and instrumentation, selection-induced changes in the flora responsible for hospital-acquired infections, and the prolonged survival of immunocompromised hosts (HIV, steroids) have changed the incidence and bacterial spectrum of purulent pericarditis. Pericardial involvement often is unrecognized when it complicates systemic infection; unusually high fever and white blood cell counts are clues to the presence of pericarditis. Children and immunosuppressed patients of all ages are most vulnerable, and the characteristic features of acute pericarditis are frequently absent. The course of bacterial pericarditis is fulminant, often presenting with cardiac tamponade; adhesive and constrictive pericarditis are common sequelae in survivors and may develop suddenly and early.[40] However, pericarditis complicating systemic infection and sepsis may go unrecognized and misdiagnosed. Many patients lack the typical findings of pericarditis, and the diagnosis of purulent pericarditis often is made either at autopsy or after cardiac tamponade develops; empyema is a common antecedent.[40] The threshold for echocardiography in the septic patient should be low, and whenever purulent pericarditis is suspected, the pericardial space should be explored. Purulent pericarditis is rarely caused by anaerobic bacteria, and the few reported cases resulted from contiguous infection or hematogenous seeding. Bacterial pericarditis is treated with surgical exploration and drainage and appropriate systemic antibiotics. Fibrinolytics may be used to lyse fibrous adhesions, liquefy purulent exudate, and prevent constrictive pericarditis.[37]

Legionella infections account for approximately 10 percent of community-acquired pneumonias and may be associated with pericarditis more often than previously was appreciated. Studies suggest that patients with pericardial involvement tend to be younger and healthier than are those without it.[41] Recurrent pericarditis, effusion, and chronic constriction occur in approximately 20 percent of cases. Pericarditis is an early complication of Lyme disease.

Mycobacterial and Fungal Pericarditis

Tuberculosis is a major cause of pericarditis in nonindustrialized countries but an uncommon cause in the United States. Nevertheless, its incidence is increasing because of HIV infection; consequently, tuberculosis should be considered in the differential diagnosis of pericardial heart disease. Tuberculous pericarditis results from hematogenous spread of primary tuberculosis or from the breakdown of infected mediastinal lymph nodes, with the result that affected individuals generally lack the typical symptoms and signs of pulmonary tuberculosis. Fever, weight loss, and night sweats occur early; pericardial pain and friction rubs are often absent. Patients may present with tamponade or constriction, which may be subacute. A fibrinous pericarditis with caseating necrosis and mononuclear infiltrate gives rise to an effusive phase, which is often voluminous and hemodynamically significant. An adhesive phase follows resolution of the effusion and eventuates in dense, calcific adhesions with clinical constriction in nearly 50 percent of patients.[1]

Mycobacteria are difficult to culture from pericardial fluid, which is diagnostic in only one-third of cases; The diagnosis of tuberculous pericarditis is based on (1) histologic identification, (2) culture of *Mycobacterium tuberculosis*, (3) pericarditis with proven extracardiac tuberculosis, or (4) pericardial effusion responsive to antituberculosis therapy. PCR-detected *M. tuberculosis* DNA, high adenosine deaminase activity, and interferon-γ concentration in the pericardial fluid are also diagnostic. A presumptive diagnosis generally requires a history of contact and/or purified protein derivative conversion (although the latter lacks sensitivity and specificity). Gadolinium-enhanced MRI may be useful in early diagnosis.

Early pericardiectomy has been recommended by some researchers in all cases of tuberculous pericarditis, but the long-term (16 years) prognosis of patients without cardiac compression during the acute illness who are treated with medical therapy alone is excellent.[42] Fluid should be removed, cultured, and antituberculous therapy begun. Depending on the echocardiographic appearance, subxiphoid drainage may be necessary. Multiple-drug therapy and corticosteroids are effective in tuberculous pericarditis, whereas atypical mycobacterial infections (especially *Mycobacterium avium-intracellulare*) may be resistant to treatment. Patients with tuberculous pericarditis should receive triple-drug therapy (isoniazid, rifampin, and either streptomycin or ethambutol) for a minimum of 9 months. Corticosteroids (prednisone 1–2 mg/kg/d) may be useful if pericardial effusion persists or recurs during therapy, and are beneficial acutely in reducing morbidity and mortality, but definitive data supporting their use to prevent constriction in primary pericardial effusion are lacking.[43] Pericardiectomy may be necessary for recurrent cardiac tamponade.

It is unclear whether open drainage or corticosteroid use prevents the progression to constrictive pericarditis. Nevertheless, patients should be observed for constriction, as up to half of these patients will require pericardiectomy. Failure to improve or worsening over 1 to 2 months, pericardial thickening, or evidence of constriction require urgent pericardiectomy.[2,44] For patients with hemodynamics consistent with effusive–constrictive pericarditis, plans for visceral and parietal pericardiectomy after a few weeks of chemotherapy should be made. Persistent hypotension may signify tuberculous adrenal insufficiency.

In contrast, pericarditis complicating deep fungal infection (histoplasmosis, coccidioidomycosis) may be immunologic, resolve spontaneously, and not require specific therapy. Surgical decompression and specific antifungal therapy may be necessary for disseminated infection with *Candida, Aspergillus, Actinomycetes*, and *Nocardia*.

HIV Pericarditis

Human immunodeficiency virus (HIV) is an important cause of pericardial heart disease. HIV-associated pericardial effusions are increasingly more common, especially in urban referral centers. A retrospective survey at one inner-city medical center revealed that of 122 patients admitted with pericardial effusion over a 9-year period, 40 (33 percent) had associated HIV infection.[45] Among those patients with HIV-associated effusions, 16 (40 percent) presented with cardiac tamponade, and the presence of a pericardial effusion predicted a poor prognosis in HIV-infected individuals. Typically, pericardial effusions are small and asymptomatic in outpatients, but large effusions and tamponade are common in hospitalized patients with acquired immunodeficiency syndrome (AIDS). Indeed, in one study, a moderate or large effusion was present in more patients with symptomatic than asymptomatic

HIV infection (17 vs. 2 percent), and most of these cases were clinically unsuspected.[46] The incidence and prevalence of pericardial effusion in a prospective, 5-year followup study of AIDS patients were high (11 percent per year and 5 percent, respectively). A literature review of echocardiographic and autopsy series found an average incidence of pericardial disease of 21 percent.[47]

Pericardial involvement may be a result of associated malignancies (e.g., lymphoma and Kaposi sarcoma), viruses (including HIV), and opportunistic infections (e.g., mycobacteria, cytomegalovirus, *Nocardia*, and cryptococci) and, irrespective of its cause, predicts a poor prognosis in patients with HIV infection.[45] Large, symptomatic pericardial effusion in patients with HIV infection should be aggressively investigated, as two-thirds of these cases have an identifiable cause.[47] Tamponade in patients with HIV is mycobacterial (*M. tuberculosis* or *M. avium-intracellulare*) in origin in approximately one-third of patients.[47]

[ ] NEOPLASTIC PERICARDITIS

Metastatic neoplasia remains the leading cause of pericardial disease in hospitalized patients, most often in patients with lung or breast cancer, melanoma, lymphoma, and acute leukemia. Many cases are asymptomatic and are found only incidentally at autopsy, but others cause symptoms and may progress to cardiac tamponade. Primary cardiac tumors may invade the pericardium directly.

Primary mesothelioma of the pericardium is a rare and highly lethal tumor. Signs and symptoms are nonspecific, and chest radiography and echocardiography are insensitive for its detection; CT and MRI are the most promising diagnostic tests. Other primary tumors of the pericardium are quite rare.

In patients with elevated jugular pressure and an intrathoracic mass, an important inclusion in the differential diagnosis is the superior vena cava syndrome. In this disorder, the characteristic pulsations of the jugular veins are not observed and pulsus paradoxus is not present. However, in a patient with respiratory distress, pulsus alternans, arrhythmia, and/or tachycardia, pulsus paradoxus may be obscured.

The pericardium may be thickened and cause constriction; less commonly, effusive–constrictive pericarditis occurs. Echocardiography rapidly and accurately detects pericardial effusion, identifies metastatic lesions, and provides evidence for cardiac compression. MRI is particularly useful in evaluating pericardial mass lesions. In many cases, neoplastic cells can be recovered from the pericardial fluid, which is usually bloody. However, it is important to remember that more than half of pericardial effusions in cancer patients are a result of causes other than metastatic disease, such as infections, radiation, and drug therapy; thus the presence of pericarditis in cancer patients does not imply imminent death.

In almost every case, fluid should be removed if large effusions are refractory or if tamponade ensues.[48] The specific approach depends on the patient's expected longevity and medical condition. Pericardiocentesis is associated with a high recurrence rate and does not provide tissue for biopsy. Subtotal pericardiectomy is most effective, but should only be performed in carefully selected patients. Balloon pericardiotomy avoids the discomfort and risk of surgery and will likely replace surgical subxiphoid pericardiotomy in critically ill patients with predictably limited survival.

[ ] POSTMYOCARDIAL INFARCTION PERICARDITIS

Pericarditis is common in the first few days after an MI, occurring in as many as 28 to 43 percent of fatal infarctions, but it is clinically apparent in as few as 7 percent of cases.[49] When a friction rub is required for diagnosis, there is an underestimation of the incidence of postinfarction pericarditis. On average, pericarditis was diagnosed by rub alone in 14 percent of patients compared with in 25 percent of patients when classic symptoms, a rub, or both were used as diagnostic criteria. The detection of atypical T-wave evolution on ECG (i.e., either persistent positivity or temporally late positivity) may be a more sensitive and objective means of diagnosing postinfarction pericarditis.[50]

Pericardial involvement is related to infarct size and is associated with a poor prognosis. An important clinical problem is the extent to which acute pericarditis in MI influences management with anticoagulants. A pericardial friction rub occurring in the first 2 or 3 days without an associated pericardial effusion should not influence clinical decisions, but pericarditis occurring later in the course or accompanied by pericardial effusion or tamponade is a contraindication to anticoagulant therapy.

In a prospective, consecutive series of 174 patients with acute MI, pericarditis occurred in 24 percent and was associated with anterior infarct location, heparin therapy, and pericardial effusion.[31] Cardiac tamponade seldom occurs except in patients who receive systemic anticoagulants or have cardiac rupture.

Treatment of infarct pericarditis is seldom indicated, but when symptomatic, infarct pericarditis responds to acetylsalicylic acid (ASA) (up to 650 mg every 4 hours by mouth for 5 to 10 days); corticosteroids should be avoided because of concerns with impaired infarct healing, steroid dependency, and toxic side effects.

Thrombolytic therapy almost invariably precedes the development of pericarditis; therefore clinical decision making usually is not affected. Surprisingly, thrombolytic therapy reduces the incidence of postinfarction pericarditis by approximately half.[51] However, when acute pericarditis is mistaken for acute MI, thrombolytic therapy can have calamitous consequences.

Dressler syndrome (post-MI syndrome) consists of pleuropericardial chest pain, friction rub, fever, leukocytosis, and pulmonary infiltrates. It usually occurs weeks or months (>10 days to 2 weeks) after the causative infarction. Dressler syndrome may be caused by a combination of viral activation and myocardial antibodies and is clinically and pathogenetically similar to the postpericardiotomy syndrome; controversy exists, however, regarding the significance of these antibodies and their relationship with the severity of myocardial injury. Cardiac tamponade and late constriction may occur. For reasons that are not entirely clear, thrombolytic therapy has helped render post-MI pericarditis nearly extinct. Together with posttraumatic pericarditis these disorders constitute the postpericardial syndrome, which is characterized by latency between the inciting pericardial event and pericarditis, tendency to recurrence, and fever and markers of systemic inflammation. Treatment of postpericardial syndrome consists of ASA, NSAIDs, colchicine (which may also be preventative), and, if necessary, a short course of steroids (which are not preventative). Therapy with intrapericardial instillation of triamcinolone appears promising but requires further investigation.

RADIATION-INDUCED PERICARDIAL DISEASE

Radiation injury to the pericardium is said to occur after exposure in excess of 4000 rads; the incidence also is dependent on the use of subcarinal blocks, the nature of the radiation source, and the duration and fractionation of the radiation regimen.

Acute pericarditis occurring early during therapy is uncommon and most likely a result of the radiation-induced effects on the tumor rather than a direct toxic effect of the radiation on the pericardium. In this instance, therapy should not be disrupted, although a reduction in dose may be necessary. A delayed (usually less than 1 year but highly variable) form of pericardial injury may present as acute pericarditis or effusion (often with some degree of cardiac compression). The reaction of the pericardium to radiation is fibrinous inflammation, often with an effusion. Although the acute lesion usually subsides within 2 years without sequelae, constrictive and effusive–constrictive pericarditis may become manifest only after many years.

The incompletely understood pathophysiology of radiation pericarditis involves, in part, extensive damage to the pericardial microcirculation and pericardial lymphatics with resultant ischemic injury. The incidence increases when anteriorly weighted field techniques are employed and is more common in patients who have also received adjunctive chemotherapy.

In the effusive stage, the differential diagnosis includes recurrence of the neoplasm; examination of pericardial fluid is then helpful, as the fluid is positive in approximately 30 percent of cases. Effusion may be a result of the hypothyroid state induced by radiation therapy. Cytology is reliable in breast and lung cancer but less so in lymphoma and leukemia, where pericardial biopsy may be needed. Acute radiation-induced pericarditis can be managed symptomatically as acute idiopathic pericarditis. Hemodynamically insignificant pericardial effusion can also be managed conservatively, as spontaneous resolution is the rule; however, pericardiectomy should be offered to symptomatic patients with large, recurrent pericardial effusions. Constrictive pericarditis requires pericardiectomy unless the biopsy reveals significant endomyocardial fibrosis.

TRAUMATIC PERICARDIAL DISEASE

Blunt trauma and penetrating trauma are important causes of pericarditis, particularly among young men. Acute tamponade beginning very soon after trauma (pericardial injury syndrome), recurrent pericardial effusion, and recurrent acute pericarditis (postpericardial syndrome), and chronic constrictive pericarditis, are well-recognized complications. The application of echocardiography in the trauma unit rapidly and accurately diagnoses hemopericardium in patients with potentially penetrating cardiac wounds. Failure to repair the injury responsible for tamponade is associated with a poor clinical outcome. Constrictive pericarditis may be delayed, presenting weeks or years after the injury.

CHYLOPERICARDIUM

Chylopericardium is a milky-white pericardial effusion comprised of chyle, the normal content of the lacteals (lymphatics of the small intestine) and thoracic duct; the composition is variable but generally has a high content of chylomicrons, protein, and lymphocytes. The disorder is rare, but morbidity (a result of nutritional, metabolic, and immunologic abnormalities) and mortality are considerable. Although the majority of cases are asymptomatic, cardiac tamponade can occur. Acute pericarditis and chronic constriction may result from the irritant effects of chyle.

Chylous pericardial effusions generally follow traumatic (blunt or penetrating) or surgical injury (thoracic or cardiac) to the thoracic duct but may result from neoplastic obstruction of the thoracic duct (secondary chylopericardium); less commonly, they may be idiopathic (primary). Drainage and dietary manipulation is effective in approximately 55% of cases.[52] Failure to respond to a diet rich in medium-chain triglycerides and pericardiocentesis warrants ligation of the thoracic duct and pericardiectomy. In cases deemed inappropriate for aggressive therapy, implantation of a valved pericardioperitoneal conduit has been helpful.

NEPHROGENIC PERICARDIAL DISEASE

Pericarditis complicates both uremia and dialytic therapy (hemo- and peritoneal dialysis) and may be clinically silent. The clinical manifestation of nephrogenic pericardial disease may be acute fibrinous pericarditis, pericardial effusion, or cardiac tamponade; classic constrictive pericarditis is rare.

The clinical manifestations of cardiac tamponade may be atypical and difficult to distinguish from cardiovascular deterioration in patients undergoing hemodialysis. Cardiac tamponade remains one of the principal causes of hemodialysis-associated morbidity and terminates fatally in 20 percent of cases.

Although intensification of dialysis is an accepted treatment modality for hemodynamically insignificant disease, considerable controversy exists regarding the optimal management of large, persistent, or recurrent pericardial effusion. Tamponade is an indication for pericardial drainage, and large, resistant chronic effusion warrants pericardiocentesis. A conservative approach, such as intensification of dialysis and nonsteroidal anti-inflammatory agents, may suffice in less-severe cases. The instillation of nonabsorbable steroids (triamcinolone 50 mg every 6 hours for 2 to 3 days) directly into the pericardial space has been advocated,[53] but randomized controlled data about this form of therapy are absent. If needle drainage is necessary, an indwelling catheter should be left in the pericardial space for at least 2 to 3 days. Dialysis-associated effusive pericarditis usually responds to intensification of dialysis and regional heparinization, or by changing to peritoneal dialysis. Pericardiectomy may be necessary for intractable effusions.

MYXEDEMA PERICARDIAL DISEASE

Pericarditis with effusion (sometimes containing cholesterol) occurs in about one-third of patients with myxedema. Effusions develop slowly and may reach a prodigious size; slow resolution usually follows the institution of thyroid replacement therapy. Pericardial drainage is generally not indicated, because myxedema effusions seldom cause tamponade.

CONNECTIVE TISSUE DISEASE-RELATED PERICARDIAL DISEASE

Pericarditis may accompany virtually any connective tissue disease and may present as either acute or chronic pericarditis with or without an effusion. Although tamponade, effusive–constrictive disease, and constrictive pericarditis are recognized complications, most cases are subclinical and in many instances are recognized only at autopsy. Rheumatoid pericardial disease is more common in middle-age men in whom the onset of arthritis is acute. Serologic tests for rheumatoid disease are usually positive, and typical rheumatoid nodules are common. Rheumatoid arthritis is one of the causes of cholesterol pericarditis. Constrictive pericarditis is usually subacute and seldom calcific. Pericardiectomy may be required within months of the first diagnosis of acute pericarditis and is almost always required within 5 years.

Effusions are common in patients with SLE, and recurrent pericarditis, adhesion, and constriction may eventuate; indeed, pericardial disease develops in nearly all patients with SLE when life is prolonged by steroid treatment. The pericardial fluid usually has high protein content and normal or slightly reduced glucose content; lupus erythematosus cells may be found. As in rheumatoid arthritis, the complement level is low.

Pericardial involvement may be found in systemic sclerosis (scleroderma), often in association with cardiomyopathy and diffuse scleroderma. Dermatomyositis may be associated with pericardial involvement, including tamponade. Pericarditis is a rare complication in a wide variety of connective tissue disorders and arteritides (see Table 84–3).

IATROGENIC PERICARDIAL DISEASE

Iatrogenic pericardial disease results from both the calculated complications and the unanticipated misadventures of diagnostic and therapeutic procedures. Radiation pericarditis is one type of iatrogenic pericardial disease and was discussed earlier. Postcardiotomy syndrome, which complicates 5 to 30 percent of cardiac operations, usually appears in 2 or 3 weeks to 2 months after cardiac surgery; affected patients frequently have high titers of antiheart and antiviral antibodies and may develop cardiac tamponade.

Cardiac perforation complicating diagnostic cardiac catheterization and pacemaker insertion, complications of endoscopic sclerotherapy of esophageal varices, and automatic defibrillator electrode placement are other causes of iatrogenic pericardial disease. Specific management depends on the particular procedure; for example, although transeptal punctures may require rescue pericardiocentesis, perforation of a coronary artery by a guidewire may require only withdrawal of the wire and watchful waiting. Coronary artery transections during coronary interventional procedures are treated with either a covered stent or perfusion balloon. Routine echocardiography is recommended after myocardial biopsy and pacemaker lead implantation.[5]

A wide variety of drugs (the more important of which are hydralazine, procainamide, and daunorubicin) and toxins may cause pericardial heart disease (see Table 84–3), by producing either drug-induced lupus, a hypersensitivity or idiosyncratic reaction, pericardial irritation, or hemorrhage.

CONGENITAL PERICARDIAL HEART DISEASE

ABSENCE AND PARTIAL ABSENCE OF THE PERICARDIUM

Congenital absence of the pericardium is an uncommon anomaly, usually involving a part or all of the left parietal pericardium. Its presence usually is suspected from the chest radiogram, which shows a leftward shift of the cardiac silhouette, elongation of the left-heart border, and radiolucencies between the aortic knob and the pulmonary artery and between the left hemidiaphragm and the base of the heart (Fig. 84–24). This anomaly may be associated with congenital malformations of the heart and lungs.[54]

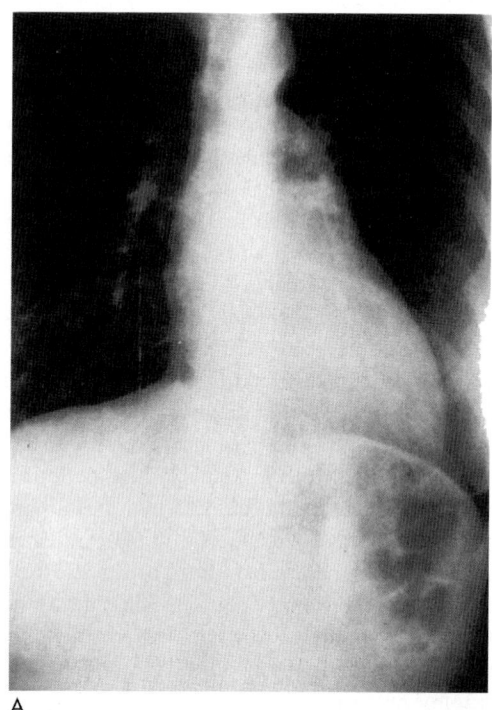

A

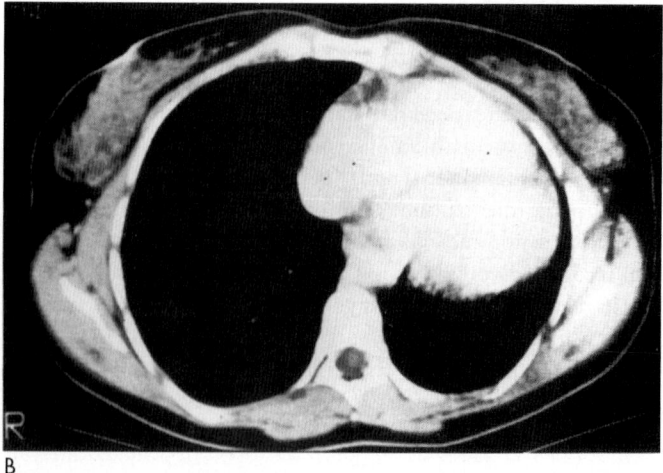

B

FIGURE 84–24. A. Posteroanterior chest radiogram of a patient with congenital absence of the pericardium. **B.** Computed tomography scan of the same patient. *Source: Reproduced with permission from Hoit BD. Imaging the pericardium. Cardiol Clin 1990;8:598.*

Although most of these patients are asymptomatic, chest pain may result from torsion of the great vessels, and recurrent pulmonary infections may be a significant feature. Physical findings are not often helpful, but a conspicuous LV heave may be found when the deficiency is substantial. Systolic and diastolic murmurs have been described.

The ECG in patients with complete absence of the left side of the pericardium usually shows an incomplete right bundle-branch block. Echocardiographic changes consist of RV enlargement and paradoxical septal motion. Contrast-enhanced CT and MRI detect lesions missed by chest radiography and echocardiography and reliably establish the anatomy of the defect.[55]

Total and very small defects are not associated with pathophysiologic changes, whereas medium-size defects may allow herniation of the left atrium. Strangulation requires surgical closure or enlargement of the defect to reduce the herniation; this may be accomplished with a thoracoscope.

[ ] PERICARDIAL CYSTS

Pericardial cysts are rare remnants of defective embryologic development of the pericardium. Cysts usually present as a prominent round, sharply demarcated opacity seen on chest radiography in an asymptomatic patient. They vary greatly in size and are most commonly found in the right cardiophrenic angle, although hilar and mediastinal locations are observed occasionally. Cysts are benign and produce no local or general symptoms; their importance lies in differentiation from neoplasm. Although they can be demonstrated on echocardiography, the nature of the lesion usually is confirmed by CT. A case of video-assisted surgical excision of a recurrent pericardial cyst has been reported.[56]

REFERENCES

1. Shabetai R. *The pericardium*. Norwell, MA: Kluwer Academic, 2003.
2. Spodick DH. *The Pericardium. A Comprehensive Textbook.* New York: Marcel Dekker, 1997.
3. Tanaka T, Hasegawa K, Fujita M, et al. Marked elevation of brain natriuretic peptide levels in pericardial fluid is closely associated with left ventricular dysfunction. *J Am Coll Cardiol* 1998;31(2):399–403.
4. Laham RJ, Rezaee M, Post M, et al. Intrapericardial administration of basic fibroblast growth factor: myocardial and tissue distribution and comparison with intracoronary and intravenous administration. *Catheter Cardiovasc Interv* 2003;58:375–381.
5. Maisch B, Seferovic PM, Ristic AD, et al. Guidelines on the diagnosis and management of pericardial diseases executive summary: the task force on the diagnosis and management of pericardial diseases of the European Society of Cardiology. *Eur Heart J* 2004;25:587–610.
6. Bonnefoy E, Godon P, Kirkorian G, et al. Serum cardiac troponin I and ST-segment elevation in patients with acute pericarditis. *Eur Heart J* 2000;21:832–836.
7. Maisch B, Ristic AD, Pankuweit S. Intrapericardial treatment of autoreactive pericardial effusion with triamcinolone: the way to avoid side effects of systemic corticosteroid therapy. *Eur Heart J* 2002;23:1503–1508.
8. Marcolongo R, Russo R, Laveder F, et al. Immunosuppressive therapy prevents recurrent pericarditis. *J Am Coll Cardiol* 1995;26(5):1276–1279.
9. Adler Y, Finkelstein Y, Guindo J, et al. Colchicine treatment for recurrent pericarditis: a decade of experience. *Circulation* 1998;97(21):2183–2185.
10. Maisch B. Pericardial diseases, with a focus on etiology, pathogenesis, pathophysiology, new diagnostic imaging methods, and treatment. *Curr Opin Cardiol* 1994;9(3):379–388.
11. Weitzman LB, Tinker WP, Kronzon I, et al. The incidence and natural history of pericardial effusion after cardiac surgery—an echocardiographic study. *Circulation* 1984;69:506–511.
12. Kuvin JT, Harati NA, Pandian NG, et al. Postoperative cardiac tamponade in the modern surgical era. *Ann Thorac Surg* 2002;74:1148–1153.
13. Tsang TS, Barnes ME, Hayes SN, et al. Clinical and echocardiographic characteristics of significant pericardial effusions following cardiothoracic surgery and outcomes of echo-guided pericardiocentesis for management: Mayo Clinic experience 1979–1998. *Chest* 1999;116(2):322–331.
14. Mueller XM, Tevaearai HT, Hurni M, et al. Etiologic diagnosis of pericardial disease: the value of routine tests during surgical procedures. *J Am Coll Surg* 1997;184(6):645–649.
15. Sagrista-Sauleda J, Merce J, Permanyer-Miralda G, et al. Clinical clues to the causes of large pericardial effusions. *Am J Med* 2000;109:95–101.
16. Iacobellis G, Leonetti F. Epicardial adipose tissue and insulin resistance in obese subjects. *J Clin Endocrinol Metab* 2005;90:6300–6302.
17. Rifkin RD, Mernoff DB. Noninvasive evaluation of pericardial effusion composition by computed tomography. *Am Heart J* 2005;149:1120–1127.
18. Hoit BD. Management of effusive and constrictive pericardial heart disease. *Circulation* 2002;105:2939–2942.
19. Merce J, Sagrista-Sauleda J, Permanyer-Miralda G, et al. Should pericardial drainage be performed routinely in patients who have a large pericardial effusion without tamponade? *Am J Med* 1998;105(2):106–109.
20. Fejka M, Dixon SR, Safian RD, et al. Diagnosis, management, and clinical outcome of cardiac tamponade complicating percutaneous coronary intervention. *Am J Cardiol* 2002;90:1183–1186.
21. Heidenreich PA, Stainback RF, Redberg RF, et al. Transesophageal echocardiography predicts mortality in critically ill patients with unexplained hypotension. *J Am Coll Cardiol* 1995;26(1):152–158.
22. Merce J, Sagrista-Sauleda J, Permanyer-Miralda G, et al. Correlation between clinical and Doppler echocardiographic findings in patients with moderate and large pericardial effusion: Implications for the diagnosis of cardiac tamponade. *Am Heart J* 1999;138(4):759–764.
23. Hoit BD. Pericarditis. In: Antman E, ed. *Cardiovascular Therapeutics,* 2nd ed. Philadelphia: WB Saunders, 2002:1113–1122.
24. Tsang TS, Enriquez-Sarano M, Freeman WK, et al. Consecutive 1127 therapeutic echocardiographically guided pericardiocentesis: clinical profile, practice patterns, and outcomes spanning 21 years. *Mayo Clin Proc* 2002;77:429–436.
25. Tsang TS, Barnes ME, Gersh BJ, et al. Outcomes of clinically significant idiopathic pericardial effusion requiring intervention. *Am J Cardiol* 2003;91:704–707.
26. Allen KB, Faber LP, Warren WH, et al. Pericardial effusion: subxiphoid pericardiostomy versus percutaneous catheter drainage. *Ann Thorac Surg* 1999;67(2):437–440.
27. Chen EP, Miller JI. Modern approaches and use of surgical treatment for pericardial disease. *Curr Cardiol Rep* 2002;4(1):41–46.
28. Talreja DR, Edwards WD, Danielson GK, et al. Constrictive pericarditis in 26 patients with histologically normal pericardial thickness. *Circulation* 2003;108:1852–1857.
29. Palka P, Lange A, Donnelly JE, et al. Differentiation between restrictive cardiomyopathy and constrictive pericarditis by early diastolic Doppler myocardial velocity gradient at the posterior wall. *Circulation* 2000;102(6):655–662.
30. Ha JW, Ommen SR, Tajik AJ, et al. Differentiation of constrictive pericarditis from restrictive cardiomyopathy using mitral annular velocity by tissue Doppler echocardiography. *Am Heart J* 2004;94:316–319.
31. Madias J, Perdoncin R, Bartoszyk O. Pericarditis and pericardial effusion in patients with acute myocardial infarction. *Am J Noninvas Cardiol* 1994;8:270–277.
32. Kutcher MA, King SB III, Alimurung BN, et al. Constrictive pericarditis as a complication of cardiac surgery: recognition of an entity. *Am J Cardiol* 1982;50:742–748.
33. Sagrista-Sauleda J, Permanyer-Miralda G, Candell RJ, et al. Transient cardiac constriction: an unrecognized pattern of evolution in effusive acute idiopathic pericarditis. *Am J Cardiol* 1987;59:961–966.
34. Haley JH, Tajik AJ, Danielson GK, et al. Transient constrictive pericarditis: causes and natural history. *J Am Coll Cardiol* 2004;43:271–275.
35. Ling LH, Oh JK, Schaff HV, et al. Constrictive pericarditis in the modern era: evolving clinical spectrum and impact on outcome after pericardiectomy. *Circulation* 1999;100:1380–1386.
36. Bertog SC, Thambidorai SK, Parakh K, et al. Constrictive pericarditis: etiology and cause-specific survival after pericardiectomy. *J Am Coll Cardiol* 2004;43:1445–1452.
37. Ustunsoy H, Celkan MA, Sivrikoz MC, et al. Intrapericardial fibrinolytic therapy in purulent pericarditis. *Eur J Cardiothorac Surg* 2002;22:373–376.

38. Sagrista-Sauleda J, Angel J, Sanchez A, Permanyer-Miralda G, et al. Effusive–constrictive pericarditis. *N Engl J Med* 2004;350:469–475.

39. Hancock EW. A clearer view of effusive-constrictive pericarditis. *N Engl J Med* 2004;350:435–437.

40. Sagrista-Sauleda J, Barrabes JA, Permanyer-Miralda G, et al. Purulent pericarditis: review of a 20-year experience in a general hospital. *J Am Coll Cardiol* 1993;22(6):1661–1665.

41. Puelo J, Matar F, McKeown P, et al. *Legionella* pericarditis diagnosed by direct fluorescent antibody staining. *Ann Thorac Surg* 1995;60:444–446.

42. Long R, Younes M, Patton N, et al. Tuberculous pericarditis: long-term outcome in patients who received medical therapy alone. *Am Heart J* 1989;117(5):1133–1139.

43. Ntsekhe M, Wiysonge C, Volmink JA, et al. Adjuvant corticosteroids for tuberculous pericarditis: promising, but not proven. *QJM* 2003;96:593–599.

44. Trautner BW, Darouiche RO. Tuberculous pericarditis: optimal diagnosis and management. *Clin Infect Dis* 2001;33:954–961.

45. Chen Y, Brennessel D, Walters J, et al. Human immunodeficiency virus-associated pericardial effusion: report of 40, cases and review of the literature. *Am Heart J* 1999;137(3):516–521.

46. Silva-Cardoso J, Moura B, Martins L, et al. Pericardial involvement in human immunodeficiency virus infection. *Chest* 1999;115(2):418–422.

47. Estok L, Wallach F. Cardiac tamponade in a patient with AIDS. A review of pericardial disease in patients with HIV infection. *Mt Sinai J Med* 1998;65(1):33–39.

48. Tsang TS, Seward JB, Barnes ME, et al. Outcomes of primary and secondary treatment of pericardial effusion in patients with malignancy. *Mayo Clin Proc* 2000;75:248–253.

49. Widimsky P, Gregor P. Pericardial involvement during the course of myocardial infarction: a long-term clinical and echocardiographic study. *Chest* 1995;108(1):89–93.

50. Oliva P, Hammill S, Edwards W. Electrocardiographic diagnosis of postinfarction regional pericarditis: Ancillary observations regarding the effect of reperfusion on the rapidity and amplitude of T-wave inversion after acute myocardial infarction. *Circulation* 1993;88:896–904.

51. Correale E, Maggioni AP, Romano S, et al. Pericardial involvement in acute myocardial infarction in the post-thrombolytic era: clinical meaning and value. *Clin Cardiol* 1997;20(4):327–331.

52. Chan BB, Murphy MC, Rodgers BM. Management of chylopericardium. *J Pediatr Surg* 1990;25:1185.

53. Wood JE, Mahnensmith RL. Pericarditis associated with renal failure: evolution and management. *Semin Dial* 2001;14:61–66.

54. Nasser W. Congenital absence of the left pericardium. *Am J Cardiol* 1970;26:466–478.

55. Gassner I, Judmaier W, Fink C, et al. Diagnosis of congenital pericardial defects, including a pathognomonic sign for dangerous apical ventricular herniation, on magnetic resonance imaging. *Br Heart J* 1995;74:60–66.

56. Horita K, Sakao Y, Itoh T. Excision of a recurrent pericardial cyst using video-assisted thoracic surgery. *Chest* 1998;114(4):1203–1204.

CHAPTER 85

Infective Endocarditis

Saptarsi M. Haldar / Patrick T. O'Gara

INTRODUCTION

Infective endocarditis (IE) is a disease caused by microbial infection of the endothelial lining of intracardiac structures and is invariably fatal if untreated. Infection most commonly resides on one or more heart valve leaflets, but may involve mural endocardium, chordal structures, myocardium, and pericardium. The presence of an intracardiac or endovascular device provides a nidus for infection, as well as a barrier to eradication. Despite significant advances in the diagnosis and treatment of IE, 6-month mortality rates still approach 25 percent.[1] Changes in both patient demographics and microbial biology have challenged conventional wisdom. Prompt recognition, triggered by a high index of clinical suspicion in susceptible patients, early diagnosis, and aggressive treatment are the critical components of a successful management strategy. Combined medical and surgical interventions can lead to improved outcomes for selected patients. Patient education and the appropriate use of prophylactic antibiotics are the mainstays of prevention.

HISTORY

The earliest description of the vegetative lesion of IE is attributed to Lazarus Riverius (1589–1655).[2] During his tenure as Vatican physician to Pope Clement XI, Giovanni Lancisi (1654–1720) recorded additional observations in *De Subitaneis Mortibus* (1709).[3] Despite these descriptions, it was not until the mid-19th century that a connection was made between vegetative lesions, systemic inflammation (Boullard, 1841), and embolic phenomena (Virchow, 1847, and Kirkes 1852).[4] Sir William Osler made several important advances in the understanding of IE, as summarized in his famed Gulstonian lectures of 1885.[5] He defined IE as a primary "mycotic" process and provided the first formal description of two clinical variants of the disease—an acute and fulminating form versus a chronic and insidious form. Despite his extensive knowledge of the disease, Osler was also the first to acknowledge the reality of diagnostic uncertainty in many cases.

EPIDEMIOLOGY

In the first half of the 20th century, IE was predominantly a complication of rheumatic heart disease and poor dentition. In developing countries, rheumatic heart disease remains the most frequent predisposing cardiac condition.[6] However, the epidemiologic features of IE in developed countries have changed considerably. The aging of the population has been paralleled by increases in the prevalence of degenerative heart valve disease, and in the use of implanted heart valve substitutes and intracardiac devices. The numbers of patients with chronic, predisposing medical comorbidities, such as diabetes, HIV infection, and end-stage renal disease, have also increased, as has the commensurate risk of exposure to nosocomial bacteremia, often with antibiotic resistance.[7-9] These changing demographics are reflected in two observations: First, the median age of patients with IE has gradually increased from 30 to 40 years in the preantibiotic era to 47 to 69 years in the late 20th century.[10,11] Second, the incidence of IE in developed countries has remained unchanged, despite the dramatic reduction in the incidence of rheumatic heart disease over the last half-century.

The incidence of IE in developed countries has been difficult to estimate principally because of the challenges of accurate case definition and identification of representative populations at risk (e.g., urban vs. rural, injection drug users, young vs. elderly). Since 1995, several well-designed epidemiologic studies have attempted to address these problems[8,10,12-16] and are summarized in Table 85–1. A number of these studies suggest that the incidence of IE is increasing among the elderly.[8,10,15,16] Increased patient longevity and the explosive use of healthcare interventions predict that the incidence of IE throughout the world will continue to rise.[17]

IE IN SELECTED PATIENT POPULATIONS

The Elderly

The incidence of IE among the elderly, often a result of nosocomial infection, appears to be rising. A heightened index of suspicion is required to make the diagnosis in this population because its presentation may be atypical.[18] There is a higher incidence of degenerative, calcific valve disease, which can decrease the specificity of echocardiographic imaging. Transesophageal echocardiography (TEE) imaging is often required for more accurate delineation of valve pathology.[19] IE caused by *Enterococcus faecalis* appears to

TABLE 85–1

Studies of Infective Endocarditis Incidence

STUDY	POPULATION STUDIED	IE INCIDENCE (CASES PER 100,000 PERSON-YEARS)	COMMENTS
Hogevik et al. 1995[10]	Well-defined urban population in Goteborg, Sweden, followed prospectively from 1994–1998.	5.9	IE incidence was age- and gender-adjusted. Crude incidence was 6.2. In the oldest age group (80–89 years), the annual incidence was 22.
Berlin et al. 1995[12]	Retrospective analysis of IE cases in metropolitan Philadelphia from 1988–1990.	11.6	The population studied had a high proportion of injection drug users, a population whose rate of IE was 5.2 cases/per 100,000 person-years.
Delahaye et al. 1995[13]	Retrospective analysis of 415 IE cases collected from a combined urban and rural population from three regions in France in 1991.	2.4	IE incidence was age- and gender-adjusted. The study population had only 5% injection drug users.
Tleyjeh et al. 2005[14]	Retrospective analysis of 107 IE cases occurring in Olmsted County, Minnesota between 1970 and 2000.	5.0 – 7.0	IE incidence was age- and gender-adjusted. Increasing temporal trend was observed for PVE and for cases associated with mitral valve prolapse.
Hoen et al. 2002[8]	Retrospective analysis of 390 IE cases in six regions of France in 1999.	3.1	IE incidence was age- and gender-adjusted. There was a high incidence of IE in the elderly–14.5 cases per 100,000 patient-years.
Cabell et al. 2002[15]	Retrospective analysis of IE incidence in the United States Medicare database, reflecting more than 16,000 cases from 1986–1991.	20.4	This study reported a 13.7 percent increase in IE incidence in the Medicare population from 1986 to 1998.
Morellion and Que, 2004[16]	Review of 26 publications between 1993 and 2003 encompassing 3784 cases of IE.	Median incidence of IE among all studies of 3.6.	In subjects older than age 65 years, the median incidence was >15 cases per 100,000 person-years, nearly three times that of subjects younger than 50 years of age.

IE, infective endocarditis; PVE, prosthetic valve endocarditis.

be more common among the elderly.[20] Although there are conflicting reports, advanced age appears to predict mortality in IE,[21–23] particularly with *Staphylococcus aureus* infection.[24]

Injection Drug Users

IE is one of the most severe complications of injection (i.e., intravenous or subcutaneous) drug use. The incidence of IE among injection drug users (IDUs) is approximately 2 to 5 percent per year, and is responsible for 5 to 20 percent of hospital admissions and 5 to 10 percent of overall mortality in this group.[25] The incidence of IE and the causative agents in this population are likely related to contaminated injection technique (e.g., sharing or licking of hypodermic needles), the injection of unsterile particulate material (e.g., talcum) and the high prevalence of HIV infection. *S. aureus* is the most common etiologic agent and causes more than 60 percent of IE in IDUs.[25] IE caused by gram-negative bacilli (notably *Pseudomonas aeruginosa*) and fungi is also more common among IDUs. The distinctive feature of IE in IDU is that it is a predominantly a disease of the right heart, with 60 to 70 percent of cases involving the tricuspid valve. The tricuspid valve may be particularly susceptible to bacterial infection because of chronic degenerative changes caused by the repetitive injection of irritants (e.g., talcum) into peripheral veins. Septic pulmonary emboli are common. Despite the high frequency of *S. aureus* infection, isolated right-heart involvement in IDUs partially explains the lower mortality in this population (4 percent) compared to other IE patient subsets. Nevertheless, left-sided infection does occur and can result in major complications, such as systemic emboli, paravalvular abscess, and severe valvular destruction. IDUs with uncomplicated right-sided IE may be eligible for short-course parenteral antibiotic therapy (2 to 4 weeks), a regimen that would not be considered in patients with left-sided IE.[26] Because the administration of a 4-week parenteral antibiotic regimen in IDUs can be challenging, combination oral therapy with ciprofloxacin plus rifampin can be used safely and effectively in selected patients with uncomplicated right-sided staphylococcal IE.[27] Given the relative efficacy of antibiotic cure for isolated right-sided IE in IDUs, surgical therapy is uncommon and is reserved for cases of severe right-heart failure because of tricuspid regurgitation and refractory septic pulmonary emboli. IDU is not an absolute contraindication to surgery for patients with IE and studies show that surgery can be performed in these patients safely and with acceptable outcomes.[28]

Human Immunodeficiency Virus Infection and the Immunocompromised Host

Although HIV infection and intravenous drug use commonly coexist, HIV infection appears to be an independent risk factor for the development of IE.[29] Patients with low CD4 counts (<200 cells/µL) tend to have an increased risk of IE,[30] as well as a higher associated mortality.[25,31] IDUs who are HIV-positive have a higher incidence of left-sided valvular involvement and complications than do HIV-negative IDUs.[31] Although they are a rare cause of IE, *Bartonella* species may result in opportunistic infections, including IE, in patients with AIDS.[32] There is a paucity of data on the characteristics of IE in the non–HIV-infected immunocompromised host. However, immunocompromised patients with gram-negative bacteremia or fungemia may be at risk for IE caused by these organisms.

Hemodialysis Patients

There are approximately 300,000 patients in the United States who are receiving hemodialysis (HD). Infectious complications of vascular access are a major cause of morbidity and mortality in HD patients. In this population, there is an alarming rate of bacteremia approaching nearly 1.0 episodes per 100 patient-care months. Few other medical conditions, with the exception of chemotherapy-induced neutropenia and intravenous drug use, are associated with such high rates of bacteremia. As a result, IE occurs in approximately 2 to 6 percent of patients receiving HD. Staphylococcal species are the predominant organisms and gain access to the bloodstream via infected central venous catheters, atrioventricular (AV) grafts or AV fistulas. Primary AV fistulas have the lowest rates of infections and are the access of choice whenever vascular anatomy allows. Indwelling central venous catheters have the highest rate of infections and are often associated with more serious metastatic complications.[33] Access-related infections are the most common cause for the loss of dialysis vascular access and cause nearly 10 percent of deaths (second to only ischemic heart disease) in this patient population.[34] Patients with end-stage renal disease have a high incidence of calcific degeneration of the aortic and mitral valves,[35] which may promote bacterial colonization of the endocardium. Such degenerative valvular disease may render echocardiographic detection of vegetations extremely challenging.[19] Vancomycin is often used as a first-line agent because of the high incidence of methicillin-resistant *S. aureus* (MRSA) in the HD population and the ease of administration of this drug. Treatment of catheter-related bloodstream infections with antibiotics alone yields poor results and removal of infected catheters or grafts is necessary in most circumstances.[36] Effective prevention of bacteremia in the HD population hinges on early referral for primary AV fistula placement (preferably before dialysis is necessary) and strict adherence to sterile technique with access manipulation.

Pacemaker/Intracardiac Cardioverter-Defibrillator–Related Endocarditis

The rate of pacemaker and intracardiac cardioverter-defibrillator placement has dramatically increased in the past 10 years, given the growing number of evidence-based indications for the implantation of these devices. The increasing rate of device infection appears to be disproportionate to the increased rate of implantation.[37] Staphylococcal species are the causative organisms in more than 70 percent of device infections.[38] The large majority of cardiac device infections are likely caused by pocket site contamination at the time of device placement. Hematogenous seeding from a distant focus of infection, particularly one caused by *S. aureus*, can cause late-onset infection. There are several important imaging considerations in patients with suspected intracardiac device infections. It can be difficult to differentiate infected vegetations from noninfected thrombotic or calcific debris using transthoracic echocardiography (TTE); TEE is often required for adequate visualization. Echocardiographic data must be integrated with clinical and microbiologic data. It is essential to image the implanted device throughout its entire course in the cardiac chambers and proximal veins with special attention to its relationship with the tricuspid valve. Device leads that track through the superior vena cava should be visualized as close to the origin of the generator as possible.[17] Although no prospective studies have been conducted, management with parenteral antibiotics and complete device removal are the standards of care.[38] Increased experience with percutaneous lead-extraction techniques may aid in the management of infected devices.[39] When there is documented valvular IE in a patient with an implanted device, there is high likelihood of concomitant device infection which may necessitate extraction.

PATHOGENESIS

The hallmark of IE is persistent endocardial or endovascular infection causing continuous bacteremia. Importantly, IE is a relatively uncommon consequence of transient bacteremia and not all organisms can effectively colonize or invade the endovascular space. It is apparent that complex series of host–pathogen interactions conspire in the development of IE lesions, including the integrity of the vascular endothelium, the host immune system, hemostatic mechanisms, cardiac anatomical characteristics, microbial properties, and the peripheral events that cause the bacteremia.[17,40] There are substantial experimental data to suggest that host endothelial damage is the key predisposing insult, with subsequent platelet and fibrin deposition and creation of a receptive milieu for bacterial colonization during episodes of transient bacteremia. That endothelial damage is the inciting event is further supported by the observation that vegetations are most likely to form in areas where blood-flow injury is likely to occur—on the ventricular side of semilunar valves and the atrial side of AV valves.[41] Jet lesions from regurgitant valves or intracardiac shunts may also damage endothelium, and vegetations may form on such sites of injury, including the mitral chordae with aortic regurgitation, the mural left atrial endocardium with mitral regurgitation, and the septal leaflet of the tricuspid valve with ventricular septal defect.[17,41] Figure 85–1 illustrates the classic locations of endocardial flow injury that are associated with vegetation formation in IE.[41]

Once endothelial injury has occurred, bacteria must gain access to the intravascular space to seed the lesion. Common sources of bacteremia include skin, surgical wounds, the periodontal space, indwelling intravascular catheters, and the urinary and gastrointestinal tracts. Bacteria that have entered the bloodstream must be able to adhere to the damaged endothelium, exposed extracellular matrix, or areas of fibrin deposition.[42] This adherence is mediated by microbial surface components recognizing adhesive matrix molecules, which recognize a variety of host proteins such as fibronectin, collagen, and integrins. Certain organisms appear to preferentially express these molecules, enabling them to adhere more effectively and colonize the injured endocardium.[40,43] The fact that S. aureus can induce endothelial tissue factor expression may partially explain why this organism can adhere to relatively normal heart valves.[44] Particulate material that may be injected may also promote S. aureus adherence by stimulating matrix protein expression on valvular endothelium.[42] Another factor in microbial pathogenesis of device-related intravascular infections is biofilm formation, which impedes microbial clearance and often mandates device removal for eradication of the infection. Staphylococcus epidermidis and S. aureus have been studied most extensively in this regard,

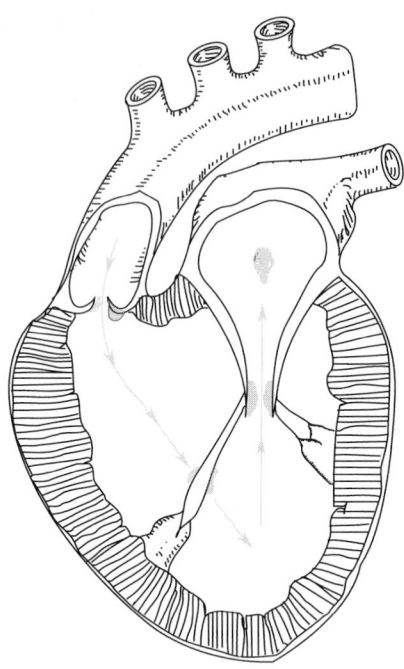

FIGURE 85–1. Sites of typical endocardial flow-related injury and associated vegetation formation in infective endocarditis (IE). Flow injury from aortic regurgitation is typically associated with vegetations on the ventricular side of the aortic valve or on the anterior mitral leaflet and its subvalvular apparatus. Flow injury from mitral regurgitation is associated with vegetation formation on the left atrial surface of the mitral leaflets or on the mural surface of the left atrial endocardium (the MacCallum patch). Flow injury from a ventricular septal defect (not shown) with left-to-right shunting is associated with vegetation formation on the septal leaflet of the tricuspid valve. *Source: Adapted from Rodbard S. Blood velocity and endocarditis. Circulation 1963;27:18–28.*

with characterization of a responsible intercellular adhesin and its gene cluster.[45] Once adherent, certain strains of bacteria are able to evade the host immune system, destroy host tissue, or occasionally enter the cytosolic compartment of endothelial cells. Repetitive cycles of bacterial proliferation, fibrin-platelet deposition, and host tissue destruction create an infected vegetation, within which bacteria can reach extremely high concentrations (10^9 to 10^{11} organisms per gram of tissue). These dense vegetations are a source of continuous bacterial seeding of the bloodstream. Figure 85–2 shows a gross pathologic specimen of the heart with large, complex vegetation attached to the left atrial surface of the anterior mitral leaflet. After successful antimicrobial therapy, vegetations will resolve completely or contract in size and persist indefinitely as a sterile mass adherent to valve tissue.

MICROBIOLOGY OF IE

A wide range of microorganisms can cause IE, but only a few species account for the vast majority of cases. Streptococci and staphylococci are the cause of more than 80 percent of IE cases in which a responsible organism is identified. Streptococcal species were historically the most common group of pathogens, but more recent data identify S. aureus as the most frequently isolated agent worldwide.[24] Moreover, the rate of antibiotic resistance among causative organisms is increasing.[24,46]

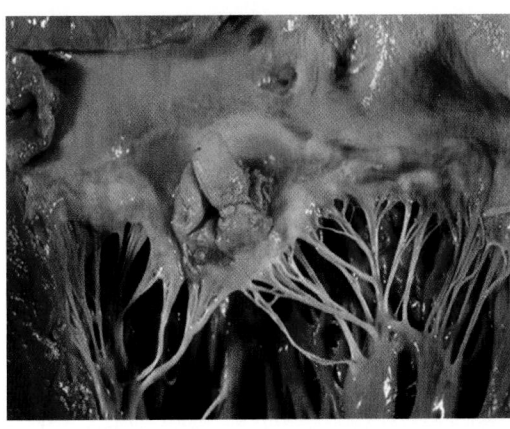

FIGURE 85–2. Large, complex vegetation attached to the left atrial surface of the anterior mitral valve leaflet from a patient with *Staphylococcus lugdunensis* IE. *Source: Image courtesy of Richard Mitchell, MD, PhD, Department of Pathology, Brigham and Women's Hospital, Boston, MA.*

【 】 NATIVE VALVE ENDOCARDITIS

Streptococci

Viridans group streptococci, or α-hemolytic streptococci, are a frequent cause of community-acquired native valve endocarditis (NVE). Viridans streptococci are responsible for 30 to 65 percent of cases of NVE in older children and adults. They are normal residents of the oropharynx and easily gain access to the circulation following dental or gingival trauma. The viridans streptococci comprise several species, of which *Streptococcus sanguis, Streptococcus bovis, Streptococcus mutans,* and *Streptococcus mitior* are most commonly isolated in cases of IE. The viridans streptococci are usually highly sensitive to penicillin, as defined by a minimum inhibitory concentration (MIC) of ≤0.1 µg/mL, and thus can often be eradicated with penicillin monotherapy.[47]

S. bovis, a normal inhabitant of the human gastrointestinal tract, is noteworthy as IE caused by this organism is strongly suggestive of GI malignancy,[48] polyp formation, or diverticular disease. Colonoscopy should be performed when this organism is detected in the blood. When meticulously investigated, GI pathology is discovered in as many as 60 percent of patients with *S. bovis* IE.[48]

Nutritionally deficient streptococci, now known as *Abiotrophia* spp. and *Granulicatella* spp., require specialized isolation and culture techniques for growth (supplemental thiol compounds or active forms of vitamin B_6) and now account for approximately 5 to 7 percent of streptococcal IE cases.[47,49] IE caused by these organisms is virtually always indolent in onset and associated with preexisting heart disease. Therapy remains difficult and prognosis is poor as these organisms are generally less sensitive to penicillin than the viridans group streptococci. Treatment often requires synergistic therapy with an aminoglycoside.

The *Enterococcus* spp., formerly classified as group D streptococci, are now defined as a distinct genus. They are responsible for 5 to 18 percent of cases of native valve IE, the vast majority of which are caused by *E. faecalis* (80 percent) or *E. faecium* (10 percent). These organisms are normal inhabitants of the GI and genitourinary tracts and may enter the bloodstream after manipulation of the colon, urethra or bladder (e.g., Foley catheterization, colonoscopy). The incidence of enterococcal endocarditis appears

to be rising, likely because of the increased genitourinary and gastrointestinal instrumentation in older adults, and the increased use of indwelling central venous catheters and prosthetic implants. These organisms can infect both normal and diseased heart tissue, as well as prosthetic materials. Indeed, among the most relevant risk factors for development of enterococcal IE is the presence of an implanted device. The pathogenesis of such infections is poorly understood, but several virulence factors have been proposed. The ability to form biofilm was recently shown to be a prominent feature of this microorganism, allowing colonization of inert and biologic surfaces and preventing antibiotic penetrance. The disease typically runs an indolent course, and cure is challenging as the organism has limited susceptibility to many antibiotics, including β-lactam drugs. There is an alarming incidence of nosocomial bacteremia with these organisms and a growing problem with drug resistance to both vancomycin and aminoglycosides. Although synergistic antibiotic therapy, as predicated by susceptibility testing, should be considered,[46] there is some debate regarding its efficacy.[50]

Group A streptococcus rarely cause IE. *Streptococcus pyogenes,* the causative organism in childhood pharyngitis, scarlet fever, impetigo, cellulitis, erysipelas, fasciitis, and myositis is not associated with IE in adults. Before 1945, *Streptococcus pneumoniae* caused approximately 10 percent of IE cases; the current incidence of pneumococcal IE, however, is very low. *S. pneumoniae* bacteremia often begins with respiratory infection and nearly half of patients with pneumococcal IE suffer from chronic alcoholism.[51] *S. pneumoniae* can infect normal valve tissue and usually results in an acute, fulminant illness often associated with severe valve damage, perivalvular extension, embolic complications, pericarditis, meningitis, and high mortality (25 to 50 percent).[51]

Group B streptococci (e.g., *Streptococcus agalactiae*) are chiefly responsible for infections in the neonate and parturient, although this organism can also be isolated from diabetic foot ulcers. Risk factors for group B streptococcal bacteremia in adults include obstetric complications,[52] diabetes, carcinoma, liver failure, alcoholism, and IDU.[53] These organisms are generally less sensitive to penicillin than group A isolates and require higher doses for treatment.

Staphylococci

S. aureus causes 80 to 90 percent of staphylococcal IE and is the most common cause of "acute" IE. Emerging data from the International Consortium on Endocarditis (ICE) suggest that *S. aureus* has become the leading cause of IE worldwide.[24] The mucous membranes of the anterior nasopharynx are the most common sites of colonization and approximately 30 percent of normal persons carry *S. aureus.* Carrier rates are higher among persons with more frequent exposures to the organism and those who are at risk for breakdown of the normal mucocutaneous barrier. Rates of *S. aureus* infection, particularly bacteremia associated with healthcare contact, have increased in hospitalized patients and among those receiving outpatient medical therapy.[54,55] Although only a fraction of patients with *S. aureus* bacteremia develop NVE,[56] populations at increased risk include patients on dialysis,[34] type I diabetics, burn victims, persons with HIV,[29] IDUs,[25] patients with certain chronic dermatologic conditions, and patients with recent surgical incisions (including median sternotomy for valve replacement). Despite the frequency of nosocomial *S. aureus* acquisition, community-acquired infection appears to be an independent risk factor for the development of IE and metastatic disease.[24,57] *S. aureus* is respected as a highly virulent organism and has the capacity to infect and destroy normal endocardial surfaces. A number of virulence factors help this organism enter the bloodstream, adhere to endothelial and prosthetic surfaces, and evade host defense.[43] *S. aureus* IE is frequently fulminant when it involves left-sided cardiac valves and often results in major complications such as heart failure, perivalvular extension with conduction disturbances, embolization and metastatic infection.[58] Unsurprisingly, *S. aureus* as a causative organism is an independent predictor of poor prognosis in IE[59] and is associated with a 25 to 30 percent mortality.[1,24] As many as 50 percent of patients with left-sided NVE caused by *S. aureus* require surgery. Right-sided (tricuspid valve) IE with *S. aureus*, by contrast, is most frequently associated with IDU and a high incidence of septic pulmonary embolization, but only a 2 to 4 percent fatality rate. The detection of *S. aureus* bacteremia should prompt echocardiography to look for evidence of IE, especially if bacteremia is persistent. Although most patients undergo TTE first, an initial TEE should be considered for patients with catheter-associated *S. aureus* bacteremia as a cost-effective means of determining the duration of antibiotic therapy (i.e., 2 weeks vs. 4 weeks).[60] Antibiotic resistance can be a particular challenge with *S. aureus* as more than 90 percent of clinical isolates produce β-lactamase and are thus penicillin-resistant. Semisynthetic penicillin analogues that are unaffected by β-lactamase, such as methicillin, oxacillin, and nafcillin, are first-line agents. Unfortunately, increasing rates of methicillin resistance (MRSA) in both hospital and community settings[24] and the recovery of clinical *S. aureus* isolates resistant to vancomycin[61] have complicated the treatment of *S. aureus* IE. Increasing hospital use of vancomycin for the treatment of MRSA is likely one additional reason for the growing incidence of vancomycin resistance among enterococci. Vancomycin, although the best available antibiotic for treatment of MRSA, is only weakly bactericidal and likely only bacteriostatic. A semisynthetic β-lactamase–resistant penicillin (e.g., nafcillin) is always preferred for treatment of susceptible *S. aureus* in nonallergic individuals.

The coagulase-negative staphylococci are constituents of normal human skin flora and are much less likely to infect normal endocardial surfaces. *S. epidermidis* is an important causative agent in prosthetic valve and device-related endocarditis. Native valve endocarditis caused by coagulase-negative staphylococci occurs mainly in patients with preexisting valvular heart disease,[62] although exceptions to this generalization do occur (see Fig. 85–2). NVE caused by coagulase-negative staphylococci has historically been regarded as an indolent disease; however, recent data from the ICE has demonstrated equal rates of heart failure and death for coagulase-negative staphylococci and *S. aureus* NVE.[62] *S. epidermidis* infections of prosthetic implants are extremely difficult to eradicate and the addition of adjunctive rifampin therapy is often recommended. Rare cases of IE caused by other coagulase-negative staphylococci (e.g., *Staphylococcus saprophyticus*, *Staphylococcus capitis*) have been reported.[63,64] A growing number of reports of IE caused by community-acquired *Staphylococcus lugdunensis* have also been reported.[65] This organisms may cause a more virulent form of IE with high morbidity despite uniform in vitro susceptibility to most antibiotics.

Gram-Negative Bacilli

IE caused by gram-negative bacilli is uncommon and tends to occur in IDUs, immunocompromised patients, patients with advanced liver disease and prosthetic heart valve recipients. The fastidious gram-negative rods of the HACEK group (*Haemophilus* spp., *Actinobacillus*, *Cardiobacterium hominis*, *Eikenella corrodens*, and *Kingella* spp.) reside normally in the oropharynx and are responsible for a very small (approximately 1 percent) proportion of cases of NVE, usually involving abnormal valve tissue. Because of their growth requirements (CO_2), they may take 3 to 4 weeks to grow in culture and have gained notoriety for their implicated role in certain cases of culture-negative IE. The *Haemophilus* species (*H. parainfluenzae*, *H. aphrophilus*, *H. paraphrophilus*) are the most common etiologic agents from this group. They typically form large and friable vegetations that have a tendency to embolize. There are numerous case reports of IE caused by other members of the HACEK group.[66] The Enterobacteriaceae (*Escherichia coli*, *Klebsiella*, *Enterobacter*, *Serratia*, etc.) are rare causes of IE. *Salmonella* species have a particular predilection for atherosclerotic plaque and may infect arterial aneurysms.[67] The vast majority of patients with *P. aeruginosa* endocarditis are intravenous drug users.[68] The source of *Pseudomonas* appears to be from standing water that contaminates needles and other drug paraphernalia. Left-sided endocarditis caused by *P. aeruginosa* is difficult to eradicate with antibiotics alone, has a high rate of complications, and often requires early surgery.[68]

The rickettsial organism, *Coxiella burnetii,* is the causative agent of Q fever and is a relevant cause of IE in areas where cattle, sheep, and goat farming are common. Cases of IE caused by *C. burnetii* are well documented in the developed world.[69] The aortic valve is affected in more than 80 percent of cases and the infection is difficult to eradicate with antibiotics. As the organism is extremely difficult to culture, the diagnosis is best made serologically using antibody titers.[66] *Bartonella* species (*B. quintana*, *B. henselae*, *B. elizabethae*), the etiologic agent in cat scratch disease, were recently described as an important cause of IE among both homeless men and HIV-infected patients. The diagnosis can be suspected serologically and confirmed with special culture or polymerase chain reaction (PCR) techniques.[70] *Brucella* spp. have been implicated in approximately 4 percent of cases of IE in Spain. These organisms are usually ingested in unpasteurized milk or cheese, and are occupational hazards for veterinarians, shepherds, and livestock handlers. IE is the most common cause of death in patients with brucellosis and surgery is usually required for cure.[71]

Fungal IE

Fungal endocarditis is a relatively new syndrome and is associated with an exceedingly high mortality (survival rates of <20 percent). Patients who develop fungal IE have multiple predisposing conditions, including an immunocompromised state, the use of endovascular devices, and previous reconstructive cardiac surgery. *Candida* and *Aspergillus* species are the most common causes of fungal IE and are associated with large, bulky vegetations that can obstruct native or prosthetic valve orifices and that can embolize to large vessels (e.g., the femoral artery). Blood cultures are usually positive in cases of *Candida* IE, whereas they are rarely positive with *Aspergillus*. Fungal endocarditis is an indication for surgical replacement of an infected valve. Cure usually requires combination fungicidal (amphotericin) and surgical treatment, followed by long-term suppressive therapy with an oral antifungal agent.[46]

Culture-Negative IE

Blood cultures are negative in up to 20 percent of patients with IE diagnosed by strict criteria.[72] Failure to isolate a microorganism may be the result of inadequate culture technique, a highly fastidious organism or a nonbacterial pathogen as the causative agent, or previous administration of antimicrobial therapy prior to blood culture acquisition. The latter is an extremely important consideration as the administration of antibiotics prior to drawing blood cultures can reduce the recovery rate of bacterial pathogens by nearly one-third.[73,74] There are numerous noninfectious causes of endocarditis that may behave like culture-negative IE, including those that are related to neoplasia (nonbacterial thrombotic endocarditis), autoimmune diseases (antiphospholipid antibody syndrome, systemic lupus erythematosus), or the postcardiac surgery state (thrombi, stitches).[74] Empiric therapy for culture-negative IE remains extremely challenging as the patient may be exposed to potentially toxic antimicrobial therapy while awaiting what is often delayed identification of a causative organism, if one is identified at all. Consultation with an infectious disease specialist to define the most appropriate therapy is recommended.[46]

【 】 PROSTHETIC VALVE ENDOCARDITIS

Prosthetic valve endocarditis (PVE) represents approximately 10 to 30 percent of all IE cases.[8,14,40] Although many of the general principles applicable to native valve IE are relevant, there are important considerations specific to PVE. After valve replacement, the incidence of PVE is approximately 1 to 3 percent at 1 year and 3 to 6 percent at 5 years. Although the current evidence is not definitive, PVE can be broadly divided into two groups based on the time of onset after valve surgery: early PVE and late PVE. Early PVE is defined as endocarditis that develops within the first 2 months to 1 year after valve surgery. During this period, the vast majority of causative organisms are nosocomially acquired with a predominance of staphylococci, notably coagulase-negative species (*S. epidermidis*). Gram-negative bacilli, diphtheroids, and fungal species, although very uncommon causes of IE overall, have a predilection to cause PVE during this early period. Late PVE is defined as that occurring beyond 1 year after operation. In contrast to early PVE, the spectrum of causative organisms in late PVE resembles that of native valve endocarditis. In late PVE, there is an emergence of cases caused by streptococci and enterococci, a significant decrease in the rate of coagulase-negative staphylococci, and a continued rate of infection with *S. aureus*. Between 2 and 12 months after valve replacement surgery, there is a gradual transition between the early and late microbiologic causes of PVE. TEE imaging is recommended in cases of suspected PVE (see below). In some cases, both TTE and TEE are performed to provide optimal characterization of the infection. Empiric therapy for suspected PVE is similar to that for NVE; however, staphylococcal coverage should always be provided with particular attention to the likelihood of antibiotic resistance (MRSA). Complication rates with PVE are high and surgery is often required even in the absence of

documented perivalvular extension. For example, *S. aureus* PVE is rarely eradicated with antibiotics alone, and retrospective analyses suggest that combined medical and surgical therapy is more effective than medical therapy alone.[75] With proper timing of antibiotic therapy and surgery, the imputed risk of reinfection of a newly implanted valve is only 2 to 3 percent.[76]

APPROACH TO THE PATIENT WITH SUSPECTED IE

The history should focus on predisposing factors such as IDU, a prior history of IE, recent exposures, the presence of an intracardiac device or indwelling central venous catheter, congenital or acquired valvular heart disease, and other congenital heart disease. The patient may report fever, fatigue, anorexia, weight loss, night sweats, joint pain, or back pain. Often, the nature of the presenting symptoms reflects the severity and type of infection. Patients with *S. aureus* infection, for example, are likely to have a fulminant course with high fever and systemic sepsis, whereas some infections with streptococcal organisms may have a more protracted course. Features on clinical examination that raise suspicion for IE include fever, a new heart murmur indicative of valvular insufficiency, signs of heart failure, and vascular phenomena. Examples of classic IE-related findings include major arterial emboli with pulse deficits, septic pulmonary emboli (with right-sided IE), mycotic brain aneurysms with intracranial hemorrhage, mucosal or conjunctival petechiae, splinter hemorrhages of the nail beds, palpable purpuric skin rashes (Fig. 85–3), Janeway lesions (small, flat, irregular erythematous spots on the palms and soles), Osler nodes (tender, erythematous nodules occurring in the pulp of the fingers), Roth spots (cytoid bodies and associated hemorrhage caused by microinfarction of retinal vessels), and urinary red cell casts suggestive of glomerulonephritis (Fig. 85–4).

Although the history and physical examination are useful, the diagnosis of IE rests on the ability to demonstrate endocardial involvement of infection and persistent bacteremia. The proper acquisition of blood cultures prior to initiation of antimicrobial therapy is essential. In hospitalized patients, the presence of bacteremia with a typical causative organism (e.g., *S. aureus*) often provides initial suspicion for IE and prompts further diagnostic evalu-

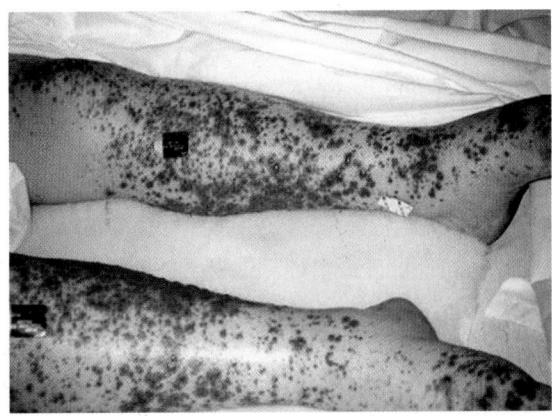

FIGURE 85–3. Cutaneous purpura fulminans in a patient with *S. abiotrophia* native valve endocarditis of the mitral and aortic valves.

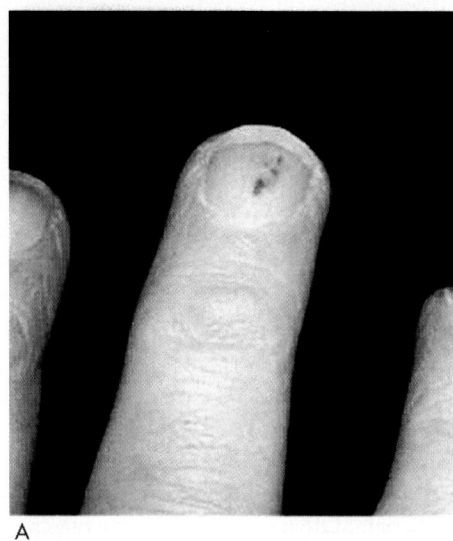

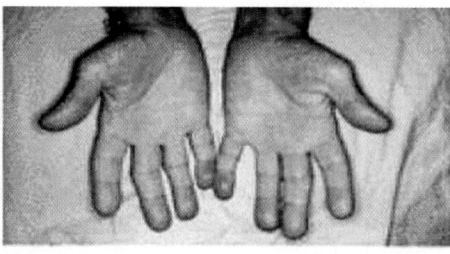

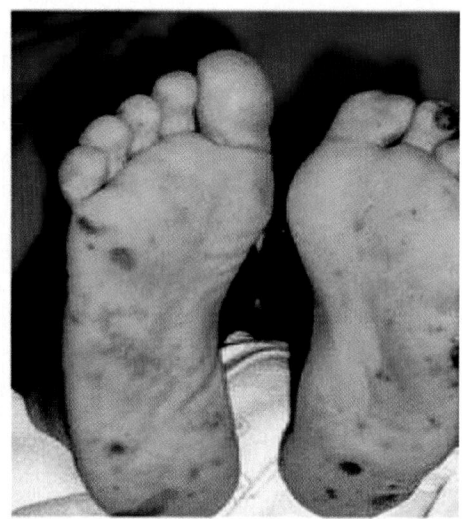

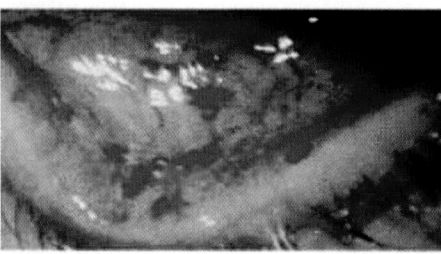

FIGURE 85–4. Selected peripheral manifestations of IE. **A.** Splinter hemorrhages are linear hemorrhages under the nails that do not reach the nail margin. They are often red for the first 2 days and brownish thereafter. **B.** Conjunctival hemorrhages. **C.** Osler nodes are tender, erythematous nodules often occurring in the pulp of the fingers. **D.** Janeway lesions are small, flat, irregular spots found on the palms and soles. They are typically erythematous and nontender. *Source: Adapted with permission from Mylonakis E, Calderwood SB. Infective endocarditis in adults. N Engl J Med 2001;18:345.*

the completion of therapy, a TTE may be performed to establish a new "post-IE baseline."[46] After successful therapy, patients with IE should be followed longitudinally for progressive valvular and ventricular dysfunction. Patients with successfully treated IE are at high risk for the development of future episodes of IE and should receive antibiotic prophylaxis for procedures, as recommended by current guidelines (see Prevention of Infective Endocarditis below).[78,79]

DIAGNOSIS OF INFECTIVE ENDOCARDITIS

IE is defined as an infection on any structure within the heart, including on normal or damaged endothelial surfaces (e.g., myocardium and valvular structures), prosthetic heart valves, and implanted devices (e.g., pacemakers, intracardiac cardioverter-defibrillators, ventricular assist devices, and surgical shunts).[17] The diagnosis of IE relies chiefly on the following factors: (1) an initial clinical suspicion, especially in a patient with identifiable risk factors, (2) microbiologic data (blood cultures demonstrating continuous bacteremia or cultures of vegetative emboli removed surgically), and (3) the results of echocardiographic imaging. Diagnosis is straightforward in only a minority of patients who present with a defined predisposing condition and the classic manifestations of fever, evidence of active valvulitis, peripheral emboli, immunologic or vascular phenomena, and bacteremia. In the majority of patients, however, IE has an extremely variable clinical presentation.[47]

CLINICAL CRITERIA

Pelletier and Petersdorf published the first formal case definition based on their 30-year experience caring for patients with IE in Seattle, Washington.[80] Although this first case definition was specific for the diagnosis of IE, it lacked sufficient sensitivity. Subsequently, von Reyn and colleagues developed the first stratified diagnostic schema in which cases were placed into four categories (rejected, possible, probable, and definite). This approach eventually proved inadequate because of overclassification of cases as "possible" and "probable," overreliance on pathologic specimens and the lack of incorporation of any echocardiographic data.[81] In 1994, Durack et al. published the Duke Criteria[82] for the diagnosis of IE that incorporated additional clinical factors and echocardiographic data. These criteria were revised in 2000 to increase the sensitivity for detection of cases related to *S. aureus* bacteremia, as well as to account for culture-negative IE.[77] The modified Duke criteria (see Tables 85–2 and 85–3) are the current standard for di-

ation. Echocardiography should be used to assess for the presence of endocardial involvement (vegetations, abscess formation, and new valvular regurgitation). These clinical, microbiologic, and echocardiographic features are the foundation for the Modified Duke Criteria, a set of integrated findings that has become the standard for diagnosis of IE (Tables 85–2 and 85–3).[77] These criteria are discussed in detail below.

Once the diagnosis is made and appropriate therapy initiated, the patient is monitored closely for complications, especially during the first week of therapy. All patients should have repeat blood cultures after institution of antibiotics to ensure sterility. Persistent fever beyond 1 week of appropriate therapy should raise suspicion for intracardiac extension or satellite abscess formation. In the absence of complications, the first several days of intravenous antibiotics are administered in the hospital and the remaining course provided via a percutaneously inserted central venous catheter (PICC line) as an outpatient with careful followup. Patients should be maintained on telemetry while in the hospital; the need for surveillance ECGs during outpatient therapy is dictated by the location of the infection and the predicted likelihood of conduction disturbances. Patients are monitored for antimicrobial toxicity, particularly with aminoglycoside use. Routine surveillance echocardiography during therapy is unnecessary unless complications develop or cardiac surgery is considered (see Echocardiography for Infective Endocarditis below). At

TABLE 85–2

Definition of Terms in the Proposed Modified Duke Criteria for the Diagnosis of Infective Endocarditis

MAJOR CRITERIA
Blood culture positive for IE
- Typical microorganisms consistent with IE from two separate blood cultures:
   Viridans streptococci, *Streptococcus bovis*, HACEK group, *Staphylococcus aureus*; or
   Community-acquired enterococci in the absence of a primary focus; or
- Microorganisms consistent with IE from persistently positive blood cultures, defined as follows:
   At least two positive cultures of blood samples drawn more than 12 h apart; or
   All of three or a majority of greater than four separate cultures of blood (with first and last sample drawn at least 1 h apart)
- Single positive blood culture for *Coxiella burnetti* or antiphase 1 IgG antibody titer greater than 1:800

Evidence of endocardial involvement
- Echocardiogram positive for IE (TEE recommended in patients with prosthetic valves, rated at least "possible IE" by clinical criteria, or complicated IE [paravalvular abscess]; TTE as first test in other patients), defined as follows:
   Oscillating intracardiac mass on valve or supporting structures, in the path of regurgitant jets, or on implanted material in the absence of an alternative anatomic explanation; or
   Abscess; or
   New partial dehiscence of prosthetic valve
- New valvular regurgitation (worsening or changing of preexisting murmur not sufficient)

MINOR CRITERIA
- Predisposition, predisposing heart condition, or injection drug use
- Fever, temperature greater than 100.4°F (38°C)
- Vascular phenomena, major arterial emboli, septic pulmonary infarcts, mycotic aneurysm, intracranial hemorrhage, conjunctival hemorrhages, and Janeway lesions
- Immunologic phenomena; glomerulonephritis, Osler nodes, Roth spots, and rheumatoid factor
- Microbiologic evidence: positive blood culture but does not meet a major criterion,[a] or serologic evidence of active infection with organism consistent with IE
- Echocardiographic minor criteria eliminated

HACEK, *Haemophilus aphrophilus, Actinobacillus actinomycetemcomitans, Cardiobacterium hominis, Eikenella corrodens,* and *Kingella*; IE, infective endocarditis; Ig, immunoglobulin; TEE, transesophageal echocardiography; TTE, transthoracic echocardiography.
[a]Excludes single positive cultures for coagulase-negative staphylococci and organisms that do not cause endocarditis.
SOURCE: Reprinted with permission from Li JS, Sexton DJ, Mick N, et al. Proposed modifications to the Duke criteria for diagnosis of infective endocarditis. Clin Infect Dis 2000;30:8.

agnosis and clinical research and have been validated in numerous studies.[83–85] A diagnosis of "definite IE" is established clinically by evidence of two major criteria, one major plus three minor criteria, or five minor criteria. Patients identified with "possible IE" (one major plus one minor criterion or three minor criteria) should be treated for IE until the diagnosis is satisfactorily excluded. Application of these criteria in clinical practice will capture the vast majority of cases of IE and render the possibility of missing a potential case quite remote. The criteria are both clinically and biologically sound, relying on microbiologic data and evidence of endocardial involvement, with attention to predisposing factors and early complications of a vascular or immunologic nature. Table 85–2 details the definitions of specific criteria and terms used in the Modified Duke Criteria.[79]

The importance of obtaining blood cultures by appropriate methods, prior to the institution of antibiotics, cannot be overemphasized. Three separate sets of blood cultures obtained from different venipuncture sites over 24 hours are recommended. For the most commonly encountered bacterial pathogens (staphylococci, streptococci, enterococci), the first two sets of blood cultures will be positive in the vast majority of cases.[86] Culture-negative IE is most commonly associated

TABLE 85–3

Definition of Infective Endocarditis According to the Proposed Modified Duke Criteria

DEFINITE INFECTIVE ENDOCARDITIS
Pathologic criteria
1. Microorganisms demonstrated by culture or histologic examination of a vegetation, a vegetation that has embolized, or an intracardiac abscess specimen; or
2. Pathologic lesions; vegetation, or intracardiac abscess confirmed by histologic examination showing active endocarditis

Clinical criteria
1. Two major criteria; or
2. One major criterion and three minor criteria; or
3. Five minor criteria

POSSIBLE INFECTIVE ENDOCARDITIS
1. One major criterion and one minor criterion; or
2. Three minor criteria

REJECTED
1. Firm alternate diagnosis explaining evidence of infective endocarditis; or
2. Resolution of infective endocarditis syndrome with antibiotic therapy for less than 4 days; or
3. No pathologic evidence of infective endocarditis at surgery or autopsy, with antibiotic therapy for less than 4 days; or
4. Does not meet criteria for possible infective endocarditis, as noted above

SOURCE: Reprinted with permission from Li JS, Sexton DJ, Mick N, et al. Proposed modifications to the Duke criteria for the diagnosis of infective endocarditis. Clin Infect Dis 2000;30:633–638.

with antecedent antibiotic use, but may be a result of fastidious (e.g., HACEK) or intracellular organisms that are not readily detected using standard culture techniques,[66] especially if the laboratory has not been alerted to the possibility of IE and the need to perform additional testing. Identification of the offending pathogen may require special culture media and prolonged incubation times (>2 weeks).[16] Additional indirect measures of active infection with difficult-to-culture organisms (e.g., *Bartonella, Brucella, Legionella*) include positive results of serology, agglutination, immunofluorescence, and PCR amplification assays.[47,66] It should be noted that many of these indirect diagnostic tests may be nonspecific and careful interpretation is needed to avoid erroneous or false-positive results.

【 】 ECHOCARDIOGRAPHY IN INFECTIVE ENDOCARDITIS

All patients with suspected IE should undergo prompt echocardiographic assessment. There are several TTE findings suggestive of endocarditis, including vegetations, evidence of periannular tissue destruction (i.e., abscess formation), aneurysms or fistula formation, leaflet perforation, or prosthetic valve dehiscence.[17] Table 85–4 provides specific definitions of these findings.[87] The echocardiographic definition of a vegetation is an irregular shaped, discrete echogenic mass that must be adherent to, yet distinct from, the endothelial surface. The presence of a vegetation is strongly supported if the suspected mass oscillates at a high frequency, independent of other intracardiac structures.

Although there remains some debate regarding the optimal initial approach, the vast majority of patients undergo TTE imaging first because of its immediate availability. A low threshold to pursue TEE imaging is appropriate, as dictated by the clinical circumstances, the adequacy of the TTE images, and the potential need for early surgical planning and intervention. It is well established that TTE has limited sensitivity for the detection of vegetations (approximately 65 percent) and intracardiac abscesses (approximately 30 percent).[19,88] The technique, however, is safe, portable, readily available, and provides useful information regarding ventricular size and function, estimated pulmonary artery systolic pressure, and the appearance and function of uninvolved valves. Another important strength of TTE is its high specificity for the detection of vegetations (approaching 98 percent).[88] When visualized, vegetations can be characterized further by their size, mobility, texture, and point of attachment. Any associated valvular dysfunction (regurgitation or stenosis) can be assessed with Doppler interrogation and a baseline established against which future comparisons could be made. Nevertheless, as many as one-fifth of patients have technically inadequate TTE images for proper resolution of valvular and endocardial structures.[9,17] TTE does not provide adequate visualization of prosthetic heart valves (especially in the mitral position) because of acoustic shadowing, a situation in which its diagnostic sensitivity is reduced to 15 to 35 percent.[89] Finally, TTE has limited ability to delineate perivalvular extension of infection under most clinical circumstances.[19,89,90]

TABLE 85–4

Typical Echocardiographic Findings in Infective Endocarditis

FINDING	DESCRIPTION
Vegetation	Irregularly shaped, discrete echogenic mass. Adherent to, yet distinct from endocardial surface. High-frequency oscillation of the mass with motion that is independent of that of normal cardiac structures is a supportive, but not mandatory finding.
Abscess	Thickened area or mass within the myocardium or annular region. Appearance is nonhomogeneous often with both echogenic and echolucent areas in the lesion. Evidence of flow (by Doppler interrogation) within the area is strongly supportive, but not mandatory.
Aneurysm	Echolucent space that is contiguous with the cavity of origin and that is completely bounded by a thin layer of tissue extending from the cavity of origin.
Fistula	Connection between two distinct cardiac blood spaces through a nonanatomic channel.
Leaflet perforation	Defect in the body of a cardiac valve leaflet with evidence of blood flow through the defect.
Prosthetic valvular dehiscence	Rocking motion of a prosthetic valve with excursion of more than 15 degrees in any single plane.

SOURCE: Adapted from Sachdev M, Peterson GE, Jollis JG. Infect Dis Clin North Am 2002;16:319–337.

TEE is now performed with increasing regularity in the assessment of patients with suspected or proven IE. Although TEE is invasive and requires conscious sedation, the procedure is generally well tolerated and has low complication rates.[90] TEE has excellent specificity and offers better sensitivity for the detection of vegetations (85 to 95 percent) and intracardiac abscesses (87 percent), and has greater spatial resolution.[19,88,89] The sensitivity of TEE for the detection of vegetations in patients with suspected PVE is 82 to 96 percent[89] and TEE should be considered a first-line imaging modality in cases of suspected PVE. TEE, combined with spectral and color-flow Doppler analysis, also provides excellent definition of intracardiac fistulas, valve leaflet perforations, and false aneurysms. Table 85–5 summarizes the performance characteristics of TTE and TEE. TEE should be performed expeditiously in patients with high-risk clinical features at presentation (e.g., suspected *S. aureus* infection of the

TABLE 85–5

Aggregate Performance Characteristics of TTE and TEE in the Diagnosis of IE

	SENSITIVITY	SPECIFICITY
TTE	60–65%	98%
TEE	85–95%	85–98%

TEE, transesophageal echocardiography; TTE, transthoracic echocardiography.
SOURCE: *Data compiled from references 88, 89, and 91–96.*

aortic valve and root), known congenital heart disease, or suboptimal TTE images. For patients undergoing cardiac surgery for IE, intraoperative TEE is routine. TEE should also be considered for patients with catheter-associated S. *aureus* bacteremia to predict the indicated duration of antibiotic therapy (i.e., 2 weeks vs. 4 weeks).[60] Other analyses have suggested that in patients with an intermediate pretest likelihood of IE, an initial TEE is a cost-effective means of diagnosis.[97]

Because of its superior performance characteristics, it is tempting to pursue TEE in all cases of suspected or proven IE. In several circumstances, however, TTE is sufficient for both diagnosis and clinical decision making. For example, in a patient with mitral valve endocarditis caused by a highly penicillin-sensitive S. *viridans* spp., an isolated posterior leaflet vegetation of less than 1 cm in length and mild mitral regurgitation, antibiotic therapy can be initiated with careful followup. If clinically indicated, a repeat TTE can be performed to assess for complications or response to therapy. A similar approach could be adopted for an IDU with tricuspid valve IE and no clinical or TTE evidence of left-sided involvement at presentation. Thus, the choice of echocardiographic modality can be tailored to the clinical situation. Tables 85–6 and 85–7 list the indications for TTE and TEE in patients with IE.[79] Figure 85–5 presents an algorithm for the use of echocardiography in IE.[47]

Although diagnostic echocardiography is recommended for all patients with suspected IE, some studies suggest that in very-low-risk subgroups, echocardiography may be avoided without loss of diagnostic accuracy. Kuruppu et al. showed that 53 percent of echocardiograms could have been avoided without loss of diagnostic accuracy by using a simple algorithm in patients with a low pretest probability of disease.[98] In another analysis, Greaves et al. showed that the negative predictive value of TEE was 1.0 in the absence of five simple clinical criteria: vasculitic/embolic phenomena, presence of central venous access, recent history of injection drug use, presence of a prosthetic valve, and positive blood cultures.[99] These studies suggest that routine echocardiographic imaging may not be indicated in many low-risk patients.

The findings on echocardiography alone do not definitively establish or exclude the diagnosis of IE. Infective vegetations may be difficult to distinguish from other intracardiac masses, such as calcified debris, torn chordae, thrombus, fibroelastoma, and the nonbacterial lesions associated with healed IE, adenocarcinoma (marantic endocarditis), antiphospholipid antibody syndrome, and systemic lupus erythematosus (Libman-Sacks).

TABLE 85–6

Indications for Transthoracic Echocardiography in Endocarditis

Class I
1. Transthoracic echocardiography to detect valvular vegetations with or without positive blood cultures is recommended for the diagnosis of infective endocarditis. *(Level of Evidence: B)*
2. Transthoracic echocardiography is recommended to characterize the hemodynamic severity of valvular lesions in known infective endocarditis. *(Level of Evidence: B)*
3. Transthoracic echocardiography is recommended for assessment of complications of infective endocarditis (e.g., abscesses, perforations, and shunts). *(Level of Evidence: B)*
4. Transthoracic echocardiography is recommended for reassessment of high-risk patients (e.g., those with a virulent organism, clinical deterioration, persistent or recurrent fever, new murmur, or persistent bacteremia). *(Level of Evidence: C)*

Class IIa
Transthoracic echocardiography is reasonable to diagnose infective endocarditis of a prosthetic valve in the presence of persistent fever without bacteremia or a new murmur. *(Level of Evidence: C)*

Class IIb
Transthoracic echocardiography may be considered for the reevaluation of prosthetic valve endocarditis during antibiotic therapy in the absence of clinical deterioration. *(Level of Evidence: C)*

Class III
Transthoracic echocardiography is not indicated to reevaluate uncomplicated (including no regurgitation on baseline echocardiogram) native valve endocarditis during antibiotic treatment in the absence of clinical deterioration, new physical findings, or persistent fever. *(Level of Evidence: C)*

SOURCE: *Bonow RO, Carabello BA, Chatterjee K, et al. ACC/AHA 2006 Guidelines for the Management of Patients with Valvular Heart Disease: a Report of the American College of Cardiology/American Heart Association Task Force on Practice Guidelines (Writing Committee to Develop Guidelines for the Management of Patients With Valvular Heart Disease). Available at American College of Cardiology website: http://www.acc.org/clinical/guidelines/valvular/index.pdf.*

In addition, an initially nondiagnostic TEE (despite its high negative predictive value) does not exclude the possibility of IE and a repeat study is indicated in 3 to 5 days if the clinical index of suspicion remains high.[100] Accurate diagnosis, therefore, relies on an integrated assessment of clinical, microbiologic, and echocardiographic data.

In uncomplicated cases of IE, a single echocardiographic study is usually sufficient. However, with complex IE, serial echocardiographic examinations may help determine prognosis and guide surgical intervention. Rohmann et al. performed serial TEE studies in 83 patients with echocardiographic evidence of IE and followed them prospectively for a mean duration of 6

SOURCE: Bonow RO, Carabello BA, Chatterjee K, et al. ACC/AHA 2006 Guidelines for the Management of Patients with Valvular Heart Disease: A Report of the American College of Cardiology/American Heart Association Task Force on Practice Guidelines (Writing Committee to Develop Guidelines for the Management of Patients With Valvular Heart Disease). Available at American College of Cardiology Website: http://www.acc.org/clinical/guidelines/valvular/index.pdf.

TABLE 85–7

Indications for Transesophageal Echocardiography in Endocarditis

Class I

1. Transesophageal echocardiography is recommended to assess the severity of valvular lesions in symptomatic patients with infective endocarditis, if transthoracic echocardiography is nondiagnostic. (Level of Evidence: C)
2. Transesophageal echocardiography is recommended to diagnose infective endocarditis in patients with valvular heart disease and positive blood cultures, if transthoracic echocardiography is nondiagnostic. (Level of Evidence: C)
3. Transesophageal echocardiography is recommended to diagnose complications of infective endocarditis with potential impact on prognosis and management (e.g., abscesses, perforation, and shunts). (Level of Evidence: C)
4. Transesophageal echocardiography is recommended as first-line diagnostic study to diagnose prosthetic valve endocarditis and assess for complications. (Level of Evidence: C)
5. Transesophageal echocardiography is recommended for preoperative evaluation in patients with known infective endocarditis, unless the need for surgery is evident on transthoracic imaging and unless preoperative imaging will delay surgery in urgent cases. (Level of Evidence: C)
6. Intraoperative transesophageal echocardiography is recommended for patients undergoing valve surgery for infective endocarditis. (Level of Evidence: C)

Class IIa

Transesophageal echocardiography is reasonable to diagnose possible infective endocarditis in patients with persistent staphylococcal bacteremia without a known source. (Level of Evidence: C)

Class IIb

Transesophageal echocardiography might be considered to detect infective endocarditis in patients with nosocomial staphylococcal bacteremia. (Level of Evidence: C)

months; they found that vegetations that increased in size were associated with a significantly increased risk of complications. Both the 2003 Update to the American College of Cardiologists/American Heart Association/American Society of Echocardiography (ACC/AHA/ASE) *Guidelines for the Application of Clinical Echocardiography*[90] and the 2006 Update to the ACC/AHA *Valvular Heart Disease Guidelines*[79] recommend, as a class I indication, reevaluation echocardiographic studies in complex IE. Complex IE is defined as infection with virulent organisms (e.g., *S. aureus*), severe hemodynamic compromise, aortic valve involvement, persistent fever or bacteremia, clinical change during therapy, or symptomatic deterioration. The use of reevalua-

tion studies in uncomplicated IE is less well established (class IIb recommendation).[90] In the vast majority of cases, no additional diagnostic information is provided after a second echocardiogram.[101]

ACUTE COMPLICATIONS

Complication rates with IE have remained relatively unchanged despite advances in diagnosis and antimicrobial therapy. Complications can generally be related to local extension of infection (e.g., valve ring abscess, fistulae, conduction block), destruction of or interference with intracardiac structures (e.g., leaflet perforation or valvular obstruction), embolization (e.g., stroke, septic pulmonary emboli), bacteremia/sepsis (e.g., multisystem organ failure), and immune complex disease (e.g., glomerulonephritis).

HEART FAILURE

Heart failure is the most frequent major complication of IE[102]; its development portends an adverse outcome with medical therapy alone[1] and is an indication for surgical intervention in most instances.[79,103] Reduced left ventricle (LV) systolic function is the most powerful predictor of an adverse outcome following surgery.[104] Heart failure in IE is most often related to acute, severe valvular dysfunction owing either to leaflet destruction or interference with normal coaptation. It may also occur from rupture of infected mitral chordae, obstruction caused by bulky vegetations, the development of intracardiac shunts, or prosthetic valve dehiscence.[47] Heart failure may also develop more gradually, over the intermediate- to long-term, as a function of continued valve incompetence and worsening ventricular function, following otherwise successful antibiotic treatment.

Heart failure is most commonly associated with aortic valve IE (29 percent), followed by mitral valve (20 percent), and then tricuspid valve (8 percent) involvement.[105] In acute severe aortic regurgitation, the LV operates on the steep portion of its diastolic pressure-volume relationship. The sudden delivery of a large regurgitant volume is met with a marked increase in LV diastolic and left atrial pressures. Forward stroke volume falls, related in part to the inability of the ventricle to dilate acutely. Tachycardia develops, but is usually not adequate to protect the cardiac output. Patients may present with pulmonary edema and shock. Examination findings may be masked. The pulse pressure is not widened, the first heart sound is soft, and the diastolic murmur is of relatively short duration. The rapid decrease in coronary driving pressure, represented by the aortic–left ventricular pressure gradient, may result in diminished coronary blood flow and myocardial ischemia even with normal epicardial coronary arteries. Inappropriate bradycardia, which can develop if the infection extends into the conduction system leading to atrioventricular block (Fig. 85–6) or if the patient receives a β blocker, can be catastrophic. Patients with acute severe mitral regurgitation may present with pulmonary edema, low output, and/or rapid atrial fibrillation. They can usually be stabilized with intensive medical management and, in contrast to patients with acute severe aortic regurgitation, surgery can be deferred into the nonacute setting. Patients with acute tricuspid regurgitation may show signs of right-heart failure; medical management is the rule rather than the exception. Premorbid

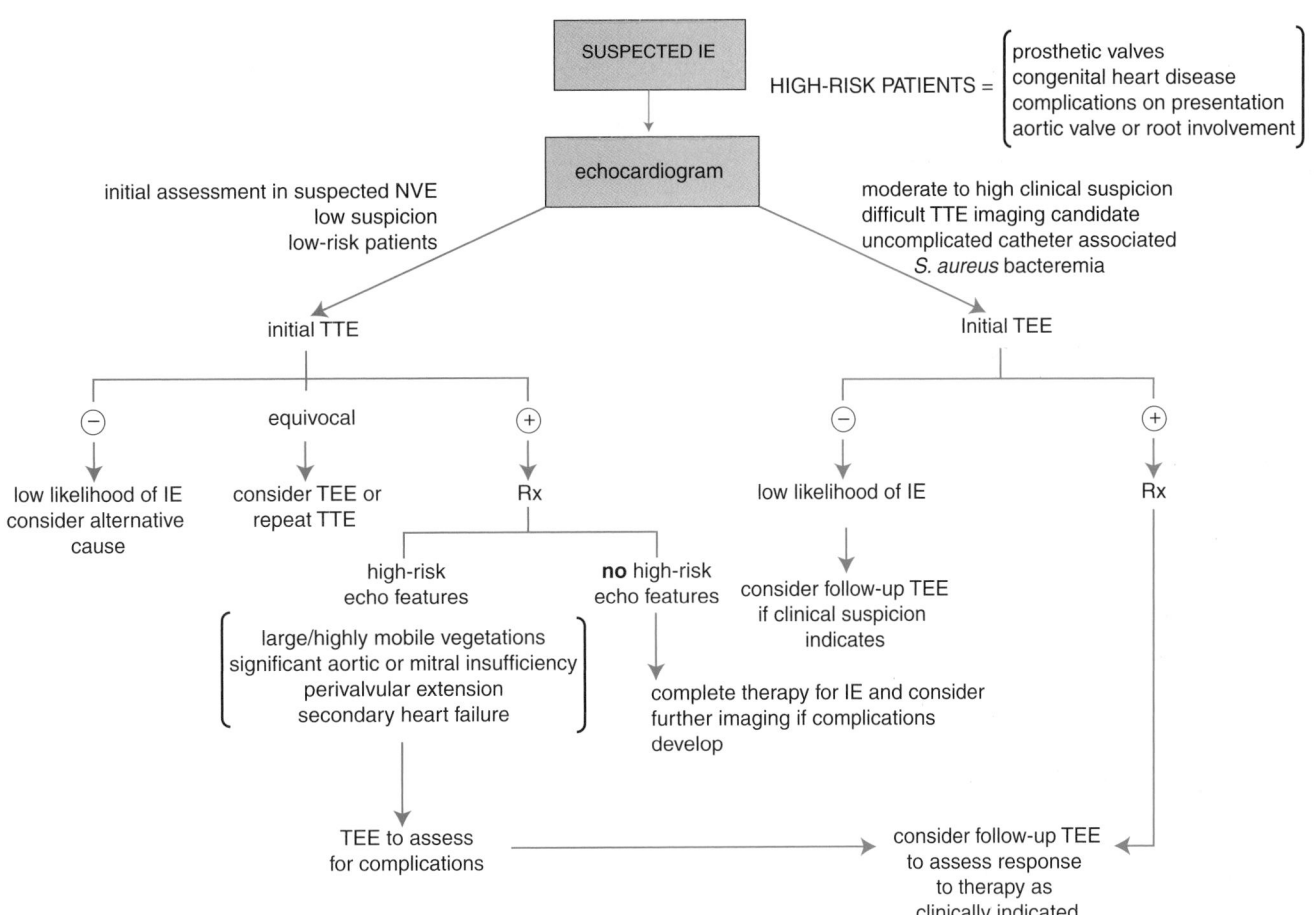

FIGURE 85–5. Use of echocardiography in diagnosis and management of IE. IE, infective endocarditis; NVE, native valve endocarditis; TEE, transesophageal echocardiography; TTE, transthoracic echocardiography. *Source: Adapted with permission from Bayer AS, Bolger AF, Taubert KA, et al. Diagnosis and management of infective endocarditis and its complications. Circulation 1998;98:2936–2950.*

heart disease, including antecedent valvular disease, coronary artery disease, cardiomyopathy, and arrhythmia, may also increase the likelihood that heart failure will develop, even with lesser degrees of acute valvular dysfunction.

【 】 EMBOLIZATION

Embolization is a dreaded complication of IE. Central nervous system (CNS) involvement is most common; stroke comprises up to 65 percent of embolic events and may be the presenting sign of IE in up to 14 percent of cases.[106] CNS embolization can present with subtle neurologic abnormalities, as seen with microembolization, or with sudden hemiplegia and obtundation, as seen with a ruptured mycotic aneurysm and intracranial hemorrhage (Fig. 85–7) or with a large embolic stroke. Up to 90 percent of CNS emboli lodge in the distribution of the middle cerebral artery, and carry a high mortality rate.[107] Any patient with suspected or definite IE who develops neurologic symptoms should promptly undergo neurologic imaging and be considered to have CNS embolization until proved otherwise.

Emboli may also involve other organ systems, including the liver, spleen, kidneys, and lungs. Metastatic sites of infection may appear in the spine and/or paraspinous space, and may be the cause of prolonged fever or bacteremia despite appropriate antimicrobial therapy. Septic pulmonary emboli are present in the major-

ity of cases of right-sided IE related to IDU.[108] On rare occasions, discrete coronary emboli can cause myocardial infarction. Although discrete coronary embolization is relatively rare, it has long been appreciated that patients with IE can develop scattered areas of myocardial "microinfarctions" in the absence of epicardial vessel occlusion. Such areas have been attributed to microembolization, hypoperfusion, and immunologic phenomena.[109] Janeway lesions are vascular phenomena indicative of embolization of vegetative material (see Fig. 85–4D).

In various series, systemic embolization occurred in 22 to 50 percent of IE cases.[80,110] Given the varied incidence of systemic embolization among patients with IE, the ability to assess patients for embolic risk is of great interest and may help identify patients who may benefit from alternative therapies, including earlier cardiac surgery. However, the prediction of individual patient risk for embolization has proven difficult. Embolization risk appears to decrease precipitously following 2 weeks of appropriate antibiotic therapy, from 13 to 1.2 embolic events per 1000 patient-days.[111] In most series, a prior embolic event has not been a predictor of recurrent embolization. An exception to this observation was noted in the report from Vilacosta et al.[112] In many series, the risk of embolization appeared to be higher for mitral than for aortic valve endocarditis (approximately 25 percent vs. 10 percent, respectively), particularly with anterior leaflet involvement.[113–115] A number of echocardiographic studies demonstrated a trend toward

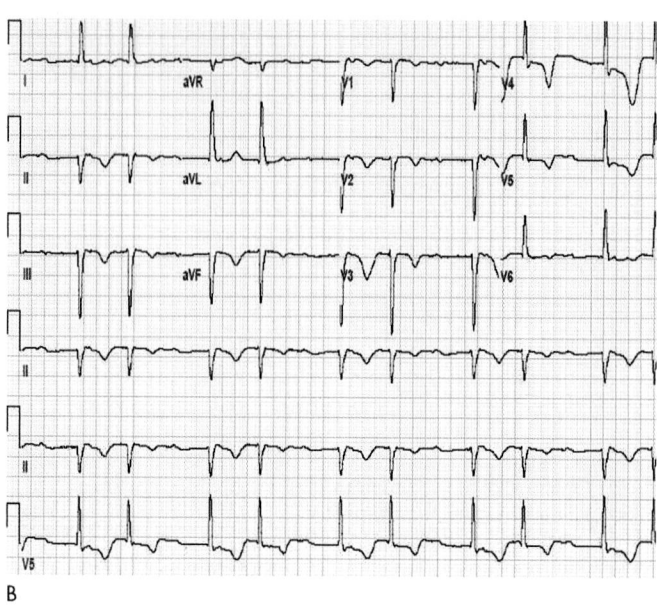

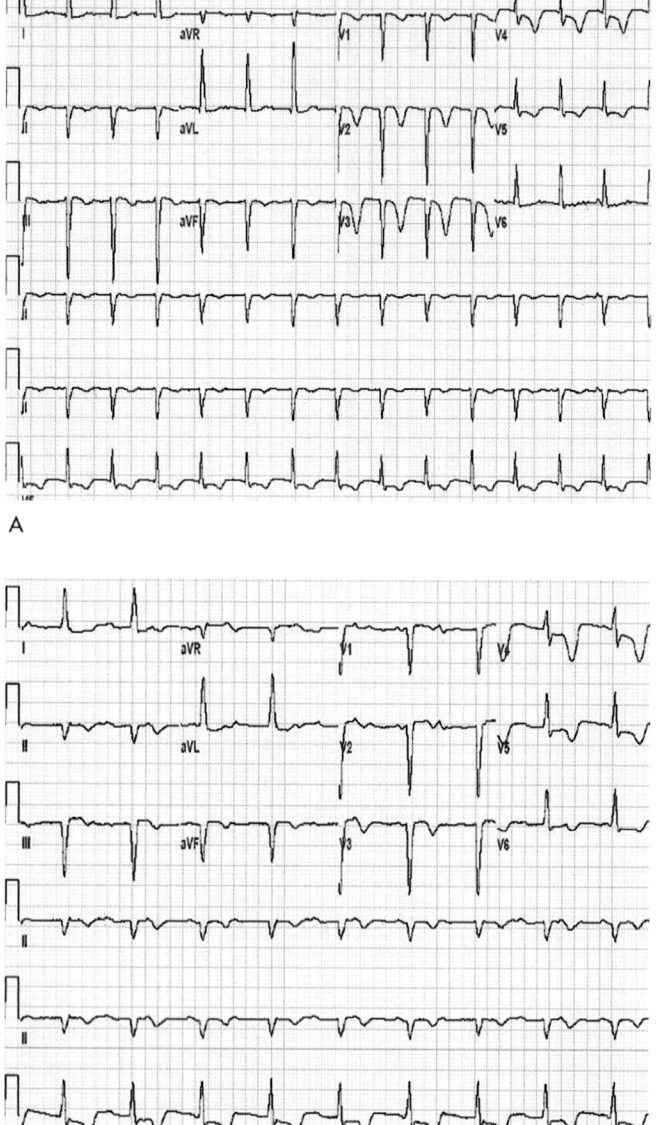

FIGURE 85-6. Serial electrocardiograms obtained in a patient with methicillin-resistant *Staphylococcus aureus* (MRSA) aortic valve endocarditis complicated by root abscess and ventricular septal rupture. Note progressive degrees of high grade atrioventricular (AV) block. **A**, first-degree AV block; **B**, second-degree AV block; **C**, complete heart block.

higher embolic rates with left-sided vegetations that are >1 cm in diameter,[91,116] and more recent work suggests that vegetation size >1.5 cm is a predictor of IE-related mortality.[117] Increasing or static vegetation size with antimicrobial therapy seen on serial TEE is associated with higher embolic rates.[118] One interesting report suggested an interaction between vegetation size and the presence of patient-specific antiphospholipid antibodies.[119] The risk of embolization may also derive from microbial-specific features and is consistently higher with *S. aureus*, *S. lugdunensis*, certain streptococcal strains, *Haemophilus influenzae*, and fungi.

【 】 MYCOTIC ANEURYSMS

Mycotic aneurysms represent a small, but extremely dangerous subset of embolic complications. They occur most frequently in the intracranial arteries and have a particular predilection for the middle cerebral artery and its branches (see Fig. 85–7).[120] They result from septic embolization to the arterial vas vasorum, with subsequent spread of infection and weakening of the vessel wall. Mycotic aneurysms tend to develop at arterial branch points, which are a common site of embolic impaction. The overall mortality rate among IE patients with intracranial mycotic aneurysms is 60 percent and approaches 80 percent if rupture occurs.[121] The presenting symptoms of intracranial mycotic aneurysms are highly variable and can range from a localized headache (as seen with a small sentinel bleed) to dense neurologic deficits resulting from sudden intracranial hemorrhage.[121] Screening patients with definite IE for the presence of intracranial mycotic aneurysms is not currently recommended and neurologic imaging is reserved for symptomatic patients. In such patients, a contrast-enhanced CT will provide useful information as it is highly sensitive for the detection of intracranial hemorrhage and may thus indirectly identify the location of the mycotic aneurysm.[47] Magnetic resonance angiography is an evolving technique for the detection of intracranial mycotic aneurysms, although its sensitivity for small aneurysms remains inferior to conventional four-vessel cerebral angiography.[122] Although many intracranial mycotic

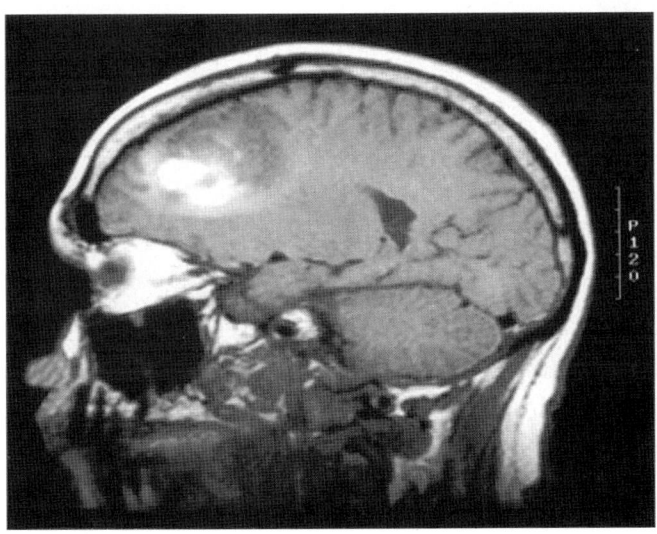
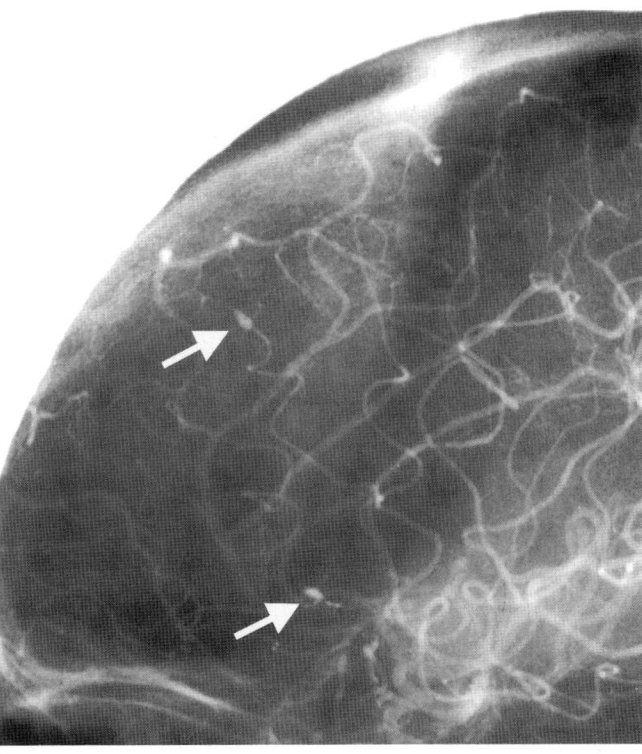

FIGURE 85–7. A. Large right frontal hemorrhage in a patient with *S. aureus* mitral valve endocarditis. **B.** Mycotic aneurysms (*arrows*) along the course of the branches of the middle cerebral artery. *Source: Adapted with permission from Mauri L, de Lemos JA, O'Gara PT. Infective endocarditis. Curr Probl Cardiol 2001;26(9):562–610.*

aneurysms often heal with medical therapy, a subset may rupture unpredictably. Given the complex risks of prophylactic neurosurgical intervention, decisions concerning medical versus surgical therapy must be individualized.[47] Percutaneous neuroradiologic intervention is preferred whenever allowed by the anatomic characteristics of the mycotic aneurysm.[123] Mycotic aneurysms may less commonly develop in other arteries (e.g., splenic, mesenteric) and remain clinically silent or rupture spontaneously.

[ ] PERIANNULAR EXTENSION OF INFECTION

Extension or spread of infection beyond the valve annulus is a very concerning development that usually presages the need for surgical therapy. Findings such as persistent fever and bacteremia despite antibiotic therapy, heart failure, or new conduction block should raise suspicion for this complication. Although a relatively insensitive sign, the development of new AV block in the setting of aortic valve IE has a high positive predictive value for the presence of perivalvular abscess formation.[124] Periannular extension may occur in 10 to 40 percent of all native valve IE, and complicates aortic valve IE more commonly than either mitral or tricuspid valve IE. Periannular extension is more common with prosthetic valve IE (occurring in >50 percent of patients),[124] as the prosthetic sewing ring is often the primary site of infection (Fig. 85–8).[125] Perivalvular extension sets the stage for abscess formation, perforation, fistula development, and hemodynamic deterioration. The aortic annular segment adjacent to the membranous septum and AV node is particularly vulnerable to abscess formation and may explain the occurrence of conduction block seen in some patients with aortic valve IE (see Fig. 85–6).[124,126] Patients with suspected periannular extension of infection and intracardiac abscess formation should undergo prompt TEE, which is both sensitive and specific for detection of this complication.[126–128] Surgical therapy is directed toward complete eradiche supporting annular structures is required.

[ ] RENAL DYSFUNCTION

Renal dysfunction is a common complication of IE and is often multifactorial in nature given the high incidence of preexisting renal disease, immune complex disease, drug-induced nephrotoxicity, and hemodynamic perturbations. A recent necropsy and biopsy study of 62 patients with IE revealed that localized renal infarction (often caused by septic emboli) was present in 31 percent, acute glomerulonephritis in 26 percent, acute interstitial nephritis (likely antibiotic related) in 10 percent, and renal cortical necrosis in 10 percent of patients.[129] Glomerulonephritis, as suggested by the appearance of red cell casts, is caused by immune complex deposition and complement activation. Similar examples of immune complex disease include Osler nodes, Roth spots, nonseptic arthritis, and palpable purpuric skin lesions with findings of leukocytoclastic vasculitis on biopsy.

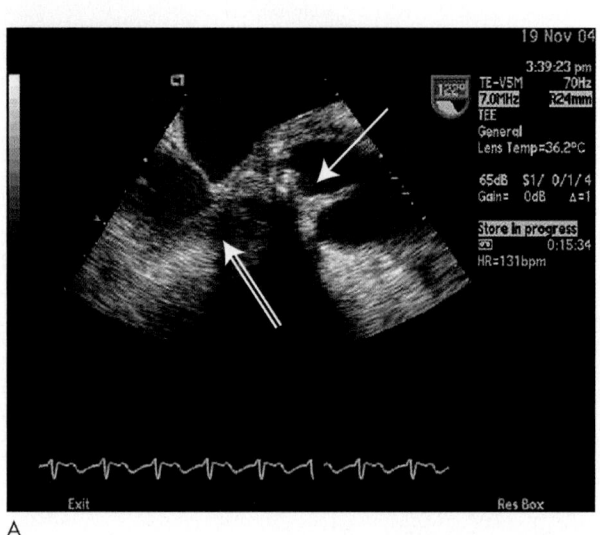
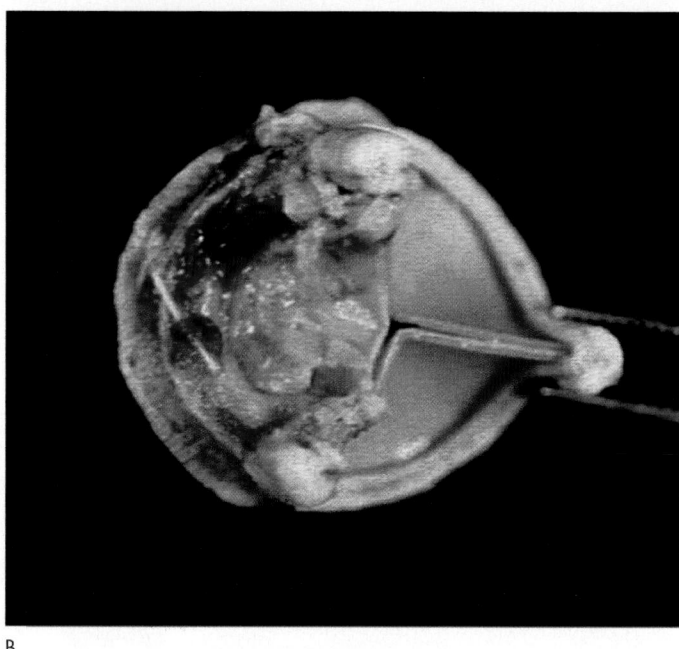

FIGURE 85-8. A. Transesophageal echocardiographic image of bioprosthetic aortic valve with large vegetation (*arrow*) and annular abscess (*double arrow*) from a patient with *Staphylococcus aureus* prosthetic valve endocarditis. **B.** Excised surgical specimen.

ANTIMICROBIAL THERAPY

【 】 GENERAL PRINCIPLES

Rapid institution of appropriate parenteral antibiotic therapy is the single most important initial intervention in the treatment of suspected or proven IE. Given the rising rate of antimicrobial resistance among causative organisms,[46] therapy is predicated on the identification of the causative isolate and delineation of its antibiotic sensitivities. An infectious disease specialist should supervise the dose, duration, and method of delivery (IV or IM) of antimicrobial therapy with longitudinal followup. Serum antibiotic levels should be monitored where appropriate and renal and hepatic function assayed when indicated. A recent American Heart Association Scientific Statement,[46] addresses antimicrobial therapy in IE in detail (Tables 85-8 to 85-14).

【 】 CHOICE OF ANTIBIOTICS

The lesions of IE are extremely difficult to eradicate, as the infection exists in a sequestered area of impaired host defense. Thus, IE requires weeks of parenteral antibiotic therapy, preferably with a drug that has bactericidal activity against the offending organism. Combination antimicrobial therapy may provide more rapid bactericidal effect and in certain circumstances acts synergistically to accelerate sterilization of the blood.[130] All patients should have surveillance blood cultures obtained 2 to 3 days after the initiation of antibiotic therapy to ensure efficacy. Most patients will require long-term venous access via a PICC or Hickman line for a 4- to 6-week course of antibiotics. Patients should remain in an inpatient setting during the initial phase of treatment when complications are most likely, after which selected low-risk patients can be considered for outpatient parenteral antibiotic therapy.[131]

【 】 EMPIRIC ANTIBIOTIC THERAPY

Initial empiric antibiotic therapy (i.e., before blood culture results are available) should cover *S. aureus*, the many species of streptococci that can cause IE, and *E. faecalis*. Thus, a combination of a β-lactamase–resistant penicillin (nafcillin), or vancomycin for penicillin-allergic patients, and gentamicin, is often used. The tempo of infection is a valuable clue; *S. aureus* endocarditis often presents with an acute and fulminant course with high-grade bacteremia. Other risk factors for *S. aureus* IE include chronic hospitalization, indwelling central venous catheters or prosthetic devices, surgical wounds, and intravenous drug use. Vancomycin should also be used if the patient is at risk for MRSA infection. Oral rifampin is added to nafcillin and gentamicin for staphylococcal infections of prosthetic materials (see Table 85-12). The duration of gentamicin therapy will vary as a function of the offending microorganism, but is usually 2 weeks or less.

【 】 ANTIPLATELET AND ANTITHROMBIN THERAPY

Despite their theoretical benefit, there are no human studies that support the use of either antiplatelet or antithrombin therapy to prevent embolic complications or to hasten antibiotic cure.[132] Moreover, small uncontrolled studies suggest that antithrombin therapy actually increases the risk of intracranial hemorrhage following CNS embolization.[133,134] For patients who require anticoagulation for either chronic atrial fibrillation or a mechanical heart valve, warfarin should be discontinued on admission and unfrac-

TABLE 85–8

Therapy of Native Valve Endocarditis Caused by Highly Penicillin-Susceptible Viridans Group Streptococci and *Streptococcus bovis*

REGIMEN	DOSAGE[a] AND ROUTE	DURATION (WK)	COMMENTS
Aqueous crystalline penicillin G sodium	12–18 million U per 24 h IV either continuously or in 4 to 6 equally divided doses	4	Preferred in most patients older than 65 y of age and in patients with impairment of 8th cranial nerve function or renal function
or Ceftriaxone sodium	2 g per 24 h IV/IM in 1 dose Pediatric dose[b]: penicillin 200,000 U/ kg per 24 h IV in 4 to 6 equally divided doses; ceftriaxone 100 mg per 24 h IV/IM in 1 dose	4	
Aqueous crystalline penicillin G sodium	12–18 million U per 24 h IV either continuously or in 6 equally divided doses	2	Two-week regimen not intended for patients with known cardiac or extracardiac abscess or for those with creatinine clearance of less than 20 mL per min, impaired 8th cranial nerve function, or *Abiotrophia, Granulicatella,* or *Gemella* spp. infection. Gentamicin dosage should be adjusted to achieve peak serum concentration of 3–4 μg/mL and trough serum concentration of less than 1μg/mL when 3 divided doses are used; nomogram used for single daily dosing.
or Ceftriaxone sodium *plus*	2 g per 24 h IV/IM in 1 dose	2	
Gentamicin sulfate[c]	3 mg/kg per 24 h IV/IM in 1 dose Pediatric dose: penicillin 200,000 U/kg per 24 h IV in 4 to 6 equally divided doses; ceftriaxone 100 mg/ kg per 24 h IV/IM in 1 dose; gentamicin 3/mg per kg per 24 h IV/IM in 1 dose or 3 equally divided doses[d]	2	
Vancomycin hydro-chloride[e]	30 mg/kg per 24 h IV in 2 equally divided doses not to exceed 2 g per 24 h unless concentrations in serum are inappropriately low Pediatric dose: 40 mg/kg per 24 h IV in 2 to 3 equally divided doses	2	Vancomycin therapy recommended only for patients unable to tolerate penicillin or ceftriaxone; vancomycin dosage should be adjusted to obtain peak (1 h after infusion completed) serum concentration of 30–45 μg/mL and a trough concentration range of 10–15 μg/ mL

IM, intramuscular; IV, intravenous.
Minimum inhibitory concentration less than or equal to 0.12 μg/per mL.
[a]Dosages recommended are for patients with normal renal function.
[b]Pediatric dose should not exceed that of a normal adult.
[c]Other potentially nephrotoxic drugs (e.g., nonsteroidal antiinflammatory drugs) should be used with caution in patients who are receiving gentamicin therapy.
[d]Data for once-daily dosing of aminoglycosides for children exist, but no data for treatment of infective endocarditis exists.
[e]Vancomycin dosages should be infused during course of at least 1 h to reduce risk of histamine-release "red man" syndrome.
SOURCE: *Modified from Baddour LM, Wilson WR, Bayer AS, et al. Infective endocarditis: diagnosis, antimicrobial therapy, and management of complications: a statement for healthcare professionals from the Committee on Rheumatic Fever, Endocarditis, and Kawasaki Disease, Council on Cardiovascular Disease in the Young, and the Councils on Clinical Cardiology, Stroke, and Cardiovascular Surgery and Anesthesia, American Heart Association. Circulation 2005;111:e394–e434.*

tionated intravenous heparin substituted. Because of its extended therapeutic effect and attenuated response to protamine reversal, low-molecular-weight heparin should be avoided when anticoagulation is needed in hospitalized patients with IE. Warfarin should

not be resumed until (1) it is clear that the patient has not had a CNS complication and (2) all invasive procedures are completed. For patients with mechanical valves, there is only a small risk of thromboembolism incurred by withholding anticoagulation for a

TABLE 85–9

Therapy of Native Valve Endocarditis Caused by Strains of Viridans Group Streptococci and *Streptococcus bovis* Relatively Resistant to Penicillin

REGIMEN	DOSAGE[a] AND ROUTE	DURATION (WK)	COMMENTS
Aqueous crystalline penicillin G sodium	24 million U per 24 h IV either continuously or in 4 to 6 equally divided doses	4	Patients with endocarditis caused by penicillin-resistant (MIC greater than 0.5 μg/mL) strains should be treated with regimen recommended for enterococcal endocarditis
or Ceftriaxone sodium *plus*	2 g per 24 h IV/IM in 1 dose	4	Recommended for enterococcal endocarditis (see Table 85–8)
Gentamicin sulfate[b]	3 mg/kg per 24 h IV/IM in 1 dose Pediatric dose[c]: penicillin 300,000 U per 24 h IV in 4 to 6 equally divided doses; ceftriaxone 100 mg/ kg per 24 IV/IM in 1 dose; gentamicin 3 mg/kg per 24 h IV/IM in 1 dose or 3 equally divided doses	2	
Vancomycin hydrochloride[c]	30 mg/kg per 24 h IV in 2 equally divided doses not to exceed 2 g per 24 h, unless serum concentration's are inappropriately low Pediatric dose: 40 mg/kg per 24 h in 2 or 3 equally divided doses	4	Vancomycin[d] therapy is recommended only for patients unable to tolerate penicillin or ceftriaxone therapy

Minimum inhibitory concentration (MIC) greater than 0.12 μg/mL to less than or equal to 0.5 μ/mL.
[a]Dosages recommended are for patients with normal renal function.
[b]See Table 85–7 for appropriate dosages of gentamicin.
[c]Pediatric dose should not exceed that of a normal adult.
[d]See Table 85–7 for appropriate dosages of vancomycin.
SOURCE: Modified from Baddour LM, Wilson WR, Bayer AS, et al. Infective endocarditis: diagnosis, antimicrobial therapy, and management of complications: a statement for healthcare professionals from the Committee on Rheumatic Fever, Endocarditis, and Kawasaki Disease, Council on Cardiovascular Disease in the Young, and the Councils on Clinical Cardiology, Stroke, and Cardiovascular Surgery and Anesthesia, American Heart Association. Circulation 2005;111:e394–e434.

short period of time. Thus, even when anticoagulation is indicated, it should be administered with caution as the acute phase of IE is a period of high hemorrhagic risk. If neurologic symptoms develop, any and all anticoagulant therapy should be stopped until CNS imaging is performed. A CNS or major visceral bleed may necessitate the discontinuation of all forms of anticoagulation for a longer period of time, depending on the clinical course and the risk-to-benefit analysis regarding the timing of reexposure. In the event of a CNS bleed, neurosurgical and interventional neuroradiologic consultation should be sought, especially as major intracranial hemorrhage is often caused by rupture of a mycotic aneurysm. CNS hemorrhage will delay the performance of cardiac surgery (if indicated) for up to 1 month. If cardiac surgery is eventually performed, a tissue valve would be preferable to avoid the need for chronic postoperative anticoagulation.[135]

SURGICAL THERAPY

The decision to undertake cardiac surgery for the treatment IE can be extremely challenging and there are no randomized clinical tri-

als to guide practice. Tables 85–15 and 85–16 summarize the most recent ACC/AHA guidelines for surgery in IE.[79]

For native valve endocarditis, the primary indication for surgery in the active phase of infection is the development of clinical heart failure from either valve stenosis or regurgitation. Evidence of elevated LV end-diastolic or left atrial pressures by either invasive (catheter) or noninvasive (echo-Doppler) assessment may also prompt surgery. Valve surgery is indicated for treatment of fungal or other highly resistant organisms, and for treatment of intracardiac abscess, perforation, fistulous tracts, and false aneurysms. Surgery is reasonable for patients with recurrent emboli and persistent vegetations and for patients with persistent bacteremia despite several days (5 to 7) of appropriate antibiotic therapy in the absence of a metastatic focus of infection. Surgery to prevent embolization can be considered for treatment of large (>1.0 cm), mobile vegetations, particularly in large-volume centers with expertise in primary valve repair. This latter issue remains controversial, although improvements in repair techniques and surgical outcomes have warranted reevaluation. Most echocardiographic studies have shown a relationship between vegetation size and the risk of embolization,

TABLE 85–10

Therapy for Native Valve or Prosthetic Valve Enterococcal Endocarditis Caused by Strains Susceptible to Penicillin, Gentamicin, and Vancomycin

REGIMEN	DOSAGE[a] AND ROUTE	DURATION (WK)	COMMENTS
Ampicillin sodium	12 g per 24 h IV in 6 equally divided doses	4–6	Native valve: 4-wk therapy recommended for patients with symptoms of illness less than or equal to 3 mo; 6-wk therapy recommended for patients with symptoms longer than 3 mo
or Aqueous crystalline penicillin G sodium	18–30 million U per 24 h IV either continuously or in 6 equally divided doses	4–6	Prosthetic valve or other prosthetic cardiac material: minimum of 6 wk of therapy recommended
plus Gentamicin sulfate[b]	3 mg/kg per 24 h IV/IM in 3 equally divided doses Pediatric dose[c]: ampicillin 300 mg per kg per 24 h IV in 4 to 6 equally divided doses; penicillin 300, 000 U/kg per 24 h IV in 4 to 6 equally divided doses; gentamicin 3 mg/kg per 24 h IV/IM in 3 equally divided doses	4–6	
Vancomycin hydro-chloride[d]	30 mg/kg per 24 h IV in 2 equally divided doses	6	Vancomycin therapy is recommended only for patients unable to tolerate penicillin or ampicillin
plus Gentamicin sulfate	3 mg/kg per 24 h IV/IM in 3 equally divided doses Pediatric dose: vancomycin 40 mg/kg per 24 h IV in 2 or 3 equally divided doses; gentamicin 3 mg/kg per 24 h IV/IM in 3 equally divided doses	6	6 wk of vancomycin therapy recommended because of decreased activity against enterococci

[a]Dosages recommended are for patients with normal renal function.
[b]Dosage of gentamicin should be adjusted to achieve peak serum concentration of 3 to 4 μg/mL and a trough concentration of less than 1μ/mL. Patients with a creatinine clearance of less than 50 mL/min should be treated in consultation with an infectious diseases specialist.
[c]Pediatric dose should not exceed that of a normal adult.
[d]See Table 85–7 for appropriate dosing of vancomycin.
SOURCE: Modified from Baddour LM, Wilson WR, Bayer AS, et al. Infective endocarditis: diagnosis, antimicrobial therapy, and management of complications: a statement for healthcare professionals from the Committee on Rheumatic Fever, Endocarditis, and Kawasaki Disease, Council on Cardiovascular Disease in the Young, and the Councils on Clinical Cardiology, Stroke, and Cardiovascular Surgery and Anesthesia, American Heart Association. Circulation 2005;111:e394–e434.) See full document for treatment regimens for resistant organisms.

particularly for lesions affecting the anterior mitral valve leaflet. In these studies, embolization risk increases significantly for vegetation size greater than 1.0 cm.[91,136] Because embolization risk appears to decrease precipitously following institution of appropriate antibiotic therapy,[111] prophylactic surgery to prevent embolization should be performed early in the course of the infection. Prior to undertaking such surgery, the members of an experienced surgical team should concur that the likelihood of successful repair is high. In many instances, repair constitutes vegetectomy and pericardial patch repair of the un-

derlying defect. Leaflet resection, placement of an annular ring, or both might be required, as dictated by the intraoperative findings.

In an attempt to clarify the benefit of surgery, Vikram et al. retrospectively analyzed 513 cases of complicated left-sided NVE from 7 Connecticut hospitals.[103] Complicated IE was defined by the presence of one of the following features for which valve surgery would be considered in current clinical practice: heart failure, new valvular regurgitation, refractory infection, systemic embolization to vital organs, or presence of a vegeta-

TABLE 85–11

Therapy for Endocarditis Caused by Staphylococci in the Absence of Prosthetic Materials

REGIMEN	DOSAGE[a] AND ROUTE	DURATION	COMMENTS
Oxacillin-susceptible strains			
Nafcillin or oxacillin[b]	12 g per 24 h IV in 4 to 6 equally divided doses	6 wk	For complicated right-sided IE and for left-sided IE; for uncomplicated right-sided IE, 2 wk
with			
Optional addition of gentamicin sulfate[c]	3 mg/kg per 24 h IV/IM in 2 or 3 equally divided doses Pediatric dose[d]: Nafcillin or oxacillin 200 mg/kg per 24 h IV in 4 to 6 equally divided doses; gentamicin 3 mg/kg per 24 h IV/IM in 3 equally divided doses	3–5 d	Clinical benefit of aminoglycosides has not been established
For penicillin-allergic (nonanaphylactoid type) patients:			Consider skin testing for oxacillin-susceptible staphylococci and questionable history of immediate-type hypersensitivity to penicillin
Cefazolin	6 g per 24 h IV in 3 equally divided doses	6 wk	Cephalosporins should be avoided in patients with anaphylactoid-type hypersensitivity to beta lactams; vancomycin should be used in these cases[d]
with			
Optional addition of gentamicin sulfate	3 mg/kg per 24 h IV/IM in 2 or 3 equally divided doses Pediatric dose: cefazolin 100 mg/kg per 24 h IV in 3 equally divided doses; gentamicin 3 mg/kg per 24 h IV/IM in 3 equally divided doses	3–5 d	Clinical benefit of aminoglycosides has not been established
Oxacillin-resistant strains			
Vancomycin[e]	30 mg/kg per 24 h IV in 2 equally divided doses Pediatric dose: 40 mg/kg per 24 h IV in 2 or 3 equally divided doses	6 wk	Adjust vancomycin dosage to achieve 1-h serum concentration of 30–45 µg/mL and trough concentration of 10–15 µg/mL

IE, infective endocarditis.

[a]Dosages recommended are for patients with normal renal function.

[b]Penicillin G 24 million U per 24 h IV in 4 to 6 equally divided doses may be used in place of nafcillin or oxacillin if strain is penicillin susceptible (minimum inhibitory concentration less than or equal to 0.1 µg/mL) and dose does not produce β-lactamase.

[c]Gentamicin should be administered in close temporal proximity to vancomycin, nafcillin, or oxacillin dosing.

[d]Pediatric dose should not exceed that of a normal adult.

[e]For specific dosing adjustment and issues concerning vancomycin, see Table 85–7 footnotes.

SOURCE: Modified from Baddour LM, Wilson WR, Bayer AS, et al. Infective endocarditis: diagnosis, antimicrobial therapy, and management of complications: a statement for healthcare professionals from the Committee on Rheumatic Fever, Endocarditis, and Kawasaki Disease, Council on Cardiovascular Disease in the Young, and the Councils on Clinical Cardiology, Stroke, and Cardiovascular Surgery and Anesthesia, American Heart Association. Circulation 2005;111:e394–e434.

tion on echocardiography. In this nonrandomized study, 45 percent of patients underwent valve surgery and 55 percent received medical therapy alone. In the unadjusted analysis, valve surgery was associated with a significant reduction in 6-month mortality (16 percent vs. 33 percent; p <0.001). In their propensity analysis, performed to account for confounding as a result of selection bias, surgical therapy remained significantly associated with a lower 6-month mortality (hazard ratio: 0.40; 95 percent confidence interval [CI]: 0.18 to 0.91; p = 0.03). The

association between valve surgery and reduced mortality was apparent *only* for those patients with moderate or severe heart failure (Fig. 85–9). These data corroborate the current ACC/AHA guidelines, which recommend heart failure as a class I indication for surgery.[79]

Indications for surgery in patients with PVE are similar. Heart failure, a poorly responsive microorganism, perivalvular extension, or an unstable prosthesis are class I indications for surgery. Prosthetic valve dehiscence is defined as a rocking mo-

TABLE 85–12

Therapy for Prosthetic Valve Endocarditis Caused by Staphylococci

REGIMEN	DOSAGE[a] AND ROUTE	DURATION (WK)	COMMENTS
Oxacillin-susceptible strains			
Nafcillin or oxacillin	12 g per 24 h IV in 6 equally divided doses	At least 6	Penicillin G 24 million U per 24 h IV in 4 to 6 equally divided doses may be used in place of nafcillin or oxacillin if strain is penicillin susceptible (minimum inhibitory concentration less than or equal to 0.1 µg/mL) and does not produce β-lactamase; vancomycin should be used in patients with immediate-type hypersensitivity reactions to β-lactam antibiotics (see Table 85–3 for dosing guidelines); cefazolin may be substituted for nafcillin or oxacillin in patients with nonimmediate-type hypersensitivity reactions to penicillins
plus Rifampin	900 mg per 24 h IV/PO in 3 equally divided doses	At least 6	
plus Gentamicin[b]	3 mg/kg per 24 h IV/IM in 2 or 3 equally divided doses	2	
	Pediatric dose[c]: nafcillin or oxacillin 200 mg/kg per h IV in 4 to 6 equally divided doses; rifampin 20 mg/kg per 24 h IV/PO in 3 equally divided doses; gentamicin 3 mg/kg per 24 h IV/IM in 3 equally divided doses		
Oxacillin-resistant strains			
Vancomycin	30 mg/kg per 24 h in 2 equally divided doses	At least 6	Adjust vancomycin to achieve 1-h serum concentration of 30–45 µg/mL and trough concentration of 10–15 µg/mL
plus Rifampin	900 mg/kg per 24 h IV/PO in 3 equally divided doses	At least 6	
plus Gentamicin	3 mg/kg per 24 h IV/IM in 2 or 3 equally divided doses	2	
	Pediatric dose: vancomycin 40 mg/kg per 24 h IV in 2 or 3 equally divided doses; rifampin 20 mg/kg per 24 h IV/PO in 3 equally divided doses (up to adult dose); gentamicin 3 mg/kg per 24 h IV or IM in 3 equally divided doses		

[a]Dosages recommended are for patients with normal renal function.
[b]Gentamicin should be administered in close proximity to vancomycin, nafcillin, or oxacillin dosing.
[c]Pediatric dose should not exceed that of a normal adult.
SOURCE: Modified from Baddour LM, Wilson WR, Bayer AS, et al. Infective endocarditis: diagnosis, antimicrobial therapy, and management of complications: a statement for healthcare professionals from the Committee on Rheumatic Fever, Endocarditis, and Kawasaki Disease, Council on Cardiovascular Disease in the Young, and the Councils on Clinical Cardiology, Stroke, and Cardiovascular Surgery and Anesthesia, American Heart Association. Circulation 2005;111:e394–e434.

TABLE 85–13

Therapy for Both Native and Prosthetic Valve Endocarditis Caused by HACEK[a] Microorganisms

REGIMEN	DOSAGE AND ROUTE	DURATION (WK)	COMMENTS
Ceftriaxone sodium	2 g per 24 h IV/IM in 1 dose[b]	4	Cefotaxime or another third- or fourth-generation cephalosporin may be substituted
or Ampicillin-sulbactam[c]	12 g per 24 h IV in 4 equally divided doses	4	
or Ciprofloxacin[c,d]	1000 mg per 24 h PO or 800 mg per 24h IV in 2 equally divided doses Pediatric dose[e]: ceftriaxone 100 mg/kg per 24 h IV/IM once daily; ampicillin-sulbactam 300 mg/kg per 24 h IV divided into 4 or 6 equally divided doses; ciprofloxacin 20–30 mg/kg per 24 h IV/PO in 2 equally divided doses	4	Fluoroquinolone therapy recommended only for patients unable to tolerate cephalosporin and ampicillin therapy; levofloxacin, gatifloxacin, or moxifloxacin may be substituted; fluoroquinolones generally not recommended for patients younger than 18 y old. Prosthetic valve: patients with endocarditis involving prosthetic cardiac valve or other prosthetic cardiac material should be treated for 6 wk

[a]*Haemophilus parainfluenzae, H aphrophilus, Actinobacillus actinomycetemcomitans, Cardiobacterium hominis, Eikenella corrodens,* and *Kingella kingae.*
[b]Patients should be informed that intramuscular injection of ceftriaxone is painful.
[c]Dosage recommended for patients with normal renal function.
[d]Fluoroquinolones are highly active in vitro against HACEK microorganisms. Published data on use of fluoroquinolone therapy for endocarditis caused by HACEK are minimal.
[e]Pediatric dose should not exceed that of a normal adult.
SOURCE: *Modified from Baddour LM, Wilson WR, Bayer AS, et al. Infective endocarditis: diagnosis, antimicrobial therapy, and management of complications: a statement for healthcare professionals from the Committee on Rheumatic Fever, Endocarditis, and Kawasaki Disease, Council on Cardiovascular Disease in the Young, and the Councils on Clinical Cardiology, Stroke, and Cardiovascular Surgery and Anesthesia, American Heart Association. Circulation 2005;111:e394–e434.*

TABLE 85–14

Therapy for Culture-Negative Endocarditis Including *Bartonella* Endocarditis

REGIMEN	DOSAGE[a] AND ROUTE	DURATION (WK)	COMMENTS
Native Valve Ampicillin-sulbactam	12 g per 24 h IV in 4 equally divided doses	4–6	Patients with culture-negative endocarditis should be treated in consultation with an infectious diseases specialist
plus Gentamicin sulfate[b]	3 mg/kg per 24 h IV/IM in 2 equally divided doses	4–6	
Vancomycin[c]	30 mg/kg per 24 h IV in 2 equally divided doses	4–6	Vancomycin recommended only for patients unable to tolerate penicillins
plus Gentamicin sulfate	3 mg/kg per 24 h IV/IM in 3 equally divided doses	4–6	
plus Ciprofloxacin	1000 mg per 24 h PO or 800 mg per 24 h IV in 2 equally divided doses Pediatric dose[d]: ampicillin-sulbactam 300 mg/kg per 24 h IV in 4 to 6 equally divided doses; gentamicin 3 mg/kg per 24 h IV/IM in 3 equally divided doses; vancomycin 40 mg/kg per 24 h in 2 or 3 equally divided doses; ciprofloxacin 20–30 mg/kg per 24 h IV/PO in 2 equally divided doses	4–6	

TABLE 85–14

Therapy for Culture-Negative Endocarditis Including *Bartonella* Endocarditis *(continued)*

REGIMEN	DOSAGE[a] AND ROUTE	DURATION (WK)	COMMENTS
Prosthetic valve (early— ≤ 1 y) Vancomycin *plus*	30 mg/kg per 24 h IV in 2 equally divided doses	6	
Gentamicin sulfate *plus*	3 mg/kg per 24 h IV/IM in 3 equally divided doses	2	
Cefepime *plus*	6 g per 24 h IV in 3 equally divided doses	6	
Rifampin	900 mg per 24 h PO/IV in 3 equally divided doses Pediatric dose: vancomycin 40 mg/kg per 24 h IV in 2 or 3 equally divided doses; gentamicin 3 mg/kg per 24 h IV/IM in 3 equally divided doses; cefepime 150 mg/kg per 24 h IV in 3 equally divided doses; rifampin 20 mg/kg per 24 h PO/IV in 3 equally divided doses	6	
Prosthetic valve (late—>1 y)		6	Same regimens as listed above for native valve endocarditis
Suspected *Bartonella*, culture negative Ceftriaxone sodium	2 g per 24 h IV/IM in 1 dose	6	Patients with *Bartonella* endocarditis should be treated in consultation with an infectious diseases specialist
plus Gentamicin sulfate	3 mg/kg per 24 h IV/IM in 3 equally divided doses	2	
with/without Doxycycline	200 mg/kg per 24 h IV/PO in 2 equally divided doses		
Documented *Bartonella* culture positive Doxycycline	200 mg per 24 h IV or PO in 2 equally divided doses	6	If gentamicin cannot be given, then replace with rifampin, 600 mg per 24 h PO/IV in 2 equally divided doses
plus Gentamicin sulfate	3 mg/kg per 24 h IV/IM in 3 equally divided doses Pediatric dose: ceftriaxone 100 mg/kg per 24 h IV/IM once daily; gentamicin 3 mg/kg per 24 h IV/IM in 3 equally divided doses; doxycycline 2–4 mg/kg per 24 h IV/PO in 2 equally divided doses; rifampin 20 mg/kg per 24 h PO/IV in 2 equally divided doses	2	

[a]Dosages recommended are for patients with normal renal function.
[b]See Table 85–7 for appropriate dosing of gentamicin.
[c]See Table 85–7 for appropriate dosing of vancomycin.
[d]Pediatric dose should not exceed that of a normal adult.

SOURCE: *Modified from Baddour LM, Wilson WR, Bayer AS, et al. Infective endocarditis: diagnosis, antimicrobial therapy, and management of complications: a statement for healthcare professionals from the Committee on Rheumatic Fever, Endocarditis, and Kawasaki Disease, Council on Cardiovascular Disease in the Young, and the Councils on Clinical Cardiology, Stroke, and Cardiovascular Surgery and Anesthesia, American Heart Association. Circulation 2005;111:e394–e434.*

TABLE 85–15

Indications for Surgery for Native Valve Endocarditis

Class I
1. Surgery of the native valve is indicated in patients with acute infective endocarditis who present with valve stenosis or regurgitation resulting in heart failure. (Level of Evidence: B)
2. Surgery of the native valve is indicated in patients with acute infective endocarditis who present with AR or MR with hemodynamic evidence of elevated LV end-diastolic or left atrial pressures (e.g., premature closure of MV with AR, rapid decelerating MR signal by continuous-wave Doppler [v-wave cutoff sign], or moderate to severe pulmonary hypertension). (Level of Evidence: B)
3. Surgery of the native valve is indicated in patients with infective endocarditis caused by fungal or other highly resistant organisms. (Level of Evidence: B)
4. Surgery of the native valve is indicated in patients with infective endocarditis complicated by heart block, annular or aortic abscess, or destructive penetrating lesions (e.g., sinus of Valsalva to right atrium, right ventricle, or left atrium fistula; mitral leaflet perforation with aortic valve endocarditis; or infection in annulus fibrosa). (Level of Evidence: B)

Class IIa
Surgery of the native valve is reasonable in patients with infective endocarditis who present with recurrent emboli and persistent vegetations despite appropriate antibiotic therapy. (Level of Evidence: C)

Class IIb
Surgery of the native valve may be considered in patients with infective endocarditis who present with mobile vegetations in excess of 10 mm with or without emboli. (Level of Evidence: C)

AR, aortic regurgitation; LV, left ventricular; MR, mitral regurgitaion; MV, mitral valve.
SOURCE: Bonow RO, Carabello BA, Chatterjee K, et al. ACC/AHA 2006 Guidelines for the Management of Patients with Valvular Heart Disease: A Report of the American College of Cardiology/American Heart Association Task Force on Practice Guidelines (Writing Committee to Develop Guidelines for the Management of Patients With Valvular Heart Disease). Available at American College of Cardiology website: http://www.acc.org/clinical/guidelines/valvular/index.pdf.

TABLE 85–16

Indications for Surgery for Prosthetic Valve Endocarditis

Class I
1. Consultation with a cardiac surgeon is indicated for patients with infective endocarditis of a prosthetic valve. (Level of Evidence: C)
2. Surgery is indicated for patients with infective endocarditis of a prosthetic valve who present with heart failure. (Level of Evidence: B)
3. Surgery is indicated for patients with infective endocarditis of a prosthetic valve who present with dehiscence evidence by cine fluoroscopy or echocardiography. (Level of Evidence: B)
4. Surgery is indicated for patients with infective endocarditis of a prosthetic valve who present with evidence of increasing obstruction or worsening regurgitation. (Level of Evidence: C)
5. Surgery is indicated for patients with infective endocarditis of a prosthetic valve who present with complications, for example, abscess formation. (Level of Evidence: C)

Class IIa
1. Surgery is reasonable for patients with infective endocarditis of a prosthetic valve who present with evidence of persistent bacteremia or recurrent emboli despite appropriate antibiotic treatment. (Level of Evidence: C)
2. Surgery is reasonable for patients with infective endocarditis of a prosthetic valve who present with relapsing infection. (Level of Evidence: C)

Class III
Routine surgery is not indicated for patients with uncomplicated infective endocarditis of a prosthetic valve caused by first infection with a sensitive organism. (Level of Evidence: C)

SOURCE: Bonow RO, Carabello BA, Chatterjee K, et al. ACC/AHA 2006 Guidelines for the Management of Patients with Valvular Heart Disease: A Report of the American College of Cardiology/American Heart Association Task Force on Practice Guidelines (Writing Committee to Develop Guidelines for the Management of Patients With Valvular Heart Disease). Available at American College of Cardiology website: http://www.acc.org/clinical/guidelines/valvular/index.pdf.

tion of the valve with excursion of 15 degrees or more in at least one plane. As noted, perivalvular abscess formation is more common with PVE than with NVE because the infection typically involves the interface between the sewing ring and surrounding tissue at inception (see Fig. 85–8).[124] Early surgery may be considered for selected patients with PVE without perivalvular extension or heart failure. For example, S. aureus PVE is rarely eradicated with antibiotics alone, and retrospective analyses suggest that combined medical and surgical therapy is more effective than medical therapy alone.[75] Relapse of PVE after appropriate antibiotic therapy should lead to a careful search for perivalvular extension or for metastatic foci of infection.[9]

Some patients with relapsed PVE may respond to a second course of antimicrobial therapy, but the majority will require surgery for cure. Despite the frequent need for surgery, medical cure with antibiotic therapy should be initially attempted for uncomplicated PVE caused by first infection with a sensitive organism (e.g., enterococci, streptococci).

The timing of surgery following CNS embolization in either native or prosthetic valve endocarditis is problematic because of the risk of hemorrhagic transformation. It is generally advisable to wait up to 5 to 7 days after bland CNS infarction, and as long as 4 weeks after primary CNS hemorrhage (e.g., from a ruptured mycotic aneurysm) before undertaking cardiac surgery. Prior to contemplating cardiac surgery for IE, mycotic an-

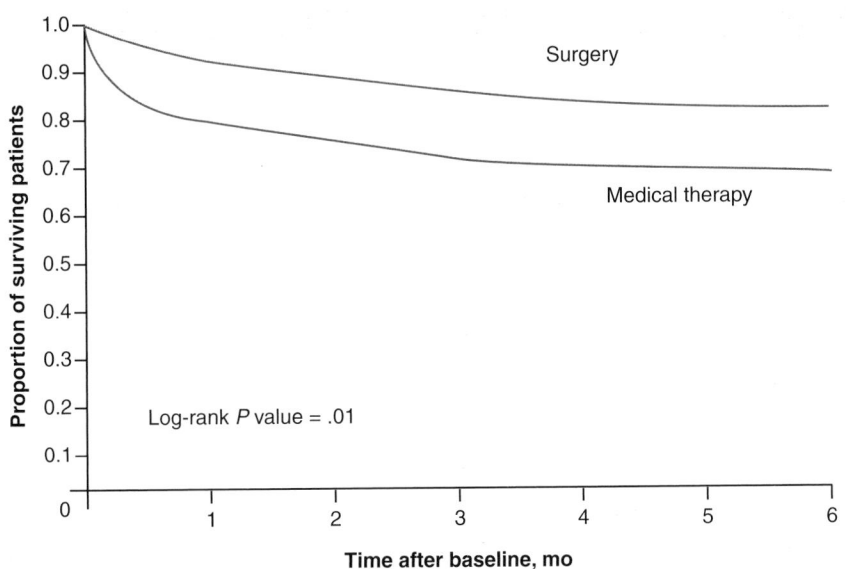

FIGURE 85–9. Survival curves for patients with complicated left-sided native valve endocarditis and moderate-to-severe heart failure managed with medical therapy alone or combined medical–surgical therapy. In this retrospective propensity analysis, there was a clear advantage with surgical therapy for this indication (hazard ratio: 0.22; 95 percent CI 0.08 to 0.53; p = 0.01). *Source: Adapted from Vikram HR, Buenconsejo J, Hasbun R, et al. Impact of valve surgery on 6-month mortality in adults with complicated, left-sided native valve endocarditis: a propensity analysis. JAMA 2003;290:24.*

eurysms require primary attention and exclusion with either percutaneous or surgical techniques.[135,137,138]

PROGNOSIS

Patients with IE are an extremely heterogeneous group with varying comorbidities, causative organisms, and complications. Accurate prognostic classification may help inform individual treatment decisions. Chu et al.[59] analyzed 267 consecutive cases of definite IE with an overall mortality of approximately 20 percent and found the following factors to be independently predictive of death: diabetes mellitus, S. aureus as a causative organism, an embolic event, and increased APACHE (Acute Physiology and Chronic Health Evaluation) II score. Data obtained from ICE has corroborated the finding that diabetes mellitus is independently associated with higher mortality in IE.[139] Hasbun et al.[1] derived and externally validated a prognostic classification system for adults presenting with complicated left-sided native valve IE. In both a derivation and validation cohort, the 6-month mortality rate was approximately 25 percent. Five baseline clinical features were significantly associated with 6-month mortality: increased Charlson comorbidity score, abnormal mental status, moderate to severe heart failure, causative organism other than S. viridans, and medical therapy without valve surgery. Using these prognostic features, the authors derived a weighted scoring system that classified patients into four groups with progressively increasing 6-month mortality risk, ranging from 5 to 59 percent. In a separate analysis, Fowler et al.[24] analyzed 300 cases of definite IE caused by S. aureus unrelated to injection drug use; these patients were enrolled in the International Collaboration on Endocarditis–Prospective Cohort Study and found the following factors to be independently associated with inhospital death: advanced age, stroke, and persistent bacteremia. Another study

of S. aureus NVE from the ICE-merged database found advanced age, heart failure, periannular abscess formation, and absence of surgical therapy to be associated with higher mortality.[140] Thuny et al. performed TEE in 384 consecutive patients with IE. Embolism occurred in 34.1 percent of patients before and 7.3 percent of patients after initiation of antibiotics. In addition to age, female gender, serum creatinine >2.0 mg/dL, moderate or severe heart failure, and infection with S. aureus, vegetation length >1.5 cm was an independent predictor of 1-year mortality. Total mortality at 1 year was 20.6 percent in this study.[117] Although the decision to undertake early surgery for the treatment of IE must be made on an individual basis, these data provide a useful means to target aggressive medical and surgical interventions to high-risk patient groups.[141]

PREVENTION OF IE

Antibiotic prophylaxis for IE remains challenging, as there is little evidence from well-designed human trials regarding its efficacy. Furthermore, as endocarditis is a rare complication of medical and dental procedures, it is extremely difficult to estimate the true risk of IE associated with these procedures. Recommendations for antibiotic prophylaxis for IE prevention have been developed are currently under revision.[78,79] The decision to provide antibiotic prophylaxis depends on two variables: patient-specific factors that predispose to IE (e.g., prosthetic valves) and the procedure-specific risk of IE.[78] It is agreed that certain groups of patients are at increased risk for the acquisition of IE (Table 85–17). Patients at high or moderate risk should generally receive antibiotic prophylaxis for procedures associated with a significant risk of bacteremia from oral, respiratory, gastrointestinal, or genitourinary sources. High-risk patients include those with any type of valve prosthesis (including bioprosthetic and homograft valves), patients with a prior history of IE, complex cyanotic congenital heart disease, and surgical pulmonary–systemic shunts (e.g., Fontan). Moderate risk patients include those with mitral valve prolapse with regurgitation and myxomatous leaflets, hypertrophic obstructive cardiomyopathy, significant acquired valvular heart disease (including rheumatic or degenerative disease of the mitral and aortic valves), and other congenital malformations (ventricular septal defect, patent ductus arteriosus, bicuspid aortic valve, aortic coarctation). Patients at negligible risk (i.e., risk no greater than the general population) include those with mitral valve prolapse without murmur or regurgitation or myxomatous/thickened leaflets, physiologic murmurs, isolated secundum atrial septal defect, 6 to 12 months after surgically repaired atrial septal defect/ventricular septal defect/patent ductus arteriosus, previous coronary artery bypass graft, cardiac pacemakers or intracardiac cardioverter-defibrillators, and history of rheumatic fever or Kawasaki disease without valvular dysfunction. Table 85–17 lists the procedures that necessitate antibiotic prophylaxis for IE in high- and moderate-risk patient subsets. These procedures generally cause trauma and bleeding in the oral/periodontal, respiratory, gastrointestinal, or genitourinary tissues. Procedures for which prophylaxis is not recommended are also listed. Importantly, endocar-

○ **TABLE 85–17**

Patients and Procedures for which Antibiotic Prophylaxis is Recommended

Patient-Specific Risk

High risk	All prosthetic heart valves (including bioprosthetic and homograft valves)
	History of prior bacterial endocarditis
	Complex cyanotic congenital heart disease
	Surgical pulmonary shunts
Moderate risk	Mitral valve prolapse with significant regurgitation, or leaflet thickening
	Hypertrophic cardiomyopathy
	Acquired valvular heart disease including stenosis, regurgitation and rheumatic
	Other congenital malformations (ostium primum ASD, VSD, PDA, bicuspid aortic valve, coarctation)
Low risk	Mitral valve prolapse without evidence of regurgitation or myxomatous leaflets
	Physiologic murmurs
	Isolated secundum ASD
	6 months after surgical repair of ASD/VSD/PDA
	Cardiac pacemakers or ICDs
	Previous CABG
	History of rheumatic fever or Kawasaki disease without evidence of valvular dysfunction

	PROPHYLAXIS[a] RECOMMENDED	PROPHYLAXIS[a] NOT RECOMMENDED	NOTES
Procedure-Specific Risk			
Dental	Extractions	Restorative dentistry	Antiseptic rinse prior to any procedure
	Periodontal procedures	Nonligamentary anesthesia	
	Initial placement of bands	Rubber dam placement	
	Intraligamentary local anesthesia	Suture removal	If unanticipated bleeding occurs, give antibiotics within 2 hours
	Dental implants	Shedding of primary teeth	
	Root canal	Endodontic therapy other than root canal	
Respiratory	Tonsillectomy/adenoidectomy	Endotracheal intubation	Antibiotics are optional for flexible bronchoscopy in high-risk patients
	Rigid bronchoscopy	Flexible bronchoscopy	
	Surgery involving respiratory mucosa	Tympanostomy tube insertion	
Gastrointestinal	Sclerotherapy for varices	Endoscopy (even with biopsy)	Antibiotics optional for endoscopy or TEE in high-risk patients
	Esophageal stricture dilation	TEE	
	Bile tract surgery or ERCP		
	Any surgery involving intestinal mucosa		
Genitourinary	Prostate surgery	Vaginal hysterectomy	Antibiotics are optional for vaginal procedures in high-risk patients
	Cystoscopy	Vaginal delivery	
	Urethral dilatation	Cesarean section	
		If uninfected: D&C, urethral catheterization, therapeutic abortion, IUD insertion and removal	
Cardiovascular		Cardiac catheterization including coronary angioplasty and stenting	
		Pacemaker and ICD placement	

ASD, atrial septal defect; CABC, coronary artery bypass graft; D & C, dilation and curettage; ERCP, endoscopic retrograde cholangiopancreatography; ICD, intracardiac cardioverter-defibrillator; IUD, intrauterine device; PDA, patent ductus arteriosus; TEE, transesophageal echocardiography; VSD, ventricular septal defect.

[a]Prophylaxis is recommended in high-and moderate-risk patients only.

SOURCE: Adapted from Dajani AS, Taubert KA, Wilson W, et al. Prevention of bacterial endocarditis: recommendations of the American Heart Association. Circulation 1997;96:358–66.

TABLE 85–18

Endocarditis Prophylaxis Regimens for Dental, Oral, Respiratory Tract, and Esophageal Procedures

SITUATION	AGENT	REGIMEN[a]
Standard general prophylaxis	Amoxicillin	*Adults:* 2.0 g; *children:* 50 mg/kg PO 1 h before procedure
Unable to take oral medication	Ampicillin	*Adults:* 2.0 g IM or IV; *children:* 50 mg/kg IM or IV within 30 min before procedure
Penicillin-allergic	Clindamycin or	*Adults:* 600 mg; *children:* 20 mg/kg PO 1 h before procedure
	Cephalexin or	*Adults:* 2.0 g; *children:* 50 mg/kg PO 1 h before procedure
	Cefadroxil or	*Adults:* 2.0 g; *children:* 50 mg/kg PO 1 h before procedure
	Azithromycin or	*Adults:* 500 mg; *children:* 15 mg/kg PO 1 h before procedure
	Clarithromycin	*Adults:* 500 mg; *children:* 15 mg/kg PO 1 h before procedure
Penicillin-allergic and unable to take oral medications	Clindamycin or	*Adults:* 600 mg; *children:* 20 mg/kg IV within 30 min before procedure
	Cefazolin[b]	*Adults:* 1.0 g; *children:* 25 mg/kg IM or IV within 30 min before procedure

[a]Total children's dose should not exceed adult dose.
[b]Cephalosporins should not be used in individuals with immediate-type hypersensitivity reaction (urticaria, angioedema, or anaphylaxis) to penicillins.
Source: Reprinted with permission from Dajani AS, Taubert KA, Wilson W, et al. Prevention of bacterial endocarditis: recommendations by the American Heart Association. Circulation 1997;96:358–66.

ditis prophylaxis is not recommended for cardiac catheterization, balloon angioplasty, vascular stenting, and pacemaker/intracardiac cardioverter-defibrillator placement. Tables 85–18 and 85–19 provide recommendations for procedure-specific antibiotic prophylaxis regimens. As expert committees continue to review emerging data, these recommendations will continue to evolve and it is anticipated that prophylactic therapy will be provided less often to lower-risk patients.

FUTURE DIRECTIONS

There are a number of developments in the field of IE that should improve preventative, diagnostic and therapeutic strategies. New molecular diagnostic methods, bacterial vaccines, antimicrobial agents (e.g., daptomycin for *S. aureus* IE[142]), and colonization-resistant biomaterials are under constant development. There is much interest in the disruption of microbial biofilm production as a means to prevent infection of intravascular devices. In addition, novel antimicrobial strategies targeted toward drug-resistant staphylococcal and en-

TABLE 85–19

Antibiotic Prophylaxis Regimens for Genitourinary or Gastrointestinal (Excluding Esophageal) Procedures

SITUATION	AGENT(S)[a]	REGIMEN[b]
High-risk patients	Ampicillin plus gentamicin	*Adults:* ampicillin 2.0 g IM/IV plus gentamicin 1.5 mg/kg (not to exceed 120 mg) within 30 min of starting the procedure. Six hours later, ampicillin 1 g IM/IV or amoxicillin 1 g PO. *Children:* ampicillin 50 mg/kg IM or IV (not to exceed 2.0 g) plus gentamicin 1.5 mg/kg within 30 min of starting the procedure. Six hours later, ampicillin 25 mg/kg IM/IV or amoxicillin 25 mg/kg PO.
High-risk patients allergic to ampicillin/amoxicillin	Vancomycin plus gentamicin	*Adults:* vancomycin 1.0 g IV over 1–2 h plus gentamicin 1.5 mg/kg IV/IM (not to exceed 120 mg). Complete injection/infusion within 30 min of starting the procedure. *Children:* vancomycin 20 mg/kg IV over 1–2 h plus gentamicin 1.5 mg/kg IV/IM. Complete the injection/infusion within 30 min of starting the procedure.
Moderate-risk patients	Amoxicillin or ampicillin	*Adults:* amoxicillin 2.0 g PO 1 h before procedure, or ampicillin 2.0 g IM/IV within 30 min of starting the procedure. *Children:* amoxicillin 50 mg/kg PO 1 h before procedure, or ampicillin 50 mg/kg IM/IV within 30 min of starting the procedure.
Moderate-risk patients allergic to ampicillin/amoxicillin	Vancomycin	*Adults:* vancomycin 1.0 g IV over 1–2 h. Complete infusion within 30 min of starting the procedure. *Children:* vancomycin 20 mg per kg IV over 1–2 h. Complete infusion within 30 min of starting the procedure.

[a]No second dose of vancomycin or gentamicin is recommended.
[b]Total children's dose should not exceed adult dose.
Source: Reprinted with permission from Dajani AS, Taubert KA, Wilson W, et al. Prevention of bacterial endocarditis: recommendations by the American Heart Association. Circulation 1997;96:358–66.

terococcal species are essential. Definitive studies of IE are extremely challenging because of the low incidence of disease at any one center and the heterogeneous characteristics of both the host and causative organisms. Most studies of IE have been small retrospective analyses or case series from a single center. To address some of these limitations, the International Collaboration on Endocarditis[143] was formed and is collecting prospective data from a large cohort of IE patients at multiple international centers.[24,62,139–141,144–148] Large, randomized clinical trials of IE management may become possible. Prospective data are needed to characterize further the role of surgery in the management of IE.

REFERENCES

1. Hasbun R, Vikram HR, Barakat LA, et al. Complicated left-sided native valve endocarditis in adults: risk classification for mortality. *JAMA* 2003;289:15.
2. Laennec R. *A Treatise on Mediate Auscultation, and on Diseases of the Lungs and Heart.* London: Cornil V, 1846.
3. Lancisi G. *De Subitaneis Mortibus.* Rome: 1709.
4. Levy DM. Centenary of William Osler's 1885 Gulstonian lectures and their place in the history of bacterial endocarditis. *JR Soc Med* 1985;78:12.
5. Osler W. Gulstonian lectures on malignant endocarditis. *Br Med J* 1885;i:467–579.
6. Jalal S, Khan KA, Alai MS, et al. Clinical spectrum of infective endocarditis: 15 years experience. *Indian Heart J* 1998;50:5.
7. Cabell CH, Jollis JG, Peterson GE, et al. Changing patient characteristics and the effect on mortality in endocarditis. *Arch Intern Med* 2002;162:1.
8. Hoen B, Alla F, Selton-Suty C, et al. Changing profile of infective endocarditis: results of a 1-year survey in France. *JAMA* 2002;288:1.
9. Mylonakis E, Calderwood SB. Infective endocarditis in adults. *N Engl J Med* 2001;345:18.
10. Hogevik H, Olaison L, Andersson R, et al. Epidemiologic aspects of infective endocarditis in an urban population. A 5-year prospective study. *Medicine (Baltimore)* 1995;74:6.
11. Watanakunakorn C, Burkert T. Infective endocarditis at a large community teaching hospital, 1980–1990. A review of 210 episodes. *Medicine (Baltimore)* 1993;72:2.
12. Berlin JA, Abrutyn E, Strom, BL, et al. Incidence of infective endocarditis in the Delaware Valley, 1988–1990. *Am J Cardiol* 1995;76:12.
13. Delahaye F, Goulet V, Lacassin F, et al. Characteristics of infective endocarditis in France in 1991. A 1-year survey. *Eur Heart J* 1995;16:3.
14. Tleyjeh IM, Steckelberg JM, Murad HS, et al. Temporal trends in infective endocarditis: a population-based study in Olmsted County, Minnesota. *JAMA* 2005;293:24.
15. Cabell C Jr, Fowler VG Jr, Engemann J. Endocarditis in the elderly: incidence, surgery, and survival in 16,921 patients over 12 years. *Circulation* 2002;106:19.
16. Moreillon P, Que YA. Infective endocarditis. *Lancet* 2004;363:9403.
17. Bashore TM, Cabell C, Fowler V Jr. Update on infective endocarditis. *Curr Probl Cardiol* 2006;31:4.
18. Dhawan VK. Infective endocarditis in elderly patients. *Curr Infect Dis Rep* 2003;5:4.
19. Werner GS, Schulz R, Fuchs JB, et al. Infective endocarditis in the elderly in the era of transesophageal echocardiography: clinical features and prognosis compared with younger patients. *Am J Med* 1996;100:1.
20. Fernandez-Guerrero ML, Herrero L, Bellver M, et al. Nosocomial enterococcal endocarditis: a serious hazard for hospitalized patients with enterococcal bacteraemia. *J Intern Med* 2002;252:6.
21. Netzer RO, Altwegg SC, Zollinger E, et al. Infective endocarditis: determinants of long term outcome. *Heart* 2002;88:1.
22. Netzer RO, Zollinger E, Seiler C, et al. Infective endocarditis: clinical spectrum, presentation and outcome. An analysis of 212 cases 1980–1995. *Heart* 2000;84:1.
23. Wallace SM, Walton BI, Kharbanda RK, et al. Mortality from infective endocarditis: clinical predictors of outcome. *Heart* 2002;88:1.
24. Fowler VG Jr, Miro JM, Hoen B, et al. *Staphylococcus aureus* endocarditis: a consequence of medical progress. *JAMA* 2005;293:24.
25. Miro JM, del Rio A, Mestres CA. Infective endocarditis in intravenous drug abusers and HIV-1 infected patients. *Infect Dis Clin North Am* 2002;16:2.
26. Fortun J, Navas E, Martinez-Beltran J, et al. Short-course therapy for right-side endocarditis due to *Staphylococcus aureus* in drug abusers: cloxacillin versus glycopeptides in combination with gentamicin. *Clin Infect Dis* 2001;33:1.
27. Heldman AW, Hartert TV, Ray SC, et al. Oral antibiotic treatment of right-sided staphylococcal endocarditis in injection drug users: prospective randomized comparison with parenteral therapy. *Am J Med* 1996;101:1.
28. Mathew J, Abreo G, Namburi K, et al. Results of surgical treatment for infective endocarditis in intravenous drug users. *Chest* 1995;108:1.
29. Manoff SB, Vlahov D, Herskowitz A, et al. Human immunodeficiency virus infection and infective endocarditis among injecting drug users. *Epidemiology* 1996;7:6.
30. Wilson LE, Thomas DL, Astemborski J, et al. Prospective study of infective endocarditis among injection drug users. *J Infect Dis* 2002;185:12.
31. Cicalini S, Forcina G, De Rosa FG. Infective endocarditis in patients with human immunodeficiency virus infection. *J Infect* 2001;42:4.
32. Resto-Ruiz S, Burgess A, Anderson BE. The role of the host immune response in pathogenesis of *Bartonella henselae*. *DNA Cell Biol* 2003;22:6.
33. Butterly DW, Schwab SJ. Dialysis access infections. *Curr Opin Nephrol Hypertens* 2000;9:6.
34. Sexton DJ. Vascular access infections in patients undergoing dialysis with special emphasis on the role and treatment of *Staphylococcus aureus*. *Infect Dis Clin North Am* 2001;15:3.
35. Umana E, Ahmed W, Alpert MA. Valvular and perivalvular abnormalities in end-stage renal disease. *Am J Med Sci* 2003;325:4.
36. Saad TF. Central venous dialysis catheters: catheter-associated infection. *Semin Dial* 2001;14:6.
37. Cabell CH, Heidenreich PA, Chu VH, et al. Increasing rates of cardiac device infections among Medicare beneficiaries: 1990–1999. *Am Heart J* 2004;147:4.
38. Chambers ST. Diagnosis and management of staphylococcal infections of pacemakers and cardiac defibrillators. *Intern Med J* 2005;35(Suppl 2):63–71.
39. Kutalek SP. Pacemaker and defibrillator lead extraction. *Curr Opin Cardiol* 2004;19:1.
40. Karchmer A. Infective endocarditis. In: Zipes D, Libby P, Bonow RO, et al., eds. *Heart Disease,* 7th ed. Philadelphia: Elsevier, 2005:1633–1656.
41. Rodbard S. Blood velocity and endocarditis. *Circulation* 1963;27:18–28.
42. Widmer E, Que YA, Entenza JM, et al. New concepts in the pathophysiology of infective endocarditis. *Curr Infect Dis Rep* 2006;8:4.
43. Moreillon P, Que YA, Bayer AS. Pathogenesis of streptococcal and staphylococcal endocarditis. *Infect Dis Clin North Am* 2002;16:2.
44. Drake TA, Pang M. *Staphylococcus aureus* induces tissue factor expression in cultured human cardiac valve endothelium. *J Infect Dis* 1988;157:4.
45. Cramton SE, Gerke C, Schnell NF, et al. The intercellular adhesion (ica) locus is present in *Staphylococcus aureus* and is required for biofilm formation. *Infect Immun* 1999;67:10.
46. Baddour LM, Wilson WR, Bayer AS, et al. Infective endocarditis: diagnosis, antimicrobial therapy, and management of complications: a statement for healthcare professionals from the committee on Rheumatic Fever, Endocarditis, and Kawasaki Disease, Council on Cardiovascular Disease in the Young, and the Councils on Clinical Cardiology, Stroke, and Cardiovascular Surgery and Anesthesia, American Heart Association—executive summary: endorsed by the Infectious Diseases Society of America. *Circulation* 2005;111:23.
47. Bayer AS, Bolger AF, Taubert KA, et al. Diagnosis and management of infective endocarditis and its complications. *Circulation* 1998;98:25.
48. Klein RS, Recco RA, Catalano MT, et al. Association of *Streptococcus bovis* with carcinoma of the colon. *N Engl J Med* 1977;297:15.
49. Sharaf MA, Shaikh N. Abiotrophia endocarditis: case report and review of the literature. *Can J Cardiol* 2005;21:14.
50. Falagas ME, Matthaiou DK, Bliziotis IA. The role of aminoglycosides in combination with a beta-lactam for the treatment of bacterial endocarditis: a meta-analysis of comparative trials. *J Antimicrob Chemother* 2006;57:4.
51. Lefort A, Mainardi JL, Selton-Suty C, et al. Streptococcus pneumoniae endocarditis in adults. A multicenter study in France in the era of penicillin resistance (1991–1998). The Pneumococcal Endocarditis Study Group. *Medicine (Baltimore)* 2000;79:5.
52. Crespo A, Retter AS, Lorber B. Group B streptococcal endocarditis in obstetric and gynecologic practice. *Infect Dis Obstet Gynecol* 2003;11:2.
53. Sambola A, Miro JM, Tornos MP, et al. *Streptococcus agalactiae* infective endocarditis: analysis of 30 cases and review of the literature, 1962–1998. *Clin Infect Dis* 2002;34:12.

54. Friedman ND, Kaye KS, Stout JE, et al. Health care-associated bloodstream infections in adults: a reason to change the accepted definition of community-acquired infections. *Ann Intern Med* 2002;137:10.

55. Wisplinghoff H, Bischoff T, Tallent SM, et al. Nosocomial bloodstream infections in U.S. hospitals: analysis of 24,179 cases from a prospective nationwide surveillance study. *Clin Infect Dis* 2004;39:3.

56. Fowler VG Jr, Olsen MK, Corey GR, et al. Clinical identifiers of complicated *Staphylococcus aureus* bacteremia. *Arch Intern Med* 2003;163:17.

57. Lesens O, Hansmann Y, Storck D, et al. Risk factors for metastatic infection in patients with *Staphylococcus aureus* bacteremia with and without endocarditis. *Eur J Intern Med* 2003;14:4.

58. Roder BL, Wandall DA, Espersen F, et al. A study of 47 bacteremic *Staphylococcus aureus* endocarditis cases: 23 with native valves treated surgically and 24 with prosthetic valves. *Scand Cardiovasc J* 1997;31:5.

59. Chu VH, Cabell CH, Benjamin DK Jr, et al. Early predictors of in-hospital death in infective endocarditis. *Circulation* 2004;109:14.

60. Rosen AB, Fowler VG Jr, Corey GR, et al. Cost-effectiveness of transesophageal echocardiography to determine the duration of therapy for intravascular catheter-associated *Staphylococcus aureus* bacteremia. *Ann Intern Med* 1999;130:10.

61. Ruef C. Epidemiology and clinical impact of glycopeptide resistance in *Staphylococcus aureus*. *Infection* 2004;32:6.

62. Chu VH, Cabell CH, Abrutyn E, et al. Native valve endocarditis due to coagulase-negative staphylococci: report of 99 episodes from the International Collaboration on Endocarditis Merged Database. *Clin Infect Dis* 2004;39:10.

63. Singh VR, Raad I. Fatal *Staphylococcus saprophyticus* native valve endocarditis in an intravenous drug addict. *J Infect Dis* 1990;162:3.

64. Lina B, Celard M, Vandenesch F, et al. Infective endocarditis due to *Staphylococcus capitis*. *Clin Infect Dis* 1992;15:1.

65. Anguera I, Del Rio A, Miro, JM, et al. *Staphylococcus lugdunensis* infective endocarditis: description of 10 cases and analysis of native valve, prosthetic valve, and pacemaker lead endocarditis clinical profiles. *Heart* 2005;91:2.

66. Brouqui P, Raoult D. Endocarditis due to rare and fastidious bacteria. *Clin Microbiol Rev* 2001;14:1.

67. Fernandez Guerrero ML, Aguado JM, Arribas A, et al. The spectrum of cardiovascular infections due to *Salmonella enterica*: a review of clinical features and factors determining outcome. *Medicine (Baltimore)* 2004;83:2.

68. Komshian SV, Tablan OC, Palutke W, et al. Characteristics of left-sided endocarditis due to *Pseudomonas aeruginosa* in the Detroit Medical Center. *Rev Infect Dis* 1990;12:4.

69. Peter O, Flepp M, Bestetti G, et al. Q fever endocarditis: diagnostic approaches and monitoring of therapeutic effects. *Clin Investig* 1992;70:10.

70. Maguina C, Gotuzzo E. Bartonellosis. New and old. *Infect Dis Clin North Am* 2000;14:1.

71. Solera J. Treatment of human brucellosis. *J Med Liban* 2000;48:4.

72. Werner M, Andersson R, Olaison L, et al. A clinical study of culture-negative endocarditis. *Medicine (Baltimore)* 2003;82:4.

73. Hoen B, Selton-Suty C, Lacassin F, et al. Infective endocarditis in patients with negative blood cultures: analysis of 88 cases from a one-year nationwide survey in France. *Clin Infect Dis* 1995;20:3.

74. Berbari EF, Cockerill FR 3rd, Steckelberg JM. Infective endocarditis due to unusual or fastidious microorganisms. *Mayo Clin Proc* 1997;72:6.

75. John MD, Hibberd PL, Karchmer AW, et al. *Staphylococcus aureus* prosthetic valve endocarditis: optimal management and risk factors for death. *Clin Infect Dis* 1998;26:6.

76. Karchmer A, Stinson E. The role of surgery in infective endocarditis. In: Remington J, Swartz M, eds. *Current Topics in Infectious Diseases.* New York: McGraw-Hill, 1998:124–157.

77. Li JS, Sexton DJ, Mick N, et al. Proposed modifications to the Duke criteria for the diagnosis of infective endocarditis. *Clin Infect Dis* 2000;30:4.

78. Dajani AS, Taubert KA, Wilson W, et al. Prevention of bacterial endocarditis: recommendations by the American Heart Association. *Clin Infect Dis* 1997;25:6.

79. Bonow RO, Carabello BA, Kanu C, et al. ACC/AHA 2006 guidelines for the management of patients with valvular heart disease: a report of the American College of Cardiology/American Heart Association Task Force on Practice Guidelines (writing committee to revise the 1998 Guidelines for the Management of Patients With Valvular Heart Disease): developed in collaboration with the Society of Cardiovascular Anesthesiologists: endorsed by the Society for Cardiovascular Angiography and Interventions and the Society of Thoracic Surgeons. *Circulation* 2006;114:5.

80. Pelletier LL Jr, Petersdorf RG. Infective endocarditis: a review of 125 cases from the University of Washington Hospitals, 1963–72. *Medicine (Baltimore)* 1977;56:4.

81. von Reyn CF. Infective endocarditis: an analysis based on strict case definitions. *Ann Intern Med* 1981;94:505–518.

82. Durack DT, Lukes AS, Bright DK. New criteria for diagnosis of infective endocarditis: utilization of specific echocardiographic findings. Duke Endocarditis Service. *Am J Med* 1994;96:3.

83. Olaison L, Hogevik H. Comparison of the von Reyn and Duke criteria for the diagnosis of infective endocarditis: a critical analysis of 161 episodes. *Scand J Infect Dis* 1996;28:4.

84. Cecchi E, Parrini I, Chinaglia A, et al. New diagnostic criteria for infective endocarditis. A study of sensitivity and specificity. *Eur Heart J* 1997;18:7.

85. Hoen B, Selton-Suty C, Danchin N, et al. Evaluation of the Duke criteria versus the Beth Israel criteria for the diagnosis of infective endocarditis. *Clin Infect Dis* 1995;21:4.

86. Fefer P, Raveh D, Rudensky B, et al. Changing epidemiology of infective endocarditis: a retrospective survey of 108 cases, 1990–1999. *Eur J Clin Microbiol Infect Dis* 2002;21:6.

87. Sachdev M, Peterson GE, Jollis JG. Imaging techniques for diagnosis of infective endocarditis. *Cardiol Clin* 2003;21:2.

88. Shively BK, Gurule FT, Roldan CA, et al. Diagnostic value of transesophageal compared with transthoracic echocardiography in infective endocarditis. *J Am Coll Cardiol* 1991;18:2.

89. Daniel WG, Mugge A, Grote J, et al. Comparison of transthoracic and transesophageal echocardiography for detection of abnormalities of prosthetic and bioprosthetic valves in the mitral and aortic positions. *Am J Cardiol* 1993;71:2.

90. Cheitlin MD, Armstrong WF, Aurigemma GP, et al. ACC/AHA/ASE 2003 guideline update for the clinical application of echocardiography: summary article. A report of the American College of Cardiology/American Heart Association Task Force on Practice Guidelines (ACC/AHA/ASE Committee to Update the 1997 Guidelines for the Clinical Application of Echocardiography). *J Am Soc Echocardiogr* 2003;16:10.

91. Mugge A, Daniel WG, Frank G, et al. Echocardiography in infective endocarditis: reassessment of prognostic implications of vegetation size determined by the transthoracic and the transesophageal approach. *J Am Coll Cardiol* 1989;14:3.

92. Jaffe WM, Morgan DE, Pearlman AS, et al. Infective endocarditis, 1983–1988: echocardiographic findings and factors influencing morbidity and mortality. *J Am Coll Cardiol* 1990;15:6.

93. Burger AJ, Peart B, Jabi H, et al. The role of two-dimensional echocardiology in the diagnosis of infective endocarditis [corrected]. *Angiology* 1991;42:7.

94. Pedersen WR, Walker M, Olson JD, et al. Value of transesophageal echocardiography as an adjunct to transthoracic echocardiography in evaluation of native and prosthetic valve endocarditis. *Chest* 1991;100:2.

95. Sochowski RA, Chan KL. Implication of negative results on a monoplane transesophageal echocardiographic study in patients with suspected infective endocarditis. *J Am Coll Cardiol* 1993;21:1.

96. Shapiro SM, Young E, De Guzman S, et al. Transesophageal echocardiography in diagnosis of infective endocarditis. *Chest* 1994;105:2.

97. Heidenreich PA, Masoudi FA, Maini B, et al. Echocardiography in patients with suspected endocarditis: a cost-effectiveness analysis. *Am J Med* 1999;107:3.

98. Kuruppu, JC, Corretti M, Mackowiak P, et al. Overuse of transthoracic echocardiography in the diagnosis of native valve endocarditis. *Arch Intern Med* 2002;162:15.

99. Greaves K, Mou D, Patel A, et al. Clinical criteria and the appropriate use of transthoracic echocardiography for the exclusion of infective endocarditis. *Heart* 2003;89:3.

100. Ryan EW, Bolger AF. Transesophageal echocardiography (TEE) in the evaluation of infective endocarditis. *Cardiol Clin* 2000;18:4.

101. Vieira ML, Grinberg M, Pomerantzeff PM, et al. Repeated echocardiographic examinations of patients with suspected infective endocarditis. *Heart* 2004;90:9.

102. Hollanders G, De Scheerder I, De Buyzere M, et al. A six years review on 53 cases of infective endocarditis: clinical, microbiological and therapeutical features. *Acta Cardiol* 1988;43:2.

103. Vikram HR, Buenconsejo J, Hasbun R, et al. Impact of valve surgery on 6-month mortality in adults with complicated, left-sided native valve endocarditis: a propensity analysis. *JAMA* 2003;290:24.

104. Stinson EB. Surgical treatment of infective endocarditis. *Prog Cardiovasc Dis* 1979;22:3.

105. Mills J, Utley J, Abbott J. Heart failure in infective endocarditis: predisposing factors, course, and treatment. *Chest* 1974;66:2.

106. Jones HR Jr, Siekert RG Neurological manifestations of infective endocarditis. Review of clinical and therapeutic challenges. *Brain* 1989;112(Pt 5):1295–1315.

107. Pruitt AA, Rubin RH, Karchmer AW, et al. Neurologic complications of bacterial endocarditis. *Medicine (Baltimore)* 1978;57:4.

108. Mathew J, Addai T, Anand A, et al. Clinical features, site of involvement, bacteriologic findings, and outcome of infective endocarditis in intravenous drug users. *Arch Intern Med* 1995;155:15.

109. Roberts WC, Buchbinder NA. Right-sided valvular infective endocarditis. A clinicopathologic study of twelve necropsy patients. *Am J Med* 1972;53:1.

110. De Castro S, Magni G, Beni S, et al. Role of transthoracic and transesophageal echocardiography in predicting embolic events in patients with active infective endocarditis involving native cardiac valves. *Am J Cardiol* 1997;80:8.

111. Steckelberg JM, Murphy JG, Ballard D, et al. Emboli in infective endocarditis: the prognostic value of echocardiography. *Ann Intern Med* 1991;114:8.

112. Vilacosta I, Graupner C, San Roman JA, et al. Risk of embolization after institution of antibiotic therapy for infective endocarditis. *J Am Coll Cardiol* 2002;39:9.

113. Anderson DJ, Goldstein LB, Wilkinson WE, et al. Stroke location, characterization, severity, and outcome in mitral vs aortic valve endocarditis. *Neurology* 2003;61:10.

114. Cabell CH, Pond KK, Peterson GE, et al. The risk of stroke and death in patients with aortic and mitral valve endocarditis. *Am Heart J* 2001;142:1.

115. Rohmann S, Erbel R, Gorge G, et al. Clinical relevance of vegetation localization by transoesophageal echocardiography in infective endocarditis. *Eur Heart J* 1992;13:4.

116. Di Salvo G, Habib G, Pergola V, et al. Echocardiography predicts embolic events in infective endocarditis. *J Am Coll Cardiol* 2001;37:4.

117. Thuny F, Di Salvo G, Belliard O, et al. Risk of embolism and death in infective endocarditis: prognostic value of echocardiography: a prospective multi-center study. *Circulation* 2005;112:1.

118. Rohmann S, Erbel R, Darius H, et al. Prediction of rapid versus prolonged healing of infective endocarditis by monitoring vegetation size. *J Am Soc Echocardiogr* 1991;4:5.

119. Kupferwasser LI, Hafner G, Mohr-Kahaly S, et al. The presence of infection-related antiphospholipid antibodies in infective endocarditis determines a major risk factor for embolic events. *J Am Coll Cardiol* 1999;33:5.

120. Wilson W, Lie J, Houser O, et al. The management of patients with mycotic aneurysm. *Curr Clin Top Infect Dis* 1981;2:151–183.

121. Bohmfalk GL, Story JL, Wissinger JP, et al. Bacterial intracranial aneurysm. *J Neurosurg* 1978;48:3.

122. Huston J 3rd, Nichols DA, Luetmer PH, et al. Blinded prospective evaluation of sensitivity of MR angiography to known intracranial aneurysms: importance of aneurysm size. *AJNR Am J Neuroradiol* 1994;15:9.

123. Chan YC, Morales JP, Taylor PR. The management of mycotic aortic aneurysms: is there a role for endoluminal treatment? *Acta Chir Belg* 2005;105:6.

124. Blumberg EA, Karalis DA, Chandrasekaran K, et al. Endocarditis-associated paravalvular abscesses. Do clinical parameters predict the presence of abscess? *Chest* 1995;107:4.

125. Karchmer A, Gibbons G. Infections of prosthetic heart valves and vascular grafts. In: Bisno A, Waldvogel F, eds. *Infections Associated with Indwelling Medical Devices*, 2nd ed. Washington DC: American Society for Microbiology, 1994:213–249.

126. Rohmann S, Seifert T, Erbel R, et al. Identification of abscess formation in native-valve infective endocarditis using transesophageal echocardiography: implications for surgical treatment. *Thorac Cardiovasc Surg* 1991;39:5.

127. Erbel R, Rohmann S, Drexler M, et al. Improved diagnostic value of echocardiography in patients with infective endocarditis by transoesophageal approach. A prospective study. *Eur Heart J* 1988;9:1.

128. Daniel WG, Mugge A, Martin RP, et al. Improvement in the diagnosis of abscesses associated with endocarditis by transesophageal echocardiography. *N Engl J Med* 1991;324:12.

129. Majumdar A, Chowdhary S, Ferreira MA, et al. Renal pathological findings in infective endocarditis. *Nephrol Dial Transplant* 2000;15:11.

130. Le T, Bayer AS. Combination antibiotic therapy for infective endocarditis. *Clin Infect Dis* 2003;36:5.

131. Andrews MM, von Reyn CF. Patient selection criteria and management guidelines for outpatient parenteral antibiotic therapy for native valve infective endocarditis. *Clin Infect Dis* 2001;33:2.

132. Chan KL, Dumesnil JG, Cujec B, et al. A randomized trial of aspirin on the risk of embolic events in patients with infective endocarditis. *J Am Coll Cardiol* 2003;42:5.

133. Tornos P, Almirante B, Mirabet S, et al. Infective endocarditis due to *Staphylococcus aureus*: deleterious effect of anticoagulant therapy. *Arch Intern Med* 1999;159:5.

134. Steckelberg JM. Does aspirin prevent emboli in infective endocarditis? *Curr Infect Dis Rep* 2004;6:4.

135. Gillinov AM, Shah RV, Curtis WE, et al. Valve replacement in patients with endocarditis and acute neurologic deficit. *Ann Thorac Surg* 1996;61:4.

136. Sanfilippo AJ, Picard MH, Newell JB, et al. Echocardiographic assessment of patients with infectious endocarditis: prediction of risk for complications. *J Am Coll Cardiol* 1991;18:5.

137. Eishi K, Kawazoe K, Kuriyama Y, et al. Surgical management of infective endocarditis associated with cerebral complications. Multi-center retrospective study in Japan. *J Thorac Cardiovasc Surg* 1995;110:6.

138. Parrino PE, Kron IL, Ross SD, et al. Does a focal neurologic deficit contraindicate operation in a patient with endocarditis? *Ann Thorac Surg* 1999;67:1.

139. Kourany WM, Miro JM, Moreno A, et al. Influence of diabetes mellitus on the clinical manifestations and prognosis of infective endocarditis: a report from the International Collaboration on Endocarditis Merged Database. *Scand J Infect Dis* 2006;38:8.

140. Miro JM, Anguera I, Cabell CH, et al. *Staphylococcus aureus* native valve infective endocarditis: report of 566 episodes from the International Collaboration on Endocarditis Merged Database. *Clin Infect Dis* 2005;41:4.

141. Cabell CH, Abrutyn E, Fowler VG Jr, et al. Use of surgery in patients with native valve infective endocarditis: results from the International Collaboration on Endocarditis Merged Database. *Am Heart J* 2005;150:5.

142. Fowler VG Jr, Boucher HW, Corey GR, et al. Daptomycin versus standard therapy for bacteremia and endocarditis caused by *Staphylococcus aureus*. *N Engl J Med* 2006;355:7.

143. Cabell CH, Abrutyn E. Progress toward a global understanding of infective endocarditis. Lessons from the International Collaboration on Endocarditis. *Cardiol Clin* 2003;21:2.

144. Benjamin DK Jr, Miro JM, Hoen B, et al. Candida endocarditis: contemporary cases from the International Collaboration of Infectious Endocarditis Merged Database (ICE-mD). *Scand J Infect Dis* 2004;36:6–7.

145. Chirouze C, Cabell CH, Fowler VG Jr, et al. Prognostic factors in 61 cases of *Staphylococcus aureus* prosthetic valve infective endocarditis from the International Collaboration on Endocarditis merged database. *Clin Infect Dis* 2004;38:9.

146. Lalani T, Kanafani ZA, Chu VH, et al. Prosthetic valve endocarditis due to coagulase-negative staphylococci: findings from the International Collaboration on Endocarditis Merged Database. *Eur J Clin Microbiol Infect Dis* 2006.

147. Wang A, Pappas P, Anstrom, KJ, et al. The use and effect of surgical therapy for prosthetic valve infective endocarditis: a propensity analysis of a multi-center, international cohort. *Am Heart J* 2005;150:5.

148. Anderson DJ, Olaison L, McDonald JR, et al. Enterococcal prosthetic valve infective endocarditis: report of 45 episodes from the International Collaboration on Endocarditis-merged database. *Eur J Clin Microbiol Infect Dis* 2005;24:10.

PART 14 Anesthesia, Surgery, and the Heart

CHAPTER (86)

Perioperative Evaluation and Management of Patients with Known or Suspected Cardiovascular Disease Who Undergo Noncardiac Surgery

Debabrata Mukherjee / Kim A. Eagle

Each year in the United States, approximately 27 million patients undergo noncardiac surgery.[1] Of these patients, approximately 50,000 suffer perioperative myocardial infarction, and more than half of the 40,000 perioperative deaths are caused by cardiac events.[2,3] As the population of the United States continues to age over the next several decades, both the total number and the percentage of patients who are older than 65 years of age will increase. These patients represent the largest group in whom surgeries are performed, a group in whom approximately a quarter of surgeries are associated with significant risk of cardiac morbidity and death, and a group at increased risk for the presence of cardiac disease. As such, the number of patients with significant perioperative risk undergoing noncardiac surgery can be expected to increase.

Most perioperative cardiac morbidity and deaths are related to myocardial ischemia, congestive heart failure, or arrhythmias. Therefore, preoperative evaluation and perioperative management to reduce morbidity and mortality rates emphasize the detection, characterization, and treatment of coronary artery disease, left ventricular systolic dysfunction, and significant arrhythmias. However, not all patients with underlying cardiac disease are at significantly increased perioperative risk of a morbid cardiac event. The broader purpose of preoperative evaluation is not to clear patients for surgery but to assess medical status and cardiac risks posed by the surgery planned, and recommend strategies to reduce risk. Evaluation must be tailored to the circumstances that have prompted the consultation and to the nature of the surgical illness. There are two specific goals of the preoperative evaluation: first, to identify patients who are at increased risk of an adverse perioperative cardiac event and, second, to identify patients with a poor long-term prognosis as a result of cardiovascular disease who come to medical attention only because of the problem requiring noncardiac surgery. In this sense, the preoperative evaluation represents an opportunity to identify and treat patients, thereby affecting long-term prognosis, even though their risk at the time of noncardiac surgery may not be prohibitive.

Preoperative evaluation can identify many patients who are at increased risk of an adverse cardiac event, and appropriate perioperative management can reduce that risk. The internist and cardiologist play a vital role in the evaluation and management of patients before, during, and after noncardiac surgery. This chapter reviews available data and recommendations for the preoperative evaluation and perioperative management of patients with known or suspected cardiovascular disease undergoing noncardiac surgery. The nature of preoperative evaluation and perioperative management should be individualized to the patient and the clinical scenario surrounding surgery. Patients presenting with an acute surgical emergency require only a rapid preoperative assessment, with subsequent management directed at preventing or minimizing cardiac morbidity and death. Among such patients, a more thorough evaluation can often be performed after surgery. In contrast, patients undergoing an elective procedure with no surgical urgency can undergo a more thorough preoperative evaluation. Among patients presenting for cardiac evaluation prior to "same-day" elective surgery, perioperative risk to the patient must be weighed against the impact of additional testing and cancellation or delay of the surgical procedure.

CLINICAL DETERMINANTS OF PERIOPERATIVE CARDIOVASCULAR RISK

The majority of patients who are at increased risk of adverse perioperative cardiac events can be identified using a simple bedside or office assessment. A careful history, physical examination, and review of the resting 12-lead electrocardiogram (ECG) are usually sufficient to allow stratification of most patients into low, intermediate, or high risk for an adverse perioperative cardiac event. A number of investigators have established readily accessible clinical markers that predict increased perioperative risk of myocardial infarction, congestive heart failure, or death.[4–12] Some investigators have used a quantitative scoring system to rank the importance of individual risk factors.[6,13,14] The advantage of such systems rests with the observation that some clinical features are stronger predictors of perioperative risk than are others. Current recommendations of the American College of Cardiology (ACC) and the American Heart Association (AHA)[15] designate risks factors as belonging to three groups: major, intermediate, and minor (Table 86–1). In the guidelines, greater weight is given to active than to quiescent disease, and the severity of disease is used to modify its importance.

[ ] HISTORY

Historical features are important in the identification of patients at increased perioperative cardiac risk. Because most perioperative morbidity and deaths are related to myocardial ischemia, congestive heart failure, and arrhythmias, the assessment of historical risk factors relies heavily on the recognition of coronary artery disease, left ventricular dysfunction, and significant arrhythmias. Risk factors recognized as predictive of increased perioperative risk[15] include advanced age, poor functional capacity, and prior history of coronary artery disease, congestive heart failure, arrhythmia, valvular heart disease, diabetes mellitus, uncontrolled systemic hypertension, renal insufficiency, and stroke. Coronary artery disease is a major risk factor in the setting of recent myocardial infarction or unstable or severe angina pectoris

TABLE 86–1

Clinical Predictors of Increased Perioperative Cardiovascular Risk

Major predictors
  Acute or recent myocardial infarction[a] with evidence of ischemia based on symptoms or noninvasive testing
  Unstable or severe[b] angina (Canadian class III or IV)
  Decompensated heart failure
  High-grade atrioventricular block
  Symptomatic ventricular arrhythmias with underlying heart disease
  Supraventricular arrhythmias with uncontrolled ventricular rate
  Severe valvular heart disease
Intermediate predictors
  Mild angina pectoris (class 1 or 2)
  Prior myocardial infarction by history or Q waves on ECG
  Compensated or prior heart failure
  Diabetes mellitus (particularly insulin-dependent)
  Renal insufficiency (creatinine ≥2.0 mg/dL)
Minor predictors
  Advanced age
  Abnormal ECG (left ventricular hypertrophy, left bundle-branch block, ST-T abnormalities)
  Rhythm other than sinus (e.g., atrial fibrillation)
  Low functional capacity (inability to climb one flight of stairs with a bag of groceries)
  History of stroke
  Uncontrolled systemic hypertension

[a]Recent myocardial infarction is defined as greater than 7 days but less than or equal to 1 month; acute myocardial infarction is within 7 days.
[b]May include stable angina in patients who are usually sedentary.
SOURCE: Adapted from Eagle KA, Berger PB, Calkins H, et al. ACC/AHA guideline update for perioperative cardiovascular evaluation for noncardiac surgery—executive summary: a report of the American College of Cardiology/American Heart Association Task Force on Practice Guidelines.[15] Reprinted with permission.

and an intermediate risk factor in the setting of mild stable angina pectoris or remote myocardial infarction. Similarly, congestive heart failure is a major risk factor if decompensated and an intermediate risk factor if compensated. A history of arrhythmias may be a major, intermediate, or minor risk factor, depending on the nature and severity of the arrhythmia, as well as the presence of underlying heart disease.

A patient's preoperative functional capacity significantly influences the assessment of perioperative cardiac risk. Good functional capacity in an asymptomatic patient predicts low perioperative risk despite the presence of other risk factors. Impaired functional capacity is important in three regards in the assessment of perioperative cardiac risk. First, among patients with chronic coronary artery disease and among those who have experienced an acute cardiac event, poor functional capacity is associated with an increased risk of subsequent cardiac morbidity and death independent of surgery. Second, many of the historical features that predict increased perioperative risk assume physical activity. Because most symptoms of cardiac disease are either associated exclusively with or exacerbated by increased physical activity, significant noncardiac limitations in physical capacity are associated with inherent problems in the ability to detect symptoms of underlying cardiac diseases and thereby to diagnose them. Finally, poor functional capacity is associated with impaired conditioning and therefore a lesser ability to accommodate the cardiovascular stresses that may accompany noncardiac surgery. Because the ability to perform tasks in daily activities correlates well with maximal oxygen uptake on treadmill testing, the assessment of functional capacity on preoperative history is an important feature in the assessment of perioperative risk.

PHYSICAL EXAMINATION

Features on physical examination may be useful in assessing perioperative risk. Patients with uncontrolled systemic hypertension should be identified and treated. Because congestive heart failure[6,15] and valvular heart disease[6,15,16] are associated with increased risk, physical findings suggestive of these diagnoses should be sought. The physical examination should include general appearance (cyanosis, pallor, dyspnea during conversation/minimal activity, Cheyne-Stokes respiration, poor nutritional status, obesity, skeletal deformities, tremor, and anxiety), blood pressure in both arms, and carotid pulses and extremity pulses. In selected patients, ankle-brachial indices may be used to determine the severity of peripheral arterial disease. Jugular venous pressure and positive hepatojugular reflux are reliable signs of hypervolemia in chronic heart failure; pulmonary rales and chest radiography evidence of pulmonary congestion correlate better with acute heart failure. Patients with aortic stenosis can be identified by a typical murmur with diminished and delayed upstroke of the carotid or brachial pulse. Patients with mitral stenosis, mitral regurgitation, or aortic regurgitation may be at increased perioperative risk of developing congestive heart failure in the setting of sufficiently severe disease and are at increased risk of infective endocarditis. Finally, the presence of carotid or other vascular bruits may help identify patients at increased risk of occult coronary artery disease.

COMORBID DISEASES

A patient's overall health affects perioperative cardiovascular risk; associated medical conditions may exacerbate risk or complicate perioperative cardiac management. Patients with diabetes mellitus have an increased risk of concomitant coronary artery disease, and the possibility of silent ischemia complicates both the preoperative recognition of coronary artery disease and the perioperative recognition of ischemia. Patients with either restrictive or obstructive pulmonary disease are at increased risk of perioperative respiratory complications, and the associated hypoxemia, acidosis, and increased work of breathing can exacerbate cardiac stress and precipitate myocardial ischemia. Patients with preexisting renal dysfunction may be predisposed to volume retention in the perioperative period, and hypovolemia may lead to renal hypoperfusion, which can exacerbate renal dysfunction. Patients with anemia of any cause are at increased risk of myocardial ischemia and congestive heart failure, mediated by increased cardiac stress and increased cardiac work. Optimal management of noncardiac conditions may therefore reduce the risk of cardiac morbidity in the perioperative period.

SURGERY-SPECIFIC RISKS

Perioperative cardiac risk is related in two ways to the type of noncardiac surgery being performed. First, some types of noncardiac surgery identify a group of patients at increased risk for concomitant cardiac disease based on shared risk factors that predispose patients to both noncardiac and cardiac disease. The most notable example of this relationship is seen with vascular surgery and coronary artery disease. In this case, the same factors that result in clinical peripheral arterial occlusive disease also predispose to the development of coronary artery disease. Among such patients, coronary artery disease may be known or occult, with no symptoms because of the physical limitations associated with significant peripheral vascular disease. Second, the nature of noncardiac surgery may be associated with variable degrees of cardiac stress, mediated by fluctuations in heart rate, blood pressure, intravascular volume, and oxygenation, as well as the cardiac stresses associated with the duration of the procedure, pain, and neurohumoral activation.[4,5,17] Emergency procedures are associated with a two- to fivefold increase in perioperative cardiac risk compared with elective procedures.[3,16] Other types of noncardiac surgery associated with high perioperative risk include aortic and peripheral vascular surgery and prolonged abdominal, thoracic, or head and neck procedures with large fluid shifts. The ACC/AHA *Task Force Report on Perioperative Cardiovascular Evaluation*[15] stratifies noncardiac surgical procedures as involving high, intermediate, and low cardiac risk (Table 86-2).

TABLE 86-2

Cardiac Risk Stratification for Different Types of Surgical Procedures

High risk (reported cardiac risk[a] >5 percent)
  Emergency major operations, particularly in the elderly
  Aortic, major vascular, and peripheral vascular surgery
  Extensive operations with large volume shifts and/or blood loss
Intermediate risk (reported cardiac risk <5 percent)
  Intraperitoneal and intrathoracic
  Carotid endarterectomy
  Head and neck surgery
  Orthopedic
  Prostate
Low risk[b] (reported cardiac risk <1 percent)
  Endoscopic procedures
  Superficial biopsy
  Cataract
  Breast surgery

[a]Combined incidence of cardiac death and nonfatal myocardial infarction.
[b]Does not generally require further preoperative cardiac testing.
SOURCE: Adapted from Eagle KA, Berger PB, Calkins H, et al. ACC/AHA guideline update for perioperative cardiovascular evaluation for noncardiac surgery—executive summary: a report of the American College of Cardiology/American Heart Association Task Force on Practice Guidelines.[15] Reprinted with permission.

The perioperative administration of anesthesia may also affect perioperative cardiac risk. Although there is no one best myocardial protective anesthetic technique,[18,19] differences in anesthetic techniques may favor the use of one over another for individual patients. Opioid-based general anesthesia generally does not affect cardiovascular function,[20] although the commonly employed inhalational agents cause afterload reduction and decreased myocardial contractility. Spinal anesthesia results in sympathetic blockade, with decreases in both preload and afterload and the potential for shifts in both systemic blood pressure and intravascular volume.[21] In general, hemodynamic effects are minimal when spinal anesthesia is used for infrainguinal procedures, whereas higher dermatomal levels of spinal anesthesia, as required for abdominal procedures, may be associated with significant hemodynamic effects, including hypotension and reflex tachycardia. No study has clearly demonstrated any beneficial change in outcome from the use of pulmonary artery catheters, ST-segment monitoring, or transesophageal echocardiography. Decisions regarding specific anesthetic technique and intraoperative monitoring are best left to the anesthesiologists involved in the patient's care (see Chap. 87).

PREOPERATIVE TESTING

Patients at very low risk and patients at high risk of an adverse perioperative cardiac event can typically be identified using clinically available features described above. Patients at low risk generally require no additional testing prior to noncardiac surgery. Among patients undergoing elective noncardiac surgery in whom risk is determined to be intermediate or high, additional testing may be useful to better define risk.[15] It is well to employ a stepwise approach to the preoperative assessment of cardiac risk (Fig. 86–1). Testing usually includes noninvasive testing and, albeit rarely, coronary angiography to assess for the presence and significance of coronary artery disease, left ventricular function, and/or valvular heart disease.

[ ] RESTING LEFT VENTRICULAR FUNCTION

Impaired left ventricular systolic or diastolic function is predictive of perioperative congestive heart failure. The greatest risk of complications occurs among patients with left ventricular ejection fraction of less than 35 percent; among critically ill patients, severely impaired left ventricular systolic function is associated with a higher risk of death. Preoperative left ventricular systolic function can be assessed noninvasively using radionuclide ventriculography or echocardiography, or it may be assessed invasively using contrast ventriculography. Unless recently defined, preoperative assessment of left ventricular systolic function should be performed among patients with poorly controlled congestive heart failure and should be considered among patients with prior congestive heart failure and among patients with dyspnea of unknown cause.

[ ] FUNCTIONAL TESTING AND RISK OF CORONARY ARTERY DISEASE

Exercise Testing

Preoperative cardiac stress testing is useful in the objective assessment of functional capacity, to help identify patients who are at risk of perioperative myocardial ischemia or cardiac arrhythmias, and to aid in the assessment of both long-term and perioperative prognosis. In general, poor functional capacity may be a result of advanced age, deconditioning, myocardial ischemia or other causes of reduced cardiac reserve, or poor pulmonary reserve. Reduced functional capacity identifies patients who are at increased risk of subsequent cardiac morbidity and death.[22] The clinical history can be effectively used to estimate functional capacity. In addition, preoperative exercise testing is a useful tool to objectively assess functional capacity, as well as to assess hemodynamic response to stress and the potential for stress-induced myocardial ischemia or cardiac arrhythmias.

In a general population, the mean sensitivity and specificity of exercise electrocardiographic studies for the detection of coronary artery disease are 68 and 77 percent, respectively, with reported ranges of sensitivity from 23 to 100 percent and specificity from 17 to 100 percent.[23] The accuracy of exercise electrocardiographic studies for the detection of coronary artery disease is influenced by the prevalence of disease in the population studied, the degree of exercise achieved, and the number, location, and severity of diseased vessels. The mean sensitivity and specificity for the detection of multivessel disease is 81 and 66 percent, respectively.[24] In addition to assessment for the presence of coronary artery disease, exercise testing is useful for the assessment of prognosis. In a large cohort of 4083 medically treated patients in the Coronary Artery Surgery Study (CASS),[25] exercise testing was useful for identifying both high- and low-risk subgroups of patients. The mortality rate was 5 percent per year or greater among a high-risk subset comprising 12 percent of the total population who were unable to achieve an exercise workload greater than Bruce stage I and who had an abnormal exercise electrocardiogram. In contrast, mortality was less than 1 percent per year among a low-risk subset comprising 34 percent of the total population who were able to achieve at least Bruce stage III with a normal exercise electrocardiogram. Preoperative exercise testing is useful in the prediction of perioperative cardiac risk among patients who are undergoing peripheral vascular surgery, abdominal aortic aneurysm repair, or other major noncardiac surgery.[26,27] In these published reports, the negative predictive value for perioperative death or myocardial infarction was 91 to 100 percent, with a positive predictive value of 0 to 81 percent.

Nonexercise Stress Testing

Many patients who are undergoing noncardiac surgery are unable to exercise. Approximately 30 to 50 percent of patients who are undergoing noncardiac surgery are unable to achieve an adequate exercise workload for a diagnostic study. This is especially problematic among patients with peripheral vascular occlusive disease, in whom the same factors that cause peripheral disease predispose to coronary atherosclerosis; significant peripheral vascular disease severely limits exercise tolerance and therefore the ability to perform diagnostic exercise stress testing. For this reason, pharmacologic stress testing may offer advantages in the preoperative testing of some patients undergoing peripheral vascular surgery as well as of other patients who are not able to perform adequate physical exercise because of noncardiac limitations.

Pharmacologic stress testing for the detection of coronary artery disease can be performed using one of several methods. Infusion of

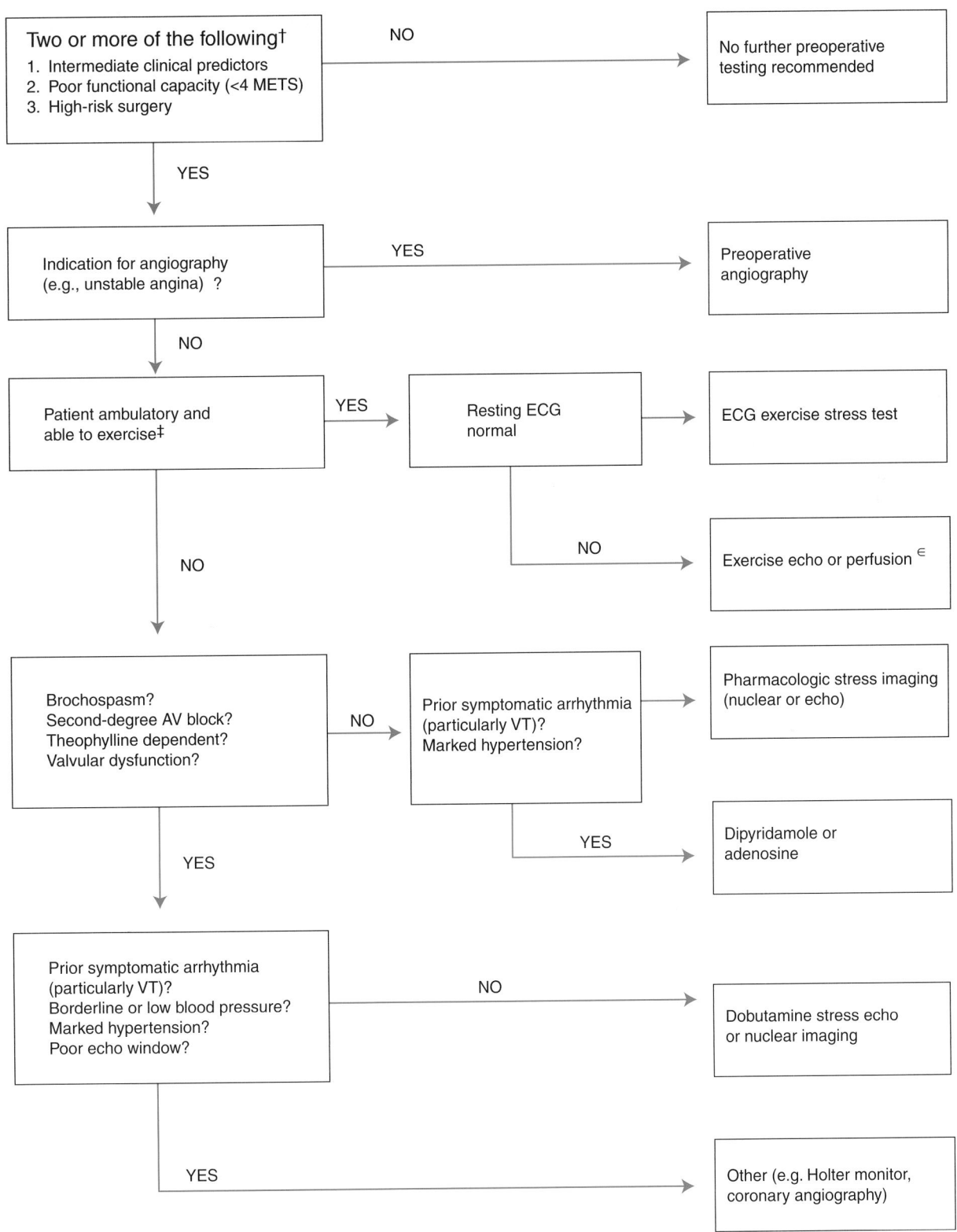

FIGURE 86–1. Supplemental preoperative evaluation: when and which test? †Testing is indicated only if the results will affect care. Refer to Table 86–1 for a list of clinical predictors and to Table 86–2 for the definition of high-risk surgical procedures. ‡Able to achieve greater than or equal to 85 percent maximum predicted heart rate (MPHR). ∈In the presence of left bundle-branch block, vasodilator perfusion imaging is preferred. AV, atrioventricular; ECG, electrocardiogram; METS, metabolic equivalents; VT, ventricular tachycardia. *Source: Adapted from Eagle KA, Berger PB, Calkins H, et al.[15] Reprinted, with permission.*

the adrenergic agonist dobutamine leads to increases in heart rate, myocardial contractility, and, to a lesser degree, blood pressure, resulting in increased myocardial oxygen demand. In the setting of a limited oxygen supply, increased demand causes myocardial ischemia. Dobutamine infusion is typically used in conjunction with echocardiographic imaging, and the failure of wall motion to augment with dobutamine or for it to become frankly dyskinetic indicates of ischemia. Alternatively, pharmacologic "stress" can be achieved using the coronary vasodilators dipyridamole or adenosine. Nuclear perfusion imaging, such as thallium scintigraphic imaging, is typically used in conjunction with dipyridamole and adenosine. Coronary artery disease is detected as heterogeneity of perfusion in response to maximal coronary vasodilation. Stress imaging using rapid multislice CT or MRI is likely to be used more often in the coming years.

Dipyridamole-thallium scintigraphy has been extensively studied for the assessment of coronary artery disease and perioperative risk among patients undergoing vascular,[5,28,29] and other noncardiac surgery.[30–32] Published reports found a uniformly high negative predictive value for perioperative morbidity associated with normal dipyridamole-thallium scintigraphic results, with values ranging from 95 to 100 percent and an average value of approximately 99 percent. The positive predictive value of dipyridamole-thallium redistribution for myocardial infarction or death from cardiac causes has been reported to be from 4 to 20 percent among studies including more than 100 patients. There is also an important long-term prognostic value associated with preoperative nuclear perfusion imaging,[33,34] suggesting that late postoperative risk after uncomplicated noncardiac surgery can also be predicted by preoperative testing. Although any abnormality on dipyridamole-thallium scintigraphy is suggestive of coronary artery disease and is associated with a higher perioperative cardiac risk compared with patients with a normal scan, perioperative cardiac risk associated with a fixed perfusion defect is substantially lower than that associated with perfusion redistribution. In addition, the size of a perfusion defect is directly related to perioperative cardiac risk.[35]

Dobutamine stress echocardiography is well established for the noninvasive detection and characterization of coronary artery disease,[36–38] with an overall predictive accuracy equivalent to that of dipyridamole-thallium scintigraphy. Several studies have evaluated the usefulness of dobutamine stress echocardiography for preoperative assessment of patients who are undergoing vascular or other noncardiac surgery.[39–41] Negative predictive values for perioperative events ranged from 93 to 100 percent. Positive predictive values were 17 to 43 percent for any cardiac event and 7 to 23 percent for predicting myocardial infarction or death. As was seen with studies using nuclear perfusion imaging, most studies of dobutamine stress echocardiography did not blind treating physicians to stress test results, and subsequent alteration of patient management based on abnormal noninvasive test results presumably contributed to a low event rate despite a positive test result. A meta-analysis of preoperative pharmacologic stress tests[42] demonstrated that dobutamine stress echocardiography and dipyridamole thallium scintigraphy are of similar power as regards predicting adverse cardiac events after noncardiac surgery.

Because clinical factors are usually able to identify patients who are at low or high risk of an adverse cardiac event after noncardiac surgery,[15,17] preoperative stress testing typically has the greatest usefulness among patients at intermediate risk. Exercise electrocardiographic study allows assessment of functional capacity, as well as evaluation for

evidence of coronary artery disease based on ST-segment analysis and hemodynamics. Performance of exercise echocardiographic testing or exercise nuclear perfusion imaging should be considered in the presence of significant resting ECG abnormalities that preclude diagnostic testing for coronary artery disease, such as left bundle-branch block, left ventricular hypertrophy with strain, or digitalis effect. Nonexercise stress testing, such as dobutamine stress echocardiographic or dipyridamole-thallium scintigraphic studies, should be considered among patients who are unable to perform adequate physical exercise.

Financial Implications of Noninvasive Testing

The performance of preoperative noninvasive testing should be based on an assessment of risk and benefit to the patient. In this setting, benefit is defined as the likelihood that testing may alter management and improve outcome because of an adverse perioperative or long-term prognosis. Risk to the patient should include risk associated with additional procedures precipitated by noninvasive testing, as well as any risk associated with the noninvasive testing. With the high costs associated with many evaluation strategies, development and implementation of evidence-based guidelines may lead to more efficient and cost-effective use of appropriate noninvasive testing (see Chap. 11).

As noted above, clinical features can be used to identify patients who are at very low risk of an adverse perioperative cardiac event, including asymptomatic patients who have undergone coronary revascularization within 5 years and patients without specific clinical markers for increased risk. Additional testing of selected patients at intermediate or higher risk can potentially reduce the cost of testing without affecting patients' outcomes. Based on a previous study validating the use of selective noninvasive testing before major aortic surgery,[43] the cost implications of selective testing were assessed in the ACC/AHA Task Force report.[15] In the earlier study, the application of a clinical algorithm resulted in only 29 percent of 201 patients undergoing noninvasive testing prior to aortic surgery, with an associated 0.5 percent perioperative cardiac mortality rate. Using estimated costs, the use of selected testing was associated with a total cost of $32,886 for 58 patients, compared with an estimated total cost of $113,967 if all 201 had undergone noninvasive screening. Froehlich et al. and Almanseer et al. demonstrated that implementation of the ACC/AHA cardiac risk-assessment guidelines appropriately reduced resource use and costs in patients who underwent elective aortic surgery without affecting outcomes.[44,45] Preoperative stress testing (88 to 47 percent; $p < 0.00001$), cardiac catheterization (24 to 11 percent; $p < 0.05$), and coronary revascularization (25 to 2 percent; $p < 0.00001$) were all significantly reduced with appropriate use of the ACC/AHA guidelines.[44,45] The low perioperative mortality rate associated with the use of a clinical algorithm and selected noninvasive testing suggest that substantial cost can be avoided without compromising patients' safety.

PREOPERATIVE THERAPY FOR CORONARY ARTERY DISEASE

Coronary artery disease is responsible for the majority of adverse perioperative cardiac events. Once disease is recognized, specific therapy should be instituted to minimize the risk of perioperative myocardial ischemia, myocardial infarction, or death.

CORONARY REVASCULARIZATION

There is limited information regarding the impact of either preoperative coronary artery bypass grafting or percutaneous coronary intervention on perioperative cardiac morbidity and mortality rates. Several retrospective studies suggest that patients with successful prior coronary revascularization have a low risk of perioperative cardiac events during noncardiac surgery and that the risk of death is comparable to that among patients with no clinical evidence of coronary artery disease.[11,46–48]

Although these studies support the theory that coronary artery revascularization lowers the risk of adverse cardiac events associated with noncardiac surgery, they do not address the overall effect on morbidity and mortality rates associated with the surgical coronary revascularization. In the assessment of patients undergoing noncardiac surgery, the well-established long-term benefits of coronary artery bypass surgery or percutaneous coronary intervention should be considered, as should any impact on noncardiac surgical morbidity and mortality rates. There may be an occasional patient for whom coronary artery bypass grafting should be performed prior to noncardiac surgery only because of an otherwise prohibitive perioperative cardiac risk. However, there are many more patients with advanced coronary artery disease who are candidates for surgical coronary revascularization, based on long-term prognosis, who are identified only during preoperative cardiac assessment. Among such patients, elective noncardiac surgery of intermediate or high risk should generally be postponed for the performance of coronary artery bypass surgery.

Several small, retrospective studies[46,48,50] suggest that there is a low risk of perioperative myocardial infarction or death following preoperative percutaneous coronary intervention. One study of 1049 noncardiac surgeries performed among 1829 patients enrolled in the Bypass Angioplasty Revascularization Investigation (BARI) trial demonstrated a low incidence of myocardial infarction or death among patients who underwent either coronary artery bypass surgery or percutaneous coronary intervention, with an event rate of 1.6 percent among patients in both groups.[51] The absence of any evident difference between groups suggests that previous percutaneous coronary intervention confers protection from perioperative cardiac events that is similar to that conferred by surgical revascularization, assuming that patients have been followed closely and that recurrent ischemia has been effectively treated. The Coronary Artery Revascularization Prophylaxis (CARP) randomized trial demonstrated that coronary artery revascularization using either bypass surgery or percutaneous coronary intervention before elective vascular surgery did not alter long-term survival.[52] Although the study was not powered to detect a beneficial effect in the short-term, there was no reduction in the number of postoperative myocardial infarctions, deaths, or days in the hospital. The results mirror those of other randomized clinical trials in the nonoperative setting that have shown that elective coronary revascularization in "low-risk" patients who have stable coronary artery disease does not provide a survival benefit and does not reduce the risk of late myocardial infarction as compared with

excellent medical and preventive therapies. On the basis of these data, coronary artery revascularization before elective vascular surgery among patients with stable cardiac symptoms cannot be routinely recommended.

Overall, indications for coronary revascularization among patients undergoing preoperative evaluation should be considered the same as for the general population (see Chap. 64).[15] These include patients who have poorly controlled angina pectoris despite maximal medical therapy and patients with one of several high-risk coronary characteristics—that is, clinically significant stenosis (>50 percent) of the left main coronary artery; severe two- or three-vessel coronary artery disease (>70 percent stenosis) with involvement of the proximal left anterior descending coronary artery; easily induced myocardial ischemia on preoperative stress testing; and/or left ventricular systolic dysfunction at rest.

Coronary stents are now used in more than 80 percent of coronary interventions and use of stents presents unique challenges because of the risk of coronary thrombosis and bleeding during the initial recovery phase. In a cohort of 40 patients who received stents prior to noncardiac surgery, all 8 deaths and 7 myocardial infarctions, as well as 8 of 11 bleeding episodes, occurred in patients who had undergone surgery within 14 days after stent placement.[53] The complications appeared to be related to serious bleeding resulting from postprocedural antiplatelet therapy or to coronary thrombosis in those who did not receive 4 full weeks of dual antiplatelet therapy after stenting. Wilson et al. demonstrated that 4.0 percent of patients undergoing surgery 6 weeks after stent placement died or suffered a myocardial infarction or stent thrombosis with no events in the patients undergoing surgery 7 to 9 weeks after stent placement.[54] These data suggest that, whenever possible, noncardiac surgery should be delayed 6 weeks after bare metal stent placement, by which time stents are generally endothelialized, and a course of antiplatelet therapy to prevent stent thrombosis has been completed.[54] Poststenting therapy currently includes a combination of aspirin and clopidogrel for at least 4 weeks, followed by aspirin for an indefinite period. Drug-eluting stents (DESs) should not be implanted prior to planned noncardiac surgery unless surgery can be safely performed on dual antiplatelet therapy or elective noncardiac surgery can be delayed for 3 to 6 months to allow effective post-DES antiplatelet therapy.

MEDICAL THERAPY FOR CORONARY ARTERY DISEASE

β Blockers

Several nonrandomized studies have addressed the effect of antiischemic medical therapy on perioperative prognosis.[55–61] Although data are lacking to support the empiric use of nitroglycerin or calcium channel blockers, there is substantial evidence that the use of perioperative β blockers may reduce the risk of an adverse cardiac event. Three small retrospective studies suggested that perioperative therapy with β blockers may result in fewer episodes of myocardial ischemia detectable on ECG[60,62] and of acute myocardial infarction.[59] One randomized study among 112 high-risk patients who underwent vascular surgery demonstrated a reduction in risk of perioperative myocardial infarction or death from 34 to 3 percent with the use of empiric β-blocker therapy.[63] Another randomized, placebo-controlled study used atenolol in 200 high-risk patients who were scheduled to undergo noncardiac surgery.[64] Atenolol was administered either intravenously or orally 2 days preoperatively and continued for 7 days postoperatively. The incidence of perioperative ischemia was significantly lower in the atenolol group than in the placebo group.[65,66] There was no difference in the incidence of perioperative myocardial infarction or death from cardiac causes, but the rate of event-free survival at 6 months was higher in the atenolol group.

Poldermans et al. reported on the perioperative use of bisoprolol in elective major vascular surgery.[63] Bisoprolol was started at least 7 days preoperatively, the dose being adjusted to achieve a resting heart rate of less than 60 beats/min, and it was continued for 30 days postoperatively. The study was confined to patients who had at least one clinical risk marker for an adverse cardiac event in the perioperative period (a history of congestive heart failure, prior myocardial infarction, diabetes, angina pectoris, heart failure, age >70 years, or poor functional status) and evidence of inducible myocardial ischemia on dobutamine echocardiography. Patients with extensive regional wall motion abnormalities were excluded. Bisoprolol was associated with a 91 percent reduction in the perioperative risk of myocardial infarction or death from cardiac causes in this high-risk population. Urban et al. evaluated the role of prophylactic β blockers in patients who were undergoing elective total knee arthroplasty.[67] A total of 107 patients were preoperatively randomized into two groups, control and β blockers, and were given postoperative esmolol infusions on the day of surgery and metoprolol for the next 48 hours to maintain a heart rate less than 80 beats/min. The number of ischemic events and total ischemic time were significantly lower with esmolol than in the control group.[67]

A meta-analysis of 6 randomized trials involving 694 surgical patients showed that β blockers were associated with a 75 percent reduction in the risk of perioperative death from cardiac causes.[68] However, not all studies have reported consistently favorable results for β blockers. The DIPOM (Diabetic Postoperative Mortality and Morbidity) trial, involving 921 patients with diabetes who were undergoing noncardiac surgery, showed that metoprolol did not significantly decrease the risk of death and cardiac complications.[69] Lindenauer et al. assessed the association between perioperative use of β blockers and inhospital mortality in an observational study.[70] The study compared outcomes among 119,632 patients who received β blockers during a surgical admission with outcomes among patients who did not receive β blockers and who were matched according to the Revised Cardiac Risk Index (RCRI) score. This index, developed by Lee et al.,[71] stratifies the risk of perioperative cardiac events according to the type of surgery and the presence or absence of a history of ischemic heart disease, congestive heart failure, cerebrovascular disease, preoperative treatment with insulin, and a preoperative serum creatinine level greater than 2.0 mg/dL (176.8 μmol/L). Scores range from 0 to 5, and the likelihood of major perioperative complications increases with increasing scores. Overall, β-blocker use was not associated with a reduced risk of death.[70] However, a gradient of benefit was observed in relation to the risk score. β-Blocker use was associated with a 43 percent increase in the risk of death among patients with a score of 0 and a 13 percent increase among patients with a score of 1, but was associated with a reduction in the risk of death (rang-

ing from 10 percent to 43 percent) among patients with a score of 2, 3, or 4 or greater. Thus, β blockers appeared to be harmful in low-risk patients, neutral in patients at intermediate risk, and beneficial in high-risk patients.[70]

The beneficial effect of β blockers in high-risk surgical patients supports the routine use of β blockers in these patients undergoing noncardiac surgery. Two ongoing randomized trials may help further clarify the role of β blockers in low-risk and intermediate-risk patients.[72,73] Based on available data it is appropriate to continue β-blocker therapy in patients who are at low or intermediate risk, given the potential cardiac risks associated with the sudden interruption of β-blocker therapy, but whether β-blocker therapy should be initiated in such patients in the perioperative period needs further study. It is important to recall that β blockers are indicated for patients with angina pectoris or its equivalent, recent myocardial infarction, distant myocardial infarction, dilated cardiomyopathy, and/or hypertension. Thus, when one or more of these conditions are identified for the first time in a preoperative assessment, initiation of β-blocker therapy is warranted. The ACC/AHA 2006 *Guideline Update on Perioperative Cardiovascular Evaluation for Noncardiac Surgery: Focused Update on Perioperative Beta-Blocker Therapy* recommends as a class I indication that β blockers be continued in patients undergoing surgery who are receiving β blockers to treat angina, symptomatic arrhythmias, hypertension, or other current ACC/AHA class I guideline indications.[74] β Blockers should also be given to patients who are undergoing vascular surgery at high cardiac risk based on the finding of ischemia on preoperative testing.[74]

Statins

Several studies now suggest that treatment with statins may significantly reduce the incidence of cardiovascular events after noncardiac surgery. In a case-controlled study, Poldermans et al. showed that statin use reduces perioperative mortality in patients who are undergoing major vascular surgery.[75] Use of statins was also protective against perioperative cardiac complications in patients who were undergoing vascular surgery in another retrospective study.[76] Durazzo et al. performed a small, prospective, randomized, placebo-controlled, double-blind clinical trial of 100 patients to analyze the effect of atorvastatin compared with placebo on the occurrence of a 6-month composite of cardiovascular events after vascular surgery.[77] They reported that short-term treatment with atorvastatin significantly reduces the incidence of major adverse cardiovascular events after vascular surgery.[77] A large retrospective cohort study based on hospital discharge and pharmacy records of 780,591 patients showed that treatment with lipid-lowering agents may reduce risk of death following major noncardiac surgery.[78] Overall, the data suggests that the use of lipid-lowering medications in the perioperative period is associated with reduced mortality among patients undergoing major noncardiac surgery, particularly vascular surgery. Larger clinical trials are required to confirm this observation and to determine the optimal timing and duration of therapy.

α₂ Agonists

There is some evidence for the perioperative use of α_2 agonists like clonidine to reduce perioperative cardiovascular events in patients undergoing noncardiac surgery. Wijeysundara et al. performed a meta-analysis to investigate the effects of α_2 adrenergic agonists on perioperative mortality and cardiovascular complications in adults undergoing surgery.[79] Twenty-three trials comprising 3395 patients were included. The analysis showed that α_2 adrenergic agonists reduce mortality and myocardial infarction following vascular surgery. During cardiac surgery, they reduce ischemia and may also have effects on mortality and myocardial infarction.[79] Wallace et al. conducted a prospective, double-blinded, clinical trial of 190 patients with or at risk for coronary artery disease with a 2:1 ratio (clonidine, n = 125 vs. placebo, n = 65) to test the hypothesis that prophylactic clonidine reduces the incidence of perioperative myocardial ischemia and postoperative death in patients undergoing noncardiac surgery. They reported that perioperative administration of clonidine for 4 days to patients who are at risk for coronary artery disease significantly reduces the incidence of perioperative myocardial ischemia and postoperative death.[80] Clonidine may be particularly attractive for patients undergoing noncardiac surgery who are unable to tolerate β blockers.

MANAGEMENT OF SPECIFIC CONDITIONS

Patients with a variety of medical conditions known to increase cardiovascular risk may require noncardiac surgery. For these patients, appropriate perioperative medical management may prevent the occurrence or minimize the impact of an adverse cardiovascular event. Factors that contribute to increased perioperative risk include interruptions in routine medical therapy, as well as physical and mental stresses associated with the surgical procedure and convalescent period. As such, cardiovascular stresses include alteration in normal medications during the preoperative period; fluctuation in heart rate, blood pressure, intravascular volume, and oxygenation during surgery; dynamic fluid shifts; pain; and limitations in the use of oral medications in the postoperative period. It is important to note that the period of maximum cardiac risk appears to occur in the postoperative period.[60] Because, cardiovascular risk is not limited to the intraoperative period, appropriate emphasis should be placed on the treatment of specific conditions throughout all phases of the perioperative period.

[ ] CORONARY ARTERY DISEASE

Among patients with known coronary artery disease who are undergoing noncardiac surgery, perioperative management should include monitoring for evidence of myocardial ischemia, therapy to prevent and treat ischemia, and postoperative surveillance to ensure that the patient did not experience an ischemic event that could mandate an alteration in therapy.

Monitoring can be accomplished with surveillance of ECG ST segments,[9,64] and transesophageal echocardiographic assessment of regional and global left ventricular wall motion,[81] or invasive measurement of pulmonary arterial and pulmonary capillary wedge pressures, although no studies have demonstrated improved outcomes with their use. Therapy to prevent ischemia should be individualized to the patient and the surgical procedure but should include β-adrenergic antagonists. Among many patients with known coronary artery disease, the prevention of ischemia can involve the

simple continuation of a routine antiischemic regimen or conversion of a regimen to a similar one available for topical or intravenous delivery during periods in which the patient is unable to take medications orally. Nitroglycerin compounds can be administered topically or via intravenous infusion. Several β-adrenergic antagonists and calcium channel-blocking agents are available for administration via intravenous bolus or infusion. In some patients, oral medications can be crushed and delivered through a nasogastric tube that is then clamped for 30 minutes to allow absorption in the upper intestine. Because of the adverse effects associated with rapid withdrawal of β-blocking medications, as well as the demonstrated benefit associated with their perioperative use,[59,60,63,65,66] every effort should be made to continue these medications during the perioperative period among patients who receive them preoperatively. Current data suggest that attempts to keep the patient's resting heart rate between 50 and 60 beats/min and a stress-related heart rate after surgery under 80 beats/min may be particularly effective.

At a minimum, an antiischemic regimen used prior to surgery should be continued during the perioperative period. Additional antiischemic medications can be used empirically and should be used in the event that ischemia is detected during the perioperative period. Intravenous nitroglycerin and/or β blockers can be titrated to specific end points of heart rate or blood pressure, or to resolution of the observed ischemia. In addition, pain relief and correction of any underlying anemia are helpful in reducing tendencies to postoperative ischemia.

Because patients with known coronary artery disease or risk factors for disease are at risk of acute myocardial infarction complicating noncardiac surgery, assessment for change in status is appropriate following a surgical procedure. A simple 12-lead ECG preoperatively, immediately postoperatively, and daily for 2 days is generally sufficient to evaluate for change if there has been no evidence of perioperative ischemia or infarction. Alternative means of assessing for perioperative infarction include assessment of serum creatine kinase, creatine kinase myocardial band isoenzyme fractions, and troponin; echocardiographic assessment of left ventricular wall motion; and nuclear perfusion studies.

At the conclusion of the perioperative period, it is important to resume antiischemic medications used by the patient prior to undergoing noncardiac surgery. In addition, antiplatelet agents such as aspirin, which may have been temporarily discontinued prior to surgery, should be reinitiated when no longer contraindicated.

[ ] HYPERTENSION

Among patients who are treated for hypertension, preoperative evaluation should include a review of present medications and any history of intolerance to previous antihypertensive medications, as well as assessment for adequacy of antihypertensive therapy. Brief evaluation for rare but potentially treatable causes of secondary hypertension should include assessment for an abdominal bruit, suggestive of renal artery stenosis; for radial–femoral delay, indicative of aortic coarctation; and for hypokalemia in the absence of diuretic use, which could suggest hyperaldosteronism.

Blood pressure should be well controlled prior to elective surgery,[60,82–84] and antihypertensive medications should be continued throughout the perioperative period. If there is a period in which the patient is unable to receive oral medications, topical or intravenous equivalents should be substituted. Rapid withdrawal of β-blocking medications has associated adverse effects on heart rate and blood pressure, may precipitate myocardial ischemia, and should be avoided.

Mild or moderate preoperative hypertension in the absence of associated cardiovascular or metabolic abnormalities should not necessitate delay of surgery.[84,85] However, severe hypertension (e.g., diastolic blood pressure of 110 mmHg or greater) should be controlled prior to an elective surgical procedure. If surgery is urgent, then preoperative blood pressure control can usually be achieved rapidly with the use of intravenous β blockers, calcium channel blockers, nitroglycerin, or nitroprusside. Finally, patients with preoperative hypertension appear to be predisposed to the development of intraoperative hypotension.[83] Because the potential for blood pressure lability, with associated ischemia and hypoperfusion, exists among patients with preoperative hypertension, blood pressure should be carefully monitored and, if necessary, treated.[86,87]

CONGESTIVE HEART FAILURE

Congestive heart failure is associated with increased cardiovascular risk during noncardiac surgery.[4,9] A careful history and physical examination should include efforts to identify evidence of congestive heart failure, and every effort should be made to treat it prior to surgery.

Congestive heart failure may be the result of a variety of cardiac abnormalities, including left ventricular systolic dysfunction, diastolic dysfunction, and valvular heart disease. Although congestive heart failure is an independent risk factor for adverse perioperative cardiac outcome, specific underlying causes of congestive heart failure may each be associated with specific independent risks, and the specific nature of the risk may be determined by the nature of the underlying disease. For these reasons, the cause of the underlying process responsible for congestive heart failure should be identified when possible. If left ventricular systolic function is not known, it is generally prudent to establish whether it is normal or abnormal prior to surgery. Similarly, evaluation of left ventricular diastolic dysfunction or valvular heart disease may help in perioperative management. If there are risk factors for coronary artery disease, further evaluation for coronary disease as a cause of left ventricular systolic dysfunction may be appropriate (see Chap. 25).

CARDIOMYOPATHY

Patients with dilated and hypertrophic cardiomyopathies are predisposed to develop perioperative congestive heart failure. Among patients with preoperative signs or symptoms of congestive heart failure, preoperative evaluation should include assessment of left ventricular systolic and diastolic function, as well as valve function. Systolic function can be determined noninvasively using either echocardiographic or radionuclide techniques. Echocardiographic imaging offers additional information reflecting diastolic function and valvular function, which could also contribute to congestive heart failure. If not previously performed, preoperative echocardiographic imaging should be strongly considered among patients with congestive heart failure.

Patients with hypertrophic cardiomyopathy require special consideration during the perioperative period. Hypertrophic cardio-myopathy can affect hemodynamics by means of dynamic left ventricular outflow obstruction or may precipitate congestive heart failure mediated by diastolic dysfunction. Left ventricular noncompliance can make patients with hypertrophic cardiomyopathy extremely sensitive to even small amounts of excess intravascular volume, while an underfilled left ventricle can exacerbate dynamic left ventricular outflow obstruction, with a resulting decrease in stroke volume and systemic hypotension. Therefore perioperative management should be directed at maintaining intravascular volume within a potentially narrow range and controlling periprocedural heart rate. These maneuvers reduce the likelihood of congestive heart failure and minimize left ventricular outflow obstruction. Catecholamines as a class should be avoided because of their potential to exacerbate dynamic left ventricular outflow obstruction (see Chap. 77).

VALVULAR HEART DISEASE

Most valvular heart disease in an adult population is acquired and therefore increasingly common among older patients undergoing noncardiac surgery. Although most elective noncardiac surgery need not be delayed, some types of valvular heart disease can pose excessive risk to the patient and may need to be addressed prior to an elective surgical procedure.[49]

Antibiotic prophylaxis should be used to reduce the risk of infective endocarditis among patients with organic valvular heart disease whenever noncardiac surgery involves a risk of bacteremia. Such procedures include oral, dental, gastrointestinal, and genitourologic procedures, in which normal bacterial flora may gain transient access to the bloodstream. Specific recommendations for prophylactic antibiotic regimens are published for specific types of noncardiac surgery in which there exists an increased risk of infective endocarditis.[88]

Aortic Stenosis

Severe aortic stenosis presents the greatest valve-associated cardiovascular risk for patients undergoing noncardiac surgery.[6] The presence of fixed obstruction to left ventricular outflow dramatically limits functional cardiac reserve and may be associated with intracavitary left ventricular pressures in excess of 300 mmHg. Accompanying left ventricular hypertrophy predisposes the patient to diastolic dysfunction and pulmonary congestion. In general, severe or symptomatic aortic stenosis should be addressed prior to the initiation of elective noncardiac surgery. In most cases, aortic valve replacement is indicated as the definitive therapy of choice.[89–91] If cardiac surgery is contraindicated, percutaneous aortic balloon valvotomy can be used to mitigate left ventricular outflow obstruction, even if only as a temporizing measure (see Chap. 75). When neither surgery nor percutaneous aortic valvotomy is considered feasible, noncardiac surgery with careful hemodynamic assessment may still be appropriate, albeit with a heightened risk of perioperative death. In such patients, avoidance of intraoperative or postoperative hypotension is particularly important.

Mitral Stenosis

The hemodynamic impact associated with mitral stenosis is affected by heart rate. The central problem with tachycardia in mitral stenosis is that increases in heart rate are associated with shortening of the diastolic portion of the cardiac cycle and a resultant rise in left atrial pressure. As a result, pulmonary congestion can be precipitated by tachycardia of even moderate degree. For this reason, heart rate should be well controlled in the perioperative period among patients with mitral stenosis of any severity. Patients with severe mitral stenosis who are undergoing high-risk noncardiac surgery may benefit from surgical or percutaneous intervention.[49,92] The relative risks and benefits and the likelihood of success associated with percutaneous balloon mitral valvotomy, surgical commissurotomy, or mitral valve replacement must be weighed in the context of mitral valve anatomy and other patient-specific factors (see Chap. 77).

Aortic Regurgitation and Mitral Regurgitation

Patients with significant aortic regurgitation are predisposed to volume overload in the perioperative period, and volume status should be carefully monitored to prevent pulmonary congestion. In addition, patients with severe aortic regurgitation may benefit from afterload reduction in the form of angiotensin-converting enzyme inhibitors, calcium channel blockers, nitroglycerin, or hydralazine.[93,94] Just as patients with mitral stenosis are sensitive to tachycardia, patients with significant aortic regurgitation are sensitive to excessive bradycardia. Prolongation of the diastolic interval associated with bradycardia increases the time during which aortic regurgitation occurs and increases total regurgitant volume.

Mitral regurgitation can be a result of a variety of underlying causes. As for patients with congestive heart failure, establishing the cause of mitral regurgitation may help define other associated perioperative risks, especially if mitral regurgitation occurs as a manifestation of coronary artery disease. Patients with significant mitral regurgitation may develop volume overload and pulmonary congestion. Diuretics and afterload-reducing therapy should be used to optimize hemodynamic status preoperatively in patients with severe mitral regurgitation who are undergoing major noncardiac surgery.

Special attention should be paid to left ventricular function in patients with severe mitral regurgitation. The left atrium and pulmonary venous system serve as a low-impedance system that effectively reduces the afterload on the left ventricle. Because of this, even a mild decrease in left ventricular ejection fraction in the setting of severe mitral regurgitation should be taken as evidence of significant impairment in systolic function and reduced left ventricular functional reserve (see Chap. 76).

Prosthetic Heart Valves

Patients with either tissue or mechanical heart valve prostheses should receive appropriate antibiotic prophylaxis when undergoing noncardiac surgery with an accompanying potential for bacteremia.[88] Patients with mechanical heart valve prostheses also require careful management of anticoagulation in the perioperative period. As a general rule, anticoagulation can be discontinued when necessary for safe performance of noncardiac surgery and should be reinstituted when it is no longer contraindicated for hemostasis. The risk of valve thrombosis or thromboembolism is related to the location and type of valve prosthesis, the length of time during which the patient is not fully anticoagulated, and the level of anticoagulation maintained during that period. A mechanical prosthesis in the mitral position is at greater risk of thrombus formation than is a similar valve in the aortic position because of lower pressure gradients and associated lower velocities of flow. Similarly, anticoagulation titrated to a subtherapeutic level maintains more protection against thrombus formation than does no anticoagulation. Finally, the risk of thrombus formation is cumulative and increases with time as the patient receives less than therapeutic anticoagulation.

Patients who require minimally invasive procedures with a low hemorrhagic risk may be managed by allowing long-term anticoagulation to decrease to a subtherapeutic range and resuming the normal dose of warfarin immediately following the procedure.[95,96] Among patients with mechanical heart valves who are undergoing major noncardiac surgery and in whom anticoagulation is contraindicated at the time of surgery, it is usually prudent to discontinue oral anticoagulation several days prior to surgery and to administer intravenous heparin to maintain anticoagulation until the time of surgery. The short half-life of heparin allows the patient to safely undergo surgery within a few hours of its discontinuation. Reestablishing therapeutic anticoagulation usually requires several days after warfarin is initiated; consequently, the patient should receive heparin in the postoperative period until oral anticoagulation is fully therapeutic. Heparin should be reinitiated when the risk of bleeding is no longer prohibitive and may be started with either a bolus followed by intravenous infusion or with intravenous infusion alone, which course being dictated by the risk of postoperative hemorrhage (see Chap. 80). Low-molecular-weight heparins are increasingly used in this situation although their overall safety and efficacy compared to unfractionated heparin have not been extensively studied for this purpose.

☐ ☐ ARRHYTHMIA AND CONDUCTION DISTURBANCES

Supraventricular and ventricular arrhythmias typically do not represent a serious risk to the patient who is undergoing noncardiac surgery. However, the arrhythmia may herald the presence of underlying cardiopulmonary disease, and any increased perioperative risk associated with ventricular and supraventricular arrhythmias[6] is most likely related to the underlying disease. The finding of an arrhythmia in the perioperative period should prompt a search for underlying cardiopulmonary disease, drug toxicity, or metabolic derangement that could be both responsible for the arrhythmia and present a risk to the patient.

An otherwise benign arrhythmia can be more risky if it unmasks a silent cardiac disease. For example, a rapid supraventricular tachycardia can provoke myocardial ischemia in the presence of minimal coronary artery disease and similarly can precipitate significant pulmonary congestion in the setting of only mild or moderate mitral stenosis. Ventricular ectopy—including isolated ventricular premature complexes, complex ectopy, and nonsustained ventricular tachycardia—usually does not require specific therapy unless there is evidence of associated hypoperfusion. Thus, hypotension or ongoing myocardial ischemia associated with an arrhythmia warrants therapy directed at the arrhythmia more than would the presence of the arrhythmia alone.

Perioperative atrial fibrillation is common, especially following intrathoracic surgical procedures (where there can be direct atrial irritation), as well as among patients with underlying cardiac or pulmonary diseases. Because of the high catecholamine state early following major surgery, it may not be possible to establish and maintain normal sinus rhythm in the setting of postoperative atrial fibrillation, and therapy should first be directed at rate control and anticoagulation when feasible. Cardioversion of atrial fibrillation in the early postoperative period should be limited to patients with evidence of hemodynamic compromise and hypoperfusion associated with the arrhythmia. For most patients, rate control can be accomplished with the use of β-adrenergic antagonists and/or calcium channel-blocking agents administered orally or intravenously. Although digoxin can also be administered, it is typically not as effective for rate control in patients with a high catecholamine state. Because of the risk of atrial thrombus formation and associated thromboembolic events, patients with atrial fibrillation, including postoperative atrial fibrillation, should be anticoagulated when feasible particularly when fibrillation persists more than 48 hours. Many patients with postoperative atrial fibrillation spontaneously revert to sinus rhythm when perioperative stresses have sufficiently decreased. If a patient does not spontaneously return to sinus rhythm, elective cardioversion should be considered prior to discharge or a few weeks later. Any form of cardioversion from atrial fibrillation—whether chemical, electrical, or spontaneous—carries an associated risk of subsequent thromboembolism ascribed to a period of atrial mechanical dysfunction following cardioversion.[97,98] For this reason, patients should receive therapeutic anticoagulation for 3 to 4 weeks following successful cardioversion.

Patients with evidence of intraventricular conduction delay on ECG but without a history of symptoms or electrical evidence of advanced heart block do not appear to be at substantial risk of progressing to complete heart block in the perioperative period. If high-grade conduction block develops, treatment can usually be managed in the short-term with transthoracic pacing units. Special note should be made of the presence of a left bundle-branch block among patients undergoing right heart catheterization for hemodynamic monitoring. Because of the risk of inducing transient right bundle-branch block during catheter manipulation through the right ventricle, the possibility of complete heart block exists, and measures to provide temporary pacing should be available.

SUMMARY OF KEY ELEMENTS OF ACC/AHA GUIDELINES

- It is important to determine the urgency of noncardiac surgery. In many cases patient- or surgery-specific factors dictate immediate surgery and may not allow further cardiac assessment or treatment. Perioperative medical management, surveillance, and postoperative risk stratification is appropriate in these cases.
- Patients with coronary revascularization in the past 5 years and who remain free of clinical evidence of ischemia generally have a low risk of cardiac complications from surgery and may proceed without further testing, particularly if they are functionally very active and asymptomatic.
- Patients with favorable invasive/noninvasive testing in the past 2 years generally require no further cardiac workup if they have been asymptomatic since the test and are functionally active.

- Patients with an unstable coronary syndrome, decompensated heart failure, symptomatic arrhythmias, or severe valvular heart disease scheduled for elective noncardiac surgery should have surgery canceled or delayed until the cardiac problem is clarified and treated (class I recommendation).
- Patients with <1 intermediate clinical predictor of cardiac risk for adverse perioperative events (see Table 86–1) and moderate or excellent functional capacity can generally undergo low- or intermediate-risk surgery with low event rates.
- Poor functional capacity or a combination of high-risk surgery and moderate functional capacity in a patient with intermediate clinical predictors of cardiac risk for adverse perioperative events (see Table 86–1; especially if ≥2) often requires further noninvasive cardiac testing (class I recommendation).
- Patients with minor or no clinical predictors of risk and moderate or excellent functional capacity can safely undergo noncardiac surgery.
- Results of noninvasive testing can be used to define further management, including intensified medical therapy or proceeding directly with surgery or cardiac catheterization. Cardiac catheterization may lead to coronary revascularization and is especially justifiable when it is likely to improve the patient's long-term prognosis (class IIa recommendation).

CONCLUSIONS

Appropriate preoperative evaluation and therapy may significantly improve periprocedural and long-term outcomes. Successful management of high-risk patients requires an integrated team approach between surgeons, anesthesiologists, cardiologists, and internists. In general, indications for further cardiac testing and revascularization are the same as in the nonoperative setting. In the absence of contraindications, β-blocker therapy should be considered in all high-risk patients who are scheduled to undergo noncardiac surgery and continued in patients undergoing surgery who are receiving β blockers to treat angina, symptomatic arrhythmias, hypertension, or other current guideline indications. For many patients, evaluation prior to noncardiac surgery may be the first comprehensive assessment of their short- and long-term cardiac risk and provides an opportunity not only to decrease their immediate periprocedural risk, but also to improve their long-term outcomes with appropriate evidence-based therapies.

REFERENCES

1. Poldermans D, Boersma E. Beta-blocker therapy in noncardiac surgery. *N Engl J Med* 2005;353:412–414.
2. National Center for Health Statistics. *Vital Statistics of the United States: 2003*. Washington, DC: NCHS U.S. Public Health Services, 2004.
3. Mangano DT. Perioperative cardiac morbidity. *Anesthesiology* 1990;72:153–184.
4. Ashton CM, Petersen NJ, Wray NP, et al. The incidence of perioperative myocardial infarction in men undergoing noncardiac surgery. *Ann Intern Med* 1993;118:504–510.
5. Eagle KA, Coley CM, Newell JB, et al. Combining clinical and thallium data optimizes preoperative assessment of cardiac risk before major vascular surgery. *Ann Intern Med* 1989;110:859–866.
6. Goldman L, Caldera DL, Nussbaum SR, et al. Multifactorial index of cardiac risk in noncardiac surgical procedures. *N Engl J Med* 1977;297:845–850.
7. Hollenberg M, Mangano DT, Browner WS, London MJ, Tubau JF, Tateo IM. Predictors of postoperative myocardial ischemia in patients undergoing

noncardiac surgery. The Study of Perioperative Ischemia Research Group. *JAMA* 1992;268:205–209.

8. Lette J, Waters D, Bernier H, et al. Preoperative and long-term cardiac risk assessment. Predictive value of 23 clinical descriptors, 7 multivariate scoring systems, and quantitative dipyridamole imaging in 360 patients. *Ann Surg* 1992;216:192–204.

9. Mangano DT, Browner WS, Hollenberg M, London MJ, Tubau JF, Tateo IM. Association of perioperative myocardial ischemia with cardiac morbidity and mortality in men undergoing noncardiac surgery. The Study of Perioperative Ischemia Research Group. *N Engl J Med* 1990;323:1781–1788.

10. Mukherjee D, Eagle KA. Cardiac risk in noncardiac surgery. *Minerva Cardioangiol* 2002;50:607–619.

11. Mukherjee D, Eagle KA. A common sense approach to perioperative evaluation. *Am Fam Physician* 2002;1826;66:1824.

12. Mukherjee D, Eagle KA. Perioperative cardiac assessment for noncardiac surgery: eight steps to the best possible outcome. *Circulation* 2003;107:2771–2774.

13. Cooperman M, Pflug B, Martin EW Jr, Evans WE. Cardiovascular risk factors in patients with peripheral vascular disease. *Surgery* 1978;84:505–509.

14. Detsky AS, Abrams HB, McLaughlin JR, et al. Predicting cardiac complications in patients undergoing non-cardiac surgery. *J Gen Intern Med* 1986;1:211–219.

15. Eagle KA, Berger PB, Calkins H, et al. ACC/AHA guideline update for perioperative cardiovascular evaluation for noncardiac surgery—executive summary: a report of the American College of Cardiology/American Heart Association Task Force on Practice Guidelines (Committee to Update the 1996, Guidelines on Perioperative Cardiovascular Evaluation for Noncardiac Surgery). *J Am Coll Cardiol* 2002;39:542–553.

16. Detsky AS, Abrams HB, Forbath N, Scott JG, Hilliard JR. Cardiac assessment for patients undergoing noncardiac surgery. A multifactorial clinical risk index. *Arch Intern Med* 1986;146:2131–2134.

17. Hertzer NR. Fatal myocardial infarction following peripheral vascular operations. A study of 951 patients followed 6 to 11 years postoperatively. *Cleve Clin Q* 1982;49:1–11.

18. Baron JF, Bertrand M, Barre E, et al. Combined epidural and general anesthesia versus general anesthesia for abdominal aortic surgery. *Anesthesiology* 1991;75:611–618.

19. Christopherson R, Beattie C, Frank SM, et al. Perioperative morbidity in patients randomized to epidural or general anesthesia for lower extremity vascular surgery. Perioperative Ischemia Randomized Anesthesia Trial Study Group. *Anesthesiology* 1993;79:422–434.

20. Hemmerling TM, Le N, Olivier JF, Choiniere JL, Basile F, Prieto I. Immediate extubation after aortic valve surgery using high thoracic epidural analgesia or opioid-based analgesia. *J Cardiothorac Vasc Anesth* 2005;19:176–181.

21. Introna RP, Blair JR, Thrush DN. Cardiac sympathetic blockade during spinal anesthesia involves both efferent and afferent pathways. *Anesthesiology* 2000;92:1850–1851.

22. Morris CK, Ueshima K, Kawaguchi T, Hideg A, Froelicher VF. The prognostic value of exercise capacity: a review of the literature. *Am Heart J* 1991;122:1423–1431.

23. Gianrossi R, Detrano R, Mulvihill D, et al. Exercise-induced ST depression in the diagnosis of coronary artery disease. A meta-analysis. *Circulation* 1989;80:87–98.

24. Detrano R, Gianrossi R, Mulvihill D, Lehmann K, Dubach P, Colombo A, Froelicher V. Exercise-induced ST segment depression in the diagnosis of multivessel coronary disease: a meta analysis. *J Am Coll Cardiol* 1989;14:1501–1508.

25. Weiner DA, Ryan TJ, McCabe CH, et al. Prognostic importance of a clinical profile and exercise test in medically treated patients with coronary artery disease. *J Am Coll Cardiol* 1984;3:772–779.

26. Sgura FA, Kopecky SL, Grill JP, Gibbons RJ. Supine exercise capacity identifies patients at low risk for perioperative cardiovascular events and predicts long-term survival. *Am J Med* 2000;108:334–336.

27. Yokoshima T, Honma H, Kusama Y, Munakata K, Takano T, Nakanishi K. Improved stratification of perioperative cardiac risk in patients undergoing noncardiac surgery using new indices of dobutamine stress echocardiography. *J Cardiol* 2004;44:101–111.

28. Mangano DT, London MJ, Tubau JF, et al. Dipyridamole thallium-201 scintigraphy as a preoperative screening test. A reexamination of its predictive potential. Study of Perioperative Ischemia Research Group. *Circulation* 1991;84:493–502.

29. Shaw LJ, Hendel R, Borges-Neto S, et al. Prognostic value of normal exercise and adenosine (99m)Tc-tetrofosmin SPECT imaging: results from the multicenter registry of 4,728 patients. *J Nucl Med* 2003;44:134–139.

30. Bry JD, Belkin M, O'Donnell TF Jr, et al. An assessment of the positive predictive value and cost-effectiveness of dipyridamole myocardial scintigraphy in patients undergoing vascular surgery. *J Vasc Surg* 1994;19:112–121; discussion 121–114.

31. Younis L, Stratmann H, Takase B, Byers S, Chaitman BR, Miller DD. Preoperative clinical assessment and dipyridamole thallium-201, scintigraphy for prediction and prevention of cardiac events in patients having major noncardiovascular surgery and known or suspected coronary artery disease. *Am J Cardiol* 1994;74:311–317.

32. Eddinger J, Cohen MC. Advances in nuclear imaging for preoperative risk assessment. *Curr Cardiol Rep* 2005;7:143–147.

33. Hendel RC, Whitfield SS, Villegas BJ, Cutler BS, Leppo JA. Prediction of late cardiac events by dipyridamole thallium imaging in patients undergoing elective vascular surgery. *Am J Cardiol* 1992;70:1243–1249.

34. Stratmann HG, Tamesis BR, Younis LT, Wittry MD, Miller DD. Prognostic value of dipyridamole technetium-99m sestamibi myocardial tomography in patients with stable chest pain who are unable to exercise. *Am J Cardiol* 1994;73:647–652.

35. Brown KA, Rowen M. Extent of jeopardized viable myocardium determined by myocardial perfusion imaging best predicts perioperative cardiac events in patients undergoing noncardiac surgery. *J Am Coll Cardiol* 1993;21:325–330.

36. Marwick T, Willemart B, D'Hondt AM, et al. Selection of the optimal nonexercise stress for the evaluation of ischemic regional myocardial dysfunction and malperfusion. Comparison of dobutamine and adenosine using echocardiography and 99mTc-MIBI single photon emission computed tomography. *Circulation* 1993;87:345–354.

37. Ritchie JL, Bateman TM, Bonow RO, et al. Guidelines for clinical use of cardiac radionuclide imaging. Report of the American College of Cardiology/American Heart Association Task Force on Assessment of Diagnostic and Therapeutic Cardiovascular Procedures (Committee on Radionuclide Imaging), developed in collaboration with the American Society of Nuclear Cardiology. *J Am Coll Cardiol* 1995;25:521–547.

38. Marwick TH, Lauer MS, Lobo A, Nally J, Braun W. Use of dobutamine echocardiography for cardiac risk stratification of patients with chronic renal failure. *J Intern Med* 1998;244:155–161.

39. Davila-Roman VG, Waggoner AD, Sicard GA, Geltman EM, Schechtman KB, Perez JE. Dobutamine stress echocardiography predicts surgical outcome in patients with an aortic aneurysm and peripheral vascular disease. *J Am Coll Cardiol* 1993;21:957–963.

40. Eichelberger JP, Schwarz KQ, Black ER, Green RM, Ouriel K. Predictive value of dobutamine echocardiography just before noncardiac vascular surgery. *Am J Cardiol* 1993;72:602–607.

41. Poldermans D, Fioretti PM, Forster T, et al. Dobutamine stress echocardiography for assessment of perioperative cardiac risk in patients undergoing major vascular surgery. *Circulation* 1993;87:1506–1512.

42. Shaw LJ, Eagle KA, Gersh BJ, Miller DD. Meta-analysis of intravenous dipyridamole-thallium-201 imaging (1985 to 1994) and dobutamine echocardiography (1991 to 1994) for risk stratification before vascular surgery. *J Am Coll Cardiol* 1996;27:787–798.

43. Cambria RP, Brewster DC, Abbott WM, et al. The impact of selective use of dipyridamole-thallium scans and surgical factors on the current morbidity of aortic surgery. *J Vasc Surg* 1992;15:43–50; discussion 51.

44. Froehlich JB, Karavite D, Russman PL, et al. American College of Cardiology/American Heart Association preoperative assessment guidelines reduce resource utilization before aortic surgery. *J Vasc Surg* 2002;36:758–763.

45. Almanaseer Y, Mukherjee D, Kline-Rogers EM, et al. Implementation of the ACC/AHA guidelines for preoperative cardiac risk assessment in a general medicine preoperative clinic: improving efficiency and preserving outcomes. *Cardiology* 2005;103:24–29.

46. Allen JR, Helling TS, Hartzler GO. Operative procedures not involving the heart after percutaneous transluminal coronary angioplasty. *Surg Gynecol Obstet* 1991;173:285–288.

47. Diehl JT, Cali RF, Hertzer NR, Beven EG. Complications of abdominal aortic reconstruction. An analysis of perioperative risk factors in 557 patients. *Ann Surg* 1983;197:49–56.

48. Huber KC, Evans MA, Bresnahan JF, Gibbons RJ, Holmes DR Jr. Outcome of noncardiac operations in patients with severe coronary artery disease successfully treated preoperatively with coronary angioplasty. *Mayo Clin Proc* 1992;67:15–21.

49. Konstadt S. Anesthesia for non-cardiac surgery in the patient with cardiac disease. *Can J Anaesth* 2005;52:R1–R7.

50. Elmore JR, Hallett JW Jr, Gibbons RJ, et al. Myocardial revascularization before abdominal aortic aneurysmorrhaphy: effect of coronary angioplasty. *Mayo Clin Proc* 1993;68:637–641.

51. Hassan SA, Hlatky MA, Boothroyd DB, et al. Outcomes of noncardiac surgery after coronary bypass surgery or coronary angioplasty in the Bypass Angioplasty Revascularization Investigation (BARI). *Am J Med* 2001;110:260–266.

52. McFalls EO, Ward HB, Moritz TE, et al. Coronary-artery revascularization before elective major vascular surgery. *N Engl J Med* 2004;351:2795–2804.

53. Kaluza GL, Joseph J, Lee JR, Raizner ME, Raizner AE. Catastrophic outcomes of noncardiac surgery soon after coronary stenting. *J Am Coll Cardiol* 2000;35:1288–1294.

54. Wilson SH, Fasseas P, Orford JL, et al. Clinical outcome of patients undergoing non-cardiac surgery in the two months following coronary stenting. *J Am Coll Cardiol* 2003;42:234–240.

55. Coriat P, Daloz M, Bousseau D, Fusciardi J, Echter E, Viars P. Prevention of intraoperative myocardial ischemia during noncardiac surgery with intravenous nitroglycerin. *Anesthesiology* 1984;61:193–196.

56. Dodds TM, Stone JG, Coromilas J, Weinberger M, Levy DG. Prophylactic nitroglycerin infusion during noncardiac surgery does not reduce perioperative ischemia. *Anesth Analg* 1993;76:705–713.

57. Gallagher JD, Moore RA, Jose AB, Botros SB, Clark DL. Prophylactic nitroglycerin infusions during coronary artery bypass surgery. *Anesthesiology* 1986;64:785–789.

58. Godet G, Coriat P, Baron JF, et al. Prevention of intraoperative myocardial ischemia during noncardiac surgery with intravenous diltiazem: a randomized trial versus placebo. *Anesthesiology* 1987;66:241–245.

59. Pasternack PF, Imparato AM, Baumann FG, et al. The hemodynamics of beta-blockade in patients undergoing abdominal aortic aneurysm repair. *Circulation* 1987;76:III1–III7.

60. Stone JG, Foex P, Sear JW, Johnson LL, Khambatta HJ, Triner L. Risk of myocardial ischaemia during anaesthesia in treated and untreated hypertensive patients. *Br J Anaesth* 1988;61:675–679.

61. Thomson IR, Mutch WA, Culligan JD. Failure of intravenous nitroglycerin to prevent intraoperative myocardial ischemia during fentanyl-pancuronium anesthesia. *Anesthesiology* 1984;61:385–393.

62. Pasternack PF, Grossi EA, Baumann FG, et al. Beta blockade to decrease silent myocardial ischemia during peripheral vascular surgery. *Am J Surg* 1989;158:113–116.

63. Poldermans D, Boersma E, Bax JJ, et al. The effect of bisoprolol on perioperative mortality and myocardial infarction in high-risk patients undergoing vascular surgery. Dutch Echocardiographic Cardiac Risk Evaluation Applying Stress Echocardiography Study Group. *N Engl J Med* 1999;341:1789–1794.

64. Mangano DT, Hollenberg M, Fegert G, et al. Perioperative myocardial ischemia in patients undergoing noncardiac surgery--I: Incidence and severity during the 4, day perioperative period. The Study of Perioperative Ischemia (SPI) Research Group. *J Am Coll Cardiol* 1991;17:843–850.

65. Mangano DT, Layug EL, Wallace A, Tateo I. Effect of atenolol on mortality and cardiovascular morbidity after noncardiac surgery. Multicenter Study of Perioperative Ischemia Research Group. *N Engl J Med* 1996;335:1713–1720.

66. Wallace A, Layug B, Tateo I, et al. Prophylactic atenolol reduces postoperative myocardial ischemia. McSPI Research Group. *Anesthesiology* 1998;88:7–17.

67. Urban MK, Markowitz SM, Gordon MA, Urquhart BL, Kligfield P. Postoperative prophylactic administration of beta-adrenergic blockers in patients at risk for myocardial ischemia. *Anesth Analg* 2000;90:1257–1261.

68. Stevens RD, Burri H, Tramer MR. Pharmacologic myocardial protection in patients undergoing noncardiac surgery: a quantitative systematic review. *Anesth Analg* 2003;97:623–633.

69. Juul AB, Wetterslev J, Kofoed-Enevoldsen A, Callesen T, Jensen G, Gluud C. The Diabetic Postoperative Mortality and Morbidity (DIPOM) trial: rationale and design of a multicenter, randomized, placebo-controlled, clinical trial of metoprolol for patients with diabetes mellitus who are undergoing major noncardiac surgery. *Am Heart J* 2004;147:677–683.

70. Lindenauer PK, Pekow P, Wang K, Mamidi DK, Gutierrez B, Benjamin EM. Perioperative beta-blocker therapy and mortality after major noncardiac surgery. *N Engl J Med* 2005;353:349–361.

71. Lee TH, Marcantonio ER, Mangione CM, et al. Derivation and prospective validation of a simple index for prediction of cardiac risk of major noncardiac surgery. *Circulation* 1999;100:1043–1049.

72. Devereaux PJ, Yusuf S, Yang H, Choi PT, Guyatt GH. Are the recommendations to use perioperative beta-blocker therapy in patients undergoing noncardiac surgery based on reliable evidence? *CMAJ* 2004;171:245–247.

73. Schouten O, Poldermans D, Visser L, et al. Fluvastatin and bisoprolol for the reduction of perioperative cardiac mortality and morbidity in high-risk patients undergoing non-cardiac surgery: rationale and design of the DECREASE-IV study. *Am Heart J* 2004;148:1047–1052.

74. Fleisher L, Beckman J, Brown K, et al. ACC/AHA 2006 guideline update on perioperative cardiovascular evaluation for noncardiac surgery: focused update on perioperative beta-blocker therapy. A report of the American College of Cardiology/American Heart Association Task Force on Practice Guidelines (Writing Committee to Update the 2002 Guidelines on Perioperative Cardiovascular Evaluation for Noncardiac Surgery). *J Am Coll Cardiol* 2006;47:2343–2355.

75. Poldermans D, Bax JJ, Kertai MD, et al. Statins are associated with a reduced incidence of perioperative mortality in patients undergoing major noncardiac vascular surgery. *Circulation* 2003;107:1848–1851.

76. O'Neil-Callahan K, Katsimaglis G, Tepper MR, et al. Statins decrease perioperative cardiac complications in patients undergoing noncardiac vascular surgery: the Statins for Risk Reduction in Surgery (StaRRS) study. *J Am Coll Cardiol* 2005;45:336–342.

77. Durazzo AE, Machado FS, Ikeoka DT, et al. Reduction in cardiovascular events after vascular surgery with atorvastatin: a randomized trial. *J Vasc Surg* 2004;39:967–975; discussion 975–966.

78. Lindenauer PK, Pekow P, Wang K, Gutierrez B, Benjamin EM. Lipid-lowering therapy and in-hospital mortality following major noncardiac surgery. *JAMA* 2004;291:2092–2099.

79. Wijeysundera DN, Naik JS, Beattie WS. Alpha-2, adrenergic agonists to prevent perioperative cardiovascular complications: a meta-analysis. *Am J Med* 2003;114:742–752.

80. Wallace AW, Galindez D, Salahieh A, et al. Effect of clonidine on cardiovascular morbidity and mortality after noncardiac surgery. *Anesthesiology* 2004;101:284–293.

81. Watters TA, Botvinick EH, Dae MW, et al. Comparison of the findings on preoperative dipyridamole perfusion scintigraphy and intraoperative transesophageal echocardiography: implications regarding the identification of myocardium at ischemic risk. *J Am Coll Cardiol* 1991;18:93–100.

82. Cucchiara RF, Benefiel DJ, Matteo RS, DeWood M, Albin MS. Evaluation of esmolol in controlling increases in heart rate and blood pressure during endotracheal intubation in patients undergoing carotid endarterectomy. *Anesthesiology* 1986;65:528–531.

83. Goldman L, Caldera DL. Risks of general anesthesia and elective operation in the hypertensive patient. *Anesthesiology* 1979;50:285–292.

84. Prys-Roberts C, Meloche R, Foex P. Studies of anaesthesia in relation to hypertension. I. Cardiovascular responses of treated and untreated patients. *Br J Anaesth* 1971;43:122–137.

85. Magnusson J, Thulin T, Werner O, Jarhult J, Thomson D. Haemodynamic effects of pretreatment with metoprolol in hypertensive patients undergoing surgery. *Br J Anaesth* 1986;58:251–260.

86. Bedford RF, Feinstein B. Hospital admission blood pressure: a predictor for hypertension following endotracheal intubation. *Anesth Analg* 1980;59:367–370.

87. Slogoff S, Keats AS. Does perioperative myocardial ischemia lead to postoperative myocardial infarction? *Anesthesiology* 1985;62:107–114.

88. Dajani AS, Bisno AL, Chung KJ, et al. Prevention of bacterial endocarditis. Recommendations by the American Heart Association. *JAMA* 1990;264:2919–2922.

89. Bernard Y, Etievent J, Mourand JL, et al. Long-term results of percutaneous aortic valvuloplasty compared with aortic valve replacement in patients more than 75, years old. *J Am Coll Cardiol* 1992;20:796–801.

90. Lieberman EB, Bashore TM, Hermiller JB, et al. Balloon aortic valvuloplasty in adults: failure of procedure to improve long-term survival. *J Am Coll Cardiol* 1995;26:1522–1528.

91. Logeais Y, Langanay T, Roussin R, et al. Surgery for aortic stenosis in elderly patients. A study of surgical risk and predictive factors. *Circulation* 1994;90:2891–2898.

92. Reyes VP, Raju BS, Wynne J, et al. Percutaneous balloon valvuloplasty compared with open surgical commissurotomy for mitral stenosis. *N Engl J Med* 1994;331:961–967.

93. Grayburn PA. Vasodilator therapy for chronic aortic and mitral regurgitation. *Am J Med Sci* 2000;320:202–208.

94. Scognamiglio R, Rahimtoola SH, Fasoli G, Nistri S, Dalla Volta S. Nifedipine in asymptomatic patients with severe aortic regurgitation and normal left ventricular function. *N Engl J Med* 1994;331:689–694.

95. Stein PD, Alpert JS, Copeland J, Dalen JE, Goldman S, Turpie AG. Antithrombotic therapy in patients with mechanical and biological prosthetic heart valves. *Chest* 1992;102:445S-455S.

96. Stein PD, Alpert JS, Copeland J, Dalen JE, Goldman S, Turpie AG. Antithrombotic therapy in patients with mechanical and biological prosthetic heart valves. *Chest* 1995;108:371S–379S.

97. Black IW, Fatkin D, Sagar KB, et al. Exclusion of atrial thrombus by transesophageal echocardiography does not preclude embolism after cardioversion of atrial fibrillation. A multicenter study. *Circulation* 1994;89:2509–2513.

98. Fatkin D, Kuchar DL, Thorburn CW, Feneley MP. Transesophageal echocardiography before and during direct current cardioversion of atrial fibrillation: evidence for "atrial stunning" as a mechanism of thromboembolic complications. *J Am Coll Cardiol* 1994;23:307–316.

CHAPTER 87

Anesthesia and the Patient with Cardiovascular Disease

David L. Reich / Alexander Mittnacht / Joel A. Kaplan

INTRODUCTION

Anesthetizing patients with cardiovascular disease is one of the greatest challenges facing the anesthesiologist. The constellation of anesthetic drug effects, the physiologic stresses of surgery, and underlying cardiovascular diseases complicate and limit the choice of anesthetic techniques for any particular procedure. Generally speaking, the anesthesiologist's approach to the patient with cardiovascular disease is to select agents and techniques that would optimize the patient's cardiopulmonary function. The perioperative management of a patient with cardiovascular disease requires close cooperation between the cardiologist/internist and the anesthesiologist. Each specialist has a unique knowledge base that complements that of the others. The approach should emphasize a continuum of care from the preoperative evaluation through the extended postoperative period.

PREOPERATIVE EVALUATION

The assessment of cardiac risk and preoperative optimization of the patient's cardiovascular status are the traditional goals of the preoperative evaluation of patients with cardiovascular disease. In 1977, Goldman et al. introduced the Cardiac Risk Index Score (CRIS) to guide more quantitatively the assignment of cardiac risk in patients undergoing noncardiac surgery.[1] This study had a major impact, because clinicians concluded that improvements in factors such as congestive heart failure symptoms and general medical condition would decrease cardiac risk. While the predictive value of the CRIS remains controversial,[2] the emphasis on preoperative optimization continues and is reviewed in Chap. 86. The American College of Cardiology/American Heart Association Task Force on Practice Guidelines published *Guidelines for Perioperative Cardiovascular Evaluation for Noncardiac Surgery,* which were last updated in 2002.[3] The algorithmic approach to preoperative evaluation described in these guidelines and that advocated by Mangano and Goldman[4] are valuable in that more consistent clinical approaches have emerged.

The information derived from the cardiac evaluation that is of particular value to the anesthesiologist can be summarized by answers to the following seven questions:

1. What is (are) the clinically significant pathologic condition(s) affecting the cardiovascular system?
2. Are further diagnostic studies required prior to elective surgery?
3. Will the patient derive benefit from delaying surgery in order to optimize preoperative medical therapy?
4. Will the patient derive benefit from preoperative myocardial revascularization as part of the patient's overall cardiovascular disease management?
5. Should there be perioperative antithrombotic therapy?
6. What is the regimen of preoperative cardiovascular medications that should be continued through the perioperative period? Should β blockers or statins be started if the patient is not already taking them?

7. What is the specific device information on the patient's pacemaker or automatic implantable cardioverter-defibrillator?

The ideal "medical clearance" consultation for the anesthesiologist consists of a cogent and legible summary of the pertinent clinical, laboratory, radiologic, echocardiographic, radionuclide, and cardiac catheterization data. With the benefit of this information, the two specialties can make intelligent decisions regarding the patient's preoperative therapy and the optimal timing of surgery.[5]

ANTICOAGULANT AND ANTIPLATELET THERAPY

As cardiovascular disease management increasingly includes anticoagulants, antiplatelet agents, and percutaneous coronary interventions, new challenges have arisen in the perioperative management of these patients. Elective surgery and neuraxial anesthesia require the withdrawal of anticoagulant and antiplatelet therapy during the immediate perioperative period.

Recent percutaneous myocardial revascularization is strongly associated with perioperative cardiac events.[6–8] These observations are likely related to the perioperative hypercoagulability associated with surgical stress in the setting of nonendothelialized stent surfaces where anticoagulant/antiplatelet medications have been discontinued to facilitate surgical hemostasis. A retrospective study by Posner et al.,[9] found that adverse cardiac outcomes after noncardiac surgery among 686 patients with prior percutaneous transluminal coronary angioplasty (PTCA) were increased. Patients with prior PTCA had twice the rate of adverse cardiac outcomes as normal subjects, seven times the rate of angina, almost four times the rate of myocardial infarction, and twice the rate of congestive heart failure. Patients who underwent PTCA within 90 days of noncardiac surgery had twice the rate of perioperative myocardial infarction compared to patients with uncorrected coronary artery disease (CAD).

The American College of Cardiology (ACC) and the American Heart Association (AHA) recommend a delay of at least 2 weeks, and ideally 4 to 6 weeks, between percutaneous myocardial revascularization and noncardiac surgery.[10] Nevertheless, these recommendations are based mainly on experience with bare metal stents. The period of risk for acute stent thrombosis may extend to several months following drug-eluting stent placement.[11] Consequently, the optimal timing of elective surgery following drug-eluting stent implantation has yet to be determined.[12,13] Ideally, elective noncardiac surgery is delayed until full completion of antiplatelet therapy.[14]

In emergency procedures, patients on long-acting antiplatelet drugs have increased risk of hemorrhage, and platelet transfusions may be necessary to achieve hemostasis. One strategy that is possible for urgent surgery is switching to short- or intermediate-acting intravenous antiplatelet agents during the perioperative period to minimize the interval during which patients are exposed to the risk of acute stent thrombosis.

In addition to the implications for perioperative cardiovascular events and surgical hemostasis, anticoagulant and antiplatelet therapy are associated with neurologic complications following neuraxial anesthesia that are described below in the section devoted to regional anesthesia.

PERIOPERATIVE MONITORING

The American Society of Anesthesiologists established standards for basic intraoperative monitoring in 1986.[15] The intraoperative monitoring that is required based upon these guidelines includes: (1) heart rate, (2) ECG, (3) blood pressure, (4) pulse oximetry, (5) capnometry, and (6) body temperature. The indications for the use of more invasive monitors, such as intraarterial and central venous monitoring, vary by institution and practitioner (Tables 87–1 and 87–2).[16] The indications for pulmonary arterial catheter (PAC) monitoring are especially controversial. There are data from the intensive care setting suggesting that the PAC is harmful,[17] whereas other data indicate that it may provide prognostic information in the perioperative period.[18] Large randomized prospective studies of PAC use in various clinical settings have failed to demonstrate improved patient outcomes.[19–22] Thus current evidence argues against specific indications for perioperative PAC monitoring. It must be recognized that the PAC is a monitoring device only, and thus, will not alter clinical outcome unless effective treatment is initiated based on its measurements. Furthermore, the caregiver's competency in interpreting PAC-derived data is essential in order to derive maximal benefit from PAC use, and to avoid potential complications.[23–25] The American Society of Anesthesiologists has published practice parameters to guide prac-

TABLE 87–1

Indications for Intraarterial Monitoring

- Major surgical procedures involving large fluid shifts and/or blood loss
- Surgery requiring cardiopulmonary bypass
- Surgery of the aorta
- Patients with pulmonary disease requiring frequent arterial blood gases
- Patients with recent myocardial infarctions, unstable angina, or severe coronary artery disease
- Patients with decreased left ventricular function (congestive heart failure) or significant valvular heart disease
- Patients in hypovolemic, cardiogenic, or septic shock, or with multiple-organ failure
- Procedures involving the use of deliberate hypotension or deliberate hypothermia
- Massive trauma
- Patients with right heart failure, chronic obstructive pulmonary disease, pulmonary hypertension, or pulmonary embolism
- Patients requiring inotropes or intraaortic balloon counterpulsation
- Patients undergoing surgery of the aorta requiring cross-clamping
- Patients with massive ascites
- Patients with electrolyte or metabolic disturbances requiring frequent blood samples
- Inability to measure arterial pressure noninvasively (e.g., morbid obesity)

TABLE 87-2

Indications for Central Venous Line Placement

- Major operative procedures involving large fluid shifts and/or blood loss in patients with good left ventricular function
- Intravascular volume assessment when urine output is not reliable or unavailable (renal failure or major urologic surgery)
- Patients with tricuspid stenosis
- Major trauma
- Surgical procedures with a high risk of air embolism, such as sitting-position craniotomies
- Frequent blood sampling in patients who do not require an intraarterial line
- Venous access for vasoactive or irritating drugs
- Chronic drug administration
- Inadequate peripheral IV access
- Rapid infusion of IV fluids (using large cannulae)

titioners in the appropriate use of this technology.[26] Specific indications are avoided in these guidelines. The decision to employ perioperative PAC monitoring should be based on a combination of patient risk factors, surgical risk, and experience of the practitioner. Despite the lack of supporting evidence, many practitioners believe that certain patient populations benefit from PAC monitoring. Perioperative PAC monitoring continues to be used in selected patients undergoing complex procedures, such as cardiac surgery and liver transplantation, and also in selected patients with clinically significant pulmonary hypertension and other severe cardiac conditions.

Transesophageal echocardiography (TEE) is minimally invasive and has acquired a much larger role in intraoperative management in recent years. The availability of high-frequency transducers and color-flow Doppler mapping has enhanced the ability of anesthesiologists, cardiologists, and surgeons to make intraoperative diagnoses, evaluate hemodynamic aberrations, and assess the quality of cardiac surgical interventions. Standardized intraoperative examination guidelines for multiplane transesophageal echocardiography[27] and training guidelines[28] have been published, and the National Board of Echocardiography administers a certifying examination. The American Society of Anesthesiologists has published practice guidelines for intraoperative transesophageal echocardiography.[29,30] These are guidelines only, and the practitioner should decide on intraoperative TEE monitoring based on the practitioner's level of experience, as well as patient- and surgery-related factors. In selected patients who are at high risk, the combined use of PAC and intraoperative TEE allows for optimal monitoring of hemodynamic parameters.

Various forms of proprietary electroencephalographic analysis technology have been developed for the purpose of monitoring depth of sedation and loss of consciousness.[31] Incomplete amnesia leading to intraoperative awareness is rare with current anesthetic techniques, with a reported incidence of 0.1 to 0.2 percent.[32,33] In a recently published practice advisory, the American Society of Anesthesiologists does not recommend routine brain function monitoring of patients who are undergoing general anesthesia.[34]

Increased risk of intraoperative awareness is associated with a prior history of intraoperative awareness, as well as morbid obesity, substance abuse, chronic pain patients with opioid tolerance, and certain procedures (e.g., trauma surgery). Brain function monitoring should be employed on a case-by-case basis.

CHOICE OF ANESTHETIC TECHNIQUE

The choice of anesthetic technique is inherently a difficult one because multiple factors must be considered, such as the desires of the patient, the requirements of the surgical procedure, and the patient's underlying medical condition. Although a specific anesthetic technique is occasionally desirable for a particular procedure (e.g., spinal anesthesia for transurethral resection of prostate), it is extremely difficult to find scientific evidence that any particular anesthetic approach is superior to reasonable alternatives or that anesthetic technique per se influences patient outcome.

There is long-standing controversy regarding the effects of regional anesthesia (with postoperative epidural analgesia) on cardiovascular morbidity/mortality in high-risk patients. While some studies suggest that regional anesthesia and epidural analgesia have salutary effects in vascular surgical patients,[35] the issue is unresolved because of the limited and conflicting clinical evidence.[36–39] In certain defined sets of endovascular, orthopedic, and genitourinary procedures, there is evidence that local and regional anesthesia techniques are associated with better outcomes compared with general anesthesia.[40,41] These data are not applicable in all circumstances, however, and clinical judgment must be exercised to make the best choices in individual circumstances.

Regional anesthetics and monitored anesthesia care, however, are not infrequently converted to general anesthetics intraoperatively because of unexpectedly long surgery, patient discomfort, or changes in the surgical plan. No anesthesiologist can be certain that a particular technique will be adequate for the surgical procedure, given the unpredictability of the situation, and the anesthesiologist must have flexibility to alter the technique as needed. Consequently, it is essential that the cardiologist/internist does not specifically exclude any anesthetic technique during a preoperative consultation.

REGIONAL ANESTHESIA

Cushing coined the term *regional anesthesia* for operations where local anesthetics were used to operate on localized areas of the body without loss of consciousness. The advantages of regional anesthesia include simplicity, low cost, and minimal equipment requirements. Many of the adverse effects of general anesthesia are avoided, such as myocardial and respiratory depression. The potential disadvantages include patients' reluctance to be awake in the operating room, local anesthetic agents of insufficient or excessive duration, local anesthetic toxicity, and the risk of neuraxial hematoma in anticoagulated patients.

The cardiovascular side effects of regional anesthesia vary depending on the technique chosen. Regional anesthesia may also be combined with general anesthesia in adults and children so as to decrease the requirements for the general anesthetic agents and for postoperative analgesia. The institution of analgesia prior to surgical stimulation (preemptive analgesia) may have salutary effects on postoperative pain control.

Local Anesthetic Agents

Local anesthetics are classified on the basis of their chemical structure as esters or amides. The esters are hydrolyzed by esterases in the plasma, and the amides are metabolized in the liver. The duration of action of local anesthetic agents is affected by the protein-binding characteristics of the molecule and the addition of vasoconstrictors to the local anesthetic solution. Toxic reactions to local anesthetics are generally characterized by central nervous system excitation (seizures), which may be followed by central nervous system depression and cardiovascular collapse. Table 87–3 gives an overview of commonly used local anesthetics in today's practice.

Epinephrine and phenylephrine may be added in very small doses to local anesthetic solutions to prolong their duration of action by local vasoconstriction. The systemic absorption of epinephrine occurs very slowly, and the β-adrenergic effects predominate. This results in slight tachycardia and diastolic hypotension, which is undesirable in patients with certain cardiovascular diseases.

Spinal Anesthesia

The injection of a relatively small dose of local anesthetic into the subarachnoid space that produces profound motor and sensory blockade is known as spinal anesthesia. Spinal anesthesia also produces blockade of preganglionic sympathetic fibers resulting in a sympathetic blockade that is generally two dermatomal segments higher than the sensory dermatomal level. A high level of sympathetic blockade results in hypotension through profound arterial and venous vasodilatation, which can be prevented or treated by intravenous hydration with crystalloid solutions. If the dermatomal level of sympathetic blockade reaches T1, then a complete sympathectomy is present until the block recedes. The loss of cardiac accelerator fiber function may lead to bradycardia. Complete sympathectomy always occurs with a "total spinal" that also produces respiratory insufficiency as a result of intercostal and phrenic nerve root blockade.

Spinal anesthesia must be undertaken cautiously, and with more intensive monitoring, in patients whose cardiovascular stability depends upon the maintenance of a high preload and afterload. Patients with conditions including significant cardiac valvular disease, hypertrophic obstructive cardiomyopathy, or tetralogy of Fallot are prone to hemodynamic decompensation during spinal anesthesia. Patients with CAD usually tolerate spinal anesthesia well, so long as diastolic arterial pressure is maintained at an appropriate level to preserve coronary perfusion pressure.

Epidural Anesthesia

The epidural space, which is filled with loose areolar tissue and a venous plexus, lies immediately external to the dura mater. An indwelling catheter is usually placed percutaneously for intermittent bolus injections or continuous infusions of local anesthetic and/or opioids. The epidural space may be entered by thoracic, lumbar, or caudal approaches.

The hemodynamic effects of epidural anesthesia are essentially similar to those of spinal anesthesia, except that the onset of sympathetic blockade is more gradual. Thus, with appropriate monitoring, cautious administration of epidural anesthetics has been safely done even in patients with mitral valvular disease, aortic stenosis, or hypertrophic obstructive cardiomyopathy. It should be emphasized, though, that more invasive monitoring such as intra-arterial catheters and PACs may be required to monitor and treat changes in preload and afterload that occur with epidural anesthesia in patients with severe cardiovascular disease. In patients with known coronary artery disease, epidural anesthesia and analgesia, especially thoracic epidural catheters, have been shown to reduce intraoperative and early postoperative ischemia events.[42,43] Patient outcome data, however, were inconclusive when epidural anesthesia was compared with general anesthesia in patients at risk for perioperative cardiac events undergoing vascular surgery.[44,45]

When compared with spinal anesthesia, epidural anesthesia requires higher doses of local anesthetic, which increase the potential for complications and side effects such as inadvertent intravascular or intrathecal injections of a high dose of local anesthetic, which potentially can cause cardiovascular collapse, seizures, or a "total

TABLE 87–3

Local Anesthetics

GENERIC	CLASS	USES	NOTES/SIDE EFFECTS
Cocaine	Ester	T	Central nervous system toxicity, arrhythmias, myocardial ischemia
Procaine	Ester	S, I	Vasoconstriction
Chloroprocaine	Ester	E, S, C, I	
Tetracaine	Ester	S, I, T	
Lidocaine	Amide	E, S, C, I, T	Antiarrhythmic properties
Mepivacaine	Amide	E, S, C, I	
Prilocaine	Amide	E, C, I	Methemoglobinemia
Bupivacaine	Amide	E, S, C, I	High cardiotoxicity, cardiovascular collapse
Levobupivacaine	Amide	E, S, C, I	Less cardiotoxicity compared to bupivacaine
Ropivacaine	Amide	E, S, C, I	Less cardiotoxicity compared to bupivacaine

C, caudal; E, epidural; I, infiltration; S, spinal; T, topical.

spinal" (see above). The hemodynamic consequences of inadvertent intravenous injections of epinephrine-containing solutions may be significant for patients who cannot tolerate tachycardia. Epidural infusions of opioids for postoperative analgesia may be complicated by pruritus, nausea, urinary retention, somnolence, and respiratory depression. Thus, appropriate monitoring and nursing care are required.

Combined Spinal–Epidural Anesthesia

The injection of intrathecal anesthetic agents via a fine-bore needle that is placed through the epidural catheter-introducing large-bore needle followed by epidural catheter placement constitutes combined spinal–epidural anesthesia. The spinal anesthetic provides rapid onset of anesthesia, while the epidural catheter permits the administration of agents for continued intraoperative anesthesia and postoperative analgesia.

Nerve Blocks and Infiltration of Local Anesthetic

Nerve blocks and local anesthetic infiltration may be performed to facilitate surgery of localized areas of the body. The brachial plexus may be blocked by various approaches. The lower extremity may be anesthetized by blocking the femoral, obturator and sciatic nerves. Local anesthetic infiltration ("field block") is performed in defined regions, such as the inguinal area to facilitate open herniorrhaphies. These blocks, when properly performed, have minimal cardiovascular effects. They do, however, require large volumes of local anesthetic solution, which result in toxic reactions if inadvertent intravascular injection occurs. Intercostal blocks are associated with high blood concentrations even without intravascular injection, because the neurovascular bundle enhances absorption of the local anesthetic and multiple blocks are required for clinical efficacy.

Regional Anesthesia and Anticoagulation Therapy

Intraoperative central neuraxial anesthesia (e.g., spinal and epidural) and postoperative neuraxial analgesia are contraindicated in patients with significant anticoagulation or antiplatelet therapy. The increasing use of anticoagulation and antiplatelet therapy in the management of cardiovascular disease and perioperative thromboembolic prophylaxis has complicated the application of neuraxial techniques, and appropriate patient selection is essential. Very rare, but potentially catastrophic hematomas within the neuraxial space are associated with perioperative anticoagulation. A careful drug history and bleeding diathesis history is more effective than laboratory investigation, because low-molecular-weight heparins and antiplatelet drugs confer higher risk (especially in combination), but will not be detected by standard preoperative coagulation tests.[46]

The establishment of guidelines for the use of neuraxial anesthesia and analgesia in patients who have or will receive anticoagulants is an evolving process. The American Society of Regional Anesthesia and Pain Medicine publishes consensus statements on neuraxial anesthesia and anticoagulation that were updated as recently as 2003.[47] These include recommendations for appropriate withdrawal of anticoagulant and antiplatelet therapy prior to neuraxial anesthesia and are found on the Internet at www.asra.com. Table 87–4 summarizes these guidelines and the current literature.[48] It is prudent to avoid neuraxial anesthesia in patients who are on a combination of newer potent antiplatelet drugs that include GP IIb/IIIa antagonists, adenosine diphosphate-inhibitors, and low-molecular-weight heparins. For patient safety, it is crucial to monitor neurologic status carefully after administration of spinal or epidural anesthesia; rapid diagnosis and treatment of neuraxial hematoma probably improves outcome.[49]

GENERAL ANESTHESIA

General anesthesia is defined as a reversible state consisting of amnesia, analgesia, immobility, and the prevention of undesirable reflexes. The general anesthetics include many drugs, almost all of which have cardiovascular side effects. Intravenous agents are nearly always used for the induction of anesthesia in adults. Anesthesia is maintained using inhalational agents, intravenous agents, or a combination of the two.

Neuromuscular blocking drugs (muscle relaxants) are commonly used to facilitate tracheal intubation, to lower the requirements for anesthetic agents, and to prevent involuntary muscular activity in surgical cases where complete paralysis is mandatory. In children, the induction of anesthesia is highly individualized according to patient needs, practitioner, and institution. With the exception of brief operations, most general anesthetics include tracheal intubation and mechanical ventilation. As an alternative to tracheal intubation, devices such as the laryngeal mask airway may be used to secure a patient's airway. The loss of consciousness is usually accompanied by a decrease in sympathetic tone. This, as well as the effects of positive pressure ventilation, and the cardiac depressant properties of inhalational and most intravenous anesthetic agents, causes a moderate decrease in cardiac output.

The patient with cardiovascular disease presents major concerns for the anesthesiologist. General anesthesia masks many of the symptoms of cardiovascular decompensation, such as angina, dyspnea, dizziness, and palpitations. Other signs of cardiovascular disease, such as tachycardia, are nonspecific and may be misinterpreted as hypovolemia or light anesthesia. Fluid shifts, obstructed venous return, and varying levels of noxious stimulation are other variables related to surgery that are unpredictable. It is for these reasons that appropriate monitoring and selection of anesthetic agents is vital to the intraoperative management of the patient with cardiovascular disease.

INTRAVENOUS ANESTHETICS

Intravenous anesthetic induction drugs are composed of lipophilic molecules that have an affinity for neuronal tissue or specific receptors. Their action is generally terminated by redistribution from the vessel-rich tissues (brain, heart, liver, and kidneys) to other tissues (muscle, fat, and skin). Elimination occurs via hepatic metabolism and takes place over several hours. With the exception of ketamine, all intravenous anesthetics exhibit some degree of cardiovascular depression in the form of myocardial depression and/or vasodilation. Reduced doses and slower injection of the drug will markedly decrease these cardiovascular effects. Table 87–5 summarizes commonly used intravenous anesthetics.

TABLE 87–4

Neuraxial Anesthesia and Antithrombotics

DRUG	CLINICAL TESTS	RECOMMENDATIONS
Unfractionated heparin	Activated partial thromboplastin time	1. NA should be avoided in fully anticoagulated patients 2. Standard subcutaneous UH: no increased risk unless used for prolonged periods; IV heparin infusion safe if started >1 h after needle placement; catheter removal 1 h before subsequent dose and >2–4 h following last heparin dose
Low-molecular-weight heparins and heparinoids	Not useful	1. Increased risk for NA, especially when used in conjunction with antiplatelet therapy 2. 12 h interval between last dose and NA 3. Catheter removal 10–12 h after last LMWH dose; next dose 2 h after catheter removed 4. If blood appears during placement of NA, surgery does not need to be postponed, but next dose of LMWH should be delayed for another 24 h
Warfarin	Prothrombin time	1. Warfarin should be discontinued 4–5 days prior to the planned procedure and normal PT/INR measured before administration of regional anesthesia (chronic oral anticoagulation) 2. PT and INR should be checked prior to neuraxial anesthesia if first dose was given >24 h before surgery or a second dose had been administered 3. Neuraxial catheters should be removed when the INR is <1.5
Lepirudin Hirudin Bivalirudin	Ecarin clotting time	No recommendations available at present
Aspirin	Not useful	Very low risk unless used in conjunction with a second drug that affects the coagulation system
Other NSAIDs	Not useful	No indication for increased risk unless used in conjunction with a second drug that affects the coagulation system
Clopidogrel Ticlopidine	Not useful	1. At present, insufficient clinical data about safe time interval between drug administration and NA 2. Recommend discontinuing clopidogrel 7 days prior to NA 3. Recommend discontinuing ticlopidine 10–14 days prior to NA
Tirofiban	Not useful	Recommend 8-h interval between drug administration and safe NA
Abciximab	Not useful	Recommend 48-h interval between drug administration and safe NA
Eptifibatide	Not useful	Recommend 8-h interval between drug administration and safe NA
Fondaparinux	Antifactor Xa assay with fondaparinux controls	No recommendations available at present

INR, international normalized ratio; LMWH, low-molecular-weight heparin; NA, neuraxial anesthesia; PT, prothrombin time; UH, unfractionated heparin.

【 】 INHALATIONAL ANESTHETICS

Inhalational anesthetics include nitrous oxide and the potent volatile agents. Nitrous oxide has analgesic properties, but it is not a very potent anesthetic. Concentrations up to 75 percent may be given safely (so as to maintain an adequate FiO_2 [fraction of inspired oxygen]), but incomplete amnesia and movement in response to painful stimuli are likely. Thus, nitrous oxide is nearly always administered with other anesthetic agents, such as opioids or potent volatile agents, and neuromuscular blockers.

The use of inhalational anesthesia with potent volatile agents is the most common anesthetic technique because of its relatively low cost, reliable amnesia, and bronchodilatation as well as the low blood solubility and overall safety record of these agents. The effect of these agents is rapidly changed when the inspiratory concentration is adjusted. The ability to titrate inhalational anesthesia is an advantage compared to intravenous drugs, because the duration of surgical procedures and the degree of surgical stimulation are often unpredictable. For this reason, low doses of volatile anesthetics may be added as supplements to nitrous oxide- or intravenous-based anesthetic techniques for the control of hypertension and the prevention of awareness (incomplete amnesia). All volatile agents are myocardial depressants and vasodilators and produce some degree of hypotension. The appearance of nodal (junctional) rhythm is also common to these agents. The loss of atrial systole may be poorly tolerated, particularly in patients with aortic stenosis, hypertrophic cardiomyopathies, or mitral stenosis.

There is robust evidence that inhalational anesthetics offer some degree of myocardial protection from ischemic insult. This effect is seen at lower doses, and the mechanism is possibly related to myocar-

TABLE 87–5

Intravenous Anesthetics

GENERIC NAME	CLASS	CARDIOVASCULAR EFFECTS				NOTES/SIDE EFFECTS
		BP	HR	SVR	CO	
Thiopental	Thiobarbiturate	↓	↑	–/↓	–/↓	Venodilation, cerebral vasoconstriction
Methohexital	Oxybarbiturate	↓	↑	–/↓	–/↓	Venodilation, cerebral vasoconstriction
Midazolam	Benzodiazepine	–/↓	–/↑	–/↓	–/↓	Anxiolysis, sedation, amnesia
Morphine	Opioid	↓	↓	↓	–/↓	Histamine release
Fentanyl	Opioid	–/↓	↓	–/↓	–/↓	Chest wall rigidity
Sufentanil	Opioid	–/↓	↓	–/↓	–/↓	Chest wall rigidity
Remifentanil	Opioid	–/↓	↓	–/↓	–/↓	Chest wall rigidity
Meperidine	Opioid	↓	↑			Histamine release, antishivering
Ketamine	Phencyclidine	↑	↑	↑	↑	Dissociative anesthesia, analgesia
Etomidate	Imidazole derivative	–/↓	–/↓	–/↓	–	Adrenocortical suppression
Propofol	Phenol derivative	↓	–	↓	↓	Rapid recovery
Dexmedetomidine	α_2-Agonist	↓	↓	↓	↓	Sedation, sympatholysis, anxiolysis, analgesia
Clonidine	α_2-Agonist	↓	↓	↓	↓	Sedation, sympatholysis, anxiolysis, analgesia

–, No or minimal change; ↓, down; ↑, up; BP, arterial blood pressure; CO, cardiac output; HR, heart rate; SVR, systemic vascular resistance.

dial ischemic preconditioning.[50] Experimental evidence of reduced myocardial infarct size following periods of ischemia,[51] and clinical evidence of protection against postischemic left ventricular dysfunction,[52] have been reported. Prospective, controlled studies are necessary to determine whether inhalational agents improve patient outcomes in patients at risk for perioperative cardiac events. The use of isoflurane was considered controversial in patients with coronary artery anatomy that predisposes to coronary steal. Isoflurane has been shown to induce myocardial ischemia with collateral-dependent myocardial blood flow in canine models[53] and in humans.[54] The tachycardia and hypotension associated with isoflurane, as well as evidence of maldistributed myocardial blood flow, might suggest that it should not be used. Nevertheless, a prospective clinical study in patients with "steal-prone anatomy"[55] did not find intraoperative myocardial ischemia or poorer outcome with isoflurane anesthesia. A reasonable conclusion would be that isoflurane should be used with caution and appropriate monitoring in patients suspected of having "steal-prone" coronary artery anatomy. In light of the evidence that volatile anesthetics protect myocardium, the concerns regarding coronary steal have become negligible in clinical practice. Table 87–6 summarizes commonly used inhalational anesthetics in today's practice.

[ ] NEUROMUSCULAR BLOCKADE

Two major classes of nondepolarizing neuromuscular blocking drugs are used today: benzylisoquinolinium compounds and aminosteroid derivatives. The benzylisoquinolinium series of nondepolarizing neuromuscular blockers are all derivatives of the curare molecule. Atracurium and mivacurium are associated with clinically important histamine release following the administration of bolus doses to facilitate tracheal intubation. Cisatracurium is not associated with histamine release, even when large doses are given. Atracurium and cisatracurium undergo a unique form of spontaneous degradation that is organ-independent (Hofmann elimination). Mivacurium undergoes enzyme-dependent ester hydrolysis; consequently, prolonged duration of neuromuscular blockade can be seen in patients with pseudocholinesterase deficiency.

TABLE 87–6

Inhalational Anesthetics

INHALATIONAL AGENT	CARDIOVASCULAR EFFECTS				NOTES
	BP	HR	SVR	CO	
Nitrous oxide	–	–	–	–	Rapidly diffuses into closed air spaces
Halothane	↓	↓	–	↓	Hepatotoxicity; useful in tetralogy of Fallot hypercyanotic episodes, dysrhythmias especially when used in combination with epinephrine
Isoflurane	↓	↑	↓	–	Coronary steal clinically not significant
Desflurane	↓	–/↑	↓	–	Rapid induction and emergence, sympathomimetic during rapid induction
Sevoflurane	↓	–	↓	–	Preferred inhalational induction agent for children, nonpungent, potential nephrotoxicity

–, No or minimal change; ↓, down; ↑, up; BP, arterial blood pressure; CO, cardiac output; HR, heart rate; SVR, systemic vascular resistance.

Pancuronium is the classic aminosteroid nondepolarizing neuromuscular blocking drug. The atropine-like molecular structure contains two quaternary nitrogen groups. The tachycardia and hypertension associated with pancuronium have been linked to myocardial ischemia during coronary artery bypass surgery.[56] The anticholinergic effects of pancuronium, however, can be useful (e.g., in patients with mitral regurgitation) for preventing the increase in vagal tone that occurs with high-dose opioid anesthetic inductions. Vecuronium is structurally very similar to pancuronium, however, with a much shorter duration of action. Vecuronium does not have clinically significant cardiovascular side effects. Rocuronium has a more rapid onset of action because of its lower potency and slightly increases heart rate. Whereas pancuronium elimination is almost entirely renal, the newer compounds are mainly degraded by the liver.

Succinylcholine is a depolarizing short-acting neuromuscular blocker that is still used because of its low cost, rapid onset, and short duration of action. Its cardiovascular effects depend on whether nicotinic or muscarinic receptor effects predominate in a given patient. Thus tachycardia and hypertension or bradycardia and hypotension may occur. Vagal effects tend to predominate with repeated doses or in children. In patients with various disorders (including neuromuscular diseases, recent burns, and massive trauma), hyperkalemic cardiac arrest may occur with succinylcholine administration because of exaggerated release of intracellular potassium from myocytes.

THE POSTOPERATIVE PERIOD AND CARDIAC COMPLICATIONS

Emergence from anesthesia is frequently accompanied by hypertension and tachycardia, which is most often a result of incomplete analgesia, but may also be related to withdrawal from antihypertensive drugs, hypoxemia, delirium, or bladder distension. If an underlying modifiable cause is not identified, then intravenous drugs—such as nitroglycerin, labetalol, or esmolol—are frequently used to control hemodynamics in patients with cardiovascular disease. Shivering is another phenomenon that may occur as a consequence of hypothermia or emergence from volatile anesthetics. Shivering results in severe increases in oxygen consumption, which may be poorly tolerated by patients with cardiovascular disease. Although the mechanism is unknown, low doses of meperidine decrease or eliminate shivering.[57]

In patients with risk factors, there is a high incidence of postoperative complications, such as myocardial infarction, pulmonary edema, malignant ventricular arrhythmia, and cardiac death.[58] Pain, high catecholamine levels, hypercoagulability, hypovolemia, anemia, intravascular volume shifts, drug effects, and a lower level of monitoring all probably contribute to this phenomenon. There is increasing evidence from large meta-analysis and prospective studies, that the perioperative use of β-adrenergic blocking drugs,[59–63] the use of statins,[64–67] and α₂ agonists,[68,69] may decrease the incidence of these complications in high-risk patients.

Traditionally, the anesthesiologist has not played a major role in postoperative management following discharge from the postanesthesia care unit. This situation has changed with the development of multidisciplinary pain services that administer epidural analgesia and patient-controlled analgesia. As noted above, it remains controversial whether regional anesthesia and intensive postoperative analgesia are capable of reducing morbidity and mortality. It is conceivable that more effective postoperative analgesia decreases the deleterious effects of the stress response. Future efforts to reduce perioperative risk likely will concentrate on assessing the effects of more intensive perioperative hemodynamic, analgesic, and anticoagulation management.

CONCLUSIONS

The optimal perioperative care of patients with cardiovascular disease is the joint responsibility of anesthesiologists, surgeons, and cardiologist/internists. Any anesthetic agent or technique has the potential for producing adverse effects, and the margin of safety is reduced in patients with cardiovascular disease. It is the anesthesiologist's role to acquire accurate and relevant information from the preoperative evaluation, to apply appropriate monitoring technology, to select an anesthetic technique that is suited to the planned procedure and the condition of the patient, and to manage hemodynamic alterations and analgesic requirements in the perioperative period. As cardiovascular disease continues to become more prevalent in the surgical population and preoperative testing and intraoperative monitoring become more sophisticated, the need for effective communication between the specialties of cardiology and anesthesiology will become even more important.

REFERENCES

1. Goldman L , Caldera DL, Nussbaum SR, et al. Multifactorial index of cardiac risk in noncardiac surgical procedures. *N Engl J Med* 1977;297:845–850.
2. Gilbert K, Larocque BJ, Patrick LT. Prospective evaluation of cardiac risk indices for patients undergoing noncardiac surgery. *Ann Intern Med* 2000;133(5):356–359.
3. ACC/AHA guideline update for perioperative cardiovascular evaluation for noncardiac surgery—executive summary. A report of the American College of Cardiology/American Heart Association Task Force on Practice Guidelines (Committee to Update the 1996 Guidelines on Perioperative Cardiovascular Evaluation for Noncardiac Surgery). *Circulation* 2002;105(10):1257–1267.
4. Mangano DT, Goldman L. Preoperative assessment of patients with known or suspected coronary disease. *N Engl J Med* 1995;333:1750–1756.
5. Katz RI, Barnhart JM, Ho G, et al. A survey on the intended purposes and perceived utility of preoperative cardiology consultations. *Anesth Analg* 1998;87(4):830–836.
6. Kaluza GL, Joseph J, Lee JR, et al. Catastrophic outcome of noncardiac surgery soon after coronary stenting. *J Am Coll Cardiol* 2000;35:1288–1294.
7. Wilson SH, Fasseas P, Orford JL, et al. Clinical outcome of patients undergoing non-cardiac surgery in the two months following coronary stenting. *J Am Coll Cardiol* 2003;42:234–240.
8. Van Norman GA, Posner K. Coronary stenting or percutaneous transluminal coronary angioplasty prior to noncardiac surgery increases adverse perioperative cardiac events: the evidence is mounting. *J Am Coll Cardiol* 2000;36:2351.
9. Posner KL, Van Norman GA, Chan V. Adverse outcomes after noncardiac surgery in patients with prior percutaneous transluminal coronary angioplasty. *Anesth Analg* 1999;89:553.
10. Eagle KA, Berger PB, Calkins H, et al. ACC/AHA Guideline update for perioperative cardiovascular evaluation for noncardiac surgery—executive summary. A report of the American College of Cardiology/American Heart Association Task Force on Practice Guidelines (Committee to Update the 1996 Guidelines on Perioperative Cardiovascular Evaluation for Noncardiac Surgery). *Anesth Analg* 2002;94:1052–1064.
11. McFadden EP, Stabile E, Regar E, et al. Late thrombosis in drug-eluting coronary stents after discontinuation of antiplatelet therapy. *Lancet* 2004;364:1519–1521.

12. Sharma AK, Ajani AE, Manias P, et al. Coronary angioplasty with stenting preceding major noncardiac surgery: when is it safe to operate? *J Am Coll Cardiol* 2003;63:141–145.

13. Satler LF. Recommendations regarding stent selection in relation to the timing of noncardiac surgery postpercutaneous coronary intervention. *Catheter Cardiovasc Interv* 2004;63:146–147.

14. Mendoza CE, Virani SS, Shah N, et al. Noncardiac surgery following percutaneous coronary intervention. *Catheter Cardiovasc Interv* 2004;63:267–273.

15. American Society of Anesthesiologists. *Standards for Basic Intraoperative Monitoring* (Approved by House of Delegates on October 21, 1986 and last amended on October 21, 1998). Park Ridge, IL. Available at: http://www.asahq.org/publicationsAndServices/standards/02.html.

16. Reich DL, Mittnacht A, London M, Kaplan JA. Monitoring of the heart and vascular system. In: Kaplan JA, Reich DL, Lake CL, Konstadt SL, eds. *Kaplan's Cardiac Anesthesia*, 5th ed. Philadelphia: Elsevier, 2006:385–436.

17. Connors AF, Speroff T, Dawson NV, et al. The effectiveness of right heart catheterization in the initial care of critically ill patients. *JAMA* 1996;276:889–897.

18. Reich DL, Bodian CA, Krol M, et al. Intraoperative hemodynamic predictors of mortality, stroke and myocardial infarction following coronary artery bypass surgery. *Anesth Analg* 1999;88:814–822.

19. Sandham JD, Hull RD, Brant RF, et al. Canadian Critical Care Clinical Trials Group. A randomized, controlled trial of the use of pulmonary-artery catheters in high-risk surgical patients. N Engl J Med 2003;348:5–14.

20. Harvey S, Harrison DA, Singer M, et al. Assessment of the clinical effectiveness of pulmonary artery catheters in management of patients in intensive care (PAC-Man): a randomised controlled trial. Lancet 2005;366:472–477.

21. Shah MR, Hasselblad V, Stevenson LW, et al. Impact of the pulmonary artery catheter in critically ill patients: meta-analysis of randomized clinical trials. JAMA 2005;294:1664–1670.

22. Binanay C, Califf RM, Hasselblad V, et al. Evaluation study of congestive heart failure and pulmonary artery catheterization effectiveness: the ESCAPE trial. JAMA 2005;294:1625–1633.

23. Jacka M, Cohen MM, To T, et al. Pulmonary artery occlusion pressure estimation: how confident are anesthesiologists? Crit Care Med 2002;30:1197–1203.

24. Squara P, Bennett D, Perret C. Pulmonary artery catheter: does the problem lie in the users? Chest 2002;121:2009–2015.

25. Iberti TJ, Fischer EP, Leibowitz AB, et al. A multicenter study of physicians' knowledge of the pulmonary artery catheter. JAMA 1990;264:2928–2932.

26. American Society of Anesthesiologists. *Practice Guidelines For Pulmonary Artery Catheterization* (Approved by House of Delegates on October 21, 1992 and last amended October 16, 2002). American Society of Anesthesiologists, Park Ridge, IL. Available at: http://www.asahq.org/publicationsAndServices/pulm_artery.pdf.

27. Shanewise JS, Cheung AT, Aronson S, et al. ASE/SCA guidelines for performing a comprehensive intraoperative multiplane transesophageal echocardiography examination: recommendations of the American Society of Echocardiography Council for Intraoperative Echocardiography and the Society of Cardiovascular Anesthesiologists Task Force for Certification in Perioperative Transesophageal Echocardiography. *Anesth Analg* 1999;89:870–884.

28. Cahalan MK, Abel M, Goldman M, et al. American Society of Echocardiography and Society of Cardiovascular Anesthesiologists Task Force guidelines for training in perioperative echocardiography. *Anesth Analg* 2002;94:1384–1388.

29. American Society of Anesthesiologists. Practice guidelines for perioperative transesophageal echocardiography. *Anesthesiology* 1996;84:986–1006.

30. Cheitlin MD, Armstrong WF, Aurigemma GP, et al. ACC/AHA/ASE 2003 guideline update for the clinical application of echocardiography: summary article. A report of the American College of Cardiology/American Heart Association Task Force on Practice Guidelines (ACC/AHA/ASE Committee to Update the 1997 Guidelines for the Clinical Application of Echocardiography). *J Am Soc Echocardiogr* 2003;16:1091–1110.

31. Schmidt GN, Bischoff P, Standl T, et al. Comparative evaluation of Narcotrend, Bispectral Index, and classical electroencephalographic variables during induction, maintenance, and emergence of a propofol/remifentanil anesthesia. *Anesth Analg* 2004;98:1346–1353.

32. Sandin RH, Enlund G, Samuelsson P, et al. Awareness during anaesthesia: a prospective case study. *Lancet* 2000;355:707–711.

33. Sebel PS, Bowdle TA, Ghoneim MM, et al. The incidence of awareness during anesthesia: a multicenter United States study. *Anesth Analg* 2004;99:833–839.

34. Practice advisory for intraoperative awareness and brain function monitoring. A report by the American Society of Anesthesiologists Task Force on intraoperative awareness. *Anesthesiology* 2006;104:847–864.

35. Tuman KJ, McCarthy RJ, March RJ, et al. Effects of epidural anesthesia and analgesia on coagulation and outcome after major vascular surgery. *Anesth Analg* 1991;73:696–704.

36. Baron JF, Bertrand M, Barre E, et al. Combined epidural and general anesthesia versus general anesthesia for abdominal aortic surgery. *Anesthesiology* 1991;75:611–618.

37. Bode RH Jr, Lewis KP, Zarich SW, et al. Cardiac outcome after peripheral vascular surgery: comparison of general and regional anesthesia. *Anesthesiology* 1996;84:3–13.

38. Christopherson R, Beattie C, Frank SM, et al. Perioperative morbidity in patients randomized to epidural or general anesthesia for lower extremity vascular surgery. *Anesthesiology* 1993;79:422–434.

39. Mofidi R, Nimmo AF, Moores C, et al. Regional versus general anaesthesia for carotid endarterectomy: impact of change in practice. *Surgeon* 2006;4:158–162.

40. Verhoeven EL, Cina CS, Tielliu IF, et al. Local anesthesia for endovascular abdominal aortic aneurysm repair. *J Vasc Surg* 2005;42:402–409.

41. Parra JR, Crabtree T, McLafferty BB, et al. Anesthesia technique and outcomes of endovascular aneurysm repair. *Ann Vasc Surg* 2005;19:123–129.

42. Limberi S, Markou M, Sakayianni K, et al. Coronary artery disease and upper abdominal surgery: impact of anesthesia on perioperative myocardial ischemia. *Hepatogastroenterology* 2003;50:1814–1820.

43. Matot I, Oppenheim-Eden A, Ratrot R, et al. Preoperative cardiac events in elderly patients with hip fracture randomized to epidural or conventional analgesia. *Anesthesiology* 2003;98:156–163.

44. Bode RH Jr, Lewis KP, Zarrich SW, et al. Cardiac outcome after peripheral vascular surgery. Comparison of general and regional anesthesia. *Anesthesiology* 1996;84:3–13.

45. Christopherson R, Beattie C, Frank SM, et al. Perioperative morbidity in patients randomized to epidural or general anesthesia for lower extremity vascular surgery. Perioperative Ischemia Randomized Anesthesia Trial Study Group. *Anesthesiology* 1993;79:422–434.

46. Horlocker T, Wedel D. Neuraxial block and low molecular weight heparin: balancing perioperative analgesia and thromboprophylaxis. *Reg Anesth Pain Med* 1998;23:164–177.

47. Horlocker TT, Wedel DJ, Benzon H, et al. Regional Anesthesia in the anticoagulated patient: defining the risks (the second ASRA Consensus Conference on Neuraxial Anesthesia and Anticoagulation). *Reg Anesth Pain Med* 2003;28:172–197.

48. American Society of Regional Anesthesia. *Recommendations for Neuraxial Anesthesia and Anticoagulation*. Available at: http://www.asra.com/items_of_interest/consensus_statements/.

49. Lawton MT, Porter RW, Heiserman JE, et al. Surgical management of spinal epidural hematoma: relationship between surgical timing and neurological outcome. *J Neurosurg* 1995;83:1–7.

50. De Hert SG, Turani F, Mathur S, Stowe DS. Cardioprotection with volatile anesthetics: mechanisms and clinical implications. *Anesth Analg* 2005;100:1584–1593.

51. Cope DK, Impastato WK, Cohen MV, Downey JM. Volatile anesthetics protect the ischemic rabbit myocardium from infarction. *Anesthesiology* 1997;86:699–709.

52. De Hert SG, ten Broecke PW, Mertens E, et al. Sevoflurane but not propofol preserves myocardial function in coronary surgery patients. *Anesthesiology* 2002;97:42–49.

53. Buffington CW, Romson JL, Levine A, et al. Isoflurane induces coronary steal in a canine model of chronic coronary occlusion. *Anesthesiology* 1987;66:280–292.

54. Reiz S, Balfors E, Sorensen MB, et al. Isoflurane: a powerful coronary vasodilator in patients with coronary artery disease. *Anesthesiology* 1983;59:91–97.

55. Pulley DD, Kirvassilis GV, Kelermenos N, et al. Regional and global myocardial circulatory and metabolic effects of isoflurane and halothane in patients with steal-prone coronary anatomy. *Anesthesiology* 1991;75:756–766.

56. Thomson IR, Putnins CL. Adverse effects of pancuronium during high-dose fentanyl anesthesia for coronary artery bypass grafting. *Anesthesiology* 1985;62:708–713.

57. De Witte J, Sessler DI. Perioperative shivering: physiology and pharmacology. *Anesthesiology* 2002;96:467–484.

58. Mackey WC, Fleisher LA, Haider S, et al. Perioperative myocardial ischemic injury in high-risk vascular surgery patients: incidence and clinical significance in a prospective clinical trial. *J Vasc Surg* 2006;43:533–538.

59. Fleisher LA, Beckman JA, Brown KA, et al. ACC/AHA 2006 guideline update on perioperative cardiovascular evaluation for noncardiac surgery: focused update on perioperative beta-blocker therapy. A report of the Ameri-

can College of Cardiology/American Heart Association Task Force on Practice Guidelines (Writing Committee to Update the 2002 Guidelines on Perioperative Cardiovascular Evaluation for Noncardiac Surgery) developed in collaboration with the American Society of Echocardiography, American Society of Nuclear Cardiology, Heart Rhythm Society, Society of Cardiovascular Anesthesiologists, Society for Cardiovascular Angiography and Interventions, and Society for Vascular Medicine and Biology. *Circulation* 2006;113:2662–2674.

60. Mangano DT, Layug EL, Wallace A, et al. Effect of atenolol on mortality and cardiovascular morbidity after noncardiac surgery. Multicenter Study of Perioperative Ischemia Research Group. *N Engl J Med* 1996;335:1713–1720.

61. Poldermans D, Boersma E, Bax JJ, et al. The effect of bisoprolol on perioperative mortality and myocardial infarction in high-risk patients undergoing vascular surgery. Dutch Echocardiographic Cardiac Risk Evaluation Applying Stress Echocardiography Study Group. *N Engl J Med* 1999;341:1789–1794.

62. Schouten O, Shaw LJ, Boersma E, et al. A meta-analysis of safety and effectiveness of perioperative beta-blocker use for the prevention of cardiac events in different types of noncardiac surgery. *Coron Artery Dis* 2006;17:173–179.

63. Devereaux DJ, Beattie WS, Choi PT, et al. How strong is the evidence for the use of perioperative beta blockers in non-cardiac surgery? Systematic review and meta-analysis of randomised controlled trials. *BMJ* 2005;331:313–321.

64. Hindler K, Eltzschik HK, Fox AA, et al. Influence of statins on perioperative outcomes. *Cardiothorac Vasc Anesth* 2006;20:251–258.

65. Kertai MD, Boersma E, Westerhout CM, et al. A combination of statins and beta-blockers is independently associated with a reduction in the incidence of perioperative mortality and nonfatal myocardial infarction in patients undergoing abdominal aortic aneurysm surgery. *Eur J Vasc Endovasc Surg* 2004;28:343–352.

66. Durazzo AE, Machado FS, Ikeoka DT, et al. Reduction in cardiovascular events after vascular surgery with atorvastatin: a randomized trial. *J Vasc Surg* 2004;39:967–975.

67. O'Neil-CallahanK, Katsimaglis G, Tepper MR, et al. Statins decrease perioperative cardiac complications in patients undergoing noncardiac vascular surgery: the Statins for Risk Reduction in Surgery (StaRRS) study. *J Am Coll Cardiol* 2005;45:336–342.

68. Oliver MF, Goldman L, Julian DG, Holme I. Effect of mivazerol on perioperative cardiac complications during non-cardiac surgery in patients with coronary heart disease: the European Mivazerol Trial (EMIT). *Anesthesiology* 1999;91:951–961.

69. Wijeysundera DN, Naik JS, Beattie WS. Alpha-2 adrenergic agonists to prevent perioperative cardiovascular complications: a meta-analysis. *Am J Med* 2003;114:742–752.

PART 15 Miscellaneous Conditions and Cardiovascular Disease

CHAPTER (88)

The Connective Tissue Diseases and the Cardiovascular System

Jose F. Roldan / Robert A. O'Rourke / William C. Roberts

The term *connective tissue disease* includes both a group of heritable conditions and a group of nonheritable acquired disorders. The heritable disorders of connective tissue associated with cardiovascular disease include the Marfan syndrome, Loeys-Dietz syndrome, Ehlers-Danlos syndrome (EDS), pseudoxanthoma elasticum (PXE), osteogenesis imperfecta, annuloaortic ectasia, and familial aneurysms.[1] The nonheritable disorders of connective tissue that may involve the cardiovascular system include systemic lupus erythematosus (SLE), polyarteritis nodosa, rheumatoid arthritis (RA), ankylosing spondylitis (AS), systemic sclerosis, polymyositis and dermatomyositis, giant-cell arteritis, Churg-Strauss syndrome, antiphospholipid syndrome, and possibly syphilis.

HERITABLE CONNECTIVE TISSUE DISEASES

【 】 MARFAN SYNDROME

Epidemiology

The prevalence of classic Marfan syndrome approximates 5 per 100,000 persons worldwide, without gender, racial, or ethnic predilection. Considering the great heterogeneity of the syndrome, the actual prevalence may be considerably greater, at about 1 per 10,000 persons.[2] Marfan syndrome has an autosomal dominant inheritance with high penetrance. In one-third of patients, the disorder occurs with no positive family history and is likely caused by a new mutation.

Molecular Genetics

Marfan syndrome is associated with defects in the fibrillin-1 gene (FBN1) on chromosome 15, where more than 125 reported and unreported mutations (of several types) have been described (see Chap. 81).[3–6] More recently, a mutation of the transforming growth factor (TGF) β receptor 2 (TGFBR2) and TGFβ receptor 1 (TGFBR1) has been identified in 10 percent of the cases.[7,8] Nearly every genotyped family has a unique mutation in the fibrillin genes, with the most common single mutation identified in just four unrelated pedigrees. This intragenic heterogenicity and the large size of the gene have precluded the routine screening of mutations to establish the diagnosis of the Marfan syndrome. Genetic testing is most helpful if (1) a mutation is detected in either of the two genes and (2) informative data are available about the phenotype of the patient's family.

Clinical Features

Considerable variation in the clinical manifestations of Marfan syndrome occurs even within the same family. The ocular, skeletal, and cardiovascular systems are usually involved. The four major manifestations include a positive family history, ectopia lentis, aortic root dilatation or dissection, and dural ectasia (see Chap. 12). Other relatively mild characteristics of Marfan syndrome occur with a relatively high prevalence in the general population. These features include mitral valve prolapse (MVP), early myopia, scoliosis, and joint hypermobility. Other findings in Marfan syndrome

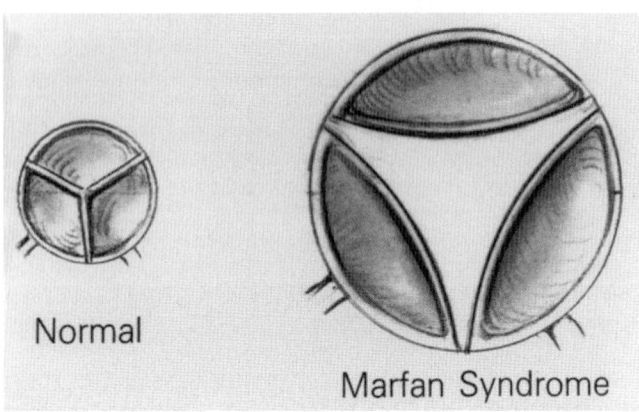

FIGURE 88–1. Mechanism of aortic regurgitation in the Marfan syndrome.

include anterior chest deformity, especially asymmetric pectus excavatum or carinatum; long, thin extremities with arachnodactyly; tall stature with increased lower body height; high, narrowly arched palate; myopia; fusiform ascending aortic aneurysm (*anuloaortic ectasia*) with aortic regurgitation (Fig. 88–1); and/or aortic dissection. Mitral regurgitation is caused by MVP, dilatation of the mitral annulus, mitral annular calcium, rupture of mitral chordae tendineae, papillary muscle dysfunction, infective endocarditis, or the combination of two or more.[1–3]

In the absence of an unequivocally affected first-degree relative, requirements for the diagnosis include at least one major manifestation with involvement of the skeleton and at least two other systems.[6–8] In the presence of at least one unequivocally affected first-degree relative, there should be involvement of at least two systems; the presence of a major manifestation is still preferred, but this can vary depending on the family's phenotype.[9]

By echocardiogram, MVP occurs in 60 percent or more and aortic root enlargement in approximately 70 percent of adults with the Marfan syndrome. It has been suggested that the Marfan syndrome and MVP are part of a phenotypic continuum.

General Evaluation

In addition to carefully recording the personal and family history and physical examination, the patient's height, arm span, and floor-to-pelvis distance should be measured. A slit-lamp ophthalmic examination and an electrocardiograph (ECG) should be obtained. Patients with Marfan syndrome should be evaluated at least yearly, and a transthoracic echocardiogram (TTE) should be obtained annually. Usually a transesophageal echocardiogram (TEE) or magnetic resonance imaging (MRI) will be obtained at least once.[10] If the diagnosis is definite or probable, screening of first-degree relatives by TTE is recommended. Genetic counseling should be offered to all patients. Psychiatric counseling also is often useful. If a patient develops suggestive widening of the proximal aorta, repeat TTE or, in some instances, TEE should be performed more frequently. Patients with possible or definite Marfan syndrome and evidence of mitral valve abnormality should receive standard antibiotic prophylaxis prior to any surgical procedure (see Chap. 88).

Management

Patients with Marfan syndrome should avoid isometric, abrupt, or strenuous exertion; contact sports; scuba diving; and trauma. Pa-

tients with aortic dilatation and aortic or mitral regurgitation should avoid competitive sports.[11,12] Patients without aortic dilatation and aortic or mitral regurgitation should be allowed to perform low-to-moderate intensity static and low-intensity dynamic sports, including bowling, golf, and archery. β-Adrenergic blockade therapy should be used in all patients, including in children with Marfan syndrome, to retard the rate of dilatation of the aortic root.[12–14] Although the optimal dose has not been established, some have suggested giving the largest dose that is clinically tolerated. Selective β$_1$-adrenergic blocking agents are preferred, although no randomized studies have been performed.

In asymptomatic patients, repair of aortic aneurysms has been recommended at different degrees of enlargement. Thus, some have advocated repair when the aortic diameter is 55 mm or greater, when it is 60 mm or greater,[15] or when the aortic diameter increases to twice that of the uninvolved distal aorta. Some patients develop aortic dissection with aortic root dimensions less than 50 to 55 mm.[15] Surgical repair is generally recommended when the diameter reaches 55 to 60 mm (see Chap. 105) and probably earlier if there is rapid progression or a family history of aortic dissection or rupture.[16] The asymmetry of the aortic root as visualized by MRI might be of clinical importance in the diagnosis of unexpected aortic root dissection.[17]

Factors resulting in earlier surgical intervention include a positive family history for aortic dissection or rupture, severe aortic or mitral regurgitation, progressive dilatation of the aortic root on serial echocardiograms, need for other major abdominal aortic or spinal surgical procedures, and planning for a pregnancy. In most patients, the ascending aorta and aortic valve are replaced, and the portion of the aorta containing the coronary ostia is reimplanted,[18] but there are exceptions.[19] Coronary ostial aneurysms have been observed in 43 percent of 40 patients with Marfan syndrome after coronary artery implantation.[20] Postoperatively annual assessment of the entire aorta by MRI may be useful (see Chap. 105).

When a mitral valve procedure is necessary, valve repair is usually preferred to replacement, although repair often may not be possible because of a large number of ruptured chordae tendineae, extensive annular calcium, or greatly dilated annuli.

Prognosis

Although earlier studies indicated that the average patient's lifetime is decreased by approximately 35 percent,[2] β-blocker therapy, endocarditis prophylaxis, and aorta and aortic valve surgery have probably improved longevity. The most common causes of death of adolescents or adults with Marfan syndrome are rupture of a fusiform aneurysm of the ascending aorta without longitudinal dissection (Fig. 88–2), ascending aortic dissection with rupture, or congestive heart failure from aortic and/or mitral regurgitation (Fig. 88–3).[15] The major histologic feature in the media of the wall of an aortic aneurysm is a massive loss of elastic fibers (Fig. 88–4).[15] Factors that can predispose to either aortic aneurysm or aortic dissection include systemic arterial hypertension, coarctation of the aorta, pregnancy, and trauma. In children with Marfan syndrome, the most common cause of death is severe mitral regurgitation (Fig. 88–5). In a longitudinal study of 70 patients with Marfan syndrome followed for 24 years, no patient died of aortic dissection whereas 4 percent died of arrhythmias.[21] Athletes with Marfan syndrome must be counseled about the type of exercise that is permitted (Table 88–1).[22]

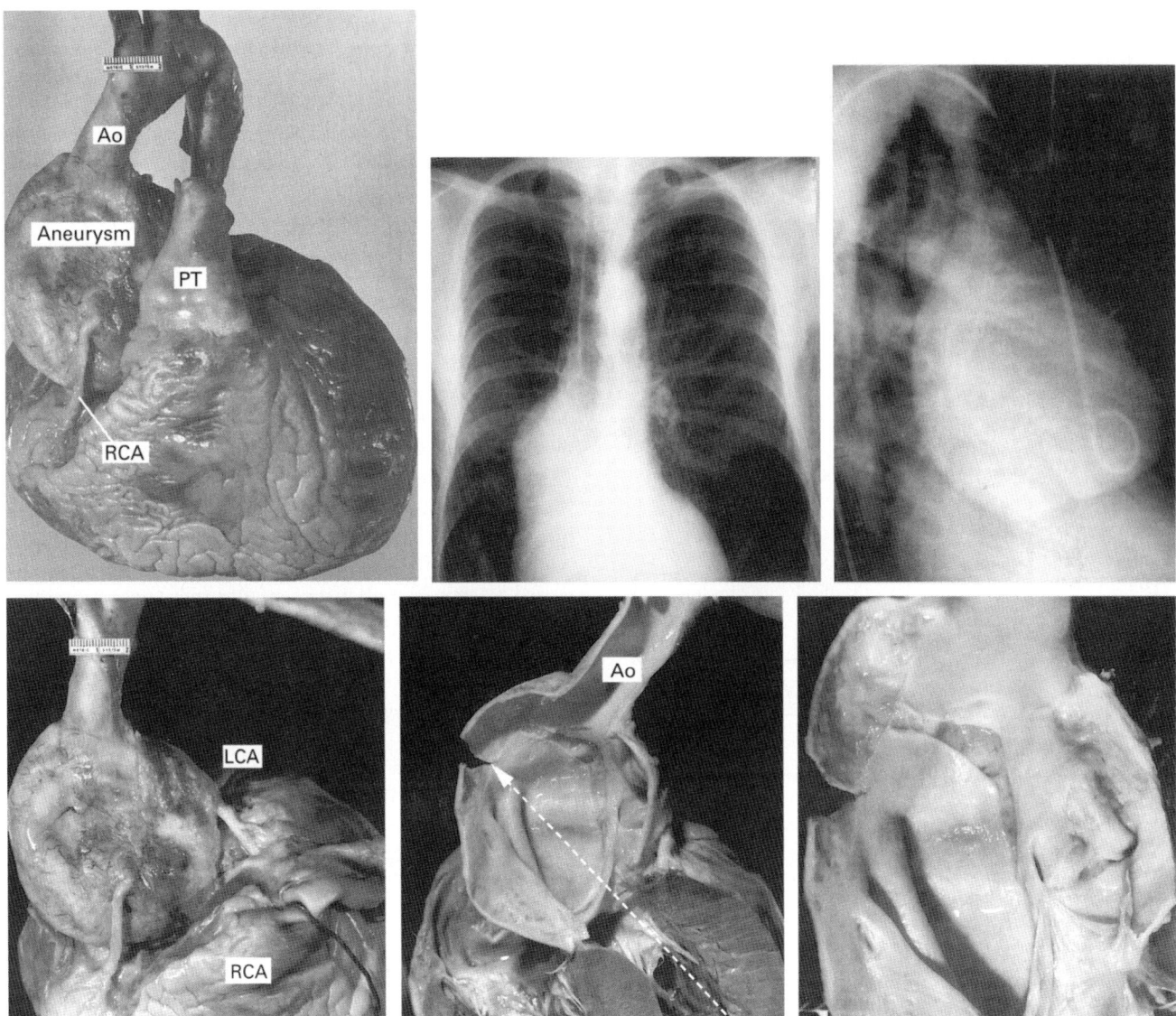

FIGURE 88–2. Heart and aorta of a 38-year-old man who was asymptomatic until exertional dyspnea appeared 5 months before death. *Top left:* Exterior view. Ao, ascending aorta; PT, pulmonary trunk; RCA, right coronary artery. *Bottom left:* Closer view of the massive aortic aneurysm after retracting the pulmonary trunk. LCA, left main coronary artery. The aneurysm does not involve the distal portion of the ascending aorta. *Bottom middle:* View of heart and aorta after removing their anterior half. Death resulted from rupture of the right lateral wall of the aorta at a point where blood ejected from the left ventricle contacts the aortic wall (*arrow*). The aneurysmal bulge is mainly to the right. *Bottom right:* Close-up of the multiple healed tears in the ascending aorta. One of the previously incomplete tears ruptured through and through. Posteroanterior chest roentgenogram (*top middle*) and lateral aortogram (*top right*) show massive dilatation of the ascending aorta. *Source: From Roberts WC, Honig HS. The spectrum of cardiovascular disease in the Marfan syndrome: a clinico-morphologic study of 18 necropsy patients and comparison to 151 previously reported necropsy patients. Am Heart J 1982;104:115–135. Reproduced with permission of the publisher and authors.*

Pregnancy

Women with Marfan syndrome should be counseled regarding the up to 50 percent risk of genetic transmission of the condition. If the woman has moderate or severe aortic regurgitation or an aortic root diameter exceeding 40 mm, she should be advised against pregnancy. Women with an aortic root diameter of less than 40 mm usually tolerate pregnancy well, but the chance of aortic dissection is still increased by pregnancy. β-Adrenergic blockers should be administered at least from the midtrimester onward.

During pregnancy, TEE should be performed every 6 to 10 weeks, depending on the initial findings. Using epidural anesthesia, vaginal delivery in the lateral decubitus position is preferred, and forceps or vacuum delivery is recommended to shorten the second stage of la-

bor. The increases in systemic blood pressure during uterine contractions should be prevented with β-blocking agents. Postpartum hemorrhage should be anticipated. If fetal maturity can be confirmed in a patient who requires aortic surgery during pregnancy, a cesarean section can be done before or concomitantly with thoracic surgery.

LOEYS-DIETZ SYNDROME

Mutations in the genes encoding TGFβ receptors 1 and 2 (TGFBR1 and TGFBR2, respectively) were recently found in association with a continuum of clinical features. On the mild end, the mutations were found in association with a presentation similar to that of Marfan syndrome or with familial thoracic aortic aneurysm

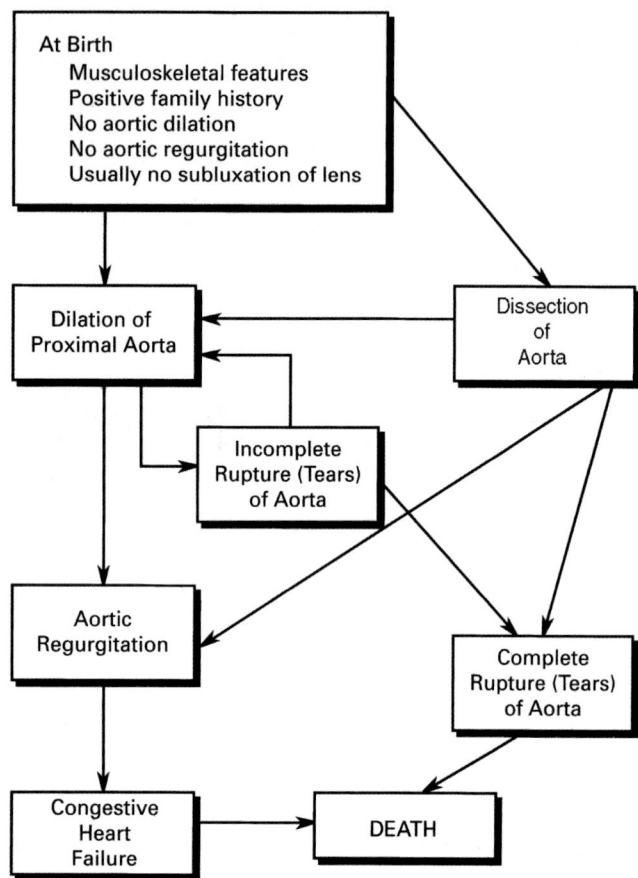

FIGURE 88–3. Scheme of development of cardiovascular complications in the Marfan syndrome. *Source: From Roberts WC, Honig HS. The spectrum of cardiovascular disease in the Marfan syndrome: a clinico-morphologic study of 18 necropsy patients and comparison to 151 previously reported necropsy patients. Am Heart J 1982;104:115–135. Reproduced with permission of the publisher and authors.*

and dissection,[23,24] and, on the severe end, they are associated with a complex phenotype in which aortic dissection or rupture commonly occurs in childhood.[25] This complex phenotype is characterized by the triad of hypertelorism; a bifid uvula, cleft palate, or both; and generalized arterial tortuosity with widespread vascular aneurysm and dissection. Previously described in 10 families, the phenotype has been classified as the Loeys-Dietz syndrome.

The disease is caused by heterozygous mutations in the genes encoding TGFBR1 and TGFBR2. Loeys et al.[26] undertook the clinical and molecular characterization of 52 affected families. Forty probands presented with typical manifestations of the Loeys-Dietz syndrome. In view of the phenotypic overlap between this syndrome and vascular Ehlers-Danlos syndrome, the investigators screened an additional cohort of 40 patients who had vascular Ehlers-Danlos syndrome without the characteristic type III collagen abnormalities or the craniofacial features of the Loeys-Dietz syndrome.

A mutation in TGFBR1 or TGFBR2 was found in all probands with typical Loeys-Dietz syndrome (type I) and in 12 probands presenting with vascular Ehlers-Danlos syndrome (Loeys-Dietz syndrome type II). The natural history of both types was characterized by aggressive arterial aneurysms (mean age at death: 26.0 years) and a high incidence of pregnancy-related complications (in 6 to 12 women). Patients with Loeys-Dietz syndrome type I, as compared with those with type II, underwent cardiovascular surgery earlier (mean age: 16.9 years vs. 26.9 years) and died earlier (22.6 years vs. 31.8 years). There were 59 vascular surgeries in the cohort, with 1 death during the procedure. This low rate of intra-operative mortality distinguishes the Loeys-Dietz syndrome from vascular Ehlers-Danlos syndrome.

Mutations in either TGFBR1 or TGFBR2 predispose patients to aggressive and widespread vascular disease. The severity of the clinical presentation is predictive of the outcome. Genotyping of patients presenting with symptoms like those of vascular Ehlers-Danlos syndrome may be used to guide therapy, including the use and timing of prophylactic vascular surgery.

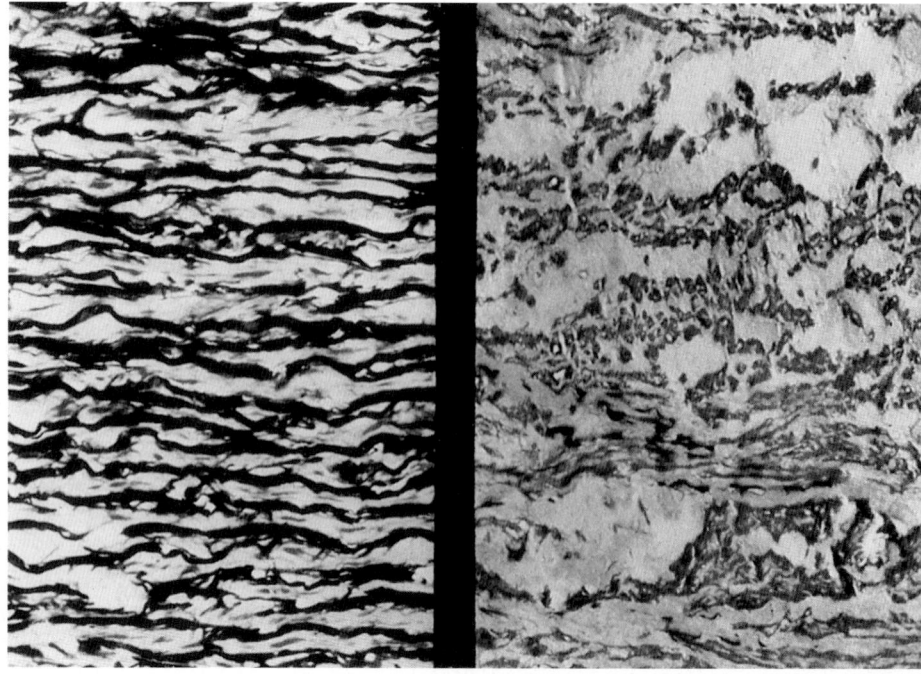

FIGURE 88–4. *Left:* Photomicrograph of the wall of the ascending aorta from a normal subject. *Right:* A similar histologic study (Movat stains) of the wall of an ascending aortic aneurysm in a 35-year-old woman with the Marfan syndrome. Note the virtual absence of elastic fibers. *Source: From Roberts WC, Honig HS. The spectrum of cardiovascular disease in the Marfan syndrome: a clinico-morphologic study of 18 necropsy patients and comparison to 151 previously reported necropsy patients. Am Heart J 1982;104:115–135. Reproduced with permission of the publisher and authors.*

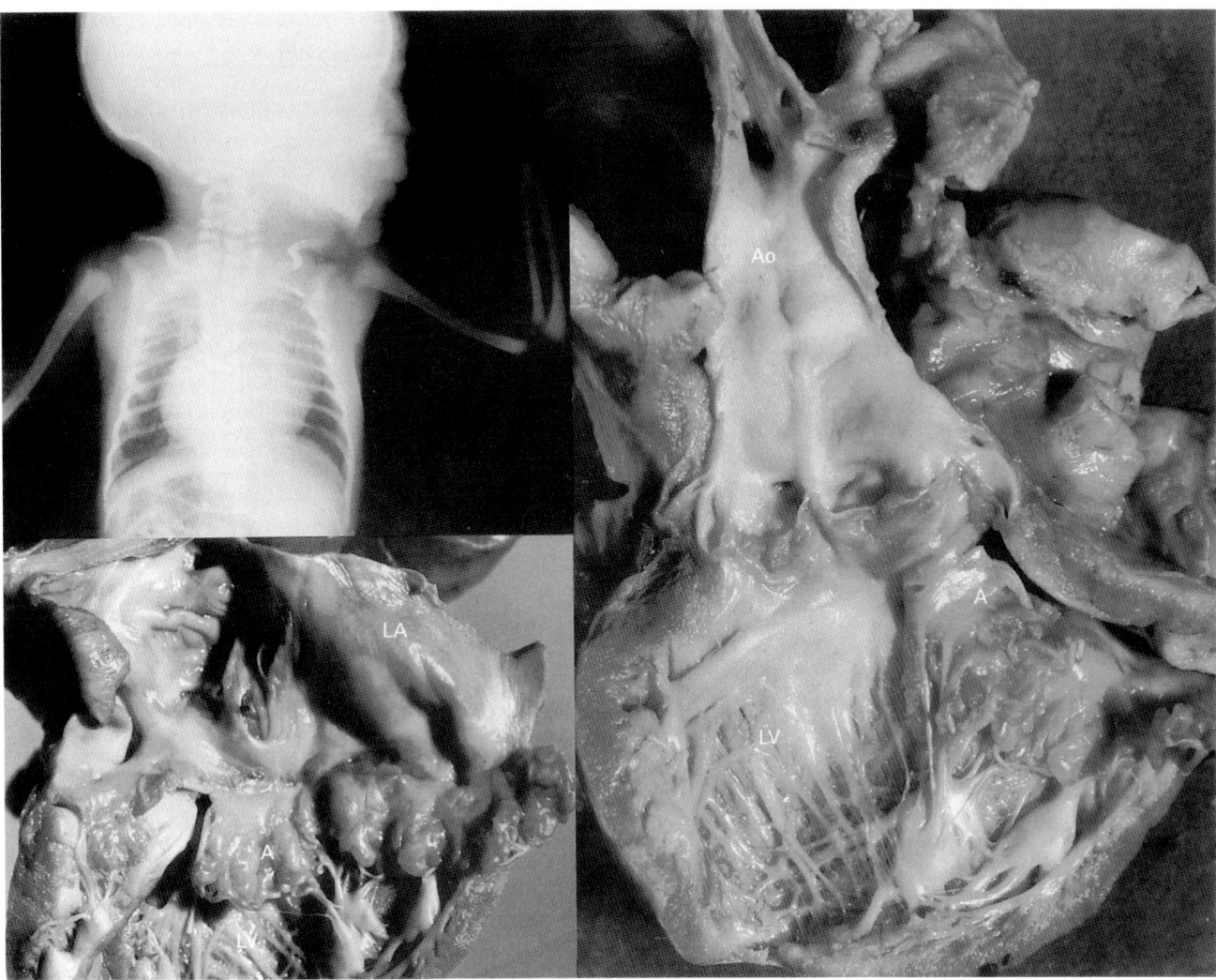

FIGURE 88-5. Congenital floppy mitral valve and floppy tricuspid valve in a 2-day-old boy who had long toes and fingers, a high-arched palate, and a grade 3/6 precordial systolic murmur typical of mitral regurgitation. The heart was enlarged (*top left*), and he died of congestive cardiac failure. At necropsy, the intima of the ascending aorta (Ao) was wrinkled (*right*), suggesting that the underlying media was abnormal at this early stage. Shown here are the opened aorta, aortic valve, and left ventricle (LV). A, anterior mitral leaflet. *Bottom left:* Opened left atrium (LA), mitral valve, and LV. The mitral leaflets are considerably elongated in both longitudinal and transverse dimensions. The left atrium is dilated. *Source: From Roberts WC, Honig HS. The spectrum of cardiovascular disease in the Marfan syndrome: a clinico-morphologic study of 18 necropsy patients and comparison to 151 previously reported necropsy patients. Am Heart J 1982;104:115–135. Reproduced with permission of the publisher and author.*

Affected patients have a high risk of aortic dissection or rupture at any early age and at aortic diameters that ordinarily would not be predictive of these events. Surgical intervention is generally successful, and this characteristic distinguishes patients with the Loeys-Dietz syndrome from those with vascular Ehlers-Danlos syndrome, a differential diagnosis often considered in patients with mutations in TGFBR1 and TGFBR2. The importance of careful clinical and molecular characterization to identify patients and families at risk for arterial dissection and rupture cannot be overemphasized, because it allows the use of a structured approach to intervention and leads to informed counseling regarding the risk of recurrence, concerns related to pregnancy, and guidelines for clinical management.

【 】 EHLERS-DANLOS SYNDROME

EDS is a heterogeneous group of several disorders of connective tissue that are characterized primarily by skin fragility, easy bruising, "cigarette paper" scars, skin hyperextensibility, multiple ecchymoses,

and joint hypermobility.[1] Because of the complexity of previous classifications, in 1997 a new simplified classification divided EDS into 6 clinical types[27]: (1) classical, (2) hypermobility, (3) vascular, (4) kyphoscoliosis, (5) arthrochalasia, and (6) dermatosparaxis.

The numerous types of the EDS have different clinical manifestations, modes of inheritance, and natural history (see Chap. 81). In vascular type III EDS, the heart, heart valves, great vessels, and larger conduit arteries may be involved. Cardiovascular abnormalities in the EDS include spontaneous rupture of the aorta or large arteries, coronary or intracranial aneurysms, arteriovenous fistulae, mitral and tricuspid valve prolapse, dilatation of the aortic root, ectasia of the sinuses of Valsalva, aortic regurgitation, renal artery aneurysms, systemic arterial hypertension, and myocardial infarction.[28–30]

【 】 PSEUDOXANTHOMA ELASTICUM

PXE is a rare heritable disorder that is characterized by the progressive accumulation of mineral precipitates within elastic fibers, particularly

TABLE 88-1

Task Force 4 Recommendations for Athletes with Marfan Syndrome

1. Athletes with Marfan syndrome can participate in low and moderate static/low dynamic competitive sports (classes IA and IIA) if they do not have one or more of the following:
   (a) An aortic root dilatation (i.e., transverse dimension 40 mm or greater in adults, or more than 2 standard deviations from the mean for body surface area in children and adolescents; z-score of 2 or more);
   (b) Moderate-to-severe mitral regurgitation;
   (c) Family history of dissection or sudden death in a Marfan relative.
   It is recommended, however, that these athletes have an echocardiographic measurement of aortic root dimension repeated every 6 months, for close surveillance of aortic enlargement.
2. Athletes with unequivocal aortic root dilatation (transverse dimension 40 mm or greater in adults or greater than 2 standard deviations beyond the mean for body surface area in children and adolescents; z-score of 2 or more), prior surgical aortic root reconstruction, chronic dissection of aorta or other artery, moderate-to-severe mitral regurgitation, or family history of dissection or sudden death can participate only in low-intensity competitive sports (class IA).
3. Athletes with Marfan syndrome, familial aortic aneurysm or dissection, or congenital bicuspid aortic valve with any degree of ascending aortic enlargement (as defined in 1 and 2 above) also should not participate in sports that involve the potential for bodily collision.

SOURCE: *From Maron BJ. Heart disease and other causes of sudden death in young athletes. Curr Probl Cardiol 1998;23:477–529 with permission.*

those of the skin, Bruch's membrane, and blood vessels. It is transmitted either as an autosomal recessive or as an autosomal dominant trait.[1,31] The estimated prevalence is 1 in 160,000 (see Chap. 81).

The elastic fiber changes cause skin, eye, gastrointestinal, and cardiovascular manifestations. The skin lesions have been described as resembling a "plucked chicken." Typically, there are yellow macules or papules that produce a rough, cobblestone texture and are maximal in the flexures of the lateral neck, axillae, antecubital fossae, groins, and popliteal spaces. They may form redundant folds of skin.[1] The retinal changes include mottled *peau d'orange* hyperpigmentation, angioid streaks, and an increased incidence of retinal hemorrhage and disk drusen. Angioid streaks, caused by breaks in the Bruch membrane behind the retina, are present in 85 percent of patients with PXE and usually develop after the second decade of life. They can be found in numerous other conditions, including Marfan syndrome, EDS, Paget disease, and sickle cell anemia, although PXE is the most common.

It is now recognized that a mutation in the gene ABCC6 (R1141X) is associated with an increased incidence of coronary artery disease (CAD) in patients with PXE. In a study of 441 patients a significant odds ratio for a coronary event was 4.23.[31]

There may be calcific deposits in the media of medium-size arteries. Both vascular deposits similar to Mönckeberg arteriosclerosis and intimal plaques similar to typical atherosclerotic plaques occur in the coronary, cerebral, gastrointestinal, renal, and peripheral arteries. Angina pectoris and myocardial infarction may occur.

Infrequent but fairly specific lesions in PXE are calcific deposits in the mural endocardium of the cardiac ventricles, atria, and atrioventricular valves. Both mitral stenosis and MVP have been described in PXE. Surgery to remove mural endocardial calcific deposits has been performed with fair results. Bleeding may occur in the gastrointestinal system, uterus, joints, and urinary bladder and may be prevented by avoiding aspirin. Coronary artery bypass surgery arterial grafts should not be used because of possible calcification of the internal elastic laminae.

OSTEOGENESIS IMPERFECTA

Osteogenesis imperfecta, also known as *brittle bone disease* because of susceptibility to sustain fractures from mild trauma, is a rare heritable disorder of connective tissue. The gene prevalence of osteogenesis imperfecta is calculated as 4 to 5 per 100,000 persons; it is inherited in an autosomal dominant fashion with variable penetrance. More than 80 different mutations have been identified in the genes for either of the two chains that form type I collagen, which is the major structural protein of the extracellular matrix of bone, skin, and tendon. There is a wide variation in its clinical severity, from some forms that are lethal in the perinatal period to other forms that may not be detected.[32] Most manifestations of osteogenesis imperfecta are bony, ocular, otologic, cutaneous, and dental. The bony changes may result in short stature, in utero fractures, severe osteoporosis, and severe bone fragility, with repeated fractures and bowing of long bones. The ocular and otologic changes include blue sclerae, angioid streaks in the retina, and hearing loss. Cutaneous and dental changes result in easy bruising and occasional dentinogenesis imperfecta. An increased risk of bleeding may also be present. A major advance in the treatment of bone manifestations of osteogenesis imperfecta is the use of cyclic administration of biphosphonates.[33]

The cardiovascular manifestations include aortic regurgitation,[32] aortic root dilatation,[32] aortic dissection, and mitral regurgitation.[34] Mitral valve repair and reconstruction are occasionally feasible for patients with severe mitral regurgitation, although most patients require valve replacement. Mitral valve replacement or any cardiac surgery is difficult because of weakness and friability of the tissues and poor wound healing. In addition, some patients have increased bleeding despite normal preoperative coagulation tests and bleeding times.[35]

ANNULOAORTIC ECTASIA

Annuloaortic ectasia, a pear-shaped enlargement of the sinus and the proximal tubular portions of the ascending aorta, is often part of Marfan syndrome, where it usually results in aortic regurgitation, partial or complete ascending aortic tears, or both. In some patients, annuloaortic ectasia is familial and no other stigmata of Marfan syndrome are present. The genetic and molecular changes in these patients are not established. Microscopically, there is severe loss of elastic fibers in the media of the ascending aorta.

❲ ❳ FAMILIAL ANEURYSMS

Various types of familial aneurysms involving cardiovascular structures have been reported, including familial aortic dissection, familial aneurysms of the ventricular septum, familial aneurysms of the carotid arteries, and familial intracranial aneurysms. At this time, it is not established that these are heritable disorders of connective tissue.

❲ ❳ HOMOCYSTINURIA

See Chap. 51.

NONHERITABLE CONNECTIVE TISSUE DISEASES

The acquired or nonheritable autoimmune or connective tissue diseases are a subset of the arthritides and rheumatic disorders. These disorders are systemic in nature, are commonly linked by a diffuse abnormality of vasculature, and are characterized by inflammatory lesions in skin, joints, muscles, and connective tissue linings such as pleura and pericardium. Involvement of the kidneys, brain, and heart is usually responsible for the fatal and most serious consequences. Specific acquired connective tissue diseases that may have major cardiac involvement include SLE, polyarteritis nodosa, giant cell arteritis, RA, ankylosing spondylitis, polymyositis and dermatomyositis, systemic sclerosis, and, possibly, syphilis (Table 88–2). Although certain immunogenetic factors have been identified, their etiology remains uncertain.

❲ ❳ SYSTEMIC LUPUS ERYTHEMATOSUS

SLE is found worldwide and affects all races, is more common among blacks, Asians, Hispanic Americans and females of childbearing age, and is usually more severe in blacks than in whites. SLE is more common among females than among males; in patients younger than 40 years of age, the female-to-male ratio is about 8:1. In pediatric and older patients, the female-to-male ratio is 2:1. In the United States, the annual incidence of SLE is about 8 per 100,000 persons, and the prevalence is approximately 1 per 2,000 persons. The following genes of the human leukocyte antigen (HLA) are associated with an increased risk for SLE: HLA-B8, HLA-DR2, HLA-DR3, HLA-DR5, HLA-DR7, HLA-DQ, and

null alleles at the C2 and/or C4 loci. Genetic deficiencies of the complement system—that is, deficiencies of C1q, C2, C4, and C8—predispose individuals to SLE and SLE-like disorders. Homozygous C4a deficiency is present in 80 percent of people with SLE irrespective of the ethnic background.[36]

The inflammatory process of SLE involves multiple organ systems, including skin, joints, kidneys, brain, heart, and virtually all serous membranes. Its clinical presentation is varied and depends on the organ systems involved. Fever, arthritis and arthralgias, skin rashes (see Fig. 12–21), and pleuritis are common early signs of SLE.

The immunologic abnormalities of SLE have been well characterized and enable it to be diagnosed despite the diversity of clinical presentations. Typical serologic abnormalities include the presence of antinuclear antibodies (ANAs), positive serum anti-DNA antibodies, positive anti-Smith antibodies, positive anti-ribonucleoprotein (anti-RNP) antibodies, and a falsely reactive Venereal Disease Research Laboratory (VDRL) test. Low C3 and C4 serum complement levels are usually markers of disease activity, especially of renal disease. Other connective tissue diseases, such as rheumatoid arthritis and scleroderma, may present with normal or elevated complement levels. Disseminated infections usually present with elevated complement levels. Low C3 and C4 complement levels have been described in gram-negative sepsis. Careful interpretation of abnormal serologic test is always of extreme importance. ANA testing is very sensitive for SLE but lacks specificity. It is estimated that 8 percent of the normal population may have a positive ANA test, with a positive result being more frequent in the elderly, patients with Hashimoto thyroiditis, hepatitis C, hepatitis B, primary biliary cirrhosis, leukemia, lymphoma, melanoma, lung cancer, kidney cancer, ovary cancer, and breast cancer. Idiopathic pulmonary fibrosis, multiple sclerosis, polymyositis, Sjögren syndrome, scleroderma, and rheumatoid arthritis may also present with a positive ANA test. Certain patients with SLE are more likely to have elevated levels of antiphospholipid antibody (aPL), particularly those with recurrent venous thrombosis, thrombocytopenia, recurrent fetal loss, hemolytic anemia, livedo reticularis, leg ulcers, arterial occlusions, transverse myelitis, or pulmonary hypertension.[37] Cardiac abnormalities may occur more frequently in patients with increased aPL or anticardiolipin antibody titers.[38]

Although it may have an acute, fulminating course, SLE most often is characterized by a chronic course marked with exacerba-

TABLE 88–2

Primary Cardiac Manifestations of the Nonhereditary Connective Tissue Diseases

DISEASE	PERICARDIUM	MYOCARDIUM	ENDOCARDIUM (VALVES)	CORONARY ARTERIES
Systemic lupus erythematosus	++	+	++	+
Systemic sclerosis	+	++	0	++
Polyarteritis nodosa	+/−	+	0	++
Ankylosing spondylitis	0	+/−	++	0
Rheumatoid arthritis	++	+	+	+
Polymyositis/dermatomyositis	++	++	+/−	+/−

+, may be involved, but less frequently; ++, major site of involvement; +/−, rarely involved; 0, not involved.

tions and remissions; the 10-year survival rate exceeds 80 percent. Nephritis and seizures decrease survival approximately twofold.[39] When patients die of SLE, it is most often in the setting of acute renal failure, central nervous system disease, associated infection, infective endocarditis, or coronary artery disease.

Cardiac Involvement

Approximately 25 percent of patients with SLE have cardiac involvement.[40–42] In addition to the valvular thickening or verrucae and mitral or aortic regurgitation (or occasional stenosis), there may be pericardial thickening and/or effusion, left ventricular regional or global systolic or diastolic dysfunction, or evidence of pulmonary hypertension. Either valvular regurgitation or stenosis as a consequence of SLE can require valve replacement. It is unclear whether cardiac abnormalities are significantly more frequent in patients with elevated titers of aPL.[40–42] In general, valve disease in SLE is frequent but apparently independent of the presence or absence of aPL.

Pericarditis

SLE may cause a pancarditis with abnormalities of pericardium, endocardium, myocardium, and coronary arteries. Pericardial involvement is the most frequent, as observed clinically, by echocardiography, or at autopsy.[40] Pericardial effusions occur at some point in more than half of the patients with active SLE. Signs of active or acute pericardial disease may precede (approximately 5 percent) the other clinical signs of SLE.[40] In most SLE patients, the pericardial involvement is clinically silent and, when present, runs a benign course. Pericardial tamponade may occur and should be considered in patients with unexplained signs of venous congestion. On rare occasions, SLE pericardial disease may lead to pericardial constriction or to acute cardiac tamponade. Although the size of the pericardial effusion usually is not sufficiently large to allow aspiration, serologic studies of the pericardial fluid can be useful in diagnosing pericardial effusions because of SLE.

The most common type of pericardial disease in SLE is the presence of diffuse or focal adhesions or fibrinous deposits.[36] The pericardial fluid in SLE may be consistent to either an exudate or transudate. The mean white blood cell count, is 30,000 cells/mL; usually the neutrophil percentage is 98 percent.[43] Presence of low complement levels, ANA, and lupus erythematosus cells has also been reported.

In patients with long-standing SLE who are treated with antiinflammatory agents, the frequency of pericardial abnormalities is no different than in patients who are not receiving these agents. However, at autopsy the involvement is less extensive and more likely to be fibrous rather than fibrinous. SLE patients with fibrinous pericardial disease, particularly those with severe debilitation or renal failure, are at increased risk for purulent pericarditis, which is usually fatal.

Endocarditis and Valve Disease

The cardiovascular lesion of SLE that has received the most attention is the *atypical verrucous endocarditis* first described by Libman and Sacks in 1924,[44] long before SLE was recognized as a systemic disease. The lesions, as they were first described and subsequently attributed to SLE, consist almost entirely of fibrin, and although they may occur on both surfaces of any of the four cardiac valves, they are now most frequently found on the left-sided valves, particularly the ventricular surface of the posterior mitral leaflet (Fig. 88–6). These *verrucae* are similar histologically to those of nonbacterial thrombotic noninfective endocarditis, the valve lesion that occurs most frequently in patients with debilitating illnesses or cancer, except that occasionally hematoxylin bodies, considered the histologic counterpart of lupus erythematosus cells, may be found within Libman-Sacks lesions. Although valvular verrucae in SLE (Libman-Sacks lesions) are usually clinically silent, they can be dislodged and embolize, and can also become infected, producing infective endocarditis.[42] It is prudent to recommend antibiotic prophylaxis against infective endocarditis when patients with SLE undergo procedures that may be associated with bacteremia (see Chap. 85).

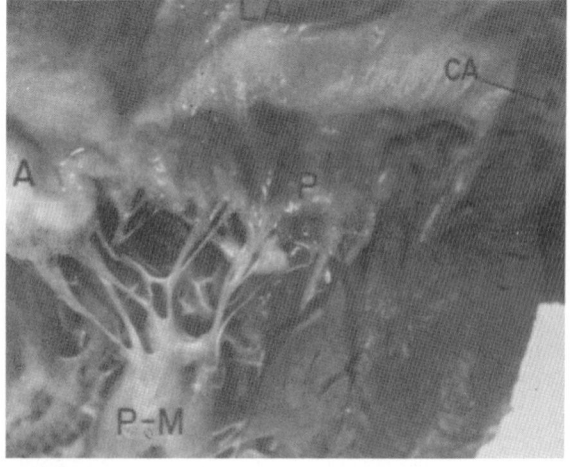
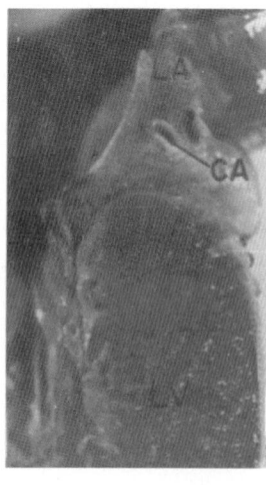
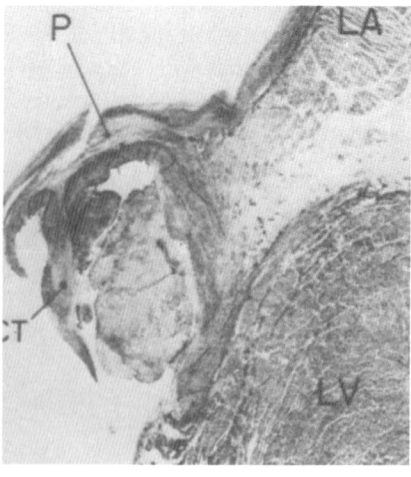

A   B   C

FIGURE 88–6. An example of Libman-Sacks endocarditis in systemic lupus erythematosus. **A** and **B.** The left atrium (LA) and left ventricle (LV) are open. **B** and **C.** Fibrofibrinous verrucae, present on the undersurface of the posterior leaflet (P) of the mitral valve, are often clinically silent. A, anterior leaflet of mitral valve; CA, left circumflex coronary artery; CT, chorda tendineae; P-M, posteromedial papillary muscle. Hematoxylin and eosin (H&E) stain, × 8. *Source: From Bulkley BH, Roberts WC. The heart in systemic lupus erythematosus and the changes induced in it by corticosteroid therapy: a study of 36 necropsy patients. Am J Med 1975;58:243–264. Reproduced with permission from the publisher and the author.*

Echocardiographically, SLE has a characteristic appearance, with leaflet thickening and valve masses (see Chap. 16). The end-stage or healed form of the verrucous endocarditis of SLE is a fibrous plaque. In some instances, if the thrombotic lesions are extensive enough, their healing may be accompanied by focal scarring and deformity of the underlying valve tissue. This healed form of SLE "endocarditis" may cause valvular dysfunction, particularly mitral and/or aortic regurgitation.[45] Verrucous endocarditis is associated with the presence of the antiphospholipid syndrome.

Myocarditis

It is unclear whether infiltration of the myocardial interstitium with acute and/or chronic inflammatory cells and focal myocardial necrosis (i.e., myocarditis) occurs as a natural part of SLE, unassociated with antiinflammatory drug therapy (glucocorticoid treatment). Several reports describe clinical features consistent with myocarditis, but actual visualization of interstitial myocardial inflammatory cells with associated myofiber necrosis has not been demonstrated histologically. Hemodynamic and echocardiographic studies, however, have shown abnormalities in both systolic and diastolic ventricular function in some SLE patients.

T1 spin-echo and T2 relaxation time cardiac MRI is being studied extensively in patients with SLE, and its use for the diagnosis of myocarditis is promising, but standards are still lacking (see Chap. 21). A recent case series of 11 consecutive patients with SLE reported an increased relaxation time by cardiac MRI (index of soft-tissue signal). Clinical improvement correlated very well with improvement of the parameters by MRI.[46]

Whether these abnormalities result from an *autoimmune attack* on the myocardium or from the effects of systemic arterial hypertension, coronary artery disease, or coexisting pericardial disease is unclear.

Coronary Artery Disease

Both fatal and nonfatal acute myocardial infarction and sudden coronary death (without demonstrable infarction) from CAD may occur early in the course of SLE, particularly among young women. In a landmark report by Manzi et al., the incidence of myocardial infarction in women with SLE (third and fourth decades of life) was found to be increased by 50-fold when compared to patients from the Framingham cohort. Two-thirds of the coronary events occurred in women younger than 55 years of age. Older age at the lupus diagnosis, longer disease duration, and the use of steroids, as well as hypercholesterolemia and postmenopausal status, were more common in the patients with coronary events (Fig. 88–7).[47]

Studies of hearts in patients with fatal SLE have demonstrated a high incidence of CAD in patients who received treatment with glucocorticoids for more than 2 years.[48,49] Accelerated CAD is increasingly recognized as a leading cause of morbidity and mortality among young women with SLE who receive long-term glucocorticoid administration.[48,49]

Although the causes of this premature CAD are uncertain, both glucocorticoid treatment and aPL have been incriminated. It has been speculated that SLE itself may induce an underlying vasculopathy that may facilitate premature atherogenesis from long-term

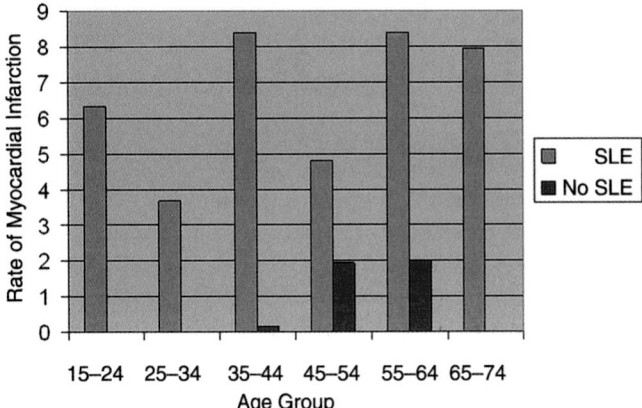

FIGURE 88–7. Comparison of rates of myocardial infarction in women with systemic lupus erythematosus (SLE) versus patients from the Framingham cohort. Rate ratio in the 35- to 44-year-old age group was 52.43 times higher in women with SLE (95 percent confidence interval 21.6–98.5). *Source: Data from Manzi S, Meilahn EN, Rairie JE, et al. Age-specific incidence rates of myocardial infarction and angina in women with systemic lupus erythematosus: comparison with the Framingham study. Am J Epidemiol 1997;145:408–415.*

glucocorticoid treatment. Premature coronary artery atherosclerosis determined by electron-beam computed tomography (coronary artery calcification) has been reported in patients with SLE.[50]

In one study, the presence of elevated aPL antibodies in patients with SLE correlated with left ventricular (global or segmental) dysfunction, verrucous valvular (aortic or mitral) thickening, and global valvular (mitral or aortic) thickening and dysfunction, as well as mitral and aortic regurgitation. Coronary thrombi may occur in patients with active lupus. Acute myocardial infarction may occur in the presence of angiographically normal coronary arteries. SLE also may cause coronary aneurysm; aPL antibodies are known to promote platelet aggregation and to be associated with the presence of a clotting tendency, the so-called *lupus anticoagulant syndrome*.[40,41]

Inflammation (arteritis) of the wall of the sinus node artery in association with scarring of both sinus and atrioventricular nodes may account for some of the rhythm and conduction disturbances seen in these patients.

Pregnancy and the Neonatal Lupus Syndrome

Neonatal lupus erythematosus is a rare disorder that arises when the so-called *anti-Ro*, or *Sjögren* (SSA), autoantibodies—mostly immunoglobulin G (IgG)—are formed and circulate in pregnant patients, cross the placenta, and cause a lupus-like syndrome in newborns with the appearance of a skin rash and transient cytopenias from passively acquired maternal autoantibodies. Because the half-life of IgG antibodies is approximately 21 to 25 days, the neonatal lupus syndrome in newborn babies is self-limiting; it usually resolves in 3 to 6 months when all of the IgG-containing anti-Ro maternal autoantibodies have been cleared from the neonate's circulation. An unfortunate exception is complete congenital heart block, which may require the implantation of a pacemaker. Once complete heart block occurs, it is usually irreversible. One neonate with first-degree heart block at birth that resolved 6 months later has been described. Antibodies to the Ro (SSA) ribonucleoprotein complexes are present in more than 85 percent of sera from mothers of infants with complete congenital heart block. A recent study found that the presence of complete heart block is strongly dependant on a specific antibody profile to Ro 52-kd; this may be a useful tool to identify pregnant women who are at risk of delivering babies with a complete heart block.[51] In many patients, antibodies reactive to the La (SSB) antigen, as well as the U1RNP protein particle, are found in association with anti-Ro (SSA) antibodies.

In most cases, the neonatal lupus syndrome is a benign disorder, and most babies of mothers with anti-Ro (SSA), anti-La (SSB), or anti-U1RNP antibodies do not develop neonatal lupus. *A pregnant woman with SLE with positive anti-Ro, anti-La, or anti-RNP antibodies has a less than 3 percent risk of having a child with neonatal lupus and congenital heart block. The risk that this patient might have an infant with neonatal lupus syndrome but without congenital heart block may be as high as 1 in 3.* The neonatal lupus syndrome mediated by the presence of maternal anti-Ro antibodies can occur in babies of mothers who do not have overt SLE, who may or may not meet criteria for a diagnosis of SLE, and who may or may not have a positive test for ANA.[52]

Neonatal lupus syndrome with congenital heart block can be diagnosed by the appearance of fetal bradycardia around week 23 of gestation.[52] The cardiac damage with conduction abnormalities in a neonate may result from binding of the passively transferred pathogenic anti-Ro antibodies to Ro (SSA)/La (SSB) antigens present in the fetal heart. All mothers of neonates with complete congenital heart block have been HLA-DR3 positive. If a mother is HLA-DR3 positive and has circulating IgG anti-Ro antibodies, her neonate is at risk regardless of the neonate's HLA-DR status.

Other cardiac abnormalities reported in neonatal lupus syndrome include right bundle-branch block, second-degree atrioventricular block, 2:1 atrioventricular block, patent ductus arteriosus, patent foramen ovale, coarctation of the aorta, tetralogy of Fallot, atrial septal defect, hypoplastic right ventricle, ventricular septal defect, dysplastic pulmonic valve, mitral and tricuspid regurgitation, pericarditis, and myocarditis. Most of these patients eventually have a pacemaker inserted.

Pregnant women with SLE should have a serum anti-Ro (SSA) antibody determination as early in pregnancy as possible. Prenatal treatment of established congenital heart block has consisted of the administration of prednisone or dexamethasone and plasmapheresis from week 23 on, although heart block has persisted in most cases.[52] It is unclear whether aggressive antiinflammatory therapy, in an effort to diminish the generalized fetal insult and to lower the titers of circulating anti-Ro (SSA) antibodies, makes a difference in fetal cardiac outcome. Fetal echocardiography is useful in following the progression of the disease and also in helping to identify decreased left ventricular contractility, increased cardiac size, tricuspid regurgitation, and pericardial effusion.

Neither dexamethasone nor plasmapheresis has had much success in reversing intrauterine third-degree heart block. Glucocorticoids, however, may be helpful in suppressing an associated inflammatory response producing pleuropericardial effusions or ascites in the fetus. Close monitoring of the clinical course in the prospective mother is also essential because of the risk of exacerbation of the SLE. If fetal bradycardia is present, an *intrauterine therapeutic approach* for as long as possible is recommended to allow for fetal maturation to occur. Ultrasound images can be useful for assessing the degree of cardiac dysfunction present. Following delivery, the neonatologist should be prepared to have a cardiac pacemaker implanted. Otherwise, all of the other clinical and laboratory features of the neonatal lupus syndrome should slowly and gradually disappear over the first few months of the baby's life. In one study, one-third of the children with autoantibody-associated congenital heart block died in the early neonatal period[53]; most survivors required a pacemaker.

Women with SLE who are anti-Ro positive should be closely monitored during pregnancy, as should mothers of previous babies born with congenital complete heart block. Pregnant patients should be reminded that congenital complete heart block is rare and that the neonatal cutaneous lupus syndrome is benign and transient. The long-term prognosis of mothers of children born with congenital heart block is generally fairly good. In these mothers, the risk of congenital heart block in children of subsequent pregnancies is low. Newborns of mothers with SLE who have a normal pulse rate are unlikely to have significant abnormalities in atrioventricular conduction.

A higher incidence of clinical evidence of myocarditis and conduction defects is found in adult anti-Ro-positive patients with SLE than it is in patients who are anti-Ro negative or in healthy controls.[52] The role of the anti-Ro antibody in inducing heart blocks in adult patients with SLE is unclear.

Secondary Effects on the Heart

Most of the clinically significant cardiac problems occurring in patients with SLE are secondary. Systemic arterial hypertension is common in patients with SLE, particularly those with renal disease and long-standing glucocorticoid therapy, in whom it is a major cause of cardiac enlargement and heart failure.[40] Pulmonary hypertension is also common, approaching 50 percent in a 5-year followup study. Uremic pericarditis may occur, of course, in patients with severe renal failure. Premature or accelerated atherosclerosis is increasingly recognized in young women with SLE who are receiving long-term glucocorticoid treatment.[40]

Therapy

Therapy of cardiovascular SLE is the treatment of the underlying disease and includes nonsteroidal antiinflammatory drugs (NSAIDs), glucocorticoids, and, in severe cases, cytotoxic agents such as azathioprine, mycophenolate mofetil, and cyclophosphamide. Systemic arterial hypertension, congestive heart failure, and arrhythmias should be treated with standard therapeutic measures. SLE-induced valve disease can require valve replacement.[40,54] Pericardial tamponade may require either high-dose steroids (prednisone 1 mg/kg), pericardiocentesis, or placement of a pericardial window, but recurrent effusions or pericardial thickening may develop. A mild to moderate pericardial effusion can be treated with NSAIDs or prednisone at a dose of 20 to 40 mg/d. Premature cardiovascular events from accelerated atherosclerosis may result in sudden death or myocardial infarction. The antimalarial agent hydroxychloroquine lowers serum cholesterol levels in patients with SLE and may decrease myocardial ischemic damage. An antimalarial such as hydroxychloroquine may be beneficial as a prophylactic agent to prevent premature or accelerated atherosclerosis in young women with SLE who are receiving long-term treatment with glucocorticoids. Although there are no studies documenting benefit, low-dose aspirin and hydroxychloroquine are often used in SLE patients receiving long-term glucocorticoid therapy.

【 】 RHEUMATOID ARTHRITIS

RA is the most common connective tissue disease. Its prevalence is 1.5 percent in males and 2.5 percent in females. It is characterized by its deforming erosions of the joints; these erosions result from chronic synovial inflammation and proliferation. Joint symptoms dominate its course, and symmetric involvement of the hands and wrists is most common. Other joints of the upper and lower extremities and the temporomandibular and sternoclavicular joints also may be affected. The most common systemic or extraarticular manifestations of RA include subcutaneous rheumatoid nodules, weight loss, anemia of chronic inflammation, and serositis. Less frequently, pneumonitis and a necrotizing vasculitis occur in patients with severe long-standing disease. Contrary to prior epidemiologic studies, new data support increased mortality in RA.[55]

A prospective cohort study comparing the incidence of myocardial infarction and cerebrovascular events between RA patients and non-RA patients with known CAD found that the RA patients had a greater incidence of vascular events and mortality.[56]

Atherosclerosis also appears to occur at an accelerated rate in RA. There is a strong correlation between the presence of inflammatory biochemical markers and carotid atherosclerotic plaques.[57] Coronary artery calcification determined by electron-beam computed tomography or multislice CT is significantly higher in patients with RA than in healthy individuals. The presence of coronary artery calcifications is highly dependent on disease duration. Patients with RA who smoke and have an elevated erythrocyte sedimentation rate have a higher incidence of coronary artery calcification.[58] In a population-based retrospective study of patients followed for 46 years, a significant excess risk of congestive heart failure (CHF) (hazard ratio [HR] 1.87; 95 percent confidence interval [CI] 1.47–2.39) was found in patients with RA.[59] CHF, rather than ischemic heart disease, contributes to the excess overall mortality among patients with RA.[60]

Pericardial Involvement

Although cardiac involvement is uncommon in RA, it does exist in a variety of forms. A diffuse, nonspecific fibrofibrinous pericarditis occurs in approximately 50 percent of patients with RA; it is usually clinically silent and is overshadowed by pleuritis or joint pain.[53] The pericardial disease tends to be benign, but sizable effusions can occur and require pericardiocentesis; however, pericardial constriction rarely necessitates pericardiectomy. Constrictive pericarditis occurred in 4 of 47 patients with RA whose cases were followed over a 10-year period. The histopathologic findings after pericardiectomy were consistent with chronic fibrosing pericardial disease. In another report, RA patients with constrictive pericarditis had a longer disease course, more severe disease, worse functional class, and more extraarticular features when compared with RA patients without cardiac constriction. The presenting clinical features of cardiac constriction included dyspnea, edema, chest pain, and pulsus paradoxus. Chronic, symptomatic pericarditis may require glucocorticoid therapy. RA pericardial disease may

shorten survival, especially in older patients. Lymphocytic infiltrates of the CD8-positive type may occur in the pericardium of patients with rheumatoid pericardial disease, suggesting that these cells may play a role in the development of the pericardial disease (see Chap. 84).

Myocardial and Endocardial Involvement

Rarely, rheumatoid nodules focally infiltrate the heart, including the myocardium and the four cardiac valves (Fig. 88–8).[53] These nodules may produce no symptoms, but, if extensive enough or strategically located, they can compromise cardiac function. A rheumatoid nodule may extend from the mural endocardium into a chamber to present as an intracavitary mass. Rheumatoid nodules developing within the valve leaflets may result in mild valvular regurgitation; if the nodule becomes necrotic, perforation of the leaflet can occur and lead to severe valvular regurgitation. The incidence of such valvular infiltration has been estimated at 1 to 2 percent in autopsy studies of patients with RA. Although distinctly uncommon, arrhythmias and conduction disturbances, including complete heart block, and congestive heart failure can also result from RA involvement of the heart. One echocardiographic study of 39 patients with RA detected left ventricular abnormalities in 25 percent of the patients.

Therapy

Methotrexate appears to reduce cardiovascular mortality.[61] However, other traditional disease-modifying antirheumatic drugs such as sulfasalazine, azathioprine, and hydroxychloroquine do not.

The outcome of patients with rheumatoid arthritis has improved dramatically since the introduction of the antitumor necrosis factor (TNF) α blockers. They are now approved for the treatment of early RA. However, they should not be used in patients with New York Health Association (NYHA) class III or IV heart failure (see Table 88–2) because of the potential risk of worsening the CHF.[62] The treatment of cardiac constriction from rheumatoid pericardial disease may include a trial of a high-dose intravenous glucocorticoid (e.g., methylprednisolone) and/or surgical therapy. Pericardiocentesis should be performed only as a lifesaving procedure. An uncomplicated asymptomatic pericardial effusion does not require any treatment.

【 】 ANKYLOSING SPONDYLITIS

Ankylosing spondylitis is the prototypical example within the group of the seronegative spondyloarthropathies. It is characterized by a progressive inflammatory lesion of the spine, leading to chronic back pain, deforming dorsal kyphosis, and, in its advanced stage, fusion of the costovertebral and sacroiliac joints with immobilization of the spine. This condition is much more frequent in men than it is in women (9:1), generally first occurring early in life but with a chronic progressive course of 20 to 30 years. The HLA-B27 histocompatibility antigen is found in 90 percent of whites and in 50 percent of black patients with ankylosing spondylitis. A spondyloarthropathy associated with an HLA-B27 is seen frequently in patients with reactive arthritis (formerly called Reiter syndrome), Crohn disease, ulcerative colitis, and psoriatic arthritis.

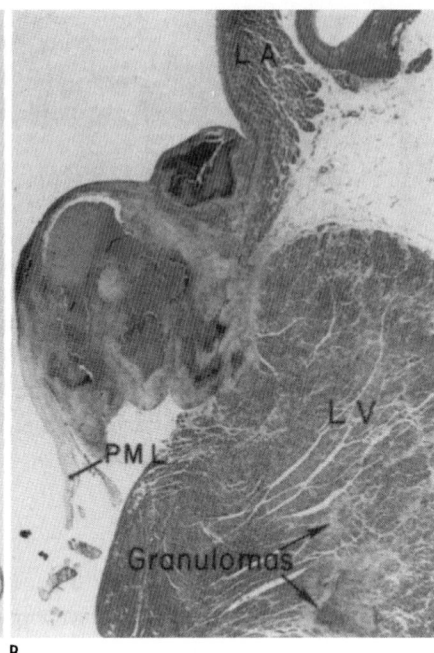

FIGURE 88–8. Rheumatoid arthritis. **A.** A tricuspid valve (TV) infiltrated by rheumatoid nodules. **B.** A mitral valve infiltrated by rheumatoid nodules. In addition, granulomas are present within the left ventricular (LV) wall. LA, left atrium; PML, posterior mitral leaflet; RV, right ventricle. Hematoxylin and eosin (H&E) stain: **A,** × 12; **B,** × 65. *Source: From Roberts WC, Dangel JC, Bulkley BH. Nonrheumatic valvular cardiac disease: a clinicopathologic survey of 27 different conditions causing valvular dysfunction. Cardiovasc Clin. Copyright 1973 by F.A. Davis Company; used by permission of F.A. Davis Company.*

Cardiac Involvement

Cardiovascular disease in ankylosing spondylitis, seen typically in patients with severe peripheral joint involvement and long-standing disease, takes the form of a sclerosing inflammatory lesion that is generally limited to the aortic root area. The inflammatory process, which extends immediately above and below the aortic valve, typically causes aortic regurgitation[63] (Fig. 88–9). As the inflammatory process extends below the aortic valve, it can infiltrate the basal portion of the mitral valve (which is contiguous with the aortic valve) and cause mitral regurgitation. Extension of the inflammatory lesion into the cephalad portion of the ventricular septum, immediately caudal to the aortic valve, accounts for the associated conduction disturbances. Ventricular diastolic dysfunction may also occur.

The major clinical manifestation of ankylosing spondylitis is aortic regurgitation, which occurs in approximately 5 percent of patients with this condition. Among patients with signs of spondylitis for 10 years, only 2 percent have clinical evidence of aortic regurgitation; by 30 years, that number increases fivefold. Ankylosing spondylitis may be associated with aortic root inflammatory lesions, as may other seronegative spondyloarthropathies such as Reiter syndrome and psoriatic arthropathy.

Therapy

Drug therapy for ankylosing spondylitis used to be directed primarily at relief of the back pain and discomfort. NSAIDs and methotrexate, in addition to physical therapy, remain the first line of therapy. Glucocorticoids do not have a role in the treatment of ankylosing spondylitis except for the treatment of uveitis. The treatment with anti-TNFα drugs is now the standard of care. Patients with long-standing disease tend to be less responsive. Whether the natural history of the disease could be improved with early anti-TNFα therapy is unknown.[64]

The inflammatory lesion of the heart generally runs a clinically silent course until aortic regurgitation develops. Not infrequently, however, the aortic regurgitation of ankylosing spondylitis may become severe enough to warrant aortic valve replacement (see Chap. 75).

[ ] CARDIOVASCULAR SYPHILIS

Although traditionally not considered to be a connective tissue disorder, cardiovascular syphilis has histologic features nearly identical to those of ankylosing spondylitis, and spirochetes have never been identified in the aorta of a patient with cardiovascular syphilis.

The distribution of the lesions, however, is distinctly different in these two conditions.[53] In cardiovascular syphilis, the process is usually limited to the tubular portion of the ascending aorta (i.e., that portion up to the origin of the innominate artery). Because the process as a rule does not extend into the wall of aorta behind the sinuses of Valsalva, aortic regurgitation is infrequent in syphilis. Exactly what percentage of patients with cardiovascular syphilis develop aortic regurgitation is unclear, but it is probably less than 15 percent and only those patients in whom the process extends into the wall of aorta behind the sinuses of Valsalva. In syphilis, the process *never* involves the aortic valve cusps and never extends below (caudal to) the aortic valve. In contrast, in ankylosing spondylitis, the process *always* involves basal portions of the aortic valve cusps and always extends into the membranous ventricular septum, the basal portion of the anterior mitral leaflet, or both. Thus, because the process in syphilis never extends below the aortic valve, bundle branch or complete heart block and mitral regurgitation never develop in cardiovascular syphilis. Cardiovascular syphilis characteristically involves the entire tubular portion of the aorta, which may become either diffusely or focally dilated. In contrast, in ankylosing spondylitis, the process involves only the proximal 1 cm of the tubular portion of the ascending aorta and then usually in the areas of the aortic valve commissures. Accordingly, aneurysms of the tubular portion of the ascending aorta do not occur in ankylosing spondylitis. Syphilitic aneurysms can become so large that they burrow into the sternum or compress adjacent structures such as the right atrium, superior vena cava, or pulmonary trunk. Rupture into the adjacent structures or into the pericardial sac may also occur.

Histologically, the aortic lesions in both cardiovascular syphilis and ankylosing spondylitis are characterized by extensive thickening by fibrous tissue of the adventitia, with collections of plasma

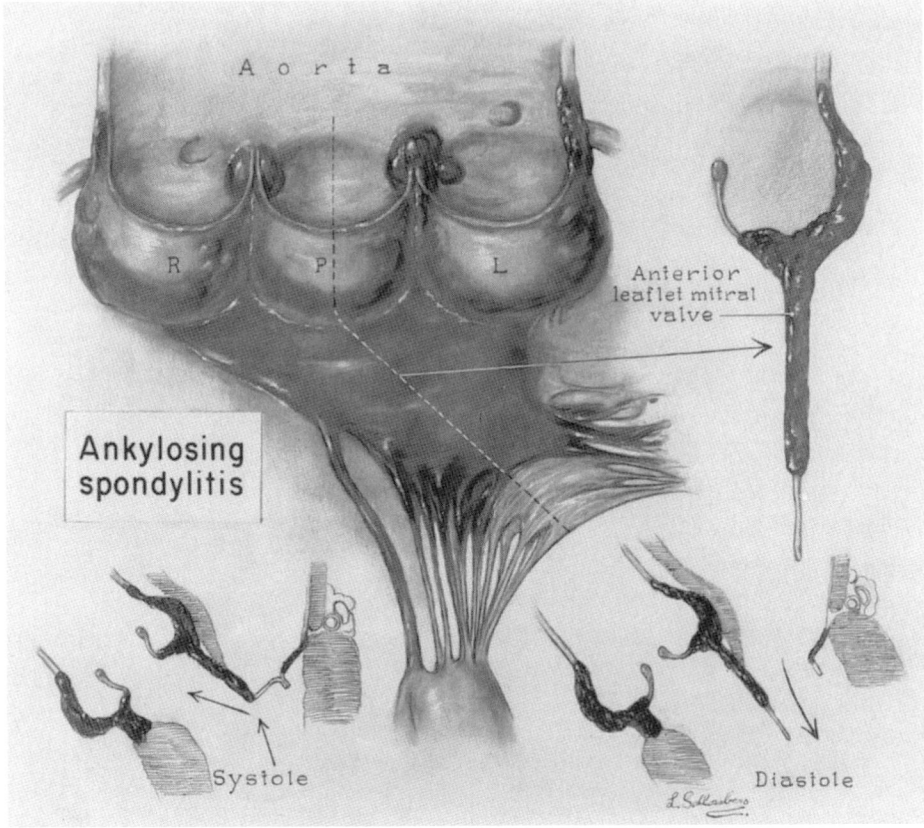

FIGURE 88–9. Diagram showing the characteristic features of ankylosing spondylitis of the heart. The aorta and aortic valve are opened, showing the thickening of the aorta in the vicinity of the aortic valve commissures and the thickening of the anterior mitral leaflet. The small diagrams at the bottom of the figure show the thickening in the wall of the aorta behind the sinuses extending below the aortic valve into the membranous ventricular septum and anterior mitral leaflet. In the patient whose heart was portrayed by this diagram, there was also some thickening in the posterior mitral leaflet.

cells and some lymphocytes within these tissues. The vasa vasorum are larger than normal, their walls are thickened, and their lumens may be severely narrowed. The inflammatory infiltrates are located primarily in the perivascular locations. The media is thinner than normal and contains scars that are generally located transversely to the long axis of the aorta. Within the scars, elastic fibers may be absent. The overlying intima is thickened, and the intimal process has the "tree bark" appearance of typical atherosclerotic plaques. Patients with cardiovascular syphilis, with or without associated aortic regurgitation, usually live into their 70s or 80s.

【 】 SYSTEMIC SCLEROSIS (SCLERODERMA)

Systemic sclerosis, which was first identified more than two centuries ago, is characterized by its striking skin manifestations; hence the name *scleroderma*. In 1943, when Weiss et al.[65] described a pattern in the cardiac dysfunction of nine patients with scleroderma and correlated these changes with abnormalities in the heart at autopsy in two patients, they recognized that the cardiac disease was a manifestation of an underlying primary vascular disorder.

Systemic sclerosis is characterized by fibrous thickening of the skin and fibrous and degenerative alterations of the fingers and of certain target organs, particularly the esophagus, small and large bowels, kidneys, lung, and heart. Central to this degenerative pro-

cess are diffuse vascular lesions. Functionally, the vascular disorder is characterized by Raynaud phenomenon, which is a prominent feature of systemic sclerosis. Raynaud disease of the digits is present in almost all patients with systemic sclerosis and is the first clinical symptom in most. Structurally, the vascular lesions show intimal and adventitial thickening of small- and medium-size vessels, including arterioles. The underlying pathophysiology of scleroderma that links structure and function is a Raynaud-type phenomenon of visceral vasculature that leads to focal vascular lesions and parenchymal necrosis and fibrosis. This concept is supported by findings in the heart, the lungs and kidneys. The underlying cause of the vascular disease in systemic sclerosis and the role of the immune system in its pathophysiology remain unclear. Systemic sclerosis may be related to increased activity of endothelial cells, mast cells, and fibroblasts, perhaps under the influence of immigrant cells, such as T cells, macrophages, or platelets.

Like most connective tissue diseases, systemic sclerosis may have a variable clinical expression. Some patients may have skin involvement predominantly; others have minimal skin abnormalities but severe visceral disease that may therefore evade diagnosis. Limited scleroderma (formerly called CREST syndrome) is most of the time a more benign form of scleroderma that presents with relatively mild skin changes limited to the face and fingers, *c*alcinosis, *R*aynaud phenomenon, *e*sophageal dysmotility, *s*clerodactyly, and *t*elangiectasia. Patients with limited scleroderma have a high incidence of pulmonary hypertension. *Overlap syndromes* are seen when a patient with typical features of systemic sclerosis also has features of SLE, polymyositis, or RA. Although systemic sclerosis may run a long and benign course, the involvement of inner organs, such as kidney, lung, and cardiovascular system, is associated with increased morbidity and mortality.

The Cardiovascular System

Cardiovascular disease in patients with systemic sclerosis can be a result of either a primary involvement of the heart by the sclerosing disease or a secondary involvement from disease of the kidney or lungs.

【 】 PRIMARY SYSTEMIC SCLEROSIS OF THE HEART

Myocardial involvement is a major determinant of survival in systemic sclerosis. When the heart is involved directly by sclero-

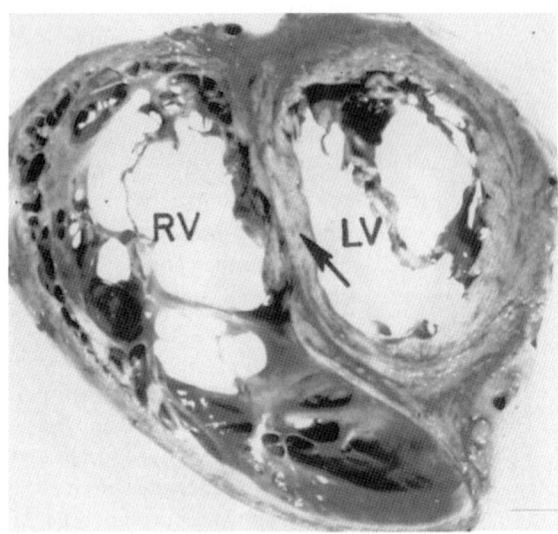

A

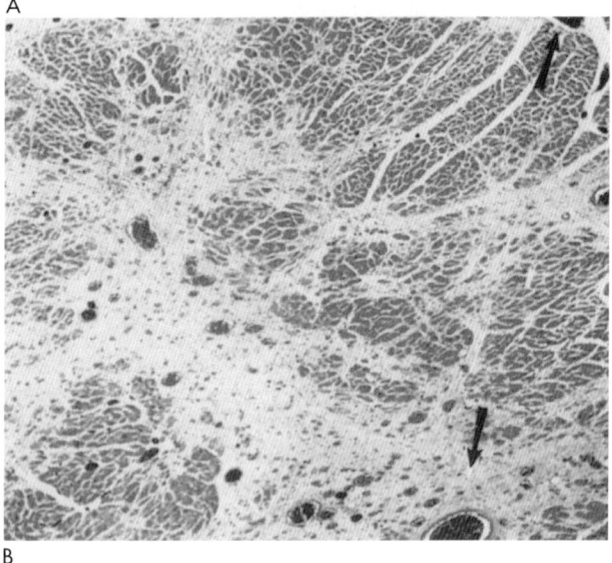

B

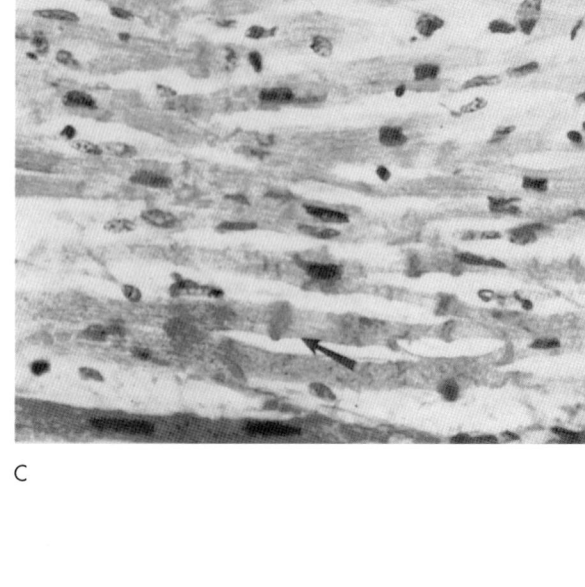

C

FIGURE 88-10. Systemic sclerosis. **A:** Cross-section through the dilated right (RV) and left (LV) ventricle of a patient with cardiac systemic sclerosis. Marked fibrous scarring of both ventricles is especially evident in the ventricular septum (*arrow*). **B:** Photomicrograph of myocardium showing replacement fibrosis with patent intramural coronary arteries (*arrows*). **C:** Higher-power magnification showing contraction-band necrosis of many fibers surrounding the areas of scar. Hematoxylin and eosin (H&E) stain, × 45 and × 60. *Source: From Bulkley BH. Progressive systemic sclerosis: cardiac involvement. Clin Rheum Dis 1979;5:131. Reproduced with permission from the publisher and author.*

derma, a myocardial fibrosis occurs that bears no direct relation to large- or small-vessel occlusions or other anatomic abnormalities. Fibrosis tends to be patchy, involving all levels of the myocardium unpredictably and the right ventricle as often as the left. Focal patchy myocardial cell necrosis may also be evident, and at autopsy over three-quarters of patients with myocardial systemic sclerosis have foci of necrosis. The type of necrosis is myofibrillar degeneration, or contraction-band necrosis (Fig. 88–10). This lesion is characteristic of myocardium that is subjected to transient occlusion followed by reperfusion. This could occur with vascular spasm and also may be induced experimentally by exposing myocardium to high concentrations of catecholamine. Thus, the morphologic characteristics of the myocardial lesions of primary cardiac systemic sclerosis are very similar to the ones seen in Raynaud phenomenon. There is increased incidence of scleroderma renal crisis during cold weather months. Thus, it is likely that the major visceral manifestations of systemic sclerosis in the heart, lungs, and kidneys are related to the vascular spasm that is evident and readily detectable in the digits. Changes that are comparable to the necrosis and scarring of the fingertips can also develop in the viscera.

Current evidence suggests that the vascular system and particularly the smaller arteries and arterioles are the primary target organ of systemic sclerosis. Also the cardiac sclerosis of scleroderma may be a consequence of focal, intermittent, and progressive ischemic injury.

Several functional studies suggest that microvascular spasm occurs in patients with cardiac scleroderma. Transient perfusion defects identified by thallium-201 radionuclide imaging in the setting of patent coronary arteries also have been identified in patients with systemic sclerosis and symptomatic cardiac disease.[66]

Clinical Manifestations

The clinical features of myocardial systemic sclerosis include biventricular congestive heart failure, atrial and ventricular arrhythmias, myocardial infarction, angina pectoris, and sudden cardiac death.[67] These clinical manifestations reflect the underlying conditions of myocardial necrosis and fibrosis and may at times mimic ischemic heart disease caused by CAD. If the myocardial injury is extensive enough, hypodynamic ventricles, a syndrome resembling idiopathic dilated cardiomyopathy (see Chap. 29) may be simulated. Patients with systemic sclerosis may have cardiac involvement but no cardiac symptoms.[68] One study examined 18 systemic sclerosis patients by electrocardiography (ECG), ambulatory ECG, radionuclide ventriculography, myocardial scintigraphy, and echocardiography and found a high rate of cardiac abnormalities, including ventricular tachyarrhythmias, supraventricular tachycardias, depressed left or right ventricular function, and reversible myocardial perfusion abnormalities. In other studies of patients with limited scleroderma, noninvasive cardiac techniques such as Doppler echocardiography and thallium-201 perfusion scintigraphy after a cold-stress test or radionuclide ventriculography have found a number of cardiovascular abnormalities, such as mild mitral regurgitation, thickening of papillary muscles, abnormal left and right ventricular diastolic function, and systolic pulmonary arterial hypertension.[69,70]

Skeletal muscle myositis can complicate systemic sclerosis, and such patients may have an increased likelihood of developing myocarditis, heart failure, and symptomatic arrhythmias, and often die suddenly.[70] Accordingly, it has been suggested that serum creatine kinase with myocardial band fractionation and studies of left ventricular function be undertaken in patients with systemic sclerosis who have skeletal myositis. Autopsy studies suggest that up to 50 percent of patients with systemic sclerosis have increased myocardial scar tissue and that up 30 percent of patients have extensive disease. Some clinical evidence of cardiac abnormalities may occur in approximately 40 percent of patients with systemic sclerosis.

Pericardial and Endocardial Disease

Pericardial involvement may occur in approximately 20 percent of patients with systemic sclerosis. Although the pericardial involvement is a result of renal failure in as many as two-thirds of patients, some develop a fibrofibrinous or fibrous pericarditis for which no other cause is evident. Exudative pericardial effusions may accompany scleroderma pericardial disease and can be massive.[71] Most cases of pericardial effusion in scleroderma have a benign course. Rarely, pericardial tamponade may occur and may precede cutaneous thickening. Rarely, constrictive pericardial disease may result from the pericardial sclerosis. Mitral regurgitation is common in patients with systemic sclerosis.[72] Tricuspid regurgitation occurs in patients with very dilated right ventricular cavities.

Secondary Cardiovascular Disease

Ventricular hypertrophy and congestive heart failure may be associated with long-standing systemic arterial hypertension and renal disease. Uremic pericarditis may occur. Pulmonary hypertension with marked right ventricular hypertrophy and right-sided heart failure may result from long-standing severe pulmonary scleroderma. Mortality as a consequence of scleroderma renal crisis and malignant hypertension has dramatically decreased with the use of angiotensin-converting enzyme inhibitors.

Pulmonary Hypertensive Disease

Although the pulmonary fibrosis of scleroderma had been known for years, the recognition of a pulmonary hypertensive lesion independent of parenchymal disease evolved later. Such patients tend to develop rapidly progressive dyspnea and right-sided heart failure in the setting of clear lungs. Morphologically, the pulmonary arterial lesions show the range of advanced alterations (medial and intimal thickening and plexiform lesions) as seen in the Eisen-menger syndrome and primary pulmonary hypertension. Arterial vasospasm is believed to be a major component of systemic sclerosis pulmonary hypertension, and the association is supported by angiographic studies. That Raynaud phenomenon of the digits accompanies idiopathic pulmonary hypertension in about one-third of patients suggests that vascular hyperreactivity may be a common link between this disease and scleroderma (see Chap. 71).

Pulmonary hypertension portends a poor prognosis. Sudden unexpected death occurs, and hypotension and death can occur precipitously in the setting of what would appear to be relatively benign procedures such as pericardiocentesis or cardiac catheterization.

Treatment

No uniform therapy is effective for the cardiovascular disease of systemic sclerosis. Treatment consists of standard therapy for congestive heart failure and arrhythmias.[72] Malignant ventricular arrhythmias in systemic sclerosis seemingly have responded well to insertion of an implantable cardioverter defibrillator (see Chap. 46). Captopril improves myocardial perfusion.[73] Unlike Raynaud disease secondary to lupus, the beneficial response to nifedipine when it is associated with scleroderma is marginal. Prazosin and hydralazine have been used with mixed results. There is growing experience with the use of angiotensin receptor blockers and their use is reasonable if there is no contraindication. The role of sympathectomy for severe Raynaud disease refractory to medical treatment is highly controversial; most patients obtain only temporary relief of their symptoms. Avoiding cool temperatures is mandatory. The use of continuous intravenous infusion of epoprostenol[74] or the inhaled prostacyclin analogue iloprost[75] have improved dramatically the symptoms and mortality caused by pulmonary hypertension (see Chap. 71). A study with the oral endothelin-receptor antagonist bosentan showed promising results.[76] The use of d-penicillamine, which until recently was standard therapy, has not been proven to be efficacious.

The use of high-dose glucocorticoids should be avoided in scleroderma and doses of prednisone higher than 30 mg daily have been associated with an increased risk of normotensive renal failure.

【 】 POLYMYOSITIS AND DERMATOMYOSITIS

These idiopathic autoimmune inflammatory myopathies are rare in the United States, with an estimated annual incidence of about 5 to 10 new patients per million. The clinical features include a typical heliotrope rash in dermatomyositis (DM), with periorbital edema (see Chap. 12) and proximal muscle weakness present in both polymyositis (PM) and DM. Typical laboratory findings reflect the presence of muscle breakdown from the inflammatory process. Creatine kinase, myoglobulin, and serum aldolase levels are commonly elevated during acute states. The former is more sensitive in those patients who present with normal, or mildly increased, creatine kinase levels. The so-called anti-Jo-1 antibody, directed against histidyl-tRNA (transfer ribonucleic acid) synthetase, is detectable in the serum of 20 percent of patients with PM/DM. Its presence has been correlated with erosive arthritis, Raynaud phenomenon, interstitial lung disease, and excess mortality, mostly as a result of respiratory failure. Another marker of disease severity is the anti–signal-recognition-particle (anti-SRP) antibody. Typical electromyogram changes include shortwave potentials, low-amplitude polyphasic units, and increased spontaneous activity with muscle fibrillation. A positive skeletal muscle biopsy of a proximal muscle such as the deltoid is often confirmatory.

In addition to skeletal muscle involvement, up to 40 percent of patients may have cardiac abnormalities. A small study of 16 autopsied patients with PM/DM suggests a poor correlation between the degree of skeletal involvement and myocarditis; however, in a study of 55 patients with PM, Behan et al. reported mild diffuse myocarditis, severe inflammation, or fibrosis of the cardiac conduction system in 70 percent of the patients. Also, anti-SSA (anti-Ro) antibody, which is classically associated with an increased risk of infant cardiac conduction abnormalities in the neonatal lupus syndrome, was present in 69 percent of patients with evidence of cardiovascular involvement.

Myocarditis leading to congestive heart failure is an uncommon but severe manifestation of PM/DM. Contrast enhancement and hypokinesia detected by cardiac MRI is reduced after treatment with corticosteroids and immunosuppressive therapy.[77]

The role of gadolinium-diethylenetriaminepentaacetic acid (DTPA)–enhanced MRI appears promising in diagnosing myocarditis in polymyositis (see Chap. 21).

Although coronary arteritis has been reported in few case reports, there are no controlled studies showing evidence of increased incidence of CAD in PM/DM. Glucocorticoids represent the mainstay of therapy. The usual practice is to begin treatment with 40 to 80 mg/d of oral prednisone or its equivalent. Methylprednisolone boluses of 500 to 1000 mg/d for 3 days is reserved for severe and acute cases. Azathioprine (Imuran) and methotrexate are used mostly as steroid-sparing agents. Intravenous immunoglobulin given in monthly boluses is an expensive therapy that is reserved for patients with severe disease (neuromuscular respiratory involvement, dysphagia) and poor response to conventional immunosuppressive therapy. Response can be seen as early as 2 weeks, but typically best effects are seen only after 3 months.

【 】 POLYARTERITIS NODOSA

Polyarteritis nodosa is an uncommon disease with an annual incidence that ranges from 4.6 to 9.0 per 100,000. Polyarteritis nodosa affects predominantly males with a male-to-female sex ratio of 2:1.[77]

Polyarteritis nodosa is characterized by segmental necrotizing inflammation of the medium- to small-size arteries, resulting in dysfunction of multiple organ systems. The commonly involved organs are the skin, kidneys, and gastrointestinal tract. Polyarteritis nodosa rarely involves the central nervous system, eyes, testes, and heart. Lungs are usually spared. A variety of cutaneous lesions may occur: livedo reticularis, palpable purpura, ulcerations, infarcts of distal digits, and nodules. Evidence of glomerulonephritis ranges from low-grade proteinuria to malignant hypertension and acute renal failure.

There is a recognized association between polyarteritis nodosa and hepatitis B infection. Hepatitis B surface antigen has been found in 15 percent of the patients. Laboratory tests are nonspecific and reflect mainly an inflammatory state. Common findings are elevated erythrocyte sedimentation rate, normochromic anemia, thrombocytosis, and low albumin. Typically, rheumatoid factor and ANA are not present and complement levels are decreased only in 5 percent of the cases. A subset of patients with microscopic polyarteritis nodosa have antineutrophil cytoplasmic antibodies directed against myeloperoxidase. The final clinical diagnosis of polyarteritis nodosa rests on the combination of multisystem disease and biopsy evidence of active arteritis of medium-size vessels. In polyarteritis nodosa, mesenteric vessel angiograms may show aneurysmal dilatation that mimics mycotic aneurysm in infective endocarditis.

Cardiac Involvement

The heart and coronary arteries are infrequent targets of polyarteritis nodosa. Most often this involvement is a vasculitis of the distal subepicardial coronary arteries just as they penetrate the myocardium (Fig. 88–11). The lesions are characterized by inflammatory infiltrates in the media and adventitia and occasionally by necrosis of the full thickness of the vessel wall, with prominent involvement of the surrounding perivascular connective tissue (Fig. 88–11). The lumens of the involved vessels may contain thrombi, and the walls may be aneurysmal. The latter is responsible for the nodular appearance of the arteries deemed characteristic of this disorder. An even later stage of the vasculitis process is evident as the lesions heal, first showing the formation of granulation tissue and subsequently fibrous tissue replacement of the original components of the artery. In this healing phase, intimal proliferation leading to coronary artery luminal narrowing is evident.

The CAD of polyarteritis nodosa may lead to myocardial infarction. The myocardial necrosis and subsequent replacement fibrosis tend to be focal and patchy throughout the left ventricular wall. This is in contrast to the large areas of grossly visible, regional, subendocardial, or transmural necrosis typically seen in the myocardial infarction caused by CAD (see Chap. 57).

Conduction system abnormalities have been identified in the heart of patients with polyarteritis nodosa. The size and location of the sinoatrial node and atrioventricular node arteries make them prime targets for polyarteritis. Atrial and ventricular conduction disturbances may be a primary manifestation of polyarteritis nodosa, despite minimal involvement of vessels elsewhere in the heart.

Other cardiac abnormalities seen in patients with polyarteritis nodosa are those that are likely secondary to the underlying systemic arterial hypertension and renal disease. Cardiomegaly and left ventricular hypertrophy most often represent secondary cardiac manifestations of this disease. Similarly, pericardial disease may develop in a patient with polyarteritis nodosa, but this is most often a consequence of renal insufficiency.

Clinical Manifestations of Cardiac Disease

Despite the dramatic involvement of coronary arteries that may accompany polyarteritis nodosa, the most frequent cardiovascular abnormalities seen in patients with polyarteritis nodosa are unrelated to the coronary arteries per se. Systemic arterial hypertension occurs in approximately 90 percent of these patients and, in combination with chronic renal failure, is the most likely cause of congestive heart failure, which may develop in up to 60 percent of patients. Those with polyarteritis nodosa also may develop acute

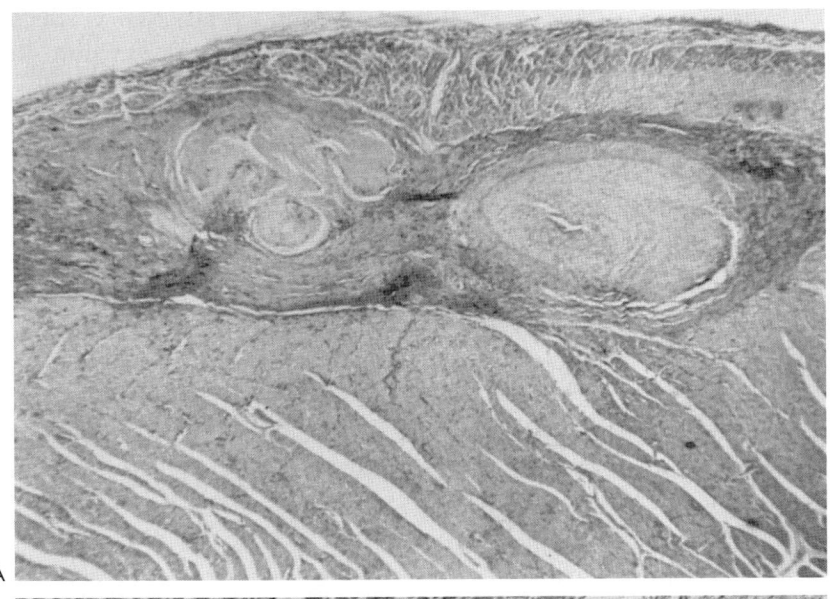

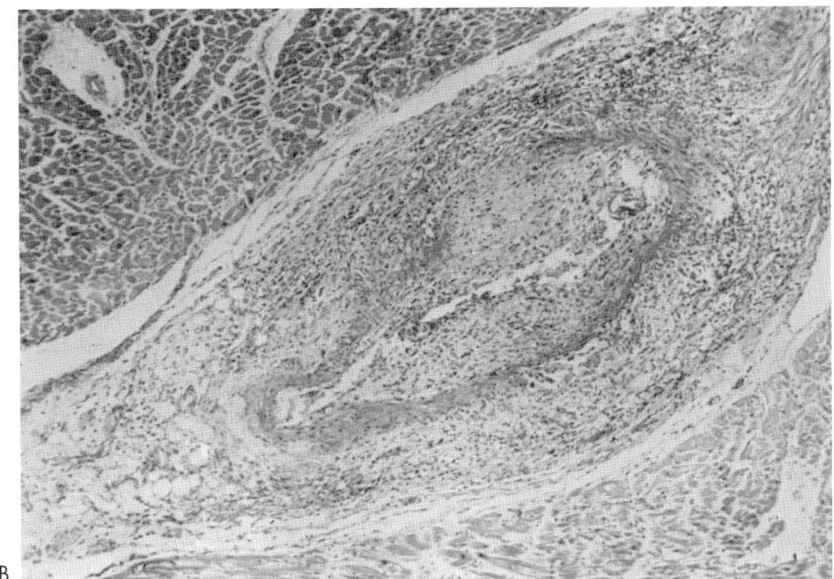

FIGURE 88–11. Polyarteritis nodosa. Examples of the necrotizing vasculitis affecting the extramural and intramural coronary arteries in polyarteritis. **A.** Extramural coronary arteries. **B.** Intramural coronary arteries. The intramural artery shows a necrotizing arteritis with inflammation involving the full thickness of the vessel. Hematoxylin and eosin (H&E) stain: *top*, × 7; *bottom*, × 22.

myocardial infarction, which poses the diagnostic question of whether the myocardial injury is caused by coronary arteritis with secondary thrombosis or to atherosclerosis.

Therapy

Polyarteritis nodosa has a poor prognosis. Treatment of the heart disease in polyarteritis nodosa is directed at the specific cardiac dysfunction. Glucocorticoids are still the initial mainstay of therapy. Early use of cyclophosphamide in severe disease with involvement of major organs has been associated with decreased mortality.

Case reports of improvement of hepatitis B virus-related polyarteritis nodosa with concomitant immunosuppressive and antiviral therapy are encouraging.[78]

The use of warfarin remains controversial; low-dose aspirin, however, is usually recommended.

【 】 GIANT CELL (CRANIAL, TEMPORAL, GRANULOMATOUS) ARTERITIS

Temporal arteritis is a systemic inflammatory vasculitis of unknown etiology that primarily involves extracranial vessels, especially branches of the external carotid artery, but can involve almost any artery in the body including the aorta. Giant cell arteritis occurs almost exclusively in patients older than 55 years of age. Common symptoms include headaches, scalp tenderness, jaw claudication, visual disturbances including blindness and diplopia, weight loss, anemia, and, in approximately 50 percent of patients, musculoskeletal symptoms attributable to polymyalgia rheumatica. Uncommon presentations of giant cell arteritis include fever of unknown origin, chest pain from aortitis or myocardial infarction, aortic aneurysm, peripheral gangrene, peripheral neuropathies, and large-vessel involvement with limb claudication, aortic regurgitation, or stroke. Typical physical findings include tenderness of the temporal or occipital arteries, nodulations of the artery, a pulseless artery, and a tender scalp.

Most giant cell arteritis patients have a greatly elevated erythrocyte sedimentation rate. The only specific diagnostic test is a temporal artery biopsy that demonstrates granulomatous arterial inflammation with disruption of the internal elastica lamina. Giant cells need not be present. Unfortunately, the positive yield for giant cell arteritis in unilateral temporal artery biopsies is no greater than 60 percent, and a contralateral biopsy may be necessary.

Because the occurrence of *skip* lesions in histologic samples is well known in giant cell arteritis, ideally a 5-cm section of artery should be examined. Angiography is generally not helpful in diagnosis or in selecting a biopsy site. A negative or inconclusive biopsy report should not prompt the clinician to stop the steroids if the clinical picture is consistent with giant cell arteritis. High-dose prednisone (1 mg/kg) should be started promptly. Not starting steroids until the temporal artery biopsy report is available, may result in serious complications including visual loss.

【 】 CHURG-STRAUSS SYNDROME

Churg-Strauss syndrome, or allergic granulomatosis and angiitis, is a systemic vasculitis that develops in the setting of allergic rhinitis, asthma, and eosinophilia. Sinusitis and pulmonary infiltrates may cause confusion with Wegener granulomatosis; the absence of cavitating pulmonary nodules or the presence of gastrointestinal involvement is often a helpful distinguishing feature. Peripheral neuropathy, cutaneous involvement, and renal disease are common clinical findings.

Pathologic studies show inflammatory lesions rich in eosinophils with intra- and extravascular granuloma formation. The major morbidity and mortality of Churg-Strauss syndrome result from cardiac involvement which is the cause of death in 48 percent of the cases. Eosinophilic endomyocarditis, coronary vasculitis, valvular lesions and pericarditis are the typical cardiovascular manifestations of Churg-Strauss syndrome.[79,80]

This may be associated with left ventricle dilatation and a reduced ejection fraction, as well as mitral regurgitation, which may require valve replacement. Left ventricular systolic function may improve significantly with glucocorticoid therapy.[81,82] Intravenous immunoglobulin infusion is reserved for severe disease unresponsive to steroids.

【 】 ANTIPHOSPHOLIPID ANTIBODY SYNDROME

The aPL syndrome is defined by the presence of aPLs in moderate titers on two or more occasions 12 weeks apart and less than 5 years prior to a venous or arterial thrombotic event or unexplained recurrent fetal losses after the 10th week of pregnancy.[83-88]

Livedo reticularis, nonhealing leg ulcers, thrombocytopenia and Coombs-positive hemolytic anemia may be also present. Clinically, the terms *anticardiolipin syndrome, antiphospholipid syndrome,* and *lupus anticoagulant syndrome* are usually considered equivalent, although some individuals may have one antibody but not the other. A false-positive Venereal Disease Research Laboratory test may also be detected in patients with aPL syndrome; aPLs, however, may be present in asymptomatic individuals. Often, anticardiolipin antibodies cross-react with β_2-glycoprotein 1 (B2GP1) antibodies. The mechanisms whereby anticardiolipin or aPLs promote intravascular thrombosis remain uncertain, but recent data suggest an important roll of complement activation.[89]

The presence of a prolonged activated partial thromboplastin time should prompt the clinician to rule out the presence of aPL.

These antibodies may react with lipid antigens on endothelial cells and/or platelets. The precise nature of the antigen recognized by B2GP1-dependent anticardiolipin antibodies is under active investigation. SLE is present frequently in patients with aPL syndrome.

An increased incidence of aortic or mitral regurgitation in association with the primary aPL syndrome also has been reported in patients with SLE who have aPLs.[90,91]

The term *catastrophic antiphospholipid antibody syndrome* is now used to classify a subset of patients with thrombosis of the small vasculature (microangiopathy) and involvement of at least three major organs. The mortality in this case approaches 50 percent.[92,93]

Therapy depends on the clinical setting. Patients with positive aPLs but without evidence of thrombosis or recurrent fetal loss should be given low-dose aspirin only. Patients with aPL syndrome who have had thrombotic events or habitual abortions should be anticoagulated for life. Anticoagulation and antithrombotic therapy in these patients has included unfractionated heparin, low-molecular-weight heparin, warfarin.

The intensity of the anticoagulation is still controversial. A recent study showed no significant difference in the recurrence of thrombotic events in a group of patients treated with high-level anticoagulation (international normalized ratio [INR] 3.1 to 4.0) versus low-level anticoagulation (INR 2.0 to 3.0). The high-level anticoagulation group had a significantly higher incidence of hemorrhagic events. Because this study did not include patients with history of recurrent thrombosis and was not powered to assess differences in patients with arterial thrombosis, the treatment in those cases remains controversial.[94]

REFERENCES

1. Beighton P, ed. *McKusick's Heritable Disorders of Connective Tissue,* 5th ed. St. Louis: Mosby-Year Book, 1993.
2. Pyeritz PE, McKusick VA. The Marfan syndrome: diagnosis and management. *N Engl J Med* 1979;300:772–777.
3. Ramirez F, Gayraud B, Pereira L. Marfan syndrome: new clues to genotype-phenotype correlations. *Ann Med,* 1999;31(3):202–207.
4. Loeys BL, Schwarze U, Holm T, et al. Aneurysm syndromes caused by mutation in the TGF-β receptor. *N Engl J Med* 2006;355:788–798.
5. Ramirez F. Fibrillin mutations in Marfan syndrome and related phenotypes. *Curr Opin Genet Dev* 1996;6:309–315.
6. Burn J, Camm J, Davies MJ, et al. The phenotype/genotype relation and the current status of genetic screening in hypertrophic cardiomyopathy, Marfan syndrome, and the long QT syndrome. *Heart* 1997;78:110–116.
7. Mizuguchi, T, Collod-Beroud, G, Akiyama, T, et al. Heterozygous TGFBR2 mutations in Marfan syndrome. *Nat Genet* 2004;36:855.
8. Loeys, BL, Chen, J, Neptune, ER, et al. A syndrome of altered cardiovascular, craniofacial, neurocognitive and skeletal development caused by mutations in TGFBR1 or TGFBR2. *Nat Genet* 2005;37:275.
9. De Paepe A, Devereux RB, Dietz HC, et al. Revised diagnostic criteria for the Marfan syndrome. *Am J Med Genet* 1996;62:417–426.
10. Wexler L, Higgins CB. The use of magnetic resonance imaging in adult congenital heart disease. *Am J Cardiac Imaging* 1995;9:15–28.
11. David TE. Current practice in Marfan's aortic root surgery: Reconstruction with aortic valve preservation or replacement? What to do with the mitral valve. *J Cardiovasc Surg* 1997;12(Suppl 2):147–150.
12. Maron BJ. Heart disease and other causes of sudden death in young athletes. *Curr Probl Cardiol* 1998;23:477–529.
13. Shores J, Berger KR, Murphy EA, Pyeritz RE. Progression of aortic dilation and the benefit of long-term beta-adrenergic blockade in Marfan's syndrome. *N Engl J Med* 1994;30:1335–1341.
14. Salim MA, Alpert BS, Ward JC, Pyeritz RE. Effect of beta-adrenergic blockade on aortic root rate of dilation in the Marfan syndrome. *Am J Cardiol* 1994;74:629–633.
15. Roberts WC, Honig HS. The spectrum of cardiovascular disease in the Marfan syndrome: a clinico-morphologic study of 18 necropsy patients and comparison to 151 previously reported necropsy patients. *Am Heart J* 1982;104:115–135.
16. Gott, VL, Greene, PS, Alejo, DE, et al. Replacement of the aortic root in patients with Marfan's syndrome. *N Engl J Med* 1999;340:1307.
17. Meijboom LJ, Groenink M, van der Wall EE, et al. Aortic root asymmetry in marfan patients; evaluation by magnetic resonance imaging and comparison with standard echocardiography. *Int J Card Imaging* 2000;16(3):161–168.
18. Hayashi J, Moro H, Namura O, et al. Surgical implication of aortic dissection on long-term outcome in Marfan patients. *Surg Today* 1996;26:980–984.
19. LeMaire SA, Coselli JS. Aortic root surgery in Marfan syndrome: current practice and evolving techniques. *J Cardiovasc Surg* 1997;12(Suppl 2):137–141.
20. Meijboom LJ, Nollen GJ, Merchant N, et al. Frequency of coronary ostial aneurysms after aortic root surgery in patients with the Marfan syndrome. *Am J Cardiol* 2002;89(9):1135–1138.
21. Yetman AT, Bornemeier RA, McCrindle BW. Long-term outcome in patients with Marfan syndrome is aortic dissection the only cause of sudden death? *J Am Coll Cardiol* 2003;41(2):329–332.
22. Maron BJ, Ackerman MJ, Nishimura RA, et al. Task Force 4: HCM and other cardiomyopathies, mitral valve prolapse, myocarditis, and Marfan syndrome. *J Am Coll Cardiol* 2005;45(8):1340–1345.

23. Mizuguchi T, Collod-Beroud G, Aklyama T, et al. Heterozygous TGFBR2 mutations in Marfan syndrome. *Nat Genet* 2004;36:855–860.

24. Pannu H, Fadulu VT, Chang J, et al. Mutations in transforming growth factor-beta receptor type II cause familial thoracic aortic aneurysms and dissections. *Circulation* 2005;112:513–520.

25. Loeys BL, Chen J, Neptune ER, et al. A syndrome of altered cardiovascular, craniofacial, neurocognitive and skeletal development caused by mutations in TGFBR1 or TGFBR2. *Nat Genet* 2005;37:275–281.

26. Loeys BL, Schwarze U, Holm T, et al. Aneurysm syndromes caused by mutation in the TGF-β receptor. *N Engl J Med* 2006;355:788–798.

27. Beighton P, De Paepe A, Steinmann B, Tsipouras P, et al. Ehlers-Danlos syndromes: revised nosology, Villefranche, 1997. Ehlers-Danlos National Foundation (USA) and Ehlers-Danlos Support Group (UK). *Am J Med Genet* 1998;77(1):31–37.

28. Slade AKB, John RM, Swanton RH. Pseudoxanthoma elasticum presenting as myocardial infarction. *Br Heart J* 1990;63:372–373.

29. Walker DEL. Overview of inherited metabolic disorders causing cardiovascular disease. *J Inherit Metab Dis* 2003;26:245–257.

30. Takahashi T, Koide T, Yamaguchi H, et al. Ehlers-Danlos syndrome. *Ann Thorac Surg* 1994;58:1180–1182.

31. Trip MD, Smulders YM, et al. Frequent mutation in the ABCC6 gene (R1141X) is associated with a strong increase in the prevalence of coronary artery disease. *Circulation* 2002;106(7):773–775.

32. Wong RS, Follis FM, Shively BK, Wenly JA. Osteogenesis imperfecta and cardiovascular diseases. *Ann Thorac Surg* 1995;60:1439–1443.

33. Gloriex FH, Bishop NJ, Plotkin H, et al. Cyclic administration of pamidronate in children with severe osteogenesis imperfecta. *N Engl J Med* 1998;339:947.

34. Fowler NO, Van der Bel-Kahn JM. Indications for surgical replacement of the mitral valve with particular reference to common and uncommon causes of mitral regurgitation. *Am J Cardiol* 1979;44:148–156.

35. Hortop J, Tsipouras P, Hanley JA, et al. Cardiovascular involvement in osteogenesis imperfecta *Circulation* 1986;73:54–61.

36. *Primer on the Rheumatic Diseases*, 12th ed. Arthritis Foundation, 2001.

37. Moder KG, Miller TD, Tazelaar HD. Cardiac involvement in systemic lupus erythematosus. *Mayo Clin Proc* 1999;74:275–284.

38. Wallace DJ, Hahn BH, eds. *Dubois' Lupus Erythematosus*, 4th ed. Philadelphia: Lea & Febiger, 1993.

39. Ward MM, Pyun E, Studenski S. Mortality risks associated with specific clinical manifestations of systemic lupus erythematosus. *Arch Intern Med* 1996;156:1337–1344.

40. Nihoyannopoulous P, Gomez PM, Joshi J, et al. Cardiac abnormalities in systemic lupus erythematosus. *Circulation* 1990;82:369–375.

41. O'Rourke RA. Antiphospholipid antibodies: a marker of lupus carditis? *Circulation* 1990;82:636–638.

42. Roldan CA, Shively BK, Crawford MH. An echocardiographic study of valvular heart disease associated with systemic lupus erythematosus. *N Engl J Med* 1996;335:1424–1430.

43. Mandell BF. Pericardial effusion in patients with systemic lupus erythematosus: comment on the article by Kahl. *Arthritis Rheum* 1993;36(7):1029–1030.

44. Libman E, Sacks B. A hitherto undescribed form of valvular and mural endocarditis. *Arch Intern Med* 1924;33:701–737.

45. Roldan CA, Shively BK, Lau CC, Gurule FT, Smith EA, Crawford MH. Systemic lupus erythematosus valve disease by transesophageal echocardiography and the role of antiphospholipid antibodies. *J Am Coll Cardiol* 1992;20(5):1127–1134.

46. Singh JA, Woodard PK, Davila-Roman VG, et al. Cardiac magnetic resonance imaging abnormalities in systemic lupus erythematosus: a preliminary report. *Lupus* 2005;14:137–144.

47. Manzi S, Meilahn EN, Rairie JE, et al. Age-specific incidence rates of myocardial infarction and angina in women with systemic lupus erythematosus: comparison with the Framingham study. *Am J Epidemiol* 1997:145:408–415.

48. Sturfelt G, Eskilsson J, Nived O, et al. Cardiovascular disease in systemic disease in systemic lupus erythematosus: a study from a defined population. *Medicine (Baltimore)* 1992;71:216–223.

49. Petri M, Spence D, Bone LR, Hochberg MC. Coronary risk factors in the Johns Hopkins lupus cohort: prevalence by patients, and preventive practices. *Medicine (Baltimore)* 1992;71:291–302.

50. Asanuma Y, Oeser A, Shintani AK, et al. Premature coronary-artery atherosclerosis in systemic lupus erythematosus. *N Engl J Med* 2003;349(25):2407–2415.

51. Salomonsson S, Dorner T, Theander E, et al. A serologic marker for fetal risk of congenital heart block. *Arthritis Rheum* 2002;46(5):1233–1241.

52. Cimaz R, Spence DL, Hornberger L, et al. Incidence of neonatal lupus erythematosus: a prospective study of infants born to mothers with anti-Ro antibodies. *J Pediatrics* 2003;142:678–683.

53. Roberts WC, Dangel JC, Bulkley BH. Nonrheumatic valvular cardiac disease: a clinicopathologic survey of 27 different conditions causing valvular dysfunction. *Cardiovasc Clin* 1973;4:333–446.

54. Morin AM, Boyer JC, Nataf P, Gandjbakhch I. Mitral insufficiency caused by systemic lupus erythematosus requiring valve replacement: three case reports and a review of the literature. *Thorac Cardiovasc Surg* 1996;44:313–316.

55. Navarro-Cano G, Del Rincon I, Pogosian S, et al. Association of mortality with disease severity in rheumatoid arthritis, independent of comorbidity. *Arthritis Rheum* 2003;48:2425–2433.

56. del Rincon ID, Williams K, Stern MP, et al. High incidence of cardiovascular events in a rheumatoid arthritis cohort not explained by traditional cardiac risk factors. *Arthritis Rheum* 2001;44(12):2737–2745.

57. Park YB, Ahn CW, Choi HK, et al. Atherosclerosis in rheumatoid arthritis: morphologic evidence obtained by carotid ultrasound. *Arthritis Rheum* 2002;46(7):1714–1719.

58. Chung CP, Oeser A, Raggi P, et al. Increased coronary-artery atherosclerosis in rheumatoid arthritis: relationship to disease duration and cardiovascular risk factors. *Arthritis Rheum* 2005;52(10):3045–3053.

59. Nicola PJ, Maradit-Kremers H, Roger VL, et al. The risk of congestive heart failure in rheumatoid arthritis: a population-based study over 46 years. *Arthritis Rheum* 2005;52(2):412–420.

60. Nicola PJ, Crowson CS, Maradit-Kremers H, et al. Contribution of congestive heart failure and ischemic heart disease to excess mortality in rheumatoid arthritis. *Arthritis Rheum* 2006;54(1):60–67.

61. Choi HK, Hernan MA, Seeger JD, et al. Methotrexate and mortality in patients with rheumatoid arthritis: a prospective study. *Lancet* 2002;359(9313):1173–1177.

62. Sarzi-Puttini P, Atzeni F, Shoenfeld Y, et al. TNF-alpha, rheumatoid arthritis, and heart failure: a rheumatological dilemma. *Autoimmun Rev* 2005;4(3):153–161.

63. Roberts WC, Hollingsworth JR, Bulkley BH, et al. Combined mitral and aortic regurgitation in ankylosing spondylitis: angiographic and anatomic features. *Am J Med* 1974;56:237–243.

64. Gorman JD, Sack KE, Davis JC Jr. Treatment of ankylosing spondylitis by inhibition of tumor necrosis factor alpha. *N Engl J Med* 2002;346(18):1349–1356.

65. Weiss S, Stead EA, Warren JV, Bailey OT. Scleroderma heart disease: with a consideration of certain other visceral manifestations of scleroderma. *Arch Intern Med* 1943;71:749–776.

66. Bulkley BH, Klacsmann PG, Hutchins GM. Angina pectoris, myocardial infarction and sudden death with normal coronary arteries: a clinicopathologic study of 9 patients with progressive systemic sclerosis. *Am Heart J* 1978;95:563–569.

67. Follansbee WP, Curtiss EI, Medsger TA Jr, et al. Physiologic abnormalities of cardiac function in progressive systemic sclerosis with diffuse scleroderma. *N Engl J Med* 1984;310:142–148.

68. Clements PJ, Furst DE. Heart involvement in systemic sclerosis. *Clin Dermatol* 1994;12:267–275.

69. Candell-Riera J, Armandans-Gil L, Simeon CP, et al. Comprehensive noninvasive assessment of cardiac involvement in limited systemic sclerosis. *Arthritis Rheum* 1996;39:1138–1145.

70. Lekakis J, Mavrikakis M, Emmanuel M, et al. Cold-induced coronary Raynaud's phenomenon in patients with systemic sclerosis. *Clin Exp Rheumatol* 1998;16(2):135–140.

71. Satoh M, Tokuhira M, Hama N, et al. Massive pericardial effusion in scleroderma: a review of five cases. *Br J Rheumatol* 1995;34:564–567.

72. Martinez-Taboada V, Olalla J, Blanco R, et al. Malignant ventricular arrhythmia in systemic sclerosis controlled with an implantable cardioverter defibrillator. *J Rheumatol* 1994;21:2166–2167.

73. Kazzam E, Caidahl K, Hallgren R, et al. Noninvasive evaluation of long-term effects of captopril in systemic sclerosis. *J Intern Med* 1991;230:203–212.

74. Badesch DB, Tapson VF, McGoon MD, et al. Continuous intravenous epoprostenol for pulmonary hypertension due to the scleroderma spectrum of disease: a randomized, controlled trial. *Ann Intern Med* 2000;132:425–434.

75. Hoeper MM, Schwarze M, Ehlerding S, et al. Long-term treatment of primary pulmonary hypertension with aerosolized iloprost, a prostacyclin analogue. *N Engl J Med* 2000;342:1866–1870.

76. Rubin L, Badesch DB, et al. The Bosentan Randomized Trial of Endothelin Antagonist Therapy. *N Engl J Med* 2002;346:896–903.

77. Allanore Y, Vignaux O, Arnaud L, et al. Effects of corticosteroids and immunosuppressors on idiopathic inflammatory myopathy related myocarditis evaluated by magnetic resonance imaging. *Ann Rheum Dis* 2006;65(2):249–252.

78. Erhardt A, Sagir A, Guillevin L, et al. Successful treatment of hepatitis B virus associated polyarteritis nodosa with a combination of prednisolone, alpha-interferon and lamivudine. *J Hepatol* 2000;33(4):677–683.

79. Conron M, Beynon LC. Churg-Strauss syndrome. *Thorax* 2000;55:870–877.

80. Pela G, Tirabassi G, Pattoneri P, Pavone L, Garini G, Bruschi G. Cardiac involvement in the Churg-Strauss syndrome. *Am J Cardiol* 2006;97(10):1519–1524.

81. Hasley PB, Follansbee WP, Coulehan JL. Cardiac manifestations of Churg-Strauss syndrome: report of a case and review of the literature. *Am Heart J* 1990;120:996–999.

82. Renaldini E, Spandrio S, Cerudelli B, et al. Cardiac involvement in Churg-Strauss syndrome: a follow-up of three cases. *Eur Heart J* 1993;14(12):1712–1716.

83. Abu-Shakra M, Gladman DD, Urowitz MB, Farewell V. Anticardiolipin antibodies in systemic lupus erythematosus: clinical and laboratory correlations. *Am J Med* 1995;99:624–628.

84. Khamashta MA, Cudrado MJ, Mujic F, et al. The management of thrombosis in the antiphospholipid-antibody syndrome. *N Engl J Med* 1995;332:993–997.

85. Beynon HLC, Walport MJ. Antiphospholipid antibodies and cardiovascular disease. *Br Heart J* 1992;67:281–284.

86. Cervera R, Asherson RA, Lie JT. Clinicopathologic correlations of the antiphospholipid syndrome. *Semin Arthritis Rheum* 1995;24:262–277.

87. Nesher G, Ilany J, Rosenmann D, Abraham AS. Valvular dysfunction in antiphospholipid syndrome: Prevalence, clinical features, and treatment. *Semin Arthritis Rheum* 1997;27:27–35.

88. Miyakis, S, Lockshin, MD, Atsumi, T, et al. International consensus statement on an update of the classification criteria for definite antiphospholipid syndrome (APS). *Thromb Haemost* 2006;4(2):295–306.

89. Pierangeli SS, Girardi G, Vega-Ostertag M, Liu X, Espinola RG, Salmon J. Requirement of activation of complement C3 and C5 for antiphospholipid antibody-mediated thrombophilia. *Arthritis Rheum* 2005;52(7):2120–2124.

90. Hojnik M, George J, Ziporen L, Shoenfeld Y. Heart valve involvement (Libman-Sacks endocarditis) in the antiphospholipid syndrome. *Circulation* 1996;93:1579–1987.

91. Ziporen L, Goldberg I, Arad M, et al. Libman-Sacks endocarditis in the antiphospholipid syndrome: immunopathologic findings in deformed heart valves. *Lupus* 1996;5(3):196–205.

92. Cervera R, Font J, Gomez-Puerta JA, et al. Validation of the preliminary criteria for the classification of catastrophic antiphospholipid syndrome. *Ann Rheum Dis* 2005;64(8):1205–1209.

93. Asherson RA, Cervera R, Piette JC, et al. Catastrophic antiphospholipid syndrome: clinical and laboratory features of 50 patients. *Medicine (Baltimore)* 1998;77:195–207.

94. Crowther MA, Ginsberg JS, Julian J, et al. A comparison of two intensities of warfarin for the prevention of recurrent thrombosis in patients with the antiphospholipid antibody syndrome. *N Engl J Med* 2003;349(12):1133–1138.

CHAPTER 89

The Diagnosis and Management of Cardiovascular Disease in Cancer Patients

Edward T.H. Yeh / Daniel J. Lenihan / Michael S. Ewer

INTRODUCTION

With the advent of more effective cancer treatments and the increasing likelihood of an earlier cancer diagnosis, patients with many forms of cancer can expect to be either cured of their disease or have their disease stabilized by maintenance therapy. Many forms of cancer should now be thought of as chronic and slowly progressive diseases. Regardless of whether the patient is in the active treatment stage, the chronic maintenance stage, or in complete remission, the cardiovascular specialist is assuming a much greater role in the management of cancer patients. In the active treatment phase, the cardiovascular consultant should manage the acute and chronic cardiovascular complications of cancer therapy such as blood pressure fluctuations, acute coronary syndromes, congestive heart failure, thromboembolism, and pericardial effusion. Also in this phase, patients who are at high risk for cardiovascular complications during complex cancer surgery can be identified and cardiovascular complications managed in the perioperative period. In the chronic maintenance stage, cardiologists are frequently asked to diagnose potential cardiovascular complications of cancer therapy or manage other developing risk factors for vascular disease. With the development of specific targeted cancer therapy, such as antiangiogenesis therapy and vascular disrupting agents, new cardiovascular complications have emerged.

The incidence of patients afflicted with both heart disease and cancer is rising, primarily because of the aging population and the length of time that cancer patients survive. Accordingly, cardiologists are increasingly involved in the care of patients with concomitant cardiovascular problems and cancer.

There are several considerations that do not pertain to the care of patients without cancer. A cardiovascular symptom that occurs during cancer treatment may be caused by the administered agent or agents, whether it is a result of an underlying cardiovascular condition or of a progressive malignancy. Frequently, a combination of chemotherapy agents are used, that adds to the complexity in determining which drug is responsible for a particular cardiac problem; causal relationships between particular agents and a cardiovascular symptom may not yet be firmly established.

Cardiologists must make every effort to optimize the management of any underlying cardiovascular risk factor such as hypercholesterolemia or hypertension and minimize any thrombogenic condition. Cardiologists must also manage cardiovascular complications that arise acutely as the result of cancer treatment. Also, long-term followup of cancer patients with regard to evolving cardiac dysfunction is an important part of such surveillance. This chapter discusses the classic and emerging cardiovascular complications of cancer therapy and describes suggested patterns for managing cancer-related cardiac issues. For this chapter, the cardiotoxicities of chemotherapy and antibody-based therapy are grouped by symptom clusters: heart failure, ischemia, blood pressure changes, and dysrhythmia (Table 89–1). This organization allows for the development of useful guidelines when dealing with cancer patients who have cardiovascular symptoms.[1–4]

FACTORS THAT CONTRIBUTE TO THE DEVELOPMENT OF CARDIOTOXICITY

Many factors contribute to the development of cardiotoxicity in patients being treated for cancer and may include the dose of the drug administered during each chemotherapy cycle, the cumulative dose, the schedule of delivery, the route of administration, the combination of drugs given, and the sequence of administration of these drugs. The age and sex of the patient, the underlying cardiovascular status, and the concomitant or sequential delivery of radiation therapy may also predispose a patient to cardiotoxicity.

Some chemotherapeutic agents induce cardiotoxicity only when administered at high doses. For example, "platinum" drugs (such as cis-platinum), can induce heart failure and pericarditis only at higher doses. Anthracyclines potentially can induce cardiac damage with the first administration, but more typically affect cardiac myocytes at higher cumulative doses. Additionally, ifosfamide can induce low-grade arrhythmias at doses of 1.2 to 2 g/m^2/d for 5 days, but may result in heart failure when administered at a higher dose of 10 to 18 g/m^2/d for 5 days.

For some agents, the cardiac side effects depend on the schedule of administration. Interleukin (IL)-2, a T-cell growth factor, causes weight gain when given in a continuous (low-dose) fashion at the rate of 9×10^6 IU/m^2/d, but hypotension when given as a bolus at a dose of 600,000 IU/kg every 8 hours. Anthracyclines and cyclophosphamide also have cardiac side effects, which depend on the schedule of administration. Administering anthracyclines by continuous infusion over 24 to 96 hours rather than by rapid intravenous infusion probably reduces the cardiotoxicity of these drugs. Similarly, parenteral but not oral busulfan can result in tachyarrhythmias, hypertension, or hypotension, as well as left ventricular (LV) systolic dysfunction.

TABLE 89–1

Cardiotoxicity of Chemotherapy and Antibody-Based Therapy

Heart failure
  Anthracyclines
  Mitoxantrone (Novantrone)
  Cyclophosphamide (Cytoxan)—high dose
  Mitomycin (Mutamycin)
  Trastuzumab (Herceptin)
  Alemtuzumab (Campath)
  Imatinib (Gleevec)
Ischemia
  Fluorouracil (5-FU; Adrucil)
  Cisplatin (Platinol)
  Capecitabine (Xeloda)
  Interleukin-2
  Vascular disrupting agents
Hypotension
  Etoposide (VePisid)
  Alemtuzumab (Campath)
  Cetuximab (Erbitux)
  Rituximab (Rituxan)
  Interleukin-2
  Denileukin (Ontak)
  Interferon-α
  All-trans-retinoic acid (ATRA; Tretinoin)
  Homoharringtonine
  Vascular disrupting agents
Hypertension
  Bevacizumab (Avastin)
  Cisplatin (Platinol)
  Interferon-α
  Angiogenesis inhibitors
Bradycardia
  Paclitaxel (Taxol)
  Thalidomide (Thalomid)
Edema
  Imatinib mesylate (Gleevec)
  Thalidomide (Thalomid)
QT prolongation or torsade de pointes
  Arsenic trioxide (Trisenox)
Thromboembolism
  Bevacizumab (Avastin)
  Thalidomide (Thalomid)
  Cyclooxygenax-2 inhibitors

Changing the sequence in which drugs are administered can also influence the risk or severity of cardiotoxicity. For example, the combination of IL-2 and interferon given simultaneously produces pronounced hypotension, but interferon treatment alone for 2 weeks followed by IL-2 treatment has less effect on blood pressure.

There are many practical ways to reduce cardiotoxicity, including altering the route of administration or the dosing schedule, as well as by avoiding the concomitant administration of agents known to synergistically enhance cardiotoxicity.

PATHOPHYSIOLOGY OF CARDIOTOXICITIES

Among the various cardiac complications of cancer therapy, the most prominent one is LV systolic dysfunction as a direct result of myocardial damage. A large number of cancer therapeutics can cause direct myocardial damage (see Appendix at end of chapter). More recently, trastuzumab (Herceptin), an antibody directed against the HER2-neu receptor, in the treatment of selected patients with breast cancer, has also been associated with an increased incidence of LV systolic dysfunction. Not all forms of cardiac dysfunction related to anticancer treatments are identical and it is likely that many forms will be identified as newer agents are developed (Table 89–3).[5,6]

Among the anthracyclines, doxorubicin, daunorubicin, epirubicin, and idarubicin are approved by the United States Food and Drug Administration for the treatment of a variety of hematologic malignancies and solid tumors. All anthracyclines are associated with both early and late toxicity. Early toxicity may be manifested as a myopericarditis with nonspecific ST-segment and T-wave abnormalities on the electrocardiogram; arrhythmias may be part of the clinical presentation. Late anthracycline cardiotoxicity is cumulative dose-related, and, at sufficiently high dosages, may result in LV dysfunction leading to life-threatening heart failure. The mechanism is thought to be direct myocardial injury because of free radical formation. The incidence of cardiomyopathy increases significantly for patients who receive cumulative doses of doxorubicin that exceed 450 mg/m^2; it can occur at lower cumulative doses.[7] The mortality rate in patients with advanced stages of heart failure secondary to anthracycline cardiotoxicity is as high as 30 to 60 percent. In addition, the prognosis can be greatly altered if cardiac dysfunction is recognized early, the offending agent is eliminated, and optimal treatment is instituted. Anthracyclines cause a unique pattern of histologic cardiac changes, including the vacuolization of myocardial cells, myofibrillar disarray and loss, and necrosis.[8] A direct relationship between biopsy grade of histopathologic change, the cumulative dose of the drug, and the clinical symptoms has been shown. Free radicals cause cardiotoxicity by injuring lipid structures in the myocardial cells, resulting in peroxidation that impairs the function of the sarcoplasmic reticulum and mitochondria, resulting in cellular necrosis. Histopathologic and pathogenic information regarding the cardiotoxicity of other anticancer drugs is sparse.

Considering other classes of agents, the reported incidence of LV dysfunction and heart failure in patients who receive trastuzumab appears to depend on whether or not the drug is given alone or in combination with other cardiotoxic agents.[9] The incidence of cardiotoxicity is also increased in older patients, those with preexisting cardiac disease, and those who previously received chemotherapy and radiation therapy. The incidence of toxicity associated with trastuzumab has been much lower, however, in more recent trials with closer monitoring and avoiding trastuzumab and anthracyclines simultaneously.[10]

HEART FAILURE AND LEFT VENTRICULAR DYSFUNCTION

The basic pathophysiology of heart failure is essentially the same in both cancer and noncancer patients. The neurohor-

---

TABLE 89–2

Causes of Left Ventricular Systolic Dysfunction or Heart Failure in Cancer Patients

Preexisting risk factors or underlying disease
    Coronary artery disease and ischemia
    Hypertension
    Alcohol-related cardiomyopathy
    Diabetes
    Nutritional deficiencies
    Cardiac cachexia
    Thyrotoxicosis or hypothyroidism
Related to cancer diagnosis
    Amyloidosis
    Myocarditis
    Cardiotoxic chemotherapy
    Radiation
    Sepsis
    Capillary leak phenomenon
    Carcinoid
Other
    Arterial venous fistula
    Endocarditis
    Pericardial disease including constrictive pericarditis
    Pulmonary emboli
    Pulmonary hypertension
    Hemochromatosis and iron overload (frequent transfusions)

---

monal hypothesis that forms the basis of the diagnosis of heart failure, and shapes the strategies for effective treatment, is applicable in both groups of patients. Heart failure and cancer progression also share pathophysiologic characteristics. It is imperative to understand the etiology of heart failure in these patients, as this is one of the most important comorbidities that affects the life span of a cancer patient. Frequently multifactorial scenarios exist, and while the triggering event may be defined, the contribution of preexisting and coexisting additive factors are difficult to quantitate (Fig. 89–1).

STRATEGIES FOR DIAGNOSING HEART FAILURE AND LEFT VENTRICULAR DYSFUNCTION

Patients who are undergoing therapy for cancer may have many stresses in their life, any one of which could contribute to the overall excess catecholamine state that further promotes LV systolic dysfunction (see Fig. 89–1). Table 89–2 summarizes the typical causes of LV systolic dysfunction and heart failure in cancer patients. All of the major contributors to heart failure need to be investigated and treated appropriately in order to optimally affect the course of illness.

It must be kept in mind that diagnosing heart failure can be a challenge, as evidenced by a recent study in a group of patients undergoing chemotherapy in which the examining physician failed to

TABLE 89–3

Different Types of Cancer Therapy-Induced Cardiomyopathy

	TYPE I	TYPE II	TYPE III
Characteristic agent	Doxorubicin	Trastuzumab	Imatinib
Clinical course, response to therapy	Appears to be irreversible	Likely to be reversible	Could be reversible, however experience is limited
Dose effects	Cumulative, dose related	Not dose related	Not dose related
Mechanism	Free radical formation, oxidative stress/damage	Blocked ErbB2 signaling	Activation of the endoplasmic reticulum stress response
Ultrastructure	Vacuoles; myofibrillar disarray and dropout; necrosis	No apparent ultrastructural abnormalities	Mitochondrial abnormality, Accumulation of membrane whorls
Effect of rechallenge	High probability of recurrent dysfunction that is progressive	Increasing evidence for the relative safety of rechallenge; additional data needed	Possible safety of rechallenge, additional data needed

SOURCE: Modified from Ewer MS and Lippman SM,[5] and Kerkela R, et al.[6]

identify shortness of breath 77 percent of the time and failed to identify fatigue 38 percent of the time.[11] Furthermore, in patients with only suspected heart disease, correct documentation of manifestations that establish the diagnosis were present only 50 percent of the time.[12] Thus, techniques other than history alone must be used to support the diagnosis of heart failure. Recent observations suggest that certain monoclonal antibodies may also produce unexpected heart failure and this is proposed to be the result of interfering with cellular mechanisms that have protean effects. The importance of the physical examination in confirming the presence of heart failure and LV systolic dysfunction in cancer patients cannot be overemphasized (see Chap. 25). Certain physical findings, such as a third heart sound, pulsus paradoxus, or jugular venous distension, can be highly predictive of heart failure (see Chap. 12).

Among basic laboratory studies, the electrocardiogram (ECG) does not discern heart failure or LV dysfunction, although it can confirm suspected abnormalities or indicate potential underlying cardiac disease, such as ischemia or conduction abnormalities. Additional laboratory testing is commonly necessary to identify those at increased risk for cardiomyopathy or to confirm a diagnosis of heart failure. The most commonly used serologic tests include a complete lipid panel to indicate a risk for vascular disease and blood glucose monitoring to screen for diabetes, both clinical predictors for heart failure. Anemia, especially common in cancer patients, has been directly correlated with outcomes in heart failure patients and should be part of a basic laboratory screen (see Chap. 26). Other specific biomarkers that are crucial in the evaluation of patients with suspected heart failure, especially those with cancer, include troponins (I and T) as well as B-type natriuretic peptide (BNP). Troponins, in conjunction with creatine kinase myocardial band, are the standard markers for confirming myocardial infarction (MI). These biomarkers may be of value in screening for LV systolic dysfunction that may occur during chemotherapy.[4] In the noncancer population, BNP has also shown promise as a biomarker to detect early cardiotoxicity. Recent data suggests that markedly elevated BNP values do not always correlate with volume overload or LV dysfunction in this population. A careful physical examination is still the most reliable means of determining the presence or absence of volume overload.

Other specific cardiac testing is frequently necessary to evaluate the extent of underlying heart disease that may be present in a patient with cancer. Exercise or pharmacologic stress testing can help confirm that coronary artery disease is present (see Chap. 14), and cardiac catheterization demonstrates angiographically the extent of coronary artery disease, LV systolic dysfunction, valvular abnormalities and other hemodynamic disturbances (see Chap. 17). A myocardial biopsy may be appropriate when it is necessary to

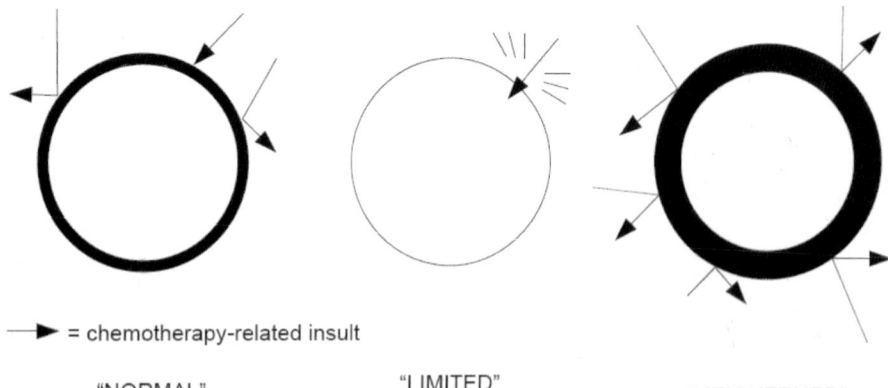

→ = chemotherapy-related insult

"NORMAL" Cardiac Reserve (Patient with minimal risk factors to develop cardiomyopathy)

"LIMITED" Cardiac Reserve (Patient with myocardial cell integrity disruption (structural or functional) due to cardiomyopathy)

"HEIGHTENED" Cardiac Reserve (Patient with minimal risk for cardiomyopathy and genetic resistance)

FIGURE 89–1. Chemotherapy-related insults.

confirm a diagnosis of amyloidosis or myocarditis. In addition, a myocardial biopsy may reveal the acute changes related to anthracycline administration. The typical histologic changes associated with the anthracyclines dissipate over time. Thus, a myocardial biopsy is not useful in evaluating patients months or years after exposure to an anthracycline. An invasive hemodynamic assessment may be extremely useful in determining the presence or absence of constrictive pericarditis or other causes of heart failure that may be difficult to discern noninvasively.

【 】 THE PRINCIPLES OF THERAPY FOR HEART FAILURE

The principles of therapy for heart failure and LV dysfunction in a cancer patient are similar to those in a noncancer patient. An often overlooked management component is the education of both the patient and family members. This is especially important in the cancer patient where noncancer issues are often considered noncrucial. One area to be emphasized is compliance with medication prescriptions. Additionally, education is necessary regarding the symptoms of cardiac decompensation.

Guidelines for the management of heart failure are very explicit regarding how to manage chronic congestive heart failure, and the evidence-based approach is detailed in these guidelines. There is no reason to suspect that the standard medical therapy would not be effective in most cancer patients as well. Table 89–4 outlines the therapeutic options for these patients. Angiotensin-converting enzyme (ACE) inhibitors remain the cornerstone of therapy in conjunction with β-adrenergic blocking agents. Loop diuretics remain a mainstay for controlling volume overload. In addition, risk factors for heart failure should also be aggressively treated, such as statins for hyperlipidemia. Other therapies that are recommended in special situations include aldosterone inhibitors, which are indicated in patients with either severe heart failure and in patients who recently suffered an MI (see Chap. 26). The usefulness of angiotensin receptor blockers as alternatives to ACE inhibitors for the treatment of heart failure is well established. The combination of nitrates and hydralazine is of special benefit in African American patients, as well as in patients with renal insufficiency.

There are important concerns with regard to patients who are undergoing active treatment for cancer that incorporates multiple agents, because treatment for heart failure can heighten the risk for drug–drug interactions. It is imperative with these patients that unnecessary medications are avoided and that the addition of a potentially beneficial heart failure medication is carefully weighed against the risk of possible interactions with anticancer agents. Aspirin is generally recommended for patients with heart failure, but there is little data to support its use unless a patient has significant vascular disease. Clopidogrel, a more potent antiplatelet agent, is also commonly recommended. However, these agents may pose a substantial bleeding risk, particularly in patients who have thrombocytopenia. Several pharmacotherapeutic agents are being developed that may be particularly appropriate for use in cancer patients with heart failure. Among these, erythropoietin to stimulate red blood cell production and reduce anemia is effective and is an area of investigation for treating heart-failure patients. Preliminary evidence suggests benefit, but formal acceptance as treatment for anemia in cancer patients awaits the completion of a definitive

TABLE 89–4

Therapeutic Options That May be Valuable in Cancer Patients with Heart Failure

MEDICATIONS	DEVICES
Angiotensin-converting enzyme inhibitors	Permanent pacemaker
β Blockers	Biventricular pacemaker
Loop diuretics	Implantable cardiac defibrillator
Angiotensin receptor blockers	Ultrafiltration
Aldosterone antagonists	
Vasopressin antagonists	
Aspirin	
Clopidogrel (Plavix)	
Hydroxymethylglutaryl coenzyme A (HMG-CoA) reductase inhibitors (statins)	
Nitrates/hydralazine	
Erythropoietin	

trial. Stem cell therapy for LV dysfunction may become an important strategy in the future; methods of delivery and the enhancement of engraftment remain subjects of intense investigation. There are a variety of other potentially useful agents for treating heart failure in cancer patients. Intravenous immunoglobulin, which is used in patients who have immune deficiencies or even an excessive graft-versus-host response after bone marrow transplantation, may have important future implications. One randomized, controlled study did not show any clear benefit. Other therapies that appear promising include sildenafil for right-heart failure because of pulmonary hypertension. Other medications of potential value include a newer class of diuretics, the vasopressin antagonists (such as conivaptan and tolvaptan). These agents produce a water diuresis without a significant solute loss. This therapy may be particularly advantageous in patients with hyponatremia who have significant volume overload.

Cardiac devices are an integral part of modern heart-failure management, including heart failure in patients with cancer. Bradycardic pacing is appropriate if a patient is unable to tolerate β-blocker therapy because of a low heart rate or disease of the conduction system. The use of a biventricular pacemaker to lessen symptomatic heart failure in patients with a wide QRS complex is an accepted therapy and should not be denied to appropriate cancer patients; the benefit of biventricular pacing devices, however, occurs after 6 months, thus their use is not warranted in patients with end-stage malignancy. Similar considerations pertain to the use of implantable cardiac defibrillators (see Chap. 26); indications include symptomatic ventricular arrhythmias in patients with severe LV dysfunction with or without a prior MI. In patients who are at high risk for life-threatening ventricular arrhythmias, such as those with marked amyloidosis, implantable cardiac defibrillators should be considered more liberally. There are other device-related treatments that may be especially useful in the management of heart failure in cancer patients. One example includes ultrafiltration, which physically removes volume in patients with significant volume overload. Ultrafiltration devices are especially useful in patients with evidence of cardiac decompensation who have not responded initially to diuretics.

Surgical therapy for heart failure has been intensely investigated, but as yet, there is no clearly established surgical technique for the management of heart failure (see Chap. 26). Coronary bypass grafting for the treatment of severe ischemic heart disease may be appropriate in cases where dysfunctional yet viable myocardium can be revascularized, thereby restoring function. Other surgical techniques may be appropriate in selected situations resulting in heart failure, such as pericardial stripping for constrictive pericarditis or removal of intracardiac masses. Ethical concerns are also important when deciding on the appropriate therapy for a cancer patient with heart failure. One must consider to what extent the two entities interplay and to what extent they affect overall prognosis. It is important to openly address end-of-life issues with patients so that the treatment approach incorporates the wishes of the patient as well as the reality of the clinical condition into consideration. The diagnosis of cancer should not imply that the heart failure cannot or should not be aggressively treated.

【 】 FUTURE DEVELOPMENTS

The ability to detect a cardiotoxic insult continues to be a major challenge. Recent use of established biomarkers, such as BNP and troponin, in patients receiving chemotherapy, has shown promise as an effective tool for identifying toxicity at its earliest stages. Future research will include mapping genetic polymorphisms to identify cancer patients who are at increased risk for cardiomyopathy as a consequence of chemotherapy or serve as a marker of an impaired ability to recover from a cardiotoxic insult. This may be especially important when considering antiangiogenic therapy, where the main goal is to decrease microvascular blood flow to a tumor.

MYOCARDIAL ISCHEMIA

Chest pain is a common symptom in cancer patients who are undergoing various forms of anticancer therapy. Chest pain often necessitates the interruption of chemotherapy while serial cardiac enzyme assessments and ECGs are performed. If non–ST-segment elevation MI or Q-wave MI is confirmed, patients should be managed according to the current American College of Cardiology and American Heart Association guidelines (see Chaps. 12, 59, and 61). However, thrombocytopenia and brain metastases pose a particular problem for cancer patients with an acute coronary syndrome because anticoagulation therapy is contraindicated under these circumstances. Invasive cardiac procedures cannot easily be performed in patients with thrombocytopenia.

It is well established that radiation therapy to the mediastinum promotes an increased risk for infarction, and it appears more prevalent in patients with left-sided chest radiation. Additionally, several chemotherapy agents are known to precipitate or exacerbate an ischemic response. Cisplatin infusions can cause chest pain, palpitations, and, occasionally, elevated cardiac enzyme levels indicative of a myocardial infarction. Cisplatin can also cause cardiovascular complications such as hypertension, LV hypertrophy, myocardial ischemia, and infarction as long as 10 to 20 years after the remission of metastatic testicular cancer.[13] 5-Fluorouracil (5-FU) can also

cause an ischemic syndrome that may range from subclinical ischemia to acute myocardial infarction. Subsequent rechallenge with 5-FU frequently reproduces the initial ischemic event. Nevertheless, the ischemia is usually reversed when 5-FU treatment is stopped and antiischemic therapy implemented. In some patients, pretreatment with nitrates and calcium channel-blocking agents has allowed therapy deemed crucial to be continued. Capecitabine is currently used in the treatment of breast and gastrointestinal cancers and is believed to be less toxic than 5-FU, but is associated with cardiotoxic effects that include ischemic phenomena[14] arrhythmias, ECG changes, and, rarely, cardiomyopathy. Vinca alkaloids, such as vinorelbine, also have been reported to cause angina associated with ECG changes and arrhythmias, as well as MI. These cardiac events may present with Prinzmetal angina with reversible ECG changes. Angina and myocardial infarction are serious, but relatively rare, consequences of interferon-α therapy. Fatal MI and thrombosis have also been noted after the use of all-*trans*-retinoic acid (ATRA). Bevacizumab, a recombinant humanized monoclonal IgG$_1$ antibody that binds to and inhibits the activity of human vascular endothelial growth factor (VEGF), was recently shown to be associated with an increased risk of angina and MI, in addition to serious arterial thromboembolic events, including cerebrovascular accident and transient ischemic attacks. It is used for the treatment of metastatic colon carcinoma and is generally used in combination with other agents. A new class of chemotherapy agents, termed *vascular disrupting agents*, are currently undergoing clinical evaluation, and have been noted to cause asymptomatic creatine kinase myocardial band release and may be associated with acute coronary syndromes.

BLOOD PRESSURE FLUCTUATIONS

The classic malignancy that causes hypertension that is often paroxysmal or episodic in nature is pheochromocytoma (see Chap. 61); pheochromocytomas are usually benign but are malignant in approximately 10 percent of cases. They may be isolated tumors but can also be associated with multiple endocrine neoplasia (MEN) syndromes of the type 2 variety, in particular the MEN 2A and MEN 2B syndromes. Bilateral pheochromocytomas are also associated with von Hippel-Lindau disease (see Chap. 12) and neurofibromatosis. Benign pheochromocytomas usually can be resected surgically, but patients with such tumors require special anesthetic considerations, including pretreatment with phenoxybenzamine followed by the administration of a β-adrenergic blocking agent. Other tumors may also cause hypertension including hyperthyroidism associated with thyroid tumors. Among the common treatments used in cancer patients that cause blood pressure fluctuations are the antirejection regimens; cyclosporine A, especially when it is used in conjunction with corticosteroids is associated with hypertension; the incidence may be greater than 50 percent. Often antihypertensive therapy is required. Cyclosporine-associated hypertension may be refractory and diastolic pressure elevations are especially troublesome. The entire class of antiangiogenesis drugs, can cause a significant rise in blood pressure. BAY43–9006 is a potent inhibitor of the VEGFR-2, VEGFR-3, FLT-3, c-kit, and platelet-derived growth factor receptor in vitro and may affect the regulation of endothelial cell proliferation and survival. These blood pressure increases are especially troublesome because they may persist after discontinuation of the agent. The usual antihypertensive medications are often effective in bevacizumab-associated hypertension.

Blood pressure variations that are unrelated to tumor products are much more common in cancer patients; the combination of malnutrition and dehydration is one of the most common causes of hypotension. Other complications of malignancy, most notably sepsis, can be accompanied by profound and refractory hypotension.

Hypotension is the most common side effect of etoposide. The infusion of monoclonal antibodies commonly causes hypotension as a result of the massive release of cytokines (an acute transfusion reaction); these agents can also cause fever, dyspnea, hypoxia, and even death. Careful monitoring for hypotension is especially important for patients with preexisting cardiac disease. Cetuximab, a human/mouse chimeric monoclonal antibody that binds to the human epidermal growth factor receptor, can cause severe, potentially fatal infusion reactions characterized by hypotension, bronchospasm, and urticaria; this phenomenon occurs in approximately 3 percent of patients.[15–16] Rituximab, a chimeric murine/human monoclonal antibody directed against the CD20 antigen, can cause infusion-related side effects that occur within the first few hours of the start of infusion. Supportive measures that are usually effective include intravenous fluids, vasopressors, bronchodilators, diphenhydramine, and acetaminophen. Interferon-α usually causes acute symptoms during the first 2–8 hours after treatment; these include flu-like symptoms, hypotension, tachycardia, and nausea, and vomiting.[17] The retinoic acid syndrome appears in approximately 26 percent of patients who receive ATRA, typically within the first 21 days of treatment. This syndrome includes fever, dyspnea, hypotension, and pericardial and pleural effusions.[18] High-dose treatment with IL-2 can result in adverse cardiovascular and hemodynamic effects similar to those of septic shock[17] and can lead to hypotension, vascular leak syndrome (hypotension, edema, hypoalbuminemia), and respiratory insufficiency requiring pressor agents and mechanical ventilation support.

Homoharringtonine, a natural product that is used in the treatment of some forms of leukemia, is associated with severe hypotension and may require elimination of the drug from the regimen. The hypotension may be related to homoharringtonine's calcium channel-blocking activity.

ARRHYTHMIAS

Arrhythmia in the cancer patient may be a consequence of cardiotoxic anticancer therapies, a response to an altered environment wherein the chemical, metabolic, or mechanical abnormalities promote abnormal impulse formation or propagation or a manifestation of tumor spread. Cancer patients often require strategies for managing their arrhythmias that take into account the underlying condition responsible for the arrhythmia. Additionally, cancer-related arrhythmias encompass the spectrum from trivial to life-threatening.

【 】 TYPES OF ARRHYTHMIA

Supraventricular Arrhythmias

Supraventricular arrhythmias are a common occurrence in cancer patients. Atrial premature complexes are a well-recognized mani-

festation of early anthracycline cardiotoxicity and may be a harbinger of the more serious late LV dysfunction. More sustained supraventricular arrhythmias are seen commonly in patients with a chest malignancy, especially lung cancer, which is often associated with increased pulmonary artery pressure. Pulmonary hypertension often precedes atrial flutter or fibrillation. Mechanical effects of an expanding tumor mass, as well as atelectasis and/or infection in areas distal to occluded bronchi, further increase right-sided pressures and cause arrhythmias. Hypoxia confounds the problem. Supraventricular arrhythmias are especially frequent early in the postoperative period following lung resection. Supraventricular arrhythmias also occur in association with high-dose chemotherapy and stem cell transplantation. Various specific chemotherapeutic agents also have been associated with atrial fibrillation, and include 5-FU, gemcitabine, docetaxel, and alemtuzumab. Radiation to the heart has a well-known association with arrhythmia; however, radiation to sites distant from the heart also has been associated with supraventricular arrhythmia. Other forms of sustained supraventricular tachycardia, including reentrant supraventricular tachycardia and multifocal atrial tachycardia, are also seen commonly in the cancer patient.

Intracardiac masses, including benign tumors and malignant processes such as primary cardiac lymphomas and cardiac metastases from lung, breast, or melanoma, often present with supraventricular arrhythmias. Atrial fibrillation is often associated with acute pulmonary embolism and pericarditis, conditions frequently encountered in cancer patients.

An important risk factor for sustained supraventricular arrhythmias is intrinsic cardiac disease. In particular, conditions resulting in increased atrial size or that are associated with inflammation contribute to elevated atrial pressure and result in atrial rhythm disturbances. Age, hypertension, lung disease, thyrotoxicosis, surgery, and other states that trigger increased catecholamine levels may all also contribute to elevated atrial pressure.

Ventricular Arrhythmias

Cancer patients are more prone to ventricular arrhythmias than the noncancer population. These patients are exposed to stressful and potentially cardiotoxic anticancer treatments, the increased ingestion of multiple noncancer medicines that may be proarrhythmic, and coexisting hormonal and metabolic abnormalities. Hypokalemia, alkalotic states, hypomagnesemia, thyrotoxicosis, pheochromocytomas, and the mediator release associated with the carcinoid syndrome are all associated with potentially life-threatening ventricular tachycardia.

Prolonged QT Interval and Torsade de Pointes

Torsade de pointes, a form of ventricular tachycardia associated with prolongation of the QT interval, is related to an increasing list of medications, many of which are used in the management of malignancy and in their supportive care. Prolongation of the QT interval may also occur in association with the supplements that cancer patients sometimes ingest, among them cesium chloride, which is commonly used as an alternative therapy for various types of malignancies. Several anticancer agents are of especial interest. Arsenic trioxide is associated with QT prolongation in more than 50 percent of treated patients.[19] Other cardiac side effects include sinus tachycardia, nonspecific ST-T changes, and *torsade de pointes*.[19] In one study, the most common acute side effect was fluid retention with pleural and pericardial effusions. Complete heart block and sudden cardiac death[20] have also been reported in patients receiving arsenic trioxide. It is important to monitor the QT interval with serial ECGs, with particular attention to patients who are simultaneously receiving other drugs that have the potential to prolong the QT interval.

Bradyarrhythmias and Atrioventricular Heart Block

Thalidomide, may cause sinus bradycardia that may be mitigated by adjusting the dosage; sinus bradycardia associated with thalidomide is often asymptomatic, but occasionally permanent pacing may be required. Paclitaxel, is used extensively in the treatment of many solid tumors, and has been reported to cause sinus bradycardia, heart block, premature ventricular contractions, and ventricular tachycardia.

The conduction system of the heart can be interrupted at all levels by primary and metastatic tumors or by infiltrative processes such as amyloidosis. Pheochromocytomas, thymomas, high-dose chemotherapy, and stem cell transplantation are all associated with block at the level of the atrioventricular node. Individual chemotherapy agents associated with transient atrioventricular block include paclitaxel and octreotide.

【 】 TREATMENT OF ARRHYTHMIAS

In managing arrhythmias in the cancer patient, one must first consider possible cancer-related etiologies for the rhythm disturbance. In many instances, correcting metabolic abnormalities or removing arrhythmogenic agents is the most successful approach. The arrhythmia may be sufficiently serious that the permanent elimination of the offending agent from the treatment regimen must be recommended. In some settings, the arrhythmia may be controlled by the use of standard medications or procedures thereby permitting completion of highly effective anticancer treatment. The use of implanted devices should not be denied to patients who have malignancy.

THROMBOEMBOLISM
【 】 GENERAL CONSIDERATIONS

The incidence of thrombosis is higher in patients with cancer than in the general population; thrombosis in these patients portends a worse prognosis. The prevention, recognition, and treatment of thromboembolism are clinical challenges for physicians treating patients with cancer. A venous thromboembolism (VTE) occurs in 5 to 7 percent of patients with malignancy, an incidence that is much greater than that for the general population, in which the incidence is approximately 0.1 percent. Patients with cancer constitute nearly 20 percent of all cases of thrombosis. Approximately 10 percent of all noncancer patients with VTE will be diagnosed with malignancy within 2 years. The incidence of arterial thromboembolism is less than that of VTE in cancer patients; they, too, occur at a much higher incidence than in the general population. The source of arterial thromboembolism is most likely atherosclerosis, but the general inflammatory condition observed in patients with cancer and treatment with the new antiangiogenic agents are also important determinants. With the more widespread use of such agents, the incidence of arterial thrombosis likely will increase in cancer patients. Thrombotic events, such as deep venous thrombosis (DVT), pulmonary embolism, and arterial thrombosis have also been observed in approximately 11 percent of patients treated with IL-2.[21] The risk of death for cancer patients diagnosed with a DVT or pulmonary embolism is substantially higher than that in cancer patients without such an event. The same is true for arterial thrombi. The inhospital mortality may approach 20 to 30 percent, especially in those with pulmonary emboli. Nonbacterial endocarditis (marantic endocarditis) and disseminated intravascular coagulation are additional examples of life-threatening thrombotic conditions associated with cancer.

【 】 PATHOPHYSIOLOGY OF THROMBOSIS

The pathophysiology of thrombosis is discussed in Chaps. 52, 53, and 72, and varies somewhat depending on the underlying etiology. This section focuses on venous and arterial thrombosis in the cancer patient. However, there is an incomplete understanding of the initial triggers for thrombosis and no single explanation pertains to all conditions in which thrombosis occurs (Table 89–5).

VTE in cancer patients occurs as a result of the classic triad: stasis, endothelial disruption, and hypercoagulability. In each situation, one component may predominate and, if identified, can be effectively treated. If, for example, a patient has an abdominal tumor that is compressing the inferior vena cava causing stasis, and this tumor can be removed or reduced by chemotherapy or radiation, then the likelihood of VTE may be markedly reduced. Indwelling intravenous catheters may cause thrombus formation (Fig. 89–2). Removal of an indwelling central catheter is also likely to be very effective in reducing the risk of subsequent recurrence or progression of a thrombus once the stimulus for hypercoagulability has been removed.

TABLE 89–5

Risks for Thrombolic Events in Cancer Patients

Immobilization
Genetic
   Inherited coagulopathy
   Polymorphism(s) at risk for thrombosis
Surgery
Trauma
Heart failure
Estrogen therapy
Prior thrombosis
Indwelling catheters
Chemotherapy or other agents
   Tamoxifen
   Thalidomide
   Bevacizumab
   Cyclooxygenase-2 inhibitors (Rofecoxib)
Mechanical effects of cancer itself

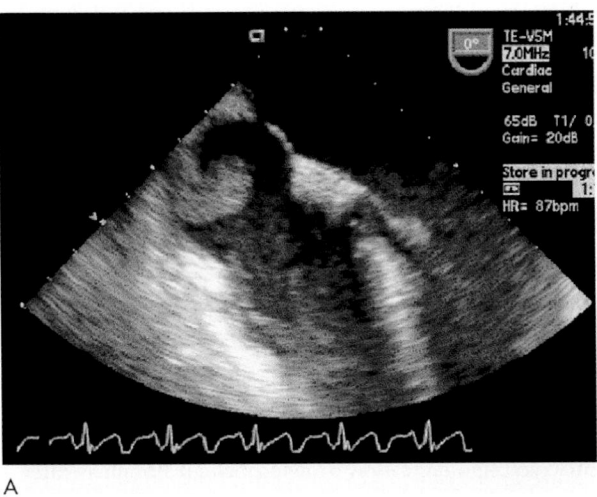

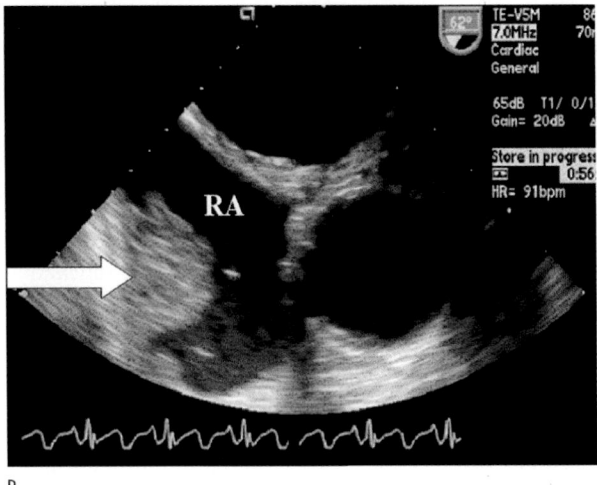

FIGURE 89–2. **A** and **B.** Two views from a transesophageal echocardiogram showing a large thrombus in the right atrium associated with an indwelling catheter. RA, right atrium.

Arterial thrombosis in cancer patients is most commonly associated with platelet activation either in the presence or absence of atherosclerosis. There are many ways platelets can be activated, including by generalized inflammatory conditions and by the malignancy itself. The exact mechanism also may include microvessel constriction and platelet activation.

CLINICAL MANIFESTATIONS

The location of a thrombosis is of paramount importance with regard to how the thrombus will manifest itself. The extent and position of collateral vessels is also crucial in determining how the thrombus will affect the patient. A deep venous thrombosis in a lower extremity, for example, is likely to cause pain, swelling, and erythema of that extremity. A deep venous thrombosis of an arm may be revealed by unilateral arm swelling that develops fairly suddenly or a bluish discoloration because of poor venous return. Arterial thrombi usually result in pain, pallor, and pulselessness in an extremity. An arterial thrombosis of an internal organ may be manifested by an episode of unstable angina, an acute coronary syndrome, a cerebral vascular accident, or intestinal ischemia that may be difficult to detect.

The most common presentation of VTE is unilateral leg edema. This can be associated with erythema, but typically it is difficult to discern VTE from cellulitis. Unilateral extremity swelling is, therefore, a hallmark of VTE. Bilateral lower-extremity edema may be caused by a proximal venous thrombosis or even congestive heart failure, malnutrition, or other causes of edema. Pulmonary emboli are most commonly manifested by the sudden onset of shortness of breath, chest discomfort, and tachypnea. In addition, patients may report hemoptysis and tachycardia. Syncope, hypotension, and sudden cardiac death are manifestations of larger pulmonary emboli. Long-term effects of pulmonary embolus and DVT include pulmonary hypertension and the postphlebitic syndrome (see Chaps. 71 and 72).

The diagnostic approaches used to detect thrombosis, either venous or arterial, in cancer patients are similar to those used in patients without malignancy; these techniques are highlighted elsewhere. Computed tomographic (CT) angiography (see Chap.

22) is a reliable and sensitive tool for detecting pulmonary embolus and peripheral extremity ultrasound remains important in the evaluation of venous flow and/or thrombus (Fig. 89–3). The techniques used to detect arterial thrombus may vary and are determined mainly by the location of the arterial insufficiency. A combination of ultrasound, sequential pressure measurements, angiography, computerized tomography, and magnetic resonance imaging (MRI), form the basis of diagnostic testing for patients with suspected arterial insufficiency.

TREATMENT OF THROMBOEMBOLISM

The optimal treatment of VTE is a challenge in cancer patients. Typically, these patients are at increased risk for bleeding; they may be anemic so that the effects of bleeding are disproportionate. There may be associated thrombocytopenia or hepatic or renal dysfunction, or perhaps the malignancy is associated with the thrombus in a location that may predispose to bleeding complications. Antithrombotic therapy may consist of medications to prevent or limit the propagation of a thrombus or perhaps throm-

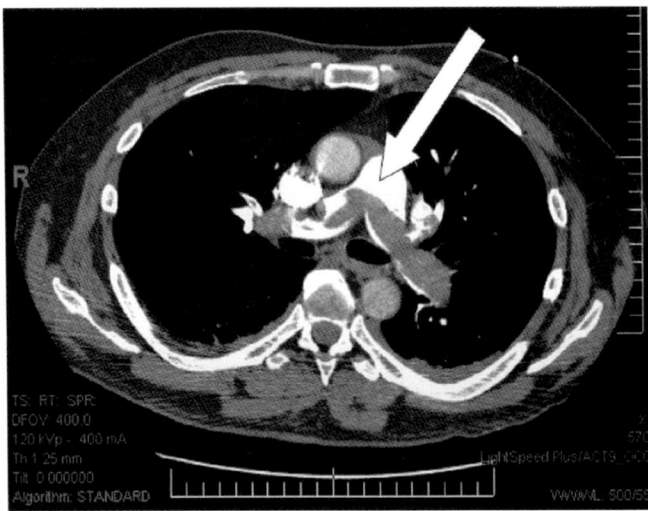

FIGURE 89–3. A contrast-enhanced CT scan showing a massive pulmonary embolus (*white arrow*).

bolytic agents to enhance the removal of a thrombus. Furthermore, the risks associated with thrombus extension, embolization, or recurrence of the thrombus must be weighed against the risks of hemorrhage as part of the decision-making process.

Guidelines for antithrombotic therapy for VTE have been published by the Seventh ACCP Conference on Antithrombotic and Thrombolytic Therapy.[22] Standard treatment for VTE traditionally consists of low-molecular-weight heparin (LMWH), unfractionated intravenous heparin, or adjusted-dose subcutaneous heparin, followed by long-term therapy with an oral anticoagulant. Unfractionated heparin has been superseded by LMWH as the initial treatment in most cancer patients with VTE in both inpatients and outpatients. Long-term treatment with warfarin may be complicated by several problems, including drug–drug interactions, malnutrition, nausea, and/or vomiting during chemotherapy, and thrombocytopenia. Additionally, hepatic dysfunction in cancer patients may lead to unpredictable levels of anticoagulation, and result in increased bleeding complications. LMWH is more effective than oral anticoagulant therapy with warfarin for the prevention of recurrent VTE in patients with cancer who have had acute, symptomatic proximal DVT, pulmonary embolism, or both.[23] Further advantages of LMWH are that the doses are more easily adjusted, the pharmacokinetic properties are more predictable, laboratory monitoring is minimized, and fewer drug interactions occur than is the case with oral anticoagulants. Also in favor of heparin therapy in cancer patients are reports that the heparins have antiproliferative, antiangiogenetic, and anti metastatic effects, and that LMWH may increase the response to chemotherapy, thereby prolonging the survival of cancer patients.[24] For these several reasons, secondary prophylaxis with LMWH may be more effective and feasible than oral anticoagulant therapy in cancer patients with VTE, although the risk of bleeding is the same for both treatment approaches. More recently, low-dose aspirin was safely used to prevent thrombotic complications in patients with polycythemia vera, and has been advocated as an alternative option in patients with cancer presenting with paraneoplastic thrombocytosis.

Certain anticoagulants might also improve cancer survival rates independent of their effect on thromboembolism. Such agents include new antithrombotic agents such as oral direct thrombin or long-acting synthetic factor Xa inhibitors. Furthermore, mechanical treatments, such as compression stockings used to prevent postthrombotic syndrome, have value in the treatment of cancer patients with thromboembolism, as do selected surgical techniques to treat venous ulceration. Venacaval filters may be employed instead of anticoagulation in patients with recurrent pulmonary embolisms who also have a high risk of serious bleeding.

PERICARDIAL CONSIDERATIONS

Both cancer and the treatment of cancer affect the pericardium more than other cardiac structures. Both primary and metastatic tumors occur in the pericardium, and the sequelae of radiation therapy may cause both acute pericardial inflammation and chronic alteration of the pericardial membranes. These processes may ultimately progress to constrictive pericarditis that can result in a life-threatening low-output state (see Chap. 84).

Tumors are found to have spread to the pericardium in approximately 9 percent of cancer patients who come to autopsy. In the general population, approximately 7 percent of all patients who experience acute pericarditis either have a history of malignancy or are later found to have a malignancy related to their pericardial inflammation. Not surprisingly, therefore, 35 percent of invasive pericardial interventions are performed on cancer patients.

BENIGN AND MALIGNANT PRIMARY PERICARDIAL TUMORS

Among primary pericardial tumors, approximately 25 percent are malignant. Benign tumors present more frequently in infancy and childhood, and malignant tumors are more common after the age of 30 years; lipoma, a slow-growing benign tumor, is often seen later in life. Pericardial cysts, the most common pericardial tumor, are usually small, and are most frequently seen along the right ventricular border. Pericardial cysts often are discovered as incidental findings at autopsy, but they may present with chest pain or arrhythmias or as a finding on a chest roentgenogram obtained for other purposes. Their presence can be confirmed by ultrasound, CT scanning, or MRI. These lesions are not malignant, and patients have an excellent prognosis.

Pericardial teratomas are usually benign, usually occur in children, and are more common in females. Compression of the right atrium is sometimes seen with these tumors, and large associated pericardial effusions are not infrequent. Surgery is the treatment of choice, and the prognosis is usually good when teratomas are benign.

The most common primary malignant tumor of the pericardium is *mesothelioma*; it usually presents in middle-aged adults, and males are afflicted more often than females. It is uncertain if this sex-related difference is linked to toxic exposure. Pericardial mesothelioma may present with pericardial effusion, pericarditis, constriction, and constitutional symptoms.

Angiosarcomas are the second most-common primary pericardial malignancy; these tumors may originate in the right atrium or the pericardium, are usually seen in young adults, and are more common in males. As with mesothelioma, presentation may include pericarditis and pericardial effusion. Pericardial effusion is usually hemorrhagic; surgical treatment may be successful. When surgery is not possible, treatment options are limited; palliation with radiation and chemotherapy is suboptimal.

Pericardial lipomas are usually benign and surgically resectable; transformation to malignant liposarcoma is possible. These tumors may also be surgically resected, and sometimes repeated surgical resection is necessary. *Thymomas* may arise from the parietal pericardium without evidence of anterior mediastinal involvement and may be benign or malignant; they are not associated with myasthenia gravis.

Metastatic spread of tumors to the *pericardium* is common; it has been estimated that 10 percent of all malignancies spread to some portion of the heart, and 85 percent of these eventually involve the pericardium. Lung cancer, breast cancer, and hematologic malignancies together account for approximately two-thirds of the cases of metastatic disease to the pericardium. Melanoma is the tumor most likely to spread to the pericardium, with 70 percent of patients with metastatic melanoma having pericardial involvement at death. *Metastatic breast cancer* invades the pericardial space in approximately 21 percent of cases, and lung cancer in approximately 19 percent.

The clinical presentation of metastatic disease to the pericardium is variable. Sometimes pericardial involvement is an incidental finding at autopsy. It may also present as a catastrophic and life-threatening pericardial tamponade. More commonly, however, patients present with acute pericarditis, chronic effusion, and constrictive disease.

Cardiac ultrasound is the most helpful test for evaluating such patients (see Chap. 16), but CT scanning and MRI (see Chaps. 16, 21, and 22) are helpful adjuncts. The diagnosis is often confirmed by cytologic analysis of pericardial fluid removed for diagnostic or therapeutic pericardiocentesis; however, cytologic findings are not always positive in patients with malignant effusions and not all pericardial effusions in cancer patients are malignant Effusions in these patients may be the result of congestive heart failure, renal failure, inflammation, interruption of lymphatic or venous drainage, infection, hypoalbuminemia, toxicities of chemotherapeutic agents, and chest irradiation.

[ ] MALIGNANT PERICARDIAL EFFUSION

The hemodynamic consequences of malignant pericardial effusion depend on the pressure under which the fluid is contained within the pericardial space. When fluid accumulates over a time sufficient to allow expansion, the pressure may remain low and symptoms may be minimal. In contrast, even small accumulations over short periods of time may lead to cardiac tamponade requiring urgent resolution (see Chap. 84).

The indications for percutaneous pericardial drainage depend on whether cardiac tamponade is imminent, or whether material is deemed crucial for diagnostic purposes. Such specimens provide important and sometimes vital cytological, bacterial, and chemical information. Because pericardial biopsy may be important in seeking a diagnosis, open surgical drainage may be the procedure of choice. When the quantity of fluid is sufficient, the initial procedure of choice may be transthoracic needle drainage.

Cardiac tamponade may be diagnosed by cardiac ultrasound (see Chap. 16). A transthoracic echocardiogram can demonstrate the size

and location of the pericardial effusion but additionally provides information regarding hemodynamic alterations (Fig. 89–4). One of the earliest ultrasound findings associated with cardiac tamponade is compression of the right atrium during systole; as tamponade progresses, right ventricular compression during diastole may be evident (see Chap. 84). In more advanced cases of tamponade, the inferior vena cava is usually shown by ultrasound to be dilated and to fail to collapse with inspiration. Doppler echocardiography (see Chap. 16) can reveal respiratory variation in ventricular filling velocities that corresponds to pulsus paradoxus, an exaggeration of the normal decrease in systemic systolic blood pressure during inspiration; findings consistent with a >25 percent decrease in mitral inflow velocities or a >50 percent decrease in tricuspid inflow velocities with respiration are suggestive of tamponade (Fig. 89–5). Real-time two-dimensional, as well as M-mode, echocardiograms may demonstrate the to-and-fro rocking motion of the heart that is responsible for electrical alternans, a phenomenon resulting from movement of the heart within the pericardial space. The electrocardiogram may show electrical alternans; pulsus paradoxus is also a very useful sign.

Treatment of impending or actual cardiac tamponade encompasses removal of the fluid, urgent or emergent pericardiocentesis may be required. Pericardiocentesis under echocardiographic guidance is a rapid and effective intervention in these patients (see Chap. 84). For cancer patients, the drainage catheter may be left in the pericardial space for several days, during which recurrent or residual fluid is drained daily. The catheter may be removed when the daily aliquot of fluid has fallen below 50 mL. Sclerosing agents are rarely used. Antibiotics or antineoplastic agents have been used in most of the reported series.

Other strategies for the management of the cancer patient with a large pericardial effusion or cardiac tamponade include surgical drainage, which should be considered when fluid has reaccumulated following percutaneous drainage or when the prognosis based on the natural history of the underlying malignancy suggests survival for at least 3 to 6 months.

[ ] ACUTE PERICARDITIS

Pericarditis in the cancer patient may be related to either the malignancy or its treatment. Interestingly, approximately 2 percent of

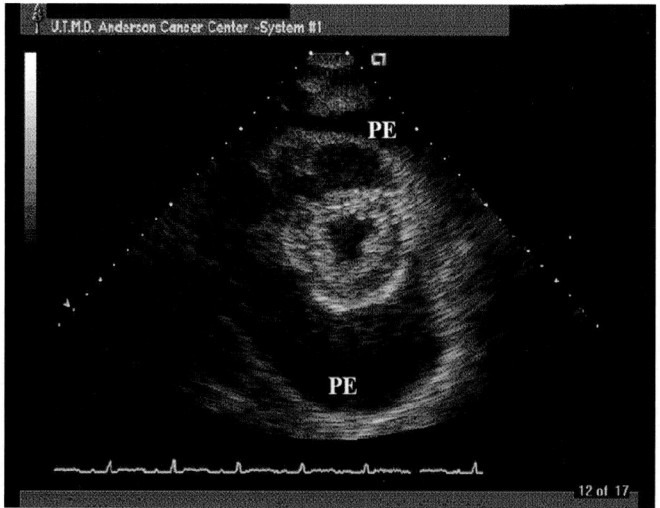
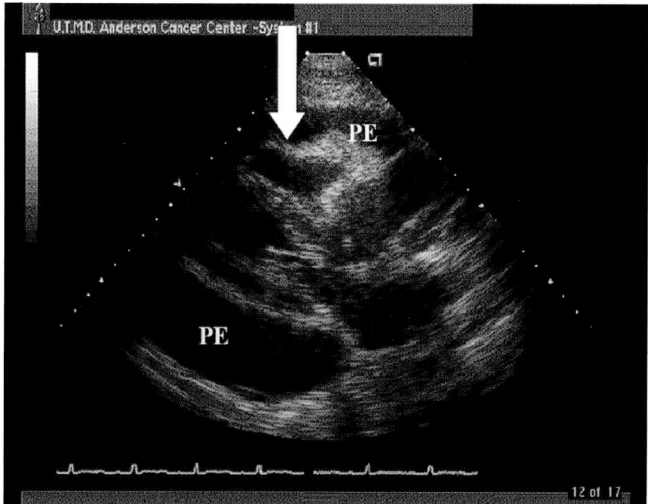

FIGURE 89–4. Large circumferential pericardial effusion. *White arrow* indicates right ventricular diastolic collapse. PE, pericardial effusion.

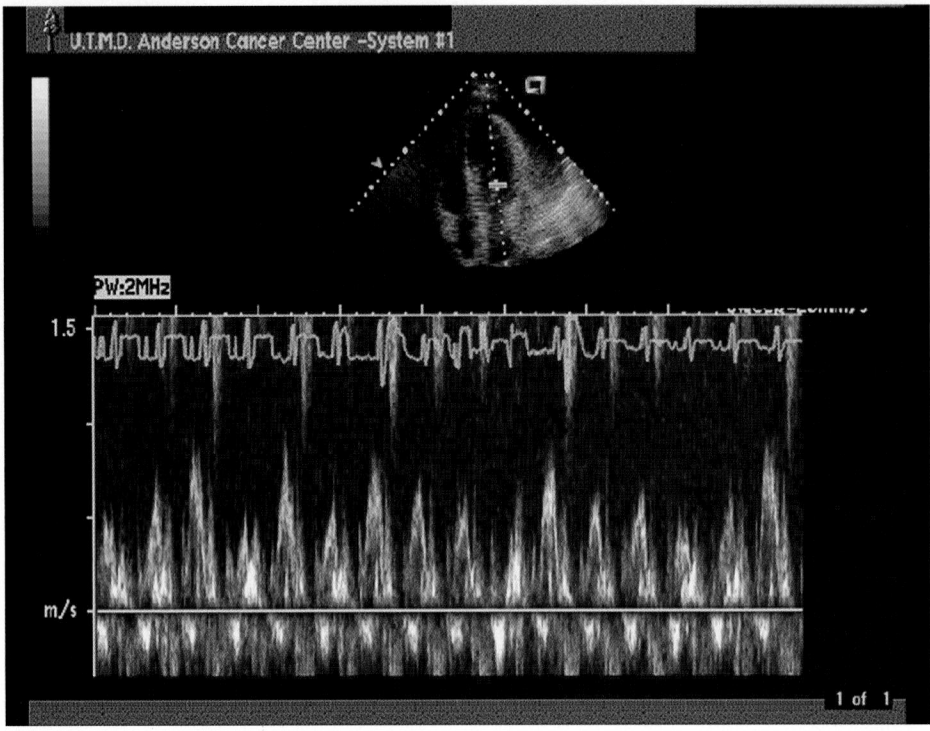

FIGURE 89–5. Peak mitral inflow velocities indicative of excessive variation seen with tamponade.

carditis that presents with signs and symptoms that are clinically similar to those associated with acute pericarditis of other etiologies (see Chap. 93). The onset may be abrupt or gradual, the discomfort well-localized or diffuse, and the intensity can range from being so mild as to be barely perceptible to being so severe that patients are acutely uncomfortable and incapacitated. The pain of acute radiation-related pericarditis is often augmented by recumbency, and it is more likely to increase with deep inspiration or movement. Radiation-associated pericarditis should be considered in the differential diagnosis of any patient presenting with chest pain for whom acute infarction has been excluded and in whom prior or ongoing radiation therapy included a portal that exposed the heart to radiation.

The finding of a pericardial friction rub can help to establish the diagnosis, but these rubs are not always present; friction rubs also may be found in patients with acute infarction (see Chap. 12). The ECG characteristically shows ST-segment elevations in diffuse leads; these are especially prominent in leads I, II, and the left precordial leads. A normal ECG does not rule out acute radiation-associated pericarditis. The changes appear over a period of days and then dissipate. A chest roentgenogram is usually normal unless a large pericardial effusion is manifested as an increased cardiac silhouette. When pericardial fluid is present, a cardiac ultrasound study (see Chap. 16) can quantify the extent, but in the absence of fluid, an echocardiogram may be entirely normal.

The treatment of acute radiation-associated pericarditis is usually rewarding. Patients may respond dramatically to nonsteroidal antiinflammatory agents; ibuprofen in a dose of 400 mg three times daily is often sufficient. Corticosteroid treatment should be reserved for those individuals who do not respond to nonsteroidal agents. When patients respond well to treatment for their pericarditis, and when radiation therapy is deemed important for tumor control, rechallenge or continuation is reasonable. However, it seems prudent to continue treatment with the antiinflammatory agent during the remainder of the radiation exposure and into the postexposure period.

A chronic effusive form of pericarditis develops in some patients following irradiation and usually is followed by exacerbations and spontaneous or pharmacologically induced remissions. The treatment of patients with chronic effusive radiation-related pericarditis is the same as that for the acute form of radiation-associated pericarditis described above.

Radiation exposure also may lead to constrictive pericarditis. This condition is associated with low cardiac output, venous distension, fluid retention, and, ultimately, cardiac death. The chest roentgenogram may show pericardial calcification, and the echocardiogram (see Chap. 16) often shows pericardial thickening. The hemodynamic sequelae of constriction are similar to those seen with cardiac

patients evaluated for acute pericarditis are found to have a malignancy as the cause. When pericarditis is deemed to be caused by malignancy, other sites of metastatic involvement should be sought, as the pericardium is seldom the only metastatic focus. Radiation, chemotherapy, renal failure, the postpericardiotomy syndrome, and sequelae of biologic therapies are all possible etiologies in the appropriate clinical setting, but infections are more likely in these patients given the immunosuppressive state that may exist.

THE EFFECTS OF RADIATION THERAPY ON THE HEART

The various cardiac tissues respond differently to ionizing radiation. The characteristics of the radiation therapy and the mass of cardiac tissue included in the radiation portal influence the response of cardiac tissue to radiation.

Cardiac manifestations of irradiation may be seen even before completion of the anticipated exposure or may occur years or decades later. Patients treated for both Hodgkin and non-Hodgkin lymphoma, and patients treated for left-sided breast cancer, are the most likely to show these manifestations, as treatment for these tumors sometimes involve portals that overlie the heart. However, patients with any malignancy requiring mediastinal or thoracic irradiation may demonstrate cardiac sequelae from their radiation exposure.

[ ] RADIATION EFFECTS ON THE PERICARDIUM

The pericardium is the most sensitive cardiac structure with regard to irradiation because it consists of tissue with rapid cell turnover. Initially, exposure can cause an acute radiation-associated peri-

tamponade, in the respect that both conditions demonstrate increased venous pressure and a low cardiac output. Cardiac catheterization may demonstrate the classic "square root" sign consisting of a dip and plateau, but differentiating constrictive pericarditis from infiltrative (i.e., restrictive) processes such as amyloidosis, a common condition in cancer patients, remains problematic even when invasive techniques are employed (see Chap. 84). Pressure measurements often demonstrate equalization and elevation of diastolic right and left ventricular pressures. Figure 89–6 depicts typical pressure measurements for a patient with restrictive physiology.

The treatment of postradiation constrictive pericarditis must be individualized. Surgical intervention consisting of pericardial stripping carries a significant risk, and mortality may be as high as 25 percent; cardiopulmonary bypass is required in many patients who undergo this procedure. In cancer patients, the decision with regard to the timing of intervention should be based on the estimated progression of the constrictive process, the underlying prognosis in the patient based on the type of malignancy and the likelihood that it has been cured, and the expertise of the available surgical team (see Chap. 84).

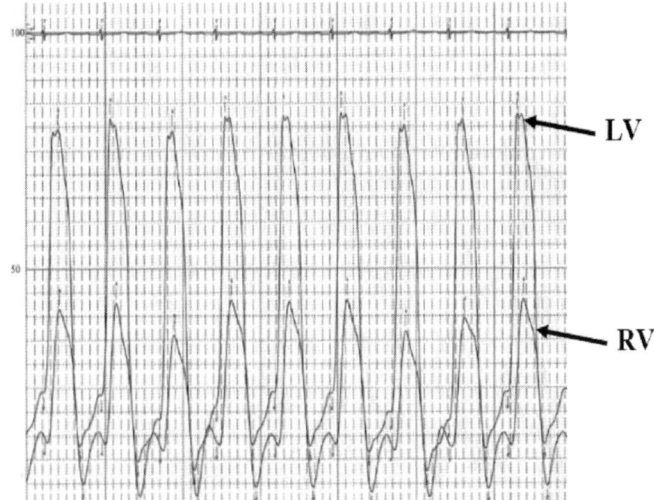

FIGURE 89–6. Simultaneous left ventricular (LV) and right ventricular (RV) pressures in a patient with restrictive physiology. The diastolic pressures are elevated and nearly equalized.

RADIATION EFFECTS ON THE MYOCARDIUM, THE HEART VALVES, AND THE CARDIAC VASCULATURE

The myocardium, the heart valves, the conduction system, and the cardiac vasculature are all less frequently affected by radiation than is the pericardium. Rarely, congestive heart failure from myocardial fibrosis or ischemia stemming from small-vessel injury; valve sclerosis with or without calcification; and conduction abnormalities that include prolongation of the PR interval and other degrees of atrioventricular nodal dysfunction, as well as intraventricular conduction delays, can all occur in the cancer patient treated with radiation. Clinically, cardiac muscle responds to radiation with a progressive decline over time that correlates with the dose of radiation.

Radiation-associated vascular injury is a well-described autopsy finding and is also frequent in young patients in the form of premature coronary occlusion. Radiation can also induce thickening of the arterial wall related to intimal thickening, thereby reducing the luminal area. Additionally, radiation can accelerate atherosclerosis and enhance cholesterol deposition and luminal ulceration.

PREOPERATIVE AND POSTOPERATIVE CARDIOVASCULAR CONSIDERATIONS IN PATIENTS UNDERGOING NONCARDIOVASCULAR SURGERY

Extensive literature has been published over the past 30 years on identifying and minimizing the risks for cardiac complications related to noncardiac surgery (see Chap. 86). Because the surgical treatment of cancer can involve lengthy and complicated procedures, the attendant risks of surgery are often increased.

PREOPERATIVE EVALUATION

The overall preoperative risk assessment for cancer patients being considered for noncardiac surgery is largely similar to that applied to other groups of patients. The American Heart Association and the American College of Cardiology guidelines (see Chaps. 11 and 86) that have been developed and updated over the last decade are sufficiently extensive and detailed in this regard. However, these guidelines have been modified to include the assessment of cancer patients and the surgical risks in this population; Table 89–6 summarizes these modifications.

A similar approach to the basic laboratory testing and stress testing for risk stratification is used in both patients with and without cancer. However, patients who are undergoing surgery for cancer may be much weaker and thus may not be able to exercise adequately. Consequently, pharmacologic stress imaging (see Chap. 79) must be used more frequently in these patients. Although this can provide important information, it may be suboptimal in assessing the overall physical capacity of these patients. This information may be relevant after surgery, as a poor functional state will likely contribute to a protracted recovery.

Special considerations in determining the perioperative risks in cancer patients include a review of the recent chemotherapy they may have received (Table 89–7). Chemotherapy affects the immune system and also results in significant thrombocytopenia or neutropenia, which may predispose the patient to infection or bleeding. Also, chemotherapy can result in ECG prolongation of the QT interval and the associated increase in ventricular arrhythmia. It is important to acquire information on such interactions preoperatively because of the bearing it can have intraoperatively and postoperatively. Radiation therapy can have an impact on surgical outcome as well.

Cancer surgery is a particular challenge in patients who have coexisting coronary artery disease. Preoperative coronary revascularization does not reduce the risk of the surgical procedure and may actually make patients more prone to complications. This is especially true with regard to the placement of drug-eluting stents, as catastrophic stent occlusion may occur following cessation of the antiplatelet regimen necessary during the intraoperative and early postoperative periods. Aggressive medical therapy to control coronary artery disease is therefore often preferable in these patients. The pre-

TABLE 89–6

Risk Assignments at M.D. Anderson Cancer Center[a]

HIGH RISK	INTERMEDIATE RISK	MINIMAL RISK
PATIENT RISK ASSIGNMENTS		
Decompensated HF	Compensated HF	Advanced age (>70 years)
Unstable coronary syndromes	Prior HF	Low functional capacity
Recent MI (<30 days)	Stable CAD	Uncontrolled hypertension (except in endocrine
Unstable angina	Post CABG	tumor where considered intermediate risk)
Large "area of risk" by noninvasive	Post PCI	Cerebrovascular disease
study	Stable angina	Abnormal ECG
Recent stent <12 weeks	Prior MI	Rhythm other than sinus
Significant arrhythmia	Diabetes	
High-grade AV block	Renal insufficiency	
Ventricular arrhythmias with concomi-	History of cardiotoxic	
tant heart disease	chemotherapy	
Uncontrolled ventricular rate in	History of chest wall irradiation	
supraventricular arrhythmia		
Severe valvular disease		
SURGICAL RISK ASSIGNMENTS		
Emergent surgery	Intraperitoneal surgery	Endoscopic procedures
Long surgery (>6 hours)	Intrathoracic surgery	Superficial procedures
Expected blood loss >25% blood volume	Head/neck surgery	Breast surgery
Large fluid shift expected	Carotid surgery	Wide local excision
Aortic or other major vascular surgery	Orthopedic surgery	Tandem and ovoid insertion
Peripheral vascular surgery	Radical prostate surgery	Cervical procedures
	Pelvic tumor reduction surgery	Brain biopsy
	Free-flap reconstruction	Nonreconstructive eye surgery

AV, atrioventricular; CABG, coronary artery bypass grafting; CAD, coronary artery disease; MI, myocardial infarction; PCI, percutaneous coronary intervention (either simple angioplasty or stent replacement).
[a]Criteria have been adapted from the (American College of Cardiology/American Heart Association) Guideline Update for Perioperative Cardiovascular Evaluation for Noncardiac Surgery that has been used at the Preoperative Consultation Center at The University of Texas M.D. Anderson Cancer Center
SOURCE: Adapted from Eagle KA, Berger PB, Caulkins H, et al. ACC/AHA guideline update for perioperative cardiovascular evaluation for noncardiac surgery. Circulation 2002;105:1257–1267.

TABLE 89–7

Preoperative Evaluation of the Cancer Patient Undergoing Noncancer Surgery

Risk assessment as per American Heart Association guidelines and modifications
Identify if chemotherapy was recently administered
Clarify location and intensity of radiation therapy
Careful consideration of a patient with established coronary artery disease
  Was a stent recently placed?
  Was optimal treatment with cardioprotective medications given?
Device management
  Recommended preoperative check of device
  Establish whether patient is pacemaker dependent
  Check device postoperatively
Cancer-specific concerns
  Pheochromocytoma (preoperative α and β blockers)
  Carcinoid (consideration of transesophageal echo to guide volume replacement)
  Assess whether there is a possible mass extension or thrombus present

operative administration of statins, β blockers, or ACE inhibitors for blood pressure control should be strongly considered. In patients with LV dysfunction, optimal management of their volume status perioperatively is equally necessary.

The perioperative management of implanted cardiac devices in patients undergoing surgery for cancer is another important consideration. The physical distance between the location of the surgery and the device is important, with a greater likelihood of problems occurring in patients undergoing procedures in the face or neck, because of the proximity of a subclavian pacemaker. Distances of less than 20 cm may be especially problematic, but longer distances may also create problems. Expertise in the management of such devices must be an integral part of the perioperative team to ensure appropriate preoperative assessment of the device including battery reserve and reprogramming.

Patients with certain tumors with a predilection for mediator release present major preoperative challenges that concern cardiologists. Specific strategies are required in patients with pheochromocytomas to prevent potentially life-threatening blood pressure elevations during the perioperative period, as noted above. Patients with carcinoid tumors may also demonstrate wide fluctuations in blood pressure during surgical resection, albeit through the release of different mediators. The volume status in these patients may also be difficult to discern, especially if concomitant tricuspid regurgitation is present. Transesophageal ultrasound (see Chap. 16) during surgery may be particularly useful in assessing the intracardiac volume status in patients who are undergoing surgery to remove these challenging tumors.

【 】 POSTOPERATIVE CARE

The postoperative management of patients who undergo cancer surgery is similar to that of the noncancer population. For some surgeries, the incidence of postoperative atrial fibrillation, estimated to be as high as 33 percent, is disproportionately higher than is the case in the noncancer population[25]; a number of these patients have persistent arrhythmia. The goal is to restore sinus rhythm within as short period of time as possible so as to minimize the need for anticoagulation (see Chap. 36). It is also imperative to reinitiate preoperative cardioprotective medications as early as possible in the postoperative period to preserve stable cardiovascular status. The general principles of early ambulation and "pulmonary toilet" remain standard postoperative surgical principles that should be employed aggressively in cancer patients as well.

CANCER SURVIVORSHIP

According to an Institute of Medicine of the National Academies report published in 2005, the number of cancer survivors has tripled in the last 30 years to 10 million. More than 6 million of these cancer survivors are older than age 65 years. Many of the potential cardiovascular complications can develop late (defined as >2 years following treatment completion), similar to cardiovascular diseases in noncancer patients. Nonetheless, 1 month following the completion of chemotherapy, radiation therapy, or cancer surgery, patients with significant underlying cardiac disease should be carefully evaluated by a cardiologist. Furthermore, traditional cardiovascular risk factors should be managed if present. Blood tests should include complete blood count, platelet count, a lipid panel, and HbA1c (glycosylated hemoglobin) and BNP measurements. Body mass index should be assessed, and an ECG and echocardiogram should be obtained if not performed recently. At this juncture, it is important to review the medical regimen of the patient and to restart or adjust cardiac medications that may have been temporarily interrupted during cancer treatment or perioperative period. If a cancer survivor has identifiable cardiac risk factors and cardiovascular diseases at the 1-month evaluation, subsequent followup should be dictated by many guidelines that have been established. In cancer survivors who were treated with mediastinal, chest, mantle, or left breast radiation, particular attention must be paid to the vasculature, cardiac valves, and pericardium, because of potential late manifestations of radiation-induced damage to these structures. In cancer survivors who received head and neck radiation, a thorough carotid evaluation is important and likely needs to include duplex imaging because of the ability of this technique to detect asymptomatic but significant carotid disease.

GENERAL MANIFESTATIONS AND LIST OF CARDIAC TUMORS

This final section provides additional clinical information on primary and secondary tumors of the heart. Table 89–8 lists the general manifestations of neoplastic heart disease are listed in and Table 89–9 enumerates the incidence of tumors and cysts of the heart and pericardium. More specific information about cardiac myxomas is included.

CARDIAC MYXOMAS

Intracardiac myxoma is the most frequent benign tumor of the heart. While most (75 percent) are located in the left atrium (LA), myxomas are also found in the right atrium (18 percent), right ventricle (4 percent), and left ventricle (3 percent). Cardiac myxomas usually originate from the region of the fossa ovalis but may arise from a variety of locations within the atria. Approximately 75 percent occur in the LA. The DNA genotype of sporadic myxomas is normal in 80 percent of patients. Tumors are likely to be associated

TABLE 89–8

General Manifestations of Neoplastic Heart Disease

Pericardial involvement
    Pericarditis and pain
    Pericardial effusion
    Radiographic enlargement
    Arrhythmia, predominantly atrial
    Tamponade
    Constriction

Myocardial involvement
    Arrhythmias, ventricular and atrial
    Electrocardiographic changes
    Radiographic enlargement
        Generalized
        Localized
    Conduction disturbances and heart block
    Congestive heart failure
    Coronary involvement
        Angina, infarction
    Intracavitary tumor
        Cavity obliteration
        Valve obstruction and valve damage
        Embolic phenomena: systemic, neurologic, and
           coronary
        Constitutional manifestations

TABLE 89–9

Tumors and Cysts of the Heart and Pericardium

TYPE	NUMBER	PERCENTAGE
Benign		
Myxoma	130	24.4
Lipoma	45	8.4
Rhabdomyoma	36	6.8
Fibroma	17	3.2
Hemangioma	15	2.8
Teratoma	14	2.6
Mesothelioma of the atrioventricular node	12	2.3
Granular cell tumor	3	
Neurofibroma	3	
Lymphangioma	2	
Subtotal	319	59.8
Pericardial cyst	82	15.4
Bronchogenic cyst	7	1.3
Subtotal	89	16.7
Malignant		
Angiosarcoma	39	7.3
Rhabdomyosarcoma	26	4.9
Mesothelioma	19	3.6
Fibrosarcoma	14	2.6
Malignant lymphoma	7	1.3
Extraskeletal osteosarcoma	5	
Neurogenic sarcoma	4	
Malignant teratoma	4	
Thymoma	4	
Leiomyosarcoma	1	
Liposarcoma	1	
Synovial sarcoma	1	
Subtotal	125	23.5
Total	533	100.0

SOURCE: Reproduced from McAllister H, Hall R, Cooley D. Tumors of the heart and pericardium. Curr Probl Cardiol 1992;24:57–116 with permission.

red blood cells, communicate from the surface to deep within the tumor and are lined by endothelial-like cells resembling multipurpose mesenchymal cells, from which the tumor is purported to arise. Similar endothelial cells line the surface of the tumor; however, fibrin, erythrocytes, and organized thrombi also may be present on the surface. Cystic areas; focal or gross hemorrhage; calcification; glandular elements; rarely, bone formation; and even hematopoietic tissue constitute the multiple, less common, variations.

Although asymptomatic patients with myxoma have been reported, most present with one or more effects of a *triad* of constitutional, embolic, and obstructive manifestations. Cardiac myxomas provoke systemic manifestations in 90 percent of the patients, characterized by weight loss, fatigue, fever, anemia (often hemolytic), elevated sedimentation rate, and elevated serum immunoglobulin concentration formed in response to tumor embolization, degenerative changes within the tumor, or overproduction of IL-6 by the tumor.

Constitutional manifestations and embolic potential are relatively common in patients with myxoma in any intracavitary location. The cardiac manifestations, symptoms, and physical findings are the consequence of the intracavitary mass and the particular location of the tumor. Myxomas of the LA may obstruct either the mitral or pulmonary venous orifices and produce pulmonary venous hypertension, secondary pulmonary hypertension, and right-sided heart failure. The clinical symptoms include dyspnea on exertion, orthopnea, paroxysmal nocturnal dyspnea, acute pulmonary edema, cough, and hemoptysis, along with palpitations, chest pain, fatigue, and peripheral edema. Episodes of syncope or dizziness are frequent, and sudden death may occur. A marked change in the severity of any symptom caused by a change in position of the patient, especially if recumbency relieves dyspnea, is suggestive of myxoma.

with other abnormal conditions and have a low recurrence rate. Approximately 5 percent of myxoma patients show a familial pattern of tumor development based on autosomal dominant inheritance; 20 percent of those with sporadic myxoma have an abnormal DNA genotype chromosomal pattern. Most true myxomas arise only from the mural endocardium despite isolated reports that they arise from the cardiac valves, pulmonary vessels, and vena cava.

PATHOLOGY OF CARDIAC MYXOMAS

Attached to the endocardium by a broad base, myxomas are usually pedunculated, polypoid, and friable, although some may have a smooth surface and are rounded. A myxoma appears as a soft, gelatinous, mucoid, usually gray-white mass, often with areas of hemorrhage or thrombosis. Myxomas vary from 1 to 15 cm in diameter, with most measuring 5 to 6 cm.

On microscopic examination, the myxoma consists of an acid mucopolysaccharide myxoid matrix in which polygonal cells and occasional blood vessels are embedded. Channels, often containing

Physical Examination

On physical examination, the S_1 is loud and frequently split, with the second component corresponding to the tumor's expulsion from the mitral orifice (see Chap. 12). P_2 is accentuated, and an early diastolic sound, the "tumor plop," is usually heard 80 to 120 milliseconds after the A_2, resembling an opening snap. The tumor plop may be confused with either an opening snap or a third heart sound and follows A_2 at an intermediate interval between these events.

The value of transthoracic echocardiography in the noninvasive diagnosis of intracavitary tumors is well documented (see Chap.

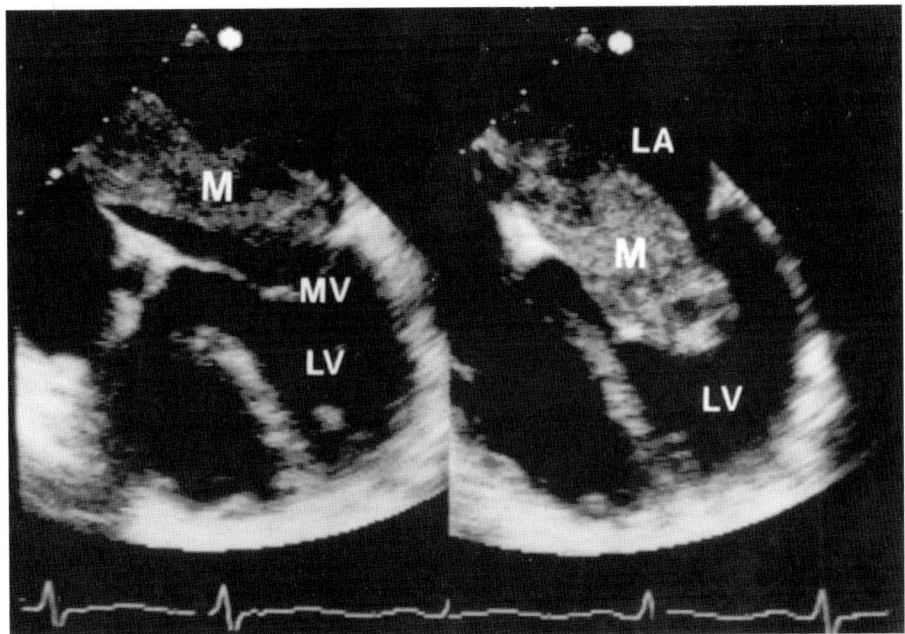

FIGURE 89–7. Transesophageal echocardiogram in the four-chamber view from a 50-year-old man who presented with exertional dyspnea and syncope. A large left atrial myxoma (M) attached to the interatrial septum is seen prolapsing across the mitral valve (MV) into the left ventricle (LV) in diastole (*right panel*). *Source: Courtesy of Susan Wilansky, MD, Medical Director, Noninvasive Imaging, St. Luke's Episcopal Hospital, Houston, Texas.*

16). M-mode recordings in patients with a prolapsing LA myxoma typically demonstrate a diminished ejection fraction slope of the anterior leaflet of the mitral valve, behind which a dense array of wavy tumor echoes is seen (see Chap. 16). The tumor plop coincides with the completion of this anterior movement of tumor echoes (see Fig. 16–132). A similar array of tumor echoes may be seen in the LA during ventricular systole. Transthoracic echocardiography and transesophageal echocardiography identify the size, shape, point of attachment, and motion characteristics of LA atrial myxomas. Transesophageal echocardiography permits superior imaging of the posterior cardiac structures and LA myxomas, especially their point of attachment. Visualization of all four chambers permits recognition of multiple tumors, as well as tumors in less common locations. Doppler assessment of the flow patterns of the mitral valve and pulmonary vein provides further information regarding the hemodynamic consequences of LA myxomas (Fig. 89–7).

Surgical resection of a myxoma is the only acceptable therapy and, in view of the dangers of embolization and sudden death, should be performed promptly. For complete removal of LA myxoma, we use a biatrial approach, excising a full thickness of interatrial septum if the tumor is attached to the region of the fossa ovalis. Right atrium myxomas are commonly attached to the fossa ovalis and, with right-sided tumors, a full thickness of atrial septum should also be resected. If a large portion of the septum is removed, a patch of knitted Dacron cloth should be used for repair to avoid distortion, arrhythmias, or possible atrial septal defect. Ventricular standstill with cardioplegia solution is induced before manipulating the heart so as to reduce the possibility of fragmentation of the gelatinous tumor. LA myxomas have been removed successfully during pregnancy, utilizing cardiopulmonary bypass, with subsequent uncomplicated completion of a full-term pregnancy. Surgical re-

moval of a right ventricle myxoma in a neonate has been reported.[26]

REFERENCES

1. Yeh ET. Cardiotoxicity induced by chemotherapy and antibody therapy. *Annu Rev Med* 2006;57:485–498.
2. Ewer M, Yeh ET. *Cancer and the Heart.* Hamilton, Ont: BC Decker, 2006:395.
3. Ewer M, Yeh ET, Benjamin RS. Cardiac complications. In: Kufe DW, et al., eds. *Cancer Medicine,* 7th ed. Hamilton, Ont: BC Decker, 2006:2131.
4. Yeh ET, et al. Cardiovascular complications of cancer therapy: diagnosis, pathogenesis, and management. *Circulation* 2004;109(25):3122–3131.
5. Ewer MS, Lippman SM. Type II chemotherapy-related cardiac dysfunction: time to recognize a new entity. *J Clin Oncol* 2005;23(13):2900–2902.
6. Kerkela R, et al. Cardiotoxicity of the cancer therapeutic agent imatinib mesylate. *Nat Med* 2006;12(8):908–916.
7. Swain SM, Whaley FS, Ewer MS. Congestive heart failure in patients treated with doxorubicin: a retrospective analysis of three trials. *Cancer* 2003;97(11):2869–2879.
8. Billingham ME, et al. Anthracycline cardiomyopathy monitored by morphologic changes. *Cancer Treat Rep* 1978;62(6):865–872.
9. Seidman A, et al. Cardiac dysfunction in the trastuzumab clinical trials experience. *J Clin Oncol* 2002;20(5):1215–1221.
10. Perez EA, Rodeheffer R. Clinical cardiac tolerability of trastuzumab. *J Clin Oncol* 2004;22(2):322–329.
11. Fromme EK, et al. How accurate is clinician reporting of chemotherapy adverse effects? A comparison with patient-reported symptoms from the Quality-of-Life Questionnaire C30. *J Clin Oncol* 2004;22(17):3485–3490.
12. St Sauver JL, et al. Agreement between patient reports of cardiovascular disease and patient medical records. *Mayo Clin Proc* 2005;80(2):203–210.
13. Meinardi MT, et al. Cardiovascular morbidity in long-term survivors of metastatic testicular cancer. *J Clin Oncol* 2000;18(8):1725–1732.
14. Frickhofen N, et al. Capecitabine can induce acute coronary syndrome similar to 5-fluorouracil. *Ann Oncol* 2002;13(5):797–801.
15. Tallman MS, et al. Clinical description of 44 patients with acute promyelocytic leukemia who developed the retinoic acid syndrome. *Blood* 2000;95(1):90–95.
16. Saltz LB, et al. Phase II trial of cetuximab in patients with refractory colorectal cancer that expresses the epidermal growth factor receptor. *J Clin Oncol* 2004;22(7):1201–1208.
17. Vial T, Descotes J. Immune-mediated side-effects of cytokines in humans. *Toxicology* 1995;105(1):31–57.
18. Frankel SR, et al. The "retinoic acid syndrome" in acute promyelocytic leukemia. *Ann Intern Med* 1992;117(4):292–296.
19. Barbey JT, Pezzullo JC, Soignet SL. Effect of arsenic trioxide on QT interval in patients with advanced malignancies. *J Clin Oncol* 2003;21(19):3609–3615.
20. Westervelt P, et al. Sudden death among patients with acute promyelocytic leukemia treated with arsenic trioxide. *Blood* 2001;98(2):266–271.
21. Olsen E, et al. Pivotal phase III trial of two dose levels of denileukin diftitox for the treatment of cutaneous T-cell lymphoma. *J Clin Oncol* 2001;19(2):376–388.
22. Hirsh J, et al. The Seventh ACCP Conference on Antithrombotic and Thrombolytic Therapy: evidence-based guidelines. *Chest* 2004;126(3 Suppl):172S–173S.
23. Lee AY, et al. Low-molecular-weight heparin versus a coumarin for the prevention of recurrent venous thromboembolism in patients with cancer. *N Engl J Med* 2003;349(2):146–153.
24. Smorenburg SM, Van Noorden CJ. The complex effects of heparins on cancer progression and metastasis in experimental studies. *Pharmacol Rev* 2001;53(1):93–105.
25. Vaporciyan AA, et al. Risk factors associated with atrial fibrillation after noncardiac thoracic surgery: analysis of 2588 patients. *J Thorac Cardiovasc Surg* 2004;127(3):779–786.
26. McAllister H, Hall R, Cooley D. Tumors of the heart and pericardium. *Curr Probl Cardiol* 1999;24:57–116.

Cardiotoxic Effects of Cancer Therapy Drugs

DRUG CLASS/NAME (GENERIC [BRAND])	CARDIAC ADVERSE EVENTS	RELATIVE FREQUENCY OF SPECIFIC ADVERSE EFFECT[a]	RELATIVE FREQUENCY OF THERAPEUTIC USE[b]	COMMENT
Anthracyclines/Anthraquinolones				
Doxorubicin (Adriamycin) Daunorubicin (Cerubidine) Epirubicin (Ellence, Pharmorubicin)	CHF/LV dysfunction	+++	+++	Risk of CHF is cumulative dose, and schedule dependent. LV dysfunction is secondary to free radical production.
Mitoxantrone (Novantrone)	CHF/LV dysfunction	++	+	Anthraquinone derivative. Low propensity for free radical production. Myocarditis and arrhythmia occurs acutely with infusion.
Alkylating Agents				
Busulfan (Myleran)	Endomyocardial fibrosis Cardiac tamponade	+ +	+	
Cisplatin (Platinol)	Ischemia Hypertension CHF	++ ++ ++	+++	CHF risk is increased in elderly, after chest XRT. Rare incidence of hemorrhagic myocarditis, more common in high dose.
Cyclophosphamide (Cytoxan)	Pericarditis/myocarditis CHF	+ ++	+++	CHF risk is increased with cumulative dose, in elderly, after chest XRT, after prior anthracyclines.
Ifosfamide (Ifex)	CHF Arrhythmias	++ ++	++	CHF risk is increased with cumulative dose, prior anthracyclines.
Mitomycin (Mutamycin)	CHF	++	+	CHF risk is increased with cumulative dose, prior anthracyclines, chest XRT.
Antimetabolites				
Capecitabine (Xeloda)	Ischemia	+	+++	More common in those with CAD. Mechanism is potentially vasospasm or thrombosis.
Cytarabine, Ara-C (Cytosar)	Pericarditis CHF	+ +	+++	Rare cases of cardiomyopathy following high-dose therapy.
Fluorouracil (Adrucil)	Ischemia Cardiogenic shock	++	+++	Risk increased in CAD, prior chest XRT, concomitant cisplatin therapy. Rate and dose dependent. Vasospasm is possible mechanism.

				Comments
Antimicrotubules				
Paclitaxel (Taxol)	Sinus bradycardia, AV block, ventricular tachycardia	+		
	Orthostatic hypotension	++		
	CHF	++	+++	Often seen with hypersensitivity; long-term hypotension likely a result of peripheral neuropathy; CHF possible if given with doxorubicin.
Vinca alkaloids	Ischemia	++	++	Increased risk with CAD or prior chest XRT.
Biologic Agents				
Monoclonal Antibodies				
Alemtuzumab (Campath)	Hypotension	+++	+	In setting of infusion reactions.
	CHF	+		LV dysfunction rarely seen in patients with mycosis fungoides.
Bevacizumab (Avastin)	Hypertension	+++	++	Severe hypertension seen in 16% of patients in a recent trial.
	CHF	++		CHF occurred in 14% of patients receiving concurrent anthracyclines.
	Deep vein thrombosis			
Cetuximab (Erbitux)	Hypotension	+	++	In setting of severe infusion reactions (bronchospasm, stridor, urticaria).
Rituximab (Rituxan)	Hypotension	++	++	Usually in setting of infusion reactions (hypotension, hypoxia, bronchospasm). Severe hypotension and angioedema estimated at 1%.
	Angioedema			
	Arrhythmias	++		Rare fatal cardiac failure. Patients with arrhythmias and CAD should be monitored during and after infusion.
Trastuzumab (Herceptin)	CHF/LV dysfunction	++	++	LV dysfunction is uncommon when given as a single agent but there is an increased incidence when given with cyclophosphamide, anthracyclines, and/or paclitaxel.
Interleukins				
Interleukin-2	Hypotension	++++	+	Usually seen at higher doses, associated with capillary leak syndrome. Severe hypotension in 3% of patients. Transient LV dysfunction seen during infusion.
	Arrhythmias	++		
Denileukin diftitox (Ontak)	Hypotension	++++	+	In the setting of a vascular leak syndrome.
Interferon α	Hypotension	+++		Increased risk with preexisting cardiac dysfunction or prior cardiotoxic therapy.
	Ischemia	++	+++	Rare cases of LV dysfunction/arrhythmia.
	LV dysfunction	+		

(continued)

Cardiotoxic Effects of Cancer Therapy Drugs (continued)

Miscellaneous

All-*trans*-retinoic acid, (ATRA; Tretinoin)	CHF	++	May occur in the setting of ATRA syndrome (respiratory distress, fever, pulmonary infiltrates).
	Hypotension	++	+
	Pericardial effusion	+	
Arsenic trioxide (Trisenox)	QT prolongation	++++	+ Important to maintain normal electrolytes and to discontinue QT-prolonging drugs. Fatal torsade de pointes has been reported.
Imatinib (Gleevec)	Pericardial effusion	++	+++ Severe fluid retention can rarely be fatal. Dose related, occurring in 50–70% of patients receiving >300 mg/d.
	CHF	+	+++
	Edema	+++	
Pentostatin (Nipent)	CHF	++	+ Rare fatal cardiac toxicity reported after high-dose cyclophosphamide prior to bone marrow transplant.
Thalidomide (Thalomid)	Edema	++	+ Known severe congenital defects in fetuses. Prescribers should be registered in STEPS program. Patients with multiple myeloma are routinely given low-dose Coumadin for DVT prophylaxis.
	Hypotension	+	
	DVT	++	
	Bradycardia	++	
Etoposide (VePesid)	Hypotension	++	++ Usually seen with rapid infusion.
Bortezomib (Velcade)		++	
Vascular-disrupting agents	Ischemia	Phase I	

AV, atrioventricular; CAD, coronary artery disease; CHF, congestive heart failure; LV, left ventricular; XRT, radiation therapy.
[a]Relative frequency of specific adverse effect: +, rare (<1%); ++, uncommon (1–5%); +++, common (6–10%); ++++, frequent (>10%).
[b]Relative frequency of therapeutic use: +, infrequent; ++, common; +++, very frequent.

CHAPTER (90)

Diabetes and Cardiovascular Disease

Michael E. Farkouh / Elliot J. Rayfield / Valentin Fuster

EPIDEMIOLOGY

Globally, diabetes mellitus is a major threat to human health. The number of people with diabetes has increased alarmingly since 1985 and the rate of new cases is escalating. In 1985, an estimated 30 million people worldwide had diabetes; by 2003, it was estimated that approximately 194 million people had diabetes, and this figure is expected to rise to almost 350 million by 2025.[1]

The prevalence of diabetes is higher in developed countries than in developing countries, but the developing world will be hit hardest by the diabetes epidemic in the future. Increased urbanization, westernization, and economic growth in developing countries have already contributed to a substantial rise in diabetes. Although diabetes is most common among the elderly in many populations, prevalence rates are rising among young populations in the developing world.

Diabetes mellitus, whether type 1 or type 2, is a very strong risk factor for the development of coronary artery disease (CHD) and stroke[2] (Table 90–1). Eighty percent of all deaths among diabetic patients are as a result of atherosclerosis, compared with approximately 30 percent among nondiabetic persons. A large National Institutes of Health (NIH) cohort study revealed that heart disease mortality in the general U.S. population is declining at a much greater rate than it is in diabetic subjects. In fact, diabetic women suffered an increase in heart disease mortality over that period.[2] Among all hospitalizations for diabetic complications, more than 75 percent are a consequence of atherosclerosis. An increase in the prevalence of diabetes has been noted, which, in part, can be attributed to the aging of the population and an increase in the rate of obesity and the sedentary lifestyle in the United States.

Diabetes accelerates the natural course of atherosclerosis in all groups of patients and involves a greater number of coronary vessels with more diffuse atherosclerotic lesions (Fig. 90–1).[3] Cardiac catheterizations in diabetic patients have shown significantly more severe proximal and distal CHD. In addition, plaque ulceration and thrombosis have been found to be significantly higher in diabetic patients.[3] Cardiovascular complications include CHD, peripheral artery disease, nephropathy, retinopathy, cardiomyopathy, and possible neuropathy (involvement of vasa vasorum). These observations underscore the heightened risks of a diabetic patient to develop vascular disease and compel the physician to monitor and correct all the risk factors (Table 90–2). By understanding the mechanisms underlying all these risks, physicians will be poised to prevent them.

TABLE 90–1

Clinical Evaluation of Risk Factors for the Development of Cardiovascular Disease in Diabetic Patients

Cigarette smoking
  Assess pack-years
Blood pressure
  Duration (if known), current and previous medications, assess presence of orthostatic hypertension
Serum lipids and lipoproteins
  Dietary habits, alcohol intake, amount of exercise and whether aerobic
  Family history of dyslipidemia, eruptive xanthoma, lipemia, retinalis, xanthelasma, thyroid function tests
  LDL, HDL, cholesterol, fasting triglycerides
Spot albumin/creatinine ratio (in micro- and macroalbuminuria)
  Serum creatinine
  Do not rely on dipstick protein, as negative results may reflect lack of sensitivity of test
Glycemic status
  Duration of diabetes; family history of diabetes; vascular, renal, and retinal complications
  Laboratory: FPG, hemoglobin A1c q 3 months: diagnosis FPG >126 × 2: impaired fasting glucose 110–126 × 2; when in doubt, have patient undergo 2-h oral glucose tolerance test

FPG, fasting blood glucose; HDL, high-density lipoprotein; LDL, low-density lipoprotein.

MECHANISMS LINKING DIABETES AND CARDIOVASCULAR DISEASE

[ ] MOLECULAR AND ENZYMATIC MECHANISMS

The spectrum of metabolic disturbances associated with diabetes and insulin resistance extends beyond hyperglycemia and includes dyslipidemia, hypercoagulability, and inflammation.

[ ] ADIPOKINES[4]

Adipose tissue is an active organ that produces multiple adipokines, which play an important role in the development and progression of atherosclerosis. Table 90–3 shows the prominent adipokines with their actions.

[ ] ENDOTHELIAL DYSFUNCTION[5]

The normal endothelium regulates vasomotor tone, and keeps the coagulation cascade in balance. Insulin resistance, itself, appears to be an endothelial dysfunction risk equivalent (Fig. 90–2).

In healthy endothelium, the stimulation of insulin receptors activates the phosphoinositol-3 kinase (PI3-K) pathway. The production of nitric oxide by endothelial cells stimulated by this pathway leads to a host of antiinflammatory and antithrombotic effects which are antiatherogenic. The endothelial dysfunction of insulin resistance is a result of decreased levels of nitric oxide and thus impaired blood flow due to a down regulation of the PI3-K pathway.

A parallel pathway downregulates the production of endothelin-1. In response to hyperglycemia, endothelial cells secrete endothelin-1 which induces proatherogenic effects such as vasoconstriction, increased vascular permeability, and VSMC proliferation. Elevated glucose levels stimulate the production of interleukin-6 by endothelial cells and monocytes and increased proteoglycan synthesis by VSMCs.

[ ] VASCULAR SMOOTH MUSCLE CELL MIGRATION AND PROLIFERATION[6]

The insulin receptors on VSMCs are structurally and functionally similar to those in skeletal muscle and adipocytes. Insulin signaling in VSMCs initiates proatherogenic cellular events such as proliferation and migration. Insulin acts synergistically with other atherogenic growth factors such as platelet-derived growth factor to promote the proliferation and migration of bovine aortic smooth muscle cells.

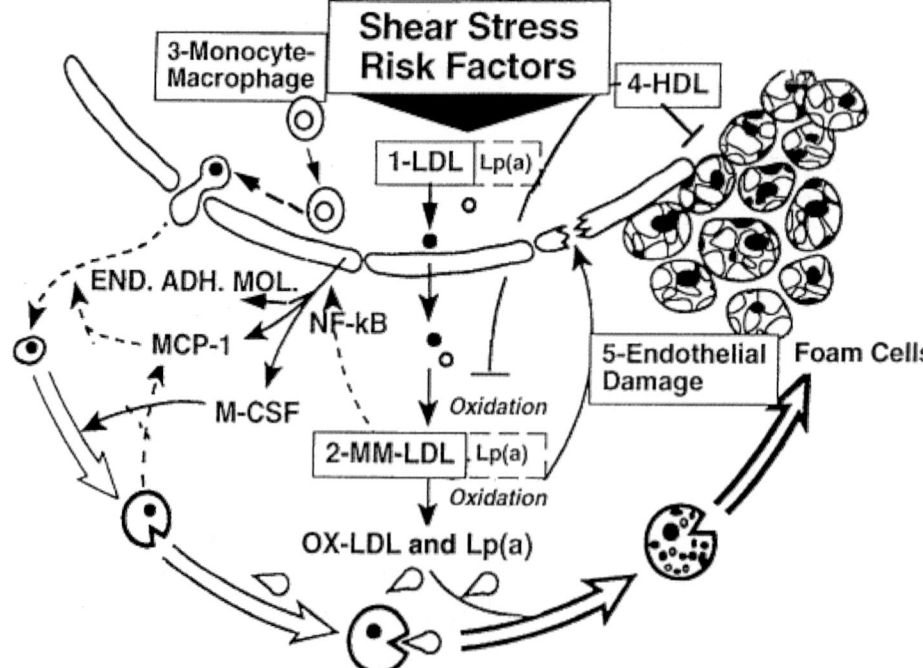

FIGURE 90–1. Schematic of staging (phases and lesion morphology of the progression of coronary atherosclerosis according to the gross pathologic and clinical findings). See text for more details. END.ADH.MOL., endothelial adhesion molecule; HDL, high-density lipoprotein; LDL, low-density lipoprotein; Lp(a), lipoprotein a; MCP-1, monocyte chemoattractant protein; M-CSF, macrophage colony-stimulating factor; MM-LDL, minimally modified low-density lipoprotein; NF-κB, nuclear factor kappa B; Numbers 1–5, stages of progression of coronary atherosclerosis; OX-LDL, oxidized low-density lipoprotein.

TABLE 90–2

Assessment of Predisposing Risk Factors in Diabetic Patients

Body weight and fat distribution
  History: Age of onset of overweight, family history of obesity
  Physical examination: Measure body weight (kg), height (m); calculate BMI (kg/m²): BMI of 25–29.9 = overweight, >30.0 = obese; BMI >27 in a diabetic patient should be treated as high risk; measure waist circumference (abdominal obesity is >40 in. in men and >36 in. in women)

Physical activity:
  History: job, activity in sports, walking, aerobics; in women, childcare, housework
  Physical examination: assess level of cardiovascular fitness in cardiac rehabilitation facility

Family history
  History of heart disease, sudden death, elevated cholesterol level, cigarette smoking; hypertension; diabetes, especially in first-degree relatives

Laboratory
  Measure fasting glucose and lipids in first-degree relatives

BMI, body mass index.

【 】 MONOCYTE/MACROPHAGES ADHESION AND MIGRATION[7]

Circulating monocytes are important inflammatory cells involved in the immune response. Insulin and insulin-like growth factor-1 receptors are present on circulating monocytes and macrophages. Defective insulin signaling is implicated in macrophage foam cell formation. Under conditions of insulin resistance, the protective effect of insulin to reduce macrophage apoptosis may be lost. Macrophage apoptosis in atherosclerotic lesions may contribute to further monocyte recruitment by the release of cytokines and may thus accelerate the development of the vascular lesion and contribute to plaque rupture.

【 】 INSULIN RESISTANCE

The insulin resistance syndrome, is a composite of dyslipidemia, hypertension, and hypercoagulability.[8] It is only now being recognized that insulin resistance (IR) is the predominant defect in more than 90 percent of type 2 diabetes patients, and the major pathologic mechanism for the susceptibility to premature cardiovascular disease. Insulin resistance and hyperinsulinemia accelerate the development of atherosclerosis. Hyperinsulinemia is an independent risk factor when adjusted for lipid profile, hypertension, and family history. Studies of multiple ethnic groups show increased carotid intima-medial thickness (a reliable marker for coronary disease) in subjects with insulin resistance. Impaired glucose tolerance (IGT), can increase the risk of heart disease. Because insulin resistance

TABLE 90–3

Adipokines

ADIPOKINE	ACTIONS
Adiponectin	• Antiinflammatory and antiatherogenic properties • Low levels characteristic of persons at increased risk of diabetes • Decreases foam cell formation • Decreases uptake of oxidized LDL • Decreases monocyte adhesion to endothelial cells • Decreases expression of adhesion molecules • Decreases proliferation and migration of vascular smooth muscle cells
Leptin	• Regulates energy intake and expenditure • Enhances cellular immune responses • Increases blood pressure levels
Angiotensinogen and angiotensin II	• Vasoconstrictive • Enhances the formation of foam cells • Stimulates intracellular adhesion molecule-1, vascular cell adhesion molecule-1, MCP-1, and M-CSF expression in the cells of the vessel wall • Increases monocyte–macrophage platelet activity in the vessel wall • Endothelial dysfunction
Tumor necrosis factor (TNF)	• Expression of adhesion molecules on the surface of the endothelial cells and VSMC
Plasminogen activator inhibitor-1 (PAI-1)	• Inhibits the breakdown of fibrin clots • Promotes thrombus formation

LDL, low density lipoprotein; MCP, monocyte chemotactic protein; M-CSF, monocyte colony-stimulating factor; VSMC, vascular smooth muscle cell.

precedes clinically diagnosed type 2 diabetes by 10 to 15 years in as many as 90 percent of patients, this extensive period of atherogenic exposure may account for the higher rates of cardiovascular disease in type 2 diabetics.[9]

Although the euglycemic-insulin clamp remains the gold standard for the measurement of IR, simpler formulae are employed clinically to quantify IR using the Homeostasis Model Assessment (HOMA IR = Serum Insulin × Serum Glucose / 22.5).[9] Insulin resistance as assessed by HOMA (HOMA-IR) also has been shown to be predictive of cardiovascular disease. In long-term followup of type 2 diabetic patients, insulin resistance was independently predictive of cardiovascular disease, with a 1-unit increase in HOMA-IR associated with a 5.4 percent increased risk of cardiovascular disease.[9] The Insulin Resistance and Atherosclerosis Study (IRAS) also demonstrated the relationship between insulin resistance and atherosclerosis in the carotid artery.

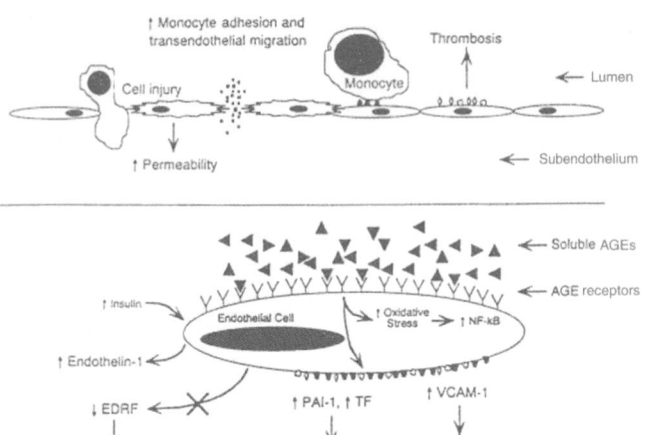

FIGURE 90–2. Generation of a dysfunctional endothelium caused by diabetes. See text for further details. AGE, advanced glycosylation end-product; EDRF, endothelium-derived relaxing factor; NF-κB, nuclear factor kappa B; PAI-1, plasminogen-activator inhibitor-1; TF, tissue factor; VCAM, vascular cell adhesion molecule. *Source: From Aronson D, Bloomgarden Z, Rayfield EJ. Potential mechanisms promoting restenosis in diabetes mellitus. J Am Coll Cardiol 1996;27:528–535, with permission.*

CLINICAL MANIFESTATIONS OF DIABETES

[ ] DYSGLYCEMIA

The San Antonio Heart Study showed a proportional increase in cardiovascular-related deaths with higher fasting blood glucose levels in type 2 diabetics.[10] Although there are abundant data linking both fasting glucose and impaired glucose tolerance to adverse events, the data demonstrating an improvement in cardiovascular outcomes with an aggressive glucose lowering treatment strategy have been lacking among patients with type 2 DM. Although data from United Kingdom Prospective Diabetes Study (UKPDS)[11] clearly demonstrated a reduction in microvascular complications with intensive glucose control, there was not a concomitant significant reduction in macrovascular complications, despite a disproportionate 25 percent risk of suffering a nonfatal myocardial infarction (MI) or stroke (compared with a 3.4 percent incidence of developing blindness or a 1 percent incidence of developing renal failure) during a 10-year period. However, it is important to remember that UKPDS only studied patients with new onset diabetes mellitus (DM). Recent data from the PROACTIVE study failed to show a significant reduction in the composite macrovascular outcomes with glucose reduction (Fig. 90–3), although the secondary outcome of MACCE was reduced by a significant 16 percent.[12]

Whether glucose management reduces macrovascular events remains unclear (Table 90–4).

Postprandial glycemia may also be an important factor in predicting future cardiovascular risk in epidemiologic studies. The DECODE study showed that an elevated 2-hour postprandial glucose level was independently associated with an increased mortality (Fig. 90–4).[13]

[ ] DYSLIPIDEMIA

Lipid disorders constitute one of the cornerstones in the cardiovascular management of diabetic patients. Many factors influence the lipid profile in these patients, including glycemic control, whether the diabetes is type 1 or type 2, and the presence of diabetic nephropathy.

In type 1 diabetes mellitus, the major determinant of the lipid profile is the level of glycemic control. Low-density lipoprotein (LDL) is moderately increased, triglycerides are markedly increased, and high-density lipoprotein (HDL) is decreased when the level of glycemic control is impaired. For patients with type 2 diabetes, lipid abnormalities are related not only to hyperglycemia but also to the interplay of the insulin-resistant state. Patients with type 2 diabetes may have normal LDL levels but elevated levels of the very-low-density lipoprotein (VLDL) triglycerides moiety and reduced HDL levels. The expected elevation in VLDL triglyceride is usually no more than 100 percent.

Low-Density Lipoprotein Cholesterol[14,15]

Although LDL levels in patients with controlled type 1 or type 2 diabetes may be normal, the atherogenic properties of LDL are increased. There is glycosylation of both apoprotein B[8] and the phospholipid component of LDL, which changes LDL

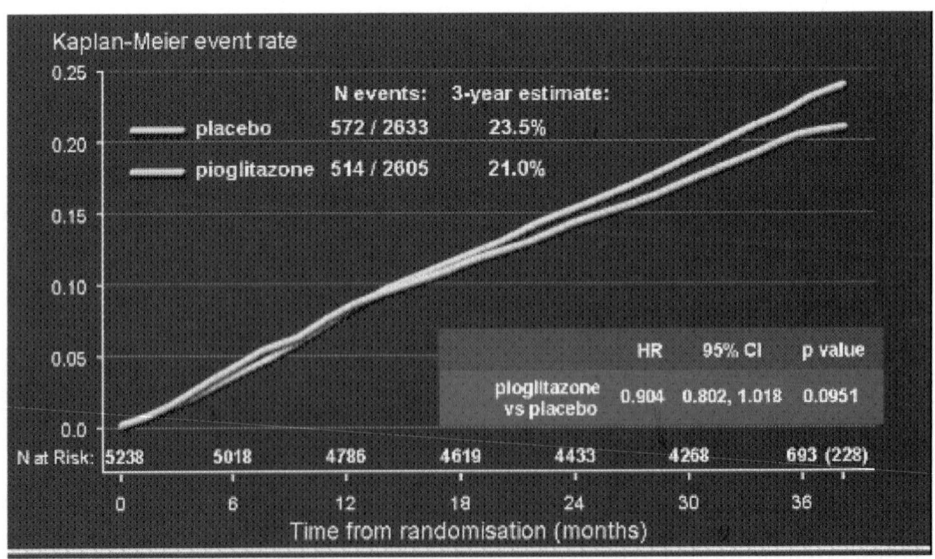

FIGURE 90–3. Time to primary composite end point curves during followup in patients receiving pioglitazone and in the control group in the PROACTIVE cohort. Absolute reduction in risk was 10.6 percent; relative risk was 0.904 (0.802 to 1.018); p, 0.0951. *Source: From Dormandy JA, Charbonnel B, Eckland DJ, et al. Secondary prevention of macrovascular events in patients with type 2 diabetes in the PROactive Study (PROspective pioglitAzone Clinical Trial In macroVascular Events): a randomised controlled trial. Lancet 2005;366(9493):1279–1289, with permission.*

TABLE 90–4

Glycemic Control

TRIAL	TREATMENT	OUTCOME	EVENTS CONTROL GROUP	EVENTS TREATMENT GROUP	RELATIVE RISK REDUCTION (%)	NUMBER NEEDED TO TREAT	P
Type 1 DM DCCT[197] n = 1441 patients[a] free of cardiac disease, HTN, and dyslipidemia	Intensive glycemic control versus conventional therapy	Macrovascular events	40/730 (5.5%)	23/711 (3.2%)	42	43	.08
Type 2 DM UKPDS[192–195] In newly diagnosed diabetes mellitus n = 3867	Sulfonylurea or insulin versus conventional therapy	Diabetes-related outcomes	438/1138 (38.4%)	963/2729 (35.2%)	8.3	31	.029

DCCT, the Diabetes Control and Complications Trial Research Group; DM, diabetes mellitus; HTN, hypertension; MI, myocardial infarction; UKPDS, United Kingdom Prospective Diabetes Study.
[a]n, total number of patients.

clearance and susceptibility to oxidative modifications. Glycosylation of apoprotein B occurs mainly in the LDL receptor-binding area and is directly related to glucose levels. As a result, there is impairment in the LDL receptor-mediated uptake, and therefore clearance of LDL. Glycosylation also makes LDL more susceptible to oxidative modification. The product generated by the combined glycosylation and oxidation of LDL is more atherogenic than is either glycosylated or oxidized LDL alone. Such LDL molecules are taken up more easily by the aortic intimal cells and macrophages, resulting in the formation of foam cells.

Type 2 diabetic patients with insulin resistance have LDL particles that are small and rich with triglycerides but have little cholesterol in them (small, dense LDL). These LDL particles increase the risk of CHD independent of the total LDL level, probably because of their increased susceptibility to oxidative modification. Therefore, even though LDL levels may be normal in these patients, high levels of small, dense LDL may contribute to the increased risk of CHD in such patients.

Very-Low-Density Lipoprotein Cholesterol[16,17]

Diabetic patients have elevated levels of VLDL as a result of increased free fatty acid mobilization and high glucose levels. There is an increase in triglyceride production by the liver, which results in large, triglyceride-rich VLDL particles. The size of these VLDL particles, which is dependent primarily on the amount of triglycerides available, is an important factor in determining their eventual fate. The conversion of large VLDL particles to LDL is inefficient; consequently, they are cleared from circulation by other pathways. Because the removal of VLDL by lipoprotein lipase also is affected, the level of VLDL triglyceride rises. Furthermore, the abundance of large triglyceride-rich VLDL is associated with an increase in small, dense, atherogenic LDL particles. Numerous studies show that elevated triglyceride levels are associated with increased risk for CHD

in diabetic patients. In contrast, elevated triglycerides are not associated with CHD risk in nondiabetic patients.

High-Density Lipoprotein Cholesterol[17,18]

A low HDL level is a strong risk factor for the development of CHD in the diabetic patient. There is decreased production and increased catabolism of HDL in diabetes. The decreased HDL production is a result of decreased lipoprotein lipase activity. The failure of lipoprotein lipase to efficiently catabolize VLDL results in reduced availability of surface components for HDL production. By contrast, increased catabolism of HDL results from the hypertriglyceridemia of diabetes, producing triglyceride-rich HDL_2 that is prone to catabolism by liver enzymes.

[ ] HYPERTENSION

The presence of hypertension in diabetic patients significantly increases their risk of micro- and macrovascular complications. It is estimated that 11 million Americans have both diabetes and hypertension. This "deadly duo" increases the cardiovascular event rate twofold.[19] Furthermore, hypertension among diabetic patients has been linked with numerous other vascular complications such as nephropathy, retinopathy, the development of cerebrovascular disease, and significant decline in cognitive function in middle aged diabetic hypertensive patients.

[ ] METABOLIC SYNDROME

The metabolic syndrome is considered to be an aggregation of various established cardiovascular risk factors. Multiple attempts have been made to define the metabolic syndrome encompassing what each investigator deems the relevant clusters. The most widely used definitions come from the National Cholesterol Education Program Adult Treatment Panel

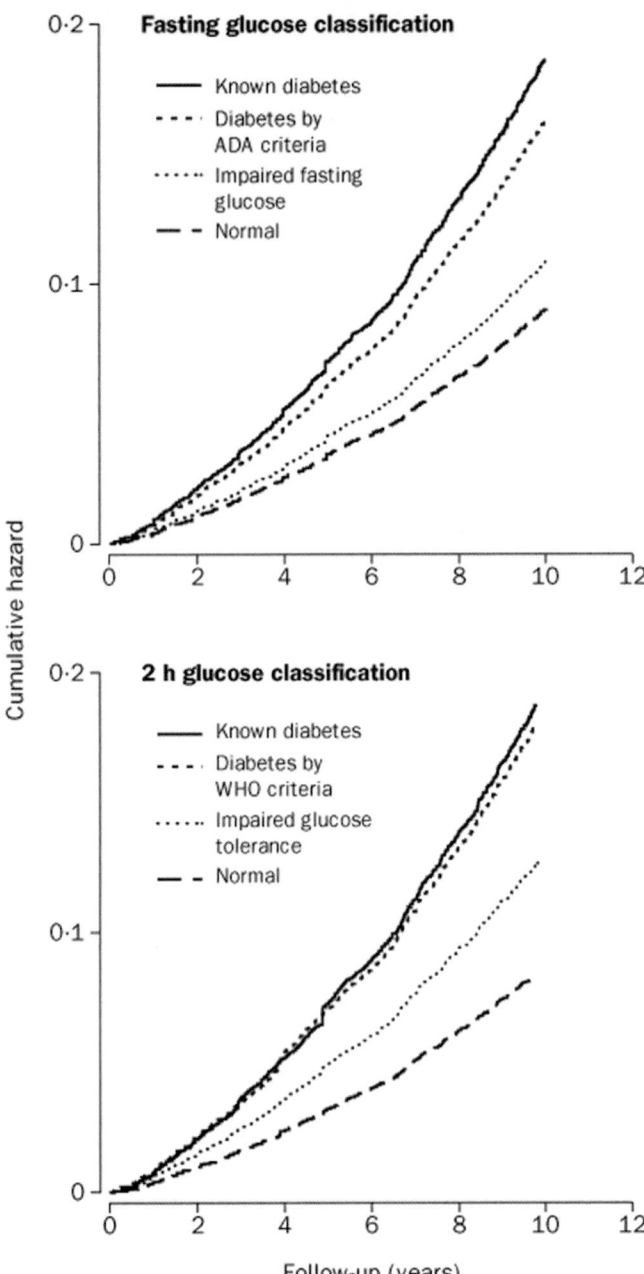

FIGURE 90–4. Cumulative hazard curves for American Diabetes Association fasting glucose criteria and the World Health Organization 2-h glucose criteria adjusted by age, sex, and study center. *Source: From the DECODE study group. Glucose tolerance and mortality: comparison of WHO and American Diabetes Association diagnostic criteria. Lancet 1999;354:617–621, with permission.*

(NCEP-ATP) III and the World Health Organization (WHO).[20,21] The ATP III criteria require any three of the following five: a triglyceride level ≥150 mg/dL or receiving a triglyceride lowering agent; HDL cholesterol <40 mg/dL in men and <50 mg/dL in women or receiving a HDL raising agent; blood pressure ≥130/≥85 mmHg or receiving antihypertensive therapy; fasting glucose ≥100 mg/dL; and a waist circumference in men >40 inches and in women >35 inches, with some variations for different ethnicities. The WHO definition requires the identification of insulin resistance by one of the following: type 2 diabetes; impaired fasting glucose, impaired glu-

cose tolerance, or for those with normal fasting glucose levels <110 mg/dL, glucose uptake below the lowest quartile for background populations under investigation under hyperinsulinemic, euglycemic conditions; plus any two of the following: antihypertensive medication and/or high blood pressure (≥140 mmHg systolic or ≥90 mmHg diastolic), plasma triglycerides ≥150 mg/dL, HDL cholesterol <35 mg/dL in men or <39 mg/dL in women, body mass index >30 kg/m² and/or waist-to-hip ratio >0.9 in men or >0.85 in women, and urinary albumin excretion rate ≥20 μg/min or albumin-to-creatinine ratio ≥30 mg/g. Other definitions from the IDF and AACE have also been proposed.[22,23] Isomaa et al. showed, using WHO criteria, a cardiovascular mortality of 12 percent in patients with metabolic syndrome versus 2 percent in patients without metabolic syndrome over a 6.9-year followup.[24] In the National Health and Nutritional Examination Surveys (NHANES) III study, metabolic syndrome was identified in 5 percent of normal weight, 22 percent of overweight, and 60 percent of obese individuals.[25] In the Framingham study, an increase in weight of 2.25 kg (5 lb) over 16 years was associated with a 21 to 45 percent increase in risk of developing metabolic syndrome. A large waist circumference identifies 46 percent of individuals who are at risk of developing metabolic syndrome in next 5 years. The 10-year risk of a cardiovascular event (per Framingham data) in men with metabolic syndrome ranged from 10 to 20 percent, and was 10 percent in women. The diagnosis of metabolic syndrome was associated with a significant threefold increase in risk of coronary heart disease and stroke and a highly significant increase in cardiovascular mortality.[26]

Five landmark studies[27–31] have established beyond any reasonable doubt the strong relationship between metabolic syndrome and cardiovascular disease. The Strong Heart Study of 890 Pima Indians showed that 144 (16.2 percent) developed DM type 2 over 4 years and that metabolic syndrome increased the risk for DM type 2 by 2.1-fold (ATP) and 3.6-fold (WHO). The Beaver Dam Study involved 4423 non-DM type 2 white patients with metabolic syndrome, showing 9- to 34-fold increase in DM type 2 at 5-year followup. The WOSCOPS study evaluated 5974 non-DM type 2 patients. At 5-year followup, patients with 4 to 5 metabolic syndrome features had DM type 2 risk increased 24.5-fold and their CHD risk was 3.7-fold higher. The Finland Study of 1200 patients and an 11-year followup demonstrated that patients with metabolic syndrome had a 4.2-fold increased relative risk of coronary artery disease and a twofold increase in all-cause mortality. Finally, the Air Force/Texas Coronary Atherosclerosis Prevention Study (AFCAPS/TexCAPS) study confirmed a 1.5-fold increase in major adverse cardiovascular events in metabolic syndrome patients.

COMPLICATIONS OF DIABETES

【 】 MICROVASCULAR COMPLICATIONS

Renal

Nephropathy occurs in 40 percent of patients with type 1 and type 2 diabetes. Risk factors include poor glycemic control, hypertension, and ethnicity (blacks, Mexicans, Pima Indians).[32] Table 90–5 summarizes the key points for the assessment of renal status in a diabetic patient. The earliest clinical finding of diabetic kidney disease is microalbuminuria, which may occur at a time when renal histology is essentially normal (Fig. 90–5). The Diabetes Control and Complications Trial (DCCT) and the UKPDS showed that the development and progression of microalbuminuria can be prevented through strict glycemic control.

The UKPDS of type 2 diabetics and studies of patients with type 1 diabetes using captopril have shown that control of hypertension slows the progression of nephropathy. The blood pressure should be maintained at <130/85 mmHg, and angiotensin-converting enzyme (ACE) inhibitors are the preferred antihypertensive agents. The UKPDS, however, showed no difference in blood pressure control with captopril versus atenolol. The benefit of antihypertensive therapy with an ACE inhibitor in type 1 diabetes can be shown early in the course of disease, when microalbuminuria is the only abnormality.[33]

There is insufficient evidence to recommend ACE inhibitors in normotensive patients without microalbuminuria. Nonetheless, physicians should still recommend screening on at least a yearly basis, since the risk-to-benefit ratio of diagnosing microalbuminuria justifies treatment with an ACE inhibi-

TABLE 90–5
Evaluation of Renal Status

Urine albumin and protein
  Yearly screen for microalbumin in type 1 and type 2 diabetes; microalbumin to creatinine ratio collected in a spot urine, ideally first morning urine specimen (normal <30 mg/g creatinine); must rule out other diseases that cause proteinuria.
  If urine albumin/creatinine is >300 mg/g in first morning specimen, macroalbuminuria is present and is usually not reversible with ACE inhibitors; nephrology consult.
  Nephrotic syndrome: urine protein >3 g/d; nephrology consult.
  Other reasons to consult nephrologists are diabetic patients with increasing creatinine from 1.4 to >2.0, elevated creatinine and symptoms of uremia, microalbuminuria not responding to ACE inhibitor.
Urinalysis
  Red cells, pyuria, casts require nephrology consult.
Blood pressure evaluation
  If hypertension is present, exclude secondary causes, including with advancing renal insufficiency.
  Treatment with an ACE inhibitor is preferred first choice even in African Americans (except if precluded by hyperkalemia or other complications).
Blood urea nitrogen, serum creatinine, and glomerular filtration rate
  Yearly creatinine clearance should be obtained with 24-h urine collection and serum creatinine; most accurate way to estimate kidney function without using a radioisotope.

ACE, angiotensin-converting enzyme.

tor, if not for renal disease alone, then for reducing the incidence of myocardial infarction.

Patients on ACE inhibitors should be monitored for potassium, as they may develop hyperkalemia in the presence of a type 4 renal tubular acidosis. Sodium restriction reduces hypertension and therefore is advised. Dietary protein should be adjusted to 0.8 g/kg/d to decrease intraglomerular pressure.

More recently, clinical trials evaluating angiotensin receptor blockers (ARBs), including losartan and irbesartan, have demonstrated a significant renal protective effect in the diabetic patient with nephropathy. There were no differences between the ARB and usual care groups with regard to cardiovascular outcomes.[34]

An optimal approach toward diabetic nephropathy combines control of hypertension, preferably with an ACE inhibitor or ARB, glycemic control, sodium restriction, and adjustment of protein intake.

If increasing macroalbuminuria occurs or if renal insufficiency is progressive despite these measures, the patient should be referred to a nephrologist. It is strongly recommended that renal arteriography be avoided. Dietary protein restriction in patients who have progressive renal insufficiency will reduce accumulation of nitrogen-containing waste products and can have a beneficial influence on progression of renal insufficiency.

OPHTHALMOLOGIC

Diabetic retinopathy is the most prevalent microvascular complication affecting nearly 50 percent of the diabetic population at a given time and eventually occurring in all diabetic patients. Diabetes remains the leading cause of visual loss in adults. Visual loss from diabetes occurs either as a result of proliferative retinopathy or macular edema.[35]

MACROVASCULAR MANIFESTATIONS
Coronary Heart Disease

CHD is strongly associated with type 2 diabetes mellitus and is the leading cause of death regardless of the duration of disease. There is a two- to fourfold increase in the relative risk ratio of cardiovascular disease in type 2 diabetes patients compared to the general population. This increase is particularly disproportionate in diabetic women when compared with diabetic men. The protection that premenopausal women have against CHD is not seen if they suffer from diabetes. The degree and duration of hyperglycemia are a strong risk factor for the development of microvascular complications, but in type 2 diabetes, macrovascular complications have not been documented to be associated with the length or severity of a patient's diabetes. Even impaired glucose tolerance increases cardiovascular risk, although there is minimal hyperglycemia.[36–38]

The first detectable sign of a problem in people genetically prone to develop type 2 diabetes is insulin resistance, which can be seen as long as 15 to 25 years before the onset of diabetes. Several atherogenic factors are associated with insulin resistance,[39] which can start the atherosclerotic process years before clinical hyperglycemia ensues. It is unclear whether the compensatory hyperinsulinemia plays a role in atherosclerosis generation in insulin-resis-

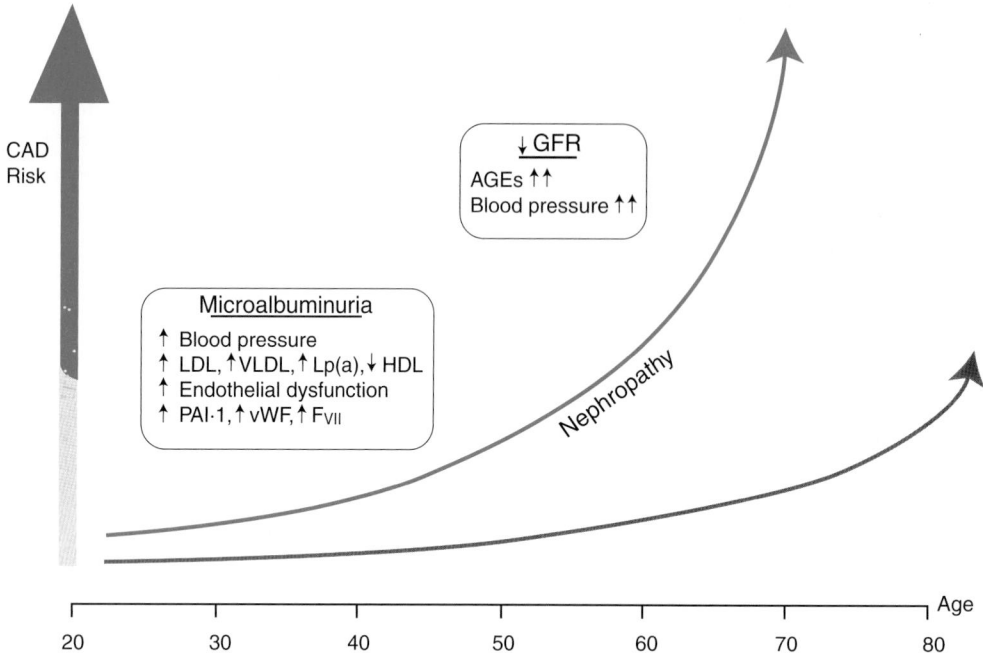

FIGURE 90–5. Coronary artery disease risk in patients with diabetes mellitus. A subset of genetically predisposed patients develops diabetic nephropathy. In these patients, the risk for coronary artery disease (CAD) increases dramatically. AGE, advanced glycosylation end-product; GFR, glomerular filtration rate; HDL, high-density lipoprotein; LDL, low-density lipoprotein; Lp(a), lipoprotein(a); PAI, plasminogen activator inhibitor; VLDL, very-low-density lipoprotein; vWF, von Willebrand factor. *Source: From Aronson D, Bloomgarden Z, Rayfield EJ. Potential mechanisms promoting restenosis in diabetes mellitus. J Am Coll Cardiol 1996;27:528–535, with permission.*

tant patients. A number of prospective studies have shown an association between fasting or postprandial hyperinsulinemia and the future development of CHD. However, this association has been demonstrated in middle-aged white men, but not in women or in other ethnic groups.[40,41]

Hyperglycemia itself plays an important role in enhancing the progression of atherosclerosis in type 2 diabetes. The threshold above which hyperglycemia becomes atherogenic is not known but may be in the range defined as impaired glucose tolerance (i.e., fasting plasma glucose level <126 mg/dL with 30-, 60-, or 90-minute plasma glucose concentrations >200 mg/L and a 2-hour plasma glucose level of 140 to 200 mg/dL during an oral glucose tolerance test). Population-based studies show that the degree of hyperglycemia increases the risk for CHD and cardiovascular events.[42]

Acute Coronary Syndromes

Diabetic patients represent a high-risk group for developing and surviving acute myocardial infarction. In particular, patients with type 1 diabetes have a worse outcome than do patients with type 2 disease, and diabetic women have almost twice the risk of mortality of diabetic men.[43]

Reperfusion therapy is the cornerstone of the management of acute myocardial infarction. In a meta-analysis of all major thrombolytic trials, diabetic patients had a nonsignificant trend toward increased reductions in 35-day mortality rates compared with nondiabetic patients.[44] The potential advantage of angioplasty over thrombolytic therapy has not been addressed in the diabetic population.

New treatment strategies are emerging. The use of insulin and glucose infusion for at least 24 hours after admission followed by intensive long-term insulin was compared with usual care in the DIGAMI trial. A total of 620 diabetic patients were randomized, and the trial demonstrated a 30 percent reduction in mortality at 12 months for the group treated under the intensive program.[45]

However the followup DIGAMI-2 trial, which compared three strategies—intensive insulin infusion followed by long-term insulin therapy, intensive insulin infusion followed by long-term standard glucose control, and regular metabolic control—in 1253 patients was unable to show a difference in short- and long-term mortality and morbidity between any of the arms. DIGAMI-2 concluded that intensive glucose control was of great importance in the periischemic period irrespective of the strategy used to achieve it.[46]

Chronic Coronary Artery Disease

The association between CHD and diabetes is strong and has led to screening strategies in diabetic patients even before they are symptomatic. In addition, diabetic patients often are unaware of myocardial ischemic pain, and so silent myocardial infarction and ischemia are markedly increased in this population. There is a heightened concern for the development of sudden cardiac death in those with diabetes. Therapeutic modalities in diabetic patients with CHD revolve around standard therapy with aspirin, β blockers, calcium channel blockers, and nitrates.

Epidemiologic evidence from the Bezafibrate Infarction Prevention Study registry shows almost a 50 percent reduction in mortality for type 2 patients with chronic CHD who were treated with β blockers, compared with controls. Other randomized trial evidence has demonstrated that diabetes is a strong predictor of death and that diabetic patients may benefit more from β-blocker therapy than do nondiabetics. In general, β blockers are extremely well tolerated, and masking or prolonging of hypoglycemic symptoms appears to be highly infrequent, particularly with cardioselective β blockers.[47]

Diabetic Cardiomyopathy

Diabetic cardiomyopathy is a term used by clinicians to encompass the multifactorial etiologies of diabetes-related left ventricular failure characterized by both systolic and diastolic function.[48] The Framingham Heart Study showed that men with diabetes who have congestive heart failure were twice as common as their nondiabetic counterpart, and that females with diabetes had a fivefold increase, in the rate of congestive heart failure. The spectrum of heart failure ranges from asymptomatic to overt systolic failure. Diabetes complicated by hypertension represents a particularly high-risk group for the development of congestive heart failure.[49] Diastolic dysfunction is exceedingly common (>50 percent prevalence in some studies) and may be linked to diabetes without the presence of concomitant hypertension.

The etiology of impaired left ventricular function may involve any of the following mechanisms: (1) coronary atherosclerotic disease, (2) hypertension, (3) left ventricular hypertrophy, (4) obesity, (5) endothelial dysfunction, (6) coronary microvasculature disease, (7) autonomic dysfunction, and (8) metabolic abnormalities.

The diabetes and cardiovascular communities have embraced the concept of diabetic cardiomyopathy as a distinct entity independent of ischemic heart disease and hypertension. This was first described in the early 1970s when autopsy specimens of diabetic patients with nephropathy demonstrated a myopathic process in the absence of epicardial CHD.

Echocardiographic studies confirm that diastolic abnormalities occur in young diabetic patients who have no known diabetic complications.[50] Diabetic patients who are hypertensive have increased left ventricular mass when compared to their nondiabetic counterparts and left ventricular function may in fact be hyperdynamic. An Australian group has confirmed that diabetic patients demonstrate early findings of systolic dysfunction preceding any change in the left ventricular ejection fraction. The management of heart failure with preserved left ventricular systolic function usually includes β blockers and ACE inhibitors, but evidence for this is sparse.

Once CHD develops in the diabetic patient, the left ventricular systolic dysfunction that ensues responds to all the same therapies as in the nondiabetic population. The findings of the HOPE (Heart Outcomes Prevention Evaluation) trial suggest that early initiation of ACE inhibition retards the progression to overt congestive heart failure.[51]

Cerebrovascular Disease

Compared to nondiabetic subjects, the mortality from stroke in diabetic patients is almost threefold higher. The small paramedial penetrating arteries are the most common sites of cerebrovascular disease. In addition, diabetes increases the likelihood of severe carotid atherosclerosis. Diabetic patients are likely to suffer increased brain damage with carotid emboli that would result in a transient ischemic attack in a nondiabetic individual.[52,53]

MANAGEMENT OF DIABETES AND ITS COMPLICATIONS

【 】 THERAPEUTIC LIFESTYLE CHANGES

STENO-2[54]

STENO-2 demonstrated that a comprehensive multifactorial strategy (including lifestyle and pharmacologic interventions) to reduce cardiovascular risk in type 2 diabetic patients with microalbuminuria was highly effective (hazard ratio: 0.47; 95 percent confidence interval: 0.24 to 0.73) when compared to usual care after a mean time of 7.8 years (Table 90–6 and Fig. 90–6). The number needed to treat to prevent a major cardiovascular event was only five patients. The approach included targets of HbA1c less than 6.5 percent, blood pressure less than 130/80 mmHg, total cholesterol less than 175 mg/dL, and triglycerides below 150 mg/dL. Patients were prescribed aspirin and an ACE inhibitor or ARB. This study validates the multidisciplinary approach to the cardiovascular care of the diabetic patient.

Weight loss is an important therapeutic strategy in all overweight or obese individuals who have type 2 diabetes or are at risk for developing diabetes.[55] The primary approach for achieving weight loss, in the vast majority of cases, is therapeutic lifestyle change, which includes a reduction in energy intake and an increase in physical activity. A moderate decrease in caloric balance

TABLE 90–6

STENO-2 Study

TRIAL	TREATMENT	OUTCOME	EVENTS CONTROL GROUP	EVENTS TREATMENT GROUP	RELATIVE RISK REDUCTION (%)	NUMBER NEEDED TO TREAT	P
STENO-2[136] n = 160	Intensive, comprehensive (includes hypertension, dyslipidemia, and glycemic control) therapy versus standard therapy	Macrovascular events: death, myocardial infarction, stroke, vascular ischemia	42/78 (53.8%)	26/77 (33.7%)	37.3	5	.03

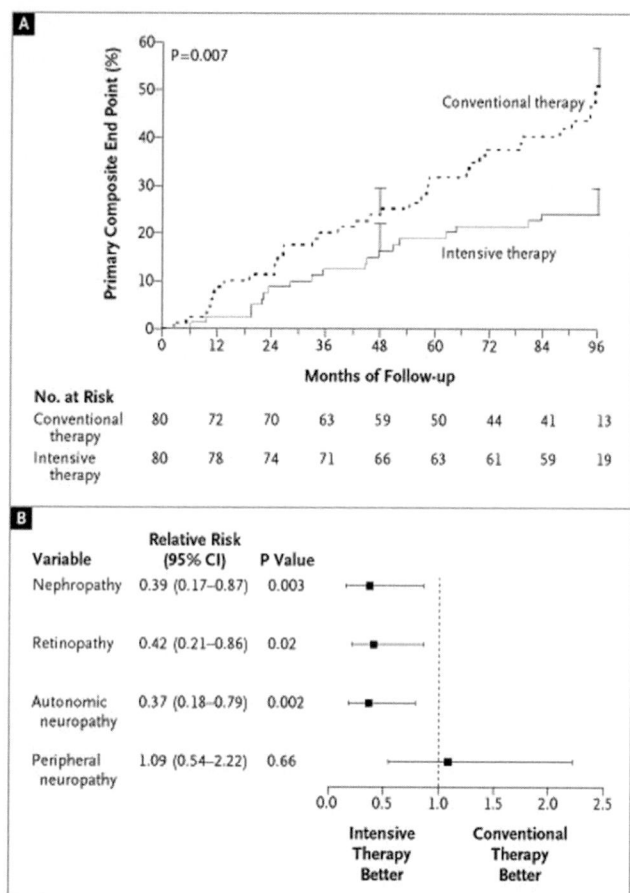

FIGURE 90–6. Kaplan-Meier estimates of the composite end point of death from cardiovascular causes, nonfatal myocardial infarction, coronary artery bypass grafting, percutaneous coronary intervention, nonfatal stroke, amputation, and surgery for peripheral atherosclerotic artery disease in the Conventional-Therapy Group and the Intensive-Therapy Group (**A**) and the relative risk of the development or progression of nephropathy, retinopathy, and autonomic and peripheral neuropathy during the average followup of 7.8 years in the Intensive-Therapy Group, as compared with the Conventional-Therapy Group (**B**). *Source: From Gaede P, Vedel P, Larsen N, et al. Multifactorial intervention and cardiovascular disease in patients with type 2 diabetes. N Engl J Med 2003;348:383–393, with permission.*

(500 to 1000 kcal/d) will result in a slow but progressive weight loss (1 to 2 lb/wk). For most patients, weight-loss diets should supply at least 1000 to 1200 kcal/d for women and 1200 to 1600 kcal/d for men. In selected patients, drug therapy to achieve weight loss as an adjunct to lifestyle change may be appropriate. However, it is important to note that regain of weight commonly occurs on discontinuation of medication.

Physical activity is an important component of a comprehensive weight management program. Regular moderate-intensity physical activity enhances long-term weight maintenance. Regular activity also improves insulin sensitivity, glycemic control, and selected risk factors for cardiovascular disease (i.e., hypertension and dyslipidemia), and increased aerobic fitness decreases the risk of CHD. Initial physical activity recommendations should be modest, based on the patient's willingness and ability, gradually increasing the duration and frequency to 30 to 45 minutes of moderate aerobic activity, 3 to 5 days per week, when possible. Greater activity levels of at least 1 hour per day of moderate (walking) or

30 minutes per day of vigorous (jogging) activity may be needed to achieve successful long-term weight loss. The American College of Sports Medicine now recommends resistance training be included in fitness programs for adults with type 2 diabetes. Resistance exercise improves insulin sensitivity to about the same extent as aerobic exercise.

In patients with severe/morbid obesity, surgical options, such as gastric bypass and gastroplasty, may be appropriate and allow significant improvement in glycemic control with reduction or discontinuation of medications. It is important to fully evaluate the patient for existing or risk for cardiovascular disease and improve glycemic control preoperatively so as to decrease the risk of complications. It is important to counsel patients on the risks of surgery, including mortality, depression, hypoglycemia, nutritional deficiencies, osteoporosis, and weight regain over the long-term. Very little data are currently available on the long-term consequences of surgery for weight loss in people with diabetes. The potential benefits should be weighed against short- and long-term risks.[55]

DYSGLYCEMIA MANAGEMENT

The medical community has progressively become more and more aggressive about risk factor modification. Multiple trials in cardiovascular prevention have shown that modification of traditional risk factors show more benefit than glycemic control. Practitioners, however, must realize that because of the importance of glycemic control in preventing microvascular complications cardiologists have adopted measures to control blood glucose levels.

The American Heart Association and the American Diabetes Association have come to consensus for goals of targets. The HbA1c goal for patients in general is an A1c goal of <7 percent.[138] The American College of Clinical Endocrinology goal is an A1c of <6.5 percent.[56] However, the ideal A1c goal for the individual patient is an A1c as close to normal (<6 percent) as possible without significant hypoglycemia. The debate presently is also whether getting to the goal is enough or whether how one gets there is important as well. The BARI (Bypass Angioplasty Revascularization Investigation) 2D study will provide more data on whether management of insulin resistance with insulin-sensitizing therapies leads to better outcomes than insulin-replacing therapies.[57]

The guidelines currently recommend treating to target and acknowledge that most type 2 diabetic patients may require more than one antidiabetic agent. Most agents have been studied to measure efficacy as monotherapy and across the board demonstrate a 40 to 60 percent reduction in fasting plasma glucose level. The following discussion outlines the mechanisms, advantages, and disadvantages of each of these therapies as individual agents (Fig. 90–7).

Traditional Medications

Insulin Insulin is used in the management of type 1 diabetes mellitus (T1DM) or type 2 diabetes mellitus (T2DM) as monotherapy or in combination with oral agents. Insulins currently available are synthetic human insulins or analogues of human insulin, which differ in their rate of absorption and duration of action. There are also products that are mixtures rapid short-acting and

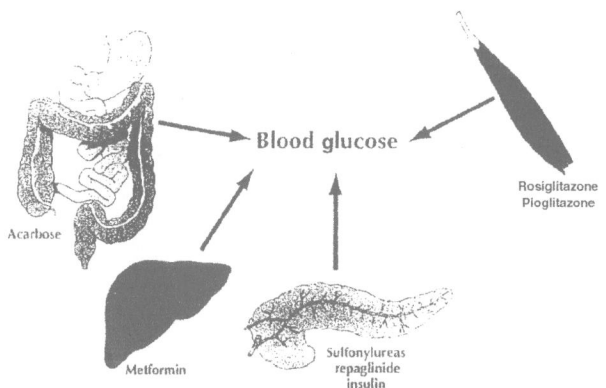

FIGURE 90–7. Mechanism of action of hypoglycemic agents.

intermediate-acting insulins (Table 90–7). Purified animal insulins are no longer used.

Recombinant human insulin (RHI) is structurally identical to human insulin and is synthesized by *Escherichia coli* bacteria. It consists of zinc insulin crystals dissolved in clear fluid. There are four rapid-acting insulins currently available. Insulin lispro is a rapid-acting insulin analogue in which the amino acids at positions 28 and 29 on the human insulin B chain are reversed. Insulin aspart is a second rapid-acting insulin analogue with a substitution of aspartic acid for proline in position 28 on the B chain. Insulin glulisine is the newest rapid-acting analogue in which the asparagine at position 3 on the B chain is replaced by glutamic acid. These amino acid changes result in a reduced propensity for insulin molecules to form aggregates (dimers and hexamers), providing a more rapid onset and shorter duration of action than RHI. These insulins are used to cover carbohydrates at mealtime to correct for an elevated glucose level, and in insulin pumps. The latest rapid-acting insulin is Exubera (a human insulin of rDNA origin), which is inhaled and has an intermediate duration of action (387 minutes) that is faster than lispro and comparable to regular insulin.[58]

Exubera comes in "blisters" of 1 mg and 3 mg, with each 1 mg of the powder approximately equal to 3 units of injected regular insulin. When the blister is placed into an inhaler, a cloud of aerosolized insulin is inhaled.[59]

Neutral pH protamine Hagedorn (NPH) is an intermediate-acting insulin that is a suspension of RHI with protamine thus delaying its absorption. NPH can be used at bedtime to normalize fasting glucose and in combination with rapid-acting insulins during the daytime to provide primarily basal coverage.

Insulin glargine is an insulin analogue in which the asparagine residue at position A21 is replaced with glycine and two arginine residues are added to the B chain C terminus. Insulin glargine has a pH of 4 in solution, but after subcutaneous injection has a pH of 7.4 microprecipitates, which delays its absorption. It is essentially peakless with a 24-hour duration of action. Insulin detemir is a soluble long-acting human insulin analogue with the elimination of the threonine in position B30 and the addition of a 14-carbon fatty acid chain at position B29. Insulin detemir is absorbed slowly from the injection site and it is more than 98 percent reversibly bound to albumin in the blood. The basal insulins are used once or twice daily to provide broad coverage.

The most physiologic way of administering insulin therapy is to give a basal insulin once or twice daily, as well as a bolus of insulin prior to each meal based on carbohydrate counting and a correction factor to bring the glucose down to premeal levels by 2 hours after eating. This basal–bolus regimen provides better glycemic control than the control obtained using mixed insulin preparations. There is less hypoglycemia with bedtime administration of insulin glargine or detemir than with NPH, because the glucose-lowering effect is slow and sustained over a period approximating 24 hours.[60]

Insulin allergies are uncommon with the recombinant preparations of insulins. Unused insulin vials, cartridges, and pens should be kept refrigerated and will stay potent until the expiration date. Once opened, Insulin glargine must be changed every 28 days, regardless of whether or not it is refrigerated. Mixed analogues in a pen should be discarded after 10 to 14 days.

Use of Insulin Pumps and Continuous Glucose Monitoring Systems[61]

Insulin pumps are devices with a subcutaneous catheter which deliver continuous subcutaneous insulin infusion. One or more basal rates are preprogrammed by the user and boluses are taken as needed whenever carbohydrates are ingested. The catheter is changed every 2 to 3 days and abdominal infusion sites are most commonly used. In a motivated patient, better glycemic control can be achieved with continuous subcutaneous insulin infusion—compared with multiple subcutaneous insulin injections—because continuous subcutaneous insulin infusion can provide multiple basal rates of insulin. Pumps are generally used in patients with T1DM but can also be used in patients with T2DM. A meta-anal-

TABLE 90–7

Insulins

TYPE	NAME	ONSET OF ACTION	TIME TO PEAK ACTIVITY	DURATION OF ACTION
Rapid acting	Aspart	15 minutes	1 hour	3–4 hours
	Glulisine	15 minutes	30–90 minutes	3–5 hours
	Lispro	15 minutes	1 hour	3–4 hours
Short acting	Regular	30–60 minutes	2–4 hours	6–8 hours
Intermediate acting	NPH	1–3 hours	6–8 hours	12–16 hours
Long acting	Detemir	1 hour	No peak	About 12 hours
	Glargine	1–2 hours	No peak	About 24 hours

NPH, neutral protamine Hagedorn.

TABLE 90–8

Commercially Available (Other Than Insulin) Agents Used to Treat Type 2 Diabetes Mellitus

DRUG CLASS	GENERIC NAME	MECHANISM OF ACTION	EXPECTED A1c REDUCTION (%)	DAILY DOSE
Biguanides	Metformin	Decreases hepatic glucose output	1.0–2.0	500 mg qd to 1000 mg bid to 850 mg tid
Thiazolidinedione	Pioglitazone	PPAR-α and-γ agonist	1.0–1.5	15–45 mg qd
	Rosiglitazone	PPAR-γ agonist	1.0–1.5	2 mg qd–bid, 8 mg qd
Sulfonylurea	Glipizide	↑ β-cell insulin synthesis and release	1.0–2.0	2.5–20 mg qd–bid
	Glyburide	↑ β-cell insulin synthesis and release		1.25–10 mg qd–bid
	Glimepiride	↑ β-cell insulin synthesis and release		0.5–8 mg qd
Meglitinides	Repaglinide	↑ β-cell insulin synthesis and release	1.0–2.0	0.5–4 mg tid
	Nateglinide	↑ β-cell insulin synthesis and release	0.5–1.0	60–120 mg tid
α-Glucosidase inhibitors	Acarbose	α-Glucosidase inhibition (decreased carbohydrate absorption)	0.5–1.0	50–100 mg tid
	Miglitol	α-Glucosidase inhibition	0.5–1.0	50–100 mg tid
Incretin mimetic	Exenatide	Increasing postprandial insulin, decreasing postprandial glucagon, increasing satiety and delaying gastric emptying	0.5–0.9	5–10 μg bid

PPAR, peroxisome proliferator-activated receptor.

ysis by Weissberg-Benchell et al. of 52 studies concluded that continuous subcutaneous insulin infusion is associated with improved A1c and mean blood glucose levels. Bode et al. demonstrated that mean A1c levels decreased from 8.3 to 7.5 percent, with a significant reduction in severe hypoglycemia, in comparison to multiple insulin injections during the first year of therapy. Patients who counted carbohydrates, checked their glucoses three or more times a day, and recorded their glucoses in a logbook had better glycemic control than those who did not.

Continuous glucose monitoring systems (CGMS) that use a glucose sensor to provide up to 3 days of continuous glucose monitoring in the subcutaneous tissue are available. The record shows glucose patterns and trends that can help in the recognition and prevention of hypoglycemia, hyperglycemia, postprandial glucose excursions, and the effects of exercise. However, "normal" interstitial glucose values may be lower than realized, including some values in the "hypoglycemic range." Also, the CGMS may not always read the glucose concentrations consistently accurately. Recently, two systems for real-time continuous glucose monitoring system became available: the Dex Com and the Guardian RT. Outcome data with these devices should be available soon.

Multiple other agents are used in the management of diabetes. Table 90–8 summarizes them; they are described in detail below.

Metformin[62] Metformin has been used in Europe for several decades but has been marketed in the United States since 1995. The mechanism of action of metformin is to decrease hepatic glucose output by inhibiting glucose-6-dehydrogenase activity and stimulating the insulin-induced component of glucose uptake into skeletal muscle and adipocytes.

The starting dose for metformin is 500 mg orally with dinner for 1 week then 500 mg orally with breakfast and dinner. A sus-

tained-release preparation is available that allows once-daily dosing. Because of its mechanism of action, there is minimal risk for hypoglycemia. This drug should not be used in renal failure or potential hypoxic states, such as congestive heart failure and severe pulmonary disease, because of the risk of lactic acidosis. The risk of lactic acidosis is low and is estimated to be 9 per 100,000 person-years. The most common side effects are gastrointestinal—nausea, diarrhea and abdominal pain—and a metallic taste. It should not be used in patients with impaired renal function (serum creatinine >1.5 mg/dL in men and >1.4 mg/dL in women). Caution should be exercised in prescribing metformin to the elderly. If used in patients older than age 80 years, then a normal glomerular filtration rate should be documented. Metformin should be discontinued on the day patients receive an iodinated contrast material for radiographic studies, which can temporarily impair renal function, as well as prior to any surgical procedure. The metformin dose can be resumed 48 hours later if the serum creatinine is in the normal range. Metformin lowers the A1c by 1 to 2 percent. Metformin can be used to treat the metabolic syndrome since it lowers serum concentrations of triglycerides, plasminogen activator inhibitor-1 activity, and body weight.

Thiazolidinediones[63,64] These agents induce peroxisome proliferator-activated receptor (PPAR)-γ binding to nuclear receptors in muscle and adipocytes, allowing insulin-stimulated glucose transport (Fig. 90–8). Three PPARs have been identified to date: PPARα, PPARδ (also known as PPARβ), and PPARγ. After ligand binding, PPARs change their conformation to permit the recruitment of one or more coactivator proteins. The first mechanism, transactivation, is DNA-dependent and consists of binding PPAR components with target genes and heterodimerization with the retinoid X receptor. The second mechanism, transrepression, interferes with other transcription factor pathways that are not DNA-depen-

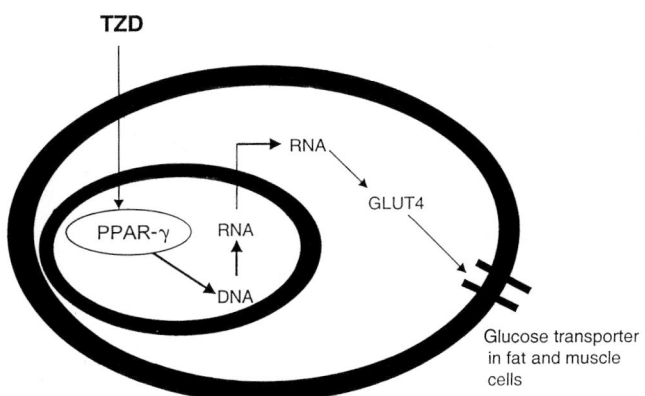

FIGURE 90–8. Mechanism of action of thiazolidinediones. GLUT, glucose-transport protein.

dent. The protein kinase C signaling pathway functions as a molecular switch that dissociates with transactivation and transrepression properties of PPARα. PPARα resides mainly in the liver, heart muscle, and vascular endothelium; when it is activated, it controls genes that regulate lipoprotein levels and confers antiinflammatory effects. PPARγ is located mainly on adipocytes, but is also found in pancreatic β cells, vascular endothelium, and macrophages.

Thiazolidinediones (TZDs) lower fasting and postprandial glucose levels, as well as free fatty acid levels. A first-generation TZD, troglitazone, is no longer available because of its hepatotoxicity. The second-generation TZDs, rosiglitazone and pioglitazone, may be used as monotherapy or in combination with insulin, sulfonylureas, or metformin, and have not been found to be hepatotoxic. TZDs are associated with weight gain caused by fluid retention and proliferation of adipose tissue. However, the TZDs increase fat in the subcutaneous adipose tissue and decrease visceral adipose tissue and fat in the liver. The dose for rosiglitazone is 2 to 8 mg/d; for pioglitazone, it is 15 to 45 mg/d. Two side effects to be noted are peripheral tissue edema and, less frequently, congestive heart failure. TZDs are contraindicated in patients with congestive heart failure and should be used cautiously in at-risk patients.

TZDs decrease A1c levels by 1 to 1.5 percent. These agents decrease insulin resistance and possibly preserve β-cell function. The Troglitazone in the Prevention of Diabetes (TRIPOD)[65] study was designed to investigate the preservation of pancreatic β-cell function with TZD. Hispanic women with a prior medical history of gestational diabetes were randomized to receive troglitazone 400 mg daily or a placebo. Women who did not develop diabetes were asked to return 8 months after the trial for an oral glucose tolerance test and an intravenous glucose tolerance. The median followup was 30 months. The troglitazone group had a 56 percent reduction in the incidence of T2DM for as long as 8 months after the medications were stopped. This protection against earlier development of diabetes was associated with a reduction in insulin resistance. Pioglitazone acts like a partial PPARα agonist and has beneficial effects on the lipid profile increasing high-density lipoprotein-cholesterol, decreasing triglycerides, and improving low-density lipoprotein-cholesterol subtypes. Dual PPARα/γ agonists have not been U.S. Food and Drug Administration (FDA) approved to date because of safety concerns.

Sulfonylureas[66] Sulfonylureas are the oldest class of treatment for T2DM. The mode of action is by stimulating β-cell insulin se-

cretion (see Fig. 90–7). The β-cell sulfonylurea receptor (SUR) is functionally linked to an adenosine triphosphate (ATP)-sensitive K+ channel (K+-ATP) on the cell membrane. In the basal state, the K+-ATP channel shifts K+ from the inside of the β cell to the extracellular space and maintains the resting potential of the β-cell membrane. When the sulfonylurea binds to the SUR, K+ efflux diminishes and the membrane depolarizes. This depolarization opens a voltage-dependent calcium channel in the same membrane, which enables extracellular calcium to enter the cell. The resultant increase in intracellular calcium triggers insulin-containing secretory granule exocytosis.

The first-generation sulfonylureas have a long half-life and bind ionically to plasma proteins, making them easily displaced. The major concern with these agents is hypoglycemia. The second-generation sulfonylureas have a shorter half-life and bind to plasma proteins nonionically, making them less easily displaced from proteins and available for binding to receptors. Commercially available second-generation sulfonylureas are glyburide (1.25 to 20 mg/d), glipizide (2.5 to 40 mg/d), and glimepiride (1 to 8 mg/d). Sulfonylureas decrease the A1c by 1 to 2 percent.

Meglitinides[58] Repaglinide is a member of the meglitinide group of insulin secretagogues with a relatively short half-life of 3.7 hours. The binding site on the SUR is distinct from the binding site for sulfonylureas. The drug is taken up to 30 minutes prior to each meal. Repaglinide is particularly useful in the elderly, patients with chronic renal insufficiency, and patients who are erratic eaters. The dose varies between 0.5 and 4 mg before meals. Repaglinide results in a 1 to 2 percent decrease in A1c.

Nateglinide, a derivative of phenylalanine, is structurally distinct from both sulfonylureas and repaglinide. It has a quicker onset and shorter duration of action than repaglinide. Nateglinide is available as 60- and 120-mg tablets, taken with each meal. It is effective for lowering postprandial glucose levels. Nateglinide results in a 0.5 to 1.0 percent decrease in A1c. As with repaglinide, the dose of nateglinide should be omitted if a meal is skipped.

α-Glucosidase Inhibitors[67] These agents inhibit α-glucosidases in the brush border of the small intestine, delaying the absorption of complex carbohydrates, and are not systemically absorbed. They are most effective in reducing postprandial blood glucose elevations and can be used as adjunctive therapy with other oral agents. The two available agents are acarbose, given 50 to 100 mg with meals, and miglitol, given 50 mg with meals. The side effects are flatulence and gastrointestinal discomfort. One study noted that the prophylactic use of acarbose delayed the development of T2DM in patients with IGT. These medications result in a 0.5 to 1.0 percent decrease in A1c levels and may be useful as an adjunct to other oral hypoglycemic agents with high-carbohydrate meals.

Amylin[68] Synthetic human amylin, pramlintide, is available as an adjunctive treatment for patients who remain uncontrolled with T1DM or T2DM with mealtime insulin use. Amylin is synthesized by pancreatic β cells and cosecreted with insulin in response to food intake. Pramlintide has been shown to decrease glucose fluctuations, improve long-term glycemic control, reduce mealtime insulin requirements, and reduce body weight. Empiric reductions in mealtime insulin doses are recommended at the initia-

TABLE 90–9

Incretins, Incretin Mimetics, and DPP-4 Inhibitors

AGENT	SITE OF PRODUCTION	PHYSIOLOGICAL ACTION	THERAPEUTIC POTENTIAL
GLP-1	L cells in ileum and proglucagon derived	Stimulates glucose-dependent insulin secretion and B-cell proliferation and cytoprotection; decreases gastric emptying, and postprandial glucagon suppression; increases satiety	Increase insulin secretion in T2DM
GIP	K cells in duodenum and proximal jejunum	Stimulates glucose-dependent insulin secretion and B-cell proliferation and cytoprotection; does not inhibit gastric emptying, glucagon secretion, or food intake	Increase insulin secretion in T2DM
Exenatide (Biretta)	Synthetic peptide	GLP-1 agonist that potentiates insulin secretion, inhibits glucagon secretion, slows gastric emptying and promotes satiety; increases growth of pancreatic cells in animals; not known if similar action exists in humans	Increase insulin secretion in T2DM, promotes weight loss
DDP-4 inhibitors	Synthetic peptides	Delays degradation of GLP-1, extending the action of insulin and suppressing release of glucagon	Increases insulin secretion in T2DM

T2DM, type 2 diabetes mellitus.

tion of pramlintide therapy to decrease the risk of hypoglycemia. Pramlintide is available in vials, but not in pen devices thus far. The package insert states that mixing pramlintide in the same syringe with insulin could change the pharmacokinetics of pramlintide and should not be done, but a study found no clinically significant effect when 30 μg of pramlintide was mixed in the same syringe with various doses of short- and long-acting insulin.

Incretins[69–71] The newest agents available for the treatment of T2DM belong to the class of incretin hormones (Table 90–9). The first pharmacologic agent available in this class is the glucagon-like peptide-1 (GLP-1) analogue, exenatide (see Table 90–9). The two key incretins are GLP-1 and GIP, both secreted in the small intestine by the L cells and K cells, respectively. Both GLP-1 and GIP are decreased in T2DM, and when given pharmacologically to animals, these hormones stimulate β-cell proliferation and can prevent or delay the onset of diabetes.

Exenatide (Byetta) is a synthetic peptide that is a GLP-1 agonist (incretin mimetic). It potentiates insulin secretion and decreases glucagons secretion postprandially. Exenatide delays gastric emptying and promotes satiety resulting in weight loss. Exenatide is FDA approved as an adjunctive treatment for patients with T2DM who have not achieved optimal glycemic control on metformin, or a sulfonylurea, or both. It can cause nausea, diarrhea, and vomiting, especially when the drug is started and hypoglycemia when added to a sulfonylurea. Exenatide is available in a prefilled pen at a dose of 5 or 10 μg bid 1 hour before breakfast and dinner. A once-weekly administered preparation is being developed. The enzyme, dipeptidyl peptidase IV (DPP-IV), rapidly degrades GLP-1 and GIP to inactive forms. DPP-IV inhibitors retard peptide degradation of these incretins allowing therapeutic efficacy. Sitagliptin has been approved by the FDA; vildagliptin (LAF 237) is nearing approval as well. The DPP-IV inhibitors are given orally and are weight neutral.

DIABETIC EDUCATION

Every patient with diabetes should be provided with diabetes education. Recommendations for glucose testing varies among individuals and depends on the current degree of control and whether the patient is taking a medication that would potentially cause hypoglycemia. It is often useful to have patients test at different times on different days, such as in the morning prior to eating ("fasting glucose"), at bedtime, before lunch or dinner, 2 hours after meals, and when the patient feels sick. The patient will want to know the reason for frequent testing because, unlike patients with T1DM, insulin cannot be administered to acutely lower blood glucose levels if they are receiving oral hypoglycemic agents. For patients to adhere to frequent testing regimens, they must understand what foods, exercise, and circumstances will have an impact on blood glucose levels, as well as how they should modify their behaviors for optimal glycemic control (Table 90–10 and Fig. 90–9).

NEWER THERAPIES
Islet Cell Transplants[72]

Whole pancreas transplants have successfully restored insulin secretion in people with advanced diabetes but are usually limited to those who are also undergoing kidney transplantation. In 2000, Shapiro et al. developed the Edmonton Protocol for islet transplantation, which used a larger quantity of islet cells with drugs that were less toxic to the immune system. This method infuses islet cells through a small tube into the portal vein of the liver. Patients whose islet cells fail to continue secreting insulin can be retransplanted. Islet cell transplants are still experimental and are available to people who are willing to participate in a study protocol. Also, only a small percentage of islet cell transplant recipients achieve normal blood glucose levels. It is unclear whether the islet

TABLE 90-10

Guide to Comprehensive Risk Reduction for Patients with Coronary and Other Vascular Disease Who Have Diabetes

RISK INTERVENTION	RECOMMENDATIONS
Smoking Goal: complete cessation	Urge smoking cessation Try NicoDerm patches or Zyban; enroll in smoking cessation program
Blood pressure control Goal: <135/85 mmHg	Initiate lifestyle modification; weight reduction, increased physical activity; alcohol moderation; sodium restriction in all patients with blood pressure >135/85 Add BP medication if BP not below above goal
Lipid management Primary goal: LDL ≤100 mg/dL	Start AHA Step II Diet in all patients: ≤30 percent fat, <7 percent saturated fat, <200 mg/dL cholesterol Assess fasting lipid profile. Immediately start cholesterol-lowering drugs when baseline LDL >130 mg/dL

Secondary goals: HDL >35 mg/DL, TG <200 mg/dL

LDL<100 mg/dL—no drug therapy	LDL 100–129 mg/dL—consider adding drug therapy to diet as follows:	LDL ≥130 mg/dL—add drug therapy as follows:	HDL<35 mg/dL—weight management, physical activity, and smoking cessation

Suggested drug therapy

TG <200 mg/dL	TG 200–400 mg/dL	TG >400 mg/dL
Statin or resin	Statin or fibrate	Consider combined drug therapy (statin + fibrate)

RISK INTERVENTION	RECOMMENDATIONS

Glucose control
  Goal: nearly normal fasting glucose
  Goal: HbA1c ≤1% above normal
	First-step therapy: lifestyle modifications
	Second-step therapy: oral hypoglycemic agents (see algorithm)
	
	Third-step therapy: insulin therapy (see algorithm)

Physical activity Goal: minimum 30 min, 3–4 times a week	Assess risk, preferably with exercise test, to guide prescription Encourage minimum of 30 to 60 min of moderate-intensity activity 3–4 times weekly (walking, jogging, cycling, etc.) supplemented by an increase in daily lifestyle activities (e.g., walking breaks at work, using stairs, household work) Maximum benefit: 5 to 6 h a week Advise medically supervised programs for moderate- to high-risk patients
Weight management	Start intensive dietary therapy and appropriate physical activity, as outlined above, in patients whose body mass index is ≥25 kg/m² Particularly emphasize need for weight loss in patients with hypertension, elevated triglycerides, or elevated glucose levels
Antiplatelet agents/anticoagulants	Start aspirin 325 mg/d if not contraindicated Manage warfarin to INR of 2–3.5 for post-MI patients not able to take aspirin
ACE inhibitors in post-MI patients	Start early post-MI in stable high-risk patients (anterior MI, previous MI, Killip class II [S₃ gallop, rales, radiographic congestive heart failure]) Continue indefinitely for all with LV dysfunction (ejection fraction ≤40%) or symptoms of failure Use as needed to manage blood pressure or symptoms in all other patients
β Blockers	Start in high-risk post-MI patients (arrhythmia, LV dysfunction, inducible ischemia) at 5 to 28 days; continue 6 months minimum; observe usual contraindications; appropriate use of β blockers not contraindicated in patients with diabetes; use as needed to manage angina, rhythm, or blood pressure in all other patients
Estrogen	Observational studies (but not clinical trials) suggest benefit in regard to osteoporosis but not CAD, individualize recommendation consistent with other health risks

AHA, American Heart Association; BP, blood pressure; CAD, coronary heart disease; HDL, high-density lipoproteins; INR, international normalized ratio; LDL, low-density lipoprotein; LV, left-ventricle; MI, myocardial infarction; TG, triglycerides.

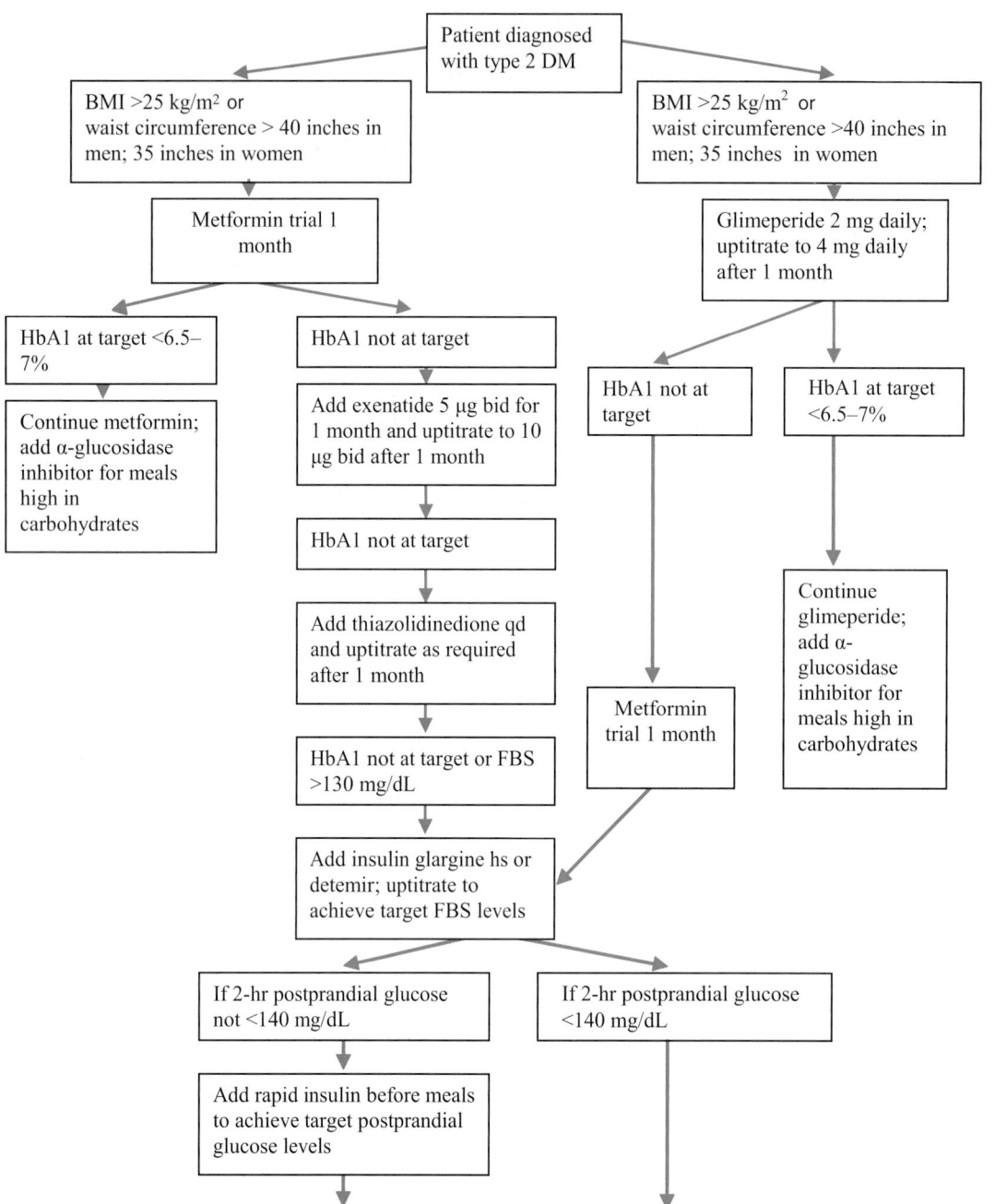

FIGURE 90–9. Algorithm for the management of type 2 diabetes. BMI, body mass index; DM, diabetes mellitus; FBS, fasting blood sugar; HbA1c, glycosylated hemoglobin.

transplants will stop or reverse secondary complication related to diabetes. It is also unclear whether islet cell transplantation will ultimately extend a patient's long-term survival.

Pancreas Transplantation[73]

Ten percent of pancreas transplantations are performed in nonuremic patients with very labile and problematic diabetes. The negative aspect of whole pancreas transplantation is the need for immunosuppression, which increases the risk of viral and fungal infections and some types of malignancy. Recipients of a pancreas

transplant alone have an average 1-year pancreas graft survival rate as high as 78 to 83 percent.

Successful pancreas transplantation will reverse the thickening of glomeruli and tubular basement membranes, and the increase in mesangial volume. Motor sensory and autonomic neuropathy are reversed within 12 to 24 months after transplantation.

Gene Therapy[74]

T1DM is caused by T-cell–mediated destruction of pancreatic insulin-producing β cells. Tian et al. found a novel way to restore central tolerance in nonobese diabetic mice using hematopoietic stem cells retrovirally transduced to express a protective form of the MHC class II β chain. As a result, autoreactive T cells will be killed in the thymus and never get to the pancreatic β cells. Central tolerance refers to mechanisms of tolerance acting in the thymus or bone marrow, in contrast to peripheral tolerance, which occurs in immune cells after they have left the primary lymphoid organs. Preclinical studies must be completed before stem cells can be successfully given to humans with T1DM. Some drugs may be synthesized so that they exert their effect only within the areas of inflammation. One example is an engineered transforming growth factor-1β that can become activated locally within areas of β-cell inflammation.

Stem Cells[75]

Stem cells are a potential source of β cells, which may restore the deficient β-cell mass found in diabetes. This concept would assume the source of β-cell destruction could be abated. Ianus et al. found an extra pancreatic source of pancreatic β cells in bone marrow–derived cells in a mouse model. Pancreatic endocrine and exocrine cells both originate from epithelial cells from early gut endoderm. A second source of stem cells is in the pancreas from progenitor epithelial cells in the pancreatic duct. Much more work is required to translate the potential that stem cells have to produce insulin on demand clinically.

Mechanical Closed-Loop Sensors[76]

Mechanical closed-loop systems are currently under development. They consist of a continuous glucose sensor and an insulin pump that can either infuse insulin subcutaneously or directly into the portal circulation. Such a device would not require immune suppression but would be potentially subject to mechanical breakdowns. In theory, these devices could provide both "basal" and synchronized "bolus" insulin requirements.

[ ] DYSLIPIDEMIA MANAGEMENT

Medical therapy for hyperlipidemia is similar in diabetic and nondiabetic patients, but diabetic patients require special considerations.

The hypertriglyceridemia of diabetes can be treated effectively with fibric acid derivatives without an adverse effect on glucose metabolism. Type 2 diabetic patients experience a reduction in the cardiovascular event rate when treated with gemfibrozil.[77] These drugs cause a 5- to 15-percent drop in LDL levels in patients with normal triglyceride levels, but in patients with hypertriglyceridemia, LDL levels go up. This elevation probably is caused by the catabolism of the atherogenic LDL particle, resulting in less atherogenic LDL.

The recently published FIELD (Fenofibrate Intervention and Event Lowering in Diabetes) trial studied 9795 patients with diabetes at risk for CHD, and showed that fenofibrate was not associated with a difference in the primary composite end point of CHD death or nonfatal MI compared with placebo at 5 years of followup. The treatment effect differences, however, may have been attenuated as a consequence of the more frequent use of statins as lipid-lowering therapy in the placebo arm.[78]

Although nicotinic acid lowers both cholesterol and triglyceride levels while raising HDL levels, it generally is not indicated in diabetes. It has an adverse effect on glycemic control, which results from the induction of insulin resistance. The NIH has initiated a multicenter, randomized study called AIM-HIGH[79] to enroll 3300 subjects with the atherogenic dyslipidemia and established cardiovascular disease to test whether the drug combination of extended-release niacin plus simvastatin is superior to simvastatin alone in delaying time to first major cardiovascular event.

Hydroxymethylglutaryl coenzyme A (HMG-CoA) reductase inhibitors—statins—are another group of drugs that are useful in lowering cholesterol levels in type 2 diabetes patients without having an adverse effect on glycemic control. In a study assessing the effectiveness of a cholesterol-lowering drug for secondary prevention of morbidity and mortality in patients with angina or prior myocardial infarction, simvastatin was found to be more efficacious in diabetic patients than it was in the overall group.[80]

Bile acid resins can decrease the levels of LDL in diabetic patients, but they can cause a significant rise in triglyceride levels, especially if VLDL levels are already high or if the diabetes is poorly controlled. In patients with high levels of both LDL and VLDL, bile acid resins can be used in low doses in combination with fibric acid derivatives.[81]

The NCEP-ATP III reported its executive summary on the treatment of hyperlipidemia.[82] One of the most striking modifications was the raising of patients with diabetes without CHD to the same risk level as someone with CHD. As stated previously, the goal for LDL cholesterol is <100 mg/dL for all those with diabetes regardless of CHD. Patients with a metabolic syndrome were also targeted for aggressive lifestyle modification in this document.

The management of diabetic patients with lipid abnormalities is a unique challenge to the cardiologist. Important evidence from large randomized trials of lipid-lowering therapies is based on subgroup analyses in which diabetic patients represented less than 10 percent of all the patients enrolled; however, more recently studies have been done exclusively in diabetic patients (Table 90–11). The 4S (Scandinavian Simvastatin Survival Study) study enrolled 202 diabetic patients with a prior history of CHD.[80] Although this number was too small, the comparison of simvastatin with a placebo showed almost a 50 percent reduction in coronary events in favor of simvastatin (45 vs. 23 percent; p = not significant). Similar trends were observed in the Cholesterol and Recurrent Events (CARE) Trial, which compared pravastatin with a placebo in secondary prevention. In the CARE trial, the baseline mean LDL concentration in diabetic patients was 136 mg/dL. LDL was reduced 27 percent in the group receiving pravastatin, which translated into a 25 percent reduction in coronary events over 5 years compared with that of the control group.[83] The Heart Protection Study (HPS), with a subgroup of 5963 diabetic patients, showed a 28 percent reduction in total CHD (nonfatal myocardial infarction and CHD death), nonfatal and fatal strokes, coronary and noncoronary revascularizations, and major vascular events (total CHD, total stroke, or revascularizations) with simvastatin therapy.[84] Table 90–5 demonstrates the relatively low number needed to treat (NNT) to prevent a major cardiovascular complication in three of the main lipid-lowering trials. These therapies are the cornerstone of diabetic management in the current era.

TABLE 90–11

Hyperlipidemia

TRIAL	TREATMENT	OUTCOME	EVENTS CONTROL GROUP	EVENTS TREATMENT GROUP	RELATIVE RISK REDUCTION (%)	NUMBER NEEDED TO TREAT	P
4S[158] (secondary prevention) n = 4444; 202 DM	Simvastatin	Death, nonfatal MI, revascularization	44/97 (45%)	24/105 (23%)	49	5	<.05
HPS[a] (primary and secondary prevention) n = 5963 DM	Simvastatin	Coronary death, nonfatal MI	748/n (25.1%)	601/n (20.2%)	20	20	<0.0001
CARE[159] (primary prevention) n = 4159; 586 DM	Pravastatin	Death, nonfatal MI, revascularization	112/304 (37%)	81/282 (29%)	21	12	.05
Helsinki Heart Study[b] (primary prevention) n = 4081 135 DM	Gemfibrozil	Death, nonfatal MI, revascularization	8/76	2/59 (3.4%)	67	14	<.02
CARDS[186] (primary prevention) n = 2838	Atorvastatin	Acute coronary event, stroke, revascularization	(10.5%) 127/ 1410 (9%)	83/1428 (5.8%)	37	31	<0.001
4D[187] (primary and secondary prevention) diabetic pts on dialysis n = 1255	Atorvastatin	CV death, nonfatal MI stroke	243/636 (38%)	226/619 (37%)	8	NA	0.37

CARDS, Collaborative Atorvastatin Diabetes Study; CARE, cholesterol and current events trial; DM, diabetes mellitus patients; 4D, Die Deutsche Diabetes Dialyse study; 4S, Scandinavian Simvastatin Survival Study; HPS, Heart Protection Study; MI, myocardial infarction; n, total number of patients.

[a]Heart Protection Study Collaborative Group. MRC/BHF Heart Protection Study of cholesterol-lowering with simvastatin in 5963 people with diabetes: a randomized placebo-controlled trial. *Lancet* 2003;361:2003–2016.

[b]Koskinen P, Manttari M, Manninen V, et al. Coronary heart disease incidence in NIDDM patients in the Helsinki Heart Study. *Diabetes Care* 1992;15:820–825.

In the trials of statin therapy with hyperlipidemia, the relative benefit appears similar between diabetic patients and nondiabetic patients. The CARDS trial showed that among 2838 diabetic subjects with at least one heart disease risk factor, but without elevated cholesterol levels, randomized to atorvastatin versus placebo and followed up for 3.9 years, statin therapy was associated with a 37 percent reduction in the primary composite end point of CHD death, fatal MI, hospitalized unstable angina, resuscitated cardiac arrest, coronary revascularization, and stroke.[85]

The 4D study (Deutsche Diabetes Dialysis Study) in contrast, studied 1255 diabetic patients on maintenance hemodialysis, but was unable to show a significant reduction in CHD death, on fatal MI and stroke with atorvastatin compared with placebo.[86]

[ ] HYPERTENSION MANAGEMENT

Patients with diabetes should be treated to a systolic blood pressure of 130 mmHg and a diastolic blood pressure of 80 mmHg. Patients with a blood pressure ≥140/90 mmHg should receive drug therapy in addition to lifestyle and behavioral therapy. Multiple drug therapy (two or more agents at proper doses) is generally required to achieve blood pressure targets. All patients with diabetes and hypertension should be treated with a regimen that includes either an ACE inhibitor or an ARB. If one class is not tolerated, the other should be substituted. If needed to achieve blood pressure targets, a thiazide diuretic should be added as second line therapy based upon the ALLHAT (Antihypertensive and Lipid-lowering Treatment to Prevent Heart Attack Trial) results. The use of calcium channel blockers is not considered frontline therapy in the current recommendations. They may be used particularly in patients who are intolerant to other first-line therapies.[87]

Multiple studies have attempted to outline the optimal strategy for the management of hypertension in the diabetic patient (Table 90–12). Compared with nondiabetic subjects, diabetic patients in the SHEP (Systolic Hypertension in the Elderly Program cooperative research group) study experienced a more pronounced benefit from treatment with chlorthalidone (Fig. 90–10).[88]

The UKPDS demonstrated no advantage of captopril over atenolol in reducing macrovascular complications.[89] Clearly, this illustrates the significant role lowering of blood pressure plays in reducing adverse events independent of the agent used. The role of further blood pressure reduction even when high-risk patients such as diabetic patients are in the normal range needs to be delineated further. The Hypertension Optimal Treatment (HOT) study showed that the risk of major cardiovascular events in diabetic patients was halved if they had a target diastolic pressure ≤80 mmHg compared with those with a diastolic pressure ≤90 mmHg (p for trend = .005).[90] There was a lower but still significant decrease in the risk of silent myocardial infarction and approximately a 30 percent risk reduction in the rate of stroke in the ≤80 mmHg group compared with the ≤90 mmHg group.

The Captopril Prevention Projects (CAPPP) trial showed significant lowering of cardiovascular events in hypertensive patients treated with captopril instead of standard therapy with beta-blockers or diuretics (see Table 90–9).[91] Approximately 5 percent of the patients had diabetes in this trial, and in these patients, similar trends in favor of captopril were observed. The use of nondihydropyridine calcium channel blockers is acceptable but not frontline therapy.

The HOPE trial evaluated over 9000 high-risk patients with evidence of vascular disease or diabetes in a randomized trial comparing ramipril with placebo over a 5-year period.[92] A total of 3578 of these patients had diabetes. This study demonstrated a 22 percent reduction in primary cardiovascular end points of death, myocardial infarction, and stroke in favor of ramipril. The beneficial effect of ramipril was observed over all predefined subgroups. Interestingly, there was a 30 percent reduction in the diagnosis of new diabetic patients in the ramipril-treated arm. This result also was observed in the CAPPP study. Ramipril lowered systolic blood pressure by a mean of only 6 mmHg. This would account for only approximately 40 percent of the reduction in the rate of stroke and approximately a 25 percent reduction in the rate of myocardial infarction. Therefore, there is some benefit to using ramipril independent of the blood pressure-lowering effect that accounts for the impressive cardiovascular protective effect. HOPE provides level 1 evidence supporting the frontline use of ACE inhibitors in the treatment of diabetic patients who are at risk for cardiovascular events, regardless of whether they are hypertensive. In the diabetic subgroup, there was even a greater relative risk reduction in primary cardiovascular events (25 percent).

β Blockers are generally underused in diabetic patients despite convincing evidence dating back to the prethrombolytic era that demonstrated both an early and late survival benefit that was more impressive than that observed in the nondiabetic cohort. The GEMINI study[93] demonstrated the superiority of carvedilol and metoprolol in achieving a more stabilized glycemic control and reduced insulin resistance in diabetic patients with hypertension who were taking a renin–angiotensin system blocker. The standard contraindications to β blockers still apply; namely, atrioventricular conduction disturbances and bronchospasm.

TABLE 90–12

Hypertension

TRIAL	TREATMENT	OUTCOME	CONTROL GROUP	TREATMENT GROUP	RELATIVE RISK REDUCTION (%)	P
CAPPP[210] n = 10985; 572 DM[a]	Captopril versus conventional therapy	Cardiac death, nonfatal MI, stroke	263	309	33	.03

CAPPP, Captopril Prevention Projects; DM, diabetes mellitus patients; MI, myocardial infarction.
[a]n, total number of patients.

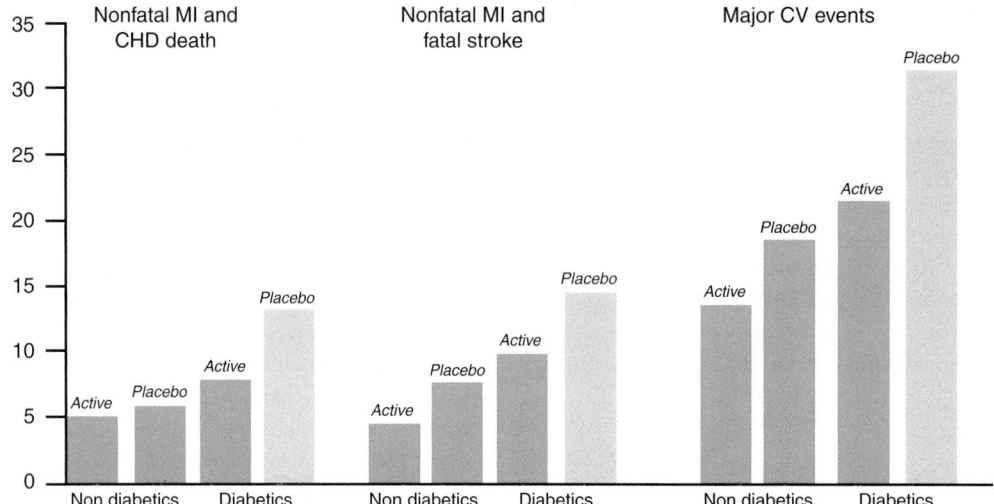

FIGURE 90–10. Five-year rates of nonfatal myocardial infarction (MI) and coronary heart disease (CHD) death, stroke, and major cardiovascular (CV) events by diabetes status and treatment (chlorthalidone vs. placebo) in the Systolic Hypertension in the Elderly Program. *Source: Data from Curb et al.*[208] *and from Furberg CD. Hypertension and diabetes: current issues. Am Heart J 1999;138:5401, with permission.*

The ongoing NIH/NHLBI (National Heart, Lung, and Blood Institute) sponsored ACCORD (Action to Control Cardiovascular Risk in Diabetes) trial shall attempt to establish the definitive role of intensive glycemic control, intensive blood pressure control and intensive lipid management together as a strategy to prevent major cardiovascular events (CHD death, nonfatal MI, or stroke) (Fig. 90–11).[94]

【 】 CORONARY REVASCULARIZATION

The management of diabetic patients with CHD entails both pharmacologic and revascularization strategies. Over the past several years, there have been many advances in the medical management of the diabetic patient with CHD. Aspirin, β blockers, statins, and ACE inhibitors are routinely administered. These agents may provide clinical benefit not only by treating ischemia, but also by stabilizing atherosclerotic plaque and inhibiting endovascular thrombosis, thereby preventing acute coronary events.

Coronary revascularization procedures have become a mainstay of therapy for CHD patients, providing both symptomatic relief and mortality reduction in certain anatomic subsets. Several studies have attempted to rationalize the use of different revascularization techniques by comparing them to medical therapy and to each other in various clinical settings.[95,96] Evidence from well-designed, prospective, randomized clinical trials suggests that surgical revascularization provides a survival advantage compared to medical therapy alone in patients with obstructive left main CHD and in patients with multivessel CHD with decreased left ventricular ejection fraction. In addition, surgical revascularization provides symptomatic improvement compared to medical therapy in patients with multivessel CHD and

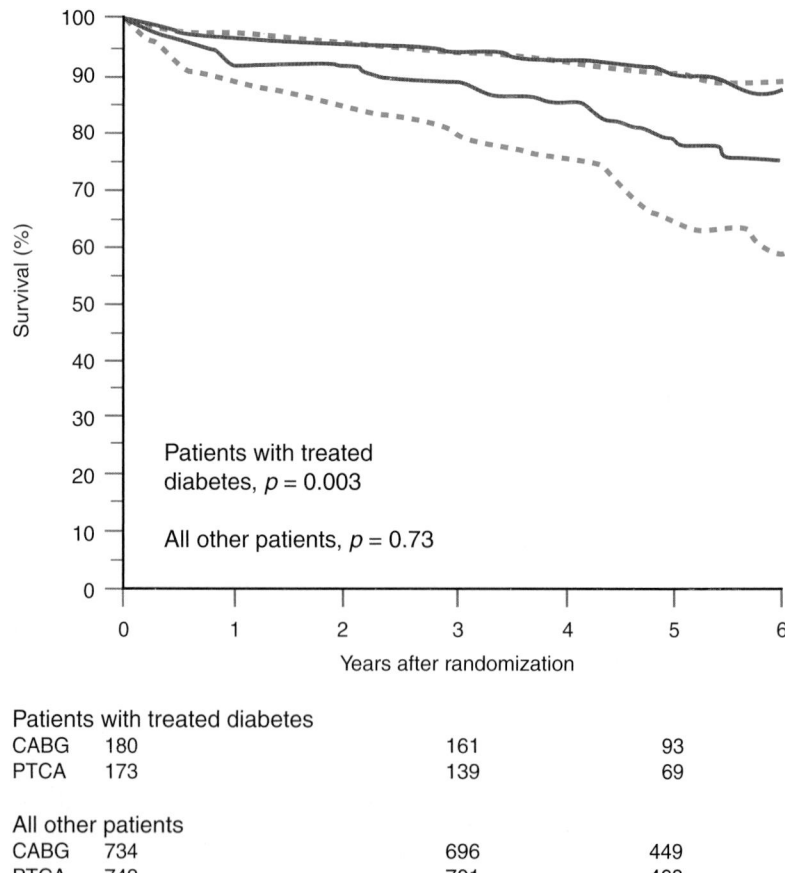

Patients with treated diabetes, *p* = 0.003

All other patients, *p* = 0.73

Patients with treated diabetes
CABG	180	161	93
PTCA	173	139	69

All other patients
CABG	734	696	449
PTCA	742	701	468

FIGURE 90–11. Survival among patients who were being treated for diabetes at baseline (*heavy lines*) and all other patients (*light lines*). Patients assigned to coronary artery bypass graft (CABG) are indicated by *solid lines*, and those assigned to percutaneous transluminal coronary angioplasty (PTCA) by *dashed lines*. The numbers of patients at risk are shown below the graph at baseline, 3 years, and 5 years. *Source: From the Bypass Angioplasty Revascularization Investigation (BARI) Investigators. N Engl J Med 1996;335:217–225 with permission.*

normal left ventricular systolic function.[97] Although none of the preceding studies was specifically conducted in diabetic patients, subgroup analyses of these studies indicated that diabetic patients (1) are at greater risk for cardiac death and ischemic complications than nondiabetic patients and (2) despite a greater surgical risk, diabetic patients indeed may derive a greater long-term benefit from revascularization than do nondiabetic patients (Table 90–13).

Options for Revascularization in Diabetic Patients: Coronary Artery Bypass Graft Surgery versus Balloon Angioplasty

For the past two decades, the question of preferred revascularization strategies—surgery versus percutaneous intervention (PCI), mostly as balloon angioplasty—in patients with obstructive coronary artery disease has led to 13 important randomized clinical trials. There is general consensus that both surgery and percutaneous interventional therapies result in similar death and MI frequency for the overall patient populations evaluated in these studies. The major departure from this observation was highlighted in the BARI trial substudy, wherein there was a clinically meaningful and statistically significant survival benefit favoring coronary artery bypass grafting (CABG) in diabetic patients. Specifically, in the BARI randomized trial (n = 1829 patients in total), diabetics on oral agent or insulin (n = 347) undergoing CABG had a 5-year survival rate of 80.6 percent compared with 65.5 percent in the balloon angioplasty arm.[98] In addition, the CABG group had

fewer repeat revascularization procedures and less angina. Although this was not a prespecified subgroup analysis according to the BARI protocol, these striking results led to the NIH recommending CABG as the revascularization strategy of choice in diabetics with multivessel coronary artery disease.[99] On the other hand, the BARI Registry showed no difference in overall long-term survival between CABG and angioplasty patients.[100] In the Northern New England Cardiovascular Disease Study, diabetic patients demonstrated a significant mortality benefit in favor of CABG.[101] Using Cox proportional hazards methods, the hazards ratio was 1.49 ($p = 0.04$) for PCI versus CABG, after adjusting for differences in baseline characteristics. Patients with three-vessel disease had the greatest benefit from CABG.

Theoretical Explanation for the Advantage of Coronary Artery Bypass Graft Over Balloon Angioplasty in Patients with Treated Diabetes

When compared with balloon angioplasty, CABG provides a greater likelihood of "complete revascularization" because it can treat total chronic occlusions, left main stem stenosis, complex bifurcation disease, and diffuse disease. In diabetic patients, balloon angioplasty is associated with high rates of reocclusion and restenosis, which may provide the mechanistic basis for the BARI randomized trial results. Van Belle et al.[102] reported that in diabetic patients this higher reocclusion and restenosis rate after balloon angioplasty was associated with higher mortality. In addition, balloon angioplasty strategies may be associated with a higher rate of

TABLE 90–13

Coronary Revascularization

TRIAL	TREATMENT	OUTCOME	EVENTS CONTROL GROUP	EVENTS TREATMENT GROUP	RELATIVE RISK REDUCTION (%)	NUMBER NEEDED TO TREAT	P
BARI[237] Multivessel CAD n = 1829[a]	CABG vs. PTCA	Mortality from all cause	PTCA 131/ 915 (14.3%)	CABG 111/ 914 (12.1%)	15.3	45	.19
Diabetics n = 353 CABG 180 PTCA 173	Same	Same	34.5%	19.4%	43.7	7	.003
EPISTENT[273] n = 2399 Diabetics[274] n = 335	Stent + abciximab versus stent + placebo	Death and nonfatal MI at 6 months	Stent + placebo 22/ 173 (12.7%)	Stent + abciximab 10/ 162 (6.2%)	51.2	15	.041
n = 318	Stent + abciximab versus PTCA + abciximab	Same	PTCA + abciximab 12/156 (7.8%)	Stent + abciximab 10/ 162 (6.2%)	20.5	62	.13

BARI, Bypass Angioplasty Revascularization Investigation; CABG, coronary artery bypass graft; CAD, coronary artery disease; EPISTENT, Evaluation of Platelet IIb/IIIa Inhibition of Stenting; MI, myocardial infarction; PTCA, percutaneous transluminal coronary angioplasty.
[a]n, total number of patients.

progression of native coronary atherosclerosis in treated (or non-treated) vessels, or with less protection from ischemic events when new atherosclerotic lesions appear or rupture, both of which may be important factors in long-term morbidity and mortality associated with CHD and diabetes mellitus.[103] In contrast, CABG surgery also has limitations, in particular, higher perioperative morbidity and mortality in diabetic patients than in nondiabetic patients. CABG surgery is more invasive by nature than angioplasty, with general involvement of multiple organs. Therefore, excessive comorbidity may be prohibitive for CABG in certain patient cohorts. Finally, CABG surgery is associated with prolonged rehabilitation and may significantly degrade neuropsychiatric function, either transiently or permanently.[104]

Modern Percutaneous Coronary Intervention Techniques (Before Drug-Eluting Stents)

Bare Metal Stents Many of the technical limitations of balloon angioplasty have been overcome by coronary stent implantation during PCI. Stenting is more predictable, giving a more reliable angiographic result in a wide variety of lesion types and is associated with lower restenosis in many lesion subsets. In the STRESS trial, patients with relatively simple de novo lesions randomized to stent implantation had a 31.6 percent rate of restenosis compared to 42.1 percent in the balloon angioplasty group (p <0.05).[105] Similarly, in the BENESTENT (Belgium Netherlands Stent) trial, patients with relatively simple de novo native lesions randomized to stent implantation had a 22 percent rate of restenosis, compared to 32 percent in the angioplasty group (p = 0.02).[106] This initial clinical benefit shown in the BENESTENT trial was sustained for 5 years during followup assessments. Sustained patency of the target vessel is associated with superior clinical results, including less angina and improved regional left ventricular wall motion, compared to vessels with recurrent restenosis or reocclusion. The advantage of stent implantation versus percutaneous transluminal coronary angioplasty alone with respect to angiographic restenosis and the need for repeat revascularization procedures has also been applicable to diabetic patients. This was evident from subgroup analyses from the stent versus angioplasty trials, as none of the studies was specifically conducted exclusively in diabetic patients. What is clear is that diabetic patients are at significantly higher risk for restenosis after either balloon angioplasty or stent implantation compared to nondiabetic patients, as shown in all previous clinical studies on restenosis.[107]

The introduction and generalized application of stenting with bare metal stents gave promise that by reducing restenosis and preventing repeat revascularizations, diabetic patients may further benefit from a PCI approach, thus achieving parity with CABG as a revascularization strategy. The Arterial Revascularization Trial Study (ARTS) randomized trial compared the clinical outcomes of aggressive stenting versus CABG surgery in 1205 patients with multivessel coronary disease and demonstrated no important differences in death, myocardial infarction, or stroke at 1 year.[108] However, there was still a 14 percent difference, favoring CABG, in 1-year repeat revascularization rates. The diabetes subset from the ARTS revealed that multivessel stenting had a poorer 1-year major adverse cardiac event rate than did CABG (63.4 vs. 84.4 percent; p <0.001); the results were mainly driven by the higher incidence of repeat revascularization after stenting than after CABG (8 percent repeat of CABG and 14.3 percent repeat of PCI vs. no repeat CABG and 3.1 percent repeat PCI, respectively).[109]

A quantitative analysis of the 1-year clinical outcomes of patients in ARTS-I, ERACI, SOS (Stent or Surgery), and MASS (Medicine, Angioplasty, or Surgery Study)-2 trials showed that percutaneous coronary intervention with multiple stenting and coronary artery bypass graft surgery provided a similar degree of protection against death, myocardial infarction, or stroke.[110]

ARTS and other studies (the SOS trial),[108,111] which have indicated a benefit of CABG surgery versus PCI with stenting, have been limited by (1) the absence of an effective antirestenotic agent in conjunction with stent implantation, and (2) the absence of routine use of platelet glycoprotein IIb/IIIa inhibitors, which have been shown to reduce ischemic complications after angioplasty and stent procedures and to potentially reduce mortality after intracoronary stent implantation procedures in diabetic patients.

Advances in Antithrombotic Therapy Before the use of stents and glycoprotein IIb/IIIa antagonists, the rate of restenosis after angioplasty in diabetic patients was shown to be as high as 71 percent. The mechanism of restenosis is believed to be related to neointimal hyperplasia, which is tightly linked to the interplay between platelet-thrombus deposition, various growth factors present after injury, and endothelial dysfunction.[112]

A large body of evidence from prospective, randomized, double-blinded clinical trials supports the use of platelet glycoprotein IIb/IIIa inhibitors during PCI; this evidence was derived mainly from the abciximab clinical trials.[113] A prespecified analysis of clinical outcomes in diabetic patients was included in the EPISTENT (Evaluation of Platelet IIb/IIIa Inhibitors of Stenting) trial (20 percent of total cohort or 491 patients with diabetes).[114] Patients were assigned to a strategy of stent implantation plus placebo, stent implantation plus abciximab, or angioplasty plus abciximab. For diabetic patients who received stent and abciximab, compared to stent alone, there was a >50 percent reduction in death, nonfatal myocardial infarction, and urgent revascularization rate at 6-month followup (Fig. 90–12). In addition, diabetic patients were less likely to require repeat target-vessel revascularization, if they were treated with stent plus abciximab (8.1 percent), compared with either stent plus placebo (16.6 percent; p = 0.02) or angioplasty plus abciximab (18.4 percent; p = 0.008). Thus, it appears that the benefit of abciximab is additive to the benefit of stent implantation in diabetic patients. One-year mortality was also marginally lower with stent plus abciximab versus stent plus placebo (1.2 vs. 4.1 percent; p = 0.11).

Restenosis Prevention Treatments directed at reducing neointimal proliferation and/or geometric arterial remodeling after PCI procedures should reduce the incidence of restenosis after balloon angioplasty and the need for repeat revascularization procedures. Because stent implantation eliminates the remodeling process, the single target to prevent in-stent restenosis is prevention of neointimal hyperplasia. After arterial injury, multiple mitogenic and proliferative factors have been identified as triggers leading to vascular smooth muscle cell (VSMC) activation.[115] The neointimal proliferation process is markedly exaggerated specifically in diabetic patients, as assessed by serial intravascular ultrasound imaging, and

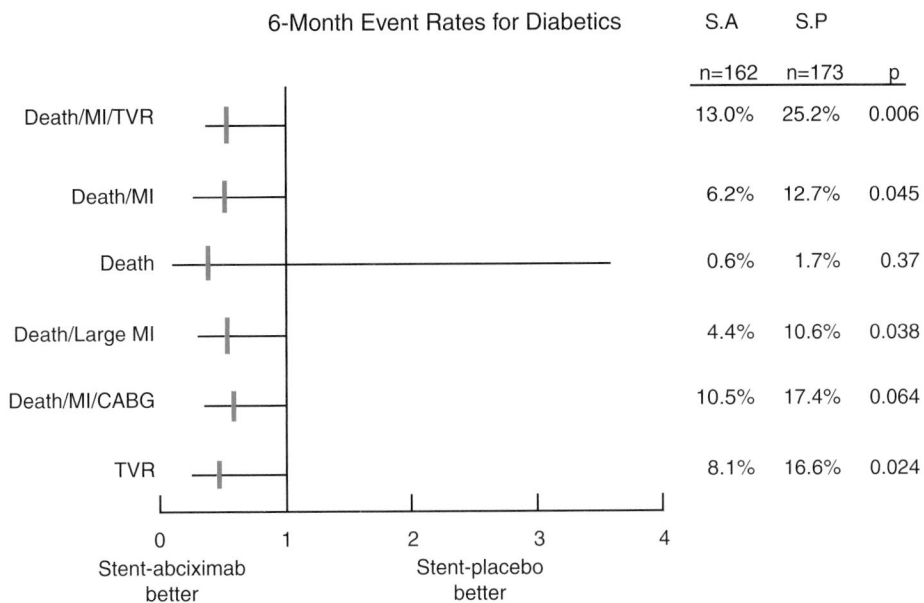

6-Month Event Rates for Diabetics

	S.A	S.P	
	n=162	n=173	p
Death/MI/TVR	13.0%	25.2%	0.006
Death/MI	6.2%	12.7%	0.045
Death	0.6%	1.7%	0.37
Death/Large MI	4.4%	10.6%	0.038
Death/MI/CABG	10.5%	17.4%	0.064
TVR	8.1%	16.6%	0.024

FIGURE 90–12. Absolute percentage of events, 95 percent confidence limits, and point estimates of listed end points for diabetic patients randomized to stenting-abciximab (S-A) or stenting-placebo (S-P). *Source: From Marso SP, Lincoff AM, Ellis SG, et al. Optimizing the percutaneous interventional outcomes for patients with diabetes mellitus: results of the EPISTENT (Evaluation of Platelet IIb/IIIa Inhibitor for Stenting Trial) diabetic substudy. Circulation 1999;100:2477–2484, with permission.*

diabetes mellitus has been identified as an independent predictor of recurrent in-stent restenosis.[116] In the past, pharmacologic therapies for the prevention of restenosis have been generally unsuccessful. Although numerous animal studies have identified agents that can reduce intimal hyperplasia associated with balloon angioplasty or after stent implantation, clinical results using systemic agents or after local catheter administration have been disappointing. A possible reason for the repeated failure is that agents given systemically or via local catheters cannot reach sufficient therapeutic levels at the injured site within the artery to inhibit significantly the localized restenotic process without producing serious systemic side effects.[117]

Clinical studies have demonstrated that intravascular treatment with catheter-based ionizing radiation (intravascular brachytherapy) is efficacious in reducing in-stent restenosis, but does not prevent restenosis as an adjunct to stent implantation in de novo lesions.[118]

Multiple randomized trials, meta-analysis of trials, and epidemiologic studies confirm the superiority of drug-eluting stents over bare metal stents in reducing restenosis and late repeat revascularization. There has also been some preliminary data forthcoming on the use of thiazolidinediones in reducing neointimal volume and restenosis rates.[119]

Drug-Eluting Stents

Sustained local delivery of an antiproliferative therapeutic agent will provide higher tissue concentrations than will systemic administration. The combination of mechanical scaffolding provided by stent implantation (to reverse arterial remodeling) with the sustained high-dose local drug delivery (via the stent) of an agent that effectively inhibits neointimal hyperplasia could provide a unique method to improve target lesion patency after PCI.

This delicate balance incorporating a highly deliverable stent platform, a drug carrier vehicle (such as a nonreactive encapsulating polymer), and an effective antiproliferative agent has been achieved with the very effective clinical application of the drug-eluting stents, predominantly sirolimus-eluting stents (SES) and paclitaxel-eluting stents (PES).[120]

Multiple other drug-eluting stents have entered experimental animal or clinical evaluations. Therapeutic agents currently undergoing assessment include taxane derivatives, actinomycin D, batimastat, tacrolimus, dexamethasone, and c-myc antisense. Drug delivery from the stent can be accomplished by a variety of means, including direct application, using either nonerodable or erodable polymers (which encapsulate the stent), phosphorylcholine coatings, and ceramic coatings. Newer delivery platforms and stent strut structures also are under investigation.[121]

Clinical Studies with Drug-Eluting Stents The advent of drug-eluting stents (DESs) has revolutionized the field of percutaneous interventions, especially in the diabetic patient. While DESs have not had a major impact on hard cardiovascular end points such as death and MI, they have been successful in reducing angiographic restenosis and the rates of target-vessel revascularizations. A recent meta-analysis of DES studies showed that for patients with diabetes the number needed to treat to reduce major adverse cardiac events were four patients for the SES and six patients for the PES.[122] Table 90–14 shows the data for the diabetic patient subset in the major interventional DES trials with SES and DES.

Sirolimus- versus Paclitaxel-Eluting Stents in Diabetic Patients With the superiority of DESs being established in the diabetic population, the next challenge has become the choice of which DES delivers better results—SES or PES. Few studies have compared these major DESs head to head. The ISAR-DIABETES[123] study enrolled 250 patients with diabetes and coronary disease and randomized patients in a 1:1 ratio to SES and PES. The in-segment late luminal loss was 0.24 mm greater in the PES group compared to the SES group ($p = 0.002$). Angiographic restenosis was identified in 16.5 percent of the PES group versus in 6.9 percent in the SES group ($p = 0.03$). Also the target lesion revascularization trended toward being higher in the PES group at 12 percent versus 6.4 percent in the SES group ($p = 0.13$). However, a meta-analysis of 10 DES trials[124] failed to show a difference in any of the above-mentioned end points in diabetic patients. A recent analysis of a registry of 1320 diabetic patients treated with DESs also concluded that SES and PES are associated with similar rates of revascularization, MACE and stent thrombosis.[125] The question of which DES is superior for the treatment of diabetic patients remains unclear.

TABLE 90–14

Incidence Rate Ratios from Trials of Sirolimus- and Paclitaxel-Eluting Stents and Ratio of Incidence Rate Ratios Comparing Sirolimus with Paclitaxel in Patients with Diabetes

STUDY	IRR (95% CONFIDENCE INTERVAL)		
	IN-STENT RESTENOSIS	TLR	MACE
Sirolimus trials			
SIRIUS (2003)	0.17 (0.08 to 0.37)	0.31 (0.15 to 0.64)	0.37 (0.19 to 0.70)
E-SIRIUS (2003)	0.13 (0.03 to 0.57)	0.21 (0.05 to 0.91)	0.27 (0.08 to 0.94)
C-SIRIUS (2004)	0.06 (0.003 to 1.02)	1.00 (0.06 to 15.99)	1.00 (0.06 to 15.99)
DIABETES (2005)	0.15 (0.06 to 0.39)	0.24 (0.10 to 0.59)	0.31 (0.15 to 0.66)
RAVEL (2002)	0.06 (0.003 to 0.97)	0.07 (0.004 to 1.19)	0.22 (0.05 to 0.98)
SES-SMART (2004)	NA	NA	NA
Combined IRR	0.15 (0.09 to 0.25)	0.27 (0.16 to 0.45)	0.33 (0.21 to 0.51)
Heterogeneity[a]	(0.0 percent, p, 0.92)	(0.0 percent, p, 0.73)	(0.0 percent, p, 0.89)
Paclitaxel trials			
TAXUS I (2003)	NA	0 events	0 events
TAXUS II (2003)	NA	0.16 (0.02 to 1.25)	NA
TAXUS IV (2004)	0.16 (0.05 to 0.48)	0.36 (0.19 to 0.70)	NA
TAXUS VI (2005)	0.20 (0.05 to 0.68)	0.20 (0.04 to 0.90)	0.55 (0.21 to 1.43)
Combined IRR	0.18 (0.08 to 0.40)	0.31 (0.18 to 0.56)	0.55 (0.21 to 1.43)
Heterogeneity[a]	0.0 percent, p, 0.80	0.0 percent, p, 0.62	NA
RIRR (sirolimus vs. paclitaxel)	0.82 (0.31 to 2.18) p, 0.694	0.86 (0.40 to 1.86) p, 0.703	0.60 (0.21 to 1.71) p, 0.336

IRR, incidence rate ratio; RIRR, ratio of incidence rate ratio.
[a]I^2, test of heterogeneity.
SOURCE: Stettler C, Allemann S, Egger M, Windecker S, Meier B, Diem P. Efficacy of drug eluting stents in patients with and without diabetes mellitus: indirect comparison of controlled trials. Heart 2006 May; 92(5):650–657.

Bypass Outcomes

CABG with use of an internal mammary artery (IMA) as a bypass conduit has been shown to be more advantageous to CABG with saphenous vein bypass conduits because of greater long-term durability of the arterial conduit.[126] The internal mammary artery is significantly stenosed or occluded in approximately 8 percent of patients early after CABG surgery but has 90 to 95 percent long-term patency; sustained patency of the IMA conduit also is associated with prolonged patient survival. Bypass conduits attrition rates are higher in diabetic patients than they are in nondiabetic patients. Bilateral IMA grafting provides even further survival advantage than left IMA plus saphenous vein grafts; these data have led to an increased application of CABG with total arterial revascularization.[127] Nonetheless, the use of bilateral IMA grafting in diabetic patients remains controversial because of the potentially increased risk for sternal wound infection.[128]

Neurologic dysfunction remains a devastating complication of CABG, especially in diabetics. Diabetes is the single greatest predictor of mortality during ischemic stroke and diabetes is an important risk factor for stroke during coronary artery bypass surgery.[129] Analysis of the Arterial Revascularization Study Group demonstrated a 6.3 percent incidence of stroke in diabetic patients undergoing coronary bypass surgery compared to 1.2 percent in nondiabetic patients.[130] Stent revascularization showed no increased rate of stroke complications, with an incidence of 1.8 percent in diabetics and 1.4 percent in nondiabetics. Therefore, if drug-eluting stenting for diabetic patients with multivessel coronary artery disease proves to be equivalent to coronary bypass surgery in achieving successful revascularization of the coronary arteries, a significant advantage for stenting may be a reduction in stroke morbidity. Measures that may decrease the risk of stroke after CABG include carotid artery stenosis screening, the intraoperative assessment of the ascending aorta with epiaortic ultrasonography, in the case of conventional CABG, the use of a soft-flow aortic cannula, precise management of cardiopulmonary bypass, and, most importantly, reconstruction of distal and proximal anastomosis using a single cross-clamp technique.[131]

Coronary artery bypass grafting using a median sternotomy approach on a beating heart (off-pump CABG) is now a well-accepted alternative for myocardial revascularization and offers the potential for lower perioperative ischemic and neurologic complications than conventional CABG. Clinical reports have particularly emphasized the benefit of off-pump CABG in the elderly and in patients with associated comorbidities. Recently, a broader application of off-pump CABG has been observed in patients with multivessel CHD because of the development of new mechanical stabilizers and positioning devices, resulting in reported lower rates of perioperative mortality and major complications.[132]

Multivessel Stenting with DESs versus Coronary Artery Bypass Graft in Patients with Treated Diabetes Mellitus

Inadequate data exists for us to be able to evaluate the definitive impact of DES for diabetic patients on long-term outcomes. Percutaneous coronary intervention using DES is being compared to contemporary CABG in multivessel disease patients with diabetes against the background of aggressive medical therapy in the ongoing NIH-NHLBI-sponsored Future Revascularization Evaluation in Patients With Diabetes Mellitus: Optimal Management of Multivessel Disease (FREEDOM) trial.[133] The CARDIA[134] and VA-CARDS[135] trials are smaller trials addressing the question of stenting with DES compared to CABG in diabetic patients.

DIABETES PREVENTION

Increasing evidence suggests that an atherogenic prediabetic state exists prior to the development of diabetes. In the San Antonio Heart Study, patients converting to overt diabetes had significantly higher blood pressure, body mass index, waist circumference, and triglyceride levels, and lower HDL cholesterol levels at baseline compared to nonconvertors.[136]

Investigators from Finland conducted a randomized trial of 522 middle-aged, overweight subjects with impaired glucose tolerance (350 women, mean age: 55 years).[137] Patients were randomized to a control group or an intervention group that consisted of individualized counseling aimed at reducing weight, total intake of fat, and intake of saturated fat and increasing intake of fiber and physical activity. Over 4 years of followup, the cumulative incidence of diabetes was 11 percent in the intervention group and 23 percent in the control group (58 percent reduction; $p < 0.001$; Fig. 90–13). The authors concluded that type 2 diabetes indeed could be prevented with an intensive lifestyle modification program (Table 90–15).

The Diabetes Prevention Program evaluated more than 3000 nondiabetic subjects with impaired fasting, and postglucose loading plasma glucose levels showed that when compared to placebo, a lifestyle intervention reduced the incidence of developing diabetes by 58 percent (95 percent confidence interval: 48 to 66 percent, and NNT of 7) whereas metformin reduced the incidence by 31 percent (95 percent confidence interval: 17 to 43 percent, and NNT of 14).[138] When compared head to head, the intervention group fared better than did the metformin group.

Evidence from large clinical trials has emerged to suggest that treatments that modify cardiovascular risk may also reduce the incidence of developing type 2 diabetes (Table 90–16).

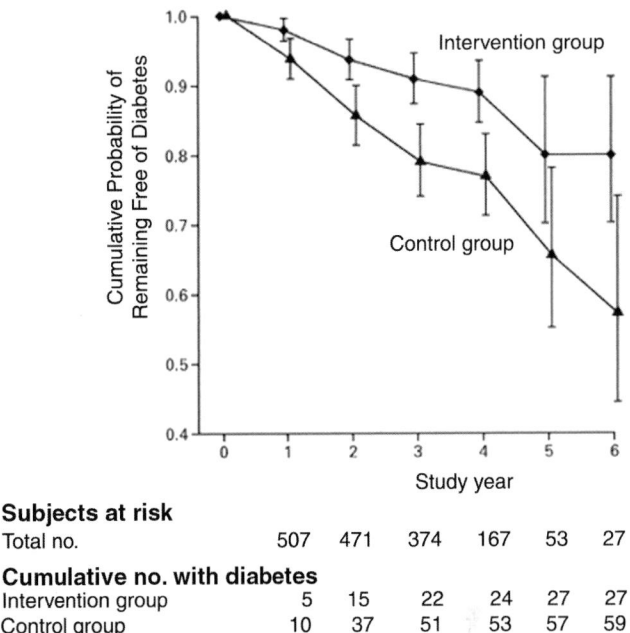

FIGURE 90–13. Finnish Trial of Lifestyle Modification in Preventing Diabetes. Proportion of subjects without diabetes during the trial. *Source: From Tuomilehto J, Lindstrom J, Eriksson JG, et al. Prevention of type 2 diabetes mellitus by changes in lifestyle among subjects with impaired glucose tolerance. N Engl J Med 2001;344:1343–1350, with permission.*

Subjects at risk						
Total no.	507	471	374	167	53	27
Cumulative no. with diabetes						
Intervention group	5	15	22	24	27	27
Control group	10	37	51	53	57	59

The WOSCOPS investigators reported on 5974 patients who were not diabetic or glucose intolerant on entry into the pravastatin primary prevention study. Therapy with pravastatin as compared with placebo was associated with a 30 percent relative reduction risk for developing overt type diabetes.[139]

Treatment with ramipril in nondiabetic patients with known vascular disease in the HOPE trial was associated with a 34 percent reduction in the development of type 2 diabetes.[140] This effect may be mediated by a potential antiinflammatory effect as well as by improved insulin sensitivity.

The DREAM (Diabetes Reduction Assessment with Ramipril and Rosiglitazone Medication) trial has randomized 5269 patients with either IGT or impaired fasting glucose (IFG) in a factorial design to ramipril and/or rosiglitazone to determine whether such therapy prevents the onset of new type 2 diabetes. Rosiglitazone therapy led to a highly significant reduction in incident diabetes (hazard ration 0.04, 95 percent CI 0.35–0.46; $p < 0.0001$), while ramipril failed to show a reduction in incident diabetes compared to placebo over 3 years of followup (hazard ration 0.91; 95 percent CI 0.81–1.03; $p = 0.15$). This study was not powered to look at cardiovascular outcomes.[148,149]

The NAVIGATOR (Nateglinide and Valsartan in Impaired Glucose Tolerance Outcomes Research) trial, the largest diabetes prevention clinical trial to date, aims to determine whether long-term administration of nateglinide or valsartan reduces

TABLE 90–15

Success in Achieving the Goals of the Intervention by 1 Year, According to Treatment Group[a]

GROUP	INTERVENTION GROUP (%)	CONTROL GROUP (%)	P VALUE[b]
Weight reduction.5%	43	13	0.001
Fat intake <30% of energy intake	47	26	0.001
Saturated-fat intake <10% of energy intake	26	11	0.001
Final intake >15 g/1000 kcal	25	12	0.001
Exercise >4 h/week[c]	86	71	0.001

[a]Nutrient intakes were calculated from 3-day food records.
[b]P values were determined by the chi-square test for the difference between the groups.
[c]Exercise frequency was reported by the subjects who chose one of the four categories. The goal identified here was a frequency category 2 or higher.

TABLE 90–16

Prevention Study

TRIAL	TREATMENT	OUTCOME	EVENTS CONTROL GROUP	EVENTS TREATMENT GROUP	RELATIVE RISK REDUCTION (%)	NUMBER NEEDED TO TREAT	P
HOPE[202] 3578 DM $n = 9297^a$	Ramipril (10 mg qd)	Cardiac death, nonfatal MI, stroke	351/1769 (19.8%)	277/1808 (15.3%)	25	22	.0004

DM, diabetes mellitus patients; HOPE, Heart Outcomes Prevention Evaluation Study; MI, myocardial infarction.
^{a}n, total number of patients

or delays the development of type 2 diabetes and cardiovascular disease in 9150 subjects who have IGT and are at high cardiovascular risk.[142]

The new endocannabinoid receptor inhibitor drug Rimonabant will be tested as a diabetes prevention agent in patients with IGT or IFG in the RAPSODI study initiated in 2006.[143]

EARLY DETECTION OF CARDIOVASCULAR DISEASE IN THE DIABETIC PATIENT

The significant increase in major micro- and macrovascular complications makes it important to begin screening for diabetes at an age younger than 45 years.[144] It has become necessary to implement aggressive screening strategies to be able to identify populations at the highest risk of developing diabetes.[145]

Current measures of cardiovascular surveillance for coronary artery disease in asymptomatic diabetic patients focus on routine stress testing in accordance with the American College of Cardiology/American Heart Association (ACC/AHA) guidelines (Table 90–17).[146] Exercise testing in diabetic patients is more likely to be accurate when combined with echocardiography or radionuclide imaging. Diabetic patients are less likely to have an appropriate blood pressure and heart rate response to exercise and less likely to experience any pain corresponding to ST-segment changes caused in part by autonomic dysfunction. The AHA recommends that the finding of subclinical coronary artery disease should prompt clinicians to initiate more aggressive preventative measures. The DIAD (Detection of Ischemia in Asymptomatic Diabetics) study has shown that the prevalence of silent ischemia in the diabetic population without known or suspected coro-

TABLE 90–17

Detection of Clinical and Subclinical Cardiovascular Disease in Diabetic Patients

A. Stress testing for coronary heart disease
   Consult AHA guidelines for exercise treadmill testing
   Considerations for testing in diabetic patients
      Blunting of heart rate and blood pressure responses
      Painless ST-segment depression common in diabetic patients (autonomic neuropathy)
      Diagnostic specificity of ST-segment depression may be reduced (previous silent myocardial infarction, etc.)
      Exercise or pharmacologic testing (^{99m}Tc) perfusion scintography favorable for exercise testing in diabetic patients
      Ambulatory ECG monitoring may be helpful in special instances in diabetic patients to diagnose silent ischemia, but not routinely
B. Noninvasive evaluation of cardiac function
   Echocardiography (Doppler) and radionuclide ventriculography issues in diabetic patients
      Diastolic dysfunction commonly and often precedes systolic dysfunction
      Left ventricular wall motion abnormalities suggest diabetic cardiomyopathy
C. Evaluation of autonomic dysfunction
   In bedside evaluation two or more of these tests are abnormal
      Resting heart rate (supine), 100 beats/min
      Excess diastolic blood pressure response to handgrip exercise
      Abnormal expiratory-to-inspiratory RR-interval ratio
      Postural hypotension
   Significance of autonomic dysfunction in diabetic patients
      50% 5-year mortality
      Sudden death common; consider electrophysiologic study
      Greater complications after elective surgery
      Increased danger with general anesthesia
D. Diagnosis of subclinical cardiovascular disease
   History: symptoms of claudication, angina, dyspnea on exertion, cerebrovascular disease
   Physical examination: routine checkup with evaluation of carotid and femoral bruits, peripheral arterial pulses, ratio of ankle-to-brachial artery systolic blood pressure (marker of subclinical peripheral vascular disease)
   Laboratory: urinary creatinine to albumin ratio (See Table 90–1)
   ECG: left ventricular hypertrophy a strong predictor of CAD morbidity and mortality
   Electron-beam CT: coronary calcium score highly correlated with total coronary atherosclerosis burden
   Carotid ultrasound: detects subclinical carotid atherosclerosis.

AHA, American Heart Association; CAD, coronary heart disease.

nary artery disease is 22 percent.[147] Whether the detection of silent ischemia will result in a reduction in cardiovascular events in this study will be reported in 2007.

FUTURE DIRECTIONS

On the clinical front, there are still many challenges in the prevention and management of diabetic cardiovascular complications. Glycemic control appears to be the mainstay of long-term diabetes management. Thus, development of better therapies and devices (e.g., closed-loop pumps, islet and pancreatic transplants) for achieving and maintaining HbA1c at not only <7 percent, but in the normal range of <6 percent, will be a primary goal in the next decade. The emphasis will also be on getting to appropriate targets faster. Clarification of the best glycemic control strategy in preventing CHD is required in order to validate the hypothesis that an insulin-sensitization strategy may be more cardioprotective than an insulin-providing strategy. The advent of drug-eluting stents during coronary percutaneous revascularization has led to a reevaluation of the need for coronary bypass surgery in multivessel disease. Finally, the role of gene therapy in the management of diabetic atherosclerotic vascular disease needs to be addressed within the context of all other advances.

REFERENCES

1. *Diabetes Atlas*, 2nd ed. International Diabetes Federation, Belgium, 2003.
2. Gu K, Cowie CC, Harris MI. Diabetes and decline in heart disease mortality in US adults. *JAMA* 1999;281:1291–1297.
3. Waller BF, Palumbo PJ, Lie JT, Roberts WC. Status of the coronary arteries at necropsy in diabetes mellitus after age 30 years: analysis of 229 diabetic patients with and without evidence of coronary heart disease and comparison to 183 control subjects. *Am J Med* 1980;69:498–506.
4. Nigro J, Osman N, Dart AM, Little PJ. Insulin resistance and atherosclerosis. *Endocr Rev* 2006;27(3):242–259.
5. Kim JA, Montagnani M, Koh KK, Quon MJ. Reciprocal relationships between insulin resistance and endothelial dysfunction: molecular and pathophysiological mechanisms. *Circulation* 2006;113(15):1888–1904.
6. Imai Y, Clemmons DR Roles of phosphatidylinositol 3-kinase and mitogen-activated protein kinase pathways in stimulation of vascular smooth muscle cell migration and deoxyribonucleic acid synthesis by insulin-like growth factor-I. *Endocrinology* 1999;140:4228–4235.
7. Sampson MJ, Davies IR, Braschi S, Ivory K, Hughes DA. Increased expression of a scavenger receptor (CD36) in monocytes from subjects with type 2 diabetes. *Atherosclerosis* 2003;167:129–113.
8. Gray RS, Fabsitz RR, Cowan LD, et al. Risk factor clustering in the insulin resistance syndrome: the Strong Heart Study. *Am J Epidemiol* 1998;148:869–878.
9. Hanley AJ, Williams K, Stern MP, Haffner SM. Homeostasis model assessment of insulin resistance in relation to the incidence of cardiovascular disease: the San Antonio Heart Study. *Diabetes Care* 2002;25(7):1177–1184.
10. Wei M, Gaskill SP, Haffner SM, Stern MP. Effects of diabetes and level of glycemia on all-cause and cardiovascular mortality. The San Antonio Heart Study. *Diabetes Care* 1998;21(7):1167–1172.
11. UK Prospective Diabetes Study Group. Effect of intensive blood glucose control with metformin on complications in overweight patients with type-2 diabetes. UKPDS 34. *Lancet* 1998;352:854–865.
12. Dormandy JA, Charbonnel B, Eckland DJ, et al. PROactive investigators. Secondary prevention of macrovascular events in patients with type 2 diabetes in the PROactive Study (PROspective pioglitAzone Clinical Trial In macroVascular Events): a randomised controlled trial. *Lancet* 2005;366(9493):1279–1289.
13. The DECODE study group. Glucose tolerance and mortality: comparison of WHO and American Diabetes Association diagnostic criteria. *Lancet* 1999;354:617–621.
14. Lyons TJ. Glycation and oxidation: a role in the pathogenesis of atherosclerosis. *Am J Cardiol* 1993;71:26B–31B.
15. Austin MA, Mykkanen L, Kuusisto J, et al. Prospective study of small LDLs as a risk factor for non-insulin-dependent diabetes mellitus in elderly men and women. *Circulation* 1995;92:1770–1778.
16. Goldschmid MG, Barrett-Connor E, Edelstein SL, et al. Dyslipidemia and ischemic heart disease mortality among men and women with diabetes. *Circulation* 1994;89:991–997.
17. Laasko M, Lehto S, Penttila I, Pyorala K. Lipids and lipoproteins predicting coronary heart disease mortality and morbidity in patients with non–insulin-dependent diabetes. *Circulation* 1993;88:1421–1430.
18. Ginsberg HN. Diabetic dyslipidemia: basic mechanisms underlying the common hypertriglyceridemia and low HDL cholesterol levels. *Diabetes* 1996;45(Suppl):27S–30S.
19. American Diabetes Association. Standards of medical care in diabetes—2006. *Diabetes Care* 2006;29(Suppl 1):S4–S42.
20. Executive Summary of The Third Report of The National Cholesterol Education Program (NCEP) Expert Panel on Detection, Evaluation, and Treatment of High Blood Cholesterol in Adults (Adult Treatment Panel III). *JAMA* 2001;285:2486–2497.
21. Alberti KG, Zimmet PZ for the WHO Consultation. Definition, diagnosis and classification of diabetes mellitus and its complications. Part I, diagnosis and classification of diabetes mellitus. Provisional report of a WHO consultation. *Diabet Med* 1998;15:539–553.
22. International Diabetes Federation. *The IDF Consensus Worldwide Definition of the Metabolic Syndrome 2005*. Available at: www.idf.org/webdata/docs/IDF_metasyndrome_definition.pdf.
23. Bloomgarden ZT. American Association of Clinical Endocrinologists (AACE) consensus conference on the insulin resistance syndrome: 25–26 August 2002 Washington, DC. *Diabetes Care* 2003;26(4):1297–1303.
24. Isomaa B, Almgren P, Tuomi T, et al. Cardiovascular morbidity and mortality associated with the metabolic syndrome. *Diabetes Care* 2001;24(4):683–689.
25. Ford ES, Giles WH, Dietz WH. Prevalence of the metabolic syndrome among US adults: findings from the third National Health and Nutrition Examination Survey. *JAMA* 2002;287(3):356–359.
26. Rutter MK, Meigs JB, Sullivan LM, D'Agostino RB Sr, Wilson PW. Insulin resistance, the metabolic syndrome, and incident cardiovascular events in the Framingham Offspring Study. *Diabetes* 2005;54(11):3252–3257.
27. Resnick HE, Jones K, Ruotolo G, et al. Strong Heart Study. Insulin resistance, the metabolic syndrome, and risk of incident cardiovascular disease in nondiabetic American Indians: the Strong Heart Study. *Diabetes Care* 2003;26(3):861–867.
28. Klein BE, Klein R, Lee KE. Components of the metabolic syndrome and risk of cardiovascular disease and diabetes in Beaver Dam. *Diabetes Care* 2002;25(10):1790–1794.
29. Sattar N, Gaw A, Scherbakova O, Ford I, et al. Metabolic syndrome with and without C-reactive protein as a predictor of coronary heart disease and diabetes in the West of Scotland Coronary Prevention Study. *Circulation* 2003;108(4):414–419.
30. Lakka HM, Laaksonen DE, Lakka TA, et al. The metabolic syndrome and total and cardiovascular disease mortality in middle-aged men. *JAMA* 2002;288(21):2709–2716.
31. Girman CJ, Rhodes T, Mercuri M et al. 4S Group and the AFCAPS/TexCAPS Research Group. The metabolic syndrome and risk of major coronary events in the Scandinavian Simvastatin Survival Study (4S) and the Air Force/Texas Coronary Atherosclerosis Prevention Study (AFCAPS/TexCAPS). *Am J Cardiol* 2004;93(2):136–141.
32. Cooper ME. Pathogenesis, prevention, and treatment of diabetic nephropathy. *Lancet* 1998;352:213–219.
33. Lewis EJ, Hunsicker LG, Bain RP, Rohde RD. The effect of angiotensin-converting-enzyme inhibition on diabetic nephropathy: The Collaborative Study Group. *N Engl J Med* 1993;329:1456–1462.
34. Brenner BM, Cooper ME, de Zeeuw D, et al. Effects of losartan on renal and cardiovascular outcomes in patients with type 2 diabetes and nephropathy. *N Engl J Med* 2001;345:861–869.
35. Fong DS, Aiello L, Gardner TW, et al. Retinopathy in diabetes. *Diabetes Care* 2004;27 Suppl 1:S84–S87.
36. Barrett-Connor E, Cohn B, Wingard D, Edelstein SL. Why is diabetes mellitus a stronger risk factor for fatal ischemic heart disease in women than in men? The Rancho Bernardo Study. *JAMA* 1991;256:627–631.
37. Nathan DM. Long-term complications of diabetes mellitus. *N Engl J Med* 1993;328:1676–1685.

38. American Diabetes Association. Consensus statement: role of cardiovascular risk factors in prevention and treatment of macrovascular disease in diabetes. *Diabetes Care* 1993;16:72–78.

39. Zavaroni I, Bonora E, Pagliara M, et al. Risk factors for coronary artery disease in healthy persons with hyperinsulinemia and normal glucose tolerance. *N Engl J Med* 1989;320:702–706.

40. Despres J-P, Lamarche B, Mauriege P, et al. Hyperinsulinemia is an independent risk factor for ischemic heart disease. *N Engl J Med* 1996;334:952–957.

41. Ferrara A, Barrett-Connor E, Edelstein SL. Hyperinsulinemia does not increase the risk of fatal cardiovascular disease in elderly men and women without diabetes: the Rancho Bernardo Study, 1984 to 1991. *Am J Epidemiol* 1994;140:857–869.

42. Gerstein HC, Yusuf S. Dysglycemia and risk of cardiovascular disease. *Lancet* 1996;347:949–950.

43. Stone PH, Muller JE, Hartwell T, et al. The effect of diabetes mellitus on prognosis and serial left ventricular function after acute myocardial infarction: contribution of both coronary disease and left ventricular dysfunction to the adverse prognosis. *J Am Coll Cardiol* 1989;14:49–57.

44. Fibrinolytic Therapy Trialists (FTT) Collaborative Group. Indications for fibrinolytic therapy in suspected acute myocardial infarction: collaborative overview of early mortality and major morbidity results from all randomized trials of more than 1000 patients. *Lancet* 1994;343:311–322.

45. Malmberg K, for the DIGAMI Study Group. Prospective randomised study of intensive insulin treatment on long-term survival after acute myocardial infarction in patients with diabetes mellitus. *BMJ* 1997;314:1512–1515.

46. Malmberg K, Ryden L, Wedel H, et al. DIGAMI 2 Investigators. Intense metabolic control by means of insulin in patients with diabetes mellitus and acute myocardial infarction (DIGAMI 2): effects on mortality and morbidity. *Eur Heart J* 2005;26(7):650–661.

47. Jonas M, Reicher-Reiss H, Boyko V, et al. Usefulness of beta-blocker therapy in patients with non-insulin-dependent diabetes mellitus and coronary heart disease. *Am J Cardiol* 1996;77:1273–1277.

48. Jain A, Avendaro G, Dharamsey S, et al. Left ventricular diastolic dysfunction in hypertension and role of plasma glucose and insulin: comparison with diabetic heart. *Circulation* 1996;93:1396–1402.

49. Palmieri V, Bella JN, Arnett DK, et al. Effect of type 2 diabetes mellitus on left ventricular geometry and systolic function in hypertensive subjects. *Circulation* 2001;103:102–107.

50. Fang ZY, Yuda S, Anderson V, et al. Echocardiographic detection of early diabetic myocardial disease. *J Am Coll Cardiol* 2003;41:611–617.

51. Arnold JM, Yusuf S, Young J, et al. Prevention of heart failure in patients in the Heart Outcomes Prevention Evaluation (HOPE) study. *Circulation* 2003;107(9):1284–1290.

52. Stamler J, Vaccaro O, Neaton JD, Wentworth D. Diabetes, other risk factors, and 12-year cardiovascular mortality for men screened in the Multiple Risk Factor Intervention Trial (MRFIT). *Diabetes Care* 1993;16:434–444.

53. O'Leary DH, Polak JF, Kronmal RA, et al. Distribution and correlates of sonographically detected carotid artery disease in the Cardiovascular Health Study. *Stroke* 1992;23:1752–1760.

54. Gæde P, Vedel P, Larsen N, et al. Multifactorial intervention and cardiovascular disease in patients with type 2 diabetes. *N Engl J Med* 2003;348:383–393.

55. Klein S, Sheard NF, Pi-Sunyer X et al. Weight management through lifestyle modification for the prevention and management of type 2 diabetes: rationale and strategies: a statement of the American Diabetes Association, the North American Association for the Study of Obesity, and the American Society for Clinical Nutrition. *Diabetes Care* 2004:(8):27:2067–2073.

56. ACE Consensus Development Conference on Guidelines for Glycemic Control. *Endocr Pract* Suppl. Nov/Dec 2001.

57. Brooks MM, Frye RL, Genuth S et al. Hypotheses, design, and methods for the Bypass Angioplasty Revascularization Investigation 2 Diabetes (BARI 2D) trial. *Am J Cardiol* 2006;97(12A):9G–19G.

58. Rayfield EJ. Pathophysiology and clinical management of diabetes and prediabetes. In: Mechanick J, Brett E, eds. *Nutritional Strategies for the Diabetic/Prediabetic Patient (Nutrition and Disease Prevention)*. Boca Raton, FL: CRC Taylor & Francis, 2006.

59. Inhaled insulin (Exubera). *Med Lett* 2006;1239:57.

60. Riddle MC, Rosenstock J, Gerich J, Insulin Glargine 4002 Study Investigators. The treat-to-target trial: randomized addition of glargine or human NPH insulin to oral therapy of type-2 diabetic patients. *Diabetes Care* 2003;26:3080–3086.

61. Bode BW, Tamborlane W, Davidson PC. Insulin pump therapy in the 21st century. *Postgrad Med* 2002;111:69–77.

62. Klip A, Leiter LA. Cellular mechanism of action of metformin. *Diabetes Care* 1990;13:696–704.

63. Yki-Jarvinem H. Thiazolidinediones. *N Engl J Med* 2004;351:1106–1118.

64. Barbier O, Torra IP, Duguay Y, et al. Pleiotropic actions of peroxisome proliferator-activated receptors in lipid metabolism and atherosclerosis. *Arterioscler Thromb Vasc Biol* 2002;22(5):717–726.

65. Nolan JJ, Ludvik B, Beerdsen P, Joyce M, Olefsky J. Improvement in glucose tolerance and insulin resistance in obese subjects treated with troglitazone. *N Engl J Med* 1994;331(18):1188–1193.

66. Schmid-Antomarchi H, De Weille J, Fosset M, Lazdunski M. The receptor for antidiabetic sulfonylureas controls the activity of the ATP-modulated K⁺ channel in insulin-secreting cells. *J Biol Chem* 1987;262(33):15840–15844.

67. Chiasson JL, Josse RG, Gomis R, Hanefeld M, Karasik A, Laakso M; STOP-NIDDM Trial Research Group. Acarbose for prevention of type 2 diabetes mellitus: the STOP-NIDDM randomised trial. *Lancet*. 2002;359(9323):2072–2077.

68. Pramlintide (Symlin) for diabetes. *Med Lett* 2005;47:1209:41–43.

69. Drucker DJ. Enhancing incretin action for the treatment of type 2 diabetes. *Diabetes Care* 2003;26(10):2929–2940.

70. Green BD, Gault VA, O'Harte FP, Flatt PR. Structurally modified analogues of glucagon-like peptide-1 (GLP-1) and glucose-dependent insulinotropic polypeptide (GIP) as future antidiabetic agents. *Curr Pharm Des* 2004;10(29):3651–3662.

71. Raz I, Hanefeld M, Xu L, et al. Sitagliptin monotherapy improved glucemic control with beta cell function after 18 weeks in patients with type 2 diabetes. ADA 2006 Annual Scientific Sessions Abstract-PO, 1996.

72. Shapiro AM, Lakey JR, Ryan EA, et al. Islet transplantation in seven patients with type 1 diabetes mellitus using a glucocorticoid-free immunosuppressive regimen. *N Engl J Med* 2000;343(4):230–238.

73. Gruessner AC, Sutherland DE. Pancreas transplant outcomes for United States (US) and non-US cases as reported to the United Network for Organ Sharing (UNOS) and the International Pancreas Transplant Registry (IPTR) as of June 2004. *Clin Transplant* 2005;19(4):433–455.

74. Tian C, Bagley J, Cretin N, et al. Prevention of type 1 diabetes by gene therapy. *J Clin Invest* 2004;114(7):969–978.

75. Zulewski H, Abraham EJ, Gerlach MJ, et al. Multipotential nesting-positive stem cells isolated from adult pancreatic islets differentiate ex vivo into pancreatic endocrine, exocrine, and hepatic phenotypes. *Diabetes* 2001;50(3):521–533.

76. Renard E. Implantable closed-loop glucose-sensing and insulin delivery: the future for insulin pump therapy. *Curr Opin Pharmacol* 2002;2(6):708–716.

77. Koskinen P, Manttrai M, Manninen V, et al. Coronary heart disease incidence in NIDDM patients in the Helsinki Heart Study. *Diabetes Care* 1992;15:820–825.

78. Keech A, Simes RJ, Barter P, et al. FIELD study investigators. Effects of long-term fenofibrate therapy on cardiovascular events in 9795 people with type 2 diabetes mellitus (the FIELD study): randomised controlled trial. *Lancet* 2005;366(9500):1849–1861.

79. http://accelerator.axioresearch.com/aim-high. Aim-High Clinical Study, 2007.

80. Scandinavian Simvastatin Survival Study Group. Randomized trial of cholesterol lowering in 4444 patients with coronary heart disease: Scandinavian Simvastatin Survival Study (4S). *Lancet* 1994;344:1383–1389.

81. Garg A, Grundy SM. Cholestyramine therapy for dyslipidemia in non-insulin-dependent diabetes mellitus. *Ann Intern Med* 1994;121:416–422.

82. Expert Panel ATP III. Executive summary of the NCEP expert panel on the detection, evaluation, and treatment of high blood cholesterol in adults (ATP III). *JAMA* 2001;285:2486–2497.

83. Goldberg RB, Mellies MJ, Sacks FM, et al. Cardiovascular events and their reduction with pravastatin in diabetic and glucose-intolerant myocardial infarction survivors with average cholesterol levels: Subgroup analyses in the cholesterol and recurrent events (CARE) trial: the Care investigators. *Circulation* 1998;98:2513–2519.

84. Collins R, Armitage J, Parish S, et al. Heart Protection Study Collaborative Group. Effects of cholesterol-lowering with simvastatin on stroke and other major vascular events in 20536 people with cerebrovascular disease or other high-risk conditions. *Lancet* 2004 6;363(9411):757–767.

85. Colhoun HM, Betteridge DJ, Durrington PN, et al. CARDS investigators. Primary prevention of cardiovascular disease with atorvastatin in type 2 diabetes in the Collaborative Atorvastatin Diabetes Study (CARDS): multicentre randomised placebo-controlled trial. *Lancet* 2004;364(9435):685–696.

86. Wanner C, Krane V, Marz W, et al. German Diabetes and Dialysis Study Investigators. Atorvastatin in patients with type 2 diabetes mellitus undergoing hemodialysis. *N Engl J Med* 2005;353(3):238–248.

87. American Diabetes Association. Treatment of hypertension in adults with diabetes. *Diabetes Care* 2003;25(Suppl 1):S71–S73.

88. Curb JD, Pressel SL, Cutler JA, et al. Effect of diuretic-based antihypertensive treatment on cardiovascular disease risk in older diabetic patients with isolated systolic hypertension: Systolic Hypertension in the Elderly Program Cooperative Research Group. *JAMA* 1996;276:1886–1892.

89. UK Prospective Diabetes Study Group. Tight blood pressure control and risk of macrovascular and microvascular complications in type-2 diabetes. UKPDS 38. *BMJ* 1998;317:703–713.

90. Hansson L, Zanchetti A, Carruthers SG, et al. Effects of intensive blood-pressure lowering and low-dose aspirin in patients with hypertension: principal results of Hypertension Optimal Treatment (HOT) randomized trial. *Lancet* 1998;351:1755–1762.

91. Hansson L, Lindholm LH, Niskanen L, et al. Effect of angiotensin-converting-enzyme inhibition compared with conventional therapy on cardiovascular morbidity and mortality in hypertension: the Captopril Prevention Project (CAPPP) randomised trial. *Lancet* 1999;353:611–616.

92. Heart Outcomes Prevention Evaluation Study Investigators. Effects of ramipril on cardiovascular and microvascular outcomes in people with diabetes mellitus: results of the HOPE study and MICRO-HOPE sub-study. *Lancet* 2000;355:253–259.

93. Bakris GL, Fonseca V, Katholi RE, et al. Metabolic effects of carvedilol vs metoprolol in patients with type 2 diabetes mellitus and hypertension: a randomized controlled trial. *JAMA* 2004;292(18):2227–2236.

94. www.clinicaltrials.gov/ct/show/NCT00000620 (ACCORD).

95. Granger CB, Califf RM, Young S, et al. Outcome of patients with diabetes mellitus and acute myocardial infarction treated with thrombolytic agents. The Thrombolysis and Angioplasty in Myocardial Infarction (TAMI) Study Group. *J Am Coll Cardiol* 1993;21:920–925.

96. Stein B, Weintraub WS, Gebhart SP, et al. Influence of diabetes mellitus on early and late outcome after percutaneous transluminal coronary angioplasty. *Circulation* 1995;91:979–989.

97. Barzilay JI, Kronmal RA, Bittner V, et al. Coronary artery disease and coronary artery bypass grafting in diabetic patients aged > or = 65 years (report from the Coronary Artery Surgery Study [CASS] Registry). *Am J Cardiol* 1994;74:334–339.

98. BARI Investigators. Influence of diabetes on 5-year mortality and morbidity in a randomized trial comparing CABG and PTCA in patients with multivessel disease: the Bypass Angioplasty Revascularization Investigation (BARI). *Circulation* 1997;96:1761–1769.

99. Ferguson JJ. NHLI BARI clinical alert on diabetics treated with angioplasty. *Circulation* 1995;92:3371.

100. Feit F, Brooks MM, Sopko G, et al. Long-term clinical outcome in the Bypass Angioplasty Revascularization Investigation Registry: comparison with the randomized trial. BARI Investigators. *Circulation* 2000;101:2795–2802.

101. Niles NW, McGrath PD, Malenka D, et al. Survival of patients with diabetes and multivessel coronary artery disease after surgical or percutaneous coronary revascularization: results of a large regional prospective study. Northern New England Cardiovascular Disease Study Group. *J Am Coll Cardiol* 2001;37:1008–1015.

102. Van Belle E, Ketelers R, Bauters C, et al. Patency of percutaneous transluminal coronary angioplasty sites at 6- month angiographic followup: a key determinant of survival in diabetics after coronary balloon angioplasty. *Circulation* 2001;103:1218–1224.

103. Kuntz RE. Importance of considering atherosclerosis progression when choosing a coronary revascularization strategy: the diabetes-percutaneous transluminal coronary angioplasty dilemma. *Circulation* 1999;99:847–851.

104. Newman MF, Kirchner JL, Phillips-Bute B, et al. Longitudinal assessment of neurocognitive function after coronary- artery bypass surgery. *N Engl J Med* 2001;344:395–402.

105. Fischman DL, Leon MB, Baim DS, et al. A randomized comparison of coronary-stent placement and balloon angioplasty in the treatment of coronary artery disease. Stent Restenosis Study Investigators. *N Engl J Med* 1994;331:496–501.

106. Serruys PW, de Jaegere P, Kiemeneij F, et al. A comparison of balloon-expandable-stent implantation with balloon angioplasty in patients with coronary artery disease. Benestent Study Group. *N Engl J Med* 1994;331:489–495.

107. Holmes DR Jr, Vietstra RE, Smith HC, et al. Restenosis after percutaneous transluminal coronary angioplasty (PTCA): a report from the PTCA Registry of the National Heart, Lung and Blood Institute. *Am J Cardiol* 1984;53:77C–81C.

108. Serruys PW, Unger F, Sousa JE, et al. Comparison of coronary-artery bypass surgery and stenting for the treatment of multivessel disease. *N Engl J Med* 2001;344:1117–1124.

109. Abizaid A, Costa MA, Centemero M, et al. Clinical and economic impact of diabetes mellitus on percutaneous and surgical treatment of multivessel coronary

disease patients: insights from the Arterial Revascularization Therapy Study (ARTS) trial. *Circulation* 2001;104:533–538.

110. Mercado N, Wijns W, Serruys PW, et al. One-year outcomes of coronary artery bypass graft surgery versus percutaneous coronary intervention with multiple stenting for multisystem disease: a meta-analysis of individual patient data from randomized clinical trials. *J Thorac Cardiovasc Surg* 2005;130(2):512–519.

111. The SOS Investigators. Coronary artery bypass surgery versus percutaneous coronary intervention with stent implantation in patients with multivessel coronary artery disease (the Stent or Surgery trial): a randomized controlled trial. *Lancet* 2002;360:965–970.

112. Aronson D, Bloomgarden Z, Rayfield EJ. Potential mechanisms promoting restenosis in diabetes mellitus. *J Am Coll Cardiol* 1996;27:528–535.

113. Lincoff AM, Califf RM, Moliterno DJ, et al. for the Evaluation of Platelet IIb/IIIa Inhibition in Stenting Investigators. Complementary clinical benefits of coronary-artery stenting and blockade of platelet glycoprotein IIb/IIIa receptors. *N Engl J Med* 1999;341:319–327.

114. Marso SP, Lincoff AM, Ellis SG, et al. Optimizing the percutaneous interventional outcomes for patients with diabetes mellitus: results of the EPISTENT (Evaluation of Platelet IIb/IIIa Inhibitor for Stenting Trial) diabetic substudy. *Circulation* 1999;100:2477–2484.

115. Lansky AJ, Mintz GS, Mehran R, et al. Insights into the mechanism of restenosis after PTCA and stenting. *Indian Heart J* 1998;50(Suppl 1):104–108.

116. Mintz GS, Popma JJ, Pichard AD, et al. Intravascular ultrasound predictors of restenosis after percutaneous transcatheter coronary revascularization. *J Am Coll Cardiol* 1996;27:1678–1687.

117. Dangas G, Fuster V. Management of restenosis after coronary intervention. *Am Heart J* 1996;132:428–436.

118. Teirstein PS, Massullo V, Jani S, et al. Catheter-based radiotherapy to inhibit restenosis after coronary stenting. *N Engl J Med* 1997;336:1697–1703.

119. Choi D, Kim SK, Choi SH, et al. Preventative effects of rosiglitazone on restenosis after coronary stent implantation in patients with type 2 diabetes. *Diabetes Care* 2004;27(11):2654–2660.

120. Kipshidze NN, Tsapenko MV, Leon MB, Stone GW, Moses JW. Update on drug-eluting coronary stents. *Expert Rev Cardiovasc Ther* 2005;3(5):953–968.

121. Popma JJ, Lansky AJ, Ito S, et al. Contemporary stent designs: technical considerations, complications, role of intravascular ultrasound, and anticoagulation therapy. *Prog Cardiovasc Dis* 1996;39:111–128.

122. Stettler C, Allemann S, Egger M, Windecker S, Meier B, Diem P. Efficacy of drug eluting stents in patients with and without diabetes mellitus: indirect comparison of controlled trials. *Heart* 2006;92(5):650–657.

123. Dibra A, Kastrati A, Mehilli J et al. ISAR-DIABETES Study Investigators. Paclitaxel- or sirolimus-eluting stents to prevent restenosis in diabetic patients. *N Engl J Med* 2005 ;353(7):663–670.

124. Roiron C, Sanchez P, Bouzamondo A, Lechat P, Montalescot G. Drug eluting stents: an updated meta-analysis of randomised controlled trials. *Heart* 2006 ;92(5):641–649.

125. Kuchulakanti PK, Chu WW, Torguson R, et al. Sirolimus-eluting stents versus Paclitaxel-eluting stents in the treatment of coronary artery disease in patients with diabetes mellitus. *Am J Cardiol* 2006;98(2):187–192.

126. Loop FD, Lytle BW, Cosgrove DM, et al. Influence of the internal-mammary-artery graft on 10-year survival and other cardiac events. *N Engl J Med* 1986;314:1–6.

127. Tatoulis J, Buxton BF, Fuller JA, Royse AG. Total arterial coronary revascularization: techniques and results in 3,220 patients. *Ann Thorac Surg* 1999;68:2093–2099.

128. Lytle BW, Cosgrove DM, Loop FD, et al. Perioperative risk of bilateral internal mammary artery grafting: analysis of 500 cases from 1971 to 1984. *Circulation* 1986;74:III37–III41.

129. Stamou SC, Hill PC, Dangas G, et al. Stroke after coronary artery bypass: incidence, predictors, and clinical outcome. *Stroke* 2001;32:1508–1513.

130. Abizaid A, Costa MA, Centemero M, et al. Clinical and economic impact of diabetes mellitus on percutaneous and surgical treatment of multivessel coronary disease patients: insights from the Arterial Revascularization Therapy Study (ARTS) trial. *Circulation* 2001;104:533–538.

131. Wareing TH, Davila-Roman VG, Daily BB, et al. Strategy for the reduction of stroke incidence in cardiac surgical patients. *Ann Thorac Surg* 1993;55:1400–1407; discussion 1407–1408.

132. Magee MJ, Dewey TM, Acuff T, et al. Influence of diabetes on mortality and morbidity: off-pump coronary artery bypass grafting versus coronary artery bypass grafting with cardiopulmonary bypass. *Ann Thorac Surg* 2001;72:776–780; discussion 780–781.

133. www.clinicaltrials.gov/ct/gui/show/NCT00086450 (FREEDOM).

134. Kapur A, Malik IS, Bagger JP, et al. The Coronary Artery Revascularisation in Diabetes (CARDia) trial: background, aims, and design. *Am Heart J* 2005;149(1):13–19.

135. http://clinicaltrials.gov/ct/show/NCT00326196 (VA–CARDS).

136. Haffner SM, Mykanen L, Festa A, et al. Insulin-resistant pre-diabetic subjects have more atherogenic risk factors than insulin-sensitive pre-diabetic subjects: implications for preventing coronary heart disease during the pre-diastolic state. *Circulation* 2000;101:975–980.

137. Tuomilehto J, Lindstrom J, Eriksson JG, et al. Prevention of type 2 diabetes mellitus by changes in lifestyle among subjects with impaired glucose tolerance. *N Engl J Med* 2001;344:1343–1350.

138. Diabetes Prevention Program Research Group. Reduction in the incidence of type 2 diabetes with lifestyle modification or metformin. *N Engl J Med* 2002;346:393–403.

139. Freeman DJ, Norrie J, Sattar N, et al. Pravastatin and the development of diabetes mellitus: Evidence for a protective treatment effect in the West of Scotland Coronary Prevention Study. *Circulation* 2001;103:357–362.

140. Hope investigators. Effects of an angiotensin converting enzyme inhibitor, ramipril, on cardiovascular events in high-risk patients. *N Engl J Med* 2000;342:145–153.

141. Gerstein HC, Yusuf S, Holman R, Bosch J, Pogue J, The DREAM Trial Investigators. Rationale, design and recruitment characteristics of a large, simple international trial of diabetes prevention: the DREAM trial. *Diabetologia* 2004;47(9):1519–1527.

142. http://clinicaltrials.gov/ct/show/NCT00097786 (NAVIGATOR).

143. http://clinicaltrials.gov/ct/show/NCT00325650 (RAPSODI).

144. The cost-effectiveness of screening for type 2 diabetes. CDC Diabetes Cost-Effectiveness Study Group, Centers for Disease Control and Prevention. *JAMA* 1998;280:1757–1763.

145. Grundy SM, Benjamin IJ, Burke GL, et al. Diabetes and cardiovascular disease: a statement for healthcare professionals from the American Heart Association. *Circulation* 1999;100:1134–1146.

146. Gibbons RJ, Balady GJ, Beasley JW, et al. ACC/AHA guidelines for exercise testing: executive summary: a report of the American College of Cardiology/American Heart Association Task Force on Practice Guidelines (Committee on Exercise Testing). *Circulation* 1997;96:345–354.

147. Baxter CG, Boon NA, Walker JD; DIAD study. Detection of silent myocardial ischemia in asymptomatic diabetic subjects: the DIAD study. *Diabetes Care* 2005;28(3):756–757.

148. DREAM (Diabetes REduction Assessment with ramipril and rosiglitazone Medication) Trial Investigators, Gerstein HC, Yusuf S, Bosch J, et al. Effect of rosiglitazone on the frequency of diabetes in patients with impaired glucose tolerance or impaired fasting glucose: a randomized controlled trial. *Lancet* 2006;368(9541):1096–1105.

149. DREAM Trial Investigators, Bosch J, Yusuf S, Gerstein HC, et al. Effect of ramipril on the incidence of diabetes. *N Engl J Med* 2006;355(15):1551–1562.

CHAPTER (91)

Metabolic Syndrome, Obesity, and Diet

Scott M. Grundy / Sidney C. Smith, Jr.

The rise in the prevalence of obesity in the United States and worldwide is threatening to undo recent advances in prevention of atherosclerotic cardiovascular disease (ASCVD). Among the complications, cardiovascular events produce the greatest morbidity and mortality. A significant portion of the latter occurs in persons in whom obesity precedes type II diabetes. But diabetes is only one of several conditions that associate strongly with obesity. Others include dyslipidemia, hypertension, systemic inflammation, and a thrombotic tendency. Recently there has been a trend in the cardiovascular field to group all of these factors together under the heading of *metabolic syndrome*.[1] In this sense, metabolic syndrome can be taken to represent a multiplex cardiovascular risk factor. This syndrome does not include, but is strongly associated with, other complications of obesity, for example, fatty liver, cholesterol gallstones, obstructive sleep apnea, and polycystic ovarian syndrome. The current definition generally regards hyperglycemia in the range of type II diabetes to be one of the components of metabolic syndrome.[1] This is because approximately 85 percent of persons classified as having type II diabetes will meet current criteria for metabolic syndrome. Even so, many investigators in the diabetes field prefer to separate metabolic syndrome from diabetes and to view it largely as a *prediabetic* condition besides being a cardiovascular risk factor.[2,3] This is a semantic argument. Regardless of viewpoint, type II diabetes must be viewed as one of the complications of obesity and strongly associated with risk for ASCVD. This chapter will focus primarily on metabolic syndrome as a cardiovascular risk factor with obesity being the primary exogenous factor driving its development. But it will further discuss other exogenous factors, such as physical inactivity and dietary excesses, as well as endogenous susceptibility factors.

Metabolic syndrome represents a clustering of cardiovascular risk factors that are amalgamated into a single multiplex risk factor for ASCVD (Fig. 91–1).[4] When the concept of metabolic syndrome was introduced into the National Cholesterol Education Program (NCEP) Adult Treatment Panel III Report (ATP III),[1] it was considered as a partner of elevated low-density lipoprotein (LDL) in the causation of cardiovascular disease (CVD). The *metabolic risk factors* that make up the syndrome include atherogenic dyslipidemia, elevated blood pressure, dysglycemia, a prothrombotic state, and a proinflammatory state. Several reports indicate that this clustering of metabolic risk factors cannot be explained by chance alone.[5–18] This suggests that there is a common, underlying etiology of this clustering. Individuals with metabolic syndrome have an approximate doubling of risk for ASCVD and approximately fourfold higher risk for developing type II diabetes compared to those without the syndrome.

LOW-DENSITY LIPOPROTEIN AND METABOLIC SYNDROME: PARTNERS IN ATHEROGENESIS

The development of atherosclerosis can be considered to occur in two stages: injury and response to injury. The primary injurious agents include LDL and other apolipoprotein B (apo B)-contain-

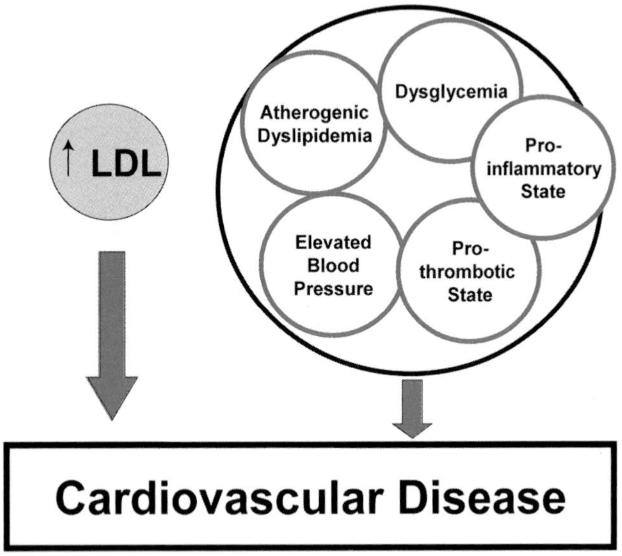

FIGURE 91–1. Risk factor partners: elevated low-density lipoprotein (LDL) and metabolic syndrome. The latter is a multiplex risk factor for arteriosclerotic cardiovascular disease (ASCVD) and a clustering of atherogenic dyslipidemia, elevated blood pressure, dysglycemia, a prothrombotic state, and a proinflammatory state.

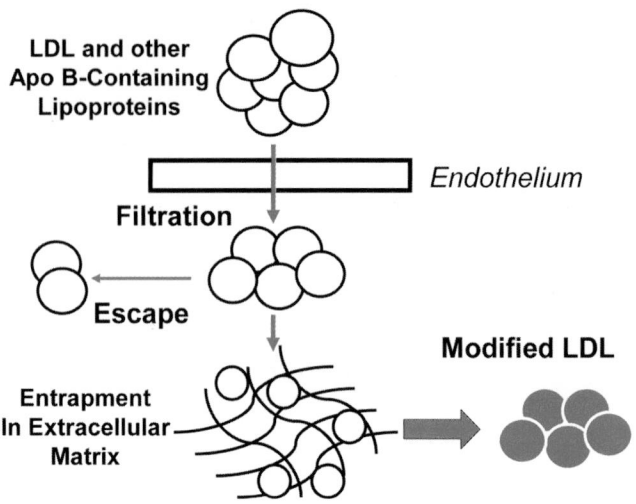

FIGURE 91–2. Details of arterial injury produced by low-density lipoprotein (LDL) and other apolipoprotein B (apo B)-containing lipoprotein. Circulating lipoproteins filter into the arterial intima through the endothelium. A portion of LDL escapes back into the circulation. Other LDL particles however become entrapped in extracellular matrix. Here they become modified in several ways; this modification occurs in ways that turn the LDL into proinflammatory agents.

ing lipoproteins. The response to injury makes up a process called inflammation. Metabolic syndrome exacerbates atherogenesis by enhancing the inflammatory response to LDL injury. The key steps in both processes can be reviewed briefly.

The first step in the pathogenesis of atherosclerosis is the infiltration of plasma LDL into the arterial intima (Fig. 91–2). The rate of infiltration of LDL depends on two factors: (1) the concentration of LDL in the circulation and (2) the permeability of the arterial wall.[19] Several mechanisms have been proposed for transport into the subendothelium: vesicular ferrying through endothelial cells, passive sieving through endothelial-cell pores, and passage between cells. Not all that enters the arterial wall stays there. Some escapes by a reversal of the same process. However, a portion of the LDL becomes entrapped into the extracellular matrix.[20] When this occurs, LDL is ripe for modification. Several types of modification have been proposed: aggregation, fusion of lipoproteins, proteolysis, lipolytic degradation such as hydrolysis of cholesterol esters, phospholipids, and triglyceride, oxidation and glycation.[21] When LDL is modified in various ways, it acquires inflammatory potential. The consequences of LDL modification include the activation of various types of cells—endothelial cells, monocyte/macrophages, and smooth muscle cells.[20,22] All of these changes come under the category of *inflammation* (Fig. 91–3). Key changes are endothelial dysfunction, which allows for a more rapid infiltration of LDL into the arterial wall and adherence to circulating monocytes, movement of monocytes into the arterial wall and their activation, proliferation of smooth muscle cells, and enhanced fibrosis. Macrophages are a key player in atherogenesis.[22] They first accumulate lipid and then undergo apoptosis—releasing their excess lipid into lipid pools. Macrophages further produce enzymes, such as metalloproteinases, that degrade the extracellular matrix. These latter two changes seemingly create unstable plaques that are prone to rupture and to causation of acute ASCVD events.

METABOLIC SYNDROME AND ARTERIAL INFLAMMATION

Whereas excess LDL initiates atherogenesis and promotes its progression, metabolic syndrome exacerbates the inflammatory process. This leads to a worsening acceleration of atherosclerosis. Each of the components of metabolic syndrome appears to worsen inflammation in plaques. First, in the case of hypertension, an increased hydrostatic pressure in elevated blood pressure can enhance influx of LDL into the arterial wall. Further, hypertension is associated with endothelial dysfunction.[23] Hypertension can be accompanied by increased angiotensin II (A-II), which can enhance leukocytal vascular adhesion molecule (VCAM)-1 on endothelial cells and cause release of proinflammatory cytokines (e.g., interleukin-6 [IL-6] and monocyte chemotactic protein-1 [MCP-1]).[24,25] A-II can also increase the expression by arterial SMCs of proinflammatory cytokines such as IL-6 and MCP-1 and of the leukocyte adhesion molecule VCAM-1 on endothelial cells.[24,25] Second, dysglycemia, particularly diabetic hyperglycemia, has been implicated in several ways in the exacerbation of inflammation—formation of inflammatory advanced glycation products, glycation of extracellular matrix enhancing retention of LDL, glycoxidative modification of LDL, and activation of protein kinase C (enhancing the inflammatory response).[26] Third, a key component of atherogenic dyslipidemia is a low high-density lipoprotein (HDL). HDL is believed to be a protective lipoprotein, and if so, most likely exerts its antiinflammatory effects at multiple levels: it transports excess cholesterol out of macrophages, reducing their atherogenic potential; it prevents conversion of LDL into proinflammatory modified LDL; and it inhibits cytokine-induced expression of cellular adhesion molecules on endothelial cells.[27] At present the role of HDL in the inflammatory process is still under intense investigation.[28,29] The protective actions of HDL are reduced in persons with ath-

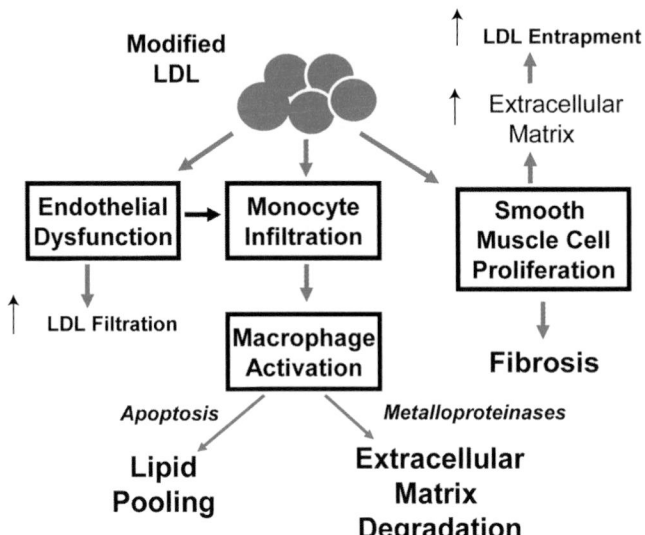

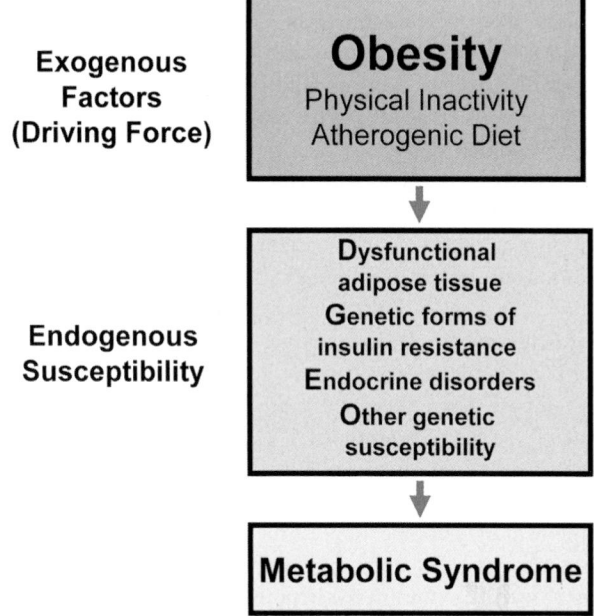

FIGURE 91–3. Details of the inflammatory process evoked by modified low-density lipoprotein (LDL). Three cellular systems are affected by modified LDL: endothelial cells, monocytes/macrophages, and smooth muscle cells. Modified LDL causes endothelial dysfunction, allowing increased amounts of LDL to filter into the arterial wall and enhanced attachment of monocytes to the endothelium. It also acts as a chemoattractant to pull monocytes into the arterial wall; at the same time it promotes transformation of monocytes into macrophages and activates them. Activated macrophages ingest modified LDL, become transformed into foam cells, undergo apoptosis to form large lipid pools and release metalloproteinases to degrade the extracellular matrix. The latter two effects lead to destabilization of arteriosclerotic plaques, plaque rupture, and acute cardiovascular events. Finally, modified LDL stimulate smooth muscle cell proliferation for production of collagen fibers leading to fibrosis of the plaque.

FIGURE 91–4. Pathogenic scheme for development of the metabolic syndrome. The syndrome develops as a result of the interaction of exogenous and endogenous factors. The major exogenous factor is obesity, but physical inactivity and atherogenic diet play an important role. Endogenous factors include dysfunctional adipose tissue, genetic forms of insulin resistance, various endocrine disorders, and other genetic susceptibility.

erogenic dyslipidemia. Fourth, in metabolic syndrome, there is an increase in circulating cytokines.[30,31] These cytokines likely act at the level of the arterial wall to enhance the inflammatory response to modified LDL. And finally, a prothrombotic state is characterized by a series of abnormalities that can enhance coagulation, inhibit fibrinolysis, and alter platelet function. Among these factors are increases in plasminogen activator inhibitor-1 (PAI-1), fibrinogen, factor VII, factor VIII, factor X, prothrombin fragments F1+2, and von Willebrand factor (vWF).[32,33] These factors can not only promote inflammation within arteriosclerotic plaques, but they can enhance thrombus propagation following a ruptured plaque.

PATHOGENESIS OF METABOLIC SYNDROME

A simple way to visualize the pathogenesis of metabolic syndrome is illustrated in Fig. 91–4. This view identifies an interaction between exogenous and endogenous factors. Obesity is the major exogenous factor, but physical inactivity and excess dietary factors can play a role. Endogenous factors include inherent insulin resistance, dysfunctional adipose tissue, endocrine disorders, and various genetic aberrations. The endogenous factors can be grouped together under the heading of *metabolic susceptibility.* To develop the syndrome, most individuals must be metabolically susceptible. But even in the presence of susceptibility, the full blown metabolic syndrome generally will not develop in

【 】 OBESITY: THE DRIVING FORCE OF METABOLIC SYNDROME

The high prevalence of metabolic syndrome in the United States[34] and worldwide[35] is secondary to a rising prevalence of obesity.[36–39] Metabolic syndrome prevalence rises in parallel with increasing obesity.[40] Physical inactivity also is associated with a higher prevalence of metabolic syndrome.[41–48] Part of this association can be related to the greater obesity accompanying a sedentary lifestyle; nevertheless it is likely that physical activity provides a protective role against metabolic syndrome independently of the obesity. Further, high-carbohydrate diets, particularly those rich in simple carbohydrates or high-glycemic index foods, have been claimed to worsen metabolic syndrome.[49–52] The literature nonetheless is mixed on the ideal diet composition for prevention and treatment of the syndrome.[49]

The mechanisms whereby obesity results in metabolic syndrome are being increasingly understood.[1] Adipose tissue releases several products that appear to worsen metabolic syndrome.[53] The most important is a key fuel source, nonesterified fatty acids (NEFA). During the fasting state, adipose tissue triglyceride undergoes lipolysis and releases NEFA into the circulation. The major enzyme involved in lipolysis is *hormone sensitive lipase* (HSL); the activity of this enzyme is enhanced by catecholamines and suppressed by insulin. When insulin levels are low during fasting, lipolysis is high as is NEFA release. NEFA is the major energy source during fasting. But if NEFA supply exceeds needs for energy utilization, they accumulate in muscle and liver. This accumulation is called *ectopic fat.* When fat accumulates in muscle and the liver, insulin resistance is increased. This change plus other metabolic alterations predisposes to the metabolic syndrome.[53]

Beyond excess fatty acids, other products of adipose tissue are released in abnormal amounts from adipose tissue. One category of products includes the *inflammatory cytokines*, for example, tumor necrosis factor-α (TNF-α) and IL-6.[54] This excess release of cytokines appears to be secondary to infiltration of adipose tissue with activated macrophages, which can produce these cytokines.[55] The result is a high level of circulating cytokines. These can have several systemic effects: enhancement of insulin resistance in muscle, production of acute phase reactants (C-reactive protein [CRP] and fibrinogen) by the liver, and exacerbation of inflammation in arteriosclerotic lesions. Both of the latter can predispose to major cardiovascular events. These cytokines play a key role in the causation of the proinflammatory state of metabolic syndrome.

The adipose tissue likewise can predispose to a prothrombotic state by release of excess amounts of *PAI-1*, which is released from adipose tissue in response to obesity.[56] Adipose tissue further secretes *leptin*, an appetite suppressant. Leptin levels are high in obesity and seemingly do not suppress the appetite of obese individuals, a condition called *leptin resistance*. Leptin can have systemic actions as well as actions in the hypothalamus. One such systemic action is to enhance fatty-acid oxidation by the liver, preventing steatosis.[57] Several other bioactive *adipokines* have been reported to be produced by adipose tissue: resistin, *angiotensinogen*, tissue factor, transforming growth factor-β, nitric oxide synthase, acylation stimulating protein, adipophilin, adipoQ, adipsin, monobutyrin, and agouti protein. Their role in the causation of metabolic syndrome remains to be fully elucidated.

In adipose tissue, 11β-hydroxysteroid dehydrogenase type 1 (11β-HSD1) converts inactive cortisone to *active cortisol*. Overexpression of 11β-HSD1 induced in mice produces central obesity and insulin resistance.[58] It also has been reported that obesity in humans is accompanied by overexpression of 11β-HSD1.[59]

Finally, the release of another substance, *adiponectin*, actually reduced with obesity.[60–63] Adiponectin can protect against insulin resistance, metabolic risk factors, and atherogenesis. The mechanisms whereby adiponectin exerts this protective effect is a topic of intense research at present.

【 】 BEYOND OBESITY: ENDOGENOUS METABOLIC SUSCEPTIBILITY

Only a portion of patients with obesity develop metabolic syndrome. It appears that an individual must be metabolically susceptible to developing the syndrome, and when obesity is acquired, the syndrome becomes manifest. Several factors seemingly contribute to endogenous susceptibility. Among these are dysfunctional adipose tissue, genetic forms of insulin resistance, various endocrine disorders, and other genetic factors. Of particular importance appears to be a dysfunction of adipose tissue.

Metabolic Susceptibility: Dysfunctional Adipose Tissue

There are at least four potential disorders that can contribute to dysfunctional adipose tissue, which in turn will accentuate metabolic syndrome. These include a deficiency of subcutaneous adipose tissue, genetic forms of insulin resistance, dysfunctional adipocytes, and inflammation of adipose tissue (Fig. 91–5).

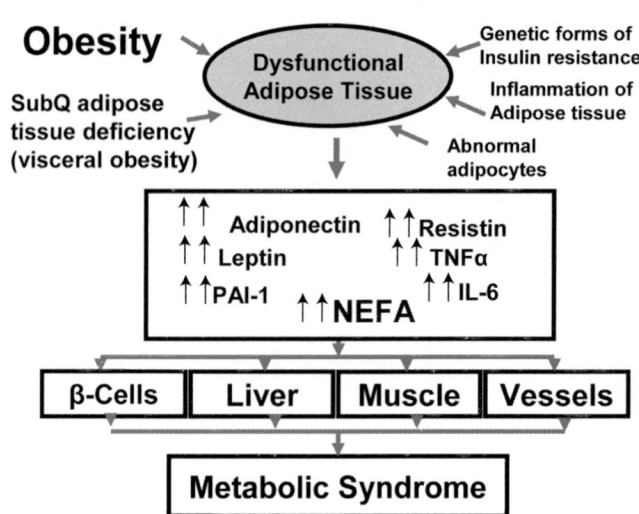

FIGURE 91–5. The role of obesity and dysfunctional adipose tissue in causation of the metabolic syndrome. When adipose tissue becomes overloaded with lipid (obesity), it produces abnormal amounts of nonesterified fatty acids (NEFA) and other adipokines. Among the latter are adiponectin, leptin, plasminogen activator inhibitor-1 (PAI-1), resistin, tumor necrosis factor-α (TNF-α), interleukin-6 (IL-6), and other inflammatory cytokines. The *protective* adiponectin is produced in subnormal amounts in obese persons. These abnormal products of adipose tissue flood various key tissues—pancreatic β cells, liver, muscle, and vessels; their effects in turn give rise to metabolic syndrome or accelerate the development of atherosclerosis at the level of the arterial wall. Additional causes of dysfunctional adipose tissue include a deficiency of subcutaneous adipose tissue, leading to visceral obesity, genetic forms of insulin resistance, abnormal adipocytes, and inflammation of adipose tissue. In the presence of these factors, defects in production of NEFA and adipokines is accentuated, worsening the metabolic syndrome.

One of the most important of these is a deficiency of subcutaneous adipose tissue. This abnormality is seen in an extreme form in a condition called lipodystrophy. Several metabolic defects can cause lipodystrophy—a severe deficiency of adipose tissue.[64] In patients with lipodystrophy, who have little adipose tissue for storage of extra energy, fat becomes deposited ectopically in the liver and muscle; the result is the development of severe metabolic syndrome. Less severe forms of adipose-tissue deficiency are manifest by an abnormal body fat distribution. Differences in body fat distribution can typically be seen between obese women and men.[65] Women normally have considerable quantities of subcutaneous adipose tissue in the lower body. Only when they are more severely obese does fat begin to accumulate in the upper body. It first enters upper body subcutaneous adipose tissue and only later does it accumulate in visceral adipose tissue beds. As a result, substantial ectopic fat accumulation is relatively rare. In contrast, men typically have a paucity of lower-body subcutaneous adipose tissue; as a result, they tend to develop upper-body obesity including considerable amounts of visceral fat as well as ectopic fat. This pattern of fat distribution is called *abdominal obesity*; it is complicated by larger amounts of ectopic fat, which predisposes to metabolic syndrome.[66] There is considerable variation in these trends in both men and women, and some individuals are particularly prone to development of ectopic fat and metabolic syndrome when they become obese.[65] The causes of a relative deficiency of subcutaneous adipose tissue are not known, although because of male/female differences, endocrine factors can contribute. The net result of adipose tissue deficiency is a shift of fat away from adipose tissue and into ectopic stores, which will worsen metabolic syndrome. In addition, the normal release of other adipokines appears to be impaired.[67]

Dysfunctional forms of adipose tissue further can result from genetic forms of insulin resistance. Insulin is a major regulator of adipose tissue metabolism. When genetic defects occur in insulin-signaling in adipocytes, suppression of lipolysis and other products is impaired.[68] In addition, adiponectin release is reduced.[68] All of these will accentuate ectopic fat distribution and metabolic syndrome. Moreover, defective insulin signaling in other tissues such as muscle and liver most likely will accentuate metabolic syndrome.[69,70] A good example of a genetic form of insulin resistance is found in many persons of South Asian origin. Insulin-resistant South Asians have multiple signs of dysfunctional adipose tissue—elevated NEFA levels, high CRP and leptin levels, and low adiponectin concentrations—even when they are not obese.[68] These persons are prone to metabolic syndrome and to premature type II diabetes and CVD.

It is likely dysfunction within adipocytes contributes to failure to store fat, to suppress lipolysis, or to suppress release of other adipokines. Defects in adipocyte function might occur at several levels including conversion of mesenchymal stem cells into preadipocyte, further conversion into various adipocyte populations, and to adipocyte cell death.[71] A variety of key pathways have been described in adipocytes in which defects potentially could lead to abnormalities in product release.[72–77]

Finally, in obese persons, the adipose tissue is invaded with macrophages.[55,78–81] The possibility has been raised that activation of these macrophages will result in the production of cytokines that will derange the function of adipocytes. In particular, these cytokines can cause insulin resistance, and the same defects are noted in persons with genetic forms of insulin resistance. Thus, *inflammation* of adipose tissue can be yet another factor contributing to dysfunctional adipose tissue and metabolic syndrome.

Genetic Forms of Insulin Resistance

In the preceding discussion the effects of genetic forms of insulin resistance on adipose tissue were reviewed. One hypothesis holds that genetic forms of insulin resistance are the major cause of metabolic syndrome.[82,83] According to this hypothesis, resistance to the action of insulin is widespread and causes a gross metabolic disturbance in many tissues. This disturbance can account for the multiple metabolic risk factors characteristic of the syndrome. This hypothesis is provocative and has provided a basis for many studies the causation of metabolic syndrome. The effects of insulin resistance in adipose tissue provides the most direct evidence for the mechanism linking resistance to insulin to metabolic syndrome. Nevertheless, it is certainly possible that widespread metabolic disturbance contributes beyond adipose tissue abnormalities.[82] Just how much of metabolic syndrome can be attributed to genetic forms of insulin resistance is uncertain. However, the close association between obesity and dysfunctional adipose tissue and the syndrome suggests that in the overall picture, genetic forms of insulin resistance are not dominant. Nonetheless, insulin resistance can be a particularly important contributor to the syndrome if it is present in conjunction with obesity.[83]

Other Genetic and Metabolic Abnormalities

In view of metabolic differences in men and women, it is likely that endocrine factors play a role in causation of metabolic syndrome. This possibility is heightened by the observation that women with polycystic ovary syndrome are prone to metabolic syndrome.[84–86] Because patients with hypercorticoidism manifest many of the features of the syndrome, abnormalities in cortisol metabolism also has been implicated.[87]

Manifestations of metabolic syndrome vary from individual to individual and also between populations. For example Asians and Hispanics appear to be particularly susceptible to diabetes, African Americans to hypertension, and Caucasians to dyslipidemia. Certainly all of the features of metabolic syndrome can occur in all of these populations, but prominent features suggest that genetic variation exists and affects manifestations of the syndrome. Research on the genetic basis of ethnic differences has been increasing the past few years and promises to provide new insights into the causes of variation in expression of the syndrome.

〖 〗 CLINICAL DIAGNOSIS OF METABOLIC SYNDROME

In 2005, the American Heart Association (AHA) and the National Heart, Lung, and Blood Institute (NHLBI) updated the ATP III criteria[1]. The essential criteria of ATP III were retained. Of note, however, they lowered the threshold for impaired fasting glucose to 100 mg/dL from the previous 110 mg/dL, in accord with current ADA recommendations.[88] The International Diabetes Federation (IDF)[89,90] recently published similar criteria for the diagnosis of metabolic syndrome. Updated ATP III criteria are shown in Table 91–1.

In IDF criteria,[89,90] for Asian populations, except for Japan, waist circumference thresholds were ≥90 cm in men and ≥80 cm in women; for Japanese they were ≥80 cm for men and ≥90 cm for women. The ATP III update accepted these same criteria for Asians including those living in the United States.[1]

〖 〗 METABOLIC SYNDROME AND RISK FOR ARTERIOSCLEROTIC CARDIOVASCULAR DISEASE

Long-Term (Lifetime) Risk

In populations at risk, metabolic syndrome is accompanied by an increase in relative risk for ASCVD.[91–100] In prospective epidemiologic studies, the relative risk for ASCVD events is essentially doubled. It is likely that the twofold increase in risk seen in short-term, prospective studies underestimates the long-term impact of the syndrome. The reason is that metabolic risk factors tend to worsen with time. Lipid levels and blood pressure rise with advancing age, and normal glucose levels advance to prediabetes or frank diabetes. Consequently, the earlier metabolic syndrome can be detected and managed, the slower will be the progression.

Short-Term (10-Year) Risk

At present, more intense clinical intervention is driven by short-term risk for ASCVD.[4] This risk usually is identified as 10-year

TABLE 91–1

Criteria for Clinical Diagnosis of Metabolic Syndrome

MEASURE (ANY THREE OF FIVE CONSTITUTE A DIAGNOSIS OF METABOLIC SYNDROME)	CATEGORICAL CUTPOINTS
Elevated waist circumference[a,b]	≥102 cm in males
	≥88 cm in females
Elevated triglycerides	≥150 mg/dL (1.7 mmol/L)
	or
	Drug treatment for elevated triglyceride[c]
Reduced HDL cholesterol	<40 mg/dL (0.9 mmol/L) in males
	<50 mg/dL (1.1 mmol/L) in females
	or
	Drug treatment for reduced HDL-C[c]
Elevated blood pressure	≥130 mmHg systolic blood pressure
	or
	≥85 mmHg diastolic blood pressure
	or
	Antihypertensive drug treatment in a patient with a history of hypertension is an alternate indicator
Elevated fasting glucose	≥100 mg/dL
	or
	Drug treatment of elevated glucose

HDL, high-density lipoprotein; HDL-C, HDL cholesterol; in, inches; TG, triglyceride.

[a]To measure waist circumference, locate the top of the right iliac crest. Place a measuring tape in a horizontal plane around the abdomen at the level of the iliac crest. Before reading the tape measure, ensure that the tape is snug, but does not compress the skin, and is parallel to the floor. The measurement is made at the end of a normal expiration.

[b]A lower waist circumference cutpoint (e.g., ≥94 cm [37 in] in men and ≥80 cm in women) appears to be appropriate for persons of Asian origin. Moreover, some persons of non-Asian origin with a marginally increased waist circumference (e.g., 94–102 [37–39 in] in men and 80–88 cm [31–35 in] in women) can have a strong genetic contribution to insulin resistance; they should benefit from changes in life habits, similarly to men with categorical increases in waist circumference.

[c]The most commonly used drugs for elevated TG and reduced HDL-C are fibrates and nicotinic acid. A patient on one of these drugs can be presumed to have high TG and low HDL.

risk for coronary heart disease (CHD). According to ATP III guidelines, risk can be stratified into four categories.

1. *High risk* is a 10-year risk for CHD >20 percent and includes patients with clinically evident ASCVD, diabetes, or enough other major risk factors to raise the risk to this level.
2. *Moderately high risk* consists of two or more major risk factors and a 10-year risk of 10 to 20 percent.
3. *Moderate risk* exhibits two or more risk factors, but a 10-year risk <10 percent.
4. *Lower-risk* individuals have 0 to 1 risk factor and a 10-year risk <10 percent.

Most persons with metabolic syndrome can be considered to be at least a moderate risk; but many will have risk >10 percent.

Framingham risk scoring should be used to estimate 10-year risk in metabolic syndrome patients without established ASCVD or type II diabetes mellitus (T2DM).[4] Because metabolic syndrome is only one part of overall risk assessment for ASCVD, *it is not an adequate tool to estimate 10-year risk for CHD*. These pa-

tients must be considered to be at higher lifetime risk for ASCVD, but metabolic syndrome alone is inadequate to guide clinical management for short-term risk reduction.

Although Framingham risk scoring provides a good first-step risk for estimating risk, other considerations can be brought into play both for confirmation of metabolic syndrome and for estimating 10-year risk in affected patients (Fig. 91–6). Besides the simple clinical measures proposed by ATP III,[1,4] other *emerging risk factors* are commonly present in patients with metabolic syndrome.[1] Identification of abnormalities in these factors can help to confirm the presence of the syndrome.[1] Although these emerging risk factors are not required for diagnosis, the presence of several of them will give strong confirmation of the presence of a systemic metabolic disorder. Therefore, their measurement is optional. In addition, confirmation of a higher risk status can be obtained by the finding of significant subclinical atherosclerosis.[4] For example, if a patient with metabolic syndrome found to be at moderate risk by Framingham risk scoring is found to have a higher coronary artery calcification (CAC) score, this patient might be elevated to a category of moderately high risk if the CAC score is >100 Agatston units.

【 】 MANAGEMENT OF UNDERLYING CAUSES

Overweight and Obesity

Because obesity is the major driving force behind metabolic syndrome it is a reasonable primary target of therapy.[1,4] Clinical guidelines for management of overweight and obesity have been published by the NHLBI and National Institute of Diabetes and Digestive and Kidney Diseases (NIDDK).[101] They distinguish between overweight and obesity by body mass index (BMI) ranges of 25 to 29.9 kg/m² and ≥30 kg/m², respectively. These guideline defined abdominal obesity a waist circumference ≥102 cm (>40 inches) in men and ≥88 cm (>35 inches) in women. These thresholds were used by ATP III as one of the clinical criteria for metabolic syndrome; but the recent update diagnostic criteria indicated that some persons can develop metabolic syndrome at lesser waist circumferences. This is particularly the case in certain ethnic groups, for example, the populations of South and Southeast Asia.

The initial goal for obesity management is to reduce the body weight by 10 percent per year; an ultimate goal is to achieve a BMI <25 kg/m² over a longer period of time. Obesity guidelines[101] recommend caloric intake and behavioral change as first-line therapies

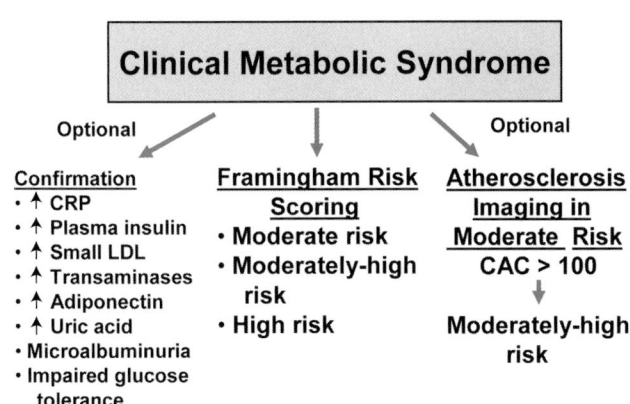

FIGURE 91–6. Approaches to cardiovascular risk assessment in patients with clinical evidence of the metabolic syndrome. All such patients should undergo Framingham risk scoring to determine 10-year risk for coronary heart disease (CHD). In addition, as an option, a series of biomarkers can be identified to support and confirm the presence of the metabolic syndrome. Another option is to use atherosclerosis imaging to bolster risk assessment carried out with Framingham scoring. Atherosclerosis imaging in patients with the metabolic syndrome is most appropriate for those found to be at moderate risk (10-year risk for CHD <10%) by Framingham scoring.

to achieve weight loss. Behavioral change should include increased physical activity as one of its components. The weight-reduction diet should not be a *crash* diet; they invariably fail in the long run. Extreme diets that allow for little variety in foods should be avoided. Many popular diets are of this type. Experience shows that they cannot be tolerated for a lifetime. Neither can their caloric adequacy be ensured. Instead, a *heart-healthy* diet of reduced caloric content can be recommended. A reduction of 500 to 1000 calories will achieve the desired 10 percent reduction in weight, depending on baseline weight.

A diet that is appropriate for long-term weight reduction should be consistent with current recommendations for a healthy diet in general. Emphasis should be given to reducing consumption of saturated and *trans-fatty* acids and cholesterol, reduced intake of simple sugars, and ample intakes of fruits, vegetables, and whole grains. Some investigators favor a relatively higher intake of unsaturated fatty acids at the expense of carbohydrates. This dietary pattern is similar to that of the *Mediterranean diet*. Avoidance of high-carbohydrate intakes will improve atherogenic dyslipidemia and will reduce postprandial rises in glucose and insulin. As mentioned before, extremes of high-fat or low-fat intakes should be avoided.

Behavioral change is the second major requirement for successful weight reduction. Without behavioral change, long-term weight loss will not be possible. It is rarely easy to reverse the lifetime of behavior that resulted in obesity. The earlier in life that obesity (or overweight) can be identified, the more effective will be the intervention. A few behavioral techniques to achieve a long-term weight loss include:

- Establishing weight goals (e.g., 10 percent loss of body weight in 1 year)
- Establishing physical activity (e.g., exercise 30 minutes daily)
- Learning to avoid situations where overeating is likely to occur
- Identifying circumstances leading to eating binges and avoiding them

- Establishing a regular eating schedule
- Avoiding eating or snacking between meals (eating on schedule)
- Taking smaller portions
- Eating slowly
- Keeping a diet diary (self-monitoring)
- Developing a social support structure
- Learning to manage stressful situations that foster overeating
- Developing a regular schedule for physical activity

Useful information on dietary change and behavioral modification can be obtained from the Web sites of the AHA (www.americanheart.org) and NHLBI (www.nhlbi.nih.gov).

Successful weight reduction will reduce all of metabolic syndrome risk factors—atherogenic dyslipidemia, blood pressure, plasma glucose, coagulation and fibrinolytic factors, and the proinflammatory state. The Diabetes Prevention Program (DPP)[102] and other studies showed that even moderate weight reduction will delay the conversion of impaired glucose tolerance (IGT)/impaired fasting glucose (IFG) into T2DM. In patients with IGT/IFG, it will reduce severity of metabolic syndrome.

Physical Inactivity

An extremely high portion of the United States population is sedentary.[103] There are multiple social trends leading to sedentary life habits. Among these are urbanization, mechanized transportation, reduced manual labor, and a variety of *labor-saving* devices. Physical inactivity is a major contributing cause of metabolic syndrome; moreover, regular physical activity and attaining physical fitness will improve most of metabolic risk factors. Increased physical fitness has been reported to reduce several chronic diseases including cardiovascular disease.

It is currently recommended that everyone engage in 30 minutes daily of moderate-intensity physical activity.[1] Even more benefit is achieved by increasing activity to 60 minutes daily.[1] The following are examples of moderate-intensity activity:

- Brisk walking, jogging, swimming, biking, golfing, team sports
- Using simple exercise equipment (e.g., treadmills)
- Several short (10 to 15 minutes) bouts of activity (brisk walking)
- Substituting more active leisure activities for sedentary ones (television watching and computer games)

【 】 MANAGEMENT OF METABOLIC RISK FACTORS

Lifestyle therapies are first-line therapies for metabolic syndrome and will improve all of the metabolic risk factors. But in higher risk patients, it can be necessary to turn to drug therapies to control the risk factors (Tables 91–2 and 91–3). The choice and intensity of drug therapy depends largely on the short-term risk of a patient. Also, the presence of metabolic syndrome itself can influence the particular drugs that are to be chosen.

Atherogenic Dyslipidemia

This condition is recognized clinically by an increase in serum triglyceride and a reduction in high-density lipoprotein-cholesterol (HDL-C). When triglycerides are elevated this is usually a sign of an increase in apo B-containing lipoproteins. The primary target

TABLE 91–2

Therapeutic Goals and Recommendations for Clinical Management of Metabolic Syndrome

THERAPEUTIC TARGET AND GOALS OF THERAPY	THERAPEUTIC RECOMMENDATIONS
Lifestyle Risk Factors Abdominal obesity Goal Reduce body weight by 7%–10% during first year of therapy. Continue weight loss thereafter to the extent possible with a goal to ultimately achieve desirable weight (BMI <25 kg/m²)	Long-term prevention of CVD and prevention (or treatment) of type II diabetes Consistently encourage weight maintenance/reduction through an appropriate balance of physical activity, caloric intake, and formal behavioral programs when indicated to maintain/achieve a waist circumference of <40 inches in men and <35 inches in women. Aim initially at a slow reduction of approximately 7%–10% from baseline weight. Even small amounts of weight loss are associated with significant health benefits.
Physical inactivity Goal Regular moderate-intensity physical activity. At least 30 minutes of continuous or intermittent (and preferably 60 or more minutes) 5 days/week, but preferably daily	In patients with established CVD, assess risk with a detailed physical activity history and/or an exercise test, to guide prescription. Encourage 30 to 60 or more minutes of moderate intensity aerobic activity such as brisk walking, preferably daily, supplemented by an increase in daily lifestyle activities (e.g., pedometer step tracking, walking breaks at work, gardening, household work). Higher exercise times can be achieved by accumulating exercise throughout the day. Encourage resistance training 2 days/week. Advise medically supervised programs for high-risk patients (e.g., recent acute coronary syndrome or revascularization, CHF).
Atherogenic diet Goal Reduced intakes of saturated fat, trans-fat, and cholesterol	Recommendations: saturated fat <7% of total calories; reduce trans-fat; dietary cholesterol <200 mg/dL; total fat 25%–35% of total calories. Most dietary fat should be unsaturated and simple sugars should be limited.
Metabolic Risk Factors Atherogenic dyslipidemia Goals Primary target: elevated LDL-C (see Table 91–3 for details) Secondary target: elevated non–HDL-C High-risk patientsª: (<130 mg/dL (3.4 mmol/L) (optional: <100 mg/dL for very high risk patientsᵇ) Moderately high-risk patientsᶜ: <160 mg/dL (4.1 mmol/L) Therapeutic option: <130 mg/dL (3.4 mmol/L) Moderate-risk patientsᵈ: <160 mg/dL 4.1 mmol/L) Lower-risk patientsᵉ <190 mg/dL (4.9 mmol/L) Tertiary target: reduced HDL-C No specific goal: raise HDL-C to extent possible with standard therapies for atherogenic dyslipidemia	Shorter-term prevention of CVD or treatment of type II diabetes Elevated LDL-C Elevated non–HDL-C Follow strategy outlined in Table 91–2 to achieve goal for LDL-C First option to achieve non–HDL-C goal: intensify LDL-lowering therapy Second option: add fibrate (preferably fenofibrate) or nicotinic acid if non–HDL-C remains relatively high after LDL-lowering drug therapy Give preference to adding fibrate or nicotinic acid in high-risk patients Give preference to avoiding addition of fibrate or nicotinic acid in moderately high risk or moderate risk patients All patients: If TG is ≥500 mg/dL, initiate fibrate or nicotinic acid (before LDL lowering therapy; treat non-LDL-C to goal after TG-lowering therapy). Reduced HDL-C Maximize lifestyle therapies: weight reduction and increased physical activity Consider adding fibrate or nicotinic acid after LDL-C lowering drug therapy as outlined for elevated non–HDL-C
Elevated BP	For BP ≥120/80 mm: initiate or maintain lifestyle modification—weight control, increased physical activity, alcohol moderation, sodium reduction, and emphasis on increased consumption of fresh fruits vegetables and low fat dairy products — in all patients with metabolic syndrome.

TABLE 91-2

Therapeutic Goals and Recommendations for Clinical Management of Metabolic Syndrome *(continued)*

THERAPEUTIC TARGET AND GOALS OF THERAPY	THERAPEUTIC RECOMMENDATIONS
Goals Reduce BP to at least achieve a BP of <140/90 mmHg (or <130/80 mmHg if diabetes present). Reduce BP further to the extent possible through lifestyle changes.	For BP ≥140/90 mm Hg (or ≥130/80 mm Hg for individuals with chronic kidney disease or diabetes): as tolerated, add blood pressure medication as needed to achieve goal blood pressure.
Elevated glucose Goals For IFG, delay progression to type II diabetes For diabetes, HbA_{1c} <7.0%	For IFG, encourage weight reduction and increased physical activity. For type II diabetes, lifestyle therapy, and pharmacotherapy, if necessary, should be used to achieve near normal HbA_{1c} (<7%). Modify other risk factors and behaviors (e.g., abdominal obesity, physical inactivity, elevated blood pressure, lipid abnormalities).
Prothrombotic state Goals: Reduce thrombotic and fibrinolytic risk factors	High-risk patients: initiate and continue low-dose aspirin therapy; in patients with ASCVD, consider clopidogrel if aspirin is contraindicated. Moderately high-risk patients: consider low-dose aspirin prophylaxis
Proinflammatory state	Recommendations: no specific therapies beyond lifestyle therapies

ASCVD, arteriosclerotic cardiovascular disease; BP, blood pressure; BMI, body mass index; CHF, congestive heart failure; CVD, cardiovascular disease; HbA_{1c}, glycosylated hemoglobin; HDL-C, high-density lipoprotein-cholesterol; IFG, impaired fasting glucose; LDL-C, low-density lipoprotein-cholesterol; TG, triglyceride; TIA, transient ischemic attack.

[a]High-risk patients: those with established arteriosclerotic cardiovascular disease, diabetes, or 10-year risk for coronary heart disease >20%. For cerebrovascular disease, high-risk condition includes TIA or stroke of carotid origin or >50% carotid stenosis.

[b]Very high-risk patients are those who are likely to have major CVD events in the next few years, and diagnosis depends on clinical assessment. Factors that can confer very high risk include recent acute coronary syndromes, and established CHD+ any of the following: multiple major risk factors [especially diabetes], severe and poorly controlled risk factors [especially continued cigarette smoking] and metabolic syndrome.

[c]Moderately high-risk patients: those with 10-year risk for coronary heart disease 10%–20%. Factors that favor the therapeutic option of non–HDL-C <100 mg/dL are those that can raise persons to the upper range of moderately high risk: multiple major risk factors, severe and poorly controlled risk factors (especially continued cigarette smoking), metabolic syndrome, and documented advanced subclinical arteriosclerotic disease [e.g., coronary calcium or carotid intimal-medial thickness >75th percentile for age and sex].

[d]Moderate-risk patients: those with 2+ major risk factors and 10-year risk <10%.

[e]Lower-risk patients: those with 0–1 major risk factor and 10-year risk <10%.

of lipid-lowering therapy in all patients is low-density lipoprotein-cholesterol (LDL-C),[4] which normally contains most of the apo B (see Table 91–3 for ATP III recommendations for management of elevated LDL-C.[1,4,104] In patients with metabolic syndrome who have high triglycerides, a sizable portion of apo B can be in very-low-density lipoprotein (VLDL). For this reason, it is useful to make LDL and VLDL a secondary target of therapy. An increase in LDL and VLDL is most readily identified by an elevation of non–HDL-C.[4] Total apo B is an alternate secondary target, but non–HDL-C is strongly correlated with total apo B. The goals for non–HDL-C are 30 mg/dL higher than those for LDL-C. A low level of HDL-C can be considered a tertiary target. After the goals for LDL-C and non–HDL-C have been achieved, consideration can be given to therapies that can raise HDL-C levels.

Clinical trials have been carried out to determine the efficacy of reducing apo B-containing lipoproteins for reducing risk for cardiovascular events. The most effective drugs for reducing these lipoproteins are statins; most of the trials have used statins as the therapeutic intervention. These trials have not specifically targeted patients with metabolic syndrome, but several of them have included subgroups with either metabolic syndrome or type II diabetes. Most of

the statin trials can be classified as secondary prevention trials, although several have been performed in patients without established ASCVD (primary prevention). The following statin trials have examined outcomes in subgroups with metabolic syndrome or type II diabetes: the Air Force Coronary Atherosclerosis Prevention Study (AFCAPS)/Texas Coronary Atherosclerosis Prevention Study (TEXCAPS), WOSCOPS, Scandinavian Simvastatin Survival Study (4S), CARE, and LIPID, HPS, Anglo-Scandinavian Cardiac Outcomes Trial (ASCOT), and Treating to New Targets (TNT).[104–113] In virtually all of these trials, patients with either metabolic syndrome or type II diabetes benefitted from statin therapy. These trials support the use of drugs that reduce apo B-containing lipoprotein in the treatment of patients with metabolic syndrome. Two clinical trials with statin therapy have specifically targeted type II diabetes. In the Collaborative Atorvastatin Diabetes Study (CARDS) trial,[114] statin treatment showed a 37 percent reduction in major coronary events by reduction of apo B-containing lipoproteins with a statin. In the Atorvastatin Study for Prevention of Coronary Heart Disease Endpoints in Noninsulin-Dependent Diabetes Mellitus (ASPEN) trial,[115] statin therapy showed a trend toward benefit in reduction of ASCVD events, although results for the primary composite ASCVD out-

TABLE 91–3

Elevated LDL Cholesterol: Primary Target of Lipid-Lowering Therapy in Persons at Risk for Arteriosclerotic Cardiovascular Disease

GOALS OF THERAPY	THERAPEUTIC RECOMMENDATIONS
High-risk patients[a]: <100 mg/dL (2.6 mmol/L) (for very high risk patients,[b] in this category, optional goal <70 mg/dL) Moderately high-risk patients[c]: <130 mg/dL (3.4 mmol/L) (for higher risk patients[d] in this category, optional goal is <100 mg/dL (2.6 mmol/L) Moderate-risk patients[e]: <130 mg/dL (3.4 mmol/L) Low-risk patients[e]: <160 mg/dL (4.9 mmol/L)	High-risk patients: lifestyle therapies[g] plus LDL-C lowering drug to achieve recommended goal. If baseline LDL-C ≥100 mg/dL, initiate LDL-lowering drug therapy If on-treatment LDL-C ≥100 mg/dL, intensify LDL-lowering drug therapy (can require LDL-lowering drug combination) If baseline LDL-C <100 mg/dL, initiate LDL-lowering therapy based on clinical judgment, i.e. assessment that the patient is at very high risk Moderately high-risk patients: lifestyle therapies + LDL-lowering drug if necessary to achieve recommended goal when LDL-C ≥130 mg/dL (3.4 mmol/L) after lifestyle therapies If baseline LDL-C is 100–129 mg/dL, LDL-lowering therapy can be introduced if patient's risk is assessed to be in the upper ranges of this risk category Moderate-risk patients: lifestyle therapies + LDL-C lowering drug if necessary to achieve recommended goal when LDL-C ≥160 mg/dL (4.1 mmol/L) after lifestyle therapies Lower-risk patients: lifestyle therapies + LDL-C lowering drug if necessary to achieve recommended goal when LDL-C ≥190 mg/dL after lifestyle therapies (for LDL-C 160–189 mg/dL, LDL-lowering drug is optional)

CHD, coronary heart disease; CVD, cardiovascular disease; LDL-C, low-density lipoprotein-cholesterol; TIA, transient ischemic attack.
[a]High-risk patients: those with established arteriosclerotic cardiovascular disease, diabetes, or 10-year risk for coronary heart disease >20%. For cerebrovascular disease, high-risk condition includes TIA or stroke of carotid origin or >50% carotid stenosis.
[b]Very high-risk patients are those who are likely to have major CVD events in the next few years, and diagnosis depends on clinical assessment. Factors that can confer very high risk include recent acute coronary syndromes, and established CHD + any of the following: multiple major risk factors (especially diabetes), severe and poorly controlled risk factors (especially continued cigarette smoking), and multiple risk factors of the metabolic syndrome.
[c]Moderately high-risk patients: those with 10-year risk for coronary heart disease 10%–20%.
[d]Factors that can raise persons to the upper range of moderately high risk are multiple major risk factors, severe and poorly controlled risk factors (especially continued cigarette smoking), metabolic syndrome, and documented advanced subclinical arteriosclerotic disease [e.g., coronary calcium or carotid intimal-medial thickness >75th percentile for age and sex]).
[e]Moderate-risk patients: those with 2+ major risk factors and 10-year risk <10%.
[f]Lower-risk patients: those with 0–1 major risk factor and 10-year risk <10%.
[g]Lifestyle therapies include weight reduction, increased physical activity, and antiatherogenic diet (see Table 91–2 for details).

come were not statistically significant. However, this trial appeared to suffer from inadequate statistical power to allow for a robust testing of the primary hypothesis.

Two other classes of drugs have been used for treatment of atherogenic dyslipidemia. These are nicotinic acid and fibrates. Their primary actions are to reduce triglyceride-rich lipoproteins and to raise HDL.[4] Both lower triglycerides similarly, whereas nicotinic acid raises HDL more than do fibrates. Several clinical trials have been performed with these classes of agents.[4] Again metabolic syndrome has not been the primary target of therapy. However, subgroup analyses strongly suggest that the greatest reduction in cardiovascular events occurs in patients who have many of the features of metabolic syndrome. The trials (and drugs used) include the Helsinki Heart Study (gemfibrozil),[116] VA-HIT (gemfibrozil),[117] the Stockholm study (clofibrate + nicotinic acid),[118] BIP (bezafibrate),[119,120] FIELD (fenofibrate),[121] and the Coronary Drug Project (nicotinic acid).[122,123] The results of these studies provide a rationale for using either nicotinic acid or a fibrate as *add-on* therapy to statins or other LDL-lowering drugs.[124,125]

For secondary prevention, that is, in patients with established ASCVD, the first goal of therapy is to reduce LDL-C to <100 mg/ dL and non–HDL-C to <130 mg/dL. These goals are strongly supported by clinical trial evidence.[4,104] Recent studies suggest lowering of LDL-C to well below 100 mg/dL will further reduce risk for future cardiovascular events in patients with established ASCVD.[104,126,127] Although the database supporting this lower goal is not as strong as for an LDL-C <100 mg/dL (non–HDL-C <130 mg/dL), the evidence is mounting that "the lower, the better" for apo B-containing lipoproteins in these patients who are at very high risk for future ASCVD events. For ASCVD patients with either metabolic syndrome or type II diabetes, subgroup analysis of clinical trials suggest that further lowering of LDL-C to <70 mg/dL (non–HDL-C to <100 mg/dL) is reasonable.[104,111,112,128]

For primary prevention, the therapeutic goals for lipids depend on the absolute risk of patients. Any patient who has metabolic syndrome with type II diabetes deserves to have the LDL-C reduced to <100 mg/dL (non–HDL-C <130 mg/dL).[4,129] The same would be true for patients with metabolic syndrome who have a 10-year risk for major coronary events by Framingham scoring of >20 percent.[1,4] In fact, it is reasonable to reduce LDL-C to <100 mg/dL (non–HDL-C <130 mg/dL) in metabolic syndrome patients whose 10-year risk for CHD is 10 to 20 percent.[104]

If a decision is made to drive the LDL-C (and non–HDL-C) to the lower ranges, which is considered reasonable for the higher risk patients with metabolic syndrome, the choice of therapies becomes important. Several alternative approaches are available.[104,128] For example, it is possible to increase the intensity of statin therapy from standard doses to high doses. The efficacy of this approach has recently been shown for the TNT trials in patients with metabolic syndrome with or without type II diabetes.[111,112] Besides increasing statin therapy, lower LDL levels can be obtained by combining a standard dose of statins with either ezetimibe or a bile acid sequestrant. To date, the added benefit of such combinations has not been documented through clinical trials. Another alternative is to combine a standard dose of statin with either nicotinic acid or fibrate.[104,128] Again however, clinical trials have not been carried out to demonstrate added efficacy.

Finally, the question of whether to specifically target a low HDL level in patients with metabolic syndrome has not been resolved. The only drug that has a substantial HDL-raising potential is nicotinic acid; but because this drug also lowers apo B-containing lipoproteins, it is not possible to attribute any benefit from nicotinic acid therapy specifically to HDL raising. Other drugs are in development that are more selective in HDL raising; therefore, in the next few years, it will be known whether raising HDL has utility beyond reduction in the known atherogenic lipoproteins.

Elevated Blood Pressure

Most patients with metabolic syndrome have mild elevation in blood pressure. ATP III defined elevated blood pressure as a component of metabolic syndrome when the blood pressure level is ≥130 mmHg systolic or ≥85 mmHg diastolic. The Seventh Report of the Joint National Committee (JNC 7) provides useful guidelines for management of blood pressure.[130] JNC 7 emphasized lifestyle therapy as first-line therapy. When lifestyle changes do not reduce the blood pressure to <140/90 mmHg, drug therapy must be considered. These guidelines do not identify a priority in choice of drugs. JNC 7 gave priority to diuretics and β blockers because of proven clinical and cost effectiveness. However, high doses of these drugs can increase insulin resistance and raise the plasma glucose. Because of the latter, they can convert prediabetes into categorical diabetes. These side effects must be taken into account when diuretics and β blockers are used in patients with metabolic syndrome and diabetes. Doses of these drugs should be kept as low as possible. Use of aldosterone receptor blockers (eplerenone or spironolactone) is one alternative to thiazides.

Some investigators propose that angiotensin-converting enzyme inhibitors (ACEIs) or angiotensin-receptor blockers (ARBs) should be first-line therapy in patients with metabolic syndrome.[131–133] The rationale for this position is based on results of some but not all clinical trials. The combination of ACEI (or ARB) plus low-dose thiazide is especially efficacious and appears to be preferable to a high dose of diuretic. Other antihypertensive drugs (calcium channel blockers, α_1 blockers and central α_2 blockers) seemingly have no adverse metabolic effect in patients with metabolic syndrome.[130] It is well known that multiple anti-hypertensive drugs in combination can be required to achieve goals for blood pressure lowering.

In patients with metabolic syndrome, but without type II diabetes or chronic renal failure, the goal is to reduce blood pressure to <140/90 mmHg.[130] When type II diabetes or renal failure is present, lowering the pressure to <130/80 mmHg appears to provide added risk reduction.[130]

Elevated Plasma Glucose

Approximately one-half of all patients with metabolic syndrome have prediabetes (impaired glucose tolerance and/or impaired fasting glucose).[3] Another one-third with metabolic syndrome have type II diabetes. At the same time, approximately three-fourths of persons with prediabetes have metabolic syndrome, and approximately 85 percent of those with diabetes have the syndrome.[3] Therefore, there is a high prevalence of dysglycemia in patients with metabolic syndrome and vice versa.[2] One of the goals for treatment of prediabetes is to curtail progression to type II diabetes. Ample clinical trial evidence shows that progression can be retarded or prevented. The DPP[102] demonstrated that lifestyle change (weight reduction and increased physical activity) will reduce progression of prediabetes to diabetes by approximately 60 percent. By comparison, the DPP further showed that metformin therapy will reduce conversion by approximately 40 percent. A thiazolidinedione (TZD) named troglitazone also was used in the DPP; but it was withdrawn because of liver toxicity. Even so, post hoc analysis of the preliminary data obtained with this drug indicated a strong trend toward reduction in conversion of prediabetes to diabetes.[134] Another smaller study, TRIPOD, showed a similar trend.[135] Recently the Diabetes Reduction Assessment with Ramipril and Rosiglitazone Medication (DREAM) study[136] demonstrated that another TZD, rosiglitazone, will also decrease conversion by approximately 60 percent. The DREAM study confirms trends noted in previous results with TZDs. At present TZDs are commonly used for treatment of hyperglycemia in type II diabetes. The question raised by DPP and DREAM is whether drug therapy is warranted to slow progression of prediabetes to diabetes. There is universal agreement that prevention of prediabetes to diabetes with lifestyle therapies is warranted. But whether drugs such as metformin and thiazolidinediones are safe and cost effective for the same purpose has not been resolved. This is particularly the case because treatment of prediabetes with these drugs has not been shown to reduce the risk for cardiovascular disease in patients with prediabetes.

Patients with type II diabetes are at high risk for developing ASCVD. This high risk is largely caused by the coexistence of metabolic syndrome.[3] Therefore, the therapeutic goal for reduction of ASCVD events in patients with type II diabetes is to treat all of the risk factors associated with metabolic syndrome. In addition, the LDL-C should be reduced to <100 mg/dL (non–HDL-C to <130 mg/dL); if ASCVD is present simultaneously, further reduction of these lipids to even lower levels is reasonable. The therapeutic options to achieve lower lipid levels were considered previously under the Atherogenic Dyslipidemia section. Blood pressure should be lowered to <130/80 mmHg, and to <120/80 mg/dL if safe. Every effort should be made to achieve smoking cessation, if the patient with diabetes is a smoker. Finally, the glycosylated hemoglobin (HbA$_{1c}$) levels should be reduced to the range of 6 to 7 percent. Choice of hypoglycemic drugs should be individualized according to available therapies and clinical judgment.

Prothrombotic State

The only widely used therapy currently available for the routine treatment of a prothrombotic state is aspirin. Other antiplatelet drugs or anticoagulants generally are reserved for special clinical circumstances. Current guidelines indicate that aspirin prophylaxis is indicated when the 10-year risk for CHD is ≥10 percent as determined by Framingham risk scoring or when patients have established ASCVD.[137] This recommendation seems appropriate for patients with metabolic syndrome who are known to have increases in prothrombotic factors.

Proinflammatory State

Metabolic syndrome is characterized by increases in circulating cytokines (e.g., TNF-α and IL-6). Secondarily elevations in acute phase reactants (high sensitivity [hs]-CRP and fibrinogen) can be present.[138] Measurement of hs-CRP is a widely accepted way to identify the presence of a proinflammatory state. The AHA/Center for Disease Control (CDC)[139] report outlined recommendations for use of hs-CRP as a marker for a proinflammatory state in clinical practice. The hs-CRP can be measured at physician discretion but is generally most useful in patients whose 10-year risk for CHD is in the range of 10 to 20 percent. If the hs-CRP level is ≥3 mg/L, therapeutic lifestyle changes should be emphasized. Whether to modify drug therapy based on hs-CRP levels is uncertain. Some investigators also believe that for patients who have metabolic syndrome plus an elevated hs-CRP, the LDL-C goal should be lower (e.g., <100 mg/dL).

CONCLUSIONS

The cardiovascular specialist and other healthcare providers must place increased emphasis on the diagnosis and early treatment of patients with metabolic syndrome. Left unchecked the sharp rise in obesity and its concomitant metabolic risk both in the United States and worldwide will result in a major worldwide increase in cardiovascular events and mortality. Unfortunately, in no country is the healthcare system prepared to deal with this emerging medical crisis. Perhaps a focus on metabolic syndrome will encourage public heath efforts to give more priority to the promotion of weight control and physical activities in their societies. This will require a reconfiguration of healthcare systems to invest more on preventive medicine. Failure to take the obesity/metabolic syndrome epidemic seriously will result in a social catastrophe, not to mention enormous personal suffering in the 21st century.

REFERENCES

1. Grundy SM, Cleeman JI, Daniels SR, Donato KA, Eckel RH, Franklin BA, et al for the American Heart Association; National Heart, Lung, and Blood Institute. Diagnosis and management of the metabolic syndrome: an American Heart Association/National Heart, Lung, and Blood Institute Scientific Statement. *Circulation.* 2005;112(17):2735–2752.
2. Grundy SM. Metabolic syndrome: connecting and reconciling cardiovascular and diabetes worlds. *J Am Coll Cardiol.* 2006;47(6):1093–1100.
3. Alexander CM, Landsman PB, Grundy SM. Metabolic syndrome and hyperglycemia: congruence and divergence. *Am J Cardiol.* 2006;98(7):982–985.
4. National Cholesterol Education Program (NCEP) Expert Panel on Detection, Evaluation, and Treatment of High Blood Cholesterol in Adults (Adult Treatment Panel III). Third Report of the National Cholesterol Education Program (NCEP) Expert Panel on Detection, Evaluation, and Treatment of High Blood Cholesterol in Adults (Adult Treatment Panel III) final report. *Circulation.* 2002;106(25):3143–3421.
5. Meigs JB, D'Agostino RB Sr, Wilson PW, Cupples LA, Nathan DM, Singer DE. Risk variable clustering in the insulin resistance syndrome. The Framingham Offspring Study. *Diabetes.* 1997;46(10):1594–1600.
6. Hoffmann IS, Cubeddu LX. Clustering of silent cardiovascular risk factors in apparently healthy Hispanics. *J Hum Hypertens.* 2002;16(suppl 1):S137–S141.
7. Hanley AJ, Karter AJ, Festa A, D'Agostino R Jr, Wagenknecht LE, Savage P, et al. Factor analysis of metabolic syndrome using directly measured insulin sensitivity: the Insulin Resistance Atherosclerosis Study. *Diabetes.* 2002;51(8):2642–2647.
8. Choi KM, Lee J, Kim KB, Kim DR, Kim SK, Shin DH, et al. Factor analysis of the metabolic syndrome among elderly Koreans—the South-West Seoul study. *Diabet Med.* 2003;20(2):99–104.
9. Shen BJ, Todaro JF, Niaura R, McCaffery JM, Zhang J, Spiro A 3rd, et al. Are metabolic risk factors one unified syndrome? Modeling the structure of the metabolic syndrome X. *Am J Epidemiol.* 2003;157(8):701–711.
10. Novak S, Stapleton LM, Litaker JR, Lawson KA. A confirmatory factor analysis evaluation of the coronary heart disease risk factors of metabolic syndrome with emphasis on the insulin resistance factor. *Diabetes Obes Metab.* 2003;5(6):388–396.
11. Tang W, Miller MB, Rich SS, North KE, Pankow JS, Borecki IB, et al. Linkage analysis of a composite factor for the multiple metabolic syndrome: the National Heart, Lung, and Blood Institute Family Heart Study. *Diabetes.* 2003;52(11):2840–2847.
12. Goodman E, Dolan LM, Morrison JA, Daniels SR. Factor analysis of clustered cardiovascular risks in adolescence: obesity is the predominant correlate of risk among youth. *Circulation.* 2005;111(15):1970–1977.
13. Aizawa Y, Kamimura N, Watanabe H, Aizawa Y, Makiyama Y, Usuda Y, et al. Cardiovascular risk factors are really linked in the metabolic syndrome: this phenomenon suggests clustering rather than coincidence. *Int J Cardiol.* 2006;109(2):213–218.
14. Girman CJ, Dekker JM, Rhodes T, Nijpels G, Stehouwer CD, Bouter LM, et al. An exploratory analysis of criteria for the metabolic syndrome and its prediction of long-term cardiovascular outcomes: the Hoorn study. *Am J Epidemiol.* 2005;162(5):438–447.
15. Esmaillzadeh A, Mirmiran P, Azizi F. Clustering of metabolic abnormalities in adolescents with the hypertriglyceridemic waist phenotype. *Am J Clin Nutr.* 2006;83(1):36–46.
16. Zanolin ME, Tosi F, Zoppini G, Castello R, Spiazzi G, Dorizzi R, et al. Clustering of cardiovascular risk factors associated with the insulin resistance syndrome: assessment by principal component analysis in young hyperandrogenic women. *Diabetes Care.* 2006;29(2):372–378.
17. Tang W, Hong Y, Province MA, Rich SS, Hopkins PN, Arnett DK, et al. Familial clustering for features of the metabolic syndrome: the National Heart, Lung, and Blood Institute (NHLBI) Family Heart Study. *Diabetes Care.* 2006;29(3):631–636.
18. Pladevall M, Singal B, Williams LK, Brotons C, Guyer H, Sadurni J, et al. A single factor underlies the metabolic syndrome: a confirmatory factor analysis. *Diabetes Care.* 2006;29(1):113-122.
19. Nielsen LB. Transfer of low density lipoprotein into the arterial wall and risk of atherosclerosis. *Atherosclerosis.* 1996;123(1–2):1–15.
20. Williams KJ, Tabas I. Lipoprotein retentionóand clues for atheroma regression. *Arterioscler Thromb Vasc Biol.* 2005;25(8):1536–1540.
21. Oorni K, Pentikainen MO, Ala-Korpela M, Kovanen PT. Aggregation, fusion, and vesicle formation of modified low density lipoprotein particles: molecular mechanisms and effects on matrix interactions. *J Lipid Res.* 2000;41(11):1703–1714.
22. Libby P, Ridker PM, Maseri A. Inflammation and atherosclerosis. *Circulation.* 2002;105(9):1135–1143.
23. van Zonneveld AJ, Rabelink TJ. Endothelial progenitor cells: biology and therapeutic potential in hypertension. *Curr Opin Nephrol Hypertens.* 2006;15(2):167–172.
24. Hernandez-Presa M, Bustos C, Ortego M, et al. Angiotensin-converting enzyme inhibition prevents arterial nuclear factor-B activation, monocyte chemoattractant protein-1 expression, and macrophage infiltration in a rabbit model of early accelerated atherosclerosis. *Circulation.* 1997;95:1532–1541.

25. Tummala PE, Chen XL, Sundell CL, et al. Angiotensin II induces vascular cell adhesion molecule-1 expression in rat vasculature: a potential link between the renin-angiotensin system and atherosclerosis. *Circulation.* 1999;100:1223–1229.

26. Aronson D, Rayfield EJ. How hyperglycemia promotes atherosclerosis: molecular mechanisms. *Cardiovasc Diabetol.* 2002;1:1.

27. Brewer HB Jr, Santamarina-Fojo S. Clinical significance of high-density lipoproteins and the development of atherosclerosis: focus on the role of the adenosine triphosphate-binding cassette protein A1 transporter. *Am J Cardiol.* 2003;92(4B):10K–16K.

28. von Eckardstein A, Hersberger M, Rohrer L. Current understanding of the metabolism and biological actions of HDL. *Curr Opin Clin Nutr Metab Care.* 2005;8(2):147–152.

29. Navab M, Anantharamaiah GM, Fogelman AM. The role of high-density lipoprotein in inflammation. *Trends Cardiovasc Med.* 2005;15(4):158–161.

30. Matsuzawa Y. The metabolic syndrome and adipocytokines. *FEBS Lett.* 2006;580(12):2917–2921.

31. Piche ME, Lemieux S, Weisnagel SJ, Corneau L, Nadeau A, Bergeron J. Relation of high-sensitivity C-reactive protein, interleukin-6 tumor necrosis factor-alpha, and fibrinogen to abdominal adipose tissue, blood pressure, and cholesterol and triglyceride levels in healthy postmenopausal women. *Am J Cardiol.* 2005;96(1):92–97.

32. Kohler HP. Insulin resistance syndrome: interaction with coagulation and fibrinolysis. *Swiss Med Wkly.* 2002;132(19–20):241–252.

33. Schneider DJ. Abnormalities of coagulation, platelet function, and fibrinolysis associated with syndromes of insulin resistance. *Coron Artery Dis.* 2005;16(8):473–476.

34. Ford ES, Giles WH, Dietz WH. Prevalence of the metabolic syndrome among U.S. adults. Findings from the Third National Health and Nutrition Survey. *JAMA.* 2002;287:356–359.

35. Eckel RH, Grundy SM, Zimmet PZ. The metabolic syndrome: epidemiology, mechanisms, and therapy. *Lancet.* 2005;365:1415–1428.

36. Silventoinen K, Sans S, Tolonen H, et al. WHO MONICA Project. Trends in obesity and energy supply in the WHO MONICA Project. *Int J Obes Relat Metab Disord.* 2004;28:710–718.

37. Wang Y, Monteiro C, Popkin BM. Trends of obesity and underweight in older children and adolescents in the United States, Brazil, China, and Russia. *Am J Clin Nutr.* 2002;75:971–977.

38. Rennie KL, Jebb SA. Prevalence of obesity in Great Britain. *Obes Rev.* 2005;6:11–12.

38a. Luo J, Hu FB. Time trends of obesity in preschool children in China from 1989 to 1997. *Int J Obes Relat Metab Disord.* 2002;26:553–558.

39. Ogden CL, Carroll MD, Curtin LR, McDowell MA, Tabak CJ, Flegal KM. Prevalence of overweight and obesity in the United States, 1999–2004. *JAMA.* 2006;295(13):1549–1555.

40. Park YW, Zhu S, Palaniappan L, Heshka S, Carnethon MR, Heymsfield SB. The metabolic syndrome: prevalence and associated risk factor findings in the U.S. population from the Third National Health and Nutrition Examination Survey, 1988–1994. *Arch Intern Med.* 2003;163(4):427–436.

41. Ford ES, Kohl HW 3rd, Mokdad AH, Ajani UA. Sedentary behavior, physical activity, and the metabolic syndrome among U.S. adults. *Obes Res.* 2005;13(3):608–614.

42. Kelishadi R, Razaghi EM, Gouya MM, Ardalan G, Gheiratmand R, Delavari A, et al. Association of physical activity and the metabolic syndrome in children and adolescents: CASPIAN Study. *Horm Res.* 2006;67(1):46–52.

43. Platat C, Wagner A, Klumpp T, Schweitzer B, Simon C. Relationships of physical activity with metabolic syndrome features and low-grade inflammation in adolescents. *Diabetologia.* 2006;49(9):2078–2085.

44. Bauduceau B, Baigts F, Bordier L, Burnat P, Ceppa F, Dumenil V, et al for the Epimil group. Epidemiology of the metabolic syndrome in 2045 French military personnel (EPIMIL study). *Diabetes Metab.* 2005;31(4 pt 1):353–359.

45. Misra KB, Endemann SW, Ayer M. Leisure time physical activity and metabolic syndrome in Asian Indian immigrants residing in northern California. *Ethn Dis.* Autumn 2005;15(4):627–634.

46. Mohan V, Gokulakrishnan K, Deepa R, Shanthirani CS, Datta M. Association of physical inactivity with components of metabolic syndrome and coronary artery disease—the Chennai Urban Population Study (CUPS no. 15). *Diabet Med.* 2005;22(9):1206–1211.

47. Slentz CA, Aiken LB, Houmard JA, Bales CW, Johnson JL, Tanner CJ, et al. Inactivity, exercise, and visceral fat. STRRIDE. a randomized, controlled study of exercise intensity and amount. *J Appl Physiol.* 2005;99(4):1613–1618.

48. Ekelund U, Brage S, Franks PW, Hennings S, Emms S, Wareham NJ. Physical activity energy expenditure predicts progression toward the metabolic syndrome independently of aerobic fitness in middle-aged healthy Caucasians: the Medical Research Council Ely Study. *Diabetes Care.* 2005;28(5):1195–1200.

49. Grundy SM, Abate N, Chandalia M. Diet composition and the metabolic syndrome: what is the optimal fat intake? *Am J Med.* 2002;113(suppl 9B):25S–29S.

50. McKeown NM, Meigs JB, Liu S, Saltzman E, Wilson PW, Jacques PF. Carbohydrate nutrition, insulin resistance, and the prevalence of the metabolic syndrome in the Framingham Offspring Cohort. *Diabetes Care.* 2004;27(2):538–546.

51. Reaven GM. The insulin resistance syndrome: definition and dietary approaches to treatment. *Annu Rev Nutr.* 2005;25:391–406.

52. Volek JS, Feinman RD. Carbohydrate restriction improves the features of metabolic syndrome. Metabolic syndrome may be defined by the response to carbohydrate restriction. *Nutr Metab (Lond).* 2005;2:31.

53. Bergman RN, Van Citters GW, Mittelman SD, Dea MK, Hamilton-Wessler M, Kim SP, et al. Central role of the adipocyte in the metabolic syndrome. *J Investig Med.* 2001;49(1):119–126.

54. Trayhurn P, Wood IS. Adipokines: inflammation and the pleiotropic role of white adipose tissue. *Br J Nutr.* 2004;92(3):347–355.

55. Weisberg SP, McCann D, Desai M, Rosenbaum M, Leibel RL, Ferrante AW Jr. Obesity is associated with macrophage accumulation in adipose tissue. *J Clin Invest.* 2003;112(12):1796–1808.

56. Juhan-Vague I, Alessi MC, Mavri A, Morange PE. Plasminogen activator inhibitor-1 inflammation, obesity, insulin resistance and vascular risk. *J Thromb Haemost.* 2003;1(7):1575–1579.

57. Lee Y, Wang MY, Kakuma T, Wang ZW, Babcock E, McCorkle K, et al. Liporegulation in diet-induced obesity. The antisteatotic role of hypoleptinemia. *J Biol Chem.* 2001;276(8):5629–5635.

58. Morton NM, Paterson JM, Masuzaki H, Holmes MC, Staels B, Fievet C, et al. Novel adipose tissue-mediated resistance to diet-induced visceral obesity in 11 beta-hydroxysteroid dehydrogenase type 1-deficient mice. *Diabetes.* 2004;53(4):931–938.

59. Kannisto K, Pietiläinen KH, Ehrenborg E, Rissanen A, Kaprio J, Hamsten A, et al. Overexpression of 11 beta-hydroxysteroid dehydrogenase-1 in adipose tissue is associated with acquired obesity and features of insulin resistance: studies in young adult monozygotic twins. *J Clin Endocrinol Metab.* 2004;89(9):4414–4421.

60. Hara T, Fujiwara H, Shoji T, Mimura T, Nakao H, Fujimoto S. Decreased plasma adiponectin levels in young obese males. *J Atheroscler Thromb.* 2003;10(4):234–238.

61. Kern PA, Di Gregorio GB, Lu T, Rassouli N, Ranganathan G. Adiponectin expression from human adipose tissue: relation to obesity, insulin resistance, and tumor necrosis factor-alpha expression. *Diabetes.* 2003;52(7):1779–1785.

62. Trujillo ME, Scherer PE. Adiponectin—journey from an adipocyte secretory protein to biomarker of the metabolic syndrome. *J Intern Med.* 2005;257(2):167–175.

63. Berg AH, Scherer PE. Adipose tissue, inflammation, and cardiovascular disease. *Circ Res.* 2005;96(9):939–949.

64. Garg A. Acquired and inherited lipodystrophies. *N Engl J Med.* 2004;350(12):1220–1234.

65. Vega GL, Adams-Huet B, Peshock R, Willett D, Shah B, Grundy SM. Influence of body fat content and distribution on variation in metabolic risk. *J Clin Endocrinol Metab.* 2006;91(11):4459–4466.

66. Browning JD, Szczepaniak LS, Dobbins R, et al. Prevalence of hepatic steatosis in an urban population in the United States: impact of ethnicity. *Hepatology.* 2004;40(6):1387–1395.

67. Matsuzawa Y. The metabolic syndrome and adipocytokines. *FEBS Lett.* 2006;580(12):2917–2921.

68. Abate N, Chandalia M, Snell PG, Grundy SM. Adipose tissue metabolites and insulin resistance in nondiabetic Asian Indian men. *J Clin Endocrinol Metab.* 2004;89(6):2750–2755.

69. Petersen KF, Befroy D, Dufour S, Dziura J, Ariyan C, Rothman DL, et al. Mitochondrial dysfunction in the elderly: possible role in insulin resistance. *Science.* 2003;300(5622):1140–1142.

70. Yki-Jarvinen H. Fat in the liver and insulin resistance. *Ann Med.* 2005;37(5):347–356.

71. Agarwal AK, Garg A. Genetic disorders of adipose tissue development, differentiation, and death. *Annu Rev Genomics Hum Genet.* 2006;7:175–199.

72. Tong Q, Dalgin G, Xu H, Ting CN, Leiden JM, Hotamisligil GS. Function of GATA transcription factors in preadipocyte-adipocyte transition. *Science.* 2000;290(5489):134–138.

73. Liu J, Farmer SR. Regulating the balance between peroxisome proliferator-activated receptor gamma and beta-catenin signaling during adipogenesis. A glycogen synthase kinase 3-beta-phosphorylation-defective mutant of beta-

catenin inhibits expression of a subset of adipogenic genes. *J Biol Chem.* 2004;279(43):45020–45027.

74. Hara-Chikuma M, Sohara E, Rai T, Ikawa M, Okabe M, Sasaki S, et al. Progressive adipocyte hypertrophy in aquaporin-7-deficient mice: adipocyte glycerol permeability as a novel regulator of fat accumulation. *J Biol Chem.* 2005;280(16):15493–15496.

75. Langin D, Dicker A, Tavernier G, Hoffstedt J, Mairal A, Ryden M, et al. Adipocyte lipases and defect of lipolysis in human obesity. *Diabetes.* 2005;54(11):3190–3197.

76. Zimmermann R, Strauss JG, Haemmerle G, Schoiswohl G, Birner-Gruenberger R, Riederer M, et al. Fat mobilization in adipose tissue is promoted by adipose triglyceride lipase. *Science.* 2004;306(5700):1383–1386.

77. Lass A, Zimmermann R, Haemmerle G, Riederer M, Schoiswohl G, Schweiger M, et al. Adipose triglyceride lipase-mediated lipolysis of cellular fat stores is activated by CGI-58 and defective in Chanarin-Dorfman syndrome. *Cell Metab.* 2006;3(5):309–319.

78. Curat CA, Wegner V, Sengenes C, Miranville A, Tonus C, Busse R, et al. Macrophages in human visceral adipose tissue: increased accumulation in obesity and a source of resistin and visfatin. *Diabetologia.* 2006;49(4):744–747.

79. Lumeng CN, Deyoung SM, Saltiel AR. Macrophages block insulin action in adipocytes by altering expression of signaling and glucose transport proteins. *Am J Physiol Endocrinol Metab.* 2007;292:166–174.

80. Yu R, Kim CS, Kwon BS, Kawada T. Mesenteric adipose tissue-derived monocyte chemoattractant protein-1 plays a crucial role in adipose tissue macrophage migration and activation in obese mice. *Obesity (Silver Spring).* 2006;14(8):1353–1362.

81. Kanda H, Tateya S, Tamori Y, Kotani K, Hiasa K, Kitazawa R, et al. MCP-1 contributes to macrophage infiltration into adipose tissue, insulin resistance, and hepatic steatosis in obesity. *J Clin Invest.* 2006;116 (6):1494–1505.

82. Reaven GM. Insulin resistance/compensatory hyperinsulinemia, essential hypertension, and cardiovascular disease. *J Clin Endocrinol Metab.* 2003;88(6):2399–2403.

83. Abbasi F, Brown BW Jr, Lamendola C, McLaughlin T, Reaven GM. Relationship between obesity, insulin resistance, and coronary heart disease risk. *J Am Coll Cardiol.* 2002;40(5):937–943.

84. Pasquali R, Gambineri A, Anconetani B, Vicennati V, Colitta D, Caramelli E, et al. The natural history of the metabolic syndrome in young women with the polycystic ovary syndrome and the effect of long-term oestrogen-progestogen treatment. *Clin Endocrinol (Oxf).* 1999;50(4):517–527.

85. Essah PA, Nestler JE. The metabolic syndrome in polycystic ovary syndrome. *J Endocrinol Invest.* 2006;29(3):270–280.

86. Ehrmann DA, Liljenquist DR, Kasza K, Azziz R, Legro RS, Ghazzi MN for the PCOS/Troglitazone Study Group. Prevalence and predictors of the metabolic syndrome in women with polycystic ovary syndrome. *J Clin Endocrinol Metab.* 2006;91(1):48–53.

87. Arnaldi G, Mancini T, Polenta B, Boscaro M. Cardiovascular risk in Cushing's syndrome. *Pituitary.* 2004;7(4):253–256.

88. Expert Committee on the Diagnosis and Classification of Diabetes Mellitus. Follow-up report on the diagnosis of diabetes mellitus. *Diabetes Care.* 2003;26:3160–167.

89. Alberti KG, Zimmet P, Shaw J for the IDF Epidemiology Task Force Consensus Group. The metabolic syndrome—a new worldwide definition. *Lancet.* Sept. 24–30 2005;366(9491):1059–1062.

90. Alberti KG, Zimmet P, Shaw J. Metabolic syndrome—a new world-wide definition. A consensus statement from the International Diabetes Federation. *Diabet Med.* 2006;23(5):469–480.

91. Lakka HM, Laaksonen DE, Lakka TA, Niskanen LK, Kumpusalo E, Tuomilehto J, et al. The metabolic syndrome and total and cardiovascular disease mortality in middle-aged men. *JAMA.* 2002;288:2709–2716.

92. Sattar N, Gaw A, Scherbakova O, Ford I, O'Reilly DS, Haffner SM, et al. Metabolic syndrome with and without C-reactive protein as a predictor of coronary heart disease and diabetes in the West of Scotland Coronary Prevention Study. *Circulation.* 2003;108:414–419.

93. Girman CJ, Rhodes T, Mercuri M, Pyorala K, Kjekshus J, Pedersen TR, et al. The metabolic syndrome and risk of major coronary events in the Scandinavian Simvastatin Survival Study (4S) and the Air Force/Texas Coronary Atherosclerosis Prevention Study (AFCAPS/TEXCAPS). *Am J Cardiol.* 2004;93:136–141.

94. Malik S, Wong ND, Franklin SS, Kamath TV, L'Italien GJ, Pio JR, et al. Impact of the metabolic syndrome on mortality from coronary heart disease, cardiovascular disease, and all causes in United States adults. *Circulation.* 2004;110:1245–1250.

95. Olijhoek JK, van der Graaf Y, Banga JD, Algra A, Rabelink TJ, Visseren FL for the SMART Study Group. The metabolic syndrome is associated with advanced vascular damage in patients with coronary heart disease, stroke, peripheral arterial disease or abdominal aortic aneurysm. *Eur Heart J.* 2004;25:342–348.

96. Alexander CM, Landsman PB, Teutsch SM, Haffner SM. Third National Health and Nutrition Examination Survey (NHANES III), National Cholesterol Education Program (NCEP). NCEP-defined metabolic syndrome, diabetes, and prevalence of coronary heart disease among NHANES III participants age 50 years and older. *Diabetes.* 2003;52:1210–1214.

97. Ninomiya JK, L'Italien G, Criqui MH, et al. Association of the metabolic syndrome with history of myocardial infarction and stroke in the Third National Health and Nutrition Examination Survey. *Circulation.* 2004;109:42–46.

98. McNeill AM, Rosamond WD, Girman CJ, Golden SH, Schmidt MI, East HE, et al. The metabolic syndrome and 11-year risk of incident cardiovascular disease in the atherosclerosis risk in communities study. *Diabetes Care.* 2005;28:385–390.

99. Solymoss BC, Bourassa MG, Lesperance J, Levesque S, Marcil M, Varga S, et al. Incidence and clinical characteristics of the metabolic syndrome in patients with coronary artery disease. *Coron Artery Dis.* 2003;14:207–212.

100. Turhan H, Yasar AS, Basar N, Bicer A, Erbay AR, Yetkin E. High prevalence of metabolic syndrome among young women with premature coronary artery disease. *Coron Artery Dis.* 2005;16:37–40.

101. [No authors listed] Clinical Guidelines on the Identification, Evaluation, and Treatment of Overweight and Obesity in Adults—The Evidence Report. National Institutes of Health. *Obes Res.* 1998;6(suppl 2):51S-209S.

102. Knowler WC, Barrett-Connor E, Fowler SE, Hamman RF, Lachin JM, Walker EA, et al for the Diabetes Prevention Program Research Group. Reduction in the incidence of type 2 diabetes with lifestyle intervention or metformin. *N Engl J Med.* 2002;346:393–403.

103. Thompson PD, Buchner D, Pina IL, Balady GJ, Williams MA, Marcus BH, et al for the American Heart Association Council on Clinical Cardiology Subcommittee on Exercise, Rehabilitation, and Prevention; American Heart Association Council on Nutrition, Physical Activity, and Metabolism Subcommittee on Physical Activity. Exercise and physical activity in the prevention and treatment of atherosclerotic cardiovascular disease: a statement from the Council on Clinical Cardiology (Subcommittee on Exercise, Rehabilitation, and Prevention) and the Council on Nutrition, Physical Activity, and Metabolism (Subcommittee on Physical Activity). *Circulation.* 2003;107:3109–3116.

104. Grundy SM, Cleeman JI, Merz CN, Brewer HB Jr, Clark LT, Hunninghake DB, et al for the National Heart, Lung, and Blood Institute; American College of Cardiology Foundation; American Heart Association. Implications of recent clinical trials for the National Cholesterol Education Program Adult Treatment Panel III guidelines. *Circulation.* 2004;110:227–239.

105. Sacks FM, Tonkin AM, Craven T, Pfeffer MA, Shepherd J, Keech A, et al. Coronary heart disease in patients with low LDL-cholesterol: benefit of pravastatin in diabetics and enhanced role for HDL-cholesterol and triglycerides as risk factors. *Circulation.* 2002;105(12):1424–1428.

106. Girman CJ, Rhodes T, Mercuri M, Pyorala K, Kjekshus J, Pedersen TR, et al for the 4S Group and the AFCAPS/TEXCAPS Research Group. The metabolic syndrome and risk of major coronary events in the Scandinavian Simvastatin Survival Study (4S) and the Air Force/Texas Coronary Atherosclerosis Prevention Study (AFCAPS/TEXCAPS). *Am J Cardiol.* 2004;93(2):136–141.

107. Sattar N, Gaw A, Scherbakova O, Ford I, O'Reilly DS, Haffner SM, et al. Metabolic syndrome with and without C-reactive protein as a predictor of coronary heart disease and diabetes in the West of Scotland Coronary Prevention Study. *Circulation.* 2003;108(4):414–419.

108. Collins R, Armitage J, Parish S, Sleigh P, Peto R for the Heart Protection Study Collaborative Group. Related MRC/BHF Heart Protection Study of cholesterol-lowering with simvastatin in 5963 people with diabetes: a randomised placebo-controlled trial. *Lancet.* 2003;361(9374):2005–2016.

109. Keech A, Colquhoun D, Best J, Kirby A, Simes RJ, Hunt D, et al for the LIPID Study Group. Secondary prevention of cardiovascular events with long-term pravastatin in patients with diabetes or impaired fasting glucose: results from the LIPID trial. *Diabetes Care.* 2003;26(10):2713–2721.

110. Tonelli M, Keech A, Shepherd J, Sacks F, Tonkin A, Packard C, et al. Effect of pravastatin in people with diabetes and chronic kidney disease. *J Am Soc Nephrol.* 2005;16(12):3748–3754.

111. Shepherd J, Barter P, Carmena R, Deedwania P, Fruchart JC, Haffner S, et al. Effect of lowering LDL cholesterol substantially below currently recommended levels in patients with coronary heart disease and diabetes: the Treating to New Targets (TNT) study. *Diabetes Care.* 2006;29(6):1220–1226.

112. Deedwania P, Barter P, Carmena R, Fruchart JC, Grundy SM, Haffner S, et al for the Treating to New Targets Investigators. Reduction of low-density lipoprotein cholesterol in patients with coronary heart disease and metabolic syndrome: analysis of the Treating to New Targets study. *Lancet.* 2006;368(9539):919–928.

113. Sever PS, Poulter NR, Dahlof B, Wedel H, Collins R, Beevers G, et al. Reduction in cardiovascular events with atorvastatin in 2,532 patients with type 2 diabetes: Anglo-Scandinavian Cardiac Outcomes Trial—Lipid-Lowering Arm (ASCOT-LLA). *Diabetes Care.* 2005;28(5):1151–1157.

114. Colhoun HM, Betteridge DJ, Durrington PN, Hitman GA, Neil HA, Livingstone SJ, et al for the CARDS investigators. Primary prevention of cardiovascular disease with atorvastatin in type 2 diabetes in the Collaborative Atorvastatin Diabetes Study (CARDS): multicentre randomised placebo-controlled trial. *Lancet.* Aug. 21–27 2004;364(9435):685–696.

115. Knopp RH, d'Emden M, Smilde JG, Pocock SJ. Efficacy and safety of atorvastatin in the prevention of cardiovascular end points in subjects with type 2 diabetes: the Atorvastatin Study for Prevention of Coronary Heart Disease Endpoints in Noninsulin-Dependent Diabetes Mellitus (ASPEN). *Diabetes Care.* 2006;29(7):1478–1485.

116. Tenkanen L, Manttari M, Kovanen PT, Virkkunen H, Manninen V. Gemfibrozil in the treatment of dyslipidemia: an 18-year mortality follow-up of the Helsinki Heart Study. *Arch Intern Med.* 2006;166(7):743–748.

117. Robins SJ. Targeting low high-density lipoprotein cholesterol for therapy: lessons from the Veterans Affairs High-Density Lipoprotein Intervention Trial. *Am J Cardiol.* 2001;88(12A):19N–23N.

118. Carlson LA, Rosenhamer G. Reduction of mortality in the Stockholm Ischaemic Heart Disease Secondary Prevention Study by combined treatment with clofibrate and nicotinic acid. *Acta Med Scand.* 1988;223(5):405–418.

119. Tenenbaum A, Motro M, Fisman EZ, Tanne D, Boyko V, Behar S. Bezafibrate for the secondary prevention of myocardial infarction in patients with metabolic syndrome. *Arch Intern Med.* 2005;165(10):1154–1160.

120. Tenenbaum A, Fisman EZ, Motro M, Adler Y. Atherogenic dyslipidemia in metabolic syndrome and type 2 diabetes: therapeutic options beyond statins. *Cardiovasc Diabetol.* 2006;5:20–28.

121. Keech A, Simes RJ, Barter P, Best J, Scott R, Taskinen MR, et al for the FIELD study investigators. Effects of long-term fenofibrate therapy on cardiovascular events in 9795 people with type 2 diabetes mellitus (the FIELD study): randomised controlled trial. *Lancet.* 2005;366(9500):1849–1861.

122. Canner PL, Furberg CD, McGovern ME. Benefits of niacin in patients with versus without the metabolic syndrome and healed myocardial infarction (from the Coronary Drug Project). *Am J Cardiol.* 2006;97(4):477–479.

123. Canner PL, Furberg CD, Terrin ML, McGovern ME. Benefits of niacin by glycemic status in patients with healed myocardial infarction (from the Coronary Drug Project). *Am J Cardiol.* 2005;95 (2):254–257.

124. Vega GL, Ma PT, Cater NB, Filipchuk N, Meguro S, Garcia-Garcia AB, Grundy SM. Effects of adding fenofibrate (200 mg/day) to simvastatin (10 mg/day) in patients with combined hyperlipidemia and metabolic syndrome. *Am J Cardiol.* 2003;91(8):956–960.

125. Grundy SM, Vega GL, Yuan Z, Battisti WP, Brady WE, Palmisano J. Effectiveness and tolerability of simvastatin plus fenofibrate for combined hyperlipidemia (the SAFARI trial). *Am J Cardiol.* 2005;95(4):462–468. Erratum: *Am J Cardiol.* 2006;98(3):427–428.

126. Cannon CP, Steinberg BA, Murphy SA, Mega JL, Braunwald E. Meta-analysis of cardiovascular outcomes trials comparing intensive versus moderate statin therapy. *J Am Coll Cardiol.* 2006;48(3):438–445.

127. Amarenco P, Bogousslavsky J, Callahan A 3rd, Goldstein LB, Hennerici M, Rudolph AE, et al for the Stroke Prevention by Aggressive Reduction in Cholesterol Levels (SPARCL) Investigators. High-dose atorvastatin after stroke or transient ischemic attack *N Engl J Med.* 2006;355(6):549–559.

128. Smith SC Jr, Allen J, Blair SN, Bonow RO, Brass LM, Fonarow GC, et al for the AHA/ACC; National Heart, Lung, and Blood Institute. AHA/ACC guidelines for secondary prevention for patients with coronary and other atherosclerotic vascular disease: 2006 update: endorsed by the National Heart, Lung, and Blood Institute. *Circulation.* 2006;113(19):2363–2372.

129. Grundy SM. Diabetes and coronary risk equivalency: what does it mean? *Diabetes Care.* 2006;29(2):457–460.

130. Chobanian AV, Bakris GL, Black HR, Cushman WC, Green LA, Izzo JL Jr, et al for the National Heart, Lung, and Blood Institute Joint National Committee on Prevention, Detection, Evaluation, and Treatment of High Blood Pressure; National High Blood Pressure Education Program Coordinating Committee. The Seventh Report of the Joint National Committee on Prevention, Detection, Evaluation, and Treatment of High Blood Pressure: the JNC 7 report. *JAMA.* 2003;289:2560–2572.

131. Nashar K, Nguyen JP, Jesri A, Morrow JD, Egan BM. Angiotensin receptor blockade improves arterial distensibility and reduces exercise-induced pressor responses in obese hypertensive patients with the metabolic syndrome. *Am J Hypertens.* 2004;17(6):477–482.

132. Abuissa H, Jones PG, Marso SP, O'Keefe JH Jr. Angiotensin-converting enzyme inhibitors or angiotensin receptor blockers for prevention of type 2 diabetes: a meta-analysis of randomized clinical trials. *J Am Coll Cardiol.* 2005;46(5):821–826.

133. Kurata A, Nishizawa H, Kihara S, Maeda N, Sonoda M, Okada T, et al. Blockade of angiotensin II type-1 receptor reduces oxidative stress in adipose tissue and ameliorates adipocytokine dysregulation. *Kidney Int.* 2006;70(10):1717–1724.

134. Knowler WC, Hamman RF, Edelstein SL, Barrett-Connor E, Ehrmann DA, Walker EA, et al for the Diabetes Prevention Program Research Group. Prevention of type 2 diabetes with troglitazone in the diabetes prevention program. *Diabetes.* 2005;54:1150–1156.

135. Buchanan TA, Xiang AH, Peters RK, Kjos SL, Marroquin A, Goico J, et al. Preservation of pancreatic beta-cell function and prevention of type 2 diabetes by pharmacological treatment of insulin resistance in high-risk Hispanic women. *Diabetes.* 2002;51:2796–2803.

136. Diabetes Reduction Assessment with Ramipril and Rosiglitazone Medication (DREAM) Trial Investigators, Gerstein HC, Yusuf S, Bosch J, Pogue J, Sheridan P, et al. Effect of rosiglitazone on the frequency of diabetes in patients with impaired glucose tolerance or impaired fasting glucose: a randomised controlled trial. *Lancet.* 2006;368(9541):1096–1105.

137. Pearson TA, Blair SN, Daniels SR, Eckel RH, Fair JM, Fortmann SP, et al. AHA guidelines for primary prevention of cardiovascular disease and stroke: 2002 update: Consensus panel guide to comprehensive risk reduction for adult patients without coronary or other atherosclerotic vascular diseases. American Heart Association Science Advisory and Coordinating Committee. *Circulation.* 2002;106:388–391.

138. Ridker PM, Wilson PW, Grundy SM. Should C-reactive protein be added to metabolic syndrome and to assessment of global cardiovascular risk? *Circulation.* 2004;109:2818–2825.

139. Pearson TA, Mensah GA, Alexander RW, Anderson JL, Cannon RO 3rd, Criqui M, et al for the Centers for Disease Control and Prevention; American Heart Association. Markers of inflammation and cardiovascular disease: application to clinical and public health practice: A statement for healthcare professionals from the Centers for Disease Control and Prevention and the American Heart Association. *Circulation.* 2003;107:499–511.

CHAPTER (92)

HIV/AIDS and the Cardiovascular System

William Lewis / Peter F. Currie

INTRODUCTION

【 】 EPIDEMIOLOGY

The acquired immunodeficiency syndrome (AIDS) was first recognized in 1981 and is caused by the human immunodeficiency virus (HIV-1). HIV-2 causes a similar illness to HIV-1 but is less aggressive and has so far been restricted mainly to western Africa. HIV is acquired through exposure to infected body fluid, particularly blood and semen; the most common modes of spread are sexual, parenteral (blood or blood product transfusion, injection drug use, and occupational injury) and vertical (mother to fetus).

By the end of 2005 more than 40 million people worldwide were infected with HIV, and more than 20 million have died since the pandemic began.[1] The vast majority of deaths have occurred in sub-Saharan Africa where more than 13 million children have been orphaned. In the United States more than 1 million people are now HIV positive[2], and infection rates are rising rapidly in many parts of the world, notably Asia and eastern Europe.[3]

A variety of cultural and social factors have determined the regional patterns of HIV disease. In the United States and northern Europe the epidemic has predominantly been in men who have sex with men. In southern and eastern Europe, Vietnam, Malaysia, Northeast India and China the incidence has been greatest in injection drug users; in Africa, the Caribbean and much of Southeast Asia the dominant route of transmission has been heterosexual and from mother to child.

The epidemic in industrialized nations is changing and in these countries heterosexual transmission is now the dominant route of infection; in the United Kingdom, for example, 58 percent of new infections in 2003 were acquired heterosexually. The disease is therefore increasingly seen in women, and in the United States the proportion of female HIV/AIDS patients increased from 7 percent in 1985 to 23 percent in 1998.[4]

【 】 HIV-RELATED CARDIOVASCULAR DISEASE

Some form of heart disease is demonstrable at autopsy in approximately 40 percent of cases and by echocardiography in approximately 25 percent of patients with AIDS (Centers for Disease Control [CDC] category C disease–see below). Many of these le-

TABLE 92–1

Cardiac Manifestations of HIV/AIDS

Pericardial effusion	• Idiopathic • Infectious (viral, bacterial especially tuberculous, and fungal) • Neoplastic (Kaposi sarcoma and non-Hodgkin lymphoma)
Heart muscle disease	• Myocarditis (idiopathic/lymphocytic, specific infections, toxins) • Dilated cardiomyopathy & LV dysfunction
Endocarditis	• Marantic (nonbacterial thrombotic endocarditis) • Infective
Tumors	• Kaposi sarcoma • Lymphoma
Right ventricular dysfunction & pulmonary hypertension	• Primary • Secondary (recurrent chest infections, thromboembolism)
Premature atherosclerosis and coronary artery disease	
Adverse drug effects	• Hyperlipidemia • Proarrhythmia
Vascular disease	
Autonomic dysfunction	

with advanced immunodeficiency, such as heart muscle disease, pericardial effusion and pulmonary hypertension, continue to predominate in resource-poor countries where less than 5 percent of patients are able to access antiretroviral drugs.

⬛ ⬜ NATURAL HISTORY AND BIOLOGY OF HIV INFECTION

HIV is a single-stranded RNA retrovirus from the lentivirus in the Retroviridae family that invades cells containing specific membrane receptors and incorporates a DNA copy of itself into the host's genome. Immune deficiency is the result of virus and immune-mediated destruction of CD4 lymphocytes caused by continuous high-level HIV replication. The reduction in the number of CD4 cells circulating in peripheral blood is tightly correlated with the plasma viral load. Both CD4 count and viral load can be monitored and are used as measures of disease progression. Virus-specific CD8 cytotoxic T-cell lymphocytes develop rapidly after infection and can lyse infected CD4 cells. They play a crucial role in controlling HIV replication after infection and can therefore determine the rate of disease progression.

Any depletion in CD4 cells renders the body susceptible to opportunistic infections and oncogenic virus-related tumors. The predominant opportunist infections seen in HIV disease are intracellular parasites (e.g., *Mycobacterium tuberculosis*) or pathogens susceptible to cell-mediated rather than antibody-mediated immune responses.

After the initial infection there is a dormant period before symptoms and disease supervenes (Fig. 92–1). In the absence of HAART, the mean length of life after infection is approximately

sions are mild, and HIV-related heart disease probably causes symptoms in less than 10 percent and death in less than 2 percent of all patients with HIV infection. The common cardiovascular manifestations of HIV infection are listed in Table 92–1.

At the beginning of the epidemic, heart muscle disease was the dominant cardiac complication of HIV infection in the developed world, and tuberculous pericarditis was the most important cardiac manifestation of the disease in Africa. The advent of highly active antiretroviral therapy (HAART) has changed the pattern of disease in developed countries where premature coronary artery disease and other manifestations of atherosclerosis are now the most common cardiovascular disorder. This is partly caused by HAART-induced metabolic problems, particularly insulin resistance and hyperlipidemia, but also reflects a high prevalence of conventional cardiovascular risk factors such as smoking. Cardiovascular problems associated

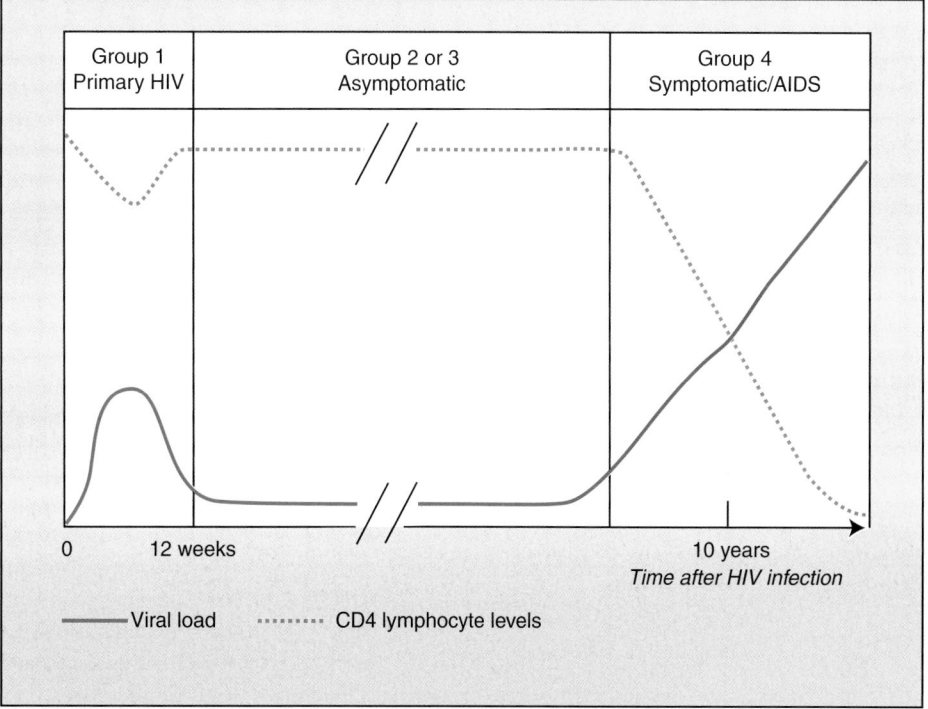

FIGURE 92–1. The natural history of HIV infection. *Source: Reprinted with permission from Mindel A, Tenant-Flowers M. ABC of AIDS—Natural history and management of early HIV infection. BMJ. 2001;322:1290–1293.*

TABLE 92–2

Centers for Disease Control and Prevention Classification of HIV Infection

Category A	Asymptomatic patients; progressive lymphadenopathy
Category B	Symptomatic patients without AIDS defining illness
Category C	Symptomatic patients with AIDS defining illness

10 years.[5] In contrast, HAART can eliminate the virus from the peripheral blood and transform a patient's prognosis.[6]

Primary Infection

Primary infection is usually established 2 to 6 weeks after exposure. Most (70 to 80 percent) patients experience a self-limiting illness, similar to infectious mononucleosis, characterized by fever, fatigue, pharyngitis, lymphadenopathy, and maculopapular rash.[7] In many patients the illness is mild and only identified by retrospective enquiry at later presentation. More than 95 percent of patients seroconvert (i.e., become HIV positive) within 6 months. This usually coincides with a surge in plasma HIV RNA levels to >1 million copies/mL (peak between 4 and 8 weeks), and a fall in the CD4 count to 300 to 400 cells/mm³. Symptomatic recovery is accompanied by a rise in the CD4 count and a fall in viral load; nevertheless, the CD4 count rarely recovers to its original value (see Fig. 92–1).

A simple classification scheme of the CDC has been used to describe the subsequent phases of disease (Table 92–2). Premature coronary disease, infective endocarditis, and drug-related problems can supervene at any time, whereas pericardial effusion and heart muscle disease are usually only seen in late stage (CDC category C) disease.

Asymptomatic Infection (CDC Category A Disease)

Viral replication takes place in the lymphoid tissue throughout this stage; there is sustained viremia, and the CD4 count falls steadily (typically by between 50 and 150 cells per year). Although there can be persistent generalized lymphadenopathy, the patient remains well.

Mildly Symptomatic Disease (CDC Category B Disease)

The median interval from infection to the development of symptoms is approximately 7 to 10 years. A variety of diseases known as AIDS-related complex conditions (e.g., oral hairy leukoplakia, weight loss, night sweats, chronic diarrhea) can supervene but by definition are not AIDS-defining.

AIDS (CDC Category C Disease)

AIDS is defined by the development of one or more specified opportunistic infections, tumors, and other conditions. These include esophageal candidiasis, cytomegalovirus (CMV) retinitis, pulmonary or extrapulmonary tuberculosis, Kaposi sarcoma, and

HIV-associated dementia. Most forms of HIV-related heart muscle and pericardial disease occur at this stage.

CARDIOVASCULAR ASSESSMENT OF THE HIV/AIDS PATIENT

It is increasingly common for HIV/AIDS patients to be seen by cardiologists,[8] and cardiovascular disease in HIV/AIDS is becoming increasingly recognized in the developing world.[9] Despite this, heart disease can be overlooked in HIV-positive patients, because symptoms of breathlessness, fatigue, and poor exercise tolerance are frequently ascribed to other conditions associated with HIV infection.[10] Echocardiographic assessment of HIV patients is extremely useful[11] and can be used to identify those cardiac conditions common in HIV-positive patients that can be associated with a poor outcome: pericardial effusion,[9] left ventricular (LV) systolic dysfunction/heart muscle disease,[10] and intracardiac masses.[12] Echocardiography also can provide useful information about the appearance of the right ventricle, provide an indirect assessment of pulmonary pressures, and detect regional wall-motion abnormalities suggestive of coronary artery disease.

Any HIV-positive patient at high risk of developing or with any potential clinical manifestation of cardiovascular disease should have a baseline echocardiogram performed with serial echocardiography every 1 to 2 years.[13] It can be justifiable to perform a baseline study at the time of diagnosis of HIV/AIDS with annual to biannual examination of asymptomatic patients (Table 92–3),[14] but more aggressive monitoring can be guided by the cardiologist on discovery of abnormalities or in those patients with significant, potentially cardiotropic viral infections or unexplained pulmonary symptoms.

HIV/AIDS AND THE PERICARDIUM

Pericardial effusion and pericarditis were the most common cardiac abnormalities found in early HIV/AIDS autopsy studies. Pericardial effusion was found in up to 38 percent of patients particularly in association with generalized fluid retention and advanced disease.[15] Small effusions are still found frequently in patients with heart failure or malignant infiltration of the pericardium, but cardiac tamponade may rarely occur. Therefore, the finding of cardiomegaly on a chest radiograph should prompt early echocardiographic assessment.[16]

Clinically significant pericardial effusions are usually caused by viral or bacterial infection or malignant infiltration particularly with Kaposi sarcoma (KS) or non-Hodgkin lymphoma (NHL). In Africa, pericardial effusion itself is suggestive of HIV infection, and here up to 72 percent of patients with serosanguineous effusions have been found to be HIV positive. Pericarditis caused by *Mycobacterium tuberculosis* or *Mycobacterium avium–intracellulare* is a pressing problem in Africa[17] but has also been reported as the first manifestation of AIDS in mainland Europe.[18]

Other unusual pathogens, including *Nocardia asteroides* and herpes simplex virus (HSV), should be considered along with CMV, which remains prevalent in the HIV population often without a definite anatomic site of infection. Appropriate antituberculous and antiviral therapies can therefore be helpful in this situation.

TABLE 92–3

Indications for Echocardiographic Assessment of HIV-Positive Patients

Possible baseline assessment at time of diagnosis of HIV infection

Baseline assessment and 1–2 yearly monitoring of patient with:

  Clinical manifestation of possible cardiac involvement
    unexplained dyspnea/hypoxia
    third heart sound inappropriate tachycardia
    raised jugular venous pressure
    peripheral edema/right heart failure
    radiographic evidence of cardiomegaly

  Viral coinfection
    cytomegalovirus
    Epstein-Barr virus
    Coxsackievirus
    adenovirus

  History of preexisting cardiac disease
    left ventricular systolic dysfunction (all cause)
    valvular heart disease
    suspicion of infective endocarditis in intravenous drug user

  High-risk HIV patients with:
    wasting
    encephalopathy
    CD4 count <100 cells/mm^3 or AIDS
    potentially cardiotoxic medication
    multiple hospitalizations

Possible 1–2 yearly monitoring of asymptomatic HIV-positive patients

Frequent assessment of HIV-positive patients with cardiovascular involvement (as guided by cardiologist)

Surgical intervention is not always beneficial in AIDS patients with large pericardial effusions.[19] However, there are no data on the long-term outcome of such measures in patients at an earlier stage of HIV/AIDS. Pericardiocentesis and pericardiectomy were used to treat a *Staphylococcus aureus* pericardial tamponade in an HIV-positive drug user who remained well for more than 5 years.[20] Culture of pericardial biopsy or fluid from symptomatic effusions can also be useful in identifying treatable opportunistic infections or malignancy.

HIV/AIDS AND THE MYOCARDIUM

【 】 MYOCARDITIS

Numerous pathologic studies have confirmed the presence of varying histologic patterns of lymphocytic myocarditis in HIV patients,[21] although many do not fulfill the Dallas criteria formulated to secure the histopathologic diagnosis (see Chap. 32).[22] Clinical correlation with myocarditis has been described in AIDS series,[23] and opportunistic infections were occasionally prominent

comorbid conditions. However, interstitial mononuclear infiltrates have also been reported in other forms of cardiomyopathy and in noncardiomyopathic conditions.[24] The apparent difference in the prevalence of myocarditis in different studies can therefore relate to clinical factors, sampling errors, and possibly the effect of HAART. As such, estimates of the prevalence of myocarditis in HIV/AIDS varies from 53 percent[25] in the pre-HAART era to much lower levels today[26] in the developed world.

Myocarditis can be precipitated by a variety of viral infections, and the inflammatory reaction can progress even after virus is no longer evident in the heart. An immune reaction, either to viral antigen or to altered myocardial protein, can precipitate myocardial necrosis and inflammatory cell infiltration.[27] However, simple histopathologic methods alone can be insufficient to exclude the diagnosis of myocarditis in AIDS patients. Infiltrating CD8 and CD45 lymphocytes have been found in association with increased MHC class I antigen expression in histologically normal endomyocardial biopsies from HIV-positive patients with cardiac failure.[28]

It is therefore possible that a subgroup of AIDS patients can have immune-mediated heart disease despite normal biopsies, and an inflammatory process remains the likeliest substrate for the development of cardiac dysfunction in HIV-positive patients. There are several hypotheses regarding the etiology of myocarditis in AIDS including: (1) primary HIV myocarditis, (2) secondary HIV myocarditis, (3) opportunistic infection, and (4) autoimmunity.

Primary HIV Infection of the Myocardium

HIV has neither been universally accepted nor unambiguously proven a causative agent of myocarditis in AIDS. The virus gains entry into cells by binding CD4 receptors with its envelope glycoprotein group 120. CD4 receptors are found on T4 (helper) lymphocytes and some other cell types. Although HIV can clearly infect monocytes/macrophages and myocardial interstitial cells, evidence proving that HIV can infect human cardiac myocytes, which do not possess CD4 receptors, is less clear.

Some reports of cardiac infection by HIV[29] utilized in situ hybridization (ISH), which did not require extraction of target sequences, and thus preserved the histologic architecture. However, the origin of the detected HIV sequences would be masked by the dense silver reaction that occurs as part of that technique, and precise localization to the myocyte was therefore lacking. Cell culture and polymerase chain reaction (PCR) were equally limited in that tissue under investigation could be contaminated by the patient's own infected blood cells and that as little as one HIV contaminant virion (e.g., from an infected and anatomically proximate interstitial cell) could confuse interpretation (Fig. 92–2). Examination of simian immunodeficiency virus (SIV) infected macaques using similar methods confirmed that SIV infected the cardiac monocytes rather than actual myocytes.[30]

Despite this, HIV gene sequences have been detected by PCR in microdissected endomyocardial biopsies from HIV-positive patients, some of whom had cardiac symptoms.[31] HIV has also been shown to gain entry into the human fetal cardiac myocyte by ingestion through a specific crystallizable fragment (of immunoglobulin) (Fc) receptor, and it remains possible that this or other, unidentified mechanisms can promote HIV entry into the myocyte and facilitate a primary HIV myocarditis.[32]

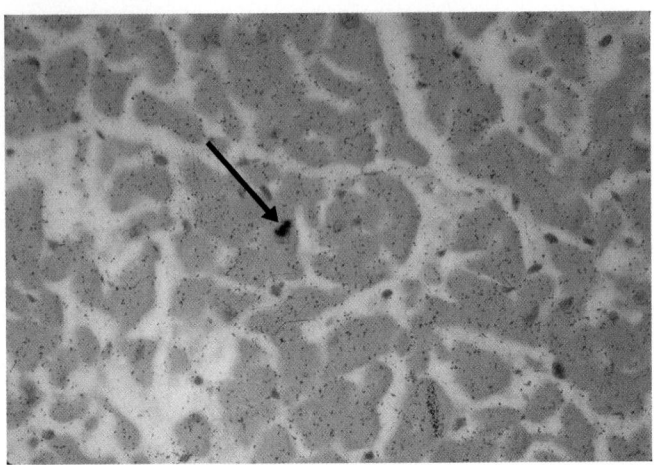

FIGURE 92–2. In situ hybridization of HIV in the heart of an AIDS patient. *Arrow* points to solitary positive cell nucleus in the field ([^{35}S]-riboprobe for HIV; counterstain H&E; original magnification × 400).

Secondary HIV Myocarditis

Immune responses are implicated in Chagas cardiomyopathy in which noninfected myocytes are damaged by the host response to *Trypanosoma cruzi*. Interstitial lymphocytes and macrophages can form contact with myocytes causing a focal loss of basement membrane through a local reaction.[33] A similar process can be involved in the pathogenesis of HIV myocarditis. Proteolytic enzymes released through HIV replication in the interstitium could also damage myocytes. Such "innocent bystander destruction"[34] can be particularly relevant to the myocardium as increased numbers of infected interstitial cells have been found in HIV-positive subjects with active myocarditis.

The HIV envelope glycoprotein group 120 can induce tumor necrosis factor-α (TNF-α) expression from macrophages and has been shown to enhance interleukin (IL)-1 induced nitric oxide production in neonatal rat cardiac myocytes.[35] Cytokine IL-6, which has some effect on immune response and viral replication in murine myocarditis models, has been found in excess in a small number of HIV-positive patients with biopsy proven myocarditis.[36] Therefore, just as cytokines can have a role in the development of congestive cardiac failure in absence of HIV/AIDS, they seem likely to be important in the course of HIV/AIDS myocarditis and heart muscle disease.

Myocardial Opportunistic Infections in HIV/AIDS

Autopsy has confirmed a variety of opportunistic infections of the myocardium in patients with AIDS. Infectious agents included *Toxoplasma gondii* in the hearts of both adults and children, Cryptococcus species, CMV, *Candida* species, *Pneumocystis carinii*, *Microsporidium*, *Histoplasma capsulatum*, atypical mycobacteria, and *Aspergillus* organisms involving the myocardium. The majority have been part of a disseminated infection and are infrequently associated with localized myocarditis.

Acute Chagas myocarditis in AIDS has also been reported and can be associated with a more frequent rate of myocarditis in up to 30 percent of cases in AIDS patients.[37] Despite this, a clear etiologic link between opportunistic infection and myocarditis in AIDS has yet to be established.

Clinical Features of Myocarditis in HIV/AIDS

Myocarditis can be diagnosed clinically based on symptoms and physical findings, although this is often difficult in the HIV patient. The symptoms are protean and include fatigue, dyspnea, and pleuritic chest pain, which can wrongly be ascribed to other conditions. The finding of an unexplained tachycardia, third heart sound, or a friction rub should alert the physician to the possibility of myocarditis and guide investigation (see Chap. 32).

The ECG can be helpful, possibly demonstrating nonspecific conduction defects, repolarization abnormalities, and ST–T wave changes, although these are not invariable. The chest radiograph can be normal or suggest cardiac enlargement with pulmonary congestion. Echocardiography is usually nondiagnostic but can show hyperdynamic LV function in HIV-positive children with myocarditis[38] or occasionally LV dyskinesia in adult AIDS patients with myocarditis. The question of whether a myocardial biopsy is helpful remains problematic. Sampling errors can reduce the diagnostic yield from this invasive procedure and finding a treatable cause of biopsy-proven myocarditis is rare.

⟦ ⟧ DILATED CARDIOMYOPATHY AND LEFT VENTRICULAR DYSFUNCTION IN HIV/AIDS

Dilated cardiomyopathy as a complication of HIV infection was first described in 1986 and was identified frequently thereafter. The pathogenesis remains obscure, but features of HIV-related heart muscle disease (HMD) are similar to idiopathic dilated cardiomyopathy in HIV-negative individuals, and an association between cardiac dysfunction and the lymphocytic myocarditis reported in AIDS postmortem series seems plausible. Isolated LV dysfunction in HIV-positive patients can resolve spontaneously, suggesting a self-limiting myocarditis, and reflects current thinking on the pathogenesis of non-HIV dilated cardiomyopathy. However, there is only a loose correlation between the histologic abnormalities found in HIV studies and clinical evidence of LV dysfunction.

Studies involving HIV-negative control groups made up of patients with hematologic malignancy, high-risk lifestyles,[39] or matched HIV-positive patients suggest that HIV HMD is not merely the result of high-risk activities or a nonspecific manifestation of a chronic illness.[10,39] However, it is not unreasonable to assess the impact of and role of any comorbid conditions or risk behavior before attributing cardiomyopathy solely to AIDS. The differential diagnosis of HIV-related cardiomyopathy includes LV dysfunction secondary to ischemic heart disease, diabetes or hypertension, hypersensitivity reactions to drugs, or foreign injected material and coronary spasm secondary to cocaine use.[40]

The prevalence of HMD appears to be approximately 4.4 percent for dilated cardiomyopathy and 6.4 percent for isolated LV dysfunction, and the condition can cause symptoms in up to 5.5 percent of HIV/AIDS patients.[10] The presence of dilated cardiomyopathy is ominous and associated with poor survival compared to patients with structurally normal hearts. This poor outlook remained true, even after correcting for CD4 counts (Figs. 92–3 and 92–4). A 1-year consecutive enrollment study of patients admitted to the intensive care unit in an urban center revealed 6 percent of

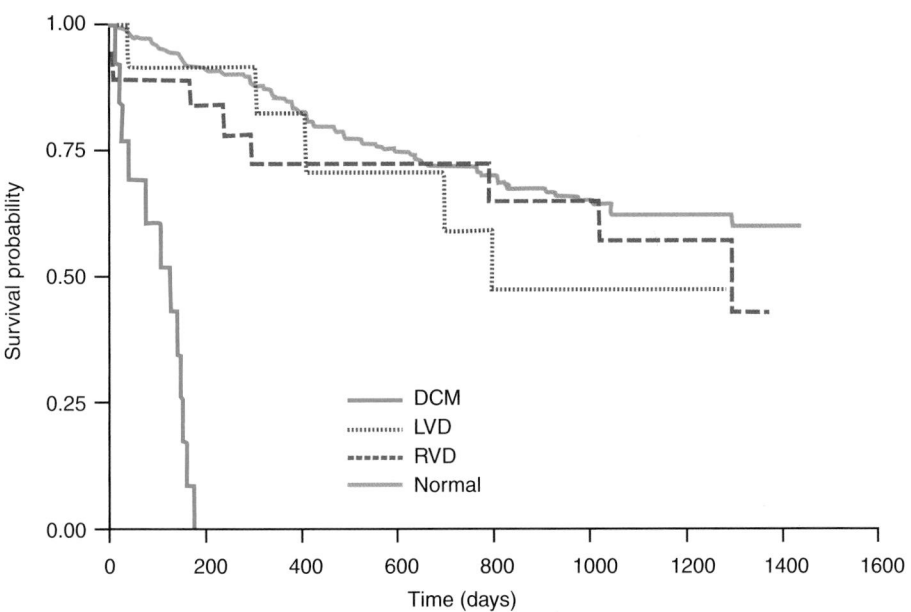

FIGURE 92–3. Kaplan-Meier survival curves for HIV-positive patients with structurally normal hearts and evidence of cardiac dysfunction. DCM, dilated cardiomyopathy; LVD, left ventricular dysfunction; RVD, right ventricular dysfunction. *Source: Currie PF, Jacob AJ, Foreman AR, et al. Heart muscle disease related to HIV infection: Prognostic implications. Br Med J. 1994;309:1605.*

admissions with either HIV infection or AIDS had echocardiographically documented cardiomyopathy, and the short-term mortality was 25 percent.[41]

Mechanisms of Cardiomyopathy in HIV/AIDS

The mechanisms for the development of LV dysfunction, cardiomyopathy, and myocarditis in AIDS remain unclear. In addition to the role of HIV, lymphocytic myocarditis, and cytokines, the contributions of autoimmune responses, illicit and prescribed medications, nutritional deficiencies, and other factors also appear to be pathogenetically or pathophysiologically important.[21]

Autoimmunity and HIV-Related Heart Muscle Disease Many autoimmune processes have been described in association with HIV/AIDS infection. Although some of these can be the result of opportunistic infection, HIV infection can itself trigger autoimmune phenomena in susceptible patients.[42]

The significance of some autoantibodies such as antineutrophil cytoplasmic autoantibody or antiphospholipid antibodies, which have been reported in AIDS patients remains unclear. However, their presence along with hypergammaglobulinemia, and elevated circulating immune complexes that are also well described suggests that, as yet undefined, autoimmune processes can take place in HIV-positive patients.[43]

Autoantibodies against β-myosin have been identified in small numbers of HIV-positive patients with cardiomyopathy and histologically proven active myocarditis. Antibodies to α-myosin, which are more highly cardiac specific, have also been found more frequently and in higher levels in patients' heart muscle disease compared to those with normal hearts or HIV-negative controls.[39]

These findings support a possible autoimmune process in the pathogenesis of HIV/AIDS heart muscle disease and have been further emphasized by experimental models in which susceptible mice developed dilated cardiomyopathy with antimyosin antibodies after exposure to Coxsackievirus B3 infection or immunization with α-myosin. Common, cardiotropic viruses could facilitate development of cardiac autoimmunity in HIV-positive patients by modifying myocyte surface antigens. CMV infection is a common opportunistic infection in AIDS patients, but has been described only infrequently as a cause of myocarditis in HIV.[15] Although this might suggest that CMV is not strongly implicated, ISH studies have identified transcripts of CMV-specific DNA within the myocytes of HIV-positive patients with myocarditis and cardiomyopathy in the absence of typical histologic features such as inclusion bodies.[28] As such CMV or some other factor could be responsible for the ongoing inflammation and cardiac injury seen in many cases of myocarditis.

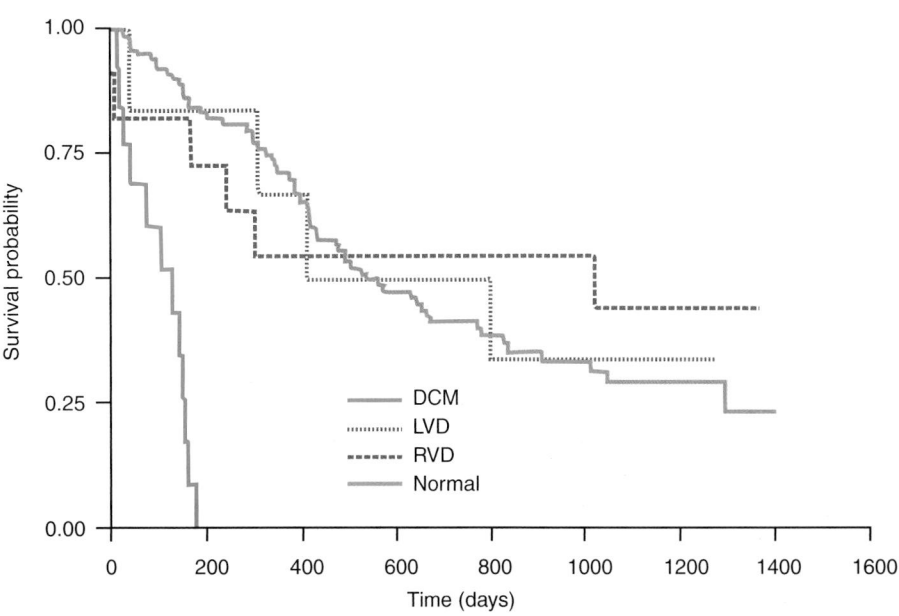

FIGURE 92–4. Survival probability for patients with CD4 <100 cells/mm³. DCM, dilated cardiomyopathy; LVD, left ventricular dysfunction; RVD, right ventricular dysfunction. *Source: Currie PF, Jacob AJ, Foreman AR, et al. Heart muscle disease related to HIV infection: Prognostic implications. Br Med J. 1994;309:1605.*

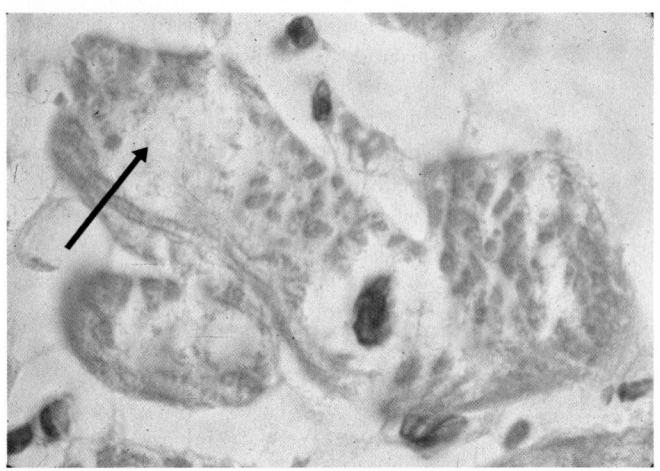

FIGURE 92–5. Cardiac myocyte with lytic change from endomyocardial biopsy from patient with zidovudine treatment and dilated cardiomyopathy. Myocytolysis (*arrow*) is found (H&E; original magnification × 400).

Drug-Induced Heart Muscle Disease Nucleoside reverse transcriptase inhibitors (NRTIs) are key elements of HAART. However, zidovudine (azidothymidine) and other NRTIs can be implicated in the development of some cases of HIV-related heart muscle disease. In addition to inhibiting HIV reverse transcriptase, the drug causes a dose-dependent reversible skeletal myopathy by altering mitochondrial DNA replication.[44] Specific histologic changes have been noted in human and animal studies and include focal necrosis, (Fig. 92–5) cytoplasmic bodies, mitochondrial abnormalities, and ragged, red fibers. Similar changes have also been discovered in the myocardium of rodents fed zidovudine.[45]

The exact role of zidovudine in the pathogenesis of HIV-related heart muscle disease in humans remains unclear, and evidence for its existence is limited, however, small numbers of HIV-positive patients who have developed cardiac dysfunction while taking the drug were seen to improve following its discontinuation.[46] It seems reasonable to discontinue zidovudine therapy for 1 month in those patients who develop cardiac dysfunction while receiving the drug. However, this should be followed by reassessment and possible reintroduction of zidovudine if no improvement in cardiac function is noted.[39] The cardiac and other side effects of NRTIs can become more common through improved AIDS survival and increasing cumulative doses of HAART.

Other drugs used in the treatment of HIV patients also can result in cardiac dysfunction (Table 92–4). Foscarnet, indicated for CMV infection in adult AIDS patients, has been associated with episodes of reversible congestive cardiac failure as has doxorubicin and interferon-α therapy for Kaposi sarcoma.

The effect of recreational drugs on myocardial function is not well delineated in patients with AIDS in whom the prevalence of substance abuse is high. Cocaine use has been associated with myocarditis and a possibly reversible dilated cardiomyopathy in non-AIDS patients and thus should be considered in the HIV population.[47]

Nutritional Deficiencies and Cardiac Dysfunction in HIV/AIDS HIV/AIDS patients with evidence of LV systolic dysfunction should be assessed for micronutrient deficiency, which is common in HIV-infected individuals. Abnormally low levels of selenium and antioxidant vitamins have been demonstrated, and *oxidative stress* can be an important mechanism for cellular damage in AIDS.[48] Selenium deficiency is implicated in the pathogenesis of Keshan disease, a specific form of dilated cardiomyopathy seen in China, which can respond to dietary supplementation. In the same way, decreased selenium content has been demonstrated in the hearts of AIDS patients,[49] and selenium replacement was associated with an improvement in LV dysfunction in a small group of HIV-positive patients. L-Carnitine deficiency has also been described in HIV patients, possibly in association with cardiac symptoms, and in whom supplementation can be advantageous.[50] Experimentally, carnitine administration reversed myopathic changes induced by zidovudine (AZT) in vitro, but the clinical effects have yet to be established.[50]

Echocardiographic Features of HIV-Related Heart Muscle Disease

Characteristic echocardiographic features of dilated cardiomyopathy are detailed elsewhere and remain relevant to HIV/AIDS (see Chap. 29). The hallmark is global LV systolic dysfunction with the consistent feature of reduced ejection fraction. Examination of adults most frequently reveals a reduced or normal ventricular wall thickness in association with systolic dysfunction, whereas in children LV hypertrophy with cavity dilation is well-recognized.[51]

LV dilation can result in mitral valve distortion and lead to regurgitation. In AIDS patients, mitral regurgitation has also been described in association with infective endocarditis.[52] In these circumstances mitral regurgitation itself can cause secondary pulmonary hypertension and right ventricular dilation, although these features are more frequently seen as part of a generalized cardiomyopathic process.[10]

Abnormalities of mitral flow, specifically reduced early mitral peak velocity (E) and other indices of diastolic dysfunction have been noted early in the course of HIV/AIDS with normal ejection fraction and in association with LV systolic dysfunction.[53] The importance of these Doppler findings requires clarification, however, the utility of echocardiography should not be underestimated, particularly as ECG and chest x-ray can be unrewarding in these patients.

Treatment of Left Ventricular Dysfunction in HIV/AIDS

No randomized controlled trials have been reported that examine effectiveness of current heart failure therapies in people with HIV/AIDS. However, the prognostic significance of LV dysfunction, either in isolation or as part of a global cardiomyopathic process cannot be overlooked in these patients (see Figs. 92–3 and 92–4).[10] Evidence-based treatment for non-HIV individuals can prove applicable to HIV/AIDS patients with respect to morbidity and mortality improvements. Therefore, despite a seemingly poor prognosis, HIV patients with LV dysfunction should be offered generally accepted treatment.

Common agents such as diuretics, aldosterone antagonists, and digoxin can improve well being. Angiotensin-converting enzyme inhibitors, however, can be poorly tolerated, possibly because many patients already have a low systemic vascular resistance.[54]

TABLE 92-4

Cardiovascular Side Effects of Specific HIV Therapies

DRUG CLASS	EXAMPLES	POTENTIAL CARDIOVASCULAR SIDE EFFECT
Protease inhibitors (PI)	Amprenavir Atazanavir Fosamprenavir Indinavir Lopinavir Nelfinavir Ritonavir Saquinavir Tipranavir Zalcitabine	Lipodystrophy/dyslipidemia Insulin resistance/diabetes mellitus Hypertension/premature atherosclerosis, angina, myocardial infarction
Nucleoside reverse transcriptase inhibitors	Abacavir Didanosine Emtricitabine Lamivudine Stavudine Tenofovir Zalcitabine Zidovudine	Hypotension (Abacavir) Skeletal myopathy/(?) myocarditis/cardiomyopathy (zidovudine) Lactic acidosis Congestive heart failure/cardiomyopathy/hypertension/chest pain (zalcitabine)
Nonnucleoside reversible transcriptase inhibitors	Capravirine Delavirdine Efavirenz Nevirapine	Dyslipidemia (efavirenz)
Antiviral agents	Foscarnet Ganciclovir	Electrolyte disturbances/heart failure (foscarnet) Ventricular tachycardia (ganciclovir)
Antiparasitic agents	Pentamidine	QT prolongation/torsade de pointes Hypotension Sudden death

The side effects of blockade can also be problematic in end-stage AIDS patients with heart muscle disease, although information on the use of these agents is lacking.

If LV dilation and hypokinesis are found with or without clinical evidence of heart failure, consideration should be given to stopping all drugs that are not absolutely essential. If a 2-week followup echocardiography reveals improvement, the suspected drug should be eliminated.

Immunomodulatory therapy for HIV patients remains largely unproven. Etanercept, a tumor necrosis factor (TNF) antagonist, and pentoxifylline, a TNF-α inhibitor, have been used in non-HIV patients with severe heart failure with some success.[55,56] Intravenous immunoglobulin therapy has been used successfully in children with symptomatic HIV heart muscle disease and can be protective against the development of LV dysfunction in that group. The mode of action is not clear, but the treatment should be considered in pediatric patients with deteriorating cardiac function. The use of cardiac resynchronization has not been described in the HIV population, although case reports of the successful use of LV assist devices[57] and orthotopic heart transplant[58] exist, although these are uncommon.

ENDOCARDIAL DISEASE IN HIV/AIDS

Endocarditis is the principal endocardial lesion identified pathologically in AIDS, and both infectious and noninfectious forms have been described. At present, the prevalence of noninfectious endocarditis is lower than originally reported, and HIV itself has not emerged as a significant risk factor for infectious endocarditis. Nonetheless, these conditions remain a potential cause of significant morbidity in the AIDS population.

NONBACTERIAL THROMBOTIC ENDOCARDITIS

Marantic or nonbacterial thrombotic endocarditis (NBTE) is a condition in which friable clumps of platelets and red cells adhere to the cardiac valves. Unlike bacterial endocarditis, these lesions are not infective and show no evidence of an inflammatory reaction. NBTE was found in a homosexual male receiving chemotherapy for KS in 1982 and was reported in approximately 10 percent of adult AIDS patients in autopsy series from that time.[59]

The pathogenesis of NBTE is not fully understood, but hypercoagulability, immune complex deposition, or specific vitamin deficiency can be important in conjunction with endothelial damage from intracardiac catheters or injected particulate matter. Any heart valve can be affected, and frequently multiple lesions are found on different valves.[59] Systemic thromboembolism is a common sequel and contributes to the morbidity and mortality associated with the condition. However, the incidence of NBTE in AIDS patients appears to be falling,[60] which is surprising given the growing interest in the cardiac manifestations of AIDS and the continuing echocardiographic surveillance of these patients.[61] The reasons for this decline are not clear, but it can be related to improvements in nutrition and HIV therapy including HAART.

INFECTIVE ENDOCARDITIS

The immunologic abnormalities associated with HIV render patients susceptible to bacterial infections. Despite this, there are few reports of infective endocarditis (IE) complicating AIDS, and IE rarely complicates HIV infection outside the setting of injecting drug use.[62] The clinical presentation of bacterial endocarditis is the same for both HIV positive and negative patients but runs a more fulminant course in the late stages of AIDS.[63] However, asymptomatic HIV infection appears to have little effect on the susceptibility to, or the mortality from, the condition.[63]

As with IE in HIV-negative intravenous drug users, the most common valve involved is the tricuspid valve although left-sided valves can also be affected.[63] The most frequently isolated organisms are *S. aureus* and *Streptococcus viridans* but *Aspergillus fumigatus*, *Pseudallescheria boydii,* and other forms of fungal endocarditis can occur in end-stage AIDS.

Clearly, there is a need for adequate bacteriological investigations in cases of suspected IE in HIV-positive individuals just as for the non-AIDS population. However, the initial best guess for antimicrobial treatment may have to be widened, particularly if fungal endocarditis is a suspected complication of end-stage AIDS. Valvular heart surgery has been used in cases of IE in HIV-positive intravenous drug users, and although the lymphopenia associated with cardiopulmonary bypass was not associated with AIDS progression,[64] prognosis was poor and related to other factors such as continued drug use (see Chap. 85).[65]

CARDIAC TUMORS IN HIV/AIDS

Primary and metastatic tumors of the heart are relatively uncommon, but the advent of AIDS has changed both their prevalence and their appreciation in some ways.

【 】 KAPOSI SARCOMA INVOLVING THE HEART IN AIDS

Kaposi sarcoma (KS) is the most common AIDS-related neoplasia, and in contrast to the classic dermatologic form of the disease, there is often widespread and potentially fatal visceral involvement in HIV-positive individuals. Therefore, although KS involving the heart is rare outside this setting, it is now well recognized in patients with AIDS. The prevalence of cardiac KS in HIV/AIDS appears to have decreased significantly since early reports.[54]

The tumor is an endothelial cell neoplasia and shows a predilection for the subpericardial fat around coronary arteries, which it can infiltrate along with the parietal pericardium or myocardium. KS is not usually associated with symptoms of cardiac dysfunction; but cases of fatal tamponade associated with the tumor have been reported, and heart failure without ventricular dilation can occur in cases with extensive myocardial infiltration.

KS can be treated with daunorubicin, doxorubicin, or related anthracyclines, although care is required as these drugs can in themselves cause a drug-related cardiomyopathy. Liposomal-encapsulated daunorubicin has an improved pharmacokinetic profile and can therefore be preferred in patients with KS and AIDS, although there are few reports of these treatments being used specifically for cardiac involvement.[66]

【 】 CARDIAC LYMPHOMA IN HIV/AIDS

Primary cardiac lymphoma is extremely rare in HIV-negative individuals, accounting for less than 10 percent of all primary malignant cardiac tumors. Disseminated lymphoma can involve the myocardium more frequently but usually only as part of widespread tumor involvement. However, both patterns of malignant cardiac involvement occur in AIDS patients.

NHL can involve the pericardium or myocardium, and echocardiography is useful to detect intracavity masses and concomitant pericardial effusions. Radionuclide and MRI scans can be required to detect more diffuse cardiac involvement. In contrast to KS, cardiac lymphoma commonly gives rise to clinical symptoms of tamponade, heart failure, and conduction abnormalities and should be considered in AIDS patients whose cardiovascular symptoms progress rapidly. Primary lymphoma involving the heart alone is uncommon in AIDS, but surgical resection of a right atrial lymphoma was reported in an HIV-positive patient with limited short-term success.[67]

RIGHT VENTRICULAR DYSFUNCTION AND PULMONARY HYPERTENSION IN HIV/AIDS

Right ventricular dysfunction can occur as part of HIV-related heart muscle disease and in these circumstances should be treated as described previously. Isolated right ventricular dysfunction without pulmonary hypertension is of unknown significance[10] and can be related to changes in the pulmonary circulation. Therefore, bronchopulmonary infections should be treated aggressively, and intravenous drug use, which can result in microvascular pulmonary emboli, should be discouraged.

Isolated pulmonary hypertension is a rare and more serious complication of HIV infection, although it occurs more frequently than primary pulmonary hypertension in the non-HIV population.[68] The condition has a grave prognosis with an approximate 50 percent survival at 1 year despite having little correlation with CD4 counts or history of pulmonary infections.[69]

Although pulmonary hypertension in HIV/AIDS can be related to the action of viral proteins[70,71] or the action of cytokines on the endothelial cell, characteristic pulmonary arteriopathy is found in HIV-related pulmonary hypertension. The pathologic lesions include intimal fibrosis remodeling and plexiform lesions confirming its similarity to primary pulmonary hypertension and thus guides possible therapies.[68]

Right heart catheterization can be worthwhile to determine if pulmonary hypertension can be reversed and has been used in HIV patients.[72] Continuous or intermittently delivered home oxygen therapy, calcium channel antagonists, and nitric oxide therapy can be as useful for the HIV patient as for primary pulmonary hypertension patients, although their use is largely unproven. The use of anticoagulation therapies can be limited by concurrent thrombocytopenia that heightens bleeding risk.[73] HAART itself can be beneficial in terms of outcome from pulmonary hypertension,[74] but agents such as oral bosentan (Tracleer), intravenous epoprostenol (Flolan),[72] subcutaneous treprostinil,[75] or sildenafil can improve feeling of well being without necessarily altering prognosis. However, sildenafil and bosentan should be used with care in HIV patients because of potential drug interactions with antiretroviral therapy (Table 92–5).

TABLE 92–5

Major Potential Cardiovascular Drug Interactions of Specific HIV Therapies

DRUG CLASS	EXAMPLES	POSSIBLE CARDIOVASCULAR DRUG INTERACTIONS	POTENTIAL RISK
Protease inhibitors (PI)	Amprenavir Atazanavir Fosamprenavir Indinavir Lopinavir Nelfinavir Ritonavir Saquinavir Tipranavir Zalcitabine	Antiarrhythmics (amiodarone/flecainide/propafenone/quinidine/lignocaine/mexiletine/disopyramide) Anticoagulants (warfarin) Antimicrobials (erythromycin/clarithromycin) CCB HMG CoA Reductase Inhibitors (statins) PDVI (sildenafil) Vasodilators (bosentan)	↑ plasma concentration of antiarrhythmic drug. Enhanced proarrhythmic effect) Enhanced/reduced anticoagulant effect ↑ risk of torsade de pointes ↑ plasma concentration of CCB. Enhanced antihypertensive effect ↑ risk of myopathy/rhabdomyolysis (avoid simvastatin/lovastatin) Possible ↑ plasma concentration of PDVI (avoid use with ritonavir) ↑ plasma concentration of bosentan (use with care with ritonavir)
Nucleoside reverse transcriptase inhibitors	Abacavir Didanosine Emtricitabine Lamivudine Stavudine Tenofovir Zalcitabine Zidovudine	Few major cardiovascular drug interactions reported but clinical data limited	
Nonnucleoside reversible transcriptase inhibitors	Capravirine Delavirdine Efavirenz Nevirapine	Antiarrhythmics Anticoagulants (warfarin) CCB Statins PDVI	↑ plasma concentration/proarrhythmic effect Can enhance/reduce anticoagulant effect Delavirdine ↑ plasma concentration/CCB toxicity ↓ or ↑ plasma concentration of statins ↓ or ↑ plasma concentration of PDVI
Fusion Inhibitors	Enfuvirtide	No major cardiovascular drug interaction reported but clinical data limited	

CCB, calcium channel blocker; PDVI, phosphodiesterase V inhibitor.

NOTE: As major interactions are common with many HIV-specific therapies, clinicians are advised to review specific drug information and prescribe cardiovascular medications in close liaison with an HIV specialist.

VASCULAR DISEASES AND HIV/AIDS

[ ] LIPODYSTROPHY AND METABOLIC SYNDROME IN HIV/AIDS

HIV lipodystrophy is an ill-defined syndrome comprising central fat accumulation and peripheral lipoatrophy in association with dyslipidemia and insulin resistance.[76] The prevalence of these abnormalities can be dependent on the type and duration of antiretroviral therapy but can be up to 35 percent after 12 months of protease inhibitor (PI) or nucleoside analogue therapies.[77]

The metabolic features of lipodystrophy in HIV patients closely resembles that of the non-HIV metabolic syndrome and specifically include hypertriglyceridemia, hypercholesterolemia, (particularly raised total and low-density lipoprotein [LDL] cholesterol), insulin resistance, type II diabetes mellitus, lactic acidemia, and hepatic dysfunction.[78] Concerns are therefore raised over the risk of accelerated cardiovascular disease in affected individuals.

The pathogenesis of HIV lipodystrophy is not known but can include lipid and adipocyte regulatory protein dysfunction through PI binding[78] or NRTI-induced mitochondrial toxicity.[79] The syndrome does not appear to be a direct effect of

HIV itself, because lipodystrophy appears to occur exclusively in patients receiving antiretroviral therapy.[80] Similarly, whereas the dyslipidemia noted in these patients can merely be a consequence of insulin resistance and lipodystrophy, PI therapy in non-HIV patients results in abnormal cholesterol, triglyceride, apolipoprotein B, and lipoprotein levels and rapidly induces insulin resistance.[81]

Therapy for Lipodystrophy and Related Conditions in HIV/AIDS

Dietary therapy for dyslipidemia in HIV disease remains contentious and has not been fully evaluated, although healthy diets rich in fruit, vegetables, and fish oils (possibly through supplementation) are encouraged. Drug therapy can also be necessary, particularly if antiretroviral treatment cannot be changed or interrupted. Bile acid sequestrants, although attractive from the point of view of drug interactions, can have adverse effects on serum triglyceride levels or impair absorption of antiretrovirals.

Most hydroxymethylglutaryl coenzyme A (HMG-CoA) reductase inhibitors (statins) are metabolized in the liver through the cytochrome P450 system. Simvastatin, lovastatin, and atorvastatin use the cytochrome P450 enzyme (CYP)3A4 whereas fluvastatin metabolizes through CYP2C9. Pravastatin is unique in that its breakdown takes place outside this enzyme system. Given that PI and nonnucleoside transcriptase inhibitor metabolism is also CYP3A4 dependent, coprescription of some statins can be associated with increased risk of myopathy and rhabdomyolysis through competitive inhibition and significantly increased plasma statin levels.

For this reason it is recommended that hypercholesterolemia in HIV patients treated with PIs be treated initially with pravastatin 20 milligrams (mg) daily with careful monitoring of virological parameters and serum creatine kinase levels. Low-dose atorvastatin (10 mg/day) can be used with care although fluvastatin is an acceptable alternative. Simvastatin and lovastatin are not recommended. For patients who do not respond or are intolerant of statins, or in whom nondrug therapy has failed to correct significant hypertriglyceridemia, gemfibrozil 600 mg twice daily or fenofibrate 200 mg once daily can be used in isolation, although combination of fibrates and statins are not recommended.[76] Other potential major cardiovascular drug interactions with specific HIV therapies are noted in Table 92–5.

Lipodystrophy, Glucose Intolerance, and HIV/AIDS

Treatment of glucose intolerance and diabetes also requires care, but if healthy diet and exercise are insufficient, drug treatment can again be necessary. Metformin can cause lactic acidosis, and some glitazones are also metabolized through the CYP3A4 system thus presenting an increased risk of myositis and hepatitis if coprescribed with PIs.[13] Rosiglitazone, which is not metabolized through the P450 system, can therefore become an attractive option.

[ ] ACCELERATED ATHEROSCLEROSIS AND CORONARY HEART DISEASE IN HIV/AIDS

HAART has clear beneficial effects on both mortality and morbidity in HIV/AIDS, however, concern remains over the significant changes in lipid metabolism noted previously and raises the possibility of an epidemic of premature atherosclerotic disease in these patients.

The first cases of acute myocardial infarction in treated HIV patients emerged in the late 1990s. Although initially there was no evidence of increased cardiovascular mortality in this population,[82] a two- to threefold increase in the incidence of acute coronary syndromes (ACSs) has recently been noted in HAART-treated HIV patients compared with controls. Moreover, in comparison to national registries, coronary heart disease (CHD) in HIV patients occurred mostly in males and at a younger age suggesting that the age adjusted incidence can be significantly higher.[83]

HIV patients with CHD tend to be older than HIV patients without coronary symptoms, and the majority will have been diagnosed with AIDS.[83] This raises the intriguing possibility that opportunistic infections such as *Cytomegalovirus* or *Chlamydiae pneumoniae* can play a role in the development of accelerated atherosclerosis.[84] However, ACS are not clearly related to HIV replication, because HIV RNA can be undetectable in up to one-third of patients at the time of presentation.[83]

Traditional risk factors in this patient group should not be overlooked. Prevalence of cigarette smoking in HIV infected patients can be as high as 50 percent in certain populations,[85] diabetes mellitus requiring treatment is common,[86] and HIV patients can be at higher risk of developing hypertension at a younger age than the general population.[87]

Acute myocardial infarction (AMI) appears to be the most common presentation of CHD, and a high ratio of AMI to stable angina exists in HIV populations.[83] Because these ACSs involve low volume, lipid rich plaques, the metabolic syndrome of HIV lipodystrophy can promote development of vulnerable lesions or influence important plaque rupture. However, it remains difficult to establish an absolute link between PI exposure and CHD, and further long-term studies are required.

Coronary angiography can be carried out in HIV patients safely and frequently reveals patterns of coronary disease similar to young non-HIV patients, such as proximal vessel involvement and single vessel disease.[83] Coronary artery bypass surgery has been carried out with reasonable survival rates, and fibrinolysis can be used successfully in the setting of acute ST elevation myocardial infarction.[83]

Although percutaneous coronary intervention is also described,[88] some concerns have been raised regarding the risk of aggressive restenosis in HIV patients.[89] For this reason the use of drug-eluting stents with a lower potential risk of restenosis should be considered.[90] However, it remains reasonable that the clinical situation should determine the use of invasive and noninvasive coronary investigations as for the non-HIV population.

[ ] VASCULITIS IN HIV/AIDS

Vascular changes, particularly vasculitis and endothelial cell structural changes have been documented in HIV/AIDS. Examination of aortic endothelial cells from HIV-infected patients showed a disturbed intima, increased leukocyte adherence, and upregulation of vascular cell adhesion molecules.[91]

This indicated profound and repeated activation of aortic endothelial cells in AIDS, and it is possible that some HIV structural proteins can play an integral role in the process.

The clinical importance of such findings is not clear, and lesions affecting small and medium sized arteries are usually only evident by microscopy. However, fusiform aneurysms of the right coronary artery were found in a child who died suddenly.[92] These lesions were histologically distinct from other arteriopathies, but other vascular abnormalities in children have been reported in the brain, thymus, spleen, and lymph nodes. Kawasaki disease, which can have a similar presentation, should be considered in the differential diagnosis.

DISORDERS OF RHYTHM ASSOCIATED WITH HIV INFECTION

Sudden death and rhythm abnormalities are common in HIV infection and account for up to 20 percent of cardiac-related deaths in this group of patients. These can be secondary to other cardiac pathology, or be a consequence of some forms of treatment. For example, pentamidine, used in the treatment and prophylaxis of *P. carinii* infection, is structurally similar to procainamide and can cause torsade de pointes ventricular tachycardia when used intravenously or intramuscularly. Ganciclovir, an acyclic nucleoside used in the treatment of severe CMV infection, can also be arrhythmogenic.

Concomitant electrolyte disturbance can be important in the development of cardiac arrhythmia, and careful evaluation of the QT interval and magnesium concentration should be used as a guide to cardiac toxicity. ECG abnormalities and rhythm disturbances are not uncommon findings in HIV-positive patients with myocarditis or heart muscle disease, and ectopic beats, ventricular tachycardia, and sudden death have all been reported.

Autonomic dysfunction is common in patients with HIV infection, and this can predispose to syncopal events and even death. Dysrhythmias caused by excessive sympathetic tone are also recognized.[93] Conduction abnormalities and arrhythmias have been demonstrated in HIV-positive children with ECG abnormalities, possibly related to small vessel vasculitis, neural tissue fibrosis, or myocarditis.[94]

HEALTHCARE WORKERS, CARDIOVASCULAR INTERVENTION, AND HIV/AIDS

There is continuing anxiety that healthcare workers can become infected with HIV, or, if infected, they can infect other patients. At the same time, cardiovascular intervention has the potential to accelerate the disease process through poorly understood immune mechanisms. In general therefore it seems sensible to avoid complex procedures associated with potential morbidity and mortality in patients with a limited life span. However, patients with HIV/AIDS are surviving significantly longer, and clearly difficult decisions regarding invasive treatment will arise.

Fear of becoming infected with HIV is understandable, but universal precautions should limit potential risk to healthcare workers and as such should not preclude the HIV/AIDS patient from possible therapies should they be felt appropriate.[95]

REFERENCES

1. Zarocostas J. Number of people infected with HIV worldwide reaches 40m. *Br Med J* 2005;331:1224.
2. Steinbrook R. The AIDS epidemic in 2004. *N Engl J Med* 2004;351:115–117.
3. Ruxrungtham K, Brown T, Phanuphak P. HIV/AIDS in Asia. *Lancet* 2004;364:69–82.
4. Fauci AS. The AIDS epidemic—considerations for the 21st century [see comments]. *N Engl J Med* 1999;341:1046–1050.
5. Pinching AJ. Factors affecting the natural history of human immunodeficiency virus infection. *Immunodefic Rev* 1988;1:23–38.
6. Deeks S, Volberding P. An approach to antiretroviral treatment of HIV disease. Combined antiretroviral therapy: the emerging role. *Hosp Pract* 1995;(30 suppl)1:23–31.
7. Schacker T. Primary HIV infection. Early diagnosis and treatment are critical to outcome. *Postgrad Med* 1997;102:143–146, 149–151.
8. Hsue PY, Waters DD. What a cardiologist needs to know about patients with human immunodeficiency virus infection. *Circulation* 2005;112:3947–3957.
9. Ntsekhe M, Hakim J. Impact of human immunodeficiency virus infection on cardiovascular disease in Africa. *Circulation* 2005;112:3602–3607.
10. Currie PF, Jacob AJ, Foreman AR, et al. Heart muscle disease related to HIV infection: prognostic implications. *Br Med J* 1994;309:1605–1607.
11. Corallo S, Mutinelli MR, Moroni M, et al. Echocardiography detects myocardial damage in AIDS. Prospective study in 102 patients. *Eur Heart J* 1988;9:887–892.
12. Pollock BH, Jenson HB, Leach CT, et al. Risk factors for pediatric human immunodeficiency virus-related malignancy. *JAMA* 2003;289:2393–2399.
13. Volberding PA, Murphy RL, Barbaro G, et al. The PAVIA consensus statement. *AIDS* 2003;17(suppl 1):S170–S179.
14. Lipshultz SE, Fisher SD, Lai WW, et al. Cardiovascular risk factors, monitoring, and therapy for HIV-infected patients. *AIDS* 2003;17(suppl 1):S96–122.
15. Lewis W. AIDS. cardiac findings from 115 autopsies. *Prog Cardiovasc Dis* 1989;32:207–215.
16. Monsuez JJ, Kinney EL, Vittecoq D, et al. Comparison among acquired immune deficiency syndrome patients with and without clinical evidence of cardiac disease. *Am J Cardiol* 1988;62:1311–1313.
17. Mayosi BM, Wiysonge CS, Ntsekhe M, et al. Clinical characteristics and initial management of patients with tuberculous pericarditis in the HIV era: the Investigation of the Management of Pericarditis in Africa (IMPI Africa) registry. *BMC Infect Dis* 2006;6:2.
18. Dalli E, Quesada A, Juan G, et al. Tuberculous pericarditis as the first manifestation of acquired immunodeficiency syndrome. *Am Heart J* 1987;114:905–906.
19. Flynn DR, McGinn JT, Tyras DH. The role of the pericardial window in AIDS. *Chest* 1995;107:1522–1525.
20. Currie PF, Wright RA, Campanella C, et al. Long-term survival following pericardiectomy for Staphylococcus aureus pericarditis in an HIV-positive drug user. *Eur Heart J* 1997;18:526–527.
21. Lewis W. Cardiomyopathy in AIDS. a pathophysiological perspective. *Prog Cardiovasc Dis* 2000;43:151–170.
22. Aretz HT. Myocarditis: the Dallas criteria. *Hum Pathol* 1987;18:619–624.
23. Reilly JM, Cunnion RE, Anderson DW, et al. Frequency of myocarditis, left ventricular dysfunction and ventricular tachycardia in the acquired immune deficiency syndrome. *Am J Cardiol* 1988;62:789–793.
24. Tazelaar HD, Billingham ME. Leukocytic infiltrates in idiopathic dilated cardiomyopathy. A source of confusion with active myocarditis. *Am J Surg Pathol* 1986;10:405–412.
25. Levy WS, Simon GL, Rios JC, et al. Prevalence of cardiac abnormalities in human immunodeficiency virus infection. *Am J Cardiol* 1989;63:86–89.
26. Pugliese A, Isnardi D, Saini A, et al. Impact of highly active antiretroviral therapy in HIV-positive patients with cardiac involvement. *J Infect* 2000;40:282–284.
27. Magnani JW, Dec GW. Myocarditis: current trends in diagnosis and treatment. *Circulation* 2006;113:876–890.
28. Herskowitz A, Wu TC, Willoughby SB, et al. Myocarditis and cardiotropic viral infection associated with severe left ventricular dysfunction in late-stage

infection with human immunodeficiency virus. *J Am Coll Cardiol* 1994;24:1025–1032.

29. Grody WW, Cheng L, Lewis W. Infection of the heart by the human immunodeficiency virus. *Am J Cardiol* 1990;66:203–206.

30. Shannon RP, Simon MA, Mathier MA, et al. Dilated cardiomyopathy associated with simian AIDS in nonhuman primates. *Circulation* 2000;101:185–193.

31. Rodriguez ER, Nasim S, Hsia J, et al. Cardiac myocytes and dendritic cells harbor human immunodeficiency virus in infected patients with and without cardiac dysfunction: detection by multiplex, nested, polymerase chain reaction in individually microdissected cells from right ventricular endomyocardial biopsy tissue. *Am J Cardiol* 1991;68:1511–1520.

32. Herskowitz A, Willoughby S, Wu TC, et al. Immunopathogenesis of HIV-1 associated cardiomyopathy. *Clin Immunol Immunopatho* 1993;68:234–241.

33. Andrade LO, Machado CR, Chiari E, et al. Trypanosoma cruzi: role of host genetic background in the differential tissue distribution of parasite clonal populations. *Exp Parasitol* 2002;100:269–275.

34. Ho DD, Pomerantz RJ, Kaplan JC. Pathogenesis of infection with human immunodeficiency virus. *N Engl J Med* 1987;317:278–286.

35. Kan H, Xie Z, Finkel MS. HIV gp120 enhances NO production by cardiac myocytes through p38 MAP kinase-mediated NF-B activation. *Am J Physiol Heart Circ Physiol* 2000;279:H3138–143.

36. Herskowitz A, Vlahov D, Willoughby S, et al. Prevalence and incidence of left ventricular dysfunction in patients with human immunodeficiency virus infection. *Am J Cardiol* 1993;71:955–958.

37. Rocha A, de Meneses AC, da Silva AM, et al. Pathology of patients with Chagas' disease and acquired immunodeficiency syndrome. *Am J Trop Med Hyg* 1994;50:261–268.

38. Lipshultz SE, Chanock S, Sanders SP, et al. Cardiovascular manifestations of human immunodeficiency virus infection in infants and children. *Am J Cardiol* 1989;63:1489–1497.

39. Currie PF, Goldman JH, Caforio AL, et al. Cardiac autoimmunity in HIV related heart muscle disease. *Heart* 1998;79:599–604.

40. Zimmerman FH, Gustafson GM, Kemp HG. Recurrent myocardial infarction associated with cocaine abuse in a young man with normal coronary arteries: evidence for coronary artery spasm culminating in thrombosis. *J Am Coll Cardiol* 1987;9:964–968.

41. De Palo VA, Millstein BH, Mayo PH, et al. Outcome of intensive care in patients with HIV infection. *Chest* 1995;107:506–510.

42. Del Prete G, Maggi E, Pizzolo G, et al. CD 30 Th2 cytokines and HIV infection: a complex and fascinating link. *Immunol Today* 1995;16:76–80.

43. de Larranaga GF, Forastiero RR, Carreras LO, et al. Different types of antiphospholipid antibodies in AIDS. A comparison with syphilis and the antiphospholipid syndrome. *Thromb Res* 1999;96:19–25.

44. Brinkman K, Smeitink JA, Romijn JA, et al. Mitochondrial toxicity induced by nucleoside-analogue reverse- transcriptase inhibitors is a key factor in the pathogenesis of antiretroviral-therapy-related lipodystrophy [comment]. *Lancet* 1999;354:1112–1115.

45. Lewis W, Grupp IL, Grupp G, et al. Cardiac dysfunction occurs in the HIV-1 transgenic mouse treated with zidovudine. *Lab Invest* 2000;80:187–197.

46. Herskowitz A, Willoughby SB, Baughman KL, et al. Cardiomyopathy associated with antiretroviral therapy in patients with HIV infection: a report of six cases. *Ann Intern Med* 1992;116:311–313.

47. Karch SB, Billingham ME. The pathology and etiology of cocaine-induced heart disease. *Arch Pathol Lab Med* 1988;112:225–230.

48. Fuchs J, Ochsendorf F, Schofer H, et al. Oxidative imbalance in HIV infected patients. *Med Hypotheses* 1991;36:60–64.

49. Dworkin BM, Antonecchia PP, Smith F, et al. Reduced cardiac selenium content in the acquired immunodeficiency syndrome [see comments]. *JPEN J Parenter Enteral Nutr* 1989;13:644–647.

50. De Simone C, Tzantzoglou S, Jirillo E, et al. L-carnitine deficiency in AIDS patients. *AIDS* 1992;6:203–205.

51. Moorthy LN, Lipshultz SE. Cardiovascular monitoring of HIV-infected patients. In: Lipshultz SE, eds. *Cardiology in AIDS.* New York: Chapman & Hall; 1998:345–384.

52. Werneck GL, Mesquita ET, Romeo LJ, et al. Doppler echocardiographic evaluation of HIV-positive patients in different stages of the disease. *Arq Bras Cardiol* 1999;73:163–168.

53. Coudray N, de Zuttere D, Force G, et al. Left ventricular diastolic function in asymptomatic and symptomatic human immunodeficiency virus carriers: an echocardiographic study. *Eur Heart J* 1995;16:61–67.

54. Currie PF, Boon AB. Prospective adult cardiovascular morbidity and mortality studies: the world. In Lipshultz SE, eds. *Cardiology in AIDS.* New York: Chapman & Hall; 1998:59–76.

55. Deswal A, Misra A, Bozkurt B. The role of anti-cytokine therapy in the failing heart. *Heart Fail Rev* 2001;6:143–151.

56. Sliwa K, Woodiwiss A, Candy G, et al. Effects of pentoxifylline on cytokine profiles and left ventricular performance in patients with decompensated congestive heart failure secondary to idiopathic dilated cardiomyopathy. *Am J Cardiol* 2002;90:1118–1122.

57. Brucato A, Colombo T, Bonacina E, et al. Fulminant myocarditis during HIV seroconversion: recovery with temporary left ventricular mechanical assistance. *Ital Heart J* 2004;5:228–231.

58. Calabrese LH, Albrecht M, Young J, et al. Successful cardiac transplantation in an HIV-1-infected patient with advanced disease. *N Engl J Med* 2003;348:2323–2328.

59. Cammarosano C, Lewis W. Cardiac lesions in acquired immune deficiency syndrome (AIDS). *J Am Coll Cardiol* 1985;5:703–706.

60. Lewis W, Grody WW. AIDS and the heart: review and consideration of pathogenetic mechanisms. *Cardiovasc Pathol* 1992;1:53–64.

61. Currie PF, Sutherland GR, Jacob AJ, et al. A review of endocarditis in acquired immunodeficiency syndrome and human immunodeficiency virus infection. *Eur Heart J* 1995;16(suppl B):15–18.

62. Cicalini S, Forcina G, De Rosa FG. Infective endocarditis in patients with human immunodeficiency virus infection. *J Infect* 2001;42:267–271.

63. Nahass RG, Weinstein MP, Bartels J, et al. Infective endocarditis in intravenous drug users: a comparison of human immunodeficiency virus type 1-negative and -positive patients. *J Infect Dis* 1990;162:967–970.

64. Aris A, Pomar JL, Saura E. Cardiopulmonary bypass in HIV-positive patients. *Ann Thorac Surg* 1993;55:1104–1107.

65. Lemma M, Vanelli P, Beretta L, et al. Cardiac surgery in HIV-positive intravenous drug addicts: influence of cardiopulmonary bypass on the progression to AIDS. *Thorac Cardiovasc Surg* 1992;40:279–282.

66. Harrison M, Tomlinson D, Stewart S. Liposomal-entrapped doxorubicin: an active agent in AIDS-related Kaposi's sarcoma. *J Clin Oncol* 1995;13:914–920.

67. Horowitz MD, Cox MM, Neibart RM, et al. Resection of right atrial lymphoma in a patient with AIDS. *Int J Cardiol* 1992;34:139–142.

68. Petitpretz P, Brenot F, Azarian R, et al. Pulmonary hypertension in patients with human immunodeficiency virus infection. Comparison with primary pulmonary hypertension. *Circulation* 1994;89:2722–2727.

69. Mesa RA, Edell ES, Dunn WF, et al. Human immunodeficiency virus infection and pulmonary hypertension: two new cases and a review of 86 reported cases. *Mayo Clin Proc* 1998;73:37–45.

70. Schecter AD, Berman AB, Yi L, et al. HIV envelope gp120 activates human arterial smooth muscle cells. *Proc Natl Acad Sci U S A* 2001;98:10142–10147.

71. Kanmogne GD, Primeaux C, Grammas P. Induction of apoptosis and endothelin-1 secretion in primary human lung endothelial cells by HIV-1 gp120 proteins. *Biochem Biophys Res Commun* 2005;333:1107–1115.

72. Recusani F, Di Matteo A, Gambarin F, et al. Clinical and therapeutical follow-up of HIV-associated pulmonary hypertension: prospective study of 10 patients. *AIDS* 2003;17(suppl 1):S88–95.

73. Saidi A, Bricker JT. Pulmonary hypertension in patients infected with HIV. In: Lipshultz SE, eds. *Cardiology in AIDS.* New York: Chapman & Hall; 1998:187–194.

74. Pugliese A, Gennero L, Vidotto V, et al. A review of cardiovascular complications accompanying AIDS. *Cell Biochem Funct* 2004;22:137–141.

75. Cea-Calvo L, Escribano Subias P, Tello de Menesses R, et al. Treatment of HIV-associated pulmonary hypertension with treprostinil. *Rev Esp Cardiol* 2003;56:421–425.

76. Dube MP, Sprecher D, Henry WK, et al. Preliminary guidelines for the evaluation and management of dyslipidemia in adults infected with human immunodeficiency virus and receiving antiretroviral therapy: recommendations of the Adult AIDS. Clinical Trial Group Cardiovascular Disease Focus Group. *Clin Infect Dis* 2000;31:1216–1224.

77. Bogner JR, Vielhauer V, Beckmann RA, et al. Stavudine versus zidovudine and the development of lipodystrophy. *J Acquir Immune Defic Syndr* 2001;27:237–244.

78. Carr A. Cardiovascular risk factors in HIV-infected patients. *J Acquir Immune Defic Syndr* 2003;34(suppl 1):S73–78.

79. Lewis W, Day BJ, Copeland WC. Mitochondrial toxicity of NRTI antiviral drugs: an integrated cellular perspective. *Nat Rev Drug Discov* 2003;2:812–822.

80. Miller RF, Shahmonesh M, Hanna MG, et al. Polyphenotypic expression of mitochondrial toxicity caused by nucleoside reverse transcriptase inhibitors. *Antivir Ther* 2003;8:253–257.

81. Noor MA, Lo JC, Mulligan K, et al. Metabolic effects of indinavir in healthy HIV-seronegative men. *AIDS* 2001;15:F11–18.

82. Bozzette SA, Ake CF, Tam HK, et al. Cardiovascular and cerebrovascular events in patients treated for human immunodeficiency virus infection. *N Engl J Med* 2003;348:702–710.

83. Vittecoq D, Escaut L, Chironi G, et al. Coronary heart disease in HIV-infected patients in the highly active antiretroviral treatment era. *AIDS* 2003;17(suppl 1):S70–76.

84. Nieto FJ. Infective agents and cardiovascular disease. *Semin Vasc Med* 2002;2:401–15.

85. Gritz ER, Vidrine DJ, Lazev AB, et al. Smoking behavior in a low-income multi-ethnic HIV/AIDS population. *Nicotine Tob Res* 2004;6:71–77.

86. Hadigan C. Diabetes, insulin resistance, and HIV. *Curr Infect Dis Rep* 2006;8:69–75.

87. Aoun S, Ramos E. Hypertension in the HIV-infected patient. *Curr Hypertens Rep* 2000;2:478–481.

88. Varriale P, Saravi G, Hernandez E, et al. Acute myocardial infarction in patients infected with human immunodeficiency virus. *Am Heart J* 2004;147:55–59.

89. Hsue PY, Giri K, Erickson S, et al. Clinical features of acute coronary syndromes in patients with human immunodeficiency virus infection. *Circulation* 2004;109:316–319.

90. Huang L, Quartin A, Jones D, et al. Intensive care of patients with HIV infection. *N Engl J Med* 2006;355:173–181.

91. Zietz C, Hotz B, Sturzl M, et al. Aortic endothelium in HIV-1 infection: chronic injury, activation, and increased leukocyte adherence. *Am J Pathol* 1996;149:1887–1898.

92. Joshi VV, Gadol C, Connor E, et al. Dilated cardiomyopathy in children with acquired immunodeficiency syndrome: a pathologic study of five cases. *Hum Pathol* 1988;19:69–73.

93. Lipshultz SE, Fisher SD, Lai W, et al. Cardiac monitoring and therapy for HIV-infected patients. *Ann NY Acad Sci.* 2001;946:236–273.

94. Bharati S, Joshi VV, Connor EM, et al. Conduction system in children with acquired immunodeficiency syndrome. *Chest* 1989;96:406–413.

95. Hughes JM. Universal precautions: CDC perspective. *Occup Med* 1989;4(suppl):13–20.

CHAPTER (93)

Effect of Noncardiac Drugs, Electricity, Poisons, and Radiation on the Heart

Andrew L. Smith / Wendy M. Book

This chapter deals with a number of deleterious side effects of treatments and environmental agents on the heart. Toxic effects can occur acutely and require emergent intervention or can be chronic and not be manifest until days or years after exposure.

NONCARDIAC DRUGS

【 】 CHEMOTHERAPEUTIC AGENTS

Chemotherapeutic agents can result in acute or chronic cardiovascular toxicity. The heart, composed of nonproliferating myocytes, was traditionally thought to be protected from the effects of drugs on rapidly dividing cells. A number of these agents are now recognized to cause cardiovascular complications including cardiomyopathy, myocarditis, pericarditis, myocardial ischemia, arrhythmias, and peripheral hypotension or vasospasm.[1]

Cardiovascular alterations in the patient receiving chemotherapy can be the result of a specific drug or combination of drugs or be related to tumor-associated factors such as hypercoagulability or release of myocardial depressant factors. Correlating a specific therapy with a particular adverse event can be difficult; however, knowledge of side effects of each agent should be considered when prescribing therapy.[1–3]

Anthracyclines

The anthracycline antineoplastics—doxorubicin, daunorubicin, and epirubicin—are the leading cause of chemotherapy-related heart disease. These agents can cause cardiac problems during therapy, weeks after completion of therapy, or, unexpectedly, years later.[4] During acute therapy, electrocardiogram (ECG) changes occur in approximately 30 percent of patients and usually regress within weeks. Findings include ST-T wave changes, decreased QRS voltage, prolongation of the QT interval, and atrial and ventricular ectopy. Sustained atrial or ventricular arrhythmias are rare. The occurrence of early ECG abnormalities does not predict cardiomyopathy and is not an indication to discontinue therapy.[1] The development of persistent sinus tachycardia in an otherwise stable oncology patient (although nonspecific), however, can raise the suspicion of ventricular dysfunction and impending congestive heart failure. Congestive heart failure is related to the cumulative dose of the anthracycline administered. The incidences of heart failure at specific doses of doxorubicin include 0.4 percent at 400 mg/m² of body surface area, 7 percent at 550 mg/m², and 18 percent at 700 mg/m² (Fig. 93–1).[5] Traditionally, the cardiac limiting dose has been described as 550 mg/m² because of the acute rise in heart failure seen above this dose. There is great individual variability, however, with reports of heart failure occurring with doses less than 100 mg/m² and, conversely, with some patients tolerating greater than 1000 mg/m² without cardiac compromise.[5,6] Risk factors for anthracycline-induced cardiomyopathy are debated but include prior chest radiation, young age (0 to 12 years of age), age older than 70 years, and preexisting heart disease.[5–7] Young females can be at particularly increased risk for late cardiac dysfunction.[7] Rapid infusion schedules associated with higher peak drug concentration appear to result in greater cardiotoxicity. Combination therapy with cyclophosphamide is an additional risk factor,[1] with cardiotoxicity noted at doses of 300 mg/m². The pathogenesis of anthracycline-induced cardiotoxicity is not known. Theories generally implicate free radical damage.[8,9] The average time to clinical development of heart failure symptoms is 1 month from the end of anthracycline therapy but can occur anytime within 1 year. There is increased recognition of symptomatic heart failure occurring years after therapy. Patient presentation is similar to that for other dilated cardiomyopathies (see Chap. 29).

Noninvasive assessment of left ventricular function has been used to guide anthracycline dosing and prevent cardiac toxicity. Serial echocardiography and/or radionuclide angiography (see Chaps. 16 and 19) are most commonly used.[10,11] The most commonly used parameter is resting left ventricular ejection fraction. Recognition that resting left ventricular ejection fraction is relatively insensitive for detecting early cardiotoxicity has resulted in the investigation of other variables (exercise or dobutamine echocardiography measurement of isovolumetric relaxation time and myocardial performance index (Tei index) in assessing this problem.[10] These methods have generally been evaluated in small-sized studies and have not gained widespread acceptance in current therapy guidelines. Adult guidelines for serial assessment have been developed. A drop in left ventricular ejection fraction greater than 10 percent (ejection fraction [EF] units) and to below a normal value of 50 percent is an indication to discontinue therapy. A baseline left ventricular ejection fraction less than 30 percent has generally been considered a contraindication to initiating anthracycline therapy.[12–14]

There is growing recognition of the occurrence of cardiac dysfunction years after completion of anthracycline therapy. Clinical strategies for preventing anthracycline cardiotoxicity have had to balance the need for antineoplastic efficacy. Lower clinical toxicity in adults has been noted with prolonged infusions of doxorubicin over 48 to 96 hours to avoid high-peak concentrations.[15] In contrast, continuous infusion schedules in children do not offer a cardioprotective advantage.[16] Several antioxidants have been evaluated but with inconclusive results.[9,17]

Other Chemotherapeutic Agents

Mitoxantrone, an anthracenedione lacking the amino sugar of anthracyclines, causes cardiotoxicity with features similar to anthracycline-induced cardiomyopathy.[1] This drug appears to have less cardiotoxicity than doxorubicin at equal myelotoxic doses. Cumulative doses above 160 mg/m² are associated with an increasing incidence of congestive heart failure. There has been increasing concern that mitoxantrone in high doses and particularly when combined with other chemotherapeutic agents can result in a high incidence of delayed myocardial toxicity.[18] High-dose *cyclophosphamide* (120 to 240 mg/kg over several days) used in bone marrow transplantation can cause acute cardiac toxicity.[1,19] Symptomatic systolic dysfunction, usually reversible with drug discontinuation, is associated with decreased QRS voltage on the ECG. Pericardial effusions have been noted, and a hemorrhagic myocarditis can result in death. Necropsy data demonstrate endothelial injury with resultant interstitial fibrin deposition and capillary microthrombosis. The cardiotoxicity of cyclophosphamide is likely caused by damage from its biologically active metabolites. Rapid metabolizers of cyclophosphamide appear to be prone to cardiotoxicity. The metabolites cause toxic endothelial damage leading to muscle damage.[19] Cyclophosphamide can also potentiate the cardiotoxic effects of the anthracyclines.[1,18] Ifosfamide is an alkylating agent that can cause toxicity similar to cyclophosphamide.[2]

5-Fluorouracil can occasionally cause angina, electrocardiographic changes, and rarely myocardial infarction.[1,20] The majority of episodes occur during the first cycle of therapy and resolve spontaneously after discontinuation. Arrhythmias and systolic dysfunction have been observed. The understanding of 5-fluorouracil toxicity is complicated because combination chemotherapy is generally used, patients can be systemically ill, and many receiving this medication have preexisting coronary artery disease.[20] The incidence of cardiac toxicity is uncertain but ranges from 1 to 8 percent.[21] Patients with known coronary artery disease are at higher risk for serious cardiotoxicity. The mechanism of toxicity remains unclear, although coronary vasospasm has been suspected. Coronary catheterization has generally failed to demonstrate vasomotor hyperreactivity with 5-fluorouracil or ergonovine challenge.

Amsacrine (AMSA P-D) has been associated with prolongation of the QT interval. Malignant ventricular arrhythmias can occur in <1 percent of patients and are exacerbated by hypokalemia.[22]

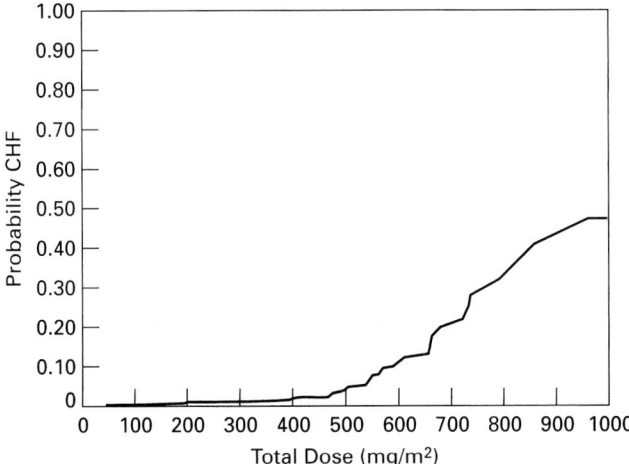

FIGURE 93–1. The development of doxorubicin-induced heart failure is related to cumulative dose. Toxicity can occur at any dose, but at 550 mg/m² the probability increases significantly. CHF, congestive heart failure. *Source: Von Hoff, Layard, Basa, et al.[5]*

Paclitaxel (Taxol) is used to treat many types of cancer. The most common cardiovascular effect is the development of transient asymptomatic bradycardia, occurring in more than 10 percent of patients.[3]

Trastuzumab (recombinant humanized anti-human epidermal growth receptor 2 [HER-2] antibody) is a relatively new treatment for breast cancer that has had favorable antitumor effects when added to standard chemotherapy in selected patients. A retrospective review described a 27 percent incidence of cardiotoxicity when this agent was given with an anthracycline and cyclophosphamide, a 13 percent incidence in combination with paclitaxel, and a 3 to 7 percent incidence given alone. The majority of these patients had received prior anthracycline therapy.[23] The pathophysiology of trastuzumab cardiotoxicity is uncertain, but unlike anthracycline cardiotoxicity ultrastructural changes have not been noted on cardiac biopsy. Clinically symptoms occur more acutely than anthracycline toxicity, and left ventricular dysfunction is often reversible with removal of the agent.[23–25]

【 】 IMMUNOMODULATING AGENTS

Interferon alpha can cause supraventricular tachyarrhythmias. A reversible cardiomyopathy has been described.[1,19,26,27]

【 】 PSYCHOTROPIC AGENTS

Psychiatric illness, particularly depression, is common in patients with cardiovascular disease (see Chap. 95). Morbidity and mortality following cardiac events are increased in patients with depression, particularly if untreated.[28,29] A variety of psychotropic agents have conduction or vascular effects. A thorough understanding of these therapeutic, but potentially toxic, agents is necessary in the treatment of patients with preexisting cardiac disease. Intentional overdose with these drugs can result in serious cardiac manifestations.

【 】 TRICYCLIC ANTIDEPRESSANTS

The tricyclic antidepressants have several properties that account for the majority of cardiovascular effects. These drugs inhibit uptake of both norepinephrine and serotonin, resulting in greater toxicity compared to the selective serotonin reuptake inhibitors (SSRIs). A hyperadrenergic state can result in tachycardia. α Blockade occurs at higher drug levels and can cause marked hypotension in the setting of overdose. The anticholinergic effects result in tachycardia, dry mouth, and constipation, and in overdose[30] they can delay gastrointestinal absorption of the drug. Sodium channel blockade, typical of the type IA antiarrhythmic compounds, results in conduction abnormalities and the potential to suppress ventricular function.[31]

The most common electrocardiographic changes include nonspecific ST-T changes and prolongation of the QT interval, PR interval, and QRS duration. PR prolongation is caused by prolonged infranodal conduction. Patients with preexisting conduction disease, particularly bundle-branch block, are at increased risk of toxicity.[32] The tricyclic antidepressants have type IA antiarrhythmic properties including the potential for a proarrhythmic effect for these drugs at therapeutic doses in patients with serious structural heart disease.[30] Tricyclic antidepressants are generally contraindicated in the recovery phase following myocardial infarction. Although tricyclic antidepressant therapy can be indicated in the treatment of severely depressed patients, the threshold for use should rise as the severity of heart disease increases or when there is QT prolongation.[30] These issues are discussed in detail in Chap. 95.

Tricyclic antidepressants can impair left ventricular function in patients with severe systolic dysfunction; however, decreases in left ventricular ejection fraction have generally not been noted in patients with moderately impaired function.

Tricyclic antidepressant overdose carries a mortality of 2 to 3 percent, which is generally related to cardiac complications. Clinical status at initial presentation and serum drug levels are not predictive of prognosis. QRS prolongation is a sign of toxicity but can be absent in the patient with serious cardiac complications. Rightward deviation of the terminal 40 millisecond (msec) of the frontal plane QRS axis is a more sensitive marker.[33] Aggressive support measures in tricyclic antidepressant overdose should be initiated immediately and include airway maintenance, gastric lavage, and repeated dosing of activated charcoal. Alkalinization with intravenous sodium bicarbonate decreases unbound drug and reverses cardiac and central nervous system conduction defects. Alkalinization is indicated in cardiac arrest, hypotension, arrhythmias, acidosis, and QRS prolongation. Hypotension refractory to volume loading and bicarbonate therapy should be treated with vasopressors, including norepinephrine or phenylephrine. Class I antiarrhythmics (quinidine, procainamide, disopyramide) are contraindicated and class III agents are potentially proarrhythmic in this setting because of prolongation of QT interval. Sodium bicarbonate is the initial therapy for ventricular dysrhythmias.[34,35]

【 】 OTHER ANTIDEPRESSANTS

SSRIs have not been studied extensively in patients with cardiac disease. Case reports of cardiac toxicity are rare, despite the increasing popularity of these agents in the treatment of depression. These agents have rarely been associated with orthostatic hypotension and with bradycardia. Cardiac function does not appear to be depressed by these agents.[36] The SSRIs can affect the cytochrome P450 system and can therefore alter the metabolism of a variety of drugs, including agents used in cardiovascular disease such as antiarrhythmic medications, β blockers, calcium channel blockers, and warfarin.[35–37]

The monoamine oxidase (MAO) inhibitors have little effect on cardiac conduction or myocardial contractility. Orthostatic hypotension is common, particularly in elderly patients. The major concern with these agents is interaction with other drugs or tyramine-containing substances, resulting in hypertensive crisis. Lithium, used commonly in the treatment of bipolar disorder, is generally well tolerated in patients with cardiac disease. Suppression of sinus node automaticity, resulting in bradycardias, is the most common complication.[38] In patients free of known heart disease, clinically significant sinus node dysfunction occurs in fewer than 1 percent of patients and is reversible with discontinuation of lithium therapy. Preexisting sinus node disease or concomitant therapy with drugs altering sinus node function, however, can result in sinus bradycardia. Lithium-induced hypothyroidism can be a contributing factor.[39] Pacemaker therapy can be required to allow continuation of lithium therapy. Lithium therapy has been associated with electrocardiographic changes simulating hypokalemia. T-wave inversion, prominent U waves, and QT prolongation can occur. PR prolongation, bundle-branch block, and complete heart block are rare.[38] Overdose with lithium can result in severe bradycardias requiring temporary pacemaker therapy. A low anion gap can suggest the presence of lithium toxicity.[40]

Antipsychotic Agents

The phenothiazine antipsychotic agents have potential cardiac toxicity similar to that of the tricyclic antidepressants. These drugs can cause sinus tachycardia, PR and QT prolongation, and disturbances of intraventricular conduction. Chlorpromazine and thioridazine[41] are the most commonly implicated phenothiazines as causes of torsade de pointes. The butyrophenone, haloperidol, is also associated with torsade de pointes at high doses given intravenously.[42]

Clozapine, an atypical antipsychotic agent, has been associated with myocarditis in rare case reports.[43]

[ ] NONCARDIAC DRUGS AND TOXIC ANTIDEPRESSANTS CAUSING TORSADE DE POINTES

As discussed earlier, tricyclic, phenothiazine, and other psychotropic agents can prolong the QT interval and induce torsade de pointes. A variety of antiarrhythmic agents, particularly the type I agents, are most strongly associated with this potentially fatal arrhythmia. Other toxic causes of torsade de pointes[44] are listed in Table 93–1.

The QT prolongation and torsade de pointes reported with the antihistamines terfenadine and astemizole and with cisapride have been associated with high drug levels from excessive dosing or altered metabolism.[45,46] These drugs have been removed from the

TABLE 93–1

Drugs That Can Cause Torsade de Pointes

Drugs commonly involved
Dofetilide
Ibutilide
Procainamide
Quinidine
Sotalol
Bepridil

Other drugs (<1 % incidence)
Amiodarone
Arsenic trioxide
Cisapride
Antiinfective agents: clarithromycin, erythromycin, halofantrine, pentamidine, sparfloxacin
Antiemetic agents: domperidone, droperidol
Antipsychotic agents: chlorpromazine, haloperidol, mesoridazine, thioridazine, pimozide
Methadone

SOURCE: Adapted from Roden.[44]

market in the United States. Terfenadine-, astemizole-, and cisapride-induced prolongation of the QT interval is caused by the electrophysiologic activity of blocking human ether-a-go-go-related gene (HERG), the ion channel that is responsible for the rapid component of the delayed rectifier current for potassium (I_{Kr}).[46] These drugs are metabolized by cytochrome P450 3A. A variety of agents inhibit this isoenzyme including antifungals (ketoconazole, fluconazole, itraconazole), erythromycin or clarithromycin (not azithromycin), SSRIs (fluvoxamine, nefazodone, fluoxetine, sertraline), quinine, and grapefruit juice. Serious cardiac arrhythmias have been reported in patients taking terfenadine, astemizole, or cisapride with drugs that inhibit cytochrome P450 3A isoenzyme.

[ ] DRUG-RELATED VALVULAR HEART DISEASE

Valvular heart disease, resembling that seen with carcinoid syndrome has been associated with antimigraine drugs methysergide and ergotamine, the weight loss medications dexfenfluramine and fenfluramine, and in several instances to pergolide mesylate used to treat Parkinson disease and restless leg syndrome.[47–55] The incidence of valvular abnormalities is more common with methysergide compared to ergotamine and appears to be greater with the chronic use of dexfenfluramine and the combination of fenfluramine and phentermine. Dexfenfluramine and fenfluramine were withdrawn from the market in 1997 when up to 30 percent of users were reported to develop asymptomatic valve regurgitation.[50,51,52,53]

[ ] ANTIMIGRAINE DRUGS

In addition to ergotamine and methysergide, sumatriptan is used to treat migraines. Sumatriptan, a selective serotonin type I agonist, can cause coronary artery vasospasm. Sumatriptan should not be taken within 24 hours of treatment with ergotamine-like medications because of the risk of prolonged vasoconstriction.[56]

Ergotamine, methysergide, and sumatriptan are generally contraindicated in patients with obstructive coronary artery disease because of vasoconstrictor effects and the possibility of precipitating angina.[57]

[ ] CHLOROQUINE

The antimalarial agent, chloroquine, is commonly used to treat collagen vascular and dermatologic disorders. Irreversible retinal damage is the primary concern with long-term or high-dose therapy. Skeletal myopathy and less commonly cardiomyopathy can occur. With cardiac involvement, features of restrictive cardiomyopathy are most common. Myocardial biopsy with analysis by electron microscopy showing curvilinear and myeloid bodies is diagnostic. These findings can be seen on skeletal muscle biopsy. The ECG can demonstrate T-wave changes and conduction abnormalities. Acute chloroquine poisoning results in hypotension, tachycardia, and prolongation of the QRS and is often fatal.[58,59]

[ ] ANABOLIC STEROIDS

Illicit use of androgens has been identified as a problem in competitive athletes and body builders. It is estimated that 300,000 persons in the United States have had recent steroid use and more than 1 million have had prior use.[60–62] Anabolic steroids, including testosterone, stanozolol, and nandrolone, are frequently used in combination and at high doses for intermittent periods of several weeks to months. Doses commonly exceed 100 times the doses used for medical purposes.[60] Animal data indicate that these agents can cause abnormal lipids, left ventricular hypertrophy, increased blood volume, and hypertension. Data on human toxicity related to vascular or myocardial abnormalities are inconclusive.[63] Stanozolol and nandrolone reduce total high-density lipoprotein levels by more than 50 percent and increase low-density lipoprotein levels by more than 30 percent.[64] Isolated reports of young men (<35 years of age) developing severe coronary atherosclerosis, myocardial infarctions, or stroke exist in the literature.[60,65] Because of the secrecy surrounding the use of these agents, the full clinical significance of abuse is not known.

【 】 COCAINE

Cocaine has a generalized sympathomimetic effect and has local anesthetic properties. Cocaine blocks the reuptake of norepinephrine and dopamine on preganglionic sympathetic nerve terminals. This produces sympathetic stimulation both centrally and peripherally. These catecholamine effects acutely result in tachycardia, hypertension, increased myocardial contractility, and vascular constriction. The local anesthetic effect, occurring through blockade of the fast sodium channel, results in slowed conduction in myocardial tissues. This can result in electrocardiographic abnormalities including prolongation of the PR, QRS, and QT intervals similar to that seen with toxicity from type I antiarrhythmic agents. These effects increase the vulnerability to reentrant ventricular arrhythmias.[66–68]

Cocaine can result in increased thrombogenicity.[69] Platelet aggregations is enhanced, and endothelial function is altered, resulting in the potential for development of coronary thrombosis in the absence of coronary atherosclerosis.[70] Chronic use of cocaine is associated with premature coronary atherosclerosis.[71] Cocaine indirectly causes constriction of both diseased and nondiseased coronary artery segments, but its effect is more marked in diseased vessels. Up to one-third of reported cases of patients with cocaine-induced myocardial infarctions have normal coronary arteries.[67] The combined cardiac effects, including early coronary atherosclerosis, coronary vasospasm, increased thrombogenicity, increased myocardial oxygen demands, and proarrhythmic effects, make this drug a lethal threat to users of all ages.

Chest pain is the most common reason for cocaine users to seek medical attention. More than 64,000 patients are evaluated annually for cocaine-related chest pain, of whom more than one-half are admitted to the hospital. The evaluation of cocaine-related chest pain is difficult.[72,73] Prospective studies demonstrate that approximately 6 percent of patients presenting to the emergency room with cocaine-related chest pain have myocardial infarction. These patients are often young men without other risk factors for coronary artery disease except for tobacco smoking. The duration and quality of discomfort does not readily distinguish those eventually noted to have enzyme documentation of infarction. Many young patients have early repolarization patterns, with ST elevation in leads V_1 to V_3, a normal variant that can be confused with acute infarction. Infarction has been noted in patients with normal or nonspecific ECGs. Because of the difficulty in excluding myocardial infarctions, patients are often monitored for a period of at least 12 hours until enzymes have excluded infarction.[72]

Treatment strategies for cocaine-induced myocardial ischemia have been developed based on the known cardiac and nervous system toxicity of the drug.[66,70] Randomized prospective trials of therapy do not exist. Patients presenting with anxiety, tachycardia, or hypertension can respond well to benzodiazepines. Nitroglycerin can reverse coronary vasoconstriction induced by cocaine. Aspirin can prevent thrombus formation. Patients not responding to these measures can benefit from the α-adrenergic antagonist phentolamine or from calcium channel blocker therapy with verapamil.[66] β-Adrenergic antagonists have been avoided because of the potential of enhanced coronary vasoconstriction and for unopposed α-mediated hypertensive crisis. Combined α and β blockade with labetalol has been used to treat tachyarrhythmias but is not an accepted therapy for myocardial ischemia.[70] However, the bias against β blockade is undergoing clinical reevaluation with recognition that β blockers can block the hyperadrenergic effects that result in thrombosis and vasospasm.[74]

In documented myocardial infarction, thrombolytic therapy is highly effective; however, more than 40 percent of patients without infarction will meet accepted electrocardiographic criteria for use of lytic therapy.[75] The early repolarization pattern common in young men makes diagnosis difficult, particularly when a prior ECG is not available. Thrombolytic therapy carries increased risk of hemorrhagic stroke in patients with recently uncontrolled hypertension. Therefore, emergent coronary angiography can be necessary to document coronary occlusion and direct strategies such as primary angioplasty or thrombolysis (see Chap. 62).

Management of supraventricular or ventricular tachyarrhythmias can be facilitated by administration of benzodiazepines. Rhythm disturbances can be exacerbated by acidosis or electrolyte disorders. Intravenous sodium bicarbonate and magnesium can be beneficial. Lidocaine should be used cautiously because of concerns of lowered seizure threshold and potential proarrhythmic effects following recent cocaine use.[70] Patients with cocaine-associated chest pain not related to myocardial infarction have a favorable 1-year prognosis, particularly if cocaine use is discontinued. Urgent diagnostic cardiac evaluation is not generally recommended. Unfortunately, recurrent cocaine use after cocaine-associated chest pain occurs in more than 60 percent of cases.[66]

【 】 METHAMPHETAMINES

The biologic effects of methamphetamines are similar to that of cocaine, but vasoconstriction is less.[76] Cardiovascular toxicity is common and includes tachycardia, hypertension, and arrhythmias. Chest pain and myocardial infarction are less common than with cocaine.[77] Chronic use can result in a catecholamine-mediated dilated cardiomyopathy.[78]

【 】 ETHANOL

See Chap. 76.

ELECTRICITY INJURY

【 】 ENVIRONMENTAL ACCIDENTS

Accidental contact with electricity can occur in the home, where young children are particularly vulnerable.[79] Job-related electrical injuries are most common in construction and electrical workers but also on any job in which electrical equipment is used, including the healthcare setting. Approximately 1200 deaths related to domestic electrical injury occur each year in the United States.[80] There are two to three times as many serious injuries, including burns and neurologic complications.[80,81] Lightning kills at least 100 people per year in the United States, representing a 30 percent mortality rate in reported cases. Lightning injuries generally occur between May and September in the late afternoon hours and affect predominantly young people involved in outdoor recreational activities.[82] Death following electrical shock is usually secondary to immediate cardiac rhythm disturbances, although later cardiac complications secondary to internal injury can occur.

【 】 PATHOPHYSIOLOGY

The degree of total body injury from electricity is determined by the amount of current delivered, tissue resistance, and duration of contact.[81] Specific organs or tissues injured are in part determined by the path of the current. Electrical injuries are classified as high voltage (>1000 V) or low voltage (< 1000 V). High-voltage electrical wires and household current (120 or 220 V) are alternating currents (AC) that can result in prolonged exposure because of tetatanic muscle contractions and inability of the victim to "let go." The frequencies of domestically generated AC (50 to 60 cycles per second) result in an increased risk for ventricular fibrillation even at household voltages.[80] Sources of domestic direct current (DC) are usually low voltage (3 to 24 V), including batteries, appliance transformers, and portable emergency generators and are less likely to cause injury. Lightning is an extremely high-voltage, direct current of brief duration.

Heat injury tissue necrosis is more severe with high-voltage AC. These burns are often internal and can mimic crush injuries.[83] Tissue resistance to current flow is least in nervous and vascular tissues, and therefore the heart and neurovascular bundles can serve as conduits for electrical current through the thorax.[84] Arm-to-arm pathway of current is associated with greater risk for cardiac injury, followed by arm-to-leg pathways determined by entry and exit sites. A stride potential, leg-to-leg, is infrequently associated with cardiac effects.[80]

【 】 CARDIOVASCULAR EFFECTS

Cardiac damage in electrical injury can occur as a result of contusion injury or myocardial necrosis or can be in part related to massive release of catecholamines. Typical symptoms or signs of myocardial damage can be absent.[85] Lightning injuries result from brief, high-voltage direct current. Immediate death can be secondary to asystole or ventricular fibrillation or result from apnea secondary to injury of the central respiratory centers. Lightning strikes can occur by a direct hit, side splash, or ground strike. Direct hits cause mechanical trauma to organs secondary to dissi-

pated energy.[81] Strikes to the chest can result in severe, often reversible global myocardial dysfunction or localized myocardial contusion. Electrocardiographic abnormalities, including QT prolongation and ST-T abnormalities, can be the result of cardiac or neurologic injury. ST elevation has been noted with direct strikes. Conduction abnormalities, including right bundle-branch block and complete heart block, have been noted.[82] Pericardial effusions can develop following direct strikes. Elevated levels of creatine kinase-myocardial band (CK-MB) are generally noted.[81,82] Splash strikes in which a tree or other object is hit prior to the victim being hit are associated with CK-MB release in less than two-thirds of patients. Severe myocardial injury is unlikely unless there is a short distance between the directly hit object and the victim. Ground strikes generally do not cause a significant cardiac injury but can be associated with nonspecific ST-T abnormalities.[82]

Domestic AC accidents can cause myocardial necrosis and conduction abnormalities. An injury pattern mimicking infarction can be seen on the ECG but is generally related to direct myocardial injury and not from coronary thrombosis.[80] Household voltages (120 to 220 V) can cause sudden death, particularly when they involve arm-to-arm pathways or low skin resistance in a wet victim. Serious myocardial damage is rare.[79]

Treatment for cardiac arrest should be initiated immediately after the patient is disconnected from the current source. Resuscitation efforts should be continued for a prolonged period. In lightning strikes involving multiple victims, attention should be directed first to those who are "apparently dead."[84] This is because there is a higher resuscitation rate for these individuals compared to those with medical cardiac arrest. Of note, lightning victims with vital signs generally survive without immediate medical attention.

Patients surviving high-voltage injuries generally require hospital admission, usually for attention to neurologic complications and internal or external burn injuries and less commonly for cardiac monitoring. An initially normal ECG carries a favorable cardiac prognosis leading some clinicians to question the need for 24-hour electrocardiographic monitoring. Patients with arm-to-arm or arm-to-leg passage of current can be at risk for postadmission rhythm disturbances, and a higher index of suspicion is required in such patients.[85]

Adults and children presenting to the emergency department following low-voltage shocks of less than 240 V have a low incidence of myocardial injury, and most do not require further monitoring.[79]

【 】 ELECTROCONVULSIVE THERAPY

Electroconvulsive therapy (ECT) is accepted therapy for a variety of psychiatric illnesses including depression resistant to pharmacologic therapy, severe suicidal ideation with vegetative signs, acute mania, and depression with intolerance to medication side effects secondary to cardiac problems.[86] ECT is performed with a brief unilateral or bilateral electrical stimulus to the brain while the patient is under short-acting anesthesia with a hypnotic drug and a muscle depolarizing agent. ECT produces brief, intense stimulation of the central nervous system. Cardiovascular complications can result from this stimulation or from the drugs used to modify the response.

Initially, the ECT stimulus activates the vagus nerve and can produce bradycardia, hypotension, and rarely asystole.[87] Sympathetic discharge occurs, which is amplified by a 15-fold rise in epinephrine and threefold rise in norepinephrine levels, resulting in tachycardia and hypertension. Transient atrial and ventricular tachyarrhythmias can occur in approximately 10 percent of patients with known or suspected cardiovascular disease.[88] Transient electrocardiographic alterations, including ST-T–wave changes, QRS changes, QT prolongation, and peaked T waves, can occur. Transient decrease in left ventricular function has been documented in more than one-fourth of patients but appear to be transient and not associated with cumulative deterioration with followup ECT sessions.[89]

The mortality rate of ECT is less than 3 in 10,000, and the complication rate is approximately 0.3 percent. Patients with severe heart disease can successfully undergo ECT with acceptable risk.[90] Prior to ECT, electrolyte abnormalities should be corrected, and systemic hypertension should be controlled. Patients with pulmonary disease require special evaluation because hypoxia and respiratory acidosis can precipitate cardiovascular events. Following ECT, hypertension and tachycardia can be controlled with adrenergic blockade with intravenous labetalol or esmolol.[91] Other antihypertensive agents such as clonidine or calcium channel blockers can be used. Sustained ventricular arrhythmias are treated with lidocaine, but pretreatment with lidocaine is not indicated. Patients with cardiac pacemakers can safely undergo ECT.[92]

POISONS

[ ] COMPLEMENTARY AND ALTERNATIVE MEDICINES

Many people now use complementary and alternative therapies including herbal medicines, acupuncture, and meditation (see Chap. 114). Most physicians are unaware that their patients are using these therapies in conjunction with orthodox medicine. Few physicians are knowledgeable about potential side effects and drug interactions of botanical medication. In addition, because these products are considered dietary supplements, they are not subject to government regulations mandating safety and efficacy. Therefore, quality and purity of these products cannot be assured.[93,94]

Concerns have been raised regarding the safety of ephedra, a dietary supplement used for weight loss and enhancement of athletic performance. Ephedra and ephedrine-alkaloid containing products have been associated with palpitations, cerebrovascular accidents, myocardial infarction, and death.[95]

[ ] HERBAL–MEDICATION INTERACTIONS

St. John's wort is commonly used by patients to treat mild depression. Hypericin and hyperforin, two components of St. John's wort are responsible for its antidepressant effects. Hyperforin acts as an inducer of the cytochrome P450 CYP3A4 and therefore can lower serum levels of medications metabolized by this pathway.[96] St. John's wort has been shown to decrease plasma cyclosporine levels, protease inhibitors such as indinavir, and the effectiveness of oral contraceptives.[96,97] St. John's wort can also decrease the effectiveness of warfarin.[97] Other herbal therapies that interact with the cytochrome P450 system and thus can interfere with metabolism of medication through these pathways include milk thistle (*Silymarin marianum*), ginseng, garlic, danshen, and licorice.[96]

[ ] ARSENIC

Arsenic, at higher concentrations, increases production of reactive oxygen species and inhibits nitric oxide synthase resulting in endothelial dysfunction. Arsenic also upregulates inflammatory cytokines tumor necrosis factor-α and interleukin-8. Prothrombotic effects contribute to atherosclerosis and arterial thrombosis. Arsenic toxicity can result from occupational exposure, water contamination, or treatment of malignancies. Cardiovascular effects of chronic arsenic exposure include peripheral vascular disease (Blackfoot disease) and coronary atherosclerosis.[98] Acute arsenic toxicity can cause QT prolongation, heart block, and ventricular arrhythmias.[99]

VENOMS AND TOXINS

Snakebites are a rare cause of death in the United States but account for more than 40,000 deaths worldwide. The majority of these fatal bites occur in Asia, South America, and Africa. Scorpion stings are a common problem in India, Southeast Asia, Mexico, Israel, and Southwestern United States.[100–107]

HALOGENATED HYDROCARBONS

Halogenated hydrocarbons are used in fire extinguishers, solvents, and refrigerants and in the manufacture of pesticides and plastics. Heavy acute exposure to these compounds can result in cardiac arrhythmias and sudden death.[108] Direct cardiac effects include depression of myocardial contractility[109] and sensitization to the arrhythmogenic effects of catecholamines. Indirect cardiotoxicity can result from hypoxia or central nervous system toxicity.

ORGANOPHOSPHATES

Organophosphates, used commercially in pesticides, are powerful inhibitors of acetylcholinesterase, and this inhibition can result in parasympathetic overstimulation. Suicide attempts account for the majority of fatalities associated with ingestion of large doses of organophosphates. Signs and symptoms of ingestion include respiratory depression, bronchospasm and secretion, and pulmonary edema. Deaths are generally related to respiratory failure. Cardiac toxicity is generally associated with QT prolongation. Both bradycardia and tachycardia can occur. Torsade de pointes, atrioventricular conduction disturbances, and ST-T abnormalities have been noted. Cardiac arrhythmias have been noted up to 15 days after exposure. Direct myocardial toxicity has been postulated, in addition to cholinergic hyperactivity.[110]

The *nerve gas* sarin (isopropyl methylphosphonofluoridate) has been used by terrorists to poison populations in public areas, with most fatalities caused by cardiopulmonary or respiratory arrest.[111] Signs and symptoms of sarin inhalation include miosis, nausea, vomiting, cough, headache, hypokalemia, hypocapnia, and seizure activity followed by low-grade fever and dysesthesia.[111] Cardiac manifestations of sarin exposure include premature ventricular contractions, QT prolongation, and rarely cardiomyopathy.[111] Treatment for nerve gas inhalation involves supportive care. Treatment for ingestion associated with bradycardia includes continued atropine administration at doses sufficient to dry mucous membranes and increase heart rate to 100 beats per minute. Oximes (obidoxime and pralidoxime) have been studied in severe ingestions, but can increase mortality and have no role in organophosphate poisoning.[112]

SMALLPOX VACCINATION

Postvaccinial myocarditis or pericarditis is a rare complication of smallpox vaccination, which typically presents with chest pain and ECG abnormalities. Myocarditis appears to be immunologically mediated, rather than caused by direct viral infection of the myocardium (see Chap. 32).[113]

CARBON MONOXIDE

Toxicity from carbon monoxide is related to tissue hypoxia. Carbon monoxide has a much higher affinity for hemoglobin than does oxygen, preventing adequate oxygen exchange. Carbon monoxide exposure worsens angina pectoris and increases the risk of myocardial infarction.[114] Carbon monoxide poisoning results in electrocardiographic abnormalities, including sinus tachycardia, atrial fibrillation, atrioventricular block, and ST-T abnormalities. Cardiac enzyme elevation can occur. Severe exposure can result in myocardial necrosis and cardiomyopathy. Myocardial injury is common and predicts a poor long-term outcome.[115] Long-term exposure to ambient air pollution is associated with an increased risk of cardiovascular events, which is in part related to carbon monoxide and particulate matter from motor vehicle exhaust.[116]

RADIATION

Mediastinal radiation—commonly used to treat Hodgkin disease, lung cancer, breast cancer, and seminoma—can result in acute or late cardiac sequelae. Prior to the 1960s, the heart was thought to be resistant to the effects of clinical radiation. It is now known that radiation can lead to acute or chronic pericarditis, coronary artery disease, systolic and diastolic ventricular dysfunction, conduction defects, and valvular dysfunction.[117,118] Many cancer patients now have improved long-term survivals, and thus are more prone to late complications of mediastinal irradiation (see Chap. 89). Risk factors for the development of radiation-induced heart disease include total radiation dose >35 Gy, high fractionated dose (>2.0 Gy/d), volume of heart irradiated, young age at exposure, long time from exposure, mediastinal tumor, traditional cardiovascular risk factors, and concomitant anthracycline administration.[117] Routine screening for conduction system abnormalities, valvular disease, and ischemic coronary disease should be undertaken in all

high-risk patients previously treated with mediastinal irradiation. Disease can manifest 20 years or more after radiation treatment, therefore ongoing screening is necessary.

BREAST CANCER

Modern adjuvant radiotherapy for breast cancer does not seem to be associated with an increased risk of late hospitalizations for major cardiac events such as ischemia, valvular heart disease, conduction abnormalities, and heart failure.[119] However, radiation for left-sided breast cancer can lead to perfusion defects of the left ventricle included in the radiation field. The long-term significance of these perfusion abnormalities is not known.[119] By contrast, in a study of Hodgkin disease survivors, the majority of whom received more than 36 Gy of mediastinal irradiation, late cardiovascular complications were common (see Chap. 89).

PERICARDIAL DISEASE

Acute pericarditis, constrictive pericarditis and effusive-constrictive pericarditis can follow radiation therapy. Although up to 40 percent of patients treated with older techniques developed pericarditis, the incidence with modern techniques (total dose <30 Gy, subcarinal blocking and daily fraction size <2 Gy) is approximately 2.5 percent.[120] Clinically apparent pericarditis can occur 4 to 12 months after radiation therapy. Acute pericarditis, asymptomatic pericardial effusion, or pericardial tamponade can occur. Other etiologies of pericarditis should be considered, particularly malignant involvement of the pericardium. Pericarditis occurring during treatment of a mediastinal mass contiguous to the heart is generally secondary to tumor effect and does not correlate with late pericardial complications.[121,122]

Radiation can cause an exudative pericarditis followed by pericardial fibrosis caused by fibroblast proliferation and collagen deposition. Although the majority of patients with pericardial effusion recover spontaneously, up to 20 percent can develop chronic and/or constrictive pericarditis 5 to 10 years after therapy.[117]

Treatment for acute pericarditis is based on relief of symptoms including antipyretics, antiinflammatory agents, and pericardiocentesis when indicated. Surgical mortality in patients with constrictive pericarditis can be as high as 20 to 40 percent.[123,124] Extensive mediastinal and pericardial fibrosis make pericardiectomy technically challenging. Radiation-induced constriction is often associated with coronary artery disease, valvular heart disease, and/or myocardial dysfunction. Long-term survival after pericardiectomy for radiation-induced constrictive pericarditis is significantly lower than for other etiologies.[124] Candidates for pericardiectomy should be carefully selected.

MYOCARDIAL DYSFUNCTION

Radiation causes diffuse interstitial fibrosis, which more commonly leads to diastolic dysfunction. Diastolic dysfunction can be detected in 14 percent of patients late after mediastinal radiation, increases with age, and is associated with poorer outcomes, in part caused by ischemia.[125] Microcirculatory damage leading to ischemia can also contribute to myocardial cell death and fibrosis.[117] Systolic dysfunction is rare and is usually associated with prior anthracycline treatment. Asymptomatic patients can have varying degrees of myocardial fibrosis that can be patchy or diffuse. Low peak oxygen consumption on cardiopulmonary exercise testing can be found in the absence of echocardiographic evidence of myocardial dysfunction and is typically associated with symptoms of exercise intolerance.[117]

[ ] CORONARY ARTERY DISEASE

Premature coronary artery disease can result from prior radiation therapy. The coronary ostia and left main coronary artery are frequently involved in radiation-induced coronary artery disease. Microscopically, these lesions demonstrate intimal proliferation and fibrosis.[117] In one study, 23 percent of patients undergoing cardiac surgery for radiation-related valvular disease also had left main disease.[123] Mediastinal and pericardial fibrosis make surgical revascularization more difficult. In addition, the left internal mammary artery, which is often used as a graft, is often included in the radiation field. The long-term patency of the internal mammary graft in radiation-related coronary artery disease is not known, but early occlusion has been reported.[125,126] Noncoronary atherosclerotic vascular disease can occur in up to 7 percent of patients at 20 years.[127] Routine assessment of cardiovascular risk factors is indicated in all patients, regardless of age, who have received radiation therapy to the chest. Annual measurement of lipid profiles, high sensitive C-reactive protein, and thyroid function are recommended. Modifications of traditional risk factors including smoking cessation, blood pressure control, weight maintenance, and treatment of diabetes are important. Exercise electrocardiography or stress perfusion testing should be considered in high-risk individuals who may not develop anginal chest pain even in the presence of significant coronary stenosis.[117] Spiral CT can detect early vascular and valvular calcifications in survivors of Hodgkin disease, but the clinical utility of routine CT screening has yet to be proven.[128]

[ ] CONDUCTION DISTURBANCES AND ARRHYTHMIAS

Radiation can result in fibrosis of the nodal and infranodal pathways causing all levels of atrioventricular block. Right bundle-branch block is more common than left. Sick sinus syndrome has been reported as well. Persistent tachycardia can also occur, similar to the denervated heart and can be related to autonomic nervous system dysfunction. Radiation-related conduction abnormalities are associated with a total dose >40 Gy, a delay of 10 years or more since therapy, interval abnormal ECG (bundle-branch block), and prior pericardial involvement.[117]

[ ] VALVULAR DISEASE

Echocardiographic evidence of at least mild regurgitation of both right- and left-sided valves can be found in more than 40 percent of survivors of Hodgkin disease treated with mediastinal irradiation.[117] Clinically significant valvular heart disease secondary to radiation is rare, but when present, usually involves the aortic or mitral valves. Coexisting pericardial disease is the rule. At autopsy fibrous thickening of the valves is seen. This most commonly leads to asymptomatic aortic and mitral regurgitation. Stenotic lesions

are rare. Echocardiographic studies have demonstrated characteristic thickening and fibrotic changes of the aortic-mitral curtain, distinct from the appearance of rheumatic valvular disease.[129,130] Successful surgical replacement of symptomatic regurgitant valves depends on the absence of concomitant constrictive pericarditis. Overall surgical mortality for radiation-induced valvular disease was 12 percent in one single-center study[131] with most deaths occurring in patients with constrictive pericarditis. Surgical morbidity was significant, including respiratory failure (18 percent), need for pacemaker implantation caused by conduction abnormalities (10 percent), bleeding (10 percent), mechanical circulatory support, infection, and stroke.[131] The most common cause of late death after valve replacement is malignancy, followed by heart failure and complications of ischemia.[131]

DIAGNOSTIC RADIATION

With the widespread availability of multislice spiral computed tomography (MSCT) for coronary angiography, concerns have been raised about the risk of radiation exposure. MSCT coronary angiography exposes patients to approximately 11 to 15 millisievert (mSV) per scan, in comparison to 5.6 to 6.4 mSV for conventional diagnostic coronary angiography.[132] The primary concern regarding MSCT currently is the estimated 0.07 percent lifetime risk of radiation-related malignancy with each scan.[133] Similar concerns have been raised in pediatric patients undergoing cardiac catheterizations, intervention, and electrophysiological studies involving prolonged fluoroscopy times.[134] The risk of repeated, chronic exposure to relatively low does of radiation on the heart is unknown at this time.

REFERENCES

1. Frishman WH, Sung HM, Yee HCM, et al. Cardiovascular toxicity with cancer chemotherapy. *Curr Probl Cardiol.* 1996;21:225–288.
2. Floyd JD, Nguyen DT, Lobins RL, et al. Cardiotoxicity of cancer therapy. *J Clin Oncol.* 2005;23:7685–7696.
3. Yeh ETH, Tong AT, Lenihan DJ, et al. Cardiovascular complications of cancer therapy: diagnosis, pathogenesis, and management. *Circulation.* 2004;109:3122–3131.
4. Shan K, Lincoff AM, Young JB. Anthracycline-induced cardiomyopathy. *Ann Intern Med.* 1996;125:47–58.
5. Von Hoff DD, Layard MW, Basa P, et al. Risk factors for doxorubicin-induced congestive heart failure. *Ann Intern Med.* 1979;91:710–717.
6. Bristow MR, Mason JW, Billingham ME, Daniels JR. Doxorubicin cardiomyopathy: evaluation of phonocardiography, endomyocardial biopsy, and cardiac catheterization. *Ann Intern Med.* 1978;88:168–175.
7. Lipschultz SE, Lipsitz SR, Mone SM, et al. Female sex and higher drug dose as risk factors for late cardiotoxic effects of doxorubicin therapy for childhood cancer. *N Engl J Med.* 1995;332:1738–1743.
8. Wouters KA, Kremer LCM, Miller TL, et al. Protecting against anthracycline-induced myocardial damage: a review of the most promising strategies. *Br J Haematol.* 2005;131:561–578.
9. Singal PK, Iliskovic N. Doxorubicin-induced cardiomyopathy. *N Engl J Med.* 1998;339:900–905.
10. Youssef G and Links M. The prevention and management of cardiovascular complications of chemotherapy in patients with cancer. *Am J Cardiovasc Drugs.* 2005;5:233–243.
11. Steinherz J, Graham T, Hurwitz R, et al. Guidelines for cardiac monitoring of children during and after anthracycline therapy: report of the Cardiology Committee of the Children's Cancer Study Group. *Pediatrics.* 1992;89:942–949.
12. Schwartz RG, McKenzie WB, Alexander J, et al. Congestive heart failure and left ventricular dysfunction complicating doxorubicin therapy: seven-year experience using radionuclide angiocardiography. *Am J Med.* 1987;82:1109–1118.

13. Steinherz LJ, Steinherz PG, Tan CTC, et al. Cardiac toxicity 4 to 20 years after completing anthracycline therapy. *JAMA.* 1991;266: 1672–1677.

14. Kramer LC, Van Dalen EC, Offringam, et al. Anthracycline-induced clinical heart failure and a cohort of 607 children: long-term followup study. *J Clin Oncol.* 2001;19:191–196.

15. Legha SS, Benjamin RS, MacKay B, et al. Reduction of doxorubicin cardiotoxicity by prolonged continuous intravenous infusion. *Ann Intern Med.* 1982;89:133–139.

16. Lipshultz SE, Giantris, AL, Lipsitz SR, et al. Doxorubicin administration by continuous infusion is not cardioprotective: Dana-Farber 91–01 acute lymphoblastic leukemia protocol. *J Clin Oncol.* 2002;20:1677–1682.

17. Schuchter LM, Hensley ML, Meropol NJ, et al. 2002 Update of recommendations for the use of chemotherapy and radiotherapy protectants: clinical practice guidelines of the American Society of Clinical Oncology. *J Clin Oncol.* 2002;20:2895–2903.

18. Gralow JR, Livingston RB. University of Washington high dose cyclophosphamide, mitoxantrone, etoposide experience in metastatic breast cancer: unexpected cardiac toxicity. *J Clin Oncol.* 2001;19: 3903–3904.

19. Feenstra J, Grobbee DE, Remme WJ, Stricker BH. Drug induced heart failure. *J Am Coll Cardiol.* 1999;3:1152–1162.

20. Robben NC, Pippas AW, Moore JO. The syndrome of 5-fluorouracil cardiotoxicity: an elusive cardiopathy. *Cancer.* 1993;71:493–509.

21. Akhtar SS, Salim KP, Bano ZA. Symptomatic cardiotoxicity with high dose 5-fluorouracil infusion: a prospective study. *Oncology.* 1993;50: 441–445.

22. Weiss RB, Grillo-Lopez AJ, Marsoni S, et al. Amsacrine-associated cardiotoxicity: an analysis of 82 cases. *J Clin Oncol.* 1986;4:918–928.

23. Sideman A, Hudis C, Pierri N. Cardiac dysfunction in the trastuzumab. *J Clin Oncol.* 2002;20:1215–1221.

24. Spire J. Cardiac dysfunction in the trastuzumab clinical experience. *J Clin Oncol.* 2002;20:1156–1157.

25. Perez EA, Rodeheffer R. Clinic Cardiac tolerability of trastuzumab. *J Clin Oncol.* 2004;2:322–329.

26. DuBois JS, Udelson JE, Atkins B. Severe reversible, global and regional ventricular dysfunction associated with high-dose interleukin-2 immunotherapy. *J Immunother.* 1995;18:119–123.

27. Kuwatu A, Ohashi M, Sugiyama M, et al. A case of reversible dilated cardiomyopathy after α interferon therapy in a patient with renal cell carcinoma. *Am J Med Sci.* 2002;324:331–334.

28. Roose SP, Dalak GW. Treating the depressed patient with cardiovascular problems. *J Clin Psychiatry.* 1992;53(9 suppl):25–31.

29. Fraser-Smith N, Lesperance F, Talajic M. Depression following myocardial infarction: Impact on 6-month survival. *JAMA.* 1993;270: 1819–1825.

30. Glassman AH, Roose SP, Bigger JT. The safety of tricyclic antidepressants in cardiac patients—risk benefit reconsidered. *JAMA.* 1993;269: 2673–2675.

31. Franco-Bronson K. The management of treatment-resistant depression in the medically ill. *Psychiatr Clin North Am.* 1996;19:329–348.

32. Roose SP, Glassman AH, Gardina EGV, et al. Tricyclic antidepressants in depressed patients with cardiac conduction disease. *Arch Gen Psychiatry.* 1987;44:273–275.

33. Wolfe TR, Caravati EM, Rollin DE. Terminal 40-ms frontal plane QRS axis as a marker for tricyclic antidepressant overdose. *Ann Emerg Med.* 1989;18:348–351.

34. Kerr GW, McGuffie AC, Wilkie S. Tricyclic antidepressant overdose: a review. *Emerg Med J.* 2001;18:236–241.

35. Ciraulo DA, Shader RI. Fluoxetine drug-drug interactions: I. Antidepressants and antipsychotics. *J Clin Psychopharmacol.* 1990;48:1990.

36. Sheline YI, Freedland KE, Carney RM. How safe are serotonin reuptake inhibitors for depression in patients with coronary heart disease? *Am J Med.* 1997;102:54–59.

37. Witchel HJ, Hancox JC, Nutt DJ. Psychotropic drugs, cardiac arrhythmia, and sudden death. *J Clin Psychopharmacol.* 2003;23:58–77.

38 Rosenqvist M, Bergfeldt L, Aili H, Mathe AA. Sinus node dysfunction during long-term lithium treatment. *Br Heart J.* 1993;70:371–375.

39. Numata T, Abe H, Terao T, Nakashima Y. Possible involvement of hypothyroidism as a cause of lithium-induced sinus node dysfunction. *PACE.* 1999;22:954–957.

40 Simard M, Gumbiner B, Lee A, et al. Lithium carbonate intoxication: A case report and review of the literature. *Arch Intern Med.* 1989;149:36–46.

41. Kemper AJ, Dunlap R, Pietro DA. Thioridazine-induced torsade de pointes. Successful therapy with isoproterenol. *JAMA.* 1983;249: 2931–2934.

42. Di Salvo TG, O'Gara PT. Torsade de pointes caused by high-dose intravenous haloperidol in cardiac patients. *Clin Cardiol.* 1995;18:285–290.

43. Merrill DB, Dec GW, Goff DC. Adverse cardiac effects associated with clozapine. *J Clin Psychopharmacol.* 2005;25:32–41.

44. Roden DM. Drug therapy: drug- induced prolongation of the QT interval. *N Engl J Med.* 2004;350:1013–1022.

45. Vitola J, Vukanovic J, Roden D. Cisapride-induced torsade de pointes. *J Cardiovasc Electrophysiol.* 1998;9:1109–1113.

46. Priori SG. Exploring the hidden danger of noncardiac drugs. *J Cardiovasc Electrophysiol.* 1998;9:1114–1116.

47. Redfield MM, Nicholson WJ, Edwards WD, Tajik AJ. Valve disease associated with ergot alkaloid: echocardiographic and pathologic correlations. *Ann Intern Med.* 1992;117:50–52.

48. Mason JW, Billingham ME, Friedman JP. Methysergide-induced heart disease: a case of multivalvular and myocardial fibrosis. *Circulation.* 1977;56:889–890.

49. Connolly HM, Crary JL, McGoon MD, et al. Valvular heart disease associated with fenfluramine-phentermine [published correction appears in *N Engl J Med.* 1997;337:1783]. *N Engl J Med.* 1997;337:581–588.

50. Cardiac valvulopathy associated with exposure to fenfluramine or dexfenfluramine: US Department of Health and Human Services interim public health recommendations, November 1997. *MMWR Morb Mortal Wkly Rep.* 1997;46:1061–1066.

51. Weissman NJ, Tighe JF Jr, Gottdiener JS, Gwynne JT. Sustained-Release Dexfenfluramine Study Group. An assessment of heart valve abnormalities in obese patients taking dexfenfluramine, sustained-release dexfenfluramine, or placebo. *N Engl J Med.* 1998;339: 725–732.

52. Hensrud DD, Connolly HM, Grogan M, et al. Echocardiographic improvement over time after cessation of use of fenfluramine and phentermine. *Mayo Clin Proc.* 1999;74:1191–1197.

53. Shively BK, Roldan CA, Gill EA, et al. Prevalence and determinants of valvulopathy in patients treated with dexfenfluramine. *Circulation.* 1999;100:2161–2167.

54. Pritchett AM, Morrison JF, Edwards WD. Valvular heart disease in patients taking pergolide. *Mayo Clin Proc.* 2002;77:1280–1286.

55. Rahimtoola MB. Drug-related valvular heart disease: here we go again: Will we do better this time? *Mayo Clin Proc.* 2002;77:1275–1277.

56. Liston H, Bennett L, Usher B, Nappi J. The association of the combination of sumatriptan and methysergide in myocardial infarction in a premenopausal woman. *Arch Intern Med.* Mar 1999;159:511–513.

57. VanDenBrink AM, Reekers M, Bax W, et al. Coronary side-effect potential of current and prospective antimigraine drugs. *Circulation.* 1998;98:25–30.

58. Cubero GI, Reguero JJ, Ortega JM. Restrictive cardiomyopathy caused by chloroquine. *Br Heart J.* 1993;69:451–452.

59. Ratliff NB, Estes ML, Myles JL et al. Diagnosis of chloroquine cardiomyopathy by endomyocardial biopsy. *N Engl J Med.* 1987;316:191–193.

60. Bagatell CJ, Bremner WJ. Androgens in men—uses and abuses: *N Engl J Med.* 1996;334:707–714.

61. Yesalis CE, Kennedy NK, Kopstein AN, Bahrke MS. Anabolic-androgenic steroid use in the United States. *JAMA.* 1993;270:1217–1221.

62. Nieminen MS, Ramo MP, Viitasalo M, Heikkila P, et al. Serious cardiovascular side effects of large doses of anabolic steroids in weight lifters. *Eur Heart J.* 1996;17:1576–1583.

63. Payne JR, Kotwinski PJ, Montgomery HE. Cardiac effects of anabolic steroids. *Heart.* 2004;90:473–475.

64. Glazer G. Atherogenic effects of anabolic steroids on serum lipid levels: a literature review. *Arch Intern Med.* 1991;151:1925–1933.

65. Mewis C, Spyridopulous I, Kuhlkamp V, Seipel L. Manifestation of severe coronary heart disease after anabolic drug abuse. *Clin Cardiol.* 1996;19:153–155.

66. Hollander JE. The management of cocaine-associated myocardial ischemia. *N Engl J Med.* 1995;333:1267–1272.

67. Kloner RA, Hale S, Alker Rezkalla S. The effects of acute and chronic cocaine use on the heart. *Circulation.* 1992;85:407–419.

68. Pirwitz MJ, Willard JE, Landau C, et al. Influence of cocaine, ethanol, or their combination epicardial coronary arterial dimensions in humans. *Arch Intern Med.* 1995;155:1186–1191.

69. Moliterno DJ, Willard JE, Lange RA, et al. Coronary-artery vasoconstriction induced by cocaine, cigarette smoking, or both. *N Engl J Med.* 1994;330:454–459.

70. Om A, Ellahham S, Disciascio G. Management of cocaine-induced cardiovascular complications. *Am Heart J.* 1993;125:469–475.

71. Hollander JE, Hoffman RS, Burstein JL, et al. Cocaine-associated myocardial infarction: mortality and complications. *Arch Intern Med.* 1995;155:1081–1086.

72. Weber JE, Shofer FS, Larkin GL, et al. Validation of a brief observation period for patients with cocaine-associated chest pain. *N Engl J Med.* 2003;348:510–517.

73. Kloner RA, Rezkalla SH. Cocaine and the heart. *N Engl J Med.* 2003;348:487–488.

74. Leikin JB. Cocaine and B-adrenergic blockers: a remarriage after a decade-long divorce? *Crit Care Med.* 1999;27:688–689.

75. Gitter MJ, Goldsmith SR, Dunbar DN, Sharkey SW. Cocaine and chest pain: clinical features and outcome of patients hospitalized to rule out myocardial infarction. *Ann Intern Med.* 1991;115:277–282.

76. Pitts DK, Marwah J. Cocaine and central monoaminergic neurotransmission: a review of electrophysiologic studies and comparison to amphetamine and antidepressants. *Life Sci.* 1988;42:949–968.

77. Derlet RW, Rice P, Horowitz BZ, Lord RV. Amphetamine toxicity: experiences with 127 cases. *J Emerg Med.* 1989;7:157–161.

78. Hong R, Matsuyama E, Nur K. Cardiomyopathy associated with the smoking of crystal amphetamine. *JAMA.* 1991;265:1152–1154.

79. Bailey B, Gaudreauh HP, Thivierge RL, Turgeon JP. Cardiac monitoring of children with household electrical injuries. *Ann Emerg Med.* 1995;25:612–617.

80. Carleton SC. Cardiac problems associated with electrical injury. *Cardiol Clin.* 1995;13:263–277.

81. Browne BJ, Gaasch WR. Electrical injuries and lightning. *Emerg Med Clin North Am.* 1992;10:211–229.

82. Lichtenberg R, Dries D, Ward K, et al. Cardiovascular effects of lightning strikes. *J Am Coll Cardiol.* 1993;21:531–536.

83. Artz CP. Electrical injury simulates crush injury. *Surg Gynecol Obstet.* 1967;125:1316.

84. Jain S, Bandi V. Electrical and lightning injuries. *Crit Care Clin.* 1999;15:319–331.

85. Jenson PJ, Thomsen PEB, Bagger JP, et al. Electrical injury causing ventricular arrhythmias. *Br Heart J.* 1987;57:279–283.

86. Banazak DA. Electroconvulsive therapy: A guide for family physicians. *Am Fam Physician.* 1996;53:273–278.

87. Gerring JP, Shields HM. The identification and management of patients with a high risk for cardiac arrhythmias during modified ECT. *J Clin Psychiatry.* 1982;43:140–143.

88. Gould L, Copalaswamy C, Chandy F, Kim B. Electroconvulsive therapy induced ECG changes simulating a myocardial infarction. *Arch Intern Med.* 1983;143:1786–1787.

89. McCully RB, Karon BL, Rummans TA, et al. Frequency of left ventricular dysfunction after electroconvulsive therapy. *Am J Cardiol.* 2003;91:1147–1150.

90. Zielinski RJ, Roose SP, Devanand DP, et al. Cardiovascular complications of ECT in depressed patients with cardiac disease. *Am J Psychiatry.* 1993;150:904–909.

91. Leslie JB, Kalayjiam RW, Sirgo MA, et al. Intravenous labetalol for the treatment of postoperative hypertension. *Anesthesiology.* 1987;67:413–421.

92. Abiusa P, Dunkelman R, Proper M. Electroconvulsive therapy in patients with pacemakers. *JAMA.* 1978;240:2459–2462.

93. Lin MC, Gershwin ME, Linghurst JC, Wu KK. State of complementary and alternative medicine in cardiovascular, lung, and blood research. *Circulation.* 2001;103:2038.

94. Hermann DD. Nutraceutical agents and cardiovascular medicine: the hope, the hype and the harm. *ACC Current Journal Review* 1999;Sept/Oct:53–57.

95. Shekelle PG, Hardy ML, Morton SC, et al. Efficacy and safety of ephedra and ephedrine for weight loss and athletic performance: a meta-analysis. *JAMA.* 2003;289:1537–1545.

96. Ioannides C. Pharmacokinetic interactions between herbal remedies and medicinal drugs. *Xenobiotica.* 2002;32:451–478.

97. DeSmet PAGM. Herbal remedies. *N Engl J Med.* 2002;347:2046–2056.

98. Navas-Acien A, Sharrett A, Silbergeld E, et al. Arsenic exposure and cardiovascular disease: a systematic review of the epidemiologic evidence. *Am J Epidemiol.* 2005;162:1037–1049.

99. Unnikrishnan D, Dutcher J, Garl S, et al. Cardiac monitoring of patients receiving arsenic trioxide therapy. *Br J Haematol.* 2004;124:610–617.

100. Karalliedde L. Animal toxins. *Br J Anaesth.* 1995;75:319–327.

101. Meki AAM, El-Deen ZMM, El-Deen HMM. Myocardial injury in scorpion envenomed children: significance of assessment of serum troponin I and Interleukin-8. *Neuroendocrinology Letters* 2002;23:133–140.

102. Gueron M, Ilia R, Margulis G. Arthropod poisons and the cardiovascular system. *Am J Emerg Med.* 2000;18:708–714.

103. Church JE, Hodgson WC. Adrenergic and cholinergic activity contributes to the cardiovascular effects of lionfish (*Pterois volitans*). *Toxicon.* 2001;40:787–796.

104. Brown CK, Shepherd SM. Marine trauma, envenomations and intoxications. *Emerg Med Clin North Am.* 1992;10:385–408.

105. Grinda J, Bellenfant F, Brivet F, et al. Biventricular assist device for scombroid poisoning with refractory myocardial dysfunction: a bridge to recovery. *Crit Care Med.* 2004;32:1957–1959.

106. Currie B, Jacups S. Prospective study of *Chironex fleckeri* and other box jellyfish stings in the "Top End" of Australia's Northern Territory. *Med J Aust* 2005;183:631–636.

107. Grady J, Burnett J. Irukandji-like syndrome in south Florida divers. *Ann Emerg Med.* 2003;42:763–766.

108. Weill H. Cardiorespiratory effects of inhalant occupational exposures. *Circulation.* 1981;63:250A–252A.

109. Zakhari S, Aviado DM. Cardiovascular toxicology of aerosol propellants, refrigerants, and related solvents. In: Van Stee EW, ed. *Cardiovascular Toxicology*. New York: Raven; 1982:281–314.

110. Karki P, Ansari J, Bhandary S, et al. Cardiac and electrocardiographical manifestations of acute organophosphate poisoning. *Singapore Med J.* 2004;45:385–389.

111. Okudera, H. Clinical features of nerve gas terrorism in Matsumoto. *J Clin Neurosci.* 2002;9:17–21.

112. Rahimi R, Shekoufeh N, Abdollahi M. Increased morbidity and mortality in acute human organophosphate-poisoned patients treated by oximes: a meta-analysis of clinical trials. *Hum Exp Toxicol.* 2006;25:157–162.

113. Eckart R, Love S, Atwood J, et al. Incidence and follow-up of inflammatory cardiac complications after smallpox vaccination. *J Am Coll Cardiol.* 2004;44:201–205.

114. Marius-Nunez AL. Myocardial infarction with normal coronary arteries after acute exposure to carbon monoxide. *Chest.* 1990;97:491–494.

115. Henry C, Satran D, Lindgren B, et al. Myocardial injury and long-term mortality following moderate to severe carbon monoxide poisoning. *JAMA.* 2006;295:398–402.

116. von Klot S, Peters A, Aalto P, et al. Ambient air pollution is associated with increased risk hospital cardiac readmission of myocardial infarction survivors in five European cities. *Circulation.* 2005;112:3073–3079.

117. Adams MJ, Hardenbergh PH, Constine LS, Lipshultz SE. Radiation-associated cardiovascular disease. *Crit Rev Oncol Hematol.* 2003;45:55–75.

118. Adams MJ, Lipsitz S, Colan SD, et al. Cardiovascular status in long-term survivors of Hodgkin's disease treated with chest radiotherapy. *J Clin Oncol.* 2004;22:3139–3148.

119. Patt D, Goodwin JS, Kuo YF, et al. Cardiac morbidity of adjuvant radiotherapy for breast cancer. *J Clin Oncol.* 2005;23:7475–7482.

120. Arsenian MA. Cardiovascular sequelae of therapeutic thoracic radiation. *Pro Cardiovasc Dis.* 1991;33:299–311.

121. Ni Y, Von Segesser LK, Turina M. Futility of pericardiectomy for postirradiation constrictive pericarditis. *Ann Thorac Surg.* 1990;49:445–448.

122. Shapiro CL, Hardenbergh PH, Gelman R, et al. Cardiac effects of adjuvant doxorubicin and radiation therapy in breast cancer patients. *J Clin Oncol.* 1998;16:3493–3501.

123. Handa N, McGregor CGA, Danielson GK, et al. Valvular heart operation in patients with previous mediastinal radiation therapy. *Ann Thorac Surg.* 2001;71:1980–1884.

124. Bertog S, Thambidorai S, Parakh K, et al. Constrictive pericarditis: etiology and cause-specific survival after pericardiectomy. *J Am Coll Cardiol.* 2004;43:1445–1452.

125. Heidenreich P, Hancock SL, Vangelos R, et al. Diastolic dysfunction after mediastinal irradiation. *Am Heart J.* 2005;150:977–982.

126. Khan MH, Ettinger SM. Post mediastinal radiation coronary artery disease and its effects on arterial conduits. *Catheter Cardiovasc Interv.* 2001;52:242–248.

127. Hull M, Morris C, Pepine C, et al. Valvular dysfunction and carotid, subclavian, and coronary artery disease in survivors of Hodgkin lymphoma treated with radiation therapy. *JAMA.* 2003;290:2831–2837.

128. Apter S, Shemesh J, Raanani P, et al. Cardiovascular calcifications after radiation therapy for Hodgkin lymphoma: computed tomography detection and clinical correlation. *Coron Artery Dis.* 2006;17:145–151.

129. Brand MD, Abadi CA, Aurigemma GP, et al. Radiation-associated valvular heart disease in Hodgkin's disease is associated with characteristic thickening and fibrosis of the aortic-mitral curtain. *J Heart Valve Dis.* 2001;10:681–685.

130. Hausleiter J, Mayer T, Hadamitzky M, et al. Radiation dose estimates from cardiac multislice computed tomography in daily practice: impact of different scanning protocols on effective dose estimates. *Circulation.* 2006;113:1305–1310.

131. Nobuhiro H, Christopher G., McGregor, MB, et al. Valvular heart operation in patients with previous mediastinal radiation therapy. *Ann Thorac Surg.* 2001;71:1880–1884.

132. Coles D, Smail M, Negus I, et al. Comparison of radiation doses from multislice computed tomography coronary angiography and conventional diagnostic angiography. *J Am Coll Cardiol.* 2006;47:1840–1845.

133. Zanzonico P, Rothenberg L, Strauss W. Radiation exposure of computed tomography and direct intracoronary angiography; risk has its rewards. *J Am Coll Cardiol.* 2006;47:1846–1849.

134. Bacher K, Bogaert E, Lapere R, De Wolf D, Thierens H. Patient-specific dose and radiation risk estimation in pediatric cardiac catheterization circulation. 2005;111:83–89.

CHAPTER (94)

Adverse Cardiovascular Drug Interactions and Complications

Michael D. Faulx / Ileana L. Piña / Gary S. Francis

INTRODUCTION

Adverse drug reactions (ADRs) are the fourth leading cause of death in patients hospitalized in the United States.[1] ADRs are responsible for approximately 1 of every 16 hospital admissions in Western countries and occur in as many as 20 percent of hospitalized patients.[1,2] The cost of these events in financial terms is huge—estimates of the financial burden of ADRs range from $30 billion to more than $130 billion annually.[3]

The World Health Organization defines an adverse drug reaction as "a response to a drug that is noxious and unintended and occurs at doses normally used in man for the prophylaxis, diagnosis and therapy of disease, or for modification of physiologic function."[4] ADRs are commonly classified as either type A (augmented) or type B (bizarre) reactions.[5] Type A reactions are predictable and based on the pharmacologic characteristics of the drug(s). Type B reactions are unpredictable and idiosyncratic. Although alternative classification schemes have been proposed, much of the literature concerning drug-related adverse events still uses this simple classification system.[6] Most of the ADRs discussed in this chapter are Type A reactions because they are fairly common and often preventable.

Individuals with heart disease comprise a population with a particular high risk for ADRs. Certain cardiovascular disease states such as heart failure can influence drug metabolism and elimination by altering perfusion of the kidneys, liver, and skeletal muscles.[7] Patients with heart disease are often elderly, and advanced age is associated with higher ADR risk because of age-related alterations in renal and hepatic function, multiple medical comorbidities, and a high prevalence of polypharmacy.[8] Dementia can influence medication compliance, and confusion regarding the indications for and doses of prescription drugs is common among older patients. ADR risk increases exponentially with the number of medications prescribed and correlates with the binomial coefficient of the total number of drugs taken by an individual patient.[9] For example, a patient taking seven medications has the potential for $6 + 5 + 4 + 3 + 2 + 1 = 21$ possible drug-drug interactions. The average nursing home patient takes seven medications, most of which are prescribed to treat cardiovascular diseases.[10] Lastly, patients with heart disease often require periodic hospitalization, and medication changes at the time of hospital admission or discharge contribute to ADR risk.[9] When patients are discharged, appropriate communication with primary care givers concerning medications is critical.

We provide an overview of the adverse reactions and interactions associated with the use of cardiovascular drugs. Disease states are emphasized rather than drug classes to highlight the clinical relevance of each interaction. The potential for an ADR with a specific drug varies depending on the indication for its use and the patient using it. For example, when flecainide is used to treat a supraventricular tachycardia in an otherwise healthy 40-year-old patient the drug is generally efficacious and well tolerated. The same dose of flecainide used to treat nonsustained ventricular tachycardia in a 75-year-old patient with ischemic cardiomyopathy is potentially lethal and entirely inappropriate.

CLINICAL PHARMACOLOGY

Drug interactions are classified as being either *pharmacokinetic* or *pharmacodynamic*. Pharmacokinetic interactions alter the delivery of a drug to its site of action. Pharmacodynamic interactions alter the effect of a drug at its site of action. Clinically relevant interactions between drugs can be pharmacokinetic, pharmacodynamic, or both. For example, patients who are taking both amiodarone and digoxin are at increased risk for symptomatic bradycardia. Amiodarone inhibits the clearance of digoxin.[11] This increases the bioavailability of digoxin and results in greater digoxin delivery to cardiac tissue, a pharmacokinetic interaction. Amiodarone also blocks the atrioventricular (AV) node. This augments the effect of digoxin on AV nodal conduction, a pharmacodynamic interaction.

[ ] PHARMACOKINETIC INTERACTIONS

The effective delivery of a drug to its biological target depends on its absorption, distribution, metabolism, and elimination. Pharmacokinetic interactions can occur at any of these levels, leading to either magnification or diminution of the drug's primary effect or side effects.

Absorption

Absorption determines drug *bioavailability*. Most orally administered drugs are absorbed by the small intestine, so agents that influence gastrointestinal (GI) metabolism, motility, or pH have the potential to interact with numerous drugs. Drugs that increase GI motility tend to reduce the bioavailability of other drugs, whereas those that decrease motility (anticholinergic drugs) can increase drug bioavailability by allowing for a longer period of absorption.[12] Drugs can also bind to one another in the GI tract and reduce bioavailability, and the bioavailability of other agents can be altered by food ingestion. The effects of food ingestion on drug absorption are usually found in the drug labeling.

Distribution

Once absorbed (or injected) many drugs bind to high-affinity sites on plasma proteins such as albumin and establish some degree of equilibrium between free and protein-bound states. The volume of distribution (Vd) is a theoretical measure that reflects how well a drug is removed from the plasma and distributed in tissue and is related to the serum concentration of a drug by the formula $Vd = D/C$, where D is the drug dose and C is the serum concentration. The pharmacologic effect of a drug is proportional to its concentration in the free state. The extent to which a drug binds plasma proteins and equilibrates between the free and bound states varies depending on the biochemical characteristics of the drug. Alterations in protein binding can influence the delivery of a drug to its site of action by influencing the proportion of free drug in the plasma. However, the clinical relevance of changes in drug distribution is frequently offset by reciprocal changes in drug elimination. For example, heparin has been shown to displace digoxin from protein-binding sites, thereby increasing the concentration of free digoxin.[13] However, the increase in free digoxin can be accompanied by a concomitant increase in digoxin elimination by the kidneys.

Drug distribution can also be influenced by the behavior of membrane transport proteins located in cells that comprise the blood-tissue interface of various organs. P-glycoprotein (Pgp) is an ATP-dependent efflux membrane transporter that was originally isolated from multidrug resistant cancer cells.[14] Pgp has also been isolated from the small intestine, liver, and blood–brain barrier, where it is thought to regulate the passage of xenobiotic substances in and out of cells. Cardiac drugs known to interact with digoxin, such as verapamil and amiodarone, have also been shown to inhibit the activity of Pgp.[15]

Metabolism

Most drugs undergo hepatic metabolism. The liver receives absorbed drugs from the small intestine by means of the portal vein and through a series of enzymatic reactions converts these relatively hydrophobic agents into water soluble compounds that are more readily eliminated from the body. Hepatic metabolism consists of two phases, biotransformation and conjugation (Fig. 94–1). During biotransformation (phase I) drugs are rendered more hydrophilic by oxidation, reduction, or hydrolysis. Phase I is typically followed by conjugation (phase II) during which drugs receive a molecular attachment such as a glucuronate that can facilitate drug transport within the body. Most drug-drug or drug-nutrient interactions involve the induction or inhibition of phase 1 metabolic enzymes. The majority of these interactions involve cytochrome P450 enzyme (CYPs) isozymes.

CYP is an iron-dependent oxidative enzyme found within the sarcoplasmic reticulum of hepatocytes and, to a lesser extent, the small intestine, kidneys, and brain. Six CYP isoenzymes are responsible for more than 90 percent of human oxidative drug metabolism and one, CYP3A4, is involved in the oxidation of one-half of *all* drugs[16] (Table 94–1; see Fig. 94–1). CYP inhibition or induction causes the serum concentrations of substrate drugs to increase or decrease, respectively. Many drugs are metabolized by more than one CYP isozyme. CYP induction also increases with hepatic blood flow and decreases with age.[17]

Elimination

Most drugs are eliminated by the kidneys, either through glomerular filtration, active tubular secretion, or passive tubular reabsorption.[12] Substances that interfere with the function of the kidneys at any of these levels can precipitate a pharmacokinetic drug interaction. Pgp, mentioned previously, is found in secretory organs such as the liver, kidney, and small intestine. Inhibition or induction of these proteins can also influence drug elimination.

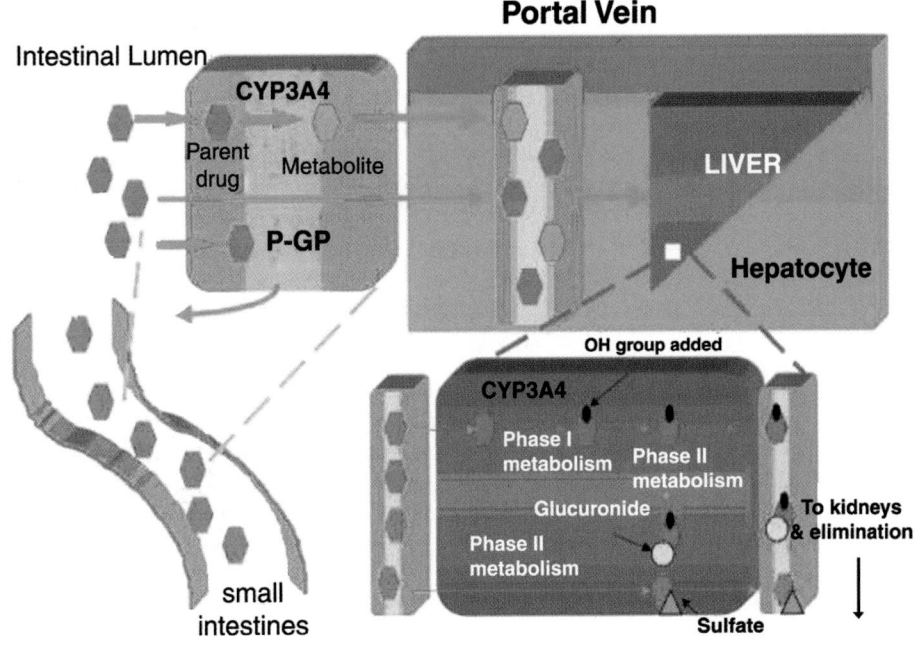

Portal Vein

Intestinal Lumen

CYP3A4

Parent drug   Metabolite

P-GP

LIVER

Hepatocyte

OH group added

CYP3A4

Phase I metabolism   Phase II metabolism

Glucuronide

Phase II metabolism

To kidneys & elimination

small intestines

Sulfate

FIGURE 94–1. Drug metabolism. Parent drugs enter the portal circulation using protein transport systems such as P-glycoprotein. Phase 1 metabolism facilitates systemic drug distribution and involves hydrolysis, reduction, or oxidation by enzymes such as cytochrome P450 (CYP) 3A4. Phase 2 metabolism facilitates drug elimination and involves sulfonation and glucuronidation. P-GP, P-glycoprotein. *Source: Illustration courtesy of Page RL, Miller GG, Lindenfeld J,[51] with permission.*

【 】 PHARMACODYNAMIC INTERACTIONS

Pharmacodynamic interactions occur commonly in the treatment of cardiovascular disease because many cardiac drugs have overlapping physiologic effects. Heart-failure therapy provides a useful example. State-of-the-art management of New York Heart Association (NYHA) class III heart failure recommends treatment with a β blocker, angiotensin-converting enzyme inhibitor/angiotensin II receptor blocker, and aldosterone-receptor antagonist is some cases, in others, a combination of hydralazine and nitrates, and in many cases a loop diuretic. All of these drugs can reduce blood pressure, so the development of symptomatic hypotension in such a patient would be considered a pharmacodynamic interaction. Although the clinician should endeavor to avoid antagonistic interactions such as drug-induced hypotension, some pharmacodynamic interactions are synergistic. For example, the diuretic metolazone enhances sodium delivery to the loop of Henle and increases the diuretic effectiveness of loop-acting drugs such as furosemide.[18]

OTHER CONTRIBUTORS TO ADVERSE DRUG REACTIONS

【 】 GENETIC FACTORS

Human genetic diversity influences the pharmacokinetics and pharmacodynamics of cardiovascular drugs. The frequency of genetic polymorphisms involving CYP isozymes varies by ethnic group (Fig. 94–2), although the clinical relevance of these polymorphisms is not uniform. For example, one third of whites carry at least one variant allele for the gene encoding CYP2C9, which is involved in the metabo-

lism of warfarin.[19] The presence of this polymorphism increases the anticoagulant effect of warfarin, and affected individuals require lower doses and more frequent monitoring. However, although patients with deactivating polymorphisms involving CYP2D6 experience up to a fivefold increase in serum metoprolol levels, adverse events and poor tolerability generally do not occur.[20] Polymorphisms involving the expression of α- and β-adrenergic receptor subunits appear to influence responsiveness to antihypertensive drug therapy.[21] Susceptibility to drug-induced torsade de pointes can be affected by polymorphisms involving ion channel genes.[22]

【 】 DIET

Dietary behavior can influence the pharmacokinetics and pharmacodynamics of certain cardiac drugs. Grapefruit juice is a popular beverage and potent CYP3A4 inhibitor that significantly increases serum levels of drugs such as simvastatin and felodipine.[23] The anticoagulant effects of warfarin can be substantially reduced in patients who consume vitamin K-rich foods such as lettuce, spinach, avocado, asparagus, and canola oil.[24] Herbal remedies have become enormously popular in recent years. Relatively few adverse herb-drug interactions have been described in the literature, but this can reflect the fact that patients seldom report the use of herbal products and physicians seldom ask.[25] *Hypericum perforatum* (St. John's wort) decreases plasma levels of digoxin, possibly because of Pgp transport induction. *H. perforatum* also reduces cyclosporin levels and has been implicated as a contributor to acute rejection of a transplanted heart.[26] Black licorice (*Glycyrrhiza glabra*) causes hypertension and pharmacodynamically competes with aldosterone antagonists for binding at the mineralocorticoid receptor.[27]

【 】 AGE

Drug pharmacokinetics can change with advancing age for several reasons. Body-fat percentage tends to increase with age and can increase the volume of distribution of fat-soluble drugs. Conversely, cachexia can increase serum levels of drugs with a large volume of distribution such as digoxin.[28] If an elderly patient is anorectic, certain medications can be more rapidly absorbed in the absence of food ingestion. Alterations in hepatic blood flow can reduce the first-pass metabolism of highly extracted drugs.[28] Glomerular filtration and renal tubular secretion decreases with increasing age and can influence drug clearance.[28] Drug pharmacodynamics are also influenced by age. β-adrenergic receptor sensitivity decreases with age and can reduce the efficacy of β-blocker therapy. Age-related changes in baroreceptor reflex sensitivity increases the risk of orthostatic hypotension in elderly patients taking antihypertensive medications.[28]

TABLE 94-1

Common CYP450 Isozyme Substrates, Inhibitors, and Inducers

	CYP ISOZYME					
FUNCTION	**CYP1A2**	**CYP2C19**	**CYP2C9**	**CYP2D6**	**CYP2E1**	**CYP3A4**
Substrate	Caffeine	Amitriptyline	Amitriptyline	Amitriptyline	Acetaminophen	Alprazolam
	Clozapine	Citalopram	Celecoxib	Clomipramine	Chlorzoxazone	Astemizole
	Cyclobenzaprine	Clomipramine	Diclofenac	Codeine	Dapsone	Buspirone
	Fluvoxamine	Cyclophosphamide	Flurbiprofen	Desipramine	Enflurane	CCB
	Imipramine	Diazepam	Ibuprofen	Dextromethor-	Ethanol	Carbamaze-
	Mexiletine	Imipramine	Losartan	phan	Halothane	pine
	Olanzapine	Lansoprazole	Naproxen	Imipramine	Isoflurane	Cisapride
	Pimozide	Nelfinavir	Phenytoin	Metoprolol	Isoniazid	Cyclosporine
	Propranolol	Omeprazole	Piroxicam	Nortriptyline		Doxorubicin
	Tacrine	Phenytoin	SMX	Oxycodone		Erythromycin
	Theophylline		Tolbutamide	Paroxetine		Etoposide
	Warfarin		Warfarin	Propafenone		Fentanyl
				Risperidone		HIV PI
				Thioridazine		Iphosphamide
				Timolol		Lovastatin
				Tramadol		Midazolam
				Venlafaxine		Pimozide
						Quinidine
						Quinine
						Simvastatin
						Tacrolimus
						Terfenadine
						Triazolam
Inhibitor	Cimetidine	Cimetidine	Amiodarone	Amiodarone	Disulfiram	Amiodarone
	Ciprofloxacin	Felbamate	Fluconazole	Chlorpheniramine	Water cress	Cimetidine
	Citalopram	Fluoxetine	Fluoxetine	Fluoxetine		Cyclosporine
	Diltiazem	Fluvoxamine	Fluvastatin	Haloperidol		Danazol
	Enoxacin	Ketoconazole	Isoniazid	Indinavir		Diltiazem
	Erythromycin	Lansoprazole	Metronidazole	Paroxetine		Fluconazole
	Fluvoxamine	Omeprazole	Paroxetine	Propafenone		Grapefruit juice
	Mexiletine	Paroxetine	Phenylbutazone	Quinidine		HIV PI
	Ofloxacin	Ticlopidine	SMX/TMP	Ritonavir		Itraconazole
	Tacrine		Sulfaphenazole	Sertraline		Ketoconazole
	Ticlopidine		Ticlopidine	Thioridazine		Macrolides
				Ticlopidine		Miconazole
						Nefazodone
						Omeprazole
						Quinidine
						Ritonavir
						Verapamil
Inducer	Carbamazepine	Carbamazepine	Phenobarbital	Ethanol	Tobacco	Carbamaze-
	Tobacco	Norethindrone	Rifampin	Isoniazid		pine
			Secobarbital			Rifabutin
						Rifampin
						Ritonavir

CCB, calcium channel blockers; HIV PI, HIV protease inhibitors; SMX, sulfamethoxazole; TMP, trimethoprim.

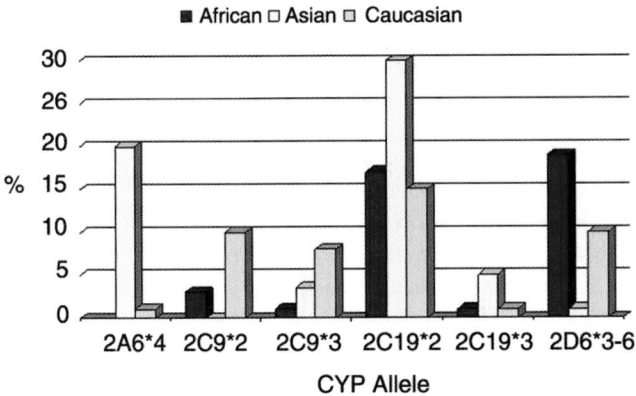

FIGURE 94–2. Prevalence of inactive cytochrome P450 (CYP) alleles within various ethnic groups. *Source: Adapted from Bjornsson TD, et al. J Clin Pharmacol. 2003;43:943–967.*

【 】 SMOKING

Cigarette smoking can influence the metabolism of cardiovascular drugs by increasing phase I hepatic enzyme activities. Heavy smoking has been shown to increase the activity of CYP2D6 fourfold when compared to nonsmokers.

HEART FAILURE AND TRANSPLANTATION

【 】 HEART FAILURE

The number of patients treated for heart failure is expected to increase as the population ages.[29] Heart failure is the classic *add-on-therapy* syndrome. In addition, the majority of patients with heart failure have comorbid conditions that are likely to require their own pharmacotherapies. The impaired cardiac output that is characteristic of advanced heart failure can slow GI transit time, affecting drug absorption and influencing hepatic blood flow. Renal dysfunction is also common in patients with heart failure (~ 30 percent) and can affect drug elimination. Therefore, heart failure patients should be considered at high risk for ADRs. The following sections highlight some of the more commonly encountered ADRs in heart failure.

Thiazolidinediones in Heart Failure

Heart failure is common in patients with advanced diabetes.[30] The American College of Cardiology/American Heart Association (ACC/AHA) Practice Guidelines for the treatment of chronic heart failure have identified diabetes as one of the risk factors for the development of heart failure.[31] Therefore, the concomitant disorders of heart failure and diabetes will challenge many clinicians. Among the advances of diabetes treatment has been the emergence of the thiazolidinediones (TDZ). These agents improve insulin sensitivity for more effective glycemic control. Troglitazone, the first on the market, was withdrawn because of liver toxicity. Rosiglitazone and pioglitazone are approved as monotherapy and in combination with other oral hypoglycemic agents; pioglitazone is also approved in combination with insulin. When compared to glyburide, rosiglitazone can decrease diastolic blood pressure.[32] Pioglitazone has been shown to improve endothelial function, which could be ultimately beneficial in heart failure.[33] Despite these potential benefits the TZDs often cause

fluid retention and worsening edema in patients with heart failure. The fluid retention appears to be worse with concomitant insulin use.[34] The mechanism for this is unclear, but warnings about TDZ use in patients with NYHA class III and IV heart failure appear in the prescribing information (rosiglitazone, SmithKline Beecham Pharmaceuticals, May 1999; pioglitazone, Eli Lilly and Company, July 1999). Therefore, these agents need to be used with caution in advanced heart failure, and patients should be closely monitored for weight gain. Additional diuretic use is frequently required.

Aldosterone Antagonists

The Randomized Aldactone Evaluation Study (RALES) trial showed that the addition of an aldosterone antagonist to standard therapy dramatically improved survival in severe heart failure patients[35,36] (see Chap. 26). However, the extension of spironolactone use to patients with less severe heart failure has resulted in an increase in the occurrence of hyperkalemia and its consequences.[37] The advent of the angiotensin II receptor blockers (ARBs) and their use as *add-on* therapy in patients treated with angiotensin-converting enzyme inhibitors (ACEIs) significantly increases the likelihood of pharmacodynamic drug interactions with spironolactone, making serious hyperkalemia even more likely.[38] Such *triple therapy* is currently not recommended. The addition of spironolactone must be done with close monitoring of renal function and serum potassium levels. Until additional evidenced-based data are published that suggest otherwise the use of spironolactone in patients with chronic heart failure outside the setting of acute myocardial infarction should be limited to patients who fit the entry criteria of the RALES trial.

β Adrenergic Receptor Blockers (β Blockers)

Once thought to be contraindicated in patients with left ventricular (LV) systolic dysfunction, certain β blockers have since been shown to dramatically reduce morbidity and mortality in patients with heart failure[39] (see Chap. 26). The benefits extend from patients with NYHA class II symptoms to those with advanced disease. In spite of these consistently positive trials, the administration and dosing of β blockers requires some careful attention to avoid giving "the right drug at the wrong time." β blockers are negative inotropic agents that acutely reduce heart rate and ventricular contractility.[40] These are the pharmacologic effects of the drug. However, their beneficial biologic effects (possible reverse remodeling) are more time dependent. Therefore, heart-failure patients should be carefully examined to assure euvolemia prior to initiating β-blocker therapy. If administered to a markedly volume overloaded patient β blockers can contribute to volume excess and precipitate heart failure decompensation. A mild increase in intravascular volume is common when β blockers are started or when doses are increased. This volume increase is usually transient and can often be controlled with additional diuretics, although patients should be followed at frequent intervals until their volume is adequately controlled. Caution should be used when beginning these agents in patients with advanced heart failure although their use in this population is strongly recommended.

Angiotensin-Converting Enzyme Inhibitors

Angiotensin-converting enzyme (ACE) inhibitors are powerful drugs that have been proven to increase survival and decrease hospitalizations in patients with NYHA Class II to IV heart failure.[41,42] In spite of these benefits clinicians continue to underuse and underdose these agents. Some of the concerns arise from inappropriate timing of administration. Patients with clinical hypovolemia, often caused by overly aggressive diuresis, can experience acute renal failure when ACE inhibitors are initiated or increased. However, the low blood pressure changes are usually transient and respond to leg elevation. Rather than remove the ACE inhibitor entirely, the diuretics should be discontinued or temporarily reduced. Avoiding the impulse to rapidly and aggressively diurese the patient will usually allow successful introduction and uptitration of these important agents. A similar rationale should be applied to ARB administration in heart failure, either alone or in combination with ACE inhibitors.[43]

Aspirin

Concerns have been raised about the loss of effectiveness with the concomitant use of ACE inhibitors and aspirin. This issue is particularly relevant because more than 50 percent of patients with heart failure have coronary artery disease and are likely to be prescribed aspirin. Much of the controversy surrounding aspirin has been generated by review of large randomized trials.[44] This important question was one of the objectives addressed by the Warfarin and Antiplatelet Therapy in Heart Failure (WATCH) trial.[45] The trial was stopped early because of poor recruitment and futility. However, a retrospective analysis did show 27 percent fewer patients were hospitalized for worsening heart failure in the warfarin group compared to the aspirin group ($p = 0.01$).[46] In spite of this observation, the aspirin group did not have increased adverse outcomes such as subsequent death, myocardial infarction (MI), or stroke. The issue of how aspirin interacts in patients with heart failure remains unresolved. The Warfarin Versus Aspirin in Patients with Reduced Cardiac Ejection Fraction (WARCEF) trial is an ongoing NIH-funded study comparing aspirin and warfarin in patients with heart failure.[47]

Doxazosin

α Blockers have been used for years to treat hypertension. Prazosin was developed for hypertension but its effect on both afterload and preload reduction made it an attractive drug for the treatment of heart failure. Reports of pharmacodynamic tachyphylaxis and fluid accumulation made the drug challenging to use with heart failure patients (see Chap. 26). More recently the α blocker, doxazosin, was tested as an arm of the Antihypertensive and Lipid-lowering Treatment to Prevent Heart Attack Trial (ALLHAT) and found to be associated with excess cases of heart failure.[48] Doxazosin is still used frequently for symptomatic treatment of prostatic hypertrophy and urinary hesitancy and is approved for use in hypertension. In patients with advanced heart failure, this drug must be used cautiously because of its inherent fluid accumulation potential and its tendency to cause orthostatic hypotension. If α blockers and diuretics are used together, diuretics should be adjusted to control volume excess as needed.

Inotropic Agents

Intravenous inotropic drugs are indicated for short-term inhospital use in patients with severe decompensated systolic heart failure who do not have mechanical outflow obstruction such as aortic stenosis or hypertrophic cardiomyopathy. Although short-term use of inotropic drugs often improves symptoms and hemodynamics in patients with advanced heart failure, long-term oral or intravenous inotrope therapy has been associated with increased mortality.[49]

Dobutamine Dobutamine stimulates β_1 adrenergic receptors on the myocyte surface, resulting in increased contractility and heart rate. The drug has a short elimination half life (2 minutes) and is metabolized by the liver and in the peripheral circulation. Dobutamine can interact pharmacodynamically with β blockers resulting in hypertension. Similar pressor responses can occur when dobutamine is given in conjunction with monoamine oxidase inhibitors, reserpine, methyldopa, and tricyclic antidepressants. Dobutamine can also cause reversible eosinophilia.[50]

Milrinone Milrinone is a phosphodiesterase inhibitor that undergoes minor hepatic metabolism and is excreted by active tubular secretion. Hypotension and ventricular tachycardia can occur as a result of reduced drug clearance in patients with renal dysfunction. Appropriate milrinone dose reduction for these patients is recommended.

Nesiritide Nesiritide is a recombinant human B-type natriuretic peptide (h-BNP) that binds to the guanylate cyclase receptor on vascular endothelial and smooth muscle cells and facilitates vaso- and venodilation. Nesiritide is used for the short-term inpatient management of acute decompensated NYHA class IV heart failure without hypotension; use in patients with systolic blood pressure (SBP) <90 mmHg is contraindicated. Recent concerns have been raised regarding potential adverse effects of nesiritide on kidney function and mortality.[51] Nesiritide has the potential to cause pharmacodynamic hypotension (sometimes prolonged) when used with other vasodilators such as ACE inhibitors (see Chap. 26).

[ ] CARDIAC TRANSPLANTATION

Cardiac transplant recipients are at unique danger of drug-drug interactions because of general unfamiliarity with immunosuppressive drugs by most nontransplant clinicians and because of the narrow therapeutic window these drugs possess. Following transplantation patients will require a variety of immunosuppressant and nonimmunosuppressant drugs. Interactions can be inevitable. Interactions with cyclosporine are numerous and can lead to increased serum levels with subsequent hypertension and renal failure or conversely, to graft rejection if levels drop significantly. This section selects the most common and potentially dangerous ADRs involving transplant patients.

Cyclosporine and Tacrolimus

Cyclosporine (CSA) and tacrolimus (TAC) belong to the family of calcineurin inhibitors that undergo metabolism by means of hepatic and intestinal CYP3A4. Oral CSA and TAC have incomplete, irregular absorption that varies from patient to patient. Table 94–2 depicts a variety of interactions with commonly used agents after transplantation. It is important to remember that after transplantation, hypertension and hyperlipidemia are common. Careful monitoring of CSA and TAC levels is critical to avoid rejection or alternatively excessive levels and side effects.

TABLE 94-2

Pharmacokinetic Interactions with Cyclosporine and Tacrolimus

DRUG CLASS	EXAMPLES	EFFECT	ONSET	MANAGEMENT
Antihyper-tensives	Amlodipine Diltiazem Felodipine Nifedipine Verapamil	Increased TAC/CSA effect	Delayed	Monitor TAC/CSA levels 3 times per week. Reduce TAC/CSA dose by 20%–50% with diltiazem or verapamil.
Lipid-lowering agents	Atorvastatin Fluvastatin Lovastatin Pravastatin Rosuvastatin Simvastatin Ezetimibe Gemfibrozil Fenofibrate	Increased statin effect with risk for myopathy or rhab-domyolysis Increased ezetimibe effect Decreased TAC/CSA effect	Delayed	Use lowest possible statin dose Consider fluvastatin or pravastatin Use lowest possible ezetimibe dose Monitor TAC/CSA 2–3 times weekly for first week then weekly for one month
Antiplatelet agents	Clopidogrel Ticlopidine	Decreased clopidogrel metabolite	Delayed	Monitor TAC/CSA levels closely for several months. Monitor for abnormal clotting.
Azole antifungals	Clotrimazole Fluconazole Itraconazole Ketoconazole	Increased TAC/CSA effect Increased TAC/CSA effect Increased TAC/CSA effect. Nephrotoxicity Increased TAC/CSA effect. Nephrotoxicity and hepa-totoxicity	Delayed Delayed Rapid Rapid	Monitor CSA/TAC levels 2–3 times for first week. Monitor CSA/TAC levels 2–3 times for first week Monitor CSA/TAC levels 2–3 times for first week; reduce initial dose of CSA/TAC by 50%. Monitor CSA/TAC levels 2–3 times for first week; reduce initial dose of CSA/TAC by 50%. Monitor renal and hepatic functions closely.

CSA, cyclosporine; TAC, tacrolimus.
SOURCE: Adapted from Page RL, Miller GG, Lindenfeld J. Circulation. 2005;111:230–239.

Antihypertensive Agents Diltiazem is a commonly used antihypertensive because of a positive effect on transplant arteriopathy in a small randomized study.[52] Diltiazem inhibits both CYP3A4 and Pgp and raises CSA levels 1.5- to 6-fold, requiring a reduction in cyclosporine dosing by 20 to 75 percent. A similar dose reduction is necessary for TAC.

Lipid-Lowering Agents Atorvastatin, simvastatin, and lovastatin are all substrates for CYP3A4 that can pharmacokinetically interact with CSA and TAC, resulting in myopathy or even rhabdomyolysis.[53] Fluvastatin is metabolized primarily by CYP2C9 and pravastatin through other pathways, which do not fully involve the CYP system. Rosuvastatin exhibits minimal metabolism by means of the CYP system.[54] With the exception of fluvastatin, all the statins have been associated with rhabdomyolysis when used in concomitantly with CSA (see Chap. 51).[53] The lowest effective dose should be initiated, and monitoring for myopathy should follow.

Antibiotics Antibiotics are frequently prescribed for patients after cardiac transplantation, particularly during the first posttransplant year where the delicate balance between rejection and overimmunosuppression exists. Depending on the structure and metabolism of antibiotics, both CSA and TAC are likely to be affected because many antibiotics are also metabolized by the CYP system (Fig. 94-3). An-

other example would be the use of fluoroquinolones such as ciprofloxacin, norfloxacin, or levofloxacin, which are also metabolized by the P450 system.

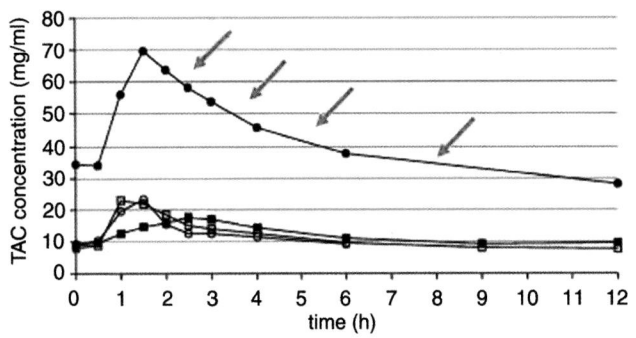

FIGURE 94-3. Significant interaction between tacrolimus (TAC) and clarithromycin (CLA). Pharmacokinetic profiles are shown for various TAC doses before CLA (8 mg/day, ◇ and 6 mg/day, ○), with CLA (4 mg/day, ●) and 2 months after CLA (4 mg/day, ■). Note the marked increase in serum TAC levels in the presence of CLA despite lower TAC dosing (arrows). *Source: Courtesy of Kunicki PW, Sobieszczanska-Malek M. Ther Drug Monit. 2005;29(1):107–108, with permission.*

Sirolimus and Everolimus

The *target of rapamycin (TOR)* inhibitors have become more commonly used in heart transplant recipients. Sirolimus (SIR) was the first introduced in the market and now everolimus (EVER) has been approved for use in cardiac transplant patients. Both of these agents are macrolide immunosuppressants. Sirolimus is extensively metabolized by CYP3A4 and therefore drug interactions are likely. Both of these agents exacerbate hyperlipidemia and therefore statin use requires the same precautions as with the calcineurin inhibitors (CI).[54]

Antihypertensives In one study diltiazem, at a dose of 120 milligrams (mg) daily, increased sirolimus levels in healthy subjects.[55] The increase in sirolimus bioavailability was attributed to inhibition of CYP3A4 by diltiazem. Thus far, by observation from efficacy data, everolimus levels have not been affected by potential CYP3A4 inhibitors such as the dihydropyridines, diltiazem, or verapamil.[56]

Other Agents In current posttransplant practice it is common to use combinations of agents with the CI drugs. The administration time of CSA with sirolimus can affect sirolimus pharmacokinetics. When CSA and sirolimus are administered together sirolimus levels increase, possibly because of inhibition of first-pass metabolism. Therefore sirolimus should be administered 4 hours after CSA dosing.[57]

Antifungal Agents The azole-derived antifungal agents should be used carefully in combination with sirolimus or everolimus. See Table 94–3.

Mycophenolate Mofetil

Mycophenolate mofetil (MMF) is an antiproliferative drug that is well absorbed after oral administration and converts to its active metabolite mycophenolic acid (MPA). MPA is metabolized by glucuronyl transferase and excreted in the urine and bile. When cyclosporine and MMF are given in combination, the result can be lower plasma MMF levels secondary to cyclosporine-induced alterations in biliary clearance. The effects of concurrent tacrolimus administration on MPA exposure are less clear.[58]

Lipid-Lowering Agents Cholestyramine can decrease MMF active compound levels. This decrease is probably because of binding of the recirculating conjugated active compound by cholestyramine, preventing enterohepatic circulation of MMF and loss of the secondary peak.[59] Package labeling recommends that MMF and cholestyramine not be coadministered.

Other Agents The absorption of MMF can be impaired by antacids or iron preparations because of possible chelation-complex formation. Therefore, it is advisable to stagger any antacids or iron supplements 2 to 4 hours with MMF administration.

Azathioprine

Azathioprine is not as widely used today as it was in the 1990s as an antiproliferative agent. The reader is referred to in-depth discussion of the pharmacokinetics of azathioprine and its potential ADRs.[60]

CORONARY ARTERY DISEASE

Major technologic and pharmacologic advances over the past two decades have substantially improved outcomes in patients with acute and chronic coronary artery disease. The widespread utilization of fibrinolytic, antiplatelet, and catheter-based therapies has dramatically improved the morbidity and mortality of coronary disease at every level, with increasingly fewer patients requiring surgical coronary revascularization.

【 】 FIBRINOLYTIC THERAPY

Although urgent catheter-based coronary revascularization has been shown to be superior to fibrinolytic therapy in patients presenting with ST-segment elevation myocardial infarction (STEMI), lack of proximity to interventional cardiology services often precludes this treatment option. Fibrinolysis thus remains an essential component to STEMI management for many patients. All fibrinolytic drugs work by either directly or indirectly promoting the conversion of plasminogen to plasmin, a nonspecific serum protease that lyses fibrin clot and degrades certain clotting factors. The risk for potentially fatal bleeding complications with the use of any fibrinolytic agent is self evident, and full knowledge of the absolute and relative contraindications of fibrinolytic drugs is mandatory prior to their use (see Chap. 60).

TABLE 94–3

Pharmacokinetic Interactions with Sirolimus and Everolimus

DRUG	EFFECT	ONSET	MANAGEMENT
Diltiazem	Increased SIR effect	Delayed	Monitor SIR levels 3 times per week in first week
Fluconazole	Increased SIR/EVER effect	Delayed	Monitor SIR/EVER levels for 1–2 weeks
Itraconazole	Increased SIR/EVER effect	Delayed	Monitor SIR/EVER levels for 1–2 weeks
Ketoconazole	Increased SIR/EVER effect	Delayed	Avoid combination
Voriconazole	Increased SIR/EVER effect	Delayed	Avoid combination
Cyclosporine	Increased SIR/EVER effect	Rapid	Administer SIR 4 hours after cyclosporine

EVER, everolimus; SIR, sirolimus.
Source: Adapted from Page RL, Miller GG, Lindenfeld J.[54]

The risk for significant pharmacokinetic interactions involving fibrinolytic drugs is thankfully low. Fibrinolytics are not dependent on CYP metabolism and are relatively immune to the effect of inhibitors and inducers of this enzyme. Agents such as alteplase and saruplase are highly cleared by the liver and thus are theoretically susceptible to reduced hepatic blood flow, which might occur in patients receiving β blockers, nitrates, or with cardiogenic shock. However, the only reported interaction of this kind involves reduced alteplase activity in the presence of nitroglycerin.[61]

There are a few potential pharmacodynamic interactions to consider when using fibrinolytic drugs. Concomitant use of heparin does increase the potential for serious bleeding in patients treated with fibrinolytic agents; however in general this increased risk does not offset the additive benefit of these drugs with respect to maintaining vessel patency. The activated partial thromboplastin time (aPTT) should be frequently monitored when heparin is used in conjunction with a fibrinolytic agent and should be maintained between 1.5 to 2.0 times the upper limit of normal.[62] Aspirin does not appear to increase the risk of bleeding when given with fibrinolytic therapy and in fact improves mortality. There is a concern that glycoprotein (GP) IIb/IIIa inhibitors can result in an unacceptably high risk for bleeding when given with full dose fibrinolytic therapy (Chap. 60).

[ ] ANTIPLATELET THERAPY

Aggressive platelet inhibition has revolutionized the medical and percutaneous management of coronary artery disease. Indeed, the broad success of intracoronary stenting is due largely to the development of potent antiplatelet agents, which prevent catastrophic early and late stent thrombosis and improve long-term stent patency rates.

Aspirin

Aspirin plays a broad role in the secondary prevention of coronary artery disease and its use is essential, along with clopidogrel or ticlopidine, to prevent intracoronary stent thrombosis and maintain stent patency (see Chap. 60). Like other inhibitors of cyclooxygenase-1 aspirin reduces prostaglandin production, which can attenuate the effects of many antihypertensive drugs, although this phenomenon is more likely to occur at higher (>100 mg) aspirin doses. Aspirin hypersensitivity, although rare, can result in life-threatening bronchospasm and anaphylaxis. Patients with true aspirin hypersensitivity who have a strong indication for the drug can undergo rapid desensitization within a few hours, preferably under the watchful eye of an allergist.[63] Aspirin use in conjunction with anticoagulants can increase the likelihood for significant bleeding complications. The phenomenon of aspirin resistance has been observed in some patients, but the true prevalence of this condition is unknown, and there is currently no accepted standard technique by which to measure it.

Thienopyridines

The thienopyridines (ticlopidine and clopidogrel) inhibit platelet function by binding to platelet surface adenosine diphosphate (ADP) receptors. Both ticlopidine and clopidogrel, alone or in combination with aspirin, have been shown to reduce the likelihood of recurrent myocardial ischemia or infarction in at-risk populations, and thienopyridine therapy is essential following intracoronary stenting.

Ticlopidine Ticlopidine use has been associated with adverse hematologic events including aplastic anemia and thrombotic thrombocytopenic purpura.[64] Although uncommon these adverse events are potentially dangerous, and the drug should be discontinued if absolute neutrophil and/or platelet counts fall below $1200/m^3$ and $80,000/m^3$, respectively. Ticlopidine is a potent inhibitor of CYP2D6 and CYP2C19 and thus carries a risk for pharmacokinetic interactions with drugs metabolized by these enzymes. Such is the case with phenytoin, which can reach toxic levels when administered with ticlopidine.

Clopidogrel Clopidogrel is associated with fewer adverse reactions than ticlopidine and is administered once daily. Hematologic abnormalities associated with clopidogrel use are rare, and rashes are uncommon (see Chap. 60). Clopidogrel is activated by CYP3A4, and its antiplatelet effects can be lessened by concurrent use of CYP3A4 promoters such as amiodarone. Pharmacodynamically, clopidogrel use is associated with an increased risk for significant bleeding when given with anticoagulants or other antiplatelet agents including aspirin. The relevance of this interaction depends on the clinical entity being treated. In patients with acute coronary syndromes the combination of aspirin and clopidogrel has been shown to significantly reduce recurrent adverse cardiac events to a greater degree than it promotes major bleeding (see Chap. 59). Thus, in this population *dual* antiplatelet therapy is preferred. The same cannot be said for patients presenting with stroke.[65] A consensus opinion regarding the most appropriate approach to the biochemical diagnosis of clopidogrel resistance is presently lacking, as are outcomes data supporting its treatment.[66]

Dipyridamole

Dipyridamole is a potent vasodilator with antiplatelet activity that is often used as the vasodilator in pharmacologic myocardial perfusion imaging studies. It also has a role as an adjunctive antiplatelet agent in patients with vascular disease (see Chaps. 59 and 60).

Glycoprotein IIb/IIIa Antagonists

The GP IIb/IIIa antagonists are parenteral drugs that have been shown to reduce ischemic event rates in patients with acute coronary syndromes and in patients receiving intracoronary stents (see Chap. 59). These molecularly diverse agents are potent inhibitors of the platelet GP IIb/IIIa receptor and as a group are associated with an increased absolute risk for significant bleeding and thrombocytopenia on the order of approximately 1 percent.[67]

Abciximab

Abciximab (see Chap. 59) is uniquely suited for use in patients with acute myocardial infarction and vessel thrombus who require intracoronary stenting. The role of abciximab outside the catheterization laboratory is limited; its benefit in patients with acute coronary syndromes who do not receive percutaneous coronary intervention has not been clearly demonstrated.[68]

Tirofiban

Tirofiban is a small, nonpeptide tyrosine derivative that reversibly binds to the GP IIb/IIIa receptor (see Chap. 59). Tirofiban appears to benefit high-risk patients with acute coronary syndromes irrespective of their need for percutaneous coronary intervention.[69]

Eptifibatide

Eptifibatide is a small synthetic peptide fashioned after barbourin, a disintegrin found in snake venom. Eptifibatide is efficacious in patients with acute coronary syndromes regardless of the need for percutaneous coronary intervention (see Chap. 59).

[ ] ANTITHROMBOTIC THERAPY

Therapeutic anticoagulation with heparin derivatives and direct thrombin inhibitors has dramatically improved outcomes in patients with coronary artery disease, particularly acute coronary syndromes (see Chaps. 59 and 60). The risk for potentially serious bleeding with antithrombin therapy is obvious, however, with appropriate monitoring the benefit these drugs provide to patients with unstable coronary syndromes far outweighs their collective risk.

Unfractionated Heparin

Heparin potentiates the effect of antithrombin III, which leads to inactivation of thrombin. Heparin also inactivates several clotting factors and prevents the conversion of fibrinogen to fibrin. Heparin has a half life of approximately 90 minutes and is metabolized by the liver and reticuloendothelial system. Pharmacokinetic drug interactions involving heparin are rare, and most pharmacodynamic interactions with heparin involve the concurrent use of drugs with antiplatelet or anticoagulant properties such as aspirin or warfarin. Life-threatening bleeding complications involving heparin can be treated with its antidote, protamine sulfate. Early, abrupt cessation of heparin therapy in patients treated for acute coronary syndromes has been associated with rebound ischemia.[70] Monitoring these individuals for at least 24 hours after heparin cessation is advisable.

One potentially dangerous adverse event associated with heparin use is heparin-induced thrombocytopenia (HIT) (see Chap. 61). HIT occurs in 1 to 5 percent of heparin-exposed patients and is associated with significant thrombocytopenia (<100,000/mm^3) that typically occurs several days after exposure to any amount of heparin, although cases of delayed-onset HIT have been described.[71] HIT is caused by autoantibodies directed against the complex of heparin and platelet factor 4 (PF4). HIT management includes discontinuation of heparin and in some cases anticoagulation with direct thrombin inhibitors and warfarin.

Low Molecular Weight Heparin

Low molecular weight heparin (LMWH) is produced by chemical or enzymatic depolymerization of the unfractionated heparin molecule. This process produces small (4,000–6,500 dalton) molecules that maintain activity against factor Xa with less potential to interact with other molecules including PF4.[72] The LMWH enoxaparin has established efficacy in the management of patients with acute coronary syndromes superior to that of heparin, with the advantage of subcutaneous administration and fixed dosing that does not require adjustment or serial monitoring (see Chap. 61).

Direct Thrombin Inhibitors

The direct thrombin inhibitor bivalirudin has established efficacy as an alternative to heparin in patients with acute coronary syndromes who require percutaneous revascularization, particularly in the setting of renal insufficiency.[73]

Adverse Drug Reactions Related to Cardiac Catheterization

Many patients presenting with acute coronary syndromes will benefit from early invasive management of their disease, and the catheterization laboratory is often the site of first exposure to potentially hazardous pharmacologic agents.[73]

[ ] RADIOCONTRAST MEDIA

Iodinated contrast agents are associated with several potential adverse reactions. Hypersensitivity reactions occur in approximately 1 percent of catheterization laboratory–treated patients and can range in severity from a mild rash to airway compromise and hemodynamic collapse. Most severe contrast reactions are anaphylactoid (non-immunoglobulin E [IgE] mediated) reactions that involve the release of molecules such as histamines and leukotrienes from mast cells and tend to occur within minutes of contrast exposure (see Chap. 17). Pretreatment of patients with a known contrast allergy with oral corticosteroids at least 6 hours prior to catheterization and antihistamines just prior to catheterization can reduce the likelihood of contrast reactions. The efficacy of intravenous corticosteroid administration just prior to catheterization has not been established. Acute management of hemodynamically unstable patients or those with airway compromise can include intravenous epinephrine or methylene blue. Contrast agents can also produce contrast-induced nephropathy (CIN), which can lead to permanent kidney damage or dialysis in a minority of patients. Underlying kidney disease appears to be the greatest risk factor for CIN, and prophylactic hydration and treatment with N-acetylcysteine appears to reduce the risk for CIN significantly (see Chap. 17). Lastly, patients taking metformin for diabetes are at risk for rare but potentially lethal lactic acidosis. It is advisable to withhold metformin for 48 hours following catheterization as this is the period when CIN typically occurs.[74]

[ ] DRUG-ELUTING STENTS

The introduction of sirolimus- and paclitaxel-coated coronary stents has significantly reduced in-stent restenosis rates and drug-eluting stents (DES) have grown to dominate the market since their debut (see Chap. 62).

RHYTHM DISORDERS

Despite the recent attention given to nonpharmacologic rhythm management options such as device therapy and catheter-based ablation procedures most patients with rhythm disorders will require antiarrhythmic medication.[75] The potential for significant adverse drug interactions involving antiarrhythmic drugs is enormous, for reasons related not only to the drugs themselves but also to the patients taking them. Antiarrhythmic drugs *in general* function within a narrow therapeutic spectrum; minor alterations in serum levels can result in loss of efficacy or overt toxicity. Many of these agents are dependent on oxidative metabolism by means of subtypes of CYP, thus allowing for possible interactions with the ever-growing list of inducers and inhibitors of these enzymes.

【 】 CLASS IA ANTIARRHYTHMICS

All class IA antiarrhythmic drugs block membrane sodium channel activity and moderately depress phase 0 of the action potential, slowing conduction and prolonging repolarization.[76] These drugs have utility in treating both atrial and ventricular tachyarrhythmias. A number of cardiac and noncardiac drugs also prolong repolarization, which is manifest electrocardiographically as QT-interval prolongation (Table 94–4). QT prolongation increases the risk for potentially fatal arrhythmias such as *torsade de pointes* (Fig. 94–4), therefore the use of QT-prolonging drugs in combination with class IA agents is contraindicated.

Quinidine

Quinidine inhibits CYP2D6 and CYP3A4 and has the potential to interact with a number of cardiac and noncardiac drugs. Coadministration of quinidine with digoxin can result in a rapid, threefold increase in digoxin levels, likely caused by quinidine-induced reduction in digoxin clearance and displacement of tissue-bound digoxin. Reducing the digoxin dose by one-half is recommended.

Procainamide

Procainamide is acetylated by the liver to form the active metabolite N-acetyl-procainamide (NAPA) and has the distinction of being the only class 1 antiarrhythmic that does not depend on CYP for its metabolism. Procainamide use can result in positive antinuclear antibod-

ies and a drug-induced lupus syndrome in 50 percent and 30 percent of patients, respectively.[77] Development of lupuslike symptoms should prompt discontinuation of the drug.

TABLE 94–4

Drugs That Prolong the QT Interval

Cardiovascular Drugs

Class IA Antiarrhythmics	*Class III Antiarrhythmics*	*Other Cardiac Drugs*
Disopyramide[a]	Amiodarone	Bepridil[a]
Procainamide[a]	Bretylium[a]	Diltiazem
Quinidine[a]	Dofetilide[a]	Indapamide
	Ibutilide[a]	Isradipine[a]
	Sotalol[a]	Moexipril/HCTZ
		Nicardipine[a]
		Ranolazine
		Triamterene

Antimicrobial Drugs

Macrolides	*Quinolones*	*Other Antimicrobial Drugs*
Azithromycin	Gatifloxacin	Chloroquine
Clarithromycin	Grepafloxacin	Foscarnet
Clindamycin	Levofloxacin	Halofantrine
Erythromycin	Moxifloxacin	Itraconazole
Roxithromycin	Ofloxacin	Ketoconazole
Telithromycin	Sparfloxacin	Trimethoprim/Sulfamethoxazole
		Voriconazole

Psychiatric Drugs

Antipsychotics	*Antidepressants*	*Other Psychiatric Drugs*
Haloperidol[a]	Amitriptyline[a]	Chloral Hydrate
Lithium	Bupropion	Felbamate
Mesoridazine	Citalopram	Fosphenytoin
Olanzapine	Clomipramine	Levomethadyl
Pimozide[a]	Desipramine[a]	Methadone
Quetiapine	Doxepin	
Risperidone	Fluoxetine[a]	
Thioridazine[a]	Imipramine	
Ziprasidone	Maprotiline	
	Nortriptyline	
	Paroxetine	
	Trazodone	
	Venlafaxine	

Other Drugs

Gastrointestinal	*Pulmonary/Allergy*	*Other Agents*
Cisapride[a]	Albuterol[a]	Amantadine
Dolasetron	Astemizole[a]	Arsenic trioxide[a]
Domperidone[a]	Fenoterol[a]	Enflurane
Droperidol	Fexofenadine	Halothane
Famotidine	Salmeterol[a]	Organophosphates (insecticide)
Granisetron	Terfenadine[a]	Pentamidine
Octreotide		Propofol
Ondansetron[a]		Quinine
		Tamoxifen
		Tacrolimus
		Vincamine

HCTZ, hydrochlorothiazide.
[a]Drugs associated with an increased risk for torsades de pointes.

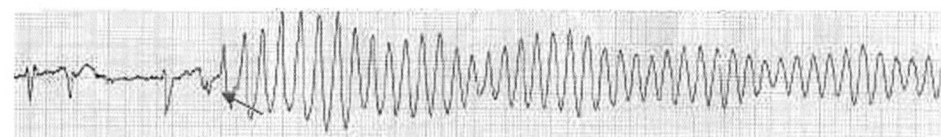

FIGURE 94–4. Torsade de pointes. The tachycardia is preceded by a short R-R interval followed by a long R-R interval with a ventricular premature complex (VPC) falling during repolarization; the *R on T* phenomenon (*arrow*).

Disopyramide

Disopyramide is metabolized by CYP3A4. This drug frequently causes anticholinergic side effects such as dry mouth, urinary retention, and constipation. Disopyramide is also a potent negative inotrope and should be used with extreme caution in patients with LV dysfunction. Coadministration of disopyramide with β blockers can result in profound bradycardia and can precipitate heart failure. Disopyramide also interacts with a number of antimicrobial agents.

【 】 CLASS IB ANTIARRHYTHMICS

The class IB antiarrhythmics block membrane sodium channels and have little effect on phase 0 of the action potential in normal cardiac tissue. These agents do depress phase 0 in abnormal cardiac tissue and can shorten repolarization. Class IB agents are useful for the treatment of arrhythmias but also have analgesic properties.

Lidocaine

Lidocaine inhibits CYP1A2 and depends on CYP1A2 and CYP3A4 for its oxidative metabolism. Amiodarone is an inhibitor of CYP3A4, and in patients already receiving intravenous lidocaine the addition of amiodarone can increase lidocaine levels and result in lidocaine toxicity.[78] Because lidocaine is often used to treat ventricular arrhythmias in patients with ischemic heart disease, particularly postmyocardial infarction ventricular tachycardia, the likelihood of using lidocaine in patients receiving β-blocker therapy is reasonably high. β Blockers as a class can reduce hepatic blood flow and therefore decrease lidocaine clearance. Some features of lidocaine toxicity include seizure activity, confusion, strokelike signs and symptoms, respiratory arrest, sinus node inhibition, nausea, and vomiting.

Mexiletine

Mexiletine-like lidocaine inhibits CYP1A2 and depends on this enzyme for oxidative metabolism, along with CYP2D6. Mexiletine levels can fall substantially in the presence of P450 inducers such as rifampicin and phenytoin, and patients can require higher mexiletine doses to achieve efficacy.[79]

【 】 CLASS IC ANTIARRHYTHMICS

Class IC antiarrhythmic drugs block membrane sodium channels and markedly reduce phase 0 of the action potential, slowing conduction with little effect on repolarization. These drugs can be used to treat ventricular arrhythmias, albeit in a select group of patients. The Cardiac Arrhythmia Suppression Trial (CAST) documented higher arrhythmic death rates in patients who were treated with certain class IC agents following myocardial infarction, illustrating the proarrhythmic potential of these drugs.

Flecainide

Flecainide inhibits the enzyme responsible for its oxidation, CYP2D6, and dose reduction should be considered when flecainide is used in conjunction with CYP2D6 inhibitors such as amiodarone and the selective serotonin reuptake inhibitors (see Chap. 43). Flecainide is also an AV nodal blocker and negative inotrope with the potential for pharmacologic interactions with agents such as β blockers and calcium-channel antagonists. In general, flecainide should not be used in patients with known structural heart disease because of its proarrhythmic potential.

Propafenone

Propafenone inhibits CYP2A6 and undergoes oxidative metabolism to variable degrees by means of CYP3A4, CYP1A2, and CYP2A6. This metabolic diversity gives propafenone the potential to interact with a broad array of agents, several of which can conceivably be used in the same patient (see Chap. 43).

【 】 CLASS II ANTIARRHYTHMIC DRUGS

The class II agents are β-adrenergic receptor blockers, ubiquitous in cardiovascular medicine because of their broad clinical utility. The pharmacokinetic profiles of these agents are discussed in detail in the Hypertension section of this chapter (see also Chap. 70). The pharmacodynamic relationships between β blockers and other antiarrhythmic drug classes are more clinically relevant, as they tend to have both positive and negative qualities. Clinical trial data suggest that combining β blockers with class III agents in patients with ischemic heart disease can improve outcomes when compared to either class alone, however such combinations also carry an increased risk for clinically significant bradycardia, especially among the elderly.

【 】 CLASS III ANTIARRHYTHMIC DRUGS

The class III antiarrhythmic drugs prolong repolarization and alter membrane potassium channel function (Chap. 43). Several class III drugs have sodium-channel antagonist properties and some have β-blocker activity. The class III drugs are used to treat both supraventricular and ventricular rhythm disorders in a diverse population of patients with a broad array of comorbid medical issues. Awareness of the potential for adverse interactions, especially QT prolongation, with the use of these drugs is mandatory. Because they prolong repolarization all class III drugs have the potential to lengthen the QT interval, which increases the risk for *torsade de pointes* (see Fig. 94–4). Therefore the use of class III antiarrhythmic agents in combination with drugs known to prolong the QT interval is contraindicated (see Table 94–4). Similarly, because both hypokalemia and hypomagnesemia can contribute to the development of torsade de pointes, the concurrent use of any class III drug with a thiazide or loop diuretic necessitates close monitoring of serum electrolyte levels.

Amiodarone

Amiodarone is arguably the most widely used antiarrhythmic agent available, but its propensity to interact with other drugs deserves special attention. The potential adverse effects of amiodarone therapy are discussed in Chap. 43.

Bretylium

Bretylium has been used to treat ventricular tachyarrhythmias, but its clinical utility has recently been called into question. Bretylium is excreted unmetabolized in the urine and thus most adverse interactions with this drug are pharmacodynamic. As mentioned above, agents that prolong the QT interval should not be used with bretylium or other class III drugs.[80]

Dofetilide

Dofetilide undergoes oxidative metabolism via CYP3A4 and is excreted in the urine by the renal cation transport system. Potent inhibitors of CYP3A4 such as cimetidine and ketoconazole can increase serum dofetilide levels and precipitate toxicity, and the use of these drugs with dofetilide is contraindicated.[81] Drugs that inhibit the renal cation transport system are also contraindicated with dofetilide and include ketoconazole, cimetidine, trimethoprim, prochlorperazine, and megestrol. Diuretics can alter the renal clearance of dofetilide and reduce serum potassium and magnesium concentrations; both risk factors to dofetilide toxicity. Verapamil use is therefore contraindicated in patients taking dofetilide. Because it requires close monitoring

and has the potential to interact with so many medications, dofetilide can only be initiated in an inpatient setting by physicians who have been specifically trained to monitor the drug.[82]

Ibutilide

Ibutilide is used acutely for the conversion of atrial fibrillation or flutter to sinus rhythm. This drug is not metabolized by CYP2D6 or CYP3A4 and does not appear to interact significantly with other drugs.[83]

Sotalol

Sotalol is a class III antiarrhythmic agent with nonselective β-adrenergic antagonist properties. Most of the administered dose is excreted unchanged in the urine. Sotalol has been observed to interact with α-adrenergic antagonists such as prazosin and clonidine. The converse has been observed with sotalol and clonidine; significant *hyper*tension has been described. Antacids containing magnesium or aluminum salts can decrease the bioavailability of sotalol and should not be given for at least 2 hours following sotalol ingestion.

【 】 CLASS IV ANTIARRHYTHMIC DRUGS

The class IV antiarrhythmic drugs block calcium channels and include verapamil and diltiazem. Verapamil interacts with several drugs including several antiarrhythmic agents (Table 94–5). Like the class II drugs (β blockers), many of the adverse interaction involving class IV antiarrhythmic drugs are pharmacodynamic.

TABLE 94–5

Significant Drug-Drug Interactions Involving Verapamil

DRUG	INTERACTION		EFFECT	RECOMMENDATION
Amiodarone	PK PD	⊗ CYP3A4	Bradycardia Hypotension Reduced cardiac output	Close clinical monitoring
Azole antifungals	PK	⊗ CYP3A4	Increased verapamil effects	Avoid concurrent use
Barbiturates	PK	⊕ CYP3A4	Reduced verapamil effects	Increase verapamil dose
β Blockers	PD	AV node	Bradycardia Hypotension Reduced cardiac output	Close clinical monitoring
Calcium	PD		Reduced verapamil effect	Increase verapamil dose
Carbamazepine	PK	⊕ CYP3A4	Reduced verapamil effects Carbamazepine toxicity	Avoid concurrent use
Cyclosporine	PK	⊗ CYP3A4	Increased cyclosporine levels, toxicity, renal failure	Avoid concurrent use
Digoxin	PK PD	⊗ CYP3A4	Bradycardia Digoxin toxicity	Reduce digoxin dose
Grapefruit juice	PK	⊗ CYP3A4	Increased verapamil effects	Avoid concurrent use
HMG-CoA reductase inhibitors	PK	⊗ CYP3A4	Increased HMG-CoA Reductase Inhibitor levels and toxicity	Use pravastatin or fluvastatin
Midazolam	PK	⊗ CYP3A4	Increased midazolam	Close clinical monitoring
Phenytoin	PK	⊕ CYP3A4	Reduced verapamil effect	Increase verapamil dose
Rifampin	PK	⊕ CYP3A4	Reduced verapamil effect	Increase verapamil dose
Tacrolimus	PK		Increased tacrolimus levels	Avoid concurrent use

CYP, cytochrome P450 enzyme; HMG-COA, hydroxymethylglutaryl coenzyme A; ⊕, induction; ⊗, inhibition; PD, pharmacodynamic; PK, pharmacokinetic.

Adenosine

Adenosine enhances permeability of acetylcholine-sensitive muscarinic potassium (K^+) channels, $I_{K(ACh)}$, in cardiac tissue and vascular smooth muscle. The drug is metabolized within a few seconds of intravenous administration by adenosine deaminase, a fact that has some practical significance. Adenosine can be both diagnostic and therapeutic in the management of supraventricular tachyarrhythmias (Chap. 43), however if the drug is pushed slowly through a small gauge peripheral (i.e., placed in the patient's hand or wrist) intravenous catheter the dose can undergo complete metabolism before it reaches the patient's heart. Thus, it is advisable to push adenosine quickly through a large caliber venous catheter placed in a proximal vein. Adenosine is also useful as a vasodilator in pharmacologic cardiac imaging.

HYPERTENSION

Hypertension perhaps more than any other medical diagnosis is associated with an increased risk for adverse drug reactions. One reason for this fact is that hypertension is quite common. The prevalence of hypertension among adults in Western societies approaches 30 percent, and the incidence of hypertension is increasing. Another reason for adverse drug reactions is the frequent need for multidrug therapy to adequately control blood pressure. Although the risk of significant pharmacodynamic interactions (principally hypotension) with a multidrug approach to hypertension is obvious, in general the consequences of untreated hypertension are graver than the risk of adverse drug reactions. Hypertension is associated with substantially increased morbidity and mortality across all age strata, and adequate blood pressure control is achieved in only a minority of treated hypertensive patients.[84] Current management guidelines recommend an aggressive approach to the initiation and titration of antihypertensive therapy. Finally, by virtue of their collective influence on cardiac output and systemic vascular resistance antihypertensive drugs can alter hepatic and renal blood flow and set the stage for adverse pharmacokinetic interactions (Chap. 70). Awareness of potential adverse drug interactions is therefore mandatory for the safe and appropriate management of hypertension.

[ ] DIURETIC THERAPY
Thiazide Diuretics

Thiazide-type diuretics are considered first-line agents in hypertension management because of their efficacy and favorable effects on cardiovascular and all-cause mortality (Chap. 70). These agents are most effective at lower doses; higher doses do not result in a substantial increase in antihypertensive effect but have been associated with class-specific adverse events such as hyperlipidemia, insulin resistance, erectile dysfunction, and a small but nonetheless concerning increase in the relative risk for renal cell carcinoma, particularly in middle aged women.[85] Thiazide diuretics have the potential to induce clinically relevant hypovolemia and electrolyte disturbances such as hypokalemia and hypomagnesemia; when severe the latter can result in life threatening ventricular arrhythmias such as torsades de pointes (see Fig. 94–4). Hyponatremia is an-

other potential risk of diuretic therapy. Although uncommon, significant hyponatremia secondary to thiazide diuretic use has been associated with permanent neurotoxicity.[86] Thiazide diuretics can also promote hyperuricemia and precipitate gout, this is a significant problem among solid organ transplant recipients. The antihypertensive efficacy of thiazide diuretics is reduced by the concurrent use of nonsteroidal antiinflammatory drugs (NSAIDs), including cyclooxygenase-2 (COX-2) inhibitors.[87] Given the increasing prevalence of hypertension and degenerative arthritis with age this is a potentially common interaction in elderly patients. As a result of their influence on plasma volume and glomerular filtration, thiazide diuretics can interfere with the pharmacokinetics of renally-excreted drugs, particularly lithium carbonate. Lithium levels can increase by as much as 40 percent with the introduction of a thiazide diuretic, potentially resulting in lithium toxicity.

Loop Diuretics

Concerning their risk for potential adverse drug reactions the loop diuretics are similar to thiazide diuretics in many respects. One significant difference between these drug classes is that loop diuretics promote renal calcium *excretion*, which can potentially promote nephrolithiasis. Loop diuretics are also used extensively in patients with heart failure and renal insufficiency. These higher risk patients are susceptible to diuretic-induced hypovolemia and can experience hypotension and worsening renal function with the administration of drugs such as ACE inhibitors and ARBs.[88] Loop diuretic–induced renal insufficiency, hypokalemia, and hypomagnesemia can also precipitate digitalis toxicity.[89]

Potassium-Sparing Diuretics

Triamterene and amiloride are mild potassium-sparing diuretics that are often coadministered with thiazide diuretics for the treatment of hypertension. This combination substantially reduces the risk of thiazide-induced hypokalemia. Although not commonly associated with adverse events these drugs do promote potassium retention, and so their use in patients with renal insufficiency or with agents known to potentiate hyperkalemia such as ACE inhibitors, ARBs and trimethoprim should be approached with extreme caution. The aldosterone receptor antagonists spironolactone and eplerenone, commonly used to treat heart failure, also promote potassium retention and thus possess the same potential for adverse drug reactions as other potassium sparing diuretics. Spironolactone is discussed more extensively in the heart failure section.

[ ] ADRENERGIC ANTAGONISTS
β-Adrenergic Blockers

Adrenergic receptor antagonists (β blockers) are commonly used as first-line agents in hypertension and have substantial clinical benefits in patients with heart failure and ischemic heart disease (Chaps. 64 and 70). β Blockers promote peripheral vasodilation, reduce myocardial contractility, and slow electrical conduction through the AV node and thus have the potential for significant pharmacodynamic interactions with drugs of similar design. Synergistic hypotension and bradycardia can also occur when β blockers are given in conjunction with antiarrhythmic drugs such as amiodarone.[90] β-Blocker therapy can result in significant, sometimes life threatening *hyper*tension through unopposed α-adrenergic stimulation in patients who are beginning therapy with clonidine or methyldopa or who abuse stimulant drugs, particularly cocaine.[91] Previous concerns regarding the risk of β-blocker therapy in patients with lung diseases such as asthma and chronic obstructive pulmonary disease (COPD) have been largely dismissed, in part because of the introduction of β_1-specific agents such as metoprolol. As is the case with many drugs, the antihypertensive effects of β blockers can be attenuated by the concurrent use of NSAIDs.

The potential for adverse pharmacokinetic interactions with β blockers depends in part on the mode of metabolism of the β blocker in question. All β blockers can reduce hepatic blood flow and can therefore interfere with hepatic drug metabolism. Many commonly used β blockers (carvedilol, metoprolol, propranolol, and labetalol) are metabolized by hepatic CYP2D6 and are therefore susceptible to hepatic pharmacokinetic changes imposed by other drugs. Cimetidine and verapamil inhibit the oxidative metabolism of these β blockers, leading to increased serum levels and exaggerated clinical effects. In contrast the hydrophilic, renally-excreted β blockers atenolol, nadolol, and sotalol are not influenced by hepatic pharmacokinetic interactions.

α-Adrenergic Receptor Blockers

The α-adrenergic receptor antagonists (α blockers) currently play a limited role in hypertension management, largely because of the established efficacy of other agents and concerns regarding the safety of α blockers in patients with cardiovascular disease.[92] Nonetheless these drugs still play a role as adjunctive agents in refractory hypertension and in the management of patients with symptomatic benign prostatic hyperplasia (BPH). Not unexpectedly the major pharmacodynamic limitation of α-blocker therapy is postural hypotension, and this can be exacerbated by other antihypertensive agents.[93] Additionally, because BPH, hypertension, and erectile dysfunction become increasingly more common with age, one needs to be particularly cautious when using α blockers in men taking phosphodiesterase 5 (PDE5) inhibitors.[94] Verapamil alters the pharmacokinetics of terazosin and prazosin resulting in increased drug bioavailability.

Calcium Channel Blockers

Calcium channel blockers are used extensively for the treatment of hypertension and other cardiovascular diseases. Although diverse with respect to mechanism of action, these drugs are uniform with respect to metabolism; all calcium channel blockers are metabolized by means of hepatic CYP3A4.[95] Therefore as a drug class calcium channel blockers are sensitive to pharmacokinetic alterations in CYP3A4 activity. Grapefruit juice, a known CYP3A4 inhibitor, increases plasma concentrations of calcium channel blockers, which can lead to significant hypotension.[96] Patients requiring treatment with calcium channel blockers should be advised to select an alternative breakfast drink.

Verapamil

Verapamil is useful for the treatment of hypertension and angina. It also has therapeutic benefit in disorders associated with labile arterial tone such as vasospastic angina, migraines, and Raynaud phenomenon.[97] Verapamil reduces AV nodal conduction, myocardial contractility, and systemic arterial tone and so can act synergistically with β blockers to

induce hypotension, heart failure, and bradycardia as previously described. Similar pharmacodynamic interactions have been observed between verapamil and antiarrhythmic agents such as amiodarone and flecainide, and the coadministration of verapamil and clonidine can result in serious hypotension and atrioventricular block.[98]

Verapamil is oxidized in the liver by CYP3A and inhibits the Pgp-mediated drug transport. This drug also enhances hepatic blood flow and can potentially alter the first-pass metabolism of hepatically-modified drugs.

These pharmacokinetic properties make verapamil a frequent culprit with respect to adverse drug interactions. Verapamil has a profound effect on the pharmacokinetics of digoxin, likely because of its influence on Pgp.[99] Digoxin levels can increase by as much 50 percent to 90 percent in the presence of verapamil, and digoxin dosing should be proportionately reduced if both drugs are required, as is sometimes the case in supraventricular tachyarrhythmias. Although verapamil and digoxin can be effective in combination when dosed appropriately, the use of intravenous verapamil in the presence of known or suspected digoxin toxicity is potentially fatal and should be considered absolutely contraindicated. Other significant drug-drug interactions involving verapamil are listed in Table 94–5.

Diltiazem

Diltiazem is similar to verapamil in most respects, especially regarding the potential for pharmacodynamic interactions with drugs such as β blockers. Diltiazem does not appear to have the same effect on Pgp as verapamil and thus does not influence digoxin levels appreciably. Diltiazem, along with verapamil does reduce the hepatic clearance of cyclosporine. This interaction can be exploited in hypertensive solid organ transplant patients where diltiazem therapy permits lower cyclosporine doses. Another potentially significant pharmacokinetic interaction involves hydroxymethylglutaryl coenzyme A (HMG-CoA) reductase inhibitors (statins). Diltiazem increases serum levels of simvastatin, lovastatin, and atorvastatin; closer monitoring for clinical and biochemical signs of statin toxicity and lower statin dosing are advised.[100]

Dihydropyridines

The dihydropyridine-type calcium channel blockers are potent vasodilators with minimal direct effect on myocardial contractility or conduction, and these agents are quite useful in the management of hypertension and angina. Because of their collective potency dihydropyridines have the propensity for pharmacodynamic interactions with blood pressure-lowering drugs, leading to significant hypotension. Dihydropyridines, as a consequence of vasodilation-induced intercompartment fluid shifts produce significant leg edema in up to 20 percent of users.[101] This type of edema can be substantially improved or avoided by coadministration of an ACE inhibitor, allowing for balanced venodilation with removal of sequestered fluid. The pharmacokinetic profile for the dihydropyridines is similar to that of diltiazem.

Angiotensin-Converting Enzyme Inhibitors

ACE inhibitors have widespread applicability in cardiovascular disease and are commonly used in the management of hypertension, heart failure, and coronary artery disease prevention. The likelihood of encountering an ACE inhibitor–related adverse event in clinical practice is reasonably high.

All ACE inhibitors have the potential to provoke a chronic, nonproductive cough in anywhere from 5 percent to 35 percent of patients.[102] The cough associated with ACE inhibitor use can be mediated by bradykinin-induced sensitization of airway sensory nerves (bradykinin in the lung is degraded by ACE) and typically resolves on discontinuation of the drug. Another rare but potentially fatal adverse reaction to ACE inhibitor therapy is oropharyngeal angioedema. ACE inhibitor–related angioedema is considered a contraindication to future ACE inhibitor use, and recent data suggest that patients who experience angioedema with ACE inhibitors are at increased risk for subsequent angioedema if treated with an ARB. ARB use in patients with a history of ACE inhibitor–related angioedema should be approached with caution.

ACE inhibitors interfere with the pharmacokinetics of lithium, and concurrent use of both agents results in increased serum lithium levels, occasionally leading to lithium toxicity.[103] If the need for ACE inhibitor therapy in a patient taking lithium is compelling, one needs to monitor lithium levels frequently to avoid this potentially dangerous interaction. ACE inhibitors should be used cautiously with potassium supplements or potassium-sparing diuretic agents to avoid significant hyperkalemia.[104] Similarly patients with hypovolemia, often a consequence of diuretic therapy, are at increased risk for ACE inhibitor–related acute renal failure, thus appropriate clinical assessment of intravascular volume is mandatory prior to initiation or titration of ACE inhibitor therapy. The use of NSAIDs can attenuate the antihypertensive effects of ACE inhibitors, and NSAIDs in combination with diuretic and ACE inhibitor use carry a substantial risk for renal failure.[105] The issue of aspirin use in combination with ACE inhibitors is controversial. Many patients in clinical practice have class 1 indications for both agents so the implications of any adverse interactions between these drugs are far reaching. Many of hemodynamic benefits of ACE inhibitors are believed to be mediated by prostaglandins, and aspirin is a potent inhibitor of prostaglandin synthesis. Finally, the ACE inhibitor, captopril, can increase digoxin levels by as much as 20 percent. This interaction has not been consistently observed with other ACE inhibitors.

Angiotensin Receptor Blockers

ARBs are effective antihypertensive agents that also have benefit in patients with heart failure.[106] ARBs are associated with few adverse reactions relative to other antihypertensive drug classes, possibly because of the limited role of the angiotensin receptor outside the cardiovascular system. Unlike the ACE inhibitors the ARBs carry little risk for cough, and angioedema with ARB therapy is extraordinarily rare. However, as mentioned previously there does appear to be some risk for ARB-induced angioedema in patients with a history of ACE inhibitor–related angioedema. The degree to which individual ARBs interact with other drugs appears to depend on agent-specific affinity for CYP.

Losartan and irbesartan have strong affinity for CYP2C9 and interact to some degree with CYP3A4 and CYP1A2. As a result the effects of these drugs can be magnified or attenuated in the presence of known inhibitors or inducers, respectively, of these P450 enzyme subtypes. Although changes in serum concentration and clearance have been observed for losartan and irbesartan in response to agents such as cyclosporine, warfarin, and grapefruit juice, the clinical relevance of these observations remains unclear.

In contrast to losartan and irbesartan, valsartan appears to depend little on oxidative metabolism, but valsartan bioavailability is reduced by approximately one-half when the drug is taken with food.[107] Patients should be advised to take valsartan 1 to 2 hours before or after meals. Candesartan cilexetil is converted to its active form within the GI tract and is eliminated unchanged in the urine and feces. Eprosartan has a similar pharmacokinetic profile, and neither drug appears to result in clinically significant interactions with commonly coprescribed agents such as warfarin, digoxin, or hydrochlorothiazide. Telmisartan is the most lipophilic ARB. Although telmisartan can increase digoxin concentrations by 50 percent this change appears to be of little clinical concern.

Vasodilators

Direct vasodilators such as hydralazine and minoxidil are generally reserved for use in patients with refractory hypertension or in heart-failure patients who do not tolerate ACE inhibitors or ARBs. Hydralazine in combination with long-acting nitrates has been recently shown to improve survival in African Americans with heart failure.[108]

Hydralazine is a direct arteriolar vasodilator that, like the dihydropyridine calcium channel blockers can produce peripheral edema in a minority of patients. Hydralazine can also induce a lupus-like syndrome with fever, malar rash, malaise, and positive antinuclear antibodies, particularly antihistone antibodies. The syndrome typically resolves several weeks after discontinuation of the drug. Abrupt cessation of hydralazine therapy can trigger a significant reflex tachycardia that can precipitate heart failure or myocardial ischemia in susceptible patients. Gradual withdrawal of hydralazine in these patients is advisable. Hydralazine is acetylated by the liver and is a weak inhibitor of CYP3A4; it can alter hepatic blood flow and increase levels of shorter acting hepatically-metabolized β blockers such as propranolol and metoprolol. Minoxidil is a potent peripheral arteriolar vasodilator that is pharmacodynamically similar to hydralazine and thus the same precautions regarding peripheral edema and reflex tachycardia apply. Minoxidil can cause hypertrichosis, a unique side effect that has been exploited for the benefit of those suffering from certain forms of alopecia. Rare cases of pericardial effusion and Stevens-Johnson syndrome have been reported with minoxidil.

PREVENTIVE CARDIOLOGY

Aggressive risk-factor modification plays a crucial role in our ongoing attempt to reduce cardiovascular event rates. In parallel with advances in catheter-based technology, advances in biotechnology have allowed us to better understand and modify cardiovascular risk at the molecular level.

【 】 HMG-COA REDUCTASE INHIBITORS

The HMG-CoA reductase inhibitors (statins) have revolutionized preventive cardiology since their introduction in the mid 1980s, and the mortality and morbidity benefits of statins have been firmly established in primary and secondary prevention trials. However, widespread public concern exists regarding the potential for statin-induced liver and muscle toxicity, a fact that can limit their use in patients who could derive significant benefit from them (Chap. 51).

Hepatotoxicity

All statins have the potential to cause asymptomatic elevation of serum hepatic aminotransferases levels. Significant (>3× the upper limit of normal) elevations in serum aminotransferase levels occur in 1 to 3 percent of statin-treated patients. Drug-induced liver injury related to statin use is an exceedingly rare, idiosyncratic reaction that occurs in less than one in one million patient years of treatment.[109]

Myotoxicity

Statin use is associated with diffuse myalgias in a minority of patients, but clinically significant muscle injury occurs in only 0.5 percent of statin-treated patients. The mechanism of statin-induced myotoxicity is unknown but can be related to the depletion of metabolic intermediaries such as ubiquinone (coenzyme-Q). However, serum coenzyme-Q levels do not appear to reflect intracellular concentration or activity, and mitochondrial activity does not appear to change in the muscles of patients after beginning statin therapy.

Drug-Drug Interactions

Most statins are dependent on CYP3A4 for metabolism and are thus subject to pharmacokinetic interactions with agents that inhibit or induce CYP3A4 (Chap. 51). One notable exception to this rule is pravastatin, which undergoes hepatic metabolism primarily by means of non-CYP dependent mechanisms. Despite the potential for adverse events relatively few drug-drug interactions involving statins have been described. Statin levels can increase substantially in the presence of potent CYP3A4, and the use of grapefruit juice in patients taking statins should be avoided. Cases of statin toxicity have also been reported in patients taking cyclosporin. Thus, pravastatin is preferred for the primary and secondary prevention of cardiovascular disease in solid organ transplant patients.

【 】 OTHER ANTILIPEMIC AGENTS

Ezetimibe

Ezetimibe is a novel inhibitor of Niemann-Pick C1-like protein, a small-bowel transport protein that facilitates the absorption of dietary and biliary cholesterol.[110] Ezetimibe preferentially blocks the absorption of cholesterol and allows the absorption of triglycerides and fat-soluble vitamins. The drug is metabolized through hepatic glucuronidation and is excreted predominantly in the feces. Ezetimibe does not interact with CYP450 isozymes or Pgp and so it results in relatively few significant pharmacokinetic interactions. Cholestyramine can bind to ezetimibe in the bowel and reduce its oral bioavailability by roughly one-half; thus these drugs should not be taken at the same time.[111] Ezetimibe can also increase serum cyclosporin levels, although the clinical significance of this is not known. Ezetimibe does not interact with statins and does not appear to be affected by food.

Niacin

Nicotinic acid (niacin) has a favorable influence on lipid profiles, but drug tolerance is poor secondary to bothersome cutaneous reactions including flushing and pruritus. These reactions are somewhat common and can be caused by prostaglandin release. Supporting this is the observation that 325 mg of oral aspirin given with niacin greatly attenuates these cutaneous effects (Chap. 51). Niacin is associated with more serious reactions, however. Sustained-release niacin is associated with an increased risk for elevated serum aminotransferases, and fulminant hepatic failure has been described.

Fibrates and Bile-Acid Sequestrants

Use of fibric-acid derivatives is associated with a number of mild complaints including GI upset, headache, and skin reactions such as increased photosensitivity. These drugs can also cause transient elevation of hepatic aminotransferase levels, but overt liver injury is rare. Fibrates can cause myopathy, especially when combined with statins or ezetimibe. Bile-acid sequestrants such as cholestyramine are associated with GI bloating and discomfort and can interfere with the absorption of other drugs, particularly warfarin.

Smoking Cessation

Cigarette smoking directly contributes to one of every five deaths in the United States and is a potent modifiable risk factor for cardiovascular disease (Chap. 51). In addition to direct end-organ toxicity cigarette smoking induces hepatic CYP1A2 and CYP2D6, potentially reducing the biologic effect of drugs metabolized by these enzymes. Conversely, smoking cessation can lessen enzyme induction with a resultant increase in the effect of CYP1A2 and CYP2D6-dependent drugs. Lasting abstinence from cigarette use can be difficult to achieve without the help of pharmacotherapy.

Nicotine Replacement Nicotine patches can cause local skin irritation although this is usually treatable with rotating patch placement and topical triamcinolone cream.

Bupropion Bupropion hydrochloride is a novel antidepressant that modulates the activity of several neurotransmitters including serotonin, norepinephrine, and dopamine. Bupropion, like nicotine replacement therapy (NRT) increases the likelihood for sustained smoking cessation by approximately twofold compared to placebo controls, and bupropion and NRT are frequently used in combination.[112] Bupropion is metabolized by CYP2B6 and thus has the potential for pharmacokinetic interactions with CYP2B6 inducers and inhibitors. Because it can lower the seizure threshold, bupropion use should be avoided in patients with a history of seizures.[113]

PERIPHERAL VASCULAR DISEASE

Vascular disease is a systemic illness. Significant coronary artery disease is therefore a strong predictor of the presence of underlying peripheral vascular disease and vice versa. Although pharmacotherapies targeting the primary and secondary prevention of coronary artery disease also benefit peripheral vascular beds, certain agents such as the phosphodiesterase (PDE) inhibitors are used specifically to treat noncoronary arterial disease. PDE inhibits the degradation of cyclic adenosine monophosphate (cAMP), a ubiquitous molecule responsible for the intracellular signal transduction of numerous cell surface receptors in a variety of tissue types including myocytes, platelets, and vascular smooth muscle cells.[114] The discovery of tissue-specific PDE subtypes has led to the development of PDE inhibitors that target individual vascular beds with reasonable specificity. PDE inhibitors are presently used to treat leg claudication and erectile dysfunction.

【 】 INTERMITTENT CLAUDICATION

Two PDE III inhibitors are currently approved for the management of moderate-to-severe leg claudication (Chap. 108). The precise mechanism of action of these agents in claudication is not known but is likely caused by cAMP-mediated dilation of vascular smooth muscle and inhibition of platelet aggregation.

Cilostazol

Cilostazol is metabolized by CYP3A4 and CYP2C19 in addition to other isozymes. Moderate inhibitors of CYP3A4 such as erythromycin and diltiazem can increase cilostazol levels by greater than 50 percent, and for this reason the coadministration of these agents with cilostazol is contraindicated in Europe; in the United States it is recommended that the cilostazol dose be reduced to 50 mg twice daily.[115] Such is also the case the CYP2C19 inhibitor omeprazole.[116] Cilostazol influences platelet function so its concurrent use with antiplatelet agents and anticoagulants can theoretically increase the risk for bleeding. Similarly, because other PDE inhibitors have been shown to increase mortality in patients with heart failure the use of cilostazol in patients with heart failure of any severity level is contraindicated.[116]

Pentoxifylline

Pentoxifylline is a xanthine derivative and its use in patients who require theophylline can result in increased theophylline levels and toxicity.[117] Pentoxifylline also influences platelet function and thus can interact pharmacodynamically with antiplatelet drugs and systemic anticoagulants. Closer monitoring of these patients for abnormal bleeding is advisable.

Erectile Dysfunction

PDE5 is highly concentrated in vascular smooth muscle cells, particularly the cells of the corpora cavernosa. There are currently three PDE5 inhibitors indicated for use in patients with erectile dysfunction: sildenafil, vardenafil, and tadalafil. The PDE5 inhibitors are generally well tolerated, but like many vasodilators these drugs can produce mild flushing and systolic hypotension.[118] The systemic vasodilator effects of PDE5 inhibitors can be dramatically amplified by the coadministration of drugs that inhibit the degradation of cyclic 3',5'-guanosine monophosphate (cGMP) such as organic nitrates. This interaction can produce dramatic increases in cAMP levels that can precipitate potentially life-threatening hypotension. For this reason PDE5 inhibitor use in patients taking any nitrate preparation is contraindicated. Concern has also been raised regarding the potential interaction between PDE5 inhibitors and α-adrenergic blockers.

DRUGS WITH HIGH INTERACTION POTENTIAL
【 】 AMIODARONE

Amiodarone has been referred to as a broad-spectrum antiarrhythmic because of its multiple mechanisms of action, established effi-

cacy in treating both ventricular and supraventricular tachyarrhythmias, and applicability across patient populations regardless of LV function. The propensity of amiodarone for end-organ toxicity and significant drug-drug interactions is equally broad (Chap. 43).

Organ Toxicity

Amiodarone has a biologic half-life of approximately 100 days, and clearance after amiodarone discontinuation can take months. The drug is extremely lipophilic and continues to accumulate in tissues after stable plasma levels have been achieved. The likelihood for end-organ toxicity is therefore greater in patients taking higher (≥ 400 mg daily) doses for longer periods on time. Periodic monitoring for end-organ toxicity in amiodarone-treated patients is recommended (Table 94–6).

Pulmonary Toxicity

The most feared complication of amiodarone therapy is amiodarone-induced pulmonary toxicity (APT). APT is directly related to the total cumulative amiodarone dose and thus tends to present after months or years of drug therapy.[119] Data from placebo controlled trials suggest that the annual incidence of severe APT is approximately 1 percent for patients taking lower (150–300 mg/day) maintenance doses of amiodarone. The incidence of APT among patients taking high dose (>400 mg/day) amiodarone is more difficult to gauge but can be as high as 5 to 10 percent. The precise pathophysiology of APT is unknown, but direct pulmonary phospholipidosis and immune-mediated hypersensitivity likely play causative roles. The symptoms and signs of APT are nonspecific and include a nonproductive cough, dyspnea, and diffuse inspiratory crackles; findings that are often attributed to underlying

---

TABLE 94–6

Recommended Approach to Monitoring for Amiodarone Toxicity

AMIODARONE MONITORING IN CLINICAL PRACTICE
Baseline
Complete history and physical exam
Ophthalmologic exam
Liver function panel
Thyroid function panel
Renal function panel with electrolytes
ECG
CXR
Pulmonary function tests (including $D_{L_{CO}}$)
Every 6 Months
Liver function panel
Thyroid function panel
Every Year
ECG
CXR
As Clinically Indicated
Any of the above at any time

CXR, chest x-ray; $D_{L_{CO}}$, carbon monoxide diffusing capacity.
SOURCE: Adapted from Goldschlager N, et al. Arch Intern Med. 2000;160:1741–1748.

heart disease. The only consistent physiologic alteration in patients with APT is a reduction of the carbon monoxide diffusing capacity (DL_{CO}), although moderate (20 percent) decreases in DL_{CO} can occur in amiodarone-treated patients without symptoms of overt lung toxicity.[120] The treatment of choice for APT is the discontinuation of amiodarone. High-dose corticosteroid therapy can be of benefit in patients with severe APT although this has not been firmly established in clinical trials.

Hepatic Toxicity

Mild, transient serum-aminotransferase elevation is not uncommon during initiation of amiodarone therapy, although amiodarone should be discontinued in patients who experience more than a twofold rise in aminotransferase levels. Overt hepatitis related to amiodarone treatment occurs in fewer than 3 percent of patients, and rare cases of hepatic failure and cirrhosis have been described.

Thyroid Toxicity

Amiodarone-induced thyroid disease is not uncommon (Chap. 43). Abnormal thyroid function is detected in approximately 5 to 20 percent of amiodarone-treated patients, and the risk for thyroid toxicity is dose dependent.[121] The features of amiodarone-induced thyroid disease depend on the mechanism of thyroid injury and the presence or absence of underlying thyroid dysfunction, thus patients can present with clinical and biochemical hyper- or hypothyroidism.[122] Amiodarone can directly injure the thyroid gland resulting in thyroiditis and clinical hyperthyroidism. Amiodarone can also influence thyroid hormone production vis-à-vis its high iodine content. Amiodarone metabolism re-

leases approximately 3 mg of iodine for every 100 mg of ingested drug. This resultant iodine excess can inhibit thyroid hormone production and the conversion of thyroxine (T4) to triiodothyronine (T3) in normal or hypoactive thyroid glands, producing clinical hypothyroidism. Conversely, autologously functioning thyroid nodules are not subject to feedback inhibition and will use the excess iodine to produce more thyroid hormone, resulting in thyrotoxicosis. Discontinuation of amiodarone often results in normalization of thyroid function, however, this can occur slowly secondary to the long elimination half-life of amiodarone. In patients who cannot safely discontinue amiodarone therapy, hypothyroidism can be successful treated with thyroid hormone replacement. Amiodarone-induced hyperthyroidism can respond to treatment with methimazole and steroids.

Ocular and Skin Manifestations

Corneal microdeposits are highly prevalent in amiodarone-treated patients but only 10 percent experience visual disturbances, usually described as halos during night vision. The presence of corneal microdeposits is not a reason to discontinue amiodarone. Skin reactions are common with long-term amiodarone therapy and can present as photosensitivity or bluish skin discoloration, often involving the face (Fig. 94–5). Patients with photosensitivity should be advised to avoid the sun and use sun block.

Pharmacokinetic Interactions

Amiodarone is metabolized by CYP3A4 and inhibits many hepatic oxidative enzymes including CYP1A2, CYP2C9, CYP2D6, and

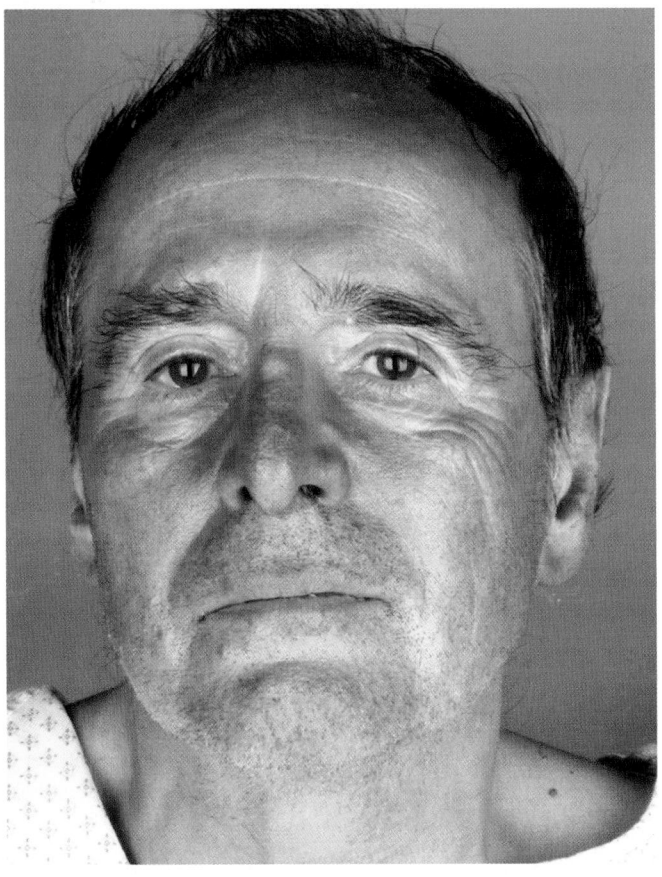
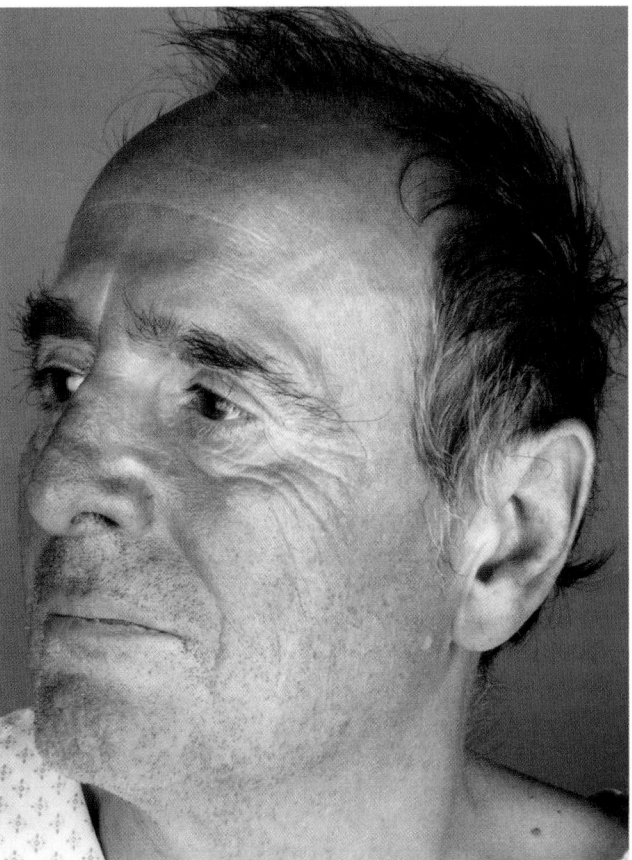

FIGURE 94–5. Amiodarone skin discoloration. *Photo courtesy of Enseleit F, et al. Images in cardiovasular medicine: The blue man. Circulation. 2006;113(5):e63, with permission.*

CYP3A4. Amiodarone also inhibits the activity of the Pgp transport system. The ability to inhibit so many enzyme systems gives amiodarone enormous potential for pharmacokinetic drug interactions. Cyclosporin levels can increase in the presence of amiodarone because of the inhibition of extrahepatic CYP3A4 activity. Similarly, serum digoxin levels can double when the drug is coadministered with amiodarone, possibly secondary to amiodarone-induced inhibition of Pgp transport in the GI tract. Periodic monitoring of cyclosporin and digoxin levels with appropriate dose reduction is recommended for patients who require amiodarone. Antimicrobial agents can also interact with amiodarone. Fluoroquinolone antibiotics can prolong the QT interval and should be avoided in patients taking amiodarone. The HIV–protease inhibitors amprenavir, nelfinavir, and ritonavir inhibit CYP3A4 and can precipitate amiodarone cardiotoxicity. Amiodarone use should be avoided in patients taking protease inhibitors. The coadministration of amiodarone and warfarin is common in patients with atrial fibrillation and mechanical heart valves. The anticoagulant effect of warfarin is enhanced by amiodarone secondary to CYP3A4 inhibition, increasing the prothrombin time by more than 40 percent. This effect can be offset by reducing the warfarin dose by 25 to 50 percent. Hypothyroidism attenuates the anticoagulant effect of warfarin, whereas thyrotoxicosis potentiates it, and cases of indirect amiodarone-warfarin interaction with thyroid disease as an intermediary have been described.

Pharmacodynamic Interactions

Amiodarone possesses the pharmacodynamic properties of several drug classes including the β blockers and calcium channel blockers. Severe sinus bradycardia and atrioventricular block can result from the concurrent use of amiodarone with β blockers such as atenolol and metoprolol. Similar pharmacodynamic interactions have been described between amiodarone and the calcium channel blockers, diltiazem and verapamil. As is the case with all class III antiarrhythmic drugs the concurrent use of amiodarone with agents known to cause QT interval prolongation is contraindicated (Chap. 43).

【 】 DIGOXIN

Digoxin is a cardiac glycoside derived from the foxglove plant (*Digitalis purpurea*) that inhibits the sodium/potassium adenosine triphosphatase (ATPase) pump on the myocyte surface. This increases the rate of sodium and calcium transport into the myocyte in exchange for potassium, and the subsequent increase in intracellular calcium improves myocardial contractility. Digoxin also reduces conduction through the sinoatrial node (SAN) and atrioventricular node (AVN). These properties make digoxin a useful drug for the management of supraventricular tachyarrhythmia such as atrial fibrillation and LV failure (Chap. 43).

Digoxin Toxicity

Digoxin toxicity can result in lethal cardiac arrhythmias and should be considered a medical emergency. Ideal serum digoxin levels are those in the range of 0.5 to 0.9 ng/mL; digoxin toxicity is more likely to occur when the serum digoxin level is 1.2 ng/mL or greater. Predisposing factors for digoxin toxicity include impaired renal function, hypokalemia, hypercalcemia, hypothyroidism, and advanced age.

The symptoms of digoxin toxicity are fairly nonspecific and include fatigue, nausea, vomiting, diarrhea, dizziness, and confusion. Bradycardia is a hallmark feature of digoxin toxicity, and the surface electrocardiogram can be diagnostic in some cases. Digoxin at therapeutic levels produces fairly characteristic ECG changes including PR-segment prolongation and lateral ST-segment depression with a *scooped* or *hockey stick* pattern (Fig. 94–6A). Atrial and ventricular ectopy and variable AVN block represent early electrocardiographic manifestations of digoxin toxicity. Another characteristic ECG finding in digoxin toxicity is atrial fibrillation with a slow ventricular response (Fig. 94–6B). The presence of a junctional escape rhythm in a patient taking digoxin is highly suggestive of digoxin toxicity, and the presence of bidirectional ventricular tachycardia is practically pathognomonic for digoxin toxicity (Fig. 94–6C, D). Complete heart block, ventricular tachycardia, and ventricular fibrillation can occur in late-stage digoxin toxicity. Discontinuation of digoxin along with supportive measures such as telemetry monitoring, electrolyte repletion, and correction of renal insufficiency can suffice in milder cases. More severe cases of digoxin toxicity can require temporary transvenous pacing, intravenous lidocaine, or the infusion of digoxin-specific fragment antigen binding (Fab) fragments.

Pharmacokinetic Interactions

Digoxin is metabolized in the stomach and small intestine by hydrolysis and eliminated by the kidneys. Anaerobic GI bacteria contribute to digoxin metabolism in approximately one-third of American patients, although the contribution of gut flora to digoxin metabolism can vary by ethnicity or geography. Verapamil and quinidine increase serum digoxin levels by 60 to 90 percent by decreasing the renal and extrarenal clearance of the drug.[123] Digoxin doses in patients taking these agents should be reduced by approximately one-half. Cholestyramine interferes with digoxin absorption by the gut, so patients should be advised to take these agents several hours apart.[124] Erythromycin increases serum digoxin levels by killing the gut bacteria responsible for digoxin hydrolysis.

Pharmacodynamic Interactions

Digoxin can produce significant bradycardia when given in conjunction with other drug classes with AVN blocking properties such as calcium channel blockers, β blockers, and amiodarone. Spironolactone can interact with digoxin indirectly by promoting hyperkalemia, with subsequent attenuation of digoxin's effect at its binding site on the ATPase pump.[125] Conversely thiazide-type and loop diuretics can promote digoxin toxicity by causing hypokalemia.

【 】 WARFARIN

Warfarin is a vitamin K antagonist that binds to several serum clotting factors including factors II, VII, IX, and X.[126] Warfarin has established efficacy in the prevention and treatment of thrombosis in a number of disease states including atrial fibrillation and venous thromboembolic disease, and it is also indicated for thrombosis prevention in patients with mechanical heart valve prostheses. Despite its widespread use warfarin has a very narrow therapeutic window and carries a substantial risk for bleeding if the drug is not closely monitored.

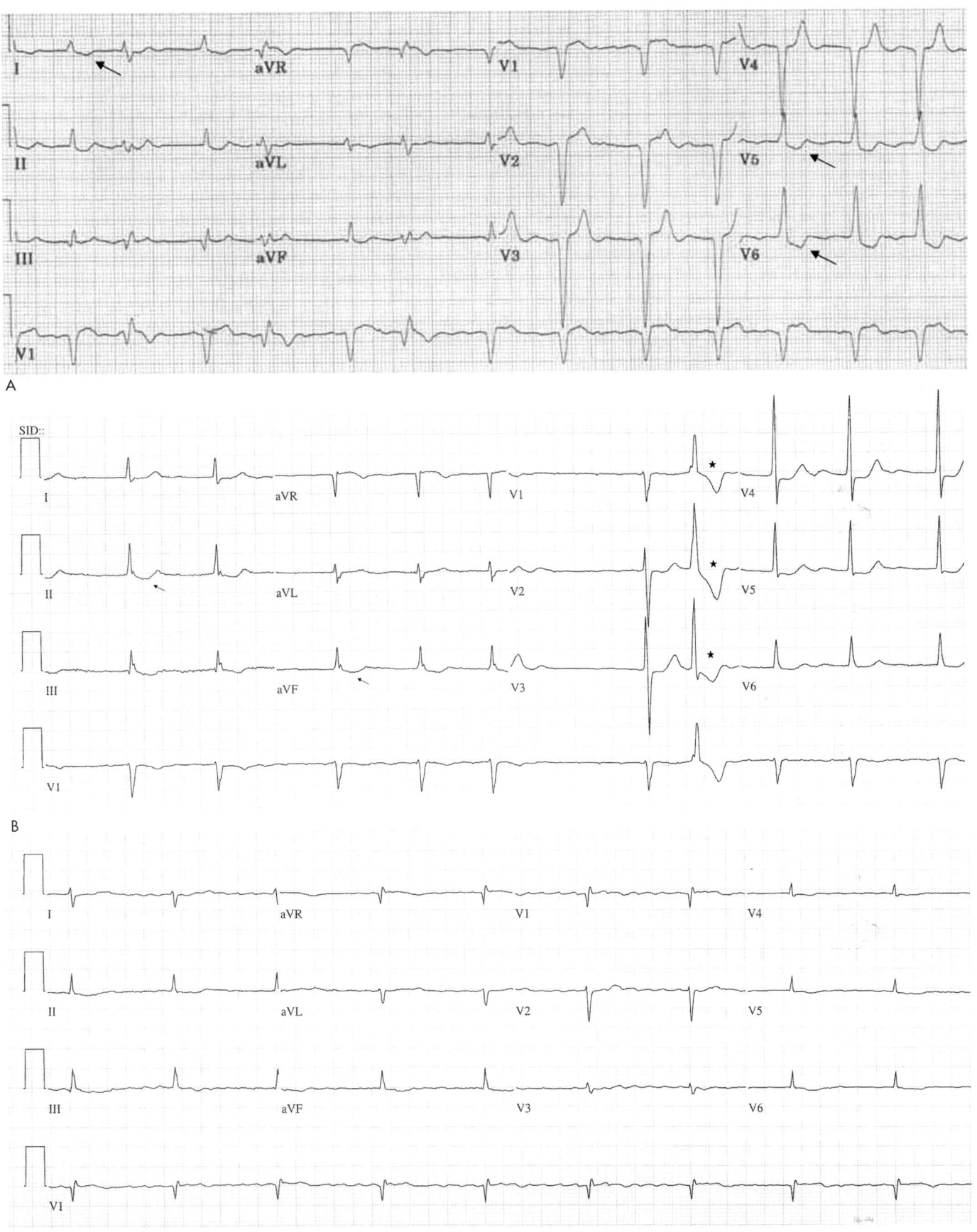

FIGURE 94–6. The electrophysiologic effects of digoxin. **A.** Digoxin effect. Please note the scooped ST segment depressions (*arrows*). **B.** Atrial fibrillation with a slow ventricular response. Note the scooped ST segments (*arrows*) and ventricular premature contraction (VPC) (*star*). **C.** Atrial fibrillation with a junctional bradycardia. **D.** Bidirectional ventricular tachycardia. Note the wide QRS duration and undulating QRS axis (*arrows*). *Source: ECG tracing courtesy of Kummer JL, et al. Images in cardiovascular medicine. Circulation. 2006;113:e156–157, with permission.* (continued)

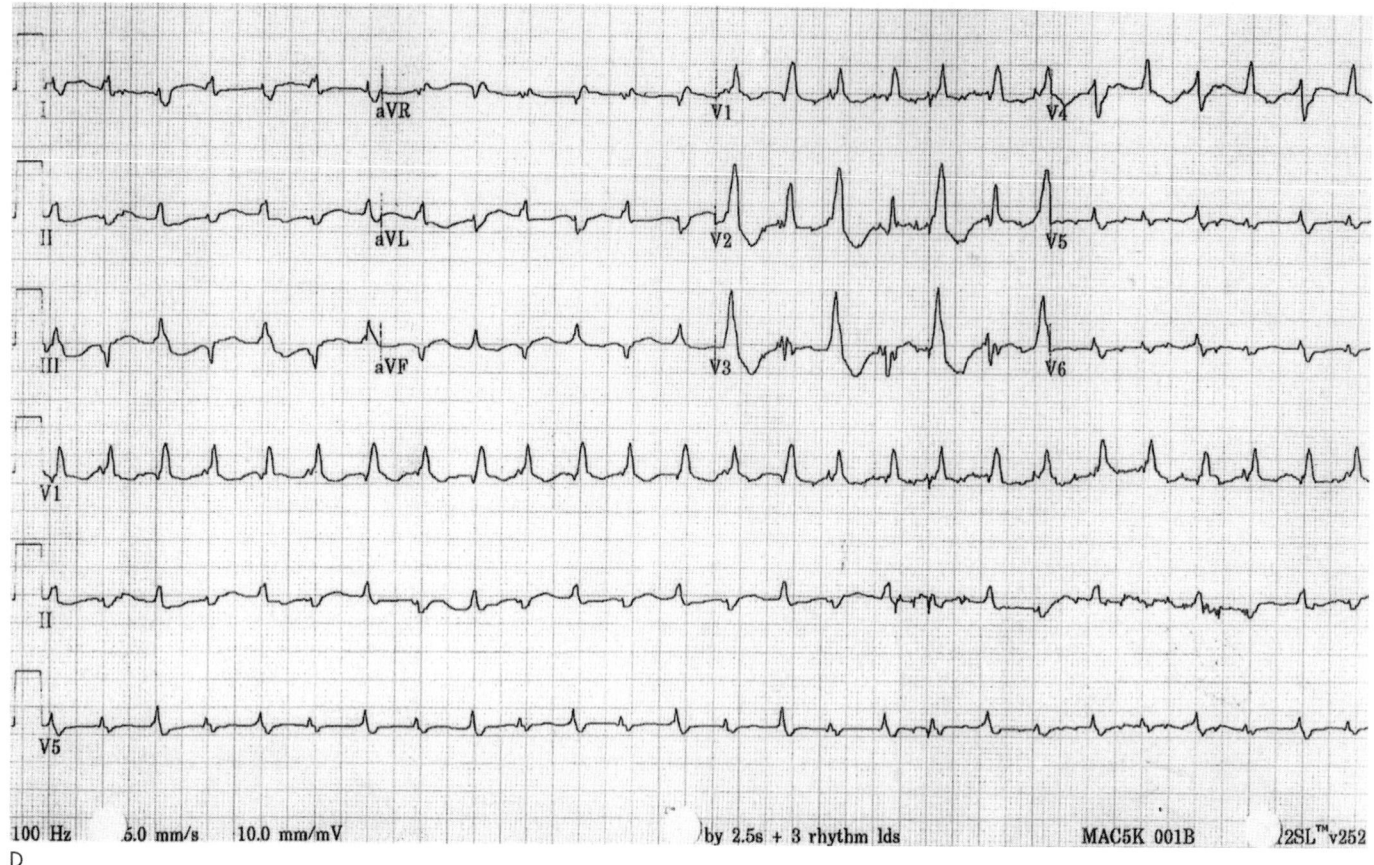

D

FIGURE 94–6. *(Continued)*

Warfarin Toxicity

The primary manifestation of warfarin overdosage is pathologic bleeding. Patients with international normalized ratios (INR) >4 are at increased risk for significant bleeding compared to those with lower INR levels, although the incidence of serious bleeding in warfarin-treated patients presenting with INRs in the range of 5 to 9 was recently shown to be approximately 1 percent.[127] One rare complication of warfarin therapy is warfarin skin necrosis, which tends to occur more commonly in women treated for deep vein thrombosis than in other patient populations.[128]

Pharmacokinetic Interactions

Warfarin exists as a racemic mixture of two isomers, although the potency of the S-enantiomer is fivefold greater than that of the R-enantiomer. The S-enantiomer undergoes oxidative metabolism through CYP2C9 whereas the R-enantiomer is dependent on CYP1A2 and CYP3A4 for metabolism. Thus, warfarin has the potential to interact with a wide range of CYP inhibitors and inducers. Potent inhibitors of CYP2C9 such as amiodarone, fluconazole, fluvastatin, sertraline, isoniazid, and lovastatin reduce warfarin metabolism and contribute to bleeding risk.[128,129] Closer monitoring of the INR and dose reduction is generally required. Quinolone and macrolide antibiotics also potentiate the effects of warfarin by inhibiting CYP1A2 and CYP3A4, respectively.[126,130,131] Although warfarin has the potential to interact with a seemingly endless list of drugs and food products, the likelihood and clinical significance of potential warfarin interacts can be difficult to predict. Holbrook and colleagues recently examined the medical literature to document which warfarin-drug and warfarin-food interactions are most probable based on published reports (Table 94–7).[126]

Pharmacodynamic Interactions

The anticoagulant properties of warfarin can be attenuated by increased dietary vitamin K intake. Foods that contain significant amounts of vitamin K include kale, spinach, lettuce, broccoli, liver, avocado, and soy beans. Concurrent use of warfarin with drugs that alter platelet function (aspirin, clopidogrel, NSAIDs) or systemic thrombostasis (heparin, direct thrombin inhibitors) can result in pharmacodynamic bleeding.

CONCLUSION

Adverse drug interactions are common in patients with cardiovascular disease, and these events are associated with substantial morbidity and mortality. As the population ages and more powerful and efficacious drugs are introduced into practice, clinicians can expect to deal with ADRs with increasing regularity. The potential numbers of adverse reactions and interactions involving cardiac drugs are overwhelming, and no physician can be expected to know every adverse drug interaction. We have described a framework that emphasizes the underlying elements that result in adverse drug interactions and highlights the more common or potential serious ADRs encountered in cardiology practice. Clinicians are encouraged to use every resource available to recognize and avoid ADRs, including the electronic medical record, on-line reference material, and routine consultation with pharmacists.

TABLE 94–7

Probability of Drug-Drug Interactions with Warfarin

LEVEL OF CAUSATION	ANTI-INFECTIVES	CARDIOVASCULAR DRUGS	ANALGESICS, ANTI-INFLAMMATORIES AND IMMUNOLOGICS	CNS DRUGS
POTENTIATION				
I (Highly probable)	Ciprofloxacin Cotrimoxazole Erythromycin Fluconazole Isoniazid Metronidazole Miconazole oral gel Miconazole vaginal suppositories Voriconazole	Amiodarone Clofibrate Diltiazem Fenofibrate Propafenone Propranolol Sulfinpyrazone (biphasic with later inhibition)	Phenylbutazone Piroxicam	Alcohol (if concomitant liver disease) Citalopram Entacapone Sertraline
II (Probable)	Amoxicillin/clavulanate Azithromycin Clarithromycin Itraconazole Levofloxacin Ritonavir Tetracycline	Acetylsalicylic acid Fluvastatin Quinidine Ropinirole Simvastatin	Acetaminophen Acetylsalicylic acid Celecoxib Dextropropoxyphene Interferon Tramadol	Disulfiram Choral hydrate Fluvoxamine Phenytoin (biphasic with later inhibition)
III (Possible)	Amoxicillin Amoxicillin/tranexamic rinse Chloramphenicol Gatifloxacin Miconazole topical gel Nalidixic acid Norfloxacin Ofloxacin Saquinavir Terbinafine	Amiodarone-induced toxicosis Disopyramide Gemfibrozil Metolazone	Celecoxib Indomethacin Leflunomide Propoxyphene Rofecoxib Sulindac Tolmetin Topical salicylates	Felbamate
IV (Highly improbable)	Cefamandole Cefazolin Sulfisoxazole	Bezafibrate Heparin	Levamisole Methylprednisolone Nabumetone	Fluoxetine/diazepam Quetiapine
INHIBITION				
I (Highly probable)	Griseofulvin Nafcillin Ribavirin Rifampin	Cholestyramine	Mesalamine	Barbiturates Carbamazepine
II (Probable)	Dicloxacillin Ritonavir	Bosentan	Azathioprine	Chlordiazepoxide
III (Possible)	Terbinafine	Telmisartan	Sulfasalazine	
IV (Highly improbable)	Cloxacillin Nafcillin/dicloxacillin Telcoplanin	Furosemide		Propofol

(continued)

TABLE 94–7

Probability of Drug-Drug Interactions with Warfarin (continued)

LEVEL OF CAUSATION	GI DRUGS AND FOOD	HERBAL SUPPLEMENTS	OTHER DRUGS
		POTENTIATION	
I (Highly probable)	Cimetidine Fish oil Mango Omeprazole	Boldo-fenugreek Guilinggao	Anabolic steroids Zileuton
II (Probable)	Grapefruit juice	Danshen Dong quai Lycium barbarum L PC-SPES	Fluorouracil Gemcitabine Levamisole/fluorouracil Paclitaxel Tamoxifen Tolterodine
III (Possible)	Cranberry juice Orlistat	Danshen/methyl salicylate	Acarbose CMF (cyclophosphamide/methotrexate/ fluorouracil) Curbicin Danazol Ifosfamide Trastuzumab
IV (Highly improbable)			Etoposide/carboplatin Levonorgestrel
		INHIBITION	
I (Highly probable)	High vitamin K content foods/enteral feeds Avocado (large amounts)		Mercaptopurine
II (Probable)	Soy milk Sucralfate	Ginseng	Chelation therapy Influenza vaccine Multivitamin supplement Raloxifene hydrochloride
III (Possible)	Sushi containing seaweed		Cyclosporine Etretinate Ubidecarenone
IV (Highly improbable)		Green tea	

CNS, central nervous system; GI, gastrointestinal.

SOURCE: Courtesy of Holbrook AM, et al. Systematic overview of warfarin and its drug and food interactions. Archives Int Med 2005;165(10):1095–1106, with permission. See this source for citations to published data on which this table is based.

REFERENCES

1. Lazarou, J, Pomeranz BH, Corey PN. Incidence of adverse drug reactions in hospitalized patients: a meta-analysis of prospective studies. *JAMA.* 1998;279(15):1200–1205.
2. Pirmohamed M, et al. Adverse drug reactions. *BMJ.* 1998;316(7140):1295–1298.
3. Johnson JA, Bootman JL. Drug-related morbidity and mortality. A cost-of-illness model. *Arch Intern Med.* 1995;155(18):1949–1956.
4. World Health Organization. International drug monitoring: the role of national centres. Report of a WHO meeting. *World Health Organ Tech Rep Ser.* 1972;498:1–25.
5. Rawlins TJ. Pathogenesis of adverse drug reactions. In: Davis DM, ed. *Textbook of Adverse Drug Reactions.* Oxford: Oxford University Press; 1981.
6. Aronson JK, Ferner RE. Clarification of terminology in drug safety. *Drug Saf.* 2005;28(10):851–870.
7. Woosley RL. Pharmacokinetics and pharmacodynamics of antiarrhythmic agents in patients with congestive heart failure. *Am Heart J.* 1987;114(5):1280–1291.
9. Kohler GI, et al. Drug-drug interactions in medical patients: effects of in-hospital treatment and relation to multiple drug use. *Int J Clin Pharmacol Ther.* 2000;38(11):504–513.
10. Landi F, et al. Comorbidity and drug use in cognitively impaired elderly living in long-term care. *Dement Geriatr Cogn Disord.* 1998;9(6):347–356.
11. Matheny CJ, et al. Pharmacokinetic and pharmacodynamic implications of P-glycoprotein modulation. *Pharmacotherapy.* 2001;21(7):778–796.
12. Anderson JR, Nawarskas JJ. Cardiovascular drug-drug interactions. *Cardiol Clin.* 2001;19(2):215–234.
13. Hooymans PM, Merkus FW. Current status of cardiac glycoside drug interactions. *Clin Pharm.* 1985;4(4):404–413.
14. Ichikawa M, et al. Modulators of the multidrug-transporter, P-glycoprotein, exist in the human plasma. *Biochem Biophys Res Commun.* 1990;166(1):74–80.

15. Funakoshi S, et al. Role of organic anion transporting polypeptide 2 in pharmacokinetics of digoxin and beta-methyldigoxin in rats. *J Pharm Sci.* 2005;94(6):1196–1203.

16. Michalets EL. Update: clinically significant cytochrome P-450 drug interactions. *Pharmacotherapy.* 1998;18(1):84–112.

17. Salem SA, et al. Reduced induction of drug metabolism in the elderly. *Age Ageing.* 1978;7(2):68–73.

18. Gunstone RF, et al. Clinical experience with metolazone in fifty-two African patients: synergy with frusemide. *Postgrad Med J.* 1971;47(554):789–793.

19. Daly AK, King BP. Pharmacogenetics of oral anticoagulants. *Pharmacogenetics.* 2003;13(5):247–252.

20. Johnson JA, Cavallari LH. Cardiovascular pharmacogenomics. *Exp Physiol.* 2005;90(3):283–289.

21. Johnson JA, et al. Beta 1-adrenergic receptor polymorphisms and antihypertensive response to metoprolol. *Clin Pharmacol Ther.* 2003;74(1):44–52.

22. Napolitano C, et al. Evidence for a cardiac ion channel mutation underlying drug-induced QT prolongation and life-threatening arrhythmias. *J Cardiovasc Electrophysiol.* 2000;11(6):691–696.

23. Lilja JJ, Kivisto KT, Neuvonen PJ. Grapefruit juice-simvastatin interaction: effect on serum concentrations of simvastatin, simvastatin acid, and HMG-CoA reductase inhibitors. *Clin Pharmacol Ther.* 1998;64(5):477–483.

24. Sorensen JM. Herb-drug, food-drug, nutrient-drug, and drug-drug interactions: mechanisms involved and their medical implications. *J Altern Complement Med.* 2002;8(3):293–308.

25. Aggarwal A, Ades PA. Interactions of herbal remedies with prescription cardiovascular medications. *Coron Artery Dis.* 2001;12(7):581–584.

26. Ruschitzka F, et al. Acute heart transplant rejection due to Saint John's wort. *Lancet.* 2000;355(9203):548–549.

27. Olukoga A, Donaldson D. Liquorice and its health implications. *J R Soc Health.* 2000;120(2):83–89.

28. Sear JW, Higham H. Issues in the perioperative management of the elderly patient with cardiovascular disease. *Drugs Aging.* 2002;19(6):429–451.

29. Croft JB, et al. Heart failure survival among older adults in the United States: a poor prognosis for an emerging epidemic in the Medicare population. *Arch Intern Med.* 1999;159(5):505–510.

30. Giles TD, Sander GE. Diabetes mellitus and heart failure: basic mechanisms, clinical features, and therapeutic considerations. *Cardiol Clin.* 2004;22(4):553–568.

31. Hunt SA, et al. ACC/AHA 2005 guideline update for the diagnosis and management of chronic heart failure in the adult: a report of the American College of Cardiology/American Heart Association Task Force on Practice Guidelines (Writing Committee to Update the 2001 Guidelines for the Evaluation and Management of Heart Failure): developed in collaboration with the American College of Chest Physicians and the International Society for Heart and Lung Transplantation: endorsed by the Heart Rhythm Society. *Circulation.* 2005;112(12):e154–235.

32. St. John Sutton M, et al. A comparison of the effects of rosiglitazone and glyburide on cardiovascular function and glycemic control in patients with type 2 diabetes. *Diabetes Care.* 2002;25(11):2058–2064.

33. Kotchen TA, et al. Effect of pioglitazone on vascular reactivity in vivo and in vitro. *Am J Physiol.* 1996;270(3 pt 2):R660–666.

34. Parulkar AA, et al. Nonhypoglycemic effects of thiazolidinediones. *Ann Intern Med.* 2001;134(1):61–71.

35. Pitt B, et al for the Randomized Aldactone Evaluation Study Investigators. The effect of spironolactone on morbidity and mortality in patients with severe heart failure. Randomized Aldactone Evaluation Study Investigators. *N Engl J Med.* 1999;341(10):709–717.

36. Masoudi FA, et al. Adoption of spironolactone therapy for older patients with heart failure and left ventricular systolic dysfunction in the United States, 1998–2001. *Circulation.* 2005;112(1):39–47.

37. Juurlink DN, et al. Rates of hyperkalemia after publication of the Randomized Aldactone Evaluation Study. *N Engl J Med.* 2004;351(6):543–551.

38. McMurray JJ et al. Effects of candesartan in patients with chronic heart failure and reduced left-ventricular systolic function taking angiotensin-converting-enzyme inhibitors: the CHARM-Added Trial. *Lancet.* 2003;362(9386):767–771.

39. Packer M, et al. Effect of carvedilol on the morbidity of patients with severe chronic heart failure: results of the carvedilol prospective randomized cumulative survival (COPERNICUS) study. *Circulation.* 2002;106(17):2194–2199.

40. Eichhorn EJ. The paradox of beta-adrenergic blockade for the management of congestive heart failure. *Am J Med.* 1992;92(5):527–538.

41. SOLVD Investigators. Effect of enalapril on survival in patients with reduced left ventricular ejection fractions and congestive heart failure. *N Engl J Med.* 1991;325(5):293–302.

42. CONSENSUS Trial Study Group. Effects of enalapril on mortality in severe congestive heart failure. Results of the Cooperative North Scandinavian Enalapril Survival Study (CONSENSUS). *N Engl J Med.* 1987;316(23):1429–1435.

43. McMurray J, et al. Practical recommendations for the use of ACE inhibitors, beta-blockers, aldosterone antagonists and angiotensin receptor blockers in heart failure: putting guidelines into practice. *Eur J Heart Fail.* 2005;7(5):710–721.

44. Nguyen KN, Aursnes I, Kjekshus J. Interaction between enalapril and aspirin on mortality after acute myocardial infarction: subgroup analysis of the Cooperative New Scandinavian Enalapril Survival Study II (CONSENSUS II). *Am J Cardiol.* 1997;79(2):115–119.

45. Massie BM, et al. The warfarin and antiplatelet therapy in heart failure trial (WATCH): rationale, design, and baseline patient characteristics. *J Card Fail.* 2004;10(2):101–112.

46. Massie BM. Aspirin use in chronic heart failure: what should we recommend to the practitioner? *J Am Coll Cardiol.* 2005;46(6):963–966.

47. Pullicino P, et al. Warfarin versus aspirin in patients with reduced cardiac ejection fraction (WARCEF): rationale, objectives, and design. *J Card Fail.* 2006;12(1):39–46.

48. Messerli FH. Implications of discontinuation of doxazosin arm of ALLHAT. Antihypertensive and Lipid-Lowering Treatment to Prevent Heart Attack Trial. *Lancet.* 2000;355(9207):863–864.

49. Packer M, et al. Effect of oral milrinone on mortality in severe chronic heart failure. The PROMISE Study Research Group. *N Engl J Med.* 1991;325(21):1468–1475.

50. El-Sayed OM, et al. Dobutamine-induced eosinophilia. *Am J Cardiol.* 2004;93(8):1078–1079.

51. Sackner-Bernstein JD, et al. Short-term risk of death after treatment with nesiritide for decompensated heart failure: a pooled analysis of randomized controlled trials. *JAMA.* 2005;293(15):1900–1905.

52. Schroeder JS, et al. A preliminary study of diltiazem in the prevention of coronary artery disease in heart-transplant recipients. *N Engl J Med.* 1993;328(3):164–170.

53. Ballantyne CM, et al. Risk for myopathy with statin therapy in high-risk patients. *Arch Intern Med.* 2003;163(5):553–564.

54. Page RL 2nd, Miller GG, Lindenfeld J. Drug therapy in the heart transplant recipient: part IV. Drug-drug interactions. *Circulation.* 2005;111(2):230–239.

55. Bottiger Y, et al. Pharmacokinetic interaction between single oral doses of diltiazem and sirolimus in healthy volunteers. *Clin Pharmacol Ther.* 2001;69(1):32–40.

56. Kovarik JM, et al. Pharmacokinetic and pharmacodynamic assessments of HMG-CoA reductase inhibitors when coadministered with everolimus. *J Clin Pharmacol.* 2002;42(2):222–228.

57. Kaplan B, et al. The effects of relative timing of sirolimus and cyclosporine microemulsion formulation coadministration on the pharmacokinetics of each agent. *Clin Pharmacol Ther.* 1998;63(1):48–53.

58. van Gelder T, Shaw LM. The rationale for and limitations of therapeutic drug monitoring for mycophenolate mofetil in transplantation. *Transplantation.* 2005;80(2 suppl):S244–253.

59. Bullingham RE, Nicholls A, Hale M. Pharmacokinetics of mycophenolate mofetil (RS61443): a short review. *Transplant Proc.* 1996;28(2):925–929.

60. Lennard L. Clinical implications of thiopurine methyltransferase--optimization of drug dosage and potential drug interactions. *Ther Drug Monit.* 1998;20(5):527–531.

61. Romeo F, et al. Concurrent nitroglycerin administration reduces the efficacy of recombinant tissue-type plasminogen activator in patients with acute anterior wall myocardial infarction. *Am Heart J.* 1995;130(4):692–697.

62. Antman EM, et al. ACC/AHA guidelines for the management of patients with ST-elevation myocardial infarction: a report of the American College of Cardiology/American Heart Association Task Force on Practice Guidelines (Committee to Revise the 1999 Guidelines for the Management of Patients with Acute Myocardial Infarction). *Circulation.* 2004;110(9):e82–292.

63. Silberman S, Neukirch-Stoop C, Steg PG. Rapid desensitization procedure for patients with aspirin hypersensitivity undergoing coronary stenting. *Am J Cardiol.* 2005;95(4):509–510.

64. Dunlop H, Siu K. Serious hematologic reactions associated with ticlopidine—update. *CMAJ.* 1999;161(7):867–868.

65. Lutsep HL. MATCH results: implications for the internist. *Am J Med.* 2006;119(6):526 e1–7.

66. Michos ED, et al. Aspirin and clopidogrel resistance. *Mayo Clin Proc.* 2006;81(4):518–526.

67. Biaggioni I et al. Cardiovascular effects of adenosine infusion in man and their modulation by dipyridamole. *Life Sci.* 1986;39(23):2229–2236.

68. Simoons ML. Effect of glycoprotein IIb/IIIa receptor blocker abciximab on outcome in patients with acute coronary syndromes without early coronary revascularisation: the GUSTO IV-ACS randomised trial. *Lancet.* 2001;357(9272):1915–1924.

69. Morrow DA et al. Usefulness of tirofiban among patients treated without percutaneous coronary intervention (TIMI high risk patients in PRISM-PLUS). *Am J Cardiol.* 2004;94(6):774–776.

70. Bijsterveld NR, et al. Recurrent cardiac ischemic events early after discontinuation of short-term heparin treatment in acute coronary syndromes: results from the Thrombolysis in Myocardial Infarction (TIMI) 11B and Efficacy and Safety of Subcutaneous Enoxaparin in Non-Q-Wave Coronary Events (ESSENCE) studies. *J Am Coll Cardiol.* 2003;42(12):2083–2089.

71. Rice L, et al. Delayed-onset heparin-induced thrombocytopenia. *Ann Intern Med.* 2002;136(3):210–215.

72. Heit, JA. Low-molecular-weight heparin: the optimal duration of prophylaxis against postoperative venous thromboembolism after total hip or knee replacement. *Thromb Res.* 2001;101(1):V163–173.

73. Chew DP, et al. Bivalirudin provides increasing benefit with decreasing renal function: a meta-analysis of randomized trials. *Am J Cardiol.* 2003;92(8):919–923.

74. Cannon CP, et al. Comparison of early invasive and conservative strategies in patients with unstable coronary syndromes treated with the glycoprotein IIb/IIIa inhibitor tirofiban. *N Engl J Med.* 2001;344(25):1879–1887.

75. Trujillo TC, Nolan PE. Antiarrhythmic agents: drug interactions of clinical significance. *Drug Saf.* 2000;23(6):509–532.

76. Vaughan Williams EM. A classification of antiarrhythmic actions reassessed after a decade of new drugs. *J Clin Pharmacol.* 1984;24(4):129–147.

77. Ellenbogen KA, Wood MA, Stambler BS. Procainamide: a perspective on its value and danger. *Heart Dis Stroke.* 1993;2(6):473–476.

78. Siegmund JB, Wilson JH, Imhoff TE. Amiodarone interaction with lidocaine. *J Cardiovasc Pharmacol.* 1993;21(4):513–515.

79. Begg EJ, et al. Enhanced metabolism of mexiletine after phenytoin administration. *Br J Clin Pharmacol.* 1982;14(2):219–223.

80. Cardiac Arrhythmia Suppression Trial (CAST) Investigators. Preliminary report: effect of encainide and flecainide on mortality in a randomized trial of arrhythmia suppression after myocardial infarction. *N Engl J Med.* 1989;321(6):406–412.

81. Tikosyn [product information]. New York: Pfizer; 1999.

82. Freeland S, Worthy C, Zolnierz M. Initiation and monitoring of class III antiarrhythmic agents. *J Cardiovasc Electrophysiol.* 2003;14(12 suppl):S291–295.

83. Cropp JS, Antal EG, Talbert RL. Ibutilide: a new class III antiarrhythmic agent. *Pharmacotherapy.* 1997;17(1):1–9.

84. Lloyd-Jones DM, Evans JC, Levy D. Hypertension in adults across the age spectrum: current outcomes and control in the community. *JAMA.* 2005;294(4):466–472.

85. Opie LH. Diuretic downsides—but in low doses they still seem among the best authenticated antihypertensives. *Cardiovasc Drugs Ther.* 2000;14(4):407–409.

86. Greenberg A. Diuretic complications. *Am J Med Sci.* 2000;319(1):10–24.

87. Houston MC. Nonsteroidal anti-inflammatory drugs and antihypertensives. *Am J Med.* 1991;90(5A):42S-47S.

88. Mignat C, Unger T. ACE inhibitors. Drug interactions of clinical significance. *Drug Saf.* 1995;12(5):334–347.

89. Crippa G, et al. Magnesium and cardiovascular drugs: interactions and therapeutic role. *Ann Ital Med Int.* 1999;14(1):40–45.

90. Boutitie F, et al for the EMIAT and CAMIAT Investigators. Amiodarone interaction with beta-blockers: analysis of the merged EMIAT (European Myocardial Infarct Amiodarone Trial) and CAMIAT (Canadian Amiodarone Myocardial Infarction Trial) databases. *Circulation.* 1999;99(17):2268–2275.

91. Lange RA, Hillis LD. Cardiovascular complications of cocaine use. *N Engl J Med.* 2001;345(5):351–358.

92. Messerli FH. Doxazosin and congestive heart failure. *J Am Coll Cardiol.* 2001;38(5):1295–1296.

93. Sica DA. Doxazosin and congestive heart failure. *Congest Heart Fail.* 2002;8(3):178–184.

94. Kloner RA. Pharmacology and drug interaction effects of the phosphodiesterase 5 inhibitors: focus on alpha-blocker interactions. *Am J Cardiol.* 2005;96(12B):42M–46M.

95. Abernethy DR, Schwartz JB. Calcium-antagonist drugs. *N Engl J Med.* 1999;341(19):1447–1457.

96. Bailey DG, et al. Interaction of citrus juices with felodipine and nifedipine. *Lancet.* 1991;337(8736):268–269.

97. Opie LH. Calcium channel antagonists should be among the first-line drugs in the management of cardiovascular disease. *Cardiovasc Drugs Ther.* 1996;10(4):455–461.

98. Jaffe R, Livshits T, Bursztyn M. Adverse interaction between clonidine and verapamil. *Ann Pharmacother.* 1994;28(7–8):881–883.

99. Verschraagen M, et al. P-glycoprotein system as a determinant of drug interactions: the case of digoxin-verapamil. *Pharmacol Res.* 1999;40(4):301–306.

100. Bellosta S, Paoletti R, Corsini A. Safety of statins: focus on clinical pharmacokinetics and drug interactions. *Circulation.* 2004;109(23 suppl 1):III50–57.

101. Pedrinelli R, et al. Heterogeneous effect of calcium antagonists on leg oedema: a comparison of amlodipine versus lercanidipine in hypertensive patients. *J Hypertens.* 2003;21(10):1969–1973.

102. Dicpinigaitis PV. Angiotensin-converting enzyme inhibitor-induced cough: ACCP evidence-based clinical practice guidelines. *Chest.* 2006;129(1 suppl):169S-173S.

103. Finley PR, O'Brien JG, Coleman RW. Lithium and angiotensin-converting enzyme inhibitors: evaluation of a potential interaction. *J Clin Psychopharmacol.* 1996;16(1):68–71.

104. Perazella MA. Drug-induced hyperkalemia: old culprits and new offenders. *Am J Med.* 2000;109(4):307–314.

105. Conlin PR, et al. Effect of indomethacin on blood pressure lowering by captopril and losartan in hypertensive patients. *Hypertension.* 2000;36(3):461–465.

106. Cohn JN, Tognoni G. A randomized trial of the angiotensin-receptor blocker valsartan in chronic heart failure. *N Engl J Med.* 2001;345(23):1667–1675.

107. Israili ZH. Clinical pharmacokinetics of angiotensin II (AT1) receptor blockers in hypertension. *J Hum Hypertens.* 2000;14(suppl 1):S73–86.

108. Taylor AL. The African American Heart Failure Trial: a clinical trial update. *Am J Cardiol.* 96(7B):44–48.

109. Tolman KG. The liver and lovastatin. *Am J Cardiol.* 2002;89(12):1374–1380.

110. Altmann SW, et al. Niemann-Pick C1 like 1 protein is critical for intestinal cholesterol absorption. *Science.* 2004;303(5661):1201–1204.

111. Kosoglou T, et al. Ezetimibe: a review of its metabolism, pharmacokinetics and drug interactions. *Clin Pharmacokinet.* 2005;44(5):467–494.

112. Hughes JR, et al. Recent advances in the pharmacotherapy of smoking. *JAMA.* 1999;281(1):72–76.

113. Ross S, Williams D. Bupropion: risks and benefits. *Expert Opin Drug Saf.* 2005;4(6):995–1003.

114. von der Leyen H. Phosphodiesterase inhibition by new cardiotonic agents: mechanism of action and possible clinical relevance in the therapy of congestive heart failure. *Klin Wochenschr.* 1989;67(12):605–615.

115. Chapman TM, Goa KL. Cilostazol: a review of its use in intermittent claudication. *Am J Cardiovasc Drugs.* 2003;3(2):117–138.

116. Suri A, Bramer SL. Effect of omeprazole on the metabolism of cilostazol. *Clin Pharmacokinet.* 1999;37(suppl 2):53–59.

117. Tjon JA, Riemann LE. Treatment of intermittent claudication with pentoxifylline and cilostazol. *Am J Health Syst Pharm.* 2001;58(6):485–493; quiz 494–496.

118. Rashid A. The efficacy and safety of PDE5 inhibitors. *Clin Cornerstone.* 2005;7(1):47–56.

119. Martin WJ 2nd, Rosenow EC 3rd. Amiodarone pulmonary toxicity. Recognition and pathogenesis (part I). *Chest.* 1988;93(5):1067–1075.

120. Gleadhill IC, et al. Serial lung function testing in patients treated with amiodarone: a prospective study. *Am J Med.* 1989;86(1):4–10.

121. Vorperian VR, et al. Adverse effects of low dose amiodarone: a meta-analysis. *J Am Coll Cardiol.* 1997;30(3):791–798.

122. Trip MD, Wiersinga W, Plomp TA. Incidence, predictability, and pathogenesis of amiodarone-induced thyrotoxicosis and hypothyroidism. *Am J Med.* 1991;91(5):507–511.

123. Pedersen KE. Digoxin interactions. The influence of quinidine and verapamil on the pharmacokinetics and receptor binding of digitalis glycosides. *Acta Med Scand.* 1985;(suppl)697:1–40.

124. Miura T, et al. Impairment of absorption of digoxin by acarbose. *J Clin Pharmacol.* 1998;38(7):654–657.

125. Paladino JA, Davidson KH, McCall BB. Influence of spironolactone on serum digoxin concentration. *JAMA.* 1984;251(4):470–471.

126. Holbrook AM, et al. Systematic overview of warfarin and its drug and food interactions. *Arch Intern Med.* 2005;165(10):1095–1106.

127. Garcia DA, et al. The risk of hemorrhage among patients with warfarin-associated coagulopathy. *J Am Coll Cardiol.* 2006;47(4):804–808.

128. Schwartz M. [Hemorrhagic necrosis of skin in dicumarol therapy]. *Nord Med.* 1957;58(34):1264–1266.

129. Haimovici H. The ischemic forms of venous thrombosis. 1. *Phlegmasia cerulea dolens.* 2. Venous gangrene. *J Cardiovasc Surg (Torino).* 1965;(suppl):164–173.

130. Ravnan SL, Locke C. Levofloxacin and warfarin interaction. *Pharmacotherapy.* 2001;21(7):884–885.

131. Foster DR, Milan NL. Potential interaction between azithromycin and warfarin. *Pharmacotherapy.* 1999;19(7):902–908.

CHAPTER 95

Effects of Mood and Anxiety Disorders on the Cardiovascular System

Dominique L. Musselman / Monica Kelly Cowles /
William M. McDonald / Charles B. Nemeroff

DEPRESSION AND COMORBID MEDICAL ILLNESS

The influence of personality traits, psychiatric syndromes, and psychological stressors has long intrigued investigators interested in the variables that contribute to the development and progression of coronary artery disease (CAD). Differences in rates of CAD in various populations remain largely obscure, even after accounting for well-established risk factors. For example the *type A* personality pattern has been intensely scrutinized as a risk factor for CAD,[1] but a consistent association between type A behavior and the subsequent development of CAD has not been shown. Researchers have examined other possible links such as the contribution of hostility,[2] and major depression. Evidence does suggest that major depression (Table 95–1),[3]—a common mood disorder—is associated with drastically elevated morbidity and mortality after an index myocardial infarction (MI) and also acts as an independent risk factor in the development of CAD.

Depressive syndromes and major depression are exceedingly common. The most recent comprehensive studies conducted in the United States, the National Comorbidity Study Replication (NCS-R) and its predecessor, the National Comorbidity Study, reported lifetime and 12-month prevalence rates of major depression[4] of 16.2 and 6.6 percent, respectively. Point prevalence rates in primary care outpatients range from 2 to 16 percent for major depression, and 9 to 20 percent for all depressive disorders.[5] The rates are even higher among medical inpatients: 8 percent for major depression and 15 to 36 percent for all depressive disorders.[6]

Minor depressive disorder (depressive symptoms subthreshold in severity compared with major depression and dysthymia) is also common in the community[7] and in primary care clinics.[8] The Epidemiologic Catchment Area Study of more than 18,500 individuals reported the lifetime prevalence rate of subthreshold depressive symptoms to be 23 percent in comparison to 6 percent, the sum of the prevalence rates of major depression and dysthymia.[7] Recognition and treatment of major depression is crucial, especially for patients after an MI. Not only do depressed patients experience greater difficulties in problem solving and coping with challenges, but depression adversely affects adherence to medical therapy[9] and rehabilitation,[10] as well as the quality of medical care received.[11] Minor depressive disorder is also associated with significant functional impairment and substantial increases in healthcare utilization.[7] Since the 1960s, multiple studies, both cross-sectional and longitudinal in design, have examined the association of cardiovascular disease (CVD), especially CAD and congestive heart failure (CHF), with depressive symptoms and major depression.

DSM-IV Diagnostic Criteria for Depressive Disorders

MAJOR DEPRESSIVE DISORDER

- Five (or more) of the following symptoms have been present during the same 2-week period and represent a change from previous functioning; at least one of the symptoms is either (1) depressed mood or (2) loss of interest or pleasure.
  (1) Depressed mood
  (2) Markedly diminished interest or pleasure
  (3) Significant weight loss or weight gain, or decrease or increase in appetite
  (4) Insomnia or hypersomnia
  (5) Psychomotor agitation or retardation (observable by others)
  (6) Fatigue or loss of energy nearly every day
  (7) Feelings of worthlessness or excessive or inappropriate guilt
  (8) Diminished concentration or indecisiveness
  (9) Recurrent thoughts of death (not just fear of dying) or suicide
- The symptoms cause clinically significant distress or impairment in social, occupational, or other important areas of functioning.
- The symptoms are not because of the direct physiologic effects of a substance or a general medical condition.
- The symptoms are not better accounted for by bereavement.

DYSTHYMIC DISORDER

A. Depressed mood for most of the day, for more days than not, for at least 2 years
B. Presence, while depressed, of two (or more) of the following:
  (1) Poor appetite or overeating
  (2) Insomnia or hypersomnia
  (3) Low energy or fatigue
  (4) Low self-esteem
  (5) Poor concentration or difficulty making decisions
  (6) Feelings of hopelessness
C. The disturbance is not better accounted for by chronic major depressive disorder.

SOURCE: *Reprinted with permission from the Diagnostic and Statistical Manual of Mental Disorders, 4th ed. (DSM-IV) Copyright 1994, American Psychiatric Association.*

EPIDEMIOLOGY

Relatively consistent point prevalence rates of depression have been documented in patients with CAD, ranging from 15 to 23 percent, despite the potential methodologic weaknesses of some of the studies.[12] A recent large-scale community (Hungarian) survey of 11,122 randomly selected participants identified an even more striking relationship between comorbid CVD and depressive symptomatology.[13] More than 20 percent of the survey participants were either receiving treatment for hypertension or had experienced a MI or stroke. Of those in this "cardiovascular" subgroup, 52 percent experienced depressive symptoms, and 30 percent fulfilled criteria for major depression. Furthermore, results indicated that the comorbidity of clinical depression among those with CVD, but no past history of MI or stroke, was similar to those subjects who were post-MI (27 percent and 31 percent respectively). This finding suggests that multiple factors mediate the relationship between CVD and depression in addition to disease severity and the negative emotional consequences of a decline in health.

The presence of depression in patients with preexisting cardiovascular disease is a risk factor for subsequent cardiovascular events and death. The seminal studies of Frasure-Smith and colleagues[14] demonstrated that post-MI depression was a significant predictor of mortality in patients both 6 and 18 months post-MI. Depression remained a significant predictor of mortality even after multivariate statistical methodology was used to factor out the effects of left ventricular dysfunction and previous MI. Multiple logistic regression analyses revealed that depression was significantly related to 18-month cardiac mortality even after controlling for other predictors. More recent studies are concordant with these results.[15,16] A meta-analysis analyzing 22 studies conducted from 1975 to 2003 calculated that post-MI depression is associated with a 2- to 2.5-fold increased risk of a poor outcome, including mortality and future cardiovascular events.[17] Depression severity had as great a detrimental impact on survival as did left ventricular dysfunction or diabetes.[12]

Depression also exerts a negative impact on patients with CHF[18–20] or recent coronary artery bypass grafting (CABG) surgery.[21,22] Indeed, evidence suggests that these patients also exhibit elevated prevalence rates of major depression. Blumenthal and colleagues[22] conducted a large, prospective study of 817 patients undergoing CABG with a 12-year follow-up period. Prior to CABG, 38 percent of patients fulfilled criteria for clinical depression; 12 percent experienced moderate to severe depression. The patients with moderate to severe depression prior to surgery had a greater than twofold risk of death post-CABG when compared to nondepressed patients, even after controlling for ethnicity, diabetes, obesity, left ventricular ejection fraction, history of cigarette smoking, number of grafts, or history of MI. Furthermore, patients with depression that persisted from baseline to 6 months, regardless of severity, had higher rates of death than those without depression.

Epidemiologic studies use self-report instruments rather than clinical interviews to evaluate the importance of psychological factors in predicting CVD. Assessments of this type typically are added to large, multiple-risk-factor studies in which population-based samples are prospectively followed.[1] The advantage of using *dimensional* measures of depression (rather than a categorical diagnosis of major depression) lies in the increased statistical power that allows these studies to detect smaller effects. Moreover, several studies have demonstrated graded relative risks (RR) for cardiac events with increasing depression severity,[23,24] providing further evidence that depression plays a causal role.

A number of these studies of antecedent depression and cardiovascular risk were included in a meta-analysis.[25] Taken as a group, the RR of developing heart disease in patients who were initially depression-free was 1.64 (95 percent confidence interval 1.29–2.08 $p < 0.001$). Lett and colleagues found that "depression confers a RR between 1.5 and 2.0 for the onset of CAD in healthy individuals, whereas depression in patients with existing CAD confers a RR between 1.5 and 2.5 for cardiac morbidity and mortality."[26] These data strongly suggest that depression is an independent risk factor in the pathophysiologic progression of CAD, rather than merely a secondary emotional response to cardiovascular illness.

PATHOPHYSIOLOGY

Advances in biological psychiatry have included the discovery of numerous neurochemical, neuroendocrine, and neuroanatomic alterations in unipolar depression, some of which likely contribute to the increased vulnerability of depressed patients to CVD. These biologic changes include immune-system activation with increased secretion of proinflammatory cytokines, endothelial dysfunction, hypothalamic-pituitary-adrenocortical (HPA) system and sympathoadrenal hyperactivity, diminished heart rate variability, alterations in platelet receptors and/or reactivity, and ventricular instability and myocardial ischemia in reaction to mental stress (Fig. 95–1).

【 】 IMMUNE SYSTEM ACTIVATION

Activation of inflammatory pathways has been implicated in the pathogenesis of both cardiovascular illness and mood disorders (Table 95–2). It has been clearly established that atherosclerosis is primarily an inflammatory disease[30,37] (see Chap. 52). Similarly, there is now unequivocal evidence that depression is associated with an activated innate immune response, although it is unclear if this activation is the etiology of depression or a consequence of the mood disorder.[43]

A key component of the inflammatory response involves the secretion of proinflammatory cytokines by activated cells such as endothelial cells, fibroblasts, macrophages, and monocytes. Cytokines coordinate immune responses and provide communication between multiple sites, including sites of infection, atherosclerotic plaques, adipose tissue, the liver, and the CNS. In addition to their biologic activity, acute-phase proteins also induce neurocognitive and behavioral changes known as *sickness* behavior. Sickness behavior, a constellation of nonspecific signs and symptoms that accompanies the physiologic response to infection and inflammation, includes fatigue, anorexia, anhedonia, decreased psychomotor activity, and disappearance of body-care activities,[43,48] all of which overlap with symptoms of major depression.

The Relationship Between Depression and Cardiovascular Disease

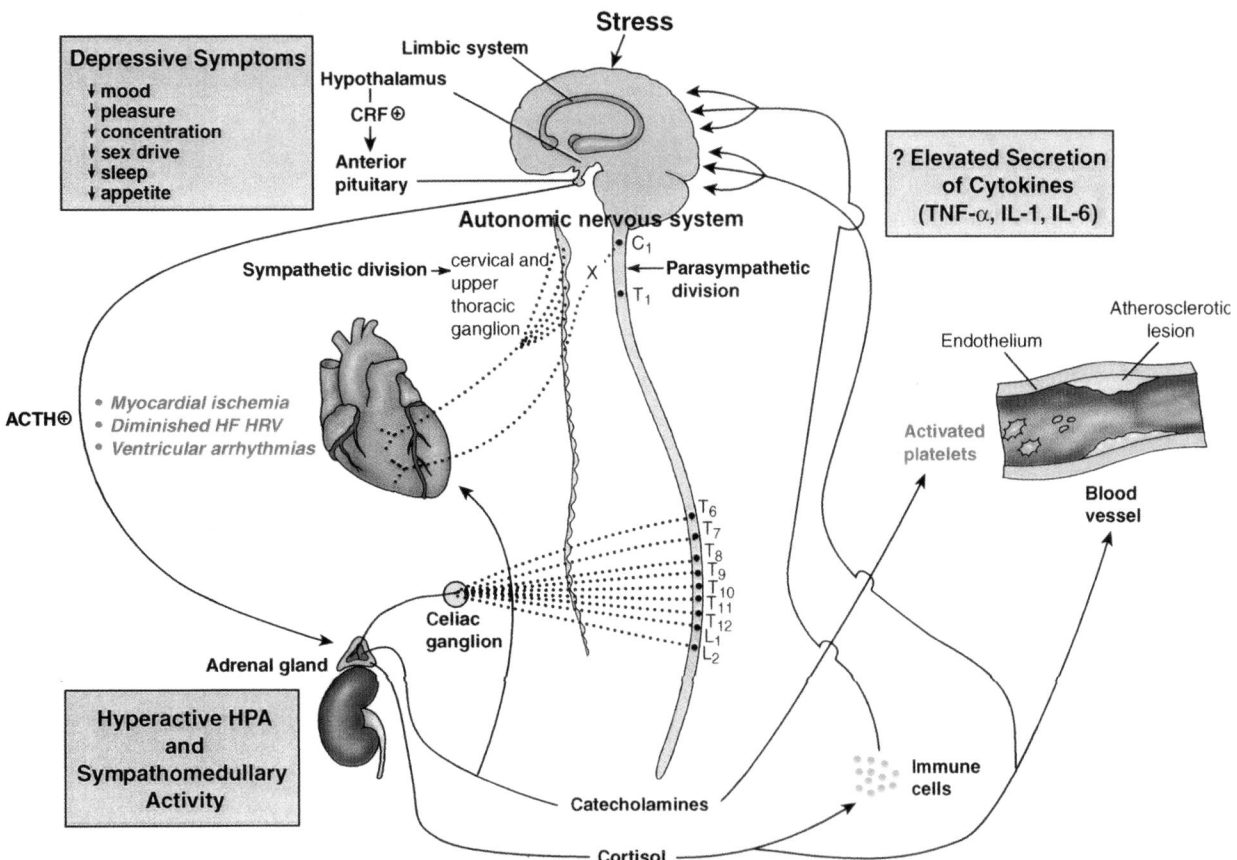

FIGURE 95–1. Hypothetical schema of pathophysiologic findings associated with depression that probably contributes to increased susceptibility to cardiovascular disease. Autonomic nervous system innervation of the heart via the parasympathetic vagus (X) nerve and sympathetic (postganglionic efferents from the cervical and upper thoracic paravertebral ganglia) nerves is shown. ACTH, corticotropin; CRF, corticotropin-releasing factor; HRV, heart rate variability; HPA, hypothalamic-pituitary-adrenocortical axis; IL-1, interleukin-1; IL-6, interleukin-6; TNF-α, tumor necrosis factor-α. *Source: Arch Gen Psychiatry. July 1998;55:583. Copyright (1998), American Medical Association.*

TABLE 95–2

Activated Markers of Inflammation in Depression and Cardiovascular Disease

DEPRESSION	CARDIOVASCULAR DISEASE	ROLE IN INFLAMMATION
CRP[27–29]	CRP[30–32]	Amplifies inflammatory and procoagulant responses[33]
		Induces expression of cellular adhesion molecules, which mediates adhesion of leukocytes to the vascular endothelium[33]
		Induces monocyte expression of tissue factor[33]
IL-1β[34,35]	IL-1β[36]	Induces expression of cellular adhesion molecules, which mediates adhesion of leukocytes to the vascular endothelium[33]
		Augments MMP expression, which is involved in the degradation of the subendothelial basement membrane[37]
IL-6[28,29]	IL-6[36,38,39]	Principal procoagulant cytokine[33]
		Stimulates hepatic production of CRP and fibrinogen[40]
	IL-7[41]	Regulates T-cell homeostasis[42]
		Stimulates monocyte production of chemokines[41]
IL-8[34]	IL-8[36]	
Interferon-γ[43]	Interferon-γ[30]	Augments synthesis of TNF-α and IL-1[44]
TNF-α[28,34]	TNF-α[36]	Induces expression of cellular adhesion molecules, which mediates adhesion of leukocytes to the vascular endothelium[33]
		Augments MMP expression, which is involved in the degradation of the subendothelial basement membrane[37]
	Nuclear factor-κB[45]	Induces transcription of the VCAM-1 gene[45]
Fibrinogen[46]	Fibrinogen[40]	Key component of the coagulation cascade
	Soluble CD-40 ligand	Augments MMP expression, which is involved in the degradation of the subendothelial basement membrane[37]
	VCAM-1[47]	Mediates early adhesion of mononuclear leukocytes to arterial endothelium[37]

CRP, C-reactive protein; IL, interleukin; MMP, matrix metalloproteinases; TNF, tumor necrosis factor; VCAM, vascular cell adhesion molecule.

Depression, in otherwise medically healthy individuals, is associated with increased production of proinflammatory cytokines, other cytokines, and acute-phase reactants, including interleukin (IL)-1β, IL-2 IL-6, IL-8, interferon-γ (IFN-γ), tumor necrosis factor-α (TNF-α), monocyte chemotactic protein-1 (MCP-1), fibrinogen, and C-reactive protein (CRP).[27,28,34,43,46] There is also evidence that plasma concentrations of IL-1β and IL-6 correlate strongly with depression severity.[35,43]

In the multiple studies examining the relationship between CRP and depression, the evidence supports a definitive association. In an analysis of 4218 individuals older than 65 years of age and free of cardiovascular disease, investigators evaluated the presence of exhaustion and depressive symptoms with respect to levels of CRP, albumin, white blood cell count, various coagulation factors, and fibrinogen. Depressive symptomatology was associated with elevated markers of low-grade inflammation including CRP and fibrinogen.[46] This relationship held true after adjusting for some control variables (age, gender, race, height, weight, diabetes mellitus, smoking, and systolic blood pressure), but not others (grip strength, 15-feet walk time, and activity level). Douglas and colleagues also found that depression scores correlated positively with serum concentrations of CRP in active duty U.S. Army personnel undergoing routine physicals,[49] but not if adjusted for body mass index (BMI). Other investigators have obtained similar results linking BMI with depression and levels of CRP.

There are gender differences with respect to depression and elevated cytokine levels. Ford and colleagues studied 6914 young adults between the ages of 18 to 39 using data from the Third National Health and Nutrition Examination Survey.[27] After adjustment for numerous potential confounders there was a significant relationship between a lifetime history of major depression and elevated CRP levels in men, but not in women. This gender difference with respect to elevated CRP levels and depression is particularly interesting given that both men and women have a similar RR of CAD related to depression.[25] An earlier study by Danner and colleagues evaluated the same patient population as the Ford group with similar results,[50] suggesting that a sustained inflammatory response can result after a depressive episode.

Further supporting this notion of a depression-induced sustained inflammatory response is a study of 119 older adults, immediately before and 2 weeks after, an annual influenza vaccination.[51] Among all participants, those with more depressive symptoms at baseline had higher levels of IL-6 before vaccination and experienced a subsequent increase in IL-6 after vaccination. Those patients with fewer depressive symptoms had lower baseline levels of IL-6 and exhibited little change in IL-6 levels after vaccination.

Exogenous cytokine therapy has also been shown to be associated with the onset of behavioral changes including major depressive episodes. IL-2 and IFN-α are both used in the treatment of melanoma and hepatitis C. In individuals free of depression, cardiovascular illness, or other systemic inflammatory diseases, the administration of cytokine therapy has been shown to induce the cytokine network, causing subsequent elevations in serum levels of IFN-γ, IL-6, IL-8, and IL-10.[52,53] Furthermore, elevations in IL-6 and IL-8 correlate with symptoms of depression and anxiety.[52] When exposed to a stressor, medically healthy patients with current depression exhibit resistance to molecules that normally terminate the inflammatory cascade. This suggests that patients with depression may exhibit an impaired ability to regulate inflammation.

Despite the evidence implicating inflammation in the pathophysiology of both cardiovascular disease and depression, it remains controversial whether inflammation, and cytokines in particular, is a critical etiologic link between the two. The majority of studies have evaluated small numbers of subjects and yielded equivocal results.[54–58] However, the few larger studies investigating the immune response in patients with both CVD and depression were consistent.[59,60] One study using population-based surveys in Germany, revealed that in healthy men, a depressed mood increased the power of a concurrently elevated serum level of CRP to predict a subsequent MI.[60] In this study of 3021 subjects, a baseline CRP and assessment of depressive symptoms were obtained. Three groups were formed based on the initial CRP level: low risk, medium risk, and high risk based on recent American Heart Association/Centers for Disease Control (AHA/CDC) guidelines.[61] The prevalence of a depressed mood was equal among the groups. Subjects were followed for a median of 7.7 years, with a combined end point of either fatal or nonfatal MI. Patients with both high-risk levels of CRP and a depressed mood were found to have a hazard ratio of 2.69 compared to that of 1.55 in the group with elevated CRP alone.

In the Prospective Study of Myocardial Infarction (PRIME) study of healthy middle-aged men from France and Belfast there was an association between depressive mood and CAD, which persisted after adjusting for inflammatory markers.[59] This study compared 335 future cases of CAD to 670 matched controls. Subjects were followed for a minimum of 5 years. There was a statistically significant correlation, independent of social characteristics and classic cardiovascular risk factors, between depression scores and levels of IL-6, CRP and intercellular adhesion molecule-1 (ICAM-1), but not fibrinogen. Furthermore, men with depressed mood had a 50 percent increase in the odds ratio of CAD.

【 】 ENDOTHELIAL DYSFUNCTION

Vascular endothelial dysfunction is a known risk factor for the development and progression of atherosclerosis, hypertension, and CHF. It is defined as a diminished vasoactive, anticoagulant, and antiinflammatory status. Multiple prospective studies have confirmed that in patients with CVD, the presence of endothelial dysfunction is an independent predictor of cardiovascular events.[62] Furthermore, recent studies have demonstrated a significant relationship between impaired endothelial function and both untreated and treated depression.[63,64]

One of the most common modalities used in the assessment endothelial function is through measurement of brachial artery flow or flow-mediated dilation (FMD). Two small case-controlled studies comparing depressed patients without risk factors for CAD to age, gender, and risk-factor matched controls suggest that endothelial function, as determined by FMD, is abnormal in depressed pa-

tients.[63,64] Broadley and coworkers evaluated patients with treated depression who were without risk factors for CAD, stable on antidepressant therapy for a minimum of 3 months, and free of depressive symptoms. This cohort showed abnormal FMD despite remission of their depressive symptoms. Sherwood and colleagues[65] assessed endothelial function inpatients with documented CAD; brachial artery FMD revealed a significantly higher incidence of endothelial dysfunction in patients with depressive symptomatology. The use of antidepressant medication was associated with an improved FMD, although the duration of antidepressant use was not reported. Rybakowski and coworkers[66] evaluated endothelial function in controls and psychiatric patients during an acute depressive episode before and after treatment of their mood disorder. Arterial endothelial dysfunction was independent of the diagnosis (major depressive disorder [MDD] versus bipolar affective disorder [BPAD]), intensity of depression, and type of depression, suggesting that endothelial dysfunction can be a marker of mood disorders.

【 】 HYPOTHALAMIC-PITUITARY-ADRENOCORTICAL AND SYMPATHOMEDULLARY HYPERACTIVITY

Two primary components that are central to the *fight or flight* stress response are the HPA system and the sympathoadrenal system. In response to stress, hypothalamic neurons containing corticotropin-releasing factor (CRF) increase the synthesis and release of corticotropin (adrenocorticotropic hormone [ACTH]), β-endorphin, and other proopiomelanocortin (POMC) products from the anterior pituitary gland. Many studies have documented evidence of HPA system hyperactivity in medication-free patients with major depression: blunting of the ACTH response to CRF administration, nonsuppression of cortisol secretion after dexamethasone administration, hypercortisolemia, and pituitary and adrenal gland enlargement, and direct evidence of increased numbers of hypothalamic CRF neurons in postmortem brain tissue from depressed patients compared with controls.[67] Administered corticosteroids have long been known to induce hypercholesterolemia, hypertriglyceridemia, and hypertension. Other atherosclerosis-inducing actions of steroids include injury to vascular endothelial cells and intima and the inhibition of normal healing. Indeed, elevated morning plasma cortisol concentrations have been significantly correlated with moderate-to-severe coronary atherosclerosis in young and middle-aged men.

Many patients with major depression also exhibit dysregulation of the sympathoadrenal system, which consists of the adrenal medulla and sympathetic nervous system (SNS). Although CNS regulation of the sympathoadrenal system has been only partially characterized, hypothalamic CRF-containing neurons provide stimulatory input to several autonomic centers that are involved in regulating sympathetic activity. Nerve impulses from regulatory centers in the CNS control catecholamine release from the sympathoadrenal system. Physiologic and pathologic conditions causing sympathoadrenal activation include physical activity, coronary artery ischemia, heart failure, and mental stress. Epinephrine in plasma is derived from the adrenal medulla, whereas plasma norepinephrine (NE) concentrations reflect the secretion of NE largely from sympathetic nerve terminals, with the remaining NE provided by the adrenal medulla and extraadrenal chromaffin cells.

Peripheral plasma NE concentrations are determined not only by the rate of release from sympathetic nervous system nerve terminals but also by reuptake into presynaptic terminals, local metabolic degradation, and redistribution into multiple physiologic compartments. Hypersecretion of NE in unipolar depression has been documented by elevated plasma NE and NE metabolite concentrations[68] and elevated urinary concentrations of NE and its metabolites,[69,70] although discordant reports exist.[71] Not only do depressed patients exhibit higher basal plasma concentrations of NE, those with melancholia exhibit even greater elevations in plasma NE concentrations when subjected to orthostatic challenge than do normal control subjects and depressed patients *without* melancholia.[72] Furthermore, depressed patients who are dexamethasone (DST) nonsuppressors exhibit significantly higher basal and cold-stimulated plasma concentrations of NE than do depressed patients who are dexamethasone suppressors.[72] After treatment with tricyclic antidepressants (TCAs), urinary excretion of NE and its metabolites diminish together with plasma NE concentrations,[73] although Veith and colleagues[68] reported that chronic treatment with desipramine increased plasma concentrations of NE. Thus, sympathoadrenal hyperactivity seems to represent a state rather than a trait marker of depression, possibly reflecting increased CRF release within the CNS.

【 】 DIMINISHED HEART RATE VARIABILITY

Alterations in autonomic nervous system activity, as demonstrated by exaggerated responses in heart rate to orthostatic challenge[71] or reduction in heart rate variability (HRV), represent another mechanism of diminished survival of depressed patients with CVD. Beat-to-beat fluctuations in hemodynamic parameters reflect the dynamic response of cardiovascular control systems to a myriad of naturally occurring physiologic perturbations. Therefore, HRV can provide a sensitive measure of the functioning of the rapidly reacting sympathetic, parasympathetic, and renin-angiotensin systems.

HRV is often decreased in patients with severe CAD or heart failure.[74] Moreover, the risk of sudden death after an acute MI is significantly higher in patients with decreased HRV.[75] Although positive predictive accuracy is not high when HRV is considered alone, in combination with other prognostic factors, clinically useful levels of negative predictive accuracy can be achieved.[76]

Reduced high-frequency HRV has been observed in depressed patients in comparison with nondepressed groups,[77] although discrepant reports exist.[78] In patients with angiographically confirmed CAD, diminished HRV during 24-hour Holter monitoring was significantly more common in depressed patients than in matched nondepressed patients.[79] Diminished high-frequency HRV is thought to reflect decreased parasympathetic tone. Diminished HRV in patients with major depression can also be secondary to a deficiency of omega-3 fatty acids.[80] These polyunsaturated lipids possess antiarrhythmic properties and reduce the risk of ventricular arrhythmias.[81,82] Multiple studies have documented a deficiency of omega-3 fatty acids in patients with major depression.[83]

HRV is also reduced in patients with depression and comorbid CAD. In a comparison of 311 depressed with 367 nondepressed patients, all with recent acute MIs, patients with depression had reduced HRV and were at higher risk for all-cause mortality.[84] Studies have yet to show improvement of HRV after effective depression treatment, either after antidepressant or cognitive behavioral psychotherapy (CBT).[85]

【 】 ALTERATIONS IN PLATELET RECEPTORS AND REACTIVITY

The adverse effects of depression on cardiovascular disease have been posited to be mediated by platelet mechanisms.[86] Markovitz and Matthews[87] first proposed that enhanced platelet responses to psychological stress can trigger adverse coronary artery ischemic events. Musselman and coworkers, using fluorescence-activated flow cytometric analysis, found that in comparison to normal controls, young, medically healthy, depressed patients without any other risk factors for CAD exhibited enhanced baseline platelet activation as well as increased platelet responsiveness.[88] Moreover, in another study, depressed patients with one or more traditional risk factors for CAD exhibited, under basal conditions, increased number of circulating platelets that had proceeded to irreversible degranulation.[89]

Indeed patients suffering from comorbid CVD and major depression also exhibit increased platelet activation as measured by markedly elevated plasma concentrations of the platelet secretion products platelet factor 4 (PF4) and β-thromboglobulin (β-TG) compared with *non*depressed, age-matched patients with CVD.[90] Increased platelet activation has also been documented in CVD patients with the negative emotion, hostility, in comparison to healthy controls.[91] Although the mechanism or mechanisms responsible remain unknown, heightened susceptibility to platelet activation and secretion can contribute, at least in part, to the increased vulnerability of depressed patients to CVD and/or mortality after an MI.

Serotonin secreted by platelets induces both platelet aggregation and coronary vasoconstriction, both of which are mediated by 5-hydroxytryptamine (5-HT$_2$) receptors. Vasoconstriction occurs especially when normal endothelial cell counterregulatory mechanisms of vascular relaxation are defective, as often occurs in patients with CAD.[92] Indeed, essential hypertension, elevated plasma cholesterol levels, older age, and smoking, which are well-known predisposing factors for the development of CVD, all contribute to 5-HT-mediated platelet activation. Moreover, alterations in platelet 5-HT-mediated activation have also been described in affective disorders, including major depression. Alterations in both CNS and platelet serotonergic function occur in depressed patients.[93]

Serotonin-mediated platelet activation can contribute to the development of atherosclerosis, thrombosis, and vasoconstriction. Even though 5-HT is a weak platelet agonist, it markedly amplifies platelet reactions to a variety of other agonists such as adenosine diphosphate (ADP), thromboxane A$_2$, catecholamines, and thrombin. Several investigators have reported increases in platelet 5-HT$_2$ binding density in depressed patients.[94] Moreover, the changes appear to be state-dependent in that 5-HT$_2$-binding-site density returned to control values only in patients who showed clinical improvement. Depressed patients have been found to exhibit significant reductions in the number of platelet and brain 5-HT transporter sites. The increased 5-HT$_2$-receptor-binding density and decreased 5-HT-transporter sites suggest that depressed patients can be particularly susceptible to 5-HT-mediated platelet activation and coronary artery vasoconstriction. Decreased numbers of platelet 5-HT transporters would potentially hinder the uptake and storage of periplatelet serotonin, exposing the increased numbers of 5-HT$_2$ receptors to 5-HT.[95]

Platelets from depressed patients also exhibit significantly increased elevations of intracellular free calcium concentration, $[Ca^{2+}]_i$, after 5-HT-induced stimulation, in comparison to controls.[96] Small increases in intraplatelet calcium *prime* the platelet secretion and aggregation response to stimulation by 5-HT or in response to increased blood flow. Thus, platelets with elevated $[Ca^{2+}]_i$, as are observed in depressed patients, probably would exhibit increased activation in comparison with normal comparison subjects under basal conditions or in response to shear-induced aggregation (e.g., after an orthostatic challenge). More recently, antidepressants that inhibit the reuptake of serotonin into neurons (and platelets) have been shown to normalize the abnormally heightened platelet activation and secretion observed in patients with depression, without[89] and with CVD.[97]

[ ] MYOCARDIAL ISCHEMIA AND VENTRICULAR INSTABILITY IN REACTION TO MENTAL STRESS AND DEPRESSION

The combination of a vulnerable myocardium after MI, acute ischemia, and negative emotional arousal has long been thought to trigger fatal ventricular arrhythmias. Jiang and colleagues[98] followed 126 patients with CAD over a 5-year period. Mental stress-induced myocardial ischemia at baseline in CAD patients was associated with significantly higher rates of subsequent fatal and nonfatal cardiac events independently of age, baseline left ventricular ejection fraction (LVEF), and previous MI. They proposed that the relation between psychological stress and adverse cardiac events is mediated by myocardial ischemia. Although myocardial ischemia is probably the most significant factor predisposing to ventricular instability, other factors also contribute. Psychological stress in humans with CAD increases ventricular ectopic activity and increases the risk of ventricular fibrillation.[99] There are several similarities between the stress response and major depression: both can be characterized by increased blood pressure and heart rate as well as increased arousal and increased mobilization of energy stores. Particularly relevant to both the stress response and depression are the critical brain structures—the locus ceruleus and the central nucleus of the amygdala—both innervated by CRF-containing cell bodies or nerve terminals.[100] The stress response and major depression differ in some respects, however. In depression, some aspects of the normal stress response escalate to a pathologic state that fails to respond appropriately to usual counterregulatory responses, resulting in a sustained version of a usually transient phenomenon (i.e., hyperactivity of the HPA system or the sympathoadrenal system). Although many studies have linked stressful life events to the onset of major depression,[101] some depressions are clearly *endogenous* (i.e., they have no obvious environmental precipitant).

Frasure-Smith and colleagues[14] proposed that depression worsens the prognosis after an MI through another mechanism: premature ventricular contractions (PVCs). Though the frequency of arrhythmias in depressed and nondepressed patients with CAD was similar, depressed patients with 10 or more PVCs per hour were at higher risk for sudden cardiac death than their nondepressed counterparts. Patients who were not depressed experienced lit-

tle increase in risk associated with PVCs even in the presence of a low LVEF.[14] Thus, the prognostic impact of PVCs can be related more to depression than to PVCs per se. In the Cardiac Arrhythmia Suppression Trial (CAST),[102] suppression of PVC frequency in post-MI patients did not reduce and actually increased mortality (even though PVCs are associated with increased mortality after an MI). Thus, treatment of depression can be necessary to improve survival in depressed patients with PVCs.

Another electrocardiographic abnormality observed in patients with depression, as well as panic disorder, is increased QT variability. Multiple studies have shown that increased QT variability in patients with CVD is predictive of arrhythmic events and sudden cardiac death.[103] Increased QT intervals have been observed in medically healthy individuals with depression[104] as well as depressed patients post-MI.[105] Carney and colleagues[105] compared QT intervals between two groups within 28 days of an acute MI. One group's participants met criteria for either major or minor depression, whereas the other group only included patients free of depressive symptoms. The QT interval variability was consistently higher at each of the eight sampling times over a 24-hour period in the depressed group; however the differences were significant only at midnight and 6:00 AM. Given the circadian variability of sudden cardiac death (with a peak incidence in the early morning hours) there can be a greater susceptibility to arrhythmias and sudden death in depressed, post-MI patients in the early morning.

ANXIETY DISORDERS AND CARDIOVASCULAR DISEASE

[ ] EPIDEMIOLOGY

Anxiety disorders are the most prevalent psychiatric disorders in the United States (Tables 95–3 and 95–4), but remain largely undiagnosed and undertreated.[107] A survey of adult primary care patients (n = 637) enrolled in a health maintenance organization revealed that 10 percent had untreated anxiety disorders.[108] Stereotyped as the "worried well," patients with anxiety disorders have substantially higher rates of health service use, increased social and role disability, diminished quality of life, and poor health outcomes.[108,109] Moreover, the comorbidity of anxiety and affec-

TABLE 95–3

12-Month Prevalence of DSM-III-R Disorders in the National Comorbidity Survey (NCS)[106]

DISORDER	PERCENT
Any anxiety disorder	19.3
Any addictive disorder	11.3
Any mood disorder	11.3
Nonaffective psychosis	0.3
Any NCS disorder	30.9

DSM-III-R, Diagnostic and Statistical manual of Mental Disorders. 3rd ed, revised; NCS, National Comorbidity Survey.
Source: Kessler, McGonagle, Zhao, et al.[96]

tive disorders is substantial. Sixty percent of patients with major depression in both the National Comorbidity Survey and the NCS-R suffered with a comorbid anxiety disorder,[4,106] and they experienced greater emotional disability and social dysfunction in comparison to patients with either condition alone.[108]

The prevalence of anxiety disorders in patients with CVD has been largely understudied, with most studies focusing on patients with mitral valve prolapse or individuals referred for evaluation of chest pain. Substantial numbers of patients each year undergo coronary angiography because of chest pain, yet are found to have normal coronary arteries. These patients are subsequently categorized as having "atypical chest pain," and often experience chest pain in response to anxiety and/or hyperventilation. In a study evaluating patients 1 year after elective catheterization, the physical disability of patients with CAD was associated with the severity of these patients' anxiety and depressive symptoms at catheterization, not with the number of main coronary vessels stenosed.[107]

A large, multi-city survey of 875 primary care outpatients revealed that patients with CHF or MI exhibited a point prevalence rate of at least one anxiety disorder (panic disorder, phobia, or generalized anxiety disorder) of 18 percent.[109] Whether the prevalence of anxiety disorders is elevated in patients who are hospitalized for CAD (e.g., elective coronary catheterization, post-MI, or unstable angina) remains to be determined.

A small number of prospective epidemiologic studies (which control for many of the commonly accepted risk factors for CAD) indicate an increased RR of nonfatal and fatal CVD events in patients with anxiety symptoms, even among those individuals who have *simple* phobias such as claustrophobia and fear of illness, heights, crowds, or going out alone.[110–112] A graded response relationship has been demonstrated in these studies, with minimal symptoms of anxiety sufficient to elevate risk, suggesting that nonclinical, or *normal* levels of anxiety can play some role in the development of CAD.[113] Moreover, an ancillary study of 348 CAST and CAST II participants who had asymptomatic ventricular arrhythmias after MI, revealed that

TABLE 95–4

Diagnostic Criteria of the Most Common DSM-IV Anxiety Disorders

DSM-IV CRITERIA OF SIMPLE PHOBIA

Marked and persistent fear that is excessive or unreasonable, cued by the presence or anticipation of a specific object or situation (e.g., flying, heights, animals, receiving an injection, seeing blood).

Exposure to the phobic stimulus almost invariably provokes an immediate anxiety response, which can take the form of a situationally bound or situationally predisposed panic attack.

The person (adults only) recognizes that the feature is excessive or unreasonable.

The phobic situation is avoided or else is endured with intense anxiety or distress.

The avoidance, anxious anticipation, or distress in the feared situations interferes significantly with the person's normal routine, occupational (or academic) functioning, or social activities or relationships.

Or there is marked distress about having the phobia.

DSM-IV DIAGNOSTIC CRITERIA OF SOCIAL PHOBIA

Marked fear of being focus of attention; avoidance of meeting unfamiliar people and close scrutiny by others.

Fear of behaving in embarrassing or humiliating way.

Extreme anticipatory anxiety, which can manifest itself as a panic attack.

DSM-IV DIAGNOSTIC CRITERIA OF POSTTRAUMATIC STRESS DISORDER

Experience of a traumatic event.

Reexperienced by intrusive and distressing recollection, dreams, flashbacks, distress in similar situations.

Persistent avoidance of stimuli associated with trauma.

Persistent symptoms of increased arousal.

Duration of disturbance of at least 1 month.

DSM-IV DIAGNOSTIC CRITERIA OF PANIC DISORDER

Recurrent and unexpected panic attacks.

Plus one or more of the following:
- Persistent concern about having additional attacks (anticipatory anxiety) or
- Worry about the consequences of the attacks or
- A significant change in behavior related to the attacks (phobic avoidance)

Not caused by a substance, medical condition, or mental illness.

At least two unexpected panic attacks for diagnosis.

DEFINITION OF PANIC ATTACK

A period of intense fear or discomfort in which at least four of the following symptoms develop suddenly:
- Palpitations or increased heart rate
- Sweating
- Trembling or shaking
- Sensations of shortness of breath or smothering
- Feeling of choking
- Nausea or abdominal distress
- Chest pain or discomfort
- Dizziness, light-headedness, or faintness
- Derealization or depersonalization
- Fear of losing control or going crazy
- Chills or hot flashes
- Paresthesia (numbness or tingling)
- Fear of dying

TABLE 95–4

Diagnostic Criteria of the Most Common DSM-IV Anxiety Disorders *(continued)*

DSM-IV CRITERIA OF GENERALIZED ANXIETY DISORDER

Excessive anxiety and worry for more days than not for past 6 months.
Difficulty controlling worry.
Functional impairment and/or distress.
Symptoms not attributable to other causes.

Physical symptoms
- Restlessness or feeling keyed up/on edge
- Fatigue
- Muscle tension

Psychological symptoms
- Excessive anxiety or worry
- Difficulty controlling worry
- Irritability
- Difficulty concentrating or mind going blank
- Sleep disturbance

SOURCE: *American Psychiatric Association.*[3]

---

higher levels of anxiety and stressful life events during the initial 4 months of study participation were predictive of mortality (independent of variables such as diabetes and ejection fraction).[114]

PATHOPHYSIOLOGY OF ANXIETY

The neurocircuitry of anxiety has been postulated to arise from the amygdala, the brain area that registers the emotional significance of environmental stimuli and stores emotional memories. The efferent pathways from the central nucleus of the amygdala travel to a multitude of critical brain structures, including the parabrachial nucleus (resulting in dyspnea and hyperventilation), the dorsomedial nucleus of the vagus nerve and nucleus ambiguous (activating the parasympathetic nervous system), and the lateral hypothalamus (resulting in SNS activation).[115] Through reciprocal neuronal pathways connecting the amygdala to the medial prefrontal cortex, cognitive experience of the specific anxiety disorder differs, although fear symptoms can overlap. During panic attacks, the fear is of imminent death; in social phobia, the fear is of embarrassment; in posttraumatic stress disorder, the traumatic memory is remembered or reexperienced; in obsessive-compulsive disorder, obsessional ideas recur and intrude; and in generalized anxiety disorder, anxiety is *free-floating* (i.e., not conditioned to specific situations or triggers).[116]

Described in the past with terms such as *cardiac neurosis, irritable heart syndrome, battle fatigue,* and *soldier's heart;* panic disorder is the anxiety disorder most often associated with cardiovascular symptoms of chest pain, tachycardia, and dyspnea. Discrete panic attacks can be induced in the laboratory setting, especially in patients with panic disorder, by a variety of stimuli: sodium lactate, caffeine, isoproterenol, serotonin receptor agonist m-chlorophenylpiperazine (m-CPP), cholecystokinin tetrapeptide (CCK-4), inhalation of CO_2-enriched air, and voluntary acute hyperventilation of room air. The common element among these disparate inducers can be their ability to stimulate the respiratory rate with the induction of an accompanying subjective sense of breathlessness.[117] Although some researchers have proposed that patients with panic disorder have only a heightened sensitivity to and develop a learned intolerance of tachypnea,[118] the higher concordance rate of panic disorder observed in monozygotic as compared with dizygotic twins[119] and evidence of altered respiratory rhythm during sleep[120] provide proof of a genetic diathesis and a biological abnormality, respectively, underlying the phenotype of panic disorder.[120]

[ ] A FOCUS ON THE CARDIOVASCULAR SYSTEM

Although the neurobiology of specific anxiety disorders has not been explored as fully as that of unipolar depression, potential neurochemical, neuroendocrine, and neuroanatomic alterations have been identified. Patients with major depression or anxiety disorders can experience common symptoms such as alterations in psychomotor activity, impairment of sleep, increased appetite, and reduced concentration. Moreover, there are several shared neurobiologic findings between patients with certain common syndromal anxiety disorders and those with depression, although differences also exist.

Although limited and inconsistent evidence suggests that alterations of HPA system activity occur across the anxiety disorder spectrum,[121,122] altered HPA system activity has been most consistently documented in individuals with posttraumatic stress disorder (PTSD). In nearly all controlled studies of PTSD, alterations of HPA system hyperactivity have been documented, including elevations of cerebrospinal fluid (CSF)-CRF concentrations[123] and blunting of the ACTH response to CRF stimulation.[124] In comparison to control subjects, however, PTSD patients generally exhibit reduced plasma cortisol concentrations, diminished 24-hour urinary cortisol concentrations, and a greater suppression of plasma cortisol concentrations in response to low doses (e.g., 0.5 mg) of dexamethasone.[124,125] However the two studies that measured CSF-CRF concentrations in PTSD[123,126] found elevated CSF-CRF concentrations identical to those repeatedly reported in depression. Whether patients with PTSD experience an increased (or decreased) RR of CVD is not known, in part because of the confounding prevalence of substance abuse, alcoholism, and tobacco abuse in PTSD patients. Patients with panic disorder do not appear to exhibit alterations in HPA system function consistently; few data are available for patients with social phobia, generalized anxiety disorder, and obsessive-compulsive disorder.

Sympathomedullary function has been investigated intensively in patients with panic disorder. SNS activity is similar under basal conditions in panic patients and control subjects[127] and increases to a similar degree in both groups under laboratory mental stress.[127] Panic patients do, however, exhibit significantly higher cardiac-derived epinephrine (EPI) under basal conditions, increased whole-body EPI secretion during laboratory mental stress, and surges of EPI during panic attacks. Such increases in EPI in panic patients presumably are due to "loading" of sympathetic neuronal stores by uptake from plasma during surges of EPI secretion during panic attacks.[127] Further investigation of cardiac and/ or systemic sympathomedullary activation during spontaneous or pharmacologically provoked panic attacks is needed to confirm these findings, along with prospective investigations of the cardiac-related risk of patients with panic disorder. However, multiple prospective cohort studies (which control for other accepted risk factors for CAD) report that increasing severity of anxiety is associated with an increased risk for developing elevated systolic blood pressure or hypertension.[128] Given the comorbidity between anxiety and depressive symptoms and syndromes, further studies are required to determine whether the evidence of increased risk for the development of CAD (or hypertension) in anxiety disorder patients is independent of the contribution of depression.[113]

In contrast to major depression, alterations of platelet 5-HT transporters and platelet 5-HT$_2$ receptors have not been detected in patients with panic disorder. However, like those with depression, patients with panic disorder have been shown to exhibit increased plasma concentrations of PF4 and β-TG, thus providing evidence of increased platelet secretion. Moreover, after treatment with alprazolam, plasma concentrations of these α granule-specific proteins were reduced significantly.[129] The presence of anxiety disorders has been hypothesized to trigger coronary events through atherosclerotic plaque rupture, coronary vasospasm, ventricular arrhythmias, or atrial arrhythmias.[113] Panic-induced hyperventilation is a well-known precipitant of coronary spasm,[130] which in turn can induce ventricular arrhythmias and MI.

Emergency room physicians and cardiologists are well acquainted with the challenges of evaluating patients with an acute onset of chest discomfort, combined with painful and overwhelming anxiety symptoms, which may or may not be associated with clinically significant cardiovascular disease (Table 95–5). The most compelling evidence regarding the association of anxiety disorders and cardiovascular dysfunction comes from reports of abnormal

cardiac autonomic control.[113] Examination of HRV in patients with anxiety disorders has revealed that patients with panic disorder[131] and patients with generalized anxiety disorder[132] exhibit reductions in high-frequency HRV.[133] Diminished HRV increases the risk of arrhythmias and sudden cardiac death. Indeed, patients with panic disorder or agoraphobia exhibit a higher density of PVCs in comparison to patients with other anxiety disorders[134] and normal comparison subjects.[135] Whether patients with panic disorder (or other anxiety disorders) exhibit increased rates of sudden cardiac death remains to be determined.

Although so-called *mental disorders* can produce effects on cardiovascular function, perhaps less well understood are the cardiovascular contributions to certain anxiety disorders. Whether cardiovascular abnormalities or dysfunction reliably produce symptoms of anxiety is an intriguing area of investigation. In comparison to gender- and age-matched controls, individuals with cardiac arrhythmias exhibited significantly higher self-reported anxiety scores.[136] Whether a causal biological mechanism exists between PVCs and anxiety symptoms or disorders is unknown.[137]

❴ ❵ TREATMENT OF MAJOR DEPRESSION AND ANXIETY DISORDERS IN PATIENTS WITH CARDIOVASCULAR DISEASE

Effective treatment of major psychiatric illnesses such as major depression and panic disorder requires patient access to informed healthcare practitioners, accurate diagnosis, and affordable, safe, and effective treatments. Factors hampering psychiatric treatment include patient reluctance, social stigma, managed care restrictions, and a dearth of psychiatrists and psychologists, particularly in rural areas. Although the safety and efficacy of anxiolytic and antidepressant treatment in patients with cardiovascular disease have not been extensively established in randomized clinical trials, these agents are prescribed routinely to patients with heart disease. This seems appropriate given the drastic reduction in psychosocial function associated with anxiety or depressive disorders, the safety and efficacy of these psychotropic agents in generally healthy populations, and existing data from psychopharmacologic treatment of medically ill patients.

Many cardiac patients believe that their persistent "worry," "lack of enjoyment of life," or "loss of interest" constitutes an understandable yet untreatable condition. However, given the prevalence of major depression in patients with heart disease, the astute clinician's index of suspicion should be high. Third-party information (particularly from a spouse or other caregiver) is often more revealing of the true extent of a patient's symptoms, including attempts to "self-medicate" through abuse of alcohol, prescription medication, or illicit substances. A thorough evaluation of anxiety, panic attacks (if any), and depressive symptoms should be performed, including queries regarding feelings of pessimism, hopelessness, and the wish not to continue living. Although patients' preferences should be respected, cardiac patients and their families should always be informed of the risks of untreated depression and the options of psychotherapeutic and/or psychopharmacologic treatment. Consultation with a knowledgeable mental health provider can assist in the discrimination of depressive disorders from complicated or pathologic grief, delirium, coexisting anxiety disorders, intoxication or withdrawal syndromes, and appropriate emotional reactions.

▌ TABLE 95–5

Medical Conditions Associated with Anxiety Symptoms

- Cardiovascular disorders: mitral valve prolapse, coronary artery disease, paroxysmal tachycardia, hypertension, hypotension
- Endocrinopathies: hyperthyroidism, hypothyroidism, diabetes, hypoglycemia, hypocalcemia, porphyria, endocrine tumors
- Neurologic disorders: migraine headaches, transient ischemic attacks, temporal lobe seizures
- Pulmonary disease: asthma, chronic obstructive pulmonary disease, pulmonary embolus
- Vestibular dysfunction: Ménière's disease
- Infectious diseases: tuberculosis, brucellosis, human immunodeficiency virus or acquired immunodeficiency syndrome
- Drug effects: cocaine abuse, alcohol or sedative withdrawal, sympathomimetics, caffeine, monosodium glutamate, akathisia

The efficacy and safety of psychotherapeutic and psychopharmacologic treatment of major depression or any of the anxiety disorders in post-MI patients is being investigated intensively. In two large-scale, randomized, multicenter studies, the Montreal Heart Attack Readjustment Trial (M-HART)[138] and the Enhancing Recovering in Coronary Heart Disease (ENRICHD) Patients Study,[139] psychosocial interventions were not superior to routine care in reducing cardiac events or prolonging survival. Whereas the individual and group CBT of ENRICHD was effective in reducing depressive symptoms and improving social support, patients receiving home-based telephone monitoring and psychosocial nursing intervention of M-HART showed no improvement in either domain.[138] Older, smaller studies have reported successful psychological interventions with post-MI patients[140] targeted primarily to diminish "psychological distress"[141] or alter type A personality traits.[142]

Since the introduction of fluoxetine and citalopram, more than a decade of clinical information has been gleaned regarding the selective serotonin reuptake inhibitor (SSRI) class of antidepressants. Furthermore, during the 1990s, the SSRIs superseded the benzodiazepines as the first-line treatment of choice for anxiety disorders.[143] These newer agents provide significant reduction of anxiety symptoms in approximately 60 percent of medically healthy patients without having a potential for addiction. SSRIs have been approved by the U.S. Food and Drug Agency (FDA) for the treatment of panic disorder, social anxiety disorder, obsessive-compulsive disorder, and generalized anxiety disorder (Table 95–6). It is important to note that although all SSRIs are potent 5-HT reuptake inhibitors, they also exert unique effects on other neurotransmitter systems. Notably, paroxetine is a very potent inhibitor of NE reuptake in vitro, whereas sertraline is a potent inhibitor of dopamine (DA) reuptake. The clinical sequelae of these pharmacologic properties remain obscure.

During the time (often 6 to 8 weeks) before the onset of an antidepressant's anxiolytic effect, benzodiazepines such as lorazepam, alprazolam, and clonazepam can be used. These agents are rapidly effective but should be used only for short-term treatment (6- to 8-week duration) of disabling anxiety symptoms. Benzodiazepines are sedating, produce gait instability, impair memory, can induce behavioral disinhibition, are ineffective in the treatment of coexisting depressive syndromes, and place patients at risk of physiologic and psychologic dependence.

The use of tricyclic and structurally related antidepressants should be limited in patients with CVD because of the myriad of side effects of these drugs on the cardiovascular system, including orthostatic hypotension, tachycardia, reduction in HRV, and slowing of intraventricular conduction. These antidepressants should never be prescribed for patients with bifascicular and left fascicular block.[152] Examination of prescription databases has revealed an increased risk of MI with administration of TCAs in comparison to SSRIs and atypical antidepressants.[153,154] Monoamine oxidase inhibitors and trazodone are generally free of effects on cardiac conduction but, like the TCAs, can cause postural hypotension.[155] Because of their fewer potential adverse effects on the cardiovascular system and the lack of lethality from an overdose, pharmacotherapeutic treatment with SSRIs or other atypical antidepressants such as bupropion, nefazodone, and mirtazapine can offer significant advantages in depressed or anxious patients with CVD.

Recent evidence suggests that venlafaxine and other serotonin-norepinephrine reuptake inhibitors (SNRIs) such as duloxetine and milnacipran should be avoided in cardiovascular patients. Several investigators[156] have noted severe cardiovascular sequelae after venlafaxine overdose, and Oslin and coworkers[157] reported an unacceptably high rate of cardiac arrhythmia in elderly patients treated with venlafaxine. Like TCAs, venlafaxine has also been shown to decrease heart rate variability, the degree of which correlates with the magnitude of norepinephrine transporter inhibition.[158] Finally, several studies[159] placed venlafaxine in a separate class with respect to toxicity in overdose, safer than TCAs, but less safe than SSRIs. This has now been confirmed in a recent study in Finland.[160] These data, taken together, led the FDA to recently change the package insert for venlafaxine, warning about the observed adverse events including tachycardia, hypotension, angina pectoris, arrhythmia, extrasystoles, and MI (rare).

The only known negative cardiac effect of SSRIs is severe sinus node slowing, which to date has been reported in only a few cases.[161] There are case reports of altered hemostasis[162] with SSRI treatment. Clinical studies have also indicated that SSRIs reduce platelet activation in patients with major depression, without[88,163] and with,[97] CAD. Although potentially advantageous in patients with heightened platelet activation such as smokers,[164] retrospective examinations of large-scale medication databases revealed no such cardioprotective effect.[165] Recently however, Serebruany and colleagues conducted a randomized, double-blind study in a group of depressed patients, identified during hospitalization for acute coronary syndromes (unstable angina or acute MI).[166] Patients were treated with sertraline or placebo with measurement of platelet/endothelial biomarkers at baseline, 6 weeks, and 16 weeks. Treatment with sertraline was associated with reductions in platelet/endothelial activation. This association held true despite concurrent treatment with other antiplatelet regimens including aspirin and clopidogrel. Thus, the antiplatelet and endothelium protective properties of SSRIs can provide an additional clinical advantage for the treatment of depression in patients with comorbid CVD.

Because of inhibition of some cytochrome P450 isoenzymes, certain SSRIs can alter the metabolism of medications often used in patients with heart disease. SSRIs that inhibit the P450 2D6 isoenzyme (fluoxetine, paroxetine, fluvoxamine, and higher doses of sertraline) should be used with caution in patients receiving medications metabolized by the same pathway, such as lipophilic β blockers and type 1C antiarrhythmics: flecainide, mexiletine, propafenone. SSRIs that inhibit the P450 3A4 isoenzyme (fluoxetine, fluvoxamine, nefazodone) can increase plasma concentrations of calcium channel blockers and warfarin.[167] Although the antidepressants citalopram and mirtazapine exhibit minimal hepatic P450 enzyme inhibition, their safety remains to be established in patients with CVD who have comorbid depression or anxiety disorders.

After short-term treatment with buproprion,[149] fluoxetine,[168] paroxetine, fluvoxamine,[78] or paroxetine,[147] depressed patients exhibit no changes in HRV. A randomized, double-blind, multicenter study compared the efficacy of nortriptyline and paroxetine in depressed patients with CAD.[147] Both antidepressants were effective in the treatment of depression, however there were more dropouts because of general and cardiac-related effects with the TCA. The Sertraline Antidepressant Heart Attack Randomized Trial (SADHART), a

TABLE 95-6

Cardiac-Related Side Effects of Psychotropic Agents Commonly Used for Treatment of Anxiety and Depression

CLASS	CARDIOVASCULAR SIDE EFFECTS	LIKELY MECHANISM OF SIDE EFFECT	OTHER EFFECTS AND BENEFITS
Tricyclic and related cyclic antidepressants			
Nortriptyline (Pamelor)	Orthostatic hypotension	Postsynaptic α_1-receptor blockade	Nortriptyline with lowest incidence of orthostatic hypotension[144,145]
Imipramine (Tofranil)			
Amitriptyline (Elavil)	Tachycardia	Secondary to hypotension	Urinary retention, dry mouth, constipation, confusion, exacerbation of narrow-angle glaucoma
Desipramine (Norpramin)			
Clomipramine (Anafranil)			
Doxepin (Sinequan)	Decreased heart rate variability	Postsynaptic cholinergic-receptor blockade	
Trimipramine (Surmontil)			
Protriptyline (Vivactil)	Slowing of intraventricular conduction	Quinidine-like effects	Avoid in patients with bifascicular block, left bundle-branch block, QTc >44 msec, or QRS >11 msec
Monoamine oxidase inhibitors			
Phenelzine (Nardil)	Orthostatic hypotension	Inhibition of metabolism of serotonin and catecholamines	Fatal in overdose
Tranylcypromine (Parnate)	Hypertensive crisis		Requires adherence to tyramine-free diet, and avoidance of other antidepressants, and sympathomimetics
Isocarboxazid (Marplan)			
SSRIs		Postsynaptic serotonin-receptor blockade	Fatal in overdose
			Typical SSRI side effects: nausea, insomnia, sexual dysfunction, nervousness
Fluoxetine (Prozac)	Sinus bradycardia[146]	Unknown	Requires 8 weeks for complete washout
			Inhibitor of CYP IID6 and CYP IIIA4 enzymes
			Also FDA-approved for treatment of adult and pediatric OCD, bulimia, pediatric depression
Paroxetine (Paxil)	Clinically insignificant decreases in heart rate[147]	Unknown	Inhibitor of CYP IID6 enzyme
			Also FDA-approved for treatment of social phobia, panic disorder, OCD, GAD
Sertraline (Zoloft)	None known		In high doses, inhibitor of CYP IID6 enzyme
			Also FDA-approved for treatment of panic disorder, adult and pediatric OCD, PTSD
Fluvoxamine (Luvox)	None known		Potent inhibitor of multiple CYP enzymes
			Also FDA-approved for treatment of adult and pediatric OCD
Citalopram (Celexa)	None known		

Drug	Mechanism	Cardiovascular effects	Comments
Escitalopram (Lexapro)	Unknown	None known	SSRI with most selective binding to serotonin transporter; No significant inhibition of CYP enzymes
Venlafaxine (Effexor)	Presynaptic inhibition of norepinephrine reuptake	Arrhythmia or cardiac block in overdose[148]; Decreased HRV; Increased diastolic blood pressure in doses >300 mg/d[143]	Also FDA-approved for treatment of GAD; Side-effect profile similar to SSRIs
Presynaptic α_2-receptor antagonist			
Mirtazapine (Remeron)	Postsynaptic histamine$_1$-receptor blockade	None known	Very sedating in low doses; Weight gain; Minimal sexual side effects; No significant inhibition of CYP enzymes
Dopamine and norepinephrine reuptake inhibitor			
Bupropion (Wellbutrin, Zyban)	Presynaptic inhibition of norepinephrine reuptake	Significant increases in blood pressure in patients with preexisting hypertension (rare)[149]	No significant inhibition of CYP enzymes; Minimal sexual side effects; Not proven effective in the treatment of anxiety disorders; FDA-approved for treatment of nicotine dependence
Atypical serotonergic agents			
Trazodone (Desyrel)	Postsynaptic α_1-receptor blockade	Orthostatic hypotension; Cardiac arrhythmias rare[150]; Sinus bradycardia[151]	Sedation, confusion, dizziness; Rare cases of priapism
Nefazodone (Serzone)	Unknown; Unknown		Similar side-effect profile as trazodone (except without priapism); Minimal sexual side effects; Potent inhibitor of multiple CYP enzymes; Liver failure rare
Psychostimulants			
Dextroamphetamine (Dexedrine)	Release of dopamine and catecholamines	Rarely increases blood pressure or induces tachycardia in therapeutic doses	Avoid in patients with hyperthyroidism, severe hypertension, severe angina, tachyarrhythmias
Methylphenidate (Ritalin)			
Benzodiazepines			
Alprazolam (Xanax); Clonazepam (Klonopin)	Allosteric alteration of GABA$_A$ receptors		Rapid relief of anxiety symptoms
Lorazepam (Ativan)	Muscle relaxation of GABA$_A$ spinal cord receptors	Hypotension	Can cause fatigue, ataxia, drowsiness, amnesia, and behavioral dyscontrol; Relatively safe in overdose; Physiologic and psychologic dependence and withdrawal symptoms if dosage not gradually tapered
Oxazepam (Serax)			

(continued)

TABLE 95-6

Cardiac-Related Side Effects of Psychotropic Agents Commonly Used for Treatment of Anxiety and Depression   (continued)

CLASS	CARDIOVASCULAR SIDE EFFECTS	LIKELY MECHANISM OF SIDE EFFECT	OTHER EFFECTS AND BENEFITS
Partial 5-HT$_{1A}$-receptor agonist Buspirone (BuSpar)	None known		FDA-approved for treatment of GAD Nonaddictive
Omega1-receptor agonist Zolpidem (Ambien)	None known	Potentiation of GABA$_A$ receptor	Sedating Nonaddictive
Zaleplon (Sonata)	None known		
Lithium	Sinus node dysfunction Sinoatrial block T-wave inversion or flattening, particularly in patients >60 years of age Arrhythmias and sudden death in patients with cardiac disease	Unknown	Narrow therapeutic index (.6–1.2 mmol/L) Many medications alter lithium plasma levels[a] Fatal in overdose Mood stabilizer for patients with bipolar disorder Yearly ECG in patients older than 50 years of age

CYP, cytochrome P450 enzyme; FDA, Food and Drug Administration; GABA, gamma-aminobutyric acid; GAD, generalized anxiety disorder; HRV, heart rate variability; OCD, obsessive-compulsive disorder; PTSD, posttraumatic stress disorder; SSRI, selective serotonin reuptake inhibitor.

[a]Medications that increase lithium levels: nonsteroidal antiinflammatory drugs, diuretics (thiazides, ethacrynic acid, spironolactone, triamterene), angiotensin converting enzyme inhibitors, metronidazole, tetracycline. Medications that decrease lithium levels: acetazolamide, theophylline, aminophylline, caffeine, osmotic diuretics.[148]

randomized, multicenter, double-blind placebo controlled trial, evaluated the safety and efficacy of sertraline in the treatment of patients hospitalized for unstable angina or MI. Sertraline exerted no significant effect on LVEF, PVCs, QT interval, or other cardiac parameters. Depressed individuals with at least one prior episode of depression exhibited a significant improvement in symptoms on sertraline. The SADHART sertraline efficacy data are generally congruent with efficacy of other oral antidepressants in medically healthy patients with major depression. That is, any of the available oral antidepressants will usually produce a therapeutic response (defined as an improvement in depressive symptoms by 50 percent or more) in 60 to 70 percent of depressed patients, provided the antidepressant is administered in sufficient dosage over a treatment duration of 5 to 6 weeks.[169] Although there is limited, case-control evidence suggesting a role for SSRIs in decreasing the likelihood of MI in smokers,[164] there are as yet no prospective, randomized, controlled trials demonstrating that treatment with SSRIs diminishes future cardiac morbidity or mortality.

Electroconvulsive therapy (ECT), is effective in up to 80 percent of patients with either unipolar or bipolar depression.[170] ECT has several advantages over medication management of depression. The response time for ECT is 1 to 3 weeks compared to the 4 to 8 weeks needed for antidepressants, and ECT is clearly the most effective treatment for depression. The most recent trial of ECT in middle-aged and older adults with severe treatment-resistant depression found that more than 80 percent had complete remission of their depressive symptoms,[171] whereas treatment with antidepressants would be expected to have a remission rate of no better than 30 to 40 percent.

ECT is the treatment of choice in depressed patients who are severely ill and require a rapid clinical response. ECT also should be considered for patients who have experienced a previous positive response to ECT, do not respond to oral antidepressants, or cannot tolerate the associated side effects of antidepressants. Patient variables associated with a positive response include increasing age[171] and the presence of psychotic and catatonic symptoms.[170]

The morbidity and mortality associated with ECT have decreased dramatically over the past 60 years. The use of short-acting paralytic agents has made orthopedic complications rare. Complications related to cognitive dysfunction, such as delirium and amnesia, also have been decreased through the use of brief pulse- and unilateral ECT.

ECT produces a seizure by providing a brief pulse (approximately 1 to 2 seconds in duration) of electrical charge over the scalp in either the area of the right parietal lobe or over both temples. This pulse elicits a generalized seizure that lasts approximately 30 to 60 seconds. The patient is anesthetized during the procedure with a short-acting barbiturate, propofol or etomidate, and paralyzed with a muscle relaxant such as succinylcholine. Respirations are controlled by masked ventilation, and intubation is not required unless there have been recurrent episodes of aspiration.

Structural brain studies using magnetic resonance imaging have shown no evidence of brain damage from ECT.[172] Patients typically do experience transient amnesia. Memory loss is increased with the use of bilateral rather than unilateral ECT and is directly correlated with the number of treatments administered and higher stimulus intensity.[173] Evidence for amnesia should be monitored carefully during ECT as some patients can experience permanent retrograde memory loss.[174] More commonly however, anterograde and retrograde memory problems occur in a temporal gradient around the time of ECT and clear completely within 6 months of the ECT treatment period.

ECT-related delirium is relatively rare, but the risk for delirium increases in patients who are older, have comorbid neurologic disorders with associated brain pathology, and/or receive more than 8 to 10 treatments. The delirium usually clears within 24 hours and can be minimized by changing the intensity and frequency of the treatment parameters.

As recently as the 1980s, deaths from ECT were estimated to be approximately 1 per 10,000 treatments (most patients receive 6 to 10 treatments per ECT trial), primarily as a result of cardiac complications. Although patients are paralyzed, the ECT electrode directly stimulates the vagus nerve and can cause asystole. Within seconds of vagal stimulation, an adrenergic discharge related to the onset of a generalized seizure causes the release of EPI with tachycardia, hypertension, and the potential for myocardial ischemia or arrhythmias. The tachycardia is relatively brief (1 to 2 minutes).

Certain cardiovascular conditions increase the risk of complications from a course of ECT: a cerebrovascular accident during the previous 6 months, a cerebral or aortic aneurysm, MI, severe valvular heart disease, high-grade atrioventricular block, symptomatic ventricular arrhythmias, and supraventricular arrhythmias with an uncontrolled ventricular rate.[175] Implanted cardiac pacemakers and defibrillators are usually not problematic during ECT.[176] Some practitioners choose to convert a demand pacemaker to a fixed mode, and inhibit a defibrillator's function during each ECT treatment. Electroconvulsive therapy is also well-tolerated by cardiac transplant patients who have normal cardiac function.[177]

Electroconvulsive therapy can induce peak heart rates of 120 to 140 beats per minute. Because of general anesthesia, the patient cannot report symptoms such as chest pain, nor can the seizure stimulating the tachycardia be terminated abruptly. Therefore, a pre-ECT workup should include a complete review of systems and screen for exercise intolerance, angina, evidence of congestive heart failure (patients will receive approximately 1 liter of fluid per ECT treatment) or diabetes, smoking, hypercholesterolemia, and other cardiac risk factors. The basic pre-ECT screening includes measuring serum electrolytes (with particular attention to hydration status and potassium) and hemoglobin and obtaining an electrocardiogram (ECG). A chest radiograph is obtained to rule out CHF or pulmonary disease, patients with a history of back pain require spine films, and those with neurologic dysfunction require neuroimaging to evaluate for a recent cerebrovascular accident or increased intracranial pressure. Although β blockers are used during ECT treatment, cardiovascular screening should determine whether the patient can tolerate transient tachycardia and hypertension. Patients with evidence of CAD should undergo a stress test.

Modern ECT suites are equipped with continuous ECG, blood pressure and heart-rate monitors as well as pulse oximetry and an electroencephalograph to record seizure activity. In addition to usual ECT medications, patients with hypertension, CAD, valvular heart disease, and CHF routinely receive prophylactic medication to prevent cardiac complications from the ECT-induced transient hypertension and tachycardia.[178] A "cardiac-modified" ECT protocol[179] should be used for elderly patients and those with cardiac disease. Typically, labetalol or esmolol is used to reduce maximal heart rate, mean arterial pressure, and arrhythmia frequency during ECT. If elderly patients pretreated with a β blocker continue to exhibit transient increases in blood pressure, a calcium channel blocker can be added. Nicardipine has replaced nifedipine as the calcium channel blocker of choice because nicardipine can be administered intravenously and has a shorter duration of action. Continuous blood pressure and ECG monitoring should be performed during all treatments, along with monitoring for shortness of breath or chest pain.

Orthostatic hypotension is common after ECT, particularly in elderly, debilitated patients and patients with medical conditions associated with autonomic dysfunction. Consideration should be given to the use of shorter-acting β blockers that have less α-adrenoreceptor blockade and/or shorter-acting calcium channel blockers.

The risks associated with ECT are approximately equivalent to those of general anesthesia. Cardiac complications are not uncommon with ECT but are reduced significantly with a cardiac ECT protocol. Although generally a safe and effective treatment, ECT in elderly patients or those with cardiovascular disease requires a multispecialty coordinated effort including a specially trained ECT-nursing service, psychiatrist, anesthesiologist, and cardiologist.

REFERENCES

1. Hayward C. Psychiatric illness and cardiovascular disease risk. *Epidemiol Rev.* 1995;17:129–138.
2. Williams R, Schneiderman N. Resolved: psychosocial interventions can improve clinical outcomes in organic disease. *Psychosom Med.* 2002;64:552–557.
3. American Psychiatric Association. *Diagnostic and Statistical Manual of Mental Disorders.* 4th ed. Washington, DC: American Psychiatric Association; 1994.
4. Kessler R, Berglund P, Demler O, et al. The epidemiology of major depressive disorder: results from the National Comorbidity Survey Replication (NCS-R). *JAMA.* 2003;289:3095–3105.
5. Cohen-Cole SA, Kaufman KG. Major depression in physical illness: diagnosis, prevalence, and antidepressant treatment (a 10-year review: 1982–1992). *Depression.* 1993;1:181–204.
6. Feldman E, Mayou R, Hawton K, Ardern M, Smith EB. Psychiatric disorder in medical inpatients. *Q J Med.* 1987;63:405–412.
7. Johnson J, Weissman MM, Klerman GL. Service utilization and social morbidity associated with depressive symptoms in the community. *JAMA.* 1992;267:1478–1483.
8. Ormel J, Koeter MWJ, van den Brink W, van de Willige G. Recognition, management, and course of anxiety and depression in general practice. *Arch Gen Psychiatry.* 1991;48:700–706.
9. DiMatteo MR, Lepper HS, Croghan TW. Depression is a risk factor for noncompliance with medical treatment: meta-analysis of the effects of anxiety and depression on patient adherence. *Arch Int Med.* 2000;160:2101–2107.
10. Mayou R, Foster A, Williamson B. Medical care after myocardial infarction. *J Psychosom Res.* 1979;23:23–26.
11. Druss BG, Bradford D, Rosenheck RA, Radford JJ, Krumholz HM. Quality of medical care and excess mortality in older patients with mental disorders. *Arch Gen Psychiatry.* 2001;58:565–572.
12. Lesperance F, Frasure-Smith N, Talajic M, Bourassa MG. Five-year risk of cardiac mortality in relation to initial severity and one-year changes in depression symptoms after myocardial infarction. *Circulation.* 2002;105:1049–1053.
13. Purebl G, Birkas E, Csoboth C, Szumska I, Kopp MS. The relationship of biological and psychological risk factors of cardiovascular disorders in a large-scale national representative community survey. *Behav Med.* 2006;31:133–9.
14. Frasure-Smith N, Lesperance F, Talajic M. Depression and 18-month prognosis after myocardial infarction. *Circulation.* 1995;91:999–1005.
15. Bush D, Ziegelstein R, Tayback M, et al. Even minimal symptoms of depression increase mortality risk after acute myocardial infarction. *Am J Cardiol.* 2001;88:337–341.
16. Frasure-Smith N, Lesperance F, Juneau M, Talajic M, Bourassa MG. Gender, depression, and one-year prognosis after myocardial infarction. *Psychosom Med.* 1999;61:26–37.
17. van Melle JP, de Jonge P, Spijkerman TA, et al. Prognostic association of depression following myocardial infarction with mortality and cardiovascular events: a meta-analysis [see comment]. *Psychosom Med.* 2004;66:814–822.
18. Jiang W, Hasselblad V, Krishnan RR, O'Connor CM. Patients with CHF and depression have greater risk of mortality and morbidity than patients without depression [comment]. *J Am Coll Cardiol.* 2002;39:919–21.
19. Vaccarino V, Kasl SV, Abramsom J, Krumholz H. Depressive symptoms and risk of functional decline and death in patients with heart failure. *J Am Coll Cardiol.* 2001;38:199–205.
20. Barth J, Schumacher M, Herrmann-Lingen C. Depression as a risk factor for mortality in patients with coronary heart disease: a meta-analysis [see comment]. *Psychosom Med.* 2004;66:802–813.
21. Connerney I, Shapiro PA, McLaughlin JS, Bagiella E, Sloan RP. Relation between depression after coronary artery bypass surgery and 12 month outcome: a prospective study. *Lancet.* 2001;358:1766–1771.
22. Blumenthal JA, Williams RS, Wallace AG, Williams RB, Needles TL. Physiological and psychological variables predict compliance to prescribed exercise therapy in patients recovering from myocardial infarction. *Psychosom Med.* 1982;44:519–527.
23. Ferketich AK, Schwartzbaum JA, Frid DJ, Moeschberger JL. Depression as an antecedent to heart disease among women and men in the NHANES I study. *Arch Intern Med.* 2000;160:1261–1268.
24. Pennix BWJH, Beekman ATF, Honig A, et al. Depression and cardiac morbidity: results from a community-based longitudinal study. *Arch Gen Psychiatry.* 2001;58:221–227.
25. Rugulies R. Depression as a predictor for coronary heart disease. A review and meta-analysis. *Am J Prev Med.* 2002;23:51–61.
26. Lett HS, Blumenthal JA, Babyak MA, et al. Depression as a risk factor for coronary artery disease: evidence, mechanisms, and treatment. *Psychosom Med.* 2004;66:305–315.
27. Ford DE, Erlinger TP. Depression and C-reactive protein in U.S. adults: data from the Third National Health and Nutrition Examination Survey. *Arch Intern Med.* 2004;164:1010–1014.
28. Penninx BW, Kritchevsky SB, Yaffe K, et al. Inflammatory markers and depressed mood in older persons: results from the Health, Aging and Body Composition study. *Biol Psychiatry.* 2003;54:566–572.
29. Miller GE, Stetler CA, Carney RM, Freedland KE, Banks WA. Clinical depression and inflammatory risk markers for coronary heart disease. *Am J Cardiol.* 2002;90:1279–1283.
30. Hansson GK. Inflammation, atherosclerosis, and coronary artery disease [see comment]. *N Engl J Med.* 2005;352:1685–1695.
31. Lindahl B, Toss H, Siegbahn A, Venge P, Wallentin L. Markers of myocardial damage and inflammation in relation to long-term mortality in unstable coronary artery disease. Fragmin during Instability in Coronary Artery Disease (FRISC) Study Group [see comment]. *N Engl J Med.* 2000;343:1139–1147.
32. Danesh J, Wheeler JG, Hirschfield GM, et al. C-reactive protein and other circulating markers of inflammation in the prediction of coronary heart disease [see comment]. *N Engl J Med.* 2004;350:1387–1397.
33. Willerson JT, Ridker PM. Inflammation as a cardiovascular risk factor. *Circulation.* 2004;109:II2–10.
34. Suarez EC, Krishnan RR, Lewis JG. The relation of severity of depressive symptoms to monocyte-associated proinflammatory cytokines and chemokines in apparently healthy men. *Psychosom Med.* 2003;65:362–368.
35. Thomas AJ, Davis S, Morris C, et al. Increase in interleukin-1beta in late-life depression. *Am J Psychiatry.* 2005;162:175–7.
36. Wu JT, Wu LL. Linking inflammation and atherogenesis: Soluble markers identified for the detection of risk factors and for early risk assessment. *Clin Chim Acta.* 2006;366:74–80.
37. Libby P. Inflammation in atherosclerosis. *Nature.* 2002;420:868–874.
38. Yudkin JS, Juhan-Vague I, Hawe E, et al. Low-grade inflammation may play a role in the etiology of the metabolic syndrome in patients with coronary heart disease: the HIFMECH study. *Metabolism.* 2004;53:852–857.
39. Arner P. The adipocyte in insulin resistance: key molecules and the impact of the thiazolidinediones. *Trends Endocrinol Metab.* 2003;14:137–145.
40. Paramo JA, Beloqui O, Roncal C, Benito A, Orbe J. Validation of plasma fibrinogen as a marker of carotid atherosclerosis in subjects free of clinical cardiovascular disease. *Haematologica.* 2004;89:1226–1231.
41. Damas JK, Waehre T, Yndestad A, et al. Interleukin-7-mediated inflammation in unstable angina: possible role of chemokines and platelets. *Circulation.* 2003;107:2670–2676.
42. Fry TJ, Mackall CL. Interleukin-7: master regulator of peripheral T-cell homeostasis? [see comment]. *Trends Immunol.* 2001;22:564–571.

43. Schiepers OJ, Wichers MC, Maes M. Cytokines and major depression [erratum appears in *Prog Neuropsychopharmacol Biol Psychiatry*. 2005;29(4):637–638]. *Prog Neuropsychopharmacol*. 2005;29:201–217.

44. Szabo SJ, Sullivan BM, Peng SL, Glimcher LH. Molecular mechanisms regulating Th1 immune responses. *Ann Rev Immunol*. 2003;21:713–758.

45. Collins T, Cybulsky MI. NF-B: pivotal mediator or innocent bystander in atherogenesis? *J Clin Invest*. 2001;107:255–264.

46. Kop WJ, Gottdiener JS, Tangen CM, et al. Inflammation and coagulation factors in persons > 65 years of age with symptoms of depression but without evidence of myocardial ischemia. *Am J Cardiol*. 2002;89:419–424.

47. Cybulsky MI, Iiyama K, Li H, et al. A major role for VCAM-1 but not ICAM-1 in early atherosclerosis [see comment]. *J Clin Invest*. 2001;107:1255–1262.

48. Dantzer R. Cytokine-induced sickness behavior: mechanisms and implications. *Ann N Y Acad Sci*. 2001;933:222–234.

49. Douglas KM, Taylor AJ, O'Malley PG. Relationship between depression and C-reactive protein in a screening population. *Psychosom Med*. 2004;66:679–683.

50. Danner M, Kasl SV, Abramson JL, Vaccarino V. Association between depression and elevated C-reactive protein. *Psychosom Med*. 2003;65:347–356.

51. Glaser R, Robles TF, Sheridan J, Malarkey WB, Kiecolt-Glaser JK. Mild depressive symptoms are associated with amplified and prolonged inflammatory responses after influenza virus vaccination in older adults. *Arch Gen Psychiatry*. 2003;60:1009–1014.

52. Bonaccorso S, Puzella A, Marino V, et al. Immunotherapy with interferon-alpha in patients affected by chronic hepatitis C induces an intercorrelated stimulation of the cytokine network and an increase in depressive and anxiety symptoms. *Psychiatry Res*. 2001;105:45–55.

53. Capuron L, Ravaud A, Gualde N, et al. Association between immune activation and early depressive symptoms in cancer patients treated with interleukin-2-based therapy. *Psychoneuroendocrinology*. 2001;26:797–808.

54. Appels A, Bar FW, Bar J, Bruggeman C, de Baets M. Inflammation, depressive symptomatology, and coronary artery disease. *Psychosom Med*. 2000;62:601–605.

55. Lesperance F, Frasure-Smith N, Theroux P, Irwin M. The association between major depression and levels of soluble intercellular adhesion molecule 1 interleukin-6 and C-reactive protein in patients with recent acute coronary syndromes [see comment]. *Am J Psychiatry*. 2004;161:271–277.

56. Lyness JM, Moynihan JA, Williford DJ, Cox C, Caine ED. Depression, medical illness, and interleukin-1beta in older cardiac patients. *Int J Psychiatry Med*. 2001;31:305–310.

57. Miller GE, Freedland KE, Carney RM. Depressive symptoms and the regulation of proinflammatory cytokine expression in patients with coronary heart disease. *J Psychosom Res*. 2005;59:231–236.

58. Schins A, Tulner D, Lousberg R, et al. Inflammatory markers in depressed post-myocardial infarction patients.[erratum appears in *J Psychiatr Res*. 2005;39(6):633]. *J Psychiatry Res*. 2005;39:137–144.

59. Empana JP, Sykes DH, Luc G, et al. Contributions of depressive mood and circulating inflammatory markers to coronary heart disease in healthy European men: the Prospective Epidemiological Study of Myocardial Infarction (PRIME). *Circulation*. 2005;111:2299–2305.

60. Ladwig KH, Marten-Mittag B, Lowel H, Doring A, Koenig W. C-reactive protein, depressed mood, and the prediction of coronary heart disease in initially healthy men: results from the MONICA-KORA Augsburg Cohort Study 1984–1998. *Eur Heart J*. 2005;26:2537–2542.

61. Pearson TA, Mensah GA, Alexander RW, et al. Markers of inflammation and cardiovascular disease: application to clinical and public health practice: A statement for healthcare professionals from the Centers for Disease Control and Prevention and the American Heart Association [see comment]. *Circulation*. 2003;107:499–511.

62. Mancini GB. Vascular structure versus function: is endothelial dysfunction of independent prognostic importance or not? [comment]. *J Am Coll Cardiol*. 2004;43:624–628.

63. Rajagopalan S, Brook RA, Rubenfire M, Pitt E, Young E. Abnormal brachial artery flow-mediated vasodilation in young adults with major depression. *Am J Cardiol*. 2001;88:196–198.

64. Broadley AJ, Korszun A, Jones CJ, Frenneaux MP. Arterial endothelial function is impaired in treated depression [see comment]. *Heart*. 2002;88:521–523.

65. Sherwood A, Hinderliter AL, Watkins LL, Waugh RA, Blumenthal JA. Impaired endothelial function in coronary heart disease patients with depressive symptomatology. *J Am Coll Cardiol*. 2005;46:656–659.

66. Rybakowski J, Wykretowicz A, Heymann-Szlachcinska A. Impairment of endothelial function in unipolar and bipolar depression. *Biol Psychiatry*. 2006;60:889–891.

67. Raadsheer FC, van Heerikhuize JJ, Lucassen PJ, et al. Corticotropin-releasing hormone mRNA levels in the paraventricular nucleus of patients with Alzheimer's disease and depression. *Am J Psychiatry*. 1995;152:1372–1376.

68. Veith RC, Lewis L, Linares OA, et al. Sympathetic nervous system activity in major depression: basal and desipramine-induced alterations in plasma NE kinetics. *Arch Gen Psychiatry*. 1994;51:411–422.

69. Hughes JW, Watkins L, Blumenthal JA, Kuhn C, Sherwood A. Depression and anxiety symptoms are related to increased 24-hour urinary norepinephrine excretion among healthy middle-aged women. *J Psychosom Res*. 2004;57:353–358.

70. Grossman F, Potter WZ. Catecholamines in depression: a cumulative study of urinary norepinephrine and its major metabolites in unipolar and bipolar depressed patients versus healthy volunteers at the NIMH. *Psychiatry Res*. 1999;87:21–27.

71. Carney RM, Freedland KE, Veith RC, et al. Major depression, heart rate, and plasma norepinephrine in patients with coronary heart disease. *Biol Psychiatry*. 1999;45:458–463.

72. Roy A, Guthrie S, Pickar D, Linnoila M. Plasma NE responses to cold challenge in depressed patients and normal controls. *Psychiatry Res*. 1987;21:161–168.

73. Golden RN, Markey SP, Risby ED, et al. Antidepressants reduce whole-body norepinephrine turnover while enhancing 6-hydroxymelatonin output. *Arch Gen Psychiatry*. 1988;45:150–154.

74. Dalack GW, Roose SP. Perspectives on the relationship between cardiovascular disease and affective disorder. *J Clin Psychiatry*. 1990;51(7 suppl):4–9; discussion 10–11.

75. Bigger JT, Kleiger RE, Fleiss JL, et al. Components of HR variability measured during healing of acute myocardial infarction. *Am J Cardiol*. 1988;61:208–215.

76. Viskin S, Belhassen B. Noninvasive and invasive strategies for the prevention of sudden death after myocardial infarction. Value, limitations and implications for therapy. *Drugs*. 1992;44:336–355.

77. Stein PK, Carney RM, Freedland KE, et al. Severe depression is associated with markedly reduced heart rate variability in patients with stable coronary artery disease. *J Psychosom Res*. 2000;48:493–500.

78. Rechlin T, Weis M, Claus D. Heart rate variability in depressed patients and differential effects of paroxetine and amitriptyline on cardiovascular autonomic functions. *Pharmacopsychiatry*. 1994;27:124–128.

79. Carney RM, Saunders RD, Freedland KE, et al. Association of depression with reduced heart rate variability in coronary artery disease. *Am J Cardiol*. 1995;76:562–564.

80. Severus WE, Ahrens B, Stoll AL. Omega-3 fatty acids—the missing link? (letter). *Arch Gen Psychiatry*. 1999;56:380–381.

81. Christensen JH, Korup E, Aaroe J, et al. Fish consumption, n-3 fatty acids in cell membranes, and heart rate variability in survivors of myocardial infarction with left ventricular dysfunction. *Am J Cardiol*. 1997;79:1670–1673.

82. Albert CM, Hennekens CH, O'Donnell CJ, et al. Fish consumption and risk of sudden cardiac death. *JAMA*. 1998;279:23–28.

83. Edwards R, Peet M, Shay J, Horrobin D. Omega-3 polyunsaturated fatty acid levels in the diet and in red blood cell membranes of depressed patients. *J Affect Disord*. 1998;48:149–155.

84. Carney RM, Freedland KE, Veith RC. Depression, the autonomic nervous system, and coronary heart disease. *Psychosom Med*. 2005;1991;67(suppl 1):S29–33.

85. Carney RM, Freedland KE, Stein PK, et al. Change in heart rate and heart rate variability during treatment for depression in patients with coronary heart disease. *Psychosom Med*. 2000;62:639–647.

86. Bruce EC, Musselman DL. Depression, alterations in platelet function, and ischemic heart disease. *Psychosom Med*. 2005;67(suppl 1):S34–36.

87. Markovitz JH, Matthews KA. Platelets and coronary heart disease: potential psychophysiologic mechanism. *Psychosom Med*. 1991;53:643–668.

88. Musselman DL, Tomer A, Manatunga AK, et al. Exaggerated platelet reactivity in major depression. *Am J Psychiatry*. 1996;153:1313–1317.

89. Musselman DL, Marzec UM, Manatunga A, et al. Platelet reactivity in depressed patients treated with paroxetine: preliminary findings. *Arch Gen Psychiatry*. 2000;57:875–882.

90. Kuijpers PMJC, Hamulyak K, Strik JJMH, Wellens HJJ, Honig A. Beta-thromboglobulin and platelet factor 4 levels in post-myocardial infarction patients with major depression. *Psychiatry Res*. 2002;109:207–210.

91. Markovitz JH, Matthews KA, Kiss J, Smitherman TC. Effects of hostility on platelet reactivity to psychological stress in coronary heart disease patients and healthy controls. *Psychosom Med*. 1996;58:143–149.

92. Laghrissi-Thode F, Wagner WR, Pollock BG, Johnson PC, Finkel MS. Elevated platelet factor 4 and b-thromboglobulin plasma levels in depressed patients with ischemic heart disease. *Biol Psychiatry*. 1997;42:290–295.

93. Owens MJ, Nemeroff CB. Role of serotonin in the pathophysiology of depression: focus on the serotonin transporter. *Clin Chem.* 1994;40:288–295.

94. Pandey GN, Pandey SC, Janicak PG. Platelet serotonin-2 binding sites in depression and suicide. *Biol Psychiatry.* 1990;28:215–222.

95. Cerrito F, Lazzaro MP, Gaudio E, Arminio P, Aloisi G. 5HT2-receptors and serotonin release: their role in human platelet aggregation. *Life Sci.* 1993;53:209–215.

96. Plein H, Berk M, Eppel S, Butkow N. Augmented platelet calcium uptake in response to serotonin stimulation in patients with major depression measured using Mn^{2+} influx and $^{45}Ca^{2+}$ uptake. *Life Sci.* 1999;66:425–431.

97. Pollock BG, Laghrissi-Thode F, Wagner WR. Evaluation of platelet activation in depressed patients with ischemic heart disease after paroxetine or nortriptyline treatment. *J Clin Psychopharmacol.* 2000;20:137–140.

98. Jiang W, Babyak M, Krantz DS, et al. Mental stress-induced myocardial ischemia and cardiac events. *JAMA.* 1996;21:1651–1656.

99. Follick MJ, Gorkin L, Capone RJ, et al. Psychological distress as a predictor of ventricular arrhythmias in a post-myocardial infarct population. *Am Heart J.* 1988;116:32–36.

100. Curtis AL, Pavcovich LA, Grigoriadis DE, Valentino RJ. Previous stress alters corticotropin-releasing factor neurotransmission in the locus coeruleus. *Neuroscience.* 1995;65:541–550.

101. Kendler KS, Kessler RC, Neale MC, Heath AC, Eaves LJ. The prediction of major depression in women: toward an integrated etiologic model. *Am J Psychiatry.* 1993;150:1139–1148.

102. Echt DS, Liebson PR, Mitchell LB, et al for the Investigators. Mortality and morbidity in patients receiving encainide, flecainide, or placebo: the Cardiac Arrhythmia Suppression Trial. *N Engl J Med.* 1991;324:781–788.

103. Haigney MC, Zareba W, Gentlesk PJ. QT interval variability and spontaneous ventricular tachycardia or fibrillation in the Multicenter Automatic Defibrillator Implantation Trial (MADIT) II patients. *J Am Coll Cardiol* 2004;44:1481–1487.

104. Yeragani VK, Pohl R, Jampala VC, et al. Increased QT variability in patients with panic disorder and depression. *Psychiatry Res.* 2000;93:225–235.

105. Carney RM, Blumenthal JA, Catellier D, et al. Depression as a risk factor for mortality after acute myocardial infarction. *Am J Cardiol.* 2003;92:1277–1281.

106. Kessler RC, McGonagle KA, Zhao S, et al. Lifetime and 12-month prevalence of DSM-III-R psychiatric disorders in the United States. *Arch Gen Psychiatry.* 1994;51:8–19.

107. Sullivan MD, LaCroix AZ, Baum C, Grothaus LC, Katon WJ. Functional status in coronary artery disease: a one-year prospective study of the role of anxiety and depression. *Am J Med.* 1997;103:348–356.

108. Fifer SK, Mathias SD, Patrick DL, et al. Untreated anxiety among adult primary care patients in a health maintenance organization. *Arch Gen Psychiatry.* 1994;51:740–750.

109. Sherbourne CD, Jackson CA, Meredith LS, Camp P, Wells KB. Prevalence of comorbid anxiety disorders in primary care outpatients. *Arch Fam Med.* 1996;5:27–34.

110. Kawachi I, Colitz GA, Ascherio A. Prospective study of phobic anxiety and risk of coronary heart disease in men. *Circulation.* 1994;89:1992–1997.

111. Kubzansky LD, Kawachi I, Spiro III A, et al. Is worrying bad for your heart? A prospective study of worry and coronary heart disease in the Normative Aging Study. *Circulation.* 1997;95:818–824.

112. Herrmann C, Brand-Driehorst S, Buss U, Ruger U. Effects of anxiety and depression on 5-year mortality in 5057 patients referred for exercise testing. *J Psychosom Res.* 2000;48:455–462.

113. Kubzansky LD, Kawachi I, Weiss ST, Sparrow D. Anxiety and coronary heart disease: a synthesis of epidemiological, psychological, and experimental evidence. *Ann Behav Med.* 1998;20:47–58.

114. Thomas SA, Friedmann E, Wimbush F, Shron E. Psychosocial factors and survival in the Cardiac Arrhythmia Suppression Trial (CAST): A reexamination. *Am J Crit Care.* 1997;6:116–126.

115. Davis M. The role of the amygdala in fear-potentiated startle: implications for animal models of anxiety. *Trends Pharmacol Sci.* 1992;13:35–41.

116. Ninan PT. The functional anatomy, neurochemistry, and pharmacology of anxiety. *J Clin Psychiatry.* 1999;60(suppl 22):12–17.

117. Stein MB, Uhde TW. Biology of anxiety disorders. In: Schatzberg AF, Nemeroff CB, eds. *The American Psychiatric Association Textbook of Psychopharmacology.* 2nd ed. Washington, DC: American Psychiatric Association; 1998:609–628.

118. McNally RJ, Eke M. Anxiety sensitivity, suffocation fear, and breath-holding duration as predictors of response to carbon dioxide challenge. *J Abnorm Psychol.* 1996;105:146–149.

119. Torgersen S. Twin studies in panic disorder. In: Ballenger J, ed. *Neurobiology of Panic Disorder.* New York: Alan R. Liss; 1990:51–58.

120. Stein MB, Millar TW, Larsen DK, Kryger MH. Irregular breathing during sleep in patients with panic disorder. *Am J Psychiatry.* 1995;152:1168–1173.

121. Condren RM, O'Neill A, Ryan MC, Barrett P, Thakore JH. HPA axis response to a psychological stressor in generalised social phobia. *Psychoneuroendocrinology.* 2002;27:693–703.

122. Marshall RD, Blanco C, Printz D, et al. A pilot study of noradrenergic and HPA axis functioning in PTSD vs. panic disorder. *Psychiatry Res.* 2002;110:219–230.

123. Baker DG, West SA, Nicholson WE, et al. Serial CSF corticotropin-releasing hormone levels and adrenocortical activity in combat veterans with posttraumatic stress disorder. *Am J Psychiatry.* 1999;156:585–588.

124. Yehuda R, Boisoneau D, Lowy MT, Giller ELJ. Dose-response changes in plasma cortisol and lymphocyte glucocorticoid receptors following dexamethasone administration in combat veterans with and without posttraumatic stress disorder. *Arch Gen Psychiatry.* 1995;52:583–593.

125. Stein MB, Yehuda R, Koverola C, Hanna C. Enhanced dexamethasone suppression of plasma cortisol in adult women traumatized by childhood sexual abuse. *Biol Psychiatry.* 1997;42:680–686.

126. Bremner JD, Randall P, Vermetten E, et al. Magnetic resonance imaging-based measurement of hippocampal volume in posttraumatic stress disorder related to childhood physical and sexual abuse--a preliminary report. *Biol Psychiatry.* 1997;41:23–32.

127. Wilkinson DJC, Thompson JM, Lambert GW, et al. Sympathetic activity in patients with panic disorder at rest, under laboratory mental stress, and during panic attacks. *Arch Gen Psychiatry.* 1998;55:511–520.

128. Rutledge T, Hogan BE. A quantitative review of prospective evidence linking psychological factors with hypertension development. *Psychosom Med.* 2002;64:758–766.

129. Sheehan DV, Coleman JH, Greenblatt DJ, et al. Some biochemical correlates of panic attacks with agoraphobia and their response to a new treatment. *J Clin Psychopharmacol.* 1984;4:66–75.

130. Freeman IJ, Nixon PGF. Are coronary artery spasm and progressive damage to the heart associated with the hyperventilation syndrome? *Br Med J.* 1985;291:851–852.

131. Sloan EP, Natarajan M, Baker B, et al. Nocturnal and daytime panic attacks—comparison of sleep architecture, heart rate variability, and response to sodium lactate challenge. *Biol Psychiatry* 1999;45:1313–1320.

132. Lyonsfield JD. *An Examination of Image and Thought Processes in Generalized Anxiety.* New York: Association for the Advancement of Behavior Therapy. 1991.

133. Thayer JF, Friedman BH, Borkovec TD. Autonomic characteristics of generalized anxiety disorder and worry. *Biol Psychiatry.* 1996;39:255–266.

134. Shear MK, Kligfield P, Harshfield G, et al. Cardiac rate and rhythm in panic patients. *Am J Psychiatry.* 1987;144:633–637.

135. Chignon J-M, Lepine J-P, Ades J. Panic disorder in cardiac outpatients. *Am J Psychiatry.* 1993;150:780–785.

136. Katz C, Martin RD, Landa B, Chadda KD. Relationship of psychologic factors to frequent symptomatic ventricular arrhythmia. *Am J Med.* 1985;78:589–594.

137. Follick MJ, Ahern DK, Gorkin L, et al. Relation of psychosocial and stress reactivity variables to ventricular arrhythmias in the Cardiac Arrhythmia Pilot Study (CAPS). *Am J Cardiol.* 1990;66:63–67.

138. Frasure-Smith N, Lesperance F, Prince RH, et al. Randomised trial of home-based psychosocial nursing intervention for patients recovering from myocardial infarction. *Lancet.* 1997;350:473–470.

139. Kandzari DE, Kay J, O'Shea JC, et al. Highlights from the American Heart Association annual scientific sessions 2001: November 11 to 14, 2001. *Am Heart J.* 2002;143:217–228.

140. Jones DA, West RR. Psychological rehabilitation after myocardial infarction: multicentre randomised controlled trial. *Br Med J.* 1996;313:1517–1521.

141. Frasure-Smith N. In-hospital symptoms of psychological stress as predictors of long-term outcome after acute myocardial infarction in men. *Am J Cardiol.* 1991;67:121–127.

142. Friedman M, Thoresen CE, Gill JJ, et al. Alteration of type A behavior and its effect on cardiac recurrences in post myocardial infarction patients: summary results of the recurrent coronary prevention project. *Am Heart J.* 1986;112:653–665.

143. Feighner JP. Cardiovascular safety in depressed patients: focus on venlafaxine. *J Clin Psychiatry.* 1995;56:574–579.

144. Roose SP, Glassman AH, Siris SG, et al. Comparison of imipramine- and nortriptyline-induced orthostatic hypotension: a meaningful difference. *J Clin Psychopharmacol.* 1981;1:316–319.

145. Thayssen P, Bjerre M, Kragh-Sorensen P. Cardiovascular effects of imipramine and nortriptyline in elderly patients. *Psychopharmacology (Berl).* 1981;1981:360–364.

146. Feder R. Bradycardia and syncope induced by fluoxetine (Letter). *J Clin Psychiatry.* 1991;52:139.

147. Roose SP, Laghriss-Thode F, Kennedy JS, et al. Comparison of paroxetine and nortriptyline in depressed patients with ischemic heart disease. *JAMA.* 1998;279:287–291.
148. Franco-Bronson K. The management of treatment-resistant depression in the medically ill. *Psychiatr Clin North Am.* 1996;19:329–350.
149. Roose SP, Dalack GW, Glassman AH, et al. Cardiovascular effects of bupropion in depressed patients with heart disease. *Am J Psychiatry.* 1991;148:512–516.
150. Hyman SE, Arana GW, Rosenbaum JF. *Handbook of Psychiatric Drug Therapy.* Boston: Little, Brown and Company; 1995.
151. Robinson DS, Roberts DL, Smith JM, et al. The safety profile of nefazodone. *J Clin Psychiatry.* 1996;57(suppl 2):31–38.
152. Roose SP, Dalack GW. Treating the depressed patient with cardiovascular problems. *J Clin Psychiatry.* 1992;53:25–31.
153. Cohen HW, Gibson G, Alderman MH. Excess risk of myocardial infarction in patients treated with antidepressant medications: association with use of tricyclic agents. *Am J Med* 2000;108:2–8.
154. Hippisley-Cox J, Pringle M, Hammersley V, et al. Antidepressants as risk factor for ischaemic heart disease: case-control study in primary care. *Br Med J.* 2001;323:666–669.
155. Arana GW, Hyman SE. *Handbook of Psychiatric Drug Therapy.* 2nd ed. Boston: Little, Brown and Company; 1995:61.
156. Drent M, Singh S, Gorgels AP, et al. Drug-induced pneumonitis and heart failure simultaneously associated with venlafaxine. *Am J Respir Crit Care Med.* 2003;167:958–961.
157. Oslin DW, Ten Have TR, Streim JE, et al. Probing the safety of medications in the frail elderly: evidence from a randomized clinical trial of sertraline and venlafaxine in depressed nursing home residents. *J Clin Psych.* 2003;64:875–882.
158. Davidson JR, Watkins L, Owens M, et al. Effects of paroxetine and venlafaxine-XR on heart rate variability in depression and the role of norepinephrine transport inhibition. *Annual Meeting of the American College of Neuropsychopharmacology* 2003;105.
159. Cheeta S, Schifano F, Oyefeso A, Webb L, Ghodse AH. Antidepressant-related deaths and antidepressant prescriptions in England and Wales, 1998–2000. *Br J Psychiatry.* 2004;184:41–47.
160. Koski A, Vuori E, Ojanpera I. Newer antidepressants: evaluation of fatal toxicity index and interaction with alcohol based on Finnish postmortem data. *Int J Legal Med.* 2005;119:344–348.
161. Enemark B. The importance of ECG monitoring in antidepressant treatment. *Nord J Psychiatry.* 1993;47(suppl 30):57–65.
162. Alderman CP, Moritz CK, Ben-Tovim DI. Abnormal platelet aggregation associated with fluoxetine therapy. *Ann Pharmacother.* 1992;26:1517–1519.
163. Markovitz JH, Shuster JL, Chitwood WS, May RS, Tolbert L. Platelet activation in depression and effects of sertraline treatment: an open-label study. *Am J Psychiatry.* 2000;157:1006–1008.
164. Sauer WH, Berlin J, Kimmel SE. Selective serotonin reuptake inhibitors and myocardial infarction. *Circulation.* 2001;104:1894–1898.
165. Meier CR, Schlienger RG, Jick H. Use of selective serotonin reuptake inhibitors and risk of developing first-time acute myocardial infarction. *Br J Clin Pharmacol.* 2001;52:179–184.
166. Serebruany VL, Glassman AH, Malinin AI, et al. Platelet/endothelial biomarkers in depressed patients treated with the selective serotonin reuptake inhibitor sertraline after acute coronary events: the Sertraline Antidepressant Heart Attack Randomized Trial (SADHART) Platelet Substudy. *Circulation.* 2003;108:939–944.
167. Callahan AM, Marangell LB, Ketter TA. Evaluating the clinical significance of drug interactions: a systematic approach. *Harv Rev Psychiatry.* 1996;4:153–158.
168. Roose SP, Glassman AH, Attia E, et al. Cardiovascular effects of fluoxetine in depressed patients with heart disease. *Am J Psychiatry.* 1998;155:660–665.
169. Glassman AH, O'Connor CM, Califf RM, et al. Sertraline treatment of major depression in patients with acute MI or unstable angina. *JAMA.* 2002;288:701–709.
170. Petrides G, Fink M, Husain MM, et al. ECT remission rates in psychotic versus nonpsychotic depressed patients: a report from CORE. *J ECT.* 2001;17:244–253.
171. O'Connor MK, Knapp R, Husain M, et al. The influence of age on the response of major depression to electroconvulsive therapy: a report from C.O.R.E. *J ECT.* 2001;17.
172. Weiner RD. Does electroconvulsive therapy cause brain damage? *Behav Brain Sci.* 1984;7:1–53.
173. American Psychiatric Association Task Force on Electroconvulsive Therapy (APATFoET). The practice of electroconvulsive therapy: recommendations for treatment, training, and privileging. Washington, DC: American Psychiatric Association Press; 2001.
174. Sackheim HA. Memory and ECT. from polarization to reconciliation. [editorial; comment]. *J ECT.* 2000;16:87–96.
175. Applegate RJ. Diagnosis and management of ischemic heart disease in the patient scheduled to undergo electroconvulsive therapy. *Convuls Ther.* 1997;13:128–144.
176. Pornnoppadol C, Isenberg K. ECT and the implantable converter defibrillator. *Journal of Electroconvulsive Therapy.* 1998;14:124–126.
177. Block M, Admon D, Bonne O, Lerer B. Electroconvulsive therapy in depressed cardiac transplant patients. *Convuls Ther.* 1992;8:290–293.
178. Maneksha FR. Hypertension and tachycardia during electroconvulsive therapy: to treat or not to treat. *Convuls Ther.* 1991;70:28–35.
179. Figiel GD, McDonald L, LaPlante R. Cardiac modified ECT in the elderly (letter). *Am J Psychiatry.* 1994;151:790–791.

CHAPTER 96

Heart Disease and Pregnancy

John H. McAnulty / Craig S. Broberg / James Metcalfe

An understanding of the remarkable cardiovascular changes during a normal pregnancy is important for optimal care. Failure to recognize and treat heart disease, when it exists, can adversely affect both the mother and the child.

HEART DISEASE ISSUES UNIQUE TO PREGNANCY

【 】 HEALTH PRIORITIES

The health of the developing fetus is predominantly determined by the health of the mother. When treating heart disease, the health of the fetus should be considered, but the safety of the mother is the highest priority. Ideally, treatment of the mother with drugs, diagnostic studies, or surgery should be avoided unless required for maternal safety.

【 】 MATERNAL FRAGILITY

Heart disease is the second most common cause of maternal death in Western countries (suicide is first).[1] Sometimes the risk is sufficient to recommend avoidance or interruption of pregnancy (Table 96–1).[2,3] Apprehension about heart disease is common; it can be lessened by keeping a pregnant woman and her family informed.

【 】 FETAL VULNERABILITY

The maternal commitment to the fetus is exceptional, but if the mother requires a redistribution of blood flow for her own safety, blood is preferentially diverted away from the uterus. This subjects the fetus to an insufficient supply of oxygen and nutrients and in-

TABLE 96-1

Cardiovascular Abnormalities Placing a Mother and Infant at Extremely High Risk

ADVISE AVOIDANCE OR INTERRUPTION OF PREGNANCY

Pulmonary hypertension
Dilated cardiomyopathy with congestive failure
Marfan syndrome with dilated aortic root
Cyanotic congenital heart disease

PREGNANCY COUNSELING AND CLOSE CLINICAL FOLLOW-UP REQUIRED

Prosthetic valve
Coarctation of the aorta
Marfan syndrome
Dilated cardiomyopathy in asymptomatic women
Obstructive lesions

SOURCE: Modified from McAnulty JH, Morton MJ, Ueland K. The heart and pregnancy. Curr Probl Cardiol. 1988;13:589–665. Reproduced with permission from the publisher and authors.

effective removal of metabolic waste and heat. Uterine blood flow can already be compromised in a woman with heart disease increasing the possibility of inadequate uterine perfusion. Treatment of maternal heart disease can also jeopardize the fetus. Diagnostic studies, drugs, or surgery can increase fetal loss, result in teratogenicity, or alter fetal growth.

NEWBORN INFANT VULNERABILITY

The health of a newborn infant is a concern when the mother has heart disease. This fragility can be caused by a marginal uterine blood flow during pregnancy or to lingering effects of the medications used to treat the mother. Additionally, there will be an increased incidence of congenital heart disease among the live-born infants of parents with congenital heart disease. Early infant nourishment can be jeopardized if maternal heart disease is severe enough to interfere with breast-feeding. Even if the mother is capable of breast-feeding, cardiovascular medications can be transmitted to the infant in breast milk. Finally, the infant is at risk of losing a parent because life expectancy with many forms of heart disease is significantly reduced.

EFFECTS OF PREVIOUS TREATMENT

Although new information has been acquired about hearts that have been altered by surgery (or a catheter), there is still much that remains unknown, particularly as it relates to pregnancy. It is best not to consider a previous lesion to have been mechanically *corrected*, because there is always some residual disease.

A WARNING

Heart disease and pregnancy exceeds the expertise of most care providers and in fact, exceeds the capabilities of any single provider. When possible, care before, during, and after pregnancy is best given by an experienced team—counselors, primary care providers, cardiologists, anesthesiologists, and pediatricians. Any woman contemplating pregnancy should be educated by experienced providers before conception.

CLINICAL CONSIDERATIONS

Preconception

Antenatal care should include a discussion of the vulnerability issues explored above. The patient should be told which medications to avoid during pregnancy. Warfarin, angiotensin-converting enzyme (ACE) inhibitors and angiotensin II receptor blockers (ARBs) should be stopped (see discussion of drugs below). Any needed diagnostic tests or interventions should be performed before the risk to the fetus becomes a factor.

First Trimester

Organ development in the fetus begins at 3 weeks, before some women even know they are pregnant. As soon as pregnancy is confirmed, drug use should be assessed, again avoiding warfarin, ACE inhibitors, and ARBs. Aspirin should be started in cyanotic patients. If not already done, referral to an appropriate center of expertise with heart disease and pregnancy should begin. Issues to address include warning symptoms, need for scheduled imaging, optimal site for delivery, and type of delivery.

Second and Third Trimester

The expected hemodynamic changes associated with pregnancy reach their peak near the 20th week. Women should be advised of the likely sensation of dyspnea. An obstetrician should monitor fetal growth and determine the need for fetal echocardiography.

Labor and Delivery

This is a time of great demands on the cardiovascular system, and management must be optimized. Vaginal delivery is usually optimal in most patients with heart disease. However, if the second stage of labor is excessively painful or prolonged, the obstetricians should plan on assisted delivery (forceps or vacuum suction) to shorten the second stage, and consider an assisted delivery depending on the severity of the mother's heart disease. Induced labor or caesarean section should be reserved for obstetrical indications, or worsening cardiovascular function. Exceptions to this include patients with extremely high-risk heart disease including Eisenmenger syndrome and Marfan syndrome with aortic root dilation, where an appropriately planned early delivery can be performed when the fetus is adequately mature. Oxytocin should be avoided because of potential hypotension.

In most cases, lumbar epidural anesthesia using low-dose techniques for cardiostability with a pudendal nerve block to minimize pain is effective and least likely to result in hemodynamic compromise[4] and should be favored over general anesthesia. Antibiotic prophylaxis against bacterial endocarditis is practiced by most experienced centers although not formally recommended.[5]

Postpartum

Successful delivery does not mean the mother is out of danger; a large proportion of maternal deaths occur more than 1 week post delivery.[6] Hemodynamic and ECG monitoring should be continued for 48 to 72 hours in those with severe abnormalities (e.g., pulmonary hypertension, cyanotic lesions, severe obstructive lesions, or a severe cardiomyopathy). Important changes in clotting factors normally prevent excessive uterine bleeding, but these changes can disrupt the fragile thrombostasis in cyanotic patients. Warfarin can be reinstated carefully when necessary.

CARDIOVASCULAR ADJUSTMENTS DURING A NORMAL PREGNANCY

Maternal adaptation to pregnancy includes remarkable cardiovascular changes. These explain in part why some cardiac abnormalities are poorly tolerated during pregnancy (see Table 96–1).

Resting cardiac output (CO) increases by more than 40 percent during pregnancy reaching its highest levels by the 20th week (Fig. 96–1). Its early increase is caused mainly by an increase in stroke volume[7–10] with heart rate increasing gradually throughout pregnancy (Fig. 96–2). In the third trimester, CO is significantly affected by body position (see Fig. 96–1), as the enlarged uterus reduces venous return from the lower extremities.[7–12] Compared with measurements made when the woman is in the left lateral position near term, CO is lower by an average of 0.6 L/min when a woman is supine and by 1.2 L/min when she assumes the upright position.[11] In general, this results in few or no symptoms; but in some women, maintenance of the supine position can result in symptomatic hypotension, particularly when collateral vessels are not well developed.[12] Symptoms of this *supine hypotensive syndrome of pregnancy* can be corrected by having the woman turn onto her side.

Blood pressure (BP) falls slightly in early pregnancy. Systemic vascular resistance falls until the 20th week, then gradually increases through the remainder of pregnancy (see Fig. 96–2). The mother's oxygen consumption (which includes that of her fetus) increases by 20 percent within the first 20 weeks of pregnancy and increases steadily to a level that is approximately 30 percent above the nonpregnant levels by the time of delivery.[10] This increase is caused by both the metabolic needs of the fetus and the increased metabolic needs of the mother. These changes are better tolerated in patients with volume overload lesions (valvular regurgitation or shunts), than in patients with fixed output (obstructive valves, coarctation, or pulmonary hypertension).

At the beginning of labor, CO measured in the supine position increases to more than 7 L/min. This increases to more than 9 L/min with each uterine contraction because of extrusion of approximately 500 mL of blood into the central venous system and to an increase in heart rate. Administration of epidural anesthesia reduces this CO to approximately 8 L/min, and the use of general anesthesia reduces it still further. Following delivery, the CO

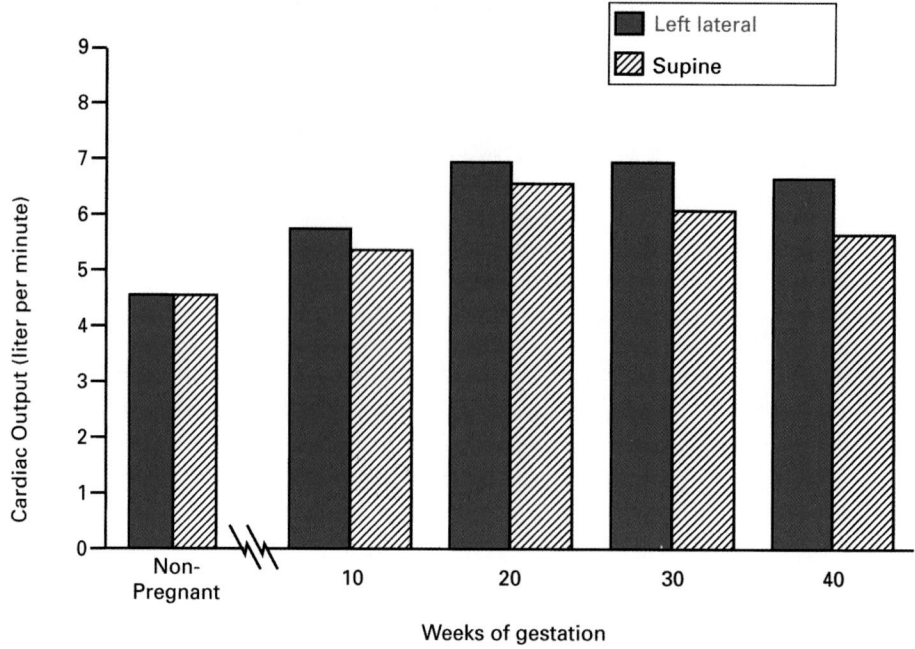

FIGURE 96–1. Cardiac output values during normal pregnancy when measured in the supine and left lateral positions. The values are derived from measurements made in many studies.[7–11]

briefly approaches 10 L/min[13] (7 to 8 L/min with cesarean section)[14]; it then falls rapidly to near-normal, nonpregnant values within a few weeks after delivery. A slight elevation in CO can persist for as long as a year.[15] The increase in maternal CO in women with twins or triplets is only slightly greater than that in women with single pregnancies.[13]

Pregnancy results in a redistribution of blood flow (Fig. 96–3). In the nonpregnant woman, uterine blood flow is approximately 100 mL/min (2 percent of the CO); it increases to approximately 1200 mL/min at term, a value approaching the mother's blood flow to her own kidneys.[16,17] During pregnancy, uterine blood vessels are maximally dilated; flow can increase, but this must result from increased maternal arterial pressure and flow. Excitement, heat, anxiety,[18] exercise, and decrease in venous return all decrease uterine blood flow. Vasoconstriction caused by endogenous catecholamines, vasoconstrictive drugs, maternal mechanical pulmonary ventilation, and some anesthetics as well as that associated with preeclampsia and eclampsia can decrease perfusion of the uterus.

〖 〗 HEMODYNAMIC CHANGES WITH EXERCISE

Pregnancy changes the hemodynamic response to exercise.[19] For any given level of exercise in the sitting position, the CO is greater than in nonpregnant women, and maximum CO is reached at lower exercise levels. During pregnancy, expected effects of conditioning or training on stroke volume are not seen, possibly because of uterine compression of the inferior vena cava or the increased venous dispensability.[20]

Exercise during pregnancy is not clearly any more dangerous or beneficial to the mother with heart disease than when she is not pregnant. The fetus is affected. In animal models, maternal exercise has been associated with a decrease in uterine blood flow. In humans, the type of exercise affects maternal hemodynamics and

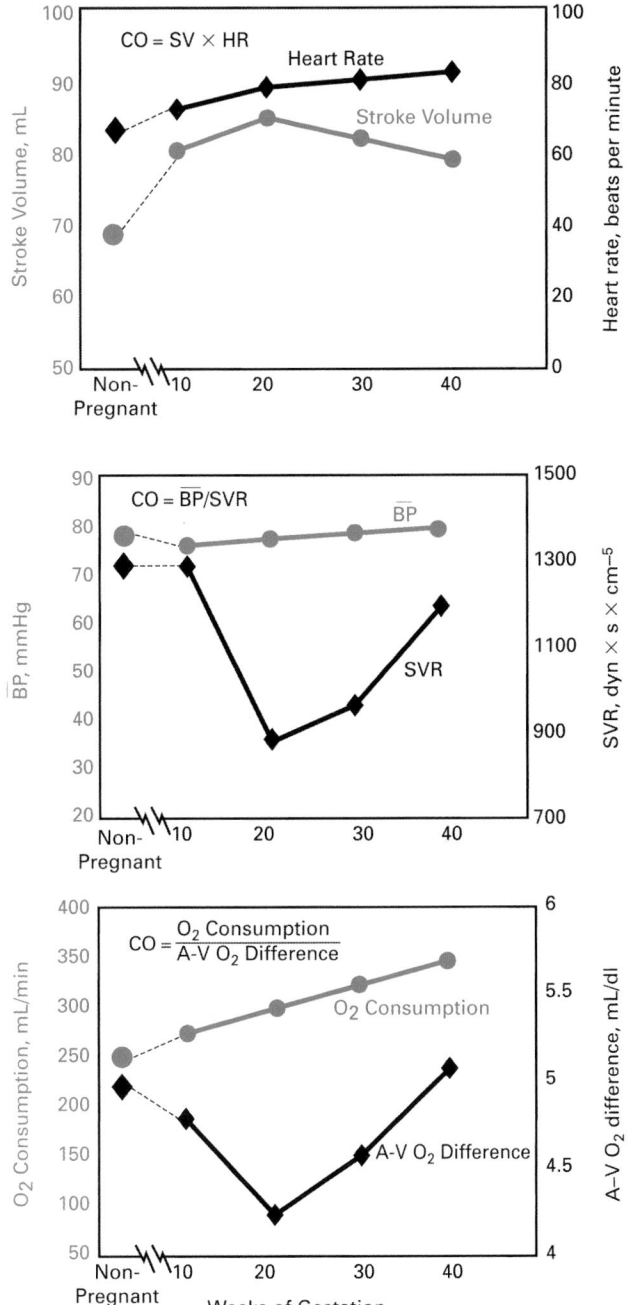

FIGURE 96–2. The cardiac output (CO) can be determined from other parameters in at least three ways: CO = heart rate (HR) × stroke volume (SV); CO = 5 mean arterial pressure (BP) minus the right atrial (RA) pressure/systemic vascular resistance (SVR); CO = 5 oxygen (O_2) consumption/arteriovenous (AV) O_2 difference. The expected values for these parameters measured in the supine position during pregnancy are based on information acquired from many studies.[7–11]

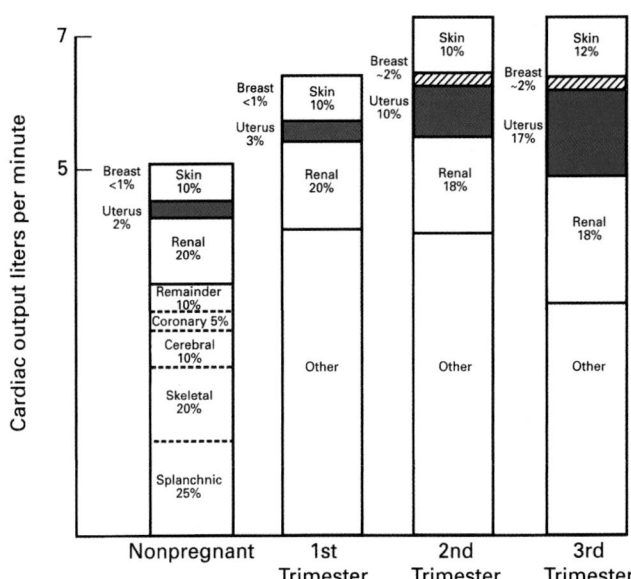

FIGURE 96–3. The changes in cardiac output and its distribution at rest in nonpregnant women. Data used in this graph are fragmentary, especially early in pregnancy.

uterine perfusion.[21,22] As an example, maximal exercise by swimming causes less fetal bradycardia (a marker of uterine blood flow) than the same level of cycling.[23] Additionally, regular aerobic endurance exercise during pregnancy has been associated with a reduction in birth weight. It is not clear if this is detrimental.[24]

Infants born to mothers who work in a standing position can be abnormally small at birth.[25] Although the long-term effects of this are not clear, the implications in relation to exercise and work in the upright position are likely greater for women with heart dis-

ease.[26–28] There is enthusiasm for recreational exercise in the United States. Although there is an insufficient amount of data to suggest that the healthy pregnant woman should avoid recreational exercise, an argument can be made for advising the woman with heart disease to keep the exercise level below that which causes symptoms.[29]

【 】 MECHANISMS FOR HEMODYNAMIC CHANGES

The mechanisms involving this adaption to pregnancy are not totally understood. They can in part be caused by volume change. Total body water increases steadily throughout pregnancy by 6 to 8 liters (L) (most is extracellular).[30] Sodium retention results in an excess accumulation of 500 to 900 mEq by the time of delivery. As early as 6 weeks after conception, plasma volume increases, approaching its maximum of 1.5 to 2 times normal by the second trimester, where it stays throughout the pregnancy.[31] The red blood cell mass also increases, but not to the same degree. Thus, the hematocrit decreases, although rarely to less than 30 percent.

Intrinsic cardiac changes can also explain some of the hemodynamic changes.[32–34] The stroke volume increases by approximately 25 percent. The ejection fraction does not change. Because the increases in left ventricular (LV) end-diastolic and systolic volumes are small and not adequate to explain the constant ejection fraction, the heart must become reconfigured as well. There is some evidence to suggest that in some disease states this remodeling persists after pregnancy.[35]

Vascular alterations also contribute to the hemodynamic changes of pregnancy. Arterial compliance is increased.[36,37] Venous capacitance increases as well, although there is an increase in venous vascular tone.[38] These changes are advantageous in maintaining the hemodynamics of a normal pregnancy. There can be disadvantages as well; vascular accidents, when they occur in women, frequently do so during pregnancy.[39,40] Additionally, the venous changes can explain, in part, the increase in thromboemboli during pregnancy.[41]

The ultimate cause of these recognized changes is uncertain. Complex interactions of the renin-angiotensin-aldosterone system[42] prostaglandins, nitric oxide, and atrial natriuretic factor contribute to the fluid and sodium changes. Currently, the effects of the increased level of circulating reproductive hormones seem to satisfactorily explain the vascular and myocardial changes.

DIAGNOSIS OF HEART DISEASE
【 】 CLINICAL EVALUATION

In a normal pregnancy, symptoms (dyspnea, fatigue) and signs (a third heart sound [S_3], pedal edema) mimic those of heart disease, making diagnosis difficult. Symptoms that should alert a caregiver to the possibility of heart disease include limiting dyspnea or orthopnea, hemoptysis, syncope with exertion, or chest pain clearly related to effort. On examination, cyanosis or clubbing, a loud systolic murmur (grade 3 or louder) or any diastolic murmur suggest heart disease. Venous hums or internal mammary flow sounds (the mammary souffle), which have diastolic components, are findings during a normal pregnancy.

【 】 DIAGNOSTIC STUDIES

Echocardiography is safe (no known risk to the mother or fetus) and is so diagnostically useful that overuse, expense, and potential misinterpretation are the only significant concerns. Chamber dimensions and velocity measurements need to be interpreted considering the hemodynamic changes outlined above.

Electrocardiography is safe, although pregnancy makes interpretation of ST-T wave variations even more difficult than usual. Inferior ST-segment depression is common enough to possibly be the result of a normal pregnancy. There is a leftward shift of the QRS axis during pregnancy, but true axis deviation (−30 degrees) implies heart disease.

Cardiac MRI is also generally safe during pregnancy, although administration of gadolinium is contraindicated.

All radiation procedures, including computed tomography, nuclear scans, and catheterization, should be avoided unless absolutely necessary. They increase the risk of abnormal fetal organogenesis or of a subsequent malignancy in the child, particularly leukemia. Although estimated exposure to the fetus from a chest x-ray (10–1400 microgray [µGy]) or radionuclide scan is low (400 µGy),[43] even these should be avoided unless necessary. If a study is required, it should be delayed to as late in pregnancy as possible, the radiation dose should be kept to a minimum, and shielding of the fetus should be optimal.

CARDIOVASCULAR DRUGS AND PREGNANCY

Nearly all cardiac drugs cross the placenta and are secreted in breast milk. Because information about the use of any drug is incomplete, it is best to avoid drug use but, if required for maternal safety, drugs should not be withheld.

【 】 DIURETICS

Diuretics can and should be used for treatment of congestive heart failure that is uncontrolled by sodium restriction, and for the treatment of hypertension.[42,44] This should not be used for prophylaxis against toxemia or for treatment of pedal edema.

【 】 INOTROPIC AGENTS

The indications for the use of digitalis are not changed by pregnancy. The same dose of digoxin in general will yield lower maternal serum levels during pregnancy than in the nonpregnant state. Fetal serum levels approximate those in the mother. The drug is often given to mothers to treat fetal arrhythmia.

When intravenous inotropic or vasopressor agents are required, the standard agents (dopamine, dobutamine, and norepinephrine) can be used, but the fetus is jeopardized because all such agents increase resistance to uterine blood flow and can stimulate uterine contractions. Ephedrine is an appropriate initial vasopressor drug because, at least in animal models, it does not adversely affect uterine blood flow.

There is little information about the efficacy or safety of the phosphodiesterase inhibitors (amrinone, milrinone) in pregnancy.

【 】 ADRENERGIC-RECEPTOR-BLOCKING AGENTS

Observations that β blockers can decrease umbilical blood flow, initiate premature labor, and result in a small and infarcted placenta with the potential for low–birth-weight infants have led to concerns about their use. However, these drugs have been used in a large number of pregnant women without adverse effects. Their use for the usual clinical indications is reasonable.[45] If these agents are used during pregnancy, it is appropriate to monitor fetal heart rate as well as, the newborn infant's heart rate, blood sugar, and respiratory status.

Experience with the α-blocking agents phenoxybenzamine and phentolamine is sparse. Clonidine, prazosin, and labetalol, with their mixed α- and β-blocking effects, have been used for the treatment of hypertension during pregnancy without clear detrimental effects.[46]

【 】 CALCIUM CHANNEL BLOCKING DRUGS

The dihydropyridine agents are effective antihypertensive and afterload-reducing agents that have been used without any adverse effect on the fetus or newborn infant. If a nondihydropyridine agent is required, verapamil is the drug of choice. The calcium channel blockers cause relaxation of the uterus; nifedipine has been used for this purpose.

【 】 ANTIARRHYTHMIC AGENTS

When atrioventricular (AV) node blockade is required during pregnancy, β blockers, calcium blockers, adenosine, or digoxin can be used.[47] As a general rule, it is preferable to avoid the standard antiarrhythmic drugs in any patient. This is true during pregnancy as well. When such drugs are essential for the treatment of recurrent arrhythmias or for maternal safety, they should be used.[47,48] If intravenous drug therapy is required, lidocaine or procainamide provide reasonable first-line therapy; there is *no reported* experience with intravenous *amiodarone or ibutilide.*

If oral antiarrhythmic therapy is necessary, flecainide and sotalol are as likely to be as effective as other drugs and fetal safety is reasonable; they are often given to the mother to treat the fetus. Quinidine has also been used frequently without clear adverse fetal effects.[47] Information about procainamide, disopyramide, mexiletine, and dofetilide is sparse. The early available information concerning amiodarone indicates a 10 percent chance of fetal thyroid abnormalities and an increased likelihood of fetal loss and deformity.[49] Thus it should be avoided unless its use is essential for maternal or fetal safety.

[ ] VASODILATOR AGENTS

When needed for a true hypertensive crisis or emergency afterload and preload reduction, nitroprusside is the vasodilator drug of choice. It is highly effective, works instantly, is easily titrated and its effects dissipate immediately when the drug is stopped. A concern is that its metabolite, cyanide, can be detected in the fetus. This has not been demonstrated to be a significant problem in humans.[50,51] The appearance of this metabolite is a reason to limit the duration of use of this drug whenever possible. Intravenous hydralazine, nitroglycerin, or labetalol are alternative options for parenteral therapy.

Chronic afterload reduction to treat hypertension, aortic or mitral regurgitation, or ventricular dysfunction during pregnancy has been achieved with the calcium blocking drugs, hydralazine and methyldopa. Adverse fetal effects have not been reported.

The ACE inhibitors increase the risk of major congenital abnormality and are *contraindicated in pregnancy.*[52,53] A series of case reports of similar problems with the ARBs suggest that their use should be avoided until more data are available.[54,55]

[ ] ANTITHROMBOTIC AGENTS

Warfarin is contraindicated during the first 3 months (particularly weeks 7 to 12) because it crosses the placenta and is associated with a 5 to 25 percent incidence of malformations that comprise the *warfarin embryopathy syndrome* (facial abnormalities, optic atrophy, digital abnormalities, epithelial changes, and mental impairment).[56,57] The syndrome can be dose-related, with one study suggesting that it occurs only with doses greater than 5 mg/day.[58] The use of warfarin at any time during pregnancy increases the risk of fetal and maternal bleeding.

Heparin does not cross the placenta; fetal risk is minimal although maternal bleeding can occur. If heparin is used, sufficient dosing is essential to present thromboemboli. Self-administered subcutaneous high-dose unfractionated heparin (200–300 U/kg subcutaneously every 12 hours) or low-molecular-weight heparin, (e.g., enoxaparin 1 mg/kg subcutaneously every 12 hours) are reasonable options. If used, a factor Xa level should be assessed initially, titrating the drug to achieve trough levels (11 hours after dose) of >0.6 units/mL. Although peak levels (1 to 2 hours after a dose) relate to bleeding risk, the emphasis should be on avoiding insufficient trough levels (particularly when using this therapy in women with a prosthetic heart valve—see below). The activated partial thromboplastin time (aPTT) is not reliable for managing heparin use during pregnancy.

When anticoagulation is required, unfractionated heparin and, more recently, low-molecular weight (LMW) heparin have been advocated for the first trimester, switching to warfarin for the next 5 months, with a return to heparin therapy prior to and through labor and delivery[57-59] (Table 96–2). Although LMW heparin has been proven effective for the prophylaxis of venous thrombosis, its value in preventing thromboemboli in patients with mechanical prostheses has not yet been extensively evaluated.[60]

Antiplatelet agents increase the chance of maternal bleeding, and they cross the placenta. Aspirin has been associated with an increased incidence of abortion and fetal growth retardation. Its inhibition of prostaglandin synthesis can result in closure of the ductus arteriosus during fetal life.[61] Still, it has frequently been used and even recommended by some as prophylaxis against preeclampsia. These trade-offs are difficult to evaluate; we suggest aspirin should be used when needed for maternal safety. Data on the effects of dipyridamole, clopidogrel, or the IIb, IIIa glycoprotein platelet-receptor inhibitors during pregnancy are anecdotal and minimal.

MANAGEMENT OF CARDIOVASCULAR SYNDROMES

Cardiovascular complications can occur with any form of heart disease. The management of each patient must be individualized, but some recommendations are applicable in most cases.

[ ] LOW-CARDIAC-OUTPUT SYNDROME

A low CO is ominous in any patient, and this is particularly true in pregnancy. Although potentially treatable causes such as tamponade, severe valvular stenosis, or cardiomyopathy should be considered, low CO is most often caused by intravascular volume depletion. This is particularly dangerous in those with lesions that limit blood flow, such as pulmonary hypertension, aortic or pulmonic valve stenosis, hypertrophic cardiomyopathy, or mitral stenosis. Measures to prevent or treat a fall in central blood volume are outlined in Table 96–3.

[ ] CONGESTIVE HEART FAILURE

The management of congestive heart failure during pregnancy should not differ greatly from that at other times *except* that the ACE inhibitors and ARBs should not be used. Congestive heart failure is one situation where maintaining a woman in the supine position can be beneficial by causing preload reduction with obstruction of return of blood from the inferior vena cava to the heart.

[ ] THROMBOEMBOLIC COMPLICATIONS

The risk of venous thromboemboli increases fivefold during and immediately after pregnancy,[62] and there is arguably an increase in arterial emboli as well. Both can be the result of a woman's hypercoagulable status during pregnancy, and the likelihood of venous

TABLE 96–2

Therapeutic Guidelines for Pregnant Patients with Mechanical Prosthetic Valves

CLASS I

1. All pregnant patients with mechanical prosthetic valves must receive continuous therapeutic anticoagulation with frequent monitoring (see Section 9.2). *(Level of Evidence: B)*
2. For women requiring long-term warfarin therapy who are attempting pregnancy, pregnancy tests should be monitored with discussions about subsequent anticoagulation therapy, so that anticoagulation can be continued uninterrupted when pregnancy is achieved. *(Level of Evidence: C)*
3. Pregnant patients with mechanical prosthetic valves who elect to stop warfarin between weeks 6 and 12 of gestation should receive continuous intravenous UFH, dose-adjusted UFH, or dose-adjusted subcutaneous LMWH. *(Level of Evidence: C)*
4. For pregnant patients with mechanical prosthetic valves, up to 36 weeks of gestation, the therapeutic choice of continuous intravenous or dose-adjusted subcutaneous UFH, dose-adjusted LMWH, or warfarin should be discussed fully. If continuous intravenous UFH is used, the fetal risk is lower, but the maternal risks of prosthetic valve thrombosis, systemic embolization, infection, osteoporosis, and heparin-induced thrombocytopenia are relatively higher. *(Level of Evidence: C)*
5. In pregnant patients with mechanical prosthetic valves who receive dose-adjusted LMWH, the LMWH should be administered twice daily subcutaneously to maintain the anti-Xa level between 0.7 and 1.2 U per mL 4 h after administration. *(Level of Evidence: C)*
6. In pregnant patients with mechanical prosthetic valves who receive dose-adjusted UFH, the aPTT should be at least twice control. *(Level of Evidence: C)*
7. In pregnant patients with mechanical prosthetic valves who receive warfarin, the INR goal should be 3.0 (range 2.5 to 3.5). *(Level of Evidence: C)*
8. In pregnant patients with mechanical prosthetic valves, warfarin should be discontinued and continuous intravenous UFH given starting 2 to 3 weeks before planned delivery. *(Level of Evidence: C)*

CLASS IIA

1. In patients with mechanical prosthetic valves, it is reasonable to avoid warfarin between weeks 6 and 12 of gestation owing to the high risk of fetal defects. *(Level of Evidence: C)*
2. In patients with mechanical prosthetic valves, it is reasonable to resume UFH 4 to 6 h after delivery and begin oral warfarin in the absence of significant bleeding. *(Level of Evidence: C)*
3. In patients with mechanical prosthetic valves, it is reasonable to give low-dose aspirin (75 to 100 mg per day) in the second and third trimesters of pregnancy in addition to anticoagulation with warfarin or heparin. *(Level of Evidence: C)*

CLASS III

1. LMWH should not be administered to pregnant patients with mechanical prosthetic valves unless anti-Xa levels are monitored 4 to 6 h after administration. *(Level of Evidence: C)*
2. Dipyridamole should not be used instead of aspirin as an alternative antiplatelet agent in pregnant patients with mechanical prosthetic valves because of its harmful effects on the fetus. *(Level of Evidence: B)*

aPTT, activated partial thromboplastin time; INR, international normalized ratio; LMWH, low molecular weight heparin; UFH, unfractionated heparin.
SOURCE: Bonow RO, et al.[59]

thrombosis is increased by venous stasis. Prevention is optimal. Prophylactic full-dose heparin or low-molecular-weight heparin[63] is indicated in those at high risk for a thromboembolic complication including women with thromboemboli during a previous pregnancy (percent risk of thrombus/embolus is 4 to 15 percent), antithrombin III deficiency (70 percent), protein C deficiency (33 percent), protein S deficiency (17 percent), and the anticardiolipin antibody syndrome. Prothrombin gene mutations and factor V mutation resulting in the resistance to activated protein C (found in 3 to 5 percent of the population) may eventually be shown to be a reason for prophylaxis as well.[64,65]

If a thrombus or embolus is identified, 5 to 10 days of intravenous heparin therapy followed by full-dose subcutaneous heparin is recommended. If a thromboembolus is life-threatening (e.g., a massive pulmonary embolus or a thrombosed prosthetic valve), thrombolytic therapy can be used.[4]

HYPERTENSION

Hypertension can be present before pregnancy (in 1 to 5 percent) and persist throughout pregnancy, or it can develop with pregnancy.[66–68] When normotensive women become pregnant, 5 to 7 percent will develop hypertension. Because of the marked early fall in systemic vascular resistance, hypertension often does not occur until the second half of pregnancy. It has been identified as *pregnancy-induced* or *gestational hypertension* or *toxemia*. When associated with proteinuria, pedal edema, CNS irritability, elevation of liver enzymes, and coagulation disturbances, the hypertension syndrome is called *preeclampsia*. If convulsions occur, the diagnosis is *eclampsia*. It is not clear that hypertension alone puts the mother or fetus at risk during pregnancy, but preeclampsia increases maternal risk (1 to 2 percent chance of CNS bleed, convulsions, or other severe systemic illness) and can cause fetal growth retardation (10 to 15 percent). Maternal and fetal morbidity and mortality increase still further with eclampsia.

Guidelines for the level of BP control are not well established.[69] Keeping the systolic BP below 160 mmHg and the

TABLE 96-3

Measures to Protect Against a Decrease in Central Blood Volume

Acute
  Position
  - 45–60° left lateral
  - 10° Trendelenburg
  Volume administration—glucose free saline
  Drugs—Ephedrine if unresponsive to fluid replacement
  Anesthetics (if required)
  - Regional: serial small boluses
  - General: emphasis on benzodiazepines and narcotics, low-dose inhalation agents

Chronic
  Full leg stockings
  Avoid vasodilatation drugs

diastolic BP below 100 mmHg provides a margin of safety against severe hypertensive episodes. Unless the patient has previously demonstrated salt-sensitive hypertension, sodium restriction is inadvisable because pregnant women with hypertension have lower plasma volumes than normotensive women. Concern about hypovolemia is a reason to bypass a thiazide diuretic as first-line therapy. A dihydropyridine calcium blocker seems the optimal alternative, for example, sustained-release nifedipine. Large experience with α methyldopa shows it is effective without adverse effects on the fetus. β_1-selective blockers or labetalol have been proven to be effective. Again, ACE inhibitors and ARBs *should not be used.*

❙ ❫ PULMONARY HYPERTENSION

Whether pulmonary hypertension (PH) is primary, or secondary to prolonged left-to-right shunting (Eisenmenger syndrome), to drug abuse, to a vascular disease syndrome, or to recurrent pulmonary emboli, maternal mortality ranges from 30 to 70 percent.[70] Even with maternal survival, fetal loss exceeds 40 percent. The mother is most vulnerable during the time of labor and delivery and in the first postpartum week. If PH is recognized early in pregnancy, interruption of the pregnancy is advised. If this is declined or if the PH is recognized late in pregnancy, close followup is required. Intravascular volume depletion puts these patients at greatest risk. Systemic vascular resistance and pressure must be maintained in patients with PH who have a right-to-left shunt, and meticulous attention to intravenous catheters is essential to avoid systemic emboli. At the time of labor and delivery, a central venous line allows adequate fluid administration, and a radial artery catheter makes determinations of BP and oxygen saturation easier. These lines should be used for 48 to 72 hours postdelivery.

❙ ❫ ARRHYTHMIAS

In the woman with dizziness, palpitations, and light-headedness, pregnancy offers many other explanations, but arrhythmias should be considered as a possible cause. The rules for treatment should be the same as in the nonpregnant patient with the possible exception that a rhythm causing hemodynamic instability should be treated somewhat more rapidly because of concern about diversion of blood flow away from the uterus. As always, if a potentially reversible cause can be identified, it should be corrected.

Tachyarrhythmias are common during pregnancy. The presence of *atrial* or *ventricular premature beats* or of *sinus tachycardia* is a reason to identify and correct the cause but not a reason to institute treatment.

Paroxysmal supraventricular tachycardia is the most common sustained abnormal rhythm occurring with pregnancy.[71,72] Initial treatment with vagal maneuvers is as appropriate as at other times. If urgent treatment is required, intravenous adenosine or verapamil is effective. Cardioversion can be used if required.[73] If recurrent episodes necessitate a daily drug, verapamil or a β blocker is often effective.

Management of *atrial fibrillation* and *flutter* should be as in the nonpregnant woman. If these rhythms occur in a woman with mitral stenosis, severe left ventricular dysfunction, or a previous thromboembolic event, antithrombotic therapy is indicated.

If necessary for refractory arrhythmias, radiofrequency catheter ablation can be performed, optimally later in pregnancy and with radiation shielding.

Ventricular tachycardia can occur during pregnancy. If it is suggestive of a right ventricular outflow tract tachycardia (a left bundle-branch block with vertical axis morphology), β-blocker therapy can be effective. Emergency management of rapid ventricular tachycardia or ventricular fibrillation should be as recommended for the nonpregnant woman. If possible, during acute management, the women should be rolled to her left side to enhance blood return from the lower extremities. If pregnancy has proceeded beyond 24 weeks and maternal survival is in question, emergency cesarean section should be considered. Pregnancies have been successful in women with implanted cardioverter/defibrillators; treatment shocks have no demonstrated adverse effects on the baby.

Repolarization abnormalities that predispose young adults to ventricular fibrillation are not well characterized during pregnancy. Most is known about the prolonged QT-interval syndrome.[74] If this is recognized (usually from transient arrhythmia symptoms) and it is an acquired form, the presumed cause (usually a drug) should be eliminated. If the syndrome is congenital, β-blocker therapy during pregnancy is recommended although unproven.[75] Implantable defibrillators have been used with recurrent ventricular arrhythmias, but their value remains unproven in this syndrome even when it is unrelated to pregnancy. In patients with a congenital syndrome, transmission with autosomal dominance can affect the child. Arrhythmogenic right ventricular dysplasia and Brugada syndrome are even less well characterized with little information related to pregnancy.

Bradyarrhythmias can occur during pregnancy. Although they are a reason to look for a reversible cause, treatment is generally not required unless the patient has clear hemodynamic compromise. Complete heart block, which in this age group is most likely to be congenital in origin, is consistent with a successful pregnancy.[76] If required, a permanent pacemaker can be inserted.

❙ ❫ LOSS-OF-CONSCIOUSNESS SPELLS

Pregnancy makes an assessment of a loss-of-consciousness spell even more difficult than usual. If a seizure disorder cannot be excluded as a cause, appropriate evaluation with electroencephalography is indicated. If a seizure is unlikely or excluded, the syndrome of syncope should include a consideration of the usual causes, most of which are caused by an imbalance of vascular volume and tone or to cardiac arrhythmias.

【 】 ENDOCARDITIS

The clinical presentation of endocarditis is the same during pregnancy as at other times.[77] *Streptococcus* is the most common cause. Intravenous drug abusers are more likely to have staphylococcal infections, and women with genitourinary tract infections are more likely to have gram-negative infections, most commonly because of *Escherichia coli*. Optimal management includes prevention. Although it is not the recommendation of the American Heart Association committee addressing this issue, most physicians caring for women with heart disease recommend antibiotic prophylaxis at the time of dental or surgical procedures or at labor and delivery. If endocarditis does occur, it should be treated aggressively with medical therapy, and the usual indications for surgery are appropriate during pregnancy. If open-heart surgery is required late in pregnancy, simultaneous cesarean section should be considered.

SPECIFIC FORMS OF HEART DISEASE

Other sections of this book discuss specific cardiovascular abnormalities in detail. The remainder of this chapter relates these to pregnancy.

【 】 VALVULAR HEART DISEASE

Worldwide, rheumatic valvular heart disease remains the most common form of heart disease during pregnancy.[78,79] It is less common in Western countries. Definition of valve morphology by echocardiography can help to clarify the etiology. Other causes of valvular heart disease can of course be seen in pregnant women, in particular congenital, although the management through pregnancy is largely the same regardless of etiology. An exception is that those with rheumatic fever as the cause should be advised of antibiotic prophylaxis against a recurrence, even during pregnancy.[80]

【 】 MITRAL STENOSIS

The most common valve disease complicating pregnancy (worldwide), mitral stenosis is often the most poorly tolerated. The increased CO, tachycardia, and fluid retention of pregnancy can double the resting pressure gradient across a stenotic mitral valve. Symptoms attributable to an increase in left atrial pressure occur in up to 25 percent of patients with mitral stenosis (MS) during pregnancy.[81–83] They usually become apparent by the 20th week and can be aggravated still further at the time of labor and delivery. Maternal death is rare when there is careful attention to the management of congestive heart failure. Although potentially at risk from the elevated left atrial pressure, the patient with MS also depends on this pressure to fill the LV. Preservation of an adequate intravascular volume is essential to prevent a dramatic fall in CO.

If a woman contemplating pregnancy has symptomatic MS, balloon dilation or valve surgery should be performed before conception. If MS is first recognized during pregnancy and symptoms develop, standard medical therapy is appropriate. If this does not control symptoms, balloon valvuloplasty can be performed (with appropriate radiation shielding of the fetus).[83] Mitral valve surgical commissurotomy or valve replacement has been performed, but fetal loss exceeds 30 percent. Atrial fibrillation is of particular concern during pregnancy. Emergency treatment of a rapid ventricular response should include intravenous verapamil or cardioversion.

【 】 MITRAL REGURGITATION

In general mitral regurgitation is well tolerated during pregnancy.[83] If it is severe, symptomatic, or associated with LV dysfunction, valve repair before pregnancy is recommended. Afterload reduction is an important component of therapy, remembering that ACE inhibitors and ARBs should not be used. One cause of mitral regurgitation is *mitral valve prolapse*. Pregnancy can alter examination findings but rare associated arrhythmias, endocarditis, cerebral emboli, and hemodynamically significant regurgitation are no more likely to occur during pregnancy than at other times.[84]

【 】 AORTIC STENOSIS

The diagnostic criteria for aortic valve stenosis (AS) are the same during pregnancy as at other times. Pregnancy in the presence of AS can be successful, but if stenosis is severe, maternal deaths have occurred (1 to 2 percent) and congestive heart failure is common.[83,85] The offspring can have an incidence of congenital heart disease as high as 20 percent, a value that interestingly can be reduced by correcting the outflow tract obstruction prior to pregnancy.[86]

If severe AS is recognized before pregnancy, balloon valvotomy or a surgical commissurotomy is recommended prior to conception. If pregnancy does occur in the presence of severe aortic stenosis, measures to avoid hypovolemia are particularly important. If congestive heart failure develops, it can be treated as previously described. If severe symptoms persist, a balloon valvuloplasty or aortic valve surgery can be performed during pregnancy,[83] the latter being associated with increased fetal loss.

【 】 AORTIC REGURGITATION

Aortic regurgitation is a reason to consider Marfan syndrome as a cause (see below)—otherwise it is generally well tolerated during pregnancy. If it is severe, symptomatic, or associated with LV dysfunction, valve surgery should be considered before pregnancy.[82,83] If congestive heart failure occurs with pregnancy, treatment should include afterload reduction. *ACE inhibitors and ARBs should be avoided.* If endocarditis should occur and the infection is not rapidly controlled, mortality with medical therapy is high, and surgical therapy is indicated. If this occurs late in pregnancy, consideration of associated cesarean section is appropriate.

【 】 PULMONIC VALVE DISEASE

Many women with pulmonic valve disease will have had previous valve commissurotomy or balloon valvuloplasty for valve stenosis or as part of the correction of tetralogy of Fallot. The residual stenosis and invariable regurgitation are potential concerns but in general do not adversely affect the outcome of pregnancy. The occasional patient with significant pulmonic valve stenosis who has not been treated appears to tolerate pregnancy well. Intravascular volume depletion should be avoided. If severe symptoms (recurrent syncope, uncontrolled dyspnea, and chest pain) occur, balloon valvuloplasty can be performed.

【 】 TRICUSPID VALVE DISEASE

Significant tricuspid valve disease is also uncommon during pregnancy, although still encountered in patients with Ebstein anomaly (see below). The incidence of regurgitation has increased because of intravenous drug use, with its resultant right-sided endocarditis. This regurgitation usually requires no specific therapy during pregnancy. Tricuspid stenosis is rare. If it is encountered, avoidance of intravascular volume depletion would seem to be important.

【 】 PROSTHETIC VALVE DISEASE

An artificial valve can perhaps be considered the ultimate form of valve disease. Although many have benefited from these valves, all are left with *prosthetic heart valve disease*. One or more of its major associated complications—thromboemboli, bleeding (from anticoagulation), endocarditis, valve dysfunction, reoperation, or death—affects patients at a rate of greater than 5 percent per year throughout their lives. Pregnancy increases the risk of each of these complications, and the prosthetic valve and its treatment can adversely affect the fetus.[87] All these are reasons that a prosthetic valve is a relative contraindication to pregnancy. Still, women with prosthetic valves often become pregnant. When a prosthetic valve is required before pregnancy, valve choice should consider future pregnancies. There is no consensus about the optimal valve choice.

Anticoagulation is required in those with a *mechanical* prosthesis. There are insufficient data to reliably predict or compare clinical outcomes or to confirm the safety of enoxaparin, unfractionated heparin, or warfarin with mechanical heart valves Although debate exists over the optimal means of anticoagulation, that recommended in the American College of Cardiology/American Heart Association (ACC/AHA) guidelines is presented in Table 96–2.[59] In essence, it suggests heparin for the first trimester, then warfarin until the 35th week, then a return to heparin through labor and delivery. Full-dose subcutaneous heparin should be dose-adjusted to maintain a "high therapeutic level" by following factor Xa levels. Low-molecular-weight heparin is an appealing alternative but has not been extensively evaluated in patients with prosthetic valves,[59] and complications have occurred because of insufficient dosing.

It is imperative to overlap heparin and warfarin during the transition phases, particularly postpartum, when hypercoagulability is at its peak.

A *heterograft* or *homograft* prosthesis is an alternative to a mechanical prosthesis. The trade-off, however, of using these valves to avoid anticoagulation is durability. The rate of heterograft degeneration is high in young women, resulting in the need for early valve replacement On balance, when choosing a prosthetic valve for a woman of childbearing age, we usually recommend a mechanical prosthesis for those capable of heparin and warfarin management. If the safe use of anticoagulation is questionable, a bioprosthesis can be preferable.

【 】 CONGENITAL HEART DISEASE

Congenital heart disease is now the most common heart disease encountered in women of childbearing age in the United States.[2,3,88] In many, it has been altered by surgery. Each abnormality is unique, but some issues apply to all. First, some abnormalities significantly increase the risk of maternal morbidity and mortality during pregnancy (Table 96–4). Second, there is an increased risk of fetal death,[3] which

TABLE 96–4

Maternal and Fetal Mortality with Congenital Heart Abnormalities

CHD LESION	MOTHERS	PREGNANCIES	MATERNAL DEATHS (%)	CV COMPLICATIONS (%)	LIVE BIRTHS (%)
All CHD	710	1011	1.3	13	85
Left-to-right shunt	128	269	0	5	82
Any obstructive lesion	179	354	4.0	4	91
All cyanotic	120	303	3.0	14	48
Eisenmenger syndrome	42	53	24.0	—	54
Transposition	54	128	0	11	79
Fontan repair	21	33	0	6	54
Ebstein anomaly	44	111	0	—	82
Marfan syndrome	21	45	4.0	11	74
HOCM	227	371	1.0	—	—

CHD, congenital heart disease; CV, cardiovascular; HOCM, hypertrophic obstructive cardiomyopathy.
The maternal deaths and CV complications are reported as percentage of pregnancies: Live births assumes hospital discharge of an infant.
SOURCE: *Reproduced and modified from Broberg C, et al. Chapter 32. In: Wenger NK and Collins P, eds. Women and Heart Disease. 2nd ed. London: Taylor and Francis; 2006. Used with the permission of the authors and the publisher. The data are from studies referenced in that chapter.*

increases with the severity of the maternal lesions (see Table 96–4). Third, the presence of a congenital cardiac abnormality in either parent or in a sibling increases the risk of cardiac and other congenital abnormalities in the fetus. Congenital heart disease is recognized in 0.8 percent of all live births in the United States.[89] Its presence in a parent increases this risk to 2 to 15 percent with generally a higher recurrence rate from an affected mother rather than father.[88,90,91] There is a 50 percent chance of recurrence from autosomal dominant traits, namely Marfan syndrome, the congenital long-QT syndrome, or hypertrophic cardiomyopathy. Although most lesions are identified in childhood occasionally defects will be diagnosed for the first time during a maternal visit. Nearly all forms of congenital heart disease, corrected with surgery or not, carry some risk for a pregnancy-related complication; the need for preconception referral to an appropriate center cannot be overstated.

【 】 LEFT-TO-RIGHT SHUNTS

Some women with left-to-right shunts reach adulthood and become pregnant without previous recognition of their disease. Although left-to-right shunting increases the chances of PH, right ventricular (RV) failure, arrhythmias, and emboli, it is not certain that these complications are accentuated by a pregnancy. The degree of shunting is generally not affected by pregnancy because the resistances of the systemic and pulmonary vascular circuits fall to a similar degree.[92] The RV volume overload associated with the shunts is generally well tolerated during pregnancy.

Atrial septal defects are the most common cause of left-to-right shunts and can occasionally be first diagnosed at the time of pregnancy. Even if the shunt is large, giving more than a 2:1 pulmonic/systemic flow ratio, pregnancy is generally well tolerated as long as pulmonary vascular resistance is normal (<3.0 Wood units). Transcutaneous closure with an occluder device should make pregnancy even safer, but there is rarely a need to offer this if the woman is already pregnant.

Ventricular septal defects are the most common congenital abnormality in children. *Patent ductus arteriosus* is also common. In adults, these lesions will most likely have either closed spontaneously, been closed surgically, or be small, restrictive lesions without hemodynamic effect (though a loud murmur will be audible). A large, unclosed defect will most likely have resulted in Eisenmenger physiology, highly dangerous for pregnancy as discussed above. Otherwise, these lesions are very well tolerated in pregnancy, with a small risk of arrhythmia or endocarditis.

【 】 RIGHT-TO-LEFT SHUNT (*CYANOTIC* HEART DISEASE)

Right-to-left shunting can occur through septal defects when pulmonary vascular resistance exceeds systemic vascular resistance (Eisenmenger physiology) or when there is an obstruction to RV outflow and pulmonary vascular resistance is normal (most often tetralogy of Fallot or pulmonary atresia). All are forms of *cyanotic* heart disease. The presence of cyanosis, especially when sufficient to result in elevated hemoglobin levels, is associated with high fetal loss, prematurity, and reduced infant birth weights.[2,3,93,94] When pulmonary hypertension is not present, maternal mortality is significantly less, but women are at increased risk of heart failure (ap-

proximately 15 percent) thromboemboli, arrhythmias, and endocarditis (4.5 percent). Providers should consider aspirin as antiplatelet therapy, and early delivery if fetal maturity allows.

Eisenmenger syndrome, or cyanosis caused by reversed or bidirectional shunting from elevated pulmonary vascular resistance, carries a 30 to 50 percent risk of maternal death and a 74 percent risk of fetal loss if the mother survives.[95] Pregnancy is therefore contraindicated, and it is advisable to offer interruption of pregnancy early on if conception occurs. A woman who opts to continue should be put on bedrest, heparin, and oxygen for at least the third trimester, and be monitored closely in the postpartum period without premature hospital discharge.

Tetralogy of Fallot is the most common form of right-to-left shunting resulting from obstruction to pulmonary flow when pulmonary vascular resistance is normal. If it is uncorrected, successful pregnancy can be achieved, but maternal mortality is high, and fetal loss can exceed 50 percent. After surgical correction of the defect, maternal mortality does not clearly exceed that of a woman without heart disease.[96,97]

Women with pulmonary atresia that has been corrected by a Fontan procedure in childhood will, like those who had surgery for tetralogy of Fallot, no longer be cyanotic. The most common issues will be pulmonic valve regurgitation, RV-pulmonary artery (PA) conduit stenosis (in pulmonary atresia), or ventricular tachycardia (see below).

【 】 OBSTRUCTIVE LESIONS

Two recommendations apply in women with any obstructive cardiac lesions. First, volume depletion should be avoided because it can result in a significant fall in CO whether the obstruction is on the left or right side of the heart. Second, surgical or catheter treatment for a left- or right-sided obstructive lesion is recommended prior to pregnancy. During pregnancy, these procedures should only be reserved for patients with severe congestive failure or fetal distress.

Congenital bicuspid aortic stenosis is likely the most common obstructive lesion encountered in pregnancy, and its management is described above. Two other LV obstructive disease processes warrant further discussion: coarctation of the aorta and hypertrophic obstructive cardiomyopathy.

Coarctation of the Aorta

Many women with corrected coarctation will reach childbearing age and conceive. Maternal mortality rates range from 2 to 8 percent.[2] Surgical correction prior to pregnancy reduces the risk of aortic dissection or rupture.[98] If pregnancy occurs in a woman with a coarctation, BP control with β blockers is mandatory, although it can result in reduced placental circulation and needs to be monitored closely. The effects of catheter dilation of a coarctation on subsequent pregnancies are uncertain, but they are as likely to decrease the risks associated with pregnancy as the surgical procedure. It is not clear whether mechanical treatment decreases the rate of rupture of associated intracranial aneurysms.

Hypertrophic Obstructive Cardiomyopathy

Hypertrophic obstructive cardiomyopathy (HOCM) is inherited as an autosomal dominant trait with variable penetrance; offspring of a parent with HOCM have a 50 percent chance of having the abnormality, although phenotypes can vary. It can occur with or without an LV outflow tract obstruction. The fall in peripheral vascular resistance and peripheral pooling of blood during pregnancy can cause hypotension, and the intermittent high catecholamine state of pregnancy can increase LV outflow tract obstruction. An increase in the symptoms of dyspnea, chest discomfort, and palpitations has been noted.[99] It is not clear that pregnancy increases the approximately 1 to 3 percent chance per year of sudden death, but deaths with pregnancy can exceed 1 percent.[99] This is another obstructive lesion where it is important to avoid hypovolemia. β-Blocker therapy is recommended at the time of labor and delivery.

【 】 COMPLEX CONGENITAL LESIONS

Maternal and fetal morbidity and mortality are high, particularly when complex abnormalities result in maternal cyanosis or marked functional limitation. Still, surgery has made pregnancy a consideration.

Transposition of the Great Vessels

Women with dextro (D)-transposition of the great arteries (some with single ventricles) can become pregnant. The little available information available indicates a very poor maternal and fetal outcome.[3,94] Partial or complete surgical correction of the lesion prior to pregnancy improves the outcome for the mother as well as the fetus.[100,101] If l-transposition (*corrected* transposition) is not complicated by cyanosis, ventricular dysfunction, or heart block, pregnancy should be well tolerated.[102]

Ebstein Anomaly of the Tricuspid Valve

This condition encompasses a spectrum that can be mild and unrecognized during pregnancy or severe and associated with other abnormalities. Increasing problems of RV dysfunction, obstruction to right-sided heart flow, and right-to-left shunting resulting in cyanosis increase the risk to the woman during pregnancy. Maternal morbidity and mortality are low if the patient does not have severe disease, and fetal loss is approximately 25 percent: Significant right-to-left shunting is a reason to avoid pregnancy.[103]

Single Ventricle/Fontan

Often patients with a single functional ventricle will have been palliated in childhood with some variant of the Fontan procedure, where venous blood flows passively to the pulmonary capillary bed. Such patients are now reaching adulthood in increasing numbers and are at risk for venous thromboembolism, atrial arrhythmia, and low-output heart failure, as well as complications related to chronic elevation of central venous pressure including hepatic congestion and protein losing enteropathy. Because cardiac output remains relatively fixed because of limitations of pulmonary blood flow, cardiovascular complications, usually heart failure symptoms or arrhythmia, occur in 10 to 20 percent of pregnant patients. There is a high risk of fetal loss (approximately 30 to 50 percent) and prematurity (38 percent).[94,100]

Marfan Syndrome

Women with Marfan syndrome require specialized attention to best address several issues. First, the risk of death from aortic rupture or dissection during pregnancy is high in women with Marfan syndrome, particularly if the aortic root is enlarged (greater than 40 mm by echocardiography).[104] Second, the expected life span of the woman with Marfan syndrome is reduced to approximately one-half of normal, implying that her years of motherhood will be limited. Third, half of the offspring will be affected with the syndrome. Should the parents elect to continue the pregnancy, regular monitoring of the aortic root diameter is required, and activity should be restricted and hypertension prevented. Although unproven, prophylactic use of β blockers during pregnancy seems reasonable. This is the one cardiovascular syndrome where cesarean delivery is recommended to avoid the hemodynamic stresses of labor.

MYOCARDIAL DISEASE
【 】 DILATED CARDIOMYOPATHY

The cause of a dilated cardiomyopathy is often unclear, but up to 30 to 50 percent of these cases are familial.[105,106] Its occurrence is a reason to suggest that pregnancy should be avoided. This recommendation is given because myocardial dysfunction is the feature associated with increased maternal and fetal mortality in many forms of heart disease. It also comes from the observations of those who develop this problem in the third trimester or first 6 weeks postpartum. This *peripartum cardiomyopathy* can simply be a dilated cardiomyopathy occurring in pregnancy, but given the timing of onset, it can be a unique entity.[107,108] Mortality in a group of these young women was 9 percent in one series, most within 2 years of delivery. In the woman with a dilated cardiomyopathy during pregnancy, standard treatment for heart failure, thromboemboli, and arrhythmias is appropriate. If ventricular function does not return to normal after pregnancy, subsequent pregnancies have been associated with maternal mortality rates of 19 to 50 percent.[108] Even in those whose LV function returns to normal, deaths have been reported with subsequent pregnancies.

【 】 HYPERTROPHIC CARDIOMYOPATHY

HOCM with *nonconcentric* hypertrophic cardiomyopathy (HCM) has been discussed as an obstructive or nonobstructive lesion. A concentric HCM can be the result of aortic stenosis or hypertension. If the cause is unexplained, there is little information about its significance during pregnancy.

ISCHEMIC HEART DISEASE

Chest discomfort is common during a normal pregnancy and for the most part is caused by abdominal distension or gastroesophageal reflux. Coronary artery disease (CAD) is an uncommon but possible cause. CAD in pregnancy can result from atherosclerosis, particularly in those with familial hyperlipidemia, diabetes, hypertension, or a smoking history.[109] Other explanations have been dissection of the coronary artery, spasm, emboli, vasculitis, or anomalous origin of a left coronary artery. An ECG and exercise stress test can help with the diagnosis.[110] If essential, MRI of the proximal coronary arteries can be worthwhile. Thallium imaging or angiography can be performed if absolutely necessary. When it is suspected or demonstrated, CAD should be treated with standard medical therapy; angioplasty or bypass surgery can be performed at an experienced center.

PREGNANCY FOLLOWING CARDIAC TRANSPLANTATION

Many cardiac transplant recipients are women of childbearing age. Successful pregnancies after transplantation have been reported,[111] but the potential hazards to the mother and fetus—which include maternal heart failure, immunosuppressive therapy, maternal infections, and serial diagnostic studies—have already been recognized as causing problems in the fetus and in newborns. A shortened maternal life span must also be considered when a patient is counseled about the advisability of pregnancy.

REFERENCES

1. Lewis G, Drife JO. Why mothers die, 2000–2002, 6th report of confidential enquiries into maternal deaths in the UK.
2. Siu SC, Sermer M, Coleman JM, et al. Prospective multicenter study of pregnancy outcomes in women with heart disease. *Circulation.* 2001;104(5):515–521.
3. Siu SC, Colman JM, Sorensen S, et al. Adverse neonatal and cardiac outcomes are more common in pregnant women with cardiac disease. *Circulation.* 2002;105(18):2179–2184.
4. McAnulty JH. Anesthesia during pregnancy in the patient with heart disease. In: Bonica JJ, McDonald JS, eds. *Principles and Practice of Obstetric Analgesia and Anesthesia.* Philadelphia: Lea & Febiger; 1994:1013–1039.
5. Dajani AS, Taubert KA, Wilson W, et al. Prevention of bacterial endocarditis: Recommendations by the American Heart Association. *JAMA.* 1997;277:1794–1801.
6. Monnery L, Nanson J, Charlton G. Primary pulmonary hypertension in pregnancy; a role for novel vasodilators. *Br J Anaesth.* 2001;87(2):295ñ298.
7. Ueland K, Novy MJ, Peterson EN, Metcalfe J. Maternal cardiovascular dynamics: IV. The influence of gestational age on the maternal cardiovascular response to posture and exercise. *Am J Obstet Gynecol.* 1969;104:856–864.
8. Capeless EL, Clapp JF. Cardiovascular changes in early phase of pregnancy. *Am J Obstet Gynecol.* 1989;161:1449–1453.
9. Easterling TR, Benedetti TJ, Schmucher BC, Millard SP. Maternal hemodynamics in normal and preeclamptic pregnancies: A longitudinal study. *Obstet Gynecol.* 1990;76:1061–1069.
10. Robson SC, Hunter S, Boys RJ, Dunlop W. Serial study of factors influencing changes in cardiac output during human pregnancy. *Am J Physiol.* 1989;256:H1060–H1065.
11. Clark SL, Cotton DB, Pivarnik JM, et al. Position change and central hemodynamic profile during normal third-trimester pregnancy and postpartum. *Am J Obstet Gynecol.* 1991;164:883–887.
12. Kinsella SM, Lohmann G. Supine hypotensive syndrome (review). *Obstet Gynecol.* 1994;83:774–788.
13. Robson S, Dunop W, Boys R, Hunter S. Cardiac output during labor. *BMJ.* 1987;295:1169–1172.
14. James C, Banner T, Caton D. Cardiac output in women undergoing cesarean section with epidural or general anesthesia. *Am J Obstet Gynecol.* 1989;160:1178–1183.
15. Clapp JF III, Capeless E. Cardiovascular function before, during, and after the first and subsequent pregnancies. *Am J Cardiol.* 1997;80:1469–1473.
16. Thoresen M, Wesche J. Doppler measurements of changes in human mammary and uterine blood flow during pregnancy and lactation. *Acta Obstet Gynecol Scand.* 1988;67:741–745.
17. Thaler I, Manor D, Itskovitz J, et al. Changes in uterine blood flow during human pregnancy. *Am J Obstet Gynecol.* 1990;162:121–125.
18. Teixerira JM, Fisk NM, Glover V. Association between maternal anxiety in pregnancy and increased uterine artery resistance index: Cohort based study. *BMJ.* 1999;318:1288–1289.
19. Sady MA, Haydon BB, Sady SP, et al. Cardiovascular response to maximal cycle exercise during pregnancy and at two and seven months postpartum. *Am J Obstet Gynecol.* 1990;162:1181–1185.
20. Morton MJ, Paul MS, Campos GR, et al. Exercise dynamics in late gestation: effects of physical training. *Am J Obstet Gynecol.* 1985;152:91–97.
21. Veille JC, Hellerstein HK, Bacevice AE. Maternal left ventricular performance during bicycle exercise. *Am J Cardiol.* 1992;69:1506–1508.
22. Rauramo I, Forss M. Effect of exercise on maternal hemodynamics and placental blood flow in healthy women. *Acta Obstet Gynecol Scand.* 1988;67:21–25.
23. Watson WJ, Katz VL, Hackney AC, et al. Fetal responses to maximal swimming and cycling exercise during pregnancy. *Obstet Gynecol.* 1991;77:382–386.
24. Clapp JF III, Capeless EL. Neonatal morphometrics after endurance exercise during pregnancy. *Am J Obstet Gynecol.* 1990;163:1805–1811.
25. Naeye RL, Peters EC. Working during pregnancy: effects on the fetus. *Pediatrics.* 1982;69:724–727.
26. Clapp JF III. Pregnancy outcome: Physical activities inside versus outside the workplace. *Semin Perinatol.* 1996;20(1):70–76.
27. Sternfeld B. Physical activity and pregnancy outcome: review and recommendations. *Sports Med.* 1997;23(1):33–47.
28. Campbell MK, Mottola MF. Recreational exercise and occupational activity during pregnancy and birth weight: a case-control study. *Am J Obstet Gynecol.* 2001;184(3):403–408.
29. Practice ACO. ACOG Committee opinion. Number 267 January 2002: exercise during pregnancy and the postpartum period. *Obstet Gynecol.* 2002;99(1):171–173.
30. Lindheimer MC, Katz AL. Sodium and diuretics in pregnancy. *N Engl J Med.* 1973;299:891–894.
31. Chesley LC. Plasma and red cell volumes during pregnancy. *Am J Obstet Gynecol.* 1972;112:440–450.
32. Katz R, Karliner JS, Resnik R. Effects of a natural volume overload state (pregnancy) on left ventricular performance in normal human subjects. *Circulation.* 1978;58:434–441.
33. Sadaniantz A, Kocheril AG, Emans SP, et al. Cardiovascular changes in pregnancy evaluated by two-dimensional and Doppler echocardiography. *J Am Soc Echo.* 1992;5:253–258.
34. Veille JC, Kitzman DW, et al. Left ventricular diastolic filling response to stationary bicycle exercise during pregnancy and the postpartum period. *Am J Obstet Gynecol.* 2001;185(4);822–827.
35. Uebing, A, et al. Pregnancy and congenital heart disease. *BMJ.* 2006;332(7538):401–406.
36. Hart MV, Morton MJ, Hosenpud JD, Metcalfe J. Aortic function during normal human pregnancy. *Am J Obstet Gynecol.* 1986;154:887–891.
37. Poppas A, Shroff SG, Korcarz CE, et al. Serial assessment of the cardiovascular system in normal pregnancy: role of arterial compliance and pulsatile arterial load. *Circulation.* 1997;95:2407–2415.
38. Edouard DA, Pannier BM, London GM, et al. Venous and arterial behavior during normal pregnancy. *Am Physiol.* 1998;274:H1605–H1612.
39. Anderson RA, Fineron PW. Aortic dissection in pregnancy: importance of pregnancy-induced changes in the vessel wall and bicuspid aortic valve in pathogenesis. *Br J Obstet Gynaecol.* 1994;101:1085–1088.
40. Nolte JE, Rutherford RB, Nawaz S, et al. Arterial dissections associated with pregnancy (review). *J Vasc Surg.* 1995;21:515–520.
41. Toglia MR, Weg JH. Venous thromboembolism during pregnancy. *N Engl J Med.* 1996;335:108–113.
42. Collins R, Yusuf S, Peto R. Overview of randomized trials of diuretics in pregnancy. *BMJ.* 1985;290:17–23.
43. Damilakis J, Theocharopoulos N, Perisinakis K, et al. Conceptus radiation dose and risk from cardiac catheter ablation procedures. *Circulation.* 2001;104(8):893–897.
44. Antihypertensive and Lipid-lowering Treatment to Prevent Heart Attack Trial (ALLHAT) Collaborative Research Group. Major outcomes in high-risk hypertensive patients randomized to angiotensin-converting enzyme inhibitor or calcium channel blocker vs. diuretic. *JAMA.* 2002;2888:2981–2997.
45. Magee LA, Elran E, Bull SB, et al. Risks and benefits of beta-receptor blockers for pregnancy hypertension: overview of the randomized trials. *Eur J Obstet Gynecol Reprod Biol.* 2000;88(1):15–26.
46. Sibai BM. Treatment of hypertension in pregnant women (review). *N Engl J Med.* 1996;335:257–265.
47. Tan HL, Lie KI. Treatment of tachyarrhythmias during pregnancy and lactation. *Eur Heart J.* 2001;22(6):458–464.
48. Oudijk MA, Michon MM, Kleinman CS, et al. Sotalol in the treatment of fetal dysrhythmias. *Circulation.* 2000;101(23):2721–2726.
49. Magee LA, Downar E, Sermer M, et al. Pregnancy outcome after gestational exposure to amiodarone in Canada. *Am J Obstet Gynecol.* 1995;172:1307–1311.

50. Stempel JE, O'Grady JP, Morton MJ, Johnson KA. Use of sodium nitroprusside in complications of gestational hypertension. *Obstet Gynecol.* 1982;60:533–538.

51. Shoemaker CT, Meyers M. Sodium nitroprusside for control of severe hypertensive disease of pregnancy: a case report and discussion of potential toxicity. *Am J Obstet Gynecol.* 1984;149:171–173.

52. Hanssens M, Keirse MJ, Vankelecom F, et al. Fetal and neonatal effects of treatment with angiotensin converting enzyme inhibitors in pregnancy. *Obstet Gynecol.* 1991;78:128–135.

53. Cooper WD, Hernandez-Diaz, S, Arbogast PQ, et al. Major congenital malformations after first-trimester exposure to ACE inhibitors. *N Engl J Med.* 2006;354:2443–2451.

54. Lambot MA, Vermeylen D, Noel JC. Angiotensin-II-receptor inhibitors in pregnancy. *Lancet.* 2001;357(9268):1619–1620.

55. Martinovic J, Benachi A, Laurent N, et al. Fetal toxic effects and angiotensin-II-receptor antagonists. *Lancet.* 2001;358:241.

56. Hall JT, Pauli RM, Wilson KM. Maternal and fetal sequelae of anticoagulation during pregnancy. *Am J Med.* 1980;68:122.

57. Hung L, Rahimtoola SH. Prosthetic heart valves and pregnancy. *Circulation.* 2003;107:1240–1246.

58. Vitale N, De Feo M, De Santo LS, et al. Dose-dependent fetal complications of warfarin in pregnant women with mechanical heart valves. *J Am Coll Cardiol.* 1999;33:1637–1641.

59. Bonow RO, et al. ACC/AHA 2006 guidelines for the management of patients with valvular heart disease: a report of the American College of Cardiology/American Heart Association Task Force on Practice Guidelines (writing Committee to Revise the 1998 guidelines for the management of patients with valvular heart disease) developed in collaboration with the Society of Cardiovascular Anesthesiologists endorsed by the Society for Cardiovascular Angiography and Interventions and the Society of Thoracic Surgeons. *J Am Coll Cardiol.* 2006;48(3):e1–e148.

60. Ginsberg JS, Chan WS, Bates SM, et al. Anticoagulation of pregnant women with mechanical heart valves. *Arch Intern Med.* 2003;163:694–698.

61. Werler MM, Mitchell AA, Shapiro S. The relation of aspirin use during the first trimester of pregnancy to congenital cardiac defects. *N Engl J Med.* 1989;321:1639–1642.

62. Haemostatis and Thrombosis Task Force. Guidelines on the prevention, investigation and management of thrombosis associated with pregnancy: Maternal and neonatal haemostasis working papers of the Haemostasis and Thrombosis Task Force. *J Clin Pathol.* 1993;46:489–496.

63. Sturridge F, de Swiet M, Letsky E. The use of low molecular weight heparin for thrombophylaxis in pregnancy. *Br J Obstet Gynaecol.* 1994;101:69–71.

64. Hellgren M, Svensson PJ, Dahlback B. Resistance to activated protein C as a basis for venous thromboembolism associated with pregnancy and oral contraceptives. *Am J Obstet Gynecol.* 1995;173:210–213.

65. Gerhart A, Scharf RE, Beckmann MW, et al. Prothrombin and factor V mutations in women with a history of thrombosis during pregnancy and the puerperium. *N Engl J Med.* 2000;342:374–380.

66. Rey E, LeLorier J, Burgess E, et al. Report of the Canadian Hypertension Society Consensus Conference: 3. Pharmacologic treatment of hypertensive disorders in pregnancy. *Can Med Assoc J.* 1997;157:1245–1254.

67. Witlin AG, Sibai BM. Hypertension. *Clin Obstet Gynecol.* 1998;41:533–544.

68. Churchill D. The new American guidelines on the hypertensive disorders of pregnancy. *J Hum Hypertens.* 2001;15:583–585.

69. Abalos E, Duley L, Steyn DW, Henderson-Smart DJ. Antihypertensive drug therapy for mild to moderate hypertension during pregnancy. *Cochrane Database Syst Rev.* 2007 update; CD002252.

70. Weiss BM, Hess OM. Pulmonary vascular disease and pregnancy: current controversies, management strategies, and perspectives. *Eur Heart J.* 2000;21:104–115.

71. Widerhorn J, Widerhorn AL, Rahimtoola SH, Elkayam U. WPW syndrome during pregnancy: increased incidence of supraventricular arrhythmias. *Am Heart J.* 1992;123:796–798.

72. Lee SH, Chan SA, Wu TJ, et al. Effects of pregnancy on first onset and symptoms of paroxysmal supraventricular tachycardia. *Am J Cardiol.* 1995;76:675–678.

73. Rosemond RL. Cardioversion during pregnancy. *JAMA.* 1993;269:3167.

74. Rashba EJ, Zareba W, Moss AJ, et al. Influence of pregnancy on the risk for cardiac events in patients with hereditary long QT syndrome. LQTS Investigators. *Circulation.* 1998;97:451–456.

75. Hobbs JB, et al. Risk of aborted cardiac arrest or sudden cardiac death during adolescence in the long-QT syndrome. *JAMA.* 2006;296(10):1249ñ1254.

76. Dalvi BV, Chaudhuri A, Kulkarni HL, Kale PA. Therapeutic guidelines for congenital complete heart block presenting in pregnancy. *Obstet Gynecol.* 1994;79:802–804.

77. Ebrahimi R, Leung CY, Elkayam U, Reid CL. Infective endocarditis. In: Gleicher N, ed. *Principles and Practice of Medical Therapy in Pregnancy,* 2d ed. Norwalk, CT: Appleton & Lange; 1992:795–801.

78. McAnulty JH. Rheumatic heart disease. In: Gleicher N, Gall SA, Sibai BM, et al. eds. *Principles and Practice of Medical Therapy in Pregnancy,* 2d ed. Norwalk, CT: Appleton & Lange; 1992:783–788.

79. Avila WS, Rossi EG, Ramires JA, et al. Pregnancy in patients with heart disease: experience with 1,000 cases. *Clin Cardiol.* 2003;26:135–142.

80. Dajani AS, Bisno AL, Chung KJ, et al. Prevention of rheumatic fever. *Circulation.* 1988;78:1082–1086.

81. Desai DK, Adanlawo M, Naidoo DP, et al. Mitral stenosis in pregnancy: a four-year experience at King Edward VIII Hospital, Durban, South Africa. *Br J Obstet Gynaecol.* 2000;107(8):953–958.

82. Hameed A, Karaalp IS, et al. The effect of valvular heart disease on maternal and fetal outcome of pregnancy. *J Am Coll Cardiol.* 2001;37(3):893–899.

83. Elkayam U, Bitar F. Valvular heart disease and pregnancy part I. Native valves. *J Am Coll Cardiol.* 2005;46(2):223ñ230.

84. Nishimura RA, McGoon MD. Perspectives on mitral-valve prolapse. *N Engl J Med.* 1999;341(1):48–59.

85. Silversides CK, Coleman JM, Sermaer M, Farine D, Siu S. Early and intermediate term outcomes of pregnancy with congenital aortic stenosis. *Am J Cardiol.* 203;91:1386–1389.

86. Whittemore R, Hobbins JC, Engle MA. Pregnancy and its outcome in women with and without surgical treatment of congenital heart disease. *Am J Cardiol.* 1982;50:641–651.

87. North RA, Sadler L, Stewart AW, et al. Long-term survival and valve-related complications in young women with cardiac valve replacements. *Circulation.* 1999;99:2669–2676.

88. Broberg, CEA. Women and congenital heart disease. In: Wenger NK and Collins P, eds. *Women and Heart Disease.* London: Taylor & Francis; 2005:459–460.

89. Nora JJ, Nora AH. The evolution of specific genetic and environmental counseling in congenital heart disease. *Circulation.* 1978;57:205–213.

90. Morris CD, Menashe VD. Evidence for maternal transmission of congenital heart defects. *Circulation.* 1993;88(suppl):1–98.

91. Whittemore R, Wells JA, Castellsagne X. A second-generation study of 427 probands with congenital heart defects and their 837 children. *J Am Coll Cardiol.* 1994;23:1459–1467.

92. Metcalfe J, Ueland K. Maternal cardiovascular adjustments to pregnancy. *Prog Cardiovasc Dis.* 1974;16:363–374.

93. Neill CA, Swanson S. Outcome of pregnancy in congenital heart disease. *Circulation.* 1961;24:1003–1011.

94. Presbytero P, Sommerville J, Stone S, et al. Pregnancy and cyanotic congenital heart disease, outcome of mother and fetus. *Circulation.* 1994;89:2673–2676.

95. Yentis SM, Steer PJ, Plaat F. Eisenmenger's syndrome in pregnancy: maternal and fetal mortality in the 1990s. *Br J Obstet Gynaecol.* 1998;105:921–922.

95a. Avila WS, Grinberg M, Snitcowsky R, et al. Maternal and fetal outcome in pregnant women with Eisenmenger's syndrome. *Eur Heart J.* 1995;16:460–464.

96. Morris CD, Manashe VD. 25-year mortality after surgical repair of congenital heart defect in childhood: a population-based cohort study. *JAMA.* 1991;266:3447–3452.

97. Veldtman GR, Connolly HM, Grogan M, Ammash NM, Warnes CA, Outcomes of pregnancy in women with tetralogy of Fallot. *J Am Coll Cardiol.* 2004;44(1):174–180.

98. Beauchesne LM, Connolly HM, Ammash NM, et al. Coarctation of the aorta: outcome of pregnancy. *J Am Coll Cardiol.* 2001;38(6):1728–1733.

99. Autore C, Conte MR, Piccininno M, et al. Risk associated with pregnancy in hypertrophic cardiomyopathy. *J Am Coll Cardiol.* 2002;40:1864–1869.

100. Conobbio MM, Mair DD, Velde M, Koos BJ. Pregnancy outcomes after the Fontan repair. *J Am Coll Cardiol.* 1996;28:763–767.

101. Clarkson PM, Wilson NJ, Neutze JM, et al. Outcome of pregnancy after the Mustard operation for transposition of the great arteries with intact ventricular septum. *J Am Coll Cardiol.* 1994;24:190–193.

102. Connolly H, Grogan M, Warnes CA. Pregnancy among women with congenitally corrected transposition of great arteries. *J Am Coll Cardiol.* 1999;33:1692–1695.

103. Connolly HM, Warnes CA. Ebstein's anomaly: outcome of pregnancy. *J Am Coll Cardiol* 1994;23:1194–1198.

104. Lipscomb KJ, Smith JC, Clarke B, et al. Outcome of pregnancy in women with Marfan's syndrome. *Br J Obstet Gynecol.* 1997;104(2):201–206.

105. Grunig E, Tasman JA, Kucherer H, et al. Frequency and phenotypes of familial dilated cardiomyopathy. *J Am Coll Cardiol.* 1998;31:86–94.

106. Olson TM, Michels VV, Thibodeau SN, et al. Actin mutations in dilated cardiomyopathy, a heritable form of heart failure. *Science.* 1998;280:750–752.

107. O'Connell JB, Costanzo-Mordin MR, Surbranian R, et al. Peripartum cardiomyopathy: Clinical, hemodynamic, histologic and prognostic characteristics. *J Am Coll Cardiol.* 1986;8:52–56.

108. Elkayam U, Tummala PP, Rao K, et al. Maternal and fetal outcomes of subsequent pregnancies in women with peripartum cardiomyopathy. (comment) [erratum appears in *N Engl J Med* 2001;345(7):552]. *N Engl J Med.* 2001;344(21):1567–1571.

109. Roth A, Elkayam U. Acute myocardial infarction associated with pregnancy. *Ann Intern Med.* 1996;125:751–762.

110. Garry D, Leikin E, Fleisher AG, Tejani N. Acute myocardial infarction in pregnancy with subsequent medical and surgical management. *Obstet Gynecol.* 1996;87(5 pt 2):802–804.

111. Morini A, Spina V, Aleandri V, et al. Pregnancy after heart transplant: update and case report. *Hum Reprod* 1998;13:749–757.

CHAPTER (97)

Traumatic Heart Disease

Panagiotis N. Symbas

Accidental or intentional trauma is the leading cause of death, hospitalization, and loss of working days among young people in American society.[1–3] Cardiac and great vessel injuries are a major contributor to this mortality and morbidity.[4]

The heart and/or great vessels are usually injured from penetrating and nonpenetrating trauma. Other causes of cardiac injuries include iatrogenic trauma caused by the various diagnostic, therapeutic, and resuscitative procedures[5–7] and ionizing radiation[8] and electric currents.[9]

Many nonpenetrating injuries and an occasional penetrating injury of the heart are well tolerated. In addition, frequently these cardiac injuries are overshadowed by the more overt manifestations of cerebral, abdominal, or musculoskeletal trauma. As a result, they can be overlooked unless a high index of suspicion is maintained, and specific studies are obtained.

PENETRATING INJURIES

Penetrating injuries usually are observed with wounds of the precordium but also can be associated with wounds elsewhere in the chest, neck, or upper abdomen. They usually are caused by missile or knife wounds but occasionally are caused by a missile embolus reaching the heart through the venous system.

▌▌ PENETRATING CARDIAC TRAUMA

Although penetrating cardiac trauma frequently involves only the free cardiac wall, injury to cardiac valves, chordae tendineae, papillary muscles, atrial or ventricular septum, coronary arteries, and the conduction system can occur. The multiplicity of heart and great vessel lesions that can be produced by penetrating wounds is indicated in Table 97–1.

The relative frequency of a single penetrating wound of the free cardiac wall is caused by its area of exposure on the anterior chest wall. In decreasing order of frequency, the structures affected are the right ventricle, left ventricle, right atrium, and left atrium.[10] Cardiac wounds can be single or multiple; the latter more commonly are caused by missiles.[11–13]

The pathophysiologic consequences and clinical manifestations of penetrating injuries to the heart depend on the size and site of the wound, the mode of injury, and especially the state of the pericardial wound. When the pericardial wound remains open and bleeding occurs freely into the pleural space, there are signs and symptoms of hemothorax and loss of circulating blood volume. When there is intrapericardial hemorrhage with a sealed pericardial wound, cardiac tamponade (see Chap. 80) is the presenting clinical picture. The diagnosis of cardiac injury should be suspected in a patient with chest, lower neck, epigastric, or especially precordial penetrating wounds and with symptoms and signs of cardiac tamponade and/or hemothorax and loss of circulating blood volume. The management of penetrating wounds of the heart consists of immediate thoracotomy and cardiorrhaphy.[10,12,14] When this cannot be done or while appropriate arrangements are made for thoracotomy, the patient's blood volume should be expanded; pericardiocentesis is performed only to provide time for a safe operation.

Although the management of symptomatic patients with a suspected penetrating cardiac wound is clearly defined, the management of the asymptomatic patients with penetrating precordial wounds presented a considerable dilemma in the past, when the op-

TABLE 97-1

Penetrating Wounds of the Heart

I. Pericardial damage
  A. Laceration or perforation
  B. Hemopericardium with or without cardiac tamponade
  C. Serofibrinous or suppurative pericarditis
  D. Pneumopericardium
  E. Constrictive pericarditis
II. Myocardial damage
  A. Laceration
  B. Penetration or perforation
  C. Retained foreign body
  D. Structural defects
    1. Aneurysm formation
    2. Septal defects
    3. Aortocardiac fistula
III. Valvular injury
  A. Leaflet or cusp injury
  B. Papillary muscle or chordae tendineae laceration
IV. Coronary artery injury
  A. Laceration or thrombosis with or without myocardial infarction
  B. Arteriovenous fistula
  C. Aneurysm
V. Embolism
  A. Foreign body
  B. Thrombus (septic or sterile)
VI. Infective endocarditis
VII. Rhythm or conduction disturbances

SOURCE: Courtesy of Loren F. Parmley, MD and Thomas W.E. Mattingly.

tions were either exploratory surgery or observation. Currently, the immediate use of echocardiography makes the treatment of these patients safer by avoiding unnecessary surgery or observation, with its accompanying risk of sudden deterioration and even death.[15]

【 】 RESIDUAL OR DELAYED SEQUELAE OF PENETRATING CARDIAC TRAUMA

Patients with penetrating cardiac wounds should be observed closely immediately postoperatively and after discharge for the clinical manifestations of residual or delayed sequelae. Such sequelae can include (1) ventricular or atrial septal defect; (2) injury of the valve cups, leaflets, or chordae tendineae; (3) aortocardiac or aortopulmonary communication, or communication from the coronary artery to the coronary vein or the cardiac chamber; (4) ventricular aneurysms; (5) posttraumatic or postoperative pericarditis; and (6) electrocardiographic abnormalities.[16,17] When symptoms and signs of a structural defect are detected, echocardiography and/or cardiac catheterization should be performed to define the lesion and its hemodynamic significance and determine the proper mode of therapy.

Posttraumatic pericarditis, which is similar to the postcardiotomy syndrome seen after cardiac surgery, occurs in approximately 20 percent of all cases of penetrating heart wounds. Medical management is the treatment of choice for this syndrome unless car-

diac tamponade or other sequelae, such as purulent or constrictive pericarditis, require surgical intervention.

Missile wounds also can result in the presence of a projectile within the heart after either a direct injury to the heart or an injury to a systemic vein with subsequent migration of the missile to the heart. The missile or the thrombus associated with it can embolize into the systemic or pulmonary arteries.[18–20] Bacterial endocarditis also can occur if the projectile is not completely embedded in the myocardium.[21] Rarely, a patient with a projectile in the heart can develop cardiac neurosis.[22] In many patients, however, the retained missile in the heart results in no ill effects over a long period of observation.[23,24] Therefore, the treatment for missiles in the heart should be individualized according to the patient's clinical course and the location, size, and shape of the missile.[23,24] Missiles that cause symptoms should be removed. Similarly, missiles that are free or partially protruding into a left cardiac chamber should be removed, because their embolization to the systemic arterial system can have serious consequences.[23,24] Missiles in the right side of the heart can be removed or left to embolize to the pulmonary vascular bed, from which they can be retrieved easily.[19] Intramyocardial and intrapericardial bullets and pellets are generally well tolerated and can be left in place.

A missile that has embolized to the systemic arterial bed should be removed without delay unless it has resulted in a significant neurologic deficit.[20] Projectiles adjacent to or embedded within the wall of one of the great or coronary arteries should be extracted to prevent subsequent erosion and bleeding.

【 】 CORONARY ARTERY PENETRATING TRAUMA

Coronary artery injuries can result in cardiac tamponade and varying degrees of myocardial ischemia or myocardial infarction. The management of these wounds is dependent on the amount of myocardium at risk. Wounds of major branches of the coronary arterial system are repaired or bypassed, whereas small terminal vessels are ligated. Coronary artery aneurysms and arteriovenous fistulas are rare sequelae of injury, and their treatment should be individualized.[25]

【 】 PENETRATING TRAUMA OF THE AORTA AND GREAT VESSELS

The pathophysiology of penetrating wounds to the great vessels is quite similar to that of penetrating wounds to the heart and depends on whether the site of the wound is intra- or extrapericardial.[26,27] In addition to the obvious results of immediate or delayed hemorrhage, a penetrating wound of a great vessel can result in the formation of a false aneurysm, with possible subsequent rupture, or an arteriovenous fistula, producing immediate or latent signs and symptoms of congestive heart failure.[28] Traumatic arteriovenous fistulas occasionally are complicated by the development of bacterial endarteritis and endocarditis.[29] These traumatic vascular lesions should be detected and repaired as soon as possible.

NONPENETRATING INJURIES

The vast majority of blunt injuries to the heart are caused by automobile accidents, although other forms of blunt trauma also can result in this type of injury. The cardiac injury usually is caused by direct compressing or decelerating forces delivered to the chest or rarely by an indirect force delivered to the abdomen that results in a marked increase in intravascular pressures. A wide variety of injuries are produced by nonpenetrating trauma (Table 97–2).

CARDIAC CONTUSION

Contusion of the heart usually refers to blunt injury that causes identifiable histopathologic changes within the myocardium. The pathologic lesions of myocardial contusion vary considerably, ranging from small areas of petechiae or ecchymosis to contusion of the full thickness of the myocardial wall with or without rupture of the heart.[1]

The forces that produce nonpenetrating lesions of the heart are such that external evidence of chest injury can be meager or undetectable. This lack of evidence of chest wall injury and the frequent absence of symptoms from the cardiac injury, along with the common presence of other, more obvious injuries to the body, can impede the early diagnosis of cardiac contusion.

Patients with contusions of the heart are commonly asymptomatic, but they can occasionally complain of pain that is identical to myocardial ischemia and/or myocardial infarction.[30] The pain is usually transient unless there is concomitant coronary artery injury or occult atherosclerotic coronary heart disease.[31] Coronary thrombosis can result from nonpenetrating trauma, but this is rare and usually is associated with existing atherosclerotic coronary artery disease.[32] Dyspnea and hypotension are rarely presenting symptoms. In mild or moderate myocardial contusion, these signs can be transient and are usually absent. Cardiac failure is relatively rare; when it is present, the possibility of an associated cardiac injury, such as rupture of the ventricular septum or of one of the cardiac valves, is high. The diagnosis of cardiac contusion should be suspected in all patients with significant blunt trauma, particularly to the precordium. Unfortunately, none of the currently available diagnostic tests for myocardial contusion can conclusively establish the diagnosis in all patients. The appropriate use and interpretation of the available tests, however, can assist in the diagnosis of myocardial contusion with reasonable accuracy.

Electrocardiography has been the most widely used test for the diagnosis of contusion of the heart. Various electrocardiographic abnormalities have been considered suggestive of cardiac contusion, such as nonspecific ST-T or Q-wave changes, supraventricular tachyarrhythmias, and ventricular arrhythmias, including fibrillation, which is usually the cause of death at the time of the traumatic impact.[33,34] However, a variety of other clinical conditions[35–37] that are frequently present in traumatized patients (i.e., pain, anxiety, hemorrhage, hypoxia, hypokalemia, head trauma, or alcohol or cocaine toxicity) can cause many of these abnormalities. Therefore, the presence of these other causes must be excluded before the electrocardiographic abnormalities are attributed to contusion of the heart.[38,39]

Elevation of the serum level of the myocardial band (MB) fraction of creatinine kinase (CK) has been extrapolated from its use in acute myocardial infarction as a diagnostic aid in patients with cardiac contusion. Other clinical conditions that cause elevation in the level of this enzyme (i.e., tachyarrhythmias and skeletal muscle diseases, including trauma; see Chap. 52) must be excluded before an abnormal level is ascribed to contusion of the heart.[38,39]

TABLE 97–2

Nonpenetrating Trauma of the Heart

1. Pericardial injury
   a. Hemopericardium
   b. Rupture or laceration
   c. Serofibrinous pericarditis
   d. Constrictive pericarditis
2. Myocardial injury
   a. Contusion
   b. Rupture of free cardiac wall, early or delayed
   c. Rupture of septum
   d. Aneurysm
   e. Laceration
3. Disturbances of rhythm or conduction
4. Valve injury
   a. Rupture of valve leaflets, cusp, or chordae tendineae
   b. Contusion of papillary muscle
5. Coronary artery injury
   a. Thrombosis with or without myocardial infarction
   b. Arteriovenous fistula
   c. Laceration with or without myocardial infarction
6. Great vessel injury
   a. Rupture
   b. Aneurysm formation
   c. Aorta-cardiac chamber fistula
   d. Thrombotic occlusion

Two-dimensional transthoracic and transesophageal echocardiography (TTE and TEE) are useful in the diagnosis of cardiac contusion, particularly of the structural lesions associated with cardiac contusion.[40,41] The sensitivity and specificity of these tests for diagnosing contusion of the heart, however, have not been clearly defined (see Chap. 15).

Circulating cardiac troponin I has been measured in many blunt trauma victims, with contradictory conclusions as to its diagnostic value of cardiac contusion.[2,43]

The treatment of myocardial contusion is symptomatic. Prevention and early treatment of arrhythmias are the most important therapeutic measures. Appropriate antiarrhythmic agents (see Chap. 35) should be used to control ectopic rhythms, and congestive heart failure should be treated with angiotensin-converting enzyme (ACE) inhibitors. If the myocardial contusion is severe, support with inotropic drugs (see Chap. 25) can be necessary. When all these measures fail, balloon counterpulsation[4] or even a left ventricular assist device[5] can be used.

CARDIAC RUPTURE

Although minor, insignificant myocardial contusion of the right ventricle is the most common blunt cardiac injury; the most fatal lesion is rupture of the heart. The rupture can occur in the free cardiac wall or the ventricular septum. Rupture of the free cardiac wall is extremely difficult to diagnose and treat in a timely manner because of the frequently rapid demise of the patient and because traumatic cardiac rupture is often only one of many severe bodily injuries. As a result, rupture of the heart has not usually been amenable to therapy. The immediate use of echocardiography in emergency rooms, however, can increase the number of successfully treated patients.[46]

【 】 RESIDUAL OR DELAYED SEQUELAE OF BLUNT INJURY TO THE HEART

Contusion of the heart usually heals with little or no obvious scarring or impairment of cardiac function. Large contusions, however, can cause a decrease in cardiac function, and extensive necrosis can lead to rupture or, rarely, congestive heart failure and the formation of a true or false aneurysm.[47] Cardiac aneurysms can cause arrhythmias, congestive heart failure, rupture, and mural thrombosis with embolism. Because of these complications, surgical repair of a traumatic aneurysm is advisable. Localized areas of necrosis and hemorrhage involving the cardiac conduction system can produce various conduction defects.

The most commonly injured valve in surviving patients is the aortic valve, with aortic regurgitation characteristically causing the rapid development of congestive heart failure. Injury of the atrioventricular valves is an uncommon result of nonpenetrating cardiac injury and usually occurs in the presence of severe cardiac trauma, resulting in death. Rupture of the mitral valve leaflet can have hemodynamic consequences somewhat similar to those of aortic valve injury but rarely is encountered clinically. In contrast, tricuspid valve injury can be tolerated for years before surgical correction is required.

Rupture of the papillary muscle or chordae tendineae occurs more frequently than does rupture of valve leaflets. Cardiac contusion also can cause papillary muscle dysfunction with secondary mitral or tricuspid regurgitation.[48] The clinical outcome depends on whether the structures involved are on the right side of the heart, where the lesion can be well tolerated, or the left side, where the high-pressure system can lead to more serious hemodynamic sequelae. The murmurs produced by these lesions are generally typical of valvular regurgitation, but unusual high-pitched systolic and diastolic murmurs of variable loudness also can result (see Chap. 12). Tricuspid regurgitation can be present despite the absence of a detectable murmur.[49] Prompt and correct diagnosis by echocardiographic, hemodynamic, and angiographic studies is important. Patients with hemodynamically significant valvular injury should undergo valve repair or replacement.

Pericardial lesions often are overlooked and frequently heal without incident. Hemopericardium can occur but usually is caused by the coexisting myocardial injury. Posttraumatic pericarditis develops less frequently with blunt than with penetrating cardiac injuries. The symptoms and signs of posttraumatic pericarditis are similar to those of pericarditis produced by a wide variety of causes (see Chap. 80). When hemopericardium or hydropericardium is suspected, echocardiography can confirm the diagnosis. Pericardial laceration usually is well tolerated, but herniation of the heart can occur, leading to more serious consequences and death.[50]

【 】 AORTIC RUPTURE

Rupture of the aorta is the most common blunt injury of the great vessels. Rupture or avulsion of the innominate, carotid, or left subclavian arteries or the venae cavae also has been observed. Because of the variety of mechanical forces produced by blunt trauma (Fig. 97–1), combined with anatomic factors, the most common sites of rupture

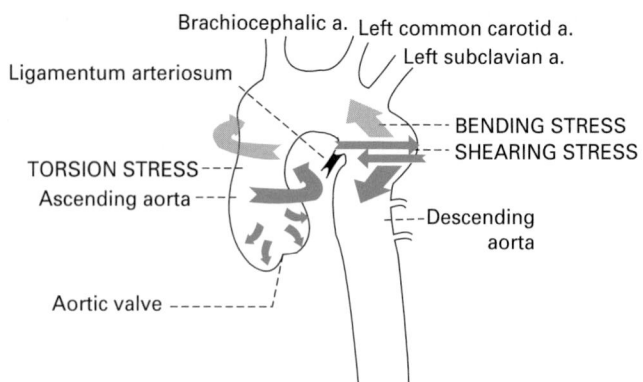

FIGURE 97–1. Diagrammatic illustration of the forces acting on the aortic wall during rupture of the aorta from blunt trauma. a., artery. *Source: Symbas PN. Traumatic Injuries of the Heart and Great Vessels. Springfield, IL: Charles C Thomas; 1971:153. Courtesy of Charles C Thomas, Publisher, Springfield, Illinois.*

of the aorta from blunt injury are the descending aorta just distal to the origin of the left subclavian artery (aortic isthmus) and the ascending aorta commonly just above the aortic valve.[51–53] Because of the high incidence of severe cardiac injury in patients with rupture of the ascending aorta, most of the patients who survive aortic rupture long enough to receive definitive surgical correction are those who have sustained rupture of the aortic isthmus. This is most commonly produced by deceleration injuries suffered in automobile accidents. Approximately 20 percent of patients with aortic rupture survive the original injury. A false aneurysm is formed in these patients at the site of rupture, the wall of which consists of adventitia and/or parietal pleura and other mediastinal structures. The intactness of these structures maintains continuity of the circulation.

The clinical manifestations of traumatic rupture of the aorta can include chest and/or midscapular pain, a new murmur, increased pulse amplitude, and hypertension of the upper extremities. Some patients, however, are surprisingly free of any major symptoms or signs from the aortic rupture. Although there are occasionally no obvious signs of external injury, patients with rupture of the aorta usually have associated injuries of the skeleton, abdominal viscera, or central nervous system that can mask the signs of aortic rupture. For this reason, *any patient who has sustained severe blunt trauma or has been exposed to major deceleration forces should be suspected of having aortic rupture if there is an increased pulse pressure, upper extremity hypertension, and especially widening of the upper mediastinal silhouette.*

Chest roentgenography is of great diagnostic value in patients with aortic rupture. Widening of the superior mediastinal shadow, depression of the left main bronchus, displacement of the trachea and esophagus to the right, and especially obliteration of the aortic knob shadow are common roentgenographic abnormalities associated with injury at the aortic isthmus (Fig. 97–2). Widening of the mediastinum also has been observed in all cases with rupture of the aortic arch and in approximately 79 percent with rupture of the ascending aorta (Fig. 97–3).[53] The most definitive procedure to establish the diagnosis of aortic rupture is aortography, which should be performed immediately in all patients whose history, physical examination, and, particularly, chest roentgenogram suggest the possibility of this injury. Contrast computed tomography scanning also is used widely to evaluate and treat patients with a widened mediastinum.[54–56] TEE

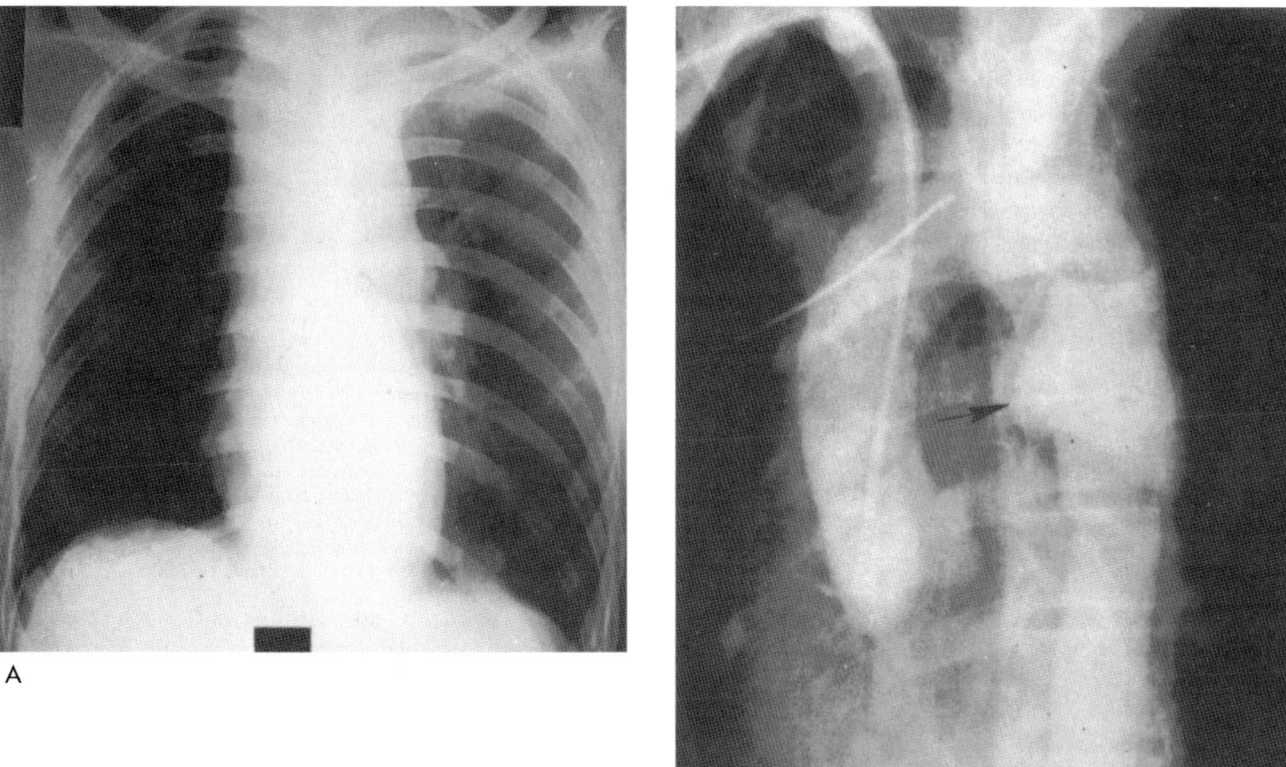

FIGURE 97–2. A. Chest roentgenogram of a young man who shortly before admission was involved in an automobile accident. Note the mediastinal widening. **B.** Aortogram the same day showing a false aneurysm distal to the origin of the left subclavian artery and two filling defects, one proximal and one distal to the aneurysm.

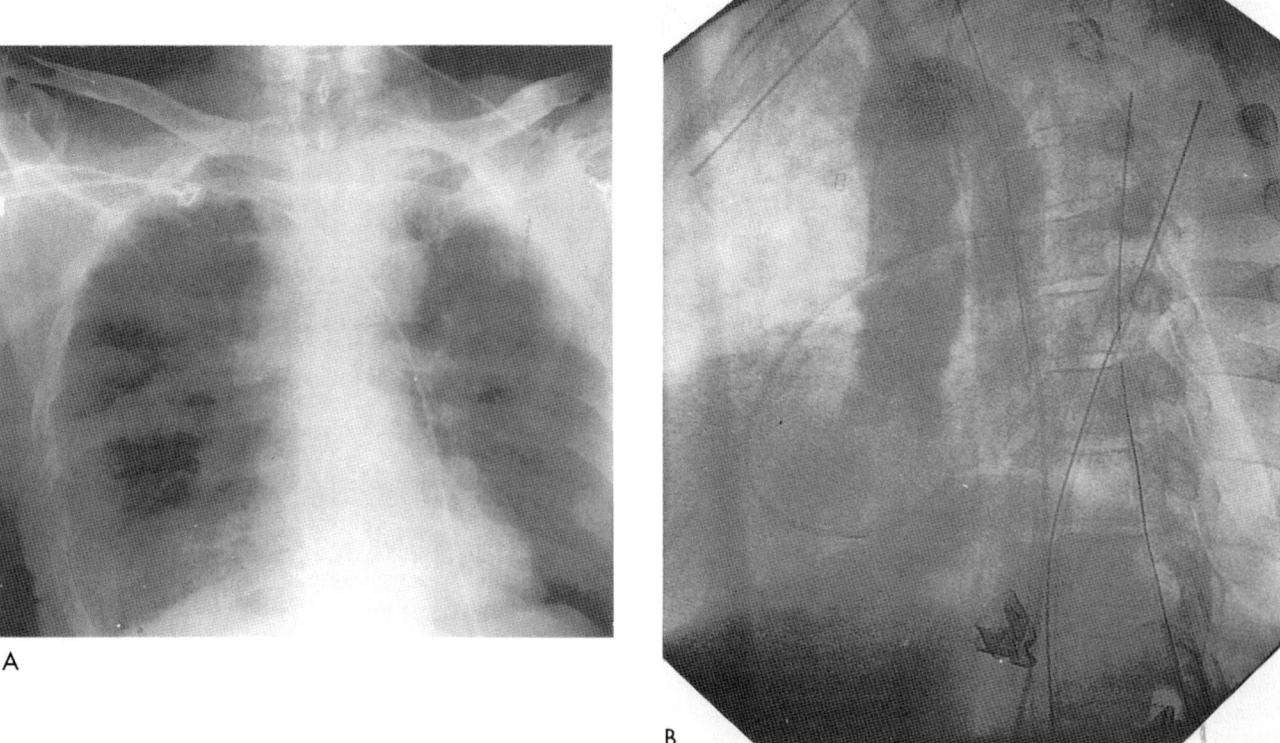

FIGURE 97–3. A. Chest roentgenogram of a young man shortly after a vehicular accident. **B.** Aortogram showing rupture of the ascending aorta.

appears to be a useful diagnostic test (see Chap. 15), but there has been no comprehensive study of its diagnostic value for aortic rupture. Until further experience is gained, caution should be exercised when it is used as the sole technique for establishing the diagnosis.

The treatment of aortic rupture is individualized. Patients with no other organ injuries that add unacceptable risk to the surgical treatment are operated on as soon as possible. The remaining patients, such as those with trauma to the central nervous system, contaminated wounds, respiratory insufficiency from lung contusion or other causes, body surface burns, blunt cardiac injury, tears of solid organs that will undergo nonoperative management, retroperitoneal hematoma, and medical comorbidities are treated either with percutaneous endovascular stenting of the tear or medical therapy to be followed by delayed surgical repair. The medical management consists of maintaining the mean systemic blood pressure below 70 mmHg to control the aortic wall tension and is continued until the other injuries or complications cease to add unacceptable risk to the surgical treatment.[57]

REFERENCES

1. Symbas PN. *Cardiothoracic Trauma*. Philadelphia, PA: Saunders; 1989.
2. James S. Injury mortality. In: *National Summary of Injury Mortality Data, 1987–1993*. Washington, DC: U.S. Department of Health and Human Services, Public Health Service, Centers for Disease Control and Prevention; June 1996.
3. Price PR, Mackenzie EJ. Cost of injury—United States: a report to Congress. *JAMA*. 1989;262:2803–2804.
4. Kemmerer WT, Eckert WG, Gathwright JB, et al. Patterns of thoracic injuries in fatal traffic accidents. *J Trauma*. 1961;1:595–599.
5. Bredlau CE, Roubin GS, Leimgruber PP, et al. In-hospital morbidity and mortality in patients undergoing elective coronary angioplasty. *Circulation*. 1985;72:1044.
6. Nobuyoshi M, Hamasaki N, Kimura T, et al. Indications, complications and short-term clinical outcome of percutaneous transvenous mitral commissurotomy. *Circulation*. 1989;80:782–792.
7. Salehian O, Teoh K, Mulji A. Blunt and penetrating cardiac trauma: a review. *Can J Cardiol*. 2003;19:1054–1059.
8. Cohn KE, Stewart JR, Fajardo LF, Hancock EW. Heart disease following radiation. *Medicine (Baltimore)*. 1967;46:281–298.
9. Jackson SH, Parry DJ. Lightning and the heart. *Br Heart J*. 1980;43:454–527.
10. Symbas PN, Harlaftis N, Waldo WJ. Penetrating wounds: a comparison of different therapeutic methods. *Ann Surg*. 1976;183:377–381.
11. Symbas PN. *Cardiothoracic Trauma: Current Problems in Surgery*. St. Louis: Mosby Year Book; 1991:742.
12. Thourani VH, Filiciano DV, Cooper WA, et al. Penetrating cardiac trauma at an urban trauma center: a 22-year experience. *Am Surg*. 1999;65:811–818.
13. Trinkle JK, Toon RS, Franz JL, et al. Affairs of the wounded heart: penetrating cardiac wounds. *J Trauma*. 1979;19:467–472.
14. Mitchell ME, Muakkassa FF, Poole GV, et al. Surgical approach of choice for penetrating cardiac wounds. *J Trauma*. 1993;34:17–20.
15. Rozycki GS, Feliciano DV, Schmidt JA, et al. The role of surgeon-performed ultrasound in patients with possible cardiac wounds. *Ann Surg*. 1996;224:1–8.
16. Symbas PN, DiOrio DA, Tyras DH, et al. Penetrating cardiac wounds: significant residual and delayed sequelae. *J Thorac Cardiovasc Surg*. 1973;6:526–532.
17. Symbas PN. *Traumatic Heart Disease: Current Problems in Cardiology*. St Louis: Mosby Year Book; 1991:539.
18. Bland EF, Beebe GW. Missiles in the heart: a 20-year follow-up report of world war cases. *N Engl J Med* 1966;274:1039–1046.
19. Symbas PN, Hatcher CR Jr, Mansour KA. Projectile embolus of the lung. *J Thorac Cardiovasc Surg*. 1968;56:97–103.
20. Symbas PN, Harlaftis N. Bullet emboli in the pulmonary and systemic arteries. *Ann Surg*. 1977;185:318–320.
21. Decker HR. Foreign bodies in the heart and pericardium: should they be removed? *J Thorac Surg*. 1939;9:62.
22. Turner GG. Bullets in the heart for 23 years. *Surgery*. 1942;9:832–852.
23. Symbas PN, Picone AL, Hatcher CR Jr, Vlasis SE. Cardiac missiles: a review of the literature and personal experience. *Ann Surg*. 1990;211:639–648.
24. Symbas PN, Vlasis SE, Picone AL, Hatcher CR Jr. Missiles in the heart. *Ann Thorac Surg*. 1989;48:192–194.
25. Konecke LL, Spitzer S, Mason D, et al. Traumatic aneurysm of the left coronary artery. *Am J Cardiol*. 1971;27:221–223.
26. Symbas PN, Schdava JS. Penetrating wounds of the thoracic aorta. *Ann Surg*. 1970;171:441–450.
27. Symbas PN, Kourias E, Tyras DH, Hatcher CR Jr. Penetrating wounds of the great vessels. *Ann Surg*. 1974;179:757–762.
28. Symbas PN, Schlant RC, Logan WD Jr, et al. Traumatic aorticopulmonary fistula complicated by postoperative low cardiac output treated with dopamine. *Ann Surg*. 1967;165:614–619.
29. Parmley LF Jr, Orbison JA, Hughes CW, Mattingly TW. Acquired arteriovenous fistulas complicated by endarteritis and endocarditis lenta due to *Streptococcus faecalis*. *N Engl J Med*. 1954;250:305–309.
30. Kissane RW. Traumatic heart diseases, especially myocardial contusion. *Postgrad Med*. 1954;15:114–119.
31. Stern T, Wolf RY, Reichart B, et al. Coronary artery occlusion resulting from blunt trauma. *JAMA*. 1974;230:1308–1309.
32. Levy H. Traumatic coronary thrombosis with myocardial infarction: postmortem study. *Arch Intern Med*. 1949;84:261–276.
33. Louhimo I. Heart injury after blunt thoracic trauma: An experimental study on rabbits. *Acta Chir Scand Suppl*. 1968;380:1–60.
34. Dolara A, Morando P, Pampaloni M. Electrocardiographic findings in 98 consecutive nonpenetrating chest injuries. *Dis Chest*. 1967;52:50–56.
35. Potkin RT, Werner JA, Trobaugh GB, et al. Evaluation of noninvasive tests of cardiac damage in suspected cardiac contusion. *Circulation*. 1982;66:627–631.
36. Marriott HJ, Nizet PM. Physiologic stimuli simulating ischemic heart disease. *JAMA*. 1967;200:715.
37. Tindall GT, Iwata K, McGraw CP, Vanderveer RW. Cardiorespiratory changes associated with intracranial pressure waves: evaluation of these changes in 27 patients with head injuries. *South Med J*. 1975;68:407–412.
38. Manor A, Alpan G. Specificity of creatine kinase MB isoenzyme for myocardial injury. *Clin Chem*. 1978;24:2206.
39. Snow N, Richardson JD, Flynt LM Jr. Myocardial contusion: Implication for patients with multiple traumatic injuries. *Surgery*. 1982;92:744–750.
40. Miller FA Jr, Seward JB, Gersh BJ, et al. Two-dimensional echocardiographic findings in cardiac trauma. *Am J Cardiol*. 1982;50:1022–1027.
41. Shapiro NG, Yanofsky SD, Trapp I, et al. Cardiovascular evaluation in thoracic blunt trauma using transesophageal echocardiography (TEE). *J Trauma*. 1991;131:835–839.
42. Velmahos GC, Karaiskakis M, Salima et al. Normal electrocardiography and serum troponin levels preclude the presence of clinically significant blunt cardiac injury. *J Trauma*. 2003;54:46–51.
43. Ferjani M, Droc G, Dreux S, et al. Circulating cardiac troponin T in myocardial contusion. *Chest*. 1997;111:427–433.
44. Snow N, Luca A E, Richardson JD. Intra-aortic balloon counterpulsation for cardiogenic shock from cardiac contusion. *J Trauma*. 1982;22:426–429.
45. Chavanon O, Dutheil V, Hacini R, et al. Treatment of severe cardiac contusion with a left ventricular assist device in a patient with multiple trauma. *J Thorac Cardiovasc Surg*. 1999;118:189–190.
46. Symbas NP, Bongiorno PF, Symbas PN. Blunt cardiac rupture: the utility of emergency department ultrasound. *Ann Thorac Surg*. 1999;67:1274–1276.
47. Singh R, Nolan SP, Schrank JP. Traumatic left ventricular aneurysm: two cases withnormal coronary angiograms. *JAMA*. 1975;234:412–414.
48. Schroeder JS, Stinson EB, Bieber CP, et al. Papillary muscle dysfunction due to nonpenetrating chest trauma, recognition in a potential cardiac donor. *Br Heart J*. 1972;34:645–647.
49. Marvin RF, Schrank JP, Nolan SP. Traumatic tricuspid insufficiency. *Am J Cardiol*. 1973;32:723–726.
50. Anderson M, Fredens M, Olesson KH. Traumatic rupture of the pericardium. *Am J Cardiol*. 1971;27:566–569.
51. Feczko JD, Lynch L, Pless JE, et al. An autopsy case review of 142 nonpenetrating (blunt) injuries of the aorta. *J Trauma*. 1992;33:846–849.
52. Symbas PN, Tyras DH, Ware RE, DiOrio DA. Traumatic rupture of the aorta. *Ann Surg*. 1973;178:6–12.
53. Symbas PJ, Horsley SW, Symbas PN. Rupture of the ascending aorta caused by blunt trauma. *Ann Thorac Surg*. 1998;66:113–117.
54. Fenner MN, Fisher KS, Sergel NL, et al. Evaluation of possible traumatic thoracic aortic injury using aortography and CT. *Am Surg*. 1990;56:497–499.
55. Miller FB, Richardson JD, Thomas HA, et al. Role of CT in diagnosis of major arterial injury after blunt thoracic trauma. *Surgery*. 1989;106:596–603.
56. Downing SW, Sperling JS, Mirvis SE, Cardarelli MG, et al. Experience with spiral computed tomography as the diagnostic method for traumatic aortic rupture. *Ann Thorac Surg*. 2001;72:495–501.
57. Symbas PN, Sherman AS, Silver JM, et al. Traumatic rupture of the aorta immediate or delayed repair? *Ann Surg*. 2002;235:796–802.

DEFINITION OF KIDNEY DISEASE
【 】 CHRONIC KIDNEY DISEASE

There is broad acceptance of a definition for chronic kidney disease (CKD) based on the persistence for 3 or more months of structural and/or functional abnormalities of the kidney.[1] The persistent structural abnormalities that define CKD are (1) microalbuminuria or macroalbuminuria (overt proteinuria); (2) an abnormal urinary sediment including the presence of red blood cells (RBCs), RBC casts, white blood cells (WBCs), WBC casts, tubular cells, cellular casts, granular casts, oval fat bodies, fatty casts, free fat; or (3) abnormal imaging tests includes ultrasound, intravenous pyelogram, computer tomogram, magnetic resonance image and nuclear scans. *Microalbuminuria* is defined as urinary albumin excretion of 20 to 200 µg/ minute (30–300 mg/24 hours), or a spot albumin-to-creatinine ratio of 30 to 300 mg/g in a first morning urine sample, and anything above this level of excretion is called *macroalbuminuria.*[2] The func-

tional measurements that define CKD use creatinine-based estimates of the glomerular filtration rate (GFR) based on either the Modification of Diet in Renal Disease (MDRD) estimating equations or the Cockcroft-Gault estimating equation for creatinine clearance.[3] One of these multivariate GFR estimation equations is strongly recommended, and clinicians should choose a method that is appropriate for the population for which they care. The GFR estimated using one of these equations is imprecise, and the accuracy improves as kidney function declines. This imprecision is accommodated by assigning patients to CKD stages based on (a) persistent structural, and (b) functional abnormalities as shown in Table 98–1.

Utility of Staging Chronic Kidney Disease: Improved Diagnostic and Prognostic Information

Table 98–2 illustrates the substantial diagnostic and prognostic information about their patients provided to clinicians by identification and staging of CKD. As the stage of CKD worsens the preva-

TABLE 98–1

Stages and Prevalence of Chronic Kidney Disease in U.S. Adults

STAGE	DESCRIPTION	GFR (ML/MIN/1.73 M²)	PREVALENCE[a] N (1000S)	PERCENT
Stage 1	Kidney damage with normal or ↑ GFR	≥90	5,900	3.3
Stage 2	Kidney damage with mild ↓ GFR	60–89	5,300	3.0
Stage 3	Moderate ↓ GFR	30–59	7,600	4.3
Stage 4	Severe ↓ GFR	15–29	400	0.2
Stage 5	Kidney failure	<15 or dialysis	300	0.1

GFR, glomeruler filtration rate; MDRD, Modification of Diet in Renal Disease; NHANES, National Health Nutrition Examination Survey; USRDS, United States Renal Data Systems.
[a]Data for stages 1–4 from NHANES III (1988–1994) Masoudi, Plomondon, Magid, et al. Population of 177 million adults age ≥20 years. Data for stage 5 from USRDS (1998) include approximately 230,000 patients treated by dialysis, and assume 70,000 additional patients not on dialysis. GFR estimated from serum creatinine by abbreviated MDRD equation based on age, sex, race, and calibration of serum creatinine. For stage 1 and 2, kidney damage was assessed by spot albumin-to-creatinine ratio >17 mg/g (men) or >25 mg/g (women) on two measurements.
SOURCE: Cooper, O'Brien, Thourani, et al.[9]

lence of hypertension, diabetes, and anemia increase, as well as the inflammatory burden as measured by C-reactive protein increases.[1,4,5] The 5-year risks of progression to end-stage renal disease (ESRD) and mortality and the 3-year risk of cardiovascular disease (CVD) all increase substantially as CKD stage worsens.[6,7]

CKD is highly prevalent among patients with incident coronary artery disease and is associated with substantial increased short- and intermediate-term mortality.[8] Knowledge of CKD stage also provides substantial information about the risk of postoperative mortality and morbidity among patients with CVD.[9]

TABLE 98–2

Impact of Chronic Kidney Disease on Cardiovascular Risks and Outcomes According to the Severity of Kidney Disease

DESCRIPTION	NORMAL TO MILD DECREASE IN GFR	MODERATE GFR LOSS	SEVERE GFR LOSS
CKD Stage	1–2	3	4
eGFR mL/min/1.73 m²	≥60	30–59	15–29
Cardiovascular risk factors			
Hypertension[1]	40%	55%	77%
Diabetes[11]	3.1–6.5%	16.8%	22.8%
C-reactive protein >0.21 mg/dL[11]	25–30%	48.7%	57.7%
Hemoglobin <13 g/dL[10]	4%	7%	29%
Outcomes			
Five-year ESRD rate[12]	1.1%	1.3%	19.9%
Five-year mortality rate[12]	19.5%	24.3	45.7%
Three-year CVD event rate[13]	2.1%	4.8%	11.4%
Acute coronary syndrome[14]			
Prevalence among patients	59.3%	31.9%	8.8%
Risk of 7-month mortality AMI	1	2.1 (1.04, 4.3)[a]	4.6 (2.1, 9.9)[a]
Risk of 7-month mortality UA	1	8.8 (1.2, 67.2)[a]	24.6 (3.0, 202.4)[a]
Acute myocardial infarction[15]			
Prevalence among patients	28.5%	43.5%	30%
Risk of 1 year mortality AMI	2.3%	9.4%	24.2%
Coronary artery bypass surgery[18]			
Prevalence among patients	73.9%	24.1%	2.0%
Risk of 30-day postop mortality	1.3–1.8%	4.3%	9.3%
Postop stroke	0.9–1.3%	2.4%	3.5%
Prolonged ventilation	5.3–6.1%	11.1%	19.7%
Deep sternal infection	0.4%	0.6%	0.9%

AMI, acute myocardial infarction; CVD, cardiovascular disease; eGFR, estimated glomerular filtration rate; ESRD, end-stage renal disease; UA, unstable angina.
[a]Odds ratios (95% confidence interval).

ASSOCIATION BETWEEN CHRONIC KIDNEY DISEASE AND CARDIOVASCULAR DISEASE

【 】 RISK OF INCIDENT CARDIOVASCULAR DISEASE AMONG CHRONIC KIDNEY DISEASE PATIENTS

Cardiovascular disease is the number one cause of death in patients with ESRD.[10] The cardiovascular mortality rate in ESRD patients on dialysis is approximately 10 to 20 times higher than in the general population (Fig. 98–1).[11] Acute myocardial infarction accounted for 14 deaths per 1000 patient-years whereas arrhythmia and sudden death accounted for 46.5 deaths per 1000 patient-years.[12,13]

There is substantial evidence that CKD is an independent risk factor for incident CVD and cardiovascular mortality. A recent American Heart Association scientific statement on kidney disease as a cardiovascular risk factor by Sarnak and colleagues provides an accessible summary of this evidence.[14] The authors identified 49 studies that examined the association between decreased GFR and risk of cardiovascular disease published between 1989 and 2003, 80 percent of those came out between 2000 and 2003. Of note, associations between cardiovascular disease and/or all-cause mortality were reported in all but two of these diverse populations. Similar associations were noted both for patients with microalbuminuria in general population.[15] In

populations at low risk for CVD, in contrast, the relationship between GFR and outcomes was less clear and was not seen in either the Framingham Study or the National Health and Nutrition Examination Survey (NHANES) I followup studies.[14] In contrast, CKD was an independent risk factor for CVD outcomes in the Atherosclerotic Risk in Communities Study (ARIC). However, the impact of CKD diminished after adjusting for traditional CVD risk factors.[16]

【 】 RISK OF CHRONIC KIDNEY DISEASE AMONG INDIVIDUALS WITH PREVALENT AND INCIDENT CARDIOVASCULAR DISEASE

Patients undergoing coronary angiography, patients treated with percutaneous coronary intervention (PCI) and coronary artery bypass grafting (CABG), and participants in clinical trials of atherosclerotic disease are at increased risk of CKD.[14] The reported prevalence of CKD is highly variable and can vary from less than 10 percent to more than 60 percent of a population of CVD patients with an average prevalence of 30 percent.[17] The presence of CVD increases the risk of developing ESRD.[18] For example, hypertensive male veterans are at a twofold increased risk of developing ESRD following a new myocardial infarction and fivefold increased risk following incident heart failure.[19] Finally, there are anatomic correlations between kidney function and extent of atherosclerosis.[20]

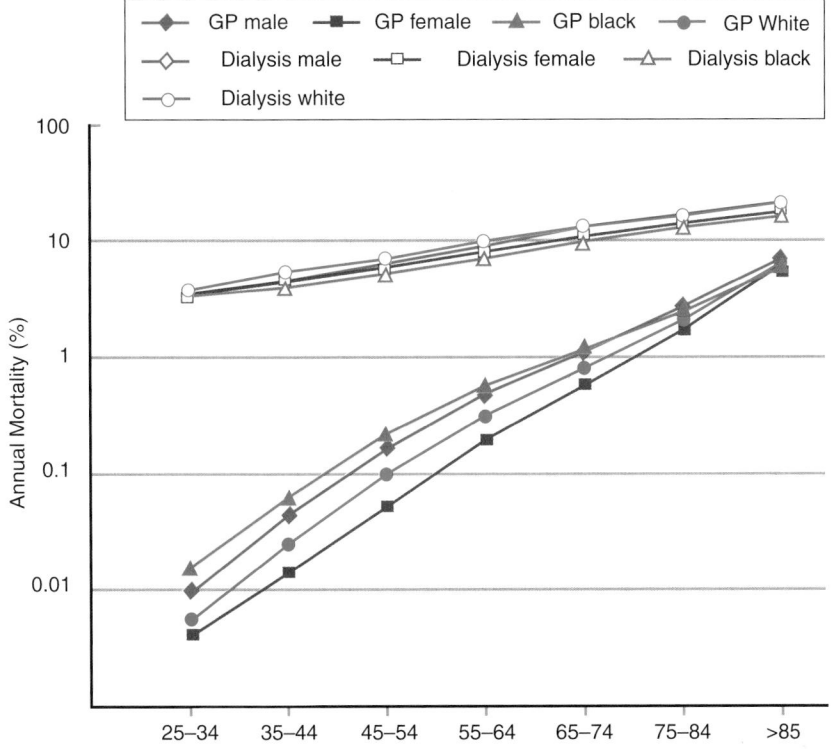

FIGURE 98–1. Cardiovascular mortality defined as death because of arrhythmias, cardiomyopathy, cardiac arrest, myocardial infarction, atherosclerotic heart disease, or pulmonary edema in the general population (GP) is compared to end-stage renal disease (ESRD) patients treated by dialysis. Data are stratified by age, race, and gender. *Source: Foley RN, Pafrey PS, Sarnack MJ.[11] Reproduced with permission from the Am J Kidney Dis. Copyright 1998 by the National Kidney Foundation.*

ACUTE KIDNEY INJURY

【 】 DEFINITION OF ACUTE KIDNEY INJURY AND RISK STRATIFICATION

The definition of acute kidney injury (AKI), in contrast to CKD, has not yet been fully standardized and is typically defined by a functional component that includes arbitrary increments of serum creatinine to dialysis-dependent kidney failure over a variable time period that reflects a period of observation in a clinical or hospital setting.[21,22] Identification of acutely impaired kidney function, typically is based on a change in serum creatinine and/or urine output. The Acute Dialysis Quality Initiative (ADQI) has recently addressed this diagnostic disarray by proposing a consensus-based definition of AKI known as RIFLE.[23,24] Recent studies have shown that the stages or levels of AKI defined by the RIFLE criteria are predictive of increased risk of mortality and dialysis-dependent kidney failure in critically ill patients and those undergoing cardiac surgery.[25,26]

The risk of AKI among patients with CVD include presence of CKD, older age, diabetes mellitus, proteinuria, heart failure, exposure to radiocontrast dye, surgical and percutaneous revascularization, and admission to acute care units. At present there are no risk stratification equations that predict risk of AKI that have been extensively validated and thus clinicians must maintain a low threshold for the identification of at-risk patients for AKI. The risk of renal damage following radiocontrast dye is a particular concern for patients with CVD undergoing diagnostic and therapeutic angiography (see discussion below).

CARDIOVASCULAR RISK FACTORS AND THE KIDNEY

CKD and cardiovascular diseases share common risk factors. The higher prevalence of CVD in patients with renal disease can be the consequence of the high prevalence of hypertension, diabetes, aging, and dyslipidemias. There are other explanations for the association between kidney disease and risk of CVD other than shared traditional and nontraditional risk factors. Patients with CKD may have survived exposure to shared cardiovascular risk factors, and this differential survival can contribute to the increased prevalence and risk of CVD.[27] Finally, there is increasing concern that interventions to reduce the risk of incident and recurrent CVD, including agents blocking renin–angiotensin-aldosterone system (RAAS), ß blockers, aspirin, platelet inhibitors, thrombolytics, or percutaneous intervention, can be underused among patients with CKD, an important omission as these interventions clearly benefit this patient population.[28] It is also possible that the association between cardiovascular risk and kidney disease can be modified among different population groups. A recent report that pooled data from the ARIC Study, Cardiovascular Health Study, Framingham Heart Study, and Framingham Offspring Study found that the increased risk for coronary heart disease differed among blacks and whites in the U.S. population, with blacks with kidney disease experiencing a 76 percent increased risk of CVD compared to a 13 percent increased risk among whites.[29] This interaction between race and kidney disease was observed for all components of the end point other than stroke.

[ ] SYSTEMIC ARTERIAL HYPERTENSION

Kidney is central to regulation of arterial pressure and increased prevalence of hypertension begins in CKD stage 3, and almost 80 percent of CKD patients have systemic hypertension before beginning dialysis therapy.[30,31] Following the onset of dialysis therapy, hypertension is almost universal among ESRD patients. The pathogenesis of hypertension includes both an expanded extracellular fluid volume (ECV) and increased peripheral vascular resistance mediated by overactivity of the sympathetic nervous system and the renin–angiotensin axis.[32] It has been proposed that circulating inhibitors of sodium-potassium-adenosine triphosphatase (Na^+-K^+-ATPase) increase peripheral vascular resistance by causing an increase in intracellular sodium, resulting in an increase in intracellular calcium and, hence, contraction of vascular smooth muscle cells.[33] Other proposed mechanisms include impaired endothelium-dependent vasodilatation because of impaired nitric oxide production caused by high plasma levels of asymmetric dimethylarginine, hyperhomocysteinemia, and secondary hyperparathyroidism by facilitating calcium entry into smooth muscle cells of the arterial wall.[34,35] Although elevated blood pressure usu-

ally resolves when the ECV is reduced by intradialytic fluid removal among ESRD patients, additional mechanisms play a role in the hypertension that many of patients experience. These factors can include a high peripheral vascular resistance in a small group (~10 percent) of ESRD patients who exhibit dialysis-resistant hypertension and high levels of plasma-renin activity, seasonal and diurnal variations, erythropoietin (EPO) therapy, and high dialysate sodium concentration.[36]

Drug therapy for hypertension in CKD stages 1 to 4 is based on strong evidence that inhibiting RAAS axis is effective even in advanced CKD,[37] is cardioprotective,[38] and reduces risk of CKD progression in both diabetic and nondiabetic CKD and is effective in African Americans.[39,40] Use of angiotensin-converting enzyme inhibitors (ACEIs) or angiotensin receptor blockers (ARBs) is associated with rises in serum creatinine and/or potassium levels that can lead to reluctance to use these agents in patients with CKD.[41] A meta-analysis of 12 randomized clinical trials found that participants with CKD often experienced an increase in serum creatinine of up to 30 percent that was not associated with progressive loss of kidney function, and it did not attenuate the renal protection of these agents.[42] Hyperkalemia can usually be managed by reduction in RAAS-blocker dose, dietary potassium restriction, avoiding dietary and prescription potassium supplement, minimizing use of nonsteroidal antiinflammatory agents, and cautious use of potassium-sparing diuretics.

It is recommended that blood pressure treatment targets in both diabetic and nondiabetic CKD be lower than those for individuals without kidney disease. Both the Seventh Report of the Joint National Committee on Hypertension and American Diabetic Association recommend a therapeutic target of 130/80 mm/Hg.[43,44] Achieving this degree of blood-pressure reduction in individuals with CKD typically entails the use of two to three antihypertensive agents including RAAS blocker and a diuretic.[45] It should be noted that thiazide diuretics retain their efficacy in CKD stage 3.[46] The cornerstone of correcting hypertension in dialysis patients must be to reduce ECV (i.e., to lower the patient's *dry weight* assignment). The dry weight of a dialysis patient is defined as that weight at which there is no ECV expansion (e.g., edema or effusions), and blood pressure is normal. Unfortunately, achieving a dry weight is difficult because patients can become symptomatically hypotensive or develop leg cramps, and these symptoms make it difficult to establish a *true* dry weight. In patients who have persistent hypertension despite control of ECV, antihypertensive medications that block RAAS or β blockers are the logical choice. If they are ineffective, calcium channel blockers, clonidine or minoxidil, can be used, but again the best medicine is to reduce the ECV. The dosage of antihypertensive drugs (like other medicines) must be adjusted for the degree of renal failure. Antihypertensive drugs are generally withheld on hemodialysis (HD) treatment days so that more ECV can be removed without causing hypotension. Bilateral nephrectomy has rarely been used to treat malignant or treatment-resistant hypertension.[47]

[ ] ANEMIA OF CHRONIC KIDNEY DISEASE

Anemia begins early in the course of CKD and is almost uniform among CKD stage 5 patients treated with dialysis.[30] An association between lower hemoglobin and risk of CVD among stage 3 and higher CKD patients is increasingly well characterized.[48] Anemia is also a risk factor for stroke and heart failure, and these associations persist after controlling for other risk factors.[49,50]

There is little evidence from clinical trials to support a cardioprotective effect of complete correction of anemia in CKD stage 3 and 4 patients.[51] Recently, in the CHOIR trial, a higher target hemoglobin value (13.5 g/dL vs 11.3 g/dL) was associated with increased risks of death, myocardial infarction, hospitalization for heart failure, and stroke without improvement in quality of life.[52] However, partial correction of anemia in CKD patients with heart failure resulted in significant improvements in New York Heart Association (NYHA) class and cardiac function.[53] Moreover, there is growing evidence from small randomized trials that correction of anemia can be beneficial with respect to improved functional status, reduced hospitalization, and improved survival among individuals with CKD.[54]

METABOLIC SYNDROME, OBESITY, AND DIABETES MELLITUS

Approximately, one-third of individuals with type I and II diabetes will develop diabetic kidney disease, and approximately 45 percent of all CKD patients who begin maintenance dialysis have diabetes, and it is predicted that this percentage will continue to increase.[30,55] As in the general population, diabetic dialysis patients have more cardiovascular morbidity and mortality and all-cause mortality compared to dialysis patients without diabetes.[30] There is strong evidence, translated into clinical practice guidelines, that tight glycemic control in type I and type II diabetes mellitus, reduction of blood pressure to below 130/80 mmHg, with either ACEIs or ARBs, and dietary protein restriction to the recommended daily allowance of 0.8 g/kg/day reduce the risk of progressive kidney disease and risk of cardiovascular disease, and these therapeutic principles should be considered when managing cardiovascular risk in patients with type I and II diabetes mellitus.[44]

There is growing interest in the role of obesity, insulin resistance, and the metabolic syndrome as mediators of progressive kidney disease, similar to the role of these as risk factors for cardiovascular disease.[56,57] Further, patients with CKD stage 5 have an increased prevalence of obesity, which is also associated with increased risk of ESRD.[58] There is some evidence that weight reduction decreases the hyperfiltration and renal blood flow associated with obesity and that it can ameliorate risk of progressive kidney disease.[59] Weight reduction should be a standard component of the dietary prescription of obese patients with CKD and CVD. However, caution should be exercised in caloric restriction among ESRD patients on hemodialysis where obesity has been associated with decreased mortality following the onset of renal replacement therapy.[60]

DYSLIPIDEMIAS

One of the important CVD risk factors in uremic patients is the presence of dyslipidemias. Serum-lipid abnormalities are more common in patients with CKD than it is in the general population, but the pattern differs.[61] All patients with CKD manifest a secondary form of dyslipidemia that mimics the atherogenic dyslipidemia of insulin-resistant patients.[62] This is characterized by an increase in serum triglyceride (TG), very low-density lipoprotein (VLDL) and low-density lipoprotein (LDL) with unchanged total cholesterol (TC) and low high-density lipoprotein (HDL). However, in patients with nephrotic syndrome, LDL and TC are markedly elevated.[63] HD patients usually have *normal* TC and LDL levels whereas higher HDL and serum TG levels. Patients treated with chronic peritoneal dialysis (CPD) have similar pattern of dyslipidemias except they are more likely to have elevated LDL levels. The usual lipid profile of a renal transplant patient shows elevated TC, LDL, and TG levels, but HDL is usually normal.[61]

Large-scale randomized trials have clearly demonstrated that lowering LDL concentration with 3-hydroxy-3-methylglutaryl coenzyme A reductase inhibitors (statins) significantly reduces the risk of coronary events and strokes.[64] However, patients with CKD have generally been excluded, or they have been the subject of subgroup secondary analysis, thus limiting the extrapolation of beneficial effects of statins on cardiovascular outcomes from those studies to patients with CKD.[65,66] Although fewer than 20 percent of HD patients worldwide are prescribed statins, observational studies have suggested that statin use in this population is associated with a reduction in cardiac and total mortality.[67,68] Recent prospective randomized clinical trials conducted exclusively on CKD patients, on the role of statins therapy in lowering CVD risk have produced equivocal results.[65,69] Until the results are available from the two ongoing large-scale randomized trials,[70,71] the National Kidney Foundation, Kidney Disease Outcomes Quality Initiative (K/DOQI) clinical practice guidelines for managing dyslipidemias are recommended for classifying and treating lipid abnormalities in patients with CKD.[61,72]

HOMOCYSTEINE

Plasma levels of total homocysteine (Hcy) in patients with CKD are often two to eight times that of the general population.[73,74] The kidneys account for approximately 70 percent of plasma clearance of Hcy.[10] However, the etiology of hyperhomocysteinemia in renal failure is still debated, that is, whether this effect is the result of a decrease in the renal clearance or a result of extrarenal metabolic changes.[75] Results from prospective, case-control studies have led to the conclusion that there is an association between an elevated Hcy level and adverse cardiovascular events in dialysis and renal transplant patients.[76–78] Results of the two ongoing multicenter clinical trials are expected to be completed by 2007 and will provide more conclusive evidence whether lowering Hcy levels in renal patients with folic acid or vitamin B supplementation reduces the risk of CVD.[79,80] Current expert opinion suggests that it is prudent to supplement, rather than risk the deficiency, especially when supplementation is safe at the recommended levels.[10]

HEMODIALYSIS-ASSOCIATED HYPOTENSION

Clinically significant hypotension occurs in approximately 10 to 30 percent of HD treatments.[81] Intradialytic hypotension (IDH) is often defined as a systolic blood pressure <100 mmHg or a blood pressure drop of >20 mmHg during a dialysis session with concomitant symptoms of dizziness, blurred vision, cramps, and fatigue.[82] Usually the consequences are minor, but cerebrovascular insufficiency and/or cardiovascular instability (myocardial ischemia and arrhythmias) can occur.[83,84] These complications of hypotension can account at least in part for the *U-shaped* relation between systolic blood pressure and cardiovascular mortality in HD patients. The relative death rate for patients with postdialysis systolic blood pressures below 110 mmHg was double than those with a postdialysis blood pressure of 140 to 149 mmHg.[85]

The main cause of intradialytic hypotension is hypovolemia caused by an imbalance between the amount of fluid removed and the refilling capacity of the intravascular compartment. Several methods have been employed to reduce the incidence of hypotension during dialysis session. Those are withholding antihypertensive medications on dialysis days, restricting interdialytic weight gain, avoiding eating on dialysis, profiling dialysate sodium concentration, and cooling of dialysate.[86] Other strategies for preventing hypotension are to remove ECV at a slower rate and use of on-line hematocrit monitoring to detect sudden decrease in blood volume.[87] For patients unresponsive to the above measures, midodrine 2.5 to 10 mg given 15 to 30 minutes before dialysis appears to be safe and effective.[82]

HYPERPHOSPHATEMIA, VITAMIN D, AND CORONARY ARTERY CALCIFICATION

Calcium phosphate deposition, in the form of bioapatite, is the hallmark of vascular calcification and can occur in blood vessels, myocardium, and cardiac valves.[88,89] There are two distinct types of arterial calcification, intimal calcification occur in atherosclerotic lesions, and medial calcification, or Mönckeberg sclerosis, that is associated with vascular stiffening and arteriosclerosis often observed with aging, diabetes, and ESRD.[90] Vascular calcification is considered an actively regulated process that can arise by several different mechanisms. A detailed discussion on these mechanisms is beyond the scope of this chapter, interested readers are referred to an excellent review on this topic.[90] Cross-sectional studies in patients with advanced CKD have clearly shown that the presence of arterial calcification is associated with adverse clinical outcomes, including myocardial infarction, congestive heart failure, endocarditis, valvular heart disease, and death.[91–93] Screening electron-beam computed tomography as well as multidetector-row computed tomography scanners are being used for detection and quantification of coronary artery calcification in general population. However, the utility of these tests as a marker of severity of vascular disease or as a predictor of adverse cardiovascular outcomes in patients with advanced CKD disease has yet to be established.[94]

The increase incidence and severity of vascular calcification in uremia is attributed to the abnormalities of mineral metabolism, which are common in CKD patients, especially those on dialysis. Observational studies have shown a strong association between cardiac death in HD patients and high serum phosphorus, high serum calcium-phosphorus product, or high serum parathyroid hormone (PTH) levels in patients with ESRD.[95,96] The regulation of calcium and phosphate homeostasis depends on two major regulatory hormone systems, PTH and active 1,25-dihydroxyvitamin D (calcitriol). As GFR decreases, there is reduction in the amount of filtered and excreted phosphate, resulting in elevation of serum phosphate concentration. This in turn leads to stimulation of parathyroid glands (secondary hyperparathyroidism). Any increase in serum phosphorus levels reduces ionized calcium, which in turn

stimulates secretion of PTH, resulting in improved phosphorus excretion. This general scheme, known as the *tradeoff hypothesis*, explains how secondary hyperthyroidism develops.[97] Once GFR declines to 25 percent of normal, however, elevated PTH levels can no longer maintain normal serum phosphorus and calcitriol levels.[98] Other mechanisms that increase PTH secretion in CKD patients include nutritional vitamin D deficiency and decreased renal production of calcitriol, which under normal circumstances is a potent inhibitor of pre-pro PTH mRNA transcription.[99] Apart from alterations in phosphorus metabolism in CKD, several therapeutic interventions, such as the use of oral calcium salts as a phosphate-binding agent and the administration of large doses of vitamin D sterols to treat secondary hyperparathyroidism, contribute to episodes of hypercalcemia and/or hyperphosphatemia, changes that can aggravate soft-tissue and vascular calcification.[100,101]

Adequate control of serum phosphorus remains a cornerstone in the clinical management of patients with CKD and ESRD, not only to attenuate the progression of secondary hyperparathyroidism but also possibly to reduce the risk for vascular calcification. However, phosphate binders are often necessary to limit dietary absorption of phosphorus. For patients with high serum calcium-phosphorus product, a noncalcium-containing phosphate binder, such as sevelamer hydrochloride or lanthanum carbonate should be selected to reduce the amount of ingested calcium. However, these agents are significantly more expensive than calcium salts, which can contribute to patient noncompliance. In contrast, if the serum calcium is low, both calcium carbonate or calcium acetate are cheaper and effective binders. Calcimimetics, are a new class of agent that binds the calcium-sensing receptor of the parathyroid gland, resulting in diminished PTH secretion without increasing serum calcium and phosphorus levels.[102]

INFLAMMATION AND SERUM ALBUMIN

In dialysis patients, low serum albumin level is closely associated with the prevalence of coronary artery disease (CAD), which is defined as the presence of angina, history of admission for CAD, and cardiac ischemic signs on electrocardiography.[103] Hypoalbuminemia is the strongest independent predictor of total and cardiovascular mortality in ESRD patients.[104,105] Perhaps, low albumin might not by itself be an independent risk factor of CVD and mortality but rather a reflection of cytokine activation and ongoing interleukin-6 (IL-6)–mediated subclinical inflammation.[106] It has been proposed that inflammation per se plays a key role in the development of atherosclerosis and, hence, the increased risk of cardiovascular death in the general population.[107] The evidence for inflammation in these reports is the finding of a high C-reactive protein (CRP). Similar associations between a high CRP and increased mortality have been reported from cross-sectional evaluations of both HD and CPD patients.[108,109] Specific therapies directed at controlling the degree of inflammation, such as blocking cytokines or their effects will have to be tested for safety and efficacy in CKD patients.

CORONARY HEART DISEASE

CAD is common among CKD patients and is the major factor in the pathogenesis of cardiac disease. Its prevalence rates are 5 to 20 times greater in ESRD patients than those for the general population.[11] Moreover, CAD is the major cause of morbidity and mortality in ESRD patients.[110] Case-fatality rates after acute myocardial infarction (AMI) are several fold greater in dialysis patients than in the general population, and mortality rates are nearly 60 percent in the year following a first AMI.[111] Even mild renal disease, as assessed by the estimated GFR, regardless of the underlying cause, is considered a major risk for mortality after an acute coronary event.[112,113] Microalbuminuria, even with preserved GFR is a strong and independent determinant of coronary heart disease and death.[15] The contributing factors to higher mortality are older age, presence of comorbidities, and receiving fewer effective therapies (less reperfusion, glycoprotein IIb/IIIa receptor inhibitors, early angiography, and less aggressive medical therapies).[114,115] The risk of AMI is understandably related to the high prevalence of hypertension, inflammation, ECV overload, anemia, hypotension and hypoxia during HD, and increased blood flow through the arteriovenous (AV) fistula.[116]

❰ ❱ DIAGNOSIS OF CORONARY ARTERY DISEASE IN RENAL PATIENTS

Evaluation of CKD patients with suspected CAD should begin with a detailed history and physical examination. However, the clinical symptoms as well as the cardiovascular risk profile are not valid predictors for the presence of CAD in ESRD diabetics.[117] In this study the symptom of angina has sensitivity of 43 percent and specificity of 82 percent to detect CAD. The classic ECG changes of acute myocardial ischemia or infarction are similar to patients without renal disease. However, HD-induced changes in serum potassium, serum calcium and fluid volume can affect changes in ECG, complicating its interpretation. HD increases the QT interval and dispersion, P-wave duration, and the amplitude of the QRS complex, especially in patients with left ventricular hypertrophy.[118–120] The ST-segment depression on resting ECG is considered an unreliable marker of coronary ischemia in the dialysis patient. It is notable that 25 to 30 percent of ESRD patients will have abnormalities on ECG or perfusion scans indicating CAD, even in the absence of significant narrowing of a major coronary artery.[117,121] In addition, asymptomatic severe CAD is not a uncommon finding because of uremic or diabetic autonomic neuropathy and a sedentary lifestyle.[122]

Serial measurements of biochemical markers of myocardial ischemia such as creatine-kinase MB isoenzyme and/or lactic dehydrogenase are useful in diagnosing AMI in dialysis patients, but they all have poor specificity.[123] Troponin-I is considered the most accurate serum biochemical marker for diagnosing acute myocardial injury in patients with ESRD.[124,125] When serum troponin-I levels are above 0.8 ng/mL, the sensitivity and specificity for the diagnosis of acute myocardial injury in patients with renal failure is reported to be 83 and 91 percent, respectively.[126] Consequently, a minimal increase in serum troponin-I should be interpreted with caution in dialysis patients.

Exercise stress ECG and thallium scintigraphy tests, are limited by the presence of an abnormal resting ECG, blunted or absent tachycardia (autonomic neuropathy) during the test, or more commonly by a markedly reduced exercise capacity in dialysis patients.[127] Dipyridamole–thallium scintigraphic test for screening

of CAD in dialysis patients has limited value because of a sensitivity of 37 to 86 percent, a specificity near 75 percent, and a positive predictive value of approximately 70 percent.[128] Dobutamine echocardiography reportedly has a sensitivity in the range of 69 to 95 percent and a specificity of approximately 95 percent in patients with chronic renal disease, making this test a better choice for detecting CAD in patients with suspicious symptoms or those awaiting a kidney transplant.[129,130] However, it should be cautioned that the risk of transient atrial fibrillation in dialysis patients with this method is approximately 2 to 4 percent, compared to only 0.5 percent in general population.[131]

❰ ❱ CARDIAC ASSESSMENT FOR RENAL TRANSPLANT CANDIDATES

Pretransplant cardiovascular disease is a major risk factor for developing posttransplant cardiovascular disease.[132] The CVD rates peak during the first 3 months following transplantation and decrease subsequently compared to those patients who are listed for transplantation but remain on dialysis, this is true for living and deceased donor recipients, irrespective of diabetic status.[133]

Screening for CAD for the risk stratification for perioperative cardiac events and long-term cardiac prognosis after transplantation is warranted. Screening all patients listed for transplantation is expensive, time-consuming, and impractical. Patients at high risk for posttransplant cardiac ischemic events are listed in Table 98–3. Patients with diabetes mellitus (DM) require special attention as they have the lowest 5-year survival on dialysis; approximately 40 percent of the renal transplants are performed in patients with DM, and approximately one-third of those have clinically silent coronary artery disease.[110] There is no consensus on the optimal screening test for the detection of CAD in these high-risk patients. Current guidelines recommend pharmacologic stress echocardiography or nuclear imaging testing as initial screening tests and reserve coronary angiography only for those whom screening tests are positive for ischemia.[10] However, patients with symptomatic ischemic heart disease should be tested directly by coronary angiography.[134] Similar screening guidelines are applicable for dialysis patients who require other types of major surgical procedures. For patients who have negative initial evaluations but remain on the transplant waiting list, repeat evaluation for CAD is recommended every 12 months if patients are classified as *high risk* as described

---

TABLE 98–3

Renal Transplant Recipients at High Risk for Posttransplant Cardiac Ischemic Events

Previous history of CAD, PCI, or CABG
CHF (LV ejection fraction <40 percent)
Diabetics
Males >45 years
Females >55 years
Abnormal resting ECG
Smokers

CABG, coronary artery bypass grafting; CAD, coronary artery disease; CHF, congestive heart failure; LV, left ventricle; PCI, percutaneous coronary intervention.

above. If patients are nondiabetic but classified as high risk then evaluation for CAD is repeated in 24 months.[10]

At present, coronary angiography is considered the gold standard for defining the presence and extent of CAD in CKD patients but, as in other patients, this invasive procedure should be reserved for those in whom an intervention (i.e., CABG or PCI) is contemplated. The dose of contrast agent used in patients should be minimized to avoid loss of residual renal function (see discussion below). For patients undergoing invasive coronary procedures, it is important to avoid internal jugular sites and to preserve brachial and radial arteries for future dialysis access.[10]

【 】 MANAGEMENT OF RENAL PATIENT WITH CORONARY ARTERY DISEASE

The medical management of acute coronary syndrome (ACS) in patients with renal disease is similar to that used for patients with no kidney disease except that the drug dosages should be adjusted appropriately (Table 98–4). These therapies include nitrates, antiplatelet agents, β blockers, ACEIs, ARBs, thrombolytic therapy, and lipid-lowering agents as discussed in Chap. 61. Usefulness of antiplatelet therapy and anticoagulation for the treatment of ACS in patients with renal disease is uncertain.[10] ESRD patients are far less likely than non-ESRD patients to be treated with aspirin after AMI.[135] The overwhelming evidence for a beneficial effect of low-dose aspirin in preventing AMI in the general population outweighs the theoretical concerns about impaired platelet function and increased risk of bleeding in dialysis patients.[10,136] A combination of aspirin plus clopidogrel should be used with caution, one randomized controlled trial of aspirin plus clopidogrel versus placebo to prevent AV graft thrombosis was terminated early because of GI bleeding.[137] Fractionated low-molecular-weight heparin exerts an unpredictable activity in renal patients because they accumulate small peptides, and should only be used with dose adjustments and close monitoring of antifactor-Xa activity.[138] Abciximab and tirofiban (glycoprotein platelet [GP] II/IIIa inhibitors) can be used as adjunctive therapy in ACS; these drugs require no dose changes in dialysis patients.[10] Bivalirudin, a direct thrombin

TABLE 98–4

Cardiovascular Drugs That Need Special Attention in Renal Patients

MEDICATIONS	PRECAUTION
Anticoagulants	
Warfarin	Close monitoring of INR and other OTC medications
Clopidogrel (Plavix) and aspirin	Increased risk of bleeding with combination use[138]
Low-molecular-weight heparins	Dose adjustment and monitoring of antifactor Xa[139]
ACEI and ARB	AKI when used with aggressive diuretic regimen[162]
	Hyperkalemia when used with potassium sparing diuretics[167]
	Risk of anaphylactoid reaction with ACEI in patients dialyzed with AN69 membranes[205]
	All ACEI except fosinopril, need dose adjusted for renal impairment, no need for dose reduction for ARB[206]
Aldosterone receptor antagonists	
Spironolactone and eplerone	Hyperkalemia when used along with ACEI/ARB and blockers[167]
Adrenergic agents	
α-Adrenergic blockers	Methyldopa, doxazosin, prazosin, and reserpine active metabolite can accumulate in CKD[207]
β Blockers	Acebutolol, nadolol, and sotalol need dose reduction in CKD[207]
Calcium channel blockers	No need for dose reduction in CKD[207]
	Verapamil, diltiazem, amlodipine, and nicardipine can significantly increase cyclosporine and tacrolimus levels in transplant recipients[208]
Vasodilators	
Nitroprusside	Risk of thiocyanate toxicity in CKD, limit exposure
Hydralazine	Need dose reduction for eGFR less than 50 mL/min[208]
Lipid-lowering drugs	Statins when used in combination with cyclosporine can increase risk of rhabdomyolysis[208]
Antiarrhythmics	Bretylium, digoxin, flecainide, procainamide need dose adjustments in CKD[207]

ACEI, angiotensin converting enzyme inhibitor; AKI, acute kidney insufficiency; ARB, angiotensinII receptor antagonist; CKD, chronic kidney disease; eGFR, estimated GFR; INR, international normalized ratio; OTC, over-the-counter.

inhibitor, when used with PCI in patients with CKD, resulted in lower death rate, lower myocardial infarction (MI) rate, or need for urgent revascularization, as well as lower risk of bleeding compared with heparin.[139]

Occurrence of ACS during a dialysis session requires treatment to be stopped and the patient evaluated by a physician promptly.

For those patients with known stable angina during dialysis, treatment can be continued with the following modifications: (1) stopping or decreasing the rate of ultrafiltration to avoid ECV depletion; (2) reducing blood flow through the dialyzer to limit cardiac oxygen demand; and (3) administering oxygen. If hypotensive, the patient should be immediately placed in the Trendelenburg position while saline is infused. Other long-term management strategies for prevention of cardiovascular complications in CKD patients are directed toward control of ECV, electrolyte disturbances, and anemia. The usual concentration of potassium in the dialysate fluid is 2 mmol/L, but this can be increased to 3 to 3.5 mmol/L for a cardiac patient to avoid hypokalemia to prevent risk of arrhythmias in patients with CAD (or those receiving digoxin). Anemia caused by renal disease, requires the use of EPO and an appropriate amount of iron to increase the hemoglobin level to at least 11 g/dL.[54] Increasing hemoglobin levels to 13 g/dL or greater does not benefit the survival of ESRD patients and could have adverse cardiovascular outcomes.[140,141]

Regarding the relative merits of medical therapy and revascularization by surgery or PCI with or without stenting, no data from large-scale prospective randomized trials exists. Retrospective data from large national databases and registries suggest that patients with ESRD and CAD who receive conservative medical management tend to fare worst among all treatment groups.[142] Dialysis patients undergoing CABG face a 4.4 times greater inhospital mortality, a 3.1 times greater risk of mediastinitis, and a 2.6 times greater risk of stroke compared to patients without renal disease.[143] These data emphasize that the physician recommending this operation should be convinced of an improved quality of life after CABG. The long-term survival of ESRD patients after CABG surgery is better than PCI (2-year all cause, 56 percent versus 48 percent with or without stenting).[144] For nondiabetic ESRD patients who underwent PCI with stent, the risk of all-cause death was 10 percent lower, compared with those who got PCI without stent, but this advantage was not seen for diabetic patients.[144] In patients with CKD and ACS, requiring acute coronary revascularization, PCI with stenting has improved the 2-year survival rate over medical therapy alone, and results were comparable to those who underwent CABG.[145] In general, PCI provides excellent angiographic success but is associated with increased restenosis and the need for revascularization.[146] Therefore, provocative stress imaging should be considered to detect clinically silent restenosis 12 to 16 weeks after PCI.[147] There are currently no data on the impact of coronary brachytherapy or drug-eluting stents on the restenosis rates after PCI in dialysis patients.

CONGESTIVE HEART FAILURE

In congestive heart failure (CHF), enhanced sympathetic activity and activation of the RAAS promote sodium and water reabsorption by the kidney. These responses expand the ECV leading to edema and increased end-diastolic volume.[148] Moreover, plasma arginine vasopressin (AVP) concentrations are usually elevated in patients with heart failure and correlate, in general, with the clinical and hemodynamic severity of the disease.[149] These responses coupled with increased water intake (possibly related to angiotensin-II–stimulated central thirst receptors) cause hyponatremia, an

important indicator of a poor prognosis.[150] Impaired renal function is independently associated with heightened risk for all-cause death, cardiovascular death, and hospitalization for heart failure in patients with CHF with both preserved as well as reduced left ventricular ejection fraction (LVEF).[151,152] Anemia at baseline and changes in hemoglobin are inversely associated with subsequent risk of morbidity and mortality in patients with CHF.[153] Albuminuria as detected by urine albumin-to-creatinine ratio is an independent baseline risk factor for the development of CHF in patients with diabetes.[154]

Echocardiograms in ESRD patients reveal a high prevalence of *hypertrophic cardiomyopathy* characterized by left ventricular hypertrophy, asymmetric septal hypertrophy, and/or impaired contractility, as well as dilated cardiomyopathy.[155] Risk factors for developing CHF in patients with renal disease include hypertension, diabetes, persistent ECV expansion, anemia, AV fistula, ischemic heart disease, metabolic acidosis, electrolyte disturbances, hypercalcemia, hyperphosphatemia, and possibly the uremic state per se.[156] A successful HD regimen can improve cardiac function dramatically, the suggested mechanisms include controlling hypertension, correcting volume overload, removing uremic toxins, and normalizing blood pH and electrolyte levels (particularly, ionized calcium and potassium).[157] The prevention of CHF in dialysis patients requires strict control of ECV and hypertension. Consequently, dietary restriction of salt and fluid are critical so that the patient's weight can be kept as close as possible to the estimated dry weight. High-output cardiac failure is a rare complication of high-flow AV fistula. When suspected of this complication, the blood-flow rate through the AV fistula should be measured by ultrasound dilution techniques. Currently, there are no guidelines for when and at what access flow to intervene. Most of the banding and surgical closure of AV fistula in the literature has occurred when patients develop frank symptoms of CHF with a corresponding ratio of blood flow through the fistula over the cardiac output was greater than 40 percent.[158]

Management of CHF in predialysis CKD patients is multifactorial and similar to the one recommended for general population (see Chap. 26). There is limited data on the use of β blockers in patients with CHF and renal disease. Given the clear benefit of β blockers in nonrenal patients with mild to moderate CHF, it seems likely these agents will also prove to be beneficial for kidney-disease patients. Here we will discuss topics related to or have consequences on renal disease.

【 】 DIURETIC USAGE IN CONGESTIVE HEART FAILURE

Use of diuretics to relieve pulmonary congestion symptoms have been the cornerstone of management of patients with CHF since the early times of modern medicine. However, the effect of diuretics use in CHF on survival has never been rigorously tested, mainly, because diuretics were introduced before the advent of large clinical trials with mortality end points. Some observational studies have pointed toward an association between the use of diuretics and worsening of renal failure.[159,160] However, these studies can only be reflective of the severity of symptoms and a precarious hemodynamic state rather than the effect of diuretics. In congested patients with CHF, diuretics are extremely effective in relieving symptoms, reducing intracardiac pressures by decreasing preloading, and reducing the increased pulmonary vascular pressures. However, like all other potent therapeutic agents, diuretics can induce undesirable effects. Administration of furosemide in noncongested patients results in a further increase in angiotensin II, and as the veins are unable to dilate further, the arterial vasoconstrictor effect predominates.[160] Volume-depletion-induced activation of the RAAS, can compromise GFR and limit the natriuretic response of the kidney.[161] Moreover, metabolic effects of diuretics, such as alterations in lipids and impairment in glucose metabolism, and therefore, the occurrence of type II diabetes can have a negative impact on the cardiovascular risk profile of patients with CHF. These metabolic effects may not translate into greater frequency of cardiovascular events in the relatively short-term followup of patients in studies such as the Antihypertensive and Lipid-lowering Treatment to Prevent Heart Attack Trial (ALLHAT).[162] The diuretic response to a given dose of diuretic also depends on whether the patient has the predominant systolic or diastolic dysfunction. Isolated diastolic dysfunction is mainly caused by impaired myocardial relaxation or rarely infiltrative disease of myocardium, but as cardiac output and blood pressure are dependent on high filling pressures, patients with this condition are more prone to the adverse consequences of volume depletion with the use of diuretics.[160]

【 】 EFFECTS OF BLOCKING RENIN–ANGIOTENSIN-ALDOSTERONE SYSTEM ON RENAL FUNCTION IN CHF

The glomerular filtration in CHF, as in any other hypoperfusion state, is dependent on angiotensin-II–induced vasoconstriction of the efferent glomerular arteriole, and blocking this response with ACEI or ARB can markedly decrease the GFR. Therefore, initiating treatment with these agents can increase the risk of diuretic-associated renal impairment in patients with CHF.[163] However, ACEI/ARB therapy should not be discontinued unless serum creatinine level increases above 30 percent over the baseline during the first 2 months after initiation of therapy or hyperkalemia (serum potassium level ≥5.6 mmol/L) develops.[164] The predictors of the development of worsening renal function in patients treated with ACEI are higher baseline serum creatinine levels, older age, and a higher dose of loop diuretics.[164] Patients taking ACEI or ARB should also be warned not to use nonsteroidal antiinflammatory drugs (NSAIDs) and to report to their physician for the development of diarrhea, vomiting, or fever, these conditions can cause dehydration and precipitate worsening of renal function. To prevent significant decline in kidney function, it is important to measure serum creatinine and serum potassium within 10 to 14 days after starting ACEI/ARB in patients with any degree of preexisting renal insufficiency. African Americans with NYHA class II or higher disease, who are unable to tolerate ACEI/ARB, can benefit from combination hydralazine and isosorbide dinitrate therapy to achieve "after-load reduction."[165] The role of ACEIs or ARBs in treating CHF patients with moderate or severe renal failure (serum creatinine >3.0 mg/dL) is not so well studied. However, dialysis patients who were treated with ACEI for 3 years had a decrease in left ventricular mass, in comparison with patients who had the same degree of blood pressure control, hemoglobin concentration, and adequacy of dialysis.[166]

In patients with CHF (NYHA class III/IV), already receiving a diuretic and ACEI, spironolactone improved survival and reduced hospital admissions, compared to placebo, irrespective of etiology.[167] However, many subsequent reports highlighted much higher risk for the development of life-threatening hyperkalemia and AKI.[168–170] Many of the problems encountered were caused by misuse of spironolactone, that is, prescription in inappropriate patients, use of unnecessary high doses of the drug, and failure to closely monitor blood chemistry.[168] It is important to note that, there is no evidence for benefit to add both an ARB and spironolactone in addition to an ACEI, for the treatment of CHF, triple combination is more likely to result in renal dysfunction and hyperkalalemia.[171]

Nesiritide, a recombinant human B-type natriuretic peptide, has been shown to be beneficial in the treatment of acute decompensated heart failure (ADHF).[172,173] Unfortunately, the safety of nesiritide is now questioned based on two meta-analyses suggesting that nesiritide can be responsible for a worsening of renal function and an increased mortality.[174,175] Recently, an ultrafiltration device for fluid removal in diuretic-resistant ADHF patients, has shown to decrease length of stay and rehospitalizations.[176] This device has received FDA approval for use in high-risk heart failure patients. A prospective randomized study comparing ultrafiltration with standard therapy for ADHF is ongoing to identify effects specifically attributable to ultrafiltration.[176] Another promising therapeutic agent for the treatment of heart failure is the development of vasopressin receptor antagonists. Selective vasopressin V_2-receptor antagonist, target the cause of abnormal water retention by producing an increase in electrolyte-free water excretion and could thus provide highly specific therapy against renal water retention and dilutional hyponatremia associated with chronic CHF. Currently, various new orally active combined V_1 and V_2 and selective V_2-receptor antagonists are undergoing clinical testing for their utility in the treatment of CHF.[177]

PERICARDIAL DISEASE

Before dialysis was widely available, pericarditis was regarded as a pre-terminal event in uremic patients. At present, the incidence of clinically apparent pericarditis has decreased from 50 percent to approximately 5 to 20 percent.[178] In general, both uremic and dialysis pericarditis have occurred more frequently in younger than in older persons and have occurred more commonly in women than in men.[179] The cause of uremic pericarditis is unknown but most likely is related to accumulation of uremic toxins because vigorous dialysis is generally associated with its resolution. The term *dialysis pericarditis* is applied to patients who develop clinical features of pericarditis after being stabilized on dialysis (usually ≥8 weeks after its initiation).[180] This type of pericarditis is less responsive to intensive dialysis therapy.

The primary treatment for uremic pericarditis is intensive dialysis (e.g., daily HD for 1 to 2 weeks). Heparin is eliminated to avoid hemorrhage into the pericardial space. Use of indomethacin and steroid therapy is of no proven benefit in uremic or dialysis pericarditis.[181]

Pericardial effusion is even more frequent in dialysis patients because it is linked to ECV expansion. Although an effusion often complicates pericarditis, cardiac tamponade is rare. *An important clue to the presence of impending cardiac tamponade is the occurrence of repeated and/or severe hypotension during dialysis.* Pericardiocentesis with or without catheter drainage should be reserved for cases of circulatory collapse associated with cardiac tamponade. In most other cases, there is sufficient time to initiate safer and more effective surgical options for retrieving pericardial fluid.[181]

INFECTIVE ENDOCARDITIS

The incidence of bacteremia in HD patients ranges from 0.7 to 1.2 episodes per 100 patient months, and close to 10 percent of these bacteremic episodes are complicated by infective endocarditis (IE).[182] *Staphylococcus aureus* is the causative organism in 60 to 80 percent cases of IE diagnosed in HD patients. Methicillin-resistant *S. aureus* has recently been reported as more common than methicillin-susceptible *S. aureus* (67 vs. 33 percent).[183] Other causative organisms causing IE are *Staphylococcus epidermidis, Streptococcus viridans,* enterococci, and gram-negative organisms.[184] Bacteremia in patients receiving HD is primarily the result of access-site infections, followed by access manipulation and procedures such as dental work.[184] The mitral valve is more often infected than aortic valve, and together both are more often infected than the right-sided valves in HD population.[184,185]

Typically, a bacteremic patient presents with abrupt onset fever and chills, especially during the dialysis session. The growth of *S. aureus* in blood cultures, persistence of signs or symptoms of infection despite antibiotics and/or access removal, or the development of septic arthritis or other metastatic infections, should raise the suspicion of IE. Transesophageal echocardiography (TEE) is the procedure of choice for the diagnosis of endocarditis in a dialysis patient with bacteremia (sensitivity of 100 percent compared to 33 percent with transthoracic echocardiography).[186] Specific organism sensitivity should guide antimicrobial therapy, current guidelines recommend a minimum of 4 weeks of antimicrobial therapy after a diagnosis of IE is made in an HD patient.[184] Surgical indications and contraindications for acute IE in ESRD patients are similar to those for general population.[187]

CARDIAC ARRHYTHMIAS

Risk factors for cardiac arrhythmias in dialysis patients include ischemic heart disease, calcification of the conduction system from secondary hyperparathyroidism, pericarditis, dialysis-associated hypotension, dialysis-induced acid-base and electrolyte disturbances (hyper- and hypokalemia, hyper- and hypocalcemia, and hypermagnesemia), and hypoxemia.[188] Fortunately, serious arrhythmias are uncommon except in patients with underlying heart disease, those receiving digitalis, or those with severe hypokalemia.[189] The risk for atrial and ventricular arrhythmias in dialysis patients receiving digitalis increases sharply during dialysis because of rapid shifts of potassium. Therefore, digitalis should be prescribed with the lowest therapeutic dosage. Notably, the potassium concentration in the dialysate can be increased to decrease the risk of digitalis-toxic arrhythmias but, in such patients, dietary potassium must be rigidly restricted to prevent hyperkalemia. However, it has been questioned whether the occurrence of complex ventricular arrhythmia is influenced by dialysate potassium concentration.[190]

RENAL FAILURE FOLLOWING CARDIAC CATHETERIZATION

【 】 CONTRAST-INDUCED NEPHROPATHY

Contrast-induced nephropathy (CIN) is the third most common cause of hospital-acquired acute renal failure.[191] The risk of CIN is a particular concern for patients with cardiovascular disease undergoing diagnostic and therapeutic angiography.[192] Typically serum creatinine begins to increase within 24 to 72 hours following a radiocontrast study, and renal dysfunction is typically brief (approximately 5 to 7 days) unless there is preexisting renal damage. Fewer than 1 percent of those who develop CIN with baseline GFR of >60 mL/min/1.73 m^2 require dialysis, but in patients with GFR of 30 mL/min/1.73 m^2 or less, the need for dialysis approaches 2 to 8 percent.[193]

To prevent the development of CIN, patients at risk for this complication need to be identified before the planned contrast administration. The categories of high-risk patients are those with established CKD stage 3 or higher (estimated GFR <60 mL/min/1.73 m^2), diabetes mellitus, multiple myeloma, heavy proteinuria, volume depletion, congestive heart failure, and in those patients whom large amounts of contrast dye use is anticipated. For these high-risk patients, the Consensus Panel for CIN recently published a list of recommendations for prevention and management of CIN as listed in Table 98–5.[194]

A standardized protocol of hydration with 0.45 percent saline, 12 hours before and 6 hours after contrast exposure has been proven effective in reducing the risk of CIN and should be used routinely. Superiority of hydration with isotonic saline compared to half-normal saline on the incidence of CIN (0.7 vs 2.0 percent) has been claimed in a recent trial, but the patient population is this study was at low risk for development of CIN.[195] In another trial, hydration with sodium bicarbonate, given as a bolus for 1 hour prior to examination followed by an infusion for 6 hours af-

---

TABLE 98–5

Six Steps for the Prevention of Contrast-Induced Nephropathy

---

1. Before contrast administration all patients should be evaluated for their risk of CIN.
2. Patients should be in optimal volume status at the time of exposure to contrast.
3. High-risk patients should be considered for pharmacologic prophylaxis with therapies supported by clinical evidence.
4. Low osmolality contrast agents should be used in all patients.
5. Drugs that adversely affect renal function should be withheld prior to and immediately following contrast exposure.
6. In all high-risk patients, a follow-up serum creatinine should be obtained at not less than 24 hours or more than 72 hours following contrast exposure.

CIN, contrast-induced nephropathy.
SOURCE: Adapted from the Consensus Panel for CIN. McCullough, Soman.[193]

ter examination, was more effective than hydration with sodium chloride for the prophylaxis of CIN.[196] Multiple pharmacologic agents have been tested for the prevention of CIN in high-risk patients, not a single agent came out as of proven benefit in randomized trials.[197] N-acetyl-L-cysteine (NAC), a potent antioxidant that scavenges a wide variety of oxygen-derived free radicals is the most investigated drug for the prevention of CIN. There were 10 reviews on randomized clinical trials (meta-analyses) published on this subject between August 2003 and March 2005.[198] Five reviews, recommended routine, or almost routine, use of NAC in the prevention of CIN. However, the other five find NAC of equivocal benefit and called for further well-designed randomized control trials on this subject. Therefore, despite the low cost and low side-effect profile of NAC, the lack of compelling evidence in favor of a beneficial effect prevents a firm recommendation from the Consensus Panel for CIN to use this agent.[194] However, they also found no evidence to prevent NAC use at the discretion of the physician, provided its use should not substitute for the application of appropriate volume-expansion strategies to prevent CIN. There are not good controlled studies available to justify the practice of immediate hemodialysis post–contrast-media administration for ESRD patients. However, in certain clinical situations patients, such as those who have preserved substantial urine output in spite of being on dialysis, or who develop pulmonary congestion or hyperkalemia following contrast administration, would need immediate dialysis.

[ ] ATHEROEMBOLIC RENAL DISEASE

Acute renal insufficiency as a result of atheroembolic renal disease (AERD) is caused by cholesterol emboli to the kidneys and is most commonly observed after invasive vascular procedure, such as manipulation of the aorta during angiography or vascular surgery or after anticoagulant and fibrinolytic therapy. The reported incidence of AERD following coronary angiography is less than 2 percent.[199] Of those who develop AERD, 37 percent require dialysis therapy and of those only one-third recover enough renal function to come off dialysis.[200] In this study, mortality risk was associated with older age, diabetes, and presence of ESRD. Atheroembolization to other organs such as the eyes (cholesterol plaques seen by funduscopy), pancreas (pancreatitis), and skin (livedo reticularis or gangrene) is commonly associated with this condition.[201] AERD can activate inflammation yielding an *active* urinary sediment with hematuria and cellular casts, hypocomplementemia, eosinophilia, and a high sedimentation rate.[202] There is no specific treatment for this condition; patients whose renal insufficiency progress to the stage of dialysis can still hope for 30 percent chance of delayed recovery from dialysis.[203]

CARDIAC DRUGS IN RENAL FAILURE

Drug regimens in patients with cardiovascular disease are frequently complex. In one study cardiovascular-related medicines accounted for 29.7 percent of medication-related problems.[204] The lack of dose adjustments in patients with CKD is an often overlooked, yet preventable, cause of drug-dosing error. Drug clearance in dialysis patient is affected by the water solubility, pro-

tein binding, distribution volume, and diffusion across the dialysis membrane. Peritoneal dialysis is less efficient at removing drugs than HD and is most effective for smaller molecular weight drugs that are not extensively bound to serum proteins. Another complicating factor of drug administration in CKD patients is the potential for adverse events caused by reduced renal function (e.g., hyperkalemia, platelet dysfunction) and drug-drug interaction altering efficacy or inducing toxicity of an agent (e.g., addition of verapamil causes an increase in cyclosporine levels).

Table 98–4 lists cardiovascular drugs that are commonly used in renal patients that need special attention. We covered the issues concerning the use of ACEI, ARB, and spironolactone in patients with CKD. Readers are advised to consult drug manufacturer's renal dose adjustment recommendations, as secondary sources of drug information are remarkably inconsistent in their advice on adjusting dosages to account for impaired kidney function. This is the worrying conclusion of a systematic comparison of four widely used and hitherto well-respected publications.[205]

REFERENCES

1. K/DOQI clinical practice guidelines for chronic kidney disease: evaluation, classification, and stratification. *Am J Kidney Dis.* 2002;39(2 suppl 1):S1–266.
2. Keane WF, Eknoyan G. Proteinuria, albuminuria, risk, assessment, detection, elimination (PARADE): a position paper of the National Kidney Foundation. *Am J Kidney Dis.* 1999;33(5):1004–1010.
3. Stevens LA, Coresh J, Greene T, et al. Assessing kidney function—measured and estimated glomerular filtration rate. *N Engl J Med.* 2006;354(23):2473–2483.
4. Astor BC, Muntner P, Levin A, et al. Association of kidney function with anemia: the Third National Health and Nutrition Examination Survey (1988–1994). *Arch Intern Med.* 2002;162(12):1401–1408.
5. Eustace JA, Astor B, Muntner PM, et al. Prevalence of acidosis and inflammation and their association with low serum albumin in chronic kidney disease. *Kidney Int.* 2004;65(3):1031–1040.
6. Keith DS, Nichols GA, Gullion CM, et al. Longitudinal follow-up and outcomes among a population with chronic kidney disease in a large managed care organization. *Arch Intern Med.* 22 2004;164(6):659–663.
7. Go AS, Chertow GM, Fan D, et al. Chronic kidney disease and the risks of death, cardiovascular events, and hospitalization. *N Engl J Med.* 2004;351(13):1296–1305.
8. Masoudi FA, Plomondon ME, Magid DJ, et al. Renal insufficiency and mortality from acute coronary syndromes. *Am Heart J.* 2004;147(4):623–629.
9. Cooper WA, O'Brien SM, Thourani VH, et al. Impact of renal dysfunction on outcomes of coronary artery bypass surgery: results from the Society of Thoracic Surgeons National Adult Cardiac Database. *Circulation.* 2006;113(8):1063–1070.
10. K/DOQI clinical practice guidelines for cardiovascular disease in dialysis patients. *Am J Kidney Dis.* 2005;45(4 suppl 3):S1–153.
11. Foley RN, Parfrey PS, Sarnak MJ. Clinical epidemiology of cardiovascular disease in chronic renal disease. *Am J Kidney Dis.* 1998;32(5 suppl 3):S112–119.
12. Herzog CA. Sudden cardiac death and acute myocardial infarction in dialysis patients: perspectives of a cardiologist. *Semin Nephrol.* 2005;25(6):363–366.
13. Bleyer AJ, Hartman J, Brannon PC, et al. Characteristics of sudden death in hemodialysis patients. *Kidney Int.* 2006;69(12):2268–2273.
14. Sarnak MJ, Levey AS, Schoolwerth AC, et al. Kidney disease as a risk factor for development of cardiovascular disease: a statement from the American Heart Association Councils on Kidney in Cardiovascular Disease, High Blood Pressure Research, Clinical Cardiology, and Epidemiology and Prevention. *Hypertension.* 2003;42(5):1050–1065.
15. Klausen K, Borch-Johnsen K, Feldt-Rasmussen B, et al. Very low levels of microalbuminuria are associated with increased risk of coronary heart disease and death independently of renal function, hypertension, and diabetes. *Circulation.* 2004;110(1):32–35.
16. Manjunath G, Tighiouart H, Ibrahim H, et al. Level of kidney function as a risk factor for atherosclerotic cardiovascular outcomes in the community. *J Am Coll Cardiol.* 2003;41(1):47–55.

17. McClellan WM. Epidemiology and risk factors for chronic kidney disease. *Med Clin North Am.* 2005;89(3):419–445.

18. McClellan WM, Langston RD, Presley R. Medicare patients with cardiovascular disease have a high prevalence of chronic kidney disease and a high rate of progression to end-stage renal disease. *J Am Soc Nephrol.* 2004;15(7):1912–1919.

19. Perry HM, Jr., Miller JP, Fornoff JR, et al. Early predictors of 15-year end-stage renal disease in hypertensive patients. *Hypertension.* 1995;25(4 pt 1):587–594.

20. Bax L, van der Graaf Y, Rabelink AJ, et al. Influence of atherosclerosis on age-related changes in renal size and function. *Eur J Clin Invest.* 2003;33(1):34–40.

21. Kellum JA, Levin N, Bouman C, et al. Developing a consensus classification system for acute renal failure. *Curr Opin Crit Care.* 2002;8(6):509–514.

22. Mehta RL, Chertow GM. Acute renal failure definitions and classification: time for change? *J Am Soc Nephrol.* 2003;14(8):2178–2187.

23. Kellum JA, Ronco C, Mehta R, et al. Consensus development in acute renal failure: The Acute Dialysis Quality Initiative. *Curr Opin Crit Care.* 2005;11(6):527–532.

24. Bellomo R, Ronco C, Kellum JA, et al. Acute renal failure—definition, outcome measures, animal models, fluid therapy and information technology needs: the Second International Consensus Conference of the Acute Dialysis Quality Initiative (ADQI) Group. *Crit Care.* 2004;8(4):R204–212.

25. Hoste EA, Clermont G, Kersten A, et al. RIFLE criteria for acute kidney injury are associated with hospital mortality in critically ill patients: a cohort analysis. *Crit Care.* 2006;10(3):R73.

26. Kuitunen A, Vento A, Suojaranta-Ylinen R, et al. Acute renal failure after cardiac surgery: evaluation of the RIFLE classification. *Ann Thorac Surg.* 2006;81(2):542–546.

27. Muntner P, Coresh J, Powe NR, et al. The contribution of increased diabetes prevalence and improved myocardial infarction and stroke survival to the increase in treated end-stage renal disease. *J Am Soc Nephrol.* 2003;14(6):1568–1577.

28. Ezekowitz J, McAlister FA, Humphries KH, et al. The association among renal insufficiency, pharmacotherapy, and outcomes in 6,427 patients with heart failure and coronary artery disease. *J Am Coll Cardiol.* 2004;44(8):1587–1592.

29. Weiner DE, Tighiouart H, Amin MG, et al. Chronic kidney disease as a risk factor for cardiovascular disease and all-cause mortality: a pooled analysis of community-based studies. *J Am Soc Nephrol.* 2004;15(5):1307–1315.

30. U.S. Renal Data System. Excerpts from the USRDS 2005 annual data report. *Am J Kidney Dis.* 2005;47(suppl 1):S1–S286.

31. Bongartz LG, Cramer MJ, Doevendans PA, et al. The severe cardiorenal syndrome: "Guyton revisited." *Eur Heart J.* 2005;26(1):11–17.

32. Remuzzi G, Perico N, Macia M, et al. The role of renin-angiotensin-aldosterone system in the progression of chronic kidney disease. *Kidney Int Suppl.* 2005;(99):S57–65.

33. Glatter KA, Graves SW, Hollenberg NK, et al. Sustained volume expansion and [Na,K]ATPase inhibition in chronic renal failure. *Am J Hypertens.* 1994;7(11):1016–1025.

34. Baylis C. Nitric oxide deficiency in chronic renal disease. *Eur J Clin Pharmacol.* 2006;2004;62(suppl 13):123–130.

35. Kamycheva E, Sundsfjord J, Jorde R. Serum parathyroid hormone levels predict coronary heart disease: the TROMSO Study. *Eur J Cardiovasc Prev Rehabil.* 2004;11(1):69–74.

36. Horl MP, Horl WH. Hemodialysis-associated hypertension: pathophysiology and therapy. *Am J Kidney Dis.* 2002;39(2):227–244.

37. Hou FF, Zhang X, Zhang GH, et al. Efficacy and safety of benazepril for advanced chronic renal insufficiency. *N Engl J Med.* 2006;354(2):131–140.

38. Mann JF, Gerstein HC, Pogue J, et al. Renal insufficiency as a predictor of cardiovascular outcomes and the impact of ramipril: the HOPE randomized trial. *Ann Intern Med.* 2001;134(8):629–636.

39. Brenner BM, Cooper ME, de Zeeuw D, et al. Effects of losartan on renal and cardiovascular outcomes in patients with type 2 diabetes and nephropathy. *N Engl J Med.* 2001;345(12):861–869.

40. Agodoa LY, Appel L, Bakris GL, et al. Effect of ramipril vs amlodipine on renal outcomes in hypertensive nephrosclerosis: a randomized controlled trial. *JAMA.* 2001;285(21):2719–2728.

41. Mann JF, Yi QL, Sleight P, et al. Serum potassium, cardiovascular risk, and effects of an ACE inhibitor: results of the HOPE study. *Clin Nephrol.* 2005;63(3):181–187.

42. Bakris GL, Weir MR. Angiotensin-converting enzyme inhibitor-associated elevations in serum creatinine: is this a cause for concern? *Arch Intern Med.* 2000;160(5):685–693.

43. Chobanian AV, Bakris GL, Black HR, et al. The Seventh Report of the Joint National Committee on Prevention, Detection, Evaluation, and Treatment of High Blood Pressure: the JNC 7 report. *JAMA.* 2003;289(19):2560–2572.

44. American Diabetes Association: clinical practice recommendations. *Diabetes Care.* 2005;28(suppl 1):S1–S79.

45. Bakris GL, Williams M, Dworkin L, et al. Preserving renal function in adults with hypertension and diabetes: a consensus approach. National Kidney Foundation Hypertension and Diabetes Executive Committees Working Group. *Am J Kidney Dis.* 2000;36(3):646–661.

46. Dussol B, Moussi-Frances J, Morange S, et al. A randomized trial of furosemide vs hydrochlorothiazide in patients with chronic renal failure and hypertension. *Nephrol Dial Transplant.* 2005;20(2):349–353.

47. Zazgornik J, Biesenbach G, Janko O, et al. Bilateral nephrectomy: the best, but often overlooked, treatment for refractory hypertension in hemodialysis patients. *Am J Hypertens.* 1998;11(11 pt 1):1364–1370.

48. Leeder SR, Mitchell P, Liew G, et al. Low hemoglobin, chronic kidney disease, and risk for coronary heart disease-related death: the Blue Mountains Eye Study. *J Am Soc Nephrol.* 2006;17(1):279–284.

49. Abramson JL, Jurkovitz CT, Vaccarino V, et al. Chronic kidney disease, anemia, and incident stroke in a middle-aged, community-based population: the ARIC Study. *Kidney Int.* 2003;64(2):610–615.

50. Sandgren PE, Murray AM, Herzog CA, et al. Anemia and new-onset congestive heart failure in the general Medicare population. *J Card Fail.* 2005;11(2):99–105.

51. Drueke TB, Locatelli F, Clyne N, et al. Normalization of hemoglobin level in patients with chronic kidney disease and anemia. *N Engl J Med.* 2006;355(20):2071–2084.

52. Singh AK, Szczech L, Tang KL, et al. Correction of anemia with epoetin alfa in chronic kidney disease. *N Engl J Med.* 2006;355(20):2085–2098.

53. Silverberg DS, Wexler D, Blum M, et al. Effects of treatment with epoetin Beta on outcomes in patients with anaemia and chronic heart failure. *Kidney Blood Press Res.* 2005;28(1):41–47.

54. KDOQI clinical practice guidelines and clinical practice recommendations for anemia in chronic kidney disease. *Am J Kidney Dis.* 2006;47(5 suppl 3):S11–145.

55. Ritz E, Orth SR. Nephropathy in patients with type 2 diabetes mellitus. *N Engl J Med.* 1999;341(15):1127–1133.

56. El-Atat FA, Stas SN, McFarlane SI, et al. The relationship between hyperinsulinemia, hypertension and progressive renal disease. *J Am Soc Nephrol.* 2004;15(11):2816–2827.

57. Chen J, Muntner P, Hamm LL, et al. The metabolic syndrome and chronic kidney disease in U.S. adults. *Ann Intern Med.* 2004;140(3):167–174.

58. Kramer HJ, Saranathan A, Luke A, et al. Increasing body mass index and obesity in the incident ESRD population. *J Am Soc Nephrol.* 2006;17(5):1453–1459.

59. Praga M. Therapeutic measures in proteinuric nephropathy. *Kidney Int Suppl.* 2005;(99):S137–141.

60. Kalantar-Zadeh K, Abbott KC, Salahudeen AK, et al. Survival advantages of obesity in dialysis patients. *Am J Clin Nutr.* 2005;81(3):543–554.

61. K/DOQI clinical practice guidelines for management of dyslipidemias in patients with kidney disease. *Am J Kidney Dis.* 2003;41(4 suppl 3):I–IV, S1–91.

62. Trevisan R, Dodesini AR, Lepore G. Lipids and renal disease. *J Am Soc Nephrol.* 2006;17(4 suppl 2):S145–147.

63. Vaziri ND. Molecular mechanisms of lipid disorders in nephrotic syndrome. *Kidney Int.* 2003;63(5):1964–1976.

64. Third Report of the National Cholesterol Education Program (NCEP) Expert Panel on Detection, Evaluation, and Treatment of High Blood Cholesterol in Adults (Adult Treatment Panel III) final report. *Circulation.* 2002;106(25):3143–3421.

65. Baigent C, Landray M, Warren M. Statin therapy in kidney disease populations: potential benefits beyond lipid lowering and the need for clinical trials. *Curr Opin Nephrol Hypertens.* 2004;13(6):601–605.

66. Tonelli M, Moye L, Sacks FM, et al. Effect of pravastatin on loss of renal function in people with moderate chronic renal insufficiency and cardiovascular disease. *J Am Soc Nephrol.* 2003;14(6):1605–1613.

67. Seliger SL, Weiss NS, Gillen DL, et al. HMG-CoA reductase inhibitors are associated with reduced mortality in ESRD patients. *Kidney Int.* 2002;61(1):297–304.

68. Mason NA, Bailie GR, Satayathum S, et al. HMG-coenzyme a reductase inhibitor use is associated with mortality reduction in hemodialysis patients. *Am J Kidney Dis.* 2005;45(1):119–126.

69. Jardine AG, Holdaas H, Fellstrom B, et al. fluvastatin prevents cardiac death and myocardial infarction in renal transplant recipients: post-hoc subgroup analyses of the ALERT Study. *Am J Transplant.* 2004;4(6):988–995.

70. Baigent C, Landry M. Study of Heart and Renal Protection (SHARP). *Kidney Int Suppl.* 2003;(84):S207–210.

71. Fellstrom BC, Holdaas H, Jardine AG. Why do we need a statin trial in hemodialysis patients? *Kidney Int Suppl.* 2003;(84):S204–206.

72. Kasiske B, Cosio FG, Beto J, et al. Clinical practice guidelines for managing dyslipidemias in kidney transplant patients: a report from the Managing Dyslipidemias in Chronic Kidney Disease Work Group of the National Kidney Foundation Kidney Disease Outcomes Quality Initiative. *Am J Transplant.* 2004;(4 suppl 7):13–53.

73. Bostom AG, Lathrop L. Hyperhomocysteinemia in end-stage renal disease: prevalence, etiology, and potential relationship to arteriosclerotic outcomes. *Kidney Int.* 1997;52(1):10–20.

74. Pernod G, Bosson JL, Golshayan D, et al. The Diamant Alpin Dialysis cohort study: clinico-biological characteristics and cardiovascular genetic risk profile of incident patients. *J Nephrol.* 2004;17(1):66–75.

75. Garibotto G, Sofia A, Valli A, et al. Causes of hyperhomocysteinemia in patients with chronic kidney diseases. *Semin Nephrol.* 2006;26(1):3–7.

76. Ducloux D, Motte G, Challier B, et al. Serum total homocysteine and cardiovascular disease occurrence in chronic, stable renal transplant recipients: a prospective study. *J Am Soc Nephrol.* 2000;11(1):134–137.

77. Pernod G, Bosson JL, Golshayan D, et al. Phenotypic and genotypic risk factors for cardiovascular events in an incident dialysis cohort. *Kidney Int.* 2006;69(8):1424–1430.

78. Mallamaci F, Zoccali C, Tripepi G, et al. Hyperhomocysteinemia predicts cardiovascular outcomes in hemodialysis patients. *Kidney Int.* 2002;61(2):609–614.

79. Homocysteine-lowering trials for prevention of cardiovascular events: a review of the design and power of the large randomized trials. *Am Heart J.* 2006;151(2):282–287.

80. Bostom AG, Carpenter MA, Kusek JW, et al. Rationale and design of the Folic Acid for Vascular Outcome Reduction In Transplantation (FAVORIT) trial. *Am Heart J.* 2006;152:448.e1–e7.

81. Perazella MA. Pharmacologic options available to treat symptomatic intradialytic hypotension. *Am J Kidney Dis.* 2001;38(4 suppl 4):S26–36.

82. Prakash S, Garg AX, Heidenheim AP, et al. Midodrine appears to be safe and effective for dialysis-induced hypotension: a systematic review. *Nephrol Dial Transplant.* 2004;19(10):2553–2558.

83. Hung SY, Hung YM, Fang HC, et al. Cardiac troponin I and creatine kinase isoenzyme MB in patients with intradialytic hypotension. *Blood Purif.* 2004;22(4):338–343.

84. Brouns R, De Deyn PP. Neurological complications in renal failure: a review. *Clin Neurol Neurosurg.* 2004;107(1):1–16.

85. Zager PG, Nikolic J, Brown RH, et al. "U" curve association of blood pressure and mortality in hemodialysis patients. Medical Directors of Dialysis Clinic, Inc. *Kidney Int.* 1998;54(2):561–569.

86. Sherman RA. Modifying the dialysis prescription to reduce intradialytic hypotension. *Am J Kidney Dis.* 2001;38(4 suppl 4):S18–25.

87. Rodriguez HJ, Domenici R, Diroll A, et al. Assessment of dry weight by monitoring changes in blood volume during hemodialysis using Crit-Line. *Kidney Int.* 2005;68(2):854–861.

88. Burke AP, Taylor A, Farb A, et al. Coronary calcification: insights from sudden coronary death victims. *Z Kardiol.* 2000;89(suppl 2):49–53.

89. Edmonds ME, Morrison N, Laws JW, et al. Medial arterial calcification and diabetic neuropathy. *Br Med J (Clin Res Ed).* 1982;284(6320):928–930.

90. Giachelli CM. Vascular calcification mechanisms. *J Am Soc Nephrol.* 2004;15(12):2959–2964.

91. He ZX, Hedrick TD, Pratt CM, et al. Severity of coronary artery calcification by electron beam computed tomography predicts silent myocardial ischemia. *Circulation.* 2000;101(3):244–251.

92. Blacher J, Guerin AP, Pannier B, et al. Arterial calcifications, arterial stiffness, and cardiovascular risk in end-stage renal disease. *Hypertension.* 2001;38(4):938–942.

93. Horton KM, Post WS, Blumenthal RS, et al. Prevalence of significant noncardiac findings on electron-beam computed tomography coronary artery calcium screening examinations. *Circulation.* 2002;106(5):532–534.

94. Dellegrottaglie S, Saran R, Rajagopalan S. Vascular calcification in patients with renal failure: culprit or innocent bystander? *Cardiol Clin.* 2005;23(3):373–384.

95. Block GA, Klassen PS, Lazarus JM, et al. Mineral metabolism, mortality, and morbidity in maintenance hemodialysis. *J Am Soc Nephrol.* 2004;15(8):2208–2218.

96. Ganesh SK, Stack AG, Levin NW, et al. Association of elevated serum PO(4), Ca x PO(4) product, and parathyroid hormone with cardiac mortality risk in chronic hemodialysis patients. *J Am Soc Nephrol.* 2001;12(10):2131–2138.

97. Slatopolsky E, Bricker NS. The role of phosphorus restriction in the prevention of secondary hyperparathyroidism in chronic renal disease. *Kidney Int.* 1973;4(2):141–145.

98. Malluche HH, Monier-Faugere MC. Hyperphosphatemia: pharmacologic intervention yesterday, today and tomorrow. *Clin Nephrol.* 2000;54(4):309–317.

99. Coburn JW. An update on vitamin D as related to nephrology practice. *Kidney Int Suppl.* 2003(87):S125–130.

100. Goodman WG, London G, Amann K, et al. Vascular calcification in chronic kidney disease. *Am J Kidney Dis.* 2004;43(3):572–579.

101. Block GA, Port FK. Re-evaluation of risks associated with hyperphosphatemia and hyperparathyroidism in dialysis patients: recommendations for a change in management. *Am J Kidney Dis.* 2000;35(6):1226–1237.

102. Block GA, Martin KJ, de Francisco AL, et al. Cinacalcet for secondary hyperparathyroidism in patients receiving hemodialysis. *N Engl J Med.* 2004;350(15):1516–1525.

103. Beddhu S, Kaysen GA, Yan G, et al. Association of serum albumin and atherosclerosis in chronic hemodialysis patients. *Am J Kidney Dis.* 2002;40(4):721–727.

104. Foley RN, Parfrey PS, Harnett JD, et al. Hypoalbuminemia, cardiac morbidity, and mortality in end-stage renal disease. *J Am Soc Nephrol.* 1996;7(5):728–736.

105. Lowrie EG, Lew NL. Death risk in hemodialysis patients: the predictive value of commonly measured variables and an evaluation of death rate differences between facilities. *Am J Kidney Dis.* 1990;15(5):458–482.

106. Reuben DB, Ferrucci L, Wallace R, et al. The prognostic value of serum albumin in healthy older persons with low and high serum interleukin-6 (IL-6) levels. *J Am Geriatr Soc.* 2000;48(11):1404–1407.

107. Ross R. Atherosclerosis—an inflammatory disease. *N Engl J Med.* 1999;340(2):115–126.

108. Wang AY, Woo J, Lam CW, et al. Associations of serum fetuin-A with malnutrition, inflammation, atherosclerosis and valvular calcification syndrome and outcome in peritoneal dialysis patients. *Nephrol Dial Transplant.* 2005;20(8):1676–1685.

109. Zimmermann J, Herrlinger S, Pruy A, et al. Inflammation enhances cardiovascular risk and mortality in hemodialysis patients. *Kidney Int.* 1999;55(2):648–658.

110. Collins AJ, Kasiske B, Herzog C, et al. Excerpts from the United States Renal Data System 2004 annual data report: atlas of end-stage renal disease in the United States. *Am J Kidney Dis.* 2005;45(1 suppl 1):A5–7.

111. Chertow GM, Normand SL, Silva LR, et al. Survival after acute myocardial infarction in patients with end-stage renal disease: results from the cooperative cardiovascular project. *Am J Kidney Dis.* 2000;35(5):1044–1051.

112. Anavekar NS, McMurray JJ, Velazquez EJ, et al. Relation between renal dysfunction and cardiovascular outcomes after myocardial infarction. *N Engl J Med.* 2004;351(13):1285–1295.

113. Gibson CM, Pinto DS, Murphy SA, et al. Association of creatinine and creatinine clearance on presentation in acute myocardial infarction with subsequent mortality. *J Am Coll Cardiol.* 2003;42(9):1535–1543.

114. Schiele F, Legalery P, Didier K, et al. Impact of renal dysfunction on 1-year mortality after acute myocardial infarction. *Am Heart J.* 2006;151(3):661–667.

115. Winkelmayer WC, Charytan DM, Levin R, et al. Poor short-term survival and low use of cardiovascular medications in elderly dialysis patients after acute myocardial infarction. *Am J Kidney Dis.* 2006;47(2):301–308.

116. Ori Y, Korzets A, Katz M, et al. The contribution of an arteriovenous access for hemodialysis to left ventricular hypertrophy. *Am J Kidney Dis.* 2002;40(4):745–752.

117. Koch M, Gradaus F, Schoebel FC, et al. Relevance of conventional cardiovascular risk factors for the prediction of coronary artery disease in diabetic patients on renal replacement therapy. *Nephrol Dial Transplant.* 1997;12(6):1187–1191.

118. Ojanen S, Koobi T, Korhonen P, et al. QRS amplitude and volume changes during hemodialysis. *Am J Nephrol.* 1999;19(3):423–427.

119. Szabo Z, Kakuk G, Fulop T, et al. Effects of haemodialysis on maximum P wave duration and P wave dispersion. *Nephrol Dial Transplant.* 2002;17(9):1634–1638.

120. Covic A, Diaconita M, Gusbeth-Tatomir P, et al. Haemodialysis increases QT(c) interval but not QT(c) dispersion in ESRD patients without manifest cardiac disease. *Nephrol Dial Transplant.* 2002;17(12):2170–2177.

121. Rostand SG. Coronary heart disease in chronic renal insufficiency: some management considerations. *J Am Soc Nephrol.* 2000;11(10):1948–1956.

122. Goldsmith DJ, Covic A. Coronary artery disease in uremia: Etiology, diagnosis, and therapy. *Kidney Int.* 2001;60(6):2059–2078.

123. George SK, Singh AK. Current markers of myocardial ischemia and their validity in end-stage renal disease. *Curr Opin Nephrol Hypertens.* 1999;8(6):719–722.

124. Al Badr W, Mukherjee D, Kline-Rogers E, et al. Clinical association between renal insufficiency and positive troponin I in patients with acute coronary syndrome. *Cardiology.* 2004;102(4):215–219.

125. Martin GS, Becker BN, Schulman G. Cardiac troponin-I accurately predicts myocardial injury in renal failure. *Nephrol Dial Transplant.* 1998;13(7):1709–1712.

126. Ikeda J, Zenimoto M, Kita M, et al. [Usefulness of cardiac troponin I in patients with acute myocardial infarction]. *Rinsho Byori.* 2002;50(10):982–986.

127. Logar CM, Herzog CA, Beddhu S. Diagnosis and therapy of coronary artery disease in renal failure, end-stage renal disease, and renal transplant populations. *Am J Med Sci.* 2003;325(4):214–227.

128. Murphy SW, Foley RN, Parfrey PS. Screening and treatment for cardiovascular disease in patients with chronic renal disease. *Am J Kidney Dis.* 1998;32(5 suppl 3):S184–199.

129. Reis G, Marcovitz PA, Leichtman AB, et al. Usefulness of dobutamine stress echocardiography in detecting coronary artery disease in end-stage renal disease. *Am J Cardiol.* 1995;75(10):707–710.

130. Sharma R, Pellerin D, Gaze DC, et al. Dobutamine stress echocardiography and cardiac troponin T for the detection of significant coronary artery disease and predicting outcome in renal transplant candidates. *Eur J Echocardiogr.* 2005;6(5):327–335.

131. Herzog CA, Marwick TH, Pheley AM, et al. Dobutamine stress echocardiography for the detection of significant coronary artery disease in renal transplant candidates. *Am J Kidney Dis.* 1999;33(6):1080–1090.

132. European best practice guidelines for renal transplantation. Section IV. Long-term management of the transplant recipient. IV 5.1. Cardiovascular risks. Cardiovascular disease after renal transplantation. *Nephrol Dial Transplant.* 2002;17(suppl 4):24–25.

133. Meier-Kriesche HU, Schold JD, Srinivas TR, et al. Kidney transplantation halts cardiovascular disease progression in patients with end-stage renal disease. *Am J Transplant.* 2004;4(10):1662–1668.

134. Pilmore H. Cardiac assessment for renal transplantation. *Am J Transplant.* 2006;6(4):659–665.

135. McCullough PA, Sandberg KR, Borzak S, et al. Benefits of aspirin and beta-blockade after myocardial infarction in patients with chronic kidney disease. *Am Heart J.* 2002;144(2):226–232.

136. Livio M, Benigni A, Vigano G, et al. Moderate doses of aspirin and risk of bleeding in renal failure. *Lancet.* 1986;1(8478):414–416.

137. Kaufman JS, O'Connor TZ, Zhang JH, et al. Randomized controlled trial of clopidogrel plus aspirin to prevent hemodialysis access graft thrombosis. *J Am Soc Nephrol.* 2003;14(9):2313–2321.

138. Lim W, Dentali F, Eikelboom JW, et al. Meta-analysis: low-molecular-weight heparin and bleeding in patients with severe renal insufficiency. *Ann Intern Med.* 2006;144(9):673–684.

139. Chew DP, Bhatt DL, Kimball W, et al. Bivalirudin provides increasing benefit with decreasing renal function: a meta-analysis of randomized trials. *Am J Cardiol.* 2003;92(8):919–923.

140. Besarab A, Bolton WK, Browne JK, et al. The effects of normal as compared with low hematocrit values in patients with cardiac disease who are receiving hemodialysis and epoetin. *N Engl J Med.* 1998;339(9):584–590.

141. Parfrey PS, Foley RN, Wittreich BH, et al. Double-blind comparison of full and partial anemia correction in incident hemodialysis patients without symptomatic heart disease. *J Am Soc Nephrol.* 2005;16(7):2180–2189.

142. McCullough PA. Evaluation and treatment of coronary artery disease in patients with end-stage renal disease. *Kidney Int Suppl.* 2005(95):S51–58.

143. Opsahl JA, Husebye DG, Helseth HK, et al. Coronary artery bypass surgery in patients on maintenance dialysis: long-term survival. *Am J Kidney Dis.* 1988;12(4):271–274.

144. Herzog CA, Ma JZ, Collins AJ. Comparative survival of dialysis patients in the United States after coronary angioplasty, coronary artery stenting, and coronary artery bypass surgery and impact of diabetes. *Circulation.* 2002;106(17):2207–2211.

145. Keeley EC, Kadakia R, Soman S, et al. Analysis of long-term survival after revascularization in patients with chronic kidney disease presenting with acute coronary syndromes. *Am J Cardiol.* 2003;92(5):509–514.

146. Tadros GM, Herzog CA. Percutaneous coronary intervention in chronic kidney disease patients. *J Nephrol.* 2004;17(3):364–368.

147. Herzog CA. How to manage the renal patient with coronary heart disease: the agony and the ecstasy of opinion-based medicine. *J Am Soc Nephrol.* 2003;14(10):2556–2572.

148. Schrier RW, Abraham WT. Hormones and hemodynamics in heart failure. *N Engl J Med.* 1999;341(8):577–585.

149. Abraham WT, Shamshirsaz AA, McFann K, et al. Aquaretic effect of lixivaptan, an oral, non-peptide, selective V2 receptor vasopressin antagonist, in New York Heart Association functional class II and III chronic heart failure patients. *J Am Coll Cardiol.* 2006;47(8):1615–1621.

150. Klein L, O'Connor CM, Leimberger JD, et al. Lower serum sodium is associated with increased short-term mortality in hospitalized patients with wors-

151. ening heart failure: results from the Outcomes of a Prospective Trial of Intravenous Milrinone for Exacerbations of Chronic Heart Failure (OPTIME-CHF) study. *Circulation.* 2005;111(19):2454–2460.

151. Hillege HL, Nitsch D, Pfeffer MA, et al. Renal function as a predictor of outcome in a broad spectrum of patients with heart failure. *Circulation.* 2006;113(5):671–678.

152. Smith GL, Lichtman JH, Bracken MB, et al. Renal impairment and outcomes in heart failure: systematic review and meta-analysis. *J Am Coll Cardiol.* 2006;47(10):1987–1996.

153. Anand IS, Kuskowski MA, Rector TS, et al. Anemia and change in hemoglobin over time related to mortality and morbidity in patients with chronic heart failure: results from Val-HeFT. *Circulation.* 2005;112(8):1121–1127.

154. Carr AA, Kowey PR, Devereux RB, et al. Hospitalizations for new heart failure among subjects with diabetes mellitus in the RENAAL and LIFE studies. *Am J Cardiol.* 2005;96(11):1530–1536.

155. McMahon LP, Roger SD, Levin A. Development, prevention, and potential reversal of left ventricular hypertrophy in chronic kidney disease. *J Am Soc Nephrol.* 2004;15(6):1640–1647.

156. Stack AG, Bloembergen WE. A cross-sectional study of the prevalence and clinical correlates of congestive heart failure among incident U.S. dialysis patients. *Am J Kidney Dis.* 2001;38(5):992–1000.

157. Hung J, Harris PJ, Uren RF, et al. Uremic cardiomyopathy--effect of hemodialysis on left ventricular function in end-stage renal failure. *N Engl J Med.* 1980;302(10):547–551.

158. MacRae JM, Pandeya S, Humen DP, et al. Arteriovenous fistula-associated high-output cardiac failure: a review of mechanisms. *Am J Kidney Dis.* 2004;43(5):e17–22.

159. de Silva R, Nikitin NP, Witte KK, et al. Incidence of renal dysfunction over 6 months in patients with chronic heart failure due to left ventricular systolic dysfunction: contributing factors and relationship to prognosis. *Eur Heart J.* 2006;27(5):569–581.

160. Gupta S, Neyses L. Diuretic usage in heart failure: a continuing conundrum in 2005. *Eur Heart J.* 2005;26(7):644–649.

161. Greenberg A. Diuretic complications. *Am J Med Sci.* 2000;319(1):10–24.

162. Salvetti A, Ghiadoni L. Thiazide diuretics in the treatment of hypertension: an update. *J Am Soc Nephrol.* 2006;17(4 suppl 2):S25–29.

163. Knight EL, Glynn RJ, McIntyre KM, et al. Predictors of decreased renal function in patients with heart failure during angiotensin-converting enzyme inhibitor therapy: results from the studies of left ventricular dysfunction (SOLVD). *Am Heart J.* 1999;138(5 pt 1):849–855.

164. Ahmed A. Use of angiotensin-converting enzyme inhibitors in patients with heart failure and renal insufficiency: how concerned should we be by the rise in serum creatinine? *J Am Geriatr Soc.* 2002;50(7):1297–1300.

165. Franciosa JA, Taylor AL, Cohn JN, et al. African-American Heart Failure Trial (A-HeFT): rationale, design, and methodology. *J Card Fail.* 2002;8(3):128–135.

166. Paoletti E, Cassottana P, Bellino D, et al. Left ventricular geometry and adverse cardiovascular events in chronic hemodialysis patients on prolonged therapy with ACE inhibitors. *Am J Kidney Dis.* 2002;40(4):728–736.

167. Pitt B, Zannad F, Remme WJ, et al. The effect of spironolactone on morbidity and mortality in patients with severe heart failure. Randomized Aldactone Evaluation Study Investigators. *N Engl J Med.* 1999;341(10):709–717.

168. Juurlink DN, Mamdani MM, Lee DS, et al. Rates of hyperkalemia after publication of the Randomized Aldactone Evaluation Study. *N Engl J Med.* 2004;351(6):543–551.

169. Tamirisa KP, Aaronson KD, Koelling TM. Spironolactone-induced renal insufficiency and hyperkalemia in patients with heart failure. *Am Heart J.* 2004;148(6):971–978.

170. Witham MD, Gillespie ND, Struthers AD. Tolerability of spironolactone in patients with chronic heart failure—a cautionary message. *Br J Clin Pharmacol.* 2004;58(5):554–557.

171. McMurray J, Cohen-Solal A, Dietz R, et al. Practical recommendations for the use of ACE inhibitors, beta-blockers, aldosterone antagonists and angiotensin receptor blockers in heart failure: putting guidelines into practice. *Eur J Heart Fail.* 2005;7(5):710–721.

172. Intravenous nesiritide vs nitroglycerin for treatment of decompensated congestive heart failure: a randomized controlled trial. *JAMA.* 2002;287(12):1531–1540.

173. Colucci WS, Elkayam U, Horton DP, et al. Intravenous nesiritide, a natriuretic peptide, in the treatment of decompensated congestive heart failure. Nesiritide Study Group. *N Engl J Med.* 2000;343(4):246–253.

174. Sackner-Bernstein JD, Skopicki HA, Aaronson KD. Risk of worsening renal function with nesiritide in patients with acutely decompensated heart failure. *Circulation.* 2005;111(12):1487–1491.

175. Sackner-Bernstein JD, Kowalski M, Fox M, et al. Short-term risk of death after treatment with nesiritide for decompensated heart failure: a pooled analysis of randomized controlled trials. *JAMA*. 2005;293(15):1900–1905.

176. Costanzo MR, Saltzberg M, O'Sullivan J, et al. Early ultrafiltration in patients with decompensated heart failure and diuretic resistance. *J Am Coll Cardiol*. 2005;46(11):2047–2051.

177. Greenberg A, Verbalis JG. Vasopressin receptor antagonists. *Kidney Int*. 2006;69(12):2124–2130.

178. Ganukula SR SD. Pericardial disease in renal patients. *Semin Nephrol*. 2001;21:52–56.

179. Wood JE, Mahnensmith RL. Pericarditis associated with renal failure: evolution and management. *Semin Dial*. 2001;14(1):61–66.

180. Renfrew R, Buselmeier TJ, Kjellstrand CM. Pericarditis and renal failure. *Annu Rev Med*. 1980;31:345–360.

181. Alpert MA, Ravenscraft MD. Pericardial involvement in end-stage renal disease. *Am J Med Sci*. 2003;325(4):228–236.

182. Ireland JH, McCarthy JT. Infective Endocarditis in Patients with Kidney Failure: Chronic Dialysis and Kidney Transplant. *Curr Infect Dis Rep*. 2003;5(4):293–299.

183. Chang CF, Kuo BI, Chen TL, et al. Infective endocarditis in maintenance hemodialysis patients: fifteen years' experience in one medical center. *J Nephrol*. 2004;17(2):228–235.

184. Maraj S, Jacobs LE, Maraj R, et al. Bacteremia and infective endocarditis in patients on hemodialysis. *Am J Med Sci*. 2004;327(5):242–249.

185. Nori US, Manoharan A, Thornby JI, et al. Mortality risk factors in chronic haemodialysis patients with infective endocarditis. *Nephrol Dial Transplant*. 2006.

186. Fowler VG, Jr., Li J, Corey GR, et al. Role of echocardiography in evaluation of patients with Staphylococcus aureus bacteremia: experience in 103 patients. *J Am Coll Cardiol*. 1997;30(4):1072–1078.

187. Olaison L, Pettersson G. Current best practices and guidelines. Indications for surgical intervention in infective endocarditis. *Cardiol Clin*. 2003;21(2):235–251.

188. Weber H, Schwarzer C, Stummvoll HK, et al. Chronic hemodialysis: high risk patients for arrhythmias? *Nephron*. 1984;37(3):180–185.

189. Kyriakidis M, Voudiclaris S, Kremastinos D, et al. Cardiac arrhythmias in chronic renal failure? Holter monitoring during dialysis and everyday activity at home. *Nephron*. 1984;38(1):26–29.

190. Locatelli F, Covic A, Chazot C, et al. Optimal composition of the dialysate, with emphasis on its influence on blood pressure. *Nephrol Dial Transplant*. 2004;19(4):785–796.

191. Nash K, Hafeez A, Hou S. Hospital-acquired renal insufficiency. *Am J Kidney Dis*. 2002;39(5):930–936.

192. Gupta R, Gurm HS, Bhatt DL, et al. Renal failure after percutaneous coronary intervention is associated with high mortality. *Catheter Cardiovasc Interv*. 2005;64(4):442–448.

193. McCullough PA, Soman SS. Contrast-induced nephropathy. *Crit Care Clin*. 2005;21(2):261–280.

194. Solomon R, Deray G. How to prevent contrast-induced nephropathy and manage risk patients: practical recommendations. *Kidney Int Suppl*. 2006(100):S51–53.

195. Mueller C, Buerkle G, Buettner HJ, et al. Prevention of contrast media-associated nephropathy: randomized comparison of 2 hydration regimens in 1620 patients undergoing coronary angioplasty. *Arch Intern Med*. 2002;162(3):329–336.

196. Merten GJ, Burgess WP, Gray LV, et al. Prevention of contrast-induced nephropathy with sodium bicarbonate: a randomized controlled trial. *JAMA*. 2004;291(19):2328–2334.

197. Briguori C, Marenzi G. Contrast-induced nephropathy: pharmacological prophylaxis. *Kidney Int Suppl*. 2006(100):S30–38.

198. Biondi-Zoccai GG, Lotrionte M, Abbate A, et al. Compliance with QUOROM and quality of reporting of overlapping meta-analyses on the role of acetylcysteine in the prevention of contrast associated nephropathy: case study. *BMJ*. 2006;332(7535):202–209.

199. Saklayen MG, Gupta S, Suryaprasad A, et al. Incidence of atheroembolic renal failure after coronary angiography. A prospective study. *Angiology*. 1997;48(7):609–613.

200. Scolari F, Ravani P, Pola A, et al. Predictors of renal and patient outcomes in atheroembolic renal disease: a prospective study. *J Am Soc Nephrol*. 2003;14(6):1584–1590.

201. Scolari F, Tardanico R, Zani R, et al. Cholesterol crystal embolism: a recognizable cause of renal disease. *Am J Kidney Dis*. 2000;36(6):1089–1109.

202. Modi KS, Rao VK. Atheroembolic renal disease. *J Am Soc Nephrol*. 2001;12(8):1781–1787.

203. Theriault J, Agharazzi M, Dumont M, et al. Atheroembolic renal failure requiring dialysis: potential for renal recovery? A review of 43 cases. *Nephron Clin Pract*. 2003;94(1):c11–18.

204. Manley HJ, Cannella CA, Bailie GR, et al. Medication-related problems in ambulatory hemodialysis patients: a pooled analysis. *Am J Kidney Dis*. 2005;46(4):669–680.

205. Vidal L, Shavit M, Fraser A, et al. Systematic comparison of four sources of drug information regarding adjustment of dose for renal function. *BMJ*. 2005;331(7511):263.

206. Song JC, White CM. Pharmacologic, pharmacokinetic, and therapeutic differences among angiotensin II receptor antagonists. *Pharmacotherapy*. 2000;20:130–139.

207. Gabardi S, Abramson S. Drug dosing in chronic kidney disease. *Med Clin North Am*. 2005;89:649–687.

208. Danovitch GM. Immunosuppressive medications and protocols for kidney transplantation. In: Danovitch GM, ed. *Handbook of Kidney Transplantation*. 3rd ed. Philadelphia: Lippincott Williams & Wilkins; 2001:62–110.

CHAPTER 99

Exercise in Health and Cardiovascular Disease

Gerald F. Fletcher / Thomas R. Flipse / Keith R. Oken / Robert E. Safford

Exercise benefits healthy individuals and those at high risk for cardiovascular disease, as well as those with manifest cardiovascular disease. This chapter addresses the hemodynamics and health benefits of exercise and exercise conditioning programs, both in healthy individuals and those with or at risk for cardiovascular disease.

ACUTE HEMODYNAMICS

During physical activity, energy expenditure increases, and the compensatory cardiovascular response represents an integration of neural, biochemical, and physiologic factors. The cardiovascular *control center* is believed to reside in the ventrolateral medulla of the brain and to respond to both central and peripheral inputs. Central impulses arise from somatomotor centers of the brain. Peripheral impulses are generated by mechanoreceptors, found in muscles, joints, and the vascular system; chemoreceptors, found in the muscles and the vascular system; and baroreceptors, found in the vascular system. These impulses are transmitted by autonomic afferent fibers. The central control center regulates cardiac output (CO) and its distribution to organs and tissues according to metabolic demand.

The *feed-forward* command system, located in the motor cortex provides a coordinated and rapid cardiovascular response to optimize tissue perfusion and maintain central blood pressure. This central command provides the greatest control over heart rate (HR)

during exercise[1] and is also involved in the preexercise anticipatory response.[2] Stimulation of the central control center by the higher command centers leads to alteration of autonomic tone. Such can explain the influence of "emotions" on the cardiovascular response.

The cardiovascular control center also receives input from peripheral receptors. Stretch and tension of muscular and articular mechanoreceptors trigger afferent impulses that are important in the regulation of the circulatory response to dynamic exercise.[3] Muscle chemoreceptors stimulated by products of metabolism influence the control center as well. This reflex neural input (termed the *exercise pressor reflex*) provides rapid feedback modifying the autonomic outflow in response to physical activity.[4]

Vascular baroreceptors are located in the aortic arch and carotid sinuses. They respond to changes in arterial blood pressure and regulate HR by eliciting reciprocal changes in both sympathetic and parasympathetic activity.[5] The arterial baroreceptors protect the cardiovascular system from relatively short-term changes in blood pressure, as seen during physical exercise. Cardiopulmonary mechanoreceptors in the atria, ventricles, and pulmonary vessels aid in regulation of the circulatory response. An increase in blood pressure elicits reflex slowing of the heart, and the converse applies during hypotension. During physical activity, this feedback mechanism is altered so that blood pressure can rise. The aortic and carotid bodies contain chemoreceptors sensitive to arterial oxygen, carbon dioxide, and hydrogen ion concentrations. Decreased arterial oxygen levels trigger an increase in arterial pressure, whereas changes in carbon dioxide and hydrogen ion concentration have a relatively small effect.

CIRCULATORY ADJUSTMENTS WITH EXERCISE

The circulatory response to exercise involves a complex series of adjustments resulting in an increase in CO proportional to metabolic demands. These changes ensure that the metabolic needs of exercising muscles are met, that hyperthermia does not occur, and that blood flow to essential organs is protected. Adequate blood flow is delivered to exercising muscles through increased CO and redistribution of blood flow away from the viscera. CO is defined as the product of stroke volume (SV) and HR. The average CO at rest is approximately 5 L/min for both trained and untrained men. In women the value is approximately 25 percent lower.

Resting CO increases immediately before the onset of physical exercise as a result of *anticipatory changes* in the autonomic nervous system resulting in tachycardia and increased venous return. After the onset of exercise, CO increases rapidly until steady-rate exercise is reached. CO then rises gradually until a plateau is achieved. The magnitude of the hemodynamic response during physical activity depends on the intensity and the muscle mass involved. In sedentary individuals, CO during maximal exercise increases approximately four times, to an average of 20 to 22 L/min. In elite-class athletes the CO can rise eightfold, to values of 35 to 40 L/min.

HEART RATE RESPONSE TO EXERCISE

From rest to strenuous exercise, HR rapidly increases to levels of 160 to 180 beats per minute. During short periods of maximal exercise, rates of 240 beats per minute have been recorded. The initial rapid increase is likely the result of central command influences or a rapid reflex from muscle mechanoreceptors. The instant acceleration in heart rate is largely caused by vagal withdrawal. Later increases result from reflex activation of the pulmonary stretch receptors, which trigger increased sympathetic tone and more parasympathetic withdrawal. Increased circulating catecholamines play a role as well. During exercise, changes in HR account for a greater percent of the increase in CO than does SV. SV plateaus when the CO has increased to only one-half of its maximum. Further increases in CO occur by increases in the HR, although HR response in older subjects can be *blunted*.

STROKE VOLUME CHANGES WITH EXERCISE

Two physiologic mechanisms influence SV. Increased venous return elicits enhanced diastolic filling and more forceful systolic contraction. Neurohormonal influences also enhance contractility through direct effects.[6]

ENHANCED DIASTOLIC FILLING

Diastolic ventricular filling (preload) is enhanced by slower HR or increased venous return. Increased end-diastolic volume stretches

myocardial fibers enhancing overlap of sarcomere myofilaments and improving ventricular compliance. This in turn results in enhanced contractility and greater SV. It is believed that this mechanism is responsible for increased SV during transition from rest to exercise or from the upright to the supine position. Resting CO and SV are highest in the supine position. Supine SV is nearly maximal at rest and increases only slightly during exercise. In the normal supine individual, increased CO with exercise results predominantly from an increase in HR, with little increase in SV. Venous return to the heart is lower in the upright position resulting in a lower resting SV and CO. During upright exercise, however, SV can approach maximum SV observed in the recumbent position, usually without an increase in ventricular diastolic dimensions.[6,7]

IMPROVED SYSTOLIC EMPTYING

Increases in SV during upright exercise most likely occur through the combined effect of enhanced diastolic filling and more complete emptying during systole. Exercise-induced increases in circulating catecholamines enhance myocardial contractility. In the early phase of upright exercise, CO rises because of a simultaneous increase in SV and HR. In the later phases of exercise, increases in HR are primarily responsible for further increases in CO.

DISTRIBUTION OF CARDIAC OUTPUT DURING EXERCISE

Blood flow to tissues is generally proportional to metabolic activity. At rest, approximately 20 percent of CO is distributed to the skeletal muscle. However, during physical activity, the majority (up to 85 percent) of the increased CO is diverted to the working muscles. This represents an increase from 4 to 7 to 50 to 75 mL blood per minute per 100 grams of muscle. Even within active muscle, the increased blood flow is highly regulated with the greatest amount of blood being delivered to the oxidative portions of the muscle at the expense of the tissue with high glycolytic capacity. Local metabolic conditions as well as neural and hormonal regulation of vasomotor tone control the shunting of blood to active muscles. The local response is primarily caused by the buildup of vasodilatory metabolites in exercising muscle.

During exertion, parasympathetic activity is withdrawn, and sympathetic discharge is maximal, which results in increased release of norepinephrine from sympathetic postganglionic nerve endings. Plasma epinephrine levels are also increased. As a result, most vascular beds constrict, except those in exercising muscles, influenced by vasodilating metabolites. Blood flow to the skin increases during light and moderate exercise, favoring body cooling. Further increases in workload cause a progressive decrease in skin flow as the rising cutaneous sympathetic vascular tone overcomes the thermoregulatory vasodilatory response.[2] The kidneys and splanchnic tissues extract only 10 to 25 percent of the oxygen available in their blood supply. Consequently, considerable reductions in blood flow to these tissues can be tolerated through increased oxygen extraction.[7] At rest, the heart extracts approximately 75 percent of the oxygen in the coronary blood flow. Because of limited margin of reserve and increased myocardial demands, coronary blood flow increases fourfold during exercise. Cerebral blood flow also increases during exercise by approximately 25 to 30 percent.[8] During maximal exercise, however, cerebral flow can decrease because of hyperventilation and respiratory alkalosis.

On cessation of exercise, there is an abrupt decrease in HR and CO secondary to withdrawal of sympathetic tone and reactivation of vagal activity. In contrast, systemic vascular resistance remains lower for some time because of persistent vasodilatation in the muscles. As a result, arterial pressure falls, often below preexercise levels, for periods up to 12 hours into recovery.[9] Blood pressure is then stabilized at normal levels by baroreceptor reflexes.

【 】 EXERCISE TYPE AND CARDIOVASCULAR RESPONSE

Different types of exercise impose different loads on the cardiovascular system. Isotonic (dynamic) exercise is defined as muscular contraction of large muscle groups resulting in movement, which induces a volume load to the heart. Isometric (static) exercise is defined as a constant muscular contraction of a smaller muscle group without movement. It provokes more pressure than volume load to the heart. Significant increases in both CO and oxygen consumption (VO_2) and a decrease in systemic vascular resistance characterize the load posed by isotonic exercise. In contrast, isometric exercise increases systemic vascular resistance while producing only minimal changes in CO and VO_2.[10] A third type of exercise is resistance exercise. This is a combination of isometric and isotonic exercise evoked by using muscular contraction with movement, as in free-weight lifting. Most activities, such as sports or those that are employment-related, combine all three types of exercise (Table 99–1).

Isotonic (Dynamic) Exercise

The response to isotonic exercise is mediated through central and peripheral adaptations that increase oxygen delivery to exercising muscles. In normal sedentary individuals, VO_2 typically increases tenfold from rest to maximal exertion,[11] whereas in world-class athletes the increase is significantly greater. Maximal VO_2 is therefore considered an indicator of the level or degree of conditioning.[12]

During isotonic exercise, such as running, peripheral vascular resistance falls, and marked vasodilatation of vessels in exercising muscles occurs in conjunction with vasoconstriction of the splanchnic and renal vessels. In active muscles, local autoregula-

tion in response to hypoxia, decreasing pH, and increased local temperature results in vasodilatation.

During prolonged dynamic exercise, skeletal muscle metabolism is primarily aerobic and requires a significant increase in oxygen supply to meet the increased demand for adenosine triphosphate (ATP). The increased oxygen requirements are met by an augmentation of the local blood flow and improved oxygen extraction.

Isometric (Static) Exercise

The cardiovascular response to isometric exercise is different. Less oxygen is required to sustain the contraction of smaller muscle groups. With isometric exercise, the necessary VO_2 is maintained with a smaller increase in CO. Increases in regional blood flow are limited by mechanical compression of blood vessels during sustained muscular contraction,[13] and regional blood flow can actually decrease. To maintain regional perfusion, a pressor response is evoked, which is mediated, at least in part, by reflexes originating in the contracting muscles.[14] The increase in blood pressure is proportional both to the relative muscle tension and the mass of the muscle groups involved.

Stroke volume usually declines as a result of increased left ventricular afterload and the absence of augmented venous return. In its *pure state*, static exercise represents a pressure, or systolic, load. To maintain the higher CO, the HR must increase, often out of proportion to the metabolic needs of the active muscle groups.

Resistance (Resistive) Exercise

Resistance exercises are activities that use repetitive movements against a resistance, generating a low-to-moderate rise in muscle tension. The response to resistance exercise is determined by the extent of both the isotonic and isometric components. Physiologic responses are described relative to the percent of maximal voluntary contraction (MVC). Static contractions (<15 to 25 percent MVC) do not fully occlude intramuscular blood flow, and oxygen can still be delivered to active muscles. If one can perform >30 percent MVC with no occlusion of blood flow there is increased VO_2, thus the aerobic or isotonic component of resistance exercise.[15]

Weight lifting is considered the prototype resistance exercise and is thought to have a high isometric component. Blood pressure and HR responses during weight lifting are proportional to the relative intensity of muscle contraction, the mass of the muscle groups involved, and the duration of the contraction.[16] Weight-

TABLE 99–1

Types of Exercises

	ISOTONIC	ISOMETRIC	RESISTANCE
Alternative terminology	Dynamic	Static	Resistive
Example	Running	Static hand grip	Weight lifting
Oxygen uptake	Greatest	Least	Intermediate
CO	Greatest	Least	Intermediate
Peripheral resistance	Greatest decrease	Least decrease	Intermediate
Blood pressure	Decreases	Increases	Increases

CO, cardiac output.

training exercises have been shown to cause a significant increase in blood pressure.[17] This is thought to be the result of restricted muscle perfusion and a centrally mediated pressor response caused by enhanced muscle tension. The HR response during maximal upper body resistance exercise is lower than that seen during maximal isotonic exercise.[18] This contributes to a lower heart rate–blood pressure product during maximal resistance exercise compared to maximal dynamic exercise.

Previous concerns regarding the safety of resistance training have been rebutted by several reports that reveal that moderate resistance training programs are safe even in subjects with cardiac disease.[19,20] At this time, it is believed that resistance training (done on a regular schedule) is useful for promoting muscle strength, flexibility, and functionality but probably contributes less significantly than does isotonic exercise to overall cardiovascular health and longevity. Resistance exercise should be done with care and in moderation in subjects with aorta or aortic valve disease.

CONDITIONING TRAINING

Physical conditioning affects the cardiovascular and musculoskeletal systems in a variety of ways that improve work performance and exercise capacity. Maximal VO_2 can increase two- to threefold through conditioning induced by repetitive periods of dynamic exercise. Increased CO and peripheral adaptations that improve oxygen extraction contribute equally.[21] Conditioning alters cardiac structure and function,[22] enhancing exercise-induced increases in stroke volume.

At rest, CO is similar for both trained and untrained individuals. Endurance training induces an increase in resting parasympathetic tone[23] and reduces resting sympathetic activity. Heart rates below 30 beats per minute have been recorded for some healthy athletes. Cardiac output is maintained in such individuals by increased SV.[22] Training-induced increase in blood volume and intrinsic myocardial factors have been cited as the source of this enhanced resting and exercise SV (Table 99–2). During exercise, trained individuals achieve a larger maximal CO than do sedentary persons. In the untrained person, there is only a small increase in SV during the transition from rest to exercise, and the major augmentation in CO is induced by tachycardia. The improved cardiac performance after conditioning is secondary to both the Frank-Starling mechanism and augmented myocardial contraction and relaxation.

In previously sedentary individuals, 8 weeks of aerobic training increases SV. This change is associated with increased left ventricular end-diastolic dimension with preservation or even reduction of the end-systolic size.[24] The enhanced end-diastolic dimensions are, however, much lower than those of well-trained athletes.[25] It is not known whether this discrepancy results from prolonged training, genetic factors, or a combination of both. After cessation of training, changes largely regress within only 3 weeks, which is of great concern in adherence to exercise programs. Unfortunately cardiovascular conditioning is more easily lost than gained, which accounts for the effort dyspnea often experienced by subjects with resumption of activity after a long absence.

Several factors contribute to the cardiac adaptations of exercise training. Parasympathetically mediated bradycardia prolongs dia-

TABLE 99–2

Clinical Effects of Exercise Training

Increase in oxygen consumption
Increase in cardiac stroke volume
Increase in maximal exercise CO
Increase in resting parasympathetic tone
Decrease in resting sympathetic tone
Decrease in resting heart rate

CO, cardiac output.

stolic filling time and expanded plasma volume also increases preload.[26] These changes enhance contractility through Frank-Starling mechanisms. Some studies have shown that endurance training results in increased compliance of the left ventricle,[27] which is probably secondary to enhanced early diastolic filling and increased peak myocardial lengthening during exercise (see Table 99–2).[28,29] These physiologic changes are accompanied by biochemical and ultrastructural alterations of the myocardial fibers, which have been demonstrated in the hearts of physically conditioned animals. There is an increase in lactic dehydrogenase and pyruvate kinase activity, which enhances the respiratory capacity of the cardiac myocytes. Myocytes enlarge and manifest more mitochondria and myofibrils. Observed ultrastructural changes in the sarcolemma and sarcoplasmic reticulum probably influence intracellular calcium homeostasis and can explain the improved diastolic function of the conditioned heart. Myocardial fibrosis and resultant impairment of ventricular filling related to aging contribute to exercise intolerance.

The cross-sectional area of the epicardial coronary arteries increases in response to exercise. Alterations in the coronary microcirculation have also been identified. Animal studies reveal increased capillary density and capillary-to-fiber ratio with training. Decreased diffusion distance between the capillaries and myocytes has also been observed.[30] Some data suggest that training can promote coronary collateral formation in ischemic vascular beds.[31] These adaptations may enable the heart to better tolerate transient ischemia and to function at a lower percentage of its total oxidative capacity during exercise.[32] Thus, training-induced myocardial adaptations appear to protect against myocardial ischemia.

Skeletal muscle also adapts to long-term training with changes that enhance oxygen extraction. Capillary density and capillary-to-fiber ratio increase.[33] The number of mitochondria increases, as do mitochondrial concentrations of oxidative enzymes. Other cellular adaptations include increases in myoglobin levels, increased concentrations of enzymes involved in lipid metabolism, and enhanced adenosine triphosphatase (ATPase) activity.[34]

GENDER DIFFERENCES

Available data suggest qualitatively similar responses to dynamic and static exercise in both women and men. Some quantitative differences have been demonstrated in teenage girls who manifest a 5 to 10 percent greater CO than boys of similar ages at any level of submaximal oxygen uptake.[35] This is likely related to a 10 percent lower hemoglobin concentration in women. To deliver the same amount of oxygen, there is a proportionate increase in CO. The gross maximal aerobic capacity in women is approximately 50 percent lower than it is in men,[36] but when adjusted to lean body mass, the difference is only 10 to 15 percent, a more accurate reflection of gender-related differences. The absolute number of skeletal muscle fibers and the fiber-type distribution are similar in women and men[37]; however, for reasons that are unclear, muscle fibers in men are hypertrophied relative to those in women, resulting in greater cross-sectional muscle mass. Although strength adjusted to cross-sectional muscle area is similar in men and women, men's increased muscle mass usually yields greater isometric strength.[38]

Exercise-induced increases in SV also differ between the sexes. Men manifest a progressive increase in ejection fraction with little or no increase in end-diastolic volume, and in contrast, women tend to increase end-diastolic volume without a significant increase in ejection fraction.[39] This results in a plateau of the ejection fraction during exercise in women compared to a progressive increase in men.

AGING DIFFERENCES

Special considerations must be addressed when prescribing exercise for the elderly. In these subjects, maximal end-diastolic volume increases, whereas maximal HR, left ventricular ejection fraction, and CO are all lower than they are in the young individuals. Coronary disease is common in the elderly and can affect the cardiac response to exercise. In addition, the increased potential for exercise-related myocardial ischemia and arrhythmias can increase the risk of adverse events. A critical factor in an elderly (older than 65 years of age) person's ability to function independently is mobility. The overall focus for exercise training should be to enhance health-related fitness, reduce the risk of various chronic diseases, and improve overall quality of life. Considerable evidence demonstrates that physical activity, both endurance and resistance-type exercise, can significantly improve these indices and facilitate functional independence and overall well-being.[40–46]

Studies in community-dwelling older adults have revealed benefits in those who are physically active. One observational study[47] involved 3075 adults (52 percent women, 42 percent black), age 70 to 79 years, who performed a long distance corridor walking test. Those who could complete the test with no difficulty walking had less overall mortality and less cardiovascular disease as well as less limitation of mobility and disability. Another smaller study[48] evaluated free-living activity expenditure including walking, climbing stairs, care giving and working for pay. Total energy expenditure was assessed using doubly labeled water and indirect calorimetry in 302 community dwellings of older adults (70 to 82 years of age) followed over a mean of 6 to 15 years. Results revealed that objectively measured free-living activity is strongly associated with lower mortality in healthy older adults. Therefore, credible data exist to support the benefits of a physically active lifestyle in the aging population.

Elderly persons should ideally undergo a medical evaluation before initiating an exercise program. This assessment should include not only a *focused* physical examination but should identify psychosocial limitations to participation, which are prevalent in this age group.[42,49–53] For older, apparently healthy persons desiring to participate in a low-to-moderate intensity activity such as walking,

an exercise test is usually not required. However, for more vigorous activities and for all cardiac patients, an exercise test is appropriate. A review of the individual's medication regimen for possible interactions with activity programs should also be performed.[54]

As with young persons, the combination of endurance and resistance exercise is best for achieving the health and fitness goals in the elderly.[55–58] However, some specific comments regarding intensity, frequency, duration, progression and mode of exercise for the elderly are required. The exercise capacity of the elderly, both before and after exercise training, is usually lower.[41,59,60] Furthermore, because many in this age group have been sedentary for years, specific muscle groups are often markedly deconditioned. In addition, musculoskeletal limitations, particularly arthritis, can be severely limiting. Thus it is important to prescribe an exercise program with low-level energy expenditure, particularly during the first few weeks, with gradual increases thereafter. In these instances, however, participants can be encouraged to increase the frequency of exercise (with shorter duration), even to perhaps 3 or 4 times per day. Higher intensity training must be recommended with caution in this age group because of the potential for musculoskeletal injury.

Those whose exercise duration is limited (<15 minutes per session) because of physical or psychosocial limitations should attempt to exercise more frequently or intermittently. Certain subjects can benefit more because of this intermittent activity. One study supporting this was done in overweight women assigned to the same caloric restriction but randomized in an exercise program to either 40 minutes of continuous exercise or to four 10-minute "bouts" or periods. At the end of the activity program those in the intermittent (bouts) group lost 8.9 kg of weight versus 6.4 in the continuous group. In the intermittent group there was also improved adherence and a higher VO_2, compared to the continuous exercise group.[61] Conversely, for those who are not limited, increasing the duration of activity to as much as 45 to 60 minutes per session is valuable for increasing caloric expenditure and improvement of risk factors, including obesity, lipid abnormalities, hypertension, and elevated blood glucose.

Many elderly persons have symptomatic concomitant medical and physical limitations (orthopedic, neurologic, and vascular) that can be exacerbated by weight-bearing exercise, especially higher impact activities such as jogging. Even walking can be difficult for the elderly person. Thus, even seemingly innocent activities should be carefully considered for potential adverse effects in this age group, especially when the activity requires individuals to bear their entire weight. Cycle and water exercise can be better tolerated by these subjects.

IMPLEMENTATION OF EXERCISE TRAINING

The type of activity, frequency, duration, intensity, and progression determine the effect of an exercise training program. Epidemiologic studies suggest that moderate-intensity activities, such as brisk walking, performed on a regular basis confer cardioprotection to both men and women.[62–66] More vigorous activity can confer greater cardioprotection, but the majority of the benefit is accrued with moderate levels of exertion.[63,64,67] Moreover, fitness appears to be a powerful, independent predictor of cardiovascular risk.[68,69] High-intensity exercise programs are often associated with poor adherence rates and more musculoskeletal injuries. Thus, a highly structured program of vigorous exercise, especially in the elderly, is not generally recommended.

Current guidelines recommend that persons of all ages perform exercise of moderate intensity for 30 to 60 minutes, 4 to 6 times weekly or at least 30 minutes of moderate-intensity physical activity on a daily basis.[70–73] At the present, only 10 to 20 percent of the population meets this recommendation.[73,74] Because only a small percentage of the population is employed in a physically demanding occupation, most need to perform this activity in their leisure time. Examples of recommended activities include brisk walking, cycling, swimming, and active yard work. The duration of any period of activity should be at least 10 minutes, and the accumulated daily duration should be at least 30 minutes. Those who choose shorter exercise periods can benefit (as discussed previously) from the effects of intermittent exercise on improved adherence and greater increases in VO$_2$. In addition, during the recovery period ([or periods] in the intermittent [discontinuous] exercise program) additional calories are expended in the postexercise state while the body returns to the resting metabolic state. These calories are not usually counted with those expended with the activity and amount to 20 to 30 kilocalories per exercise session, which could be doubled if one exercised twice daily.[75]

Those who are sedentary should be encouraged to initially perform a duration of activity that is "comfortable" and to gradually increase to 30 to 60 minutes of daily activity. People who meet these daily standards and who wish to increase their activity further should be encouraged to do so. Fig. 99–1 displays a protocol for an effective training program. Resistance exercises should be added to the activity program to increase muscle strength. Resistance training using 8 to 10 different exercise sets with 10 to 15 repetitions each (arms, shoulders, chest, trunk, back, hips, and legs) performed at a moderate to high intensity (e.g., 10 to 15 pounds of free weight) for a minimum of 2 days per week is recommended.

Physicians and other health professionals should encourage the general public and their patients to follow these guidelines. Incor-

porating preventive services into medical practice is challenging because of time and financial constraints. To address these issues, the Centers for Disease Control and Prevention developed the Physician-Based Assessment and Counseling for Exercise (PACE) project.[76] This system includes a simple discussion of physical activity counseling and illustrates how a clinician can efficiently incorporate physical activity counseling into a busy clinical practice through the use of paramedical personnel.

As the problem with overweight and obesity continues to increase worldwide, new physical activity guidelines have been developed to hopefully combat this problem more effectively. A consensus conference was held in Bangkok with experts in exercise, energy expenditure, and body weight reduction in attendance.[77] It was concluded that 60 to 90 min/day of moderate intensity exercise is needed for prevention of weight regain (lesser amounts of vigorous activity). To prevent transition of overweight to obesity, 45 to 60 min/day of moderate intensity exercise is needed. The 2005 U.S. government recommendation[78] is for 60 minutes of exercise on most days to prevent weight gain and 60 to 90 minutes on most days for the previously overweight who have lost weight.

【 】 TRAINING IN INDIVIDUALS WITH CARDIOVASCULAR DISEASE (SECONDARY PREVENTION)

Historical Perspective

Exercise training has assumed a prominent role in contemporary prevention and management of cardiovascular disease.[70,72,73,79–87] In the 1950s, traditional management of acute myocardial infarction (MI) did not include physical exertion of any kind. Hospitalization and strict bedrest were recommended for at least 6 weeks following acute MI.[88] In 1951, Levine and Lown described reductions in post-MI morbidity and mortality associated with limited early mobilization.[89] This "chair treatment" involved progressive periods of sitting in an armchair starting 1 day after MI. By the end of that same decade, early inpatient mobilization was codified into detailed programs of physical activity.[90] By the 1970s, a series of small randomized, controlled trials of exercise training (typically starting 3 to 6 months post-MI) suggested significant benefit following myocardial infarction. Although these studies were individually underpowered to demonstrate survival advantage, meta-analysis suggested a 24 percent reduction in cardiovascular disease (CVD) mortality with exercise-based cardiac rehabilitation.[65,91]

Early rehabilitation programs focused almost exclusively on exercise training. As the discipline matured, patient education, risk factor management, psychological screening/intervention, and dietary, vocational and smoking cessation counseling were integrated to forge the comprehensive cardiac rehabilitation programs that we know today. In the past three decades the benefits of comprehensive cardiac rehabilitation programs have become widely recognized.[70,82,92,93] Further, the population deemed appropriate for this intervention continues to expand, incorporating higher risk individuals including those with left ventricular systolic dysfunction, valvular heart disease, and recipients of surgical or percutaneous revascularization (Table 99–3).

More recently, secondary prevention of cardiovascular events through optimizing proven pharmacologic therapies has been

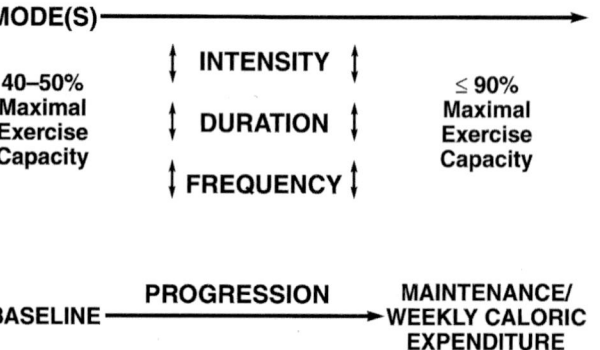

FIGURE 99–1. Exercise training model protocol. *Mode* refers to the type of exercise, such as jogging, swimming, or biking. *Maximal exercise capacity* refers to that achieved at peak exercise testing and can be expressed in terms of oxygen consumption, metabolic units, caloric expenditure, or perceived exertion. Intensity, duration, and frequency are each increased or decreased appropriately to ultimately achieve a maintenance level of total weekly caloric expenditure.

TABLE 99–3

Center for Medicare/Medicaid Services Recognized Indications for Cardiac Rehabilitation

PRIOR TO 2006	ADDED IN 2006
Post MI[a]	Post-PTCA or intracoronary stent implantation[a]
Post CABG[a]	Post valve surgery[a]
Chronic stable angina	Post cardiac transplantation[a]
Intermittent claudication	

CABG, coronary artery bypass surgery; MI, myocardial infarction; PTCA, percutaneous transluminal coronary angioplasty.
[a]Within 1 year prior to initiating cardiac rehabilitation.

woven into the fabric of contemporary cardiac rehabilitation programs.[82,92]

Exercise and Secondary Prevention

Acute and chronic therapy of coronary artery disease (CAD) has evolved significantly since early meta-analyses[65,91] suggested survival benefit from exercise-based cardiac rehabilitation. Major advances in the therapy of CAD over the past quarter century call into question the validity of those potentially dated conclusions. However, more contemporary meta-analyses of randomized, controlled trials of exercise-based cardiac rehabilitation have largely confirmed the findings of the 1980s.[94,95] One study added more than 4000 additional patients enrolled in studies of comprehensive and exercise-only rehabilitation programs for CAD published through March, 2003.[95] A most recent update included 48 trials enrolling nearly 9000 individuals. Although the older studies enrolled primarily low-risk, middle-aged, white men, this review included a larger number of females (20 percent), elderly people (≥65 years of age) and recipients of coronary revascularization. In this analysis, cardiac rehabilitation was associated with a 20 percent reduction in all cause mortality (odds ratio [OR] = 0.80; 95 percent confidence interval [CI]: 0.68–0.93) and a 26 percent reduction in CVD mortality (OR = 0.74; 95 percent CI: 0.61–0.96)

when compared to usual care (Table 99–4). Based on data from a limited number of trials, they also noted significant improvements in total cholesterol, triglycerides, systolic blood pressure, and self-reported smoking rates. As also shown in Table 99–4, there was a favorable trend in the rates of MI and revascularization that failed to meet statistical significance. Cardiac rehabilitation did not yield significant reductions in high- or low-density lipoprotein cholesterol or diastolic blood pressure. Contrary to their previous review,[94] subgroup analysis did not reveal a discrepancy in mortality rates between exercise-only programs and comprehensive cardiac rehabilitation programs. Similarly, there was no distinction between studies published pre- and post-1995.

Exercise and Functional Capacity

Exertional intolerance is one of the principal clinical features of symptomatic CVD even in the absence of heart failure. Exercise-based cardiac rehabilitation is consistently associated with improvements in functional capacity that significantly impact quality of life.[93,96] Exercise training reduces heart rate and blood pressure at submaximal workloads, improves the metabolic efficiency of both skeletal and cardiac muscle, enhances the mechanical performance of the myocardium, favorably influences autonomic tone, and prolongs the time to angina and ischemic ECG changes during treadmill exercise.[70,97] These physiologic adaptations translate into improved ability to perform activities of daily living with fewer symptoms and fewer limitations. Furthermore, enhanced exercise capacity is associated with significantly lower CVD mortality and fewer nonfatal CVD events.[69,98,99]

The landmark Agency for Health Care Policy and Research (AHCPR) practice guideline of 1995 summarized the results of 114 scientific reports on the effect of exercise-based cardiac rehabilitation on measures of exercise tolerance. These included 46 randomized controlled trials, of which 35 compared exercise-based rehabilitation with a no-exercise control group. Of these 35 trials, 30 demonstrated statistically significant improvement in exercise capacity in those assigned to exercise intervention.[93] Supervised exercise programs lasting 3 to 6 months have been associated with an 11 to 36 percent improvement in peak VO_2. The most deconditioned derive the greatest benefit.[82]

TABLE 99–4

Effects of Exercise-Based Cardiac Rehabilitation on Study End Points

OUTCOME	MEAN DIFFERENCE (%)	95% CONFIDENCE LIMIT	STATISTICAL DIFFERENCE
Total mortality	−20	−7% to −32%	$p = 0.005$
Cardiac mortality	−26	−10% to −29%	$p = 0.002$
Nonfatal MI	−21	−43% to 9%	$p = 0.150$
CABG	−13	−35% to 16%	$p = 0.400$
PTCA	−19	−51% to 34%	$p = 0.400$

Note: Mean difference is the percentage of difference between exercise-trained and usual-care control group.
CABG, coronary artery bypass graft; MI, myocardial infarction; PTCA, percutaneous coronary angioplasty.
SOURCE: Leon AS, Franklin BA, Costa F, et al. Cardiac rehabilitation and secondary prevention of coronary heart disease: an American Heart Association scientific statement from the Council on Clinical Cardiology (Subcommittee on Exercise, Cardiac Rehabilitation, and Prevention) and the Council on Nutrition, Physical Activity, and Metabolism (Subcommittee on Physical Activity), in collaboration with the American association of Cardiovascular and Pulmonary Rehabilitation. Circulation. 2005;11:369-376

Exercise and Risk Factor Modification

Coronary artery disease is a chronic, progressive condition associated with numerous metabolic, toxic, and hemodynamic precipitants, most of which respond favorably to exercise training. Consensus guidelines emphasize the role of exercise in managing hypertension,[100] diabetes,[101] hyperlipidemia,[102] the metabolic syndrome,[80] and obesity.[103]

Blood Pressure

Meta-analyses of randomized controlled trials of exercise in both hypertensive and normotensive individuals suggest a 3 to 4 mmHg decline in systolic blood pressure and a 2 to 3 mmHg decline in diastolic blood pressure with both aerobic and resistive exercise training.[104,105] From a public health perspective, even such modest effects on blood pressure significantly impact CVD mortality.[100]

Blood Glucose (Diabetes)

When combined with dietary intervention, exercise lowers the incident rate of new diabetes in high-risk individuals by 42 percent.[106–108] Further, it is superior to metformin in the prevention of type II diabetes,[106] and at least a portion of its beneficial effects appear to be independent of weight loss.[107]

Lipids

The effect of exercise on blood lipids varies among available studies.[109] Despite these mixed results, it appears that exercise can lower plasma triglycerides, very-low-density lipoprotein (VLDL) cholesterol, and, in some individuals, low-density lipoprotein (LDL) cholesterol. It also raises high-density lipoprotein (HDL) cholesterol. A meta-analysis of 51 studies of "moderate to hard" intensity aerobic exercise on blood lipids[109] involved approximately 4700 participants. Nearly all studies involved exercise 3 to 5 times per week, lasting at least 12 weeks. The estimated weekly exercise expenditure during structured programs ranged from 500 to >5,000 kcal/week, with a mean of 1,408.8 ± 824.7 kcal/week. On average, LDL cholesterol decreased 5.0 percent ($p < 0.05$), and triglycerides decreased 3.7 percent ($p < 0.05$). HDL cholesterol increased by 4.6 percent ($p < 0.05$).

The HERITAGE Family Study prospectively evaluated serial blood lipids in a diverse population of 675 healthy, sedentary, normolipidemic individuals undergoing 20 weeks of supervised cycle-ergometer exercise.[110] They demonstrated a 3.6 percent increase in HDL cholesterol (1.1 mg/dL in men and 1.4 mg/dL in women). The improvement in HDL cholesterol levels was primarily caused by an increase in the HDL$_2$ subfraction with an associated increase in apolipoprotein (apo) A-1 ($p < 0.001$). They noted only a transient reduction in plasma total and VLDL triglycerides, reflecting the acute effects of the last training session. There were no significant changes in total, LDL, and VLDL cholesterol or apo B.

As is the case for managing hypertension, diabetes, and weight, combining diet and exercise appears to be more effective in lowering LDL cholesterol. One significant study randomized 377 men and postmenopausal women with low HDL cholesterol and moderately elevated LDL cholesterol to aerobic exercise, the National Cholesterol Education Program Step 2 diet, combined diet and exercise, or no intervention.[111] Serial lipids revealed significant reductions in LDL cholesterol in both men and women only in the group assigned to combined diet and exercise. Along with other studies,[109] this study suggests that exercise mitigates the reduction in HDL cholesterol typically seen with low fat diets.

Weight

Weight loss is also associated with improvements in blood pressure, lipid profile, and glycemic control in those with type II diabetes.[103] As little as a 10-pound (4.5 kg) weight loss reduces blood pressure.[100] Weight loss by dietary means improves plasma triglyceride levels by 2 to 44 percent, total cholesterol by 0 to 18 percent, and LDL cholesterol by 3 to 22 percent.[103] Although exercise is an important component of weight-management strategies, exercise alone is a rather inefficient method of achieving weight loss. A meta-analysis of 28 studies of exercise compared to diet or control groups calculated an average weight loss of 3 kg in men and 1.4 kg in women assigned to exercise-intervention compared to controls.[112] On average, diet alone yields 3 kg greater weight loss than exercise alone.[103] The combination of diet and exercise is most effective and on average yields 8.5 kg of weight loss.[113]

Contrary to its role in initial weight loss, exercise plays a leading role in weight-loss maintenance. Six randomized controlled trials examining the effects of exercise on weight-loss maintenance concluded that higher levels of exercise were significantly more successful in maintaining weight-loss over an average followup interval of 2.7 years.[114] Those performing higher levels of physical activity maintained 54 percent of their initial weight loss, twice that of those assigned to lower levels of physical activity. Thus, exercise is an important component of strategies for weight management and offers synergistic benefits to weight loss itself in risk factor control. This is particularly important in the management of metabolic syndrome, a constellation of metabolic risk factors associated with increased risk for diabetes and CVD.[80,115] The components of the metabolic syndrome all respond favorably to aerobic exercise, making exercise a mainstay in its management.[80]

[ ] OTHER EFFECTS OF EXERCISE IN SECONDARY PREVENTION

Progression of Coronary Artery Disease

A number of studies have investigated the effect of exercise on progression of atherosclerotic disease. The majority of these studies incorporated exercise into a multifaceted intervention including diet. Four trials demonstrated significant slowing of angiographic progression and/or enhanced regression on serial angiographic studies (Table 99–5). A significant study reported long-term followup of one of these carefully controlled trials of diet and exercise in 113 men with stable CAD.[120] The men were randomized to an intensive diet and exercise intervention or limited diet and exercise advice. After 6 years, 66 patients underwent followup angiography. The exercise group was encouraged to perform 30 minutes of daily cycle-ergometer exercise at home and attend at least two supervised 60-minute group-exercise sessions weekly. The intervention group improved their physical work capacity by 28 percent, whereas the control group remained unchanged. There was no distinction between the two groups in temporal changes in total cholesterol, triglycerides, or body mass index. Analyzing serial quanti-

TABLE 99-5

Randomized Controlled Trials Examining the Effects of Exercise Training, with or without Additional Lifestyle Changes, on Angiographic Progression of Coronary Artery Disease

STUDY	N	MEN (%)	INTER	F/U (YEARS)	ANGIO PROGRESSION/ REGRESSION
Ornish[116]	48	88	M	1	↓
Schuler[117]	92	100	E	1	↓
Hambrecht[118]	88	100	E	1	↓
Haskell[119]	300	86	M	4	↓

↓, statistically significant decrease favoring intervention; angio, angiographic; E, exercise training only; Inter, intervention; M, multifactorial.

tative coronary angiograms on a per patient basis, these investigators found significantly less progression (59 percent vs. 74 percent) and significantly more regression (19 percent vs. 0 percent) in the intervention group compared to control.

Systemic Inflammation

Systemic inflammation is emerging as a significant predictor of cardiovascular risk.[122] Elevated serum levels of interleukin-6, tumor necrosis factor-α, high-sensitivity C-reactive protein (hs-CRP), and a number of other cytokines, acute-phase reactants, and soluble cytokine receptors have been associated with increased risk of CVD events and diabetes.[122–128] Modest elevation of CRP, in particular, has been associated with CVD risk in observational studies.[127] Further, lowering hs-CRP with hydroxymethylglutaryl coenzyme A (HMG-CoA) reductase inhibitor therapy has been shown to reduce risk beyond the benefits accrued from LDL cholesterol lowering alone.[121] Obesity and visceral adiposity are associated with increased levels of CRP and diet-induced weight loss reduces CRP levels.[122] Physical inactivity also correlates with elevated CRP levels in observational studies. Randomized, controlled trials examining the effect of exercise on CRP levels are limited.[123] Three, small prospective trials of the impact of exercise training on inflammatory markers have enrolled only 104 participants. Two of the three included a control group and showed significantly greater reductions in CRP with exercise training. One small, noncontrolled prospective trial demonstrated a trend toward lower CRP after 6 months of supervised exercise.

Endothelial Function

Exercise training enhances endothelium-dependent coronary and peripheral arterial vasodilatation in individuals with CAD, peripheral arterial disease, heart failure (HF), diabetes, and hypertension.[124–131] The effect of exercise on vascular function in individuals free of atherosclerotic risk factors has been mixed.[126,132] Exercise's influence on vascular function appears to be mediated through increased arterial wall shear stress, which promotes enhanced expression and activation of endothelial nitric oxide synthase (eNOS) by means of Akt-dependent phosphorylation.[125,127] In addition to influencing vascular tone, nitric oxide also conveys significant antiatherogenic and antithrombotic effects, as well.[133]

Exercise also has beneficial effects of thrombotic tendencies and autonomic function in secondary prevention, but further discussion will not be included herein.

Exercise in the Patient with Heart Failure

There is a daily increase in the millions of people diagnosed with HF, creating a significant impact on the healthcare system.[134] Exercise endurance is limited in these subjects in spite of advanced drug therapy.[135,136] Based on substantial data exercise training can improve both cardiac and noncardiac indices.[135] Recommendations based on randomized controlled trials encourage exercise training for individuals with HF to impact both functional and symptomatic improvement.[137–140] Exercise training can improve physiologic indices including exercise tolerance, ventricular function, skeletal muscle function, peripheral blood flow, endothelial function, and quality of life.[135,141] Experience has revealed that exercise in HF is safe and well tolerated if appropriately prescribed. Clinical trials are underway to further elucidate the role of exercise in patients with HF.

Components of Contemporary Cardiac Rehabilitation

Historically, cardiac rehabilitation has been arbitrarily divided into successive phases, typically starting during hospitalization for an acute event (Table 99-6). As clinical care and medical economics have evolved, these traditional phases have lost much of their relevance. Contemporary cardiac rehabilitation emphasizes a continuum of care. The American Association of Cardiovascular and Pulmonary Rehabilitation recommends a more descriptive paradigm incorporating three levels of intervention, inpatient, early outpatient and lifetime cardiac rehabilitation.[142]

Inpatient Rehabilitation

The contemporary management of acute coronary syndromes focuses on timely reperfusion, risk stratification, and introduction of proven pharmacotherapy in appropriately selected individuals. The timeline of this intervention has become quite truncated with many patients discharged within 3 days of an acute ST-elevation myocardial infarction.[143] Accordingly, inpatient cardiac rehabilitation has assumed an introductory role. It is focused on early mobilization, starting as soon as patients are hemodynamically stable

TABLE 99–6

Phases of Traditional Cardiac Rehabilitation

PHASE	LOCATION/TIMING	DESCRIPTION	DURATION
I	Inpatient Starting as soon as clinically stable	Gradual progressive activity and introductory education, i.e., disease process, cardiovascular symptoms, risk-factor management and lifestyle changes	Days
II	Outpatient Shortly after discharge	Multidisciplinary intervention including progressive exercise, exercise prescription, psychological screening/intervention, smoking cessation, dietary counseling, verification of optimal pharmacologic and device therapy for secondary prevention and functional status, in-depth education, i.e., disease process, risk-factor management medications and weight loss	2–12 weeks
III	Outpatient Immediately after Phase II is complete	Supervised exercise and reinforcement of the principles promulgated during Phase II. Implementation of progressive exercise prescription. Transitional to independent exercise venue. Can serve as a long-term exercise facility for those lacking alternatives.	6–12 months following Phase II
IV	Outpatient	Maintenance Focus on adherence to exercise prescription, healthy eating, weight management, tobacco abstinence, medications, and cardiovascular symptom surveillance	Indefinite

SOURCE: Squires RW, Gau GT, Miller TD, Allison TG, Lavie CJ. Cardiovascular rehabilitation: status, 1990. Mayo Clin Proc. 1990;65:731–755; Pasternak RC. Comprehensive rehabilitation of patients with cardiovascular disease. In Braunwald E, Zipes DP, Libby P, Bonow RO, eds. Braunwald's Heart Disease: A Textbook of Cardiovascular Medicine, 7th ed. Philadelphia, PA: Elsevier Saunders; 2005:1085.

and free of symptoms of ischemia, arrhythmia, or heart failure. As the patient progresses to an ECG telemetry environment, progressive ambulation is appropriate, initially with assistance and hemodynamic assessment before, during, and after exercise.

Patients are often unable to assimilate the large amount of information that needs to be introduced. Therefore, providing written information for the patient and family, ensuring stable clinical status with activities of daily living and referring to an appropriate comprehensive cardiac rehabilitation program is the current emphasis. In addition, ensuring that patients are discharged from the hospital on appropriate medical therapy is an important part of the initial intervention. A number of practice tools are available to help address the gap between recommended therapy and that which is delivered in practice.[144,145] Patients are usually more adherent to drug therapy when initiated in the inpatient environment.

Early Outpatient Rehabilitation

When formal cardiac rehabilitation programs first evolved in the 1960s and 1970s, the primary concern was the safety of *early* exercise. As such, ECG telemetry *monitoring* was incorporated as a means of surveillance for significant arrhythmias. Currently, this monitoring goes beyond telemetry and includes surveillance of symptoms, hemodynamics, glycemic response to exercise (in diabetics), weight, tobacco use, emotional status, and adherence with medications, diet, and home exercise. It also includes review of each individuals pharmacologic and device therapy to ensure ad-

herence with consensus guidelines. This monitored phase is an intensive, multidisciplinary intervention focused on educating the individual about the disease, its manifestations, and all aspects of its treatment. The goal is to provide each participant with the tools needed to slow disease progression, maintain optimal functional status, and become an informed and active participant in managing his or her condition.

Maintenance

The distinction between traditional phase III (medically supervised) and IV (nonmedically supervised) cardiac rehabilitation has been unclear for some time. Most participants progress to independent exercise without a transitional "phase III." Nonetheless, some patients are concerned by the prospect of continuing exercise in unfamiliar surroundings and elect to continue exercising at a cardiac rehabilitation facility where they feel safe and are familiar with personnel, protocol, facilities, and clientele. Clinical features occasionally mandate closer supervision than an unmonitored independent exercise program, either because of adherence, cognitive limitations, serious comorbidities, hemodynamics, or arrhythmias that require medical supervision during exercise. Unfortunately, continuing cardiac rehabilitation services under such circumstances are generally not reimbursed by third-party payers. Regardless of the venue and the degree of medical surveillance, the goal of this maintenance phase is exercise independence and adherence to exercise prescription, healthy diet, weight management, tobacco abstinence, and medications.

REFERENCES

1. Williamson JW, Nobrega AC, Garcia JA, Friedman DB, Mitchell JH. Cardiovascular responses at the onset of static exercise in patients with dual-chamber pacemakers. *J Appl Physiol*. 1995;79:1668–1672.

2. Rowell LB. *Human Cardiovascular Control*. New York: Oxford University Press; 1993:xv, 500.

3. Strange S, Secher NH, Pawelczyk JA, et al. Neural control of cardiovascular responses and of ventilation during dynamic exercise in man. *J Physiol (Lond)*. 1993;470:693–704.

4. Rowell LB, O'Leary DS. Reflex control of the circulation during exercise: chemoreflexes and mechanoreflexes. *J Appl Physiol*. 1990,69:407–418.

5. Carter JB, Banister EW, Blaber AP. Effect of endurance exercise on autonomic control of heart rate. *Sports Med*. 2003;33:33–46.

6. Vella CA, Roberggs RA. A review of the stroke volume response to upright exercise in healthy subjects. *Br J Sports Med*. 2005;39:190–195.

7. Musch TI, Haidet GC, Ordway GA, Longhurst JC, Mitchell JH. Training effects on regional blood flow response to maximal exercise in foxhounds. *J Appl Physiol*. 1987;62:1724–1732.

8. Thomas SN, Schroeder T, Secher NH, Mitchell JH. Cerebral blood flow during submaximal and maximal dynamic exercise in humans. *J Appl Physiol*. 1989;67:744–748.

9. Pescatello LS, Fargo AE, Leach CN Jr, Scherzer HH. Short-term effect of dynamic exercise on arterial blood pressure. *Circulation*. 1991;83:1557–1561.

10. Bechuza GR, Lenser MC, Hanson PG, Nagle FJ. Comparison of hemodynamic responses to static and dynamic exercise. *J Appl Physiol*. 1982;53:1589–1593.

11. Bruce RA, Kusumi F, Hosmer D. Maximal oxygen intake and normographic assessment of functional aerobic impairment in cardiovascular disease. *Am Heart J*. 1973;85:546–562.

12. Saltin B, Astrand PO. Maximal oxygen uptake in athletes. *J Appl Physiol*. 1967;23:353–358.

13. Asmussen E. Similarities and dissimilarities between static and dynamic exercise. *Circ Res*. 1981;48:I3–10.

14. Hanson P, Nagle F. Isometric exercise: Cardiovascular responses in normal and cardiac populations. In: Hanson P, ed. *Exercise and the Heart, Cardiology Clinics*. Philadelphia, PA: W.B. Saunders; 1987:157–170.

15. Plowman SA, Smith DL. *Exercise Physiology for Health, Fitness, and Performance*. 2nd ed. San Francisco: Benjamin Cummings; 2003:372–373.

16. Seals DR, Washburn RA, Hanson PG, Painter PL, Nagle FJ. Increased cardiovascular response to static contraction of large muscle groups. *J Appl Physiol*. 1983;54:434–437.

17. Wescott W, Howeff B. Blood pressure response during weight training exercises. *NSCA J*. 1983;5:67–71.

18. DeBusk RF, Valdez R, Houston N, Haskell W. Cardiovascular responses to dynamic and static effort soon after myocardial infarction. Application to occupational work assessment. *Circulation*. 1978;58:368–375.

19. Ghilarducci LE, Holly RG, Amsterdam EA. Effects of high resistance training in coronary artery disease. *Am J Cardiol*. 1989;64:866–870.

20. Sparling PB, Cantwell JD, Dolan CM, Niederman RK. Strength training in a cardiac rehabilitation program: a six-month follow-up. *Arch Phys Med Rehabil*. 1990;71:148–152.

21. Rowell LB. Human cardiovascular adjustments to exercise and thermal stress. *Physiol Rev*. 1974;54:75–159.

22. Stickland MK, Welsh RC, Petersen SR, et al. Does fitness level modulate the cardiovascular hemodynamic response to exercise? *J Appl Physiol*. 2006;100:1895–1901.

23. Ueno LM, Moritani T. Effects of long-term exercise training on cardiac autonomic nervous activities and baroreflex sensitivity. *Eur J Appl Physiol*. 2003;89:109–114.

24. Ehsani AA, Hagberg JM, Hickson RC. Rapid changes in ventricular dimensions and mass in response to physical conditioning and deconditioning. *Am J Cardiol*. 1972;42:52–56.

25. Saltin B. Physiologic effects on physical conditioning. *Med Sci Sports*. 1969;1:50–56.

26. Convertino VA. Blood volume: its adaptation to endurance training. *Med Sci Sports Exerc*. 1991;23:1338–1348.

27. Levy WC, Cerqueira MD, Abrass IB, Schwartz RS, Stratton JR. Endurance exercise training augments diastolic filling at rest and during exercise in healthy young and older men. *Circulation*. 1993;88:116–126.

28. Granger CB, Karimeddini MK, Smith VE, et al. Rapid ventricular filling in left ventricular hypertrophy: I. Physiologic hypertrophy. *J Am Coll Cardiol*. 1985;5:862–868.

29. Matsuda M, Sugishita Y, Koseki S, et al. Effect of exercise on left ventricular diastolic filling in athletes and nonathletes. *J Appl Physiol*. 1983;55:323–328.

30. Anversa P, Levicky V, Beghi C, McDonald SL, Kikkawa Y. Morphometry of exercise-induced right ventricular hypertrophy in the rat. *Circ Res*. 1983;52:57–64.

31. Froelicher V, Jensen D, Atwood JE, et al. Cardiac rehabilitation: evidence for improvement in myocardial perfusion and function. *Arch Phys Med Rehabil*. 1980;61:517–522.

32. Starnes JW, Bowles DK. Role of exercise in the cause and prevention of cardiac dysfunction. *Exerc Sport Sci Rev*. 1995;23:349–373.

33. Hermansen L, Wachtlova M. Capillary density of skeletal muscle in well-trained and untrained men. *J Appl Physiol*. 1971;30:860–863.

34. Holloszy JO, Booth FW. Biochemical adaptations to endurance exercise in muscle. *Annu Rev Physiol*. 1976;38:273–291.

35. Bar-Or O, Shephard RJ, Allen CL. Cardiac output of 10- to 13-year-old boys and girls during submaximal exercise. *J Appl Physiol*. 1971;30:219–223.

36. Drinkwater BL. Women and exercise: physiological aspects. *Exerc Sport Sci Rev*. 1984;12:21–51.

37. Costill DL, Daniels J, Evans W, et al. Skeletal muscle enzymes and fiber composition in male and female track athletes. *J Appl Physiol*. 1976;40:149–154.

38. Astrand PO, Rodahl K. *Textbook of Work Physiology, Physiological Basis of Exercise*. New York: McGraw-Hill; 1986:756.

39. Higginbotham MB, Morris KG, Coleman RE, Cobb FR. Sex-related differences in the normal cardiac response to upright exercise. *Circulation*. 1984;70:357–366.

40. Brown M, Holloszy JO. Effects of a low intensity exercise program on selected physical performance characteristics of 60- to 71-year olds. *Aging (Milano)*. 1991;3:129–139.

41. Elia EA. Exercise and the elderly. *Clin Sports Med*. 1991;10:141–155.

42. Emery CF, Hauck ER, Blumenthal JA. Exercise adherence or maintenance among older adults: 1-year follow-up study. *Psychol Aging*. 1992;7:466–470.

43. King AC, Haskell WL, Taylor CB, Kraemer HC, DeBusk RF. Group- vs home-based exercise training in healthy older men and women. A community-based clinical trial. *JAMA*. 1991;266:1535–1542.

44. King AC, Haskell WL, Young DR, Oka RK, Stefanick ML. Long-term effects of varying intensities and formats of physical activity on participation rates, fitness, and lipoproteins in men and women aged 50 to 65 years. *Circulation*. 1995;91:2596–2604.

45. Shephard RJ. Exercise and aging: extending independence in older adults. *Geriatrics*. 1993;48:61–64.

46. Stewart AL, King AC, Haskell WL. Endurance exercise and health-related quality of life in 50–65 year-old adults. *Gerontologist*. 1993;33:782–789.

47. Newman AB, Simonsick EM, Naydeck BL, et al. Association of long-distance corridor walk performance with mortality, cardiovascular disease, mobility limitation, and disability. *JAMA*. 2006;295:2018–2026.

48. Manini TM, Everhart JE, Patel KV, et al. Daily activity energy expenditure and mortality among older adults. *JAMA*. 2006;296:171–179.

49. Barry HC, Eathorne SW. Exercise and aging. Issues for the practitioner. *Med Clin North Am*. 1994;78:357–376.

50. Courneya KS. Understanding readiness for regular physical activity in older individuals: an application of the theory of planned behavior. *Health Psychol*. 1995;14:80–87.

51. Hassmen P, Ceci R, Backman L. Exercise for older women: a training method and its influences on physical and cognitive performance. *Eur J Appl Physiol Occup Physiol*. 1992;64:460–466.

52. King AC, Taylor CB, Haskell WL. Effects of differing intensities and formats of 12 months of exercise training on psychological outcomes in older adults. *Health Psychol*. 1993;12:292–300.

53. Marcus BH, Simkin LR. The stages of exercise behavior. *J Sports Med Phys Fitness*. 1993;33:83–88.

54. Rich MW, Palmeri S, McCluskey ER, Schwartz JB. Calcium channel blockers for hypertension in older patients. *Cardiovasc Rev Rep*. 1991;12:11–14.

55. Brown M, Holloszy JO. Effects of walking, jogging and cycling on strength, flexibility, speed and balance in 60- to 72-year olds. *Aging (Milano)*. 1993;5:427–434.

56. Franklin BA, Whaley MH, Howley ET. *ACSM's Guidelines for Exercise Testing and Prescription*. Philadelphia, PA: Lippincott Williams & Wilkins; 2000.

57. McAuley E. Self-efficacy and the maintenance of exercise participation in older adults. *J Behav Med*. 1993;16:103–113.

58. Rogers MA, Evans WJ. Changes in skeletal muscle with aging: effects of exercise training. *Exerc Sport Sci Rev*. 1993;21:65–102.

59. Williams MA, Maresh CM, Esterbrooks DJ, Harbrecht JJ, Sketch MH. Early exercise training in patients older than age 65 years compared with that in younger patients after acute myocardial infarction or coronary artery bypass grafting. *Am J Cardiol*. 1985;55:263–266.

60. Woo JS, Derleth C, Stratton JR, Levy WC. The influence of age, gender, and training on exercise efficiency. *J Am Coll Cardiol*. 2006;47:1049–1057.

61. Jakicic JM, Wing RR, Butler BA, Robertson RJ. Prescribing exercise in multiple short bouts versus one continuous bout: effects on adherence, cardiorespiratory fitness, and weight loss in overweight women. *Int J Obes Relat Metab Disord*. 1995;19:893–901.

62. Berlin JA, Colditz GA. A meta-analysis of physical activity in the prevention of coronary heart disease. *Am J Epidemiol*. 1990;132:612–628.

63. Lee IM, Rexrode KM, Cook NR, Manson JE, Buring JE. Physical activity and coronary heart disease in women: is "no pain, no gain" passe? *JAMA*. 2001;285:1447–1454.

64. Manson JE, Greenland P, LaCroix AZ, et al. Walking compared with vigorous exercise for the prevention of cardiovascular events in women. *N Engl J Med*. 2002;347:716–725.

65. O'Connor GT, Buring JE, Yusuf S, et al. An overview of randomized trials of rehabilitation with exercise after myocardial infarction. *Circulation*. 1989;80:234–244.

66. Powell KE, Thompson PD, Caspersen CJ, Kendrick JS. Physical activity and the incidence of coronary heart disease. *Annu Rev Public Health*. 1987;8:253–287.

67. Lee IM, Hsieh CC, Paffenbarger RS, Jr.: Exercise intensity and longevity in men. The Harvard Alumni Health Study. *JAMA*. 1995;273:1179–1184.

68. Laukkanen JA, Lakka TA, Rauramaa R, et al. Cardiovascular fitness as a predictor of mortality in men. *Arch Intern Med*. 2001;161:825–831.

69. Myers J, Prakash M, Froelicher V, et al. Exercise capacity and mortality among men referred for exercise testing. *N Engl J Med*. 2002;346:793–801.

70. Fletcher GF, Balady GJ, Amsterdam EA, et al. Exercise standards for testing and training: a statement for healthcare professionals from the American Heart Association. *Circulation*. 2001;104:1694–1740.

71. NIH Consensus Development Panel: Physical activity and cardiovascular health. *JAMA*. 1996;276:241–246.

72. Pate RR, Pratt M, Blair SN, et al. Physical activity and public health. A recommendation from the Centers for Disease Control and Prevention and the American College of Sports Medicine. *JAMA*. 1995;273:402–407.

73. U. S. Department of Health and Human Services. *Physical activity and health: A report of the Surgeon General*. Edited by CoDCaP US Department of Health and Human Services, National Center for Chronic Disease Prevention and Health Promotion. Pittsburgh, PA: President's Council on Physical Fitness and Sports; 1996:278.

74. Caspersen CJ, Christenson GM, Pollard RA. Status of the 1990 physical fitness and exercise objectives—evidence from NHIS 1985. *Public Health Rep*. 1986;101:587–592.

75. Plowman SA, Smith DL. *Exercise Physiology for Health, Fitness, and Performance*. 2nd ed. San Francisco: Benjamin Cummings; 2003:96–98.

76. Patrick K, Calfas KJ, Sallis JF, Long B. Basic principles of physical activity counseling: Project PACE. In: Thomas R, ed. *The Heart and Exercise*. New York: Igaku-Shoin; 1996:33–50.

77. Saris WH, Blair SN, van Baak MA, et al. How much physical activity is enough to prevent unhealthy weight gain? Outcome of the IASO 1st Stock Conference and consensus statement. *Obes Rev*. 2003;4:101–114.

78. Executive Office of the President, U.S. Department of Health and Human Services. Available at: www.healthierus.gov.

79. Gibbons RJ, Abrams J, Chatterjee K, et al. ACC/AHA 2002 guideline update for the management of patients with chronic stable angina—summary article: a report of the American College of Cardiology/American Heart Association Task Force on practice guidelines (Committee on the Management of Patients With Chronic Stable Angina). *J Am Coll Cardiol*. 2003;41:159–168.

80. Grundy SM, Hansen B, Smith SC, Jr., Cleeman JI, Kahn RA. Clinical management of metabolic syndrome: report of the American Heart Association/National Heart, Lung, and Blood Institute/American Diabetes Association conference on scientific issues related to management. *Circulation*. 2004;109:551–556.

81. Hunt SA, Abraham WT, Chin MH, et al. ACC/AHA 2005 guideline update for the diagnosis and management of chronic heart failure in the adult: a report of the American College of Cardiology/American Heart Association Task Force on Practice Guidelines (Writing Committee to Update the 2001 Guidelines for the Evaluation and Management of Heart Failure): developed in collaboration with the American College of Chest Physicians and the International Society for Heart and Lung Transplantation: endorsed by the Heart Rhythm Society. *Circulation*. 2005;112:e154–235.

82. Leon AS, Franklin BA, Costa F, et al. Cardiac rehabilitation and secondary prevention of coronary heart disease: an American Heart Association scientific statement from the Council on Clinical Cardiology (Subcommittee on Exercise, Cardiac Rehabilitation, and Prevention) and the Council on Nutrition, Physical Activity, and Metabolism (Subcommittee on Physical Activity), in collaboration with the American association of Cardiovascular and Pulmonary Rehabilitation. *Circulation*. 2005;111:369–376.

83. Mosca L, Appel LJ, Benjamin EJ, et al. Evidence-based guidelines for cardiovascular disease prevention in women. *Circulation*. 2004;109:672–693.

84. Pearson TA, Blair SN, Daniels SR, et al. AHA Guidelines for Primary Prevention of Cardiovascular Disease and Stroke: 2002 Update: Consensus Panel Guide to Comprehensive Risk Reduction for Adult Patients without Coronary or Other Atherosclerotic Vascular Diseases. American Heart Association Science Advisory and Coordinating Committee. *Circulation*. 2002;106:388–391.

85. Pina IL, Apstein CS, Balady GJ, et al. Exercise and heart failure: a statement from the American Heart Association Committee on exercise, rehabilitation, and prevention. *Circulation*. 2003;107:1210–1225.

86. Smith SC Jr, Allen J, Blair SN, et al. AHA/ACC guidelines for secondary prevention for patients with coronary and other atherosclerotic vascular disease: 2006 update: endorsed by the National Heart, Lung, and Blood Institute. *Circulation*. 2006;113:2363–2372.

87. Thompson PD, Buchner D, Pina IL, et al. Exercise and physical activity in the prevention and treatment of atherosclerotic cardiovascular disease: a statement from the Council on Clinical Cardiology (Subcommittee on Exercise, Rehabilitation, and Prevention) and the Council on Nutrition, Physical Activity, and Metabolism (Subcommittee on Physical Activity). *Circulation*. 2003;107:3109–3116.

88. Squires RW, Gau GT, Miller TD, Allison TG, Lavie CJ. Cardiovascular rehabilitation: status, 1990. *Mayo Clin Proc*. 1990;65:731–755.

89. Levine SA, Lown B. The "chair" treatment of acute thrombosis. *Trans Assoc Am Physicians*. 1951,64:316–327.

90. Hellerstein HK, Ford AB. Rehabilitation of the cardiac patient. *J Am Med Assoc*. 1957;164:225–231.

91. Oldridge NB, Guyatt GH, Fischer ME, Rimm AA. Cardiac rehabilitation after myocardial infarction. Combined experience of randomized clinical trials. *JAMA*. 1988;260:945–950.

92. American Association of Cardiovascular & Pulmonary Rehabilitation. *Guidelines for Cardiac Rehabilitation and Secondary Prevention Programs: Promoting Health and Preventing Disease*. 3rd ed. Champaign, IL: Human Kinetics; 1999.

93. Wenger NK, Froehler ES, Smith LK. *Cardiac Rehabilitation: Clinical Practice Guideline No. 17*. Rockville, MD: Lung and Blood Institute, U.S. Dept of Health and Human Services; 1995. AHCPR Publication 96–0672.

94. Jolliffe JA, Rees K, Taylor RS. *Exercise-based rehabilitation for coronary heart disease*. Cochrane Database Syst Rev. 2001.

95. Taylor RS, Brown A, Ebrahim S, et al. Exercise-based rehabilitation for patients with coronary heart disease: systematic review and meta-analysis of randomized controlled trials. *Am J Med*. 2004;116:682–692.

96. Gibbons RJ, Balady GJ, Bricker JT, et al. ACC/AHA 2002 guideline update for exercise testing: summary article: a report of the American College of Cardiology/American Heart Association Task Force on Practice Guidelines (Committee to Update the 1997 Exercise Testing Guidelines). *Circulation*. 2002;106:1883–1892.

97. La Rovere MT, Bersano C, Gnemmi M, Specchia G, Schwartz PJ. Exercise-induced increase in baroreflex sensitivity predicts improved prognosis after myocardial infarction. *Circulation*. 2002;106:945–949.

98. Kavanagh T, Mertens DJ, Hamm LF, et al. Prediction of long-term prognosis in 12 169 men referred for cardiac rehabilitation. *Circulation*. 2002;106:666–671.

99. Mark DB, Lauer MS. Exercise capacity: the prognostic variable that doesn't get enough respect. *Circulation*. 2003;108:1534–1536.

100. Chobanian AV, Bakris GL, Black HR, et al. Seventh report of the Joint National Committee on Prevention, Detection, Evaluation, and Treatment of High Blood Pressure. *Hypertension*. 2003;42:1206–1252.

101. American Diabetes Association: Clinical practice recommendations. *Diabetes Care*. 2004;27:S1-S45.

102. Expert Panel on Detection Evaluation and Treatment of High Blood Cholesterol in Adults. Executive summary of the third report of the National Cholesterol Education Program (NCEP) Expert Panel on Detection, Evaluation, and Treatment of High Blood Cholesterol in Adults (Adult Treatment Panel III). *JAMA*. 2001;285:2486–2497.

103. NHLBI Obesity Education Initial Expert Panel. *Clinical Guidelines on the Identification, Evaluation, and Treatment of Overweight and Obesity in Adults: The Evidence Report*. Rockville, MD: National Heart Lung and Blood Institute in cooperation with the National Institutes of Diabetes and Digestive and Kidney Diseases, U.S. Dept of Health and Human Services; 1998.

104. Kelley GA, Kelley KS. Progressive resistance exercise and resting blood pressure: A meta-analysis of randomized controlled trials. *Hypertension*. 2000;35:838–843.

105. Whelton SP, Chin A, Xin X, He J. Effect of aerobic exercise on blood pressure: a meta-analysis of randomized, controlled trials. *Ann Intern Med*. 2002;136:493–503.

106. Knowler WC, Barrett-Connor E, Fowler SE, et al. Reduction in the incidence of type 2 diabetes with lifestyle intervention or metformin. *N Engl J Med.* 2002;346:393–403.

107. Laaksonen DE, Lindstrom J, Lakka TA, et al. Physical activity in the prevention of type 2 diabetes: the Finnish diabetes prevention study. *Diabetes.* 2005;54:158–165.

108. Tuomilehto J, Lindstrom J, Eriksson JG, et al. Prevention of type 2 diabetes mellitus by changes in lifestyle among subjects with impaired glucose tolerance. *N Engl J Med.* 2001;344:1343–1350.

109. Leon AS, Sanchez OA. Response of blood lipids to exercise training alone or combined with dietary intervention. *Med Sci Sports Exerc.* 2001;33:S502–515; discussion S528–509.

110. Leon AS, Rice T, Mandel S, et al. Blood lipid response to 20 weeks of supervised exercise in a large biracial population: the HERITAGE Family Study. *Metabolism.* 2000;49:513–520.

111. Stefanick ML, Mackey S, Sheehan M, et al. Effects of diet and exercise in men and postmenopausal women with low levels of HDL cholesterol and high levels of LDL cholesterol. *N Engl J Med.* 1998;339:12–20.

112. Garrow JS, Summerbell CD. Meta-analysis: effect of exercise, with or without dieting, on the body composition of overweight subjects. *Eur J Clin Nutr.* 1995;49:1–10.

113. Blair SN. Evidence for success of exercise in weight loss and control. *Ann Intern Med.* 1993;119:702–706.

114. Anderson JW, Konz EC, Frederich RC, Wood CL. Long-term weight-loss maintenance: a meta-analysis of U.S. studies. *Am J Clin Nutr.* 2001;74:579–584.

115. Grundy SM, Brewer HB Jr, Cleeman JI, Smith SC Jr, Lenfant C. Definition of metabolic syndrome: Report of the National Heart, Lung, and Blood Institute/American Heart Association conference on scientific issues related to definition. *Circulation.* 2004;109:433–438.

116. Ornish D, Brown SE, Scherwitz LW, et al. Can lifestyle changes reverse coronary heart disease? The Lifestyle Heart Trial. *Lancet.* 1990;336:129–133.

117. Schuler G, Hambrecht R, Schlierf G, et al. Regular physical exercise and low-fat diet. Effects on progression of coronary artery disease. *Circulation.* 1992;86:1–11.

118. Hambrecht R, Niebauer J, Marburger C, et al. Various intensities of leisure time physical activity in patients with coronary artery disease: effects on cardiorespiratory fitness and progression of coronary atherosclerotic lesions. *J Am Coll Cardiol.* 1993;22:468–477.

119. Haskell WL, Alderman EL, Fair JM, et al. Effects of intensive multiple risk factor reduction on coronary atherosclerosis and clinical cardiac events in men and women with coronary artery disease. The Stanford Coronary Risk Intervention Project (SCRIP). *Circulation.* 1994;89:975–990.

120. Niebauer J, Hambrecht R, Velich T, et al. Attenuated progression of coronary artery disease after 6 years of multifactorial risk intervention: role of physical exercise. *Circulation.* 1997;96:2534–2541.

121. Ridker PM, Cannon CP, Morrow D, et al. C-reactive protein levels and outcomes after statin therapy. *N Engl J Med.* 2005;352:20–28.

122. Nicklas BJ, You T, Pahor M. Behavioural treatments for chronic systemic inflammation: effects of dietary weight loss and exercise training. *CMAJ.* 2005;172:1199–1209.

121. Kasapis C, Thompson PD. The effects of physical activity on serum C-reactive protein and inflammatory markers: a systematic review. *J Am Coll Cardiol.* 2005;45:1563–1569.

124. Brendle DC, Joseph LJ, Corretti MC, Gardner AW, Katzel LI. Effects of exercise rehabilitation on endothelial reactivity in older patients with peripheral arterial disease. *Am J Cardiol.* 2001;87:324–329.

125. Dimmeler S, Zeiher AM. Exercise and cardiovascular health: get active to "AKTivate" your endothelial nitric oxide synthase. *Circulation.* 2003;107:3118–3120.

126. Gaenzer H, Neumayr G, Marschang P, et al. Flow-mediated vasodilation of the femoral and brachial artery induced by exercise in healthy nonsmoking and smoking men. *J Am Coll Cardiol.* 2001;38:1313–1319.

127. Hambrecht R, Adams V, Erbs S, et al. Regular physical activity improves endothelial function in patients with coronary artery disease by increasing phosphorylation of endothelial nitric oxide synthase. *Circulation.* 2003;107:3152–3158.

128. Hambrecht R, Wolf A, Gielen S, et al. Effect of exercise on coronary endothelial function in patients with coronary artery disease. *N Engl J Med.* 2000;342:454–460.

129. Higashi Y, Sasaki S, Kurisu S, et al. Regular aerobic exercise augments endothelium-dependent vascular relaxation in normotensive as well as hypertensive subjects: role of endothelium-derived nitric oxide. *Circulation.* 1999;100:1194–1202.

130. Linke A, Schoene N, Gielen S, et al. Endothelial dysfunction in patients with chronic heart failure: systemic effects of lower-limb exercise training. *J Am Coll Cardiol.* 2001;37:392–397.

131. Maiorana A, O'Driscoll G, Cheetham C, et al. The effect of combined aerobic and resistance exercise training on vascular function in type 2 diabetes. *J Am Coll Cardiol.* 2001;38:860–866.

132. Maiorana A, O'Driscoll G, Dembo L, et al. Exercise training, vascular function, and functional capacity in middle-aged subjects. *Med Sci Sports Exerc.* 2001;33:2022–2028.

133. Niebauer J, Cooke JP. Cardiovascular effects of exercise: role of endothelial shear stress. *J Am Coll Cardiol.* 1996;28:1652–1660.

134. American Heart Association. *Heart Disease and Stroke Statistics—2006 Update.* Dallas, TX: American Heart Association; 2005.

135. Afzal A, Brawner CA, Keteyian SJ. Exercise training in heart failure. *Prog Cardiovasc Dis.* 1998;41:175–190.

136. Ferrari R. Physical training in chronic heart failure: much more than training. *Eur Heart J.* 2002;23:1803–1804.

137. *Guidelines for Cardiac Rehabilitation Programs*, 2nd ed. Champaign, IL: Human Kinetics; 1995:1–154.

138. Coats AJ, Adamopoulos S, Meyer TE, Conway J, Sleight P. Effects of physical training in chronic heart failure. *Lancet.* 1990;335:63–66.

139. Giannuzzi P, Temporelli PL, Corra U, et al. Attenuation of unfavorable remodeling by exercise training in postinfarction patients with left ventricular dysfunction: results of the Exercise in Left Ventricular Dysfunction (ELVD) trial. *Circulation.* 1997;96:1790–1797.

140. Giannuzzi P, Temporelli PL, Tavazzi L, et al. EAMI—exercise training in anterior myocardial infarction: an ongoing multicenter randomized study. Preliminary results on left ventricular function and remodeling. The EAMI Study Group. *Chest.* 1992;101:315S-321S.

141. Braith RW, Edwards DG. Neurohormonal abnormalities in heart failure: impact of exercise training. *Congest Heart Fail.* 2003;9:70–76.

142. American Association of Cardiovascular & Pulmonary Rehabilitation. *Guidelines for Cardiac Rehabilitation and Secondary Prevention Programs.* 4th ed. Champaign, IL: Human Kinetics, 2004.

143. Antman EM, Anbe DT, Armstrong PW, et al. ACC/AHA guidelines for the management of patients with ST-elevation myocardial infarction: a report of the American College of Cardiology/American Heart Association Task Force on Practice Guidelines (Committee to Revise the 1999 Guidelines for the Management of Patients with Acute Myocardial Infarction). *Circulation.* 2004;110:e82–292.

144. LaBresh KA, Ellrodt AG, Gliklich R, Liljestrand J, Peto R. Get with the guidelines for cardiovascular secondary prevention: pilot results. *Arch Intern Med.* 2004;164:203–209.

145. Montoye CK, Eagle KA. An organizational framework for the AMI ACC-GAP Project. *J Am Coll Cardiol.* 2005;46:1–29.

CHAPTER (100)

The Athlete and the Cardiovascular System

N. A. Mark Estes III / Mark S. Link / Barry J. Maron

INTRODUCTION

Although athletes are considered to be symbols of the healthiest segment of our society, they are occasionally affected by cardiovascular conditions that can manifest tragic consequences. The incongruity of the seemingly healthy and invulnerable individual being burdened with cardiac disease can be perplexing to the medical community and the public. The physician can be challenged by clinical judgments related to evaluation of symptoms such as chest discomfort, or signs such as a murmur which can be either benign or a manifestation of an underlying cardiac condition. In this setting there is considerable risk of unnecessarily treating and restricting sports activity in an athlete misdiagnosed as having an underlying cardiac condition. It is evident that consequences of missing an important cardiac diagnosis can be life-threatening.

The cardiovascular conditions that predispose to life-threatening complications with athletic activity are now well characterized.[1,2] Recommendations for evaluation, management, and athletic participation are also available to guide clinicians.[3,4] This chapter will review cardiovascular disease in the athlete from multiple perspectives. These include distinguishing physiologic cardiovascular adaptations to exercise from true cardiac disease, clinical evaluation of the athlete with suspected cardiovascular disease, arrhythmias in athletes, commotio cordis, guidelines for athletic restriction and performance-enhancing substances.

THE ATHLETE'S HEART

The *athlete's heart*, refers to the clinical syndrome of cardiac chamber enlargement, hypertrophy, and normal or augmented ventricular systolic function in association with sinus arrhythmia, sinus bradycardia, and a systolic flow murmur (Fig. 100–1).[5–9] The notion that the cardiovascular system differentiates structurally and functionally in response to athletic training was introduced more than a century ago.[5] Using only cardiac auscultation and percussion, Henschen initially described enlargement of the heart caused by athletic activity in cross-country skiers. He reported that right and left heart physiologic dilation and hypertrophy resulted from cross-country skiing and that these athletic hearts could perform more work than a normal heart.[5] Debate has ensued about whether these adaptations to exercise are physiologic and benign or pathologic and the potential harbinger of disease and disability. The heart of the trained athlete was considered by some to be enlarged and weakened because of the strain of endurance training with the potential to progress to deterioration of cardiac function and a clinical syndrome of heart failure.[7] However, it is now accepted that the athlete's heart represents a benign increase in cardiac mass, with specific circulatory and cardiac morphologic alterations, representing a physiologic adaptation to systematic training.[9] These cardiac changes represent unique physiologic cardiovascular adaptations to dynamic exercise, also known as isotonic or aerobic training. Thus, the clinical components of the athlete's heart are typically limited to athletes

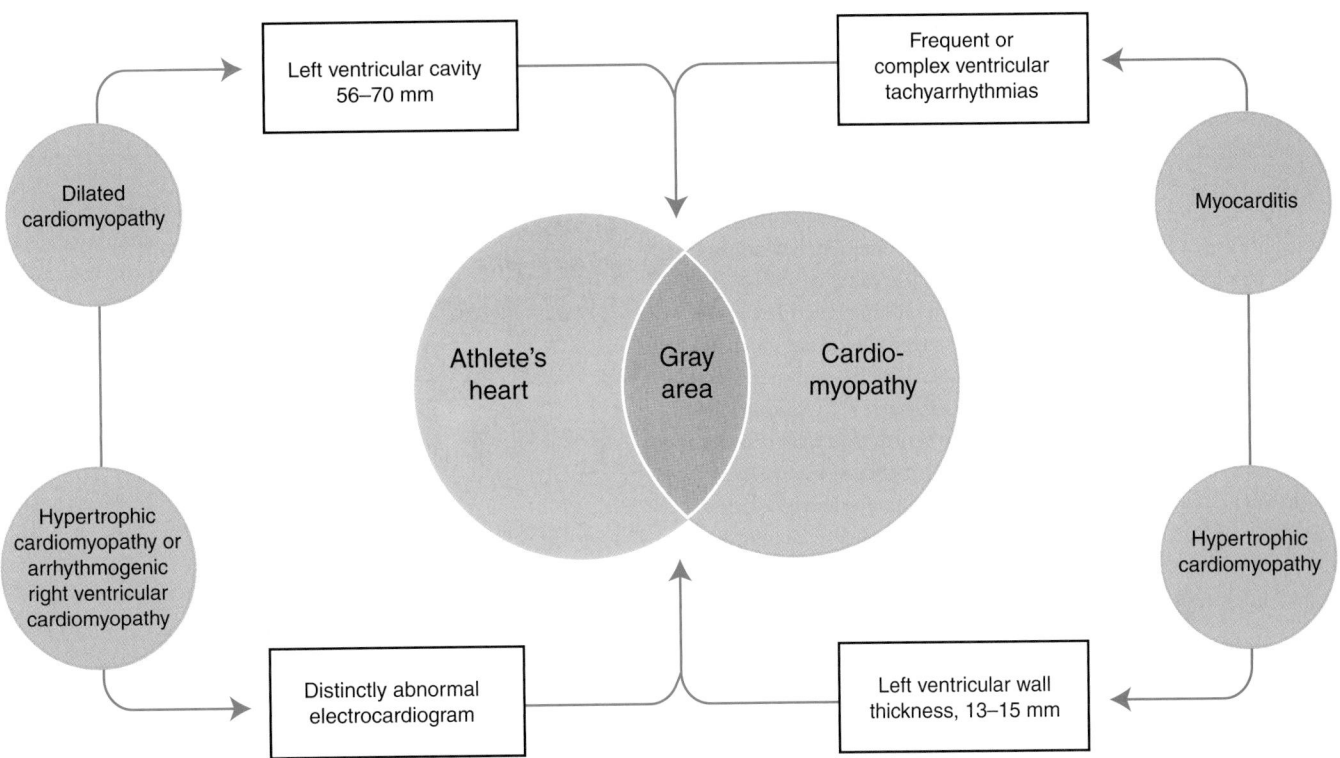

FIGURE 100–1. Gray area of overlap between athlete's heart and cardiomyopathies, including myocarditis, hypertrophic cardiomyopathy, and arrhythmogenic right ventricular cardiomyopathy. The important diagnostic features compatible with both physiologically based adaptations to athletic training (athlete's heart) and the pathologic conditions are shown. *Source: Maron.*[1]

involved in sports that involve a considerable endurance or aerobic exercise component.

The acute response to training for such athletic activities as cross-country skiing, long-distance running, swimming, or bicycling include substantial increases in maximum oxygen consumption, cardiac output, stroke volume, and systolic blood pressure, associated with decreased peripheral vascular resistance.[9] With prolonged endurance training, the chronic adaptations to training include increased maximal oxygen uptake from augmented stroke volume and cardiac output and increased arteriovenous oxygen difference. Thus, the response to endurance exercise predominantly produces a volume load on the left ventricle.

Over the last several decades, the morphologic adaptations to endurance training have been quantitatively characterized by multiple studies, largely relying on echocardiography.[9–16] The cardiac changes of athletes in response to systematic conditioning is somewhat variable with some degree of cardiac remodeling in approximately one-half of trained athletes. These changes include alterations in ventricular chamber dimensions including increased left and right ventricular and left atrial cavity size (and volume), associated with normal systolic and diastolic function.[9] Enlargement of the left ventricular (LV) chamber (≥60 mm) occurs in approximately 15 percent of highly trained athletes.[9–12] Occasionally this enlargement of the left ventricle is accompanied by a mild increase in absolute LV wall thickness exceeding upper normal limits (range 13 to 15 mm).[10–12] Remodeling of LV mass is dynamic and develops after the initiation of vigorous conditioning. Because these changes are reversible with cessation of training, restriction from exercise and reassessment of LV size and wall thickness can be used to distinguish physiologic changes from those associated with cardiovascular conditions such as hypertrophic cardiomyopathy (HCM).[9]

Differentiating the physiologic changes that occur from habitual exercise in the Athletic Heart syndrome with HCM or dilated cardiomyopathy can be difficult (see Fig. 100–1). Physiologic cardiac adaptation secondary to regular exercise can lead to an increase in LV wall thickness, which can be difficult to distinguish from pathologic changes of hypertrophic cardiomyopathy. Criteria favoring HCM include a high degree of LV hypertrophy (wall thickness, >16 mm) with an unusual distribution (heterogeneous, asymmetric, or sparing the anterior septum); a small LV cavity (<45 mm); the presence of striking ECG abnormalities; and the persistence of hypertrophy after deconditioning. Although many athletes have increased intracavitary dimensions, LV end-diastolic diameter (EDD) >70 mm is distinctly unusual as a manifestation of the athlete's heart. Additionally, LV wall thickness >12 mm is very unusual even in elite athletes. LV wall thickness >16 mm and values above this range raise the possibility of HCM. Hypertrophy (>12 mm) above the normal range is very uncommon in female athletes. Athletes with wall hypertrophy have increased cavity dimensions, which is not seen in diseases with pathologic wall thickening.

Arrhythmias commonly noted in athletes include sinus arrhythmia, sinus bradycardia, and junctional rhythm. They are frequently accompanied by other manifestations of enhanced parasympathetic tone and modulation of sympathetic tone. Atrioventricular (AV) conduction delays with first degree and Wenckebach or Mobitz type I second degree AV block are common in endurance athletes and attributable to enhanced vagal tone.[17–20] Ambulatory monitoring of athletes has demonstrated ventricular arrhythmias including frequent premature beats, couplets, and nonsustained ventricular tachycardia. These arrhythmias can be within the spectrum of physiologic athlete's heart.[21,22] Such arrhythmias are generally not associated with symptoms or an increased risk of sudden cardiac death, and are reduced with exercise or deconditioning.[21,22]

A spectrum of abnormal 12-lead ECG patterns are present in up to one-half of trained athletes, more commonly in men and in endurance athletes (Table 100–1).[17–21] The most frequent alterations are early repolarization patterns, increased QRS voltages, diffuse T-wave inversion and deep Q waves. ECGs in endurance athletes can show mildly increased P-wave amplitude suggesting atrial enlargement, incomplete right bundle-branch block (RBBB), and increased voltages consistent with right and LV hypertrophy.[17–21] Among endurance athletes, voltage criteria for right ventricular hypertrophy are present in a substantial proportion. Abnormal and bizarre ECG patterns suggestive of cardiac disease are noted in a minority of elite athletes.[17–21] Most such ECGs represent only extreme manifestations of physiologic athlete's heart.

SUDDEN CARDIAC DEATH IN THE ATHLETE

The underlying cardiovascular conditions that predispose to the rare and tragic sudden deaths in young athletes are known.[1,2,23–30] Available population-based data show that these events occur with an incidence of 2.3 per 100,000 athletes (12–35 years of age) per year.[1,2,23] The frequency of sudden death in female athletes is lower than males (2.6 in males versus 1.1:100,000 per year in females). Although this predominance of fatal events in male athletes has been attributed to the higher participation rate of males in competitive athletics, there is some evidence that the male gender can represent itself as a risk factor for sports-related sudden death. Greater prevalence in males of cardiovascular diseases such as cardiomyopathies or premature coronary artery disease potentially resulting in cardiac arrest can contribute to this observation. In athletes younger than 35 years of age inherited diseases such as HCM, arrhythmogenic right ventricular cardiomyopathy/dysplasia, and congenital coronary artery abnormalities of wrong sinus origin are the most common causes of sudden death (Table 100–2). In athletes older than 35 years, coronary artery disease is most commonly cause of sudden death.[1,2,23–30]

HCM is the principal cause of sudden cardiac arrest on the athletic field in the United States, accounting for up to one-third of sport-related cardiac fatalities (Fig. 100–2).[1,23,28] HCM is a genetically transmitted disease characterized by genotypic and phenotypic heterogeneity. Usually the characteristic hypertrophied, nondilated left ventricle with increased wall thickness manifests during adolescence.[1,23,28] Usually, hypertrophy is asymmetric with disproportionate septal thickening, and reduction in LV chamber size.[1,23,28] Decrease in LV compliance can contribute to increased wall stress and inadequate intramural coronary blood filling with exercise. Dynamic LV outflow tract obstruction at rest or with exercise is demonstrable in a most patients.

The characteristic histopathologic marker of HCM is myocardial disarray, with disorganized patterns of myocytes in association with increased interstitial fibrosis and often replacement scarring. These latter fibrotic changes are considered an acquired phenomenon related to microvascular-based myocardial ischemia. This

TABLE 100–1

Electrocardiographic Abnormalities Found in Various Disease States

DIAGNOSIS OF HEART DISEASE	ECG ABNORMALITIES
Arrhythmogenic right ventricular dysplasia	T-wave inversions anteriorly Epsilon wave RBBB (complete or incomplete) Rarely normal
Hypertrophic cardiomyopathy (HCM)	Left ventricular hypertrophy Pseudoinfarct with Q-waves T-wave inversion Rarely normal
Idiopathic dilated cardiomyopathy	LBBB Prolonged QT Can be normal
Long QT syndrome	Prolonged QT Abnormal appearance of ST segment
Brugada syndrome	RBBB (complete or incomplete) ST elevation anteriorly Changes can vary with time
Anomalous coronary artery	Typically no abnormalities
Coronary artery disease	Typically no abnormalities Q ST
Wolff-Parkinson-White	Short PR interval Delta waves Pseudoinfarct patterns

LBBB, left bundle-branch block; RBBB, right bundle-branch block.
SOURCE: Adapted from Link MS, Wang PJ, Estes NAM III. Ventricular arrhythmias in the athlete. Curr Opin Cardiol. 2001;16:30–39.

small-vessel disease in HCM involves the intramural coronary arteries, which commonly show dysplasia of the tunica media often with luminal obstruction.[1,23,28]

Sudden cardiac arrest in athletes with HCM is attributable to ventricular tachyarrhythmias mediated by multiple factors. Myocardial damage observed in athletes dying suddenly, supports the notion that acute episodes of myocardial ischemia can trigger life-threatening cardiac arrhythmias. Alternate potential mechanisms of cardiac arrest include hemodynamic compromise or primary ventricular arrhythmias.

Arrhythmogenic right ventricular dysplasia (ARVD) is an inherited heart muscle disorder characterized pathologically by fibrofatty replacement of right ventricular myocardium.[26,30,31,32] It represents the leading cause of sudden death on the athletic field in the Veneto region of Italy, accounting for approximately 25 percent of cardiovascular sudden death in young competitive athletes.[26,30,31,32] Clinical manifestations include ECG depolarization and repolarization abnormalities commonly localized to right precordial leads. Cardiac imaging techniques demonstrate right ventricular global or regional morphologic and functional abnormalities. Commonly, premature ventricular contractions or sustained

TABLE 100–2

Causes of Sudden Death in 387 Young Athletes[a]

CAUSE	NO. OF ATHLETES	PERCENT
Hypertrophic cardiomyopathy	102	26.4
Commotio cordis	77	19.9
Coronary-artery anomalies	53	13.7
Left ventricular hypertrophy of indeterminate causation[b]	29	7.5
Myocarditis	20	5.2
Ruptured aortic aneurysm (Marfan syndrome)	12	3.1
Arrhythmogenic right ventricular cardiomyopathy	11	2.8
Tunneled (bridged) coronary artery[c]	11	2.8
Aortic-valve stenosis	10	2.6
Atherosclerotic coronary artery disease	10	2.6
Dilated cardiomyopathy	9	2.3
Myxomatous mitral valve degeneration	9	2.3
Asthma (or other pulmonary condition)	8	2.1
Heat stroke	6	1.6
Drug abuse	4	1.0
Other cardiovascular cause	4	1.0
Long QT syndrome[d]	3	0.8
Cardiac sarcoidosis	3	0.8
Trauma involving structural cardiac injury	3	0.8
Ruptured cerebral artery	3	0.8

[a]Data are from the registry of the Minneapolis Heart Institute Foundation.[6,28]
[b]Findings at autopsy were suggestive of hypertrophic cardiomyopathy but were insufficient to be diagnostic.
[c]Tunneled coronary artery was deemed the cause in the absence of any other cardiac abnormality.
[d]The long QT syndrome was documented on clinical evaluation.
SOURCE: Maron,[1] with permission.

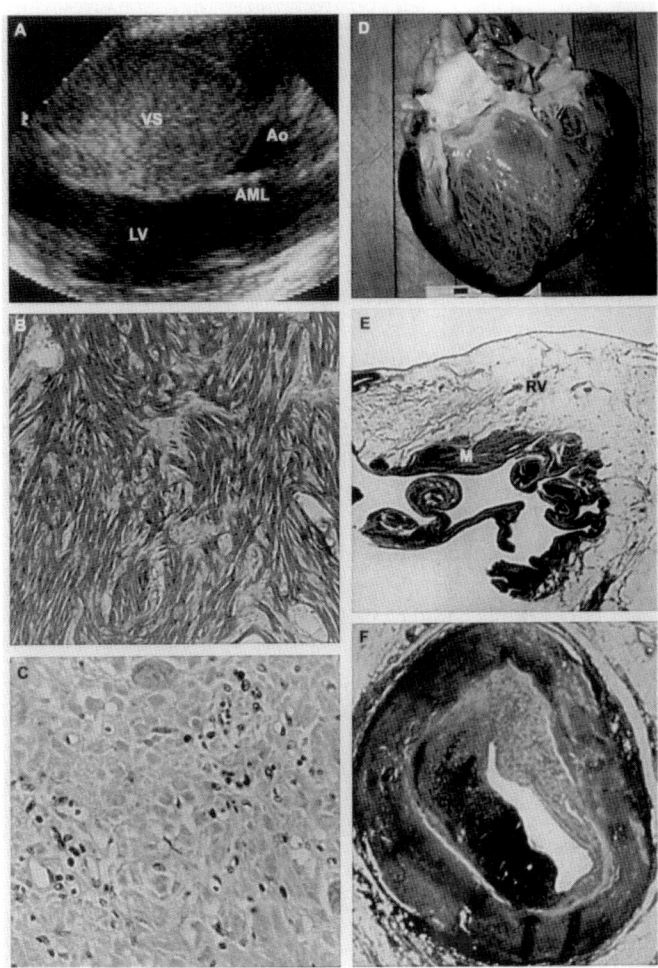

FIGURE 100–2. Some cardiac causes of sudden death in young competitive athletes: hypertrophic cardiomyopathy (panels **A** and **B**), myocarditis (panel **C**), dilated cardiomyopathy (panel **D**), arrhythmogenic right ventricular cardiomyopathy (panel **E**), and premature coronary artery disease (panel **F**). **A.** A two-dimensional echocardiogram in the parasternal long-axis view shows extreme asymmetric thickening of the ventricular septum (53 mm), diagnostic of hypertrophic cardiomyopathy. **B.** Histopathologic analysis shows a substrate of disorganized cardiac-muscle cells and a chaotic architectural pattern (hematoxylin and eosin, ×40). **C.** An area of left ventricular myocardium with clusters of inflammatory mononuclear cells, diagnostic of myocarditis (hematoxylin and eosin, ×400). **D.** A greatly enlarged left ventricular cavity in a patient with dilated cardiomyopathy. **E.** Arrhythmogenic right ventricular cardiomyopathy with extensive fatty replacement of the wall of the right ventricle adjacent to a small area of residual myocytes (hematoxylin and eosin, ×8). **F.** A portion of the right coronary artery shows atherosclerotic narrowing and ruptured plaque in a patient with premature coronary artery disease. Ao, aorta; AML, anterior mitral leaflet; LV, left ventricle; M, myocytes; RV, right ventricle; VS, ventricular septum. *Source: Maron.[1]*

monomorphic ventricular tachycardia with left bundle morphology originate from the right ventricle are associated with exercise.[26,30,31,32] Aneurysmal dilations are localized to the posterobasal, apical, and outflow tract regions resulting in the clinical characterization of these regions as the triangle of dysplasia. Sudden death during physical exercise is likely related to hemodynamic factors, increased right ventricular volume and wall stress, and enhanced sympathetic tone that culminate in ventricular tachycardia.[26,31,32] Physical exercise can acutely increase right ventricular afterload and cavity enlargement, which in turn, can trigger ventricular arrhythmias by stretching the diseased right ventricular musculature.

Anomalies of coronary artery origin can precipitate sudden and unexpected cardiac arrest in athletes probably related to acute ischemia.[1,2,23,33] Most commonly the anatomic findings at the time of autopsy is the left main coronary artery arising from the right

coronary sinus. The acute angle with the aorta taken by the anomalous coronary artery leaves a narrowed and compromised lumen, frequently characterized as "slit-like," which limits coronary blood flow and myocardial perfusion with exercise. Evidence of myocardial ischemia caused by anomalous origin of the coronary artery is not present on 12-lead ECG and are rarely elicited with stress testing. Therefore, false negative exercise stress tests are common in athletes who have subsequently died suddenly from the above coronary anomaly.[33] The diagnosis of anomalous origin of the coronary artery requires a high index of suspicion in young people presenting with exertional chest pain and/or syncope.[33] Once diagnosed, anomalous origins of the coronary arteries are treated with coronary artery bypass grafting.

Because sudden cardiac death in those older than 35 years of age participating in athletic activity most commonly occurs because of atherosclerotic coronary artery disease,[1,2,23] it is recommended that a careful history for coronary risk factors or symptoms be taken. If an athlete is identified as being at risk for coronary artery disease or if symptoms suggest ischemia, an exercise stress test should be performed. Stress testing is also recommended in males older than 40 years of age or females older than 50 years of age in whom coronary artery disease is suspected based on the presence of at least two risk factors other than age and gender or one marked abnormal finding.[34] In older athletes without chest pain and risk factors, the routine use of exercise testing is limited by its low specificity and pretest probability.

Myocarditis, either acute or healed, is also associated with sudden death in the athlete presumptively by resulting in an inflammatory or fibrotic pathologic substrate predisposing to ventricular arrhythmias.[2,35–37] Life-threatening ventricular arrhythmias in athletes can be associated with focal myocarditis that is clinically silent and not reliably detected by endomyocardial biopsy.

Approximately 10 percent of young athletes who die suddenly with exercise have no evidence of structural heart diseases. In many such patients the cause of sudden death is likely a primary electrical heart disease. Conditions such as ventricular preexcitation (Wolff-Parkinson-White [WPW] syndrome), inherited cardiac ion channelopathies including long-QT syndrome, Brugada syndrome, and catecholaminergic polymorphic ventricular tachycardia are the likely underlying causes of sudden death.[38,39]

COMMOTIO CORDIS

In the absence of underlying cardiovascular disease, blunt nonpenetrating chest blows during athletic or recreational activities that cause sudden cardiac death are known as commotio cordis.[1,40,41] Although first noted a century ago,[40,42] it is only in the last 10 years that commotio cordis has been recognized as a not uncommon occurrence in youth sports.[43] It has now regarded as the second leading cause of sudden cardiac death in youth sports.[1] The most common sports are those in which projectiles are integral to the game (youth baseball and softball, ice hockey, football, and lacrosse). Ages range from 1 to 50 years, although the mean age of individuals experiencing commotio cordis is only 14 years with approximately 30 percent of individuals older than 18 years. Collapse is instantaneous in one-half of individuals and within 10 to 20 seconds in the others. Cardiac arrhythmias documented soon after collapse are generally ventricular fibrillation (VF); however, as the time to first documented arrhyth-

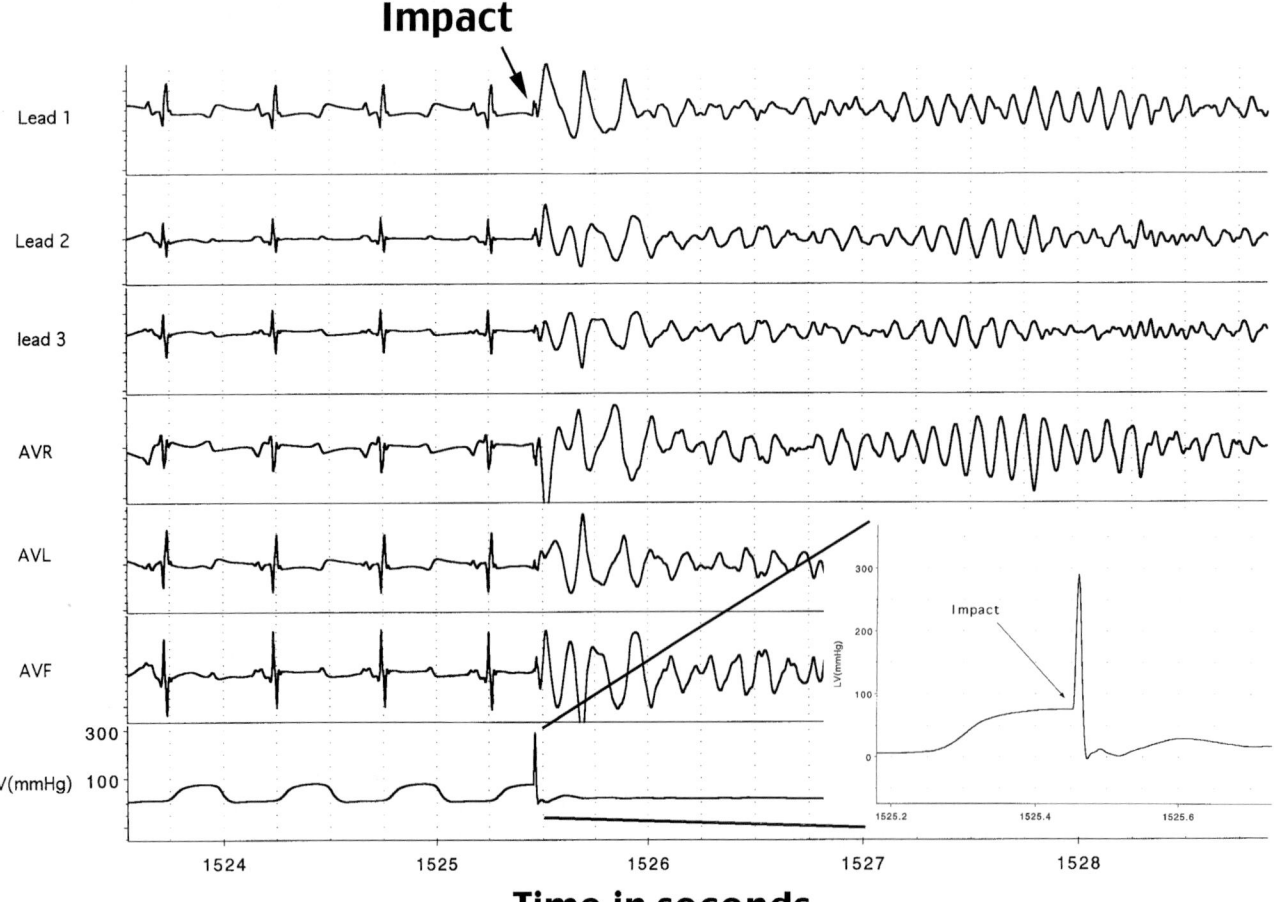

FIGURE 100–3. Six-lead electrocardiogram from a 12-kg swine undergoing chest wall impact with a 30 mph baseball. Note the immediate generation of ventricular fibrillation and the acute rise in left ventricular (LV) pressure. *Source: Link, Maron, VanderBrink.*[48]

mia increases, asystole is more frequently present. Early reports of resuscitated commotio cordis showed dismal survival, although similar to other causes of sudden cardiac death. Yet, there remains a possibility that resuscitation is more difficult in commotio cordis despite a structurally normal heart.[44-46]

Recently, a porcine model was developed for the study of this syndrome, which demonstrated that the immediate cause of collapse was VF (Fig. 100–3).[47] Use of this model has allowed the elaboration of several important determinants of VF following a chest blow, including impact delivered directly over the heart,[48] and timing within the vulnerable phase of repolarization (a narrow 10-to-30-millisecond [msec] window just prior to the T-wave peak, equivalent to only 1 to 2 percent of the cardiac cycle).[47] Furthermore, impact velocity appears to have a Gaussian distribution with 40 miles per hour (mph) the most prone to cause VF.[49] In addition, the hardness of the impact object correlated directly with the risk of VF.[47,50] These variables can be united by two predominant physiologic properties: timing of impact relative to the cardiac cycle and the peak LV pressures caused by the blow. Indeed, in multiple experiments both of these two characteristics are associated with the risk of VF.[47-50] The importance of timing and pressure risk have also been demonstrated in a recent Langendorff preparation.[51] The timing variable is likely critical because of the dispersion in repolarization present during this narrow time window, whereas the pressure variable can be related to optimal pressure rises to activate specific ion channels.

Sudden cardiac death (SCD) in commotio cordis appears to be a primary electrical event. The cellular determinants of VF induced by chest-wall blows likely include ion channel activation caused by increased LV pressure.[52-54] The potassium-adenosine triphosphate (I_{K-ATP}) ion channel mediates the initiation of VF in the swine model,[55] and has also been shown to be activated by atrial stretch.[56] It is possible that more stretch-activated ion channels are also involved.

Efforts to minimize the risk of SCD because of commotio cordis have centered on the impact object, chest protectors, and changes in rules of the sport. Softer than standard baseballs have been demonstrated to reduce the risk of commotio cordis.[47,50] Chest wall protectors intuitively should reduce the risk of commotio cordis. However, in the Commotio Cordis registry approximately one-third of the victims suffering commotion cordis in organized sports were wearing chest protectors, and in the laboratory model chest protectors did not appear to reduce the risk of VF.[57] Ongoing efforts to develop more effective chest protectors can decrease the risk of SCD in vulnerable athletes. The 36th Bethesda Conference promote the use of age-appropriate soft balls to reduce the risk of commotion cordis, as well as the timely availability of automated external defibrillators (AEDs).[58]

CLINICAL EVALUATION OF THE ATHLETE WITH SYMPTOMS

Arrhythmias can be nonsustained or sustained and hemodynamically significant or not. Thus, arrhythmia-related symptoms range from brief palpitations, to syncope and resuscitated sudden death. The severity of the symptoms, the presence or absence of structural heart disease, and the family medical history determine the extent of the workup. As a general rule the severity of the symptoms are related to the risk of subsequent sudden death. Thus, palpitations are frequently benign; presyncope and certainly syncope are more concerning, and resuscitated sudden death is of utmost worry.

Palpitations can be caused by atrial or ventricular premature depolarizations, nonsustained arrhythmias such as atrial tachycardia or nonsustained ventricular tachycardia, or even on occasion by sustained arrhythmias such as supraventricular or ventricular tachycardias that do not cause hemodynamic collapse. The critical element in the workup is to capture an ECG recording during symptoms. A 24-hour ambulatory Holter or event loop recorder can be used in the athlete with daily or frequent symptoms. Subsequent cardiac workup and treatment depend on the specific arrhythmia found.

Syncope is a common symptom in young people and in athletes. Syncope without prodromal symptoms or occurring at peak exercise are more concerning and are likely to represent underlying cardiac disease (Table 100–3). Injury secondary to syncope is more often seen in arrhythmic disorders and rarely seen in neurocardiogenic syncope. Athletes with syncope should at a minimum be tested with a resting 12-lead electrocardiogram and an echocardiogram. In athletes older than 35 years of age and those with syncope during exertion, an exercise tolerance test should be performed for an evaluation for cardiac ischemia and exercise-induced arrhythmias.

Unfortunately, we evaluate only a small fraction of athletes with SCD as the minority are resuscitated.[45] In those fortunate to survive an episode of cardiac arrest a complete cardiovascular assessment is necessary. Thus, ECGs, long-term telemetry monitoring, echocardiography, and stress tests are generally warranted. These tests will identify most of individuals with HCM, exercise-induced polymorphic ventricular tachycardia, long QT syndrome (LQTS), Brugada syndrome, and possibly arrhythmogenic right ventricular cardiomyopathy (ARVC). Cardiac catheterization, cardiac MRI and computed tomography should be considered if underlying heart disease is not found with this initial workup. Specific electrophysiologic tests

TABLE 100–3

Clinical Characteristics Helpful in Differentiating Arrhythmic from Nonarrhythmic Syncope

	NEUROCARDIOGENIC OR NONARRHYTHMIC	ARRHYTHMIC
Prodrome	Lightheadedness, warmth, nausea	None or brief lightheadedness
Number of episodes	Multiple	Few or 1
Situational factors	Fear, fright, upright posture	Exertional Unrelated to posture
Post syncopal symptoms	Frequently fatigue	Usually none
Injury	Unusual	Common
Underlying heart disease	Unusual	Common

SOURCE: Adapted from Link MS, Wang PJ, Estes NAM III. Ventricular arrhythmias in the athlete. Curr Opin Cardiol. 2001;16:30–39.

for primary electrical diseases (LQTS, Brugada syndrome, WPW syndrome) are often warranted if the diagnosis is not clear.

Because many of the cardiac diseases that predispose to sudden death in athletes are inherited, the family medical history is important. Therefore, the presence of early sudden death or hereditary cardiac abnormality in the family of an athlete should prompt a thorough cardiac workup regardless of the presenting symptoms.

ELIGIBILITY GUIDELINES

Consensus recommendations regarding the eligibility of athletes with cardiovascular conditions for competition in organized sports are available to guide clinicians.[3,4,59] The competitive athlete is defined as one who participates in an organized team or individual sport that requires regular competition against others as a central component, places a high premium on excellence and achievement, and requires some form of systematic and frequently intense training. Because of the considerable pressures of competitive sports, athletes are commonly unable to exercise judgment and control their level of exertion or reliably discern or respond appropriately to cardiac symptoms.

Although these guidelines are focused on the competitive athlete, other recommendations are useful for the clinician evaluating recreational athletes.[36] These recommendations are based on the best available data and the consensus of an expert panel regarding a variety of genetic and acquired cardiovascular diseases that can cause athletic field deaths or place the athlete at increased risk for sudden and unexpected death or disease progression. Specific recommendations are available according to cardiovascular condition and the type of athletic activity.[3,36] Recently, the European recommendations for participation in competitive athletics assessing eligibility criteria for competitive athletes with cardiovascular disease have been modeled after the Bethesda Conference.[3,59] Although these guidelines are similar in many respects, they are more restrictive in disqualifying those with LQTS, HCM, and Marfan syndrome, particularly when diagnostic cardiac findings are borderline.[59]

Although restricting the competitive athletes from sports is reasonable and intuitively justified, these recommendations are not evidence-based. Although these guidelines are largely formulated based on expert opinion, there is support for this approach from the uniquely rigorous screening and disqualification program in Italy. A decline in the rate of athletic sudden deaths has been attributed to the systematic national preparticipation screening program. A dramatic reduction approaching 90 percent in the annual incidence of sudden cardiovascular death in competitive athletes was documented in association with implementation of nationwide screening and the increasing identification of athletes with heart disease who were then disqualified from competitive sports.[60]

PREPARTICIPATION SCREENING

Because the vast majority of athletes dying suddenly have preexisting and underlying heart disease, screening for these conditions allows for identification of at-risk athletes. Those identified at high risk for SCD can be withdrawn from vigorous training or competition and thus potentially reduce the risk of SCD.[61,62] Although never subjected to a randomized trial there is anecdotal evidence that cardiac

risk for SCD is increased by vigorous training. The most compelling evidence for this assertion comes from Italy where all athletes engaged in organized sports (approximately 10 percent of the Italian population) are mandated to undergo annual screening in a government-sponsored supported program.[22] This unique system served as the impetus for a proposal in 2005 by the European Society of Cardiology (ESC) for a common European protocol for preparticipation athlete screening.[61] Central to these recommendations are medical screening, performed prior to the onset of athletic training, by specially trained physicians, consisting of personal and family history, physical examination, and routine 12-lead ECGs. The guidelines recommend repeated screening for the duration of exposure to athletic activity annually to identify progressive traits of potential cardiac pathology. Further diagnostic evaluations (both invasive and noninvasive) can be obtained when appropriate based on abnormal cardiac findings. If abnormalities are detected that are compatible with conditions known to elevate risk of SCD, the ESC recommends exclusion of the individual from athletic activity, as further delineated by the newly revised 36th Bethesda Conference guidelines.[63]

However, in the United States, with a large and geographically dispersed population, preparticipation evaluations of high school and college athletes has traditionally been limited to a history and physical examination (Table 100–4). The issue regarding routine use of ECG is a complex one and not solely limited to economic concerns. Evidence suggests that the preparticipation screening process currently used at many U.S. colleges can have limited potential to detect cardiovascular abnormalities associated with SCD in student athletes.[64] In a large survey reported by Pfister and colleagues, 97 percent of 879 colleges and universities surveyed required some form of preparticipation screen-

---

TABLE 100–4

American Heart Association Consensus Panel Recommendations for Preparticipation Athletic Screening

Family History
  1. Premature sudden cardiac death
  2. Heart disease in surviving relatives younger than 50 years old
Personal History
  3. Heart murmur
  4. Systemic hypertension
  5. Fatigue
  6. Syncope/near-syncope
  7. Excessive/unexplained exertional dyspnea
  8. Exertional chest pain
Physical Examination
  9. Heart murmur (supine/standing[a])
  10. Femoral arterial pulses (to exclude coarctation of aorta)
  11. Stigmata of Marfan syndrome
  12. Brachial blood pressure measurement (sitting)

[a]In particular, to identify heart murmur consistent with dynamic obstruction to left ventricular outflow.
SOURCE: Maron BJ, et al. Circulation. 1996;94:850–856, reprinted with permission from American Heart Association.

ing.[65] However, only approximately 25 percent of these schools used preparticipation screening forms that contained at least 9 of the recommended 12 American Heart Association (AHA) screening guidelines (judged to be adequate), whereas 24 percent contained ≥4 of these parameters and were considered inadequate. A wide range of medical and nonmedical personnel were responsible for preparticipation screening. It is therefore clear that, at least at the collegiate level, little semblance of a uniform screening process presently exists. Maron has speculated that adoption of a formalized screening process in the United States such as that proposed by the ESC is unlikely.[66] Although such an endeavor is indeed praiseworthy, with the potential to save young lives, it may not be readily applicable within the U.S. healthcare system; competing healthcare interests and heightened concerns for medical-legal liability are cited. Indeed, the medico-legal aspect has recently been the focus of a review by Paterick and coworkers providing practice guidelines for physicians performing the medical evaluations of competitive athletes by clarifying the standard of care, potential pitfalls, and the evolving legal framework associated with this clinical practice.[67]

PERFORMANCE-ENHANCING SUBSTANCES

Athletes commonly use drugs and dietary supplements because they are considered to enhance athletic performance.[63,68] These performance-enhancing substances include stimulants, anabolic steroids, and peptide hormones. Studies assessing the risks and benefits of these substances are very limited, but clinical observations indicate that some have the potential for serious side effects. Despite aggressive marketing and user testimonials, systematic studies assessing the benefits and risks of any of these substances have not been conducted. Clinical observations indicate some supplements can have serious side effects including fatal adverse reactions. Athletes should make informed decisions regarding the use of drugs and dietary supplements with careful consideration to what is known. The dietary supplement ephedra (ma huang), for example, is associated with life-threatening toxicity and death, which ultimately resulted in a ban on its sale in many countries.[69] Anabolic steroids are associated with premature coronary disease and sudden death. Recreational drugs including cocaine are associated with fatal myocardial infarction, sudden death, and stroke. Peptide hormones and analogues such as recombinant erythropoietin (EPO) are used as a pharmacologic alternative to the procedure of *blood doping* or autotransfusion steroids, peptide hormones, and others that can have life-threatening toxicity. Comprehensive lists of prohibited drugs and dietary supplements are now available from governing athletic bodies. A rigorous approach to prevent performance-enhancing and recreational drug and dietary supplement is needed to reduce the risk of these substances triggering sudden death. The important elements of programs to discourage drug performance-enhancing substances include education in ethical principles inherent in athletic participation. Healthcare professionals should ask athletes about drug and dietary supplements and serve as an educational resource for athletes and athletic organizations.[63,68]

CONCLUSION

Sudden cardiac death in athletes presents several challenges to the medical professional and healthcare system alike, including diagnosis

of cardiac abnormalities associated with SCD, management of these cardiac disorders, and the evolution of universally applicable screening protocols aimed at reducing exposure of susceptible individuals to risk of death. Significant advances have been made internationally in each of these areas. Current clinical focus rests on identification of underlying cardiac disease by noninvasive means, application of intracardiac cardioverter-defibrillator (ICD) therapy where indicated, and reduction of risk by provision of safety equipment and, where necessary, exclusion from competitive sports participation.

REFERENCES

1. Maron BJ. Sudden death in young athletes. *N Engl J Med.* 2003;349:1064–1075.
2. Van Camp SP, Bloor CM, Mueller FO, Cantu RC, Olsen HG. Nontraumatic sports death in high school and college athletes. *Med Sci Sports Exerc.* 1995;27:641–647.
3. Maron BJ, Zipes DP. Introduction: eligibility recommendations for competitive athletes with cardiovascular abnormalities-general considerations. *J Am Coll Cardiol.* 2005;45:1318–1321.
4. Estes NA 3rd, Link MS, Cannom D, et al. Report of the NASPE policy conference on arrhythmias and the athlete. *J Cardiovasc Electrophysiol.* 2001;12:1208–1219.
5. Henschen S. Skilanglauf und Skiwettlauf. Eine medizinische Sportstudie. *Mitt Med Klin Upsala (Jena).* 1899;2:215–218.
6. Thompson PD. Bruce Dill Historical lecture. Historical concepts of the athlete's heart. *Med Sci Sports Exerc.* 2004;36:363–370.
7. Rost R. The athlete's heart. Historical perspectives—solved and unsolved problems. *Cardiol Clin.* 1997;15:493–512.
8. Wharton J. "Athlete's Heart": The medical debate over athleticism, 1870–1920. In: Berryman JW, Park RJ, eds. *Sport and Exercise Science, Essays in the History of Sports Medicine.* Urbana, IL: University of Illinois Press; 1992:109–135.
9. Maron BJ, Pelliccia A. The heart of trained athletes: cardiac remodeling and the risks of sports including sudden death. *Circulation.* 2006;114:1633–1644.
10. Pelliccia A, Maron BJ, Spataro A, Proschan MA, Spirito P. The upper limit of physiologic cardiac hypertrophy in highly trained elite athletes. *N Engl J Med.* 1991;324:295–301.
11. Pelliccia A, Maron BJ, Culasso F, Spataro A, Caselli G. Athlete's heart in women. Echocardiographic characterization of highly trained elite female athletes. *JAMA.* 1996;276:211–215.
12. Pelliccia A, Culasso F, Di Paolo FM, Maron BJ. Physiologic LV cavity dilatation in elite athletes. *Ann Intern Med.* 1999;130:23–31.
13. Douglas PS, O'Toole ML, Katz SE, et al. LV hypertrophy in athletes. *Am J Cardiol.* 1997;80:1384–1388.
14. Abernethy WB, Choo JK, Hutter AM Jr. Echocardiographic characteristics of professional football players. *J Am Coll Cardiol.* 2003;41:280–284.
15. Scharhag J, Schneider G, Urhausen A, et al. Athlete's heart: right and LV mass and function in male endurance athletes and untrained individuals determined by magnetic resonance imaging. *J Am Coll Cardiol.* 2002;40:1856–1863.
16. Maron BJ, Gardin JM, Flack JM, et al. Prevalence of hypertrophic cardiomyopathy in a general population of young adults. Echocardiographic analysis of 4111 subjects in the CARDIA Study. Coronary Artery Risk Development in (Young) Adults. *Circulation.* 1995;92:785–789.
17. Estes NAM III, Link MS, Homoud MK, Wang PJ. Electrocardiographic variants and cardiac rhythm and conduction disturbances in the athlete. In: Thompson PD, ed. *Exercise and Sports Cardiology.* New York: McGraw Hill; 2000.
18. Link MS, Wang PJ, Estes NAM III. Cardiac arrhythmias and electrophysiologic observations in the athlete. In: Williams RA, ed. *The Athlete and Heart Disease: Diagnosis, Evaluation & Management.* Philadelphia: Lippincott Williams & Wilkins, 1999:2196.
19. Serra-Grima R, Estorch M, Carrio I, et al. Marked ventricular repolarization abnormalities in highly trained athletes' electrocardiograms: clinical and prognostic implications. *J Am Coll Cardiol.* 2000;36:1310–1316.
20. Chapman J. Profound sinus bradycardia in the athletic heart syndrome. *J Sports Med Physical Fitness.* 1981;22:294–298.
21. Biffi A, Pelliccia A, Verdile L, et al. Long-term clinical significance of frequent and complex ventricular tachyarrhythmias in trained athletes. *J Am Coll Cardiol.* 2002;40:446–452.

22. Biffi A, Maron BJ, Verdile L, et al. Impact of physical deconditioning on ventricular tachyarrhythmias in trained athletes. *J Am Coll Cardiol.* 2004;44:1053–108.

23. Maron BJ, Shirani J, Poliac LC, et al. Sudden death in young competitive athletes: clinical, demographic, and pathologic profiles. *JAMA.* 1996;276:199–204.

24. Corrado D, Basso C, Schiavon M, Thiene G. Screening for hypertrophic cardiomyopathy in young athletes. *N Engl J Med.* 1998;339:364–369.

25. Corrado D, Basso C, Rizzoli G, Schiavon M, Thiene G. Does sports activity enhance the risk of sudden death in adolescents and young adults? *J Am Coll Cardiol.* 2003;42:1959–1963.

26. Priori SG, Aliot E, Blomstrom-Lundqvist C, et al. Task force report on sudden cardiac death of the European Society of Cardiology. *Eur Heart J.* 2001;22:1374–1450.

27. Basso C, Calabrese F, Corrado D, Thiene G. Postmortem diagnosis in sudden cardiac death victims: macroscopic, microscopic and molecular findings. *Cardiovasc Res.* 2001;50:290–300.

28. Maron BJ. Hypertrophic cardiomyopathy; A systemic review. *JAMA.* 2002;287:1308–1320.

29. Basso C, Thiene G, Corrado D, et al. Hypertrophic cardiomyopathy and sudden death in the young: pathologic evidence of myocardial ischemia. *Hum Pathol.* 2000;31:988–998.

30. Corrado D, Basso C, Thiene G, et al. Spectrum of clinicopathologic manifestations of arrhythmogenic right ventricular cardiomyopathy/dysplasia: a multicenter study. *J Am Coll Cardiol.* 1997;30:1512–1520.

31. Corrado D, Leoni L, Link MS, et al. Implantable cardioverter-defibrillator therapy for prevention of sudden death in patients with arrhythmogenic right ventricular cardiomyopathy/dysplasia. *Circulation.* 2003;108:3084–3091.

32. Nava A, Bauce B, Basso C, et al. Clinical profile and long-term follow-up of 37 families with arrhythmogenic right ventricular cardiomyopathy. *J Am Coll Cardiol.* 2000;36:2226–2233.

33. Basso C, Maron BJ, Corrado D, Thiene G. Clinical profile of congenital coronary artery anomalies with origin from the wrong aortic sinus leading to sudden death in young competitive athletes. *J Am Coll Cardiol.* 2000;35:1493–1501.

34. Zipes DP, Ackerman MJ, Estes NA 3rd, et al. Task Force 7: arrhythmias. *J Am Coll Cardiol.* 2005;45:1354–1363.

35. Priori SG, Aliot E, Blomstrom-Lundqvist C, et al. Task Force on Sudden Cardiac Death, European Society of Cardiology. *Europace.* 2002;4:3–18.

36. Maron BJ, Chaitman BR, Ackerman MJ, et al. Recommendations for physical activity and recreational sports participation for young patients with genetic cardiovascular diseases. *Circulation.* 2004;109:2807–2816.

37. Basso C, Corrado D, Thiene G. Congenital coronary artery anomalies as an important cause of sudden death in the young. *Cardiol Rev.* 2001;9:312–317.

38. Corrado D, Basso C, Thiene G. Sudden cardiac death in young people with apparently normal heart. *Cardiovasc Res.* 2001;50:399–408.

39. Wilde AA, Antzelevitch C, Borggrefe M, et al. Proposed diagnostic criteria for the Brugada syndrome: consensus report. *Circulation.* 2002;106:2514–2519.

40. Maron BJ, Doerer JJ, Haas TS, Estes NA 3rd, Link MS. Historical observation on commotio cordis. *Heart Rhythm.* 2006;3:605–606.

41. Maron BJ, Gohman TE, Kyle SB, Estes NA 3rd, Link MS. Clinical profile and spectrum of commotio cordis. *JAMA.* 2002;287:1142–1146.

42. Nesbitt AD, Cooper PJ, Kohl P. Rediscovering commotio cordis. *Lancet.* 2001;357:1195–1197.

43. Maron BJ, Poliac LC, Kaplan JA, Mueller FO. Blunt impact to the chest leading to sudden death from cardiac arrest during sports activities. *N Engl J Med.* 1995;333:337–342.

44. Maron BJ, Wentzel DC, Zenovich AG, Estes NA 3rd, Link MS. Death in a young athlete due to commotio cordis despite prompt external defibrillation. *Heart Rhythm.* 2005;2:991–993.

45. Drezner JA, Rogers KJ. Sudden cardiac arrest in intercollegiate athletes: detailed analysis and outcomes of resuscitation in nine cases. *Heart Rhythm.* 2006;3:755–759.

46. Link MS. Resuscitation in athletes: a sobering tale. *Heart Rhythm.* 2006;3:760–761.

47. Link MS, Wang PJ, Pandian NG, et al. An experimental model of sudden death due to low-energy chest-wall impact (commotio cordis). *N Engl J Med.* 1998;338:1805–1811.

48. Link MS, Maron BJ, VanderBrink BA, et al. Impact directly over the cardiac silhouette is necessary to produce ventricular fibrillation in an experimental model of commotio cordis. *J Am Coll Cardiol.* 2001;37:649–654.

49. Link MS, Maron BJ, Wang PJ, et al. Upper and lower limits of vulnerability to sudden arrhythmic death with chest-wall impact (commotio cordis). *J Am Coll Cardiol.* 2003;41:99–104.

50. Link MS, Maron BJ, Wang PJ, et al. Reduced risk of sudden death from chest wall blows (commotio cordis) with safety baseballs. *Pediatrics.* 2002;109:873–877.

51. Bode F, Franz MR, Wilke I, et al. Ventricular fibrillation induced by stretch pulse: implications for sudden death due to commotio cordis. *Heart Rhythm.* 2006;27:2196–2200.

52. Link MS. Mechanically induced sudden death in chest wall impact. *Prog Biophys Molecular Biol.* 2003;82:175–186.

53. Kohl P, Nesbitt AD, Cooper PJ, Lei M. Sudden cardiac death by Commotio cordis: role of mechanico-electrical feedback. *Cardiovasc Res.* 2001;50:280–289.

54. Kohl P, Ravens U. Cardiac mechano-electric feedback: past, present, and prospect. *Prog Biophys Mol Biol.* 2003;82:3–9.

55. Link MS, Wang PJ, VanderBrink BA, et al. Selective activation of the K(+)(ATP) channel is a mechanism by which sudden death is produced by low-energy chest-wall impact (Commotio cordis). *Circulation.* 1999;100:413–418.

56. Van Wagoner DR. Mechanosensitive gating of atrial ATP-sensitive potassium channels. *Circ Res.* 1993;72:973–983.

57. Weinstock J, Maron BJ, Song C, et al. Failure of commercially available chest wall protectors to prevent sudden cardiac death induced by chest wall blows in an experimental model of commotio cordis. *Pediatrics.* 2006;117:e656–662.

58. Maron BJ, Estes NA 3rd, Link MS. Task Force 11: Commotio cordis: 36th Bethesda Conference: Eligibility Recommendations for Competitive Athletes with Cardiovascular Abnormalities. *J Am Coll Cardiol.* 2005;45:1371–1373.

59. Pelliccia A, Fagard R, Bjornstad HH, et al. Recommendations for competitive sports participation in athletes with cardiovascular disease: a consensus document from the Study Group of Sports Cardiology of the Working Group of Cardiac Rehabilitation and Exercise Physiology and the Working Group of Myocardial and Pericardial Diseases of the European Society of Cardiology. *Eur Heart J.* 2005;26:1422–1445.

60. Pelliccia A, Di Paolo FM, Corrado D, et al. Evidence for efficacy of the Italian national pre-participation screening programme for identification of hypertrophic cardiomyopathy in competitive athletes. *Eur Heart J.* 2006;27(18):2152–2153.

61. Corrado D, Pelliccia A, Bjornstad HH, et al. Cardiovascular pre-participation screening of young competitive athletes for prevention of sudden death: proposal for a common European protocol. Consensus Statement of the Study Group of Sport Cardiology of the Working Group of Cardiac Rehabilitation and Exercise Physiology and the Working Group of Myocardial and Pericardial Diseases of the European Society of Cardiology. *Eur Heart J.* 2005;26:516–524.

62. Pelliccia A, Maron BJ. Preparticipation cardiovascular evaluation of the competitive athlete: perspectives from the 30-year Italian experience. *Am J Cardiol.* 1995;75:827–829.

63. Dhar R, Stout CW, Link MS, et al. Cardiovascular toxicities of performance-enhancing substances in sports. *Mayo Clin Proc.* 2005;80:1307–1315.

64. Maron BJ, Douglas PS, Graham TP, Nishimura RA, Thompson PD. Task Force 1: preparticipation screening and diagnosis of cardiovascular disease in athletes. *J Am Coll Cardiol.* 2005;45:1322–1326.

65. Pfister GC, Puffer JC, Maron BJ. Preparticipation cardiovascular screening for US collegiate student-athletes. *JAMA.* 2000;283:1597–1599.

66. Maron BJ. How should we screen competitive athletes for cardiovascular disease? *Eur Heart J.* 2005;26:428–430.

67. Paterick TE, Paterick TJ, Fletcher GF, Maron BJ. Medical and legal issues in the cardiovascular evaluation of competitive athletes. *JAMA.* 2005;294:3011–3018.

68. Estes NA 3rd, Kloner R, Olshansky B, Virmani R. Task Force 9: drugs and performance-enhancing substances. *J Am Coll Cardiol.* 2005;45:1368–1369.

69. Stout CW, Weinstock J, Homoud MK, et al. Herbal medicine: beneficial effects, side effects, and promising new research in the treatment of arrhythmias. *Curr Cardiol Rep.* 2003;5:395–401.

CHAPTER (101)

Aging and Cardiovascular Disease in the Elderly

Edward G. Lakatta / Samer S. Najjar /
Steven P. Schulman / Gary Gerstenblith

INTRODUCTION

The world population in both industrialized and developing countries is aging. In the United States, 35 million people are older than the age of 65 years, and the number of older Americans is expected to double by the year 2030. The clinical and economic implications of this demographic shift are staggering, because age is the most powerful risk factor for cardiovascular diseases.

The incidence and prevalence of hypertension, coronary artery disease, congestive heart failure, and stroke, the quintessential diseases of Western society, increase steeply with advancing age (Fig. 101–1). Al-though epidemiologic studies have discovered that some aspects of life-style and genetics are risk factors for these diseases, age, per se, confers the major risk. There is a continuum of age-related alterations of cardiovascular structure and function in healthy humans.[1-4] These changes appear to influence the steep increases in hypertension, athero-sclerosis, stroke, left ventricular hypertrophy, chronic heart failure, and atrial fibrillation with increasing age. Specific pathophysiologic mecha-nisms that underlie these diseases become superimposed on cardiac and vascular substrates that have been modified by an "aging process," and the latter modulates disease occurrence and severity. In other words, age-associated changes in cardiovascular structure and function

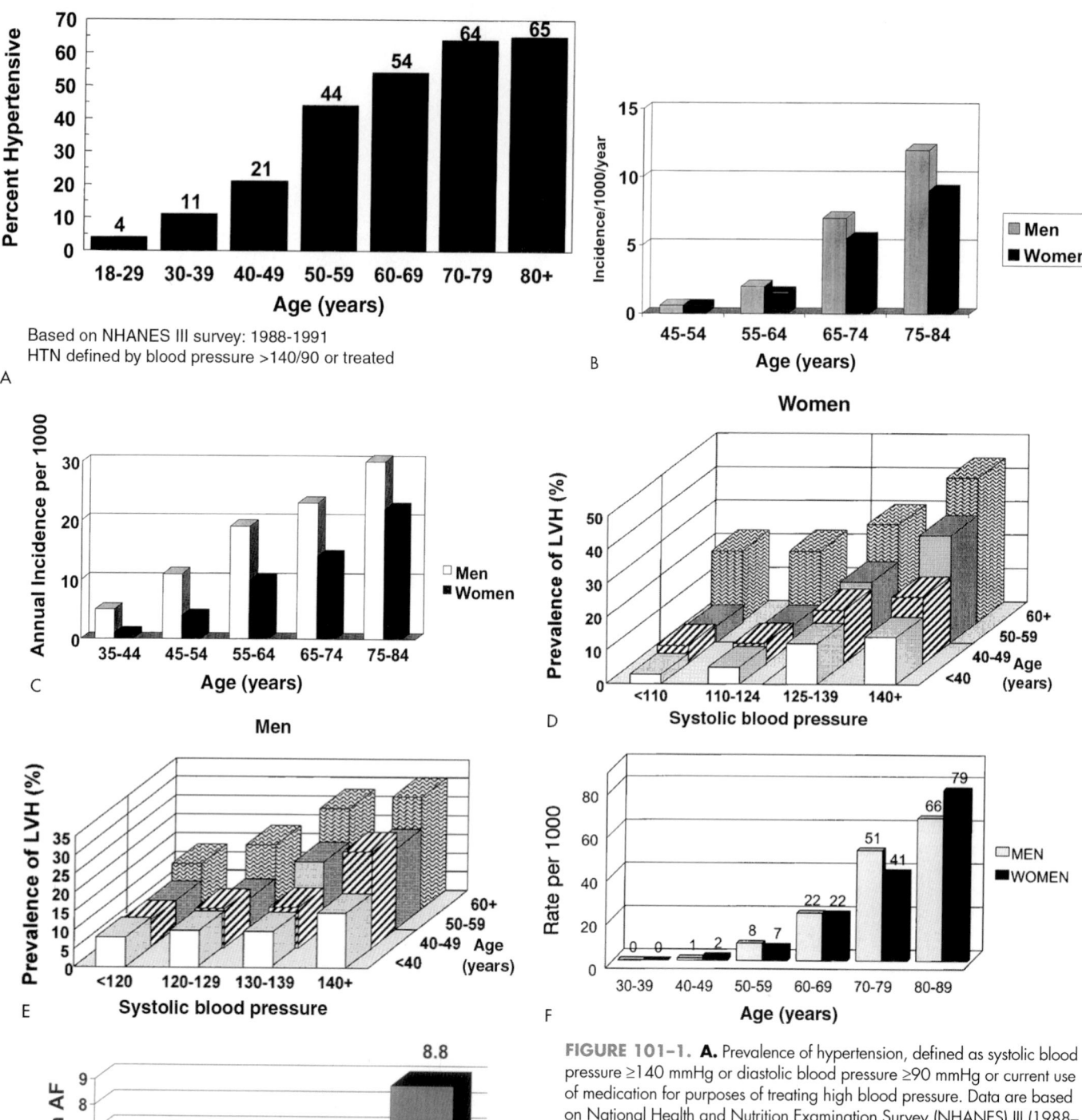

FIGURE 101–1. **A.** Prevalence of hypertension, defined as systolic blood pressure ≥140 mmHg or diastolic blood pressure ≥90 mmHg or current use of medication for purposes of treating high blood pressure. Data are based on National Health and Nutrition Examination Survey (NHANES) III (1988–1991). **B.** Incidence of atherothrombotic stroke (per 1000 subjects per year) by age in men (*light bars*) and women (*dark bars*) from the Framingham Heart Study. **C.** Incidence of coronary heart disease by age in men (*light bars*) and women (*dark bars*) from the Framingham Heart Study. **D.** Prevalence of echocardiographic left ventricular hypertrophy (LVH) in women according to baseline age and systolic blood pressure. **E.** Prevalence of echocardiographic left ventricular hypertrophy in men according to baseline age and systolic blood pressure. **F.** Prevalence of heart failure by age in Framingham Heart Study men (*light bars*) and women (*dark bars*). **G.** Prevalence of atrial fibrillation (AF) by age in subjects from the Framingham Heart Study. *Source: A, B, and C from Lakatta EG, Levy D. Arterial and cardiac aging: major shareholders in cardiovascular disease enterprises. Part I. Aging arteries: a "set-up" for vascular disease. Circulation 2003;107:129–146. With permission. D, E, F, and G from Lakatta EG, Levy D. Arterial and cardiac aging: major shareholders in cardiovascular disease enterprises. Part II: the aging heart in health: links to heart disease. Circulation 2003;107:346–354. With permission.*

become "partners" with pathophysiologic disease mechanisms, lifestyle, and genetics in determining the threshold, severity, prognosis, and therapeutic response of cardiovascular disease in older persons.

The nature of age–disease interactions is complex and involves mechanisms of aging, multiple defined disease risk factors, and as yet undefined risk factors. The role of specific age-associated changes in cardiovascular structure and function in such age–disease interactions has not been considered in most epidemiologic studies of cardiovascular disease.

Quantitative information on age-associated alterations in cardiovascular structure and function in health is essential to unravel age–disease interactions and to target the specific characteristics of cardiovascular aging that render it such a major risk factor for cardiovascular diseases. Such information is also of practical value, to differentiate between the limitations of an older person that relate to disease, and those that might be expected, within limits, to accompany advancing age or a sedentary lifestyle. During the past three decades, a sustained effort has been applied to characterize the effects of aging in health on multiple aspects of cardiovascular (CV) structure and function in a single study population, the Baltimore Longitudinal Study on Aging (BLSA). These community-dwelling volunteers are rigorously screened to detect both clinical and occult CV disease and are characterized with respect to lifestyle (e.g., exercise habits) in an attempt to clarify the interactions of disease, risk factors, and aging itself. Perspectives gleaned from these studies are emphasized throughout this chapter.

SUCCESSFUL VS. UNSUCCESSFUL CARDIOVASCULAR AGING

To define why age (or an aging process × exposure time) is so risky, the specific components of the risk associated with age must be identified. Two complementary approaches have evolved. Epidemiologists search for novel measures of "subclinical disease" (in addition to the more established risk factors that are already well characterized) in large, unselected cohorts composed of persons both with and without cardiovascular disease. In contrast, gerontologists attempt to develop quantitative information on cardiovascular structure and function in apparently healthy individuals to define the specific characteristics of aging that render it such a major risk factor for cardiovascular disease, even in the absence of clinically apparent comorbidity. The latter approach consists of identifying and selecting community-dwelling individuals who do not have (or have not yet experienced) clinical disease and who do not have occult disease that can be detected by noninvasive methods. These individuals are then grouped by age and stratified according to the level of a given variable, which may include some of the novel measures of subclinical disease identified by the epidemiologists. If the variable is perceived as beneficial or deleterious with respect to cardiovascular structure or function, those with extreme measures are considered to be aging "successfully" or "unsuccessfully," respectively. "Unsuccessful" aging in this context is not synonymous with having clinical disease, as individuals with defined overt or occult clinical disease have been excluded from consideration a priori. Instead, unsuccessful aging, that is, falling within the poorest category with respect to the measure viewed as deleterious, may be viewed as a risk factor for future clinical cardiovascular disease. In this regard, unsuccessful aging is a manifestation of the interaction of the cardiovascular aging process and specific aspects of vascular disease pathophysiology. Thus, gerontologists and epidemi-

ologists have become part of a joint effort in the quest to define why aging confers enormous risk for cardiovascular disease.

AGE-ASSOCIATED CHANGES IN ARTERIAL STRUCTURE AND FUNCTION

Close examination of the age-associated changes in arterial structure and function may help explain why aging is such a strong predictor of adverse events. Findings from clinical studies show that the age-associated changes in arterial structure and function, previously not defined as clinical or subclinical diseases, are themselves risk factors for cardiovascular diseases. These novel risk factors, including intimal-medial thickness, arterial stiffness and endothelial dysfunction, alter the substrate upon which the cardiovascular diseases are superimposed; therefore, they affect the development, manifestation, severity, and prognosis of these diseases.

Many age-associated changes are seen in the large arteries of humans. Cross-sectional studies show that central elastic arteries dilate with age, leading to an increase in lumen size[5] (Fig. 101–2A), which results in increased inertance. In addition, postmortem studies have indicated an age-associated increase in arterial wall thickening, which is caused mainly by an increase in intimal thickening. In cross-sectional studies, carotid intimal-medial thickening increases nearly threefold between the ages of 20 and 90 years[6] (Fig. 101–2B). Note in Fig. 101–2B that both the average and range of intimal-medial thickness values is greater at higher ages, suggesting heterogeneity in the magnitude of the age-associated thickening process among older individuals. The increase in arterial wall thickening is accompanied by an increase in arterial stiffening (reduction in compliance)[7] (Fig. 101–2C), which is due to several structural changes in the arterial wall.[8] These changes include an increase in collagen content, cross-linking of adjacent collagen molecules to form advanced glycation end products, fraying of elastin, a decrease in the amount of elastin, and deposition of calcium in the medial layer. In addition to structural changes, functional alterations include an age-associated deterioration in vascular endothelial vasoreactivity.[9]

【 】 BLOOD PRESSURE

Both systolic and pulse pressures increase with age in all adults, whereas diastolic blood pressure increases until the fifth decade of life and then levels off before decreasing after 60 years of age (Fig. 101–3A to C). These age-dependent changes in systolic, diastolic, and pulse pressures are consistent with the idea that in younger people, blood pressure is determined largely by peripheral vascular resistance, whereas in older people blood pressure is determined mainly by the stiffness of central conduit vessels.[8]

In older individuals, isolated systolic hypertension (ISH) is the most common form of hypertension. ISH is defined as a systolic blood pressure >140 mmHg and a diastolic blood pressure <90 mmHg (i.e., a widened pulse pressure), and it could be described as a disease related, in part, to arterial stiffening. Even mild isolated systolic hypertension (stage 1) is associated with an appreciable increase in cardiovascular disease risk,[10] and is an indication for treatment. Although the initial cut-off value for normal systolic pressure was 160 mmHg, the value was adjusted downward when

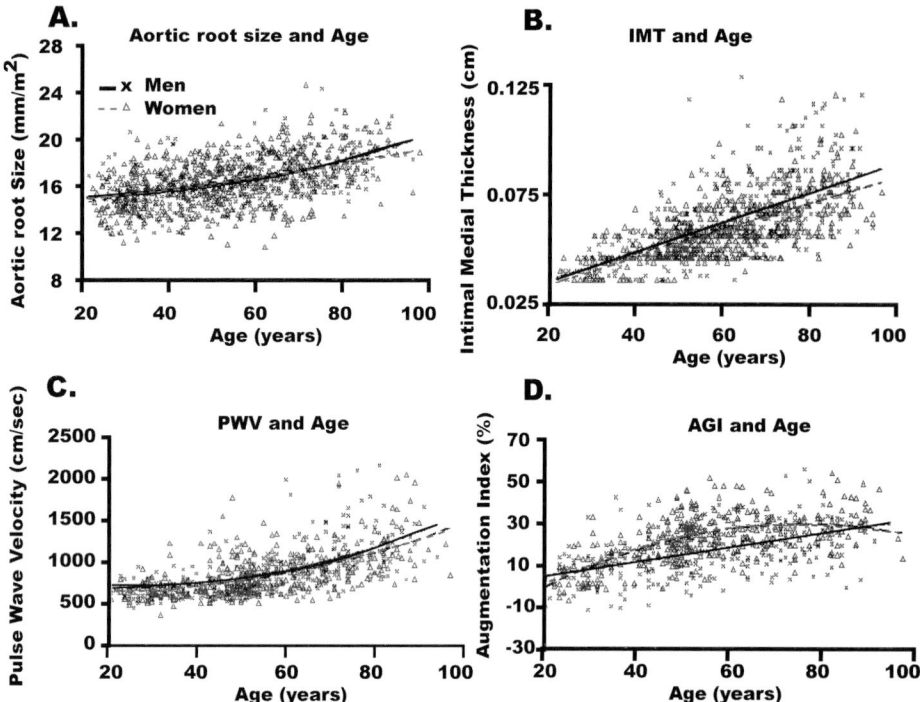

FIGURE 101–2. Age-associated changes in arterial structure and function in healthy Baltimore Longitudinal Study of Aging volunteer men (x) and women (Δ). Best fit regression lines (quadratic or linear) are shown for men (*solid lines*) and women (*dotted lines*). **A.** Aortic root size, measured via M-mode echocardiography. **B.** Common carotid intimal-medial thickness (IMT) as a function of age and gender. Note that the range of values for intimal medial thickness is much greater in older individuals than in younger ones **C.** Carotid–femoral pulse wave velocity (PWV). **D.** Carotid arterial augmentation index (AGI), which is defined as the ratio of the distance from the inflection point to the peak of the arterial waveform, over the pulse pressure. Note that unlike PWV which increases quadratically with age, the age-associated increase in AGI is linear in men and convex shape in women, suggesting that factors other than stiffness also modulate the origin of reflected waves and the amplitude of AGI. *Source: From Najjar SS, Scuteri A, Lakatta EG. Arterial aging: is it an immutable cardiovascular risk factor? Hypertension 2005;46:454–462. With permission.*

uals rigorously screened for the absence of clinical cardiovascular disease, excessive intimal-medial thickening at a given age predicts silent coronary artery disease[6] (Fig. 101–4A), which, in turn, progresses to symptomatic ischemic heart disease. In the Atherosclerosis Risk In Communities (ARIC) study, which comprised middle-aged adults, intimal-medial thickening was associated with a greater prevalence of cardiovascular diseases and was an independent predictor of stroke.[15] In the Cardiovascular Health Study (CHS), which comprised individuals older than the age of 65 years, intimal-medial thickening was an independent predictor of future myocardial infarction and stroke.[16] In the CHS study, subjects were grouped according to quintiles of intimal-medial thickening, and the results indicated a nonlinear gradation in risk, with higher quintiles conferring a greater risk for cardiovascular diseases (Fig. 101–4B). Compared to the lowest quintile, the 5th quintile had a 3.15 relative risk for cardiovascular events, even after adjusting for traditional risk factors. In fact, the strength of intimal-medial thickening as a risk factor for cardiovascular diseases equals or exceeds that of most other traditional risk factors (Fig. 101–4C).

Thus intimal-medial thickening is not a manifestation of atherosclerosis but is associated with it. Intimal-medial thickening is an aging-related process that is separate from the pathophysiologic process of atherosclerosis, yet intimal thickening is a risk factor for atherosclerosis.

Studying the relationship between primary age-associated vascular wall remodeling and cardiovascular diseases has led researchers to search for new phenotypic manifestations of arterial remodeling to explore their clinical and prognostic significance. For example, the various carotid geometric patterns that are derived by combining the measurements of vascular mass with wall-to-lumen ratio were recently associated with unique functional and hemodynamic profiles that are largely independent of age and hypertension.[17] These patterns were recently found to have differing prognostic implications.[18]

studies showed that pressures between 140 and 160 mmHg conferred added risk. The systolic value was recently pushed further down to 130 mmHg for patients with diabetes mellitus.[11]

[ ] INTIMAL-MEDIAL THICKNESS

Studies of morphologic, cellular, enzymatic, and biochemical changes in animal models have increased our understanding of age-associated arterial remodeling in humans. For example, the age-associated intimal-medial thickening seen in humans is often ascribed to "subclinical" atherosclerosis.[12] This idea has become so well accepted that intimal-medial thickening is used by some investigators as a surrogate measure of atherosclerosis. However, intimal-medial thickening, which is usually measured in areas devoid of atherosclerotic plaque, is only weakly associated with the extent and severity of coronary artery disease.[13] Furthermore, findings in rodent[4] and nonhuman primate models of aging clearly indicate that intimal-medial thickening is an age-related process that is separate from atherosclerosis, because atherosclerosis is absent in both of these animal models. Thus, excessive intimal-medial thickening is not necessarily synonymous with early or subclinical atherosclerosis.

Nonetheless, an association between intimal-medial thickening and atherosclerosis[14] has been documented in humans. In individ-

[ ] ARTERIAL STIFFNESS

In addition to intimal-medial thickening, increased arterial stiffness has been observed with advancing age in humans and in animal models of aging.[4] Strictly speaking, stiffness and its inverse, distensibility, depend on intrinsic structural properties of the blood vessel wall that relate a change in pressure with a corresponding change in volume. However, in this chapter, the terms *stiffness* and *compliance* are used in a broader sense, to denote the

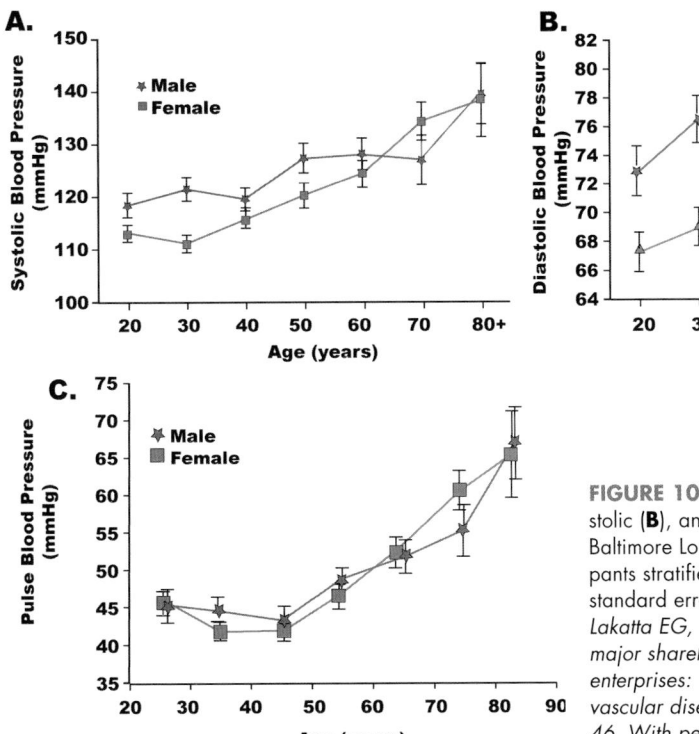

FIGURE 101-3. Average systolic (**A**), diastolic (**B**), and pulse (**C**) pressures and age, in Baltimore Longitudinal Study of Aging participants stratified by gender. Values are mean ± standard error of mean (SEM). *Source: From Lakatta EG, Levy D. Arterial and cardiac aging: major shareholders in cardiovascular disease enterprises: Part I: aging arteries: a "set up" for vascular disease. Circulation 2003;107:139–46. With permission.*

overall lumped stiffness and compliance, which include the additional effects of vascular tone, blood pressure, and other modulating factors, all of which impact left ventricular (LV) afterload. Of note, in contrast to central arteries, the stiffness of muscular arteries does not increase with advancing age. Thus, the manifestations of arterial aging may vary among the different vascular beds, reflecting differences in the structural compositions of the arteries and, perhaps, differences in the age-associated signaling cascades that modulate the arterial properties, or differences in the response to these signals across the arterial tree.

【 】 PULSE WAVE VELOCITY

With each systolic contraction of the ventricle, a propagation wave that is generated in the arterial wall travels down the arterial tree. This propagation wave accompanies (and slightly precedes) the luminal flow wave generated during systole. The velocity of propagation of this wave is determined by the intrinsic stress–strain relationship of the vascular wall, and by the smooth muscle tone, reflected by the mean arterial pressure.

The availability of noninvasive measures of the velocity of this pulse wave allow for large-scale epidemiologic studies. Pulse wave velocity was assessed in BLSA participants who were rigorously screened for the absence of overt or silent cardiovascular disease[7] and in other populations with varying degrees of prevalence of cardiovascular disease.[19] In all these studies, a significant age-associated increase in pulse wave velocity has been observed in both men and women.

Several clinical studies have recently shown the adverse cardiovascular effects of accelerated vascular stiffening. In the ARIC study, several indices of arterial compliance were predictors of hypertension.[20] In hypertensive patients, pulse wave velocity was a marker of cardiovascular risk[21] and coronary events[22] and was an

independent predictor of mortality.[23] In addition, pulse wave velocity was an independent predictor of mortality in population based studies,[24,25] in subjects older than 70 years of age[26] and in patients with end-stage renal disease[27] (Fig. 101–5A). Other noninvasive indices of vascular compliance, including stroke volume divided by pulse pressure[28] and the incremental modulus of elasticity,[29] are also independent predictors of adverse outcomes. Thus arterial stiffening, like intimal-medial thickening, should be viewed as another marker of aging, which, when accelerated, also becomes a risk factor for cardiovascular diseases.

The interaction between vascular wall stiffening and cardiovascular diseases may set in motion a vicious cycle. Pulse wave velocity is determined, in part, by smooth muscle cell tone, which, in turn, is partially regulated by endothelial cells. Moreover, endothelial dysfunction occurs early in several cardiovascular disorders including atherosclerosis, diabetes, and hypertension. Thus, in this cycle, alterations in the mechanical properties of the vessel wall contribute to endothelial cell dysfunction and, ultimately, vascular stiffening.

【 】 REFLECTED WAVES

In addition to the forward pulse wave, each cardiac cycle generates a reflected wave, which travels back up the arterial tree toward the central aorta. This reflected wave, which probably originates in the smaller arteries and arterioles, alters the arterial pressure waveform and is modulated, in part, by nitric oxide.[30] The velocity of the reflected flow wave is proportional to the stiffness of the arterial wall. Thus, in young individuals whose vascular wall is compliant, the reflected wave does not reach the large elastic arteries until diastole. With advancing age and increasing vascular stiffening, the velocity of the reflected wave increases, and the wave reaches the central circulation earlier in the cardiac cycle, during the systolic phase.

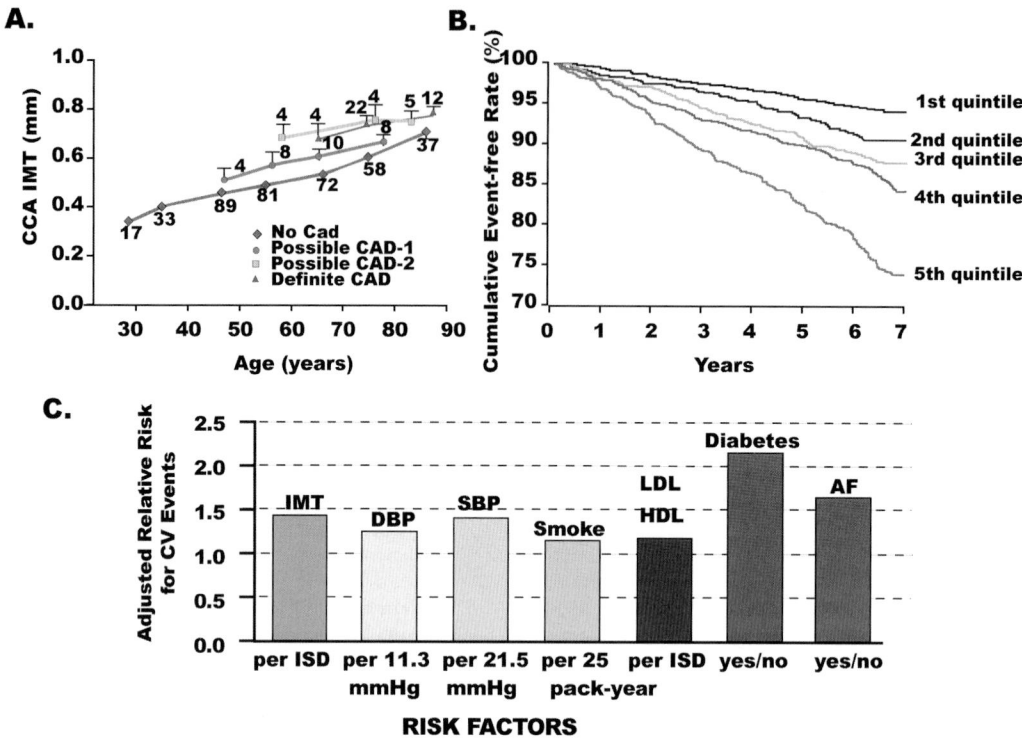

FIGURE 101–4. Carotid intimal-medial thickness and cardiovascular diseases. **A.** Common carotid artery intimal-medial thickness (CCA-IMT) as a function of age, stratified by coronary artery disease (CAD) classification, in Baltimore Longitudinal Study of Aging subjects. CAD-1 denotes a subset with positive exercise electrocardiogram (ECG) but negative thallium scans; CAD-2 represents a subset with concordant positive exercise ECG and thallium scans. **B.** Common carotid intimal-medial thickness as a predictor of future cardiovascular events in the Cardiovascular Health Study (CHS). Note the nonlinear increase in the risk for cardiovascular event rates with increasing quintiles. **C.** Comparisons of the associations of age- and sex-adjusted cardiovascular risk factors with the combined events of stroke or myocardial infarction in the CHS study, using Cox proportional hazards models. Note that intimal-medial thickness is a potent risk factor for future cardiovascular events. AF, atrial fibrillation; CCA, common carotid artery; CV, cardiovascular; DBP, diastolic blood pressure; HDL, high-density lipoprotein; IMT, intimal-medial thickness; 1 SD, one standard deviation; LDL, low-density lipoprotein; SBP, systolic blood pressure. *Source: B and C, From O'Leary DH, Polak JF, Kronmal RA, et al. Carotid artery intima and media thickness as a risk factor for myocardial infarction and stroke in older adults. Cardiovascular Health Study Collaborative Research Group. N Engl J Med 1999;340:14–22. With permission.*

This reflected wave can be noninvasively assessed from recordings of the carotid[31] or radial[32] arterial pulse waveforms by arterial applanation tonometry and high-fidelity micromanometer probes. Inspection of the recorded arterial pulse wave contour shows an inflection point, which heralds the arrival of the reflected wave. The difference in pressures between those at the inflection point and at the peak of the arterial waveform is the pressure pulse augmentation that is due to the early arrival of the reflected wave. Dividing this augmentation by the distance from the peak to the trough of the arterial waveform (corresponding to the pulse pressure) yields the augmentation index. The augmentation index, like the pulse wave velocity, increases with age[7,12,31] (see Fig. 101–2D).

Because reflected waves originate in small arteries and arterioles, the age-associated changes in this index are also probably determined, in part, by the age-associated changes in the structure and function of distal vessels, and by age-associated alterations in the structure and function of large elastic arteries. Although attention has focused on the transmission velocity of reflected waves as an index of arterial stiffness, evaluation of the pulse wave contour may provide valuable insight into the characteristics and the pathology of more distal vessels, where reflected waves originate.[33]

The pressure pulse augmentation provided by the early return of the reflected wave is an added load against which the ventricle must contract. Furthermore, the loss of the diastolic augmentation present in compliant vessels caused by the late return of the reflected waves decreases diastolic blood pressure and thus has the potential to reduce coronary blood flow as most coronary flow occurs during diastole. These considerations suggest that excessively early return of the reflected waves may be detrimental to the cardiovascular system. In fact, the augmentation index has been shown to be a predictor of adverse events in end-stage renal disease patients[34] (Fig. 101–5B). Thus, this index is another marker of vascular aging that is a risk factor for cardiovascular diseases.

【 】 PULSE PRESSURE

The combination of arterial wall stiffening and early return of the reflected waves widens the pulse pressure. Age-associated decreased elasticity also increases the systolic pressure for any given volume of ejected blood and lowers diastolic pressure by diminishing elastic recoil. Thus, pulse pressure is a useful hemodynamic marker of the vascular stiffness of conduit arteries. Clinical and epidemiologic studies in several different populations with varying prevalences of cardiovascular diseases

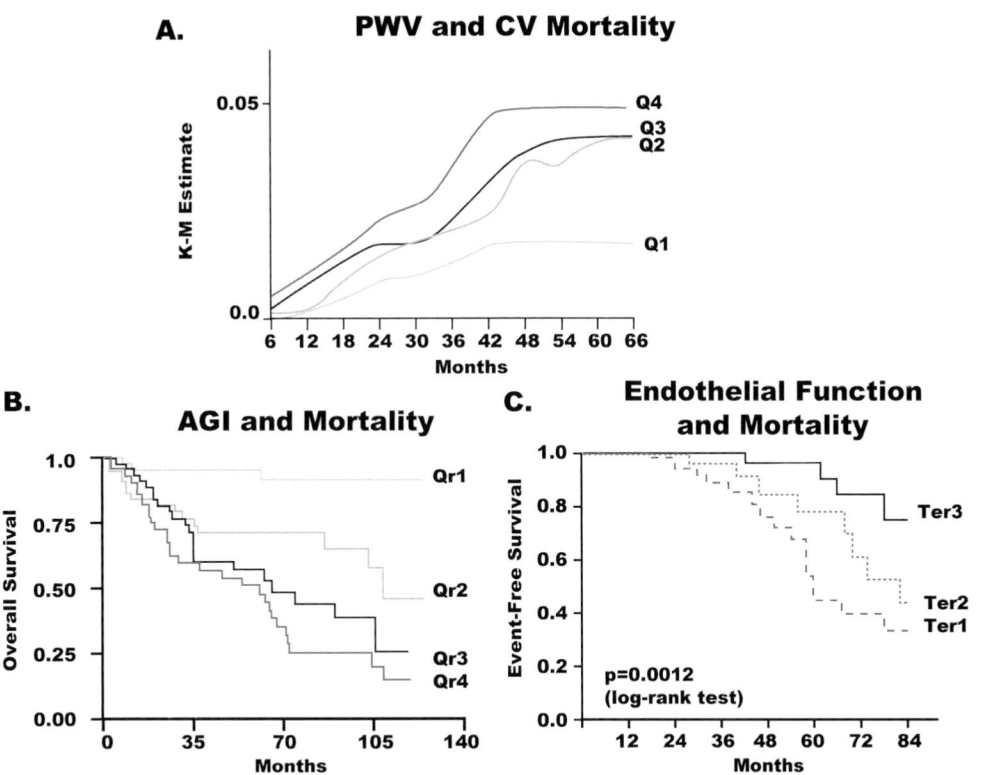

FIGURE 101–5. Markers of arterial aging are risk factors for adverse cardiovascular outcomes. **A.** Pulse wave velocity (PWV) is a predictor of cardiovascular (CV) mortality in community-dwelling older subjects. This association remained significant after adjusting for age, gender, race, systolic blood pressure, known cardiovascular disease, and other variables related to events. Q, quartile. **B.** Probability of overall survival in patients with end-stage renal failure, stratified by quartiles of augmentation index. Qr, quartile. **C.** Probability of event-free survival in never treated hypertensive patients, stratified by tertiles of endothelial dysfunction. Ter, tertile. *Source: A, From Sutton-Tyrrell K, Najjar SS, Boudreau RM, et al. Health ABC Study. Elevated aortic pulse wave velocity, a marker of arterial stiffness, predicts cardiovascular events in well-functioning older adults. Circulation 2005;111:3384–3390. With permission. B, From London GM, Blacher J, Pannier B, et al. Arterial wave reflections and survival in end-stage renal failure. Hypertension 2001;38:434–438. C, From Perticone F, Ceravolo R, Pujia A, et al. Prognostic significance of endothelial dysfunction in hypertensive patients. Circulation 2001;104(2):191–196. With permission.*

have confirmed the prognostic importance of pulse pressure.[35] Furthermore, in several studies pulse pressure was a stronger predictor of outcome than were systolic or diastolic blood pressures. This suggests the need for studies to evaluate whether pulse pressure should replace systolic or diastolic pressures as a screening criterion or as a therapeutic end point in the treatment of hypertension.

【 】 ARTERIAL STIFFNESS AND HYPERTENSION

Recent studies showing that increased vascular stiffness may precede the development of hypertension have underscored the relationship between hypertension and arterial wall stiffening.[36] An increase in mean arterial pressure (or peripheral resistance) can lead to a secondary increase in large-artery stiffness; however, the primary age-associated increase in large-artery stiffness can lead to an increase in arterial pressures. Thus, hypertension can be defined as a disease that is, in part, determined or modulated by properties of the arterial wall.

【 】 ENDOTHELIAL FUNCTION

Endothelial cells are extremely important and powerful regulators of the vasculature (see Chap. 7). Several cardiovascular conditions and

risk factors are associated with endothelial dysfunction, including hypercholesterolemia, insulin resistance, cigarette smoking, and heart failure. Endothelial cell dysfunction contributes to the pathogenesis of hypertension and atherosclerosis.[37] In addition, endothelial cells play a pivotal role in regulating several arterial properties, including vascular tone, vascular permeability, angiogenesis, and the response to inflammation. Several features of these arterial properties undergo age-associated alterations in function. Endothelial-derived substances (e.g., nitric oxide [NO] and endothelin-1) are determinants of large-artery compliance,[38] suggesting that endothelial cells may modulate arterial stiffness. Endothelial function in central arteries, however, has not been directly assessed in humans. In the brachial artery, endothelial function, as assessed by agonist- or flow-mediated vasoreactivity, declines with advancing age.[9] Several studies have demonstrated that impaired endothelial vasoreactivity, in both the coronary and peripheral arterial beds, is an independent predictor of future cardiovascular events (Fig. 101–5C).

【 】 VASOREACTIVITY

With advancing age, nitric oxide-dependent mechanical and agonist-mediated endothelial vasodilatation is reduced in humans and animals. This vasoreactivity depends on nitric oxide generated by endothelial nitric oxide synthase (eNOS). In aging rats,[39] activity of the eNOS isoform is markedly reduced. In addition, the bioavailability of nitric oxide may be reduced to age-associated increases in the amounts of superoxide and nitrated tyrosine residues of proteins.[40]

INFLAMMATION

Aging is associated with increased expression of adhesion molecules in rats and increased adherence of monocytes to the endothelial surface in rabbits.[4] Adhesion molecules on the luminal surface of endothelial cells mediate leukocyte binding to endothelial cells and subendothelial migration. This process is probably facilitated by the actions of matrix metalloproteases (MMPs).[41] Serum levels of adhesion molecules show age-associated alterations in humans.[42] In patients with hypercholesterolemia and ischemic heart disease, serum levels of soluble vascular cell adhesion molecule-1, but not soluble intercellular adhesion molecule-1 (ICAM-1), are positively associated with aging.[43]

PERMEABILITY

In rat aortae, aging is associated with increased permeability to albumin.[4] Moreover, glycosaminoglycans, which help regulate several arterial properties including vascular permeability, accumulate in greater number in the intima of older rabbits. Within hours of an acute arterial balloon injury to the rabbit carotid artery, the pericellular distribution of glycosaminoglycans is significantly reduced in the arterial wall, and this loss is associated with a significant expansion of the extracellular space. The glycosaminoglycans are rapidly replaced in the media but not in the developing neointima by smooth muscle cells.[44]

ENDOTHELIAL DYSFUNCTION AND CELLULAR SENESCENCE

Telomeres are specialized DNA–protein complexes that form the ends of chromosomes, and which may be may be good indicators of biologic, as opposed to chronologic aging. Telomeres shorten with each replicative cell division, unless they are rescued by the enzyme telomerase reverse transcriptase. When telomere length reaches a critical size, reflecting numerous cycles of attrition, no further cellular replication is possible and the cell becomes senescent. Telomere length has been shown to be inversely associated with atherosclerotic grade[45] and with chronologic age in endothelial cells from human abdominal aorta, iliac arteries, and iliac veins.[46] In a study of Danish twins, telomere length of chromosomes in white blood cells was negatively associated with pulse pressure.[47] In a normotensive French cohort, telomere length of chromosomes in white blood cells was longer in women than in men, but was associated with variations in pulse pressure and pulse wave velocity only in men.[48] Loss of telomere function induces endothelial dysfunction in vascular endothelial cells, whereas inhibition of telomere shortening suppresses age-associated dysfunction in these cells.[49] The impact of telomere-induced vascular senescence may be accentuated in older individuals, in whom studies indicate that the number[50] and activity[51] of progenitor cells is reduced, suggesting an age-associated diminution in regenerative capacity, which may contribute to the age-associated impairment in angiogenesis.[52]

ENDOTHELIAL DYSFUNCTION AND ANGIOGENESIS

Endothelial cells play a pivotal role in angiogenesis, in which new vessels grow from the existing microvasculature. Angiogenesis requires the migration and proliferation of endothelial cells in response to cytokines. The age-associated impairment in angiogenesis is partly a result of changes in the levels of extracellular enzymes, matrix proteins, and growth factors that affect endothelial cell migration.

ARTERIAL AGING IN CARDIOVASCULAR DISEASES

Although the aforementioned changes in arterial structure and function with aging were previously thought to be part of normative aging, this concept was challenged when data emerged showing that these changes are accelerated in the presence of cardiovascular diseases and, as noted above, that they are risk factors for cardiovascular morbidity and mortality.

Patients with hypertension exhibit greater carotid wall thickness,[53] central arterial stiffness,[54] and central pressure augmentation,[55] than do normotensive subjects, even after adjusting for age. They are thought to have higher central arterial diameters,[56] although this is presently debated.[57,58] Hypertensive individuals exhibit endothelial dysfunction, and the mechanisms underlying their endothelial dysfunction are similar to the ones that occur with normotensive aging, albeit they appear at an earlier age.[59] The normotensive offsprings of hypertensives also exhibit endothelial dysfunction,[60] suggesting that endothelial dysfunction may precede the development of clinical hypertension. Among hypertensive men, shorter telomere length of circulating white blood cells is associated with greater arterial stiffness.[48] The metabolic syndrome, which is quite prevalent among older individuals,[61] is associated with elevated carotid arterial thickness and stiffness.[62] Diabetics also exhibit higher carotid intimal medial thickness than non-diabetics and accelerated progression of intimal-medial thickness (IMT).[63] Even though their central arterial stiffness is increased,[54] this is not accompanied by an increase in the central pressure augmentation.[64] Diabetics also exhibit endothelial dysfunction,[65] which is also present in their first-degree relatives with insulin resistance.[66]

The circulating white blood cells of insulin-dependent diabetics have shorter telomere lengths than those from normoglycemic controls or non–insulin-dependent diabetics.[67] Patients with atherosclerosis have increased thickness[6,14] and stiffness[68] of their central arterial walls, greater central pressure augmentation,[69] and shorter telomere lengths on their circulating white blood cells.[70] They also exhibit endothelial dysfunction, which has been implicated in the pathogenesis of atherosclerosis and is one its earliest pathologic manifestations.

AGE-ASSOCIATED CHANGES IN CARDIAC STRUCTURE AND FUNCTION IN PERSONS WITHOUT A HEART DISEASE DIAGNOSIS

Cross-sectional studies of sedentary BLSA volunteer subjects without CV disease indicate that the LV wall thickness, measured via

M-mode (one-dimensional) echocardiography, increases progressively with age in both sexes (Fig. 101–6A).[71] This is mostly the result of an increase in average myocyte size. In older, hospitalized patients without apparent CV disease, autopsy studies indicate that overall LV mass and end-diastolic volume decreased with age, and cardiac myocyte enlargement was observed concurrently with an estimated decrease in myocyte number. The observed frequency of apoptotic myocytes is higher in older male hearts than in female hearts.[72] An increase in the amount and a change in the physical properties of collagen (purportedly because of nonenzymatic cross-linking) also occur within the myocardium with aging.

However, the cardiac myocyte-to-collagen ratio in the older heart either remains constant or increases.

【 】 LEFT VENTRICULAR FILLING AND PRELOAD

The early diastolic filling rate progressively slows after age 20 years, so that by age 80 years the rate is reduced up to 50 percent (Fig. 101–6B). This reduction in filling rate is likely attributable either to structural (fibrous) changes within the LV myocardium or to residual myofilament Ca^{2+} activation from the preceding systole.

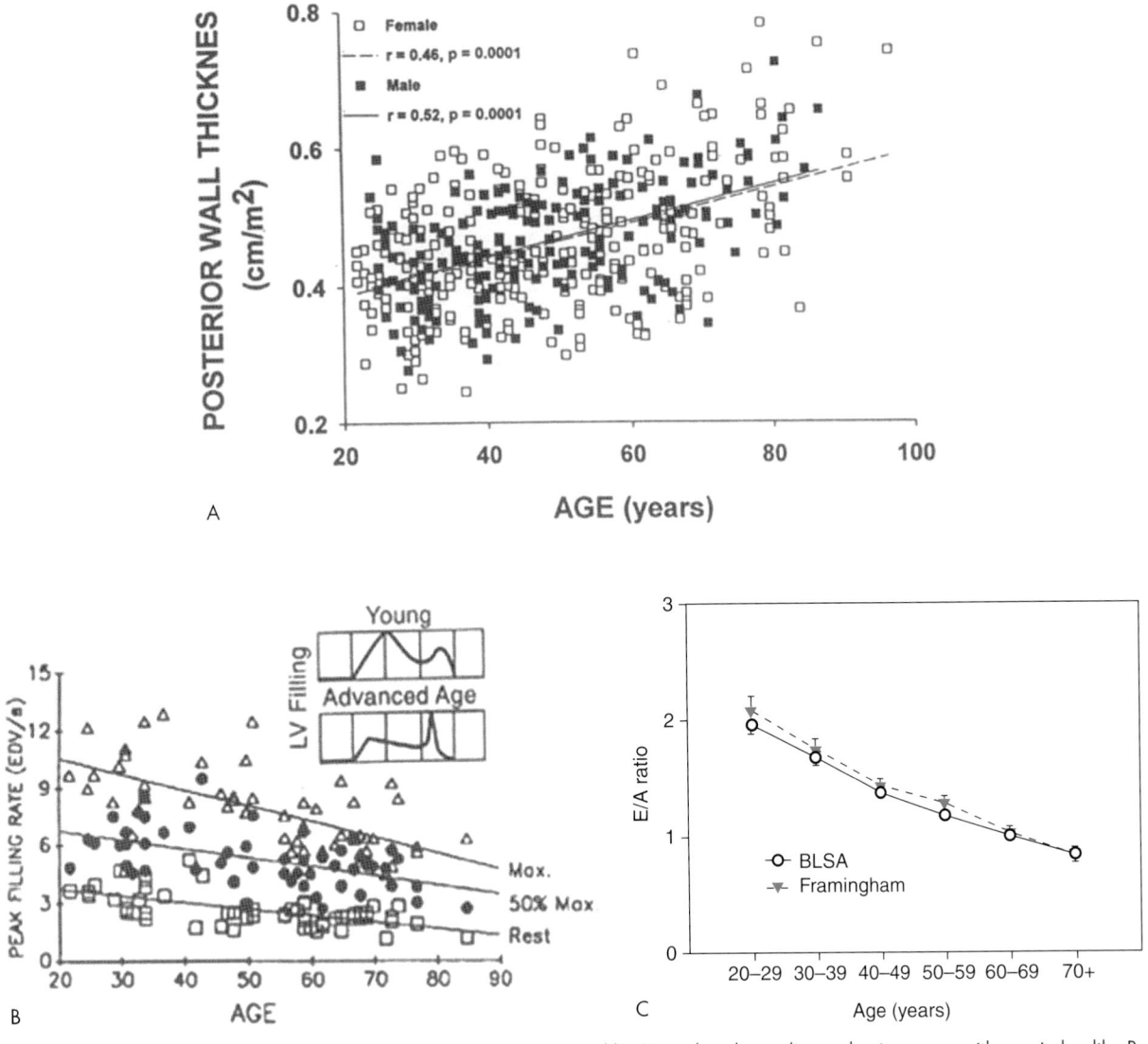

FIGURE 101–6. A. Left ventricular posterior wall thickness, measured by M-mode echocardiography, increases with age in healthy Baltimore Longitudinal Study on Aging (BLSA) men and women. Note that the marked age-associated increase in left ventricular wall thickness in these healthy BLSA participants is within what is considered to be the clinically "normal" range. **B.** Maximum left ventricular (LV) filling rate at rest and during vigorous cycle exercise assessed via equilibrium gated blood-pool scans in healthy volunteers from the BLSA. EDV, end-diastolic volume. **C.** The ratio of early left ventricular diastolic filling rate (E) to the atrial filling component (A) declines with aging, and the extent of this E/A decline with aging in healthy BLSA volunteers is identical to that in participants of the Framingham Study. *Source: A, From Gerstenblith G, Frederiksen J, Yin FC. Echocardiographic assessment of a normal adult aging population. Circulation 1977;56:273–278. With permission. B, From Schulman SP, Lakatta EG, Fleg JL, et al. Age-related decline in left ventricular filling at rest and exercise. Am J Physiol 1992;263:H1932–H1938. With permission. C, From Lakatta EG, Levy D. Arterial and cardiac aging: major shareholders in cardiovascular disease enterprises: Part II: the aging heart in health: links to heart disease. Circulation 2003;107(2):346–354.*

Despite the slowing of LV filling early in diastole, more filling occurs in late diastole, partly as a result of a more vigorous atrial contraction. Hence the ratio of early to late LV filling decreases with age (Fig. 101–6C). The augmented atrial contraction is accompanied by atrial enlargement, and the blood filling a stiff, hypertrophied ventricle in late diastole is manifested by a fourth heart sound (atrial gallop) on auscultation. Despite the age-associated changes in the diastolic filling pattern in older men, their LV end-diastolic volume index (EDVI)—that is, normalized for body surface area in the supine position at rest—does not substantially differ from that in their younger counterparts (Fig. 101–7A).

The acute reserve capacity of specific functions (e.g., end-diastolic volume [EDV]) that determine cardiac performance can be conveniently illustrated by depicting these over a wide range of demand for blood flow and pressure regulation—for example, assumption of the sitting posture and during submaximal and exhaustive (maximal) upright exercise (Fig. 101–7). Assumption of the sitting position reduces EDVI in younger, but not in older, individuals (Fig. 101–7A); the age-associated decline in the maximum LV filling rate observed at rest persists. During submaximal cycle-seated exercise, EDVI increases equivalently at all ages; but during exhaustive exercise, EDVI drops to the seated rest level in young men but remains elevated in older men (Fig. 101–7A). Thus, for EDVI, the average, acute, dynamic EDV reserve range during the postural change and during graded upright exercise is moderately greater at age 85 years than at age 20 years. This does not support the widely held concept that the dynamic range of filling volumes is compromised in older hearts despite a reduction in LV early diastolic filling rate (see Fig. 101–6B). In fact, during vigorous (maximal) exercise, the LV at end-diastole becomes acutely dilated in healthy, older persons, but not in younger persons.

[ ] LEFT VENTRICULAR EJECTION

Figure 101–7B illustrates a remarkable age-associated reduction in the range of reserve in the end-systolic volume index (ESVI): in younger men, the ESVI becomes progressively reduced with increasing demands for CV perfusion from supine rest to maximum upright exercise, but the range of acute ESV reserve at age 85 is only about one-fifth of that at age 20. The age-associated failure in end-systolic volume (ESV) regulation across the various levels of demand depicted in Fig. 101–7B causes a similar age-associated loss of ejection fraction regulation (Fig. 101–7C).

The net result of the age-associated changes in EDVI and ESVI regulation depicted in Fig. 101–7A and B is that the stroke volume index (SVI) in older persons is preserved at the level achieved by younger persons over a wide range of performance (Fig. 101–7D).

Specifically, the Frank-Starling mechanism is used in older men with the assumption of an upright, seated posture at rest (Fig. 101–7A) to produce a modest age-associated increase in SVI (Fig. 101–7D). During progressive exhaustive exercise, however, the failure of older men to reduce ESVI (Fig. 101–7B) impairs the ejection fraction (Fig. 101–7C), and SVI is not augmented in older men when compared with younger men, as would be anticipated on the basis of their augmented EDVI.

[ ] HEART RATE

In the supine position at rest, the heart rate in healthy BLSA men is not age-related (Fig. 101–7E). In other populations, a reduction in the spontaneous and respiratory variations in resting heart rate is observed and reflects altered autonomic modulation with aging (see Sympathetic Modulation below). With assumption of the seated resting position, heart rate increases slightly less in older men than in younger men (Fig. 101–7E). The magnitude of this age-associated reduction increases progressively during exercise. The net result is that maximum acute dynamic reserve range of heart rate is reduced by about one-third between 20 and 85 years of age.

[ ] CARDIAC OUTPUT

The cardiac index, as expected from the behavior of the SVI and heart rate functions in Fig. 101–7D and E, does not vary with age in either posture at rest (Fig. 101–7E) but is reduced at maximal exercise in older men. This reduction is entirely a consequence of a reduction in heart rate reserve, as SVI at maximal exercise is preserved in healthy men rigorously screened to exclude occult coronary disease at older age. The loss of acute cardiac output reserve from seated rest to exhaustive, seated cycle exercise averages approximately 30 percent in healthy, community-dwelling BLSA volunteer men. Alternatively stated, subjects at the older end of the age range can augment their cardiac index 2.5-fold over seated rest, whereas those at the younger end of the spectrum can increase their cardiac index 3.5-fold.

The same pattern of age-associated endogenous deficits depicted in BLSA subjects during graded, upright exercise in Fig. 101–7 is observed during prolonged exercise (>1 hour) at a fixed (70 percent of maximal oxygen consumption [VO$_2$max]) relative submaximal workload.[73]

In summary, Fig. 101–7 illustrates that when CV function in adult volunteer community-dwelling subjects ranging in age from 20 to 85 years is compared, impaired cardioacceleration and LV ejection reserve capacity are the most dramatic health changes in cardiac function with aging. Impaired ejection reserve, indicated by the failure of older persons to regulate ESV (Fig. 101–7B) as effectively as younger persons do, is accompanied by LV dilation at end-diastole (Fig. 101–7A) and an altered diastolic filling pattern (see Fig. 101–6B,C).

MECHANISMS OF IMPAIRED LV EJECTION WITH AGING IN PERSONS WITHOUT CLINICAL CV DISEASE

[ ] MYOCARDIAL CONTRACTILITY

Information as to how aging affects factors that regulate intrinsic myocardial contractility in humans is incomplete because the intrinsic myocardial contractility in the intact circulation is difficult to separate from loading and autonomic modulatory influences on contractility. A deficit in maximal intrinsic contractility of older persons might be expected on the basis of the reduced maximum heart rate (see Fig. 101–7), as the heart rate per se is a determinant of the myocardial contractile state. Additional supporting evidence for reduced LV contractility with aging comes from studies in

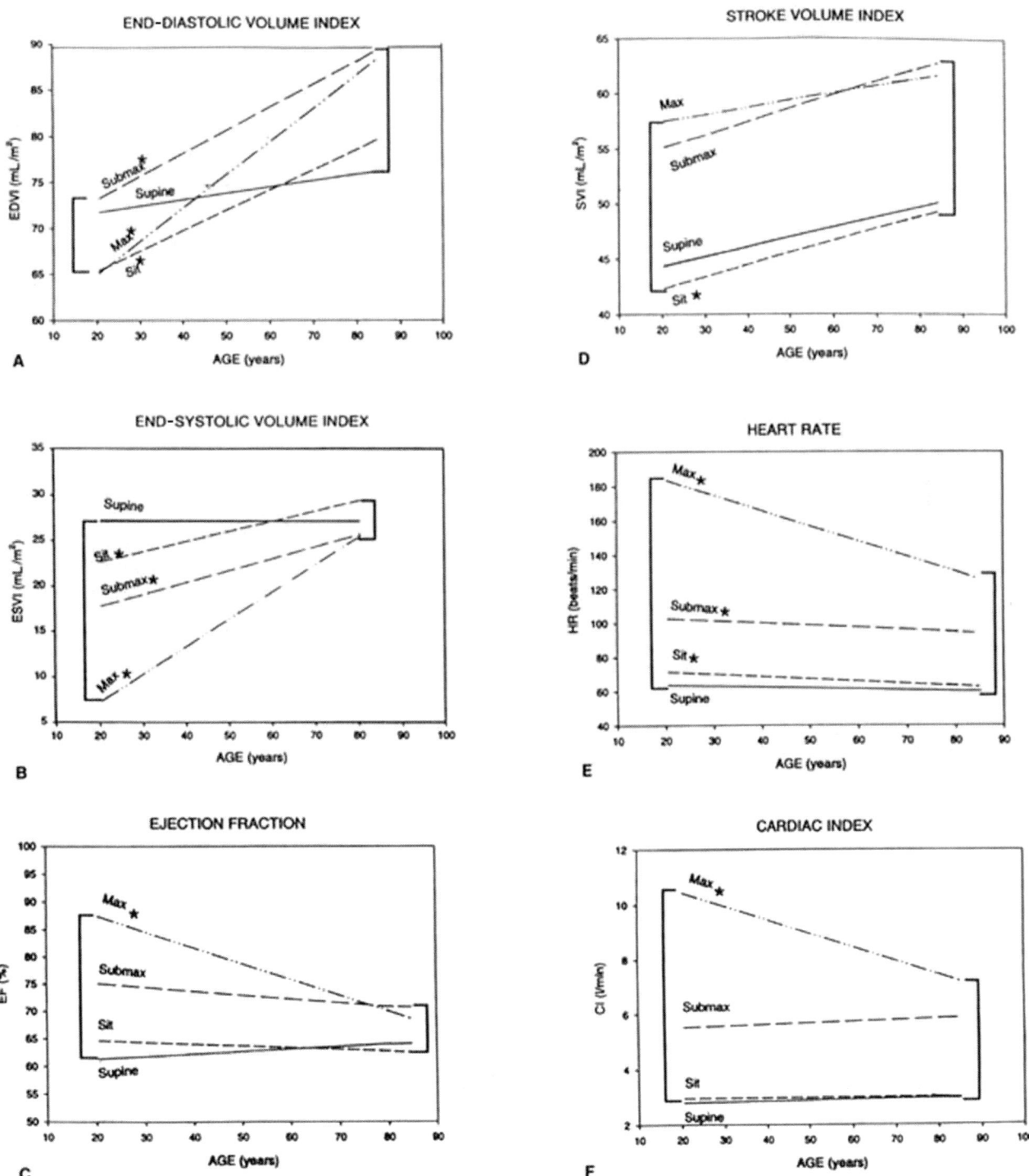

FIGURE 101–7. Least-squares linear regression on age of left ventricular (LV) volumes, ejection fraction (EF), heart rate (HR), and cardiac index (CI) at rest and during graded cycle exercise in 149 healthy males from the Baltimore Longitudinal Study on Aging (BLSA) who exercised to at least a 100-W workload. The *asterisk* indicates that regression on age is statistically significant. The overall magnitude of the acute, dynamic range of reserve of a given function in younger compared with older subjects can quickly be gleaned from the length of the brackets depicted at the extremes of the regression lines. For end-diastolic volume index (EDVI), the average, acute, dynamic end-diastolic volume (EDV) reserve range during the postural change and during graded upright exercise is moderately greater at age 85 years than at age 20 years (**A**). There is a remarkable age-associated reduction in the range of reserve in the ESVI (**B**), which causes a similar age-associated loss of *EF* regulation (**C**). The stroke volume index (SVI) is preserved in older persons over a wide range of performance (**D**). During progressive exhaustive exercise, however, the failure to reduce ESVI (**B**) impairs the EF in older men (**C**). Thus, SVI is not augmented in older men when compared with younger men, as would be anticipated on the basis of their augmented EDVI. The maximum acute dynamic reserve range of HR is reduced by about one-third between 20 and 85 years of age (**E**). The loss of acute cardiac output reserve from seated rest to exhaustive, seated cycle exercise averages approximately 30 percent in healthy, community-dwelling BLSA volunteer men (**F**). This reduction is entirely caused by a reduction in HR reserve, as SVI at maximal exercise is preserved. At maximal exercise, the age-associated increase in EDVI is of borderline statistical significance in women, but the change in EDVI from rest to maximal exercise in a given individual (not shown) significantly increases with age and is nearly identical in both men and women. *Source: From Fleg JL, O'Connor FC, Gerstenblith G, et al. Impact of age on the cardiovascular response to dynamic upright exercise in healthy men and women. J Appl Physiol 1995;78:890–900. With permission.*

which the LV of older but not younger healthy BLSA men dilates during β-adrenergic blockade, both at end-systole and end-diastole, in response to a given increase in afterload.[74]

The most reliable estimate of myocardial systolic stiffness or elastance, the slope of the end-systolic pressure (ESP)/ESV coordinates measured across a range of ESVs at rest, has not been estimated in a homogeneous, healthy study population across a broad age range, and by convention cannot be assessed during exercise. A single point, depicting ESP/ESV as a contractility index at each overall CV level of performance in Fig. 101–7, presents an age-associated pattern of myocardial contractile reserve that is nearly identical to the age-associated change in the pattern of ejection fraction in Fig. 101–7.[75]

LEFT VENTRICULAR AFTERLOAD

Cardiac afterload has two components—one generated by the heart itself and the other by the vasculature. The cardiac component of afterload during exercise can be expected to increase slightly with age because the heart's size increases in older persons throughout the cardiac cycle during exercise.[75] The vascular load on the heart has four components: conduit artery compliance characteristics, reflected pulse waves, resistance, and inertance. Inertance is determined by the mass of blood in the large arteries that requires acceleration prior to LV ejection. As the central arterial diastolic diameter increases with aging (see Fig. 101–2A), the inertance component of afterload also likely increases. Thus, each of the pulsatile components of vascular load, measured at rest, increase with age. Hence, the aortic impedance, a composite function of the determinants of vascular afterload, increases with age.

Increased vascular loading on the heart is a likely cause of the increase in LV wall thickness with aging (see Fig. 101–6A). Studies in large populations of broad age range demonstrate that arterial pressure, which varies directly with vascular loading, is a major determinant of LV mass, and that the relative impact of age and arterial pressure on LV wall thickness varies with the manner in which study subjects are screened with respect to hypertension.[76] The increase in LV wall thickness with aging reduces the expected increase in cardiac afterload caused by increased LV volume in older persons during stress.[75]

ARTERIAL/VENTRICULAR LOAD MATCHING

Optimal and efficient ejection of blood from the heart occurs when ventricular and vascular loads are matched. (Note that in this context, *stiffness* refers to time-varying cardiac elastance throughout the cardiac cycle as a result of combined effects of active contractile and "passive" structural properties and to the interaction of both of these.) It has been suggested that the precise cardiac and vascular load matching that is characteristic in younger persons is preserved at older ages, at least at rest, because the increased vascular stiffness in older persons at rest is matched by increased resting ventricular stiffness.[77]

During exercise, in order for the ejection fraction to increase, the LV end-systolic elastance (E_{LV}), that is, end-systolic pressure-to-end-systolic volume ratio, must increase to a greater extent than the effective vascular elastance (E_A), that is, end-systolic pressure-to-stroke volume ratio. With increasing age, however, E_{LV} fails to

increase in proportion to the increase in E_A; hence the E_A/E_{LV} during exercise in older persons decreases to a lesser extent than it does in younger persons (Fig. 101–8A).[78] This altered arterial–ventricular load matching in older versus younger persons during exercise is a mechanism for the deficit in the acute left ventricular ejection fraction (LVEF) reserve that accompanies advancing age in many individuals. Thus the LVEF, often attributed by cardiologists to a measure of LV pump function, is in fact determined by both cardiac and vascular properties, and both change with age. An acute pharmacologic reduction in both cardiac and vascular components of LV afterload by sodium nitroprusside (SNP) infusions in older, healthy BLSA volunteers augments LVEF (Fig. 101–8B) in these subjects (at rest and exercise).[79] Because of concomitant reductions in preload and afterload during SNP infusion, the LV of older persons delivers the same stroke volume, stroke work and cardiac output while working at a smaller size (Fig. 101–8C).

SYMPATHETIC MODULATION

The essence of sympathetic modulation of the CV system is to increase the heart rate, augment myocardial contractility and relaxation, and redistribute blood to working muscles and to skin so as to dissipate heat. All of the factors that have been identified to play a role in the deficient CV regulation with aging—that is, heart rate (and thus filling time), afterload (both cardiac and vascular), myocardial contractility, and redistribution of blood flow—exhibit a deficient sympathetic modulatory component.

SYMPATHETIC NEUROTRANSMITTERS

Apparent deficits in sympathetic modulation of cardiac and arterial functions with aging occur in the presence of exaggerated neurotransmitter levels.

During any perturbation from the supine basal state, plasma levels of norepinephrine and epinephrine increase to a greater extent in older than in younger, healthy humans. The age-associated increase in plasma levels of norepinephrine results from an increased spillover into the circulation and, to a lesser extent, to reduced plasma clearance. Increased spillover occurs within the heart, probably because of deficiency of norepinephrine reuptake at nerve endings. During prolonged exercise, however, diminished neurotransmitter reuptake might also be associated with depletion, and reduced release.[80] Thus depending on the duration of the stress, deficient neurotransmitter release might be a basis for apparent impairment of sympathetic CV regulation with aging (see Fig. 101–6B).

DEFICITS IN CARDIAC β-ADRENERGIC RECEPTOR SIGNALING

The age-associated increase in neurotransmitter spillover into the circulation during acute stress implies a greater heart and vascular receptor occupancy by these substances. Experimental evidence indicates that this leads to desensitization of the postsynaptic signaling components of sympathetic modulation. Indeed, multiple lines of evidence support the idea that the efficiency of postsynaptic β-adrenergic signaling declines with aging (see Ref. 81 for a review).

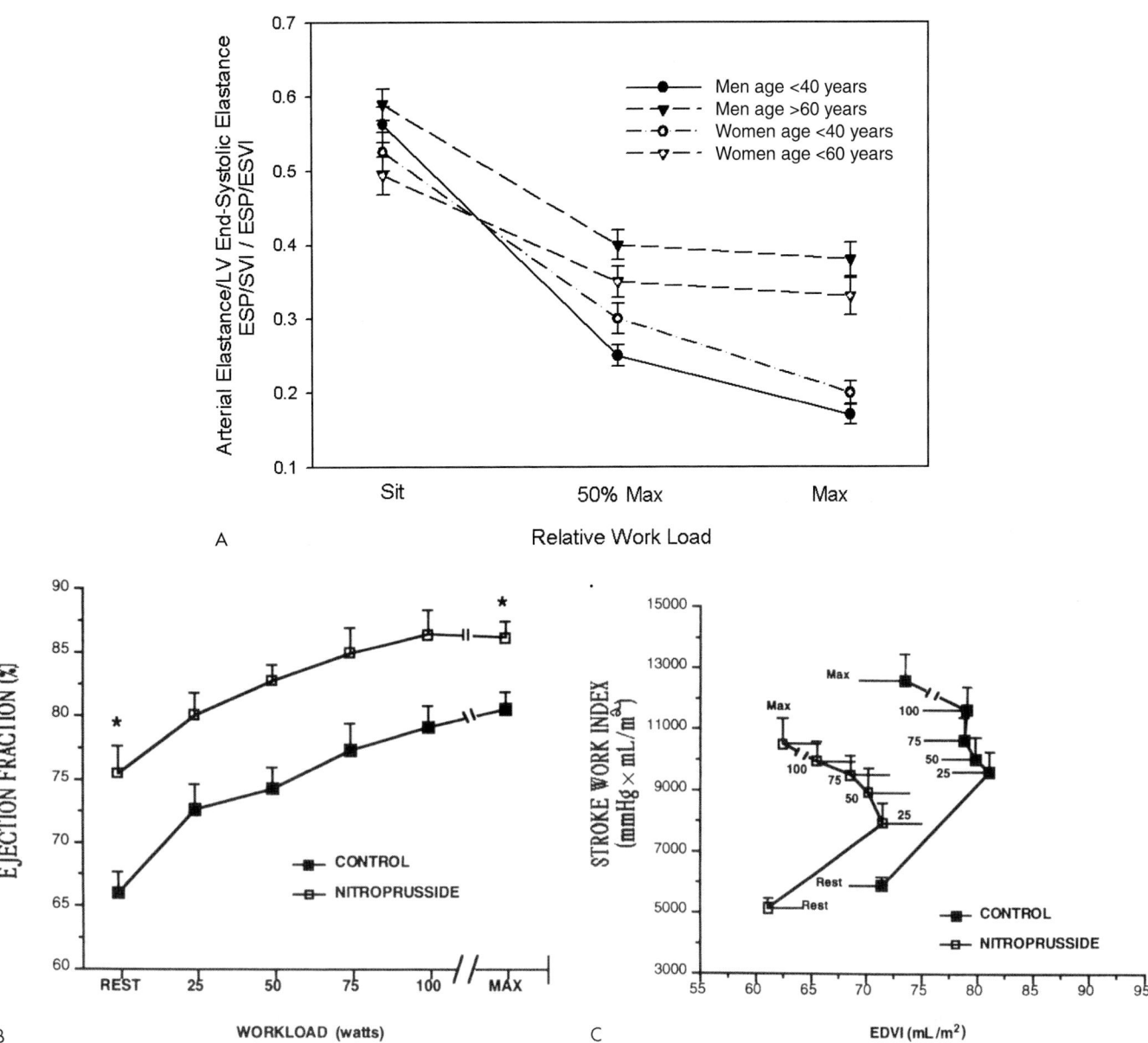

FIGURE 101-8. A. Load mismatch during exercise. **B.** Ejection fraction at seated, at upright rest, at intermediate common submaximal workloads, and at maximum effort in healthy volunteers aged 71 ± 7 years prior to and during sodium nitroprusside (SNP) infusion. At any level of effort, ejection fraction is substantially increased by SNP. **C.** Ventricular function, depicted as stroke work index versus end-diastolic volume index (EDVI) relationship at upright, at seated rest, and during exercise in the presence and absence of SNP. The relationship is shifted leftward and downward with SNP, indicating a smaller EDVI and lower stroke work index at any exercise load. ESP, end-systolic pressure; ESVI, end-systolic volume index; SVI, stroke volume index. *Source: A, From Najjar SS, Schulman SP, Fleg JL, et al. Relationship of age and sex on ventricular-vascular coupling at rest and exercise. Circulation 2000(Suppl);102:II-602. With permission. B and C, From Nussbacher A, Gerstenblith G, O'Connor FC, et al. Hemodynamic effects of unloading the old heart. Am J Physiol 1999;277:H1863–H1871. With permission.*

One line of evidence stems from the observation that acute β-adrenergic receptor blockade changes the exercise hemodynamic profile of younger persons to resemble that of older ones (Fig. 101–9). The reduction in heart rate during exercise in the presence of acute β-adrenergic blockade is greater in younger than in older subjects (Fig. 101–9B), and significant β-adrenergic blockade–induced LV dilatation occurs only in younger subjects (Fig. 101–9A). The age-associated deficits in LV early diastolic filling rate both at rest and during exercise (Fig. 101–9C) also are abolished by acute β-adrenergic blockade.[82] Note, however, that β-adrenergic blockade in younger individuals in Fig. 101–9 causes SVI to increase to a greater extent than does β-adrenergic blockade in older individ-

uals, suggesting that mechanisms other than deficient β-adrenergic regulation compromise LV ejection. One potential mechanism is an age-associated decrease in maximum intrinsic myocardial contractility. Another likely mechanism is enhanced vascular afterload caused by the structural changes in compliance arteries and possibly also by impaired vasorelaxation during exercise. In this regard, it has been observed that the increase in aortic impedance during exercise in old dogs is abolished by β-adrenergic blockade.[83]

The second type of evidence for a diminished efficacy of synaptic β-adrenergic receptor signaling is that CV responses at rest to β-adrenergic agonist infusions decrease with age.

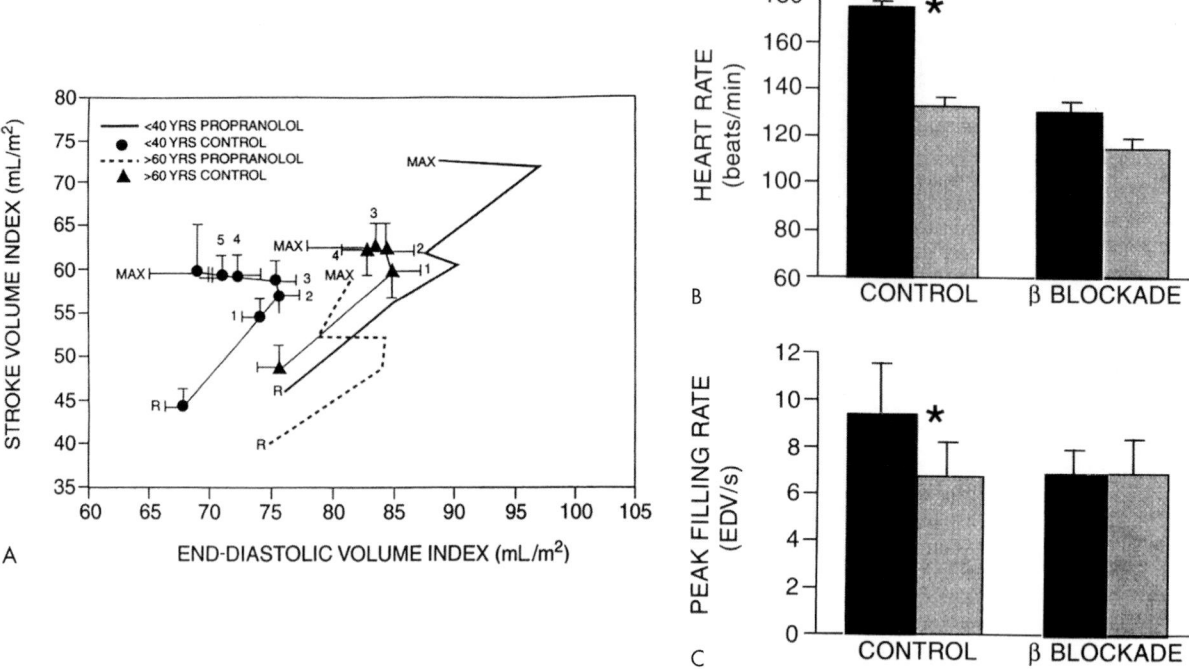

FIGURE 101–9. A. Stroke volume index as a function of end-diastolic volume (EDV) index at rest (R) and during graded cycle workloads in the upright seated position in healthy men from the Baltimore Longitudinal Study on Aging (BLSA), in the presence and absence (*dashed line*) of β-adrenergic blockade. 1 to 4 or 5, Graded submaximal workloads on cycle ergometer; max, maximum effort; R, seated rest. Stroke volume/end-diastolic functions with symbols are those measured in the absence of propranolol; *dashed* and *solid line* functions without symbols are the stroke volume compared with end-diastolic function measured in the presence of propranolol. Note that, in the absence of propranolol, the stroke volume versus EDV relationship in older persons is shifted rightward from that in younger persons. This indicates that the left ventricle of older persons in the sitting position, compared with that of younger persons, operates from a greater preload both at rest and during submaximal and maximal exercise. Propranolol markedly shifts the stroke volume-to-EDV relationship in younger persons (*solid line without points*) rightward but does not markedly offset the curve in older persons (*dashed line without points*). Thus, with respect to this assessment of ventricular function curve, β-adrenergic blockade with propranolol makes younger men appear to be older men. The abolition of the age-associated differences in the left ventricular (LV) function curve after propranolol are accompanied by a reduction or abolition of the age-associated reduction in heart rate, which, at maximum, is shown in (**B**). Note, however, that β-adrenergic blockade in younger individuals in this figure causes the stroke volume index to increase to a greater extent than during β blockade in older persons, suggesting that mechanisms other than deficient β-adrenergic regulation compromise LV ejection. One potential mechanism is an age-associated decrease in maximum intrinsic myocardial contractility. Another likely mechanism is enhanced vascular afterload due to the structural changes in compliance arteries noted above and possibly also to impaired vasorelaxation during exercise. **B.** Peak exercise heart rate in the same subjects as in (**A**) in the presence and absence of acute β-adrenergic blockade by propranolol. **C.** The age-associated reduction in peak LV diastolic filling rate at maximum exercise in healthy BLSA subjects is abolished during exercise in the presence of β-adrenergic blockade with propranolol. Solid, younger than 40 years old; light = older than 60 years old. *Source: A, From Fleg JL, Schulman S, O'Connor F, et al. Effects of acute β-adrenergic receptor blockade on age-associated changes in cardiovascular performance during dynamic exercise. Circulation 1994;90:2333–2341. With permission. B and C, From Schulman SP, Lakatta EG, Fleg JL, et al. Age-related decline in left ventricular filling at rest and exercise. Am J Physiol 1992;73:H1932–H1938. With permission.*

【 】 PHYSICAL DECONDITIONING

Because a marked reduction in physical activity accompanies advancing age in a majority of adults,[84,85] it may be hypothesized that a reduction in physical conditioning status might be implicated as a factor in the reduced CV reserve of older, healthy, sedentary individuals.

【 】 MAXIMUM OXYGEN CONSUMPTION

The international standard for cardiorespiratory fitness is VO_2max. The extent to which the maximum aerobic capacity declines with aging, as well as its suspected underlying mechanisms, vary among studies. Aerobic capacity in persons of varying age, estimated by either peak oxygen consumption or work capacity, accompanying the hemodynamic pattern at maximal exercise across

the age range (which is illustrated in Fig. 101–7) declines approximately 50 percent (Fig. 101–10A). In this study population, rigorously prescreened to exclude disease, the age-associated reduction in the cardiac component, exclusively a result of a reduced ability to accelerate the heart rate (Fig. 101–10B), accounts for roughly half of the age-associated decline in aerobic capacity, the remainder being attributable to age-associated differences in O_2 use. Such reductions in O_2 use during vigorous exercise result from age-associated reduction in muscle mass and from a reduction in the shunting of blood from viscera to working muscles during exercise, as well as the amount of O_2 use.

Cross-sectional studies, for example, those in Fig. 101–10, have been largely interpreted to indicate that the VO_2max declines linearly as a function of age. The longitudinal rate of decline in peak VO_2 in healthy adults, however, is not constant across the age span in healthy persons, as assumed by cross-sectional studies, but ac-

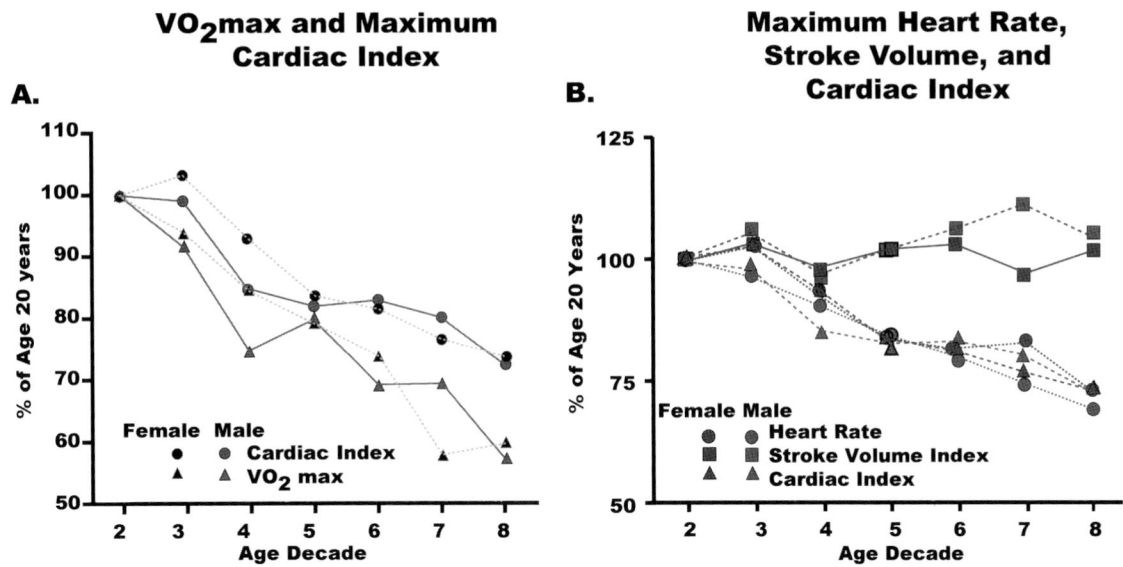

FIGURE 101-10. A. Peak oxygen consumption and cardiac index at exhaustion during upright cycle exercise. The age-associated reduction in peak VO_2 in both males and females is twofold greater than the decline in maximum cardiac index. This indicates, via the Fick Principle, that O_2 extraction declines by approximately 25% over this age range. **B.** The age-associated decline in maximum cardiac index is entirely a result of a decline in maximum heart rate. Maximum stroke volume varies little with aging in healthy persons. Data in A and B are from the same BLSA participants depicted in Fig. 101–7. *Source: From Fleg JL, O'Connor FC, Gerstenblith G, et al. Impact of age on the cardiovascular response to dynamic upright exercise in healthy men and women. J Appl Physiol 1995;78:890–900. With permission.*

celerates markedly with each successive age decade, especially in men, regardless of physical activity habits (Fig. 101–11). When the components of peak VO_2 were examined, the rate of longitudinal decline of the oxygen pulse (i.e., the O_2 use per heart beat) mirrored that of peak VO_2, whereas the longitudinal rate of heart rate decline averaged only 4 to 6 percent per 10 years, and accelerated only minimally with age (Fig. 101–11). The accelerated rate of decline of peak aerobic capacity has substantial implications

with regard to functional independence and quality of life, not only in healthy older persons, but particularly when disease-related deficits are superimposed.

Metabolic debts associated with the performance of dynamic exercise increase with aging. For several minutes after an acute bout of exercise, the body continues to consume oxygen at a rate in excess of the basal rate. This continued increased VO_2 during recovery from exercise, sometimes referred to as an *oxygen debt*,

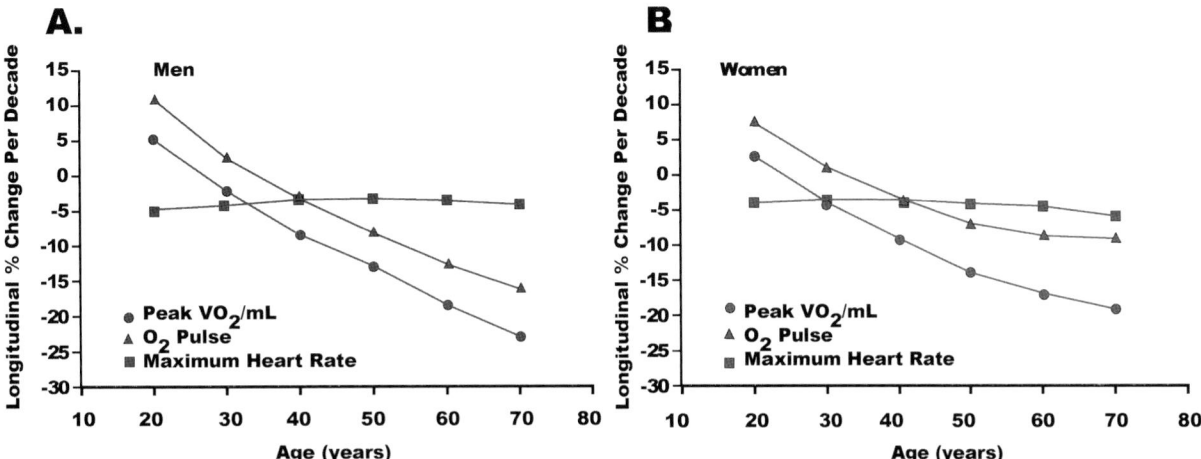

FIGURE 101-11. Longitudinal changes in maximal heart rate, O_2 pulse, and peak VO_2 by gender, predicted from the mixed-effects model, and separated by gender into panels **A** and **B**. Peak VO_2/FFM (fat free mass) declines progressively more steeply with advancing age, with similar declines in men and women. Note that peak VO_2 per kg FFM is only slightly higher in men than women at younger ages, converging by old age. Declines in heart rate are similar across age in men but steepen modestly with age in women. O_2 pulse declines progressively more steeply with age, especially in men, leading to near convergence of O_2 pulse in elderly men and women. Note the similarity of these plots to those of peak VO_2 in Fig. 101–1A. The longitudinal percent change per decade in maximal heart rate is only 4 to 5 percent per decade across the age span in both genders. In contrast, longitudinal decline in O_2 pulse accelerates progressively with age, especially in men. Note the similarity in the shape and magnitude of the decline in O_2 pulse to that of peak VO_2. *Source: From Fleg JL, Morrell CH, Bos AG, et al. Accelerated longitudinal decline of aerobic capacity in healthy older adults. Circulation 2005;112:674–682.*

when expressed relative to work performed during the exercise, can range from 14 to 21 percent of the total VO_2 associated with the performance of and recovery from exercise.[86] This oxygen debt, paid during recovery from exercise, often has not been factored into estimates of exercise efficiency (calories expended for work performed) and reduces efficiency, because it contributes to the total O_2 cost associated with the exercise but contributes no external work.

Although work performed and VO_2 during the exercise are lower in most older persons than in younger persons, the VO_2 during the exercise, per unit work performed, does not change with age.[86] VO_2 during recovery (metabolic debt) from exercise in older subjects, however, exceeds that in younger persons by >30 percent. This debt, paid during recovery from exercise is likely attributable to an inability of the older body to adapt to the energy requirements of exercise. Specific factors include reductions in muscle mass and strength, inadequate blood flow to muscles, and a reduced efficiency of muscle respiration. Excessive elevation of catecholamines and core temperature occurs during exercise in older persons, as do other less well-characterized factors (e.g., excessive reactive O_2 species and an exaggerated elevation of inflammatory cytokines). These factors cause muscle fatigue and a shift to anaerobic metabolism. During recovery, excessive catecholamine concentrations, and incomplete waning of cell responses to catecholamine drive during exercise, might continue to stimulate both muscle respiration in the absence of continued demand for muscle work and the cardiovascular system to dissipate lactate and heat generated during exercise. The physiologic significance of this metabolic debt incurred during exercise is that its underlying factors collectively reduce exercise capacity, with all the attendant health and performance drawbacks of such a reduction.

The issue arises as to whether physical conditioning via aerobic training of sedentary older persons can affect deficits in CV reserve capacity as a consequence of the aging process per se. It has been amply documented that physical conditioning of older persons can substantially increase their maximum aerobic work capacity and peak oxygen consumption. The extent to which this conditioning effect results from enhanced central cardiac performance or from augmented peripheral circulatory and O_2 use mechanisms, including changes in skeletal muscle mass, varies with the characteristics of the population studied, the type and degree of conditioning achieved, gender, body position during study, and likely genetic factors. A longitudinal study of older men in the upright position indicates that an enhanced physical conditioning status increases O_2 consumption and work capacity, in part by increases in the maximum cardiac output by increasing the maximum stroke volume, and in part by increasing the estimated total body arteriovenous O_2 use.[87] There is no strong evidence that physical conditioning of older persons can offset the deficiency in sympathetic modulation. Rather, conditioning effects to increase LV ejection appear to relate to the reduction in vascular afterload, as reflected in a reduced pulse wave velocity,[88] and to carotid augmentation index (AGI) in older athletes compared with sedentary controls, as well as possibly to an augmentation of the maximum intrinsic myocardial contractility.

Aerobic exercise training in older persons not only improves exercise work capacity but also increases muscle mass; improves capillary density, muscle respiration, mitochondrial enzymes, and muscle oxidative capacity; reduces plasma lactate during exercise; and reduces the O_2 debt. Thus the good news is that the exercise training benefits on exercise efficiency of O_2 use are more pronounced in older than younger subjects, irrespective of gender. For example, in older subjects, an exercise-conditioning program reduced the metabolic debt following exercise by nearly 30 percent, which translated into an 18 percent increase in exercise efficiency; but efficiency did not change in younger persons.[86]

HEART CONDUCTION AND RHYTHM

There is an increase in elastic and collagenous tissue in all parts of the conduction system with advancing age. Fat accumulates around the sinoatrial node, sometimes producing a partial or complete separation of the node from the atrial musculature. There may be a pronounced decrease in the number of pacemaker cells in the sinoatrial node beginning at age 60 years, and by age 75 years the sinoatrial node cell number may become substantially reduced. A variable degree of calcification of the left side of the cardiac skeleton, which includes the aortic and mitral annuli, the central fibrous body, and the summit of the interventricular septum, also occurs with aging. Because of their proximity to these structures, the atrioventricular (AV) node, AV bundle, bifurcation, and proximal left and right bundle branches may be affected by this process.

The P-R interval increases with aging as a result of a prolongation of the A-H time with no change in the H-V time.[89] While the supine basal heart rate is not affected by aging, beat-to-beat fluctuation of heart rate, commonly known as heart rate variability, declines steadily with age.[90] Reduced heart rate variability is an indicator of altered cardiac autonomic regulation commonly found in older people and has been linked to increased risk for morbid and fatal outcomes.[90]

An increase in the prevalence and complexity of both supraventricular and ventricular arrhythmias—whether detected by resting ECG, ambulatory monitoring, or exercise testing—occurs in otherwise healthy older, as opposed to younger, persons. Isolated atrial premature beats (APBs) appear on the resting ECG in 5 to 10 percent of subjects older than 60 years of age and are generally not associated with heart disease. Isolated APBs are detected in 6 percent of resting healthy BLSA volunteers older than 60 years of age, in 39 percent during exercise testing, and in 88 percent during ambulatory 24-hour monitoring.[91] Over a 10-year mean followup period, isolated APBs, even if frequent, are not predictive of increased cardiac risk in these individuals.[92]

Short bursts of paroxysmal supraventricular tachycardia (PSVT) are observed in 1 to 2 percent of apparently healthy individuals older than 65 years of age who were rigorously screened to exclude disease. Several 24-hour ambulatory monitoring studies have demonstrated short runs of this PSVT (usually 3 to 5 beats) in 13 to 50 percent of clinically healthy older subjects.[91,93] Although the presence of nonsustained PSVT did not predict an increase in risk of a future coronary event in BLSA subjects, 15 percent with PSVT later developed de novo atrial fibrillation, compared with fewer than 1 percent of subjects without PSVT. The incidence of PSVT during exercise, typically asymptomatic three- to five-beat salvos, increases with age, from nil in the youngest age group to approximately 10 percent in the ninth decade.[94] Although those individuals with exercise-induced PSVT were not at a greater risk for coronary events over a multiyear follow up, 10 percent developed a spontaneous atrial tachyarrhythmia, compared with only 2 percent of the control group. Thus, PSVT at rest or induced by exercise is an early clue that some healthy individuals are at increased risk for future atrial fibrillation (AF). Another risk factor for AF may be the increase in left atrial size that accompanies advancing age in otherwise healthy persons.[5]

In older subjects without apparent heart disease, the limited data available support a marked age-associated increase in the prevalence and complexity of ventricular ectopy (VE), both at rest and during exercise, at least in men. A steep increase in the prevalence of VE with advancing age occurs both in those clinically free of heart disease and in unselected populations. In healthy BLSA volunteers with a normal ST-segment response to treadmill exercise, isolated VE occurred at rest in 8.6 percent of men older than age 60 years compared to only 0.5 percent in those 20 to 40 years of age. Interestingly, the prevalence of VE at rest was not age-related in women. Among 98 carefully screened asymptomatic BLSA participants older than 60 years of age, 35 percent had multiform isolated VE, 11 percent had ventricular couplets, and 4 percent had short runs of ventricular tachycardia on 24-hour monitoring[91]; all occurred substantially more commonly in older than in healthy younger persons. Neither the prevalence nor the complexity of resting VE was a determinant of future coronary events over a 10-year mean followup period.[92] Isolated VE during or after maximal treadmill exercise increased in prevalence fivefold, from 11 to 57 percent, between the third and ninth decades in apparently healthy BLSA volunteers.[95]

Many of the age-associated changes in cardiac and arterial structure or function that have been observed in humans also occur across a wide range of other species. Insights gained from cellular and molecular studies in these animal models may hold clues that will assist in directing future efforts toward developing novel therapies for age-associated arterial structural and functional remodeling in humans. The results of studies have been reviewed.[2,4,96]

[ ] SUMMARY

In summary, there is a growing body of evidence that increased large-artery thickening and stiffness and endothelial dysfunction in apparently otherwise healthy older persons and the ensuing increase in systolic and pulse pressure, formerly thought to be part of "normal" aging, precede clinical disease and predict a higher risk for developing clinical atherosclerosis, hypertension, and stroke (Table 101–1). There is also evidence of a vicious cycle: altered mechanical properties of the vessel wall influence the development of atherosclerosis, and the latter, via endothelial cell dysfunction and other mechanisms, influences vascular stiffness. Some of the vascular changes that occur with aging in normotensive humans, including endothelial dysfunction, have been observed in hypertensives at an earlier age and are more marked than in normotensives. Such otherwise asymptomatic individuals might be considered to manifest "unsuccessful" vascular aging. When stated in this context, "unsuccessful vascular aging" becomes the risk factor for eventual clinical disease manifestations. Combinations of age-associated endothelial dysfunction, intimal-medial thickening, arterial stiffening, and arterial pulse pressure widening occurring to vary-

ing degrees determine the overall vascular aging profile of a given individual. Worse combinations may lead to a vessel wall with the most "unsuccessful" aging.

WHAT TO DO NOW ABOUT "UNSUCCESSFUL" AGING OF THE HEART AND BLOOD VESSELS

Extreme age-associated changes in CV structure/function that are perceived as deleterious aspects of CV aging in otherwise healthy persons ought to be interpreted to reflect "unsuccessful" CV aging. Indeed, data emerging from epidemiologic studies indicate that specific aspects of cardiac and vascular aging in otherwise apparently healthy persons confer an increased risk for CV events.

If cardiac and vascular aging are risk factors for disease, they represent potential targets for treatment and prevention. Lifestyle intervention or pharmacotherapy, to retard the rate of progression of subclinical disease, might be considered before clinical disease becomes manifest. With respect to lifestyle, the risk factor of lack of vigorous exercise increases dramatically with age in otherwise healthy persons.[84] It is noteworthy that the pulse pressure, pulse wave velocity, and carotid augmentation index are lower[7,88] and baroreceptor reflex function is improved[97] in older persons who are physically conditioned than in those who are sedentary. Exercise conditioning also improves endothelial function in older persons.[98]

There is also evidence to indicate that diets low in sodium are associated with reduced arterial stiffening with aging.[99] Exercise conditioning improves LV reserve function. Intriguingly, it was recently shown in the rat model, as well as in elderly patients, that physical activity and exercise training restore the cardiac protective effects of ischemic preconditioning and preinfarction angina that are otherwise lost during aging.[100]

With respect to pharmacotherapy, angiotensin-converting enzyme (ACE) inhibitors have been shown to retard vascular aging in rodents.[101] An emerging concept in the treatment of hypertension recognizes that progressive vascular damage can continue to occur even when arterial pressure is controlled. It is conceivable that drugs that retard or reverse age-associated vascular wall remodeling and increased stiffness will be preferable to those that lower pressure without affecting the vascular wall properties. In this regard, a novel drug that breaks such crosslinks has been shown to reduce indices of arterial stiffness measures in rodents, dogs, and nonhuman primates, as well as in humans.[102–105] Retardation or reduction in IMT in humans has been achieved by drug/diet intervention.[106,107] It is thus far unproved if such treatment can "prevent" unsuccessful aging of the vasculature in individuals of early middle age who exhibit excessive subclinical evidence of unsuccessful aging.

Accelerated cardiac and vascular aging in apparently healthy younger and middle-aged adults—that is, those who exhibit measurements of heart or vascular aging that usually occur later in life—may indicate the need for interventions designed to decrease the occurrence and/or manifestations of CV disease at later ages. Similarly, exaggerated heart or vascular aging in older persons, such as those with age-associated vascular measurements in the upper tertile, may merit similar consideration. Such a strategy would thus advocate treating "unsuccessful" aging. However, additional studies of the effectiveness of treatment regimens to delay or prevent each change are required for this strategy to be put into practice.

TABLE 101–1

Relationship of Cardiovascular Human Aging in Health to Cardiovascular Diseases

AGE-ASSOCIATED CHANGES	PLAUSIBLE MECHANISMS	POSSIBLE RELATION TO HUMAN DISEASE
Cardiovascular Structural Remodeling		
↑ Vascular intimal thickness	↑ Migration of and ↑ matrix production by VSMC Possible derivation of intimal cells from other sources	Promotes development of atherosclerosis
↑ Vascular stiffness	Elastin fragmentation ↑ Elastase activity ↑ Collagen production by VSMC and cross-linking of collagen Altered growth factor regulation/tissue repair mechanisms	Systolic hypertension Left ventricular wall thickening Stroke Artherosclerosis LVH ??
↑ LV wall thickness	↑ LV myocyte size with altered Ca²⁺ handling ↓ Myocyte number (necrotic and apoptotic death) Altered growth-factor regulation Focal matrix collagen deposition	Retarded early diastolic cardiac filling ↑ Cardiac filling pressure Lower threshold for dyspenea ↑ Likelihood of heart failure with relatively normal systolic function
↑ Left atrial size	↑ Left atrial pressure/volume	↑ Prevalence of atrial fibrillation and other atrial arrhythmias
Cardiovascular Function Changes		
Altered regulation of vascular tone	↓ NO production/effects	Vascular stiffening; hypertension Early atherosclerosis
Reduced threshold for cell Ca²⁺ overload	Changes in gene expression of proteins that regulate Ca²⁺ handling; increased ω6:ω3 polyunsaturated fatty acids in ration in cardiac membranes	Lower threshold for atrial and ventricular arrhythmia Increased myocyte death Increased fibrosis Reduced diastolic and systolic function
↓ Cardiovascular reserve	↑ Vascular load ↓ Intrinsic myocardial contractility Ventricular–vascular load mismatch during stress ↑ Plasma levels of catecholamines ↓ β-Adrenergic modulation of heart rate, myocardial contractility, and vascular tone as a result of postsynaptic signaling deficits	Lower threshold for heart failure and increased severity of heart failure
Reduced Physical Activity		
	Learned lifestyle	Exaggerated age Δ in some aspects of cardiovascular structure and function, e.g., arterial stiffening Negative impact on atherosclerotic vascular disease, hypertension, and heart failure

LV, left ventricular; LVH, left ventricular hypertrophy; VSMC, vascular smooth muscle cell; Δ, changes; ω6:ω3, ratio of omega 6 to omega 3.

THERAPEUTIC CONSIDERATIONS IN OLDER PATIENTS WITH CLINICAL CARDIOVASCULAR DISEASES

[ ] ISCHEMIC HEART DISEASE

Increasing age is the most powerful predictor of future coronary artery disease in asymptomatic individuals. Autopsy studies dem-onstrate that the prevalence of obstructive coronary disease in-creases from approximately 10 to 20 percent in the fourth decade to 50 to 70 percent in the eighth decade. Advancing age is also as-sociated with more severe, diffuse atherosclerosis and more dam-age to the left ventricle, with the prevalence of triple vessel and left main coronary disease doubling between ages 40 and 80 years. El-evated end-diastolic pressure and wall motion abnormalities on left ventriculography are also more common in the elderly patient with coronary artery disease. Therefore, almost all clinical manifestations of ischemic heart disease have a higher mortality rate and a worse outcome in the older population. Finally, the clinical assessment of the elderly patient with coronary artery disease is often limited by the coexistence of diseases that make interpretation of ischemic symptoms difficult. Coexisting comorbidities, such as chronic kidney disease, also make certain cardiovascular therapies and diagnostic tests more challenging in the elderly.

【 】 ACUTE CORONARY SYNDROMES

The incidence of myocardial infarction appears to be increasing in the elderly over the last 15 years, particularly in older women.[108] Despite increased use of therapies shown to be effective in acute myocardial infarction patients, 5-year survival has not changed over the last 15 years in acute infarct patients who are at least 75 years of age.[108] Older patients with acute myocardial infarction are more likely to be female, have a preexisting history of angina, heart failure, hypertension, and diabetes, and experience a non–ST-segment elevation myocardial infarction. Older patients are also more likely to present with atypical symptoms of acute myocardial ischemia and infarction such as shortness of breath, confusion, and failure to thrive. Furthermore, nearly one-half of myocardial infarctions in the elderly are unrecognized clinically. The frequent atypical presentation of acute coronary syndrome results in delay in diagnosis and initiation of treatment in this age group and likely contributes to the high in-hospital mortality in the elderly patient presenting with an acute coronary syndrome.

Age is a powerful independent predictor of short- and long-term mortality in patients with non–ST-segment elevation acute coronary syndromes,[109,110] and ST-segment elevation acute myocardial infarction. In the Platelet Glycoprotein IIb/IIIa in Unstable Angina: Receptor Suppression Using Integrilin (eptifibatide) Therapy (PURSUIT) trial of 9461 patients with unstable angina or non–ST-segment elevation myocardial infarction, age was the most powerful predictor of short-term mortality. The 6-month death rate increased from 2 percent in patients with non–ST-segment elevation acute coronary syndrome who were younger than 50 years of age to 11 percent in those patients 70–79 years of age and 19 percent in those patients 80 years of age and older.[110] In patients admitted with a first ST-segment elevation myocardial infarction and treated with thrombolytic therapy, in-hospital mortality increases exponentially as a function of age from 1.9 percent among patients age 40 years or younger to 31.9 percent among patients older than age 80 years. Similarly, in the Global Utilization of Streptokinase and Tissue Plasminogen Activator for Occluded Arteries (GUSTO-1) trial, 30-day mortality following an ST-segment elevation myocardial infarction increased from 3 percent in patients younger than 65 years of age to 19.6 percent in patients 75 to 85 years of age and to 30.3 percent in patients older than 85 years of age. Age was the most powerful predictor of in-hospital and 30-day mortality in this trial.

Elderly acute infarct patients experience a much greater incidence of heart failure, atrial fibrillation, and cardiogenic shock in spite of the fact that indices of infarct size, such as creatinine phosphokinase levels and QRS scores, do not change with age. Age is a powerful predictor of cardiogenic shock in both ST-segment and non–ST-segment elevation acute coronary syndromes. The risks of heart failure and shock increase three- to fourfold in patients older than age 85 years compared to those younger than age 65 years. The higher incidence of heart failure and shock may result from age-related changes in diastolic filling, aortic compliance, and a decrease in sensitivity to catecholamine stimulation resulting in diminished cardiac reserve and afterload mismatch following ischemic damage. The worse outcome with acute myocardial infarction is also contributed by fewer angiographic collateral vessels to an occluded infarct vessel in older patients with an acute ST-segment elevation myocardial infarction compared to younger infarct patients.[111] This age-related decrease in collateral vessels predicts mortality in elderly infarct patients and may result in less recovery of left ventricular function, especially if the timing of reperfusion therapy is delayed. Endothelial repair and angiogenesis arise from bone marrow endothelial progenitor cells.[112] Increasing age is a powerful predictor of a decreased number and function of endothelial progenitor cells.[50,113] This age-associated decrease in endothelial progenitor cell number and function likely contributes to the progression of atherosclerosis; impaired ability to heal following acute myocardial infarction, decreased collateral blood vessel development, and poor prognosis in the setting of coronary disease.[114]

Mortality in older patients with myocardial infarction is less likely to result from ventricular fibrillation compared to younger patients, but the former are much more likely to have electromechanical dissociation and cardiac rupture on autopsy. The latter age-associated risk is particularly notable in patients receiving fibrinolytic therapy.[115] In addition to the high in-hospital mortality risk in the elderly patient with acute coronary syndrome, the risk of death following hospital discharge also increases by almost 6 percent per year.[116]

The high morbidity and mortality associated with acute ischemic syndromes in the elderly dictates an aggressive approach to management, but the evidence to guide care is limited by the low number of patients older than 75 years of age enrolled in clinical trials. Even in acute coronary syndrome trials without age restrictions, elderly patients with a comorbidity, such as renal insufficiency or cerebrovascular disease, are usually excluded. Consequently, treatment guidelines for the elderly acute coronary syndrome patient are often based on limited information (see Chap. 11).

【 】 REPERFUSION IN ST-SEGMENT ELEVATION MYOCARDIAL INFARCTION

Prompt reperfusion of the infarct-related artery is critical to reducing the high mortality in the elderly patient with acute ST-segment elevation myocardial infarction. Unfortunately, the delay in presenting to the hospital and in diagnosing acute ST-segment elevation infarction, along with increased comorbidity, make the elderly patient less likely to be eligible for reperfusion therapy. Large registry data in the United States show that fibrinolytic eligible patients older than 75 years of age are significantly less likely to receive reperfusion therapy than are patients younger than age 65 years.[117] Fibrinolytic therapy in acute myocardial infarction reduces mortality, and data suggest a benefit in the elderly. In a meta-analysis of large randomized trials of fibrinolytic therapy, subset analyses of the nearly 5800 patients older than age 74 years showed a nonsignificant trend toward treatment benefit, with a net saving of 1.0 life per 100 patients treated at 35 days after infarction. The benefit for fibrinolytic therapy is even more apparent in patients older than the age of 75 years when this meta-analysis is confined to patients presenting within 12 hours of symptom onset with ST-segment elevation or left bundle-branch block on their admission electrocardiogram (34 lives saved per 1000 patients treated).[118] It is difficult to draw conclusions about the risk-to-benefit ratio of fibrinolytic therapy in patients 85 years of age and older, even with no contraindications, given that so few patients in this age group were enrolled into randomized trials and observational database studies that show no benefit or even harm compared to no treatment in patients 85 years of age and older.[119]

Use of fibrinolytic agents in the elderly is limited by the risk of intracranial hemorrhage, which rises with age. This increased hemorrhagic risk of reperfusion strategies in the elderly was demonstrated in recent reperfusion trials, which evaluated half-dose fibrinolytic therapy with glycoprotein IIb/IIIa inhibitors compared to full-dose fibrinolytic therapy, and studies comparing fibrinolytic therapy with low-molecular-weight heparin compared with unfractionated heparin.[120] Careful dose adjustment of anticoagulation is necessary to limit the bleeding risk in the elderly. In considering fibrinolytic therapy, careful risk stratification of the patient with an ST-segment elevation infarction who is older than the age of 75 years needs to be considered. These factors include the age and weight of the patient, other comorbidities, the number of leads with ST-segment elevation, the duration of symptoms, as well as the proximity of the hospital to a high volume center with onsite percutaneous coronary intervention.

Primary angioplasty has been compared with fibrinolytic therapy in several trials with beneficial effects on mortality, recurrent myocardial infarction, and recurrent ischemia for percutaneous coronary intervention. Subgroup analyses suggest that there is a large survival advantage for percutaneous coronary intervention compared to fibrinolytic therapy in patients 70 years of age and older with an ST-segment elevation myocardial infarction.[121] Patients treated with direct angioplasty have a lower overall stroke and hemorrhagic stroke risk compared to fibrinolytic treated patients. Patients with ST-segment elevation myocardial infarction and a high-risk profile, which includes advanced age, have a greater benefit from percutaneous intervention compared with fibrinolytic therapy than do low-risk patients.[122]

Older patients have a higher risk of cardiogenic shock than do younger subjects. In a randomized study of early revascularization compared to initial medical stabilization, mean 6-year survival was significantly greater with an early revascularization strategy.[123] Survival curves show an absolute 13 percent long-term survival advantage for an early revascularization strategy. Because there was no age (<75 years versus >75 years) treatment interaction over the long-term, these data suggest that elderly acute myocardial infarction patients with cardiogenic shock should receive emergent revascularization therapy if possible.

[ ] MEDICAL THERAPY FOR ACUTE MYOCARDIAL INFARCTION

β-Blocker therapy is greatly underprescribed in older postmyocardial infarction patients, despite overwhelming data showing a significant survival advantage with this therapy. In the Cooperative Cardiovascular Project database of more than 200,000 Medicare beneficiaries who suffered a myocardial infarction, only 34 percent of this elderly cohort was discharged home on a β blocker. Of ideal postinfarct patients older than 65 years of age with no contraindications to β-blocker therapy, only one-half leave hospital on this therapy. Confirming older randomized trials, all subgroups of patients in this database had a large survival advantage with β-blocker therapy. Benefits extended to subjects with Q-wave and non–Q-wave infarction, age younger than 70 years to older than 80 years, and all categories of left ventricular function. The benefits of chronic β-blocker therapy after myocardial infarction in the Cardiovascular Cooperative Project database are similar to subgroup analyses of the placebo-controlled trials of chronic β-blocker therapy following stabilization from myocardial infarction. In the large, randomized trials, the majority of the long-term benefit of β-blockers was driven by the survival advantage in those patients older than age 65 years.

Aspirin therapy decreases mortality and reinfarction in elderly infarct subjects.[124] Nevertheless, among 10,000 Medicare beneficiaries with an acute myocardial infarction and no contraindication to receive aspirin therapy, only 61 percent of patients received it within the first two hospital days.[121] Aspirin therapy in this large group of elderly infarct patients was independently associated with a lower 30-day mortality. Furthermore, only 76 percent of elderly subjects without any contraindications were discharged home on aspirin following a myocardial infarction. Aspirin use was independently associated with improved 6-month outcomes. In a randomized, placebo-controlled trial of 45,852 medically treated patients with acute ST-segment elevation myocardial infarction, clopidogrel therapy added to aspirin reduced the short-term composite end point of death, reinfarction, or stroke, as well as mortality alone.[125] On subgroup analysis, all age groups benefited from this therapy. Therefore, in elderly infarct patients with a low bleeding risk, dual antiplatelet therapy should be considered. ACE inhibitor therapy following acute myocardial infarction reduces morbidity and mortality. In the randomized, placebo-controlled clinical trials that involved high-risk patients with left ventricular dysfunction or clinical heart failure, there was a large survival benefit in older patients randomized to ACE inhibitor therapy compared to placebo. A meta-analysis of these trials involving 5966 patients with left ventricular dysfunction (ejection fraction <40 percent) or heart failure was reported.[126] Significant reductions in mortality, heart failure, and recurrent myocardial infarction were comparable among subjects age <55 years, 55 to 75 years, or >75 years.

For lower-risk elderly patients without heart failure or left ventricular dysfunction postmyocardial infarction, the benefits of ACE inhibitors are clearly less, and individualized treatment that takes into account the risks of hypotension and renal insufficiency needs to be considered. Aggressive ACE inhibitor blockade on arrival to the hospital should be avoided in the elderly. The resultant hypotension may result in ischemia and worsen outcomes in this age group.

In older postinfarction patients with left ventricular dysfunction, clinical heart failure, or both, who are intolerant of ACE inhibition (such as cough), high-dose angiotensin receptor blockade is an equivalent alternative.[127] The combination of an ACE inhibitor plus receptor blocker does not benefit these patients compared to either alone, and results in a higher incidence of side effects.

Randomized trial data show that in patients with left ventricular dysfunction plus heart failure in the coronary care unit, the addition of an aldosterone antagonist to standard postinfarction therapy decreases cardiovascular morbidity and mortality, with similar efficacy among subjects <65 years of age or >65 years of age. These data suggest that in appropriate older patients with left ventricular dysfunction and heart failure following a large transmural myocardial infarction, one should consider the addition of an aldosterone antagonist to standard postinfarction therapy. An important caveat to adding an aldosterone antagonist to an ACE inhibitor or receptor blocker in the older postinfarct patient with left ventricular dysfunction and heart failure is the frequent occurrence of renal insufficiency. Creatinine clearance should be calculated in this age group. Renal function and potassium levels should be followed particularly closely in the elderly when these agents are used (see Chap. 61).

[ ] NON–ST-SEGMENT ELEVATION ACUTE CORONARY SYNDROME

Large cohort studies show that the majority of patients admitted with non–ST-segment elevation acute coronary syndromes are 65 years of age and older, and that more than 10% of patients are 85 years of age and older. With advancing age, guideline-recommended medication contraindications are more frequent, especially for glycoprotein IIb/IIIa antagonists. Even in patients without stated contraindications, in-hospital use of aspirin, β blockers, and anticoagulants decrease with increasing age. An early invasive approach to management of non–ST-segment elevation acute coronary syndrome is reduced with advancing age as well, with only 40 percent of patients older than 75 years of age proceeding to early catheterization. This decreased use of medications and procedures in the elderly patient with acute coronary syndrome is mirrored by an escalating in-hospital mortality that is 2.5- to 3-fold greater in patients 75 to 84 years of age and 85 years of age and older, respectively, compared to patients younger than 65 years of age. As guideline-recommended therapies are used more commonly (aspirin, heparin, β blockers, glycoprotein IIb/IIIa antagonists, and cardiac catheterization), the risk of in-hospital death is lowered in patients 75 years of age and older. Greater adherence to guideline-recommended therapies in the elderly acute coronary syndrome patient during hospitalization and at discharge can result in a decrease risk of short-term mortality and morbidity in this high-risk group of patients.

In elderly patients with non–ST-segment elevation acute coronary syndromes, antiplatelet therapy decreases adverse events. Studies show that the addition of a parenteral glycoprotein IIb/IIIa inhibitor to standard antiischemic therapy that includes aspirin and heparin, reduces short-term risks of death, myocardial infarction, and refractory angina. There is no heterogeneity of effect of a glycoprotein IIb/IIIa antagonist across age subgroups. Importantly, creatinine clearance should be calculated prior to dosing these agents in the elderly because of the frequent need for dose adjustments, but age should not exclude the addition of a glycoprotein IIb/IIIa inhibitor to standard antiischemic therapy for unstable angina or non–ST-segment elevation myocardial infarction, particularly in higher risk elderly patients proceeding to coronary revascularization.

Clopidogrel was evaluated in 12,562 patients with non–ST-segment elevation acute coronary syndrome patients, all treated with aspirin.[125] The primary end point of cardiovascular mortality, nonfatal myocardial infarction, or stroke was reduced 20 percent compared to placebo following a mean of 9 months of therapy. This benefit was evident in the 6208-patient subgroup of patients older than the age of 65 years. Thus in low-bleeding-risk elderly patients with non–ST-segment acute coronary syndromes, the addition of clopidogrel to aspirin reduces future cardiovascular events.

Several randomized trials have assessed the impact of a conservative medical strategy versus an invasive approach on short-term outcomes of death, myocardial infarction, and recurrent ischemic events in patients with non–ST-segment elevation acute coronary syndromes.

Most studies, including a recent meta-analysis,[128] show decreased death or nonfatal myocardial infarction for an initial invasive strategy when compared to a conservative strategy. The benefit of an invasive approach was much more evident in higher-risk patients, including those with positive troponin, ST-segment depression on electrocardiography, and, importantly, the large subgroup of patients older than the age of 65 years in these studies. Subgroup analysis of the randomized elderly patients with non–ST-segment elevation acute coronary syndromes show a large absolute and relative reduction in death or nonfatal myocardial infarction at 6 months with an invasive strategy when compared to a conservative approach.[129] These data suggest that because older patients with acute coronary syndromes are often at increased risk for adverse outcomes, an early invasive approach should be considered for many older patients with acute coronary syndromes.

[ ] CHRONIC CORONARY DISEASE

The use of coronary revascularization, both percutaneous coronary intervention and coronary artery bypass surgery, has increased in patients 75 years of age and older, with a decline in short-term mortality with both revascularization modalities.[130] The use of percutaneous coronary intervention has increased significantly, along with improved outcomes in elderly patients with chronic coronary artery disease.

Use of bypass surgery has also increased in the very elderly. In-hospital mortality is significantly greater in octogenarians undergoing coronary artery bypass surgery than in younger patients.[131] In a large cohort of patients undergoing coronary artery bypass surgery, in-hospital mortality was 8.1 percent in octogenarians, in addition to an increased incidence of postoperative stroke (4 percent) and renal failure (7 percent). In a subset of octogenarians without significant comorbidity and undergoing elective coronary artery bypass surgery, in-hospital mortality was only 4.2 percent. These data suggest that octogenarians can undergo coronary artery bypass surgery with relatively low short-term mortality, especially if the surgery is elective, it is the first coronary artery bypass procedure, and comorbidity is low. In spite of the higher short-term morbidity and mortality in elderly bypass patients compared to younger subjects, the 3-year mortality rate of this group was similar to the general octogenarian population.

Recent data also suggest that older age is a powerful predictor of both short-term and 5-year cognitive decline following coronary artery bypass surgery.[132] An important addition to the treatment of the elderly patient with critical multivessel coronary artery disease and aortic atherosclerosis may be off-pump coronary artery bypass surgery. Because emboli are the main source of strokes following coronary artery bypass surgery, off-pump bypass may theoretically reduce intraoperative cerebral emboli, resulting in a decrease in perioperative stroke and cognitive decline. A meta-analysis of 9 observational studies comparing conventional coronary bypass surgery with off-pump surgery in subjects 70 years of age and older suggests that the stroke risk may be lower with off-pump surgery.[133] These data contrast with a recent trial in low-risk patients (mean age: 61 years) randomized to standard versus off-pump bypass showing no difference in short-term or 1-year stroke, death, myocardial infarction, or coronary reintervention.[134] A recent randomized study in older subjects (mean age: 76 years) undergoing coronary artery bypass surgery showed that cognitive function 3 months following surgery was similar in subjects randomized to conventional coronary artery bypass surgery to those subjects randomized to off-pump coronary artery bypass surgery.[135] Ongoing prospective randomized trials address the best method of coronary artery bypass grafting in the elderly patient with multivessel coronary disease requiring revascularization.

Previous randomized trials of medical versus revascularization therapy in patients with stable coronary artery disease excluded the elderly. An important recent trial prospectively randomized patients age 75 years and older (mean age: 80 years) with moderate angina despite at least two antianginal drugs to coronary angiography and revascularization versus optimal medical therapy.[136] The primary end point of this trial was quality of life scores at 6 months. Seventy-four percent of patients randomized to the invasive arm had anatomy appropriate for either percutaneous intervention (54 percent) or coronary artery bypass surgery (20 percent).

Although quality of life improved in both groups by 6 months, the group randomized to invasive therapy had significantly better quality of life compared to medically treated patients. Secondary end points at 6 months, including death, myocardial infarction, or hospitalization for unstable angina, were significantly lower in those elderly patients randomized to invasive therapy (19 percent) versus medical therapy (49 percent). Furthermore, one-third of patients in the medical arm crossed over to revascularization as a consequence of refractory symptomatology. Four-year survival was similar between the two groups as was nonfatal myocardial infarction. Rehospitalization was significantly greater in those patients randomized to initial medical therapy.[137] This important study suggests that age alone is not a contraindication to proceed with an invasive approach to the treatment of moderate to severe angina that is present despite antianginal therapy.

Although several trials have randomized patients with stable coronary artery disease to percutaneous coronary intervention versus coronary artery bypass surgery, the elderly were generally excluded. A recent randomized trial of 454 high-risk military veterans with medically refractory angina were randomized to percutaneous coronary intervention with or without stents or coronary artery bypass surgery.[138] High risk included patients older than age 70 years, prior coronary bypass, left ventricular ejection fraction <35 percent, recent myocardial infarction, or need for intraaortic balloon pump. Survival at 30 days was excellent in both groups (95 percent vs. 97 percent for bypass and angioplasty, respectively). Survival up to 3 years remained similar in the two groups. These data suggest that high-risk patients with medically

refractory angina, including the elderly, can undergo revascularization with angioplasty or bypass surgery with excellent survival as well as relief of angina.

【 】 CONGESTIVE HEART FAILURE

In contrast to other cardiovascular disorders, the prevalence of congestive heart failure (CHF) is dramatically increasing (see Fig. 101–1F). Approximately 5 million Americans have CHF and each year 550,000 new cases are diagnosed.[139] The incidence of heart failure doubles with each decade of life and the prevalence rises to almost 10 percent of those older than age 80 years. In part this is because heart failure represents a final common pathway for most other cardiac disorders, and in part because of the more successful treatments of heart failure,[140] as well as ischemic and valvular disease. These successes increase the numbers surviving, albeit with, or at increased risk for, heart failure.

Evaluation of the older patient presenting with failure symptoms should include a noninvasive study to determine whether the primary problem is systolic dysfunction. Although systolic dysfunction is present in at least half of CHF cases, the presence of a normal, or elevated, ejection fraction is more common in the older group, particularly in women and those with atrial fibrillation and hypertension. Although the existence of this entity is sometimes questioned, these patients do experience significant limitations in exercise duration and quality of life, increases in neurohormonal activation and CHF markers such as natriuretic peptide,[141] as well as increased mortality, hospitalization rates, and healthcare costs when compared with the general population, and mortality and rehospitalization rates similar to those with heart failure and systolic dysfunction.[142] The etiology is not clear, although in addition to abnormalities in diastolic filling, hypertension is almost invariably present and increased pulse pressure with exercise suggests increased central vascular stiffness. It should be noted that evidence of long-standing volume overload and an S_3 gallop are less likely in patients with preserved systolic function, and that in the general, older, heart-failure population, exertional symptoms are less common whereas those related to fatigue and mental status changes are more common. The diagnosis of heart failure with preserved systolic function is primarily one of exclusion in patients with objective evidence of pulmonary vascular congestion without findings of an ischemic, hypertensive, or valvular etiology. Amyloid should also be considered in older patients presenting with heart failure symptoms in the absence of another identifiable cause.

It is often helpful to investigate reversible precipitants in older individuals who present with new-onset or worsening heart-failure symptoms, including anemia, infection, thyroid disease, atrial fibrillation, and dietary or medication noncompliance. Investigation for common comorbidities is also useful as they are common and associated with increased hospitalizations and adverse clinical outcomes.[143] Diuretics are particularly useful in older patients with increased vascular stiffness who present with acute congestive symptoms, as significant reductions in pressure occur with relatively small changes in intravascular volume. In patients with systolic dysfunction, sinus rhythm, and congestive heart failure, digitalis might improve signs and symptoms of heart failure. However, the maintenance dose should generally be no higher than 0.125 mg/d because of the age-associated decreased volume of distribution and creatinine clearance. ACE inhibitors are a cornerstone of therapy in patients with systolic dysfunction and their benefit extends to the elderly. Studies indicating the value of the β blockers,[144] as well as the value of aldosterone antagonists,[145] in patients with continued symptoms despite ACE inhibitor therapy probably are extendable to the older population. There are few controlled, randomized trials of interventions in the patient population with preserved systolic function. Increasing vascular and LV chamber stiffness increase the likelihood of significant pressure shifts with relatively small changes in volume. Thus diuretics, although extremely useful in the acute setting, may be associated with symptomatic hypotension in the absence of volume overload. Careful control of blood pressure is also important, as is control of ventricular rate in patients with atrial fibrillation.

New devices may also significantly improve outcomes in patients with persistent failure despite medical therapy. The use of atrial-synchronized, biventricular pacing, left ventricular assist devices, and implantable defibrillators are being used with increased frequency in the elderly, and appropriate indications are evolving.

【 】 ARRHYTHMIAS

Supraventricular and ventricular arrhythmias increase in frequency with aging, and hospitalization rates for these arrhythmias are increasing more than the growth in this population.[146] Age-associated changes in both passive and active state diastolic properties, as well as decreased systolic reserve (see Fig. 101–7) may increase the likelihood that the older individual will develop hemodynamic compromise and/or ischemia during an arrhythmic episode. Evaluation of the older patient presenting with symptomatic or asymptomatic arrhythmias, therefore, should include a search for concomitant illnesses as well as other presenting triggers, such as chest pain, exercise, smoking, caffeine, electrolyte abnormalities, and medicine and alcohol ingestion. Ambulatory electrocardiographic monitoring during the patient's normal activities is most likely to determine the nature and severity of the arrhythmia. Invasive electrophysiology studies can be used to not only diagnose the arrhythmia, but also to determine its mechanism, obtain prognostic information, and determine the suitability of different therapeutic approaches.

Atrial flutter and fibrillation are common in the elderly[147] (see Chap. 37). Both are often associated with structural heart disease, and patients with newly diagnosed atrial tachyarrhythmias should undergo echocardiographic evaluation. In addition to identification and treatment of any precipitating factors, patients with atrial flutter who are at increased stroke risk, which includes those older than 75 years of age, should receive anticoagulation therapy unless there are contraindications. If the flutter is symptomatic, cardioversion should be attempted. If flutter recurs, catheter ablation was demonstrated to be more successful than pharmacologic therapy in the maintenance of sinus rhythm.[148]

Atrial fibrillation is the most common arrhythmia in the elderly, and is associated with increasing age, heart failure, valvular heart disease, stroke, diabetes, and hypertension. Older individuals are more likely to experience hemodynamic compromise resulting from the increased ventricular rate and loss of atrial–ventricular synchrony accompanying the arrhythmia, because of the age-associated changes in relaxation properties and increased dependence

on atrial contribution. Because of the increased likelihood of coronary disease, the higher rate is also more likely to be associated with myocardial ischemia. Atrial fibrillation may also result in atrial remodeling, which increases the likelihood of maintenance of the arrhythmia, cardiomyopathy because of the rapid rate, and lower output related to the irregularity of the rhythm. The risk of embolic stroke in atrial fibrillation also increases with age. The Framingham Study reported that the risk of stroke attributed to atrial fibrillation rose from 7.3 percent in those 60 to 69 years of age to 30.8% in those age 80 to 89 years.

Therapeutic goals in patients with atrial fibrillation include stroke prevention, rate control, and possibly rhythm control. In randomized trials, anticoagulation therapy prevents embolic strokes in most patients with atrial fibrillation, including those older than age 75 years. This benefit of anticoagulation therapy is greater than aspirin therapy in the elderly, although there is a higher rate of intracranial hemorrhage. Careful monitoring of the international normalized ratio (INR) is important as most embolic strokes in the elderly occur when the ratio is under 2.0 and most cerebral hemorrhages occur when the ratio is above 3.0. Although the benefits of aspirin are less significant, aspirin can be used in older patients who have a contraindication to warfarin therapy, including an inability to carefully monitor the INR. Rate control in patients without systolic dysfunction may be attempted with diltiazem, verapamil, and β blockers; in patients with systolic dysfunction, amiodarone or digitalis may be used. A useful goal is a rate of <80 beats/min at rest and <110 beats/min on a 6-minute walk test. If patients are intolerant of medical therapy, or if medical therapy is ineffective, AV node ablation and pacemaker insertion,[149] or AV node modification, which results in slowed AV conduction, but not complete heart block, should be considered. Cardioversion should be attempted in patients who are hemodynamically compromised, in acute atrial fibrillation, and for those in whom there is a low likelihood of reversion to atrial fibrillation if conversion does occur. This can be attempted with electrical or pharmacologic approaches.

Several studies compared rate control and rhythm control strategies in primarily older (mean ages: 70 and 68 years) patients with atrial fibrillation,[150,151] and found that rate control is a reasonable strategy in older patients with atrial fibrillation that is not associated with significant symptoms or hemodynamic compromise. Anticoagulation therapy should be maintained regardless of a rate or rhythm control strategy. If rhythm control is attempted, flecainide and propafenone may be used in patients without ischemic or structural heart disease.

In those patients with ischemic disease, sotalol may be used. In patients with heart failure, dofetilide increases the likelihood of conversion to and maintenance of sinus rhythm[152] without the increase in mortality associated with some other anti-arrhythmic agents in patients with heart failure. Amiodarone is useful in nearly all patient populations and in a randomized trial was more effective than sotalol or propafenone in preventing recurrences of atrial fibrillation.[153]

About one-half of pacemakers are placed because of sinus node dysfunction with bradycardia. The use of programmable pacemakers to appropriately time atrial and ventricular systoles may be particularly useful in older patients because diastolic filling and cardiac output are more dependent on atrial contribution. In the

Medicare population, dual-chamber pacing is associated with improved 1- and 2-year survival, when compared with single-chamber pacing, after adjustment for confounding patient characteristics. In a randomized trial comparing the two pacing modalities in patients with sinus node dysfunction, there was no difference in stroke-free mortality, but the risk of new and chronic atrial fibrillation and signs and symptoms of heart failure were significantly reduced and quality of life was higher in patients assigned to dual-chamber pacing.[154]

Ventricular arrhythmias in the elderly are to be approached in the same fashion as in younger individuals, that is, arrhythmias that are asymptomatic and unassociated with evidence of cardiac disease can be viewed as less serious than those associated with evidence of left ventricular dysfunction and/or ischemia. Both older and younger postmyocardial infarction patients benefit from β-blocker therapy with a reduction in sudden death. Life-threatening ventricular arrhythmias are common in the elderly patient with severe coronary disease and left ventricular dysfunction. As in younger subjects, aggressive management of elderly survivors of cardiac arrest and of those with hypotensive ventricular tachycardia is justified. In the Multicenter Automatic Defibrillator Implantation Trial (MADIT)-II, patients with an ejection fraction of <30 percent and a prior myocardial infarction randomized to an implantable defibrillator experienced improved survival as compared to those randomized to conventional therapy. For those older than 70 years of age, the hazard ratio of death was decreased by more than 30 percent.[155] In the DEFINITE study of prophylactic implantable defibrillators in patients with nonischemic dilated cardiomyopathy, an ejection fraction of <35 percent, and premature ventricular complexes, the magnitude of the decrease in the outcome of death from any cause was similar in those older and younger than 65 years of age.[156]

[ ] VALVULAR HEART DISEASE

The most frequent valvular heart disease in the elderly is calcific aortic stenosis (see Chap. 75). The development of clinically significant aortic stenosis may be very rapid in this age group, as calcification and severe scarring occur rather abruptly. In addition, animal studies demonstrate that there is less compensatory hypertrophy in response to increased impedance to left ventricular ejection in the aged heart, which could also contribute to the development of heart failure.

The most helpful study one can perform in detailing the extent of aortic stenosis in an elderly subject is a Doppler echocardiogram to assess aortic valve calcification, mobility, aortic valve area, and the transvalvular gradient. The presence of left ventricular hypertrophy can be assessed as well as left ventricular function. It appears that asymptomatic elderly patients with significant aortic stenosis by echocardiography can be followed carefully without surgical intervention until the first symptoms appear.[157] It should be noted, however, that if the older patient is limited by other disease, for example, arthritis, they may not be able to exercise to the point at which symptoms occur despite the presence of significant disease requiring surgery. In the presence of asymptomatic severe stenosis, or if the assessment of symptoms is difficult because of concomitant diseases, physician-supervised exercise testing is safe in patients with moderate to severe asymptomatic aortic stenosis and can identify those who would benefit from surgery.[158] As in younger patients, a low calculated valve area in the presence of a low cardiac output may be caused by incomplete valve opening, rather than severe stenosis. Calculation of the valve area during dobutamine administration in these instances will provide a more accurate assessment of valvular stenosis. Because significant coronary stenosis increases valvular surgical risk, coronary angiography is usually performed in patients being considered for surgery. A recent report suggests that multislice computed tomography may serve as an alternative to the invasive diagnostic procedure in these patients.[159]

Aortic valve replacement often results in marked improvement in symptoms and left ventricular function, as well as expected survival in the older patient. Predictors of surgical mortality with aortic valve replacement include low ejection fraction and congestive heart failure, atrial fibrillation, associated surgical procedures, and an emergency procedure, suggesting that aortic valve replacement for symptomatic aortic stenosis should not be delayed merely because the patient is elderly.[160] Percutaneous aortic valvuloplasty in the elderly is associated with poor outcomes, including early restenosis, aortic regurgitation, stroke, high mortality, and heart failure. It is useful only for palliation and as a "bridge" to valve replacement in very ill patients. Preliminary results of the use of a percutaneous aortic valve stent inserted within a balloon-expandable stent in patients with inoperable severe aortic stenosis also have been reported.[161]

Chronic aortic regurgitation may occur in elderly individuals secondary to aortic root dilatation related to long-standing hypertension. Symptoms include angina, even in patients without significant coronary disease, and congestive heart failure. It is important to recognize, however, that symptoms may not occur until significant left ventricular dysfunction is present; consequently, the onset of dysfunction is sufficient to prompt surgery, rather than await the occurrence of symptoms. Although vasodilator therapy was reported to delay the occurrence of systolic dysfunction, results of prospective studies are conflicting and further studies are required before the value of this therapy is well defined.[162] Best operative results occur in individuals with no or minimal symptoms, mild to moderate ventricular dysfunction, and a brief duration of left ventricular dysfunction.

The most common cause of mitral stenosis in the elderly is rheumatic disease, which at times may not result in symptoms until the patient reaches old age. Mitral valve obstruction may also result from extensive mitral annular calcification. The diagnosis of mitral stenosis may be more difficult in the elderly because calcification of the valve may decrease the intensity of the first heart sound and the opening sound, and diminished cardiac output may decrease the intensity of the diastolic rumble. Doppler echocardiography is very useful in diagnosing the presence of significant disease. If symptoms are more than mild, or if pulmonary hypertension develops, surgery or balloon mitral valvuloplasty should be considered. Atrial fibrillation often triggers functional deterioration in older individuals because the dependence of filling on atrial contribution is exaggerated in the presence of mitral stenosis. Balloon mitral valvuloplasty compares favorably with open surgical commissurotomy in appropriate candidates, and should be considered for elderly patients with symptomatic mitral stenosis.

Mitral regurgitation in the elderly is most often related to ischemic heart disease and to myxomatous degeneration of the mitral valve. As is true for aortic insufficiency, symptoms may be recognized only after significant left ventricular dysfunction and cavity dilatation have occurred, and intervention should be considered on the basis of these factors, rather than await symptom onset. For elderly patients with mitral regurgitation, mitral valve repair is associated with a lower operative mortality and eliminates the need for anticoagulation in patients without atrial fibrillation and results in excellent long-term results. Thus repair, rather than replacement, should be performed if possible. If repair is not possible, chordal preservation should be attempted.[163] Numerous percutaneous approaches also are being investigated in phase 1 and early phase 2 studies.[164]

For elderly patients requiring valve replacement, the choice of a mechanical valve with the bleeding risk of lifelong anticoagulation must be balanced against a bioprosthetic valve and the risk of structural deterioration. Additional factors in the choice include candidacy for anticoagulation and other requirements for anticoagulation such as atrial fibrillation, age, and valve position. In a series of elderly subjects receiving aortic or mitral mechanical valve replacements, freedom from major anticoagulant-related hemorrhage was 76 percent at 10 years.[165] A bioprosthetic valve in the mitral position deteriorates more rapidly than in the aortic position. In a large series of elderly patients receiving porcine bioprostheses, freedom from structural deterioration at 10 years for the aortic valve bioprostheses was 98 percent and for the mitral valve bioprosthesis was 79 percent; with excellent long-term survival free of major morbidity (see Chap. 79).[166]

REFERENCES

1. Lakatta EG. Cardiovascular regulatory mechanisms in advanced age. *Physiol Rev* 1993;73:413–465.
2. Lakatta EG. Cellular and molecular clues to heart and arterial aging. *Circulation* 2003;107:490–497.
3. Najjar SS, Lakatta EG. Vascular aging: from molecular to clinical cardiology. In: *Principles of Molecular Cardiology*. Totowa, NJ: Humana Press, 2002:517–567.
4. Wang M, Lakatta EG. Arterial stiffness in hypertension. In: Safar M (ed). *Handbook of Hypertension*. The Netherlands: Elsevier, 2006.
5. Gerstenblith G, Frederiksen J, Yin FC, et al. Echocardiographic assessment of a normal adult aging population. *Circulation* 1977;56:273–278.
6. Nagai Y, Metter EJ, Earley CJ, et al. Increased carotid artery intimal-medial thickness in asymptomatic older subjects with exercise-induced myocardial ischemia. *Circulation* 1998;98:1504–1509.
7. Vaitkevicius PV, Fleg JL, Engel JH, et al. Effects of age and aerobic capacity on arterial stiffness in healthy adults. *Circulation* 1993;88:1456–1462.
8. Lakatta EG, Levy D. Arterial and cardiac aging: major shareholders in cardiovascular disease enterprises: part I. Aging arteries: a "set up" for vascular disease. *Circulation* 2003;107:139–146.
9. Celermajer DS, Sorensen KE, Spiegelhalter DJ, et al. Aging is associated with endothelial dysfunction in healthy men years before the age-related decline in women. *J Am Coll Cardiol* 1994;24:471–476.
10. Kannel WB. Elevated systolic blood pressure as a cardiovascular risk factor. *Am J Cardiol* 2000;85:251–255.
11. Chobanian AV, Bakris GL, Black HR, et al. National Heart, Lung, and Blood Institute Joint National Committee on Prevention, Detection, Evaluation, and Treatment of High Blood Pressure; National High Blood Pressure Education Program Coordinating Committee. The seventh report of the Joint National Committee on Prevention, Detection, Evaluation, and Treatment of High Blood Pressure: the JNC 7 report. *JAMA* 2003;289:2560–2572.
12. Woo KS, Chook P, Raitakari OT, et al. Westernization of Chinese adults and increased subclinical atherosclerosis. *Arterioscler Thromb Vasc Biol* 1999;19:2487–2493.
13. Adams MR, Nakagomi A, Keech A, et al. Carotid intima-media thickness is only weakly correlated with the extent and severity of coronary artery disease. *Circulation* 1995;92:2127–2134.

14. Graner M, Varpula M, Kahri J, et al. Association of carotid intima-media thickness with angiographic severity and extent of coronary artery disease. *Am J Cardiol* 2006;97:624–629.
15. Chambless LE, Folsom AR, Clegg LX, et al. Carotid wall thickness is predictive of incident clinical stroke: the Atherosclerosis Risk in Communities (ARIC) study. *Am J Epidemiol* 2000;151:478–487.
16. O'Leary DH, Polak JF, Kronmal RA, et al. Carotid artery intima and media thickness as a risk factor for myocardial infarction and stroke in older adults. Cardiovascular Health Study Collaborative Research Group. *N Engl J Med* 1999;340:14–22.
17. Scuteri A, Chen CH, Yin FC, et al. Functional correlates of central arterial geometric phenotypes. *Hypertension* 2001;38:1471–1475.
18. Scuteri A, Manolio TA, Marino EK, et al. Prevalence of specific variant carotid geometric patterns and incidence of cardiovascular events in older persons. The Cardiovascular Health Study (CHS E-131). *J Am Coll Cardiol* 2004;43:187–193.
19. Sutton-Tyrrell K, Newman A, Simonsick EM, et al. Aortic stiffness is associated with visceral adiposity in older adults enrolled in the study of health, aging, and body composition. *Hypertension* 2001;38:429–433.
20. Liao D, Arnett DK, Tyroler HA, et al. Arterial stiffness and the development of hypertension. The ARIC study. *Hypertension* 1999;34:201–206.
21. Blacher J, Pannier B, Guerin AP, et al. Carotid arterial stiffness as a predictor of cardiovascular and all-cause mortality in end-stage renal disease. *Hypertension* 1998;32:570–574.
22. Boutouyrie P, Tropeano AI, Asmar R, et al. Aortic stiffness is an independent predictor of primary coronary events in hypertensive patients: a longitudinal study. *Hypertension* 2002;39:10–15.
23. Laurent S, Boutouyrie P, Asmar R, et al. Aortic stiffness is an independent predictor of all cause and cardiovascular mortality in hypertensive patients. *Hypertension* 2001;37:1236–1241.
24. Willum-Hansen T, Staessen JA, Torp-Pedersen C, et al. Prognostic value of aortic pulse wave velocity as index of arterial stiffness in the general population. *Circulation* 2006;113:664–670.
25. Mattace-Raso FU, van der Cammen TJ, Knetsch AM, et al. Arterial stiffness as the candidate underlying mechanism for postural blood pressure changes and orthostatic hypotension in older adults: the Rotterdam Study. *J Hypertens* 2006;24:339–344.
26. Sutton-Tyrrell K, Najjar SS, Boudreau RM, et al. Health ABC study. Elevated aortic pulse wave velocity, a marker of arterial stiffness, predicts cardiovascular events in well-functioning older adults. *Circulation* 2005;111:3384–3390.
27. Blacher J, Guerin AP, Pannier B, et al. Impact of aortic stiffness on survival in end-stage renal disease. *Circulation* 1999;99:2434–2439.
28. de Simone G, Roman MJ, Koren MJ, et al. Stroke volume/pulse pressure ratio and cardiovascular risk in arterial hypertension. *Hypertension* 1999;33:800–805.
29. Blacher J, Asmar R, Djane S, et al. Aortic pulse wave velocity as a marker of cardiovascular risk in hypertensive patients. *Hypertension* 1999;33:1111–1117.
30. McVeigh GE, Allen PB, Morgan DR, et al. Nitric oxide modulation of blood vessel tone identified by arterial waveform analysis. *Clin Sci (Lond)* 2001;100:387–393.
31. Kelly R, Hayward C, Avolio A, et al. Noninvasive determination of age-related changes in the human arterial pulse. *Circulation* 1989;80:1652–1659.
32. Chen CH, Nevo E, Fetics B, et al. Estimation of central aortic pressure waveform by mathematical transformation of radial tonometry pressure. Validation of generalized transfer function. *Circulation* 1997;95:1827–1836.
33. McVeigh GE, Hamilton PK, Morgan DR. Evaluation of mechanical arterial properties: clinical, experimental and therapeutic aspects. *Clin Sci (Lond)* 2002;102:51–67.
34. London GM, Blacher J, Pannier B, et al. Arterial wave reflections and survival in end-stage renal failure. *Hypertension* 2001;38:434–438.
35. Sesso HD, Stampfer MJ, Rosner B, et al. Systolic and diastolic blood pressure, pulse pressure, and mean arterial pressure as predictors of cardiovascular disease risk in men. *Hypertension* 2000;36:801–807.
36. Dernellis J, Panaretou M. Aortic stiffness is an independent predictor of progression to hypertension in nonhypertensive subjects. *Hypertension* 2005;45:426–431.
37. Toborek M, Kaiser S. Endothelial cell functions. Relationship to atherogenesis. *Basic Res Cardiol* 1999;94:295–314.
38. Wilkinson IB, Franklin SS, Cockcroft JR. Nitric oxide and the regulation of large artery stiffness: from physiology to pharmacology. *Hypertension* 2004;44:112–116.

39. Cernadas MR, Sanchez de Miguel L, et al. Expression of constitutive and inducible nitric oxide synthases in the vascular wall of young and aging rats. *Circ Res* 1998;83:279–286.

40. Csiszar A, Ungvari Z, Edwards JG, et al. Aging-induced phenotypic changes and oxidative stress impair coronary arteriolar function. *Circ Res* 2002;90:1159–1166.

41. Rosenberg GA, Estrada EY, Dencoff JE. Matrix metalloproteinases and TIMPs are associated with blood–brain barrier opening after reperfusion in rat brain. *Stroke* 1998;29:2189–2195.

42. Blann AD, Daly RJ, Amiral J. The influence of age, gender and ABO blood group on soluble endothelial cell markers and adhesion molecules. *Br J Haematol* 1996;92:498–500.

43. Morisaki N, Saito I, Tamura K, et al. New indices of ischemic heart disease and aging: studies on the serum levels of soluble intercellular adhesion molecule-1 (ICAM-1) and soluble vascular cell adhesion molecule-1 (VCAM-1) in patients with hypercholesterolemia and ischemic heart disease. *Atherosclerosis* 1997;131:43–48.

44. Bingley JA, Hayward IP, Campbell GR, et al. Relationship of glycosaminoglycan and matrix changes to vascular smooth muscle cell phenotype modulation in rabbit arteries after acute injury. *J Vasc Surg* 2001;33:155–164.

45. Okuda K, Khan MY, Skurnick J, et al. Telomere attrition of the human abdominal aorta: relationships with age and atherosclerosis. *Atherosclerosis* 2000;152:391–398.

46. Chang E, Harley CB. Telomere length and replicative aging in human vascular tissues. *Proc Natl Acad Sci U S A* 1995;92:11190–11194.

47. Jeanclos E, Schork NJ, Kyvik KO, et al. Telomere length inversely correlates with pulse pressure and is highly familial. *Hypertension* 2000;36:195–200.

48. Benetos A, Okuda K, Lajemi M, et al. Telomere length as an indicator of biological aging: the gender effect and relation with pulse pressure and pulse wave velocity. *Hypertension* 2001;37:381–385.

49. Minamino T, Miyauchi H, Yoshida T, et al. Endothelial cell senescence in human atherosclerosis: role of telomere in endothelial dysfunction. *Circulation* 2002;105:1541–1544.

50. Rauscher FM, Goldschmidt-Clermont PJ, Davis BH, et al. Aging, progenitor cell exhaustion, and atherosclerosis. *Circulation* 2003;108:457–463.

51. Conboy IM, Conboy MJ, Wagers AJ, et al. Rejuvenation of aged progenitor cells by exposure to a young systemic environment. *Nature* 2005;433:760–764.

52. Edelberg JM, Reed MJ. Aging and Angiogenesis. *Front Biosci* 2003;8:s1199–s1209.

53. Arnett DK, Tyroler HA, Burke G, et al. Hypertension and subclinical carotid artery atherosclerosis in blacks and whites. The Atherosclerosis Risk in Communities Study. ARIC Investigators. *Arch Intern Med* 1996;156:1983–1989.

54. Amar J, Ruidavets JB, Chamontin B, et al. Arterial stiffness and cardiovascular risk factors in a population-based study. *J Hypertens* 2001;19:381–387.

55. Nichols WW, Nicolini FA, Pepine CJ. Determinants of isolated systolic hypertension in the elderly. *J Hypertens Suppl* 1992;10:S73–S77.

56. Laurent S, Lacolley P, Girerd X, et al. Arterial stiffening: opposing effects of age- and hypertension-associated structural changes. *Can J Physiol Pharmacol* 1996;74:842–849.

57. O'Rourke MF, Nichols WW. Aortic diameter, aortic stiffness, and wave reflection increase with age and isolated systolic hypertension. *Hypertension* 2005;45:652–658.

58. Mitchell GF, Lacourciere Y, Ouellet JP, et al. Determinants of elevated pulse pressure in middle-aged and older subjects with uncomplicated systolic hypertension: the role of proximal aortic diameter and the aortic pressure-flow relationship. *Circulation* 2003;108:1592–1598.

59. Taddei S, Virdis A, Mattei P, et al. Hypertension causes premature aging of endothelial function in humans. *Hypertension* 1997;29:736–743.

60. Taddei S, Virdis A, Mattei P, et al. Defective L-arginine-nitric oxide pathway in offspring of essential hypertensive patients. *Circulation* 1996;94:1298–1303.

61. Scuteri A, Najjar SS, Morrell CH, et al. The metabolic syndrome in older individuals: prevalence and prediction of cardiovascular events: the Cardiovascular Health Study. *Diabetes Care* 2005;28:882–887.

62. Scuteri A, Najjar SS, Muller DC, et al. Metabolic syndrome amplifies the age-associated increases in vascular thickness and stiffness. *J Am Coll Cardiol* 2004;43:1388–1395.

63. Wagenknecht LE, Zaccaro D, Espeland MA, et al. Diabetes and progression of carotid atherosclerosis: the insulin resistance atherosclerosis study. *Arterioscler Thromb Vasc Biol* 2003;23:1035–1041.

64. Lacy PS, O'Brien DG, Stanley AG, et al. Increased pulse wave velocity is not associated with elevated augmentation index in patients with diabetes. *J Hypertens* 2004;22:1937–1944.

65. Schofield I, Malik R, Izzard A, et al. Vascular structural and functional changes in type 2, diabetes mellitus: evidence for the roles of abnormal myogenic responsiveness and dyslipidemia. *Circulation* 2002;106:3037–3043.

66. Balletshofer BM, Rittig K, Enderle MD, et al. Endothelial dysfunction is detectable in young normotensive first-degree relatives of subjects with type 2 diabetes in association with insulin resistance. *Circulation* 2000;101:1780–1784.

67. Jeanclos E, Krolewski A, Skurnick J, et al. Shortened telomere length in white blood cells of patients with IDDM. *Diabetes* 1998;47:482–486.

68. van Popele NM, Grobbee DE, Bots ML, et al. Association between arterial stiffness and atherosclerosis: the Rotterdam Study. *Stroke* 2001;32:454–460.

69. Weber T, Auer J, O'Rourke MF, et al. Arterial stiffness, wave reflections, and the risk of coronary artery disease. *Circulation* 2004;109:184–189.

70. Samani NJ, Boultby R, Butler R, et al. Telomere shortening in atherosclerosis. *Lancet* 2001;358:472–473.

71. Lakatta EG, Levy D. Arterial and cardiac aging: major shareholders in cardiovascular disease enterprises: part II. The aging heart in health: links to heart disease. *Circulation* 2003;107(2):346–354.

72. Olivetti G, Giordano G, Corradi D, et al. Gender differences and aging: Effects in the human heart. *J Am Coll Cardiol* 1995;26:1068.

73. Correia LC, Lakatta EG, O'Connor FC, et al. Attenuated cardiovascular reserve during prolonged submaximal cycle exercise in healthy older subjects. *J Am Coll Cardiol* 2002;40:1290–1297.

74. Yin FCP, Raizes GS, Guarnieri T, et al. Age-associated decrease in ventricular response to haemodynamic stress during beta-adrenergic blockade. *Br Heart J* 1978;40:1349–1355.

75. Fleg JL, O'Connor FC, Gerstenblith G, et al. Impact of age on the cardiovascular response to dynamic upright exercise in healthy men and women. *J Appl Physiol* 1995;78:890–900.

76. Chen C-H, Ting C-T, Lin S-J, et al. Which arterial and cardiac parameters best predict left ventricular mass? *Circulation* 1998;98:422.

77. Chen C-H, Nakayama M, Talbot M, et al. Verapamil acutely reduces ventricular-vascular stiffening and improves aerobic exercise performance in elderly individuals. *J Am Coll Cardiol* 1999;33:1602–1609.

78. Najjar SS, Schulman SP, Gerstenblith G. Age and gender affect ventricular-vascular coupling during aerobic exercise. *J Am Coll Cardiol* 2004;44(3):611–617.

79. Nussbacher A, Gerstenblith G, O'Connor F, et al. Hemodynamic effects of unloading the old heart. *Am J Physiol* 1999;277:H1863–H1871.

80. Seals DR, Dempsey JA. Aging, exercise and cardiopulmonary function. In: Lamb DR, Gisolfi CV, Nadel E, eds. *Perspectives in Exercise Science and Sports Medicine*. Vol 8. Carmel, IN: Cooper Publishing Group, 1995:237–304.

81. Lakatta EG. Deficient neuroendocrine regulation of the cardiovascular system with advancing age in healthy humans (point of view). *Circulation* 1993;87:631.

82. Fleg JL, Schulman S, O'Connor F, et al. Effects of acute β-adrenergic receptor blockade on age-associated changes in cardiovascular performance during dynamic exercise. *Circulation* 1994;90:2333.

83. Yin FCP, Weisfeldt ML, Milnor WR. Role of aortic input impedance in the decreased cardiovascular response to exercise with aging in dogs. *J Clin Invest* 1981;68:28–38.

84. Talbot LA, Metter EJ, Fleg JL. Leisure-time physical activities and their relationship to cardiorespiratory fitness in healthy men and women 18–95 years old. *Med Sci Sports Exerc* 2000;32:417–425.

85. Fleg JL, Morrell CH, Bos AG, et al. Accelerated longitudinal decline of aerobic capacity in healthy older adults. *Circulation* 2005;112:674–682.

86. Woo JS, Derleth C, Stratton JR, et al. The influence of age, gender, and training on exercise efficiency. *J Am Coll Cardiol* 2006;47(5):1049–1057.

87. Schulman SP, Fleg JL, Goldberg AP, et al. Continuum of cardiovascular performance across a broad range of fitness levels in healthy older men. *Circulation* 1996;94:359–367.

88. Tanaka H, DeSouza CA, Seals DR. Absence of age-related increase in central arterial stiffness in physically active women. *Arterioscler Thromb Vasc Biol* 1998;18:127–132.

89. Das DN, Fleg JL, Lakatta EG. Effect of age on the components of atrioventricular conduction in normal man. *Am J Cardiol* 1982;49(2):1031.

90. Tsuji H, Larson MG, Venditti FJ, et al. Impact of reduced heart rate variability on risk for cardiac events. *Circulation* 1996;94:2850–2855.

91. Fleg JL, Kennedy HL. Cardiac arrhythmias in a healthy elderly population: detection by 24-hour ambulatory electrocardiography. *Chest* 1982;81:302–307.

92. Fleg JL, Kennedy HL. Long-term prognosis significance of ambulatory electrocardiographic findings in apparently healthy subjects 60 years of age. *Am J Cardiol* 1992;70:748–751.

93. Manolio TA, Furberg CD, Rautaharju PM, et al. Cardiac arrhythmias on 24-hour ambulatory electrocardiography in older women and men: the Cardiovascular Health Study. *J Am Coll Cardiol* 1994;23:916–925.

94. Maurer MS, Shefrin EA, Fleg JL. Prevalence and prognostic significance of exercise-induced supraventricular tachycardia in apparently healthy volunteers. *Am J Cardiol* 1995;756:788–792.

95. Busby MJ, Shefrin EA, Fleg JL. Prevalence and long-term significance of exercise-induced frequent or repetitive ventricular ectopic beats in apparently healthy volunteers. *J Am Coll Cardiol* 1989;14(7):1659–1665.

96. Lakatta EG, Sollott SJ. The "heartbreak" of older age. *Mol Interv* 2002;2(7):431–446.

97. Hunt BE, Farquhar WB, Taylor JA. Does reduced vascular stiffening fully explain preserved cardiovagal baroreflex function in older, physically active men? *Circulation* 2001;103:2424–2427.

98. Rywik TM, Blackman R, Yataco AR, et al. Enhanced endothelial vasoreactivity in endurance trained older men. *J Appl Physiol* 1999;87:2136–2142.

99. Avolio AP, Clyde KM, Beard TC, et al. Improved arterial distensibility in normotensive subjects on a low salt diet. *Arteriosclerosis* 1986;6:166–169.

100. Abete P, Ferrara N, Cacciatore F, et al. High level of physical activity preserves the cardioprotective effect of preinfarction angina in elderly patients. *J Am Coll Cardiol* 2001;38:1357–1365.

101. Michel JB, Heudes D, Michel O, et al. Effect of chronic ANG I-converting enzyme inhibition on aging processes. II. Large arteries. *Am J Physiol* 1994;267:R124–R135.

102. Wolfenbuttel BHR, Boulanger CM, Crijns FRL, et al. Breakers of advanced glycation end products restore large artery properties in experimental diabetes. *Proc Natl Acad Sci U S A* 1998;95:4630–4634.

103. Asif M, Egan J, Vasan S, et al. An advanced glycation end product cross-link breaker can reverse age-related increases in myocardial stiffness. *Proc Natl Acad Sci U S A* 2000;97:2809–2813.

104. Vaitkevicius PV, Lane M, Spurgeon HA, et al. A cross-link breaker has sustained effects on arterial and ventricular properties in older rhesus monkeys. *Proc Natl Acad Sci U S A* 2001;98:1171–1175.

105. Kass DA, Shapiro EP, Kawaguchi M, et al. Improved arterial compliance by a novel advanced glycation end-product crosslink breaker. *Circulation* 2001;104:1464–1470.

106. Glynn RJ, Chae CU, Guralnik JM, et al. Pulse pressure and mortality in older people. *Arch Intern Med* 2000;160:2765–2772.

107. Fagard RH, Pardaens K, Staessen JA, et al. The pulse pressure-to-stroke index ratio predicts cardiovascular events and death in uncomplicated hypertension. *J Am Coll Cardiol* 2001;38:227–231.

108. Roger VL, Jacobsen SJ, Weston SA, et al. Trends in the incidence and survival of patients with hospitalized myocardial infarction, Olmstead County, Minnesota 1979 to 1994. *Ann Intern Med* 2002;136:341–348.

109. Eagle KA, Lim MJ, Dabbous OH, et al. A validated prediction model for all forms of acute coronary syndrome. *JAMA* 2004;291:2727–2733.

110. Hasdai D, Holmes DR, Criger DA, et al. Age and outcome after acute coronary syndromes without persistent ST-segment elevation. *Am Heart J* 2000;139:858–866.

111. Kurotobi T, Sato H, Kinjor K, et al. Reduced collateral circulation to the infarct-related artery in elderly patients with acute myocardial infarction. *J Am Coll Cardiol* 2004;44:28–34.

112. Szmitko PE, Fedak PWM, Weisel RD, et al. Endothelial progenitor cells. New hope for a broken heart. *Circulation* 2003;107:3093–3100.

113. Scheubel RJ, Zorn H, Rolf-Edgar S, et al. Age-dependent depression in circulating endothelial progenitor cells in patients undergoing coronary artery bypass grafting. *J Am Coll Cardiol* 2003;42:2073–2080.

114. Werner N, Kosiol S, Schiegl T, et al. Circulating endothelial progenitor cells and cardiovascular outcomes. *N Engl J Med* 2005;353:999–1007.

115. Bueno H, Martinez-Selles M, Perez-David E, et al. Effect of thrombolytic therapy on the risk of cardiac rupture and mortality in older patients with first acute myocardial infarction. *Eur Heart J* 2005;26:1705–1711.

116. Maggioni AP, Maseri A, Fresco C, et al. Age-related increase in mortality among patients with first myocardial infarctions treated with thrombolysis. *N Engl J Med* 1993;329:1442–1448.

117. Eagle KA, Goodman SG, Avezum A, et al. Practice variation and missed opportunities for reperfusion in ST-segment-elevation myocardial infarction: findings from the Global Registry of Acute Coronary Events (GRACE). *Lancet* 2002;359:373–377.

118. White HD. Thrombolytic therapy in the elderly. *Lancet* 2000;356:2028–2030.

119. Thiemann DR, Coresh J, Schulman SP, et al. Lack of benefit of thrombolysis in patients with myocardial infarction who are older than 75 years. *Circulation* 2000;101:2239–2246.

120. GUSTO V Investigators. Reperfusion therapy for acute myocardial infarction with fibrinolytic therapy or combination reduced fibrinolytic therapy and platelet glycoprotein IIb/IIIa inhibition: the GUSTO V randomised trial. *Lancet* 2001;357:1905–1914.

121. Mehta RH, Granger CB, Alexander KP, et al. Reperfusion strategies for acute myocardial infarction in the elderly. *J Am Coll Cardiol* 2005;45:471–478.

122. Thune JJ, Hoefsten DE, Lindholm MG, et al. Simple risk stratification at admission to identify patients with reduced mortality from primary angioplasty. *Circulation* 2005;112:2017-2021.

123. Hochman JS, Sleeper LA, Webb JG, et al. Early revascularization and long-term survival in cardiogenic shock complicating acute myocardial infarction. *JAMA* 2006;295:2511–2515.

124. Antithrombotic Trialists' Collaboration. Collaborative meta-analysis of randomised trials of antiplatelet therapy for prevention of death, myocardial infarction, and stroke in high risk patients. *BMJ* 2002;324:71–86.

125. The Clopidogrel in Unstable Angina to Prevent Recurrent Ischemia Events Trial Investigators. Effects of clopidogrel in addition to aspirin in patients with acute coronary syndromes without ST segment elevation. *N Engl J Med* 2001;345:494–502.

126. Flather MD, Yusuf S, Køber L, et al. Long-term ACE-inhibitor therapy in patients with heart failure or left-ventricular dysfunction: a systematic overview of data from individual patients. *Lancet* 2000;355:1575–1581.

127. Pfeffer MA, McMurray JJV, Velazquez EJ, et al. Valsartan, captopril, or both in myocardial infarction complicated by heart failure, left ventricular dysfunction, or both. *N Engl J Med* 2003;349:1893–1906.

128. Mehta SR, Cannon CP, Fox KAA, et al. Routine versus selective invasive strategies in patients with acute coronary syndrome: a collaborative meta-analysis of randomized trials. *JAMA* 2005;292:2908–2917.

129. Bach RG, Cannon CP, Weintraub WS, et al. The effect of routine, early invasive management on outcome for elderly patients with non-ST-segment elevation acute coronary syndromes. *Ann Intern Med* 2004;141:186–195.

130. Peterson ED, Alexander KP, Malenka DJ, et al. Multicenter experience in revascularization of very elderly patients. *Am Heart J* 2004;148:486–492.

131. Alexander KP, Anstrom KJ, Muhlbaier LH, et al. Outcomes of cardiac surgery in patients age > 80, years: results from the National Cardiovascular Network. *J Am Coll Cardiol* 2000;35:731–738.

132. Newman MF, Kirchner JL, Phillips-Bute B, et al. for the Neurological Outcome Research Group and the Cardiothoracic Anesthesiology Research Endeavors Investigators. Longitudinal assessment of neurocognitive function after coronary artery bypass surgery. *N Engl J Med* 2001;344:395–402.

133. Athanasiou T, Al-Ruzzeh S, Kumar P, et al. Off-pump myocardial revascularization is associated with less incidence of stroke in elderly patients. *Ann Thorac Surg* 2004;77:745–753.

134. Nathoe HM, van Dijk D, Jansen WEL, et al. A comparison of on-pump and off-pump coronary bypass surgery in low-risk patients. *N Engl J Med* 2003;348:394–402.

135. Jensen BO, Hughes P, Rasmussen LS, et al. Cognitive outcomes in elderly high-risk patients after off-pump versus conventional coronary artery bypass grafting. *Circulation* 2006;113:2790–2795.

136. The TIME Investigators. Trial of invasive versus medical therapy in elderly patients with chronic symptomatic coronary-artery disease (TIME): a randomised trial. *Lancet* 2001;358:951-957.

137. Pfisterer M. Long-term outcome in elderly patients with chronic angina managed invasively versus by optimized medical therapy. Four year quality of life scores improved over time in both groups. *Circulation* 2004;110:1213–1218.

138. Morrison DA, Sethi G, Sacks J, et al. Percutaneous coronary intervention versus coronary artery bypass graft surgery for patients with medically refractory myocardial ischemia and risk factors for adverse outcomes with bypass: a multicenter, randomized trial. *J Am Coll Cardiol* 2001;38:143–149).

139. American Heart Association. *Heart Disease and Stroke Statistics—2006 Update*. Dallas, TX: American Heart Association, 2006.

140. Levy D, Kenchaiah S, Larson MG, et al. Long-term trends in the incidence of and survival with heart failure. *N Engl J Med* 2002;347:1397–1402.

141. Kitzman DW, Little WC, Anderson RT, et al. Pathophysiological characterization of isolated diastolic heart failure in comparison to systolic heart failure. *JAMA* 2002;288:2144–2150.

142. Bhatia RS, Tu JV, Lee DS, et al. Outcome of heart failure with preserved ejection fraction in a population-based study. *N Engl J Med* 2006;355:260–269.

143. Braunstein JB, Anderson GF, Gerstenblith G, et al. Noncardiac comorbidity increases preventable hospitalizations and mortality among Medicare beneficiaries with chronic heart failure. *J Am Coll Cardiol* 2003;42:1226–1233.

144. Packer M, Coats AJS, Fowler MB, et al. Effect of carvedilol on survival in severe chronic heart failure. *N Engl J Med* 2001;344:1651–1658.

145. Pitt B, Zannad F, Remme WJ, et al. for the Randomized Aldactone Study Investigators. The effect of spironolactone on morbidity and mortality in patients with severe heart failure. *N Engl J Med* 1999;341:709–717.

146. Baine WB, Yu W, Weis KA. Trends and outcomes in the hospitalization of older Americans for cardiac conduction disturbances or arrhythmias 1991–1998. *J Am Geriatr Soc* 2001;49:763–770.

147. Granda J, Uribe W, Chyou PH, et al. Incidence and predictors of atrial flutter in the general population. *J Am Coll Cardiol* 2004;36:2242–2246.

148. Natale A, Newby KH, Pisano E, et al. Prospective randomized comparison of antiarrhythmic therapy versus first-line radiofrequency ablation in patients with atrial flutter. *J Am Coll Cardiol* 2000;335:1898–1904.

149. Ozcan C, Zahangir A, Friedman PA, et al. Long-term survival after ablation of the atrioventricular node and implantation of a permanent pacemaker in patients with atrial fibrillation. *N Engl J Med* 2001;344:1043–1051.

150. The Atrial Fibrillation Follow-Up Investigation of Rhythm Management (AFFIRM) Investigators. A comparison of rate control and rhythm control in patients with atrial fibrillation. *N Engl J Med* 2002;347:1825–1833.

151. Van Gelder IC, Hagens VE, Hosker HA, et al. A comparison of rate control and rhythm control in patients with recurrent persistent atrial fibrillation. *N Engl J Med* 2002;347:1834-1840.

152. Torp-Pedersen C, Moller M, Bloch-Thomsen PE, et al. for the Danish Investigations of Arrhythmia and Mortality on Dofetilide Study Group. Dofetilide in patients with congestive heart failure and left ventricular dysfunction. *N Engl J Med* 1999;341:857–865.

153. Roy D, Talajic M, Dorian P, et al. Amiodarone to prevent recurrence of atrial fibrillation. *N Engl J Med* 2000;342:913–920.

154. Lamas GA, Lee KL, Sweeney MO, et al. Ventricular pacing or dual-chamber pacing for sinus node dysfunction. *N Engl J Med* 2002;346:1854–1862.

155. Moss AJ, Zareba W, Hall, J, et al. Prophylactic implantation of a defibrillator in patients with myocardial infarction and reduced ejection fraction. *N Engl J Med* 2002;346:877–883.

156. Kadish A, Dyer A, Daubert JP. Prophylactic defibrillator implantation in patients with nonischemic dilated cardiomyopathy. *N Engl J Med* 2004;350:2151–2158.

157. Bonow RO, Carabello BA, Chatterjee K, et al. ACC/AHA 2006 guidelines for the management of patients with valvular heart disease: a report of the American College of Cardiology/American Heart Association Task Force on Practice Guidelines (Writing Committee to Develop Guidelines for the Management of Patients With Valvular Heart Disease). *Circulation* 2006;114:c86–c231.

158. Carabello BA. Aortic stenosis. *N Engl J Med* 2002;346:677–682.

159. Gilard M, Cornily J-C, Pennee P-Y, et al. Accuracy of multislice computed tomography in the preoperative assessment of coronary disease in patients with aortic valve stenosis. *J Am Coll Cardiol* 2006;47:2020–2024.

160. Ambler G, Omar RZ, Royston P, et al. Generic, simple risk stratification model for heart valve surgery. *Circulation* 2005;112:224–231.

161. Cribier A, Eltchanioff H, Tron, et al. Early experience with percutaneous transcatheter implantation of heart valve prosthesis for the treatment of end-stage inoperable patients with calcific aortic stenosis. *J Am Coll Cardiol* 2004;43:698–703.

162. Carabello BA. Vasodilators in aortic regurgitation—where is the evidence of their effectiveness? *N Engl J Med* 2005;353:1400–1402.

163. Otto CM. Evaluation and management of chronic mitral regurgitation. *N Engl J Med* 2001;345:740–746.

164. Mack MJ. Percutaneous mitral valve repair. A fertile field of innovative treatment strategies. *Circulation* 2006;113:2269–2271.

165. Holper K, Ottke M, Lewe T, et al. Bioprosthetic and mechanical valves in the elderly: benefits and risks. *Ann Thorac Surg* 1995;60:S443–S446.

166. Burr LH, Jamieson RE, Munro AI, et al. Porcine bioprostheses in the elderly: clinical performance by age groups and valve positions. *Ann Thorac Surg* 1995;60:S264–S269.

CHAPTER 102

Women and Coronary Artery Disease

Pamela Charney

Cardiovascular (CV) mortality continues at similar or increasing rates for American women, whereas it is decreasing in men (Fig. 102–1). The importance of coronary artery disease (CAD) and its prevention in women is gradually receiving increased physician and public attention.[1–4] Evidence-based guidelines have been published following an expert panel review of the literature for the prevention of CAD in women.[2] Yet, an online survey of primary care physicians, gynecologists, and cardiologists[4] found that fewer than 20 percent of physicians were aware that more women than men die annually of CAD. Intermediate-risk women, defined by Framingham criteria, were more likely to be defined as low risk by the physicians surveyed. Similarly, among >1000 American women telephone interviewed in 2005, only 55 percent identified heart attack and heart disease as the major cause of mortality for women; an improvement from 30 percent of women surveyed in 1997[3] (Fig. 102–2). In contrast, 61 percent of the women reported heart disease as the leading cause of mortality in men. There were substantial ethnic variation among the women surveyed in 2005 (white 62 percent, black 38 percent, and Hispanic women 34 percent). Interestingly, the most frequent reason women had not discussed heart health with their physician was that their provider did not bring up this issue (38 percent).

PREVENTION: GENDER-SPECIFIC ISSUES

TOBACCO

Tobacco exposure is the single most important coronary artery risk factor for women and men.[1,5,6] In epidemiologic studies greater tobacco exposure in amount and duration is related to higher CAD events in a dose-related fashion.[5–7] In 2005 21.9 percent of Americans smoked (>45 million people), 23.9 percent of men and 18.1 percent of women.[8] Among women, more Native American women smoke (26.8 percent) than white (20 percent) or black women (17.3 percent), with lower rates among Hispanic (11.1 percent) and Asian women (6.1 percent).[8,9] Cigarette smoking has been associated with an earlier age of first myocardial infarction (MI) (see also Chap. 51) and menopause.[5] Because middle-aged women experience less symptomatic CAD than middle-aged men, the increased risk of MI and sudden death related to tobacco use is greater for women than men. There is a dose-response relationship for CAD in diabetic women who smoke, as discussed further below, in the Diabetes section.[7]

Over the last several decades, American women's personal use of cigarettes has not decreased as dramatically as it has among men (Fig. 102–3). The prevalence of cigarette use among women reflects both higher initiation rates and lower initial and long-term

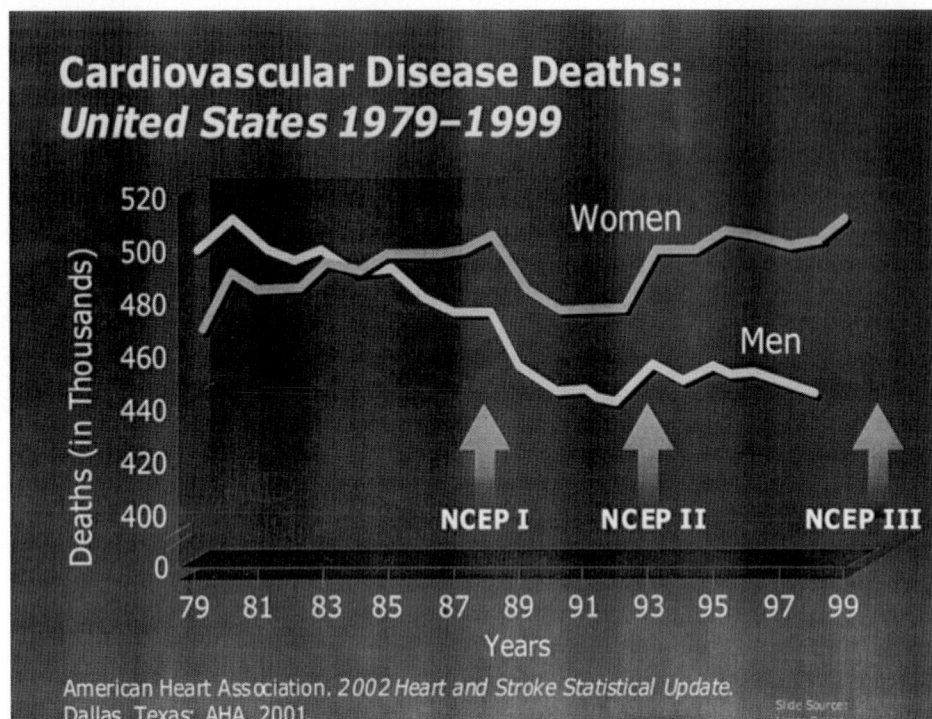

FIGURE 102–1. Graph comparing rates of coronary artery disease for women and men over two decades, with marks when cholesterol guidelines were released. NCEP, National Cholesterol Education Program. *Source: American Heart Association as adapted at http://www.lipidsonline.org. With permission.*

cessation rates.[5,6] However, successful tobacco cessation for women, as for men, dramatically decreases the risk of further coronary events.[5–7] Black smokers also have low both short- and long-term cigarette cessation rates.[5,10]

Women contemplating smoking cessation are often concerned about potential weight gain, a common consequence of efforts to stop smoking.[5,11] Weight gain with tobacco cessation is on average 7 to 10 pounds, with fewer than 10 percent gaining >20 pounds. Weight gain tends to be higher among women, blacks, and smokers who inhale more than 25 cigarettes per day. Women smokers report that they are unwilling to experience any or minimal weight increase as a result of smoking cessation.[5,9] Yet, smokers trying to lose weight are still interested in discontinuing the use of tobacco.[11]

To avoid weight gain with tobacco cessation, several types of interventions have been recommended.[5] Realistic expectations may be helpful as well as exercise, careful choice of snacks, and appropriate pharmacotherapy. Increasing physical activity contributes to success in smoking cessation, as does an increased expenditure of calories, even if it does not modify weight gain.[12]

Multiple pharmacologic therapies are available.[5,6,10,13–15] Success with nicotine replacement products is approximately double tobacco cessation compared with tobacco cessation groups alone.[4,5,13] The patch has the highest compliance rate and provides smoother levels than the gum, spray, or lozenge. However, in a meta-analysis comparing the efficacy of nicotine products in women and men, efficacy was similar up to 6 months followup only.[13] Bupropion has been found to be effective in improving tobacco cessation rates in both white and black smokers[14] and is reported to minimize weight gain while it is used.[5,14] Although bu-

propion is an antidepressant, it has been effective in smokers who are not depressed. Bupropion is contraindicated in patients with a history of seizures, head trauma or heavy alcohol consumption (since it lowers the seizure threshold). Bupropion can exacerbate symptoms related to anorexia and bulimia and should be avoided if there is a history of these disorders or recent use of a monoamine oxidase inhibitor. It has been observed that black smokers may have more trouble giving up tobacco than white smokers.[14,15] Physiologic addiction in black smokers may previously have been underestimated, resulting in undertreatment of nicotine addiction. In a comparison of black and white smokers consuming similar amounts of tobacco, black smokers were found to have higher blood levels of cotinine than white smokers.[15]

Many surveys reveal that physicians can have a powerful effect on smoking cessation, even with minimal effort.[5,6] Programs that promote activities to minimize weight gain and stress social support may be more effective for women. There is substantial evidence that avoiding tobacco exposure is important for women.[1,2,5–8] Additional research about sex and racial differences is needed.

【 】 DIABETES

Diabetic individuals have higher mortality rates from CAD than nondiabetics[16–21] (see also Chap. 90). In the last decade, coronary heart disease (CHD) mortality rates have increased by 23 percent in diabetic women, whereas they have decreased by 27 percent in nondiabetic women. This is in comparison to diabetic men, where mortality rates have declined by 13 percent; but they have de-

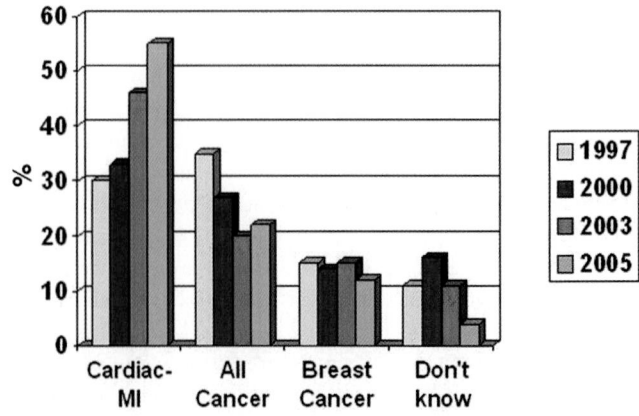

FIGURE 102–2. Trends in American women's knowledge of coronary artery disease. MI, myocardial infarction.

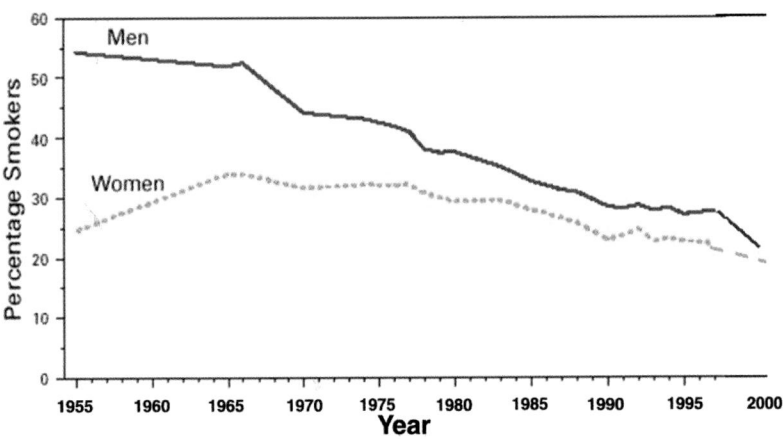

FIGURE 102–3. Prevalence of smoking among men and women age 18 years and under in the United States. Before 1992, current smokers were defined as persons who reported having smoked more than 100 cigarettes and who currently smoked. Since 1992, current smokers are defined as persons who reported having smoked more than 100 cigarettes during their lifetime and who reported now smoking every day or some days. *Sources: 1955 Current Population Survey; 1965-1997 National Health Interview Survey.*

creased by 36 percent in nondiabetic men.[16] A prospective 25-year follow up from Scotland revealed highest mortality rates among those with both diabetes and known CHD with the hazard ratios (HRs) especially high for women 1.97 (95 percent confidence interval [CI] 1.27–3.08, *p* = 0.003) compared with women with neither risk factor[17] (Fig. 102–4). The higher CAD risk for diabetic women has been noted in multiple population studies.[18,19] It has been postulated that sex differences in endothelial function, especially endothelial-dependent vasodilation, may play a pathophysiologic role.[19] Diabetic women have CAD rates similar to those of diabetic men, so the *female advantage* is lost.

Diabetes confers substantial increased relative risk (RR) of first, incident, and admission for MI for women (1.5–4.5 increased RR) compared with age-to-sex matched controls younger than age 65 years over 20 years followup in Copenhagen City Heart Study.[18] This was less dramatic for men (1.5–2.0 increased RR). Diabetic women also have higher in-hospital mortality after MI and an increased incidence of congestive heart failure (CHF) than do diabetic men.[16] In a review of data from the National Registry of Myocardial Infarction (NRMI) II, women's increased post-MI mortality was not associated with glycemic control but rather with hypertension and hyperlipidemia.[20] Additional study may determine whether these observations reflect gender differences in risk factors, natural history, or how less aggressive CAD prevention in diabetic women plays a role. In telephone interviews of diabetic patients with cardiovascular disease (CVD) in 2001, aspirin use was reported by 54.7 percent of women and 82.7 percent of men (RR 0.81, 95 percent CI 0.70–0.90).[21]

Diabetic women and men with hypertension have especially high rates of CAD.[16,20] Native Americans, Mexican Americans, and black populations have a higher prevalence of both diabetes and hypertension than American white populations.[9] Women and men generally have similar incidence rates of diabetes, but more women become hypertensive with increasing age.

Lipid abnormalities are common in diabetic patients. At the time of diagnosis of type II diabetes, women have substantially lower high-density lipoprotein (HDL) cholesterol than age-matched nondiabetic women.[22] Other lipid abnormalities are also present, including elevated triglycerides. Subgroup analysis of diabetic patients treated with hydroxymethylglutaryl coenzyme A (HMG-CoA) reductase inhibitors documented improved lipoprotein patterns with treatment and fewer CAD events.[16] Studies including more women diabetics are in progress.

For diabetic women the dose-response hazards of tobacco use have been documented in the Nurses' Health Study with 20 years of followup.[7] The relative risk for a CAD event was 2.68 for current diabetic smokers of >15 cigarettes daily, 1.66 for current diabetic smokers of <15 cigarettes daily, and 1.21 for past diabetic smokers, all compared with women who had never smoked (*p* <0.001 for trend). Diabetic women who had not smoked for 10 years had a risk similar to that of nonsmoking diabetic women.

Women at risk for developing diabetes include obese women and those who have experienced gestational diabetes (compared with women who have had a pregnancy without glucose intolerance).[16] Greater weight is associated with greater insulin resistance as well as a higher rate of glucose intolerance. Even a moderate increase in physical activity (such as walking 3 hours per week) and avoiding weight gain decreases the risk of developing diabetes.[16]

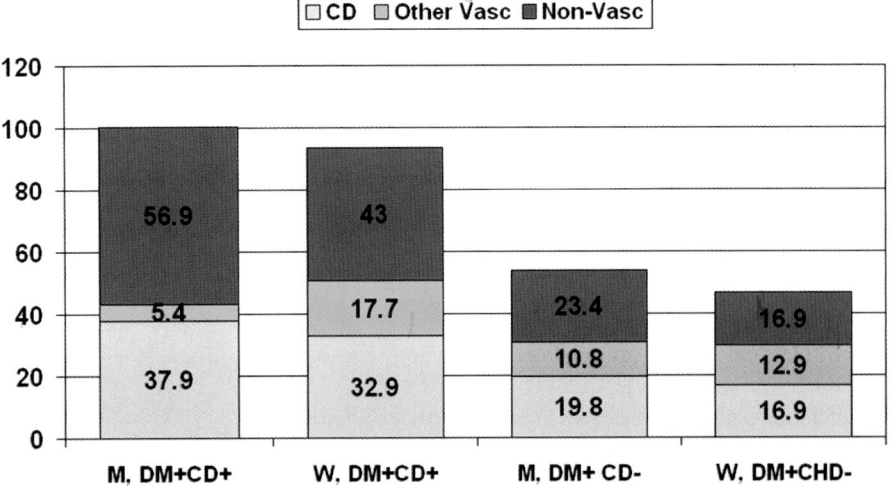

FIGURE 102–4. Mortality in diabetic patients followed prospectively for 25 years. Mortality (deaths per 1000 patient-years) from coronary heart disease (CD), other vascular disease, and nonvascular causes in men (M) and women (W) with and without diabetes (DM+ and DM-) and known coronary heart disease (CD+ and CD-). *Source: Whiteley L, Padmanabhan S, Hole D, Isles C.[17]*

Women with insulin resistance, characterized by elevated levels of circulating insulin often have associated glucose intolerance, higher levels of free fatty acids, central obesity, and hypertension are also at greater risk of developing diabetes.[16] The *metabolic syndrome* was defined in the Third Report of the National Cholesterol Education Program Expert Panel on Detection, Evaluation, and Treatment of High Blood Cholesterol[23] to include obesity, glucose intolerance, hypertension, and lipid abnormalities occurs in women and men at greater rates with increasing age (see Chap. 91). The metabolic syndrome is increasingly diagnosed at an early age[24,25]; tobacco exposure during 12 to 19 years of age dramatically increases the risk of having the metabolic syndrome.[24] Polycystic ovarian syndrome (PCOS) with increased androgens, lower HDL, and higher triglycerides and higher rates of CAD may affect as many as 10 to 20 percent of women of childbearing age.[25,26] In a retrospective chart review of PCOS, patients at an endocrine clinic also had a 43 percent prevalence of the metabolic syndrome (twice the rate of metabolic syndrome for age-matched women without PCOS) once assessed.[27] Pharmacologic and lifestyle interventions may improve prognosis (see Chap. 91). Aggressive management of tobacco use,[7] lipoprotein abnormalities,[16,22] and hypertension[16] is beneficial. Regular exercise can also improve glucose and blood pressure control[16] as well as insulin resistance.[16]

[ ] HYPERTENSION

The prevalence of hypertension also increases with advancing age; and because life expectancy is greater for women than men, there are more elderly women with hypertension.[28] Although women are more likely to be hypertensive than men, there are substantial race and ethnicity variations in hypertension prevalence rates reported in Americans older than age 19 years with black, non-Hispanic women (43.4 percent) and men (40.4 percent) having higher rates than white, non-Hispanic women (28.4 percent) and men (27.5 percent) as well as Mexican American women (27.8 percent) and men (26.7 percent) in 1999 to 2002.[29] Generally, women are more likely to have controlled blood pressure than men. However, sex differences in autonomic nervous system function may explain difficulties in blood pressure modulation in some premenopausal women when exposed to stress or vasoactive drugs.[30]

Both systolic and diastolic blood pressures have been found in population, cohort, and treatment studies to predict coronary events. Framingham data revealed that with a systolic blood pressure >180, the annual incidence of CHD (angina, coronary insufficiency, MI, or death from these diagnoses) in women older than 65 years of age is >30 percent, whereas for men older than age 65 years, it is approximately 50 percent.[31] In other epidemiologic studies, higher diastolic blood pressure also predicts greater rates of clinical CAD.[32] Through Framingham data analysis predictors of new-onset isolated systolic hypertension included female sex, increasing age, and body mass index (BMI) during followup but not initial BMI.[33]

Although treatment trials have also documented that lower blood pressure decreases the incidence of a first MI and sudden death, this effect has been less dramatic than the decrease in stroke occurrence with blood pressure control.[28,33,34] Especially when older subjects were included in clinical trials, the benefit of treating hypertension to prevent coronary events received greater recognition.

Gender-specific information about pharmacologic therapy of hypertension with angiotensin-converting enzyme (ACE) inhibi-

tors and thiazide diuretics continues to evolve. ACE inhibitors should be used cautiously in women of reproductive age as teratogenic effects have been documented in the first as well as second trimester.[35] Potentially fertile women must understand the potential risk to the fetus before initiating therapy. Infants with only first trimester ACE inhibitor exposure had increased risk of CV and central nervous system malformations (RR 2.71 with CI 1.72–4.27) compared with infants not exposed to antihypertensive medications; other antihypertensive medications did not increase risk for congenital abnormalities. Cough, a common side effect of first-generation ACE inhibitors, but not the angiotensin receptor blockers (ARBs), occurred substantially more frequently in women than in men.[36] Thiazide diuretics are a preferred first choice in the treatment of hypertension in women as well as men (Chap. 70) and are also beneficial for bone health. Epidemiologic studies have documented a reduction of approximately one third in hip fracture with the use of thiazide diuretics. In a randomized, double-blind, placebo-controlled trial, thiazides were associated with preservation of hip and spine bone mineral density.[35]

[ ] LIPIDS

There are sex differences in lipoprotein profiles and the impact of lipids on CV risk.[37,38] Many experts consider HDL more predictive for women than any other lipoprotein component, with the strongest correlation between low HDL levels and CAD events. Low-density lipoprotein (LDL) levels increase with increasing age for both women and men and are especially predictive of events in men. Triglyceride levels may be especially important in women. In fact, one group of researchers suggest that enlarged waist (>88 cm) combined with elevated triglycerides (≥1.45 mmol/L) best prospectively identified postmenopausal women at CV risk followed over 8 years.[39]

Although secondary prevention with pharmacologic treatment of hyperlipidemia decreases CAD events in women as well as men,[37,40] these agents are underprescribed for women after MI and target treatment levels are often not reached.[40] Primary prevention trials for hyperlipidemia in women with HMG-CoA reductase inhibitors (which simultaneously decrease LDL and increase HDL) on careful review to do document evidence of benefit with approximately 3 to 6 years of followup, perhaps related to low event rates.[37] With the latest cholesterol treatment guidelines, diabetic women are candidates for primary prevention with aggressive treatment of lipid abnormalities.[23] There is still controversy about the cost-to-benefit ratio for aggressive treatment in the woman at low risk for vascular disease.[37] Treatment of hyperlipidemia is discussed in detail in Chaps. 51 and 91 and the risks and potential benefits of hormonal therapy are discussed under Menopause and Hormonal Therapy.

[ ] OBESITY

The prevalence of obesity has been steadily increasing with a doubling among Americans older than age 20 years from 1980 to 2002.[41] Ethnic and racial differences in obesity are more marked among women than men (Fig. 102–5). Racial differences in BMI, as well as glycosylated hemoglobin, start in childhood, with black and Mexican American girls having less favorable profiles than white girls.[9]

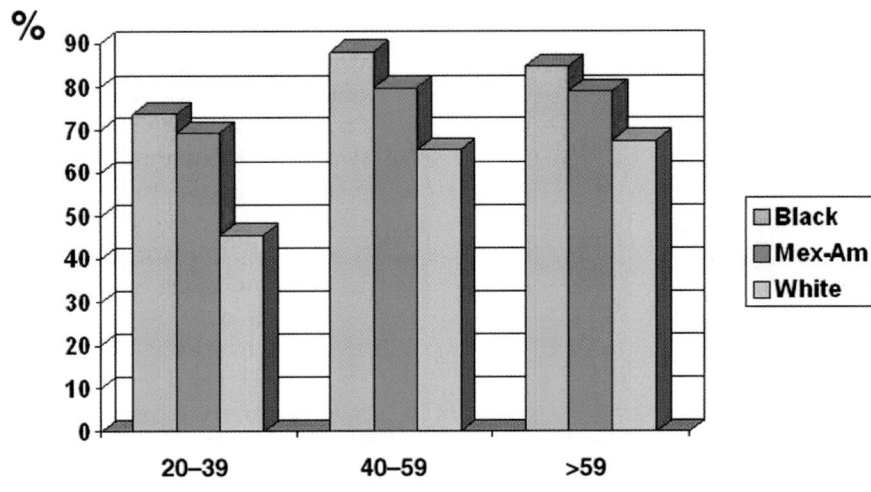

FIGURE 102–5. Prevalence of obesity or overweight by race and age, 2003–2004. *Source: Adapted from Ogden CL, Carroll MD, Curtin LR, McDowell MA, Tabak CJ, Flegal KM.*[39]

Obesity is linked to multiple cardiac risk factors (including insulin resistance, diabetes, hypertension, and hyperlipidemia) and independently associated with coronary artery event rates.[41] The pattern of weight distribution is also predictive of coronary events, with more events among women with the *apple* shape, with a greater central or abdominal girth, than among those with the *pear* shape, with more weight on the hips and buttocks.[42,43] A greater waist circumference increases health risk regardless of BMI.[39,44]

Increased physical activity or limited weight loss is associated with a decreased risk of CAD events.[42,43] Behavioral interventions to decrease weight have been most successful when there is a physical activity component. A study of obese twins revealed that lack of physical activity correlated with the more obese twin.[42] In the Nurses' Health Study, both BMI >25 and physical activity were important predictors of CHD in 20-year followup (Fig. 102–6).[43] Although new pharmacologic treatments for obesity have been developed, many have been documented to be hazardous.[44]

PHYSICAL ACTIVITY AND EXERCISE

Women's physiologic response to exercise includes a lower work capacity and oxygen uptake than men.[1] This occurs because women's cardiac output is increased by raising heart rate. Men, in comparison, accomplish an increase in cardiac output by increasing stroke volume.

Physical activity is important for primary and secondary prevention. Historically, physical activity data collection has focused on leisure-time activity and excluded housework and child care. In 2004 leisure-time physical inactivity was reported by 25.9 percent of women compared with 21.4 percent men, which was an improvement from a decade earlier (31.5 percent for women and 27.9 percent for men).[45] Leisure-time activity reports may greatly underestimate the actual amount of energy expended daily, especially by women. In observing women health professionals over an average of 5 years, women who walked at least 1 hour each week had half the CHD rate as women who did not walk regularly.[46] Both women and men benefit from referral to cardiac rehabilitation programs after

MI; however, fewer women than men are referred for cardiac rehabilitation.[1]

MENOPAUSE AND HORMONAL THERAPY

The importance of the menstrual cycle and menopause as risk factors for CAD in women is still being defined.[47,48] Women with early menopause after gynecologic surgery have been considered at higher risk for CAD and osteoporosis on the basis of less hormonal exposure.[49] However, a 1999 analysis from the Nurses' Health Study found only women smokers with a younger age of menopause have a greater risk of CAD.[48]

Although population surveys suggested hormonal therapy after menopause may decrease the risk of CAD, the women using hormones reported less tobacco exposure, greater levels of exercise, and readier access to medical care; they also tended to be healthier and wealthier.[50–52] The Women's Health Initiative (WHI), a prospective randomized clinical trial of women 50 to 79 years of age, revealed the combination of estrogen and progestin after menopause increases CAD risk[50]; and estrogen alone in women without a uterus, does not decrease CAD risk.[51] Estrogen alone is contraindicated in women with a uterus because of the associated increased risk of endometrial cancer. In the WHI subgroup analysis of women ages 50 to 59 years with 7-year followup conjugated equine estrogen also was not protective.[51] In contrast the observational Nurses' Health Study noted that women beginning hormonal therapy soon after menopause had lower CHD risk (RR 0.72, 95 percent CI 0.56–0.92 for estrogen and progesterone and RR 0.6, 95 percent CI 0.54–0.80 for estrogen alone) than women beginning treatment 10 years after menopause.[53]

The earlier Heart and Estrogen Progestin Replacement Study (HERS)[54] was the first secondary prevention clinical trial of hormonal therapy that also did not demonstrate CV benefit. These postmenopausal women had evidence of CAD (MI, coronary artery bypass grafting [CABG], percutaneous transluminal coronary angioplasty [PTCA] for occlusion >50 percent, or angiography with more than one major coronary artery). Not only was there no overall reduction in CAD events, substantially more venous thrombotic events occurred in the group receiving hormonal therapy. Also remarkable in HERS was the lack of secondary prevention reported in these women with known heart disease (Fig. 102–7).

National guidelines have reflected WHI and HERS results and emphasize other modalities for the prevention of heart disease in women.[3,52] In counseling menopausal women, CV prevention should be a focus. Hormonal therapy is used to control severe vasomotor symptoms.

PSYCHOSOCIAL RISK FACTORS

Both socioeconomic and psychological factors affect the prevalence and outcome of CAD[55,56] (see Chap. 95). Coronary disease morbidity and mortality are greater among those of lower socio-

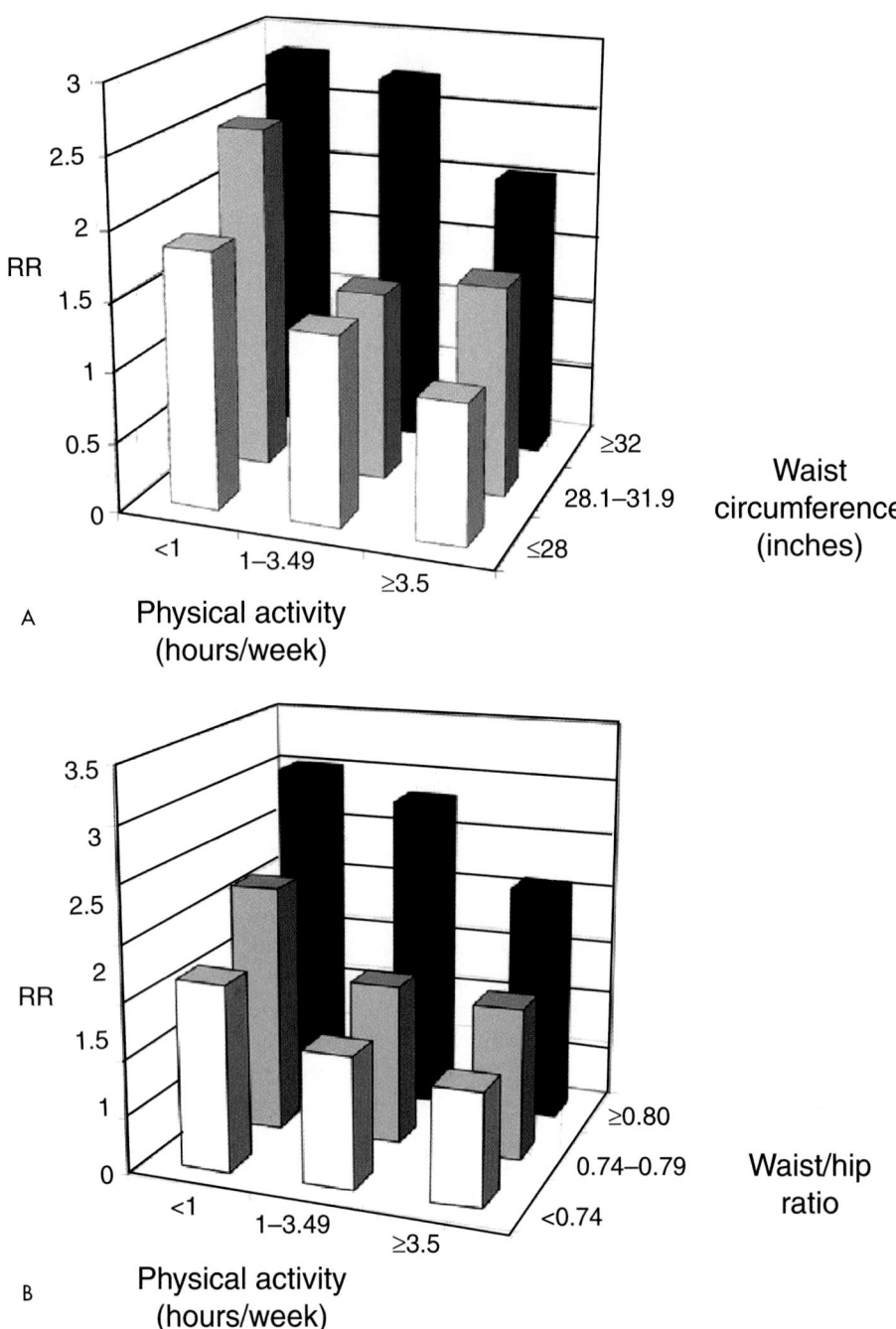

FIGURE 102–6. Physical activity compared with obesity (waist circumference and waist/hip ratio) in predicting risk of coronary heart disease. RR, relative risk. *Source: Li TY, Rana JS, Manson JE, et al.*[43]

sion, and self-reported diabetes were especially prevalent in black women. Although obesity levels did not vary by educational level, as in white and Mexican American women rates of hypertension and self-reported diabetes were more common in those who had not completed high school[57] (Fig. 102–8). Similarly, the Coronary Artery Risk Development in Young Adults Study education level was significantly inversely associated to baseline smoking, BMI, and systolic blood pressure. Furthermore, positive CT coronary artery calcium levels evaluated at age 15 years, mean age 25.2 years, was also inversely related to education (not completing high school odds ratio [OR] 4.4, 95 percent CI 2.33–7.35) overall and in both sexes and races (black and white).[58]

Depression is diagnosed twice as often in women as in men and affects outcomes in CAD.[57,59,60] Depressive symptoms were common within the prior week in the women in the observational arm of the WHI study, which did not include participants with major depression (15.8 percent). There was variation by race and ethnicity ranging from 27 percent for Hispanic women, 26 percent for American Indian Alaskan Native women, 19 percent for black women, 15 percent for white women, and only 11 percent for Asian Pacific Islander American women.[61] There were even larger differences by educational level with 30 percent prevalence among women with less than an eighth-grade education compared with 13 percent for women with a college degree. History of CAD symptoms and diagnoses increased the risk of depression to a greater degree than a history of cancer. For women without CAD history followed for over 4 years, depressive symptoms adjusted for age and race was independently associated with 58 percent higher CVD mortality (RR, 1.58, 95 percent CI 1.19–2.10). In multivariate analysis even including pharmacologic treatment of depression, the increased risk persisted.

economic status (SES).[55,56] Markers for SES have included years of formal education, owning a car, income defined by absolute or relative amount, sex, parental status, and more recently race and ethnicity independent of other issues.[55–58]

Some researchers have used years of formal education, sex, and race to explore disparities.[57,58] The prevalence of common CV risk factors were analyzed in white, black, and Mexican Americans comparing individuals with self-reported completion of high school education or fewer years of formal education. As in other population studies, white women had the highest prevalence of smoking, especially those with less education. Obesity, hyperten-

Depressive symptoms screened for at hospitalization in the Prospective Registry Evaluation Outcomes After Myocardial Infarction: Events and Recovery (PREMIER) study were common (40 percent of women and 22 percent of men 60 years old or younger compared with 21 percent of women and 15 percent of men older than age 60 years).[62] In this cohort the depressed young women had more comorbidity and less favorable health and socioeconomic status. Only 18 percent of those depressed were discharged

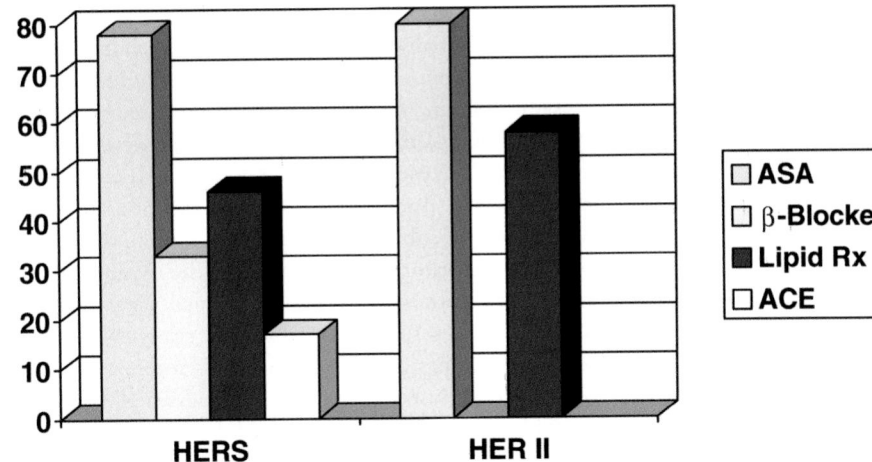

FIGURE 102-7. Preventive medication use (%) among women enrolled in HERS. ACE, angiotensin-converting enzyme; ASA, acetylsalicylic acid; HERS, Heart and Estrogen Progestin Replacement Study; Rx, medication. *Source: Adapted from Grady D, Herrington D, Bittner V, et al.[54] With permission.*

malities in 64.3 percent. Cardiac biomarkers were abnormal in 86.2 percent. The left ventricular dysfunction on admission included ejection fraction means of 20 to 49 percent. Inpatient mortality was only 1.1 percent, and patients generally did well with supportive treatment.

【 】 RACE, WOMEN, AND CORONARY ARTERY DISEASE

Racial differences in mortality, risk factors, physiology have also begun to be considered (see Chap. 103). Black women's CAD mortality rates are related to traditional CAD risk factors as well as racial and socioeconomic issues.[56] Combined analysis of data from the 1986 National Mortality Feedback Survey, the 1985 National Health Interview Survey, and the U.S. Bureau of the Census revealed that black women younger than age 55 years had more than twice the rate of CAD mortality (sudden and nonsudden) as young white Americans.[65] CAD death rates for young black women in this study exceeded rates for young men and white women. Importantly, family income, educational level, and occupational status accounted for more of this observed difference than traditional coronary risk factors.[65] In HERS, a large secondary prevention trial of estrogen and progestin, black women were at increased risk for coronary events at 6 years of followup (relative hazard 2.05 with CI 1.52 to 2.77, $p < 0.001$).[67]

with antidepressant medication. Although an adequate pharmacologic interventional trial of depression diagnosed after MI in women has not yet been reported, the selective serotonin reuptake inhibitors have been found to be clinically safe in the presence of cardiac disease.[60]

Emotional stress, besides depression, has also been related to CV outcomes in women. Acute and reversible cardiomyopathy has been documented after profound stress.[63,64] In the Nurses' Health Study, phobic anxiety has been associated with increased risk of sudden death (discussed in the later section, Sudden Death).[65]

An acute and reversible severe cardiomyopathy was first described in Japan as *tako-tsubo* and more recently in a series of 22 women in the United States.[63] The characteristics are the development of acute symptoms including substernal chest pain most often associated with ST-segment elevation or T wave inversion, or dyspnea, with profound systolic dysfunction and the absence of significant luminal narrowing at angiography. In this initial report, just before developing symptoms each patient experienced either severe emotional or physical distress. Severe left ventricular systolic dysfunction and wall-motion abnormalities described as a ballooning appearance of the mid- and apical left ventricle with a hypercontractile left ventricular base were documented and resolved over as little as 5 days or as long as over 2 months. In a literature review from Europe,[66] 14 studies were identified and 81.6 percent of the patient had ST-segment elevation with T wave abnor-

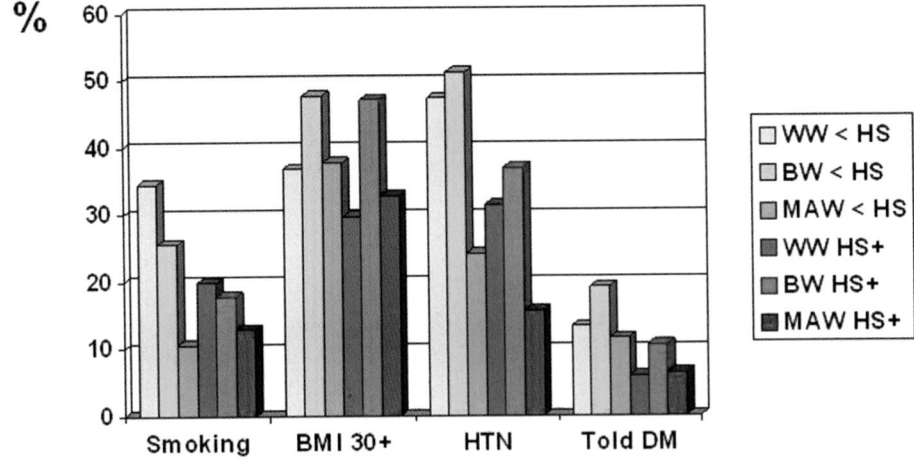

FIGURE 102-8. Selected cardiovascular risk factors for women by self-reported race and high school completion (less years of formal schooling or at least high school graduation). Smoking and *told diabetes* data from the Behavioral Risk Factor Surveillance System and Obesity (BMI ≥30) or hypertension defined by blood pressure >140/90 mmHg or self-reported current use of antihypertensive medication or having been told hypertension diagnosis by a health professional at least twice from National Health and Nutrition Survey 1999–2002. BMI, body mass index; DM, diabetes mellitus; HTN, hypertension; WW, white women; BW, black women; MAW, Mexican-American women. *Source: Adapted from Mensah G, Mokadad A, Ford E, Greenlund K, Croft J.[57]*

With the application of careful methodology, Mexican American women have CHD mortality rates higher or equal to those of non-Hispanic white American women.[68] This observation is consistent with the higher rates of obesity, hypertension, and diabetes among Mexican American women than among white women, even if tobacco use is less frequent.[57] There are less data available on Asian Indian immigrants and those living in India, but preliminary publications report high CAD rates at a young age in both men and women.[69]

【 】 SIGNIFICANT COMORBIDITIES: LUPUS, RHEUMATOID ARTHRITIS, AND MIGRAINE HEADACHES

The potential relationship between medical illness associated with inflammation and the development of CAD has been highlighted because there has been increasing attention to the potential role of inflammation as an etiology of CAD. A case-control evaluation using population-based data from the United Kingdom-based General Practice Research Database compared 8688 patients with MI with matched controls.[70] Higher risk of MI was seen in systemic lupus erythematosus (SLE) 2.67 (95 percent CI 1.34 to 5.34) and rheumatoid arthritis (RA) 1.47 (95 percent CI 1.23–1.76).

The risk of MI in SLE is known to be increased at least fivefold.[71] Coronary risk has been assessed by screening SLE patients with electron-beam CT[71] and carotid ultrasound.[72] When electron-beam cardiac CT was provided to 65 consecutive patients with SLE (91 percent female) as well as age-, race-, and sex-matched controls, coronary calcification was more often seen (31 percent vs. 9 percent, $p = 0.002$) with after adjustment for risk factors and OR 9.8 ($p = 0.001$). There was a substantial effect of increasing age with a prevalence of coronary calcification of 7 percent in the small number of subjects younger than 40 years, 35 percent in the fourth decade, 78 percent in the fifth decade and 100 percent in those older than age 60 years.[71] When carotid ultrasound was completed on 197 SLE patients and matched controls, carotid plaques were present among 37.1 percent of those with SLE compared with hypertensive controls (RR 2.4, 95 percent CI 1.7–3.6, $p < 0.001$). This contrast was seen in each age group, but was most remarkable among patients younger than age 40 (RR 5.6). SLE patients with carotid plaques were generally older than age 40, with a longer duration of SLE and less likely to be treated with prednisone, cyclophosphamide, or hydroxychlorquine.[72]

Rheumatoid arthritis has also been associated with increased CV mortality and morbidity. CAD may occur a decade earlier.[70,73,74] Assessment for preclinical evidence of atherosclerosis among 98 women with RA through carotid ultrasonography documented carotid atherosclerosis in 44 percent of those with RA compared to 15 percent of age matched hypertensive controls ($p < 0.001$). Interestingly, the greatest increase in carotid atherosclerosis was seen in those in their fourth decade.[74] Methotrexate, which decreases the inflammatory process in RA, is also associated with lower rates of CAD.[73]

Although 18 percent of American women report migraine headaches, compared with 6 percent of men, the CV implications of this diagnosis are unclear, especially when associated with aura. Within the Atherosclerosis Risk in the Communities Studies, where women and men ages 45 to 64 years were assessed and followed, a lifetime history of headaches with aura

was more often associated with angina symptoms but not CHD events.[75] In the Women's Health Study developed to assess low-dose aspirin for primary prevention, there was a 10-year follow up of women initially age 45 years or older. Among the participants 18.4 percent reported migraines, and 39.6 percent of those with migraine headaches had an associated aura. Over 10 years of followup, the women with migraines with aura had more major CVD events including angina, MI, coronary revascularization, and death from CAD.[76] Less robust results were provided when a subset of 905 women who answered a single query about a history of migraines in the Women's Ischemic Syndrome Evaluation (WISE), a National Heart, Lung, and Blood Institute prospective, multicenter study. Women with a history of migraines (24 percent) had less severe CAD at catheterization than those women without migraines, even after adjustment for age and other cardiac risk factors. Over 4.4 years of followup, there was no increase in cardiac events or all-cause mortality.[77] The evidence to date suggests that with long-term followup, patients with migraine headaches and aura may be at higher risk for coronary events.

DIAGNOSIS OF CORONARY ARTERY DISEASE IN WOMEN

Because CAD is often diagnosed clinically by a careful history, preconceived biases can affect perception of CAD risk.[1,3,78] A web-based survey of attending cardiologists, primary care physicians, and gynecologists revealed that intermediate-risk women were more often rated as low risk compared with men with the same risk factors ($p < 0.0001$) by primary care physicians, with a similar trend among cardiologists and gynecologists.[3] When physicians were recruited to view a video of different actors (black and white women and men) accompanied by the same written information, the black woman was least likely to be referred for cardiac catheterization.[79] Adequately assessment of CAD risk and severity is required for appropriate evaluation and management to occur. The clinical history typical for angina and acute coronary syndromes is reviewed in Chaps. 59 and 64.

Once CAD is considered as a diagnosis, further evaluation is required to assess disease presence and severity. Noninvasive stress testing can help assess disease control and determine which patients with an intermediate risk for CAD will benefit from further interventions.[80] More extensive discussion can be found in Chap. 14, but potential gender differences in noninvasive testing are discussed briefly here. Unfortunately, each noninvasive technique has limitations in women.[80–84]

Exercise stress testing was the earliest noninvasive way to assess CAD risk. However, women have lower sensitivity and specificity with exercise stress testing than men, in part related to lower ECG voltage. In multiple populations women have been noted to have more frequent ST-T-wave abnormalities.[81] Gender-specific criteria for exercise stress testing interpretation have been proposed to compensate for the generally smaller ST-segment changes seen in women.[82–84] A negative exercise stress test with adequate exertion is often helpful because it decreases the need to consider cardiac catheterization.[80] After exercise stress testing, the maximal exercise capacity and heart rate recovery in women are important prognostically.[80] Among asymptomatic women with low risk Framingham scores, those with lower exercise capacity and slower heart rate recovery were at increased risk for CV death.[82,83] Stress imaging techniques are often favored in assessing symptomatic woman for severity of CAD.[80] Local expertise is an important consideration in deciding between nuclear medicine and echocardiography techniques. Nuclear stress perfusion testing in women can be potentially hindered by soft tissue attenuation from breast tissue with the use of thallium, so technetium may be preferred. Stress echocardiography is highly dependent on operator expertise and may be technically difficult in obese patients. Many authors prefer stress imaging tests, with their lower false-positive rates, to exercise stress tests for women.[80,82]

Patterns of referral for cardiac catheterization may vary by gender, with some appropriate differences.[1,82] Because cardiac catheterization is less likely to reveal CAD in women, many clinicians initially evaluate women at intermediate risk with stress-imaging techniques. For example, anginal symptoms are less predictive of abnormal coronary anatomy in women than men (Fig. 102–9).[85] Direct referral to cardiac catheterization should occur with a high suspicion of significant CAD that might benefit from intervention or after an abnormal noninvasive stress test. Outcome differences in a registry of patients in Alberta, Canada, undergoing cardiac catheterization from 1995 to 2000 revealed women were 29.9 percent of the cohort. Women were older with more comorbid conditions; women had a higher 1-year mortality (5.6 percent vs. 4.6 percent; $p < 0.001$) that occurred early after PTCA or catheterization.[86]

MANAGEMENT OF CAD IN WOMEN
[ ] ASYMPTOMATIC WOMEN

Some individuals are truly asymptomatic with respect to CAD. Others may have had atypical symptoms undiagnosed as possible CAD. In several population studies over 25 percent of MIs are not clinically recognized and a history of angina was lacking. After 34 years of Framingham followup, 34 percent of women and 26 percent of men had MIs unidentified by their physicians. Of these patients, 33 percent of women and 24 percent of men had a prior history of angina compared with 45 percent of women and 53 percent of men with recognized MI. Morality for women is similar after an unrecognized or recognized MI.[87]

For truly asymptomatic women, national guidelines for prevention are gradually developing.[2] Counseling for asymptomatic women about CAD should include a review of the common risk factors and symptoms of CAD as well as encouragement for implementing a healthy lifestyle.[1,2] The single most important intervention for prevention is avoiding exposure to tobacco.[1,2,5] Finally, a randomized control trial of aspirin for primary prevention of CVD in women age 45 years or older is complete.[88] In the Women's Health Study, >39,000 women professionals received 100 mg aspirin on alternating days or placebo with 10 years of followup. Overall, there was an insignificant decrease in CV risk, and no decrease in MI. However, stroke reduction occurred (0.83, 95 percent CI 0, 69–0.99, $p = 0.04$) from a decrease in ischemic strokes (RR 0.76, 95 percent CI 0.63–0.93, $p = 0.009$) without a statistically increased risk of hemorrhagic stroke. In subgroup analysis, aspirin at 100 mg every other day decreased MI, ischemic

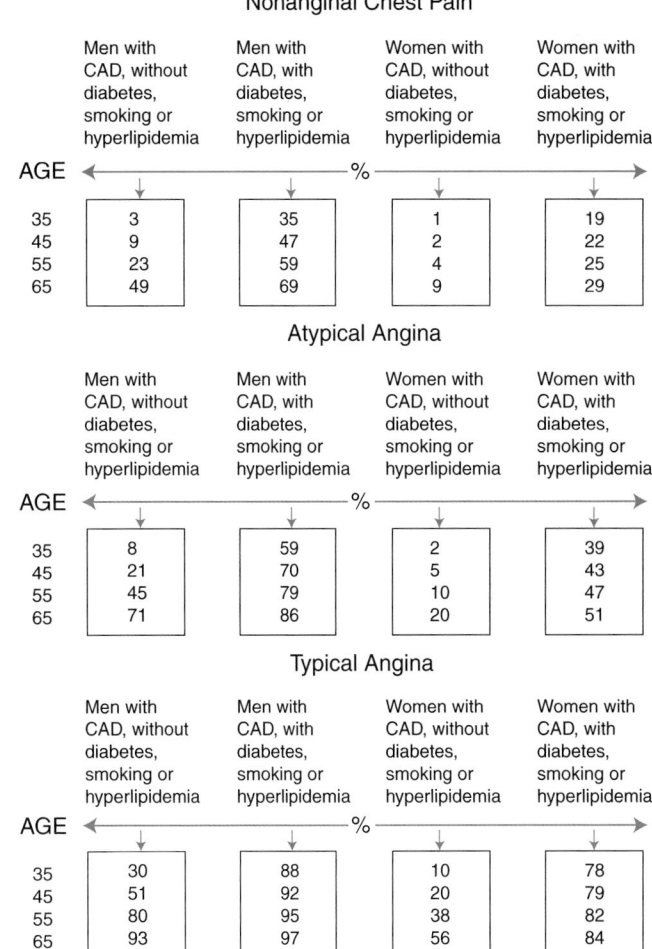

FIGURE 102–9. Comparison of chest pain clinical scenarios and risk of having coronary artery disease on testing. *Source: From Snow V, Barry P, Fihn SD, et al.[85]*

stroke, and major CV events among women at least age 65 years. In a meta-analysis of international primary prevention data, aspirin decreased the RR of MI in men and of stroke in women, but did not alter the RR of MI among all women (Fig. 102–10).

Prospective cohort studies have been used to develop models predicting the impact of one or more risk factors on the likelihood of future coronary artery events.[2,22,89] When multiple individual risk factors are present; the cumulative risk of CAD is greater than the sum of its parts. The prevalence and impact of risk factors has been explored for women in several studies including the Third National Health and Nutrition Examination Survey[9] as well as the Framingham Heart Study.[89,90]

Clustering risk factors was an important predictor in the Framingham Offspring Study (patients ages 30 to 74 years at enrollment), where 17 percent of all participants had three of the six risk factors (lowest-quintile HDL cholesterol, highest-quintile cholesterol, BMI, systolic blood pressure, triglycerides, and glucose).[90] With 16 years of followup for coronary artery events (MI or sudden death), there were 79 first coronary artery events among the 1818 women who were initially free of symptomatic CAD, compared with 229 events among the 1759 men. However, CAD events were associated with three or more risk factors for 48 percent of the CAD events in women and 20 percent of the CAD events in men.

Long-term CV outcome has also been considered among white women with a low risk-factor profile in the Chicago Heart Association Detection Project in Industry.[91] A low risk-factor profile was defined as not a current smoker, blood pressure ≤120/80 mmHg, total cholesterol <200, no history of diabetes or MI, and no ECG abnormalities. At entry, only 6.8 percent of the cohort ages 40 to 59 years met these criteria. However, these women had substantially lower CAD mortality with a mean follow up of 22 years (3.5 compared with 14.5 age-adjusted mortality rate per 10,000 person-years, RR 0.21, 95 percent; CI 0.05 to 0.84).

【 】 ANGINA

As described from Framingham data, the first presentation of symptomatic CAD is typically angina in women and MI in men.[92] The prevalence of angina in women and men is similar, but women less often have angiographic documented CAD.[92]

The clinical diagnosis of angina can be challenging. Women generally visit physicians more often than men and report more symptoms, including chest pain. Women compared with men with angina more frequently report angina with emotional or mental stress.[1] Too often, older women ascribe their decreased ability to complete housework or walk to *getting old*. Therefore it is essential

to explore a patient's exercise tolerance and if a decrease occurs, consider CAD in the differential.

The prognosis after the clinical diagnosis of angina has been elucidated in two recent studies. National registry data from Finland was reviewed data from January 1996 through December 1998 with an overall prevalence of angina similar to the United States (with 5.4 percent men and 6.3 percent of women).[92] Those who received prescriptions for nitrates in any form were compared with those who were certified to receive special compensation because of specific ECG or catheterization abnormalities. Although the total incidence of angina was similar in men, women were less likely to have abnormal catheterization than men in each age group. Mortality rates were similar for women and men using nitrates; but in women who had evaluations revealing possible CAD, mortality rates were higher[92] (Fig. 102–11).

The evaluation and medical care of 3779 men and women diagnosed with stable angina has been explored between March and December 2002 in patients who were seen by cardiologists throughout study centers in Europe for the first time, or for the first consultation in at least 1 year.[93] Women were 42 percent of this cohort, and less often received antiplatelet or statin medications, referral for exercise stress test (0.81; 95 percent CI 0.69–0.95), or coronary angiogram (0.59; 95 percent CI 0.48–0.73). Managing angina in women is complicated by the observation that anginal symptoms in women are less predictive of

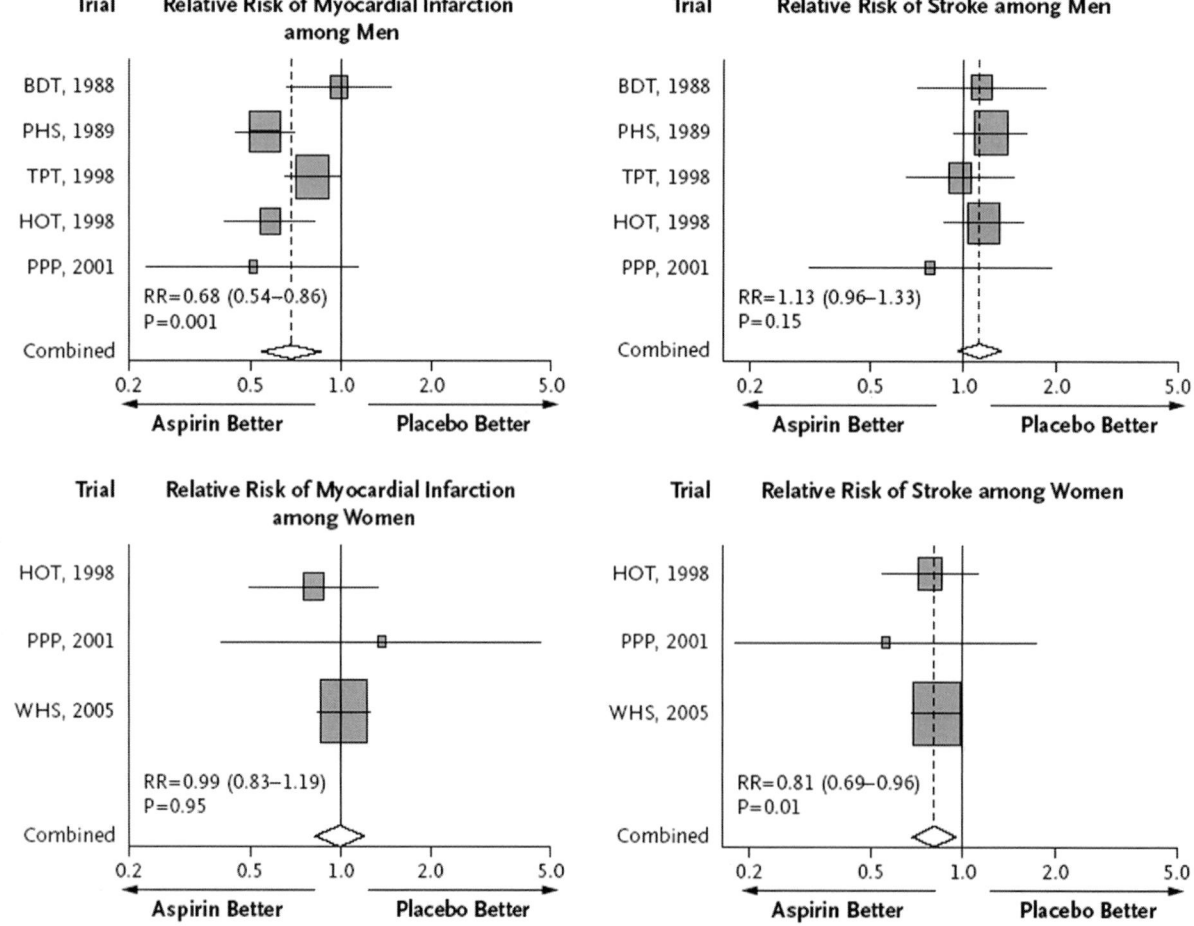

FIGURE 102–10. Relative risk of MI and stroke among men and women with aspirin as primary prevention. RR, relative risk. *Source: From Hemingway H, McCallum A, Shipley M, Manderbacka K, Matikainen P, Keskimaki I.[92]*

abnormal coronary anatomy than in men[85] (see Fig. 102–9). Coronary angiography was completed in 34 percent of women and 47 percent of men; even after adjustment for multiple clinical factors, women were 40 to 50 percent less likely to undergo angiography. Results of the completed angiography revealed coronary disease among 63 percent of women compared with 87 percent of men catheterized.[93] Women had less revascularization and more death and nonfatal MI during 1 year of followup (2.09; 95 percent CI 1.13–3.85). Major clinical events after 1 year occurred at higher rates among those with CAD on angiography than those with a clinical diagnosis of angina (Fig. 102–11).

The relationship between the menstrual cycle and vascular spasm is beginning to receive attention.[47,92] The menstrual cycle can be divided into menstrual, follicular (from menses to ovulation, high estrogen levels), and luteal (ovulation to menses, low estrogen, and high progesterone levels) phases using historical timing, basal body temperature, bleeding patterns, and laboratory results. An important study of 10 women with vasospastic angina throughout the menstrual cycle has added to our understanding.[47] Participants were premenopausal women with a history of vasospastic angina (all with a normal cardiac catheterization followed by intracoronary acetylcholine infusion leading to both symptoms and typical ST-segment elevation). All cardiac medication was held for a full menstrual cycle, with every other morning estrogen and progesterone levels, ST-Holter monitoring, and flow-mediated dilation measurement of the brachial artery (Doppler study of the brachial artery before and after blood pressure cuff elevation above systolic pressure). The average number of ischemic episodes inversely correlated with flow-mediated vasodilatation of the brachial artery. In contrast to hormonal stimuli, similar amounts of vasodilatation in different parts of the menstrual cycle occurred after nitroglycerin exposure. Other studies have also raised speculation about the importance of documenting when in the menstrual cycle a stress test is completed. More research is required in this area.[47,92]

Secondary prevention should be initiated with the diagnosis of angina, including control of risk factors and appropriate pharmacologic therapies (aspirin and lipid-lowering agents but usually not hormone replacement therapy). Underuse of these agents in women is discussed in the Acute Coronary Ischemia Including Acute Myocardial Infarction section. In one Swiss study, elderly women with angina had a less favorable 6-month outcome and reported a lower quality of life than men despite less frequent coronary obstruction at cardiac catheterization.[93]

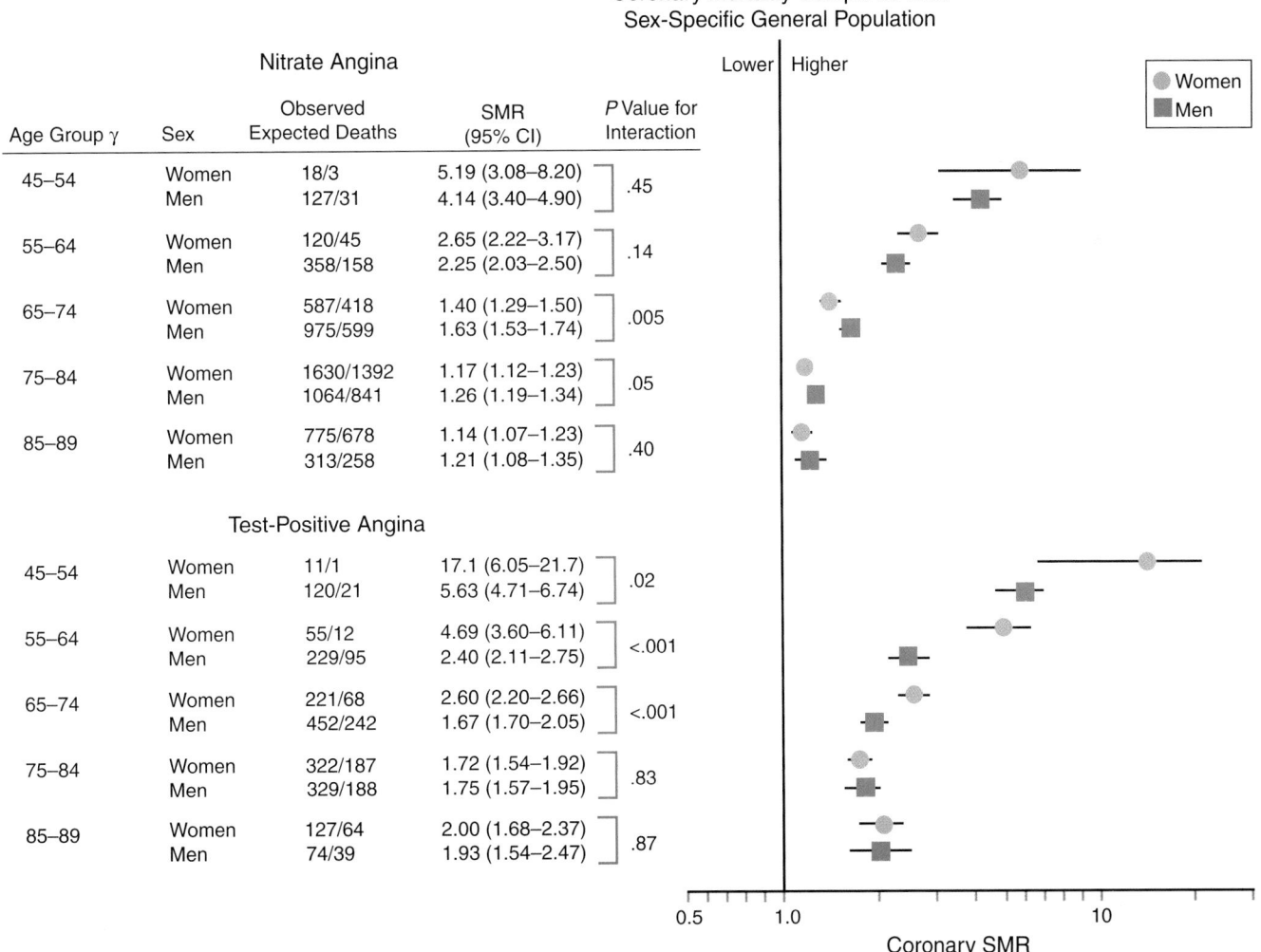

FIGURE 102–11. Incidence of major clinical events occurring in 1 year followup in patients with chronic angina enrolled in 2002. *Source: Adapted from Daly C, Clemens F, Sendon JLL, et al.[93]*

【 】 ACUTE CORONARY ISCHEMIA INCLUDING ACUTE MYOCARDIAL INFARCTION

There are substantial gender differences in the presentation and natural history of acute coronary ischemia (including both unstable angina and MI). Extensive general discussions of acute coronary ischemia syndromes can be found in other chapters. Potential physiologic differences such as sex differences in vascular tone and microvascular or endothelial dysfunction have been postulated as possible explanations why anatomic lesions are less common in women.[94] Women with acute ischemia may present with upper abdominal symptoms (nausea, discomfort), neck or jaw pain, or shortness of breath rather than the more classical crushing chest pain.[1,95] Atypical symptoms are more common in all patients who are older or diabetic. Therefore, coronary ischemia should be considered in the differential diagnosis for women who present acutely ill even if there is no associated crushing chest pain.

Sex differences in the spectrum of acute coronary ischemic events, natural history and 5-year prognosis were explored in Alberta Canada from 1993 through 2000.[95] Unstable angina admissions were defined as coronary ischemia admissions without any acute MI admissions for the same patient during the entire study period. These admissions had a lower crude 1-year mortality than patients with MI during any admission. Women were 33.7 percent of those hospitalized, had a median age of 6 to 7 years older, and more comorbid diagnoses. More women than men were diagnosed with unstable angina (32.3 percent compared with 24.1 percent, $p < 0.001$). Women had lower rates of inpatient angiography within 6 months. Crude mortality rates for women and men with unstable angina were similar, whereas in multivariate analysis women had a survival advantage (HR 0.81, 95 percent CI 0.72–0.92). The female survival advantage was noted only in women older than 65 years of age.

Unstable angina natural history and prognosis was also explored in a 6-year follow up of patients seen for the first time with unstable angina in the emergency department in Olmsted County, Minnesota.[96] Women were older and more often had atypical angina and a history of hypertension. Fewer noninvasive and invasive procedures were completed on women; yet after adjustment for confounders, women had fewer cardiac events with 6 years of followup.

Gender differences with MI and during follow up have been increasingly explored.[1,95–99] In the Alberta Canada study from 1993 through 2000 described above, women with MI were also older and had more comorbidities.[95] Hospital length of stay was longer for women and less often included care in cardiac or intensive care units. Women received less catheterization and CABG. Five-year mortality was higher overall among women than men (38.8 percent compared with 26.8 percent, $p < 0.001$), but multivariate analysis did not confirm sex was key (HR 0.91, 95 percent CI 0.93–1.05). In subgroup analysis by age, women younger than age 65 years had a lower survival advantage. Similar rates of interventions were found in data from 33 U.S. hospitals from 1995 to 2001.[98] After MI women were nearly as likely to have cardiac catheterization, angioplasty, or stenting; but still underwent CABG less often (adjusted prevalence ratio [PR], 0.78; 95 percent CI, 0.77 to 0.79). Through the 1990s in the Worcester, Massachu-

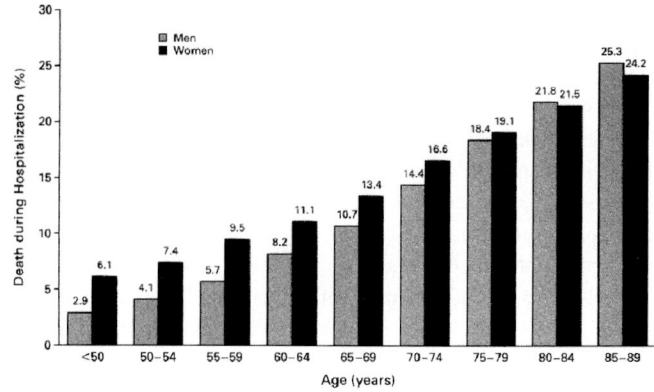

FIGURE 102–12. Mortality after myocardial infarction: sex differences by age. *Source: From Vaccarino V, Parsons L, Every NR, et al.[100] With permission.*

setts, metropolitan area, there has been increased use of catheterization and percutaneous coronary interventions after MI with greater increases for women than men.[99]

The interaction of gender and age was explored with data available from the NRMI II.[100] Again it was found that women with MI are often older and have more comorbid conditions than do men. Although overall there was a 14 percent early mortality in women after hospitalization for MI compared with 10 percent in men, when age was further considered, the picture became more complex. Analysis of the interaction of gender and age revealed that the 30-day mortality after MI was approximately twice as great for women ages 30 to 50 years compared with men of the same age and progressively decreased with increasing age until reaching unity at age 75 years (Fig. 102–12).

Acute MI in pregnancy was reviewed among a 2000 to 2002 Nationwide Inpatient Survey; the rate was 6.2 per 100,000 deliveries in the United States (three to four times higher than nonpregnant women in the same age range).[101] Most MI occurred during an admission for pregnancy (73 percent), but 27 percent occurred during a postpartum admission. The most substantial risk factor was increasing age older than 20 years. In multivariate analysis, the most prominent risk factors were thrombophilia, hypertension, age 35 years and older compared with age younger than 20 years, smoking, requiring blood transfusion, diabetes, and black race. Of women with pregnancy-related MI, 45 percent had cardiac catheterization and 45 percent had subsequent intervention (angioplasty, stent placement, or surgery). Coronary artery dissection as a complication may occur. Among women with an MI during pregnancy, the mortality rate was 5.1 percent.

Although medical therapy that provides survival advantage after MI has been well defined, women have historically received these treatments less and not reached goal as often (achieving blood pressure or lipid control).[1,54,67,98,102,103] Community-wide trends have shown some gradual improvement in compliance in women as well as men with the use of β blockers after MI.[103] The intervention was order sets and a special hospital discharge tool (including patient education about treatment goals, medications, and lifestyle modification provided by an inpatient nurse and signed by both nurse and patient). These measures improved clinician compliance with guidelines for aspirin and β blocker use in both women and men. Interestingly, use of the discharge tool was associated with higher lipid-lowering medication use in women and a 50 percent lower risk of death at 1 year even though the discharge tool was only used for 27.9 percent of women (compared with 34 percent of men).[98]

In long-term followup after MI, women tend to have more angina and congestive heart failure despite better systolic left ventricular function.[100] Women, as well as men, most often develop congestive heart failure from ischemic heart disease.[1] Further study is indicated.

Aggressive management of associated risk factors after MI may especially benefit women. The natural history of women and men after hospitalization for MI from 1990 to 1998 was explored in Olmsted County, Minnesota, with a mean follow up of 3.7 years. As in other populations, women were older (age 73 years vs. men 64 years, $p < .001$). For women only the presence of hypertension, diabetes, and hypercholesterolemia increased risk of a second ischemic event.[91] In the Third National Health and Nutrition Survey a focus on secondary prevention revealed women, blacks, and those ages 46 to 65 years were more likely to have more than two poorly controlled major risk factors.[104] Cardiac rehabilitation is equally effective for women; but historically, more men than women have participated.

【 】 INTERVENTIONS FOR CORONARY ARTERY DISEASE

Gender differences in the prevalence and complications of percutaneous coronary interventions (PCIs) and CABG surgery are evolving.[1,105] There is controversy over whether women are undertreated or men overtreated. Historically, after MI, evaluation has been less aggressive for women than men. Data from 33 U.S. hospitals from 1995 to 2001 revealed that after MI women were nearly as likely to have cardiac catheterization, angioplasty, or stenting but still underwent CABG less often (adjusted PR, 0.78; 95 percent CI, 0.77–0.79).[97] From 1990 to 1999 among those with acute MI hospitalized in the Worcester, Massachusetts, area, the gap between cardiac catheterization and PCI use in women and men narrowed.[99]

Currently, approximately 33 percent of the PCIs are performed in women.[106] Primary angiography is superior to fibrinolytic therapy when available within 3 hours of symptoms, even with the higher procedure complication rate for women. The development of smaller coronary artery catheters only partially decreased the sex difference in complications.[106,107] Most experts note that the higher short- and long-term complication rates in women are probably also related to older age, more comorbidities, and longer duration of symptoms compared with men. Vascular complications at the access site, retroperitoneal, or requiring transfusion are more common in women than men.[106,107] In a clinical trial comparing PCI balloon versus stenting with or without the addition of abciximab, overall women received treatment after a longer delay and had higher 1-year mortality, revascularization, and adverse cardiac events. Women benefited most from stenting with lower revascularization and adverse cardiac events. In women, less revascularization in the first 30 days was required without an increased bleeding risk with the addition of abciximab, but no difference was found at 1 year.[108] CABG surgery is also more commonly performed in men than women.[107,108]

Among the population in Ontario, Canada, from 1991 to 2002, only 22 percent of those to undergo CABG were women. Older age and socioeconomic status as well as more severe symptoms were noted in the women compared with the men. The conduit selected is less often the internal mammary artery in women than in men, but this graft is associated with the best short- and long-term results.[109] Reasons for this might include smaller size, higher rates of diabetes in women undergoing CABG, and the decreased use of internal mammary artery grafting in the setting of osteoporosis. After hospital discharge women had a lower mortality but more readmissions.[109] The hospitalization including CABG was not explored in this study; but among 9218 Michigan Medicare beneficiaries who had CABG from 1997 to 1998, 37.6 percent were women.[110] During the CABG hospitalization, 12.2 percent had an infection, most often respiratory followed by urinary tract, gastrointestinal, and skin. For women the infection rate was 16.1 percent compared with 9.8 percent for men ($p < 0.001$). Mortality was higher for both women and men with infection, during hospitalization as well as at 30 and 100 days after CABG. Of interest 96 percent of the sex difference at 100 day mortality was related to infection.

Experience over a decade with off-pump CABG revealed women were older and had a smaller surface area. After controlling for these differences and other comorbidities, women had more wound infections and longer hospitalization but similar mortality.[111] Among patients at least 75 years old at time of CABG in the Society of Thoracic Surgeons' voluntary data base, women were 38.9 percent of the sample and were older with smaller body surface area. Women were more likely to have emergency surgery and had higher operative mortality, more pulmonary and vascular complications, and longer hospitalizations.[112]

【 】 SUDDEN DEATH

Sudden death occurs 30 percent less in American women than men.[113] However, from 1989 to 1998 the rate of sudden death for women 35 to 44 years of age increased 21 percent compared with a 2.8 percent decrease in men.[113] In the Nurses' Health Cohort 636 women or 57.3 percent of the cohort died out of the hospital or in the emergency department. There was no prior history of heart disease in 69 percent of the women with sudden death. At least one coronary risk factor was present in 94 percent of those who died. The strongest associations were with cigarette smoking, diabetes, and hypertension.[113] The Nurses' Health Study assessed phobic anxiety, which is more common in women than men, and found it correlated with higher smoking rates, hypertension, diabetes, hypercholesteremia, and BMI ≥ 30 kg/m^2. Similar to prior results in men, high levels of phobic anxiety in women were associated with an increased risk of fatal CAD including sudden death, even after controlling for these comorbidities in women with no CVD initially.[64] Out-of-hospital arrest survival is similar for women and men; however, men had higher rates of ventricular fibrillation.[114]

The prognosis of silent MI still requires further exploration; sudden death is one possible sequela, as documented in an autopsy study where clinical history was obtained after sudden death ($n = 51$) or death after trauma ($n = 15$).[115] On autopsy, only 2 of 51 women had a documented prior MI, but 35 percent of the sample had evidence of a prior MI. The acute thrombus associated with plaque erosion (often noted in early atherosclerosis) occurred more often in younger women smokers without obesity, high cholesterol, or elevated glycohemoglobin. In comparison, plaque rupture was more often found in older women with elevated cholesterol.

ARRHYTHMIAS

Women generally have a higher heart rate than men and respond to increasing cardiac demand by increasing heart rate rather than increasing stroke volume.[1] Women in their seventh decade with a heart rate >77 beats/min had substantially higher CV (>77 beats/min, ROR, 13.99, 95 percent CI 1.93–101.16) and all-cause mortality rates (>77 beats/min, ROR, 3.71, 95 percent CI 1.41–9.80) than women with slower pulses with 6 years of followup after controlling for potential confounders such as prior CVD, smoking, hypertension, activity level, and anemia.[116] When women exposed to β blockers were excluded, the results were more dramatic. This association was not statistically significant in men within the same cohort.

Gender differences in the incidence and management of arrhythmias have been noted. There is a female predominance of atrioventricular node reentrant tachycardia and orthodromic supraventricular tachycardia, but men are more likely to have atrial and ventricular fibrillation associated with Wolff-Parkinson-White syndrome.[36,117] Although in the treatment of supraventricular reentrant tachycardias there has been increasing use of radiofrequency catheter ablation therapy, limited data has focused on gender differences. In a meta-analysis of implantable cardioverter defibrillators as primary prevention, there was only a 12 percent reduction in death from any cause compared with 24 percent in men.[118]

Overall, women have a higher risk of dying of atrial fibrillation.[119] In an important clinical randomized control trial comparing rate and rhythm control in patients with atrial fibrillation despite prior electrical cardioversion, the primary endpoints (composite of death from CVD, heart failure, thromboembolism complications, bleeding, the need for pacemaker implantation, or severe adverse effects of antiarrhythmic agents) had important sex differences.[117] For women, rhythm control had substantially worse outcomes with an absolute difference of 21.5, 95 percent (CI 30.8 to 2.1) compared with results for men revealing only a trend with an absolute difference of 3.9, 95 percent (CI 3.2 to 11.1). Therefore, for women it may be beneficial to focus on rate rather than rhythm control in persistent atrial fibrillation. Whenever possible these patients are anticoagulated to prevent embolism, but women are less likely to be anticoagulated than men.[120] Anticoagulation may be especially important for women; a recent prospective study of patients with atrial fibrillation found that for those not on warfarin sodium (Coumadin) women had higher embolism rates than men (3.5 percent compared with 1.8 percent, RR 1.6, 95 percent CI 1.3–1.9) after multivariable analysis. Interestingly, in this study women on warfarin sodium (Coumadin) developed less intracranial bleeding than men, but women are at greater risk of intracranial bleeding with stroke than men.[120] Sex differences in pacemaker placement have been studied in two retrospective studies. In a single Canadian center there were not sex differences; however, a pacemaker registry retrospective review from Germany

(with 31,913 entries) found that when pacemakers are implanted, women are more likely to receive a single-chamber pacer, whereas men are more likely to receive a dual-chamber pacer.[121]

Drug-induced torsade de pointes occurs more commonly in women than men.[36,122] As this sex difference is noticed after puberty, a prospective study explored the impact of the menstrual cycle on the development of torsade de pointes.[122] After infusion of low-dose ibutilide, the greatest increase in QT interval was seen in women during menses and in their ovulatory phase compared with women during the luteal phase of menstruation and men.[122] Current QT interval standards were developed in the white population. Exploration of QT intervals among women without CVD in the WHI suggests the Asian women have a QTrr that is 10 msec longer than other ethic groups.[123]

SUMMARY

Significant differences in individual patient factors that affect diagnosis and management are under investigation. As these differences are further defined and explored, the care of individual patients can be improved. Identification of CAD in women can be improved by assessing possible angina symptoms and screening high-risk women as well as men. All physicians and patients must focus on primary and secondary prevention for both women and men.

REFERENCES

1. Charney P, ed. *Coronary Artery Disease in Women: Prevention, Diagnosis and Management.* Philadelphia: American College of Physicians; 1999.
2. Mosca L, Appel L, Benjamin E, et al. Evidence-based guidelines for cardiovascular disease prevention in women. *Circulation* 2004;109:672–693.
3. Mosca L, Linfante A, Benjamin E, et al. National Study of Physician Awareness and Adherence to Cardiovascular Disease Prevention Guidelines. *Circulation* 2005;111:499–510.
4. Mosca L, Mochari H, Christian A, et al. National Study of Women's Awareness, Preventive Action, and Barriers to Cardiovascular Health. *Circulation* 2006;113:525–534.
5. Ockene JK, Bonollo DP, Adams A. Smoking. In: Charney P, ed. *Coronary Artery Disease in Women.* Philadelphia: American College of Physicians; 1999.
6. Centers for Disease Control and Prevention. Women and Smoking: A Report of the Surgeon General (Executive Summary). *MMWR Morb Mortal Wkly Rep* 2002;51(RR 12):1–13.
7. Al-Delaimy WK, Manson JE, Solomon CG, et al. Smoking and the risk of coronary heart disease among women with type 2 diabetes mellitus. *Arch Intern Med* 2002;162:273–279.
8. Centers for Disease Control and Prevention. Tobacco use among adults—United States, 2005. *MMWR Morb Mortal Wkly Rep* 2006;55(42):1145–1148.
9. Winkleby MA, Robinson TN, Sundquist J, Kraemer HC. Ethnic variations in cardiovascular disease risk factors among children and young adults: findings from the third National Health and Nutrition Examination Survey, 1988–1994. *JAMA* 1999;281:1006–1013.
10. Perez-Stable EJ, Herrera B, Jacob P, Benowitz NL. Nicotine metabolism and intake in black and white smokers. *JAMA* 1998;280:152–156.
11. Wee CC, Rigotti N, Davis RB, et al. Relationship between smoking and weight control efforts among adults in the United States. *Arch Intern Med* 2001;161:546–550.
12. Marcus BH, Albrecht AE, King TK, et al. The efficacy of exercise as an aid for smoking cessation in women: a randomized controlled trial. *Arch Intern Med* 1999;159:1229–1234.
13. Cepeda-Benito A, Reynoso J, Erath S. Meta-analysis of the efficacy of nicotine replacement therapy for smoking cessation: differences between men and women. *J Consult Clin Psychol* 2004;72(4):712–722.
14. Ahluwalia JS, Harris KJ, Catley D, et al. Sustained-release bupropion for smoking cessation in African Americans: a randomized controlled trial. *JAMA* 2000;288:468–474.

15. Carballo RS, Giovino GA, Perchaeck TF, et al. Racial and ethnic differences in serum cotinine levels for cigarette smokers: Third National Health and Nutrition Examination Survey, 1988–1991. *JAMA* 1998;280:135–139.

16. Rennert NJ, Charney P. Preventing cardiovascular disease in diabetes and glucose intolerance: evidence and implications for care. *Prim Care* 2003;30:569–592.

17. Whiteley L, Padmanabhan S, Hole D, Isles C. Should diabetes be considered a coronary heart disease equivalent? Results from 25 years of follow-up in the Renfrew and Paisley Survey. *Diabetes Care* 2005;28:1588–1593.

18. Almdal T, Scharling H, Jensen J, Vestergaard H. The independent effect of type 2 diabetes mellitus on ischemic heart disease, stroke and death. *Arch Intern Med* 2004;164:1422–1426.

19. Barrett-Conner E, Giardina E, Gitt A, Gudat U, Steinberg H, Tschoepe D. Women and heart disease: the role of diabetes and hyperglycemia. *Arch Intern Med* 2004;164:934–942.

20. Vaccarino V, Parsons L, Every N, et al. Impact of history of diabetes mellitus on hospital mortality in men and women with first acute myocardial infarction. *Am J Cardiol* 2000;85:1486–1489.

21. Persell S, Baker D. Aspirin use among adults with diabetes. *Arch Intern Med* 2004;164:2492–2499.

22. Prospective Diabetes Study Group. United Kingdom Prospective Diabetes Study 27: Plasma lipids and lipoproteins at diagnosis of NIDDM by age and sex, UK: *Diabetes Care* 1997;20(11):1683–1687.

23. Expert Panel on Detection, Evaluation, and Treatment of High Blood Cholesterol in Adults. Executive Summary of the Third Report of the National Cholesterol Education Program (NCEP) Expert Panel on Detection, Evaluation, and Treatment of High Blood Cholesterol in Adults (Adult Treatment Panel III). *JAMA* 2001;285:2486–2497.

24. Weitman M, Cook S, Auinger P, et al. Tobacco smoke exposure is associated with the metabolic syndrome in adolescents. *Circulation* 2005;112:862–869.

25. Schneider JG, Tompkins C, Blumenthal RS, Mora S. The metabolic syndrome in women. *Cardiol Rev* 2006;14:286–291.

26. Wild R. Polycystic ovary syndrome: a risk for coronary artery disease? *Am J Obstet Gynecol* 2002;186(1):35–43.

27. Aoridonidze T, Essah P, Iuorno M, Nestler J. Prevalence and characteristics of the metabolic syndrome in women with polycystic ovary syndrome. *J Clin Endocrinol Metab* 2005;90(4):1929–1935.

28. The Women's Caucus, Working Group on Women's Health of the Society of General Internal Medicine. Hypertension in women: what is really known? *Ann Intern Med* 1991;115:287–293.

29. National Center for Health Statistics. QuickStats: percentage of persons aged ≥ 20 years with hypertension, by race/ethnicity—United States, 1999–2002. *MMWR Morb Mortal Wkly Rep* 2005;54(33):826.

30. Christou D, Jones P, Jordan J, Diedrich A, Robertson D, Seals D. Women have lower tonic autonomic support of arterial blood pressure and less effective baroreflex buffering than men. *Circulation* 2005;111:494–498.

31. Sagie A. The natural history of borderline isolated systolic hypertension. *N Engl J Med* 1993;329:1912–1917.

32. Franklin SS, Pio JR, Wong ND, et al. Predictors of new-onset diastolic and systolic hypertension: the Framingham Heart Study. *Circulation* 2005;111:1121–1127.

33. Stamler J, Stamler R, Neaton JD, et al. Blood pressure, systolic and diastolic, and cardiovascular risks: U.S. population data. *Arch Intern Med* 1993;153:598–615.

34. Kannel WB. Blood pressure as a cardiovascular risk factor: prevention and treatment. *JAMA* 1996;275:1571–1576.

35. Cooper WO, Hernandez-Diaz S, Arbogast PG. Major congenital malformations after first-trimester exposure to ACE inhibitors. *N Engl J Med* 2006;354:2443–2451.

36. Schaefer BM, Caracciolo V, Frishman WH, Charney P. Gender, ethnicity and genetics in cardiovascular disease: Part II. Implications for pharmacotherapy. *Heart Dis* 2003;5:202–214.

37. Walsh JME, Pignone M. Drug treatment of hyperlipidemia in women. *JAMA* 2004;291:2243–2252.

38. Mosca L. Management of dyslipidemia in women in the post-hormone therapy era. *J Gen Intern Med* 2005;20:297–305.

39. Ogden CL, Carroll MD, Curtin LR, McDowell MA, Tabak CJ, Flegal KM. Prevalence of overweight and obesity in the United States, 1999–2004. *JAMA* 2006;295:1549–1555.

40. Tanko L, Bagger Y, Qin G, Alexandersen P, Larsen P, Christiansen C. Enlarged waist combined with elevated triglycerides is a strong predictor of accelerated atherogenesis and related cardiovascular mortality in postmenopausal women. *Circulation* 2005;111:1883–1890.

41. Wilson PF, D'Agostino RB, Sullivan L, Parise H, Kannel WB. Overweight and obesity as determinants of cardiovascular risk: the Framingham experience. *Arch Intern Med* 2002;162:1867–1872.

42. Samaras K, Kelly PJ, Chiano MN, et al. Genetic and environmental influences on total-body and central abdominal fat: the effect of physical activity in female twins. *Ann Intern Med* 1999;130:873–882.

43. Li TY, Rana JS, Manson JE, et al. Obesity as compared with physical activity in predicting risk of coronary heart disease in women. *Circulation* 2006;113:499–506.

44. Yanoviski SZ, Yanoviski JA. Obesity. *N Engl J Med* 2002;346:591–602.

45. Centers for Disease Control and Prevention. Trends in leisure-time physical inactivity by age, sex, and race/ethnicity: United States, 1994–2004. *MMWR* 2005;54(39):991–994.

46. Lee I, Rexrode KM, Cook NR, Manson JE, Burling JE. Physical activity and coronary heart disease in women: is "no pain, no gain" passé? *JAMA* 2001;285:1447–1454.

47. Charney P. Coronary artery disease in young women: the menstrual cycle and other risk factors. *Ann Intern Med* 2001;135(11):1002–1004.

48. Hu FB, Grodstein F, Hennekens CH, et al. Age at natural menopause and risk of cardiovascular disease. *Arch Intern Med* 1999;159:1061–1066.

49. Oliver MF, Boyd GS. Effect of bilateral ovariectomy on coronary artery disease and serum lipid levels. *Lancet* 1959;2:690.

50. Women's Health Initiative Steering Committee. Effects of conjugated equine estrogen on postmenopausal women with hysterectomy: the Women's Health Initiative randomized controlled trial. *JAMA* 2004;291:1701–1712.

51. Hsia J, Langer RD, Manson JE, et al. Conjugated equine estrogens and coronary heart disease: the Women's Health Initiative. *Arch Intern Med* 2006;166:357–365.

52. U.S. Preventive Task Force. Postmenopausal hormone replacement therapy for primary prevention of chronic conditions: recommendations and rationale. *Ann Intern Med* 2002;137:834–839.

53. Goldstein F, Manson J, Stampfer M. Hormone therapy and coronary heart disease: the role of time since menopause and age at hormone initiation. *J Womens Health* 2006;15(1):35–44.

54. Grady D, Herrington D, Bittner V, et al. Cardiovascular disease outcomes during 6.8 years of hormone therapy: Heart and Estrogen/Progestin Replacement Study Follow-Up (HERS II). *JAMA* 2002;288:49–57.

55. Jacobs SC, Stone PH. Psychosocial issues. In: Charney P, ed. *Coronary Artery Disease in Women*. Philadelphia: American College of Physicians; 1999:496–534.

56. Charney P. Future directions. In: Charney P, ed. *Coronary Artery Disease in Women: Prevention, Diagnosis and Management*. Philadelphia: American College of Physicians; 1999:575–593.

57. Mensah G, Mokdad A, Ford E, Greenlund K, Croft J. State of disparities in cardiovascular health in the United States. *Circulation* 2005;111:1233–1241.

58. Yan LL, Liu K, Daviglus ML, et al. Education, 15-year risk factor progression, and coronary artery calcium in young adulthood and early middle age: the Coronary Artery Risk Development in Young Adults Study. *JAMA* 2006;295:1793–1800.

59. Riolo SA, Nguyen TA, Greden JF, King CA. Prevalence of depression by race/ethnicity: findings from the National Health and Nutrition Examination Survey III. *Am J Public Health* 2005;95:998–1000.

60. Carney RM, Jaffe AS, ed. Treatment of depression following acute myocardial infarction. *JAMA* 2002;288:750–752.

61. Wassertheil-Smoller S, Shumaker S, Ockene J, et al. Depression and cardiovascular sequelae in postmenopausal women. *Arch Intern Med,* 2004;164:289–298.

62. Mallik S, Spertus JA, Reid KJ, et al. Depressive symptoms after acute myocardial infarction: evidence for higher rates in younger women. *Arch Intern Med* 2006;166:876–883.

63. Sharkey SW, Lesser JR, Zenovich AG, et al. Acute and reversible cardiomyopathy provoked by stress in women from the United States. *Circulation* 2005;111(4):472–479.

64. Albert CM, Chae CU, Rexrode KM, Manson JE, Kawachi I. Phobic anxiety and risk of coronary heart disease and sudden cardiac death among women. *Circulation* 2005;111(4):480–487.

65. Escobedo LG, Giles WH, Anda RF. Socioeconomic status, race, and death from coronary heart disease. *Am J Prev Med* 1997;13:123–130.

66. Gianni M, Dentali F, Grandi AM, Sumner G, Hiralal R, Lonn, E. Apical ballooning syndrome or tako-tsubo cardiomyopathy: a systematic review. *Eur Heart J* 2006. 27(13):1523–1529.

67. Vittinghoff E, Shlipak MG, Varosy PD, et al. Risk factors and secondary prevention in women with heart disease: the Heart and Estrogen/Progestin Replacement Study. *Ann Intern Med* 2003:138:81–89.

68. Pandey DK, Labarthe DR, Goff DC Jr, et al. Community-wide coronary heart disease mortality in Mexican Americans equals or exceeds that in Non-Hispanic whites: the Corpus Christi Heart Project. *Am J Med* 2001;110:81–87.

69. Vallapuri S, Gupta D, Talwar KK, et al. Comparison of atherosclerotic risk factors in Asian Indian and American Caucasian patients with angiographic coronary artery disease. *Am J Cardiol* 2002;90(10):1147–50.

70. Fischer LM. Schlienger RG. Matter C. Jick H. Meier CR, Effect of rheumatoid arthritis or systemic lupus erythematosus on the risk of first-time acute myocardial infarction. *Am J Cardiol* 2004;93(2):198–200.

71. Asanuma Y, Oeser A, Shintani AK, et al. Premature coronary-artery atherosclerosis in systemic lupus erythematosus. *N Engl J Med* 2003;349:2407–2415.

72. Roman MJ, Shanker BA, Davis A, et al. Prevalence and correlates of accelerated atherosclerosis in systemic lupus erythematosus. *N Engl J Med* 2003;349:2399–2406.

73. Kaplan MJ. Cardiovascular disease in rheumatoid arthritis. *Curr Opin Rheumatol* 2006;18(3):289–297.

74. Roman MJ, Moeller AB, Davis A, et al. Preclinical carotid atherosclerosis in patients with rheumatoid arthritis. *Ann Intern Med* 2006;144:249–156.

75. Rose KM, Carson AP, Snaford CP, et al. Migraine and other headaches: associations with Rose angina and coronary heart disease. *Neurology* 2004;63:2233–2239.

76. Kurth T. Migraine and risk of cardiovascular disease in women *JAMA* 2006;296:283–291.

77. Ahmed B, Bairey Merz CN, McClure C, et al. WISE Study Group: migraines, angiographic coronary artery disease and cardiovascular outcomes in women. *Am J Med* 2006;119(8):670–675.

78. Birdwell BG, Herbers JE, Kroenke K. Evaluating chest pain: the patient's presentation style alters the physician's diagnostic approach. *Arch Intern Med* 1993;153:1991–1995.

79. Schulman KA, Berlin JA, Harless W, et al. The effect of race and sex on physician's recommendations for cardiac catheterization. *N Engl J Med* 1999;340:618–626.

80. Mieres JH, Shaw LJ, Arai A, et al. Role of noninvasive testing in the clinical evaluation of women with suspected coronary artery disease. *Circulation* 2005;111:682–696.

81. De Bacquer D, De Backer G, Kornitzer. Prevalence of ECG findings in large population based samples of men and women. *Heart* 2000;84:625–633.

82. Roger V, Jacobsen SJ, Weston SA, et al. Sex differences in evaluation and outcome after stress testing. *Mayo Clin Proc* 2002;77:638–645.

83. Mora S, Redberg RF, Cui Y, et al. Ability of exercise testing to predict cardiovascular and all-cause death in asymptomatic women. *JAMA,* 2003;290:1600–1607.

84. Nasir K, Redberg RF, Budoff MJ, Hui E, Post WS, Blumenthal RS. Utility of stress testing and coronary calcification measurement for detection of coronary artery disease in women. *Arch Intern Med* 2004;164:1610–1620.

85. Snow V, Barry P, Fihn SD, et al. Evaluation of primary care patients with chronic stable angina: guidelines from the American College of Physicians. *Ann Intern Med* 2004;141:57–64.

86. King KM, Ghali WA, Faris PD, et al. Sex differences in outcomes after cardiac catheterization: effect modification by treatment strategy and time. *JAMA* 2004;291:1220–1225.

87. Sheifer SE, Manolio TA, Gersh BJ. Unrecognized myocardial infarction. *Ann Intern Med* 2001;135:801–811.

88. Ridker PM, Cook NR, Lee IM, et al. A randomized trial of low-dose aspirin in the primary prevention of cardiovascular disease in women. *N Engl J Med* 2005;352; 1293–1304.

89. Wilson PWF, Kannel WB, Silbershatz H, D'Agostino RB. Clustering of metabolic factors and coronary heart disease. *Arch Intern Med* 1999;159:1104–1109.

90. Hubert HB, Eaker ED, Garrison R, Castelli WP. Life-style correlates of risk factor change in young adults: an eight-year study of coronary heart disease risk factors in the Framingham offspring. *Am J Epidemiol* 1987;125(5):812–831.

91. Stamler J, Stamler R, Neaton JD, et al. Low risk-factor profile and long-term cardiovascular and noncardiovascular mortality and life expectancy: findings for 5 large cohorts of young adults and middle-aged men and women. *JAMA* 1999;282:2012–2018.

92. Hemingway H, McCallum A, Shipley M, Manderbacka K, Matikainen P, Keskimaki I. Incidence and prognostic implications of stable angina pectoris among women and men. *JAMA* 2006;295:1404–1411.

93. Daly C, Clemens F, Sendon JLL, et al. Gender differences in the management and clinical outcome of stable angina. *Circulation* 2006;113:490–498.

94. Jacobs AK. Coronary vascularization in women in 2003: sex revisited. *Circulation* 2003;107(3):375–377.

95. Chang W, Kaul P, Westerhout CM, et al. Impact of sex on long-term mortality from acute myocardial infarction vs unstable angina. *Arch Intern Med,* 2003;163:2476–2484.

96. Roger VL, Farkouh ME, Weston SA, et al. Sex differences in evaluation and outcome of unstable angina. *JAMA* 2000;283:646–652.

97. Bertoni AG, Bonds DE, Lovato J, Goff DC, Brancati FL. Sex disparities in procedure use for acute myocardial infarction in the United States, 1995 to 2001. *Am Heart J* 2004;147(6):1054–1060.

98. Jani SM, Montoye C, Mehta R, et al. Sex differences in the application of evidence-based therapies for the treatment of acute myocardial infarction. *Arch Intern Med* 2006;166:1164–1170.

99. Harrold LR, Esteban J, Lessard K, et al. Narrowing gender differences in procedure use for acute myocardial infarction: insights from the Worcester Heart Attack Study. *J Gen Intern Med* 2003;18:423–431.

100. Vaccarino V, Parsons L, Every NR, et al. Sex-based differences in early mortality after myocardial infarction. *N Engl J Med* 1999;341:217–225.

101. James AH, Jamison MG, Biswas MS, Brancazio LR, Swamy GK, Myers ER. Acute myocardial infarction in pregnancy. *Circulation* 2006;113:1564–1571.

102. Qureshi AI, Suri FK, Guterman LR, et al. Ineffective secondary prevention in survivors of cardiovascular events in the U.S. population: Report from the Third National Health and Nutrition Examination Survey. *Arch Intern Med* 2001;161:1621–1628.

103. Silvet H, Spencer F, Yarzebski J, Lessard D, Gore JM, Goldberg RJ. Communitywide trends in the use and outcomes associated with beta-blockers in patients with acute myocardial infarction. *Arch Intern Med* 2003;163:2175–2183.

104. Gerber Y, Weston SA, Killian JM, Jacobsen SJ, Roger VL. Sex and classic risk factors after myocardial infarction: a community study. *Am Heart J* 2006;152(3):461–468.

105. Gahli WA, Faris PD, Galbraith D, et al. Sex differences in access to coronary revascularization after cardiac catheterization: importance of detailed clinical data. *Ann Intern Med* 2002;136:723–732.

106. Lansky AJ, Hochman JS, Ward PA, et al. Percutaneous coronary intervention and adjunctive pharmacotherapy in women. *Circulation* 2005;111:940–953.

107. Argulian E, Patel AD, Abramson JL, et al. Gender differences in short-term cardiovascular outcomes after percutaneous coronary interventions. *Am J Cardiol* 2006;98(1):48–53.

108. Lansky AJ, Pietras C, Costa RA, et al. Gender differences in outcomes after primary angioplasty versus primary stenting with and without abciximab for acute myocardial infarction. *Circulation* 2005 111:1611–1618.

109. Guru V, Fremes SE, Austin PC, Blackstone EH, Tu JV. Gender differences in outcomes after hospital discharge from coronary artery bypass grafting. *Circulation* 2006;113:507–513.

110. Rogers MA, Langa KM, Kim C, et al. Contribution of infection to increased mortality in women after cardiac surgery. *Arch Intern Med* 2006;116:437–443.

111. Patel S, Smith JM, Engel AM. Gender differences in outcomes after off-pump coronary artery bypass graft surgery. *Am Surg* 2006;72(4):310–313.

112. Haan CK, Chiong JR, Coombs LP, et al. Comparison of risk profiles and outcomes in women versus men ≥ 75 years of age undergoing coronary artery bypass grafting. *Am J Cardiol* 2003;91:1255–1258.

113. Albert CM, Chae CU, Grodstein F, et al. Prospective study of sudden cardiac death among women in the United States. *Circulation* 2003;107(16):2096–2101.

114. Kim C, Fahrenbruch CE, Eisenberg MS. Out-of-hospital arrest in men and women. *Circulation* 2001;104:2699–2703.

115. Oparil S. Pathophysiology of sudden coronary death in women: implications for prevention. *Circulation* 1998:97:2103–2104.

116. Perk G, Stessman J, Ginsberg G, Bursztyn M. Sex differences in the effect of heart rate on mortality in the elderly. *J Am Geriatr Soc* 2003;51:1260–1264.

117. Van Gelder IC, Hagens VE, Bosker HA, et al. A comparison of rate control and rhythm control in patients with recurrent persistent atrial fibrillation. *N Engl J Med* 2002;347:1834–1840.

118. Henyan NN, White CM, Gillespie EL, et al. The impact of gender on survival among patients with implantable cardioverter defibrillators for primary prevention against sudden cardiac death. *J Intern Med* 2006;260(5):467–473.

119. Benjamin EJ, Wolf PA, D'Agostino RB, et al. Impact of atrial fibrillation on the risk of death: the Framingham Heart Study. *Circulation* 1998;98:946–952.

120. Fang MC, Singer DR, Change Y, et al. Gender differences in the risk of ischemic stroke and peripheral embolism in atrial fibrillation: the Anticoagulation and Risk factors In Atrial fibrillation (ATRIA) study. *Circulation* 2005;112:1687–1691.

121. Raj SR, Brennan FJ, Abdollah H. Is there a sex bias in the selection of permanent pacemaker implantations? *Can J Cardiol* 1996;12(4):375–378.

122. Rodriquez I, Kilborn MJ, Liu X, Pezzullo JC, Woosley RL. Drug-induced QT prolongation in women during the menstrual cycle. *JAMA* 2001;285:1322–1326.

123. Rautaharju PM, Kadish PRJ, Kadish A, Larson JC, Hsia J, Lund B. Normal standards for QT and QT subintervals derived from a large ethnically diverse population of women aged 50 to 79 years (the Women's Health Initiative). *Am J Cardiol* 2006;97(5):730–737.

CHAPTER (103)

Cardiovascular Disease and Ethnicity

S. Carolina Masri / Anne L. Taylor

INTRODUCTION

Although race, ethnicity, and geographic ancestry have been associated with differences in disease prevalence, expression, and outcomes, the public and academic discourse surrounding the role of race in health and disease has been both intense and complex. In the United States and many parts of the world, racial and ethnic differences have been used for social and political purposes to confer advantage to some and disadvantage to others based on presumed natural superiority or inferiority. Because of this, an intellectual goal of the late twentieth century has been to eliminate use of inherent racial and ethnic differences for purposes of societal stratification and advantage. However, recent advances in genetics and pharmacogenetics have resulted in renewed discussion of biologic and genetic correlates of racial and geographic ancestry, igniting a highly polarized discussion about the nature and meaning of race in healthcare.[1–4] Factors adding complexity to the analysis of the health impact of race and ethnicity are the high prevalence of racial misclassification and the admixture of populations typical of the United States. Despite the recent genetic data, it remains true that African Americans and other non-European minorities have had societally imposed disadvantages in economics, education, access to healthy environments, and barriers to adequate health care, all of which increase disease prevalence, morbidity, and mortality. Thus, discussions about cardiovascular health by racial and ethnic groups require the context that environmental factors in their broadest sense and perhaps some ge-

netic factors are operative in determining health risk among different racial and ethnic groups. In this chapter we accept that race, ethnicity, and geographic descent includes clustering of some common genetic characteristics but also social, environmental, and lifestyle variables, which have a huge impact on cardiovascular health. A critical challenge for multidisciplinary researchers is to define the relative contributions of each variable to cardiovascular health and disease as well as to discover how to use knowledge from biologic and social sciences to bring equity in cardiovascular health outcomes across racial and ethnic populations.

CORONARY HEART DISEASE MORTALITY BY RACE AND ETHNICITY

Cardiovascular disease (CVD) has been recognized as the dominant cause of death in the United States for at least 50 years, with heart disease ranking first and stroke third.[5–6] Fig. 103–1A and Fig. 103–1B show the prevalence and percent of deaths attributable to cardiovascular disease by major U.S. ethnic groups. Although coronary heart disease (CHD) death rates in all major demographic groups have declined in the United States, the decline in CHD has not been uniform across racial and ethnic groups. For example, in African American men, it has declined by 33.3 percent between 1979 and 1998, compared to 46.1 percent in white men. At the same time, CHD death rates decreased by 26.6 percent in African American women compared to 40.1 percent in white women. Analysis of annual rates

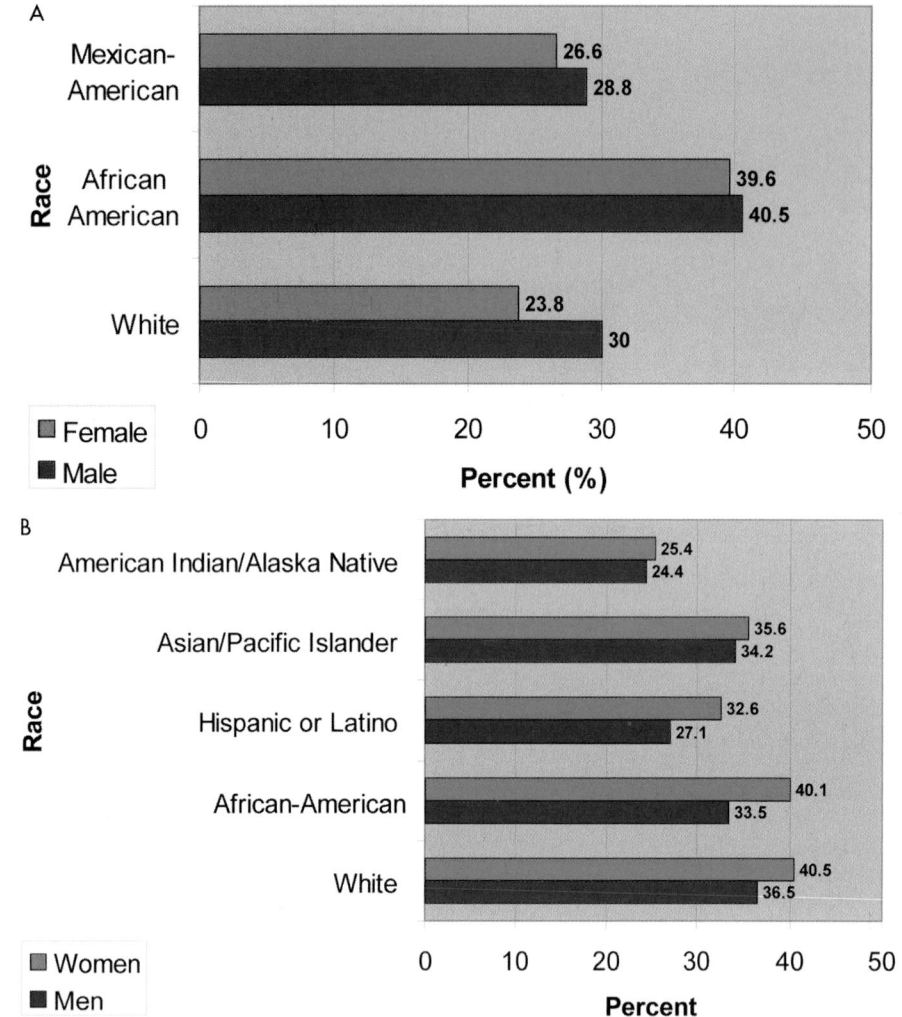

A. Prevalence of cardiovascular disease.
Female / Male
Percent (%)

Mexican-American: 26.6 / 28.8
African American: 39.6 / 40.5
White: 23.8 / 30

B.
Women / Men
Percent

American Indian/Alaska Native: 25.4 / 24.4
Asian/Pacific Islander: 35.6 / 34.2
Hispanic or Latino: 32.6 / 27.1
African-American: 40.1 / 33.5
White: 40.5 / 36.5

FIGURE 103–1. A. Prevalence of cardiovascular disease. From NHANES III (1988–94), CDC/NCHS. Data for white and black males and females are for non-Hispanics. Total population data include children; percentages for racial/ethnic groups are age-adjusted for Americans ages 20 years and older. **B.** Percent of total deaths attributed to cardiovascular disease (from CDC/NCHS). CDC, Centers for Disease Control and Prevention; NCHS, National Center for Health Statistics; NHANES, National Health and Nutrition Examination Survey. *Source: Adapted from American Heart Association.*[6]

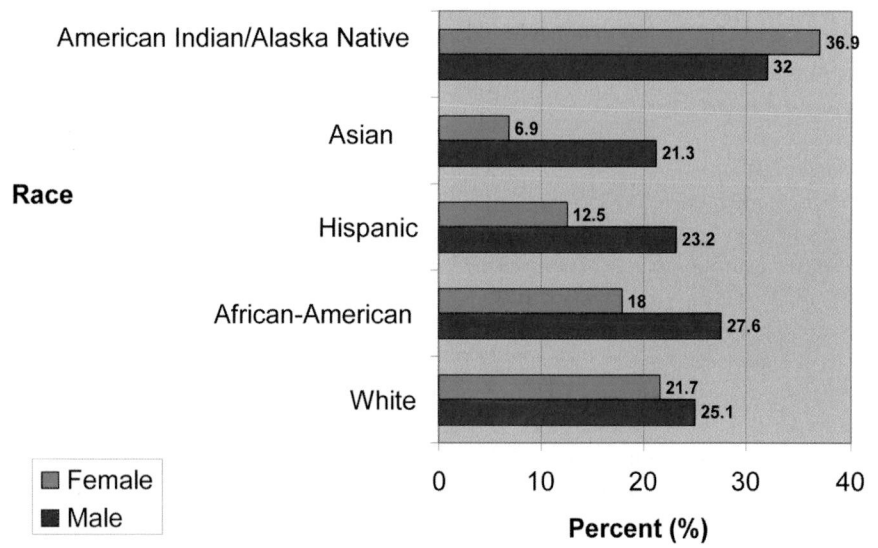

Female / Male
Percent (%)

American Indian/Alaska Native: 36.9 / 32
Asian: 6.9 / 21.3
Hispanic: 12.5 / 23.2
African-American: 18 / 27.6
White: 21.7 / 25.1

FIGURE 103–2. Prevalence of tobacco use in 2001. From CDC, National Center for Health Statistics. *Source: Adapted from American Heart Association.*[6]

of first heart attack, first cerebral infarction, and first cerebral hemorrhage by age, sex, and African American or white race demonstrates higher rates of all three entities in African Americans compared to whites.[6]

CARDIOVASCULAR RISK FACTORS BY RACE AND ETHNICITY

A differential prevalence of risk factors for CVD exists by ethnicity and may contribute to a portion of the differences in outcomes by ethnicity[7] either by virtue of the number of risk factors clustered by ethnicity and/or to differences in the intensity of treatment of risk factors by ethnicity. Approximately 25 percent of the overall U.S. population continues to smoke on a daily basis. Smoking prevalence rates vary markedly by racial and ethnic group as well as sex. Native Americans seem to have the highest prevalence rates and African American men without high school diplomas have the next highest smoking prevalence. The lowest rates of smoking are found in Hispanic and Asian women (Fig. 103–2).

Current estimates of body mass index (BMI) from National Health and Nutrition Examination Survey (NHANES) III for U.S. adults ages 20 to 74 years identify approximately 60 percent of men and approximately 50 percent of women as overweight, with 20 percent of men and 25 percent of women as obese,[8] with significant variation by ethnicity (Fig. 103–3).

With respect to physical activity, data from 1996 suggests that only 28 percent of adults meet the recommended levels of moderate or vigorous physical activity and 29 percent report no physical activity outside of their work. The prevalence of physical inactivity increases with age, is higher in women than men, and highest in African Americans and Hispanics[6,9–10] (Fig. 103–4).

Diabetes mellitus, a major contributor to CVD morbidity and mortality in the United States has increased in incidence by 49 percent in the past decade, closely coupled to the rapidly increasing incidence of obesity. Among people age 20 years or older, the prevalence of diabetes in the United States is highest in American Indians and Alaska Natives followed by African Americans. On average African Americans are 1.6 times more likely to have diabetes than non-Hispanic whites of similar age. Hispanic/Latino Americans are 1.5 times more likely to have diabetes than non-Hispanic whites. Mexican Americans, the largest Hispanic/Latino subgroup, are over twice as likely to have diabetes as non-Hispanic whites of similar age[6,11–12] (Fig. 103–5).

Hypertension, an important risk factor for CHD, heart failure (HF), stroke, and renal disease affects more than 43 million Americans with an estimated age-adjusted prevalence of 26 percent in all adult males and of 22 percent of all adult females.[6] African Americans have the highest prevalence, earliest age at onset, and most severe target organ damage at all ages and in both sexes (Fig. 103–6).

According to the Behavioral Risk Factor Surveillance System, the prevalence of hypercholesterolemia was generally high among white and Mexican American men as well as white women in all education groups, with lesser prevalence in African Americans.[11] However, African Americans and Hispanics with dyslipidemia are less likely to be treated to guideline recommended goals[13] (Fig. 103–7).

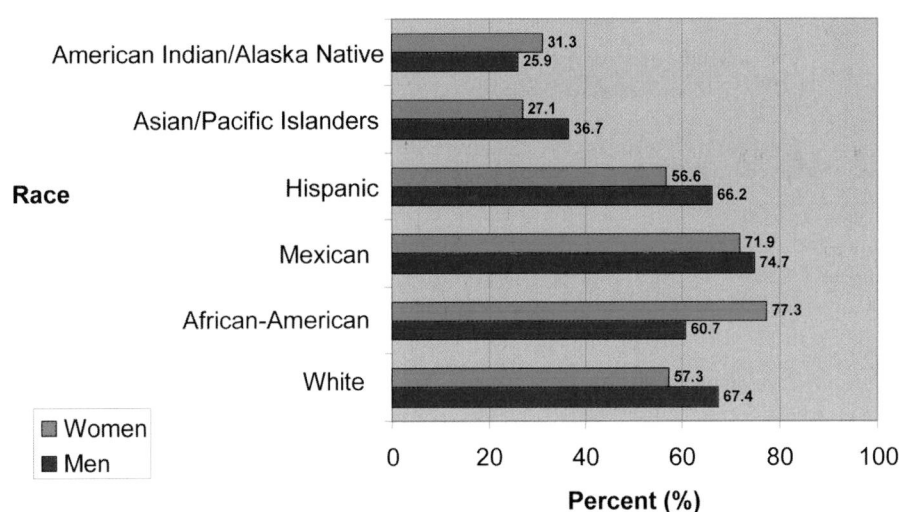

FIGURE 103–3. Prevalence of overweight and obesity in adults. From National Health and Nutrition Examination Survey IV (1999–2000), CDC/NCHS. Data in adults are for age 20 and older. *Source: Adapted from American Heart Association.*[6]

ASPECTS OF CARDIOVASCULAR DISEASE BY HIGH-RISK POPULATION GROUPS

[ ] AMERICAN INDIANS AND ALASKA NATIVES

Recently, data indicated that CVD is the leading cause of death among American Indians with variation in mortality by tribal affiliation. The Northern Plains Indians have higher rates of coronary heart disease whereas the Southwestern Indians have lower rates.[14] Data from the Strong Heart Study[15] suggest that CVD incidence rates among Native Americans are increasing and that CVD may more often be fatal in American Indians. A total of 4549 participants, ages 47 to 74 years old were subjected to surveillance (average 4.2 years). CVD morbidity and mortality were higher in men than in women. The CHD incidence rates among American Indian men and women were almost twofold higher than those of subjects of European descent in the Atherosclerosis Risk In Communities Study.[15] A large contributor to the high rate of CVD in American Indians is the high prevalence of smoking and diabetes in these communities. Seventy percent of American In-

dian individuals in Arizona and >40 percent in Oklahoma and South and North Dakota have diabetes. In a study of 75,993 death certificates in Montana from 1991 to 1995 and 1996–2000, analysis of heart disease and stroke death rates (per 100,000) for American Indians and whites was done.[16] There were striking differences in premature death from heart disease among American Indians compared to whites. In American Indians 40 percent of men and 29 percent of women who died of heart disease during these years were younger than 65 years old compared to only 21 percent of white men and 8 percent of white women. The percentage of the population with two or more risk factors for heart disease in American Indian adults increased from 34 percent in 1999 to 44 percent in 2003. These data showed a significant increase in CVD risk and mortality among middle-aged American Indians and a growing disparity in CVD mortality compared with the general population.[17]

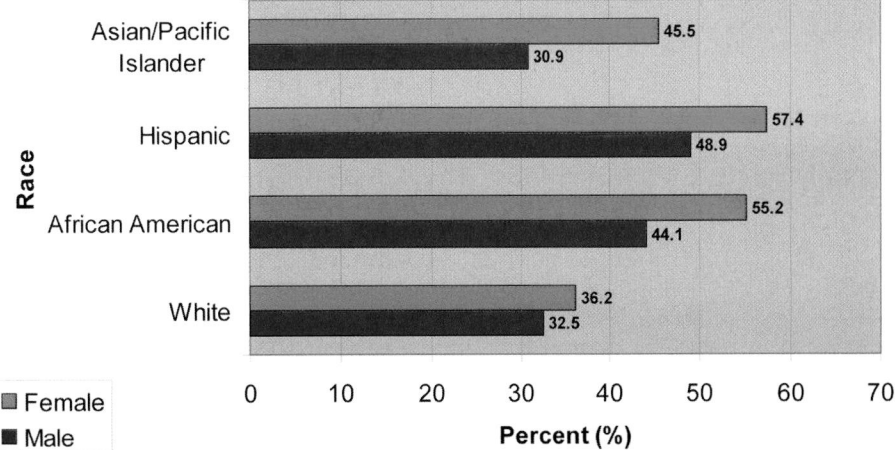

FIGURE 103–4. Prevalence of physical inactivity 1998. Prevalence is the percentage of population who reported no leisure-time physical activity. Data are age-adjusted for Americans age 18 and older. *Source: From National Health Interview Survey (1997–1998), CDC, National Center for Health Statistics. Adapted from American Heart Association.*[6]

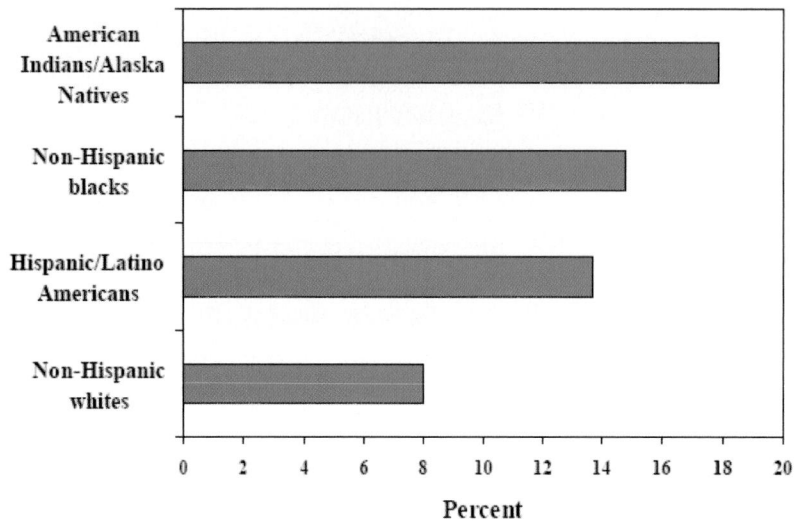

FIGURE 103–5. Estimated age-adjusted total prevalence of diabetes in U.S. people aged 20 years or older, by race/ethnicity in 2005. For American Indians/Alaska Natives, the calculation is based on the estimate of diagnosed diabetes from the 2003 outpatient database of the Indian Health Service, and the estimate of undiagnosed diabetes from the 1999–2002 NHANES. For the other groups, 1999–2002 NHANES estimates of total prevalence was projected to year 2005. *Source: From CDC. National Diabetes Fact Sheet: General Information and National Estimates on Diabetes in the United States, 2005.*

【 】 HISPANICS

Hispanic or Latino is considered a designation of ethnicity, not race; and people of Hispanic or Latino origin may be of Cuban, Mexican, Puerto Rican, South or Central American, or other Spanish culture or origin, regardless of race.[18] The U.S. Hispanic population has become the fastest growing and largest minority group in the country. In the year 2000, there were an estimated 35.3 million Hispanics, (12.5 percent of the total U.S. population) with Mexican Americans being the largest ethnically distinct subgroup of Hispanics.

On average, Hispanics have more risk factors for CHD than non-Hispanic whites, including higher body mass indices, more central obesity, lower high-density lipoprotein (HDL) cholesterol, and higher triglyceride levels.[19] Diabetes is more prevalent in Hispanics, whereas the prevalence of hypertension is similar to that in whites. In addition, Hispanics have lower socioeconomic levels, less health insurance coverage, and use fewer preventative services compared to non-Hispanic whites.[19] Previous observational population-based studies suggest that despite the fact that Hispanics have higher rates of diabetes and obesity as well as barriers to healthcare, they have lower all-cause and cardiovascular mortality rates than do non-Hispanic whites.[20–21] This phenomenon has been dubbed the *Hispanic Paradox.*

In the CRUSADE study,[22] data was evaluated regarding the management of non–ST-segment elevation acute coronary syndrome in Hispanic patients. Hispanics were younger and had less hyperlipidemia, but they were more likely to be hypertensive and diabetic. During hospitalization, Hispanics were more often managed conservatively, undergoing stress testing more frequently and interventional procedures (cardiac catheterization [48.7 percent vs. 55.5 percent; $p < 0.001$] or angioplasty [39.6 percent vs. 46.4 percent; $p < 0.001$]) less frequently than non-Hispanic whites. Adjusted in-hospital mortality was the same for the two groups. Data from the second National Registry of Myocardial Infarction showed no significant differences in in-hospital mortality between Hispanics and non-Hispanic whites.[23] However, data from the San Antonio Heart Study has raised the question of the validity of the Hispanic Paradox.[24–25] After 15 years of followup it was observed that Mexican Americans compared with non-Hispanic whites had more than a 50 percent greater risk of all-cause mortality, a 70 percent greater risk of cardiovascular mortality, and a 60 percent greater risk of CHD mortality. Similarly, data from the Corpus Christi Heart Project[26–27] a community-based surveillance program, has shown both greater rates of hospitalization for CHD and worse in-hospital survival after myocardial infarction among Mexican Americans compared with non-Hispanic whites. Thus, although Hispanics with acute coronary syndrome appear to have equivalent short-term outcomes compared to whites in some studies, long-term follow-up studies suggest that outcomes are poorer.

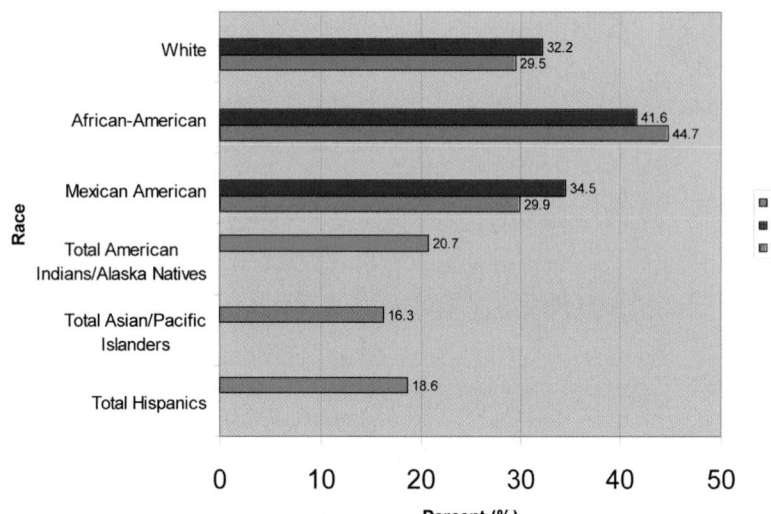

FIGURE 103–6. Prevalence of high blood pressure in 2001. Data are age adjusted for ages 20 and older. Rates are for white only and African American only. From National Health and Nutrition Examination Survey IV (1999–2000), CDC, National Center for Health Statistics. *Source: Adapted from American Heart Association.*[6]

【 】 SOUTH ASIANS

Multiple studies of immigrants of South Asian ethnicity (India and Pakistan) have found a three- to fivefold increase in the risk for myocardial infarction and cardiovascular death as compared with other ethnic groups. In an analysis of age-standardized CHD mortality in Canada over a 15-year period, South Asians had the highest CHD mortality compared to individuals of Chinese or European descendent.[28] In addition, South Asians tend to develop CHD at younger ages (often before age 40) and are more likely to have significant left main, multivessel and distal coronary artery disease.[29]

The INTERHEART study[30] demonstrated that traditional risk factors play an important role in the prediction of myocardial infarction in populations around the world including South Asians. The use of tobacco is lower among South Asian men and almost nonexistent among South Asian women. The levels of low-density lipoprotein (LDL) cholesterol are comparable to other populations, but the LDL-cholesterol particle size tends to be the smaller, more atherogenic particles in South Asians. South Asians also have the lowest HDL-cholesterol levels. The prevalence of diabetes is higher in South Asians than other populations. Compared with European populations, South Asians have increased abdominal visceral fat and greater insulin resistance at similar levels of BMI including BMI levels that are considered ideal (< 25 kg/m²). In the Study of Health Assessment and Risk in Ethnic Groups (SHARE) trial,[31] South Asians were found to have a higher prevalence of subclinical atherosclerosis and South Asian ethnicity was an independent predictor of CVD. More aggressive screening has been suggested for this population.[32]

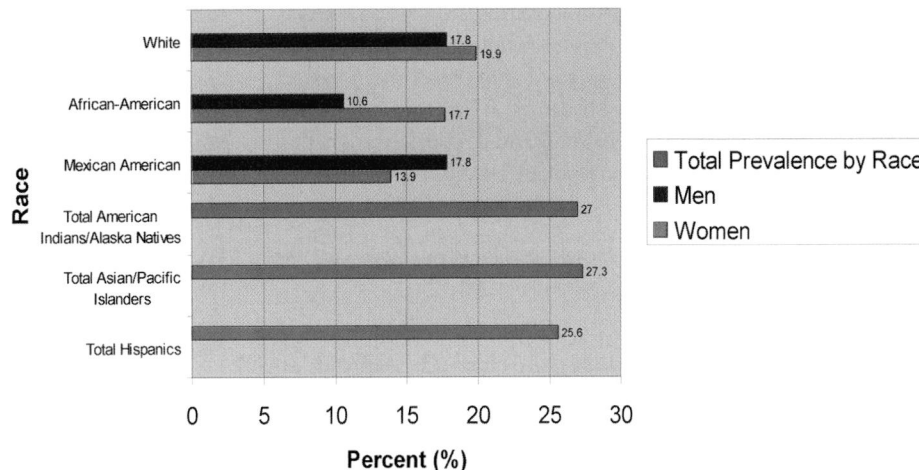

FIGURE 103–7. Prevalence of Total Cholesterol 240 mg/dL or higher in 2001. *Source: From CDC, National Center for Health Statistics. Adapted from American Heart Association.*[6]

【 】 AFRICAN AMERICANS

In the United States the African American population has the highest rate of overall mortality caused by CHD of any ethnic group.[33] The risk of sudden death is higher and the onset occurs approximately 6 years earlier than in whites. Interestingly, despite the increased cardiovascular mortality, the presence of obstructive epicardial coronary artery disease by angiography is less than that in white patients[34–35] as is the prevalence of coronary artery calcification.[36–38] However, the presence of left ventricular hypertrophy (LVH) is greater.[39] In the Dallas Heart Study,[39] 1335 African Americans and 858 whites underwent cardiac MRI to measure left ventricular (LV) mass. The prevalence of LVH measured by cardiac MRI was two- to threefold significantly higher in African Americans compared to whites. As defined by body surface area, LVH prevalence was 14 percent in African American men and 6 percent in white men, 14 percent in African American women and 3.4 percent in white women. These ethnic differences in LV mass persisted in multivariable models despite adjustment for body mass, systolic blood pressure, age, gender, and measures of socioeconomic status. When hypertensive African Americans and whites were compared, the association of African American race and LVH was strong. Thus, LVH coupled to more severe hyper-

tension may contribute to the higher mortality from CHD despite the lesser extent of epicardial coronary disease observed in African Americans.[39]

The prevalence of having two or more concomitant risk factors was higher among African Americans (48.7 percent) as well as American Indians and Alaska natives (46.7 percent) and lowest among Asians (25.9 percent).[40] The differential prevalence of the cardiac risk factors in African Americans compared with whites is evident from childhood. Data from NHANES, which included 2769 African American children and young adults, ages 6 to 24 years, revealed that the BMIs were significantly higher for African Americans and Mexican Americans, with ethnic differences evident by the ages of 6 to 9 years and widening thereafter.[41] Percentage of energy from dietary fat paralleled these findings and was also significantly higher for African Americans than for white boys. Blood pressure was higher for African American girls than for white girls in every age group and glycosylated hemoglobin (HbA₁c) was significantly higher for African American and Mexican American girls and boys at every age group. In the Bogalusa Heart Study,[42] systolic and diastolic blood pressures in adolescents were 3.4 mmHg and 1.9 mmHg higher in African American boys and girls respectively. Total cholesterol tends to be lower and HDL-cholesterol levels higher in African Americans, but in the Multi-Ethnic Study of Atherosclerosis (MESA) study it was observed that African Americans with elevated cholesterol were less likely to be treated and controlled.[11]

Studies of the association between race and outcomes in acute coronary syndrome have yielded conflicting results, with some studies suggesting higher rates of adverse cardiovascular events and others equivalent or lower rates of events. Data from the CRUSADE study,[43] of patients presenting with non–ST-segment elevations acute coronary syndrome showed that African American patients were younger; more likely to be female; and more likely to have hypertension, renal insufficiency, history of smoking, congestive HF, and stroke. African American patients were less likely to present with ST-segment depression or positive cardiac markers but more likely to present with signs of HF when compared to white subjects. Acute risk-adjusted outcomes were similar in African Americans and whites, despite the fact that African Americans were less likely to receive revascularization procedures or newer acute coronary syndrome therapies. Several trials and databases[35,43–62] have demonstrated differences in procedure use in African Americans and Hispanics. These groups are less likely to receive cardiac catheterization and revascularization procedures and a negative impact on outcomes has been reported.[35]

RACE, ETHNICITY, AND HEART FAILURE

In the United States an estimated 4.8 million individuals have HF and approximately 550,000 new cases develop each year, with associated substantial morbidity, mortality, and economic impact. There is more data comparing African Americans and whites with HF than other ethnic groups, so this will constitute the focus of this section.

The overall incidence of HF within the non-black U.S. population is 2 percent, but occurs in 3 percent of the African American population. HF occurs at earlier ages in African Americans compared to whites,[63–64] and is more frequently attributable to hypertension than to ischemic heart disease.[65–68]

[ ] HOSPITALIZATION FOR HEART FAILURE

Although detailed data regarding HF morbidity for most minority/ethnic groups are sparse, there are data from analysis of Medicare enrollees showing that HF hospitalization was 1.5 times greater for African Americans, 1.2 times higher for Hispanics, but 0.5 times less likely for Asian patients.[69] African Americans with HF have a higher risk for hospitalization and readmission compared to whites.[70–76] Observed racial differences in morbidity in HF may be related to differences in comorbid conditions (such as hypertension, diabetes, or renal disease), effectiveness of treatment, socioeconomic factors (i.e., access to specialty care), lifestyle, and healthcare-seeking behaviors (i.e., time between symptom onset and presentation for care).[76] For example, in a retrospective cohort study from the Veterans Affairs system where patients should have *equal access* to cardiovascular care, it was observed that African American patients more frequently had uncontrolled hypertension at the time of hospital admission for HF.[72,77] Nonclinical factors contributing to hospitalization such as nonadherence with medications or diet, inadequate patient followup, and poor social support, may also vary by ethnicity.[77]

[ ] HEART FAILURE MORTALITY

African Americans with HF have been reported to have similar,[75] higher,[78] and lower mortality than whites.[73,77] Conflicting reports may be in part caused by differences in study period, method (registries, observational databases, administrative databases, or clinical trials), population studied (HF with preserved or decreased LV function), statistical modeling and age of patients studied.

[ ] RACIAL DIFFERENCES IN RESPONSE TO DRUG TREATMENT IN HEART FAILURE

The considerable current controversy regarding the efficacy of some pharmacologic treatments in African Americans is a result of the fact that there are few randomized clinical trials of HF treatment that have *prespecified* a subgroup analysis of outcomes by ethnicity. However, there are retrospective analyses that suggest that there may be differences between African Americans and majority populations in response to some HF pharmacotherapy.

Angiotensin-Converting Enzyme Inhibitors

Pooled data from the Studies of Left Ventricular Dysfunction (SOLVD) prevention and treatment trials[79] found that enalapril therapy was associated with a significant reduction in the risk of hospitalization for HF among white patients but not among African American patients. African American patients randomly assigned to receive enalapril had 7.9 more hospitalizations per 100 persons per years of followup than matched white patients.[80] Analysis of this same database from both the SOLVD prevention and treatment study showed no significant difference in the risk of death associated with enalapril treatment in African American and matched white patients,[79] but African American patients overall had higher rates of all cause mortality and mortality from pump failure. In whites treated with enalapril, a significant reduction in both systolic blood pressure (5 ± 17.1 mmHg) and diastolic blood pressure (3.6 ± 10.6 mmHg) was observed, whereas no reduction in blood pressure was shown in African Americans treated with enalapril. However, in both SOLVD prevention and treatment studies, African Americans were at higher risk for all cause mortality as well as death from pump failure despite standardized treatment in both African American and white subjects.[80] In a post hoc analysis of the SOLVD prevention arm only,[81] it was demonstrated that enalapril delayed the progression of asymptomatic left ventricular dysfunction (ALVD) to symptomatic HF in both African American and white subjects. However, despite the comparable relative reduction in risk for the development of symptomatic HF associated with enalapril, the differences in the baseline magnitude of risk were such that African Americans randomized to enalapril remained at higher risk than whites randomized to placebo for the development of HF. The differences between African American and white subjects in the risk of progression of ALVD remained after adjusting for potential confounders including ejection fraction, New York Heart Association class, serum sodium, and etiology of LV dysfunction.[81]

β Blockers

Several large multicenter trials have proven the beneficial effects of β blockers in HF; however, all have had small numbers of African Americans and the analyses by ethnicity were post hoc[82–84]; however, these post hoc analyses show a trend toward a beneficial effect in African Americans. Therefore, the interpretation of these data is that African American patients are likely to have comparable risk reduction as white patients treated with metoprolol, bisoprolol, or carvedilol, despite the small numbers in the trials and failure of hazard ratios to reach statistical significance.

In the Beta-Blocker Evaluation of Survival Trial (BEST), the only trial prospectively stratified by African American or white race, the β blocker bucindolol significantly reduced the risk of death or hospitalization among white patients but was associated with a nonsignificant increase in the risk of serious clinical events in African American patients.[85] Taken together, the data would support the use of β-blocker therapy (metoprolol or carvedilol but *not* bucindolol) combined with angiotensin-converting enzyme (ACE) inhibitors in the management of HF in African Americans.

Vasodilator Drugs

Two of the most important clinical trials providing the bases for contemporary HF treatment were the Vasodilator-Heart Failure Trials (VHeFTs).[86–87] VHeFT I[86] compared the effects on mortality of vasodilator therapy consisting of either combined hydralazine-isosorbide dinitrate or prazosin versus placebo. Although hemodynamic variables were similar in the two vasodilator arms, mortality was favorably impacted only by treatment with combined hydralazine/isosorbide dinitrate. This suggested that therapeutic targets beyond hemodynamic improvement were responsive to the hydralazine isosorbide dinitrate combination. VHeFT II[87] compared two treatments, the ACE-I enalapril versus combined hydralazine/isosorbide dinitrate. In this study, overall mortality was lower in the enalapril treatment arm. Fortuitously and uniquely, these two trials had nearly 28 percent African American men, thus providing a database which could be retrospectively analyzed for the effects of ethnicity on treatment responses to enalapril and isosorbide dinitrate.

Retrospective analyses of these two seminal HF trials comparing African-Americans to whites in the trial cohorts revealed significant ethnic differences in response to treatment,[88] suggesting that consideration of ethnicity in HF therapy might have some role. Analysis by ethnicity of both VHeFTs[88] revealed the following: In VHeFT-I, comparing a combination of hydralazine/isosorbide dinitrate to prazosin or placebo, a significant mortality benefit was observed in African American but not in white patients treated with hydralazine/isosorbide dinitrate. In the VHeFT II, comparing treatment with enalapril to hydralazine/isosorbide dinitrate, a significant survival advantage of enalapril was observed only in white patients, with no survival advantage of enalapril over hydralazine/isosorbide dinitrate observed in African Americans. The recent African American Heart Failure Trial (A-HeFT) tested the hypothesis derived from the retrospective analyses of the VHeFTs, that addition of combined isosorbide dinitrate and hydralazine to background neurohormonal blockade would improve HF outcomes in African American patients with low ejection fractions and advanced symptoms.[68] Importantly, 40 percent of the trial cohort were women, thus providing the only clinical trial data of this treatment strategy in women.[89] Although patients in both arms of the trial were well treated with background neurohormonal blockade, there were some baseline clinical differences between men and women, but no differences in baseline HF medications.[89]

A-HeFT demonstrated that therapy with fixed dose combined isosorbide dinitrate and hydralazine added to neurohormonal blockade significantly improved survival in self-identified African American men and women with advanced HF receiving background neurohormonal blockade.[68,89] The incremental improvement in outcomes in the setting of neurohormonal blockade strongly suggested additional or alternative mechanisms of HF progression responsive to combined isosorbide dinitrate/hydralazine. Identification of the specific mechanism of benefit as well as markers to identify responsiveness in other population groups will be important for future research directions.

SUMMARY

Differences in cardiovascular healthcare outcomes amongst populations of differing race, ethnicity, or geographic ancestry are critically important challenges for American medicine. Although causes of these differences are many (including biologic, genetic, environmental, and social factors) and complexly interrelated, effective multidisciplinary research provides insights into pathophysiologic variations in disease mechanisms as well as contributes to a reduction in health care disparities. Clearly needed are more precise predictors of disease risk, expression, and treatment response (such as specific genotypes, biomarkers, or metabolic phenotypes), which should transcend usage of the conventional racial/ethnic/geographic ancestry descriptors. Continued collection of data on health status in racial and ethnic populations, assessment of differences in disease patterns, design of clinical trials with the inclusion of adequate numbers of diverse populations to probe for differences in pathophysiology (including biologic, environmental, and social factors), and potential differential responses to treatment are essential. Finally, where differences are observed among population segments, clinical trials focused in these population groups are essential to define optimal evidence based therapeutic strategies.[4]

REFERENCES

1. Root M. How we divide the world. Philosophy of Science, 6th Proceedings, 2000;67:S628–S639.
2. Tang H, Quertermous T, Rodriguez B, et al. Genetic structure, self-identified race/ethnicity, and confounding in case-control association studies. *Am J Hum Genet* 2005;76:268–275.
3. Risch N. Dissecting racial and ethnic differences. *N Engl J Med* 2006;354(4):408–412.
4. Taylor AL, Wright JT, Cooper RS, Psaty BM. Should ethnicity serve as the basis for clinical trial design? Importance from the African-American Heart Failure Trial (A-HeFT), the African-American Study of Kidney Disease and Hypertension (AASK), and the Antihypertensive and Lipid-Lowering Treatment to Prevent Heart Attack Trial (ALLHAT) and Diversity and Inclusiveness Should Remain the Guiding Principles for Clinical Trials. *Circulation* 2005;112:3654–3666.
5. Ford E, Giles W, Mokdad A. The distribution of 10-year risk for coronary heart disease among U.S. adults. *J Am Coll Cardiol* 2004;43(10):1791–1796.
6. American Heart Association. *Heart Disease and Stroke Statistics: 2004 Update.* Dallas: American Heart Association, 2003.
7. Cooper R, Cutler J, Desvigne-Nickens P, et al. Trends and disparities in coronary heart disease, stroke, and other cardiovascular diseases in the United States: findings of the national conference on cardiovascular disease prevention. *Circulation* 2000;102:3137–3147.
8. Gregg E, Cheng Y, Cadwell B, et al. Secular trends in cardiovascular disease risk factors according to body mass index in U.S. adults. *JAMA* 2005;293(15):1868–1874.
9. Pratt M, Macera CA, Blanton C. Levels of physical activity and inactivity in children and adults in the United States: current evidence and research issues. *Med Sci Sports Exerc* 1999;11:S526–S533.
10. U.S. Department of Health and Human Services. *Physical Activity and Health: A Report of the Surgeon General.* Atlanta: U.S. Department of Health and Human Services, Centers for Disease Control and Prevention, National Center for Chronic Disease Prevention and Health Promotion, 1996.
11. Centers for Disease Control and Prevention. *National Diabetes Fact Sheet: General Information and National Estimates on Diabetes in the United States, 2003.* Rev ed. Atlanta: U.S. Department of Health and Human Services, Centers for Disease Control and Prevention, 2004.
12. Burrows N, Geiss L, Engelgau M, Acton K. Prevalence of diabetes among Native Americans and Alaska Natives, 1990–1997. *Diabetes Care* 2000;23(12)1786–1790.
13. Goff D, Bertoni A, Kramer H, et al. Dyslipidemia prevalence, treatment, and control in the Multi-Ethnic Study of Atherosclerosis (MESA): gender, ethnicity, and coronary artery calcium. *Circulation* 2006;113:647–656.

14. Howard BV, Lee ET, Cowan LD, et al. Coronary heart disease prevalence and its relation to risk factors in American Indians. The Strong Heart Study. *Am J Epidemiol* 1995;142:254–268.

15. Howard B, Lee E, Cowan L, et al. Rising tide of cardiovascular disease in American Indians. The Strong Heart Study. *Circulation* 1999;99:2389–2395.

16. Harwell TS, Oser CS, Okon NJ, Fogle CC, Helgerson SD, Gohdes D. Defining disparities in cardiovascular disease for American Indians: trends in heart disease and stroke mortality among American Indians and whites in Montana, 1991 to 2000. *Circulation* 112:2263–2267.

17. Rhoades D. Racial misclassification and disparities in cardiovascular disease among American Indians and Alaska Natives. *Circulation* 2005;111:1250–1256.

18. Centers for Disease Control and Prevention. Use of race and ethnicity in public health surveillance: summary of the CDC/ATSDR Workshop. *MMWR Recomm Rep* 1993;42(RR-10)1–16.

19. Winkleby M, Kraemer H, Ahn D, Varady A. Ethnic and socioeconomic differences in cardiovascular disease risk factors: findings for Women from the Third National and Nutrition Examination Survey, 1988–1994. *JAMA* 1998;280(4):356–362.

20. Liao X, Cooper R, Cao G, et al. Mortality from coronary heart disease and cardiovascular disease among adult U.S. Hispanics: findings from the National Health Interview Survey (1986–1994). *J Am Coll Cardiol* 1997;30(5):1200–1205.

21. Sorlie P, Backlund E, Johnson N, Rogot E. Mortality by Hispanic status in the United States. *JAMA* 1993;270(20):2464–2468.

22. Cohen M, Roe M, Mulgund J, et al. Clinical characteristics, process of care, and outcomes of Hispanic patients presenting with non-ST-segment elevation acute coronary syndromes: results from Can Rapid Risk Stratification of Unstable Angina Patients Suppress Adverse Outcomes with Early Implementation of the ACC/AHA Guidelines (CRUSADE). *Am Heart J* 2006;152(1):110–117.

23. Vaccarino V, Rathore S, Wenger N, et al. Sex and racial differences in the management of acute myocardial infarction. *N Engl J Med* 2005;353(7):671–682.

24. Mitchell B, Hazuda H, Haffner S, Patterson J, Stern M. Myocardial infarction in Mexican-American and non-Hispanic whites. The San Antonio Heart Study. *Circulation* 1991;83(1):45–51.

25. Hunt K, Resendez R, Williams K, Haffner S, Stern M, Hazuda H. All-cause and cardiovascular mortality among Mexican-American and Non-Hispanic white older participants in the San Antonio Heart Study: evidence against the "Hispanic Paradox." *Am J Epidemiol* 2003;158:1048–1057.

26. Goff DC, Nichaman MZ, Chan W, Ramsey DJ, Labarthe DR, Ortiz C. Greater incidence of hospitalized myocardial infarction among Mexican Americans than non-Hispanic whites. The Corpus Christi Heart Project, 1988–1992. *Circulation* 1997;95:1433–1440.

27. Goff DC, Varas C, Ramsey DJ, Wear ML, Labarthe DR, Nichaman MZ. Mortality after hospitalization for myocardial infarction among Mexican Americans and non-Hispanic whites. The Corpus Christi Heart Project. *Ethn Dis* 1993;3(1):55–63.

28. Sheth T, Nair C, Nargundkar M, et al. Cardiovascular and cancer mortality among Canadians of European, South Asian, and Chinese origin from 1979 to 1993: an analysis of 1.2 million deaths. *Can Med Assoc J* 1999;161:132–138.

29. Enas EA, Garg A, Davidson MA, et al. Coronary heart disease and its risk factors in first-generation immigrant Asian Indians to the United States of America. *Indian Heart J* 1996;48:343–353.

30. Yusuf S, Hawken S, Ounpuu S, et al. Effect of potentially modifiable risk factors associated with myocardial infarction in 52 countries (the INTERHEART study): case-control study. *Lancet* 2004;364:937–952.

31. Anand S, Yusuf S, Vuksan V, et al. Differences in risk factors, atherosclerosis, and cardiovascular disease between ethnic groups in Canada: the Study of Health Assessment and Risk in Ethnic Groups (SHARE). *Lancet* 2000;356:279–284.

32. Gupta M, Singh N, Verma S. South Asians and cardiovascular risk: what clinicians should know. *Circulation* 2006;113:e924–e929.

33. Gillum R. The epidemiology of cardiovascular disease in Black Americans. *N Engl J Med* 1996;335:1597–1599.

34. Okelo SO, Taylor AL, Wright JT, et al. Race and the decision to refer for coronary revascularization: effect of physician awareness of patient ethnicity. *J Am Coll Cardiol* 2001;38:698–704.

35. Peterson E, Shaw L, DeLong E, Pryor D, Califf R, Mark D. Racial variation in the use of coronary-revascularization procedures: are the differences real? Do they matter? *N Engl J Med* 1997:336(7):480–486.

36. Eggen DA, Strong JP, McGill HC. Coronary calcification: relationship to clinically significant coronary lesions and race, sex, and topographic distribution. *Circ* 1965;32:948–955.

37. McCleland R, Chung H, Detrano R, Post W, Kronmal R. Distribution of coronary artery calcium by race, gender, and age: results from the Multi-Ethnic Study of Atherosclerosis (MESA). *Circulation* 2006;113:30–37.

38. Bild D, Detrano R, Peterson D, et al. Ethnic differences in coronary calcification. The Multi-Ethnic Study of Atherosclerosis (MESA). *Circulation* 2005;111:1313–1320.

39. Drazner M, Dries D, Peshock R, et al. Left ventricular hypertrophy is more prevalent in blacks than whites in the general population. The Dallas Heart Study. *Hypertension* 2005;46:124–129.

40. Centers for Disease Control. Weekly morbidity and mortality report. February 11, 2005;54(05);113–117. Available at: http://www.cdc.gov/mmwr/preview. Accessed September 2006.

41. Winkleby M, Robinson T, Sundquist J, et al. Ethnic variation in cardiovascular disease risk factors among children and young adults: finding from the Third National Health and Nutritional Examination Survey, 1988–1994. *JAMA* 1999;281(11)1006–1013.

42. Cruickshank J, Mzayek F, Liu L, et al. Origins of the "black/white" difference in blood pressure: roles of birth weight, postnatal growth, early blood pressure, and adolescent body size. The Bogalusa Heart Study. *Circ* 2005;111:1932–1937.

43. Sonel A, Good C, Mulgund J, et al. Racial variations in treatment and outcomes in black and white patients with high-risk non-ST-elevation acute coronary syndromes: insights from CRUSADE. *Circulation* 2005;111:1225–1232.

44. Ford ES, Cooper RS. Racial/ethnic differences in health care utilization of cardiovascular procedures: a review of the evidence. *Health Serv Res* 1995;30:237–252.

45. Gonzalez-Klayman N, Barnhart JM. Racial differences in the utilization of coronary revascularization: a review of the literature. *CVD Prevention* 1998;1:114–122.

46. Rumsfeld J, Plomondon M, Peterson E, et al. The impact of ethnicity on outcomes following coronary artery bypass graft surgery in the Veterans Health Administration. *J Am Coll Cardiol* 2002;40(10):1786–1793.

47. Vaccarino V, Rathore S, Wenger N, et al. Sex and racial differences in the management of acute myocardial infarction. *N Engl J Med* 2005;353(7):671–682.

48. Cohen M, GrangerC, Ohman E, et al. Outcome of Hispanic patients treated with thrombolytic therapy for acute myocardial infarction: results from the GUSTO-I and III Trials. *J Am Coll Cardiol* 1999;34(6):1729–1737.

49. Laouri M, Kravitz RL, French WJ, et al. Underuse of coronary revascularization procedures: application of a clinical method *J Am Coll Cardiol* 1997;29:891–897.

50. Leape LL, Hilborne LH, Bell R, Kamberg C, Brook RH. Underuse of cardiac procedures: do women, ethnic minorities, and the uninsured fail to receive needed revascularization? *Ann Intern Med* 1999;130:183–92.

51. Sedlis SP, Fisher VJ, Tice D, Esposito R, Madmon L, Steinberg EH. Racial differences in performance of invasive cardiac procedures in a Department of Veterans Affairs Medical Center *J Clin Epidemiol* 1997;50:899–901.

52. Lightner S, Groman R, Ginsburg J, et al. Racial and ethnic disparities in health care: a position paper of the American College of Physicians. *Ann Intern Med* 2004;141:226–232.

53. Lillie-Blanton M, Maddox T, Rushing O, et al. Disparities in cardiac care: rising to the challenge of healthy people 2010. *J Am Coll Cardiol* 2004;44(3):503–508.

54. Sabatine M, Blake G, Drazner M, et al. Influence of race on death and ischemic complications in patients with non-ST elevation acute coronary syndromes despite modern, protocol-guided treatment. *Circulation* 2005;111:1217–1224.

55. Canto J, Allison J, Kiefe C, et al. Relation of race and sex to the use of reperfusion therapy in medicare beneficiaries with acute myocardial infarction. *N Engl J Med* 2000;342(15):1094–1100.

56. LaVeist T, Arthur M, Morgan A, et al. The Cardiac Access Longitudinal Study: a study of access to invasive cardiology among African American and white patients. *J Am Coll Cardiol* 2003;41(7):1159–1166.

57. Chen J, Rathore S, Radford M, Wang Y, Krumholz H. Racial differences in the use of cardiac catheterization after acute myocardial infarction. *N Engl J Med* 2001;344(19):1443–1449.

58. Maynard C, Fisher LD, Passamani ER, Pullum T. Blacks in the Coronary Artery Surgery Study (CASS): race and clinical decision making *Am J Public Health* 1986;76:1446–1448.

59. Schulman K, Berlin J, Harless W, et al. The effect of face and sex on physicians' recommendations for cardiac catheterization. *N Engl J Med* 1999;340:618–626.

60. Bach P, Pham H, Schrag D, Tate R, Hargraves J. Primary care physicians who treat blacks and whites. *N Engl J Med* 2004;351(6):575–584.

61. Trivedi A, Sequist T, Zyanian J. Impact of hospital volume on racial disparities in cardiovascular procedure mortality. *J Am Coll Cardiol* 2006;47(2):417–424.

62. Rumsfeld J, Epstein A. Racial disparities in cardiovascular procedure outcomes: turn down the volume. *J Am Coll Cardiol* 2006;47(2):425–426.

63. Yancy C. Heart failure in African Americans: a cardiovascular enigma. *J Card Fail* 2000;6(3):183–186.

64. Yancy C. Heart failure in African Americans: pathophysiology and treatment. *J Card Fail* 2003;9(5):S210–S215.

65. Philbin E, Weil H, Francis C, Marx H, et al. Race-related differences among patients with left ventricular dysfunction: observations from a biracial angiographic cohort. *J Card Fail* 2000;6(3):187–193.

66. Afzal A, Ananthasubramaniam K, Sharma N, et al. Racial differences in patients with heart failure. *Clin Cardiol* 1999;22:791–794.

67. Mathew J, Davidson S, Narra L, et al. Etiology and characteristics of congestive heart failure in blacks. *Am J Cardiol* 1996;78:1447–1450.

68. Taylor A, Ziesche S, Yancy C, et al. Combination of isosorbide dinitrate and hydralazine in blacks with heart failure. *N Engl J Med* 2004;351(20):2049–2057.

69. Brown D, Haldeman G, Croft J, Giles W, Mensah G. Racial or ethnic differences in hospitalization for heart failure among elderly adults: Medicare, 1990–2000. *Am Heart J* 2005;150(3):448–454.

70. Vaccarino V, Gahbauer E, Kasl SV, et al. Differences between African Americans and whites in the outcome of heart failure: evidence for a greater functional decline in African Americans. *Am Heart J* 2002;143(6):1058–1067.

71. Lafata JE, Pladevall M, Divine G, et al. Are there race/ethnicity differences in outpatient congestive heart failure management, hospital use, and morality among an insured population? *Med Care* 2004;42(7):680–689.

72. Deswal A, Petersen NJ, Urbauer DL, et al. Racial variations in quality of care and outcomes in an ambulatory heart failure cohort. *Am Heart J* 2006;152(2):348–354.

73. Rathore S, Foody J, Wang Y, et al. Race, quality of care, and outcomes of elderly patients hospitalized with heart failure. *JAMA* 2003;289(19):2517–2524.

74. Philbin EF, Di Salvo TG. Influence of race and gender on care process, resource use, and hospital based outcomes in congestive heart failure. *Am J Cardiol* 1998;82(1):76–81.

75. Mathew J, Wittes J, McSherry F, et al. Racial differences in outcome and treatment effect in congestive heart failure. *Am Heart J* 2005;150(5):968–976.

76. Ghali J. Race, Ethnicity, and Heart Failure. *J Card Fail* 2002;8(6):387–389.

77. Singh H, Gordon H, Deswal A. Variation by race in factors contributing to heart failure hospitalizations. *J Card Fail* 2005;11(1):23–29.

78. Agoston I, Cameron C, Yao D, DeLa Rosa A, Mann D, Deswal A. Comparison of outcomes in white versus black patients hospitalized with heart failure and preserved ejection fraction. *Am J Cardiol* 2004;94:1003–1007.

79. Exner D, Dries D, Domanski M, Cohn J. Lesser response to angiotensin-converting enzyme inhibitor therapy in black as compared with white patients with left ventricular dysfunction. *N Engl J Med* 2001;344(18):1351–1357.

80. Dries D, Exner D, Gersh B, Cooper H, Carson P, Domanski M. Racial differences in the outcome of left ventricular dysfunction. *N Engl J Med* 1999;340(8):609–616.

81. Dries D, Strong M, Cooper R, Drazner M. Efficacy of angiotensin-converting enzyme inhibition in reducing progression from asymptomatic left ventricular dysfunction to symptomatic heart failure in black and white patients. *J Am Coll Cardiol* 2002;40(2):311–317.

82. Goldstein S, Deedwania P, Gottlieb S, et al. Metoprolol CR/XL in black patients with heart failure. *Am J Cardiol* 2003;92:478–480.

83. Yancy C, Fowler M, Colucci W, et al. Race and the response to adrenergic blockade with carvedilol in patients with chronic heart failure. *N Engl J Med* 2001;344(18):1358–1365.

84. Eichhorn E, Domanski M, Krause-Steinrauf H, Bristow M, Lavori P, for the Beta-Blocker Evaluation of Survival Trial Investigators: a trial of the beta-blocker bucindolol in patients with advanced chronic heart failure. *N Engl J Med* 2001;344(22):1659–1667.

85. Shekelle P, Rich M, Morton S, et al. Efficacy of angiotensin-converting enzyme inhibitors and beta-blockers in the management of left ventricular systolic dysfunction according to race, gender, and diabetic status. *J Am Coll Cardiol* 2003;41(9):1529–1538.

86. Cohn JN, Archibald DG, Ziesche S, et al. Effect of vasodilator therapy on mortality in chronic congestive heart failure: results of a Veterans Administration Cooperative Study. *N Engl J Med* 1986;314:1547–1552.

87. Cohn JN, Johnson G, Ziesche S, et al. A comparison of enalapril with hydralazine-isosorbide dinitrate in the treatment of chronic congestive heart failure. *N Engl J Med* 1991;325:303–310.

88. Carson P, Ziesche S, Johnson G, Cohn J, for the Vasodilator-Heart Failure Trial Study Group. Racial differences in response to therapy for heart failure: analysis of the Vasodilator-Heart Failure Trials. *J Card Fail* 1999;5(3):178–187.

89. Taylor AL, Lindenfeld J, Ziesche S, et al. Outcomes by gender in the African-American Heart Failure Trial. *J Am Coll Cardiol* 2006;48(11):2263–2267.

CHAPTER (104)

Air Pollution and Heart Disease

Robert D. Brook / Qinghua Sun /
Sanjay Rajagopalan

INTRODUCTION

Air pollution is a complex heterogeneous mixture of gases (e.g., ozone, CO, NO_2) and particulate matter (PM) varying in surface area, size, chemical composition, and source of origin. Although particulate and gaseous air pollutants coexist and are both linked to adverse health effects, there is compelling and consistent evidence implicating PM as a major mediator of cardiorespiratory disease.[1-3] In urban societies the major source of PM exposure not caused by environmental tobacco smoke is from fossil fuel combustion (e.g., automobiles, power plants, industry). PM can be broadly categorized according to aerodynamic diameter.[1] Fine PM <2.5 μm in size ($PM_{2.5}$) is capable of penetrating the depths of the tracheobronchial tree, whereas ultrafine PM (<0.1 μm) or soluble constituents of $PM_{2.5}$ (e.g., metals) may translocate directly into the systemic circulation. The current focus of research as well as regulatory measures has been on $PM_{2.5}$, because a wealth of epidemiologic data and mechanistic studies implicate the latter in cardiovascular morbidity and mortality. Once thought to pose detrimental effects on the lungs alone, the totality of evidence now indicates that most adverse health effects of PM (in terms of both relative and absolute morbidity and mortality) are on the cardiovascular system.[1-3]

EPIDEMIOLOGIC STUDIES

Associations between total mortality and PM have been established for more than half a century. The relationship between level of $PM_{2.5}$ and CV mortality appears to be linear, without any lower *safe* threshold.[1] Epidemiological studies linking PM with cardiovascular disease can be broadly divided into long-term (years), short-term (days to months), and ultra-rapid (hours) air pollution exposure studies. Table 104–1 outlines several major studies. Short-term studies (typically time series analyses of the change in

daily rate of cardiovascular [CV] morbidity/mortality in relation to alteration in PM levels) have consistently, but not uniformly, revealed increases in daily cardiovascular mortality averaging approximately 0.5 to 1.0 percent per 10 $\mu g/m^3$ increase in PM.[4-8]

There have been fewer studies prospectively investigating the chronic impact of PM exposure. These studies demonstrate an increase in relative risk in the range of 4 to 20 percent for cardiovascular events (including mortality) for every 10 $\mu g/m^3$ increase in long-term PM exposure.[9,10] Ultra-rapid CV effects following acute PM exposure have also been documented. One-hour $PM_{2.5}$ levels have been shown to increase the relative risk for myocardial infarction (MI), in studies performed in the United States, Japan, and Germany.[11-13] Other observations show that ambient PM can very rapidly promote myocardial ischemia on stress testing,[14] increase blood pressure,[15,16] promote alterations in heart rate variability,[1-3] and trigger acute arrhythmias.[1,17] Several additional conclusions regarding PM and cardiovascular events can be made based on the body of epidemiologic evidence thus far:

- Air pollution increases the risk for many types of events including stroke,[18] arrhythmia,[17] sudden death,[2,10] heart failure,[4] aneurysmal disease, and peripheral atherosclerotic disease.[2,10]
- Susceptible individuals, such as diabetics, patients with lower levels of education, the elderly, and possibly those with preexisting heart and lung diseases seem to be at higher relative risk.[1-3]
- Air pollution does not simply expedite the inevitable mortality of very frail people destined to die within days (harvesting effect). Rather, the evidence from cohort studies suggests that PM exposure may reduce overall life expectancy of the general population by 2 to 4 years.[19,20]

❙ ❙ PROPOSED BIOLOGICAL MECHANISMS

Inhalation of PM has been consistently shown to increase pulmonary inflammation and oxidative stress that could then secondarily impact

TABLE 104–1

Summary of Selected Major Epidemiologic Studies Linking Air Pollution with Cardiovascular Disease

STUDY	DESCRIPTION	EXPOSURE	FINDINGS
Short-Term Studies			
NMMAPS[4]	50 million people in 20 large U.S. cities	20 µg/m³ PM_{10}	• Cardiopulmonary mortality (RR 1.06)
APHEA-2[5]	29 European cities	20 µg/m³ PM_{10}	• CV mortality (RR 1.15)
Long-Term Studies			
Harvard 6 cities study[9]	8111 adults originally followed for 14–16 y (extended 8 more y until 1998)	10 µg/m³ $PM_{2.5}$	• Extended followup: CV mortality (1.28)
			• Reduced PM exposure leads to reduced CV events
ACS[10]	16-y followup of approximately 500,000 people throughout U.S.	10 µg/m³ $PM_{2.5}$	• Mortality for CV disease (RR 1.12)
			• Mortality for MI (RR 1.18)
			• Absolute numbers of mortality greatest for MI
			• Smoking increases RR for events caused by PM
			• RR (1.49) increase even greater because of PM gradient within single city (Los Angeles)
Ultra-Rapid Effects			
MI onset (U.S.)[11]	772 patients (PM level 1 h before MI)	25 µg/m³ $PM_{2.5}$	• Increase in risk for MI (RR 1.48)
KORA Augsburg registry (Germany)[13]	691 patients (Exposure 1 h before MI)	Traffic exposure	• Increase in risk for MI (RR 2.73)

ACS, American Cancer Society study; APHEA-2, Air Pollution and Health: a European Approach; CV, cardiovascular; MI, myocardial infarction; NMMAPS, National Mortality Morbidity Air Pollution Study; PM, particulate matter; RR, relative risk; WHI, Women's Health Initiative.

the systemic and coronary circulation.[1,2] These effects include endothelial dysfunction/vasoconstriction, increased platelet aggregation, and thrombosis. However, some vascular responses (impaired vasomotion) have been shown to occur without or with only minimal pulmonary inflammation, suggesting possible direct effects. PM constituents such as ultrafine particles may directly impact the systemic circulation.[21,22] In support of a rapid direct effect on the systemic circulation, acute endothelial dysfunction,[23] vasoconstriction,[24] increases in markers of systemic oxidative stress/inflammation,[25,26] hypercoagulability,[21–23] and alteration in autonomic tone[1,25] have all been demonstrated, either in human or animal models following the inhalation of PM. Studies in fat-fed apolipoprotein E mice have shown that long-term exposure to relevant levels of PM leads to the acceleration of atherosclerosis concomitant with reduced endothelial-dependent nitric oxide mediated dilatation and enhanced vasoconstrictor responsiveness.[27] These findings are supported by evidence linking air pollution levels to increased carotid intima-media progression in humans measured by ultrasonography.[28] Therefore, there is strong biological plausibility that both acute and chronic PM exposure could trigger rapid and long-term adverse CV health effects.

SUMMARY

PM-related air pollution is a serious public health problem because of the tremendous numbers of individuals exposed through-

out the world on a daily basis. Both epidemiologic and mechanistic studies strongly implicate PM and propensity for future cardiovascular events. Because of the rapid urbanization of cultures on a global scale, the problems of air pollution may only compound in the years to come despite current efforts to curb PM concentrations. Renewed attempts to further reduce PM levels globally and an effort to understand the mechanisms of air pollution mediated cardiovascular disease are urgently warranted.

REFERENCES

1. Brook RD, Franklin B, Cascio W, et al. Air pollution and cardiovascular disease: a statement for healthcare professionals from the Expert Panel on Population and Prevention Science of the American Heart Association. *Circulation* 2004;109:2655–2671.
2. Pope CA, Dockery DW. Health effects of fine particulate air pollution: lines that connect. *J Air Waste Manage Assoc* 2006;56:709–742.
3. U.S. Environmental Protection Agency. Air quality criteria for particulate matter. Washington, DC: U.S. Environmental Protection Agency; 2004. EPA publication EPA/600/P-99/002aF.
4. Dominici F, Daniels M, McDermott A, et al. Shape of the exposure-response relation and mortality displacement in the NMMAPS database. In: *Revised Analyses of Time-Series of Air Pollution and Health. Special Report.* Boston: Health Effects Institute; 2003:91–96.
5. Analitis A, Katsouyanni K, Dimakopoulou K, et al. Short-term effects of ambient particles on cardiovascular and respiratory mortality. *Epidemiology* 2006;17:230–233.
6. Zanobetti A, Schwartz J. The effect of particulate air pollution on emergency admissions for myocardial infarction: a multicity case-crossover analysis. *Environ Health Perspect* 2005;113:978–982.

7. von Klot S, Peters A, Aalto P, et al. Ambient air pollution is associated with increased risk of hospital cardiac readmissions of myocardial infarction survivors in five European cities. *Circulation* 2005;112:3073–3079.

8. Dominici F, Peng RD, Bell ML, et al. Fine particulate air pollution and hospital admission for cardiovascular and respiratory diseases. *JAMA* 2006;295:1127–1134.

9. Laden F, Schwartz J, Speizer FE, et al. Reduction in fine particulate air pollution and mortality: extended follow-up of the Harvard Six Cities Study. *Am J Respir Crit Care Med* 2006;173:667–672.

10. Pope CA, Burnett RT, Thurston GD, et al. Cardiovascular mortality and long-term exposure to particulate air pollution: epidemiological evidence of general pathophysiological pathways of disease. *Circulation* 2004;109:71–77.

11. Peters A, Dockery DW, Muller JE, et al. Increased particulate air pollution and the triggering of myocardial infarction. *Circulation* 2001;103:2810–2815.

12. Murakami Y, Ono M. Myocardial infarction deaths after high level exposure to particulate matter. *J Epidemiol Community Health* 2006;60:262–266.

13. Peters A, von Klot S, Heier M, et al. Exposure to traffic and the onset of myocardial infarction. *N Engl J Med* 2004;351:1721–1730.

14. Pekkanen J, Peters A, Hoek G, et al. Particulate air pollution and risk of ST-segment depression during repeated submaximal exercise tests among subjects with coronary heart disease: the exposure and risk assessment for fine and ultrafine particles in ambient air (ULTRA) study. *Circulation* 2002;106:933–938.

15. Zanobetti A, Canner MJ, Stone PH, et al. Ambient pollution and blood pressure in cardiac rehabilitation patients. *Circulation* 2004;110:2184–2189.

16. Urch B, Silverman F, Corey P, et al. Acute blood pressure responses in healthy adults during controlled air pollution exposures. *Environ Health Perspect* 2005;113(8):1052–1055.

17. Peters A, Liu E, Verrier RL, et al. Air pollution and incidence of cardiac arrhythmias. *Epidemiology* 2000;11:11–17.

18. Hong YC, Lee JT, Kim H, et al. Air pollution: a new risk factor in ischemic stroke mortality. *Stroke* 2002;33:2165–2169.

19. Pope CA III, Epidemiology of fine particulate air pollution and human health: biologic mechanisms and who's at risk? *Environ Health Perspect* 2000;108:713–723.

20. Kunzli N, Medina S, Kaiser R, et al. Assessment of deaths attributable to air pollution: should we use risk estimates based on time series or on cohort studies? *Am J Epidemiol* 2001;153:1050–1055.

21. Nemmar A, Hoylaerts MF, Hoet PH, et al. Ultrafine particles affect experimental thrombosis in an in vivo hamster model. *Am J Respir Crit Care Med* 2002;166(7):998–1004.

22. Nemmar A, Hoet PH, Dinsdale D, Vermylen J, Hoylaerts MF, Nemery B. Diesel exhaust particles in lung acutely enhance experimental peripheral thrombosis. *Circulation* 2003;107(8):1202–1208.

23. Mills NL, Tornqvist H, Robinson SD, et al. Diesel exhaust inhalation causes vascular dysfunction and impaired endogenous fibrinolysis. *Circulation* 2005;112:3930–3936.

24. Brook RD, Brook JR, Urch B, et al. Inhalation of fine particulate air pollution and ozone causes acute arterial vasoconstriction in healthy adults. *Circulation* 2002;105:1534–1536.

25. Rhoden CR, Wellenius GA, Ghelfi E, et al. PM-induced cardiac oxidative stress and dysfunction are mediated by autonomic stimulation. *Biochim Biophys Acta* 2005;1725:305–313.

26. Sorensen M, Daneshvar B, Hansen, et al. Personal $PM_{2.5}$ exposure and markers of oxidative stress in blood. *Environ Health Perspect* 2003;111:161–165.

27. Sun Q, Wang Am Jin X, et al. Long-term air pollution exposure and acceleration of atherosclerosis and vascular inflammation in an animal model. *JAMA* 2005;294:3003–3010.

28. Kunzli N, Jerrett M, Mack WJ, et al. Ambient air pollution and atherosclerosis in Los Angeles. *Environ Health Perspect* 2005;113:201–206.

PART 16 · Diseases of the Great Vessels and Peripheral Vessels

CHAPTER (105

Diseases of the Aorta

John A. Elefteriades / Jeffrey W. Olin /
Jonathan L. Halperin

THE NORMAL AORTA

The aorta has a complex intrinsic biology and sophisticated mechanical properties involving intrinsic relaxation and contraction that interact with left ventricular ejection to enhance hemodynamic function. The major conductance vessel of the body, the aorta is an elastic artery with a trilaminar wall: the tunica intima, tunica media, and tunica adventitia (Fig. 105–1).[1,2] The innermost lining of the tunica intima is the endothelium, resting on a thin basal lamina. The subendothelial tissue comprises fibroblasts, collagen fibers, elastic fibers, and mucoid ground substance. An internal elastic membrane forms the outer lining of the tunica intima. The tunica media is approximately 1 mm thick, comprising elastin, smooth muscle cells, collagen, and ground substance. The predominance of elastic fibers in the aortic wall and their arrangement as circumferential lamellae distinguish this elastic artery from the smaller muscular arteries. A lamellar unit comprises two concentric elastic lamellae and the smooth muscle cells, collagen, and ground substance contained within.[3,4] The thoracic aorta incorporates 35 to 56 lamellar units and the abdominal aorta about 28 units.[5] Surrounding the tunica media is the tunica adventitia, which is composed of loose connective tissue, including fibro-

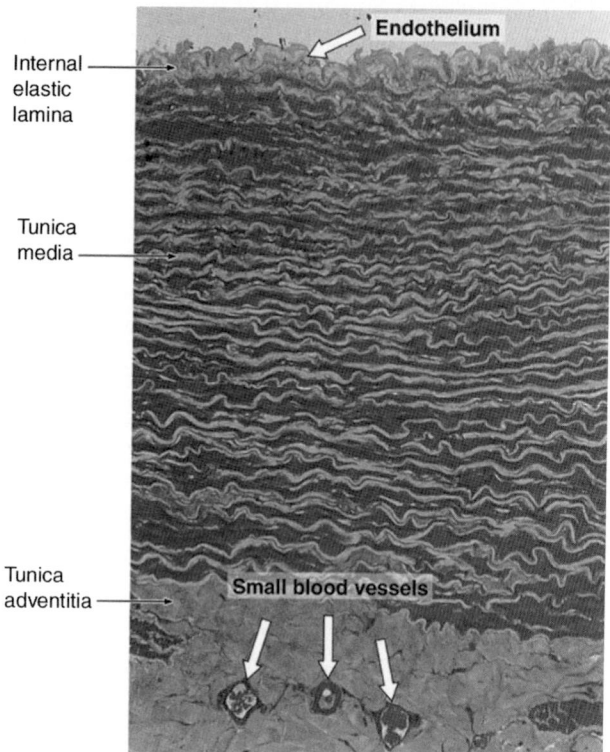

FIGURE 105–1. Transverse section of the wall of a large elastic artery demonstrating the well-developed tunica media containing elastic lamellae. Pararosaniline–toluidine blue stain; medium magnification. *Source: Reproduced with permission from: The circulatory system. In: Junqueira LC, Carneiro J, eds. Basic Histology: Text and Atlas, 11th ed. New York: McGraw-Hill Access Medicine (electronic format), 2005.*

blasts, relatively small amounts of collagen fibers, elastin, and ground substance. The adventitia is known to surgeons as the "strength" layer of the aorta, essential for secure suturing of aortic tissues. Within the tunica adventitia lie the nervi vasorum and vasa vasorum. The arteries arising along the course of the aorta give rise to the vasa vasorum, which develop into a capillary network supplying the adventitia and media of the thoracic aorta. The vasa vasorum do not supply the media of the abdominal aorta. Unlike the elastic fibers of the arterial wall, which are highly distensible, collagen is inelastic and provides the tensile strength required to prevent deformation or rupture of the aortic wall.

The ascending aorta is approximately 3 cm in diameter, depending on age, gender, and body surface area. The diameter of the aortic arch is similar. Descending in the posterior mediastinum, the thoracic aorta tapers slightly to about 2 to 2.3 cm. The abdominal aorta narrows to 1.7 to 1.9 cm in its distal portion. The aortas of males are larger than those of females, and aortic root dimension increases with age, height, and weight. The gender difference in aortic root dimension is not entirely explained by body surface area.[5]

【 】 HEMODYNAMIC FUNCTION OF THE AORTA

The force of left ventricular (LV) ejection creates a pressure wave that traverses the aorta, producing radial expansion and contraction of the arterial walls.[6] Potential energy derived from myocardial contraction and stored in the aortic wall during systole is transformed during diastolic recoil into kinetic energy, which drives blood into the peripheral vessels (see Chap. 12).[7] The pressure wave is conducted at an approximate velocity of 5 milliseconds, increasing in amplitude as it traverses the aorta.

Forward blood flow in the aorta begins when the aortic valve opens, and systolic pressure rises as the pressure wave courses along the length of the aorta. Flow velocity rises rapidly to a peak and then gradually decreases. With aortic valve closure there is a transient period of backward flow before forward flow resumes during diastole, particularly in the descending thoracic and abdominal aorta, albeit at considerably less than systolic velocity. The incisura, present in the arterial waveform in the proximal portion of the thoracic aorta, gradually disappears and is generally absent in the abdominal aorta.[8]

【 】 CHANGES WITH AGE AND DISEASE

Each of the four components of the aortic wall—elastic tissue, collagen fibers, smooth muscle cells, and mucoid ground substance—change with age (Fig. 105–2).[8] Elastic fibers fragment, collagen becomes more prominent at the expense of smooth muscle cells, and glycosaminoglycans accumulate. As a result, the aorta becomes less distensible, reducing its capacity to absorb the forces derived form left ventricular contraction.[9] Weakening of the aortic wall leads to dilatation of the lumen, as well as elongation and uncoiling of the aortic arch, collectively producing ectasia.

The elderly aorta is characterized by dilatation and elongation. Accompanying these changes are alterations in aortic wall structure, with fragmentation of elastic fibers, loss of smooth muscle cell nuclei (medionecrosis), accumulation of collagenous tissue, and deposition of basophilic ground substance. As the aorta dilates because of disease of the medial layer, tension on the aortic wall increases shear stress. This process is accelerated by hypertension, particularly when pulsatile forces are high (see Precipitation of Aortic Dissection). Under conditions of increased peripheral vascular resistance, a reflected wave has an impact additive to that of antegrade pulsatile flow. The combination of inherited, degenerative, mechanical, and hemodynamic factors adversely affects the medial layer of the aortic wall, leading to dilatation and setting the stage for the catastrophes of aortic dissection or rupture (see Chap. 12).

DEFINITIONS AND CATEGORIES

The aorta can be affected by a variety of pathologic processes leading to *aneurysm, dissection,* or *ischemic* syndromes (Fig. 105–3A). The term *aneurysm*—derived from the Greek *aneurysma,* referring to dilatation—is distinguished from *ectasia,* which refers to the modest generalized dilatation and elongation of the aorta that occurs with aging.[10] The criterion for definition of small aneurysms is controversial. Although the size of the normal aorta varies with gender and body size, most would agree that maximum diameter of the thoracic aorta should not exceed 4 cm. For the abdominal aorta, which normally has a smaller diameter than the thoracic segments, it has been suggested that the term *aneurysm* be restricted to situations where the diameter exceeds 3 cm.[11] Another proposed definition depends on the affected segment having a diameter more than 1.5 to 2 times normal.[12]

Aneurysms may be classified according to morphology, location, or etiology. In *true* aneurysms, the wall of the aneurysm is

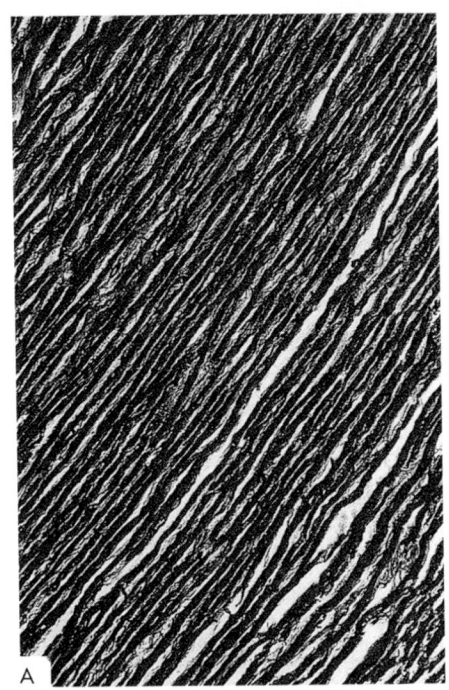
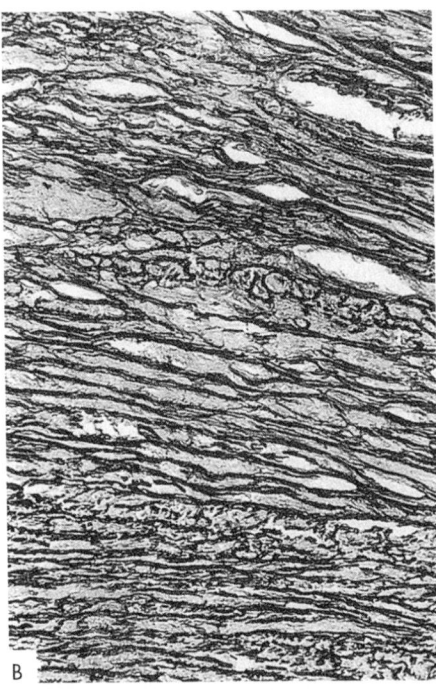

FIGURE 105–2. Histology of the normal aorta of a child (**A**) and an elderly adult (**B**). With aging, elastic fibers fragment, collagen becomes more prominent, smooth muscle cells diminish, and acid mucopolysaccharide ground substance accumulates. Weakening of the aortic wall leads to dilation of the lumen as well as elongation and uncoiling of the aortic arch. Orcein and van Gieson stain, magnification ×414. *Source: From Nichols WW, O'Rourke MF. McDonald's Blood Flow in Arteries: Theoretic, Experimental and Clinical Principles, 3d ed. Philadelphia: Lea & Febiger, 1990, with permission.*

composed of the normal histologic components of the aorta. A *false* aneurysm, on the other hand, represents a contained rupture, and the wall does not contain the normal histologic components of the aorta. It is a fibrous peel that has formed from a small perforation of the aorta, initially controlled by adherence of surrounding tissues, and gradually enlarging over time.

The gross morphologic classification distinguishes true aneurysms as *fusiform* (most common) or *saccular*. A fusiform aneurysm is roughly cylindrical and affects the entire circumference of the aorta; a saccular aneurysm is an outpouching of only a portion of the aortic circumference. Frequently, a small neck provides continuity between the aortic lumen and the saccular aneurysm.

Aortic dissection refers to splitting of the layers of the aortic wall (within the media) permitting longitudinal propagation of a blood-filled space within the aortic wall (Fig. 105–3B). Aortic dissection is considered the most common cause of death as a result of human aortic disease.[13] *Atherosclerosis of the aorta* can narrow the ostia of the great vessels or produce mobile intraaortic atheromatous masses capable of embolization to the brain or other organs.

Several additional entities should be distinguished (Fig. 105–4A to C). *Acute aortic transection* is a consequence of trauma and involves localized disruption of the aortic wall, which is intrinsically normal and resistant to propagating dissection. A *ruptured* aortic aneurysm is self-explanatory unless an acute aortic transection or acute aortic dissection happens to rupture, which are com-

mon developments. *Acute aortic dissection* refers to the separation of layers of the aortic wall discussed fully below. *Intramural aortic hematoma* is akin to circumferential rather than longitudinal dissection, such that there is no identifiable flap separating true and false lu-

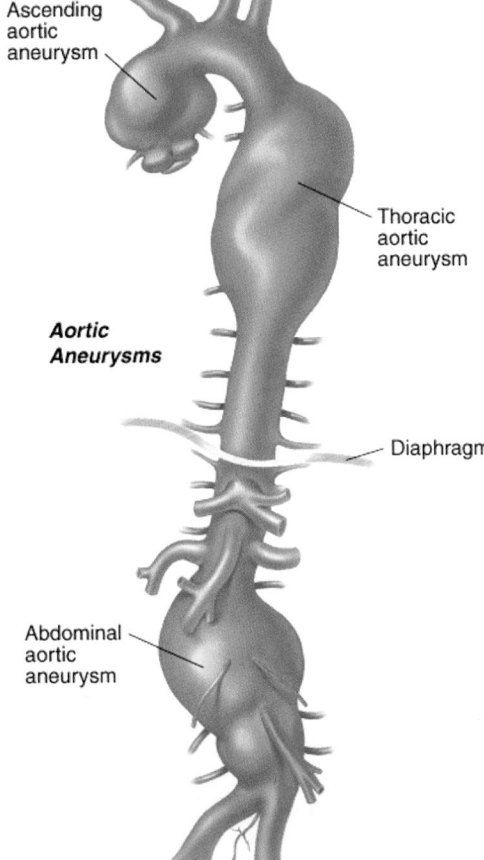
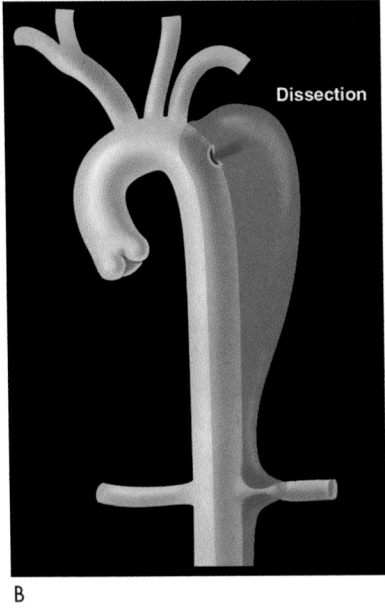

FIGURE 105–3. Artist's rendition of (**A**) aortic aneurysms at various locations and (**B**) type B aortic dissection.

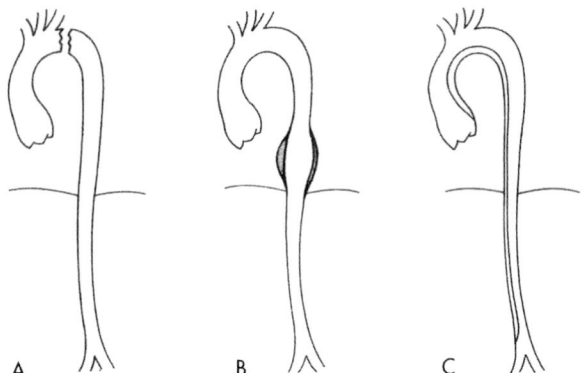

FIGURE 105–4. Three commonly confused aortic disorders. **A.** Acute aortic transection. **B.** Degenerative aneurysm of the descending aorta. **C.** Type A acute aortic dissection. *Source: Reprinted with permission from Elefteriades JA, Geha AS, Cohen LS. House Officer Guide to ICU Care. Raven Press, 1994.*

mens. *Penetrating aortic ulcer* involves localized perforation of the medial layer of the aortic wall at the site of an atherosclerotic plaque.

Aortic aneurysms may also be classified according to the segment involved—as thoracic, thoracoabdominal, or abdominal. Aneurysm formation can be considerably more widespread along the length of the aorta (Fig. 105–5) than obstructive atherosclerotic disease, potentially affecting almost the entire vessel, whereas obstruction tends to involve only the abdominal portion of the aorta, when the iliac arteries are commonly affected as well. Dilatation of the aorta may occur as a consequence of atherosclerosis alone, as well as of aging, infection, inflammation, trauma, congenital anomalies, and medial degeneration, or in combinations of pathologic states. The pathologic changes that accompany these conditions cause the aorta to thicken, thin, bulge, tear, rupture, narrow, or dissect, or to be altered by combinations of these conditions.

Over the course of normal aging, degenerative changes occur throughout most of the length of the aorta, leading to a mild form of what is termed *cystic medial necrosis*. Although essentially a normal physiologic process of aging, cystic medial necrosis develops more rapidly in patients with bicuspid aortic valve, during pregnancy, and very markedly in the Marfan syndrome. The mechanism by which the medial layer of the aorta is subject to this accelerated rate of degeneration is a subject of active molecular genetic investigation. Severe elastic fiber degeneration, necrosis of muscle cells, and cystic spaces filled with mucoid material is most often encountered in the ascending aorta from the region of the valve to the brachiocephalic artery (see Fig. 105–5). Because of the dilatation of the aortic root, aortic regurgitation may be a secondary feature, although the valve leaflets themselves are histologically unaffected.

Cystic medial necrosis is the most common cause of ascending aortic aneurysm,[13] and although this type of aortic pathology is typical of patients with the Marfan syndrome, it may also occur in the absence of any clinical Marfan stigmata (see Chap. 88).

ANEURYSMS

【 】 ASCENDING AORTIC ANEURYSMS

Ascending aortic aneurysms occur more frequently in men than in women, are typically fusiform, and extend into the aortic arch. Consequently, aneurysms of the aortic arch are often contiguous with aneurysms in the ascending aorta. Ascending aortic aneurysms are divisible into three categories according to the pattern of involvement of the aortic root (Fig. 105–6), with direct implications for surgical treatment. The most common type is *supracoronary aneurysm*, in which the aortic annulus is normal in size, as is the short segment of aorta between the annulus and the coronary ostia. This type is well-treated by a tube graft, starting above the coronary arteries and extending cephalad to the end of the aneurysm. The second category is termed *annuloaortic ectasia*, calling attention to the enlargement of both the aortic annulus and the proximal portion of the aorta. This type of aneurysm is typical of Marfan syndrome and other related disorders characterized by cystic medial necrosis of the aortic wall (see Chap. 88).[15] Because the annulus and proximal aorta are the most dilated portions, the aneurysmal ascending aorta takes on a "flask-like" shape, requiring replacement of the entire aortic root and valve, usually with a prefabricated composite graft that includes a prosthetic valve and aortic graft in an integrated unit. The third category, the *tubular* type of ascending aortic aneurysm, has features midway between the other two configurations. In patients with tubular aortic aneurysms, the annulus and proximal aorta are mildly dilated and the caliber of the ascending aorta is more uniform. When surgical repair is necessary, either a supracoronary tube graft or total aortic root replacement may be appropriate based on such considerations as patient age. In younger individuals, composite grafting may confer greater protection against late dilatation of the proximal portion of the aortic root.

【 】 DESCENDING THORACIC AORTIC ANEURYSMS

In contrast to the ascending aorta, the majority of aneurysms of the descending thoracic aorta are atherosclerotic.[16] These are typically fusiform, may extend to the level of the abdominal aorta, and often begin distal to the origin of the left subclavian artery. Descending thoracic aneurysms may also develop in patients with aortic coarctation.

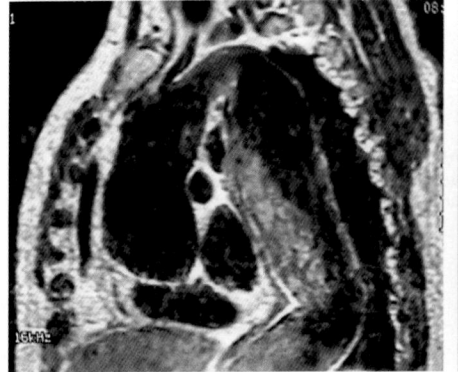
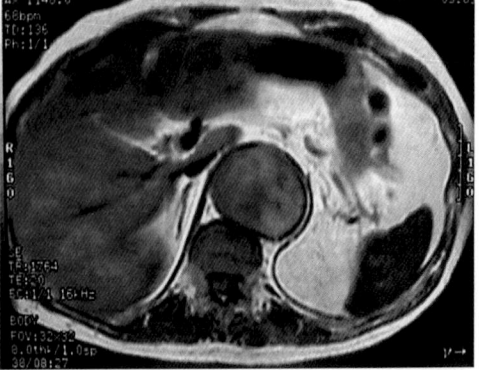

FIGURE 105–5. Magnetic resonance imaging demonstrating aneurysm of the entire aorta viewed in the sagittal thoracic and axial abdominal views.

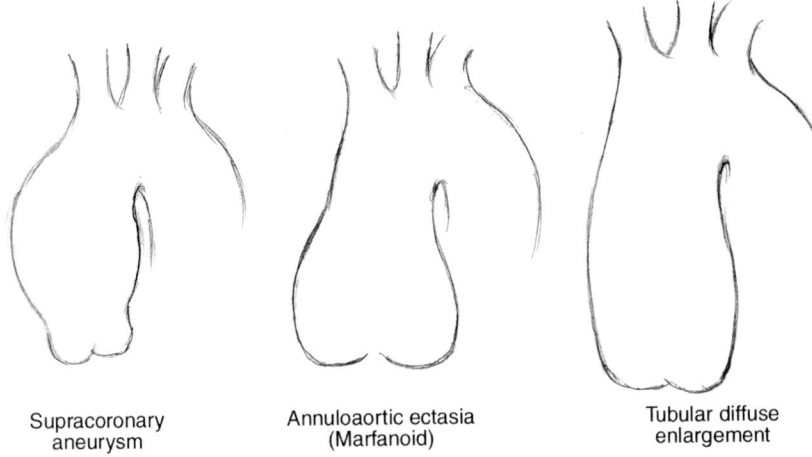

FIGURE 105-6. Three common patterns of ascending aortic aneurysmal disease: supracoronary, annuloaortic ectasia, and tubular. See text for details.

【 】 ABDOMINAL AORTIC ANEURYSMS

In more than 90 percent of cases, the superior margins of abdominal aneurysms are distal to the renal arteries. Atherosclerosis has been held responsible for the majority, although some authors suggest that atherosclerosis may be a secondary phenomenon in aneurysmal disease.

【 】 THORACOABDOMINAL AORTIC ANEURYSMS

As suggested by the nomenclature, thoracoabdominal aortic aneurysms have features of both thoracic and abdominal aortic aneurysms (Fig. 105-7). Although they constitute only approximately 3 percent of all aortic aneurysms, thoracoabdominal aneurysms are considered as a separate class because of the diffuse and extensive aortic involvement in the disease process (usually atherosclerosis) and special considerations for surgical repair, which may entail reimplantation of the origins of visceral arteries.[17] Crawford and colleagues delineated four types of thoracoabdominal aortic aneurysms, according to the segment and extent of aorta involved, and which are described in Fig. 105-7.[18]

EPIDEMIOLOGY OF ANEURYSMAL DISEASE

The epidemiology of aortic aneurysms and their corresponding acute aortic syndromes presents methodologic challenges because of confusion in terminology, referral bias, unknown inci-

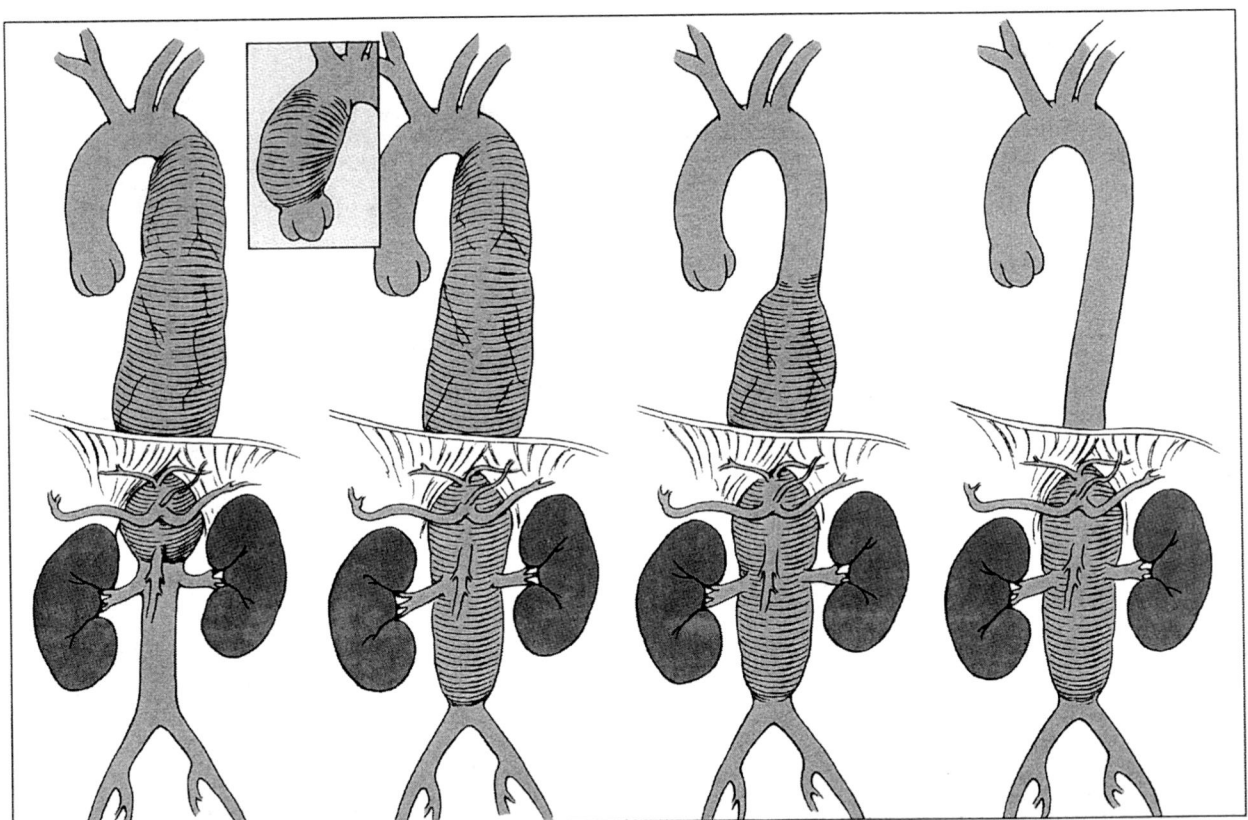

FIGURE 105-7. Classification of thoracoabdominal aortic aneurysms. Type I aneurysms involve most of the descending aorta from near the origin of the left subclavian artery to the abdominal vessels, but the renal arteries are not involved. Type II aneurysms also begin near the origin of the left subclavian artery but extend below the origins of the renal arteries. Type III aneurysms arise more distally and involve less of the descending thoracic aorta but often more of the abdominal aorta than types I and II aneurysms. Type IV aneurysms arise at the level of the diaphragm and typically extend below the origins of the renal arteries. *Source: From Crawford ES, Coselli JS. Thoracoabdominal aortic aneurysms. Thorac Cardiovasc Surg 1991;3:302, with permission.*

dence of asymptomatic cases, misdiagnosis of aortic rupture or dissection as myocardial infarction, and limitations of administrative databases. Despite these considerable limitations, multiple studies have assessed the epidemiology of abdominal and thoracic aortic aneurysms.[19–21] The most recent data available from the Centers for Disease Control and Prevention lists aneurysmal disease as the 17th most common cause of death in all individuals and the 15th most common in individuals older than 65 years of age.[20]

Abdominal aortic aneurysm affects approximately 5 percent of individuals older than age 65 years, and the prevalence is considerably higher in men than women.[21] The annual incidence of ruptured abdominal aortic aneurysm is approximately 10 per 100,000 population, and is similar in men and women. However, age at diagnosis is a decade higher in women.[22,23] For men in their sixties, the rate rises to approximately 50 per 100,000, and for those in their seventies, the rate exceeds 1 in 1000 men suffering rupture of abdominal aortic aneurysm each year.

The incidence of thoracic aortic aneurysm is also approximately 10 per 100,000 population, and is similar in women and men, but the age at diagnosis is a decade higher in women (seventies). The yearly incidence of rupture or dissection of an existing thoracic aortic aneurysm is approximately 7 percent, divided equally between rupture and dissection. A curious and as yet unexplained finding is that 79 percent of thoracic aortic aneurysm ruptures occur in women.[22,23]

Aortic aneurysm and its acute complications are recognized with increasing frequency. These trends during the last three decades have been confirmed by the Centers for Disease Control and Prevention for the United States as a whole, Scotland, the Netherlands, and for England and Wales as well.[24]

【 】 SCREENING FOR ABDOMINAL AORTIC ANEURYSM

The epidemiologic implications of screening for abdominal aortic aneurysms have been extensively studied.[21] Screening programs based on abdominal ultrasonography clearly detect aneurysms effectively and reduce the number of aneurysm-related deaths. The cost of medical care per single aneurysm-related death prevented is about $10,000. One important benefit of screening is that a single negative ultrasonogram at 65 years of age suffices: patients without aneurysms at this age simply will not die of aneurysm rupture.[21]

Cost-effective screening of the general population is focused on family history of aneurysmal disease, age, male gender, history of cigarette smoking, coronary artery disease, cerebrovascular disease, and hypercholesterolemia as factors linked with incremental risk for aneurysm development. Abdominal aortic aneurysm is five times more common in smokers, in whom 89 percent of all aneurysm ruptures occur.[21]

The U.S. Preventive Services Task Force recommends a one-time screening for abdominal aortic aneurysm by ultrasonography in men age 65 to 75 years who have ever smoked. There is no recommendation (for or against) screening in men age 65 to 75 who have never smoked, and an explicit recommendation against routine screening for abdominal aortic aneurysm in women, based on the relatively low yield.

ETIOLOGY AND PATHOPHYSIOLOGY

【 】 AORTIC ANEURYSM AS AN INHERITED DISEASE

The Marfan Syndrome

This inherited disorder, described in 1896, is characterized primarily by dolichostenomelia (long, thin extremities), ligamentous redundancy, ectopia lentis, ascending aortic dilatation, and incompetence of the aortic or mitral valves, or both.[25] A large number of specific mutations (more than 600) produce the Marfan phenotype, thus reducing the clinical usefulness of genetic testing in the diagnosis of Marfan syndrome.[26] Diagnosis is made largely on a clinical basis, using the criteria summarized in Table 105–1. The syndrome is linked to an autosomal dominant anomaly in the genes regulating synthesis of fibrillin type 1, a large glycoprotein that helps direct and orient elastin in the developing aorta.[27] Mutations have been identified both on chromosome 15 and on chromosome 5. It is not clear whether these mutations lead to a qualitative or quantitative defect of elastin, or both, but there is a link between the pathology of the aortic media and the identification of specific genetic mutations involving these two chromosomes.[26,27]

In patients with the Marfan syndrome, the aortic root tends to enlarge in fusiform fashion in association with aortic valvular regurgitation, and about half of the patients also have mitral insufficiency (Fig. 105–8). Aneurysms involve the sinuses of Valsalva and the tubular portion of the ascending aorta, producing annuloaortic ectasia characterized by degeneration of elastic fibers and accumulation of mucoid material within the medial layer of the aortic wall (Fig. 105–9). Abnormalities associated with the Marfan syndrome typically affect the entire length of the aorta, although dissection most often involves the thoracic portion.[28]

Ehlers-Danlos Syndrome

Another inherited connective tissue disorder associated with aneurysm formation in the *Ehlers-Danlos syndrome*. This disease is seen in clinical practice much less frequently than Marfan syndrome (see Chap. 88).

Loeys-Dietz Syndrome

A recently recognized syndrome is the development of aneurysms caused by mutations in the transforming growth factor (TGF)-β receptor (*Loeys-Dietz syndrome*; see Chap. 88). This has a phenotypic overlap with the vascular form of Ehlers-Danlos syndrome and individuals with this mutation develop aneurysms that enlarge rapidly and are prone to rupture; in one series, the mean age at death was 26 years.[29]

Bicuspid Aortic Valve

Patients born with bicuspid aortic valve have structural abnormalities of the ascending aorta predisposing to aneurysm and dissection.[30–33] Some have aortic coarctation as part of this syndrome as well. It is important to recognize that aneurysmal enlargement of the aorta in patients with bicuspid aortic valve may occur before the onset of aortic stenosis or regurgitation and is not, therefore, predominantly a result of poststenotic dilatation (Table 105–2). Because bicuspid valve disease is so common (affecting approxi-

TABLE 105–1

Quick Guide to Diagnosis of Marfan Disease

	CARDIOVASCULAR SYSTEM	SKELETAL SYSTEM	OCULAR SYSTEM	PULMONARY SYSTEM	SKIN AND INTEGUMENT	DURA	FAMILY HISTORY/ GENETICS
Major criteria	One required: • Dilatation of Asc Ao (+ AI), involving sinuses of Valsalva • AAD	Four required: • Pectus carinatum • Pectus excavatum (requiring surgery) • Reduced upper-to-lower segment ratio or increased arm span-to-height ratio • Positive wrist and thumb signs • Elbow extension reduced below 170° • Pes planus • Protrusion acetabulae	• Ectopia lentis	None	None	• Dural ectasia	• Parent, child, or sibling with Marfan disease • FBN1 mutation
Minor criteria	• MVP (± prolapse) • Dilation main PA (patients younger than 40 years old)	• Pectus excavatum (mod) • Hypermobile joints • Crowding of teeth or highly arched palate	• Flat corneas • Increased axial length of globe • Hypoplastic iris or ciliary muscles, causing decreased meiosis	• Spontaneous pthx • Apical blebs	• Striae • Recurrent or incisional hernias	None	None
Involvement (required to say organ system involved)	One major or one minor criterion	Two major or one major and one minor criteria	One major or two minor criteria	One minor criterion	One minor criterion	Major criterion	Major criterion

AAD, ascending aortic dissection; AI, aortic insufficiency; Ao, aorta; Asc, ascending; MVP, mitral valve prolapse; PA, pulmonary artery; pthx, pneumothorax.

Diagnosis requires:
• For index case (without documented mutation)
  > Major criteria in two organ systems, plus
  > Involvement of another organ system
• For index case (with documented mutation)
  > Major criterion in one organ system, plus
  > Involvement of another organ system
• For a relative of a known case
  > Major criterion in the family history, plus
  > Major criterion in one organ system, plus
  > Involvement of another organ system

Definitions and normals:
Upper-to-lower segment = distance from top of head to symphisis pubis/distance symphisis pubis to floor (normal 0.89–0.95)
Arm span-to-height ratio (normal <1.05)
Wrist sign = positive if a person's thumb and little finger overlap when gripping own wrist
Thumb sign = positive if the entire nail of a person's thumb projects beyond the border of the hand when their fist is closed around their thumb

SOURCE: Table compiled from Tsipouras P, Silverman DI. The genetic basis of aortic disease: Marfan syndrome and beyond. Cardiol Clin 1999;17:683–696, and from National Library of Health of National Health Services at: http://www.library.nhs.uk/genepool/ViewResource.aspx?resID=126262. Last accessed September 28, 2006.

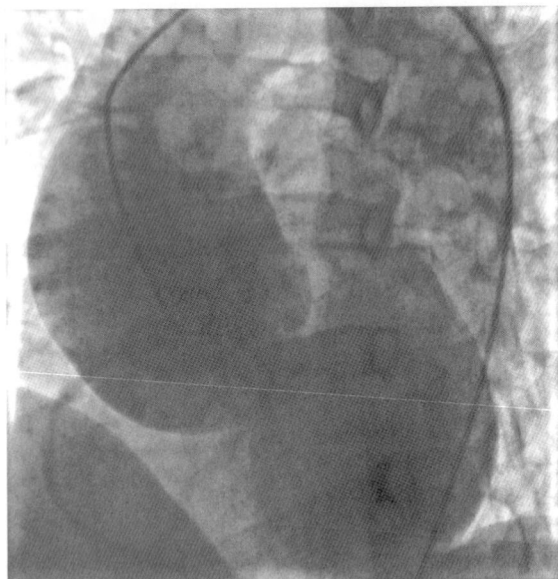

FIGURE 105–8. Aortogram of a patient with the Marfan syndrome. Aortic aneurysms in this disorder are characterized by annuloaortic ectasia involving the sinuses of Valsalva and the ascending aorta produced by degeneration of elastic fibers and the accumulation of mucoid material within the medial layer of the aortic wall, grossly resembling cystic medial necrosis.

mately 2 percent of the population), the associated aortic disease is responsible for more cases of dissection than the more commonly appreciated Marfan syndrome (which affects 1 in 10,000 people).

Familial Aortic Aneurysm

Many cases that were once considered idiopathic or attributed to atherosclerosis can be traced to genetic and/or metabolic abnormalities affecting the aortic wall. In many cases of nonmarfanoid aortic aneurysm, there is a family history of aneurysmal disease. When the proband has a thoracic aortic aneurysm, the chance that a relative has an aortic aneurysm is 1 in 5.[34] An autosomal dominant pattern of inheritance predominates with reduced penetrance, but other genetic patterns also are manifest (Fig. 105–10). Probands with ascending aortic aneurysm are more likely to have family members with ascending aneurysm and those with aneurysms involving the descending aorta are more likely to have family members with abdominal aneurysms.

Multiple genetic mutations have been linked with familial aortic aneurysms,[35,36] including the thoracic aortic aneurysm and dissection 1 (TAAD1) mutation, which accounts for 20 to 30 percent of familial cases, the transforming growth factor beta receptor 2 (TGFBR2) mutation, which accounts for approximately 5 percent of cases, the familial aortic aneurysm 1 (FAA1) mutation, and the myosin heavy chain 11 (MYH11) mutation. Much attention is currently focused on the TGF-β pathway and its potential inhibition by losartan, the angiotensin-II receptor blocker.[37]

❪ ❫ MOLECULAR PATHOPHYSIOLOGY

Although in many patients genetic mutations establish the propensity for aneurysm development, gene substitution may set the stage while lytic *matrix metalloproteinase* (MMP) enzymes degrade the structural proteins of the aortic wall leading to aneurysm formation and dissection (Fig. 105–11). These enzymes are normally regulated by tissue

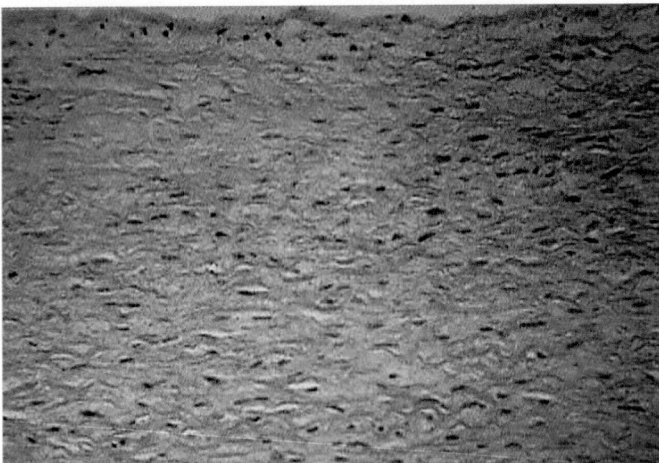

A

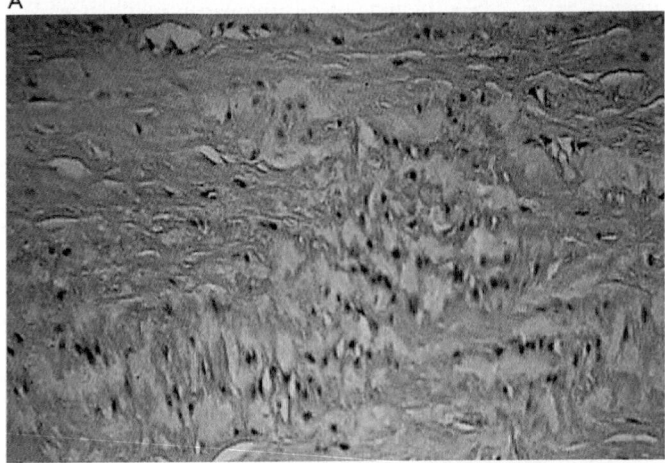

B

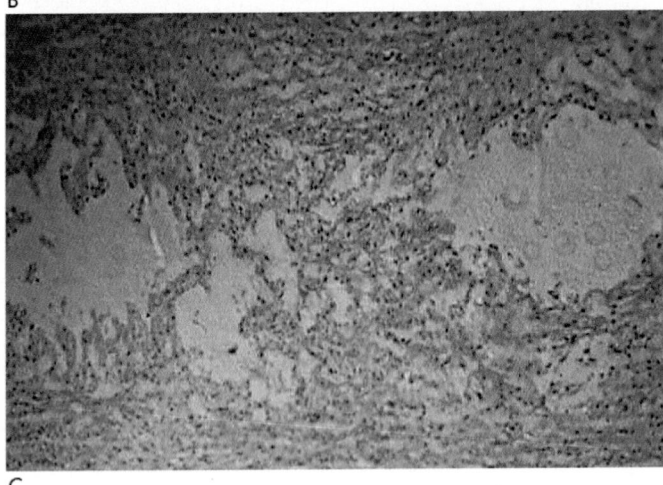

C

FIGURE 105–9. **A, B,** and **C** show cystic medial necrosis of progressive severity. Blood gaining access to one of the cystic spaces through a defect in the intimal layer of the aortic wall can propagate longitudinally along the aorta, initiating dissection.

inhibitor of metalloproteinase (TIMP), which antagonizes the lytic action of the MMP. An uncertain proportion of patients with aortic aneurysms manifest excessive MMP activity, but such activity has been documented in cases of abdominal aortic aneurysm,[38,39] as well as in cases of ascending aortic aneurysm and aortic dissection.[40] Several dozen specific MMP enzymes and certain TIMPs have been implicated in the pathogenesis of aneurysm disease.[41]

In addition to proteolysis of the extracellular matrix, the pathogenesis of aortic aneurysms involves inflammation, cytokine activity, and loss of smooth muscle cells. Together, these processes undermine the integrity of the aortic wall and set the stage for aneurysm formation, growth, and rupture. Inflammatory cells participate in the genesis of aneurysms.[41-43] Smooth muscle cells of the aortic wall are charged with repairing damaged proteins, and substantial (approximately 75 percent) reduction in the number of smooth muscle cells in the walls of abdominal aortic aneurysms impair this function. Aneurysmal smooth muscle cells display a threefold increase in apoptosis, and impaired growth capacity. Fig. 105–12 illustrates the interaction of proteolysis, inflammation, cytokine activation, and deficient smooth muscle cell function in the pathophysiology of aneurysm formation.

Many patients with ascending aortic aneurysms, which are typically nonatherosclerotic, display relatively little evidence of systemic atherosclerotic disease. A study comparing patients with ascending aortic aneurysm associated with annuloaortic ectasia or aortic dissection with age- and sex-matched controls found significantly less arterial calcification as detected by CT imaging in those with aneurysms. This implies that the mutation responsible for ascending aortic aneurysm may have protective value against atherosclerosis, and certain MMPs that exert dilatory effects on the aortic wall may have antiatherogenic properties as well.

◖ TABLE 105–2

Comparison of Epidemiology of Marfan Disease and Bicuspid Aortic Valve (BAV) with Special Reference to Number of Cases of Aortic Dissection Brought on by Disease[a]

	INCIDENCE	AAD LIKELIHOOD (LIFETIME)	AADS CAUSED (AS % OF POPULATION)
Marfan Disease	1/10,000 (0.01%)	40%	0.004%
Bicuspid aortic valve	2/100 (2%)	5%	0.1%

AAD, acute aortic dissection.
[a]Note that BAV causes 25 times more acute aortic dissections than Marfan disease.

CLINICAL MANIFESTATIONS
【 】 AORTIC ANEURYSMS

Unfortunately, the vast majority of thoracic and abdominal aortic aneurysms are clinically silent, with rupture constituting the first manifestation.[44] A minority of patients (5 to 10 percent) experience symptoms, permitting earlier detection of the aneurysm. Aneurysms of any kind can produce pain arising from stretching of the aortic tissue or impingement on adjacent structures. Pain originating in the ascending aorta is usually felt retrosternally. Pain from the descending aorta is characteristically located between the scapulae. Pain in the lateral or posterior chest can occur when the aneurysm compresses surrounding structures or erodes into adjacent ribs or vertebrae. Pain from the abdominal aorta may occur in the abdomen, left flank, or lower part of the back. It is often difficult to distinguish aneurysm pain from that resulting from other causes, but patients may distinguish deep visceral pain from superficial or musculoskeletal pain. The interscapular location of pain caused by descending aortic enlargement or dissection is less often caused by musculoskeletal disease.

Rupture of the aorta in any location produces acute symptoms, usually severe pain followed by loss of consciousness or death as a result of internal hemorrhage. Rupture of an abdominal aortic aneurysm usually produces the clinical picture of extreme distress as a result of an abdominal catastrophe. Despite surgical advances, mortality is still the most frequent outcome because abrupt circulatory collapse prevents timely intervention except in unusual circumstances. Patients frequently have severe abdominal or back pain, but

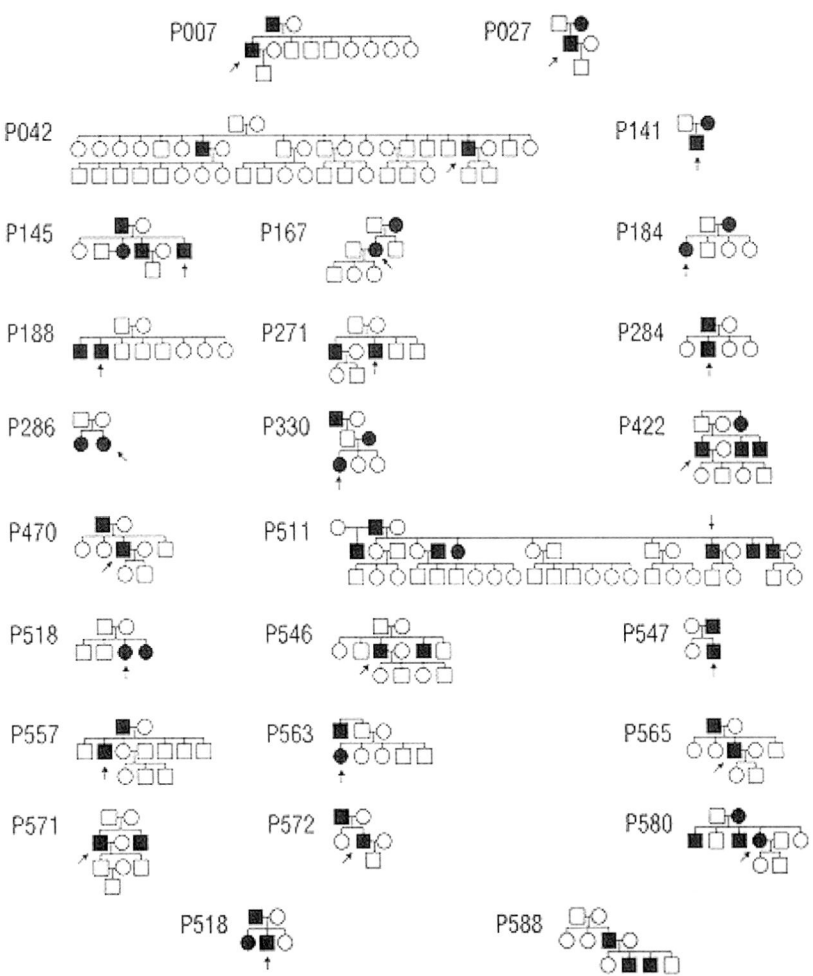

FIGURE 105–10. In a series of 100 family pedigrees of patients with thoracic aortic aneurysm or dissection, 21 suggested genetic transmission. Autosomal-dominant inheritance predominates, but other patterns of transmission also are evident.

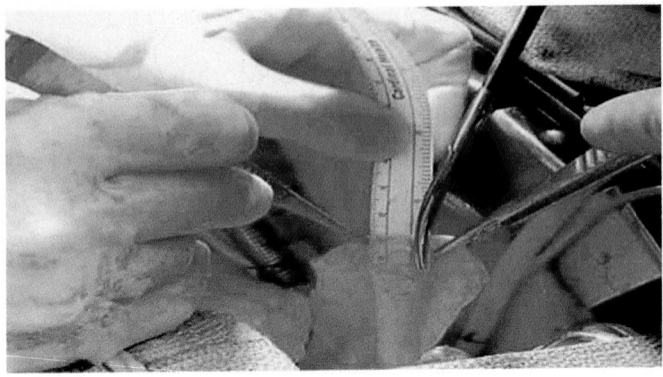

FIGURE 105–11. The proteins in the wall of this ascending aortic aneurysm were degraded, presumably by matrix metalloproteinase (MMP)-related activity, to the extent that the aortic wall became so thin that the markings on a ruler are visible through the aortic wall.

the pattern varies considerably. The aneurysm may rupture into the retroperitoneum or into the peritoneal or pleural cavities, leading to tachycardia, hypotension, diaphoresis, pallor, or shock, depending on the extent of rupture and associated blood loss into the extravascular space. On occasion, rupture occurs directly into the duodenum, causing an aortoduodenal fistula and acute gastrointestinal bleeding. This possibility should be considered when gastrointestinal bleeding is evident along with signs of an aneurysm on physical examination. Rupture may also occur into the inferior vena cava or iliac veins, producing an arteriovenous fistula; this is suggested by rapid development of leg swelling or high-output heart failure in the presence of an abdominal aortic aneurysm. Rupture of a descending or thoracoabdominal aortic aneurysm produces similar physiologic derangements, with the associated pain typically located higher in the trunk, consistent with the anatomical location of the disease process.

Aside from pain, ascending aortic aneurysms may produce heart failure on the basis of incompetence of the aortic valve. As the aortic root enlarges, diastolic coaptation of the aortic valve leaflets progressively falters, causing regurgitation of blood through the resultant central gap. Aneurysms of the sinuses of Valsalva may rupture directly into the right ventricular cavity, right atrium, or pulmonary artery, causing heart failure associated with a continuous murmur (see Chap. 12). Ascending aortic aneurysms can distort or obstruct the trachea, producing respiratory symptoms. Compression of the superior vena cava may produce venous congestion in the head, neck, and upper extremities. Aortic arch aneurysms or descending thoracic aortic aneurysms may produce hoarseness or dysphagia ("dysphagia lusoria") from distortion of the recurrent laryngeal nerve or direct impingement on the esophagus. Descending thoracic aortic aneurysms may cause hemoptysis from direct erosion into the lung parenchyma or bronchi, or hematemesis from esophageal erosion. Because mural thrombosis is so common in atherosclerotic aneurysms, they may be the source of peripheral embolism of thrombus or atherosclerotic debris causing occlusion of distal vessels or clinical features of atheroembolism. Occasionally, patients with abdominal aortic aneurysms may become aware of prominent abdominal pulsation. Nausea and vomiting may occur if an aneurysm compresses the duodenum. Compression of the left iliac vein may cause left leg swelling, compression of the left ureter may cause hydronephrosis, compression of testicular

veins may cause varicocele, or compression of bladder may cause urinary frequency or urgency.

Thoracic or abdominal aortic aneurysms are most commonly diagnosed not on the basis of symptoms, but incidentally by imaging procedures carried out for another reason. Occasionally, chest roentgenograms obtained to evaluate pulmonary symptoms or for general screening suggests an aortic aneurysm, which may then be confirmed by computerized tomographic or magnetic resonance imaging.

【 】 AORTIC DISSECTION

Aortic dissection typically produces sudden intense pain, often described as tearing or shearing in quality. Ascending aortic dissection usually causes anterior, substernal chest pain, whereas dissection of the descending aorta causes posterior, interscapular pain. Pain may migrate inferiorly to the flank or pelvis as the dissection propagates distally. Impending aortic rupture should be considered when pain subsides and later recurs.[43]

Painless dissection occurs in as many as 15 percent of patients,[44] and is not uncommonly detected as an asymptomatic finding on elective CT scans obtained for another purpose. By convention, aortic dissection is considered acute when identified within 2 weeks of onset, and chronic when symptoms or other markers of dissection have been present longer.

Clinically, the inciting event responsible for aortic dissection is an intimal tear that permits blood to pass from the true lumen into the middle or outer layer of the aortic media, forming a second or false lumen separated by an intimal flap.[45] In some cases, intramural hematoma precedes perforation of the intima, possibly related to rupture of a vasa vasorum.[46] The dissection may propagate distally (antegrade) or proximally (retrograde) to narrow or occlude the origin of any branch artery arising from the aorta. Antegrade propagation is more common and the dissection usually has a spiral morphology, leaving some aortic branches supplied by the true lumen and others in continuity with the false lumen (see Fig. 105–11).

The intimal tear originates in the ascending aorta in 65 percent of cases, and transverse arch in 10 percent, upper descending aorta just beyond the origin of the left subclavian artery in 20 percent, and more distally in 5 percent of cases. The false lumen may ter-

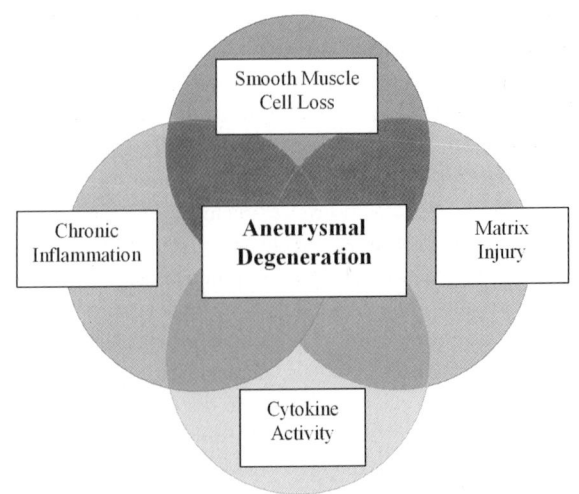

FIGURE 105–12. Factors involved in the pathogenesis of aortic aneurysms.

minate at any point along the length of the aorta or in the iliac or femoral arteries, and there are sometimes multiple flaps and several sites of reentry. The false lumen can undergo retrograde dissection, thrombotic occlusion, pseudoaneurysm formation, compression, or rupture.

Aortic dissection occurs more often in men than in women, with a 2–5:1 preponderance,[44] usually in the sixth or seventh decades of life. Systemic hypertension is the major predisposing risk factor. In the International Registry of Acute Aortic Dissection, 194 of 289 patients (69 percent) with proximal dissections and 132 of 175 (77 percent) with distal dissections had a history of hypertension; similar ratios were reported by investigators at the Mayo Clinic.[44] Other predisposing conditions include the Marfan syndrome, Ehlers-Danlos syndrome, Loeys-Dietz syndrome, bicuspid aortic valve, aortic aneurysm, and annuloaortic ectasia associated with cystic medial necrosis. The most common causes of aortic dissection in patients younger than 40 years of age are the Marfan syndrome and pregnancy. Iatrogenic trauma resulting from intravascular catheterization is the cause in approximately 5 percent of cases, and may involve the ascending, descending, or abdominal aorta. Cocaine abuse is increasingly recognized as a factor predisposing to acute aortic dissection.[47]

Aortic dissection is often fatal unless early diagnosis is made and aggressive treatment implemented. Because the presenting symptoms and signs are myriad and nonspecific, dissection may be initially overlooked in up to 40 percent of cases. The diagnosis is made only at postmortem examination in a disturbingly large fraction of cases. Few other conditions demand such prompt diagnosis and treatment, since the mortality rate of untreated aortic dissection approaches 1 to 2 percent per hour during the first 48 hours, reaching 90 percent at 3 months, and most deaths directly related to dissection occur within the first 14 days after onset.[48,49] Up to 20 percent of victims die before reaching hospital.[48] With expert care, however, survival of approximately 70 percent of patients reaching the hospital with acute aortic dissection has been reported. Most patients require intensive medical therapy, either as the sole treatment or as a stabilizing measure until surgical therapy is undertaken. Even if the patient survives an aortic dissection, the aneurysm then expands more rapidly than the nondissected aortic aneurysm, contributing to shortened survival.

Dissections of the thoracic aorta may occur in the ascending (type A) or descending (type B) segments, determined by the location of the inciting intimal tear. Tears generally occur in two specific locations: the ascending aorta, 2 to 3 cm above the coronary arteries and in the descending aorta, 1 to 2 cm beyond the origin of the left subclavian artery. The first type produces ascending dissection and the second descending dissection, but dissections originating in the ascending aorta commonly extend along the aortic arch to involve the descending and abdominal portions of the aorta as well.

Aortic dissection can cause death in four main ways (Fig. 105–13):

- Hemopericardium with cardiac tamponade caused by retrograde dissection of an ascending aortic dissection
- Acute aortic insufficiency caused by retrograde dissection of an ascending aortic dissection
- Rupture of a descending aortic dissection into the pleural space
- Occlusion of a branch artery with consequent tissue ischemia

Fig. 105–14 illustrates the mechanism of branch occlusion and the benefits of spontaneous or surgical fenestration.

Most patients with aortic dissection present with hypertension, but 3 to 18 percent present with shock, sometimes secondary to extension of dissection into the coronary arteries, acute myocardial infarction, left ventricular failure, acute severe aortic insufficiency, cardiac tamponade, or aortic rupture. Coronary perfusion may be compromised by retrograde dissection, compression by the false lumen, or hypotension. In one series, differential pulse volume and blood pressure between the right and left upper extremities was detected in 38 percent of patients with ascending aortic dissection. An abrupt loss of pulse can affect the carotid, subclavian, axillary, radial, ulnar, or femoral arteries, and acute limb ischemia has been reported in 20 percent of patients. Branch vessel occlusion results from compression by the distended false lumen of the true lumen of the branch vessel.

Approximately 15 to 20 percent of patients with aortic dissection develop neurologic deficits, with transient cerebral ischemia or stroke in up to 10 percent of cases resulting from extension of dissection into the carotid or vertebral arteries. In such cases, brain imaging and neurologic or neurosurgical consultation may be helpful to determine whether cerebral infarction has occurred; surgery is best avoided in such cases for fear of inducing intracerebral bleeding or otherwise extending the zone of infarction. When cerebral infarction is absent or incomplete, urgent operation is generally indicated, as repair of the dissection may restore brain perfusion. Similarly, urgent surgical intervention is indicated when interruption of spinal circulation by a dissection of the descending aorta threatens to cause paraplegia.

Aortic rupture is the most common cause of death in patients with aortic dissection. After aortic rupture, the second most common cause of death is acute, severe aortic regurgitation, which has been reported in 44 percent of patients with dissection of the ascending aorta and is poorly tolerated hemodynamically, compared to chronic aortic insufficiency, because sudden volume overload allows no time for LV adaptation; cardiogenic shock typically ensues.

[ ] VARIANTS OF AORTIC DISSECTION: INTRAMURAL HEMATOMA AND PENETRATING AORTIC ULCER

Intramural aortic hematoma differs from typical dissection in that there is no flap delineating the true and false lumens, and the hematoma is located circumferentially around the aortic lumen, rather than obliquely (Fig. 105–15).[50] Whether the intramural hematoma arises from a small intimal tear that is not radiographically detected or from a rupture of a vasa vasorum within the aortic wall remains controversial. The clinical course is variable; the hematoma may persist, resorb (returning the aorta to a normal appearance), leave an aneurysm with the possibility of rupture, or later result in dissection.

Penetrating aortic ulcer involves disruption of the internal elastic lamina and erosion of the medial layer of the aortic wall, resulting in local penetration at the site of an atherosclerotic plaque. This lesion may mimic or result in aortic dissection, pseudoaneurysm formation, intramural hematoma, or rupture (Figs. 105–15 to 105–17).[51]

It is important to recognize that intramural hematoma and penetrating aortic ulcer are diseases associated with advanced age, characteristically occurring in patients older than those with

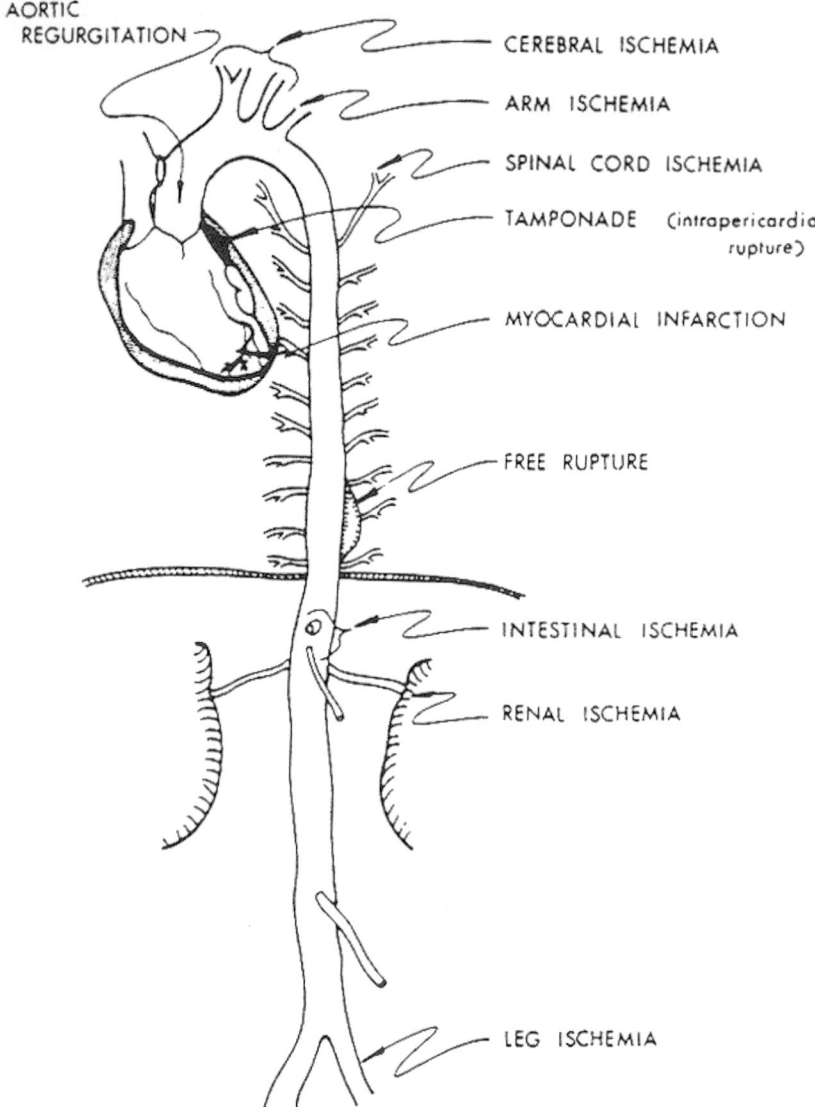

AORTIC
REGURGITATION

CEREBRAL ISCHEMIA

ARM ISCHEMIA

SPINAL CORD ISCHEMIA

TAMPONADE (intrapericardial rupture)

MYOCARDIAL INFARCTION

FREE RUPTURE

INTESTINAL ISCHEMIA

RENAL ISCHEMIA

LEG ISCHEMIA

FIGURE 105-13. The mechanisms by which acute aortic dissection cause death: (1) intrapericardial rupture and tamponade, (2) acute aortic insufficiency, (3) free rupture into left pleural space, (4) occlusion of a branch of the aorta.

dramatic case in which a penetrating ulcer ruptured through the posterior wall of the ascending aorta, mimicking "cryptogenic" pericardial effusion until surgical exploration made the diagnosis clear.

PHYSICAL EXAMINATION

Ascending aortic aneurysms are usually not detected by physical examination (see Chaps. 12 and 88) unless they produce the characteristic diastolic blowing murmur of aortic regurgitation, heard best at the upper right or left sternal border. Descending aortic aneurysms are seldom detectable on physical examination, except in rare instances when they can be palpated through an attenuated chest wall. In contrast, the abdominal aorta is easily palpable in most patients.

Dissection of the aorta is typically associated with physical signs, including the murmur of aortic regurgitation, decrement or loss of peripheral (most commonly one of the femoral) pulses. Of course, a substantial difference in blood pressure between the two arms in the appropriate clinical setting should raise suspicion of acute or chronic aortic dissection as well.

DIAGNOSTIC STUDIES

For evaluation of patients with known or suspected aortic disease, pertinent imaging studies should be selected to identify aneurysm formation and delineate zones of dissection or rupture. Plain chest roentgenography (chest radiography) is useful for screening for thoracic aortic disease (see Chap. 13). In the International Registry of aortic dissection, chest radiography was abnormal in 87.6 percent of patients.

Multiple three-dimensional imaging modalities are applicable to patients with aortic aneurysmal disease, including transesophageal echocardiography (TEE), computed tomography (CT), and magnetic resonance (MR) imaging, each of which offers high sensitivity and specificity. While CT or MR imaging shows the three-dimensional structure of the aorta along its entire course, TEE may not fully delineate the aortic arch[53] or the abdominal aorta; conversely, TEE provides more detailed information about the pericardium, aortic valve, and left ventricular function. Both the ascending and descending portions of the aorta are well visualized by TEE, and the abdominal aorta can be examined by ultrasonography as well as by CT or MR. The primary advantage of TEE is that it can be rapidly performed in the emergency department while the patient is receiving intensive medical support.

The primary criterion for diagnosis of aortic dissection by CT is demonstration of two contrast-filled lumens separated by an intimal flap.[54] Inaccuracy may result from inadequate contrast opacification, nonvisualization of the intimal flap, artifacts extending

type B aortic dissection. In addition, although branch vessel occlusion is commonly associated with aortic dissection, this does not occur as a consequence of penetrating aortic ulcer or intramural hematoma.

The management of patients with penetrating aortic ulcer or intramural hematoma is controversial. When the descending aorta is involved, most authorities advocate medical management with pharmacologic therapy aimed at plaque stabilization and reducing systolic arterial wall stress. Others take a more aggressive stance, operating on all patients except the very old and infirm, based on observational followup of unoperated patients, many of whom die of aortic rupture within 1 to 2 years.

For intramural hematoma involving the ascending aorta, there is more unanimity favoring immediate surgical intervention, although the Japanese literature challenges the need for routine surgery, even in this anatomic location.[52] Penetrating aortic ulcers usually involve the descending aorta distal to the origin of the left subclavian artery, and for those associated with persistent pain stent grafting is the treatment of choice. Fig. 105–16 illustrates a

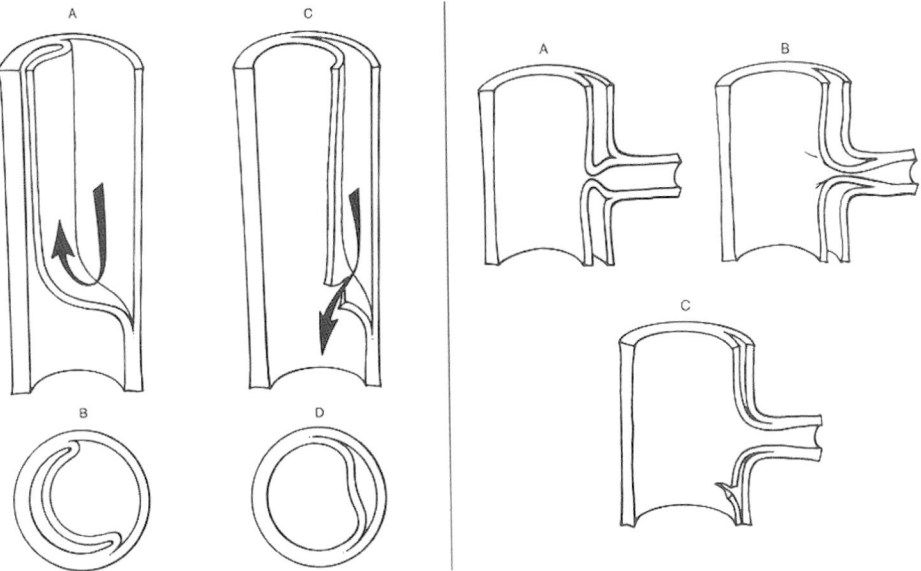

FIGURE 105–14. Schematic representation of the distended false channel in a case of aortic dissection impinging on the lumen of a branch vessel. *Left:* main aortic trunk, with A and B before fenestration, and C and D after fenestration. *Right:* anatomic events at branch vessel; A and B show impingement by a false lumen, and C shows relief by fenestration. *Source: From Crawford and Crawford,[14] with permission.*

across the aortic lumen that simulate an intimal flap, misinterpretation of adjacent vessels or a prominent sinus of Valsalva as a flap, atelectasis or pleural thickening, or thrombosis of the false lumen. Modern multidetector-row CT scanners offer rapid image acquisition, variable section thickness, three-dimensional rendering, diminished helical artifacts, and smaller contrast requirements, overcoming many of these pitfalls. The sensitivity and specificity of CT and MR imaging for diagnosis of aortic dissection currently approach 100 percent, and TEE does not lag far behind. Contrast aortography is more invasive and does not provide the three-dimensional anatomic information afforded by CT, MR, or TEE imaging. Intravascular ultrasonography using high-frequency transducers may be a useful adjunct in cases where other imaging studies are not definitive. It can provide an accurate determination

of the location and extent of aortic dissection and assessment of branch vessels.

DIFFERENTIAL DIAGNOSIS

The imaging studies discussed above provide specific information that may establish or exclude the diagnosis of aortic aneurysm or dissection. Aortic dissection may masquerade as other acute cardiovascular, pulmonary, musculoskeletal, neurologic or gastrointestinal disorders because it can produce symptoms related to almost any organ. The diagnosis is most strongly suggested by migratory chest and back pain of less than 24 hours duration arising in a patient with a history of hypertension. Prompt diagnosis is essential, as the clinical course may evolve rapidly to a catastrophic outcome unless appropriate therapy is instituted. In particular, aortic dissection should be considered in all patients presenting with chest pain without another obvious cause, and the thoracic aorta should be imaged routinely in such cases.

Other conditions frequently confused with aortic dissection are musculoskeletal chest pain, mediastinal tumors, pericarditis, pleuritis, pneumothorax, pulmonary embolism, cholecystitis, ureteral colic, appendicitis, mesenteric ischemia, pyelonephritis, stroke, transient ischemic attack, and primary limb ischemia. Especially troublesome are patients with abdominal symptoms and signs who display no apparent abdominal cause, and it is important to consider aortic dissection in this situation. Given the extensive differential diagnosis, prompt objective diagnostic testing is necessary once the possibility of aortic dissection is raised. Consider aortic dissection and ruptured thoracic or abdominal aneurysm in the differential diagnosis of chest, abdominal or back pain.

- *Obtain appropriate imaging to exclude acute aortic pathology:* 64-row multidetector CT angiography can effectively exclude the major forms of life-threatening thoracic pathology, includ-

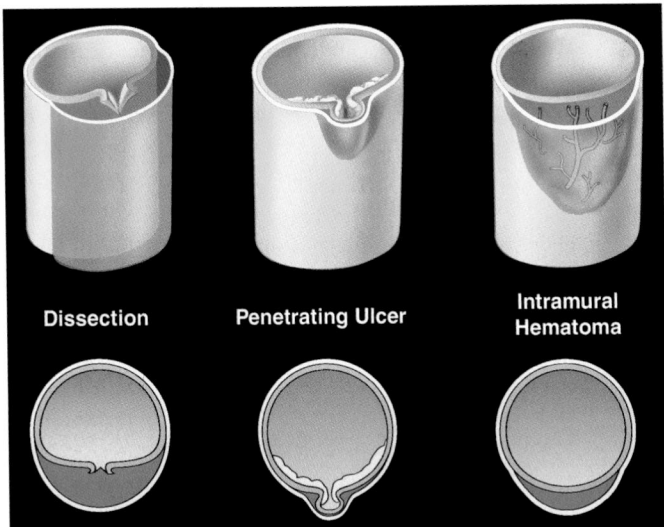

FIGURE 105–15. Variant forms of aortic dissection. Typical dissection, penetrating aortic ulcer (PAU), and intramural hematoma (IHA).

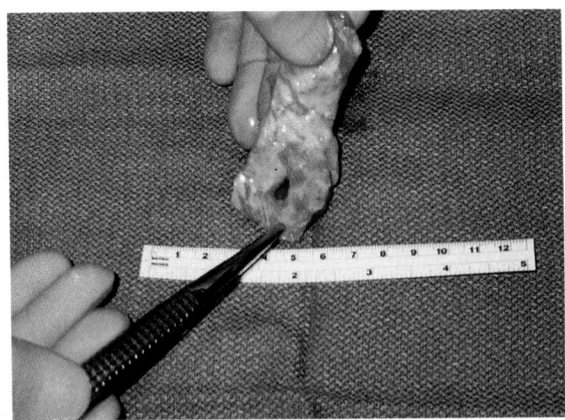

FIGURE 105–16. Gross specimen of a removed segment of aortic wall harboring a penetrating aortic ulcer (PAU).

ing coronary atherosclerosis, pulmonary thromboembolism, and aortic aneurysm or dissection, intramural hematoma and penetrating aortic ulcer, but the threshold at which this technology can be most cost-effectively applied has not yet been established.

- *Employ appropriate biomarkers indicating activation of the coagulation system:* The D-dimer assay not only helps evaluate patients with suspected acute pulmonary embolism but, when negative, also effectively excludes acute aortic dissection. Thrombosis of the false lumen in cases of aortic dissection typically raises D-dimer levels substantially in the peripheral blood.

- *Examine the aorta carefully* in cases whenever a CT scan is obtained in search of other thoracic or abdominal pathology.

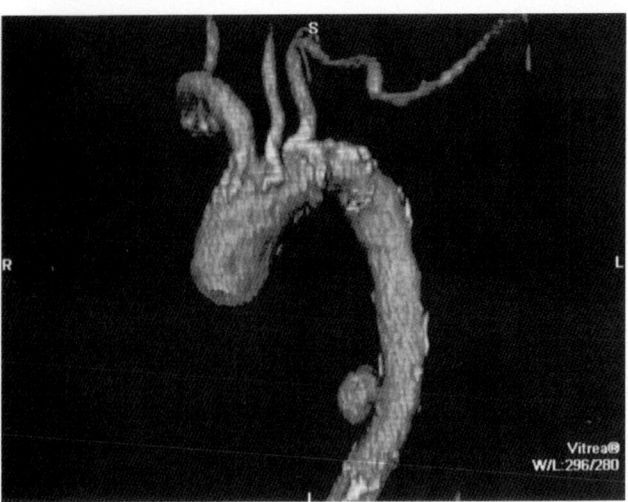

FIGURE 105–17. Magnetic resonance angiogram with surface-shaded rendering demonstrating a penetrating aortic ulcer in the distal portion of the descending thoracic aorta. Note severe generalized aortic arteriosclerosis.

NATURAL HISTORY, PROGNOSIS, AND CLINICAL DECISION-MAKING

Studies of the natural history of thoracic aortic aneurysms using large databases involving thousands of patient-years of observation have established that thoracic aortic aneurysm is associated with approximately 50% mortality over 5 years, but not all deaths in these cohorts are directly attributable to aneurysm. On average, aneurysms of the aorta expand at a rate of about 0.1 cm annually, the descending aorta enlarging somewhat more rapidly than the ascending aorta. Such aneurysms usually develop over decades, so imaging is seldom necessary more often than once a year, and often only every 2 or 3 years, depending on the initial diameter and other factors. Rapid expansion of a thoracic aneurysm in the absence of dissection is rare, and usually reflects measurement error. One common source of error is oblique measurement of the aorta at the arch or near the diaphragm, where an ectatic aorta may take a sharp turn (Fig. 105–18). Current CT and MR technology can correct for most of these problems in measurement. More important than frequent imaging is to compare the most recent images with the *earliest* image available for a given patient, to avoid underestimation of total growth over time.

[ ] INDICATIONS FOR SURGERY

Asymptomatic, Intact Thoracic Aortic Aneurysms

When viewed in terms of cumulative lifetime risk, the natural history of thoracic aortic aneurysms is characterized by an abrupt increment in the incidence of dissection or rupture at maximum diameter of 6 cm for the ascending aorta; these events tend to occur at a larger dimension at the level of the descending aorta (Fig. 105–18). Yearly risks of rupture, dissection, or death reflect a stepwise increment in risk as the aorta expands, rising most dramatically to 14.1 percent at a dimension of 6 cm. Based on this observation, patients without overwhelming comorbidities should undergo resection of thoracic aortic aneurysm before the maximum diameter reaches 5.5 to 6 cm (Table 105–3). For patients with the Marfan syndrome or a family history of this disease, a criterion of 5 cm is usually applied, as they are more prone to rupture or dissection. Patients

with ascending aortic aneurysms associated with bicuspid aortic valve are probably at intermediate risk, and operation is generally recommended at a diameter of 5.5 cm. Intervention is generally recommended at larger diameters for patients with aneurysms of the descending aorta, based upon both the different risk of rupture and the greater associated cardiovascular comorbidities that characterize the typically older individuals who often have advanced atherosclerotic disease.[55–57]

Asymptomatic, Intact Thoracoabdominal Aortic Aneurysms

No randomized trials have addressed the size at which suprarenal, juxtarenal, or type IV thoracoabdominal aortic aneurysms should be repaired to prevent rupture. Because of the high risk of postoperative death, renal insufficiency, and other surgical complications, however, elective intervention is generally recommended for these aneurysms at slightly larger diameter than for infrarenal abdominal aortic aneurysms. In the absence of contraindications to surgery or comorbidities associated with a life expectancy less than 2 years, intervention is generally indicated in patients with suprarenal or type IV thoracoabdominal aortic aneurysms larger than 5.5 to 6.0 cm.

As for aortic aneurysms confined to the chest or abdomen, the dimensional criteria for surgical intervention criteria apply only to asymptomatic aneurysms. *Symptomatic aortic aneurysms at any level should be resected regardless of size.* The development of symptoms frequently portends rupture and mandates surgical or endovascular repair.

Asymptomatic, Intact Abdominal Aortic Aneurysms

Multiple studies have addressed the appropriate size for resection of abdominal aortic aneurysms, including randomized trials in the United Kingdom and the United States[58,59] and meta-analyses (Table 105–4). Small aneurysms, less than 4 cm in diameter, pose a low risk of rupture and should be managed with periodic surveillance for enlargement and symptoms. Abdominal aortic aneurysms between 4.0 and 5.0 cm in diameter

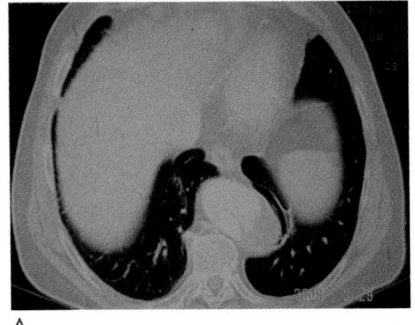
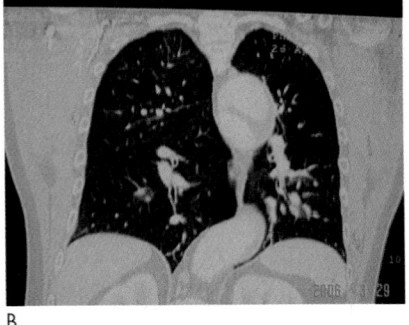

A   B

FIGURE 105–18. Spurious calculation of large aortic dimension (**A**), due to measuring an oblique cross-section across a tortuous portion of the thoracic aorta (**B**).

are associated with a 1 percent per year risk of rupture, and decisions regarding surveillance or surgery should be individualized based on age, familial features and an assessment of surgical risk. Aneurysms 5.5 cm in diameter or larger carry a substantial risk of rupture and should be repaired. As for thoracic aneurysms, the occurrence of symptoms supersedes diameter as a basis for intervention. In general, patients with infrarenal or juxtarenal abdominal aortic aneurysms measuring 4.0 to 5.4 cm in diameter should be monitored by ultrasonography or CT scans every 6 months to detect expansion. Repair may be beneficial in selected patients with aneurysms of 5.0 to 5.4 cm in diameter at this level. For patients with aneurysms smaller than 4.0 cm in diameter, monitoring by ultrasonograph examination every 2 to 3 years is reasonable. Intervention is not recommended for patients with asymptomatic infrarenal or juxtarenal smaller than 5.0 cm in diameter in men or 4.5 cm in women.

PRECIPITATION OF AORTIC DISSECTION

Matrix metalloproteinases and other factors leading to degeneration of the aortic wall play an important role in aneurysm formation. Mechanical studies of human aortas in vivo have shown loss of elasticity when expanded to a diameter of 6 cm, beyond which systolic forces cannot be dissipated by further aortic distension and instead accelerate disruption of the integrity of the aortic wall.[60] In addition to diameter, blood pressure plays a major role in determining wall tension. Without aortic enlargement, hypertension alone cannot generate sufficient wall stress to overcome the tensile strength of aortic tissue.

There are case reports of young, ostensibly healthy, athletic men suffering aortic dissection during isometric weight training or other extreme exertion.[61] All had unknown moderate enlargement of the aorta and all experienced acute onset of dissection pain during effort; aortic dissection proved fatal in one-third of these cases. The magnitude of hypertension during weight lifting contributes excess wall stress that exceeds the tolerable aortic load limit, resulting in acute dissection. Nearly three-fourths of patients report either extreme emotion or exertion at the onset of symptomatic dissection, again suggesting a link with hemodynamic forces. Based on these considerations, some authors recommended that individuals embarking on programs involving heavy weight-lifting or extreme physical training first undergo echocardiography to exclude ascending aortic aneurysm.

TABLE 105–3

The Yale Center for Thoracic Aortic Disease Recommended Surgical Intervention Criteria for Thoracic Aortic Aneurysms

1. Rupture
2. Acute aortic dissection
   a. Ascending requires urgent operation
   b. Descending requires a "complication specific approach"
3. Symptomatic states
   a. Pain consistent with rupture and unexplained by other causes
   b. Compression of adjacent organs, especially trachea, esophagus, or left main stem bronchus
   c. Significant aortic insufficiency in conjuction with ascending aortic aneurysm
4. Documented enlargement
   a. growth ≥1 cm/yr or substantial growth and aneurysm is rapidly approaching absolute size criteria
5. Absolute size (cm)

	MARFAN	NON-MARFAN
Ascending	5.0 cm	5.5 cm
Descending	6.0 cm	6.5 cm

TREATMENT OF ANEURYSM AND DISSECTION

The modern era in the treatment of aneurysms and dissections was ushered in by the pioneering innovations of Cooley and DeBakey, which were first reported in 1952.[62]

TABLE 105–4

Decision Making for Abdominal Aortic Aneurysms

HSTAT meta-analysis of surgical intervention criteria for AAA leads to the following conclusions:

3.0–3.9 cm AAA	Very low risk of rupture	Periodic surveillance
4.0–5.4 cm AAA	Yearly rupture rate ≈1%	Surgery or surveillance
5.5 cm or larger AAA	Substantial rupture risk	Surgery advised

SOURCE: *Adapted from Elefteriades JA, Rizzo JA. Epidemiology: incidence, prevalence, trends. In: Elefteriades J, ed. Acute Aortic Conditions. New York: Taylor & Francis, 2007, and Health Services/Technology Assessment Text (HSTAT). Guide to Clinical Preventative Services, 3rd ed. Evidence syntheses, formerly systematic evidence reviews. National Library of Medicine and NCBI. Available at http://hstat.nlm.nih.gov. Last accessed September 24, 2006. Reproduced with permission.*

MEDICAL TREATMENT OF CHRONIC ANEURYSMS

Patients with aortic aneurysms are commonly treated with β-adrenergic antagonist drugs to decrease systolic arterial wall stress, but the effectiveness of this strategy has been validated only in one long-term study of 70 patients with clinical features of the Marfan syndrome,[63–65] and its value in patients without Marfan syndrome is controversial. Among the concerns, in addition the potential for side effects, is evidence that β blockers decrease the elasticity of the aortic wall.

The antibiotic agent doxycycline, an MMP inhibitor, has shown promise in large-scale clinical trials in patients with abdominal aortic aneurysms.[66] Other drugs that have undergone animal or clinical testing, including cyclooxygenase (COX) 2 inhibitory antiinflammatory agents, hydroxymethylglutaryl coenzyme A (HMG-CoA) reductase inhibitors (statins), the immunosuppressive agent rapamycin, and the angiotensin-receptor inhibitor losartan,[67–69] have not been proven to produce clinical benefit. Impressive suppression of aneurysmal disease was achieved with losartan in an animal model of Marfan syndrome, and clinical trials are underway to investigate this potential avenue of treatment.

MEDICAL TREATMENT OF ACUTE AORTIC SYNDROMES (DISSECTION, RUPTURE, AND IMPENDING RUPTURE)

Aortic dissection propagates more vigorously when either blood pressure or the force of cardiac contraction is elevated.[49,70] Accordingly, control of blood pressure is an important aspect of treatment in patients with acute aortic syndromes, including dissection, rupture or impending rupture. Intravenous nitroglycerin or sodium nitroprusside are commonly used for this purpose. Lowering blood pressure by administration of vasodilator drugs alone may increase the sheer stress on the aortic wall; however, this can be ameliorated by decreasing the force of cardiac contraction. The objective is to reduce the rate of rise of arterial pressure (*dP/dt*), reflected in attenuation of the upslope of the aortic pulse wave,[70] by administering a short-acting β-blocking drug like esmolol or the β- and α-adrenergic antagonist labetalol by intravenous infusion. When β-blocking drugs are contraindicated, the nondihydropyridine calcium channel blockers diltiazem and verapamil are reasonable alternatives.

SURGICAL THERAPY

Specific surgical procedures have been developed for resection and graft replacement of aneurysms involving the ascending aorta, transverse (arch), descending thoracic, thoracoabdominal, and abdominal aortic segments. The Dacron grafts employed are durable and do not require long-term anticoagulant therapy. The risks of such surgery include bleeding, stroke, paralysis, myocardial infarction, renal failure, death and other complications; safety is greatest when surgery is performed electively, prior to aortic rupture or dissection.

Ascending aortic (type A) dissection requires urgent surgery to avoid death as a consequence of intrapericardial rupture, aortic regurgitation, or myocardial infarction. Repair involves reapproximation of the aortic wall between layers of Teflon felt. At experienced centers, survival is approximately 85 percent.[71] Patients with descending aortic (type B) dissections face a better prognosis with initial medical management ("anti-impulse" therapy with β blockers and vasodilator drugs), withholding surgery unless specific complications develop.

Following corrective surgery for type A aortic dissection or stabilization on medication therapy for type B dissection, close observation is necessary with serial aortic imaging during the first month and periodically thereafter. Some patients eventually develop enlargement of the dissected aorta requiring resection,[72] and in these cases the dimensional criteria for surgical intervention are the same as those employed for intact aneurysms.

AORTIC ROOT

The morphology of the aortic root dictates the surgical procedure required for correction of aneurysmal pathology. For supracoronary aneurysms, tube graft replacement is typically employed, unless stenosis or insufficiency of the aortic valve requires concomitant valve replacement. In patients with annuloaortic ectasia, composite graft replacement of the aortic root and the aortic valve with a prefabricated unit is preferred. This more complex procedure requires meticulous reimplantation of the coronary arteries, with "buttons" of surrounding aortic tissue. Recently, Yacoub and David have advocated techniques for "valve-sparing" aortic root replacement, but these require further followup to determine long-term efficacy compared to composite graft replacement.[73,74]

AORTIC ARCH

Surgery for aneurysms of the aortic arch requires methods for cerebral protection during attachment of the cerebral arteries (great vessels) to the aortic graft. For attachment of the great vessels, Carrel patches (with a rim of aorta carrying the innominate, left carotid, and left subclavian arteries) are commonly employed or, alternatively, prefabricated branched grafts that permit individual anastomosis of each great vessel. At 64.4°F (18°C), the temperature commonly employed, the metabolic rate is below 15 percent of normal, permitting 30 to 45 minutes for manipulation of the aortic arch. When longer periods of circulatory arrest are necessary, direct cerebral perfusion can be provided through cannulae placed individually in the great vessels.

THORACOABDOMINAL AORTA

The key issues in surgery of the thoracoabdominal aorta involve protection of the lower body organs and spinal cord during the period of aortic cross-clamping and attachment of the visceral arteries (superior mesenteric artery, celiac axis, and renal arteries). The arterial supply of the spinal cord is segmental, and viability of spinal cord cells is highly dependent on the artery of Adamkiewicz or arteries arising from the low intercostal or lumbar territory (T8-L2), which are excluded during thoracoabdominal aortic surgery. Intraoperative perfusion of the lower body by blood aspirated from the left atrium helps prevent paraplegia,[75,76] one of the most worrisome complications of this procedure. Other protective techniques include mild systemic hypothermia, aspiration of cerebrospinal fluid to decrease ambient pressure on the spinal cord, and implantation of the intercostal arteries.

The technical challenge of attaching all the important branch vessels of the abdominal aorta has been met by technical advances, most specifically by the implementation of reimplantation of the branch arteries on pedicles of surrounding aorta, often by the inclusion technique (in which the pedicle is not mobilized completely from its bed). Current rates of mortality or paraplegia for this type of surgery are below 10 percent, reflecting technical improvements in graft technology, surgical techniques, perfusion, anesthesia, and perioperative care.

CONCOMITANT CORONARY ARTERY DISEASE

The most important risk factor for cardiac events and death in patients undergoing aneurysm surgery is coronary artery disease. Because operative mortality is related mainly to myocardial ischemia, it has been suggested that coronary revascularization be performed in selected patients prior to abdominal aortic aneurysm resection.[77–79] No well-designed studies are available, however, comparing the outcome of serial myocardial revascularization and abdominal or thoracic aortic aneurysm repair with aneurysm surgery alone. Even so, an effort should be made to identify preoperatively those patients at highest cardiac risk using noninvasive diagnostic methods. Findings of extensive myocardial ischemia may prompt angiography to define the coronary pathoanatomy and LV function. Thereafter, decisions regarding coronary revascularization must be based on symptoms, angiographic findings, and other elements of risk. One anticipates a survival advantage imparted by surgical revascularization in patients with left main coronary artery disease or stenosis greater than 70 percent involving each of the three major coronary arteries in patients with substantial zones of ischemia. In those with severe discrete proximal stenosis of a first-order coronary artery and either symptomatic or extensive ischemia or reversible left ventricular dysfunction amenable to catheter-based myocardial revascularization, clinical decision making must balance the long-term advantages of drug-eluting intracoronary stents against the need for potent platelet inhibitor therapy that may be difficult to administer in the days prior to and following aortic aneurysmectomy. Furthermore, in patients soon to undergo aortic reconstructive surgery, coronary balloon angioplasty or bare-metal stenting may be preferred, even though the potential for coronary restenosis may later require a second revascularization procedure after aortic surgery has been completed.

Diagnostic cardiac catheterization and angiography are routinely performed as part of the preoperative evaluation of patients undergoing surgical repair of ascending aortic aneurysms to evaluate the morphology of the ascending aorta, function of the aortic valve, and coronary anatomy. Based on the angiographic findings, myocardial revascularization can be readily incorporated into the reparative surgical procedure if warranted. If severe proximal coronary artery disease is found, then options include staged percutaneous or surgical coronary revascularization followed after an interval of several weeks by resection of the aneurysm.

ENDOVASCULAR THERAPY FOR AORTIC ANEURYSMS

Parodi et al., in 1991, first reported the technique of transfemoral catheter-based repair of infrarenal abdominal aortic aneurysms as an alternative to open repair for patients at high risk of complications with conventional surgical treatment.[80] Over the ensuing years, a variety of stent grafts and delivery systems have been introduced, and endovascular repair has become a valuable alternative for elderly patients and those with advanced cardiopulmonary disease.

Most stent graft devices involve a modular construction consisting of a metallic exoskeleton surrounding an intimal fabric graft to maintain linear stability and prevent kinking.

Stent-graft therapy has a valid role in the management of patients with ruptured aortic aneurysm[81,82] traumatic transaction of the aorta,[83] and penetrating aortic ulcers.[84] The role of endograft therapy in typical, fusiform degenerative aneurysms is more controversial. An important limiting complication of stent-graft therapy is the propensity for *endoleak*,[85] in which blood flow continues into the excluded aneurysm sac after stent graft deployment. Type I endoleaks are caused by incompetent proximal or distal attachments, producing high intrasac pressures that can lead to rupture, and require repair using intraluminal extension cuffs or open surgery. Type II endoleaks resulting from retrograde flow from branch vessels (e.g., intercostal, lumbar, or inferior mesenteric arteries) occur in as many as 40 percent of patients after endograft implantation. Over half of these seal spontaneously, but when persistent, they can be corrected by selective arterial embolization, and do not appear to cause rupture over short-term followup. Type III endoleaks are caused by fabric defects, tears or disruption of modular graft components. These carry the same potential for delayed aneurysm rupture as Type I endoleaks and should be promptly repaired. Type IV endoleaks, the least common variety, result from graft porosity and diffuse leakage through interstices, and usually develop within 30 days of implantation.

Other complications of stent-graft repair of abdominal aortic aneurysms include occlusion of the iliac limbs of bifurcation endografts and migration from the proximal attachment as a result of progressive aortic expansion, which can be detected in at least 1 in 5 cases. Technical improvements in graft design and deployment techniques are reducing implant complications, but because of the potential for endoleak, graft migration or graft limb occlusion, periodic followup imaging at intervals of 6–12 months is recommended after endovascular stent-graft repair.[85,86]

The effectiveness of endograft therapy in preventing aneurysm growth, rupture, and aneurysm-related mortality compared to open surgical repair remains controversial.[87] Although often ultimately lethal, thoracic aortic aneurysm is an indolent disease, and years may elapse between diagnosis of a small or moderate-size aneurysm and aneurysm-related death. The EUROSTAR survey of endograft repair of abdominal aortic aneurysms exposed cases of late mortality and rupture even after initially successful intervention. Information regarding late outcomes following endograft repair of abdominal aortic aneurysms are more comprehensive than for thoracic aortic aneurysm, but it appears that the risk of endoleak is ongoing over at least 5 years (Fig. 105–19). Endoleak predicted rupture, surgical intervention or death in 13 percent, 14 percent, and 27 percent of patients by 5 years postprocedure in patients originally presenting with large aneurysms (Fig. 105–20). These concerns about long-term effectiveness support the view that endograft therapy should be reserved for patients in whom comorbidity precludes direct open surgical repair and emphasize the need for lifelong surveillance.[88–91] Randomized trials of thoracic endografting versus open surgical repair will be required to provide conclusive evidence regarding the relative merits; in the

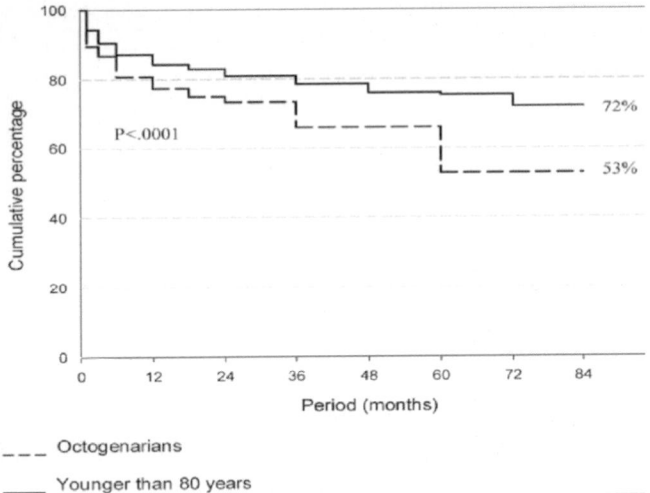

FIGURE 105–19. Kaplan-Meier graph represents cumulative freedom from any endoleak in patients operated on for abdominal aortic aneurysm with endovascular aneurysm repair. *Source: Reprinted with permission from Lange C, Leurs LJ, Buth K, et al. Endovascular repair of abdominal aortic aneurysm in octogenarians: An analysis based on EUROSTAR data. J Vasc Surg 2005;42:624–630.*

mean time, open surgical repair remains the current standard in terms of both efficacy and durability.

ATHEROSLEROSIS OF THE AORTA

【 】 PATHOLOGIC ANATOMY

Atherosclerosis of the aorta is common in western society. The usual risk factors are tobacco smoking, diabetes mellitus, hypertension, hypercholesterolemia, obesity, and sedentary lifestyle, while the contribution of elevated levels of plasma homocysteine

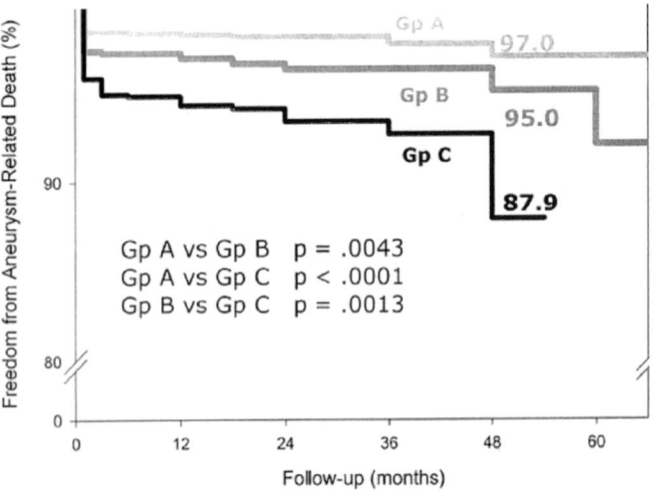

FIGURE 105–20. Cumulative freedom from aneurysm-related death following endovascular repair of abdominal aortic aneurysm in the EUROSTAR registry. Note low attrition during first 3 years of followup followed by rapid attrition in the fourth year. *Gp* denotes groups defined by increasing initial aneurysm size: Gp A = 4.0 to 5.4 cm, Gp B = 5.5 to 6.4 cm, Gp C ≥ 6.5 cm. *Source: Reprinted from Peppelenbosch N, Buth J, Harris PL, et al. Diameter of abdominal aortic aneurysm and outcome of endovascular aneurysm repair: Does size matter? A report from EUROSTAR. J Vasc Surg 2004;39:288–297, with permission.*

and C-reactive protein has more recently been suggested. The pathogenesis of atherosclerosis is discussed in Chap. 52.

Atherosclerosis most commonly develops in the infrarenal aorta and may be asymptomatic or produce intermittent claudication, critical limb ischemia, or atheromatous embolism. Atherosclerosis typically involves the aortic arch and the origins of the brachiocephalic, carotid and subclavian vessels, and the descending thoracic aorta.

【 】 ATHEROMATOUS EMBOLISM

Embolism of cholesterol-laden atheromatous material and thrombus from the surface of the aorta occurs commonly in patients with severe aortic atherosclerosis.[92] Atheroembolism may be spontaneous, although it more frequently occurs after surgical or arteriographic manipulation, such as catheter-based coronary or peripheral interventions. In a retrospective study of 71 autopsies, the incidence of cholesterol embolism in patients who had undergone arteriography before death was 27 percent, compared to 4.3 percent in an age- and disease-matched control group who did not undergo angiography.[93]

Whether or not anticoagulant and thrombolytic drugs can exacerbate atheroembolism associated with the "blue-toe syndrome" is controversial.[94–95] Few cases of this complication were reported in clinical trials of anticoagulation in high-risk patients with atrial fibrillation, despite the frequent finding of morphologically complex aortic plaque in this population.[96]

Patients with atheromatous embolism typically have a history of angina pectoris, myocardial infarction, transient ischemic attack, stroke, intermittent claudication, or peripheral gangrene. Clinical signs and symptoms are variable, depending on the amount, size, and location of origin of the atheromatous material as well as on the tissue affected. Macroembolism may present catastrophically as an acute ischemic limb, whereas patients with microembolism may have milder localized signs or a clinical picture suggesting systemic illness, including fever, weight loss, anorexia, myalgia, headache, nausea, vomiting, or diarrhea. Occasionally, the presentation may suggest vasculitis, infective endocarditis, or malignancy. Cutaneous manifestations are the most frequent findings[97] and include cyanotic toes, gangrenous digits, livedo reticularis, or nodules (Fig. 105–21).[98] When atheroembolism affects both lower extremities, the source is generally the aorta, but when only one extremity is involved, it may be difficult to determine whether the origin is a diseased ipsilateral iliofemoral artery or a more proximal or distal site.

Atheroembolism originating from the suprarenal aorta may involve the kidneys, producing occlusion of multiple small arteries and segmental ischemic atrophy. This small-vessel occlusive disease may cause accelerated hypertension, microscopic hematuria, or renal failure. Pathologically, biconvex cholesterol crystals occlude the interlobular and afferent arterioles (150 to 200 μm in diameter). A foreign-body reaction leads to small-vessel occlusion, reducing glomerular filtration rate, activating the renin–angiotensin–aldosterone system, and accelerating hypertension. Various patterns of renal insufficiency may develop and progress over weeks or months to irreversible renal failure requiring dialysis.[99] The differential diagnosis includes renal artery stenosis, renal artery thrombosis, infective endocarditis, vasculitis such as polyarteritis nodosa, and other causes of acute renal failure. No single laboratory test is diagnostic, as acceleration of the erythrocyte sedimentation rate, leukocytosis with eosinophilia, and anemia are common in many systemic illnesses.[100] Blood urea nitrogen and creatinine elevations may be early manifestations of renal involvement, and the urine sediment may be abnormal. Elevated serum amylase or hepatic transaminase levels may indicate pancreatic or hepatic involvement, and creatine phosphokinase and aldolase arise from affected muscle. Renal biopsy is rarely required but may reveal pathognomonic needle-shaped cholesterol clefts within small vessels. Atheroembolic renal disease carries a poor prognosis, with a mortality rate of 81 percent (179 of 221 patients) in one series; the most common causes of death were cardiac, renal, or multiorgan failure.[100]

【 】 ATHEROSCLEROSIS OF THE AORTIC ARCH

Atherosclerosis of the thoracic aorta is a strong predictor of initial and recurrent stroke, coronary events, and death.[101] The thickness and morphology (protrusion, ulceration, or mobility) of atheromatous plaque correlate with the prevalence of stroke. Whether this association has a direct atheroembolic mechanism or reflects associated cerebrovascular pathology has not been conclusively determined.

Atheromatous embolism arising from the aortic arch or the carotid and vertebral arteries may cause stroke, transient ischemic attack, amaurosis fugax, blindness, headache, confusion, organic brain syndromes, dizziness or spinal cord infarction. Retinal artery occlusion may be identified by Hollenhorst plaque visible on ophthalmoscopic examination as yellow, highly refractile atheromatous material at an arteriolar bifurcation.

TREATMENT

Because treatment of atheroembolism seldom reverses damage, emphasis is on prevention of subsequent ischemic events. When the source of embolism can be confirmed, it is often feasible to isolate or replace a discrete segment of the aorta by surgery, angioplasty, or stent-graft insertion. Treatment should include symptomatic care of affected ischemic tissue and risk-factor modification to prevent progression of atheromatous disease and promote plaque stabilization. If embolism affects the lower extremities, this involves local care of ischemic ulcers; when gangrene is present, amputation may be required. The role of sympathectomy is controversial, but this may be helpful when pain is intractable. In cases of renal atheroembolism, dialysis should be performed as necessary, and blood pressure controlled pharmacologically.

Optimum antithrombotic therapy (anticoagulants, platelet inhibitors, or a combination of both) for atheromatous embolism has not been defined, but platelet inhibitor drugs generally lessen the risk of cardiovascular ischemic events. Anticoagulation therapy is far from protective, however, with a recurrence rate of cerebral events of 26 percent in patients with plaques more than 4 mm in thickness, despite antiplatelet or warfarin therapy. Case reports of improvement with lipid-lowering therapy are supported by observations in non-randomized series and evidence in coronary disease that HMG-CoA-reductase inhibitor ("statin") drugs improve plaque stabilization.[102]

The role of surgical therapy for patients with localized atheromata in the aortic arch and cerebral ischemia is controversial, as it

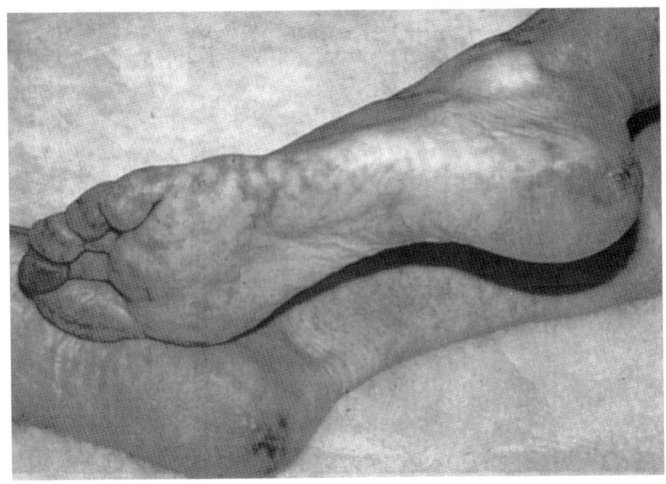

FIGURE 105–21. Typical appearance of atheromatous embolism involving the feet. There are cyanotic toes, livedo reticularis along the lateral portion of the foot, and ischemic lesions on both heels, indicating that the source of embolism is proximal to the aortic bifurcation. *Source: Reproduced from Bartholomew JR, Olin JW. Atheromatous embolization. In: Bartholomew JR, ed. Peripheral Vascular Diseases, 2d ed. St. Louis: Mosby, 1996, with permission.*

is seldom possible to determine conclusively whether the cause of symptoms is the aorta or associated cerebrovascular disease.[103]

【 】 AORTOILIAC OCCLUSIVE DISEASE

Atherosclerotic occlusive disease of the infrarenal aorta and iliac arteries may occur with or without atherosclerosis of the infrainguinal vessels.[104,105] When isolated, aortoiliac atherosclerosis typically occurs in younger individuals who smoke cigarettes. Almost half the cases are women, many of whom angiographically exhibit the "hypoplastic aortic syndrome," with small-caliber aortic, iliac, and femoropopliteal arteries. The disease in these cases is usually confined to the aortic bifurcation. Disease localized to the distal aorta and common iliac arteries (type I) rarely produces limb-threatening ischemia because of extensive collateral vessels. The classic presentation is the Leriche syndrome, a clinical triad of intermittent claudication involving the low back, buttocks, hip or thigh, which is often mistaken for degenerative joint disease of the low back or hips, impotency (which occurs in 30 to 50 percent of males with aortoiliac occlusive disease), and "global atrophy" of the lower extremities, reflecting the chronicity of low-grade ischemia.[106] The femoral pulses are often weak or absent, but the ankle-brachial index may be normal at rest. A decline in ankle systolic pressure following exercise confirms hemodynamically significant stenosis.

MANAGEMENT

Treatment of patients with occlusive atherosclerosis of the aorta should include measures directed at improving symptoms (e.g., claudication or limb ischemia) and thus quality of life, as well as reduction of overall cardiovascular risk. The latter involves the same measures as management of other manifestations of systemic atherosclerosis or peripheral arterial disease (see Chaps. 52 and 108).[107] Catheter-based intervention to relieve aortic obstruction should be considered in lifestyle interfering claudication or critical limb ischemia. Although this point is controversial, there is general consensus that patients with aortoiliac occlusive disease do not respond as well to exercise or medications (pentoxifylline or cilostazol) as do patients with infrainguinal peripheral arterial disease. Most cases of aortoiliac occlusive disease requiring treatment are now treated with endovascular devices.

The Transatlantic Inter-Societal Consensus (TASC) II[6] classifies patients with aortoiliac occlusive disease into four categories. There have been modifications from TASC I because of technological advances, but the overall principles are similar. Endovascular therapy was favored for patients with type A lesions; surgery was preferred for those with type D lesions. Although the evidence available was insufficient to support firm recommendations for type B or C aortoiliac lesions, subsequent advances justify an attempt at angioplasty and stenting, with most cases meeting clinical criteria for revascularization, unless obstructive disease extends into the common femoral artery. Surgical revascularization of aortoiliac lesions is associated with patency rates of 74 to 95 percent over 5 years,[108] similar, but not superior, to results with catheter-based interventions.[109]

ACUTE OBSTRUCTION OF THE TERMINAL AORTA

【 】 ETIOLOGY

Sudden occlusion of the terminal aorta may result from a large "saddle" embolus,[110] trauma, dissection or in situ thrombosis superimposed on aneurysmal or atherosclerotic disease. Most emboli large enough to occlude the terminal aorta (saddle embolism) originate in the heart in patients with mitral stenosis, atrial fibrillation, acute anterior myocardial infarction, infective endocarditis, or paradoxical embolism through a right-to-left intracardiac shunt from a peripheral venous source. When thrombotic occlusion of the aorta develops at a point of atherosclerotic narrowing, collateral perfusion is usually sufficient to prevent acute limb ischemia. Acute aortic occlusion related to thrombosis of an abdominal aortic aneurysm is considerably less common than thrombosis of popliteal aneurysms.

【 】 CLINICAL FEATURES

Unlike gradually progressive obstruction, abrupt total or near-total interruption of flow through the terminal aorta or common iliac arteries poses an immediate threat to life and limb. Although the clinical picture varies depending on collaterals, the full-blown syndrome is characterized by abrupt onset of pain, typically severe, in the lumbar area, buttocks, perineum, abdomen, and legs. Diffuse cyanosis may be present from the umbilicus to the feet and the lower limbs may be pale and cold. Numbness, paresthesiae, and paralysis dominate the picture. Pulses are absent in the lower limbs and, unless circulation is restored promptly, muscle necrosis may produce myoglobinuria, renal failure, acidosis, hyperkalemia and death.

【 】 MANAGEMENT

In contrast to chronic aortoiliac occlusion, acute aortic occlusion calls for immediate revascularization. The optimum procedure depends on etiology and the strategy for prevention of recurrent embolism. Transfemoral catheter-based embolectomy can extract even large amounts of embolic material from the distal aorta. Even after circulation has been restored, however, mortality is high, related to the underlying disease.

AORTITIS

Inflammation of the aortic wall may occur in noninfectious diseases, such as Takayasu disease, giant cell arteritis, the spondyloarthropathies, Behçet syndrome, relapsing polychondritis, Cogan syndrome, rheumatoid arthritis, systemic lupus erythematosus, sarcoidosis, idiopathic retroperitoneal fibrosis, and other disorders. Only the most common of these uncommon entities are discussed in detail.

【 】 TAKAYASU DISEASE

The prototypical nonspecific aortitis, Takayasu arteritis was named for the Japanese ophthalmologist who first called attention to the funduscopic findings (see Chap. 88).[111,112] Because of its predilection for the brachiocephalic vessels, this arteritis has been labeled *pulseless disease* and *aortic arch syndrome*. The classic form occurs with greatest frequency in Asian countries, but patients with a similar nonspecific aortitis are encountered worldwide. The etiology is unknown; no infectious agent has been identified, and identification of endothelial antibodies in 18 of 19 patients with this disease supports an autoimmune mechanism. This finding is nonspecific.

Histopathology

Histologic examination during active stages of the disease discloses a granulomatous arteritis similar to giant cell arteritis and to the aortitis associated with the seronegative spondyloarthropathies and Cogan syndrome. In later stages, medial degeneration, fibrous scarring, intimal proliferation, and thrombosis result in narrowing of the vessel, yet there remains a lack of adequate histopathologic criteria for the differential diagnosis of noninfectious arteritides, including Takayasu disease and giant cell aortitis.[113] Aneurysm formation is less common than stenosis, but aneurysm rupture is an important cause of death in patients with Takayasu arteritis. Angiographically, the left subclavian artery is narrowed in approximately 90 percent of patients. The right subclavian artery, left carotid artery, and brachiocephalic trunk follow closely in frequency of stenosis. Thoracic aortic lesions occur in 66 percent of patients, the abdominal aorta is involved in 50 percent, and aortoiliac involvement is seen in approximately 12 percent. Pulmonary arteritis occurs in about half the patients and may be associated with pulmonary hypertension.

Clinical Features

In 70 to 80 percent of cases, clinical manifestations of the illness appear during the second or third decade of life, but onset in childhood and in middle life have been reported. Women are affected eight to nine times more often than men. During the early or "prepulseless" phase, symptoms include fever, night sweats, malaise, nausea, vomiting, weight loss, rash, arthralgia, and Raynaud phenomenon. Splenomegaly may occur and laboratory findings may include acceleration of the erythrocyte sedimentation rate, elevated levels of C-reactive protein, anemia, and plasma protein abnormalities.

Once arterial obstruction develops, upper-extremity claudication may occur as a consequence of subclavian artery stenosis. Stroke, transient cerebral ischemia, dizziness, or syncope usually indicates narrowing of the brachiocephalic arteries or subclavian steal. The retinopathy that first drew the attention of Takayasu is believed to result from retinal ischemia. Hypertension, observed in over half the cases, is sometimes malignant and suggests narrowing of the aorta proximal to the renal arteries or involvement of the renal arteries themselves.[114]

Cardiac manifestations result from severe hypertension, dilatation of the aortic root producing valvular insufficiency, or coronary artery stenosis (Fig. 105–22). Angina pectoris, myocardial infarction, and heart failure have been reported. Clinical pericarditis has been observed infrequently, but healed pericarditis is often encountered at necropsy. Involvement of the visceral arteries may result in splanchnic ischemia, and aortoiliac obstruction may produce intermittent claudication in the lower limbs.

Patients in whom severe aortitis is evident at the time of diagnosis face a 25 to 30 percent risk of ischemic events or death over the next 5 years. Those without ischemic complications at presentation tend to fare better over 5 to 10 years. Severe hypertension and cardiac involvement are associated with shortened life expectancy.

Diagnosis

The American College of Rheumatology has identified six major criteria for the diagnosis of Takayasu arteritis.[115] Onset of illness by age 40 years avoids overlap with giant cell arteritis. Other criteria include upper-extremity claudication, diminished brachial pulses, greater than 10 mmHg difference between systolic blood pressure in the arms, subclavian or aortic bruit, and narrowing of the aorta or a major branch. The presence of three of these six criteria carries high diagnostic accuracy.

Arteriography typically shows long areas of smooth narrowing interspersed with areas that appear normal. Aneurysm and occlusions are also common. CT scans may show wall thickening resulting from inflammation of the media and adventitia, and MRI may disclose arterial wall edema as a marker of active disease (see Chap. 88). MR or CT angiography of the aorta, arch vessels, and iliac vessels is generally recommended for all patients with suspected

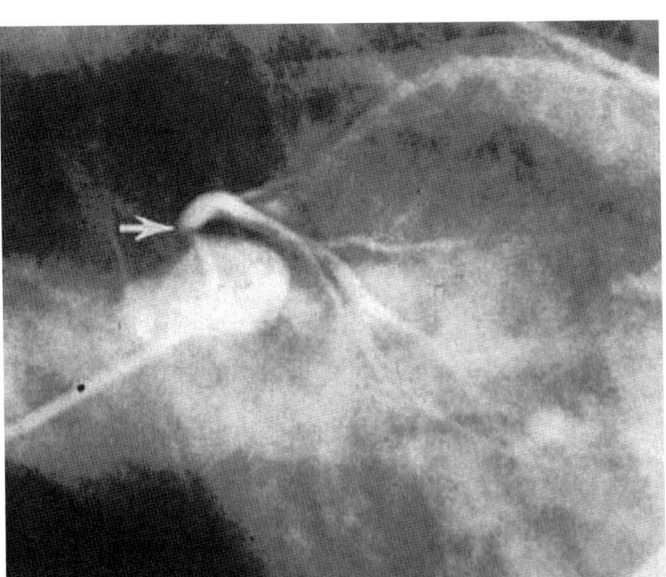

FIGURE 105–22. *Typical angiographic appearance of Takayasu arteritis, showing focal ostial stenosis of the left main coronary artery. Source: From Jolly M, Bartholomew JR, Flamm S, Olin JW. Angina and ostial lesions in a young woman as a presentation of Takayasu's arteritis. J Cardiovasc Surg 1999;7:443–446, with permission.*

Takayasu disease to define the extent of disease, identify aneurysms, and estimate the activity of disease.

Management

Corticosteroid therapy appears effective in suppressing inflammation during the active phase, and favorable results have been reported with immunosuppressive and cytotoxic agents (see Chap. 88).[115] Operative treatment may be employed to relieve symptoms caused by arterial obstruction, and percutaneous angioplasty and stenting are associated with favorable results. These procedures are best reserved for patients in whom the acute inflammatory stage of the disease has been controlled.[8]

GIANT CELL ARTERITIS

Giant cell arteritis (temporal arteritis, polymyalgia rheumatica) involves extracranial arteries, including the aorta, in 10 to 13 percent of cases. A peak incidence late in life sets giant cell arteritis apart from other nonspecific arteritides. Like Takayasu disease, giant cell arteritis may produce narrowing of the brachiocephalic arteries, aneurysms of the ascending aorta, aortic dissection, and aortic regurgitation.[116] Despite clinical, angiographic, and pathologic similarities to Takayasu arteritis, giant cell arteritis almost always occurs in individuals older than 50 years of age. Although the most common presentation involves polymyalgia rheumatica with temporal arteritis, any large artery may be involved.

Treatment of giant cell arteritis usually involves oral prednisone in an initial dose of 40 to 60 mg daily. Induction therapy with intravenous steroids has been found beneficial in a randomized trial. During clinical followup, MRI can be of value in monitoring improvement in arterial abnormalities with therapy. In unresponsive cases (<10 percent) or in those who relapse as the dose is tapered, cytotoxic agents such as cyclosporine, azathioprine, and methotrexate may be helpful. One randomized double-blind trial found a significant reduction in the rate of relapse and the cumulative mean does of corticosteroid medication with methotrexate compared to placebo in corticosteroid-treated patients,[117] but another study did not.[118]

HLA-B27-ASSOCIATED SPONDYLOARTHROPATHIES

Aortitis is present in a substantial portion of patients with ankylosing spondylitis and Reiter syndrome; more than 90 percent have the histocompatibility antigen HLA-B27. Aortic involvement is most common in those with spondylitis of long duration, peripheral joint complaints in addition to spondylitis, and iritis.[119] Inflammation of the aortic root and surrounding tissues manifest by aortic valve regurgitation or cardiac conduction abnormalities in patients with the HLA-B27 histocompatibility antigen may also occur without spondyloarthropathies. Histologically, the aortic lesion in this setting resembles the inflammation seen in syphilis, with focal destruction of medial elastic tissue and thickening of the intima and adventitia. Aortic dissection has been reported.[120]

INFECTIOUS AORTITIS

Primary infection of the aortic wall is a rare cause of aortic aneurysms, which are more often saccular than fusiform. Infectious or "mycotic" aneurysms may arise secondarily from an infection occurring in a pre-existing aneurysm of another etiology. *Staphylococcus, Salmonella,* and *Pseudomonas* species are the most frequent pathogens causing primary aortic infections.[120] Many cases arise as complications of infective endocarditis or arterial catheterization. An intrinsically abnormal aorta, however, may become infected as a consequence of bacteremia. Such infection produces suppurative aortitis, leading to weakness of a portion of the aortic wall. In these cases, aneurysms are typically saccular, yet there is a comparatively high propensity to rupture.

SYPHILITIC AORTITIS

Treponemal infection produces chronic aortitis in approximately 10 percent of patients with untreated tertiary syphilis and is the primary cause of death in about the same proportion of cases, but there is evidence of the process at autopsy in about half of patients who have had untreated syphilis for more than 10 years.[121] During the spirochetemic phase of primary syphilis, *Treponema pallidum* organisms lodge in the adventitia of the vasa vasorum and initiate an inflammatory response characterized by perivascular lymphocytic and plasma cell infiltrate. This is followed by obliterative endarteritis, resulting in patchy medial necrosis, elastic fiber fragmentation, weakening of the aortic wall, and aneurysm formation. The intima of the aorta has a characteristic wrinkled appearance, frequently with superimposed atherosclerotic plaques. Because the infection is seeded through the vasa vasorum, the process is most severe in the ascending aorta and the arch, where the density of these vessels is greatest. Luetic aneurysms are typically saccular and involve the ascending aorta whether or not the transverse and descending portions are also affected. Aortic aneurysms resulting from cardiovascular syphilis follow interruption of the elastic fibers as a result of periaortitis and mesoaortitis, which thicken but weaken the aortic wall. Rupture is the major complication, but the enlarging aneurysm may also compress or erode adjacent structures of the mediastinum. Because the inflammatory process tends to interrupt the medial layer by transverse scars, dissection is distinctly uncommon.

Aortic involvement may be asymptomatic or associated with aortic regurgitation, coronary ostial stenosis, or aortic aneurysm. Asymptomatic aortitis may sometimes be identified by linear calcification of the ascending aorta, evident on chest radiographs. Valvular regurgitation, present in 20 to 30 percent of patients with syphilitic aortitis, is mainly a consequence of aortic root dilatation. Syphilitic coronary ostial stenosis, only a century ago more common than coronary atherosclerosis as a cause of angina pectoris, occurs in 25 to 30 percent of such patients, most of whom also have aortic regurgitation. Myocardial infarction is rare. The least frequent manifestation of syphilitic aortitis is aneurysm formation, which occurs in 5 to 10 percent of affected patients. While the prognosis for patients with uncomplicated syphilitic aortitis is comparable to that of the general population, the outlook is poor when syphilitic aneurysms of the aorta are large enough to produce symptoms. The diagnosis of cardiovascular syphilis may be difficult in patients older than age 50 years, when hypertensive and atherosclerotic disease often coexist.

The frequency of cardiovascular syphilis has fallen dramatically over recent decades as a consequence of early identification and treatment of the disease. Adequate antimicrobial therapy of early syphilis is the most important preventive measure, though whether such treatment retards the progression of disease once aortitis has developed has not been clearly established. Without surgical intervention, symptomatic syphilitic aortic aneurysms are associated with a high mortality rate.

TUBERCULOUS AORTITIS

Tuberculous aneurysms usually result from direct extension of infection from hilar lymph nodes and subsequent granulomatous destruction of the medial layer, leading to loss of aortic wall elasticity. The posterior or posterolateral aortic wall is usually the site of saccular aneurysm formation in these cases. Caseating granulomatous lesions affecting the medial layer of the aortic wall characterize the histology. Pseudoaneurysm formation,[122] perforation, or aortoenteric fistula may result. Infection may occasionally invade the aortic valve ring and adjacent structures, producing a caseating paravalvular abscess. Rupture of tuberculous aortic lesions can occur.

FUTURE PROSPECTS

As the familial nature of aneurysmal diseases becomes familiar to a broader array of physicians, testing of relatives of affected individuals is likely to become standard practice and reimbursable by insurers. Recognizing an aneurysm in advance of symptoms is the optimal method to enhance survival, and family members represent the most cost-effective candidates for diagnostic testing.

Greater knowledge of the pathogenesis of aneurysm formation and rupture at the molecular level will open new avenues for directed drug therapy. Clinical trials with MMP antagonists and drugs that influence the TGF-β pathways are currently in progress. Directed drug development will be feasible when enhanced genetic and proteomic profiling of susceptible individuals leads to better appreciation of exactly how aortic wall proteins are deficient.

More than 100 years ago, Sir William Osler stated that "There is no disease more conducive to clinical humility than aneurysm of the aorta." This is still true today, as aneurysms and dissections remain virulent processes that challenge the skill and experience of physicians and surgeons.

REFERENCES

1. The circulatory system. In: Junqueira LC, Carneiro J, eds. *Basic Histology: Text and Atlas,* 11th ed. McGraw-Hill Access Medicine (electronic format), 2005.
2. Sanz J, Einstein AJ, Fuster V. Acute aortic dissection: anti-impulse therapy. In: Elefteriades J. *Acute Aortic Conditions.* New York: Taylor & Francis; 2007.
3. Glagov S, Wolinsky H. New concepts of the relation of structure to function in the arterial wall. *Proc Inst Med Chicago.* 1968;27:106.
4. Wolinsky H. Glagov S. Comparison of abdominal and thoracic aortic, medial structure in mammals: Deviation of man from the usual pattern. *Circ Res.* 1969;25:677–686.
5. Wolinsky H, Glagov S. A lamellar unit of aortic medial structure and function in mammals. *Circ Res.* 1967;20:99–111.
6. Caro CG. *The Mechanics of the Circulation,* New York: Oxford University Press; 1978.
7. Slater EE, DeSanctis RW, Diseases of the aorta, In: Braunwald E, ed. *Heart Disease,* Philadelphia: Saunders; 1984:1540–1571.
8. Nichols WW, O'Rourke MF. *McDonald's Blood Flow in Arteries: Theoretic, Experimental and Clinical Principles,* 3d ed. Philadelphia: Lea & Febiger; 1990.
9. Avolio AP et al, Effects of aging on changing arterial compliance and left ventricular load in a northern Chinese urban community. *Circulation.* 1983;68:50–58.
10. Becker AE. Medionecrosis aortae. *Pathol Microbiol.* 1975;43:124.

11. Weintraub AM, Gomes MN. Clinical manifestations of abdominal aortic aneurysm and thoracoabdominal aneurysm. In: Lindsay J Jr, Hurst JW, eds. *The Aorta*. New York: Grune & Stratton; 1979:131–168.

12. Crawford ES, Hess KR. Abdominal aortic aneurysm (editorial). *N Engl J Med*. 1989;321:1040–1042.

13. Anagnostopoulos CE. *Acute Aortic Dissections*. Baltimore: University Park Press; 1975.

14. Campbell CD. Aneurysms of the ascending aorta. In: Campbell D, ed. *Aortic Aneurysms: Surgical Therapy*. Mount Kisco, NY: Futura; 1981: 19–46.

15. Becker AE. Medionecrosis aortae. *Pathol Microbiol*. 1975;43:124.

16. Dillon ML, Young WG, Sealy WC. Aneurysms of the descending thoracic aorta. *Ann Thorac Surg*. 1967;3;430–438.

17. Crawford ES, Snyder DM, Cho GC, et al. Progress in treatment of 8 thoracoabdominal and abdominal aortic aneurysms involving celiac, superior mesenteric and renal arteries. *Ann Surg*. 1978: 188:404–421.

18. Crawford ES, Coselli JS. Thoracoabdominal aortic aneurysms. *J Thorac Cardiovasc Surg*. 1991;3:302.

19. Elefteriades JA, Rizzo JA. Epidemiology: incidence, prevalence, trends. In: Elefteriades J. *Acute Aortic Conditions*. New York: Taylor & Francis; 2007.

20. Centers for Disease Control. National Center for Injury Prevention and Control. http://webapp.cdc.gov/cgi-bin/broker.exe.

21. Health Services/Technology Assessment Text (HSTAT). Guide to Clinical Preventative Services, 3rd Ed. Evidence Syntheses, formerly Systematic Evidence Reviews. National Library of Medicine and NCBI. hstat.nlm.nih.gov (accessed 9/24/06).

22. Acosta S, Ogren M, Bengtsson H, Bergqvist D, Lindblad B, Zdanowski Z. Increasing incidence of ruptured abdominal aortic aneurysm: a population-based study. *J Vasc Surg*. 2006;44:237–243.

23. Clouse WWE, Hallett JW Jr., Schaff HV, Gayari MM, Ilstrup DM, Melton LJ 3rd. Improved prognosis of thoracic aortic aneurysms: a population-based study. *JAMA*. 1998;280:1926–1929.

24. Filopvic M, Goldacre MJ, Roberts SE, et al. Trends in mortality and hospital admission rates for abdominal aortic aneurysm in England and Wales. 1979–1999.

25. Marfan AB. Un cas de deformation congenitale des quatre membres, plus prononce des extremites, caracterise par r allongement des coeur avec un certain degre d' amincissement. *Bull Mem Soc Med Hop Paris*. 1896;13:220–226.

26. Milewicz DM, Hariyadarshi P, Avidan N, Guo D, Tran-Fadulu V. The genetic basis of thoracic aortic aneurysms and dissections. In: Elefteriades J. *Acute Aortic Conditions*. New York: Taylor & Francis; 2007.

27. Jondeau G, Delorme G, Guiti C. [Marfan syndrome]. *Rev Prat*. 2002;52:1089–1093.

28. Finkbohner R, Johnston D, Crawford ES, et al. Marfan syndrome: Long-term survival and complications after aortic aneurysm repair. *Circulation*. 1995;91:728–733.

29. Loeys BL, Chen J, Neptune ER, et al. A syndrome of altered cardiovascular, craniofacial, neurocognitive and skeletal development caused by mutations in TGFBR1 or TGFBR2. *Nat Genet*. 2005;37:275–281.

30. Ward C. Clinical significance of the bicuspid aortic valve. *Heart*. 2000;83:81–85.

31. Fedak WM, David TE, Borger M, Verma S, Butany J, Weisel RD. Bicuspid aortic valve disease: recent insights in pathophysiology and treatment. *Expert Rev Cardiovasc Ther*. 2005;3:295–308.

32. Braverman AC, Guven H, Beardslee MA, Makan M, Kates AM, Moon MR. The bicuspid aortic valve. *Curr Probl Cardiol*. 2005;30:470–522.

33. Gleason TG. Heritable disorders predisposing to aortic dissection. *Semin Thorac Cardiovasc Surg*. 2005;17:274–281.

34. Coady MA, Davies RR, Roberts M, et al. Familial patterns of thoracic aortic aneurysms. *Arch Surg*. 1999;134:361–367.

35. Milewicz DM, Hariyadarshi P, Avidan N, Guo D, Tran-Fadulu V. The genetic basis of thoracic aortic aneurysms and dissections. In: Elefteriades J. *Acute Aortic Conditions*. New York: Taylor & Francis; 2007.

36. Milewicz DM, Michael K, Fisher N, Coselli JS, Markello T, Biddinger A. Fibrillin-1 (FBN1) mutations in patients with thoracic aortic aneurysms. *Circulation*. 1996;94:2708–2711.

37. Habashi JP, Judge DP, Holm TM, et al. Losartan, an AT1 antagonist, prevents aortic aneurysm in a mouse model of Marfan syndrome. *Science* 2006. 7;312:117–21.

38. Mao D, Lee JK, VanVickle SJ, Thompson RW. Expression of collagenase-3 (MMP-13) in human abdominal aortic aneurysms and vascular smooth muscle cells in culture. *Biochem Biophys Res Commun*. 1999; 261:904–910.

39. Thompson RW, Parks WC. Role of matrix metalloproteinases in abdominal aortic aneurysms. *Ann NY Acad Sci*. 1996; 800:157–174.

40. Koullias G, Korkolis D, Ravichandran P, Tranquilli M, Kopf G, Elefteriades JA. Increased tissue microarray MMP expression favors proteolysis in thoracic aortic aneurysms and dissections. *Ann Thorac Surg*. 2004;78:2106–2111.

41. Hackmann AE, LeMaire SA, Thompson RW. Long-term suppressive therapy: clinical reality and future prospects. In: Elefteriades J. *Acute Aortic Conditions*. New York: Taylor & Francis; 2007.

42. Schonbeck U, Sukhova GK, Gerdes N, Libby P. T(H)2 predominant immune responses prevail in human abdominal aortic aneurysm. *Am J Pathol* 2002;161:499–506.

43. Tang PC, Yakimov AO, Teesdale MA, et al. Transmural inflammation by interferon-gamma-producing T cells correlates with outward vascular remodeling and intimal expansion of ascending thoracic aortic aneurysms. *Faseb J*. 2005;19:1528–1530.

44. Barrat-Boyes BG. Symptomatology and prognosis of abdominal aortic aneurysm. *Lancet*. 1957;2:716–720.

45. DeSanctis RW, Doroghazi RM, Austen WG. Buckley MJ. Aortic dissection. *N Engl J Med*. 1990;317:1060–1067.

46. Wilson SK, Hutchins GM. Aortic dissecting aneurysms: Causative factors in 204 subjects. *Ann Pathol Lab Med*. 1982;106: 175–180.

47. Perron AD, Gibbs M. Thoracic aortic dissection secondary to crack cocaine ingestion. *Am J Emerg Med*. 1997;12:507–509.

48. Meszaros I, Morocz J, Szlavi J, et al. Epidemiology and clinicopathology of aortic dissection. *Chest*. 2000;117:1271–1278.

49. Sanz J, Einstein AJ, Fuster V. Acute aortic dissection: anti-impulse therapy. In: Elefteriades J. *Acute Aortic Conditions*. New York: Taylor & Francis; 2007.

50. Coady MA, Rizzo JA, Elefteriades JA. Pathologic variants of thoracic aortic dissections. In: Elefteriades JA (Ed.) Diseases of the Aorta. *Cardiol Clin*. 999;17:637–657.

51. Cooke JP, Kazmier FJ, Orszulak. TA. The penetrating aortic ulcer: Pathologic manifestations, diagnosis, and management. *Mayo Clin Proc*.1988;63:718–725.

52. Motoyoshi N, Moizumi Y, Komatsu T, Tabayashi K. Intramural hematoma and dissection involving ascending aorta: the clinical features and prognosis. *Eur J Cardiothorac Surg*. 2003; 24:237–222; discussion: 242.

53. Keren A, Kim CB, Hu BS, et al. Accuracy of biplane and multiplane transesophageal echocardiography in diagnosis of typical acute aortic dissection and intramural hematoma. *J Am Coll Cardiol*. 1996;28:627–636.

54. Cigarroa IE, Isselbacher EM, DeSanctis RW, Eagle KA. Diagnostic imaging in the evaluation of suspected aortic dissection—Old standards and new directions. *N Engl J Med*. 1993; 128:35–43.

55. Coady MA, Rizzo JA, Hammond GL, Kopf GS, Elefteriades JA. Surgical intervention criteria for thoracic aortic aneurysms: a study of growth rates and complications. Ann Thorac Surg. 1999;67:1922–1926.

56. Davies RR, Goldstein LJ, Coady MA, et al. Yearly rupture or dissection rates for thoracic aortic aneurysms: simple prediction based on size. *Ann Thorac Surg*. 2002;73:17–27.

57. Davies RR, Gallo A, Coady MA, et al. Novel measurement of relative aortic size predicts rupture of thoracic aortic aneurysms. *Ann Thorac Surg*. 2006;81:169–177.

58. Powell IT, Greenhalgh RM, Ruckley CV, Fowkes FG. The UK Small Aneurysm Trial. *Ann N Y Acad Sci*. 1996;800:249–251.

59. Lederle FA WS, Johnson GR, Reinke DB, et al. Immediate repair compared with surveillance of small abdominal aortic aneurysms. *N Engl J Med*. 2002;346:1437–1444.

60. Koullias G, Modak R, Tranquilli M, Korkolis DP, Barash P, Elefteriades JA. Mechanical deterioration underlies malignant behavior of aneurysmal human ascending aorta. *J Thorac Cardiovasc Surg*. 2005;130:677–683.

61. Elefteriades JA, Hatzaras I, Tranquilli MA, et al. Weight lifting and rupture of silent aortic aneurysms. *JAMA*. 2003;290:2803.

62. Cooley DA, DeBakey ME. Surgical considerations of intrathoracic aneurysms of the aorta and great vessels. *Ann Surg*. 1952;135:660–680.

63. Shores J, Berger K, et al. Progression of aortic dilatation and the benefit of long term beta blockade in Marfan's syndrome. *N Engl J Med*. 1994;330:1335–1341.

64. Haouzi A, Pelikn P, et al. Are beta blockers beneficial in the Marfan's patients. *Circulation*. 1991;86(Suppl):I–662.

65. Yin FCP, Brin KP, et al. Arterial hemodynamic indexes in Marfan's syndrome. *Circulation*. 1989;79:854.

66. Hackmann AE, LeMaire SA, Thompson RW. Long-term suppressive therapy: clinical reality and future prospects. In: Elefteriades J. *Acute Aortic Conditions*. New York: Taylor & Francis; 2007.

67. Kalyanasundaram A, Elmore JR, Manazer JR, et al. Simvastatin suppresses experimental aortic aneurysm expansion. *J Vasc Surg*. 2006;43:117–124.

68. Cipollone F, Prontera C, Pini B, et al. Overexpression of functionally coupled cyclooxygenase-2 and prostaglandin E synthase in symptomatic atherosclerotic plaques as a basis of prostaglandin E(2)-dependent plaque instability. *Circulation*. 2001;104:92–107.

69. Wheat MW, Jr., Palmer RF. Drug therapy for dissecting aneurysms. *Dis Chest*. 1968;54:62–67.

70. Wheat MW Jr, Palmer RF, Bartley TD, et al. Treatment of dissecting aneurysms of the aorta without surgery. *J Thorac Cardiovasc Surg*. 1965;50:364–373.

71. Elefteriades JA. What operation for acute Type A dissection? *J Thorac Cardiovasc Surg*. 2002;123:201–203.

72. Elefteriades JA, Hartleroad J, Gusberg RJ, et al. Long-term experience with descending aortic dissection: The complication-specific approach. *Ann Thorac Surg*. 1992;53:11–21.

73. Yacoub MH, Gehle P, Chandrasekaran V, Birks EJ, Child A, Radley-Smith R. Late results of a valve-sparing operation in patients with aneurysms of the ascending aorta and root. J Thorac Cardiovasc Surg. 1998.

74. David TE, Ivanov J, Armstrong S, Feindel CM, Webb GD. Aortic valve-sparing operations in patients with aneurysms of the aortic root or ascending aorta. Ann Thorac Surg. 2002;74:S1758–S1761.

75. Hilgenberg AD. Spinal cord protection for thoracic aortic surgery. In: Elefteriades JA (Ed.) Diseases of the Aorta. *Cardiol Clin*. 1999;17:i–850.

76. Elefteriades JA, Coady MA, Nikas DJ, Kopf GS, Gusberg RJ. "Cobrahead" graft for intercostal artery implantation during descending aortic replacement. *Ann Thorac Surg*. 2000;69:1282–1284.

77. Hertzer NR, et al. Coronary artery disease in peripheral vascular patients. *Ann Surg*. 1984;199:223–233.

78. Tomatis LA, Fierens EE, Verbrugge GP. Evaluation of surgical risk in peripheral vascular disease by coronary arteriography: A series of 100 cases. *Surgery*. 1972;71:429–435.

79. McCollum CH, et al. Myocardial revascularization prior to subsequent major surgery in patients with coronary artery disease. *Surgery*. 1977;81:302–304.

80. Parodi JC, Palamz JC, Barone HD. Transfemoral intraluminal graft implantation for abdominal aortic aneurysms. *Ann Vasc Surg*. 1991;5:491–499.

81. Veith FJ, Gargiulo NJ, Ohki T. Endovascular treatment of ruptured infrarenal aortic and iliac aneurysms. *Acta Chir Belg*. 2003;103:555–562.

82. Brinster DR, Szeto WY, Bavaria JE. Endovascular thoracic aortic stent grafting in acute aortic catastrophes. In: Elefteriades JA (Ed.) Diseases of the Aorta. *Cardiol Clin*. 1999;17:i–850.

83. Tehrani HY, Peterson BG, Katariya K, et al. Endovascular repair of thoracic aortic tears. *Ann Thorac Surg*. 2006;82:873–877.

84. Kaya A, Heijmen RH, Overtoom TT, et al. Thoracic stent grafting for acute aortic pathology. *Ann Thorac Surg*. 2006;82:560–565.

85. Veith FJ, Johnston KW. Endovascular treatment of abdominal aortic aneurysms: An innovation in evolution and under evaluation. *J Vasc Surg*. 2002;35:183.

86. Sapirstein W, Chandeysson P, Wentz C. The Food and Drug Administration approval of endovascular grafts for abdominal aortic aneurysm: An 18-month retrospective. *J Vasc Surg*. 2001;34:180–183.

87. Elefteriades JA. "Endograft therapy of thoracic aneurysms: wave of the future, or the emperor's new clothes." *J Thorac Cardiovasc Surg*. In press.

88. Peppelenbosch N, Buth J, Harris PL, et al. Diameter of abdominal aortic aneurysm and outcome of endovascular aneurysm repair: Does size matter? A report from EUROSTAR. *J Vasc Surg*. 2004;39:288–297.

89. Laheij RJ, Buth J, Harris PL, Moll FL, Stelter WJ, Verhoeven EL. Need for secondary interventions after endovascular repair of abdominal aortic aneurysm. Intermediate-term follow-up results of a European collaborative registry (EUROSTAR). *Br J Surg*. 2000;87:1666–1673.

90. Hobo R, Roth J, and the EUROSTAR investigators. Secondary interventions following endovascular abdominal aortic aneurysm repair using current endografts. A EUROSTAR report. J VascSurg. 2006;43:896–902.

91. Leurs LJ, Bell R, Degrieck Y, et al. Endovascular treatment of thoracic aortic diseases: Combined experience from the EUROSTAR and United Kingdom Thoracic Endograft registries. *J Vasc Surg*. 2004;40:670–680.

92. Khatibzadeh M, Mitusch R, Stierle U, et al. Aortic atherosclerotic plaques as a source of systemic embolism. *J Am Coll Cardiol*. 1996;27:664–669.

93. Ramirez G, O'Neill WM Jr, et al. Cholesterol embolization: A complication of angiography. *Arch Intern Med*. 1978;138:1430–1432.

94. Hyman BT, Landas SK, Ashman RF. Warfarin-related purple toes syndrome and cholesterol microembolization. *Am J Med*. 1987;82:1233–1237.

95. Bruns FJ, Segel DP, Adler S. Control of cholesterol embolization by discontinuation of anticoagulant therapy. *Am J Med Sci*. 1978;275:105–108.

96. Eggebrecht H, Oldenburg O, Dirsch O, et al. Potential embolization by atherosclerotic debris dislodged from aortic wall during cardiac catheterization: Histologic and clinical findings in 7621 patients. *Catheter Cardiovasc Interv*. 2000;49:389–394.

97. Pennington M, Yeager J, Skelton J, Smith KJ. Cholesterol embolization syndrome: Cutaneous histopathological features and the variable onset of symptoms in patients with different risk factors. *Br J Dermatol*. 2002;146:511–517.

98. Fine MJ, Kapoor WN, Falanga V. Cholesterol crystal embolization: A review of 221 cases in the English language. *Angiology*. 1987;38:769–784.

99. Scolari F, Tardanico R, Zani R, et al. Cholesterol crystal embolism: A recognizable cause of renal disease. *Am J Kidney Dis*. 2000;36:1089–1109.

100. Fine MJ, Kapoor WN, Falanga V. Cholesterol crystal embolization: A review of 221 cases in the English language. *Angiology*. 1987;38:769–784.

101. The French Study of Aortic Plaques in Stroke Group. Atherosclerotic disease of the aortic arch as a risk factor for recurrent ischemic stroke. *N Engl J Med*. 1996;334:1216–1221.

102. Pitt B, Waters D, Brown WV, et al. Aggressive lipid-lowering therapy compared with angioplasty in stable coronary artery disease. *N Engl J Med*. 1999;341:70–76.

103. Cohen AP. Atherosclerosis of the thoracic aorta: From risk stratification to treatment. *Am J Cardiol*. 2002;90:1333–1335.

104. Brewster DC. Clinical and anatomical considerations for surgery in aortoiliac disease and results of surgical treatment. *Circulation*. 1991;83(suppl 1):1-42–1-52.

105. Debakey ME, Lawrie GM, Glaeser DH. Patterns of atherosclerosis and their surgical significance. *Ann Surg*. 1985;201:115–131.

106. Leriche R, Morel A. The syndrome of thrombotic obliteration of the aortic bifurcation. *Ann Surg*. 1948;127:193–204.

107. Diethrich EB. Endovascular treatment of abdominal aortic occlusive disease: the impact of stents and intravascular ultrasound imaging. *Eur J Vasc Surg*. 1993;7:228–236.

108. Johnston KW. Balloon angioplasty: Predictive factors for long-term success. *Semin Vasc Surg*. 1989;3:117–122.

109. Sullivan TM, Childs MB, Bacharach JM, et al. Percutaneous transluminal angioplasty and primary stenting of the iliac arteries in 288 patients. *J Vasc Surg*. 1997;25:829–839.

110. Busuttil RW, Keehn G, Milliken J, et al. Aortic saddle embolus: A twenty-year experience. *Ann Surg*. 1983;197:698–706.

111. Ito I. Aortitis syndrome (Takayasu's arteritis): A review. *Jpn Heart J*. 1995;36:273–281.

112. Kerr GS, Hallahan CW, Giordano J, et al. Takayasu arteritis. *Ann Intern Med*. 1994;120:919–929.

113. Tavora F, Burke A. Review of isolated ascending aortitis: differential diagnosis, including syphilitic, Takayasu's and giant cell aortitis. *Pathology*. 2006;38:302–308.

114. Wolak T, Szendro G, Goleman L, Paran E. Malignant hypertension as a presenting symptom of Takayasu arteritis. *Mayo Clin Proc*. 2003;78:231–236.

115. Arend WP, Michel BA, Bloch DA, et al. The American College of Rheumatology 1990 criteria for the classification of Takayasu arteritis. *Arthritis Rheum*. 1990;33:1129–1134.

116. Evans JM, O'Fallon WM, Hunder GG. Increased incidence of aortic aneurysm and dissection in giant cell (temporal) arteritis. *Ann Intern Med*. 1995;122:502–507.

117. Jover JA, Hernandez-Garcia C, Morado IC, et al. Combined treatment of giant-cell arteritis with methotrexate and prednisolone. A randomized, double-blind, placebo-controlled trial. *Ann Intern Med*. 2002;46:1309–1318.

118. Hoffman GS, Cid MC, Hellmann DB, et al. A multicenter randomized double blind, placebo-controlled trial of adjuvant methotrexate treatment for giant cell arteritis. *Arthritis Rheum*. 2002;46:1309–1318.

119. Roldan CA, Chavez J, Wiest PW, et al. Aortic root disease and valve disease associated with ankylosing spondylitis. *J Am Coll*. 1998;32:1397–1404.

120. Takagi H, Kato T, Matsuno Y, et al. Aortic dissection without Marfan's syndrome in ankylosing spondylitis. *J Thorac Cardiovasc Surg*. 2004;127:600–602.

121. Jackman JD, Radolf JD. Cardiovascular syphilis. *Am J Med*. 1989;87:425–433.

122. Hagino RT, Clagett GP, Valentine RJ. A case of Pott's disease of the spine eroding into the suprarenal aorta. *J Vasc Surg*. 1996;24:482–486.

CHAPTER (106)

Cerebrovascular Disease and Neurologic Manifestations of Heart Disease

Megan C. Leary / Louis R. Caplan

Many vascular diseases affect both the heart and the brain. Heart diseases often lead to lesions and dysfunction within the brain, and central nervous system (CNS) diseases can influence the heart and its function.

BRAIN AND CEREBROVASCULAR COMPLICATIONS OF HEART DISEASE

Stroke is a common and devastating disease, the third leading cause of death and the leading cause of disability in the United States. Cardiogenic stroke can occur when (1) the heart pumps unwanted materials into the circulation that reach the brain (embolism), (2) pump function fails and the brain is hypoperfused, and (3) drugs given to treat cardiac disease have neurologic side effects.

【 】 DIRECT CARDIOGENIC BRAIN EMBOLISM
Etiology

Diagnostic criteria for cardiogenic embolism were formerly very restrictive. Previously, embolism was diagnosed when sudden focal neurologic signs, maximal at onset, developed in patients with peripheral systemic embolism and recent myocardial infarction (MI) or rheumatic mitral stenosis.[1] Using these criteria, cardioembolic infarcts were diagnosed in only 3 to 8 percent of stroke patients.[2–5] In various stroke registries, however, approximately 10 to 20 percent of patients diagnosed with cardioembolic strokes did not have maximal symptoms at onset.[5–7] Additionally, certain cardiac arrhythmias are now well-accepted sources of embolic stroke. Lastly, only about 2 percent of patients with cardiogenic brain embolism have clinically recognized peripheral emboli. Although necropsy studies of patients with brain embolism note that infarcts are commonly found in the spleen and kidneys and other organs, the symptoms of peripheral embolism are often so minor and nonspecific (transient abdominal discomfort, leg cramp, etc.) that they are seldom diagnosed correctly.

Cardiogenic cerebral embolism is responsible for approximately 20 percent of ischemic strokes.[7–11] However, because many patients have coexisting cardiac and extracranial vascular disease,[11] criteria for the diagnosis of cardiac embolism remain controversial even today. As more advanced diagnostic techniques have been developed, more causative cardiac abnormalities (and their association with stroke) have been recognized. Cardiac sources of brain emboli can be divided into three groups[1]:

1. *Cardiac wall and chamber abnormalities*: cardiomyopathies, hypokinetic and akinetic ventricular regions after MI, atrial septal aneurysms, ventricular aneurysms, atrial myxomas, papillary fibroelastomas and other tumors, septal defects, and patent foramen ovale
2. *Valve disorders*: rheumatic mitral and aortic disease, prosthetic valves, bacterial endocarditis, fibrous and fibrinous endocardial lesions, mitral valve prolapse, and mitral annulus calcification
3. *Arrhythmias*: especially atrial fibrillation (AF) and *sick-sinus* syndrome

Some cardiac sources have much higher rates of initial and recurrent embolism. The Stroke Data Bank[12] divided potential sources into *strong sources* (prosthetic valves, AF, sick-sinus syndrome, ventricular aneurysm, akinetic segments, mural thrombi, cardiomyopathy, and diffuse ventricular hypokinesia) and *weak sources* (myocardial infarct more than 6 months old, aortic and mitral stenosis and regurgitation, congestive failure, mitral valve prolapse, mitral annulus calcification, and hypokinetic ventricular segments). The risk of embolism varies within individual cardiac abnormalities depending on many factors. For example, in patients with AF, associated heart disease, patient age, duration, chronic versus intermittent fibrillation, and atrial size all influence embolic risk. The presence of a potential cardiac source of embolism does not mean that a stroke was caused by an embolus from the heart. Coexistent occlusive cerebrovascular disease is common. In the Lausanne Stroke Registry, among patients with potential cardiac embolic sources, 11 percent of patients had severe cervicocranial vascular occlusive disease (>75 percent stenosis) and 40 percent had mild to moderate stenosis proximal to brain infarcts.[11]

Atrial Fibrillation Persistent and paroxysmal AF is a potent predictor of first and recurrent stroke, with >75,000 attributed cases annually. In patients with brain emboli caused by a cardiac source, there is a history of nonvalvular AF in roughly one half of all cases, of left ventricular thrombus in almost one third, and of valvular heart disease in one fourth.[7,13]

Intracavitary Thrombus Intracavitary thrombus caused by acute MI occurs in an estimated one third of patients within the first 2 weeks after anterior MI and in an even greater proportion of those with large left ventricular apex infarcts.[8,13] Ventricular thrombi can also occur in patients with chronic ventricular dysfunction caused by coronary disease, hypertension, and dilated cardiomyopathy. Stroke is less common among uncomplicated MI patients but can occur in up to 12 percent of patients with acute MI complicated by a left ventricular thrombus. The rate of stroke is higher in patients with anterior rather than inferior infarcts and may reach up to 20 percent in those with large anteroseptal MI. The incidence of embolism is highest during the period of active thrombus formation in the first 1 to 3 months, with substantial risk remaining even beyond the acute phase in patients with persistent myocardial dysfunction, congestive heart failure, or AF.[13,14]

Congestive Heart Failure Congestive heart failure affects >4 million Americans and increases stroke risk by a factor of 2 to 3, accounting for an estimated 10 percent of ischemic strokes.[9,13] In patients with nonischemic dilated cardiomyopathy, the rate of stroke is similar to that of cardiomyopathy caused by ischemic heart disease. An estimated 72,000 initial strokes annually are associated with left ventricular systolic dysfunction, and the 5-year recurrent stroke rate in patients with cardiac failure has been reported as high as 45 percent.[13,15]

Valvular Heart Disease

Rheumatic Mitral Valve Disease Recurrent embolism occurs in 30 to 60 percent of patients with rheumatic mitral valve disease and a history of a previous embolic event.[13,16–19] Between 60 and 65 percent of these recurrences develop the first year, many within the first 6 months.[13,16,17] Mitral valvuloplasty does not appear to eliminate the risk of embolism.[13,20,21]

Mitral Valve Prolapse Mitral valve prolapse (MVP) is the most common form of valve disease in adults and is generally benign.[22,23] MVP as a source of embolic stroke continues to be controversial.[1] Several small clinical series have reported cerebral embolism in MVP patients who lacked other possible embolic sources.[24–27] Patients with MVP also may have other disorders such as AF, syncope, and migraine. The rate of recurrent stroke in patients with MVP as the only known cause is very low.[26,27] Given the very high incidence of MVP, the frequency of MVP-related stroke is extremely low.[27]

Mitral Annulus Calcification Mitral annulus calcification (MAC) is an important, often unrecognized cause of embolism. Several series show a convincing relation between MAC and brain emboli and stroke.[1,28–30] Bacterial endocarditis can also develop on the MAC. Anticoagulation does not prevent calcific emboli. The decision to use antiplatelet agents versus anticoagulants should include consideration of other potential comorbid factors such as AF, which can occur 12 times more often in patients with MAC than it would in those without MAC.[23,31]

Aortic Valve Disease Aortic valve disease, in isolation, is not often associated with systemic embolism. Although there are isolated case reports of patients who had strokes from spontaneous aortic valve calcific emboli, few trials of selected patients with stroke and aortic valve disease exist at present.[13,32] One prospective analysis of 815 patients with calcification of the aortic valve (with or without stenosis) did not show any association between either of the two aortic valvular lesions and stroke.[33] Current treatment recommendations in these cases are based on larger antiplatelet trials of stroke and transient ischemic attack (TIA) patients.[13]

More patients may have cardiogenic embolism than are now diagnosed. Clinical features and brain investigations such as CT, MRI, and angiography (CT, magnetic resonance [MR], and digital subtraction angiography) may suggest emboli; but often a clear source is unidentified. These cases, which are termed *infarcts of unknown causes* in the Stroke Data Bank,[6,34,35] include as many as 40 percent of patients.

Fibrous and fibrinous lesions of the heart valves and endocardium are associated with certain medical conditions.[1] Valve lesions occur in patients with systemic lupus erythematosus (Libman-Sacks endocarditis[36]), antiphospholipid antibody syndrome,[37] and cancer and other debilitating diseases (nonbacterial thrombotic endocarditis). Mobile fibrous strands are also often found during echocardiography.[1,38–40] Fibrin-platelet aggregates may attach to these fibrous and fibrinous lesions.

Embolic complications are common in patients who have *infective endocarditis*.[1,41] Mycotic aneurysms can cause fatal subarachnoid bleeding. Bleeding can also result from vascular necrosis as a result of an infected embolus.[41] Embolization usually stops when infection is controlled.[38] Warfarin does not prevent embolization and is probably contraindicated unless there are other important lesions such as prosthetic valves or life-threatening pulmonary embolism. In children and young adults with congenital heart defects, especially those with right-to-left shunts and polycythemia, brain abscess is an important complication.

Emboli often arise from sources other than the heart, such as the *aorta, proximal arteries (intraarterial or so-called* local embolism*), leg veins (paradoxical emboli), fat in the liver or bones (fat embolism), and materials* introduced by the patient or physician (drug particles or air).[1] The types of embolic material also vary (Table 106–1).[1,42] *Atheromatous plaques in the aortic arch and ascending* aorta are an important and previously neglected source of embolism to the brain (Fig. 106–1 and Fig. 106–2). Ulcerated atheromatous plaques are often found at necropsy in patients with ischemic strokes, especially in those in whom the stroke etiology was not determined during life.[43] Transesophageal echocardiography (TEE) often shows these atheromas, but technical factors limit visualization of the entire arch.[44] Large (>4 mm), protruding mobile aortic atheromas are especially likely to cause embolic strokes and are associated with a high rate of recurrent strokes.[45,46] Use of oral anticoagulants rather than antiplatelet agents is recommended in these patients.[23,47,48]

Clinical Onset and Course

Warning signs of stroke can include sudden hemiparesis, hemisensory loss, confusion, trouble speaking or understanding, visual loss, diplopia, ataxia, vertigo, or sudden severe headache with no known cause. Most embolic events occur during activities of daily living but some embolic strokes have their onset during rest or sleep. Sudden coughing, sneezing, or arising at night to urinate can precipitate embolism.[1,5] Although the deficit is most often maximal at outset, 11 percent of embolic stroke patients in the Harvard Stroke

Registry had a stuttering or stepwise course, whereas 10 percent had fluctuations or progressive deficits. Later progression, if it occurs, is usually within the first 48 hours. Progression is usually caused by distal passage of emboli. *Nonsudden* embolism is explained by an embolus moving from its initial location, as demonstrated by angiography, to a more distal branch.[1,49] Early angiography has a very high rate of showing intracranial emboli,[6,50] but angiography after 48 hours shows a much lower rate of blockage. More recently, transcranial Doppler (TCD) sonography has shown a high incidence of middle cerebral artery (MCA) blockage acutely in patients with sudden-onset hemispheric strokes; but later, recanalization of the MCA and normalization of the intracranial blood velocities occur.[1,51] As in all large infarcts, brain edema and swelling may develop during the 24 to 72 hours after stroke with headache, decreased alertness, and worsening of neurologic signs. The edema is often cytotoxic (inside cells) and usually does not respond to corticosteroid treatment.

Diagnostic Testing

Emboli usually cause occlusion of distal branches and produce surface infarcts that are roughly triangular, with the apex of the tri-

TABLE 106–1

Embolic Materials

CARDIAC	INTRAARTERIAL
1. Red fibrin-dependent thrombi	1. Red fibrin-dependent thrombi
2. White platelet-fibrin nidi	2. White platelet-fibrin nidi
3. Material from marantic endocarditis	3. Combined fibrin-platelet and fibrin-dependent clots
4. Bacteria from vegetations	4. Cholesterol crystals
5. Calcium from valves and mitral annulus calcification	5. Atheromatous plaque debris
6. Myxoma cells and debris	6. Calcium from vascular calcifications
	7. Air
	8. Mucin from tumors
	9. Talc or microcrystalline cellulose from injected drugs

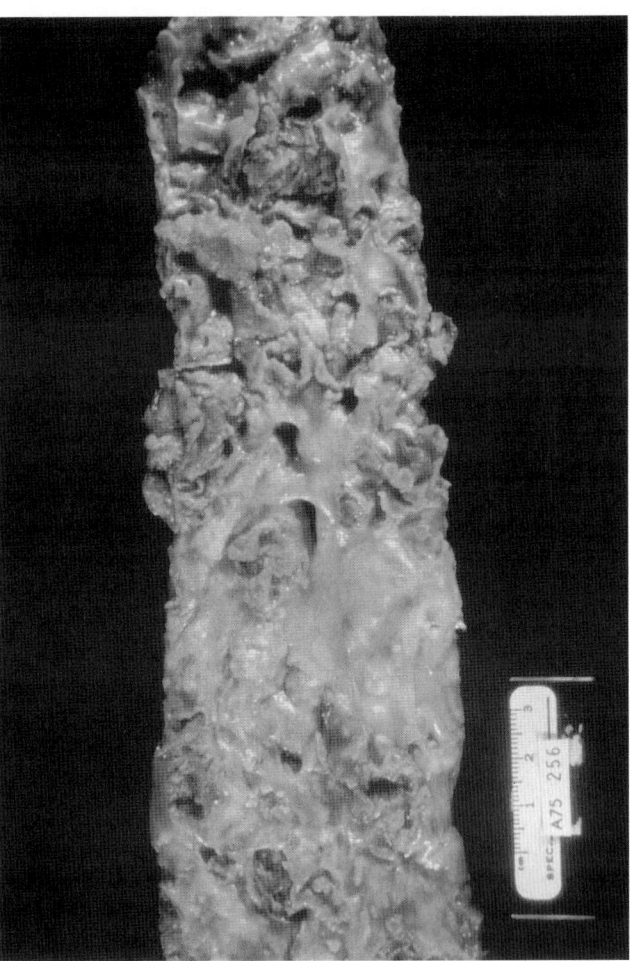

FIGURE 106–1. Descending aorta at necropsy from a patient whose transesophageal echocardiography before surgery showed severe disease of the ascending aorta and aortic arch with mobile protruding plaques. This patient died after coronary artery bypass grafting surgery having never awakened after the procedure. Submitted by Denise Barbut. *Source: From Caplan LR.[5] With permission.*

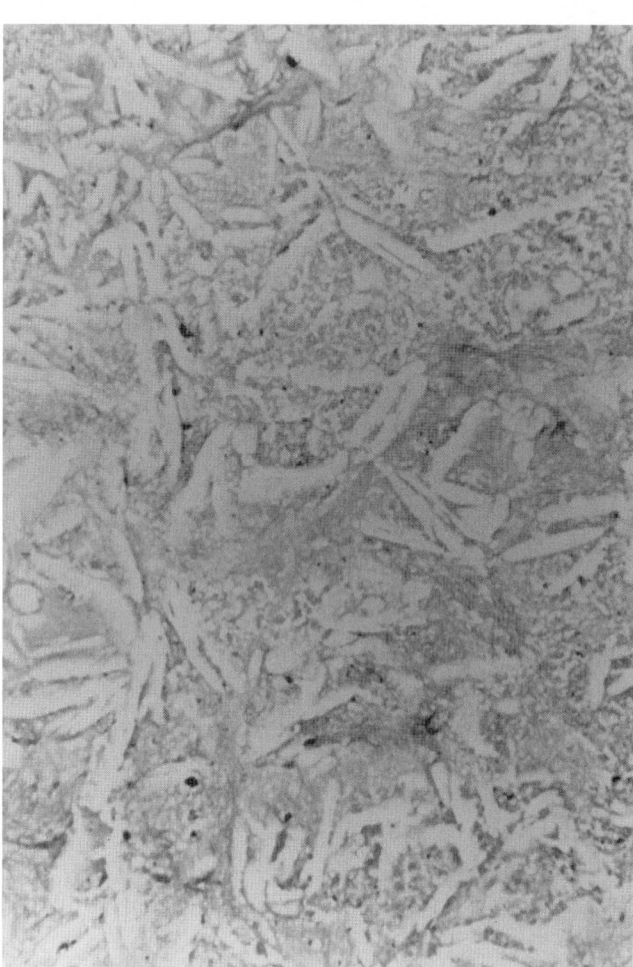

FIGURE 106–2. Cholesterol crystals and other particulate debris are caught in a filter placed in the aorta at the time that aortic clamps are removed. Submitted by Denise Barbut. *Source: From Caplan LR.[5] With permission.*

angle pointing inward. CT and MRI findings can suggest the presence of embolism by the location and shape of the lesion,[52] presence of superficial wedge-shaped infarcts in multiple different vascular territories, and hemorrhagic infarction, as well as visualization of thrombi within arteries. Among 60 patients with cardiogenic sources of embolism studied by CT in whom occlusive atherosclerotic cerebrovascular disease had been excluded, 56 had superficial large or small cortical or subcortical infarcts and only 4 had deep infarcts.[52] Emboli can block the MCA and occasionally cause solely deep infarcts because the superficial territory has good collateral flow; these infarcts are called *striatocapsular* because they involve the internal capsule and the adjacent basal ganglia, which are supplied by lenticulostriate branches of the MCA.[1,5,53] Tiny emboli may cause small deep or superficial infarcts.

MRI, particularly with the use of MR diffusion-weighted and MR gradient recall echo (GRE) imaging, is more sensitive for detection of acute brain infarcts than is CT and is also superior in detecting hemorrhagic infarction by imaging hemosiderin. Hemorrhagic infarction has long been considered characteristic of embolism, especially when the artery leading to the infarct is patent.[54] The mechanism of hemorrhagic infarction is reperfusion of ischemic zones, which occurs with spontaneous passage of the embolus, after iatrogenic opening of an occluded artery (e.g., endar-

terectomy, fibrinolytic treatment), or after restoration of the circulation after a period of systemic hypoperfusion. Hemorrhage occurs into proximal reperfused regions of brain infarcts.[1,5,55] At times, it is also possible to image the acute embolus on CT.[1,56,57]

In unselected series of stroke patients, transthoracic echocardiography (TTE) has been variably useful in detecting sources.[1,58–60] TTE is useful in patients with known cardiac disease to clarify potential embolic sources and heart function,[5] in young patients without stroke risk factors, and in stroke patients who do not have lacunar infarction or ultrasound evidence of intrinsic atherostenosis of a major extracranial and intracranial artery. Transesophageal echocardiography (TEE) provides much better visualization of the aorta, atria, cardiac valves, and septal regions. Reports of TEE suggest that the diagnostic yield is 2 to 10 times that of TTE.[61–64] Aortic plaques, atrial septal aneurysms, and atrial septal defects are also much better seen with TEE (Fig. 106–3). The use of an echo-enhancing agent such as agitated saline helps detect intracardiac shunts.

Echocardiography has definite limitations. Particles the size of 2 mm can block major brain arteries but are beyond the imaging resolution of current echocardiographic technology.[65] Also, thromboembolism is a dynamic process. When a clot forms in the heart and embolizes, there may be no residual evidence until a clot reforms.[1,42] Cardiac thrombi are imaged differently on sequential echocardiograms[1,66]; even large thrombi seen on one echocardiogram can disappear later.[66] Platelet scintigraphy using platelets labeled with radionuclides may be helpful in localizing cardiac and intraarterial sources, but its sensitivity and specificity are undefined.[67]

Cerebral embolic signals are now detected by monitoring with TCD.[1,68,69] Embolic particles passing under TCD probes produce transient, short-duration, high-intensity signals referred to as HITSs (high-intensity transient signals). Examples of HITSs are shown in Fig. 106–4 and Fig. 106–5. TCD monitoring of patients with AF,[70] cardiac surgery,[71] prosthetic valves, left ventricular assist devices,[72] carotid artery disease, and carotid endarterectomy have shown a relatively high frequency of embolic signals. Monitoring of emboli with TCD may help guide treatment decisions.

Prevention and Treatment

Early studies showed that warfarin was effective in preventing brain embolism in patients with both rheumatic mitral stenosis and AF. Previously, the intensity of anticoagulation was higher than that currently used, and brain hemorrhages and other bleeding complications were common. Trials have now shown that low-dose warfarin (international normalized ratio [INR] 2.0–3.0) is also effective in preventing brain emboli in patients with nonrheumatic AF.

In the Copenhagen Atrial Fibrillation, Aspirin, Anticoagulation (AFASAK) study, 1007 patients (median age 74.2 years) with chronic, nonrheumatic AF were assigned to warfarin (INR 2.8–4.2), aspirin (75 mg/d), or placebo.[73] The study was halted prematurely when analysis of effectiveness reached a predetermined level of significance in favor of warfarin treatment. The principal outcome was the composite of ischemic or hemorrhagic stroke, TIA, and systemic embolism. The observed reduction for warfarin compared to placebo was 64 percent, an absolute risk reduction of 3.5 percent per year. An analysis by intention to treat, which excluded

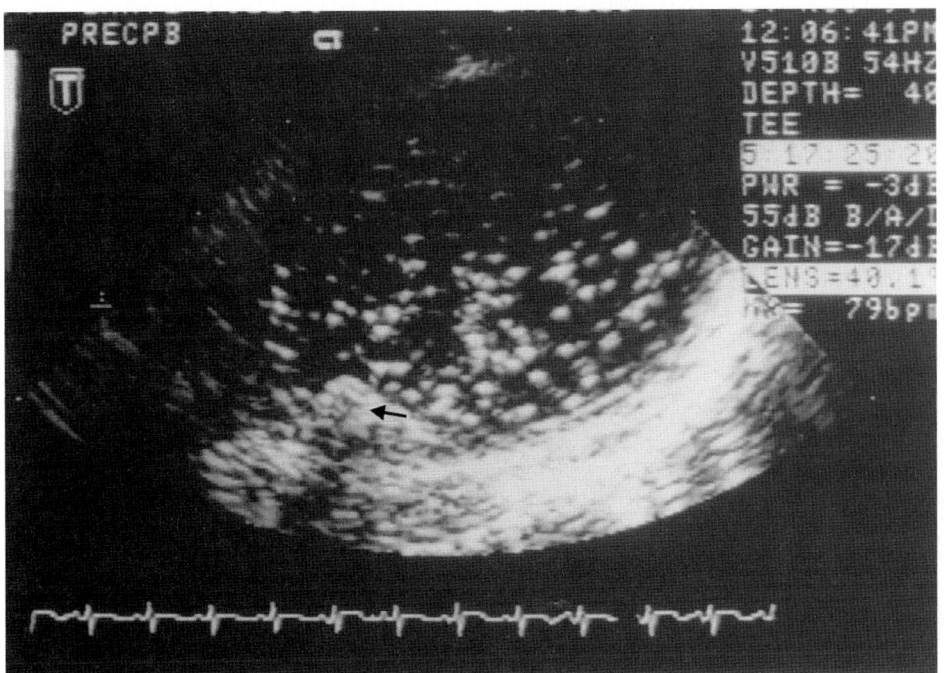

FIGURE 106–3. Transesophageal echocardiography recording during cardiac surgery from the aorta at the level of the origin of the left subclavian artery. A mobile plaque is seen protruding into the aortic lumen (*small black arrow*). This recording was taken after the release of aortic clamps and shows a *shower* of emboli within the aortic lumen beyond where the aorta was previously clamped. Submitted by Denise Barbut. *Source: From Caplan LR.⁵ With permission.*

TIA and minor stroke, indicated a risk reduction of about 50 percent (*p* < 0.05) and an absolute reduction of about 1.5 percent per year.

The Stroke Prevention in Atrial Fibrillation (SPAF) study investigators evaluated warfarin and aspirin in patients with nonrheumatic AF.[74,75] The study evaluated two groups of patients on the basis of their eligibility for warfarin. In the first group, 627 patients judged eligible for warfarin were randomized to open label warfarin (INR 2.8–4.5; prothrombin time [PT], 1.3–1.8 times control) or, in a double-blinded fashion, to either aspirin (325 mg daily, enteric coated) or a matching placebo. In the second group, 703 patients ineligible for warfarin were randomized (double blind) to aspirin (325 mg daily, enteric coated) or placebo. The principal outcome, a composite of ischemic stroke and systemic embolism, was significantly decreased during a mean follow up of 1.3 years. The outcome of disabling ischemic stroke or vascular death was reduced by warfarin by 54 percent (*p* = 0.11), an absolute reduction of 2.6 percent per year. The outcome of disabling stroke or death was reduced 22 percent by aspirin (*p* = 0.33), an absolute reduction of about 1 percent per year. The SPAF investigators later compared low-intensity, fixed-dose war-

farin (INR 1.2–1.5) plus aspirin (325 mg/d) with adjusted-dose warfarin (INR 2.0–3.0) in elderly patients with one or more risk factors for embolism.[76] Ischemic stroke and systemic embolism were present in 7.9 percent of patients on fixed-dose warfarin plus aspirin versus only 1.9 percent on adjusted-dose warfarin. SPAF investigators later studied the effectiveness of 325 mg aspirin in patients with low risk and found that the rate of ischemic stroke was low (2 percent per year).[77]

The SPAF study identified three risk factors for thromboembolism: 1) recent congestive heart failure, 2) history of hypertension, and 3) previous thromboembolism[78,79]; and it suggested that anticoagulation with warfarin was not indicated in patients with none of the three risk factors who were at low risk for thromboembolism (2.5 percent per year). In such patients the dangers of anticoagulant therapy may outweigh its benefits. Aspirin (325 mg daily) is probably reasonable and safe therapy for patients with lone, nonrheumatic AF who are younger than 60 years of age and have none of the three identified risk factors.[78–80] In all other patients with AF, long-term oral warfarin therapy (INR 2.0–3.0) should be used unless contraindicated.[77,80,81]

In the Boston Area Anticoagulation Trial for Atrial Fibrillation (BAATAF), 420 patients with nonrheumatic AF, mean age 68

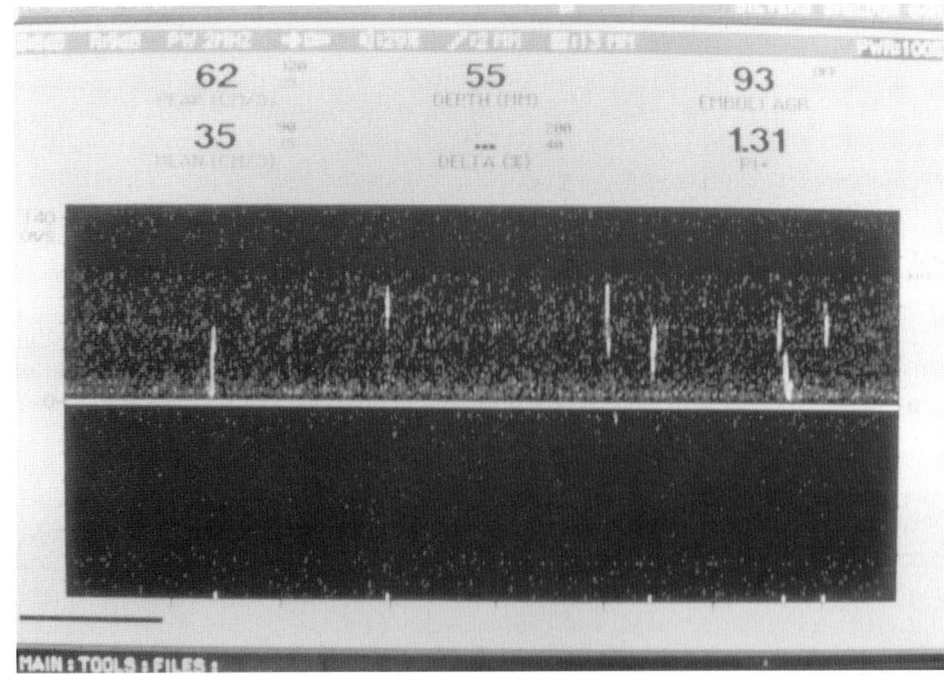

FIGURE 106–4. Transcranial Doppler recording from the middle cerebral arteries during steady-state cardiac bypass surgery at a time when the aorta was manipulated. The white streaks represent microemboli. Submitted by Denise Barbut. *Source: From Caplan LR.⁵ With permission.*

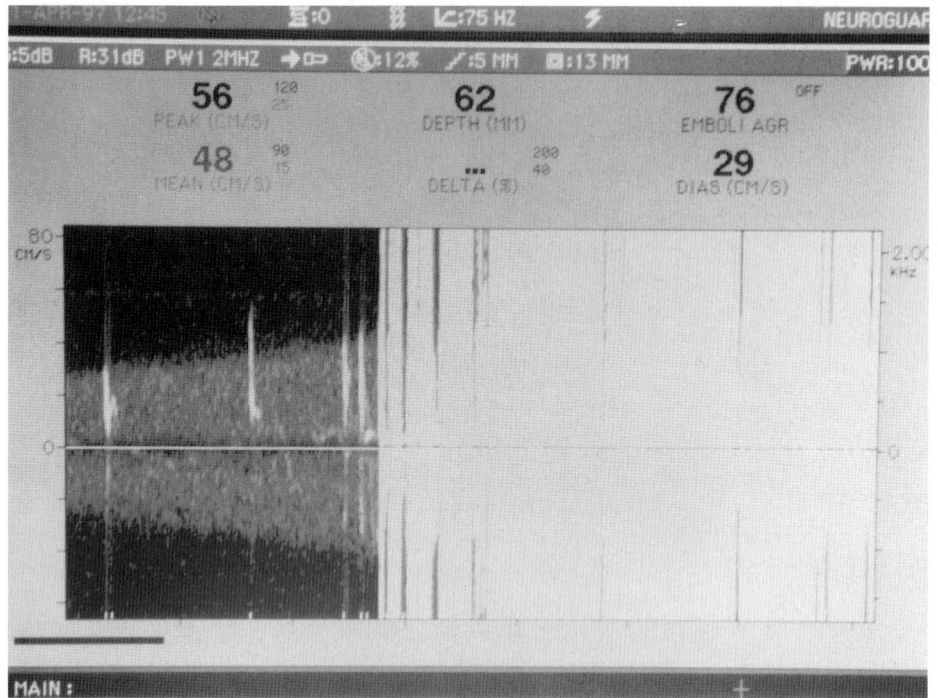

FIGURE 106–5. Transcranial Doppler recording from the middle cerebral arteries during cardiac bypass surgery. A few distinct emboli (*white streaks* in the left of the figure) are followed by a massive shower of emboli (*whiteout*) at the time of the release of aortic clamps. Submitted by Denise Barbut. *Source: From Caplan LR.[5] With permission.*

years, were randomized unblinded to warfarin (target PT ratio, 1.2:1.5 × control; INR 1.5–2.7) or to a control group who were allowed to take aspirin.[82] The principal outcome was ischemic stroke or systemic embolism, and the mean follow up was 2.2 years. The incidence of stroke was reduced by 86 percent in the warfarin group compared to control ($p = .002$), equivalent to an absolute risk reduction of 2.6 percent per year. There was no demonstrable benefit of aspirin, but the study was not designed to test aspirin.

In the Canadian Atrial Fibrillation Anticoagulation (CAFA) study, 187 patients were randomized to warfarin (INR target range 2.0–3.0) and 191 to placebo.[83] The principal outcome was the composite of nonlacunar stroke, non-CNS embolism, and fatal or intracranial hemorrhage. The relative risk reduction for warfarin was 37 percent ($p = .17$). The study was ended prematurely when the results of the Copenhagen AFASAK and SPAF studies became known.

The European Atrial Fibrillation Trial (EAFT) Study Group addressed the question of the optimal level of anticoagulation by reviewing the results of their own trial.[84] No treatment effect was found with anticoagulation responses less than INRs of 2.0. The rate of thromboembolic events was lowest at INRs from 2 to 3.9; most major hemorrhages occurred at INRs of 5.0 and above. The EAFT group recommended a target of 3.0 with a range from 2 to 5.0.[84] Fixed-dose warfarin with a target of 1.3 to 1.5 was not as effective as standard adjusted-dose warfarin at an average INR of 2.4, even when aspirin 325 mg/d was added to the low fixed-dose warfarin in another study.

Warfarin is approximately 50 percent more effective than aspirin in preventing stroke in patients with AF who do not have valvular disease. Data suggest that the optimal intensity of oral anticoagula-

tion for stroke prevention in patients with AF appears to be a target INR of 2.0 to 3.0. However, the narrow therapeutic margin of warfarin, in addition to associated food and drug interactions, requires frequent INR testing and dosage adjustments. These liabilities likely contribute to underuse of warfarin, and alternative therapies are needed. An ongoing study, Atrial Fibrillation Clopidogrel Trial with Irbesartan for Prevention of Vascular Events (ACTIVE), is evaluating the safety and efficacy of the combination of aspirin plus clopidogrel in AF patients. Additional studies have assessed ximelagatran's efficacy in stroke prevention.[13]

Ximelagatran is a direct thrombin inhibitor that is orally administered, has stable pharmacokinetics independent of the hepatic P450 enzyme system, and has a low potential for food and drug interactions. Two large studies, Stroke Prevention Using the Oral Thrombin Inhibitor in Atrial Fibrillation (SPORTIF) III and V compared fixed-dose ximelagatran (36 mg BID) with dose-adjusted warfarin (INR 2.0–3.0) in 7329 high-risk patients with AF. In both trials ximelagatran was noninferior to warfarin and had fewer major and minor bleeding complications. However, serum alanine-aminotransferase levels rose transiently to >3 times normal in 6 percent of patients with ximelagatran (usually within the first 6 months). At the time of this publication, the Food and Drug Administration (FDA) has not yet approved ximelagatran.[13,85]

The effectiveness of anticoagulation on embolic stroke prevention from other cardiac conditions has not been well studied. The concurrent use of aspirin plus warfarin in MI patients with left ventricular thrombus is based on American College of Cardiology/ American Heart Association (ACC/AHA) guidelines for patients with ST-segment elevation MI.[13,86] The rate of recurrent stroke in patients with MVP is so low that warfarin is not recommended for prophylaxis except when a thrombus is seen on echocardiography. Warfarin may not be effective in preventing calcific, myxomatous, bacterial, and fibrin-platelet emboli; and warfarin has been posited to worsen cholesterol crystal embolization.[87]

The timing of the initiation of warfarin anticoagulation after embolic stroke remains controversial. Embolic brain infarcts often become hemorrhagic, and serious brain hemorrhage has occurred after anticoagulation.[88–92] Large infarcts, hypertension, large bolus doses of heparin, and excessive anticoagulation have been associated with hemorrhage. Because most hemorrhagic transformations occur within 48 hours, the recommendations of the Cerebral Embolism Task Force were to avoid early anticoagulation in patients with large infarcts or hemorrhagic transformation on repeat CT.[93,94] Studies of patients with cerebral and cerebellar hemorrhagic infarction show that, in the vast majority, the cause is embolic, hemorrhagic infarction occurs equally with and without anticoagulation, and the development of hemorrhagic infarction is rarely accompanied by clinical worsening.[95,96] Patients with hemorrhagic transformation who were continued on anticoagulants did not worsen. The risk of re-embolism must be balanced against the small but definite risk of important bleeding. However, if the patient has a large brain infarct, heparin should be delayed and bolus heparin infusions should be avoided. If the risk for re-embolism is high, immediate heparinization is advisable; whereas if the risk seems low, it is prudent to delay anticoagulants for at least 48 hours. One study showed that patients with AF with embolic strokes who were treated with well-controlled heparin anticoagulation soon after stroke onset fared better than did patients treated later.[97,98]

[ ] PARADOXICAL EMBOLISM

Although once considered rare, emboli entering the systemic circulation through right-to-left shunting of blood are now often recognized with the advent of newer diagnostic technologies. By far the most common potential intracardiac shunt is a residual patent foramen ovale (PFO). The high frequency of PFOs in the normal adult population has made it difficult to be certain in an individual stroke patient with a PFO whether paradoxical embolism through the PFO was the cause of the stroke or whether the PFO was merely an incidental finding. Autopsy series have shown that about 30 percent of adults have a probe patent foramen ovale at necropsy.[99] Hagen and colleagues studied 956 patients with clinically and pathologically normal hearts and found a PFO in 27.3 percent.[99] The frequency of PFOs declined with age: 34.3 percent during the first 3 decades of life, 25.4 percent during the fourth to eighth decades, and 20.2 percent during the ninth and tenth decades. The average diameter of PFOs was 4.9 mm and the size tended to increase with age.[99] Echocardiographic studies have shown that PFOs are more common in patients with an undetermined cause of stroke than in those in whom another etiology has been defined.[100–102] Lechat and coworkers, using transthoracic echocardiography with contrast injection during Valsalva maneuver, demonstrated right-to-left shunting through a PFO in 56 percent of patients with cryptogenic stroke, in comparison to 10 percent of the patients in the control group.[100] Webster and colleagues, in a study of stroke patients younger than 40 years of age, found a PFO in 50 percent of patients with stroke using contrast echocardiography.[103] Di Tullio and coworkers demonstrated the presence of a PFO in 42 percent of patients with a cryptogenic stroke, compared with 7 percent in those with a determined etiology of stroke. This was observed in the younger (47 percent compared with 4 percent) and in the older (38 percent compared with 8 percent) age subgroups.[101]

Neuroimaging studies are not conclusive with regard to the link between patent foramen ovale and embolic stroke. However, in 1998, Steiner and colleagues reported on a series of 95 patients with first stroke and who had PFOs.[104] Those with large PFOs had more features of embolic strokes with brain imaging than did patients with small PFOs.

Review of series of patients with paradoxical embolism[105–107] through a PFO and the authors' experience allows the derivation of five criteria that, when four or more are met, establish the presence of paradoxical embolism with a high degree of certainty[1]:

1. A situation that promotes thrombosis of leg or pelvic veins (e.g., long sitting in one position, such as prolonged airplane flight, or recent surgery)

2. Increased coagulability (e.g., the use of oral contraceptives, presence of V Leiden factor, dehydration, etc.)
3. The sudden onset of stroke during sexual intercourse, straining at stool, or other activity that includes a Valsalva maneuver or that promotes right-to-left shunting of blood
4. Pulmonary embolism within a short time before or after the neurologic ischemic event
5. The absence of other putative causes of stroke after thorough evaluation

Current treatment options for future stroke prevention in patients with PFO and ischemic stroke include medical therapy, open or minimally invasive cardiac surgical closure, and transcatheter closure. With regard to medical therapies, antiplatelet therapy is reasonable for future stroke prevention in cryptogenic stroke patients with a first ischemic stroke/TIA plus an isolated PFO. Warfarin is considered to be an appropriate treatment option in the subgroup of PFO/ischemic stroke patients with concomitant hypercoagulable state or venous thrombosis. With regard to surgical closure, there is no clear evidence at present that it is superior to medical therapy for secondary stroke prevention. Transcatheter closure may ultimately demonstrate a benefit to medical therapy for future stroke prevention: A recent review of 10 nonrandomized unblended transcatheter closure studies for secondary stroke prevention reported a 1-year rate of recurrent neurologic events of 0 to 4.9 percent in transcatheter closure patients versus 3.8 to 12.0 percent in medically treated patients. The incidence of minor and major procedural complications was 7.9 percent and 1.45 percent, respectively. Other randomized trials evaluating the efficacy of transcatheter closure devices are ongoing.[13,108] At the time of this publication, transcatheter closure is not FDA approved for use after a first ischemic stroke in PFO patients; however, in PFO patients who fail medical therapy and have a second ischemic cerebral event, it is a treatment option to consider.

[ ] BRAIN HYPOPERFUSION (CARDIAC PUMP FAILURE)

After cardiopulmonary resuscitation (CPR), the heart often recovers in individuals whose brain has been irreversibly damaged by ischemic-anoxic damage.[109] Cardiologists must become very familiar with the pathology, signs, and prognosis of brain dysfunction after periods of circulatory failure.

Different brain regions have selective vulnerability to hypoxic-ischemic damage. Regions that are most remote and at the edges of major vascular supply are more liable to hypoperfusion injury. These zones are usually referred to as *border zones* or *watersheds*. The cerebral cortex and hippocampus are particularly vulnerable to injury.[110–113] In the cerebral cortex, the border zone regions are between the anterior cerebral artery (ACA) and MCA and between the MCA and posterior cerebral artery (PCA). Damage is usually most severe in the posterior parieto-temporo-occipital region and in frontal areas most remote from the heart and thus called *distal fields*. The basal ganglia and thalamus are most involved if hypoxia is severe but some circulation is preserved. This situation applies most to hanging, strangulation, drowning, and carbon monoxide exposure.[114] Cerebellar neurons may also be selectively injured.[115]

When circulatory arrest is complete and abrupt, brainstem nuclei are especially vulnerable to necrosis in young humans and experimental animals.[116] When hypoxia and ischemia are especially severe, the spinal cord may also be damaged.[117,118] When cortical damage is severe and protracted, cytotoxic edema causes massive brain swelling, with cessation of blood flow and brain death.

Clinical Findings

Very severe hypoxic-ischemic damage can lead to mortal injury to the cortex and brainstem, irreversible coma, and brain death. When initially examined, such patients have no brainstem reflexes and no response to stimuli except perhaps a decerebration response. These findings do not improve, and respiratory control is absent or lost.

When cerebral cortical damage is very severe but brainstem reflexes are preserved, there is no meaningful response to the environment. Automatic facial movements such as blinking, tongue protrusion, and yawning usually persist. The eyes may rest slightly up and move from side to side. When this state does not improve, it is referred to as the *persistent vegetative state*[109,112,119,120] or *wakefulness without awareness*. Laminar cortical necrosis can cause seizures: multifocal myoclonic twitches or jerks of the facial and limb muscles, which are difficult to control with anticonvulsants.

With severe hypoperfusion ACA-MCA border-zone injury, there is weakness of the arms and proximal lower extremities with preservation of face, leg, and foot movement (the "man in a barrel" syndrome). With MCA-PCA ischemia, the symptoms and signs are predominantly visual. Patients describe difficulty seeing and inability to integrate the features of large objects or scenes despite retained capacity to see small objects in some parts of their visual fields. Reading is impossible. There are features of Balint syndrome.[109,121] Apathy, inertia, and amnesia are also common. Patients cannot make new memories and have patchy, retrograde amnesia for events during and before hospitalization. This Korsakoff-type syndrome is caused by hippocampal damage and may not be fully reversible. Amnesia may be accompanied by visual abnormalities, apathy, and confusion, or may be isolated.

Action myoclonus (the Lance-Adams syndrome)[115] is thought to be caused by cerebellar damage.[115] This disorder is characterized by arrhythmic fine or coarse jerking, especially on attempted movement. Reaching for an object may be accompanied by gross oscillation and tremor-like movements. Gait ataxia is also common.

Prognosis

Shortly after resuscitation or arrest, patients with less severe cerebral injuries show some reactivity to the environment. Eye opening and restless limb movements develop. The eyes may fixate on objects. Noise, a flashlight, or a gentle pinch may arouse patients to react to stimuli. Soon patients awaken fully and may begin to speak. Cognitive and behavioral abnormalities may be detected after the patient awakens, depending on the degree of injury.

Prognostic signs and variables have been extensively studied.[109,122–125] The initial neurologic findings and their course are helpful in predicting outcome. Among patients who have meaningful responses to pain at 1 hour, almost all survivors have preserved intellectual function. Patients who do not respond to pain

by 24 hours typically either die or remain in a vegetative state. Being comatose predicts a poor prognosis.[124,125] *Thus, two simple observations—the presence or absence of coma and the response to pain—predict neurologic outcome very early.*[125] Recurrent myoclonus is also a poor prognostic sign. Wijdicks, Parisi, and Sharbrough reported that in the setting of diffuse, persistent myoclonus in comatose survivors of cardiac arrest, all patients in myoclonus status died.[126]

In a study in Seattle of out-of-hospital cardiac arrests, patients who did not awaken died on average 3.5 days after arrest.[127,128] Of 459 patients, 183 never awakened (40 percent). Among those who did awaken, 91 (33 percent) had persistent neurologic deficits.[127] Prognosis could be made by analysis of pupillary light reflexes, eye movements, and motor responses.[128] It is unclear whether bystander initiation of CPR is significantly related to awakening.[128,129] After in-hospital CPR, pneumonia, hypotension, renal failure, cancer, and a housebound state before hospitalization were significantly related to death in the hospital.[130]

Diagnostic Testing

Neuroimaging and other tests have proved to be relatively unhelpful in contrast to the neurologic examination.[109] CT is used to exclude other causes of coma such as brain hemorrhage. Electroencephalography (EEG) is helpful in studying cortical activity in unresponsive patients. TCD may be helpful in the evaluation of brain death.[131–133]

Treatment

Other than maintaining adequate circulation and oxygenation, treatment has not helped improve outcome. Increased blood sugar correlates with poor outcome,[134] and experimental animals subjected to circulatory arrest do worse if they have been fed glucose before the arrest.[135,136] Blood calcium, the presence of free radicals, and excitatory neurotoxins have all been postulated to affect neuronal cell death.[136–138] A multifaceted approach to therapy has been most successful.[139]

【 】 NEUROLOGIC EFFECTS OF CARDIAC DRUGS AND CARDIAC ENCEPHALOPATHY

Drugs given to patients with cardiac disease often have neurologic side effects.[140] Digitalis can cause visual hallucinations, yellow vision, and general confusion.[141,142] Digitalis levels need not be excessively elevated; the symptoms disappear with drug cessation. Quinidine can cause delirium, seizures, coma, vertigo, tinnitus, and visual blurring.[143] Similar toxicity has been seen with lithium. Patients may become acutely comatose while being treated with intravenous lidocaine. This effect has been associated with the accidental administration of very large doses; more common CNS effects of less extreme toxicity include sedation, irritability, and twitching. The latter may progress to seizures accompanied by respiratory depression. Amiodarone can cause ataxia, weakness, tremors, paresthesias, visual symptoms, a Parkinsonian-like syndrome, and occasionally delirium.[140]

Patients with congestive heart failure often develop an encephalopathy characterized by decreased alertness, sleepiness, decrease in all intellectual functions, asterixis, and variability of alertness and cognitive functions from hour to hour.[140] These patients may not have pulmonary, liver, or renal failure or electrolyte abnormalities. This cardiac encephalopathy is probably multifactoral.[140]

NEUROLOGIC AND CEREBROVASCULAR COMPLICATIONS OF ENDOVASCULAR CARDIAC PROCEDURES AND CARDIAC SURGERY

Patients with heart disease are diagnosed, treated, and at times even cured with a variety of cardiac procedures. Although the implicit goal with any cardiac intervention (diagnostic or therapeutic) is to improve a patient's quality of life, these procedures often carry risk as well as the possibility of benefit.

【 】 ENDOVASCULAR CARDIAC DIAGNOSTIC AND THERAPEUTIC PROCEDURES

Cardiac Catheterization

Stroke and TIA are known complications of heart catheterization. In 1977, Dawson and Fischer reported cerebrovascular complications in 10 of 1000 consecutive cardiac catheterizations. Nine out of 10 of these events were determined to be embolic.[144,145] Similarly, Mendez Dominguez, and colleagues reported thromboembolic neurologic complications in 7 patients in a series of 2178 consecutive cardiac catheterizations. In all cases the cerebrovascular impairment occurred either during or within several minutes following the cardiac catheterization. All strokes were confirmed with CT or MRI, and the clinical profile in most cases supported an embolic mechanism.[146] Central retinal artery occlusion has been reported in association with cardiac catheterization.[147] More recently, Liu and coworkers reported 6 ischemic strokes and 1 intracerebral hemorrhage in a series of 3648 cardiac catheterizations in children. In this study the suspected catheterization-related stroke mechanisms included intracranial hemorrhage caused by intraprocedure anticoagulation as well as cerebral embolism from local clot.[148] Other potential mechanisms for cerebrovascular events during cardiac angiography may include catheter tip thromboembolism, atherosclerotic plaque or cholesterol embolism, air emboli, arterial vasospasm, and/or hypotension.[144,149–152]

Coronary Artery Angioplasty and Stenting

The stroke rate in patients undergoing percutaneous coronary interventions for both stable as well as unstable coronary artery disease (including angioplasty for acute MI) has been reported to be between 0 and 4 percent.[153–160] A combined analysis of data from 4 double-blind, placebo-controlled, randomized trials (EPIC, CAPTURE, EPILOG, EPISTENT) conducted between 1991 and 1997 assessed 8555 patients undergoing various percutaneous coronary interventions. Among the 8555 patients, there were 33 strokes in 31 patients (0.36 percent) within 30 days. Stroke occurred in 9 (0.29 percent) of 3079 patients receiving percutaneous coronary interventions alone: 6 were ischemic and 3 hemorrhagic. Stroke was diagnosed in 22 (0.41 percent) of 5476 patients who underwent percutaneous treatment in conjunction with abciximab treatment, of which there were 13 ischemic strokes and 9 hemorrhages.[153–158]

Galbreath and colleagues reported a 0.2 percent rate of focal central neurological complication in their series of 1968 percutaneous transluminal coronary angioplasties (PTCAs): 3 were ischemic strokes and 1 was a TIA. The mechanism in these cases was determined to be embolic in three cases: one patient had air inadvertently injected through the guide catheter and two had events after the ascending aorta was *scraped* with the guide catheter in search of a graft ostium. The remaining patient had an event during a period of hypotension.[159]

Electrophysiologic Procedures and Electrical Cardioversion

Thromboembolic stroke can be a complication of cardiac electrophysiologic procedures, including radiofrequency catheter ablation of arrhythmia. Multicenter data are limited; however, the stroke risk appears to be <2 percent.[144,161–164] Additionally, electrical cardioversion may be used in the treatment of AF and atrial flutter. The risk of stroke caused by direct current cardioversion has been estimated to occur in 1.3 percent of cardioverted patients.[165] Anticoagulation before and after cardioversion lowers the risk of embolism.[144,165,166]

Percutaneous Valvuloplasty

Percutaneous balloon mitral as well as aortic valvuloplasties have also been complicated by stroke. With regards to when the neurologic events occur, Letac and coworkers' 1988 series of 218 patients undergoing transcutaneous balloon aortic valvuloplasty indicates that 1 stroke occurred intraprocedure, whereas 3 additional strokes occurred during the postprocedure time period.[144,167–170]

Intraaortic Balloon Pump

Intraaortic balloon pumps (IABPs) are used in patients with severe left ventricular failure or cardiogenic shock. The IABP is inserted into the patient's midthoracic aorta to maintain adequate perfusion. Spinal cord infarcts can occur in patients with IABPs caused by local thromboembolism, aortic dissection, aortic atherosclerotic plaque rupture, or local hypoperfusion.[144,171]

【 】 CARDIOVASCULAR SURGERY

Every year, an estimated 1 million patients undergo cardiac surgery throughout the world. Coronary artery bypass graft (CABG) surgery is the most common major cardiovascular operation performed.

The frequency of abnormalities of intellectual function and behavior after cardiac surgery is high.[172,173] Preoperative diagnoses of diabetes, history of prior stroke, older age, female sex, smoking, hypertension, left main coronary disease, and mild renal impairment (defined as serum creatinine 1.47–2.25 mg/dL) have all been identified to increase perioperative stroke risk.[174–176] The cerebrovascular risk depends upon the particular procedure performed. Estimations of stroke risk for isolated CABG range from 0.8 to 3.8 percent.[177–181] Recent review of current data suggests that there may potentially be a decrease in postoperative stroke rates in patients undergoing off-pump CABG compared to patients undergoing the traditional on-pump operation, but conflicts in the literature do exist.[182–188] One potential reason for the discrepancies in data may be that most studies did not differentiate between clampless and partial clamp off-pump techniques. One study of 700 consecutive patients undergoing multiple vessel off-pump CABG demonstrated a decreased incidence of stroke (0.2 percent versus 2.2 percent) in the *aortic no-touch* group. Additionally, logistic regression identified partial aortic clamping as the only independent predictor of stroke, increasing this risk 28-fold.[189]

In one multicenter study, the incidence of stroke plus severe intellectual dysfunction from CABG has been reported to be 6 percent.[190] With regard to combined procedures, one multicenter investigation assessing 273 patients undergoing combined CABG and left-sided cardiac procedure (such as aortic or mitral valve replacement) estimated that 15.8 percent of patients had neurologic complications: 8.5 percent with stroke or TIA and 7.3 percent with new intellectual deterioration.[191] This combined procedure appears to carry a higher stroke risk than CABG performed in isolation.

It is unclear whether minimally invasive cardiac surgical procedures may potentially have a lessened stroke risk, because further data is needed. One single center's result with direct-access, minimally invasive mitral valve surgery in 106 patients demonstrates a low rate of stroke and TIA, with a total of 0.28 percent of patients having either stroke or TIA. However, a second center's results with minimally invasive, reoperative, isolated valve surgery did not demonstrate a lower stroke rate compared to patients undergoing sternotomy.[192,193]

Overall, in prospective studies, transient complications have been noted in 61 percent of cardiac surgery patients.[194] In one series in CABG patients, 16.8 percent had stroke or encephalopathy postoperatively; the encephalopathies usually cleared, and only 2 percent of patients had severe strokes.[195] The potential mechanisms of cerebral impairment in the cardiac surgery population will be explored later.

Atherothrombotic, Hemodynamically Mediated Brain Infarcts

An estimated 12 percent of patients requiring CABG also have significant carotid artery disease.[193] One major concern regarding cardiac surgery patients has been whether the hemodynamic stress of heart surgery leads to underperfusion of areas supplied by already stenotic or occluded arteries, resulting in brain infarcts. This concern underlies neck auscultation for bruits, ultrasound carotid artery testing, and cerebral angiography prior to CABG. However, hemodynamically induced infarction related to preexisting atherosclerotic occlusive cervicocranial arterial disease is a rare complication of heart surgery. Asymptomatic patients with carotid bruits have a very low rate of stroke after elective surgery.[196] However, the risk of perioperative stroke does increase with increasing severity of carotid stenosis.[178,197,198] In a retrospective study of CABG patients with known carotid disease, ipsilateral strokes occurred in 1.1 percent of arteries with 50 to 90 percent stenosis, in 6.2 percent of arteries with >90 percent stenosis, and in only 2 percent of vessels with carotid occlusion.[197,198]

Uncertainty exists about whether carotid endarterectomy (CEA) performed simultaneous or prior to CABG improves perioperative stroke risk. Stroke rates vary greatly in those undergoing combined CEA-CABG as opposed to staged procedures.[199] Definitive management of combined cervicocerebral and coronary artery disease awaits the outcome of clinical trials. One systematic review of 97 published studies of staged versus synchronous operations found no significant difference in outcomes between these two surgical groups. Unfortunately in this study, there were no comparable data for patients with combined carotid stenosis and cardiac disease *not* undergoing either staged or synchronous surgery.[200]

Most studies have relied on clinical localization of focal deficits and inference about their mechanisms. A neuroradiology study reviewed neuroimaging results from 30 patients with acute strokes in relation to CABG.[201] Only one had evidence of a hemodynamic atherostenotic mechanism, which supports the data suggesting hemodynamically induced infarction during cardiac surgery is rare. Embolism arising from cardiac and aortic sources is much more common than atherothrombotic infarcts and is of a much greater concern.[172]

Brain Embolism

One point against a hemodynamic or hypoperfusion cause of many strokes is their timing. It appears that strokes may occur more frequently *after* recovery from the anesthetic. If the mechanism of stroke were hemodynamic, the major circulatory stress would be intraoperative and patients would at least awaken from anesthesia with the deficit. In two studies in which the authors record the timing of coronary artery bypass surgery (CABS)-related strokes, only 16[202] and 17 percent[203] of patients had deficits noted immediately postoperatively. The distribution of infarcts and their multiplicity on neuroimaging scans were most consistent with embolism. Embolic infarcts may involve either the anterior or the posterior circulation.[172,195,201,202] In one series of postoperative, posterior circulation strokes, most were embolic and followed cardiac surgery.[203]

In cardiac surgery patients, the preponderance of evidence suggests that macroemboli (>200 μm in diameter) and microemboli are responsible for most neurologic complications.[190,195,200,204,205] Macroemboli (associated with atherosclerotic plaque disruption or rupture) are believed to precipitate focal deficits, whereas particulate microemboli (white blood cell and platelet aggregates, fat, or air) may be implicated in more subtle diffuse cognitive dysfunction.[190,206]

Emboli may arise from preexisting cardiac abnormalities (such as hypofunctioning ventricles, dilated atria, and aortic atheromas) or from postoperative arrhythmias.[172] Evidence links operative and postoperative embolism to aortic ulcerative atherosclerotic lesions. Crossclamping of the ascending aorta and aortotomy liberate cholesterol or calcific plaque debris.[172,207] Data from a series of 2641 consecutive cardiac surgery patients showed that left-body symptoms (right-hemispheric stroke) were twice as common as right-body symptoms, suggesting that aortic manipulation and anatomic mechanisms in the aortic arch were more likely to cause cerebrovascular accidents than effects from aortic cannula stream jets.[208] Fig. 106–1 shows the aorta of a patient who died having never awakened after CABG. Fig. 106–2 shows cholesterol crystals and other debris trapped within a filter placed in the aorta at the time of unclamping.

In one series in which embolic signals were monitored during CABG surgery, 34 percent of signals were detected as the aortic cross clamps were removed and another 24 percent as aortic partial occlusion clamps were removed.[207] The number of microemboli detected correlates with abnormalities of cognitive function studied after surgery.[172,209] Fig. 106–3 shows microemboli within the aorta shown by TEE after release of aortic clamps. Fig. 106–4 and Fig. 106–5 are TCD recordings during manipulation of the aorta and after release of aortic clamps.

Necropsy examination of patients dying after cardiac surgery has shown severe bilateral, predominantly border-zone infarcts.[210] The small arteries of the brain and other viscera (heart, kidney, spleen, pancreas) may be packed with birefringent cholesterol crystal emboli.[210] TEE makes it possible to detect protruding ulcerative plaques in the aorta preoperatively and intraoperatively.[172,211,212] In one patient with repeated peripheral emboli, a protruding atherosclerotic plaque was removed surgically.[211] Intraaortic atherosclerotic debris identified by TEE has been found to be associated with embolic events.[212] Intraoperative B-mode ultrasonography with the probe placed on the aorta has also been used to detect severe aortic atherosclerotic plaques.[213] Ultrasonic imaging showed aortic atheromas in 58 percent of patients, whereas visual examination and palpation detected plaques in only 24 percent.[213] *Atherosclerosis of the ascending aorta is a very important risk factor for post-CABS stroke.*[172,214] *In patients who are scheduled to undergo elective cardiac surgery, consideration should be given to having TEEs performed before surgery to evaluate cardiac lesions and thrombi, cardiac function, and aortic atheromas.*

Thromboembolic infarction often occurs in the days following surgery when cessation of anticoagulation is necessary. Postoperative activation of coagulation factors in cardiac surgery patients can promote hypercoagulability. Disseminated intravascular coagulation, acquired antithrombin III deficiency, and acquired protein C deficiencies are not uncommon. Activation of the coagulation-fibrinolytic system can persist for 2 months after cardiopulmonary bypass surgery.[215,216] In some patients, hypercoagulability related to surgery can precipitate occlusive thrombosis in atherostenotic arteries, and the newly formed thrombus can lead to intraarterial embolism. Cardiac, aortic, and intraarterial embolism accounts for the vast majority of cardiac-surgery-related focal neurologic deficits.

With regard to interventional treatment of cardiac surgery patients with an acute embolic stroke, unfortunately, given their recent surgery, these patients are not candidates to receive IV tissue plasminogen activator (t-PA). However, these patients may be candidates for another FDA-approved acute stroke treatment that can be used within the first 8 hours after acute ischemic stroke onset: embolectomy using the Concentric Thrombus Retriever. The device is used for mechanical clot extraction in cerebral arteries. In the multicenter prospective Mechanical Embolus Removal in Cerebral Ischemia (MERCI) trial that led to FDA clearance in August 2004, the MERCI Retriever achieved 48 percent recanalization and resulted in lower morbidity and mortality in revascularized patients.[217,218] Although use of this device is available only in certain tertiary stroke centers with Interventional Neuroradiology capability at present, it does provide an additional postoperative treatment option for surgical stroke patients in those areas.

Postoperative Encephalopathy: Microemboli and Other Causes

Gilman described a diffuse CNS disorder following open heart surgery (characterized by altered levels of consciousness and activity and confusion[219]) that is now referred to as *encephalopathy.* Clinical and imaging studies usually do not show important focal neurologic signs or large focal infarcts. The incidence of encephalopathy varies. In one series, 57 of 1669 (3.4 percent) CABG patients had postoperative mental state changes including delirium and encephalopathy.[220] In the Cleveland Clinic prospective series, 11.6 percent were *encephalopathic* on the fourth postoperative day.[185]

Encephalopathy has multiple causes. A necropsy study of patients who died after cardiopulmonary bypass or angiography has awakened interest in this subject.[221] Focal, small capillary, and arteriolar dilatations (SCADs) were commonly found in the brain.[221] About one-half of the SCADs show birefringent crystalline material within the dilated capillaries. SCADs could, at least in part, explain the decreased cerebral blood flow found during cardiopulmonary bypass. SCADs are iatrogenically generated microemboli, but as yet their origin is unknown. Their morphology is most consistent with air or fat.[221]

Other causes of encephalopathy are common. Diffuse hypoxic-ischemic insults from hypotension and hypoperfusion do occur. *Drugs are a very common cause of encephalopathy in the postoperative period. Particularly important are haloperidol, narcotics, and sedatives.* Morphine is sometimes used heavily intraoperatively, and opiate withdrawal with restlessness and hyperactivity can result. Agitation and restlessness are often early signs of organic encephalopathy and may lead to the administration of haloperidol, barbiturates, phenothiazines, or benzodiazepines for calming and sedation. When these drugs wear off and the patient begins to awaken, agitation may occur and more sedatives may be given. Haloperidol causes rigidity, restlessness, agitation, hallucinations, and confusion. In experimental animals, haloperidol delays recovery from strokes by months and its use is not advised.[222,223] Phenothiazines and sedatives are also problematic; *in general, use of sedatives and narcotics should be minimized and they should be tapered as soon as possible.*

Postoperative Intracranial Hemorrhage

Intracerebral or subarachnoid hemorrhages have occasionally been reported after cardiac surgery, most commonly in children who had repair of congenital heart disease[224] or in cardiac transplantation patients.[225] The postulated mechanism involves an abrupt increase in brain blood flow with rupture of small intracranial arteries unprepared for the new load. Usually, there is a prolonged period when cardiac output is low, and this output is suddenly increased by the surgery. Abrupt increases in brain blood flow or pressure in other situations have also been associated with intracerebral hemorrhage.[226]

Stroke Mimics: Postoperative Peripheral Nerve Complications

Brachial plexus and peripheral nerve lesions frequently develop after cardiac surgery and can be confused with CNS complications.[227] In one series, new peripheral nervous system deficits occurred in 13 percent of patients.[227] The most common deficit is a unilateral brachial plexopathy characterized by shoulder pain and usually weakness and numbness of one hand. It is probably caused by either sternal retraction or by positioning of the arm during surgery, with traction on the lower trunk of the brachial plexus.

Ulnar, peroneal, and saphenous nerve injuries are also common and are also related to positioning. Diaphragmatic and vocal cord paralyses are likely related to local effects of the cardiac surgery on the recurrent laryngeal and phrenic nerves. Postoperative Horner syndrome may be caused by manipulation of the sympathetic chain, but carotid dissection (particularly in surgical patients undergoing aortic dissection repair) should be excluded.

CARDIAC EFFECTS OF BRAIN LESIONS

Information is beginning to emerge on cardiac muscle changes (myocytolysis), arrhythmias, pulmonary edema, electrocardiogram (ECG) changes, and sudden death caused by brain disease and sudden emotional stresses.[228,229]

【 】 CARDIAC LESIONS

The two most common lesions found in the hearts of patients dying with acute CNS lesions are patchy regions of myocardial necrosis and subendocardial hemorrhage. The abnormalities range from eosinophilic staining of cells with preserved striations to transformation of myocardial cells into dense eosinophilic contraction bands. These changes have been referred to as *myocytolysis*.[228,230] Subendocardial petechiae and frank hemorrhages are also noted. These lesions were described in the 1950s[229,231] but were considered rare.[232,233] One study found a high incidence of myocardial abnormalities in patients dying of brain lesions that increase intracranial pressure rapidly.[234] Stress-related release of catecholamines and possibly corticosteroids may be responsible, at least in part, for the cardiac lesions found in patients with CNS lesions.[228,235–240] Adrenoreceptor polymorphisms can explain increased catecholamine sensitivity and so increased risk of cardiac injury in patients with subarachnoid hemorrhage and acute ischemic stroke.[241]

【 】 ELECTROCARDIOGRAPHIC AND ENZYME CHANGES

In stroke patients, especially those with subarachnoid hemorrhage (SAH), ECGs may show a prolonged QT interval; giant, wide, roller-coaster–inverted T waves; and U waves.[242] These changes are often called *cerebral T waves*. Patients with stroke undergoing continuous ECG monitoring have a high incidence of T-wave and ST-segment changes, various arrhythmias, and cardiac enzyme abnormalities. ECG changes may include a prolonged QT interval, depressed ST segments, flat or inverted T waves, and U waves.[228,242–245] Less often, tall, peaked T waves and elevated ST segments are noted. Myocardial enzyme release and echocardiographic wall motion abnormalities are associated with impaired left ventricular performance after SAH. In severely affected patients, reduction of cardiac output may elevate the risk of vasospasm-induced cerebral ischemia.[246] Cardiac and skeletal muscle enzymes, including the MB isoenzyme of creatine kinase (MB-CK), are often abnormal in stroke patients.[245,247–250] During the 4 to 7 days after stroke, there is usually a slow rise and later fall in serum MB-CK levels, a pattern quite different from that found in acute MI; the temporal pattern of cardiac isoenzyme release is

more compatible with smoldering low-grade necrosis, such as patchy, focal myocytolysis.[232,247] The ST-segment and T-wave abnormalities and cardiac arrhythmias correlate significantly with raised levels of MB-CK in stroke patients.[232]

【 】 ARRHYTHMIAS

Various cardiac arrhythmias have been found in stroke patients, most frequently sinus bradycardia and tachycardia and premature ventricular contractions.[228,243–245] Some arrhythmias are manifestations of primary cardiac problems, but others are undoubtedly secondary to the brain lesions. The incidence of sinus tachycardia and bradycardia is maximal on the first day after intracerebral hemorrhage.[250] Ventricular bigeminy, atrioventricular dissociation and block, ventricular tachycardia, AF, and bundle-branch blocks are found less often.[251] Arrhythmias are more common in patients who have primary brainstem lesions or brainstem compression.

【 】 ECHOCARDIOGRAPHIC CHANGES

Transient apical ballooning has been found after severe emotional stress, especially in women, and has occasionally been identified in stroke patients with subarachnoid hemorrhage.[252,253] This abnormality has often been referred to as *tako-tsubo left ventricular dysfunction* because the shape of the end-systolic left ventriculogram resembles an octopus catcher used in Japan.[252,254] Echocardiography shows a hyperkinetic basal region and an akinetic apical half of the ventricle in the absence of obstructed epicardial coronary arteries.[252–254] The frequency of this finding in patients with acute brain ischemic strokes and brain and subarachnoid hemorrhages is not known because few such patients have had modern echocardiographic studies and the tako-tsubo abnormality has only very recently become well known.

【 】 NEUROGENIC PULMONARY EDEMA

Acute pulmonary edema may complicate strokes, especially SAH and posterior circulation ischemia and hemorrhage.[232,255] Pulmonary edema has been found in 70 percent of patients with fatal SAH and correlates with the development of raised intracranial pressure.[256] The pulmonary edema can develop despite normal cardiac function.[232,257]

【 】 SUDDEN DEATH

Sudden death associated with stressful situations, including so-called *voodoo death*, must involve CNS mechanisms.[240,258–263] Ventricular fibrillation, the presumed mechanism of sudden death, can be reliably elicited by stimulation of cardiac sympathetic nerves in both the normal and the ischemic heart.[262] Ischemia reduces the threshold for ventricular fibrillation.[232,260,263] Stress must cause CNS stimulation that triggers autonomic activation.[240] Sudden vagotonic stimulation can cause bradycardia and cardiac standstill. The effects of vagal stimulation on the development of ventricular arrhythmias is uncertain.[262] Patients with lateral medullary and lateral pontine infarcts affecting reticular formation structures die unexpectedly and have a high incidence of various types of autonomic dysregulation, such as labile blood pressure, syncope, tachycardia, and flushing, and failure of automatic respiration.

COEXISTENT VASCULAR DISEASES AFFECTING BOTH HEART AND BRAIN

[ ] ATHEROSCLEROSIS

The most common and important vascular disease that affects both the brain and the heart is atherosclerosis. The most frequent cause of death in stroke patients is coronary artery disease,[260] and extra- and intracranial arterial atherosclerosis[261] is common in patients with coronary artery disease.

Pathology and Predominant Sites of Disease

In white men the predominant atherosclerotic lesions involve the origins of the internal carotid artery (ICA) and the vertebral artery (VA) origins in the neck.[5,264–266] Fatty streaks and flat plaques first affect the posterior wall of the common carotid artery (CCA) opposite the flow divider between the ICA and the external carotid artery (ECA), a region of low shear stress.[267,268] Atherosclerotic plaques at this site do not differ from plaques in the aorta or coronary arteries. At first, plaques expand gradually and encroach on the lumen of the ICA and sometimes the CCA (Fig. 106–6). Atheromatous plaques often develop concurrently at the VA origin or spread from the parent subclavian artery to involve the VA origin.[48,269] When plaques reach a critical size, they affect turbulence, flow, and motion of the arteries, causing complications to develop within the plaques. Cracking, ulcerations, and mural thrombi develop, and the overlying endothelium is damaged with the development of occlusive thrombi.[270] Fresh thrombi loosely adherent to vascular walls rapidly propagate and embolize. Because the ICA has no nuchal branches, the clot often propagates cranially. In the VA collateral channels from the ECA and thyrocervical trunk usually provide collateral channels that reconstitute the VA in the neck and limit propagation of thrombi. In the initial 2 to 3 weeks after the development of an occlusive thrombus, the clot gradually organizes and is much less likely to propagate or embolize. The reduction in cranial blood flow caused by severe stenosis or occlusion of the ICA or VA stimulates development of collateral circulation that usually becomes adequate.

Fig. 106–7 shows diagrammatically the sites of predilection for development of atherosclerosis in the cervicocranial circulation. Note the concentration of these sites at branch points and flow dividers. There are important race

and sex differences in the distribution of cerebral atherosclerosis.[271–274] White men usually develop lesions of the ICA and VA origins. Patients with ICA-origin disease have a high frequency of hypercholesterolemia, coronary artery disease, and peripheral vascular occlusive disease. Blacks and individuals of Chinese, Japanese, and Thai ancestry have a much higher incidence of intracranial occlusive disease and a rather low frequency of extracranial disease.[271–275] Intracranial disease is more prevalent in women and those with diabetes. Patients with intracranial occlusive disease do not have a high incidence of coronary or peripheral vascular occlusive disease.

Mechanisms of Ischemia

Ischemia in patients with atherosclerotic occlusive lesions is caused by two different mechanisms: hypoperfusion and embolism.[5,276,277] Hypoperfusion develops only when a critical reduction in luminal diameter causes reduced distal perfusion. When flow is reduced slowly, the brain vasculature has a remarkable capacity to develop collateral circulation. Patients with severe ICA-origin occlusive disease can remain asymptomatic despite marked decrease in blood flow.[278,279] Even when vascular occlusion is abrupt—as in tying neck arteries to treat brain aneurysms—surprisingly few patients develop persistent brain ischemia. In most patients within a few days or at most 2 weeks following an arterial occlusion, collateral circulation stabilizes.

Intraarterial embolism from atherosclerotic lesions is probably a much more frequent and important cause of brain infarction than hypoperfusion. However, decreased perfusion probably limits clearance (washout) of emboli.[277] In patients with anterior circulation infarcts, angiography shows a very high frequency of intraarterial

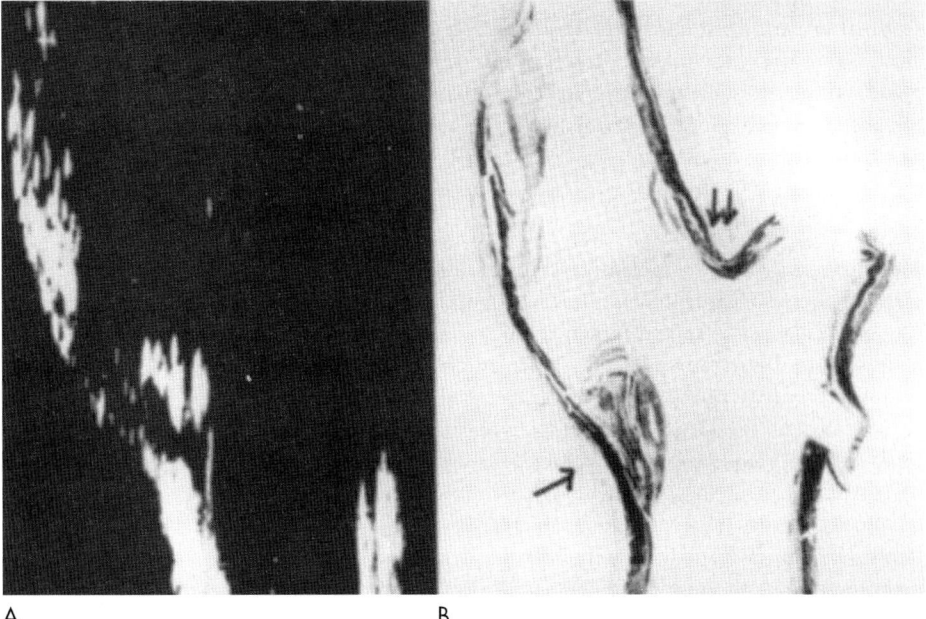

A   B

FIGURE 106–6. A. B-mode ultrasonic image showing plaque at internal carotid artery origin. **B.** A carotid specimen. The plaque (*single arrow*) is opposite the flow divider between the internal and external carotid arteries (*two arrows*). *Source: From Hennerici M, Steinke W. Abbildende ultraschallverfahren (B-scan) in duplex system. In: Durchblutungsstörungen des Gehirns—Neue Diagnostische Möglichkeiten. Gutersloh: Bertelsmann; 1987. With permission.*

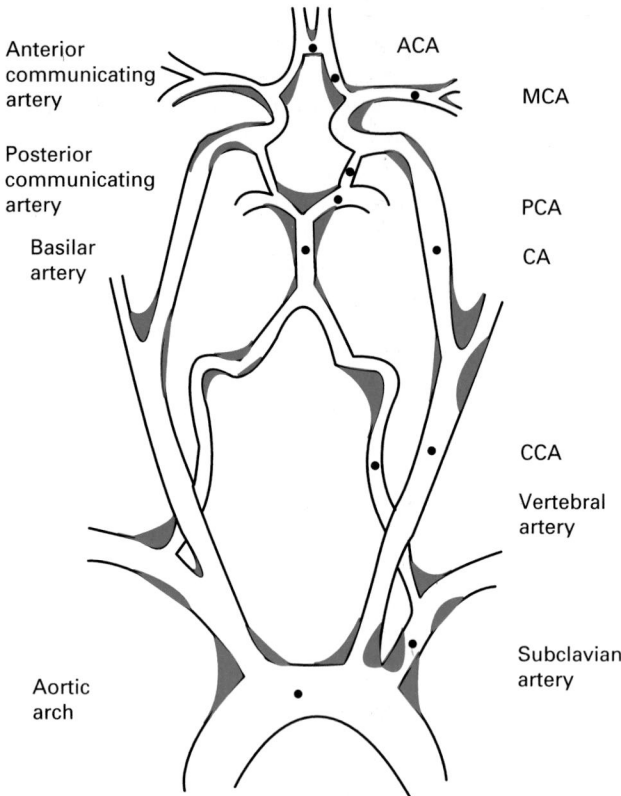

FIGURE 106–7. Sites of predilection for atherosclerotic narrowing: dark areas represent plaques. ACA, anterior cerebral artery; CCA, common carotid artery; ICA, internal carotid artery; MCA, middle cerebral artery; PCA, posterior cerebral artery. *Source: From Caplan LR.[5] With permission.*

intracranial emboli distal to an ICA thrombosis.[280] These emboli most often involve the MCA and its branches. If angiography is repeated or performed later than 48 hours after stroke, MCA occlusion is usually not present.[5,6] Intraarterial emboli often fragment and move distally. Intraarterial embolism is also common in the posterior circulation, where the most common donor sites are the VA origin and intracranial VA.[281]

Clinical Findings

Many patients with atherosclerotic occlusive disease are asymptomatic. The most frequent symptoms of hypoperfusion or embolism are headache, TIAs, and focal neurologic signs from brain infarction. Headaches are caused by vascular distension or brain swelling secondary to infarction. Unaccustomed headaches often precede strokes.[5,282] TIAs are caused by hypoperfusion or intraarterial emboli. Frequent, very brief stereotyped TIAs precipitated by postural changes suggest a hemodynamic mechanism. In contrast, emboli cause longer, less frequent attacks.[276,283] In many patients with clinical TIAs (i.e., with no lasting symptoms or signs), neuroimaging tests show brain infarcts.[284,285] Strokes may have various temporal features such as being maximal at outset, fluctuating, stepwise, or gradually progressive.

Neurologic symptoms and signs depend on the region of brain that is ischemic. Table 106–2 outlines the most frequent clinical patterns resulting from occlusions of the major extracranial and intracranial arteries.[5,266]

Diagnostic Testing

In most patients, the nature and severity of the brain and vascular lesions causing the stroke can be defined. CT and MRI should localize brain lesions, distinguish between infarcts and hemorrhages, and determine the location, extent, and size of the processes. CT or MRI is usually the first test in patients with suspected stroke because the information allows clinicians to exclude nonvascular disease such as tumor or abscess, differentiate hemorrhage from ischemia, identify the vascular territory involved, and define the extent of brain damaged.

The vascular territory involved should be inferred by the nature of the neurologic symptoms and signs and the location of brain lesions on CT or MRI. Echocardiography, especially TEE, has dramatically improved the ability to detect potential cardiac sources of emboli.

Ultrasound techniques can be used to screen for obstructive lesions in the major extracranial and intracranial arteries in both an-

TABLE 106–2

Common Signs in Cerebrovascular Occlusive Disease at Various Sites

ICA origin	Ipsilateral transient monocular blindness; MCA and ACA signs
ICA siphon (proximal to ophthalmic artery)	Same as ICA origin
ICA siphon (distal to ophthalmic artery)	MCA and ACA signs
ACA	Contralateral weakness of the lower limb and shoulder shrug
MCA	Contralateral motor, sensory, and visual loss
	Left: Aphasia
	Right: Neglect of left space, lack of awareness of deficit, apathy, impersistence
AChA	Contralateral motor, sensory, and visual loss, usually without cognitive changes
Subclavian artery (proximal to VA)	Lack of arm stamina, cool hand, transient dizziness, veering, diplopia
VA origin	Same as subclavian, but no ipsilateral arm or hand findings
VA intracranially	Lateral medullary syndrome; staggering and veering (cerebellar infarction)
BA	Bilateral motor weakness; ophthalmoplegia and diplopia
PCA	Contralateral hemianopia and hemisensory loss
	Left: alexia with agraphia
	Right: neglect of left visual space

ACA, anterior cerebral artery; AChA, anterior choroidal artery; BA, basilar artery; ICA, internal carotid artery; MCA, middle cerebral artery; PCA, posterior cerebral artery; VA, vertebral artery.

terior (carotid) and posterior (vertebrobasilar) circulation arteries. For extracranial use, the two most important are *B-mode scans* and *Doppler spectra*, both pulsed and continuous-wave (CW) Doppler. The anatomy of the carotid bifurcation (the CCA, proximal ICA, and ECA) and the proximal VAs can be imaged by high-frequency, 5- to 10-MHz, B-mode ultrasound systems, which provide images of the vessels in real time both longitudinally and in cross section (Fig. 106–8). Plaque calcifications and clot are often difficult to image. Pulsed Doppler registers frequency shifts from moving columns of blood. Doppler analysis can show the direction and velocity of blood flow. Multigated Doppler and B-mode scanning are now used together in so-called *duplex systems.*[5,286,287] The duplex system is probably >90 percent effective in separating arteries that are normal or minimally narrowed from those that have moderate disease (30–70 percent narrowing), and from those with severe narrowing (>70 percent stenosis). B-mode scanning sometimes suggests the presence of ulceration or hemorrhage in plaques that show heterogeneous images.[287] CW Doppler uses a movable probe to measure flow velocities along the carotid and vertebral arteries; the technique is less time consuming and less expensive than the duplex system and, in expert hands, is very accurate in detecting high-grade stenosis.[287,288] Ultrasound techniques cannot reliably separate complete occlusion from very high degrees of stenosis. Color-flow and power Doppler can show turbulence and altered flow dynamics.

TCD ultrasound is used to analyze the presence of intracranial arterial stenoses and provide information about the intracranial effects of extracranial occlusive lesions. The technique takes advantage of the soft spots in the temporal bones and natural foramina (the orbit and foramen magnum) that provide windows for ultrasound recording. The depth and angle of the probe recording can be varied, allowing the recording of velocities and sound spectra from all the major intracranial arteries.[5,131,289] Major obstructive lesions are reliably shown by both extracranial ultrasound and TCD. Continuous recording of intracranial arteries with TCD is a very sensitive and accurate method of detecting microemboli passing under the probes.[172,207,290,291] Examples of microembolic signals are shown in Fig. 106–4 and Fig. 106–5.

Magnetic resonance angiography (MRA) provides an additional method of imaging both the extracranial and intracranial arteries for areas of stenosis and occlusion.[5,275,292,293] computed tomography angiography (CTA), using a spiral (helical) CT machine and dye injected intravenously, can also image the major large craniocervical arteries.[293] Standard catheter angiography is warranted when ultrasound and CTA or MRA have not sufficiently defined the vascular lesion and treatment is clinically feasible.[5,275]

Treatment

For rational treatment, know the following:

- Location, nature, and severity of the occlusive lesion
- Location, extent, and reversibility of the brain lesion
- Blood constituents and coagulability[5,294]

Treatment should *not* be guided solely by the temporal pattern of the symptoms, such as TIA, progressing stroke, or so-called *completed stroke.*[5,284,294,295] These time courses do not predict the cause and mechanism of ischemia, tell if an infarct is present, or identify patients who will have further or recurrent ischemia.[295]

Physicians should first decide whether or not any specific therapy is indicated. Very severe neurologic deficits, serious intercurrent illnesses (dementia, cancer, etc.), and psychosocioeconomic considerations may make patients unsuitable for specific treatments. If treatment is feasible, two questions should be considered next: What brain tissue is at risk for further ischemia? What may be the benefit-to-risk ratio of specific treatments? To determine the

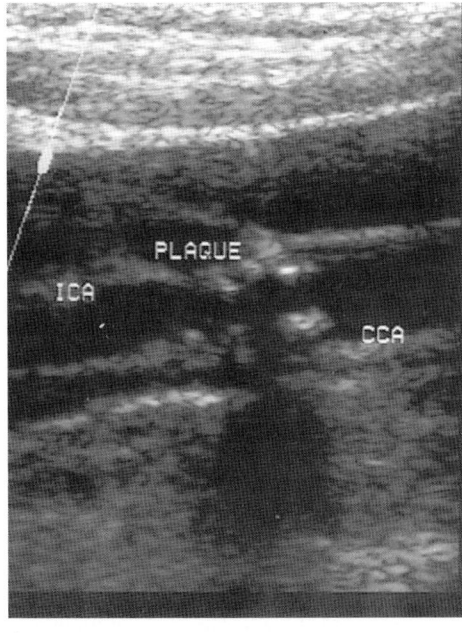
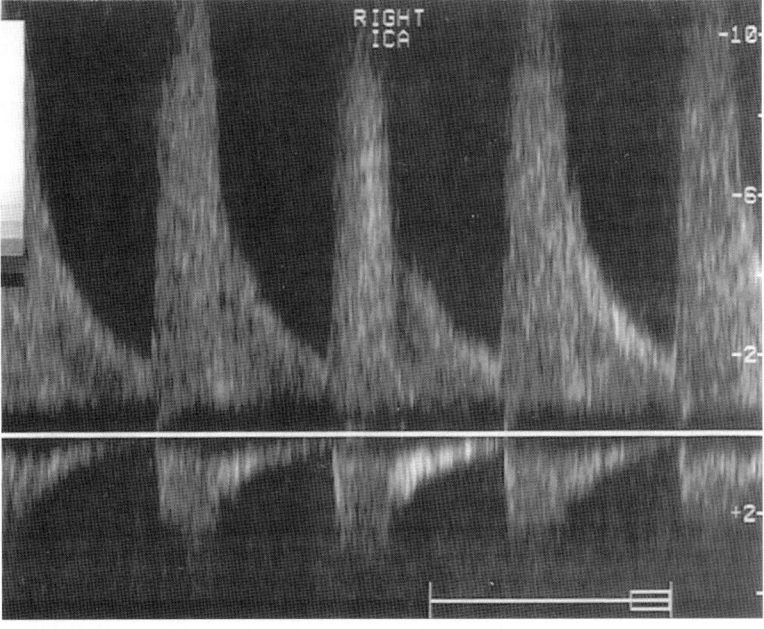

A   B

FIGURE 106–8. Duplex scan of carotid artery plaque. **A.** B-mode ultrasonic image showing plaque protruding into internal carotid artery (ICA) lumen. **B.** Doppler spectra at level of plaque showing high voltage related to stenosis.

tissue at risk, clinicians consider the cause and the deficit. For example, a man with a slight hemiplegia caused by a small lacunar infarct in the anterior limb of the internal capsule may have infarcted the entire tissue supplied by an occluded small artery. In that case treatment consists of controlling hypertension, the cause of the microvasculopathy. If, however, that same patient has a small cortical infarct in the precentral gyrus caused by ICA disease, the rest of the ICA territory is at risk for further ischemia and aggressive treatment is warranted. Newer MRI techniques, diffusion-weighted and perfusion MRI, along with MRA, can show, even very soon after symptoms begin, brain that is already infarcted, and brain tissue that is underperfused but not yet infarcted.[5,293,296,297]

Patients who have little tissue at risk are not candidates for specific interventional therapy. If there is considerable residual at-risk tissue, the guidelines in Table 106–3 are used to direct treatment,

TABLE 106–3

Suggested Use of Anticoagulants and Platelet Antiaggregants

Heparin (Standard Dose)
Short term, 2–4 weeks. Usually given by intravenous infusion, keeping APTT between 60 and 100s (1.5–2 × control APTT).
1. Immediate therapy for definite cardiac-origin cerebral embolism (large cerebral infarct, hypertension, bacterial endocarditis, or sepsis would delay or contraindicate this use).
2. Patients with severe stenosis or occlusion of the ICA origin, ICA siphon, MCA, vertebral artery, or basilar artery with less than a large clinical deficit. Subsequent treatment could consist of warfarin or surgery.

Heparin (Subcutaneous Minidose)
For prophylaxis of deep vein occlusion in patients immobilized by stroke (unless contraindicated; see Chap. 54).

Warfarin
Usually overlapped with heparin; keeping prothrombin time around INR of 2.0–3.0 (approximately 1.3–1.5 × control).
1. Long term (>3 months)
   a. Patients with cardiogenic cerebral embolization and rheumatic heart disease, atrial fibrillation with large atria or prior cerebral embolism, prosthetic valves, and some hypercoagulable states.
   b. Patients with severe stenosis of the ICA origin, ICA siphon, MCA stem, vertebral artery, and basilar artery. Used until studies show artery has been occluded for at least 3 weeks.
2. Short term (3–6 weeks)
   a. Patients with recent occlusion of the ICA, MCA, vertebral, or basilar arteries.

Platelet Antiaggregants (Aspirin, Ticlopidine, Clopidogrel)
1. Patients with plaque disease of the extracranial and intracranial arteries without severe stenosis.
2. Patients with polycythemia or thrombocytosis and related ischemic attacks.

APTT, activated partial thromboplastin time; ICA, internal carotid artery; INR, international normalized ratio; MCA, middle cerebral artery.

which depends on the location and severity of the causative vascular lesions. Carotid endarterectomy (CEA) is effective in symptomatic patients with severe ICA stenosis (>70 percent). For patients with carotid stenosis <50 percent, these trials showed there was no significant benefit from CEA. For those with carotid stenosis in the moderate category (50–69 percent), the relative and absolute risk reductions were less impressive than for those in the severely stenotic group.[298–301]

The Asymptomatic Carotid Artery Study (ACAS) suggested that carotid endarterectomy is slightly better than medical therapy in asymptomatic patients with severe carotid stenosis when the operation is executed by surgeons who have records of very low surgical morbidity and mortality.[302] To be effective, the operative mortality and morbidity of CEA must be ≥ 2 to 4 percent.[298–302] Surgery is also feasible on the extracranial vertebral artery in selected patients with intraarterial embolism from this site or with intractable posterior circulation hemodynamic ischemia, a rare occurrence.[303]

Data on carotid (artery balloon) angioplasty and stenting (CAS) is emerging. The Wallstent Trial randomized 219 symptomatic patients with 60 to 90 percent stenosis to either CEA or CAS. In this early study, CAS was performed without distal protection, without antiplatelet prophylaxis, and study design also allowed operators with limited experience to participate. The risk of perioperative stroke or death was 4.5 percent for CEA and 12.1 percent for CAS; 1-year risk of major stroke and death was 0.9 percent for CEA and 3.7 percent for CAS. The Carotid and Vertebral Artery Transluminal Angioplasty Study (CAVATAS), comparing CAS to CEA, did not find a difference in the rate of ipsilateral ischemic stroke up to 3 years after randomization. More recently, the Stenting and Angioplasty With Protection in Patients at High Risk for Endarterectomy (SAPPHIRE) trial randomized 334 patients to CAS or CEA. Distal protection devices were used, and study operators had a periprocedural stroke, death, or MI complication rate of 4 percent or less. Thirty percent of the study population was symptomatic. Results revealed that CAS did not appear to be inferior to CEA, with a benefit of lower MI risk being detected in the CAS group.[13,304–306]

With regard to medical therapy, for minor and moderate degrees of stenosis in extra- and intracranial arteries, agents that alter platelet aggregation and adhesion are recommended. The most likely mechanism of ischemia in these patients is *white clot*, or platelet fibrin emboli. Aspirin,[307,308] ticlopidine,[309,310] clopidogrel,[311] and Aggrenox (a tablet containing 25 mg aspirin and 200 mg of modified-release dipyridamole given 2 times a day)[312] have all proven effective in randomized trials that contained large numbers of patients with TIAs and minor strokes. Recently, the results of the Management of Atherothrombosis With Clopidogrel in High-Risk Patients (MATCH) with TIA or Stroke trial were reported. Patients with a prior stroke or TIA (*n* = 7599) were assigned to either clopidogrel 75 mg daily or combination therapy (clopidogrel 75 mg daily plus aspirin 75 mg daily). Primary outcomes observed included ischemic stroke, MI, vascular death, or rehospitalization caused by ischemic event. There was no significant benefit observed in the combination group compared to clopidogrel alone; the risk of major hemorrhage was also increased in the combination therapy group. Thus, although clopidogrel plus aspirin is recommended over aspirin alone for acute coronary syndromes, the MATCH results do not suggest a similar benefit for stroke and TIA patients.[13,313] Clopidogrel is as effective as ticlopidine and has fewer serious hematologic complications.[311]

For patients with severe stenosis of large intracranial arteries, we previously recommended warfarin if there were no contraindications. The randomized, double-blind, multicenter trial Warfarin-Aspirin Recurrent Stroke Study (WARSS) compared the efficacy of aspirin with warfarin (INR 1.4–2.8) for the prevention of secondary ischemic stroke caused by noncardioembolic sources (*n* = 2206). Various subgroups, including large-artery atherosclerotic lesions, were evaluated. No significant difference between aspirin and warfarin for secondary stroke prevention or death were found. However, patients treated with warfarin in whom the INRs were in target range had significantly less strokes than those treated with aspirin. Given the cost of monitoring warfarin plus the potential increase in bleeding risk with warfarin use, the authors recommended that antiplatelets be chosen over anticoagulants for stroke prevention in patients with prior noncardioembolic strokes.[13,314]

The state of the intracranial arteries can be monitored using TCD and/or MRA or CTA.[293] For patients with complete occlusions and with stump-emboli induced ischemic strokes, we still recommend heparin and then warfarin 2 to 3 months.[5] Heparin should be used without a bolus, and target INR with warfarin should be 2.0 to 3.0.

Thrombolytic drugs, especially recombinant tissue-type plasminogen activator (rt-PA) and streptokinase, have been given intravenously and intraarterially in patients with acute brain ischemia. In a study in which the arterial lesions were undefined, intravenous therapy with rt-PA given within 90 minutes and 3 hours of ischemia onset, in the aggregate, provided a statistically significant benefit.[315] Unfortunately, in this and other studies approximately 6 to 12 percent of patients treated with thrombolytic agents developed important intracranial bleeding. Uncontrolled studies show that patients with distal intracranial arterial embolic occlusions do well with intravenous thrombolytic therapy.[316–321] Patients with ICA occlusions in the neck and intracranially rarely reperfuse after intravenous thrombolytic therapy, especially if collateral circulation is poor. Intraarterially administered prourokinase thrombolysis has also been proven to be very effective in opening blocked intracranial arteries within the anterior circulation.[322] The dose, timing, mode of delivery, and target group for therapy remain unsettled. The authors believe vascular imaging should precede administration of thrombolytic agents. Brain and vascular imaging can guide physicians as to who should receive thrombolytics and by what route.[323]

Because all patients with atherosclerosis are at risk of developing more lesions, control of risk factors is very important and should be begun in the hospital. Risk factors include smoking, hyperlipidemia, obesity, inactivity, and hypertension. Blood pressure should not be excessively lowered during the acute ischemic period as this may decrease flow in collateral arteries. Blood pressure control can be instituted 3 to 4 weeks after the stroke. Rehabilitation must also begin early.

【 】 MANAGEMENT OF COEXISTING CORONARY AND CEREBROVASCULAR DISEASE

In patients considered for cardiac surgery who have symptoms of brain ischemia, it is important to define the extent of cerebrovas-

cular disease preoperatively by noninvasive means (ultrasound and/or MRA), as well as to define cardiac and coronary artery anatomy and function. In some patients with excessive surgical risks, anticoagulation may represent an alternative treatment. Clearly, optimal medical therapy should be instituted preoperatively and continued after surgery.

【 】 SYSTEMIC ARTERIAL HYPERTENSION

High blood pressure, both acute and chronic, damages deep, penetrating small intracranial arteries; accelerates the development of atherosclerosis in the extracranial and large intracranial arteries; and results in ischemic syndromes of lacunar infarction,[5,321,322] diffuse ischemic changes in white matter and basal gray matter structures (Binswanger disease[5,323]), and intracerebral hemorrhage. Hypertension is also frequent in patients with aneurysmal SAH and may contribute to enlargement and rupture of aneurysms.

Hypertension especially damages the deep arteries that penetrate perpendicularly from the major intracranial arteries (Fig. 106–9). Serial sections of these arteries in patients with hypertension show characteristic abnormalities consisting of focal microaneurysmal enlargements and small hemorrhagic extravasations through the arterial walls. The media are often considerably thickened. In places the vessels are often replaced by whorls, tangles, and wisps of connective tissue that completely obliterate the usual vascular layers, causing segmental arterial disorganization as a consequence of lipohyalinosis and fibrinoid degeneration.[5,324,325] Microaneurysms are common in patients with hypertensive intracerebral hemorrhages and in hypertensive older patients.[326–330]

The two major patterns of brain ischemia in patients with hypertension are *discrete lacunar infarcts* and a more *diffuse, patchy, white and gray matter degeneration with gliosis*. Both are caused by sclerotic changes in deep intracerebral arteries and arterioles. The term *lacune* (hole) refers to a small, deep infarct caused by lipohyalinosis of the penetrating artery feeding the ischemic brain tissue.[324,325,331,332] Amyloid angiopathy can also cause small, deep infarcts in normotensive and hypertensive patients. Single lacunes cause discrete clinical syndromes.[5,333,334] The

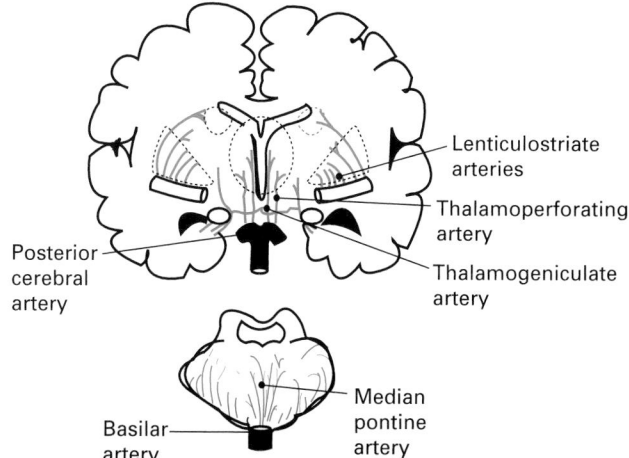

FIGURE 106–9. Deep penetrating arteries prone to the development of lipohyalinosis and microaneurysms (*dark blue*). Occlusion of these arteries causes lacunar infarcts, and rupture of these arteries causes intracerebral hemorrhage. *Source: From Caplan LR.[5] With permission.*

most common syndromes are pure motor hemiparesis,[335] pure sensory stroke,[336] ataxic hemiparesis,[337] and the dysarthria–clumsy hand syndrome.[338]

Since the advent of CT and MRI, it has become widely appreciated that hypertensive patients with lacunes often have more diffuse changes in the white matter of the brain, referred to as *leukoariosis*.[323,339] The clinical picture consists of acute strokes; subacute progression of neurologic signs; dementia, slow shuffling gait disorder; parkinsonian, pyramidal, and pseudobulbar signs.[323,340,341] The clinical signs and gross pathology are identical to those partially described by Otto Binswanger in 1894 and 1895[340] and by his students Alzheimer and Nissl.[340] The deep arteries are thickened and hyalinized and show lipohyalinosis and sometimes amyloid angiopathy in regions of white matter atrophy and gliosis. Invariably, lacunar infarcts are also found. The pathogenesis most likely is related to diffuse vascular narrowing in deep arteries and altered microvascular flow and perfusion. The diagnosis is made on the basis of the clinical findings, the CT and MRI abnormalities, and the absence of cortical infarcts, larger artery occlusive disease, or cardioembolic sources.

Hypertensive Intracerebral Hemorrhage

Intracerebral hemorrhage (ICH) accounts for about 10 percent of all strokes.[5,6] Head trauma, vascular malformations, bleeding diatheses, drugs (especially anticoagulants, amphetamines, and cocaine), amyloid angiopathy, and intracranial aneurysms account for some cases.[326,342] Traditionally, spontaneous ICH has usually been equated with hypertensive hemorrhage. Many patients, however, have no history of hypertension or associated changes of hypertensive vasculopathy at necropsy.[230,326,343,344] Acute elevations of blood pressure and/or blood flow to the brain (Table 106–4) can cause ICH by the sudden increase in blood pressure, causing breakage of capillaries and arterioles.[226,330]

Hypertensive ICH issues from the deep penetrating arteries, so the locations parallel the distribution of these arteries. Hematomas develop in the same sites as lacunes; the most frequent locations are the putamen/internal capsule (30–40 percent), caudate nu-

cleus (8 percent), lobar white matter (20 percent), thalamus (15 percent), pons (10 percent), and cerebellum (10 percent).[326] In fatal hematomas microaneurysms and lipohyalinosis are prevalent in penetrating arteries, but the hematomas obscure findings in the middle of the lesions.[345] Arterioles or capillaries rupture in the center of the lesion, suddenly increasing local tissue pressure and leading to pressure on adjacent capillaries, which then rupture. As the hematoma gradually grows on its periphery (Fig. 106–10), local tissue pressure and finally intracranial pressure increase until the hematoma is contained. Alternatively, the pressure is decompressed by the lesion emptying into the ventricular system or into the subarachnoid space on the brain surface.[5]

Clinical Findings Patients with ICH most often have a gradual evolution of neurologic signs.[326] The first neurologic signs are related to the bleeding site (e.g., left putaminal hematoma patients might first notice right arm weakness or numbness), whereas cerebellar hematoma patients feel off balance. As the hematoma grows, focal signs worsen. When and if the hematoma increases sufficiently in size to increase intracranial pressure, headache, vomiting, and decreased levels of alertness develop.[326] In the presence of small, restricted hemorrhages, headache is absent and the patient remains alert. The course and findings mimic so-called *progressing ischemic stroke.* Headache is absent or not a very prominent symptom in more than half of patients with ICH. Loss of consciousness is a bad prognostic sign when present.

Diagnosis Noncontrast CT, MR-GRE, and MR-susceptibility imaging accurately show the location, size, shape, and extent of acute intracerebral hemorrhages.[346] The presence of ventricular and surface drainage, surrounding edema, and pressure shifts in surrounding tissues are also demonstrated. Routine MRI (without MR susceptibility or GRE sequences) in the patient with an acute hematoma is more difficult to interpret. MRI is superior to CT in imaging arteriovenous malformations and cavernous angiomas. Lumbar puncture is seldom warranted. Atypical location, absence of hypertension, and abnormal vascular echoes on MRI are indications for angiography.

Prognosis and Treatment Coma, increased intracranial pressure, and large hematoma size (>3 cm in one dimension on CT) all indicate a poor prognosis.[326,347] Ordinarily, severe systemic hypertension should be reduced, but not excessively. Patients with ICH can die from raised intracranial pressure. To perfuse the brain and maintain an arteriovenous pressure gradient, the systemic arterial pressure must rise. Overzealous reduction of systemic blood

> **TABLE 106–4**
>
> **Causes of Acute Changes in Blood Pressure or Blood Flow That Can Result in Intracerebral Hemorrhage**
>
> Drugs, especially cocaine and amphetamines
> Recent onset of arterial hypertension
> Pheochromocytoma
> Cold hemorrhages (exposure to freezing ambient temperatures)
> Dental chair hemorrhages
> Intracranial operations on the fifth cranial nerve
> Stereotactic treatment of the fifth cranial nerve for trigeminal neuralgia
> Carotid endarterectomy (reflex hypertension and reperfusion)
> Cardiac transplantation, especially in children
> Surgical repair of congenital heart disease in children
> Migraine

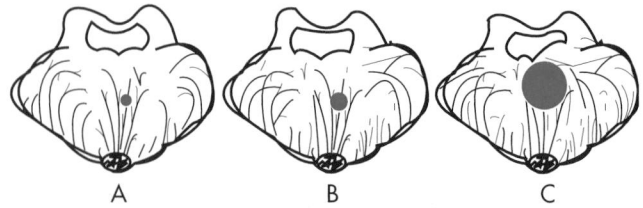

FIGURE 106–10. Gradual evolution of a hypertensive pontine intracerebral hematoma. **A.** The earliest leakage of blood from a paramedian penetrating artery. **B, C.** The hematoma has grown. *Source: From Caplan LR.[5] With permission.*

pressure can cause clinical deterioration. The patient's state of alertness and neurologic signs should be carefully monitored, together with the blood pressure.

Recent hematomas in the cerebral lobes, cerebellum, and right putamen are sometimes drained surgically without leaving a major deficit, at times using stereotactic equipment with CT guidance. The indications for drainage are increased intracranial pressure and the presence of lesions that require removal (tumor, arteriovenous malformations, aneurysm).[326] When hematomas resolve, they leave a cavity disconnecting but not destroying the overlying cortex.

Small hematomas usually resolve well without specific therapy except blood pressure control, whereas massive hematomas usually kill or maim patients before they can be treated. Medium-sized hematomas (2–4 cm), which increase intracranial pressure and cause worsening signs or decreased consciousness while patients are under observation, are indications for drainage if the hematoma is favorably located.

SUBARACHNOID HEMORRHAGE

SAH is not directly caused by hypertension in most cases, although an abrupt increase in blood pressure (e.g., caused by cocaine or amphetamines) can sometimes lead to SAH, as can a bleeding diathesis, trauma, and amyloid angiopathy. The most frequent lesions causing SAH are abnormal vessels such as aneurysms and vascular malformations on or near the surface of the brain. SAH describes bleeding directly into the subarachnoid space with rapid dissemination into the cerebrospinal fluid (CSF) pathways. Usually blood is suddenly released under systemic arterial pressure, causing an abrupt rise in intracranial pressure and producing headache, vomiting, and interruption of conscious behavior and memory, at least temporarily.[5,348] In some patients the jet and spread of blood cause neckache, backache, or sciatica instead of headache. Patients are usually agitated and restless or sleepy and have a stiff neck.

The most frequent cause of SAH is leakage from a berry aneurysm. Often there has been a past history of a *warning leak,* a sudden-onset headache unusual for the patient that lasts days and prevents normal daily activities.[348,349] Aneurysms are most often located at bifurcations of major intracranial arteries. CT can often suggest the site of rupture if blood is pooled locally near a typical site.[350] Large aneurysms are occasionally visible on contrast-enhanced CT or MRI. CTA and MRA are useful tests for screening for aneurysms.[293] Lumbar puncture is very important in the diagnosis of SAH.[351] The absence of blood in the CSF effectively excludes the diagnosis of SAH if the fluid is examined within 24 hours of the onset of the headache, but bleeds that are very small in volume or older than 72 hours can be missed. The CSF pressure, presence of xanthochromia, and quantification of the hemoglobin and bilirubin content of the CSF by spectrophotometry can help establish and date the bleeding and document increased intracranial pressure.[352]

The two most important complications of aneurysmal SAH are rebleeding and brain ischemia caused by vasoconstriction (so-called vasospasm). Once an aneurysm has ruptured either a tiny cap of platelets and fibrin seals the point of rupture or continued bleeding leads to death. Lysis of the fibrin cap initiates rebleeding. Surgical clipping of the aneurysmal sac or obliteration of the aneurysm by endovascular use of balloons or other devices should be attempted before rebleeding occurs.

Vasoconstriction of arteries is thought to be caused by blood or blood products that bathe the adventitia of arteries.[352–355] In the presence of a large accumulation of blood, there is a much higher incidence of arterial vasoconstriction and resultant brain ischemia and infarction. Delayed ischemia can also develop after surgery, as manipulation of vessels can precipitate vasoconstriction. The clinical findings in patients with vasoconstriction confirmed by angiography are often those of diffuse brain swelling, such as headache, decreased alertness, and confusion. When vasoconstriction is focal, the clinical findings are those of focal ischemia, such as hemiparesis, aphasia, hemianopia, and so on. Vasoconstriction usually has its onset 3 to 5 days after hemorrhage. The peak time for constriction is days 5 to 9; vasoconstriction usually improves after the second week unless rebleeding occurs.[356]

Vasoconstriction is detected by angiography in 30 to 70 percent of patients with SAH, depending on the timing of the study.[352,353] Severe vasoconstriction is manifested by a lumen size of <0.5 mm, delayed anterograde flow, and evidence of collateral filling distal to the vasoconstricted vessel. TCD is effective in monitoring for the presence of vasoconstriction.[357,358] Single-photon emission computed tomography (SPECT) can also show regions of poor perfusion and delayed ischemia.[359]

Many treatments have been tried to prevent or treat vasoconstriction after SAH[355]; including removal of blood by lumbar puncture and at the time of early surgery, pharmacologic agents such as calcium channel blockers to minimize contraction of the arterial wall, and hypervolemia to prevent ischemia by maintaining perfusion. At present, the most popular approaches are early surgery, nimodipine (a calcium channel blocker), and hypervolemic therapy, especially after aneurysmal clipping. Hypovolemia is common after SAH, as is hyponatremia. Hypervolemia does not reverse the vasoconstriction but helps maintain brain perfusion.

COAGULOPATHIES

Hypercoagulability and bleeding caused by decreased coagulability affect most body organs, including the brain and heart. An increased tendency for clotting can be caused by abnormalities of the formed blood elements or serologic factors.[5,360–362] Increased numbers of red blood cells and platelets and qualitative abnormalities such as sickle cell disease can cause intravascular clotting, especially in the presence of dehydration and reduced plasma volume. Excessive platelet activation, or so-called *sticky platelets,* can also explain increased coagulability but has proved hard to measure reliably in vitro.[363,364] The level of β-thromboglobulin is a good marker for platelet activation. Serologic abnormalities may be congenital or acquired. Decreased amounts of natural anticoagulants (antithrombin III, protein C, and protein S), resistance to activated protein C, and prothrombin gene mutations can cause hypercoagulability.[360–362,365] These proteins may be decreased in patients with hypoproteinemia, especially that caused by the nephrotic syndrome and urinary protein loss. Fibrinogen levels and the levels of the various coagulation factors such as factors VIII and XI may also be high in patients with a prothrombotic state. In many of these patients—those on high-dose estrogen birth control pills, pregnant women, and patients with cancer—serologic and standard coagulation tests (in vitro) do not clarify the mechanism of the excessive clotting in vivo. Stroke patients may have serologic evidence of platelet activation and increased fibrin formation but decreased natural fibrinolytic and anticoagulant activity.[361,365]

Measurement of various serum antiphospholipid antibodies elicited considerable interest. The usually measured substances are the so-called *lupus anticoagulant,*[366-368] anticardiolipin antibodies, and β_2-glycoprotein 1 antibodies. Increased activity of antiphospholipid antibodies (APLA) is found in patients with systemic lupus erythematosus, AIDS, giant cell arteritis, and Sneddon syndrome[368-371] (livedo reticularis and strokes), as well as in association with the use of some drugs (e.g., phenytoin, phenothiazines, procainamide, hydralazine, and quinidine). When the APLAs are not associated with other conditions and the patient has clinical evidence of excess clotting, the disorder is considered to be primary and is referred to as the *primary APLA syndrome.*[359-362] Patients with APLAs can have an increased incidence of spontaneous abortions, venous occlusive disease of the legs and pulmonary embolism, brain infarcts (often multiple), thrombocytopenia, and false-positive syphilis serologic tests. Older patients with APLAs often also have important risk factors for stroke.[372-375]

Patients with systemic illnesses often have elevated erythrocyte sedimentation rates, and strokes and pulmonary emboli often follow and complicate MI. Customarily, such brain infarcts have been attributed to cardiogenic embolism, but some undoubtedly are related to thromboses precipitated by increased levels of acute-phase reactant coagulation proteins. Cancer, especially mucinous adenocarcinoma, has been associated with multiple vascular occlusions, large and tiny brain infarcts, and venous and arterial occlusions.[376]

Deficient coagulability can lead to serious intracranial bleeding. The hemorrhage can be into the brain (ICH), cerebrospinal fluid (SAH), or the subdural and epidural compartments. Thrombocytopenia, hemophilia, and leukemia are common conditions leading to intracranial hemorrhage. The most common iatrogenic cause of bleeding is anticoagulation with heparin or warfarin.[326,377] Brain hemorrhage has also been described after fibrinolytic treatment of patients with coronary artery disease[378,379] and after rt-PA infusion to treat cerebrovascular occlusive disease.[315-320]

Anticoagulant-related ICH, a catastrophic complication with high morbidity and mortality, is relatively rare considering the frequency of anticoagulant use. Anticoagulant-related hemorrhages develop more insidiously and evolve more slowly and more often than do other causes of ICH.[321,373] Many are erroneously attributed to brain ischemia. Any patient taking anticoagulants who develops CNS symptoms should be considered to have anticoagulant-related ICH until CT or MRI excludes the diagnosis. The hematoma insidiously increases intracranial pressure. Many patients require surgical drainage of their hematomas to ensure survival. Anticoagulants should be stopped immediately and their effect reversed by fresh frozen plasma or vitamin K. It is probably safe to resume anticoagulation with heparin 7 days to 2 weeks after the ICH if indicated, such as for prophylaxis in patients with mechanical heart valves.[380] In patients treated with fibrinolytic agents, hemorrhages are most often lobar or cerebellar and may be multiple. ICH is more common when there is a past stroke, when

heparin or other agents that affect coagulation are given with or after fibrinolytic agents, and when there is a hemostatic defect secondary to treatment.[379,380]

【 】 ARTERIAL DISSECTION

Aortic dissections involving the innominate or common carotid arteries are a well-known cause of stroke and TIA. Less well known are the syndromes produced by dissections of the extracranial and intracranial cervicocephalic arteries, which are especially likely to occur in young, active individuals without risk factors for atherosclerosis or stroke but after trauma or chiropractic or other neck manipulations. They are also associated with fibromuscular dysplasia, α_1-antitrypsin deficiency, Marfan syndrome, pseudoxanthoma elasticum, and migraine.

Dissections start with a tear in the media and spread longitudinally (Fig. 106–11), often disrupting adventitial fibers or even rupturing through the adventitia to produce an extravascular hematoma and a false or pseudoaneurysm within muscle and connective tissue. Intracranially, such a rupture can produce SAH. Other dissections cause arterial obstruction and secondary thrombosis of the narrowed vascular lumen. Most cerebrovascular dissections occur in the extracranial vessels, particularly the pharyngeal portion of the internal carotid artery and the nuchal vertebral arteries.[5,381-386]

Extracranial dissections produce sharp pain and throbbing headache; brain and retinal ischemic episodes, which may occur in rapid-fire attacks (*carotid allegro*[386]); and pressure on adjacent structures especially cranial nerves X through XII, which exit at the skull base. Strokes, usually from embolization of clots, are common but may have a benign course. Intracranial dissections have a poorer prognosis, often with vascular rupture and SAH. The diagnosis is confirmed by angiography, CT, or MRI. Ultrasound studies can be helpful in suggesting the diagnosis of dissection in the neck.[387]

Treatment typically consists of the use of heparin acutely, followed by warfarin. In patients in whom the dissected artery is initially occluded and remains occluded, warfarin can be stopped

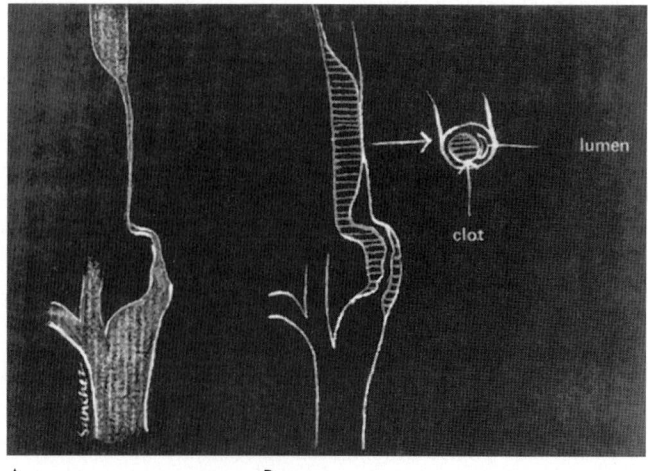

A   B

FIGURE 106–11. Diagrams of a carotid artery dissection. **A.** The intramural clot encroached on the lumen. **B.** The dissection (*crosshatched*). *Source: From Caplan LR.[5] With permission.*

after 6 to 12 weeks. The authors continue warfarin in other patients until there no longer is severe luminal narrowing, monitoring the dissected arteries by noninvasive techniques (ultrasound, CTA, or MRA). Intracranial dissections with SAH have been treated surgically.[382,388,389]

REFERENCES

1. Caplan LR. Brain embolism. In: Caplan LR, Hurst JW, Chimowitz MI, eds. *Clinical Neurocardiology*. New York: Marcel Dekker; 1999:35–185.
2. Aring C, Merritt H. Differential diagnosis between cerebral hemorrhage and cerebral thrombosis. *Arch Intern Med* 1935;56:435–456.
3. Whisnant J, Fitzgibbons J, Kurland L, Sayre GP. Natural history of stroke in Rochester, Minnesota 1945–1954. *Stroke* 1971;2:11–22.
4. Matsumoto N, Whisnant J, Kurland L, Okazaki H. Natural history of stroke in Rochester, Minnesota 1955–1969. *Stroke* 1973;4:2–29.
5. Caplan LR. *Stroke: A Clinical Approach.* 3rd ed. Boston: Butterworth-Heinemann; 2000.
6. Mohr J, Caplan LR, Melski J, et al. The Harvard Cooperative Stroke registry: a prospective study. *Neurology* 1978;28:754–762.
7. Cardiogenic brain embolism. The second report of the Cerebral Embolism Task Force. *Arch Neurol* 1989;46:727–743.
8. Fuster V, Halperin JL. Left ventricular thrombi and cerebral embolism. *N Engl J Med* 1989;320:392–394.
9. Wolf PA, Abbot RD, Kannel WB. Atrial fibrillation: a major contributor to stroke in the elderly. The Framingham study. *Archives of Internal Medicine* 1987;147:1561–1564.
10. Bogousslavsky J, Van Melle G, Regli F. The Lausanne Stroke Registry: analysis of 1000 consecutive patients with first strokes. *Stroke* 1988;19:1083–1092.
11. Bogousslavsky J, Cachin C, Regli F, et al. Cardiac sources of embolism and cerebral infarction: clinical consequences and vascular concomitants. The Lausanne Stroke Registry. *Neurology* 1991;41:855–859.
12. Kittner SJ, Sharkness CM, Sloan M, et al. Infarcts with a cardiac source of embolism in the NINDS Stroke Data Bank: neurologic examination. *Neurology* 1992;42:299–302.
13. Sacco RL, Adams R, Albers G, et al. Guidelines for prevention of stroke in patients with ischemic stroke or transient ischemic attack: a statement for healthcare professionals from the American Heart Association/American Stroke Association Council on Stroke—co-sponsored by the Council on Cardiovascular Radiology and Intervention: the American Academy of Neurology affirms the value of this guideline. *Stroke* 2006;37:577–617.
14. Visser CA, Kan G, Meltzer RS, Lie KI, Durrer D. Long-term follow-up of left ventricular thrombus after acute myocardial infarction: a two-dimensional echocardiographic study in 96 patients. *Chest* 1984;86:532–536.
15. Sacco RL, Shi T, Zamanillo, MC, Kargman DE. Predictors of mortality and recurrence after hospitalized cerebral infarction in an urban community. The Northern Manhattan Stroke Study. *Neurology* 1994;44:626–634.
16. Carter AB. Prognosis of cerebral embolism. *Lancet* 1965;2:514–519.
17. Wood P. *Diseases of the Heart and Circulation*. Philadelphia: JB Lippincott; 1956.
18. Levine HJ. Which atrial fibrillation patients should be on chronic anticoagulation? *J Cardiovasc Med (Hagerstown)* 1981;6:483–487.
19. Friedberg CK. *Diseases of the Heart*. Philadelphia: WB Saunders; 1966.
20. Deverall PB, Olley PM, Smith DR, Watson DA, Whitaker W. Incidence of systemic embolism before and after mitral valvotomy. *Thorax* 1968;23:530–536.
21. Coulshed N, Epstein EJ, McKendrick CS, Galloway RW, Walker E. Systemic embolism in mitral valve disease. *Br Heart J* 1970;32:26–34.
22. Jeresaty RM. *Mitral Valve Prolapse*. New York: Raven Press; 1979.
23. Salem DN, Hartnett Daudelin D, Levine HJ, et al. Antithrombotic therapy in valvular heart disease. *Chest* 2001;119:207S–219S.
24. Barnett HJM, Jones MW, Boughner DR, Kostuk WJ. Cerebral ischemic events associated with prolapsing mitral valve. *Arch Neurol* 1976;33:777–782.
25. Barnett HJM, Boughner DR, Taylor DW, et al. Further evidence relating mitral valve prolapse to cerebral ischemic events. *N Engl J Med* 1980;302:139–144.
26. Sandok BA, Giuliani ER. Cerebral ischemic events in patients with mitral valve prolapse. *Stroke* 1982;13:448–450.
27. Lauzier S, Barnett HJM. Cerebral ischemia with mitral valve prolapse and mitral annulus calcification. In: Furlan AJ, ed. *The Heart and Stroke*. London: Springer-Verlag; 1987:63–100.
28. deBono DP, Warlow CP. Mitral-annulus calcification and cerebral or retinal ischemia. *Lancet* 1979;2:383–385.
29. Korn D, DeSanctis RW, Sell S. Massive calcification of the mitral annulus: a clinicopathological study of fourteen cases. *N Engl J Med* 1962;267:900–909.
30. Benjamin EJ, Plehn JF, D'Agostino RB, et al. Mitral annular calcification and the risk of stroke in an elderly cohort. *N Engl J Med* 1992;327:374–379.
31. Savage DD, Garrison RJ, Castelli WP, et al. Prevalence of submitral (annular) calcium and its correlations in a general population–based sample. The Framingham study. *Am J Cardiol* 1983;51:1375–1378.
32. Debruxelles S, Sibon I, Rouanet F, Orgogozo JM. Cerebral infarction by calcified embolism: a spontaneous complication of calcified aortic stenosis. *Rev Neurol* 2004;160:582–584.
33. Boon A, Lodder J, Cheriex E, Kessels F. Risk of stroke in a cohort of 815 patients with calcification of the aortic valve with or without stenosis. *Stroke* 1996;27:847–851.
34. Sacco RL, Ellenberg JH, Mohr JP, et al. Infarcts of undetermined cause: the NINCDS Stroke Data Bank. *Ann Neurol* 1989;25:382–390.
35. Mohr JP. Infarct of unclear cause. In: Furlan AJ, ed. *The Heart and Stroke*. London: Springer-Verlag; 1987:101–116.
36. Galve E, Candell-Riera J, Pigrau C, et al. Prevalence, morphology, types and evaluation of cardiac valvular disease in systemic lupus erythematosus. *N Engl J Med* 1988;319:817–823.
37. Barbut D, Borer JS, Wallerson D, et al. Anticardiolipin antibody and stroke: possible relation of valvular heart disease and embolic events. *Cardiology* 1991;79:99–109.
38. Nighoghossian N, Derex L, Loire R, et al. Giant Lambl excrescences: an unusual source of cerebral embolism. *Arch Neurol* 1997;54:41–44.
39. Cohen A, Tzourio C, Chauvel C, et al. Mitral valve strands and the risk of ischemic stroke in elderly patients. *Stroke* 1997;28:1574–1578.
40. Caplan LR. Mitral valve strands: what are they and what is their relation to stroke? *Neurol Network Comment* 1998;2:11–14.
41. Kanter MC, Hart RG. Neurologic complications of infective endocarditis. *Neurology* 1991;41:1015–1020.
42. Caplan LR. Of birds and nests and brain emboli. *Rev Neurol (Paris)* 1991;147:265–273.
43. Amarenco P, Duyckaerts C, Tzourio C, et al. The prevalence of ulcerated plaques in the aortic arch in patients with stroke. *N Engl J Med* 1992;326:221–225.
44. Amarenco P, Cohan A, Baudrimont M, Bousser M-G. Transesophageal echocardiographic detection of aortic arch disease in patients with cerebral infarction. *Stroke* 1992;23:1056–1061.
45. Weinberger J, Azhar S, Danisi F, et al. A new noninvasive technique for imaging atherosclerotic plaque in the aortic arch of stroke patients by transcutaneous real-time B-mode ultrasonography. *Stroke* 1998;29:673–676.
46. The French Study of Aortic Plaques in Stroke Group. Atherosclerotic disease of the aortic arch as a risk factor for recurrent ischemic stroke. *N Engl J Med* 1996;334:1216–1221.
47. Dressler F, Craig W, Castello R, Labovitz AJ. Mobile aortic atheroma and systemic emboli: efficacy of anticoagulation and influence of plaques morphology on recurrent stroke. *J Am Coll Cardiol* 1998;31:134–138.
48. Ferrari E, Vidal R, Chevallier T, Baudouy M. Atherosclerosis of the thoracic aorta and systemic emboli: efficacy of anticoagulation and influence of plaque morphology on recurrent stroke. *J Am Cardiol* 1999;33:1317–1322.
49. Fisher CM, Perlman A. The nonsudden onset of a cerebral embolism. *Neurology* 1967;17:1025–1032.
50. Fieschi C, Argentino C, Lenzi GL, et al. Clinical and instrumental evaluation of patients with ischemic stroke within the first six hours. *J Neurol Sci* 1989;91:311–322.
51. Kushner MJ, Zanotte EM, Bastianiello S, et al. Transcranial Doppler in acute hemispheric brain infarction. *Neurology* 1991;41:109–113.
52. Ringlestein EB, Koschorke S, Holling A, et al. Computed tomographic patterns of proven embolic brain infarcts. *Ann Neurol* 1989;26:759–765.
53. Bladin PF, Berkovic SF. Striatocapsular infarction. *Neurology* 1984;34:1423–1430.
54. Fisher CM, Adams RD. Observations on brain embolism. *J Neuropathol Exp Neurol* 1951;10:92–94.
55. Fisher CM, Adams RD. Observations on brain embolism with special reference to hemorrhagic infarction. In: Furlan AJ, ed. *The Heart and Stroke*. London: Springer-Verlag; 1987:17–36.
56. Gacs G, Fox AJ, Barnett HJ, Vinuela F. CT visualization of intracranial arterial thromboembolism. *Stroke* 1983;14:756–763.
57. Tomsick T, Brott T, Barsan W, et al. Thrombus localization with emergency cerebral computed tomography. *Stroke* 1990;21:180.

58. Bergeron GA, Shah PM. Echocardiography unwarranted in patients with cerebral ischemic events. *N Engl J Med* 1981;304:489.

59. Greenland P, Knopman D, Mikell F, et al. Echocardiography in diagnostic assessment of stroke. *Ann Intern Med* 1981;95:51–54.

60. Donaldson R, Emmanuel R, Earl C. The role of two-dimensional echocardiography in the detection of potentially embolic intracardiac masses in patients with cerebral ischemia. *J Neurol Neurosurg Psychiatry* 1981;44:803–809.

61. Tegeler CH, Downes TR. Cardiac imaging in stroke. *Stroke* 1991;22:1206–1211.

62. Pop G, Sutherland GR, Koudstaal PJ, et al. Transesophageal echocardiography in the detection of intracardiac embolic sources in patients with transient ischemic attacks. *Stroke* 1990;21:560–565.

63. Zenker G, Ecbel R, Kramer G, et al. Transesophageal echocardiography in young patients with cerebral ischemic events. *Stroke* 1988;19:345–348.

64. Cohen A, Chauvel C. Transesophageal echocardiography in the management of transient ischemic attack and ischemic stroke. *Cerebrovasc Dis* 1996;6(suppl 1):15–25.

65. Kase CS, White R, Vinson TL, Eichelberger RP. Shotgun pellet embolus to the middle cerebral artery. *Neurology* 1981;31:458–461.

66. DeWitt LD, Pessin MS, Pandian NG, et al. Benign disappearance of ventricular thrombus after embolic stroke: a case report. *Stroke* 1988;19:393–396.

67. Ezekowitz MD, Wilson DA, Smith EO, et al. Comparison of indium-III platelet scintigraphy and two-dimensional echocardiography in the diagnosis of left ventricular thrombi. *N Engl J Med* 1982;306:1509–1513.

68. Markus HS, Droste DW, Brown MM. Detection of symptomatic cerebral embolic signals with Doppler ultrasound. *Lancet* 1994;343:1011–1012.

69. Markus HS, Harrison MJ. Microembolic signal detection using ultrasound. *Stroke* 1995;26:1517–1519.

70. Tong DC, Bolger A, Albers GW. Incidence of transcranial Doppler-detected cerebral microemboli in patients referred for echocardiography. *Stroke* 1994;25:2138–2141.

71. Barbut D, Hinton RB, Szatrowski TP, et al. Cerebral emboli detected during bypass surgery are associated with clamp removal. *Stroke* 1994;25:2398–2402.

72. Nabavi DG, Georgiadis D, Mumme T, et al. Clinical relevance of intracranial microembolic signals in patients with left ventricular assist devices: a prospective study. *Stroke* 1996;27:891–896.

73. Petersen P, Boysen G, Godtfredsen J, et al. Placebo-controlled, randomized trial of warfarin and aspirin for prevention of thromboembolic complications in chronic atrial fibrillation. The Copenhagen AFASAK Study. *Lancet* 1989;1:175–179.

74. Stroke Prevention in Atrial Fibrillation Study Group Investigators. Preliminary report of the Stroke Prevention in Atrial Fibrillation Study. *N Engl J Med* 1990;322:863–868.

75. Stroke Prevention in Atrial Fibrillation Investigators. The Stroke Prevention in Atrial Fibrillation Trial: final results. *Circulation* 1991;84:527–539.

76. Stroke Prevention in Atrial Fibrillation Investigators. Adjusted-dose warfarin versus low-intensity fixed-dose warfarin plus aspirin for high-risk patients with atrial fibrillation. Stroke Prevention in Atrial Fibrillation III randomized clinical trial. *Lancet* 1996:348:633–638.

77. Stroke Prevention in Atrial Fibrillation Investigators. Prospective identification of patients with nonvalvular atrial fibrillation at low risk during treatment with aspirin: Stroke Prevention in Atrial Fibrillation III Study [abstract]. *Circulation* 1997;96(suppl) I–28.

78. Stroke Prevention in Atrial Fibrillation Investigators. Predictors of thromboembolism in atrial fibrillation: I. Clinical features of patients at risk. *Ann Intern Med* 1992;116:1–5.

79. Stroke Prevention in Atrial Fibrillation Investigators. Predictors of thromboembolism in atrial fibrillation: II. Echocardiographic features of patients at risk. *Ann Intern Med* 1992;116:6–12.

80. Pritchett ELC. Management of atrial fibrillation. *N Engl J Med* 1992;326:1264–1271.

81. Ezekowitz MD, Bridgers SL, James KE, et al. Randomized trials of warfarin for atrial fibrillation. *N Engl J Med* 1992;327:1451–1453.

82. Boston Area Anticoagulation Trial for Atrial Fibrillation Investigators. The effect of low-dose warfarin on the risk of stroke in patients with nonrheumatic atrial fibrillation. *N Engl J Med* 1990;323:1505–1511.

83. Connolly SJ, Laupacis A, Gent M, et al. Canadian Atrial Fibrillation Anticoagulation (CAFA) study. *J Am Coll Cardiol* 1991;18:349–355.

84. European Atrial Fibrillation Trial Study Group. Optimal oral anticoagulation therapy in patients with nonrheumatic atrial fibrillation and recent cerebral ischemia. *N Engl J Med* 1995;333:5–10.

85. Halperin JL. Ximelagatran compared with warfarin for prevention of thromboembolism in patients with nonvalvular atrial fibrillation: rationale, objectives, and design of a pair of clinical studies and baseline patient characteristics (SPORTIF II and V). *Am Heart J* 2003;146:431–438.

86. Braunwald E, Antman EM, Beasley JW, et al. ACC/AHA 2002 guideline update for the management of patients with unstable angina and non-ST segment elevation myocardial infarction: summary article: a report of the American College of Cardiology/American Heart Association Task Force on Practice guidelines. *J Am Coll Cardiol* 2002;40:1366–1374.

87. Moldveen-Geronimus M, Merriam JC. Cholesterol embolization: from pathologic curiosity to clinical entity. *Circulation* 1967;35:946–953.

88. Shields RW Jr, Laureno R, Lachman T, Victor M. Anticoagulant-related hemorrhage in acute cerebral embolism. *Stroke* 1984;15:426–437.

89. Lieberman A, Hass WK, Pinto R, et al. Intracranial hemorrhage and infarction in anticoagulated patients with prosthetic heart valves. *Stroke* 1978;9:18–24.

90. Drake ME, Shin C. Conversion of ischemic to hemorrhagic infarction by anticoagulant administration: report of two cases with evidence from serial computed tomographic brain scans. *Arch Neurol* 1983;40:44–46.

91. Cerebral Embolism Study Group. Immediate anticoagulation of embolic stroke: a randomized trial. *Stroke* 1983;13:668–676.

92. Toni D, Fiorelli M, Bastianello S, et al. Hemorrhagic transformation of brain infarct. *Neurology* 1996;46:341–345.

93. Cerebral Embolism Task Force. Cardiogenic brain embolism. *Arch Neurol* 1986;43:71–84.

94. Cerebral Embolism Task Force. Cardiogenic brain embolism: the second report of the Cerebral Embolism Task Force. *Arch Neurol* 1989;46:727–743.

95. Pessin MS, Estol CJ, Lafranchise F, Caplan LR. Safety of anticoagulation after hemorrhagic infarction. *Neurology* 1993;43:1298–1303.

96. Chaves CJ, Pessin MS, Caplan LR, et al. Cerebellar hemorrhagic infarction. *Neurology* 1996;46:346–349.

97. Chamorro A, Vila N, Ascaso C, Blanc R. Heparin in acute stroke with atrial fibrillation. Clinical relevance of very early treatment. *Arch Neurol* 1999;56:1098–1102.

98. Caplan LR. When should heparin be given to patients with atrial fibrillation–related brain infarcts. *Arch Neurol* 1999;56:1059–1060.

99. Hagen PT, Scholz DG, Edwards WD. Incidence and size of patent foramen ovale during the first 10 decades of life: an autopsy study of 965 normal hearts. *Mayo Clin Proc* 1984;59:17–20.

100. Lechat PH, Mas JL, Lascault G, et al. Prevalence of patent foramen ovale in patients with stroke. *N Engl J Med* 1988;318:1148–1152.

101. Di Tullio M, Sacco RL, Gopal A, et al. Patent foramen ovale as a risk factor for cryptogenic stroke. *Ann Intern Med* 1992;117:461–465.

102. Petty GW, Khanderia BK, Chu C-P, et al. Patent foramen ovale in patients with cerebral infarction: a transesophageal echocardiographic study. *Arch Neurol* 1997;54:819–822.

103. Webster MW, Chancellor AM, Smith HJ, et al. Patent foramen ovale in young stroke patients. *Lancet* 1988;2:11–12.

104. Steiner MM, Di Tullio MR, Rundek T, et al. Patent foramen ovale size and embolic brain imaging findings among patients with ischemic stroke. *Stroke* 1998;29:944–948.

105. Jones HR, Caplan LR, Come PC, et al. Cerebral emboli of paradoxical origin. *Ann Neurol* 1983;13:314–319.

106. Biller J, Adams HP, Johnson MR, et al. Paradoxical cerebral embolism: eight cases. *Neurology* 1986;36:1356–1360.

107. Gautier JC, Durr A, Koussa S, et al. Paradoxical cerebral embolism with a patent foramen ovale: a report of 29 patients. *Cerebrovasc Dis* 1991;1:193–202.

108. Khairy P, O'Donnell CP, Landzberg MJ. Transcatheter closure versus medical therapy of patent foramen ovale and presumed paradoxical thromboemboli: a systemic review. *Ann Intern Med* 2003;139:753–760.

109. Caplan LR. Cardiac arrest and other hypoxic-ischemic insults. In: Caplan LR, Hurst JW, Chimowitz MI, eds. *Clinical Neurocardiology.* New York: Marcel Dekker; 1999:1–34.

110. Brierley J, Meldrum B, Brown A. The threshold and neuropathology of cerebral "anoxic-ischemic" cell change. *Arch Neurol* 1973;29:367–373.

111. Brierley JB, Adams JH, Graham DI, Simpson JA. Neocortical death after cardiac arrest: a clinical, neurophysiological report of two cases. *Lancet* 1971;2:560–565.

112. Dougherty JH, Rawlinson DG, Levy DE, Plum F. Hypoxic-ischemic brain injury and the vegetative state: clinical and neuropathologic correlation. *Neurology* 1981;31:991–997.

113. Cummings JL, Tomiyasu U, Read S, Benson DF. Amnesia with hippocampal lesions after cardiopulmonary arrest. *Neurology* 1984;34:679–681.

114. Dooling E, Richardson EP. Delayed encephalopathy after strangling. *Arch Neurol* 1976;33:196–199.

115. Lance J, Adams RD. The syndrome of intention and action myoclonus as a sequel to hypoxic encephalopathy. *Brain* 1963;86:111–133.

116. Gilles F. Hypotensive brainstem necrosis. *Arch Pathol* 1969;88:32–41.

117. Silver JR, Buxton PH. Spinal stroke. *Brain* 1974;97:539–550.

118. Caronna JJ, Finkelstein S. Neurological syndromes after cardiac arrest. *Stroke* 1978;9:517–520.

119. Jennett B, Plum F. Persistent vegetative state after brain damage: a syndrome in search of a name. *Lancet* 1972;1:734–737.

120. Levy DE, Knill-Jones RP, Plum F. The vegetative state and its prognosis following non-traumatic coma. *Ann NY Acad Sci* 1978;315:293–306.

121. Hecaen H, Ajuriaguerra J. Balint's syndrome and its minor forms. *Brain* 1954;77:373–400.

122. Willoughby J, Leach B. Relation of neurological findings after cardiac arrest to outcome. *BMJ* 1974;3:437–439.

123. Plum F, Caronna J. Can one predict outcome of medical coma? In: *Outcome of Severe Damage to the Central Nervous System. A CIBA Foundation Symposium*. New York: Elsevier; 1975:121–139.

124. Bell JA, Hodgson HJ. Coma after cardiac arrest. *Brain* 1974;97:361–372.

125. Levy D, Carrona JJ, Singer BH, et al. Predicting outcome from hypoxic-ischemic coma. *JAMA* 1985;253:1420–1426.

126. Wijdicks EFM, Parisi JE, Sharbrough FW. Prognostic value of myoclonus status in comatose survivors of cardiac arrest. *Ann Neurol* 1994;35:239–243.

127. Longstreth WT, Inui TS, Cobb LA, Copass MK. Neurologic recovery after out-of-hospital cardiac arrest. *Ann Intern Med* 1983;38:588–592.

128. Longstreth WT, Diehr P, Inui TS. Prediction of awakening after out-of-hospital cardiac arrest. *N Engl J Med* 1983;308:1378–1382.

129. Thompson RG, Hallstrom AP, Cobb LA. Bystander-initiated cardiopulmonary resuscitation in the management of ventricular fibrillation. *Ann Intern Med* 1979;90:737–740.

130. Bedell SE, Delbanco TG, Cook EF, Epstein FH. Survival after cardiopulmonary resuscitation in the hospital. *N Engl J Med* 1983;309:569–576.

131. Caplan LR, Brass LM, DeWitt LD, et al. Transcranial Doppler ultrasound: present status. *Neurology* 1990;40:696–700.

132. Kirkham F, Levin S, Padayachee T, et al. Transcranial pulsed Doppler ultrasound findings in brainstem death. *J Neurol Neurosurg Psychiatry* 1987;50:1504–1513.

133. Ropper A, Kehne S, Wechsler L. Transcranial Doppler in brain death. *Neurology* 1987;37:1733–1735.

134. Longstreth WT, Inui TS. High blood glucose level on hospital admission and poor neurological recovery after cardiac arrest. *Ann Neurol* 1984;15:59–63.

135. Myers C, Yamaguchi S. Nervous system effects of cardiac arrest in monkeys. *Arch Neurol* 1977;34:65–74.

136. Plum F. What causes infarction in ischemic brain. *Neurology* 1983;33:222–233.

137. Collins RC, Dobkin BH, Choi DW. Selective vulnerability of the brain: new insights into the pathophysiology of stroke. *Ann Intern Med* 1989;110:992–1000.

138. Albers G, Goldberg M, Choi D. *N*-methyl-*D*-aspartate antagonists: ready for clinical trial in brain ischemia? *Ann Neurol* 1989;25:398–403.

139. Giswold S, Safar P, Rao G, et al. Multifaceted therapy after global brain ischemia in monkeys. *Stroke* 1984;15:803–812.

140. Caplan LR. Encephalopathies and neurological effects of drugs used in cardiac patients. In: Caplan LR, Hurst JW, Chimowitz MI, eds. *Clinical Neurocardiology*. New York: Marcel Dekker; 1999:186–225.

141. Volpe BT, Soave R. Formal visual hallucinations as digitalis toxicity. *Ann Intern Med* 1979;91:868–869.

142. Closson RG. Visual hallucinations as the earliest symptom of digoxin intoxication. *Arch Neurol* 1983;40:386.

143. Gilbert GJ. Quinidine dementia. *JAMA* 1977;237:2093–2094.

144. Adams HP. Neurologic complications of cardiovascular procedures. In: Biller J, ed. *Iatrogenic Neurology*. Boston: Butterworth-Heinemann; 1998:51–61.

145. Dawson DM, Fischer EG. Neurologic complications of cardiac catheterization. *Neurology* 1977;27:496–497.

146. Mendez Dominguez A, Aguilera R, Martinez Rios MA. Cerebral ischemia: a complication in heart catheterization—an assessment in 2178 catheterizations. *Arch Inst Cardiol Mex* 1993;63:247–251.

147. Nakata A, Sekiguchi Y, Hirota S, et al. Central retinal artery occlusion following cardiac catheterization. *Jpn Heart J* 2002;43:187–192.

148. Liu XY, Wong V, Leung M. Neurologic complications due to catheterization. *Pediatr Neurol* 2001;24:270–275.

149. Colt HG, Begg RJ, Saporito JJ, et al. Cholesterol emboli after cardiac catheterization: eight cases and a review of the literature. *Medicine* 1988;67:389–400.

150. Weissman BM, Aram DM, Levinsohn MW, Ben-Shacher G. Neurologic sequelae of cardiac catheterization. *Catheter Cardiovasc Diagn* 1985;11:577–583.

151. Wijman CA, Kase CS, Jacobs AK, Whitehead RE. Cerebral air embolism as a cause of stroke during cardiac catheterization. *Neurology* 1998;51:318–319.

152. Ramirez G, O'Neill WM Jr, Lambert R, Bloomer HA. Cholesterol embolization: a complication of angiography. *Arch Intern Med* 1978;138:1430–1432.

153. Dorros G, Cowley MJ, Simpson J, et al. Percutaneous transluminal coronary angioplasty: report of complications from the National Heart, Lung, and Blood Institute PTCA Registry. *Circulation* 1983;67:723–730.

154. Akkerhuis KM, Deckers JW, Lincoff AM, et al. Risk of stroke associated with abciximab among patients undergoing percutaneous coronary intervention. *JAMA* 2001;286:78–82.

155. EPIC Investigators. Use of a monoclonal antibody directed against the platelet glycoprotein IIb/IIIa receptor in high-risk coronary angioplasty. *N Engl J Med* 1994;330:956–961.

156. CAPTURE Investigators. Ramdomised placebo-controlled trial of abciximab before and during coronary intervention in refractory unstable angina: the CAPTURE study. *Lancet* 1997;349:1429–1435.

157. EPILOG Investigators. Platelet glycoprotein IIb/IIIa receptor blockade and low-dose heparin during percutaneous coronary revascularization. *N Engl J Med* 1997;336:1689–1696.

158. EPISTENT Investigators. Randomised placebo-controlled and balloon-angioplasty-controlled access safety of coronary stenting with use of platelet glycoprotein-IIb/IIIa blockade. *Lancet* 1998;352:87–92.

159. Galbreath C, Salgado ED, Furlan AJ, Hollman J. Central nervous system complications of percutaneous transluminal coronary angioplasty. *Stroke* 1986;17:616–619.

160. Malenka DJ, O'Rourke D, Miller MA, et al. Cause of in-hospital death in 12,232 consecutive patients undergoing percutaneous transluminal coronary angioplasty. The Northern New England Cardiovascular Disease Study Group. *Am Heart J* 1999;137:632–638.

161. Borger van der Burg AE, de Groot NM, van Erven L, et al. Long-term follow-up after radiofrequency catheter ablation of ventricular tachycardia: a successful approach? *J Cardiovasc Electrophysiol* 2002;13:424–426.

162. Tanel RE, Walsh EP, Triedman JK, et al. Five-year experience with radiofrequency catheter ablation: implications for management of arrhythmias in pediatric and young adult patients. *J Pediatr* 1997;131:878–887.

163. Alvarez M, Merino JL. Spanish registry on catheter ablation: 1st official report of the working group on electrophysiology and arrhythmias of the Spanish Society of Cardiology (Year 2001). *Rev Esp Cardiol* 2002;55:1273–1285.

164. DiMarco JP, Garan H, Ruskin JN. Complications in patients undergoing cardiac electrophysiologic procedures. *Ann Intern Med* 1982;97:490.

165. Arnold AZ, Mick MJ, Mazurek RP, et al. Role of prophylactic anticoagulation for direct current cardioversion in patients with atrial fibrillation or atrial flutter. *J Am Coll Cardiol* 1992;19:851–855.

166. Ewy GA. Optimal technique for electrical cardioversion of atrial fibrillation. *Circulation* 1992;86:1645–1647.

167. Letac B, Cribier A, Koning R, Bellefleur JP. Results of percutaneous transluminal valvuloplasty in 218 adults with valvular aortic stenosis. *Am J Cardiol* 1988;15:62:598–605.

168. Eisenhauer AC, Hadjipetron P, Piemonte TC. Balloon aortic valvuloplasty revisited: the role of the Inoue balloon and transseptal antegrade approach. *Catheter Cardiovasc Interv* 2000;50:484–491.

169. Peixoto EC, de Olivera PS, Netto MS, et al. Percutaneous balloon mitral valvuloplasty. Immediate results, complications, and hospital outcome. *Arq Bras Cardiol* 1995;64:109–116.

170. Peixoto EC, de Olivera PS, Netto MS, et al. Percutaneous mitral valvuloplasty with the single balloon technique: short-term results, complications, and in-hospital follow-up. *Arq Bras Cardiol* 1996;66:267–273.

171. Ho AC, Hong CL, Yang MW, et al. Stroke after intraaortic balloon counterpulsation with mobile atheroma in thoracic aorta diagnosed using transesophageal echocardiography. *Chang Gung Med J* 2002;25:612–616.

172. Barbut D, Caplan LR. Brain complications of cardiac surgery. *Curr Probl Cardiol* 1997;22:455–476.

173. Wolman RL, Nussmeier NA, Aggarwal A, et al. Cerebral injury after cardiac surgery: identification of a group at extraordinary risk. *Stroke* 1999;30:514–522.

174. Baker RA, Hallsworth LJ, Knight JL. Stroke after coronary artery bypass grafting. *Ann Thorac Surg* 2005;80:1746–1750.

175. Ozatik MA, Gol MK, Fansa I, et al. Risk factors for stroke following coronary artery bypass operations. *J Card Surg* 2005;20:52–57.

176. Zakeri R, Freemantle N, Barnett V, et al. Relation between mild renal dysfunction and outcomes after coronary artery bypass grafting. *Circulation* 2005;112(suppl) I270–I275.

177. Bucerius J, Gummert JF, Borger MA, et al. Stroke after cardiac surgery: a risk factor analysis of 16,184 consecutive adult patients. *Ann Thorac Surg* 2003;75:472–478.

178. Naylor AR, Mehta Z, Rothwell PM, et al. Carotid artery disease and stroke during coronary artery bypass: a critical review of the literature. *Eur J Vasc Endovasc Surg* 2002;23:283–294.

179. Bypass Angioplasty Revascularization Investigation (BARI) Investigators. Comparison of coronary bypass surgery with angioplasty in patients with multivessel disease. *N Engl J Med* 1996;335:217–225.

180. King SB, Lembo NJ, Weintrub WS, et al. Emory Angioplasty versus Surgery Trial (EAST). *N Engl J Med* 1994;331:1044–1050.

181. Ricotta JJ, Char DJ, Cuadra SA, et al. Modeling stroke risk after coronary artery bypass and combined coronary artery bypass and carotid endarterectomy. *Stroke* 2003;34:1212–1217.

182. Salzberg SP, Adams DH, Filsoufi F. Coronary artery surgery: conventional coronary artery bypass grafting versus off-pump coronary artery bypass grafting. *Curr Opin Cardiol* 2005;20:509–516.

183. Lund C, Sundet K, Tennoe B, et al. Cerebral ischemic injury and cognitive impairment after off-pump and on-pump coronary artery bypass grafting surgery. *Ann Thorac Surg* 2005;80:2126–2131.

184. Wijeysundera DN, Beattie WS, Djaiani G, et al. Off pump coronary artery surgery for reducing mortality and morbidity: meta-analysis of randomized and observational studies. *J Am Coll Cardiol* 2005;46:872–882.

185. Lamy A, Farrokhyar F, Kent R, et al. The Canadian off-pump coronary artery bypass graft registry: a one-year prospective comparison with on-pump coronary artery bypass grafting. *Can J Cardiol* 2005;21:1175–1181.

186. Panesar SS, Athanasiou T, Nair S, et al. Early outcomes in the elderly: a meta-analysis of 4921 patients undergoing coronary artery bypass grafting—a comparison between off-pump and on-pump techniques. *Heart* December 2006; 92(12):1808–1816. Epub ahead of print June 27, 2006.

187. Van Dijk D, Jansen EW, Hijman R, et al. Octopus Study Group: cognitive outcome after off-pump and on-pump coronary artery bypass graft surgery—a randomized trial. *JAMA* 2002;287:1405–1412.

188. Novick RJ, Fox SA, Stitt LW, et al. Effect of off-pump coronary artery bypass grafting on risk-adjusted and cumulative sum failure outcomes after coronary artery surgery. *J Card Surg* 2002;17:520–528.

189. Lev-Ran O, Braunstein R, Sharony R, et al. No-touch aorta off-pump coronary surgery: the effect on stroke. *J Thorac Cardiovasc Surg* 2005;129:307–313.

190. Roach GW, Kanchuger MS, Mora Mangano CT, et al. Adverse cerebral outcomes after coronary bypass surgery. *N Engl J Med* 1996;335:1857–1863.

191. Gansera B, Angelis I, Weingartner J, et al. Simultaneous carotid endarterectomy and cardiac surgery: additional risk or safety procedure? *J Thorac Cardiovasc Surg* 2003;51:22–27.

192. Sharony R, Grossi EA, Saunders PC, et al. Minimally invasive reoperative isolated valve surgery: early and mid-term results. *J Card Surg* 2006;21:240–244.

193. Aklog L, Adams DH, Couper GS, et al. Techniques and results of direct-access minimally invasive mitral valve surgery: a paradigm for the future. *J Thorac Cardiovasc Surg* 1998;116:705–715.

194. Shaw PJ, Bates D, Cartlidge NEF, et al. Early neurological complications of coronary artery bypass surgery. *Br Med J* 1985;291:1384–1387.

195. Breuer AC, Furlan AJ, Hanson MR, et al. Central nervous system complications of coronary artery bypass graft surgery: prospective analysis of 421 patients. *Stroke* 1983;14:682–687.

196. Ropper AH, Wechsler LR, Wilson LS. Carotid bruit and the risk of stroke in elective surgery. *N Engl J Med* 1982;307:1388–1390.

197. Furlan AJ, Craciun AR. Risk of stroke during coronary artery bypass graft surgery in patients with internal carotid artery disease documented by angiography. *Stroke* 1985;16:797–799.

198. Sila C. Neuroimaging of cerebral infarction associated with coronary revascularization. *AJNR Am J Neuroradiol* 1991;12:817–818.

199. Hertzer NR, Loop FD, Beven EG, et al. Surgical staging for simultaneous coronary and carotid disease: A study including prospective randomization. *Vasc Surg* 1989;9:455–463.

200. Naylor AR, Cuffe RL, Rothwell PM, Bell PR. A systematic review of outcomes following staged and synchronous carotid endarterectomy and coronary artery bypass. *Eur J Vasc Endovasc Surg* 2003;25:380–389.

201. Hise JH, Nippu ML, Schnitker JC. Stroke associated with coronary artery bypass surgery. *AJNR Am J Neuroradiol* 1991;12:811–814.

202. Wijdicks EFM, Jack CR. Coronary artery bypass grafting-associated stroke. *J Neuroimag* 1996;6:20–22.

203. Tettenborn B, Caplan LR, Sloan MA, et al. Postoperative brainstem cerebellar infarcts. *Neurology* 1993;43:471–477.

204. Mills SA. Risk factors for cerebral injury and cardiac surgery. *Ann Thorac Surg* 1995;59:1796–1799.

205. Lynn GM, Stefanko K, Reed JF III, et al. Risk factors for stroke after coronary artery bypass. *J Thorac Cardiovasc Surg* 1992;104:1518–1523.

206. Mangano DT, Mora Mangano CT. Perioperative stroke encephalopathy and CNS dysfunction. *J Intensive Care Med* 1997;12:148–160.

207. Barbut D, Hinton RB, Szatrowski TP, et al. Cerebral emboli detected during bypass surgery are associated with clamp removal. *Stroke* 1994;25:2398–2402.

208. Boivie P, Edstrom C, Engstrom KG. Side differences in cerebrovascular accidents after cardiac surgery: a statistical analysis of neurological symptoms and possible implications for anatomic mechanisms of aortic particle embolization. *J Thorac Cardiovasc Surg* 2005;129:591–598.

209. Pugsley W, Paschalis C, Treasure T, et al. The impact of microemboli during cardiopulmonary bypass on neuropsychological functioning. *Stroke* 1994;25:1393–1399.

210. Price DL, Harris J. Cholesterol emboli in cerebral arteries are a complication of retrograde aortic perfusion during cardiac surgery. *Neurology* 1970;20:1207–1214.

211. Tunick PA, Culliford AT, Lamparello PJ, Kronzon I. Atheromatosis of the aortic arch as an occult source of multiple systemic emboli. *Ann Intern Med* 1991;114:391–392.

212. Karalis DG, Chandrasekaran K, Victor MF, et al. Recognition and embolic potential of intraaortic atherosclerotic debris. *J Am Coll Cardiol* 1991;17:73–78.

213. Marshall JNG, Barzilai B, Kouchoukos N, Saffitz J. Intraoperative ultrasonic imaging of the ascending aorta. *Ann Thorac Surg* 1989;48:339–344.

214. Gardner TJ, Horneffer PJ, Manolio TA, et al. Stroke following coronary artery bypass grafting: a ten-year study. *Ann Thorac Surg* 1985;40:574–581.

215. Petaja J, Peltola K, Sairanen H, et al. Fibrinolysis, antithrombin III, and protein C in neonates during cardiac operations. *J Thorac Cardiovasc Surg* 1996;112:665–671.

216. Parolari A, Colli S, Mussoni L, et al. *J Thorac Cardiovasc Surg* 2003;125:336–343.

217. Katz JM, Gobin YP. Merci Retriever in acute stroke treatment. *Expert Rev Med Devices* 2006;3:273–280.

218. Smith WS, Sung G, Starkman S, et al. Safety and efficacy of mechanical embolectomy in acute ischemic stroke: results of the MERCI trial. *Stroke* 2005;1432–1438.

219. Gilman S. Cerebral disorders after open-heart operations. *N Engl J Med* 1965;272:489–498.

220. Coffey CE, Massey EW, Roberts KB, et al. Natural history of cerebral complications of coronary artery bypass graft surgery. *Neurology* 1983;33:1416–1421.

221. Moody DM, Bell MA, Challa VR, et al. Brain microemboli during cardiac surgery or aortography. *Ann Neurol* 1990;28:477–486.

222. Feeney DM, Gonzalez A, Law WA. Amphetamine, haloperidol and experience interact to affect the rate of recovery after motor cortex injury. *Science* 1982;217:855–857.

223. Houda DA, Feeney DM. Haloperidol blocks amphetamine induced recovery of binocular depth perception after bilateral visual cortex lesions in the cat. *Proc West Pharmacol Soc* 1985;28:209–211.

224. Humphreys RP, Hoffman JH, Mustard WT, Trusler GA. Cerebral hemorrhage following heart surgery. *J Neurosurg* 1975;43:671–675.

225. Sila CA. Spectrum of neurologic events following cardiac transplantation. *Stroke* 1989;20:1586–1589.

226. Caplan LR. Intracerebral hemorrhage revisited. *Neurology* 1988;38:624–627.

227. Lederman RJ, Breuer AC, Hanson MR, et al. Peripheral nervous system complications of coronary artery bypass graft surgery. *Ann Neurol* 1982;12:297–301.

228. Caplan LR, Hurst JW. Cardiac and cardiovascular findings in patients with nervous system disease: strokes. In: Caplan LR, Hurst JW, Chimowitz MI, eds. *Clinical Neurocardiology*. New York: Marcel Dekker; 1999:303–312.

229. Natelson BH. Neurocardiology: An interdisciplinary area for the 80s. *Arch Neurol* 1985;42:178–184.

230. Schlesinger MJ, Reiner L. Focal myocytolysis of heart. *Am J Pathol* 1955;31:443–459.

231. Smith RP, Tomlinson BE. Subendocardial hemorrhages associated with intracranial lesions. *J Pathol Bacteriol* 1954;68:327–334.

232. Norris JW, Hachinski V. Cardiac dysfunction following stroke. In: Furlan AJ, ed. *The Heart and Stroke.* London: Springer-Verlag; 1987:171–183.

233. Cropp GJ, Manning GW. Electrocardiographic changes stimulating myocardial ischemia and infarction associated with spontaneous intracranial hemorrhage. *Circulation* 1960;22:25–38.

234. Kolin A, Norris JW. Myocardial damage from acute cerebral lesions. *Stroke* 1984;15:990–993.

235. Samuels MA. Electrocardiographic manifestations of neurologic disease. *Semin Neurol* 1984;4:453–459.

236. Myers MG, Norris JW, Hachinski V, Sole MJ. Plasma norepinephrine in stroke. *Stroke* 1981;12:200–204.

237. Marion DW, Segal R, Thompson ME. Subarachnoid hemorrhage and the heart. *Neurosurg Rev* 1986;18:101–106.

238. Haggendal J, Johansson G, Jonsson L, et al. Effect of propranolol on myocardial cell necrosis and blood levels of catecholamines in pigs subjected to stress. *Acta Pharmacol Toxicol (Copenh)* 1982;50:58–66.

239. Hunt D, Gore J. Myocardial lesions following experimental intracranial hemorrhage. *Am Heart J* 1972;83:232–236.

240. Samuels M. "Voodoo" death revisited: the modern lessons of neurocardiology. *Neurologist* 1997;3:293–304.

241. Zaroff JG, Pawlikowska L, Miss JC, et al. Adrenoceptor polymorphisms and the risk of cardiac injury and dysfunction after subarachnoid hemorrhage. *Stroke* 2006;37:1680–1685.

242. Burch GE, Myers R, Abildskov JA. A new electrocardiographic pattern observed in cerebrovascular accidents. *Circulation* 1954;9:719–723.

243. Dimant J, Grob D. Electrocardiographic changes and myocardial damage in patients with acute cerebrovascular accidents. *Stroke* 1977;8:448–455.

244. Rolak LA, Rokey R. Electrocardiographic features: In: Rolak LA, Rokey R, eds. *Coronary and Cerebral Vascular Disease.* Mt. Kisco, NY: Futura; 1990:139–197.

245. Goldstein DS. The electrocardiogram in stroke: relationship to pathophysiological type and comparison with prior tracings. *Stroke* 1979;10:253–259.

246. Mayer SA, Homma S, Lennihan L, et al. Myocardial injury and left ventricular performance after subarachnoid hemorrhage. *Stroke* 1999;30:780–786.

247. Puleo P. Cardiac enzyme assessment. In: Rolak L, Rokey R, eds. *Coronary and Cerebral Vascular Disease.* Mt. Kisco, NY: Futura; 1990:199–216.

248. Fabinyi G, Hunt D, McKinley L. Myocardial creatine kinase isoenzyme in serum after subarachnoid hemorrhage. *J Neurol Neurosurg Psychiatry* 1977;40:818–820.

249. Neil-Dwyer G, Cruickshank J, Stratton C. Beta-blockers, plasma total creatine kinase and creatine kinase myocardial isoenzyme, and the prognosis of subarachnoid hemorrhage. *Surg Neurol* 1986;25:163–168.

250. Myers MG, Norris JW, Hachinsky VC, et al. Cardiac sequelae of acute strokes. *Stroke* 1982;13:838–842.

251. Stober T, Sen S, Anstatt T, Bette L. Correlation of cardiac arrhythmias with brainstem compression in patients with intracerebral hemorrhage. *Stroke* 1988;19:688–692.

252. Ako J, Sudhir K, Farouque O, Honda Y, Fitzgerald PJ. Transient left ventricular dysfunction under severe stress: brain-heart relationship revisited. *Am J Med* 2006;119:10–17.

253. Kono T, Morita H, Kuroiwa T, et al. Left ventricular wall motion abnormalities in patients with subarachnoid hemorrhage: neurogenic stunned myocardium. *J Am Coll Cardiol* 1994;24:636–640.

254. Tsuchihashi K, Ueshima K, Uchida T, et al. Transient left ventricular apical ballooning without coronary artery stenosis: a novel heart syndrome mimicking acute myocardial infarction. *J Am Coll Cardiol* 2001;38:11–18.

255. Hoff JT, Nishimura M. Experimental neurogenic pulmonary edema in cats. *J Neurosurg* 1978;18:383–389.

256. Wier BK. Pulmonary edema following fatal aneurysmal rupture. *J Neurosurg* 1978;49:502–507.

257. Theodore J, Robin ED. Pathogenesis of neurogenic pulmonary edema. *Lancet* 1975;2:749–751.

258. Engel GL. Psychologic factors in instantaneous cardiac death. *N Engl J Med* 1976;294:664–665.

259. Engel GL. Psychologic stress, vasodepressor (vasovagal) syncope and sudden death. *Ann Intern Med* 1978;89:403–412.

260. Lown B. Sudden cardiac death: the major challenge confronting contemporary cardiology. *Am J Cardiol* 1979;43:313–328.

261. Lown B, Temte JV, Reich P, et al. Basis for recurring ventricular fibrillation in the absence of coronary heart disease and its management. *N Engl J Med* 1976;294:623–629.

262. Talman WT. Cardiovascular regulation and lesions of the central nervous system. *Ann Neurol* 1985;18:1–12.

263. Schwartz PJ, Stone HL, Brown AM. Effects of unilateral stellate ganglion blockage on the arrhythmias associated with coronary occlusion. *Am Heart J* 1976;92:589–599.

264. Adams H, Kassell N, Mazuz H. The patients with transient ischemic attacks: is this the time for a new therapeutic approach? *Stroke* 1984;15:371–375.

265. Hennerici M, Aulich A, Sandmann W, Freund HJ. Incidence of asymptomatic extracranial arterial disease. *Stroke* 1981;12:750–758.

266. Caplan LR. Cerebrovascular disease: Large artery occlusive disease. In: Appel S, ed. *Current Neurology.* Vol. 87. Chicago: Year Book; 1988:179–226.

267. McMillan DE. Blood flow and the localization of atherosclerotic plaques. *Stroke* 1985;16:582–587.

268. Zarins CK, Giddins DP, Bharadvaj BK, et al. Carotid bifurcation atherosclerosis. *Circ Res* 1983;53:502–514.

269. Hutchinson EC, Yates DO. The cervical portion of the vertebral artery: a clinicopathologic study. *Brain* 1956;79:319–331.

270. Fisher CM, Ojemann RG. A clinico-pathologic study of carotid endarterectomy plaques. *Rev Neurol (Paris)* 1986;142:573–589.

271. Caplan LR, Gorelick PB, Hier DB. Race, sex, and occlusive vascular disease: a review. *Stroke* 1986;17:648–655.

272. Gorelick PB, Caplan LR, Hier DB, et al. Racial differences in the distribution of posterior circulation occlusive disease. *Stroke* 1985;16:785–790.

273. Gorelick PB, Caplan LR, Hier DB, et al. Racial differences in the distribution of anterior circulation occlusive cerebrovascular disease. *Neurology* 1984;34:54–59.

274. Feldmann E, Daneault N, Kwan E, et al. Chinese-white differences in the distribution of occlusive cerebrovascular disease. *Neurology* 1990;40:1541–1545.

275. Caplan LR, Wolpert SM. Angiography in patients with occlusive cerebrovascular disease: views of a stroke neurologist and neuroradiologist. *AJNR Am J Neuroradiol* 1991;12:593–601.

276. Pessin MS, Duncan GW, Mohr JP, Poskanzer DC. Clinical and angiographic features of carotid transient ischemic attacks. *N Engl J Med* 1977;296:358–362.

277. Caplan LR, Hennerici M. Impaired clearance of emboli is an important link between hypoperfusion, embolism, and ischemic stroke. *Arch Neurol* 1998;55:1475–1482.

278. Chambers BR, Norris JW. Outcome in patients with asymptomatic neck bruits. *N Engl J Med* 1986;315:860–865.

279. Hennerici M, Hulsbomer HB, Rautenberg W, Hefter H. Spontaneous history of asymptomatic internal carotid occlusion. *Stroke* 1986;17:718–722.

280. Ringelstein EB, Zeumer H, Angelou D. The pathogenesis of strokes from internal carotid artery occlusion: diagnostic and therapeutical implications. *Stroke* 1983;14:867–875.

281. Caplan LR, Tettenborn B. Vertebrobasilar occlusive disease: review of selected aspects. 2. Posterior circulation embolism. *Cerebrovasc Dis* 1992;2:320–326.

282. Gorelick PB, Hier DB, Caplan LR, Langenberg P. Headache in acute cerebrovascular disease. *Neurology* 1986;36:1445–1450.

283. Pessin MS, Hinton RC, Davis KR, et al. Mechanism of acute carotid stroke. *Ann Neurol* 1979;6:245–252.

284. Caplan LR. TIAs: we need to return to the question, what is wrong with Mr. Jones? *Neurology* 1988;791–793.

285. Caplan LR. Significance of unexpected (silent) brain infarcts. In: Caplan LR, Shifrin EG, Nicolaides AN, Moore WS, eds. *Cerebrovascular ischaemia, investigation and management,* London: Med-Orion; 1996:423–433.

286. Hennerici M, Freund H. Efficacy of C-W Doppler and duplex system examinations for the evaluation of extracranial carotid disease. *J Clin Ultrasound* 1984;12:155–161.

287. O'Donnell TF, Erdoes L, Mackey WC, et al. Correlation of B-mode ultrasound imaging and arteriography with pathologic findings at carotid endarterectomy. *Arch Surg* 1985;120:443–449.

288. Zwiebel WJ, Zagzebski JA, Crummy AB, Hirscher M. Correlation of peak Doppler frequency with lumen narrowing in carotid stenosis. *Stroke* 1982;13:386–391.

289. Hennerici M, Rautenberg W, Sitzer G, Schwartz A. Transcranial Doppler ultrasound for the assessment of intracranial arterial flow velocity: I. Examination technique and normal values. *Surg Neurol* 1986;315:860–865.

290. Russell D, Madden KP, Clark WM, et al. Detection of arterial emboli using Doppler ultrasound in rabbits. *Stroke* 1991;22:253–258.

291. Spencer MP, Thomas GI, Nicholls SC, Sauvage LR. Detection of middle cerebral artery emboli during carotid endarterectomy using transcranial Doppler ultrasonography. *Stroke* 1990;21:415–423.

292. Edelman RR, Mattle HP, Atkinson DJ, Hoogewoud HM. MR angiography. *AJR Am J Roentgenol* 1990;154:937–946.

293. Caplan LR, DeWitt LD, Breen JC. Neuroimaging in patients with cerebrovascular disease. In: Greenberg J, ed. *Neuroimaging, A Companion to Adams and Victor's Principles of Neurology.* New York: McGraw-Hill; 1999:493–520.

294. Caplan LR. Treatment of cerebral ischemia: where are we headed? *Stroke* 1984;15:571–574.

295. Caplan LR. Are terms such as completed stroke or RIND of continued usefulness? *Stroke* 1983;14:431–433.

296. Warach S, Gaa J, Siewert B, et al. Acute human stroke studied by whole brain echo planar diffusion-weighted magnetic resonance imaging. *Ann Neurol* 1995;37:231–141.

297. Sorensen AG, Buonanno F, Gonzalez RG, et al. Hyperacute stroke: evaluation with combined multisection diffusion-weighted and hemodynamically weighted echo-planar MR imaging. *Radiology* 1996;199:391–401.

298. North American Symptomatic Carotid Endarterectomy Trial (NASCET) Collaborators. Beneficial effect of carotid endarterectomy in symptomatic patients with high-grade carotid stenosis. *N Engl J Med* 1991;325:445–453.

299. Barnett HJM, Taylor DW, Eliasziw M, et al. Benefit of carotid endarterectomy in patients with symptomatic moderate or severe stenosis. *N Engl J Med* 1998;339:1415–1425.

300. European Carotid Surgery Trialist's Collaborative Group. MRC European Carotid Surgery Trial: interim results for symptomatic patients with severe (70–99 percent) or with mild (0–29 percent) carotid stenosis. *Lancet* 1991;1:1235–1243.

301. European Carotid Surgery Trialist's Collaborative Group. Randomised trial of endarterectomy for recently symptomatic carotid stenosis: final results of the MRC European Carotid Surgery Trial (ECST) *Lancet* 1998;351:1379–1387.

302. Executive Committee for the Asymptomatic Carotid Atherosclerosis Study. Endarterectomy for asymptomatic carotid artery stenosis. *JAMA* 1995;273:1421–1428.

303. Berguer R, Caplan LR, eds. *Vertebrobasilar Arterial Disease.* St. Louis: Quality Medical Publishers; 1991:201–261.

304. Alberts MJ. Results of a multicenter prospective randomized trial of carotid artery stenting vs. carotid endarterectomy. *Stroke* 2001;32:325.

305. Endovascular versus surgical treatment in patients with carotid stenosis in the Carotid and Vertebral Artery Transluminal Angioplasty Study (CAVATAS): a randomized trial. *Lancet* 2001;357:1729–1737.

306. Yadav JS, Wholey MH, Kuntz RE, et al. Protected carotid stenting versus endarterectomy in high risk patients. *N Engl J Med* 2004;351:1493–1501.

307. Fields WS, Lemak NA, Frankowski RF, Hardy RJ. Controlled trial of aspirin in cerebral ischemia. *Stroke* 1977;8:301–314.

308. Antiplatelet Trialists' Collaboration. Collaborative overview of randomised trials of antiplatelet therapy: 1. Prevention of death, myocardial infarction, and stroke by prolonged antiplatelet therapy in various categories of patients. *BMJ* 1994;308:81–106.

309. Hass WK, Easton JD, Adams HP, et al. A randomized trial comparing ticlopidine hydrochloride with aspirin for the prevention of stroke in high risk patients. *N Engl J Med* 1989;321:501–507.

310. Warlow CP. Ticlopidine, a new antithrombotic drug: but is it better than aspirin for long term use? *J Neurol Neurosurg Psychiatry* 1990;53:185–187.

311. CAPRIE Steering Committee. A randomised, blinded, trial of clopidogrel versus aspirin in patients at risk of ischaemic events. *Lancet* 1996;348:1329–1339.

312. Diener HC, Cunha L, Forbes C, et al. European Stroke Prevention Study 2: dipyridamole and acetylsalicylic acid in the secondary prevention of stroke. *J Neurol Sci* 1996;143:1–13.

313. Diener HC, Bogousslavsky J, Brass LM, et al. Aspirin and clopidogrel compared with clopidogrel alone after recent ischaemic stroke or transient ischaemic attack in high-risk patients (MATCH): randomised, double-blind, placebo-controlled trial. *Lancet* 2004;364:331–337.

314. Mohr JP, Thompson JL, Lazar RM, et al. A comparison of warfarin and aspirin for the prevention of recurrent ischemic stroke. *N Engl J Med* 2001;345:1444–1451.

315. National Institute of Neurological Disorders and Stroke rt-PA Study Group. Tissue plasminogen activator for acute ischemic stroke. *N Engl J Med* 1995;333:1581–1587.

316. del Zoppo GJ, Poeck K, Pessin MS, et al. Recombinant tissue plasminogen activator in acute thrombotic and embolic stroke. *Ann Neurol* 1992;32:78–86.

317. Wolpert SM, Bruckmann H, Greenlee R, et al. Neuroradiologic evaluation of patients with acute stroke treated with recombinant tissue plasminogen activator. *AJNR Am J Neuroradiol* 1993;14:3–13.

318. Pessin MS, del Zoppo GJ, Furlan AJ. Thrombolytic treatment in acute stroke: review and update of selected topics. In: Moskowitz MA, Caplan LR, eds. *Cerebrovascular Diseases: Nineteenth Princeton Stroke Conference.* Boston: Butterworth-Heinemann; 1995:409–418.

319. Furlan A, Higashida R, Wechsler L, et al. Intra-arterial prourokinase for acute ischemic stroke. The PROACT II study: a randomized controlled trial—Prolyse in acute cerebral thromboembolism. *JAMA* 1999;282:2003–2011.

320. Caplan LR, Mohr JP, Kistler JP, et al. Should thrombolytic therapy be the first-line treatment for acute ischemic stroke? *N Engl J Med* 1997;337:1309–1313.

321. Caplan LR. Intracranial branch atheromatous disease. *Neurology* 1989;39:1246–1250.

322. Caplan LR. Lacunar infarction: a neglected concept. *Geriatrics* 1976;31:71–75.

323. Caplan LR. Binswanger's disease revisited. *Neurology* 1995;45:626–633.

324. Fisher CM. The arterial lesions underlying lacunes. *Acta Neuropathol (Berl)* 1969;12:1–15.

325. Fisher CM. Lacunes, small deep cerebral infarcts. *Neurology* 1965;15:774–784.

326. Kase CS, Caplan LR. *Intracerebral Hemorrhage.* Boston: Butterworth-Heinemann; 1994.

327. Rosenblum WI. Miliary aneurysms and "fibrinoid" degeneration of cerebral blood vessels. *Hum Pathol* 1977;8:133–139.

328. Cole F, Yates P. Intracerebral microaneurysms and small cerebrovascular lesions. *Brain* 1966;90:759–767.

329. Fisher CM. Pathological observations in hypertensive cerebral hemorrhage. *J Neuropathol Exp Neurol* 1971;30:536–550.

330. Fisher CM. Cerebral miliary aneurysms in hypertension. *Am J Pathol* 1972;66:314–324.

331. Fisher CM, Caplan LR. Basilar artery branch occlusion: a cause of pontine infarction. *Neurology* 1971;21:900–905.

332. Fisher CM. Bilateral occlusion of basilar artery branches. *J Neurol Neurosurg Psychiatry* 1977;40:1182–1189.

333. Mohr JP. Lacunes. *Stroke* 1982;13:3–11.

334. Fisher CM. Lacunar strokes and infarcts: a review. *Neurology* 1982;32:871–876.

335. Fisher CM. Pure motor hemiplegia of vascular origin. *Arch Neurol* 1965;13:30–44.

336. Fisher CM. Pure sensory stroke and allied conditions. *Stroke* 1982;13:434–447.

337. Fisher CW. Ataxic hemiparesis. *Arch Neurol* 1978;35:126–128.

338. Fisher CM. A lacunar stroke, the dysarthric-clumsy hand syndrome. *Neurology* 1967;17:614–617.

339. Hachinski VC, Potter P, Merskey H. Leukoariosis. *Arch Neurol* 1987;44:21–23.

340. Caplan LR, Schoene W. Subcortical arteriosclerotic encephalopathy (Binswanger disease): clinical features. *Neurology* 1978;28:1206–1219.

341. Babikian V, Ropper AH. Binswanger's disease: a review. *Stroke* 1987;18:2–12.

342. Kase CS. Intracerebral hemorrhage: non-hypertensive causes. *Stroke* 1986;17:590–594.

343. Bahemuka M. Primary intracerebral hemorrhage and heart weight: a clinicopathological case-control review of 218 patients. *Stroke* 1987;18:531–536.

344. Brott T, Thalinger K, Hertzberg V. Hypertension as a risk factor for spontaneous intracerebral hemorrhage. *Stroke* 1986;17:1078–1083.

345. Fisher CM. Pathological observations in hypertensive cerebral hemorrhages. *J Neuropathol Exp Neurol* 1971;30:536–550.

346. Linfante I, Linas RH, Caplan LR, Warach S. MRI features of intracerebral hemorrhage within 2 hours from symptoms onset. *Stroke* 1999;30:2263–2267.

347. Tuhrim S, Dambrosia JM, Price TR, et al. Prediction of intracerebral hemorrhage survival. *Ann Neurol* 1988;24:258–263.

348. Adams HP, Jergenson DD, Kassell NF, Sahs AL. Pitfalls in the recognition of subarachnoid hemorrhage. *JAMA* 1980;244:794–796.

349. Ostergaard JR. Warning leaks in subarachnoid hemorrhage. *BMJ* 1990;301:190–191.

350. Weisberg L. Computed tomography in aneurysmal subarachnoid hemorrhage. *Neurology* 1979;29:802–808.

351. Caplan LR, Flamm ES, Mohr JP, et al. Lumbar puncture and stroke. *Stroke* 1987;18:540A–544A.

352. Heros R, Zervas NT, Varsos V. Cerebral vasospasm after subarachnoid hemorrhage: an update. *Ann Neurol* 1983;14:599–608.

353. Kassell N, Sasaki T, Colohan A, Nazar G. Cerebral vasospasm following aneurysmal subarachnoid hemorrhage. *Stroke* 1985;16:562–572.

354. MacDonald RL, Weir BK. A review of hemoglobin and the pathogenesis of cerebral vasospasm. *Stroke* 1991;22:971–982.

355. Wilkins RH. Attempts at prevention or treatment of intracranial arterial spasm: an update. *Neurosurgery* 1986;18:808–825.

356. Weir B, Grace M, Hansen J, Rothberg C. Time course of vasospasm in man. *J Neurosurg* 1978;48:173–178.

357. Kwak R, Niizuma H, Ohi T, Suzuki J. Angiographic study of cerebral vasospasm following rupture of intracranial aneurysms: I. Time of the appearance. *Surg Neurol* 1979;11:257–262.

358. Sloan MA, Haley EC, Kassell NF, et al. Sensitivity and specificity of transcranial Doppler ultrasonography in the diagnosis of vasospasm following subarachnoid hemorrhage. *Neurology* 1989;39:1514–1518.

359. Davis S, Andrews J, Lichtenstein M, et al. A single-photon emission computed tomography study of hypoperfusion after subarachnoid hemorrhage. *Stroke* 1990;21:252–259.

360. Hart RG, Kanter MC. Hematologic disorders and ischemic stroke: a selective review. *Stroke* 1990;20:1111–1121.

361. Coull BM, Goodnight SH. Current concepts of cerebrovascular disease and stroke: antiphospholipid antibodies, prothrombotic states and stroke. *Stroke* 1990;21:1370–1374.

362. Feinberg WM, Bruck DC, Ring ME. Hemostatic markers in acute stroke. *Stroke* 1989;20:592–597.

363. Holliday P, Mammen E, Buday J, et al. "Sticky platelet" syndrome and cerebral infarction. *Neurology* 1983;33(suppl 2):145.

364. Wu K, Hoak J. Increased platelet aggregation in patients with transient ischemic attacks. *Stroke* 1975;6:521–524.

365. Feinberg WM. Coagulation. In: Caplan LR, ed. *Brain Ischemia: Basic Concepts and Clinical Relevance*. London: Springer-Verlag; 1995:85–96.

366. Hart R, Miller V, Coull B, Bril V. Cerebral infarction associated with lupus anticoagulants: preliminary report. *Stroke* 1984;15:114–118.

367. Levine SR, Welch KMA. The spectrum of neurologic disease associated with antiphospholipid antibodies, lupus anticoagulants, and anticardiolipin antibodies. *Arch Neurol* 1987;44:876–883.

368. Kushner M, Simonian N. Lupus anticoagulant, anticardiolipin antibodies and cerebral ischemia. *Stroke* 1989;20:225–229.

369. Levine SR, Langer SL, Albers JW, Welch KMA. Sneddon's syndrome: an antiphospholipid antibody syndrome. *Neurology* 1988;38:798–800.

370. Rebollo M, Vol JF, Garijil F, et al. Livedo reticularis and cerebrovascular lesions (Sneddon's syndrome): clinical, radiologic, and pathologic features in eight cases. *Brain* 1983;106:965–979.

371. Bruyn RP, VanderVeen JP, Donker AJ, et al. Sneddon's syndrome: case report and literature review. *J Neurol Sci* 1987;79:243–253.

372. Antiphospholipid Antibodies in Stroke Study Group (APASS). Clinical and laboratory findings in patients with antiphospholipid antibodies and cerebral ischemia. *Stroke* 1990;21:1268–1273.

373. DeWitt LD, Caplan LR. Antiphospholipid antibodies and stroke. *AJNR Am J Neuroradiol* 1991;12:454–456.

374. Asherson RA. A "primary antiphospholipid syndrome"? [editorial]. *J Rheumatol* 1988;15:1742–1746.

375. Coull BM, Boudette DN, Goodnight SH, et al. Multiple cerebral infarction and dementia associated with anticardiolipin antibodies. *Stroke* 1987;18:1107–1112.

376. Amico L, Caplan LR, Thomas C. Cerebrovascular complications of mucinous cancers. *Neurology* 1989;39:522–526.

377. Kase C, Robinson R, Stein R, et al. Anticoagulant-related intracerebral hemorrhage. *Neurology* 1985;35:943–948.

378. Bovill EG, Terrin ML, Stump DC, et al. Hemorrhagic events during therapy with recombinant tissue-type plasminogen activator, heparin, and aspirin for acute myocardial infarction. *Ann Intern Med* 1991;115:256–265.

379. Kase CS, Pessin MS, Zivin JA, et al. Intracranial hemorrhages following coronary thrombolysis with tissue plasminogen activator. *Am J Med* 1992;92:384–390.

380. Babikian V, Kase C, Pessin M, et al. Resumption of anticoagulation after intracranial bleeding in patients with prosthetic valves. *Stroke* 1988;19:407–408.

381. Hart RG, Easton JD. Dissections of cervical and cerebral arteries. *Neurol Clin* 1983;1:255–282.

382. Anson J, Crowell RM. Cervicocranial arterial dissection. *Neurosurgery* 1991;29:89–96.

383. Caplan LR, Zarins CK, Hemmati M. Spontaneous dissection of the extracranial vertebral arteries. *Stroke* 1985;16:1030–1036.

384. Mas JL, Bousser MG, Hasboun D, Laplane D. Extracranial vertebral artery dissections. *Stroke* 1987;18:1037–1047.

385. Mokri B, Houser W, Sandok B, Piepgras D. Spontaneous dissections of the vertebral arteries. *Neurology* 1988;38:880–885.

386. Ojemann RG, Fisher CM, Rich JC. Spontaneous dissecting aneurysms of the internal carotid artery. *Stroke* 1972;3:434–440.

387. Hennerici M, Steinke W, Rautenberg W. High-resistance Doppler flow pattern in extracranial carotid dissection. *Arch Neurol* 1989;46:670–672.

388. Berger MS, Wilson CB. Intracranial dissecting aneurysms of the posterior circulation. *J Neurosurg* 1984;61:882–894.

389. Friedman AH, Drake CG. Subarachnoid hemorrhage from intracranial dissecting aneurysm. *J Neurosurg* 1984;60:325–334.

CHAPTER (107)

The Nonsurgical Approach to Carotid Disease

Vivek Rajagopal / Samir R. Kapadia / Jay S. Yadav

Carotid artery stenoses, both symptomatic and asymptomatic, increase risk for ischemic cerebrovascular events. The long-standing *gold standard* for invasive treatment of these lesions has been surgical carotid endarterectomy (CEA). CEA reduces risk of stroke for both severe asymptomatic carotid stenosis[1-4] and moderate or severe symptomatic stenosis[5-7] when compared to medical management.

Surgery, however, is not without limitations. The risk of stroke associated with CEA ranged from 2.9 to 10.7 percent in major trials.[1-3,5-7] Also, the coronary artery disease (CAD) that frequently accompanies carotid atherosclerosis increases risk of perioperative myocardial infarction (MI), which can make the management of these patients difficult. Additionally, several groups of patients have an unacceptable risk for CEA secondary to comorbid conditions such as severe coronary atherosclerotic disease, a history of head or neck radiation, previous ipsilateral CEA, or contralateral carotid occlusion.

Because of these factors, along with the inherent invasiveness and recovery time associated with surgery, nonsurgical intervention was developed to treat atherosclerotic carotid stenosis.

CAROTID ANATOMY

The right carotid artery originates from the innominate (brachiocephalic) artery, typically the first branch of aortic arch. The left carotid artery arises as a second branch from the arch somewhat posterior to the innominate. A bovine arch, in which the left common carotid arises from the innominate artery, is the most common anomaly of the origins of the great vessels and occurs in approximately 20 percent of patients. Elongation of aorta with aging and atherosclerosis along with different shapes of chest cavity imparts tortuosity to arch vessels and alters relationship of their origins to descending aorta. These changes are important to recognize for an interventionalist because they determine accessibility of these vessels for percutaneous interventions. Fig. 107–1 demonstrates the commonly used anatomic classification of the origins of the great vessels. The aortic arch can be classified into three types based on the distance of the origin of the great vessels from the top of the arch. The widest diameter of the left common carotid is used as a reference unit. In a type I arch (see Fig. 107–1A), all great vessels originate within one diameter length from the top of

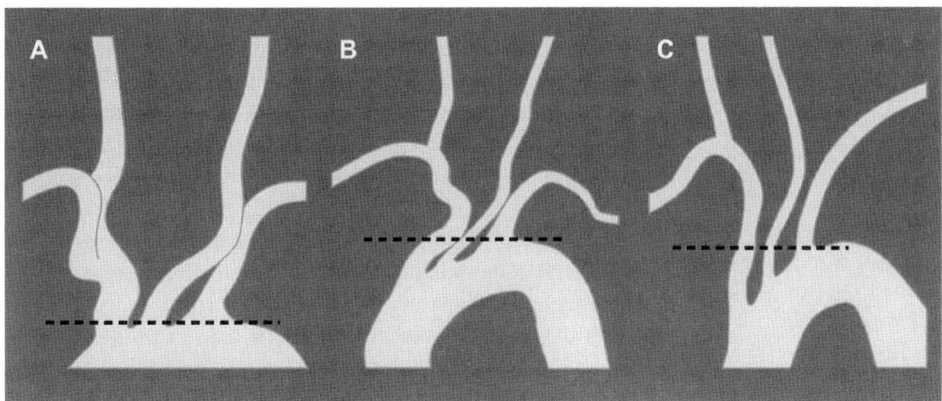

FIGURE 107–1. Aortic arch classifications.

the arch; in a type II arch (see Fig. 107–1B), all great vessels originate within two diameter lengths from the top of the arch; and in a type III arch (see Fig. 107–1C), the great vessels originate more than two diameter lengths from the top of the arch.

The common carotid artery (CCA) bifurcates into the internal carotid artery (ICA) and the external carotid artery at the level of the C4-C5 intervertebral space. The ICA continues superiorly and gives rise to its first major branch, the ophthalmic artery, in the subarachnoid space. It then bifurcates into the anterior and middle cerebral arteries. The ICA is divided into the prepetrous, petrous, cavernous, and supraclinoid segments (Fig. 107–2).

The carotid sinus is located in the ICA just distal to the bifurcation of the CCA and measures approximately 7 mm in diameter in most adults. The sinus contains mechanoreceptors, which are responsible for the carotid sinus reflex.

The external carotid artery has an extensive collateral network; therefore unilateral stenosis is rarely symptomatic. Severe stenosis or obstruction, however, may cause jaw claudication in patients with concomitant contralateral occlusion.

CAROTID ATHEROSCLEROTIC DISEASE

【 】 EPIDEMIOLOGY

Stroke is the third leading cause of death in the United States, causing >157,000 deaths in the year 2003. Overall, approximately 700,000 people experience either an initial or recurrent stoke each year, with approximately 40,000 more women than men suffering a stroke each year. In 2006 >$57 billion dollars were spent on the diagnosis and treatment of stroke. Ischemic strokes, which are closely related to vascular stenosis, account for 88 percent of all strokes. In addition to the acute clinical and financial consequences, there are significant long-term effects related to stroke. Stroke is the number one cause of long-term disability, with 20 percent of victims needing institutional care 3 months after the event. Further, nearly a quarter of all stroke patients will die within 1 year following the event, and this number is even higher for those who are above age 65.[8]

【 】 RISK FACTORS

The common and internal carotid arteries are muscular arteries similar to those in the coronary system. They consist of an in-

tima, media, and adventitia. It is not surprising, therefore, that the atherosclerotic disease in patients with carotid artery stenosis is very similar to that in CAD. Atheromatous plaque accumulates most frequently at sites of turbulent flow, such as the bifurcations. Examination of material collected after carotid stenting with distal emboli prevention devices (EPD) has demonstrated that the microemboli from these lesions contain lipid vacuoles, fibrin, platelets, and foam cells.[9] Because the disease processes are very similar, it is not surprising that concomitant CAD is a significant problem for patients with carotid coronary stenosis. However, only 5 to 10 percent of patients with CAD will also have severe carotid atherosclerosis.[10]

There are several risk factors for the development of carotid atherosclerosis and its associated clinical sequelae. Stroke rates increase in a stepwise fashion with age. Tobacco use imparts a significant risk of stroke that is correlated to usage. Heavy smokers have twice the relative risk (RR) of stroke compared to light smokers, and the risk of stroke is significantly reduced within 2 years of smoking cessation, with a return to baseline at 5 years.[11] Race has also been shown to impart risk. Blacks have twice the age-adjusted risk for stroke compared to non-Hispanic whites, and both male and female blacks are more likely to die secondary to strokes when compared to non-Hispanic whites.[8] Hypertension, diabetes, the metabolic syndrome, male gender, and hypercholesterolemia are additional risk factors that have been shown to impart an elevated risk of carotid disease.[12–14] Similar to recent work in the coronary realm, inflammation has been shown to be associated with an increased risk of both carotid atherosclerosis and carotid plaque instability.[15–17]

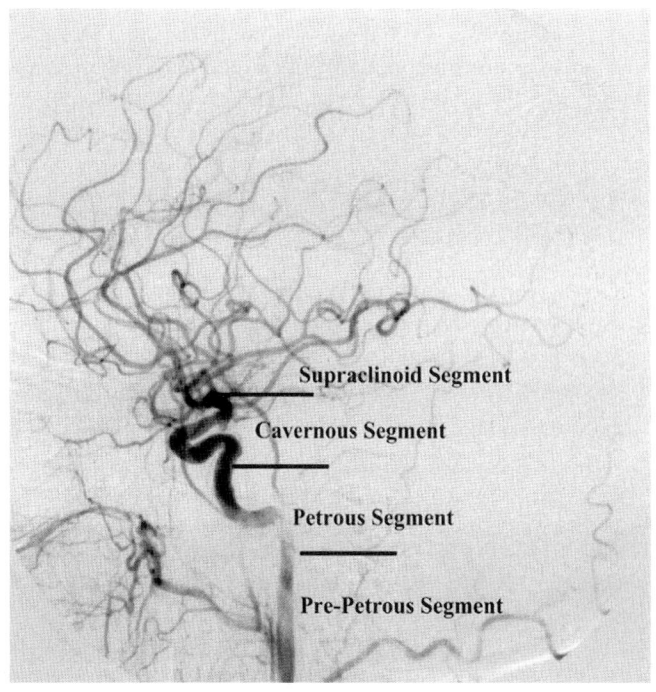

FIGURE 107–2. Segments of the internal carotid artery.

NATURAL HISTORY

The physical examination hallmark of carotid atherosclerosis is the carotid bruit. Although carotid bruits are poor predictors of the severity of atherosclerosis, they are associated with an increased risk of stroke, MI, and death.[11,18] More specifically, once carotid atheromatous lesions have formed, the severity of stenosis as well as associated symptoms are predictive of the risk of stroke.[18] In asymptomatic carotid stenosis of ≥60 percent, the yearly risk of stroke has been found to be 2.1 percent.[1] The addition of symptoms such as transient ischemic attack (TIA) significantly increases the risk of stroke in patients with even moderate stenosis, and this risk increases in a stepwise fashion with the severity of stenosis. The risk of stroke following a TIA was 40 percent in the Framingham Study, and two-thirds of these strokes occurred within the first 6 months.[13] The North American Symptomatic Carotid Endarterectomy Trial (NASCET) demonstrated the risk of ipsilateral stroke to be 18.7 percent over 5 years in medically treated patients with >50 percent symptomatic stenosis and 22.2 percent in those with 50 to 69 percent symptomatic stenosis.[19] There is also a dose-response association between the severity of stenosis and the risk of death. The adjusted RR of death for stenoses <45 percent is 1.32; for stenoses 45 to 74 percent, it is 2.22; and for stenoses 75 to 99 percent, it is 3.24.[20] Progressive carotid stenoses are more likely to be associated with adverse events.[21,22]

CLINICAL PRESENTATION

Carotid bruits can be auscultated over one or both carotid arteries and have a harsh blowing quality associated with them. Evidence of a carotid bruit on physical examination is the most common finding leading to the diagnosis of asymptomatic carotid stenosis. The severity of the bruit, however, has not been shown to be associated with the degree of stenosis.

A TIA is the most common presentation of symptomatic carotid stenosis. By definition, a TIA lasts for less than 24 h and typically resolves within 30 minutes. Symptoms from a TIA are related to the distribution affected by the area of ischemia. Importantly, TIAs caused by vertebrobasilar insufficiency must be differentiated from those secondary to carotid origin, which can be done with careful history taking and physical examination. Carotid-related symptoms include aphasia and dysarthria. Visual disturbances, such as ipsilateral amaurosis fugax or contralateral homonymous hemianopia, can also be present. Sensory and motor deficits are typically contralateral. Conversely, symptoms related to vertebrobasilar insufficiency include transient cranial nerve findings, diplopia, and dysarthria. Motor deficits are ipsilateral and visual losses are frequently bilateral.

DIAGNOSIS

NONINVASIVE TECHNIQUES

Ultrasonography

Stenosis Severity The standard noninvasive method for the evaluation of carotid artery stenosis is duplex ultrasonography. Several studies have encouraged diagnosis of the severity of carotid artery stenosis on the basis of ultrasound alone, without the need for angiography.[23–27] Results concerning the diagnostic accuracy of carotid ultrasound in the centers participating in the NASCET study, however, cast some doubt on the validity of ultrasound by showing that the sensitivity and specificity of carotid ultrasound were 68 and 67 percent, respectively.[28] This poor correlation has been attributed to many factors, including variations in patient selection, imaging device performance, and the imaging protocols used. Ultrasound evaluation fared better in the Asymptomatic Carotid Atherosclerosis Study (ACAS). In this study, centers had to show evidence of Doppler measurements and carotid arteriography correlation; a standard protocol was adopted, which played a part in the specificity of carotid ultrasound being measured above 95 percent.[29] Recent data suggest that carotid ultrasound also has a high accuracy for carotid restenosis after endarterectomy.[30] Nonetheless, despite the overall high sensitivity and specificity for carotid ultrasound, accuracy varies widely according to laboratory.[31] Therefore, properly trained sonographers and a routine quality assurance program are critical to the sensitivity and specificity of results obtained from carotid ultrasound.

Various criteria have been proposed to diagnose severe carotid stenosis with high level of accuracy. Different cutoff points for peak systolic and diastolic velocities from internal carotid and ratio of peak systolic velocity from internal and common carotid have been correlated with severe stenosis.[32] Typically, >80 percent stenosis correlates with systolic velocity greater than 300 to 400 cm/sec, diastolic velocity greater than 100 to 135 cm/sec and ratio of ICA/CCA systolic velocity of >4 to 6. Contralateral occlusion, severe left ventricular (LV) dysfunction, aortic stenosis, common carotid stenosis are some of the variables that make these measurements less reliable and should be factored in when interpreting carotid ultrasound information.

Carotid Intimal-Medial Thickness Although not as commonly measured as carotid artery stenosis, carotid intimal-medial thickness (IMT) has correlated with increased risk of MI and stroke in a wide range of patients.[33–35] Recently, carotid IMT has also shown to correlate with increased risk of stroke recurrence in ischemic stroke patients.[36,37] It is, however, unclear at this time how to integrate carotid IMT measurements with other data in risk stratification and treatment strategy.

Magnetic Resonance Angiography

Magnetic resonance angiography (MRA) has been used to evaluate the carotid bifurcation, because this segment of the carotid artery is relatively motionless, superficial, and large enough for visualization. Newer methods of MRA have addressed some of the shortcomings associated with initial techniques and have made better visualization possible with reliable imaging of the carotids from their origin to the intracranial branches.

Three-dimensional (3D) contrast-enhanced MRA of the carotid and thoracic aorta has made significant advancements for noninvasive examination of the extracranial carotid and the aortic arch. Prior to the evolution of 3D gadolinium contrast MRA as a standard part of MRA, it was routine to use 2D time-of-flight (TOF) and 3D-multislab TOF MRA alone. These techniques are complementary, making it important to use them together to diagnose stenoses accurately.[38,39] They are limited by their flow dependence and their consequent susceptibility to flow and motion artifacts. Advantages of gadolinium-enhanced MRA for carotid angiography include the ability to image plaque ulcerations, which are often not seen on TOF; lack of flow-related artifacts, which can degrade tortuous vessels by in-plane saturation; short imaging times with excellent signal-to-noise ratio; and the ability to image from the aortic arch to circle of Willis in approximately 30 seconds. The contrast-enhanced MRI technique is limited by interference from contrast in the jugular vein, which may impair visualization of the carotid artery and thereby decrease the sensitivity for measuring stenoses when a long scan time is used. Conversely, using the shorter scan time decreases the spatial resolution. It is unclear how important these differences in techniques are, and small studies have yielded conflicting data about the accuracy of 3D TOF MRI compared to contrast-enhanced MRI.[39–41]

Ignoring these differences, a study comparing the sensitivity and specificity of noninvasive imaging with angiography on 569 patients demonstrated that MRA was associated with a sensitivity of 75 percent and specificity of 88 percent. However, concordant noninvasive testing with Doppler ultrasound and MRA resulted in an improved sensitivity of 96 percent and specificity of 85 percent, suggesting that surgical decisions should be made cautiously if based solely on the results of individual noninvasive studies.[42] Furthermore, although a systematic review of the literature found better discriminatory power for MRA compared to Doppler ultrasound,[43] a recent study found that MRA significantly overestimated degree of stenosis for moderate-grade lesions.[38] Thus, concordant Doppler ultrasound and MRA may result in better sensitivity and specificity, possibly reducing the need for invasive diagnostic angiography.[44]

Computed Tomography Angiography

First-generation CT scanners obtained images by rotating the x-ray tube around the patient once, returning to the x-ray tube back to the starting position while moving the patient, and starting the process over again.[45] These scanners obtained noncontiguous single slices of patients after long scan times. *Spiral* CT scanners improved imaging by continuously rotating the x-ray tube with the patient moving, allowing contiguous slices to be obtained in less time. Initially, these scanners had single detectors, and only one slice could be captured at a time. The development of multislice detectors (from 4 to 16 to 32 to 64 slice) greatly improved resolution and scan time.

Thus, multislice computed tomography angiography (CTA) matured to become a promising form of noninvasive angiography for numerous vascular beds—coronary, peripheral, and carotid arteries. In one of the first studies evaluating CTA for carotid imaging, Sameshima and colleagues examined 128 carotid bifurcations, comparing CTA to Doppler ultrasound and MRA, using conventional angiography as the standard.[46] MRA tended to overestimate stenosis, whereas CTA strongly correlated with conventional angiography ($r = 0.987$, $p < 0.0001$).

Further data supported usefulness of CTA, and a systematic review of 43 studies found an overall sensitivity of 95 percent and specificity of 98 percent for detecting a severe (>70 percent) carotid stenosis.[47] Some of the included studies, however, had meth-odological flaws, and this analysis likely overestimates the true accuracy of CTA. In fact, another systematic review used stricter methodological criteria and found a more modest sensitivity of 85 percent and specificity of 93 percent for detecting a stenosis >70 percent.[48]

INVASIVE TECHNIQUES

Angiography

The gold standard of assessing the severity of carotid stenosis severity remains the angiogram. There are several factors that make angiography unique and attractive in its detection of atherosclerotic plaque. It provides high-resolution images of the stenosis and plaque surface and is able to distinguish easily between a high-grade stenosis and occlusion. It allows the simultaneous study of the origin of the neck vessels and intracranial circulation. This is important for the detection of tandem stenoses, which pose diagnostic problems for Doppler ultrasound. The ability to assess collateral circulation as well as the speed of blood flow is quite useful in clinical decision making, particularly in predicting the safety of temporary carotid occlusion associated with either CEA or carotid artery stenting. Additionally, angiography provides information regarding the atherosclerotic lesion and surrounding reference vessel. The risks associated with angiography include embolization and dissection, but these risks have been shown to be relatively low, particularly when angiography is performed in the cardiac catheterization laboratory.[49]

MEDICAL MANAGEMENT

Therapies with antiplatelet agents, anticoagulant agents, lipid lowering agents, and antihypertensive agents have all been studied for reducing the risk of stroke.

ANTIPLATELET THERAPIES

The long-standing foundation of antiplatelet therapy in the management of atherosclerotic disease has been aspirin. Aspirin exerts its antiplatelet effect by acetylating platelet cyclooxygenase, thereby irreversibly inhibiting the formation of platelet-dependent thromboxane. The Antithrombotic Trialists' Collaboration has documented, in its most recent meta-analysis of >200,000 patients from 287 randomized trials, the powerful effect of antiplatelet agents, primarily aspirin, in reducing both fatal and nonfatal strokes compared to control. Aspirin was found to be effective in dosages ranging from 75 to 1500 mg without a dose-associated difference in effect. There is substantially less data for doses <75 mg, which leaves uncertain the effectiveness of this small dose. The subanalysis of five CEA trials and one asymptomatic carotid disease trial demonstrated a 19 percent reduction in vascular events, which, although it did not reach statistical significance, demonstrated a consistent trend with that seen in other high-risk patient populations in the metanalysis.[50]

Clopidogrel and ticlopidine are thienopyridines, which irreversibly inhibit binding of adenosine diphosphate to the $P2Y_{12}$ receptor. Inhibition of the $P2Y_{12}$ receptor directly prevents fibrinogen receptor activation and platelet activation, along with inhibiting the action of other platelet agonists such as thrombin and thromboxane A$_2$.[51] The Ticlopidine Aspirin Stroke Study compared the use of ticlopidine and aspirin in patients with a history of TIA, reversible ischemic neurologic deficit, or minor stroke. Ticlopidine significantly reduced the risk of fatal and nonfatal stroke by 24 percent ($p = 0.011$) compared to aspirin. This effect was even greater during the first year, with a 48 percent reduction in the risk of stroke.[52] In The Canadian American Ticlopidine Study, patients with a history of previous atherothrombotic stroke were treated with ticlopidine or placebo for up to 3 years. Ticlopidine significantly reduced the RR of stroke by 24 percent over 3 years ($p = 0.017$).[53] However, secondary to complications associated with ticlopidine, such as neutropenia and thrombotic thrombocytopenic purpura, the use of a newer thienopyridine inhibitor, clopidogrel, has become standard.

The Clopidogrel Versus Aspirin in Patients at Risk of Ischemic Events (CAPRIE) trial was a randomized, double-blind trial that compared clopidogrel and aspirin in patients with a history of recent MI, ischemic stroke, or peripheral vascular disease. Clopidogrel demonstrated an 8.7 percent RR reduction for the primary outcome of stroke, MI, or vascular death ($p = 0.04$). In a subgroup analysis of patients with a history of a previous stroke, there was a trend toward reducing the risk of adverse events with a relative-risk reduction of 7.3 percent in favor of clopidogrel ($p = 0.26$).[54]

The Clopidogrel in Unstable Angina to Reduce Ischemic Events (CURE) study included patients with acute coronary syndrome without ST-segment elevation. Patients were randomized to receive clopidogrel or placebo and were treated for up to 1 year. All patients were also treated with aspirin. There was a 20 percent RR reduction in the occurrence of cardiovascular death, MI, or stroke for the clopidogrel-treated group. Similar to findings in the CAPRIE trial, there was a trend favoring clopidogrel for the reduction of ischemic stroke (1.2 percent clopidogrel vs. 1.4 percent placebo, $p = $ NS).

The Management of Atherothrombosis with Clopidogrel in High-Risk Patients (MATCH) with Recent Transient Ischaemic Attack or Ischaemic Stroke trial evaluated dual antiplatelet therapy in 7599 patients with recent stroke or TIA. All patients received clopidogrel 75 mg daily and were randomized to aspirin (75 mg daily) or placebo.[55] After a follow up of 18 months, the primary endpoint, a composite of ischemic stroke, MI, vascular death, or rehospitalization for acute ischemia, was insignificantly lower for the dual therapy (15.7 percent vs. 16.7 percent, RR reduction 6.4 percent, 95 percent confidence interval [CI] 4.6–16.3). Life-threatening bleeding, however, was higher in the dual group (2.6 percent) than the clopidogrel only group (1.3 percent) ($p < 0.0001$).

The Clopidogrel for High Atherothrombotic Risk and Ischemic Stabilization, Management and Avoidance trial (CHARISMA) evaluated dual antiplatelet therapy in patients with either clinically overt vascular disease (cardiovascular, cerebrovascular or peripheral vascular) or multiple risk factors.[56] In this study 15,603 patients were randomized to clopidogrel (75 mg daily) plus aspirin (75 to 162 mg daily) or to aspirin alone. After a median follow up of 28 months, the primary endpoint—a composite of cardiovascular death, stroke, or MI—did not differ between the aspirin plus clopidogrel group (6.8 percent) and the aspirin-only group (7.3 per-

cent), $p = 0.22$. The subgroup of patients with cerebrovascular disease similarly did not benefit. Therefore, MATCH and CHARISMA demonstrate that patients with cerebrovascular disease do not benefit from prolonged dual antiplatelet therapy.

[ ] ANTICOAGULANTS

Although there is evidence that warfarin reduces the risk of stroke in specific subsets of patients, such as those with atrial fibrillation,[57] there is no convincing evidence that it is superior to aspirin in patients with a history of ischemic stroke from a noncardioembolic source. The Stroke Prevention in Reversible Ischemia Trial evaluated the use of warfarin with a target international normalized ratio (INR) of 3.0 to 4.5 compared to aspirin for the prevention of adverse events in patients with a history of noncardioembolic TIA or stroke. Warfarin was associated with twice the risk of vascular death, stroke, MI, or major bleeding complications compared to aspirin (12.4 vs. 5.4 percent, $p < 0.05$). This poor outcome was mainly attributable to excess bleeding complications, including 27 intracranial bleeds associated with warfarin.[58] The Warfarin Aspirin Recurrent Stroke Study compared warfarin with a lower target INR of 1.4 to 2.8 and aspirin in 2206 patients with a history of ischemic, noncardioembolic stroke. The rates of complications, including major hemorrhage, were not statistically different between the two treatment groups with the more conservative dosing of warfarin, and there was no difference between aspirin and warfarin for the prevention of recurrent ischemic stroke or death (17 vs. 16 percent; $p = 0.25$).[59] The Warfarin-Aspirin Symptomatic Intracranial Disease Trial randomized symptomatic patients (TIA or stroke within 90 days) with a 50 to 99 percent major intracranial artery stenosis to warfarin (INR 2 to 3) or aspirin (1300 mg/d).[60] During a mean follow up of 1.8 years, 4.3 percent of aspirin patients died compared to 9.7 percent of warfarin patients ($p = 0.02$), resulting in early termination of the trial. Warfarin patients had a higher incidence of major hemorrhage (8.3 percent vs. 3.2 percent, $p = 0.01$) and MI or sudden death (7.3 percent vs. 2.9 percent, $p = 0.02$). Thus, current data do not support the use of warfarin over aspirin for the prevention of noncardioembolic stroke.

[ ] ANTIHYPERLIPIDEMICS

The treatment of hyperlipidemia has been confirmed in multiple studies to confer a cardiovascular and mortality benefit.[61–63] More specifically, the use of hydroxymethylglutaryl coenzyme A (HMG-CoA) reductase inhibitors (statins) has also been shown to help reduce stroke and treat carotid atherosclerosis. Several large meta-analyses have demonstrated a reduction in stroke with the use of statins. Bucher and coworkers analyzed the results from >100,000 patients treated with statins, fibrates, resins, or dietary intervention. Only statins were associated with a reduction in the risk of stroke ($p < 0.05$).[64] Cheung and colleagues examined outcomes for >47,000 patients from 10 major statin trials, finding an 18 percent risk reduction of stroke (95 percent CI 10–25 percent).[65] The Cholesterol Treatment Trialists' (CTT) Collaborators evaluated >90,000 patients from 14 randomized trials of statins, finding a 17 percent risk reduction of stroke (95 percent CI 22–12 percent).[66] This risk reduction is robust, occurring in patients with and without CAD. Briel and colleagues demonstrated this by evaluating outcomes for more than 200,000 patients from 65 trials.[67] They found risk ratio of 0.75 (95 percent CI 0.65–0.87) for patients with CAD compared to 0.77 (95 percent CI 0.62–0.95) for patients without CAD.

There is also evidence that statin therapy has a positive effect on carotid atherosclerotic lesions. A total of 35 aortic and 25 carotid artery plaques were monitored by serial MRIs of the aorta and carotid at baseline and 6 and 12 months after initiation on simvastatin. Statin therapy was associated with significant reductions in vessel wall thickness and vessel wall area over 12 months of followup in both aortic and carotid arteries ($p < 0.001$).[68] Further work by Corti and coworkers on 44 aortic and 32 carotid artery plaques detected by MRI in 21 asymptomatic hypercholesterolemic patients demonstrated not only a decrease in vessel wall thickness and vessel wall area after treatment with simvastatin but also an increase in lumen area, ranging from 4 to 6 percent at 18 and 24 months in both carotid and aortic lesions.[69]

Other trials have demonstrated changes in carotid plaque morphology. Watanabe and colleagues randomized 60 nonhypercholesteremic CAD patients to placebo or pravastatin, finding a significant increase in echogenicity of carotid plaques with pravastatin, suggesting a decrease in plaque vulnerability.[70] Similarly, when patients are on statins, carotid plaques retrieved at time of CEA have significantly fewer matrix metalloproteinases and interleukin-6, which are proteins both associated with plaque instability.[71]

Larger studies confirm statins' ability to alter carotid plaque. The Carotid Atherosclerosis Italian Ultrasound Study (CAIUS) was performed to test the effect of lipid lowering on the progression of carotid IMT in 305 asymptomatic patients. Progression of IMT was less in the pravastatin-treated group compared to the control group ($p < 0.0007$).[72] A meta-analysis of 10 trials with >3000 patients found slowing of carotid IMT progression in 8 of these studies.[73] Another meta-analysis by Amarenco and coworkers evaluated >2700 patients from 9 trials.[74] Each 10 percent reduction in low-density lipoprotein cholesterol was estimated to decrease carotid IMT by 0.73 percent per year (95 percent CI, 0.27–1.19). These studies suggest that the benefit of statin therapy in patients with carotid artery atherosclerotic disease might be related to both decreases in plaque progression and changes in plaque morphology.

HISTORY OF INVASIVE CAROTID TREATMENTS

[ ] CAROTID ENDARTERECTOMY

Historically, carotid artery stenosis has been invasively treated with CEA. The first report of this was in 1954, and its use increased steadily until the mid-1980s, when questions arose concerning its effectiveness and safety.[75] Subsequent studies, however—including NASCET, the European Carotid Surgery Trialists' (ECST) collaboration, and the VA Cooperative trial—have all demonstrated a decrease in the risk of stroke for patients with severe, symptomatic carotid stenosis treated with CEA compared to medical management.[5–7] The ACAS study showed that asymptomatic patients with >60 percent stenosis treated with CEA had a decreased risk of stroke at 5 years compared to those medically managed.[1]

Although in experienced hands CEA has been proven safe and effective for many patients with carotid stenosis, CEA has limitations in the *real world* because patients treated outside clinical trials may be at higher risk of complications than trial patients. For example, patients operated on by trial hospitals in ACAS and NASCET had a perioperative mortality of 1.4 percent, despite a mortality of 0.1 percent in ACAS and 0.6 percent in NASCET.[76] Percutaneous treatment of these patients has proven promising and provided a treatment alternative for many.

[ ] CAROTID ANGIOPLASTY

The first percutaneous transluminal angioplasty (PTA) of the carotid artery in humans was reported by both Mullan and Kerber in 1980.[77,78] This was followed by widespread controversy associated with the investigation of carotid PTA. In Kachel's 1996 review, the results of >500 carotid angioplasties are presented, demonstrating a very low event rate comparable to that of CEA.[79] Concerns such as vascular recoil, distal embolization, and dissection, however, have made stand-alone carotid artery angioplasty a historical procedure that has been supplanted by carotid artery stenting and the use of emboli prevention devices.

CAROTID ARTERY STENTING

[ ] EARLY EXPERIENCE

Significant improvements in interventional technology, including the use of stents, have allowed the field of percutaneous carotid artery intervention to grow in acceptance as an investigational procedure; recently, it has proven noninferior to CEA in select patient populations.[80] Carotid artery stenting successfully addressed many of the shortcomings of balloon angioplasty, including vessel recoil and dissection, but it introduced its own unique challenges. Because of the superficial nature of the carotid arteries and their vulnerability to external forces, balloon-expandable stents have proved to be poor choices for carotid artery stenting. These stents are easy to place; but stent deformation caused by external compression has been demonstrated with the Palmaz stents.[81] Self-expanding Elgiloy stents (Wallstent) or nitinol stents (Precise, Memotherm, Acculink, Endostent), which continue to exert outward forces, have proven to be better suited for carotid arteries. Most carotid stenting is now performed using nitinol stents because of their better conformability and radial force.

The first reports of the use of stents for the treatment of carotid artery disease were published by Mark and Mathias.[82,83] Since that time, several large-scale observational series with and without emboli protection devices have been published documenting experience with this treatment method. These are summarized in Table 107-1. Most patients included in these reports were at high surgical risk for CEA.

In 1996 Diethrich and coworkers published the first large-scale series of patients treated with carotid artery stenting. This study reported the results of 117 carotid artery stents placed in 31 symptomatic and 79 asymptomatic patients.[84] Of these, 109 (99 percent) patients were successfully treated, with 7 resultant strokes and 1 death within the first 30 days of followup. Over a mean follow up of 7.6 months, there were no additional neurologic events or deaths, and the stent patency rate was 96.6 percent.

TABLE 107-1

Carotid Artery Stenting Registries

STUDY	LESIONS	30-DAY OUTCOMES					FOLLOWUP
		SUCCESS (%)	STROKE (%)	MI (%)	DEATH (%)	RESTENOSIS (%)	
Diethrich[84]	117	99.1	8.3	0	0.9	1.7	7.6 mo
Yadav[85]	126	100	6.3	—	0.8	4.9	6 mo
Wholey—Global Experience[a,86]	12254	98.9	3.3	—	0.64	2.6	3 y
Shawl[119]	192	99.0	2.9	0	0	2.0	19 mo
Gupta[120]	100	100	1.0	—	0	1.0	12 mo
Reimers[b,121]	88	97.7	1.2	2.3	0	0	30 d
Roubin[122]	604	98.0	5.8	—	1.5	3.0	36 mo
Total	13481	99.2	3.4	—	0.66	2.6	

[a]4221 patients treated with emboli protection devices.
[b]Emboli protection (3 filters).

The first protocol-driven study with independent neurologic assessment prior to and following the procedure was published by Yadav and colleagues in 1997.[85] In 107 consecutive patients, most of whom met NASCET exclusion criteria for CEA, a total of 126 stenoses were treated with percutaneous carotid angioplasty with elective stenting. The success rate was 100 percent, and the 30-day risk of major stroke or death was 2.4 percent. Angiographic restenosis was noted in 3 of 61 patients who had follow-up angiography at 6 months.

In 2003 Wholey and coworkers published the third global review of carotid stenting.[86] In 11243 patients, 12254 carotid artery stents were placed worldwide, with a technical success rate of 98.9 percent. The risk of stroke at 30 days was 3.3 percent (2.1 percent minor and 1.2 percent major), and the mortality rate was 0.64 percent. Restenosis was 2.6 and 2.4 percent at 1 and 2 years, respectively.

▌ ▐ BRIEF REVIEW OF THE CURRENT PROCEDURE

Carotid stenting typically requires an overnight stay, but ambulatory stenting also appears to be safe.[87] The procedure is commonly performed using a 6 Fr to 8 Fr femoral sheath. Heparin is used to achieve an activated clotting time of 250 to 300 seconds. Bivalirudin has been used for carotid stenting although little data exist comparing bivalirudin to heparin.[88] A guiding catheter or a sheath is advanced to the CCA, and the lesion is crossed with an emboli prevention device. Guide catheter approach is favored for severe tortuosity where stiffness and shape of the catheter allows for better control and manipulation capabilities. The device is deployed in the ICA, and the lesion is predilated with a small coronary balloon. The lesion is then stented with a self-expanding stent, and the stent is postdilated to the appropriate diameter. The emboli prevention device is captured and removed at the end of the procedure. Routine use of a temporary pacing wire is unnecessary. Monitoring of intracardiac filling pressure is helpful in patients with severe LV dysfunction or severe aortic stenosis or in those who are hemodynamically unstable. Adjunctive treatment with IIb/IIIa inhibitors has been studied in small studies and may be beneficial, but it has been largely supplanted by emboli prevention devices.[89,90] Aspirin is continued for life and clopidogrel for at least 1 month after the procedure (Fig. 107–3 and Fig. 107–4).[91]

▌ ▐ EMBOLI PREVENTION DEVICES

The modern era of percutaneous carotid artery intervention was heralded by the development of the distal emboli prevention device. Numerous studies have demonstrated the occurrence of microemboli as detected by transcranial Doppler during carotid artery stenting and CEA.[92,93] There are data suggesting a correlation between the number of emboli and neurologic events after

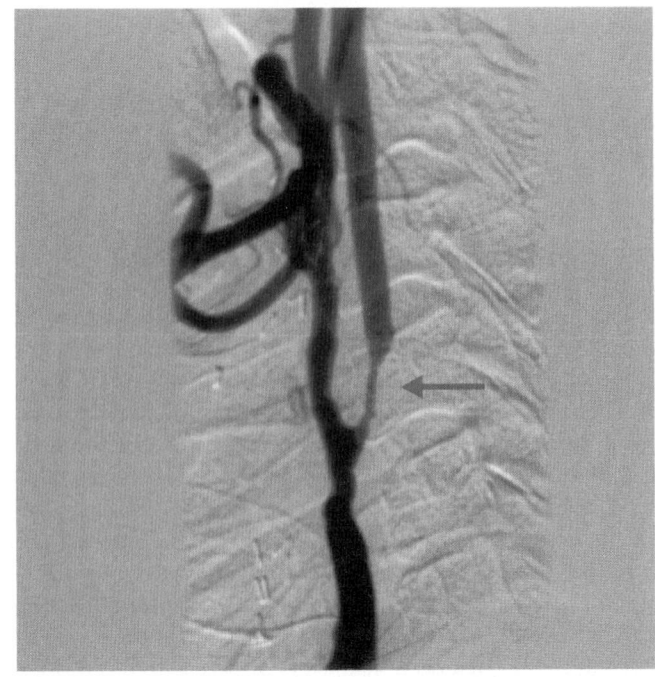

FIGURE 107–3. Internal carotid stenosis before treatment.

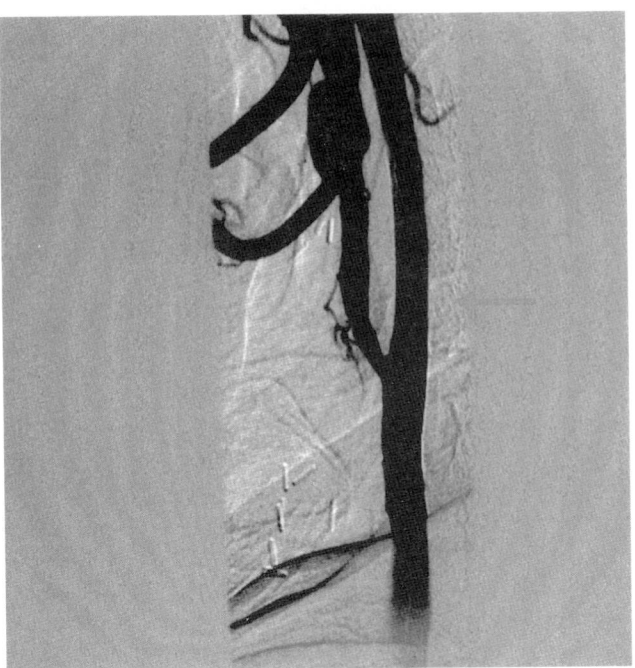

FIGURE 107-4. Internal carotid artery stenosis after stenting.

CEA.[94-96] Accordingly, numerous mechanical devices have been developed to prevent the distal embolization of debris during carotid artery stenting. There are three major types of emboli prevention devices: 1) the distal occlusive balloon, 2) the proximal occlusive balloon, and 3) the filter wire.

The PercuSurge GuardWire (Medtronic, Santa Rosa, CA) (Fig. 107–5) is the prototypical distal occlusive balloon emboli prevention device. A low-pressure balloon is located at the distal tip of a hollow wire. This balloon is inflated after the lesion is crossed and traps any debris released during the percutaneous procedure in the ICA, which is then aspirated prior to deflation of the balloon. The advantages of this system include a low crossing profile and superior wire flexibility. Disadvantages include the occlusive nature of this device, which is not well tolerated in patients without good collateral flow, as well as potential damage to the distal ICA by the device. Additionally, after inflation of the balloon, angiography to localize balloon or stent placement is difficult.

Proximal occlusion balloon systems create retrograde flow in the ICA, which prevents emboli from traveling to the cerebral circulation. Like the GuardWire device, this requires occlusive balloon inflation and can cause vessel damage. Good collateral circulation is also critical. Examples of these devices include the Parodi and Mo.Ma devices. The advantage of this approach is the fact that emboli prevention is achieved without crossing the lesion. This is particularly helpful when there is a large clot burden in the lesion.

The AngioGuard Emboli Capture Guidewire (Cordis, Miami, FL) (Fig. 107–6) was the first distal filtration wire system designed to conform to the artery and trap microemboli while maintaining distal flow through a filter umbrella with multiple perfusion pores. The major advantage of filters is the preservation of flow during the intervention and the ability to visualize the vessel with contrast material throughout the procedure. Disadvantages of filters include a larger crossing profile, which may necessitate predilatation prior to placement of the filter distal to the lesion. Many other filter devices, such as Accunet by Guidant, FilterWire EX by Boston Scientific, Sulzer-IntraGuard by IntraTherapeutics, MDT-Filter by Medtronic, Spider by EV3, Microvena-Trap by Microvena, and Emboshield by Abbott, have since been introduced. Accunet and Emboshield have been approved for carotid stenting application in the United States.

Most currently available data are from the case series using these devices to perform carotid stenting (Table 107–2). These results are very encouraging and convincing regarding the efficacy of the devices in reducing procedural stroke compared to retrospective cohorts where these devices were unavailable.

Similarly, several single-arm clinical trials evaluating carotid stenting with emboli protection devices have recently been presented or are ongoing (Table 107–3). Many of these trials evaluated patients considered high-risk for CEA but nevertheless demonstrated favorable results compared to historical controls.

Other data support results of these studies, providing a strong rationale for routine use of emboli protection devices. For example,

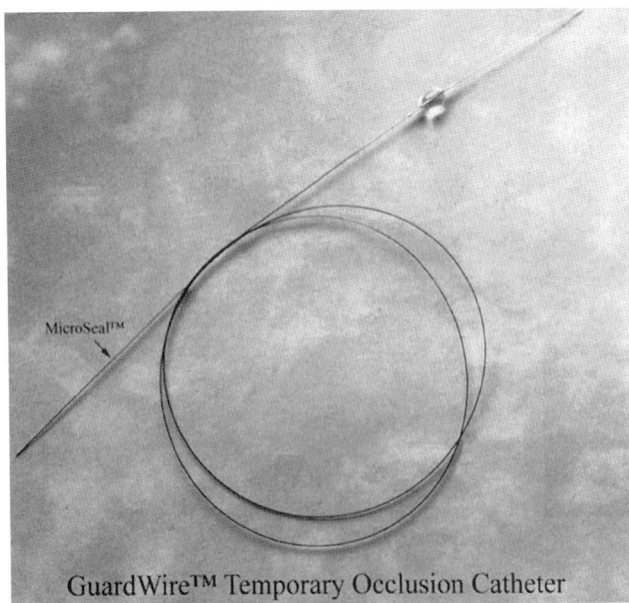

FIGURE 107-5. The PercuSurge GuardWire.

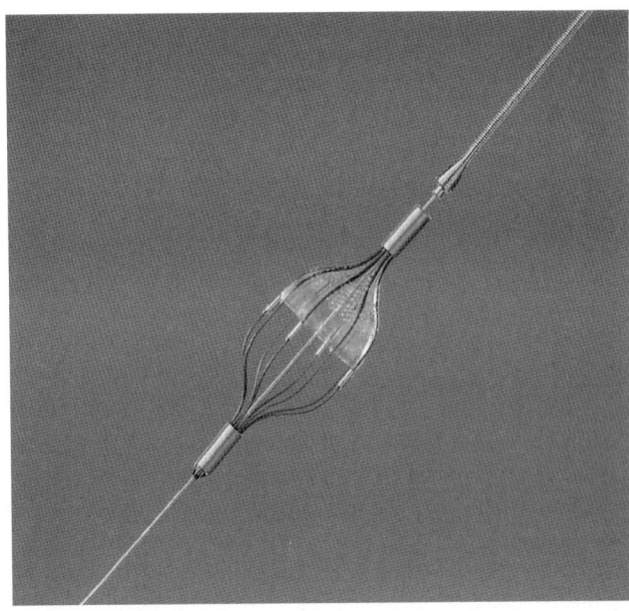

FIGURE 107-6. The AngioGuard Emboli Capture Guidewire System.

TABLE 107–2

Experience with Devices to Prevent Emboli: Case Series

STUDY	PROCEDURES (N)	DEVICE	MAJOR STROKE (%)	MINOR STROKE (%)	DEATH (%)	ALL (%)
Henry[126]	268	GuardWire	0.4	1.5	0.4	2.3
Al Mubarak[124]	164	NeuroShield	0	1.2	1.2	2.4
Whitlow[123]	75	GuardWire	0	0	0	0
Reimers[121]	88	Filters (3 types)	0	1	0	1
MacDonald[125]	50	NeuroShield	0	2	4	6
Wholey Global Registry[86]	4221	All types	0.7	1.1	0.4	2.2
All	4866		0.6	1.0	0.5	2.2

Kastrup and colleagues systematically reviewed the literature, analyzing outcomes for 896 procedures performed with emboli protection, compared to 2537 procedures performed without emboli protection.[97] Patients treated with emboli protection had a 30-day stroke or death incidence of 1.8 percent compared to 5.5 percent for patients treated without emboli protection. Likewise, the Endarterectomy versus Angioplasty in Patients with Symptomatic Severe Carotid Stenosis (EVA-3S) trial, a randomized trial comparing CEA to stenting in symptomatic patients, reported outcomes for 80 patients randomized to stenting according to use of an embolic protection device.[98] EVA-3S found a stunning incidence of stroke, 26.7 percent, for patients treated without emboli protection compared to 8.6 percent for patients treated with emboli protection. Thus, emboli prevention devices have become standard of care for carotid stenting procedure in clinical practice. At this time, there are no studies comparing safety and efficacy of different emboli prevention devices.

TABLE 107–3

Experience with Devices to Prevent Emboli: Nonrandomized Clinical Trials

STUDY	PATIENTS (N)	DEVICE	TYPE OF DEVICE	HIGH RISK	30-DAY DEATH, MYOCARDIAL INFARCTION, OR STROKE (%)
ARCHER-2	278	Accunet OTW	Filter	Yes	8.6
ARCHER-3	145	Accunet RW	Filter	Yes	8.3
BEACH	747	FilterWire EX/EZ	Filter	Yes	5.8
CABERNET	454	FilterWire EX/EZ	Filter	Yes	3.8
CAPTURE	1603 (2500 planned)	Accunet	Filter	Yes	5.1
CAPTURE 2	~10000	Accunet	Filter	Yes	Enrolling
CaRESS	143 CAS / 254 CEA	GuardWire Plus	Balloon	No	2 (CAS) vs. 3 (CEA)
CASES-PMS	1279 (1493 planned)	AngioGuard	Filter	Yes	4.8
CREATE-Pivotal	419	Spider	Filter	Yes	6.8
CREATE II	160	SpideRX	Filter	Yes	5.6
EXACT	~1500	Emboshield	Filter	Yes	Enrolling
EPIC	50	FiberNet	Filter	Yes	Enrolling
MAVErIC I	99	GuardWire	Balloon	Yes	5.1
MAVErIC II	399	GuardWire	Balloon	Yes	5.3
MAVErIC III	413	GuardWire	Balloon	Yes	Enrolling
MO.MA	157	Mo.Ma	Proximal Occlusion	No	5.7
PRIAMUS	416	Mo.Ma	Proximal Occlusion	No	4.6
RULE-Carotid	60	Rubicon	Filter	No	5.0
SECURITY	305	Emboshield	Filter	Yes	6.9
SHELTER	400	GuardWire	Balloon	Yes	Enrolling
VIVA	>500	Emboshield	Filter	Yes	Enrolling
Total (Completed)	6918				4.9

【 】 COMPLICATIONS AND THEIR MANAGEMENT

There are several important issues, some unique to carotid artery stenting and some similar to those seen in percutaneous coronary intervention, of which the physician must be mindful to avert an adverse and potentially catastrophic outcome. The major periprocedural complications of carotid artery stenting are stroke, MI, and death. The SAPPHIRE trial documented a 30-day risk of 5.8 percent in high-risk patients for these endpoints[80] (Fig 107–7). Importantly, the CREATE Pivotal trial found that independent predictors of death or stroke at 30 days included baseline renal insufficiency, symptomatic carotid stenosis, and duration of filter deployment. The lead-in phase for the Carotid Revascularization Endarterectomy versus Stent Trial (CREST) demonstrated a substantially increased risk of stroke for patients at least age 80 years (12.1 percent) compared to those younger than age 80 years (3.2 percent).[99] The recently presented CAPTURE trial confirmed the CREATE and CREST findings, demonstrating a higher incidence of 30-day death, MI, or stroke for octogenarians (8.2 percent vs. 5.7 percent for entire cohort) and for symptomatic patients (13.5 percent vs. 4.9 percent for asymptomatic patients).[100] Other associated adverse events are intracranial hemorrhage, bradycardia, hypotension, seizures, contrast nephrotoxicities, and access site complications.

Although most ischemic complications occur during the procedure, they can occur several hours later. Careful neurologic examination is essential to identify these complications. Routine use of cerebral angiography before and after stenting can help identify occluded intracranial vessels. Intraarterial thrombolytic therapy has been used to treat this complication but with very limited success, reflecting the fact that embolic materials are commonly plaque fragments and not thrombus.[101] Further, the risk of intracranial hemorrhage with this approach is substantial. Mechanical dislodgement of the embolic debris with soft wires may be the best approach to minimize the size of cerebral infraction.

The carotid sinus reflex is most often responsible for the bradycardia and hypotension associated with carotid sinus manipulation. In anticipation of this effect, antihypertensives medications are typically held the morning of the procedure, and depending on the response to stenting, may also be held until the following morning. Adequate volume expansion is the cornerstone of effective treatment. Atropine is helpful in cases of severe bradycardia. Vasopressors may be required for severe and persistent hypotension. The carotid sinus reflex is typically transient, but it may continue to be a concern for up to 24 hours after the procedure.

On the other side of the spectrum, brisk return of blood flow distal to a chronically ischemic cerebral hemisphere with disordered cerebral autoregulation can lead to problems. Hyperperfusion syndrome is a potentially deadly complication from carotid artery stenting or CEA. Severe hypertension, critical carotid stenosis, and contralateral carotid occlusion appear to be predisposing factors.[102] Strict monitoring of blood pressure with appropriate treatment is crucial to preventing this. All patients undergoing carotid artery stenting should be instructed on the importance of medication compliance as well as home blood pressure monitoring. They should be instructed to keep their systolic blood pressure (SBP) <140 mmHg. Furthermore, patients must be instructed to monitor for headaches localized to one side associated with nausea, vomiting, and photophobia. Treatment of hyperperfusion syndrome includes strict blood pressure control with the lowering of SBP to approximately 100 mmHg.

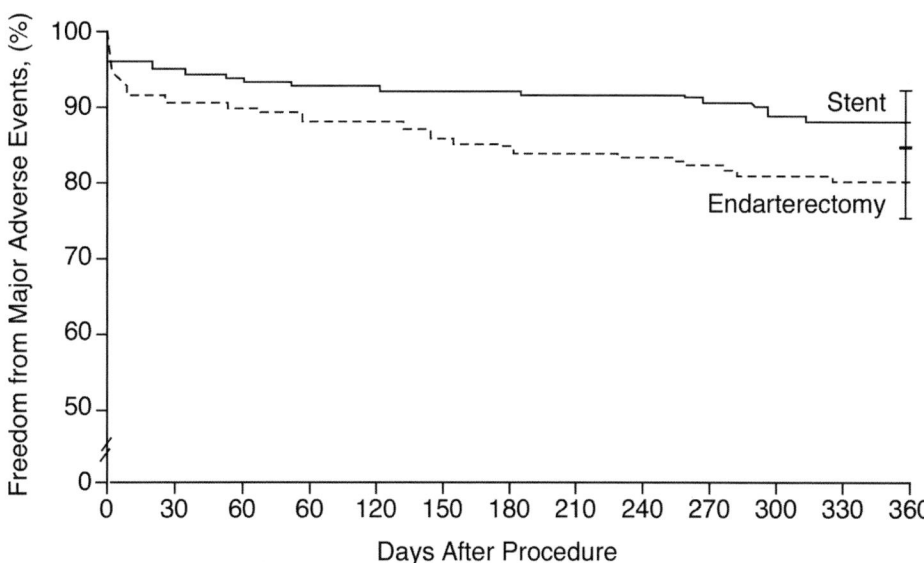

FIGURE 107–7. Stenting and Angioplasty with Protection in Patients at High Risk for Endarterectomy Trial Results. *Source: Reprinted with permission from Yadav JS, Wholey MH, Kuntz RE, et al. Protected carotid-artery stenting versus endarterectomy in high-risk patients. N Engl J Med 2004;351:1493–1501. All rights reserved.*

COMPARISONS OF CAROTID ARTERY STENTING AND CAROTID ENDARTERECTOMY

【 】 TRIALS

Although carotid artery stenting is a less invasive method of treating carotid artery stenosis compared to CEA, extensive evidence of the safety and feasibility of CEA have made it difficult to establish carotid artery stenting as a viable alternative. Two major studies comparing these procedures have been completed, however, and many more are currently enrolling.

The Carotid and Vertebral Artery Transluminal Angioplasty Study (CAVATAS) compared the outcomes of percutaneous angioplasty and stenting to surgical CEA.[103] There was no difference between the two treatment groups with regard to stroke or mortality. However, complications such as cranial neuropathy and significant hematoma formation occurred more often in the surgical group. Conversely, the percutaneous treatment group was more likely to experience restenosis. This trial demonstrated equivalent major outcomes with no significant difference at 1 year for ipsilateral neurologic complications. Minor complications such as bleed-

TABLE 107–4

One-Year Outcomes from the SAPPHIRE Trial

MAJOR OUTCOME EVENT	STENT (167 PATIENTS)	CEA (167 PATIENTS)	P VALUE
Death	7.4%	13.5%	0.08
Major ipsilateral stroke	0.6%	3.3%	0.09
Myocardial infarction	3.0%	7.5%	0.07
Cranial nerve palsy	0	4.9%	0.004
Target-vessel revascularization	0.6%	4.3%	0.04
Primary end point[a]	12.2%	20.1%	0.05

[a]Death, stroke, or myocardial infarction at 30 days plus ipsilateral stroke or death from neurologic causes within 31 days to 1 year.

ing and cranial nerve palsies were higher for CEA. This trial has been criticized for having higher than expected complication rates with CEA. However, the percutaneous method used would not be considered state of the art by current standards because only 25 percent of the patients undergoing percutaneous revascularization received stents and emboli prevention devices were not used in this study.

More recently, the SAPPHIRE trial was published in October 2004.[80] This trial randomized 334 patients to either carotid angioplasty plus stenting with emboli protection or to CEA. Patients were either asymptomatic with ≥80 percent stenosis by ultrasound or symptomatic with ≥50 percent stenosis. All patients enrolled had a comorbid condition that increased the risk of CEA. The entry inclusion criteria included previous CEA, congestive heart failure, severe CAD, previous radical neck surgery or radiation therapy, and chronic obstructive pulmonary disease. Patients who, in the opinion of a vascular surgeon, could not have surgery were enrolled in a stent registry (409 patients). Patients considered at too high a risk for percutaneous management were likewise enrolled in a surgical registry (17 patients). The primary end point was main adverse coronary events (MACEs), including death, stroke, or MI within 30 days of the procedure plus death from neurological causes or ipsilateral stroke up to 1 year. The results are shown in Table 107–4. The MACE rate was lower in the percutaneous treatment group compared to the CEA group (12.2 percent vs. 20.1 percent, $p = 0.05$). In the registry data, the 30-day MACE rate was 7.8 percent for stenting (32 of 409) and 14.3 percent (1 of 7) for CEA. There were no significant differences between the two groups with regard to either major bleeding (8.3 vs. 10.6 percent, $p = 0.56$) or TIA (3.85 vs. 2.0 percent, $p = 0.5$), but carotid stenting did have an advantage over CEA with regard to cranial nerve injury (0 vs. 5.3 percent, $p < 0.01$). Restenosis rates were not presented. This trial clearly demonstrated a reduction in risk of MACE for high-risk patients treated with carotid stenting compared to conventional CEA.

Recent trials randomizing patients to CEA or carotid stenting include the Stent-Supported Percutaneous Angioplasty of the Carotid Artery versus Endarterectomy (SPACE) Trial[104] and the EVA-3S Trial.[105] The SPACE trial randomized 1200 patients with carotid stenosis at least 70 percent by carotid duplex (correspond-

ing to ≥50 percent by NASCET criteria), and history of TIA or stroke within 180 days, to CEA or carotid stenting. Patients in SPACE were clearly lower risk than patients in SAPPHIRE. Specifically, exclusion criteria in SPACE included contralateral carotid occlusion, carotid stenosis after endarterectomy, and history of neck radiation, which were inclusion criteria for SAPPHIRE. The mean age of patients was approximately 68 years and 72 percent were men with approximately 27 percent incidence of diabetes and approximately 22 percent incidence of CAD. The primary endpoint was ipsilateral stroke or death from any cause within 30 days. Importantly, SPACE was designed as a noninferiority trial. To show noninferiority difference in the primary endpoint between groups could not exceed 2.5 percent in the 90 percent CI.

By 30 days the primary endpoint occurred in 6.84 percent of the carotid stenting group compared to 6.34 percent of the CEA group (90 percent CI: 1.89–2.91 percent). Because the upper bound of the 90 percent CI, 2.91 percent, exceeds 2.5 percent, the trial failed to prove noninferiority.

It is important to understand the context of these findings and their limitations. Specifically, SPACE *does not* prove that carotid stenting is inferior to CEA. Instead, SPACE *failed to prove noninferiority*, and it is difficult to understand the implications of this. The editorialists commented as follows:

> *Despite SPACE being the biggest trial to date, one is left with the unavoidable conclusion that it was stopped prematurely. Notwithstanding funding issues, the planned margin of noninferiority (<2.5%) was based on a power calculation of 1900 patients and this larger sample might have provided much tighter CIs and more robust statistical data.[106]*

Also, broader applicability of the results is questionable given the high incidence of stroke or death compared to other trials and registries (e.g., 30-day death, stroke, or MI was 4.8 percent for carotid stent patients in SAPPHIRE). Emboli protection devices were not mandated in SPACE, but the authors noted no difference in death or stroke for patients treated with embolic protection (7.3 percent) compared to those treated without protection (6.7 percent).

The EVA-3S trial randomized 520 patients with carotid stenosis at least 60 percent, and history of TIA or stroke within 120 days, to CEA or carotid stenting. Similar to patients in SPACE, patients in EVA-3S were not high risk. The mean age was approximately 70 years with approximately 23 percent incidence of diabetes and approximately 13 percent incidence of CAD treated by surgery or stenting. The primary endpoint was 30-day stroke or death.

EVA-3S planned to enroll 827 patients but was stopped prematurely because of a significantly higher event rate in the carotid stenting arm. Thirty-day stroke or death occurred in 3.9 percent of endarterectomy patients compared to 9.6 percent of stenting patients ($p = 0.01$), driven by a highly significant difference in nonfatal stroke (2.7 percent vs. 8.8 percent, $p = 0.004$). By 6 months, any stroke or death occurred in 6.1 percent of endarterectomy patients compared to 11.7 percent of stenting patients ($p = 0.02$). The trial also demonstrated important differences in carotid stenting patients treated with and without cerebral protection. Patients treated with embolic protection had a 30-day incidence of death or stroke of 7.9 percent compared to 25 percent for patients not treated with embolic protection ($p = 0.03$). Nonetheless, the RR of stroke or death for stenting over endarterectomy did not differ significantly for the trial before routine embolic protection (RR 2.0, 95 percent CI 0.8–5.0) or after (RR 3.4, 95 percent CI 1.1–10.0, $p = 0.50$).

Although striking, these results must be tempered by concerns about general applicability. As noted by the editorialist of EVA-3S,[107] symptomatic patients in SAPPHIRE had a much lower 30-day incidence of death, MI, or stroke than patients in EVA-3S (2.1 percent compared to 9.6 percent); this occurred despite the higher features of SAPPHIRE patients. Similarly, a systematic review of carotid stenting found a 30-day incidence of death or stroke of 1.8 percent for carotid stent patients (asymptomatic and symptomatic patients pooled).[97] Unlike SAPPHIRE investigators, who used a single embolic protection device (AngioGuard, Cordis), EVA-3S physicians used five different stents and seven different embolic protection devices. Further, only two procedures with any one device were required for use of that device. Thus, it is unclear how much a *learning-curve effect*[88] contributed to difference in endpoint between the groups and between EVA-3S carotid stenting patients and those generally described in the literature.

[ ] SPECIAL SUBGROUPS

There are several patient subgroups that have posed special challenges for the vascular surgeon contemplating a surgical approach to treatment of their carotid artery stenosis. Existing data support the treatment of these patients with carotid artery stenting instead of CEA.

[ ] CONCOMITANT CAROTID STENOSIS AND CORONARY ARTERY DISEASE

An important issue surrounding the treatment of carotid artery atherosclerosis is the optimal treatment strategy used to treat those with both significant carotid artery disease and coronary atherosclerosis. This is not an insignificant issue, as evidenced by the 50 to 60 percent of patients with carotid artery disease who also have significant coronary atherosclerosis.[10] Approaches using CEA followed by open heart surgery (OHS), OHS followed by CEA, or combined OHS and CEA have been studied. Although the stroke, MI, and death rates vary in different series, the risk is high with all strategies (Table 107–5).[108] Recent data from the SAPPHIRE trial demonstrated that treatment of carotid disease with carotid stenting is a lower-risk procedure and is associated with a lower rate of MI when compared to CEA. In the randomized patients, carotid stenting was associated with a 2.6 percent rate of MI and CEA was associated with a 7.3 percent rate of MI at 30 days ($p = 0.07$).[80] Additionally, Ziada and coworkers recently evaluated the outcomes of 64 patients with both severe carotid steno-

sis and coronary atherosclerosis who were treated with carotid stenting followed by coronary artery bypass surgery and compared them to 112 patients who underwent combined CEA and OHS. The stent group had a much higher prevalence of unstable angina, poor LV function, critical aortic valve stenosis, TIA or stroke, and history of previous OHS. Although there was no difference in mortality, the stent patients had significantly lower incidence of strokes (2 vs. 9 percent, $p = 0.05$) and strokes or MI (6 vs. 19 percent, $p = 0.02$) compared to those who received concomitant CEA and OHS.[109] Antiplatelet therapy poses a challenge for patients scheduled for immediate surgery. It is preferable if patients can wait 2 to 4 weeks after stenting and be kept on aspirin and clopidogrel during this time. Anecdotal use of short-acting IIb/IIIa inhibitors until the cardiac surgery and immediate loading with clopidogrel and aspirin after the surgery has been reported to be successful. Use of balloon angioplasty to temporize the situation prior to OHS has been tried. The availability of heparin-coated stents may reduce the need for dual antiplatelet therapy.

[ ] RADICAL NECK SURGERY AND RADIATION THERAPY

Extracranial carotid stenosis frequently occurs in patients who have had surgery and head and neck irradiation for cancer therapy. Tissue dissection is complicated by the extensive fibrosis of the arterial wall and normal tissue planes, and the difficult locations of the lesions caused by extensive involvement of long segments of the carotid artery above and below the carotid bifurcation make access difficult.[110] Carotid stenting has been reported as safe and effective in the treatment of this problem.[111–115] The procedural risks are not increased compared to stenting for conventional treatment of atherosclerotic carotid disease. Therefore, carotid stenting can be considered the treatment of choice for severe carotid stenosis requiring revascularization after cervical radiation or radical neck surgery.

There is a higher surgical risk for patients with restenotic lesions after CEA compared to those undergoing CEA for the first time. Occasionally, the lesion is also in an anatomically unfavorable location for surgery. These lesions can be successfully treated with percutaneous stenting with no increased risk. Data from a multicenter registry of 14 U.S. centers included 338 patients undergoing carotid stenting of 358 arteries for restenosis after CEA revealed an overall 30-day stroke and death rate of 3.7 percent.[116] There was one (0.3 percent) fatal and one (0.3 percent) nonfatal stroke during the follow-up period. The overall 3-year rate of free-

TABLE 107–5

Adverse Events in Patients Undergoing Carotid Endarterectomy and Coronary Artery Bypass Grafting

TREATMENT STRATEGY	STROKE	MI	DEATH	ALL EVENTS
CEA + CABG	6.2	4.7	5.6	16.5
CEA followed by CABG	5.3	11.5[a]	9.4[a]	26.2[a]
CABG followed by CEA	10.0[a]	2.8	3.6	16.4

[a]$p < 0.05$.

SOURCE: Modified from Moore WS, Barnett HJ, Beebe HJ, et al.[108] With permission.

dom from all fatal and nonfatal strokes was 96 percent. These results suggest that carotid artery stenting is an excellent treatment alternative for restenosis following CEA.

FUTURE APPLICATIONS AND TRIALS

Several trials to evaluate the percutaneous treatment of carotid artery atherosclerosis are ongoing. The updated information on these trials is available online at www.strokecenter.org. Like SAPPHIRE, the International Carotid Stenting Study (or CAVATAS-2) is randomizing high-risk symptomatic patients (>50 percent stenosis) to CEA or carotid stenting.[117] CREST is a multicenter randomized trial to compare CEA with carotid artery stenting using emboli prevention device. Unlike SAPPHIRE, the patients studied in this trial are at low risk; therefore, this trial will add insight into the use of this treatment strategy in additional patient populations.

For asymptomatic patients, the Asymptomatic Carotid Stenosis Stenting Versus Endarterectomy Trial is randomizing low-risk asymptomatic patients to carotid stenting versus CEA (3:1). Similarly, the Transatlantic Asymptomatic Carotid Intervention Trial (TACIT) is randomizing asymptomatic patients to medical therapy, carotid endarterectomy, or carotid stenting.[118]

REFERENCES

1. Executive Committee for the Asymptomatic Carotid Atherosclerosis Study. Endarterectomy for asymptomatic carotid artery stenosis. *JAMA* 1995;273(18):1421–1428.
2. Hobson RW II, Weiss DG, Fields WS, et al. Efficacy of carotid endarterectomy for asymptomatic carotid stenosis. The Veterans Affairs Cooperative Study Group. *N Engl J Med* 1993;328(4):221–227.
3. CASANOVA Study Group. Carotid surgery versus medical therapy in asymptomatic carotid stenosis. *Stroke* 1991;22(10):1229–1235.
4. Mohammed N, Anand SS. Prevention of disabling and fatal strokes by successful carotid endarterectomy in patients without recent neurological symptoms: randomized controlled trial. MRC asymptomatic carotid surgery trial (ACST) collaborative group. *Lancet* 2004;363:1491–502. *Vasc Med* February 2005;10(1):77–78.
5. North American Symptomatic Carotid Endarterectomy Trial Collaborators. Beneficial effect of carotid endarterectomy in symptomatic patients with high-grade carotid stenosis. *N Engl J Med* 1991;325(7):445–453.
6. European Carotid Surgery Trialists' Collaborative Group. MRC European Carotid Surgery Trial: interim results for symptomatic patients with severe (70–99%) or with mild (0–29%) carotid stenosis. *Lancet* 1991;337(8752):1235–1243.
7. Mayberg MR, Wilson SE, Yatsu F, et al. Carotid endarterectomy and prevention of cerebral ischemia in symptomatic carotid stenosis. Veterans Affairs Cooperative Studies Program 309 Trialist Group. *JAMA* 1991;266(23):3289–3294.
8. American Heart Association. Heart disease and stroke statistics: 2006 update.
9. Angelini A, Reimers B, Della Barbera M, et al. Cerebral protection during carotid artery stenting: collection and histopathologic analysis of embolized debris. *Stroke* 2002;33(2):456–461.
10. Hertzer NR, Beven EG, Young JR, et al. Coronary artery disease in peripheral vascular patients: a classification of 1000 coronary angiograms and results of surgical management. *Ann Surg* 1984;199(2):223–233.
11. Wolf PA, D'Agostino RB, Kannel WB, Bonita R, Belanger AJ. Cigarette smoking as a risk factor for stroke. The Framingham Study. *JAMA* February 19, 1988;259(7):1025–1029.
12. Byington RP, Furberg CD, Crouse JR III, Espeland MA, Bond MG. Pravastatin, Lipids, and Atherosclerosis in the Carotid Arteries (PLAC-II). *Am J Cardiol* September 28, 1995;76(9):54C–59C.
13. Whisnant JP, Homer D, Ingall TJ, Baker HL Jr, O'Fallon WM, Wievers DO. Duration of cigarette smoking is the strongest predictor of severe extracranial carotid artery atherosclerosis. *Stroke* 1990;21(5):707–714.
14. McNeill AM, Rosamond WD, Girman CJ, et al. Prevalence of coronary heart disease and carotid arterial thickening in patients with the metabolic syndrome. The ARIC Study. *Am J Cardiol* November 15, 2004;94(10):1249–1254.
15. Magyar MT, Szikszai Z, Balla J, et al. Early-onset carotid atherosclerosis is associated with increased intima-media thickness and elevated serum levels of inflammatory markers. *Stroke* January 2003;34(1):58–63.
16. Sangiorgi G, Mauriello A, Bonanno E, et al. Pregnancy-associated plasma protein-a is markedly expressed by monocyte-macrophage cells in vulnerable and ruptured carotid atherosclerotic plaques: a link between inflammation and cerebrovascular events. *J Am Coll Cardiol* June 6, 2006;47(11):2201–2211.
17. Redgrave JN, Lovett JK, Gallagher PJ, Rothwell PM. Histological assessment of 526 symptomatic carotid plaques in relation to the nature and timing of ischemic symptoms: the Oxford plaque study. *Circulation* May 16, 2006;113(19):2320–2328.
18. Norris JW, Zhu CZ, Bornstein NM, Chambers BR. Vascular risks of asymptomatic carotid stenosis. *Stroke* 1991;22(12):1485–1490.
19. Barnett HJ, Taylor DW, Eliasziw M, et al. Benefit of carotid endarterectomy in patients with symptomatic moderate or severe stenosis. North American Symptomatic Carotid Endarterectomy Trial Collaborators. *N Engl J Med* 1998;339(20):1415–1425.
20. Joakimsen O, Bonaa KH, Mathiesen EB, Stensland-Bugge E, Arnesen E. Prediction of mortality by ultrasound screening of a general population for carotid stenosis. The Tromso Study. *Stroke* 2000;31(8):1871–1876.
21. Taylor LM Jr, Loboa L, Porter JM. The clinical course of carotid bifurcation stenosis as determined by duplex scanning. *J Vasc Surg* 1988;8(3):255–261.
22. Fabris F, Poli L, Zanocchi M, Bo M, Fiandra U, Fonte G. A four year clinical and echographic follow-up of asymptomatic carotid plaque. *Angiology* 1992;43(7):590–598.
23. Erdoes LS, Marek JM, Mills JL, et al. The relative contributions of carotid duplex scanning, magnetic resonance angiography, and cerebral arteriography to clinical decision making: a prospective study in patients with carotid occlusive disease. *J Vasc Surg* 1996;23(5):950–956.
24. Chervu A, Moore WS. Carotid endarterectomy without arteriography. *Ann Vasc Surg* 1994;8(3):296–302.
25. Dawson DL, Zierler RE, Strandness DE Jr, Clowes AW, Kohler TR. The role of duplex scanning and arteriography before carotid endarterectomy: a prospective study. *J Vasc Surg* 1993;18(4):673–680; discussion 680–673.
26. Horn M, Michelini M, Greisler HP, Littooy FN, Baker WH. Carotid endarterectomy without arteriography: the preeminent role of the vascular laboratory. *Ann Vasc Surg* 1994;8(3):221–224.
27. Mattos MA, Hodgson KJ, Faught WE, et al. Carotid endarterectomy without angiography: is color-flow duplex scanning sufficient? *Surgery* 1994;116(4):776–782; discussion 782–773.
28. Eliasziw M, Rankin RN, Fox AJ, Haynes RB, Barnett HJ. Accuracy and prognostic consequences of ultrasonography in identifying severe carotid artery stenosis. North American Symptomatic Carotid Endarterectomy Trial (NASCET) Group. *Stroke* 1995;26(10):1747–1752.
29. Howard G, Baker WH, Chambless LE, Howard VJ, Jones AM, Toole JF. An approach for the use of Doppler ultrasound as a screening tool for hemodynamically significant stenosis (despite heterogeneity of Doppler performance): a multicenter experience. Asymptomatic Carotid Atherosclerosis Study Investigators. *Stroke,* 1996;27(11):1951–1957.
30. Telman G, Kouperberg E, Sprecher E, et al. Duplex ultrasound verified by angiography in patients with severe primary and restenosis of internal carotid artery. *Ann Vasc Surg* 2006;20(4):478–481.
31. Jahromi AS, Cina CS, Liu Y, Clase CM. Sensitivity and specificity of color duplex ultrasound measurement in the estimation of internal carotid artery stenosis: a systematic review and meta-analysis. *J Vasc Surg* June 2005;41(6):962–972.
32. Filis KA, Arko FR, Johnson BL, et al. Duplex ultrasound criteria for defining the severity of carotid stenosis. *Ann Vasc Surg* July 2002;16(4):413–421.
33. Lorenz MW, von Kegler S, Steinmetz H, Markus HS, Sitzer M. Carotid intima-media thickening indicates a higher vascular risk across a wide age range: prospective data from the Carotid Atherosclerosis Progression Study (CAPS). *Stroke* January 2006;37(1):87–92.
34. van der Meer IM, Bots ML, Hofman A, del Sol AI, van der Kuip DA, Witteman JC. Predictive value of noninvasive measures of atherosclerosis for incident myocardial infarction. The Rotterdam Study. *Circulation* March 9, 2004;109(9):1089–1094.
35. Wattanakit K, Folsom AR, Chambless LE, Nieto FJ. Risk factors for cardiovascular event recurrence in the Atherosclerosis Risk in Communities (ARIC) study. *Am Heart J* April 2005;149(4):606–612.
36. Tsivgoulis G, Vemmos K, Papamichael C, et al. Common carotid artery intima-media thickness and the risk of stroke recurrence. *Stroke* July 2006;37(7):1913–1916.
37. Staub D, Meyerhans A, Bundi B, Schmid HP, Frauchiger B. Prediction of cardiovascular morbidity and mortality: comparison of the internal carotid

artery resistive index with the common carotid artery intima-media thickness. *Stroke* March 2006;37(3):800–805.

38. Muhs BE, Gagne P, Wagener J, et al. Gadolinium-enhanced versus time-of-flight magnetic resonance angiography: what is the benefit of contrast enhancement in evaluating carotid stenosis? *Ann Vasc Surg* November 2005;19(6):823–828.

39. Fellner C, Lang W, Janka R, Wutke R, Bautz W, Fellner FA. Magnetic resonance angiography of the carotid arteries using three different techniques: accuracy compared with intraarterial x-ray angiography and endarterectomy specimens. *J Magn Reson Imaging* April 2005;21(4):424–431.

40. Nederkoorn PJ, Elgersma OE, van der Graaf Y, Eikelboom BC, Kappelle LJ, Mali WP. Carotid artery stenosis: accuracy of contrast-enhanced MR angiography for diagnosis. *Radiology* September 2003;228(3):677–682.

41. Townsend TC, Saloner D, Pan XM, Rapp JH. Contrast material-enhanced MRA overestimates severity of carotid stenosis, compared with 3D time-of-flight MRA. *J Vasc Surg* July 2003;38(1):36–40.

42. Johnston DC, Goldstein LB. Clinical carotid endarterectomy decision making: noninvasive vascular imaging versus angiography. *Neurology* 2001;56(8):1009–1015.

43. Nederkoorn PJ, van der Graaf Y, Hunink MG. Duplex ultrasound and magnetic resonance angiography compared with digital subtraction angiography in carotid artery stenosis: a systematic review. *Stroke* May 2003;34(5):1324–1332.

44. Borisch I, Horn M, Butz B, et al. Preoperative evaluation of carotid artery stenosis: comparison of contrast-enhanced MR angiography and duplex sonography with digital subtraction angiography. *AJNR Am J Neuroradiol* June–July 2003;24(6):1117–1122.

45. Traversi E, Bertoli G, Barazzoni G, Baldi M, Tramarin R. Non-invasive coronary angiography with multislice computed tomography: technology, methods, preliminary experience and prospects. *Ital Heart J* February 2004;5(2):89–98.

46. Sameshima T, Futami S, Morita Y, et al. Clinical usefulness of and problems with three-dimensional CT angiography for the evaluation of arteriosclerotic stenosis of the carotid artery: comparison with conventional angiography, MRA, and ultrasound sonography. *Surg Neurol* March 1999;51(3):301–308; discussion 308–309.

47. Hollingworth W, Nathens AB, Kanne JP, et al. The diagnostic accuracy of computed tomography angiography for traumatic or atherosclerotic lesions of the carotid and vertebral arteries: a systematic review. *Eur J Radiol* October 2003;48(1):88–102.

48. Koelemay MJ, Nederkoorn PJ, Reitsma JB, Majoie CB. Systematic review of computed tomographic angiography for assessment of carotid artery disease. *Stroke* 2004;35(10):2306–2312.

49. Fayed AM, White CJ, Ramee SR, Jenkins JS, Collins TJ. Carotid and cerebral angiography performed by cardiologists: cerebrovascular complications. *Catheter Cardiovasc Interv* 2002;55(3):277–280.

50. Collaborative meta-analysis of randomised trials of antiplatelet therapy for prevention of death, myocardial infarction, and stroke in high risk patients. *BMJ* 2002;324(7329):71–86.

51. Dorsam RT, Kunapuli SP. Central role of the P2Y12 receptor in platelet activation. *J Clin Invest* February 2004;113(3):340–345.

52. Hass WK, Easton JD, Adams HP, Jr, et al. A randomized trial comparing ticlopidine hydrochloride with aspirin for the prevention of stroke in high-risk patients. Ticlopidine Aspirin Stroke Study Group [comments]. *N Engl J Med* 1989;321(8):501–507.

53. Gent M, Blakely JA, Easton JD, et al. The Canadian American Ticlopidine Study (CATS) in thromboembolic stroke. *Lancet* 1989;1(8649):1215–1220.

54. CAPRIE Steering Committee. A randomised, blinded, trial of clopidogrel versus aspirin in patients at risk of ischaemic events (CAPRIE). *Lancet* 1996;348(9038):1329–1339.

55. Diener HC, Bogousslavsky J, Brass LM, et al. Aspirin and clopidogrel compared with clopidogrel alone after recent ischaemic stroke or transient ischaemic attack in high-risk patients (MATCH): randomised, double-blind, placebo-controlled trial. *Lancet* July 24–30, 2004;364(9431):331–337.

56. Bhatt DL, Fox KA, Hacke W, et al. Clopidogrel and aspirin versus aspirin alone for the prevention of atherothrombotic events. *N Engl J Med* March 12, 2006.

57. Risk factors for stroke and efficacy of antithrombotic therapy in atrial fibrillation: analysis of pooled data from five randomized controlled trials. *Arch Intern Med* 1994;154(13):1449–1457.

58. Stroke Prevention in Reversible Ischemia Trial (SPIRIT) Study Group. A randomized trial of anticoagulants versus aspirin after cerebral ischemia of presumed arterial origin. *Ann Neurol* 1997;42(6):857–865.

59. Mohr JP, Thompson JL, Lazar RM, et al. A comparison of warfarin and aspirin for the prevention of recurrent ischemic stroke. *N Engl J Med* 2001;345(20):1444–1451.

60. Chimowitz MI, Lynn MJ, Howlett-Smith H, et al. Comparison of warfarin and aspirin for symptomatic intracranial arterial stenosis. *N Engl J Med* March 31, 2005;352(13):1305–1316.

61. Randomised trial of cholesterol lowering in 4444 patients with coronary heart disease: the Scandinavian Simvastatin Survival Study (4S). *Lancet* 1994;344(8934):1383–1389.

62. Long-Term Intervention with Pravastatin in Ischaemic Disease (LIPID) Study Group. Prevention of cardiovascular events and death with pravastatin in patients with coronary heart disease and a broad range of initial cholesterol levels. *N Engl J Med* 1998;339(19):1349–1357.

63. Sacks FM, Pfeffer MA, Moye LA, et al. The effect of pravastatin on coronary events after myocardial infarction in patients with average cholesterol levels. Cholesterol and Recurrent Events Trial Investigators. *N Engl J Med* 1996;335(14):1001–1009.

64. Bucher HC, Griffith LE, Guyatt GH. Effect of HMGcoA reductase inhibitors on stroke: a meta-analysis of randomized, controlled trials. *Ann Intern Med* 1998;128(2):89–95.

65. Cheung BM, Lauder IJ, Lau CP, Kumana CR. Meta-analysis of large randomized controlled trials to evaluate the impact of statins on cardiovascular outcomes. *Br J Clin Pharmacol* May 2004;57(5):640–651.

66. Baigent C, Keech A, Kearney PM, et al. Efficacy and safety of cholesterol-lowering treatment: prospective meta-analysis of data from 90,056 participants in 14 randomised trials of statins. *Lancet* October 8, 2005;366(9493):1267–1278.

67. Briel M, Schwartz GG, Thompson PL, et al. Effects of early treatment with statins on short-term clinical outcomes in acute coronary syndromes: a meta-analysis of randomized controlled trials. *JAMA* May 3, 2006;295(17):2046–2056.

68. Corti R, Fayad ZA, Fuster V, et al. Effects of lipid-lowering by simvastatin on human atherosclerotic lesions: a longitudinal study by high-resolution, noninvasive magnetic resonance imaging. *Circulation* 2001;104(3):249–252.

69. Corti R, Fuster V, Fayad ZA, et al. Lipid lowering by simvastatin induces regression of human atherosclerotic lesions: two years' follow-up by high-resolution noninvasive magnetic resonance imaging. *Circulation* 2002;106(23):2884–2887.

70. Watanabe K, Sugiyama S, Kugiyama K, et al. Stabilization of carotid atheroma assessed by quantitative ultrasound analysis in nonhypercholesterolemic patients with coronary artery disease. *J Am Coll Cardiol* December 6, 2005;46(11):2022–2030.

71. Molloy KJ, Thompson MM, Schwalbe EC, Bell PR, Naylor AR, Loftus IM. Comparison of levels of matrix metalloproteinases, tissue inhibitor of metalloproteinases, interleukins, and tissue necrosis factor in carotid endarterectomy specimens from patients on versus not on statins preoperatively. *Am J Cardiol* July 1, 2004;94(1):144–146.

72. Mercuri M, Bond MG, Sirtori CR, et al. Pravastatin reduces carotid intima-media thickness progression in an asymptomatic hypercholesterolemic Mediterranean population: the Carotid Atherosclerosis Italian Ultrasound Study. *Am J Med* 1996;101(6):627–634.

73. Kang S, Wu Y, Li X. Effects of statin therapy on the progression of carotid atherosclerosis. *Atherosclerosis* December 2004;177(2):433–442.

74. Amarenco P, Labreuche J, Lavallee P, Touboul PJ. Statins in stroke prevention and carotid atherosclerosis: systematic review and up-to-date meta-analysis. *Stroke* December 2004;35(12):2902–2909.

75. Fisher C. Occlusion of the carotid arteries. *AMA Arch Neurol Psychiatry* 1954;72:187–204.

76. Wennberg DE, Lucas FL, Birkmeyer JD, Bredenberg CE, Fisher ES. Variation in carotid endarterectomy mortality in the Medicare population: trial hospitals, volume, and patient characteristics. *JAMA* April 22–29, 1998;279(16):1278–1281.

77. Mullan S, Duda EE, Patronas NJ. Some examples of balloon technology in neurosurgery. *J Neurosurg* 1980;52(3):321–329.

78. Kerber CW, Cromwell LD, Loehden OL. Catheter dilatation of proximal carotid stenosis during distal bifurcation endarterectomy. *AJNR Am J Neuroradiol* 1980;1(4):348–349.

79. Kachel R. Results of balloon angioplasty in the carotid arteries. *J Endovasc Surg* 1996;3(1):22–30.

80. Yadav JS, Wholey MH, Kuntz RE, et al. Protected carotid-artery stenting versus endarterectomy in high-risk patients. *N Engl J Med* October 7, 2004;351(15):1493–1501.

81. Mathur A, Dorros G, Iyer SS, Vitek JJ, Yadav SS, Roubin GS. Palmaz stent compression in patients following carotid artery stenting. *Cathet Cardiovasc Diagn* 1997;41(2):137–140.

82. Marks MP, Dake MD, Steinberg GK, Norbash AM, Lane B. Stent placement for arterial and venous cerebrovascular disease: preliminary experience [comments]. *Radiology* 1994;191(2):441–446.

83. Mathias K. *Stent Placement in Arteriosclerotic Disease of the Internal Carotid Artery.* Oxford: Isis Medical Media; 1997.

84. Diethrich EB, Ndiaye M, Reid DB. Stenting in the carotid artery: initial experience in 110 patients. *J Endovasc Surg* 1996;3(1):42–62.

85. Yadav JS, Roubin GS, Iyer S, et al. Elective stenting of the extracranial carotid arteries. *Circulation* 1997;95(2):376–381.

86. Wholey MH, Al-Mubarek N. Updated review of the global carotid artery stent registry. *Catheter Cardiovasc Interv* October 2003;60(2):259–266.

87. Al-Mubarak N, Roubin GS, Vitek JJ, New G, Iyer SS. Procedural safety and short-term outcome of ambulatory carotid stenting. *Stroke* 2001;32(10):2305–2309.

88. Lin PH, Bush RL, Peden EK, et al. Carotid artery stenting with neuroprotection: assessing the learning curve and treatment outcome. *Am J Surg* December 2005;190(6):850–857.

89. Kapadia SR, Bajzer CT, Ziada KM, et al. Initial experience of platelet glycoprotein IIb/IIIa inhibition with abciximab during carotid stenting: a safe and effective adjunctive therapy. *Stroke* 2001;32(10):2328–2332.

90. Hofmann R, Kerschner K, Steinwender C, Kypta A, Bibl D, Leisch F. Abciximab bolus injection does not reduce cerebral ischemic complications of elective carotid artery stenting: a randomized study. *Stroke* 2002;33(3):725–727.

91. Bhatt DL, Kapadia SR, Bajzer CT, et al. Dual antiplatelet therapy with clopidogrel and aspirin after carotid artery stenting. *J Invasive Cardiol* December 2001;13(12):767–771.

92. McCleary AJ, Nelson M, Dearden NM, Calvey TA, Gough MJ. Cerebral haemodynamics and embolization during carotid angioplasty in high-risk patients. *Br J Surg* 1998;85(6):771–774.

93. Markus HS, Clifton A, Buckenham T, Brown MM. Carotid angioplasty. Detection of embolic signals during and after the procedure. *Stroke* 1994;25(12):2403–2406.

94. Jansen C, Ramos LM, van Heesewijk JP, Moll FL, van Gijn J, Ackerstaff RG. Impact of microembolism and hemodynamic changes in the brain during carotid endarterectomy. *Stroke* 1994;25(5):992–997.

95. Gaunt ME, Martin PJ, Smith JL, et al. Clinical relevance of intraoperative embolization detected by transcranial Doppler ultrasonography during carotid endarterectomy: a prospective study of 100 patients. *Br J Surg* 1994;81(10):1435–1439.

96. Ackerstaff RG, Jansen C, Moll FL, Vermeulen FE, Hamerlijnck RP, Mauser HW. The significance of microemboli detection by means of transcranial Doppler ultrasonography monitoring in carotid endarterectomy. *J Vasc Surg* 1995;21(6):963–969.

97. Kastrup A, Groschel K, Krapf H, Brehm BR, Dichgans J, Schulz JB. Early outcome of carotid angioplasty and stenting with and without cerebral protection devices. *Stroke* March 2003;34(3):813–819.

98. Mas JL, Chatellier G, Beyssen B, et al.B Carotid angioplasty and stenting with and without cerebral protection: clinical alert from the Endarterectomy Versus Angioplasty in Patients With Symptomatic Severe Carotid Stenosis (EVA-3S) trial. *Stroke* January 2004;35(1):e18–e20.

99. Hobson RW II, Howard VJ, Roubin GS, et al. Carotid artery stenting is associated with increased complications in octogenarians: 30-day stroke and death rates in the CREST lead-in phase. *J Vasc Surg* December 2004;40(6):1106–1111.

100. Gray W. Carotid RX ACCULINK/RX ACCUNET Post-Approval Trial to Uncover Unanticipated or Rare Events (CAPTURE). Paper presented at: American College of Cardiology; 3/14/2006, 2006; Atlanta, GA.

101. Wholey MH, Tan WA, Toursarkissian B, Bailey S, Eles G, Jarmolowski C. Management of neurological complications of carotid artery stenting. *J Endovasc Ther* 2001;8(4):341–353.

102. Abou-Chebl A, Yadav JS, Reginelli JP, Bajzer C, Bhatt D, Krieger DW. Intracranial hemorrhage and hyperperfusion syndrome following carotid artery stenting: risk factors, prevention, and treatment. *J Am Coll Cardiol* May 5, 2004;43(9):1596–1601.

103. Endovascular versus surgical treatment in patients with carotid stenosis in the Carotid and Vertebral Artery Transluminal Angioplasty Study (CAVATAS): a randomised trial. *Lancet* 2001;357(9270):1729–1737.

104. Ringleb PA, Allenberg J, Bruckmann H, et al. 30 day results from the SPACE trial of stent-protected angioplasty versus carotid endarterectomy in

105. Mas JL, Chatellier G, Beyssen B, et al. Endarterectomy versus stenting in patients with symptomatic severe carotid stenosis. *N Engl J Med* October 19, 2006;355(16):1660–1671.

106. Naylor AR. SPACE: not the final frontier. *Lancet.* October 7, 2006;368(9543):1215–1216.

107. Furlan AJ. Carotid-artery stenting—case open or closed? *N Engl J Med* October 19, 2006;355(16):1726–1729.

108. Moore WS, Barnett HJ, Beebe HG, et al. Guidelines for carotid endarterectomy: a multidisciplinary consensus statement from the Ad Hoc Committee, American Heart Association. *Circulation* 1995;91(2):566–579.

109. Ziada KM, Yadav JS, Mukherjee D, et al. Comparison of results of carotid stenting followed by open heart surgery versus combined carotid endarterectomy and open heart surgery (coronary bypass with or without another procedure). *Am J Cardiol* August 15, 2005;96(4):519–523.

110. Friedell ML, Joseph BP, Cohen MJ, Horowitz JD. Surgery for carotid artery stenosis following neck irradiation. *Ann Vasc Surg* 2001;15(1):13–18.

111. Al-Mubarak N, Roubin GS, Iyer SS, Gomez CR, Liu MW, Vitek JJ. Carotid stenting for severe radiation-induced extracranial carotid artery occlusive disease. *J Endovasc Ther* 2000;7(1):36–40.

112. Alric P, Branchereau P, Berthet JP, Mary H, Marty-Ane C. Carotid artery stenting for stenosis following revascularization or cervical irradiation. *J Endovasc Ther* 2002;9(1):14–19.

113. Dangas G, Laird JR Jr, Mehran R, et al. Carotid artery stenting in patients with high-risk anatomy for carotid endarterectomy. *J Endovasc Ther* 2001;8(1):39–43.

114. Paniagua D, Howell M, Strickman N, et al. Outcomes following extracranial carotid artery stenting in high-risk patients. *J Invasive Cardiol* 2001;13(5):375–381.

115. Houdart E, Mounayer C, Chapot R, Saint-Maurice JP, Merland JJ. Carotid stenting for radiation-induced stenoses: a report of 7 cases. *Stroke* 2001;32(1):118–121.

116. New G, Roubin GS, Iyer SS, et al. Safety, efficacy, and durability of carotid artery stenting for restenosis following carotid endarterectomy: a multicenter study. *J Endovasc Ther* 2000;7(5):345–352.

117. Featherstone RL, Brown MM, Coward LJ. International carotid stenting study: protocol for a randomised clinical trial comparing carotid stenting with endarterectomy in symptomatic carotid artery stenosis. *Cerebrovasc Dis* 2004;18(1):69–74.

118. Gaines P, Randall M. Carotid artery stenting for patients with asymptomatic carotid disease (and news on TACIT). *Eur J Vasc Endovasc Surg* 2005;30(5):461–463.

119. Shawl F, Kadro W, Domansk MJ, et al. Safety and efficacy of elective carotid artery stenting in high-risk patients. *J Am Coll Cardiol* 2000;35(7):1721-1728.

120. Gupta A, Bhatia A, Ahuja A, et al. Carotid stenting in patients older than 65 years with inoperable carotid artery disease. *Cathet Cardiovasc Interv* 2000;50(1):1-8.

121. Reimers B, Corvaja N, Moshiri S, et al. Cerebral protection with filter devices during carotid artery stenting. *Circulation* 2001;104(1):12-15.

122. Roubin GS, New G, Iyer SS, et al. Immediate and late clinical outcomes of carotid artery stenting in patients with symptomatic and asymptomatic carotid artery stenosis. *Circulation* 2001;103:532.

123. Whitlow PL, Lylyk P, Londero H, et al. Carotid artery stenting protected with an emboli containment system. *Stroke* 2002;33(5):1308-1314.

124. Al-Mubarak N, Colombo A, Gaines PA, et al. Multicenter evaluation of carotid artery stenting with a filter protection system. *J Am Coll Cardiol* 2002;39(5):841-846.

125. MacDonald S, Venables GS, Cleveland TJ, et al. Protected carotid stenting: safety and efficacy of the MedNova NeuroShield filter. *J Vasc Surg* 2002;35(5):966-972.

126. Henry M, Polydorou A, Henry I, et al. Carotid angioplasty under cerebral protection with the PercuSurge GuardWire System. *Cathet Cardiovasc Interv* 2004;61(3):293-305.

CHAPTER (108)

Diagnosis and Management of Diseases of the Peripheral Arteries and Veins

Paul W. Wennberg / Thom W. Rooke

INTRODUCTION

Peripheral vascular diseases are a diverse collection of disorders that affect all organ systems. Although peripheral arterial disease (PAD) is the disease most commonly encountered by the cardiologist, disease of the lymphatics and veins is equally common (globally more so). For the cardiologist or internist with an interest in vascular disorders, a systematic and comprehensive approach is required. This chapter covers commonly encountered areas of vascular disease including lymphedema, venous disease, and peripheral arterial disease. Accompanying chapters on aortic and cerebrovascular disease address those areas in more detail.

LYMPHEDEMA

Lymphedema is an abnormal buildup of lymphatic fluid in the dermal and subcutaneous tissues. In contrast to the venous system, the superficial lymphatic vessels carry a low volume. They are a fragile, easily damaged network of vessels that drain the interstitial fluid and propel fluid proximally by peristalsis. As vessels ascend, larger conduits are formed at the inguinal level and again at the iliac level coalescing into the paraaortic lymphatic channels, which eventually empty via the thoracic duct at the left subclavian vein. Lymph nodes are located along lymphatic vessels, trauma to which affects the lymphatic vessel function. Globally, lymphedema is the most common vascular disease, affecting 90 to 120 million people.[1] Mosquito-borne infection with filarial is endemic in tropical countries. However, cases occur within the contiguous United States including *cold-weather* states.[2]

Lymphedema may be primary or secondary in etiology. Primary lymphedema may be congenital (present at birth) or, more commonly in the early teen years (lymphedema praecox). This is more common in females and often presents around menarche. Lymphedema tarda presents in later years and is a diagnosis of exclusion because a secondary cause is much more likely in this age group. Secondary lymphedema is much more common than primary. Trauma, recurrent infection, obstruction, infiltration, and radiation all cause lymphatic vessel damage. Upper extremity lymphedema may occur after axillary node dissection. Recurrent cellulitis is common in patients with lymphedema, both as an initiating, exacerbating, and complicating event. *Streptococcus* is the most common organism. It typically enters the skin through a crack in the toe webs caused by tinea pedis. The organism damages the lymphatic channels and the lymph nodes, with repeated infection eventually obliterating the vessel.[3]

DIAGNOSIS AND TESTING

History and physical exam make the diagnosis in most cases. Unlike edema and lipedema, lymphedema involves the toes, and usually the toes first. Dependent edema spares the toes because footwear does not allow the swelling to occur. Lipedema, caused by excess fatty deposits usually increased at the time of menarche, is more difficult to differentiate from lymphedema. However, with lipedema the toes are spared and there is often a ridge or fold overhanging the ankle. The skin is thickened and takes on an orange peel consistency (*peau d'orange*) (Fig. 108–1), a diffuse, flat, warty consistency that may affect the skin over time.

The techniques currently available for imaging of the lymphatic system are lymphangiography and lymphoscintigraphy. Lymphangiography is difficult to perform and carries a risk of iatrogenic lymphangitis. However, anatomic features are obtained and differentiation between primary lymphedema (absence of lymphatic structures) and secondary lymphedema (obstruction at a level by a mass, injury, or lymph node hypertrophy caused by lymphoma) can often be determined. The lymphoscintigram is based on uptake and ascent of technetium-99 (^{99}Tc)-labeled antimony trisulfide colloid after injection between the web spaces of digits. It is easier to perform than lymphangiography, has a low risk of lymphangitis, and good ability to differentiate lymphedema from other causes of edema. It cannot reliably distinguish primary from secondary lymphedema.[4,5]

TREATMENT

Treatment for lymphedema is volume reduction of the limb. Reduction in limb size by elevation, mechanical pumping, or manual massage is effective. Wrapping of the limb, distal to proximal, is required whenever the patient is up. After leg volume is decreased, an elastic compression garment, 40 to 50 mmHg in strength, should be worn daily, replaced 2 to 4 times per year as needed.[6] Early and aggressive treatment of cellulitis and fungal infections of the toes help to prevent cellulitis is required.

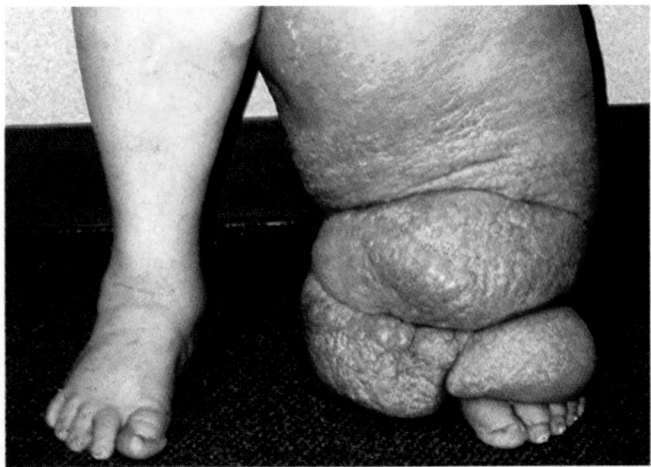

FIGURE 108–1. Left leg lymphedema with typical skin changes. Note the toes are edematous and the skin is thickened in a classic *peau d'orange* pattern with verrucal changes.

LABORATORY ASSESSMENT OF VENOUS DISEASE

IMAGING AND ANATOMIC STUDIES

Duplex ultrasound, CT, MRI, and magnetic resonance venography (MRV) are the methods available for evaluation of venous anatomy, but venography is considered the *gold standard*.[7] However, venous duplex ultrasound is the most commonly used method. It has the advantage of differentiating acute from old thrombus based on the presence or absence of venous distension (common with acute clot) and increased echogenicity (common with chronic clot). Compared to venography, duplex ultrasound is less sensitive both above the groin and below the knee.[8] MRV and CT venography are rapidly emerging technologies that are proving to be accurate and applicable in clinical practice. In addition to providing accurate information above the groin, both may be performed concurrently with pulmonary embolism studies.[9,10] A negative D-dimer profile has proven an excellent predictor for absence of acute thrombosis.[11,12]

PHYSIOLOGIC STUDIES

Continuous-Wave Doppler

Continuous-wave Doppler (CWD) provides qualitative information about blood flow. A loss of phasicity with respiration suggests venous obstruction. When a Doppler is placed over a vein and the limb distal to the probe is compressed, there should be augmentation of venous flow. If not, obstruction is present. By examining multiple levels, localization of incompetence or obstruction can be made (specificity 88 percent, sensitivity 85 percent).[13] CWD alone is a poor technique for evaluating partially obstructing thrombus or confirming acute deep venous thrombosis (DVT).

Plethysmography

Plethysmography measures the change volume in limb (due to arterial inflow, venous outflow or venous reflux) over time. The most common plethysmographic techniques are strain gauge plethysmography, air plethysmography, and impedance plethysmography. Outflow plethysmography is useful in screening for venous outflow obstruction.[14] Impedance plethysmography (IPG) is the best studied technique. Unlike venography or duplex ultrasound, IPG identifies the presence of functional rather than anatomic venous obstruction.[15] IPG screening has been replaced by Duplex ultrasound in most centers. Venous insufficiency is assessed by raising the legs to attain an empty state and then rapidly lowered. If incompetent, blood falls from the proximal veins (retrograde) and calf volume increases rapidly when the legs are lowered.[16] If the incompetence is superficial placing light tourniquets around the leg and/or directly compressing an incompetent superficial vein will normalize refilling time. Exercise plethysmography assesses *calf pump function* and subsequent refilling of the lower extremities.

CLINICAL VENOUS DISEASE

Venous disease is common with cross sectional studies demonstrating some form of venous disease present in >50 percent of the population of Edinburgh Scotland.[17–19] Venous disease is extremely variable with multiple clinical presentations and causes. The CEAP classification organizes this by the clinical manifestations, etiologic factors, anatomic involvement, pathophysiologic features[20,21] (Table 108–1). Despite the comprehensive structure of the CEAP system, the *C* or clinical classification is commonly used alone.

[ ] VARICOSE VEINS

Primary varicosities tend to be familial and without other causative events. They often first appear during pregnancy. Prolonged dependency at the place of work may also increase the risk of developing varicose veins.[22] Secondary varicosities may be caused by several etiologies including extrinsic venous compression, prior DVT, congenital lesions, arteriovenous fistulas, right heart disease, or perforator vein incompetence. History, examination, and laboratory evaluation of the deep venous system allows differentiation of primary from secondary varicosities.

Varicose veins are common.[19] *Burning, bursting, bruised,* or *aching* are just some of the sensations reported by patients.[23] Symptoms are exacerbated by prolonged standing or dependency and pregnancy or other volume overload states. Elevation relieves symptoms. If the discomfort worsens with elevation it is unlikely caused by varicosities. Episodes of superficial thrombophlebitis may occur; and if repetitive, ablation of the veins is appropriate. Symptoms and progression can be improved by graduated compression hose. Ablation of the vein should be considered if complications or discomfort interfere with occupation or lifestyle.[24] Sclerotherapy is effective for small varicosities and *spider veins.* Laser therapy is effective for small "spider veins" and telangiectasias.[25] Surgical removal is indicated for longer segments and proximal varicosities, especially if perforator vein or saphenofemoral junction incompetence is present.[26] Recently, endovascular techniques have become available including endovascular laser ablation and endovascular radiofrequency ablation.[27]

Venous ulceration is common and has a great economic impact in developed countries. Ulceration most often occurs at the medial perimalleolar region. This area has the highest venous pressure that is often well in excess of perfusion pressure resulting in chron-ically hypoxic skin prone to injury. Once ulceration has occurred successful management requires reduction of the edema by compression and conservative debridement of necrotic tissue and fibrinous slough. After skin integrity is restored control of venous hypertension with elastic support hose is required indefinitely. When venous ulceration occurs in the setting of moderate to severe PAD, treatment is difficult. Compression must be applied with a low-stretch wrap in order to avoid further reduction of arterial inflow.

[ ] VENOUS THROMBOSIS
Superficial Thrombophlebitis

Superficial thrombophlebitis (STP) presents as a tender, erythematous, indurated lesion in the course of a superficial vein. Ultrasound can differentiate thrombophlebitis from lymphangitis, erythema nodosum, and other lesions. STP often occurs in a varicose vein or at sites of indwelling catheters and recent intravenous injections. Cellulitis is common, and when present antibiotics should be used. STP is usually self-limited with recovery accelerated by rest, elevation, warm compresses, and antiinflammatory agents. There is a moderate incidence of concurrent DVT in STP.[28] Duplex ultrasound should be used to screen for DVT because management with chronic anticoagulation is then indicated. Systemic anticoagulation is appropriate for lesions that progress despite conservative care or when located proximally in the greater saphenous vein near the saphenofemoral junction where minimal extension would enter the deep system.[29] Evaluation for underlying diseases that predispose to clotting or a primary clotting abnormality should be considered in the setting of recurrent STP or those with a strong family history of thrombosis.[30]

Deep Vein Thrombosis

The morbidity and mortality of DVT are high. Risk factors for DVT and pulmonary embolism have been well defined in several studies[31,32] (Table 108–2). The signs and symptoms of DVT are nonspecific and unreliable.[33] Objective testing to confirm and define the extent of DVT should be obtained whenever the diagnosis

---

TABLE 108–1

CEAP Classification Scheme for Lower-Extremity Venous Disease[a]

CLINICAL PRESENTATION		ETIOLOGY	ANATOMY[b]	PATHOPHYSIOLOGY
C_0	No venous disease	E_C Congenital	A_S Superficial veins	P_R Reflux
C_1	Telangiectasia, or reticular veins			
C_2	Varicose veins	E_P Primary	A_D Deep veins	P_O Obstruction
C_3	Edema without skin changes			
C_{4a}	Skin pigmentation or eczema	E_S Secondary	A_P Perforator veins	$P_{R,O}$ Reflux and obstruction
C_{4b}	Lipodermatosclerosis or atrophie blanche			
C_5	Healed ulceration			
C_6	Active ulceration			

CEAP, clinical manifestation, etiologic factor, anatomic involvement and pathophysiology feature.
[a]Each category is scored independently of the others. For example, with this scheme a patient with postphlebitic syndrome, an active venous ulcer, and hemodynamic evidence of reflux but no obstruction is scored as $C_6 E_S A_D P_R$. A patient with telangiectasias and no other symptoms or findings is $C_2 E_P A_S$.
[b]The complete anatomy classification also identifies the venous 'segment(s) involved.

TABLE 108–2

Risk Factors for Deep Vein Thrombosis

TRANSIENT CAUSE	FIXED CAUSE
Recent surgery	Prior superficial vein thrombosis
Hospitalization	Prior deep venous thrombosis
Trauma	Residence in healthcare facility
Malignancy	Immobility
Hormonal therapy	Age

is entertained.[34] If the DVT is not present the cost and risks of treatment including hemorrhage, heparin-induced thrombocytopenia, and warfarin necrosis are avoided.

Treatment with heparin acutely and warfarin chronically is highly effective in preventing clot propagation and pulmonary embolism. Low-molecular weight heparins (adjusted for weight) have proven effective in treating DVT and can be used for outpatient management in uncomplicated cases.[35] Heparin-induced thrombocytopenia is not uncommon and only detected by monitoring platelets routinely. If present, hirudin or danaparoid may be used in place of heparin until warfarin effect is therapeutic.[36] Warfarin-induced necrosis, although rare, may be avoided by overlapping heparin with warfarin for 4 to 5 days.[37] The duration of treatment with warfarin for optimal risk benefit ratio following DVT is not known. Recent literature suggests treatment for a minimum of 6 to 12 months in patients with spontaneous DVT, but this decision must be individualized for each case.[38] The international normalized ratio (INR) should be followed to ensure consistency between laboratories. Patients should be urged to know and record their INR. The risk of major hemorrhage from anticoagulation is 1 to 3 percent per year when control is strict. Bleeding risk increases significantly when the INR exceeds 4.0. Catheter-directed thrombolysis or mechanical thrombectomy for DVT when performed early accelerates recovery and may reduce incidence and severity of postphlebitic syndrome.[39] Lysis appears to be most effective for ileofemoral DVT (Fig. 108–2). However, clearly defined indications for thrombolytic therapy in DVT are not yet established and individual and center experience and careful patient selection must be considered.[40] Immediate and long-term use of compression stockings to the knee or higher drastically reduces the incidence of postphlebitic syndrome, venous stasis changes, and venous ulceration.[41] Strict bedrest is not beneficial or protective in the setting of acute DVT.[42–44]

Phlegmasia Cerulea Dolens Phlegmasia cerulea dolens is a rare complication of DVT characterized by acute, massive edema, severe pain, and cyanosis in the setting of extensive iliofemoral thrombosis. A third of patients die because of pulmonary embolism, and half develop distal gangrene caused by thrombus-induced compartment syndrome. It is seen most commonly with advanced malignancy or severe infections but can occur following surgery, fractures, and other common precipitants of thrombosis. Treatment includes placement of a caval filter, heparinization, and often physical removal of the clot by thrombectomy (surgical or endovascular) and possibly thrombolysis.[45]

PERIPHERAL ARTERIAL DISEASE

PAD caused by atherosclerosis is the most common cause of lower extremity ischemic syndromes in Western societies.[46] Symptoms of PAD are variable and, unfortunately, frequently lead to incorrect diagnoses.[47] Risk factors for PAD are essentially the same as those for coronary artery disease (CAD) with tobacco and diabetes having and even greater effect[48] (Table 108–3). Tobacco use, current and past, has at 2- to 4-time increase in relative risk for PAD.[49] Diabetes mellitus has a similar increase in relative risk.[50,51] Other modifiable risk factors include hyperhomocysteinemia, hyperlipidemia, and hypertension.[52]

PREVALENCE

PAD affects a large and increasing numbers of patients not only in the United States but worldwide. Exact numbers for prevalence and incidence are confounded by varying methods of assessment and criteria for diagnosis.[53] It is estimated that 10 million people with symptomatic PAD and another 20 to 30 million with asymptomatic disease. Of patients older than age 60 years, 10 percent are affected and prevalence continues to increases with age.[54] In the Framingham Offspring Study, the prevalence of PAD was determined in 1554 males and 1759 females from 1995 to 1998.[55] The mean age was 59 years. PAD, defined as an ankle-brachial (blood pressure) index (ABI) of <0.90, was present in 3.9 percent of males and 3.3 percent of females. Yet, the prevalence of intermittent claudication was only 1.9 percent in males and 0.8 percent in females suggesting that only half of men and only a quarter of women have subjective symptoms. Lower extremity bruits were present in 2.4 percent of males, 2.3 percent of females; prior surgical intervention was 1.4 percent in males and 0.5 percent in females. The PARTNERS (PAD Awareness, Risk, and Treatment: New Resources for Survival) program assessed the prevalence of PAD in patients older than age 70 years and those ages 50 to 69 years with a smoking history or diabetes at 250 primary clinics across the United States.[56] As defined by a charted or screening ABI of <0.90, 29 percent of the population was found to have PAD. There was a high incidence (nearly half) of concurrent coronary or cerebral vascular disease.

NATURAL HISTORY

Death directly caused by peripheral arterial disease is rare. Mortality and morbidity is more often due to concomitant coronary or cerebrovascular disease. The relative risk of death for all cause mortality is 2- to 6-fold higher in PAD patients versus the general population.[57–59] The risk of death increases as the ABI decreases.[60] The 5-year mortality of an ABI less than 0.85 is 10 percent; when the ABI is <0.40 mortality approaches 50 percent mortality per year.[61] Lower extremity symptoms not associated with a decrease in the ABI do not demonstrate the increase in mortality.[62] In contrast, a decrease in ABI without symptoms still portends an increase in cardiovascular morbidity and mortality.[63]

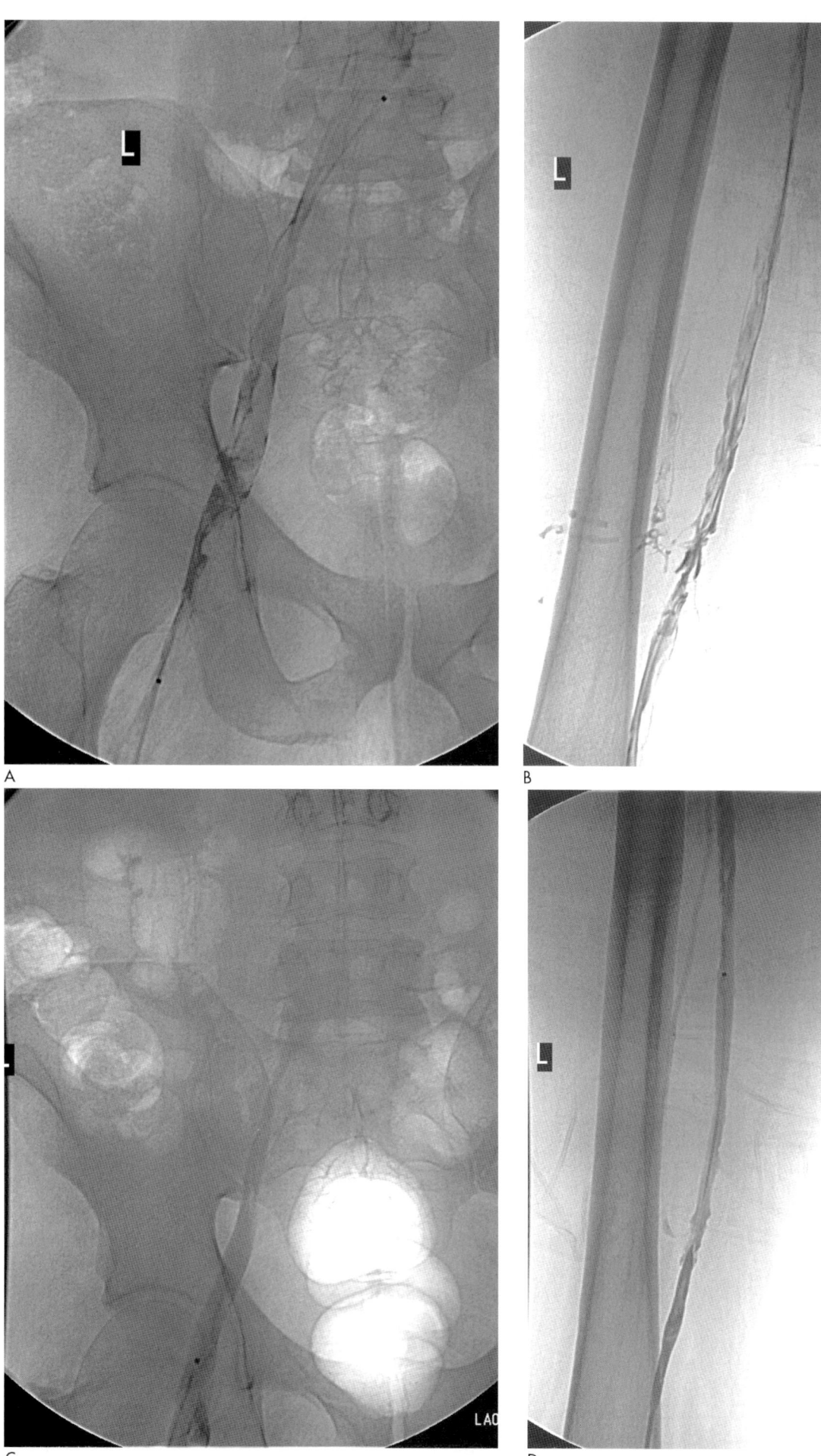

FIGURE 108-2. This series of panels demonstrates an acute left iliac vein thrombosis (**A**) with extension into the femoral vein (**B**). Following 48 hours of catheter-directed thrombolysis, the thrombus is essentially resolved at the iliac (**C**) with slight residual narrowing at the left femoral vein (**D**).

TABLE 108–3

Risk Factors for Peripheral Arterial Disease

HIGH RISK	MODERATE RISK	LOW RISK
2- to 4-fold increase	1- to 3-fold increase	1- to 2-fold increase
Smoking	Hypertension	Hypercholesterolemia
Diabetes mellitus	Homocysteinemia	

Although the cardiovascular mortality and morbidity of patients with PAD is staggering, the rate of progression of symptoms and need for limb revascularization or amputation is low.[64] Requirement for revascularization caused by imminent tissue or limb loss or rest pain approaches 5 percent per year.[53] Amputation rates are similarly low, approximately 1 percent per year.[65] The rate of progression and amputation in those who continue to smoke is more that two-fold higher than those who quit with 15 percent of those who continue smoking undergoing amputation within 5 years.[66] Historically, diabetics have an amputation rate of 25 percent over 10 years, which has changed little over time.[67,68] For those who present with acute critical limb ischemia, 30-day amputation rates are 10 to 30 percent with 1-year mortality rate of 15 percent.[69]

[ ] CLINICAL ASSESSMENT OF ARTERIAL DISEASE

History

Information including age, gender, associated medical problems (including prior trauma, vascular and orthopedic procedures, and medication use) and risk factors for atherosclerosis, should be obtained. The description of symptoms may be quite different from patient to patient, but a discomfort or pain is the common thread among patients.[47] Symptoms including onset, progression, and aggravating or alleviating factors should be rigorously clarified. Commonly, several types of discomfort caused by several etiologies are present.[70] The differential of claudication is broad; an abbreviated list is given in Table 108–4.

TABLE 108–4

Differential Diagnosis of Claudication

Atherosclerosis obliterans
Arteritis (Takayasu, giant cell)
Embolic disease/acute arterial occlusion
Degenerative joint disease (hip, back, knee)
Spinal stenosis
Myopathy
Thromboangiitis obliterans
Popliteal entrapment
Venous claudication/varicosities
Baker cyst
Deconditioning
Aortic dissection
Aortic coarctation
Retroperitoneal fibrosis

Claudication Claudication (literally *limping*) is a stereotypical, reproducible distress in single or multiple muscle groups of the lower extremity brought on by sustained exercise and relieved by rest. The distress may be described as numbness, weakness, giving way, aching, cramping, or pain.[71] The distress changes in character and/or location as the causative lesion(s) progress. When workload is increased by rapid pace, a burden, walking uphill or over rough terrain, the distance or time to onset will shorten. When the distance abruptly decreases, consider thrombosis in situ or an embolic event. In general, symptoms occur distal to the level of stenosis or occlusion. Claudication occurs in muscle groups rather than joints. Relief with rest is independent of position and is timely, usually within 5 minutes. When specific positions are required for relief, musculoskeletal or neurologic disorders should be suspected. Claudication often worsens after a period of inactivity such as hospitalization but usually returns to baseline with reconditioning. Although lifestyle limitation and changes in quality of life are an integral part of the history, quantification of disease severity by history alone is unreliable.[33] Standardized treadmill testing using ankle/brachial indices at rest and after completion of an exercise protocol confirms the diagnosis, determines the severity, and documents claudication distance for future followup.[72]

Critical Limb Ischemia Critical limb ischemia results in constant and agonizing rest pain. It is confined to affected digits, foot, or hand and less commonly the entire limb. Small, localized areas of ischemic pain can occur with vasculitis or embolization but is more often caused by trauma in an area with poor perfusion and not always as progression of chronic occlusive disease.[73] It is important to inquire about new shoes, recent nail care, and other potential sources of trauma. Rest pain is present when supine and is relieved by dependency, such as hanging the limb off the bed; sleeping in a chair; and, paradoxically, by walking. Pain may progress to constant, interrupting sleep, suppressing appetite, inducing weight loss and delirium, and requiring large doses of analgesics for pain relief.

Ischemic Neuropathy Ischemic neuropathy is an agonizing lancinating pain that affects the entire limb. Features may initially suggest a neuropathic process but the clinical setting includes severe ischemia and fairly acute onset of symptoms rather than the insidious onset of a neuropathy. In sharp contrast to this are those with insensate or poorly sensate feet from peripheral neuropathy, most commonly diabetes. The usual reflexive *avoidance of painful stimuli* is lost, resulting in higher degrees of trauma and tissue injury prior to seeking medical care. This group frequently presents at a late stage of disease with tissue loss rather than claudication.

Pseudoclaudication Pseudoclaudication is typically of neurogenic origin. The patient with neurogenic claudication describes exercise-induced distress with a dysesthetic quality that clears slowly or requires a specific posture for relief, usually with the hips flexed.[74] Clumsiness may develop as walking progresses. Symptoms occur with prolonged standing or when supine. Compression of the distal spinal cord by hypertrophic bone, disk protrusion, or tumor may be the cause. A history of back injury should be sought. Arterial and pseudoclaudication often coexist. In this situation the dominant lesion can be identified by observing symptoms with just standing and measuring the arterial indices before and after exercise.[75]

Venous Claudication

Venous claudication is described as a congestive, often *bursting*, distress of thighs and calves induced by standing, walking, and sometimes running. Relief with rest is slow and notably accelerated when the patient elevates the legs. Venous claudication occurs in the setting of iliocaval obstruction. Signs of venous hypertension of the legs and lower abdomen are often noted during examination.[76]

Arterial Examination

Sight

A red or purplish color of the forefoot during dependency (dependent rubor) is common with severe ischemia. The patient may do this to let gravity assist blood flow to the limb. Dependent rubor caused by ischemia will change to pallor with elevation.[77] Timing of onset of pallor and time to venous refilling can be performed in the exam room (Table 108–5). Loss of normal hair growth is also a marker of ischemia.

Livedo reticularis is a transient, bluish discoloration with a lacy pattern, found on the extremities and sometimes the trunk, that is variable in its extent and intensity. It is most apparent after exposure to cold or emotion, and fades with warmth and exercise. It is first seen in childhood or at puberty and is more common in women and fair-skinned individuals. It is so frequent in its milder form that it is often overlooked or considered a variant of normal skin. It is postulated that spasm of the cutaneous arterioles (with secondary dilation of the capillaries and venules) causes slow flow, increased oxygen uptake, and reduced oxygenation of hemoglobin, producing color change. Secondary livedo reticularis is patchy, focal, and asymmetric in distribution and may be complicated by local infarction or ulceration (Fig. 108–3). Embolism is a common etiology when following instrumentation. The lesions may be elevated or tender when caused by vasculitis.

Palpation

The aorta, radial, ulnar, subclavian, carotid, temporal, occipital, femoral, popliteal, posterior tibial, and dorsalis

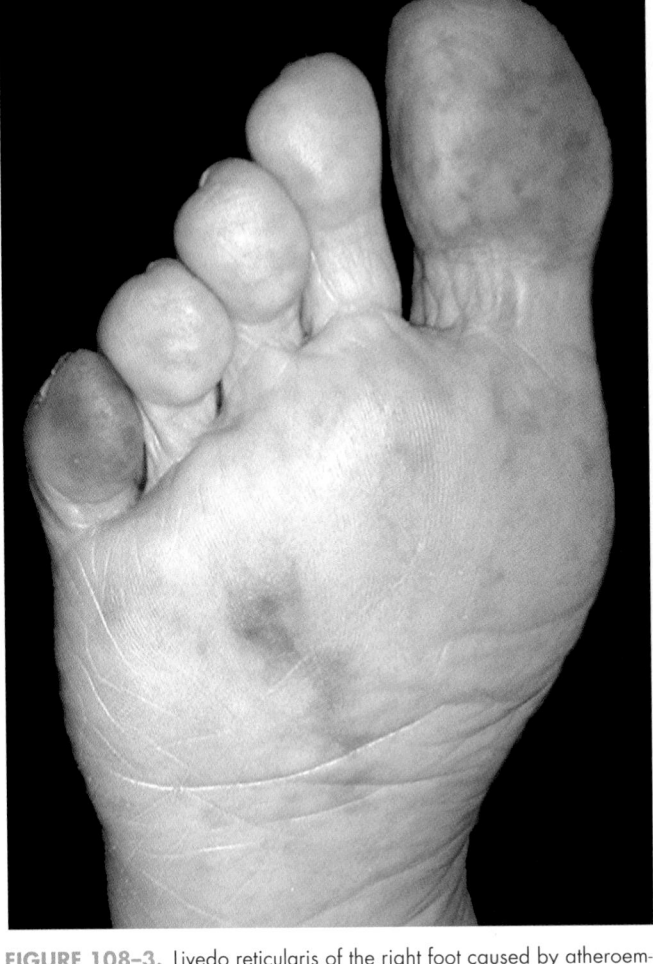

FIGURE 108-3. Livedo reticularis of the right foot caused by atheroembolism following cardiac catheterization.

pedis arteries are accessible by palpation. Pulses are graded on a scale (Table 108–6).[78] If a pulse is not palpable, Doppler examination should be performed to establish whether flow is absent or below the level of detection by palpation. Surface temperature is reduced when perfusion is compromised. Temperature

TABLE 108-5

Elevation and Dependency

GRADE	PALLOR ONSET
Elevation Pallor[a]	
Normal	None
Grade I	>60 sec
Grade II	<60 sec
Grade III	<30 sec
Grade IV	Pallor supine
Venous Refilling[b]	
Severity	Venous Refill
Normal	<15 sec
Moderate	15–30 sec
Severe	>30 sec

[a]Feet held passively at 60 degrees while supine.
[b]Legs dependent while sitting after elevation.

TABLE 108-6

Pulse Grading Scale[a]

MAYO	PHYSICAL FINDINGS	ACC/AHA
0	Absent	0
1	Severely reduced—palpable with great difficulty; unable to accurately count pulse	1
2	Moderately reduced—palpable with some difficulty; able to count pulse	1
3	Mildly reduced—easily palpable	1
4	Normal pulse—easily palpable	2
5	Enlarged—widened, possibly aneurysmal	3

ACC/AHA, American College of Cardiology/American Hearty Association.
[a]Pulse grading scale. Presence of edema and other physical barriers at time of examination must be taken into account when grading.

differences are best felt with the dorsum of the fingers; comparisons to the contra-lateral limb or proximal ipsilateral limb should be made. The sizes of paired arteries are similar in magnitude. Ectasia or aneurysm is suspected when one side is larger or more forceful than the other. Tortuosity of the carotids, abdominal aorta, and subclavian arteries can mimic an aneurysm. Ultrasound or other imaging studies are needed to clarify the findings when the diagnosis of and aneurysm is entertained.

Auscultation Blood pressure should be taken in both arms and should be similar but rarely identical, even when done simultaneously. Respiratory variation, positioning of the arm, and atrial fibrillation are just a few reasons the pressures vary. If a large difference is noted between arms (>14 mmHg) blood pressures should be rechecked. If still discrepant, simultaneous pressures are done to confirm the finding. The femoral, iliac, aortic, carotid, and subclavian arteries should be auscultated. Simultaneous palpation of a radial artery during auscultation will improve detection of subtle bruits (especially abdominal bruits when bowel sounds are vigorous) and allows accurate timing of bruits. The further a bruit extends into diastole the greater the degree of stenosis.

[ ] LABORATORY ASSESSMENT OF ARTERIAL DISEASE

Objective testing of the arterial system is done for confirmation or clarification of the clinical findings, monitoring disease progression, or assessment of outcome after intervention.

Anatomic Studies

Conventional Angiography Conventional angiography is the standard by which all other imaging techniques are judged.[78] It provides reproducible information with very high resolution not yet matched by other modalities (Fig. 108–4A). Assessment of distal vessels fine structural detail and arteriovenous shunting are still best determined by angiography. Drawbacks include risk of distal embolization and arterial damage at the puncture site. Iodinated contrast is used with small but real risk of anaphylactoid reaction and contrast nephropathy.

Computed Tomography Angiography Computed tomography angiography (CTA) provides detailed anatomic information without need of arterial access.[79] Iodinated contrast is still required (Fig. 108–5). Three-dimensional (3D) reconstructions can include or exclude bony structures and other organs in the final images and also has the advantage of being 3D, allowing the image to be rotated on an axis. CTA has become standard for assessing and planning and following endograft repair of aortic aneurysms because accurate measurement of the *landing zone* (distance between the renal arteries and the neck of the aneurysm) can be made. An argument may be made for using CTA as an initial imaging modality when percutaneous intervention is unlikely.[80]

Magnetic Resonance Angiography Magnetic resonance angiography (MRA) provides information similar to CTA without

the need for iodinated contrast. For those at risk of contrast nephropathy or anaphylactoid reaction, it is a safe and accurate alternative to CTA and conventional angiography.[81] MRA, like CTA, provides a 3D image and can include or exclude structures of interest. Patients with implantable devices such as pacemakers, automated defibrillators, recently placed arterial stents and intracranial clips cannot be safely placed into the magnetic field, limiting availability to a small extent.

Duplex Ultrasound Duplex ultrasound provides safe and reliable data of not only arterial anatomy but also of the hemodynamic effects of stenosis when Doppler flow analysis is incorporated (see Fig. 108–4B). Anatomic reconstruction is limited to two-dimensional imaging at present, but methods for reconstruction to 3D images are under development and available at some research facilities. Contrast is not required and no ionizing radiation is used. Ultrasound is portable and captures images in real time allowing both bedside and intraoperative monitoring of therapy (Fig. 108–6). However, data acquisition may be limited by body habitus, overlying structures such as bowel gas, and other tissues that interfere with imaging. Nonetheless, surgical intervention on duplex imaging alone has proven effective.[82]

Hemodynamic Studies

The hemodynamic significance of a stenosis may be assessed by multiple methods. Invasive measurement of a pressure gradient across a stenosis is still considered the *gold standard* of hemodynamic assessment. Spectral broadening, poststenotic velocity increase, and dampening of the waveform are seen at the degree of stenosis increases. CWD provides valuable information as well, at minimal cost and great portability, with the normal triphasic waveform changing to a monophasic and eventually absent as the severity of a stenosis increases to occlusion.[83] Noninvasive evaluation is most readily available by measuring segmental pressures (see below). Hemodynamic studies are frequently combined with functional assessment.

Functional Studies

The information obtained by anatomic or hemodynamic testing is often insufficient to explain or differentiate the symptoms or quantify the degree of impairment described by the patient. Therefore, functional assessment is usually appropriate. Functional studies involve some form of applied stress, such as treadmill testing, to assess claudication.

Segmental Pressures Segmental pressures and exercise testing provide a simple, reproducible, inexpensive, and accurate method of determining whether or not arterial stenosis is present, the severity of the stenosis, and the approximate location of the stenosis. Pneumatic cuffs are placed around the thigh, calf, ankle, upper or lower arm, or digits. A CWD probe is positioned over the artery at a site distal to the cuff and the systolic pressure at which arterial flow ceases and resumes is recorded. The limb pressures are divided by a reference arterial pressure (the brachial artery pressure most commonly) to create an index. The most commonly reported segmental pressure is the ABI.

A normal ABI should be ≥1.0, but >0.90 is considered normal in most laboratories. Severe disease is present when the ABI is less than 0.50 (Table 108–7).

The biggest disadvantage of segmental pressure measurement is that it is unreliable in patients with non- or poorly compressible vessels.[84] There are patients with poorly compressible vessels, particularly those with diabetes, caused by calcium deposition in the media of the arteries (Mönckeberg calcification). Many groups use the great toe index in these patients. Even when the large vessels of the limb are non-compressible the digital vessels in the toes and fingers often remain non-calcified and can be used to estimate pressure with an appropriate sized cuff. Pulse volume recording, toe-brachial indices, laser Doppler fleximetry (LFD) and transcutaneous oximetry can be effective in these patients.

Lower Extremity Arterial Exercise Testing Lower extremity arterial exercise testing is performed with treadmill and the patient is exercised at a standardized protocol.[85] Protocols may be *fixed* (e.g., 2 miles per hour at a 12 percent incline for a maximum of 5 minutes) or *graded* similar to those used in cardiac exercise studies.[86] Select parts of the lower extremity study (i.e. ankle/brachial indices or CWD at the common femoral level) are performed before and after exercise. With exercise the systolic blood pressure increases as peripheral resistance decreased resulting in a larger pressure gradient and the resultant lower ABI and abnormal Doppler signals. Therefore, a decrease in ankle/brachial index or a change in Doppler signal may be detected after exercise (see Table 108–7). Even if the resting values are normal, a decreased ABI following exercise predicts an increase in mortality.[87] Equally important, exercise studies provide ancillary data such as the walking distance to onset of symptoms, absolute walking distance, and blood pressure response during exercise. They also correlate symptoms, which may be very vague, with the data generated providing objective evidence of the patientís symptoms.[88] Toe tip exercise testing has good correlation to treadmill testing and is an excellent alternative in patients that are unable to walk safely on a treadmill.[89]

Pulse Volume Recording Pulse volume recording assesses the magnitude of the arterial impulse entering a limb or segment of a limb. A pneumatic pressure cuff placed around the limb is filled with air to a low pressure (typically 40–60 mmHg) and connected to a pressure transducer. During systole, transient distension of the arterial system causes distension of the limb. This technique has the advantage of remaining accurate in the setting of poorly compressible vessels.[90,91]

Toe-Brachial Index The toe vessels are often spared of the calcification seen in the posterior tibial and dorsalis pedis vessels. The toe-brachial pressure index is considered normal when >0.70. The great toe is most often used with the second toe as an alternative.[92]

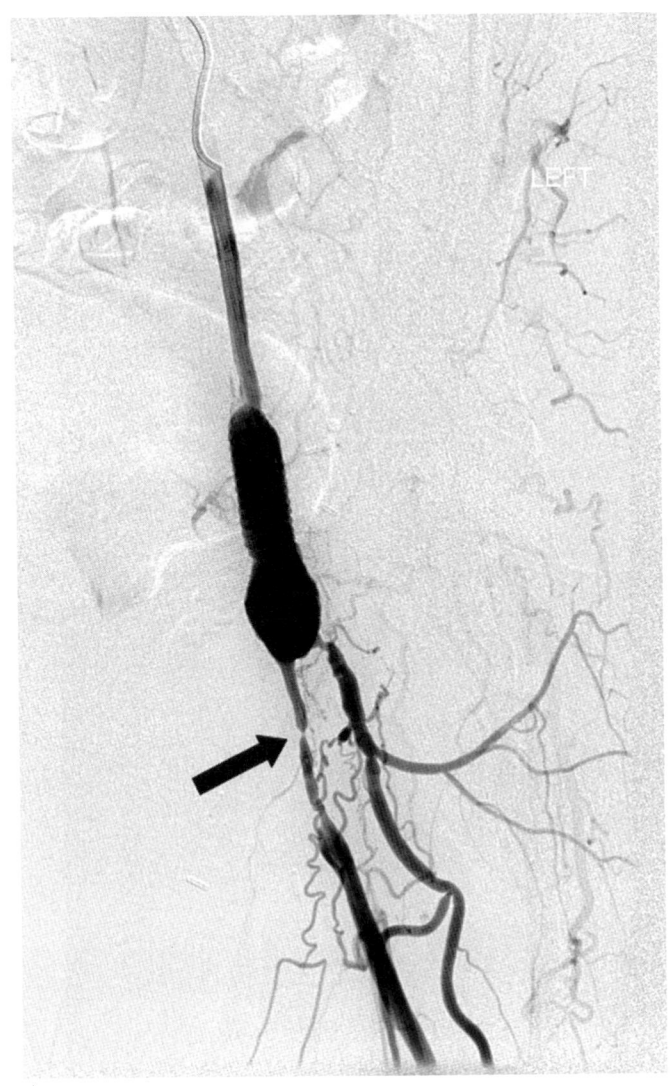

A

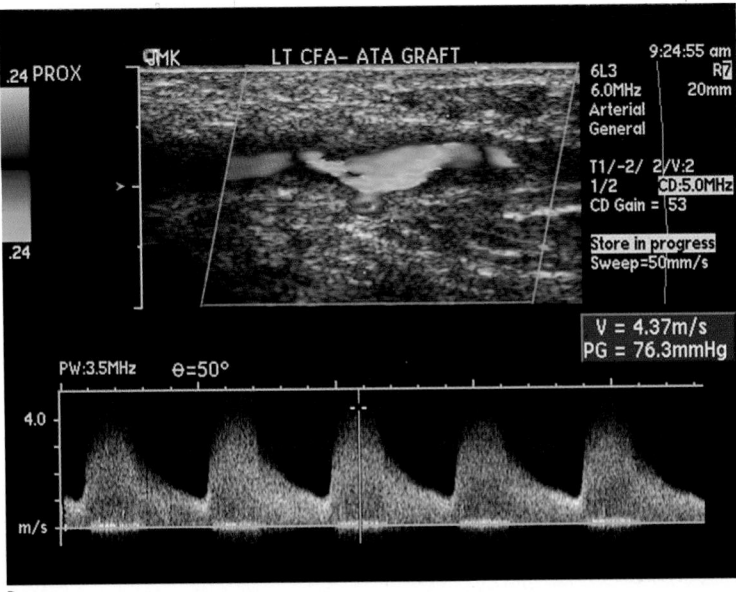

B

FIGURE 108–4. A. Conventional arteriogram showing a high grade stenosis of the common femoral artery distal to a polytetrafluoroethylene graft (*arrow*). **B.** Duplex ultrasound of the same stenosis showing velocity elevation of >400 cm/sec.

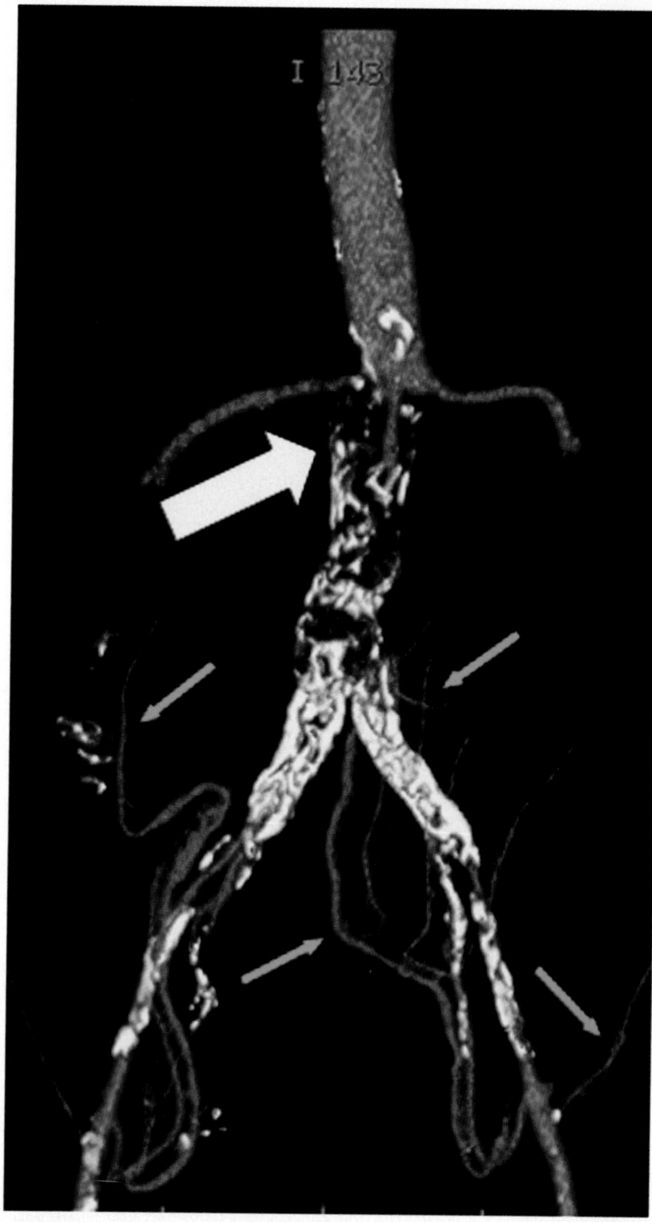

FIGURE 108–5. Computed tomography angiography of a distal aortic occlusion (*white arrow*), with numerous collaterals (*green arrows*) reconstituting the femoral vessels bilaterally.

Transcutaneous Oxygen Transcutaneous oxygen pressure measurement (TCPO$_2$) assesses the microcirculation by quantifying the amount of oxygen that diffuses out of the skin.[93] It is dependent on a number of factors including the arterial partial pressure of oxygen, cutaneous blood flow, and the rate of oxygen consumption by the skin. TCPO$_2$ can be used to monitor the effect of therapy such as sympathectomy or spinal cord stimulation.[94] It may also predict whether the cutaneous perfusion is adequate for healing at a given amputation site.[95] Values >40 mmHg are typically sufficient for healing, whereas those <20 mmHg are unlikely to heal.

Laser Doppler Fleximetry LDF is increasing in popularity for determination of cutaneous perfusion. Frequently, LDF is used to image skin flaps and burns to determine viability of the tissue. Skin perfusion pressure may be assessed locally.[96]

TREATMENT OF ARTERIAL DISEASE

Once the diagnosis of PAD has been made, aggressive risk factor modification is the cornerstone of therapy. The slow rate of progression and high incidence of cardiovascular comorbidities creates the optimal situation for modifying the underlying atherosclerotic process.

【 】 CLAUDICATION TREATMENT

The recent American College of Cardiology/American Heart Association (ACC/AHA) Practice Guidelines on lower extremity PAD nicely summarize the medical and interventional treatment option and level of evidence available[97] (Table 108–8).

Walking Programs

Walking programs should be initiated in all patients with claudication, both with typical and atypical symptoms.[98] Unfortunately, bicycling and other forms of exercise used for cardiovascular conditioning do not provide the same lower extremity benefit as walking. The effectiveness of a supervised walking program has been well demonstrated and proven more effective than nonsupervised programs.[99] Between 20 and 30 minutes, 4 to 5 days per week improves functional ability and exercise capacity and increases total and absolute walking distance from 50 to 300 percent.[100] Walking should be to near maximal tolerated pain, then rest for relief and repeated.[101] The mechanism of improvement is unclear; but increased collateral formation or recruitment, muscle training, improved oxygen uptake, and improved mechanics of walking are all likely.[102] Diligent foot care and protection must be emphasized, particularly in diabetics and those with severe reductions in ABI or TCPO$_2$ values. Footwear must be supportive and protective, and nail care should be performed regularly by professionals.[103]

Medical Therapy

Cilostazol is effective in conjunction with a walking program and increased walking distance. The effect is lost when the drug is stopped.[104] Although effective, it should always be used as part of a comprehensive program including a walking program and risk factor reduction.[105]

Antiplatelet agents including aspirin and clopidogrel are considered first-line agent for patients with PAD.[106] The Clopidogrel Versus Aspirin in Patients at Risk of Ischaemic Events (CAPRIE) trial showed a benefit of clopidogrel over aspirin in all cause cardiovascular mortality with PAD patients having the most significant improvement.[107,108]

Lipid lowering has a beneficial role in patients with PAD, and targets are identical to those for patients with CAD. Unfortunately, the aggressiveness of lipid lowering often lags that of patients with CAD.[109,110] Lipid lowering in PAD has been shown to decrease progression of claudication symptoms.[111] Hypertension control should be optimized; recognizing that pressure reduction in the setting of severe stenosis rarely worsens symptoms. Angiotensin-converting enzyme inhibitors (ACEIs) and β-blockers have proven effective in reducing cardiovascular mortality in a longitudinal study.[112] Recently, a small study suggested that ramipril improved pain free and maximal walking time.[113] β-Blockade has long been subject to medical mythology and believed to be contraindicated for patients with arteriosclerosis obliterans (ASO), but studies have refuted this idea.[114,115] Given the beneficial effects of β-blockade in patents with CAD, these agents should not be withheld in patients with peripheral ASO.

Homocysteinemia plays an independent role in development of PAD. The mechanism is at least in part related to an inborn genetic mutation affecting methylenetetrahydrofolate reductase (MTHFR) resulting in accelerated intimal damage and early atherosclerosis.[116,117] Treatment with folic acid and vitamins B_{12} and B_6 is appropriate when elevated to >14 μmol/L.[118]

Revascularization

The indication for revascularization is based on a number of factors. Comorbidities, functional status, and severity of symptoms must be considered.[119] Surgical and endovascular treatment strategies are addressed in adjacent chapters.

Critical Limb Ischemia

Revascularization should be considered for patients with rest pain, tissue loss, or lifestyle-limiting symptoms.[120] Surgical revascularization has been available for years and is effective and durable with good outcome regarding limb salvage.[121] Percutaneous transluminal angioplasty (PTA), with or without stent placement, is useful and durable for lesions of the iliac and proximal superficial femoral arteries. Distal PTA has been less durable; but for patients at high risk for limb loss who are poor surgical candidates or technically unfeasible for surgical revascularization, it is reasonable to consider distal angioplasty for limb salvage.[122] Medical treatment for critical limb ischemia has been challenging.[123] Intermittent pneumatic compression and angiogenesis with growth factors are emerging therapies.[124,125]

ACUTE ARTERIAL OCCLUSION

【 】 PRESENTATION

Acute arterial ischemia is a particularly ominous sign, with a 20-day mortality rate of 25 percent.[155] It presents suddenly as a painful, cold (polar), pale, pulseless limb that progresses to paresthesia and paralysis. Limb viability is at risk if flow is not restored quickly. Distal changes of livedo caused by microembolization may be present. If caused by arterial dissection, variability in the pulse deficit and affected area (a migration of symptoms) may cause discrepancy in findings between examiners over time. Severe ischemia is suggested by pallor at rest, profound coolness, tender or hard muscles, and loss of motor and or sensory functions.

【 】 ETIOLOGY

The etiology of acute arterial occlusions may be trauma, dissection, thrombosis in situ, or embolism from any proximal source, but most originates from the heart. Aneurysms, clotting disorders, atherosclerosis, and recent arterial manipulation may precipitate acute occlusion. Both the left ventricle and atrium may harbor thrombus and should be interrogated with transesophageal echocardiography if available.[126] Paradoxical emboli from the right heart or limbs can pass across cardiac septal defects or a patent foramen ovale and causing cerebrovascular events.

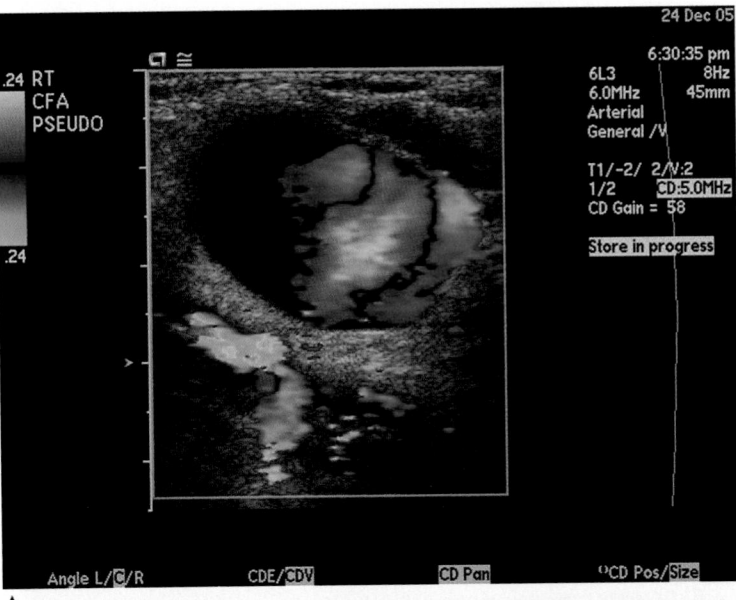

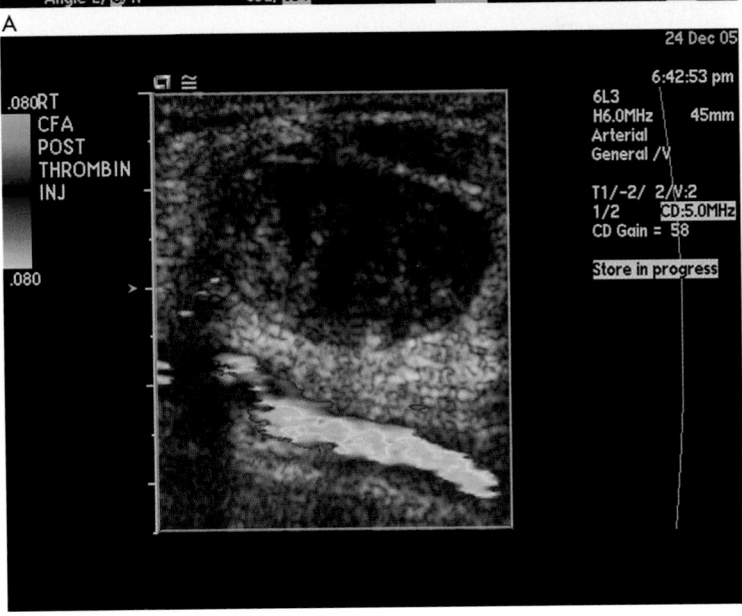

FIGURE 108–6. A. Duplex ultrasound of a femoral artery pseudoaneurysm showing flow within the aneurysm sac. **B.** Duplex following thrombin injection demonstrating no flow within the thrombosed pseudoaneurysm and preserved flow in the femoral artery.

【 】 TREATMENT

Immediate measures are needed to protect the limb and restore blood flow. Heparinization should be started to prevent clot propagation and to stabilize the embolic source(s). Angiography, conventional or other, may be required to plan repair when there is preexisting occlusive or aneurysmal disease or when the etiology is unclear. Ideally, all occlusions should be considered for reestablishment of flow, but urgency is governed by the degree of ischemia. Additional time may be taken to address ancillary problems in lesser degrees of ischemia. When critical ischemia is present, repair must occur within hours to salvage the limb, provided risks to the patient are acceptable.[127] When indicated, thrombolysis of acute occlusion can be effective although the risks of bleeding risk and stroke must be considered.[128,129] If the affected limb is not viable, amputation should be performed as quickly as possible to avoid further complications.

TABLE 108–7

Ankle/Brachial Index Criteria[a]

	PREEXERCISE	POSTEXERCISE	CLAUDICATION	WALKING TIME
Normal	>0.90[b,c]	>0.90	None	5 min
Minimal	>0.90	<0.90	None	5 min
Mild	>0.80	>0.50	Present late	5 min
Moderate	<0.80	<0.50	Present, limiting	<5 min
Severe	<0.50	<0.15	Early, limiting	<3 min

ABI, ankle-brachial index.
[a]ABI is the systolic blood pressure at the ankle measured in the supine position/systolic blood pressure of the higher arm. Postexercise values are after 5 minutes at a 10 percent grade at 2 mph (the authors' laboratory protocol; other protocols may be used). Speed may be varied if patient is unable.
[b]An ABI >1.40 (1.30 in some laboratories) is considered noncompressible and an alternative means of investigation considered.
[c]Some laboratories use 0.95 as the lower limit for normal.

ARTERIAL DISEASE OF DIVERSE ETIOLOGIES

[ ] THROMBOANGIITIS OBLITERANS

Thromboangiitis obliterans (TAO) or Buerger disease is an inflammatory vasculopathy affecting small and medium-sized arteries and veins that is caused by an inflammatory, highly cellular intraluminal thrombus.[130] TAO is always associated with tobacco use. Cannabis, either on its own or because of contamination with tobacco, may cause a similar entity and its use should also be addressed.[131] Historically, TAO was seen predominantly in males in the second through fifth decades. Incidence in women is rising reflecting the changed demographics of tobacco use but does not equal the incidence in men. Clinically, TAO differs from atherosclerosis in that involvement of the upper extremity is common

and usually present. The initial involvement is in digital, pedal, and hand vessels frequently with ulceration of one or more digits. Rare manifestations include coronary, cerebral, and mesenteric artery lesions.[132] Episodes of recurrent superficial phlebitis are common. Biopsy of acute lesions, particularly accessible veins, is diagnostic, whereas angiographic features are characteristic.[133]

Stability or improvement is variable and possible only after all exposure to tobacco ceases.[134] Spinal cord stimulation and intravenous prostacyclin analogs can accelerate healing of ischemic lesions, but amputation of ulcerated digits and limbs is often required.[135,136] Progressive tissue loss is inevitable until tobacco exposure is stopped with amputation rates approaching 50 percent in those who continue to use tobacco.[130,137]

[ ] GIANT CELL AND TAKAYASU ARTERITIS

Takayasu arteritis (TA) and giant cell (temporal) arteritis (GCA) are similar in pathologic process but affect different age groups; TA affects ages younger than 40 years and GCA usually older than the age of 50 years.[138,139] Also, TA generally involves arteries below the neck and GCA above the diaphragm. However, involvement of the aorta, subclavian, axillary, renal, iliac, femoral, and superficial femoral arteries have been described in both. Disease is usually bilateral and presents with rapidly progressive symptoms in the setting of a nonspecific systemic illness. Limb threatening ischemia is rare but does occur when diagnosed late. Both GCA and TA have characteristic clinical and laboratory findings including an elevated sedimentation rate (>90 percent but not in all) and typi-

TABLE 108–8

Treatment of PAD ACC/AHA Indications[a]

INTERVENTION	CLASS I	CLASS IIA	CLASS IIB
Smoking Cessation	Yes		
Walking Program	Supervised		Unsupervised
Lipid Treatment	Statin to LDL <100	Statin to LDL <70	Fibric acid derivative High TG/Low HDL
Antihypertensive Treatment	SBP<130; DBP<80 β blockade	ACEI (symptomatic)	ACEI (asymptomatic)
Diabetes	Proper foot care	Hb A$_{1c}$ <7%	
Homocysteinemia			Folic acid
Antiplatelet Therapy	Aspirin Clopidogrel		
Pharmacologics	Cilostazol		Pentoxifylline
Supplements			L-arginine p-L-carnitine Ginkgo biloba

ACC, American College of Cardiology; ACEI, angiotensin-converting enzyme inhibitor; AHA, American Heart Association; DBP, diastolic blood pressure; HDL, high-density lipoprotein; LDL, low-density lipoprotein; PAD, peripheral arterial disease; SBP, systolic blood pressure; TG, triglyceride.
[a]Summary of AHA/ACC level of evidence guidelines for therapies in claudication.

cal angiographic features of smooth tapered narrowing of large and medium sized arteries (Fig. 108–7).[140]

For GCA confirmatory biopsy of the temporal artery within 3 days of starting steroids is the gold standard.[141] A preceding history or polymyalgia rheumatica is present in >50 percent.[138] Visual changes in the setting of an elevated sedimentation rate, jaw claudication, or a pulse deficit should be treated as medical emergency with hospitalization and parenteral corticosteroids.[142] TA may present as a medical emergency as well. The coronary arteries may be involved resulting in unstable angina.[143] It may also affect the aortic root causing acute aortic insufficiency and pulmonary edema.[144] This should be considered in a young woman with absent pulse(s), dyspnea, and a diastolic murmur.

These diseases are unique among arteriopathies in that the acutely stenotic lesions improve rapidly with steroid therapy. Alternative immunosuppressive agents are often used, but corticosteroids remain the mainstay of treatment.[145] When required, revascularization is best performed when the inflammatory process is quiet or *burned out* and steroids have been discontinued or tapered to a maintenance dose.[146,147]

【 】 FIBROMUSCULAR DYSPLASIA

Fibromuscular dysplasia most commonly affects women in the middle years and has been described in almost all arteries. The renal artery is most commonly involved, affecting 4 to 5 percent of the general population, and is bilateral in about 10 percent of cases.[148] Treatment is angioplasty without stent use and has generally good outcomes. Surgical repair is reserved for refractory cases.[149]

【 】 RAYNAUD PHENOMENON

Raynaud phenomenon is diagnosed by history. The syndrome is classically defined as episodes of discoloration of white ischemia, then blue stasis, then red hyperemia during the recovery phase.

TABLE 108–9

Raynaud Phenomenon

	COLOR	PHYSIOLOGY
Phase 1	White	Vasospasm of arterioles with cutaneous ischemia
Phase 2	Blue	Venule dilation with stasis of deoxygenated blood
Phase 3	Red	Arteriolar dilation, hyperemic flow of oxygenated blood

However, most patients do not describe all three phases.[150] Fingers are involved more often than toes. The fingertips are affected more commonly than the palm or dorsum of the hand. Prevalence was estimated at slightly fewer than 10 percent of the population in the Framingham study.[151]

Allen and Brown defined primary Raynaud phenomenon as episodes of bilateral color changes induced by cold or emotion without evidence of ischemia or other disease for 2 years[152] (Table 108–9). This represents most cases and in some sense can be considered simply an exaggerated response of a normal reflex. The pathophysiology of the exaggerated vasoconstriction is complex but appears to involve both local and systemic pathways.[150] Secondary Raynaud phenomenon, symptoms caused by another etiology, is present in approximately 10 percent of patients at initial evaluation (Fig. 108–8). For those without a secondary cause at presentation, one is identified at a rate of 2 percent per year over a 10-year interval.[153] Causes of secondary Raynaud phenomenon are diverse (Table 108–10).

Most patients with primary Raynaud phenomenon require no therapy and quickly learn to keep not only hands but the whole body warm. For the few that have severe symptoms, treatment is similar to secondary Raynaud. Treatment of secondary Raynaud is directed at the underlying cause when feasible. Calcium channel blockers and blockers, either as monotherapy or in combination, can blunt the episodes in many patients, but may have little im-

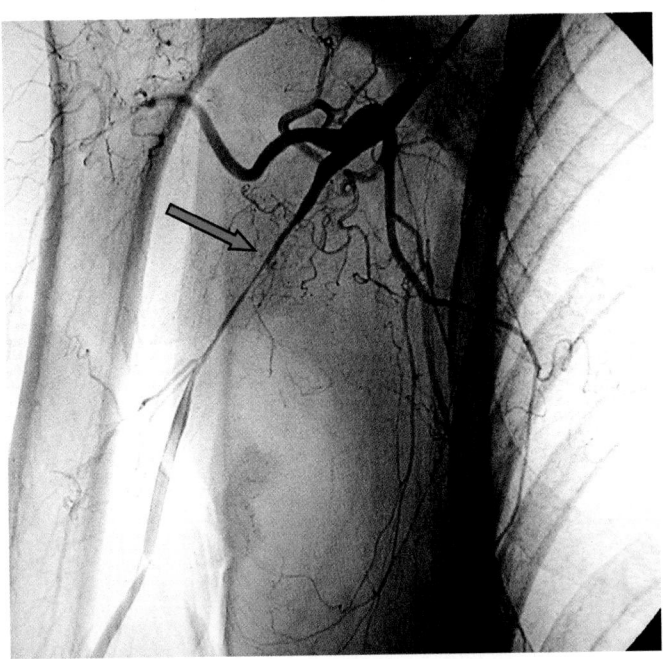

FIGURE 108–7. Extracranial giant cell arteritis affecting the brachial artery of an elderly woman. Note the smooth, tapered narrowing (*red arrow*) with normal appearing vessel proximal and distal to the affected segment.

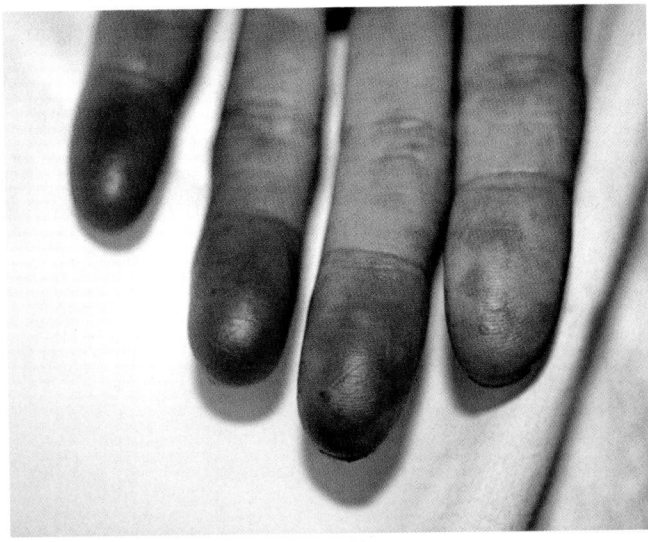

FIGURE 108–8. Hyperemic (red) phase in a patient with secondary Raynaud phenomenon. Note the pallor still present in the proximal digits.

TABLE 108–10

Raynaud Phenomenon: Secondary Causes

Collagen vascular disease
- Scleroderma
- Mixed connective tissue disease
- Rheumatoid arthritis
- Myositis
- Sjögren syndrome
- Necrotizing vasculitis

Hematologic disorders

Neurogenic
- Thoracic outlet irritation
- Carpal tunnel syndrome
- Neuropathy

Myxedema

Acromegaly

Pulmonary hypertension

Medications
- β Blockers
- Ergotamine
- Methysergide
- Vinblastine, bleomycin
- Estrogens
- Imipramine

Microcirculatory diseases

Buerger disease

Hypothenar hammer syndrome

Environmental
- Cold injury
- Vibration syndrome
- Vinyl chloride disease

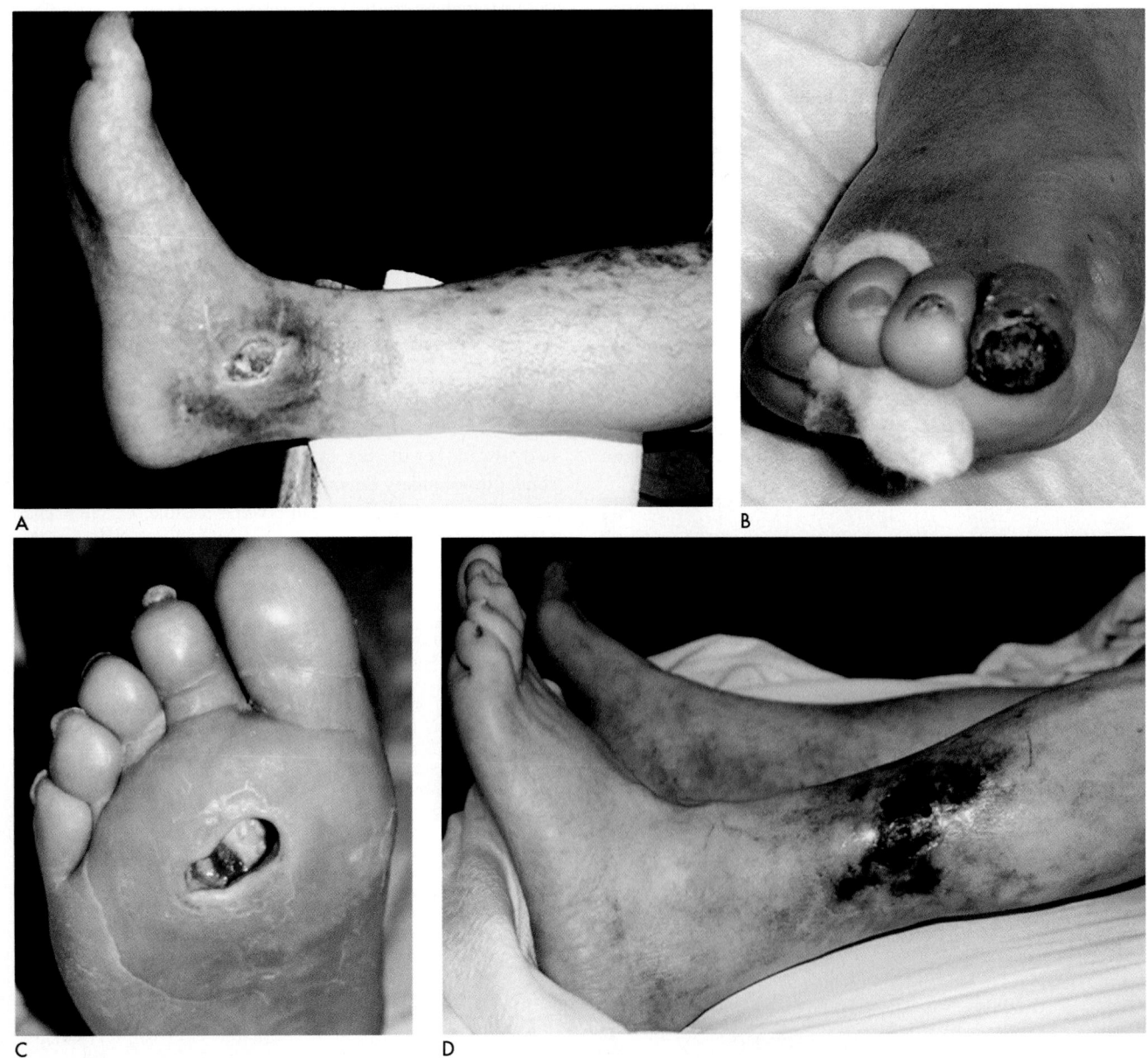

FIGURE 108–9. Ulcers caused by venous insufficiency (**A**), arterial insufficiency (**B**), neurotrophic ulceration (**C**), and small vessel (arteriolar or venular) disease (**D**).

TABLE 108-11

Recognition of Ulcers of Vascular Etiology

TYPE	VENOUS	ARTERIAL	NEUROTROPHIC	ARTERIOLAR
Location	Above medial and lateral malleoli	Shins, toes, sites of injury	Plantar surface, pressure points	Shin, calf
Pain	No, unless infected	Yes	No	Exquisite
Skin	Stasis pigmentation Thickening with lipodermatosclerosis	Shiny, pale, decreased hair, may see livido	Callous, normal to changes of ischemia	Normal or *satellite* ulcers in various stages
Edges	Clean	Smooth	Trophic, calloused	Serpiginous
Base	Wet, weeping, healthy granulation	Dry, pale with eschar	Healthy to pale depending on PAD	Dry, punched out pale, thin eschar
Cellulitis	Common	Often	Common	No
Treatment	Compression	Revascularize	Revascularize, remove pressure	Treat underlying disease and pain

pact on ischemic complications. ACEI, angiotensin II receptor inhibition and endothelin receptor inhibition are promising in the setting of scleroderma.[154]

[ ] VASCULAR ULCERS

Space does not allow adequate discussion of wound etiology and treatment. Fig. 108–9A through Fig. 108–9D and Table 108–11 provide a framework for recognition. Regardless of the etiology, treatment goals are always the same: wound healing. Treatment modalities and potential combinations of modalities are legion. Aggressive and early treatment of cellulitis should be done whenever suspected. Removal of any exacerbating forces (i.e., poorfitting shoes) can be initiated by any healthcare provider. Referral to a wound care specialist is never inappropriate.

REFERENCES

1. Moffatt CJ, Franks PJ, Doherty DC, et al. Lymphoedema: an underestimated health problem. *Q J Med* 2003;96:731.
2. Baird JB, Charles JL, Streit TG, et al. Reactivity to bacterial, fungal, and parasite antigens in patients with lymphedema and elephantiasis. *Am J Trop Med Hyg* 2002;66:163.
3. Holcomb SS. Identification and treatment of different types of lymphedema. *Adv Skin Wound Care* 2006;19:103.
4. Stanton AW, Modi S, Mellor RH, et al. A quantitative lymphoscintigraphic evaluation of lymphatic function in the swollen hands of women with lymphoedema following breast cancer treatment. *Clin Sci* 2006;110:553.
5. Szuba A, Shin WS, Strauss HW, et al. The third circulation: radionuclide lymphoscintigraphy in the evaluation of lymphedema. *J Nucl Med* 2003;44:43.
6. Tiwari A, Myint F, Hamilton G. Management of lower limb lymphoedema in the United Kingdom. *Eur J Vasc Endovasc Surg* 2006;31:311.
7. Lee AY, Gent M, Julian JA, et al. Bilateral vs. ipsilateral venography as the primary efficacy outcome measure in thromboprophylaxis clinical trials: a systematic review. *J Thromb Haemost* 2004;2:1752.
8. Zierler BK. Screening for acute DVT: optimal utilization of the vascular diagnostic laboratory. *Semin Vasc Surg* 2001;14:206.
9. Lim KE, Hsu WC, Hsu YY, et al. Deep venous thrombosis: comparison of indirect multidetector CT venography and sonography of lower extremities in 26 patients. *Clin Imaging* 2004;28:439.
10. Kluge A, Mueller C, Strunk J, et al. Experience in 207 combined MRI examinations for acute pulmonary embolism and deep vein thrombosis. *AJR Am J Roentgenol* 2006;186:1686.
11. Wells PS. Advances in the diagnosis of venous thromboembolism. *J Thromb Thrombolysis* 2006;21:31.
12. Hafner JW, Gerdes E, Aldag JC. Combining clinical risk with D-dimer testing to rule out acute deep venous thrombosis (DVT). *J Emerg Med* 2006;30:100.
13. Wheeler H, Anderson FJ. Use of noninvasive tests as the basis for treatment of deep vein thrombosis. In: Rutherford RB, ed. *Vascular Diagnosis*. 4th ed. St. Louis: Mosby; 1993:862.
14. Robinson BJ, Kesteven PJ, Elliott ST. The role of strain gauge plethysmography in the assessment of patients with suspected deep vein thrombosis. *Br J Haematol* 2002;118:600.
15. Kahn SR, Joseph L, Grover SA, et al. A randomized management study of impedance plethysmography vs. contrast venography in patients with a first episode of clinically suspected deep vein thrombosis. *Thromb Res* 2001;102:15.
16. Persson LM, Arnhjort T, Larfars G, et al. Hemodynamic and morphologic evaluation of sequelae of primary upper extremity deep venous thromboses treated with anticoagulation. *J Vasc Surg* 2006;43:1230.
17. Allan PL, Bradbury AW, Evans CJ, et al. Patterns of reflux and severity of varicose veins in the general population. Edinburgh Vein Study. *Eur J Vasc Endovasc Surg* 2000;20:470.
18. Evans CJ, Allan PL, Lee AJ, et al. Prevalence of venous reflux in the general population on duplex scanning. The Edinburgh vein study. *J Vasc Surg* 1998;28:767.
19. Evans CJ, Fowkes FG, Ruckley CV, et al. Prevalence of varicose veins and chronic venous insufficiency in men and women in the general population: Edinburgh Vein Study. *J Epidemiol Community Health* 1999;53:149.
20. Beebe HG, Bergan JJ, Bergqvist D, et al. Classification and grading of chronic venous disease in the lower limbs: a consensus statement. *Eur J Vasc Endovasc Surg* 1996;12:487.
21. Eklof B, Rutherford RB, Bergan JJ, et al. Revision of the CEAP classification for chronic venous disorders: consensus statement. *J Vasc Surg* 2004;40:1248.
22. Kroeger K, Ose C, Rudofsky G, et al. Risk factors for varicose veins. *Int Angio* 2004;23:29.
23. Andreozzi GM, Signorelli S, Di Pino L, et al. Varicose symptoms without varicose veins: the hypotonic phlebopathy, epidemiology and pathophysiology. The Acireale project. *Minerva Cardioangiol* 2000;48:277.
24. Kurz X, Lamping DL, Kahn SR, et al. Do varicose veins affect quality of life? Results of an international population-based study. *J Vasc Surg* 2001;34:641.
25. Bergan J, Pascarella L, Mekenas L. Venous disorders: treatment with sclerosant foam. *J Cardiovasc Surg (Torino)* 2006;47:9.
26. Bountouroglou DG, Azzam M, Kakkos SK, et al. Ultrasound-guided foam sclerotherapy combined with sapheno-femoral ligation compared to surgical treatment of varicose veins: early results of a randomised controlled trial. *Eur J Vasc Endovasc Surg* 2006;31:93.
27. Puggioni A, Kalra M, Carmo M, et al. Endovenous laser therapy and radiofrequency ablation of the great saphenous vein: analysis of early efficacy and complications. *J Vasc Surg* 2005;42:488.

28. Leon L, Giannoukas AD, Dodd D, et al. Clinical significance of superficial vein thrombosis. *Eur J Vasc Endovasc Surg* 2005;29:10.

29. Unno N, Mitsuoka H, Uchiyama T, et al. Superficial thrombophlebitis of the lower limbs in patients with varicose veins. *Surg Today* 2002;32:397.

30. Decousus H, Epinat M, Guillot K, et al. Superficial vein thrombosis: risk factors, diagnosis, and treatment. *Curr Opin Pulm Med* 2003;9:393.

31. O'Fallon W, Heit J, Mohr D, et al. Predictors of recurrence after deep vein thrombosis and pulmonary embolism: a population-based cohort study. *Blood* 1999;10:560.

32. Heit JA, Melton LJ III, Lohse CM, et al. Incidence of venous thromboembolism in hospitalized patients vs community residents. *Mayo Clin Proc* 2001;76:1102.

33. Khan NA, Rahim SA, Anand SS, et al. Does the clinical examination predict lower extremity peripheral arterial disease? *JAMA* 2006;295:536.

34. Wells PS, Owen C, Doucette S, et al. Does this patient have deep vein thrombosis? *JAMA* 2006;295:199.

35. Merli G. Anticoagulants in the treatment of deep vein thrombosis. *Am J Med* 2005;118(suppl 8A):13S.

36. Warkentin TE. Management of heparin-induced thrombocytopenia: a critical comparison of lepirudin and argatroban. *Thromb Res* 2003;110:73.

37. Ageno W, Steidl L, Ultori C, et al. The initial phase of oral anticoagulation with warfarin in outpatients with deep venous thrombosis. *Blood Coagul Fibrinolysis* 2003;14:11.

38. Pinede L Ninet J Duhaut P, et al. Comparison of 3 and 6 months of oral anticoagulant therapy after a first episode of proximal deep vein thrombosis or pulmonary embolism and comparison of 6 and 12 weeks of therapy after isolated calf deep vein thrombosis. *Circulation* 2001;103:2453–2460.

39. Blum A, Roche E. Endovascular management of acute deep vein thrombosis. *Am J Med* 2005;118(suppl 8A):31S.

40. Watson LI, Armon MP. Thrombolysis for acute deep vein thrombosis. *Cochrane Database Syst Rev* October 18, 2004; 4:CD002783.

41. Kahn SR. The post-thrombotic syndrome: the forgotten morbidity of deep venous thrombosis. *J Thromb Thrombolysis* 2006;21:41.

42. Junger M, Diehm C, Storiko H, et al. Mobilization versus immobilization in the treatment of acute proximal deep venous thrombosis: a prospective, randomized, open, multicentre trial. *Curr Med Res Opin* 2006;22:593.

43. Schellong SM, Schwarz T, Kropp J, et al. Bed rest in deep vein thrombosis and the incidence of scintigraphic pulmonary embolism. *Thromb Haemost* 1999;82(suppl 1):127.

44. Partsch H, Blattler W. Compression and walking versus bed rest in the treatment of proximal deep venous thrombosis with low molecular weight heparin. *J Vasc Surg* 2000;32:861.

45. Eklof B, Arfvidsson B, Kistner RL, et al. Indications for surgical treatment of iliofemoral vein thrombosis. *Hematol Oncol Clin North Am* 2000;14:471.

46. Criqui M, Denenberg J, Langer R, et al. The epidemiology of peripheral arterial disease: importance of identifying the population at risk. *Vasc Med* 1997;2:221.

47. McDermott MM, Mehta S, Greenland P. Exertional leg symptoms other than intermittent claudication are common in peripheral arterial disease. *Arch Intern Med* 1999;159:387.

48. Cimminiello C. PAD: epidemiology and pathophysiology. *Thromb Res* 2002;106:V295.

49. Willigendael EM, Teijink JA, Bartelink ML, et al. Influence of smoking on incidence and prevalence of peripheral arterial disease. *J Vasc Surg* 2004;40:1158.

50. Ogren M, Hedblad B, Engstrom G, et al. Prevalence and prognostic significance of asymptomatic peripheral arterial disease in 68-year-old men with diabetes: results from the population study of men born in 1914 from Malmo, Sweden. *Eur J Vasc Endovasc Surg* 2005;29:182.

51. Gregg EW, Sorlie P, Paulose-Ram R, et al. Prevalence of lower-extremity disease in the US adult population ≥ 40 years of age with and without diabetes: 1999–2000 national health and nutrition examination survey. *Diabetes Care* 2004;27:1591.

52. Higgins JP, Higgins JA. Peripheral arterial disease—Part I. Diagnosis, epidemiology and risk factors. *J Okla State Med Assoc* 2002;95:765.

53. Garcia LA. Epidemiology and pathophysiology of lower extremity peripheral arterial disease. *J Endovasc Surg* 2006;13(suppl 2):II3.

54. Ness J, Aronow WS, Newkirk E, et al. Prevalence of symptomatic peripheral arterial disease, modifiable risk factors, and appropriate use of drugs in the treatment of peripheral arterial disease in older persons seen in a university general medicine clinic. *J Gerontol* 2005;60:255.

55. Murabito JM, Evans JC, Nieto K, et al. Prevalence and clinical correlates of peripheral arterial disease in the Framingham Offspring Study. *Am Heart J* 2002;143:961.

56. Hirsch AT, Criqui MH, Treat-Jacobson D, et al. Peripheral arterial disease detection, awareness, and treatment in primary care. *JAMA* 2001;286:1317.

57. Criqui M, Langer R, Fronek A, et al. Mortality over a period of 10 years in patients with peripheral arterial disease. *N Engl J Med* 1992;326:381.

58. Newman AB, Tyrrell KS, Kuller LH. Mortality over four years in SHEP participants with a low ankle-arm index. *J Am Geriatr Soc* 1997;45:1472.

59. Hooi J, Stoffers H, Kester A, et al. Risk factors and cardiovascular diseases associated with asymptomatic peripheral arterial occlusive disease. The Limburg PAOD Study. Peripheral Arterial Occlusive Disease. *Scand J Prim Health Care* 1997;16:177.

60. Cleven AH, Kester AD, Hooi JD, et al. Cardiovascular outcome stratification using the ankle-brachial pressure index. *Eur J Gen Pract* 2005;11:107.

61. McKenna M, Wolfson S, Kuller L. The ratio of ankle and arm arterial pressure as an independent predictor of mortality. *Atherosclerosis* 1991;87:119.

62. Ogren M, Hedblad B, Engstrom G, et al. Leg blood flow and long-term cardiovascular prognosis in men with typical and atypical intermittent claudication. *Eur J Vasc Endovasc Surg* 2003;26:272.

63. Leng GC, Lee AJ, Fowkes FG, et al. Incidence, natural history and cardiovascular events in symptomatic and asymptomatic peripheral arterial disease in the general population. *Int J Epidemiol* 1996;25:1172.

64. McDaniel M, Cronenwett J. Basic data related to the natural history of intermittent claudication. *Ann Vasc Surg* 1989;3:273.

65. Feinglass J, Brown J, LoSasso A, et al. Rates of lower extremity amputation and arterial reconstruction in the United States, 1979–1996. *Am J Public Health* 89:1999;1222:7.

66. Dormandy J, Heeck L, Vig S. Major amputations: clinical patterns and predictors. *Semin Vasc Surg* 1999;12:154.

67. Carmona GA, Hoffmeyer P, Herrmann FR, et al. Major lower limb amputations in the elderly observed over ten years: the role of diabetes and peripheral arterial disease. *Diabetes Metab* 2005;31:449.

68. Jude EB, Oyibo SO, Chalmers N, et al. Peripheral arterial disease in diabetic and nondiabetic patients: a comparison of severity and outcome. *Diabetes Care* 2001;24:1433.

69. Dormandy J, Heeck L, Vig S. Acute limb ischemia. *Semin Vasc Surg* 1999;12:148.

70. Collins TC, Petersen NJ, Suarez-Almazor M. Peripheral arterial disease symptom subtype and walking impairment. *Vasc Med* 2005;10:177.

71. Olson KW, Treat-Jacobson D. Symptoms of peripheral arterial disease: a critical review. *J Vasc Nurs* 2004;22:72.

72. Wang JC, Criqui MH, Denenberg JO, et al. Exertional leg pain in patients with and without peripheral arterial disease. *Circulation* 2005;112:3501.

73. Matzke S, Lepantalo M. Claudication does not always precede critical leg ischemia. *Vasc Med* 2001;6:77.

74. Kavanaugh G, Svein H, Holman C, et al. "Pseudoclaudication" syndrome produced by compression of the cuada equina. *JAMA* 1968;206:2477.

75. Goodreau J, Creasy J, Flanigan D, et al. Rational approach to the differentiation of vascular and neurogenic claudication. *Surgery* 1978;84:749.

76. Delis KT, Bountouroglou D, Mansfield AO. Venous claudication in iliofemoral thrombosis: long-term effects on venous hemodynamics, clinical status, and quality of life. *Ann Surg* 2004;239:118.

77. Allen E, Barker N, Hines AJ. *Peripheral Vascular Diseases*. 1st ed. Philadelphia: W.B. Saunders; 1946:44–46.

78. Hirsch AT, Haskal ZJ, Hertzer NR, et al. ACC/AHA 2005 guidelines for the management of patients with peripheral arterial disease (lower extremity, renal, mesenteric, and abdominal aortic). *J Am Coll Cardiol* 2006;47:1239.

79. Fleischmann D, Hallett RL, Rubin GD. CT angiography of peripheral arterial disease. *J Vasc Interv Radiol* 2003;17:3.

80. Kock MC, Adriaensen ME, Pattynama PM, et al. DSA versus multi-detector row CT angiography in peripheral arterial disease: randomized controlled trial. *Radiology* 2005;237:727.

81. Sommerville RS, Jenkins J, Walker P, et al. 3-D magnetic resonance angiography versus conventional angiography in peripheral arterial disease: pilot study. *ANZ J Surg* 2005;75:373.

82. Ascher E, Hingorani A, Markevich N, et al. Lower extremity revascularization without preoperative contrast arteriography: experience with duplex ultrasound arterial mapping in 485 cases. *Ann Vasc Surg* 2002;16:108.

83. Strandness DJ, McCutcheon E, Rushmer R. Application of transcutaneous Doppler flowmeter in evaluation of occlusive arterial disease. *Surg Gynecol Obstet* 1966;122:1039.

84. Hobbs J, Yao J, Lewis J, et al. A limitation of the Doppler ultrasound method of measuring ankle systolic pressure. *Vasa* 1974;3:160.

85. Labs KH, Nehler MR, Roessner M, et al. Reliability of treadmill testing in peripheral arterial disease: a comparison of a constant load with a graded load treadmill protocol. *Vasc Med* 1999;4:239.

86. Regensteiner JG, Gardner A, Hiatt WR. Exercise testing and exercise rehabilitation for patients with peripheral arterial disease: status in 1997. *Vasc Med* 1997;2:147.

87. Feringa HH, Bax JJ, van Waning VH, et al. The long-term prognostic value of the resting and postexercise ankle-brachial index. *Arch Intern Med* 2006;166:529.

88. McDermott MM, Mehta S, Liu K, et al. Leg symptoms, the ankle-brachial index, and walking ability in patients with peripheral arterial disease. *J Gen Intern Med* 1999;14:173.

89. McPhail IR, Spittell PC, Weston SA, et al. Intermittent claudication: an objective office-based assessment. *J Am Coll Cardiol* 2001;37:1381.

90. Halperin JL. Evaluation of patients with peripheral vascular disease. *Thromb Res* 2002;106:V303.

91. Creager, MA. Clinical assessment of the patient with claudication: the role of the vascular laboratory. *Vasc Med* 1997;2:231.

92. Kroger K, Stewen C, Santosa F, et al. Toe pressure measurements compared to ankle artery pressure measurements. *Angiology* 2003;54:39.

93. Rossi M, Carpi A. Skin microcirculation in peripheral arterial obliterative disease. *Biomed Pharmacother* 2004;58:427.

94. Ubbink DT, Gersbach PA, Berg P, et al. The best $TCPO_2$ parameters to predict the efficacy of spinal cord stimulation to improve limb salvage in patients with inoperable critical leg ischemia. *Int Angio* 2003;22:356.

95. Bacharach J, Rooke T, Osmundson P, et al. Predictive value of transcutaneous oxygen pressure and amputation success by use of supine and elevation measurements. *J Vasc Surg* 1998;15:558.

96. Tsai FW, Tulsyan N, Jones DN, et al. Skin perfusion pressure of the foot is a good substitute for toe pressure in the assessment of limb ischemia. *J Vasc Surg* 2000;32:32.

97. Hirsch AT, Haskal ZJ, Hertzer NR, et al. ACC/AHA 2005 Practice Guidelines for the management of patients with peripheral arterial disease (lower extremity, renal, mesenteric, and abdominal aortic): a collaborative report from the American Association for Vascular Surgery/Society for Vascular Surgery, Society for Cardiovascular Angiography and Interventions, Society for Vascular Medicine and Biology, Society of Interventional Radiology, and the ACC/AHA Task Force on Practice Guidelines (Writing Committee to Develop Guidelines for the Management of Patients With Peripheral Arterial Disease)—endorsed by the American Association of Cardiovascular and Pulmonary Rehabilitation; National Heart, Lung, and Blood Institute; Society for Vascular Nursing; TransAtlantic Inter-Society Consensus; and Vascular Disease Foundation. *Circulation* 113:e463, 2006.

98. McDermott MM, Liu K, Greenland P, et al. Functional decline in peripheral arterial disease: associations with the ankle brachial index and leg symptoms. *JAMA* 2004;292:453.

99. Regensteiner JG. Exercise rehabilitation for the patient with intermittent claudication: a highly effective yet underutilized treatment. *Curr Drug Targets Cardiovasc Haematol Disord* 2004;4:233.

100. Degischer S, Labs KH, Hochstrasser J, et al. Physical training for intermittent claudication: a comparison of structured rehabilitation versus home-based training. *Vasc Med* 2002;7:109.

101. Gardner AW, Poehlman ET. Exercise rehabilitation programs for the treatment of claudication pain: a meta-analysis. *JAMA* 1995;274:975.

102. Hiatt WR, Regensteiner JG, Wolfel EE, et al. Effect of exercise training on skeletal muscle histology and metabolism in peripheral arterial disease. *J Appl Physiol* 1996;81:780.

103. Ali SM, Basit A, Sheikh T, et al. Diabetic foot ulcer—a prospective study. *J Pak Med Assoc* 2001;51:78.

104. Strandness DE Jr, Dalman RL, Panian S, et al. Effect of cilostazol in patients with intermittent claudication: a randomized, double-blind, placebo-controlled study. *Vasc Endovascular Surg* 2002;36:83.

105. Hiatt WR. The US experience with cilostazol in treating intermittent claudication. *Atheroscler Suppl* 2005;6:21.

106. Peripheral Arterial Diseases Antiplatelet Consensus Group. Antiplatelet therapy in peripheral arterial disease: consensus statement. *Eur J Vasc Endovasc Surg* 2003;26:1.

107. Hiatt WR. Preventing atherothrombotic events in peripheral arterial disease: the use of antiplatelet therapy. *J Intern Med* 2002;251:193.

108. Dippel DW. The results of CAPRIE, IST and CAST. Clopidogrel vs. Aspirin in Patients at Risk of Ischaemic Events. International Stroke Trial. Chinese Acute Stroke Trial. *Thromb Res* 1998;92:S13.

109. Okaa RK, Umoh E, Szuba A, et al. Suboptimal intensity of risk factor modification in PAD. *Vasc Med* 2005;10:91.

110. Hirsch AT, Gotto AM Jr. Undertreatment of dyslipidemia in peripheral arterial disease and other high-risk populations: an opportunity for cardiovascular disease reduction. *Vasc Med* 2002;7:323.

111. Giri J, McDermott MM, Greenland P, et al. Statin use and functional decline in patients with and without peripheral arterial disease. *J Am Coll Cardiol* 2006;47:998.

112. Feringa HH, van Waning VH, Bax JJ, et al. Cardioprotective medication is associated with improved survival in patients with peripheral arterial disease. *J Am Coll Cardiol* 2006;47:1182.

113. Ahimastos AA, Lawler A, Reid CM, et al. Brief communication: ramipril markedly improves walking ability in patients with peripheral arterial disease: a randomized trial. *Ann Intern Med* 2006;144:660.

114. Olin JW. Hypertension and peripheral arterial disease. *Vasc Med* 2005;10:241.

115. Hiatt W, Stoll S, Nies A. Effect of beta-adrenergic blockers in the peripheral circulation in patients with peripheral arterial disease. *Circulation* 1985;72:1226.

116. Mueller T, Furtmueller B, Aigelsdorfer J, et al. Total serum homocysteine: a predictor of extracranial carotid artery stenosis in male patients with symptomatic peripheral arterial disease. *Vasc Med* 2001;6:163.

117. Guthikonda S, Haynes WG. Homocysteine as a novel risk factor for atherosclerosis. *Current Opinion in Cardiology* 1999;14:283.

118. Voller H. Peripheral arterial disease (PAD): secondary prevention. *Dtsch Med Wochenschr* 2002;127:1870.

119. Muhs BE, Gagne P, Sheehan P. Peripheral arterial disease: clinical assessment and indications for revascularization in the patient with diabetes. *Curr Diab Rep* 2005;5:24.

120. Novo S, Coppola G, Milio G. Critical limb ischemia: definition and natural history. *Curr Drug Targets Cardiovasc Haematol Disord* 2004;4:219.

121. Chung J, Bartelson BB, Hiatt WR, et al. Wound healing and functional outcomes after infrainguinal bypass with reversed saphenous vein for critical limb ischemia. *J Vasc Surg* 2006;43:1183.

122. Bosiers M, Deloose K, Verbist J, et al. Percutaneous transluminal angioplasty for treatment of "below-the-knee" critical limb ischemia: early outcomes following the use of sirolimus-eluting stents. *J Cardiovasc Surg (Torino)* 2006;47:171.

123. Marston WA, Davies SW, Armstrong B, et al. Natural history of limbs with arterial insufficiency and chronic ulceration treated without revascularization. *J Vasc Surg* 2006;44:108.

124. Montori VM, Kavros SJ, Walsh EE, et al. Intermittent compression pump for nonhealing wounds in patients with limb ischemia. The Mayo Clinic experience (1998–2000). *Int Angio* 2002;21:360.

125. Emmerich J. Current state and perspective on medical treatment of critical leg ischemia: gene and cell therapy. *Int J Low Extrem Wounds* 2005;4:234.

126. Kroger K, Biro F, Zeeh JM, et al. Value of transesophageal echocardiography, esophagogastroduodenoscopy and retinoscopy prior to intra-arterial fibrinolytic therapy in patients with peripheral arterial disease. *Vasa* 2002;31:255.

127. Blaisdell F, Steele M, Allen R. Management of acute lower extremity arterial ischemia due to embolism and thrombosis. *Surgery* 1978;84:822.

128. Ouriel K, Vieth F, Sasahara A. Thrombolysis of Peripheral Arterial Surgery (TOPAS) Investigators. A comparison of recombinant urokinase with vascular surgery as initial treatment for acute arterial occlusion of the legs. *N Engl J Med* 1998;338:1105.

129. Giannini D, Balbarini A. Thrombolytic therapy in peripheral arterial disease. *Curr Drug Targets Cardiovasc Haematol Disord* 2004;4:249.

130. Olin JW, Shih A. Thromboangiitis obliterans (Buerger's disease). *Curr Opin Rheumatol* 2006;18:18.

131. Disdier P, Granel B, Serratrice J, et al. Cannabis arteritis revisited: ten new case reports. *Angiology* 2001;52:1.

132. Sasaki S, Sakuma M, Kunihara T, et al. Distribution of arterial involvement in thromboangiitis obliterans (Buerger's disease): results of a study conducted by the Intractable Vasculitis Syndromes Research Group in Japan. *Surg Today* 2000;30:600.

133. Allen EV. Thromboangiitis obliterans: methods of diagnosis of chronic occlusive arterial lesions distal to the wrist with illustrative cases. *Am J Med Sci* 1929;178:237.

134. Olin J, Young J, Graor R, et al. The changing clinical spectrum of thromboangiitis obliterans (Buerger's disease). *Circulation* 1990;82(suppl IV):3.

135. Chierichetti F, Mambrini S, Bagliani A, et al. Treatment of Buerger's disease with electrical spinal cord stimulation: review of three cases. *Angiology* 2002;53:341.

136. Fernandez B, Strootman D. The prostacyclin analog, treprostinil sodium, provides symptom relief in severe Buerger's disease: a case report and review of literature. *Angiology* 2006;57:99.

137. Borner C, Heidrich H. Long-term follow-up of thromboangiitis obliterans. *Vasa* 1998;27:80.

138. Gonzalez-Gay MA. Giant cell arteritis and polymyalgia rheumatica: two different but often overlapping conditions. *Semin Arthritis Rheum* 2004;33:289.

139. Hunder GG. Epidemiology of giant-cell arteritis. *Cleve Clin J Med* 2002;69(suppl 2):SII79.

140. Weyand CM, Goronzy JJ. Medium- and large-vessel vasculitis. *N Engl J Med* 2003;349:160.

141. Achkar AA, Lie JT, Hunder GG, et al. How does previous corticosteroid treatment affect the biopsy findings in giant cell (temporal) arteritis? *Ann Intern Med* 2004;120:987.

142. Danesh-Meyer H, Savino PJ, Gamble GG. Poor prognosis of visual outcome after visual loss from giant cell arteritis. *Ophthalmology* 2005;112:1098.

143. Endo M, Tomizawa Y, Nishida H, et al. Angiographic findings and surgical treatments of coronary artery involvement in Takayasu arteritis. *J Thorac Cardiovasc Surg* 2003;125:570.

144. Song JK, Jeong YH, Kang DH, et al. Echocardiographic and clinical characteristics of aortic regurgitation because of systemic vasculitis. *J Am Soc Echocardiogr* 2003;16:850.

145. Koenig CL, Langford CA. Novel therapeutic strategies for large vessel vasculitis. *Rheum Dis Clin North Am* 2006;32:173.

146. Alonso JH, Rueda E, Hernandez JM, et al. Complete percutaneous revascularization in Takayasu's disease. *Int J Cardiol* 2006;108:271.

147. Joh JH, Kim DK, Park KH, et al. Surgical management of Takayasu's arteritis. *J Korean Med Sci* 2006;21:20.

148. Andreoni KA, Weeks SM, Gerber DA, et al. Incidence of donor renal fibromuscular dysplasia: does it justify routine angiography? *Transplantation* 2003;73:1112.

149. Carmo M, Bower TC, Mozes G, et al. Surgical management of renal fibromuscular dysplasia: challenges in the endovascular era. *Ann Vasc Surg* 2005;19:208.

150. Cooke JP, Marshall JM. Mechanisms of Raynaud's disease. *Vasc Med* 2005;10:293.

151. Brand FN, Larson MG, Kannel WB, et al. The occurrence of Raynaud's phenomenon in a general population. The Framingham Study. *Vasc Med* 1997;2:296.

152. Allen E, Brown G. Raynaud's disease: a critical review of minimal requisites for diagnosis. *Am J Med Sci* 1932;183:187.

153. Hirschl M, Hirschl K, Lenz M, et al. Transition from primary Raynaud's phenomenon to secondary Raynaud's phenomenon identified by diagnosis of an associated disease: results of ten years of prospective surveillance. *Arthritis Rheum* 2006;54:1974.

154. Zandman-Goddard G, Tweezer-Zaks N, Shoenfeld Y. New therapeutic strategies for systemic sclerosis—a critical analysis of the literature. *Clin Dev Immunol* 2005;12:165.

155. Clason AE, Stonebridge PA, Duncan AJ, et al. Morbidity and mortality in acute lower limb ischaemia: a 5-year review. *Eur J Vasc Surg* 1989;3:339–343.

CHAPTER (109)

Surgical Treatment of Carotid and Peripheral Vascular Disease

Deepak G. Nair / Thomas F. Dodson

Over the past 50 years, the discipline of vascular surgery has witnessed a rapid proliferation, as well as remarkable progress, in technique, technology, and research. Advances in anesthesia and perioperative care have resulted in improved mortality and morbidity. Endovascular therapy has become a fundamental part of the vascular specialist's practice, and evidence-based studies have made certain practice patterns standard of care. The end result has been an improvement in the clinical care of patients. This chapter limits itself to three topics in vascular surgery: (1) carotid endarterectomy (CEA), (2) upper and lower extremity revascularization, and (3) upper and lower extremity venous thrombosis.

CAROTID ENDARTERECTOMY

Stroke ranks as the third leading cause of death in the United States. Nearly 5,500,000 people are afflicted by this condition. Of the 700,000 new or recurrent cases of stroke that occur every year, 500,000 are new and 200,000 are recurrent cases.[1] This problem exacts an emotional and economic toll as well. Stroke is commonly viewed as worse than death by patients.[2] It is often a life-changing event for the patient as well as their families. There exists a significant morbidity amongst the survivors: 18 percent are unable to return to work, and nearly 5 percent are completely dependent on custodial care.[3] The cost of stroke on society continues to be a significant burden with the estimated cost of stroke in 2006 being $57.9 billion.[1]

CEA is the most frequently performed surgical procedure to prevent stroke. In 2003, >117,000 CEA procedures were per-

formed.[1] This number has steadily increased over the years since CEA was first described in 1954 by Eastcott and colleagues.[4] There have been at least five randomized clinical trials of CEA for patients with symptomatic extracranial carotid artery stenosis. The North American Symptomatic Endarterectomy Trial (NASCET) was started in the mid-1980s and enrolled patients who had a hemispheric transient ischemic attack or a nondisabling stroke within 120 days and had an ipsilateral carotid artery stenosis.[5] The National Institutes of Health terminated this study early because of clear benefit in patients treated with CEA. The risk of any ipsilateral stroke at 2 years after CEA (9 percent) was lower than medical treatment (26 percent). There was also a lower risk of major or fatal strokes at 2 years with CEA (2.5 percent vs. 13.1 percent).[6] In the European Carotid Surgery Trial (ECST), 2518 patients were prospectively randomized to CEA or medical therapy. After a 3-year follow up, CEA was shown to have superior results in the incidence of ipsilateral stroke (2.8 percent vs. 16.8 percent).[7] A 10-year follow up revealed that reduced risk of stroke was maintained in patients who had undergone CEA.[8] The Veterans Administration Cooperative Trial was halted after 1 year because of the announcement of the results of the NASCET trial. The rates of stroke and transient ischemic attacks were lower in CEA patients (7.7 percent vs. 19.4 percent). Although not sufficiently powered, the trial supported the results of NASCET and ECST for symptomatic patients. A meta-analysis of the trials supported the efficacy of CEA for 70 to 99 percent symptomatic stenosis.[9] In patients with 50 to 69 percent symptomatic stenosis, the 5-year rate of ipsilateral stroke was 15.7 percent for CEA and 22.2 percent for medical therapy. In patients with <50 percent symptomatic stenosis, there was a nonsignificant difference that favored CEA at 5 years (14.9 percent vs. 18.7 percent).[10]

There have also been randomized trials assessing CEA in patients with asymptomatic extracranial internal carotid artery stenosis. The Mayo Asymptomatic Carotid Endarterectomy (MACE) trial was stopped early because of the high rate of myocardial infarctions in the CEA group (22 percent vs. 9 percent). This was attributed to the lack of platelet antiaggregants in the surgical arm of the trial.[11] In the Veterans Affairs Cooperative Study, which included patients with >50 percent asymptomatic stenosis, there was a risk of stroke with CEA at 4 years (9.4 percent vs. 4.7 percent).[12] The Asymptomatic Carotid Atherosclerosis Study (ACAS) randomized patients to medical therapy or CEA and medical therapy. The study was stopped early by the Data Safety and Monitoring Board after 2.7 years of follow up, because of a projected rate of stroke at 5 years that favored CEA (5.1 percent vs. 11 percent).[13] The current recommendation favors CEA in patients aged 40 to 75 years with an asymptomatic carotid stenosis of 60 to 99 percent if they have a 5-year life expectancy, and if the surgical stroke and death rate can be kept to <3 percent. Our current decision-making process for patients with carotid disease is outlined in Table 109–1.

The aforementioned studies have also brought to light other patient variables when it comes to CEA. Women with 50 to 69 percent symptomatic stenosis did not show a clear benefit from CEA in any of the trials. CEA also provided a greater benefit in those patients with hemispheric strokes or transient ischemic attacks as compared to retinal ischemic events. Patients with contralateral carotid occlusion deserve special attention. Asymptomatic patients with contralateral occlusion derived a much smaller benefit from CEA than those who were symptomatic. Timing of CEA is also important. Those who have a CEA performed within 2 weeks of their transient ischemic attack or mild stroke derive the greatest benefit.[10]

Arteriography, the *gold standard* of preoperative imaging of carotid disease, is used less in an effort to reduce both the risk and cost of the overall procedure. The ACAS and NASCET had 1.2 percent and 0.7 percent morbidity rates, respectively, from carotid angiography. Several studies have touted the benefits of CEA without angiography.[14,15] The consensus of opinion is that, with a dedicated, certified vascular laboratory, most patients (perhaps as many as 90 percent) can be safely evaluated with duplex ultrasound only. Indications suggesting the need for angiography include the following:

- Uncertainty about the accuracy or reliability of the vascular laboratory
- Uncertainty about possible complete occlusion of the internal carotid artery in a patient with ongoing localizing symptoms
- Concern about proximal or intrathoracic disease
- Patients with *technically difficult* studies caused by variant arterial anatomy
- Patients with symptoms and an indeterminate study

CT angiograms have been improving in their ability to accurately and descriptively describe extracranial carotid pathology, and may be a better option than angiograms for most patients in the future. There is currently no consensus of opinion on the usefulness of magnetic resonance angiograms for diagnosing carotid occlusive disease.

The operation is performed under general, cervical block, or local anesthesia. Although general anesthesia has the advantage of improved airway control and patient comfort, it does require the use of routine or selective shunting (Fig. 109–1). Selective shunting re-

TABLE 109–1

Treatment Plan for Patients with Carotid Disease

CATEGORY OF PATIENT	TREATMENT
Patients with Symptomatic Carotic Stenosis	
>80% stenosis of internal carotid artery	CEA indicated
50%–79% stenosis of carotid artery but with vascular laboratory data suggesting closer to 79%	CEA probably indicated; assess risk factors
50%–79% stenosis of carotid artery but with vascular laboratory data suggesting closer to 50%	CEA may be indicated; assess risk factors
<50% stenosis of carotid artery	Trial of medical therapy
Patients with Asymptomatic Carotid Stenosis	
>80% stenosis of carotid artery	CEA indicated
50%–79% stenosis of carotid artery but with vascular laboratory data suggesting closer to 79%	CEA may be indicated; assess risk factors
50%–79% stenosis of carotid artery but with vascular laboratory data suggesting closer to 50%	CEA not indicated
<50% stenosis of carotid artery	CEA not indicated

CEA, carotid endarterectomy.

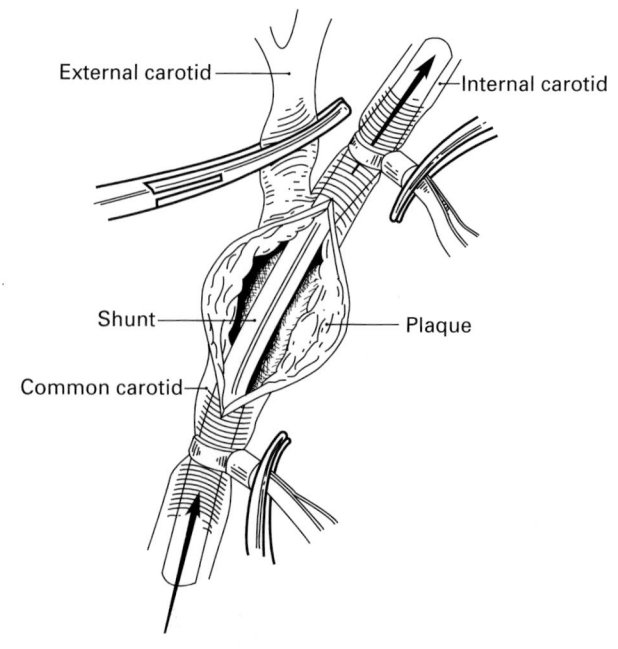

FIGURE 109–1. Indwelling shunt in place to preserve internal carotid flow during the endarterectomy.

quires the use of intraoperative electroencephalography, measurement of internal carotid stump pressures, or transcranial Doppler to assess the need for a shunt. Cervical block anesthesia has also been shown to be well tolerated in experienced hands. Carotid endarterectomy is performed through a vertical incision along the anterior border of the sternocleidomastoid muscle. The endarterectomy is carried out along a smooth plane in the media of the artery. The key to the procedure is to obtain a smooth tapering endpoint into the internal carotid artery. It is also our practice to patch the carotid after endarterectomy. In the past, indications for use of the patch were female gender and recurrent stenoses and the necessity for reoperation. Two reports that have been influential are the work of Moore and colleagues reporting on the results of the ACAS study[16] and the work of AbuRahma reporting on a prospective, randomized trial of primary closure versus patching.[17] In the former study, the authors were able to show an overall incidence of recurrent carotid stenosis of 4.5 percent in patients who underwent patch angioplasty, compared with 16.9 percent in patients undergoing primary arterial repair. The second report looked at 74 patients undergoing bilateral CEAs with primary closure on one side and patch angioplasty on the other. Not only did patch angioplasty have a lower incidence of recurrent stenosis (1 percent vs. 22 percent), but the total internal carotid occlusion rate was lower as well (0 percent vs. 8 percent with primary closure). Addition of a patch adds only a few minutes to the operation, with no significant change in the perioperative morbidity or mortality rate. It is important to note that autogenous patches have been prone to pseudoaneurysm formation. The use of a synthetic or nonautogenous biologic patch avoids this complication but has the potential (albeit a small one) for infection as it is a foreign body. With the use of a prosthetic patch, we adhere to American Heart Association guidelines[18] and recommend oral antibiotics before dental procedures or other invasive exams such as colonoscopy.

Postoperatively, the patient should be monitored carefully. Frequent neurologic assessment is essential. Hemodynamic monitoring should focus on maintaining the patient's blood pressure at its preoperative level. The patient should also be watched for development of a neck hematoma. It is our practice to routinely place a drain in the operative site, to minimize hematoma formation and, potentially, subsequent airway compromise.

The treatment of carotid artery disease represents a benchmark for many other common vascular problems. The economic milieu made a search for more cost-effective and efficient care a necessity, and the authors have responded by diminishing invasive preoperative testing and markedly shortening hospital stay, both of which were accomplished without sacrifice of quality of care.

UPPER AND LOWER EXTREMITY REVASCULARIZATION

【 】 UPPER EXTREMITY REVASCULARIZATION

Compared with lower extremity ischemia, symptomatic vascular diseases involving the upper extremity are uncommon. In the upper extremity, temperature and color changes of the digits are more common than complaints of tiredness (or claudication). Posterior circulation insufficiency of the brain may also present as a symptom caused by subclavian steal syndrome. Although atherosclerosis ac-

counts for much of lower extremity arterial disease, upper-limb ischemia can result from multiple causes. Diagnosis of the location of the occlusive disease is based on blood pressure measurements, pulse palpation, Allen test, and thoracic outlet maneuvers. Segmental blood pressure measurements of the extremity allow detection of obstruction in large arteries. Digital Doppler measurements or plethysmographic recordings) are better for small arteries. Angiography is required in most cases for definitive diagnosis. Arterial occlusive disease of the aortic arch vessels may be caused by atherosclerosis, inflammatory arteritis, or trauma. Most surgeons prefer extrathoracic procedures to intrathoracic endarterectomy or bypass procedures, unless there is occlusive disease in two or more major vessels.

Surgical reconstruction depends on the location of the disease. Innominate lesions require endarterectomy, bypass from the aorta to one of the great vessels, or axilloaxillary bypass. Common carotid lesions can also be treated with a subclavian-carotid bypass. Atherosclerotic occlusive disease of the subclavian artery is the most common lesion involving the proximal branches of the aortic arch. When the ipsilateral common carotid artery is patent and has minimal or no disease, it is frequently chosen as the site of arterial inflow. Subclavian lesions can be operatively repaired with a carotid-subclavian bypass or subclavian-carotid transposition. Patency rates in excess of 90 percent after 5 years have been demonstrated for these procedures.[19] Endovascular therapy has been applied successfully to treatment of many of these lesions. Its long-term durability and efficacy have yet to be fully elucidated; but in patients who are at high risk for a traditional vascular procedure, endoluminal angioplasty and stenting of these arteries may be preferable.

Arterial occlusive disease involving the axillary, brachial, radial, or ulnar arteries most commonly involves emboli, trauma, and iatrogenic injury. Though brachial or axillary artery occlusion following catheterization may present with minimal symptoms early on (because of collateral flow around joints), late symptoms are present in up to 45 percent of patients. Furthermore, because the operative procedure is generally straightforward, early repair is advocated. Hematomas along the course of the brachial or axillary artery require prompt decompression to prevent neurologic sequelae from pressure within the neurovascular sheath. Embolic occlusion of the brachial or axillary artery can be treated by embolectomy through the brachial artery just above the antecubital fossa. Chronic upper extremity arterial occlusions are bypassed with saphenous vein if the patient's symptoms are severe. Distal occlusive lesions tend to predominate in the arteries of the wrist and hand. Collagen vascular diseases can manifest as chronic symptoms ranging from Raynaud phenomenon to digital gangrene. Buerger disease and calciphylaxis can also manifest with distal upper extremity arterial occlusive disease. Unilateral causes of distal arterial occlusion include vibration white finger, hypothenar hammer syndrome, catheter injury, dialysis access steal, and accidental arterial drug injection.[20]

【 】 LOWER EXTREMITY REVASCULARIZATION

Claudication (derived from the Latin word claudication, meaning *to limp*) is defined classically as reproducible muscular discomfort brought on by exercise and relieved by rest. It occurs because of an increased demand for blood flow by the muscles that the diseased vasculature cannot supply. A nonoperative approach to patients with claudication is generally appropriate. Because the symptom of claudication is an ominous predictor of widespread vascular disease, risk-factor modification is the first step in the treatment of such patients.[21] Cigarette smoking, diabetes, hyperlipidemia, hyperhomocysteinemia, elevated C-reactive protein, and hypertension are factors that influence the progression of disease in these patients. Cigarette smoking is two to three times more likely to cause lower extremity peripheral arterial disease (PAD) than coronary artery disease.[22] The presence of diabetes mellitus increases the risk of PAD two to four times and it increases the risk of claudication 3.5 times in men and 8.6 times in women. Diabetic patients with lower extremity PAD are 7- to 15-fold more likely to undergo a major amputation than nondiabetics with lower extremity PAD.[23] The risk of developing lower extremity PAD increases by approximately 5 to 10 percent for each 10 mg/dL rise in total cholesterol.[24] Hyperhomocysteinemia also increases the risk of progression of PAD.[25,26] The Physician's Health Study noted that C-reactive protein levels were higher in individuals who subsequently developed lower extremity PAD and highest in those who ultimately required vascular surgery.[27] Although hypertension is associated with lower extremity PAD, its relationship is generally weaker than that with cerebrovascular and coronary artery disease. In the Framingham Heart Study, hypertension increased the risk of intermittent claudication 2.5- to 4-fold in men and women, respectively. The risk was proportional to the severity of high blood pressure.[28]

After control of risk factors, an exercise program is the next part of the effective treatment of the claudicant. Supervised exercise training should be performed for a minimum of 30 to 45 minutes, in sessions performed at least three times per week for a minimum of 12 weeks. Patients who stop smoking and take part in a regular exercise program have an approximate 70 percent likelihood of improvement in their walking distance. The next step is often pharmacologic therapy. Cilostazol (100 mg orally two times a day) is indicated as an effective therapy (in the absence of heart failure) to improve symptoms and increase walking distance in patients with intermittent claudication.[29]

Revascularization, whether endovascular or surgical, may be considered if the disease produces a serious impairment of activities important to the patient. Absence of another disease that would limit exercise even if the claudication was improved should be documented.[30] Younger patients fare worse with invasive therapy. They may have a more virulent form of atherosclerosis, resulting in a poorer response, and may require graft revisions or replacements.[31]

Initial revascularization strategies increasingly rely on endovascular techniques, with surgical intervention reserved for individuals whose arterial anatomy is unfavorable for endovascular procedures. In patients with combined inflow and outflow disease, inflow problems are corrected first. An improvement in inflow may diminish symptoms; and if distal revascularization is needed, reduce the likelihood of distal graft thrombosis from low flow. There are several patterns of aortoiliac occlusive disease and procedures for surgical repair (Table 109–2). Aortoiliac endarterectomy offers excellent long-term results for focal occlusive disease limited to the distal aorta and common iliac arteries. It is contraindicated in the presence of aneurysmal disease, aortic occlusion to the level of the renal arteries, or any significant occlusive disease in the external iliac or

TABLE 109–2

Operative Procedures for Improvement of Vascular Inflow

PROCEDURE	OPERATIVE MORTALITY (%)	5-YEAR PATENCY RATE (%)
Aortobifemoral bypass	3	88
Aortoiliac or aortofemoral bypass	1–2	90
Iliac endarterectomy	0.5	85
Femorofemoral bypass	6	71
Axillofemoral bypass	6	65
Axillofemoral-femoral bypass	5	60

femoral arteries. The 5- and 10-year patency rates are 95 percent and 85 percent, respectively. However, such focal aortoiliac disease is treated, currently, in most patients by percutaneous angioplasty and stenting. When proximal bypass is needed, aortofemoral bypass grafts are preferred to aortoiliac bypass grafts because the external iliac artery is often severely diseased. In patients with unilateral iliac disease, unilateral aortoiliac or aortofemoral bypass may be performed through a retroperitoneal approach to avoid the morbidity of a transabdominal approach. The most common approach to unilateral iliac disease, however, is the femoral-to-femoral bypass with an anticipated 71 percent patency at 5 years.

There are multiple options to improve outflow in claudicants (Table 109–3). The superficial femoral artery and proximal popliteal artery are the most common sites of stenosis or occlusion

TABLE 109–3

Operative Procedures for Improvement of Vascular Outflow

PROCEDURE	OPERATIVE MORTALITY (%)	5-YEAR PATENCY RATE (%)
Fem-AK popliteal vein	1–6	80
Fem-AK popliteal prosthetic	1–6	75
Fem-BK popliteal vein	1–6	66
Fem-BK popliteal prosthetic	1–6	56
Fem-Tib vein	1–6	74–80
Fem-Tib prosthetic	1–6	25 (at 3 years)
Composite sequential bypass	0–4	28–40
Fem-Tib blind segment bypass	2–3	64–67 (at 2 years)
Profundaplasty	0–3	50 (at 3 years)

Fem-AK, femoral, above knee; Fem-BK, femoral, below knee; Fem-Tib, femoral, tibial.

in patients with intermittent claudication. The most commonly performed operative bypass for the treatment of claudication is the femoral-popliteal artery bypass. Nearly every study that has compared vein with prosthetic conduit for arterial reconstruction of the lower extremity has demonstrated the superiority of vein. Bypass with prosthesis should rarely be necessary for the treatment of mild intermittent claudication because of the increased risk of amputation associated with failure of such grafts.

Critical limb ischemia implies an acute or chronic process that, if left untreated, may result in amputation. Prompt recognition of the signs of threatened limb loss and prompt initiation of therapy are necessary. These patients often present with rest pain, nonhealing ulcers, and/or gangrene. Although patients with claudication are often managed in a conservative or nonoperative manner,[32] patients with critical limb ischemia are evaluated for a potential operation. If the patient is ambulatory and has a reasonable operative risk (dependent on cardiac, pulmonary, and renal factors), a revascularization procedure is offered. Arteriography remains the definitive method to delineate the exact level of arterial occlusion and to define vascular anatomy before selecting an intervention. For individuals with combined inflow and outflow disease with critical limb ischemia, inflow lesions should be addressed first. If symptoms persist, an outflow procedure is warranted. Also, if infection, ischemic ulcers, or gangrenous ulcers are present, an outflow procedure that bypasses all major stenoses and occlusions should be considered. Although the greater saphenous vein is preferred as a conduit for bypass (Fig. 109–2), there are a number of alternatives. Besides prosthetic bypasses, arm and lesser saphenous vein grafts, composite sequential bypass using a vein sewn to a prosthetic graft, use of an anastomotic vein patch, umbilical vein grafts, distal venous arterialization, and cryopreserved vein allografts are all options when adequate greater saphenous vein is unavailable. Currently, there is an emphasis on detecting failing grafts before they occlude. Periodic re-evaluation (3–6 months) should focus on any recurrent symptoms and objective signs of a failing graft. These signs include a 0.15 fall in the ankle-brachial index. Important duplex ultrasound predictors of graft failure include a decrease in peak systolic flow velocity to less than 45 cm/s in the graft plus an increased peak systolic velocity across a stenotic area (two to three times the normal graft velocity). Catheter-based treatment of patients with acute limb ischemia of <14 days duration has been used successfully as a treatment to recanalize acutely occluded arteries.[33,34] A meta-analysis comparing lysis and surgery, that included randomized trials and case series, concluded that lysis improved 30-day and 6- to 12-month limb salvage and reduced mortality compared with surgery.[35] Finally, patients who have significant necrosis of the weight-bearing portions of the foot (in ambulatory patients), an uncorrectable flexion contracture, paresis of the extremity, refractory ischemic rest pain, sepsis, or a very limited life expectancy caused by comorbid conditions should be evaluated for primary amputation of the leg.

It is important to remember that atherosclerosis is a systemic disease. Patients with peripheral vascular disease have a shortened lifespan, primarily because of death from coronary artery disease. Those with severe symptomatic peripheral arterial disease are up to 15 times more likely to die from a cardiovascular cause than healthy, age-matched controls.[36] A concentrated effort should be made toward risk factor reduction in an effort to decrease cardiovascular mortality in these patients.

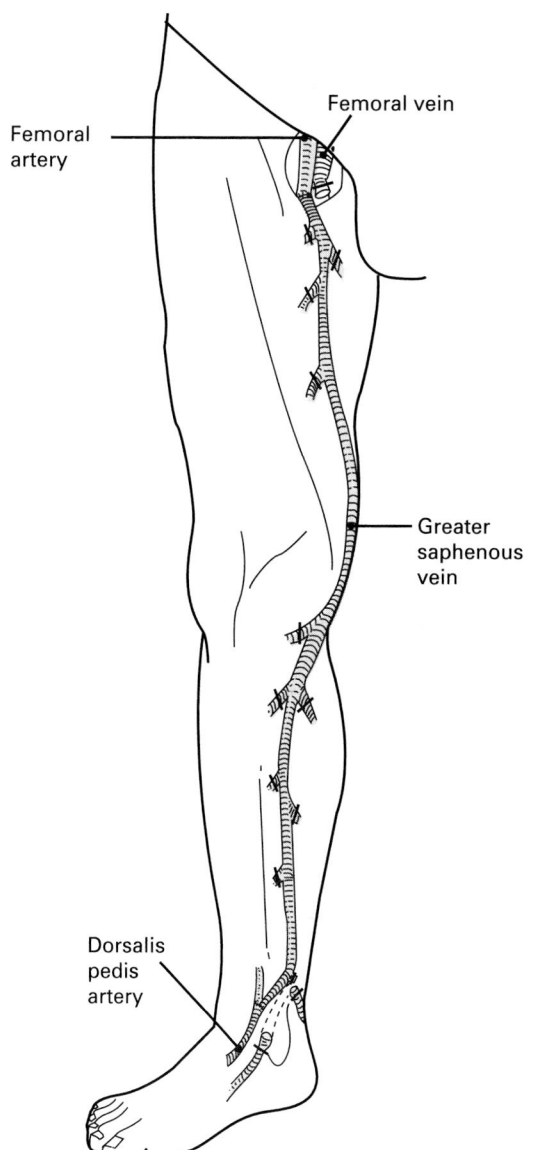

FIGURE 109–2. In situ bypass from common femoral artery to dorsalis pedis artery.

UPPER AND LOWER EXTREMITY VENOUS THROMBOSIS

【 】 UPPER EXTREMITY VENOUS THROMBOSIS

In the past deep venous thrombosis (DVT) of the upper extremity was considered a rare event with a relatively benign outcome. However, a report by Prandoni and coworkers evaluated 58 patients suspected of having upper extremity DVT,[37] 27 (47 percent) of whom had thrombosis. Central venous catheters, *thrombophilic states,* and previous lower extremity thromboses were all associated with the development of upper extremity thrombosis. Of 22 patients who underwent either perfusion lung scanning or pulmonary angiography, 8 (36 percent) were found to have *high probability* for a pulmonary embolus (PE).

Patients with primary subclavian-axillary vein thrombosis present with swelling (100 percent), venous engorgement (82 percent), pain (73 percent), and cyanosis (55 percent).[38] Often referred to as *Paget-*

Schroetter syndrome, effort thrombosis of the subclavian vein is generally seen in healthy young people after repetitive motion or exercise involving the swollen extremity. As many as 10 percent may progress to PE, but only 1 percent will develop venous gangrene. However, fewer than 10 percent of thrombi recanalize spontaneously. The thrombus burden is significantly more than in secondary subclavian-axillary vein thrombosis. The amount of swelling and discomfort is related directly to the amount of arm use (venous claudication), because the symptoms are a result of obstruction and not reflux. Currently, the first step in treatment of primary subclavian-axillary vein thrombosis is catheter-directed thrombolytic therapy followed by surgical decompression of the thoracic outlet. The latter is frequently accomplished by axillary resection of the first rib. Because these patients are often young, they more easily tolerate operative intervention and have more to gain from it over time because of the success and durability of the procedure.

Secondary venous thrombosis is caused mainly by indwelling venous catheters and the onset of signs and symptoms is more gradual and often subtle. A high index of suspicion should come with the realization that most patients with long-term indwelling catheters suffer some degree of thrombosis. Loss of access is a common presentation in these patients. Because of milder symptoms, limited longevity, and reduced activity, most patients are treated conservatively with device removal, anticoagulation therapy, avoidance of excessive use of the involved arm, arm elevation to combat swelling, and the use of an elastic support. Thrombectomy does not succeed as this is a more chronic and inflammatory process. Thrombolysis may succeed initially, but long-term follow up has not shown a sustained benefit.

Venous gangrene is a rare but devastating complication of upper extremity venous thrombosis. Many of these patients may require an amputation with an associated mortality of 33 percent.[39] Although there is no consensus on the optimal treatment of this problem, catheter-directed thrombolysis has been used successfully in the treatment of phlegmasia cerulea dolens.[40] Patients with upper extremity DVT who have contraindications to or unsuccessful use of anticoagulation have been a significant source of concern. Superior vena cava filters are often the only option in this group. Spence and associates[41] showed that superior vena cava filters can be successfully placed without undue difficulty; and in their series of 41 patients, using four different types of filters, no complications or clinical evidence of pulmonary embolism or superior vena cava syndrome were seen. The filter is, of course, inverted in the superior vena cava in comparison to its configuration in the inferior vena cava.

LOWER EXTREMITY VENOUS THROMBOSIS

It has been estimated that there are approximately 600,000 cases of venous thromboembolism in the United States each year.[42,43] Pulmonary embolism, the most serious complication of DVT, accounts for approximately 200,000 deaths per year and 10 percent of hospital deaths.[44] The pathogenesis of DVT was first described by Virchow as caused by the triad of stasis, vascular injury, and hypercoagulability. Risk factors have been detailed in multiple publications and include age older than age 40 years, past history of DVT, general anesthesia, operations, pregnancy, malignant disease, hypercoagulable states, and trauma. Most studies cite inadequate

DVT prophylaxis as a significant factor in DVT and pulmonary embolus. DVT alone can negatively impact patient outcomes and healthcare costs. Patients with multiple segment involvement of their deep veins are among those most commonly hospitalized for treatment. A long-term sequelae of DVT is postthrombotic syndrome, a clinical entity of chronic venous insufficiency. It manifests as edema, hyperpigmentation, and ulceration (Fig. 109–3) and can occur in up to one-third of patients who have had prior DVT.

There have been various treatment strategies used in the management of DVT. Conventional treatment continues to be anticoagulation. Current clinical practice recommends full anticoagulation for a duration of 3 to 6 months to a lifetime, often depending on risk of recurrence or the presence of hypercoagulable states.[45] Anticoagulation, however, only prevents clot propagation, and relies on the body's fibrinolytic system to dissolve the thrombus. In light of the morbidity of postthrombotic syndrome more aggressive treatment has been proposed. Recent reports of poor results with surgical thrombectomy have quelled much of the enthusiasm for this procedure.[46] Comerota and Aldridge reviewed 13 studies comparing thrombolysis versus anticoagulation and confirmed that thrombolysis rapidly clears thrombus from obstructed veins and reduces the chance of subsequent obstruction and reflux.[47] Multiple investigators have found that catheter-directed thrombolysis is more effective than a systemic infusion for treatment of DVT.[48] A review by Baldwin and colleagues found that catheter-directed thrombolysis decreased postthrombotic syndrome, improved quality of life, and reduced the incidence of recurrent DVT, with a risk of intracranial hemorrhage of 0.2 percent.[49]

DVT can also present as thrombosis in calf veins or superficial veins of the extremity. Although these patients are often viewed as having benign problems, more recent data suggest that this may be a false assumption. In one study investigators showed that 24 (32 percent) of 75 patients with lower extremity calf vein thrombi had propagation of their thrombi, and 11 of those 24 (46 percent) had progression into the popliteal or larger veins of the thigh.[50] Numerous reports of patients with superficial thrombophlebitis have documented a high incidence of associated hypercoagulability,

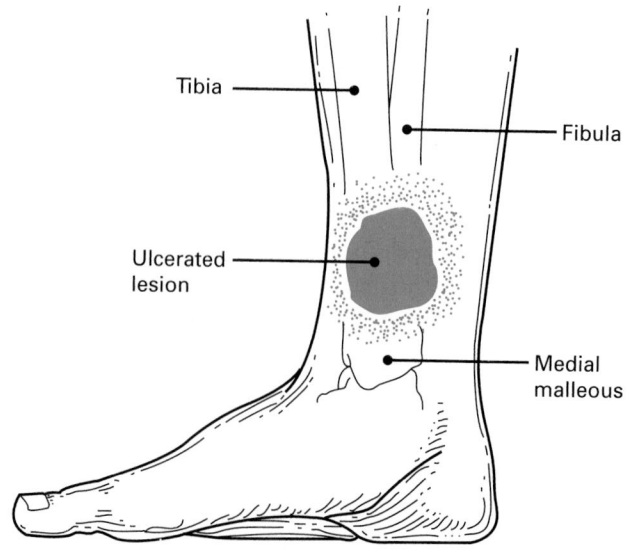

FIGURE 109–3. Venous stasis ulceration on the medial malleolus after an episode of deep venous thrombosis.

propagation into the common femoral vein, and an unexpectedly high incidence of pulmonary embolism.[51]

We have followed such patients closely, particularly those with thigh vein superficial thrombosis, with periodic duplex exams. Extension to the saphenofemoral junction (or within 2 cm) is an indication for anticoagulation or disconnection and ligation of the greater saphenous vein at its junction with the common femoral vein. In patients with DVT, the placement of a vena cava filter prevents subsequent pulmonary emboli in >90 percent of patients. Although the Greenfield filter has been the primary choice in recent years, there are now a variety of percutaneously placed devices available. Operative caval clipping or ligation is rarely performed. Our practice is to perform an inferior venacavogram to delineate the level of the renal veins and to allow safe deployment below them (usually at the L2–L3 level). If anticoagulation can be continued, it appears to reduce the risk of postthrombotic syndrome as compared to patients who have anticoagulation discontinued after filter placement.[52]

SUMMARY

The management of vascular disease has undergone a significant change since the beginning of the new millennium. Improvements in endovascular techniques and technology are at the forefront of new developments. Surgery continues to be the gold standard in all arterial segments with which endovascular therapy must be compared. Nevertheless, endovascular therapies have, at the least, provided options for patients who may not be candidates for surgery. These minimally invasive procedures may establish themselves as a step between medical management and surgical intervention in the algorithm of many vascular diseases. Prospective, randomized trials will bear out the efficacy, role, and durability of both open and endovascular procedures in the near future.

REFERENCES

1. Thom T, Haase N, Rosamond W, et al. Heart disease and stroke statistics-2006 update: a report from the American Heart Association statistics committee and stroke statistics subcommittee. *Circulation* 2006;113:85.
2. Samsa GP, Matchar DB, Goldstein L, et al. Utilities for major stroke: results from a survey of preferences among persons at increased risk for stroke. *Am Heart J* 1998;136:703.
3. Gresham GE, Fitzpatrick TE, Wolf PA, et al. Residual disability in survivors of stroke the Framingham study. *N Engl J Med* 1975;293:954.
4. Eastcott H, Pickering G, Rob C. Reconstruction of internal carotid artery. *Lancet* 1954;1:994.
5. North American Symptomatic Carotid Endarterectomy Trial. Methods, patient characteristics, and progress. *Stroke* 1991;22(6):711.
6. Barnett HJ, Taylor DW, Eliasziw M, et al. Benefit of carotid endarterectomy in patients with symptomatic moderate or severe stenosis. North American Symptomatic Carotid Endarterectomy Trial Collaborators. *N Engl J Med* 1998;339(20):1415.
7. European Carotid Surgery Trialists' Collaborative Group. MRC European Carotid Surgery Trial: interim results for symptomatic patients with severe (70–99%) or with mild (0–29%) carotid stenosis. *Lancet* 1991;337:1235.
8. Cunningham EJ, Bond R, Mehta Z, et al. Long-term durability of carotid endarterectomy for symptomatic stenosis and risk factors for late postoperative stroke. *Stroke* 2002;33:2658.
9. Goldstein LB, Hasselblad V, Matchar DB, et al. Comparison and meta-analysis of randomized trials of endarterectomy for symptomatic carotid artery stenosis. *Neurology* 1995;45:1965.

10. Chaturvedi S, Bruno A, Feasby T, et al. Carotid endarterectomy—an evidence-based review. Report of the therapeutics and technology assessment subcommittee of the American Academy of Neurology. *Neurology* 2006;65:794.
11. Mayo Asymptomatic Carotid Endarterectomy Study Group. Results of a randomized controlled trial of carotid endarterectomy for asymptomatic carotid stenosis. *Mayo Clin Proc* 1992;67:513.
12. Hobson RW, Weiss DG, Fields WS, et al. Efficacy of carotid endarterectomy for asymptomatic carotid stenosis. *N Engl J Med* 1993;328:221.
13. Executive Committee for the Asymptomatic Carotid Atherosclerosis Study. Endarterectomy for asymptomatic carotid stenosis. *JAMA* 1995;273:1421.
14. Ballotta E, Da Giau G, Abbruzzese E, et al. Carotid endarterectomy without angiography: Can clinical evaluation and duplex ultrasound scanning alone replace traditional arteriography for carotid surgery workup? *Surgery* 1999;126:20.
15. Collier PE. Changing trends in the use of preoperative carotid arteriography: the community experience. *Cardiovasc Surg* 1998;6:485.
16. Moore WS, Kempczinski RF, Nelson JJ, et al. Recurrent carotid stenosis: results of the asymptomatic carotid atherosclerosis study. *Stroke* 1998;29:2018.
17. AbuRahma AF, Robinson PA, Saiedy S, et al. Prospective randomized trial of bilateral carotid endarterectomies: primary closure versus patching. *Stroke* 1999;30:1185.
18. Committee on Rheumatic Fever, Endocarditis, and Kawasaki Disease. Prevention of bacterial endocarditis: recommendations by the American Heart Association. *JAMA* 1997;277:1794.
19. Berguer R, Morasch MD, Kline RA, et al. Cervical reconstruction of the supra-aortic trunks: a 16-year experience. *J Vasc Surg* 1999;29:239.
20. Johnston KW. Upper extremity ischemia, in Rutherford RB. *Vascular Surgery.* 5th ed. Philadelphia: W.B. Saunders; 2000:1111.
21. Rehring TF, Sandhoff BG, Stolcpart RS, et al. Atherosclerotic risk factor control in patients with peripheral arterial disease. *J Vasc Surg* 2005;41:816.
22. Price JF, Mowbray PI, Lee AJ, et al. Relationship between smoking and cardiovascular risk factors in the development of peripheral arterial disease and coronary artery disease. Edinburgh Artery Study. *Eur Heart J* 1999;20:344.
23. McDaniel MD, Cronenwett JL. Basic data related to the natural history of intermittent claudication. *Ann Vasc Surg* 1989;3:273.
24. Murabito JM, D'Agostino RB, Silbershatz H, et al. Intermittent claudication: a risk profile from the Framingham Heart Study. *Circulation* 1997;96:44.
25. Robinson K, Arheart K, Refsum H, et al. Low circulating folate and vitamin B_6 concentrations: risk factors for stroke, peripheral vascular disease, and coronary artery disease. European COMAC Group. *Circulation* 1998;97:437.
26. Taylor LM Jr, DeFrang RD, Harris EJ Jr, et al. The association of elevated plasma homocysteine with progression of symptomatic peripheral arterial disease. *J Vasc Surg* 1991;13:128.
27. Ridker PM, Cushman M, Stampfer MJ, et al. Plasma concentrations of C-reactive protein and risk of developing peripheral vascular disease. *Circulation* 1998;97:425.
28. Kannel WB, McGee DL. Update on some epidemiologic features of intermittent claudication: the Framingham Study. *J Am Geriatr Soc* 1985;33:13.
29. Regensteiner JG, Ware JE Jr, McCarthy WJ, et al. Effect of cilostazol on treadmill walking, community-based walking ability, and health-related quality of life in patients with intermittent claudication due to peripheral arterial disease: meta-analysis of six randomized controlled trials. *J Am Geriatr Soc* 2002;50:1939.
30. Dormandy JA, Rutherford RB. Management of peripheral arterial disease (PAD). TASC Working Group. TransAtlantic Intersociety Consensus (TASC). *J Vasc Surg* 31:S1, 2000.
31. Reed AB, Conte MS, Donaldson MC, et al. The impact of patient age and aortic size on the results of aortobifemoral bypass grafting. *J Vasc Surg* 2003;37:1219.
32. Dormandy J, Heeck L, Vig S. The natural history of claudication: risk to life and limb. *Semin Vasc Surg* 1999;12:123.
33. Tefera G, Hoch J, Turnipseed WD. Limb-salvage angioplasty in vascular surgery practice. *J Vasc Surg* 2005;41:988.
34. BASIL Trial Participants. Bypass versus angioplasty in severe ischaemia of the leg (BASIL): multicentre, randomized controlled trial. *Lancet* 2005;366:1925.
35. Diffin DC, Kandarpa K. Assessment of peripheral intraarterial thrombolysis versus surgical revascularization in acute lower-limb ischemia: a review of limb-salvage and mortality statistics. *J Vasc Interv Radiol* 1996;7:57.
36. Kinikini D, Sarfati MR, Mueller MT, et al. Meeting AHA/ACC secondary prevention goals in a vascular surgery practice: an opportunity we cannot afford to miss. *J Vasc Surg* 2006;43:781.

⟪2396⟫ PART 16 • Diseases of the Great Vessels and Peripheral Vessels

37. Prandoni P, Polistena P, Bernardi E, et al. Upper-extremity deep vein thrombosis: risk factors, diagnosis, and complications. *Arch Intern Med* 1997;157:57.

38. Hulbert SN, Rutherford RB. Primary subclavian-axillary vein thrombosis. *Ann Vasc Surg.* 1995;9:217.

39. Smith BM, Shield GW, Riddell DH, et al. Venous gangrene of the upper extremity. *Ann Surg* 1985;201:511.

40. Patel NH, Plorde JJ, Meissner M. Catheter-directed thrombolysis in the treatment of phlegmasia cerulea dolens. *Ann Vasc Surg* 1998;12:471.

41. Spence LD, Gironta MG, Malde HM, et al. Acute upper extremity deep venous thrombosis: safety and effectiveness of superior vena caval filters. *Radiology* 1999;210:53.

42. Weinmann EE, Salzman EW. DVT Deep-vein thrombosis. *N Engl J Med* 1994;331:1630.

43. Kyrle PA, Eichinger S. Deep vein thrombosis. *Lancet* 2005;365:1163.

44. Kim V, Spandorfor J. Epidemiology of venous thromboembolic disease. *Emerg Med Clin North Am* 2001;19:839.

45. Bates SM, Ginsberg JS. Clinical practice: treatment of deep-vein thrombosis. *N Engl J Med* 2004;351:268.

46. Augustinos P, Ouriel K. Invasive approaches to treatment of venous thromboembolism. *Circulation* 2004;110:127.

47. Comerota AJ, Aldridge SC. Thrombolytic therapy for deep venous thrombosis: a clinical review. *Can J Surg* 1993;36:359.

48. Watson LI, Armon MP. Thrombolysis for acute deep vein thrombosis. *Cochrane Database Syst Rev* 2004;CD002783.

49. Baldwin CK, Comerota AJ, Schwartz LB. Catheter-directed thrombolysis for deep venous thrombosis. *Vasc Endovascular Surg* 2004;38:1.

50. Lohr JM, Kerr TM, Lutter KS, et al. Lower extremity calf thrombosis: to treat or not to treat? *J Vasc Surg* 1991;14:618.

51. Verlato F, Zucchetta P, Prandoni P, et al. An unexpectedly high rate of pulmonary embolism in patients with superficial thrombophlebitis of the thigh. *J Vasc Surg* 1999;30:1113.

52. Wakefield TW. Treatment options for venous thrombosis. *J Vasc Surg* 2000;31:613.

CHAPTER (110)

Advances in the Minimally Invasive Treatment of Peripheral Vascular Disease

Joaquin Solis / Anjan Gupta / Tanvir K. Bajwa

INTRODUCTION

In the past 25 years, significant advances in endovascular treatment for peripheral vascular disease (PVD) have given doctors and their patients minimally invasive alternatives to major surgical procedures that carry significant morbidity and mortality. This chapter reviews current advances and explores the benefits and limitations in minimally invasive therapies for the treatment of occlusive and aneurysmal disease of the aorta and peripheral vessels.

Endovascular treatment of PVD with balloon catheters was first reported by Fogarty and coworkers in 1963.[1] The next year, Dotter and Judkins introduced the concept of percutaneous revascularization using coaxial dilating catheters, followed by Grüntzig's pioneering work that led to the evolution of percutaneous transluminal angioplasty (PTA).[2,3]

Since then, dramatic advances in balloon and guide wire technology have made it possible to cross difficult lesions and chronic occlusions. Better-designed stents have revolutionized endovascular interventions, providing an attractive, reliable alternative to vascular surgery to the point that endovascular stents are now the standard of care in peripheral vascular interventions. Marked improvement in immediate and long-term results with stent grafts now permit minimally invasive treatment of aneurysmal disease of the aorta as well as other major vascular areas. Improvements in pharmacologic agents and in catheter-based thrombectomy devices have made endovascular interventions the first-line therapy in patients who have acute limb ischemia (ALI) caused by thromboembolic disease.

OCCLUSIVE DISEASE OF AORTIC ARCH VESSELS
【 】 SUBCLAVIAN ARTERY STENTING

Although occlusive disease of the subclavian artery is most often asymptomatic, when it is symptomatic, patients may present with subclavian-steal syndrome; upper extremity claudication; or, in patients who have an internal mammary artery bypass graft, subclavian-coronary-steal syndrome.

Surgical treatment of subclavian artery stenosis (SAS) is effective; but, among other complications, it carries a mortality rate of approximately 2 percent and a stroke rate of approximately 3 percent.[4]

Although initial reports of using PTA alone showed mixed results with high restenosis rates, recent reports on subclavian artery stenting indicate high procedural success (92–100 percent) with good long-term patency (90–100 percent).[5–8]

The largest source of data is the report of a multicenter registry[8] that evaluated the results of subclavian artery stenting in 258 patients whose primary indications for intervention were arm claudication (in 43 percent), subclavian steal syndrome (25 percent), and compromised flow from the internal mammary graft to the coronary artery (24 percent) with 86 percent of the lesions involving the left subclavian artery. Overall, the rate of procedural success was 98.5 percent with a major complication rate of 1 percent. At a mean follow up of 19 ± 15 months, the primary patency rate was 89 percent and secondary patency rate was 98.5 percent. These results suggest that subclavian artery stenting should be considered the primary treatment in patients who need revascularization for SAS. (Fig. 110–1).

[ ] VERTEBROBASILAR ANGIOPLASTY/ STENTING

Patients who have occlusive disease of the vertebrobasilar artery (VBA) are at risk for posterior-circulation ischemia[9] and have an eightfold higher rate of stroke than does the normal population.[10] Surgical options are ostial vertebral endarterectomy, vein patch angioplasty, or reimplantation of the vertebral artery in the subclavian or carotid artery. In the series of 290 treated surgically patients, Berguer[11] reported no deaths; however, there was a relatively high rate of postoperative complications including Horner syndrome (15 percent), recurrent laryngeal nerve palsy (2 percent), lymphocele (4 percent), and immediate thrombosis (1 percent).

When PTA alone has been used to treat patients who have VBA stenosis,[12] vessel recoil and restenosis have resulted in unfavorable long-term results. Recent reports have indicated that stent-supported angioplasty can be performed safely and effectively with low rates of recurrence.[13–17] Jenkins and colleagues[13] reported a procedural success rate of 100 percent after vertebral artery stenting in 32 patients (38 arteries) and no deaths at a mean follow up of 10.6 months. Malek and coworkers[16] also reported high rates for procedural success (95.2 percent) and no adverse events during followup.

These reports suggest that stent-supported percutaneous revascularization can be performed in patients who have VBA stenosis with excellent immediate and long-term results and with very low rates of morbidity and mortality (Fig. 110–2).

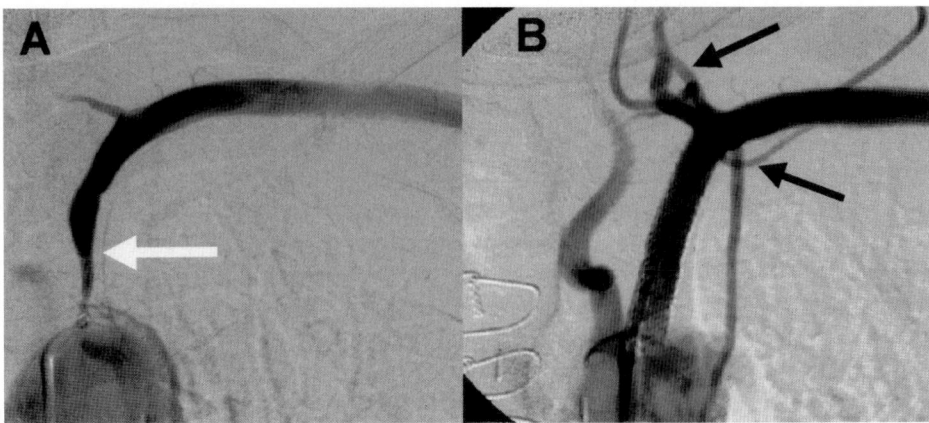

FIGURE 110–1. A 72-year-old female with dizziness and left arm claudication was found by Doppler ultrasound to have reversed flow in the vertebral artery (VA). **A.** Severe left subclavian artery stenosis (*white arrow*) with no antegrade flow in VA. **B.** After stent placement there is antegrade flow in the VA and left internal mammary artery (*black arrows*).

American Heart Association/American Stroke Association Council on Stroke Guidelines: Prevention of Stroke in Patients with Ischemic Stroke or Transient Ischemic Attack[17]

Extracranial vertebrobasilar disease

Class IIB

1. *Endovascular treatment of patients with symptomatic extracranial vertebral stenosis may be considered when patients are having symptoms despite medical therapies (antithrombotics, statins, and other treatments for risk factors) (Evidence Level C).*

OCCLUSIVE DISEASE OF AORTA AND AORTOILIAC BIFURCATION

Patients who have atherosclerotic occlusive disease of the aorta (Fig. 110–3) and the distal aortic bifurcation and proximal iliac arteries can present with lifestyle-limiting claudication, limb-threat-

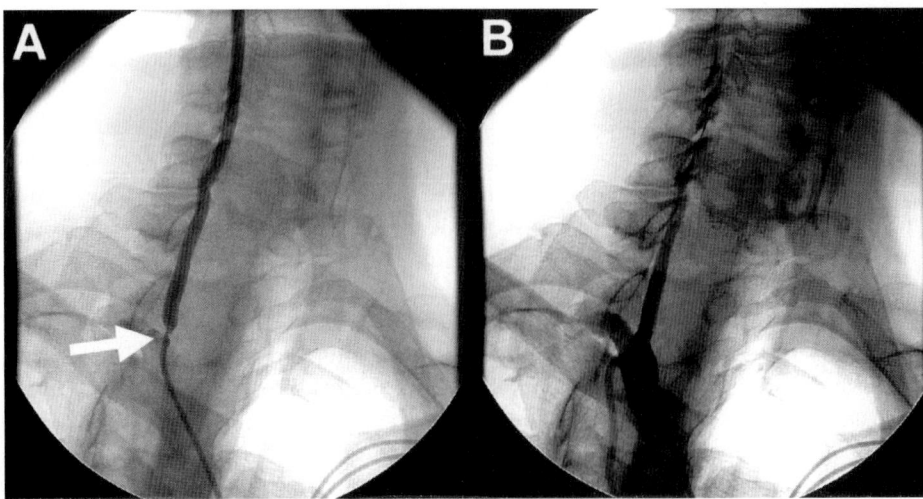

FIGURE 110–2. A 65-year-old male with a history of severe dizziness spells was diagnosed with severe right vertebral artery (VA) stenosis. **A.** Selective angiography of right VA showed a severe ostial lesion (*arrow*). **B.** After percutaneous intervention and stenting.

ening ischemia, or impotence. Traditionally, aortoiliac bifurcation disease has been treated with bypass grafting, which yields an excellent long-term outcome but has been associated with a perioperative mortality rate up to 2 to 4 percent and a rate of major early complications (including sexual dysfunction, ureteral damage, intestinal ischemia, and spinal cord injury) of 5 to 13 percent.[18] PTA of the ostium of the common iliac artery sometimes causes plaque to shift across the aortic bifurcation, producing stenosis in the contralateral iliac artery.[19]

To avoid these complications, the kissing balloon technique was developed (i.e., positioning two balloons across the origins of both iliac arteries and inflating these balloons simultaneously). This technique has good rates of procedural and clinical success, including lower mortality; however, the incidence of significant residual stenosis, dissection, thrombosis, and/or distal embolization can be up to 9 percent.[19,20] These complications can be minimized by using a kissing stent technique (i.e., simultaneous deployment of stents at the aortoiliac bifurcation). Our results and those of others have been excellent, both immediately postprocedure and long term (Fig. 110–4).[21–25] Our rate of procedural success has been 100 percent with rates for primary patency of 92 percent during followup of >18 months and for secondary patency of 100 percent. Although acute complications (distal embolization) occurred in 4 percent, our patients had no vascular complications, myocardial infarctions, or perioperative deaths.

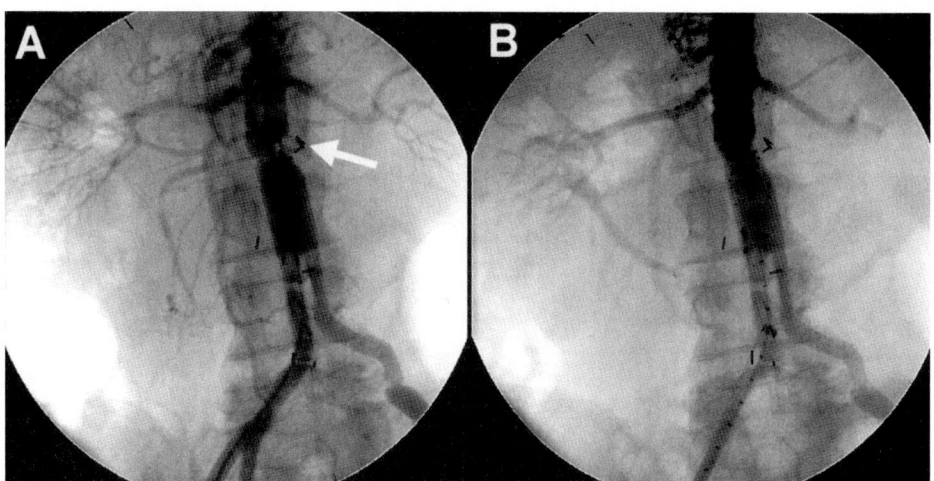

FIGURE 110–3. A 65-year-old female with a history of severe claudication and peripheral vascular disease after surgical bypass. **A.** Selective abdominal aorta angiography showed severe stenosis below the renal artery at site of surgical clamping (*white arrow*) **B.** After balloon and stenting of abdominal aorta with resolution of gradient.

OCCLUSIVE DISEASE OF ILIAC ARTERIES

Iliac arteries are best suited for percutaneous intervention because they are easily accessible and are relatively large vessels, which improves expected immediate technical results and yields excellent postprocedural rates of long-term patency. Aortofemoral bypass, the traditional surgical treatment for iliac occlusive disease, carries a mortality rate of up to 5 percent, an early graft failure rate of 5.7 percent, and a patency rate after 2 years of 92.8 percent.[26]

Indicators for good results from PTA are as follows:

• Focal lesions (< 3 cm)
• Stenosis (vs. occlusion)
• Claudication (vs. critical limb ischemia)
• Noncalcified lesions
• Absence of diabetes mellitus
• Good distal run-off vessels

In patients who fit these criteria, the initial technical success rate can be >90 percent with a 5-year primary patency rate of approximately 80 percent.[27] In those who have longer, calcified lesions or occluded arteries, the success rate may be lower, in which case, intravascular stents have been employed with excellent results.

Several studies have investigated the role of endovascular stents in treating iliac artery occlusive disease.[28–32] In a meta-analysis (14 studies, >2000 patients) of PTA versus PTA plus stenting, Bosch and Hunink concluded that PTA with stent placement lowered the risk of long-term failure by 39 percent compared with PTA alone (Table 110–1).[29]

It is also possible to compare results of a variety of stent designs. Vorwerk and colleagues,[30] using self-expanding Wallstents to treat 109 patients who had iliac artery stenoses after failed PTA, reported a primary patency rate of 82 percent and secondary patency rate of 91 percent at 4 years. In a multicenter study[31] (486 patients) using Palmaz-Schatz balloon expandable stents, the rate of technical success was 99 percent and the rate of clinical patency at 2 years was 84

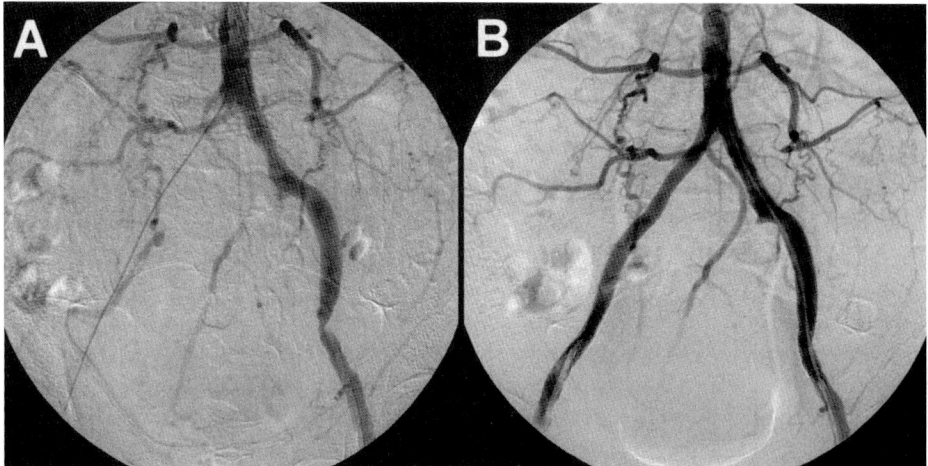

FIGURE 110–4. A 71-year-old male with severe lifestyle limiting claudication. **A.** Angiography showed occluded right common iliac artery and moderate lesion in left common iliac artery and severe lesion in left external iliac artery. **B.** Self-expanding SMART Control stents (Cordis Corp., Minneapolis, MN) deployed with kissing technique followed by postdilatation using kissing balloons.

TABLE 110-1

PTA versus PTA Plus Stenting in Iliac Occlusive Disease:
Results of Meta-analysis of 14 Studies

	PTA		PTA + STENT	
	STENOSIS	OCCLUSION	STENOSIS	OCCLUSION
Immediate technical success (%)	96	80	100	80
Primary patency (%)	65	54	77	61
Secondary patency (%)	80		80	
Major complications (%)	4.3		5.2	

PTA, percutaneous transluminal angioplasty.

percent. Current data indicates that in iliac artery interventions, the choice of stent type makes little difference with regard to technical success rates and follow-up results. Therefore, the choice can be based on such factors as location, extent, and nature of the lesion, as well as on one's experience and familiarity with a specific stent.

Scheinert and coworkers[32] recently evaluated the role of primary stenting after excimer laser-assisted recanalization in 212 patients who had chronically occluded iliac arteries. These authors reported a rate of technical success of 90 percent and a complication rate of 1.4 percent (arterial rupture or embolism) with rates of primary patency of 91 percent at 1 year, 84 percent at 2 years, and 76 percent at 4 years.

Iliac artery PTA/stenting is also used as an adjunct to peripheral vascular surgery. For example, it may help to facilitate the patency of a downstream surgical conduit during surgical revascularization for femoropopliteal disease. In patients who are at high risk for vascular surgery because of concomitant coronary artery disease, it may provide a less invasive femoral femoral bypass compared with a high-risk surgical procedure such as aortobifemoral bypass. Thus, iliac artery PTA/stenting is well supported by current data as the initial choice for treating patients who have iliac occlusive disease for its reduced invasiveness, excellent rates of technical success, and good rates of long-term patency.

OCCLUSIVE DISEASE OF FEMOROPOPLITEAL ARTERIES

Atherosclerotic occlusive disease is 2 to 5 times more frequent in femoropopliteal arteries than in iliac arteries. Patients vary in their clinical presentation from claudication to rest pain and leg ischemia. In addition, acute-onset ischemia is much more frequent than in patients who have iliac artery disease. Although choices for managing iliac artery disease are clear cut, choices for managing disease in the femoropopliteal arteries are not supported by strong evidence either for or against percutaneous intervention (i.e., PTA, atherectomy, laser, stenting, or a combination of these) or peripheral bypass surgery. Although opinions vary over how to treat patients who have claudication, some form of intervention is imperative when pulsatile flow must be restored to prevent limb loss in patients who have rest pain or leg ischemia.

Despite attempted comparisons of angioplasty and peripheral bypass surgery for femoropopliteal arterial disease, controversy remains. Hunink and colleagues[33] compiled a useful analysis of the literature to compare the outcomes of PTA with those of bypass surgery that helps identify patient subgroups that will benefit most from each treatment modality. Despite study limitations, they concluded that successful PTA depends on lesion type (i.e., stenosis vs. occlusion) and on the patient's having good distal runoff vessels. With good distal runoff vessels, the patency rate in stenotic vessels at 5 years was 56 to 63 percent, decreasing to 35 to 48 percent if the treated vessel was occluded or if runoff was poor, and to 19 percent to 22 percent if there were both an occluded vessel and poor runoff.

The BASIL (Bypass versus Angioplasty in Severe Ischemia of the Leg) trial prospectively assigned patients with severe limb ischemia caused by infrainguinal disease to undergo either angioplasty or bypass surgery. At the end of the study there was no difference between the two groups in either the rate of mortality or survival free of the need for amputation. However, in the angioplasty group rates for morbidity and length of hospital stay were significantly lower and total cost was significantly less.[34]

Improved techniques and better-designed balloon catheters and wires, especially the introduction of the hydrophilic/glide wire (Terumo wire) and such devices as the Frontrunner catheter system (LuMend Inc., Redwood City, CA) and the Outback Re-Entry Catheter (LuMend, Inc., Redwood City, CA), have raised the rate of procedural success to 95 to 100 percent for treating stenotic lesions and 70 to 80 percent for occluded lesions.[35-37] Consequently, even though rates of long-term patency are far lower than those in iliac arteries, PTA is increasingly used to treat disease in femoropopliteal arteries.

In their prospective study of PTA in 106 patients who had claudication, Pekka and coworkers[35] achieved a primary success rate of 99 percent for patients who had stenotic lesions and 80 percent for those with occlusions; however, the rate of long-term patency was only 47 percent at 1 year and 43 percent at 3 years. Others reported lower rates of primary success, i.e., 88 percent[36] and 90 percent.[37] It is likely that this wide discrepancy can be attributed to differences in patient population, in lesion characteristics, and in the experience and level of skill of the operator. In light of its challenges, PTA for occluded femoropopliteal arteries is not recommended unless claudication limits a patient's lifestyle or the patient has progressed to critical limb ischemia.

Review of the literature shows that the following indicators adversely affect the degree of patency achieved in treating femoropopliteal arteries with PTA:

• Occlusion (especially >10 cm)
• Calcified vessels
• Multiple-lesion segments
• Rest ischemia (vs. claudication)
• Poor distal runoff

Although in treating iliac artery disease intravascular stenting can be expected to yield excellent rates of long-term patency, its long-term benefits for femoropopliteal lesions are unclear, despite many studies. The small number of patients studied and differences in type of stent used make useful comparison between studies impossible.

In femoropopliteal arteries, use of balloon-expandable stents can no longer be recommended because of high rates of stent deformation from crush injury and because of poor rates of long-term patency. At present, only self-expanding stents and covered stents-grafts (VIABAHN, W.L. Gore & Associates, Inc. Flagstaff, AZ) (Fig. 110–5 and Fig. 110–6) are used for treating occlusive disease in femoropopliteal arteries, but even here one must be cautious, since not all self-expanding stents work equally well. Sapoval and coworkers[38] reported poor results with the use of a Wallstent in femoropopliteal lesions.

Long-term results with nitinol self-expandable stents have been disappointing. Using SMART stents (Cordis Corporation, Miami Lakes, FL) in the superficial femoral artery (SFA), Kazemi and colleagues showed 76 percent primary patency rate and 86 percent rate for primary assisted patency at 11 months.[39] However, during the second year of followup the primary patency rate declined to 60 percent. Similar results have been replicated by other studies. Using nitinol self-expanding stents, Mewissen and coworkers found primary patency rates of 92 percent at 6 months, 76 percent at 12 months, and 60 percent at 24 months.[40]

Because of these results with nitinol stent placement at the femoropopliteal level, the paucity of available data dissuades most investigators from recommending their routine use.[41–43] The consensus is to reserve this for bailout or for suboptimal results of PTA and to avoid stenting lesions in the popliteal artery unless essential for limb salvage. Without a large-scale prospective study, there can be no definitive answer for the best use of stents and the long-term benefits of primary stenting for patients who have femoropopliteal occlusive disease.

Recently, covered stents (VIABAHN) have been approved by the Food and Drug Administration in the treatment of long SFA lesions with a hope of reducing the rate of restenosis and improving long-term patency; however, initial reports have been mixed. When it was assessed in an

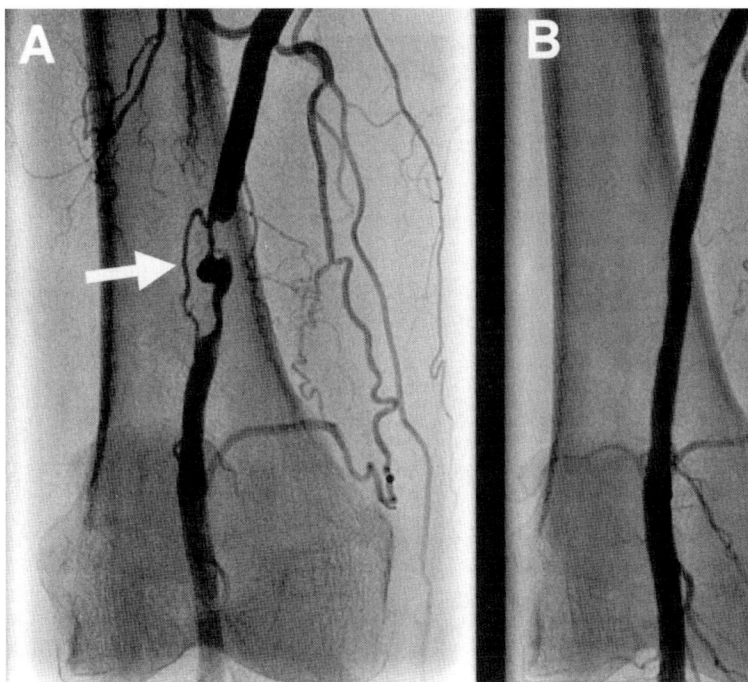

FIGURE 110–5. A 67-year-old female with resting claudication. **A.** Angiography of the right superficial femoral artery showed a subtotally occluded artery (*white arrow*). **B.** After percutaneous intervention with a self-expandable SMART stent (Cordis Corporation, Miami Lakes, FL).

international feasibility trial, the commercially available Hemobahn endoprosthesis (W.L. Gore & Associates, Flagstaff, AZ) was found to yield a 100 percent rate for technical success with a primary patency rate of 90 percent at 6 months and 79 percent at one year.[44]

Kazemi and colleagues followed 27 patients prospectively after VIABAHN stent-graft implantation in the SFA with clinical fol-

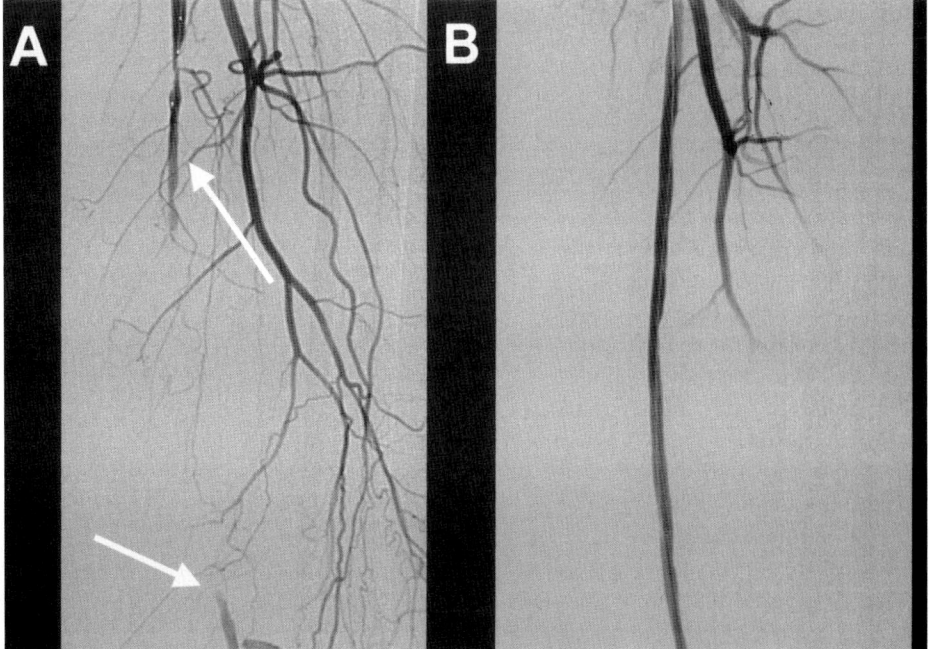

FIGURE 110–6. A 74-year-old male with a history nonhealing ulcer in the left foot. **A.** Angiography showed a 15-cm occlusion of the left superficial femoral artery (*arrows*). **B.** After percutaneous revascularization with VIABAHN stent-graft (W.L. Gore and Associates, Inc., Flagstaff, AZ).

lowup and with Doppler ultrasound scans at 1, 3, 6, and 12 months. The result showed a 100 percent primary patency rate at 6 months and 90 percent primary patency rate at 1 year.[45] If these results can be replicated by large-scale trials, minimally invasive therapy may become the treatment of choice for patients who have femoropopliteal disease.

OCCLUSIVE DISEASE OF INFRAPOPLITEAL ARTERIES

There are three main differences between PVD involving the infrapopliteal arteries and that involving other peripheral arteries:

1. When an iliac artery or SFA is occluded or has critical stenosis, the result may be lifestyle-limiting claudication or limb ischemia, whereas in isolated below-the-knee disease, having only one patent infrapopliteal artery is enough to maintain blood flow and prevent limb ischemia, in spite of disease in other infrapopliteal arteries.

2. In isolated below-the-knee disease, especially in patients with diabetes and renal failure, ankle-brachial indices (ABIs) are unreliable for assessing symptoms or for determining disease severity due to the noncompressibility of these vessels.

3. With infrapopliteal occlusion, the restenosis rate after angioplasty is reportedly as high as 40 to 60 percent, primarily related to diffuse disease and the presence of small-diameter vessels, and, frequently, to long calcified lesions.

The immediate and long-term results of arterial reconstruction for infrapopliteal disease are better in patients who have claudication than in those who have critical limb ischemia (CLI). However, tibial artery bypass surgery has traditionally been reserved for selected patients who have CLI to achieve revascularization distal to infrapopliteal obstructions. Although data have not been encouraging,[46–48] Veith and coworkers used innovative and creative techniques to improve results, dramatically decreasing rates of procedure-related amputation from 49 to 14 percent. Their distal bypass procedures, however, resulted in a coincident 30-day mortality rate of 4 percent and a 90-day graft failure rate of nearly 5 percent. These results led to acceptance of tibial artery bypass surgery as the standard of care, with success defined as clinical improvement with resolution of rest pain. All the same, use of percutaneous intervention is a more attractive alternative when graft patency deteriorates as a result of distal anastomoses to small diseased vessels, diffuse distal arterial occlusive disease produces poor runoff, or grafts have to cross a joint.

New low-profile balloons and new generation wires have greatly improved the success rate of infrapopliteal angioplasty for treating occlusions and stenotic lesions. Of several recent reports concerning angioplasty of tibioperoneal vessels for limb salvage, the largest is by Dorros and colleagues,[49] in which the procedure was technically successful in 92 percent of the tibioperoneal lesions. Rest pain was relieved or blood flow to a lower extremity was improved in 95 percent of the endangered limbs. Clinical 5-year follow up of the successfully revascularized CLI patients documented a limb salvage rate of 91 percent.

In our published study of 97 patients who had lifestyle-limiting claudication or CLI, or both, the success rate was 95 percent, including an 86 percent rate of successful limb salvage.[50] These reports demonstrate that patients who have CLI caused by infrapopliteal disease should be seriously considered for endovascular procedures as an alternative to surgery (Fig. 110–7).

More recently, varying rates of clinical success have been reported with other new devices including directional atherectomy catheters and laser assisted angioplasty. Zeller and coworkers reported successful use of the SilverHawk device in below-knee arteries. Their procedural success rate was 98 percent with significant improvement in ABIs postprocedure. The 6-month cumulative patency rate was 98 percent.[51] Laird and colleagues reported use of laser assisted angioplasty in 145 patients with 155 critically ischemic limbs. Procedural success was seen in 86 percent of the patients with limb salvage achieved in 92 percent of the patients.[52] However, the validity of this data remains controversial because of lack of randomized trials and long-term follow up.

In our view, endovascular intervention for below-the-knee disease should be considered only in patients with rest pain, limb threatening ischemia, or a nonhealing leg ulcer caused by arterial occlusive disease.

Endovascular Treatment of Claudication: Current American College of Cardiology/American Heart Association Practice Guidelines[53]

Class I

1. *Endovascular procedures are indicated for individuals with a vocational or lifestyle-limiting disability caused by*

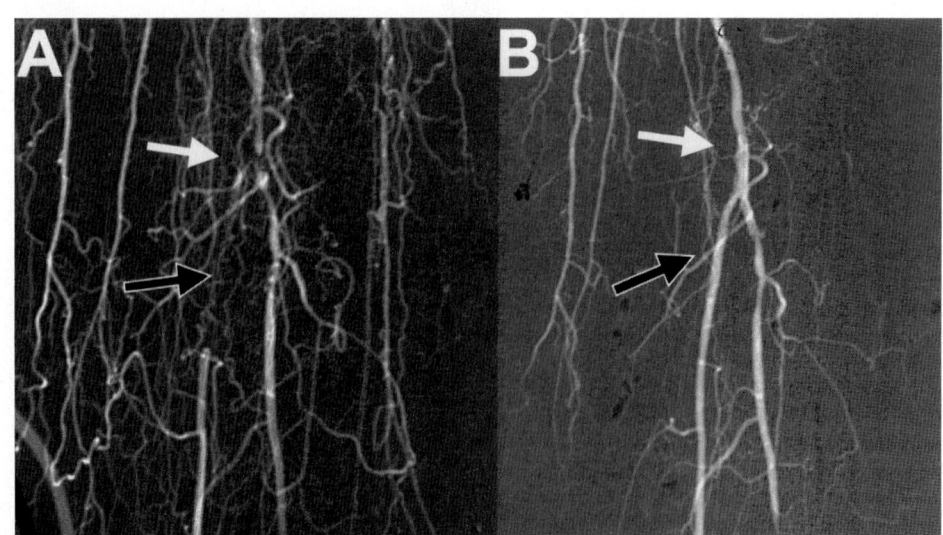

FIGURE 110–7. A 67-year-old male with a history of nonhealing ulcer in the left foot. **A.** Angiography showed severe below-the-knee disease with occluded anterior tibialis artery, severely diseased tibioperoneal trunk (*white arrow*), and occluded posterior tibial artery (*black arrow*). **B.** After percutaneous balloon angioplasty of tibioperoneal trunk and posterior tibial artery.

intermittent claudication when clinical features suggest a reasonable likelihood of symptomatic improvement with endovascular intervention and (a) there has been an inadequate response to exercise or pharmacological therapy and/or (b) there is a very favorable risk-benefit ratio (e.g., focal aortoiliac occlusive disease).

2. *Endovascular intervention is recommended as the preferred revascularization technique for TASC type A iliac and femoropopliteal arterial lesions (Table 110–2).*

3. *Stenting is effective as primary therapy for common and external iliac artery stenoses and occlusions.*

Class IIa

1. *Stents (and other adjunctive techniques such as lasers, cutting balloons, atherectomy devices, and thermal devices) can be useful in the femoral, popliteal, and tibial arteries as salvage therapy for a suboptimal or failed result from balloon dilation (e.g., persistent translesional gradient, residual diameter stenosis greater than 50 percent, or flow-limiting dissection).*

Class IIb

1. *The effectiveness of uncoated/uncovered stents, atherectomy, cutting balloons, thermal devices, and lasers for the treatment of infrapopliteal lesions (except to salvage a suboptimal result from balloon dilation) is not well established.*

Class III

1. *Endovascular intervention is not indicated if there is no significant pressure gradient across a stenosis despite flow augmentation with vasodilators.*

2. *Primary stent placement is not recommended in the femoral, popliteal, or tibial arteries.*

3. *Endovascular intervention is not indicated as prophylactic therapy in an asymptomatic patient with lower-extremity PAD.*

ENDOVASCULAR TREATMENT FOR ACUTE LIMB ISCHEMIA

Acute limb ischemia occurs when suddenly decreased blood flow to a limb threatens its viability. The etiology of acute limb ischemia commonly involves a major artery or a bypass graft that is acutely obstructed by either an embolus (often from the heart) or by thrombosis in-situ. The principal goal of treatment for acute limb ischemia is to rapidly restore blood flow to the ischemic region to forestall irreversible changes. Although surgical intervention was once the standard of care for restoring limb perfusion, now catheter-directed thrombolysis (CDT) has been shown to be useful for rapid clot dissolution, for unmasking underlying stenoses, and for helping to determine the best treatment strategy (either surgery or PTA).[54]

Studies have shown that use of CDT leads to long-term clinical outcomes equal to those of surgical revascularization in treating

TABLE 110-2

TASC Morphologic Stratification of Iliac Lesions for Treatment Purposes

TASC CLASSIFICATION	CHARACTERISTICS
A	<3-cm stenosis, single, CIA or EIA, uni/bilateral
B	3–10-cm stenosis, single <5-cm stenoses × 2, CIA or EIA occlusion, CIA, unilateral
C	5–10-cm stenosis, bilateral, of CIA or EIA (away from CFA) unilateral EIA stenosis or occlusion bilateral CIA occlusions
D	Diffuse or multiple stenoses involving CIA and EIA (total >10 cm) unilateral occlusion of both CIA and EIA bilateral EIA occlusions diffuse disease of aorta in addition to iliacs stenoses associated with aneurysmal or other A-I disease requiring surgery

A-I, aortoiliac; CFA, common femoral artery; CIA, common iliac artery; EIA, external iliac artery; TASC, transatlantic intersocietal commission.

limb-threatening ischemia.[55–57] The prospective, randomized Surgery versus Thrombolysis for Ischemia of the Lower Extremity (STILE) trial reported no difference in rates of mortality, amputation, or major morbidity in groups treated surgically and those treated with thrombolysis (urokinase or recombinant tissue-type plasminogen activator [rt-PA]).[55] The rates of limb salvage were also similar (88.2 percent in the surgical group vs. 89.4 percent in the thrombolysis group).

The Thrombolysis or Peripheral Arterial Surgery (TOPAS) studies I and II found no difference in rates for mortality and for amputation between groups treated with urokinase and those treated with surgery, but the magnitude of surgery was reduced in the thrombolysis group.[56,57] Nonrandomized trials have demonstrated that thrombolytic therapy followed by PTA may obviate bypass grafting in >50 percent of patients.[58] Accordingly, unless patients present with critical ischemia that demands immediate restoration of pulsatile blood flow by surgical embolectomy (patients with loss of motor and sensory function in a viable limb), CDT should be the initial therapy of choice.

Patients who are selected for CDT should be started on aspirin and heparin as soon as possible, followed by angiography and placement within the occluded vessel of an infusion catheter with multiple side holes. Thrombolytic agents are introduced through the infusion catheter for a period of 12 to 24 hours, after which angiography is repeated to evaluate results and identify any underlying lesions, which are then usually corrected by PTA with or without stenting (Fig. 110–8).

Thrombolytic agents currently available include streptokinase, urokinase, rt-PA, reteplase, and tenecteplase. Urokinase is the

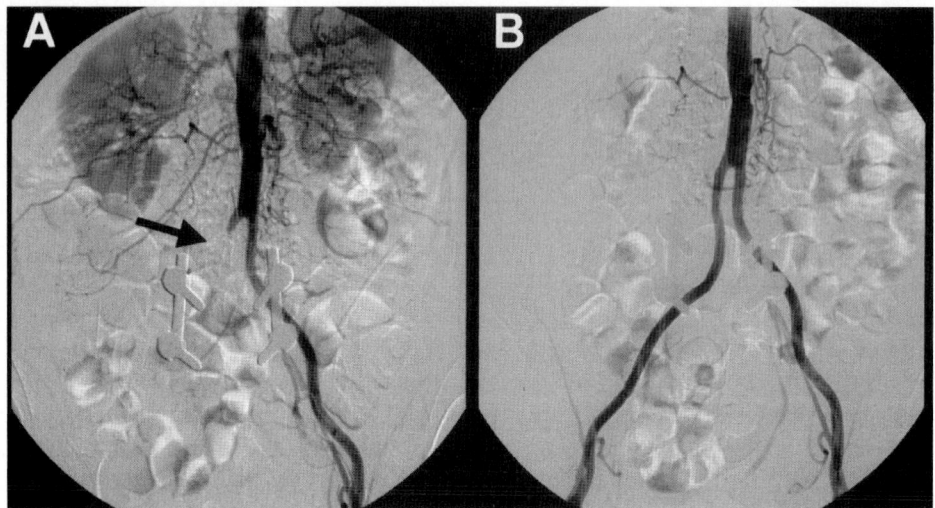

FIGURE 110–8. A 54-year-old female with a history of peripheral artery disease treated by aortofemoral bypass presented with acute onset of severe claudication in right lower extremity. **A.** Abdominal aortography showed occlusion of the right limb of the graft (*arrow*). **B.** After 16 hours of intraarterial administration of a thrombolytic through a perfusion catheter.

most studied for treatment of ALI; however, rt-PA, reteplase, and tenecteplase are now successfully used to treat patients with ALI. Recently several studies have compared the outcome after use of different thrombolytic agents. Ouriel and coworkers demonstrated similar bleeding complication rates after use of rt-PA and urokinase. However, in-hospital mortality rates were lower in the urokinase treated group even though the overall hospital costs did not differ significantly in the two groups.[59]

In addition to CDT, percutaneous mechanical thrombectomy has also been used to treat ALI patients. Of the devices developed to disrupt thrombus formation and remove freshly formed thrombus from the circulation, only the AngioJet Rheolytic Thrombectomy System (Possis Medical, Inc., Minneapolis, MN) is currently approved in the United States for use in the arterial circulation. Several studies[60,61] have shown this device to be effective in the treatment of ALI, but it is generally used as an adjunct to CDT rather than as stand-alone therapy. Used together, percutaneous mechanical thrombectomy and CDT appear to hasten reperfusion and reduce dose and duration of thrombolytic infusion, thus achieving successful reperfusion with lower rates of complications.

Endovascular Treatment for Critical Limb Ischemia (CLI): American College of Cardiology/American Heart Association Practice Guidelines[53]

Class I

1. *For individuals with combined inflow and outflow disease with CLI, inflow lesions should be addressed first.*

2. *For individuals with combined inflow and outflow disease in whom symptoms of CLI or infection persist after inflow revascularization, an outflow revascularization procedure should be performed.*

Thrombolysis for Acute and Chronic Limb Ischemia

Class I

1. *Catheter-based thrombolysis is an effective and beneficial therapy and is indicated for patients with acute limb*

ischemia (Rutherford categories I and IIa) of <14 days' duration (Level of Evidence: A).

Class IIa

1. *Mechanical thrombectomy devices can be used as adjunctive therapy for acute limb ischemia due to peripheral arterial occlusion (Level of Evidence: B).*

Class IIb

1. *Catheter-based thrombolysis or thrombectomy may be considered for patients with acute limb ischemia (Rutherford category IIb) of more than 14 days' duration (Level of Evidence: B).*

OCCLUSIVE DISEASE OF RENAL ARTERIES

Renal artery stenosis (RAS) is the most common cause of secondary hypertension. Atherosclerosis accounts for 90 percent of the cases of RAS, whereas fibromuscular dysplasia results in RAS in approximately 10 percent of cases. The incidence of atherosclerotic RAS increases with age and is more common in patients who have occlusive disease in other vascular territories. At our institution of 196 unselected patients who presented with diabetes and hypertension and underwent coronary angiography, renal angiography revealed that 18 percent had RAS >50 percent.[62] Atherosclerotic renal artery stenosis is an independent predictor of death regardless of the presence, severity, or method of revascularization of coronary arteries.[63–65]

RAS should be suspected in hypertensive patients if there are any of following conditions:

- Blood pressure difficult to control despite multiple medications
- Sudden worsening of blood pressure control
- Recurrent pulmonary edema despite a normal left ventricular systolic function
- Sudden worsening of renal function with the introduction of angiotensin-converting enzyme inhibitors (ACEIs)
- Unexplained discrepancy of >1.5 cm in size of kidneys

In most patients, atherosclerotic RAS is progressive and, in a significant number of these patients, results in renal atrophy.[66,67] Before percutaneous revascularization procedures became widely available, aortorenal bypass surgery was commonly performed to treat patients who had RAS, but rates of perioperative mortality were 2 to 6 percent with significant morbidity.[68]

Grüntzig first reported percutaneous revascularization of the renal arteries in 1978. Since then, the procedure has been refined and simplified until it has virtually replaced open surgical revascularization of renal arteries for patients who have RAS.

The two major goals of percutaneous revascularization of the renal arteries are as follows:

1. Control of blood pressure
2. Preservation of renal function

When RAS is caused by fibromuscular dysplasia, results of percutaneous transluminal renal angioplasty alone are excellent with a success rate of 82–100 percent and a restenosis rate of approximately 10 percent, making PTA the treatment of choice in patients who have uncontrolled hypertension and fibromuscular dysplasia.[69] Conversely, stand-alone PTA for atherosclerotic RAS has yielded poor results caused by high elastic recoil in the atherosclerotic ostial lesions.[69] As is the case when used in most other arteries, stents improve both immediate and long-term patency following PTA. Although not yet substantiated by reports from large randomized studies, many other reports show renal artery stenting to be highly effective.[70–75] As shown in Table 110–3, rates for immediate technical success following renal artery stenting are 97 to 100 percent, rates for procedure-related major complications are approximately 2 to 3 percent, and rates for restenosis are 5 to 21 percent.

Variations in reporting standards make it hard to judge the efficacy of renal artery stenting for patients who have hypertension and renal function. Nonetheless, renal artery stenting appears to improve control of blood pressure in 70 percent of patients. However, the procedure cures hypertension in <30 percent of the patients who have atherosclerotic RAS compared with >60 percent of patients who have fibromuscular dysplasia. Renal artery stenting improves or stabilizes renal function in approximately 70 percent of the patients. There is evidence that the procedure is more effective if performed in the early stages of RAS, i.e., before renal impairment becomes either severe (serum creatinine levels >4.0 mg/dL) or permanent.

Dorros and Jaff recently published data from the multicenter Palmaz-Stent Renal Artery Stenosis Revascularization registry on 1058 patients (1443 atherosclerotic renal arteries) in whom Palmaz-Schatz stent revascularization was successfully performed to improve poorly controlled hypertension, preserve renal function, or improve congestive heart failure.[76] At a 4-year follow up, there were significant decreases in both systolic blood pressure (168–147 mmHg) and in diastolic blood pressure (84–78 mmHg) as well as in serum creatinine levels (1.7–1.3 mg/dL). In addition, renal function was improved or stabilized in 70 percent of patients who had unilateral RAS and in 92 percent of those who had bilateral RAS.

The current consensus is to perform renal artery revascularization in patients who have RAS to preserve renal function or to improve control of hypertension.

Few randomized studies have compared results of balloon angioplasty with those of medical therapy in patients treated for renal artery stenosis and hypertension. The DRASTIC trial demonstrated significant improvement in systolic and diastolic blood pressures in 3 months in the angioplasty group. However, at 12 months there was no significant difference in blood pressures because of significant crossover from the medical therapy arm.[77] More recently, the ASPIRE study demonstrated a significant decrease in systolic and diastolic blood pressures after renal artery stenting with relative preservation of renal function.[78] There is no definite predictor of blood pressure response after renal artery stenting. Preliminary data suggests that lesion selection is improved through use of physiologic assessment (renal fractional flow reserve) or biomarkers (BNP), or both, resulting in improved clinical response rates.[79–80]

Recent concern about distal embolization of atherosclerotic debris during PTA/stenting of renal arteries is being addressed by studies to determine if devices shown to be effective in preventing distal embolization when used in the coronary and carotid arteries are equally as effective when used in renal arteries. Henry and coworkers[81] have reported the results of a pilot study evaluating feasibility and safety in 28 patients with atherosclerotic renal artery stenosis who underwent angioplasty and stenting using distal protection provided by a GuardWire temporary occlusion balloon. Visible debris was aspirated from all patients; at a 6-month follow up, renal function did not deteriorate in any patient. These beneficial effects must be confirmed by randomized studies before any general recommendation can be made for this strategy (Fig. 110–9). A recent large-scale randomized CORAL (Cardiovascular Outcomes In Renal Atherosclerotic Lesions) study will give us more insight into the benefits if any of using distal protection device during renal angioplasty.[82]

Endovascular Treatment for Renal Artery Stenosis (RAS): American College of Cardiology/American Heart Association Practice Guidelines[53]

Class I

1. *Renal stent placement is indicated for ostial atherosclerotic RAS lesions that meet the clinical criteria for intervention (Evidence Level B).*

2. *Balloon angioplasty with bailout stent placement, if necessary, is recommended for fibromuscular dysplasia (FMD) lesions (Evidence Level B) (Fig. 110–10).*

OCCLUSIVE DISEASE OF VISCERAL ARTERIES

Patients who have chronic intestinal ischemia secondary to either occlusion or stenosis of a visceral artery (i.e., celiac, superior, or inferior mesenteric artery), can present with recurrent episodes of abdominal pain (intestinal angina) caused by eating, which leads to fear of eating and pronounced weight loss.

Surgical revascularization involves transaortic endarterectomy and end-to-end aortomesenteric bypass grafting, which carries high rates of operative mortality (4–16 percent) and recurrence (long-term patency of approximately 78 percent).[83,84] Nonetheless, as late as 1980, when the first report of visceral angioplasty was published, surgery remained the only effective treatment.[85] Since then, there have been many reports of successful treatment by this means.[86,87]

As with angioplasty in most other arteries, restenosis rates after visceral angioplasty tend to be high (24 percent).[86] Intravascular stent placement in the visceral arteries has been successful in addressing this problem, as documented by several case reports and some case series of stent placement in the mesenteric arteries and the celiac trunk (Fig. 110–11).[88–90]

In their series in which stents were placed in mesenteric arteries, Sheeran and colleagues[88] reported an initial technical success rate of 92 percent for relieving ischemia, a primary patency rate of 76 percent, and a secondary patency rate at 18 months of 83 percent.

In 12 patients who underwent stenting of celiac arteries (3 patients) and superior mesenteric arteries (9 patients), Liermann and

● TABLE 110–3

Renal Artery Stenting: Results in Recent Studies

STUDY/YEAR OF PUBLICATION	PATIENTS (N)	ARTERIES (N)	FOLLOW-UP (MO)	TECHNICAL SUCCESS RATE (%)	HYPERTENSION CURED OR CONTROL IMPROVED (%)	RENAL FUNCTION IMPROVED OR STABILIZED (%)	RESTENOSIS (%)	MAJOR COMPLICATIONS (%)
Lederman[70]/2001	300	363	16	100	70	73	21	2
Burket[71]/2000	127	171	15 ± 14	100	71	67	7.8	3
Rodriguez-lopez[72]/1999	108	125	36	97.6	79	100	5.5	3.2
Rocha-Singh[73]/1999	150	180	13.1	97.3	91	92	12	1.3
Dorros[74]/1998	163	202	48	99	49	71	NR	1.8
White[75]/1997	100	133	8.7 ± 5	99	76	22	18.8	2
Pooled Results	948	1174	22.8	98.8	72.6	70.8	13.2	2.2

2406

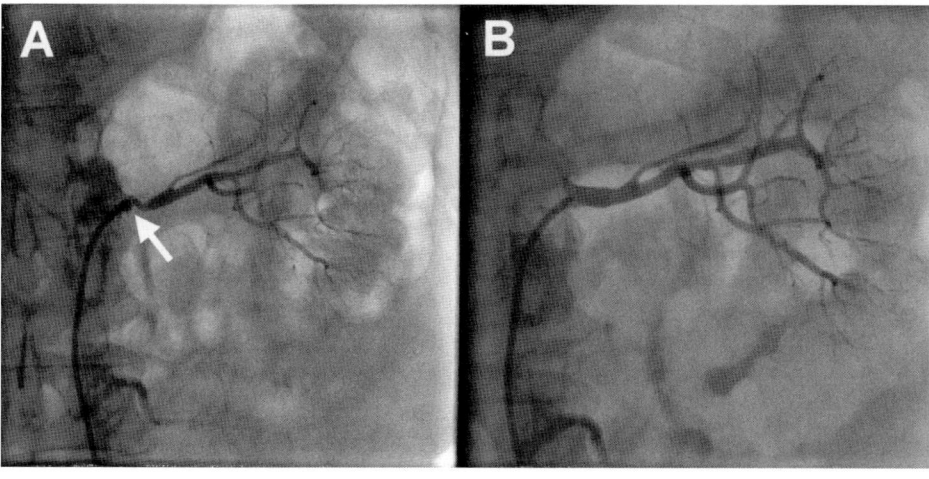

FIGURE 110–9. A 45-year-old female with a history of coronary artery disease, uncontrolled hypertension, and decreased renal function. **A.** Selective angiography showed severe ostial stenosis in the left renal artery (*white arrow*). **B.** After balloon and stent placement in left renal artery.

coworkers[89] reported a technical success rate of 100 percent. All patients reported relief of symptoms at a mean follow up of 28 months. Four patients had recurrent symptoms that were treated successfully with repeat balloon angioplasty. Given these high rates of technical success and clinical effectiveness, stent placement in the celiac and mesenteric arteries should be the method of choice for patients who have chronic mesenteric ischemia due to stenosis of a visceral artery.

Endovascular Treatment for Mesenteric Artery Disease: American College of Cardiology/American Heart Association Practice Guidelines[53]

Acute Intestinal Ischemia Caused by Arterial Obstruction

Class IIb

1. *Percutaneous interventions (including transcatheter lytic therapy, balloon angioplasty, and stenting) are appropriate in selected patients with acute intestinal ischemia caused by arterial obstructions. Patients so treated may still require laparotomy (Evidence Level C).*

Chronic Intestinal Ischemia

Class I

1. *Percutaneous endovascular treatment of intestinal arterial stenosis is indicated in patients with chronic intestinal ischemia. (Evidence Level B).*

ANEURYSMAL DISEASE OF AORTOILIAC AND FEMOROPOPLITEAL VESSELS

A true aneurysm is defined as a localized dilatation of the aorta that is 50 percent larger than the normal diameter, which includes all three layers of the vessel: intima, media, and adventitia. Arterial aneurysms share many of the same atherosclerotic risk factors and pose similar threats to life, limb, and the function of vital organs as does occlusive arterial disease.

[ ] DESCENDING THORACIC AORTIC ANEURYSM

The estimated prevalence of thoracic aortic aneurysms (TAAs) is 10 of every 100,000 elderly adults.[91] The incidence is TAA has been increasing, in part, because of better detection through the wide use of computed tomography (CT). Between 30 and 40 percent of these aneurysms occur exclusively in the descending thoracic aorta and, with time, are likely to expand and rupture.[92] Thoracic aortic aneurysms most often result from cystic medial degeneration that leads to weakening of the aortic wall. Cystic medial degeneration occurs normally with aging and is increased with hypertension. When it occurs in young patients, it is most often caused by Marfan syndrome or other, less common, connective tissue disorders, such as Ehlers-Danlos syndrome.

The risk of rupture is directly related to the size of the aneurysm, Coady and coworkers found that, in an ascending aorta an aneurysm with a diameter >6 cm increased the risk of rupture or dissection by 25 percent and in a descending aorta an aneurysm with a diameter of >7 cm increased the risk by 37 percent.[93] Davies et al. found an annual rate of rupture and dissection of 2 percent for aneurysms <5 cm, 3 percent for aneurysms 5 to 5.9 cm, and 7 percent for aneurysms >6 cm in diameter.[94] Therefore, the risk appears to rise abruptly as thoracic aneurysms reach a diameter of 6 cm.

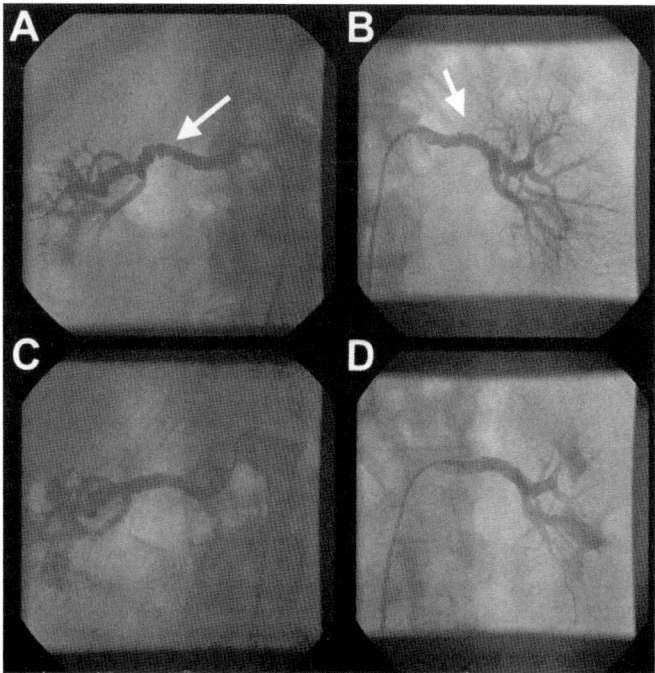

FIGURE 110–10. A 40-year-old male with severe uncontrolled hypertension over the previous year. Selective angiography of right (**A**) and left (**B**) renal arteries showed typical appearance of fibromuscular dysplasia (*arrows*). After balloon, a repeat angioplasty was performed in both renal arteries (**C, D**).

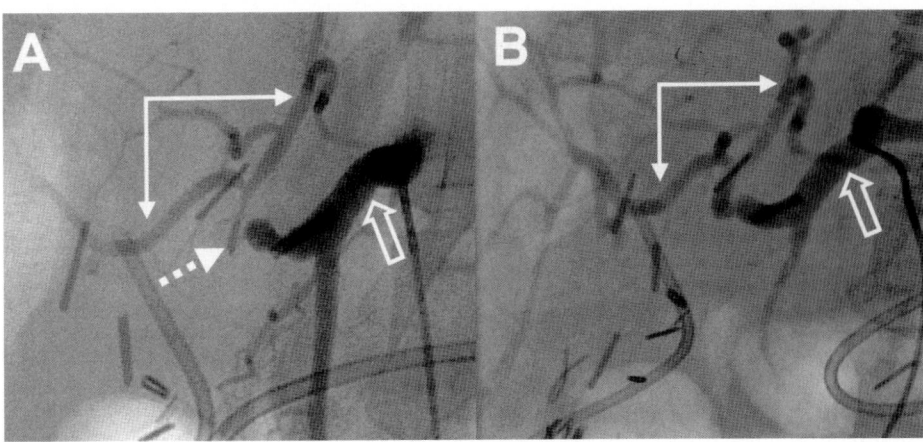

FIGURE 110–11. A 50-year-old female with liver failure 1 month after liver transplant was found by Doppler ultrasound to have increased velocity in the hepatic artery at the site of anastomosis. **A.** Selective angiography of common hepatic artery (*empty white arrow*) showed a severe stenosis in the proper hepatic artery just before the division into right and left hepatic arteries (*white arrows*). **B.** After a balloon expandable stent was placed in the proper hepatic artery the stenosis is resolved.

The indications for intervention in patients with thoracic aneurysm include the following:

- Symptoms related to the aneurysm
- Diameter of 50 mm for an aneurysm in the ascending aorta and 6 mm for an aneurysm in the descending aorta (early in some subgroups, i.e., Marfan syndrome patients)
- Growth rate >10 mm/y
- Complications associated with aneurysm that increase risk of rupture, such as dissection, leak, or ulceration

The first multicenter nonrandomized trial using GORE TAG thoracic endoprosthesis (W.L. Gore, Flagstaff, AZ) involved 17 sites in the United States, Makaroun and colleagues showed a success rate of 98 percent after the device was implanted in 142 patients, 90 percent of whom were classified as American Society of Anesthesiologists category III or IV. The only reason for failure was inadequate arterial access. The mean diameter size was 64.1 mm and mean follow up was 24.0 months. At 2 years, there has been a 97 percent rate of aneurysm-related survival and an overall survival rate of 75 percent. Three patients have undergone endovascular revisions for endoleak. No ruptures have been reported.[95] A related trial, TAG 03–03, compared results of implantation using the TAG device with those of surgical therapy and showed that endovascular repair had one-fifth the rate of paraplegia (3 percent vs. 14 percent), one-sixth the rate of operative mortality (1 percent vs. 6 percent), an average of 80 percent lower procedural blood loss (472 mL vs. 2402 mL), a lower rate of aneurysm-related death through the first year (3 percent vs. 10

percent), a shortened average stay in the intensive care unit (1 day vs. 3 days), and shortened average hospital stay (3 days vs. 10 days) (Fig. 110–12).[96]

【 】 ANEURYSMAL DISEASE OF ABDOMINAL AORTA

Abdominal aortic aneurysm (AAA) is defined as focal enlargement of the abdominal aorta (usually involving the infrarenal portion) to a diameter >50 percent larger than normal or to >3 cm in its largest true transverse dimension. Untreated, the major complication is rupture leading to death. Aneurysmal rupture is directly related to aneurysm size. A recent population-based study from the Mayo Clinic revealed that the estimated risk of rupture was 0 percent per year for an AAA diameter of <4 cm, with increases to 1 percent per year for diameters of 4.0 to 4.9 cm, 11 percent per year for diameters of 5.0 to 5.9 cm, and 25 percent per year for diameters >6 cm.[97]

At least 1 million Americans have a clinically recognized AAA, but only 70,000 to 80,000 surgical repairs are performed annually. Many of these patients are older than age 70 years and have other serious comorbidities.[98] Consequently, their operative risk is increased, prohibiting open surgical repair. Even in low-risk patients, open repair of AAA is associated with a mortality rate of up to 5 percent.[99,100] In a 36-year population-based study by Mayo Clinic in Olmstead County, Minnesota, the rate of 30-day mortality was

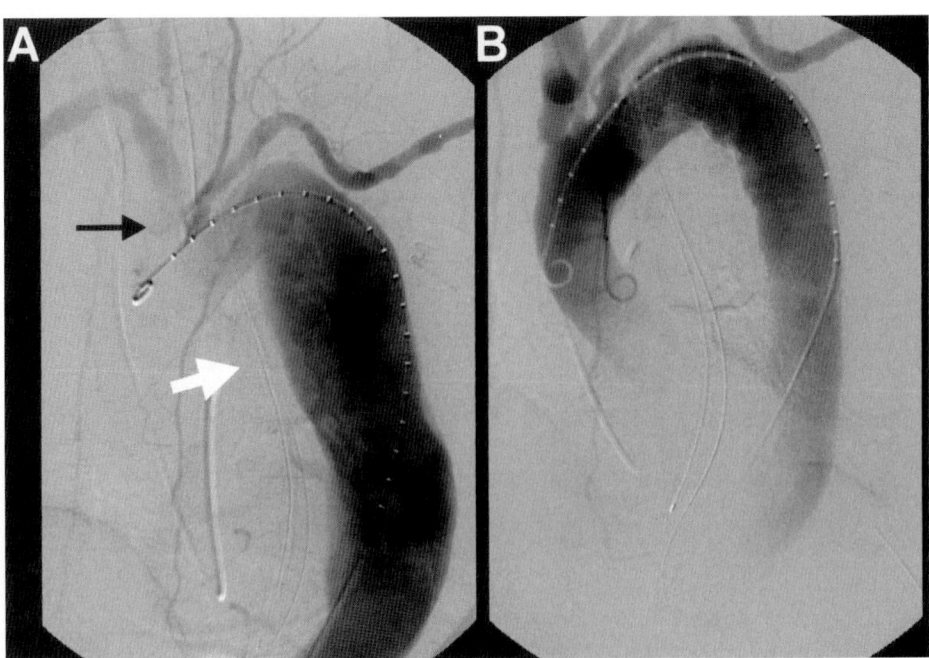

FIGURE 110–12. A 68-year-old female had a 6-cm thoracic aneurysm that surgery failed to repair. **A.** Aortic angiography showed the thoracic aneurysm (*white arrow*) distal to the left subclavian artery (*black arrow*). **B.** After percutaneous intervention with a Gore Tag device (W.L. Gore and Associates, Inc., Flagstaff, AZ).

5 percent in 307 patients who underwent elective open surgical repair for an AAA.[98] The Canadian multicenter study reported a similar rate of 5.4 percent.[101]

In 1991, Parodi described the first successful implantation of an endoluminal stent graft in a patient with an infrarenal AAA.[102] Since then, this technique has evolved to gain widespread acceptance by patients and physicians. The rationale for placing an endovascular stent graft is to exclude the aneurysm from the effects of arterial pressure that might cause further dilatation and rupture (Fig. 110–13).

In the U.S. AneuRx clinical trial (1192 patients), the rate of implant success was 98 percent, the rate of procedure-related mortality at 30 days was 1.9 percent, and the rate of conversion to open repair within the first 30 days was 1.3 percent.[103] At 4 years, the rate of aneurysm-related mortality was 2.5 percent (0.5 percent per year) and the rate of event-free survival was 97.1 percent. Investigators in the European Collaborators on Stent-Graft Techniques for AAA Repair (EUROSTAR) study[104] reported similar results following endovascular (stent) graft (EVG) implantation. In addition to reducing mortality risk, EVG repair decreases hospital stay, reduces blood loss, and speeds functional recovery.[105,106] Table 110–4 compares the mortality from endovascular repair to that of open surgical repair in patients who underwent elective AAA repair.

Multicenter randomized controlled trials of endovascular aneurysm repair (EVAR) have reported their results. EVAR 1 randomly assigned 1082 patients with abdominal aortic aneurysm to undergo either EVAR or open repair. In contrast to previous studies, patients were candidates for both procedures. At 4 years after randomization, the rate for all-cause mortality was similar in the two groups; however, there was a persistent reduction in aneurysm-related deaths in the EVAR group (3 percent ARR).[107]

A second randomized controlled trial was the DREAM (Dutch Randomized Endovascular Aneurysm Management) study, which compared open repair and endovascular repair.[108] In the study 345 patients whose abdominal aortic aneurysm had a diameter of ≥5 cm were considered suitable candidates for either of the two techniques. In the endovascular-repair group the rate of operative mortality was 1.2 percent; in the open-repair group it was 4.6 percent. In the endovascular-repair group the combined rate of operative mortality and severe complications was 4.7 percent; in the open-repair group the combined rate was 9.8 percent. Two years after randomization, endovascular repair was found to have a clear advantage over open repair that was accounted for entirely by events occurring in the perioperative period: an equally

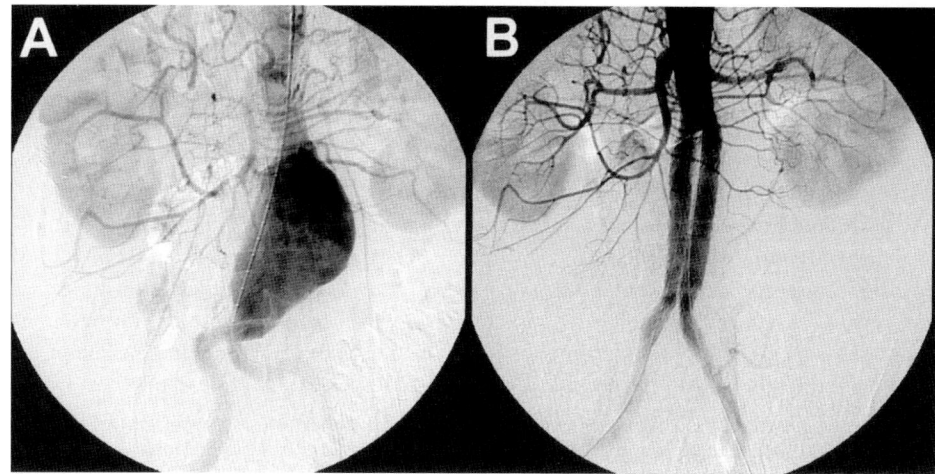

FIGURE 110–13. A 73 year-old-male with a history of coronary artery disease, congestive heart failure (ejection fraction of 30 percent), and hypertension was found to have an infrarenal AAA of 8.5 cm. **A.** Angiography showed the large infrarenal AAA. **B.** After successful EVG repair with an AneuRx stent-graft (Medtronic, Inc., Minneapolis, MN) there is no evidence of endoleak. AAA, abdominal aortic aneurysm; EVG, endovascular graft.

good cumulative survival rate (89.6 percent vs. 89.7 percent) but a much better cumulative rate of aneurysm-related death (2.1 percent vs. 5.7 percent).[109]

In our own experience, from 2000 to 2006 we have performed more than 200 cases in moderate to high risk patients with a technical success of 99.3 percent and a 30 day mortality rate of 1 percent related to vascular access complication. Hospital stay was <48 hours in 84.6 percent of patients. During a median-term follow up there was only one death related to AAA endoleak, which was not treated because of patient comorbidities. These results are consistent with the general practice.[110]

Note that it is imperative for patients who undergo EVG repair to have a close follow up with regular CT or ultrasound scans to detect any endoleaks. An endoleak is defined as any persistent blood flow outside the vascular graft but inside the original intact aneurysm. Endoleaks are classified into four types[111]:

1. Type I: Lack of complete seal between stent graft and vessel wall at attachment sites
2. Type II: Back filling of the aneurysm sac via such branch vessels as the lumbar of inferior mesenteric arteries

TABLE 110–4

Mortality Related to Open and EVG Repair of AAA

STUDY	PATIENTS (N)	FOLLOW-UP (Y)	30-DAY MORTALITY (%)	TOTAL AAA DEATHS (%)
Mayo Clinic AAA[98]	307	36 (mean 5.8)	5	7.6
Canadian AAA[101]	680	6	5.4	5.8
AneuRx I–III[103]	1192	4	1.9	2.4
EUROSTAR[104]	2955	4	1.7	2.5

AAA, abdominal aortic aneurysm; EUROSTAR, European Collaborators on Stent-Graft Techniques for AAA Repair.

3. Type III: Leaks at connections of modular components, device disruption, fabric tears
4. Type IV: Extravasation of contrast material through interstices in the grafted artery

Type I and type III endoleaks are considered to constitute a major complication, potentially leading to aortic rupture, whereas type II endoleaks appear to cause a lesser extent of aneurysm enlargement. Type IV endoleak usually disappears over time and does not pose any major clinical problem. In a recent study, Zarins and coworkers reported the incidence and clinical significance of endoleaks from the U.S. AneuRx clinical trial.[112] The incidence of any endoleak at the time of the hospital discharge was 50 percent, of which 15 percent were type I, 20 percent were type II, and another 15 percent were undetermined. The rate of endoleak decreased to 13 percent at one month and 20 percent at 1 year. However, the development of an endoleak did not always translate into aneurysm rupture, as the rupture-free survival rate was 99.7 percent at one year. At the present time, consensus opinion is to treat type I and type III endoleaks immediately and to follow type II endoleaks with close surveillance to detect any increase in aneurysm size. Fortunately, most endoleaks can be treated successfully by endovascular procedures (i.e., either deployment of additional cuffs of the stent-graft or use of coil or gel foam embolization).

[ ] ANEURYSMAL DISEASE OF ILIAC ARTERIES

Iliac artery aneurysms (IAA) are most commonly associated with AAA, accounting for up to 50 percent of all cases. It is rare to find an isolated aneurysm of the iliac artery (an incidence of 0.03–0.1 percent).[113] Although most aneurysms in this region are asymptomatic, symptoms may be caused by local compression, thrombosis, or by distal embolization of atheromatous debris. Expansive growth and subsequent rupture of iliac artery aneurysms are also well documented.[114]

The treatment of choice is for patients to undergo elective repair of IAA with these traditional criteria:

• Asymptomatic if >3.5 cm in diameter
• Rapid increase in diameter (>0.5 cm/y)
• Symptomatic

As with surgical repair of AAA, open surgical repair for IAA is a major procedure that is associated with high rates of procedure-related morbidity and mortality. Placement of an endovascular stent-graft, if technically feasible (good neck and adequate iliac artery size), provides a less invasive way to exclude an IAA.

In a report on 48 patients who underwent implantation of an endoprostheses in the iliac artery, Scheinert and colleagues[115] achieved a rate of technical success of 97.9 percent for complete exclusion of an aneurysm. Primary patency rates were 100 percent after 1 year, 97.9 percent after 2 years, 94.9 percent after 3 years, and 87.6 percent after 4 years. Sahgal and coworkers recently reported that 30 of their 31 patients had a decrease in the size of their iliac aneurysm (35 true isolated IAAs) treated with EVG repair and coil embolization of the hypogastric artery or its branches.[116]

It is thus both feasible and safe to attempt percutaneous exclusion of IAA by EVG. As a minimally invasive procedure associated with very low rates of procedure-related morbidity and mortality, we recommend it as the primary alternative to open surgical repair.

[ ] POPLITEAL ARTERY ANEURYSM

Popliteal artery aneurysms, defined as localized dilatations of the popliteal artery >2 cm in diameter, are the most common aneurysms of the peripheral arteries, with a prevalence of 1 percent in men ages 65 to 80 years.[117] Popliteal aneurysms have a well-documented natural history, tending to occur with significant comorbidity in older men. Popliteal aneurysms are often bilateral (50 percent) and associated with abdominal aorta aneurysms (40 percent). Patients usually present with acute limb ischemia caused, not by rupture, but by either thrombosis or by distal embolization. The amputation rate in patients who present with acute limb ischemia due to popliteal artery aneurysms may be as high as 15 percent.[118]

Surgery has been the procedure of choice for preventing complications. No randomized trials have been conducted to compare results of treatment of popliteal artery aneurysms by medical management with those of surgery. Dawson and colleagues, reporting on results following elective surgery for popliteal artery aneurysms, found a 90 percent rate for limb salvage and an 80 percent rate for graft patency.[119] Rates for mortality and limb loss have been reported; up to 1 percent of patients will have residual symptoms after surgery.[120]

Covered stents have been proven feasible and safe to use for popliteal artery aneurysms with several studies reporting patency rates of 60 to 70 percent at 18 months. Telliu and coworkers reported on their prospective study of 28 patients with 23 popliteal artery aneurysms, all of whom underwent endovascular repair with a self-expanding stent graft.[121] Technical success in placing the stent-graft and excluding the aneurysm was 100 percent. During a median follow up of 15 months, 5 of 23 stent-grafts became occluded, resulting in a cumulative patency rate of 74 percent. All occlusions occurred within 6 months after intervention; two occlusions were successfully recanalized; and none of the three patients with persisting occlusion required an amputation (Fig. 110–14).

> *Endovascular Treatment for Abdominal or Iliac Aneurysms: American College of Cardiology/American Heart Association Practice Guidelines*[53]
>
> *Class IIa*
>
> *Endovascular repair of infrarenal aortic and/or iliac aneurysms is reasonable in patients at high risk of complications from open operations.*
>
> *Class IIb*
>
> *Endovascular repair of infrarenal aortic and/or iliac aneurysms may be considered in patients at low or average surgical risk.*

SUMMARY

In only the last 10 years, percutaneous revascularization has revolutionized the treatment of PVD so rapidly that it is easy to forget that not long ago surgery was the only available treatment for severe PVD and was frequently held off until rest pain or gangrene forced the issue. The risks of morbidity and death from surgery were simply too high to justify earlier intervention. The unfortunate consequences of withholding early treatment ranged from

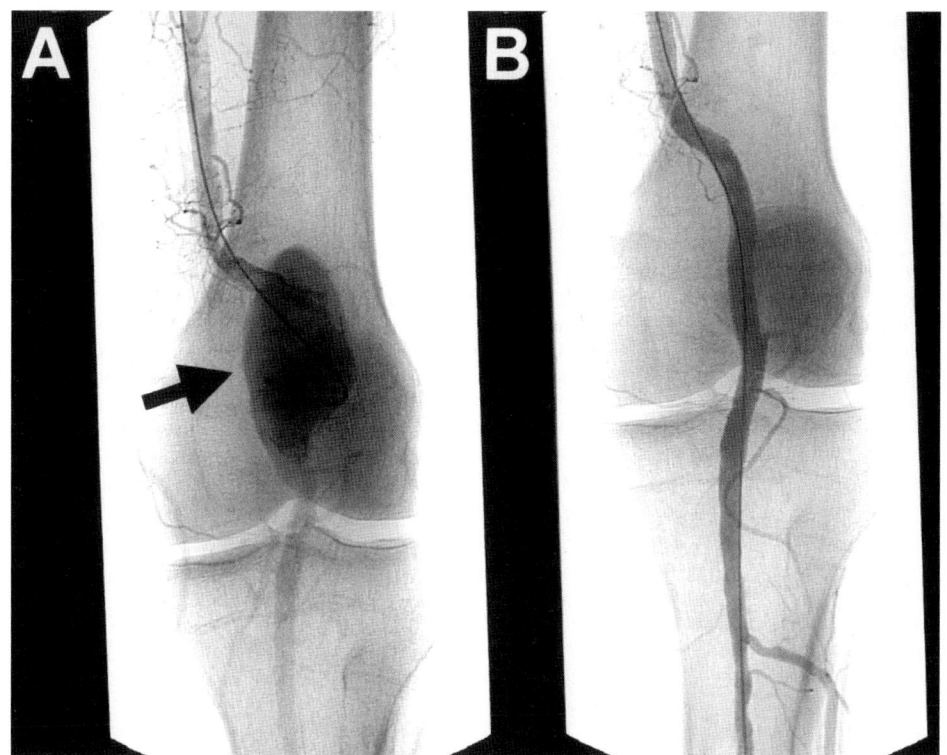

FIGURE 110–14. A 54-year-old male was found to have a unilateral popliteal aneurysm of 4 cm (*arrow*). Before (**A**) and after (**B**) intervention using a VIABAHN stent-graft (W.L. Gore and Associates, Inc., Flagstaff, AZ).

the option of percutaneous revascularization despite their diagnosis of PVD. In patients suspected of having renal artery stenosis (i.e., their blood pressure is hard to control or their renal function becomes worsen on ACEI therapy), however, we proceed with renal angiography followed by PTA and stenting.

Endovascular stent grafts have revolutionized the treatment of aneurysmal disease of thoracic, infrarenal aorta, iliac, and femoropopliteal vessels. Even patients who are high surgical risk candidates can be treated effectively by EVG repair at a much lower risk of morbidity and mortality. In the near future, the availability of fenestrated stent-grafts will make it possible to treat disease in the aortic arch as well as suprarenal aneurysm of the aorta.

In conclusion, by covering familiar ground and mapping out areas of frontier exploration, we hope that we have brought clarity to the challenging task of steering amid rapidly evolving field of minimally invasive therapies for treating PVD and of plotting the best course of treatment for each patient.

chronic, lifestyle-limiting infirmity to severe ischemia that left no choice but amputation if the patient's life was to be saved.

Thanks to vastly improved balloon catheters and guidewire systems and to the advent of endovascular stents, not only can we intervene earlier, we can now offer the benefits of intervention to many more categories of patients. In considering our treatment options (percutaneous revascularization, conservative medical treatment, or surgical revascularization), we must judiciously evaluate the scope of the problem in light of the standard question: "Does the benefit of this procedure outweigh the risk?" In answering this question, it is encouraging that the risk of endovascular interventions is much lower and our expectation of benefits is higher for so many patients who a decade or so ago would have been considered ineligible.

At our institution, we triage patients who present with PVD into those who have claudication and those who have rest pain and ischemic ulceration. (Regardless of how they are categorized, all patients are thoroughly evaluated to rule out coronary artery disease, i.e., by either cardiac angiography or by pharmacologic stress testing.)

Considering the high risk for potential loss of limb in those who have rest pain or ischemic ulcerations (especially in those who have diabetes and those who smoke), we treat these patients immediately, beginning with angiography and followed by either percutaneous or surgical revascularization so that pulsatile flow is reestablished. For patients who are at lower risk with only symptoms of claudication, the key consideration is to determine if their lifestyle and ability to earn a living are significantly limited. If so, we encourage them to undergo percutaneous revascularization. If there is no such significant limitation, we advise our patients that there is no firm basis for

REFERENCES

1. Fogarty TD, Cranley JJ, Krause RJ. Method of extraction of arterial emboli and thrombi. *Surg Gynecol Obstet* 1963;116:241–244.
2. Dotter CT, Judkins MP. Transluminal treatment of arteriosclerotic obstruction: description of a new technique and a preliminary report of its application. *Circulation* 1964;30:654–670.
3. Grüntzig A, Kumpe D. Technique of percutaneous transluminal angioplasty with the Grüntzig balloon catheter. *AJR Am J Roentgenol* 1979;132:547–552.
4. Beebe HG, Stark R, Johnson ML, et al. Choices of operation for subclavian vertebral arterial disease. *Am J Surg* 1980;139:616–623.
5. Hadjipetrou P, Cox S, Piemonte T, et al. Percutaneous revascularization of atherosclerotic obstruction of aortic arch vessels. *J Am Coll Cardiol* 1999;33:1238–1245.
6. Rodriguez-Lopez JA, Werner A, Martinez R, et al. Stenting for atherosclerotic occlusive disease of the subclavian artery. Ann Vasc Surg 1999;13:254–260.
7. Al-Mubarak N, Liu MW, Dean LS, et al. Immediate and late outcomes of subclavian artery stenting. *Catheter Cardiovasc Interv* 1999;46:169–172.
8. Jain SP, Zhang SY, Khosla S, et al. Subclavian and innominate arteries stenting: acute and long term results. *J Am Coll Cardiol* 1998;31:63A.
9. Wityk RJ, Chang HM, Rosengart A, et al. Proximal extracranial vertebral artery disease in the New England Medical Center Posterior Circulation Registry. *Arch Neurol* 1998;55:470–478.
10. Moufarrij NA, Little JR, Furlan AJ, et al. Vertebral artery stenosis: long-term follow-up. *Stroke* 1984;15:260–263.
11. Berguer R. Long-term results of vertebral artery reconstruction. In: Yao JST, Pearce WH, eds. *Long-term Results in Vascular Surgery.* Norwalk, CT: Appleton and Lange; 1993:69.
12. Motarjeme A. Percutaneous transluminal angioplasty of supra-aortic vessels. *J Endovasc Surg* 1996;3:171–181.
13. Jenkins JS, White CJ, Ramee SR, et al. Vertebral artery stenting. *Catheter Cardiovasc Interv* 2001;54:1–5.
14. Storey GS, Marks MP, Dake M, et al. Vertebral artery stenting following percutaneous transluminal angiography. *J Neurosurg* 1996;84:883–887.
15. Feldman RL, Rubin JJ, Kuykendall RC. Use of coronary Palmaz-Schatz stent in the percutaneous treatment of vertebral artery stenoses. *Cathet Cardiovasc Diagn* 1996;38:312–315.

16. Malek AM, Higashida RT, Phatouros CC, et al. Treatment of posterior circulation ischemia with extracranial percutaneous balloon angioplasty and stent placement. *Stroke* 1999;30:2073–2085.

17. Sacco RL, Adams R, Albers G, et al. Guidelines for prevention of stroke in patients with ischemic stroke or transient ischemic attack: a statement for healthcare professionals from the American Heart Association/American Stroke Association Council on Stroke. *Stroke* 2006;37(2):577-617.

18. Brewster DC. Direct reconstruction for aortoiliac occlusive disease. In: Rutherford RB, ed. *Vascular Surgery.* Philadelphia: WB Saunders; 1995:766–794.

19. Tegtmeyer CJ, Kellum CD, Irving LKK, et al. Percutaneous transluminal angioplasty in the region of the aortic bifurcation. *Radiology* 1985;157:661–665.

20. Insall RI, Loose HWC, Chamberlain J. Long-term results of double balloon percutaneous transluminal angioplasty of the aorta and iliac arteries. *Eur J Vasc Surg* 1993;7:31–36.

21. Vorwerk D, Gunther RW, Schurmann K, et al. Aortic and iliac stenoses: follow-up results of stent placement after insufficient balloon angioplasty in 118 cases. *Radiology* 1996;198:45–48.

22. Martinez R, Rodriguez-Lopez J, Diethrich EB. Stenting for abdominal aortic occlusive disease: long-term results. *Tex Heart Inst J* 1997;24:15–22.

23. Mendelsohn FO, Santos RM, Crowley JJ, et al. Kissing stents in the aortic bifurcation. Am Heart J 1998;136:600–605.

24. Haulon S, Mounier-Vehier C, Gaxotte V, et al. Percutaneous reconstruction of the aortoiliac bifurcation with the "kissing stents" technique. *J Endovasc Ther* 2002;9:363–368.

25. Mouanoutoua M, Allaqaband S, Bajwa T, et al. Endovascular intervention of aortoiliac occlusive disease in high-risk patients using the kissing stents technique: long-term results [abstract]. *J Am Coll Cardiol* 2003;41:1199–1200.

26. Ameli FM, Stein M, Provan JL, et al. Predictors of surgical outcome in patients undergoing aortobifemoral bypass reconstruction. *J Cardiovasc Surg (Torino)* 1990;30:333–339.

27. Johnson KW, Rae M, Hogg-Johnston SA, et al. Five-year results of a prospective study of percutaneous transluminal angioplasty. *Ann Surg* 1987;206:403.

28. Vorwerk D, Guenther RW, Schurmann K, et al. Primary stent placement for chronic iliac artery occlusions: follow-up results in 103 patients. *Radiology* 1995;194:745–749.

29. Bosch JL, Hunink MG. Meta-analysis of the results of percutaneous transluminal angioplasty and stent placement for aortoiliac occlusive disease. *Radiology* 1997;204:87–96.

30. Vorwerk D, Gunther RW, Schurmann K, et al. Aortic and iliac stenoses: follow-up results of stent placement after insufficient balloon angioplasty in 118 cases. *Radiology* 1996;198:45–48.

31. Palmaz JC, Laborde JC, Rivera FJ, et al. Stenting of the iliac arteries with the Palmaz stent: experience from a multicenter trial. *Cardiovasc Intervent Radiol* 1992;15:291–297.

32. Scheinert D, Schroder M, Ludwig J, et al. Stent-supported recanalization of chronic iliac artery occlusions. *Am J Med* 2001;110:708.

33. Hunink MGM, Wong JB, Donaldson MC, et al. Patency results of percutaneous and surgical revascularization for femoropopliteal arterial disease. *Med Decis Making* 1994;14:71–81.

34. Adam DJ, Beard JD, Cleveland T, et al. Bypass versus angioplasty in severe ischaemia of the leg (BASIL): multicentre, randomised controlled trial. *Lancet* 2005;3;366(9501):1925–1934.

35. Pekka JM, Hannu IM, Ritva LV, et al. Femoropopliteal angioplasty in patients with claudication: primary and secondary patency in 140 limbs with 1–3 year follow-up. *Radiology* 1994;191:727–733.

36. Johnson KW. Femoral and popliteal arteries: reanalysis of results of balloon angioplasty. *Radiology* 1992;183:767–771.

37. Capek P, McLean GK, Berkowitz HD. Femoropopliteal angioplasty factors influencing long-term success. *Circulation* 1991;83:70–80.

38. Sapoval MR, Long AL, Raynaud AC, et al. Femoropopliteal stent placement: long-term results. *Radiology* 1992;184:833–839.

39. Kazemi S, Allaqaband S, Bajwa T, et al. Percutaneous revascularization of femoropopliteal arteries with self-expanding nitinol stentsimmediate success and one-year results. *J Am Coll Cardiol* 2005;3(suppl 1):68A.

40. Mewissen MW. Self-expanding nitinol stents in the FP segment: technique and mid-term results. *Tech Vasc Interv Radiol* 2004;7(1):2-5.

41. Cikrit DF, Dalsing MC. Lower-extremity arterial endovascular stenting. *Surg Clin North Am* 1998;78:617–629.

42. Criado FJ. Endovascular treatment of occlusive lesions in the femoropopliteal territory. In: Criado FJ, ed. *Endovascular Intervention: Basic Concepts and Techniques.* Armonk, NY: Futura Publishing Company; 1999:105–114.

43. Vroegindeweij D, Vos LD, Tielbeek AV, et al. Balloon angioplasty combined with primary stenting versus balloon angioplasty alone in femoropopliteal obstructions: a comparative randomized study. *Cardiovasc Intervent Radiol* 1997;20:420–425.

44. Lammer J, Dake MD, Bleyn J, et al. Peripheral arterial obstruction: prospective study of treatment with a transluminally placed self-expanding stent-graft. International Trial Study Group. *Radiology* 2000;217:95–104.

45. Kazemi S, Gupta A, Bajwa T, et al. Intermediate patency rate of the Viabahn stent-graft for chronic total occlusion or long high-grade stenosis of the superficial femoral artery. *Am J Cardiol* 2005;96(suppl 7A):141H.

46. Veith FJ, Gupta SK, Ascer E, et al. Improved strategies for secondary operations on infrainguinal arteries. *Ann Vasc Surg* 1990;4:85–93.

47. Ascer E, Collier P, Gupta SK, et al. Reoperation for polytetrafluoroethylene bypass failure: the importance of distal outflow site and operative technique in determining outcome. *J Vasc Surg* 1987;5:298–310.

48. Veith FJ, Gupta SK, Wengerter KR, et al. Changing arteriosclerotic disease patterns and management strategies in lower-limb threatening ischemia. *Ann Surg* 1990;212:402–414.

49. Dorros G, Jafff MR, Dorros AM, et al. Tibioperoneal (outflow lesion) angioplasty can be used as primary treatment in 235 patients with critical limb ischemia: five-year follow-up. *Circulation* 2001;104:2057–2062.

50. Shalev Y, Bajwa T, Schmidt DH, et al. A modification of the peripheral angioplasty procedure to treat below-the-knee vascular disease: initial success and late outcome in 97 patients. *J Am Coll Cardiol* 1996;29:191A.

51. Zeller T, Rastan A, Schwarzwälder U, et al. Midterm results after atherectomy-assisted angioplasty of below-knee arteries with use of the Silverhawk device. *J Vasc Interv Radiol* 2004 15:1391–1397.

52. Laird, JR, Zeller, T Gray BH, et al. Limb salvage following laser-assisted angioplasty for critical limb ischemia: results of the LACI multicenter trial. *J Endovasc Ther* 2006;13;1-11.

53. American College of Cardiology/American Heart Association. ACC/AHA 2005 Guidelines for the Management of Patients With Peripheral Arterial Disease (Lower Extremity, Renal, Mesenteric, and Abdominal Aortic): A Collaborative Report From the AAVS/SVS, SCAI, SVMB, SIR, and the ACC/AHA Task Force on Practice Guidelines. Available at: www.acc.org.

54. Ouriel K. Surgery versus thrombolytic therapy in the management of peripheral arterial occlusions. *J Vasc Interv Radiol* 1995;6:48S–54S.

55. STILE Investigators. Results of a prospective randomized trial evaluating surgery versus thrombolysis for ischemia of the lower extremity. STILE trial. *Ann Surg* 1994;220:251–268.

56. Ouriel K, Veith FJ, Sasahara AA. Thrombolysis or peripheral arterial surgery (TOPAS): phase I results. *J Vasc Surg* 1996;23:64–73.

57. Ouriel K, Veith FJ, Sasahara AA. A comparison of recombinant urokinase with vascular surgery as initial treatment for acute arterial occlusion of the legs. *N Engl J Med* 1998;338:1105–1111.

58. Pilger E, Decrinis M, Stark G, et al. Thrombolytic treatment and balloon angioplasty in chronic occlusion of the aortic bifurcation. *Ann Intern Med* 1994;120:40–44.

59. Ouriel K, Kandarpa K. Safety of thrombolytic therapy with urokinase or recombinant tissue plasminogen activator for peripheral arterial occlusion: a comprehensive compilation of published work. *J Endovasc Ther* 2004;11;4;436–446.

60. Silva JA, Ramee SR, Collins TJ, et al. Rheolytic thrombectomy in the treatment of acute limb-threatening ischemia: immediate results and six-month follow-up of the multicenter AngioJet registry. Possis Peripheral AngioJet Study AngioJet Investigators. *Cathet Cardiovasc Diagn* 1998;45:386–393.

61. Wagner HJ, Mueller-Huelsbeck S, Pitton MB, et al. Rapid thrombectomy with a hydrodynamic catheter: results from a prospective, multicenter trial. *Radiology* 1997;205:675–681.

62. Jean WJ, Al-bitar I, Bajwa TK, et al. High incidence of renal artery stenosis in patients with coronary artery disease. *Catheter Cardiovasc Interv* 1994;32(1):8–10.

63. Conlon PJ, Athirakul K, Kovalik E, et al. Survival in renal vascular disease. *J Am Soc Nephrol* 1998;9:252–256.

64. Conlon PJ, Little MA, Pieper K, et al. Severity of renal vascular disease predicts mortality in patients undergoing coronary angiography. *Kidney Int* 2001;60:1490–1497.

65. Kennedy DJ, Colyer WR, Brewster PS, et al. Renal insufficiency as a predictor of adverse events and mortality after renal artery stent placement. *Am J Kidney Dis* 2003;42:926–935.

66. Caps MT, Perissinotto C, Zierler RE, et al. Prospective study of atherosclerotic disease progression in the renal artery. *Circulation* 1998;98:2866–2872.

67. Caps MT, Zierler RE, Polissar NL, et al. Risk of atrophy in kidneys with atherosclerotic renal artery stenosis. *Kidney Int* 1998;53:735–742.

68. Hansen KJ, Starr SM, Sands RE, et al. Contemporary surgical management of renovascular disease. *J Vasc Surg* 1991;16:319–331.

69. Kidney D, Deutsch LS. The indications and results of percutaneous transluminal angioplasty and stenting in renal artery stenosis. *Semin Vasc Surg* 1996;9:188–197.

70. Lederman RJ, Mendelsohn FO, Santos R, et al. Primary renal artery stenting: characteristics and outcomes after 363 procedures. *Am Heart J* 2001;142:314–323.

71. Burket MW, Cooper CJ, Kennedy DJ, et al. Renal artery angioplasty and stent placement: predictors of a favorable outcome. *Am Heart J* 2000;139:64–71.

72. Rodriguez-Lopez JA, Werner A, Ray LI, et al. Renal artery stenosis treated with stent deployment: indications, technique, and outcome for 108 patients. *J Vasc Surg* 1999;29(4):617–624.

73. Rocha-Singh KJ, Mishkel G, Katholi RE, et al. Clinical predictors of improved long-term blood pressure control after successful stenting of hypertensive patients with obstructive renal artery atherosclerosis. *Catheter Cardiovasc Interv* 1999;47:167–172.

74. Dorros G, Jaff M, Mathiak L, et al. Four-year follow-up of Palmaz-Schatz stent revascularization as treatment for atherosclerotic renal artery stenosis. *Circulation* 1998;98:642–647.

75. White CJ, Ramee SR, Collins TJ, et al. Renal artery stent placement: utility in lesions difficult to treat with balloon angioplasty. *J Am Coll Cardiol* 1997;30:1445–1450.

76. Dorros G, Jaff M, Mathiak L, et al. Multicenter Palmaz stent renal artery stenosis revascularization registry report: four-year follow-up of 1,058 successful patients. *Catheter Cardiovasc Interv* 2002;55:182–188.

77. van Jaarsveld B, Krijnen P, Pieterman H, et al. The effect of balloon angioplasty on hypertension in atherosclerotic renal artery stenosis. *N Engl J Med* 2000;342:1007–1014.

78. Rocha-Singh K, Jaff MR, Rosenfield K. Evaluation of the safety and effectiveness of renal artery stenting after unsuccessful balloon angioplasty. The ASPIRE-2 Study. *J Am Coll Cardiol* 2005;46:776-783.

79. Mitchell J, Subramanian R, Stewart R, et al. Pressure-derived renal fractional flow reserve with clinical outcomes following intervention [abstract]. *Catheter Cardiovasc Interv* 2005;65:135.

80. Silva JA, Chan AW, White CJ, et al. Elevated brain natriuretic peptide predicts blood pressure response after stent revascularization in patients with renal artery stenosis. *Circulation* 2005;111:328–333.

81. Henry M, Klonaris C, Henry I, et al. Protected renal stenting with the PercuSurge GuardWire device: a pilot study. *J Endovasc Ther* 2001;8(3):227–237.

82. Murphy TP, Cooper CJ, Dworkin LD, et al. The Cardiovascular Outcomes with Renal Atherosclerotic Lesions (CORAL) Study: rationale and methods. *J Vasc Interv Radiol* 2005;16:1295–1300.

83. Rapp JH, Reilly LM, Quarfordt PG, et al. Durability of endarterectomy and antegrade graft in the treatment of chronic visceral ischemia. *J Vasc Surg* 1986;3:799–806.

84. Moawad J, McKinsey JF, Wyble CW, et al. Current results of surgical therapy for chronic mesenteric ischemia. *Arch Surg* 1997;132:613–619.

85. Furrer J, Grüntzig A, Kugelmeier J, et al. Treatment of abdominal angina with percutaneous dilatation of an arterial mesenteric superior stenosis. *Cardiovasc Intervent Radiol* 1980;3:43–44.

86. Maspes F, Mazzetti di Pietralata G, Gandini R, et al. Percutaneous transluminal angioplasty in the treatment of chronic mesenteric ischemia: results and three years of follow-up in 23 patients. *Abdom Imaging* 1998;23:358–363.

87. Matsumoto AH, Tegtmeyer CJ, Fitzcharles EK, et al. Percutaneous transluminal angioplasty of visceral arterial stenoses: results and long-term, clinical follow-up. *J Vasc Interv Radiol* 1995;6:165–174.

88. Sheeran SR, Murphy TP, Khwaja A, et al. Stent placement for treatment of mesenteric artery stenoses or occlusions. *J Vasc Interv Radiol* 1999;10(7):861–867.

89. Liermann D, Strecker EP. Tantalum stents in the treatment of stenotic and occlusive disease of abdominal vessels. In: Liebermann DD, ed. *Stents: State of the Art and Future Developments.* Watertown, MA: Boston Scientific; 1995:127–134.

90. Nyman U, Ivancev K, Lindh M, et al. Endovascular treatment of chronic mesenteric ischemia: report of five cases. *Cardiovasc Intervent Radiol* 1998;21:305–313.

91. Clouse WD, Hallett JW Jr, Schaff HV, et al. Improved prognosis of thoracic aortic aneurysms: a population based study. *JAMA* 1998;280:1926-1929.

92. Bickerstaff LK, Pairolero PC, Hollier LH, et al. Thoracic aortic aneurysms: a population based study. *Surgery* 1982;92:1103-1108.

93. Coady MA, Rizzo JA, Hammond GL, et al. Surgical intervention criteria for thoracic aortic aneurysms: a study of growth rates and complications. *Ann Thorac Surg* 1999;67:1922-1926.

94. Davies RR, Goldstein LJ, Coady MA, et al. Yearly rupture or dissection rates for thoracic aortic aneurysms: simple prediction based on size. *Ann Thorac Surg* 2002;73:17–27.

95. Makaroun MS, Dillavou ED, Kee ST, et al. Endovascular treatment of thoracic aortic aneurysms: results of the Phase II multicenter trial of the GORE TAG thoracic endoprosthesis. *J Vasc Surg* 2005;41(1):1-9.

96. Food and Drug Administration. Summary of safety and effectiveness: GORE TAG thoracic endoprosthesis. Available at: www.fda.gov/cdrh/pdf4/p040043.html.

97. Reed WW, Hallett JW Jr, Damiano MA, et al. Learning from the last ultrasound: a population-based study. *N Engl J Med* 1989;321:1009–1014.

98. Hallett JW Jr. Management of abdominal aortic aneurysms. *Mayo Clin Proc* 2000;75:395–399.

99. Hollier LH, Taylor LM Jr, Ochsner J. Recommended indications for operative treatment of abdominal aortic aneurysms: report of a subcommittee of the Joint Council of the Society for Vascular Surgery and the International Society for Cardiovascular Surgery. *J Vasc Surg* 1992;15:1046–1056.

100. Hallett JW, Marshall DM, Petterson TM, et al. Graft-related complications after abdominal aortic aneurysm repair: reassurance from a 36-year population-based experience. *J Vasc Surg* 1997;25:277–286.

101. Johnston KW. Canadian Society for Vascular Surgery Aneurysm Study Group. Nonruptured abdominal aortic aneurysm: six-year follow-up results from the multicenter prospective Canadian aneurysm study. *J Vasc Surg* 1994;20:163–170.

102. Parodi JC, Palmaz JC, Barone HD. Transfemoral intraluminal graft implantation for abdominal aortic aneurysms. *Ann Vasc Surg* 1991;5:491–499.

103. Zarins CK, White RA, Moll FL, et al. The AneuRx stent graft: four-year results and worldwide experience 2000. *J Vasc Surg* 2001;33:S135–S145.

104. Buth J, Laheij RJF. Early complications and endoleaks after endovascular abdominal aortic aneurysm repair: report of a multicenter study. *J Vasc Surg* 2000;31:134–146.

105. Zarins CK, White RA, Schwarten D, et al. AneuRx stent graft vs. open surgical repair of abdominal aortic aneurysms: multicenter prospective clinical trial. *J Vasc Surg* 1999;29:292–308.

106. May J, White GH, Yu W, et al. Concurrent comparison of endoluminal versus open repair in treatment of abdominal aortic aneurysms: analysis of 303 patients by life-table method. *J Vasc Surg* 1998;27:213–221.

107. EVAR Trial Participants. Endovascular aneurysm repair versus open repair in patients with abdominal aortic aneurysm (EVAR trial 1): randomised controlled trial. *Lancet* 2005;365:2179–2186.

108. Prinssen M, Verhoeven EL, Buth J, et al. A randomized trial comparing conventional and endovascular repair of abdominal aortic aneurysms. *N Engl J Med* 2004;351:1607–1618.

109. Blankensteijn JD, de Jong SE, Prinssen M, et al. Two-year outcomes after conventional or endovascular repair of abdominal aortic aneurysms. *N Engl J Med* 2005;352:2398–2405.

110. Solis J, Kumar A, Bajwa T. Endovascular aneurysm repair: safer alternative to open surgical repair in high risk patients. *Catheter Cardiovasc Interv* 2005;(suppl)65:152.

111. White GH, May J, Waugh RC, et al. Type I and type II endoleaks: a more useful classification for reporting results of endoluminal AAA repair. *J Endovasc Surg* 1998;5:189–193.

112. Zarins CK, White RA, Hodgson KJ, et al. Endoleak as a predictor of outcome after endovascular aneurysm repair. AneuRx multicenter clinical trial. *J Vasc Surg* 2000;32:90–107.

113. Nachbur BH, Inderbitzi RG, Bar W. Isolated iliac aneurysms. *Eur J Vasc Surg* 1991;5:375–381.

114. Richardson JW, Greenfield LJ. Natural history and management of iliac aneurysms. *J Vasc Surg* 1988;8:165–171.

115. Scheinert D, Schroder M, Steinkamp H, et al. Treatment of iliac artery aneurysms by percutaneous implantation of stent grafts. *Circulation* 2000;102:III-253–III-258.

116. Sahgal A, Veith F, Lipsitz E, et al. Diameter changes in isolated iliac artery aneurysms 1 to 6 years after endovascular graft repair. *J Vasc Surg* 2001;33:289–295.

117. Trickett JP, Scott RAP, Tilney HS. Screening and management of asymptomatic popliteal aneurysms. *J Med Screen* 2002;9:92–93.

118. Thompson MM, Sayers RD. Arterial aneurysms: companion to specialist surgical practice. Vol. 7. In: Berard JD. *Arterial Surgery.* London: WB Saunders; 1998.

119. Dawson I, Sie RB, van Bockel JH. Atherosclerotic popliteal aneurysm. *Br J Surg* 1997;84:293–299.

120. Michaels JA, Galland RB. Management of asymptomatic popliteal aneurysms: the use of a Markov decision tree to determine the criteria for a conservative approach. *Eur J Vasc Surg* 1993;7:136–143.

121. Tielliu IFJ, Verhoeven ELG, Prins TR, et al. Treatment of popliteal artery aneurysms with the Hemobahn stent-graft. *J Endovasc Ther* 2003;10:111–116.

PART 17 Social Issues and Cardiovascular Disease

CHAPTER (111)

Cost-Effective Strategies in Cardiology

William S. Weintraub / Harlan M. Krumholz

A SOCIETAL PERSPECTIVE

Healthcare expenditures in the United States have increased dramatically. Between 1965 and 2004, public healthcare expenditures increased from $10.2 billion to $600 billion, and total national expenditures increased from $40 billion to $1.90 trillion.[1] This change represents an increase in percentage of gross national product (GNP) from 5.1 to 16 percent (Fig. 111–1). Furthermore, following a period of stabilization in the mid- to late 1990s, growth in percentage of GNP devoted to healthcare is expected to rise to 20 percent of GNP by 2015.[1] This increase in expense is focusing ever greater attention on resource allocation in healthcare.

Cardiovascular disease consumes substantial societal resources in economically advantaged countries. In the United States alone, the American Heart Association estimates that the cost of cardiovascular disease in 2006 will total $403.1 billion[2] (Table 111–1). Of this total, $257.6 billion will be related to direct consumption of medical resources, and an additional $109.9 billion will be related to lost productivity because of early death and disability. Costs related to coronary artery disease (CAD) lead the other categories at $142.5 billion, a little more than one-third of the total. Given its magnitude, there is a strong societal interest that the $257.6 billion in direct costs be spent wisely and that the $109.9 billion in lost productivity be minimized. The field of healthcare economics has developed to guide decision-making.

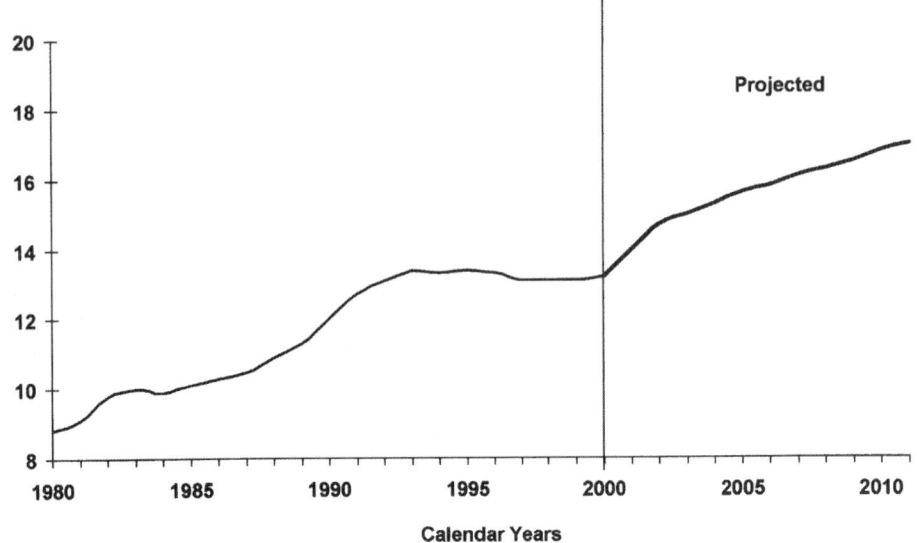

FIGURE 111-1. Increasing costs of medical services over time: national health expenditures as a share of the gross domestic product (GDP). Between 2001 and 2011, health spending is projected to grow 2.5 percent per year faster than the GDP, so that by 2011, it will constitute 17 percent of the GDP. *Source: Centers for Medicare and Medicaid Services, Office of the Actuary, National Health Statistics Group.*

BACKGROUND ON ECONOMIC ANALYSES

If resources were not limited, then medical care could be provided based on anticipated clinical effectiveness alone, no matter how small the benefit. In a world of inexhaustible resources, it would be reasonable to provide a treatment that benefited only 1 of every million or 10 million or 100 million individuals screened or treated. Because this is not the case, diagnostic testing and therapies should be justified based on their value. Within medicine, these issues are perhaps most relevant to cardiovascular care because of the vast array of diagnostic and therapeutic strategies as well as the high cost and the diversity of relevant outcomes.

Frequently, to understand the relative value of different approaches, the costs are compared between competing forms of therapeutic or diagnostic strategies.

TABLE 111-1

Estimated Direct and Indirect Costs (in Billions of Dollars) of Cardiovascular Diseases and Stroke, United States, 2006

	HEART DISEASE[a]	CORONARY HEART DISEASE	STROKE	HYPERTENSIVE DISEASE	HEART FAILURE	TOTAL CARDIOVASCULAR DISEASE[b]
Direct costs						
Hospital	$81.3	$41.8	$15.5	$6.2	$15.4	$114.8
Nursing home	20.7	10.9	14.3	4.2	3.9	42.6
Physicians/other professionals	19.7	11.1	3.1	11.0	2.0	38.3
Drugs/other medical durables	21.2	9.8	1.3	24.4	3.1	50.1
Home health care	5.2	1.6	3.1	1.7	2.4	11.8
Total Expenditures[b]	$148.1	$75.2	$37.3	$47.5[c]	$26.8	$257.6
Indirect costs						
Lost productivity/morbidity	21.9	9.6	6.4	7.7	NA[e]	35.6
Lost productivity/mortality[d]	88.5	57.7	14.2	8.3	2.8	109.9
Grand Total[b]	$258.5	$142.5	$57.9	$63.5	$29.6	$403.1

[a]This category includes coronary heart disease, congestive heart failure, part of hypertensive disease, cardiac dysrhythmias, rheumatic heart disease, cardiomyopathy, pulmonary heart disease, and other or ill-defined "heart" diseases.
[b]Totals may not add up because of rounding and overlap.
[c]Tom Hodgson and Liming Cai estimated that health care expenditures attributed to hypertension that could be allocated to cardiovascular complications and other diagnoses totaled $108 billion in 1997 (*Med Care* 2001;39:599–615).
[d]Lost future earnings of persons who will die in 2006, discounted at 3 percent.
[e]Not available.

SOURCES: Hodgson TA, Cohen AJ. Medical care expenditures for selected circulatory diseases: Opportunities for reducing national health expenditures. *Med Care.* 1999;37:994–1012.
National Health Expenditure Amounts, and Average Percent Change, by Type of Expenditure: Selected Calendar Years 1990–2013. Available at: www.hcfa.gov.
Rice DP, Hodgson TA, Kopstein AN. The economic cost of illness: a replication and update. *Health Care Finance Rev.* 1985;7:61–80.
Historic Income Tables—"People." Available at: www.census.gov.
Deaths for 358 Selected Causes by 5-Year Age Groups, Race, and Sex, United States, 2002. Available at: www.cdc.gov/nchs.
Ric DP, Max W, Michel M, Sung HY. Present value of lifetime earnings, U.S. 2003. Unpublished tables, Institute for Health and Aging, University of California, San Francisco, 2005.
All estimates by Thomas Thom, National Heart Lung, and Blood Institute.

This comparison can involve a simulation in which costs and outcome are estimated from various sources. Alternatively, an economic analysis can derive from a discrete calculation based on extensive primary data collection. For any design, the simplest type of economic study is a comparison of costs between two or more strategies, or a *cost-minimization study*. Such a study is most useful when it is reasonable to assume that two treatment or diagnostic arms offer similar outcomes.

When comparative strategies involve different costs and effects, then a different approach is required. There are three related analyses that are relevant: cost-effectiveness, cost-utility, and cost-benefit. *Cost-effectiveness analysis measures the cost per unit of effectiveness.*[3] This form of analysis assumes that there is one overall measure of effectiveness, often survival. This method is less useful when there are multiple distinct measures of effectiveness. For instance, one form of therapy increases the risk of death but improves symptomatic status. This situation can be addressed through *cost-utility analysis, in which all measures of effectiveness are incorporated into one measure called utility.*[3] Utility, however, is a very difficult parameter to measure, as discussed below. A third and somewhat less popular form of analysis is *cost-benefit analysis, in which measures of both cost and effectiveness except survival are reduced to a single measure, generally a specific currency.*[3] Although cost-benefit analysis has not been popular in medicine because of the inherent difficulty of expressing clinical outcome in monetary terms, it is, at least in theory, the most generalizable of these methods.

The perspective, or viewpoint, in these analyses can have an important impact on their structure and outcome. For example, an analysis from a hospital's perspective may not include the long-term consequences of a particular clinical strategy, whereas this issue can be the most important to the patient and the payer. Also, different stakeholders can place different values on the outcomes and costs of medical care.

To be most useful in serving societal goals, cost and cost-effectiveness analyses should be performed from a societal perspective, from which an economic analysis should attempt to measure all the costs and measures of outcome associated with a particular treatment. These costs should include those incurred by the patient, the costs of medical resources that could have been used for other patients, and any loss of income that the patient sustained because of poor health. Outcome should include events, taking into account quality of life and survival.

Although it is possible, in theory, to rank order the cost-effectiveness of multiple strategies into what are called *league tables*, limitations in data quality and variability in study design limit the wide applicability of such efforts.[4] An effort to create league tables was made in Oregon, with cost-effectiveness used to guide whether a form of therapy or a test would be funded. This experiment was criticized and finally abandoned because of the limited amount and quality of data available as well as concern over whether the approach was appropriate.[5]

Far more common are cost-effectiveness analyses that compare two alternative treatments for a single medical condition, for example, percutaneous coronary intervention (PCI) and coronary artery bypass grafting (CABG) for symptomatic angina. In addition to focusing on a single clinical condition, the analyses most commonly limit the measured costs to direct and some portion of indirect medical costs. The purpose of these analyses is usually not to dictate policy but to inform decision-making.

DETERMINING COSTS
【 】 TAXONOMY FOR COSTS

An economic perspective on cost is complex. Cost can be used to sum resource use when a procedure or test uses resources of several types, and to permit comparison of costs among services. Summing resource use to arrive at cost is done through cost accounting (Table 111–2).

Costs must be considered from one of several possible perspectives. For a hospital, the cost is the expenses to provide a service. For payers, the cost is what the providers charge, plus their administrative expenses. Cost studies often seek to determine societal costs, which should be used in cost-effectiveness analyses to gain the widest perspective. However, societal costs are never directly measurable, and thus combinations of cost proxies from one or several stakeholders, where measurable, are often used as estimates.

Costs are classified as direct or indirect. Theoretically, *direct costs* are those incurred by a stakeholder for a therapy or test, and *indirect costs* are those incurred by other societal groups. Generally, direct costs relate to the provision of medical care, whereas indirect costs are other societal costs, such as loss of productivity.

Medical costs for a major inpatient procedure such as coronary surgery can be divided into three components: inhospital direct costs, followup direct costs, and indirect costs. Inpatient costs comprise hospital costs (e.g., room, laboratory testing, pharmacy, etc.) and physician professional billings. Followup direct costs include physician office visits, outpatient testing, medications, home health providers, and additional hospitalizations. Indirect costs reflect lost patient or business opportunity and can be referred to as *productivity costs.*[6] Another way of thinking about costs is that direct costs are linked to a particular service, whereas indirect costs are not. This type of indirect cost is also called *overhead.*[7]

The appropriate length of time over which to measure costs depends on the procedures being studied and outcomes being measured. The cost of angioplasty could be considered to be the costs of the initial hospitalization and followup care for the first 6 months, when restenosis commonly would occur. Alternatively, the cost of angioplasty could be considered the initial hospitalization alone, and the costs during the initial 6 months could be considered followup

TABLE 111–2

Summary of Taxonomy for Costs

Cost perspective
    Provider, i.e., hospital or professional
    Payer, i.e., insurance carrier
    Patient
Cost category
    Direct costs
    Indirect costs
Accounting method
    Top-down
    Bottom-up
Costs per service
    Average cost
    Marginal (incremental) cost

or induced costs, which are those generated beyond the specific time of service delivery.[8] Induced costs also could be a savings. For instance, there can be savings for stents relative to balloon angioplasty in followup because of less additional revascularization.

What a hospital charges for a service is not its cost.[9] Measuring hospital cost is difficult and has been approached using what is called either *top-down* or *bottom-up accounting*.[10] Top-down costing involves dividing all the money spent on a hospitalization or procedure by the number of episodes of care of the particular type performed. In contrast, a bottom-up approach involves individually costing all resources used for a service, that is, supplies, equipment depreciation and facilities, salaries, and so on. All methods involve a set of assumptions and limitations. When the cost of a specific procedure using top-down costing is being considered, it must be assumed that costs in the department in which the procedure is provided can be separated from costs in other departments. However, it is not clear for example that the costs of the cardiac catheterization laboratory can be clearly separated from hospital maintenance costs. There can also be variability within a department. Therefore, using identical methods to calculate the costs of angioplasty and diagnostic catheterization may not be appropriate if angioplasty consumes more resources in a period of time, such as technician time. Bottom-up methods also are limited by the ability to account for all resources consumed and to appropriately apply costs.

Another issue in measuring hospital costs is average versus marginal or incremental cost.[11] Average cost is calculated by dividing all costs for a therapy or test by the number of that particular type. In contrast, the marginal cost is the cost of the next similar procedure. Average costs include all resources used, including overhead, which costs would not be decreased if not used. Marginal costing accepts fixed costs as a given and focuses only on additional resources consumed by each additional patient. Variable costs are separated analytically from fixed costs by establishing the perspective and time frame as fixed. For instance, facility cost is commonly considered fixed, but how should marginal personnel costs be assigned? If coronary surgery decreases as angioplasty becomes more common, nurses can remain on staff in the operating room, or can be assigned to other duties.

【 】 COST MEASUREMENT

There is a particularly detailed approach to top-down costing that is based on the UB92 summary of charges.[12] The UB92 is a uniform billing statement used by all third-party carriers. Charges are available for such services as the surgical suite, cardiac catheterization laboratory, intensive care unit, postoperative or postprocedural floor care, respiratory therapy, supplies, electrocardiography, telemetry, social services, and so on. Although hospitals will set their charges to maximize insurance reimbursements, the relationship between costs and charges, cost-to-charge ratios, must be developed using American Hospital Association guidelines and then filed annually with the Centers for Medicare and Medicaid Services (CMS) in the form of a hospital cost report, which is in the public domain.

An alternative approach is to use bottom-up cost accounting and assign cost weights to each type of resource used.[13] The sum of resources times their cost weights yields total cost. However, the methods are so laborious that they are rarely used.

Another approach is to use a payer perspective.[14] In the United States, Medicare diagnosis-related group (DRG) reimbursement

rates could be used to define cost. Similar methods are available in other countries. The use of DRGs to assign cost does not account for variation in cost within that DRG and may not even reflect average resource use. Although the DRG is an excellent measure of cost from the point of view of the payer, it may not represent as meaningful a proxy for societal cost as do provider-level hospital costs. Nonetheless, this approach has been used for cost-effectiveness analyses in multiple countries in international clinical trials.[15]

The assessment of professional medical costs is challenging. It is not sufficient to consider physicians' fees alone, because other professionals provide services.[16] The goal should be to capture all the professional services for a procedure. There is no cost-to-charge ratio, analogous to the situation for the hospital, available for physician fees to convert their charges to costs.

In the United States, there has been an effort to improve physician payments by developing a set of scales for the effort and complexity of skills required for each service.[17] This system, the resource-based relative value scale (RBRVS), was developed to measure the relative time, physical, and cognitive efforts associated with physician services.[17] Each service is assigned a number called the relative value unit (RVU). If the profile of physician services for a procedure or hospitalization is known, then RVUs for each service can be used to develop a proxy for the physician costs. The total RVUs can be converted to a dollar figure by the standard CMS conversion factor. The appeal of the RBRVS is that it is a relative weighting system that assigns unique weights for physician work and practice costs for each physician service by Current Procedural Terminology (CPT) code. As a result, after assigning a conversion factor, standardized estimates of the costs can be calculated and used as a gauge of physician costs. Although there is still some controversy about this approach and the values it attributes, it can overcome some of the major drawbacks of physician charge data. An alternative approach is to use published percent shares of hospital expenses by DRG for professional costs.[18]

Determining the costs of outpatient services presents different challenges in determining patient services use, including direct and indirect medical costs. Direct costs include physician office visits, medications, procedures and testing, rehabilitation, nursing-home stays, and home health services as well as patient out-of-pocket expenses, including travel. Assessment of these costs is difficult and complicated by insurance, because patients cannot be expected to report reliably exactly how much they paid out of pocket for services and how much the insurance company paid. Unless there is access to a comprehensive insurance claims database, the most reasonable approach is to have patients identify the services they have received. Costs can then be attributed to the individual services and medications. Office visits and other medical services costs can be similarly estimated. Professional services can be estimated using the Medicare fee schedule. Medication costs can be estimated by sampling pharmacies or using published wholesale pharmaceutical prices. Indirect productivity costs include missed time from work by the patient or family members. Followup indirect costs are probably the most difficult to determine and are often excluded as unmeasurable. In any case, it is not possible to measure all the indirect costs explicitly. For instance, if an executive in a company has coronary surgery and is out of work for 6 weeks, there may or may not be loss of pay, but the effect on the business cannot readily be quantified. Indirect costs, if measured at all, are often confined to family loss of income, and these numbers must be examined with both interest and skepticism.

Over a multiyear time horizon, inflation must be considered. Costs must be inflated or deflated by multiplying by a constant to convert from any one year to another, based on either the general or medical inflation rate.[19] Future costs also should be discounted to reflect the opportunity costs of current dollars, or future costs should be expressed at their present value.[20] For instance, if a policy maker were given the alternative of spending $1000 now or $1000 in 5 years to treat a given condition and obtain the same outcome, the decision should always be the latter. Costs are often discounted at a rate of 3 percent per year as a matter of convention.[20]

【 】 VARIATION IN COST

Variation in cost for a service arises from either differences in the type of measurement, as discussed earlier, or differences in resource use. Table 111–3 presents a framework for considering variation in medical costs, according to quality of care, patient, and geographic levels. These levels do not separate clearly, providing a somewhat confusing picture of the sources of variation.

Quality of care is often broken down into the subunits of process, structure, and outcome.[21] These components of quality can also be viewed as reflecting variation in cost. For process measures of access and appropriateness, the effect on cost can be less on the individual service and more at the societal level for provision of that service. Thus, if access to coronary surgery is inadequate, the initial cost to society of coronary surgery can decrease as fewer procedures are performed, but costs can increase because of lost productivity from failing to perform necessary surgery. However, if access to adequate diabetes care is inadequate, there can be an increase in the cost to society of inadequately treated diabetes. If inappropriate angioplasty is being performed, then the societal cost will increase, even if the individual service is little affected. How care is delivered will affect the individual service; variation in management will cause variation in cost.

Structure is related to cost. Facilities and supplies vary considerably in cost even within a single geographic location. Staffing can also vary in intensity. Outcome can also vary with quality of care. Complications can be iatrogenic and relate to quality of care and generally increase the cost of a service. Similarly, a patient's health status can vary with quality, which will affect induced productivity costs. Thus, if there is variation in relief from angina after revascularization because of variation in quality of care, then there can be variation in ability to return to work.

Patient-level factors—such as age, gender, and race—can affect cost as much as, or perhaps more than, quality of care. Age is similar to comorbidity, potentially raising cost. Disease severity can also affect costs. Thus it can cost more to perform coronary surgery or coronary angioplasty on patients with a recent acute myocardial infarction (MI) than on those without one.[22,23] Similarly, comorbidity can increase costs. *However, complications generally have a greater effect on costs than comorbidity or severity.*[22,23] Complications and health status outcomes related to patient-level factors are difficult to separate from complications and heath status outcomes related to quality of care.

Finally, variation in cost can be influenced by geographic and nonmedical economic factors such as land and construction costs, cost of living, and personnel availability.[24] Also, there can be variation in cost that is independent of both quality and geography. For

---

TABLE 111–3
Sources of Variation in Cost

QUALITY OF CARE

1. Process: access, appropriateness, management
2. Structure: facilities, supplies, staffing
3. Outcome: iatrogenic complications, patients' health status

PATIENT

1. Demographic: age, sex, race
2. Disease severity: extent of left ventricular dysfunction or severity of coronary atherosclerosis
3. Comorbidity: cardiac or noncardiac
4. Outcome: noniatrogenic complications, patients' health status

GEOGRAPHIC AND NONMEDICAL ECONOMIC FACTORS

1. Facilities
2. Supplies
3. Labor

---

example, hospitals organized into buying cooperatives may be able to purchase supplies at discount.

Because determining the specific cost of any service is difficult, cost estimates may not be generalizable outside the bounds of a particular study. In the same sense that effect sizes are considered subject to confidence intervals, cost estimates must be recognized as *estimates*. This limitation also applies to using cost measurements in cost-effectiveness analyses and in constructing league tables in which several cost-effectiveness analyses are compared.

COMPARING COSTS WITH OUTCOME

Determining therapeutic or diagnostic costs independent of patient outcome is not particularly helpful for making clinical decisions or setting policy. Measuring costs without considering outcomes would preclude judgments about the value of allocating resources in the healthcare system. The most extreme cost-minimization approach would be to stop offering medical services. However, the goal of the healthcare system is to optimize patient outcomes within resource constraints. Consequently, both costs and outcomes need to be considered. Although it is possible to relate cost to any measure of outcome, the most generalizable approach in medicine is cost-utility analysis based on patient preference.[25,26]

【 】 DETERMINATION OF PATIENT UTILITY AND QUALITY-ADJUSTED LIFE YEARS

In the treatment of cardiovascular diseases, it is unusual for one measurement of outcome to be sufficiently important such that all other outcome measures can be ignored. Although death overwhelms other outcome measures in importance, it is relatively infrequent over short periods of time for most conditions. Moreover, patients can consider some fates to be as unwelcome as death. Consequently, it is important to consider other outcomes such as MI, unstable angina, revascularization procedures, measures of quality of life, and return to work. In trials comparing percutaneous coronary intervention with coronary surgery, there was no difference in mortality.[27,28] Although surgery relieved angina somewhat better[29–36] at higher cost,[37] it was a disadvantage to the patient to have to undergo the surgery in the first place. Without some method to incorporate various measures of outcome, it can be difficult to make an informed choice. In principle, this task can be accomplished through the determination of patient utility.

The utility of a therapy or test is the sum of effects, both positive and negative, which accrues to a patient over time as a result of the procedure.[32] We can best consider the assessment of utility using a decision tree (Fig. 111–2). A decision tree takes a patient at a specific point and then considers all possible events up to some point in the future. In this model, branch points or nodes with squares represent choices, and nodes with circles represent chance events. In the simplified model shown, a single choice is made, and there are two possible outcomes for each choice. Each outcome is the sum of the utility of health state 1 times its probability plus the utility of health state 2 times its probability. If choices were this easy, then the ability to determine utility of diagnostic or therapeutic strategies would be simple. However, decision trees are almost never this simple. The decision trees for diagnostic tests tend to be much more complicated than those for therapeutics because a test can lead to additional tests or to a range of therapeutic alternatives. For any one treatment, there can be multiple possible health states, and the paucity of literature can make it difficult to determine the probability of different ones, much less their associated utilities.

Utility can change over time. After successful PCI, patients feel well and their utility increases, but then they can suffer restenosis, and their utility decreases. After a successful additional procedure, their utility increases again. After PCI not complicated by restenosis, their utility would be expected to increase. Ultimately, patients with or without restenosis can achieve the same utility, but patients who have the episode of restenosis will have suffered a period of decreased utility.

Utility measurement involves taking patient preference into account. One patient can dislike chest pain enough to be willing to undergo repeat procedures to relieve angina. Another patient can dislike the catheterization suite enough to be willing to put up with more angina. Utility can be measured using either a validated survey such as the Health Utilities Index[33] or the EQ-5D[34] or by directly assessing patient preference. These surveys have been validated against patient preference methods and are easy to administer. Patient preference methods ask patients directly to evaluate their current state of health and then evaluate what they would give up or risk to achieve perfect health. The patient preference

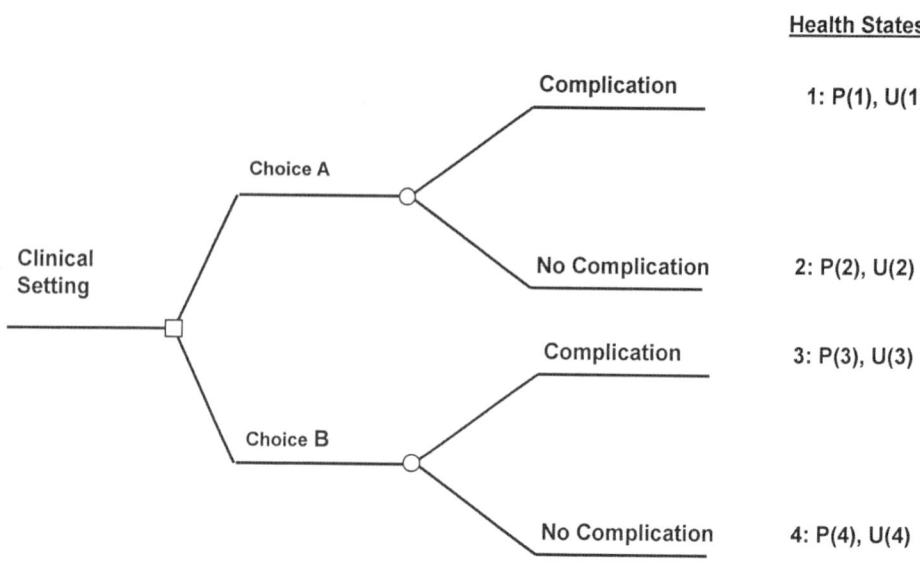

FIGURE 111–2. Idealized decision tree for a decision on diagnostic strategy or therapeutic choice. P, probability of health state; U, utility of health state.

methods are probably superior to surveys because the evaluation of a patient's view of his or her own state of health is measured directly, but patient preference methods are difficult to administer. The two patient preference methods are *time trade-off* and *standard gamble*.[3] In the time trade-off, patients weigh the fraction of expected survival they are willing to give up to live in perfect health instead of their current health. A patient with good health would presumably not trade any time whereas someone who was suffering might be willing to trade considerable time. The standard gamble is probably superior because it includes the element of risk.[3]

Utility alone does not provide a final summary measure of outcome because it does not include life expectancy. This summary measure can be determined using quality-adjusted life-years (QALYs), which are calculated by combining utility and survival.[35] Median or mean survival must be estimated from either the data set under consideration or from the literature. Survival is generally discounted, which means that patients value a year of survival at the present time more than a year of survival in the future. The appropriate discount rate for survival is unknown. Values in the literature for the discount rate have varied from 2 to 10 percent, with 3 percent being the most common.[20] *QALYs are the best summary measure of outcome in a cost-utility analysis because they incorporates patient value, risk aversion, expected survival, and a discount rate.*

COST-EFFECTIVENESS AND COST-UTILITY ANALYSIS

Once cost and a measure of outcome are available, it is relatively straightforward to determine cost-effectiveness. Fig. 111–3 offers an overview of an approach to integrate a range of outcomes including survival, health status assessment, and cost. We can begin to understand the approach of cost-effectiveness analysis by considering two competing therapies (or tests), A and B, to treat (or diagnose) the same condition (Fig. 111–4).[26] In quadrant 1, therapy A is more effective and more expensive than therapy B. In this situation, where one form of therapy or a test is both more ef-

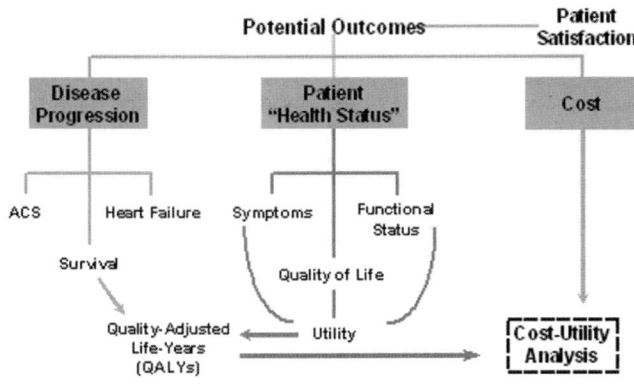

FIGURE 111–3. Integration of outcome measures, including survival, health status, and cost.

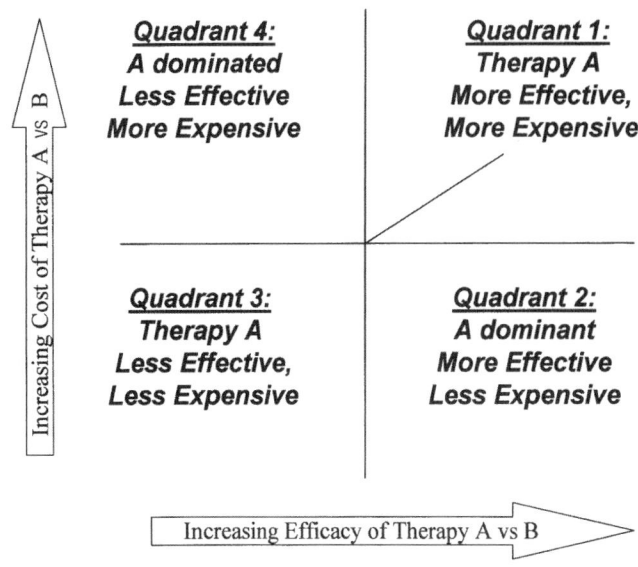

FIGURE 111–4. The cost-effectiveness plane. ICER in cost per life of QALY gained. ICER, incremental cost-effectiveness ratio; QALY, quality-adjusted life-year.

fective and more expensive than a competing therapy or test, cost-effectiveness analysis can help portray the resources required to achieve better health outcomes. In quadrant 2, A is both more effective and less expensive than B. In this setting, A is said to dominate B and is the obvious choice. In quadrant 3, B is more effective and more expensive than A. As in quadrant 1, cost-effectiveness analysis can help guide decision making. In quadrant 4, A is less effective and more expensive. In this quadrant, B would dominate. Returning to quadrant 1, the slope of the line at an acute angle represents a threshold or ceiling level in cost per unit of effectiveness. Below this line in quadrant 1 and in quadrant 2, choice A would be considered cost-effective.

Cost-effectiveness is the change in cost per unit increase in effectiveness. If the summary effectiveness measure is in QALYs—that is, a cost-utility analysis—then the marginal or incremental cost-effectiveness ratio (ICER) of therapy or test A compared with therapy or test B is described as the difference in cost between A and B divided by the difference in QALYs between A and B $[(\text{cost}_A - \text{cost}_B)/(\text{QALYs}_A - \text{QALYs}_B)]$.[36]

Cost-effectiveness analysis involves multiple assumptions in measuring both cost and outcome, which introduces uncertainty or error that is approached through sensitivity analysis. Measurements in which there is uncertainty are varied between appropriate values, and the analysis is repeated. The problem with sensitivity analysis is that the appropriate ranges for the variables may not be clear. For measurements made using several different scales, such as the multiple models for calculating marginal costs, these different scales can be used to perform the sensitivity analysis. For measurements that are continuous, such as professional charges, one standard deviation may be appropriate.

There is, however, no absolute standard for sensitivity analysis other than common sense and an intuitive feel for what is medically reasonable. If the results of a study vary significantly with changes in certain variables, then the outcome is said to be sensitive for those variables. Properly performed, sensitivity analyses should give insight into the medical decision-making process by identifying thresholds that result in changes in the process. This type of information, however, is difficult to convey to patients in actual practice.

When cost-effectiveness analysis is performed with data from clinical trials there is also stochastic error related to chance. Both measures of cost and effectiveness may not be normally distributed. The distribution of both can be assessed using *bootstrap*

methods.[31] Dual bootstraps for cost and effectiveness allow the ICER to be displayed in either the cost-effectiveness plane (Fig. 111–4), or as a cost-effectiveness acceptability curve.[26]

CURRENT AND FUTURE TRENDS AND POLICY IMPLICATIONS

To date, most cost-effectiveness analyses have been simulations. The formidable difficulties in determining cost and utility have limited the use of these tools in medical care. As the methods and science of cost-effectiveness analyses improve, these analyses can be integrated increasingly into clinical trials and observational databases. With the current changes in healthcare, accountability and cost are increasingly important, and we can expect to see more studies using these methods, and greater incorporation of cost-effectiveness analysis into the medical care delivery system.

The cost-effectiveness ratio or ICER, expressed in dollars per QALY, can be used, at least in principle, to affect societal choice regarding the use of scarce resources. A number that is often used, with inadequate justification, is that less than $50,000 per QALY, a procedure or form of therapy is economically attractive, whereas at more than $100,000 per QALY, it is expensive. These thresholds are historic and arbitrary, as society has rarely explicitly articulated levels that would guide the allocation of resources.

In addition to problems of measurement, there can be problems of the choice of the comparator; if a new therapy or test is not compared to the current standard, but to something more expensive or less efficacious, then the ICER can be artificially low. Thus, the common benchmarks should be seen as relatively rough numbers that policy makers can use; they do not represent empiric scientific levels, nor do they reflect thresholds for decisions in actual practice.

It is clear that using a single number, such as the ICER, for policy-making purposes is inappropriate because cost-effectiveness methods can vary considerably, despite recent efforts to create standards,[20] leading to different results. In addition, the cost-effectiveness ratio may not reflect the difference between small changes made for many people with an inexpensive form of therapy, and a big change for a few with expensive therapy. Finally, cost-effectiveness analysis does not adequately reflect the variability of patient populations. Policy planners, representing society, can choose to lower the threshold for a form of therapy for the young compared with the elderly, even though the impact of age is already included in the calculation of the ratio.

COST-EFFECTIVENESS IN PREVENTION, DIAGNOSIS AND THERAPY

[ ] HYPERLIPIDEMIA

Until recently, most estimates of the economic impact of lipid-lowering treatment have been based on decision-analytic models,[38–41] using data from epidemiologic studies such as the Framingham Heart Study. These models have not only incorporated certain assumptions about the effect of lipid lowering on prevention of cardiovascular events but also have had to include assumptions about resource use. However, several randomized trials have documented the benefit of lipid-lowering therapy and also analyzed its cost-effectiveness.

The advantages of lipid-lowering therapy have been clarified by several clinical trials in the United States and Europe. From the Scandinavian Simvastatin Survival Study (4S), a cost-effectiveness analysis was developed on the basis of resource use, with costs attributed to these resources.[42,43] The direct medical costs were estimated to range from approximately $4000 to $30,000 per year of life saved. Treatment was most cost-effective in older men with high baseline cholesterol levels and was least cost-effective in younger women with low baseline cholesterol levels. Inclusion of indirect costs lowered the estimated cost per life year gained (LYG) still further: the youngest patients had an estimated net savings, whereas elderly women with a baseline cholesterol level of 213 mg/dL had a cost of approximately $13,000 per year of life saved.

In the West of Scotland Coronary Prevention Study, a cost-effectiveness analysis based on outcomes data and resource use, the estimated cost per LYG (discounted 3 to 6 percent per year) ranged from $25,000 to $40,000 depending on risk group and model assumptions.[44]

With information derived from the Pravastatin Limitation of Atherosclerosis in the Coronary Arteries (PLAC I) and PLAC II studies, plus survival estimates 10 years post-MI from the Framingham study, Ashraf and colleagues[45] used a Markov decision-analytic model to estimate the cost-effectiveness of lipid-lowering therapy for secondary prevention. The cost ranged from $7124 to $12,665 for each LYG, depending on the patient's risk group.

The Heart Protection Study broadened the group of patients for whom treatment of low-density lipoprotein cholesterol (LDL-C) was appropriate.[46] Cost of preventing a major vascular event ranged from £4500 (95 percent confidence interval [CI] 2300–7400) in patients with a 42 percent 5-year major vascular event rate to £31,100 (22,900–42,500) in patients with a 12 percent rate (corresponding to 5-year major coronary event rates of 22 percent and 4 percent, respectively).[47] This study suggests that in patients at moderate risk, aggressive lipid-lowering therapy is cost-effective.

Compared with multiple clinical trials concerning low-density lipoprotein (LDL) lowering, there are less data on raising high-density lipoprotein cholesterol (HDL-C) levels and lowering triglyceride levels. In the Veterans Affairs HDL-C Intervention Trial (VA-HIT), gemfibrozil, an agent that raises HDL-C and lowers triglyceride, without affecting LDL-C, reduced major cardiovascular events (cardiovascular death, MI, and stroke) in patients with coronary heart disease, low HDL-C levels, and low LDL-C levels. The use of gemfibrozil, based on VA-HIT, was cost saving.[48] Using widely available prices, the ICER per QALY saved by gemfibrozil ranged from $6300 and $17,100.

For high-risk patients, for example, those whose LDL-C levels are increased after an acute MI, the cost-effectiveness of statin treatment is unquestioned. In lower risk groups, however, the cost-effectiveness is less clear. However, using a decision analytic model, Pignone and colleagues[49] have suggested that treatment with statins is cost-effective in patients without a prior cardiovascular event but with a 10 percent 10-year incidence of an event. Furthermore, Brandle and coworkers[50] suggested that statins would be cost-effective in patients with diabetes and LDL-C above 100 mg/dL. In none of the studies of lipid-lowering agents have the researchers considered patient preferences or QALYs.

A study by Pilote and colleagues demonstrated the issue of the economic attractiveness of lipid treatment for individuals and for society.[51] Using data from the Canadian Heart Health Survey, they showed that among those with an elevated cholesterol level, lipid-lowering therapy with simvastatin was cost-effective for 85.6 percent of men and 28.7 percent of women for primary prevention and 99.8 percent of the men and 86.1 percent of the women for secondary prevention. However, if implemented, the cost would exceed a billion dollars a year.

[ ] SMOKING CESSATION

According to the Centers for Disease Control and Prevention, cigarette smoking accounted for $75.5 billion in medical expenditures in 1998 as well as $92 billion in lost productivity.[52] Therefore, for each cigarette pack smoked, more than $2 (including approximately 90 cents derived from public funds) was spent for smoking-related medical care. These estimates are conservative as they do not consider the entire spectrum of cigarette-induced harm such as fires or smoke-related complications leading to premature childbirth.

In assessing short-term economic benefits related to a rapid decrease in acute MI and stroke after smoking cessation, Lightwood and Glantz[53] concluded that if a 7-year program reduced smoking prevalence by 1 percent per year, hospitalizations would decrease by 63,840 for acute MI and by 34,261 for stroke, saving approximately 13,000 lives and $3.2 billion.

Successful smoking-cessation programs are remarkably cost-effective relative to other medical interventions.[54,55] Cromwell and colleagues[56] found that, for smokers who successfully underwent a nonpharmatherapeutic intervention at a primary care clinic, the cost ranged from $2186 for group intensive counseling to $7922 for minimal counseling, and the cost per QALY was $1108 versus $4015 respectively. When pharmacotherapy was added, both the cost and the effectiveness of the intervention increased. With adjunctive transdermal nicotine treatment, the cost per QALY was

$1171 for group intensive counseling versus $2405 for minimal counseling. With nicotine gum, the respective costs were $1822 versus $4542. In a British decision-analytic study, Woolacott and coworkers[57] examined the cost-effectiveness of transdermal nicotine and bupropion treatment. Both methods proved both effective and cost-effective, the cost per year of life gained being £1000 to £2400 with transdermal nicotine, £640 to £1500 with bupropion, and £900 to £2000 with the combination.

For smokers with cardiovascular disease, smoking-cessation programs can be even more cost-effective than other interventions. Krumholz and colleagues[58] evaluated a nurse-based educational intervention for acute-MI survivors, finding the program's cost-effectiveness to be $220 per life year gained. Sensitivity analysis showed that the cost of a smoking-cessation program aimed at these patients would remain less than $20,000 per life year gained even if only 3 additional patients stopped smoking out of every 1000 enrolled (baseline assumption, 26 per 100 patients) or if the program cost up to $8840 for each smoker (baseline assumption, $100). These interventions should be equally valuable for other cardiovascular patients at high risk.

【 】 EXERCISE

Although exercise is widely recommended to prevent coronary artery disease, little information is available about its cost-effectiveness. In one study in this area, Jones and Eaton[59] used a decision-analytic model to construct hypothetical cohorts of sedentary 35- to 74-year-old individuals. Assuming that sedentary behavior incurs a relative risk of 1.9 for heart disease, these researchers concluded that $5.6 billion per year would be saved if 10 percent of adults started walking regularly. Moreover, if the entire sedentary population began a walking program, $4.3 billion could be saved, accounting for costs in individuals who dislike exercising. According to these baseline assumptions, walking has an economic benefit for men aged 35 to 64 years and women aged 55 to 64 years. The relative risk threshold at which walking offers an overall economic benefit is estimated to be 1.7, and for those who walk voluntarily, most adults would benefit even at a relative risk of only 1.15.

Hambrecht and Walther[60] compared PCI with exercise training in patients with stable coronary artery disease in a randomized trial of 101 male patients. The exercise training was 20 minutes of bicycle ergometry a day. The exercise program was associated with a significantly higher event-free survival at a lower cost than PCI.

【 】 DIABETES MELLITUS CONTROL

Diabetes mellitus is a major risk factor for cardiovascular disease, and glycemic control is essential to prevent complications[61] (see Chap. 90). Although the recommended glycosylated hemoglobin (HbA1c) level is less than 7 percent,[62] many patients fail to achieve this goal, incurring a need for additional medical care. According to an observational study of adults with diabetes enrolled in a large health maintenance organization, charges for medical care are strongly related to the HbA1c level[63]; for a 1 percent increase, charges can increase by 7 percent. For patients who have diabetes plus hypertension and heart disease, a 9 to 10 percent variation in the HbA1c level can entail a cost difference of more than $4000 over a 3-year period, even after adjustment for age, sex, and other chronic conditions.

Various interventions are aimed at improving glycemic control.[63] These interventions include closer monitoring, better patient education, more frequent telephone contact, increased clinical visits, and additional pharmacologic therapy, all of which entail substantial costs. The Diabetes Control and Complications trial[64] showed that in type I diabetes, intensive treatment decreased the risk of development or progression of retinopathy, nephropathy, and neuropathy by 50 to 75 percent. Over the lifetime of each patient, such treatment is approximately $30,000 more expensive than conventional therapy.[65] However, given the benefits, the cost-effectiveness of intensive intervention was estimated at $28,661 per life year gained. When quality of life is considered, the cost is reduced to $19,987 per QALY gained.

Similarly, the United Kingdom Prospective Diabetes Study, the largest and longest available study of type II diabetes, confirmed the importance of blood glucose control in preventing retinal and renal problems and perhaps also neurologic ones.[66,67] Although intensive treatment of these patients doubled the cost of their medical care, this increase was partly counterbalanced by a reduction in complications. The estimated cost-effectiveness of intensive treatment was estimated at $16,002 per QALY gained.

【 】 HYPERTENSION SCREENING AND THERAPY

Hypertension in the United States is estimated to cost $63.5 billion, including $16 billion for losses in wages and productivity.[2] The complications of hypertension drive the overall cost considerably higher. By preventing vascular events, screening for and treatment of hypertension will partially pay for themselves, yielding a favorable ICER.

More than 15 years ago, researchers at Stanford University[68] reported that screening for hypertension is economically advantageous for both men and women of all ages, comparing favorably with other widely used medical interventions in terms of cost-effectiveness. Because older adults, particularly men, tend to have high blood pressure, they have the most favorable ICERs (in 1990 dollars, $8374 per QALY for 60-year-old men). In contrast, 20-year-old women had the least favorable ICER ($44,412 per QALY). Krakoff and coworkers[69] have suggested that adding ambulatory blood pressure evaluation to office evaluation can improve diagnosis and outcome at lower cost.

Because so many strategies are available for the treatment of hypertension, the selection of a comparison group can be difficult. Among competing strategies, any one that is only more expensive than another, without showing an incremental benefit, will always be dominated. There is no proven benefit of current treatments for hypertension over inexpensive low-dose hydrochlorothiazide, and their use may be causing a waste of substantial resources.[70] The Seventh Joint National Committee report recommends diuretic agents or β blockers as initial choices for managing essential hypertension.[71] According to an economic analysis of the prior guidelines, a diuretic or β blocker can achieve and maintain blood pressure control much less expensively than a calcium-channel blocker or angiotensin-converting enzyme (ACE) inhibitor.[72] Nevertheless, ACE inhibition was particularly beneficial in the Heart Outcomes Prevention Evaluation (HOPE) trial, and the benefit appeared to extend further than blood pressure control.[73] Although an economic paper from HOPE has shown that the benefit of ACE inhibition could be achieved at no increase in costs,[74] a recent Markov model found that ACE inhibition as first-line therapy for blood pressure control never had an ICER of less than $100,000 per QALY gained.[75]

Montgomery and Fahey[76] performed an analysis that illustrated the role of underlying patient risk in the decision on how to treat hypertension. They employed a Markov decision analysis model and demonstrated that high-risk patients are the most cost-effective to treat. For low-risk patients, they suggest consideration should be given to preferences and cost.

ACUTE CORONARY SYNDROMES

[ ] REPERFUSION

The two earliest and largest trials of fibrinolytic therapy used streptokinase; this agent was the focus of early economic analyses[77,78] that found it was economically appealing over a wide spectrum of risk-benefit assumptions. According to one study, thrombolytic therapy can be cost saving because it decreases rehospitalization.[79]

After tissue plasminogen activator (t-PA) was introduced as a more costly but more effective alternative to streptokinase, investigators attempted to determine whether the incremental benefit was worth the incremental cost. According to the Global Utilization of Streptokinase and Tissue Plasminogen Activator for Occluded Arteries (GUSTO) trial results and the patients' estimated life expectancy, the additional life expectancy per t-PA recipient was 0.14 years. This yielded an ICER for t-PA versus streptokinase of $32,678 per year of life gained. However, the ICER varied, depending on the infarction site and patient age: younger and lower risk patients tended to have higher ICERs. A separate study, unrelated to GUSTO, yielded similar results.[80]

In randomized trials, percutaneous transluminal coronary angioplasty (PTCA) or percutaneous coronary intervention (PCI) with stenting has proved superior to pharmacologic thrombolysis in treating ST-segment elevation MI (STEMI). Economic analyses based on early studies showed that primary PTCA prevents death without increasing cost.[81] More recently, coronary stenting for acute STEMI was evaluated in the Primary Angioplasty in Myocardial Infarction (PAMI) Stent trial.[82] In the stent group, the index hospital costs were approximately $2000 higher, mainly because the stents were more expensive.[83] During the first year, however, fewer followup procedures were necessary, so the excess cost decreased by approximately half.

[ ] ANTITHROMBOTIC AGENTS

Aspirin reduces mortality and morbidity for patients with acute coronary syndromes (see Chap. 61). As a result of the marked benefit and the minimal cost of the therapy, no formal economic analysis of aspirin for the treatment of acute coronary syndromes has been published. However, in a decision-analytic model in patients who have not had a cardiovascular event, Pignone and colleagues[49] showed that in patients with a 7.5 percent 10-year incidence of a cardiovascular event, aspirin is cost-saving. The International Study of Infarct Survival (ISIS)-2 trial found that aspirin avoided 25 deaths for every 1000 patients with suspected acute MI.[84] In addition, the 1 month of aspirin therapy in ISIS-2 was associated with halving the risk of

stroke or reinfarction. Aspirin avoided approximately 10 reinfarctions and 3 strokes for every 1000 patients treated. The avoidance of complications would likely translate into cost savings, leading aspirin to be considered a *strongly dominant* therapy.

Heparin for the treatment of acute MI also has not been formally evaluated in an economic analysis. Given the uncertainty about its effectiveness, heparin would only be a favored therapy if there were evidence that heparin reduces cost.

Antiplatelet therapy with clopidogrel in 12,562 patients with unstable angina or non-ST elevation MI was studied in the Clopidogrel in Unstable Angina to Prevent Recurrent Ischemic Events (CURE) trial. A cost-effectiveness analysis used patient-level clinical outcomes and resource use from CURE, and estimates of life expectancy gains because of the prevention of the clinical events of death, stroke, and MI, based on data from Framingham and the Saskatchewan Health database.[85] Average total costs were $442 higher for the clopidogrel arm (95 percent CI: $62 to $820). The ICER based on Framingham is $6318 per life year gained (LYG) with clopidogrel, with 94 percent of bootstrap-derived ICER estimates less than $50,000/LYG; based on Saskatchewan, the ICER is $6475/LYG with 98 percent of estimates less than $50,000. These results were supported by a decision analytic model by Schleinitz and coworkers.[86] In the subgroup in CURE undergoing PCI, Mahoney and colleagues[87] found the incremental cost per year of life gained with clopidogrel for 1 year to range from $2856 to $4775 overall and from dominant to $935 for patients undergoing early PCI. In contrast, Gaspoz and colleagues found clopidogrel to be expensive for secondary prevention of coronary heart disease. However, the analysis was most sensitive to the price of the drug.[88]

Mark and coworkers[89] performed an economic analysis of low molecular weight heparin for a subset of patients enrolled in the Efficacy and Safety of Subcutaneous Enoxaparin in Non–Q-Wave Coronary Events (ESSENCE) study group.[89] Patients treated with enoxaparin had lower resource use during the initial hospitalization, and this benefit persisted at 30 days, with a cumulative cost savings associated with enoxaparin of $1172 ($p = 0.04$). The investigators concluded that enoxaparin both improves important clinical outcomes and saves money relative to therapy with standard unfractionated heparin, making it a strongly dominant therapy.

Platelet receptor glycoprotein IIb/IIIa inhibitors have found greatest use in patients with acute coronary syndromes undergoing PCI. An economic analysis of the EPIC trial found that the use of this therapy for high-risk patients was associated with a cost savings of $622 per patient during the initial hospitalization from reduced acute ischemic events.[90] During the 6-month followup, the therapy decreased repeat hospitalization rates by 23 percent ($p = 0.004$) and repeat revascularization by 22 percent ($p = 0.04$), producing a mean $1270 savings per patient (exclusive of drug cost) ($p = 0.018$). If the cost of the drug were less than $1270, then the strategy would be effective and cost saving.

The Randomized Efficacy Study of Tirofiban for Outcomes and Restenosis (RESTORE) trial found that in patients undergoing coronary angioplasty for acute coronary syndromes, tirofiban protects against early adverse cardiac events related to abrupt closure.[91] A subsequent economic analysis reported that the use of tirofiban (including drug costs) was not associated with an increase in healthcare costs.[92] A formal cost-effectiveness analysis of glycoprotein IIb/IIIa blockade for balloon angioplasty showed improved cost-effectiveness in higher risk patients.[93]

Neither of these studies directly examined the use of this agent in patients with acute ischemic syndromes. This was specifically addressed in the Platelet Glycoprotein IIb/IIIa in Unstable Angina: Receptor Suppression Using Integrilin Therapy (PURSUIT) trial, in which 10,948 patients with acute coronary syndromes were randomized to eptifibatide versus placebo, revealing an absolute 1.5 percent decrease in the composite of death or MI at 30 days with active therapy. In an economic analysis of 9461 patients in the United States, the costs were similar in the two arms, exclusive of drug costs. The ICER for eptifibatide therapy in U.S. PURSUIT patients was $16,491 per year of life saved and $19,693 per added quality-adjusted life-year.[94] It should be noted that in PURSUIT the clinical benefit to eptifibatide was shown only in patients who subsequently were treated with an invasive strategy, which would lower the cost-effectiveness ratios in these patients.

INVASIVE VERSUS CONSERVATIVE STRATEGIES IN NON–ST-SEGMENT ELEVATION ACUTE CORONARY SYNDROMES

The relative value of an invasive strategy with early catheterization and possible revascularization compared with a conservative strategy with exercise testing in patients with unstable angina or non–ST-segment elevation acute MI has been studied in several clinical trials, with more recent studies showing an advantage to an invasive approach.[95–98] The Treat Angina with Aggrastat and Determine Cost of Therapy with Invasive or Conservative Strategy (TACTICS) Thrombolysis in Myocardial Infarction (TIMI)-18 study found better outcome with an invasive approach with a primary end point of 19.4 percent with an conservative approach and 15.9 percent with an invasive approach. Initially the invasive approach was more costly, but at 6 months the difference was only $586 (95 percent CI: –$1087, $2486).[99] Estimated cost per life year gained for the invasive strategy, based on projected life expectancy, was $12,739, with a range of between $8371 and $25,769 depending on model assumptions.[99]

β-BLOCKER THERAPY

β-Blocker therapy has been shown to reduce mortality following an acute MI.[100] Goldman and colleagues[101] conducted the most widely cited economic analysis of the costs and effectiveness of β-blocker therapy. For a 45-year-old man with low risk, the ICER was $23,457, with medium risk it was $5890, and with high risk it was $3623.

ANGIOTENSIN-CONVERTING ENZYME INHIBITION

Several large randomized trials have demonstrated a reduction in acute MI for patients with left ventricular dysfunction after an acute MI who are treated with an ACE inhibitor.[102] Tsevat and coworkers[103] examined the cost-effectiveness of this intervention using resource use, survival, and health-related quality of life information from the Survival and Ventricular Enlargement (SAVE)

trial, a randomized trial of captopril for survivors of an anterior MI with an ejection fraction (EF) of 40 percent or less. The investigators conservatively estimated that the benefit of captopril did not persist beyond 4 years. The trial found that captopril improved survival at 3.5 years by approximately 20 percent. Costs were calculated in 1991 dollars. The ICER ranged from $60,800 per QALY gained for 50-year-old patients to $3600 for 80-year-old patients. McMurray and colleagues[104] also found that ACE inhibitors are an economically attractive intervention after MI.

REHABILITATION

In a decision-analytic model, Ades and coworkers[105] studied the cost-effectiveness of cardiac rehabilitation to coordinate exercise training and secondary prevention after acute MI (see Chap. 67). Cardiac rehabilitation participants had an incremental life expectancy of 0.202 years. In 1988, the average cost of rehabilitation and exercise testing was $1485, partially offset by averted cardiac rehospitalizations of $850 per patient. An ICER of $2130 per year of life saved was determined for the late 1980s, projected to a value of $4950 per year of life saved in 1995. A sensitivity analysis was conducted to support these findings.

Yu and colleagues evaluated the cost-effectiveness of cardiac rehabilitation for patients with a recent acute myocardial infarction (AMI) or PCI based on a randomized trial of 269 patients.[106] They compared an 8-week exercise and education program with standard therapy without an exercise program. The intervention was associated with $640 dollars saved per QALY gained.

REVASCULARIZATION
SOCIETAL BURDEN

Revascularization, either by CABG or PCI, represents an expensive form of therapy for the treatment of angina pectoris and, in some patients, the prolongation of life. The societal burden is substantial with more than 515,000 CABG and more than 657,000 PCI procedures performed in 2002.[107] PCI has increased by 324 percent since 1987. The total cost is unknown, but if CABG costs approximately $30,000 and PCI approximately $15,000, then something more than 25 billion dollars is being spent annually on revascularization in the United States alone.

TECHNICAL IMPROVEMENTS

The evaluation of cost as well as cost-effectiveness of these procedures is complicated by technological improvements and changes in the delivery of healthcare. In addition, care maps and other efforts to improve efficiency have dramatically decreased the incidence of complications, shortened length of stay, and cut costs.[19,108] Just as these improvements may not be reflected in published clinical trials concerning outcomes, the available cost-effectiveness analyses also do not entirely reflect either technologic improvements nor increased efficiency in healthcare delivery.

Coronary surgery has improved in recent years with greater use of arterial grafts, improved anesthesia and cardioplegia, and the introduction of less invasive coronary surgery. Outcome and costs in 1996 dollars in 12,266 patients undergoing coronary bypass surgery between 1988 and 1996 at Emory University were evaluated.[19] Mean hospital cost decreased from $22,689 to $15,987, and postoperative length of stay decreased from 9.2 to 5.9 days. After accounting for other variables, cost decreased by $1118 per year and length of stay by 0.55 days per year. A more recent improvement has been the introduction of off-pump coronary surgery. In the SMART trial 200 patients were randomized to on-pump versus off-pump coronary surgery, with results suggesting better outcome at lower cost with off-pump surgery.[109]

PCI also has improved, especially with the introduction of coronary stents. Stent procedures have improved with better deployment and less need for full anticoagulation. Improvements in PCI between 1990 and 1997 in 1997 dollars were investigated in 17,399 patients undergoing PTCA at Emory University.[110] Mean hospital cost decreased from $9816 to $7442 ($p < 0.0001$), and the length of stay after the procedure decreased from 2.81 to 2.00 days ($p < 0.0001$).

Some technologic improvements have been specifically subjected to economic analyses. The use of stents was compared with balloon angioplasty in the STRESS trial.[111] In this relatively early evaluation of stents, there was less additional revascularization and less restenosis with stents but no difference in survival. Costs were higher with stents, because of the prolonged hospitalization and full anticoagulation. A purely theoretical paper has suggested that a therapy costing in the range of $1000 that decreases restenosis after coronary angioplasty by 50 percent could offer a cost-effectiveness ratio of $16,000 per QALY.[112] Using data from the Controlled Abciximab and Device Investigation to Lower Late Angioplasty Complications (CADILLAC) trial, Bakhai and colleagues found that primary stenting was economically attractive compared with balloon angioplasty for patients with STEMI.[113] The cost-effectiveness ratio was $11,237 per QALY.

The major advance in preventing restenosis has been the introduction of the drug-eluting stent (DES).[114–116] In the SIRIUS trial,[115] 1058 patients undergoing elective coronary stent implantation were randomized to a bare metal stent or the sirolimus DES and then followed up for 1 year. Initial hospital costs were higher in the sirolimus stent arm ($11,345 versus $8464, $p < 0.001$), entirely caused by the difference in cost between the stents ($2900 versus $900).[117] However, because of fewer repeat revascularizations, the followup costs were lower in the Sirolimus stent arm. Thus, at 1 year there was little difference in cost, at $16,813 with the Sirolimus DES and $16,504 with bare metal ($p = 0.64$). The ICER in cost per repeat revascularization avoided was $1650. Utility was not measured in SIRIUS, but was imputed from an external source. The ICER in cost per QALY gained was $27,540, with 63 percent of estimates less than $50,000 per QALY gained. Bagust and Grayson[118] examined the cost-effectiveness of DES versus conventional stents based on data from the United Kingdom. They found that DES was not cost-effective except for a minority of the patients at high risk of needing repeat revascularization. Kaiser and colleagues,[119] in another European study using data from actual practice, also reported that the higher costs of DES were not offset by lower downstream costs and suggested that DES be restricted to high risk groups.

Antiplatelet therapy is necessary to prevent thrombosis with intracoronary stents. The Clopidogrel for the Reduction of Events During Observation (CREDO) trial found improved outcome if clopidogrel was continued for a full year.[120] The cost-effectiveness clopidogrel for 1 year was established by Beinart and colleagues,[121] using data from the CREDO trial, finding an ICER of $2929 to $4353 per LYG. This was supported by a decision-analytic model by Cowper and coworkers.[122]

[ ] CORONARY SURGERY VERSUS PERCUTANEOUS CORONARY INTERVENTION

In the Emory Angioplasty Versus Surgery Trial (EAST), Weintraub and colleagues[29] examined the inhospital and 3-year costs of patients randomized to revascularization with coronary surgery or coronary angioplasty. Although the inhospital costs of surgery were higher than those of angioplasty, there was little difference in 3-year costs. This was because of the need for additional procedures in many of the angioplasty patients.

Bypass Angioplasty Revascularization Investigation (BARI)[123] was a multicenter trial with 1829 patients and included prospective information on economic costs and quality of life in 934. The initial cost of angioplasty was $21,113 and coronary surgery was $32,247 ($p < 0.001$).[124] However, by 5 years, the costs were much closer, $56,225 for angioplasty and $58,889 for surgery ($p = 0.047$). The costs were surprisingly and disturbingly high in both treatment arms, and there was considerable overlap. The BARI trial showed that CABG dominated PTCA for treated diabetics with three-vessel disease. In the analysis at 10 to 12 years after randomization, CABG had a cost-effectiveness ratio of $14,300 per year of life saved compared with PCI.[125]

Two European randomized trials of PTCA and CABG have included economic end points: the Randomized Intervention Trial of Unstable Angina (RITA)[124,126] of 1011 patients and the German Angioplasty Bypass Surgery Investigation (GABI) trial[127] of 358 patients. In the GABI trial, the initial procedural costs were $16,562 for CABG and $5000 for PTCA. After 1 year, the authors found that there was little increase in cumulative costs in the CABG group, whereas the cumulative costs for the PTCA group were $11,250.[128] Similar results were found in the RITA trial, where initially there were much higher costs in the CABG group, but by 2 years the cumulative costs in the PTCA group were 80 percent of those for the CABG group.[129] Cost at 3 years in the Argentine Randomized Trial of Percutaneous Transluminal Coronary Angioplasty Versus Coronary Artery Bypass Surgery in Multivessel Disease (ERACI) also was higher in the CABG group than in the PTCA group but had narrowed from inhospital costs.[130]

Other than for treated diabetics in the BARI trial, there are inadequate data to perform a cost-effectiveness analysis comparing PTCA with CABG from any of the trials to date because the difference in symptomatic status makes it necessary to include utility assessment. There are three more contemporary trials comparing PCI with stents to CABG: Arterial Revascularization Therapies Study (ARTS) in Europe and Israel, ERACI II in Argentina, and Stent or Surgery (SOS) in Europe and Canada. In ARTS there was similar mortality between the two arms, but more repeat revascularization after PCI. The inhospital costs averaged $10,652 with CABG and $6441 with PCI, a difference of $4212 ($p < 0.001$). This difference narrowed because of repeat revascularization in the PCI arm to a 1-year cost of $13,638 with CABG and $10,665 with PCI, a difference of $2973 ($p < 0.001$).[131] In SOS one year mortality was 2.5 percent in the PCI arm and 0.8 percent in the CABG arm ($p = 0.05$). There was no difference in the composite of death or Q-wave MI. There were more repeat revascularizations with PCI. There was no significant difference in utility between arms at 6 months or 1 year, and QALYs were similar. Initial length of stay was longer with CABG (12.2 vs. 5.4 days, $p < 0.0001$), and initial hospitalization costs were higher (£7,321 vs. £3,884, Δ = £3,437, 95 percent CI Δ: £3,040 to £3,848). At 1 year the cost difference narrowed, but costs remained higher for CABG (£8,905 vs. £6,296, Δ = £2,609, 95 percent CI Δ: £1,769 to £3,314).[37]

[ ] PERCUTANEOUS CORONARY INTERVENTION VERSUS MEDICINE

PTCA has been compared with medicine in three randomized trials, Angioplasty Compared to Medical Therapy Evaluation (ACME),[110] Atorvastatin Versus Revascularization Treatment (AVERT),[132] and RITA II.[133] All showed less angina with PTCA. AVERT and RITA II found more cardiovascular events with angioplasty. However, these trials have been small, underpowered to examine hard end points, and have largely included low-risk patients. None included a formal cost or cost-effectiveness analysis. In the ongoing Clinical Outcomes Utilizing Aggressive Drug Evaluation (COURAGE) trial, a larger cohort of 2287 higher-risk patients, all treated with the best available medical therapy, were randomized to PCI with medicine versus medicine alone.[133a] COURAGE includes a formal cost-effectiveness analysis with utility assessment by direct patient preference. There was no difference in event rates.[134] Economic results are expected in 2007.

ELECTROPHYSIOLOGY
[ ] PATIENT MONITORING, PUBLIC ACCESS DEFIBRILLATORS

Monitoring involves multiple areas, including Holter monitoring, cardiac event recording, and monitoring in the hospital. Event recorders were compared with a 48-hour monitor in a randomized trial by Kinlay and coworkers[135] using a randomized crossover trial design in 43 patients with palpitations. Event monitors were twice as likely to provide a diagnostic rhythm strip ECG during symptoms as the 48-hour monitor. Event monitors dominated continuous monitors with cost savings.

Defibrillators in public places have become popular in recent years. Walker and colleagues[136] created a decision analytic model to determine the cost-effectiveness of putting defibrillators in all major airports, railway stations, and bus stations throughout Scotland. They found the ICERs to exceed $50,000 per QALY saved. They suggest that public defibrillators are a poor value for improving survival after prehospital cardiopulmonary arrest. Cram and colleagues examined the cost-effectiveness of in-home automated external defibrillators.[137] They found that most scenarios were not economically attractive, particularly for individuals with a 4 percent annual or lower probability of sudden cardiac death. Nichol did report that it is economically attractive to allow defibrillation by targeted nontraditional responders in high-risk settings, expanding the reach from emergency medical services personnel.[138]

Ultimately these analyses demonstrate that the economic case for these strategies is very dependent on the incidence of arrests in the areas where they are deployed.

[ ] INTRACARDIAC CARDIOVERTER-DEFIBRILLATORS

Intracardiac cardioverter-defibrillators (ICDs) have become widely used to prevent sudden cardiac death in patients at high risk (see Chap. 46). The cost-effectiveness of this therapy has been investigated with decision-analytic models as well as within the context of randomized trials. Kupersmith and coworkers[139] investigated the cost-effectiveness of ICD implantation using a decision-analytic model The ICER was $31,100 per year of life saved. At an EF of less than 25 percent and greater than or equal to 25 percent, the ICER was $44,000 and $27,200 per year of life saved. Endocardial ICDs became popular at the time of this study and decreased the cost-effectiveness ratio to $25,700 per year of life saved.

Owens and colleagues[140] also developed a decision-analytic model, but with a different construction and a somewhat different question. Specifically, ICDs were compared with amiodarone in patients at high or intermediate risk using a highly detailed model with event rates from the literature and costs estimated from published cost rates in California.[141] In high-risk patients, if an ICD reduces total mortality by 20 percent, the marginal cost-effectiveness of an ICD relative to amiodarone was $74,400 per QALY saved. If an ICD reduces mortality by 40 percent, the cost-effectiveness of ICD use was $37,300 per QALY saved, with the results sensitive to assumptions about quality of life. Decision-analytic models were noted by Larsen and coworkers[141] and Kupermann and colleagues.[142] In these studies, the cost-effectiveness of treatment with an ICD was better than that noted by Owens and coworkers[140] at $30,500[142] and $47,700[140] per LYG, adjusted to 1995 dollars. However, the study by Owens and colleagues[140] considered the more superior antiarrhythmic agent amiodarone.

In a small, randomized trial conducted by Wever and coworkers,[143] 60 consecutive postinfarct survivors of sudden cardiac death were randomly assigned either ICD as first choice or antiarrhythmic drugs and guided by electrophysiologic testing. The ICER for an ICD compared with drug therapy was $11,315 per LYG by early ICD implantation. If quality-of-life measures are taken into account, the ICER of early ICD implantation was even more favorable. A cautionary note came from O'Brien in the 430 patient Canadian Implantable Defibrillator Study (CIDS) trial, which evaluated ICD implantation in patients post–ventricular tachycardia or fibrillation, finding an ICER of Can $213,543 per life-year gained, and Can $108,484 for patients with an EF under 35 percent. However, In a more recent analysis based on the Antiarrhythmics Versus Implantable Defibrillator (AVID) trial of patients with life threatening arrhythmias, Larsen and coworkers[144] found costs at 3 years of $71,421 for a patient taking antiarrhythmic drugs and $85,522 for a patient with an ICD, which provided a 0.21-year incremental survival benefit. The base-case ICER was thus $66,677 per year of life saved.

Cost-effectiveness of ICD compared with conventional therapy from the Multicenter Automatic Defibrillator Implantation Trial (MADIT) was reported by Mushlin and colleagues,[145] based on 181 patients randomized in the United States. The discounted survival was 3.46 years for the ICD group and 2.66 years for the conventional therapy group to 4 years of followup and was associated with an ICER of $27,000 (95 percent CI, $200 to $68,200) per LYG. The results probably would have been more favorable if all patients had been treated with endocardial implants.

The potential application of ICDs was greatly expanded by MADIT-II, which demonstrated a survival in patients with an EF of 30 percent or less after an acute MI.[146] It has been estimated that this could double the potential indications for ICDs.[147] Al-Khatab and coworkers used data from GUSTO-IIb and the Duke database to estimate the ICER at $50,500 per LYG.[148] The ICER was sensitive to the efficacy of the ICD.

The indications were further expanded by the results of the Sudden Cardiac Death in Heart Failure Trial (SCD-HeFT), which showed that ICDs reduced all-cause mortality rates compared with medical therapy alone in patients with stable, moderately symptomatic heart failure. Based on SCD-HeFT, Mark and colleagues[149] found that for ICD relative to medical therapy, the ICERs (discounted at 3 percent) were $38,389 per life-year saved and $41,530 per QALY saved. ICERs of <$100,000 were obtained in 99 percent of 1000 bootstrap repetitions. For New York Heart Association class II, the ICER was $29,872 per LYG, whereas there was incremental cost without incremental benefit in class III.

Sanders and coworkers[150] summarized the data from the eight trials that evaluated whether ICD improves survival in patients at risk for sudden death because of left ventricular systolic dysfunction but who have not had a life-threatening ventricular arrhythmia using a Markov model. ICD use increased lifetime costs in every trial. Two trials, the Coronary Artery Bypass Graft (CABG) Patch trial and the Defibrillator in Acute Myocardial Infarction Trial (DINAMIT), found that an ICD did not reduce the risk of death. In six trials, the Multicenter Automatic Defibrillator Implantation Trial (MADIT) I, MADIT II, the Multicenter Unsustained Tachycardia Trial (MUSTT), the Defibrillators in Non-Ischemic Cardiomyopathy Treatment Evaluation (DEFINITE) trial, the Comparison of Medical Therapy, Pacing, and Defibrillation in Heart Failure (COMPANION) trial, and the SCD-HeFT, an ICD added 1.01 to 2.99 QALY and $68,300 to $101,500 in cost. The base-case ICER in these six studies ranged from $34,000 to $70,200 per QALY gained. Sensitivity analyses showed that the ICER was less than $100,000 per QALY gained if an ICD reduced mortality for seven or more years. ICDs are expensive, but as they are life saving with rather large gains in life years, the ICERs are from borderline to favorable.

❬ ❭ RADIOFREQUENCY ABLATION

Radiofrequency ablation (RFA) can be curative of supraventricular arrhythmias and offers the potential for dominating older forms of therapy (see Chap. 44). This was studied in a small group of patients by Kalbfleisch and colleagues.[151] The authors determined charges for radiofrequency catheter modification of the atrioventricular (AV) node in 15 patients with symptomatic AV-node reentrant tachycardia despite pharmacologic therapy and compared these charges with the estimated healthcare charges by the same patients before the catheter procedure was performed. The estimated cost of healthcare use for these 15 patients before cure of AV-node reentrant tachycardia was $7651 per patient per year. Al-

though small in scale, this study reflects the dominance of RFA. A similar costing study from Australia of RFA compared with continued medical therapy also showed the dominance of the procedure.[152] RFA in 20 patients was compared with surgical treatment in 20 patients and medical therapy in 12 patients in the nonrandomized comparison. RFA dominated medical therapy. Surgical therapy was slightly more efficacious, but at a much higher cost.[153]

A more sophisticated decision-analytic model was created by Hogenhuis and coworkers.[153] In four groups of patients with Wolff-Parkinson-White syndrome, those with (1) prior cardiac arrest, (2) paroxysmal supraventricular tachycardia or atrial fibrillation (PSVT/AF) with hemodynamic compromise, (3) PSVT/AF without hemodynamic compromise, and (4) no symptoms, the authors developed a cost-effectiveness analysis examining five clinical management strategies: (1) observation, (2) observation until a cardiac arrest dictates the need for therapy, (3) initial drug therapy guided by noninvasive monitoring, (4) initial RFA, and (5) initial surgical ablation. A model was developed that included the risks of cardiac arrest, PSVT/AF, drug side effects, procedure-related complications and mortality, the efficacy of drugs and RFA, and cost. RFA was assumed to have an overall efficacy of 92 percent in preventing cardiac arrest and arrhythmias. The model predicted that RFA would yield life expectancy greater than or equal to other strategies. In cardiac arrest survivors and patients who have had PSVT/AF with hemodynamic compromise, the model suggested that RFA would prolong survival at a lower cost. For patients with PSVT/AF without hemodynamic compromise, the ICER of attempted RFA ranged from $6600 for 20-year-olds to $19,000 for 60-year-olds per QALY gained. However, for asymptomatic patients, RFA costs ranged from $174,000 for 20-year-olds to $540,000 for 60-year-olds per QALY gained.

❬ ❭ PACEMAKERS

There is a paucity of cost-effectiveness data concerning pacemakers. This may be so because in the classic indication of heart block they are so clearly life-saving that there can be little doubt about their cost-effectiveness. Some effort has gone into resource utilization issues. Stamato and colleagues[154] performed a cost-minimization study in which they showed that charges and probably costs will be lower with implantation in a catheterization laboratory as opposed to the operating room. The cost-effectiveness of dual-chamber DDD pacing compared with single-chamber VVI pacing was studied using a decision-analytic model by Sutton and Bourgeois.[155]

Over a 10-year period, a computer model calculated the incidence and prevalence of atrial fibrillation, stroke, permanent disability, heart failure, and mortality in the following patient categories: sick sinus syndrome paced VVI, sick sinus syndrome and atrioventricular block upgraded to DDD, sick sinus syndrome paced DDD from the outset, atrioventricular block paced VVI and those upgraded to DDD, and atrioventricular block paced initially DDD. Survival and functional capacity were improved with DDD pacing both for sick sinus syndrome and for atrioventricular block. DDD pacing also was less expensive in the long term, with healthcare costs in followup being a number of times more expensive than the pacemaker. In appropriate patients, DDD pacing dominates VVI pacing.

The use of dual chamber compared to ventricular pacing has also been studied by Rinfret and coworkers.[156] Based on data from a 2010-patient randomized trial combined with a decision analytic model, dual-chamber pacing was projected to have an ICER of approximately $6800 dollars per QALY gained, with 91.9 percent of bootstrap simulations less than $50,000 dollars per QALY gained.

ATRIAL FIBRILLATION

The major risk of atrial fibrillation is embolic stroke. The cost-effectiveness of anticoagulation was considered using a decision-analytic model by Gage and coworkers.[157] The authors obtained the probabilities of adverse outcomes from trials involving anticoagulation for nonvalvular atrial fibrillation. They noted a 22 percent reduction in ischemic stroke with aspirin therapy from a metaanalysis[158] and a 68 percent reduction with warfarin therapy from the atrial fibrillation investigators' collaborative analysis of five clinical trials.[159] The authors obtained utility estimates by interviewing 74 patients with atrial fibrillation, using the time trade-off method for three degrees of severity of stroke and for daily therapy with aspirin or warfarin. Costs were estimated, based on the literature. For patients at medium risk of stroke (i.e., patients with atrial fibrillation and one additional stroke risk factor, including a history of stroke, transient ischemic attack, hypertension, diabetes, or heart disease), the ICER of warfarin therapy as compared with aspirin therapy was $8000 (range, $200 to $30,000) per QALY. Both warfarin and aspirin dominated no therapy. For patients at low risk of stroke (i.e., isolated atrial fibrillation), quality-adjusted life expectancy was 6.70 years with warfarin therapy, 6.69 years with aspirin therapy, and 6.51 years with no therapy. The ICER of warfarin over aspirin was $370,000 per QALY saved in the base case. If the annual rate of stroke were 0.5 percent higher in low-risk patients, warfarin treatment would cost $66,000 per QALY. Aspirin dominated no therapy.

In a decision-analytic model from Sweden, Gustafsson and colleagues[160] found that anticoagulation dominated no therapy, and in a decision-analytic model from the United Kingdom, Lightowlers and McGuire[161] found anticoagulation to be cost-effective and dominate no therapy in higher-risk patients.

Recent efforts have focused on strategies for managing cardioversion, antiarrhythmic therapy, and anticoagulation. Eckman and coworkers[162] constructed a decision-analytic model considering the base case of a 65-year-old man with nonvalvular atrial fibrillation. Cardioversion followed by a combination of amiodarone and warfarin was the most effective strategy, yielding a gain of 2.3 QALYs compared with no therapy. The ICER of cardioversion followed by aspirin with amiodarone was $33,800 per QALY and without amiodarone was $10,800 per QALY. Cardioversion followed by amiodarone and warfarin an ICER of $92,400 per QALY compared with amiodarone and aspirin. Catherwood[163] constructed a similar decision-analytic model considering multiple strategies involving cardioversion followed by aspirin, amiodarone, and warfarin. Strategies involving cardioversion dominated no cardioversion. For patients at high risk of stroke (5.3 percent per year), cardioversion alone followed by repeated cardioversion plus amiodarone therapy on relapse was cost-effective at $9300 per QALY compared with cardioversion alone followed by warfarin therapy on relapse. This strategy also was preferred for moderate-risk patients (3.6 percent per year), but with a higher cost-effectiveness ratio of $18,900 per QALY. In the lowest-risk patients (1.6 percent per year), cardiover-

sion alone followed by aspirin therapy on relapse was preferred. Efforts to assess cost-effectiveness of methods for cardioversion have been cast in some doubt by the Atrial Fibrillation Follow-up Investigation of Rhythm Management (AFFIRM) trial in which patients were randomized to rhythm versus rate control and then followed for 3.5 years. In AFFIRM there was no advantage or a trend to worse outcome to attempting to control rhythm for fatal and non-fatal events as well as quality of life.[164] Patients in the rate-control group used fewer resources, costing $5077 less per person than rhythm control. Rate control was less costly and more effective than rhythm control in 95 percent of bootstrap simulations over a wide range of cost assumptions.

Assuming that there is still reason to consider cardioversion, another issue concerning the care of patients with atrial fibrillation is the role of transesophageal echocardiography in avoiding prolonged anticoagulation prior to cardioversion. This was investigated using a decision-analytic model by Seto and colleagues.[165] The authors studied the cost-effectiveness of three strategies: (1) conventional therapy with transthoracic echocardiography and warfarin therapy for 1 month before cardioversion, (2) initial transthoracic echo followed by transesophageal echo and early cardioversion if no thrombus was detected, and (3) initial transesophageal echo with early cardioversion if no thrombus is detected. With strategies 2 and 3, if a thrombus was seen, a followup transesophageal echo was performed. If no thrombus was seen, cardioversion was performed. All strategies used anticoagulation before and extending for 1 month after cardioversion. Life expectancy, utilities, event probabilities, and cost were ascertained from the literature. Strategy 3 (cost, $2774; QALYS, 8.49) dominated strategy 2 (cost, $3106; QALYs, 8.48) and conventional therapy (cost, $3070; QALYs, 8.48). The study demonstrated that transesophageal echo-guided cardioversion dominated conventional therapy if the risk of stroke after transesophageal echo negative for atrial thrombus is slightly less than that after conventional therapy. Cardioversion with transesophageal echo versus Coumadin for one month was also studied in the Assessment of Cardioversion Using Transesophageal Echocardiography (ACUTE) trial, which found no difference in embolic rates between the two approaches.[166] However, the transesophageal echocardiography (TEE)-guided strategy had a shorter time to cardioversion and a lower rate of composite bleeding. Cost was evaluated in 833 of the 1222 patients from 53 U.S. sites. At 8-week followup, total mean costs did not differ significantly between the two groups, respectively ($6508 TEE-guided $6239 conventional, $p = 0.50$).

Atrial fibrillation is a frequent complication of cardiac surgery, which can prolong length of stay. Using the Emory cardiovascular database as well as the medical literature, Mahoney and coworkers[167] showed that in high risk patients, such as those undergoing combined coronary and valve surgery, pretreatment with amiodarone to prevent atrial fibrillation can be cost-effective.

HEART FAILURE
PERSPECTIVE

Heart failure differs from other areas of consideration in this chapter because it is a disease process rather than a single form of therapy or service. Patients have a baseline health state, with associated baseline continuing costs for medication and office visits as well as productivity costs. The patient can then decompensate, resulting in a hospitalization, presumably with a somewhat worse health state and associated costs. Efforts will then be made to return the patient to his or her baseline health state and maintain him or her there. Finally, patients can be considered for transplantation to try to reverse or partially reverse heart failure, also with associated cost.

SCREENING

There are few studies on screening patients for heart failure. Heidenreich and colleagues[168] constructed a decision analytic model to evaluate screening for depressed EF with B-type natriuretic peptide (BNP) followed by echocardiography for abnormal tests, finding an ICER of $22,300 per QALY gained for men and $77,700 for women.

DIGOXIN

Despite more than 200 years of experience, the role of digoxin in the treatment of congestive heart failure remains uncertain. In the absence of adequate clinical data, the cost-effectiveness data similarly will be limited. Nonetheless, Ward and coworkers[169] developed a decision-analytic model concerning digoxin withdrawal in patients with stable heart failure. The clinical sequelae of digoxin withdrawal came from the Prospective Randomized Study of Ventricular Failure and Efficacy of Digoxin (PROVED) and Randomized Assessment of Digoxin and Inhibitors of Angiotensin-Converting Enzyme (RADIANCE) trials.[170,171] Costs were estimated from hospital and Medicare data. Outcomes included treatment failures, digoxin toxicity, and healthcare costs. Continuation of digoxin therapy in patients with heart failure nationally would avoid 185,000 office visits, 27,000 emergency visits, and 137,000 hospital admissions for heart failure, but with 12,500 cases of digoxin toxicity. The net annual savings would be $406 million (90 percent confidence interval, $106 to $822 million). Sensitivity analysis showed that digoxin is cost saving if the incidence of digoxin toxicity is 33 percent or less. Thus digoxin therapy was found to dominate withdrawal of digoxin in stable heart failure.

Based on data from a large randomized trial study, the DIG trial, Eisenstein and colleagues[172] found that digoxin was cost saving compared to placebo in 27 percent of bootstrap samples using Medicare costs (mean $12,648 versus $12,362) and in 44 percent of samples using commercial carrier costs (mean $17,400 versus $17,306). Digoxin was cost saving in >50 percent of samples for several higher-risk patient subgroups.

ANGIOTENSIN-CONVERTING ENZYME INHIBITION

The efficacy of ACE inhibition in preserving left ventricular size and in prolonging survival in patients with heart failure has been well established in a series of clinical trials. Glick and coworkers[173,174] developed a decision-analytic model based on the Studies of Left Ventricular Dysfunction (SOLVD) trial, in which 2569 patients with symptomatic heart failure and EFs of 35 percent or less received either the ACE inhibitor enalapril or placebo. Costs were estimated based on CMS reimbursement rates in 1992 dollars. For patients with heart failure, enalapril dominates pla-

cebo in the short term and is highly economically attractive in the long term. Enalapril saved approximately $717 per patient over the period of the SOLVD treatment trial. When trial data were projected over a patient's lifetime, therapy with enalapril produced an ICER of $115 per QALY gained. As pointed out by Boyko and colleagues,[175] there is variation in the cost of ACE inhibitors, and as these agents become less expensive, their cost-effectiveness ratio can become even more attractive.

The cost-effectiveness of ACE inhibition also has been studied in Europe using decision-analytic techniques. In mild heart failure, Kleber[176] found ACE inhibition to be cost-effective but not cost saving. However, in the Netherlands, van Hout and coworkers[177] found ACE inhibition to dominate not using ACE. Similarly, in a study from the United Kingdom based on SOLVD, Hart and colleagues[178] found that ACE therapy potentially could dominate not using ACE therapy.

ALDOSTERONE BLOCKADE

Aldosterone blockade with spironolactone in the setting of chronic heart failure in the Randomized Aldactone Evaluation Study (RALES) trial, and eplerenone in the setting of heart failure after acute MI in the Eplerenone Post-Acute Myocardial Infarction Heart Failure Efficacy and Survival Study (EPHESUS) trial have both been shown to decrease mortality.[179,180] Spironolactone during 35 months followup in RALES increased quality-adjusted survival time without increasing costs.[181] Spironolactone therapy either dominated placebo or had an ICER unlikely to exceed $20,300 per QALY gained. In EPHESUS, 6632 patients with left ventricular systolic dysfunction and heart failure after acute MI were randomized to eplerenone or placebo and followed up for a mean of 16 months. The evaluation of resource use included hospitalizations, outpatient services, and medications. Survival beyond the trial period was estimated from data from the Framingham Heart Study, the Saskatchewan Health database, and the Worcester Heart Attack Registry. Cost was $1391 higher over the trial period in the eplerenone arm (95 percent CI, 656 to 2165) because of drug cost. The ICER was $13,718 per life-year gained with Framingham (96.7 percent under $50,000 per life-year gained), $21,876 with Saskatchewan, and $10,402 with Worcester.[182] The analysis did not include a comparison with spironolactone, which is a less expensive alternative to eplerenone.

ISOSORBIDE DINITRATE AND HYDRALAZINE

Recently isosorbide dinitrate and hydralazine therapy was found to be beneficial for the treatment of heart failure in black patients. An economic analysis by Angus and colleagues[183] revealed that within the African-American Heart Failure Trial (A-HeFT) that the combination therapy reduced costs and improved outcomes compared with placebo. The benefit was largely because of the reduction in hospitalizations.

β BLOCKADE

Recently, β blockade, especially with carvedilol, has been added to the therapeutic armamentarium for heart failure. There have been four randomized trials in 1094 patients with New York Heart Association class II to IV symptoms and left ventricular EF of 0.35 or less.[184] The series of trials was terminated early, based on a finding of a 65 percent mortality reduction in patients receiving carvedilol (95 percent CI, 39 to 82 percent). Delea and coworkers[185] constructed a decision-analytic model estimating life expectancy and healthcare costs for patients with heart failure receiving carvedilol plus conventional therapy (digoxin, diuretics, and ACE inhibitors) or conventional therapy alone. Benefit estimates were based on the carvedilol trial results, assuming either "limited benefits" persisting for 6 months, the average duration of followup in the clinical trials, or "extended benefits" persisting for 6 months and then declining gradually over 3 years. For conventional therapy alone, estimated life expectancy was 6.67 years, and for carvedilol it was 6.98 and 7.62 years, assuming limited and extended benefits, respectively. Expected lifetime costs of heart failure–related care were estimated at $28,756 for conventional therapy and $36,420 and $38,867 for carvedilol, assuming limited and extended benefits, respectively. Cost per LYG for carvedilol was $29,477 and $12,799 under limited and extended benefits assumptions, respectively. Thus the cost-effectiveness of carvedilol remains in a reasonable range but is not as attractive as ACE inhibition.

【 】 DISEASE MANAGEMENT STRATEGIES

Heart failure is particularly well suited to developing strategies, such as the development of heart failure clinics, to improve management. Despite the difficulties in mounting trials to evaluate outcome of management strategies is, several small efforts have been made. Rich and colleagues[186] conducted a randomized trial using a nurse-directed, multidisciplinary intervention on readmission rate within 90 days of hospital discharge, quality of life, and costs for elderly patients admitted to the hospital with heart failure. In a subgroup of 126 patients, quality-of-life scores at 90 days improved more from baseline in the treatment group ($p = 0.001$). Because of the reduction in hospital admissions, the total cost of care was $460 less per patient in 1994 dollars in the treatment group, confirming strong dominance for the management strategy.

Kornowski and coworkers[187] analyzed outcome of 42 patients aged 78 ± 8 years with New York Heart Association congestive heart failure class III or IV who were examined at home weekly by local internists and a trained paramedical team. This study showed improved outcome but at an uncertain tradeoff in resource use between increased home visits and decreased hospitalizations for the intervention.

West and colleagues[188] used a strategy of physician-led but nurse-managed, home-based heart failure management not involving home visits. Compared with 1 year before enrollment, hospitalization rates for heart failure and for all causes declined 87 and 74 percent ($p = 0.001$). This strategy improved clinical outcome for heart failure while reducing resource use, again suggesting strong dominance.

【 】 HEART TRANSPLANTATION AND NEW DEVICES

Heart transplantation remains sufficiently infrequent, with just 2057 in the United States in 2002, that its overall impact on cost from a public health standpoint is small. The cost of the initial hospitalization from transplantation to discharge has been estimated at $91,600, with an annual followup cost of perhaps $20,000.[107,189] Cardiac transplantation has not been subjected to rigorous cost-effectiveness analysis, perhaps because of inadequate natural history data with which to compare transplant patients. In a somewhat preliminary, and now dated study, Evans[190] showed that overall cost-effectiveness of heart transplant was estimated at $44,300 per year of life saved.

Recent clinical trial have shown the efficacy of new therapies such as left ventricular assist devices (LVADs),[191] and biventricular pacing with cardiac resynchronization therapy (CRT).[192] Nichol and coworkers developed a Markov model to assess the incremental cost-effectiveness of CRT, discounting future costs and effects 3 percent. All outcome data were from the medical literature. Compared to medical therapy, the median ICER for CRT was $107,800 (interquartile range, $79,800 to $156,500) per QALY gained. Results were sensitive to key variables, including the relative risk or death and hospitalization. Feldman and colleagues,[193] based on data from the COMPANION trial, found that CRT by means of pacemaker (CRT-P) or pacemaker-defibrillator (CRT-D) in combination with optimal pharmacologic therapy (OPT) was economically attractive compared with OPT alone. Nichol and colleagues[194] reported that resynchronization therapy had an incremental cost per QALY of approximately $100,000 per QALY.

The cost of LVADs were evaluated by Moskowitz and coworkers.[195] In "bridge-to-transplantation" patients, first-year costs averaged $222,460, which is somewhat comparable to transplantation. Establishing cost-effectiveness will require more experience and additional economic evaluations.

DIAGNOSIS AND SCREENING

Establishing the cost-effectiveness of diagnostic testing is considerably more difficult than it is for therapeutics because testing itself rarely affects outcome. Rather, diagnostics generally lead to a range of choices of therapeutic options with the potential for very different outcomes. Thus decision-analytic models with diagnostics tend to be more complicated than with therapeutics, and consequently, the uncertainty is much greater. Randomized trials with diagnostics are also quite unusual. Thus, the cost-effectiveness analyses that exist are all decision-analytic simulations.

【 】 TESTING FOR CORONARY ARTERY DISEASE

Garber and Solomon[196] evaluated the cost-effectiveness of noninvasive testing and coronary angiography without prior noninvasive testing in the diagnosis of CAD. The tests evaluated included treadmill exercise ECG, planar thallium imaging, single-photon-emission computed tomography, stress echocardiography, and positron-emission tomography, all followed by coronary angiography, if positive, and finally, direct coronary angiography. Survival was based on the medically or surgically treated patients in the Coronary Artery Surgical Study (CASS) study. Based on a meta-analysis of trials comparing angioplasty with medicine, surgery was assumed to have 1.6 times the ability of angioplasty to relieve symptoms. Sensitivities and specificities of testing were developed from a meta-analysis of the literature.

Little difference in life expectancy was noted with the various strategies, but somewhat more variation to QALYs because the calculation of QALYS gives credit to strategies that improve symptoms rapidly. Nonetheless, the differences amounted to a couple of weeks over approximately 12 years in men and 14 years in women. Costing was based on Medicare payments.

Single-photon emission computed tomography (SPECT) had higher QALYs at higher cost than stress echocardiography with a marginal cost-effectiveness ratio of $64,000 in 65-year-old men to nearly $150,000 in 45-year-old women. Positron emission tomography (PET) generally produced slightly better outcomes than SPECT but at much greater cost. Although immediate angiography dominated PET in every group, immediate angiography was more expensive than SPECT with a margin from approximately $80,000 in 65-year-old men to nearly $200,000 in 45-year-old women.

Strategies in which patients are neither tested nor treated initially are not no-cost strategies, because patients can experience an MI and undergo medical or surgical treatment in the future. Thus the cost-effectiveness of stress echocardiography compared with no testing ranges from $31,000 per QALY in 65-year-old men to $98,000 per QALY in 45-year-old women.

With a different prevalence of disease, the ranking of tests changes somewhat. For 55-year-old men with a 75 percent pretest risk for disease, initial angiography becomes more attractive (it will be chosen whenever a cost-effectiveness ratio of $45,000 is acceptable), and stress echocardiography remains preferable to exercise testing (with an ICER of $22,000 per QALY). At a 25 percent prevalence of disease, echocardiography seems to be the most attractive test under most circumstances; SPECT would be chosen over echocardiography only if an ICER of $110,000 is considered acceptable, and immediate angiography would be chosen over SPECT only an ICER of $355,000. Thus stress echocardiography remains a cost-effective strategy at a wide range of prevalence of disease, whereas immediate angiography is a cost-effective choice when the pretest probability of disease is high.

Somewhat similar analyses have been offered by Kim and colleagues[197] and Kuntz and coworkers.[198] The study by Kim and colleagues[197] specifically studied women. In a 55-year-old woman with definite angina, angiography without prior noninvasive testing was found to be appropriate, with an ICER of $17,000 per QALY. This figure increases as the probability of angina decreases, and in the midrange of probabilities, echocardiography was felt to be preferable. In the study by Kuntz and coworkers,[198] the ICER of direct coronary angiography compared with exercise echocardiography was $36,400 per QALY in a 55-year-old man. For 55-year-old men with atypical angina, exercise echocardiography compared with exercise electrocardiography at a cost of $41,900 per QALY. If exercise echocardiography was not available, exercise SPECT cost $54,800 per QALY gained compared with exercise electrocardiography. For a 55-year-old man with nonspecific chest pain, the cost-effectiveness of exercise electrocardiography compared with no testing was $57,700 per QALY gained.

These studies can be criticized easily for making multiple assumptions. However, the end result is quite reasonable. In patients with chest pain in the intermediate range of probabilities, a test that includes myocardial imaging, either echocardiography or SPECT, is appropriate, with echo more appropriate in the lower probability range and SPECT in the higher probability range. Immediate angiography is appropriate as the probability of disease rises. In lower-risk populations, a treadmill exercise test is probably appropriate, and ultimately, in very low-risk populations, in the single digits of pretest probability, reassurance and watchful waiting would be the strategy of choice.

【 】 SCREENING FOR CORONARY CALCIUM

The newest test to diagnose coronary artery disease is CT angiography. There is not yet enough experience with this test to evaluate cost-effectiveness. There is considerably more experience using calcium scoring to evaluate risk of future events. There have been several attempts to assess the cost-effectiveness of electron-beam computed tomography (EBCT). O'Malley and colleagues constructed a decision analytic model of the additional of coronary calcium scoring to the Framingham risk index.[199] The base case assumed that any coronary calcium would increase the relative risk fourfold. Multiple additional assumptions were made, most of which are uncertain. The base case offered an ICER of $86,752 for a 42-year-old subject, which was sensitive to the gain in life expectancy for early intervention, the utility of being at risk and the added prognostic value of the calcium score. This analysis was updated using the hazard ratio from the Prospective Army Coronary Calcium project, finding an ICER of $31,500.[200] This analysis also remained limited by the underlying assumptions. Shaw and coworkers[201] developed a similar decision-analytic model, finding that in individuals with risk or coronary events below 0.6 percent year the ICER approached $50,000, but was $42,339 if the event rate was 1 percent per year and $30,742 if the event rate was 2 percent per year. This model was also highly dependent on the underlying assumptions. Although the several efforts to understand the cost-effectiveness of coronary calcium scoring have been made, the models were not, and could not be sufficiently well grounded in data to offer results suitable for medical decision making or establishing public policy.

CONCLUSIONS

Healthcare economics offer a powerful set of tools for establishing cost and overall measures of outcome and relating cost to outcome. These tools have been used increasingly in cardiovascular medicine for the purposes of gaining greater insight to facilitate improved patient management but also to help guide public policy. These tools have been applied widely now in cardiovascular medicine, with peer-reviewed literature on cost and often cost-effectiveness analysis, in most areas of cardiovascular medicine. However, the methods of measurement and analysis have varied widely, limiting the ability to compare studies and thus generalize the findings. A recent effort in the United States should provide a guide to investigators performing cost-effectiveness analyses to perform them in a more standard manner.[20] The quality of data available in many areas probably poses a greater problem. Over time, however, the quality of data and of scholarship should increase, making economic studies ever more meaningful and relevant to the practice of medicine.

REFERENCES

1. Centers for Medicare and Medicaid Services. Available at: http://www.cms.hhs.gov/NationalHealthExpendData/02_NationalHealthAccountsHistorical.asp#TopOfPage.
2. Thom T, Haase N, Rosamond W, et al. Heart disease and stroke statistics—2006 update: a report from the American Heart Association Statistics Committee and Stroke Statistics Subcommittee. *Circulation.* 2006;113(6):e85–151.
3. Drummond MF, O'Brien B, Stoddart GL, Torrance GW. *Methods for the Economic Evaluation of Health Care Programmes.* Oxford: Oxford Medical Publications; 1987.
4. Winkelmayer WC, Cohen DJ, Berger ML, Neumann PJ. Comparing cost-utility analyses in cardiovascular medicine. In: Weintraub WS, ed. *Cardiovascular Health Care Economics.* Totowa, NJ: Humana Press; 2003:329–356.
5. Borna S, Sundaram S. An approach to allocating limited health resources. *J Health Soc Policy.* 1999;11(2):85–94.
6. Boccuzzi SJ. Indirect health care cost: an overview. In: Weintraub WS, ed. *Cardiovascular Health Care Economics.* Totowa, NJ: Human Press; 2003:63–79.
7. Evans D. Principles involved in costing. *Med J Aust.* 1990;153:S10–S12.
8. Hlatky MA. Analysis of costs associated with CABG and PTCA. *Ann Thorac Surg.* 1996;61(2 suppl):S30–32; discussion S33–34.
9. Finkler SA. The distinction between cost and charges. *Ann Intern Med.* 1982;96(1):102–109.
10. Finkler SA. *Essentials of Cost Accounting for Health Care Organizations.* 2nd ed. Gaithersburg, MD: Aspen Publications; 1999.
11. Hlatky MA, Lipscomb J, Nelson C, et al. Resource use and cost of initial coronary revascularization. Coronary angioplasty versus coronary bypass surgery. *Circulation.* 1990;82(5 suppl):IV208–213.
12. Weintraub WS, Mauldin PD, Talley JD, et al. Determinants of hospital costs in acute myocardial infarction. *Am J Manag Care.* 1996;2:977–986.
13. Lefebvre C, Van Der Perre T. Activity based costing. *Acta Hospitalia.* 1994;34:5–16.
14. Coulam RF, Gaumer GL. Medicare's prospective payment system: a critical appraisal. *Health Care Financ Rev Annu Suppl.* 1991;45–77.
15. Weintraub WS, Zhang Z, Mahoney EM, et al. Cost-effectiveness of eplerenone compared with placebo in patients with myocardial infarction complicated by left ventricular dysfunction and heart failure. *Circulation.* 2005;111:1106–1113.
16. Becker ER, Mauldin PD, Culler SD, et al. Applying the resource-based relative value scale to the Emory angioplasty versus surgery trial. *Am J Cardiol.* 2000;85(6):685–691.
17. Hsiao WC, Braun P, Yntema D, Becker ER. Estimating physicians' work for a resource-based relative-value scale. *N Engl J Med.* 1988;319(13):835–841.
18. Mitchell J, Burge R, Lee A, et al. *Per Case Prospective Payment for Episodes of Hospital Care.* Springfield, VA: US Department of Commerce National Technical Information Service. Publication PB95226023.
19. Weintraub WS, Craver JM, Jones EL, et al. Improving cost and outcome of coronary surgery. *Circulation.* 1998;98(19 suppl):II23–28.
20. Gold MR, Siegel JE, Russel LB, Weinstein MC. *Cost-Effectiveness in Health and Medicine.* New York: Oxford University Press; 1996.
21. Measuring and improving quality of care: a report from the American Heart Association/American College of Cardiology First Scientific Forum on Assessment of Healthcare Quality in Cardiovascular Disease and Stroke. *Circulation.* 2000;101(12):1483–1493.
22. Mauldin PD, Weintraub WS, Becker ER. Predicting hospital costs for first-time coronary artery bypass grafting from preoperative and postoperative variables. *Am J Cardiol.* 1994;74(8):772–775.
23. Ellis SG, Miller DP, Brown KJ, et al. In-hospital cost of percutaneous coronary revascularization. Critical determinants and implications. *Circulation.* 1995;92(4):741–747.
24. Topol EJ, Ellis SG, Cosgrove DM, et al. Analysis of coronary angioplasty practice in the United States with an insurance-claims data base. *Circulation.* 1993;87(5):1489–1497.
25. Harris RA, Nease RF Jr. The importance of patient preferences for comorbidities in cost-effectiveness analyses. *J Health Econ.* 1997;16(1):113–119.
26. Mahoney EM, Chu H. Cost-effectiveness analysis alongside clinical trials: statistical and methodologic issues. In: Weintraub WS, ed. *Cardiovascular Health Care Economics.* Totowa, NJ: Humana Press, Inc; 2003:123–156.
27. King SB 3rd, Lembo NJ, Weintraub WS, et al. A randomized trial comparing coronary angioplasty with coronary bypass surgery. Emory Angioplasty versus Surgery Trial (EAST). *N Engl J Med.* 1994;331(16):1044–1050.
28. Serruys PW, Unger F, van Hout BA, et al. The ARTS study (Arterial Revascularization Therapies Study). *Semin Interv Cardiol.* 1999;4(4):209–219.
29. Weintraub WS, Mauldin PD, Becker E, Kosinski AS, King SB 3rd. A comparison of the costs of and quality of life after coronary angioplasty or coronary surgery for multivessel coronary artery disease. Results from the Emory Angioplasty Versus Surgery Trial (EAST). *Circulation.* 1995;92(10):2831–2840.
30. Zhang Z, Mahoney EM, Stables RH, et al. Disease-specific health status after stent-assisted percutaneous coronary intervention and coronary artery bypass surgery: one-year results from the stent or surgery trial. *Circulation.* 2003;108:1694–1700.
31. Efron B, Tibshirani R. *An Introduction to the Bootstrap.* New York: Chapman and Hall; 1993.
32. Alchian A. The meaning of utility measurement. *Am Econ Review.* 1953;43:26–50.
33. Feeny DH, Torrance GW, Furlong W. Health utilities index. In: Spilker B, ed. *Quality of Life and Pharmacoeconomics in Clinical Trials.* Philadelphia, PA: Lippincott-Raven Press; 1996:239–252.
34. Cook TA, O'Regan M, Galland RB. Quality of life following percutaneous transluminal angioplasty for claudication. *Eur J Vasc Endovasc Surg.* 1996;11(2):191–194.
35. Loomes G, McKenzie L. The use of QALYs in health care decision making. *Soc Sci Med.* 1989;28(4):299–308.
36. Nease RF, Jr. Introduction to cost-effectiveness analysis. In: Weintraub WS, ed. *Cardiovascular Health Care Economics.* Totowa, NJ: Humana Press; 2003:111–121.
37. Weintraub WS, Mahoney EM, Zhang Z, et al. One year comparison of costs of coronary surgery versus percutaneous coronary intervention in the stent or surgery trial. *Heart.* 2004;90(7):782–788.
38. Schulman KA, Kinosian B, Jacobson TA, et al. Reducing high blood cholesterol level with drugs. Cost-effectiveness of pharmacologic management. *JAMA.* 1990;264(23):3025–3033.
39. Tosteson AN, Weinstein MC, Hunink MG, et al. Cost-effectiveness of population-wide educational approaches to reduce serum cholesterol levels. *Circulation.* 1997;95(1):24–30.
40. Goldman L, Weinstein MC, Goldman PA, Williams LW. Cost-effectiveness of HMG-CoA reductase inhibition for primary and secondary prevention of coronary heart disease. *JAMA.* 1991;265(9):1145–1151.
41. Garber AM, Browner WS, Hulley SB. Cholesterol screening in asymptomatic adults, revisited. Part 2. *Ann Intern Med.* 1996;124(5):518–531.
42. Pedersen TR, Kjekshus J, Berg K, et al. Cholesterol lowering and the use of healthcare resources. Results of the Scandinavian Simvastatin Survival Study. *Circulation.* 1996;93(10):1796–1802.
43. Johannesson M, Jonsson B, Kjekshus J, et al. Cost effectiveness of simvastatin treatment to lower cholesterol levels in patients with coronary heart disease. Scandinavian Simvastatin Survival Study Group. *N Engl J Med.* 1997;336(5):332–336.
44. Caro J, Klittich W, McGuire A, et al. The West of Scotland coronary prevention study: economic benefit analysis of primary prevention with pravastatin. *BMJ.* 1997;315(7122):1577–1582.
45. Ashraf T, Hay JW, Pitt B, et al. Cost-effectiveness of pravastatin in secondary prevention of coronary artery disease. *Am J Cardiol.* 1996;78(4):409–414.
46. MRC/BHF Heart Protection Study of cholesterol lowering with simvastatin in 20,536 high-risk individuals: a randomised placebo-controlled trial. *Lancet.* 2002;360(9326):7–22.
47. Mihaylova B, Briggs A, Armitage J, et al. Cost-effectiveness of simvastatin in people at different levels of vascular disease risk: economic analysis of a randomised trial in 20,536 individuals. *Lancet.* 2005;365(9473):1779–1785.
48. Nyman JA, Martinson MS, Nelson D, et al. Cost-effectiveness of gemfibrozil for coronary heart disease patients with low levels of high-density lipoprotein cholesterol: the Department of Veterans Affairs High-Density Lipoprotein Cholesterol Intervention Trial. *Arch Intern Med.* 2002;162(2):177–182.
49. Pignone M, Earnshaw S, Tice JA, Pletcher MJ. Aspirin, statins, or both drugs for the primary prevention of coronary heart disease events in men: a cost-utility analysis. *Ann Intern Med.* 2006;144(5):326–336.
50. Brandle M, Davidson MB, Schriger DL, Lorber B, Herman WH. Cost effectiveness of statin therapy for the primary prevention of major coronary events in individuals with type 2 diabetes. *Diabetes Care.* 2003;26(6):1796–1801.
51. Pilote L, Ho V, Lavoie F, et al. Cost-effectiveness of lipid-lowering treatment according to lipid level. *Can J Cardiol.* 2005;21(8):681–687.
52. Center for Disease Control and Prevention. Annual Smoking-Attributable Mortality, Years of Potential Life Lost, and Productivity Losses—United States, 1997–2001. *Morb Mortal Wkly Rep.* 2005;54:625–628.

53. Lightwood JM, Glantz SA. Short-term economic and health benefits of smoking cessation: myocardial infarction and stroke. *Circulation.* 1997;96(4):1089–1096.

54. Warner KE. Cost effectiveness of smoking-cessation therapies. Interpretation of the evidence-and implications for coverage. *Pharmacoeconomics.* 1997;11(6):538–549.

55. Meenan RT, Stevens VJ, Hornbrook MC, et al. Cost-effectiveness of a hospital-based smoking cessation intervention. *Med Care.* 1998;36(5):670–678.

56. Cromwell J, Bartosch WJ, Fiore MC, Hasselblad V, Baker T. Cost-effectiveness of the clinical practice recommendations in the AHCPR guideline for smoking cessation. Agency for Health Care Policy and Research. *JAMA.* 1997;278(21):1759–1766.

57. Wollacott NF, Jones L, Forbes CA, et al. The clinical effectiveness and cost-effectiveness of bupropion and nicotine replacement therapy for smoking cessation: a systematic review and economic evaluation. *Health Technology Assessment.* 2002;6:1–245.

58. Krumholz HM, Cohen BJ, Tsevat J, Pasternak RC, Weinstein MC. Cost-effectiveness of a smoking cessation program after myocardial infarction. *J Am Coll Cardiol.* 1993;22(6):1697–1702.

59. Jones TF, Eaton CB. Cost-benefit analysis of walking to prevent coronary heart disease. *Arch Fam Med.* 1994;3(8):703–710.

60. Hambrecht R, Walther C, Mobius-Winkler S, et al. Percutaneous coronary angioplasty compared with exercise training in patients with stable coronary artery disease: a randomized trial. *Circulation.* 2004;109(11):1371–1378.

61. Moss SE, Klein R, Klein BE, Meuer SM. The association of glycemia and cause-specific mortality in a diabetic population. *Arch Intern Med.* 1994;154(21):2473–2479.

62. Summary of revisions for the 2006 Clinical Practice Recommendations. *Diabetes Care.* 2006;2005;29(suppl 1):S3.

63. Gilmer TP, O'Connor PJ, Manning WG, Rush WA. The cost to health plans of poor glycemic control. *Diabetes Care.* 1997;20(12):1847–1853.

64. Diabetes Control and Complications Trial Research Group. The effect of intensive treatment of diabetes on the development and progression of long-term complications in insulin-dependent diabetes mellitus. *N Engl J Med.* 1993;329(14):977–986.

65. Diabetes Control and Complications Trial Research Group. Lifetime benefits and costs of intensive therapy as practiced in the diabetes control and complications trial. *JAMA.* 1996;276(17):1409–1415.

66. UK Prospective Diabetes Study (UKPDS) Group. Intensive blood-glucose control with sulphonylureas or insulin compared with conventional treatment and risk of complications in patients with type 2 diabetes (UKPDS 33). *Lancet.* 1998;352(9131):837–853.

67. Eastman RC, Javitt JC, Herman WH, et al. Model of complications of NIDDM. II. Analysis of the health benefits and cost-effectiveness of treating NIDDM with the goal of normoglycemia. *Diabetes Care.* 1997;20(5):735–744.

68. Littenberg B, Garber AM, Sox HC, Jr. Screening for hypertension. *Ann Intern Med.* 1990;112(3):192–202.

69. Krakoff LR. Cost-effectiveness of ambulatory blood pressure: a reanalysis. *Hypertension.* 2006;47(1):29–34.

70. Moser M. Why are physicians not prescribing diuretics more frequently in the management of hypertension? *JAMA.* 1998;279(22):1813–1816.

71. Chobanian AV, Bakris GL, Black HR, et al. The Seventh Report of the Joint National Committee on Prevention, Detection, Evaluation, and Treatment of High Blood Pressure: the JNC 7 report. *JAMA.* 2003;289(19):2560–2572.

72. Ramsey SD, Neil N, Sullivan SD, Perfetto E. An economic evaluation of the JNC hypertension guidelines using data from a randomized controlled trial. Joint National Committee. *J Am Board Fam Pract.* 1999;12(2):105–114.

73. Yusuf S, Sleight P, Pogue J, et al. Effects of an angiotensin-converting-enzyme inhibitor, ramipril, on cardiovascular events in high-risk patients. The Heart Outcomes Prevention Evaluation Study Investigators. *N Engl J Med.* 2000;342(3):145–153.

74. Lamy A, Yusuf S, Pogue J, Gafni A. Cost implications of the use of ramipril in high-risk patients based on the Heart Outcomes Prevention Evaluation (HOPE) study. *Circulation.* 2003;107(7):960–965.

75. Nordmann AJ, Krahn M, Logan AG, Naglie G, Detsky AS. The cost effectiveness of ACE inhibitors as first-line antihypertensive therapy. *Pharmacoeconomics.* 2003;21(8):573–585.

76. Montgomery AA, Fahey T, Ben-Shlomo Y, Harding J. The influence of absolute cardiovascular risk, patient utilities, and costs on the decision to treat hypertension: a Markov decision analysis. *J Hypertens.* 2003;21(9):1753–1759.

77. Krumholz HM, Pasternak RC, Weinstein MC, et al. Cost effectiveness of thrombolytic therapy with streptokinase in elderly patients with suspected acute myocardial infarction. *N Engl J Med.* 1992;327(1):7–13.

78. Midgette AS, Wong JB, Beshansky JR, et al. Cost-effectiveness of streptokinase for acute myocardial infarction: A combined meta-analysis and decision analysis of the effects of infarct location and of likelihood of infarction. *Med Decis Making.* 1994;14(2):108–117.

79. Herve C, Castiel D, Gaillard M, Boisvert R, Leroux V. Cost-benefit analysis of thrombolytic therapy. *Eur Heart J.* 1990;11(11):1006–1010.

80. Kalish SC, Gurwitz JH, Krumholz HM, Avorn J. A cost-effectiveness model of thrombolytic therapy for acute myocardial infarction. *J Gen Intern Med.* 1995;10(6):321–330.

81. Stone GW, Grines CL, Rothbaum D, et al. Analysis of the relative costs and effectiveness of primary angioplasty versus tissue-type plasminogen activator: the Primary Angioplasty in Myocardial Infarction (PAMI) trial. The PAMI Trial Investigators. *J Am Coll Cardiol.* 1997;29(5):901–907.

82. Grines CL, Cox DA, Stone GW, et al. Coronary angioplasty with or without stent implantation for acute myocardial infarction. Stent Primary Angioplasty in Myocardial Infarction Study Group. *N Engl J Med.* 1999;341(26):1949–1956.

83. Cohen DJ, Taira DA, Berezin R, et al. Cost-effectiveness of coronary stenting in acute myocardial infarction: results from the stent primary angioplasty in myocardial infarction (stent-PAMI) trial. *Circulation.* 2001;104(25):3039–3045.

84. Randomised trial of intravenous streptokinase, oral aspirin, both, or neither among 17,187 cases of suspected acute myocardial infarction: ISIS-2. ISIS-2 (Second International Study of Infarct Survival) Collaborative Group. *Lancet.* 1988;2(8607):349–360.

85. Weintraub WS, Mahoney EM, Lamy A, et al. Long-term cost-effectiveness of clopidogrel given for up to one year in patients with acute coronary syndromes without ST-segment elevation. *J Am Coll Cardiol.* 2005;45(6):838–845.

86. Schleinitz MD, Heidenreich PA. A cost-effectiveness analysis of combination antiplatelet therapy for high-risk acute coronary syndromes: clopidogrel plus aspirin versus aspirin alone. *Ann Intern Med.* 2005;142(4):251–259.

87. Mahoney EM, Mehta S, Yuan Y, et al. Long-term cost-effectiveness of early and sustained clopidogrel therapy for up to 1 year in patients undergoing percutaneous coronary intervention after presenting with acute coronary syndromes without ST-segment elevation. *Am Heart J.* 2006;151(1):219–227.

88. Gaspoz JM, Coxson PG, Goldman PA, et al. Cost effectiveness of aspirin, clopidogrel, or both for secondary prevention of coronary heart disease. *N Engl J Med.* 2002;346(23):1800–1806.

89. Mark DB, Cowper PA, Berkowitz SD, et al. Economic assessment of low-molecular-weight heparin (enoxaparin) versus unfractionated heparin in acute coronary syndrome patients: results from the ESSENCE randomized trial. Efficacy and Safety of Subcutaneous Enoxaparin in Non-Q wave Coronary Events [unstable angina or non-Q-wave myocardial infarction]. *Circulation.* 1998;97(17):1702–1707.

90. Mark DB, Talley JD, Topol EJ, et al. Economic assessment of platelet glycoprotein IIb/IIIa inhibition for prevention of ischemic complications of high-risk coronary angioplasty. EPIC Investigators. *Circulation.* 1996;94(4):629–635.

91. Effects of platelet glycoprotein IIb/IIIa blockade with tirofiban on adverse cardiac events in patients with unstable angina or acute myocardial infarction undergoing coronary angioplasty. The RESTORE Investigators. Randomized Efficacy Study of Tirofiban for Outcomes and REstenosis. *Circulation.* 1997;96(5):1445–1453.

92. Weintraub WS, Culler S, Boccuzzi SJ, et al. Economic impact of GPIIB/IIIA blockade after high-risk angioplasty: results from the RESTORE trial. Randomized Efficacy Study of Tirofiban for Outcomes and Restenosis. *J Am Coll Cardiol.* 1999;34(4):1061–1066.

93. Weintraub WS, Thompson TD, Culler S, et al. Targeting patients undergoing angioplasty for thrombus inhibition: a cost-effectiveness and decision support model. *Circulation.* 2000;102(4):392–398.

94. Mark DB, Harrington RA, Lincoff AM, et al. Cost-effectiveness of platelet glycoprotein IIb/IIIa inhibition with eptifibatide in patients with non-ST-elevation acute coronary syndromes. *Circulation.* 2000;101(4):366–371.

95. Cannon CP, Weintraub WS, Demopoulos LA, et al. Comparison of early invasive and conservative strategies in patients with unstable coronary syndromes treated with the glycoprotein IIb/IIIa inhibitor tirofiban. *N Engl J Med.* 2001;344(25):1879–1887.

96. Effects of tissue plasminogen activator and a comparison of early invasive and conservative strategies in unstable angina and non-Q-wave myocardial infarction. Results of the TIMI IIIB Trial. Thrombolysis in Myocardial Ischemia. *Circulation.* 1994;89(4):1545–1556.

97. Boden WE, O'Rourke RA, Crawford MH, et al. Outcomes in patients with acute non-Q-wave myocardial infarction randomly assigned to an invasive as compared with a conservative management strategy. Veterans Affairs

Non-Q-Wave Infarction Strategies in Hospital (VANQWISH) Trial Investigators. *N Engl J Med.* 1998;338(25):1785–1792.

98. Invasive compared with non-invasive treatment in unstable coronary-artery disease: FRISC II prospective randomised multicentre study. Fragmin and fast revascularisation during instability in coronary artery disease investigators. *Lancet.* 1999;354(9180):708–715.

99. Mahoney EM, Jurkovitz CT, Chu H, et al. Cost and cost-effectiveness of an early invasive vs conservative strategy for the treatment of unstable angina and non-ST-segment elevation myocardial infarction. *JAMA.* 2002;288(15):1851–1858.

100. Yusuf S, Peto R, Lewis J, Collins R, Sleight P. Beta blockade during and after myocardial infarction: an overview of the randomized trials. *Prog Cardiovasc Dis.* 1985;27(5):335–371.

101. Goldman L, Sia ST, Cook EF, Rutherford JD, Weinstein MC. Costs and effectiveness of routine therapy with long-term beta-adrenergic antagonists after acute myocardial infarction. *N Engl J Med.* 1988;319(3):152–157.

102. Brown NJ, Vaughan DE. Angiotensin-converting enzyme inhibitors. *Circulation.* 1998;97(14):1411–1420.

103. Tsevat J, Duke D, Goldman L, et al. Cost-effectiveness of captopril therapy after myocardial infarction. *J Am Coll Cardiol.* 1995;26(4):914–919.

104. McMurray JJ, McGuire A, Davie AP, Hughes D. Cost-effectiveness of different ACE inhibitor treatment scenarios post-myocardial infarction. *Eur Heart J.* 1997;18(9):1411–1415.

105. Ades PA, Pashkow FJ, Nestor JR. Cost-effectiveness of cardiac rehabilitation after myocardial infarction. *J Cardiopulm Rehabil.* 1997;17(4):222–231.

106. Yu CM, Lau CP, Chau J, et al. A short course of cardiac rehabilitation program is highly cost effective in improving long-term quality of life in patients with recent myocardial infarction or percutaneous coronary intervention. *Arch Phys Med Rehabil.* 2004;85(12):1915–1922.

107. American Heart Association. *Heart Disease and Stroke Statistics—2005 Update.* Dallas, TX: American Heart Association.

108. Weintraub WS, Mahoney EM, Ghazzal ZM, et al. Trends in outcome and costs of coronary intervention in the 1990s. *Am J Cardiol.* 2001;88(5):497–503.

109. Puskas JD, Williams WH, Mahoney EM, et al. Off-pump vs conventional coronary artery bypass grafting: early and 1-year graft patency, cost, and quality-of-life outcomes: a randomized trial. *JAMA.* 2004;291(15):1841–1849.

110. Parisi AF, Folland ED, Hartigan P. A comparison of angioplasty with medical therapy in the treatment of single-vessel coronary artery disease. Veterans Affairs ACME Investigators. *N Engl J Med.* 1992;326(1):10–16.

111. Cohen DJ, Krumholz HM, Sukin CA, et al. In-hospital and one-year economic outcomes after coronary stenting or balloon angioplasty. Results from a randomized clinical trial. Stent Restenosis Study Investigators. *Circulation.* 1995;92(9):2480–2487.

112. Weintraub WS. Evaluating the cost of therapy for restenosis: considerations for brachytherapy. *Int J Radiat Oncol Biol Phys.* 1996;36(4):949–958.

113. Bakhai A, Stone GW, Grines CL, et al. Cost-effectiveness of coronary stenting and abciximab for patients with acute myocardial infarction: results from the CADILLAC (Controlled Abciximab and Device Investigation to Lower Late Angioplasty Complications) trial. *Circulation.* 2003;108(23):2857–2863.

114. Morice MC, Serruys PW, Sousa JE, et al. A randomized comparison of a sirolimus-eluting stent with a standard stent for coronary revascularization. *N Engl J Med.* 2002;346(23):1773–1780.

115. Moses JW, Leon MB, Popma JJ, et al. Sirolimus-eluting stents versus standard stents in patients with stenosis in a native coronary artery. *N Engl J Med.* 2003;349(14):1315–1323.

116. Stone GW, Ellis SG, Cox DA, et al. One-year clinical results with the slow-release, polymer-based, paclitaxel-eluting TAXUS stent: the TAXUS-IV trial. *Circulation.* 2004;109(16):1942–1947.

117. Cohen DJ, Bakhai A, Shi C, et al. Cost-effectiveness of sirolimus-eluting stents for treatment of complex coronary stenoses: results from the Sirolimus-Eluting Balloon Expandable Stent in the Treatment of Patients With De Novo Native Coronary Artery Lesions (SIRIUS) trial. *Circulation.* 2004;110(5):508–514.

118. Bagust A, Grayson AD, Palmer ND, Perry RA, Walley T. Cost effectiveness of drug eluting coronary artery stenting in a UK setting: cost-utility study. *Heart.* 2006;92(1):68–74.

119. Kaiser C, Brunner-La Rocca HP, Buser PT, et al. Incremental cost-effectiveness of drug-eluting stents compared with a third-generation bare-metal stent in a real-world setting: randomised Basel Stent Kosten Effektivitats Trial (BASKET). *Lancet.* 2005;366(9489):921–929.

120. Steinhubl SR, Berger PB, Mann JT 3rd, et al. Early and sustained dual oral antiplatelet therapy following percutaneous coronary intervention: a randomized controlled trial. *JAMA.* 2002;288(19):2411–2420.

121. Beinart SC, Kolm P, Veledar E, et al. Long-Term Cost Effectiveness of Early and Sustained Dual Oral Antiplatelet Therapy with Clopidogrel Given for

Up to One Year after Percutaneous Coronary Intervention Results from the Clopidogrel for the Reduction of Events during Observation (CREDO) Trial. *J Am Coll Cardiol.* 2005;46(5):761–769.

122. Cowper PA, Udayakumar K, Sketch MH Jr, Peterson ED. Economic effects of prolonged clopidogrel therapy after percutaneous coronary intervention. *J Am Coll Cardiol.* 2005;45(3):369–376.

123. Bypass Angioplasty Revascularization Investigation (BARI) Investigators. Comparison of coronary bypass surgery with angioplasty in patients with multivessel disease. *N Engl J Med.* 1996;335(4):217–225.

124. Hlatky MA, Rogers WJ, Johnstone I, et al. Medical care costs and quality of life after randomization to coronary angioplasty or coronary bypass surgery. Bypass Angioplasty Revascularization Investigation (BARI) Investigators. *N Engl J Med.* 1997;336(2):92–99.

125. Hlatky MA, Boothroyd DB, Melsop KA, et al. Medical costs and quality of life 10 to 12 years after randomization to angioplasty or bypass surgery for multivessel coronary artery disease. *Circulation.* 2004;110(14):1960–1966.

126. Coronary angioplasty versus coronary artery bypass surgery: the Randomized Intervention Treatment of Angina (RITA) trial. *Lancet.* 1993;341(8845):573–580.

127. Hamm CW, Reimers J, Ischinger T, et al. A randomized study of coronary angioplasty compared with bypass surgery in patients with symptomatic multivessel coronary disease. German Angioplasty Bypass Surgery Investigation (GABI). *N Engl J Med.* 1994;331(16):1037–1043.

128. Bertrand ME, Simoons ML, Fox KA, et al. Management of acute coronary syndromes in patients presenting without persistent ST-segment elevation. *Eur Heart J.* 2002;23(23):1809–1840.

129. Sculpher MJ, Seed P, Henderson RA, et al. Health service costs of coronary angioplasty and coronary artery bypass surgery: the Randomised Intervention Treatment of Angina (RITA) trial. *Lancet.* 1994;344(8927):927–930.

130. Rodriguez A, Mele E, Peyregne E, et al. Three-year follow-up of the Argentine Randomized Trial of Percutaneous Transluminal Coronary Angioplasty Versus Coronary Artery Bypass Surgery in Multivessel Disease (ERACI). *J Am Coll Cardiol.* 1996;27(5):1178–1184.

131. Serruys PW, Unger F, Sousa JE, et al. Comparison of coronary-artery bypass surgery and stenting for the treatment of multivessel disease. *N Engl J Med.* 2001;344(15):1117–1124.

132. Pitt B, Waters D, Brown WV, et al. Aggressive lipid-lowering therapy compared with angioplasty in stable coronary artery disease. Atorvastatin versus Revascularization Treatment Investigators. *N Engl J Med.* 1999;341(2):70–76.

133. Coronary angioplasty versus medical therapy for angina: the second Randomised Intervention Treatment of Angina (RITA-2) trial. RITA-2 trial participants. *Lancet.* 1997;350(9076):461–468.

133a. Boden WE, O'Rourke RA, Teo KK, et al. Optimal medical therapy with or without PCI for stable coronary disease. *N Engl J Med.* 2007;356:1503–1516.

134. Weintraub WS, Barnett P, Chen S, et al. Economics methods in the Clinical Outcomes Utilizing percutaneous coronary Revascularization and Aggressive Guideline-driven drug Evaluation (COURAGE) trial. *Am Heart J.* 2006;151(6):1180–1185.

135. Kinlay S, Leitch JW, Neil A, et al. Cardiac event recorders yield more diagnoses and are more cost-effective than 48-hour Holter monitoring in patients with palpitations. A controlled clinical trial. *Ann Intern Med.* 1996;124(1 pt 1):16–20.

136. Walker A, Sirel JM, Marsden AK, Cobbe SM, Pell JP. Cost effectiveness and cost utility model of public place defibrillators in improving survival after prehospital cardiopulmonary arrest. *BMJ.* 2003;327(7427):1316.

137. Cram P, Vijan S, Katz D, Fendrick AM. Cost-effectiveness of in-home automated external defibrillators for individuals at increased risk of sudden cardiac death. *J Gen Intern Med.* 2005;20(3):251–258.

138. Nichol G, Valenzuela T, Roe D, et al. Cost effectiveness of defibrillation by targeted responders in public settings. *Circulation.* 2003;108(6):697–703.

139. Kupersmith J, Hogan A, Guerrero P, et al. Evaluating and improving the cost-effectiveness of the implantable cardioverter-defibrillator. *Am Heart J.* 1995;130(3 pt 1):507–515.

140. Owens DK, Sanders GD, Harris RA, et al. Cost-effectiveness of implantable cardioverter defibrillators relative to amiodarone for prevention of sudden cardiac death. *Ann Intern Med.* 1997;126(1):1–12.

141. Larsen GC, Manolis AS, Sonnenberg FA, et al. Cost-effectiveness of the implantable cardioverter-defibrillator: effect of improved battery life and comparison with amiodarone therapy. *J Am Coll Cardiol.* 1992;19(6):1323–1334.

142. Kuppermann M, Luce BR, McGovern B, et al. An analysis of the cost effectiveness of the implantable defibrillator. *Circulation.* 1990;81(1):91–100.

143. Wever EF, Hauer RN, Schrijvers G, et al. Cost-effectiveness of implantable defibrillator as first-choice therapy versus electrophysiologically guided, tiered strategy in postinfarct sudden death survivors. A randomized study. *Circulation.* 1996;93(3):489–496.

144. Larsen G, Hallstrom A, McAnulty J, et al. Cost-effectiveness of the implantable cardioverter-defibrillator versus antiarrhythmic drugs in survivors of serious ventricular tachyarrhythmias: results of the Antiarrhythmics Versus Implantable Defibrillators (AVID) economic analysis substudy. *Circulation.* 2002;105(17):2049–2057.

145. Mushlin AI, Hall WJ, Zwanziger J, et al. The cost-effectiveness of automatic implantable cardiac defibrillators: results from MADIT. Multicenter Automatic Defibrillator Implantation Trial. *Circulation.* 1998;97(21):2129–2135.

146. Moss AJ, Zareba W, Hall WJ, et al. Prophylactic implantation of a defibrillator in patients with myocardial infarction and reduced ejection fraction. *N Engl J Med.* 2002;346(12):877–883.

147. Coats AJ. MADIT II, the Multi-center Autonomic Defibrillator Implantation Trial II stopped early for mortality reduction, has ICD therapy earned its evidence-based credentials? *Int J Cardiol.* 2002;82(1):1–5.

148. Al-Khatib SM, Anstrom KJ, Eisenstein EL, et al. Clinical and economic implications of the Multicenter Automatic Defibrillator Implantation Trial-II. *Ann Intern Med.* 2005;142(8):593–600.

149. Mark DB, Nelson CL, Anstrom KJ, et al. Cost-effectiveness of defibrillator therapy or amiodarone in chronic stable heart failure: results from the Sudden Cardiac Death in Heart Failure Trial (SCD-HeFT). *Circulation.* 2006;114(2):135–142.

150. Sanders GD, Hlatky MA, Owens DK. Cost-effectiveness of implantable cardioverter-defibrillators. *N Engl J Med.* 2005;353(14):1471–1480.

151. Kalbfleisch SJ, Calkins H, Langberg JJ, et al. Comparison of the cost of radiofrequency catheter modification of the atrioventricular node and medical therapy for drug-refractory atrioventricular node reentrant tachycardia. *J Am Coll Cardiol.* 1992;19(7):1583–1587.

152. Kertes PJ, Kalman JM, Tonkin AM. Cost effectiveness of radiofrequency catheter ablation in the treatment of symptomatic supraventricular tachyarrhythmias. *Aust N Z J Med.* 1993;23(4):433–436.

153. Weerasooriya HR, Murdock CJ, Harris AH, Davis MJ. The cost-effectiveness of treatment of supraventricular arrhythmias related to an accessory atrioventricular pathway: comparison of catheter ablation, surgical division and medical treatment. *Aust N Z J Med.* 1994;24(2):161–167.

154. Stamato NJ, O'Toole MF, Enger EL. Permanent pacemaker implantation in the cardiac catheterization laboratory versus the operating room: an analysis of hospital charges and complications. *Pacing Clin Electrophysiol.* 1992;15(12):2236–2239.

155. Sutton R, Bourgeois I. Cost benefit analysis of single and dual chamber pacing for sick sinus syndrome and atrioventricular block. An economic sensitivity analysis of the literature. *Eur Heart J.* 1996;17(4):574–582.

156. Rinfret S, Cohen DJ, Lamas GA, et al. Cost-effectiveness of dual-chamber pacing compared with ventricular pacing for sinus node dysfunction. *Circulation.* 2005;111(2):165–172.

157. Gage BF, Cardinalli AB, Albers GW, Owens DK. Cost-effectiveness of warfarin and aspirin for prophylaxis of stroke in patients with nonvalvular atrial fibrillation. *JAMA.* 1995;274(23):1839–1845.

158. Barnett HJ, Eliasziw M, Meldrum HE. Drugs and surgery in the prevention of ischemic stroke. *N Engl J Med.* 1995;332(4):238–248.

159. Laupacis A, Feeny D, Detsky AS, Tugwell PX. Tentative guidelines for using clinical and economic evaluations revisited. *CMAJ.* 1993;148(6):927–929.

160. Gustafsson C, Asplund K, Britton M, et al. Cost effectiveness of primary stroke prevention in atrial fibrillation: Swedish national perspective. *BMJ.* 1992;305(6867):1457–1460.

161. Lightowlers S, McGuire A. Cost-effectiveness of anticoagulation in non-rheumatic atrial fibrillation in the primary prevention of ischemic stroke. *Stroke.* 1998;29(9):1827–1832.

162. Eckman MH, Falk RH, Pauker SG. Cost-effectiveness of therapies for patients with nonvalvular atrial fibrillation. *Arch Intern Med.* 1998;158(15):1669–1677.

163. Catherwood E, Fitzpatrick WD, Greenberg ML, et al. Cost-effectiveness of cardioversion and antiarrhythmic therapy in nonvalvular atrial fibrillation. *Ann Intern Med.* 1999;130(8):625–636.

164. Wyse DG, Waldo AL, DiMarco JP, et al. A comparison of rate control and rhythm control in patients with atrial fibrillation. *N Engl J Med.* 2002;347(23):1825–1833.

165. Seto TB, Taira DA, Tsevat J, Manning WJ. Cost-effectiveness of transesophageal echocardiographic-guided cardioversion: a decision analytic model for patients admitted to the hospital with atrial fibrillation. *J Am Coll Cardiol.* 1997;29(1):122–130.

166. Klein AL, Murray RD, Becker ER, et al. Economic analysis of a transesophageal echocardiography-guided approach to cardioversion of patients with atrial fibrillation: the ACUTE economic data at eight weeks. *J Am Coll Cardiol.* 2004;43(7):1217–1224.

167. Mahoney EM, Thompson TD, Veledar E, Williams J, Weintraub WS. Cost-effectiveness of targeting patients undergoing cardiac surgery for therapy with intravenous amiodarone to prevent atrial fibrillation. *J Am Coll Cardiol.* 2002;40(4):737–745.

168. Heidenreich PA, Gubens MA, Fonarow GC, et al. Cost-effectiveness of screening with B-type natriuretic peptide to identify patients with reduced left ventricular ejection fraction. *J Am Coll Cardiol.* 2004;43(6):1019–1026.

169. Ward RE, Gheorghiade M, Young JB, Uretsky B. Economic outcomes of withdrawal of digoxin therapy in adult patients with stable congestive heart failure. *J Am Coll Cardiol.* 1995;26(1):93–101.

170. Uretsky BF, Young JB, Shahidi FE, et al. Randomized study assessing the effect of digoxin withdrawal in patients with mild to moderate chronic congestive heart failure: results of the PROVED trial. PROVED Investigative Group. *J Am Coll Cardiol.* 1993;22(4):955–962.

171. Packer M, Gheorghiade M, Young JB, et al. Withdrawal of digoxin from patients with chronic heart failure treated with angiotensin-converting-enzyme inhibitors. RADIANCE Study. *N Engl J Med.* 1993;329(1):1–7.

172. Eisenstein EL, Yusuf S, Bindal V, et al. What is the economic value of digoxin therapy in congestive heart failure patients? Results from the DIG trial. *J Card Fail.* 2006;12(5):336–342.

173. Effect of enalapril on survival in patients with reduced left ventricular ejection fractions and congestive heart failure. The SOLVD Investigators. *N Engl J Med.* 1991;325(5):293–302.

174. Glick H, Cook J, Kinosian B, et al. Costs and effects of enalapril therapy in patients with symptomatic heart failure: an economic analysis of the Studies of Left Ventricular Dysfunction (SOLVD) Treatment Trial. *J Card Fail.* 1995;1(5):371–380.

175. Boyko WL, Jr., Glick HA, Schulman KA. Economics and cost-effectiveness in evaluating the value of cardiovascular therapies. ACE inhibitors in the management of congestive heart failure: comparative economic data. *Am Heart J.* 1999;137(5):S115–119.

176. Kleber FX. Socioeconomic aspects of ACE inhibition in the secondary prevention in cardiovascular diseases. *Am J Hypertens.* 1994;7(9 pt 2):112S–116S.

177. van Hout BA, Wielink G, Bonsel GJ, Rutten FF. Effects of ACE inhibitors on heart failure in The Netherlands: a pharmacoeconomic model. *Pharmacoeconomics.* 1993;3(5):387–397.

178. Hart W, Rhodes G, McMurray J. The cost effectiveness of enalapril in the treatment of chronic heart failure. *Br J Med Econ.* 1993;6:91–98.

179. Pitt B, Zannad F, Remme WJ, et al. The effect of spironolactone on morbidity and mortality in patients with severe heart failure. Randomized Aldactone Evaluation Study Investigators. *N Engl J Med.* 1999;341(10):709–717.

180. Pitt B, Remme W, Zannad F, et al. Eplerenone, a selective aldosterone blocker, in patients with left ventricular dysfunction after myocardial infarction. *N Engl J Med.* 2003;348(14):1309–1321.

181. Glick HA, Orzol SM, Tooley JF, et al. Economic evaluation of the randomized Aldactone evaluation study (RALES): treatment of patients with severe heart failure. *Cardiovasc Drugs Ther.* 2002;16(1):53–59.

182. Weintraub WS, Zhang Z, Mahoney EM, et al. Cost-effectiveness of eplerenone compared with placebo in patients with myocardial infarction complicated by left ventricular dysfunction and heart failure. *Circulation.* 2005;111(9):1106–1113.

183. Angus DC, Linde-Zwirble WT, Tam SW, et al. Cost-effectiveness of fixed-dose combination of isosorbide dinitrate and hydralazine therapy for blacks with heart failure. *Circulation.* 2005;112(24):3745–3753.

184. Packer M, Bristow MR, Cohn JN, et al. The effect of carvedilol on morbidity and mortality in patients with chronic heart failure. U.S. Carvedilol Heart Failure Study Group. *N Engl J Med.* 1996;334(21):1349–1355.

185. Delea TE, Vera-Llonch M, Richner RE, Fowler MB, Oster G. Cost effectiveness of carvedilol for heart failure. *Am J Cardiol.* 1999;83(6):890–896.

186. Rich MW, Beckham V, Wittenberg C, et al. A multidisciplinary intervention to prevent the readmission of elderly patients with congestive heart failure. *N Engl J Med.* 1995;333(18):1190–1195.

187. Kornowski R, Zeeli D, Averbuch M, et al. Intensive home-care surveillance prevents hospitalization and improves morbidity rates among elderly patients with severe congestive heart failure. *Am Heart J.* 1995;129(4):762–766.

188. West JA, Miller NH, Parker KM, et al. A comprehensive management system for heart failure improves clinical outcomes and reduces medical resource utilization. *Am J Cardiol.* 1997;79(1):58–63.

189. Hershberger RE. Clinical outcomes, quality of life, and cost outcomes after cardiac transplantation. *Am J Med Sci.* 1997;314(3):129–138.

190. Evans RW. Cost-effectiveness analysis of transplantation. *Surg Clin North Am.* 1986;66(3):603–616.

191. Rose EA, Gelijns AC, Moskowitz AJ, et al. Long-term mechanical left ventricular assistance for end-stage heart failure. *N Engl J Med.* 2001;345(20):1435–1443.

192. Abraham WT, Fisher WG, Smith AL, et al. Cardiac resynchronization in chronic heart failure. *N Engl J Med.* 2002;346(24):1845–1853.

193. Feldman AM, de Lissovoy G, Bristow MR, et al. Cost effectiveness of cardiac resynchronization therapy in the Comparison of Medical Therapy, Pacing, and Defibrillation in Heart Failure (COMPANION) trial. *J Am Coll Cardiol.* 2005;46(12):2311–2321.

194. Nichol G, Kaul P, Huszti E, Bridges JF. Cost-effectiveness of cardiac resynchronization therapy in patients with symptomatic heart failure. *Ann Intern Med.* 2004;141(5):343–351.

195. Moskowitz AJ, Rose EA, Gelijns AC. The cost of long-term LVAD implantation. *Ann Thorac Surg.* 2001;71(3 suppl):S195–198; discussion S203–194.

196. Garber AM, Solomon NA. Cost-effectiveness of alternative test strategies for the diagnosis of coronary artery disease. *Ann Intern Med.* 1999;130(9):719–728.

197. Kim C, Kwok YS, Saha S, Redberg RF. Diagnosis of suspected coronary artery disease in women: a cost-effectiveness analysis. *Am Heart J.* 1999;137(6):1019–1027.

198. Kuntz KM, Fleischmann KE, Hunink MG, Douglas PS. Cost-effectiveness of diagnostic strategies for patients with chest pain. *Ann Intern Med.* 1999;130(9):709–718.

199. O'Malley PG, Greenberg BA, Taylor AJ. Cost-effectiveness of using electron beam computed tomography to identify patients at risk for clinical coronary artery disease. *Am Heart J.* 2004;148(1):106–113.

200. Taylor AJ, Bindeman J, Feuerstein I, et al. Coronary Calcium Independently Predicts Incident Premature Coronary Heart Disease Over Measured Cardiovascular Risk Factors Mean Three-Year Outcomes in the Prospective Army Coronary Calcium (PACC) Project. *J Am Coll Cardiol.* 2005;46(5):807–814.

201. Shaw LJ, Raggi P, Berman DS, Callister TQ. Cost effectiveness of screening for cardiovascular disease with measures of coronary calcium. *Prog Cardiovasc Dis.* 2003;46(2):171–184.

CHAPTER (112)

Insurance Issues in Patients with Heart Disease

Michael B. Clark / William T. Friedewald

INSURANCE MEDICINE AND CARDIOLOGY

Physicians serve as resources for and, ultimately, rely on a variety of insurance programs (Table 112–1) for personal and professional financial security. The purpose of insurance is to provide for financial relief in the event of significant economic loss. Insurance usually takes the form of a contract, a legal agreement between insurer and insured, specifying those losses that are to be covered and the insurance benefit agreed on. This contract demands specific requirements (see Table 112–1) that once fulfilled, allow actuarial probability analysis to predict the total amount of loss for a large group of individuals over some defined period of time.[1] Employer-sponsored health insurance relies on this "law of large numbers" to determine group premiums without the need for medical evaluation. For life insurance and private health insurance, however, an analytic process termed *insurance underwriting* serves to identify the need for insurance as well as the potential risk of loss for each individual. The ultimate premium charged will be determined by need, but will be proportional to the risk assumed by the insurer, allowing for an equitable distribution of economic spread over large groups of people (see Table 112–1).

These concepts of insurance and insurance underwriting are not new; insurance for commercial ventures existed in some form by the Middle Ages, and life insurance had appeared by the seventeenth century. Private medical insurance, usually for catastrophic illnesses, was available in the 1800s.[2] Within the past 100 years, there has been an explosion in the amount of life and health insurance available and in the diversity of insurance products. Basic *whole life insurance* has been supplanted by a wide variety of *term* and *variable* financial offerings as individual policies or, more commonly, as part of employer-sponsored group life insurance (see Table 112–1).

The changes in the health insurance industry have been even more dramatic. Unique to the administration of health insurance is the concept of *shared risk* whereby the insurer, the insured, and the insured's employer (or the government) all participate in payment of premiums and claims. There can be a *copayment* for routine office visits or a residual *amount due* over and above a *reasonable and customary* reimbursement schedule. The goal is to meet expense and utilization goals that allow for maximal distribution of insurance at an affordable price. Employer and government-sponsored fee-for-service or managed care organizations provide health, disability, and long-term care insurance for the majority of the U.S. population. Within the medical community, the impact of this changing insurance climate has been enormous,[3,4] and, as medical care providers and as consultants, cardiologists will continue to play an important role in insurance underwriting evaluation.

TABLE 112–1

Insurance Frequently Asked Questions (FAQs)

Insurable Risk: Definition

The risk is definable by amount of loss and duration of coverage.

The amount of insurance does not exceed the actual financial loss.

The insured loss occurs by chance, not by intent such as suicide or homicide.

The loss occurs within a sufficiently large population at risk to allow for application of the laws of probability.

The beneficiary of the insurance must have an *insurable interest*; a genuine concern for the continued well-being of the insured.

Major Types of Insurance

Life Insurance (individual and group)
- Whole life
- Variable life
- Universal life

- Universal variable life
- *Term* life (10-year, 20-year)

Non-Life Insurance

- Property and casualty
- Malpractice
- Automobile owners insurance
- Homeowners insurance

Health Insurance (individual and group)
- Fee-for-service
- Health maintenance organizations (HMOs)
- Preferred provider organizations (PPOs)
- Disability
- Long-term care
- Critical illness

The Components of the Insurance Premium

Mortality Costs
- Excess risk of death
- Present value of ultimate benefit

Loading Costs
- Company expenses to develop and administer the product
- Commissions
- Profit

MEDICAL UNDERWRITING FOR LIFE INSURANCE

【 】 APPLICATION AND MEDICAL REQUIREMENTS

Most applicants for insurance are in excellent health and are quickly offered policies at standard or even preferred premium rates. When medical impairments are uncovered, however, each must be correlated with long-term mortality data relevant to that impairment. The process begins once the candidate for insurance completes an insurance application that often contains important *past medical history* and *review of systems* information. Authorized query to one of the national informational database exchanges can

provide additional leads. The next step, an insurance medical examination with laboratory assessment, usually includes comprehensive medical history and physical examination review, but noninvasive cardiac testing can also be considered. Stress testing, in particular, is often requested if large amounts of insurance are applied for (*age and amount* guidelines) or if the initial impression suggests intermediate or high cardiac risk (*for cause* guidelines) to permit an accurate mortality assessment. Here, the cardiology consultant serves as a member of the medical underwriting team, reviewing all of the cardiac information available, including electrocardiograms and stress test tracings.

The Attending Physician Statement

Underwriting risk assessment guidelines often direct the patient's physician to submit medical information to the insurance company in the form of the attending physician's statement (APS). This can include an outline of recent medical history and will often contain office and hospital records for review. Clinical problems identified in the APS are analyzed for severity of disease, extent of clinical evaluation, and thoroughness of clinical followup to provide data for risk assessment.

Mortality Analysis

Each medical impairment identified during the medical underwriting evaluation must be correlated with long-term population survival statistics relevant to that disease process. The number of *excess deaths* attributable to that impairment is used to derive a mortality ratio (the observed deaths in a population of impaired individuals compared to the expected deaths for an otherwise comparable standard population).[5,6] Published data relevant to mortality assessment derive from several sources. The mortality ratio serves as a useful measure for comparing mortality projections among various medical impairments. In general, the higher the mortality ratio calculated, the greater the relative risk assumed by the company to provide life insurance for individuals affected by that impairment. The mortality ratios calculated for various medical conditions are integrated into a table of risk classes or *ratings*. Applicants within a rating class are grouped together to be assessed for similar *mortality costs of insurance*. The mortality cost is an important element in premium computation, a complex calculation that varies by company and by insurance product.

Insured Populations Insurance policies are generally issued for durations (*terms*) that can continue for 20 to 30 years. The most valuable prognostic data, then, would necessarily derive from studies with extended periods of followup. Excellent long-term followup data are available for insured populations based on medical conditions, laboratory abnormalities, demographic characteristics, avocations, and personal habits identified at the time of original insurance application (Table 112–2). Results are usually expressed as mortality ratios or excess death rates in the impairment group as compared to a standard population. As might be expected, however, these data become limited where significant medical advances or transformations in demographics or lifestyles occurred during the period of study.

Clinical Studies and National Databases Important predictive data can also be derived from long-term clinical and epidemi-

TABLE 112–2

Mortality Ratios in Cardiac Impairments: Selected Data

MEDICAL FINDING OR CONDITION	AGE INTERVAL (YEARS)	NUMBER OF PATIENTS	MORTALITY RATIO (PERCENT)
ECG findings in men	40–64	21,415	
Axis deviation (symptomatic)			225
Axis deviation (asymptomatic)			139
ST depression (symptomatic)			420
ST depression (asymptomatic)			220
Heart murmurs	50–59	21,295	
Apical systolic (not transmitted to neck; presumed functional)			114
Apical systolic (transmitted)			178
Basal systolic			276
Acute myocardial infarction	30–59	1,608	145
Coronary bypass reoperation	50–59	1,608	145

SOURCE: Adapted from Medical Impairment Study 1983 [abstract]; Chait [30]; Rose, Baxter, Reid, McCartney. [34]

ologic studies published in the clinical literature. Particularly useful for mortality assessment are reports derived from the nationally maintained databases, such as the Surveillance, Epidemiology, and End Results (SEER) and United Network for Organ Sharing (UNOS). Data from these databases, in which interval survival data are usually reported (e.g., 5-year Kaplan-Meier survival curves) can be extrapolated to provide actuarial information useful to the calculation of mortality risk. At times, however, the focus or inclusion criteria of a particular study may not allow extrapolation to a larger population. Here, the conclusions of the study must be interpreted cautiously. Iacovino discusses such a situation in a review[7] of mortality analysis methodology. Clinical investigators followed 48 patients with a mean age of 36 years for approximately 6 years and noted a favorable observed mortality of 10 percent for the entire period.[8] However, reference to the U.S. Standard Life Tables (1979–1981) revealed a much lower expected mortality (approximately 1.46 percent) at this age for the same length of followup. The estimated mortality ratio of 685 percent (10 percent/1.46 percent × 100) represented a highly substandard risk level for life insurance purposes, even though it may represent good clinical results in young patients with severe cardiac disease.[9]

Health Insurance Risk Assessment

Most applicants for health insurance apply as members of a group, usually through the workplace. The basic insurance coverage is often an important part of the employee benefits package, with costs borne in large part (or entirely) by employers. Government-sponsored insurance such as Medicare also involves groups identified by age, income, or handicap. Medical risk assessment plays little role in the underwriting of these policies. In private health insurance, premium determination is based on an *experience rating* determined through historical review of medical expenses most recently incurred by the members of the group. Government-sponsored insurance premiums represent a complex interplay of mortality projection, budgetary constraints, and political considerations.

Individuals who desire additional coverage over and above that available at work or those without a workplace benefit program can choose from a variety of individual health insurance plans. On completion of the usually mandatory medical questionnaire, the risk assessment process becomes quite similar to that of life insurance underwriting.

One important difference, however, relates to exclusions and limitations for specified impairments. Certain underwriting factors, such as admitted medical impairments or claims history, can necessitate exclusion of identified impairments from insurance coverage. The limitation can apply to all related claims or only to those over and above a specified claim frequency or duration. Although seemingly restrictive, this can allow health insurance coverage for some that would otherwise be denied any coverage at all.

CORONARY HEART DISEASE: ANGINA PECTORIS AND MYOCARDIAL INFARCTION

Initial and short-term mortality following the diagnosis of coronary disease is, in general, unacceptably high for life insurance consideration (estimated at 1150 percent of standard mortality) but can be quite variable for clinical subpopulations. A plateau phase is seen following this period, during which the mortality ratio (found to be close to 390 percent of standard) is relatively stable and thus more predictable. Other studies in insured individuals have confirmed this pattern.[10,11] Common underwriting practice is to consider a life insurance applicant after a period of 6 to 12 months following the initial presentation of coronary heart disease (CHD). Aggressive revascularization strategies such as postinfarction thrombolysis and primary angioplasty with stenting have allowed for earlier life insurance consideration in selected applicants. On reaching the more predictable plateau phase, a permanent, somewhat substandard risk assessment is usually applied to correspond to the more stable but still substandard mortality rate seen in individuals with established ischemic heart disease.

To facilitate appropriate risk assessment, special attention is directed to the presence of known atherosclerosis risk factors such as high blood pressure, diabetes mellitus, hyperlipidemia, smoking history, and obesity. In addition, a strong family history of cardiovascular disease has been confirmed in studies in insured as well as in other broader-based epidemiologic populations to be an independent risk factor for CHD, with mortality ratios in insureds of 189 and 121 percent for men and women, respectively.[11]

Long-term prognosis in patients with ischemic heart disease can be influenced by intercurrent clinical interventions, such as thrombolysis, coronary angioplasty, stenting, and coronary bypass surgery.[12,13] Again, consideration for life insurance is usually postponed for a short interval to allow for review of the clinical course soon after the intervention. After this period, particular consideration would be given to the status of left ventricular function before and after intervention, the number and extent of coronary artery lesions seen on coronary angiography, and the results of electrocardiographic, echocardiographic, and radionuclide stress testing. The presence or absence of coronary artery risk factors, in particular smoking, will influence the level of the final medical assessment. The frequency and thoroughness of followup care can also influence the medical underwriter in otherwise borderline cases.

Mortality risk assessment is considerably more difficult when only limited information is available. A complaint of chest pain can be recorded as "possible angina, begin aspirin" with no further cardiac testing initiated by the time of insurance review. For purposes of risk assessment, this information would commonly be considered as "definite angina" until further clinical followup or noninvasive cardiac testing results were made available. Exercise electrocardiograms are, in general, routinely required for applicants requesting large amounts of insurance, although some insurance companies have recently discontinued this requirement. Certainly, these tests continue to be ordered when indicated by the presence of strong risk factors for CHD or by suggestive clinical presentations documented in the attending physician's medical summary forwarded to the insurance company. Substandard insurance ratings based on abnormal electrocardiographic stress testing results can be revised with supplementary evidence, particularly with cardiac imaging studies or coronary angiography.

HEALTH INSURANCE AND CORONARY HEART DISEASE

In the United States, healthcare expenditures of $351.8 billion dollars are predicted to care for an estimated 61,800,000 patients with established coronary disease.[14] The aging of the U.S. population and the frequent introduction of new medical technologies combined with the ever-present price inflation to maintain or increase this enormous cost to society. Efforts to contain these costs have led to the introduction of cumbersome, complicated, and at times restrictive reimbursement protocols from government and other health insurance providers. On the positive side, *cost-benefit* is now accepted as a valid and important end point for clinical research. A strong resolve to focus on primary prevention strategies promises to reduce the annual incidence of new coronary disease cases and should have a positive impact on healthcare expenditures.

Patients with CHD rely on health insurance providers to cover the costs of initial treatment and ongoing monitoring and therapy. Rising prescription drug costs have made the pharmaceutical benefit an increasingly important component of the overall employee health insurance coverage plan.

HIGH BLOOD PRESSURE

Since 1925, the life insurance industry has published several major comprehensive studies demonstrating increased mortality among insured populations with high blood pressure.[15–17] All show a direct, nearly linear relation between systolic and diastolic blood pressure and mortality. Most recently, the Multiple Medical Impairment Study[18] published in 1998 underscored the necessity for adequate blood pressure control. This study reviewed the insurance company mortality experience on nearly 2,400,000 policies. Persons with diastolic blood pressure readings of 90 mmHg demonstrated a mortality ratio of 101 percent at systolic blood pressure readings under 128 mmHg. Systolic determinations in men at 140 mmHg and 150 mmHg correlated with mortality ratios of 134 and 164 percent respectively when associated with a diastolic pressure of 85 mmHg, and 126, 144, and 174 percent respectively when associated with a diastolic pressure of 90 mmHg. Women exhibited a similar but less dramatic relationship between elevation of blood pressure and mortality that was limited to policies originally issued at substandard rates. The mortality risk from hypertension deteriorated further when considered in association with other impairments.[18] The mortality ratio for diabetes in this study was 236 percent, but it was further increased to 283 percent in association with elevated blood pressure readings. Similar associations were found for insureds with heart murmurs (mortality ratio with elevated blood pressure 234 percent) and abnormal ECGs (mortality ratio 251 percent in association with blood pressure elevation). Excess mortality risk, then, generally applies only to patients with untreated hypertension, those who are noncompliant with prescribed medical regimens, or where hypertension is complicated by end-organ damage (ventricular hypertrophy or cerebrovascular or renal disease), or in association with other medical impairments. These developments are often identified in the clinical record or at the time of insurance evaluation. This evaluation might include electrocardiography, urinary protein quantitation, or, occasionally, echocardiography to assess the degree of hypertensive cardiac impairment.

HYPERTENSION AND HEALTH INSURANCE

Health insurance coverage allows access to medical care and treatment for most patients with hypertension. For the uninsured, representing approximately 41 million Americans younger than 65 years of age, the cost of physician visits and antihypertensive medications remains a significant barrier to healthcare access. Particularly affected are those in fair to poor health, including smokers, diabetics, and those with hypertension and lipid disorders.

A wide range of options have been proposed to remedy this situation. These include government-sponsored universal healthcare administered at a state or federal level, as well as private insurance options with funding on an individual basis in preference to an employed-group basis. Reform of existing Medicare and Medicaid programs is being seen by many as the most realistic option at present.

VALVULAR HEART DISEASE

【 】 HISTORICAL UNDERWRITING: HEART MURMURS

In the past, information extracted from large studies of insureds with heart murmurs had been extrapolated to provide mortality projections in people with valvular heart disease (see Table 112–2). Advances in cardiac diagnostic technology since publication of these studies, particularly the development of echocardiographic and Doppler imaging systems, have allowed better definition of valvular pathology. Risk assessment can now be more realistically directed to the identified valvular pathology. However, earlier and more aggressive repair or replacement of these defective valves has made it more difficult to accumulate data concerning the natural history of unoperated cardiac valvular impairments.[19,20]

【 】 MITRAL VALVE PROLAPSE

This is, at present, the most common valve condition reported to insurance companies. Although most such patients are offered standard insurance rates, a small subset of patients with frequent chest pain, cardiac arrhythmias, and significant mitral regurgitation can be rated below standard.[21]

【 】 CONGENITAL VALVULAR HEART DISEASE

Most companies postpone consideration of life insurance for an infant with known or suspected congenital heart disease until the child reaches 1 or 2 years of age. Even then, the history must include a definitively proven diagnosis as well as successful repair of all surgically correctable lesions before the applicant can be considered insurable. After successful restoration of normal cardiac hemodynamics, most applicants with congenital defects—including those with atrial and ventricular septal defects, corrected pulmonic stenosis, patent ductus, or coarctation of the aorta (once blood pressure has returned to normal)—can be considered as standard risks.[22] Uninsurable applicants would include most cases of transposition of the great vessels, Ebstein anomaly, anomalous venous return, and Eisenmenger syndrome.

Congenital bicuspid aortic valve remains a difficult clinical and underwriting problem.[23] In the absence of associated echocardiographic evidence of left ventricular enlargement, most companies are willing to assess this risk as only mildly substandard. Left ventricular dilation or hypertrophy seen on echocardiography or the presence by Doppler analysis of any significant degree of aortic stenosis or regurgitation will usually require a more substantial rating assessment.

【 】 ACQUIRED VALVULAR HEART DISEASE

To perform risk assessment in applicants known to have acquired valvular disease, the underwriter usually first considers the clinical and electrocardiographic findings on the insurance examination. The degree of cardiac enlargement and severity of left ventricular dysfunction will also be considered and will commonly be outlined in the medical record. The medical underwriter will also give consideration to the attendant risk of anticipated surgical valve repair or replacement as well as to the risk of lifelong anticoagulation following such surgery. Applicants with valvular disease who show evidence of marked cardiomegaly, especially with prior history or physical examination findings consistent with left-sided or right-sided heart failure, cannot usually be offered life insurance. Other significant complications, such as new-onset atrial fibrillation or systemic embolization, will usually result in a postponement for up to 1 year prior to reconsideration. In most other cases, life insurance can be offered, albeit at much higher premiums.[20,23,24] Early followup studies of patients undergoing surgical procedures that preserve the native cardiac valve have demonstrated an improvement in perioperative and short-term postoperative survival.[21] One recent study at the Toronto General Hospital reported on the long-term followup of mitral valve surgery performed on 573 patients with rheumatic heart disease; 80 percent were female. Over the 17-year period of the study, the mortality ratios following valve repair, mechanical valve replacement, and bioprosthetic valve replacement were 175, 290, and 350 percent respectively as compared to a standard Canadian population. It may be that the data in patients operated on for mitral regurgitation secondary to myxomatous degeneration would be closer to standard; that on patients with ischemic valvular disease would most likely be somewhat worse than that on any of the other groups.

VALVULAR HEART DISEASE, EXERCISE PROGRAMS, AND HEALTH INSURANCE

Little information is available on the effects of exercise on patients with severe valvular disease. Considerably more evidence exists, however, in support of an exercise rehabilitation prescription following correction of the valvular impairment. Salutary effects on myocardial and respiratory function, peripheral blood flow, and quality of life are well-documented. This value has fairly recently been acknowledged by most health insurance providers after an initial resistance based on difficulty in proving long-term benefit. Reimbursement is now available for early postdischarge monitoring as well as postrecovery aerobic and isometric training programs to facilitate return to an optimal functional level.

OTHER CARDIAC DISEASES OR ABNORMAL LABORATORY FINDINGS

【 】 CARDIOMYOPATHY

Insurance risk assessment of the applicant with cardiomyopathy is based on the initial clinical presentation of the patient and the subsequent clinical and physiologic evaluation. Life insurance cannot usually be offered to those diagnosed with dilated (congestive) cardiomyopathy or amyloid heart disease. Systemic diseases with cardiac involvement, such as scleroderma and sarcoidosis, are most often assessed on the basis of overall disease activity and response to therapy. Insurance may be available to many in this latter group of patients, albeit at rates below standard.[23]

Evaluation of the asymptomatic individual with a strong family history of heart disease or in whom a heart murmur has been discovered can at times produce findings consistent with the obstructive or nonobstructive hypertrophic cardiomyopathies. Complete information concerning the natural history of these impairments is not yet available, particularly in the mild asymptomatic cases.[25] In the past, many clinical reports were of severe and fatal outcomes, leading many insurance companies to decline or rate highly any applicant with an established diagnosis of hypertrophic cardiomyopathy.[23] More recent experience in defining mortality outcomes in hypertrophic cardiomyopathy, particularly where nonobstructive, has been much more favorable[26,27] and can allow for more favorable mortality risk assessment in the future.[28]

[ ] ARRHYTHMIAS

Medical underwriters will consider applicants who give a history of paroxysmal or chronic atrial arrhythmias in the context of the presence and severity of coexisting cardiac disease. One series of insured persons with paroxysmal atrial tachycardia noted mortality rates quite similar to those of the standard population (mortality ratio 73 percent).[11] This can be contrasted with mortality ratios of 700 percent or greater in the presence of atrial fibrillation and coexisting heart disease.[29] In the apparently asymptomatic young individual with new-onset atrial arrhythmias, particular attention is paid to social history and habits such as smoking or excessive alcohol use. In the middle-aged or older applicant, the possibility of asymptomatic coronary heart disease must also be assessed.

Ventricular arrhythmias have remained a difficult risk-assessment problem. In many cases, isolated ventricular ectopy is considered in the context of the underlying cardiac impairment, such as coronary artery or valvular heart disease. Particular attention is directed during the review of the medical record to the results of clinical cardiac evaluation, including stress testing and noninvasive analysis of cardiac function.[30] Survivors of sudden death will, in most cases, be declined—a situation that can change as long-term data on the benefits of an automatic implantable cardioverter-defibrillator (AICD) become available. This change would probably apply to those patients in whom AICD implantation has been performed as prophylaxis in the setting of high clinical risk for sudden death[31] (see also Chaps. 39 and 46).

[ ] HEART TRANSPLANTATION

Heart transplantation techniques and immunosuppressive strategies have continued to evolve and have been associated with significant improvement in 5- to 10-year survival (see also Chap. 27). Longer survival durations have been problematic, particularly related to the late development of coronary arteriopathy. Most insurance companies would continue to decline such risks until additional long-term survival data became available.

[ ] LABORATORY EVALUATION OF ABNORMALITIES

Life insurance underwriting protocols generally include a clinical laboratory panel with a full lipid profile and a resting electrocardiogram. Depending on the age of the applicant and the amount of life insurance requested, additional testing, including stress testing and echocardiography, can be required. In most cases, abnormalities revealed during this laboratory evaluation are fully consistent with the clinical history as reported in the APS. In a minority of applicants, however, medical history is scanty or medical records are unavailable. In such patients, medical underwriting risk assessment is then based primarily on the findings from the insurance physical and laboratory examination. Studies in insured as well as general populations provide the necessary mortality projections for underwriting risk assessment using these parameters (see Table 112–2). The Medical Impairment Study (1983), for example, confirmed the benign prognosis of incidental bradycardia found on insurance examination (mortality ratios of 73 to 80 percent).[11] Conversely, a relative mortality of 250 percent was found for the finding of tachycardia.[11] Additional information is available to perform risk assessment for findings such as overweight and underweight,[9,32] low serum albumin,[33] and an abnormal electrocardiogram.[34,35]

HEALTH INSURANCE

Health insurance continues to evolve in terms of overall cost, quality, and availability within the current environment of healthcare reform. The delivery of healthcare under managed care plans by both governmental and employer insurance plans has begun to redefine many aspects of the traditional patient–doctor, doctor–doctor, and doctor–insurer relationships.[3,4] Recent U.S. privacy reforms (Health Insurance Portability and Accountability Act [HIPAA], Gramm-Leach-Bliley legislation) are important attempts to safeguard the privacy of medical information. However, they will almost certainly limit access to medical information for insurance underwriting, making accurate risk assessment in life and health insurance a much more difficult task.

Within this environment, cardiologists remain vitally important, functioning both as clinical consultants to primary care providers as well as professional consultants to managed care organizations and indemnity insurance plans. This latter role deserves special emphasis. Cardiologists will often be called on to provide the expertise essential to the determination of the medical necessity and appropriateness of care for health insurance case management and claim review. Assessment of new technology in its evolution from experimental procedure to accepted standard of care is a particularly important responsibility of the insurance consultant in the managed care environment.[36]

Physicians' net incomes have remained stagnant over the past several years, a trend that compares unfavorably with income trends of other professional groups.[37] Further, the continued rise in societal health costs has translated into increased financial pressures on physicians.[38] The result, according to one physician survey,[39] has been a tendency to refer complex problems to others, more difficulty in obtaining referrals to certain medical and surgical specialists, and more travel required to obtain medical care. Certainly, declining cardiology procedure-related reimbursement can be in part mitigated by technology-supported improvements in productivity. Significant issues related to payment reform and patient access to medical care remain to be resolved.

DISABILITY INSURANCE

The role of the physician in disability determination is more complex, often requiring legal interpretation of disability based on the results of medical data available. The expertise of medical specialists—including physiatrists, physical and occupational therapists, and social workers—can be required for complete evaluation and recommendations. In general, thorough analysis coupled with appropriate goal-directed therapy often allows for return to work in a supportive environment accommodated to individual needs.

For practical purposes, the patient with known heart disease of any kind is going to have difficulty in obtaining standard individual health or disability insurance. As in the case of patients with high blood pressure, however, effective subclassification of patients and effective new therapies can allow insurance to become available to more and more patients who were considered unacceptable insurance risks in the past.

MEDICAL LIABILITY INSURANCE

Most would agree that the medical malpractice system, a product of the nonlife property and casualty insurance lines, remains in need of reform. The current insurance climate has been characterized as a "liability crisis" based on increased in the median jury awards, settlement size, and legal costs related to litigation.[40] Although the primary drivers and the level of crisis remain arguable, the result has been less available and more costly malpractice insurance.[41] Insurance companies, including large carriers, continue to exit the market, and industry profitability has been reduced in recent years.[42] Physician, consumer, and governmental advocacy will hopefully arrive at an equitable solution for all in the near future.

ACKNOWLEDGMENT

We gratefully acknowledge the work of Dr. M. Irene Ferrer and Dr. Joseph A. Wilber in previous editions of this textbook, on which we drew for the current chapter.

REFERENCES

1. Morton GA. *Principles of Life and Health Insurance*. Atlanta: Life Office Management Association; 1984.
2. Brackenridge RDC, Brown AE. A historical survey of the development of life assurance. In: Brackenridge RDC, Elder WJ, eds. *Medical Selection of Life Risks*. 3rd ed. New York: Stockton Press; 1992:3–17.
3. Billi JE, Wise CG, Bills EA, Mitchell RL. Potential effects of managed care on specialty practice at a university medical center. *N Engl J Med*. 1995;333:979–983.
4. Weisbuch JB, Roberts NK. Without the denominator, where is the quality improvement paradigm in the nation's health care reform? *J Ins Med*. 1995;27:12–14.
5. Pokorski RJ. Mortality methodology and analysis seminar test. *J Ins Med*. 1995;20:20–45.
6. Seltzer F. Choosing a standard for adjusted mortality rates. *Stat Bull*. 1996;77:13–19.
7. Iacovino JR. A "quick hit" method to assess insurance mortality from a clinical article. *J Ins Med*. 1994;26:317–318.
8. Negus BH. Coronary anatomy and prognosis of young, asymptomatic survivors of myocardial infarction. *Am J Med*. 1994;96:354–358.
9. Clarke RD. Mortality of impaired lives 1964–73 [abstract]. *J Inst Act*. 1979;100 (pt 1). In: Lew EA, Gajewski J, eds. *Medical Risks: Trends in Mortality by Age and Time Elapsed*. New York: Praeger; 1990:7–120.
10. Jarvis HJ. Development of the diabetic, coronary, and blood pressure pools [abstract]. *Cooperation internationale pour les assurances des risques aggraves*, 1986. In: Lew EA, Gajewski J, eds. *Medical Risks: Trends in Mortality by Age and Time Elapsed*. New York: Praeger; 1990:7–122.
11. Medical Impairment Study 1983 [abstract]. I. Boston: Society of Actuaries and Association of Life Insurance Medical Directors of America, 1986. In: Lew EA, Gajewski J, eds. *Medical Risks: Trends in Mortality by Age and Time Elapsed*. New York: Praeger; 1990:6–78.
12. Singer RB. Comparative mortality by sex and age in residents of Rochester, Minnesota, with acute myocardial infarction during 1960–1979 (sudden deaths included). *J Ins Med*. 1995–1996;27:235–240.
13. Hutchinson R. Additional follow-up of patients with coronary bypass reoperation at Cleveland Clinic. *J Ins Med*. 1994;26:324–328.
14. Centers for Disease Control and Prevention. *A Public Health Action Plan to Prevent Heart Disease and Stroke*. U.S. Department of Health and Human Services; 2006.
15. *Build and Blood Pressure Study 1959*. Chicago: Society of Actuaries; 1959.
16. *Mortality Investigation of Declined Lives in Japan*. Tokyo: The Life Insurance Association of Japan; 1979.
17. *Blood Pressure Study 1979*. Boston: Society of Actuaries and Association of Life Insurance Medical Directors of America; 1980.
18. *Multiple Medical Impairment Study*. Westwood, MA: Center for Medico-Actuarial Statistics of MIB; 1998.
19. Borer JS, Kligfield P. Aortic regurgitation: Making management decisions. *ACC Curr J Rev*. 1995;4:30–32.
20. MacKenzie BR. Long-term mortality and complications of Bjork-Shiley spherical-disc valves—a life table analysis. *J Ins Med*. 1992;24:128–132.
21. Jeresaty RM. Mitral valve prolapse: an update. In: Arnold CB, ed. *Transactions of the American Academy of Insurance Medicine: One Hundred and First Annual Meeting*. Tampa, FL: Klay Printing; 1993:24–33.
22. Singer RB, Gajewski J. Cardiovascular diseases I. In: Lew EA, Gajewski J, eds. *Medical Risks: Trends in Mortality by Age and Time Elapsed, 1*. New York: Praeger; 1990;(6):30–38.
23. Croxson RS. Cardiovascular disorders: Part II. Other cardiovascular disorders. In: Brackenridge RDC, Elder WJ, eds. *Medical Selection of Life Risks*, 3rd ed. New York: Stockton Press; 1992:324–431.
24. Cumming GR. Survival after valve replacement. In: Arnold CB, ed. *Transactions of the America Academy of Insurance Medicine: One Hundred and First Annual Meeting*. Tampa, FL: Klay Printing; 1993:40–55.
25. Elliott PM, Saumarez RC, McKenna WJ. Recent clinical advances in hypertrophic cardiomyopathy. *Heart Failure*. 1995;11:15–25.
26. Cannan CR, Reeder GS, Bailey KR, et al. Natural history of hypertrophic cardiomyopathy: a population-based study, 1976 through 1990. *Circulation*. 1995;92:2488–2495.
27. Ten Cate FJ. Prognosis of hypertrophic cardiomyopathy. *J Ins Med*. 1996;28:42–45.
28. Iacovino JR. The nonmortality of hypertrophic cardiomyopathy in an unselected, community diagnosed and treated population. *J Ins Med*. 1996;28:51–54.
29. Gajewski J, Singer RB. Mortality in an insured population with atrial fibrillation. *JAMA*. 1981;245:1540–1544.
30. Chait L. Electrocardiography. In: Brackenridge RDC, Elder WJ, eds. *Medical Selection of Life Risks*. 3rd ed. New York: Stockton Press; 1992:433–472.
31. Gorlin R. Cost-effectiveness of ICD therapy for ventricular arrhythmias. *Prim Cardiol*. 1995;21:32–38.
32. *Build Study 1979*. Boston: Society of Actuaries and Association of Life Insurance Medical Directors of America; 1980.
33. Segel L. Serum albumin: "Phoenix" of the blood profile. *On the Risk*. 1995;11:81–83.
34. Rose G, Baxter PJ, Reid DD, McCartney P. Prevalence and prognosis of electrocardiographic findings in middle-aged men [abstract]. *Br Heart J*. 1978;40:636–643. In: Lew EA, Gajewski J, eds. *Medical Risks: Trends in Mortality by Age and Time Elapsed*. New York: Praeger; 1990.
35. Ferrer MI. A survey of 19,734 electrocardiograms obtained in insurance applicants. *J Ins Med*. 1985;16:6–13.
36. Privette M, ed. Court overrules HCFA 1986 investigational devices payment policy. *Cardiology*. 1996;25:4.

37. Tu HT, Ginsburg PB. Losing ground: physician income, 1995–2003. Community Tracking Study. *Center for Studying Health System Change.* June 2006.

38. Alper PR. The decline of the family doctor. *Policy Review.* April 2004;(124). www.hoover.org/publications/policyreview/3438846.html.

39. American Medical Association. Member connect survey. February/March 2006. www.ama-assn.org.

40. American Medical Association. Medical Liability Reform—NOW! 2005. www.ama-assn.org.

41. Mello MM. Understanding medical malpractice insurance: a primer. Research synthesis 8. Robert Wood Johnson Foundation; January 2006.

42. Hoyt RE, Powell LS. Pricing and reserving in medical malpractice insurance. Physician Insurers Association of America; April 2006. www.piaa.us.

CHAPTER (113)

Behavioral Cardiology Treatment Approaches to Heart Disease

Nina Rieckmann / Karina W. Davidson / Lynn Clemow / Daichi Shimbo / Thomas G. Pickering

Approximately 36 percent of all deaths that occurred in the United States in 2000, most of which were caused by heart disease, were attributable to behavioral or lifestyle factors, including tobacco use, poor diet, physical inactivity, and alcohol.[1] Although genetic factors undoubtedly contribute to individual susceptibility to these factors, a prime ingredient of this risk is the person's behavior. The costs of treating heart disease are escalating at an increasingly rapid pace because of the widespread use of sophisticated and increasingly expensive treatments such as drug-eluting coronary artery stents, implantable cardio-defibrillators, and gene therapy. Most efforts to contain the increase in healthcare costs have focused on limiting supply (a largely unfulfilled promise of managed care) and imposing some sort of rationing. However, as long ago as 1993, Fries and others[2] pointed out that restricting demand could achieve the same objective. They identified six factors, four of which are directly relevant to this chapter. They include the following facts:

1. Much disease is preventable.
2. Risky behavior costs money. Lifetime medical costs, which averaged $225,000 per person, have been clearly related to health behavior. For example, costs are approximately one-third higher in smokers compared to nonsmokers.
3. Self-management can result in savings. Several studies have shown that providing medical consumers with information and

guidelines about self-management can lower the use of medical services by 10 percent or more.
4. The promotion of healthy behavior at work has successfully reduced costs. This has also been documented in numerous studies.

This chapter focuses on the major behavioral and psychological factors that influence the course of coronary artery disease (CAD), and how they can be modified. The behavioral factors are smoking, diet, and obesity, and the psychological factors are depression and chronic stress.

A dramatic example of the effects of environmental and psychosocial factors on CAD is provided by an analysis of the changing mortality rates in Russia during the 1990s. Over a 4-year period following the dissolution of the Soviet Union, there was a 5-year decline in life expectancy, most of which could be attributed to increased mortality in men aged 25 to 64, as a results of accidents and cardiovascular disease. Factors that may have contributed to these changes included economic instability, stress, depression, and increased intake of alcohol and tobacco. In the middle of the 1990s, the trend reversed, and the average life expectancy increased again to the level of the early 1980s, mostly because of a reduction in the rate of deaths caused by alcohol consumption.[3]

Psychosocial factors can influence the course of chronic disease by two main pathways: first, by encouraging and inhibiting behavioral or lifestyle patterns such as smoking, and, second, by a direct effect on the disease process. Many psychosocial factors such as hostility and depression interact with both pathways—they influence how patients choose their lifestyles, and have deleterious impact on pathophysiologic mechanisms implicated in CAD progression.

Most practicing cardiologists are not involved in the primary prevention of disease. However, lifestyle and psychological factors influence not only the incidence, but also the *progression* of established CAD, as well as prognosis after acute coronary syndrome (ACS).[4]

Cardiologists need to be aware of the extent to which these factors influence a patient's prognosis, as well as the potential to modify these risks. This chapter reviews some of the interventions targeted to improve healthy behaviors and patient adherence, and to reduce psychosocial distress. We also discuss the importance of cardiologists' adherence to evidence-based guidelines in the management of existing CAD.[5]

Knowledge alone is not sufficient to change behavior: Motivation is also needed. A fundamental problem is that intervention studies commonly produce improvements in the behavior being manipulated lasting a few weeks or months, but by 1 year there is almost always some relapse. Many interventions apply a didactic, informative approach with little attention to what are now recognized as important differences in learning styles, levels of motivation to change behavior, and patient self-regulation skills. Over the past two decades, research on the *stages of change* model has yielded valuable insights regarding how, why, and when patients will change their behavior. The stages of change model suggests that behavioral change is achieved through a series of stages, defined as precontemplation, contemplation, preparation, action, and maintenance (Table 113–1).[6] For behavioral changes to be successfully implemented *permanently*, self-regulatory processes are needed to not only initiate but also maintain behavior change.

TABLE 113–1

Stages of Behavior Change

Precontemplation	Patient is not yet thinking about changing behavior
Contemplation	Patient is considering but is not yet ready to engage in behavior change
Preparation	Patient intends to take action in the next month
Action	Patient begins actual process of behavior change
Maintenance	Patient develops strategies to prevent relapse

tions, healthcare providers can and should use behavioral techniques to improve patients' self-care. These include contracting with the patient to reach specific goals; evaluating the patient's readiness for self-care; breaking self-care tasks down into small, manageable steps; providing personalized feedback to the patient; teaching the self-monitoring of health-related behaviors; enlisting social support; checking patient commitment to key tasks; and providing structure through followup appointments. One of the first tasks is to define the problem clearly. Physicians are usually concerned with items such as poor patient adherence and unhealthy lifestyle, whereas patients are more concerned about symptoms and emotional distress. Few physicians ask patients to identify the biggest problems they face in managing their illness.

Given the lack of training in behavioral techniques and the severe limitations on cardiologists' time, a team approach should ideally be employed. Behavioral interventions tend to require relatively large amounts of time, but nurses, psychologists, dietitians, and social workers can contribute to ensure that this need is met.

BEHAVIORAL INTERVENTIONS AND THE ROLE OF COLLABORATIVE MANAGEMENT OF PATIENTS WITH HEART DISEASE

Behavioral and lifestyle factors need to be addressed within a context of collaborative management. Heart disease is almost always chronic, and its successful management requires an active collaboration between the patient and healthcare providers. There is a big gap between the care prescribed and what is actually achieved. A classic example is the control of hypertension, where despite the availability of numerous powerful medications, blood pressure is adequately controlled in less than one-third of the patients.[7]

Patients often lack the knowledge and motivation to make behavioral changes, and the training of cardiologists rarely includes anything to do with behavior or behavioral intervention. Physicians generally have a low expectation of the effectiveness of behavioral interventions and no particular incentive to implement them, let alone the time to do so. And because neither patients nor physicians have pressured the healthcare system to recognize the importance of making these changes, behavioral interventions are rarely reimbursed. However, recent (2002) changes in Medicare policy have for the first time introduced the possibility of reimbursing providers such as health psychologists for assessing and treating health behaviors related to medical diagnoses. Despite these limita-

SMOKING INTERVENTIONS

Smoking kills more than 400,000 Americans every year, and more than half of these deaths are caused by cardiovascular disease and stroke. Smoking has for many years been recognized as one of the *big three* risk factors for cardiovascular disease (the others being hypertension and hyperlipidemia), and it is responsible for approximately 30 percent of cardiovascular morbidity and mortality. Smoking more than doubles the incidence of coronary artery disease, and it increases mortality by 70 percent. A dose-response relationship has been established between smoking and the severity of atherosclerosis in coronary and cerebral arteries and the aorta, particularly in men, and also between smoking status and the progression of carotid atherosclerosis. The contribution to cardiovascular disease deaths in younger smokers is particularly high, with 40 percent of cardiovascular disease (CVD) deaths in adults younger than 65 years of age being smoking related. Likewise, smoking contributes particularly strongly to increasing CVD risk in women and African Americans. In interaction with other risk factors, smoking contributes to CVD through a number of biological pathways involving the central and peripheral nervous systems, the walls of blood vessels, the coagulation system, and the immune system.

Fortunately, the cardiovascular risks associated with smoking are almost completely reversible after a patient quits. In quitting smoking a patient reduces his or her risk of a CVD-related event by half virtually immediately. It is estimated that as much as 24 percent of the decrease in CVD mortality over the past 30 years is related to reductions in cigarette smoking, and smoking cessation has been shown to be one of the most cost-effective interventions in the whole field of medicine.

Agency for Healthcare Research and Quality Guidelines

The importance and effectiveness of smoking cessation programs has been reviewed extensively by the Agency for Healthcare Research and Quality (AHRQ), which issued its guidelines in 1996 and updated them in 2000.[8] The guidelines emphasize that healthcare clinics and cardiology practices are ideal settings for the promotion of smoking cessation. More than 70 percent of smokers report that they see a physician at least once a year. The guidelines emphasize that a variety of effective strategies can be adopted, some very simple, others more complex. AHRQ recommendations are summarized in Table 113–2.

A general rule is that "more is better," or that the quit rate is proportional to the amount of effort that is put in. For example, a 5- to 7-minute brief counseling intervention using the counseling model suggested above increased cessation rates to 20 percent, over the 7 to 10 percent with advice alone. The components, which are not mutually exclusive, include counseling, which has two basic components: providing social support and boosting skills in problem solving. A state-funded telephone quit line to provide brief counseling services has also proved to be effective. Other components include the use of nicotine replacement therapy, which can be delivered in a variety of ways, including gum, skin patches, and nasal sprays. A number of clinical trials have shown that the nicotine patches can double the quit rates. Finally, the use of the antidepressant drug bupropion (Zyban) has also been found to be very effective. A recent study (published since the AHRQ guidelines were issued) found that bupropion also approximately doubled the quit rate and that the best results were obtained with a combination of counseling, nicotine patch, and bupropion treatment (see Table 113–3 for a summary).

Smoking interventions based on the AHRQ guidelines have proven effective in randomized controlled trials in primary care settings.[9] There is evidence that a healthcare system's performance can be effectively improved by provider feedback, intensive office

TABLE 113–2

Agency for Healthcare Research and Quality Smoking Cessation Guideline Overview

ACTION	COMMENTS
Identify the smokers	Adding smoking status to vital sign stamp on clinical records increases likelihood that physician will discuss smoking with the patient. Chart stickers indicating smoking status can also help.
Advise smokers to quit	Advice should be clear, strong, and personalized. Quit rate will increase from 7.9% to 10.2% with advice alone. This can seem like a small increment on an individual basis, but each smoker who quits will add 15 years to his or her life expectancy.
Assess smoker's willingness to quit and provide informational support appropriate to his or her readiness to quit	Ask about how important it seems to quit smoking at this time. Encourage patients to discuss their personal reasons why quitting might be important to them. Assess history of previous quit attempts to explore previous successful strategies and identify problem areas. Encourage discussion that builds patient's confidence in his or her ability to quit.
For patient who is *willing* to quit, develop plan for initiating treatment and followup	Assist in plans to set quit date, line up support. Consider nicotine replacement or tapering plan to minimize nicotine withdrawal symptoms, possibly other approved medications to reduce cravings. Assess needs for specialized smoking cessation services. Arrange followup plan.
For patients *unwilling* to attempt to quit, provide counseling to promote patient's readiness to quit	Emphasize the "five Rs": Personal *relevance* to the patient's medical and social situation; *Risks* associated with smoking (acute and long-term risks, and risks to others in their environment); The *rewards* of quitting; *Roadblocks* that might interfere with successfully quitting or increase risk of relapse; *Repetition* of a stop-smoking message.

staff training, and other systems interventions. An excellent recent review and meta-analysis of smoking cessation in patients with CAD[10] emphasizes that significantly better outcomes are seen with more intensive treatment, with a minimum length of 1-month of counseling, medications, if used, and followup.

Current Developments, Future Directions

The fundamentals of smoking cessation treatment have changed little in the past 10 years. Much of the recent research has focused on adapting the available technology to meet the needs of special populations, including patients with depression, attention-deficit/ hyperactivity disorder (ADHD), and chronic psychiatric illnesses. Most patients are served well by the current technology, but some have not been effectively treated. Behavior genetic studies have be-

TABLE 113-3

Drugs to Assist with Smoking Cessation[a]

Nicotine replacement	Strong evidence exists, regardless of method, that use of nicotine replacement roughly doubles the success rate for smoking cessation. Some evidence for combining patch with additional PRN doses when one method alone fails. **Patches:** Approved for OTC use since 1995, used for 16 hours/day, either in a fixed or tapering dose over 6–10 weeks. **Nicotine lozenges and gum:** Also OTC drugs, both are available in 2 and 4 mg doses. Recommend 1–2 pieces/hour. **Nicotine spray or inhaler:** Prescription items, designed to deliver nicotine more quickly than gum and patches.
Bupropion (Zyban or Wellbutrin)	A prescription drug, originally developed as antidepressant, which appears to help reduce urges to smoke. Recommended dose is 300 mg/day, started 1 week before quite date and continued for 7–12 weeks. Approximately doubles successful quit rate, regardless of depression status of patients.

PRN, as needed; OTC, over-the-counter.
[a]Best evidence suggests using both nicotine replacement and bupropion in the context of counseling.

gun to yield information identifying patients who may need different interventions and to suggest possible new treatments for some subsets of patients.[11]

In summary, physician counseling for smoking cessation has been shown to be one of the most cost-effective interventions in the whole field of medicine (Table 113–4).

DIETARY INTERVENTIONS

Dietary factors have a substantial impact on the development and progression of coronary artery disease (CAD). The intake of saturated fats and lipids is associated with increased rates of CAD-related death and all-cause mortality.[12] On the basis of epidemiologic and observational studies in men, women, African Americans, and elderly persons as well as postmortem angiographic studies in young persons, the National Institutes of Health (NIH) and the European Atherosclerosis Society have concluded that elevation of

TABLE 113-4

Example of the Cost-Benefit Ratio of Physician Counseling for Smoking Cessation

If one physician counsels 100 smokers, 95 can continue to smoke—a dispiritingly large number.
However, of the 5 who do quit, one ex-smoker will avoid a premature smoking-related death, and another will gain up to 15 years of life expectancy.
The cost of this benefit will have been a total of 3 hours and 20 minutes of the physician's time.

serum lipids is a causal factor in CAD.[12,13] Saturated fat is the principal dietary determinant of serum cholesterol levels including low-density lipoprotein. As serum cholesterol levels can be affected by dietary interventions, this has led to recommendations by the National Cholesterol Education Program (NCEP) and the American Heart Association (AHA) that dietary counseling should form the basis of lipid-regulating regimens for both the primary prevention of CAD events and the clinical management of patients with CAD.[14,15] NCEP[14] and AHA[15] guidelines recommend restricting the composition of total fat to an upper limit of 30 percent and saturated fat to an upper limit of 7 to 10 percent of the daily caloric intake.

Several diets have been examined in CAD patients. In this chapter, we discuss four dietary interventions: saturated fat reduction, very low fat diet, increased fish oil consumption, and the Mediterranean diet. For a more comprehensive discussion of these and other diets, we refer readers to a recent review.[16] Finally, although there is a dearth of information of the efficacy of the low carbohydrate diet in patients with CAD, we also briefly discuss this diet here because of its increasing controversy in the public and scientific community.

Low Fat Diets

Comprehensive reviews of dietary intervention studies[17] indicate that aggressive treatment with a diet low in total and saturated fats lowers serum lipids levels, produces positive angiographic changes, and potentially helps to improve anginal and other non–lipid-related symptoms. However, reducing fat intake alone only goes so far. Randomized controlled trials of dietary fat reduction have shown varying results on reducing cardiovascular events. A meta-analysis of 27 randomized controlled trials conducted by the Cochrane Collaboration showed that reduced or modified dietary fat was associated with a small but nonsignificant reduction in cardiovascular mortality (rate ratio 0.91; 0.77 to 1.07) and a significant reduction in cardiovascular events (0.84; 0.72 to 0.99). However, the latter reductions were attenuated (0.86; 0.72 to 1.03) in an analysis that excluded a trial that additionally included oily fish in the intervention arm.[18] In a systematic review conducted by Iestra and colleagues,[19] saturated fat reduction was not associated with a better prognosis in patients with CAD.

Very Low Fat Diets

Although NCEP and AHA both recommend an upper limit for total dietary fat (30 percent), these expert panels do not specify a lower limit. A very low fat (VLF) diet is characterized by one in which fat comprises ≤15 percent of the total calories. Typically, 15 percent and 70 percent of the total calories is comprised of protein and carbohydrates respectively. The VLF diet in combination with exercise was associated with weight loss, improvement in cholesterol and triglyceride levels, and less progression of coronary atherosclerosis by angiography at 12 months in 113 patients with stable angina.[20] Similarly, in the Ornish Lifestyle Heart Trial, a VLF diet with other lifestyle changes such as smoking cessation, exercise, and stress reduction was associated with an improvement in coronary atherosclerosis progression, and a reduction in cardiovascular events.[21] These studies were limited by small sample size and possible confounding with other lifestyle changes, which were included as part of the intervention.

Increased Fish Oil Consumption

Several epidemiologic studies have indicated that increased fish consumption is associated with a lower risk of cardiovascular mortality. The benefit of fish consumption is thought to be secondary to omega-3 fatty acids, specifically eicosapentaenoic acid (EPA) and docosahexaenoic acid (DHA), which are present in seafood. Several randomized controlled trials have indicated that omega-3 fatty acid supplementation reduces the risk of cardiovascular mortality including sudden cardiac death and nonfatal events in patients with CAD,[22] although not all studies have been positive.[23] Based on this evidence, the AHA has recommended that CAD patients intake approximately 1 gram of EPA and DHA (combined) daily, either from fish consumption or from omega-3 fatty acid capsules.[22]

The Mediterranean Diet

The Mediterranean diet consists of higher intakes of fiber-rich food (vegetables, legumes, fruits, and nuts), fish, and polyunsaturated fats in the form of olive oil; lower intakes of dairy products and meat, including red meat and poultry; and wine in low to moderate amounts. Several randomized controlled trials have shown that the Mediterranean diet reduces the risk of all-cause mortality, cardiovascular mortality, and nonfatal myocardial infarction.[16] Although the Mediterranean diet is multifaceted, some investigators hypothesize the major benefit of this diet is explained by the inclusion of omega-3 fatty acids, which are not only present in fish (EPA and DHA) but also in nuts and plant oils (alpha-linolenic acid).

Low Carbohydrate Diet

The low carbohydrate diet is comprised of 5 to 30 percent carbohydrates, >25 percent protein, and a relative increased percentage of fat 30 to 70 percent. Several small studies[16] have shown that compared with a low fat diet, a low carbohydrate diet is associated with short term weight loss (4–6 kg), a greater increase in high-density lipoprotein (HDL) cholesterol, and a greater decrease in triglycerides in obese or overweight individuals without CAD. Although these results are promising, concerns have been raised about the concomitant increase in protein intake and fat content associated with a low carbohydrate diet. Proposed adverse effects include ketosis, deficits in nutrients and fiber, reduced renal function, and increased atherogenesis.

【 】 ADHERENCE: THE KEY TO SUCCESSFUL INTERVENTIONS

No matter how efficacious an interventional strategy, it is doomed to failure unless it is implemented at the right time and the right dose, and followed through by the patient. Adherence is defined as the extent to which (1) providers follow established clinical guidelines in their treatment, and (2) patients follow the prescribed regimens of their providers, including the above described changes in lifestyle, as well as all prescribed medication. (Historically, the term "compliance" has often been used interchangeably with "adherence." Nowadays, researchers prefer the term "adherence" because it underscores the active role of both patients and caregivers as collaborators in long-term patient care.)

Thus, adherence is *the* key factor in achieving risk factor control and reducing adverse cardiovascular outcomes. Despite this obvious notion, nonadherence is one of the biggest problems in clinical practice: Reports of failure to fully adhere to a prescribed medication regimen range from 25 to 85 percent, and less than 50 percent of all patients adhere to recommended dietary changes, exercise, and smoking cessation.

Nonadherence—A Major Risk Factor for Incident and Recurrent CAD Events

Recently, data from the Health Professionals Follow-up Study showed that among initially healthy men, 62 percent of incident CAD events could have been prevented had all men adhered to five low-risk behaviors: not smoking, exercising regularly, eating prudently, consuming alcohol in moderation, and maintaining a healthy weight.[24] Importantly, men who initially reported all five risk behaviors but who adopted positive lifestyle changes in at least two areas over time also substantially decreased their risk of incident CAD events (by 27 percent).

Adherence to recommended pharmacologic and nonpharmacologic interventions is equally important in patients with manifest CAD. Rates of discontinuation of prescribed medication after hospitalization are as high as 46 percent in the first year after hospitalization.[25] Meta-analyses have shown that even partial medication nonadherence significantly increases the risk for mortality after hospitalization for a CAD event.[26] The Beta Blocker Heart trial, for example, showed that β-blocker adherence ≤75 percent was associated with a 2.6 times greater risk for mortality within 1 year.[27] Interestingly, the recent Candesartan in Heart Failure Assessment of Reduction in Mortality and Morbidity (CHARM)[28] trial showed that poor adherence to medication increased the risk for mortality in chronic heart failure (CHF) patients regardless of whether the patients were taking the study medication or a placebo. This suggests that patients who poorly adhere to their medication might be neglectful of other effective treatments and recommended behaviors; thus, nonadherence to one type of treatment might be a good indicator for general nonadherence. This notion, however, has yet to be tested empirically.

Partial nonadherence to nonpharmacologic interventions also increases the risk for adverse outcomes. For example, lower adherence to the Mediterranean diet in CAD patients was associated with a 27 percent higher all-cause mortality rate, and a 31 percent increase in cardiac deaths across an average of 3.8 years.[29]

Risk Factors for Patient Nonadherence

Nonadherence crosses age and gender groups and socioeconomic strata. Increasing age appears to be a risk factor primarily for nonadherence to pharmacologic treatments. More important are negative aspects of the pharmacologic and nonpharmacologic regimens: long duration of a prescribed intervention, complexity of the regimen, asymptomatic conditions, lack of immediate or perceived benefits, and high monetary and/or social costs.[30] Next to these impediments that are inherent to the disease or regimen, and thus are modifiable only to a limited extent, patients' mental health also plays a critical role. One of the most established risk factors for nonadherence is depression: patients with depression are up to three times more likely not to adhere to treatment recommendations than patients without any depression symptoms (see Fig. 113–1).[31,32] There is no systematic evidence to date that shows that treating depression results in improved adherence, but the large impact that this mental health problem has on nonadherence suggests so.

Adherence Needs to Be Targeted on Multiple Levels

It is widely recognized that successful interventions targeting adherence require a multilevel approach that involves the joint effort and commitment of patients, healthcare providers, and the organizations delivering care. Healthcare providers need to acknowledge the importance of adherence and their critical role in helping their patients to establish and maintain behavior change. They need to educate themselves and follow the latest guidelines, improve their communication skills, and collaborate with each other. Healthcare organizations need to educate patients and providers, provide physicians with feedback on their performance, establish and support professional networks, and minimize structural barriers to patient adherence (costs, access to care, language problems, etc.).

Interventions to Improve Adherence in Healthcare Providers

Despite the availability of published practice guidelines for secondary prevention in CAD (see Table 113–1), many patients receive inadequate treatment recommendations. The 1998 Medicare data collection showed that up to one-third of post-myocardial infarction (MI) patients did not receive the medication that was indicated for them, and smoking cessation counseling was documented in only 40 percent of cases.[33] The AHA's Get With The Guidelines (GWTG) program, an acute-care hospital-based quality improvement program, is a nationwide initiative designed to improve healthcare providers' adherence in secondary prevention. It is based on the observation that interventions to improve guideline adherence are most effective if they are implemented early on in the treatment process, while the patient is still inhospital; in addition, patients are more adherent to treatment recommendations when these are given inhospital as opposed to after discharge. A GWTG pilot study involving 24 diverse hospitals was initiated in 2000.[34] The intervention involved (1) an interactive Web-based patient management tool that takes approximately 90 seconds to complete and provides data entry, embedded reminders and guideline summaries, and online reports of quality measure per-

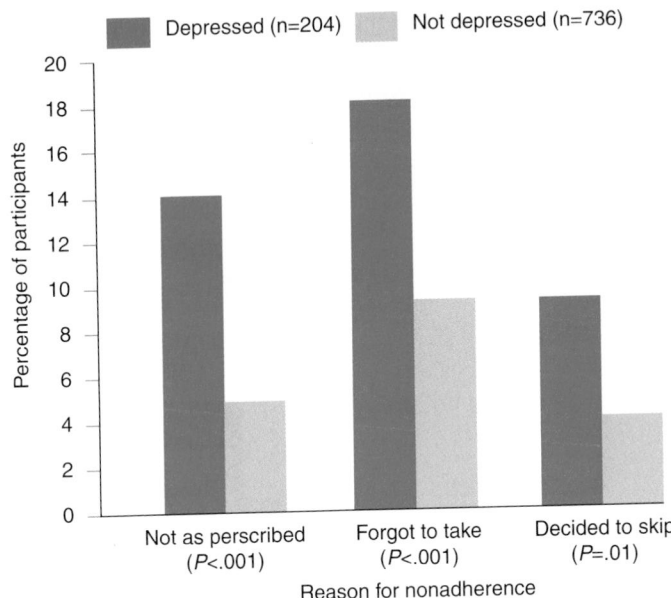

FIGURE 113–1. The impact of depression on medication adherence in 1024 stable coronary heart disease patients. *Source: Data from Gehi, Haas, Pipkin, et al.*[32]

formance (Fig. 113–2)[35]; (2) four collaborative learning sessions and monthly conference calls among multidisciplinary hospital teams; and (3) best-practices sharing and the use of an Internet tool to change systems and collect data on 1738 patients. Results were promising: Within 1 year, smoking cessation counseling increased from 48 to 87 percent, lipid treatment from 54 to 79 percent, lipid measurement from 59 to 81 percent, and cardiac rehabilitation referral from 34 to 73 percent. An improving trend was seen in blood pressure control. AHA plans to extend this program on a nationwide basis, including the rewarding of institutions that achieve evidence-based quality. Other large quality-improvement efforts include the American College of Cardiology (ACC) Guidelines Applied in Practice efforts, and the Can Rapid Risk Stratification of Unstable Angina Patients Suppress Adverse Outcomes with Early Implementation of the ACC/AHA Guidelines (CRUSADE) Quality-Improvement Initiative.

Interventions to Improve Adherence in Patients

Behavioral changes are difficult to establish and sustain. Interventions designed to improve patient adherence have largely failed to improve long-term adherence, and most did not result in improved medical outcome. The lessons learned to date are the following: (1) education alone is not effective; (2) single strategies (such as phone call reminders) are not effective, but the use of multiple strategies is needed; and (3) motivationally-based strategies (i.e., motivational interviewing) that foster internal incentives are more promising than external incentive approaches. The most promising strategy appears to be the implementation of *combinations* of interventions,[36] including patient education, contracts, reminders, counseling, reinforcement, mobilization of social support, self-efficacy enhancement and telephone followup (Table 113–5). Ideally, these interventions are initiated before the patient is discharged from hospital. Future research will show whether the integration of mental health screenings and collaborative care

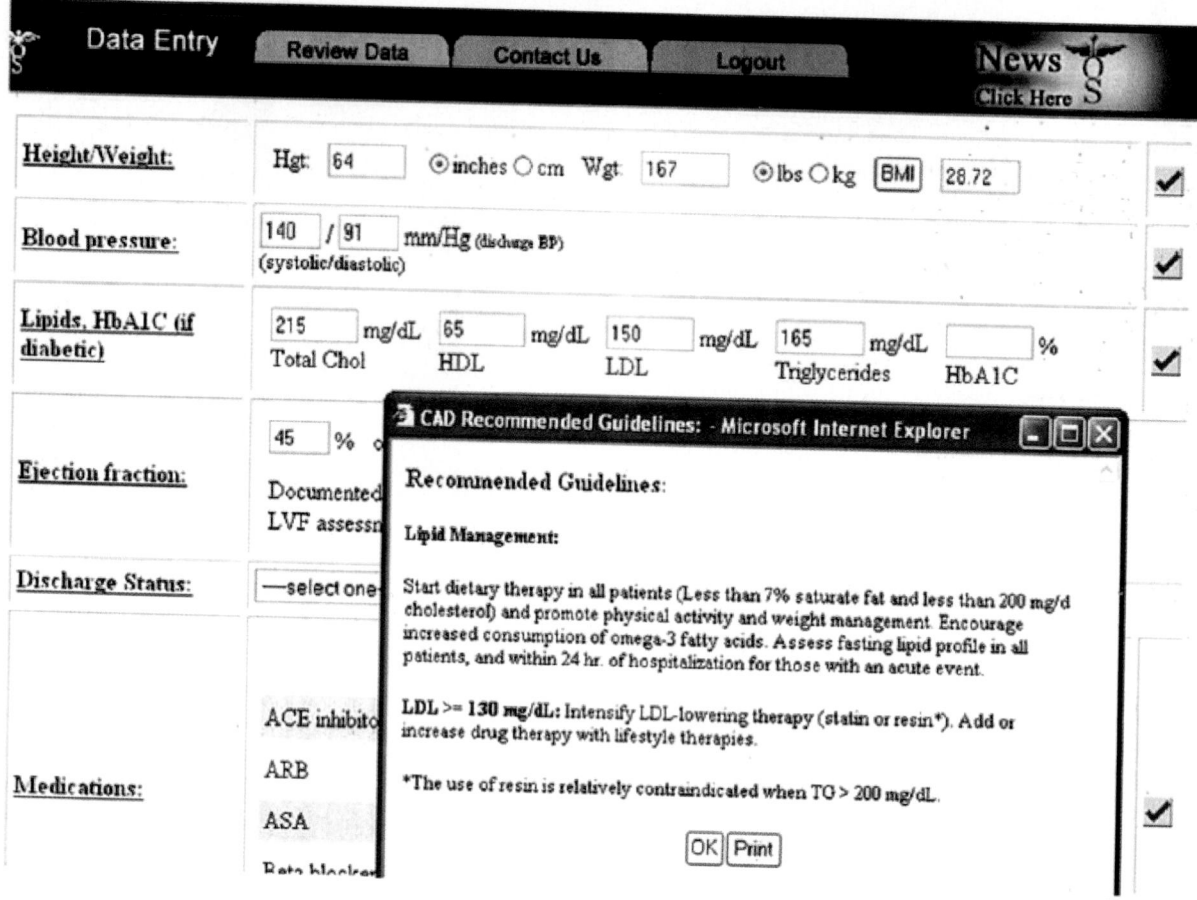

FIGURE 113–2. Example of a Web-based data entry and healthcare provider feedback tool: Simple, one-page, online form reminds the physician to evaluate adherence to AHA practice guidelines. ACE, angiotensin-converting enzyme; AHA, American Heart Association; ARB, angiotensin II receptor blocker; ASA, aspirin; HDL, high-density lipoprotein; LDL, low-density lipoprotein; HbA1C, glycosylated hemoglobin. *Source: Smaha.*[35]

TABLE 113–5

Strategies to Improve Patient Adherence in Clinical Practice

• Effective communication	Provide clear, direct messages about the importance of a recommended lifestyle change/medication. Provide verbal and written instructions.
• Signed agreements	Encourage written contract about *specific* set of behaviors (e.g., number of servings of fruits and vegetables per day, number of minutes of cardiovascular-strengthening exercise). Patient maintains behavioral logs.
• Behavioral skill training	Encourage patient to attend classes that teach healthy cooking, proper stretching techniques before and after exercise, or how to respond to an anger-provoking situation.
• Self-monitoring	Ask patient to establish a baseline for their behavior: number of cigarettes they smoke, their daily intake of fat (current packaging requirements make this relatively easy), etc.
• Self-efficacy enhancement	Assess and reinforce even small improvements in behavior.
• Telephone/mail contact	Such reminders have been shown to have a positive effect on adherence.
• Spousal/social support	Encourage the presence of a significant other/supportive person when discussing behavioral change with the patient.
• Stages of change	Tailor advice to the patient's current stage of readiness (e.g., precontemplation, contemplation, implementation phase).
• Mental health screening	Screen for mental health problems such as depression and substance abuse that pose significant barriers to adherence.
• Professional support	Develop a network of healthcare professionals who can support efforts for behavior change and to whom patients can be referred for help with specific interventional strategies.

treatment of such comorbid conditions will bring about the much needed improvements in patient adherence.

PSYCHOSOCIAL INTERVENTIONS

Given the emphasis that CVD patients place on stress and psychosocial factors contributing to their disease—as well as some of the recent evidence suggesting that psychosocial factors predict CVD recurrence and death—offering psychosocial interventions for CVD patients seems reasonable. However, there are many different types of interventions aimed at different psychosocial factors and different outcomes.

TABLE 113–6

Diagnostic and Statistical Manual-IV Depressive Disorder Categories

DEPRESSIVE DISORDERS	SYMPTOM CRITERIA	DURATION CRITERIA
Major depressive disorder	>5 depressive symptoms, including depressed mood, anhedonia, or anergia	>2 weeks
Dysthymia	2–4 symptoms	>2 years
Adjustment disorder	Depressed mood, hopelessness	3–6 months, in relation to stressor
Depression caused by a general medical condition	Depressed mood, anhedonia, with established relation to medical condition	N/A
Depression NOS	2–4 depressive symptoms	>2 weeks

NA, not applicable; NOS, not otherwise specified.
SOURCE: American Psychiatric Association. Diagnostic and Statistical Manual of Mental Disorders. 4th ed. Washington, D.C: 1994.

[ ] DEPRESSION: A CARDIOTOXIC PSYCHOSOCIAL RISK FACTOR

To the CAD patient, depression is synonymous with feelings of sadness, distress, and hopelessness, and to the cardiologist, it is an unwelcome but expected reaction to a life-changing event—that of experiencing an acute coronary syndrome (ACS). However, depression as defined within psychiatry is comprised of a number of disorders (Table 113–6), all of which are relevant to cardiologists and our patients. Briefly, adjustment disorder—a temporary emotional reaction to a major life event—is often what both patients and their treating physician expect to occur after an ACS, and if with an uncomplicated course, should resolve within 6 months without need for treatment. However, all of the other depressive disorders listed in Table 113–6 require appropriate assessment and treatment, and all, with the possible exception of a mild depressive adjustment disorder,[37] identify patients at high risk for poor cardiovascular prognosis.

Depression Is Prevalent in Coronary Artery Disease Patients

Depression, whether diagnosed as a psychiatric disorder or assessed by a patient-report of the presence of some depression symptoms, is prevalent among CAD patients. An Agency for Healthcare Research and Quality systematic review reported that up to 20 percent of hospitalized post-MI patients meet criteria for a major depressive disorder, up to 47 percent have significant patient-reported depression symptoms, and these diagnoses/symptoms remain long after discharge.[38]

Depression Predicts Important Outcomes in Coronary Artery Disease Patients

Recent meta-analyses and systematic reviews conclude that depression is a predictor of all-cause mortality (odds ratio [OR] = 2.4; confidence interval [CI] = 1.8–3.2),[39] cardiovascular mortality (OR = 2.6; CI = 1.8–3.8),[39] cardiovascular event recurrence (OR = 2.0; CI = 1.3–2.9),[39] and compromised health-related quality of life (OR = 3.1; CI = 2.2–4.6) in post-MI patients.[40] These findings occur despite using different ways to assess depression, different patient populations, different followup periods, and different covariates. This consistent finding of risk in the face of these formidable methodological obstacles has led some to consider that we can still be underestimating the impact of depression on our CAD patients.[38] Numerous mechanisms have been proposed and tested to account for the association between depression, an affective disorder, and these outcomes, including both behavioral pathways such as nonadherence to medication and other physician treatment recommendations, and pathophysiologic mechanisms such as increased chronic inflammation and platelet activation.[4]

Depression Interventions for CAD Patients

There are two recent randomized controlled trials that have examined the impact of depression treatment on various outcomes in post-MI patients, but only one of these had sufficient power (N = 2481) to determine if a depression psychotherapy intervention improved survival,[41] but no such effect was found. Calls for the next sufficiently powered trial have been issued, and current thinking is that both antidepressant and psychotherapy should be employed to successfully treat depression in CAD patients.[42]

Lack of Practice Guidelines for Depression Assessment and Treatment in Coronary Artery Disease Patients

Despite the recognition of the importance of depression assessment in the recent ACC/AHA practice guidelines for ST-elevation MI patients,[43] the guidelines offer no explicit guidance on how to conduct such an assessment, or the type of preferred depression treatment. Grissom and Phillips have identified a number of barriers that prevent cardiologists from assessing and treating depression.[44] They note that lack of training, skepticism that depression treatment will improve medical outcomes, limitations of current depression screening tools, and lack of time are all impediments to successful depression management for cardiologists.

A recent grand rounds presentation in *The Journal of the American Medical Association* offers some useful guidance for depression screening in the cardiac care unit (CCU) by a cardiologist (Fig. 113–3), or for the collection of patient-reported depression symptoms that can aid in depression management (see Table 113–7).[45]

Finally, resources for cardiologists, their staff, and patients are starting to become available over the Internet. For example, the MacArthur Initiative on Depression in Primary Care (www. depression-primarycare.org) offers manuals, patient pamphlets, and practice re-engineering tips for increasing the detection and treatment of depression in the medically ill patient. Similarly the Web site, Improving Mood—Promoting Access to Collaborative Treatment for Late Life Depression (IMPACT; http://impact-uw.org/) offers the key depression management components of their primary care-based, collaborative care depression model that was recently found to be effective for more than 1800 medical patients diagnosed with a depressive disorder.

Detecting and treating depression in CAD patients will increasingly become a priority of treating cardiologists, their patients, and the patients' family members. Systematic detection and management of depression that interdigitates with busy CCU practices, is not stigmatizing, is effective, is a goal that will improve the health and well-being of our patients, and is something to which we should aspire.

Given that depression treatment guidelines have not yet been proposed or tested for CAD patients, probably the simplest treatment regimen is that currently recommended in primary care (Table 113–8), which makes use of the Patient Health Questionnaire-9 shown below in Table 113–7 for treatment decisions.[46]

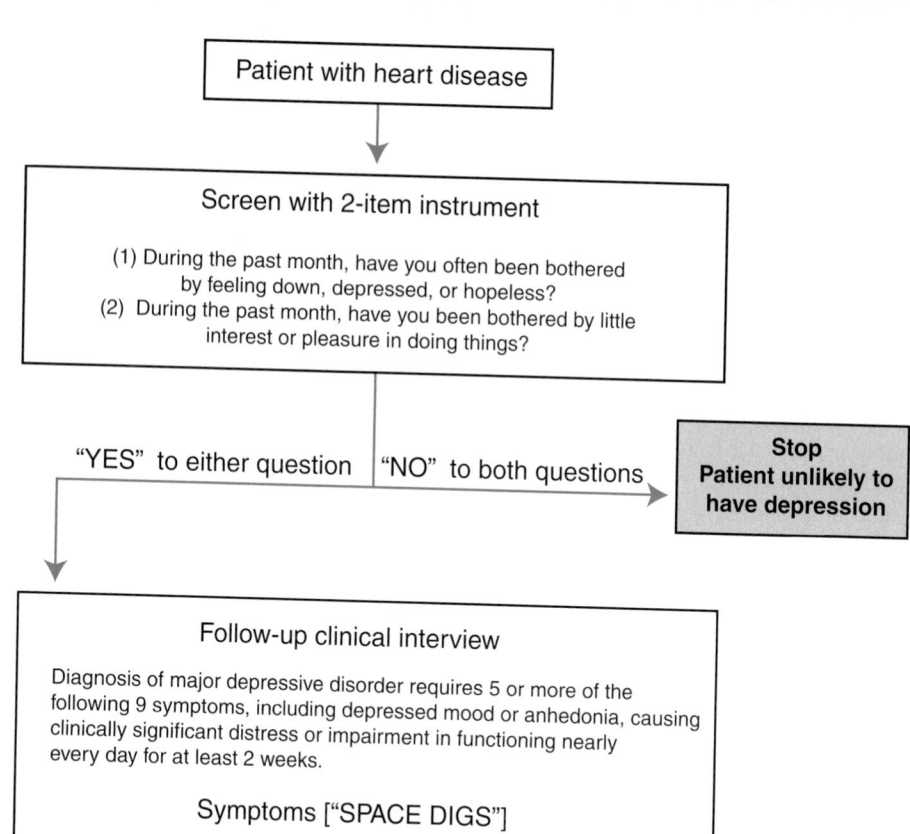

FIGURE 113–3. Depression-screening algorithm in patients with heart disease. *Source: Whooley MA.[45]*

[ ] CHRONIC STRESS: ANOTHER CORONARY ARTERY DISEASE RISK FACTOR

There are numerous psychosocial factors other than depression that have been proposed as markers for cardiovascular recurrence risk in

TABLE 113–7

The Two-Item Patient Health Questionnaire Depression Screening Instrument

Over the last 2 weeks, how often have you been bothered by any of the following problems?	Not at all	Several days	More than half the days	Nearly every day
1. Little interest or pleasure in doing things				
2. Feeling down, depressed, or hopeless				

TABLE 113-8

MaineHealth Treatment Algorithm Based on the PHQ-9 Score

PHQ-9 SCORE	SYMPTOM LEVEL	MOST LIKELY DIAGNOSIS	TREATMENT RECOMMENDATION	CARE MANAGEMENT	PSYCH CONSULT
0–9	Minimal	Minor depression, no depression	Consider other diagnoses, watchful waiting; treat if symptoms persistent or for other clinical reasons	Recommended as part of watchful waiting; otherwise not recommended	Not recommended unless needed to clarify diagnosis
10–14	Mild	Major depression, minor depression, dysthymia	Watchful waiting, medication, psychotherapy	Recommended as part of watchful waiting; otherwise optional, depending on comorbidities, social support	Not recommended unless needed to clarify diagnosis or if symptoms are persistent
15–19	Moderate	Major depression	Medication, psychotherapy, or both	Recommended	Suggested, especially if psychosocial comorbidities or persistent symptoms
20–27	Severe	Major depression	Medication with or without psychotherapy	Recommended	Recommended

Notes:
1. Self-management activities are recommended for all patients diagnosed with depression (e.g. exercise, sleep, avoid alcohol).
2. Watchful waiting is active followup of a patient at a minimum duration of monthly contacts by clinician or care manager.
3. Dysthymia is defined as a presence of symptoms of depressed mood most of the time for the last two years with at least two other symptoms and functional impairment.
4. Formal referral to specialty mental health care is also recommended for:
   • Those with any suicidal risk.
   • Those who appear to have psychiatric comorbidities such as posttraumatic stress disorder (PTSD) or active substance abuse.
   • Those for whom there is concern about possible bipolar disorder.

SOURCE: Rollman BL, Weinreb L, Korsen N, et al.[46]

CAD patients, many of which assess various aspects of chronic stress.[4] Chronic stress can result from numerous life circumstances, such as lasting social isolation, ongoing lack of control or autonomy at work, or impoverished economic circumstances.

One of the core concerns in determining if stress is a marker of risk for CAD patients is the lack of standard definition for *stress*. Stress has been used to refer to the *perception* of stress, that is, the report by the patient or person of the level of distress they experience, and it has also been used to refer to exposure to external circumstances that are consensually agreed on to be distressful. However, when exposures to stressors, such as recent life events, are assessed, patients are rarely asked if this event actually caused distress to them. Thus, the term *stress* is used in (at least) two different ways—one as a report of distress, and one as an exposure. Without a common parlance, it is difficult to know what meaning of stress—the perception of being overwhelmed? The exposure to constant daily hassles? The endurance of one major life event?—might be responsible for elevating patient risk for increased cardiovascular and quality of life outcomes. Without standard nomenclature, definitions, and measures, the field that examines the impact of stress on ACS incidence and progression has been seriously impeded.

Chronic Stress Predicts Important Outcomes in Coronary Artery Disease Patients

Excellent reviews exist detailing the evidence that various definitions of stress, including the experience of chronic negative emotions, ex-

posure to chronic stressors, and experience of social isolation or conflict, is each associated with cardiovascular disease incidence and progression.[4,47] Those factors with the most evidence of plausible independent cardiovascular disease recurrence risk include work stress, defined in differing ways, lack of social support, and lower socioeconomic circumstances.

It is an understatement to assert that incidence and prevalence are difficult to ascertain without knowledge of what is meant by stress. Nevertheless, when asked, CAD patients report that stress was the most likely reason for their heart disease,[48] but again, what is meant by patient report of stress is unclear. A recent case-control study of first-time MI patients versus healthy controls found that patients reported higher levels of general stress defined as several or permanent stress periods at work, home, or both (15.6–43.8 percent, depending on country or ethnicity sampled), compared to controls.[49] When detailing the specific source of stress, these post-MI patients reported more frequent periods of stress at work, at home, in general, with finances, and also more frequent exposure to major life events in the year prior to the MI.

Stress Interventions for Coronary Artery Disease Patients

An exciting stress management trial has been conducted with patients with documented coronary heart disease, in which stress management had been compared to both exercise and usual care (although random assignment was only to the first two conditions; those who lived too

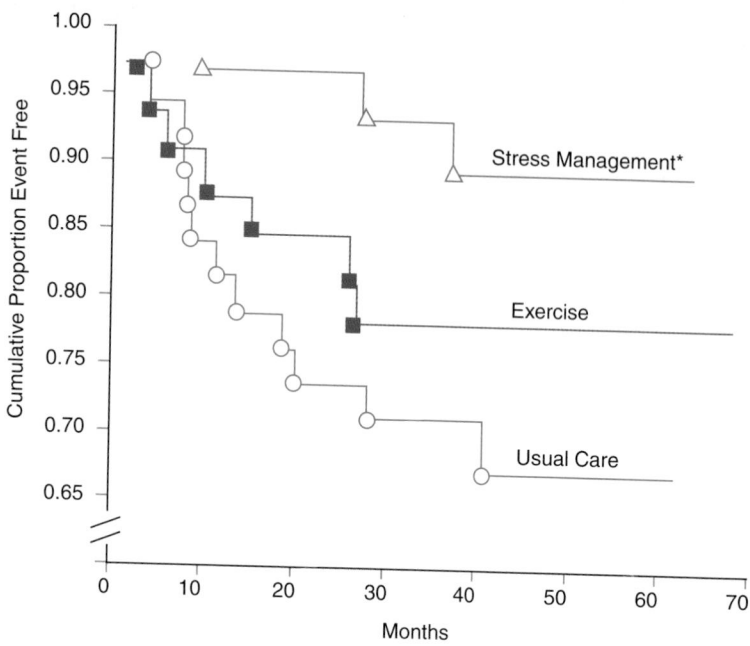

FIGURE 113–4. Impact of stress management intervention versus exercise or usual care on cardiovascular event rate. After adjusting for age, baseline left ventricular ejection fraction, and history of MI, stress management was associated with a significantly lower risk (relative risk, 0.26; P = .04) of an adverse cardiac event compared with usual care. Exercise was also associated with a lower risk compared with usual care, but this difference was not statistically significant (relative risk, 0.68; P = .34). The asterisk indicates significant difference from usual care at P <.05. *Source: Blumenthal JA, Jiang W, Babyak MA, et al.*[50]

far away to participate formed the usual care group.[50] To be eligible, the 117 patients had to have ischemia to a mental stress test, an exercise stress test, or ambulatory ECG testing. Stress management included 16 weekly 1.5-hour group sessions focused on education about the health costs of stress, ways to minimize the cognitive, physical, and emotional effects of stress, progressive muscle relaxation (a stress reduction technique) as well as other stress management components. Exercise patients received 16 weekly group supervised exercise sessions. Across an average of 38 months, there was a clear reduction in cardiovascular disease recurrence in those receiving stress management, compared to the usual control, but not for the exercise group (Fig. 113–4). These patients were then contacted after 5 years of followup, and the stress intervention was associated with fewer medical costs then either the exercise intervention or the usual care intervention groups over 2 years, and with lower costs than usual care group over 5 years.[51] Such stress management techniques clearly need to be tested in larger patient samples but hold promise for moving this field forward, without the need for a clear definition of stress.

Lack of Practice Guidelines for Stress Assessment and Treatment in Coronary Artery Disease Patients

Although there are now European guidelines on the detection and prevention of cardiovascular disease that in-

Behavioral and Medical Interventions for Psychosocial Risk Factors

TYPE OF INTERVENTION	TARGETED CONDITION	INTENSITY OF INTERVENTION	
		LESS INTENSE[a]	MORE INTENSE
Exercise training	Psychologic distress	Exercise prescription plus general guidelines	Supervised exercise
Nutritional counseling	Management of stress by overeating	Provide nutritional advice	Supervised dietary instruction, weight management, and behavior modification
Relaxation training	General stress and stress caused by specific situations	Advise patient to initiate relaxation training; provide audiotapes, videotapes, or instructional scripts	Teach muscle relaxation, imagery, autogenic training, diaphragmatic breathing, or biofeedback
Stress management	General stress and stress caused by specific situations	Recommend vacations, hobbies, yoga, relaxing music, pets, or pleasurable activities	Teach behavioral strategies (e.g., problem-solving, self-monitoring, appropriate goal-setting, relapse-prevention technique)
Social support	Poor structural or functional support	Provide specific social suggestions (e.g., join walking groups or engage in socially altruistic activities)	Use staff as a support base, enroll patient in support group, or facilitate family involvement
Health information	Specific stress situations (e.g., at work or home) or low health literacy	Provide situation-specific information in form of book, articles, pamphlet, audiotapes, videotapes, or Web sites	Discuss and answer patient questions regarding materials related to health and treatment recommendations

[a]Most amenable to direct cardiologist management.
Source: Rozanski A, Blumenthal JA, Davidson KW, et al.[4]

clude assessing and monitoring of stress and other chronic negative emotions,[52] the body of evidence is not yet sufficiently organized and coherent to warrant practice guidelines at this time. Some suggestions have been offered for physicians to consider should their patient require intervention (see Table 113–9).[4]

CLINICAL IMPLICATIONS

Although there is a dearth of large, randomly assigned psychosocial interventions showing any effect on cardiac outcomes in patients with CAD, there is ample evidence that improvement in psychosocial functioning can be obtained by standardized, empirically supported therapeutic protocols administered by mental health professionals to patients who are at psychosocial risk. Improving the quality of life and decreasing the psychological distress of cardiac patients can also have other benefits. First, many of the mechanisms proposed to account for the association between psychosocial factors and CVD are behavioral. Thus, decreasing depressive symptoms is hypothesized to decrease smoking rates, increase engagement in physical activity, and improve dietary habits.[53] Second, decreasing psychosocial distress is thought to increase patient compliance with physicians' recommendations, but the testing of these behavioral mechanisms, as well as the pathophysiologic mechanisms addressed elsewhere, again awaits larger, controlled trials.

Cardiologists should be aware of psychosocial risk factors present in their patients. Asking about social support and recent symptoms of depression will mark patients at increased risk of event recurrence or death. Referring such patients to mental health specialists for further diagnostic and intervention investigations can improve these patients' quality of life and behavioral risk-factor profile if not their cardiac outcome.

COST IMPLICATIONS

Thorough cost-effectiveness and cost-offset analyses are now being conducted in some of the recent psychosocial trials. For example, the average cost of adding a behavioral intervention to the treatment of a cardiac patient in one study was $790.[54] The longest and most comprehensive psychosocial intervention (for reducing type A behavior), the Recurrent Coronary Care Project in California, showed that MI recurrence decreases for the intervention patients, but treatment required an average of 58 hours per patient. This amount of therapy delivered in group format, as occurred in this trial, would cost on average $1200 per patient.

CONCLUSIONS

The potential applications of behavioral techniques in cardiology are enormous and largely unrealized. In principle they can help to prevent the onset of disease, to treat it once established, and to be used in conjunction with virtually any other kind of treatment. In practice few cardiologists have either the time or the interest to pay much attention to them, despite the demonstrated efficacy of many programs. Future success depends on better education of physicians, incorporation of a team approach, and recognition of the value of behavioral interventions by third-party payers.

ACKNOWLEDGMENTS

Preparation of this manuscript was supported by grants HC-25197, HL-076857, and HL-04458 from the National Heart, Lung, and Blood Institute, Bethesda, Maryland.

REFERENCES

1. Mokdad AH, Marks JS, Stroup DF, et al. Actual causes of death in the United States, 2000. *JAMA.* 2004;291(10):1238–1245.
2. Fries JF, Koop CE, Beadle CE, et al. Reducing health care costs by reducing the need and demand for medical services. The Health Project Consortium. *N Engl J Med.* 1993;329(5):321–325.
3. Shkolnikov V, McKee M, Leon DA. Changes in life expectancy in Russia in the mid-1990s. *Lancet.* 2001;357(9260):917–921.
4. Rozanski A, Blumenthal JA, Davidson KW, et al. The epidemiology, pathophysiology, and management of psychosocial risk factors in cardiac practice: the emerging field of behavioral cardiology. *J Am Coll Cardiol.* 2005;45(5):637–651.
5. Smith SC, Jr., Allen J, Blair SN, et al. AHA/ACC guidelines for secondary prevention for patients with coronary and other atherosclerotic vascular disease: 2006 update endorsed by the National Heart, Lung, and Blood Institute. *J Am Coll Cardiol.* 2006;47(10):2130–2139.
6. Prochaska JO, DiClemente CC, Norcross JC. In search of how people change. Applications to addictive behaviors. *Am Psychol.* 1992;47(9):1102–1114.
7. The sixth report of the Joint National Committee on prevention, detection, evaluation, and treatment of high blood pressure. *Arch Intern Med.* 1997;157(21):2413–2446.
8. Fiore M, Bailey W, Cohen S, et al. *Treating Tobacco Use and Dependence: Clinical Practice Guideline.* Rockville, MD: U.S. Department of Health and Human Services, 2000.
9. Katz DA, Muehlenbruch DR, Brown RL, et al. Effectiveness of implementing the agency for healthcare research and quality smoking cessation clinical practice guideline: a randomized, controlled trial. *J Natl Cancer Inst.* 2004;96(8):594–603.
10. Barth J, Critchley J, Bengel J. Efficacy of psychosocial interventions for smoking cessation in patients with coronary heart disease: a systematic review and meta-analysis. *Ann Behav Med.* 2006;32(1):10–20.
11. Lerman C, Patterson F, Berrettini W. Treating tobacco dependence: state of the science and new directions. *J Clin Oncol.* 2005;23(2):311–323.
12. Levine GN, Keaney JF Jr, Vita JA. Cholesterol reduction in cardiovascular disease. Clinical benefits and possible mechanisms. *N Engl J Med.* 1995;332(8):512–521.
13. The Lipid Research Clinics Coronary Primary Prevention Trial results. I. Reduction in incidence of coronary heart disease. *JAMA.* 1984;251(3):351–364.
14. Executive Summary of The Third Report of The National Cholesterol Education Program (NCEP) Expert Panel on Detection, Evaluation, And Treatment of High Blood Cholesterol In Adults (Adult Treatment Panel III). *JAMA.* 2001;285(19):2486–2497.
15. Krauss RM, Eckel RH, Howard B, et al. AHA dietary guidelines: revision 2000: a statement for healthcare professionals from the Nutrition Committee of the American Heart Association. *Circulation.* 2000;102(18):2284–2299.
16. Parikh P, McDaniel MC, Ashen MD, et al. Diets and cardiovascular disease: an evidence-based assessment. *J Am Coll Cardiol.* 2005;45(9):1379–1387.
17. Kromhout D, Menotti A, Kesteloot H, et al. Prevention of coronary heart disease by diet and lifestyle: evidence from prospective cross-cultural, cohort, and intervention studies. *Circulation.* 2002;105(7):893–898.
18. Hooper L, Summerbell CD, Higgins JP, et al. Reduced or modified dietary fat for preventing cardiovascular disease. *Cochrane Database Syst Rev.* 2001(3):CD002137.
19. Iestra JA, Kromhout D, van der Schouw YT, et al. Effect size estimates of lifestyle and dietary changes on all-cause mortality in coronary artery disease patients: a systematic review. *Circulation.* 2005;112(6):924–934.
20. Niebauer J, Hambrecht R, Marburger C, et al. Impact of intensive physical exercise and low-fat diet on collateral vessel formation in stable angina pectoris and angiographically confirmed coronary artery disease. *Am J Cardiol.* 1995;76(11):771–775.

21. Ornish D, Scherwitz LW, Billings JH, et al. Intensive lifestyle changes for reversal of coronary heart disease. *JAMA.* 1998;280(23):2001–2007.

22. Kris-Etherton PM, Harris WS, Appel LJ. Fish consumption, fish oil, omega-3 fatty acids, and cardiovascular disease. *Circulation.* 2002;106(21):2747–2757.

23. Burr ML, Ashfield-Watt PA, Dunstan FD, et al. Lack of benefit of dietary advice to men with angina: results of a controlled trial. *Eur J Clin Nutr.* 2003;57(2):193–200.

24. Chiuve SE, McCullough ML, Sacks FM, et al. Healthy lifestyle factors in the primary prevention of coronary heart disease among men: benefits among users and nonusers of lipid-lowering and antihypertensive medications. *Circulation.* 2006;114(2):160–167.

25. Kulkarni SP, Alexander KP, Lytle B, et al. Long-term adherence with cardiovascular drug regimens. *Am Heart J.* 2006;151(1):185–191.

26. McDermott MM, Schmitt B, Wallner E. Impact of medication nonadherence on coronary heart disease outcomes. A critical review. *Arch Intern Med.* 1997;157(17):1921–1929.

27. Horwitz RI, Viscoli CM, Berkman L, et al. Treatment adherence and risk of death after a myocardial infarction. *Lancet.* 1990;336(8714):542–545.

28. Granger BB, Swedberg K, Ekman I, et al. Adherence to candesartan and placebo and outcomes in chronic heart failure in the CHARM programme: double-blind, randomised, controlled clinical trial. *Lancet.* 2005;366(9502):2005–2011.

29. Trichopoulou A, Bamia C, Trichopoulos D. Mediterranean diet and survival among patients with coronary heart disease in Greece. *Arch Intern Med.* 2005;165(8):929–935.

30. Ockene IS, Hayman LL, Pasternak RC, et al. Task force 4—adherence issues and behavior changes: achieving a long-term solution. 33rd Bethesda Conference. *J Am Coll Cardiol.* 2002;40(4):630–640.

31. DiMatteo MR, Lepper HS, Croghan TW. Depression is a risk factor for noncompliance with medical treatment: meta-analysis of the effects of anxiety and depression on patient adherence. *Arch Intern Med.* 2000;160(14):2101–2107.

32. Gehi A, Haas D, Pipkin S, et al. Depression and medication adherence in outpatients with coronary heart disease: findings from the Heart and Soul Study. *Arch Intern Med.* 2005;165(21):2508–2513.

33. Jencks SF, Cuerdon T, Burwen DR, et al. Quality of medical care delivered to Medicare beneficiaries: a profile at state and national levels. *JAMA.* 2000;284(13):1670–1676.

34. LaBresh KA, Ellrodt AG, Gliklich R, et al. Get with the guidelines for cardiovascular secondary prevention: pilot results. *Arch Intern Med.* 2004;164(2):203–209.

35. Smaha LA. The American Heart Association Get with the Guidelines program. *Am Heart J.* 2004;148(5 suppl):S46–48.

36. McDonald HP, Garg AX, Haynes RB. Interventions to enhance patient adherence to medication prescriptions: scientific review. *JAMA.* 2002;288(22):2868–2879.

37. Lesperance F, Frasure-Smith N, Talajic M, et al. Five-year risk of cardiac mortality in relation to initial severity and one-year changes in depression symptoms after myocardial infarction. *Circulation.* 2002;105(9):1049–1053.

38. Bush DE, Ziegelstein RC, Patel UV, et al. *Post-myocardial Infarction Depression Summary.* Rockville, MD: Agency for Healthcare Research and Quality; 2005:123.

39. van Melle JP, de Jonge P, Spijkerman TA, et al. Prognostic association of depression following myocardial infarction with mortality and cardiovascular events: a meta-analysis. *Psychosom Med.* 2004;66(6):814–822.

40. Ruo B, Rumsfeld JS, Hlatky MA, et al. Depressive symptoms and health-related quality of life: the Heart and Soul Study [see comment]. *JAMA.* 2003;290(2):215–221.

41. Berkman LF, Blumenthal J, Burg M, et al. Effects of treating depression and low perceived social support on clinical events after myocardial infarction: The Enhancing Recovery in Coronary Heart Disease Patients (ENRICHD) randomized trial. *JAMA.* 2003;289(23):3106–3116.

42. Davidson KW, Kupfer DJ, Bigger JT, et al. Assessment and treatment of depression in patients with cardiovascular disease: National Heart, Lung, and Blood Institute working group report. *Psychosom Med.* 2006;68(5):645–650.

43. Antman EM, Anbe DT, Armstrong PW, et al. ACC/AHA guidelines for the management of patients with ST-elevation myocardial infarction—executive summary. A report of the American College of Cardiology/American Heart Association Task Force on Practice Guidelines (Writing Committee to revise the 1999 guidelines for the management of patients with acute myocardial infarction). *J Am Coll Cardiol.* 2004;44(3):671–719.

44. Grissom GR, Phillips RA. Screening for depression: this is the heart of the matter. *Arch Intern Med.* 2005;165(11):1214–1216.

45. Whooley MA. Depression and cardiovascular disease: healing the broken-hearted. *JAMA.* 2006;295(24):2874–2881.

46. Rollman BL, Weinreb L, Korsen N, et al. Implementation of guideline-based care for depression in primary care. *Adm Policy Ment Health.* 2006;33(1):43–53.

47. Everson-Rose SA, Lewis TT. Psychosocial factors and cardiovascular diseases. *Annu Rev Public Health.* 2005;26:469–500.

48. Strain LA. Lay explanations of chronic illness in later life. *J Aging Health.* 1996;8(1):3–26.

49. Rosengren A, Hawken S, Ounpuu S, et al. Association of psychosocial risk factors with risk of acute myocardial infarction in 11119 cases and 13648 controls from 52 countries (the INTERHEART study): case-control study [see comment]. *Lancet.* 2004;364(9438):953–962.

50. Blumenthal JA, Jiang W, Babyak MA, et al. Stress management and exercise training in cardiac patients with myocardial ischemia. Effects on prognosis and evaluation of mechanisms. *Arch Intern Med.* 1997;157(19):2213–2223.

51. Blumenthal JA, Babyak M, Wei J, et al. Usefulness of psychosocial treatment of mental stress-induced myocardial ischemia in men. *Am J Cardiol.* 2002;89(2):164–168.

52. De Backer G, Ambrosioni E, Borch-Johnsen K, et al. European guidelines on cardiovascular disease prevention in clinical practice. Third Joint Task Force of European and Other Societies on Cardiovascular Disease Prevention in Clinical Practice. *Eur Heart J.* 2003;24(17):1601–1610.

53. Davidson K, Jonas BS, Dixon KE, et al. Do depression symptoms predict early hypertension incidence in young adults in the CARDIA study? Coronary Artery Risk Development in Young Adults. *Arch Intern Med.* 2000;160(10):1495–1500.

54. Oldridge N, Furlong W, Feeny D, et al. Economic evaluation of cardiac rehabilitation soon after acute myocardial infarction. *Am J Cardiol.* 1993;72(2):154–161.

CHAPTER (114)

Complementary and Alternative Medical Therapy in Cardiovascular Care

Mitchell W. Krucoff / Rebecca Costello / Daniel Mark / John H. K. Vogel

With publication of the consensus paper on complementary and alternative medicine (CAM) practices in cardiovascular care, the American College of Cardiology has pointed cardiologists to a unique dimension of healthcare concepts, research, and practice.[1] As the trend among patients to use CAM therapies has risen exponentially,[2] growing professional interest in CAM therapies as adjuncts to the *high-tech* world of cardiovascular care has been paralleled by concerns about exaggerated claims of efficacy, quackery, and frank toxicity across the largely unregulated pantheon of CAM practices. The combination of relatively unrestricted access to Internet information and widespread cultural interest in self-empowerment and holistic paradigms of healthcare in the lay public constitute a mandate for cardiologists to become better informed about CAM therapeutics. At the very least such education will support more thoughtful, less defensive dialogue between physicians and patients. At best, cardiologists knowledgeable about CAM therapies will be better positioned to encourage and envision both the many necessary research directions and more integrated clinical strategies necessary for the advance of optimal data-driven practice in modern cardiovascular care.

Although many CAM therapies have been practiced for thousands of years in culturally based health systems, there is a growing but still very immature literature by modern standards in most of these areas. The introduction to the American College of Cardiology (ACC) consensus document observes that "Topics chosen for coverage by Expert Consensus Documents are so designed because the evidence base and experience with technology or clinical practice are not considered sufficiently well developed to be evaluated by the formal ACC/[American Heart Association] AHA Practice Guidelines process."[1] Ambiguous nomenclature, certification standards for practice methods, or profiles of active principles in consumables such as herbal remedies, still confound a systematic appreciation of actual safety and efficacy in selected heart disease populations. As with other areas of immature literature in medical practices, investigator bias, reporting bias, and publisher bias continue to impact the interpretation of what data are available.

Even more essential to the actual integration of modern medical technology and practice with CAM therapies is the challenge to engage whole new paradigms both of healing and of how research defining optimal healing might be conducted. The modern scientific tendency to articulate biochemical mechanisms and translate them into clinical practice therapeutics tested by clinical protocols is potentially fatally reductionist with regard to holistic systems that view interaction with the body as approximately 20 percent of the mind-body-spirit process that actually accomplishes the transformation of suffering called healing.[3,4] Research in CAM therapies in cardiovascular care must balance ethical and robust standards for clinical trial designs and mechanistic studies with sensitivity to the cultural metaphors of how these therapies actually work to meaningfully move the field forward.[5–8]

With the growth of the Office of Alternative Medicine into the National Center for Complementary and Alterative Medicine (NCCAM) at the National Institutes of Health, more comprehensive attention and research resources have been directed to sort through some of these issues and to develop the requisite infrastructure. With even the terms *alternative, complementary, integrative,* and others still in flux, in this chapter the authors have taken selected therapies and references from the general topical framework that NCCAM has developed for CAM therapies[9] with a focus, where possible, specifically on cardiovascular applications across NCCAM's five key treatment areas: biologically based therapies, manipulative and body-based methods, energy therapies, mind-body interventions, and alternative medical systems.

BIOLOGICALLY BASED THERAPIES: SELECTED BOTANICALS AND DIETARY SUPPLEMENTS

【 】 BOTANICALS

Herbal remedies, vitamins and food-substance derivatives, teas, alcohol, nuts, soy, and other specific dietary constituents have a long-standing place in healthcare as a predominantly culturally based pharmacopoeia. In most cases the initial scientific suggestion of benefit has come from epidemiologic comparisons of different cohorts, with interpretation limited both by different endogenous rates of disease and varied levels of consumption of the substance of interest, which itself can have varied concentrations of active compounds. Early hypothesis-generating studies are typically supported by subsequent case-control studies and, in some cases, larger prospective cohort studies. In cardiovascular applications, surrogate end points in the smaller prospective studies include effects on low-density-lipoprotein cholesterol (LDL-C), platelet function, endothelial function, and immune/inflammatory activity. In some cases larger randomized, controlled trials have been conducted using clinical outcome end points. Studies of herbal medicines have suffered from poorly characterized interventions and often studies of short duration. To improve the reporting of randomized controlled trials using herbal medicine interventions, members of the Consolidated Standards of Reporting Trials (CONSORT) group have developed a checklist to assist investigators in the design and reporting of clinical trials using herbal medicines.[10]

The medicinal use of botanicals originated more than 7000 years ago; the written history spans more than 3500 years.[11] Prescribed by great ancient physicians such as Hippocrates, Theophrastus, and Pliny, botanicals were catalogued and illustrated, with specific indications noted for each active plant. Intact botanicals were used singly or in combination until the nineteenth century, when the identification and isolation of individually active compounds was conceived and accomplished. Approximately 25 percent of pharmaceuticals prescribed today are derived from plant sources. At the same time, there has been a rekindling of consumer interest in the use of natural whole-plant products. A

significant result of this public interest and demand for access to herbal products was the passage of the Dietary Supplement Health and Education Act (DSHEA) of 1994. Herbs, vitamins, minerals, and proteins were classified as dietary supplements. Manufacturers are allowed to describe the effects of these supplements on "structure or function" of the body or the "well-being" achieved by consuming the dietary ingredient. To use these claims, manufacturers must have substantiation that the statements are truthful and not misleading, and the product label must bear the statement: "This statement has not been evaluated by the Food and Drug Administration." Furthermore, neither good manufacturing practices nor labeling requirements certifying concentrations of active ingredients or bioavailability have been required for DSHEA products. As a result, independent examination has revealed great inconsistency between product labeling and actual compound concentration.[12] In this setting safety concerns with potential adulteration of supplements with active prescription compounds, contamination of preparations, herb-herb and herb-drug interactions are significant.[13,14] Research into the safety and efficacy of botanical compounds has been hampered by this lack of standardization.[15] Recently the FDA has reconsidered these issues, and it is now moving toward requiring labeling for botanicals that specifies and certifies concentrations of active compounds.

【 】 GARLIC (*ALLIUM SATIVUM*)

Garlic has long been touted as a natural product useful for the modulation of immune system activity, in the treatment of hyperlipidemia and hypertension, as well as the primary and secondary prevention of myocardial infarction. Medicinal use of garlic can be traced back to the ancient Babylonians and Chinese, with long-term usage occurring in Western folk medicine as well.[16] Allicin is felt to be the bioactive component responsible for the potential cardiovascular activity of garlic.[17] Allicin content is determined by the nature of the garlic preparation, with raw crushed garlic having the highest concentration. Multiple mechanisms of action have been proposed, including decrease in cholesterol and fatty acid synthesis and cholesterol absorption[18] as well as potent antioxidant properties.[19] Antiplatelet and fibrinolytic activity with garlic has also been reported.[20]

Clinical studies of garlic have yielded contradictory results, with significant design flaws notable in trials designed to demonstrate garlic's effectiveness.[21–23] Short-term studies have shown some benefit in the lipid profiles of patients taking garlic, whereas long-term studies of 6 months or more fail to show sustained benefit when garlic is used as a single agent. Studies of garlic's effectiveness in hypertension have also suffered from poor methodology, and results have revealed small, mostly insignificant decreases in blood pressure.[24–26] Evidence for the supplemental intake of garlic for both the primary and secondary prevention of heart disease is not sufficient to recommend its use for this indication.

The anticoagulant properties of garlic can be problematic in the perioperative period and in combination with other anticoagulant compounds and have been reported to interact with the P450 enzyme system. Garlic will also decrease the effectiveness of some HIV drugs.[27] Side effects are minor other than occasional nausea with excessive raw intake of garlic and the development of an unpleasant odor.

HAWTHORN (*CRATAEGUS* SPECIES)

Hawthorn species are a group of small trees and shrubs found throughout North America, Asia, and Europe. Purported cardiovascular indications include congestive heart failure (CHF), angina, and arrhythmias. Hawthorn's activity is felt to be related to the presence of a number of key constituents, including flavonoids and oligomeric procyanidins.[28]

Literature review reveals significant evidence for hawthorn's efficacy in the treatment of mild to moderate CHF.[29–32] Preparations made from flowers with leaves are sold as a prescription medication in parts of Europe and Asia. Animal and in-vitro models reveal positive inotropism with a mechanism of action similar to that of digitalis through a cyclic adenosine monophosphate (AMP)-independent effect.[33,34] There is also evidence of a direct vasodilating effect.[35] Some efficacy has been documented in increasing maximal workload capacity and decreasing symptom severity in patients with CHF. One uncontrolled study also reported an increase in ejection fraction measured by angiography from 30 to 41 percent in patients with stage II to III heart failure.[36] No published studies have examined mortality effects. There are very limited data regarding actual benefit in angina, and antiarrhythmia data are present only in animal studies.

The usual dose of hawthorn for CHF is 300 to 600 milligrams three times daily of an extract standardized to contain approximately 2 to 3 percent flavonoids or 18 to 20 percent procyanidins. Full effects can take up to 6 months to develop. Combination with cardiac glycosides and CNS depressants should be avoided. Side effects are rare but include gastrointestinal upset, sedation, dizziness, vertigo, headaches, migraines, and palpitations.[37]

GINKGO BILOBA

Ginkgo extracts are derived from the leaf of the ginkgo tree, a botanical with a known history dating back 300 million years. Originally present throughout Europe, the tree died out during the Ice Age, surviving in China and Japan. Ginkgo is the most commonly purchased herbal remedy in the United States, with sales of more than $150 million.[38] (Ginkgo was the seventh most popular herb in 2004 with $113 million in sales according to the Nutrition Business Journal.) Widely used for its purported benefits in treating nondementia-related memory problems, Alzheimer disease, and vertigo, ginkgo has also been proposed as a treatment for intermittent claudication and peripheral vascular disease.

Ginkgo has been documented to inhibit platelet activation factor, decrease blood viscosity, and decrease vascular resistance.[39,40] The mechanisms responsible for ginkgo's effectiveness in peripheral vascular disease are unknown but can include its ability to scavenge free radicals, promote vasodilatation and decrease blood viscosity; it also possesses antiinflammatory and antiplatelet actions. Individual studies have revealed benefit in increasing mean pain-free walking distance.[41,42] Two meta-analyses have examined the literature and reported a statistically significant increase in walking distance averaging nearly 25 meters (82 feet).[43,44] The clinical significance of this difference is questionable, but it can provide a small benefit in the treatment of peripheral arterial disease.[13]

The usual dose of ginkgo for the treatment of claudication is 40 to 80 milligrams three times daily of a 50:1 extract standardized to contain 24 percent ginkgo-flavone glycosides. Caution must be exercised in using ginkgo, as it inhibits platelet aggregation factor and has been reported to increase both spontaneous and trauma-related bleeding, including bleeding during surgery and other procedures.[45,46] Ginkgo is considered to be relatively safe, however, caution must also be exercised in combining gingko with heparin, warfarin, clopidogrel, and other compounds that can increase the risk of bleeding. Ginkgo has been reported to decrease the metabolism of trazodone in at least one case report, perhaps by an inhibition of monoamine oxidase.[47] Side effects are common and include headaches, dizziness, gastrointestinal complaints, and skin reactions.

HORSE CHESTNUT TREE EXTRACT (*AESCULUS HIPPOCASTANUM*)

The horse chestnut tree is found worldwide. Its seeds contain active compounds known as saponins, which have mild antiinflammatory properties.[48] Aescin, a combination of triterpene saponins, appears to be the pharmacologically active component. Its mechanism of action is considered to be sensitization to Ca^{2+} ions and a sealing effect on small vessel permeability to water.[49] Traditionally, this botanical has been used for hemorrhoids, rheumatism, swellings, varicose veins, and leg ulcers. Research has focused on horse chestnut tree extract in the treatment of chronic venous insufficiency, and multiple studies have reported the superiority of horse chestnut tree extract over placebo, with equal effectiveness to compression stockings as quantified by significant improvement in objective measurements of leg edema and subjective reporting of pain and sensation of heaviness.[50–53]

The usual dose of horse chestnut tree extract is 300 milligrams twice daily, standardized to contain 50 milligrams aescin per dose, for a total daily dose of 100 milligrams aescin. Aescin binds to plasma protein and can affect the binding of other drugs. Side effects are rare, including headache, itching, and dizziness. Concerns regarding risk of renal impairment do not appear to be warranted.[54]

POLICOSANOL

Policosanol is a combination of aliphatic alcohols derived most commonly from sugar cane wax, although octacosanol, the predominant active ingredient, is also present in wheat germ oil and other vegetable oils.[55] Policosanol *inhibits cholesterol biosynthesis* in a step located between acetate and mevalonate as well as by an increase in low-density lipoprotein (LDL) receptor–dependent processing. There is no evidence for a direct inhibition of hydroxymethylglutaryl coenzyme A (HMG-CoA) reductase.[56] Policosanol has been extensively used clinically and researched in Cuba.[57] These studies suggest a lipid-lowering effect of approximately 15 percent for total cholesterol and 20 percent for LDL cholesterol, which can be increased to 30 percent with higher doses. Maximal effects are seen after only 6 to 8 weeks of use, and benefits have been demonstrated in studies lasting longer than 1 year. In a head-to-head comparison of 10 milligrams policosanol with 20 milligrams fluvastatin in women with elevated cholesterol, the lipid-lowering effects of policosanol were slightly superior to those of fluvastatin, and policosanol alone significantly inhibited the susceptibility of LDL to lipid peroxidation.[58] A recent review has noted the efficacy of policosanol and suggested a unique role for this natural compound, given the large number of patients desiring a natural alternative to synthetically derived drugs for cholesterol management.[59] There are no data on efficacy determined by clinical end points.

The typical starting dose of policosanol is 5 milligrams per day, which can be increased to a maximal dose of 20 milligrams per day. Side effects are infrequent, with weight loss, polyuria, and headache most commonly reported. There is concern that policosanol can potentiate anticoagulant activity; it should therefore be used with caution in combination with any agents known to increase the risk of bleeding. There is also a report of an increased effect of L-dopa when used in combination with policosanol, leading to dyskinesias.[60]

【 】 GUGULIPID (COMMIPHORA MUKUL)

Guggul is a substance derived from the mukul myrrh tree in India. It has played a role in traditional Indian medicine (Ayurveda) for several thousand years, used in the treatment of arthritis, digestive, skin, and menstrual problems. Today, guggul is used as a lipid-lowering agent that is believed to work by blocking the farnesoid X receptor in liver cells and as a consequence altering cholesterol metabolism.[61] Studies of guggul have demonstrated a significant reduction in total cholesterol and LDL-C of 15 to 23 percent and triglyceride reduction of 20 percent.[62,63] The usual dose is 100 milligrams of guggulsterone per day. Side effects are usually limited to mild gastrointestinal symptoms. A hypersensitivity rash was reported in a small number of healthy subjects enrolled in a randomized control trial for hypercholesterolemia.[64] There is some evidence that when guggul is used concomitantly with diltiazem or propranolol, there can be a reduction in the bioavailability of those drugs and therefore decreased clinical efficacy.[65]

【 】 RED RICE YEAST (MONASCUS PURPUREUS)

Red rice yeast is a product that is derived from a yeast that grows on rice. Red rice yeast has been a food staple and folk remedy for thousands of years in the Asia. It was noted in the 1970s that a product of the yeast, monacolin K (lovastatin), was an *inhibitor of HMG-CoA reductase*.[66] The concentration of lovastatin varies in red rice yeast but averages near 0.4 percent by weight.

In a multicenter study of 187 subjects, red rice yeast lowered total cholesterol by 16.4 percent, LDL-C by 21.0 percent, triglycerides by 24.5 percent, and the ratio of total-to-high-density lipoprotein (HDL) cholesterol by 17.7 percent; it increased high-density-lipoprotein cholesterol (HDL-C) by 14.6 percent.[67] Although the reported side effects of red rice yeast are few—including mainly gastrointestinal upset, headaches, and dizziness—red rice yeast must theoretically be considered a typical HMG-CoA reductase inhibitor, and caution is advised with regard to potential side effects, including rhabdomyolysis. Similarly, drug interactions should be considered to be identical to those with lovastatin, requiring caution when red yeast rice is combined with niacin, macrolides, cyclosporine, ketoconazole, and many other agents. Products range in their recommended dosage from 2.5 to 10 milligrams of lovastatin equivalent per day. However, red yeast rice is no longer marketed with standardized lovastatin levels in the United States, owing to legal issues, and it is now sold without lovastatin levels declared.

【 】 DIETARY SUPPLEMENTS

A number of dietary supplements have been postulated to have beneficial effects on cardiovascular disease. These include antioxidant vitamins, B vitamins, omega-3 fatty acids, plant sterols, soluble fiber, soy, nuts, alcohol, and teas.[68,69] Some of these are also discussed in other chapters of this book (e.g., Chap. 51).

Omega-3 Fatty Acids

Omega-3 polyunsaturated fatty acids (FAs) can be derived from either plant or marine sources. The principal plant-based omega-3 FA, alpha linolenic acid (ALA), is found in soy and its derivative tofu as well as in canola oil, flax seeds, and nuts. Omega-3 FAs derived from the tissues of marine animals (*fish oil*) include docosahexaenoic acid (DHA) and eicosapentaenoic acid (EPA). Typical dietary sources include mackerel, salmon, herring, sardines, anchovies, and albacore tuna. Early suggestions that fish oil might be beneficial came from epidemiologic comparisons of Greenland and Alaskan Inuits with other cohorts. The Inuits consumed a high-fat diet with a high component of omega-3 FAs from seal and whale meat. Despite this diet, they had more favorable lipid profiles and lower rates of coronary artery disease (CAD) than the comparison groups. Three followup epidemiologic studies in the 1980s found that persons who ate fish every week had a lower mortality from CAD.[70,71]

Several mechanisms of benefit have been proposed for omega-3 FAs. The reductions in sudden death observed in several studies suggest a direct antiarrhythmic effect. High-dose omega-3 FAs produce a significant reduction in serum triglyceride concentrations and a small drop in blood pressure. They also decrease platelet aggregation. Other suggested mechanisms include an antiinflammatory effect and enhanced production of nitric oxide. In addition, there are many reports of fish oil ingestion favorably affecting a variety of other intermediate targets believed to be relevant to cardiovascular disease.[72,73]

More than 40 cohort studies have now examined the effects of fish consumption on CAD outcomes.[71–74] The best of these suggest a protective effect, with a stronger effect on death (4 studies, relative risk [RR] 0.65) than on cardiovascular events (7 studies, RR 0.91). Additional reports suggest that atherosclerotic progression in native coronaries and vein grafts is slowed in men in association with fish oil ingestion.[74,75]

A systematic review of randomized trials of omega-3 FAs published 1966 to 2003 involving more than 33,000 patients found a small nonsignificant reduction in all-cause mortality with a strategy of high omega-3 intake relative to low omega-3 intake (RR 0.87, 95 percent confidence interval 0.73 to 1.03).[74] For cardiovascular events, the RR for high omega-3 was 0.95. Among these trials, the ones with the largest estimated benefit for high omega-3 intake were almost always the smallest trials. The largest of these is the Gruppo Italiano per lo Studio della Sopravvivenza nell'Infarto Miocardico (GISSI)-Prevenzione study, which randomized 5666 post-myocardial infarction (MI) patients to 1 gram per day or usual therapy.[76] The primary analysis showed a 20 percent reduction in all-cause mortality ($p = 0.01$) and a 45 percent reduction in sudden death ($p < 0.01$).[76a] One of the most recent trials, the Diet and Angina Randomized Trial (DART) 2 actually estimated borderline excess mortality from high omega-3 intake (adjusted hazard ratio 1.26, $p = 0.047$).[77] This study randomized 3114 men younger than age 70 to a factorial design involving advice to eat two portions of oily fish each week (or take 3 g of fish oil capsules daily) versus sensible eating advice. The plasma levels of omega-3 FAs increased significantly in a small subset of the fish advice arm relative to the control arm, but data on adherence to the dietary advice in this trial is inconclusive. The apparent excess mortality seen in this trial appeared to be driven by results in the subjects given fish oil capsules.

One interesting line of investigation in this area has been the use of fish oil supplements in patients with intracardiac cardioverter-defibrillators (ICDs). In a pilot study of 10 patients undergoing an electrophysiology study at baseline and again after infusion of 3.8 grams of intravenous fish oil, 5 of 7 patients with initially inducible ventricular tachycardia (VT) were no longer inducible.[78] More recently, 200 patients with an ICD and a history of sustained VT or ventricular fibrillation (VF) were randomized to fish oil (1.8 grams/day) or placebo.[79] Over a median of 718 days, recurrent VT/VF events were more common in the fish oil arm than in the placebo arm ($p < .001$). A second study randomized 546 patients with an ICD and a history of malignant ventricular arrhythmias to 2 grams per day of fish oil or placebo in a double-blind trial.[80] Over approximately a 1-year followup, death or appropriate ICD therapy for VT/VF was not significantly reduced in the fish oil arm (hazard ratio 0.86, $p = 0.33$).

Currently, there are strong recommendations for the general public to consume two servings of fish (especially fatty fish) per week as part of a heart-healthy diet.[81] In Europe, use of fish oil for secondary prevention after myocardial infarction is almost considered routine. Nonetheless, the value of supplemental fish oil for primary or secondary prevention will need significant new studies to clarify current uncertainties. One important ongoing trial is GISSI-Heart Failure, which is testing omega-3 FAs versus placebo in more than 7000 class II to IV heart failure patients over 3 years. Results are expected in 2007.[82] An additional concern is the rapid depletion of the world's fish stores by industrial overfishing. Resulting rises in prices for fish can well put this form of therapy out of reach of patients with limited means.[83]

Antioxidants and Antioxidant Vitamins

Despite a large body of epidemiologic evidence suggesting a favorable association between a diet high in antioxidants and reduced risk of coronary heart disease (CHD), the clinical trial evidence has failure to confirm the expected benefits. Most of the observational studies examined the consumption of foods and estimated the likely vitamin content, whereas a few studies have examined the supplemental consumption of vitamins.

Vitamin E refers to a group of molecules that includes four tocopherols and four tocotrienols. Alpha tocopherol is the most prevalent and most potent lipid-soluble antioxidant in plasma. Several large epidemiologic studies involving more than 170,000 subjects have assessed the association between dietary and supplement-based vitamin E and CHD outcomes.[84–86] Three of these found supplement-based vitamin E to be associated with a significant reduction in hard cardiac events, especially in doses >100 international unit (IU) for >2 years.

The Cambridge Heart Antioxidant Study (CHAOS) demonstrated that 400 to 800 IU of vitamin E given as secondary prevention reduced the combined end point of death or nonfatal MI by 47 percent.[87] However, the larger and more recent Heart Outcomes Prevention Evaluation (HOPE) trial, which tested 400 IU of vitamin E in a high-risk secondary prevention population, found no therapeutic benefit on a variety of outcome measures including disease progression as assessed by carotid ultrasound.[88] The GISSI-Prevenzione trial, which tested 300 IU of vitamin E in almost 8000 patients, also failed to detect a benefit.[89] Finally, the collaborative group of the Primary Prevention Project (PPP) found no evidence for a therapeutic benefit for 300 IU of vitamin E in 4495 subjects with one or more major cardiovascular risk factors.[90] More recently, the HOPE—The Ongoing Outcomes (TOO) trial reported on almost 4000 patients from the original HOPE study with long-term followup. As with the original HOPE analysis, there was no evidence of a benefit of vitamin E on cardiovascular outcomes, and there was actually a modest increase in heart failure with active treatment.[91] The Women's Heath Study of 39,876 apparently healthy women age 45 and older found that vitamin E (600 IU on alternate days) reduced cardiovascular death (RR 0.76, $p = 0.03$) but had no effect on total cardiovascular events, myocardial infarction or stroke.[92] At present, therefore, the preponderance of the evidence *does not support* a role for vitamin E supplements in either primary or secondary prevention of CHD.

Vitamin C (ascorbic acid) is a strong water-soluble antioxidant. In the Nurses' Health Study, 85,118 female nurses completed a detailed dietary questionnaire in 1980 and were followed for 16 years. Estimated vitamin C intake using the questionnaire data was modestly related to incident heart disease events with an adjusted RR 0.72, $p < 0.05$.[93] Several randomized trials have tested vitamin C supplements in varying doses for CHD prevention. In the Heart Protection Study, 20,536 patients with CAD or diabetes were randomized to antioxidant vitamins (600 milligrams of vitamin E, 250 milligrams of vitamin C, and 20 milligrams of beta-carotene) versus placebo.[94] Although the vitamin regimen was found to be safe, there was no evidence for a therapeutic effect after 5 years of treatment. In contrast, in the Antioxidant Supplementation in Atherosclerosis Prevention (ASAP) study, hypercholesterolemic patients were randomized to twice-daily supplements of 136 IU of vitamin E, 250 milligrams of slow-release vitamin C, both, or placebo only.[95] At 6 years among the 440 subjects completing the study, vitamin supplementation slowed carotid atherosclerosis (judged by common carotid intimal-medial thickness) by 25 percent.

B Vitamins

Moderate elevations of plasma homocysteine levels have been associated with an enhanced risk for atherosclerotic disease. The metabolism of homocysteine requires several B vitamins as cofactors, specifically vitamins B_6, B_{12}, and folate. Homocysteine levels can be decreased by the administration of supplemental folate, with or without vitamins B_6 and B_{12}. Although epidemiologic studies suggested potential cardiovascular benefit with B-vitamin supplementation, either through this or other undefined mechanisms,[96,97] most trial results have shown no such benefit. A meta-analysis of four randomized, controlled trials of B-vitamin therapy found *no evidence that B vitamin supplements slowed the progression of atherosclerosis.*[98] A randomized, placebo-controlled trial with 636 patients found that combined folate, B_6, and B_{12} therapy can increase the risk of restenosis and revascularization after coronary stenting.[99]

Chelation Therapy

The intravenous infusion of ethylenediamine-tetraacetic acid (EDTA) is a form of alternative medicine commonly used for the treatment of atherosclerotic vascular disease. The original rationale behind this therapy was that EDTA chelation would remove calcium from atheromatous arterial lesions. However, there is little empiric support for this putative mechanism, and other possible benefits such as an antioxidant effect have been proposed. The evidence base on chelation consists of case reports and case series involving a total of more than 4600 patients, largely describing the beneficial effects of EDTA chelation.

There have been four randomized trials of chelation therapy, all quite small. The most recent is the Program to Assess Alternative Treatment Strategies to Achieve Cardiac Health (PATCH),[100] which randomized 84 stable angina patients and followed them for 6 months. Event rates in this trial were quite low, and there were no differences between the chelation and the placebo arms. The investigators concluded that a much larger trial would be required.

The National Institutes of Health has funded a major randomized trial of chelation, the Trial to Assess Chelation Therapy (TACT). This study, which started enrollment in 2003, will randomize 1950 patients ≥50 years of age with a prior MI to either chelation therapy or placebo. Results are expected by 2010.

Soluble Fiber

Dietary fiber supplements have been shown to produce desirable changes in LDL-cholesterol and blood sugar levels.[101] Epidemiologic findings suggest a possible impact on coronary disease and outcome.[102,103] However, there are no prospective trials of the effect of these dietary supplements on cardiac outcomes.

Soy Protein and Isoflavones

Substitution of soy protein for animal protein can produce significant reductions in LDL-cholesterol and triglycerides.[104] Whether this reflects a unique benefit of soy or isoflavones in particular or merely a reduction in dietary animal protein and fat is unclear. Much of the most favorable evidence on this intervention is observational. For example, a recent cross-sectional study of 4680 persons 40 to 59 years of age from 4 countries found an inverse association between vegetable protein intake and blood pressure.[105] A review of the benefits of soy protein and isoflavones has been published by the AHA Nutrition Committee.[106] A total of 22 randomized trials tested the effects of soy protein and found a small decrease in LDL-cholesterol with no effects on other lipid fractions or blood pressure. Soy isoflavones were tested in 19 studies and had no effects on lipids or blood pressure.

Plant Sterols

Plant sterols and stanols have been persuasively shown to lower cholesterol and are now commercially available in margarine products.[107] Long-term outcome studies with these compounds are needed.

[ ] ALCOHOL

Mild to moderate alcohol consumption has been associated in a variety of reports with reduction in stroke and rates of MI, functional improvement with claudication, and improved cardiovascular survival.[108–111] Vasodilating and central nervous system effects, as well as antioxidant compounds in alcohol preparations such as red wine, have all been proposed as potential mechanisms of these benefits. At higher dose in susceptible individuals, alcohol is a well-known myocardial toxin, with equally deleterious potential in other end organs such as the liver, gastrointestinal tract, and central nervous system. A science advisory overview from the AHA was issued on this topic in 2001.[112] More information on the value of modest alcohol intake for primary and secondary prevention of coronary heart disease can be found in Chap. 51.

MANIPULATIVE AND BODY-BASED METHODS

Acupuncture, acupressure, and an array of massage techniques represent manipulative and body-based therapies. Of these, the most robust scientific information is available on acupuncture.

[ ] ACUPUNCTURE

The ancient Chinese medical therapy acupuncture has garnered growing interest over the course of increasing communication between the United States and China since the early 1970s. Worldwide, more than 40 percent of physicians recommend acupuncture to their patients, and more than 50 percent of physicians want to add this modality to their therapeutic armamentarium.[113] Although not required for licensed physicians, the practice of acupuncture by others, such as those trained in traditional Chinese medicine, is currently regulated by more than 35 state boards in the United States. Furthermore, the FDA regulates the use of disposable stainless steel and acupuncture needles. The National Institutes of Health has published a consensus statement indicating that many issues related to acupuncture—including efficacy, sham effects, adverse reactions, acupuncture points, training, credentialing, and mechanism of action—need further definition.[114]

Clinically, acupuncture is most accepted for the treatment of pain.[114,115] In cardiovascular care, there are three areas for which acupuncture has been explored: anginal pain from ischemia, hypertension, and arrhythmias. The rationale for using acupuncture to treat myocardial ischemia, hypertension, and arrhythmias can stem from its ability to inhibit autonomic sympathetic outflow. Acupuncture techniques can release opioids in a number of regions in the hypothalamus, midbrain, and medulla concerned with processing information that influences sympathetic neuroactivity. Other neurotransmitters that can also be associated with the cardiovascular effects of acupuncture include gamma-aminobutyric acid, serotonin, and acetylcholine.[116] Because placebo effects can occur in as many as 40 percent of the patients and because acupuncture seems to be efficacious in only approximately 70 percent of patients, actual benefit can represent a narrow window of response.[117]

Mechanistic studies suggest that catecholamine reduction with acupuncture can affect myocardial ischemia and stress-induced hypertension.[118–120] These studies indicate that acupuncture probably limits myocardial ischemia by reducing myocardial oxygen demand rather than by increasing coronary blood flow. In sham acupuncture placebo-controlled studies of moderate anginal pain and exercise tolerance, Ballegaard was unable to document a decrease in the rate of anginal attacks, consumption of nitroglycerin, or improvement in exercise tolerance,[116] whereas two other studies including patients with severe stable angina who had been treated vigorously with medical therapy showed an acupuncture-related improvement in exercise capacity and rate-pressure product, particularly when acupuncture reduced measures of sympathetic tone.[117,118] There are currently no trials showing reduction in mortality or other clinical outcomes with acupuncture in ischemic heart disease.

General vascular reactivity can be affected by acupuncture. Improvement in primary Raynaud cold-induced vasoconstriction by acupuncture compared to sham treatment has been reported.[119] Hypertension can also be improved by acupuncture, although the absolute effects on blood pressure reported are small.[120] These findings can be more profound in selected hypertensive syndromes responsive to central nervous system modulation.[114]

Reliable data on arrhythmia control with acupuncture are rare. Acupuncture can inhibit ventricular extrasystoles induced by stimulating the hypothalamus or paraventricular nucleus or following administration of $BaCL_2$.[114] Understanding patient selection and the level of incremental effect in the context of other drug or device therapies will require dedicated research.

Most authorities agree that the risk of an adverse event resulting from acupuncture is small, generally below 10 percent when performed by physicians. Pneumothorax, spinal cord lesions, hepatitis HIV infections, endocarditis, arthritis, and osteomyelitis have been reported but are rare, with an overall rate of less than 2 percent. The risk of an adverse event for nonphysician acupuncturists is higher (up to 30 percent), although the risk of serious events is low.

ENERGY THERAPIES

Bioenergetics or energy therapies are a series of healing *disciplines* that claim to harness intangible natural forces to influence physiologic, emotional, and spiritual healing. No scientific evidence has demonstrated or characterized actual bioenergy fields associated with many of these techniques, although practitioners claim to see, feel, or otherwise sense the color, alignment, intensity, and flow of such energy in practice. In several ancient Eastern practices, detailed diagrams of energy meridians and chakras are well known. Examples of bioenergy disciplines include therapeutic and healing touch, Qigong, Johrei, Reiki, crystal therapy, and magnet therapy. Energy therapies are generally administered by an active practitioner who conducts both diagnostic and therapeutic func-

tions by *sensing* or *reading* energy patterns and then manipulating or adding to those energy patterns, with the patient in a more passive role. It is quite conceivable that placebo effects, hypnosis, and other trance states can also belong to this largely metaphorically defined practice area.

Practitioners of the ancient Chinese healing tradition of Qigong use deep breathing, meditation, and body movement to capture and focus the vital life energy, Qi. In cardiovascular application, Qigong has been claimed to influence hypertension in patients with heart disease[121] as well as sudden death by accentuating vagal tone, as demonstrated by changes in heart-rate variability.[122] Qigong has also been associated with shorter hospitalization in patients after myocardial infarction and reduced mortality with stroke.[123] The reproducibility of these findings has not been established.

Healing touch[124,125] and Reiki[126] therapies conceptually involve concentration and transmission of bioenergy from healer to patient, with restoration and realignment of energy fields in the patient, either by touching the patient directly or by touching the energy fields around the body. The Vedic paradigm of energy concentrated in and through anatomically related chakras along the spine and central nervous system, with the energy flow between and around the chakras determined by paths or meridians both within the somatic body and in a field around the body, is frequently included in the conceptual constructs of these practices.

In hospitalized patients, therapeutic touch has been reported to palliate anxiety,[127] with a potential effect on serum catecholamines prior to invasive procedures.[128] In a small pilot study of healing touch prior to urgent percutaneous coronary intervention, this modality was associated with a suggestive trend toward improved short term outcomes.[129]

In the absence of known mechanisms the safety assessment of bioenergy practices is problematic. Although bioenergy approaches are widely considered safe by practitioners,[130] careful attention to both safety and efficacy in future research in these areas should be considered mandatory.

MIND-BODY INTERVENTIONS

A remarkably large and consistent observational literature provides evidence that the presence or absence of acute and chronic stress; emotional states such as obsessive behavior, depression, and hostility; spiritual attitudes such as faith and hope; and interactive support systems such as companionship and community connectedness have significant correlations to cardiovascular outcomes such as hypertension, MI, stroke, and cardiac death.[131–134] It is possible that these observations result from genetically driven physiologic responses to stress, with measurable impact on catecholamine levels, cortisol levels, glucose metabolism, autonomic tone, vascular tone, coagulability, pain perception, and immune reactivity. Teleologically the *fight-or-flight* responses are frequently recognized as physiologic survival mechanisms. However, with chronic, repetitive overstimulation or in the setting of preexistent heart disease, the roles of stress, isolation, anger, and depression can clearly reach pathologic proportions. Also, these states of mind and spirit are frequently paired with behaviors such smoking, eating disorders, obesity, diabetes, hypercholesterolemia, a sedentary lifestyle, and hypertension. Coping strategies and therapies that address this mind-body axis can be a fertile area to integrate into the current predominantly pharmacologic armamentarium. The actual ability of mind-body or mind-body-spirit therapies to benefit the natural history of cardiovascular disease, however, remains unclear.

Mind-body therapies are generally characterized by learned disciplines that affect both mind and body in a deliberately harmonious or even simultaneous way. Techniques can emphasize the mental component, such as in meditation, mindfulness, relaxation therapy, guided imagery, music, and mirthful laughter, with a *secondary* relaxation, quieting, or energizing of the body, or they can emphasize the somatic component, as in exercise, tai chi, and yoga, with a secondary quieting or energizing of the mind.[135] A strong emphasis on awareness of and control of the breath, generally with attention to moving the locus of the breath from the chest into a relaxed abdominal breathing, is common among many of these techniques. Similarly, the final objective of mind-body healing techniques is to promote or restore an equilibrium between the mental and the somatic characterized by a feeling of calm peacefulness and filled with a sense of vital energy. In culturally rooted disciplines, this equilibrium and the path leading to it are conceived of not only as wellness and healing-oriented but as frankly spiritual paths providing a source of joy, a sense of meaning in life, and even an awareness of unifying or divine principles.

Less explicitly used in mind-body practices but a topic of great interest to healing science is the *placebo effect*. Suggestion and belief have repeatedly been shown to produce measurable changes in somatic symptoms such as angina.[136] Although historically equated to neurosis or deceit, "nothing," or other negative connotations, more recently research in the placebo effect has come to be regarded as a possible window into internally mediated healing processes and human potential currently untapped in medical practice.[137]

One area of mind-body therapy that has been reported in application to cardiovascular disorders is relaxation therapy, where triggering of relative bradycardia, vasodilatation, and changes in the electroencephalogram have been described as the "relaxation response."[138] Relaxation therapies generally involve some combination of relaxed abdominal breathing, quieting of the mind with meditation or related techniques, and somatic relaxation of the body. Relaxation therapies are frequently applied for stress reduction, including just prior to invasive cardiac procedures.[139,140] Relaxation therapy has been associated with lowering of blood pressure and possibly with better outcomes in men with risk factors for coronary artery disease. Concerns with possibly unanticipated negative effects from changing vascular tone or heart rhythm must also be carefully evaluated for therapies in patients with known heart disease. Although a reduction in premature ventricular contractions (PVCs) has been observed with relaxation therapy,[141] higher mortality rates were associated with relaxation therapy in a female cohort of the MHEART study who had survived MI.[142]

Other mind-body techniques with published experience in cardiology include music and imagery. Anxiety reduction has been observed with music in coronary care unit (CCU) and MI populations, although outcomes benefit has not been established.[143,144] Imagery techniques usually encourage a patient to envision a beautiful, peaceful place from his or her life or experience, using a relaxed abdominal breath to let the mind dwell in that place. Music is used in the background in some imagery scripts. Imagery has been reported to reduce pain or the need for sedation in patients undergoing catheterization and to shorten hospital stay after bypass surgery.[145,146]

Meditation and mindfulness constitute a very broad range of disciplines providing tools that, with practice, cultivate personal access to calming of the body and quieting of the mind, with a variety of potential healing effects including reduction of angina and improved quality of life.[147] In addition to the use of these techniques in cardiac rehabilitation programs, they can have a role in lifestyle modification strategies associated with atheroregression in established coronary disease.[148] Meditative states have been demonstrated to measurably impact numerous autonomic and hormonal processes, although the precise mechanistic relationship to cardiovascular benefit is unknown.[149]

Many forms of meditation, like a number of mind-body disciplines, extend beyond mind-body into mind-body-spirit diagnostics and therapeutics, at least metaphorically. The role of spiritual attitudes, mental intentionality, spiritual intervention, and prayer in life process, disease states, and healing have been the subjects of numerous studies, from their effects on microorganisms and cell growth to human clinical trials.[129,150–153] With no insight into mechanism but consistent suggestion of effect, this area of research has slowly moved beyond the traditional separation of science and religion into the more balanced systematic exploration of intangible human potential and its impact on healing in a modern medical context. As editors at the *Lancet* reflected with regard to such "noetic" human capacities, "The contribution that…(noetic human capacities)…make to a personal understanding of illness cannot be dismissed….They are proper subjects for science, even while transcending its known bounds."[154]

The spiritual dimension and the role of spiritual attitudes or interventions across patients, family, community, and medical staff have particular relevance in cardiovascular care, as patients suffering from heart disease are very directly confronted by issues of personal mortality.[1] Although spiritual practices such as prayer have been documented at approximately 90 percent of patients undergoing elective coronary interventions,[155] little is actually known about the role of the human spirit in response to therapy, tolerance of procedures, or as an influence on outcomes per se.

To date a total of six prospective, randomized clinical trials of distant intercessory prayer in cardiovascular populations have been published in the peer review literature.[129,155–159] Data on therapeutic benefit are inconclusive. In early studies, statistical significance was shown for novel hospital severity indices in CCU patients, however the clinical relevance of these differences have neither been proven or reproduced.[156,157] Classical outcomes in a CCU population studied at the Mayo Clinic were negative.[158] The Monitoring and Actualization of Noetic Trainings (MANTRA) Study Project from Duke University published the first multicenter randomized study of noetic therapies in cardiovascular care, in which both double-blinded distant prayer and open-label bedside music-imagery-touch (MIT) therapy were applied in 750 patients undergoing elective percutaneous coronary intervention (PCI) in the MANTRA II study.[155] The 6-month composite primary clinical end point was negative, however the bedside MIT group had lower 6-month mortality ($p < 0.02$), and there was a trend toward outcome differences with different prayer methods.

Most recently, Harvard University reported the Study of Therapeutic Effects of Intercessory Prayer (STEP) in 1802 cardiac bypass surgery patients randomized in 6 centers to double-blinded placebo, double-blinded off-site prayer and open label off-site prayer.[159] Patients in the group who received distant prayer and knew about it had a significantly higher incidence of adverse outcomes, in particular postoperative atrial fibrillation, than patients in the double-blinded group. That the Mayo Clinic, Duke University, and Harvard Medical Centers have directed research efforts in the role of intangible human capacities in high tech cardiovascular care is a signal that this is no longer simply a fringe area, but one of clearly perceived unmet and poorly understood clinical practice needs. The MANTRA II and STEP studies in particular represent applications of noetic therapies in more robust multicenter, randomized, blinded study designs, and data from these studies raise key questions on the effects of patient participation as well as potential safety issues related to the use of noetic therapies in human subjects with heart disease.[160] Attempts to pool or reflect on this literature all indicate that existing data are most useful for hypothesis generation to guide future research.[1,153,154,161,162]

ALTERNATIVE MEDICAL SYSTEMS

Alternative medical systems broadly constitute approaches to diagnostic and therapeutic applications that are based on paradigms conceptually distinct from the allopathic structure of modern medical practices in the Western world. By and large, alternative medical systems are culturally based and in many cases ancient in their history. Perhaps the most notable hallmark of these systems is their holistic character. In many, the allopathic fixation on mechanical processes in the body, detailed analysis of biochemical or serologic measures, and discrete end-organ focus on individual body systems constitute the conceptual equivalent of a gross undersampling error. In traditional Chinese medicine, for instance, cardiovascular disorders are simply one feature of symptom complexes characterized across four relative states of yin deficiency or excess combined with yang deficiency or excess, where both yin and yang energies are associated with a broad range of emotional states, symbolic imagery, as well as specific body organs.[163] In Ayurvedic medical systems, the body is essentially referenced across five inorganic elements constituting the material universe—earth, water, fire, air, and ether. The body itself is envisioned as coarse material, or *maya*, that is structurally configured by vibrational energy conveyed from a collective or cosmic source, or Atma.[164] This coarse material structure rendered by vibrational influences of life energy could be conceptually compared, in a different metaphor, to the modern Western medical understanding of the genome. In both of these paradigms, wellness and illness exist in the individual human being, but they are also structurally shared across populations and beyond. Computationally demanding statistical models being developed for genomic applications might provide some intriguing approaches to novel medical paradigms in alternative medical systems.

Although alternative medical systems at first blush can seem radical in their departure from the rigorously articulate Western scientific medical model, current directions in wellness-oriented lifestyle modification strategies for both the primary and secondary prevention of cardiovascular disease represent a movement with a distinctively holistic character in the mainstream of modern practice.

CONCLUSION

CAM therapies in cardiovascular care represent an enormous area of unregulated and widely practiced therapeutics with an immature scientific literature but, in many cases, an ancient and deeply rooted cultural basis. In modern medicine, CAM therapeutics are probably best considered as adjuncts to current standard medical care, whose study provides opportunities to advance more integrative medical practice. Systematic research to uncover mechanisms of action as well as to better profile the actual safety and efficacy of CAM therapies in specific cardiac disorders is both justified and clearly necessary for new paradigms of integrative medical practice to have an impact and be widely adopted by physicians. In lieu of such research, the education and familiarity of cardiologists with CAM therapies is likely to promote better dialogue with patients and more awareness of issues of self-empowerment in dealing with heart disease, opening the door to a broadened range of options for optimizing cardiovascular care.

REFERENCES

1. Vogel JHK, Bolling SF, Costello RB, et al. Integrating complementary medicine into cardiovascular medicine: a report of the American College of Cardiology Foundation Task Force on Clinical Expert Consensus Documents (Writing Committee to Develop an Expert Consensus Document on Complementary and Integrative Medicine). *J Am Coll Cardiol.* 2005;46:184–221.
2. Eisenberg, DM, Davis R, Ettner S, et al. Trends in alternative medicine use in the United States 1990–1997: results of a follow up national survey. *JAMA.* 1998;1995;280(18):1569–1575.
3. Linde K, Jonas WB. Evaluating complementary and alternative medicine: the balance of rigor and relevance. In: Jonas W, Levin J, eds. *Essentials of Complementary and Alternative Medicine.* Philadelphia: Lippincott, Williams & Wilkins; 1999.
4. Horrigan B. Papa Henry Auwae Po'okela la'au lapa'au: Master of Hawaiian medicine. *Alt Ther Health Med.* 2000;6(1):83–88.
5. Begg C, Cho M, Eastwood S, et al. Improving the quality of reporting of randomized controlled trials. The CONSORT statement. *JAMA.* 1996;276:637–639.
6. MacPherson H, White A, Cummings M, et al. Standards for reporting interventions in controlled trials of acupuncture: the STRICTA recommendations. *Comp Ther Med.* 2001;9:246–249.
7. Dusek JA, Astin JA, Hibberd PL, Krucoff MW. Healing prayer outcomes studies: Consensus recommendations. *Alt Ther Health Med.* 2003;9(3):A44–A53.
8. Jonas WB, Linde K., Walach H. How to practice evidence-based complementary and alternative medicine. In: Jonas W, Levin J, eds. *Essentials of Complementary and Alternative Medicine.* Philadelphia: Lippincott, Williams & Wilkins; 1999.
9. National Institutes of Health. National Center for Complementary and Alternative Medicine (NCCAM). Available at: http://nccam.nih.gov.
10. Gagnier JJ, Boon H, et al. Reporting randomized, control trials of herbal interventions: an elaborated CONSORT statement. *Ann Intern Med.* 2006;144(5);364–367.
11. Sigerist HE. *A History of Medicine.* New York: Oxford University Press; 1951.
12. Abramowicz M. Problems with dietary supplements. *Med Lett Drugs Ther.* 2002;44:84–86.
13. Ernst E. Adulteration of Chinese herbal medicines with synthetic drugs: a systematic review. *J Intern Med.* 2002;252:107–113.
14. Ernst E. Harmless herbs? A review of the recent literature. *Am J Med.* 1998;104:170–178.
15. Lin MC, Nahin R, Gershwin M, et al. State of complementary and alternative medicine in cardiovascular, lung, and blood research: executive summary of a workshop. *Circulation.* 2001;103(16):2038–2041.

16. Brace LD. Cardiovascular benefits of garlic (*Allium sativum* L). *J Cardiovasc Nurs*. 2002;16(4):33–49.

17. Amagase H, Petesch BL, Matsuura H, et al. Intake of garlic and its bioactive compounds. *J Nutr*. 2001;131:955S–962S.

18. Matsuura H. Saponins in garlic as modifiers of the risk of cardiovascular disease. *J Nutr*. 2001;131:1000S–1005S.

19. Borek C. Antioxidant health effects of aged garlic extract. *J Nutr*. 2001;131:1010S–1015S.

20. Harenberg J, Giese C, Zimmermann R. Effect of dried garlic on blood coagulation, fibrinolysis, platelet aggregation and serum cholesterol levels in patients with hyperlipoproteinemia. *Atherosclerosis*. 1988;74:247–249.

21. Mulrow C, Lawrence V, Ackerman R, et al. *Garlic: Effects on Cardiovascular Risks and Disease, Protective Effects against Cancer, and Clinical Adverse Effects*. Rockville, MD: Agency for Healthcare Research and Quality; 2000. AHRQ publication 01-E023.

22. Ackermann RT, Mulrow CD, Ramirez G, et al. Garlic shows promise for improving some cardiovascular risk factors. *Arch Intern Med*. 2001;161:813–824.

23. Stevinson C, Pittler MH, Ernst E. Garlic for treating hypercholesterolemia. A meta-analysis of randomized clinical trials. *Ann Intern Med*. 2000;133(6):420–429.

24. Steiner M, Khan AH, Holbert D, Lin RIS. A double-blind crossover study in moderately hypercholesterolemic men that compared the effect of aged garlic extract and placebo administration on blood lipids. *Am J Clin Nutr*. 1996;64:866–870.

25. Adler AJ, Holub BJ. Effect of garlic and fish-oil supplementation on serum lipid and lipoprotein concentrations in hypercholesterolic men. *Am J Clin Nutr*. 1997;65:445–450.

26. Silagy CA, Neil HA. A meta-analysis of the effect of garlic on blood pressure *J Hypertens*. 1994;12(4):463–468.

27. Piscitelli SC, Burstein AH, Welden N, et al. The effect of garlic supplements on the pharmacokinetics of saquinavir. *Clin Infect Dis*. 2002;34:234–238.

28. Schulz V, Hansel R, Tyler VE. *Rational phytotherapy: A Physician's Guide to Herbal Medicine*. 4th ed. Berlin: Springer-Verlag; 2001.

29. De Smet PA. Herbal remedies. *N Engl J Med*. 2002;347(25):2046–2056.

30. Leuchtgens VH. *Crataegus* special extract WS 1442 in NYHA II heart failure. A placebo controlled randomized double-blind study. *Fortschr Med*. 1993;111:36–38.

31. Rietbrock N, Hamel M, Hempel B, et al. Efficacy of a standardized extract of fresh *Crataegus* berries on exercise tolerance and quality of life in patients with congestive heart failure (NYHA II). *Arzneimittelforschung*. 2001;51:793–798.

32. Tauchert M. Efficacy and safety of *Crataegus* extract WS 1442 in comparison with placebo in patients with chronic stable New York Heart Association class III heart failure. *Am Heart J*. 2002;143(5):910–915.

33. Schwinger RH, Pietsch M, Frank K, et al. *Crataegus* special extract WS1442 increases force of contraction in human myocardium cAMP-independently. *J Cardiovasc Pharmacol*. 2000;35:700–707.

34. Popping S, Rose H, Ionescu I, et al. Effect of a hawthorn extract on contraction and energy turnover of isolated rat cardiomyocytes. *Arzneimittelforschung*. 1995;45:1157–1161.

35. Ammon HPT, Handel M. *Crataegus*, Toxikologie und Pharmakologie. II. Pharmakodynamik. *Planta Med*. 1981;43:209–239.

36. Weikl A, Noh HS. Der Einfluss von *Crataegus* bei globaler Herzinsuffizienz. *Herz Gefasse*. 1992;11:516–524.

37. Daniele C, Mazzanti G, Pittler MH, Ernst E. Adverse-event profile of *Crataegus* spp: a systematic review. *Drug Saf*. 2006;29:523–535.

38. Blumenthal M. Herb sales down 3% in mass market retail stores. *Herbal Gram*. 2000;49:68.

39. Chatterjee SS, Gaqbard B. Studies on the mechanism of action of an extract of Gingko biloba, a drug used for treatment of ischemic vascular diseases. *Naunyn Schmiedebergs Arch Pharmacol*. 1982;320:R52.

40. Chung KF, McCusker M, Page CP, et al. Effect of a ginkgolide mixture (BN 52063) in antagonizing skin and platelet responses to platelet activating factor in man. *Lancet*. 1987;I:248–250.

41. Blume J, Kieser M, Holscher U. Placebo-controlled, double-blind study on the effectiveness of *Ginkgo biloba* special extract EGb 761 in trained patients with intermittent claudication. *Vasa*. 1996;25:265–274.

42. Peters H, Kieser M, Holscher U. Demonstration of the efficacy of *Ginkgo biloba* special extract EGb 761 on intermittent claudication—a placebo-controlled, double-blind multicenter trial. *Vasa*. 1998;27:106–110.

43. Moher D, Pham B, Ausejo M, et al. Pharmacological management of intermittent claudication: a meta-analysis of randomised trials. *Drugs*. 2000;59:1057–1070.

44. Pittler MH, Ernst E. *Ginkgo biloba* extract for the treatment of intermittent claudication: a meta-analysis of randomized trials. *Am J Med*. 2000;108:276–281.

45. Rowin J, Lewis SL. Spontaneous bilateral subdural hematomas associated with chronic *Ginkgo biloba* ingestion. *Neurology*. 1996;46:1775–1776.

46. Fessenden JM, Wittenborn W, Clarke L. Gingko biloba: A case report of herbal medicine and bleeding postoperatively from a laparoscopic cholecystectomy. *Am Surg*. 2001;67:33–35.

47. White HL, Scates PW, Cooper BR. Extracts of *Ginkgo biloba* leaves inhibit monamine oxidase. *Life Science*. 1996;58(16):1315–1321.

48. Sirtori, CR. Aescin: pharmacology, pharmacokinetics and therapeutic profile. *Pharm Res*. 2001;44(3):183–193.

49. Arnould T, Janssens D, Michiels C, Remacle J. Effect of asecin on hypoxia-induced activation of endothelial cells. *Eur J Pharmacol*. 1996,315(2):227–233.

50. Diehm C, Trampisch HJ, Lange S, et al. Comparison of leg compression stocking and oral horse-chestnut seed extract therapy in patients with chronic venous insufficiency. *Lancet*. 1996;347:292–294.

51. Neiss A, Bohm C. Demonstration of the effectiveness of the horse-chestnut-seed extract in the varicose syndrome complex. *Munch Med Wochenschr*. 1976;118:213–216.

52. Pittler MH, Ernst E. Horse-chestnut seed extract for chronic venous insufficiency. A criteria-based systematic review. *Arch Dermatol*. 1998;134:1356–1360.

53. Pittler MH, Ernst E. Horse chestnut seed extract for chronic venous insufficiency. *Cochrane Database Syst Rev*. 2006;1:CD003230.

54. Brinker FJ. *Herb Contraindications and Drug Interactions*. 2nd ed. Sandy, OR: Eclectic Medical Publications; 1998.

55. Mas R. Policosanol. *Drugs Future*. 2000;25:569–586.

56. Menéndez R, Fernández I, Del Rio A, et al. Policosanol inhibits cholesterol biosynthesis and enhances LDL processing in cultured human fibroblasts. *Biol Res*. 1994;27:199–203.

57. Canetti M, Morera M, Illnait J, et al. One year study on the effect of policosanol (5 mg twice-a-day) on lipid profile in patients with type II hypercholesterolemia. *Adv Ther*. 1995;12:245–254.

58. Fernández JC, Más R, Castaño G, et al. Comparison of the efficacy, safety and tolerability of policosanol versus fluvastatin in elderly hypercholesterolemic women. *Clin Drug Invest*. 2001;21(2):103–113.

59. Gouni-Berthold I, Berthold HK. Policosanol: clinical pharmacology and therapeutic significance of a new lipid-lowering agent. *Am Heart J*. 2002;143:356–365.

60. Snider SR. Octacosanol in parkinsonism. *Ann Neurol*. 1984;16:723.

61. Urizar NL, Liverman AB, Dodds DT, et al. A natural product that lowers cholesterol as an antagonist ligand for FXR. *Science*. 2002;296(5573):1703–1706.

62. Singh RB, Niaz MA, Ghosh S. Hypolipidemic and antioxidant effects of *Commiphora mukul* as an adjunct to dietary therapy in patients with hypercholesterolemia. *Cardiovasc Drugs Ther*. 1994;8:659–664.

63. Nityanand S, Srivastava JS, Asthana OP. Clinical trials with gugulipid. A new hypolipidaemic agent. *J Assoc Physicians India*. 1989;37:323–328.

64. Szapary PO, Wolfe ML, Bloedon LT, et al. Guggulipid for the treatment of hypercholesterolemia: a randomized control trial. *JAMA*. 2003;290:765–772.

65. Dalvi SS, Nayak VK, Pohujani SM, et al. Effect of gugulipid on bioavailability of diltiazem and propranolol. *J Assoc Physicians India*. 1994;42:454–455.

66. Heber D, Yip I, Ashley JM, et al. Cholesterol-lowering effects of a proprietary Chinese red yeast rice dietary supplement. *Am J Clin Nutr*. 1999;69:231–236.

67. Rippe J, Bonovich K, Colfer H, et al. *A multicenter, self-controlled study of Cholestin in subjects with elevated cholesterol*. 39th Annual Conference on Cardiovascular Disease Epidemiology and Prevention. Orlando, Florida; 1999.

68. Hu FB, Willett WC. Optimal diets for prevention of coronary heart disease. *JAMA*. 2002;288:2569–2578.

69. de Lorgeril M, Salen P, Martin JL, et al. Mediterranean diet, traditional risk factors, and the rate of cardiovascular complications after myocardial infarction: final report of the Lyon Diet Heart Study. *Circulation*. 1999;99:779–785.

70. Burr ML, Fehily AM, Gilbert JF, et al. Effects of changes in fat, fish, and fibre intakes on death and myocardial reinfarction: diet and reinfarction trial (DART). *Lancet*. 1989;2:757–761.

71. Kromhout D, Bosschieter EB, de Lezenne CC. The inverse relation between fish consumption and 20-year mortality from coronary heart disease. *N Engl J Med*. 1985;312:1205–1209.

72. Marckmann P, Gronbaek M. Fish consumption and coronary heart disease mortality. A systematic review of prospective cohort studies. *Eur J Clin Nutr.* 1999;53:585–590.

73. von Schacky C, Angerer P, Kothny W, et al. The effect of dietary omega-3 fatty acids on coronary atherosclerosis. A randomized, double-blind, placebo-controlled trial. *Ann Intern Med.* 1999;130:554–562.

74. Hooper L, Thompson RL, Harrison RA, et al. Risks and benefits of omega 3 fats for mortality, cardiovascular disease, and cancer: systematic review. *Brit Med J.* 2006;332:752–760.

75. Eritsland J, Arnesen H, Gronseth K, et al. Effect of dietary supplementation with n-3 fatty acids on coronary artery bypass graft patency. *Am J Cardiol.* 1996;77:31–36.

76. Marchioli R, Barzi F, Bomba E, et al. Early protection against sudden death by n-3 polyunsaturated fatty acids after myocardial infarction: time-course analysis of the results of the Gruppo Italiano per lo Studio della Sopravvivenza nell'Infarto Miocardico (GISSI)-Prevenzione. *Circulation.* 2002;105:1897–1903.

76a. Bucher HC, Hengstler P, Schindler C, Meier G. N-3 polyunsaturated fatty acids in coronary heart disease: A meta-analysis of randomized controlled trials. *Am J Med.* 2002;112:298–304.

77. Burr ML, Ashfield-Watt PAL, Dunstan FDJ, et al. Lack of benefit of dietary advice to men with angina: results of a controlled trial. *Eur J Clin Nutr.* 2003;57:193.

78. Schrepf R, Limmert T, Weber C, et al. Immediate effects of n-3 fatty acid infusion on the induction of sustained ventricular tachycardia. *Lancet.* 2004;363:1441–1442.

79. Raitt MH, Connor WE, Morris C, et al. Fish oil supplementation and risk of ventricular tachycardia and ventricular fibrillation in patients with implantable defibrillators: a randomized controlled trial. *JAMA.* 2005;293:2884–2891.

80. Brouwer IA, Zock PL, Camm AJ, et al. Effect of fish oil on ventricular tachyarrhythmia and death in patients with implantable cardioverter defibrillators: the SOFA randomized trial. *JAMA.* 2006;295:2613–2619.

81. Kris-Etherton PM, Harris WS, Appel LJ; American Heart Association. Nutrition Committee. Fish consumption, fish oil, omega-3 fatty acids, and cardiovascular disease. *Circulation.* 2002;106:2747–2757.

82. GISSI-HF Investigators. Rationale and design of the GISSI heart failure trial: a large trial to assess the effects of n-3 polyunsaturated fatty acids and rosuvastatin in symptomatic congestive heart failure. *Eur J Heart Fail.* 2004;6:635–641.

83. Brunner E. Oily fish and omega 3 fat supplements: Health recommendations conflict with concerns about dwindling supply. *Brit Med J.* 2006; 332:739–740.

84. Stampfer MJ, Hennekens CH, Manson JE, et al. Vitamin E consumption and the risk of coronary disease in women. *N Engl J Med.* 1993;328:1444–1449.

85. Rimm EB, Stampfer MJ, Ascherio A, et al. Vitamin E consumption and the risk of coronary heart disease in men. *N Engl J Med.* 1993;328:1450–1456.

86. Losonczy KG, Harris TB, Havlik RJ. Vitamin E and vitamin C supplement use and risk of all-cause and coronary heart disease mortality in older persons: the Established Populations for Epidemiologic Studies of the Elderly. *Am J Clin Nutr.* 1996;64:190–196.

87. Adams AK, Wermuth EO, McBride PE, et al. Antioxidant Vitamins and the Prevention of Coronary Heart Disease. *Am Fam Phys.* 1999;60:895–904.

88. The Heart Outcomes Prevention Evaluation Study Investigators. Vitamin E supplementation and cardiovascular events in high-risk patients. *N Engl J Med.* 2000;342:154–160.

89. GISSI-Prevenzione Investigators. Dietary supplementation with n-3 polyunsaturated fatty acids and vitamin E after myocardial infarction: results of the GISSI-Prevenzione trial. *Lancet.* 1999;354:447–455.

90. De Gaetano G. Collaboratory Group of the Primary Prevention Project: low-dose aspirin and vitamin E in people at cardiovascular risk: a randomised trial in general practice. Collaborative Group of the Primary Prevention Project. *Lancet.* 2001;357(9250):89–95.

91. HOPE and HOPE-TOO Trial Investigators. Effects of long-term vitamin E supplementation on cardiovascular events and cancer: a randomized controlled trial. *JAMA.* 2005;293:1338–1347.

92. Lee IM, Cook NR, Gaziano JM, et al. Vitamin E in the primary prevention of cardiovascular disease and cancer: the Women's Health Study: a randomized controlled trial. *JAMA.* 2005;294:56–65.

93. Osganian SK, Stampfer MJ, Rimm E, et al. Vitamin C and risk of coronary heart disease in women. *J Am Coll Cardiol.* 2003;42:246–252.

94. MRC/BHF Heart Protection Study of antioxidant vitamin supplementation in 20,536 high-risk individuals: a randomised placebo-controlled trial. *Lancet.* 2002;360:23–33.

95. Salonen RM, Nyyssonen K, Kaikkonen J, et al. Six-year effect of combined vitamin C and E supplementation on atherosclerotic progression: the Antioxidant Supplementation in Atherosclerosis Prevention (ASAP) study. *Circulation.* 2003;107:947–953.

96. Folsom AR, Nieto FJ, McGovern PG, et al. Prospective study of coronary heart disease incidence in relation to fasting total homocysteine, related genetic polymorphisms, and B vitamins: the Atherosclerosis Risk in Communities (ARIC) study. *Circulation.* 1998;98:204–210.

97. Rimm EB, Willett WC, Hu FB, et al. Folate and vitamin B6 from diet and supplements in relation to risk of coronary heart disease among women. *JAMA.* 1998;279:359–364.

98. Bleys J, Miller ER 3rd, Pastor-Barriuso R, et al. Vitamin-mineral supplementation and the progression of atherosclerosis: a meta-analysis of randomized controlled trials. *Am J Clin Nutr.* 2006;84:880–887.

99. Lange H, Suryapranata H, De Luca G, et al. Folate therapy and in-stent restenosis after coronary stenting. *N Engl J Med.* 2004;350:2673–2681.

100. Knudtson ML, Wyse DG, Galbraith PD, et al. Chelation therapy for ischemic heart disease: a randomized controlled trial. *JAMA.* 2002;287:481–486.

101. Olson BH, Anderson SM, Becker MP, et al. Psyllium-enriched cereals lower blood total cholesterol and LDL cholesterol, but not HDL cholesterol, in hypercholesterolemic adults: results of a meta-analysis. *J Nutr.* 1997;127:1973–1980.

102. Wolk A, Manson JE, Stampfer MJ, et al. Long-term intake of dietary fiber and decreased risk of coronary heart disease among women. *JAMA.* 1999;281:1998–2004.

103. Todd S, Woodward M, Tunstall-Pedoe H, Bolton-Smith C. Dietary antioxidant vitamins and fiber in the etiology of cardiovascular disease and all-causes mortality: results from the Scottish Heart Health Study. *Am J Epidemiol.* 1999;150:1073–1080.

104. Anderson JW, Johnstone BM, Cook-Newell ME. Meta-analysis of the effects of soy protein intake on serum lipids. *N Engl J Med.* 1995;333:276–282.

105. Elliott P, Stamler J, Dyer AR, et al. Association between protein intake and blood pressure: the INTERMAP Study. *Arch Intern Med.* 2006;166:79–87.

106. Sacks FM, Lichtenstein A, Van Horn L, et al. Soy protein, isoflavones, and cardiovascular health: an AHA Science Advisory for professionals from the Nutrition Committee. *Circulation.* 2006;113:1034–1344.

107. Law M. Plant sterol and stanol margarines and health. *BMJ.* 2000;320:861–864.

108. Truelsen T, Gronbaek M, Schnohr P, Boysen G. Intake of beer, wine, and spirits and risk of stroke: the Copenhagen City Heart study. *Stroke.* 1998;29:2467–2472.

109. Sacco RL, Elkind M, Boden-Albala B, et al. The protective effect of moderate alcohol consumption on ischemic stroke. *JAMA.* 1999;281:53–60.

110. Djousse L, Levy D, Murabito JM, et al. Alcohol consumption and risk of intermittent claudication in the Framingham Heart Study. *Circulation.* 2000;102:3092–3097.

111. Mukamal KJ, Maclure M, Muller JE, et al. Prior alcohol consumption and mortality following acute myocardial infarction. *JAMA.* 2001;285:1965–1970.

112. Goldberg IJ, Mosca L, Piano MR, Fisher EA. AHA Science Advisory: Wine and your heart: a science advisory for healthcare professionals from the Nutrition Committee, Council on Epidemiology and Prevention, and Council on Cardiovascular Nursing of the American Heart Association. *Circulation.* 2001;103:472–475.

113. Longhurst JC. Acupuncture's beneficial effects on the cardiovascular system. *Prev Cardiol.* 1998;1:21–33.

114. Jackson MD. Acupuncture: an evidence-based review of the clinical literature. *Annu Rev Med.* 2000;51:49–63.

115. Andersson SA, Ericson T, Holmgren E, Lindqvist G. Electro-acupuncture and pain threshold. *Lancet.* 1973;2:564.

116. Ballegaard S, Pedersen F, Pietersen A, et al. Effects of acupuncture in moderate, stable angina pectoris: a controlled study. *J Intern Med.* 1990;227:25–30.

117. Ballegaard S, Meyer CN, Trojaborg W. Acupuncture in angina pectoris: Does acupuncture have a specific effect? *J Intern Med.* 1991;229:357–362.

118. Richter A, Herlitz J, Hjalmarson A. Effect of acupuncture in patients with angina pectoris. *Eur Heart J.* 1991;12:175–178.

119. Parameswaran PG. Ischemic foot treated with acupuncture. Proceedings of the 2nd Asian Congress for Microcirculation. Beijing, China; August 17–20, 1995.

120. Chiu UJ, Chi A, Reid IA. Cardiovascular and endocrine effects of acupuncture in hypertensive patients. *Clin Exp Hypertens.* 1997;19:1047–1063.

121. Wang CX, Xu DH, Qi YH, Kuang AK. The beneficial effect of qigong on the hypertension incorporated with coronary heart disease. *J Gerontol.* 1988;8(2):83.

122. Lee MS, Ki m BG, Huh HJ, et al. Effect of Qi-training on blood pressure, heart rate, and respiration rate. *Clin Physiol.* 2000;20:173–176.

123. Kuang AK, Wang CX, Zhao GS, et al. Long-term observation on QiGong in prevention of stroke-follow up of 244 hypertensive patients for 18–22 years. *J Tradit Chin Med.* 1986;6:235–238.

124. Quinn JF. Building a body of knowledge: research on therapeutic touch, 1974–1986. *J Holist Nurs.* 1974;6:37–45.

125. Hover-Krame M, Mentgen D. *Healing Touch: A Resource for Health Care Professionals.* Albany, NY: Delmar; 1996.

126. Miles P, True G. Reiki—Review of a biofield therapy history, theory, practice and research. *Alt Ther Health Med.* 2003;9(2):62–72.

127. Heidt P. Effect of therapeutic touch on anxiety level of hospitalized patients. *Nurs Res.* 1981;30:32–37.

128. Turton MB, Deegan T, Coulshed N. Plasma catecholamine levels and cardiac rhythm before and after heart catheterization. *Br Heart J.* 1977;39:1307–1311.

129. Krucoff MW, Crater SW, Green CL, et al. Integrative noetic therapies as adjuncts to percutaneous intervention during unstable coronary syndromes: Monitoring and Actualization of Noetic Training (MANTRA) feasibility pilot. *Am Heart J.* 2001;142:760–769.

130. Zhang SX, Guo HZ, Jing BS, et al. Experimental verification of effectiveness and harmlessness of the QiGong maneuver. *Aviat Space Environ Med.* 1991;62:46–52.

131. Koenig HG. *Is Religion Good for Your Health?* New York: Haworth Press; 1997.

132. Rozanski A, Bairey CN, Krantz DS, et al. Mental stress and the induction of silent myocardial ischemia in patients with coronary artery disease. *N Engl J Med.* 1988;318(16):1005–1012.

133. Williams R. *Anger Kills.* New York: Random House; 1993.

134. Koenig HG, Hays JC, George LK, Blazer DG. Modeling the cross-sectional relationships between religion, physical health, social support, and depressive symptoms. *Am J Geriatr Psychiatry.* 1997;5(2):131–144.

135. Krucoff C, Krucoff MW. *Healing Moves.* New York: Harmony Books; 2000.

136. Benson H, McCallie DP Jr. Angina pectoris and the placebo effect. *N Engl J Med.* 1979(300):1424–1429.

137. Hrobjartsson A, Gotzsche PC. Is the placebo powerless? An analysis of clinical trials comparing placebo with no treatment. *N Engl J Med.* 2001;344:1594–1602.

138. Benson H. The relaxation response: therapeutic effect. *Science.* 1997;278(5344):1694–1695.

139. Mandle CL, Domar AD, Harrington DP, et al. Relaxation response in femoral angiography. *Radiology.* 1990;174:737–739.

140. Warner, CD, Peebles, BU, Miller J, et al. The effectiveness of teaching a relaxation technique to patients undergoing elective cardiac catheterization *J Cardiovasc Nurs.* 1992;6:66–75.

141. Benson H, Alexander S, Feldman, C. Decreased premature ventricular contractions through use of the relaxation response in patients with stable ischemic heart disease. *Lancet.* 1975;2:380–382.

142. Frasure-Smith N, Lesperance F, Prince RH, et al. Randomized trial of home-based psychosocial nursing intervention for patients recovering from myocardial infarction. *Lancet.* 1997;350(9076):473–479.

143. Zimmerman LM, Pierson MA, Marker J. Effects of music on patients' anxiety in coronary care units. *Heart Lung.* 1988;17:560–566.

144. Guzzetta C. Effects of relaxation and music therapy on patients in a coronary care unit with presumptive acute myocardial infarction. *Heart Lung.* 1989;18:609–616.

145. Lang EV, Hamilton D. Anodyne imagery: an alternative to IV sedation in interventional radiology. *AJR.* 1994;162:1221–1226.

146. Tusek DL, Cosgrove DM. Effect of guided imagery on length of stay, pain, and anxiety in cardiac surgery patients. *J Cardiovasc Mgt.* 1999;10:22–28.

147. Zamarra JW, Schneider RH, Besseghini I, et al. Usefulness of the transcendental meditation program in the treatment of patients with coronary artery diseases. *JAMA.* 1995;274:867–869.

148. Ornish DM, Brown SE, Scherwitz LZ, et al. Can lifestyle changes reverse atherosclerosis? *Lancet.* 1990;336:129–133.

149. Jevning R, Wallace RK, Beidebach M. The physiology of meditation: a review. A wakeful hypometabolic integrated response. *Neurosci Biobehav Rev.* 1992;16:415–424.

150. Benor DJ. *Healing Research.* Munich, Germany: Helix Verlag; 1992.

151. Dossey L. *Healing Words: The Power of Prayer and the Practice of Medicine.* New York: Harper Collins; 1993.

152. Schlitz M, Braud W. Distant intentionality and healing: assessing the evidence. *Alt Ther Health Med.* 1997;3:62–73.

153. Astin JA, Harkness E, Ernst E. The efficacy of "distant healing": a systematic review of randomized trials. *Ann Intern Med.* 2000;132:903–910.

154. Mantra II. Measuring the unmeasurable? [editorial]. *Lancet.* 2005;366:178.

155. Krucoff MW, Crater SW, Gallup D, et al. Music, imagery, touch and prayer as adjuncts to interventional cardiac care: the Monitoring and Actualization of Noetic Trainings (MANTRA) II randomized study. *Lancet.* 2005;366:211–217.

156. Byrd RC. Positive therapeutic effects of intercessory prayer in a coronary care unit population. *South Med J.* 1988;81:826–829.

157. Harris WS, Gowda M, Kolb JW, et al. A randomized, controlled trial of the effects of remote, intercessory prayer on outcomes in patients admitted to the coronary care unit. *Arch Int Med.* 1999;159:2273–2278.

158. Aviles JM, Whelan SE, Hernke DA, et al. Intercessory prayer and cardiovascular disease progression in a coronary care unit population: a randomized controlled trial. *Mayo Clin Proc.* 2001;76:1192–1198.

159. Benson H, Dusek JA, Sherwood JB, et al. Study of the Therapeutic Effects of Intercessory Prayer (STEP) in cardiac bypass patients: a multicenter randomized trail of uncertainty and certainty of receiving intercessory prayer. *Am Heart J.* 2006;151(4):934–42.

160. Krucoff MW, Crater SW, Lee KL. From efficacy to safety concerns: a STEP forward or a step back for clinical research and intercessory prayer? The Study of Therapeutic Effects of Intercessory Prayer (STEP). *Am Heart J.* 2006;151:762–764.

161. Krucoff MW, Crater SW. Dose response and the effects of distant prayer on health outcomes: The state of the research. *Integr Med Consult.* 2002;4(5):56–58.

162. Jonas WB, Crawford CC. Science and spiritual healing: a critical review of spiritual healing, "energy" medicine and intentionality. *Alt Ther Health Med.* 2003;9(2):56–61.

163. Lao L. Traditional Chinese medicine. In: Jonas W, Levin J, eds. *Essentials of Complementary and Alternative Medicine.* Philadelphia: Lippincott, Williams & Wilkins; 1999.

164. Ghooi C. *Spirituality and Health.* Prasanthi Nilayam: Sri Sathya Sai Boolls; 2001.

CHAPTER 115

Social and Societal Issues of Heart Disease

Roberto De Vogli / Michael Marmot

INTRODUCTION

Heart disease is a condition largely influenced by societal and social factors. Although the previous chapters have primarily focussed on clinical factors and proximal determinants, in this chapter we will examine the broader economic and social forces that determine this health condition at the population level. The chapter is divided into three parts. First, we will analyze how *societal factors* influence heart disease, with particular reference to socioeconomic development and socioeconomic gradients of heart disease and related behavioral risk factors. Then, we will examine the role of *social factors* including social organization, social relations, and chronic stress. Finally, we will discuss *prevention strategies* to reduce heart disease and the socioeconomic gradient of heart disease at the population level.

SOCIETAL FACTORS AND HEART DISEASE

The influence of societal factors on heart disease is supported by at least two major categories of scientific evidence: the epidemic changed in response to *socioeconomic development* that profoundly affected standards of living and habits; the *socioeconomic gradients* of heart disease and related behavioral risk factors varied according to the stage of socioeconomic development.

【 】 SOCIOECONOMIC DEVELOPMENT AND HEART DISEASE (ACROSS SOCIETIES)

The emergence of heart disease is associated with the advent of industrialization and urbanization that improved socioeconomic conditions and changed our way of living.[1,2] The diffusion and decline of this health condition vary according to the stage of socioeconomic development in the context of the epidemiologic transition from infectious to chronic diseases. Although heart disease has often been regarded as a disease of affluent societies, the rapid socioeconomic changes that transformed patterns of consumption and lifestyle have rapidly affected developing countries as well. Rates of coronary heart disease are still low in the poorest regions of the world including sub-Saharan Africa, and the rural areas of South America and South Asia. They have become more common in regions characterized by increasing wealth, longevity, and lifestyle changes in diet, exercise, and smoking such as India and Latin America. They are declining in Western Europe, North America (excluding some parts of Mexico), Australia, and New Zealand as changes in the way of living delay ischemic heart disease and stroke to more advanced ages.[3]

Whereas the epidemic in affluent societies increased and declined over the course of a century, the transition in the developing world has been compressed into a few decades.[4] More recently, this process of rapid diffusion of heart disease has been exacerbated by the *Westernization* of lifestyle and economic globalization that produced further changes in terms of urbanization, agricultural production, and food consumption.[5] One of the effects of globalization is what has been called the *coca-colonization* of living habits including increased consumption of fats and sweeteners.[6] As countries are more progressively integrated in the world economy, they converge to more homogeneous patterns of lifestyle and consumption leading to similar chronic diseases. The globalization of lifestyle patterns has been particularly strong among younger generations[7] with the United States leading the change[8] and exporting conditions such as obesity to less developed societies.[9]

2473

【 】SOCIOECONOMIC GRADIENT OF HEART DISEASE (WITHIN SOCIETIES)

The effect of societal factors on heart disease is also manifested as socioeconomic inequalities in the distribution of this health outcome and its related behavioral risk factors. Such patterns of inequalities change according to the stage of epidemiologic transition. People in higher socioeconomic positions are the first to be affected by the disease and related behaviors, but then they are also the first to experience a decline of both the condition and risk factors. Later in the transition, such conditions become progressively more prevalent among lower socioeconomic groups with socioeconomic gradients of heart disease and risk factors that reverse over time.

Socioeconomic Position and Heart Disease

The epidemiologic transition of heart disease from being a disease of the wealthy to one of the poor has been analyzed in the changes in the socioeconomic distribution of heart disease in developing and developed societies. Fig. 115–1 shows the unadjusted odds ratios for stroke in different regions of the world and their association with secondary and low educational strata using high education as the reference group. An inverse association with education was found in Asia, Latin America, and Eastern Europe, with the effect most pronounced in Eastern Europe and least apparent in Latin America. On the contrary, the association appeared to be positive in Africa.[10]

In developing societies, the epidemic struck the more affluent sections of society first, but as the epidemic matured, the socioeconomic gradient reversed, with socioeconomically disadvantaged groups becoming increasingly vulnerable.[11] Higher risk for coronary heart diseases among advantaged groups have not been reported only in Africa, but also in Hong Kong,[12] Puerto Rico,[13] and Pakistan.[14] In the most affluent nations, and former socialist countries, there has been a reversal in the association between coronary heart disease mortality and socioeconomic position observed during the twentieth century, with widening mortality gap over time. The

switch-over has been documented in England and Wales[15] where there has been a greater decline in coronary heart disease mortality among higher socioeconomic groups during the latter part of the century, which has increased inequalities over time.[16]

As countries develop they converge to a more homogeneous social pattern with low socioeconomic position that progressively becomes a systematic risk factor for coronary heart disease both in developed and developing societies.

Socioeconomic Position and Behavioral Risk Factors

The epidemiologic transition of heart disease across socioeconomic groups coincides with the transition of conventional coronary heart disease (CHD) risk factors including health behaviors. The most affluent social groups are the first to change their lifestyle and consumption that lead to the development of risk factors such as obesity, physical inactivity, smoking, high blood pressure, and high cholesterol levels. However, as these changes influence society as a whole, behavioral risk factors for heart disease become more common among less privileged socioeconomic groups both in affluent and less affluent societies.

Fig. 115–2 shows the age-standardized prevalence ratio for women's obesity by quartiles of years of education in low, lower-middle, and upper-middle income economies in 1992 to 2000. Results indicate that belonging to the lower socioeconomic group is a protective factor against obesity in low-income economies (gross national product [GNP] less than $745 per capita), but is a risk factor for the disease in upper-middle-income economies (GNP ≥ $2995 per capita).[17]

As countries reach the later stages of socioeconomic development, the relationships between low socioeconomic position and CHD behavioral risk factors become more homogeneous. In most developed societies the relation between low socioeconomic status and behavioral risk factors is consolidated and consistent across individual-level[17] and area-level indicators.[18,19] The poorest sectors of society, almost everywhere now, use tobacco with greater frequency than their most privileged counterparts in terms of income, education, and occupation.[20] Although behavioral risk factors become more prevalent among the lower socioeconomic groups in almost any nation, there are some exceptions to the rule. Perhaps, the most notable ones are represented by the weaker, absent, or inverse social gradients of behavioral risk factors[21,22] in southern European countries that are also characterized by lower rates of coronary heart disease compared to northern Europe, the United States, and the United Kingdom.[23] Such international differences in the transition of the social gradient of health behaviors remain largely unexplained, and further research is needed to analyze the interrelations and relative importance of social causes versus risk factors[24] in determining heart disease and the social gradient of heart disease. With regard to the latter, scientific evidence indicates that only a small proportion of the social gradient in heart disease is explained by conventional risk factors.[11]

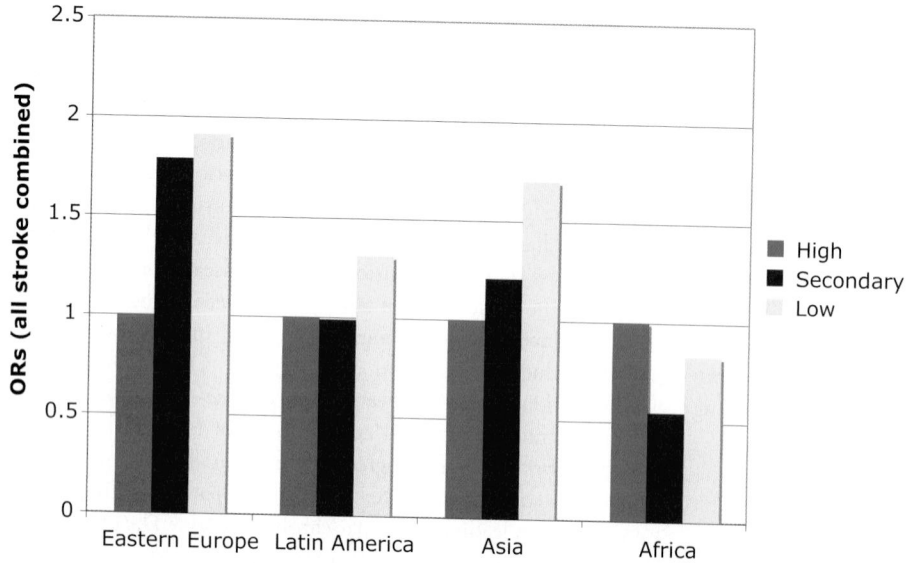

FIGURE 115–1. Unadjusted odds ratios (ORs) for all stroke combined by educational level (high, secondary, and low) in four regions. *Source: Chang C, Marmot M, Farley T, Poulter N.*[10]

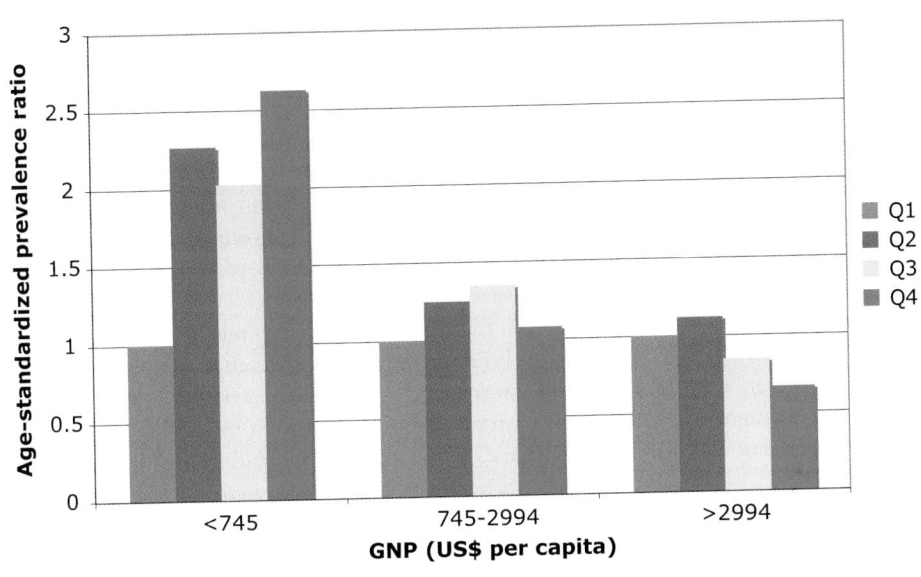

FIGURE 115–2. Age-standardized prevalence ratio for women's obesity by quartiles (Q) of years of education in low, lower-middle, and upper-middle income economies (1992–2000). *Source: Monteiro CA, Conde WL, Lu B, Popkin BM.[17]*

Fig. 115–3 shows mortality from coronary heart disease over 25 years in the first Whitehall study showing the contribution of risk factors to the social gradient. Results indicate that adjusting for traditional CHD risk factors such as smoking, blood pressure, plasma cholesterol, short height, and blood sugar accounted for less than one-third of the social gradient in mortality.

Results of the Whitehall study stimulated further investigations on the contribution of social and psychological factors in explaining the other two-thirds of the social gradient of heart disease.

SOCIAL FACTORS AND HEART DISEASE

A large body of evidence showed that social factors such as social networks and social support as well as psychological factors including chronic stress have an independent effect on coronary heart disease that cannot be explained by conventional risk factors.

【 】 SOCIAL ORGANIZATION

Although the progression from one stage of socioeconomic development to the next tends to proceed in a predictable manner, there are important differences between societies. Several hypotheses have been proposed to explain such variations including the income inequality and social cohesion hypotheses. Evidence shows that more egalitarian societies tend to have lower risks of coronary heart disease compared to highly unequal societies.[25] Furthermore, low social cohesion or social capital have been found to be predictors of coronary heart disease.[26] Japan, a country character-

ized by low inequality and high social cohesion, is unique among high-income countries, because the transition started later but proceeded much more rapidly than in other affluent nations. It is often considered a puzzle in the epidemiologic transition because, despite having one of the highest rates of smoking in the world, Japan experiences very low rates of heart attacks.[27] On the opposite side, in the former Soviet Union and other socialist countries, drastic increases of income inequality and disruption of social organization were accompanied by unprecedented increases of coronary heart disease.[28] A cross-national analysis showed that heart disease was four times higher in Lithuania than in Sweden, despite small differences in traditional risk factors.[29]

【 】 SOCIAL NETWORKS AND SOCIAL SUPPORT

Social networks and social support (emotional and practical) have been found to be relevant predictors of coronary heart disease in a number of studies.[30–32] Social networks refer to the web of social relations, including both intimate relationships with family and close friends and more formal relationships with other individuals and groups.[33] Social support refers to the social resources that persons perceive to be available or that are actually provided to them by nonprofessionals in the context of both formal support groups and informal helping relations.

Social relations provide benefits to health and heart disease in at least two major ways. According to the stress-buffering model, so-

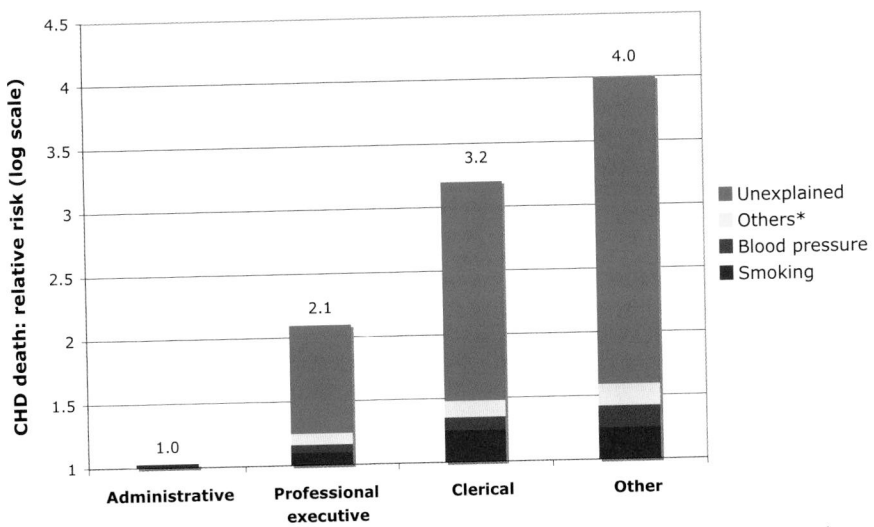

FIGURE 115–3. Relative risk of death from coronary heart disease (CHD) among British civil servants according to employment grade (proportions of differences explained by risk factors). *Source: Marmot M, Rose G, Shipley M, Hamilton J.[11]*

cial relations provide beneficial health effects because they protect individuals from the negative effects of chronic stress. According to the main or direct effect model, social resources have beneficial effects on heart disease by encouraging healthy behaviors, and positive psychological states that enhance immune function.[34]

The importance of the disruption of social ties and their effect on heart disease has been shown by changes in myocardial infarction in Roseto, a small Italian-American community in Pennsylvania. Roseto, which in the 1960s was characterized by close-knit social relations and egalitarian values, presented a rate of heart attacks approximately 40 percent lower than expected, a figure that could not be explained by the prevalence of traditional CHD risk factors including smoking, overweight, and diet. However, as community bonds weakened in the following years, Roseto caught up with the prevalence of adjacent towns and lost its protection from heart disease.[35]

The hypothesis that social ties provide benefits to health can also help to explain why in southern European countries (Spain, Portugal, Italy, France, and Greece), characterized not only by the Mediterranean diet, but also by extended systems of social relations, heart diseases remained low, despite rapid socioeconomic and lifestyle changes.

【 】 CHRONIC STRESS

A substantial body of evidence showed that heart disease is influenced by chronic stress, with particular reference to occupational stress. There are two major models of work stress in the literature: job strain and effort-reward imbalance. The job strain model showed that "lack of autonomy" (or having too little influence over the day-to-day organization of work) combined with high demand (having too much to do over a long period of time with constant imposed deadlines) is positively associated with coronary heart disease.[36] The effort-reward imbalance model showed that high effort (high levels of mental and physical energy expended to achieve an organizational goal) and low reward (perceiving too little compensation for, or acknowledgment of efforts in terms of bestowed status, financial gain, or career advancement) are conducive to heart disease.[37]

Potential mechanisms explaining why chronic stress at work is associated with coronary heart disease include behavioral risk factors and biological activation of the hypothalamic-pituitary-adrenal axis and the central nervous system.[38] A recent study found a link between job stress and the metabolic syndrome.[39]

STRATEGIES FOR PREVENTION AT THE POPULATION LEVEL

In the previous sections of this chapter, we showed that changes in the distributions of heart disease and behavioral risk factors are inextricably intertwined with societal factors. We also showed that social factors are independent predictors of this health condition. Although heart disease is mainly addressed through clinical and behavioral interventions, as underlined by Geoffrey Rose, the "high-risk" approach that seeks to understand the causes of disease of individuals is very different from the "population" approach that seeks to analyze the causes of incidence at the population level. Individual and population approaches to control heart disease are not incompatible. However, to effectively reduce heart disease and inequalities in heart disease, prior concern should always be to discover the ultimate causes of incidence at the population level.[40]

The rise of heart disease in the developing world, and the welcome decline in the developed world has often been attributed to changes in smoking, cholesterol level, high-consumption diet, physical inactivity, and obesity. However, as shown by evidence reviewed in this chapter, all these factors are socially patterned or strongly influenced by societal factors and economic development. Moreover, conventional risk factors play only a minor role in explaining the social gradient of heart disease. Therefore, even if we were able to reduce such risks, inequality in heart disease would continue.[24]

The evidence presented in this chapter provides the basis for addressing the "causes of the causes" of heart disease rather than only conventional risk factors. Societal-level approaches include measures promoting a healthy lifestyle such as restrictions of smoking in public spaces, increased availability of healthful foods, and quality and safety of recreational areas. They also require broader economic policies affecting poverty and inequality, policies regarding the agriculture, food, and tobacco industries as well as changes in urban planning, social participation, the work environment, and transportation policies.

CONCLUSIONS

Although most medical personnel see health merely as a problem of the individual,[40] in this chapter we showed the importance of societal and social factors as key determinants of heart disease and related risk factors at the population level. Although the control of immediate biological risk factors and clinical interventions are important strategies at the individual level, to reduce heart disease and inequalities in heart disease at the population level, in both developed and developing societies, we need to adopt a broader societal approach.

REFERENCES

1. Stallones R. The rise and fall of ischemic heart disease. *Sci Am.* 1980;243:53–59.
2. Sijbrands E, Westendorp R, Defesche J. Mortality over two centuries in large pedigree with familial hypercholesterolemia: family tree mortality study. *BMJ.* 2001;322:1019–1023.
3. Omran A. The epidemiologic transition: a theory of the epidemiology of population change. *Milbank Mem Fund Q.* 1971;49:509.
4. Srinath K, Reddy D. Cardiovascular disease in non-Western countries. *N Eng J Med.* 2004;350(24):2438–2440.
5. Faergeman O. The societal context of coronary heart disease. *Eur Heart J.* 2005;7(suppl):A5–A11.
6. Zimmet P. Globalization, coca-colonization and the chronic disease epidemic: can the Doomday scenario be averted? *J Intern Med.* 2000;247:301–310.
7. Adair L, Popkin B. Are child eating patterns being transformed globally? *Obes Res.* 2005;13(7):1281–1299.
8. Popkin BM, Zizza C, Siegra-Riz A. Who is leading the change? U.S. dietary quality comparison between 1965 and 1996. *Am J Prev Med.* 2003;25(1):1–8.
9. Ebrahim S, Davey-Smith G. Exporting failure? Coronary heart disease and stroke in developing countries. *Am J Epidemiol.* 2001;30:201–205.
10. Chang C, Marmot M, Farley T, Poulter N. The influence of economic development on the association between education and the risk of acute myocardial infarction and stroke. *J Clin Epidemiol.* 2002;55:741–747.
11. Marmot M, Rose G, Shipley M, Hamilton J. Employment grade and coronary heart disease in British Civil Servants. *J Epidemiol Community Health.* 1978;32:244–249.

12. Wong S, Donnan S. Influence of socioeconomic status on cardiovascular diseases in Hong Kong. *J Epidemiol Community Health.* 1992;46:148–150.

13. Solie P, Garcia-Palmieri M. Educational status and coronary heart disease in Puerto Rico: the Puerto Rico Heart Health Program. *Int J Epidemiol.* 1990;19:59–65.

14. Hameed K, Kadir M, Gibson T, et al. The frequency of know diabetes, hypertension and ischaemic heart disease in affluent and poor urban populations of Karachi. *Diabetes Med.* 1995;12:500–503.

15. Marmot M, Adelstein A, Robinson N, Rose G. Changing social class distribution of heart disease. *BMJ.* 1978;2:1109–1112.

16. Cooper R, Cutler J, Desvigne-Nickens P. Trends and disparities in coronary heart disease, stroke and other cardiovascular diseases in the United States. Findings of the National Conference on Cardiovascular Disease Prevention. *Circulation.* 2000;102:3137–3147.

17. Monteiro CA, Conde WL, Lu B, Popkin BM. Obesity and inequity in health in the developing world. *Int J Obesity.* 2004;28:1181–1186.

18. Diez-Roux A, Link B, Northridge M. A multilevel analysis of income inequality and cardiovascular disease risk factors. *Soc Sci Med.* 2000;50:673–687.

19. Gordon-Larsen P, Nelson M, Page P, Popkin B. Inequality in the built environment underlies key health disparities in physical activity and obesity. *Pediatrics.* 2006;117(2):417–424.

20. Bobak M, Prabhat J, Nguyen S. Poverty and smoking. In: Jha P, Chaloupka F, eds. *Tobacco control in developing countries.* Oxford, UK: Oxford University Press; 2000.

21. Cavelaars A, Kunst A, Geurts J, et al. Educational differences in smoking: international comparison. *BMJ.* 2000;320:1102–1107.

22. De Vogli R, Gnesotto R, Goldstein M, Andersen R, Cornia G. The lack of social gradient of health behaviors and psychosocial factors in Northern Italy. *Soz Praventivmed.* 2005;50(4):197–205.

23. Levi F, Lucchini F, Negri E, Vecchia CL. Trend in mortality from cardiovascular and cerebrovascular diseases in Europe and other areas of the world. *Heart.* 2002;88:119–124.

24. Marmot M. Commentary: risk factors or social causes? *Int J Epidemiol.* 2004;33:297–298.

25. Kennedy B, Kawachi I, Prothrow-Stith D. Income distribution and mortality: cross sectional ecological study of the Robin Hood Index in the United States. *BMJ.* 1996;312:1004–1007.

26. Sundquist J, Johansson S, Yang M, Sundquist K. Low linking social capital as predictor of coronary heart disease in Sweden: a cohort study of 2.8 million people. *Soc Sci Med.* 2006;62:954–963.

27. Gaziano T. Cardiovascular disease in the developing world and its cost-effective management. *Circulation.* 2005;112:3547–3553.

28. Marmot M, Bobak M. International comparators and poverty and health in Europe. *BMJ.* 2000;321:1124–1128.

29. Kristenson M, Orth-Gomer K, Kucinskiene Z. Attenuated cortisol response to a standardized stress test in Lithuanian versus Swedish men: the LiVicordia study. *Int J Behav Med.* 1998;5(1):17–30.

30. Kaplan G, Salonen J, Cohen R. Social connections and mortality from all causes and cardiovascular disease. *Am J Epidemiol.* 1988;128:370–380.

31. Kawachi I, Colditz G, Ascherio A, et al. A prospective study of social networks in relation to total mortality and cardiovascular disease in men in the USA. *J Epidemiol Community Health.* 1996;50:245–251.

32. Rosengren A, Wilhelmsen L, Orth-Gomer K. Coronary disease in relation to social support and social class in Swedish men: a 15-year follow-up in the study of men born in 1933. *Eur Heart J.* 2004;25(1):56–63.

33. Seeman T. Social ties and health: the benefits of social integration. *Eur Psychiatry.* 1996;6(5):442–451.

34. Cohen S, Gottlieb B, Underwood L. Social relationships and health. In: Cohen S, Underwood L, Gottlieb B, eds. *Social Support Measurement and Intervention: A Guide for Health and Social Scientists.* New York: Oxford University Press; 2000.

35. Lasker J, Egolf B, Wolf S. Community social change and mortality. *Soc Sci Med.* 1994;39(1):53–62.

36. Schnall P. Job strain and cardiovascular disease. *Annu Rev Public Health.* 1994;15:381–411.

37. Kuper H, Singh-Manoux A, Siegrist J, Marmot M. When reciprocity fails: effort-reward imbalance in relation to coronary heart disease and health functioning within the Whitehall II study. *Occup Environ Med.* 2002;59:777–784.

38. McEwen B. Protective and damaging effects of stress mediators. *N Engl J Med.* 1998;338:171–179.

39. Chandola T. Chronic stress at work and the metabolic syndrome: prospective study. *BMJ.* 2006;332:521–525.

40. Rose G. Sick individuals and sick populations. *Int J Epidemiol.* 1985;14(1):32–38.

INDEX

Note: Boldface page numbers indicate main discussions; page numbers followed by *f* indicate figures, and those followed by *t* indicate tables.